Your PDR® Supplements should be placed over this page

BEFORE PRESCRIBING OR ADMINISTERING ANY PRODUCT IN PHYSICIANS' DESK REFERENCE®, YOU SHOULD FIRST CONSULT YOUR SUPPLEMENT TO DETERMINE IF NEW OR REVISED PRODUCT INFORMATION HAS DEVELOPED SINCE THE CURRENT PDR WENT TO PRESS.

PDR

[illegible]eword to the [illegible]urth Edition

[illegible] edition of PHYSICIANS' DESK REFERENCE® went to press, it included the [illegible] [illegible] on approximately 2,500 products. During the year ahead, however, [illegible] revised information about these pr[illegible] [illegible] published periodically in a PDR® Supplement. [illegible] volume you will find instructions for convenient retention of the PDR Sup[illegible] suggested method you can use to alert yourself to revisions in a particular product [illegible] Before prescribing or administering any product described in PHYSICIANS' [illegible] ENCE, consult the latest PDR Supplement to determine if new or re[illegible] product has been published in a Supplement.

In response to the growing trend toward "self-medication" and to the lack of [illegible] information available for practitioners concerning over-the-counter drugs, the [illegible] PHYSICIANS' DESK REFERENCE will distribute a separate edition [illegible] REFERENCE for NONPRESCRIPTION [illegible]

PHYSICIANS' DESK REFERENCE is published annually by Medical Economics Company [illegible] the cooperation of the manufacturers whose products are [illegible] (White Section) and Diagnostic [illegible] physicians, PDR's purpose is to make available [illegible] products.

This edition includes information concerning [illegible] drugs. The information has been prepared [illegible] found printed inside the back cover. [illegible] page 10[illegible]

The function of the Publisher is the compilation, organization, and distribution of [illegible] information. Each product description has been prepared [illegible] approved by the manufacturer [illegible] consultant. Manufacturers have suggested [illegible] listed in the Product Classification Index (Blue Section) and in Generic and Chemical Name Index (Yellow Section). In some instances, the Publisher has deviated from the manufacturer's suggestions in an attempt to make these indices more valuable to the user. Products [illegible] in PHYSICIANS' DESK REFERENCE which have official package circulars must be in compliance with Food & Drug Administration regulations pertaining to labeling for prescription drugs. These regulations require that for PDR "indications, effects, dosages, routes, methods, and frequency and duration of administration, and any relevant warnings, hazards, contraindications, side effects, and precautions" must be the "same in language and emphasis" as the approved labeling for the product. FDA regards the words "same in language and emphasis" as requiring verbatim use of the approved labeling providing [illegible] do not have official package circulars [illegible] necessity of describing such products comprehensively [illegible] information essential for intelligent and informed prescribing. In organizing and presenting the material in PHYSICIANS' DESK REFERENCE, the Publisher is providing all the [illegible] made available to PDR by manufacturers. Additional information, on any product [illegible] obtained from the manufacturer.

In making this material available to the medical profession, it should be [illegible] Publisher is not advocating the use of any product described herein.

CHARLES E. BAKER
Publisher

Manufacturers' Index

PDR 34 EDITION

SECTION 1

The manufacturers appearing in this index (white pages) have provided information concerning their pharmaceutical products in either the Product Information or Diagnostic Product Information Section. It is through their patronage that PHYSICIANS' DESK REFERENCE® is made available to you.

Included in this index are the names and addresses of manufacturers, individuals or departments to whom you may address inquiries, a partial list of products as well as emergency telephone numbers wherever available. The symbol ◆ indicates the product shown in the Product Identification Section. The symbol ▣ indicates the product is described in PDR FOR NONPRESCRIPTION DRUGS.

Part 1

PAGE

ABBOTT LABORATORIES **403, 502**
North Chicago, IL 60064
Address inquiries to:
Medical Director (312) 688-6100
Distribution Centers
ATLANTA
Stone Mountain, GA 30302
P.O. Box 5049 (404) 491-7190
CHICAGO
Abbott Park
North Chicago, IL 60064
P.O. Box 68 (312) 937-6180
DALLAS
Dallas, TX 75265
P.O. Box 225295 (214) 387-1350
DENVER
Denver, CO 80217
P.O. Box 5466 (303) 399-7576
HONOLULU
Honolulu, HI 96819
2815 Kilihao Street (808) 833-1691
KANSAS CITY
Kansas City, MO 64141
P.O. Box 685 (816) 753-1250
LOS ANGELES
Los Angeles, CA 90060
60162 Terminal Annex (213) 921-0321
MINNEAPOLIS
Minneapolis, MN 55440
P.O. Box 271 (612) 559-5666
PHILADELPHIA
King of Prussia, PA 19406
920 Eighth Ave., East (215) 265-9100
ST. LOUIS
St. Louis, MO 63178
P.O. Box 14394 (314) 993-4066
SEATTLE
Seattle, WA 98124
P.O. Box 24064 (206) 244-5151
TOLEDO
Toledo, OH 43608
P.O. Box 327 (419) 726-2687
Products Available
Abbokinase
◆ Abbo-Pac
Abbott Unit Dose Systems
Dayalets Filmtab
E.E.S. Granules
Enduron Tablets
Enduronyl Forte Tablets
Enduronyl Tablets
Erythrocin Stearate Filmtab
Erythromycin Base Filmtab
Fero-Grad-500 Filmtab
Iberet-500 Filmtab
K-Lor
Nembutal Sodium Capsules
Oretic Tablets
Panwarfin Tablets
Placidyl Capsules
Surbex-T Filmtab
Tranxene Capsules
Acetic Acid Irrigation
Aerohalor
A-hydroCort
Alcohol, Absolute, Ampoules
Alcohol 5% & Dextrose 5% in Water
A-MethaPred
Aminophyllin 250 mg., 10 ml., Ampoule
Aminophyllin 500 mg., 20 ml., Ampoule
Aminosyn 3.5% M
Aminosyn 5%
Aminosyn 7%
Aminosyn 7% Kit
Aminosyn 7% TPN with Electrolytes Kit
Aminosyn 7% with Electrolytes
Aminosyn 10%
Ammonium Chloride
◆ A-poxide
Atropine 0.1 mg./ml., 5 ml., Abboject, Syringe
Atropine 0.1 mg./ml., 10 ml., Abboject, Syringe
Bejectal Vial
Bejectal w/Vitamin C Vial
Bejex Vial
Bupivacaine Hydrochloride Solution, 0.5%
Butesin Picrate Ointment
Butyn Dental Ointment
Calcidrine Syrup
Calcium Chloride 10%, Abboject
Calcium Gluceptate Injection Ampoule & Abboject
Cecon Solution
◆ Cefol Filmtab
Cenolate Ampoules
Clear Eyes Eye Drops
Colchicine Tablets
Covicone Cream
◆ Cylert Chewable Tablets
◆ Cylert Tablets
L-Cysteine Hydrochloride
Dayalets Filmtab
Dayalets plus Iron Filmtab
◆ Depakene Capsules & Syrup
◆ Desoxyn Gradumet Tablets
Desoxyn Tablets
Dextran 6% w/v in Dextrose 5% in Water Abbo-Vac
Dextran 6% w/v in Saline 0.9% Abbo-Vac
Dextrose 5% in Water w/Potassium Chloride 10mEq
Dextrose 5% in Water w/Potassium Chloride 20mEq
Dextrose 5% in Water w/Potassium Chloride 30mEq
Dextrose 5% in Water w/Potassium Chloride 40mEq
Dextrose 5% in ¼ Strength Saline w/Potassium Chloride 10mEq
Dextrose 5% in ¼ Strength Saline w/Potassium Chloride 20mEq
Dextrose 5% in ¼ Strength Saline w/Potassium Chloride 30mEq
Dextrose 5% in ¼ Strength Saline w/Potassium Chloride 40mEq
Dextrose 5% in ½ Strength Saline w/Potassium Chloride 10mEq
Dextrose 5% in ½ Strength Saline w/Potassium Chloride 20mEq
Dextrose 5% in ½ Strength Saline w/Potassium Chloride 30mEq
Dextrose 5% in ½ Strength Saline w/Potassium Chloride 40mEq
Dextrose 10% Injection, partial Fill
Dextrose 20% Injection, Partial Fill

Dextrose 30% Injection, Partial Fill
Dextrose 40% Injection, Partial Fill
Dextrose 50% Injection, Partial Fill
Dextrose 60% Injection, Partial Fill
Dextrose 70% Injection, Partial Fill
40% Dextrose Injection w/Electrolytes, Partial Fill
50% Dextrose Injection w/Electrolytes, Partial Fill
60% Dextrose Injection w/Electrolytes, Partial Fill
70% Dextrose Injection w/Electrolytes, Partial Fill
Diasone Sodium Enterab Tablets
Dical-D Capsules
Dical-D Wafers
Dical-D with Iron Capsules
Dical-D with Vitamin C Capsules
◆ Dicumarol Tablets
Digitoxin Tablets
◆ E.E.S. Chewable Tablets
E.E.S. Drops
E.E.S. Granules
E.E.S. 200 Liquid
◆ E.E.S. 400 Filmtab
E.E.S. 400 Liquid
Ear Drops by Murine
See Murine Ear Wax Removal System/Murine Ear Drops
Empty Evacuated Container
Endrate Solution, Ampoules
◆ Enduron Tablets
Enduronyl Forte Tablets
◆ Enduronyl Tablets
Ephedrine & Nembutal-25, Capsule
Ephedrine Sulfate, Injection
Epinephrine 1:10,000, 10 ml., Abboject
Erythrocin Lactobionate-I.V.
◆ Erythrocin Stearate Filmtab
◆ Erythromycin Base Filmtab
◆ Eutonyl Filmtab
◆ Eutron Filmtab
◆ Fero-Folic-500 Filmtab
Fero-Grad-500 Filmtab
Fero-Gradumet Filmtab
Fructose 10% in Water
Gemonil Tablets
Gerilets Filmtab
Gerix Elixir
Glycine Solution 1.5%, Irrigation/Aqualite
Halazone Tablets
Halothane, U.S.P.
◆ Harmonyl Tablets
Hydron Burn Bandage
Iberet Filmtab
◆ Iberet-500 Filmtab
Iberet-500 Liquid
◆ Iberet-Folic-500 Filmtab
Iberet-Liquid
Iberol Filmtab
Iberol-F Filmtab
Inpersol w/Dextrose 1.5% Solution
Inpersol w/Dextrose 4.25% Solution
Inpersol-K w/Dextrose 1.5% Solution
Invert Sugar 10% in Water
Ionosol B w/Dextrose 5%
Ionosol B w/Invert Sugar 10%
Ionosol D w/Invert Sugar 10%
Ionosol D-CM (Duodenal)
Ionosol D-CM w/Dextrose 5%
Ionosol G w/Dextrose 10% (Gastric)
Ionosol G w/Invert Sugar 10%
Ionosol MB w/Dextrose 5%
Ionosol T w/Dextrose 5%
Isoproterenol HCl 1:5,000 1 mg. Pintop
Isoproterenol HCl 1:5,000 2 mg. Pintop
Isoproterenol HCl 1:5,000 5 ml., Universal Add Syringe
Isoproterenol HCl 1:5,000 10 ml., Universal Add Syringe
Isoproterenol HCl 1:50,000, 10 ml., Abboject
◆ Janimine Filmtab
◆ K-Lor Powder
LMD 10% in D5-W
LMD 10% in Saline
LTA II Kit
Lactated Ringer's Injection
Lidocaine 1%, 5 ml., Abboject
Lidocaine 1%, 5 ml., Sterile Pack Abboject
Lidocaine 2%, 5 ml., Abboject
Lidocaine 2%, 5 ml., Sterile Pack Abboject
Lidocaine 20%, 5 ml., 1 gram-Pintop, U.A.S.
Lidocaine 20%, 10 ml., 2 gram-Pintop, U.A.S.
Lidocaine Hydrochloride Injection, U.S.P.
◆ Lidone Capsules
Liposyn 10%, 500 ml., 200 ml.
Lubritine
Magnesium Sulfate 12.5%, 8 ml., Pintop
Magnesium Sulfate 50% w/v Ampoules & Abboject
Mammol Ointment
Mannitol I.V. (5, 10, 15, 20%)
Murine Ear Wax Removal System/Murine Ear Drops
Murine Eye Drops
Murine Plus Eye Drops
Nembutal Elixir
◆ Nembutal Sodium Capsules
Nembutal Sodium Solution
Nembutal Sodium Suppositories
Neut Abbo-Vial & Pintop
Niacin Tablets
Norisodrine Aerotrol
Norisodrine Sulfate Aerohalor
Norisodrine w/Calcium Iodide Syrup
Normosol-M 900 CAL
Normosol-M in D5-W
Normosol-M Surbex T in D5-W
Normosol-R
Normosol-R in D5-W
Normosol-R pH 7.4
Normosol-R/K + in D5-W
◆ Ogen Tablets
◆ Ogen Vaginal Cream
◆ Optilets-500 Filmtab
◆ Optilets-M-500 Filmtab
◆ Oretic Tablets
◆ Oreticyl Tablets
◆ Oreticyl Forte Tablets
Panheprin LOK Syringe
Panheprin 2115 (Pliapak) w/attached Collection Tube & Siliconed Needle
Panheprin 2115 (Plia-Stor) w/attached Collection Tube, Siliconed Needle & Auxiliary A-C-D Supply
Panheprin SDS Syringes
Panheprin Vials
◆ Panwarfin Tablets
◆ Paradione Capsules & Oral Solution
◆ Peganone Tablets
Penthrane
Pentothal Kit
Pentothal Rectal Suspension in Abbo-Sert Syringe
Pentothal Sodium Thiopental for Injection
Pentothal, (Sterile Powder)
Pentothal Syringe
Phenobarbital Sodium Ampoules
Phenurone Tablets
Physiosol Irrigation/Aqualite
◆ Placidyl Capsules
Potassium Acetate 40 mEq Vial, Pintop & Fliptop
Potassium Chloride Injection Ampoules & Vials, Pintop & Universal Additive Syringe
Potassium Chloride 20 mEq. in D-5 W in Abbo-Vac
Potassium Phosphate 15 mM Vial, Pintop & Fliptop
Potassium Phosphate 45 mM Vial
Procaine Hydrochloride Injection 1% & 2% Vial
Quelicin Injection Ampoule & Vial, Pintop
Quelidrine Syrup
Ringer's Injection Irrigation Aqualite
Selsun Blue Lotion
Selsun Lotion
Selsun Suspension
Sodium Acetate 40 mEq Vial
Sodium Bicarbonate Ampoules, 7.5% Solution
Sodium Bicarbonate 8.4% in Abboject Disposable Syringe
Sodium Bicarbonate 5% Solution Abbo-Vac
Sodium Chloride Injection, Normal Saline 0.9%
Sodium Chloride 0.45% Irrigation/Aqualite
Sodium Chloride 5% Irrigation
Sodium Lactate, 1/6 Molar
Sodium Lactate 50 mEq, Vial
Sodium Phosphate 45 mM Vial
Sorbital-Mannitol Irrigating Solution/Aqualite
Sulfadiazine Dulcet Tablets
Surbex Filmtab
Surbex w/C Filmtab
◆ Surbex-750 with Iron Filmtab
◆ Surbex-750 with Zinc Filmtab
◆ Surbex-T Filmtab
Surbex-T Solution w/D5-W
TPN Electrolytes
Tham Solution
Tral Filmtab
Tral Gradumet
◆ Tranxene Capsules
◆ Tranxene-SD Half Strength Tablets
◆ Tranxene-SD Tablets
◆ Tridione Capsules
◆ Tridione Dulcet Tablets
Tridione Solution
Tronothane Hydrochloride Cream, Jelly
Tubocurarine Chloride Injection
Ureaphil
Urological Solution G
Vercyte Tablets
Vita-Kaps Filmtab
Vita-Kaps M Filmtab
Vitamin C Filmtab
Water for Injection, Ampoules, Vial
Water for Injection Bacteriostatic 30 ml. Fliptop
Water for Injection, Sterile, Sterile Water
Water, for Irrigation, Sterile/Aqualite
Wheat Germ Oil Capsules, Fortified

Gamma Counting Systems
Automatic and Manual
Auto-Logic 50
Auto-Logic 100
System Options
Logic 201
Logic 211
Logic 221
Hepatitis
Ausab Hepatitis B Surface Antigen ^{125}I (Human) Radioimmunoassay Diagnostic Kit
Ausab Hepatitis B Surface Antigen ^{125}I (Human) Radioimmunoassay Confirmatory Test
Auscell Antibody to Hepatitis B Surface Antigen (Guinea Pig) Reversed Passive Hemagglutination (RPHA) Diagnostic Kit
Auscell Antibody to Hepatitis B Surface Antigen (Human) Reversed Passive Hemagglutination (RPHA) Confirmatory Test Kit
Ausria II-125 Antibody to Hepatitis B Surface Antigen ^{125}I (Human) Radioimmunoassay Diagnostic Kit
Ausria II-125 Antibody to Hepatitis B Surface Antigen (Human) Radioimmunoassay Confirmatory Test
Aus-tect Test System, Rheophoresis Procedure
Thyroid
HTSH•RIA Diagnostic Kit
Prolactin RIA Diagnostic Kit
Quantisorb-125 T4N Diagnostic Kit
T3RIA (PEG) Diagnostic Kit
T4RIA (PEG) Diagnostic Kit
Thypinone (Protirelin) Synthetic TRH
Thyroscreen T4 Neonate
Triobead T3 Diagnostic Kit
Radiopharmaceuticals
Sensor [Radionuclide-Labeled (^{125}I) Fibrinogen (Human)Glofil]
Diagnostics, General
Digoxin I 125 Imusay Diagnostic Kit
Reptilase-R (Bothrops atrox) (Lyophilized) Coagulation Test
Ruba-tect Rubella Diagnostic Test Systems (Kaolin or Heparin-Manganese Chloride)
Rubacell Rubella Screening Test
Strep-tect FA Group A Beta Hemolytic Streptococcus Fluorescent Antibody Detection System
UTI-tect Bacteriuria Diagnostic Test System

ABBOTT LABORATORIES **2002**
DIAGNOSTICS DIVISION
Abbott Park
North Chicago, IL 60064
Outside Illinois call toll free (800) 323-9100
In Illinois, call collect (312) 937-6161
Address inquiries to:
Marketing Services Dept. 49B
Products Available
Thypinone

ADRIA LABORATORIES INC. **560**
Administrative Offices:
5000 Post Road
Dublin, OH 43017
Mailing Address:
P. O. Box 16529
Columbus, OH 43216
Address inquiries to:
Medical Department (614) 889-1300
Products Available
Adriamycin
Adrucil

ALBA PHARMACAL CORPORATION **562**
P.O. Box 628
Munoz Rivera 938
Penuelas, Puerto Rico 00724
(809) 836-1157
Address inquiries to:
Mr. Alberto Bartolomei, Jr.
(809) 836-1157
Products Available
Alba-3 Ointment
Alba-Ce Liquid, Drops, Capsules
Albacort Cream
Albacort Injectable
Alba-Dex Injectable, Liquid & Tablets
Albadryl Injectable
Albaform-HC Cream
Albafort Injectable
Alba-Gyn Vaginal Cream
Alba-Lybe
Albapirin Suppositories
Alba-Temp Suppositories, Liquid, Tablets & Drops
Albatussin (Sugar Free)
Albazine Injectable
Alvimin
Asmex KI Liquid
Asmex Liquid
Benzotic Ear Drops
Dramatrol Injectable
Hemogesic HC Suppositories
Hemogesic Suppositories
Myoforte Tablets

Myophen Injectable
Pasmin Injectable, Liquid, Capsules
Sedaril
Tia-Doce Injectable Univial

ALLERGAN PHARMACEUTICALS, INC. 563
2525 Dupont Drive
Irvine, CA 92713
Address inquiries to:
Dave Fancher (714) 752-4500
(See also Herbert Laboratories)
Products Available
Albalon Liquifilm ophthalmic solution
Albalon-A Liquifilm ophthalmic solution
Atropine Sulfate ½% S.O.P. ophthalmic ointment
Atropine Sulfate 1.0% S.O.P. ophthalmic ointment
Atropine Sulfate Ophthalmic Solution 1%, 2%
Bleph 10/30 Liquifilm ophthalmic solution
Blephamide Liquifilm ophthalmic suspension
Blephamide S.O.P. sterile ophthalmic ointment
Blink-N-Clean hard contact lens solution
Chloroptic ophthalmic solution
Chloroptic S.O.P. ophthalmic ointment
Chloroptic-P S.O.P. ophthalmic ointment
Clean-N-Soak hard contact lens solution
Clean-N-Soakit hard contact lens storage case
Clean-N-Stow hard contact lens storage case
Epifrin ophthalmic solution
Ethamide tablets
FML Liquifilm ophthalmic suspension
Genoptic S.O.P. Sterile Ophthalmic Ointment
Genoptic Sterile Ophthalmic Solution
Glazcote plastic eyeglass cleaner
HMS Liquifilm ophthalmic suspension
Herplex Liquifilm ophthalmic solution
Homatropine Sterile Ophthalmic Solution
LC-65 hard contact lens cleaning solution
Lacril artificial tears
Lacri-Lube S.O.P. ophthalmic ointment
Lensrins preserved saline solution
Liquifilm Forte enhanced artificial tears
Liquifilm Tears artificial tears
Liquifilm Wetting Solution hard contact lens solution
Ophthetic ophthalmic solution
P.V. Carpine Liquifilm ophthalmic solution
Polyspectrin Liquifilm ophthalmic solution
Polyspectrin S.O.P. ophthalmic ointment
Pred Forte ophthalmic suspension
Pred Mild ophthalmic suspension
Prefrin Liquifilm eye drops
Prefrin-A ophthalmic solution
Prefrin-Z Liquifilm ophthalmic solution
Pre-Sert hard contact lens cushioning solution
Scopolamine 0.2% S.O.P. ophthalmic ointment
Scopolamine 0.25% Sterile Ophthalmic Solution
Soakare hard contact lens soaking solution
Soflens Enzymatic Contact Lens Cleaner
Total all-in-one hard contact lens solution
Wet-N-Soak wetting and soaking solution for hard contact lenses

ALTO PHARMACEUTICALS, INC. 404, 563
Route 1 Box 424A
Casey Road Extensions & Otto Road
Tampa, FL 33624
Address inquiries to:
John J. Cullaro
Post Office Box 15564
Tampa, FL 33684 (813) 961-1010
Products Available
Akne Drying Lotion
Akne Kaps
Akne pH Lotion
Akne-Oral Kapsulets
Alto-Pred LA-100 Injection
Alto-Pred Soluble Injection
Anabolin IM Injection
Anabolin LA-100 Injection
Antispasmodic Elixir
Bifed-20 Capsules
D'Alpha-E Capsules
Dexamethasone Injection
Efed Tablets
Hydroxyzine Injection
Lotio-P Lotion
Microcort Lotion
Povidone Scrub
Povidone Solution
Theophylline Elixir
◆ Zinc-220 Capsules (Zinc Sulfate Capsules)

AMERICAN PHARMACEUTICAL COMPANY 563
245 Fourth Street
Passaic, NJ 07055
Address inquiries to:
Mr. Richard McNall (201) 799-5300
Products Available
Afko Ear Drops
Afko-Lube Capsules
Afko-Lube Lax Capsules
Ampicillin Trihydrate Capsules
Aphco Hemorrhoidal Ointment, Suppositories
Bacitracin Ointment
Belexon Fortified Capsules
Bisacodyl Tablets & Suppositories
Brompheniramine Elixir, Tablets
Chlorothiazide Tablets
Chlorpromazine Tablets
Codanol A&D Ointment
Codanol Malt with Hemoglobin
Cortisone Acetate Tablets
Cyclandelate Capsules
Daily Dose 1 Vitamins
B-Complex Liver & Iron Tablets
Belexa B-Complex & C Capsules
Fe-ritol Tablets
Gerifort Plus
Multiple Vitamins with Iron Tablets
Multiple Vitamins with Minerals Tablets
Nutri-Drops
Super Stress-600 Tablets
Super Stress-600 with Iron Tablets
Super Z Stress-600 Tablets
Thera-Amcaps
Thera-Amcaps M
Vitamin E Capsules
Dicyclomine HCl Capsules
Di-O-Gest Antacid Tablets
Diphenhydramine Capsules, Elixir, Expectorant
Diphenoxylate with Atropine Sulfate Tablets
Erythromycin Stearate Tablets
Fendon Tablets, Elixir
Ferrous Gluconate Tablets
Ferrous Sulfate Tablets, Capsules
Gelumina Plus Liquid
Gelumina Tablets
Gerifort Elixir, Tablets
Hydralazine Tablets
Hydrochlorothiazide Tablets
Hyrocain Cream
Iso-Lo Eye Wash, Drops
Isoxsuprine HCl Tablets
Ka-Pek Suspension
Methenamine Mandelate Tablets
Methocarbamol Tablets
Neo-Mist Nasal Spray
Neomycin Tablets
Nite-Rest Capsules
Nutri-Caps with Minerals
Papaverine Capsules, Tablets
Penicillin V Potassium Tabs.
Pertinex Cream, Spray
Phendex Elixir, Tablets
Phenylazo Tablets
Prednisolone Tablets
Prednisone Tablets
Prenacaps
Procainamide Capsules
Promethazine Tablets, Expectorant
Propylthiouracil Tablets
Quinidine Sulfate Tablets
Quinine Sulfate Capsules
Rhusticon Lotion
Romex Decongestant Cough, Cold Liquid, Capsules & Troches
SPD Analgesic Cream Lotion
Spectro-Biotic Ointment
Tetracycline Capsules
Triprolidine w/Pseudoephedrine Tablets, Syrup
Verv Alertness Capsules

AMES DIVISION 2003
Miles Laboratories, Inc.
1127 Myrtle Street
P.O. Box 70
Elkhart, IN 46515
Order/Pricing Information:
(219) 264-8645
Customer Services
(219) 264-8901
Products Available
Ames Instruments
Ames Blood Analyzer
Eyetone Reflectance Colorimeter
Urin-Tek System for Urine Specimen Collection and Transportation
Ames Tests
Dextrostix Calibration and Control Set
Dextrostix Reagent Strips
Diastix Reagent Strips
Glucola Carbonated Preparation for Postprandial & Glucose Tolerance Test
Keto-Diastix Reagent Strips
Microcult-GC
Microstix-3 Reagent Strips
Microstix-Candida
Microstix-Nitrite
N-Multistix Reagent Strips
N-Uristix Reagent Strips
Tek-Chek Controls for Dextrostix
Tek-Chek Controls for Routine Urinalysis

ARCO PHARMACEUTICALS, INC. 564
105 Orville Drive
Bohemia, NY 11716
Address inquiries to:
Professional Service Dept. (516) 567-9500
Products Available
Arco-Cee Tablets
Arco-Lase Tablets
Arco-Lase Plus Tablets
Arcoret Tablets
Arcoret w/Iron Tablets
Arcotinic Liquid
Arcotinic Tablets
C-B Time Capsules
C-B Time 500 Tablets
C-B Time Liquid
Co-Gel Tablets
Mega-B
Megadose
Spantuss Liquid
Spantuss Tablets

AR-EX PRODUCTS CO. 564
1036 West Van Buren St.
Chicago, IL 60607
Address inquiries to:
Robert W. Francke (312) 226-5241
Products Available
Ar-Ex Hypo-Allergenic Cosmetics
Bath Oil - unscented
Body Lotion - unscented
Brush-On Complexion Coloring - unscented
Brush-On Eyeshadow - unscented
Chap Cream - scented & unscented
Cleansing Cream - scented & unscented
Cold Cream - scented & unscented
Compact Powder - unscented
Cream for Dry Skin - scented & unscented
Cream for Oily Skin - unscented
Deodorant (Cream, Spray, Roll-On) - unscented
Disappear (Blemish Stick) - unscented
Eye Cream - unscented
Eye Makeup Remover Pads - unscented
Eye Pencil- unscented
Eye Shadow Stick - unscented
Face Powder - unscented
Foundation Lotion - unscented
Hair Spray - unscented
Hand Lotion - unscented
Lip Gloss & Sun Screen Stick - unscented
Moisture Cream - unscented
Moisture Lotion - unscented
Night Cream - unscented
Roll-On Mascara - unscented
Shampoo - unscented
Special Formula Lipstick - unscented
Superfatted Soap - unscented
Safe Suds - unscented

ARMOUR PHARMACEUTICAL COMPANY 404, 565
Executive Office
6991 East Camelback Road
Suite A-210
Scottsdale, AZ 85251 (602) 941-2924
P.O. Box 1849
Scottsdale, AZ 85252
Eastern Distribution Center
P.O. Box 383
South Plainfield, NJ 07080 (201) 668-0110
Midwest Distribution Center
P.O. Box 511
Kankakee, IL 60901 (815) 932-6771
Western Distribution Center
P.O. Box 63249
Los Angeles, CA 90063 (213) 263-9359
Products Available
Acthar
Alpha Chymar
◆ Armour Thyroid (Tablets)
Biopar Forté
Biozyme
Calcimar Solution
◆ Chymoral
◆ Chymoral-100
Depinar Suspension
Dialume
HP Acthar Gel
Heprinar
◆ Levothroid
◆ Nicobid
Nicolar
Nidar
◆ Pentritol-60 mg.
Posterior Pituitary Capsules
Thyrar
◆ Thyrolar
Thytropar
Tussar DM
Tussar SF
Tussar-2
Protein Reagents
Bovine Albumin
Crystallized Bovine Plasma Albumin

Bovine Albumin Powder
Protein Standard Solution
Therapeutic Blood Derivative Products
Antihemophilic Factor (Human) Dried Factorate
Immune Serum Globulin (Human) U.S.P. Gammar
Normal Serum Albumin (Human) U.S.P. 5% Albuminar-5
Normal Serum Albumin (Human) U.S.P. 25% Albuminar-25

ARNAR-STONE LABORATORIES, INC. 573
1600 Waukegan Road
McGaw Park, IL 60085
Subs. of American Hospital Supply Corp.
Address inquiries to:
Medical Director or Emergency Call: (312) 473-3000
Products Available
▣ Americaine Aerosol
Americaine Anesthetic Lubricant
▣ Americaine Hemorrhoidal Ointment
Americaine-Otic
Bretylol Injection
Hasacode Strong Tablets
Intropin Injection
Inulin Solution, Purified
Isoclor Tablets, Liquid, Timesule Capsules & Expectorant
Liqui-Cee Liquid
Sopor Tablets

ASCHER & COMPANY, INC., B.F. 577
5100 East 59th St.
Kansas City, MO 64130
Address inquiries to:
Product Information Dept. (816) 363-5900
Products Available
Anaspaz PB Tablets
Anaspaz Tablets
Ayrtab
Buren (Improved) Tablets
Converspaz Improved Capsules
Converzyme Improved Capsules
Drize M Capsules
Drotic Ear Drops
Ethaquin Tablets
Mobidin Tablets
Mobigesic Tablets
Mobisyl Creme
Nioric Elixir
Nioric Tablets
Soft'N Soothe Creme
Tolfrinic Tablets
Zestē MT Tablets
Zestē Tablets

ASTRA PHARMACEUTICAL PRODUCTS INC. 404, 577
7 Neponset St.
Worcester, MA 01606
Address inquiries to:
Professional Information Department (617) 620-0600
Products Available
◆ Bricanyl Subcutaneous Injection
◆ Bricanyl Tablets
Citanest Solutions
Duranest Solutions
Xylocaine Intramuscular Injection for Cardiac Arrhythmias
Xylocaine Intravenous Injection for Cardiac Arrhythmias
Xylocaine 2% Jelly
Xylocaine 2.5% Ointment
Xylocaine 5% Ointment
Xylocaine Solutions
Xylocaine 1.5% Solution with Dextrose 7.5%
Xylocaine 4% Topical Solution
Xylocaine 5% Solution with Glucose 7.5%
Xylocaine Suppositories
Xylocaine 2% Viscous Solution

AVICON, INC. 590
6201 South Freeway
Fort Worth, TX 76134
Address inquiries to:
Medical Department (817) 293-0450
Products Available
Avitene
Microfibrillar Collagen Hemostat

AYERST LABORATORIES 404, 591, 2004
Division of American Home Products Corp.
685 Third Ave.
New York, NY 10017
Address inquiries to:
Medical Department (212) 986-1000 Ext. 555
Divisional Sales Offices
Burlingame, CA 94010
Suite 100
840 Hinckley Road (415) 692-4258
Chamblee, GA (Atlanta) 30341
3600 American Drive (404) 457-2518
Chevy Chase, MD 20015
Suite 703
8401 Connecticut Ave. (301) 654-4884
Chicago, IL 60648
7545 N. Natchez Ave. (312) 763-0888
(Niles) (312) 647-8840-1
Lakewood, OH 44107
Suite 795
14701 Detroit Ave. (216) 226-4128
Los Angeles, CA 90061
12833 S. Spring St. (213) 321-5550
Mesquite, TX (Dallas) 75149
3601 Executive Blvd. (214) 285-8741
South Plainfield, NJ 07080
4000 Hadley Rd. (201) 754-6220 (NJ)
(212) 964-3903 (NY)
Distribution Centers
Chamblee—3600 American Drive
Chamblee, GA 30341 (404) 457-2518
Chicago—7545 N. Natchez Ave.
Chicago, IL 60648
(312) 763-0888 (Chicago)
(312) 647-8840 or 8841 (Niles)
Cleveland—15620 Industrial Parkway
Cleveland, OH 44135 (216) 267-9090
Lenexa—10700 Pflumm Road
Lenexa, KS 66210 (913) 888-4310
Los Angeles—12833 S. Spring St.
Los Angeles, CA 90061
(213) 321-5550-1-2
Mesquite—3601 Executive Blvd.
Mesquite, TX 75149 (214) 285-8741
Seattle—405 Baker Blvd., Andover Park
Seattle, WA 98188 (206) 244-1921
South Plainfield—4000 Hadley Road
South Plainfield, NJ 07080
(201) 754-6220 (NJ)
(212) 964-3903 (NY)

Products Available
A.P.L.
Almocarpine
◆ Antabuse
◆ Atromid-S
Auralgan Otic Solution
Avlosulfon
◆ Beminal-500
◆ Beminal Forte w/Vitamin C
Beminal Fortified w/Iron & Liver
Clusivol Capsules
Clusivol Syrup
Clusivol 130 Tablets
Cytoferin Hematinic Tablets
Dermoplast Aerosol Spray
◆ Diucardin
Enzactin Cream
Ayerst Epitrate
Estradurin
Estrogenic Substance (estrone) In Aqueous Suspension
Fluor-I-Strip Applicators
Fluor-I-Strip-A.T. Applicators
Fluothane
◆ Formatrix
◆ Grisactin
◆ Inderal
◆ Inderide
Kerodex Cream (water-miscible)
Kerodex Cream (water-repellent)
Larylgan Throat Spray
◆ Mediatric Capsules
Mediatric Liquid
◆ Mediatric Tablets
Mysoline Suspension
◆ Mysoline Tablets
Ophthalgan
◆ PMB 200 & PMB 400
◆ Penbritin Capsules
Penbritin for Oral Suspension
Penbritin Pediatric Drops for Oral Suspension
Penbritin-S for Injection
Peptavlon
Phospholine Iodide
◆ Plegine
Premarin Intravenous
◆ Premarin Tablets
◆ Premarin Vaginal Cream
◆ Premarin w/Methyltestosterone
Protopam Chloride for Injection
Protopam Chloride Tablets
◆ Riopan Antacid Chew Tablets
Riopan Antacid Suspension
◆ Riopan Antacid Swallow Tablets
◆ Riopan Plus Chew Tablets
Riopan Plus Suspension
Thiosulfil Duo-Pak Package
◆ Thiosulfil Forte Tablets
◆ Thiosulfil Tablets
◆ Thiosulfil-A Forte Tablets
◆ Thiosulfil-A Tablets
Turgasept Aerosol
◆ Veracillin Capsules

BAKER/CUMMINS 636
Div. Chester A. Baker Laboratories, Inc.
Subsidiary of Key Pharmaceuticals, Inc.
50 N.W. 176th Street
Miami, FL 33169 (305) 652-2276
Products Available
Acno Astringent
Acno Lotion
Acticort Lotion 25
Acticort Lotion 100
P&S Liquid
P&S Shampoo
Panscol Lotion & Ointment
Pan-Ultra Stick
Pan-Ultra Sun Lotion
Phacid Shampoo
Ultra-Derm Bath Oil
Ultra-Derm Moisturizer
Ultra-Mide Lotion
Xseb Shampoo
Xseb-T Shampoo

BARNES-HIND PHARMACEUTICALS, INC. 637
895 Kifer Road
Sunnyvale, CA 94086
Address inquiries to:
James L. Jansen (408) 736-5462
Products Available
Barnes-Hind Germicidal Solution
Barseb HC Scalp Lotion
Barseb Thera=Spray
HEB Cream Base
HEB-Cort Creams
Komed Acne Lotion
Komed HC Lotion
Komed Mild Acne Lotion
Komex
Tinver Lotion
Barnes-Hind Barium Products
Barotrast
Clysodrast
Esophotrast
Oratrast

BARRY LABORATORIES, INC. 638
461 N.E. 27th Street
Pompano Beach, FL 33064
In Florida call (1-305) 943-7722
Outside of Florida—
Toll Free WATS Line (1-800) 327-1141
Address inquiries to:
Special Services Department
Products Available
Allergenic Extracts
Autogenous Extractions
Dusts
Epidermals
Foods
Fungi (molds and smuts)
Inhalents
Insects
Poison Ivy, Oak, Sumac combined (Rhus-All Antigen)
Pollens
Stinging Insects (Stinging Insect Antigen #108)
Allergenic Extracts for Immunotherapy
Immunorex - Prescription allergy treatment sets
Rhus-All Antigen (Poison Ivy, Oak, Sumac combined)
Stinging Insect Antigen #108
Diagnostic Allergenic Extracts
Cutaneous
Intracutaneous
Diagnostic Allergenic Test Sets
"50+" - Includes a selection of perennial and seasonal allergens for each of 5 botanical zones
"60 +" - Food allergens only
Regionalized Pollen Test Set
Sensi-Test Kit (Disposable Allergy Scarifier)
Merphene Germicidal Concentrate

BAYLOR LABORATORIES, INC. 638
Post Office Drawer 277
Hurst, TX 76053
Address inquiries to:
John Q. Adams (817) 267-3906
Products Available
Airet G.G. Capsules
Airet G.G. Elixir
Airet G.G. II Liquid
Airet L.A. Tablets
Airet Liquid
Airet II Liquid
Airet 400 Tablets
Airet Tablets
Comhist L.A. Capsules
Comhist Tablets & Liquid
Entex Capsules
Entex KI Tablets
Entex LA Tablets
Entex Liquid
LāBID 250 mg Tablets
Orlex H.C. Otic
Orlex Otic

BEACH PHARMACEUTICALS 405, 640
Division of Beach Products, Inc.
Executive Office
5220 S. Manhattan Ave.
Tampa, FL 33611 (813) 839-6565
Manufacturing and Distribution
Main St. at Perimeter Rd.
Conestee, SC 29605
Toll Free 1-(800) 845-8210
Address inquiries to:
Raymond LaForge, Ph.D. (803) 277-7282
Richard Stephen Jenkins (813) 839-6565
Products Available
Beelith Tablets
Citrolith Tablets
Fer-Bid Improved
◆ K-Phos M.F. (Modified Formula) Tablets
◆ K-Phos Neutral
◆ K-Phos No. 2 Tablets
◆ K-Phos Original Formula 'Sodium Free' Tablets
K-Phos w/S.A.P.
Levo Uroqid-Acid
◆ Thiacide
◆ Uroqid-Acid
◆ Uroqid-Acid No. 2

BEECHAM PRODUCTS 641
Division of Beecham Inc.
P.O. Box 1467
Pittsburgh, PA 15230
Address inquiries to:
Ms. Dona L. Fundis,
Professional Services Dept.
(412) 928-1050
Products Available
Massengill Disposable Douche
Massengill Liquid Concentrate
Massengill Powder

BEECHAM LABORATORIES 405, 642
Division of Beecham, Inc.
Bristol, TN 37620
Address inquiries to:
Medical Director
Beecham Laboratories
501 Fifth Street
Bristol, TN 37620 (615) 764-5141
Distributing Divisions
Arlington, TX 76011
2118 E. Randol Mill Rd. (817) 261-6626
Bristol, TN 37620
501 Fifth Street (615) 764-5141
Elmhurst, IL 60126
449 West Wrightwood Avenue
Mourekson Industrial Center
(312) 530-2424
Orlando, FL 32859
P.O. Box 13770 (305) 859-9300
Piscataway, NJ 08854
101 Possumtown Road (201) 469-5441
or (201) 469-5449
Sacramento, CA 95826
5900 Warehouse Way (916) 381-4030
Products Available
Actol Expectorant Liquid
Actol Expectorant Tablets
Adrenosem Injectable, Syrup & Tablets
◆ Amoxil Capsules and For Oral Suspension
Amoxil Pediatric Drops for Oral Suspension
Anexsia w/Codeine Tablets
Anexsia-D Tablets
Baby Ointment
Bactocill Capsules
Bactocill for Injection
C M w/Paregoric
Celbenin for Injection
Cloxapen Capsules
Conar Expectorant Syrup
Conar Suspension
Conar-A Suspension
◆ Conar-A Tablets
Corrective Mixture
Corrective Mixture w/Paregoric
Cotrol-D Tablets
◆ Daricon
◆ Daricon PB
Dasikon Capsules
Dasin Capsules
Dycill Capsules
◆ Enarax Tablets
◆ Fastin Capsules
Gualfenesin Syrup
Hybephen Tablets
Hycal Liquid
Livitamin Capsules
Livitamin Capsules w/Intrinsic Factor
Livitamin Chewable Tablets
Livitamin Liquid
Livitamin Prenatal Tablets
◆ Menest Tablets
Morphine & Atropine Injectable
Moruguent Ointment
Morusan Ointment
Nucofed Capsules
Nucofed Syrup
Phe-Mer-Nite Tincture 1:3000 (Orange)
Pyopen Injectable
Semets Troches
Thalfed Tablets
Theralax Tablets & Suppositories
Ticar for Injection
◆ Tigan Capsules
Tigan Injectable
Tigan Suppositories
Totacillin Capsules
Totacillin For Oral Suspension
Totacillin-N Injectable
Trisem Suspension & Tablets

BERLEX LABORATORIES INC. 408, 662
Cedar Knolls, NJ 07927
Address inquiries to:
Professional Services
110 East Hanover Avenue
Cedar Knolls, NJ 07927 (201) 540-8700
For Medical Information
Write: Medical Department
110 East Hanover Avenue
Cedar Knolls, NJ 07927
Call: (201) 540-8700 *(Business Hours Only)*
For Medical Emergency Information
After Hours or on Weekends, call
Young W. Cho, M.D., Ph.D. (201) 879-7606
Jerome F. Grattan (201) 821-8846
Products Available
◆ Aminodur Dura-Tabs
Anodynos DHC Tablets
Deconamine Elixir
◆ Deconamine SR Capsules
Deconamine Syrup
◆ Deconamine Tablets
Elixicon Suspension
◆ Elixophyllin Capsules
Elixophyllin Elixir
◆ Elixophyllin SR Capsules
Elixophyllin-KI Elixir
Enuretrol Tablets
Ferronord Tablets
Kay Ciel Elixir
Kay Ciel Powder
L-Glutavite Capsules
Pyocidin-Otic
◆ Quinaglute Dura-Tabs
Stomaseptine
Sus-Phrine Injection
◆ Therapav Capsules
Vi-Twel

BEUTLICH, INC. 667
7006 N. Western Ave.
Chicago, IL 60645 (312) 262-7900
Products Available
Ceo-Two Rectal Suppositories
Hurricaine Oral, Topical Anesthetic Gel
Hurricaine Oral, Topical Anesthetic Liquid
Hurricaine Topical Anesthetic Spray
Mevanin-C Capsules
Mevatinic-C Tablets
Peridin-C Tablets
Pregent Tablets

BIO-DYNAMICS/bmc 2005
Diagnostic Division
9115 Haugue Road
Indianapolis, IN 46250 (317) 845-2000
Products Available
Chemstrip bG Blood Glucose Test
Chemstrip Urine Testing System
Fecscan Fecal Blood Test

Bird CORPORATION 667
92263
MARK 7
Palm Springs, CA 92263 (714) 327-1571
Products Available
microNEFRIN

BOCK PHARMACAL COMPANY 667
5435 Highland Park Drive
St. Louis, MO 63110
Address inquiries to:
Professional Services Dept. (314) 535-4060
Products Available
Amobell Capsules
Broncholate Capsules
Corodyl Forte Capsules
G-200 Capsules
Hemaspan Capsules
Hemaspan-FA Capsules
Hyscorbic Tablets
Limit Tablets
Onset-5 Tablets
Onset-10 Tablets
Pavadyl Capsules
Pavadyl-300 Capsules
Pedo-Sol Elixir
Pedo-Sol Tablets
Poly-Histine Capsules
Poly-Histine Elixir
Poly-Histine Expectorant, Plain
Poly-Histine Expectorant with Codeine
Poly-Histine-D Capsules
Poly-Histine-D Elixir
Poly-Histine-DX Capsules
Poly-Histine-DX Syrup
Theon Elixir
Theon-300 Capsules

BOEHRINGER INGELHEIM LTD. 405, 668
90 East Ridge
P.O. Box 368
Ridgefield, CT 06877
Address inquiries to:
Medical Services Dept. (203) 438-0311
Products Available
Alupent Metered Dose Inhaler
Alupent Syrup
◆ Alupent Tablets
◆ Catapres Tablets
◆ Combipres Tablets
◆ Dulcolax Suppositories
◆ Dulcolax Tablets
◆ Persantine Tablets
◆ Preludin Endurets
◆ Preludin Tablets
Serentil Ampuls
Serentil Concentrate
◆ Serentil Tablets
Torecan Ampuls
Torecan Suppositories
◆ Torecan Tablets

BOOTS PHARMACEUTICALS, INC. 675
6540 Line Avenue
Shreveport, LA 71106
Address inquiries to:
Medical Director (318) 869-3551
Products Available
Azo-Med Tablets
Diaction Tablets
F & B Capsules
F-E-P Creme
Lopurin Tablets
P-200 Tablets
Ruc-Dane Tablets
Ru-Hist Tablets
Ru-Hy-T Tablets
Ru-K-N Liquid
Ru-Lor Tablets
Ru-Lor-N Tablets
Ru-Spas #2 Tablets
Ru-Tuss Expectorant
Ru-Tuss Liquid
Ru-Tuss Plain
Ru-Tuss Tablets
Ru-Vert Liquid
Ru-Vert Tablets
Su-Tinic Liquid
Su-Tinic Tablets
Su-Ton
Su-Zol
Tetra-Bid Capsules
Twin-K

BOWMAN PHARMACEUTICALS 679
Division of Bowman, Inc.
5801 Mayfair Road, N.W.
North Canton OH 44720
Address inquiries to:
C. Richard Chaddock (216) 456-2431
Branch Office
Columbus, OH 43216
111 Liberty St. (614) 224-4157
Products Available
Al-ay Tablets
Asperbuf (Varicolor)
Bovims Improved Tablets
Bowtussin Syrup
Buffets (Haberle)
Butseco Tablets
Digoxin Tablets
Dimentabs
Guistrey Fortis Tablets
Hiserpia
Histagesic (Haberle)
Histrey Syrup & Tablets
Histrey (Time Release Capsule)
Hiwolfia Tablets
Iodized Lime Tablets
Ivy-Chex (Non-Aerosol)
Klix (Time Release Capsule)
Multagen-12 + E Bocaps
Niacal (Haberle)
Niacin Tablets
Niacinamide Tablets
Phendimetrazine Bitartrate
Phenobarbital ⅛ gr Tablets
Rhinibab (Haberle)
Rhinicomp Tablets
Sinoze Tablets
Sodium Levothyroxine
Statomin Maleate CC Improved Tablets
Stim-tab
V.M.F. Tablets (Vitamins & Minerals)

BOYLE & COMPANY 679
6330 Chalet Dr.
Los Angeles CA 90040
Address inquiries to:
Susan M. Boyle (213) 927-9766
Products Available
Citra Capsules
Citra Forte Capsules
Citra Forte Syrup

Digolase Capsules
Glytinic Liquid
Glytinic Tablets
Thera-Deimal Tablets
Triva Combination
Triva Douche Powder
Triva Jel

BREON LABORATORIES INC. 406, 680
90 Park Ave.
New York, NY 10016
Address inquiries to:
Medical Department (212) 972-6316
Main Office
90 Park Avenue
New York, NY 10016 (212) 972-4141
Branch Offices
Atlanta, GA 30336
5090 MacDougall Drive, S.W. (404) 696-4480
Dallas, TX 75235
6627 Maple Ave. (214) 357-4015
Des Plains, IL 60018
200 E. Oakton St. (312) 296-8141
Menlo Park, CA 94025
160 Scott Drive (415) 324-4721
Products Available
Alevaire Solution
Breokinase
Bronkephrine Injection
◆ Bronkodyl
Bronkolixir
Bronkometer Aerosol
Bronkosol
◆ Bronkotabs Tablets
Carbocaine Hydrochloride Injection
◆ Demerol APAP Tablets
Dextrose Solution, 10%
◆ Fergon Capsules
Fergon Elixir
Fergon Plus Caplets
◆ Fergon Tablets
Isuprel Hydrochloride Compound Elixir
◆ Isuprel Hydrochloride Glossets
Isuprel Hydrochloride 1:200 & 1:100
Isuprel Hydrochloride Injection 1:5000
Isuprel Mistometer
Kayexalate
Levophed Bitartrate 0.2% Injection
Marcaine Hydrochloride Solutions
Measurin Tablets
◆ Mebaral Tablets
Novocain for Spinal Anesthesia
Novocain Injection
Pediacof Cough Syrup
Pontocaine Hydrochloride
◆ Trancopal Caplets

BRISTOL LABORATORIES 406, 701
(Div. of Bristol-Myers Co.)
Thompson Rd., P.O. Box 657
Syracuse, NY 13201 (315) 432-2000
Address medical inquiries to:
Dept. of Medical Services (315) 432-2838
or (315) 432-2000
Orders may be placed by calling the following toll free numbers:
Within New York State 1-(800) 962-0904
All Other States 1-(800) 448-1010
(Continental U.S. only)
Mail orders and all inquiries should be sent to:
Bristol Laboratories
Order Entry Department
P.O. Box 657
Syracuse, NY 13201
Products Available
Amikin
Azotrex Capsules
◆ Betapen-VK Tablets and Oral Solution
BiCNU
Blenoxane
◆ Bristacycline Capsules
◆ Bristamycin Tablets
Bristoject Products
- Atropine Sulfate
- Calcium Chloride
- Dextrose
- Epinephrine
- Lidocaine HCl
- Magnesium Sulfate
- Metaraminol Bitartrate
- Sodium Bicarbonate

CeeNU
Cefadyl for Intramuscular or Intravenous Injection
◆ Dynapen Capsules and Powder for Oral Suspension
◆ Kantrex Capsules
Kantrex Injection and Pediatric Injection
Ketaject
Lysodren
Mexate
Mutamycin
Nafcil
◆ Naldecon Syrup, Tablets, Pediatric Drops and Pediatric Syrup
◆ Naldegesic Tablets
Platinol
◆ Polycillin Capsules, for Oral Suspension, and Pediatric Drops
Polycillin-N for Intramuscular or Injection
Polycillin-PRB (ampicillin-probenecid) for Oral Suspension
◆ Polymox Capsules, for Oral Suspension, and Pediatric Drops
◆ Prostaphlin Capsules, Oral Solution
Prostaphlin for Injection
◆ Saluron
◆ Salutensin/Salutensin-Demi
Stadol
Staphcillin Injection—Buffered
◆ Tegopen Capsules and For Oral Solution
◆ Tetrex Capsules, *bid*CAPS
Versapen Oral Suspension and Pediatric Drops
◆ Versapen-K Capsules

BRISTOL-MYERS PRODUCTS 736
(Div. of Bristol-Myers Co.)
345 Park Avenue
New York, NY 10022
Address inquiries to:
Dr. B. M. Lanman (212) 644-4287
Products Available
Ammens medicated powder
Arthritis Strength Bufferin analgesic
B.Q. cold tablets
Ban Basic antiperspirant
Ban Big Ball antiperspirant
Ban cream antiperspirant
Ban roll-on
Ban solid
Body on Tap
Bufferin analgesic
Comtrex capsules
Comtrex liquid
Comtrex tablets
Congespirin cold tablets
Congespirin cough syrup
Congespirin liquid cold medicine
Datril acetaminophen tablets
Datril 500 acetaminophen tablets
Excedrin analgesic
Excedrin P.M. analgesic
4-Way cold tablets
4-Way long acting mentholated nasal spray
4-Way long acting nasal spray
4-Way mentholated nasal spray
4-Way nasal spray
Minit-Rub analgesic balm
Monster vitamins
Monster with Iron vitamins
Multi-Scrub everyday scrubbing lotion with particles
Multi-Scrub medicated cleansing scrub
Mum cream deodorant
No Doz keep alert tablets
Pals plus iron vitamins
Pals vitamins
Pazo hemorrhoid ointment/suppositories
Sal Hepatica laxative
Score hair cream
Tickle antiperspirant
Ultra Ban roll-on
Ultra Ban II antiperspirant
Vitalis Dry Control hair groom
Vitalis Dry Texture hair groom
Vitalis hair groom liquid
Vitalis hair groom tube
Vitalis regular hold hair spray
Vitalis Super Hold hair spray

BROWN PHARMACEUTICAL COMPANY, INC., THE 406, 739
2500 West Sixth St.
Los Angeles, CA 90057
(213) 389-1394-1395
Address inquiries to:
Professional Service Department
Products Available
◆ Android-5 Buccal
◆ Android-10 Tablets
◆ Android-25 Tablets
Android-F Tablets
Android-G I.M.
Brohembione
Calphosan B-12 I.M.
Calphosan I.M.
Cerebro-Nicin Capsules
Heparin Sodium I.M., I.V.
Lipo-Nicin/100 mg.
Lipo-Nicin/250 mg. Tablets
Lipo-Nicin/300 mg. Caps Timed
Vivikon I.M.

BURROUGHS WELLCOME CO. 406, 740
3030 Cornwallis Road
Research Triangle Park, NC 27709
(919) 541-9090
Address inquiries to:
Mr. C. A. Parish, Jr. (919) 541-9090
Branch Office
Burlingame, CA 94010
1760 Rollins Rd. (415) 697-5630
Products Available
◆ Actidil Tablets & Syrup
◆ Actifed Tablets & Syrup
Actifed-C Expectorant
Aerosporin Powder
Aerosporin Otic Solution
◆ Alkeran Tablets
Ammonia Aromatic, Vaporole
Amyl Nitrite, Vaporole
Anectine Flo-Pack
Anectine Injection
◆ Antepar Syrup & Tablets
◆ Ascodeen-30
Atropine Sulfate Injection, Wellcome
Borofax Ointment
◆ Cardilate Chewable Tablets
◆ Cardilate Oral/Sublingual Tablets
◆ Cardilate-P Tablets
Cortisporin Cream
Cortisporin Ointment
Cortisporin Ointment Ophthalmic
Cortisporin Ophthalmic Suspension
Cortisporin Otic Solution
Cortisporin Otic Suspension
◆ Daraprim Tablets
Digoxin (See Lanoxin)
◆ Empirin Analgesic Tablets
◆ Empirin w/Codeine Phosphate Nos. 2, 3 & 4
◆ Empracet with Codeine Phosphate Nos. 3 & 4
◆ Emprazil Tablets
◆ Emprazil-C Tablets
Erythrityl Tetranitrate (See Cardilate)
◆ Fedrazil Tablets
Imuran Injection
◆ Imuran Tablets
◆ Kemadrin Tablets
Lanoline, Wellcome
◆ Lanoxin—Tablets, Injection & Elixir Pediatric
◆ Leukeran Tablets
Lidosporin Otic Solution
Lubafax Surgical Lubricant, Sterile
Mantadil Cream
◆ Marezine Tablets & Injection
◆ Migral Tablets
◆ Myleran Tablets
Neosporin Aerosol
Neosporin G.U. Irrigant
Neosporin Ointment
Neosporin Ointment Ophthalmic
Neosporin Ophthalmic Solution
Neosporin Topical Powder
Neosporin-G Cream
Polymyxin B Sulfate
Polysporin Ointment
Polysporin Ointment Ophthalmic
◆ Purinethol Tablets
Scopolamine Hydrobromide Injection, Wellcome
◆ Septra DS Tablets
Septra Suspension
◆ Septra Tablets
Sudafed Plus Syrup & Tablets
◆ Sudafed Pseudoephedrine Hydrochloride Syrup and Tablets
◆ Sudafed S.A. Capsules
Syncurine Injection
◆ Tabloid brand A.P.C. w/Codeine Phosphate
◆ Tabloid Brand Thioguanine
Vasoxyl Injection
Zincofax Soothing Skin Cream
◆ Zyloprim Tablets

BURTON, PARSONS & COMPANY, INC. 770
120 Westhampton Avenue
Washington, DC 20027 (301) 336-5700
Address inquiries to:
Professional Services Dept.
Products Available
Konsyl
L. A. Formula

CAMPBELL LABORATORIES, INC. 770
145 East 52nd Street, (PH #1)
New York, NY 10022 (212) 688-7684
Address inquiries to:
Richard C. Zahn, President
Post Office Box 812, FDR Station
New York, NY 10022
Products Available
Herpecin-L Cold Sore Lip Balm

CARLTON CORPORATION, THE 770
83 N. Summit Street
Tenafly, NJ 07670
Address inquiries to:
Professional Service Dept. (201) 569-0050
Products Available
Calphosan
Calphosan B-12

CARNRICK LABORATORIES, INC. 407, 771
65 Horse Hill Road
Cedar Knolls, NJ 07927 (201) 267-2670
Address inquiries to:
Medical Director (201) 267-2675
Products Available
◆ Amen
◆ Bontril PDM

◆ Capital with Codeine Suspension
◆ Capital with Codeine Tablets
◆ Hormonin No. 1
◆ Hormonin No. 2
◆ Midrin
◆ Minotal
◆ Nolamine
◆ Phrenilin
◆ Sinulin

CENTRAL PHARMACAL COMPANY, THE 407, 777
112-128 East Third St.
Seymour, IN 47274
Address inquiries to:
Norman B. Kolbe (812) 522-3915
Products Available
Analbalm, Liquid
Andronaq-50 Sterile Suspension
Asphac-G Tablets
Biotres Ointment
Bisilad
Cenac
Cenalene Elixir
Cenalene Tablets
Cenocort A-40 Sterile Suspension
Cenocort Forte Sterile Suspension
Centet-250
Codimal DH Syrup
Codimal DM Syrup
Codimal Expectorant
Codimal Injection
Codimal PH Syrup
Codimal Tablets & Capsules
◆ Codimal-L.A. Cenules
Coditrate Syrup
Coditrate Tablets
Co-Xan Syrup
Dexacen LA-8 Sterile Suspension
Dexacen-4 Injectable
Di-Est Sterile Suspension
Di-Pred Sterile Suspension
Dramocen Injectable
Estradiol Cypionate Injection
Estronol Aqueous Sterile Suspension
Feryl Injection
GG-Cen Syrup/Capsules
Glycogel Tablets
Hexalol Tablets
Lifolbex Injectable
Neocylate Tablets
Neocyten Injection
Neolax Tablets
Niferex Elixir
Niferex Tablets
Niferex w/Vitamin C Tablets
◆ Niferex-150 Capsules
◆ Niferex-150 Forte Capsules
◆ Niferex-PN Tablets
Pavacen Cenules
Phencen-50 Injectable
Prednicen-M Tablets
Prednisolone Acetate Sterile Suspension
Rep Estra Injectable
Rep-Pred 40 Sterile Suspension
Rep-Pred 80 Sterile Suspension
Rhinidrin Tablets
Rhinihist Syrup
Rubesol-1000 Injectable
Rubesol-L.A. 1000 Injectable
Synophylate Elixir
Synophylate Tablets
Synophylate-GG Syrup
Synophylate-GG Tablets
◆ Theoclear L.A.-130 Cenules
◆ Theoclear L.A.-260 Cenules
Theoclear-80 Syrup
◆ Theoclear-100 Tablets
◆ Theoclear-200 Tablets
Uritral Capsules

CENTURY PHARMACEUTICALS, INC. 780
4553 Allisonville Road
Indianapolis, IN 46205
Address inquiries to:
Ross A. Deardorff, R.Ph. (317) 547-6888
Products Available
Aceta with Codeine
B-12 Injection
Cenahist
Conest
Cortigesic Otic Drops
Hydrozide
Indogesic
Iodosone Cream
L-Caine Injection
Nil Vaginal Cream
Pavadur
Polydine Ointment
Polydine Scrub
Polydine Solution
Potassium Chloride Liquid
Potassium Chloride Powder
Rectacort Suppository
Sodium Hypochlorite
Sodium P.A.S.
Vitanate FA

CETYLITE INDUSTRIES, INC. 780
9051 River Road
Pennsauken, NJ 08110
Address inquiries to:
Mr. Stanley L. Wachman, President
(609) 665-6111
Products Available
Cetacaine Topical Anesthetic
Cetylcide Germicidal Concentrate
Protexin Oral Breath Spray
Protexin Oral Rinse Concentrate
Skin Screen Protective Skin Lotion

CIBA PHARMACEUTICAL COMPANY 408, 781
Division of CIBA-GEIGY Corporation
Address inquiries to:
556 Morris Avenue
Summit, NJ 07901
New Jersey (201) 277-5000
New York (212) 267-6615
Division Offices
Warehouse Offices and Shipping Branches
Eastern
14 Henderson Drive
West Caldwell, NJ 07006 (201) 575-6510
New York (212) 267-6640
Central
7530 No. Natchez Ave.
Niles, IL 60648 Niles (312) 647-9332
Chicago (312) 763-8700
Western
100 Rollins Road
Millbrae, CA 94030
Millbrae (415) 697-1444
San Francisco Bay Area
Dial 0 - Ask for Enterprise 16447
Products Available
◆ Antrenyl Tablets
◆ Anturane Capsules
◆ Anturane Tablets
◆ Apresazide Capsules
Apresoline Ampuls
◆ Apresoline Tablets
◆ Apresoline-Esidrix Tablets
Coramine Ampuls
Coramine Oral Solution
Desferal Vials
◆ Dialog Tablets
◆ Dianabol Tablets
◆ Esidrix Tablets
◆ Esimil Tablets
◆ Forhistal Lontabs
INH Tablets
◆ Ismelin Tablets
Locorten Cream
◆ Metandren Linguets and Tablets
◆ Metopirone Tablets
Nupercainal Cream
Nupercainal Ointment
Nupercainal Suppositories
Nupercaine Ampuls 1:200
Nupercaine Ampuls 1:1500
Nupercaine (Heavy) Ampuls
Ocular Therapeutic System
Ocusert
Percorten Pellets
Percorten pivalate Multiple-dose Vials
Priscoline Multiple-dose Vials
Priscoline Tablets & Lontabs
Privine Nasal Solution
Privine Nasal Spray
◆ Regitine hydrochloride Tablets
Regitine mesylate Vials
◆ Rimactane Capsules
Rimactane/INH Dual Pack
◆ Ritalin Tablets
◆ Ser-Ap-Es Tablets
Serpasil Ampuls
Serpasil Elixir
Serpasil Parenteral Solution
◆ Serpasil Tablets
◆ Serpasil-Apresoline Tablets
◆ Serpasil-Esidrix Tablets
◆ Slow-K Tablets
Vioform Cream
Vioform Ointment
Vioform-Hydrocortisone Cream
Vioform-Hydrocortisone Lotion
Vioform-Hydrocortisone Mild Cream
Vioform-Hydrocortisone Mild Ointment
Vioform-Hydrocortisone Ointment

CIRCLE PHARMACEUTICALS, INC. 811
4553 Allisonville Road
Indianapolis, IN 46205
Address inquiries to:
Ross A. Deardorff, R.Ph. (317) 546-8855
Products Available
Amcap
Aromatic Elixir
Circavite T
Duohist Tablet
Paxarel
Restora
Septa Ointment
Suspen
Tetracap

Tusquelin
Uropeutic

COMATIC LABORATORIES, INC. 812
Post Office Box 42300
Houston, TX 77042
Address inquiries to:
Professional Services Dept. (713) 783-2032
Evening Emergency (713) 493-5953
Products Available
Acetaminophen with Codeine Elixir
▣ Anuphen Suppositories
Aspirin Suppositories
Bisacodyl Suppositories
Dibucaine Ointment
Guaifenesin Syrup
Guaifenesin-Dextromethorphan Syrup
▣ Hepahydrin Tablets
Matropinal Elixir
Matropinal Forte Inserts
Matropinal Inserts
Matropinal Tablets
▣ Oraphen-PD (Additive Free)
Phenobarbital Elixir (Additive Free)
Pseudoephedrine Syrup
Rhinosyn Capsules
▣ Rhinosyn Syrup (Additive Free)
▣ Rhinosyn-DM Syrup (Additive Free)
▣ Rhinosyn-PD Syrup (Additive Free)
▣ Rhinosyn-X Syrup (Additive Free)

COMER PHARMACEUTICALS, INC. 812
P.O. Box 5471
Hamden, CT 06518 (203) 281-6116
Address inquiries to:
Ben Comer, R.Ph. President
Joyce B. Comer, Pharm. D. Vice-Pres.
Director of CME.
Products Available
Amoxicillin Capsules
Amoxicillin Oral Suspension
Ampicillin Capsules
Ampicillin Powder
Erythromycin Stearate Film Tabs.
Penicillin G Potassium Tablets
Penicillin VK Powder
Penicillin VK Tablets
Prednisone Tablets
Tetracycline HCl Capsules

CONNAUGHT LABORATORIES, INC. 813
Swiftwater, PA 18370
Address inquiries to:
Marketing Services Ass't (717) 839-7187
For Medical Emergencies Contact:
Medical Director (717) 839-7187
Direct orders & returns to:
Elkins-Sinn, Inc.,
Customer Services (800) 257-8349
Distributed in the Continental U.S.A. by:
Elkins-Sinn, Inc.
2 Esterbrook Lane
Cherry Hill, NJ 08034
Products Available
Diphtheria Antitoxin (Purified, Concentrated Globulin-Equine)
Diphtheria and Tetanus Toxoids and Pertussis Vaccine Adsorbed (For Pediatric Use)
Fluzone (Influenza Virus Vaccine)
Menomune (Meningococcal Polysaccharide Vaccine, Groups A and C Combined, Group A or Group C
Tetanus Toxoid
Tetanus Toxoid Adsorbed
Tetanus and Diphtheria Toxoids Adsorbed (For Adult Use)
Yellow Fever Vaccine

CONNAUGHT LABORATORIES, LTD. 813
1755 Steeles Avenue West
Willowdale, Ontario M2N5T8, Canada
Address inquiries to:
Manager, International Customer Services (416) 667-2630
For Medical Emergencies Contact:
Medical Director (416) 667-2622
Direct orders & returns to:
Elkins-Sinn, Inc.
Customer Services (800) 257-8349
Distributed in the Continental U.S.A. by:
Elkins-Sinn, Inc.
2 Esterbrook Lane
Cherry Hill, NJ 08034
Products Available
Albuconn (Normal Serum Albumin [Human], 5% & 25%
Poliomyelitis Vaccine (Purified) (For the Prevention of Poliomyelitis)
Tet-Conn-G (Tetanus Immune Globulin [Human])
Tuberculin Purified Protein Derivative (Concentrated Solution in 50% Glycerine for Sterneedle [Heaf] Multiple Puncture Test)
Tubersol (Tuberculin Purified Protein Derivative [Mantoux]

(◆ Shown in Product Identification Section) (▣ Described in PDR For Nonprescription Drugs)

CONSOLIDATED CHEMICAL, INC. 813
3224 So. Kingshighway Blvd.
St. Louis, MO 63139
Address inquiries to:
John A. Brereton (314) 772-4610
Products Available
CC-500
Consept
Consol 20
Consol Concentrate
Formula Magic
Perineal Spray Cleaner
Satin
Skin Magic
Staphoclean
Staphosan
Swirlsoft

COOK-WAITE LABORATORIES, INC. 814
90 Park Avenue
New York, NY 10016 (212) 972-4141
Products Available
Carbocaine Hydrochloride 3% Injection
Carbocaine Hydrochloride 2% with Neo-Cobefrin 1:20,000 Injection

COOPER LABORATORIES, INC. 408, 815
Internal Medicine Division
(See Berlex Laboratories, Inc.)

CUTTER BIOLOGICAL 815, 2006
Div. Cutter Laboratories, Inc
4th & Parker Sts.
Berkeley, CA 94710
Address inquiries to:
Director of Professional Services
(415) 841-0123
Branch Offices
Chattanooga, TN 37421
5910 Quintus Loop (615) 624-4661
Chicago Office
725 Golf Lane
Bensenville, IL 60106 (312) 595-3620
Dallas, TX 75240
4542 McEwen Road (214) 661-5850
Los Angeles Office
15320 East Salt Lake Avenue
City of Industry, CA 91744
(213) 968-8561
New Orleans Office
2631 Delaware St.
Kenner, LA 70062 (504) 469-8479
New York Office
40 E. Cotters Lane
East Brunswick, NJ 08816
(201) 238-0140
Ogden, UT 84404
475 W. Cutter Way (801) 393-8401
Northern California Office
2480 Baumann Avenue
San Lorenzo, CA 94580 (415) 276-8200
Seattle Office
1147 Andover Park West
Tukwila, WA 98188 (206) 575-0490
Products Available
Antihemophilic Factor (Human) (Factor VIII, AHF, AHG) Koāte
Antithrombin III Assay—ThromboScreen
Factor IX Complex (Human) (Factors II, VII, IX, and X) Konȳne
Gamastan (Immune Serum Globulin-Human)
Heparin Assay—ThromboScreen
Hepatitis B Immune Globulin (Human) HyperHep
Hyperab (Rabies Immune Globulin-Human)
HyperHep (Hepatitis B Immune Globulin-Human)
Hyper-Tet (Tetanus Immune Globulin-Human)
Hypertussis (Pertussis Immune Globulin-Human)
HypRho-D (Rh_o-D Immune Globulin-Human)
Immune Serum Globulin (Human) Gamastan
Koāte (Factor VIII, Antihemophilic Factor-Human)
Konȳne (Factor IX Complex-Human) (Factors II, VII, IX and X)
Pertussis Immune Globulin (Human) Hypertussis
Plague Vaccine (Human)
Rh_o-D Immune Globulin (Human) HypRho-D
Rabies Immune Globulin (Human) Hyperab
Tetanus Immune Globulin (Human) Hyper-Tet

DALIN PHARMACEUTICALS, INC. 815
1750 New Highway
Farmingdale, NY 11735
Address inquiries to:
Professional Services Dept. (516) 454-9282
Subsidiary:
Garden Pharmaceuticals, Inc.
DG Packaging
Branch Offices
Panamerican Pharmaceutical Distributors, Inc.
Reparada Industrial Park
Estacion #6
Ponce, Puerto Rico 00731
(809) 842-6263

Products Available
About Face Tablets
Aerosept
Aquatabs
Aquatabs Plus Iron
Audax Ear Drops
Ban Itch
Bio Slim T Capsules
Bio Slim Tablets
Celluzyme Capsules
Cremesone
Dalex Capsules & Lozenges
Dalex Pediatric Syrup
Dalex Syrup
Dalex Syrup Forte
Dalicote Lotion
Dalicreme
Daliderm Liquid & Powder
Dalidyne
Dalidyne Jel
Dalidyne Spray (Mouth and Throat)
Dalifort Tablets
Daligesic Liniment
Dalihist Nasal Spray
Dalimycin Capsules
Dalisept Ointment
Dalivim Forte Liquid & Tablets
Dermasoothe
Eez Cream
Liqui-Trim Drops
Pentarcort Cream
Phase 5 Lotion
Phase 10 Lotion
Phenagesic Syrup & Capsules
Phenatuss Expectorant
Podiaspray
Polysept Ointment
Salts of the Earth
Second Honeymoon Tablets
Slim One Capsules
Sorbutuss
Spandecon Capsules
Spasmid Elixir & Capsules
Syr Tane
Syr Tane Jr.
Tricon Syrup

DAYWELL LABORATORIES CORPORATION 815
78 Unquowa Place, Fairfield, CT 06430
Address inquiries to:
Judge J. H. Norton (203) 255-3154
Products Available
Vergo

DELCO CHEMICAL CO., INC. 815
Sellersville, PA 18960
Address inquiries to:
Mr. Mark Rosenwald (215) 723-5544
(800) 523-6542
Products Available
Delcobese Capsules
Delcobese Tablets
Delcobese T.R. Capsules

DERMIK LABORATORIES, INC. 817
500 Virginia Drive
Fort Washington, PA 19034
Address inquiries to:
Albert M. Packman, D.Sc. (215) 628-6429
Branch Offices
Fort Washington, PA 19034
500 Virginia Drive (215) 628-6550
Hammond, IN 46320
2500 165th Street (219) 845-1677
San Leandro, CA 94577
1550 Factor Avenue (415) 357-9741
Tucker, GA 30084
4660 Hammermill Road (404) 934-3091
Products Available
Anthra-Derm Ointment
10-Benzagel (Acne Gel) & 5-Benzagel (Acne Gel)
Comfortine Ointment
Drest
Fomac Foam
Hytone Cream ½%
Hytone Cream 1%
Hytone Cream 2½%
Hytone Ointment ½%, 1%
Jeri-Bath
Jeri-Lotion
Klaron Acne Lotion
Loroxide Acne Lotion
Loroxide-HC Lotion
Postacne Acne Lotion
Rezamid Acne Lotion
Shepard's Cream Lotion
Shepard's Dry Skin Cream
Shepard's Hand Cream
Shepard's Moisturizing Soap
Sulfacet-R Lotion
Vanoxide Acne Lotion
Vanoxide-HC Lotion
Vytone Cream ½%, 1%
Zetar Emulsion
Zetar Shampoo

DISTA PRODUCTS COMPANY 409, 820
Division of Eli Lilly and Company
General Offices
307 East McCarty Street, 46225
Post Office Box 1407
Indianapolis, IN 46206
For Medical Information, Write:
Medical Department
307 East McCarty Street
Post Office Box 618
Indianapolis, IN 46206 (317) 261-4000
Regional Sales Offices
Chicago, IL 60631
Suite 270, O'Hare Plaza
5735 East River Road (312) 693-8360
Norcross, GA 30091
5944 Peachtree Corners East
Post Office Box 628 (404) 449-4928
Pasadena, CA 91101
301 East Colorado Blvd. (213) 792-3197
White Plains, NY 10604
925 Westchester Ave. (914) 949-7755
Products Available
Becotin Pulvules
◆ Becotin with Vitamin C Pulvules
◆ Becotin-T Tablets
◆ Co-Pyronil Pulvules, Pediatric Pulvules, and Suspension
◆ Cordran Ointment & Lotion
◆ Cordran SP Cream
◆ Cordran Tape
Cordran-N Cream and Ointment
◆ Ilosone Chewable Tablets
Ilosone, for Oral Suspension
Ilosone Liquids, Oral Suspensions
◆ Ilosone Pulvules and Tablets
Ilosone Ready-Mixed Drops
Ilotycin Gluceptate, I.V., Ampoules
Ilotycin Ointment
Ilotycin Sterile Ophthalmic Ointment
◆ Ilotycin Tablets
◆ Mi-Cebrin Tablets
◆ Mi-Cebrin T Tablets
◆ Nalfon Pulvules and Tablets
◆ Trinsicon Pulvules
Trinsicon M Pulvules
◆ Valmid Pulvules

DOAK PHARMACAL CO., INC. 831
700 Shames Drive
Westbury, L.I., NY 11590
Address inquiries to:
Frank P. Panzarella, Ph.D. (516) 333-7222
Branch Offices
Obergfel Brothers
2660 East 37th Street
Vernon, CA 90058 (213) 583-8981
Products Available
Buro-Sol Antiseptic Powder
Diasporal Cream
Doak Oil & Doak Oil Forte
Formula 405
Lavatar
Lotio Alsulfa
Normaderm Cream
Normaderm Lotion
Petro-Phylic Soap Cake
Solar Cream
Tar Distillate "Doak"
Tar-Doak Lotion
Tarpaste
Tersaseptic
Tersa-Tar
Unguentum Bossi

DOME DIVISION 831
Miles Laboratories, Inc.
400 Morgan Lane
West Haven, CT 06516
Address inquiries to:
Director, Medical Services (203) 934-9225
Products Available
Acne-Dome Creme & Lotion
Acne-Dome Medicated Cleanser
Allpyral Allergenic Extracts
Candex Creme
Candex Lotion
Cort-Dome ⅛%, ¼%, ½%, and 1% Creme
Cort-Dome ⅛%, ¼%, ½%, and 1% Lotion
Cort-Dome Suppositories
DTIC-Dome
Daxolin C Liquid
Daxolin Capsules
Decholin Tablets
Domeboro Powder Packets, Effervescent Tablets
Dome-Paste Bandage (Unna's Boot)
Domol Bath & Shower Oil
Exzit Medicated Cleanser
Exzit Medicated Creme and Lotion
Lidaform-HC Creme
Lithane Tablets
Mithracin
Mycelex 1% Cream
Mycelex 1% Solution
Mycelex-G Tablets & Cream
Mycelex-G 1% Vaginal Cream
Nystaform Ointment

Otic Domeboro Solution
Otic Neo-Cort-Dome Suspension
Otic Tridesilon Solution
Stilphostrol Tablets and Ampuls
Sungard Lotion
Tridesilon Creme 0.05%
Tridesilon Ointment 0.05%

DOONER LABORATORIES, INC. **409, 843**
500 Virginia Drive
Fort Washington, PA 19034
Address inquiries to:
Johanna L. Roskow, Marketing Services Manager (215) 628-6314
Products Available
◆ D-Feda Gyrocaps
D-Feda Syrup
Dularin Syrup
Fedahist Expectorant
◆ Fedahist Gyrocaps
◆ Fedahist Syrup & Tablets
◆ Slo-Phyllin 60 Gyrocaps
◆ Slo-Phyllin 125 Gyrocaps
◆ Slo-Phyllin 250 Gyrocaps
◆ Slo-Phyllin Tablets
Slo-Phyllin 80 Syrup
◆ Slo-Phyllin GG Capsules
Slo-Phyllin GG Syrup

DORSEY LABORATORIES **409, 844**
Division of Sandoz, Inc.
P.O. Box 83288
Lincoln, NB 68501
Address inquiries to:
Medical Department (402) 464-6311
Products Available
Acid Mantle Creme and Lotion
◆ Asbron G Elixir and Inlay-Tabs
◆ Bellergal Tablets
◆ Bellergal-S Tablets
Calurin Tablets
◆ Cama Inlay-Tabs
Chexit Tablets
Dorcol Pediatric Cough Syrup
Dorsacaine Solution (Benoxinate Hydrochloride Ophthalmic Solution)
Glysennid Tablets
◆ Gris-PEG Tablets
◆ Kanulase Tablets
◆ Klorvess Effervescent Granules/Tablets
Klorvess 10% Liquid
MSC Triaminic Tablets
◆ Metaprel MDI, Syrup, Tablets
Neo-Calglucon Syrup
Pabirin Buffered Tablets
Rautensin Tablets
Sunbrella Sunscreen Lotion
◆ Tavist Tablets
◆ Tavist-1 Tablets
◆ Trest Tablets
Triaminic Expectorant
Triaminic Expectorant DH
Triaminic Expectorant w/Codeine
Triaminic Juvelets
Triaminic Oral Infant Drops
Triaminic Syrup
Triaminic Tablets
Triaminic-DM Cough Formula
▣ Triaminicin Chewables
▣ Triaminicin Tablets
Triaminicol Syrup
▣ Tussagesic Tablets & Suspension
Tussaminic Tablets
▣ Ursinus Inlay-Tabs
Uval Sunscreen Lotion
Vacuetts Suppositories

DOW PHARMACEUTICALS **410, 852**
The Dow Chemical Company
P.O. Box 68511
Indianapolis, IN 46268
Address inquiries to:
Director, Professional Relations (317) 873-7338
Products Available
Accurbron
Dow-Isoniazid
Dyclone 0.5%, 1%
◆ Lorelco
Neocholan
Neo-Polycin Ophthalmic
Neo-Polycin Ophthalmic Solution
Neo-Polycin Topical Antibiotic
◆ Novafed A Capsules
Novafed A Liquid
◆ Novafed Capsules
Novafed Liquid
Novahistine DH
▣ Novahistine DMX
▣ Novahistine Elixir
Novahistine Expectorant
▣ Novahistine Sinus Tablets
▣ Novahistine Tablets
Phenoxene
Quide Tablets
◆ Rifadin
◆ Rifamate
◆ Singlet
▣ 2/G
▣ 2/G-DM
Tussend Expectorant
Tussend Liquid & Tablets

DOYLE PHARMACEUTICAL CO., THE **862**
A Division of The Delmark Company, Inc.
5320 West 23rd Street
Minneapolis, MN 55416
Address inquiries to:
L. R. Eggleston (612) 925-2100
Products Available
Citrotein
Compleat-B
Controlyte
Dietene
Meritene Liquid
Meritene Powder
Precision High Nitrogen Diet
Precision Isotonic Diet
Precision LR Diet

DRUG INDUSTRIES CO., INC. **410, 864**
13700 Woodward Avenue
Detroit, MI 48203
Address inquiries to:
Howard W. Mordue, Pres. (313) 883-3784
Products Available
A-Caps
◆ Al-Vite
BC-Vite
◆ Bilax
C-Caps 500
Calfer-Vite
Day-Vite
Dee-Caps
Di-Pav
Di-Sosul
Di-Sosul Forte
E-Plus
◆ Hemo-Vite
Hemo-Vite Liquid
N-Caps 400
Pro-min-vite
Sinovan Timed
◆ Trilax
Vanodonnal Timed
Vicef

ELDER, INC., THOMAS C. **410, 865**
P.O. Box 125
Hamilton, IN 46742

ELDER, COMPANY, PAUL B. **410, 865**
705 E. Mulberry Street
Bryan, OH 43506
Address inquiries to:
P.O. Box 31
Bryan, OH (800) 537-4294
In Ohio (419) 636-1168
Products Available
Alised (Revised) Tablet
Allylgesic w/Ergotamine Tartrate Capsule
Analgesine Liquid
Ansemco #8 Tablet
Benoquin Ointment
CZO Lotion
Caleate Ointment
Chlorpheniramine Maleate Capsule
Codel Syrup
Coldate Tablet
Coryzaid Tablet
Coryztime Capsule
Danthross
Diastay Tablet
Donabarb Tablet
Eldadryl Cough Syrup
El-Da-Mint Tablet
Eldatapp Tablets
Eldecort Cream
Eldefed Tablets
Elder Cold Tabs
Elder Compound 65 Capsule
Elder Diaper Rash Ointment
Eldodram Tablets
Eldopaque Ointment
Eldopaque-Forte Ointment
Eldoquin Lotion
Eldoquin Ointment
Eldoquin-Forte Ointment
Elpetn
Elzyme 303 Tablets
FBC Tabs
HQC Kit
Hydrelt Ointment
Hyperetic
Hyperserp
Iodized Lime Tablet
Isohalant Liquid
Kamadrox Tablet
LV Penicillin Tablets
Nitrofurantoin
Noviplex Capsule
Opacedrin Capsule
Opasal Capsule
Ostrakal Tablet
◆ Oxsoralen Capsules
Oxsoralen Lotion
Pabanol Lotion
Parbocyl
Phencaset Tablet
Phendimetrazine Tartrate
Psoralite
Quadetts Tablet
Quadramoid Liquid
RVP Ointment
RVPaba Lip Stick
RVPaque Ointment
RVPlus Ointment
Statuss Capsules & Syrup
T-250 Caps
TSG Croup Liquid
TSG-KI Elixir
Teenac Ointment
◆ Trisoralen Tablets
Urostat Forte Tablets
Vagadine Suppositories
Velvet Glove Hand Cream
Vitadye Liquid
Vitamin B-12 Injectable
Volaxin Tablet

ELKINS-SINN, INC. **867**
A subsidiary of A.H. Robins Company
2 Esterbrook Lane
Post Office Box 5483
Cherry Hill, NJ 08034
(609) 424-3700
Address price and packaging inquiries to:
Customer Service
Address scientific information inquiries to:
Technical Services
Products Available
Aminophylline Injection
Ascorbic Acid Injection
Atropine Sulfate Injection
Calcium Chloride Injection
Calcium Gluconate Injection
Chlorpromazine HCl Injection
Codeine Phosphate Injection
Cyanocobalamin Injection
Dexamethasone Sodium Phosphate Injection
Dexpanthenol Injection
Dextrose Injection
Digoxin Injection
Diphenhydramine HCl Injection
Epinephrine Injection
Heparin Sodium Injection
Hep-Lock (Heparin Sodium for IV Flush)
Hydromorphone HCl Injection
Isoproterenol HCl Injection
Lidocaine HCl Injection
Lidocaine Hydrochloride Injection for Cardiac Arrhythmias
Lidocaine HCl & Epinephrine Injection
Magnesium Sulfate Injection
Meperidine HCl Injection
Metaraminol Bitartrate Injection
Methylene Blue Injection
Mineral Oil, Sterile
Morphine Sulfate Injection
Neomycin Sulfate (not sterile)
Neostigmine Methylsulfate Injection
Paraldehyde, Sterile
Pentobarbital Sodium Injection
Phenobarbital Sodium Injection
Phenobarbital Sodium, Sterile
Phenytoin Sodium Injection
Potassium Chloride Injection
Procaine HCl Injection
Promethazine HCl Injection
Scopolamine HBr Injection
Secobarbital Sodium, Sterile
Sodium Chloride Injection
Sotradecol (Sodium Tetradecyl Sulfate Injection)
Sterile Empty Vials
Thiamine HCl Injection
Water For Injection

EMKO COMPANY, THE
Note: Products formerly available from the Emko Company, are now marketed by Schering Corporation. Please refer to the Schering Corporation segment of the product information section for complete prescribing information on the following products:
Because Contraceptor Vaginal Contraceptive Foam
Emko Pre-Fil Vaginal Contraceptive Foam
Emko Contraceptor Vaginal Contraceptive Foam

ENDO LABORATORIES, INC. **410, 868**
Sub. of the DuPont Company
1000 Stewart Ave.
Garden City, NY 11530
Address inquiries to:
Director, Professional Services (516) 832-2123
Emergency No. (516) 832-2210
Branch Offices
Chicago, IL 60641
4956 W. Belmont Ave. (312) 282-0440
Los Angeles, CA 90064
11400 W. Olympic Blvd. (213) 272-7153

ENDO INC. **410, 868**
Manati, Puerto Rico 00701
Subsidiary of the DuPont Company
Address inquiries to:
Endo Laboratories, Inc.
Sub. of the DuPont Company
1000 Stewart Avenue
Garden City, NY 11530
Director, Professional Services
(516) 832-2123
Products Available
Acon Capsules
◆ Azene Capsules
◆ Coumadin Injection & Tablets
Endecon Tablets
Endotussin-NN Pediatric Syrup
Endotussin-NN Syrup
Hycodan Syrup, Tablets
◆ Hycomine Compound Tablets
Hycomine Pediatric Syrup
Hycomine Syrup
Hycotuss Expectorant Syrup
◆ Moban Tablets
Narcan Injection
Narcan Neonatal Injection
Nubain Injection
Numorphan Hydrochloride Injection, Suppositories
Percobarb Capsules
◆ Percocet-5 Tablets
◆ Percodan Tablets
◆ Percodan-Demi Tablets
Percogesic Tablets
Percogesic w/Codeine Tablets
Remsed Tablets
◆ Symmetrel Capsules and Syrup
◆ Tessalon Perles
◆ Valpin 50 Tablets
◆ Valpin 50-PB Tablets
Tin-Co-Ben Dispenser
Vio-Pramosone Cream
Vio-Pramosone Lotion

ETHICAL DATA, INC. **2006**
Post Office Box 263
West Chicago, IL 60185
Address inquiries to:
Oscar G. Rasmussen, Ph.D. (312) 293-0660
Products Available
Hair Analysis TMA-H

EVERETT LABORATORIES, INC. **880**
76 Franklin Street
East Orange, NJ 07017
Address inquiries to:
Professional Service Dept. (201) 674-8455
Products Available
Anatym Capsules
Florvite Chewable Tablets
Florvite Pediatric Drops
Florvite & Iron Pediatric Drops
Nicotym Capsules
Nitrotym Capsules
Pavatym Capsules
Repan Tablets
Vitafol Tablets

FERNDALE LABORATORIES, INC. **880**
780 W. Eight Mile Road
Ferndale, MI 48220
Address inquiries to:
Professional Service Dept. (313) 548-0900
Products Available
Adphen Capsules
Adphen Tablets
Aquaphyllin Syrup
Bellkatal Tablets
Betuline Liniment
Dapa Tablets
Dapa & Codeine Tablets
Dapase Tablets
Delaxin Tablets
Detachol Adhesive Remover
Dexasone Phosphate Injectable
Doss 300 Capsule
Ferndex Tablets
Fernisolone Injectable
Fernisolone-P-Tablets
Fernisone Injectable
Flavitab Tablets
Kronofed-A-Kronocaps
Kronohist Kronocaps
Liqui-Doss
Livonamine Tablets
Lixaminol AT Elixir
Lixaminol Elixir
Maigret Tablets
Mastisol Liquid Adhesive
Niapent Tablets
Oxychinol Tablets
Panacort R-P Injectable
Pernavit Injectable
Phenobella Tablets
Pramosone Cream
Pramosone Lotion
Procute Cream
Procute Lotion
Rauserpin Tablets
Salatin & Codeine Tablets
Strifon Forte Tablets
Strilaxin Tablets
Tin-Ben Dispenser

FERRING PHARMACEUTICALS INC. **880**
475 Park Avenue South
New York, NY 10016
Address inquiries to:
Mr. Dan Silkiss (212) 725-5665
For Medical Emergencies Contact:
Dr. J. H. Cort (212) 348-1111
(212) 725-5665
(nights) (212) 751-6384
Place orders at the following Branch Office:
Centerchem Products Inc.
475 Park Avenue South
New York, NY 10016 (212) 725-5665
Products Available
DDAVP (Desmopressin Acetate)

FISONS CORPORATION **881**
Pharmaceutical Division
Two Preston Court
Bedford, MA 01730
Address inquiries to:
Professional Services Dept. (617) 275-1000
Distribution Centers
ATLANTA
James M. Hogan Co., Inc.
1595 Mountain Industrial Blvd.
Stone Mountain, GA 30083
(404) 938-7901
BEDFORD
Fisons Corporation
2 Preston Court
Bedford, MA 01730 (617) 275-1000
LOS ANGELES
Obergfel Brothers
2660 East 37th Street
Vernon, CA 90058 (213) 583-8981
Products Available
Bacid Capsules
Ergomar
Intal
Kondremul
Kondremul with Cascara
Kondremul with Phenolphthalein
Persistin
Somophyllin Oral Liquid
Somophyllin Rectal Solution
Somophyllin-T Capsules
Tusscapine
Vapo-Iso Solution
Vaponefrin Solution
Vi-Syneral Injectable
Vi-Syneral One Caps
Vitron-C
Vitron-C-Plus

FLEET CO., INC., C. B. **887**
4615 Murray Pl.
Lynchburg, VA 24506
Address inquiries to:
William P. Ferrell (804) 528-4000
Products Available
Fleet Bisacodyl Enema
Fleet Enema
Fleet Enema Pediatric
Fleet Mineral Oil Enema
Fleet Phospho-Soda
Fleet Prep Kits

FLEMING & COMPANY **888**
1600 Fenpark Dr.
Fenton, MO 63026
Address inquiries to:
John J. Roth, M.D. (314) 343-8200
Products Available
Aerolate Liquid
Aerolate III
Aerolate Jr. T. D. Capsules
Aerolate Sr. T. D. Capsules
Alumadrine Tablets
Ectasule Minus III
Ectasule Minus Jr. T. D. Capsules
Ectasule Minus Sr. T. D. Capsules
Ectasule III
Ectasule Jr. T. D. Capsules
Ectasule Sr. T. D. Capsules
Extendryl Chewable Tablets
Extendryl Syrup
Extendryl T. D. Capsules
Impregon Concentrate
Magonate Tablets
▣ Marblen Suspension Peach/Apricot
▣ Marblen Suspension Unflavored
▣ Marblen Tablets
Menotabs Tablets
▣ Nephrox Suspension
▣ Nicotinex Elixir
Obegyn Tablets
▣ Ocean Nasal Mist
Ocean-Plus Mist
Pima Syrup
Pseudo-G T.D. Capsules
Rum-K Syrup
S-P-T "Liquid" Capsules

FLINT LABORATORIES **410, 888**
Division of Travenol Laboratories, Inc.
Deerfield, IL 60015 (312) 480-5224
(312) 480-5227
Address inquiries to:
Professional Services Dept.
Products Available
◆ Choloxin
Synthroid Injection
◆ Synthroid Tablets
◆ Travase Ointment

FLUORITAB CORPORATION **891**
P.O. Box 381
Flint, MI 48501
Address inquiries to Main Office:
M. L. Cleveland, Manager (1-313) 239-9770
Howard D. Vogt, (1-813) 439-1652
Research & Promotion
Post Office Box 263
Lake Hamilton, FL 33851
Products Available
Fluoritab Liquid
Fluoritab Tablets

FOREST LABORATORIES, INC. **891**
919 Third Avenue
New York, NY 10022
Address inquiries to:
Professional Service Dept. (212) 421-7850
Products Available
Brocon C.R. Tablets
Brocon Chewable Tablets
Sudachron CR Tablets

FRYE PHARMACEUTICALS, INC. **892**
2625 2nd Avenue, North
P.O. Box 10163
Birmingham, AL 35202
Address inquiries to:
Bill Frye, President (205) 252-5833
Products Available
C-Bid 1000 Tablets
C-Natal FA Tablets
Isor-Bid Capsules
Norcet Tablets
Novert Capsules
Obe-Nil Tablets
Obe-Nil TR Capsules
Obe-Nix 30 Capsules
Otocain
PT-300 Capsules
Polyflex Tablets
Pseudo-Bid Capsules
Pseudo-Bid A Capsules
Pseudo-Hist Capsules
Pseudo-Hist Expectorant
Pseudo-Hist Liquid
T-Lex Elixir
T-Lex Tablets
Theratinic-C Tablets
Vagi-Nil Cream

GEIGY PHARMACEUTICALS **411, 893**
Division of CIBA-GEIGY Corporation
Ardsley, NY 10502
Address inquiries to:
Medical Services Dept. (201) 277-5000
Products Available
Brethine Ampuls
◆ Brethine Tablets
◆ Butazolidin
◆ Butazolidin Alka
Eurax Cream & Lotion
◆ Lioresal Tablets
◆ Lopressor Tablets
Otrivin Nasal Spray
Otrivin Nasal Solution
Otrivin Pediatric Solution
PBZ Elixir
PBZ Expectorant w/Codeine & Ephedrine
PBZ Expectorant w/Ephedrine
PBZ Hydrochloride Cream
PBZ Hydrochloride Ointment
PBZ Lontabs
◆ PBZ Tablets
PBZ Tablets w/Ephedrine
◆ PBZ-SR Tablets
◆ Tandearil
◆ Tegretol
Tofranil Ampuls
◆ Tofranil Tablets
◆ Tofranil-PM

GERBER PRODUCTS COMPANY **912**
Fremont, MI 49412 (616) 928-2000
Address inquiries to:
Professional Communications Department
Products Available
Gerber Cereals
Barley Cereal
Cereals with Fruit
High Protein Cereal
Mixed Cereal
Oatmeal Cereal
Rice Cereal
Gerber High Meat Dinners (Strained & Junior)

(◆ Shown in Product Identification Section)

(▣ Described in PDR For Nonprescription Drugs)

943

-7687

its
s
rmula) Liquid

943

M. CORP. 912
rnpike
11001 (516) 354-1121
roducts Available
sules (sustained release)
ablets
Plus Tablets
Capsules (sustained release)
lus Tablets
Tablets
al-S Tablets
tinic Tablets
ritonic Liquid
er-O-Foam Aerosol
Gustalac Tablets
Gustase Tablets
Gustase-Plus Tablets
Iso-Bid Capsules (sustained release)
Menic Tablets
Stimulax Capsules
Testand-B Injectable

GILBERT LABORATORIES 411, 913
31 Fairmount Avenue
Chester NJ 07930
Address inquiries to:
Professional Service Dept. (201) 879-7374
Products Available
◆ Esgic

GLAXO INC. 419, 913
1900 West Commercial Blvd.
Fort Lauderdale, FL 33309
(305) 776-5300
Address inquiries to:
Professional Service Department
Products Available
Almebex Syrup
Almezyme Capsules
◆ Athemol Tablets
◆ Athemol-N Tablets
◆ Beclovent Inhaler
Bronchobid Duracap Capsules
◆ Corticaine Cream
Doctate Tablets
Doctate-P Tablets
Duragesic Tablets
◆ Ethatab Tablets
Ferrobid Duracap Capsules
◆ Histabid Duracap Capsules
Levamine Tablets
Proctalme Ointment
Renalgin Tablets
Sinacon Tablets
◆ Theobid Duracap Capsules
Theobid Jr. Duracap Capsules
◆ Tri-Cone Capsules
◆ Tri-Cone Plus Capsules
Vicon Chewable Tablets
◆ Vicon Forte Capsules
Vicon with Iron
◆ Vicon-C Capsules
◆ Vicon-Plus Capsules
Vicon-T Capsules
◆ Vi-Zac Capsules

GLENBROOK LABORATORIES 918
Division of Sterling Drug Inc.
90 Park Avenue
New York, NY 10016
Address inquiries to:
Medical Director (212) 972-4141
Products Available
Bayer Aspirin
Bayer Children's Chewable Aspirin
Bayer Children's Cold Tablets
Bayer Cough Syrup for Children
Bayer Timed-Release Aspirin
Jayne's P-W Vermifuge
Midol
Phillips' Milk of Magnesia
Vanquish

GLENWOOD LABORATORIES, INC. 919
83 North Summit Street
Tenafly, NJ 07670
Address inquiries to:
Professional Service Dept. (201) 569-0050
Products Available
Amid-Sal Tablets
Myotonachol (formerly Myocholine Chloride)
Potaba
Potaba Plus 6
Pyridoxine HCl
Yodoxin
Zinc-Glenwood

GRAY PHARMACEUTICAL CO. 920
Affiliate, The Purdue Frederick Company
50 Washington Street
Norwalk, CT 06856
Address inquiries to:
Medical Department (203) 853-0123
Products Available
G.B.-Prep Emulsion
X-Prep Bowel Evacuant Kit
X-Prep Liquid
X-Prep Powder

GUARDIAN CHEMICAL CORPORATION 921
230 Marcus Boulevard
Hauppauge, L.I., NY 11787 (516) 273-0900
Address inquiries to:
Director of Medical Research
Products Available
Clorpactin WCS-90
Clorpactin XCB
Lubrajel HC
Lubraseptic Jelly
pHos-pHaid Tablets
Renacidin
Warexin

HAUCK, INC., W.E. 921
P.O. Box 1065
Roswell, GA 30075
Address inquiries to:
Warren E. Hauck (404) 992-3918
Products Available
Besta Capsules
Cantri Vaginal Cream
Chlorafed Timecelles
Cydel Capsules
Diaqua Tablets
Dolacet Tablets
Entuss Expectorant
Entuss Tablets
G-2 Tablets
G-3 Capsules
Geravite Elixir
Histor-D Timecelles
Isotrate Chewable Tablets
Isotrate Tablets
Isotrate Timecelles
MSG-600
Meditussin
Otic-HC Ear Drops
Otic-Plain Ear Drops
Palbar Tablets
Palmiron Forte Tablets
Palmiron-C Tablets
Sinufed Timecelles
Wehless Capsules
Zetran Capsules

HEALTH CARE INDUSTRIES, INC. 921
4295 S. Ohio Street
Michigan City, IN 46360
Address inquiries to:
Walter Tuman, RPh., PhD. or
Roland C. Zagnoli, RPh. (219) 879-8227
Products Available
Allimin Filmcoated Tablets
Cosanyl Cough Syrup
Cosanyl-DM Cough Syrup
Nilcol Elixir
Nilcol Tablets
Oil-O-Sol Liquid
Oil-O-Sol Pad-ettes
Oil-O-Sol Streem-Top

HERBERT LABORATORIES 922
Dermatology Division of Allergan
Pharmaceuticals, Inc.
2525 DuPont Drive
Irvine, CA 92713 (714) 752-4500
Products Available
Aeroseb-Dex
Aeroseb-HC
⊡ Aquacare Dry Skin Cream & Lotion
⊡ Aquacare/HP Dry Skin Cream & Lotion
⊡ Bluboro Powder Astringent Soaking Solution
⊡ Danex Dandruff Shampoo
⊡ Eclipse After Sun Lotion
⊡ Eclipse Sunscreen Gel, Original
⊡ Eclipse Sunscreen Lip & Face Protectant
⊡ Eclipse Sunscreen Lotion, Original
⊡ Eclipse Sunscreen Lotion, Total
⊡ Eclipse Suntan Lotion, Partial
Exsel Lotion
Fluonid Ointment, Cream & Topical Solution
Fluoroplex Topical Solution & Cream
⊡ Vanseb Cream Dandruff Shampoo
⊡ Vanseb-T Cream Tar Shampoo
⊡ Vanseb-T Lotion Tar Shampoo

HICKAM, INC., DOW B. 924
5629 Grapevine
Houston, TX 77085
Address inquiries to:
Professional Service Dept. (713) 723-0690
Products Available
DBH-B_{12}
Granulex
Probolik
Proderm Topical Dressing

Thiolate
U-R-D Injection

HIGH CHEMICAL COMPANY 925
Div. Day & Frick, Inc.
1760 N. Howard St.
Philadelphia, PA 19122
Address inquiries to:
Professional Service Dept. (215) 634-2224
Products Available
Amo-Derm
Hy-Panthron
Klorlyptus
Mus-L-Tone
Na-Co-Al
Sarapin

HILL DERMACEUTICALS, INC. 925
3102 Corrine Drive
Orlando, Florida 32803
Address inquiries to:
Mr. Jerry S. Roth, President
(305) 896-8280
Products Available
Burdeo
Derma-Smoothe Oil
Florida Foam Improved
Hill Cortac Lotion
Hill-Shade Lotion

HOECHST-ROUSSEL PHARMACEUTICALS INC. 411, 925
Route 202-206 North
Somerville, NJ 08876
Address inquiries to:
Medical Dept. (201) 685-2000
Products Available
Doxan
◆ Doxidan
Doxinate
Doxinate Solution
Duadacin
◆ Festal
◆ Festalan
◆ Lasix Tablets/Injection/Oral Solution
Streptase
◆ Surfak
◆ Topicort

HOFFMANN-LA ROCHE INC.
(See Roche Laboratories)

HOLLAND-RANTOS COMPANY, INC. 928
Post Office Box 385
865 Centennial Avenue
Piscataway, NJ 08854
Address inquiries to:
Mr. Phillip L. Frank or
Mr. Murray H. Glantz (201) 885-5777
Products Available
H-R Sterile Lubricating Jelly
Koro-Flex Arcing Spring Diaphragm
Koro-Flex Arcing Spring Diaphragm Compact Set
Koro-Flex Fitting Rings, Set of
Koromex Coil Spring Diaphragm
Koromex Coil Spring Diaphragm Compact Set
⊡ Koromex Contraceptive Foam
Koromex Diaphragm Introducer
Koromex Fitting Rings, Set of
Koromex Jelly/Cream Applicator
⊡ Koromex[II] Contraceptive Cream
⊡ Koromex[II] Contraceptive Jelly
⊡ Koromex[II]-A Contraceptive Jelly
Korostatin (Nystatin) Vaginal Tablets
Koro-Sulf (Sulfisoxazole) Vaginal Cream
⊡ Nylmerate[II] Solution Concentrate
Rantex Personal Cloth Wipes

HOUSER PHARMACEUTICALS, INC. 929
6503 Warwick Road
P. O. Box 25756
Richmond, VA 23260
Address inquiries to:
Special Service Dept. (804) 745-3403
Products Available
Amitriptyline
Chlordiazepoxide
Diphenhydramine
Hydrochlorothiazide
Imipramine
Mayodon
Mayotapp
Meclizine
Meprobamate
Methocarbamol
Papaverine
Propoxyphene
Zymenol

HOYT LABORATORIES 929
Division of Colgate-Palmolive Co.
633 Highland Avenue
Needham, MA 02194
Address inquiries to:
Professional Services Dept. (617) 444-8610
Products Available
Luride Drops
Luride Lozi-Tabs Tablets

(◆ Shown in Product Identification Section) (⊡ Described in PDR For Nonprescription Drugs)

Orabase HCA Oral Paste
Orabase Plain Oral Protective Paste
Orabase with Benzocaine Analgesic Oral Protective Paste
PerioCal-D Tablets
Phos-Flur Oral Rinse/Supplement
Point-Two Dental Rinse
Thera-Flur Topical Gel-Drops
Thera-Flur-N Topical Gel-Drops

HYNSON, WESTCOTT & DUNNING 930
Becton Dickinson Immunodiagnostics
Division of Becton Dickinson and Co.
Charles & Chase Sts.
Baltimore, MD 21201 (301) 837-0890
Products Available
BAL in Oil Ampules
Cardio-Green Vials And Single Use Units
Indigo Carmine Ampules
▣ Lactinex Tablets & Granules
Phenolsulfonphthalein Solution Ampules
Thantis Lozenges

HYREX PHARMACEUTICALS 931
3494 Democrat Road
Memphis, TN 38118
Address inquiries to:
Professional Service Dept. (901) 794-9050
Products Available
Atropine Sulfate
C & T
Chorex
Depogen
Depotest
Depotestogen
Dermarex Cream
Efedron Nasal Jelly
Everone
Glukor Injection
Hybolin
Hylate Tablets & Syrup
Hylutin Injection
Hytinic Capsules & Elixir
Hytinic Injection
Hytuss Tablets
Hytuss-2X Capsules
Kavrin Capsules
Kestrin Injection
Kestrin Tablets
Key-Plex Capsules
Key-Pred
Key-Pred Plus
Key-Pred SP
Manacid Tablets
ND-Gesic Tablets
ND-Stat Injection
Nicozol Capsules & Elixir
Panzyme Tablets
Prorex Injection
Pylora Tablets
Solurex Injection
Trac Tablets
Trac Tablets 2X
Two-Dyne Tablets
Valergen
Valertest #1
Valertest #2

ICN PHARMACEUTICALS, INC. 931
222 N. Vincent Avenue
Covina, CA 91722
Address inquiries to:
Professional Service Dept. (213) 967-0771
Products Available
Testred Capsules

INVENEX LABORATORIES 932
5885 Lakehurst Drive
Orlando, FL 32809
Address inquiries to:
Customer Service (305) 351-1400
Branch Offices
Grand Island, NY 14072
3175 Staley Road (716) 773-6666
Products Available
Aminophyllin Injection
Ascorbic Acid Injection
Atropine Sulfate Injection
Calcium Chloride Injection
Calcium Gluconate Injection
Cyanocobalamin Injection
Dexpanthenol Injection
Dextrose Injection
Digoxin Injection
Diphenhydramine Hydrochloride Injection
Ephedrine Sulfate Injection
Ergonovine Maleate Injection
Heparin Lock Flush Solution
Heparin Sodium Injection
Isoproterenol Hydrochloride Injection
Lidocaine HCl Injection
Lidocaine HCl Injection (For Cardiac Arrhythmias)
Magnesium Sulfate Injection
Mannitol Injection
Metaraminol Bitartrate Injection
Muri-lube (Mineral Oil), Light/Heavy; Vial
Oxytocin Injection (Synthetic)
Potassium Acetate Injection
Potassium Chloride Injection
Potassium Chloride Injection (Concentrated)
Potassium Phosphate Injection
Procaine HCl Injection
Pyridoxine HCl Injection
Scopolamine Hydrobromide Injection
Sodium Acetate Injection
Sodium Bicarbonate Injection
Sodium Chloride Injection
Sodium Chloride Injection (Bacteriostatic)
Sodium Chloride Injection (Concentrated)
Thiamine HCl Injection
Water for Injection
Water for Injection (Bacteriostatic)

IVES LABORATORIES INC. 411, 932
685 Third Ave.
New York, NY 10017
Address inquiries to:
Clarence Denton, M.D. (212) 986-1000
Night Emergency (914) 769-9060
Branch Warehouses
Andover, MA 01810
7 Lowell Junction Rd. Connector (617) 475-7227
Atlanta, GA 30324
221 Armour Dr., N.E. (404) 875-8380
Baltimore, MD 21224
101 Kane St. (301) 633-4005
Buena Park, CA 90620
6530 Altura Blvd. (714) 523-5110
Dallas, TX 75247
8717 Directors Row (214) 631-7865
Denver, CO 80216
4345 Oneida St. (303) 377-0233
Honolulu, HI 96814
1013 Kawaiahao St. (808) 538-1988
N. Kansas City, MO 64116
1340 Taney St. (816) 842-3680
Memphis, TN 38127
4171 Steele Road (901) 353-5040
St. Paul, MN 55121
935 Apollo Road
Eagandale Center Indus. Pk. (612) 454-1613
Kent, WA 98031
19255 80th Ave. South (206) 854-5471
Secaucus, NJ 07094
555 Secaucus Road (201) 864-4240
(NY) (212) 736-9468
Skokie, IL 60076
3435 Madison St. (312) 267-1700
Strongsville, OH 44136
17647 Foltz Industrial Parkway (216) 238-3820
Products Available
Cerose
Cerose Compound Capsules
Cerose-DM
Cetro-Cirose
◆ Cyclospasmol Capsules & Tablets
◆ Isordil Chewable
◆ Isordil Oral Titradose Tablets
◆ Isordil Sublingual Tablets
◆ Isordil Tembids Capsules
◆ Isordil Tembids Tablets
◆ Isordil w/Phenobarbital
◆ Surmontil Capsules
◆ Synalgos Capsules
◆ Synalgos-DC Capsules
Trecator-SC Tablets

JACOBUS PHARMACEUTICAL CO., INC. 936
37 Cleveland Lane
Princeton, NJ 08540
Address inquiries to:
Professional Services (609) 921-7447
For Medical Emergencies Contact:
Medical Department (609) 921-7447
Products Available
Dapsone

JAMOL LABORATORIES INC. 937
13 Ackerman Avenue
Emerson, NJ 07630 (201) 262-6363
Products Available
Bahim Foot-Aide
Bahim Oil
Otide
Ponaris Nasal Mucosal Emollient
Prep-Aide
Roma-Nol Antiseptic

JANSSEN PHARMACEUTICA INC. 420, 937
501 George Street
New Brunswick, NJ 08903
Products Available
Droperidol, See Inapsine
Fentanyl, See Sublimaze
Inapsine Injection
Innovar Injection
Monistat I.V.
Sublimaze Injection
◆ Vermox Chewable Tablets

JAYCO PHARMACEUTICALS
890 Poplar Church Drive
Suite 305
Camp Hill, PA 17011
Address inquiries to:
Lester Jay Lifton, M.D. (717) 763
Products Available
Hydra-Lyte
Quik-Prep

JOHNSON & JOHNSON BABY PRODUCTS COMPANY 412,
Professional Products Division
220 Centennial Avenue
Piscataway, NJ 08854
Address inquiries to:
Professional Service Dept. (201) 524-8885
For Medical Emergencies Contact:
office hours — (201) 524-1403
after hours — (201) 524-0400
Distribution Offices
Piscataway, NJ 08854
240 Centennial Ave.
(P.O. Box 665) (201) 524-8731
Products Available
◆ Pancrease Capsules

JOHNSON & JOHNSON 943
Dermatological Division
501 George St.
New Brunswick, NJ 08903
(See Ortho Pharmaceutical Corporation
Dermatological Division
Raritan, New Jersey 08869
a Johnson & Johnson Company)

KENWOOD LABORATORIES, INC. 943
490-A Main Street
New Rochelle, NY 10801 (914) 632-1002
Products Available
Apatate Liquid
Bonacal Plus Tablets
Cebral Capsules
Ferrous-G Elixir
Glutofac Tablets
I.L.X. B_{12} Elixir
I.L.X. B_{12} Tablets
I.L.X. Elixir
Kenpectin
Kenpectin-P
Kenwood Therapeutic Liquid
Ominal Tablets
Papavatral L.A. Capsules
Papavatral L. A. c̄ Phenobarbital Capsules
Papavatral Tablets
Papavatral 20 Tablets
Posterisan Ointment
Posterisan Suppositories
Therapeutic Liquid
Tossecol

KESSEL LABORATORIES, INC. 944
P.O. Box 6204
Surfside, FL 33154 (305) 223-1287
Products Available
Aseptol
Bronkisan A.C.
Calcicalcium D
Dermosan
Digestol Elixir and Tablets
Diurazide
Duralina
Flavin C
Flavin Plus
Karbokof Capsules
Lipotrex
Midy H.C.
Neuro Niacin
OTO-K
Periflex
Politiosulfato
Primotest
Pro-Plan
Sulfadrin
Vicolirium Sodico
Vitafort
Vitalax
Vitar-C

KEY PHARMACEUTICALS, INC. 412, 944
50 N.W. 176th St.
Miami, FL 33169
Address inquiries to:
Professional Service Dept. (305) 652-2276
Products Available
Casafru
Genapax
Geriliquid
Guanidine HCl Tablets
Ipsatol Expectorant Syrup
Ipsatol-DM Expectorant/Antitussive
Ipsatol-P Expectorant/Decongestant
Ircon Tablets
Ircon-FA Tablets
◆ Nico-Span Capsules
◆ Nitroglyn Tablets
Pavakey Capsules
Pavakey-300 Capsules
Pil-Digis Tablets

(◆ Shown in Product Identification Section) (▣ Described in PDR For Nonprescription Drugs)

- ◆ Proternol Tablets
- Quinora Tablets
- ◆ Theo-Dur Tablets
- ◆ Theo-Nar 100 and Theo-Nar 200 Tablets
- Tyzine Nasal Solution
- Tyzine Pediatric Nasal Drops

KNOLL PHARMACEUTICAL COMPANY 412, 948
30 North Jefferson Road
Whippany, NJ 07981 (201) 887-8300
Address inquiries to:
Professional Services Department
Products Available

- Akineton Injection
- ◆ Akineton Tablets
- Codeine Phosphate Injection
- Codeine Sulfate Tablets
- ◆ Dicodid Tablets
- Dilaudid Cough Syrup
- Dilaudid Injection
- Dilaudid Multiple Dose Vials (Sterile Solution)
- Dilaudid Powder
- Dilaudid Rectal Suppositories
- ◆ Dilaudid Tablets
- Meperidine Hydrochloride Injection
- Metrazol Injection
- Metrazol Liquidum
- Metrazol Tablets
- Morphine Sulfate Injection
- Nico-Metrazol Elixir
- Nico-Metrazol Tablets
- Promethazine Hydrochloride Injection
- Quadrinal Suspension
- ◆ Quadrinal Tablets
- ◆ Santyl Ointment
- Theokin Elixir
- Theokin Tablets
- ◆ Theophyl Chewable Tablets
- ◆ Theophyl-SR Capsules
- Theophyl-225 Elixir
- ◆ Theophyl-225 Tablets
- Verequad Suspension
- Verequad Tablets
- ◆ Vicodin Tablets
- Vita-Metrazol Elixir
- Vita-Metrazol Tablets

KREMERS-URBAN COMPANY 412, 958
P.O. Box 2038
Milwaukee, WI 53201
Address inquiries to:
Professional Service Dept. (414) 354-4300
Products Available

- ◆ Calciferol Tablets
- Kremplex B_{12} 1,000
- Kudrox Suspension (Double Strength)
- Kudrox Tablets
- Kutapressin Injection
- ◆ Kutrase Capsules
- ◆ Ku-Zyme Capsules
- ◆ Ku-Zyme HP Capsules
- Levsin Drops
- Levsin Elixir
- Levsin Forte Tablets
- Levsin Injection
- ◆ Levsin Tablets
- Levsin-PB Drops
- Levsin/Phenobarbital Elixir
- ◆ Levsin/Phenobarbital Tablets
- ◆ Levsinex Timecaps
- ◆ Levsinex/Phenobarbital Timecaps
- Loryl Capsules
- Milkinol
- ◆ Nitrol Ointment
- Pre-Pen
- Ronuvex Tablets
- Salimeph Forte

LAMBDA PHARMACAL LABORATORIES 961
Sub. of A.J. Bart, Inc.
Plainview, NY 11803 (516) 931-3300
Address inquiries to:
In the United States
Mr. Tony Zimardo (516) 931-3300
In Puerto Rico
Dr. L.O. Bartolomei (809) 844-3506
Products Available

- Dextrotussin Syrup
- Feraplex Injectable
- Feraplex Liquid
- Gotas Ce Drops
- Migralam Capsules
- Neuro B-12 Forte Injectable
- Neuro B-12 Injectable
- Virilam Capsules

LANNETT COMPANY, INC., THE 961
9000 State Road
Philadelphia, PA 19136
Address inquiries to:
Medical Service Dept. (215) 333-9000
Products Available

- Acetazolamide Tablets
- ▣ Acnederm Lotion & Soap
- Adalan Lanatabs
- Alphamul Suspension
- Amtren Tablets
- Arithmin Tablets
- Baroflave Powder
- Bellafedrol AH Tablets
- Bethanechol Chloride
- Bisacodyl Suppositories and Tablets
- Brompheniramine Maleate Tablets
- Castaderm
- Chlorpromazine Tablets
- Chlorulan Tablets
- Codalan
- Diphenoxylate & Atropine Tablets
- Disanthrol Capsules
- Disolan Capsules
- Disonate Capsules & Liquid
- Efricon Expectorant
- Glutethimide Tablets
- Hydrochlorulan Tablets
- Kaylixir
- Lanacillin "400"
- Lanahex Liquid
- Lanamin Capsules
- Lanatuss Expectorant
- Lanvisone Cream
- Lofene Tablets
- Lycolan Elixir
- ▣ Magnatril Suspension & Tablets
- Nitrofurantoin Tablets
- Obalan Tablets
- Orcophen Capsules
- P-I-N Forte Tablets
- Paverolan Lanacaps
- Potasalan Elixir
- Primidone Tablets
- Probenecid Tablets
- Promethazine Expectorant
- Promethazine Tablets
- Pyrralan Expectorant DM
- Rufolex Capsules
- S-A-C Tablets
- Salatar Cream
- Sedragesic Tablets
- Trichlorex Tablets
- Trichlormethiazide Tablets
- Veltane Tablets and Expectorant

LASER, INC. 961
2000 N. Main Street
Crown Point, IN 46307
Address inquiries to:
Donald A. Laser (219) 663-1165
Products Available

- D-Sinus Capsules
- Dallergy Capsules
- Dallergy "Stat"
- Dallergy Syrup
- Dallergy Tablets
- Donatussin Pediatric Drops
- Donatussin Syrup
- Fumatinic Tablets
- KIE Syrup and Tablets
- Lactocal Tablets
- Lactocal-F Tablets
- Myobid Capsules
- Theospan SR Capsules, 130 mg. & 260 mg.
- Theospan 80 Syrup
- Theospan Tablets, 100 mg. & 200 mg.
- Trimstat Tablets

LEDERLE LABORATORIES 412, 962, 2006
Division of American Cyanamid Co.
Wayne, NJ 07470 (201) 831-1234
Address inquiries on medical matters to:
Professional Services Dept.
Lederle Laboratories
Pearl River, NY 10965 (914) 735-5000
Distribution Centers

ATLANTA
Bulk Address
Chamblee (Atlanta), GA 30341
5180 Peachtree Industrial Blvd.
Mail Address
Atlanta, GA 30302
P.O. Box 4272
(GA Only) (800) 282-0399
(All Other) (800) 241-3043
(404) 455-0320

BOSTON
Westwood, MA 02090
201 University Avenue
(617) 329-4300
(MA Only) (800) 532-9684
(All Other) (800) 225-6022

CHICAGO
Bulk Address
Rosemont, IL 60018
10401 W. Touhy Ave.
Mail Address
Chicago, IL 60666
P.O. Box 66189
(IL Only) (800) 942-1493
(All Other) (800) 323-9744
(312) 827-8871

CINCINNATI
Bulk Address
Cincinnati, OH 45241
10340 Evendale Drive
Mail Address
Cincinnati, OH 45241
P.O. Box 41316
(OH Only) (800) 582-4661
(All Other) (800) 543-4590
(513) 563-6200

DALLAS
Bulk Address
Dallas, TX 75247
7611 Carpenter Freeway
Mail Address
Dallas, TX 75265
P.O. Box 225731
(TX Only) (800) 492-4412
(All Other) (800) 527-2490
(214) 631-2130

LOS ANGELES
Bulk Address
Los Angeles, CA 90040
2300 S. Eastern Ave.
Mail Address
Los Angeles, CA 90051
T.A. Box 2202
(CA Only) (800) 372-6325
(All Other) (800) 423-4120
(213) 726-1016

PHILADELPHIA
Fort Washington, PA 19034
185 Commerce Drive
(PA Only) (800) 562-6924
(NY-NJ-MD-DE) (800) 523-6610
(CT-VA-WV-DC) (800) 523-6230
(Phila. Only) (215) 248-3900
(All Other) (215) 646-7000
Products Available

- APC w/Codeine Tablets
- ◆ Acetaminophen Capsules, Tablets, Elixir
- Achromycin Intramuscular
- Achromycin Intravenous
- Achromycin Ophthalmic Ointment 1%
- Achromycin Ophthalmic Suspension 1%
- Achromycin 3% Ointment
- ◆ Achromycin V Capsules
- Achromycin V Syrup
- ◆ Achrostatin V Capsules
- Amicar Intravenous, Syrup & Tablets
- ◆ Amitriptyline HCl
- ◆ Ampicillin Trihydrate
- Antirabies Serum
- ◆ Aristocort A Topical Cream
- ◆ Aristocort A Topical Ointment
- Aristocort Forte Parenteral
- Aristocort Intralesional
- Aristocort Syrup
- ◆ Aristocort Tablets
- ◆ Aristocort Topical Cream
- ◆ Aristocort Topical Ointment
- Aristogel
- Aristospan Suspension (Intraarticular)
- Aristospan Suspension (Intralesional)
- Artane Elixir
- ◆ Artane Sequels
- ◆ Artane Tablets
- Ascorbic Acid Tablets
- Aureomycin Ointment 3%
- Aureomycin Ointment (Ophthalmic) 1%
- B Vitamins with Vitamin C Capsules
- ◆ Bisacodyl Tablets
- ◆ Centrum
- ◆ Chloral Hydrate
- ◆ Chlordiazepoxide HCl
- Chlorothiazide
- ◆ Chlorpheniramine Maleate
- ◆ Chlorpromazine HCl
- Cholera Vaccine (India Strains)
- Cyantin Tablets
- Cyclocort
- ◆ Declomycin Capsules
- Declomycin Syrup
- ◆ Declomycin Tablets, Film-coated
- ◆ Declostatin Capsules
- ◆ Declostatin Tablets
- Dexamethasone
- Diamox Parenteral
- ◆ Diamox Sequels, Tablets
- Dicyclomine HCl
- Digitoxin Tablets
- Digoxin Tablets
- Dihydroergotoxine Methanesulfonate Sublingual Tablets
- Diluting Fluid
- ◆ Dimenhydrinate Tablets
- Diphenhydramine HCl
- Diphenoxylate HCl
- Diphtheria & Tetanus Toxoids, Combined
- Docusate Sodium, USP (DSS)
- Docusate Sodium, USP w/Casanthranol
- Dolene AP-65 Tablets
- ◆ Dolene Capsules
- ◆ Dolene Compound-65 Capsules
- Erythromycin Ethylsuccinate Oral Suspension
- ◆ Erythromycin Stearate Tablets
- ◆ Ferro-Sequels
- Ferrous Fumarate
- Ferrous Gluconate Iron Supplement
- Ferrous Sulfate
- ◆ Filibon F.A. Prenatal Vitamin Tablets
- ◆ Filibon Forte

(◆ Shown in Product Identification Section) (▣ Described in PDR For Nonprescription Drugs)

◆ Filibon OT
◆ Filibon Prenatal Vitamin Tablets
Folbesyn Tablets
Folbesyn Vitamins, Parenteral
Folvite Parenteral & Tablets
Folvron Capsules
▣ Gevrabon Liquid
Gevral Protein Powder
▣ Gevral T Tablets
▣ Gevral Tablets
Gevrite Tablets
Guaifenesin
Guaifenesin w/D-Methorphan Hydrobromide
Hetrazan Tablets
Hydralazine HCl
◆ Hydrochlorothiazide
Hydrocortisone
◆ Hydromox R Tablets
◆ Hydromox Tablets
◆ Imipramine HCl Tablets
▣ Incremin w/Iron Syrup
Isosorbide Dinitrate
Isorsorbide Dinitrate, Sublingual
Ledercillin VK Oral Solution and Tablets
▣ Lederplex Capsules, Liquid & Tablets
Leucovorin Calcium
Levoprome
Levothyroxine Sodium
Liver Injection
Loxitane C Oral Concentrate
◆ Loxitane Capsules
Loxitane I.M.
M-Vac Measles Vaccine
◆ Materna 1•60 Tablets
◆ Meclizine HCl
Meprobamate
Methenamine Mandelate
Methocarbamol
Methotrexate Tablets & Parenteral
◆ Minocin Capsules
Minocin Intravenous
Minocin Syrup
Myambutol Tablets
Neoloid Emulsified Castor Oil
Neomycin Sulfate
Neptazane Tablets
Niacin
Niacinamide
Nilstat Oral Suspension
Nilstat Oral Tablets
Nilstat Topical Cream
Nilstat Topical Ointment
Nilstat Vaginal Tablets
◆ Nitroglycerin
Nylidrin HCl
Orimune Poliovirus Vaccine, Live, Oral, Trivalent
Oxytetracycline HCl
◆ Papaverine HCl
◆ Pathibamate Tablets
Pathilon Parenteral
◆ Pathilon Sequels
◆ Pathilon Tablets
◆ Pathilon w/Phenobarbital Sequels & Tablets
Penicillin G Potassium
Penicillin V Potassium
Perihemin Capsules
Peritinic Tablets
Phenobarbital
◆ Phenytoin Sodium
Pnu-Imune
Potassium Chloride Liquid
Potassium Gluconate
Prednisone
◆ Probenecid
◆ Procainamide HCl
Promethazine HCl Expectorant, Plain
Promethazine HCl Expectorant V.C. Plain
Promethazine HCl Expectorant V.C. w/Codeine
Promethazine HCl Expectorant w/Codeine
Promethazine HCl Tablets
Pronemia Capsules
Propantheline Bromide
◆ Propoxyphene HCl
Propylthiouracil Tablets
Pseudoephedrine HCl Tablets & Syrup
Pyrazinamide Tablets
Pyridoxine HCl
◆ Quinidine Sulfate
Rauwolfia Serpentina
Recoup Hematinic Tablets
Reserpine
▣ Rhulicream
▣ Rhuligel
▣ Rhulihist Lotion
▣ Rhulispray
Staphylococcus Toxoids
▣ Stresscaps Capsules
◆ Stresstabs 600 Tablets
◆ Stresstabs 600 with Iron
◆ Stresstabs 600 with Zinc
Sulfadiazine-Sulfamerazine-Sulfamethazine
Sulfasalazine
Sulfisoxazole
Tetanus Toxoid, Adsorbed
Tetanus Toxoid Purogenated
Tetanus & Diphtheria Toxoids, Combined Purogenated
Thiamine HCl (Vitamin B-1) Tablets
Thiotepa Parenteral
Thyroid
◆ TriHemic 600 Tablets
Tri-Immunol
Tuberculin, Old, Tine Test
Tuberculin Purified Protein Derivative Tine Test (PPD)
Typhus Vaccine
Varidase Intramuscular
Varidase Oral Tablets
Varidase Topical or Local
Vi-Magna Capsules
Vitamin A, Natural
Vitamin C Chewable
Vitamin E, Natural, N.F.
Vitamin E, N.F.
▣ Zincon Dandruff Shampoo

LEEMING DIVISION 999
Pfizer Inc.
100 Jefferson Rd.
Parsippany, NJ 07054
Address inquiries to:
Research and Development Dept.
(201) 887-2100
Products Available
Ben Gay External Analgesic Products
▣ Desitin Ointment
Nytilax Tablets
Rheaban Tablets & Liquid
Unisome Nighttime Sleep-Aid
Visine Eye Drops

LEGERE & CO, INC., R. J. 999
7326 E. Evans Road
Scottsdale AZ 85260 (602) 991-4033
Address inquiries to:
Customer Service & Product Information
Toll Free 1-(800) 528-3144
Products Available
Acetaco Tablets
Allerphen 12 Tablets
Apectol Tablets
Azo-Sulfisoxazole Tablets
B Complex 100
B-Cee-50
Benzide
Brosema
Cafamine T.D. Capsules
Cee-500
Cee-500 T.D. Capsules
Cinalone 40
Cinonide 40
Dekabolin
Depo-Predate 80
Dexasone
Dextraron-50
Di-Atro Tablets
E-Cypionate
E.D.T.A.
Hydrochlor 50
Hyser Plus Tablets
Imotep
Livolex
Mag-5
Meclizine Tablets
Menaval-10
Menaval-20
Myotrol
Neucalm 50
Phenazine Tablets & Capsules
Phentermine Tablets
Predate S
Predate TBA - LASA
Predate-50-100
Probacon
Probacon II Capsules
Promet
Promochlor
Propoxy Compound Capsules
Spasgesic
Sudachlor Capsules
T-Cypionate
T.E.-Cypionate
Teramine Capsules
Teramine Tablets
Testaval 90/4
Two Estrones

LEMMON COMPANY 414, 1000
Post Office Box 30
Sellersville, PA 18960
Address inquiries to:
Professional Services Department
Toll Free (800) 523-6542
In Pennsylvania (215) 723-5544
Branch Offices
SOUTHERN BRANCH
Atlanta, GA 30303
Suite 1009
Peachtree Center, South (404) 577-1979
LEMMON SALES CORP.
Gretna, LA 70053
294 Wright Avenue, #124
(504) 367-7711
Divisions:
Claridge Laboratories
Drummer Laboratories
Haack Laboratories
Lemmon Pharmacal Export Company
Mulford Laboratories
The Pfeiffer Company
3965 Laclede Ave.
Saint Louis, MO 63108 (314) 371-3000
Sellersville, PA (215) 723-5544
Products Available
A.P.B.
Adipex Tablets
◆ Adipex-P Capsules
◆ Adipex-P Tablets
Allerstat Capsules
Aluprin Tablets
Amobarbital D•Lay Tablets
Antipress Tablets
B.P.P.-Lemmon
B.S.G Tablets
Belap Elixir
Belap SE
Belap Tablets
Bevitone Tablets
Bucacet Improved
Buffadyne-Lemmon
Codone Tablets
◆ Dexampex Capsules
◆ Dexampex Tablets
Diacin
Dipav
Donphen Tablets
Dralserp Tablets
Dralzine Tablets
Evasof Tablets
Forcold Syrup
Glucoron with B_{12} Tablets
KEFF
Laverin Tablets
Laxadane Supules
Laxadane Tablets
Lemidyne with Codeine Tablets
Lemiserp Tablets
Lemivite Tablets
Lemoquine
Lexor
Mepriam Tablets
Mequin
Methampex Tablets
Neosorb Plus Tablets
Neospect Tablets
Neothylline Elixir
Neothylline Injection
◆ Neothylline Tablets
Neothylline-GG Elixir
Neothylline-GG Tablets
▣ Neutralox Suspension
Nu'Leven Plus Tablets
Nu'Leven Tablets
Otocort Ear Drops
Oxoids Tablets
Pecto-Kalin Suspension
Phenobarbital Tablets
Phenylpropanolamine Hydrochloride Tablets
Phyldrox Tablets
Prednisolone Tablets
Prednisone Tablets
Prōmex Syrup
Prōmex w/Codeine Syrup
Pseudoephedrine Hydrochloride Tablets
Pyracort-D Nasal Spray
Pyradyne Comp. Tablets
Pyradyne Tablets
◆ Quāālude (Formerly the product of William H. Rorer, Inc.)
Racet Cream
Racet LCD Cream
Rhinex D•Lay Tablets
Rhinex DM Syrup
Rhinex DM Tablets
Rhinex Tablets
Rhinspec Tablets
Rhus Tox Antigen Injection
Rhus Tox Lotion
Ruhexatal w/Reserpine Tablets
S.B.P. Plus Tablets
Sed-Tens SE Tablets
Statobex Capsules
◆ Statobex Tablets
◆ Statobex-G Tablets
Thriocaine Lozenges
Thyroid Tablets
Trilamine Capsules
Triphed
Uristat Tablets
Vagilia Vaginal Cream
Vagilia Vaginal Suppositories

LILLY AND COMPANY, ELI 414, 1005, 2007
For Medical Information, Write
Medical Department (317) 261-2000
307 E. McCarty
Post Office Box 618, 46206
Indianapolis, IN 46225
Lilly Regional & District Offices
Albany, NY 12205
125 Wolf Road (518) 458-1585

Bellevue, WA 98004
10655 Northeast 4th St. (206) 455-3959
Birmingham, AL 35223
3300 Cahaba Road (205) 879-2441
Bloomington, MN 55420
Suite 1142, One Appletree Square (612) 854-3521
Camp Hill, PA 17011
890 Poplar Church Road (717) 761-7138
Charlotte, NC 28209
1515 Mockingbird Lane (704) 525-8905
*Chicago, IL 60631
5735 East River Road (312) 693-8740
Cincinnati, OH 45241
4015 Executive Park Dr. (513) 563-0720
Cleveland, OH 44130
16600 W. Sprague Rd. (216) 243-3600
*Dallas, TX 75234
4404 Beltwood Parkway, South (214) 661-5620
*Dedham, MA 02026
990 Washington St. (617) 329-2816
(617) 329-4320
Enfield, CT 06082
150 Freshwater Blvd. (203) 741-0761
Englewood, CO 80110
5555 South Trenton Way (303) 770-2123
Garden City, NY 11530
585 Stewart Ave. (516) 222-0360
(516) 222-0361
Grand Rapids, MI 49506
3445 Lake Eastbrook Blvd., S.E. (616) 949-0876
Hasbrouck Heights, NJ 07960
377 Route 17 South (201) 288-3321
(201) 288-3324
Honolulu, HI 96825
117 Poipu Drive (808) 395-1030
Houston, TX 77056
5050 Westheimer Rd. (713) 622-2032
Indianapolis, IN 46268
3901 West 86th Street (317) 261-2512
Kansas City, MO 64112
800 W. 47th St. (816) 561-2100
(816) 561-2101
Louisville, KY 40202
680 S. 4th St. (502) 583-7255
Memphis, TN 38104
1331 Union Ave. (901) 725-7034
Metarie, LA 70002
4900 Veterans Memorial Blvd. (504) 885-9645
Miami, FL 33143
8603 S. Dixie Highway (305) 661-2787
*Norcross, GA 30091
5944 Peachtree Corners East (404) 449-4910
Oklahoma City, OK 73112
5900 Mosteller Drive (405) 848-8886
(405) 848-8887
*Pasadena, CA 91101
301 E. Colorado Blvd. (213) 792-5121
Pittsburgh, PA 15220
1910 Cochran Rd. (412) 922-9770
Portland, OR 97205
720 S.W. Washington St. (503) 223-8298
Raleigh, NC 27625
2920 Highwoods Blvd. (919) 872-4836
St. Louis, MO 63105
7777 Bonhomme Ave. (314) 862-8788
(314) 862-8789
Sacramento, CA 95814
555 Capitol Mall (916) 444-2173
San Antonio, TX 78216
800 N.W. Loop 410 (512) 341-2211
San Diego, CA 92103
2550 Fifth Ave. (714) 234-6664
San Francisco, CA 94111
100 California St. (415) 362-0559
*Southfield, MI 48075
Suite 940, 3000 Town Center (313) 358-2206, 2207, 2208
Tampa, FL 33609
5401 W. Kennedy Blvd. (813) 870-2036
Towson, MD 21204
One Investment Place (301) 823-2242
Washington, DC 20036
1901 L Street, N.W. (202) 296-2575
*White Plains, NY 10604
925 Westchester Ave. (914) 949-7723
Williamsville, NY 14221
5820 Main St. (716) 634-0178
Worthington, OH 43085
130 E. Wilson Bridge Rd. (614) 846-5090
Wynnewood, PA 19096
Seven Wynnewood Rd. (215) 477-8739
(215) 642-2649

*Regional office also

Products Available

AD-Cebrin c̄ Fluoride Drops
A.S.A. Compound Pulvules & Tablets
◆ A.S.A. & Codeine Compound Pulvules & Tablets
A.S.A. Enseals, Pulvules, Suppositories & Tablets
Acidulin Pulvules
Aerolone Solution
Alphalin Gelseals and Pulvules
Amertan Jelly
◆ Amesec, Enseals & Pulvules
Aminophylline & Amytal Pulvules
Aminosalicylic Acid Enseals
Ammoniated Mercury Ointments
Ammonium Chloride Enseals
Amyl Nitrite Aspirols
◆ Amytal Elixir & Tablets
Amytal Sodium Ampoules
◆ Amytal Sodium Pulvules
Analgesic Balm Ointment
◆ Anhydron Tablets
Antiseptic No. 3, R. St. J. Perry, Tablets
Antiseptic Solution
Apomorphine Hydrochloride Soluble Tablets
Arnica Tincture
Aromatic Ammonia Aspirols & Spirit
Aromatic Elixir
Asafetida Tincture
Atropine Sulfate Ampoules (Vials), Sterile Ophthalmic Ointment, Tablets & Soluble Tablets
◆ Aventyl HCl Liquid & Pulvules
BCG Vaccine
Bacitracin Ointment & Sterile Ophthalmic Ointment
Belladonna Extract Tablets
Belladonna Ointment, Powdered Extract & Tincture
Benzoin Tincture
Betalin Complex Ampoules, Vials & Elixir
Betalin Complex F.C. Ampoules and Vials
Betalin Compound Pulvules
Betalin S Ampoules, Vials, Elixir & Tablets
Betalin 12 Crystalline Ampoules (Vials)
Bilron Pulvules
Bismuth Subcarbonate Tablets
Blank (Placebo) Soluble Tablets
Boric Acid Ointment & Sterile Ophthalmic Ointments
Brevital Sodium Ampoules (Vials)
Brown Mixture Solution
Buchu, Juniper & Potassium Acetate Elixir
Caffeine & Sodium Benzoate Ampoules
Calcium Carbonate Tablets, Aromatic
Calcium Gluceptate Ampoules
Calcium Gluconate Tablets
Calcium Gluconate w/Vitamin D Pulvules & Tablets
Calcium Hydroxide Powder
Calcium Lactate Tablets
Camphor & Soap Liniment
Camphor Liniment & Spirit
Capastat Sulfate Ampoules (Vials)
Capsules, Empty Gelatin
Carbarsone Pulvules
Cascara, Aromatic, Fluid Extract
Cascara Compound Tablets
Cascara Sagrada Fluid Extract
Cascara Tablets
Castor Oil Elastic Filled Capsules
◆ Ceclor Pulvules & Suspension
Cevalin Ampoules & Tablets
Citrated Caffeine Tablets
Cocaine Hydrochloride Solvets
Coco-Quinine Suspension
Codeine Phosphate Ampoules (Vials) & Soluble Tablets
Codeine Sulfate Tablets & Soluble Tablets
Colchicine Ampoules & Tablets
Cold Cream, for Compounding Prescriptions, Ointment
Cologel Liquid
Compound Benzoin Tincture
Copavin Pulvules
Crystodigin Ampoules
◆ Crystodigin Tablets
Cyanide Antidote Package
Cytellin Suspension
◆ Darvocet-N 50 Tablets
◆ Darvocet-N 100 Tablets
◆ Darvon Pulvules
◆ Darvon Compound Pulvules
◆ Darvon Compound-65 Pulvules
◆ Darvon with A.S.A. Pulvules
◆ Darvon-N Suspension & Tablets
◆ Darvon-N with A.S.A. Tablets
Deltalin Gelseals
Dextrose Ampoules
Dextrose (Buffered) Ampoules
Diamond Antiseptics Tablets
Dibasic Calcium Phosphate Tablets
Dibasic Calcium Phosphate w/Vitamin D Pulvules
Dibasic Calcium Phosphate w/Vitamin D and Iron Pulvules
Dicumarol Pulvules
Dicurin Procaine Ampoules (Vials)
Diethylstilbestrol Enseals, Tablets & Suppositories
Digiglusin Tablets
Digitalis Pulvules
◆ Dobutrex Vials
Dolophine Hydrochloride Ampoules & Tablets
Drolban Ampoules (Vials)
Duracillin A.S. Ampoules (Vials) & Hyporets
◆ Dymelor Tablets
Emetine Hydrochloride Ampoules
En-Cebrin Pulvules
En-Cebrin F Pulvules
Ephedrine & Amytal Pulvules
Ephedrine & Seconal Sodium Pulvules
Ephedrine Sulfate Ampoules, Pulvules, Solution & Syrups
Ephedrol, w/Codeine
Epragen Pulvules
Eprolin Gelseals
Ergotrate Maleate Ampoules & Tablets
Essence Pepsin Elixir
Extralin B Pulvules
Extralin F Pulvules
Extralin Pulvules
Ferrous Gluconate Pulvules
Ferrous Sulfate Enseals & Tablets
Folic Acid Tablets
Glucagon for Injection Ampoules (Vials)
Green Soap Tincture
Haldrone Tablets
Heparin Sodium Ampoules (Vials)
Hepicebrin Tablets
Hexa-Betalin Ampoules (Vials) & Tablets
Hista-Clopane Pulvules
Histadyl E.C. Syrup
Histadyl & A.S.A. Compound Pulvules
Histalog Ampoules
Histamine Phosphate (For Gastric Test)
Histamine Phosphate (Histamine Test for Pheochromocytoma)
Homicebrin
Hydriodic Acid Syrup
Hyoscyamus Tincture
Ichthammol Ointments
◆ Lente Iletin, 40, 80, & 100 units
◆ Regular Iletin, 40, 80 & 100 units
Regular Iletin, (Concentrated), 500 units
◆ Semilente Iletin, 40, 80, & 100 units
◆ Ultralente Iletin, 40, 80, & 100 units
◆ NPH Iletin, 40, 80, & 100 units
◆ Protamine, Zinc & Iletin, 40, 80, & 100 units
Beef Regular Iletin, 100 units
Beef Lente Iletin, 100 units
Beef NPH Iletin, 100 units
Beef Protamine Zinc & Iletin, 100 units
Pork Regular Iletin, 100 units
Pork Lente Iletin, 100 units
Pork NPH Iletin, 100 units
Pork Protamine, Zinc & Iletin, 100 units
Iodine, Strong, Tincture
Ipecac Syrup
I-sedrin Plain Solution
Isoniazid Tablets
Isopropyl Alcohol, Lilly, 91%
Kafocin Pulvules
Kappadione Ampoules
◆ Keflex Pulvules & Tablets
Keflex, for Oral Suspension
Keflex, for Pediatric Drops
Keflin, Neutral, Ampoules (Vials)
Kefzol Ampoules (Vials)
Lactated Pepsin Elixir
Lexavite Ampoules (Vials)
Lextron F.G. Pulvules
Lextron Ferrous Pulvules
Lextron Pulvules
Liver Ampoules (Vials)
Loridine Ampoules (Vials)
Magnesium Sulfate Ampoules
Mandol Vials
Menadione Tablets
Mercuric Oxide, Yellow, Sterile Ophthalmic Ointments
Merthiolate Aeropump, Cream, Glycerite, Sterile Ophthalmic Ointment, Powder, Solution & Tincture
◆ Methadone Hydrochloride Diskets
Methenamine Tablets
Methenamine & Sodium Biphosphate Tablets
Methyltestosterone Tablets
Metubine Iodide Ampoules (Vials)
Metycaine Hydrochloride Ampoules (Vials) & Powder
Metycaine Hydrochloride & Zinc Oxide Compound Suppositories
Milk of Bismuth
Milk of Magnesia
Morphine & Atropine Ampoules (Vials)
Morphine Sulfate Ampoules (Vials) & Soluble Tablets
Morrhuate Sodium Ampoules
Mouthwash Solution
Multicebrin Tablets
Mumps Skin-Test Antigen
Myrrh Tincture
Nebcin Ampoules (Vials) & Hyporets
Neo-Betalin 12 Crystalline Ampoules (Vials)
Neomycin Sulfate Ointment & Tablets
Neotrizine Suspension & Tablets
Niacin Ampoules & Tablets
Niacinamide Ampoules (Vials) & Tablets
Nitroglycerin Sublingual Tablets
Novacebrin Chewable Tablets
Novacebrin Drops

Novacebrin c̄ Fluoride Chewable Tablets
Novacebrin c̄ Fluoride Drops
Novrad Pulvules & Suspension
Oncovin Ampoules (Vials)
Opium (Deodorized) Tincture
Ouabain Ampoules
Ox Bile Extract Enseals
Pagitane Hydrochloride Tablets
Pancebrin Ampoules (Vials)
Pancreatin Enseals, Powder & Tablets
Pantholin Tablets
Papaverine Hydrochloride Ampoules, Vials, Powder & Tablets
Parathyroid Ampoules (Vials)
Paregoric Tincture
Paveril Phosphate Tablets
Pectocel
Penicillin G Potassium Ampoules (Vials) (Buffered)
Penicillin G Potassium, Sterile, Ampoules (Vials)
Peppermint Spirit
Phenobarbital Elixir & Tablets
Phenobarbital Sodium Ampoules
Phenobarbital & Belladonna Tablets
Posterior Pituitary Powder
Potassium Chloride Ampoules & Enseals
Potassium Iodide Enseals
Potassium Permanganate Tablets
Potassium Triplex Liquid
Powder Papers
Progesterone Ampoules (Vials)
Propylthiouracil Tablets
Protamine Sulfate Ampoules & Vials
Prunicodeine
Quinidine Gluconate Ampoules (Vials)
Quinidine Sulfate Pulvules & Tablets
Quinine Sulfate Pulvules & Tablets
Quintess
Rabies Vaccine (Duck Embryo), Dried Killed Virus
Reticulex Pulvules
Reticulogen Ampoules (Vials)
Reticulogen Fortified Ampoules (Vials)
Rhinitis, Full Strength, Tablets
Riboflavin Tablets
Rose, Soluble, for Making Artificial Rose Water
Saccharin Sodium Tablets
Sandril Ampoules (Vials) & Tablets
Scarlet Red Ointment
Scopolamine Hydrobromide Soluble Tablets
Seconal Elixir
◆ Seconal Sodium Ampoules (Vials), Pulvules & Suppositories
Sedatussin
Senna Compound Powder
◆ Seromycin Pulvules
Silver Nitrate Wax Ampoules
Soap Liquid
Soda Mint Tablets
Sodium Bicarbonate Tablets
Sodium Chloride Ampoules (Vials), Enseals & Tablets
Sodium Citrate Ampoules
Sodium Iodide Ampoules
Sodium Salicylate Enseals
Spiritex (Rubbing Alcohol)
Streptomycin Sulfate Ampoules (Vials)
Sulfadiazine Tablets
Sulfapyridine Tablets
Sulfonamides Duplex Suspension
Sulfur Ointment
Surfacaine Cream, Jelly, Ointment & Suppositories
Surfadil Cream & Lotion
Tapazole Tablets
Terpin Hydrate & Codeine Elixir
Terpin Hydrate Elixir
Tes-Tape
Testosterone Ampoules (Vials)
Testosterone Propionate Ampoules (Vials)
Theracebrin Pulvules
Thyroid Enseals & Tablets
Tolu Balsam Syrup
Trisogel Liquid & Pulvules
Tuamine Sulfate Solution
Tubocurarine Chloride Ampoules (Vials)
◆ Tuinal Pulvules
Tycopan Pulvules
Tylosterone Tablets
V-Cillin Drops
V-Cillin K for Oral Solution
◆ V-Cillin K Tablets
Valerian Tincture
Vancocin HCl, I.V.
Vancocin HCl, Oral
Vanilla Extract
Velban Ampoules (Vials)
Water for Injection Ampoules
Wheat Germ Oil
White Pine & Ammonium Chloride Compound, Mentholated, Syrup
White Pine Compound Syrup
Whitfield's Ointment (Double Strength)
Wild Cherry Syrup
Zentinic Pulvules
Zentron Chewable Tablets
Zentron Liquid
Zinc Oxide Ointments
Zinc Oxide Paste Ointment
Zinc Sulfate Compound Powder

LINCOLN LABORATORIES, INC. 1089, 2010
Post Office Box 1139
Decatur, IL 62525
Address inquiries to:
Professional Service Dept. (217) 877-2531
Products Available
A-D-R Capsules
Andesterone
Androlin
Asmolin
Bedoce
C-Ject
C-Ject w/B
Estrogenic Substances
Hexathricin Otic
Liver, B_{12} & Folic Acid
Mono-Vacc
Multi-Test
Soraden
Stemutrolin
Tuberculin, Mono-Vacc Test

LOMA LINDA FOODS 1089
Address inquiries to:
Marketing Office
Riverside, CA 92515 (714) 785-2444
(714) 785-2475
Branch Offices
Andover, NJ 07821
11 Meadow Lane, Lake Tranquility
(201) 850-0012
Atlanta, GA
P.O. Box 664
(Calhoun) 30701 (404) 629-4693
Berrien Springs, MI 49103
140 Sunset Drive (616) 473-2614
Columbus, OH
P.O. Box 388
(Mount Vernon) 43050 (614) 397-7077
Dallas, TX
P.O. Box 246
(Keene) 76059 (817) 645-8465
Denver, CO
318 Eugene Way
(Loveland) 80537 (303) 399-8041
Fresno, CA
31644 Road 144
(Visalia) 93277 (209) 798-1419
Honolulu, HI 96822
P.O. Box 22421 (808) 695-8733
New York City, NY
341 Evans Avenue
(Elmont) 11003 (516) 354-4533
Oakland, CA
1473 Doolittle Drive
(San Leandro) 94577 (415) 562-5133
Portland, OR 97211
1707 NE Argyle (503) 283-5983
Riverside, CA 92515
11503 Pierce St. (714) 785-2519
Seattle, WA
P.O. Box 101
(Lakewood) 98259 (206) 652-8775
Products Available
▣ I-Soyalac: Liquid Concentrate, Ready-to-Serve
▣ Soyalac: Liquid Concentrate, Ready-to-Serve and Powder

M² ETHICALS, INC. 1089
P.O. Box 174
West Chicago, IL 60185
Address inquiries to:
O. G. Rasmussen, Ph.D. (312) 293-0660
Products Available
Ampromin
ArtiSal
Carozyme
Complere
Desatrate
Dizyme
HM-X
Hematem
Karbozyme
KardioCaps
M² - 3 + E
M² - A & D
M² - B
M² - B 60
M² - C
M² - Calcium
M² - E 200
M² - E 400
M² - E Perles
M² - Lacto
M² -Lipotrophic
M² - Magnesium
M² - Manganese
M² -Pancreatin
M² - Potassium
M² - Zinc
Magacin
Millitrace
N-E-Time
Nertran
Plumate

MACSIL, INC. 1090
A Street & Lehigh Avenue
Philadelphia, PA 19125 (215) 423-5566
Products Available
▣ Balmex Baby Powder
▣ Balmex Emollient Lotion
▣ Balmex Ointment

MALLARD INCORPORATED 1090
3021 Wabash Ave.
Detroit, MI 48216
Address inquiries to:
Sales Department (313) 964-3910
Products Available
Allersone
Analgestine
Anaphen
Anoquan
Bexomal
Bexophene
Buffex
Chlorohist
Conhist
Coracin
Cortisone Acetate Injectable
Coryza Brengle
Dermal Rub
Dermogen
Dynosal
Ekrised
Enzobile
Estrocon
Evac-U-Lax
Fenylhist
Fenylhist-25
Ferronese
Fynex
Gelazine
Halercol
Hemalgen
Histex
Hyper-Cholate
Hysone
Iromal
Ivy-Rid
Laxinate 100
Magnagel
Malatal
Mallamint
Mallenzyme
Mallergan
Mallo-Pectin
Malotuss
Minro-Plex
Nelex-100
Neotal
Nialex
Nialexo-C
Nurosal
Palodyne
Pavased
Phenate
Phenzine
Predoxine
Prenabex
Presalin
Quan-III
Saleto
Saleto-D
Salphenyl
Secophen
Serfolia
Therabex
Trocal
Tyrobenz
Urazide
Uremide
Uro-Ves
Vera-67
Vitamin B_{12} Concentrate
Vitamin B_{12} Crystalline Injectable
Vitamin-C
Vitamin-E
Vitasol

MARION LABORATORIES, INC. 416, 1090
Pharmaceutical Division
Marion Industrial Park
10236 Bunker Ridge Rd.
Kansas City, MO 64137
Address inquiries to:
Director, Corporate Medical Services
P.O. Box 9627
Kansas City, MO 64134 (816) 761-2500
Products Available
◆ Ambenyl Expectorant
◆ Debrox Drops
Dia-Quel Liquid
◆ Ditropan
◆ Duotrate Plateau Caps
◆ Duotrate 45 Plateau Caps
◆ Gaviscon Liquid
◆ Gaviscon Tablets
◆ Gaviscon-2 Tablets
◆ Gly-Oxide Liquid
Metasep Shampoo

(◆ Shown in Product Identification Section)

(▣ Described in PDR For Nonprescription Drugs)

Napril Plateau Caps
◆ Nico-400 Plateau Caps
◆ Nitro-Bid Ointment
◆ Nitro-Bid 2.5 Capsules
◆ Nitro-Bid 6.5 Capsules
◆ Nitro-Bid 9 Capsules
◆ Os-Cal 500 Tablets
◆ Os-Cal Forte Tablets
◆ Os-Cal Plus Tablets
◆ Os-Cal Tablets
◆ Os-Cal-Gesic Tablets
◆ Pavabid Capsules
◆ Pavabid HP Capsulets
Pretts Tablets
◆ Silvadene Cream
Throat Discs Throat Lozenges
◆ Thyroid Strong Tablets
Thyroid Tablets
Triten Tablets

MARLYN PHARMACEUTICAL CO., INC. 1097
18261 Enterprise Lane, Bldg. A
Huntington Beach, CA 92648
(714) 847-4545
Products Available
C Speridin Tablets
Hep-Forte Capsules
Marbec Tablets
Marlyn Formula 50 Capsules
Nu-Natal with Fluoride
Test-Estrin Buccal Tablets
Test-Estrin Capsules
Test-Estrin Full Strength
Test-Estrin Half Strength
Test-Estrin Injectable (in aqueous susp.)

MAYRAND, INC. 1097
P.O. Box 20246
1026 E. Lindsay Street
Greensboro, NC 27420 (919) 275-9601
Products Available
Anamine Syrup
Anamine T.D. Caps
Anatuss Syrup
Anatuss Tablets
Antora T.D. Capsules
Antora-B T.D. Capsules
Asproject
Becomject-100
Benoject-10
Benoject-50
Buff-A Comp Caps
Buff-A Comp Tablets
Buff-A Comp No. 3 (with Codeine)
Buff-A Tablets
Corgonject-5
Cyanoject
Decaject
Decaject-L.A.
Dramoject
Eldercaps
Eldertonic Elixir
Estroject-2
Estroject-LA
Feryl-Vita Ovalets
Flexoject
Glytuss Tabs
Hasp Elixir
Hasp Ovalets
Histaject
Hydrotensin-25 Tablets
Hydrotensin-50 Tablets
Hydro-Z-25 Tablets
Hydro-Z-50 Tablets
K-Cillin-500 Tablets
Lidoject-1
Lidoject-2
Lifoject
Menoject
Menoject-LA
Nascobarb Ovalets
Nu-Iron Elixir
Nu-Iron 150 Caps
Nu-Iron-V Tablets
Pavatran TD Caps
Pavatran-300 TD Caps
Penalate Elixir
Phenoject-50
Predaject
Sedapap Elixir
Sedapap-10 Tablets
Soluject
Sorbide T.D. Caps
Spasmoject
Stera-Form Cream
Steramine Otic
Sterapred Tablets
Sterapred Uni-Pak
Testoject-50
Testoject-L.A.
Trimtabs
Tristoject
Vistaject

McNEIL CONSUMER PRODUCTS CO. 417, 1099
McNEILAB, INC.
Fort Washington, PA 19034
Address inquiries to:
Professional Relations Department
Fort Washington, PA 19034
Manufacturing Divisions
Fort Washington, PA 19034
Southwest Manufacturing Plant
4001 N. I-35
Round Rock, TX 78664
Distribution Centers
Arlington, TX 76010
3129 Pinewood Drive (817) 640-1167
Broadview, IL 60153
2122 Roberts Drive (312) 343-1569
Doraville, GA 30360
2801 Bankers Industrial Drive
(404) 448-0200
Glendale, CA 91201
512 Paula Avenue (213) 245-1491
Montgomeryville, PA 18936
2 Progress Drive (215) 699-7081
Products Available
◆ Children's Tylenol acetaminophen Chewable Tablets & Elixir
◆ CoTylenol Cold Formula Tablets
CoTylenol Liquid Cold Formula (with Couth Suppressant)
Extra-Strength Tylenol acetaminophen Adult Liquid Pain Reliever
◆ Extra-Strength Tylenol acetaminophen Capsules & Tablets
Infants' Tylenol acetaminophen Drops
◆ Regular Strength Tylenol acetaminophen Tablets
Sine-Aid Sinus Headache Tablets

McNEIL LABORATORIES 417, 1101
McNEILAB, INC.
Fort Washington, PA 19034
Address inquiries to:
Professional Services Department
Fort Washington, PA 19034
(215) 628-5000
Manufacturing Division
Dorado, Puerto Rico 00646
P.O. Box P
Distribution Divisions
Arlington, TX 76010
3129 Pinewood Drive (817) 265-4251
Broadview, IL 60153
2122 Roberts Drive (312) 344-3187
Doraville, GA 30360
2801 Bankers Industrial Drive
(404) 447-8600
Glendale, CA 91201
512 Paula Avenue (213) 245-0217
Montgomeryville PA 18936
2 Progress Drive (215) 699-3551
Products Available
Butibel Tablets & Elixir
Butibel-Zyme Tablets
Buticaps Capsules
Butigetic Tablets
◆ Butisol Sodium Elixir & Tablets
Carbinoxamine Maleate, see Clistin
Chlorzoxazone, see Paraflex
Clistin Elixir & Tablets
Clistin Expectorant Syrup
Clistin R-A Tablets
Clistin-D Tablets
Droperidol, see Inapsine
Fentanyl, see Sublimaze
Grifulvin V Tablets & Suspension (For Product Information, see Ortho Pharmaceutical Corporation, Dermatological Div.)
Griseofulvin Microsize, see Grifulvin V
◆ Haldol Injection, Tablets & Concentrate
Haloperidol, see Haldol
Inapsine Injection (See listing under Janssen)
Innovar Injection (See listing under Janssen)
Paraflex Tablets
◆ Parafon Forte Tablets
Sodium Butabarbital, see Butisol Sodium
Sublimaze Injection (See listing under Janssen)
◆ Tolectin Tablets & DS Capsules
Tolmetin Sodium, see Tolectin Tablets
◆ Tylenol w/Codeine Tablets and Elixir
◆ Tylox Capsules

MEAD JOHNSON NUTRITIONAL DIVISION 1107
Mead Johnson & Company
2404 W. Pennsylvania St.
Evansville, IN 47721 (812) 426-6000
Address inquiries to:
Scientific Information Section
Medical Department
Products Available
ⓄⓉⒸ Casec
ⓄⓉⒸ Ce-Vi-Sol
ⓄⓉⒸ Enfamil
ⓄⓉⒸ Enfamil Nursette
ⓄⓉⒸ Enfamil Ready-To-Use
ⓄⓉⒸ Enfamil w/Iron
ⓄⓉⒸ Enfamil w/Iron Ready-To-Use
ⓄⓉⒸ Feminins
ⓄⓉⒸ Fer-In-Sol
ⓄⓉⒸ Flexical
ⓄⓉⒸ Isocal
ⓄⓉⒸ Isocal Tube Feeding Set
ⓄⓉⒸ Lofenalac
ⓄⓉⒸ Lonalac
ⓄⓉⒸ Lytren
ⓄⓉⒸ MCT Oil
ⓄⓉⒸ Nutramigen
Poly-Vi-Flor Vitamins w/Fluoride, Chewable Tablets & Drops
Poly-Vi-Flor Vitamins w/Iron & Fluoride, Chewable Tablets & Drops
Poly-Vi-Flor 0.25 mg. Vitamins w/Fluoride, Drops
Poly-Vi-Flor 0.5 mg. Vitamins w/Fluoride, Chewable Tablets
ⓄⓉⒸ Poly-Vi-Sol Vitamins, Chewable Tablets & Drops
Poly-Vi-Sol Vitamins w/Iron, Chewable Tablets & Drops
ⓄⓉⒸ Portagen
ⓄⓉⒸ Pregestimil
ⓄⓉⒸ Probana
ⓄⓉⒸ ProSobee
ⓄⓉⒸ Sustacal
ⓄⓉⒸ Sustagen
ⓄⓉⒸ Tempra
ⓄⓉⒸ Trind
ⓄⓉⒸ Trind-DM
Tri-Vi-Flor Vitamins w/Fluoride, Chewable Tablets & Drops
Tri-Vi-Flor 0.25 mg. Vitamins w/Fluoride, Drops
Tri-Vi-Flor 0.25 mg. Vitamins w/Iron & Fluoride, Drops
ⓄⓉⒸ Tri-Vi-Sol Vitamins, Chewable Tablets & Drops
ⓄⓉⒸ Tri-Vi-Sol Vitamins w/Iron, Drops

MEAD JOHNSON PHARMACEUTICAL DIVISION 417, 1110
Mead Johnson & Company
2404 W. Pennsylvania St.
Evansville, IN 47721 (812) 426-6000
Address inquiries to:
Scientific Information Section
Medical Department
Products Available
◆ Colace
◆ Cytoxan
◆ Deapril-ST
◆ Duricef
◆ Estrace
◆ K-Lyte & K-Lyte DS
◆ K-Lyte/Cl
◆ Megace Tablets
Mucomyst
Mucomyst with Isoproterenol
◆ Natalins
◆ Natalins Rx
◆ Ovcon-35
◆ Ovcon-50
◆ Peri-Colace
Questran
◆ Quibron & Quibron-300
◆ Quibron Plus
◆ Vasodilan

MEDICAL PRODUCTS PANAMERICANA, INC. 1129
Post Office Box 771
Coral Gables, FL 33134
Address inquiries to:
Professional Service Dept. (305) 545-6524
Branch and Distribution Division
San Juan, Puerto Rico (809) 783-6736
Products Available
Aminobrain Capsules
Aminobrain Injection
Aminobrain Tablets
Aminobrain-PT Elixir
Atoximetin-B Injection
Atoximetin-B Tablets
Broncopectol Syrup
Dermaplen Ointment
Digesplen Drops
Digesplen Elixir
Digesplen Tablets
Ferlivit Capsules
Ferlivit Injection
Ferlivit Syrup
Flebomedic
Folisplen B-12 Capsules
Folisplen B-12 Injection
Medispray Aerosol
Neurodep
Novaflor Capsules
Otomedic Drops
Ovagin Inserts
Rubroben-1000 Injection
Rutiplen-C
Tempotest Caps
Tempotest 225
Trilycal-12
VG Capsules
Varidin Capsules

(◆ Shown in Product Identification Section) (ⓄⓉⒸ Described in PDR For Nonprescription Drugs)

MEDICONE COMPANY 418, 1130
225 Varick St.
New York, NY 10014
Address inquiries to:
Professional Service Dept. (212) 924-5166
Products Available
Derma Medicone
Derma Medicone-HC
DioMedicone Tablets
Medicone Dressing
Mediconet
◆ Rectal Medicone Suppositories
Rectal Medicone Unguent
◆ Rectal Medicone-HC Suppositories

MEDICS PHARMACEUTICAL CORPORATION 1131
203 Rio Circle
Decatur, GA 30030
Address inquiries to:
Marketing Director (404) 377-7160
Branch Offices & Warehouse for Puerto Rico & Central America
Post Office Box 233
Ponce, Puerto Rico 00731
(809) 842-6263
Address inquiries to:
Dir. of Sales, Puerto Rico
Products Available
Cervex Vaginal Cream
Cobalamed-100
Cobalamed-1000
Drusilate
Essential-8, Capsules
Estro-Med
Glucotropin-Forte
Hemocyte Injection
Hemocyte Plus Tabules
Hemocyte Tablets
Hemocyte-F Tablets
Isovex-100 Capsules
Medigesic Plus Capsules
Mediplex
Medizinc Tablets
Mercurasol
Norel Plus Capsules
Norel Plus Injection
Omega-P.A.
Repo-Estro Med
Testro-Med

MENLEY & JAMES LABORATORIES
Professional Products Division
a SmithKline company
P.O. Box 8082
Philadelphia, PA 19101
Address inquiries to:
Medical Department (215) 854-4000
For Products Available, see Smith Kline & French Laboratories

MERCHANT PHARMACEUTICAL CO., INC., W. F. 1131
P.O. Box 6
Mt. Rainier, MD 20822
Address inquiries to:
Professional Service Dept. (202) 635-7890
Products Available
Adatuss Cough Syrup
Adatuss D.C. Expectorant Cough Syrup
Circubid Capsules
Decubitex Ointment
Historal Capsules
Historal Liquid
Maxigesic Capsules

MERCK SHARP & DOHME 418, 1132
Division of Merck & Co., Inc.
West Point, PA 19486 (215) 699-5311
For Medical Information
Write: Professional Information
Business hours only (8:30 a.m. to 4:45 p.m. EST), call (215) 699-5848
For Medical Emergency Information after hours or on weekends, call
(215) 699-5311
Address inquiries to:
Professional Service Department
West Point, PA 19486
Branch Offices
Arlington, TX 76011
Great Southwest Industrial District
925-111th Street (817) 261-7527
Atlanta, GA 30354
3415 Empire Blvd., S.W. (404) 766-3608
Baltimore Area:
see Columbia, MD
Boston Area:
see Needham Heights, MA
Chicago Area:
see Oak Brook, IL
Columbia, MD 21045
9199 Red Branch Rd. (301) 730-8240
Columbus, OH 43228
4242 Janitrol Road (614) 276-5308
Commerce, CA 90040
6409 E. Gayhart Street (213) 723-9661
Dallas/Ft. Worth Area:
see Arlington, TX
Denver, CO 80216
4900 Jackson Street (303) 355-1601
Kansas City area:
see Overland Park, KS
Kenner, LA 70062
1431 E. Airline Highway (504) 729-4588
King of Prussia, PA 19406
1045 First Avenue (215) 278-2550
Los Angeles Area:
see Commerce, CA
Memphis, TN 38106
1980 Latham Street (901) 948-8501
Minneapolis, MN 55441
12955 State Highway 55
(612) 559-4445
Needham Heights, MA 02194
40 A Street (617) 444-5510
New Orleans Area:
see Kenner, LA
New York Area:
see Teterboro, NJ
Oak Brook, IL 60521
2010 Swift Drive (312) 920-2160
Overland Park, KS 66215
9001 Quivira Rd. (913) 888-1110
Philadelphia Area:
see King of Prussia, PA
Portland, OR 97211
717 N.E. Lombard St. (503) 285-2582
S. San Francisco, CA 94080
340 Shaw Road (415) 583-4330
Teterboro, NJ 07608
111 Central Avenue (201) 288-2275
Products Available
Albumisol
◆ Aldoclor Tablets
◆ Aldomet Tablets & Injection
◆ Aldoril Tablets
alphaREDISOL Injection
Antivenin (Black Widow Spider)
AquaMEPHYTON Injection
Aramine Injection
Attenuvax
◆ Benemid Tablets
Biavax$_{II}$
◆ Clinoril Tablets
Cogentin Injection
◆ Cogentin Tablets
◆ ColBENEMID Tablets
Cortone Saline Suspension
Cortone Tablets
Cosmegen Injection
◆ Cuprimine Capsules
Cyclaine Topical Solution
Daranide Tablets
Decaderm
Decadron Phosphate Injection
Decadron Phosphate Respihaler
Decadron Phosphate Sterile Ophthalmic Ointment
Decadron Phosphate Sterile Ophthalmic Solution
Decadron Phosphate Topical Cream
Decadron Phosphate Turbinaire
Decadron Phosphate w/Xylocaine Injection
◆ Decadron Tablets & Elixir
Decadron-La Suspension
Decaspray Topical Aerosol
◆ Diupres Tablets
◆ Diuril Tablets & Oral Suspension
◆ Edecrin Tablets
◆ Elavil Tablets & Injection
Elspar
◆ Flexeril Tablets
Floropryl Ointment
Fluax
Gammagee
Hep-B-Gammagee
Humorsol Ophthalmic Solution
Hydeltrasol Injection
Hydeltrasol—Ophthalmic Ointment, Ophthalmic Solution
Hydeltra-T.B.A., Suspension
Hydrocortone Acetate Ophthalmic Preparations
Hydrocortone Phosphate Injection
Hydrocortone Saline Suspension
Hydrocortone Tablets
Hydrocortone Topical Ointment
◆ HydroDIURIL Tablets
◆ Hydropres Tablets
◆ Indocin Capsules
Inversine Tablets
Lyo B-C w/B$_{12}$ Principal B-Complex Factors w/Ascorbic Acid
Lyo B-C Forte w/B$_{12}$
M-M-R$_{II}$
M-R-VAX$_{II}$
Mannitol
Mefoxin
Meningovax-AC
Mephyton Tablets
Meruvax II
Mintezol Chewable Tablets/Suspension
Mumpsvax
Mustargen
Myochrysine Injection
NeoDECADRON Ophthalmic Solution & Ointment
NeoDECADRON Topical Cream
NeoDECASPRAY Topical Aerosol
Neo-Hydeltrasol—Ophthalmic Ointment, Ophthalmic Solution
Normal Serum Albumin (Human)
◆ Periactin Tablets & Syrup
Pneumovax
Propadrine HCl Capsules & Elixir
Redisol, Injection & Tablets
Respihaler Decadron Phosphate
◆ Sinemet Tablets
Sodium Diuril Intravenous
Sodium Edecrin Intravenous
Sulfathalidine Tablets
T-I-Gammagee
Tetanus Toxoid, Purified, Adsorbed, MSD
Thrombolysin
Timoptic Ophthalmic Solution
◆ Triavil Tablets
Turbinaire (see Decadron Phosphate, Turbinaire)
Urecholine Injection
◆ Urecholine Tablets
◆ Vivactil Tablets

MERICON INDUSTRIES, INC. 1205
420 S.W. Washington Street
Peoria, IL 61602
Address inquiries to:
Thomas P. Morrissey (309) 676-0744
Products Available
▣ Orazinc Capsules
▣ Zinc Tablets

MERRELL-NATIONAL LABORATORIES 419, 1205
Division of Richardson-Merrell Inc.
Cincinnati, OH 45215
Address inquiries to:
Manager Professional Services
(513) 948-9111
MERRELL-NATIONAL LABORATORIES Inc.
Cayey, Puerto Rico 00633
Address inquiries to:
Manager, Professional Services
MERRELL-NATIONAL LABORATORIES
Division of Richardson-Merrell Inc.
Cincinnati, OH 45215 (513) 948-9111

Products Available
AVC Suppositories
AVC Vaginal Cream
AVC/Dienestrol Cream
AVC/Dienestrol Suppositories
Bacimycin Ointment
◆ Bendectin Tablets
◆ Bentyl 10 mg. Capsules
Bentyl 10 mg. w/Phenobarbital Capsules
Bentyl Injection
Bentyl Syrup
Bentyl w/Phenobarbital Syrup
◆ Bentyl 20 mg. Tablets
Bentyl 20 mg. Tablets w/Phenobarbital
◆ Cantil Tablets
Cantil w/Phenobarbital Tablets
Cēpacol Anesthetic Troches
Cēpacol Mouthwash/Gargle
Cēpacol Throat Lozenges
Cēpastat Mouthwash/Gargle
Cēpastat Sore Throat Lozenges
◆ Cephulac Syrup
◆ Chronulac
Clomid Tablets
Consotuss Antitussive Syrup
Cotussis Syrup
Cyanocobalamin Injection
DV Cream/DV Suppositories
Decapryn Syrup & Tablets
Delcid
Diothane Ointment
Ganatrex Elixir
Hedulin Tablets
◆ Hiprex Tablets
Imferon
Kolantyl Gel
Kolantyl Tablets
Kolantyl Wafers
Mercodol Cough Syrup w/Decapryn
◆ Metahydrin
◆ Metatensin
Nicalex
◆ Norpramin
Orenzyme
Orenzyme Bitabs
Papaverine Hydrochloride Tablets
Pyridoxine Hydrochloride Tablets
◆ Quinamm Tablets
Sedadrops
Simron Capsules
Simron Plus Capsules
Sterile Hydroxystilbamidine Isethionate
◆ TACE 12 mg. Capsules
◆ TACE 25 mg. Capsules
◆ TACE 72 mg. Capsules
◆ Tenuate Dospan Tablets

◆ Tenuate Tablets
Terpin Hydrate & Codeine Elixir
◆ Triclos Tablets & Liquid
Vanobid Vaginal Ointment
◆ Vanobid Vaginal Tablets

METABOLIC PRODUCTS CORPORATION 1222
37 Hurley Street
Cambridge, MA 02141
Address inquiries to:
Professional Services (617) 547-5900
Products Available
Melasol
Prostall Capsules
Prostex Capsules
Te Tree Foot Cream
Te Tree Oil
Te Tree Ointment

METRO MED, INC. 1223
5400 Hudson Bend Road
Austin, TX 78734
Address inquiries to:
Medical Services Dept. (512) 474-7724
Products Available
Digestamic
Digestamic #2
Digestamic Liquid
Furon
Histamic
Metrogesic
Metrogesic #2
Metrogesic #3
Span-FF
Span-RD Tabs
Tenzide
Tet-Cy

MEYER LABORATORIES, INC. 419, 1223
1900 West Commercial Blvd.
Fort Lauderdale, FL 33309
(305) 776-5300
See product listing under Glaxo Inc.

MILES LABORATORIES, INC. 1223
P.O. Box 340
Elkhart, IN 46515
Address inquiries to:
Medical Dept. (219) 262-7886
Products Available
▣ Alka-Seltzer Effervescent Antacid
▣ Alka-Seltzer Effervescent Pain Reliever and Antacid
▣ Alka-Seltzer Plus Cold Medicine
▣ Alka-2 Chewable Antacid Tablets
▣ Chocks Bugs Bunny Multivitamin Supplement
▣ Chocks Bugs Bunny Plus Iron Multivitamin Supplement
▣ Chocks Multivitamin Supplement
▣ Chocks Plus Iron Multivitamin Supplement
▣ Flintstones Multivitamin Supplement
▣ Flintstones Plus Iron Multivitamin Supplement
▣ One-A-Day Vitamins
▣ One-A-Day Vitamins Plus Iron
▣ One-A-Day Vitamins Plus Minerals

MILEX PRODUCTS, INC. 1223
5915 Northwest Highway
Chicago, IL 60631 (312) 631-6484
Shipping Offices
Milex-Western
Post Office Box 46030
Los Angeles, CA 90046 (213) 651-4301
Milex Central
1873 Grove Street
Glenview, IL 60025 (312) 729-5253
Milex Michigan
Post Office Box 20264
Ferndale, MI 48220 (313) 399-9223
Milex Puerto Rico
GPO Box 554
San Juan, Puerto Rico 00936
(809) 791-3309
Milex Hawaii
Box 6337
Honolulu, HI 96818 (808) 422-9581
Milex-Southeastern
Post Office Drawer 4647
Clearwater, FL 33518 (813) 461-1949
Milex Southern
Post Office Drawer "M"
Weatherford, TX 76086 (817) 594-6865
Milex Carolinas
Post Office Box 23060
Charlotte, NC 28212 (704) 545-4567
Milex Delaware Valley
350 White Horse Pike
Atco, NJ 08004 (609) 767-4818
Products Available
Amino-Cerv
Amniotome
Cannula Curette with Swivel Handle
Dilateria
Fertilo-Pak
Laminaria Japonica
Oligospermia Cups
Pro-Ception
Spatula
Sufamal
Tis-U-Trap
Tricho-San
Trimo-San

MILLER PHARMACAL 1224
Div. of Medical Modalities Associates, Inc.
An Akorn Co.
1425 Melody Drive
Metairie, LA 70002 (504) 835-4955
Address inquiries to:
Anthony Umbdenstock Ph.D.
(312) 231-3632
Products Available
A/G Pro
Banapp
Ca-Plus
Cu-Plus
Cardenz
Carota
Cemill (Vitamin C)
Chenatal
Dequasine
DoFus
Fe-Plus
Glutamic Acid
Hyalex
Iso-pH
Lysmins
Mg-Plus
Mg-+"C"
M-Levelose
M-Levelyte #1
Mn-Plus
M-Ultramins
Milco-B
Milco-Pro
Milco-Trim
Milco-Zyme
Niarb Super
Nuclomin
Pheryl E (Vit. E)
Ragus
Sclerex
Sust-A (Vit. A)
Wamel
Zn-Plus

MISSION PHARMACAL COMPANY 1225
1325 E. Durango
San Antonio, TX 78210
Address inquiries to:
Professional Service Dept. (512) 533-7118
Post Office Box 1676
San Antonio, TX 78296
Products Available
Calcet
Dilax-100
Dilax-250
Equilet
Ferralet
Fosfree
Iromin-G
Mission Prenatal
Mission Prenatal F.A.
Mission Prenatal H.P.
Prulet
Prulet Liquitab
Supac
Therabid

MURO PHARMACAL LABORATORIES, INC. 1227
Muro-Derm
890 East Street
Tewksbury, MA 01876
Address inquiries to:
Professional Service Dept. (617) 851-2557
(617) 851-5981
Products Available
Dermodex 5 Gel
Dermodex 10 Gel
Duolube S.O.P. Ophthalmic Ointment
Goniogel
Muro 128 Ophthalmic Ointment
Muro 128 Ophthalmic Solution
Murocel - Ophthalmic Solution
Murocoll-2 Ophthalmic Solution
Phenoptic Ophthalmic Solution
Piloptic Ophthalmic Solution
Teen 5 Lotion
Teen 10 Lotion
Teen 5 Wash

NATURE'S BOUNTY, INC. 1228
105 Orville Drive
Bohemia, NY 11716
Address inquiries to:
Professional Service Dept. (516) 567-9500
(800) 645-5412
Products Available
Acerola "C" Tablets
Acidophilus Capsules
Alfalfa Tablets
B-1 Tablets
B-2 Tablets
B-6 Tablets
B-12 Tablets
B-50 Tablets
B-100 Tablets
B-100 Time Release Tablets
B-125 Tablets
B-Complex & B-12 Tablets
B-Complex & C Time Release Capsules
B & C Liquid
Bee Pollen Tablets
Biotin Tablets with Vitamin D
Bone Meal Tablets
Brewer's Yeast Powder
Brewer's Yeast Tablets
C-1000 Tablets
C-Liquid
C-Time Time Release Tablets
Calcium Ascorbate Tablets
Calcium Lactate Tablets
Calcium Pangamate Tablets
Children's Chewable Tablets
Choline Tablets
Cod Liver Oil Capsules
Copper Tablets
Dolomite Tablets
Fructose Tablets
Garlic Oil Capsules
Garlic & Parsley Capsules
Ginseng, Manchurian Capsules
Glutamic Acid Tablets
Gotu Kola Tablets
Inositol Tablets
Kelp Tablets
L-Glutamine Tablets
L-Lysine Tablets
Lecithin Capsules & Granules
Magnesium Tablets
Manganese Tablets
Mega V & M Tablets
Multi-Mineral Tablets
Niacin Tablets
Niacinamide Tablets
Oyster Calcium Tablets
PABA Tablets
Pantothenic Acid Tablets
Potassium Tablets
Protein Capsules, Tablets, Liquid, Powder
RNA (Nucleic Acid) Tablets
Rutin Tablets
Safflower Oil Capsules
Selenium Tablets
Tryptophane Tablets
Ultra "A" Capsules & Tablets
Ultra "A & D" Tablets
Ultra "D" Tablets
Vitamin A & D
Vitamin E Capsules (D-Alpha Tocopheryl)
Vitamin E-Oil
Wheat Bran Tablets
Wheat Germ Oil Capsules
Zacne Tablets
Zinc Tablets

NEUTROGENA CORPORATION 1228
5755 West 96th Street
P.O. Box 45036
Los Angeles, CA 90045 (800) 421-6857
In CA (213) 776-5223
Products Available
Neutrogena Acne-Drying Gel
Neutrogena Baby Soap
Neutrogena Lotion for Hand and Skin
Neutrogena Norwegian Formula Hand Cream
Neutrogena Rainbath Shower Gel
Neutrogena Sesame Seed Body Oil
Neutrogena Soap for Normal-to-Dry Skin
Neutrogena Soap for Normal-to-Oily Skin
Neutrogena Soap for Skin with Acne
Neutrogena Solid Soap Shampoo
Neutrogena Vehicle/N

NORCLIFF THAYER INC. 1229
One Scarsdale Road
Tuckahoe, NY 10707 (914) 969-8383
Products Available
▣ A-200 Pyrinate Liquid, Gel
▣ Co-Salt, Salt Substitute
▣ Dicarbosil Antacid Tablets
▣ Esoterica Medicated Creams
▣ Liquiprin Acetaminophen
▣ Oxy-5 Lotion
▣ Oxy-10 Lotion
▣ Oxy-Wash
▣ Tums

NORGINE LABORATORIES, INC. 1230
420 Lexington Avenue
New York, NY 10017 (212) 697-1513
Products Available
Bilamide Tablets
Enzypan Tablets
Fybranta Tablets
Hepp-Iron Drops
Hepron Tablets
Movicol Granules
Muripsin Tablets

(◆ Shown in Product Identification Section) (▣ Described in PDR For Nonprescription Drugs)

NORTH AMERICAN PHARMACAL, INC. 1230
6851 Chase Road
Dearborn, MI 48126 (313) 846-6400
(800) 521-4686
Products Available
APAC
Barbipil
Barbita
Baumodyne
Benegyn Vaginal Cream
Bexibee
Cal Prenal
Colsalide (improved)
Digestalin
Donna Sed
Estradiol L.A.
Fumaral Spancap
Hi Bee w/C
Hypnaldyne
Oraminic Spancap
Pavarine Spancap
Spastosed
Sulfavitin
Uracel
Uranap
Uritab
Vermizine Syrup
Vio-Hydrosone Cream
Vitagett

NORWICH-EATON PHARMACEUTICALS 410, 1230
Professional Products Group
(formerly Eaton Laboratories)
Consumer Products Group
(formerly Norwich Products)
Division of Morton-Norwich Products, Inc.
13-27 Eaton Avenue
Norwich, NY 13815
Address medical inquiries to:
Medical Department
Norwich, NY 13815 (607) 335-2565
Sales Offices
CHICAGO
Elk Grove Village, IL 60007
1350 Greenleaf Avenue (312) 593-0100
DALLAS
Dallas, TX 75222
P.O. Box 5490, Terminal Annex
(214) 337-4794
GREENVILLE
Greenville, SC 29602
P.O. Box 2468 (803) 277-7110
LOS ANGELES
Los Angeles, CA 90051
P.O. Box 2171, Terminal Annex
(213) 726-0505
NEW YORK CITY
New Rochelle, NY 10801
56 Harrison Street (914) 576-3900
NORWICH
Norwich, NY 13815
13-27 Eaton Avenue (607) 335-2243
Products Available
Alphaderm Cream
Chloraseptic Preparations
Menthol Chloraseptic Mouthwash & Gargle
Cherry Chloraseptic Mouthwash & Gargle
Menthol Chloraseptic Spray
Cherry Chloraseptic Spray
Menthol Chloraseptic Lozenges
Cherry Chloraseptic Lozenges
Children's Chloraseptic Lozenges
Chloraseptic DM Cough Control Lozenges
Chloraseptic Gel
Dantrium Capsules
Dantrium Intravenous
Dopar Capsules
Duvoid Tablets
Encare
Furacin Preparations
Furacin Soluble Dressing
Furacin Soluble Powder
Furacin Topical Cream
Furadantin Oral Suspension
Furadantin Tablets
Furoxone Liquid
Furoxone Tablets
Ivadantin
◆ Macrodantin Capsules
Ocusol Eye Drops
Ocusol Eye Lotion
Vivonex Delivery System
Vivonex Flavor Packets
Vivonex HN High Nitrogen Diet
Vivonex Standard Diet

NUTRITION CONTROL PRODUCTS 1241
Division of Pharmex Inc.
2113 Lincoln Street
P.O. Box 151
Hollywood, FL 33022 (305) 923-2821
Products Available
Adenocrest Injection
Betacrest Injection
▣ Betacrest Kapules
▣ Bio-Crest Tabseals
Calcium Orotate Tablets
▣ Chelated Minerals
Crestabolic Injection
Evac-U-8 Fortified Tabseals
Evac-U-8 Tabseals
Exabese Capsules
Gel-Kote Chewettes
Gericrest Tonic (Liquid)
Hexacrest Injection
Hy-E-Plex
Kelex Tabseals
▣ Lethopherol Kapules
Levoid Injection
Levoid Tablets
Liv-O-Rex Tablets
Magnesium Orotate Tablets
Multi-Vi-Rex Capsules
NCP-500 Capsules
Natacrest Capsules
Nutra-500 Tablets
▣ Nutricol Capsules
Nutricol Injection
Plexovims Capsules
Pro-Gestive Tablets
Progiatric Tablets
Pro-Neurin
Rubicrest Crystalline B_{12}
Rubicrest Injection
Trinsicrest Capsules
Vasotherm Injection
▣ Vitacrest Capsules
▣ Zinc Sulfate
Zymacrest Tablets

OLC LABORATORIES, INC. 1241
99 N.W. Miami Gardens Dr.
Miami, FL 33169
Toll Free WATS Line 1-(800) 327-7914
Address inquiries to:
OLC Laboratories, Inc
Herman H. Orlove
6770 N. Lincoln Ave.
Lincolnwood, IL 60646
Toll Free WATS Line 1-(800) 327-7914
Branch Offices
Orlove's Lincoln Crawford
6770 N. Lincoln Ave.
Lincolnwood, IL 60646
Toll Free WATS Line 1-(800) 327-7914
Products Available
Tryptacin Tablets
L. Tryptophan Tablets

OBETROL PHARMACEUTICALS 420, 1241
(Division of Rexar Pharmacal Corp.)
396 Rockaway Avenue
Valley Stream, NY 11581
Address inquiries to:
Ellen Zivitz (516) 561-7662
Products Available
◆ Obetrol
Oby-Rex
Oby-Rex Tablets

O'NEAL, JONES & FELDMAN PHARMACEUTICALS 420, 1242
2510 Metro Blvd.
Maryland Heights, MO 63043
(314) 569-3610
Products Available
A.C.T.H. "40" & "80" Injectable
Acetycol Tablets
Adeno Injectable
Almora Tablets
Aluscop Capsules
Amonidrin Tablets
Amphenol Tablets
Anaids Tablets
Andro L.A. Injectable
Andro "50" & "100" Injectable
Androgyn L.A. Injectable
Anergan "25" & "50" Injectable
Antilirium Injectable
Antilirium Tablets
Arbon Injectable
Arbon Tablets
Ascorbic Acid "2500" Injectable
Asminyl Tablets
Atoka Tablets
B-12 Plus Injectable
B-A Tablets
Banalg Liniment
Bancap Capsules
Bancap c̄ Codeine Capsules
Banesin Tablets
Basiget Tablets
Becomco Elixir
Beesix Injectable
Belfer Tablets
Betaprone Liquid
Biamine Injectable
Blandlube Liquid
Breonex Injectable
Calcium Gluconate Injectable
Calscorbate Tablets & Injectable
Canz Tablets
Caquin Cream
Cebucap
Cellubolic Injectable
Cetane Injection
Cetane Injection (w/o preservative)
Cetane Timed Capsules
Choron Injectable
Choron "10" Injectable Pak
Codroxomin Injectable
Conex DA Tablet
Conex Liquid
Conex Lozenges
Conex Plus Tablets
Conex Tablets
Conex c̄ Codeine Liquid
Cyomin Injectable
Cytobolin Injectable
Dalalone Injectable
Dalalone L.A. Injectable
Dalalone R.P. Injectable
Dehist Capsules
Dehist Injectable
Delladec Injectable
depAndro Injectable
depAndrogyn Injectable
depGynogen Injectable
depMedalone "40" & "80" Injectable
depPredalone "40" & "80" Injectable
Derfule Capsules
Dexpanthenol Injectable
Diabismul Suspension
Diabismul Tablets
Dialixir Liquid
Disotate Injectable
Dommanate Injectable
Duradyne DHC Tablets
Duradyne Forte Tablets
Duradyne Tablets
Duranabolic Injectable
Durapav Capsules
Dureze Drops
E-ferol Acetate Capsules
E-ferol Injectable
E-ferol Ointment
E-ferol Succinate Capsules
Enzymet Tablet
Euphenex Tablets
Fellows Compound Syrup
Fellozine "25" & "50" Injectable
Femogen Tablets
Femogen Vaginal Cream (w/applicator)
Feostat Drops
Feostat Injectable
Feostat Suspension
Feostat Tablets
Feostim Tablets
Ferrospan Injectable
G.B.S. Tablets
Gest Tablets
Gesterol in Oil "100" Injectable
Gesterol L.A. "250" Injectable
Glycate Tablets
Gynogen Injectable
Gynogen L.A. "10" & "20" Injectable
Gynogen R.P. Injectable
Heparin Sodium Injectable
Heparin Sodium w/o preservative Injectable
Hista-Derfule Capsules
Hycorace "100" & "250" Monovial Injectable
Hydrochloric Acid Injectable
Iatric Injectable
Iodo-Niacin Injectable
◆ Iodo-Niacin Tablets
KBP/O Capsules
Kiddisan Chewable Cold Tablets
Lidocaine Injectable
Livroben Injectable
Magnesium Chloride Injectable
Magnesium Sulfate Injectable
Malogen Cyp "200" Injectable
Malogen L.A. "200" Injectable
Medalone R.P. Injectable
Metra Tablets
N.B.P. Ointment
Neonic Tablets
Neoquess Tablets
Neo-Rhiban Tablets
Neurogyn Injectable
Niac Capsules
Nuxaphen Tablets
Osteolate Injectable
Oxothalein Tablets
Panvitex Prenatal Tablets
Paral Injectable
Paral Liquid
◆ Pedameth Capsules
Pedameth Liquid
Pentryate "80" Capsules
Petameth Capsules
Phenobarbital Tablets
Phentermine "30" Capsules
Philject Injectable
Potassium Chloride Injectable
Predalone R.P. Injectable
Predalone T.B.A. Injectable
Predalone Tablets
Proklar Suspension
Proklar Tablets

Psychozine Injectable
Queltuss Tablets
Raurine Tablets
Rauverid Tablets
Renelate Tablets
Robam Tablets
Rogenic Injectable
Rogenic Tablets
Sarcoptic Mange Liquid
Senilex Tablets
Sodium Chloride Injectable
Solu-Eze Solvent
soluPredalone Injectable
Soniphen Tablets
Sulfaloid "500" Tablets
Sulfaloid Suspension
Tanurol Ointment
Tetracycline HCl Capsules
Tralmag Suspension
Triamolone "40" Injectable
Triamonide Injectable
Uri-Pak Unit
Urithol Tablets
Verazinc Capsules
Water USP Injectable
Wolfina "50" & "100" Tablets

ORGANON PHARMACEUTICALS 420, 1244
375 Mount Pleasant Ave.
West Orange, NJ 07052 (201) 325-4500
Address inquiries to:
Manager, Educational & Technical Services (201) 325-4665
Products Available
◆ Accelerase
◆ Accelerase-PB
Bilogen
Cortrophin Gel
Cortrophin-Zinc
Cortrosyn
◆ Cotazym
Cotazym-B
◆ Cotazym-65B
Deca-Durabolin
Doca Acetate
Dodex Injectable
Durabolin
Hexadrol Cream
Hexadrol Phosphate Injection
◆ Hexadrol Tablets
◆ Hexadrol Therapeutic Pack
Liquaemin Sodium
◆ Liquamar
◆ Maxibolin
Medache
Monosticon Dri Dot
Pavulon
Pernaemon
Pregnosticon Dri Dot
Pregnyl
Regonol
Succinylcholine
◆ Wigraine

ORTHO DIAGNOSTICS INC. 1251
Route 202
Raritan, NJ 08869
Address inquiries to:
Professional Service Div. (201) 524-1732
(201) 524-2374
Products Available
Activated Thrombofax Reagent-Optimized
Affirmagen Reagent Red Blood Cells
Fetaldex Screening Test for Fetal Red Blood Cells in the Maternal Blood Circulation
Fibrindex Thrombin (Human)
Gravindex Slide Test for Pregnancy
Gravindex Tube Test for Pregnancy
Identigen Reagent Red Blood Cells
MICRhoGAM Rh_0 (D) Immune Globulin (Human), Micro-Dose
Monospot Slide Test for Infectious Mononucleosis
Ortho A_2 Cells Reagent Red Blood Cells
Ortho Abnormal Plasma Coagulation Control
Ortho Anti-Human Serum
Ortho Antithrombin III Assay
Ortho Blood Grouping Sera
Ortho Blood Group Substances
Ortho Bovine Albumin and Ortho Polymerized Bovine Albumin
Ortho Brain Thromboplastin
Ortho Coombs Control
Ortho Papanicolaou Smear Stains
Ortho Plasma Coagulation Control
Ortho Pregnancy Test Control Urines
Ortho Reagent Confidence Sera
Ortho Rh-hr Control
Raphadex Reversed Passive Hemagglutination Test for the Detection of HB_sAg
RhoGAM Rh_0 (D) Immune Globulin (Human)
Selectogen Reagent Red Blood Cells
Sickledex Tube Test for Hemoglobin S
Thrombofax Reagent

ORTHO PHARMACEUTICAL CORPORATION 420, 1253
Raritan, NJ 08869
Address inquiries to:
Director of Medical Services, Medical Research Dept. (201) 524-0400
Products Available
Aci-Jel Therapeutic Vaginal Jelly
▣ Conceptrol Birth Control Cream
▣ Delfen Contraceptive Foam
◆ Imodium Capsules
Lippes Loop Intrauterine Double-S
◆ Micronor Tablets
◆ Modicon Tablets 21-day regimen
◆ Modicon Tablets 28-day regimen
Monistat 7 Vaginal Cream
Nickerson's Medium
Ortho Diaphragm Kit-All Flex
Ortho Diaphragm Kit-Coil Spring
Ortho Diaphragm Kit-Flat Spring
Ortho Dienestrol Cream
▣ Ortho Disposable Applicator
▣ Ortho-Creme Contraceptive Cream
▣ Ortho-Gynol Contraceptive Jelly
◆ Ortho-Novum 1/50□21
◆ Ortho-Novum 1/50□28
◆ Ortho-Novum 1/80□21
◆ Ortho-Novum 1/80□28
◆ Ortho-Novum Tablets 2 mg□21
◆ Ortho-Novum Tablets 10 mg □21
Salpix Contrast Medium
Sultrin Triple Sulfa Cream
Sultrin Triple Sulfa Vaginal Tablets

ORTHO PHARMACEUTICAL CORPORATION 1269
Dermatological Division
Raritan, NJ 08869
a Johnson & Johnson Company
(201) 524-0400
Products Available
Grifulvin V
MicaTin Brand Miconazole Nitrate Cream and Lotion
▣ Purpose Brand Dry Skin Cream
▣ Purpose Brand Shampoo
▣ Purpose Brand Soap
Retin-A Brand Tretinoin

PARKE-DAVIS 420, 1270 , 2010
Division of Warner-Lambert Company
201 Tabor Road
Morris Plains, NJ 07950 (201) 540-2000
Regional Sales Offices
Atlanta (Doraville), GA 30340
2935 Northeast Parkway (404) 449-9691
Baltimore (Hunt Valley), MD 21031
11350 McCormick Road (301) 666-7810
Dallas, TX 75247
7777 Carpenter Freeway (214) 631-2323
Detroit, MI 48207
2211 E. Jefferson (313) 393-0200
East Hartford, CT 06108
111 Founders Plaza (203) 528-9601
Memphis, TN 38138
1355 Lynnfield Road (901) 767-1921
Pittsburgh, PA 15220
Manor Oak Two
1910 Cochran Road (412) 343-9855
Schaumburg, IL 60195
1111 Plaza Drive (312) 884-6990
Seattle, WA 98188
150 Andover Park, W (206) 244-7400
Tustin, CA 92680
17822 East 17th St. (714) 731-3441
Products Available
A-R-D
A.R.D. Anoperineal Dressings
Abdec Baby Vitamin Drops
Abdec Kapseals
abdec teens
abdec teens with iron
Abdec with Fluoride Baby Vitamin Drops
Abdol with Minerals Capsules
Acetaminophen (Tapar)
Acetaminophen with Codeine Phosphate Tablets, No. 2
Acetaminophen with Codeine Phosphate Tablets, No. 3
Adrenalin Chloride Solution 1:100 and 1:1,000.
Adroyd Tablets
Agoral
Agoral, Marshmallow Flavor
Agoral, Raspberry Flavor
Albuspan (normal serum albumin [human])
Alcohol, Rubbing (Lavacol)
Alophen Pills
Ambodryl Hydrochloride Kapseals
◆ Amcill Capsules
Amcill for Oral Suspension
Amcill Pediatric Drops
Amcill-S
◆ Amitril
Amodiaquine Hydrochloride Tablets (Camoquin Hydrochloride)
Amoxicillin for Oral Suspension
◆ Amoxicillin (Utimox) Capsules
Analgesic Balm
Antibiotics
◆ Amcill Products
◆ Amoxicillin Products
◆ Chloromycetin Products
◆ Erythromycin Stearate Tablets (Erypar)
Humatin
Oxytetracycline Hydrochloride Capsules (Oxlopar)
Penicillin Products
Penicillin V Potassium Products (Penapar VK)
◆ Tetracycline Hydrochloride Capsules, (Cyclopar) (Cyclopar 500)
Antuitrin "S"
Anugesic Ointment
Anugesic Suppositories
◆ Anusol Hemorrhoidal Suppositories
Anusol Ointment
◆ Anusol-HC Cream
◆ Anusol-HC Hemorrhoidal Suppositories
Aplisol (tuberculin PPD, diluted)
Aplitest (tuberculin PPD, multiple-puncture device)
Ascorbic Acid Injection
Ascorbic Acid Tablets
Aspirin Compound Tablets
Aspirin Compound with Codeine Phosphate Tablets, No. 2 & No. 3
Aspirin Tablets
◆ Azo-Mandelamine
◆ Benadryl Capsules
Benadryl Cream
Benadryl Elixir
◆ Benadryl Kapseals
Benadryl Steri-Vials, Ampoules, and Steri-Dose Syringe
Benadryl with Ephedrine Sulfate Kapseals
Benylin Cough Syrup
Benylin DM
Benzoin Compound Tincture
Betapar
Biological Products
Biomydrin Nasal Spray - Drops
Brondecon Elixir
◆ Brondecon Tablets
Caladryl Cream, Lotion
Calcium Gluconate Injection, Tablets
Calcium Lactate Tablets
Camphorated Tincture of Opium (Paregoric)
Capsolin Ointment
◆ Carbrital Kapseals
Cascara Aromatic Fluidextract
Cascara Sagrada Extract Filmseal
Cas-Evac
Castor Oil
Celontin (Half Strength) Kapseals
◆ Celontin Kapseals
Cetacort Lotion
Cetaphil Cream
Cetaphil Lotion
Cherry Syrup
Chloral Hydrate Capsules
Chloramphenicol (Chloromycetin)
Chlordiazepoxide Hydrochloride Capsules
Chloromycetin Cream, 1%
Chloromycetin Hydrocortisone Ophthalmic
◆ Chloromycetin Kapseals
Chloromycetin Ophthalmic
Chloromycetin Ophthalmic Ointment, 1%
Chloromycetin Ophthalmic Solution (Ophthochlor)
Chloromycetin Otic
Chloromycetin Palmitate, Oral Suspension
Chloromycetin Sodium Succinate
Chloromycetin Solution, Ampoules
Chloromycetin-Polymyxin-Hydrocortisone Acetate Ophthalmic Ointment (Ophthocort)
Chloromyxin
Chlorpromazine Hydrochloride Tablets (Promapar)
Choledyl Elixir
Choledyl Pediatric Syrup
◆ Choledyl Tablets
Chorionic Gonadotropin (Antuitrin S)
Codeine Phosphate, Aspirin, Phenacetin and Caffeine Tablets
Codeine Phosphate Injection
Coly-Mycin M Parenteral
Coly-Mycin S Oral Suspension
Coly-Mycin S Otic w/Neomycin & Hydrocortisone
Combex Kapseals
Combex with Vitamin C Kapseals
Corticotropin Injection (ACTH)
Cyanocobalamin Injection (Sytobex)
Cyclopar Capsules (tetracycline hydrochloride)
Depancol
Dermovan
◆ Dilantin Infatabs
◆ Dilantin Kapseals
Dilantin, Parenteral
◆ Dilantin with Phenobarbital Kapseals
Dilantin-30 Pediatric Suspension
Dilantin-125 Suspension
Dioctyl Sodium Sulfosuccinate Capsules (D-S-S Capsules)

Dioctyl Sodium Sulfosuccinate with Casanthranol Capsules (D-D-S Plus Capsules)
Diphenhydramine Hydrochloride (Benadryl)
Duraquin
Elase
Elase Ointment
V-Applicator (for Elase Ointment)
Elase-Chloromycetin Ointment
◆ Eldec Kapseals
Ephedrine Sulfate Injection, Ampoules
Epinephrine (Adrenalin)
◆ Ergostat
◆ Erythromycin Stearate Tablets (Erypar)
Estrovis
Ethosuximide (see Zarontin)
◆ Euthroid
Ferrous Sulfate Filmseals
Fluogen (influenza virus vaccine)
Gamma Globulin (Human) (Immu-G)
Gamulin Rh
Gelusil Flavor-Pack
◆ Gelusil Liquid & Tablets
Gelusil-Lac
Gelusil-M Liquid & Tablets
◆ Gelusil-II
Geriplex Kapseals
◆ Geriplex-FS Kapseals
Geriplex-FS Liquid
Green Soap Tincture
Heparin Sodium Injection
Hexavibex
Histoplasmin, Diluted
Humafac
Humatin Capsules & Syrup
Hydrochlorothiazide Tablets, USP (Thiuretic)
Hydrogen Peroxide Solution
Hydroxocobalamin Injection, NF (Sytobex-H)
Immu-G (Immune Serum Globulin [Human])
Infatabs (Dilantin)
Influenza Virus Vaccine (Fluogen)
Initia Drops
Initia Drops with Fluoride
Ketalar
Ketamine Hydrochloride Injection (Ketalar)
Lavacol
Liver Extract for Parenteral Use
◆ Loestrin [21] 1/20
◆ Loestrin [Fe] 1/20
◆ Loestrin [21] 1.5/30
◆ Loestrin [Fe] 1.5/30
Magnesium Sulfate Injection
◆ Mandelamine
Mandelamine Granules
Mandelamine Suspension
Mandelamine Suspension Forte
Meperidine Hydrochloride Injection
Meprednisone (Betapar)
Meprobamate Tablets
Meted Shampoo
Meted 2 Shampoo
Methaqualone Hydrochloride Capsules, NF (Parest)
Methsuximide (Celontin)
Milk of Bismuth
Milk of Magnesia
Milontin (Half Strength) Kapseals
Milontin Kapseals
Milontin Suspension
Mineral Oil
Morphine Sulfate Injection
Myadec
◆ Nardil
◆ Natabec Kapseals
◆ Natabec Rx Kapseals
Natabec with Fluoride Kapseals
Natabec-FA Kapseals
Natafort Filmseal
Niacin Tablets
Nitroglycerin Tablets (Nitrostat)
◆ Nitrostat Tablets
Norethindrone Acetate and Ethinyl Estradiol Tablets (Loestrin, Norlestrin)
◆ Norlestrin [21] 1/50
◆ Norlestrin [21] 2.5/50
Norlestrin [28] 1/50
◆ Norlestrin [Fe] 1/50
◆ Norlestrin [Fe] 2.5/50
◆ Norlutate
◆ Norlutin
Normal Serum Albumin (Human), USP (Albuspan)
◆ Ophthochlor Ophthalmic Solution, 0.5%
Ophthocort Ophthalmic Ointment
Oxymetholone (Adroyd)
Oxytetracycline Hydrochloride Capsules (Oxlopar)
Oxytocin, Buccal (Pitocin Citrate, Buccal Tablets)
Oxytocin Injection (Pitocin)
Paladac
Paladac with Minerals Tablets
◆ Palaflor Tablets
◆ Papase
Paracort (prednisone)
Paregoric
◆ Parest Capsules
Paromomycin (Humatin)
Parsidol
Penicillin G Potassium for Injection, and Tablets
Penicillin G Procaine
Penicillin V Potassium for Oral Solution
◆ Penicillin V Potassium Tablets (Penapar VK)
Pentrax Tar Shampoo
◆ Peritrate Sustained Action
◆ Peritrate Tablets
Peritrate w/Nitroglycerin
◆ Peritrate w/Phenobarbital
◆ Peritrate w/Phenobarbital Sustained Action
Peroxide, Hydrogen
Persadox Acne Cream/Lotion
Persadox HP Acne Cream/Lotion
Persa-Gel 5% & 10%
Phenobarbital Elixir, Tablets
Phensuximide (Milontin)
Phenytoin Sodium (Dilantin)
Pitocin Citrate, Buccal Tablets
Pitocin Injection, Ampoules, Steri-Dose Syringes
Pitressin Ampoules
Pitressin Tannate in Oil Ampoules
Pituitrin Ampoules
Pituitrin-S Ampoules
Poison Ivy Extract
Polybrade
◆ Ponstel
Potassium Chloride Liquid
Potassium Gluconate Elixir
◆ Povan Filmseals
Povan Suspension
Prednisone Tablets (Paracort)
Prep-Aid
◆ Pre-Sate
Proct-Kit
◆ Proloid Tablets
Propoxyphene Compound 65
Propoxyphene Hydrochloride Capsules
Propylthiouracil Tablets
◆ Pyridium
◆ Pyridium Plus
Pyridoxine Hydrochloride (Hexavibex)
Pyrvinium Pamoate (Povan)
Quinidine Sulfate Tablets
Quinine Sulfate Capsules
◆ Renoquid Tablets
Rubbing Alcohol (Lavacol)
Saf-Tip Enema, Oil Retention
Saf-Tip Enema, Phosphate
Scopettes, Jr., Sterile
Scopettes, Jr. Swabs
Scopettes Proctosigmoidoscopic Swabs
Seba-Nil
Seba-Nil Cleansing Mask
Seba-Nil Towelettes
Siblin Granules
◆ Sinubid
Sinutab w/Codeine
Sodium Chloride Tablets
Sulfacytine Tablets (Renoquid)
Sulforcin Base
Sulforcin Lotion
sunSwept Cream
Surital Ampoules, Steri-Vials
Symptom 1,2,3, and Multi-Symptom
Sytobex Ampoules, Steri-Vials, and Steri-Dose Disposable Syringes
Sytobex-H Steri-Vials
◆ Tabron Filmseal
Taka-Combex Kapseals
Taka-Diastase Products
◆ Tedral
Tedral Anti-H
Tedral Elixir
◆ Tedral Expectorant
◆ Tedral SA
Tedral Suspension
◆ Tedral-25
Terpin Hydrate Elixir, and w/Codeine
Tetanus Toxoid, Adsorbed
◆ Tetracycline HCl Capsules (Cyclopar)
◆ Tetracycline HCl Capsules, (Cyclopar 500)
Texacort Scalp Lotion
Theelin Aqueous Suspensions
Theelin in Oil
Theelin R-P Steri-Vials
◆ Thera-Combex H-P Kapseals
Thera-Combex Kapseals
Therapads
Therapads Plus
Thiamine Hydrochloride Injection, and Tablets
Thiamylal Sodium (Surital)
Thiuretic (Hydrochlorothiazide Tablets)
Thrombin, Topical
Triogen
Tuberculin Aplisol and Aplitest
Tucks Cream
Tucks Cream HC
Tucks Ointment
Tucks Premoistened Pads
Tucks Saf Tip Phosphate Enema
Tucks Take-Alongs
Unibase
Utibid
◆ Uticort
V-Applicators for Elase Ointment
Vanilla Extract
Vasopressin Injection (Pitressin)
Velvachol
Verdefam Cream
Verdefam Solution
◆ Verstran Tablets
Vira-A for Infusion
◆ Vira-A Ophthalmic Ointment, 3%
Vitamin B Complex Elixir, Kapseals, and Steri-Vials
Vitamin B_1 (thiamine hydrochloride) Tablets
Vitamin C (ascorbic acid) Tablets
Vitamin E, Natural and Synthetic Capsules
Water for Injection, Bacteriostatic, Steri-Vials
◆ Zarontin
Ziradryl Lotion

PENNWALT PHARMACEUTICAL DIVISION 423, 1350
Pennwalt Corporation
755 Jefferson Road
Rochester, NY 14623

PENNWALT Rx DIVISION
755 Jefferson Road
Rochester, NY 14623
Address inquiries to:
Director of Professional Relations
P.O. Box 1766
Rochester, NY 14603 (716) 271-1000
PHARMACRAFT
755 Jefferson Road
Rochester, NY 14623
Address inquiries to:
Professional Services Department
P.O. Box 1212
Rochester, NY 14603
Products Available
◆ Adapin Capsules
◆ Biphetamine Capsules
Caldecort
Cholan HMB
Cholan V
Cholan-DH
Emul-O-Balm
◆ Ionamin Capsules
Kolyum Liquid and Powder
Nesacaine
Nesacaine-CE
Omni-Tuss Suspension
Tussionex Capsules
Tussionex Suspension
Tussionex Tablets
◆ Zaroxolyn Tablets

PERSŌN & COVEY, INC. 1354
616 Allen Avenue
Glendale, CA 91201
Address inquiries to:
Lorne V. Persōn, President (213) 240-1030
Products Available
A.C.N. Tablets
Ceebec Tablets
DHS Shampoo
DHS Tar Shampoo
DispAtabs Tablets
DOB Bath & Shower Oil (Formerly Tolakol)
Drysol
Enisyl Tablets
Solbar Sun Protective Cream
Xerac
Xerac AC
Xerac BP5
Xerac BP10
Z-Pro-C Tablets

PFIPHARMECS DIVISION 423, 1356
Pfizer Inc.
235 E. 42nd St.
New York, NY 10017
Address inquiries to:
Professional Services Dept. (212) 573-2323
Address Export inquiries to:
Pfizer International Inc. (212) 573-2323
Distribution Centers
Doraville, GA 30340
4360 Northeast Expressway (404) 448-6666
Hoffman Estates, IL 60196
2400 W. Central Road (312) 381-9500
Clifton, NJ 07012
230 Brighton Rd. (201) 546-7700
Grand Prairie, TX 75050
502 Fountain Parkway (817) 261-9131
Irvine, CA 92705
16700 Red Hill Ave. (714) 540-9180
Products Available
Bacitracin Topical Ointment
Bonine
Cortril Topical Ointment
Coryban-D Capsules
Coryban-D Cough Syrup
◆ Neobiotic Tablets
Obron-6 Tablets
◆ Pen A Capsules
Pen A Powder For Oral Suspension
◆ Pfizer-E Film Coated Tablets
Pfizerpen G Powder for Syrup
◆ Pfizerpen G Tablets

Pfizerpen VK Powder For Oral Solution
◆ Pfizerpen VK Tablets
RID Pediculicide
RoeriBeC Tablets
◆ Sterane Tablets
Terramycin Topical Ointment
◆ Tetracyn Capsules
Tetracyn Syrup
◆ Tetrastatin Capsules
Viterra C
Viterra E
Viterra High Potency Tablets
Viterra Original Formulation Tablets

PFIZER LABORATORIES DIVISION 423, 1363
Pfizer Inc.
235 E. 42nd St.
New York, NY 10017
Address inquiries to:
Professional Services Dept. (212) 573-2422
Medical Emergency Calls
(Day or Night) (212) 573-2422
Address Export inquiries to:
Pfizer International Inc. (212) 573-2323
Distribution Centers
Doraville, GA 30340
4360 Northeast Expressway
(404) 448-6666
Hoffman Estates, IL 60196
2400 W. Central Road (312) 381-9500
Clifton, NJ 07012
230 Brighton Rd. (201) 546-7700
Grand Prairie, TX 75050
502 Fountain Parkway (214) 647-0222
Irvine, CA 92714
16700 Red Hill Ave. (714) 540-9180
Products Available
Ataraxoid Tablets
Azapen for Injection
Bacitracin Sterile Powder
Bonine Chewable Tablets
Cortril Acetate Aqueous Suspension
◆ Diabinese Tablets
Hydrocortisone Powder
Isoject Permapen in Aqueous Suspension
Isoject Pfizerpen-AS in Aqueous Suspension
Isoject Streptomycin Sulfate Injection
Isoject Terramycin Intramuscular Solution
Isoject Vistaril Intramuscular Solution
◆ Minipress Capsules
◆ Moderil Tablets
Pen A/N Injectable
Pfizerpen for Injection
Pfizerpen-AS in Aqueous Suspension
Polymyxin B Sulfate Sterile
◆ Renese Tablets
◆ Renese-R Tablets
◆ Sinequan Capsules
Sinequan Oral Concentrate
Streptomycin Sulfate (Dry)
Streptomycin Sulfate Injection
Terra-Cortril Ophthalmic Suspension
Terra-Cortril Topical Ointment
Terra-Cortril Topical Spray
◆ Terramycin Capsules
Terramycin I.M. Solution
Terramycin I.V.
Terramycin Ophthalmic Ointment
Terramycin Otic Ointment
Terramycin Syrup
Terramycin Tablets (film coated)
Terramycin Topical Powder
◆ Terramycin Vaginal Tablets
◆ Terrastatin Capsules
Tetracyn Intramuscular
Tetracyn Intravenous
Vibramycin Calcium Syrup
◆ Vibramycin Hyclate Capsules
Vibramycin Hyclate Intravenous
Vibramycin Monohydrate for Oral Suspension
◆ Vistaril Capsules
Vistaril Intramuscular Solution
Vistaril Oral Suspension
◆ Vistrax Tablets

PHARMACIA LABORATORIES 424, 1379
Division of Pharmacia Inc.
800 Centennial Ave.
Piscataway, NJ 08854
Address inquiries to:
Medical Director (201) 469-1222
Products Available
◆ Azulfidine Tablets & EN-tabs
Debrisan
Hyskon Hysteroscopy Fluid
Macrodex
Rectoid
Rheomacrodex

PHARMACRAFT CONSUMER PRODUCTS 1383
Pharmaceutical Division
Pennwalt Corporation
755 Jefferson Road
Rochester, NY 14623
Address inquiries to:
Professional Service Department
P.O. Box 1212
Rochester, NY 14603 (716) 271-1000
Products Available
▣ Allerest Tablets
▣ Allerest Timed Release Allergy Capsules
▣ Caldesene Medicated Ointment
▣ Caldesene Medicated Powder
▣ Cruex Medicated Cream
▣ Cruex Medicated Powder
▣ Desenex Ointment, Powder, Soap & Solution
▣ Desenex Spray-On Foot Powder
▣ Sinarest Tablets

PHILIPS ROXANE LABORATORIES, INC. 1383
330 Oak St., Columbus, OH 43216
Address inquiries to:
Professional Services Department
P.O. Box 16532
Columbus, OH 43216
(Toll Free) (800) 848-0120
(In Ohio call) (614) 228-5403
Products Available
Acetaminophen Elixir
Acetaminophen Suppositories
Acetaminophen Tablets
Acetaminophen with Codeine Phosphate Elixir
Acetaminophen with Codeine Phosphate Tablets
Acutuss Expectorant with Codeine Phosphate
Aluminum Hydroxide Gel
Aminophylline Suppositories
Amitriptyline Hydrochloride Tablets
Aromatic Cascara Fluidextract
Ascorbic Acid Tablets
Aspirin Suppositories
Barium Enema Prep Kit
Bisacodyl Patient Pack
Bisacodyl Suppositories
Bisacodyl Tablets
Calcium Gluconate Tablets
Castor Oil
Castor Oil Flavored
Chloral Hydrate Capsules
Chloral Hydrate Syrup
Chlordiazepoxide Hydrochloride Capsules
Chlorpheniramine Maleate Tablets
Chlorpromazine Hydrochloride Tablets
Dexamethasone Tablets
Digoxin Tablets
Dihydrotachysterol Tablets
Dioctyl Sodium Sulfosuccinate Capsules
Dioctyl Sodium Sulfosuccinate Syrup
Dioctyl Sodium Sulfosuccinate with Casanthranol Capsules
Diphenhydramine Hydrochloride Capsules
Diphenhydramine Hydrochloride Elixir
Diphenoxylate Hydrochloride & Atropine Sulfate Tablets
Dovamide Capsules
Duphaston (Dydrogesterone) Tablets
Ferrous Sulfate Liquid
Ferrous Sulfate Tablets
Gentz Wipes
Geroniazol Elixir
Geroniazol T.T. Tablets
Glycerin Solution (Flavored) 50% V/V
Guaifenesin Syrup
Guaiahist T.T. Tablets
Guaiahist Tablets
Hemorrhoidal Suppositories with Hydrocortisone Acetate
Hospital Unit Dose
Hydrochlorothiazide Tablets
Imipramine Hydrochloride Tablets
Ipecac Syrup
Kaolin-Pectin Suspension
Lithium Carbonate Capsules & Tablets
Lithium Citrate Syrup
Magnesia & Alumina Oral Suspension
Meprobamate Tablets
Milk of Magnesia
Milk of Magnesia-Concentrated
Milk of Magnesia-Cascara Suspension
Milk of Magnesia-Mineral Oil Emulsion & Emulsion (Flavored)
Mineral Oil
Mineral Oil-Light Sterile
Neomycin Sulfate Tablets
Niacin Tablets
Papaverine Hydrochloride Capsules
Paregoric
Penicillin G, Potassium Tablets
Phenobarbital Elixir
Phenobarbital Tablets
Potassium Chloride for Oral Solution (Flavored)
Potassium Chloride Oral Solution
Potassium Chloride Powder Unflavored
Potassium Gluconate Elixir
Potassium Iodide Liquid
Prednisolone Tablets
Prednisone Tablets
Propantheline Bromide Tablets
Propoxyphene Hydrochloride Capsules
Propoxyphene Hydrochloride 65mg & APC Capsules
Quinidine Sulfate Tablets
Reserpine Tablets
SSKI
Sodium Chloride Solutions & Sterile Purified Water for Respiratory Therapy
Sodium Phosphate & Biphosphate Oral Solution
Sulfisoxazole Tablets
Sulfisoxazole with Phenazopyridine HCl Tablets
Terpin Hydrate & Codeine Elixir
Tetracycline Hydrochloride Capsules
Theophylline Elixir
Vitamin A Capsules (Solubilized)
Vitamin E Capsules (Natural)

POYTHRESS & CO., INC., WM. P. 424, 1389
16 N. 22nd St.
Post Office Box 26946
Richmond, VA 23261 (804) 644-8591
Address inquiries to:
Special Services Department
Products Available
Antrocol Elixir
◆ Antrocol Tablets & Capsules
Bensulfoid
▣ Bensulfoid Lotion
Mudrane GG Elixir
◆ Mudrane GG Tablets
◆ Mudrane GG-2 Tablets
◆ Mudrane Tablets
◆ Mudrane-2 Tablets
Panalgesic
◆ Solfoton Tablets, Capsules & S/C (Sugar-Coated) Tablets
◆ Trocinate Tablets
◆ Uro-Phosphate Tablets

PREMO PHARMACEUTICAL LABORATORIES, INC. 1391
111 Leuning Street
South Hackensack, NJ 07606
Address inquiries to:
Mr. Martin H. Klein (201) 343-5000
Products Available
Acti-Prem Tablets
Algemol Velvetabs
Allopurinol Tablets
Amoxicillin Capsules
Ampicillin Trihydrate Capsules
Beta-Val Cream
Cephalexin Monohydrate Capsules
Chlordiazepoxide HCl Capsules
Chlordinium Sealets
Chlorothiazide Tablets
Chlorzoxazone with APAP Tablets
Cyclandelate Capsules
Decon-Aid TR Capsules
Decon-Tuss TR Capsules
Diphenhydramine HCl Capsules
Dipyridamole Tablets
Doxine Tablets
Dynohist S.A. Tablets
Erythromycin Stearate Tablets
Fluocin Cream
Folic Acid Tablets
Hydergot Sublingual Tablets
Hydralazine HCl Tablets
Hydrap-Es Tablets
Hydrochlorothiazide Tablets
Hydrocortisone Tablets
Hydro-Serp Tablets
Hydroxyzine HCl Tablets
Hy-Pam Capsules
Imipramine HCl Tablets
Insulase Tablets
Iso-Perazine TR Capsules
Isoxsuprine HCl Tablets
Meclizine HCl Tablets
Meprobamate Tablets
Meprogesic Tablets
Mepro-Hex Tablets
Myco Triacet Cream & Ointment
Nitrofurantoin Tablets
Nylidrin HCl Tablets
Nystatin Cream, Oral Tablets & Vaginal Tablets
Oxytetracycline HCl Capsules
Papaverine HCl TR Capsules
Phenatapp Extend Tablets
Phentermine HCl Capsules
Phentermine Resin Capsules
Phenylbutazone Alka Capsules
Phenytoin Sodium Capsules
Prednisolone Tablets
Prednisone Tablets
Propoxyphene Compound-65 Capsules
Propoxyphene HCl Capsules
Pseudoephedrine HCl Tablets
Tetracycline HCl Capsules
Theophedrizine Tablets
Thioridazine HCl Tablets
Tolbutamide Tablets
Triacet Cream
Triamterene with Hydrochlorothiazide
Trifluoperazine Tablets

PROCTER & GAMBLE 424, 1392
P.O. Box 171
Cincinnati, OH 45201
Address inquiries to:
Arnold P. Austin (513) 977-5547
For Medical Emergencies Contact:
H. Patterson Mack, M.D. (513) 977-2606
Products Available
◆ Didronel
⊞ Head & Shoulders
◆ Topicycline

PURDUE FREDERICK COMPANY, THE 424, 1394
50 Washington Street
Norwalk, CT 06856 (203) 853-0123
Address inquiries to:
Medical Department
Products Available
Arthropan Liquid
Athrombin-K Tablets
Betadine Aerosol Spray
Betadine Antiseptic Gauze Pad
Betadine Douche
Betadine Douche Kit
Betadine Hēlafoam Solution
Betadine Microbicidal Bath Concentrate
Betadine Mouthwash/Gargle
Betadine Ointment
Betadine Perineal Wash Concentrate
Betadine Shampoo
Betadine Skin Cleanser
Betadine Skin Cleanser Foam
Betadine Solution
Betadine Solution Swab Aid
Betadine Solution Swabsticks
Betadine Surgical Scrub
Betadine Surgi-Prep Sponge-Brush
◆ Betadine Vaginal Gel
Betadine Viscous Formula Antiseptic Gauze Pad
Betadine Whirlpool Concentrate
◆ Cardioquin Tablets
◆ Cerumenex Drops
Parelixir Liquid
Probilagol Liquid
Senokap DSS Capsules
Senokot Suppositories
Senokot Syrup
Senokot Tablets/Granules
Senokot Tablets Unit Strip Pack
Senokot w/Psyllium Powder
Senokot-S Tablets
Sulfabid Tablets
Supertah Ointment
◆ Trilisate Tablets

BLAIR LABORATORIES, INC.
Calamatum Lotion
Calamatum Ointment
Calamatum Spray
Fungacetin Ointment
Gertlax B Granules
Gertlax B Tablets
Gertlax S Tablets
Isodine Antiseptic Solution
Isodine Concentrate Gargle/Mouthwash
Kerid Ear Drops
Saratoga Ointment

SHIELD LABORATORIES, INC.
Central Venous Catheter Dressing Change Set
Urinary Catheter Care Set

PUREPAC PHARMACEUTICAL CO. 1398
200 Elmora Ave.
Elizabeth, NJ 07207 (201) 527-9100
Products Available
A.P.C. Tablets
A.P.C. w/Butalbital Tablets
A.P.C. w/Codeine Phosphate Tablets
Acetaminophen Elixir, Tablets
Acetaminophen w/Codeine Tablets
Aminophylline Tablets & Suppositories
Amitriptyline HCl Tablets
Ampicillin For Oral Suspension
Ampicillin Trihydrate Capsules
Antispasmodic Tablets & Elixir
Aspirin Suppositories & Tablets
Azma-Aid Tablets
Belladonna Alkaloids with Phenobarbital Tablets & Elixir
Belladonna Tincture
Bisacodyl Suppositories & Tablets
Butabarbital Sodium Elixir & Tablets
Calcium Lactate Tablets
Chloral Hydrate Capsules & Syrup
Chlordiazepoxide HCl Capsules
Chlorothiazide Tablets
Chlorpheniramine Maleate Time Release Capsules
Chlorpheniramine Maleate Tablets
Chlorpromazine HCl Tablets
Codeine Sulfate Tablets
Colchicine Tablets
Conjugated Estrogens Tablets
Cortisone Acetate Tablets
Cyclandelate Capsules
Dexamethasone Tablets
Digitoxin Tablets
Digoxin Tablets
Dimenhydrinate Tablets
Diocto Capsules
Diphenhydramine HCl Capsules
Diphenhydramine HCl Elixir & Expectorant
Diphenoxylate HCl & Atropine Sulfate, Tablets & Liquid
Doctase Capsules
Doxycycline Hyclate Capsules
Ergonovine Maleate Tablets
Ergotamine Tartrate & Caffeine Tablets
Erythromycin Stearate Tablets
Estrogenic Aqueous & Oil Injectable
Estrone Aqueous Suspension Injectable
Ferrous Fumarate Tablets
Ferrous Gluconate Tablets
Ferrous Sulfate Capsules, Time Release
Ferrous Sulfate Tablets
Folic Acid Tablets
Glutethimide Tablets
Hydralazine HCl Tablets
Hydrochlorothiazide Tablets
Hydrochlorothiazide with Reserpine Tablets
Hydrochlorothiazide with Reserpine & Hydralazine Tablets
Hydrocortisone Acetate Cream, Lotion & Powder
Hydrocortisone Tablets
Imipramine HCl Tablets
Iodine Solution Strong (Lugols)
Isoniazid Tablets
Isosorbide Dinitrate Tablets (Oral & Sublingual)
Isosorbide Dinitrate TD Tablets
Meclizine Multi-Layered Tablets
Meclizine Tablets, Chewable
Meprobamate Tablets
Methenamine Mandelate Tablets
Methocarbamol Tablets
Methyltestosterone Tablets
Nitrofurantoin Tablets
Nitroglycerin Capsules, Time Release
Oxytetracycline HCl Capsules
Papaverine Hydrochloride Capsules (Time Release) & Tablets
Paregoric
Penicillin G Potassium Powdered
Penicillin G Tablets, Buffered
Penicillin V (Buffered Potassium Penicillin V Powder)
Penicillin V Potassium Tablets
Pentaerythritol Tetranitrate Capsules, Time Release
Pentaerythritol Tetranitrate Tablets
Pentrobarbital Sodium Capsules
Phenobarbital Elixir & Tablets
Phenytoin Sodium Capsules
Potassium Chloride Oral Solution (Sugar Free)
Prednisolone Tablets & Injectable
Prednisone Tablets
Probenecid & Colchicine Tablets
Procainamide HCl Capsules
Progesterone in Oil Injectable
Promethazine Expectorant VC w/Codeine
Promethazine HCl Expectorant
Promethazine HCl Expectorant w/ Codeine
Promethazine HCl Tablets
Propantheline Bromide Tablets
Propoxyphene Compound 65
Propoxyphene HCl Capsules
Propoxyphene HCl & APAP Tablets
Propylthiouracil Tablets
Puretane DC Expectorant
Puretane Expectorant
Puretane Tablets
Puretapp Elixir
Puretapp PA Tablets
Pyridoxine HCl Injectable
Quinidine Sulfate Tablets
Quinine Sulfate Capsules
Rauwolfia Serpentina Tablets
Reserpine Tablets
Secobarbital Sodium Capsules
Spironolactone Tablets
Spironolactone w/Hydrochlorothiazide
Sulfamethoxazole Tablets
Sulfisoxazole Tablets
Testosterone Aqueous Suspension Injectable
Testosterone Propionate in Oil Injectable
Tetracycline HCl Capsules
Tetracycline Syrup
Thyroid Tablets
Tolbutamide Tablets
Triamcinolone Tablets
Tridihexethyl Chloride w/Meprobamate Tablets
Triple Antibiotic Ointment
Triprolidine HCl w/Pseudoephedrine HCl Syrup & Tablets

REED & CARNRICK 424, 1399
30 Boright Ave.
Kenilworth, NJ 07033
Address inquiries to:
Professional Service Dept. (201) 272-6600
Products Available
Alphosyl Lotion, Cream
Alphosyl-HC Lotion & Cream
◆ Cortifoam
Dilatrate-SR
Epifoam
Kwell Cream
Kwell Lotion
Kwell Shampoo
Peptenzyme Elixir
◆ Phazyme
◆ Phazyme-95
◆ Phazyme-PB Tablets
◆ Proctofoam-HC
◆ proctoFoam/non-steroid
Proxigel
R&C Spray
Sebical Cream Shampoo
◆ Sidonna
Syntrogel
Tarbonis
Trichotine Liquid, Vaginal Douche
Trichotine Powder, Vaginal Douche
Trichotine-D Disposable Vaginal Douche

REID-PROVIDENT LABORATORIES, INC. 424, 1404
Scientific Affairs and Manufacturing
25 Fifth Street, N.W.
Atlanta, GA 30308
Executive Offices
640 Tenth Street, N.W.
Atlanta, GA 30318

Address inquiries to:
Medical Director

Products Available
Anduracaine Injection
Azosul
◆ Calinate-FA
Chloramate Unicelles
Coton Syrup
Crystimin-1000
Curretab Tablets
Dentavite Chewable Tablets
Dentavite Drops
Estraguard Vaginal Cream
◆ Estratab Tablets
◆ Estratest H.S.
◆ Estratest Tablets
Eugel Liquid
Eugel Tablets
Femguard Vaginal Cream
Fumatrin-Forte
G-Recillin Powdered Buffered
G-Recillin Tablets
Histalet DM Syrup
◆ Histalet Forte T.D. Tablets
Histalet Syrup
Histalet X Syrup
◆ Histalet X Tablets
Infadorm Drops
Jectasone Injection
Jectatest-L.A. Injection
◆ Melfiat Tablets
Mity-Mycin Ointment (Topical)
Mity-Quin
Mulvitab
Neo-Ferraplex Injection
Otoreid-HC Ear Drops
P-V-Tussin Syrup
◆ P-V-Tussin Tablets
Pavacap Unicelles
Polysorbin Chewable Tablets
Polysorbin Drops
Polysorbin-F Drops
Proaqua
Proval Drops
Proval #3
Proval Tablets
Provigan Injection
Prov-U-Sep
Prov-U-Sep-Forte
RP-Mycin Tablets
Reidacol
Reidamine Injection
Relutin Injection
Repen-VK Suspensions
Repen-VK Tablets
Repro Compound-65
Retet-500
Retet Capsules
Retet-S Syrup
Spalix Elixir
Spalix Tablets
Sumox Capsules
Sumox Oral Suspensions
Supen Capsules
Supen Oral Suspensions
Symptomax Suspension
Tenax Capsules
Tranmep
Trisorbin Drops
Trisorbin-F Drops
Trisureid Suspension
Tusstrol
Unifast Unicelles

◆ Unipres Tablets
Vaso-80 Unicelles
Vasoglyn Unicelles
Vasotrate Sublingual
Vasotrate Tablets

RESEARCH INDUSTRIES CORPORATION 1405
Pharmaceutical Division
1847 West 2300 South
Salt Lake City, UT 84119
(800) 453-8432
(801) 972-5500
Products Available
Rimso-50

REXALL DRUG COMPANY 1406
3901 North Kingshighway Blvd.
St. Louis, MO 63115 (314) 679-7100
Branch Offices
Columbus, OH 43228 (614) 276-2665
East Point, GA 30344 (404) 768-0123
Grand Prairie, TX 75050 (214) 647-2221
St. Louis (Lab.) MO 63115 (314) 679-7269
Sparks, NV 89431 (702) 359-1777
Products Available
A.P.C. Tablets, see Monacet Comp.
Acetaminophen (No Aspirin) Tablets
Alurex Suspension
Ampicillin Capsules
Ampicillin Powder for Oral Suspension
Antihistamine Tablets
Asma-Kets A.H. Tablets
Aspirin Tablets
Bacitracin Ointment
Bisma-Rex Antacid Powder
Bisma-Rex Chewable Antacid Tablet
Calamine Lotion
Calcium Lactate Tablets
Children's Cough Syrup
Chloral Hydrate Capsules
Cold Tablets
Dicalcium Phosphate with Calcium Gluconate and Vitamin D Capills
Erythromycin Stearate Tablets
Eudicaine Ointment
Eudicaine Suppositories
Ger-Rite High Potency Vitamins with Iron Tablets
Glycerin Suppositories
Hay Fever Allergy Capsules & Tablets
Histacalma Lotion
Hot Lemon Cold Medicine
Hydrochlorothiazide Tablets
Iron Tabs (Ferrous Sulfate)
Meprobamate Tablets
Milk of Magnesia Suspension & Tablets
Minuteman Children's Chewable Multi-Vitamin Tablets, Plain & w/Iron
Monacet (APC) w/Codeine, Tablets
Monacet Comp. A.P.C. Tablets
Nasal Decongestant Time Capsules
Nasal Spray Mist
Niacin Tablets
No Aspirin Tablets (acetaminophen)
One Tablet Daily Family Vitamins, plain, w/Iron
Pabizol with Paregoric
Papaverine Hydrochloride Timed Release Capsules
Paregoric
Penicillin G. Potassium Tablets
Penicillin V. Potassium For Oral Suspension
Penicillin V. Potassium Tablets
Phenobarbital Elixir & Tablets
Prednisolone Tablets
Prednisone Tablets
Propoxyphene Hydrochloride Capsules
Propoxyphene Hydrochloride w/A.P.C. Capsules
Quiet-Nite, Night-time Cold Formula
Quinidine Sulfate Tablets
Reserpine Tablets
Saccharin Tablets
Salt Tablets
Sinurex Tablets
Stress Formula High Potency B-Complex Vitamins w/E & C Tablets
Super Plenamins Multiple Vitamins with Minerals
Terpin Hydrate & Codeine Elixir
Terpin Hydrate and Dextromethorphan Hydrobromide Elixir
Tetracycline Hydrochloride Capsules
Tetracycline Syrup
Thru Penetrating Analgesic
Thyroid Tablets
Triple Antibiotic Ointment
Tri-Salve Ointment (w/Benzocaine)
Vitamin A Capsules
Vitamin B Complex Tabs
Vitamin B_{12} Tablets
Vitamins B & C Capsules
Vitamin C Tablets
Vitamin E Capsules
Vitamins E + C Tablets
Zinc Oxide Ointment

RIKER LABORATORIES, INC. 425, 1408
Subsidiary of 3M Company
19901 Nordhoff Street
Northridge, CA 91324
Address inquiries to:
Director, Medical Services
(213) 341-1300, Ext. 421
Products Available
Alu-Cap Capsules
Alu-Tab Tablets
Buf Acne-Cleansing Bar
Buf Beauty Bar
Buf Beauty Basics
Buf Beauty Cream
Buf Body Scrub
Buf Foot-Care Kit
Buf Foot-Care Lotion
Buf Foot-Care Soap
Buf Kit for Acne
Buf-Ped
Buf-Puf
Buf-Puf Duo
Calcium Disodium Versenate Injection
Calcium Disodium Versenate Tablets
◆ Circanol Tablets
◆ Deaner Tablets
◆ Deaner-250 Tablets
Diafen
◆ Disalcid Tablets
◆ Disipal Tablets
◆ Dorbane Tablets
◆ Dorbantyl Capsules
◆ Dorbantyl Forte Capsules
Duohaler Aerosol
Duo-Medihaler Aerosol
Duovent Tablets
Estomul-M Liquid
Estomul-M Tablets
Heparin Sodium Injection, Aqueous (Lipo-Hepin)
Lipo-Hepin (Heparin Sodium Injection, Aqueous)
Lipo-Hepin/BL
Medihaler Ergotamine Aerosol
Medihaler-Epi Aerosol
Medihaler-Iso Aerosol
Norflex Injectable
◆ Norflex Tablets
◆ Norgesic Tablets
◆ Norgesic Forte Tablets
Rauwiloid Tablets
Sedamyl Tablets
Sodium Versenate Injection
Sombulex Tablets
◆ Tepanil Tablets
◆ Tepanil Ten-tab Tablets
Theolair Liquid
◆ Theolair Tablets
◆ Theolair-SR Tablets
Titralac Liquid
◆ Titralac Tablets
Ulo Syrup
◆ Urex Tablets
Veriloid Tablets

ROBINS COMPANY, A. H. 425, 1418
1407 Cummings Drive
Richmond, VA 23220
Address inquiries to:
The Medical Dept. (804) 257-2000
Medical Emergency calls (day or night) (804) 257-2000
If no answer, call answering service (804) 257-7788
Products Available
Adabee Tablets
Adabee w/Minerals Tablets
◆ Allbee w/C Capsules
◆ Allbee-T Tablets
Arthralgen Tablets
Cough Calmers
◆ Dimacol Capsules
Dimacol Liquid
Dimetane Elixir
Dimetane Expectorant
Dimetane Expectorant-DC
◆ Dimetane Extentabs
◆ Dimetane Tablets
Dimetane-Ten Injectable
Dimetapp Elixir
◆ Dimetapp Extentabs
Donnagel
Donnagel-PG
◆ Donnatal Capsules
Donnatal Elixir
◆ Donnatal Extentabs
◆ Donnatal No. 2 Tablets
◆ Donnatal Tablets
◆ Donnazyme Tablets
Dopram Injectable
◆ Entozyme Tablets
◆ Exna Tablets
◆ Exna-R Tablets
Heparin Lock Flush Solution
Heparin Sodium Injection, USP
Imavate Tablets
◆ Pabalate Tablets
◆ Pabalate-SF Tablets
◆ Phenaphen Capsules
Phenaphen Tablets
◆ Phenaphen w/Codeine Capsules
◆ Phenaphen-650 with Codeine Tablets
◆ Pondimin Tablets
◆ Quinidex Extentabs
Reglan Injectable
Repoise Tablets
Robalate Tablets
◆ Robamox Capsules
Robamox for Oral Suspension
Robaxin Injectable
◆ Robaxin Tablets
◆ Robaxin-750 Tablets
◆ Robaxisal Tablets
Robicillin VK for Oral Solution
◆ Robicillin VK Tablets
◆ Robimycin Robitabs
◆ Robinul Forte Tablets
Robinul Injectable
◆ Robinul Tablets
◆ Robinul-PH Tablets
◆ Robinul-PH Forte Tablets
Robitet Syrup
◆ Robitet '250' Hydrochloride Robicaps
◆ Robitet '500' Hydrochloride Robicaps
Robitussin
Robitussin A-C
Robitussin-CF
Robitussin-DAC
Robitussin-DM
Robitussin-PE
Silain Tablets
Silain-Gel Liquid
Skelaxin Tablets
◆ Sulla Tablets
Tybatran Capsules
◆ Z-Bec Tablets

ROCHE LABORATORIES 426, 1445, 2013
Division of Hoffmann-La Roche Inc.
Nutley, NJ 07110 (201) 235-5000
For Medical Information
Write: Professional Services Department
Business hours only (8:30 a.m. to 5:00 p.m. EST), call (201) 235-2355
For Medical Emergency Information only after hours or on weekends, call (201) 235-2355
Branch Warehouses
Dallas, TX 75229
2727 Northaven Rd.
(P.O. Box 29009) (214) 241-8573
Decatur, GA 30031
421 DeKalb Industrial Way
(404) 296-1241
Des Plaines, IL 60018
105 E. Oakton St. (312) 299-0021
(Chicago) (312) 775-0733
San Leandro, CA 94577
1599 Factor Ave. (415) 352-1660
Somerville, NJ 08876
3070 Highway 22, West
(P.O. Box 2010) (201) 526-7650

ROCHE PRODUCTS INC. 426, 1445, 2013
Manati, Puerto Rico 00701
Address inquiries to:
Roche Laboratories (see above)
Products Available
Alurate Elixir
◆ Ancobon
Arfonad Ampuls
◆ Azo Gantanol Tablets
◆ Azo Gantrisin Tablets
◆ Bactrim DS Tablets
Bactrim Pediatric Suspension
Bactrim Suspension
◆ Bactrim Tablets
◆ Berocca Tablets
Berocca-C & Berocca-C 500
◆ Clonopin
◆ Dalmane
Efudex Cream
Efudex Solution
◆ Endep
FUDR
Fluorouracil Ampuls
◆ Gantanol DS Tablets
Gantanol Suspension
◆ Gantanol Tablets
Gantrisin Injectable
Gantrisin Ophthalmic Ointment/Solution
Gantrisin Pediatric Suspension
Gantrisin Syrup
◆ Gantrisin Tablets
Konakion
◆ Larobec
◆ Larodopa Capsules
◆ Larodopa Tablets
◆ Larotid Capsules
Larotid for Oral Suspension
Larotid Pediatric Drops
Levo-Dromoran Injectable
◆ Levo-Dromoran Tablets
◆ Librax
◆ Libritabs
◆ Librium Capsules

Librium Injectable
◆ Limbitrol Tablets
Lipo Gantrisin
Lorfan
◆ Marplan Tablets
◆ Matulane
◆ Menrium
Mestinon Injectable
Mestinon Syrup
◆ Mestinon Tablets
◆ Mestinon Timespan
Nipride
Nisentil
◆ Noludar Tablets
◆ Noludar 300 Capsules
Pantopon
Prostigmin Injectable
◆ Prostigmin Tablets
◆ Quarzan
◆ Rocaltrol Capsules
Roniacol Elixir
◆ Roniacol Tablets
◆ Roniacol Timespan
◆ Solatene
Synkayvite Injectable
◆ Synkayvite Tablets
Taractan Concentrate
Taractan Injectable
◆ Taractan Tablets
◆ Tel-E-Dose (unit dose) Products:
Bactrim Tablets
Bactrim DS Tablets
Dalmane Capsules
Endep Tablets
Gantanol DS Tablets
Gantanol Tablets
Gantrisin Tablets
Larotid Capsules
Larotid Oral Suspension
Librax Capsules
Librium Capsules
Limbitrol Tablets
Valium Tablets
Tensilon Injectable
◆ Valium Injectable
◆ Valium Tablets
◆ Valium Tel-E-Ject
◆ Vi-Penta F Chewables
Vi-Penta F Infant Drops
Vi-Penta F Multivitamin Drops
Vi-Penta Infant Drops
Vi-Penta Multivitamin Drops
Vitamin K—see Synkayvite
Vitamin K_1—see Konakion

ROERIG 428, 1488
A division of Pfizer Pharmaceuticals
235 E. 42nd St., New York, NY 10017
Address inquiries to:
Medical Department (212) 573-2187
Branch Offices
Doraville, GA 30340
4360 N.E. Expressway
(Southern Region) (404) 448-6666
Hoffman Estates, IL 60196
2400 W. Central Road (312) 381-9500
(Midwestern & Great Lakes Regions)
Clifton, NJ 07012
230 Brighton Road
(Metro Region) (201) 546-7700
Dallas, TX 75222
P.O. Box 22249
(Southwestern Region) (214) 647-0222
Irvine, CA 92705
16700 Red Hill Ave.
(Western Region) (714) 540-9180
Products Available
Antiminth Oral Suspension
◆ Antivert, Antivert/25 Tablets & Antivert/25 Chewable Tablets
◆ Atarax Tablets & Syrup
Cartrax Tablets
Emete-con Intramuscular/Intravenous
◆ Geocillin Tablets
Geopen Intramuscular/Intravenous
◆ Heptuna Plus Capsules
◆ Marax Tablets & DF Syrup
◆ Navane Capsules and Concentrate
Navane Intramuscular
◆ Sustaire Tablets
◆ Tao Capsules & Oral Suspension
◆ Urobiotic-250 Capsules

ROGER PHARMACAL, INC. 1501
P.O. Box 011022
Miami, FL 33101
1654 North West 35th Street
Miami, FL 33142
Address inquiries to:
Mr. Roger Hernandez (305) 635-2263
(305) 264-7746
Products Available
Arteril Injection
Eta-Lent Capsules
Fluxine Drops
Fluxine Tablets
Hydrex Tablets
Provein Injection
Revit-E Capsules
Venolax Tablets
Viferrin Liquid

RORER, INC., WILLIAM H. 428, 1501
500 Virginia Drive
Fort Washington, PA 19034
Address inquiries to:
Johanna L. Roskow
Marketing Services Manager
(215) 628-6314
Branch Offices
Fort Washington, PA 19034
P.O. Box 46 (215) 628-6000
Hammond, IN 46320
2500-165th Street (219) 845-1677
San Leandro, CA 94577
P.O. Box 1569
1550 Factor Avenue (415) 357-9741
Tucker, GA 30084
4660 Hammermill Road (404) 934-3091
Products Available
◆ Ananase Tablets
◆ Ascriptin Tablets
◆ Ascriptin A/D Tablets
◆ Ascriptin w/Codeine Tablets
Camalox Suspension
◆ Camalox Tablets
◆ Chardonna-2 Tablets
Emetrol Solution
◆ Fermalox Tablets
◆ Maalox No. 1 Tablets
◆ Maalox No. 2 Tablets
Maalox Plus Suspension
◆ Maalox Plus Tablets
Maalox Suspension
Maalox Therapeutic Concentrate
Neoxyn Solution
Parepectolin Suspension

ROSS LABORATORIES 428, 1504
Div. Abbott Laboratories
Columbus, OH 43216
Address inquiries to:
Henry S. Sauls, M.D., Vice President,
Medical Affairs (614) 227-3333
Products Available
Ensure
Ensure Plus
Ensure Vari-Flavors Flavor Pacs
Glucose Water 5% & 10%
Isomil 20
Osmolite
Pediaflor
Pedialyte
Pediamycin
◆ Pediamycin Chewable
Pediazole
Polycose
◆ Pramet FA
◆ Pramilet FA
Redi-Nurser System
Rondec Drops
Rondec Syrup
◆ Rondec Tablet
Rondec-DM
Ross Hospital Formula System
Similac
Advance
Isomil
Similac PM 60/40
Similac 13
Similac 20
Similac 24
Similac 24 LBW
Similac 27
Similac With Iron
Similac With Iron 13
Similac With Iron 20
Similac With Iron 24
Sterilized Water
Vi-Daylin ADC Drops
◆ Vi-Daylin Chewable
Vi-Daylin Drops
Vi-Daylin Liquid
Vi-Daylin Plus Iron ADC Drops
◆ Vi-Daylin Plus Iron Chewable
Vi-Daylin Plus Iron Drops
Vi-Daylin Plus Iron Liquid
◆ Vi-Daylin w/Fluoride Chewable
Vi-Daylin/F ADC Drops
Vi-Daylin/F ADC + Iron Drops
Vi-Daylin/F Drops
Vi-Daylin/F + Iron Drops
Vital
Volu-Feed

ROTEX PHARMACEUTICALS, INC. 1517
3102 Corrine Drive
Orlando, FL 32803
Address inquiries to:
Mr. Jerry S. Roth, President
(305) 896-8280
Products Available
Arthrogesic
Nasalspan Capsules
Nasalspan Expectorant
Podiliquid
Ropres
Rothav-150
Rovite

ROWELL LABORATORIES, INC. 1517
210 Main Street, W.
Baudette, MN 56623
Toll Free (800) 346-5040
In Minn. Call (800) 542-5012
Address inquiries to:
Professional Service Dept.
Products Available
C-Ron
C-Ron FA
C-Ron Forte
C-Ron Freckles
Cin-Quin
Colrex Capsules
Colrex Compound Capsules
Colrex Compound Elixir
Colrex Decongestant
Colrex Expectorant
Colrex Syrup
Colrex Troches
Cortenema
Dermacort Cream
Dermacort Lotion
Dexone 0.5, 0.75, 1.5, 4
Gourmase
Hydrocil Fortified
Hydrocil Plain
Lithobid
Lithonate
Lithonate-S
Lithotabs
Multivitamins Rowell
Norlac
Norlac RX
Orasone 1, 5, 10, 20, 50
Perifoam
Prednisone Tablets
Proctocort
Proctodon
Quinidine Sulfate Capsules & Tablets
Quinine Sulfate Capsules
Ro-Bile
S.A.S.-500
Vio-Bec
Vio-Bec Forte
Vio-Geric
Vio-Serpine

RYSTAN COMPANY, INC. 1521
470 Mamaroneck Avenue
White Plains, NY 10605
Address inquiries to:
Professional Service Dept. (914) 761-0044
Products Available
Chloresium Dental Ointment
Chloresium Nasal Solution
Chloresium Ointment
Chloresium Solution
Chloresium Tablets
Derifil Tablets & Powder
Panafil Ointment
Panafil-White Ointment
Prophyllin Ointment
Prophyllin Powder

SDA PHARMACEUTICALS, INC. 1521
919 Third Avenue
New York, NY 10022
Address inquiries to:
Dr. Edward L. Steinberg (212) 688-4420
Products Available
Anorexin Capsules
Anorexin One-Span Capsules

SANDOZ PHARMACEUTICALS 429, 1521
(Division of Sandoz, Inc.)
Route 10, East Hanover, NJ 07936
Address inquiries to:
William F. Westlin, M.D. (201) 386-7500
New York City (212) 349-1212
Products Available
◆ Belladenal Tablets
◆ Belladenal-S Tablets
Bellafoline
Cafergot Suppositories
◆ Cafergot Tablets
Cafergot P-B Suppositories
◆ Cafergot P-B Tablets
◆ Cedilanid Tablets
Cedilanid-D Injection
D.H.E. 45 Injection
Diapid Nasal Spray
◆ Fiogesic Tablets
Fiorinal Capsules
◆ Fiorinal Tablets
◆ Fiorinal w/Codeine Capsules
◆ Fiorinal-R Capsules
Glysennid
Gynergen Injection
Gynergen Tablets
◆ Hydergine Tablets & Sublingual Tablets
Mellaril Concentrate
Mellaril-S Suspension
◆ Mellaril Tablets
◆ Mesantoin Tablets
Methergine Injection

◆ Methergine Tablets
◆ Pamelor Capsules
Pamelor Solution
◆ Parlodel Tablets
◆ Plexonal Tablets
◆ Sanorex Tablets
◆ Sansert Tablets
Syntocinon Injection
Syntocinon Nasal Spray

SARON PHARMACAL CORP. 1533
Subsidiary of Para-medical Enterprises, Inc.
1640 Central Ave.
St. Petersburg, FL 33712
Address inquiries to:
Robert Saron, President
P.O. Box 13547
St. Petersburg, FL 33733 (813) 898-8525
Products Available
AL-R TD
AL-R TD, Pediatric
Angidil
Arthrin
Aural Acute Econopak
B O F
Beef-Amine
Butabell HMB
Butabell HMB Elixir
Cardabid TD
Cardabid-Forte TD
Cerebid TD
Cerebid-200 TD
Cerebid-300 TD
Chick-Amine
Denta-FL Chewables
Denta-FL Drops
E-Biotic
Emfabid TD
Emfaseem
Emfaseem Elixir
Fem-H
Gevizol
Gevizol Elixir
HC Creme
HC Rectal Creme
HCV Creme
Hi-Temp
Hycoff Caps
Hycoff-A NN
Hycoff-X NN
MG Blue
M.I. 30%
Mega Am-Pro
Mega Trace-L
Mega-Vita
Mega-Vita Hematinic
Mega-Vita Tonic
NICL TD
Natalets-F
Otall
Pred-5
RBC-Plus
Reserpatabs
S-Aqua
S-Aqua-D
S-Painacet
Saramp
Saro-C
Sarocycline
Sarodant
Saroflex
Sarolax
Saropen-VK
Sulfstat-Forte
Surg-C
Symptafed TD
Symptrol Injectable
Symptrol Liquid
Symptrol TD
Verstat
Vertrol

SAVAGE LABORATORIES 429, 1534
a division of Byk-Gulden, Inc.
1000 Main Street
Post Office Box 1000
Missouri City, TX 77459 (713) 499-4547
Products Available
Alpha-Ruvite
Aridose
◆ Brexin Capsules
◆ Chromagen Capsules
Chromagen Injection
Chromagen-D
Cortigel-40
Cortigel-80
Dilor Elixir
◆ Dilor Injectable
◆ Dilor Tablets
◆ Dilor-400 Tablets
Dilor-G Liquid
◆ Dilor-G Tablets
Estate
Estrone (Aqueous)
Ethiodol
Homo-Tet
Immuglobin
Libigen 10,000 & Diluent
Mepred-40
Mepred-80
Minoplex
Negatan
Neopavrin Forte Tablets
◆ Physpan
Progesterone (Aqueous)
Ruvite 1000
Savacort-50
Savacort-100
Savaplex
Spanestrin P
Testate
Testosterone (Aqueous)
Thiodyne
Tracilon
ZiPan-25 & ZiPan-50

SCHATTNER COMPANY, THE R. 1535
Pharmaceutical Division
4000 Massachusetts Ave., N.W.
Washington, DC 20016
Address inquiries to:
Dr. Robert I. Schattner, President
(202) 244-6606
Products Available
Chloraderm
Derma La Douche
Gynaseptic
Hot Lips
Oraderm
Permacide
Ristex
Sporicidin

SCHERING CORPORATION 429, 1536
Galloping Hill Road
Kenilworth, NJ 07033 (201) 931-2000
Address inquiries to:
Professional Services Department
Galloping Hill Road
Kenilworth, NJ 07033 (201) 931-2000
Branch Offices
Southeast Branch
5884 Peachtree Rd., N.E.
Chamblee, GA 30341 (404) 457-6315
Midwest Branch
7500 N. Natchez Ave.
Niles, IL 60648 (312) 647-9363
Southwest Branch
9151 King Arthur Dr.
Dallas, TX 75247 (214) 631-7880
West Coast Branch
14775 Wicks Blvd.
San Leandro, CA 94577 (415) 357-3125
Products Available
A and D Hand Cream*
A and D Ointment*
Afrin Menthol Nasal Spray, 0.05%
Afrin Nasal Spray 0.05%
Afrin Nose Drops 0.05%
Afrin Pediatric Nose Drops 0.025%
◆ Afrinol Long-Acting Decongestant Repetabs Tablets
Akrinol Cream
◆ Because Contraceptor Vaginal Contraceptive Foam
Celestone Cream
Celestone Phosphate Injection
◆ Celestone 0.6 mg. Six-Day Pack
Celestone Soluspan Suspension
Celestone Syrup
◆ Celestone Tablets
Chlor-Trimeton Allergy Syrup
◆ Chlor-Trimeton Allergy Tablets
◆ Chlor-Trimeton Decongestant Tablets
Chlor-Trimeton Expectorant
Chlor-Trimeton Expectorant w/Codeine
Chlor-Trimeton Injection
◆ Chlor-Trimeton Long-Acting Allergy Repetabs Tablets
◆ Chlor-Trimeton Repetabs Tablets
◆ Cod Liver Oil Concentrate Capsules*
◆ Cod Liver Oil Concentrate Tablets*
◆ Cod Liver Oil Concentrate Tablets w/Vitamin C*
Coricidin Children's Cough Syrup
Coricidin Cough Syrup
◆ Coricidin "D" Decongestant Tablets
Coricidin Decongestant Nasal Mist
◆ Coricidin Demilets Tablets For Children
◆ Coricidin Medilets Tablets For Children
◆ Coricidin Sinus Headache Tablets
◆ Coricidin Tablets
◆ Coriforte Capsules
Corilin Infant Liquid
◆ Demazin Repetabs Tablets
Demazin Syrup
◆ Deronil Tablets
Diprosone Aerosol 0.1% w/w
Diprosone Cream 0.05%
Diprosone Lotion 0.05% w/w
Diprosone Ointment 0.05%
◆ Disophrol Chronotab Tablets*
◆ Disophrol Tablets*
◆ Drixoral Sustained-Action Tablets
◆ Emko Pre-Fil Vaginal Contraceptive Foam
◆ Emko Vaginal Contraceptive Foam
◆ Estinyl Tablets
◆ Etrafon A Tablets (4-10)
◆ Etrafon 2-10 Tablets (2-10)
◆ Etrafon Tablets (2-25)
◆ Etrafon Forte Tablets (4-25)
◆ Fulvicin P/G Tablets
◆ Fulvicin-U/F Tablets
Garamycin Cream 0.1%
◆ Garamycin Injectable
◆ Garamycin Injectable Disposable Syringes
Garamycin Intrathecal Injection
Garamycin Ointment 0.1%
Garamycin Ophthalmic Ointment
Garamycin Ophthalmic Solution
◆ Garamycin Pediatric Injectable
◆ Gitaligin Tablets
◆ Gyne-Lotrimin Vaginal Cream 1%
◆ Gyne-Lotrimin Vaginal Tablets
◆ Gynetone Tablets
◆ Hyperstat I.V. Injection
◆ Lotrimin Cream 1%
◆ Lotrimin Solution 1%
Meticortelone Acetate Aqueous Suspension
◆ Meticorten Tablets
Meti-Derm Aerosol
Meti-Derm Cream 0.5%
Meti-Derm w/Neomycin Aerosol
Meti-Derm w/Neomycin Topical Ointment
Metimyd Ophthalmic Ointment*
Metimyd Ophthalmic Suspension*
Metreton Ophthalmic Solution
◆ Miradon Tablets
◆ Mol-Iron Chronosule Capsules*
Mol-Iron Liquid
◆ Mol-Iron Tablets*
◆ Mol-Iron w/Vitamin C Chronosule Capsules*
◆ Mol-Iron w/Vitamin C Tablets
◆ Naqua Tablets
◆ Naquival Tablets
◆ Optimine Tablets
Optimyd Ophthalmic Solution*
◆ Oreton Methyl Buccal Tablets
◆ Oreton Methyl Tablets
Oreton Pellets for Subcutaneous Implantation
◆ Oreton Propionate Buccal Tablets
Otobione Otic Suspension*
Otobiotic Otic Solution*
◆ Permitil Chronotab Tablets*
Permitil Oral Concentrate*
◆ Permitil Tablets*
Polaramine Expectorant
◆ Polaramine Repetabs Tablets
Polaramine Syrup
◆ Polaramine Tablets
◆ Prantal Tablets
◆ Proglycem Capsules
Proglycem Suspension
Progynon Pellets For Subcutaneous Implantation
◆ Rela Tablets
Sebizon Lotion
Sodium Sulamyd Ophthalmic Ointment 10%*
Sodium Sulamyd Ophthalmic Solution 10%*
Sodium Sulamyd Ophthalmic Solution 30%*
Solganal Suspension
Sunril Premenstrual Capsules
Theovent Long-Acting Capsules
Tinactin Cream 1%
Tinactin Powder 1%
Tinactin Powder 1% Aerosol
Tinactin Solution 1%
◆ Tindal Tablets
◆ Tremin Tablets
Trilafon Concentrate
Trilafon Injection
◆ Trilafon Repetabs Tablets
◆ Trilafon Tablets
Valisone Aerosol 0.15% w/w
Valisone Cream 0.1%
Valisone Lotion 0.1%
Valisone Ointment 0.1%
Valisone Reduced Strength Cream 0.01%
◆ Vanceril Inhaler
*Schering/White Product Line

SCHMID PRODUCTS COMPANY 1578
Division of Schmid Laboratories, Inc.
Route 46 West
Little Falls, NJ 07424
Address inquiries to:
Professional Service Dept. (201) 256-5500
Products Available
Ramses Bendex Flexible Cushioned Diaphragm
Ramses Contraceptive Vaginal Jelly
Ramses Flexible Cushioned Diaphragm
Saf-T-Coil 33-S, 32-S and 25-S Nullip Intra-Uterine Contraceptive Devices
Vagisec Liquid
Vagisec Plus Suppositories

SCLAVO INC. 1581, 2015
5 Mansard Court
Wayne, NJ 07470

Address inquiries to:
Francis J. O'Grady (201) 696-8300
Products Available
Antirabies Serum (equine), Purified
Cholera Vaccine
Diphtheria Antitoxin (equine), Refined
Diphtheria & Tetanus Toxoids, Adsorbed (For Pediatric Use)
Diphtheria Toxoid, Adsorbed
Diphtheria Toxoid, Adsorbed (For Adult Use)
SclavoTest-PPD, Tuberculin PPD Multiple Puncture Device
Tetanus Antitoxin (equine), Refined
Tetanus Toxoid, Adsorbed
Tetanus & Diphtheria Toxoids, Adsorbed (For Adult Use)

SCOT-TUSSIN PHARMACAL CO., INC. 1581
50 Clemence Street
Post Office Box 8217
Cranston, RI 02920
Address inquiries to:
Louis J. Scotti (401) 942-8555
Products Available
Ferro-Bob 2 Capsules
Ferro-Bob Tablets
S-T Cort Lotion
S-T Decongest "Sugar-Free & Dye-Free"
S-T Expectorant Sugar-Free & Dye-Free
S-T Expectorant w/Codeine S-F
S-T Febrol Tablets & Elixir
S-T Forte Syrup and Sugar-Free
Scot-Tussin Cough Capsules
Scot-Tussin Sugar-Free
Scot-Tussin Syrup
Sodium Nitrite Tablets
Tussirex Sugar-Free Liquid
Tussirex w/Codeine Syrup
Vita-Bob Capsules
Vita-Natal Capsules
Vita-Plus B 12
Vita-Plus D (diet) Capsules
Vita-Plus E Capsules Natural
Vita-Plus G (geriatric) Capsules
Vita-Plus H (hematinic) Capsules
Vita-Plus H (hematinic) S-F Half Strength
Vita-Plus H (hematinic) Sugar-Free, liquid full strength

SEARLE LABORATORIES 431, 1582
Division of Searle Pharmaceuticals Inc.
Box 5110
Chicago, IL 60680
Address inquiries to:
Medical Communications Department
(312) 982-7000
Products Available
Aminophyllin Injection
◆ Aminophyllin Tablets
Amodrine
◆ Anavar
◆ CU-7
◆ Comfolax
◆ Comfolax-*plus*
◆ Diulo
Dramamine Ampules
Dramamine Liquid
Dramamine Supposicones
◆ Dramamine Tablets
Dramamine Vials
Icy Hot
Ketochol
Metamucil
Metamucil, Instant Mix
◆ Norpace

SEARLE & CO. 431, 1588
San Juan, Puerto Rico 00936
Address medical inquiries to:
G.D. Searle & Co.
Medical Communications Department,
Box 5110
Chicago, IL 60680
Products Available
◆ Aldactazide
◆ Aldactone
Banthīne Tablets
◆ Demulen
Demulen-28
◆ Enovid 5 mg. & 10 mg.
◆ Enovid-E
Enovid-E 21
◆ Flagyl Tablets
Lomotil Liquid
◆ Lomotil Tablets
◆ Ovulen
Ovulen-21
Ovulen-28
◆ Pro-Banthīne Tablets
Pro-Banthīne for Injection
Pro-Banthīne w/Dartal Tablets
◆ Pro-Banthīne w/Phenobarbital Tablets

SERONO LABORATORIES, INC. 1605
11 Brooks Drive
Braintree, MA 02184

Address inquiries to:
Director, Sales and Marketing
(outside MA) (800) 255-5185
(within MA) (617) 848-8404
For Medical Emergencies Contact:
Director, Research and Development
(outside MA) (800) 255-5185
(within MA) (617) 848-8404
Products Available
Asellacrin (somatropin)
Pergonal (menotropins)
Profasi HP

SMITH KLINE & FRENCH LABORATORIES 432, 1608
Division of SmithKline Corporation
1500 Spring Garden St.
P.O. Box 7929
Philadelphia, PA 19101
Address inquiries to:
Medical Dept. (215) 854-4000
SK&F CO. 432, 1608
Carolina, Puerto Rico 00630
Subsidiary of SmithKline Corporation
Address inquiries to:
Smith Kline & French Laboratories (see above)
SK&F LAB. CO. 432, 1608
Carolina, Puerto Rico 00630
Subsidiary of SmithKline Corporation
Address inquiries to:
Smith Kline & French Laboratories (see above)
MENLEY & JAMES LABORATORIES 432, 1608
Professional Products Division
a SmithKline company
P.O. Box 8082
Philadelphia, PA 19101
Address inquiries to
Medical Department (215) 854-4000
Products Available
Acnomel Cream & Cake*
Ancef Injection
◆ Anspor Capsules
Anspor for Oral Suspension
Benzedrex Inhaler*
◆ Benzedrine Spansule Capsules
◆ Benzedrine Tablets
◆ Combid Spansule Capsules
Compazine Concentrate
Compazine Injection
◆ Compazine Spansule Capsules
◆ Compazine Suppositories
Compazine Syrup
◆ Compazine Tablets
◆ Cytomel Tablets
◆ Darbid Tablets
◆ Dexamyl Spansule Capsules
◆ Dexamyl Tablets
Dexedrine Elixir
◆ Dexedrine Spansule Capsules
◆ Dexedrine Tablets
◆ Dibenzyline Capsules
◆ Dyazide Capsules
◆ Dyrenium Capsules
◆ Ecotrin Tablets*
◆ Eskalith Capsules
◆ Eskalith Tablets
◆ Eskatrol Spansule Capsules
Feosol Elixir*
◆ Feosol Plus Capsules*
◆ Feosol Spansule Capsules*
◆ Feosol Tablets*
◆ Fortespan Capsules*
◆ Hispril Spansule Capsules
◆ Ornacol Capsules*
Ornacol Liquid*
◆ Ornade Spansule Capsules
Ornade 2 Liquid
◆ Ornex Capsules*
Paredrine 1% w/Boric Acid, Ophthalmic Solution
◆ Parnate Tablets
Pragmatar w/Sulfur & Salicylic Acid Ointment*
Quotane Ointment*
SK-APAP Elixir
SK-APAP Tablets
SK-APAP with Codeine Tablets
SK-Amitriptyline Tablets
SK-Ampicillin Capsules
SK-Ampicillin For Oral Suspension
SK-Ampicillin Tablets
SK-Ampicillin-N For Injection
SK-Bamate Tablets
SK-Bisacodyl Tablets
SK-Chloral Hydrate Capsules
SK-Chlorothiazide Tablets
SK-Dexamethasone Tablets
SK-Digoxin Tablets
SK-Diphenhydramine Capsules
SK-Diphenhydramine Elixir
SK-Diphenoxylate Tablets
SK-Erythromycin Tablets
SK-Hydrochlorothiazide Tablets
SK-Lygen Capsules
SK-Niacin Tablets
SK-Penicillin G For Oral Solution
SK-Penicillin G Tablets
SK-Penicillin VK For Oral Solution
SK-Penicillin VK Tablets
SK-Phenobarbital Tablets
SK-Pramine Tablets
SK-Prednisone Tablets
SK-Quinidine Sulfate Tablets
SK-Reserpine Tablets
SK-65 APAP Tablets
SK-65 Capsules
SK-65 Compound Capsules
SK-Soxazole Tablets
SK-Tetracycline Capsules
SK-Tetracycline Syrup
SK-Triamcinolone Tablets
◆ Selacryn Tablets
Spansule, sustained release capsules:
'Benzedrine' Spansule Capsules
'Combid' Spansule Capsules
'Compazine' Spansule Capsules
'Dexamyl' Spansule Capsules
'Dexedrine' Spansule Capsules
'Eskatrol' Spansule Capsules
'Feosol' Spansule Capsules
'Hispril' Spansule Capsules
'Ornade' Spansule Capsules
'Prydon' Spansule Capsules
'Temaril' Spansule Capsules
'Thorazine' Spansule Capsules
'Tuss-Ornade' Spansule Capsules
Stelazine Concentrate
Stelazine Injection
◆ Stelazine Tablets
Stoxil Ophthalmic Ointment & Solution
Tagamet Injection
◆ Tagamet Tablets
◆ Teldrin Timed-Release Capsules*
◆ Temaril Spansule Capsules
Temaril Syrup
◆ Temaril Tablets
Thorazine Concentrate
Thorazine Injection
◆ Thorazine Spansule Capsules
◆ Thorazine Suppositories
Thorazine Syrup
◆ Thorazine Tablets
◆ Troph-Iron Liquid & Tablets*
◆ Trophite Liquid & Tablets*
Tuss-Ornade Liquid
◆ Tuss-Ornade Spansule Capsules
◆ Urispas Tablets
Vontrol Injection
◆ Vontrol Tablets
*A product of Menley & James Laboratories, Professional Products Division, a SmithKline company

SMITH, MILLER & PATCH 1644
Div. Cooper Vision P.R., Inc.
San German, Puerto Rico 00753
Address inquiries to:
Professional Services
San German, Puerto Rico or call
(except New Jersey) (800) 631-0184
(New Jersey only) (800) 562-6925
For Medical or Contact Lens Solution Information
Write: Medical Department
455 East Middlefield Road
Mountain View, CA 94043
Call: *(Business Hours Only)*
Joseph Krezanoski, Ph.D. (415) 969-9030
For Medical Emergency Information After Hours or on Weekends, call
Jerome F. Grattan (201) 821-8846
Products Available
Argyrol Stabilized Solution 10%
Atropisol Ophthalmic Solution 1%
Catarase 1:5,000 & 1:10,000
Contactisol
Dacriose Ophthalmic Irrigating Solution
Dropperettes:
Argyrol S.S. 20%
Atropisol 0.5%, 1%, 2%
Epinephrine 1:1000
Fluorescein Sodium 2%
Homatropine HBr 2%, 5%
Phenylephrine HCl 10%
Pilocar 1%, 2%, 4%
Sulf-10 (Sodium Sulfacetamide 10%)
Tetracaine HCl 0.5%
E-Pilo Ophthalmic Solutions 1, 2, 3, 4, 6
Eserine Sulfate Ophthalmic Ointment ¼%
Funduscein-10 or -25 (Fluorescein sodium I.V.)
Glucose Ophthalmic Ointment 40%
Glyrol
Goniosol
Homatropine Hydrobromide Ophthalmic Solution 2%, 5%
Hypotears Moisturizing Eye Drops
Inflamase Forte 1% Ophthalmic Solution
Inflamase ⅛% Ophthalmic Solution
Lens Care Products:
aqua-FLOW

CLERZ
d-FILM
duo-FLOW
hy-FLOW
Lensine
Lensine Extra Strength Cleaner
Pliagel
Lipoflavonoid Vitamin Supplement (Capsule)
Lipotriad Vitamin Supplement (Capsule, Liquid)
M-Z Ophthalmic Solution
Miochol Intraocular
Phenylephrine Hydrochloride Ophthalmic Solution 10%
Phenylzin Ophthalmic Solution
Pilocar Ophthalmic Solutions 0.5%, 1%, 2%, 3%, 4%, 6%
Pilocar Ophthalmic Solutions Twin Pak 0.5%, 1%, 2%, 3%, 4%, 6%
Pilomiotin 1%, 2%, 4%
Pyocidin Ophthalmic Ointment
Sal-Fayne
Schirmer Tear Test
Sulf-10 Ophthalmic Solution
Tear-Efrin Ophthalmic Solution
Tearisol Ophthalmic Solution
Vasocidin Ophthalmic Ointment
Vasocidin Ophthalmic Solution
VasoClear Ophthalmic Decongestant Eye Drops
Vasocon Regular Ophthalmic Solution
Vasocon-A Ophthalmic Solution
Vasosulf Ophthalmic Solution

SOUTH LABORATORIES, INC. 1644
P.O. Box 341658
Coral Gables, FL 33134 (305) 266-6176
Products Available
Azo Soxazol
Betonal
Bioclasine
Broncoplumonar
Decaxone
Dee Plus
Digestolin
Diuretin
Duolax
Dyspne Inhal
Ferroanem
Matropasmol
Nasoline
Nervisan
Optisul
Otocetic
Pepanzyme
Salitron
Trofosteno
Tylophen
Vigoman

SQUIBB & SONS, INC., E.R. 433, 1644, 2015
General Offices
Post Office Box 4000
Princeton, NJ 08540 (609) 921-4000
Address inquiries to:
Squibb Professional Services Dept.
Lawrenceville-Princeton Road
Princeton, NJ 08540 (609) 921-4006
Distribution Centers
ATLANTA, GEORGIA
Post Office Box 4775
Atlanta, GA 30302
State of Ga. Customers Call (800) 282-9103
Customers in States of Ala., Fla., Miss., N.C., S.C., and Tenn. Call (800) 241-1744
All others call (800) 241-5364
CINCINNATI, OHIO
Mail or telephone orders and customer service inquiries should be directed to Atlanta, GA (see above)
State of Ky. Customers Call (800) 241-1744
All others call (800) 241-5364
CHICAGO, ILLINOIS
Post Office Box 788
Arlington Heights, IL 60006
State of IL Customers Call (800) 942-0674
All others call (800) 323-0665
KANSAS CITY, KANSAS
Mail or telephone orders and customer service inquiries should be directed to Chicago, IL (see above)
State of IL Customers Call (800) 942-0674
All others call (800) 323-0665
LOS ANGELES, CALIFORNIA
Post Office Box 428
La Mirada, CA 90637
State of CA Customers Call (800) 422-4254
All others call (800) 854-3050
SEATTLE, WASHINGTON
Mail or telephone orders and customer service inquiries should be directed to Los Angeles, CA (see above)
State of Mont. Customers Call (714) 521-7050
State of CA Customers Call (800) 422-4254
All others call (800) 854-3050
NEW YORK AREA
E. R. Squibb & Sons, Inc.
Post Office Box 2013
New Brunswick, NJ 08903
State of NJ Customers Call (800) 352-4865
N.Y. City Area Customers Call (212) 227-1371
State of N.C. Customers call (201) 469-5400
All others call (800) 631-5244
BOSTON, MASSACHUSETTS
Mail or telephone orders and customer service inquiries should be directed to the New York Area (see above)
State of ME Customers Call (201) 469-5400
All others call (800) 631-5244
HOUSTON, TEXAS
Post Office Box 1510
Houston, TX 77001
State of N. Mex. Customers Call (713) 622-4242
State of TX Customers Call (800) 392-2030
All others call (800) 231-3209
SQUIBB LABORATORIES
E. R. Squibb & Sons, Inc.
Georges Road
New Brunswick, NJ 08903
Products Available
Amitid Tablets
Aspirin Tablets USP
B Complex Vitamin Tablets
B Complex with Vitamin C Tablets
Brewer's Yeast Tablets
Broxodent Automatic-Action Toothbrush
Calcium, Phosphate and Vitamin D Tablets
Cardiografin
Castor Oil USP
Chlordiazepoxide Hydrochloride Capsules USP
Chlorothiazide Tablets USP
Cholografin Meglumine
Cholografin Meglumine for Infusion
Cod Liver Oil Capsules
Cod Liver Oil Plain & Mint Flavored
Crysticillin 300 A.S. & 600 A.S.
Cystografin
Deladumone
Deladumone OB
Delalutin
Delatestryl
Delestrogen
Diatrizoate Meglumine Injection USP 76%
Engran-HP Tablets
Epi*Clear Acne Kit
◆ Ethril '250' and Ethril '500' Tablets
Florinef Acetate Tablets
Follutein
Fungizone Cream, Lotion and Ointment
Fungizone for Tissue Culture
Fungizone Intravenous
Gastrografin
Halog Cream, Ointment & Solution
◆ Hydrea Capsules
Hydrochlorothiazide Tablets USP
Insulin, Globin Zinc Insulin
Insulin, Isophane Insulin (NPH)
Insulin, Lente
Insulin, Protamine Zinc Insulin
Insulin (Regular)
Insulin, Semilente
Insulin, Ultralente
Iron with Vitamin C Tablets
Kenacort Diacetate Syrup
Kenacort Tablets
Kenalog Cream, Lotion, Ointment, Spray
Kenalog in Orabase
Kenalog-H Cream
Kenalog-10 Injection
Kenalog-40 Injection
Kinevac
Medotopes (Radiopharmaceuticals)
A-C-D Solution Modified
Albumotope I 131 (Diagnostic Injection)
Angiotensin I Immutope Kit
Chromitope Sodium (Diagnostic Injection)
Cobatope-57 Reference Standard Solution
Cobatope-60 Reference Standard Solution
Cortisol RIA Kit (for use c̄ Gammaflo)
Digoxin Clasp RIA Kit
Digoxin RIA Kit (for use c̄ Gammaflo)
HTSH Clasp RIA Kit
Hipputope I 131 (Diagnostic Injection)
Intrinsic Factor Concentrate Capsules
Iodotope Therapeutic Capsules (I 131)
Iodotope Therapeutic Oral Solution (I 131)
Macrotec
Minitec
Phosphotec
Renotec Diagnostic Kit
Robengatope Diagnostic Injection
Rubratope-57 Diagnostic Capsules
Rubratope-57 Diagnostic Kit
Rubratope-60 Diagnostic Capsules
Rubratope-60 Diagnostic Kit
Sethotope
Tesuloid Diagnostic Kit
Thyrostat-3 Diagnostic Test Kit
T3 Clasp RIA Kit
T3 Uptake Kit (for use c̄ Gammaflo)
T4 Clasp RIA Kit
T4 RIA Kit (for use c̄ Gammaflo)
Thyrostat-FTI
Milk of Magnesia Liquid & Tablets
Mineral Oil
Mint-O-Mag
Mycolog Cream, Ointment
Mycostatin Cream, Ointment
Mycostatin Oral Suspension
◆ Mycostatin Oral Tablets
Mycostatin Powder (for laboratory use)
Mycostatin Topical Powder
◆ Mycostatin Vaginal Tablets
◆ Mysteclin-F Capsules
◆ Mysteclin-F '125' Capsules
Mysteclin-F Syrup
◆ Naturetin Tablets
Neomycin Sulfate Sterile Powder
Neomycin Sulfate Tablets USP
Niacin Tablets
Nitrazine Paper
◆ Noctec Capsules
Noctec Syrup
Nydrazid Injection, Tablets
O-V Statin
Ophthaine Solution
Oragrafin Calcium Granules
◆ Oragrafin Sodium Capsules
Ora-Testryl Tablets
Penicillin G Potassium for Injection USP
Penicillin G Sodium for Injection NF
Pentids for Syrup
Pentids '400' for Syrup
◆ Pentids '400' & '800' Tablets
◆ Pentids Tablets
◆ Principen Capsules '250' & '500'
Principen for Oral Suspension '125' & '250'
Principen with Probenecid Capsules
Principen/N
Prolixin Decanoate
Prolixin Enanthate
Prolixin Elixir
Prolixin Injection
◆ Prolixin Tablets
◆ Pronestyl Capsules and Tablets
Pronestyl Injection
Propoxyphene Hydrochloride Capsules USP
Propoxyphene Hydrochloride and APC Capsules
Protein Powder & Tablets
Quinolor Compound Ointment
◆ Raudixin Tablets
Rau-Sed
◆ Rauzide Tablets
Renografin-60
Renografin-76
Reno-M-DIP
Reno-M-30
Reno-M-60
Renovist
Renovist II
Renovue-65
Renovue-DIP
Rubramin PC
Saccharin Tablets
Serenium Tablets
Sinografin
Spec-T Sore Throat Anesthetic Lozenges
Spec-T Sore Throat/Cough Suppressant Lozenges
Spec-T Sore Throat/Decongestant Lozenges
Spectrocin Ointment
Stomahesive
Stomahesive Wafer with Sur-Fit Flange
Sucostrin Injection, for Infusion, High Potency
◆ Sumycin '250' & '500' Capsules
◆ Sumycin '250' and '500' Tablets
Sumycin Syrup
Suppositories, Glycerin
Sur-Fit Pouches
Sweeta Liquid & Tablets
Terfonyl Tablets, Oral Suspension
Teslac Injection & Tablets
◆ Theragran Hematinic Tablets
Theragran Liquid
◆ Theragran Tablets
◆ Theragran-M Tablets
Theragran-Z Tablets
Trigesic Tablets
Trigot Tablets
◆ Trimox '250' & '500' Capsules
Trimox '125' & '250' For Oral Suspension
Tubocurarine Chloride Injection USP
Valadol Liquid
◆ Valadol Tablets
Veetids '125' & '250' for Oral Solution
◆ Veetids '250' & '500' Tablets
◆ Velosef '250' & '500' Capsules
Velosef for Infusion
Velosef for Injection
Velosef '125' & '250' for Oral Suspension

◆ Velosef Tablets
Vesprin Injection, Tablets, High-Potency Suspension
Vigran Chewables
Vigran plus Iron Tablets
Vigran Tablets
Vitamin A Capsules
Vitamin B_1 Tablets
Vitamin B_{12} Capsules
Vitamin C Tablets
Vitamin E Capsules & Tablets
Wheat Germ Oil Capsules
Yeast Tablets & Flavored Powder
Zinc Oxide Ointment

STANDARD PROCESS LABORATORIES, INC. 1696
2023 West Wisconsin Avenue
Milwaukee, WI 53201 (414) 933-2100
Branch Offices
Campbell, CA 95008
501-C Vandell Way (408) 866-0707
Chilton, WI 53014
253 East Main (414) 849-9014
Columbus, OH 43227
5195 Ivyhurst Drive (614) 866-5520
Dallas, TX 75211
9103 Highway 67, South
(214) 298-1417
Denver, CO 80222
2179 South Ash (303) 758-6321
Harrisburg, PA 17112
5145 Jonestown Road (717) 545-9264
Honolulu, HI 96818
1106 Ukana Street (808) 423-1616
Kansas City, MO 64111
3711 Southwest Trafficway
(816) 561-5550
(Los Angeles)
City of Commerce, CA 90040
2401 S. Atlantic Blvd. (213) 263-6133
Oklahoma City, OK 73112
3419 Roff Ave., North (405) 943-1056
Orlando, FL 32859
7653 Currency Drive (305) 851-6610
Portland, OR 97220
10704 N.E. Wygant St. (503) 252-2405
St. Joseph, MI 49085
413 State Street (616) 983-3014
Seattle, WA 98101
930 Terminal Sales Building
(206) 622-6381
Watertown, MA 02172
76 Coolidge Hill Rd. (617) 923-2330
Products Available
Allorganic Trace Minerals-B12
Antronex
Betaine Hydrochloride
Biost Powder
Cal-Amo
Calcium Lactate (Fortified)
Cardio-Plus
Cardiotrophin (Heart)
Catalyn
Cataplex A-F & Betaris
Cataplex E-2
Cataplex F
Chlorophyll Complex Ointment (Fat Soluble)
Chlorophyll Complex Perles (Fat Soluble)
Choline
Comfrey, Pepsin—Formula E-3
Ferroplus
Inositol
Multizyme
Niacinamide B6
Ovex
Pneumotrophin (Lung)
Prost-X
Ribo-Nucleic Acid (RNA)
Thymex
Vasculin
Vitamin B-6 w/Niacinamide
Zypan Tablets

STAR PHARMACEUTICALS, INC. 1697
16499 North East 19th Avenue
North Miami Beach, FL 33160
Address inquiries to:
Scott L. Davidson,President (305) 949-1612
Products Available
Methavin Tablets
Microsul Tablets
Microsul-A
Nitrex Tablets
Prosed
Star-Otic
Uro-KP-Neutral
Urolene Blue
Vesicholine Tablets
Virilon

STERI-MED INC. 1697
P.O. Box 459
Lindenhurst, NY 11757
Address inquiries to:
Director, Professional Services Dept.
(516) 842-4209
Products Available
Aminophylline Tablets
Amoxicillin Capsules
Ampicillin Capsules
Chlordiazepoxide Capsules
Chlorothiazide Tablets
Chlorpheniramine Maleate Tablets
Chlorpromazine HCl Tablets
Conjugated Estrogen Tablets
Cortisone Acetate Tablets
Digitoxin Tablets
Dimenhydrinate Tablets
Diphenhydramine HCl Capsules
Hydralazine HCl Tablets
Hydrochlorothiazide Tablets
Hydrocortisone Cream
Hydrocortisone Tablets
Imipramine HCl Tablets
Levodopa Capsules
Meprobamate Tablets
Nitrofurantoin Tablets
Phenytoin Sodium Capsules
Pilocarpine HCl Ophthalmic Solution
Potassium Chloride Liquid
Prednisolone Tablets
Prednisone Tablets
Probenecid Tablets
Procainamid HCl Capsules
Propoxyphene HCl Compound Capsules
Propylthiouracil
Quinidine Sulfate Tablets
Reserpine Tablets
Tetracycline Capsules

STIEFEL LABORATORIES, INC. 1698
2801 Ponce de Leon Blvd.
Coral Gables, FL 33134
Address inquiries to:
Melvin Ader (305) 443-3807
Branch Offices
CALIFORNIA
P.O. Box 375
Gardena, CA 90247 (213) 321-4006
GEORGIA
Post Office Box 47789
Doraville, GA 30340 (404) 455-1896
NEW YORK
Route 145
Oak Hill, NY 12460 (518) 239-6901
PUERTO RICO
Laboratories Stiefel, Inc.
P.O. Box 387
Mayaguez, Puerto Rico 00708
(809) 832-1376
Products Available
Acne-Aid Cream
Acne-Aid Detergent Soap
Acne-Aid Lotion
AluWets Wet Dressing Crystals
Benoxyl-5 Lotion
Benoxyl-10 Lotion
Brasivol Base
Brasivol Fine
Brasivol Medium
Brasivol Rough
Duofilm
Ichthyol Ointment
LactiCare Lotion
Lasan Unguent
Oilatum Soap
PanOxyl 5, PanOxyl 10
PanOxyl AQ 2½, 5 & 10 Acne Gel
Polytar Bath
Polytar Shampoo
Polytar Soap
Salicylic Acid Soap
Salicylic Acid & Sulfur Soap
Saligel
SAStid (AL)
SAStid (Plain)
SAStid Soap
Sulfoxyl Lotion Regular
Sulfoxyl Lotion Strong
Sulfur Soap
Surfol
ZeaSorb Medicated Powder

STUART PHARMACEUTICALS 434, 1699
Div. of ICI Americas Inc.
Wilmington, DE 19897
Address inquiries to:
John W. Council, Manager
Professional Services (302) 575-2231
Products Available
ALternaGEL Liquid
◆ Bucladin-S Softab
Cari-Tab Softab
◆ Dialose Capsules
◆ Dialose Plus Capsules
Effersyllium Instant Mix
◆ Ferancee Tablets
◆ Ferancee-HP Tablets
◆ Hibiclens
◆ Hibitane
◆ Kasof Capsules
◆ Kinesed Tablets
Mucoplex Tablets
Mulvidren Softab
◆ Mulvidren-F Softab
Mylanta Liquid
◆ Mylanta Tablets
Mylanta-II Liquid
◆ Mylanta-II Tablets
◆ Mylicon (Tablets & Drops)
◆ Mylicon-80 Tablets
◆ Nolvadex Tablets
Orexin Softab
◆ Probec-T Tablets
◆ Sorbitrate Chewable Tablets
◆ Sorbitrate Oral Tablets
◆ Sorbitrate Sublingual Tablets
◆ Sorbitrate Sustained Action Tablets
Stuart Formula (liquid), The
◆ Stuart Formula (tablets), The
Stuart Hematinic Liquid
◆ Stuart Prenatal Tablets
◆ Stuart Prenatal w/Folic Acid Tablets
Stuart Therapeutic Multivitamin Tablets
◆ Stuartinic Tablets
◆ Stuartnatal 1+1 Tablets
Theron Tablets

SUGARLO COMPANY 435, 1706
3540 Atlantic Ave.
P. O. Box 1017
Atlantic City, NJ 08404
Address inquiries to:
Alan E. Kligerman (609) 348-3148
Products Available
◆ LactAid brand lactase enzyme

SURGIKOS 1706
A Johnson & Johnson Company
501 George Street
New Brunswick, NJ 08903
(201) 524-0400
Products Available
Arterial Graft (Bovine Origin) artegraft
Surgicel Absorbable Hemostat
Surgikos Artegraft

SURVIVAL TECHNOLOGY, INC. 435, 1708
7801 Woodmont Avenue
Bethesda, MD 20014 (301) 654-2303
Products Available
AtroPen Auto-Injector
(Atropine for Intramuscular Injection for organophosphorus or carbamate insecticide poisoning)
◆ LidoPen Auto-Injector
(Lidocaine Hydrochloride for Intramuscular Injection for Cardiac Arrhythmias)

SWEEN CORPORATION 1709
P.O. Box 3404
Mankato, MN 56001
(507) 278-3898
Products Available
Fordustin'
Peri-Care
Peri-Wash
Surgi-Kleen
Sween Cream
Sween Karaya Powder
Whirl-Sol
Xtracare II

SYNTEX (F.P.) INC. 435, 1710
Humacao, Puerto Rico 00661
Address inquiries to:
Syntex Laboratories, Inc.
3401 Hillview Avenue
Palo Alto, CA 94304
Products Available
◆ Brevicon 21-Day Tablets
◆ Brevicon 28-Day Tablets
◆ Norinyl 1+50 21-Day Tablets
◆ Norinyl 1+50 28-Day Tablets
◆ Norinyl 1+80 21-Day Tablets
◆ Norinyl 1+80 28-Day Tablets
◆ Norinyl 2 mg. Tablets
◆ Nor-Q.D. Tablets

SYNTEX LABORATORIES, INC. 435, 1710
3401 Hillview Ave.
Palo Alto, CA 94304
Address Medical inquiries on marketed products to:
Medical Services Dept. (415) 855-5545
Other inquiries to:
(415) 855-5050
Products Available
◆ Anadrol-50 Tablets
Carmol HC Cream
▣ Carmol 10 Lotion
▣ Carmol 20 Cream
▣ Cho-Free Formula Base
Evex Tablets
Lidex Cream
Lidex Ointment
Lidex-E Cream
▣ Methakote Diaper Rash Cream
Microsyn Acne Lotion
Mull-Soy Liquid
▣ Neo-Mull-Soy Liquid

Neo-Synalar Cream
Synalar Creams, Ointment and Topical Solution
Synalar-HP Cream
Synemol Cream
(NP) Topic Gel
Topsyn Gel
Vagitrol Cream
Vagitrol Suppositories

SYNTEX PUERTO RICO, INC. 435, 1710
Humacao, Puerto Rico 00661
Address Medical inquiries on marketed products to:
Medical Services Dept. (415) 855-5545
Other inquiries to:
(415) 855-5050
Products Available
Kato Powder
◆ Naprosyn Tablets

THEX CORPORATION 1727
202 Green St.
San Francisco, CA 94111
Address inquiries to:
Professional Service Dept. (415) 362-1700
Products Available
Cantharone
Dermolatum Cream
Dricort
Hydrocortisone Cream
Thex Forte Capsules

THOMPSON MEDICAL COMPANY, INC. 1728
919 Third Avenue
New York, NY 10022
Address inquiries to:
Dr. Edward L. Steinberg (212) 688-4420
Products Available
Appedrine, Extra Strength
Aspercreme
Control Capsules
Dexatrim
Dexatrim Extra Strength
Prolamine Capsules, Super Strength

TRAVENOL LABORATORIES, INC. 1729
Parenteral Products Division
One Baxter Parkway
Deerfield, IL 60015
Address inquiries to:
Marketing Communications (312) 480-5175
Products Available
Amigen Injection*
Travamin Injection
Travasol (Amino Acid) Injection
Travasol M, 3.5% (Amino Acid) Injection
*Available in certain states as, Travamin (Protein Hydrolysate Injection, USP casein)

TRIMEN LABORATORIES, INC. 1733
80 - 26th Street
Pittsburgh, PA 15222
Address inquiries to:
Professional Service Dept. (412) 261-0339
Branch Office
Philadelphia, PA 19107
1009 Western Savings Fund Bldg.
Products Available
Allerid-D.C. Capsules
Allerid-O.D.-8 Capsules
Allerid-O.D.-12 Capsules
Amaphen Capsules
Banatil-O.D. Capsules
Bellermine-O.D. Capsules
Delta-E Tablets
Deltamycin Capsules
Deltapen-VK Solution
Deltapen-VK Tablets
Deltavac Cream
Dialex Capsules
Dilart Capsules
Emerox-O.D. Capsules
Fe-O.D. Tablets
Flexaphen Capsules
Hydrex Tablets
Korigesic Tablets
Laxatyl Tablets
Natacomp-FA Tablets
Neurate-400 Tablets
Ovest-0.3 Tablets
Ovest-0.625 Tablets
Ovest-1.25 Tablets
Sorate-5 Chewable Tablets
Sorate-2.5 Sublingual Tablets
Sorate-5 Sublingual Tablets
Sorate-10 Tablets
Sorate-40 Capsules
Titracid Tablets
Trimedine Expectorant
Viopan-T Tablets

TUTAG PHARMACEUTICALS, INC. 435, 1733
2599 W. Midway Blvd.
Broomfield, CO 80020
Address inquiries to:
Professional Service Dept. (303) 466-8841
Products Available
Acetospan Injection
Alermine Tablets
Amitriptyline HCl Tablets
Ampicillin Capsules, Suspension
Analone Injection
Andriol Injection
◆ Aquatag Tablets
Arthrolate Injection
Asminorel Improved Tablets
◆ Bacarate Tablets
Baltron Injection
Bendylate Capsules, Elixir
Bendylate Injection
C-BE Zinc Tablets
Cino Tablets
Cino-40 Injection
Codap Tablets
Cotropic-Gel 40 Injection
Cotropic-Gel 80 Injection
Cyvaso Capsules
Depletite-25 Tablets
Dezone Injection
Dezone Tablets
Dimate Injection
Diphylets
Droxomin Injection
Dua-Pred Injection
Duo-Dezone Injection
Duoval P.A. Injection
E-Ionate P.A. Injection
Enoxa Tablets
Erca Tablets
◆ Escot Capsules
Estraval 2X Injection
Estraval 4X Injection
Estraval-P.A. Injection
Fenbutal Tablets
Ganphen Injection
Geritag Injection
Hyproval P.A. Injection
I.D. 50 Injection
Irolong Granucaps
L.A. Dezone Injection
Lo-Tussin Syrup
Meclizine HCl Tablets
Meprobamate Tablets
Methoxal Tablets
Murcil Capsules
Nandrolin Injection
Nasobid Granucaps
◆ Neotep Granucaps
Neozyl
Nitrofurantoin Tablets
◆ Normacid Tablets
Nospaz Injection
1000 BC Injection
P.S.P. IV (four) Injection
Penicillin G Tablets
Piracaps Capsules
Pre-Dep 40 Injection
Pre-Dep 80 Injection
Prednisolone Acetate Injection
Pre-Enthus F Capsules
Proco Capsules
Quadnite Tablets
◆ Quinite Tablets
Rauserpa Tablets
Ropanth Tablets
SPRX-1, SPRX-2 Tablets
SPRX-3 Capsules
Sanicide Liquid
Setamine Tablets
Sodestrin Injection
Sodestrin-H Tablets
Sonazine Tablets
Sorquad Tablets
Spasmate Tablets
◆ Suladyne Tablets
T.D. Alermine Granucaps
T.D. Therals Granucaps
T-E Ionate P.A. Injection
T-Ionate P.A. Injection
Tagafed Tablets
Tagatap Tablets & Elixir
Testostroval P.A. Injection
Tora Tablets
Tora-I & -II Capsules
Tora-30 Capsules
Trates Granucaps
Tudecon T.D. Tablets
Tumol Tablets
Tuzon Tablets
◆ Unproco Capsules
Vagimine Cream
Vasal Granucaps
Vernate II Granucaps
Viotag Cream
W.D.D. Tablets
X-Otag Injection
Zide Tablets

U.S. ETHICALS INC.
37-02 48th Avenue
Long Island City, NY 11101
Address inquiries to:
Medical Director (212) 786-8606
Products Available
Azlytal Tablets
Azmadrine Capsules & Tablets
Bellastal Capsules
Bellastal Elixir & Tablets
Capa Tablets
Eclabron Capsules & Elixir
Eclamide Capsules
Eclasufed Capsules
Etnapa Elixir
Ferbetrin Tablets
Gastrical Tablets
Geristone Capsules
Hepaferron Syrup
Histabs Tablets
Klavikordal Tablets
Natalac Capsules
Natalac Forte Capsules
Neocomplex Injection
Neodex Tablets & Syrup
Nicostrol Capsules
Niong Tablets
Nitromed
Nitronet Tablets
Nitrong Ointment (See Wharton Laboratories)
Nitrong Tablets (See Wharton Laboratories)
Supervim Drops, Tablets & Syrup
Ulcinal Tablets
Vitacoms Capsules

USV LABORATORIES, DIVISION USV PHARMACEUTICAL CORP. 436, 1736
1 Scarsdale Road
Tuckahoe, NY 10707
Address inquiries to:
Medical Department (914) 779-6300
Nights, Weekends and Holidays, call
(914) 779-6300

USV LABORATORIES Inc. 436, 1736
Manati, Puerto Rico 00701
Address inquiries to:
USV Pharmaceutical Corp. (see above)

USV (P.R.) DEVELOPMENT CORP. 436, 1736
Manati, Puerto Rico 00701
Address inquiries to:
USV Pharmaceutical Corp. (see above)
Products Available
◆ Aquasol A Capsules
Aquasol A Drops
Aquasol A Parenteral
Aquasol Body Lotion
◆ Aquasol E Capsules
Aquasol E Drops
◆ Arlidin Tablets
◆ Azolid
◆ Azolid-A
C-B Vone Capsules
◆ Cerespan Capsules
◆ Demi-Regroton
◆ Doriden
◆ Histaspan Capsules
◆ Histaspan-D Capsules
◆ Histaspan-Plus Capsules
◆ Hygroton
Lufa Capsules
◆ M.V.I. (Multi-Vitamin Infusion)
Methischol Capsules
◆ Nitrospan Capsules
◆ Oxalid
Panthoderm Lotion and Cream
◆ Pertofrane
◆ Presamine Tablets
◆ Regroton
Vi-Aqua Capsules
Vi-Aqua Forte Capsules
Vi-Aquamin Capsules
Vi-Aquamin Forte Capsules
◆ Voranil

ULMER PHARMACAL COMPANY 1749
(Division of Physicians & Hospitals Supply Co.)
2440 Fernbrook Lane
Minneapolis, MN 55441
Address inquiries to:
Professional Service Dept. (612) 559-3333
Products Available
Aerosan
Andoin Ointment
Anesta-Caine
Aspirin Tablets
Bacitracin Ointment
Bi-Amine
Bu-Lax Capsules
Bu-Lax Plus Capsules
Cal-Zo Ointment
Cardiocreme
Cardio-Pads
Chloral Methylol Ointment
Cobalin Injection
Co-Gel Tablets
Col-Vi-Nol Ointment
Decongestcaps
Dextro-Tuss GG

Gentle Shampoo
Hematovals
Hiscatabs
Iodocort Cream
Kler-ro Liquid
Kler-ro Powder
L.F.B. 12-100 Injection
Lobana Body Powder
Lobana Body Shampoo
Lobana Conditioning Shampoo
Lobana Liquid Hand Soap
Lobana Lotion
Lobana Perineal Cleanse
Milk of Magnesia
Mineral Oil
P-B-Sal
Pentazyme Tablets
Pheneen Sanitizer
Pheneen Solution
Pheneen Solution N.R.I.
Progesic Compound-65
Progesic-65
Super Ulex Injection
Surgel Liquid
Ta-Poff
Ta-Poff Aerosol
Theolixir
Tokols Capsules
Ulcort Cream
Ulcort Lotion
Ultar Cream
Ultracaine Injection
Ulvical SG
Vasospan Capsules
Vitamin A & D Ointment
Vitamin B 12 Crystalline Injection
Vitamin C Tablets
Vleminckx'
Zinc Oxide Ointment

UNITED STATES PACKAGING CORPORATION 2038
506 Clay Street
La Porte, IN 46350
Address inquiries to:
Dr. Max Ben, Medical Director
(219) 362-9782
Products Available
Gonodecten Test Kit

UPJOHN COMPANY, THE 436, 1751
7000 Portage Road
Kalamazoo, MI 49001
(616) 323-4000
Emergency Medical Information
(616) 323-6615
Pharmaceutical Sales Areas and Distribution Centers
Atlanta (Chamblee), GA 30341 (404) 451-4822
Boston (Needham Heights), MA 02194 (617) 449-0320
Buffalo (Cheektowaga), NY 14240 (716) 681-7160
Chicago (Oak Brook), IL 60680 (312) 654-3300
Cincinnati, OH 45214 (513) 242-4573
Dallas, TX 75265 (214) 824-3027
Denver, CO 80217 (303) 399-3113
Honolulu, HI 96809 (808) 538-1181
Kalamazoo, MI 49001 (616) 323-4000
Kansas City, MO 64141 (816) 361-2286
Los Angeles, CA 90051 (213) 463-8101
Memphis, TN 38122 (901) 761-4170
Miami, FL 33152 (305) 758-3317
Minneapolis, MN 55440 (612) 588-2786
New York (Hicksville), Long Island, NY 11802 (516) 747-1970
Philadelphia (Wayne) PA 19087 (215) 265-2100
Pittsburgh, PA 15220 (412) 343-9377
Portland, OR 97208 (503) 232-2133
St. Louis, MO 63177 (314) 872-8626
San Francisco (Palo Alto) CA 94304 (415) 493-8080
Washington, DC 20013 (202) 882-6163
Divisions
Laboratory Procedures-West
The Upjohn Company
Inglewood, CA 90301 (213) 887-8500
Laboratory Procedures
The Upjohn Company
Denver, CO 80602 (303) 321-6300
Laboratory Procedures-South
Atlanta, GA 30302 (404) 981-9900
Laboratory Procedures-East
The Upjohn Company
King of Prussia, PA 19406
(215) 265-6200
Laboratory Procedures-East
Great Neck, NY 11021 (516) 829-5630
Laboratory Procedures-Wilkes-Barre
Wilkes-Barre, PA 18703 (717) 822-8101
Laboratory Procedures Northwest, Inc.
The Upjohn Company
Tacoma, WA 98411
(206) 597-6681
University Laboratory Medicine, Inc.
Subsidiary of The Upjohn Company
Philadelphia, PA 19102 (215) 448-7419
Washington Representative
Washington, DC 20036 (202) 659-3657
The Upjohn Manufacturing Company
Barceloneta, Puerto Rico 00617
(809) 724-3578
The Upjohn Manufacturing Company M
Barceloneta, Puerto Rico 00617
(809) 724-3578
Products Available
◆ Adeflor Chewable Tablets
Adeflor Drops
Adeflor M Tablets
Albamycin Capsules
Alkets Tablets
Alphadrol Tablets
Aspirin Tablets
Baciguent Ointment
Baciguent, Sterile Ophthalmic Ointment
Bacitracin USP, Sterile
Berubigen Crystalline, Sterile Solution
Calcium Chloride Sterile Solution
Calcium Gluconate Flavored Wafers
Calcium Gluconate Injection, Sterile Solution
Calcium Lactate Tablets
Cardrase Tablets
Caripeptic Liquid
Casyllium
Cebefortis Tablets
Cebenase Tablets
Cebetinic Tablets
Cheracol D, Bilingual Cough Syrup (English and Spanish labeling)
Cheracol D, Cough Syrup
Cheracol Syrup
Citrocarbonate, Granular Effervescent Salt
◆ Cleocin HCl Capsules
Cleocin Pediatric Flavored Granules
◆ Cleocin Phosphate Sterile Solutions
Clocream
Colestid Granules
Cortef Acetate, Ointments
Cortef Acetate Sterile Injectable Suspension
Cortef (Intramuscular) Sterile Aqueous Suspension
Cortef, Tablets & Fluid
Cortisone Acetate Sterile Aqueous Suspension
Cortisone Acetate Tablets
Cytosar-U Sterile Powder
Delta-Cortef Tablets
◆ Deltasone Tablets
Depo-Estradiol Cypionate, Sterile Solutions
◆ Depo-Medrol Sterile Aqueous Suspension
Depo-Provera Sterile Aqueous Suspension
Depo-Testadiol Sterile Solution
Depo-Testosterone Sterile Solution
◆ Didrex Tablets
Diostate D Tablets
◆ E-Mycin E Liquid
◆ E-Mycin Tablets
Epinephricaine Ointment
Ergophene Ointment
Erythromycin Tablets (E-Mycin)
Feminone Tablets
Ferritrinsic Tablets
Ferrous Sulfate Tablets
◆ Florone Cream
◆ Florone Ointment
Gelfilm Ophthalmic, Sterile
Gelfilm, Sterile
Gelfoam, Compressed
Gelfoam Dental Packs
Gelfoam Packs
Gelfoam Prostatectomy Cones
Gelfoam Sterile Powder
Gelfoam Sterile Sponge
Gerizyme
Halodrin Tablets
◆ Halotestin Tablets
Heparin Sodium Sterile Solutions From Beef Lung
Hydriodic Acid (Upjohn), Syrup
Hydrocortisone Acetate, U.S.P.; Micronized, Nonsterile (For Prescription Compounding)
Hydrocortisone, U.S.P. Micronized, Nonsterile (For Prescription Compounding)
Hydrolose Syrup
Kaopectate
Kaopectate, Bilingual (English and Spanish labeling)
Kaopectate Concentrate
Lincocin Capsules
Lincocin Pediatric Capsules
Lincocin Sterile Solutions
Lincocin Syrup
Lipomul-Oral
◆ Loniten Tablets
◆ Maolate Tablets
Medicated Foot Powder
Medrol Acetate Ointment
Medrol Enpak Kit
Medrol Enpak Refill
◆ Medrol, 4 mg, Dosepak
Medrol, 16 mg, ADT Pak
◆ Medrol Tablets
Meroracin Tincture
◆ Motrin Tablets
Mycifradin Oral Solution
Mycifradin Sterile Powder
Mycifradin Tablets
Myciguent, Cream & Ointment
Myciguent Sterile Ophthalmic Ointment
Mycitracin Ointment
Mycitracin Sterile Ophthalmic Ointment
Myringacaine
Neo-Cortef Cream
Neo-Cortef Lotion
Neo-Cortef Ointment
Neo-Cortef Sterile Ophthalmic Ointment
Neo-Cortef Sterile Ophthalmic Suspension
Neo-Delta-Cortef Ointment
Neo-Delta-Cortef Ophthalmic Suspension
Neo-Delta-Cortef Sterile Ophthalmic Ointment
Neo-Medrol Acetate, Topical
Neo-Medrol Sterile Ophthalmic Ointment
Neo-Oxylone Ointment
Neosone Sterile Ophthalmic Ointment
Optef Eye Drops, Sterile Solution
Oral Pentacresol 1:1000
Orinase Diagnostic, Sterile
◆ Orinase Tablets
Orthoxicol Syrup
Orthoxine Hydrochloide, Tablets & Syrup
Orthoxine & Aminophylline Capsules
Oxylone Cream
P-A-C Compound, Capsules and Tablets
P-A-C Compound w/Codeine Sulfate, Capsules and Tablets
◆ Pamine Tablets
◆ Panmycin Hydrochloride Capsules
Panmycin Syrup Aqueous Suspension
◆ Panmycin Tablets
◆ Pensyn Capsules
Pensyn Oral Powder
Pentacresol Instrument Disinfecting Solution
Phenobarbital Elixir
Phenobarbital & Belladonna, No. 1, Tablets
Phenobarbital & Belladonna, No. 2, Tablets
Phenolax Wafers
Protamine Sulfate for Injection, Sterile, with Bacteriostatic Water for Injection
◆ Provera Tablets
Pyrroxate, Capsules & Tablets
Pyrroxate w/Codeine Phosphate, Capsules
Reserpoid, Tablets
Salicresin Fluid
Sigtab Tablets
Sodium Chloride (Bacteriostatic) Injection with Benzyl Alcohol, Sterile Solution
Solu-B, Sterile, Mix-O-Vial
Solu-B w/Ascorbic Acid Sterile Powder
Solu-B-Forte (S-B-F) Sterile Powder
Solu-Cortef, Sterile & Mix-O-Vial Sterile
Solu-Cortef, Sterile, with Bacteriostatic Water for Injection
◆ Solu-Medrol Sterile Powder
Special Formula, No. 2, Tablets
Sugracillin Flavored Granules
Super D Perles
Tanicaine Ointment & Suppositories
◆ Tolinase Tablets
Trobicin, Sterile
Unicap Chewable Tablets
Unicap M, Tablets
Unicap Multivitamin Capsules
Unicap Plus Iron
Unicap Senior Tablets
Unicap T Tablets
Unigesic-A Tablets
Upjohn Vitamin C Tablets, 250 mg
Upjohn Vitamin E Capsules, 200 I.U.
Uracil Mustard Capsules
Uticillin VK Flavored Granules
◆ Uticillin VK Tablets
Water for Injection w/Benzyl Alcohol, Sterile
Zinc Sulfide Compound, Lotion, Improved
Zymacap Capsules
Zymalixir
Zymasyrup

UPSHER-SMITH LABORATORIES, INC. 1793
14905 23rd Ave. North
Minneapolis, MN 55441
(612) 473-4412
Address inquiries to:
Professional Service Department
Products Available
Acetaminophen Uniserts Suppositories
Algitab Tablets
Aspirin Uniserts Suppositories
Bisacodyl Tablets
Bisacodyl Uniserts Suppositories
Cyclandelate Capsules
Dioctyl Sodium Sulfosuccinate Capsules
Dioctyl Sodium Sulfosuccinate with (Casanthranol) Capsules
Ferrous Gluconate Tablets
Ferrous Sulfate Tablets
Hemorrhoidal Uniserts Suppositories
Hemorrhoidal-HC Uniserts Suppositories
Hexavitamin Tablets
Histatapp Elixir
Histatapp T.D. Tablets

Hydrochlorothiazide Tablets
Kerasol Therapeutic Bath Oil
Klor-Con Powder
Klor-Con 20% Solution
Klor-10% Solution
Papaverine Hydrochloride T.R. Capsules
SSKI
Sorbitol Solution
Sudahist Tablets
Therapeutic B Complex with C Capsules
Therapeutic Multivitamin Tablets
Therapeutic Multivitamin & Mineral Tablets
Trofan Tablets (L-Tryptophan)
Zinc Sulfate Capsules

VALE CHEMICAL CO., INC., THE 1794
1201 Liberty St.
Allentown, PA 18102
Address inquiries to:
Thomas R. Davis (215) 433-7579
Products Available
Acedoval Tablets
Acedyne Tablets
Aluminum Hydroxide Gel, Tablets
Aminophyllin Tablets
Ammonium Chloride Tablets
Antrin Tablets
Antussal Syrup
Ascorbic Acid Tablets
Asmacol Tablets
Aspir-10 Tablets
Atrobyl Tablets
Barbeloid Tablets
Belexal Tablets
Biothesin Tablets
Bismapec Tablets
Butalix
Calcium Gluconate Tablets
Calfos-D Tablets
Coraval Improved Tablets
Dermaval Cream
Double-Sal Tablets
Duphrene Syrup & Tablets
Ephedrine & Sodium Phenobarbital Tablets
Extract of Ox Bile Tablets
Ferate-C Tablets
Glucovite Tablets
Glycofed
Glycotuss Syrup & Tablets
Glycotuss-dM Syrup & Tablets
Guiosan Syrup
Hydra-Mag Tablets
Ironco-B Tablets
Magmalin Tablets & Suspension
Mandex Tablets
Methenamine & Acid Sodium Phosphate Tablets
Methiokap Capsules
Neocet Tablets
Neofed
Neogesic Tablets
Neo-Tab Tablets
Nevrotose Capsutabs
Niacin Tablets
Nisaval Tablets
Nyral Lozenges
Obeval Tablets
Oxynitral w/Veratrum Viride Tablets
Pedric Elixir & Tablets
Pedric Senior Tablets
Phenobarbital Tablets
Potassium Iodide Tablets
Quadsul Tablets
Rauval Tablets
Rhinogesic Tablets
Rhinogesic-GG Tablets
Riboflavin Tablets
Serpate Tablets
Sodium Salicylate Tablets
Soothogel Cream
Synthetar Cream
Taurophyllin Tablets
Taystron Tablets
Terphan Elixir
Theolix Elixir
Thiamine Hydrochloride Tablets
Thyroid Tablets
Tono-B, Wafers
Trioval Tablets
Triple Sulfoid Tablets Suspension
Valacet Tablets
Valcaine Ointment
Valdeine Tablets
Valdrene Expectorant Syrup
Valdrene Tablets
Val-Tep Tablets

VICKS TOILETRY PRODUCTS DIVISION 1794
Richardson-Merrell Inc.
10 Westport Road
Wilton, CT 06897
Address inquiries to:
Director of Scientific & Regulatory Affairs
Vicks Divisions Research & Development (914) 664-5000
For Medical Emergencies Contact
Medical Director
Vicks Divisions Research & Development (914) 664-5000
Products Available
Clearasil Acne Treatment Cream
Clearasil Antibacterial Acne Lotion
Topex Acne Clearing Medication

VICKS HEALTH CARE DIVISION 1794
Richardson-Merrell Inc.
10 Westport Road
Wilton, CT 06897
Address inquiries to:
Director of Scientific & Regulatory Affairs
Vicks Divisions Research & Development (914) 664-5000
For Medical Emergencies Contact
Medical Director
Vicks Divisions Research & Development (914) 664-5000
Products Available
Daycare Daytime Colds Medicine
Formula 44 Cough Control Discs
Formula 44 Cough Mixture
Formula 44D Decongestant Cough Mixture
Nyquil Nighttime Colds Medicine
Oracin Cherry Flavor Cooling Throat Lozenges
Oracin Cooling Throat Lozenges
Sinex Decongestant Nasal Spray
Sinex Long-Acting Decongestant Nasal Spray
Vaposteam
Vatronol Nose Drops
Vicks Cough Silencers Cough Drops
Vicks Cough Syrup
Vicks Formula 44 Cough Control Discs
Vicks Formula 44 Cough Mixture
Vicks Formula 44D Decongestant Cough Mixture
Vicks Inhaler
Vicks NyQuil Nighttime Colds Medicine
Vicks Sinex Decongestant Nasal Spray
Vicks Sinex Long-Acting Decongestant Nasal Spray
Vicks Throat Lozenges
Vicks Vaporub
Vicks Vaposteam
Vicks Vatronol Nose Drops

VIOBIN CORPORATION 1797
a Subsidiary of A. H. Robins Co
226 W. Livingston St.
Monticello, IL 61856
Address inquiries to:
W. E. Melby (217) 762-2561
Products Available
Jayron Capsules
Viobin Wheat Germ Oil, Liquid & Capsules
Viokase

WALKER, CORP & CO., INC. 1798
Easthampton Pl. & N. Collingwood Ave.
Syracuse, NY 13206
Address inquiries to:
P.O. Drawer 1320
Syracuse, NY 13201 (315) 463-4511
Products Available
Evac-U-Gen

WALKER PHARMACAL COMPANY 1798
4200 Laclede Avenue
St. Louis, MO 63108
Address inquiries to:
Customer Service (314) 533-9600
Products Available
Succus Cineraria Maritima

WALLACE LABORATORIES 437, 1799
Half Acre Road
Cranbury, NJ 08512
Address inquiries to:
Professional Services (609) 655-6000
Night and Weekend Emergencies (609) 799-1167
Send all orders to:
Wallace Laboratories
Div. of Carter-Wallace, Inc.
Post Office Drawer 5
Cranbury, NJ 08512
Products Available
◆ Aquatensen Tablets
Avazyme/Avazyme-100 Tablets
Barbidonna Elixir & Tablets
Barbidonna No. 2 Tablets
Covanamine Liquid & Tablets
Covangesic Liquid & Tablets
Dainite Tablets
Dainite-KI Tablets
◆ Depen Titratabs
Deprol Tablets
Diutensen Tablets
◆ Diutensen-R Tablets
Ephed-Organidin Elixir
Luftodil
Lufyllin Elixir
◆ Lufyllin Injection
◆ Lufyllin & Lufyllin-400 Tablets
Lufyllin-EPG Elixir & Tablets
◆ Lufyllin-GG Elixir & Tablets
Maltsupex Liquid, Powder & Tablets
Meprospan Capsules
◆ Micrainin
◆ Milpath Tablets
Milprem Tablets
◆ Miltown Tablets
◆ Miltown 600 Tablets
Miltrate Tablets
Mylaxen
◆ Organidin Elixir, Solution & Tablets
Rectalad-Aminophylline
◆ Rondomycin Capsules
Ryna Liquid
Ryna-C Liquid
Ryna-Cx Liquid
Rynatan Pediatric Suspension
◆ Rynatan Tablets
Rynatuss Pediatric Suspension
◆ Rynatuss Tablets
Ryna-Tussadine Expectorant Liquid & Tablets
◆ Soma Tablets
◆ Soma Compound Tablets
◆ Soma Compound w/Codeine Tablets
Syllact Powder
Syllamalt Powder & Effervescent Powder
Theo-Organidin Elixir
Tussi-Organidin Liquid
Tussi-Organidin DM Liquid
◆ Unitensen Aqueous
◆ Unitensen Tablets
Vastran Tablets
◆ VōSol HC Otic Solution
◆ VōSol Otic Solution

WARREN-TEED LABORATORIES 438, 1827
Division of Adria Laboratories Inc.
582 W. Goodale St.
Columbus, OH 43215
Address inquiries to:
Warren Myers (614) 889-1300
Branch Offices
Dallas, TX 75229 (214) 243-2551
Los Angeles, CA 90040 (213) 726-1248
Humacao, Puerto Rico (809) 852-2595
Products Available
Axotal Tablets
Epsilan-M Capsules
Evac-Q-Kit
Evac-Q-Kwik
Ilopan Injection (Ampuls & Vials)
Ilopan Stat-Pak (Disposable Syringes)
Ilopan-Choline Tablets
Ilozyme Tablets
Kaochlor 10% Liquid
Kaochlor-Eff Tablets
Kaochlor S-F 10% Liquid
Kaon Elixir
Kaon Tablets
◆ Kaon-Cl Tabs
Kaon-Cl 20%
Magan Tablets
Modane Bulk
Modane Liquid
Modane Mild Tablets
Modane Soft
Modane Tablets
Myoflex Creme
Pektamalt
Ratio Tablets
Taloin Ointment
Thi-Cin Capsules
Tympagesic
W-T Lotion

WEBCON PHARMACEUTICALS 1833
Division of Alcon Laboratories (Puerto Rico), Inc.
Post Office Box 1629
Fort Worth, TX 76101
Address inquiries to:
Medical Department
Post Office Box 1629
Fort Worth, TX 76101 (817) 293-0450
Products Available
Alconefrin 12 Drops
Alconefrin 25 Drops
Alconefrin 50 Drops
Alconefrin 25 Spray
Anestacon Sterile Solution
Aquachloral Supprettes
Aqualin Children Supprettes
Aqualin Supprettes
Azo-Standard Tablets
B & O No. 15A & No. 16A Supprettes
Cystospaz Tablets
Cystospaz-M Capsules
Cystospaz-SR Capsules
Hexalet Tablets
Neopap Supprettes
*Oxiphen Tablets
Revac Supprettes
Urised Tablets
Urisedamine Tablets
WANS Children Supprettes
WANS No. 1 & No. 2 Supprettes
*TM The Dow Chemical Co.

(◆ Shown in Product Identification Section) **(▣ Described in PDR For Nonprescription Drugs)**

WESLEY PHARMACAL COMPANY, INC., THE 1835
4831-33 Rising Sun Avenue
Philadelphia, PA 19120
Address inquiries to:
Professional Service Dept. (215) 324-6566
Products Available
Alkaline Gargle
Allee
Aqwadril
Aqweside
Aqwesine
Atrobarbital Tablets
Auralcort
Auralgesic Drops
Avasol
Bee 12 Injection
Bilagog
Bilox Tablets
Bioplex
Calfoject Injection
Calodex Cream
Camadine Tablets
Cee w/Bee
Ceeject
Ceespan T.D. Capsules
Cetacet Capsules
Cetased
Charloid
Cinolone
Cobaldrox-12
Codasol
Codinets Tablets
Deco SPC
Deco-Disc Lozenges
Decodult Tablets
Decofed
Decogest Tablets
Decolate Tablets
Decominic
Deco-Mist Spray
Decospan
Decostat
Decotapp
Decotussin Tablets
Dexadrol
Diotabs
Duolate-Q
EDTA Injection
Eisenzucker Tablets
Eramycin
Estralate
Estrosol Forte
Flatulence Tabs
Flexon
Foli-B
Galopectin Tablets
Gasticans
Gastomins
Glycotone Tablets
Gonadoplex
Hydocaine
Hytrophen
Infer
K-Glucon
Kaogoric
Kaybiotic Cream
Kaycort H.C. Cream
Kaylog
Kaytar Cream
Kryzen Tablets
Lactoease
Liferavite
Marfonyl
Megabee
Merculyn
Metabol
Niaspan
Niazole, Improved
Nicosine
Optolow
Optozine
P.D.P. Capsules
P.D.P. Liquid
P.D.P. Powder
P.D.P. Wafers
Panitol Tablets
Panitone Liquid
Panitone Tablets
Panivon
Pecadine Tablets
Peritrol
Phenterspan
Prednasol
Prednaspan Forte
Prednoid
Protobol
Pulsaphen Tablets
Quadramin
Reposans-10
Ribozime
Robinetts
Romazine Cough Syrup
Romazine Injection
Salisicol Tablets
Sedastat
Sterozone Cream
Sweet-Ups
Tapuline Tablets
Tenalate Ointment
Tensex Tablets
Testostal
Testralate-200
Theolate
Thyrodine
Thyrodoxine
Tiniquad
Triacillin
Trimette Tablets
Trimette TD Capsules
Triptos
Trisilobarb Tablets
Uracid
Uratin Tablets
Urisal
Veresconite Tablets
Wescaldrin
Wescoid Tablets
Wescolates Tablets
Wescophen-S Tablets
Wesdex-T
Weslin
Wesmatic Forte Tablets
Wesmatic Tablets
Wesplex
Wesplex, Liver w/B_{12}
Wesper-C
Wesprin Buffered Tablets
Westrol
Westron Tablets
Z-Glucon

WESTERN RESEARCH LABORATORIES, INC. 1835
301 South Cherokee
Denver, CO 80223
Address inquiries to:
Charles Gifford (303) 733-7207
Products Available
ASC Tablets
AWSC Tablets
Ammonium Chloride Tablets
Amphetamine Tablets
Aquazide Tablets
B_1-50 Tablets
B_6-50 Tablets
BBR (B_1 B_{12}) Tablets
BCO B-Complex Tablets
Calcium Gluconate Tablets
Chlordiazepoxide HCl Capsules
Chlorphentermine HCl Tablets
Chlorpromazine HCl Tablets
Cobile Tablets
Copper Gluconate Tablets
Digitalis Leaf Tablets
EFA Tablets
Elecal Tablets
Elekap Capsules
Ferrous Gluconate Tablets
Ferrous Sulfate Tablets
Fructose & Honey Tablets
Guarsol Tablets
Hemaferrin Tablets
Hydrochlorthiazide with Reserpine Tablets
KCL Packets
Laxative Tablets
Lecithin Capsules
Lec-Kelp Capsules
Levo Thyroxine Tablets
Magnesium Gluconate Tablets
Manganese Gluconate Tablets
Methocarbamol Tablets
Methyltestosterone Tablets
Multivitamins MDRW Tablets
Nonamin Tablets
Obezine Tablets
PGA Tablets
Pepsin Tablets PGA
Pepsocoll Tablets
Phentermine HCl Tablets
Phenylpropanolamine HCl Capsules
Phenylpropanolamine HCl Injectable
Phenylpropanolamine HCl Tablets
Placebo Capsules
Placebo Tablets
Potassium Gluconate Tablets
Potassium Penicillin Tablets
Protein Tablets PRT
Pyridamide Tablets
Pyridoxine HCl Tablets
Q.S. Tablets
Reserpine Tablets
SC-Plus Tablets
S-DSS Tablets
Sodium Carboxymethylcellulose Tablets
Sodium Phenobarbital Tablets
Super Westvite Tablets
Tetracycline Capsules
Thiamine HCl Tablets
Thyroid Hard Shell Capsules, Porcine
Thyroid Hormone Tablets, Porcine
Thyroid Soft Gel Capsules, Porcine
Thyroid Tablets, Porcine
Triticoll Tablets
Vitamin C 250 mg. Chewable
Vitamin C 500 mg., Timed
Vitamin E Chewable Tablets
Vitamin E. Soft Gel Capsules
Wes B/C Capsules
Westvite Tablets
Zinc Gluconate Tablets
Zinc Sulfate Capsules

WESTWOOD PHARMACEUTICALS INC. 1836
468 Dewitt St.
Buffalo, NY 14213
Address inquiries to:
Frank R. Nero, President (716) 887-3400
Products Available
Alpha Keri Bath Oil
Alpha Keri Soap
Alpha Keri Spray
Balneol
Balnetar
Capitrol Cream Shampoo
Desquam-X 5 Gel
Desquam-X 10 Gel
Desquam-X Wash
Estar
Fostex BPO 5%
Fostex Cake
Fostex Cream & Medicated Cleanser
Fostril
Halotex Cream and Solution
Keralyt
Keri Creme
Keri Facial Soap
Keri Lotion
Lowila Cake
Pernox
Pernox Lotion
Pernox Shampoo
PreSun
Sebucare
Sebulex
Sebulex Conditioning Shampoo with Protein
Sebutone
Tacaryl Chewable Tablets
Tacaryl Syrup and Tablets
Transact
Westcort Cream

WHARTON LABORATORIES, INC. 1841
Div. U.S. Ethicals Inc.
37-02 48th Ave.
Long Island City, NY 11101
Address inquiries to:
Medical Director (212) 786-8606
Products Available
Nitrong Ointment
Nitrong Tablets

WILLEN DRUG COMPANY 1842
18 North High St.
Baltimore, MD 21202 (301) 752-1865
Products Available
Bicitra—Sugar-Free
Neutra-Phos Powder & Capsules
Neutra-Phos-K Powder & Capsules
Polycitra Syrup
Polycitra-K Syrup
Polycitra-LC—Sugar-Free

WINTHROP LABORATORIES 438, 1843, 2039
90 Park Avenue
New York, NY 10016
(212) 972-4141
Professional Services Department
(212) 972-4095
Products Available
A.P.C. w/Demerol
Amipaque
Anti-Rust Tablets
Aralen Hydrochloride Injection
◆ Aralen Phosphate Tablets
Aralen Phosphate w/Primaquine Phosphate
Atabrine Hydrochloride Tablets
◆ Bilopaque Sodium
Codeine Phosphate Carpuject
◆ Danocrine
Demerol Carpuject
Demerol Hydrochloride Injection
Demerol Hydrochloride Syrup
◆ Demerol Hydrochloride Tablets
Demerol Uni-Amps
Drisdol 50,000 Unit Capsules
Drisdol in Propylene Glycol
Hydromorphone Carpuject
Hypaque Meglumine 30%
Hypaque Meglumine 60%
Hypaque Sodium Oral Powder & Liquid
Hypaque Sodium 20%
Hypaque Sodium 25%
Hypaque Sodium 50% Injection
Hypaque-Cysto
Hypaque-M, 75% Injection
Hypaque-M, 90% Injection
Hytakerol Capsules & Liquid
Isopaque 280
Isopaque 440
Lotusate Caplets
Luminal Ovoids
Luminal Sodium Injection
Morphine Sulfate Carpuject
Mytelase Chloride Caplets

◆ NegGram Caplets
NegGram Suspension
Neo-Synephrine Hydrochloride 1% Injection
Neo-Synephrine Hydrochloride (Ophthalmic)
pHisoHex
pHisoScrub
◆ Plaquenil Sulfate Tablets
Primaquine Phosphate Tablets
Skiodan Sodium Injection
Sulfamylon Cream
◆ Talwin Compound
◆ Talwin 50 Tablets
Talwin Lactate Injectable
Talwin Uni-Amps
◆ Telepaque Tablets
Vitamins
Vitamin D, USP
Drisdol 50,000 Unit Capsules
Drisdol in Propylene Glycol
◆ Winstrol Tablets
Zephiran Chloride Aqueous Solution
Zephiran Chloride Concentrate Solution
Zephiran Chloride Spray
Zephiran Chloride Tinted Tincture
Zephiran Towelettes

CONSUMER PRODUCTS DIVISION

Astring-o-sol
Bronkaid Mist
Bronkaid Tablets
Campho-Phenique Liquid, Powder and Gel
Caroid Laxative
Caroid Tooth Powder
Creamalin Tablets
▣ Haley's M-O, Regular and Flavored
Mucilose Flakes & Granules
▣ NTZ Drops and Spray
Neocurtasal
Neo-Synephrine Cold Tablets
Neo-Synephrine Jelly
▣ Neo-Synephrine Nasal Sprays (Mentholated)
Neo-Synephrine Nose Drops
▣ Neo-Synephrine II Long Acting Nasal Spray
▣ Neo-Synephrine II Long Acting Nose Drops (Adult and Pediatric Strengths)
▣ Neo-Synephrine II Long Acting Vapor Nasal Spray
PNS Suppositories
pHisoAc
pHisoDan
▣ pHisoDerm
▣ WinGel Liquid and Tablets

WYETH LABORATORIES 438, 1860
Division of American Home Products Corporation
P.O. Box 8299
Philadelphia, PA 19101

Address inquiries to:
Professional Service (215) 688-4400

For Medical Emergency Information
Day or night call (215) 688-4400

Wyeth Distribution Centers:

Andover, MA 01810
P.O. Box 1776 (617) 475-9075
Boston (617) 423-2644

Atlanta, GA 30302
P.O. Box 4365 (404) 873-1681

Baltimore, MD 21224
101 Kane St. (301) 633-4000

Boston Distribution Center, see under Andover, MA
Buena Park, CA 90620
6530 Altura Blvd. (714) 523-5500
(Los Angeles) (213) 627-5374
Emergency (714) 523-5500
Chicago Distribution Center, see under Evanston, IL
Cleveland, OH 44101
Post Office Box 91549 (216) 238-9450

Dallas, TX 75235
P.O. Box 35213 (214) 631-4360

Denver, CO 80201
P.O. Box 2107 (303) 388-3635

Evanston, IL 60204
P.O. Box 1659 (Skokie) (312) 675-1400
(Chicago) (312) 463-2400

Honolulu, HI 96814
1013 Kawaiahao St. (808) 538-1988

Kansas City Distribution Center, see under North Kansas City, MO
Kent, WA 98031
Post Office Box 5609 (206) 852-6720

Los Angeles Distribution Center, see under Buena Park, CA

Memphis, TN 38101
P.O. Box 1698 (901) 353-4680

New York Distribution Center, see under Secaucus, NJ
North Kansas City, MO 64116
P.O. Box 7588 (816) 842-0680

Philadelphia Distribution Center
Paoli, PA 19301,
P.O. Box 61 (215) 644-8000

St. Paul, MN 55164
P.O. Box 43034 (612) 454-6270

Seattle Distribution Center, see under Kent, WA

Secaucus, NJ 07094
555 Secaucus Rd. (201) 867-0300

Products Available

A-M-T Tablets
A.P.C. Tablets, Redipak
A.P.C. with Codeine Phosphate, Tablets, Redipak
A.P.C. with Meperidine HCl, Tablets, Redipak
Alcohol Sponges
Aludrox, Suspension
Aludrox, Tablets
Aminophylline, Rectal Suppositories
Amphojel, Suspension
Amphojel, Suspension w/o Flavor
Amphojel, Tablets
Antisnakebite Serum, see Antivenin
Antivenin (Crotalidae) Polyvalent
Antivenin (Micrurus Fulvius)
Aspirin, Rectal Suppositories
Aspirin, Tablets, Redipak
◆ Ativan Tablets
Atropine Sulfate, Injection
Atropine Sulfate and Meperidine Hydrochloride Injection
Basaljel, Capsules
Basaljel, Suspension
Basaljel, Suspension, Extra Strength
Basaljel, Swallow Tablets
Benzathine Penicillin G, (see Bicillin)
Bewon, Elixir
Bicillin C-R, Injection
Bicillin C-R 900/300 Injection
Bicillin Long-Acting, Injection
Bicillin Oral Suspension
Bicillin, Tablets
Biologicals
Bisacodyl, Suppositories
Chloral Hydrate, Capsules, Redipak
Chlorpromazine Hydrochloride, Injection
Cholera Vaccine
Codeine Phosphate, Injection
Codeine Sulfate, Tablets, Redipak
Collyrium, Eye Lotion
Collyrium w/Ephedrine, Eye Drops
Cyanocobalamin, Injection
Dexamethasone Sodium Phosphate Injection
Digitoxin (See Purodigin)
Digoxin, Injection
Dimenhydrinate Injection
Diphenhydramine Hydrochloride, Injection
Diphtheria and Tetanus Toxoids Adsorbed (Adult Use), see Tetanus and Diphtheria Toxoids Adsorbed
Diphtheria & Tetanus Toxoids Adsorbed, Pediatric
Diphtheria & Tetanus Toxoids & Pertussis Vaccine Adsorbed (See Triple Antigen)
Dryvax, Dried Smallpox Vaccine
Epinephrine Injection (1:1000)
◆ Equagesic Tablets
◆ Equanil, Capsules
◆ Equanil, Tablets
◆ Equanil, Wyseals
Equanitrate 10 & 20, Tablets
Ergonovine Maleate, Injection
Erythromycin Ethylsuccinate Oral Suspension (See Wyamycin E Liquid)
Erythromycin Stearate, Tablets (See Wyamycin S Tablets)
Ethobral, Triple Barbiturate Capsules
Hep. Lock Flush Solution, U S P
Heparin Sodium, Injection USP
Hydromorphone Hydrochloride, Injection
Immune Serum Globulin (Human)
Influenza Virus Vaccine Subvirion Type
Largon, Injection
Lidocaine HCl Injection
◆ Lo/Ovral, Tablets
◆ Lo/Ovral-28, Tablets
◆ Mepergan Fortis Capsules
Mepergan Injection
Meperidine Hydrochloride, Injection
Meperidine Hydrochloride, Tablets, Redipak
Morphine Sulfate, Injection
Nursoy, Soy Protein Formula for Infants, Concentrated Liquid & Ready-to-feed
◆ Omnipen, Capsules
Omnipen, for Oral Suspension
Omnipen Pediatric Drops
Omnipen-N, Injection
Opium & Belladonna, Rectal Suppositories
◆ Ovral, Tablets
◆ Ovral-28, Tablets
◆ Ovrette, Tablets
Oxaine M, Suspension
Oxytocin, Injection, Synthetic
◆ Pathocil, Capsules
Pathocil, for Oral Suspension
Pediatric Phenergan Expectorant w/Dextromethorphan
Penicillin Preparations:
Bicillin Products
Penicillin G, Potassium, Tablets
Pen•Vee Products
Wycillin Products
Pentobarbital Sodium, Capsules, Redipak
Pentobarbital Sodium, Injection
Pen•Vee K for Oral Solution
◆ Pen•Vee K Tablets
Petrogalar, Plain
◆ Phenergan Compound, Tablets
Phenergan Expectorant, Plain
Phenergan Expectorant, w/Codeine
Phenergan Expectorant, w/Dextromethorphan, Pediatric
Phenergan Injection
Phenergan Syrup Fortis
◆ Phenergan Tablets, Syrup and Rectal Suppositories
Phenergan VC Expectorant, Plain
Phenergan VC Expectorant, w/Codeine
◆ Phenergan-D Tablets
Phenobarbital Sodium, Injection
Phenobarbital, Tablets, Redipak
Phosphaljel
Plebex, Injection
◆ Polymagma Plain, Tablets
Potassium Penicillin G Tablets, Buffered
Prochlorperazine Edisylate Injection
◆ Proketazine, Tablets
Propion Gel
Purodigin, Tablets
Redipak Unit Dose Medications (Strip Pack and/or Individually Wrapped) Products:
A.P.C. Tablets
A.P.C. with Codeine Phosphate Tablets
A.P.C. with Meperidine Hydrochloride Tablets
Aspirin, Tablets
Ativan Tablets
Chloral Hydrate, Capsules
Codeine Sulfate, Tablets
Equagesic, Tablets
Equanil, Tablets
Meperidine Hydrochloride, Tablets
Omnipen, Capsules
Penicillin G, Potassium, Tablets Buffered
Pentobarbital Sodium, Capsules
Pen•Vee K, Tablets
Phenergan Tablets
Phenobarbital, Tablets
Secobarbital Sodium Capsules
Serax Capsules
Unipen, Capsules
Wygesic Tablets
Zactirin Compound-100, Tablets
Redipak (Liquid Unit Dose) Products:
Omnipen for Oral Suspension
Pen•Vee K Solution
Redipak (Unit of Use Suppository Pack) Products:
Aminophylline Rectal Suppositories
Aspirin, Rectal Suppositories
Phenergan Rectal Suppositories
Wyanoids HC, Rectal Suppositories w/Hydrocortisone
Redipak (Respiratory Therapy Unit) Products:
Sodium Chloride 0.9% and 0.45%
Sterile Distilled Water
RediTemp-C, Disposable Cold Pack
SMA, Infant Formula, Liquid Concentrated
SMA, Infant Formula, Powder
SMA, Infant Formula, Ready-to-Feed
Saline Solution (see Sodium Chloride Injection)
Secobarbital Sodium Capsules, Redipak
Secobarbital Sodium Injection
◆ Serax Capsules
◆ Serax Tablets
Simeco Suspension
Smallpox Vaccine, Dried (see Dryvax)
Snakebite Serum (see Antivenin)
Sodium Chloride Injection, Bacteriostatic
Sopronol Ointment, Powder & Solution
Sparine, Concentrate
Sparine Injection
Sparine, Syrup
◆ Sparine, Tablets
Sulfose Tablets

(◆ Shown in Product Identification Section) (▣ Described in PDR For Nonprescription Drugs)

Tetanus Immune Globulin (Human)
Tetanus Toxoid Adsorbed, Aluminum Phosphate
Tetanus Toxoid, Fluid, Purified
Tetanus & Diphtheria Toxoids Adsorbed (Adults)
Tetracycline HCl, Capsules
Thiamine Hydrochloride Injection
Thiomerin Injection
Triple Antigen

Tubex Closed Injection System Products:
Atropine Sulfate and Meperidine HCl
Bicillin C-R
Bicillin C-R 900/300
Bicillin L-A
Chlorpromazine HCl, U.S.P.
Codeine Phosphate
Cyanocobalamin (Vitamin B_{12})
Dexamethasone Sodium Phosphate
Digoxin
Dimenhydrinate
Diphenhydramine Hydrochloride
Diphtheria & Tetanus Toxoids Adsorbed, Pediatric
Epinephrine
Ergonovine Maleate
Heparin Sodium
Heparin Sodium in Normal Saline Solution
Hydromorphone Hydrochloride
Immune Serum Globulin (Human)
Influenza Virus Vaccine, Purified, Sub-Virion
Largon
Lidocaine HCl
Mepergan
Meperidine Hydrochloride
Morphine Sulfate
Oxytocin, Synthetic
Pentobarbital Sodium
Phenergan
Phenobarbital Sodium
Prochlorperizine Edisylate
Secobarbital Sodium
Sodium Chloride, Bacteriostatic
Sparine
Tetanus Immune Globulin (Human)
Tetanus & Diphtheria Toxoids Adsorbed (Adult)
Tetanus Toxoid Aluminum Phosphate Adsorbed
Tetanus Toxoid, Fluid, Purified
Thiamine Hydrochloride
Thiomerin
Triple Antigen
Vitamin B Complex
Vitamin B Complex with B_{12}
Vitamin B_{12} (Cyanocobalamin)
Wyamine Sulfate
Wycillin
Tubex Hypodermic Syringe
Tubex Sterile Cartride-Needle Unit Empty
Typhoid Vaccine
◆ Unipen Capsules
Unipen Injection
Unipen Oral Solution
◆ Unipen, Tablets
Vitamin B Complex w/B_{12}, Injection
Vitamin B Complex w/C, Injection
Vitamin B_{12} Injection (see Cyanocobalamin)
Water for Injection, Bacteriostatic
Wyamine Sulfate, Injection
Wyamycin E Liquid
◆ Wyamycin S Tablets
Wyanoid Ointment
◆ Wyanoids HC, Rectal Suppositories w/Hydrocortisone
◆ Wyanoids, Hemorrhoidal Suppositories
Wycillin, Injection
Wycillin Injection and Probenecid Tablets
Wydase Lyophilized
Wydase, Stabilized Solution
◆ Wygesic Tablets
◆ Wymox Capsules
Wymox Oral Suspension
Wyseals (see Equanil)
Zactane, Tablets
◆ Zactirin Compound-100, Tablets
◆ Zactirin, Tablets

(◆ Shown in Product Identification Section)

(▣ Described in PDR For Nonprescription Drugs)

PDR 34 EDITION

SECTION 2

Product Name Index

In this section products are listed in alphabetical sequence by brand name or (if described) generic name. Page numbers have been included to assist you in locating additional information on described products. The symbol ◆ indicates the product is shown in the Product Identification Section. The symbol ▣ indicates the product is described in PDR FOR NONPRESCRIPTION DRUGS.

Part II

A

B

(◆ Shown in Product Identification Section) (▣ Described in PDR For Nonprescription Drugs)

C

D

E

I

(◆ Shown in Product Identification Section) (▣ Described in PDR For Nonprescription Drugs)

M

N

O

P

(◆ Shown in Product Identification Section)

(▣ Described in PDR For Nonprescription Drugs)

Q

(◆ Shown in Product Identification Section) (▣ Described in PDR For Nonprescription Drugs)

(◆ Shown in Product Identification Section) (▣ Described in PDR For Nonprescription Drugs)

(◆ Shown in Product Identification Section) (▣ Described in PDR For Nonprescription Drugs)

W

X – Z

(◆ **Shown in Product Identification Section**)

(▣ **Described in PDR For Nonprescription Drugs**)

Product Classification Index

PDR 34 EDITION

SECTION 3

Products described in the Product Information (White) or Diagnostic Product (Green) Sections are listed according to their classifications. The headings and sub-headings have been determined by the Publisher with the cooperation of the individual manufacturers. In cases where there were differences of opinion or where the manufacturer had no opinion, the Publisher made the final decision.

A

Preludin Tablets (Boehringer Ingelheim) p 405, 672
Pre-Sate (Parke-Davis) p 422, 1338
Pretts Tablets (Marion) p 1094
Prolamine Capsules, Super Strength (Thompson Medical) p 1729
Sanorex (Sandoz) p 429, 1530
Statobex Capsules (Lemmon) p 1004
Statobex Tablets (Lemmon) p 414, 1004
Statobex-G Tablets (Lemmon) p 414, 1004
Tenuate Dospan (Merrell-National) p 419, 1221
Tenuate 25 mg. (Merrell-National) p 419, 1221
Tepanil (Riker) p 425, 1415
Tepanil Ten-tab (Riker) p 425, 1415
Voranil (USV Pharmaceutical) p 436, 1749

Other
Appedrine, Extra Strength (Thompson Medical) p 1728

ANTACIDS

Antacids
ALternaGEL Liquid (Stuart) p 1699
Aludrox Oral Suspension (Wyeth) p 1861
Aludrox, Tablets (Wyeth) p 1861
Amphojel Suspension (Wyeth) p 1861
Amphojel Tablets (Wyeth) p 1861
Basaljel Capsules & Swallow Tablets (Wyeth) p 1862
Basaljel Suspension & Suspension, Extra Strength (Wyeth) p 1862
Camalox (Rorer) p 428, 1502
Delcid (Merrell-National) p 1211
Equilet (Mission) p 1225
Escot Capsules (Tutag) p 435, 1735
Gaviscon Antacid Tablets (Marion) p 416, 1092
Gaviscon Liquid Antacid (Marion) p 416, 1092
Gaviscon-2 Antacid Tablets (Marion) p 416, 1092
Gelusil (Parke-Davis) p 421, 1304
Kolantyl (Merrell-National) p 1213
Kudrox Suspension (Double Strength) (Kremers-Urban) p 958
Kudrox Tablets (Kremers-Urban) p 958
Maalox (Rorer) p 428, 1503
Maalox Therapeutic Concentrate (Rorer) p 1503
Phillips' Milk of Magnesia (Glenbrook) p 919
Riopan (Ayerst) p 405, 633
Riopan Plus (Ayerst) p 405, 633
Robalate Tablets (Robins) p 1434
Simeco (Wyeth) p 1889
Titralac (Riker) p 425, 1418
Trisogel (Lilly) p 1082

with Antiflatulents
Gelusil-M (Parke-Davis) p 1304
Gelusil-II (Parke-Davis) p 421, 1305
Maalox Plus (Rorer) p 1503
Mylanta Liquid (Stuart) p 1702
Mylanta Tablets (Stuart) p 435, 1702
Mylanta-II Liquid (Stuart) p 1702
Mylanta-II Tablets (Stuart) p 435, 1702
Riopan Plus (Ayerst) p 405, 633
Simeco (Wyeth) p 1889

ANTHELMINTICS

Antepar (Burroughs Wellcome) p 406, 745
Antiminth Oral Suspension (Roerig) p 1489
Povan Filmseals (Parke-Davis) p 422, 1338
Povan Suspension (Parke-Davis) p 1338
Vermox Chewable Tablets (Janssen) p 420, 942

ANTIALCOHOL PREPARATIONS

Antabuse (Ayerst) p 404, 591

ANTIARTHRITICS

Antiarthritics
Aristospan Parenteral 20 mg./ml (Lederle) p 971
Arthropan Liquid (Purdue Frederick) p 1394
Ascriptin (Rorer) p 428, 1501
Ascriptin A/D (Rorer) p 428, 1501
Azolid (USV Pharmaceutical) p 436, 1737
Azolid-A (USV Pharmaceutical) p 436, 1737
Bayer Timed-Release Aspirin (Glenbrook) p 919
Butazolidin (Geigy) p 411, 895
Butazolidin Alka (Geigy) p 411, 895
Cama Inlay-Tabs (Dorsey) p 409, 845
Celestone Phosphate Injection (Schering) p 1537
Celestone Soluspan Suspension (Schering) p 1539
Celestone Syrup and Tablets (Schering) p 429, 1536
Clinoril (Merck Sharp & Dohme) p 418, 1147
Cuprimine Capsules (Merck Sharp & Dohme) p 418, 1153
Decadrón Elixir (Merck Sharp & Dohme) p 1157
Decadron Phosphate Injection (Merck Sharp & Dohme) p 1161
Decadron Tablets (Merck Sharp & Dohme) p 418, 1158
Decadron-La (Merck Sharp & Dohme) p 1166
Depo-Medrol (Upjohn) p 436, 1762
Ecotrin (Smith Kline & French) p 432, 1623
Empirin (Burroughs Wellcome) p 407, 749
Empirin with Codeine (Burroughs Wellcome) p 407, 750
Gaysal (Geriatric) p 912
Gaysal-S (Geriatric) p 912
Ger-O-Foam (Geriatric) p 912
Hyalex (Miller) p 1224
Indocin Capsules (Merck Sharp & Dohme) p 418, 1182
Kenalog-10 Injection (Squibb) p 1659
Kenalog-40 Injection (Squibb) p 1656
Magan (Warren-Teed) p 1832
Medrol Tablets (Upjohn) p 437, 1776
Meticortelone Acetate Aqueous Suspension (Schering) p 1561
Meticorten Tablets (Schering) p 431, 1561
Mobidin (Ascher) p 577
Motrin Tablets (Upjohn) p 437, 1779
Myochrysine (Merck Sharp & Dohme) p 1194
Nalfon (Dista) p 409, 828
Naprosyn (Syntex) p 435, 1724
Os-Cal-Gesic (Marion) p 416, 1094
Oxalid (USV Pharmaceutical) p 436, 1742
Pabalate Tablets (Robins) p 425, 1430
Pabalate-SF Tablets (Robins) p 425, 1430
Pabirin Buffered Tablets (Dorsey) p 848
Plaquenil Sulfate (Winthrop) p 438, 1852
Solganal Suspension (Schering) p 1570
Tabloid brand A.P.C. w/Codeine (Burroughs Wellcome) p 407, 764
Tandearil (Geigy) p 411, 904
Tolectin Tablets & DS Capsules (McNeil Laboratories) p 417, 1104
Trilisate Tablets (Purdue Frederick) p 424, 1397

Antigout
Anturane Tablets & Capsules (Ciba) p 408, 783
Azolid (USV Pharmaceutical) p 436, 1737
Azolid-A (USV Pharmaceutical) p 436, 1737
Benemid Tablets (Merck Sharp & Dohme) p 418, 1144
Butazolidin (Geigy) p 411, 895
Butazolidin Alka (Geigy) p 411, 895
Clinoril (Merck Sharp & Dohme) p 418, 1147
ColBENEMID (Merck Sharp & Dohme) p 418, 1150
Colchicine Ampoules (Lilly) p 1022
Colchicine Tablets (Lilly) p 1023
Hyalex (Miller) p 1224
Indocin Capsules (Merck Sharp & Dohme) p 418, 1182
Lopurin (Boots) p 676
Oxalid (USV Pharmaceutical) p 436, 1742
Tandearil (Geigy) p 411, 904
Zyloprim (Burroughs Wellcome) p 407, 768

ANTIASTHMA

Accurbron (Dow Pharmaceuticals) p 852
Airet & Airet 400 Tablets (Baylor) p 638
Airet L.A. Tablets (Baylor) p 638
Airet II Liquid (Baylor) p 638
Amesec, Enseals & Pulvules (Lilly) p 414, 1011
Aminodur Dura-Tabs (Berlex) p 408, 662
Beclovent Inhaler (Glaxo) p 419, 913
Brethine (Geigy) p 411, 894
Brethine Ampuls (Geigy) p 894
Bronkephrine Hydrochloride Injection (Breon) p 682
Bronkodyl (Breon) p 406, 682
Bronkolixir (Breon) p 685
Bronkometer (Breon) p 684
Bronkosol (Breon) p 684
Bronkotabs (Breon) p 406, 685
Choledyl Pediatric Syrup (Parke-Davis) p 1289
Co-Xan (Improved) Syrup (Central Pharmacal) p 778
Elixicon Suspension (Berlex) p 662
Elixophyllin Capsules (Berlex) p 408, 662
Elixophyllin Elixir (Berlex) p 662
Elixophyllin SR Capsules (Berlex) p 408, 662
Elixophyllin-KI Elixir (Berlex) p 662
Historal (Merchant) p 1132
Intal (Fisons) p 881
LāBID 250 mg Tablets (Baylor) p 639
microNEFRIN (Bird) p 667
Neothylline Elixir (Lemmon) p 1001
Neothylline Injection (Lemmon) p 1001
Neothylline Tablets (Lemmon) p 414, 1001
Neothylline-GG Elixir (Lemmon) p 1002
Neothylline-GG Tablets (Lemmon) p 1002
Norisodrine Aerotrol (Abbott) p 534
Norisodrine Sulfate Aerohalor (Abbott) p 534
Slo-Phyllin Gyrocaps, Tablets (Dooner) p 409, 843
Slo-Phyllin 80 Syrup (Dooner) p 843
Slo-Phyllin GG Capsules, Syrup (Dooner) p 409, 844
Sus-Phrine (Berlex) p 666
Synophylate Tablets/Elixir (Central Pharmacal) p 778
Synophylate-GG Tablets/Syrup (Central Pharmacal) p 778
Theobid, Theobid Jr. Duracap (Glaxo) p 419, 916
Theoclear L.A.-130 & -260 Cenules (Central Pharmacal) p 408, 779
Theoclear-80 Syrup (Central Pharmacal) p 779
Theoclear-100 & Theoclear-200 Tablets (Central Pharmacal) p 408, 779
Theolair (Riker) p 425, 1416
Theovent Long-Acting Capsules (Schering) p 1571
Vanceril Inhaler (Schering) p 431, 1576

ANTIBACTERIALS & ANTISEPTICS

Antibacterial
Alba-3 Ointment (Alba) p 562
Bactrim DS Tablets (Roche) p 426, 1448
Bactrim Pediatric Suspension (Roche) p 1448
Bactrim Suspension (Roche) p 1448
Bactrim Tablets (Roche) p 426, 1448
Chloromyxin (Parke-Davis) p 1289
Declostatin for Oral Use (Lederle) p 413, 975
Furadantin Oral Suspension (Norwich-Eaton) p 1236
Furadantin Tablets (Norwich-Eaton) p 1236
Hibiclens Antimicrobial Skin Cleanser (Stuart) p 434, 1701
Hibitane Tincture (Tinted & Non-tinted) (Stuart) p 435, 1701
Ivadantin (Norwich-Eaton) p 1236
Macrodantin Capsules (Norwich-Eaton) p 410, 1237
Neo-Polycin (Dow Pharmaceuticals) p 853
Orlex Otic Solution (Baylor) p 640
Polydine Solution, Scrub, Ointment (Century Pharmaceuticals) p 780
Pyocidin-Otic (Berlex) p 665
Septra DS Tablets (Burroughs Wellcome) p 407, 762
Septra Suspension (Burroughs Wellcome) p 762
Septra Tablets (Burroughs Wellcome) p 407, 762

Antifungal
Betadine Vaginal Gel (Purdue Frederick) p 424, 1395
Betadine Viscous Formula Antiseptic Gauze Pad (Purdue Frederick) p 1396
Declostatin for Oral Use (Lederle) p 413, 975
Gyne-Lotrimin Vaginal Cream 1% (Schering) p 430, 1557
Gyne-Lotrimin Vaginal Tablets (Schering) p 430, 1557
Hibiclens Antimicrobial Skin Cleanser (Stuart) p 434, 1701
Hibitane Tincture (Tinted & Non-tinted) (Stuart) p 435, 1701
Lotrimin Cream 1% (Schering) p 431, 1561
Lotrimin Solution 1% (Schering) p 431, 1561
MicaTin Brand Miconazole Nitrate Cream and Lotion 2% (Ortho Pharmaceutical (Dermatological Div.)) p 1269
Orlex Otic Solution (Baylor) p 640
Polydine Solution, Scrub, Ointment (Century Pharmaceuticals) p 780
Racet Cream (Lemmon) p 1003
Triva Combination (Boyle) p 680
Triva Douche Powder (Boyle) p 680

Parenteral
Gantrisin Injectable (Roche) p 1456
Garamycin Injectable (Schering) p 430, 1550
Garamycin Intrathecal Injection (Schering) p 1556
Garamycin Pediatric Injectable (Schering) p 430, 1553
Ivadantin (Norwich-Eaton) p 1236
Polymyxin B Sulfate (Burroughs Wellcome) p 742

Sulfonamide Combinations
Metimyd Ophthalmic Ointment - Sterile (Schering) p 1561
Metimyd Ophthalmic Suspension (Schering) p 1561
Optimyd Ophthalmic Solution-Sterile (Schering) p 1565
Septra DS Tablets (Burroughs Wellcome) p 407, 762
Septra Suspension (Burroughs Wellcome) p 762
Septra Tablets (Burroughs Wellcome) p 407, 762
Suladyne Tablets (Tutag) p 436, 1735
Thiosulfil Duo-Pak (Ayerst) p 634
Thiosulfil-A Forte (Ayerst) p 405, 635

Sulfonamides
Azulfidine (Pharmacia) p 424, 1379

Topical

Urinary Antibacterial

Urinary Antibacterial with Analgesics

ANTIBIOTICS

Amebicides

Antifungal

Antituberculosis

Antiviral

Broad & Medium Spectrum

COUGH & COLD PREPARATIONS

Cold Preparations

Non-Narcotic

with Narcotics

Cough Preparations

Non-Narcotic

with Narcotics

Cough & Cold Preparations

Non-Narcotic

with Narcotics

D

DECONGESTANTS

Oral

I

L

M

URICOSURIC AGENTS

URINARY ACIDIFIERS

URINARY ALKALINIZING AGENTS

URINARY TRACT ANALGESIC

UROLOGICAL IRRIGANTS

UTERINE CONTRACTANTS

V - W - X

VAGINAL THERAPEUTICS

Capsules, Tablets

Creams

Douches

Inserts, Suppositories

Jellies, Ointments

Trichomonacides

VITAMINS

Geriatric

Multivitamins

PDR 34 EDITION

SECTION 4

Generic and Chemical Name Index

In this section the products described in the Product Information (White) and Diagnostic Product (Green) Sections are listed under generic and chemical name headings according to the principal ingredient(s). The headings under which products are listed have been determined by the Publisher with the cooperation of the individual manufacturers.

G

I

K

L

U

V

W–Z

Product Identification Section

Designed to help you identify products, this section contains actual size, full-color reproductions selected for inclusion by participating manufacturers. Because tablets and capsules, for the most part, are shown here, you should not infer that these are the only dosage forms. Where other dosage forms are available, the product name is preceded by the † symbol. Refer to the product's description in the PRODUCT INFORMATION (White Section) or check directly with manufacturer.

While every effort has been made to reproduce products faithfully, this section should be considered only as a quick reference identification aid.

If overdosage is suspected, the user may wish to consult Guide to Management of Drug Overdose printed inside the back cover.

A list of Poison Control Centers, their addresses and emergency telephone numbers appears on page 1900.

INDEX BY MANUFACTURER

This section is made possible through the courtesy of the manufacturers whose products appear on the following pages. Page numbers of individual products included can be found in the Alphabetical Product, Generic and Product Classification Indices.

ABBOTT

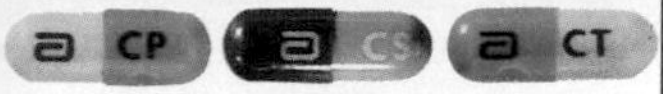
5 mg. 10 mg. 25 mg.
A-Poxide® Ⓒ IV
(chlordiazepoxide hydrochloride capsules, U.S.P.)

Abbott

2.5 mg. 5 mg.
grooved tablets
Enduron®
(methyclothiazide tablets, N.F.)

Abbott

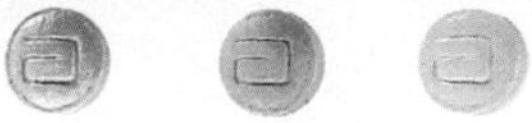
10 mg. 25 mg. 50 mg.
Eutonyl®
(pargyline hydrochloride tablets, N.F.)

Abbott Ⓒ II

30 mg. 50 mg. 100 mg.
†Nembutal® sodium
(pentobarbital sodium capsules, U.S.P.)

Abbott

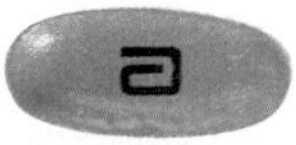
Cefol®
(high potency B-complex, folic acid, vitamin E with 750 mg. vitamin C)

Abbott

Enduronyl® **Enduronyl Forte**
grooved tablets
(methyclothiazide and deserpidine)

Abbott

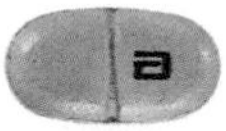
Eutron®
(pargyline hydrochloride and methyclothiazide)

Abbott

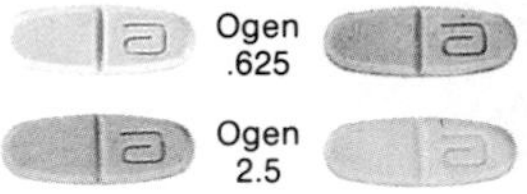
Ogen .625 Ogen 1.25
Ogen 2.5 Ogen 5
Ogen®
(piperazine estrone sulfate tablets, N.F.)

Abbott Ⓒ IV

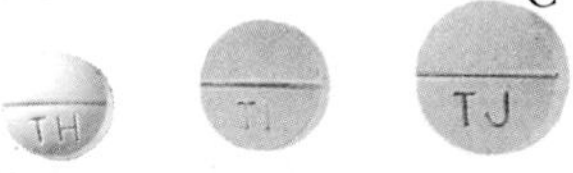
18.75 mg. 37.5 mg. 75 mg.
Cylert®
(pemoline)

Abbott

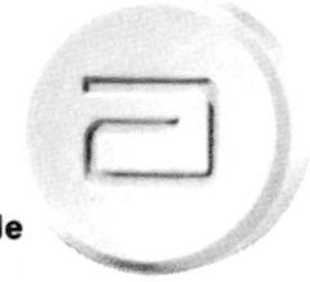
200 mg.
†E.E.S.® Chewable
(erythromycin ethylsuccinate tablets, U.S.P.)

Abbott

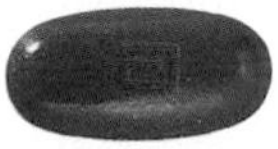
Fero-Folic-500®

Abbott
(shown smaller than actual size)

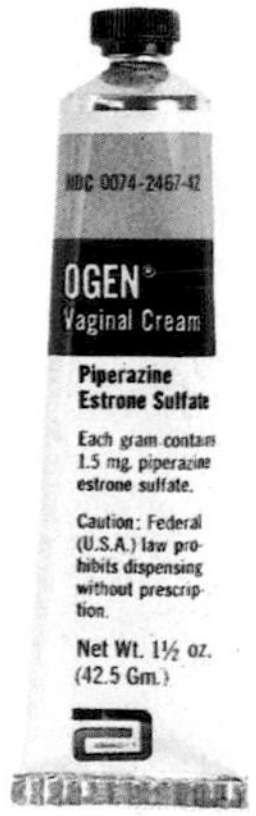

Ogen® Vaginal Cream
(piperazine estrone sulfate)

Abbott Ⓒ IV

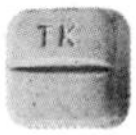
37.5 mg.
chewable tablets
Cylert®
(pemoline)

Abbott

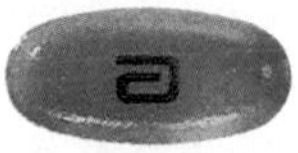
400 mg.
†E.E.S. 400® Filmtab®
(erythromycin ethylsuccinate tablets, U.S.P.)

Abbott

0.1 mg. 0.25 mg.
Harmonyl®
(deserpidine)

Abbott

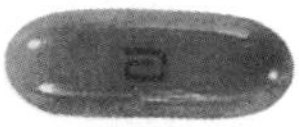
250 mg.
†Depakene®
(valproic acid)

Abbott

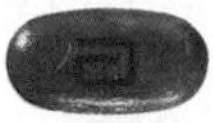
125 mg.

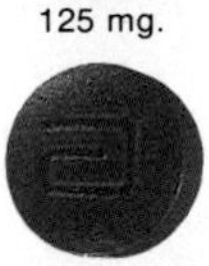
250 mg.

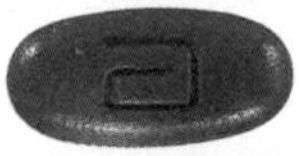
500 mg.
Erythrocin® Stearate Filmtab®
(erythromycin stearate tablets, U.S.P.)

Abbott

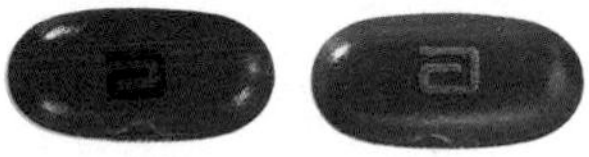
Iberet®-500 **Iberet-Folic-500®**

Abbott Ⓒ II

5 mg. 10 mg. 15 mg.
Gradumet® tablets
†Desoxyn®*
(methamphetamine hydrochloride)

Abbott

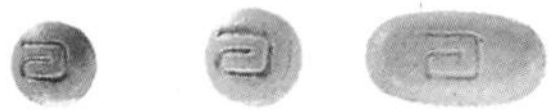
10 mg. 25 mg. 50 mg.
Janimine®
(imipramine hydrochloride tablets, U.S.P.)

Abbott

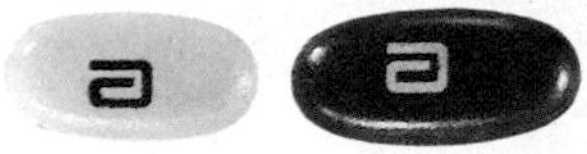
Optilets®-500 (therapeutic vitamin formulation)
Optilets-M-500® (therapeutic vitamin formulation with minerals)

Abbott

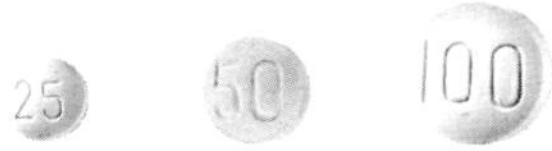
25 mg. 50 mg.* 100 mg.*
*grooved tablets
Dicumarol tablets, U.S.P.

Abbott

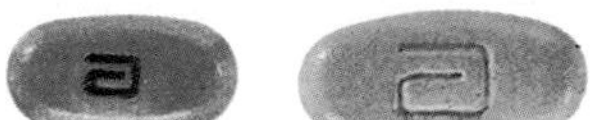
250 mg. 500 mg.
Erythromycin Base Filmtab®
(erythromycin tablets, U.S.P.)

Abbott (shown smaller than actual size)

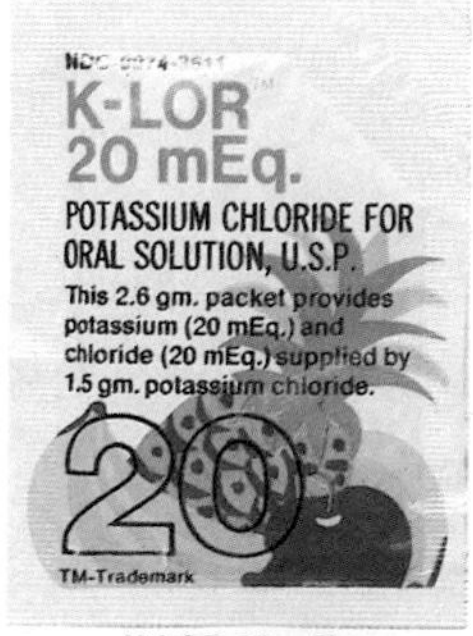

K-LOR 20 mEq.
(potassium chloride for oral solution, U.S.P.)

Abbott

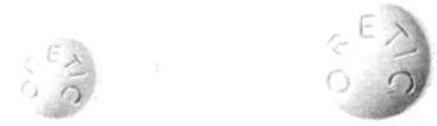
25 mg. 50 mg.
Oretic®
(hydrochlorothiazide tablets, U.S.P.)

ABBO-PAC®

EXAMPLE OF ABBO-PAC UNIT-DOSE PACKAGE

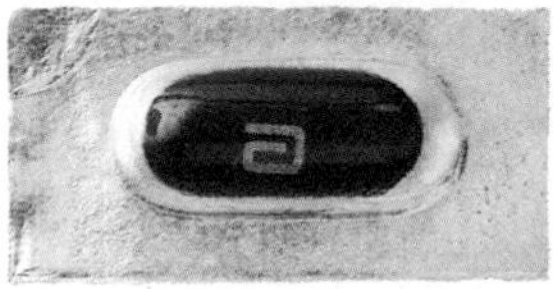

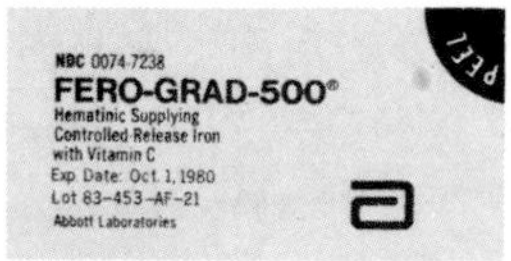

FERO-GRAD-500®
Controlled-Release Iron with Vitamin C
Many Abbott products are available to institutions in Abbo-Pac® unit-dose packaging.

Abbott

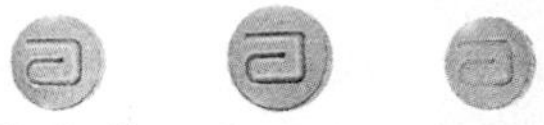
Oreticyl® 25 **Oreticyl** 50 **Oreticyl** Forte
grooved tablets
(hydrochlorothiazide and deserpidine)

Abbott

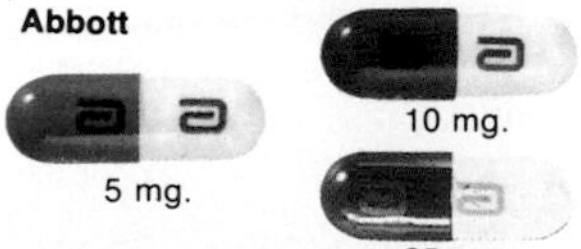
5 mg. 10 mg. 25 mg.
Lidone®
(molindone hydrochloride)

Abbott

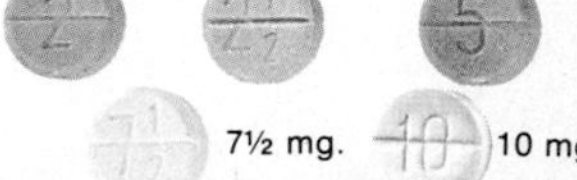
2 mg. 2½ mg. 5 mg. 7½ mg. 10 mg.
Panwarfin®
(warfarin sodium tablets, U.S.P.)

†Other dosage forms available. See Product Information section or check directly with manufacturer.
*Logo only may appear on tablet. **Logo only may appear on capsules. ®Filmtab—Film-sealed tablets, Abbott.

Abbott

150 mg. 300 mg.

†Paradione®
(paramethadione capsules, U.S.P.)

Abbott

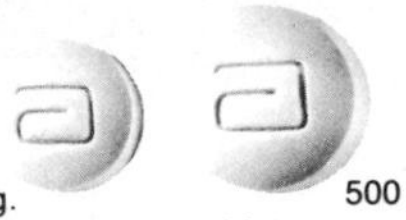

250 mg. 500 mg.
grooved tablets
Peganone®
(ethotoin)

Abbott Ⓒ IV

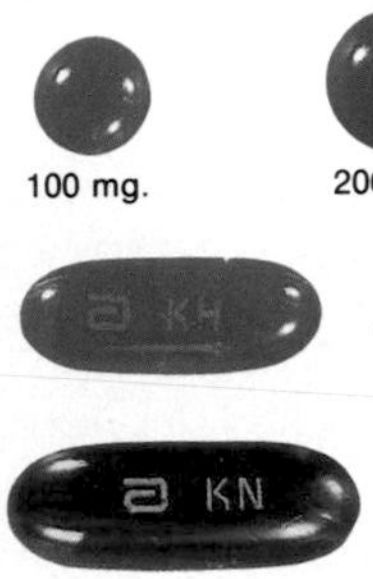

100 mg. 200 mg.

500 mg.

750 mg.

Placidyl®
(ethchlorvynol capsules, N.F.)

Abbott

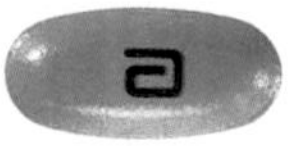

Surbex-T®
(high potency vitamin B-complex with 500 mg. of vitamin C)

Abbott

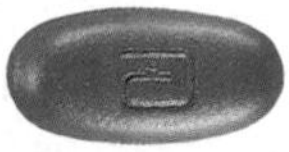

Surbex®-750 With Iron
(high potency B-complex with iron, vitamin E, and 750 mg. of vitamin C)

Abbott

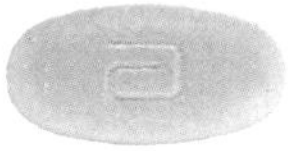

Surbex®-750 With Zinc
(zinc, vitamin B-complex and vitamins C and E)

Abbott Ⓒ IV

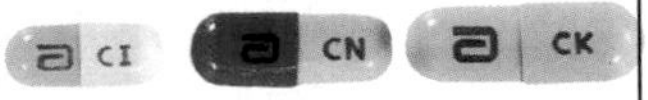

3.75 mg. 7.5 mg. 15 mg.

Tranxene®**
(clorazepate dipotassium)

Abbott Ⓒ IV

11.25 mg. **Tranxene®-SD Half Strength** 22.5 mg. **Tranxene®-SD**
(clorazepate dipotassium)

Abbott

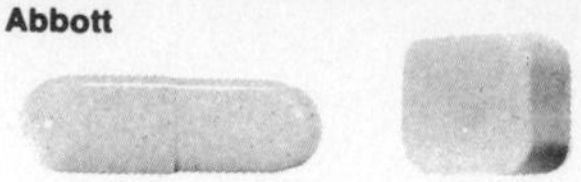

300 mg. Capsules, U.S.P. 150 mg. Dulcet® Tablet, U.S.P.
†Tridione®
(trimethadione)

ALTO

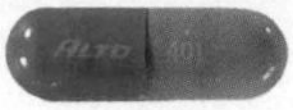

220 mg.
Zinc-220® Capsules
(zinc-sulfate)

ARMOUR

Chymoral*
50,000 Armour Units

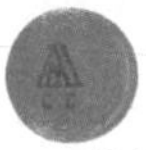

Chymoral®-100
100,000 Armour Units

(trypsin-chymotrypsin tablets, Armour)

Armour

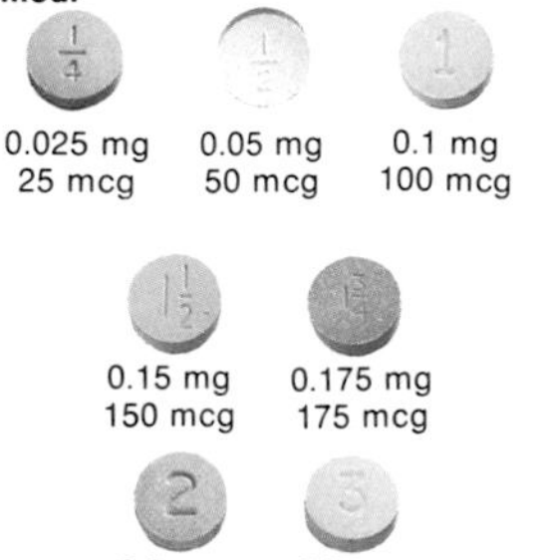

0.025 mg 25 mcg | 0.05 mg 50 mcg | 0.1 mg 100 mcg
0.15 mg 150 mcg | 0.175 mg 175 mcg
0.2 mg 200 mcg | 0.3 mg 300 mcg

Levothroid™
(sodium levothyroxine tablets, U.S.P.)

Armour

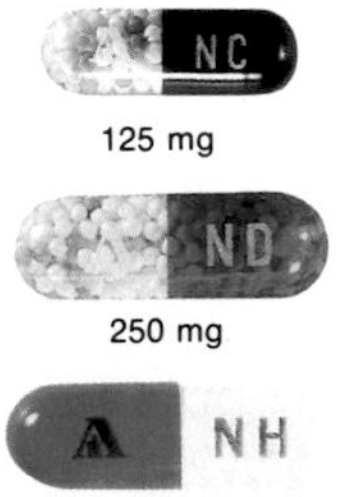

125 mg
250 mg
500 mg

Nicobid®
(niacin, Armour)
Timed Release Nicotinic Acid Tempules®

Armour

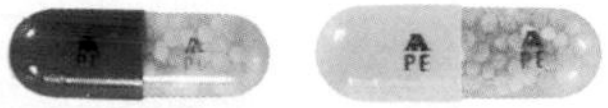

30 mg 60 mg

Pentritol®
(pentaerythritol tetranitrate)
Timed Release Tempules,® Armour

Armour

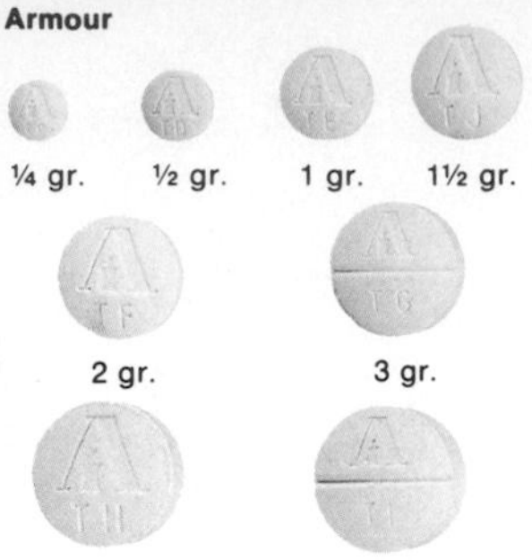

¼ gr. ½ gr. 1 gr. 1½ gr.
2 gr. 3 gr.
4 gr. 5 gr.

Armour® Thyroid

Armour

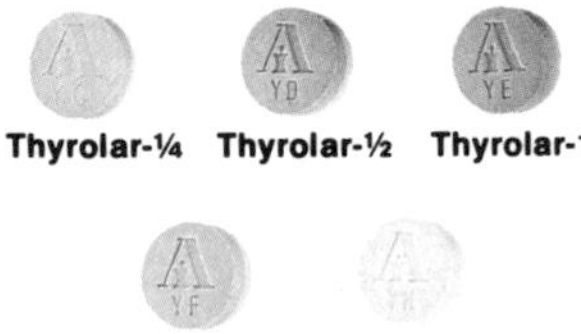

Thyrolar-¼ Thyrolar-½ Thyrolar-1
Thyrolar-2 Thyrolar-3

Thyrolar®
(liotrix, Armour) tablets

Each Thyrolar-1 tablet contains 50 mcg. T^4 and 12.5 mcg. T^3

ASTRA

(Ampule shown smaller than actual size)

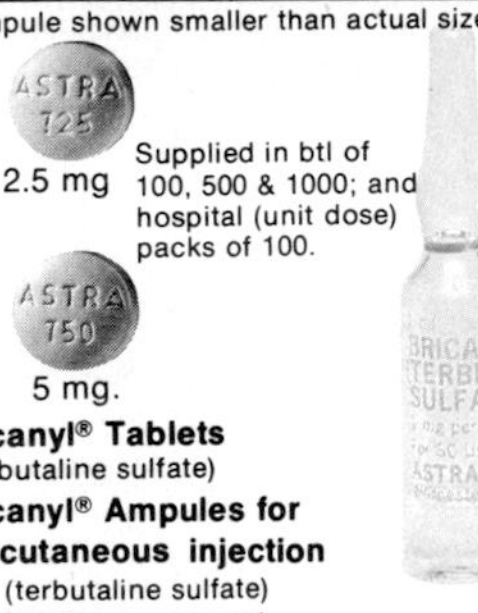

2.5 mg
5 mg.

Supplied in btl of 100, 500 & 1000; and hospital (unit dose) packs of 100.

Bricanyl® Tablets
(terbutaline sulfate)
Bricanyl® Ampules for subcutaneous injection
(terbutaline sulfate)
0.25 mg. per ml.
(1 ml./ampule)

AYERST

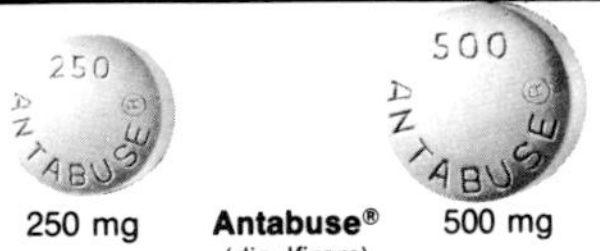

250 mg **Antabuse®** 500 mg
(disulfiram)

Ayerst

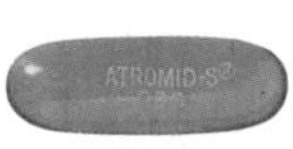

Atromid-S®
(clofibrate)

Ayerst

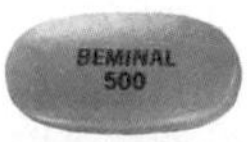

Beminal®—500

Ayerst

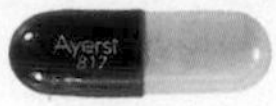

Beminal® Forte with Vitamin C

Ayerst

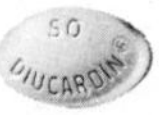

Diucardin®
(hydroflumethiazide)

Ayerst

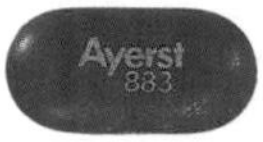

Formatrix®

Ayerst

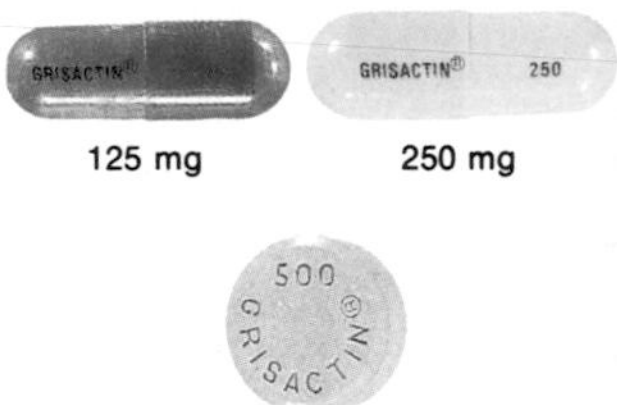

125 mg 250 mg
500 mg

Grisactin®
[griseofulvin (microsize)]

Ayerst

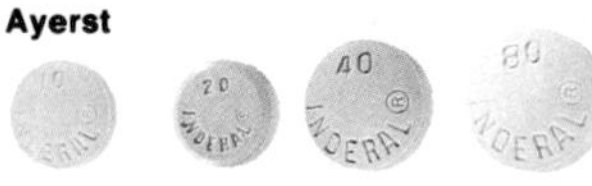

10 mg 20 mg 40 mg 80 mg

†Inderal®
(propranolol hydrochloride)

Ayerst

40/25 80/25

Inderide®
[propranolol hydrochloride (Inderal®) and hydrochlorothiazide]

Ayerst Ⓒ III

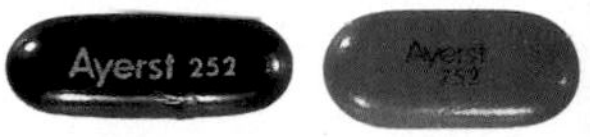

Capsule **†Mediatric®** Tablet

Ayerst

250 mg 50 mg

†Mysoline®
(primidone)

†Other dosage forms available. See Product Information section or check directly with manufacturer.
*Logo only may appear on tablet. **Logo only may appear on capsules. ®Filmtab—Film-sealed tablets, Abbott.

Ayerst

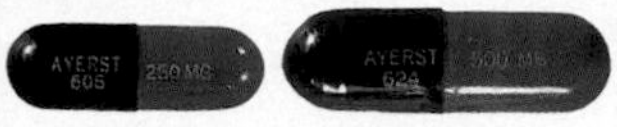

250 mg 500 mg
†Penbritin*
(ampicillin)
*Mfr. lic'd. under ®705,484

Ayerst

Plegine®
(phendimetrazine tartrate)

Ayerst

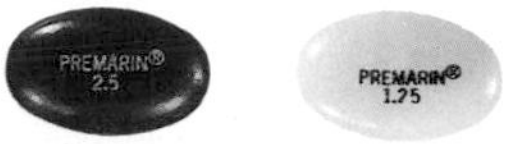

2.5 mg 1.25 mg

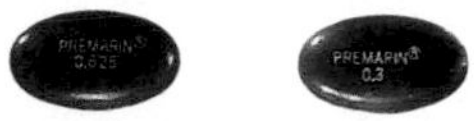

0.625 mg 0.3 mg

†Premarin®
(Conjugated Estrogens Tablets, U.S.P.)

Ayerst

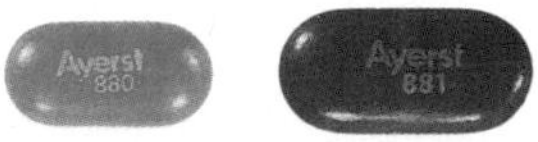

PMB® 200 **PMB® 400**
[Premarin® (Conjugated Estrogens, U.S.P.) with meprobamate]

Ayerst

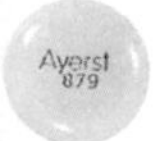

1.25 mg with 10.0 mg MT

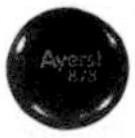

0.625 mg with 5.0 mg MT

Premarin®
(Conjugated Estrogens, U.S.P.)
with Methyltestosterone

Ayerst (Tube and applicator shown smaller than actual size)

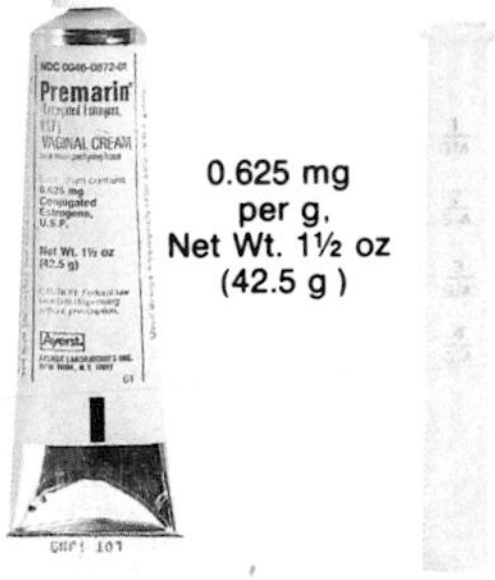

0.625 mg per g,
Net Wt. 1½ oz (42.5 g)

Premarin® Vaginal Cream
(Conjugated Estrogens, U.S.P.)

Ayerst

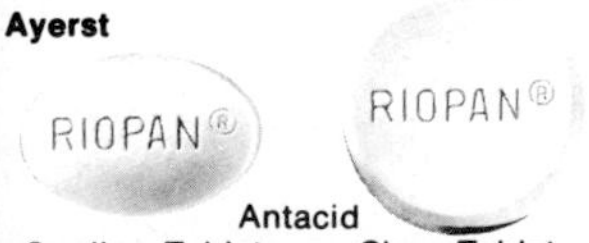

Antacid
Swallow Tablet Chew Tablet
†Riopan®
magaldrate

Ayerst

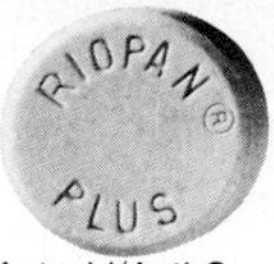

Chew Tablet
Antacid/Anti-Gas
†Riopan Plus®
magaldrate and simethicone

Ayerst

0.25 g 0.5 g
Thiosulfil® (sulfamethizole)
Thiosulfil® Forte (sulfamethizole 0.5 g)

Ayerst

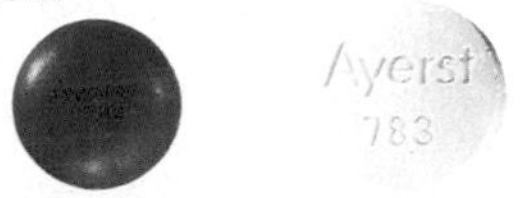

Thiosulfil®—A (sulfamethizole w/ phenazopyridine HCl)
Thiosulfil®—A Forte (sulfamethizole 0.5 g w/phenazopyridine HCl)

Ayerst

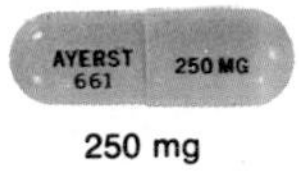

250 mg

500 mg
Veracillin*
(dicloxacillin sodium)
*Mfr. lic'd. under ®734,467

BEACH

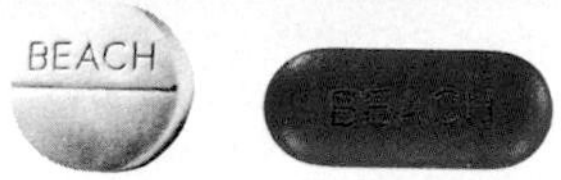

K-PHOS® M.F. (Modified Formula)
K-PHOS® No. 2

Beach

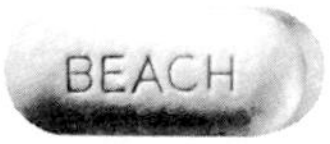

K-PHOS® NEUTRAL

Beach

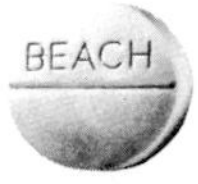

500 mg.
K-PHOS® Original (Sodium Free)
(Potassium Acid Phosphate)

Beach

THIACIDE™

Beach

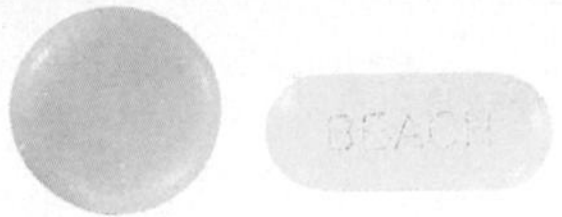

UROQID®-Acid **UROQID-Acid® No. 2**

Beecham Laboratories

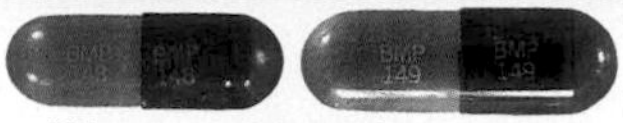

250 mg. **†Amoxil®** 500 mg.
(amoxicillin)
Available also as oral suspension, pediatric drops

Beecham Laboratories

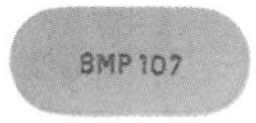

Cough Tablets
†Conar®-A Tablets
(Available also as cough syrup)

Beecham Laboratories

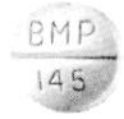

10 mg.
Daricon® Tablets
(oxyphencyclimine hydrochloride)

Beecham Laboratories

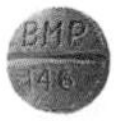

Daricon®-PB
(oxyphencyclimine hydrochloride with phenobarbital)

Beecham Laboratories

Enarax® 5 **Enarax® 10**
(oxyphencyclimine HCl and hydroxyzine HCl)

Beecham Laboratories

30 mg.
Fastin® Capsules
(phentermine hydrochloride)

Beecham Laboratories

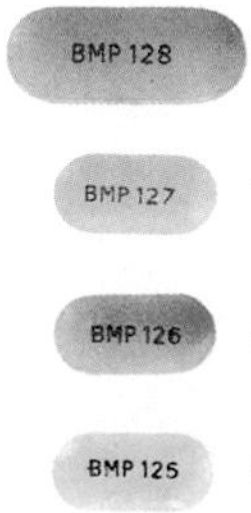

2.5 mg.
1.25 mg.
0.625 mg.
0.3 mg.
Menest™
(Esterified Estrogens, U.S.P.)

Beecham Laboratories

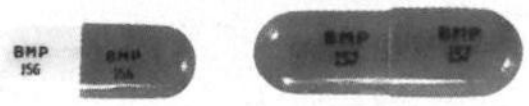

100 mg. 250 mg.
†Tigan® Capsules
(trimethobenzamide HCl)

Boehringer Ingelheim Ltd.

74* 72*

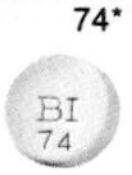

10 mg.

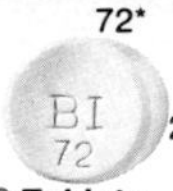

20 mg.
†Alupent® Tablets
(metaproterenol sulfate)

Boehringer Ingelheim Ltd.

6* 7* 11*

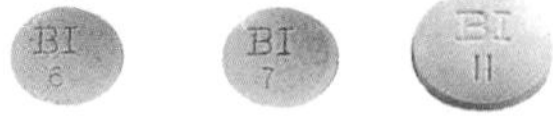

0.1 mg. 0.2 mg. 0.3 mg.
Catapres® Tablets
(clonidine hydrochloride)

Boehringer Ingelheim Ltd.

8* 9*

0.1 0.2
Combipres® Tablets
(clonidine hydrochloride, 0.1 mg. or 0.2 mg. and chlorthalidone, 15 mg.)

Boehringer Ingelheim Ltd.

12*

5 mg.
Dulcolax® Tablets
(bisacodyl USP)

Boehringer Ingelheim Ltd.

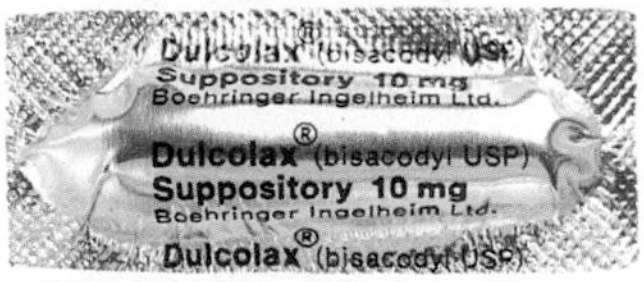

Dulcolax® Suppositories 10 mg.
(bisacodyl USP)

Boehringer Ingelheim Ltd.

17* 18* 19*

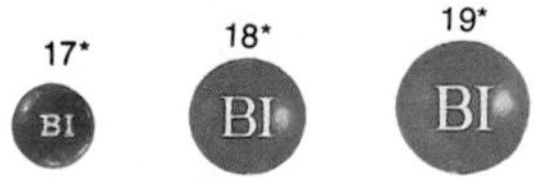

25 mg. 50 mg. 75 mg.
Persantine® Tablets
(dipyridamole)

Boehringer Ingelheim Ltd.

42*

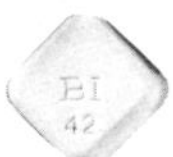

25 mg.
79* Tablets 62*

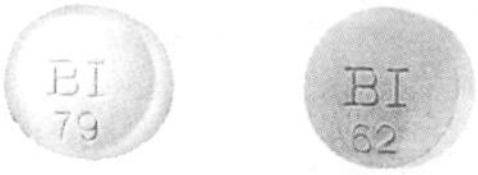

50 mg. 75 mg.
Endurets®
(prolonged-action tablets)
Preludin®
(phenmetrazine hydrochloride NF)

†Other dosage forms available. See Product Information section or check directly with manufacturer.
*Manufacturers' identification number.

Boehringer Ingelheim Ltd.

20*

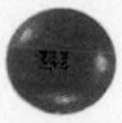

10 mg.

†Serentil® Tablets
(mesoridazine besylate NF)
Also 25 mg., 21*; 50 mg., 22*; 100 mg., 23*

Boehringer Ingelheim Ltd.

28*

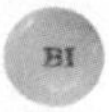

10 mg.

†Torecan® Tablets
(thiethylperazine maleate NF)

BREON

100 mg 200 mg

Bronkodyl®
(Micro-pulverized)
(theophylline, USP anhydrous)

Breon

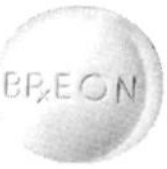

Bronkotabs®

Breon Ⓒ II

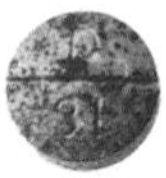

Demerol® APAP
(meperidine HCl, USP with acetaminophen)

Breon

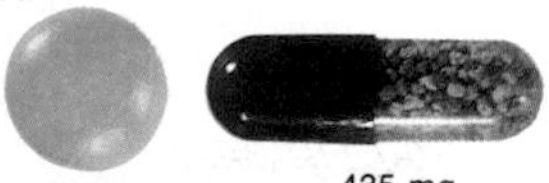

320 mg Tablets

435 mg Capsules

Fergon®
(ferrous gluconate)

Breon

10 mg 15 mg

Isuprel® Glossets®
(isoproterenol HCl tablets, USP)

Breon Ⓒ IV

32 mg 50 mg

100 mg 200 mg

Mebaral®
(mephobarbital tablets, NF)

Breon

100 mg 200 mg

Trancopal®
(chlormezanone)

BRISTOL

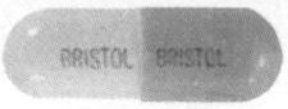

250 mg.

Bristacycline®
(tetracycline HCl)

Bristol

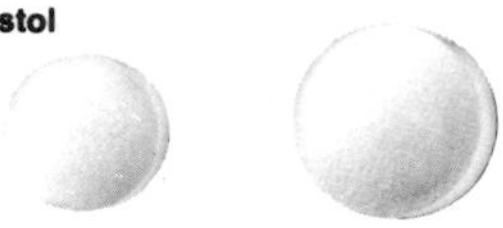

250 mg. 500 mg.

†Betapen®-VK
(penicillin V potassium)

Bristol

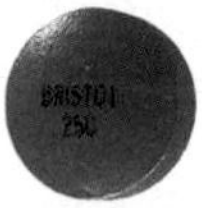

250 mg.

Bristamycin®
(erythromycin stearate)

Bristol

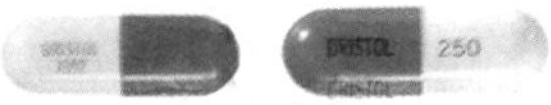

125 mg. 250 mg.

Also available: 500 mg. Capsule

†Dynapen®
(dicloxacillin sodium)

Bristol

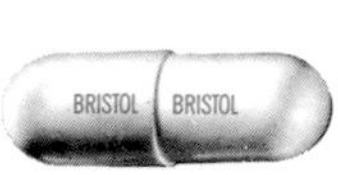

†Kantrex®
(kanamycin sulfate)

Bristol

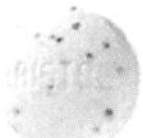

†Naldecon®
(antihistamine/decongestant)

Bristol

Naldegesic®
(decongestant/analgesic)

Bristol

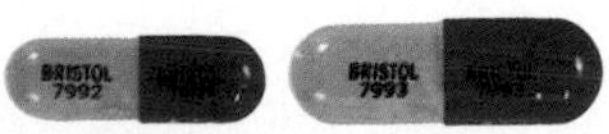

250 mg. 500 mg.

†Polycillin®
(ampicillin)

Bristol

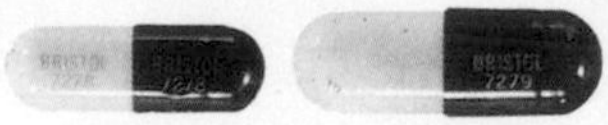

250 mg. 500 mg.

†Polymox®
(amoxicillin)

Bristol

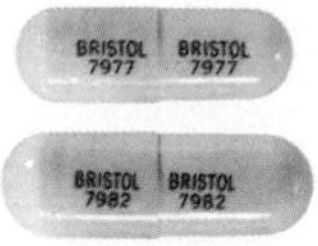

250 mg.

500 mg.

†Prostaphlin®
(oxacillin sodium)

Bristol

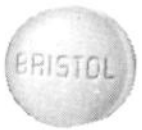

50 mg.

Saluron®
(hydroflumethiazide)

Bristol

Also available: Salutensin-Demi™

Salutensin®
(hydroflumethiazide, reserpine)

Bristol

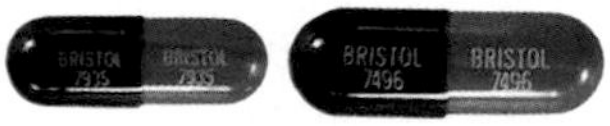

250 mg. 500 mg.

†Tegopen®
(cloxacillin sodium)

Bristol

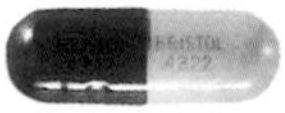

250 mg.

†Tetrex®
(tetracycline phosphate complex)

Bristol

Tetrex® bidCAPS®
(tetracycline phosphate complex, 500 mg.)

Bristol

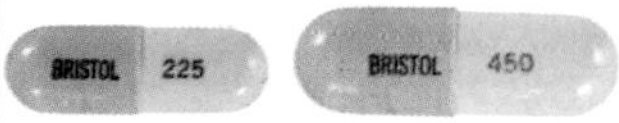

225 mg. 450 mg.

†Versapen®-K
(potassium hetacillin)

Designed to help you identify drugs, this section contains actual size, full-color reproductions of products selected for inclusion by participating manufacturers.

Brown Pharmaceutical Co.

Android® 5 Buccal Tab* **Android® 10** **Android® 25**
(methyltestosterone USP)

BURROUGHS WELLCOME

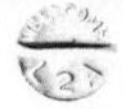

2.5 mg

†ACTIDIL® tablets
(triprolidine hydrochloride)

Burroughs Wellcome

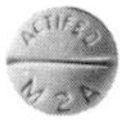

†ACTIFED® tablets
(triprolidine hydrochloride 2.5 mg and pseudoephedrine hydrochloride 60 mg)

Burroughs Wellcome

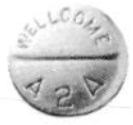

2 mg

ALKERAN® tablets
(melphalan)

Burroughs Wellcome

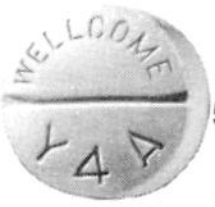

500 mg

†ANTEPAR® tablets
(piperazine citrate)

Burroughs Wellcome

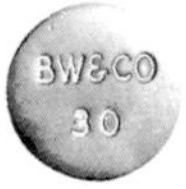

ASCODEEN-30® tablets
(codeine phosphate 30 mg and aspirin 325 mg)

Burroughs Wellcome

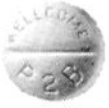

5 mg

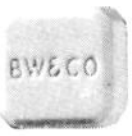

10 mg

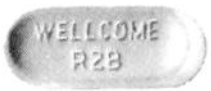

15 mg

CARDILATE® tablets
(erythrityl tetranitrate)

Burroughs Wellcome

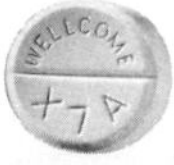

10 mg

CARDILATE® CHEWABLE tablets
(erythrityl tetranitrate)

†Other dosage forms available. See Product Information section or check directly with manufacturer.
*Manufacturers' identification number.

Burroughs Wellcome

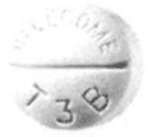

CARDILATE-P tablets
(erythrityl tetranitrate 10 mg and phenobarbital 15 mg)

Burroughs Wellcome

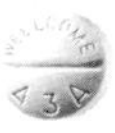

25 mg

DARAPRIM® tablets
(pyrimethamine)

Burroughs Wellcome

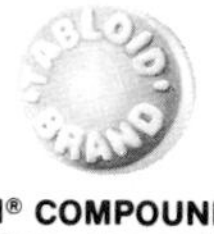

EMPIRIN® COMPOUND tablets
(aspirin 227 mg , phenacetin 162 mg , caffeine 32 mg)

Burroughs Wellcome

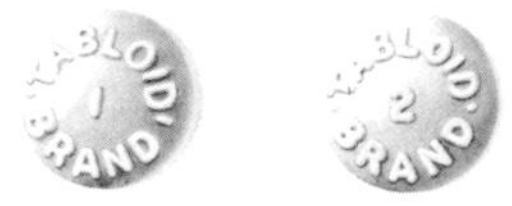

NO. 1, gr ⅛ NO. 2, gr ¼

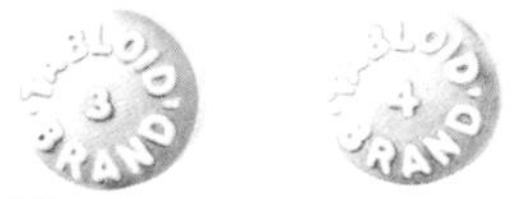

NO. 3, gr ½ NO. 4, gr 1

TABLOID® brand A.P.C. WITH CODEINE tablets
(each tablet contains the ingredients of Empirin Compound plus codeine phosphate)

Burroughs Wellcome

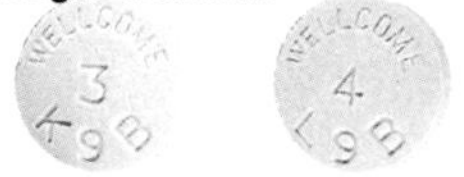

No. 3, gr ½ No. 4, gr 1

Empracet® With Codeine tablets
(each tablet contains acetaminophen 300 mg plus codeine phosphate)

Burroughs Wellcome

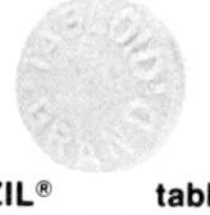

EMPRAZIL® tablets
(pseudoephedrine hydrochloride 20 mg , phenacetin 150 mg , aspirin 200 mg , caffeine 30 mg)

Burroughs Wellcome

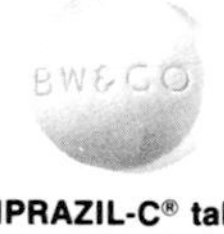

EMPRAZIL-C® tablets
(each tablet contains the ingredients of Emprazil plus 15 mg codeine phosphate)

Burroughs Wellcome

FEDRAZIL® tablets
(pseudoephedrine hydrochloride 30 mg and chlorcyclizine hydrochloride 25 mg)

Burroughs Wellcome

50 mg

IMURAN® tablets
(azathioprine)

Burroughs Wellcome

2 mg 5 mg

KEMADRIN® tablets
(procyclidine hydrochloride)

Burroughs Wellcome

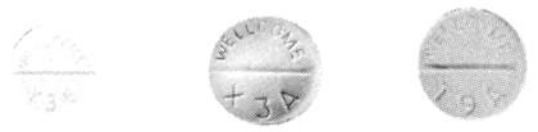

0.125 mg 0.25 mg 0.5 mg

†LANOXIN® tablets
(digoxin)

Burroughs Wellcome

2 mg

LEUKERAN® tablets
(chlorambucil)

Burroughs Wellcome

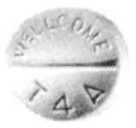

50 mg

†MAREZINE® tablets
(cyclizine hydrochloride)

Burroughs Wellcome

MIGRAL® tablets
(ergotamine tartrate 1 mg , cyclizine hydrochloride 25 mg , caffeine 50 mg)

Burroughs Wellcome

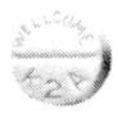

2 mg

MYLERAN® tablets
(busulfan)

Burroughs Wellcome

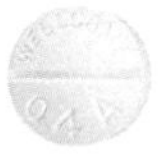

50 mg

PURINETHOL® tablets
(mercaptopurine)

Burroughs Wellcome

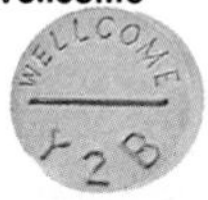

†SEPTRA® tablets
(trimethoprim 80 mg and sulfamethoxazole 400 mg)

Burroughs Wellcome

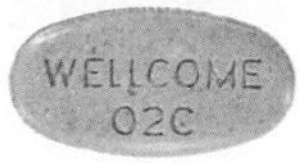

†SEPTRA® DS
(trimethoprim 160 mg and sulfamethoxazole 800 mg)

Burroughs Wellcome

30 mg 60 mg

†SUDAFED® tablets
(pseudoephedrine hydrochloride)

Burroughs Wellcome

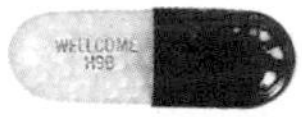

120 mg

SUDAFED® S.A. capsules
Sustained Action Capsules
(pseudoephedrine hydrochloride)

Burroughs Wellcome

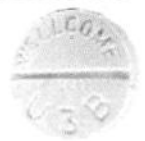

40 mg

THIOGUANINE, TABLOID® brand tablets
(thioguanine)

Burroughs Wellcome

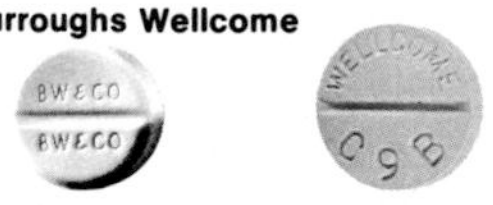

100 mg 300 mg

ZYLOPRIM® tablets
(allopurinol)

CARNRICK

AMEN®
(medroxyprogesterone acetate U.S.P. 10 mg)

Carnrick Ⓒ

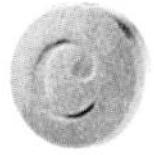

BONTRIL PDM™
(phendimetrazine tartrate 35 mg)

Carnrick

Suspension Ⓒ
Tablets Ⓒ

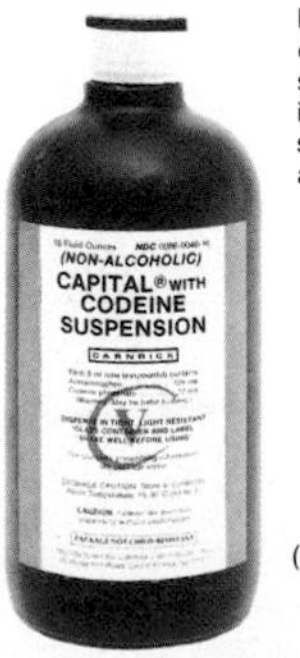

Bottle containing suspension is shown smaller than actual size

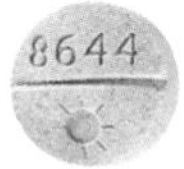

CAPITAL®
(acetaminophen)
with CODEINE

Carnrick

No. 1 No. 2

HORMONIN®
(estriol, estradiol, estrone)

Carnrick

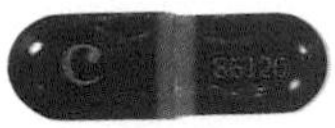

MIDRIN™
(isometheptene mucate, acetaminophen, dichloralphenazone)

Carnrick

MINOTAL®
(acetaminophen, sodium butabarbital)

Carnrick

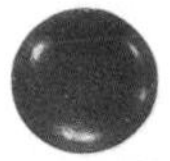

NOLAMINE™
(phenindamine tartrate, chlorpheniramine maleate, phenylpropanolamine hydrochloride)

Carnrick

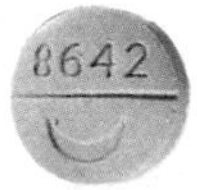

PHRENILIN®
(sodium butabarbital, acetaminophen, caffeine)

Carnrick

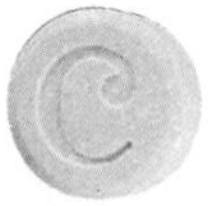

SINULIN™
(phenylpropanolamine HCl, chlorpheniramine maleate, acetaminophen, salicylamide, homatropine methylbromide)

CENTRAL

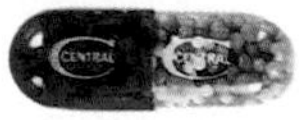

CODIMAL®-L.A. Cenules®

Central Pharmacal

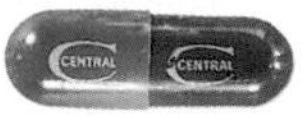

NIFEREX®-150 Capsules

Central Pharmacal

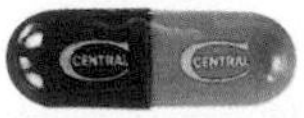

NIFEREX®-150 Forte Capsules
(polysaccharide-iron complex with folic acid and vitamin B_{12})

†Other dosage forms available. See Product Information section or check directly with manufacturer.

Central Pharmacal

NIFEREX®-PN Tablets

CIBA

129*

Apresoline®-Esidrix®
(hydralazine hydrochloride and hydrochlorothiazide)

CIBA

30* 32*

10 mg. 25 mg.
Tablets

51* 64*

5 mg. 10 mg.
Linguets

Metandren®
(methyltestosterone)

CIBA

13* 97*

#1 #2
Serpasil®-Esidrix®
(reserpine and hydrochlorothiazide)

Central Pharmacal

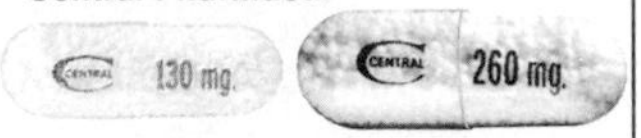

130 mg. 260 mg.
THEOCLEAR® L.A.-130 **Cenules®** **THEOCLEAR® L.A.-260**
(theophylline anhydrous)

CIBA

105*

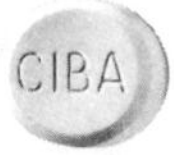

15/300
Dialog®
(allobarbital and acetaminophen)

CIBA

165*

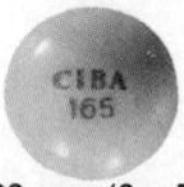

600 mg. (8 mEq)
Slow-K® slow-release tablets
(potassium chloride)

Central Pharmacal

THEOCLEAR®-100 Tablets
(Both sides of tablets shown)

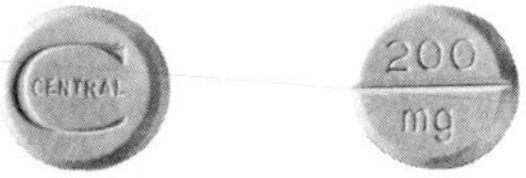

THEOCLEAR®-200 Tablets
(theophylline anhydrous)

CIBA

17* 20*

2.5 mg. 5 mg.
Dianabol®
(methandrostenolone)

CIBA

152*

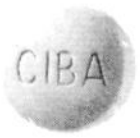

50 mg.
†Regitine® hydrochloride
(phentolamine hydrochloride)

BERLEX
(Formerly Cooper)

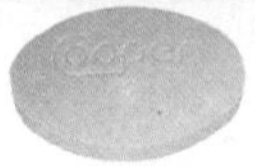

300 mg. scored dye-free tablet
(sustained release)
Aminodur® Dura-Tabs®
(aminophylline)

CIBA

47*

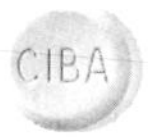

Esimil®
(guanethidine monosulfate and hydrochlorothiazide)

CIBA

154*

300 mg.
Rimactane®
(rifampin)

Berlex

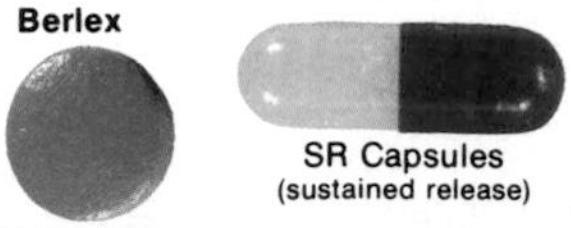

Tablets SR Capsules
(sustained release)
†Deconamine®
(chlorpheniramine maleate and d-pseudoephedrine hydrochloride)

CIBA

15*

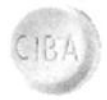

5 mg.
Antrenyl® bromide
(oxyphenonium bromide)

CIBA

22* 46*

25 mg. 50 mg.

192*

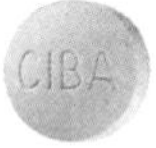

100 mg.
Esidrix®
(hydrochlorothiazide)

CIBA

7* 3*

5 mg. 10 mg.

34*

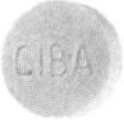

20 mg.
Ritalin® hydrochloride
(methylphenidate hydrochloride)

Berlex

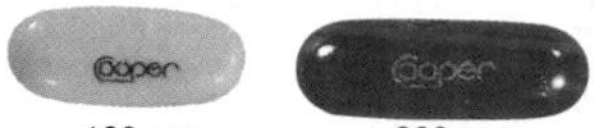

100 mg. dye-free 200 mg.
†Elixophyllin® Capsules
(anhydrous theophylline)

CIBA 41* 168*

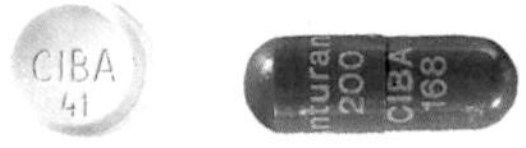

100 mg. 200 mg.
Anturane®
(sulfinpyrazone USP)

Berlex dye-free

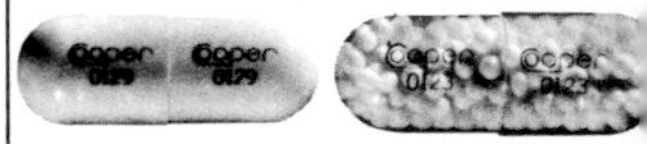

125 mg. 250 mg.
(sustained release)
†Elixophyllin® SR Capsules
(anhydrous theophylline)

CIBA 139* 149* 159*

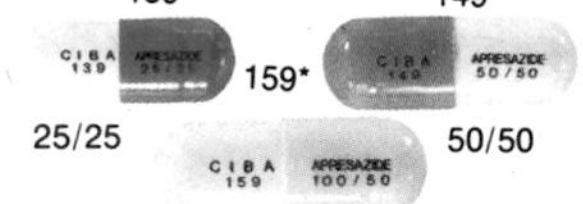

25/25 50/50 100/50
Apresazide®
(hydralazine HCl and hydrochlorothiazide)

CIBA

45*

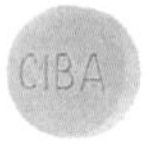

2.5 mg. Lontabs®
Forhistal® maleate
(dimethindene maleate)

CIBA

71*

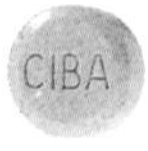

Ser-Ap-Es®

Berlex

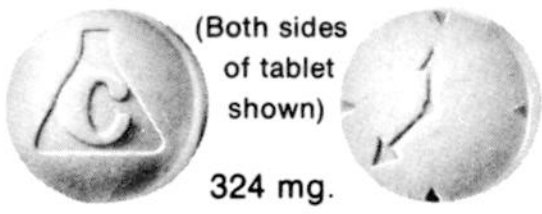

(Both sides of tablet shown)
324 mg.
Quinaglute® Dura-Tabs®
(quinidine gluconate)

CIBA

37* 39*

10 mg. 25 mg.

73* 101*

50 mg. 100 mg.
†Apresoline® hydrochloride
(hydralazine hydrochloride)

CIBA

49* 103*

10 mg. 25 mg.
Ismelin® sulfate
(guanethidine sulfate)

CIBA

35* 36*

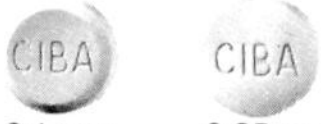

0.1 mg. 0.25 mg.
†Serpasil®
(reserpine)

Berlex

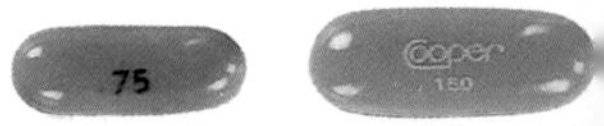

75 mg. 150 mg.
Therapav® Capsules
(papaverine hydrochloride)

CIBA

130*

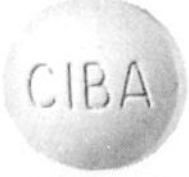

250 mg.
†Metopirone®
(metyrapone)

CIBA

40* 104*

#1 #2
Serpasil®-Apresoline
(reserpine and hydralazine hydrochloride)

Because tablets and capsules are shown in this section, do not infer that these are the only dosage forms available. Where a product name is preceded by the symbol†, refer to the description in the Product Information (White Section) for other forms.

†Other dosage forms available. See Product Information section or check directly with manufacturer.
*Manufacturers' identification number.

DISTA

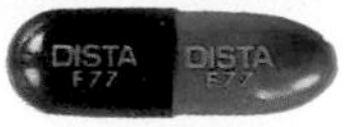

Becotin® with Vitamin C
(vitamin B complex with vitamin C)

Dista

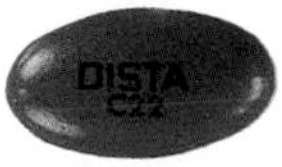

Becotin®-T
(vitamin B complex with vitamin C, therapeutic)

Dista

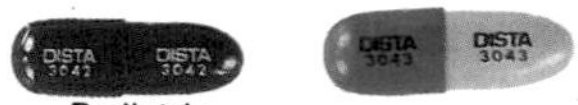

Pediatric

†Co-Pyronil®
(pyrrobutamine compound)

Dista

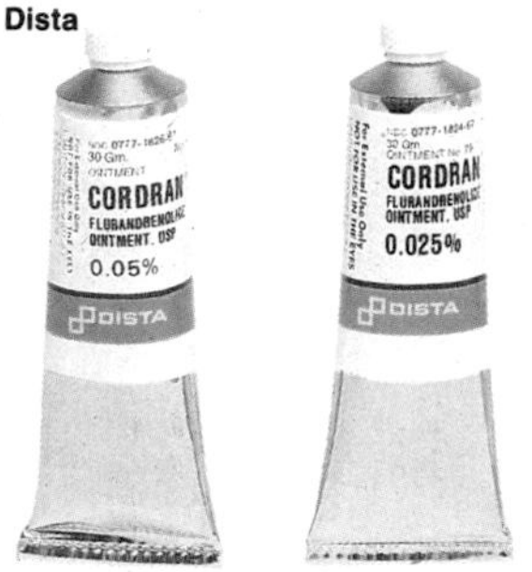

0.05% 0.025%

Cordran® Ointment
(flurandrenolide)

Dista

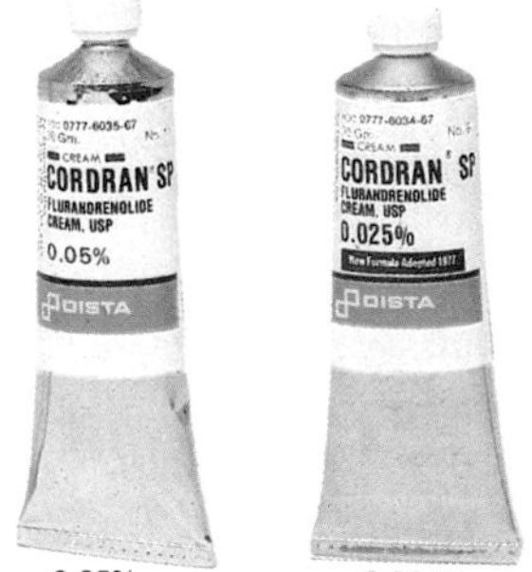

0.05% 0.025%

Cordran® SP Cream
(flurandrenolide)

Dista

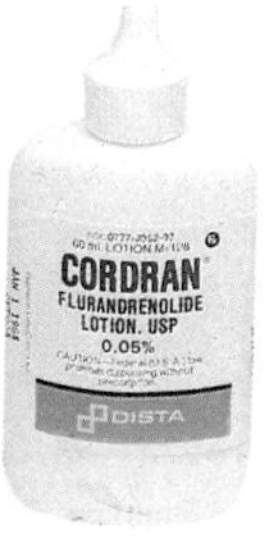

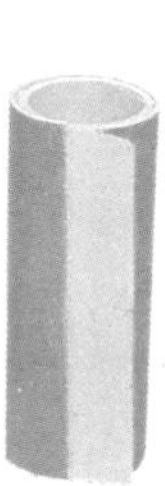

0.05% — **Cordran® Lotion** (flurandrenolide)

4 mcg per sq cm — **Cordran® Tape** (flurandrenolide tape)

IDENTI-CODE®

(formula identification code, Dista)
Provides Positive Product Identification

A letter-number symbol, a four-digit number, the name of the product, the strength of the product, or a combination of these appears on each Dista capsule and tablet and on each label of pediatric liquids and powders for oral suspension. The letter/number or four-digit number identifies the product, which is listed in the Dista IDENTI-CODE® INDEX.

For example:

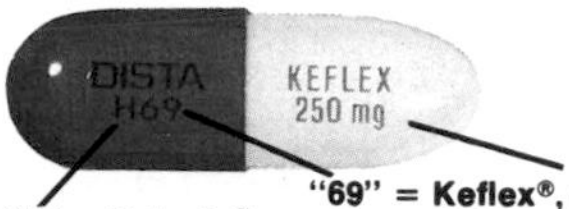

"H" = Pulvule®

"69" = Keflex®, 250 mg
(cephalexin)

The complete IDENTI-CODE® INDEX appears in the Product Information Section under Dista Products Company.

Dista

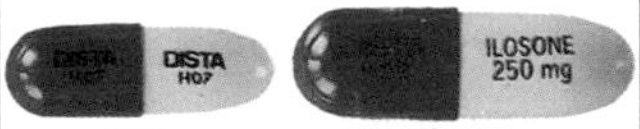

125 mg 250 mg

†Ilosone®
(erythromycin estolate)

Dista

500 mg.
Ilosone®
(erythromycin estolate)

Dista

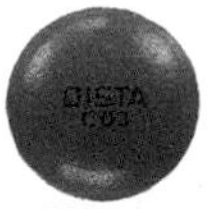

250 mg.
†Ilotycin®
(erythromycin)

Dista

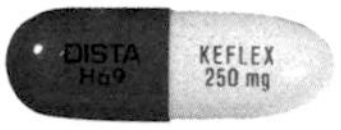

250 mg.

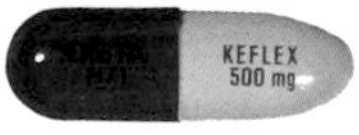

500 mg.

†Keflex®
(cephalexin)

Dista

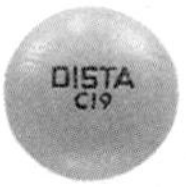

Mi-Cebrin®
(vitamins-minerals)

Dista

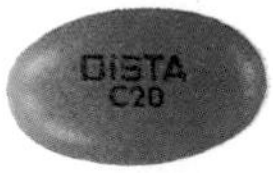

Mi-Cebrin T®
(vitamin-minerals therapeutic)

Dista

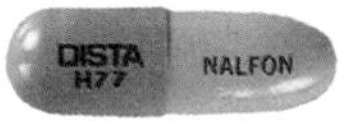

300 mg.

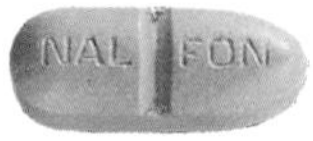

600 mg.

Nalfon®
(fenoprofen calcium)

Dista

Trinsicon®
(hematinic concentrate with intrinsic factor)

Dista C-IV

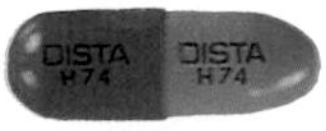

500 mg.
Valmid®
(ethinamate)

DOONER**

60 mg.

(timed release capsule)
†D-FEDA® Gyrocap®
(pseudoephedrine HCl)

Dooner

(timed release capsule)
Gyrocap®

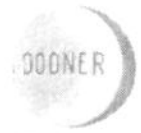

Tablet

†FEDAHIST®

Dooner

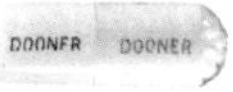

60 mg.

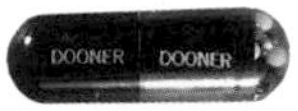

125 mg.

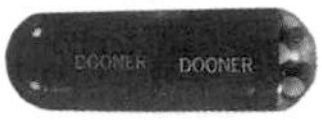

250 mg.
(timed release capsules)
†SLO-PHYLLIN® Gyrocap®
(anhydrous theophylline)

Dooner

100 mg. 200 mg.

†SLO-PHYLLIN® Tablets
(anhydrous theophylline)

Dooner

†SLO-PHYLLIN® GG Capsules
(anhydrous theophylline w/guaifenesin)

DORSEY

†ASBRON G® Inlay-Tabs®

Dorsey

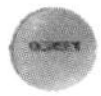

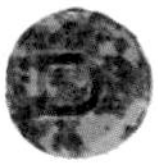

BELLERGAL® Tablets **BELLERGAL-S® Tablets**

Dorsey

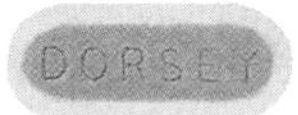

CAMA® Inlay-Tabs®

Dorsey

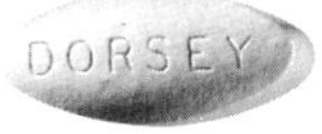

Gris-PEG® Tablets
(griseofulvin ultramicrosize)

Dorsey

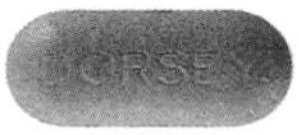

KANULASE® Tablets

†Other dosage forms available. See Product Information section or check directly with manufacturer.
**Logo only may appear on capsules.

Dorsey

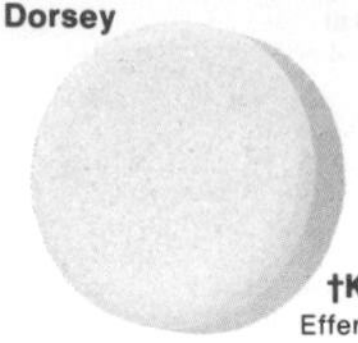

†KLORVESS®
Effervescent Tablets

Dorsey

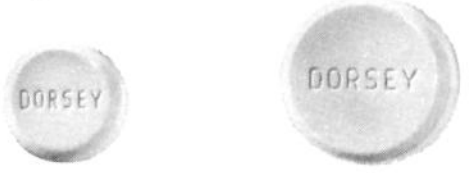

10 mg. 20 mg.
†METAPREL® Tablets
(metaproterenol sulfate)

Dorsey

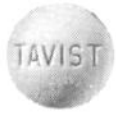

2.68 mg
TAVIST® Tablets
(clemastine fumerate)

Dorsey

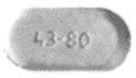

1.34 mg.
Tavist-1™
(clemastine fumurate)

Dorsey

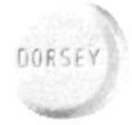

TREST® Tablets
(methixene hydrochloride)

Dorsey

TRIAMINICIN® Allergy Tablets

DOW

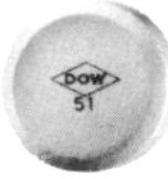

250 mg. tablets
Lorelco®
(probucol)

Dow

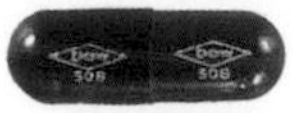

300 mg.
Rifadin® capsules
(rifampin)

Dow

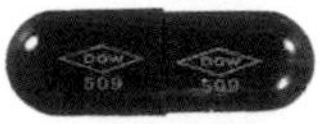

Rifamate™ capsules
(300 mg. rifampin and 150 mg. isoniazid)

Dow

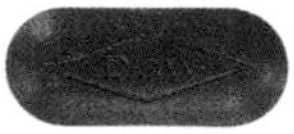

Singlet®
(phenylephrine HCl, chlorpheniramine maleate and acetaminophen)

Dow

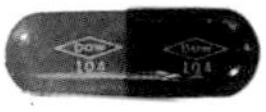

120 mg.
Novafed® capsules
(pseudoephedrine HCl)
controlled-release

Dow

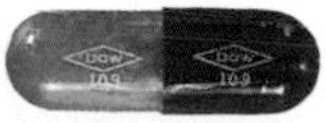

Novafed® A capsules
(120 mg. pseudoephedrine HCl and 8 mg. chlorpheniramine maleate)
controlled-release

DRUG INDUSTRIES

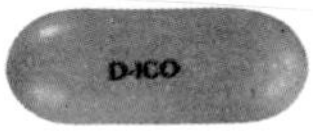

AL-VITE™

Drug Industries

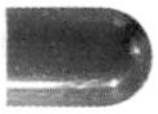

BILAX™

Drug Industries

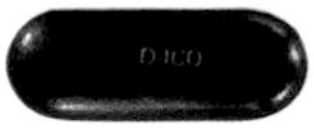

HEMO-VITE DI

Drug Industries

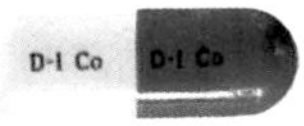

TRILAX™

EATON

Eaton Laboratories Inc.
Manati, Puerto Rico

25 mg 50 mg

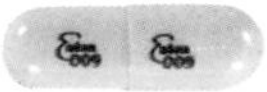

100 mg
See: Norwich-Eaton
Macrodantin® Capsules
(nitrofurantoin macrocrystals)

ELDER

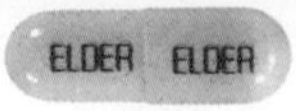

10 mg.
Oxsoralen® Capsules
(methoxsalen)

Elder

5 mg.
Trisoralen® Tablets
(trioxsalen)

ENDO

Ⓒ IV

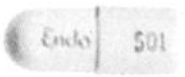

3.25 mg

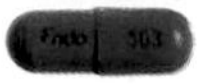

13.0 mg

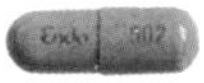

6.5 mg
AZENE® Capsules
(clorazepate monopotassium)

Endo

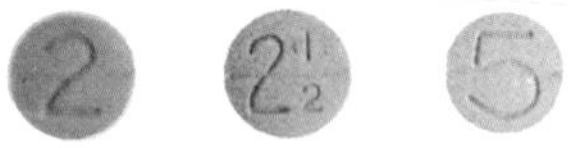

2 mg lavender; 2½ mg orange; 5 mg peach

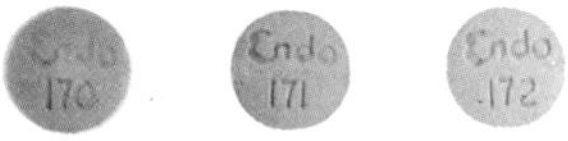

7½ mg yellow; 10 mg white

COUMADIN® Tablets
(crystalline warfarin sodium)

Endo Ⓒ III

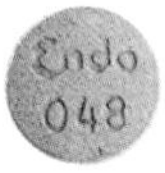

HYCOMINE® COMPOUND Tablets
[hydrocodone bitartrate 5 mg chlorpheniramine maleate 2 mg phenylephrine HCl 10 mg acetaminophen (APAP) 250 mg caffeine 30 mg]

Endo

0072 0073 0074

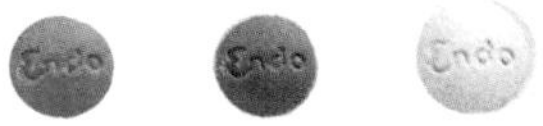

5 mg 10 mg 25 mg
MOBAN®
(molindone HCl)

Endo Inc.
Manati, Puerto Rico Ⓒ II
0060-0127

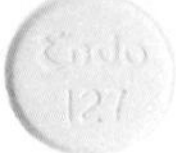

PERCOCET®-5 Tablets

Endo Inc.
Manati, Puerto Rico Ⓒ II
0060-0122

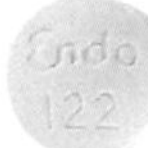

PERCODAN® Tablets

Ⓒ II
0060-0123

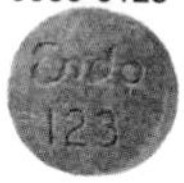

PERCODAN®-Demi Tablets

Endo

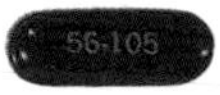

100 mg
†SYMMETREL® Capsules
(amantadine HCl)

Endo
0056-0010

100 mg
TESSALON® Perles
(benzonatate NF)

Endo
0056-0161

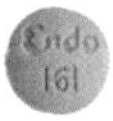

50 mg
VALPIN® 50 Tablets
(anisotropine methylbromide)

Endo
0056-0162

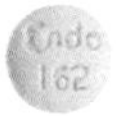

50 mg
VALPIN® 50-PB Tablets
(50 mg. anisotropine methylbromide with 15 mg. phenobarbital)

FLINT

1 mg. 2 mg.

4 mg. 6 mg.
CHOLOXIN®
(dextrothyroxine sodium, NF)

†Other dosage forms available. See Product Information section or check directly with manufacturer.

Flint

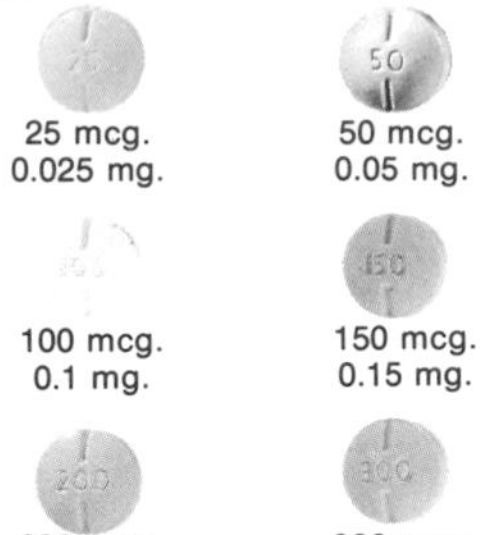

25 mcg. 0.025 mg. | 50 mcg. 0.05 mg. | 100 mcg. 0.1 mg. | 150 mcg. 0.15 mg. | 200 mcg. 0.2 mg. | 300 mcg. 0.3 mg.

†SYNTHROID®
(levothyroxine sodium, USP)

Flint

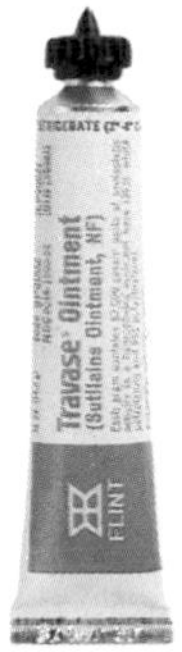

(Tube shown smaller than actual size)

TRAVASE® Ointment
(sutilains ointment, NF)

GEIGY

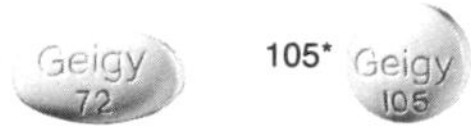

72* 2.5 mg. 105* 5 mg.

†Brethine®
(terbutaline sulfate)

Geigy

14*

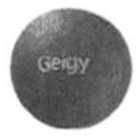

100 mg.

Butazolidin®
(phenylbutazone USP)

Geigy

02*

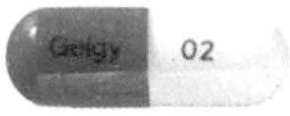

Butazolidin® alka
(phenylbutazone USP, 100 mg.; dried aluminum hydroxide gel USP, 100 mg.; magnesium trisilicate USP, 150 mg.)

Geigy

23*

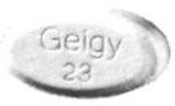

10 mg.

Lioresal®
(baclofen)

Geigy

51* 71*

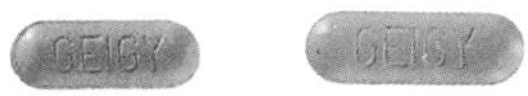

50 mg. 100 mg.

Lopressor™
(metoprolol tartrate)

Geigy

48*

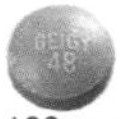

100 mg.

PBZ-SR®
(tripelennamine HCl sustained-release tablet)

Geigy

95* 43*

25 mg. 50 mg.

PBZ® Tablets
(tripelennamine HCl USP)

Geigy

24*

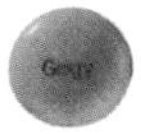

100 mg.

Tandearil®
(oxyphenbutazone NF)

Geigy

67*

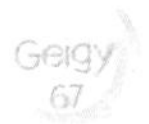

200 mg

Tegretol®
(carbamazepine USP)

Geigy

21* 11* 74*

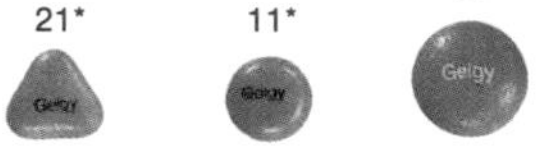

10 mg. 25 mg. 50 mg.

†Tofranil®
(imipramine hydrochloride USP)

Geigy

20* 40*

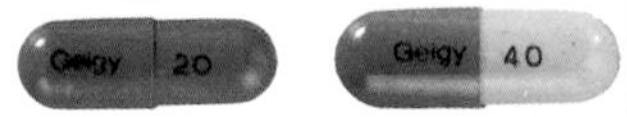

75 mg.** 100 mg.**

45* 22*

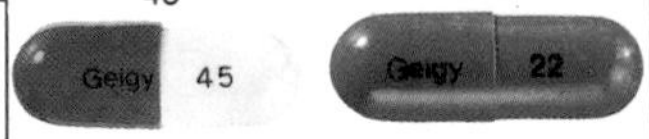

125 mg.** 150 mg.**

Tofranil-PM®
(imipramine pamoate)

**Capsules contain imipramine pamoate equivalent to 75, 100, 125 or 150 mg. of imipramine hydrochloride.

GILBERT

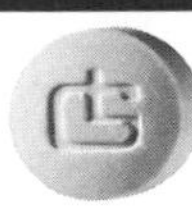

(both sides of tablet shown)

NDC # 535-11

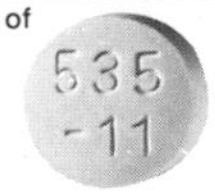

ESGIC®
(color removed—formerly **YELLOW**)

GLAXO

See page 419 for Glaxo products which were formerly shown under Meyer Laboratories.

HOECHST-ROUSSEL

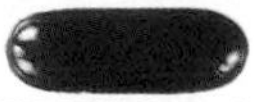

DOXIDAN® Capsules
(dioctyl calcium sulfosuccinate N.F. with danthron N.F.)

Hoechst-Roussel

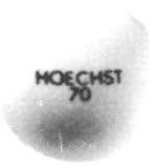

FESTAL® Tablets
(digestive enzymes with bile constituents)

Hoechst-Roussel

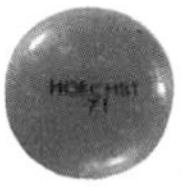

FESTALAN® Tablets
(atropine methyl nitrate with digestive enzymes and bile constituents)

Hoechst-Roussel

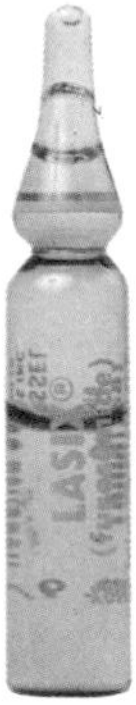

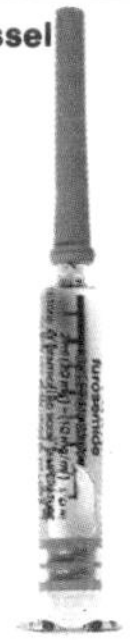

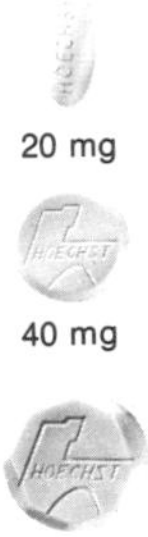

20 mg | 40 mg | 80 mg

LASIX® Tablets
(furosemide)

Ampuls
2 ml, 4 ml, & 10 ml
(10 mg/ml)
LASIX® Injection
(furosemide)

2 ml and 4 ml
(10 mg/ml)
LASIX® Prefilled Syringe
(furosemide)

(Ampul and syringe shown smaller than actual size)

Hoechst-Roussel

60 ml (with calibrated dropper)
Also available, 120 ml
(with dispensing spoon)

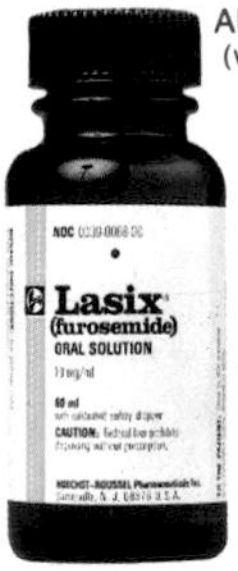

LASIX® Oral Solution
(furosemide)

(Lasix Oral Solution shown smaller than actual size)

Hoechst-Roussel

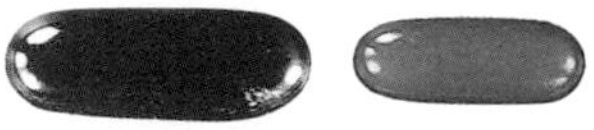

240 mg 50 mg

SURFAK® Capsules
(dioctyl calcium sulfosuccinate N.F.)

Hoechst-Roussel
(Shown smaller than actual size)

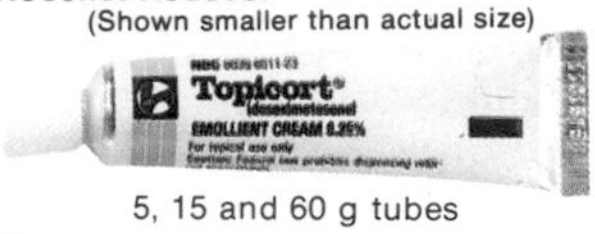

5, 15 and 60 g tubes

TOPICORT® Emollient Cream 0.25%
(desoximetasone)

IVES LABORATORIES

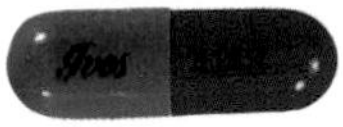

400 mg.

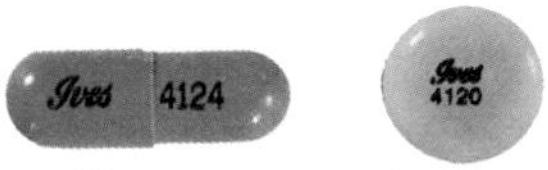

200 mg. 100 mg.

CYCLOSPASMOL®
(cyclandelate)

Ives Laboratories

Sublingual 5 mg. Sublingual 2.5 mg.

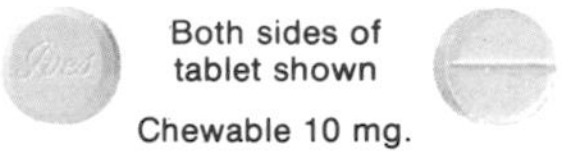

Both sides of tablet shown

Chewable 10 mg.

Oral Titradose® Dosage Forms:

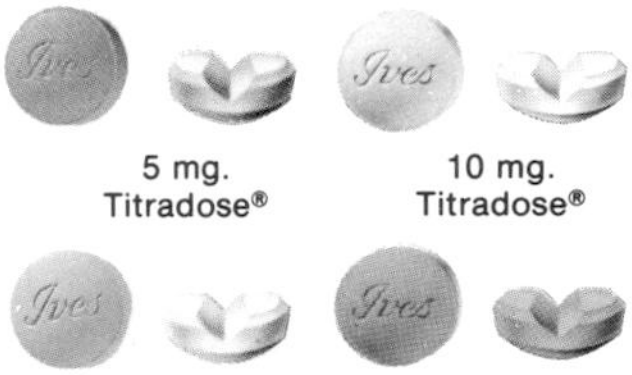

5 mg. Titradose® | 10 mg. Titradose® | 20 mg. Titradose® | 30 mg. Titradose®

Both sides of Titradose tablets shown above

ISORDIL®
(isosorbide dinitrate)

Ives Laboratories

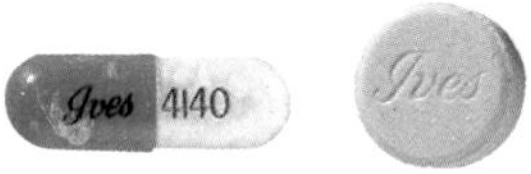

Tembids® Capsules | Tembids® Tablets
Sustained Action 40 mg.

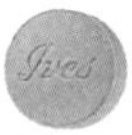

w/Phenobarbital

ISORDIL®
(isosorbide dinitrate)

Ives Laboratories

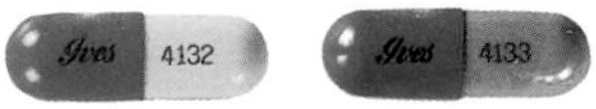

25 mg. 50 mg.

SURMONTIL®
(trimipramine maleate)

†Other dosage forms available. See Product Information section or check directly with manufacturer.
*Manufacturers' identification number.

Ives Laboratories

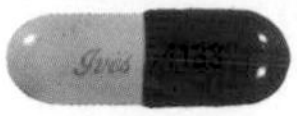

SYNALGOS®

Ives Laboratories

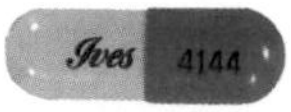

SYNALGOS®-DC

JOHNSON & JOHNSON

Baby Products Company

Enteric Coated Microspheres

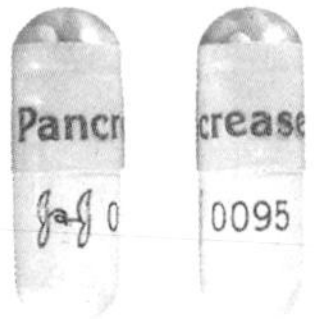

0095*

PANCREASE® Capsules
(brand of pancrelipase)
Bottles of 100 and 250

Key Pharmaceuticals

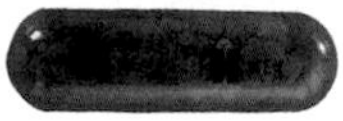

400 mg.
nico-Span®
(niacin)

Key Pharmaceuticals

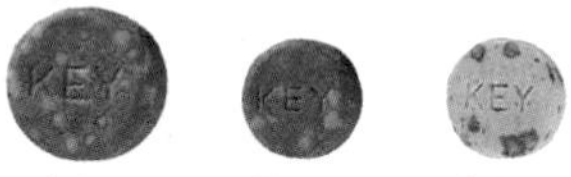

1/10 gr. 1/25 gr. 1/50 gr.
Nitroglyn® (nitroglycerin)

Key Pharmaceuticals

15 mg. 30 mg.
proTernol®
(isoproterenol HCl)

Key Pharmaceuticals

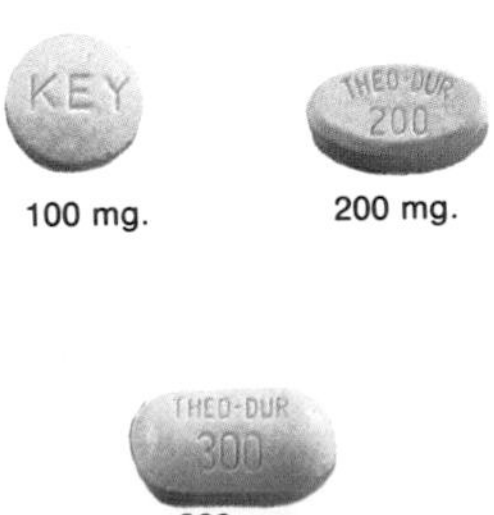

100 mg. 200 mg.

300 mg.

Theo-dur™
(theophylline, anhydrous)

Key Pharmaceuticals

"100" "200"
Theo-nar®
(theophylline, anhydrous and noscapine)

KNOLL

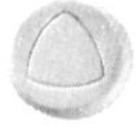

2 mg.
†Akineton®
(biperiden HCl)

Knoll Ⓒ II

Both sides of tablet shown

5 mg.
Dicodid®
(hydrocodone bitartrate)

Knoll Ⓒ II

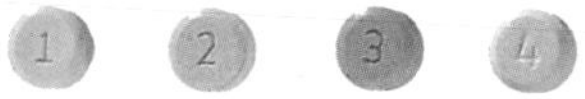

1 mg. 2 mg. 3 mg. 4 mg.
†Dilaudid®
(hydromorphone HCl)

Knoll

Both sides of tablet shown

†Quadrinal™

Knoll (Shown smaller than actual size)

Both sides of tube shown

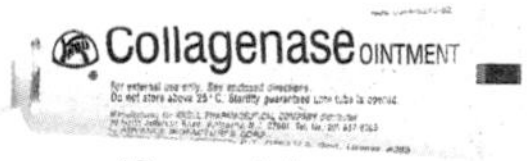

15 gram tube

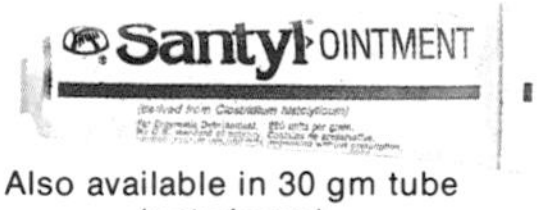

Also available in 30 gm tube
(not shown)
Santyl® Ointment
(collagenase)
250 units per gram.
No U.S. standard of potency.

Knoll

Both sides of tablet shown

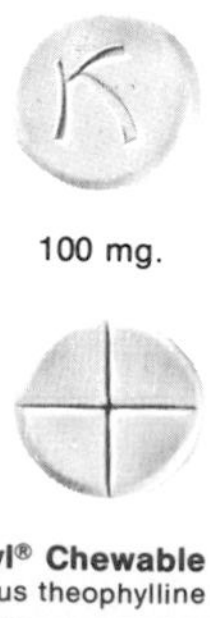

100 mg.

Theophyl® Chewable Tablet
(anhydrous theophylline U.S.P.)

Knoll

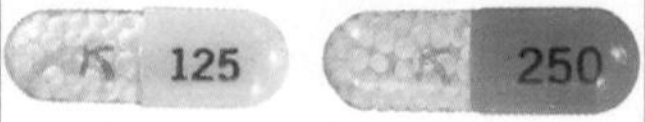

125 mg. 250 mg.
Theophyl®-SR
(anhydrous theophylline U.S.P.)

Knoll

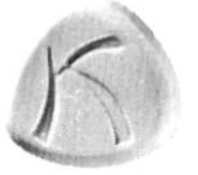

Theophyl®-225 Tablet
(theophylline anhydrous U.S.P.)

Knoll Ⓒ III

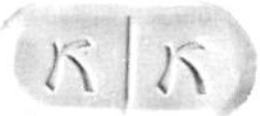

Vicodin®
(hydrocodone bitartrate 5 mg. and acetaminophen 500 mg.)

KREMERS-URBAN

531* 534*

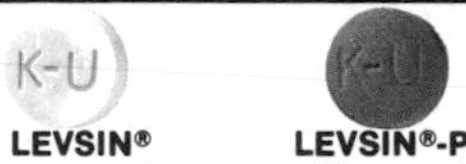

LEVSIN®
(l-Hyoscyamine sulfate, 0.125 mg.)
Oral/Sublingual Tab

LEVSIN®-PB
(l-Hyoscyamine sulfate, 0.125 mg. with Phenobarbital, 15 mg.)
Oral Tab

Kremers-Urban

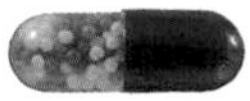

LEVSINEX™ Timecap™
(l-Hyoscyamine sulfate, 0.375 mg.)

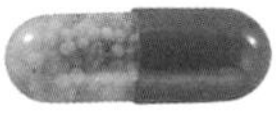

LEVSINEX™-PB Timecap™
(l-Hyoscyamine sulfate, 0.375 mg. with Phenobarbital, 45 mg.)

Kremers-Urban

522* 475*

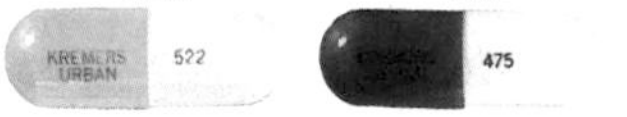

KU-ZYME®
(Amylase, Lipase, Protease, Cellulase)

KUTRASE®
(KU-ZYME plus Anti-spasmodic/ Calmative)

525*

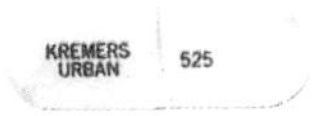

KU-ZYME® HP
(Pancrelipase Capsules, N.F.)

Kremers-Urban

50,000 Units/Tab
CALCIFEROL™
(Ergocalciferol U.S.P., Vit. D_2)

Kremers-Urban

(Shown smaller than actual size)

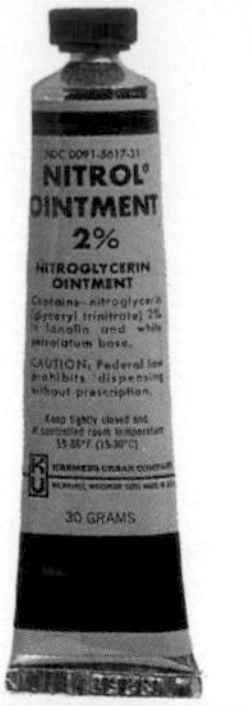

30 and 60 gram tubes

NITROL® Ointment
(Nitroglycerin 2%)

LEDERLE*

*See also LEDERLE GENERICS which follow

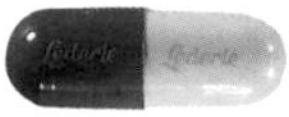

250 mg.

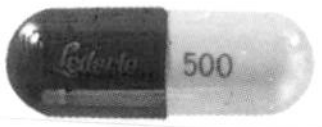

500 mg.

†ACHROMYCIN® V Capsules
(tetracycline)

Lederle

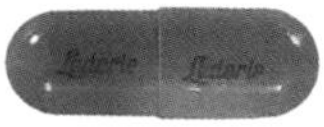

ACHROSTATIN® V Capsules
(tetracycline HCl 250 mg. and nystatin 250,000 units)

Lederle

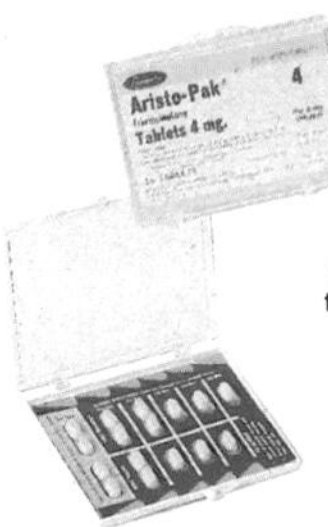

(Shown smaller than actual size)

ARISTO-PAK®
(triamcinolone, 4 mg.)
Six-Day Therapy Pack

Lederle (Tubes shown smaller than actual size)

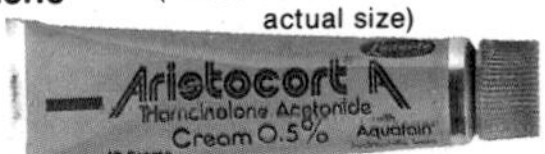

Cream 0.5% 15 Gm. Tubes and 240 Gm. Jars

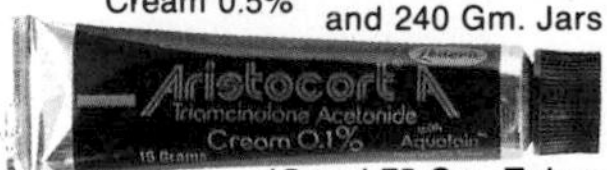

Cream 0.1% 15 and 75 Gm. Tubes and 240 Gm. Jars

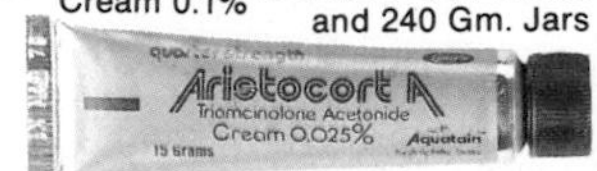

Cream 0.025% 15 and 75 Gm. Tubes

ARISTOCORT® A
(Triamcinolone Acetonide with AQUATAIN™)

†Other dosage forms available. See Product Information section or check directly with manufacturer.
*Manufacturers' identification number.

Lederle

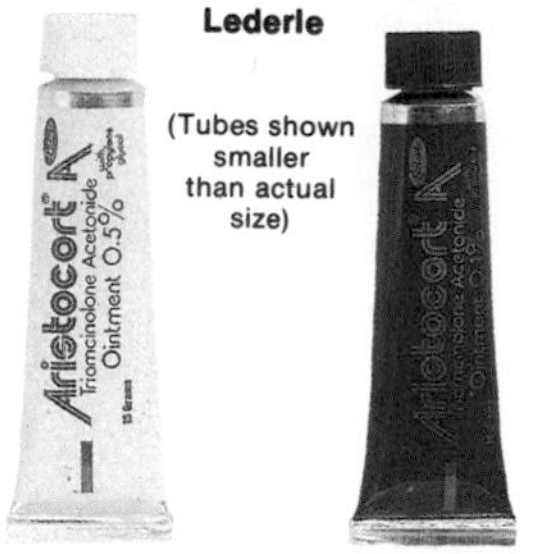

(Tubes shown smaller than actual size)

Ointment 0.5% 15 Gm. tubes | Ointment 0.1% 15 and 75 Gm. tubes

ARISTOCORT® A
(Triamcinolone Acetonide with Propylene Glycol)

Lederle

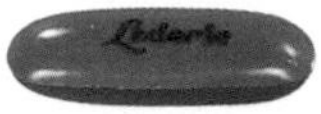

150 mg.

†DECLOMYCIN® Capsules
(demeclocycline)

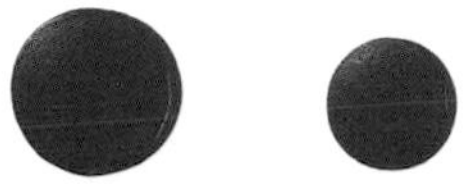

300 mg. | 150 mg.

†DECLOMYCIN® Tablets
(demeclocycline)

Lederle

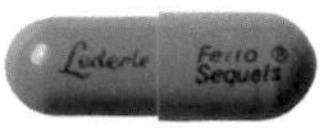

FERRO-SEQUELS® Capsules
Supplied in bottles of 80 and 100

Lederle

25 mg. **Tablets** | 25 mg. **Tablets** with Phenobarbital, 15 mg.

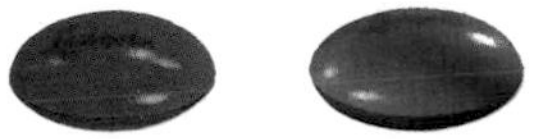

75 mg. **Sequels®** | 75 mg. **Sequels®** with Phenobarbital, 45 mg.

†PATHILON®
(tridihexethyl chloride)

Lederle

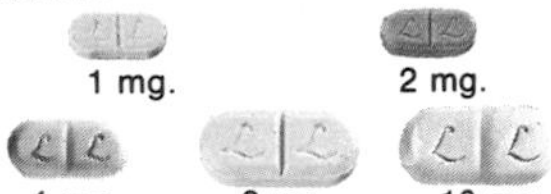

1 mg. | 2 mg. | 4 mg. | 8 mg. | 16 mg.

†ARISTOCORT® Tablets
(triamcinolone)

Lederle

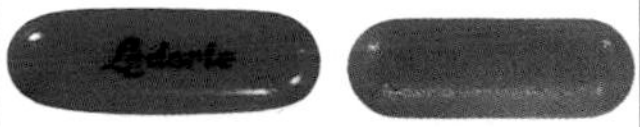

Capsules 150 mg. | Tablets 300 mg.

†DECLOSTATIN® Capsules
(demeclocycline and nystatin)

Lederle

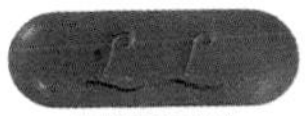

FILIBON®

FILIBON® F.A.

Supplied in bottles of 100

FILIBON® Forte
Prenatal Tablets

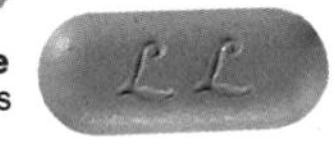

FILIBON® OT Tablets

Lederle

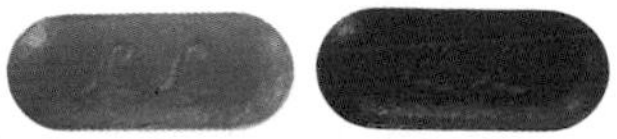

STRESSTABS® 600
(high potency stress formula vitamins)

STRESSTABS® 600 w/Iron
(high potency stress formula vitamins plus iron)

STRESSTABS® 600 w/Zinc
(high potency stress formula vitamins with zinc)

Supplied in bottles of 30 and 60

Lederle

Color Coding for
ARISTOCORT® Triamcinolone Acetonide
Dermatological Products

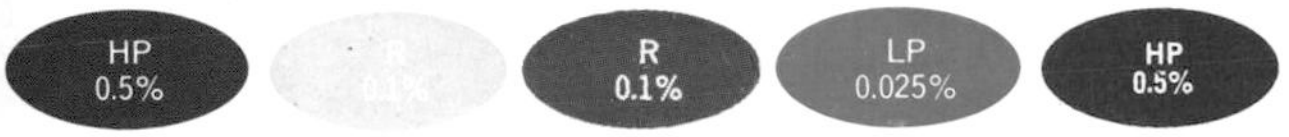

HIGH POTENCY CREAM	REGULAR POTENCY CREAM	REGULAR POTENCY OINTMENT	LOW POTENCY CREAM	HIGH POTENCY OINTMENT

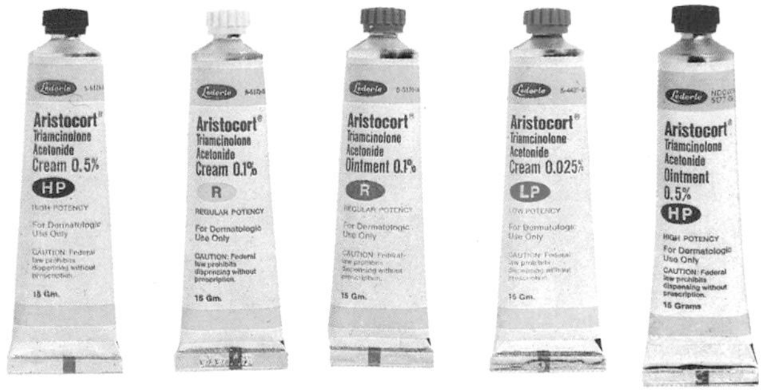

(Tubes shown smaller than actual size)

15 Gm. tubes 240 Gm. jar	15 and 75 Gm. tubes 240 Gm. and 5¼ lb. jars	15 and 75 Gm. tubes 240 Gm. and 5 lb. jars	15 and 75 Gm. tubes 240 Gm. and 5¼ lb. jars	15 Gm. tubes 240 Gm. jars

Lederle

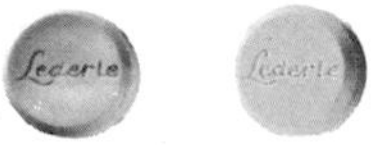

50 mg.

HYDROMOX® Tablets
(Quinethazone)

HYDROMOX® R
(Quinethazone 50 mg. with Reserpine 0.125 mg.)

Lederle

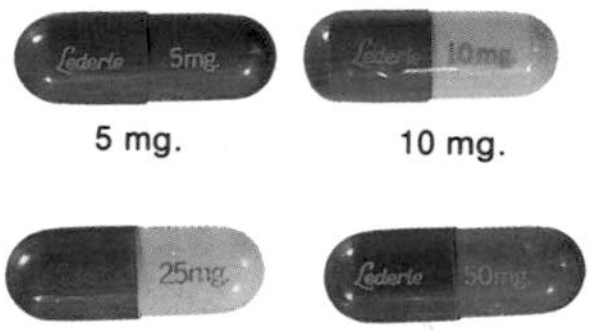

5 mg. | 10 mg. | 25 mg. | 50 mg.

LOXITANE® Capsules
(Loxapine Succinate)

Lederle

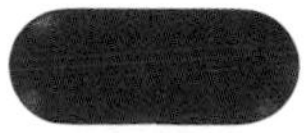

Tri-HEMIC™ 600 Tablets
(hematinic)

LEDERLE GENERICS

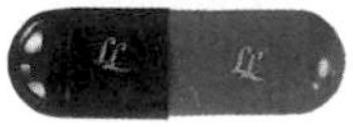

500 mg.

Acetaminophen Capsules

Lederle

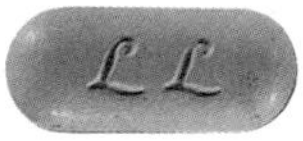

MATERNA™ 1-60
Prenatal Tablets
Supplied in bottles of 100

Lederle Generics

10 mg. | 25 mg.

50 mg. | 75 mg. | 100 mg.

Amitriptyline HCl, U.S.P. Tablets

Lederle

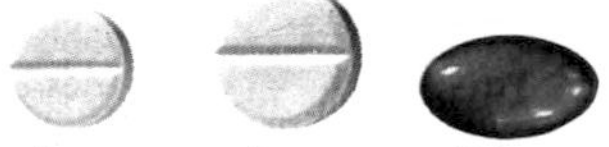

2 mg. | 5 mg. | 5 mg.

ARTANE® Tablets | **†ARTANE® Sequels®**
(trihexyphenidyl hydrochloride)

Lederle

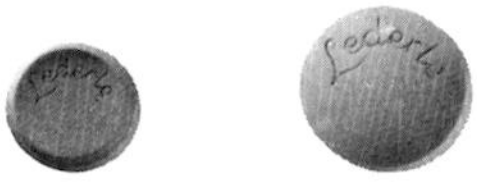

125 mg. | 250 mg.

†DIAMOX® Tablets

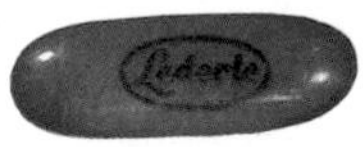

500 mg.

†DIAMOX® Sequels
(acetazolamide)

Lederle

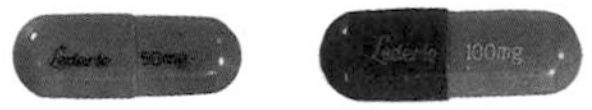

50 mg. | 100 mg.

†MINOCIN® Capsules
(minocycline HCl)

Lederle

Bottle of 100

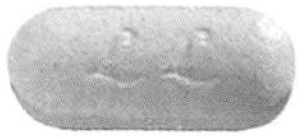

CENTRUM®
High Potency Multivitamin/ Multimineral Formula Tablets

Lederle

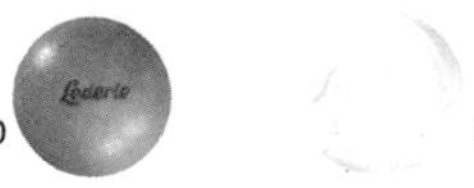

200 | 400

PATHIBAMATE® Tablets
(tridihexethyl chloride 25 mg.-meprobamate 200/400)

Lederle Generics

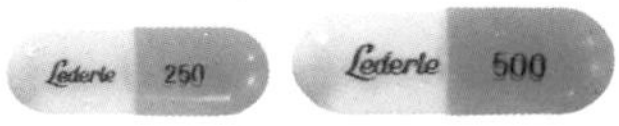

250 mg. | 500 mg.

Ampicillin Trihydrate Capsules

†Other dosage forms available. See Product Information section or check directly with manufacturer.

Lederle Generics

5 mg.

Bisacodyl Tablets, U.S.P.

Lederle Generics

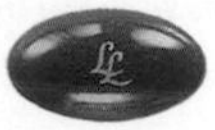

100 mg./30 mg.

Dioctyl Sodium Sulfosuccinate, U.S.P. w/Casanthranol Capsules

Lederle Generics

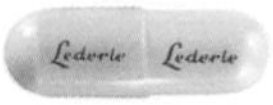

250 mg.

Procainamide HCl, U.S.P. Capsules

Lemmon

35 mg.

Statobex®-G **Statobex®**

(phendimetrazine tartrate)

Lederle Generics Ⓒ IV

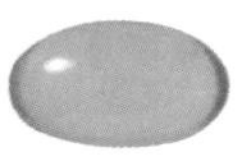

500 mg.

Chloral Hydrate, U.S.P. Capsules

Lederle Generics

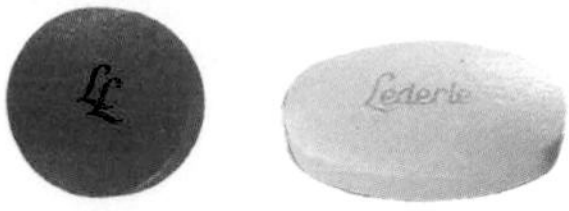

250 mg. 500 mg.

Erythromycin Stearate, U.S.P. Tablets

Lederle Generics Ⓒ IV

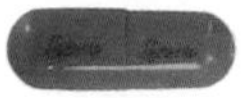

65 mg.

Propoxyphene HCl, U.S.P. Capsules

(DOLENE®)

ELI LILLY

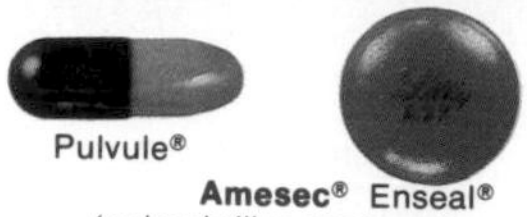

Pulvule®

Amesec® **Enseal®**

(aminophylline compound)

Lederle Generics Ⓒ IV

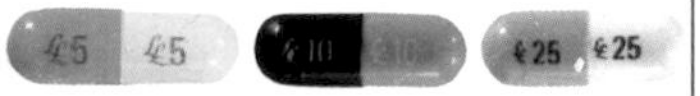

5 mg. 10 mg. 25 mg.

Chlordiazepoxide HCl, U.S.P. Capsules

Lederle Generics

25 mg. 50 mg.

Hydrochlorothiazide, U.S.P. Tablets

Lederle Generics Ⓒ IV

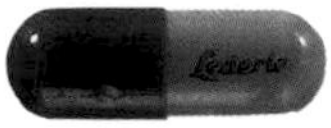

Propoxyphene HCl, U.S.P., Aspirin, Phenacetin, and Caffeine Capsules

(DOLENE® Compound-65)

Lilly Ⓒ II

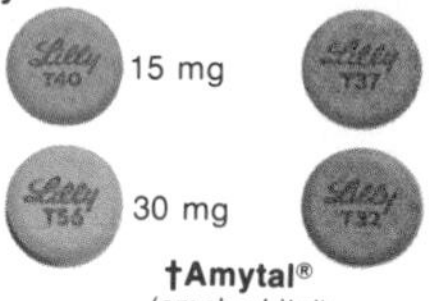

15 mg 50 mg 30 mg 100 mg

†Amytal®

(amobarbital)

Lederle Generics

4 mg. 8 mg. T.D.

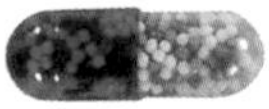

12 mg. T.D.

Chlorpheniramine Maleate, U.S.P. Tablets & Capsules

Lederle Generics

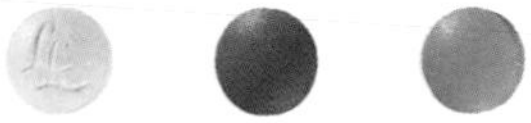

10 mg. 25 mg. 50 mg.

Imipramine HCl, U.S.P. Tablets

Lederle Generics Ⓒ IV

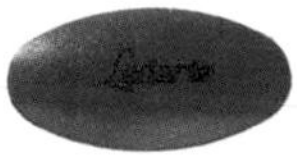

Propoxyphene HCl, U.S.P., Acetaminophen, U.S.P. Tablets

(DOLENE® AP-65)

Lilly Ⓒ II

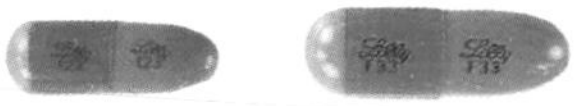

65 mg. 200 mg.

†Amytal® Sodium

(amobarbital sodium)

Lederle Generics

Lederle logo appears on reverse sides

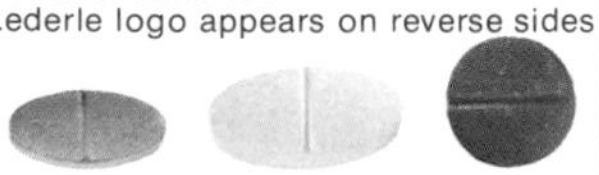

12.5 mg. 25 mg. 25 mg. (chewable)

Meclizine HCl, U.S.P.

Lederle Generics

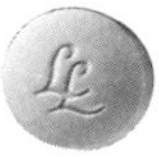

200 mg.

Quinidine Sulfate, U.S.P. Tablets

Lilly

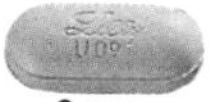

2 mg.

Anhydron®

(cyclothiazide)

Lederle Generics

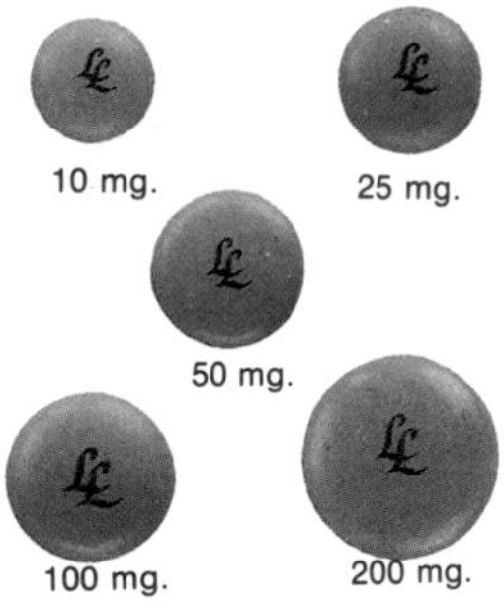

10 mg. 25 mg. 50 mg. 100 mg. 200 mg.

Chlorpromazine HCl, U.S.P. Tablets

Lederle Generics

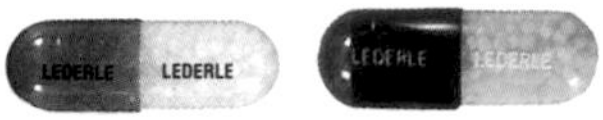

2.5 mg. T.D. 6.5 mg. T.D.

Nitroglycerin

LEMMON

Tablet Capsule

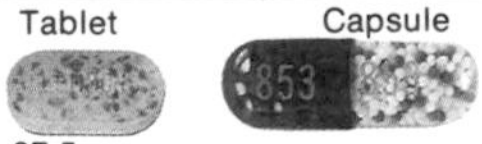

37.5 mg. 30 mg.—pelletized

Adipex-P®

(phentermine hydrochloride)

Lilly Ⓒ III

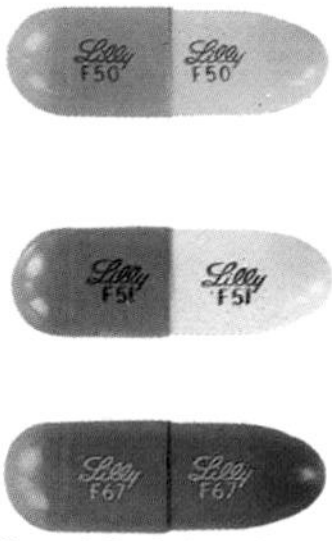

A.S.A.® and Codeine Compound

(aspirin, phenacetin, and caffeine with codeine)

Lederle Generics

150 mg. T.R.

Papaverine HCl Capsules

Lemmon

Tablets Capsule

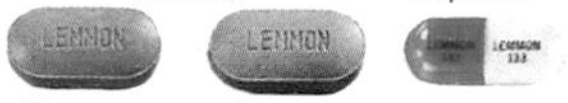

5 mg. 10 mg. 15 mg.

Dexampex™

(dextroamphetamine)

Lederle Generics

50 mg.

Dimenhydrinate, U.S.P. Tablets

Lederle Generics

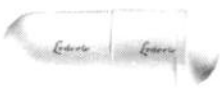

100 mg.

Phenytoin Sodium, U.S.P. Capsules

Lemmon

200 mg. 400 mg.

†Neothylline®

(dyphylline)

Lilly

10 mg. 25 mg.

†Aventyl® HCl

(nortriptyline hydrochloride)

Lederle Generics

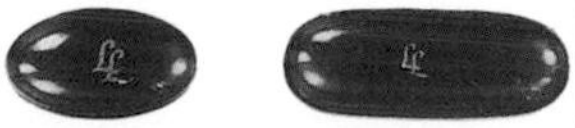

100 mg. 250 mg.

Dioctyl Sodium Sulfosuccinate, U.S.P Capsules

Lederle Generics

500 mg.

Probenecid, U.S.P. Tablets

Lemmon Ⓒ II

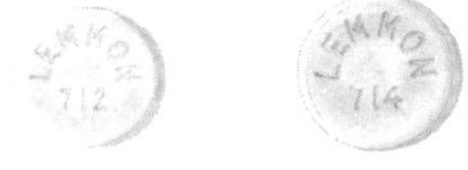

150 mg. 300 mg.

Quāālude®

(methaqualone)

Lilly

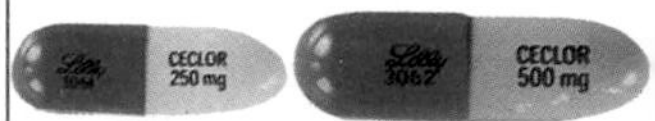

250 mg 500 mg

†Ceclor®

(cefaclor)

†Other dosage forms available. See Product Information section or check directly with manufacturer.

Lilly

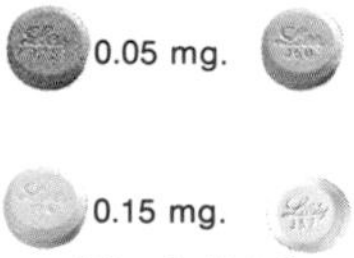

0.05 mg. 0.1 mg.

0.15 mg. 0.2 mg.

†Crystodigin®
(digitoxin)

Lilly

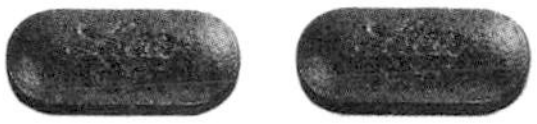

Darvocet-N® 50
(propoxyphene napsylate with acetaminophen)

Lilly

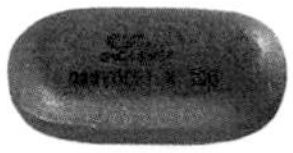

Darvocet-N® 100
(propoxyphene napsylate with acetaminophen)

Lilly

32 mg. 65 mg.

Darvon®
(propoxyphene hydrochloride)

Lilly

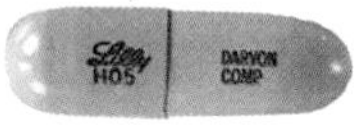

Darvon® Compound
(propoxyphene hydrochloride and APC)

Lilly

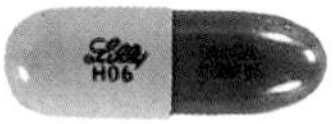

Darvon® Compound-65
(propoxyphene hydrochloride and APC)

Lilly

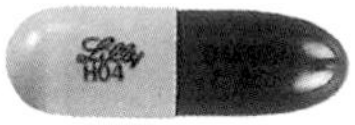

Darvon® with A.S.A.®
(propoxyphene hydrochloride and aspirin)

Lilly

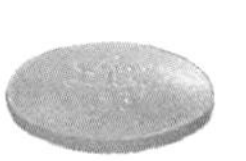

100 mg.

†Darvon-N®
(propoxyphene napsylate)

Lilly

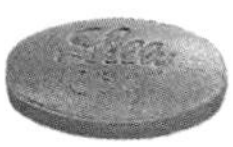

Darvon-N® with A.S.A.®
(100 mg. propoxyphene napsylate and 325 mg. aspirin)

Lilly

(Vials shown smaller than actual size)

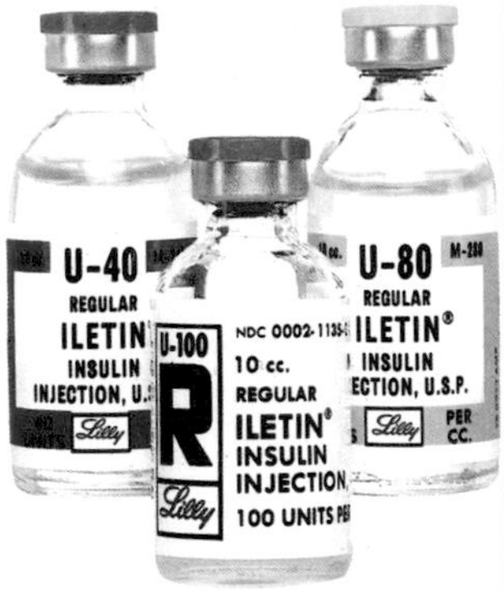

Regular Iletin®
Insulin Injection, USP

U-40, U-80, U-100

Lilly

(Vials shown smaller than actual size)

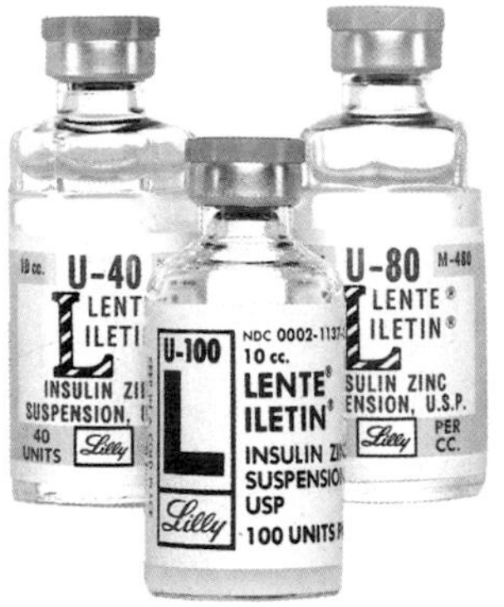

Lente® Iletin®
Insulin Zinc Suspension, USP

U-40, U-80, U-100

Lilly

(Vials shown smaller than actual size)

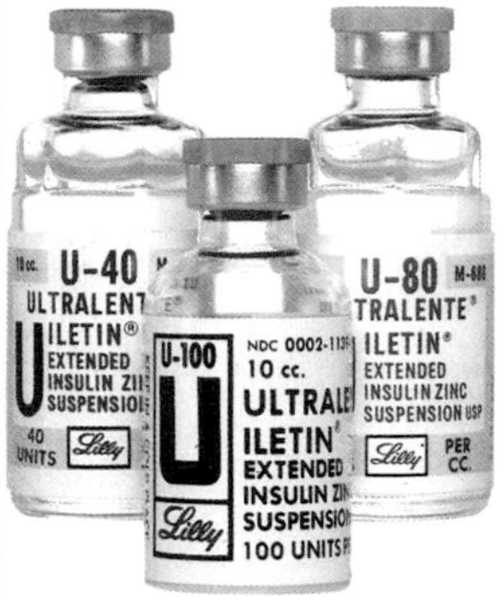

Ultralente® Iletin®
Extended Insulin Zinc Suspension, USP

U-40, U-80, U-100

Lilly

(Vials shown smaller than actual size)

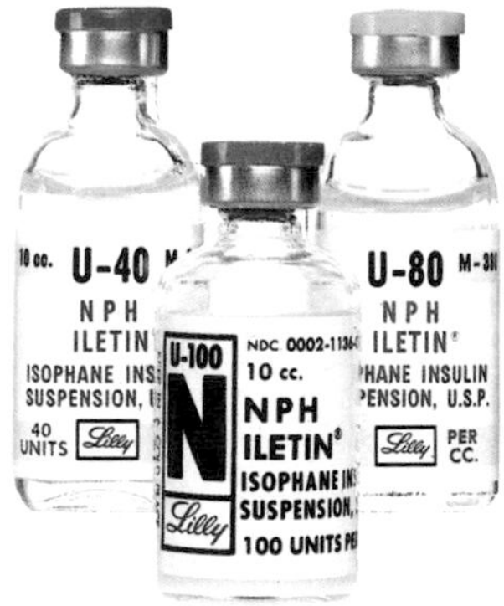

NPH Iletin®
Isophane Insulin Suspension, USP

U-40, U-80, U-100

Lilly

(Vials shown smaller than actual size)

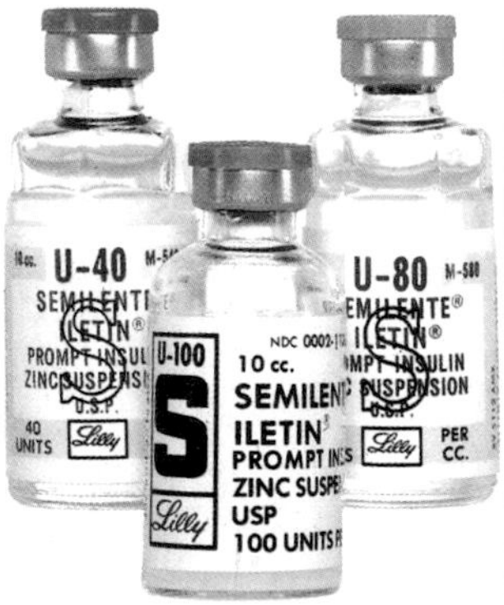

Semilente® Iletin®
Prompt Insulin Zinc Suspension, USP

U-40, U-80, U-100

Lilly

(Shown smaller than actual size)

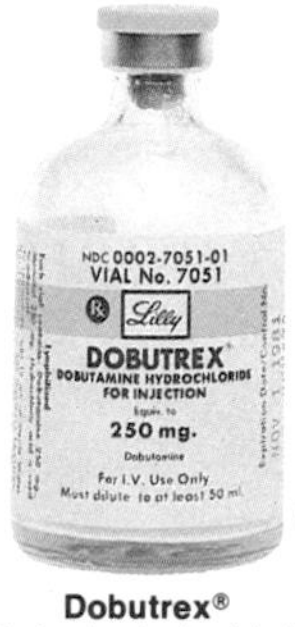

250 mg

Dobutrex®
(dobutamine hydrochloride)

Lilly

250 mg. 500 mg.

Dymelor®
(acetohexamide)

Lilly

(Vials shown smaller than actual size)

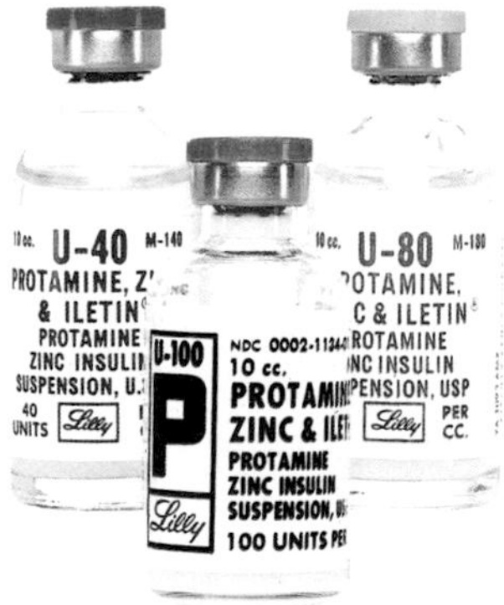

Protamine, Zinc & Iletin®
Protamine Zinc
Insulin Suspension, USP

U-40, U-80, U-100

IDENTI-CODE®

(formula identification code, Lilly)
Provides Positive Product Identification

A letter-number symbol, a four-digit number, the name of the product, the strength of the product, or a combination of these appears on each Lilly capsule and most tablets and on each label of pediatric liquids, powders for oral suspension, and suppositories. The letter/number or four-digit number identifies the product,which is listed in the Lilly IDENTI-CODE® INDEX.

For example:

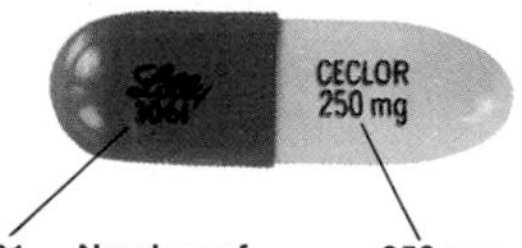

3061 = Number of product

250 mg = Strength of product

The complete IDENTI-CODE® INDEX appears in the Product Information Section under Eli Lilly and Company.

†Other dosage forms available. See Product Information section or check directly with manufacturer.

Lilly Ⓒ II

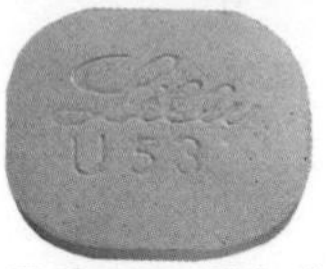

Methadone Disket®

Lilly Ⓒ II

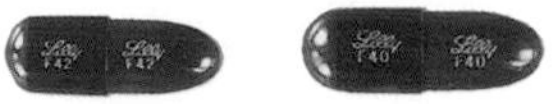

50 mg. 100 mg.

†Seconal® Sodium
(secobarbital sodium)

Lilly

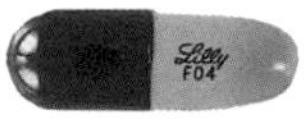

250 mg.

Seromycin®
(cycloserine)

Lilly Ⓒ II

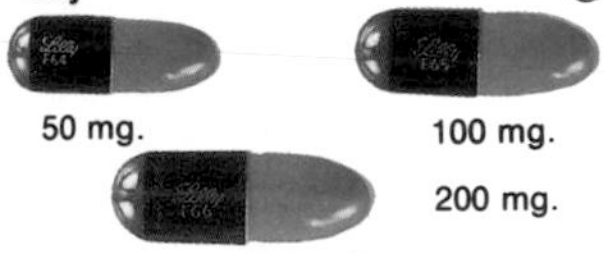

50 mg. 100 mg. 200 mg.

Tuinal®
(secobarbital sodium and amobarbital sodium)

Lilly

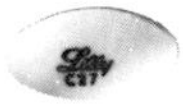

125 mg.

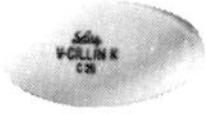

250 mg.

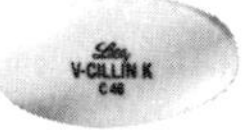

500 mg.

†V-Cillin K®
(penicillin V potassium)

Lilly

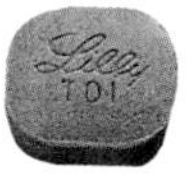

†Zentron® Chewable
(iron, vitamin B complex, and vitamin C)

Designed to help you identify drugs, this section contains actual size, full-color reproductions of products selected for inclusion by participating manufacturers.

While every effort has been made to reproduce products faithfully, this section is to be considered a quick-reference identification aid. In cases of suspected overdosage, etc., chemical analysis of the product should be done.

MARION

(shown smaller than actual size) Ⓒ V

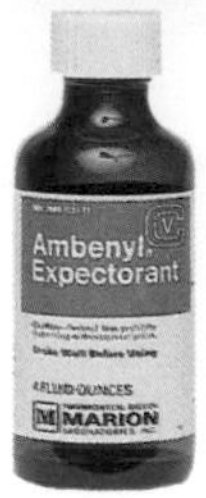

Available in 4-oz., 1-pint and 1-gallon bottles

Ambenyl® Expectorant

Marion
(shown smaller than actual size)

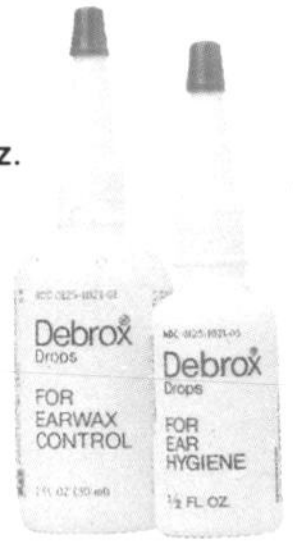

1 fl. oz. ½ fl. oz.

Debrox® Drops

Marion
(both sides of tablet shown)

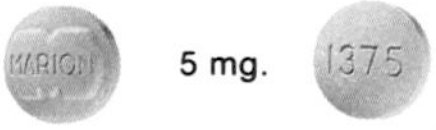

5 mg.

Ditropan® Tablets
(oxybutynin chloride)

Marion

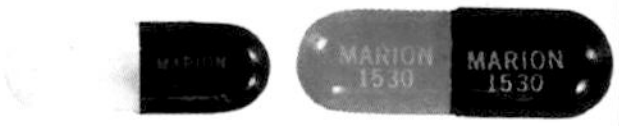

Duotrate® **Plateau CAPS®** **Duotrate® 45** **Plateau CAPS®**
(pentaerythritol tetranitrate)

Marion (both sides of tablet shown)

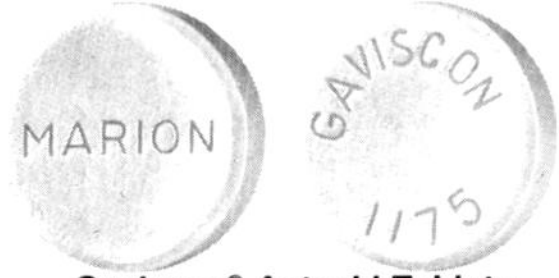

Gaviscon® Antacid Tablets

Marion (both sides of tablet shown)

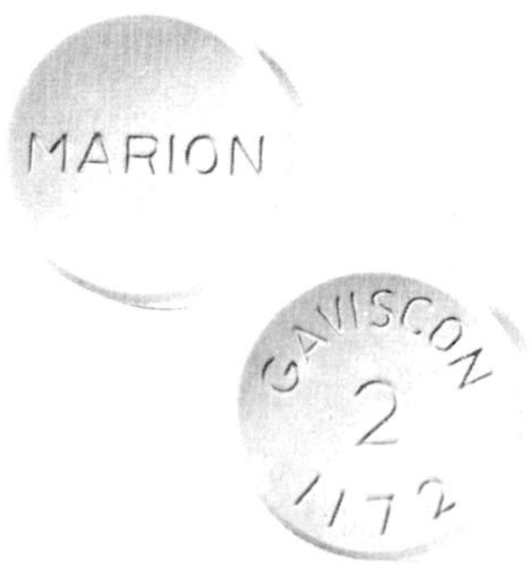

Gaviscon®-2 Antacid Tablets

Marion
(shown smaller than actual size)

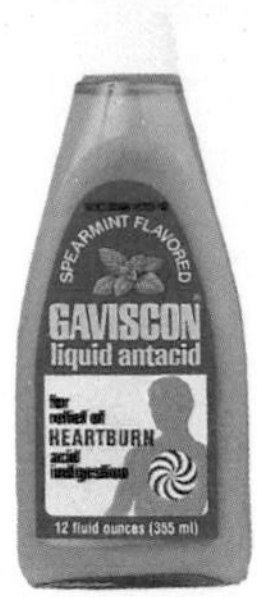

12 oz.

Gaviscon® Liquid Antacid

Marion
(shown smaller than actual size)

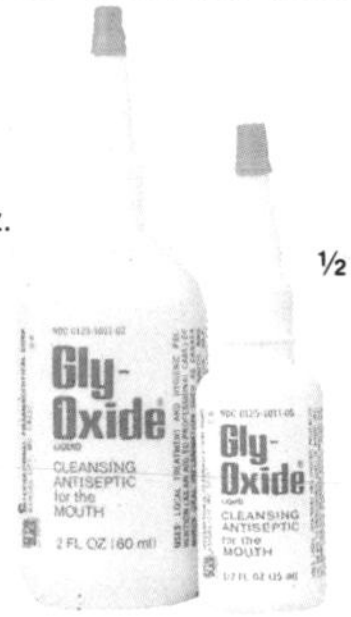

2 fl. oz. ½ fl. oz.

Gly-Oxide® Liquid

Marion

400 mg.

Nico-400® Plateau CAPS®
(nicotinic acid)

Marion

(shown smaller than actual size)

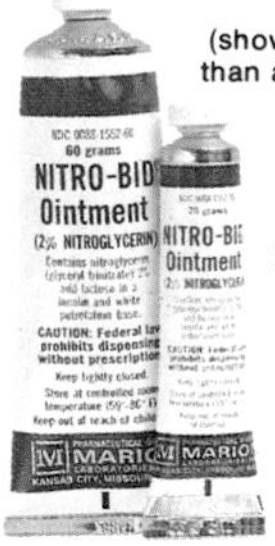

60 gm. 20 gm.

Nitro-Bid® Ointment
(nitroglycerin 2%)

Marion

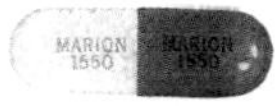

2.5 mg.

Nitro-Bid® 2.5 Plateau CAPS®
(nitroglycerin)

Marion

6.5 mg.

Nitro-Bid® 6.5 Plateau CAPS®
(nitroglycerin)

Marion

9 mg.

Nitro-Bid® 9 Plateau CAPS®
(nitroglycerin)

Marion

Os-Cal®

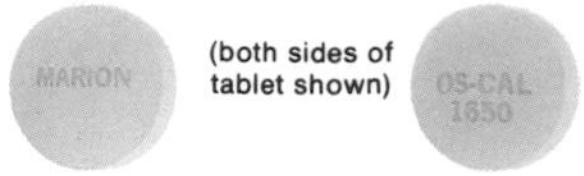

(both sides of tablet shown)

Os-Cal® 500

Os-Cal Forte®

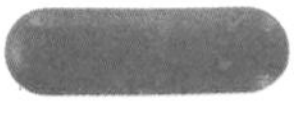

Os-Cal-Gesic®

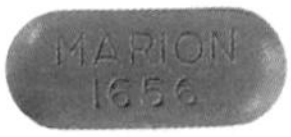

Os-Cal® Plus

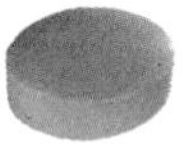

(oyster shell calcium family)

Marion

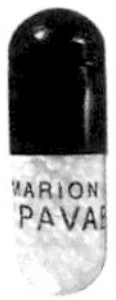

Pavabid® Plateau CAPS®
(papaverine HCl)
150 mg.

Marion (both sides of tablet shown)

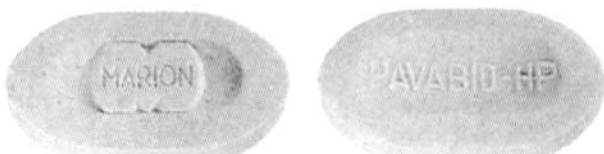

300 mg.

Pavabid® HP Capsulets
(papaverine hydrochloride)

Marion

(shown smaller than actual size)

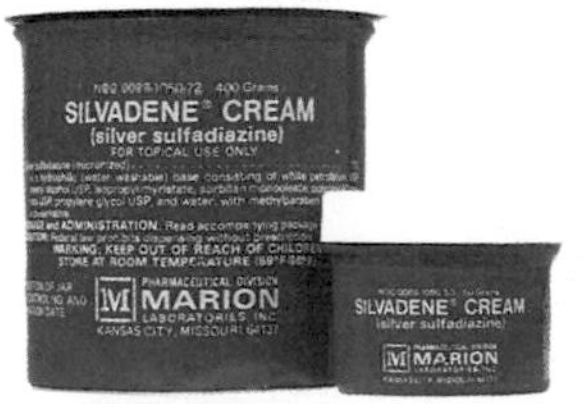

400 gm. 50 gm.

Silvadene® Cream
(silver sulfadiazine, micronized)

†Other dosage forms available. See Product Information section or check directly with manufacturer.

Marion

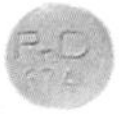

1 grain, plain
(Also available in ½-grain and 2-grain plain tablets)

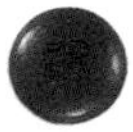

1 grain, sugar-coated
(Also available in ½-grain, 2-grain, and 3-grain sugar-coated tablets)
Thyroid Strong Tablets

McNEIL

Ⓒ III

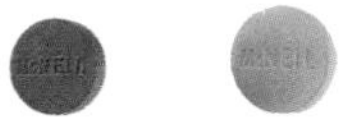

15 mg. 30 mg.
†BUTISOL SODIUM®
(sodium butabarbital)

McNeil

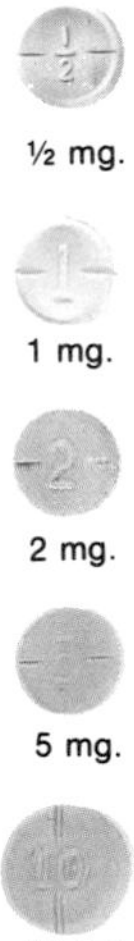

Concentrate
2 mg. per ml.

½ mg.

1 mg.

2 mg.

5 mg.

10 mg. tablets

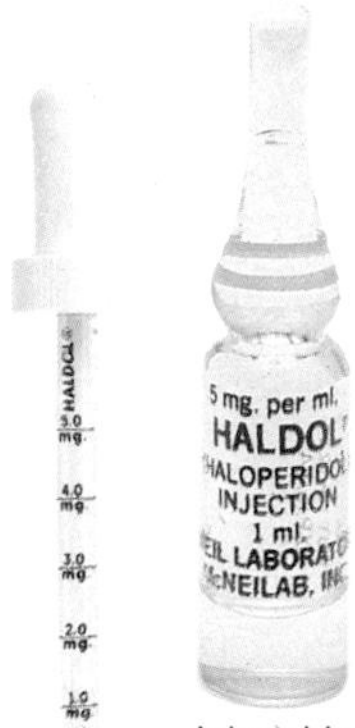

Injectable
5 mg. per ml.
(1 ml./ampul)

HALDOL®
(haloperidol)

McNeil

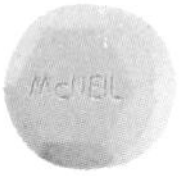

PARAFON FORTE®
tablets

McNeil

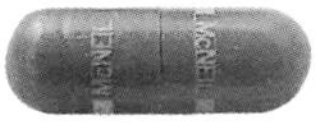

400 mg.
TOLECTIN® DS
(tolmetin sodium) capsules

McNeil

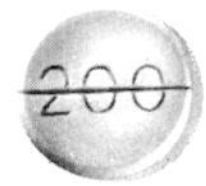

200 mg.
TOLECTIN®
(tolmetin sodium) tablets

McNeil Ⓒ III

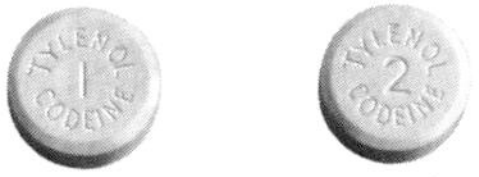

No. 1 (⅛ gr.) No. 2 (¼ gr.)

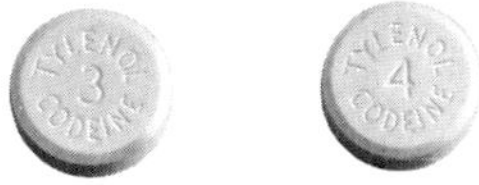

No. 3 (½ gr.) No. 4 (1 gr.)
†TYLENOL® with Codeine
tablets
also available Ⓒ V
TYLENOL® with Codeine elixir

McNeil Ⓒ II

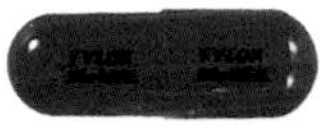

TYLOX®
capsules

McNeil Consumer Products

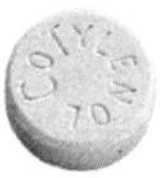

Also available: Children's CoTylenol® Liquid Cold Formula; for adults, CoTylenol® Liquid Cold Formula (with Cough Suppressant)
CoTylenol® Cold Formula Tablets

McNeil Consumer Products

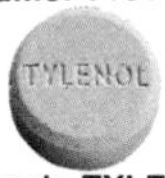

80 mg.
Children's TYLENOL® Chewable Tablets
(acetaminophen)
Also Available: Children's TYLENOL® Elixir and Infants' TYLENOL® Drops

McNeil Consumer Products

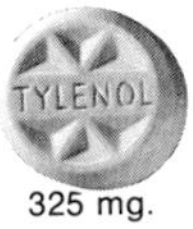

325 mg.
TYLENOL® Tablets
(acetaminophen)

McNeil Consumer Products

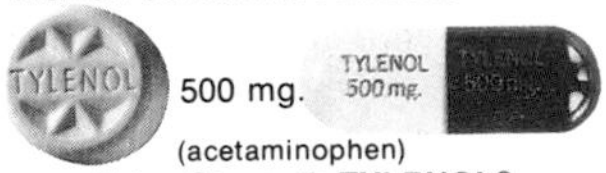

500 mg.
(acetaminophen)
Extra-Strength TYLENOL® Tablets and Capsules
Also Available: Extra-Strength TYLENOL® Adult Liquid

Because tablets and capsules are shown in this section, do not infer that these are the only dosage forms available. Where a product name is preceded by the symbol†, refer to the description in the Product Information (White Section) for other forms.

Mead Johnson Pharm. Div.

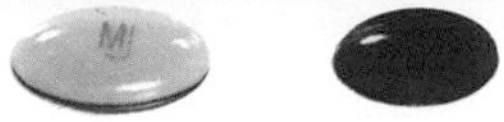

100 mg. 50 mg.
†Colace® Capsules
(docusate sodium)

Mead Johnson Pharmaceutical Division

25 mg. 50 mg.
†Cytoxan® Tablets
(cyclophosphamide)

Mead Johnson Pharmaceutical Division

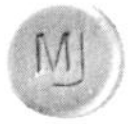

Sublingual tablet, 1.0 mg.
Deapril-ST®
(dihydroergotoxine mesylate)

Mead Johnson Pharmaceutical Division

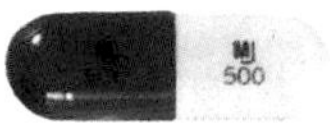

500 mg.
Capsules
Duricef®
(cefadroxil)

Mead Johnson Pharmaceutical Division

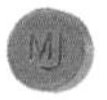

Scored Tablets

1 mg. 2 mg.
Estrace®
(estradiol)

Mead Johnson Pharmaceutical Division

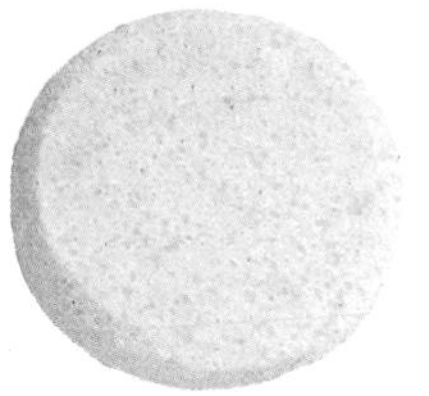

lime flavor

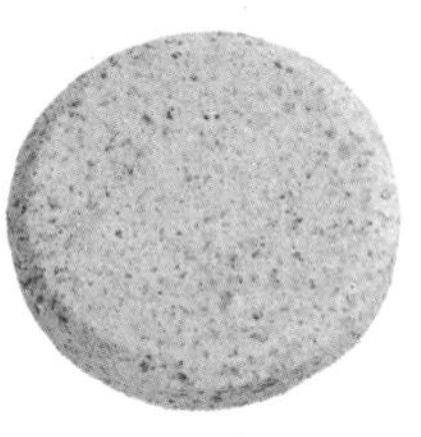

orange flavor
K-Lyte® Effervescent Tablets
Potassium Supplement

Mead Johnson Pharmaceutical Division

citrus flavor

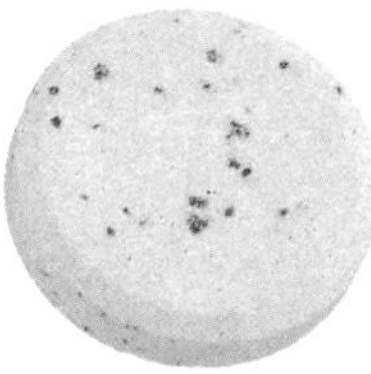

fruit punch flavor
K-Lyte/Cl® Effervescent Tablets
Potassium Chloride Supplement

Mead Johnson Pharmaceutical Division

20 mg. 40 mg.
Megace® Tablets
(megestrol acetate)

Mead Johnson Pharmaceutical Division

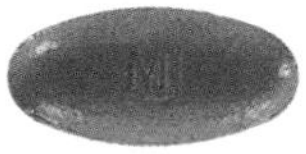

Natalins® Tablets
Multivitamin and Multimineral Supplement

Mead Johnson Pharmaceutical Division

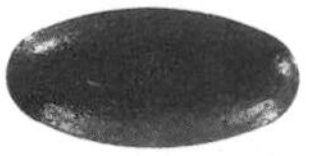

Natalins® Rx Tablets
Multivitamin and Multimineral Supplement

Mead Johnson Pharmaceutical Division

Ovcon®-50
(each yellow tablet contains 1 mg. norethindrone and 0.05 mg. ethinyl estradiol)

Mead Johnson Pharmaceutical Division

Ovcon®-35
(each tablet contains 0.4 mg. norethindrone and 0.035 mg. ethinyl estradiol)

Mead Johnson Pharmaceutical Division

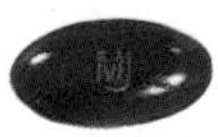

†Peri-Colace® Capsules
(casanthranol and docusate sodium)

†Other dosage forms available. See Product Information section or check directly with manufacturer.

Mead Johnson Pharmaceutical Division

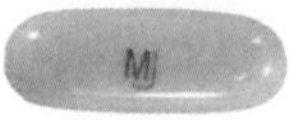

†Quibron® Capsules
(theophylline-glyceryl guaiacolate)

Mead Johnson Pharmaceutical Division

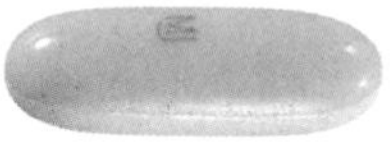

300 mg.
Quibron®-300 Capsules
(theophylline-glyceryl guaiacolate)

Mead Johnson Pharmaceutical Division

†Quibron Plus® Capsules
(theophylline-glyceryl guaiacolate-ephedrine HCl-butabarbital)

Mead Johnson Pharmaceutical Division

10 mg. 20 mg.
†Vasodilan® Tablets
(isoxsuprine HCl)

MEDICONE

Rectal Medicone® Suppository
(Gold Foil Wrapped)

Medicone

Rectal Medicone®-HC Suppository
(Pink Foil Wrapped)

Merck Sharp & Dohme

612* 634*

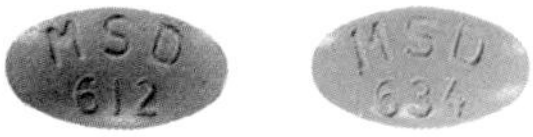

150 250
ALDOCLOR®

Merck Sharp & Dohme

423* 456*

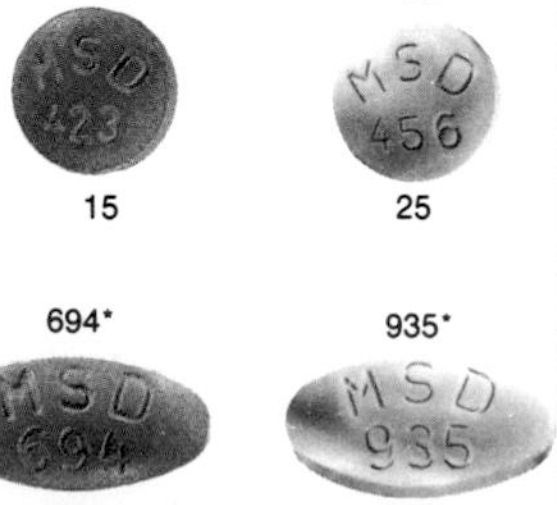

15 25

694* 935*

D30 D50
ALDORIL®

Merck Sharp & Dohme

135* 401* 516*

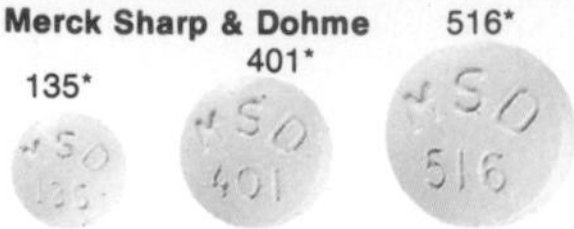

125 mg. 250 mg. 500 mg.
†ALDOMET®
(methyldopa | MSD)

Merck Sharp & Dohme

501*

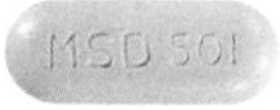

0.5 g.
BENEMID®
(probenecid | MSD)

Merck Sharp & Dohme

941* 942*

150 200
CLINORIL®
(sulindac | MSD)

Merck Sharp & Dohme

60* 635* 21*

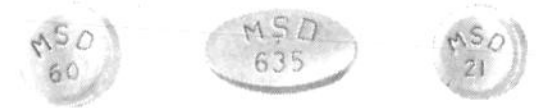

2 mg. 1 mg. 0.5 mg.
†COGENTIN®
(benztropine mesylate | MSD)

Merck Sharp & Dohme

614*

ColBENEMID®

Merck Sharp & Dohme

672* 602*

125 mg. 250 mg.
CUPRIMINE®
(penicillamine | MSD)

Merck Sharp & Dohme

20* 41*

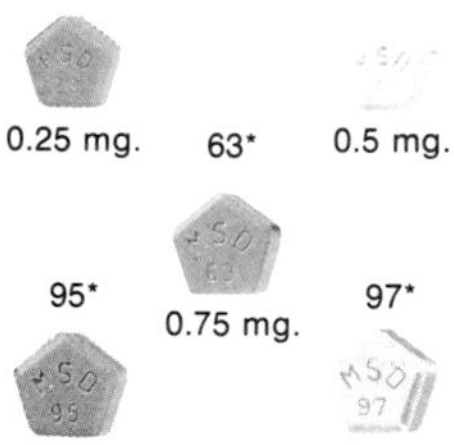

0.25 mg. 63* 0.5 mg.

95* 0.75 mg. 97*

1.5 mg. 4 mg.
†DECADRON®
(dexamethasone | MSD)

Merck Sharp & Dohme

230* 405*

250 500
DIUPRES®

MERCK SHARP & DOHME
PRODUCT IDENTIFICATION CODE

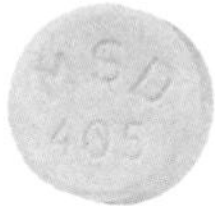

DIUPRES-500

MSD tablet and capsule products bear an identification code.
The code designation bears the initials MSD plus a code number. As illustrated above, DIUPRES-500 is identified as MSD 405.
For a complete listing of Merck Sharp & Dohme Identification Codes, see Product Information Section.

Merck Sharp & Dohme

214* 432*

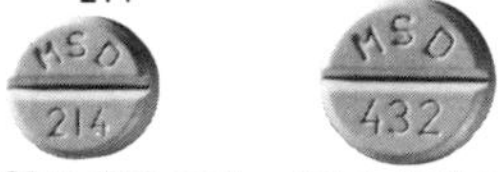

0.25 g. (250 mg.) 0.5 g. (500 mg.)
†DIURIL®
(chlorothiazide | MSD)

Merck Sharp & Dohme

65* 90*

25 mg. 50 mg.
†EDECRIN®
(ethacrynic acid | MSD)

Merck Sharp & Dohme

23* 45* 102*

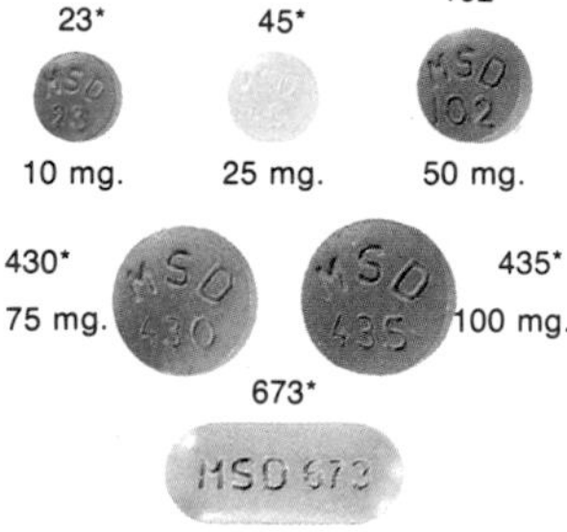

10 mg. 25 mg. 50 mg.

430* 435*
75 mg. 100 mg.

673*

150 mg.
†ELAVIL®
(amitriptyline HCl | MSD)

Merck Sharp & Dohme

931*

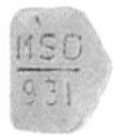

10 mg.
FLEXERIL®
(cyclobenzaprine HCl | MSD)

Merck Sharp & Dohme

42* 105* 410*

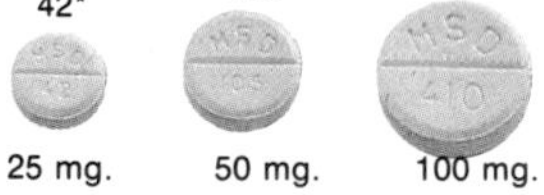

25 mg. 50 mg. 100 mg.
HydroDIURIL®
(hydrochlorothiazide | MSD)

Merck Sharp & Dohme

53* 127*

25 50
HYDROPRES®

Merck Sharp & Dohme

25* 50*

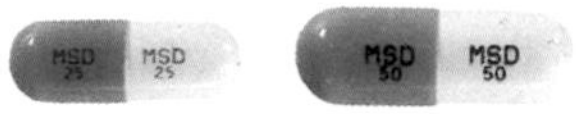

25 mg. 50 mg.
INDOCIN®
(indomethacin | MSD)

Merck Sharp & Dohme

62*

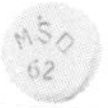

4 mg.
†PERIACTIN®
(cyproheptadine hydrochloride | MSD)

Merck Sharp & Dohme

647* 650* 654*

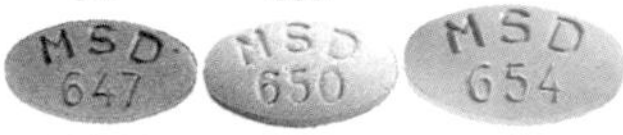

10/100 25/100 25/250
SINEMET®

Merck Sharp & Dohme

946* 921* 517*

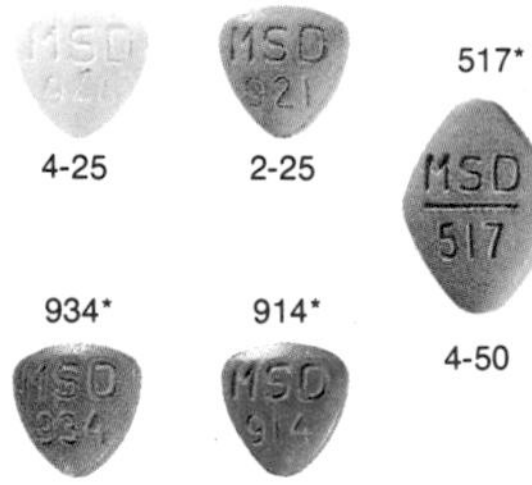

4-25 2-25

934* 914* 4-50

4-10 2-10

TRIAVIL®

Merck Sharp & Dohme

403* 412* 457*

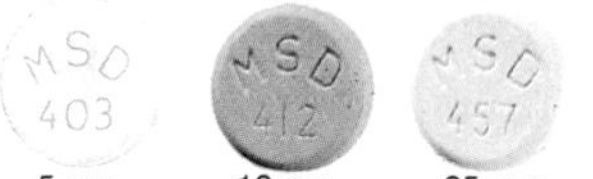

5 mg. 10 mg. 25 mg.
†URECHOLINE®
(bethanechol chloride | MSD)

Merck Sharp & Dohme

26* 47*

5 mg. 10 mg.
VIVACTIL®
(protriptyline hydrochloride | MSD)

†Other dosage forms available. See Product Information section or check directly with manufacturer.
*Manufacturers' identification number.

MERRELL-NATIONAL

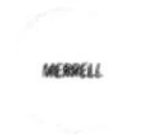

Bendectin®

Merrell-National

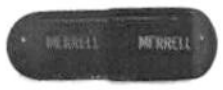

10 mg.

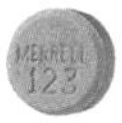

20 mg.

†Bentyl®
(dicyclomine hydrochloride USP)

Merrell-National

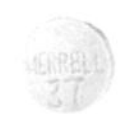

CANTIL®
(mepenzolate bromide 25 mg.)

Merrell-National

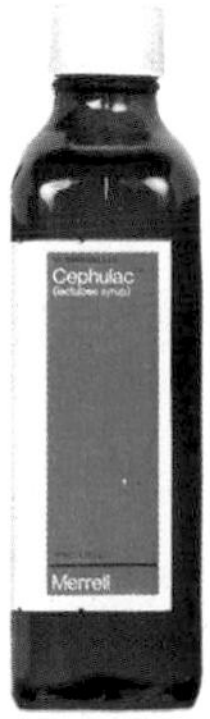

Cephulac®
(lactulose)
Syrup

(Shown smaller than actual size)

Merrell-National

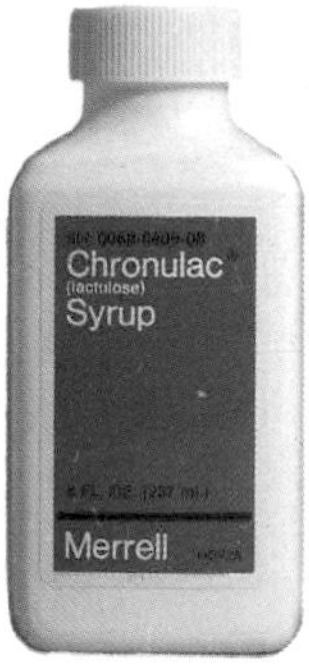

Chronulac®
(lactulose)
Syrup

(Shown smaller than actual size)

Merrell-National

1.0 Gm. Tablets
Hiprex®
(methenamine hippurate)

Merrell-National

2 mg. 4 mg.
Metahydrin®
(trichlormethiazide NF)

Merrell-National

2 mg. 4 mg.
Metatensin®
(trichlormethiazide 2 mg. or 4 mg.; reserpine 0.1 mg.)

Merrell-National

25 mg. 50 mg.

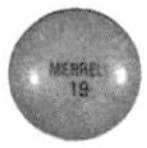

75 mg.

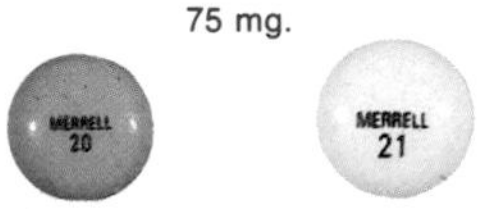

100 mg. 150 mg.
Norpramin®
(desipramine hydrochloride)

MERRELL-NATIONAL LABORATORIES Inc., Cayey, Puerto Rico

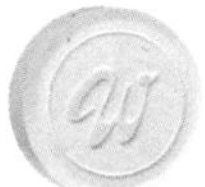

Quinamm™

Merrell-National

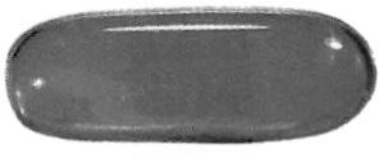

12 mg.

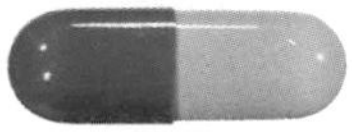

25 mg.

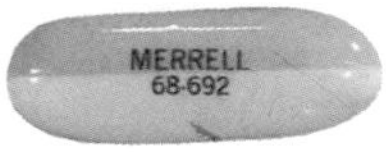

72 mg.
†TACE®
(CHLOROTRIANISENE NF)

MERRELL-NATIONAL LABORATORIES Inc., Cayey, Puerto Rico Ⓒ IV

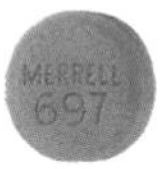

25 mg.
Tenuate®
(diethylpropion hydrochloride NF)

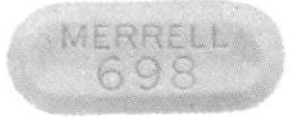

75 mg.
Tenuate Dospan®
(diethylproprion hydrochloride NF)

Merrell-National

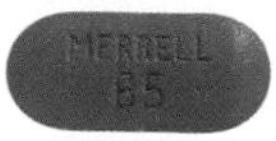

750 mg.
†Triclos®
(triclofos sodium)

Merrell-National

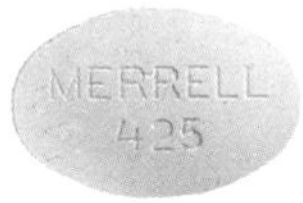

†Vanobid® Vaginal Tablets
(candicidin NF)

GLAXO

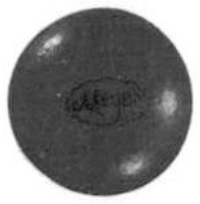

Athemol®

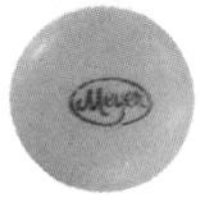

Athemol®-N*

(theobromine magnesium oleate 200 mg.)
*magnesium nicotinate 100 mg.

Glaxo
(Shown smaller than actual size)

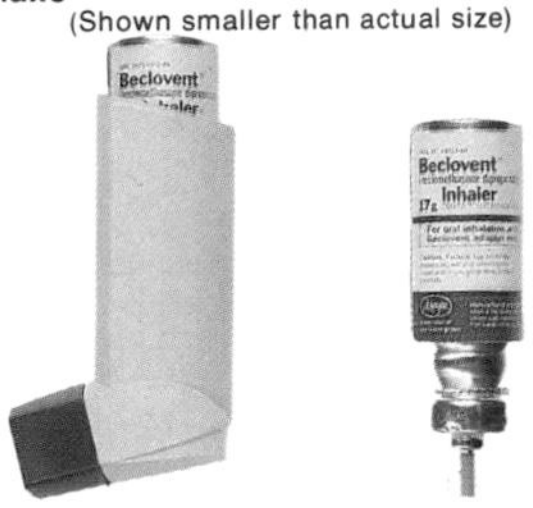

Beclovent® Inhaler
(beclomethasone dipropionate)
42 mcg. of beclomethasone dipropionate per inhalation

Glaxo

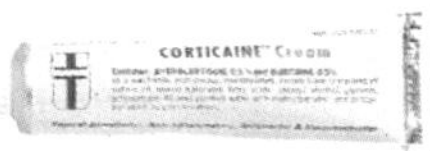

(Shown smaller than actual size)
Corticaine™ Cream
(hydrocortisone 0.5%, dibucaine 0.5%)

Glaxo

Ethatab® Tablets
(ethaverine hydrochloride 100 mg.)

Glaxo

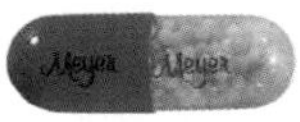

Histabid® Duracap® Capsules
(chlorpheniramine maleate 8 mg., phenylpropanolamine hydrochloride 75 mg.)

Glaxo

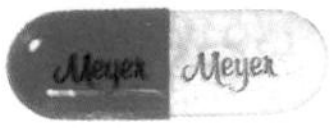

Theobid® Duracap® Capsules
(anhydrous theophylline 260 mg.)

Glaxo

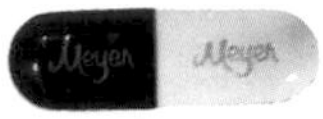

Tri-Cone® Capsules
(digestive enzymes with simethicone)

Glaxo

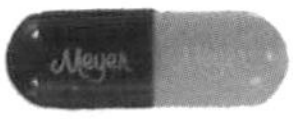

Tri-Cone® Plus
(digestive enzymes and simethicone plus hyoscyamine sulfate)

Glaxo

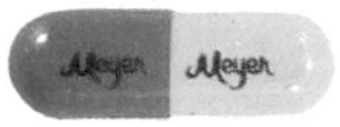

Vicon-C®
(B-Complex with Vitamin C, zinc and magnesium)

Glaxo

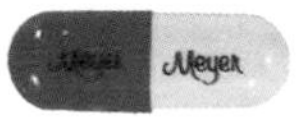

Vicon® Plus Capsules
(B-complex with Vitamin C, A, E, zinc, magnesium, and manganese)

Glaxo

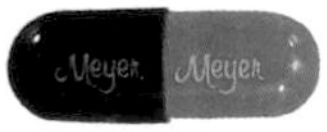

Vicon Forte® Capsules
(B-complex with C, A, E, zinc, magnesium, and manganese)

Glaxo

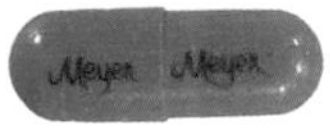

Vi-Zac® Capsules
(Vitamin A, C, and E with zinc)

Because tablets and capsules are shown in this section, do not infer that these are the only dosage forms available. Where a product name is preceded by the symbol†, refer to the description in the Product Information (White Section) for other forms.

†Other dosage forms available. See Product Information section or check directly with manufacturer.

OBETROL

Obetrol® 10 Obetrol® 20

O'Neal, Jones & Feldman

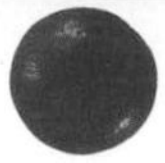

Iodo-Niacin®

O'Neal, Jones & Feldman

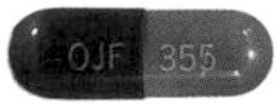

†Pedameth® Capsules
(dl-methionine, OJF)

ORGANON

391* 393*

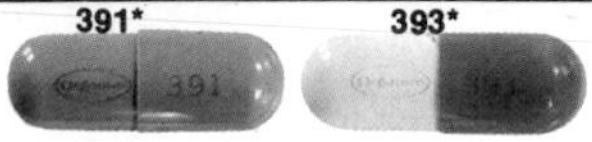

Accelerase® Accelerase® PB*
(pancrelipase N.F. with bile salts
*with phenobarbital)

Organon
381* 386*

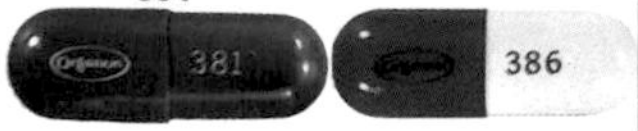

†Cotazym® †Cotazym® Cherry Flavored
(pancrelipase capsules N.F.)

Organon
384*

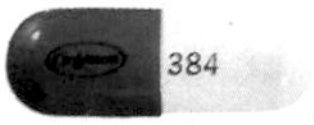

Cotazym®-65B
(pancrelipase N.F. with mixed conjugated bile salts)

Organon
798* 790* 791* 792*

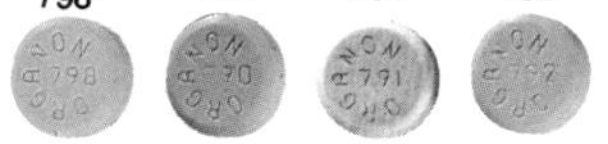

4.0 mg. 1.5 mg. 0.75 mg. 0.5 mg.
†Hexadrol®
(dexamethasone tablets, U.S.P.)

Organon
795*

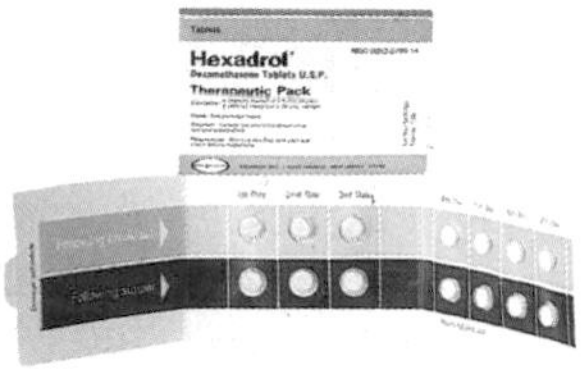

(pack shown smaller than actual size)

6 Hexadrol 1.5 mg. tablets and
8 Hexadrol 0.75 mg. tablets

Hexadrol® Therapeutic Pack
(dexamethasone tablets, U.S.P.)

Organon
821*

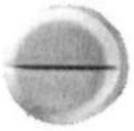

3 mg.
Liquamar®
(penprocouman tablets, N.F.)

Organon
685*

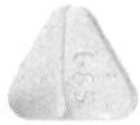

2 mg.
†Maxibolin®
(ethylestrenol)

Organon 546*

Wigraine® Suppositories

Organon
541*

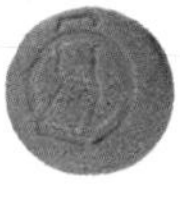

Wigraine®

ORTHO

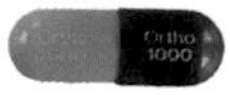

2 mg.
IMODIUM™ Capsules
(loperamide HCl)

Ortho

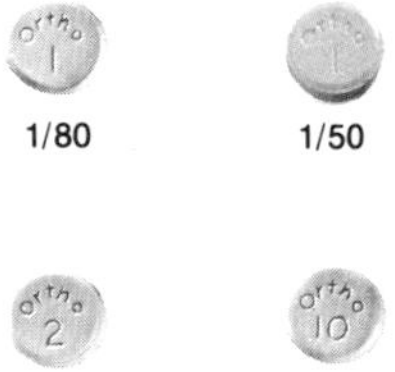

1/80 1/50
2 mg. 10 mg.
ORTHO-NOVUM™ Tablets
(norethindrone with mestranol)

Ortho

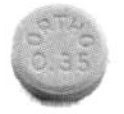

0.35 mg.
MICRONOR™ Tablets
(norethindrone)

Ortho

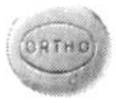

MODICON™ Tablets
(norethindrone with ethinyl estradiol)

Ortho

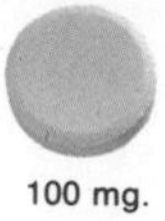

100 mg.
VERMOX™ Chewable Tablets
(mebendazole)

PARKE-DAVIS

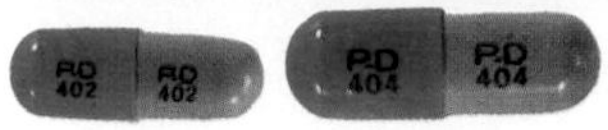

250 mg. 500 mg.
†Amcill® Capsules
(ampicillin capsules, USP) as the trihydrate

Parke-Davis

272* 273* 274*

10 mg. 25 mg. 50 mg.
275* 271* 278*

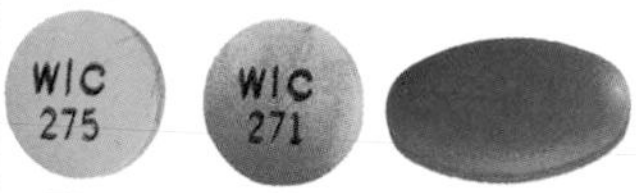

75 mg. 100 mg. 150 mg.
Amitril
(amitriptyline HCl)

Parke-Davis

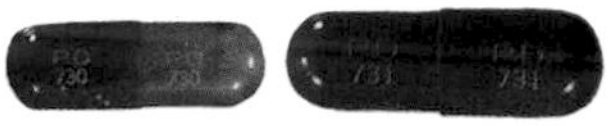

250 mg. 500 mg.
Amoxicillin
(Utimox)

Parke-Davis

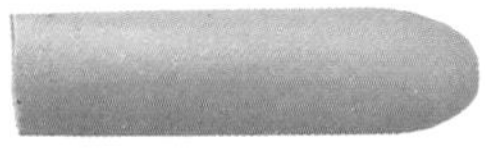

088*
Anusol® Suppositories

089*
Anusol-HC® Suppositories w/Hydrocortisone

Parke-Davis
(shown smaller than actual size)

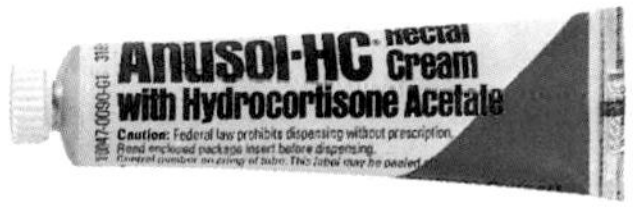

090*

28.4 gram tube

Anusol-HC®
(rectal cream with hydrocortisone acetate)

Parke-Davis

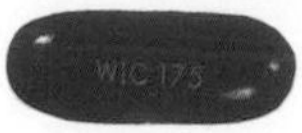

175*

Azo-Mandelamine®

Parke-Davis

50 mg. 25 mg.
Benadryl® Kapseals® Benadryl Capsules
(diphenhydramine hydrochloride capsules, USP)

Parke-Davis

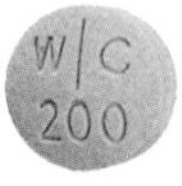

200*

†Brondecon®

Parke-Davis Ⓒ III

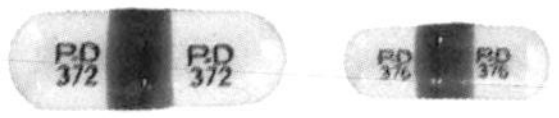

Carbrital® Kapseals® Carbrital Kapseals (Half Strength)

Parke-Davis

300 mg.
Celontin® Kapseals®
(methsuximide capsules, NF)

Parke-Davis

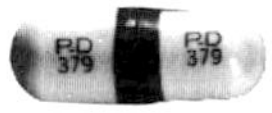

250 mg.
†Chloromycetin® Kapseals®
(chloramphenicol capsules, USP)

Parke-Davis

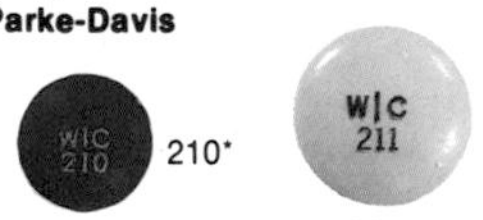

210* 211*
100 mg. 200 mg.
†Choledyl®
(oxtriphylline)

Parke-Davis

30 mg. 100 mg.
†Dilantin® Kapseals®
(phenytoin sodium capsules, USP)

Parke-Davis

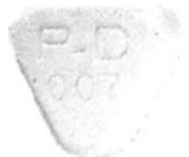

50 mg.
Dilantin® Infatabs®
(phenytoin tablets, USP)

†Other dosage forms available. See Product Information section or check directly with manufacturer.
*Manufacturers' identification number.

Parke-Davis

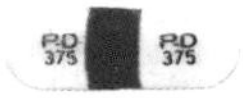

†Dilantin® (phenytoin sodium) **with ¼ gr. Phenobarbital Kapseals®**

Parke-Davis

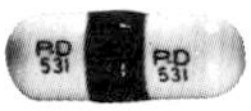

†Dilantin® (phenytoin sodium) **with ½ gr. Phenobarbital Kapseals®**

Parke-Davis

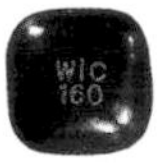

182*

Pyridium® Plus
(formerly Doloril®)

Parke-Davis

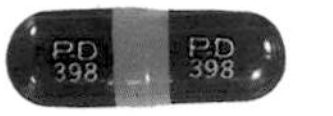

Eldec® Kapseals®

Parke-Davis

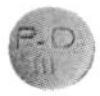

Ergostat®
(ergotamine tartrate tablets)
Sublingual Tablets, 2 mg.

Parke-Davis

250 mg.

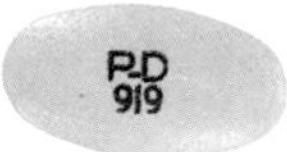

500 mg.

Erythromycin Stearate Tablets, USP
(Erypar® Filmseal®)

Parke-Davis

260*

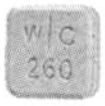

-½

261*

-1

262*

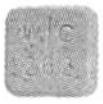

-2

263*

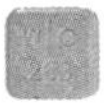

-3

Euthroid®
(liotrix)

Parke-Davis

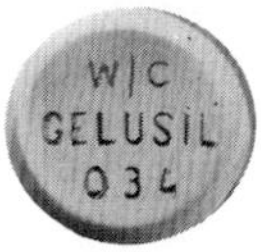

034*

†Gelusil®

Parke-Davis

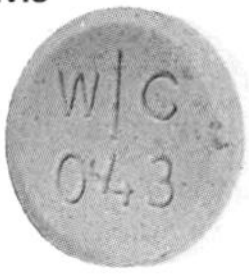

043*

†Gelusil® II

Parke-Davis

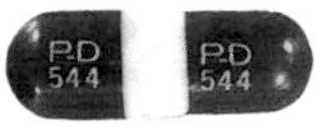

†Geriplex-FS® Kapseals®

Parke-Davis

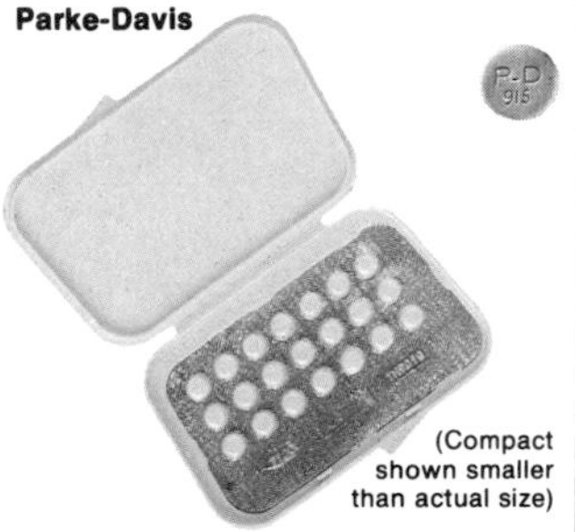

(Compact shown smaller than actual size)

Loestrin® 21 1/20
(1 mg. norethindrone acetate and 20 mcg. ethinyl estradiol tablets, USP)

Parke-Davis

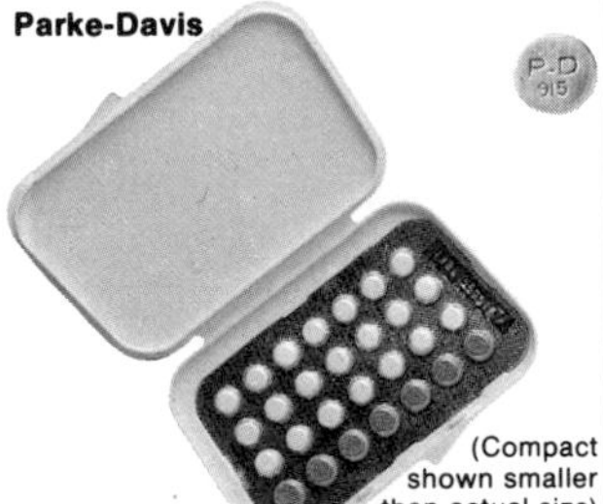

(Compact shown smaller than actual size)

Loestrin® Fe 1/20
(1 mg. norethindrone acetate and 20 mcg. ethinyl estradiol tablets, USP)
Each brown tablet contains 75 mg. ferrous fumarate, USP.

Parke-Davis

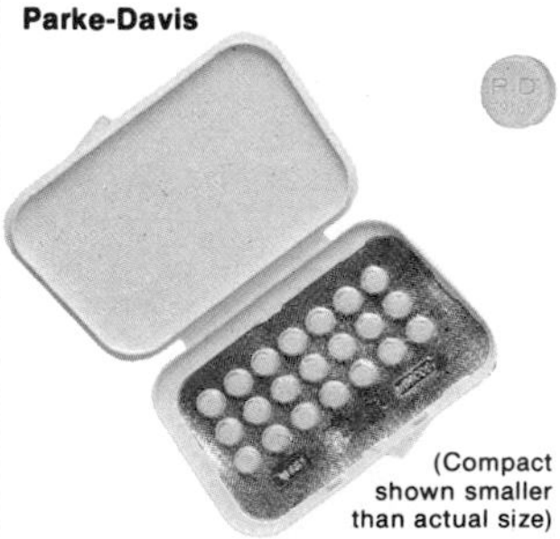

(Compact shown smaller than actual size)

Loestrin® 21 1.5/30
(1.5 mg. norethindrone acetate and 30 mcg ethinyl estradiol tablets, USP)

Parke-Davis

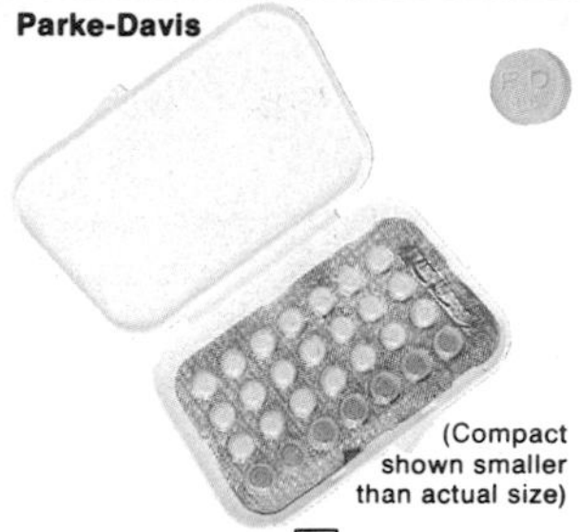

(Compact shown smaller than actual size)

Loestrin® Fe 1.5/30
(1.5 mg. norethindrone acetate and 30 mcg. ethinyl estradiol tablets, USP)
Each brown tablet contains 75 mg. ferrous fumarate, USP.

Parke-Davis

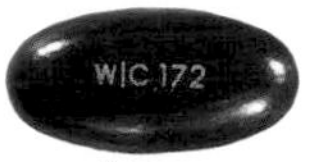

172*

1 gram
†Mandelamine®
(methenamine mandelate)

Parke-Davis

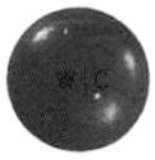

270*

15 mg.
Nardil®
(phenelzine sulfate)

Parke-Davis

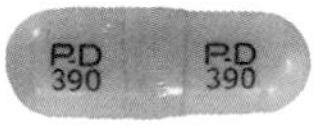

Natabec® Kapseals®

Parke-Davis

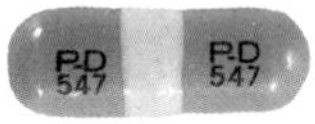

Natabec Rx® Kapseals®

Parke-Davis
(Bottles shown smaller than actual size)

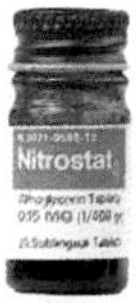

0.15 mg.

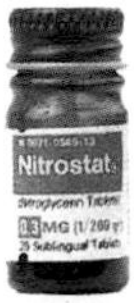

0.3 mg

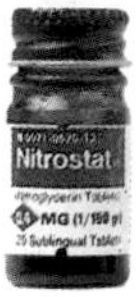

0.4 mg.

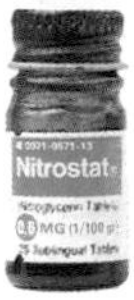

0.6 mg

Nitrostat®
(nitroglycerin tablets, USP) Sublingual Tablets

Parke-Davis

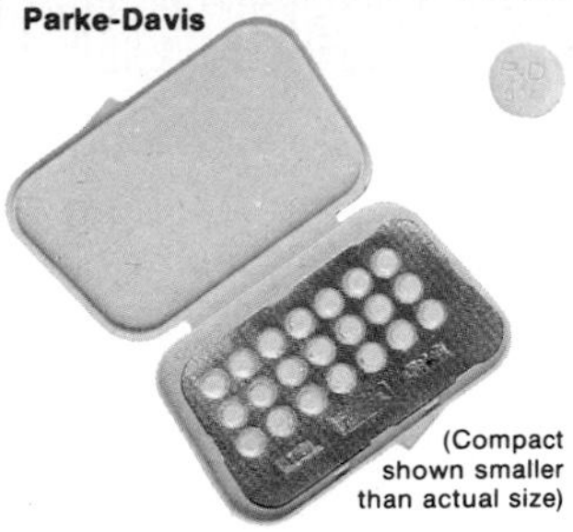

(Compact shown smaller than actual size)

Norlestrin® 21 1/50
(1 mg. norethindrone acetate and 50 mcg. ethinyl estradiol tablets, USP)

Parke-Davis

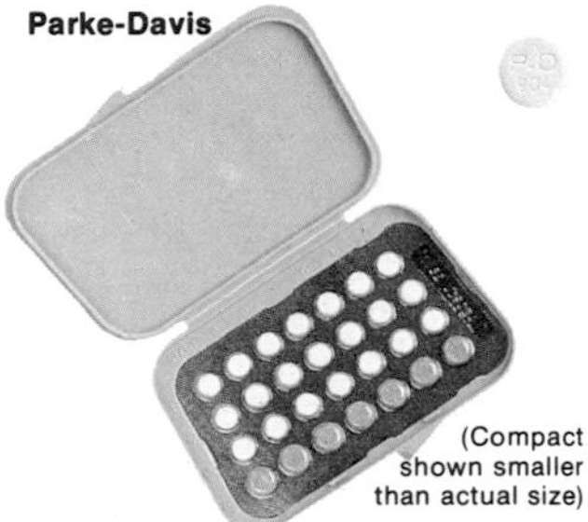

(Compact shown smaller than actual size)

Norlestrin® Fe 1/50
(1 mg. norethindrone acetate and 50 mcg. ethinyl estradiol tablets, USP)
Each brown tablet contains 75 mg ferrous fumarate USP.

Parke-Davis

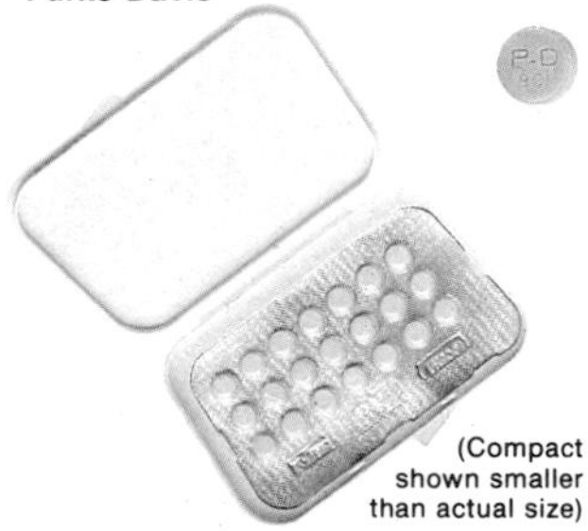

(Compact shown smaller than actual size)

Norlestrin® 21 2.5/50
(2.5 mg. norethindrone acetate and 50 mcg. ethinyl estradiol tablets, USP)

Parke-Davis

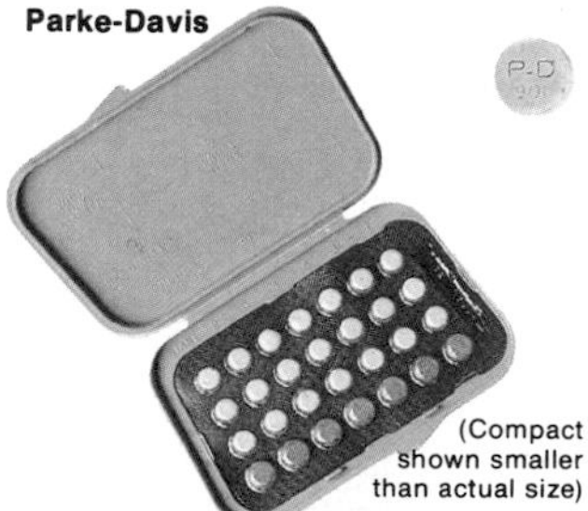

(Compact shown smaller than actual size)

Norlestrin® Fe 2.5/50
(2.5 mg. norethindrone acetate and 50 mcg. ethinyl estradiol tablets, USP)
Each brown tablet contains 75 mg. ferrous fumarate, USP.

Parke-Davis

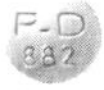

5 mg.

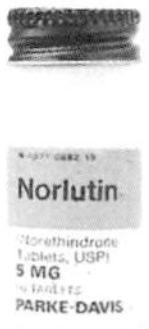

Norlutin® Tablets
(norethindrone tablets, USP)

(Bottle shown smaller than actual size)

†Other dosage forms available. See Product Information section or check directly with manufacturer.
*Manufacturers' identification number.

PARCODE® (Parke-Davis Accurate Recognition Code)

For Prompt, Accurate Product Identification

The imprinted P-D identifies the product as manufactured by Parke-Davis. The imprinted number designates the particular Parke-Davis Product.

Parke-Davis

Dilantin® Infatabs®
(phenytoin tablets, USP)
50 mg.

Amcill® Capsules
(ampicillin capsules, USP)
as the trihydrate,
500 mg.

A complete listing of PARCODE and W/C code numbers appears at the beginning of Parke-Davis Product monographs in the white section.

Parke-Davis Ⓒ III

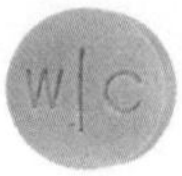

65 mg. 310*

Pre-Sate®
(chlorphentermine HCl)

Parke-Davis

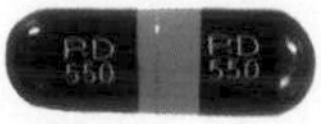

Thera-Combex H-P® Kapseals®

Parke-Davis

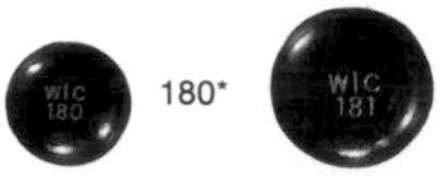

180* 181*

Pyridium® 100 mg. Pyridium® 200 mg.
(phenazopyridine hydrochloride)

Parke-Davis
(Tubes shown smaller than actual size)

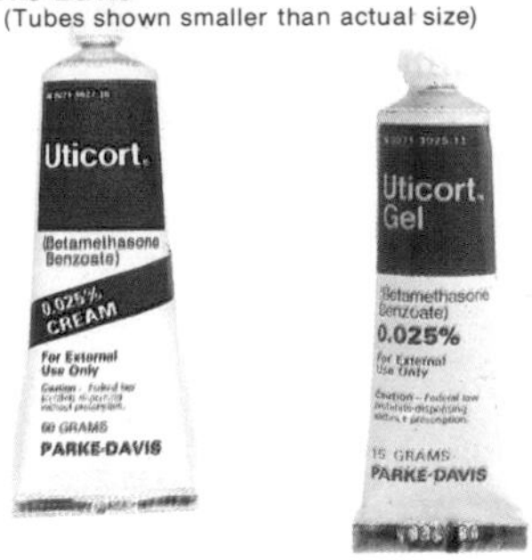

Uticort® Cream **Uticort® Gel**
(betamethasone benzoate, USP)

Parke-Davis

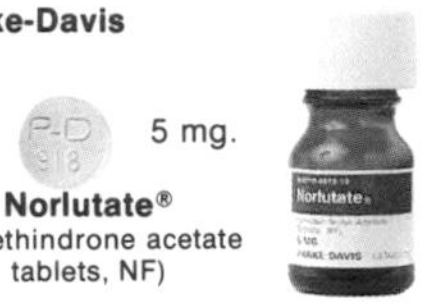

5 mg.

Norlutate®
(norethindrone acetate tablets, NF)

(Bottle shown smaller than actual size)

Parke-Davis

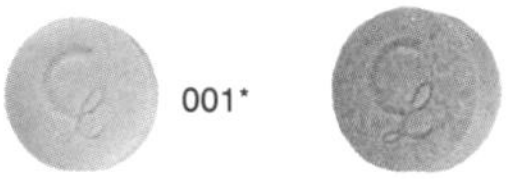

001* 004*

20 mg. Sustained Action 80 mg.

Peritrate®
(pentaerythritol tetranitrate)

40 mg. 008*

Parke-Davis
(Pack shown smaller than actual size)

250 mg.

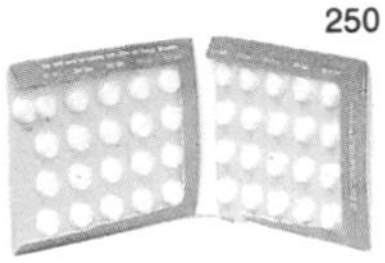

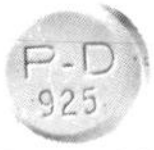

Renoquid Tablets
(sulfacytine)

Parke-Davis

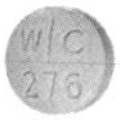

276*

10 mg.

Verstran
(prazepam)

Parke-Davis

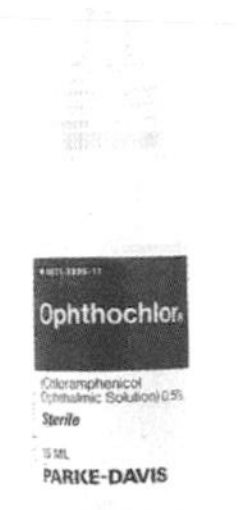

(Bottle shown smaller than actual size)

Ophthochlor® Ophthalmic Solution
(chloramphenicol ophthalmic solution) 0.5%

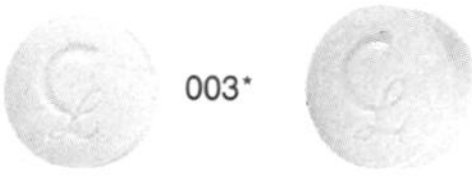

003* 005*

20 mg. Sustained Action 80 mg.

Peritrate® with Phenobarbital

Parke-Davis

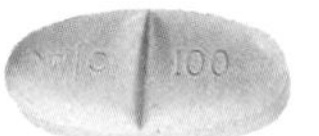

100*

Sinubid®

Parke-Davis

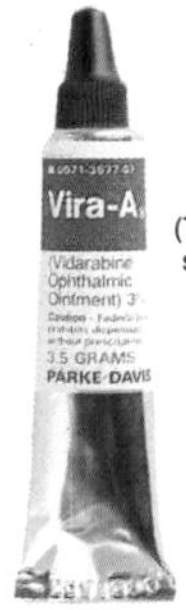

(Tube shown smaller than actual size)

VIRA-A®
(vidarabine ophthalmic ointment), 3%

Parke-Davis

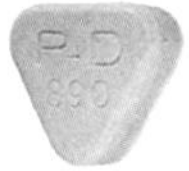

Palaflor® Tablets

Parke-Davis

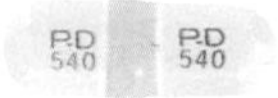

250 mg.

Ponstel® Kapseals
(mefenamic acid)

Parke-Davis

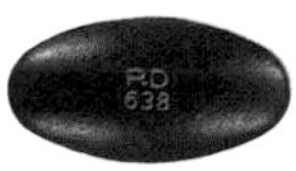

Tabron® Filmseal®

Parke-Davis

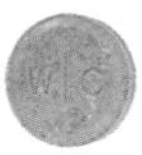

300*

Papase®
(proteolytic enzymes extracted from Carica papaya)

Parke-Davis

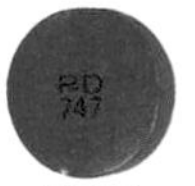

50 mg.

Povan® Filmseal
(pyrvinium pamoate)

Parke-Davis

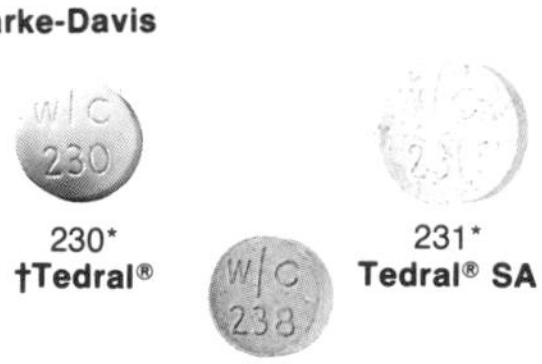

230* **†Tedral®** 231* **Tedral® SA**

238* **Tedral-25®**

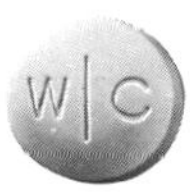

239* **†Tedral® Expectorant**

Parke-Davis

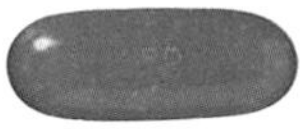

250 mg.

†Zarontin® Capsules
(ethosuximide capsules, USP)

Parke-Davis Ⓒ II

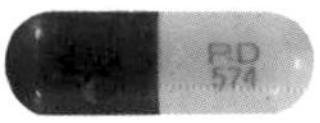

400 mg.

Parest-400™
(methaqualone hydrochloride capsules, NF)

Parke-Davis

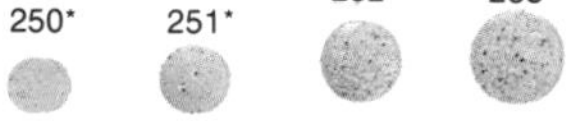

250* 251* 252* 253*

¼ grain ½ grain 1 grain 1½ grain

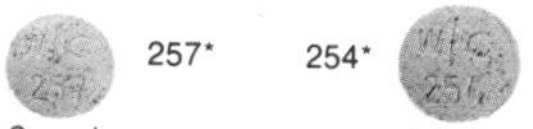

257* 254*

2 grain 3 grain

Proloid®
(thyroglobulin)

Parke-Davis

250 mg. 500 mg.

Penicillin V Potassium Tablets, USP
(Penapar VK®)

Parke-Davis

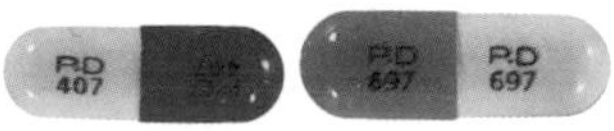

250 mg. 500 mg.

Tetracycline HCl Capsules, USP
(Cyclopar®)

Because tablets and capsules are shown in this section, do not infer that these are the only dosage forms available. Where a product name is preceded by the symbol†, refer to the description in the Product Information (White Section) for other forms.

†Other dosage forms available. See Product Information section or check directly with manufacturer.
*Manufacturers' identification number.

PENNWALT

10 mg. 25 mg.

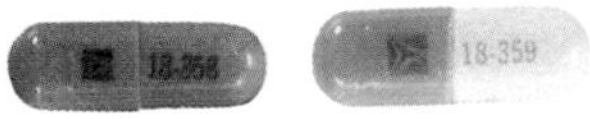

50 mg. 100 mg.

Adapin®
(doxepin hydrochloride)

Pennwalt Ⓒ II

'12½'

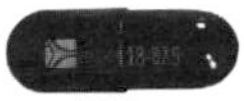

'20'

Biphetamine®
(resin complexes of amphetamine and dextroamphetamine)

Pennwalt Ⓒ IV

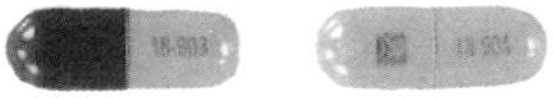

15 mg. 30 mg.
Ionamin®
(phentermine resin)

Pennwalt
Both sides of tablets shown

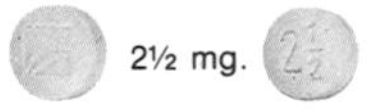

2½ mg.

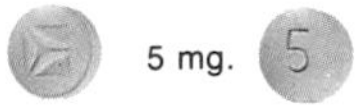

5 mg.

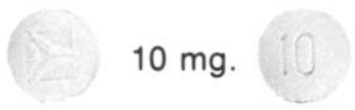

10 mg.

Zaroxolyn®
(metolazone)

PFIPHARMECS

Division of Pfizer Inc.

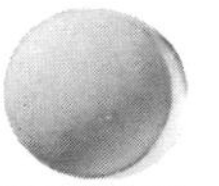

041*
500 mg.

Neobiotic®
(neomycin sulfate)

Pfipharmecs

300* 310*

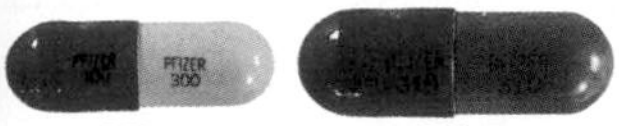

250 mg. 500 mg.
†Pen A®
(ampicillin)

Pfipharmecs
024* 028*

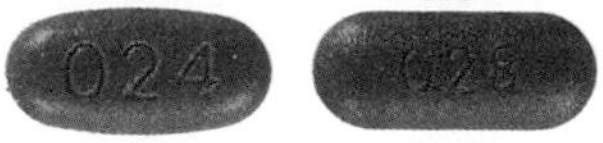

250 mg. 500 mg.
Pfizer-E®
(erythromycin stearate)

Pfipharmecs

200,000 units 046* 250,000 units 047*

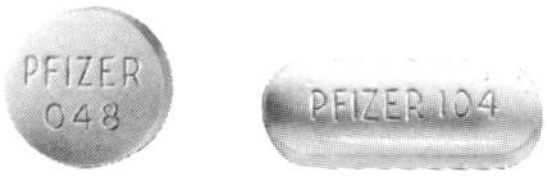

400,000 units 048* 800,000 units 104*

†Pfizerpen G®
(penicillin G potassium)

Pfipharmecs
105* 106*

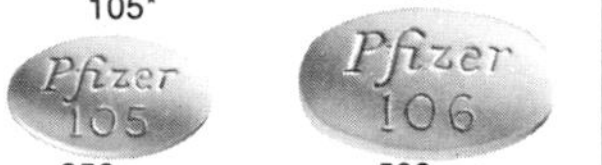

250 mg. 500 mg.
†Pfizerpen VK®
(penicillin V potassium)

Pfipharmecs

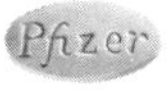

335*

5.0 mg.
†Sterane®
(prednisolone)

Pfipharmecs
015*, 175* or 166* 016* or 172*

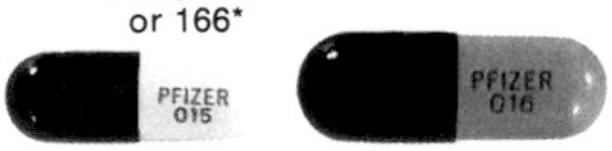

250 mg. 500 mg.
Tetracyn® **Tetracyn® 500**
(tetracycline HCl)

Pfipharmecs

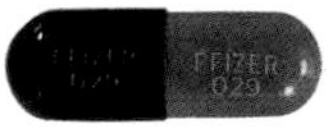

029*

Tetrastatin®
(tetracycline HCl and nystatin)

PFIZER LABORATORIES *

*see also Roerig and Pfipharmecs

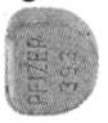

393*

100 mg.
(scored)

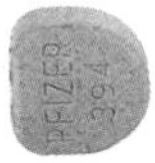

394*

250 mg.
(scored)

Diabinese®
(chlorpropamide)

Pfizer Laboratories

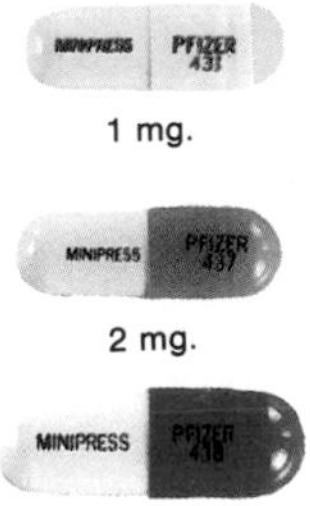

431* 1 mg.
437* 2 mg.
438* 5 mg.

Minipress®
(prazosin HCl)

Pfizer Laboratories

441*

0.25 mg.
Moderil®
(rescinnamine)

Pfizer Laboratories

442*

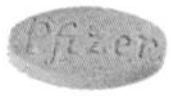

0.5 mg.
Moderil®
(rescinnamine)

Pfizer Laboratories

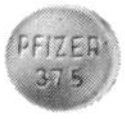

375*
1 mg.

376*
2 mg.

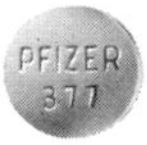

377*
4 mg.

Renese®
(polythiazide)

Pfizer Laboratories

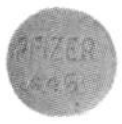

446*

Renese®-R
(polythiazide 2.0 mg. and reserpine 0.25 mg.)

Pfizer Laboratories

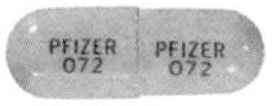

072*
125 mg.

073*
250 mg.

†Terramycin®
(oxytetracycline HCl)

Pfizer Laboratories

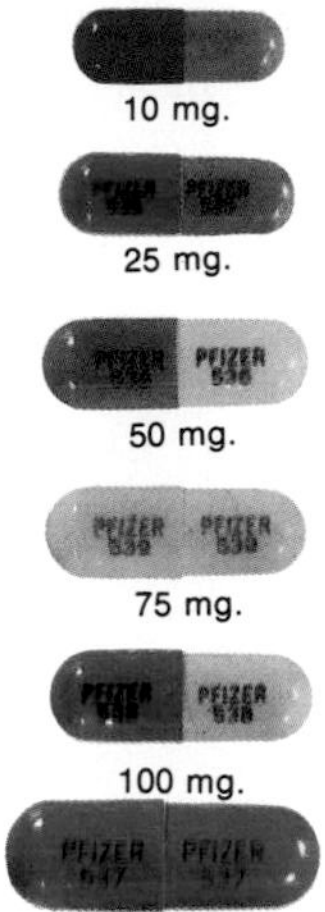

534* 10 mg.
535* 25 mg.
536* 50 mg.
539* 75 mg.
538* 100 mg.
537* 150 mg.

Sinequan®
(doxepin HCl)

Pfizer Laboratories

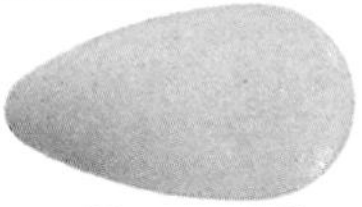

087*

†Terramycin®
(oxytetracycline HCl)
Vaginal Tablets with Polymyxin B Sulfate

Pfizer Laboratories

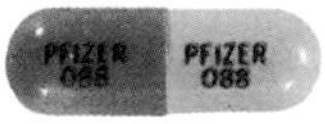

088*

Terrastatin®
(oxytetracycline 250 mg. and nystatin 250,000 units)

Pfizer Laboratories

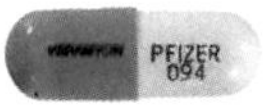

094*
50 mg.

095*
100 mg.

†Vibramycin® Hyclate
(doxycycline hyclate)

Pfizer Laboratories

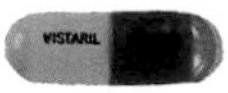

541*
25 mg.

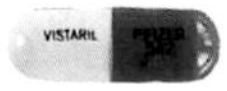

542*
50 mg.

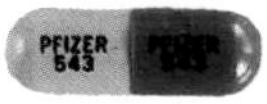

543*
100 mg.

†Vistaril®
(hydroxyzine pamoate)

†Other dosage forms available. See Product Information section or check directly with manufacturer.
*Manufacturers' identification number.

Pfizer Laboratories

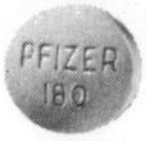

180*

Vistrax® 5
(oxyphencyclimine HCl 5 mg., and hydroxyzine HCl 25 mg.)

181*

Vistrax® 10
(oxyphencyclimine HCl 10 mg., and hydroxyzine HCl 25 mg.)

PHARMACIA

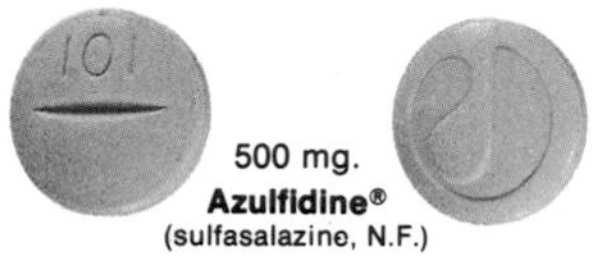

500 mg.
Azulfidine®
(sulfasalazine, N.F.)

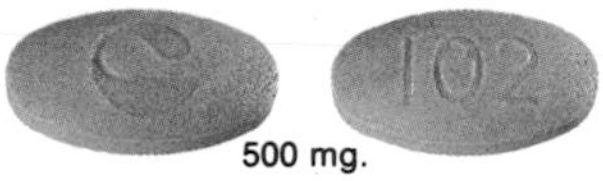

500 mg.

Azulfidine EN-Tabs®
(sulfasalazine, N.F.)

POYTHRESS

Tablets (uncoated) Capsules

Antrocol®

Poythress

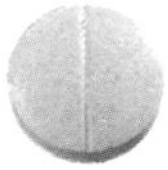

(uncoated tablets)
Mudrane®

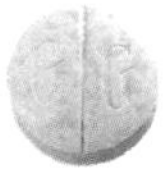

(uncoated tablets)
†Mudrane® GG

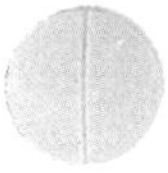

(uncoated tablets)
Mudrane®-2

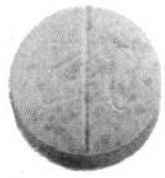

(uncoated tablets)
Mudrane® GG-2

Poythress

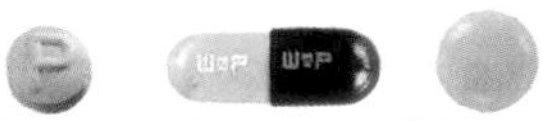

Tablets (uncoated) Capsules Tablets (sugar-coated)

Solfoton®

Poythress

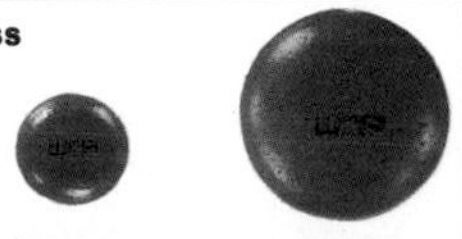

(coated) 100 mg. (coated) 400 mg.
Trocinate® Tablets
(thiphenamil hydrochloride)

Poythress

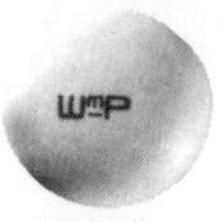

(coated)
Uro-Phosphate® Tablets

PROCTER & GAMBLE

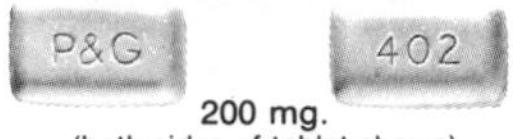

200 mg.
(both sides of tablet shown)
Didronel®
(etidronate disodium)

Procter & Gamble
(Shown smaller than actual size)

2.2 mg./ml.—
70 ml. bottle

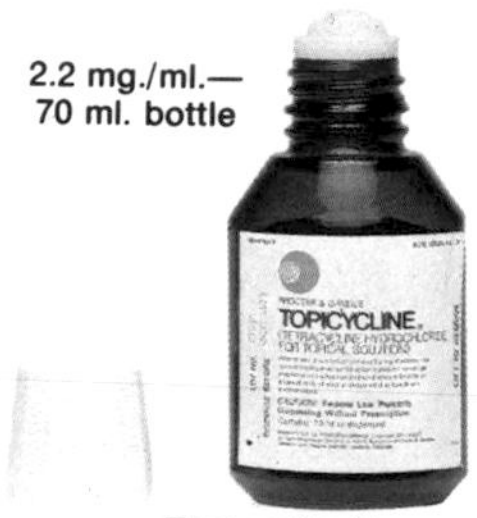

Topicycline®
(tetracycline hydrochloride for topical solution)

PURDUE FREDERICK

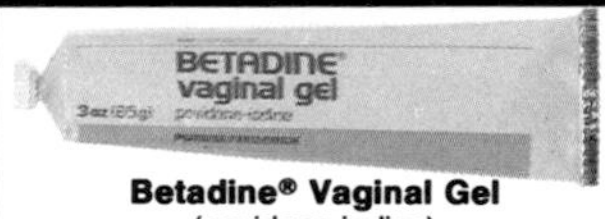

Betadine® Vaginal Gel
(povidone-iodine)
Tubes of 3 oz (85g) and 18g

Purdue Frederick
(Bottle shown smaller than actual size)

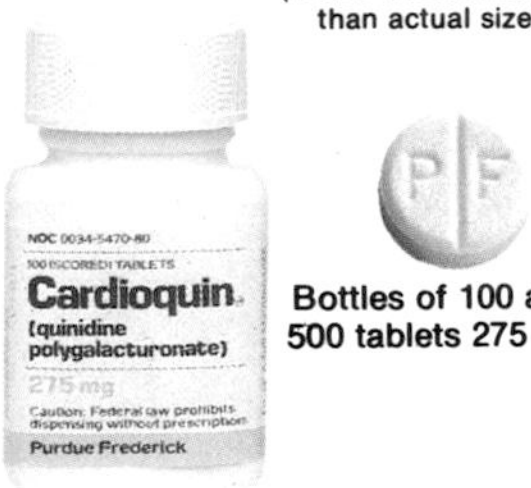

Bottles of 100 and 500 tablets 275 mg

Cardioquin® Tablets
(quinidine polygalacturonate)

Purdue Frederick
(Shown smaller than actual size)

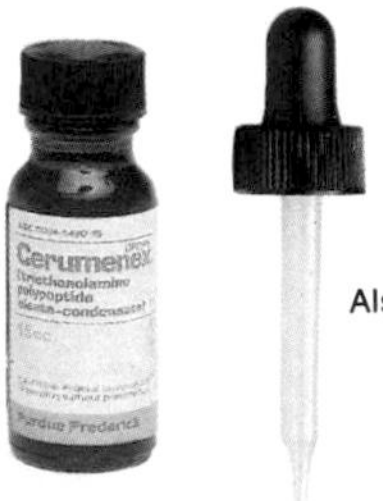

15 cc.
Also available:
8 cc.

Cerumenex®
(triethanolamine polypeptide oleate-condensate)

Purdue Frederick
(Bottle shown smaller than actual size)

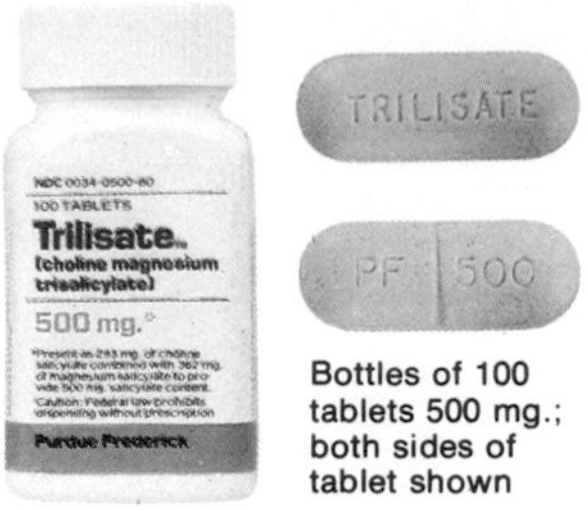

Bottles of 100 tablets 500 mg.; both sides of tablet shown

Trilisate ® Tablets
(choline magnesium trisalicylate)

REED & CARNRICK

(shown smaller than actual size)

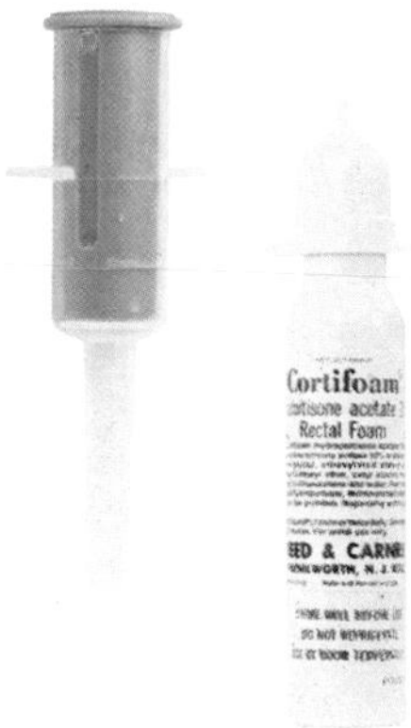

Cortifoam®
(hydrocortisone acetate 10%)

Reed & Carnrick

(shown smaller than actual size)

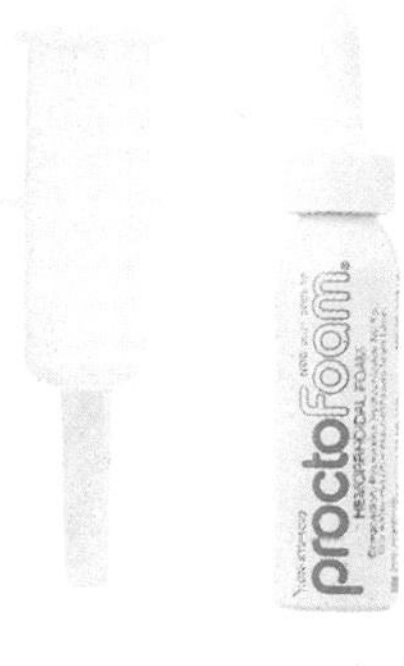

proctoFoam®
(pramoxine hydrochloride 1%)

Reed & Carnrick

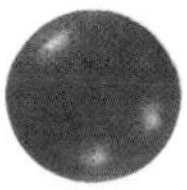

Phazyme®

Reed & Carnrick

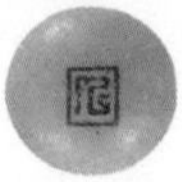

Phazyme-PB®

Reed & Carnrick

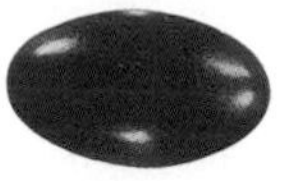

Phazyme®-95

Reed & Carnrick

(shown smaller than actual size)

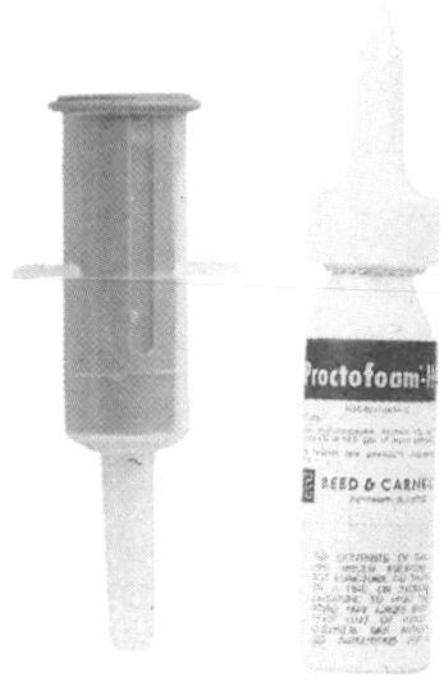

Proctofoam-HC®
(hydrocortisone acetate 1%)

Reed & Carnrick

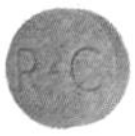

Sidonna®

REID-PROVIDENT

*1138

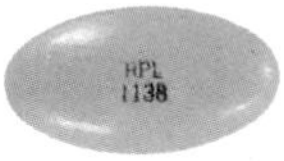

Calinate®-FA

Reid-Provident

*1022 *1024 *1025

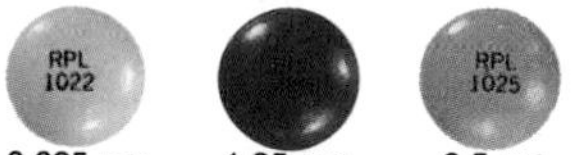

0.625 mg. 1.25 mg. 2.5 mg.
Estratab®
(esterified estrogens)

Reid-Provident

*1023

Estratest® H.S.
(esterified estrogens 0.625 mg. with methyltestosterone 1.25 mg.)

†Other dosage forms available. See Product Information section or check directly with manufacturer.
*Manufacturers' identification number.

Reid-Provident

*1026

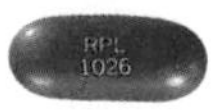

Estratest®
(esterified estrogens 1.25 mg. with methyltestosterone 2.5 mg.)

Reid-Provident

*1039

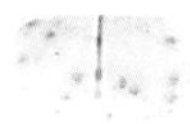

Histalet® Forte

Reid-Provident

*1046

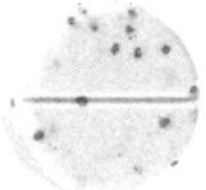

Histalet X

Reid-Provident CIII

*1079

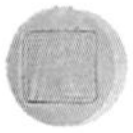

35 mg. Tablets
Melfiat®
(phendimetrazine tartrate)

Reid-Provident CIII

*1088

P-V Tussin

Reid-Provident

*1132

Unipres®
(reserpine 0.1 mg., hydralazine hydrochloride 25 mg., hydrochlorothiazide 15 mg.)

RIKER

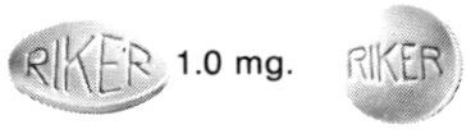

1.0 mg. 0.5 mg.
†Circanol®
(hydrogenated ergot alkaloids)

Riker

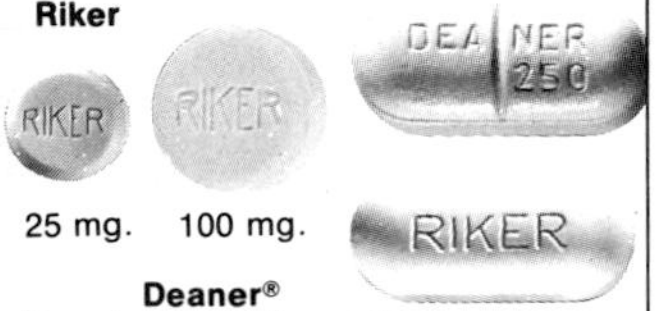

25 mg. 100 mg. 250 mg.
Deaner®
(deanol acetamidobenzoate)

Riker

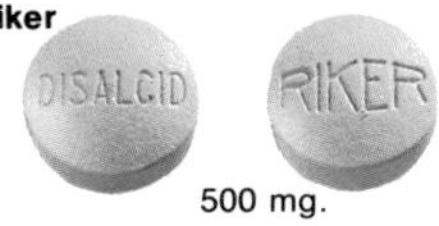

500 mg.
Disalcid®
(salsalate)

Riker

50 mg.
Disipal®
(orphenadrine hydrochloride)

Riker

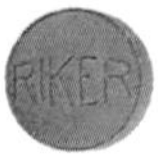

75 mg.
Dorbane®

Riker

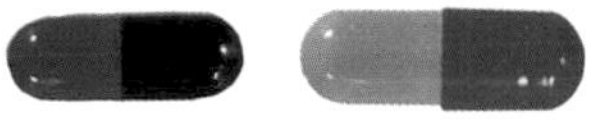

Dorbantyl® **Dorbantyl® Forte**

Riker

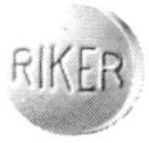

100 mg.
†Norflex®
(orphenadrine citrate)

Riker

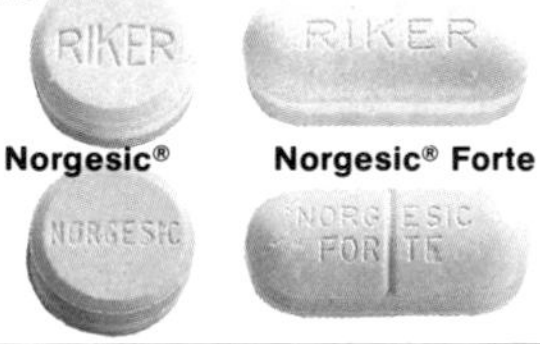

Norgesic® **Norgesic® Forte**

Riker

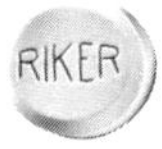

25 mg.
Tepanil®
(diethylpropion hydrochloride, N.F.)

Riker

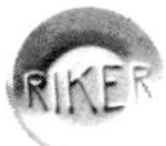

75 mg.
Reverse side reads: "Tepanil® Ten-tab®"
Tepanil® Ten-tab®
(diethylpropion hydrochloride, N.F.)

Riker

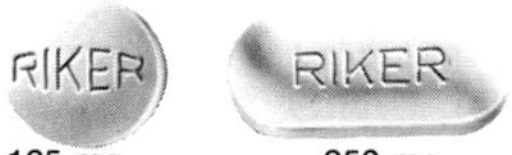

125 mg. 250 mg.
†Theolair™
(theophylline U.S.P., anhydrous)

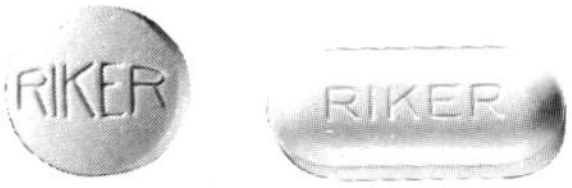

250 mg. 500 mg.
Theolair™-SR
(theophylline U.S.P., anhydrous)

Riker

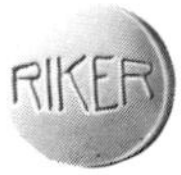

†Titralac®
Also available as Titralac® Liquid

Riker

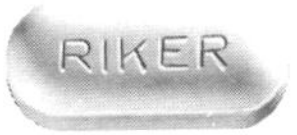

Reverse side reads: UREX
Urex®
(Methenamine hippurate, 1 Gm.)

A. H. ROBINS

Albee® with C

A. H. Robins

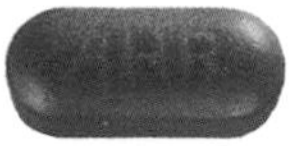

Allbee-T®

A. H. Robins

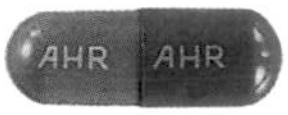

†Dimacol®

A. H. Robins

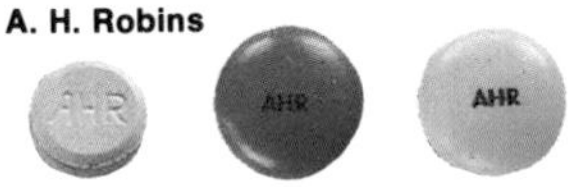

4 mg. Tablets; 8 mg. 12 mg. Extentabs®
†Dimetane®
(brompheniramine maleate, N.F.)

A. H. Robins

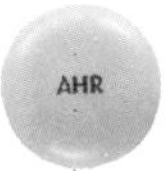

†Dimetapp Extentabs®

A. H. Robins

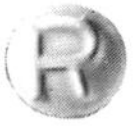

Tablets

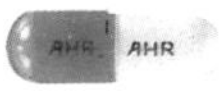

Capsules

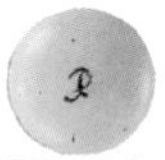

Extentabs®
†Donnatal®

A. H. Robins

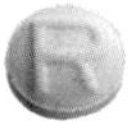

Donnatal® No. 2

A. H. Robins

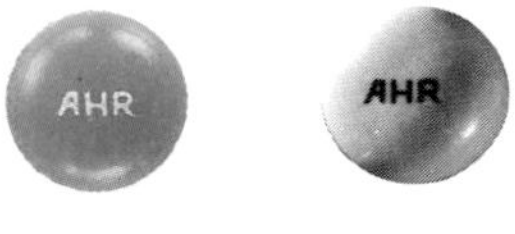

Donnazyme® **Entozyme®**

A. H. Robins

50 mg.
Exna® **Exna®-R**
(benzthiazide tablets, N. F.)

A. H. Robins

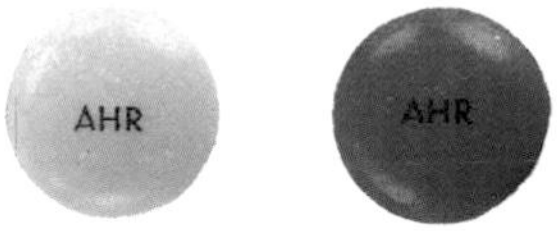

Pabalate® **Pabalate®-SF**

A. H. Robins

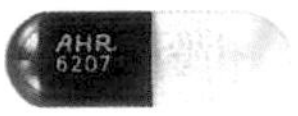

Phenaphen®
(acetaminophen, U.S.P.)

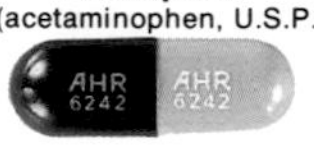

No. 2

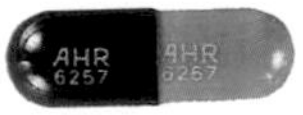

No. 3

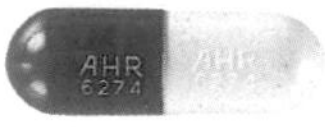

No. 4
Phenaphen® with Codeine

A. H. Robins

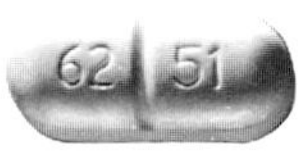

Phenaphen®-650 with Codeine

A. H. Robins

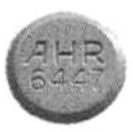

20 mg.
Pondimin®
(fenfluramine hydrochloride)

A. H. Robins

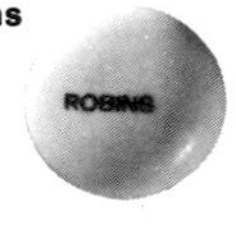

Quinidex Extentabs®
(quinidine sulfate, U.S.P.)

†Other dosage forms available. See Product Information section or check directly with manufacturer.
*Manufacturers' identification number.

A. H. Robins

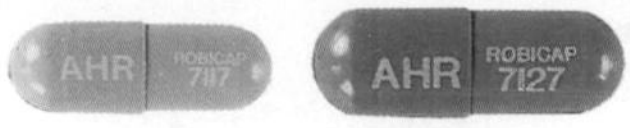

250 mg. 500 mg.
Robamox®
(amoxicillin)

A. H. Robins

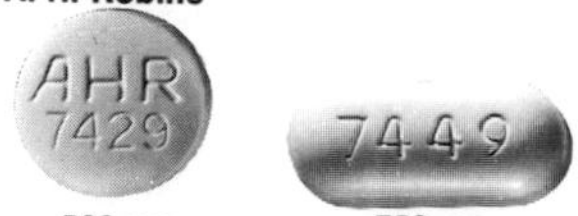

500 mg. 750 mg.
†Robaxin® **Robaxin®-750**
(methocarbamol tablets, N.F.)

A. H. Robins

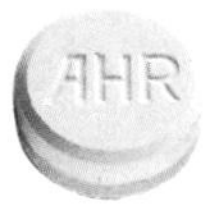

Robaxisal®

A. H. Robins

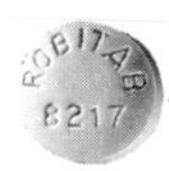

250 mg. 400,000 units

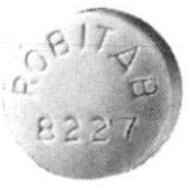

500 mg. 800,000 units

†Robicillin VK
(penicillin V potassium tablets, U.S.P.)

A. H. Robins

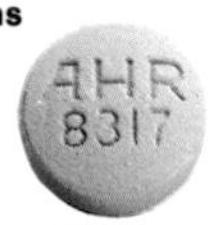

250 mg.
Robimycin
(erythromycin, U.S.P., enteric-coated tablet)

A. H. Robins

†Robinul® **Robinul® Forte**
(glycopyrrolate tablets, N.F.)

A. H. Robins

Robinul®-PH **Robinul®-PH Forte**

A. H. Robins

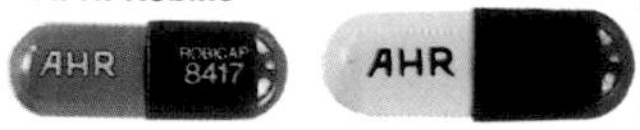

250 mg. 500 mg.
Robitet® '250' Hydrochloride
Robitet® '500' Hydrochloride
(tetracycline hydrochloride capsules, U.S.P.)

A. H. Robins

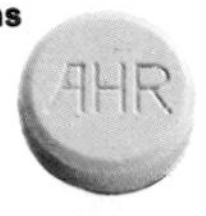

500 mg.
Sulla®
(sulfameter)

A. H. Robins

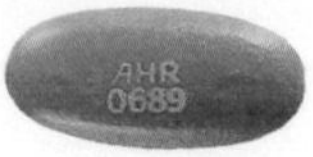

Z-BEC®

ROCHE

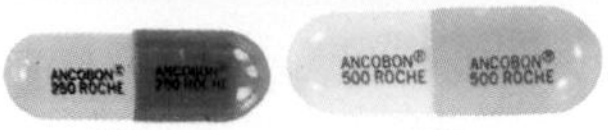

250 mg 500 mg
Ancobon®
(flucytosine)

Roche

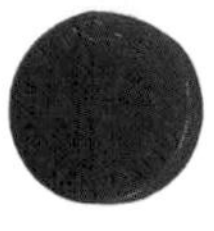

Azo Gantanol®

Roche

Azo Gantrisin®

Roche

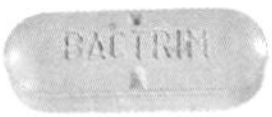

†Bactrim™

Roche

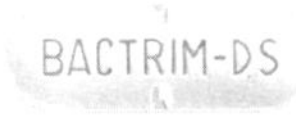

†Bactrim™ DS

Roche

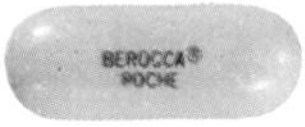

Berocca® Tablets

Roche Ⓒ IV

ROCHE 61 ROCHE 62 ROCHE 63

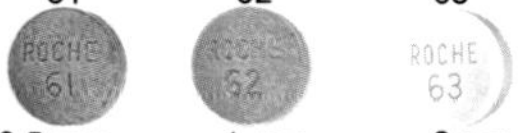

0.5 mg 1 mg 2 mg
Clonopin®
(clonazepam)

Roche Ⓒ IV

15 mg 30 mg
***Dalmane®**
(flurazepam hydrochloride)

Roche

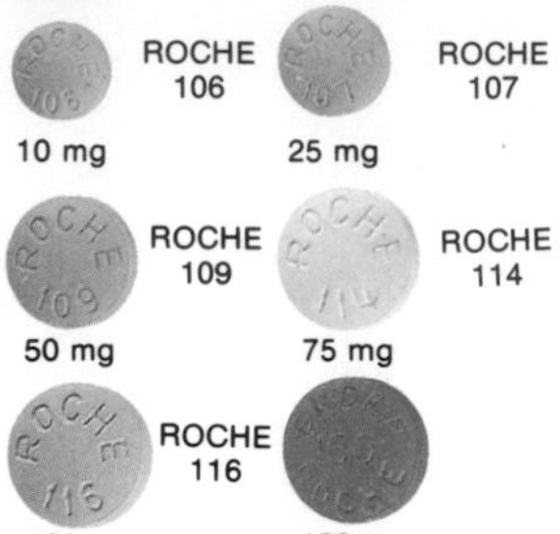

ROCHE 106 — 10 mg
ROCHE 107 — 25 mg
ROCHE 109 — 50 mg
ROCHE 114 — 75 mg
ROCHE 116 — 100 mg
150 mg
Endep®
(amitriptyline HCl)

Roche

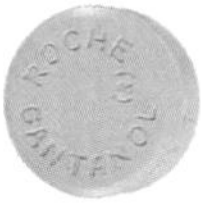

500 mg
†Gantanol®
(sulfamethoxazole)

Roche

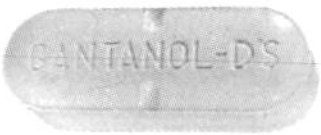

1 Gm
†Gantanol® DS
(sulfamethoxazole)

Roche

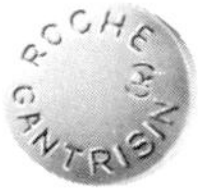

500 mg
†Gantrisin®
(sulfisoxazole)

Roche

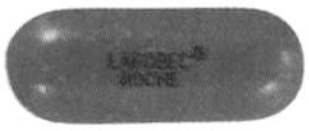

Larobec®

Roche

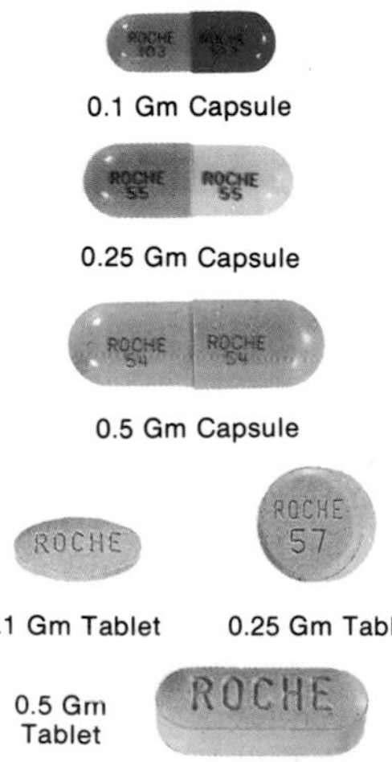

0.1 Gm Capsule
0.25 Gm Capsule
0.5 Gm Capsule
0.1 Gm Tablet 0.25 Gm Tablet
0.5 Gm Tablet
All Larodopa capsules and tablets now bear the Tel-E-Mark.
Larodopa® (levodopa)

Roche

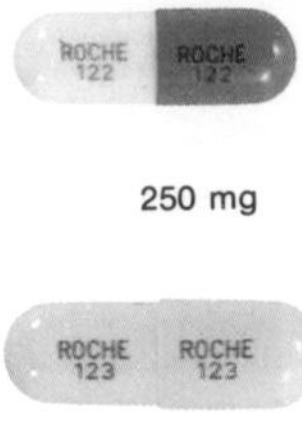

ROCHE 122
250 mg
ROCHE 123
500 mg
†Larotid®
(amoxicillin)

Roche Ⓒ II

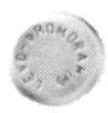

2 mg
†Levo-Dromoran®
(levorphanol tartrate)

Roche

***Librax®**

Roche Ⓒ IV

5 mg 10 mg 25 mg
***Libritabs®**
(chlordiazepoxide)

Roche Ⓒ IV

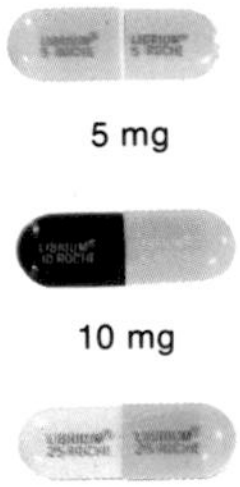

5 mg
10 mg
25 mg
***†Librium®**
(chlordiazepoxide hydrochloride)

Roche Ⓒ IV

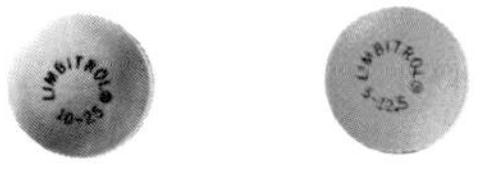

10-25 5-12.5
***Limbitrol®**

Roche

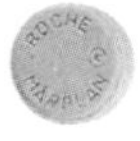

10 mg
Marplan®
(isocarboxazid)

†Other dosage forms available. See Product Information section or check directly with manufacturer.
*Dalmane, Librax, Libritabs, and Librium are products of Roche Products Inc., Manati, P.R. 00701.

ROCHE
Tel-E-Mark™ System

Example:

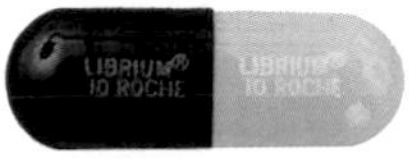

Librium® 10 mg
(chlordiazepoxide HCl)

Quick and simple product identification is provided by the Roche Tel-E-Mark, whereby product and company names and, where applicable, dosage strength are imprinted directly on the tablet or capsule. Eventually, most solid oral dosage forms of Roche products will bear the Tel-E-Mark.

ROCHE
Tel-E-Code™ System

Example:

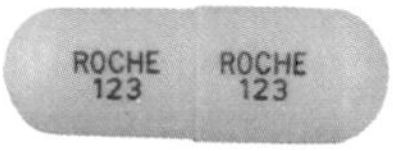

Larotid® 500 mg
(amoxicillin)

Based on the National Drug Code, the Roche Tel-E-Code marking includes the Roche name and numbers indicating product and strength. It, too, provides speedy product identification when needed. Solid oral dosage forms of Roche products not phased into the Tel-E-Mark System are marked with this Tel-E-Code.

TEL-E-DOSE® ROCHE®

Example:

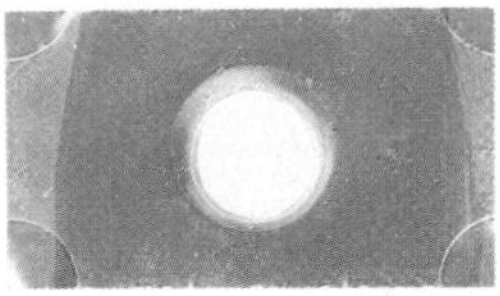

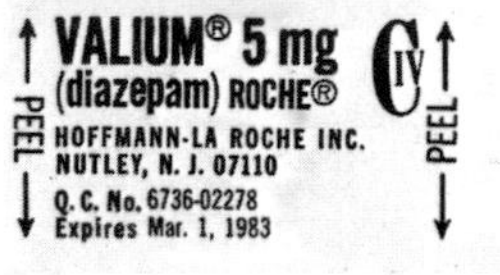

VALIUM® 5 mg
(diazepam)

Tel-E-Dose is a unit package designed by Roche for convenience in dispensing medications in the hospital and nursing home. Each unit, sealed against contamination and moisture, is clearly identified by product name and strength and carries the control number and expiration date.

Currently available in this package form are the following Roche products: Bactrim™ (80 mg trimethoprim and 400 mg sulfamethoxazole tablets; Bactrim™ DS (160 mg trimethoprim and 800 mg sulfamethoxazole) tablets; Dalmane® (flurazepam HCl) capsules, 15 mg, 30 mg; Endep® (amitriptyline HCl) tablets, 10 mg, 25 mg, 50 mg, 75 mg, 100 mg, 150 mg; Gantanol® (sulfamethoxazole) tablets, 0.5 Gm; Gantanol® DS (sulfamethoxazole) tablets, 1 Gm; Gantrisin® (sulfisoxazole) tablets, 0.5 Gm; Larotid® (amoxicillin) capsules, 250 mg, 500 mg; Larotid® (amoxicillin) Oral Suspension, 125 mg and 250 mg/5 ml.; Librax® (5 mg chlordiazepoxide HCl and 2.5 mg clidinium Br) capsules; Librium® (chlordiazepoxide HCl) capsules, 5 mg, 10 mg, 25 mg; Limbitrol® (chlordiazepoxide and amitriptyline HCl) tablets, 10-25, 5-12.5; and Valium® (diazepam) tablets, 2 mg, 5 mg, 10 mg

Roche

150 mg

†Roniacol® Timespan® Tablets
(nicotinyl alcohol)

Roche Ⓒ IV

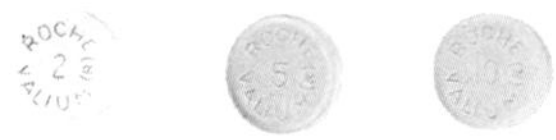

2 mg 5 mg 10 mg

†Valium®
(diazepam)

Roche

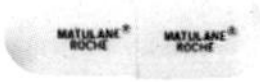

50 mg

Matulane®
(procarbazine hydrochloride)

Roche Ⓒ III

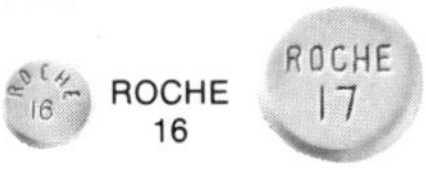

ROCHE 16 — 50 mg
ROCHE 17 — 200 mg

Noludar® Tablets
(methyprylon)

Roche

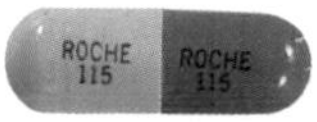

ROCHE 115

30 mg

Solatene®
(beta-carotene)

Roche Ⓒ IV

(Shown slightly smaller than actual size)

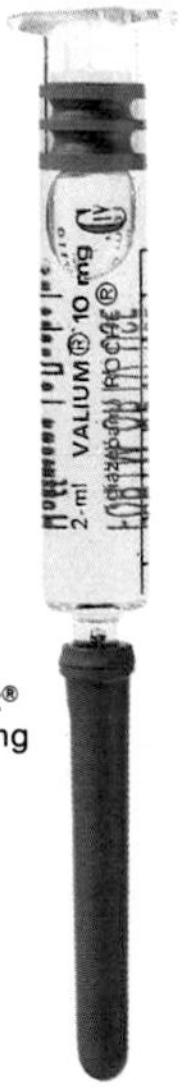

Tel-E-Ject®
2 ml = 10 mg

†Valium Injectable
(diazepam)

Roche

ROCHE 23 — ROCHE 24 — ROCHE 25

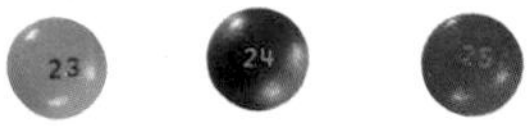

Menrium® 5-2 — **Menrium® 5-4** — **Menrium® 10-4**

Roche

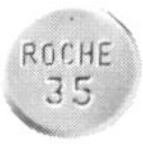

ROCHE 35

15 mg

†Prostigmin®
(neostigmine bromide)

Roche

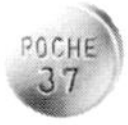

ROCHE 37

5 mg

†Synkayvite®
(menadiol sodium diphosphate)

Roche

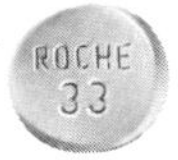

ROCHE 33

60 mg

†Mestinon®
(pyridostigmine bromide)

Roche

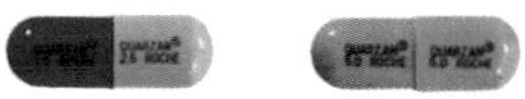

2.5 mg 5 mg

Quarzan®
(clidinium bromide)

Roche

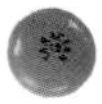

10 mg

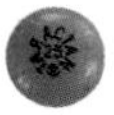

25 mg

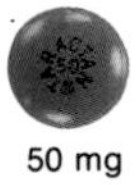

50 mg

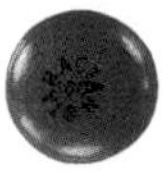

100 mg

†Taractan®
(chlorprothixene)

Roche

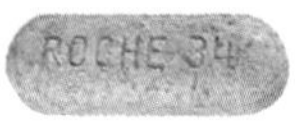

ROCHE 34

180 mg

†Mestinon® Timespan® Tablets
(pyridostigmine bromide)

Roche

ROCHE 143 — ROCHE 144

0.25 mcg — 0.5 mcg

Rocaltrol®
(calcitriol)

Roche Ⓒ III

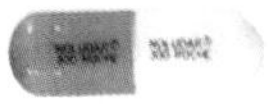

300 mg

Noludar® 300
(methyprylon)

Roche

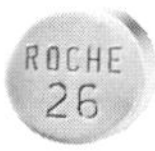

ROCHE 26

50 mg

†Roniacol® Tablets
(nicotinyl alcohol)

†Other dosage forms available. See Product Information section or check directly with manufacturer.

Roche

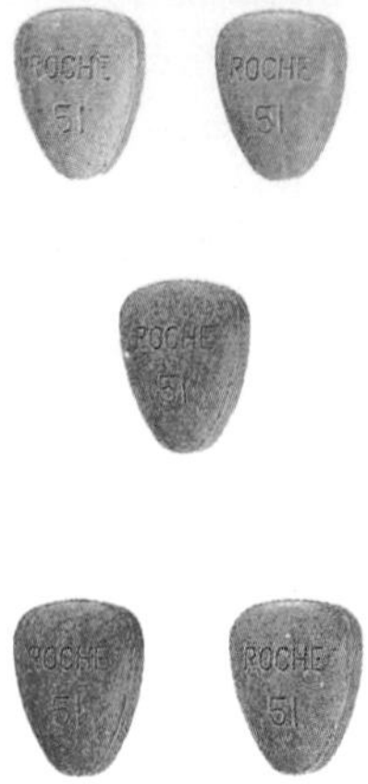

†Vi-Penta® F Chewables

ROERIG

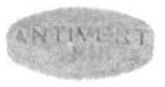

210*

12.5 mg.

Antivert®
(meclizine HCl)

Roerig

211*

25 mg.

Antivert®/25
(meclizine HCl)

Roerig

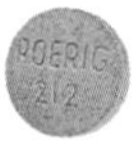

212*

25 mg.

Antivert®/25 Chewable Tablets
(meclizine HCl)

Roerig

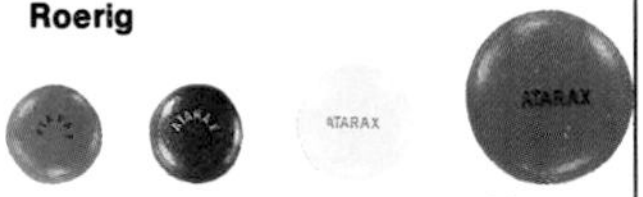

10 mg. 560* | 25 mg. 561* | 50 mg. 562* | 100 mg. 563*

†Atarax®
(hydroxyzine hydrochloride)

Roerig

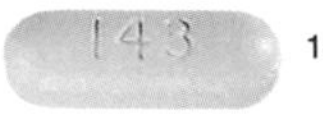

143*

Geocillin® Tablets
(carbenicillin indanyl sodium)
equivalent to 382 mg. carbenicillin

Roerig

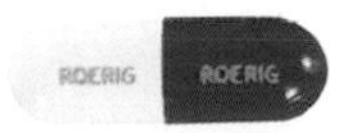

504*

Heptuna® Plus

Roerig (Both sides of tablet shown)

254*

†Marax®
(Each tablet contains ephedrine sulfate 25 mg.; theophylline, 130 mg.; and Atarax [hydroxyzine HCl], 10 mg.)

Roerig

1 mg. 571* | 2 mg. 572*

5 mg. 573* | 10 mg. 574*

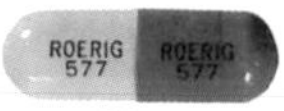

20 mg.
577*

†Navane®
(thiothixene)

Roerig

100 mg. 220* | 300 mg. 221*

Sustaire®
theophylline (anhydrous)

Roerig

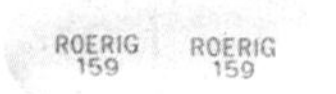

159*

250 mg.

†Tao®
(troleandomycin)

Roerig

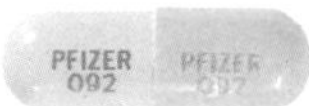

092*

Urobiotic®-250
(Each capsule contains oxytetracycline HCl 250 mg., sulfamethizole 250 mg., and phenazopyridine HCl 50 mg.)

WILLIAM H. RORER

Both sides of tablet shown

50,000 Rorer Units**

Ananase®—50 (bromelains)

Both sides of tablet shown

100,000 Rorer Units**

Ananase®—100 (bromelains)

**See prescribing information.

William H. Rorer

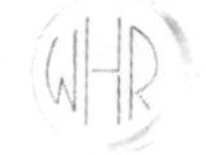

Ascriptin®
325 mg. (5 grains) aspirin, 150 mg. Maalox® (magnesium-aluminum hydroxide)

William H. Rorer

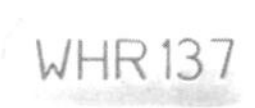

Ascriptin® A/D
325 mg. (5 grains) aspirin, 300 mg. Maalox® (magnesium-aluminum hydroxide)

William H. Rorer Ⓒ III

Both sides of tablet shown

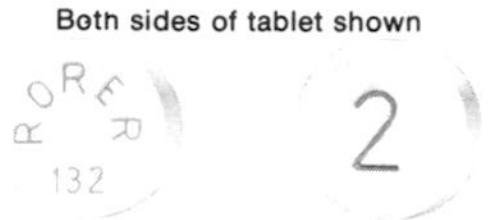

Ascriptin® with Codeine No. 2
16.2 mg. (¼ gr.) codeine

Both sides of tablet shown

Ascriptin® with Codeine No. 3
32.4 mg. (½ gr.) codeine
(each tablet contains the ingredients of Ascriptin plus codeine phosphate)

William H. Rorer

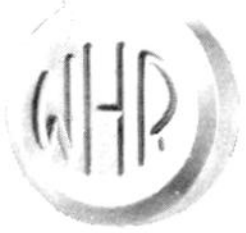

†Camalox® (magnesium and aluminum hydroxides with calcium carbonate)

William H. Rorer Ⓒ IV

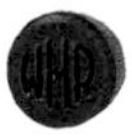

Chardonna®-2
(15 mg. phenobarbital, and 15 mg. belladonna extract)

William H. Rorer

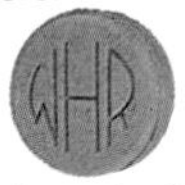

Fermalox®
[200 mg. ferrous sulfate; 200 mg. Maalox® (magnesium-aluminum hydroxide)]

William H. Rorer

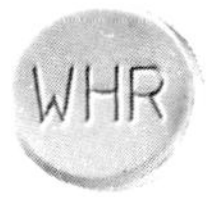

NO. 1 (400 mg.)

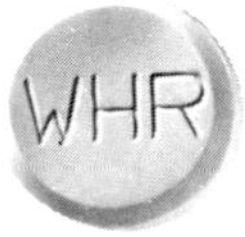

NO. 2 (800 mg.)

†Maalox®
(magnesia and alumina tablets, Rorer)

William H. Rorer

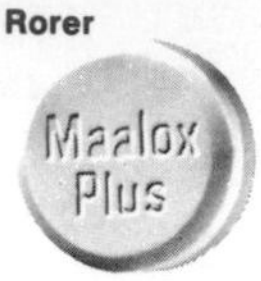

(both sides of tablet shown)

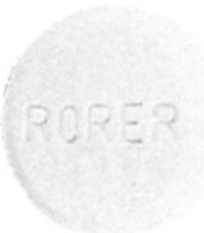

†Maalox® Plus
(400 mg. magnesium-aluminum hydroxide, 25 mg. simethicone)

ROSS

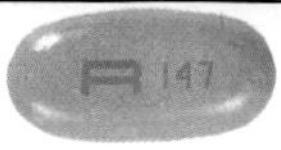

Pramet® FA
(vitamin/mineral prescription for the expectant and new mother)

Ross

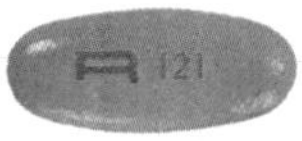

Pramilet® FA
(prenatal vitamin mineral preparation with folic acid)

Ross 200 mg.

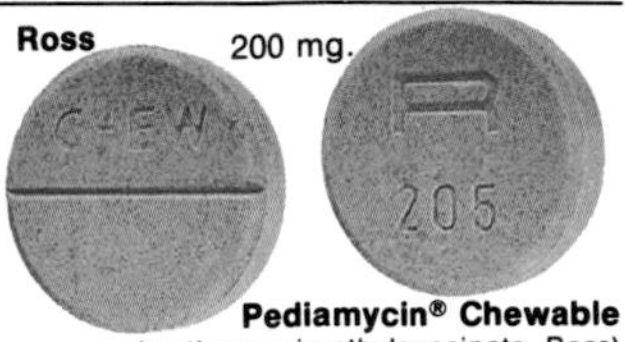

Pediamycin® Chewable
(erythromycin ethylsuccinate, Ross)

Ross

†RONDEC™ Tablet

Ross

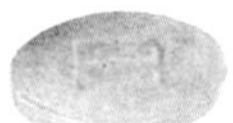

†Vi-Daylin® w/Fluoride Chewable
(multivitamins with fluoride)

Ross

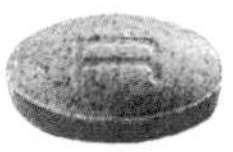

Vi-Daylin® Chewable
(multivitamin supplement for children under 4 years of age, and adults and children 4 or more years of age)

Ross

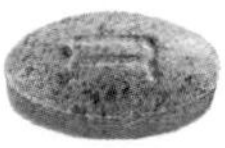

Vi-Daylin® + iron Chewable
(multivitamin supplement for children under 4 years of age, and adults and children 4 or more years of age)

†Other dosage forms available. See Product Information section or check directly with manufacturer.
*Manufacturers' identification number.

SANDOZ

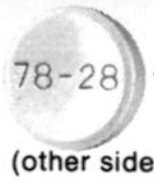

#78-28*

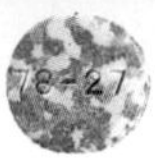
#78-27*

(other side: scored)

Belladenal® Tablets

Belladenal-S® Tablets

Sandoz

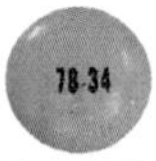

#78-34*

(other side: branded CAFERGOT)

†Cafergot® Tablets
(ergotamine tartrate and caffeine) tablets, NF

Sandoz

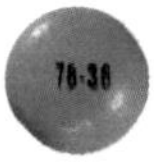
#78-36*

(other side: branded SANDOZ)

†Cafergot® P-B Tablets

Sandoz

#78-38*

(other side: branded SANDOZ)

†Cedilanid® Tablets
(lanatoside C) tablets

Sandoz

#78-65*

(other side: branded 78-65)

Fiogesic®

Sandoz

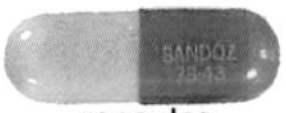

capsules
#78-43*
Fiorinal-R®

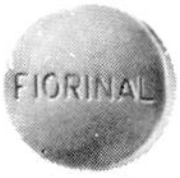

tablets
#78-44*

(other side: tablets branded 78-44; tablet also branded with product name encircled)

Fiorinal®

Sandoz

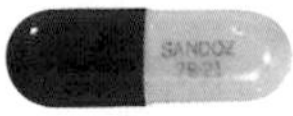
#78-21*

⅛ gr.
(#1)

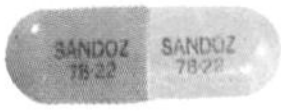

#78-22*

¼ gr.
(#2)

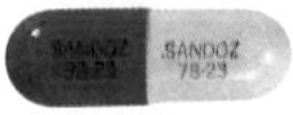
#78-23*

½ gr.
(#3)

Fiorinal® with Codeine

Sandoz

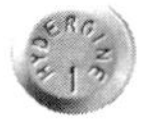

#78-70*

1 mg.
(other side: branded 78-70)

Hydergine Tablets (oral)

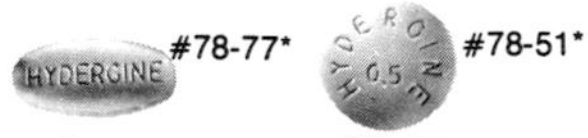

#78-77* #78-51*

1 mg. 0.5 mg.

(other side: 1 mg. tablet branded 78-77 and 0.5 mg. tablet branded 78-51)

Hydergine Sublingual Tablets

Sandoz

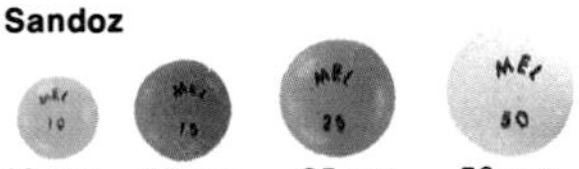

10 mg. 15 mg. 25 mg. 50 mg.

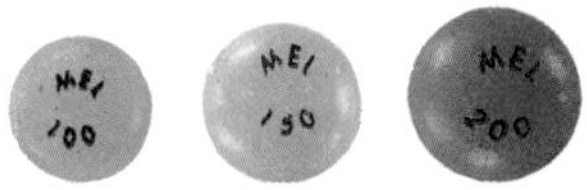

100 mg. 150 mg. 200 mg.

Other side: triangle (S)

†Mellaril® Tablets
(thioridazine) HCl tablets, USP

Sandoz

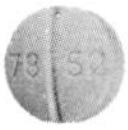
#78-52*

(other side: triangle (S) SANDOZ)

Mesantoin® Tablets
(mephenytoin) tablets, NF

Sandoz

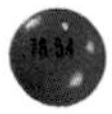
#78-54*

(other side: branded SANDOZ)

†Methergine® Tablets
(methylergonovine maleate) tablets, NF

Sandoz

#78-86 #78-87

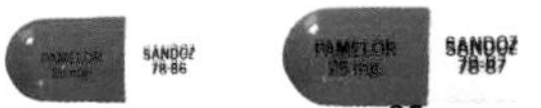
10 mg. 25 mg.

†Pamelor®
(nortriptyline HCl) capsules, NF

Sandoz

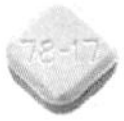
#78-17

(other side: branded SANDOZ)

Parlodel®
(bromocriptine mesylate) tablets

Sandoz

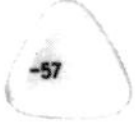
#78-57*

(other side: branded 78-)

Plexonal® Tablets

Sandoz

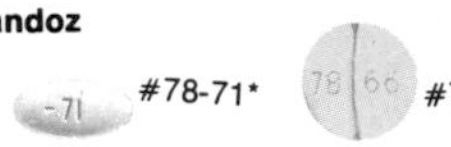
#78-71* #78-66*

1 mg. 2 mg.

(other side: 1 mg. branded 78-71 and 2 mg. branded SANDOZ; 1 mg. stamped SANOREX on reverse side)

Sanorex® (mazindol)

Sandoz

#78-58*

(other side: branded SANDOZ)

Sansert® Tablets
(methysergide maleate) tablets, USP

SAVAGE

Brexin® Capsules

Savage

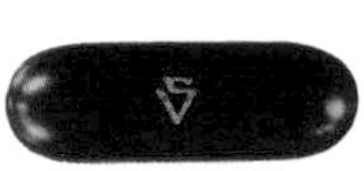

Chromagen® Capsules

Savage

Dilor®
(dyphylline)
200 mg

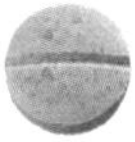

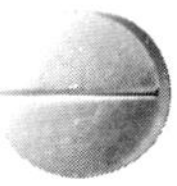

Dilor®-400
(dyphylline)
400 mg

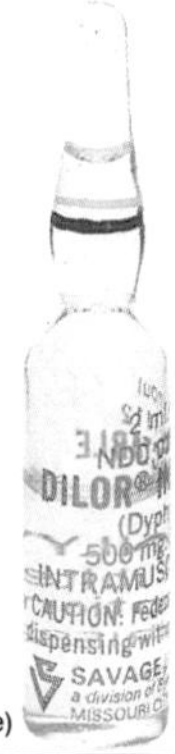

Dilor® Injectable
(dyphylline)
2 ml-250 mg/ml
(Shown smaller than actual size)

Savage

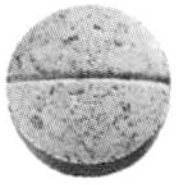

Dilor®-G

Savage

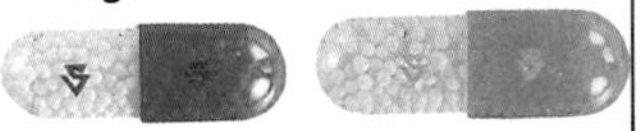
130 mg 260 mg
Physpan™-130 **Physpan™**

(theophylline USP anhydrous, sustained release)

Because tablets and capsules are shown in this section, do not infer that these are the only dosage forms available. Where a product name is preceded by the symbol†, refer to the description in the Product Information (White Section) for other forms.

SCHERING**

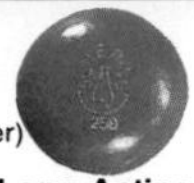
120 mg
(60 mg per layer)
258

AFRINOL™ Long-Acting Decongestant REPETABS® Tablets
(pseudoephedrine sulfate)

Schering/Emko

(Shown smaller than actual size)

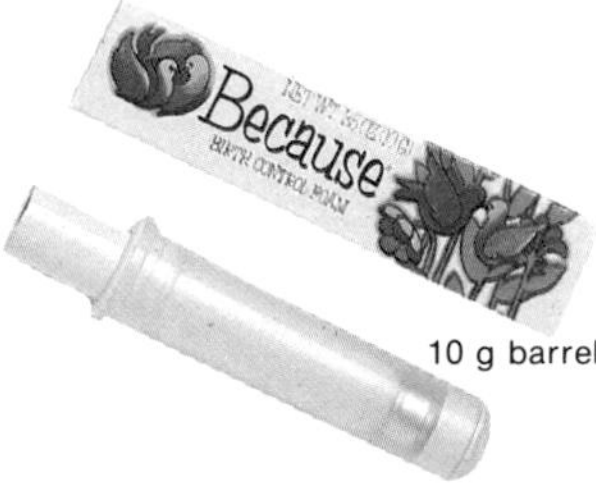

10 g barrel

BECAUSE® Contraceptor®
(nonoxynol-9)

Schering

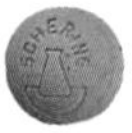
BDA
or
011

0.6 mg

†CELESTONE® Tablets
(betamethasone, NF)

Schering

(Shown smaller than actual size)

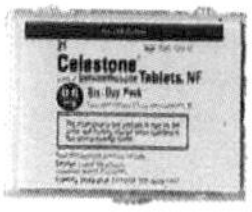

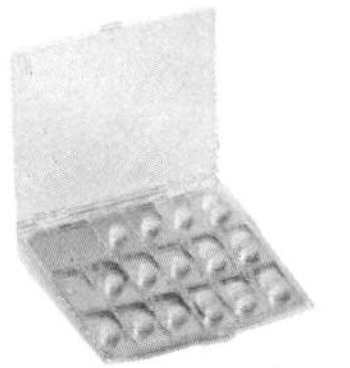
BDA
or
011

†CELESTONE® Six-Day Pack (21 Tablet Pack)
(betamethasone, NF 0.6 mg)

Schering

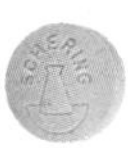
901

CHLOR-TRIMETON® Decongestant Tablets
(4 mg chlorpheniramine maleate, USP and 60 mg pseudoephedrine sulfate)

Schering

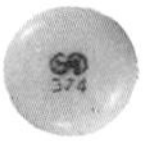
CC**
or
374

8 mg

†CHLOR-TRIMETON® Long-Acting Allergy REPETABS® Tablets
(chlorpheniramine maleate, USP)

Schering

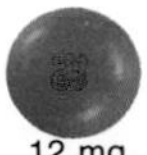
AAE**
or
009

12 mg

CHLOR-TRIMETON® REPETABS Tablets
(chlorpheniramine maleate, USP)

†Other dosage forms available. See Product Information section or check directly with manufacturer. *Manufacturers' identification number.
**During the next year, either National Drug Identification numbers or letters may be imprinted on the products.

Schering

TW** or 080

4 mg

†CHLOR-TRIMETON® ALLERGY Tablets
(chlorpheniramine maleate, USP)

Schering/White Product Line

Cod Liver Oil Concentrate Capsules

Cod Liver Oil Concentrate Tablets

Cod Liver Oil Concentrate Tablets w/Vitamin C

Schering

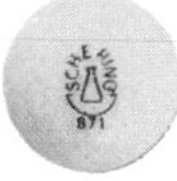

ANF or 116   871** or 524

†CORICIDIN D'® Decongestant Tablets

Schering

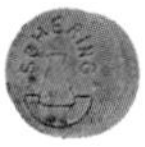

CORICIDIN® DEMILETS® Tablets   **CORICIDIN® MEDILETS® Tablets**

Schering

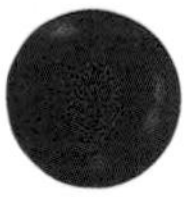

PKD ** or SN or 171

†CORICIDIN® Tablets

Schering

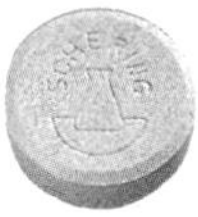

CORICIDIN® Sinus Headache Tablets

Schering

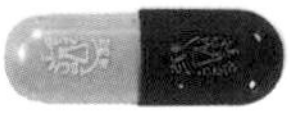

ANR ** or 432

CORIFORTE® Capsules

Schering

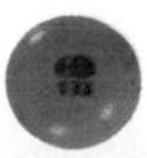

ADD ** or 133

†DEMAZIN® REPETABS® Tablets
(chlorpheniramine maleate, USP and phenylephrine hydrochloride)

Schering

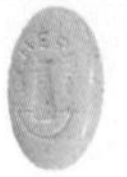

AEY ** or 420

0.75 mg

DERONIL® Tablets
(dexamethasone, USP)

Schering

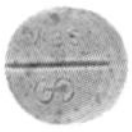

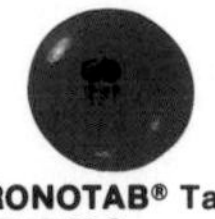

Tablets WBS ** or 866   WMH ** or 231

CHRONOTAB® Tablets
DISOPHROL®
(dexbrompheniramine maleate, NF and pseudoephedrine sulfate)

Schering

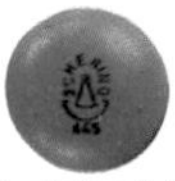

AMN ** or 445

DRIXORAL® Sustained-Action Tablets
(dexbrompheniramine maleate, NF and pseudoephedrine sulfate)

Schering/Emko
(Shown smaller than actual size)

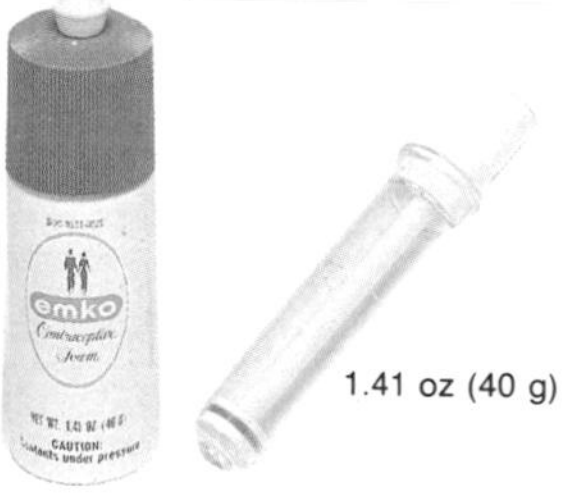

1.41 oz (40 g)

EMKO® Contraceptive Foam
(nonoxynol-9)

Schering/Emko
(Shown smaller than actual size)

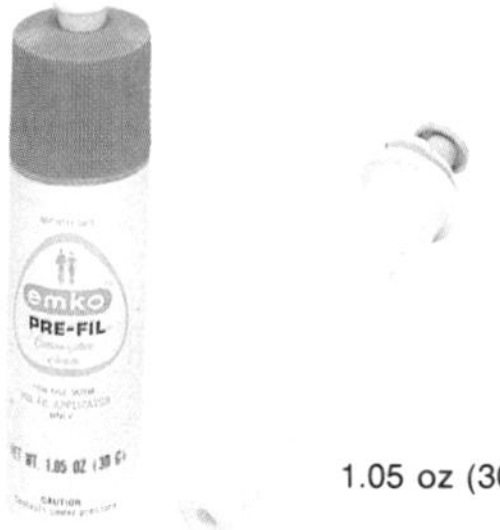

1.05 oz (30 g)

EMKO Pre-Fil® Contraceptive Foam
(nonoxynol-9)

Schering

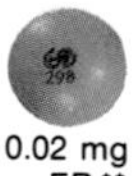

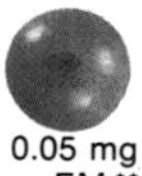

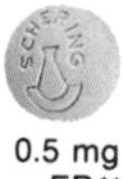

0.02 mg ER ** or 298   0.05 mg EM ** or 070   0.5 mg EP ** or 150

ESTINYL® Tablets
(ethinyl estradiol, USP)

Schering

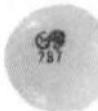

ANA ** or 287

ETRAFON® 2-10 Tablets (2-10)

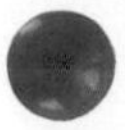

ANB ** or 119

ETRAFON-A Tablets (4-10)

ANC ** or 598

ETRAFON Tablets (2-25)

ANE ** or 720

ETRAFON-FORTE Tablets (4-25)

(perphenazine, NF and amitriptyline hydrochloride, USP)

Schering

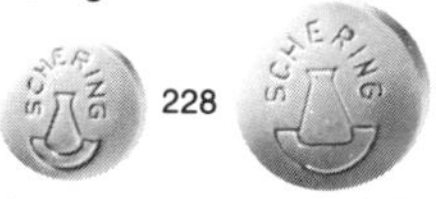

228   507

125 mg   250 mg

FULVICIN® P/G Tablets
(griseofulvin ultramicrosize)

Schering

AUH ** or 176   AUF ** or 948   AUG ** or 496

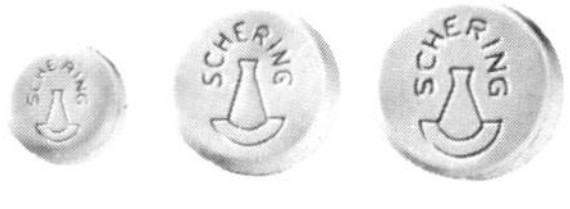

125 mg   250 mg   500 mg

FULVICIN-U/F® Tablets
[griseofulvin (microsize), USP]

Schering

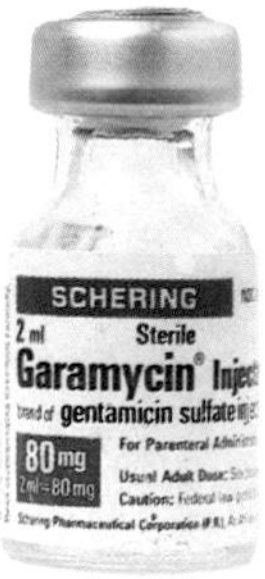

80 mg vial (40 mg per ml)

†GARAMYCIN® Injectable
(gentamicin sulfate, USP)

Schering

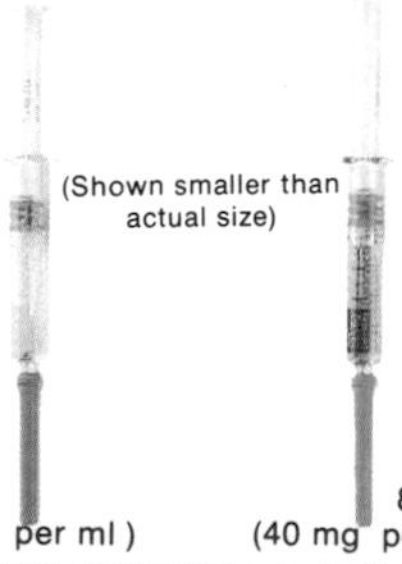

(Shown smaller than actual size)

60 mg (40 mg per ml)   80 mg (40 mg per ml)

†GARAMYCIN® Injectable Disposable Syringe
(gentamicin sulfate, USP)

Schering

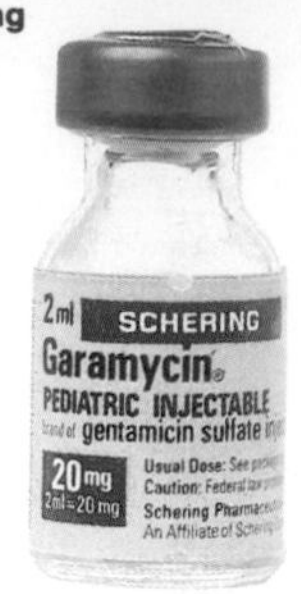

20 mg vial (10 mg per ml)

†GARAMYCIN® Pediatric Injectable
(gentamicin sulfate, USP)

Schering

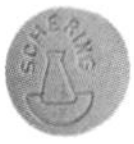

WAR or 617

0.5 mg

GITALIGIN® Tablets
(gitalin)

Schering
(Shown smaller than actual size)

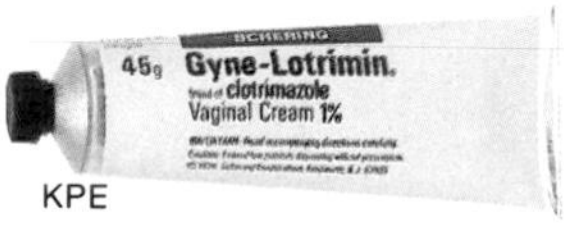

KPE

45 g tube

Applicator

Delbay labeled stocks are available

GYNE-LOTRIMIN® Vaginal Cream 1%
(clotrimazole)

Schering

734

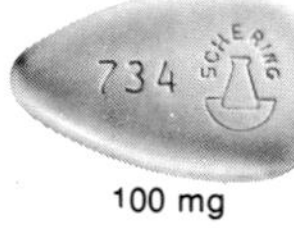

100 mg

GYNE-LOTRIMIN® Vaginal Tablets
(clotrimazole)

Schering

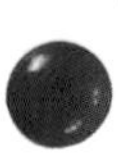

AMT ** or 800

".02"

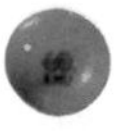

AMU ** or 490

".04"

GYNETONE® Tablets
(ethinyl estradiol, USP and methyltestosterone, USP)

†Other dosage forms available. See Product Information section or check directly with manufacturer.
**During the next year, either National Drug Identification numbers or letters may be imprinted on the products.

Schering

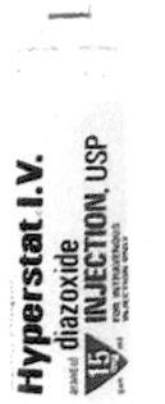

20 ml ampule
(300 mg /ampule)

HYPERSTAT® I.V. Injection

(diazoxide, USP)

Schering/White Product Line

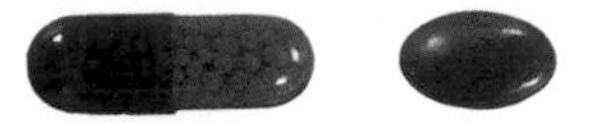

CHRONOSULE® Capsules — Tablets

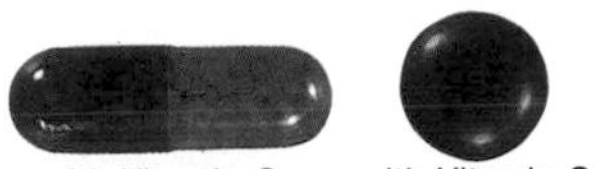

with Vitamin C **CHRONOSULE® Capsules** — with Vitamin C Tablets

†MOL-IRON®

Schering/White Product Line

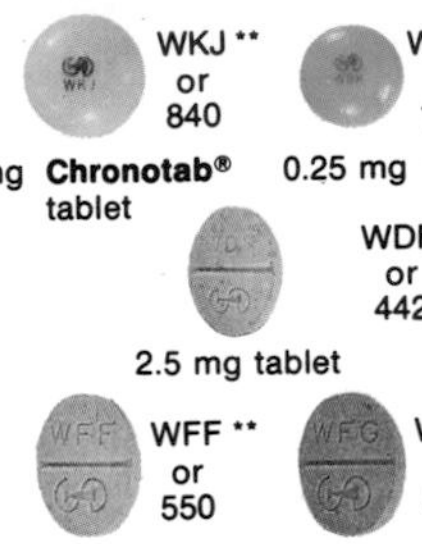

WKJ ** or 840 — 1 mg **Chronotab®** tablet

WBK ** or 122 — 0.25 mg tablet

WDR ** or 442 — 2.5 mg tablet

WFF ** or 550 — 5 mg tablet

WFG ** or 316 — 10 mg tablet

†PERMITIL®
(fluphenazine hydrochloride, USP)

Schering

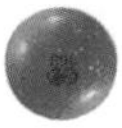
BBA or 968

20 mg

TINDAL® Tablets
(acetophenazine maleate, NF)

Schering

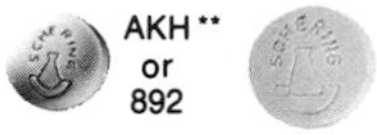

AKH ** or 892 — 2 mg

AKJ ** or 596 — 5 mg

TREMIN® Tablets
(trihexyphenidyl hydrochloride, USP)

Schering

(Shown smaller than actual size)

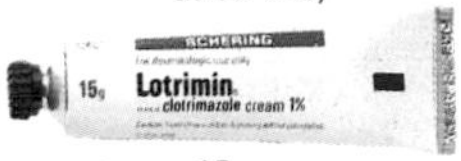

KPE

15 g

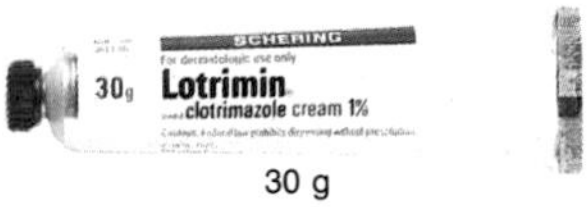

30 g

LOTRIMIN® Cream 1%
(clotrimazole)

Schering

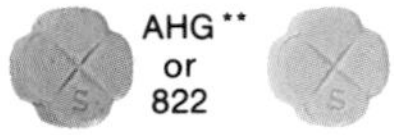

AHG ** or 822 — 2 mg

AHH ** or 547 — 4 mg

NAQUA® Tablets
(trichlormethiazide, NF)

Schering

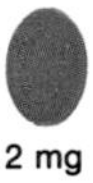
AGT ** or 820

2 mg

†POLARAMINE® Tablets
(dexchlorpheniramine maleate, NF)

Schering

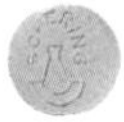
AHT ** or 394

NAQUIVAL® Tablets
(trichlormethiazide NF and reserpine USP)

Schering

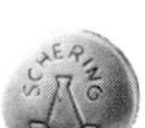
662

100 mg

PRANTAL® Tablets
(diphemanil methylsulfate, NF)

Schering

(Shown smaller than actual size)

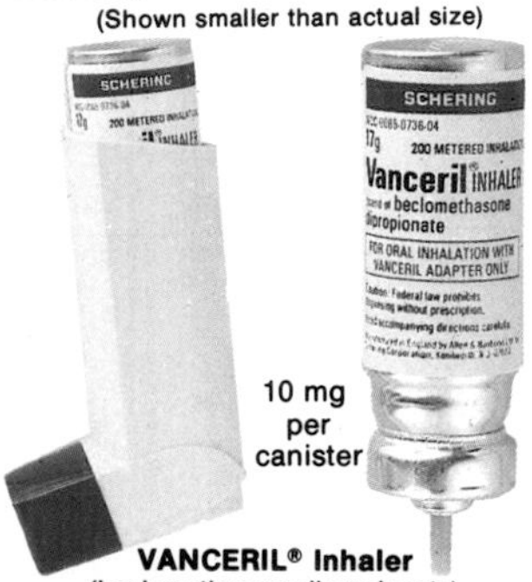

10 mg per canister

VANCERIL® Inhaler
(beclomethasone dipropionate)

Schering

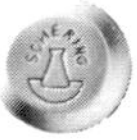
282

1 mg

OPTIMINE® Tablets
(azatadine maleate)

Schering

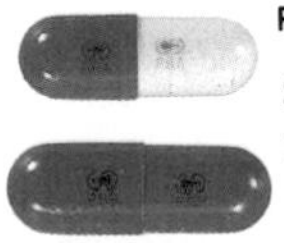

50 mg — PBA or 205

100 mg — PBB or 830

†PROGLYCEM® Capsules
(diazoxide, USP)

SEARLE

Both sides of tablet shown

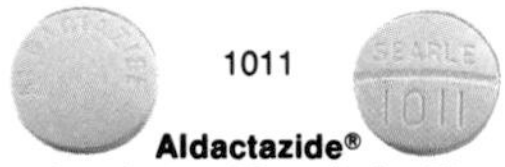

1011

Aldactazide®
(spironolactone 25 mg./hydrochlorothiazide 25 mg.)

Schering

(Shown smaller than actual size)

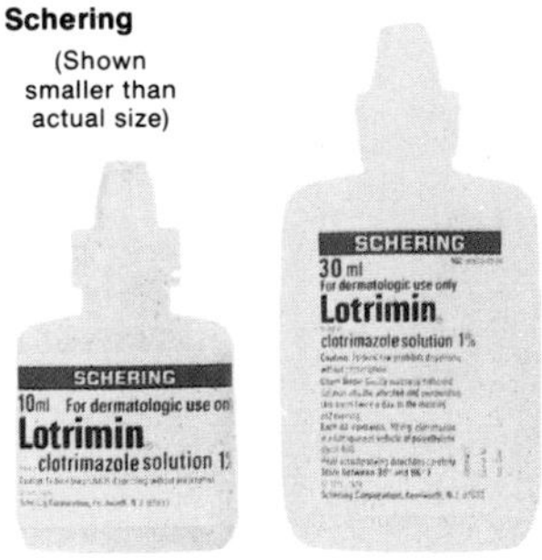

10 ml — 30 ml

LOTRIMIN® Solution 1%
(clotrimazole)

Schering

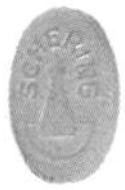
BE ** or 970

10 mg

ORETON® Methyl Buccal Tablets
(methyltestosterone, USP)

Schering

AHR or 160

350 mg

RELA® Tablets
(carisoprodol)

Searle

Both sides of tablet shown

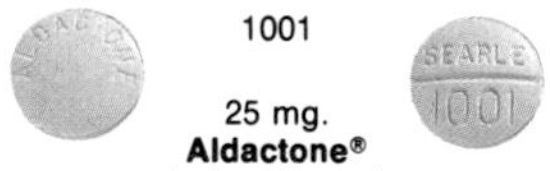

1001

25 mg.

Aldactone®
(spironolactone)

Schering

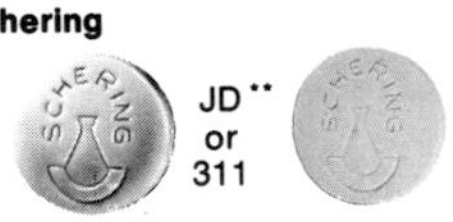

JD ** or 311 — 10 mg

JE ** or 499 — 25 mg

ORETON® Methyl Tablets
(methyltestosterone, USP)

Schering

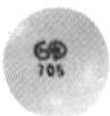
ADH ** or 705

2 mg

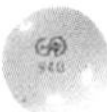
ADK ** or 940

4 mg

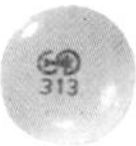
ADJ ** or 313

8 mg

ADM ** or 077

16 mg

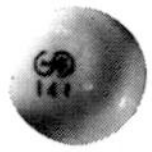
ADX ** or 141

8 mg **REPETABS®**

TRILAFON® Tablets
(perphenazine, NF)

Searle

Both sides of tablet shown

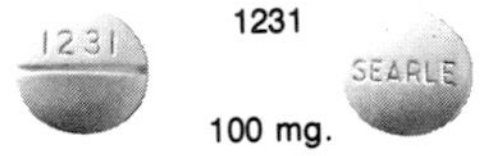

1231

100 mg.

1251

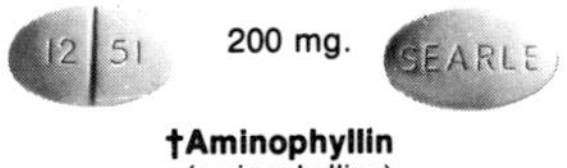

200 mg.

†Aminophyllin
(aminophylline)

Schering

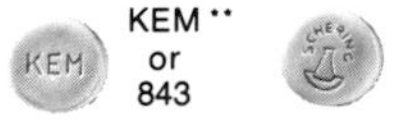

KEM ** or 843 — 1 mg

ABB ** or 172 — 5 mg

METICORTEN® Tablets
(prednisone, USP)

Schering

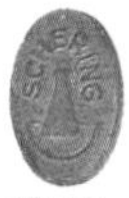
BJ ** or 675

10 mg

†ORETON® Propionate Buccal Tablets
(testosterone propionate, USP)

Schering

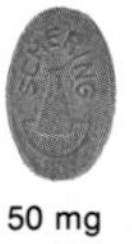
ANK ** or 795

50 mg

MIRADON® Tablets
(anisindione)

Schering

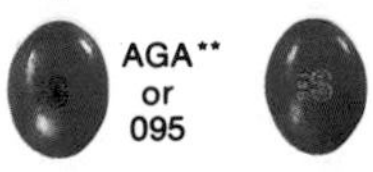

AGA ** or 095 — 4 mg

AGB ** or 148 — 6 mg

POLARAMINE® REPETABS® Tablets
(dexchlorpheniramine maleate, NF)

Searle

Both sides of tablet shown

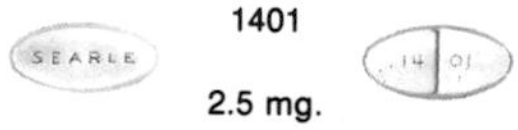

1401

2.5 mg.

Anavar®
(oxandrolone)

†Other dosage forms available. See Product Information section or check directly with manufacturer.
**During the next year, either National Drug Identification numbers or letters may be imprinted on the products.

Searle

1552

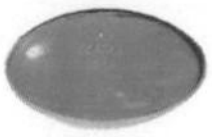

100 mg.

Comfolax®
(dioctyl sodium sulfosuccinate U.S.P.)

Searle

1572

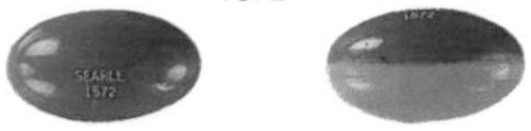

Comfolax-*plus*®
(dioctyl sodium sulfosuccinate U.S.P. 100 mg./casanthranol 30 mg.)

Searle

0708

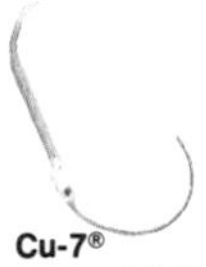

Cu-7®
(intrauterine copper contraceptive)

Searle

Both sides of tablet shown

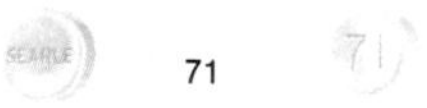

71

Demulen®
(ethynodiol diacetate 1 mg./ethinyl estradiol 50 mcg.)

Searle

501 511 521

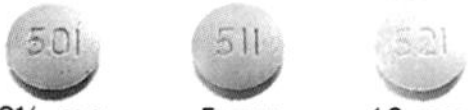

2½ mg. 5 mg. 10 mg.

(reverse side: SEARLE)

Diulo™
(metolazone)

Searle

Both sides of tablet shown

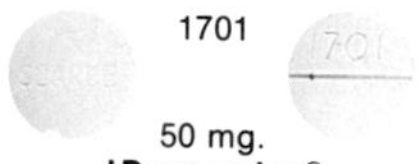

1701

50 mg.

†Dramamine®
(dimenhydrinate)

Searle

Both sides of tablet shown

51 101

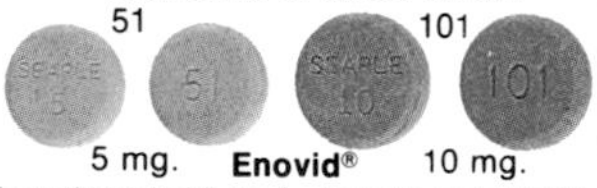

5 mg. **Enovid®** 10 mg.
(norethynodrel 5 mg./mestranol 0.075 mg.) (norethynodrel 9.85 mg./mestranol 0.15 mg.)

Searle

Both sides of tablet shown

131

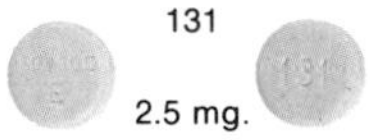

2.5 mg.

Enovid-E®
(norethynodrel 2.5 mg./with mestranol 0.1 mg.)

Searle

Both sides of tablet shown

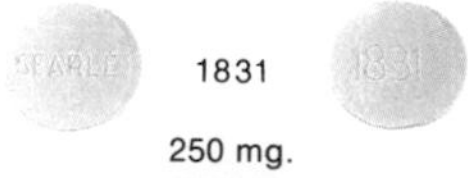

1831

250 mg.

Flagyl®
(metronidazole)

Searle

Both sides of tablet shown

61

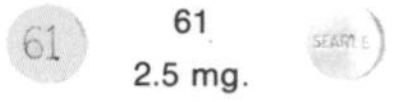

2.5 mg.

†Lomotil®
(diphenoxylate hydrochloride 2.5 mg./atropine sulfate 0.025 mg.)

Searle

2752

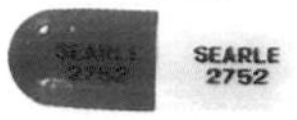

100 mg.

2762

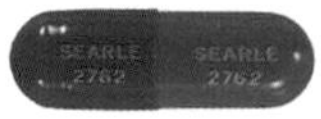

150 mg.

Norpace®
(disopyramide phosphate)

Searle

Both sides of tablet shown

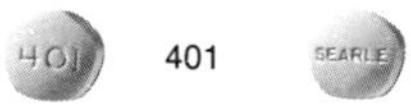

401

Ovulen®
(ethynodiol diacetate 1 mg./mestranol 0.1 mg.)

Searle

Both sides of tablets shown

611 601

7.5 mg. 15 mg.

†Pro-Banthīne®
(propantheline bromide)

Searle

Both sides of tablet shown

631

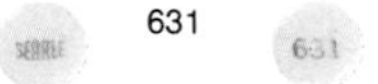

†Pro-Banthīne® with Phenobarbital
(propantheline bromide 15 mg./phenobarbital 15 mg.)

SMITH KLINE & FRENCH

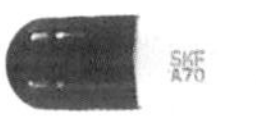

A70

250 mg.

A71

500 mg.

†Anspor® Capsules
(cephradine, SK&F)

Smith Kline & French Ⓒ II

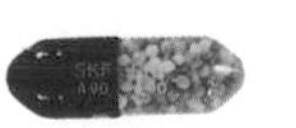

A90

15 mg.

†Benzedrine® Spansule® Capsules
(amphetamine sulfate, SK&F)

Smith Kline & French Ⓒ II

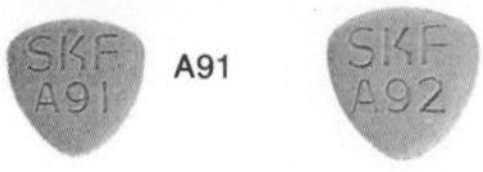

A91 A92

5 mg. **†Benzedrine® Tablets** 10 mg.
(amphetamine sulfate, SK&F)

Smith Kline & French

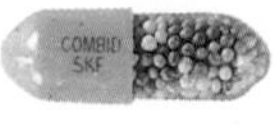

COMBID

Combid® Spansule® Capsules

Smith Kline & French

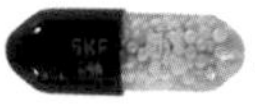

C46
15 mg.

Also 10 mg. C44, 30 mg. C47, 75 mg. C49

†Compazine® Spansule® Capsules
(prochlorperazine, SK&F)

Smith Kline & French

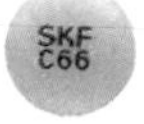

C66
5 mg.

Also 10 mg. C67, 25 mg. C69

†Compazine® Tablets
(prochlorperazine, SK&F)

Smith Kline & French

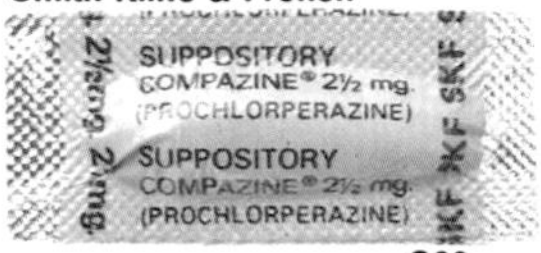

C60
2½ mg.

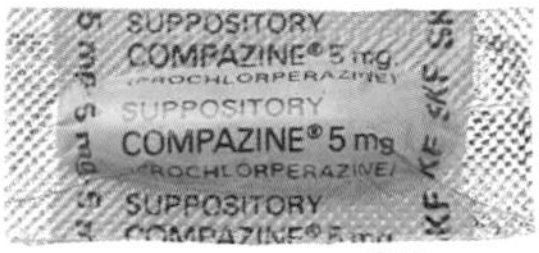

C61
5 mg.

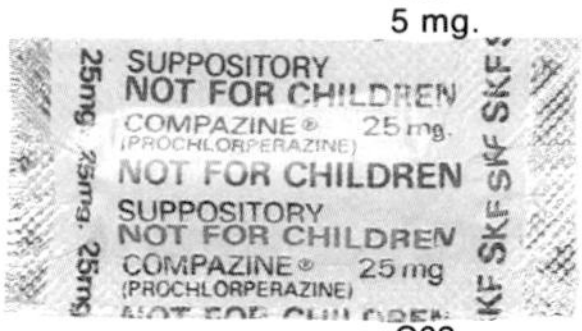

C62
25 mg.

†Compazine® Suppositories
(prochlorperazine, SK&F)

Smith Kline & French

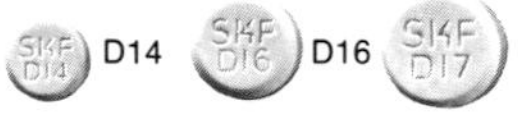

D14 D16 D17

5 mcg. 25 mcg. 50 mcg.

liothyronine as the sodium salt

Cytomel® Tablets
(brand of liothyronine sodium)

Smith Kline & French

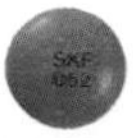

D62

5 mg.

Darbid® Tablets
(brand of isopropamide iodide)

Smith Kline & French Ⓒ II

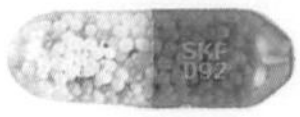

D92
No. 2

Also No. 1 D91

†Dexamyl® Spansule® Capsules

Smith Kline & French Ⓒ II

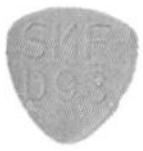

D93

†Dexamyl® Tablets

Smith Kline & French Ⓒ II

E14
15 mg.

Also 5 mg. E12, 10 mg. E13

†Dexedrine® Spansule® Capsules
(dextroamphetamine sulfate, SK&F)

Smith Kline & French Ⓒ II

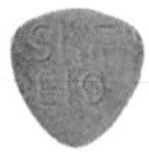

E19

5 mg.

†Dexedrine® Tablets
(dextroamphetamine sulfate, SK&F)

Smith Kline & French

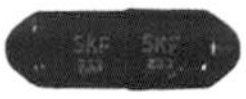

E33

10 mg.

Dibenzyline® Capsules
(phenoxybenzamine hydrochloride, SK&F)

SK & F Co.

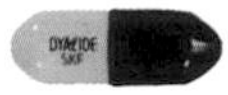

DYAZIDE

Dyazide® Capsules

SK & F Co.

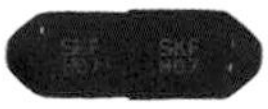

H07

100 mg.

Also 50 mg. H06

Dyrenium® Capsules
(triamterene, SK&F)

SmithKline Corp.‡

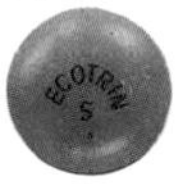

ECOTRIN

5 gr.

Ecotrin® Tablets

Smith Kline & French

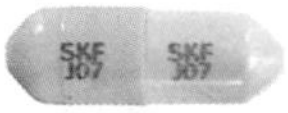

J07

300 mg.

Eskalith® Capsules
(lithium carbonate, SK&F)

†Other dosage forms available. See Product Information section or check directly with manufacturer.
‡Professional Products Division, Menley & James Laboratories.

Smith Kline & French

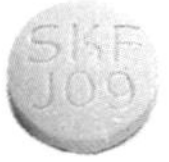

J09

300 mg.
Eskalith® Tablets
(lithium carbonate, SK&F)

Smith Kline & French

K77

5 mg.
Hispril® Spansule® Capsules
(diphenylpyraline hydrochloride, SK&F)

SK & F Co.

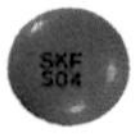

2 mg. S04
Also 1 mg. S03,
5 mg. S06, 10 mg.
S07

†Stelazine® Tablets
(trifluoperazine HCl, SK&F)

SmithKline Corp.‡

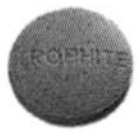

TROPHITE

†Trophite® Tablets

Smith Kline & French Ⓒ

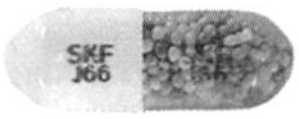

J66

Eskatrol® Spansule® Capsules

SmithKline Corp.‡

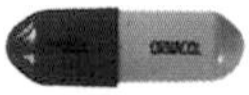

ORNACOL

†Ornacol® Capsules

SK&F Lab Co.

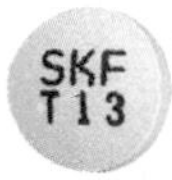

T13
300 mg.

†Tagamet® Tablets
(cimetidine, SK&F)

Smith Kline & French

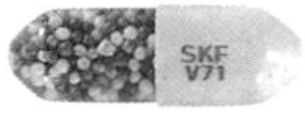

V71

†Tuss-Ornade® Spansule® Capsules

SmithKline Corp.‡

FEOSOL

†Feosol® Spansule® Capsules

Smith Kline & French

ORNADE

Ornade® Spansule® Capsules

SmithKline Corp.‡

TELDRIN
12 mg.

Also 8 mg. TELDRIN

Teldrin® Timed-Release Capsules
(chlorpheniramine maleate)

Smith Kline & French

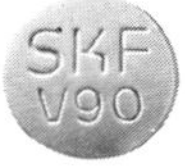

V90

100 mg.
Urispas® Tablets
(flavoxate HCl, SK&F)

SmithKline Corp.‡

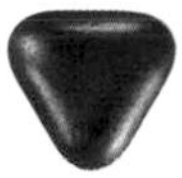

†Feosol® Tablets

SmithKline Corp.‡

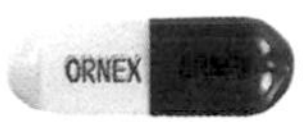

ORNEX

Ornex® Capsules

Smith Kline & French

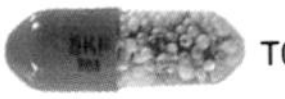

T01

5 mg.
†Temaril® Spansule® Capsules
(trimeprazine tartrate, SK&F)

Smith Kline & French

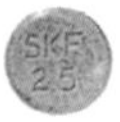

X42

25 mg.
†Vontrol® Tablets
(diphenidol as the hydrochloride, SK&F)

SmithKline Corp.‡

K33

Feosol Plus® Capsules

Smith Kline & French

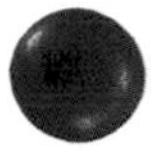

N71

10 mg.
Parnate® Tablets
(tranylcypromine sulfate, SK&F)

Smith Kline & French

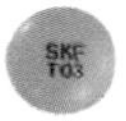

T03

2.5 mg.
Temaril® Tablets
(trimeprazine tartrate, SK&F)

E. R. SQUIBB & SONS

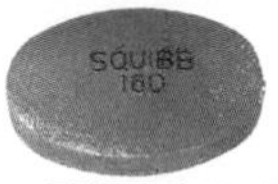

#160**
250 mg.

ETHRIL® '250'
(Erythromycin Stearate Tablets U.S.P.)

SmithKline Corp.‡

FORTESPAN

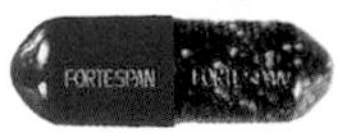

Fortespan® Capsules

Smith Kline & French

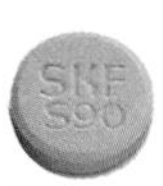

S90

250 mg.
Selacryn® Tablets
(ticrynafen, SK&F)

Smith Kline & French

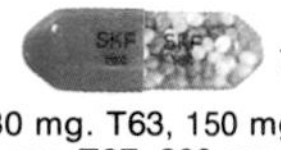

T64
75 mg.

Also 30 mg. T63, 150 mg. T66,
200 mg. T67, 300 mg. T69

†Thorazine® Spansule® Capsules
(chlorpromazine hydrochloride, SK&F)

E. R. Squibb & Sons

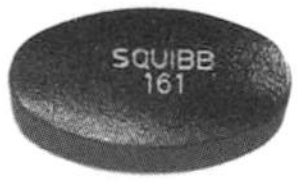

#161**

500 mg.
ETHRIL® '500'
(Erythromycin Stearate Tablets U.S.P.)

SMITH KLINE & FRENCH LABORATORIES
Division of SmithKline Corporation
TABLET & CAPSULE IDENTIFICATION

The unique "taper-end" shape of SK&F capsules is a trademark that quickly identifies them as products of Smith Kline & French Laboratories.

Product Identification Code: Each SK&F capsule and tablet bears a monogram consisting of a three-character code or the name of the specific product. An index for the SK&F Product Identification Code appears at the beginning of the Product Information Section for Smith Kline & French Laboratories.

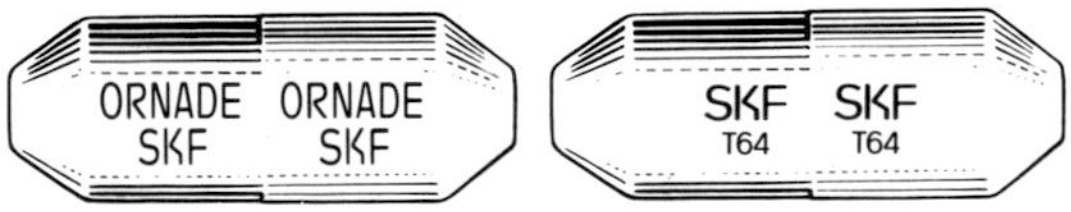

Capsule Shape: Trademark

The three-unit product identification codes or names that appear beside products in the photo blocks are the same as those imprinted on the pictured products because the codes may be difficult to read in the photo reproductions.

NOTE: Dyazide®, Dyrenium® and Stelazine® are products of SK&F Co., Carolina, P.R. 00630, a subsidiary of SmithKline Corporation. Tagamet® is a product of SK&F Lab Co.. Carolina, P.R. 00630, a subsidiary of SmithKline Corporation.

Smith Kline & French

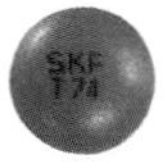

25 mg. T74

Also 10 mg. T73, 50 mg. T76,
100 mg. T77, 200 mg. T79
†Thorazine® Tablets
(chlorpromazine hydrochloride, SK&F)

E. R. Squibb & Sons

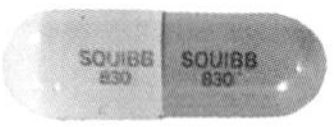

500 mg.
#830**

HYDREA®
(Hydroxyurea Capsules U.S.P.)

Smith Kline & French

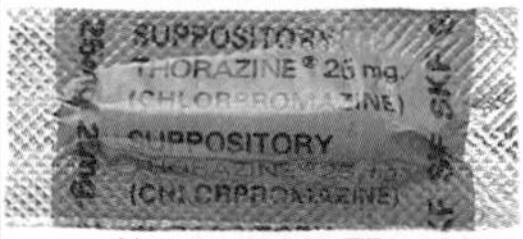

T70
25 mg.

Also available T71, 100 mg.
†Thorazine® Suppositories
(chlorpromazine, SK&F)

E. R. Squibb & Sons

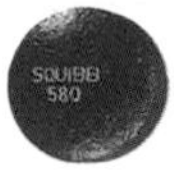

500,000 u.
#580**

†MYCOSTATIN® Oral Tablets
(Nystatin Tablets U.S.P.)

SmithKline Corp.‡

TROPH-IRON

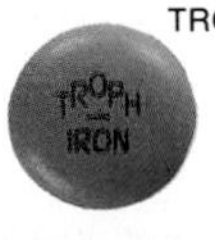

†Troph-Iron® Tablets

E. R. Squibb & Sons

100,000 u.
#457**

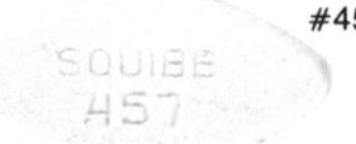

MYCOSTATIN® Vaginal Tablets
(Nystatin Vaginal Tablets U.S.P.)

†Other dosage forms available. See Product Information section or check directly with manufacturer.
‡Professional Products Division, Menley & James Laboratories. **Squibb product identification number.

E. R. Squibb & Sons

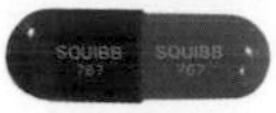

125 mg./25 mg.
#767**

250 mg./50 mg.
#779**

†MYSTECLIN-F® Capsules
(Tetracycline-Amphotericin B Capsules)

E. R. Squibb & Sons

1 mg. #863** | 2.5 mg. #864**

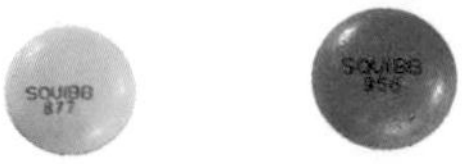

5 mg. #877** | 10 mg. #956**

†PROLIXIN®
(Fluphenazine Hydrochloride Tablets U.S.P.)

E. R. Squibb & Sons

250 mg.
#655**

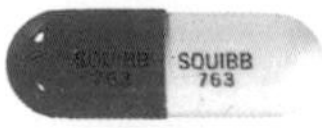

500 mg.
#763**

†SUMYCIN® CAPSULES
(Tetracycline Hydrochloride Capsules U.S.P.)

E. R. Squibb & Sons

1 g
#147**

†VELOSEF® TABLETS
(Cephradine Tablets)

STUART

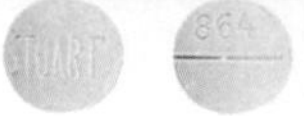

NDC 38-864

(Both sides of tablet shown)
BUCLADIN®-S Softab™
(buclizine hydrochloride 50 mg.)

E. R. Squibb & Sons

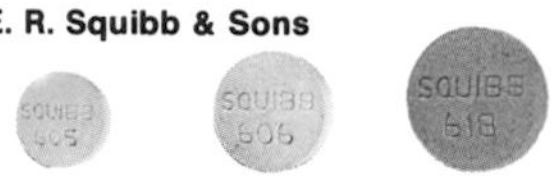

2.5 mg. #605** | 5 mg. #606** | 10 mg. #618**

NATURETIN®
(Bendroflumethiazide Tablets N.F.)

E. R. Squibb & Sons

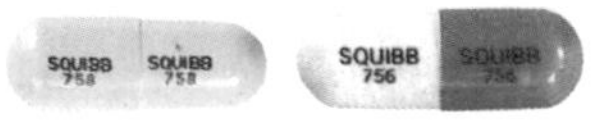

250 mg. #758** | 375 mg. #756**

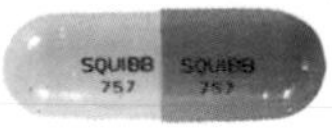

500 mg.
#757**

†PRONESTYL® CAPSULES
(Procainamide Hydrochloride Capsules U.S.P.)

E. R. Squibb & Sons

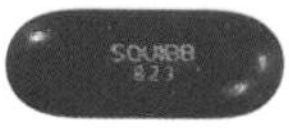

#823**

†THERAGRAN®
(High Potency Vitamin Formula)

Stuart

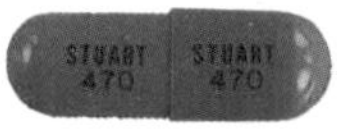

NDC 38-470

DIALOSE® capsules
(dioctyl potassium sulfo-succinate, 100 mg.)

E. R. Squibb & Sons Ⓒ

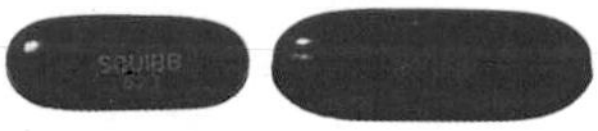

250 mg. (3¾ gr.) #623** | 500 mg. (7½ gr.) #626**

†NOCTEC®
(Chloral Hydrate Capsules U.S.P.)

E. R. Squibb & Sons

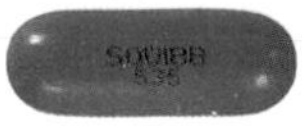

#535**

THERAGRAN® HEMATINIC
(Therapeutic Formula Vitamin Tablets with Hematinics)

Stuart

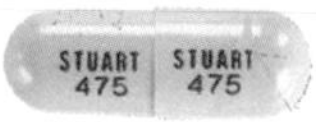

NDC 38-475

DIALOSE® PLUS capsules
(casanthranol, 30 mg.; dioctyl potassium sulfosuccinate, 100 mg.)

E. R. Squibb & Sons

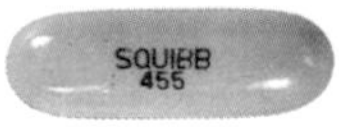

500 mg.
#455**

†ORAGRAFIN® SODIUM
(Ipodate Sodium Capsules U.S.P.)

E. R. Squibb & Sons

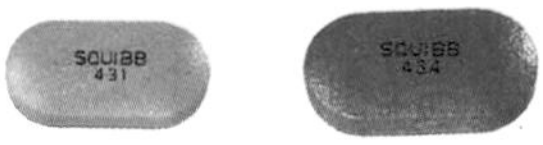

250 mg. #431** | 375 mg. #434**

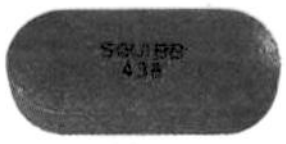

500 mg.
#438**

†PRONESTYL® TABLETS
(Procainamide Hydrochloride Tablets)

E. R. Squibb & Sons

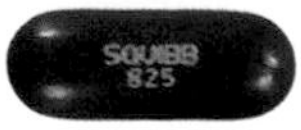

#825**

THERAGRAN®-M
(High Potency Vitamin Formula with Minerals)

Stuart (layered tablet)

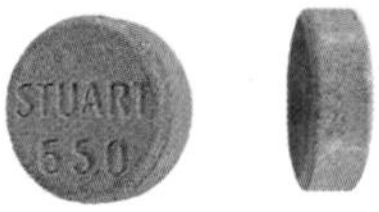

NDC 38-650

FERANCEE® chewable tablets

E. R. Squibb & Sons

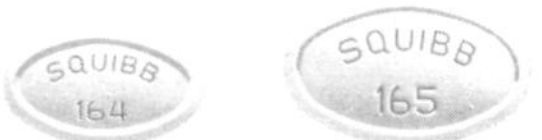

200,000 u. #164** | 400,000 u. #165**

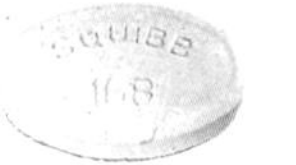

800,000 u.
#168**

†PENTIDS® Tablets
†PENTIDS® '400' Tablets
PENTIDS® '800' Tablets
(Penicillin G Potassium Tablets U.S.P.)

E. R. Squibb & Sons

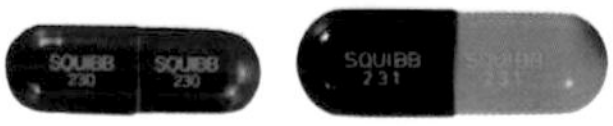

250 mg. #230** | 500 mg. #231**

†TRIMOX® CAPSULES
(Amoxicillin Capsules)

Stuart

NDC 38-863

FERANCEE®-HP tablets

E. R. Squibb & Sons

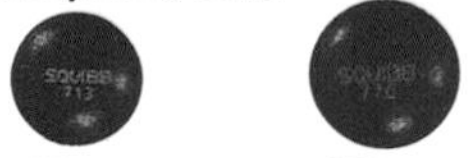

50 mg. #713** | 100 mg. #776**

RAUDIXIN®
(Rauwolfia Serpentina Tablets N.F.)

E. R. Squibb & Sons

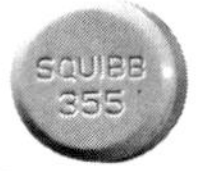

#355**

325 mg. (5 gr.)

†VALADOL®
(Acetaminophen Tablets U.S.P.)

Stuart (Shown smaller than actual size)

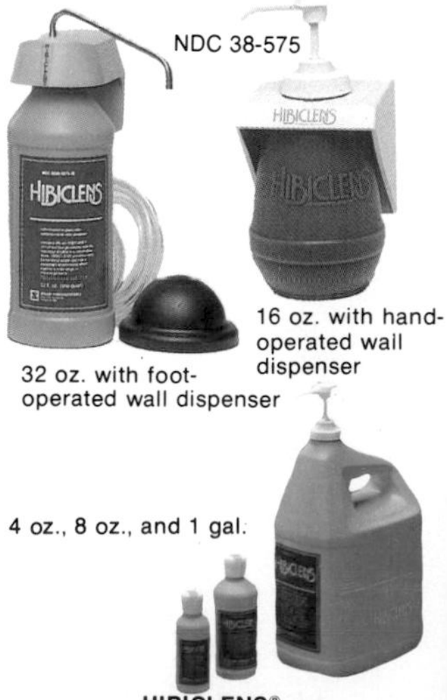

HIBICLENS®
(chlorhexidine gluconate)

E. R. Squibb & Sons

250 mg.
#971**

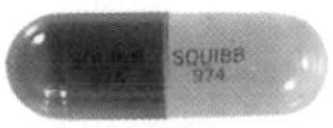

500 mg.
#974**

†PRINCIPEN®
(Ampicillin Capsules U.S.P.)

E. R. Squibb & Sons

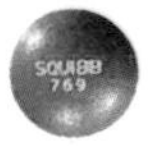

#769**

RAUZIDE®
(Powdered Rauwolfia Serpentina 50 mg. with Bendroflumethiazide 4 mg.)

E. R. Squibb & Sons

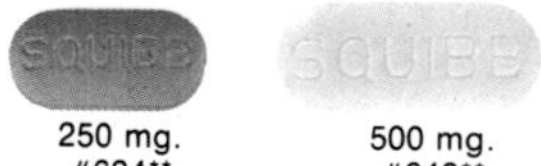

250 mg. #684** | 500 mg. #648**

†VEETIDS®
(Penicillin V Potassium Tablets U.S.P.)

E. R. Squibb & Sons

250 mg. #663** | 500 mg. #603**

†SUMYCIN® TABLETS
(Tetracycline Hydrochloride Tablets N.F.)

E. R. Squibb & Sons

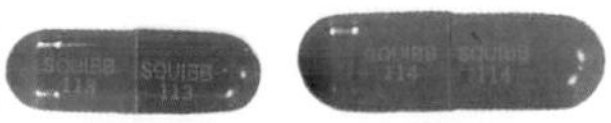

250 mg. #113** | 500 mg. #114**

†VELOSEF® CAPSULES
(Cephradine Capsules)

†Other dosage forms available. See Product Information section or check directly with manufacturer.
**Squibb product identification number.

Stuart

(Shown smaller than actual size)

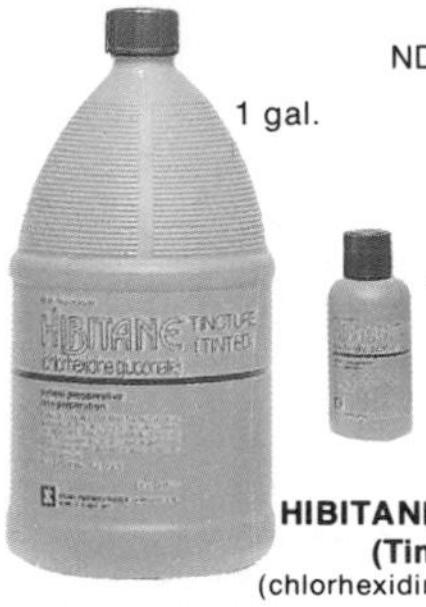

NDC 38-0580

1 gal.

4 oz.

HIBITANE® Tincture (Tinted)
(chlorhexidine gluconate)

Stuart

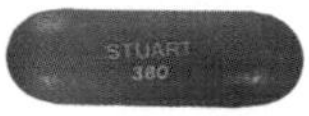

NDC 38-380

240 mg.

KASOF® capsules
(dioctyl potassium sulfosuccinate)

Stuart (Both sides of tablet shown)

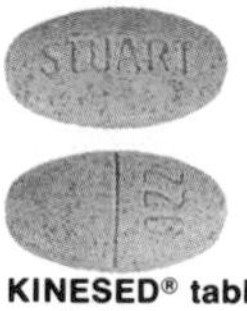

NDC 38-220

KINESED® tablets
(belladonna alkaloids and phenobarbital)

Stuart

(Both sides of tablet shown)

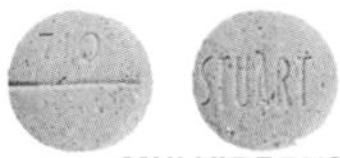

NDC 38-710

MULVIDREN®—F Softab®
(Fluoride with Multivitamins)

Stuart

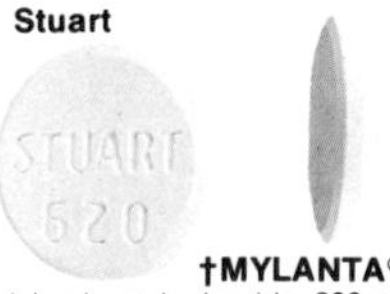

NDC 38-620

(layered tablet)

†MYLANTA® tablets
(aluminum hydroxide, 200 mg.; magnesium hydroxide, 200 mg.; simethicone, 20 mg.)

Stuart

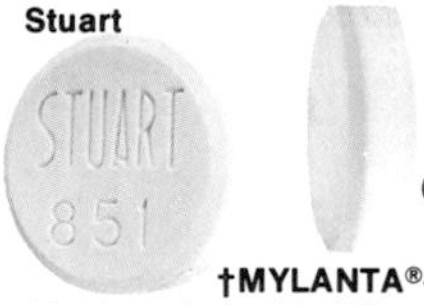

NDC 38-851

(layered tablet)

†MYLANTA®-II tablets
(aluminum hydroxide, 400 mg.; magnesium hydroxide, 400 mg.; simethicone, 30 mg.)

Stuart (Both sides of tablet shown)

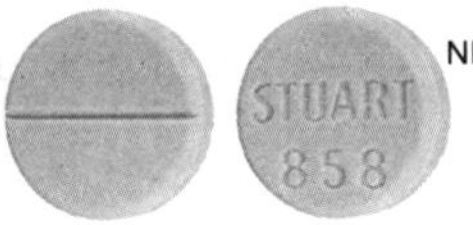

NDC 38-858

MYLICON®-80 tablets
(simethicone 80 mg.)

Stuart (Both sides of tablet shown)

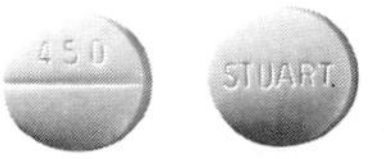

NDC 38-450

†MYLICON® tablets
(simethicone, 40 mg.)

Stuart

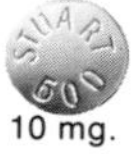

NDC 38-600

10 mg.

NOLVADEX® tablets
(tamoxifen citrate)

Stuart

NDC 38-840

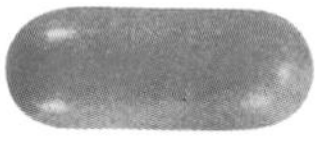

PROBEC®-T tablets

Stuart

NDC 38-810 NDC 38-815

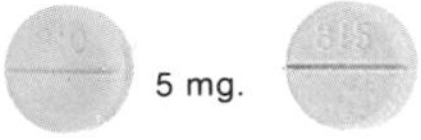

5 mg. 10 mg.

CHEWABLE SORBITRATE® tablets
(isosorbide dinitrate)

Stuart (Both sides of tablet shown)

NDC 38-770 NDC 38-780

Oral

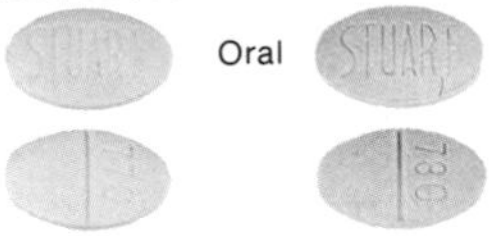

5 mg. 10 mg.

NDC 38-820

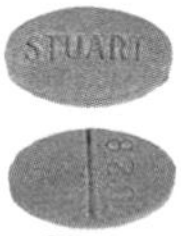

20 mg.

NDC 38-880

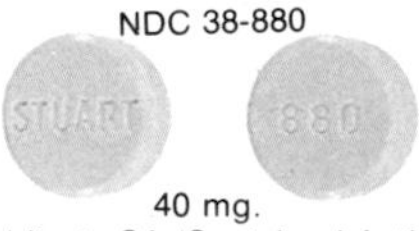

40 mg.
Sorbitrate SA (Sustained Action)

SORBITRATE® tablets
(isosorbide dinitrate)

Stuart

NDC 38-853 NDC 38-760

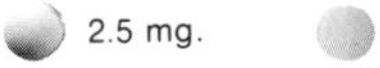

2.5 mg. 5 mg.

SORBITRATE® SUBLINGUAL tablets
(isosorbide dinitrate)

Stuart

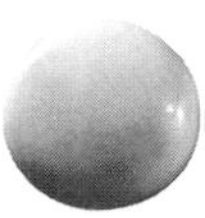

NDC 38-866

†STUART FORMULA® tablets

Stuart

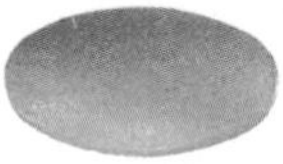

NDC 38-862

STUARTINIC® tablets

Stuart

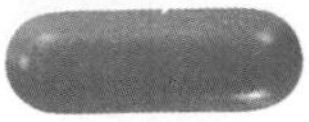

NDC 38-270

STUART PRENATAL® tablets

NDC 38-800

STUART PRENATAL® c̄ Folic Acid

NDC 38-850

STUARTNATAL® 1 + 1 tablets

SugarLo

(Shown smaller than actual size)

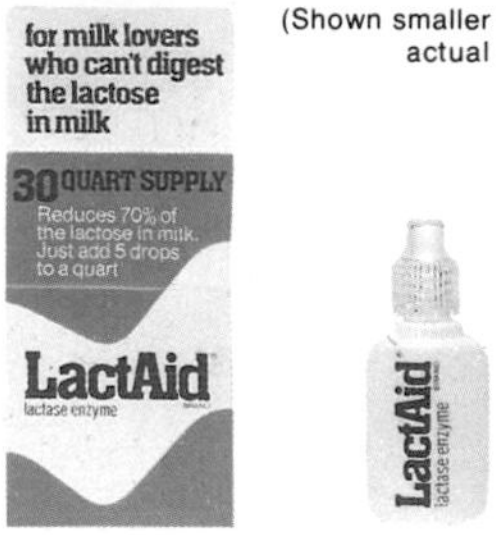

Lact-Aid®
(lactase enzyme)

Survival Technology, Inc.

(shown approximately half size)

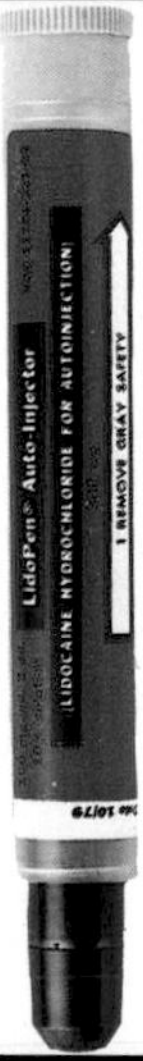

NDC 11704-221-02

300 mg. (3 ml. 10% solution)

LidoPen® Auto-Injector
(lidocaine hydrochloride for autoinjection)

SYNTEX

2902*

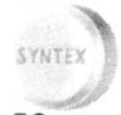

50 mg.

Anadrol®-50
(oxymetholone)

Syntex

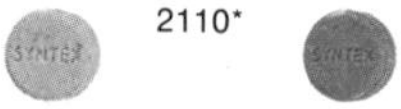

2110*

(inert tablet)

Brevicon® Tablets
(norethindrone 0.5 mg. with ethinyl estradiol 0.035 mg.) Available in 21- and 28-day (with 7 inert tablets) regimens.

Syntex

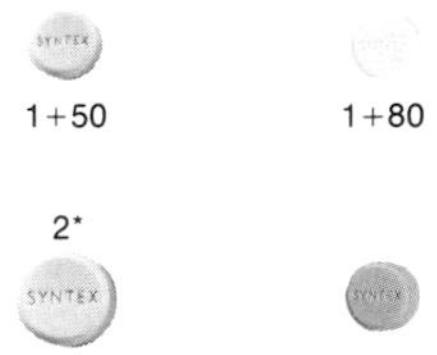

1*

1+50 1+80

2*

2 mg. (inert tablet)

Norinyl® Tablets
(norethindrone with mestranol)
Norinyl 1+50 and Norinyl 1+80 available in both 21- and 28-day (with 7 inert tablets) regimens.

Syntex

2107*

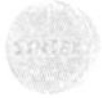

0.35 mg.

Nor-Q.D.® Tablets
(norethindrone)

Syntex

272*

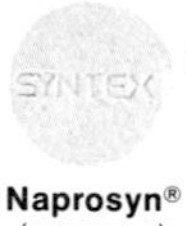

250 mg. tablets

Naprosyn®
(naproxen)

TUTAG

50 mg.

Aquatag® Tablet
(Benzthiazide, NF)

Tutag Ⓒ III

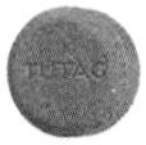

35 mg.

Bacarate® Tablet
(Phendimetrazine Tartrate)

Tutag

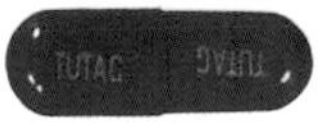

Escot® Capsule

Tutag

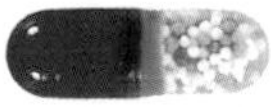

Neotep® Granucap®

Tutag

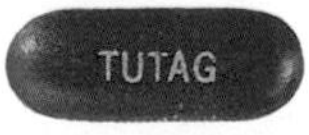

Normacid® Tablet

†Other dosage forms available. See Product Information section or check directly with manufacturer.
*Manufacturers' identification number.

Tutag

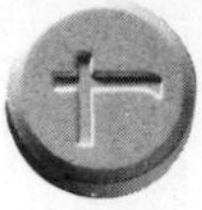

Quinite™ Tablet

Tutag

Suladyne® Tablet

Tutag

Unproco® Capsule

USV

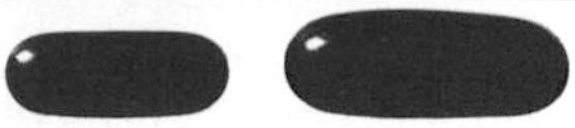

25,000 I.U. 50,000 I.U.

Aquasol® A
(water-miscible vitamin A)

USV

100 I.U.
Also available: 30 I.U., 400 I.U.

Aquasol® E
(aqueous vitamin E)

USV

6 mg. 12 mg.

****Arlidin®**
(nylidrin HCl)

USV

100 mg.

Azolid®
(phenylbutazone USP)

USV

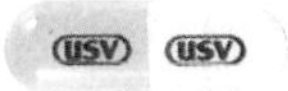

Azolid®-A
(phenylbutazone 100 mg., dried aluminum hydroxide gel 100 mg., magnesium trisilicate 150 mg.)

USV

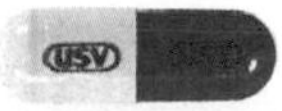

150 mg.—in micro-dialysis cells

Cerespan®
(papaverine HCl)

USV

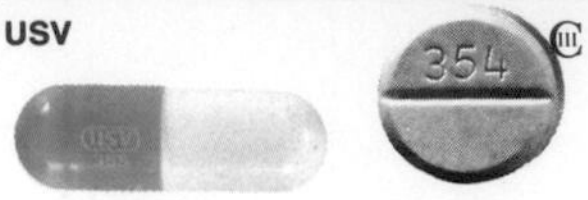

0.5 Gm. 0.5 Gm.
Also available: 0.25 Gm. tablets

*****Doriden®**
(glutethimide NF)

USV

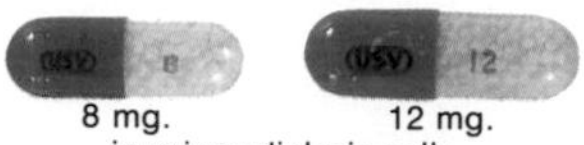

8 mg. 12 mg.
in micro-dialysis cells

Histaspan®
(chlorpheniramine maleate)

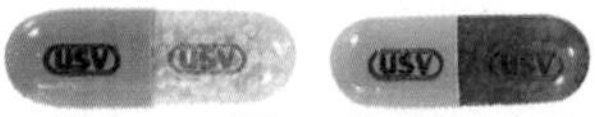

Histaspan-D®
(Histaspan [chlorpheniramine maleate] 8 mg., phenylephrine HCl 20 mg., methscopolamine nitrate 2.5 mg. in micro-dialysis cells)

Histaspan®-Plus
(Histaspan [chlorpheniramine maleate] 8 mg., and phenylephrine HCl 20 mg. in micro-dialysis cells)

USV

25 mg. 50 mg. 100 mg.

****Hygroton®**
(chlorthalidone USP)

USV
(Shown smaller than actual size)

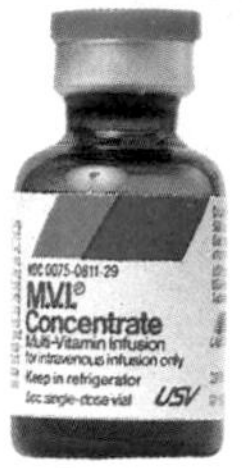

5 cc. vial
M.V.I.® Concentrate

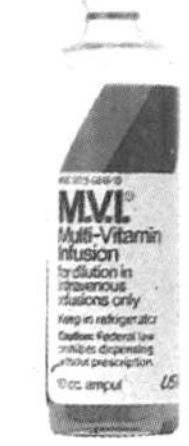

(Multi-Vitamin Infusion)

10 cc. ampul
M.V.I.®

USV

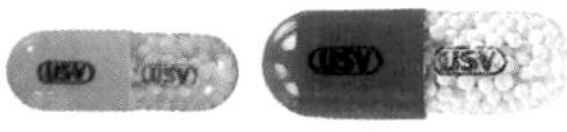

2.5 mg. 6.5 mg.

Nitrospan®
(nitroglycerin—in micro-dialysis cells)

USV

100 mg.

Oxalid®
(oxyphenbutazone)

USV

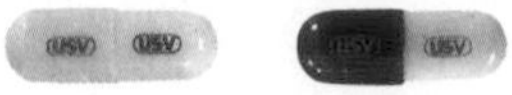

25 mg. 50 mg.

****Pertofrane®**
(desipramine HCl NF)

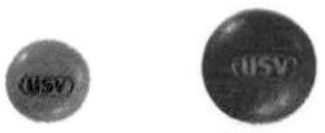

25 mg. 50 mg.

Presamine™
(imipramine HCl USP)

USV

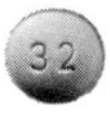

****Demi-Regroton®**
(chlorthalidone USP 25 mg., reserpine USP 0.125 mg.)

USV

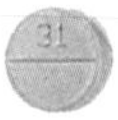

****Regroton®**
(chlorthalidone USP 50 mg. reserpine USP 0.25 mg.)

USV

50 mg.

Voranil®
(clortermine HCl)

UPJOHN

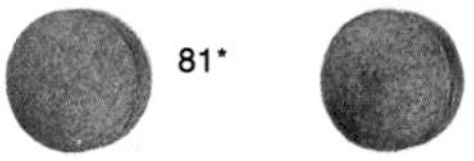

81* 92*

0.5 mg. 1 mg.

†Adeflor Chewable® Tablets

Upjohn

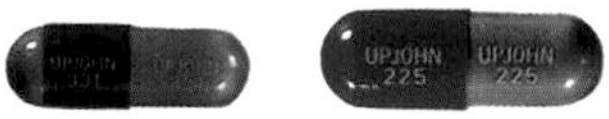

75 mg. 150 mg.
331* 225*

Cleocin HCl™ Capsules
(clindamycin HCl capsules, USP)

Upjohn

870* 2 ml ampoule (300 mg.)

(Shown smaller than actual size)

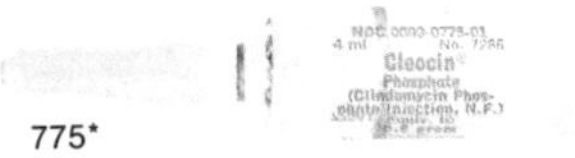

775* 4 ml ampoule (600 mg.)

Cleocin Phosphate™ Sterile Solution
(clindamycin phosphate injection, NF)

Upjohn

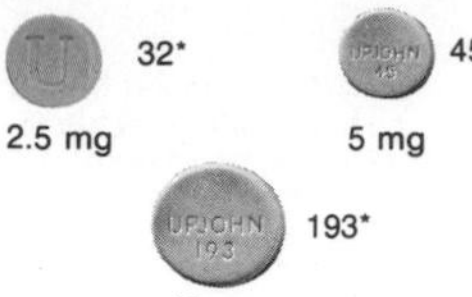

32* 45*
2.5 mg 5 mg
193*
10 mg

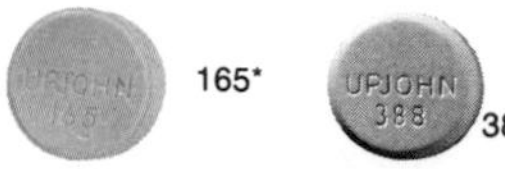

165* 388*
20 mg 50 mg

Deltasone® Tablets
(prednisone tablets, USP)

Upjohn

(shown smaller than actual size)

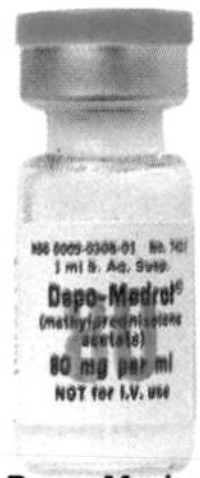

available:
20 mg
40 mg
80 mg

Depo-Medrol®
Sterile Aqueous Suspension
(sterile methylprednisolone acetate suspension, NF)
(20 mg /5 ml., 40 mg /1 ml., 40 mg /5 ml., 40 mg /10 ml., 80 mg /1 ml., 80 mg /5 ml.)

Upjohn

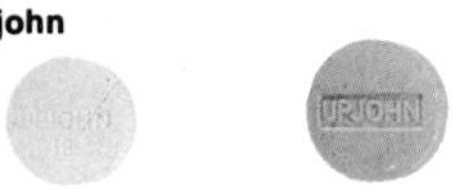

25 mg 50 mg
18* 24*

Didrex™ Tablets
(benzphetamine hydrochloride)

Upjohn

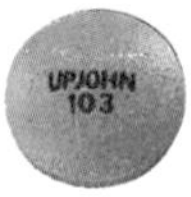

103*

250 mg

E-Mycin® Tablets
(erythromycin enteric coated tablets)

Upjohn

939* 940*

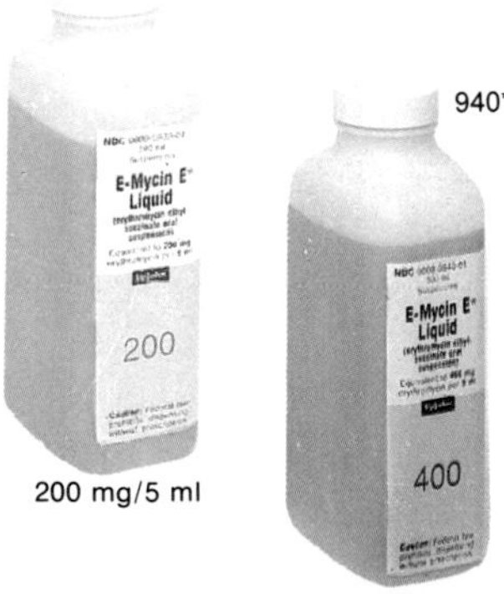

200 mg/5 ml 400 mg/5 ml

(Shown smaller than actual size)

E-Mycin E™ Liquid
(erythromycin ethylsuccinate oral suspension)

*Manufacturers' identification number. **Arlidin®, Hygroton®, Pertofrane®, Demi-Regroton™ and Regroton® are products of USV Laboratories Inc., Manati, P.R. 00701. ***Doriden® is a product of USV (P.R.) Development Corp., Manati, P.R. 00701. †Other dosage forms available. See Product Information section or check directly with manufacturer.

Upjohn

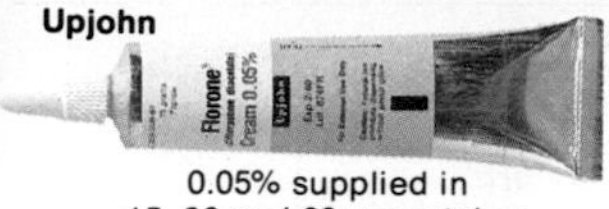

0.05% supplied in
15, 30 and 60 gram tubes
(Shown smaller than actual size)
Florone® Cream
(diflorasone diacetate)

Upjohn

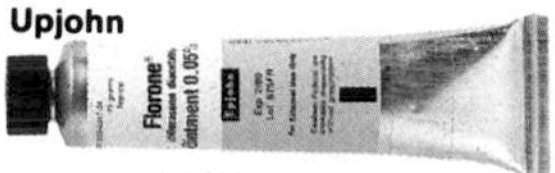

0.05% supplied in
15, 30 and 60 gram tubes
(Shown smaller than actual size)
Florone® Ointment
(diflorasone diacetate)

Upjohn

14* 2 mg | 19* 5 mg | 36* 10 mg

Halotestin® Tablets
(fluoxymesterone tablets, USP)

Upjohn

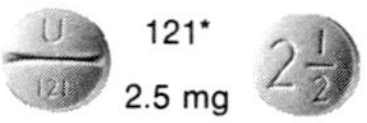

121*
2.5 mg

(Both sides of tablets shown)

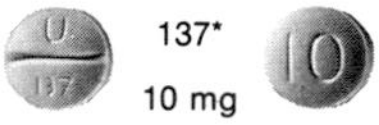

137*
10 mg

Loniten® Tablets
(minoxidil)

Upjohn

2 mg 49* | 4 mg 56* | 8 mg 22*

16 mg 73* | 24 mg 155* | 32 mg 176*

†Medrol® Tablets
(methylprednisolone tablets, NF)

Upjohn
(Shown smaller than actual size)

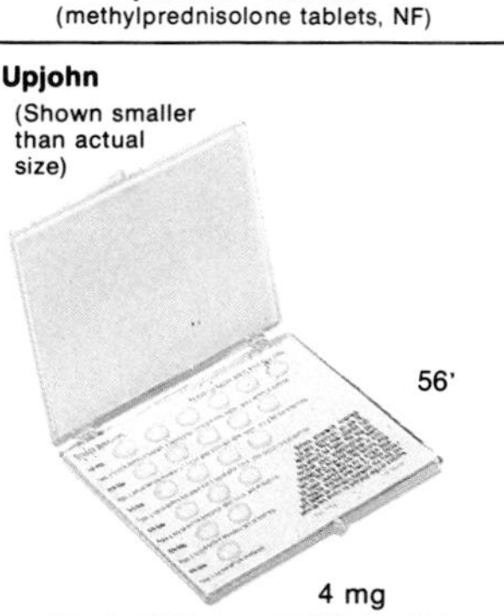

56*
4 mg
Medrol® Dosepak™ Unit of Use
(methylprednisolone tablets, NF)

Upjohn

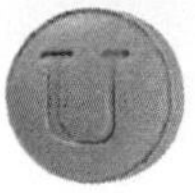

412*
400 mg
Maolate® Tablets
(chlorphenesin carbamate)

Upjohn

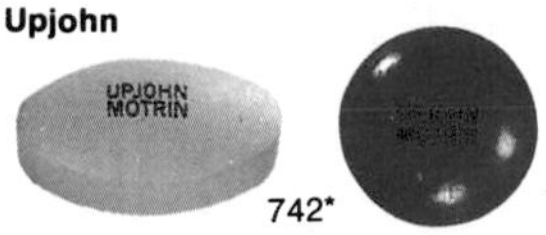

742* 600 mg | 750* 400 mg

Motrin® Tablets
(ibuprofen)

Upjohn

701*

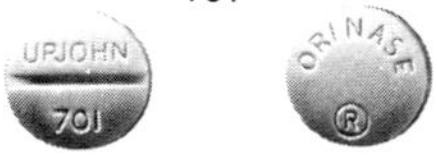

250 mg

(both sides of tablets shown)

100*

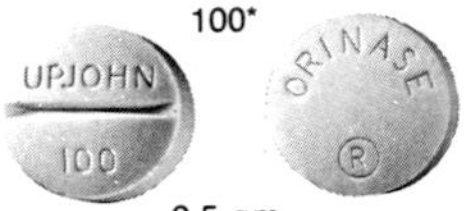

0.5 gm

Orinase® Tablets
(tolbutamide tablets, USP)

Upjohn

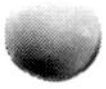

61*
2.5 mg
Pamine® Tablets
(methscopolamine bromide tablets, NF)

Upjohn

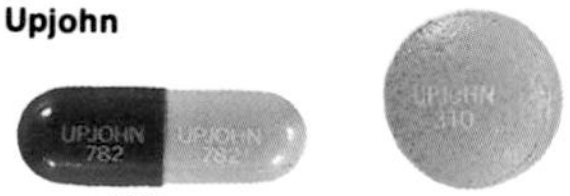

250 mg 782* | 500 mg 310*

†Panmycin® Capsules and Tablets
(tetracycline HCl)

Upjohn

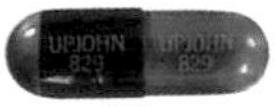

250 mg
829*

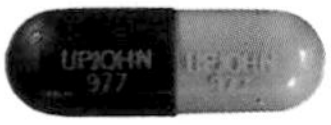

500 mg
977*

†Pensyn™ Capsules
(ampicillin capsules, USP)

Upjohn

2.5 mg 64* | 10 mg 50*

†Provera® Tablets
(medroxyprogesterone acetate tablets, USP)

Upjohn

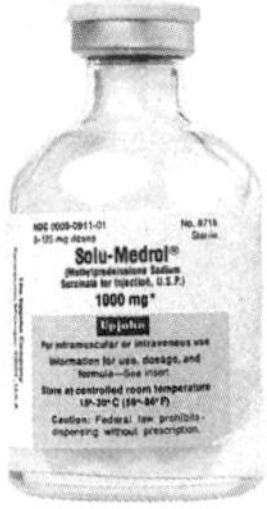

40 mg *Mix-O-Vial®*
125 mg *Mix-O-Vial®*
500 mg vial
1000 mg vial

(shown smaller than actual size)

Solu-Medrol® Sterile Powder
(methylprednisolone sodium succinate for injection, USP)

Upjohn

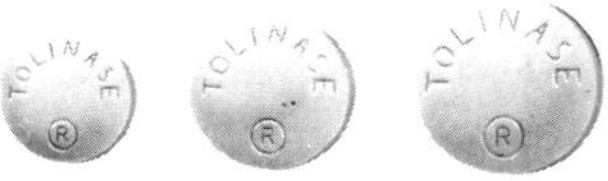

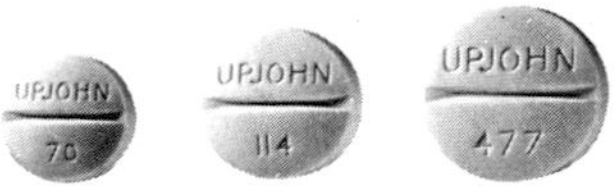

100 mg 70* | 250 mg 114* | 500 mg 477*

(Both sides of tablets shown)

Tolinase® Tablets
(tolazamide tablets, USP)

Upjohn

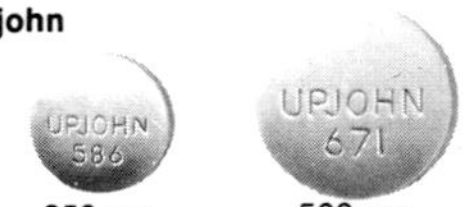

250 mg 586* | 500 mg 671*

†Uticillin VK® Tablets
(penicillin V potassium tablets, USP)

*Upjohn Product Identification Code. All products manufactured by The Upjohn Company have been assigned a National Drug Code (NDC) number. That portion of the number indicating product and strength has been or will be imprinted on each Upjohn tablet or capsule. This number along with the Upjohn imprint which also appears on the tablet or capsule will provide for prompt and positive identification. Complete NDC numbers for all listed products are included in Product Information (White Section).

WALLACE

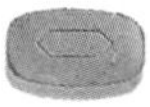

Aquatensen®
(methyclothiazide 5 mg.)

Wallace

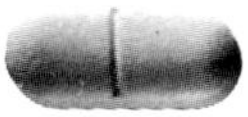

250 mg.
Depen® Titratabs™
(penicillamine)

Wallace

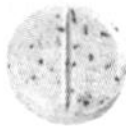

Diutensen®-R

Wallace

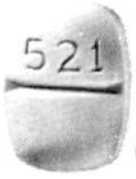

200 mg.
†Lufyllin®
(dyphylline)

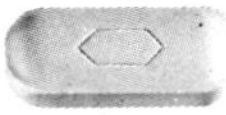

400 mg.
Lufyllin®-400
(dyphylline)

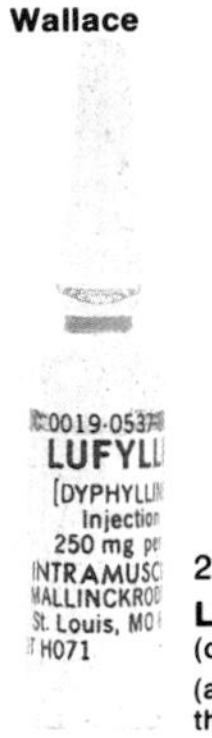

2 ml. (250 mg./ml.)
Lufyllin® Injection
(dyphylline)
(ampul shown slightly smaller than actual size)

Wallace

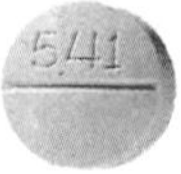

†Lufyllin®-GG

Wallace

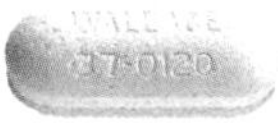

Micrainin®
(200 mg. meprobamate and 325 mg. aspirin)

Wallace

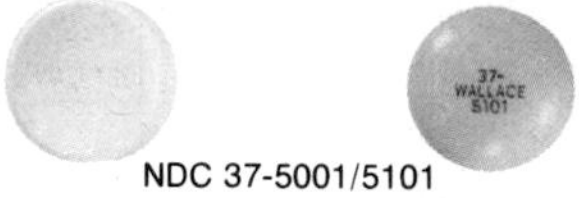

NDC 37-5001/5101
Milpath®—400 **Milpath®—200**
(meprobamate 400 mg. or 200 mg. + tridihexethyl chloride 25 mg.)

Wallace Ⓒ IV

NDC 37-1101
200 mg.

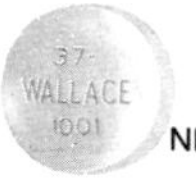

NDC 37-1001
400 mg.

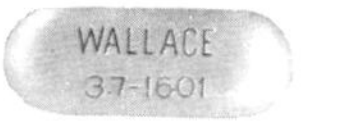

NDC 37-1601
600 mg.
Miltown
(meprobamate)

Wallace

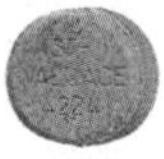

NDC 37-4224
30 mg.
†Organidin®
(iodinated glycerol)

†Other dosage forms available. See Product Information section or check directly with manufacturer.
*Manufacturers' identification number.

Wallace

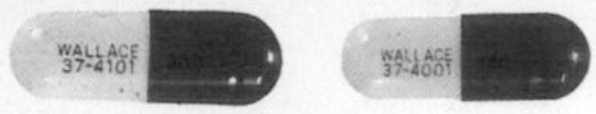

NDC 37-4101/4001

300 mg. 150 mg.

†Rondomycin®
(methacycline HCl)

Wallace

Rynatan®

Wallace

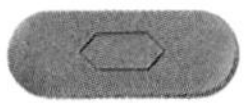

Rynatuss®

Wallace

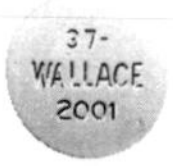

350 mg.

NDC 37-2001

Soma®
(carisoprodol)

Wallace

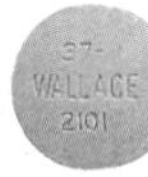

NDC 37-2101

Soma® Compound
(200 mg. carisoprodol + 160 mg. phenacetin + 32 mg. caffeine)

Wallace Ⓒ III

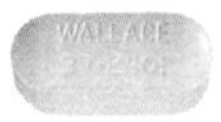

NDC 37-2401

Soma® Compound with Codeine
(200 mg. carisoprodol + 160 mg. phenacetin + 32 mg. caffeine + 16 mg. codeine phosphate)

Wallace

2 mg.

Unitensen® Tablets
(cryptenamine tannates)

Equivalent to 260 Carotid Sinus Reflex (CSR) Units

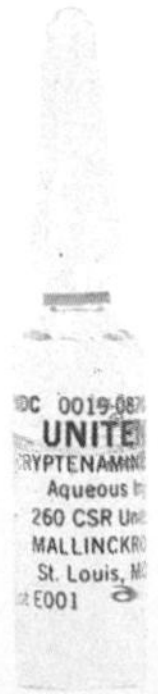

Unitensen® Aqueous Injection
(cryptenamine acetates)

260 Carotid Sinus Reflex (CSR) Units in each ml.

(ampul shown slightly smaller than actual size)

Wallace

(shown smaller than actual size)

NDC 37-3611/3811

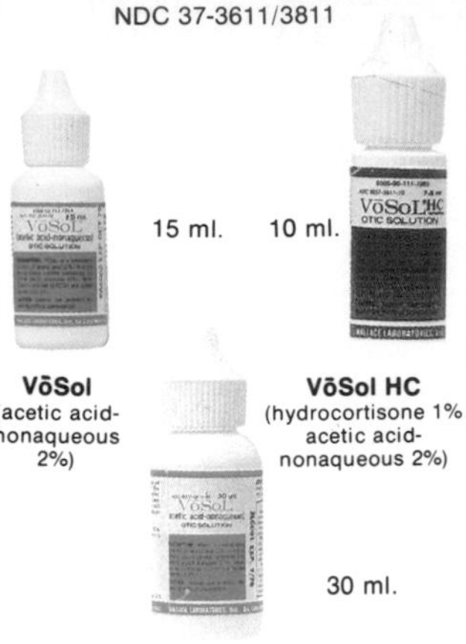

15 ml. 10 ml.

VōSol
(acetic acid-nonaqueous 2%)

VōSol HC
(hydrocortisone 1% acetic acid-nonaqueous 2%)

30 ml.

VōSol
(acetic acid-nonaqueous 2%)

WARNER/CHILCOTT

Effective October 1, 1979 products formerly marketed by Warner/Chilcott are marketed by Parke-Davis. Division of Warner-Lambert Company. Please refer to the product illustrations under Parke-Davis.

WARREN-TEED

Division of Adria Laboratories Inc.

500 mg
(6.7 mEq)

Kaon-Cl Tabs®
Controlled Release Tablets

(potassium chloride)

WINTHROP

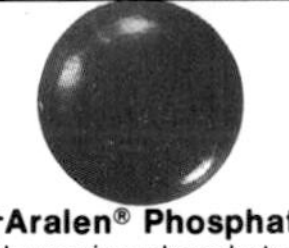

500 mg

†Aralen® Phosphate
Brand of chloroquine phosphate tablets, USP

Winthrop

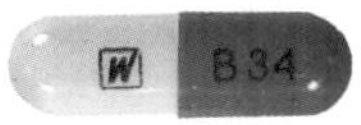

B34*

750 mg

Bilopaque® Sodium Capsules
Brand of sodium tyropanoate

Winthrop Ⓒ II

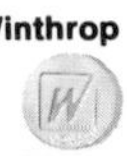

D35*

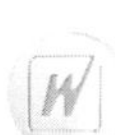

D37*

50 mg
scored tablet

100 mg

†Demerol® Hydrochloride Tablets
Brand of meperidine hydrochloride tablets, USP

Winthrop

D05*

200 mg

Danocrine®
Brand of danazol

Winthrop

N21* N22*

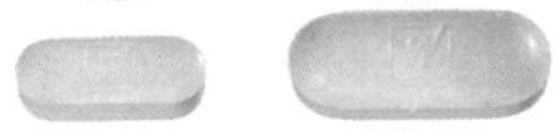

250 mg 500 mg

N23*

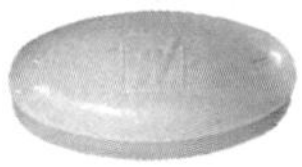

1 Gram

scored tablets

†NegGram® Caplets®
Brand of nalidixic acid tablets, NF

Winthrop

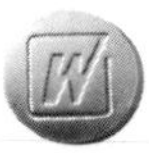

P61*

200 mg
scored tablet

Plaquenil® Sulfate Tablets
Brand of hydroxychloroquine sulfate tablets, USP

Winthrop Ⓒ IV

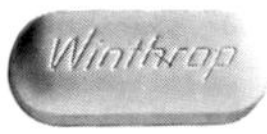

T27*

Talwin® Compound Caplets
Each tablet contains pentazocine hydrochloride, NF, equivalent to 12.5 mg base and aspirin 325 mg

Winthrop Ⓒ IV

T21*

50 mg
scored tablet

†Talwin® Tablets
Brand of pentazocine hydrochloride tablets, NF

Winthrop

T31*

500 mg
scored tablet

Telepaque®
Brand of iopanoic acid tablets, USP

Winthrop

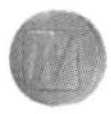

W53*

2 mg
scored tablet

Winstrol®
Brand of stanozolol tablets, NF

Because tablets and capsules are shown in this section, do not infer that these are the only dosage forms available. Where a product name is preceded by the symbol†, refer to the description in the Product Information (White Section) for other forms.

WYETH

Wyeth Product Identification Code. The process of imprinting all oral solid dosage forms manufactured by Wyeth with their respective National Drug Code numbers is at present incomplete. A list of NDC numbers for most Wyeth tablets and capsules is included in the Product Information Section.

Wyeth Ⓒ IV

81** 64** 65**

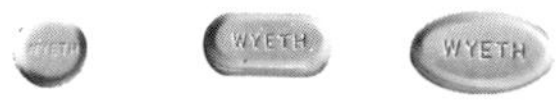

0.5 mg. 1 mg. 2 mg.

ATIVAN®
(lorazepam)

Wyeth Ⓒ IV

5

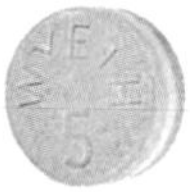

EQUAGESIC®
(meprobamate and ethoheptazine citrate with aspirin)

Wyeth Ⓒ IV

44

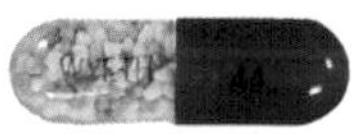

400 mg.

†EQUANIL®
(meprobamate)

Wyeth Ⓒ IV

2** 1**

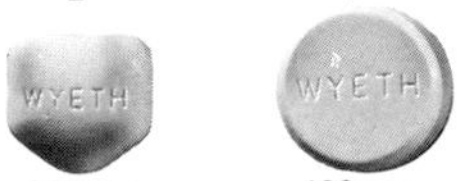

200 mg. 400 mg.

†EQUANIL®
(meprobamate)

Wyeth Ⓒ IV

33

400 mg.

†EQUANIL® WYSEALS®
(meprobamate)

Wyeth

78**

(Dispenser shown smaller than actual size)

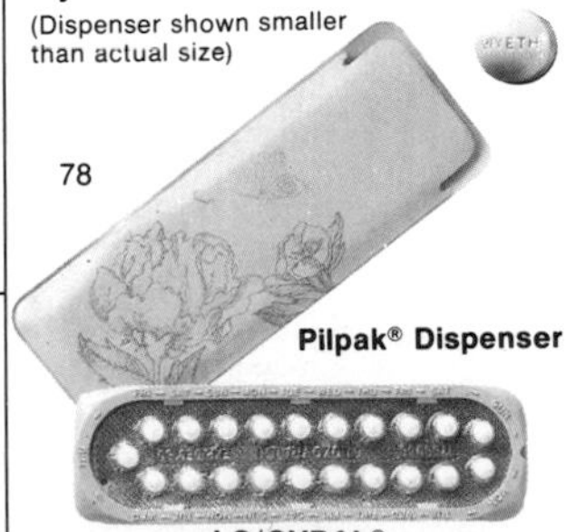

78

Pilpak® Dispenser

LO/OVRAL®
(each tablet contains 0.3 mg. norgestrel with 0.03 mg. ethinyl estradiol)

†Other dosage forms available. See Product Information section or check directly with manufacturer.
*Manufacturers' identification number. **Product identification number on reverse side of tablet.

Wyeth

486 78**

(Dispenser shown smaller than actual size)

2514

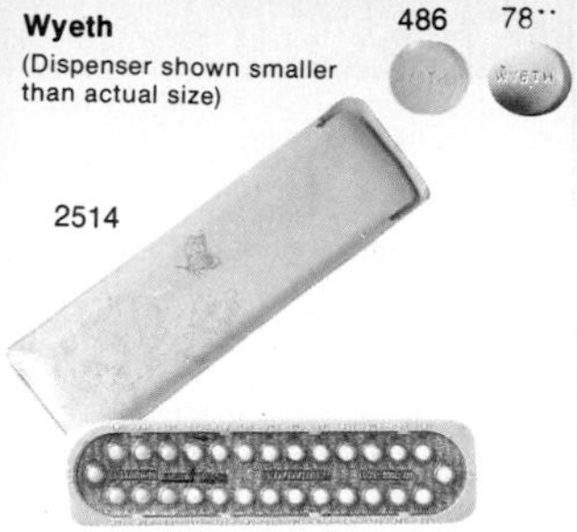

LO/OVRAL®-28 Pilpak® Dispenser
(21 white tablets, each containing 0.3 mg. norgestrel with 0.03 mg. ethinyl estradiol, and 7 pink inert tablets)

Wyeth

53 309

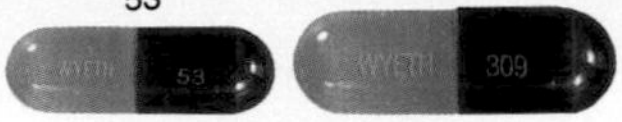

250 mg. 500 mg.

†OMNIPEN®
(ampicillin)
ampicillin anhydrous

Wyeth

360

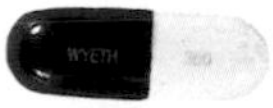

250 mg.

†PATHOCIL®
(dicloxacillin sodium monohydrate)

Wyeth

58 59

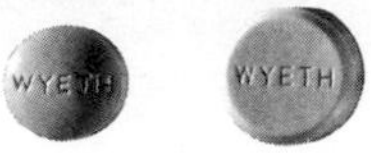

125 mg. 250 mg.

390**

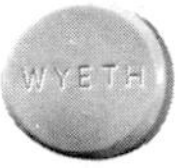

500 mg.

†PEN-VEE® K
(penicillin V potassium)

Wyeth

469 470

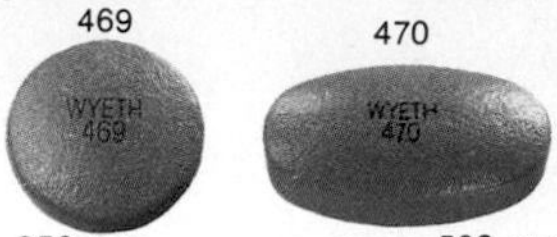

250 mg. **WYAMYCIN® S** 500 mg.
(erythromycin stearate)

Wyeth Ⓒ II

261

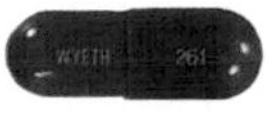

MEPERGAN® FORTIS
(meperidine HCl and promethazine HCl)

Wyeth

433

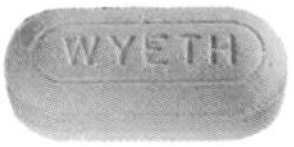

PHENERGAN® COMPOUND
(Each tablet contains 6.25 mg. promethazine hydrochloride and 60 mg. pseudoephedrine hydrochloride with 600 mg. aspirin)

Wyeth

251 252 253

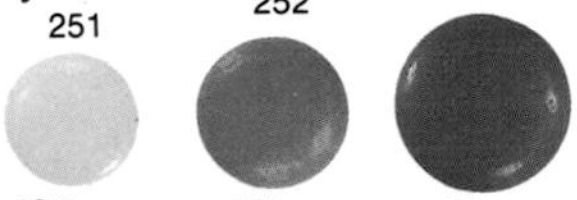

12.5 mg. 25 mg. 50 mg.

†PROKETAZINE®
(carphenazine maleate)

Wyeth

15

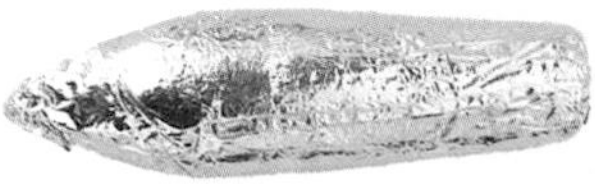

WYANOIDS®
Hemorrhoidal Suppositories
[15 mg. extract belladonna (0.19 mg. equiv. total alkaloids), 3 mg. ephedrine sulfate, zinc oxide, boric acid, bismuth oxyiodide, bismuth subcarbonate and peruvian balsam in cocoa butter and beeswax.]

Wyeth

56**

(Dispenser shown smaller than actual size)

56

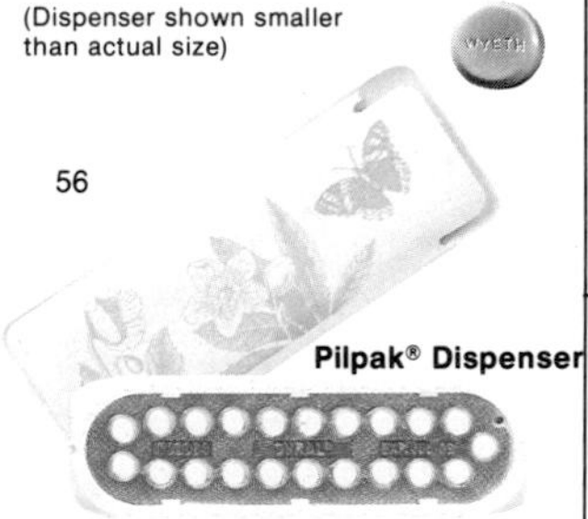

Pilpak® Dispenser

OVRAL®
(0.5 mg. norgestrel with 0.05 mg. ethinyl estradiol)

Wyeth

434

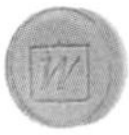

PHENERGAN®-D
(Each tablet contains 6.25 mg. promethazine hydrochloride and 60 mg. pseudoephedrine hydrochloride)

Wyeth Ⓒ IV

51

6 10 mg. 52

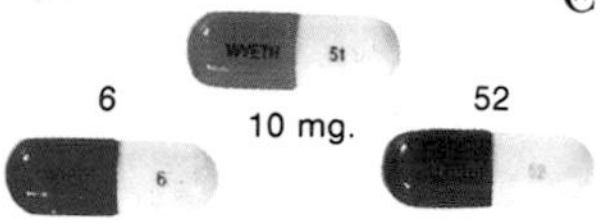

15 mg. 30 mg.

†SERAX®

Wyeth

31

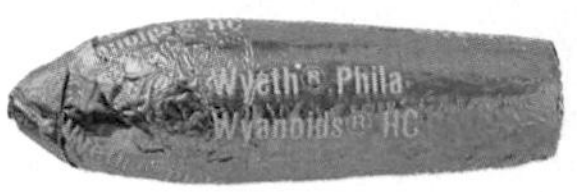

WYANOIDS® HC Rectal Suppositories with hydrocortisone
[Each suppository contains 10 mg. hydrocortisone acetate, 15 mg. extract belladonna (0.19 mg. equiv. total alkaloids), 3 mg. ephedrine sulfate, 176 mg. zinc oxide, 543 mg. boric acid, 30 mg. bismuth oxyiodide, 146 mg. bismuth subcarbonate, 30 mg. peruvian balsam in cocoa butter and beeswax.]

Wyeth

19 27

12.5 mg. 25 mg.

227

50 mg.

†PHENERGAN®
(promethazine hydrochloride)

Wyeth Ⓒ IV

317

15 mg.

†SERAX®
(oxazepam)

Wyeth

56** 445**

(Dispenser shown smaller than actual size)

2511

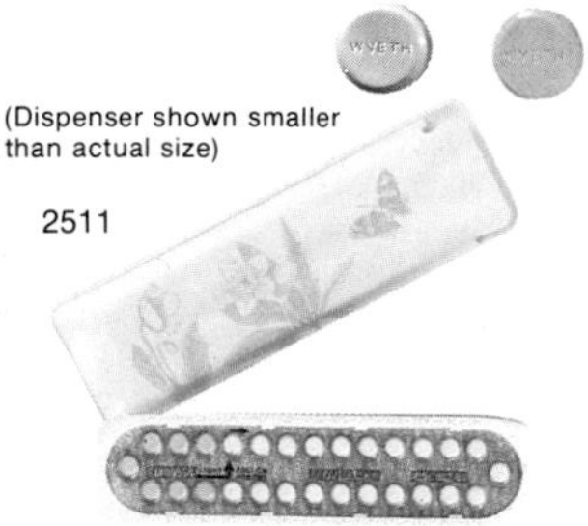

OVRAL®-28 Pilpak® Dispenser
(21 white tablets each containing 0.5 mg. norgestrel with 0.05 mg. ethinyl estradiol and 7 pink inert tablets)

Wyeth

202 29 28

10 mg. 25 mg. 50 mg.

200

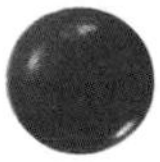

100 mg.

†SPARINE®
(promazine hydrochloride)

Wyeth Ⓒ IV

85**

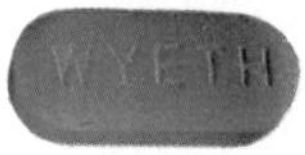

WYGESIC®
(each tablet contains 65 mg. propoxyphene HCl, U.S.P., and 650 mg. acetaminophen, U.S.P.)

Wyeth

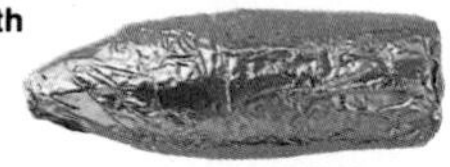

498

12.5 mg.

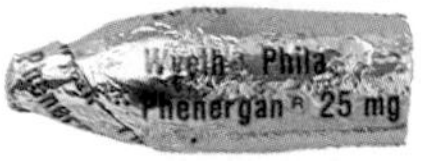

212

25 mg.

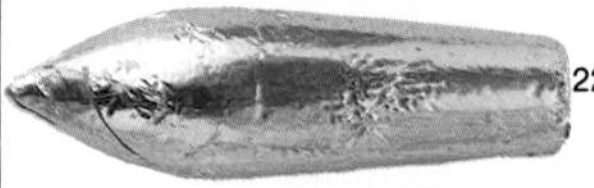

229

50 mg.

†PHENERGAN® Rectal Suppositories
(promethazine HCl)

Wyeth

559 560

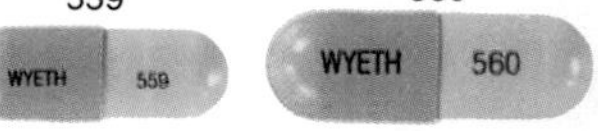

250 mg. 500 mg.

WYMOX™
(amoxicillin)

Wyeth

62

(Dispenser shown smaller than actual size)

62

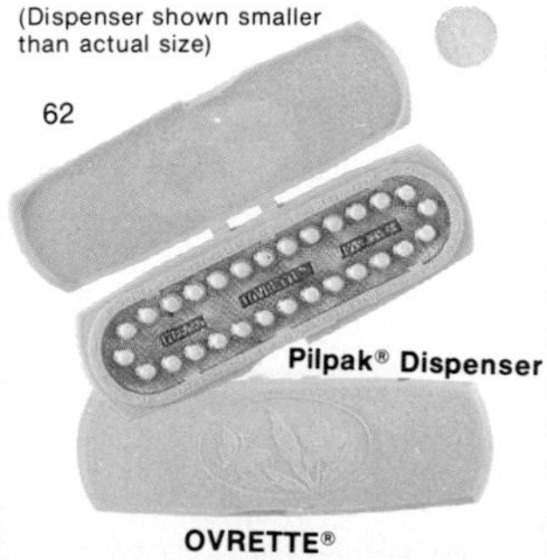

Pilpak® Dispenser

OVRETTE®
(norgestrel)

Wyeth

57

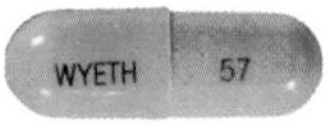

250 mg.

†UNIPEN®
(nafcillin sodium)

Wyeth

30**

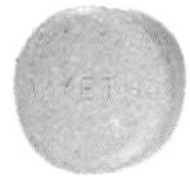

ZACTIRIN®
(ethoheptazine citrate with aspirin)

Wyeth

443

†POLYMAGMA® PLAIN
[Claysorb® (activated attapulgite) and pectin with hydrated alumina]

Wyeth

464**

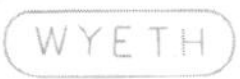

500 mg.

†UNIPEN®
(nafcillin sodium)

Wyeth

49**

ZACTIRIN® COMPOUND-100
(ethoheptazine citrate with aspirin, phenacetin and caffeine)

†Other dosage forms available. See Product Information section or check directly with manufacturer.
**Product identification number on reverse side of tablet.

Product Information

PDR
34
EDITION
SECTION 6

This section is made possible through the courtesy of the manufacturers whose products appear on the following pages. The information concerning each product has been prepared by the manufacturer, and edited and approved by the medical department, medical director, and/or medical counsel of each manufacturer.

Products described in PHYSICIANS' DESK REFERENCE® which have official package circulars must be in full compliance with Food & Drug Administration regulations pertaining to labeling for prescription drugs. These regulations require that for PDR copy, "indications, effects, dosages, routes, methods, and frequency and duration of administration, and any relevant warnings, hazards, contraindications, side effects, and precautions" must be the "same in language and emphasis" as the approved labeling for the product. FDA regards the words "same in language and emphasis" as requiring verbatim use of the approved labeling providing such information. For products which do not have official package circulars, the Publisher has emphasized to manufacturers the necessity of describing such products comprehensively so that physicians would have access to all information essential for intelligent and informed prescribing. In organizing and presenting the material in PHYSICIANS' DESK REFERENCE, the Publisher is providing all the information made available to PDR by manufacturers.

This edition of PHYSICIANS' DESK REFERENCE contains the latest product information available at press-time. During the year, however, new and revised information about the products described herein may be furnished us. This information will be published in the PDR Supplement. Therefore, before prescribing or administering any product described in the following pages, you should first consult the PDR Supplement.

In presenting the following material to the medical profession, the Publisher is not necessarily advocating the use of any product listed.

Abbott Laboratories
NORTH CHICAGO, IL 60064

ABBO-PAC®
Unit Dose Packages

Abbott's Abbo-Pac unit dose system offers a wide range of drugs in capsule and tablet form. Each individual dose is clearly identified by generic name, Abbott name, strength, NDC identification number, and expiration date. Abbo-Pac unit dose containers are designed to accommodate virtually all hospital pharmacy storage racks and to provide maximum accessibility and ease of handling.

The following is a list of Abbo-Pac tablets and capsules which are now available:

PRODUCT	*DOSAGE*
Dayalets® Filmtab® Multivitamin Supplement	
Enduron® Tablets (methyclothiazide tablets, NF)	5 mg
Enduronyl® Tablets (methyclothiazide 5 mg and deserpidine 0.25 mg)	
Enduronyl® Forte Tablets (methyclothiazide 5 mg and deserpidine 0.5 mg)	
E.E.S.® Granules (erythromycin ethylsuccinate for oral suspension, USP)	200 mg/5 ml
Erythrocin® Stearate Filmtab (erythromycin stearate tablets, USP)	250 mg
Erythromycin Base Filmtab (erythromycin tablets, USP)	250 mg
Fero-Grad-500® Filmtab Controlled-Release Iron with Vitamin C	
Iberet®-500 Filmtab Controlled-Release Iron with Vitamin C and B-complex	
K-Lor™ 20 mEq (potassium chloride for oral solution, USP) 20 mEq Potassium 20 mEq Chloride/Packet	
K-Lor™ 15 mEq (potassium chloride for oral solution, USP) 15 mEq Potassium 15 mEq Chloride/Packet	
Nembutal® Sodium Capsules Ⓒ (pentobarbital sodium capsules, USP)	50 mg
Nembutal® Sodium Capsules Ⓒ (pentobarbital sodium capsules, USP)	100 mg
Nembutal Sodium Capsules Ⓒ (pentobarbital sodium capsules, USP) Disp. Pack (20/25's)	100 mg
Oretic® Tablets (hydrochlorothiazide tablets, USP)	25 mg
Oretic® Tablets (hydrochlorothiazide tablets, USP)	50 mg
Panwarfin® Tablets (warfarin sodium tablets, USP)	2 mg
Panwarfin® Tablets (warfarin sodium tablets, USP)	2.5 mg
Panwarfin® Tablets (warfarin sodium tablets, USP)	5 mg
Panwarfin® Tablets (warfarin sodium tablets, USP)	7.5 mg
Panwarfin® Tablets (warfarin sodium tablets, USP)	10 mg
Placidyl® Capsules Ⓒ (ethchlorvynol capsules, NF)	500 mg
Placidyl® Capsules Ⓒ (ethchlorvynol capsules, NF)	750 mg
Surbex-T® Filmtab (high potency vitamin B-complex with vitamin C)	
Tranxene® Capsules Ⓒ (clorazepate dipotassium)	3.75 mg
Tranxene® Capsules Ⓒ (clorazepate dipotassium)	7.5 mg
Tranxene® Capsules Ⓒ (clorazepate dipotassium)	15 mg

[*Shown in Product Identification Section*]

ABBOKINASE® ℞
Urokinase For Injection

ABBOKINASE (urokinase for injection) should only be used by physicians with wide experience in the management of thrombotic disease in hospitals where the recommended clinical and laboratory monitoring (see WARNINGS, PRECAUTIONS and DOSAGE AND ADMINISTRATION) can be performed.

When considering treatment with urokinase, the physician should carefully assess the overall clinical status and history of the patient. The hemostatic capability of the patient is more profoundly altered and bleeding more frequent with urokinase therapy than with heparin or oral coumarin anticoagulant therapy. When bleeding occurs it is also more severe and more difficult to manage. The potential risk of serious hemorrhage relative to such factors as age, physical condition, and underlying bleeding tendency of the patient (as described under WARNINGS and PRECAUTIONS) should be weighed against the potential benefits of treating the patient with urokinase.

Description: Urokinase is an enzyme (protein) produced by the kidney, and found in the urine. It is a potent activator of the fibrinolytic system. Two molecular forms of urokinase (UK) are found in current therapeutic preparations: the 55,000 dalton High Molecular Weight (HMW) form, and the 34,000 dalton Low Molecular Weight (LMW) form. The LMW form is derived from the HMW form by proteolysis.[1] Immunologically, the two forms are similar. Depending on the method of preparation, either one or the other form (or both in varying proportions) is isolated. Kidney tissue cultures and urine are sources for urokinase.

ABBOKINASE (urokinase for injection) is a sterile, lyophilized preparation of urokinase intended for INTRAVENOUS INFUSION ONLY. It is obtained from human kidney cells by tissue culture techniques.

ABBOKINASE (urokinase for injection) is a white powder. Following reconstitution with 5.2 ml of Sterile Water for Injection, U.S.P., it is a clear, practically colorless solution; each ml contains 50,000 I.U. of urokinase activity, 0.5% mannitol, and 0.9% sodium chloride.

The pH of ABBOKINASE is adjusted with sodium hydroxide and/or hydrochloric acid prior to lyophilization.

Action: Urokinase acts on the endogenous fibrinolytic system by converting plasminogen to the proteolytic enzyme plasmin. Plasmin, in turn, degrades fibrin clots as well as fibrinogen and other plasma proteins.[2] The plasmin is rapidly inactivated by a variety of naturally occurring plasma inhibitors.[3] Since plasminogen is present in the thrombus/embolus, activation by urokinase occurs within the thrombus/embolus as well as on its surface.[4]

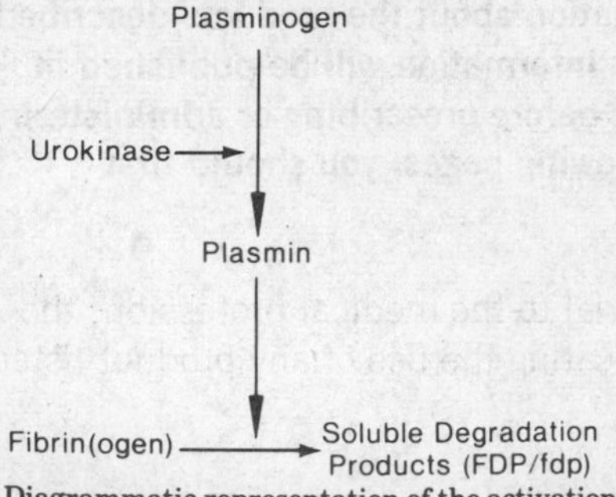

Diagrammatic representation of the activation of plasminogen by urokinase, and the degradation of fibrin(ogen) by plasmin.

Intravenous infusion of urokinase is promptly followed by increased fibrinolytic activity and its effect may persist for up to 12 hours after discontinuation. This activity is evidenced by a shortening of the euglobulin lysis time, a decrease in plasma levels of fibrinogen and plasminogen, and an increase in the amount of circulating fibrinogen and fibrin degradation products (FDP/fdp).[5] ABBOKINASE (urokinase for injection) and urokinase of urinary source have comparable fibrinolytic activities in humans.[6]

The activity of urokinase is expressed in International Units (I.U.) and is a measure of its ability to cause lysis of a fibrin clot via the plasmin system *in vitro*. The activity has been standardized, i.e., the *in vitro* measurement has been performed in a test system adjusted so that the HMW and LMW forms assay with a potency reflecting the *in vivo* effect.

The efficacy of urokinase in the lysis of pulmonary emboli has been established in controlled clinical studies by angiography, perfusion lung scans, and pulmonary arterial and right heart pressure measurements before and after treatment.[5,7–11]

Indications:

Pulmonary Embolism

ABBOKINASE (urokinase for injection) is indicated in adults:

— for the lysis of acute massive pulmonary emboli, defined as obstruction or significant filling defects involving two or more lobar pulmonary arteries or an equivalent amount of emboli in other vessels.[8]

— for the lysis of pulmonary emboli accompanied by unstable hemodynamics, i.e., failure to maintain blood pressure without supportive measures.

The diagnosis should be confirmed by objective means, preferably pulmonary arteriography. Urokinase treatment should be instituted as soon as possible after onset of pulmonary embolism, and no later than five days after onset. Under these circumstances, angiographic and hemodynamic measurements demonstrate a more rapid improvement during the first 24 hours of therapy than with heparin therapy (Table I).[7–9] However, it has not been established that treatment with urokinase decreases morbidity or mortality, when compared to heparin therapy alone.

[See table on next page].

Contraindications: Because thrombolytic therapy increases the risk of bleeding, urokinase is contraindicated in the following situations:

1. Surgery within ten days. Liver or kidney biopsy, lumbar puncture, thoracentesis or paracentesis, extensive or multiple cut-downs should be considered surgical procedures.
2. Intraarterial diagnostic procedure within ten days.
3. Ulcerative wound.
4. Recent trauma with possibility of internal injuries.
5. Visceral or intracranial malignancy.
6. Pregnancy and the first ten days of the post-partum period.
7. Ulcerative colitis, diverticulitis or an actively bleeding lesion (or one with a significant potential for bleeding) of the gastrointestinal or genitourinary tract.
8. Severe hypertension.
9. Acute or chronic hepatic or renal insufficiency.
10. Uncontrolled hypocoagulable state, including one that may be caused by a coagulation factor deficiency, thrombocytopenia, spontaneous fibrinolysis, or another purpuric or hemorrhagic disorder.
11. Chronic lung disease with cavitation, e.g., tuberculosis.
12. Subacute bacterial endocarditis or rheumatic valvular disease.
13. Recent cerebral embolism, thrombosis or hemorrhage. Treatment with urokinase is contraindicated for at least two months after cerebral embolism, thrombosis or hemorrhage because patients with cere-

bral infarction remain at risk of bleeding into the infarcted tissue.

14. Any other condition in which bleeding might constitute a significant hazard or be particularly difficult to manage because of its location.

The conditions listed above should not be regarded as absolute contraindications. Rather, the risk of hemorrhage must be weighed carefully against the anticipated benefits of urokinase therapy in an individual patient and the benefits and risks associated with the use of urokinase should be compared to the benefits and risks associated with other forms of therapy.

Warnings:

Bleeding

Activation of the fibrinolytic system with urokinase results in a more profound alteration of the hemostatic status of the patient than does anticoagulant therapy with heparin or coumarin agents. The aim of urokinase therapy is the production of sufficient amounts of plasmin for the lysis of intravascular deposits of fibrin; however, fibrin deposits which provide hemostasis, for example, at sites of needle punctures, are also destined for lysis, and bleeding from such sites may occur. The possibility of bruising or hematoma formation, especially with intramuscular injections, is high during thrombolytic therapy. Unneccessary handling of the patient should be avoided. Strict attention should be given to this section and the CONTRAINDICATIONS section in order to minimize the risk of bleeding.

Because of the high risk of hematoma formation, intramuscular injections must be avoided during urokinase therapy, as with heparin therapy. Bleeding at sites of recent invasive procedures may occur. Hence, arterial invasive procedures must also be avoided before and during treatment with urokinase. Should an arterial puncture be *absolutely* necessary, the femoral artery must be avoided and the radial or brachial artery used. It should be done carefully by a physician experienced in such a procedure. Pressure should be applied for at least 15 minutes, a pressure dressing applied, and the puncture site checked frequently for evidence of bleeding. Also, venipunctures should be performed as carefully and infrequently as possible. If the bleeding from an invasive site is not serious, treatment may be continued with appropriate clinical observation. Local measures, i.e., pressure, should be initiated immediately.

Spontaneous bleeding from internal sites (not accessible for pressure application) may also occur. The risk of spontaneous bleeding is greater in patients with pre-existing hemostatic defects, e.g., patients with histories suggestive of prior bleeding problems, with or without demonstrable abnormalities in platelet count, prothrombin time, partial thromboplastin time, or bleeding time. Such patients should be assessed carefully before initiating treatment with urokinase.

In addition to its fibrinolytic action, plasmin also degrades fibrinogen, Factor V, Factor VIII, and other proteins. The products of plasmin degradation of fibrinogen and fibrin (FDP/fdp) possess an anticoagulant effect. Bleeding may be difficult to control because of this anticoagulant effect.

Should serious spontaneous bleeding occur, the infusion of urokinase should be terminated immediately, and treatment instituted as described under ADVERSE REACTIONS.

Predisposition to Cerebral Embolism

Treatment with urokinase of patients with atrial fibrillation or other conditions in which there is possible risk of cerebral embolism may be hazardous because of the risk of bleeding into the infarcted area.

Use of Anticoagulants

Concurrent use of anticoagulants with urokinase is not recommended and may be hazardous. Before starting urokinase in patients being treated with heparin, the effects of heparin should be allowed to diminish with time. As a general rule, a thrombin time of *less than twice* the normal control value is adequate for starting urokinase infusions safely. Similarly, heparin should not be started following urokinase therapy until the thrombin time has returned to *less than twice* the normal control value.

Rethrombosis has been observed after termination of urokinase treatment. In order to minimize this risk, the use of intravenous heparin followed by oral anticoagulant therapy is considered a necessary adjunct following urokinase therapy (see DOSAGE AND ADMINISTRATION).

Use in Pregnancy

See CONTRAINDICATIONS.

Use in Children

Safety and effectiveness of urokinase therapy in children have not been established; therefore, treatment of such patients is not recommended.

Precautions:

Drug Interactions

Concurrent use of drugs that may alter platelet function, e.g., aspirin, indomethacin, and phenylbutazone, should be avoided. The interaction of ABBOKINASE (urokinase for injection) with other drugs has not been studied.

Laboratory Monitoring

In patients who have received heparin, the thrombin time should be measured prior to starting urokinase. (See WARNINGS.) Similarly, the thrombin time should be monitored following urokinase therapy prior to instituting heparin. (See DOSAGE AND ADMINISTRATION.) During urokinase administration, the levels of fibrinogen, plasminogen, Factor V, and Factor VIII are usually substantially diminished. Concomitantly, the level of fibrin(ogen) degradation products (FDP/fdp) is increased. The combination of reduced fibrinogen and increased FDP/fdp results in a prolongation of the thrombin time. While changes in any of these parameters may serve as confirmation of the existence of a lytic state, no adjustment of dosage should be made on the basis of these test results.

Adverse Reactions:

Incidence and Management

Strict observance of the contraindications, warnings, and precautions to the use of urokinase is essential to minimize the incidence and severity of adverse effects.[7]

Bleeding:

Incidence

Where thrombolytic agents (streptokinase and urokinase) were used in the same controlled clinical trial, severe bleeding (patients receiving a transfusion of greater than two units of blood) was seen in 4 and 6%, respectively. Several fatalities due to cerebral hemorrhage have occurred during urokinase therapy.

Less severe spontaneous bleeding has been observed during urokinase treatment at approximately twice the frequency as that occurring during heparin therapy. Oozing of blood from sites of percutaneous trauma is frequent; hence, all invasive procedures, especially arterial punctures and intramuscular injections must be avoided and intravenous punctures kept to a minimum before and during treatment with urokinase.

A moderate decrease in hematocrit not accompanied by clinically detectable bleeding occurred in approximately one out of five patients treated with urokinase.

Management of Severe Bleeding

In case of serious bleeding, urokinase therapy must be discontinued. If blood loss has been large, packed red cells are indicated. Plasma volume expanders (other than Dextran) are indicated to replace blood volume deficit. If only whole blood is available, it may also be used. Although the use of aminocaproic acid (ACA, AMICAR®) in humans as an antidote for urokinase has not been documented, it may be considered if the hemorrhage is unresponsive to blood replacement. (See WARNINGS.)

Allergic Reactions: Although urokinase is a protein of human origin, and *in vitro* tests with the drug, as well as intradermal tests in humans, gave no evidence of induced antibody formation, the possibility of serious allergic reactions (including anaphylaxis) occurring with its use cannot be excluded. Relatively mild allergic reactions, e.g., bronchospasm and skin rash, were reported rarely.

Fever: Febrile episodes occurred in approximately two to three out of 100 patients. A cause and effect relationship has not been established. Symptomatic treatment is usually sufficient to alleviate discomfort. The use of acetaminophen rather than aspirin is recommended.

Dosage and Administration:

Preparation

Reconstitute ABBOKINASE (urokinase for injection) by aseptically adding 5.2 ml of Sterile Water for Injection, U.S.P., to the vial. (It is important that ABBOKINASE be reconstituted *only* with Sterile Water for Injection, U.S.P., *without* preservatives. Bacteriostatic Water for Injection should not be used.) Because ABBOKINASE contains no preservatives, it should not be

Continued on next page

If desired, additional literature on any Abbott Product will be provided upon request to Abbott Laboratories.

TABLE I†

	UPET*		USPET**	
	Heparin	12-Hour Urokinase	12-Hour Urokinase	24-Hour Urokinase
Change in angiographic severity score based on 4-point system	0.54	1.78	1.66	1.76
Decrease in relative percentage perfusion defect on lung scans	8.3	24.1	20	29.2
Change in pulmonary artery pressure (mm Hg)	−1.1	−6.2	−7.28	−7.53
Change in cardiac index (l/min/m^2)	−0.05	+0.02	+0.06	+0.30

* Urokinase pulmonary embolism trial.
** Urokinase-streptokinase pulmonary embolism trial.
Evaluations were obtained between 18 and 30 hours after the start of therapy.
After several days, there were no differences between the results in the heparin treated patients and those receiving urokinase.
†Adapted from (7).

Abbott—Cont.

reconstituted until immediately before using. Any unused portion of the reconstituted material should be discarded.
Reconstituted ABBOKINASE is diluted with Normal Saline 0.9%, prior to intravenous infusion. (See Table II, Dose Preparation.)

Dosing

ABBOKINASE IS INTENDED FOR INTRAVENOUS INFUSION ONLY

A priming dose of 2,000 I.U./lb (4,400 I.U./kg) of ABBOKINASE is given as the ABBOKINASE-Normal Saline admixture over a period of ten minutes. This is followed by a continuous infusion of 2,000 I.U./lb/hr (4,400 I.U./kg/hr) of ABBOKINASE (given as the ABBOKINASE-Normal Saline admixture) for 12 hours. (See Table II, Dose Preparation.) The total volume of fluid administered should not exceed 200 ml.
Administer ABBOKINASE (urokinase for injection) by means of a constant infusion pump that is capable of delivering a total volume of 195 ml. Table II may be used as an aid in the preparation of ABBOKINASE for administration.

Anticoagulation After Terminating Urokinase Treatment

At the end of urokinase therapy, treatment with heparin by continuous intravenous infusion is recommended. Heparin treatment should not begin until the thrombin time has decreased to *less than twice* the normal control value. See manufacturer's prescribing information for proper use of heparin.
[See table below].

How Supplied: ABBOKINASE (urokinase for injection) is supplied as a sterile lyophilized preparation (**NDC** 0074-6109-05). Each vial contains 250,000 I.U. urokinase activity, 25 mg mannitol, and 45 mg sodium chloride. Store ABBOKINASE powder at 2°C to 8°C.

References:

1. Bang, N. U.: Physiology and Biochemistry of Fibrinolysis. In *Thrombosis and Bleeding Disorders* (Bang, N. U., Beller, F. K., Deutsch, E., Mammen, E. F., eds). Academic Press (1971). pp. 292–327.
2. McNicol, G. P.: The Fibrinolytic Enzyme System. Postgrad. Med. J. (August Suppl.). *49:*10–12 (1973).
3. Aoki, N., Maroi, M., Matsuda, M., Tachiya, K.: The Behavior of α_2-Plasmin Inhibitor in Fibrinolytic States. J. Clin. Invest. *60:*361–369 (1977).
4. Chesterman, C. N., Allington, M. J., Sharp, A. A.: Relationship of Plasminogen Activator to Fibrin. Nature (New Biol.) *238:*15–17 (1972).
5. Bell, W. R.: Thrombolytic Therapy: A Comparison Between Urokinase and Streptokinase. Sem. Thromb. Hemost. *2:*1–13 (1975).
6. Marder, V. J., Donahoe, J. F., Bell, W. R., Cranley, J. J., Kwaan, H. C., Sasahara, A. A., and Barlow, G. H.: Comparison of *In Vivo* Biochemical Effects of Human Urokinase Prepared from Urinary and Tissue Cultures Sources. Abstracts of the 6th International Congress on Thrombosis and Haemostasis, July 1, 1977, p. 195.
7. Fratantoni, J. C., Ness, P., Simon, T. L.: Thrombolytic Therapy: Current Status. N. Eng. J. Med., *293:*1073–1078 (1975).
8. Sasahara, A. A., Hyers, T. M., Cole, C. M., et al.: The Urokinase Pulmonary Embolism Trial. Circulation, (Suppl. II) *47:*1–108 (1973).
9. Urokinase pulmonary embolism trial study group: Urokinase-Streptokinase Embolism Trial. JAMA *229:*1606–1613 (1974).
10. Sherry, S.: Streptokinase, Urokinase: Do They Really Work? Modern Med. (November 1) 72–76 (1976).
11. Sasahara, A. A., Bell, W. R., Simon, T. L., Stengle, J. M., and Sherry, S.: The Phase II Urokinase-Streptokinase Pulmonary Embolism Trial. Thrombos. Diathes, Haemorrh. (Stuttg.). *33:*464–476 (1975).

Ref. No. 01-2912-R1

TABLE II
Dose Preparation

Weight (pounds)	Total Dose* Urokinase (I.U.)	Number Vials ABBOKINASE (urokinase for injection)	Volume of ABBOKINASE After Reconstitution (ml)** +	Volume of NaCl 0.9% (ml) =	Final Volume (ml)
81–90	2,250,000	9	45	150	195
91–100	2,500,000	10	50	145	195
101–110	2,750,000	11	55	140	195
111–120	3,000,000	12	60	135	195
121–130	3,250,000	13	65	130	195
131–140	3,500,000	14	70	125	195
141–150	3,750,000	15	75	120	195
151–160	4,000,000	16	80	115	195
161–170	4,250,000	17	85	110	195
171–180	4,500,000	18	90	105	195
181–190	4,750,000	19	95	100	195
191–200	5,000,000	20	100	95	195
201–210	5,250,000	21	105	90	195
211–220	5,500,000	22	110	85	195
221–230	5,750,000	23	115	80	195
231–240	6,000,000	24	120	75	195
241–250	6,250,000	25	125	70	195

Infusion Rate:	Priming Dose	Dose for 12-Hour Period
	15 ml/10 min	15 ml/hr/12 hr

*Priming dose + dose administered during 12-hour period.
**After addition of 5.2 ml of Sterile Water for Injection, U.S.P., per vial. (See Preparation.)

A-HYDROCORT™ ℞

(hydrocortisone sodium succinate for injection, USP)
For Intravenous or Intramuscular Use

Description: Hydrocortisone sodium succinate, USP, an adrenocortical-like steroid, is the sodium succinate ester of hydrocortisone.
It occurs as a white, or nearly white, odorless hygroscopic amorphous solid. Hydrocortisone sodium succinate is very soluble in water and in alcohol; it is insoluble in chloroform and is very slightly soluble in acetone.
Hydrocortisone sodium succinate is soluble in water and is especially well suited for intravenous use in situations in which high blood levels of hydrocortisone are required rapidly.
A-HYDROCORT (hydrocortisone sodium succinate for injection, USP) is available as:
100 mg Univial®—Each 2 ml (when mixed) contains hydrocortisone sodium succinate equivalent to 100 mg hydrocortisone; also 0.8 mg sodium biphosphate anhydrous; 8.73 mg dried sodium phosphate; and 18 mg of benzyl alcohol.
250 mg Univial—Each 2 ml (when mixed) contains hydrocortisone sodium succinate equivalent to 250 mg hydrocortisone; also 2 mg sodium biphosphate anhydrous; 21.8 mg dried sodium phosphate; and 18 mg of benzyl alcohol.
500 mg Univial—Each 4 ml (when mixed) contains hydrocortisone sodium succinate equivalent to 500 mg hydrocortisone; also 4 mg sodium biphosphate anhydrous; 44 mg dried sodium phosphate; and 36 mg benzyl alcohol.
1000 mg Univial—Each 8 ml (when mixed) contains hydrocortisone sodium succinate equivalent to 1000 mg hydrocortisone; also 8 mg sodium biphosphate anhydrous; 88 mg dried sodium phosphate; and 72 mg benzyl alcohol.
100 mg Vial with Diluent—Each 2 ml (when mixed) contains hydrocortisone sodium succinate equivalent to 100 mg hydrocortisone; also 0.8 mg sodium biphosphate anhydrous; 8.73 mg dried sodium phosphate; and 18 mg of benzyl alcohol.
The pH of each formula was adjusted with sodium hydroxide and/or hydrochloric acid.
Important: The solid contents of A-HYDROCORT should not be used with any diluent other than that provided.
Use within 3 days after mixing. Store below 86°F. Protect from light. Avoid freezing. Refrigeration not required.
When reconstituted as directed, the pH of the solutions ranges from 7–8 and the tonicities are, for the 100 mg per ml solution, 0.36 osmolar; for the 250 mg per 2 ml, 500 mg per 4 ml, and 1000 mg per 8 ml solutions, 0.57 osmolar. (Isotonic saline = 0.28 osmolar.)
Clinical Pharmacology: Hydrocortisone sodium succinate has potent anti-inflammatory effects. Because it is an adrenocortical-like steroid, hydrocortisone sodium succinate may cause profound and varied metabolic effects in addition to modifying the body's immune response to diverse stimuli.
When given parenterally and in equimolar quantitites, hydrocortisone sodium succinate and hydrocortisone are equivalent in biologic activity.
Following intravenous injection of hydrocortisone sodium succinate, demonstrable effects are evident within one hour and persist for a variable period. Excretion of the administered dose is nearly complete within 12 hours. Thus, if constantly high blood levels are required, injections should be made every four to six hours.
This preparation is also rapidly absorbed when administered intramuscularly and is excreted in a pattern similar to that observed after intravenous injection.
Indications: Sterile A-HYDROCORT (hydrocortisone sodium succinate) is indicated in situations requiring a rapid and intense hormonal effect.
Intravenous administration of A-HYDROCORT is most appropriate for the following indications:

1. **Endocrine disorders:**
   a. Acute adrenocortical insufficiency (hydrocortisone or cortisone is the drug of choice; mineralocorticoid supplementation may be necessary, particularly when synthetic analogs are used).
   b. Preoperatively and in the event of serious trauma or illness, in patients with known adrenal insufficiency or when adrenocortical reserve is doubtful.

c. Shock unresponsive to conventional therapy if adrenocortical insufficiency exists or is suspected.
2. **Collagen diseases**—During an exacerbation or as maintenance therapy in selected cases of:
a. Acute rheumatic carditis.
3. **Allergic states**—Control of severe or incapacitating allergic conditions intractable to adequate trials of conventional treatment in:
a. Bronchial asthma.
b. Serum sickness.
c. Drug hypersensitivity reactions.
d. Urticarial transfusion reactions.
e. Acute noninfectious laryngeal edema (epinephrine is the drug of first choice).
4. **Hematologic disorders:**
a. Idiopathic thrombocytopenic purpura in adults (I.M. administration is contraindicated).

Intramuscular administration of A-HYDROCORT is appropriate for the following indications:
1. **Endocrine disorders:**
a. Primary or secondary adrenocortical insufficiency (hydrocortisone or cortisone is the drug of choice; synthetic analogs may be used in conjunction with mineralocorticoids where applicable; in infancy, mineralocorticoid supplementation is of particular importance).
b. Acute adrenocortical insufficiency (hydrocortisone or cortisone is the drug of choice; mineralocorticoid supplementation may be necessary, particularly when synthetic analogs are used).
c. Preoperatively and in the event of serious trauma or illness, in patients with known adrenal insufficiency or when adrenocortical reserve is doubtful.
d. Shock unresponsive to conventional therapy if adrenocortical insufficiency exists or is suspected.
e. Congenital adrenal hyperplasia.
f. Nonsuppurative thyroiditis.
g. Hypercalcemia associated with cancer.
2. **Rheumatic disorders**—As adjunctive therapy for short-term administration (to tide the patient over an acute episode or exacerbation) in:
a. Post-traumatic osteoarthritis.
b. Synovitis of osteoarthritis.
c. Rheumatoid arthritis, including juvenile rheumatoid arthritis (selected cases may require low-dose maintenance therapy).
d. Acute and subacute bursitis.
e. Epicondylitis.
f. Acute nonspecific tenosynovitis.
g. Acute gouty arthritis.
h. Psoriatic arthritis.
i. Ankylosing spondylitis.
3. **Collagen diseases**—During an exacerbation or as maintenance therapy in selected cases of:
a. Systemic lupus erythematosus.
b. Acute rheumatic carditis.
4. **Dermatologic diseases:**
a. Severe erythema multiforme (Stevens-Johnson syndrome).
b. Exfoliative dermatitis.
c. Bullous dermatitis herpetiformis.
d. Severe seborrheic dermatitis.
e. Severe psoriasis.
f. Pemphigus.
g. Mycosis fungoides.
h. Systemic dermatomyositis (polymyositis).
5. **Allergic states**—Control of severe or incapacitating allergic conditions intractable to adequate trials of conventional treatment in:
a. Bronchial asthma.
b. Contact dermatitis.
c. Atopic dermatitis.
d. Serum sickness.
e. Seasonal or perennial allergic rhinitis.
f. Drug hypersensitivity reactions.
g. Urticarial transfusion reactions.
h. Acute noninfectious laryngeal edema (epinephrine is the drug of first choice).
6. **Ophthalmic diseases**—Severe acute and chronic allergic and inflammatory processes involving the eye, such as:
a. Herpes zoster ophthalmicus.
b. Iritis, iridocyclitis.
c. Chorioretinitis.
d. Diffuse posterior uveitis and choroiditis.
e. Optic neuritis.
f. Sympathetic ophthalmia.
g. Anterior segment inflammation.
h. Allergic conjunctivitis.
i. Allergic corneal marginal ulcers.
7. **Gastrointestinal diseases**—To tide the patient over a critical period of disease in:
a. Ulcerative colitis—(Systemic therapy).
b. Regional enteritis—(Systemic therapy).
8. **Respiratory diseases:**
a. Symptomatic sarcoidosis.
b. Berylliosis.
c. Fulminating or disseminated pulmonary tuberculosis when concurrently accompanied by appropriate antituberculous chemotherapy.
d. Aspiration pneumonitis.
e. Loeffler's syndrome not manageable by other means.
9. **Hematologic disorders:**
a. Acquired (autoimmune) hemolytic anemia.
b. Secondary thrombocytopenia in adults.
c. Erythroblastopenia (RBC anemia).
d. Congenital (erythroid) hypoplastic anemia.
10. **Neoplastic diseases**—For palliative management of:
a. Leukemias and lymphomas in adults.
b. Acute leukemia of childhood.
11. **Edematous state**—To induce diuresis or remission of proteinuria in the nephrotic syndrome, without uremia, of the idiopathic type or that due to lupus erythematosus.
12. **Miscellaneous:**
a. Tuberculous meningitis with subarachnoid block or impending block when used concurrently with appropriate antituberculous chemotherapy.
b. Trichinosis with neurologic or myocardial involvement.

Contraindications: Systemic fungal infections.

Warnings: In patients on corticosteroid therapy subjected to any unusual stress, increased dosage of rapidly acting corticosteroids before, during, and after the stressful situation is indicated.

Corticosteroids may mask some signs of infection, and new infections may appear during their use. There may be decreased resistance and inability to localize infection when corticosteroids are used.

Prolonged use of corticosteroids may produce posterior subcapsular cataracts, glaucoma with possible damage to the optic nerves, and may enhance the establishment of secondary ocular infections due to fungi or viruses.

Average and large doses of cortisone or hydrocortisone can cause elevation of blood pressure, salt and water retention, and increased excretion of potassium. These effects are less likely to occur with the synthetic derivatives except when used in large doses. Dietary salt restriction and potassium supplementation may be necessary. All corticosteroids increase calcium excretion.

While on corticosteroid therapy patients should not be vaccinated against smallpox. Other immunization procedures should not be undertaken in patients who are on corticosteroids, especially on high dose, because of possible hazards of neurological complications and a lack of antibody response.

The use of A-HYDROCORT (hydrocortisone sodium succinate) in active tuberculosis should be restricted to those cases of fulminating or disseminated tuberculosis in which the corticosteroid is used for the management of the disease in conjunction with appropriate antituberculous regimen.

If corticosteroids are indicated in patients with latent tuberculosis or tuberculin reactivity, close observation is necessary as reactivation of the disease may occur. During prolonged corticosteroid therapy, these patients should receive chemoprophylaxis.

Because rare instances of anaphylactoid reactions have occurred in patients receiving parenteral corticosteroid therapy, appropriate precautionary measures should be taken prior to administration, especially when the patient has a history of allergy to any drug.

Usage in Pregnancy: Since adequate human reproduction studies have not been done with corticosteroids, the use of these drugs in pregnancy, nursing mothers, or women of childbearing potential requires that the possible benefits of the drug be weighed against the potential hazards to the mother and embryo or fetus. Infants born of mothers who have received substantial doses of corticosteroids during pregnancy should be carefully observed for signs of hypoadrenalism.

Precautions: Drug-induced secondary adrenocortical insufficiency may be minimized by gradual reduction of dosage. This type of relative insufficiency may persist for months after discontinuation of therapy; therefore, in any situation of stress occurring during that period, hormone therapy should be reinstituted. Since mineralocorticoid secretion may be impaired, salt and/or a mineralocorticoid should be administered concurrently.

There is an enhanced effect of corticosteroids on patients with hypothyroidism and in those with cirrhosis.

Corticosteroids should be used cautiously in patients with ocular herpes simplex because of possible corneal perforation.

The lowest possible dose of corticosteroid should be used to control the condition under treatment, and when reduction in dosage is possible, the reduction should be gradual.

Psychic derangements may appear when corticosteroids are used, ranging from euphoria, insomnia, mood swings, personality changes and severe depression, to frank psychotic manifestations. Also, existing emotional instability or psychotic tendencies may be aggravated by corticosteroids.

Aspirin should be used cautiously in conjunction with corticosteroids in hypoprothrombinemia.

Steroids should be used with caution in nonspecific ulcerative colitis, if there is a probability of impending perforation, abscess or other pyogenic infection; diverticulitis; fresh intestinal anastomoses; active or latent peptic ulcer; renal insufficiency; hypertension; osteoporosis; and myasthenia gravis.

Continued on next page

Abbott—Cont.

Growth and development of infants and children on prolonged corticosteroid therapy should be carefully observed.

Adverse Reactions:

Fluid and Electrolyte Disturbances

- Sodium retention
- Fluid retention
- Congestive heart failure in susceptible patients
- Potassium loss
- Hypokalemic alkalosis
- Hypertension

Musculoskeletal

- Muscle-weakness
- Steroid myopathy
- Loss of muscle mass
- Osteoporosis
- Vertebral compression fractures
- Aseptic necrosis of femoral and humeral heads
- Pathologic fracture of long bones

Gastrointestinal

- Peptic ulcer with possible perforation and hemorrhage
- Pancreatitis
- Abdominal distention
- Ulcerative esophagitis

Dermatologic

- Impaired wound healing
- Thin fragile skin
- Petechiae and ecchymoses
- Facial erythema
- Increased sweating
- May suppress reactions to skin tests

Neurological

- Increased intracranial pressure with papilledema (pseudo-tumor cerebri) usually after treatment
- Convulsions
- Vertigo
- Headache

Endocrine

- Development of Cushingoid state
- Suppression of growth in children
- Secondary adrenocortical and pituitary unresponsiveness, particularly in times of stress, as in trauma, surgery or illness
- Menstrual irregularities
- Decreased carbohydrate tolerance
- Manifestations of latent diabetes mellitus
- Increased requirements for insulin or oral hypoglycemic agents in diabetics

Ophthalmic

- Posterior subcapsular cataracts
- Increased intraocular pressure
- Glaucoma
- Exophthalmos

Metabolic

- Negative nitrogen balance due to protein catabolism

The following additional adverse reactions are related to parenteral corticosteroid therapy:

- Hyperpigmentation or hypopigmentation
- Subcutaneous and cutaneous atrophy
- Sterile abscess

Administration and Dosage: A-HYDROCORT may be administered by intravenous injection, by intravenous infusion, or by intramuscular injection, the preferred method for initial emergency use being intravenous injection. Following the initial emergency period, consideration should be given to employing a longer acting injectable preparation or an oral preparation.

The initial dosage of A-HYDROCORT (hydrocortisone sodium succinate) may vary from 20 to 240 mg per day depending on the specific disease entity being treated. In situations of less severity, lower doses will generally suffice while in selected patients, higher initial doses may be required. The initial dosage should be maintained or adjusted until a satisfactory response is noted. If after a reasonable period of time there is a lack of satisfactory response, A-HYDROCORT should be discontinued and the patient transferred to other appropriate therapy. IT SHOULD BE EMPHASIZED THAT DOSAGE REQUIREMENTS ARE VARIABLE AND MUST BE INDIVIDUALIZED ON THE BASIS OF THE DISEASE UNDER TREATMENT AND THE RESPONSE OF THE PATIENT. After a favorable response is noted, the proper maintenance dosage should be determined by decreasing the initial drug dosage in small increments at appropriate time intervals until the lowest dosage which will maintain an adequate clinical response is reached. It should be kept in mind that constant monitoring is needed in regard to drug dosage. Included in the situations which may make dosage adjustments necessary are changes in clinical status secondary to remissions or exacerbations in the disease process, the patient's individual drug responsiveness, and the effect of patient exposure to stressful situations not directly related to the disease entity under treatment; in this latter situation, it may be necessary to increase the dosage of A-HYDROCORT for a period of time consistent with the patient's condition. If after longterm therapy the drug is to be stopped, it is recommended that it be withdrawn gradually rather than abruptly.

Preparation of Solutions:

Univial:

1. Remove protective cap, give the plunger-stopper a quarter turn and press to force diluent into lower compartment.
2. Gently agitate to effect solution. Use solution within 72 hours.
3. Sterilize top of plunger-stopper with a suitable germicide.
4. Insert needle squarely through center of plunger-stopper until tip is just visible. Invert vial and withdraw dose.

100 mg/2 ml Combination Package:

Prepare solution by aseptically adding 2 ml of Bacteriostatic Water for Injection to the vial.

For Intravenous Infusion:

The prepared solution should be added to 100 to 1000 ml (but not less than 100 ml) of the following: 5% dextrose in water (or isotonic saline solution or 5% dextrose in isotonic saline solution if patient is not on sodium restriction).

How Supplied: Sterile A-HYDROCORT (hydrocortisone sodium succinate for injection, USP) is available in the following packages:

100 mg/2 ml Univial **NDC** 0074-5671-02;
250 mg/2 ml Univial **NDC** 0074-5672-02;
500 mg/4 ml Univial **NDC** 0074-5673-04;
1000 mg/8 ml Univial **NDC** 0074-5674-08;
100 mg/2 ml Combination Package
NDC 0074-5676-02.

01-2909/R3

A-METHAPRED® ℞

(methylprednisolone sodium succinate for injection, USP)

For Intravenous or Intramuscular Use

Description: Methylprednisolone sodium succinate, USP, an adrenocortical-like steroid, is the sodium succinate ester of methylprednisolone.

It occurs as a white, or nearly white, odorless hygroscopic, amorphous solid.

Methylprednisolone sodium succinate is extremely soluble in water and is especially well suited for intravenous use in situations in which high blood levels of methylprednisolone are required rapidly.

A-METHAPRED (methylprednisolone sodium succinate for injection, USP) is available as:

40 mg Univial®—Each 1 ml (when mixed) contains methylprednisolone sodium succinate equivalent to 40 mg methylprednisolone; also 1.6 mg sodium biphosphate anhydrous; 17.46 mg dried sodium phosphate; 25 mg lactose anhydrous; and 9 mg of benzyl alcohol.

125 mg Univial—Each 2 ml (when mixed) contains methylprednisolone sodium succinate equivalent to 125 mg methylprednisolone; also 1.6 mg sodium biphosphate anhydrous; 17.4 mg dried sodium phosphate; and 18 mg of benzyl alcohol.

500 mg Vial with Diluent—Each 8 ml (when mixed) contains methylprednisolone sodium succinate equivalent to 500 mg methylprednisolone; also 6.4 mg sodium biphosphate anhydrous; 69.6 mg dried sodium phosphate; and 72 mg of benzyl alcohol.

1000 mg Vial with Diluent—16 ml (when mixed) contains methylprednisolone sodium succinate equivalent to 1000 mg methylprednisolone; also 12.8 mg sodium biphosphate anhydrous; 139.2 mg dried sodium phosphate; and 144 mg of benzyl alcohol.

The pH of each formula was adjusted with sodium hydroxide and/or hydrochloric acid.

Important: The solid contents of A-METHAPRED should not be used with any diluent other than that provided.

Use within 48 hours after mixing. Store below 86°F. Protect from light. Avoid freezing. Refrigeration not required.

When reconstituted as directed, the pH of the solutions ranges from 7–8 and the tonicities are, for the 40 mg per ml solution, 0.50 osmolar; for the 125 mg per 2 ml, 500 mg per 8 ml and 1000 mg per 16 ml solutions, 0.40 osmolar. (Isotonic saline = 0.28 osmolar).

Clinical Pharmacology: Methylprednisolone sodium succinate is a potent anti-inflammatory steroid. It has a greater anti-inflammatory potency than prednisolone and even less tendency than prednisolone to induce sodium and water retention. Like the adrenocortical steroids, methylprednisolone sodium succinate may cause profound and varied metabolic effects in addition to modifying the body's immune response to diverse stimuli.

When given parenterally and in equimolar quantities, methylprednisolone sodium succinate and methylprednisolone are equivalent in biologic activity.

The relative potency of methylprednisolone sodium succinate and hydrocortisone sodium succinate, as indicated by depression of eosinophil count, following intravenous administration, is at least four to one. This is in good agreement with the relative oral potency of methylprednisolone and hydrocortisone.

Indications: Sterile A-METHAPRED (methylprednisolone sodium succinate) is indicated in situations requiring a rapid and intense hormonal effect.

Intravenous administration of A-METHAPRED is most appropriate for the following indications:

1. **Endocrine disorders:**
   1. Preoperatively and in the event of serious trauma or illness, in patients with known adrenal insufficiency or when adrenocortical reserve is doubtful.
   b. Shock unresponsive to conventional therapy if adrenocortical insufficiency exists or is suspected.
2. **Collagen diseases**—During an exacerbation or as maintenance therapy in selected cases of:
   a. Acute rheumatic carditis.
3. **Allergic states**—Control of severe or incapacitating allergic conditions intractable to adequate trials of conventional treatment in:
   a. Bronchial asthma.
   b. Serum sickness.
   c. Drug hypersensitivity reactions.
   d. Urticarial transfusion reactions.
   e. Acute noninfectious laryngeal edema (epinephrine is the drug of first choice).
4. **Hematologic disorders:**
   a. Idiopathic thrombocytopenic purpura in adults (I.M. administration is contraindicated).

Intramuscular administration of A-METHAPRED is appropriate for the following indications:

1. **Endocrine disorders:**
   a. Preoperatively and in the event of serious trauma or illness, in patients with known adrenal insufficiency or when adrenocortical reserve is doubtful.
   b. Shock unresponsive to conventional therapy if adrenocortical insufficiency exists or is suspected.
   c. Congenital adrenal hyperplasia.
   d. Nonsuppurative thyroiditis.
   e. Hypercalcemia associated with cancer.
2. **Rheumatic disorders**—As adjunctive therapy for short-term administration (to tide the patient over an acute episode or exacerbation) in:
   a. Post-traumatic osteoarthritis.
   b. Synovitis of osteoarthritis.
   c. Rheumatoid arthritis, including juvenile rheumatoid arthritis (selected cases may require low-dose maintenance therapy).
   d. Acute and subacute bursitis.
   e. Epicondylitis.
   f. Acute nonspecific tenosynovitis.
   g. Acute gouty arthritis.
   h. Psoriatic arthritis.
   i. Ankylosing spondylitis.
3. **Collagen diseases**—During an exacerbation or as maintenance therapy in selected cases of:
   a. Systemic lupus erythematosus.
   b. Acute rheumatic carditis.
4. **Dermatologic diseases:**
   a. Severe erythema multiforme (Stevens-Johnson syndrome).
   b. Exfoliative dermatitis.
   c. Bullous dermatitis herpetiformis.
   d. Severe seborrheic dermatitis.
   e. Severe psoriasis.
   f. Pemphigus.
   g. Mycosis fungoides.
   h. Systemic dermatomyositis (polymyositis).
5. **Allergic states**—Control of severe or incapacitating allergic conditions intractable to adequate trials of conventional treatment in:
   a. Bronchial asthma.
   b. Contact dermatitis.
   c. Atopic dermatitis.
   d. Serum sickness.
   e. Seasonal or perennial allergic rhinitis.
   f. Drug hypersensitivity reactions.
   g. Urticarial transfusion reactions.
   h. Acute noninfectious laryngeal edema (epinephrine is the drug of first choice).
6. **Ophthalmic diseases**—Severe acute and chronic allergic and inflammatory processes involving the eye, such as:
   a. Herpes zoster ophthalmicus.
   b. Iritis, iridocyclitis.
   c. Chorioretinitis.
   d. Diffuse posterior uveitis and choroiditis.
   e. Optic neuritis.
   f. Sympathetic ophthalmia.
   g. Anterior segment inflammation.
   h. Allergic conjunctivitis.
   i. Allergic corneal marginal ulcers.
7. **Gastrointestinal diseases**—To tide the patient over a critical period of disease in:
   a. Ulcerative colitis—(Systemic therapy).
   b. Regional enteritis—(Systemic therapy).
8. **Respiratory diseases:**
   a. Symptomatic sarcoidosis.
   b. Berylliosis.
   c. Fulminating or disseminated pulmonary tuberculosis when concurrently accompanied by appropriate antituberculous chemotherapy.
   d. Aspiration pneumonitis.
   e. Loeffler's syndrome not manageable by other means.
9. **Hematologic disorders:**
   a. Acquired (autoimmune) hemolytic anemia.
   b. Secondary thrombocytopenia in adults.
   c. Erythroblastopenia (RBC anemia).
   d. Congenital (erythroid) hypoplastic anemia.
10. **Neoplastic diseases**—For palliative management of:
    a. Leukemias and lymphomas in adults.
    b. Acute leukemia of childhood.
11. **Edematous state**—To induce diuresis or remission of proteinuria in the nephrotic syndrome, without uremia, of the idiopathic type or that due to lupus erythematosus.
12. **Miscellaneous:**
    a. Tuberculous meningitis with subarachnoid block or impending block when used concurrently with appropriate antituberculous chemotherapy.
    b. Trichinosis with neurologic or myocardial involvement.

Contraindications: Systemic fungal infections.

Warnings: In patients on corticosteroid therapy subjected to any unusual stress, increased dosage of rapidly acting corticosteroids before, during, and after the stressful situation is indicated.

Corticosteroids may mask some signs of infection, and new infections may appear during their use. There may be decreased resistance and inability to localize infection when corticosteroids are used.

Prolonged use of corticosteroids may produce posterior subcapsular cataracts, glaucoma with possible damage to the optic nerves, and may enhance the establishment of secondary ocular infections due to fungi or viruses.

Average and large doses of cortisone or hydrocortisone can cause elevation of blood pressure, salt and water retention, and increased excretion of potassium. These effects are less likely to occur with the synthetic derivatives except when used in large doses. Dietary salt restriction and potassium supplementation may be necessary. All corticosteroids increase calcium excretion.

While on corticosteroid therapy patients should not be vaccinated against smallpox. Other immunization procedures should not be undertaken in patients who are on corticosteroids, especially on high dose, because of possible hazards of neurological complications and a lack of antibody response.

The use of A-METHAPRED (methylprednisolone sodium succinate) in active tuberculosis should be restricted to those cases of fulminating or disseminated tuberculosis in which the corticosteroid is used for the management of the disease in conjunction with appropriate antituberculous regimen.

If corticosteroids are indicated in patients with latent tuberculosis or tuberculin reactivity, close observation is necessary as reactivation of the disease may occur. During prolonged corticosteroid therapy, these patients should receive chemoprophylaxis.

Because rare instances of anaphylactoid reactions have occurred in patients receiving parenteral corticosteroid therapy, appropriate precautionary measures should be taken prior to administration, especially when the patient has a history of allergy to any drug.

There are reports of circulatory collapse following the administration of large I.V. doses of methylprednisolone sodium succinate (>0.5 gm) to recipients of renal transplants. Use of the drug for this condition is not a listed indication, but physicians should be aware of the above possibility.

Usage in Pregnancy: Since adequate human reproduction studies have not been done with corticosteroids, the use of these drugs in pregnancy, nursing mothers, or women of childbearing potential requires that the possible benefits of the drug be weighed against the potential hazards to the mother and embryo or fetus. Infants born of mothers who have received substantial doses of corticosteroids during pregnancy should be carefully observed for signs of hypoadrenalism.

Precautions: Drug-induced secondary adrenocortical insufficiency may be minimized by gradual reduction of dosage. This type of relative insufficiency may persist for months after discontinuation of therapy; therefore, in any situation of stress occurring during that period, hormone therapy should be reinstituted. Since mineralocorticoid secretion may be impaired, salt and/or a mineralocorticoid should be administered concurrently.

There is an enhanced effect of corticosteroids on patients with hypothyroidism and in those with cirrhosis.

Corticosteroids should be used cautiously in patients with ocular herpes simplex because of possible corneal perforation.

The lowest possible dose of corticosteroid should be used to control the condition under treatment, and when reduction in dosage is possible, the reduction should be gradual.

Psychic derangements may appear when corticosteroids are used, ranging from euphoria, insomnia, mood swings, personality changes and severe depression, to frank psychotic manifestations. Also, existing emotional instability or psychotic tendencies may be aggravated by corticosteroids.

Aspirin should be used cautiously in conjunction with corticosteroids in hypoprothrombinemia.

Steroids should be used with caution in nonspecific ulcerative colitis, if there is a probability of impending perforation, abscess or other pyogenic infection; diverticulitis; fresh intestinal anastomoses; active or latent peptic ulcer; renal insufficiency; hypertension; osteoporosis; and myasthenia gravis.

Growth and development of infants and children on prolonged corticosteroid therapy should be carefully observed.

Adverse Reactions:

Fluid and Electrolyte Disturbances

- Sodium retention
- Fluid retention
- Congestive heart failure in susceptible patients
- Potassium loss
- Hypokalemic alkalosis
- Hypertension

Musculoskeletal

- Muscle-weakness
- Steroid myopathy
- Loss of muscle mass
- Osteoporosis
- Vertebral compression fractures
- Aseptic necrosis of femoral and humeral heads
- Pathologic fracture of long bones

Gastrointestinal

- Peptic ulcer with possible perforation and hemorrhage
- Pancreatitis
- Abdominal distention
- Ulcerative esophagitis

Dermatologic

- Impaired wound healing
- Thin fragile skin
- Petechiae and ecchymoses
- Facial erythema

Continued on next page

Vitamin	per 10 ml	per 1 ml	U.S. RDA Multiple* per 1 ml
Thiamine Hydrochloride (B_1)	200 mg	20 mg	13.3
Riboflavin (as riboflavin-5'-phosphate sodium (B_2)	30 mg	3 mg	1.3
Niacinamide (Niacin)	750 mg	75 mg	3.8
Pyridoxine Hydrochloride (B_6)	50 mg	5 mg	2.1
Cyanocobalamin (B_{12})	20 mcg	2 mcg	0.3
d-Sodium Panthothenate (Pantothenic Acid)	50 mg	5 mg	0.5
Ascorbic Acid (C)	1 Gm	100 mg	1.7

Abbott—Cont.

Increased sweating
May suppress reactions to skin tests

Neurological

Increased intracranial pressure with papilledema (pseudo-tumor cerebri) usually after treatment
Convulsions
Vertigo
Headache

Endocrine

Development of Cushingoid state
Suppression of growth in children
Secondary adrenocortical and pituitary unresponsiveness, particularly in times of stress, as in trauma, surgery or illness
Menstrual irregularities
Decreased carbohydrate tolerance
Manifestations of latent diabetes mellitus
Increased requirements for insulin or oral hypoglycemic agents in diabetics

Ophthalmic

Posterior subcapsular cataracts
Increased intraocular pressure
Glaucoma
Exophthalmos

Metabolic

Negative nitrogen balance due to protein catabolism

The following additional adverse reactions are related to parenteral corticosteroid therapy:

Hyperpigmentation or hypopigmentation
Subcutaneous and cutaneous atrophy
Sterile abscess

Administration and Dosage: A-METHAPRED may be administered by intravenous injection, by intravenous infusion, or by intramuscular injection, the preferred method for initial emergency use being intravenous injection. Following the initial emergency period, consideration should be given to employing a longer acting injectable preparation or an oral preparation.

The initial dosage of A-METHAPRED (methylprednisolone sodium succinate) may vary from 4 to 48 mg per day depending on the specific disease entity being treated. In situations of less severity, lower doses will generally suffice while in selected patients, higher initial doses may be required. The initial dosage should be maintained or adjusted until a satisfactory response is noted. If after a reasonable period of time there is a lack of satisfactory clinical response, A-METHAPRED should be discontinued and the patient transferred to other appropriate therapy. IT SHOULD BE EMPHASIZED THAT DOSAGE REQUIREMENTS ARE VARIABLE AND MUST BE INDIVIDUALIZED ON THE BASIS OF THE DISEASE UNDER TREATMENT AND THE RESPONSE OF THE PATIENT. After a favorable response is noted, the proper maintenance dosage should be determined by decreasing the initial drug dosage in small increments at appropriate time intervals until the lowest dosage which will maintain an adequate clinical response is reached. It should be kept in mind that constant monitoring is needed in regard to drug dosage. Included in the situations which may make dosage adjustments necessary are changes in clinical status secondary to remissions or exacerbations in the disease process, the patient's individual drug responsiveness, and the effect of patient exposure to stressful situations not directly related to the disease entity under treatment; in this latter situation, it may be necessary to increase the dosage of A-METHAPRED for a period of time consistent with the patient's condition. If after long-term therapy the drug is to be stopped, it is recommended that it be withdrawn gradually rather than abruptly.

Preparation of Solutions:

Univial:

1. Remove protective cap, give the plunger-stopper a quarter turn and press to force diluent into the lower compartment.
2. Gently agitate to effect solution. Use solution within 48 hours.
3. Sterilize top of plunger-stopper with a suitable germicide.
4. Insert needle squarely through center of plunger-stopper until tip is just visible. Invert vial and withdraw dose.

500 mg (vial) with Bacteriostatic Water for Injection:
Prepare solution by aseptically adding 8 ml of Bacteriostatic Water for Injection to the vial.
1000 mg (vial) with Bacteriostatic Water for Injection:
Prepare solution by aseptically adding 16 ml of Bacteriostatic Water for Injection to the vial.
For Intravenous Infusion:
The prepared solution should be added to 100 to 1000 ml (but not less than 100 ml) of the following: 5% dextrose in water (or isotonic saline solution or 5% dextrose in isotonic saline solution if patient is not on sodium restriction).

How Supplied: Sterile A-METHAPRED (methylprednisolone sodium succinate for injection, USP) is available in the following packages:
40 mg/ml Univial **NDC** 0074-5684-01;
125 mg/2 ml Univial **NDC** 0074-5685-02;
500 mg/8 ml Combination Package **NDC** 0074-5687-08;
1000 mg/16 ml Combination Package **NDC** 0074-5689-16.
Ref. No. 01-2904/R3

A–POXIDE® ℞ ©
(chlordiazepoxide hydrochloride capsules, U.S.P.)

How Supplied: A-POXIDE (chlordiazepoxide hydrochloride capsules, U.S.P.) are supplied in three dosage strengths:
5 mg capsules (yellow and green) in bottles of 500 (**NDC** 0074-2648-53).
10 mg capsules (green and evergreen) in bottles of 500 (**NDC** 0074-2649-53).
25 mg capsules (light and dark green) in bottles of 100 (**NDC** 0074-2650-13).

[*Shown in Product Identification Section*]

Vitamin	per 10 ml	per 1 ml	U.S. RDA Multiple* per 1 ml
Thiamine Hydrochloride (B_1)	100 mg	10 mg	6.7
Riboflavin (as riboflavin-5'-phosphate sodium) (B_2)	20 mg	2 mg	0.9
Niacinamide (Niacin)	750 mg	75 mg	3.8
Pyridoxine Hydrochloride (B_6)	50 mg	5 mg	2.1
d-Sodium Pantothenate (Pantothenic Acid)	50 mg	5 mg	0.5

BEJECTAL®
BEJECTAL® with Vitamin C ℞
BEJEX®
INJECTABLE B-COMPLEX VITAMINS WITH OR WITHOUT VITAMIN C

Description: BEJECTAL is an injectable vitamin preparation containing five B-complex vitamins. It is intended for intravenous or intramuscular use only.
[See table below].
Also contains sodium formaldehyde sulfoxylate, 0.05 mg/ml, and sodium sulfide, 0.04 mg/ml, added as stabilizers; and benzyl alcohol, 9 mg/ml, added as preservative. pH adjusted with hydrochloric acid.

BEJECTAL with VITAMIN C is an injectable vitamin preparation containing six B-complex vitamins and vitamin C. It is intended for intravenous or intramuscular use only.
[See table above].
Also contains sodium formaldehyde sulfoxylate, 0.04 mg/ml, and sodium sulfide, 0.04 mg/ml, added as stabilizers; and methylparaben, 1.8 mg/ml, propylparaben, 0.2 mg/ml, and benzyl alcohol, 9 mg/ml, added as preservatives.

BEJEX is an injectable vitamin preparation containing six B-complex vitamins and vitamin C. It is intended for intravenous or intramuscular use only.
[See table on next page].
Also contains sodium formaldehyde sulfoxylate, 0.01 mg/ml, and sodium sulfide, 0.01 mg/ml, added as stabilizers; and methylparaben, 1.8 mg/ml, propylparaben, 0.2 mg/ml, and benzyl alcohol, 9 mg/ml, added as preservatives.

---

*Based on U.S. RDA for adults, and children 4 or more years of age.

Indications: For the treatment of patients with deficiencies of, or increased requirements for, certain of the water-soluble vitamins.
Parenteral administration of the B-complex vitamins and of vitamin C rapidly restores depleted tissue levels of these vitamins. Conditions that may require parenteral administration of water-soluble vitamins include: disorders adversely affecting the oral intake, gastrointestinal absorption, or the utilization of these vitamins; severe burns; chronic alcoholism; chronic diarrhea; chronic disease complicated by a deficiency of, or increased requirement for, these nutrients; many postoperative states including those involving delayed healing, particularly of the gastrointestinal tract; and other conditions that require parenteral nutrition.

Contraindications: BEJECTAL, BEJECTAL WITH VITAMIN C, and BEJEX are contraindicated in patients known to be hypersensitive to thiamine or to other components of the drugs.

Warnings: Allergic reactions including anaphylaxis may occur in patients hypersensitive to thiamine or to other components of BEJECTAL, BEJECTAL WITH VITAMIN C, or BEJEX.
Pyridoxine, even in small amounts, can decrease the efficacy of levodopa in the treatment of parkinsonism. This fact should be considered before prescribing BEJECTAL, BEJECTAL

WITH VITAMIN C, or BEJEX for patients receiving levodopa for the treatment of parkinsonism.

Precautions: Transient pain may be experienced when BEJECTAL, BEJECTAL WITH VITAMIN C, or BEJEX is administered by intramuscular injection. Intramuscular injections should be made deep into a large muscle mass to insure rapid absorption and to minimize pain.

Adverse Reactions: Occasional hypersensitivity reactions have been reported.

Pain as a result of intramuscular injection has also been reported.

Dosage and Administration: Preparation of Solutions: BEJECTAL is supplied in a 10 ml combination package containing two separate vials of sterile solution. Prior to administration, aseptically withdraw 4 ml of Bejectal Solution No. 2 and add to the vial of Bejectal Solution No. 1 BEJECTAL mixed solution is stable for 60 days when stored below 77°F (25°C).

BEJECTAL WITH VITAMIN C is supplied in a 10 ml closed, sterile, two-compartment vial as a lyophilized solid and a diluent. Prior to administration, exert simple pressure on the top rubber stopper of the vial to dislodge the plug between the two compartments and allow mixing of the ingredients. BEJECTAL WITH VITAMIN C reconstituted solution is stable for two weeks at refrigerator temperature.

BEJEX is supplied in a 5 ml closed, sterile, two-compartment vial as a lyophilized solid and a diluent. Prior to administration, exert simple pressure on the top rubber stopper of the vial to dislodge the plug between the two compartments and allow mixing of the ingredients. BEJEX reconstituted solution is stable for one week at refrigerator temperature.

Dosage and Administration: The daily dose of BEJECTAL, BEJECTAL WITH VITAMIN C, or BEJEX may range from 2 to 10 ml, depending upon the patient's condition and his therapeutic needs.

BEJECTAL, BEJECTAL WITH VITAMIN C, and BEJEX are usually administered intravenously by addition of the appropriate dose to any one of the following parenteral infusion fluids: Dextrose 5% in water, Dextrose 5% in saline, or Normal Saline 0.9%.

When intravenous infusion is not feasible, the appropriate dose of BEJECTAL, BEJECTAL WITH VITAMIN c, or BEJEX may be administered undiluted by SLOW intravenous injection or by intramuscular injection. Intravenous injection is usually preferred since intramuscular administration may cause temporary pain. If the intramuscular route is employed, the injection should be made deep into a large muscle mass to insure rapid absorption and to minimize pain. Intramuscular injections of BEJECTAL, BEJECTAL WITH VITAMIN C, or BEJEX should not exceed 2 ml at any one injection site.

How Supplied: BEJECTAL is supplied in a combination package containing 2 vials, the contents of which when mixed provide 10 ml of solution (**NDC** 0074-3285-03).

BEJECTAL WITH VITAMIN C is supplied in a 10 ml UNIVIAL ® container (**NDC** 0074-6430-02).

BEJEX is supplied in a 5 ml UNIVIAL container (**NDC** 0074-6823-02).

UNIVIAL—Sterile two-compartment vial, Abbott.

Ref. 01-2028-R7

Vitamin	per 5 ml	per 1 ml	U.S. RDA Multiple* per 1 ml
Thiamine Hydrochloride (B_1)	10 mg	2 mg	1.3
Riboflavin (as riboflavin-5'-phosphate sodium) (B_2)	10 mg	2 mg	0.9
Niacinamide (Niacin)	250 mg	50 mg	2.5
Pyridoxine Hydrochloride (B_6)	5 mg	1 mg	0.4
Cyanocobalamin (B_{12})	25 mcg	5 mcg	0.8
d-Sodium Pantothenate (Pantothenic Acid)	50 mg	10 mg	0.9
Ascorbic Acid (C)	500 mg	100 mg	1.7

BUTESIN® PICRATE

(butambem picrate)
ointment

Description: Butesin Picrate is an anesthetic ointment containing Butesin Picrate (Butamben Picrate), 1%.

Indication: For temporary relief of pain due to minor burns.

Warning: Certain persons, due to idiosyncrasy, are sensitive to this ointment and may develop a rash following its application. In such cases its use should be discontinued, and the ointment remaining on the skin removed with soap and water.

Precautions: Should not be applied repeatedly or to large areas except under a physician's instructions. As Butesin Picrate stains cannot be removed from animal fibers, contact with silk or wool fabrics and hair should be avoided.

Dosage and Administration: Spread thinly on painful or denuded lesions of the skin, if these are small. Apply a loose bandage to protect the clothing.

How Supplied: 1 oz tube (**NDC** 0074-4392-01).

Ref. 09-5413-2/R4

CALCIDRINE® SYRUP ℞ Ⓒ

Description: Each 5 ml. (teaspoonful) contains:

Codeine, N.F. .... 8.4 mg.
Warning—may be habit forming.
Calcium Iodide, anhydrous .... 152 mg.
In a palatable syrup, Alcohol 6%.

Indications: As an expectorant, and for symptomatic relief of coughs.

Contraindications: Calcidrine Syrup should not be used in patients with a history of iodism, or in patients with known hypersensitivity to iodides or codeine. Long-term use of iodide-containing preparations is contraindicated during pregnancy. Maternal ingestion of large amounts of iodides during pregnancy has been associated with the development of fetal goiter and resultant acute respiratory distress of the neonate.

Warnings: Physiological dependence may develop with the use of codeine.

Precautions: Patients who must receive prolonged iodide therapy should be evaluated periodically for possible depression of thyroid function.

Adverse Reactions: Codeine may produce nausea and vomiting. Constipation can occur with the use of codeine. Iodism can occur with the use of this drug. Symptoms of iodism include metallic taste, acneform skin lesions, mucous membrane irritation, salivary gland swelling, and gastric distress. These side effects subside quickly upon discontinuance of the iodide-containing drug. Severe and sometimes fatal skin eruptions (ioderma) occur rarely after the prolonged use of iodides.

Dosage and Administration: For adult and children over ten years of age, the usual dose is 1 to 2 teaspoonfuls every 4 hours. For children 6 to 10 years of age, ½ to 1 teaspoonful every 4 hours. Children 2 to 6 years of age, ½ teaspoonful every 4 hours.

How Supplied:

4 fl. oz.	**NDC** 0074-5763-04
1 Pint	**NDC** 0074-5763-16
1 Gallon	**NDC** 0074-5763-11

Ref. No. 02-5545-2/R1

CEFOL® FILMTAB® tablets ℞

(B-Complex, folic acid, vitamin E with 750 mg vitamin C)

Description: Each tablet provides:

Ascorbic Acid (C) (as sodium ascorbate) .... 750 mg
Niacinamide .... 100 mg
Calcium Pantothenate .... 20 mg
Thiamine Mononitrate (B_1) .... 15 mg
Riboflavin (B_2) .... 10 mg
Pyridoxine Hydrochloride (B_6) .... 5 mg
Folic Acid .... 500 mcg
Cyanocobalamin (B_{12}) .... 6 mcg
Vitamin E (as dl-alpha tocopheryl acetate) .... 30 IU

Indications: Cefol Filmtab vitamin tablets are indicated in non-pregnant* adults for the treatment of Vitamin C deficiency states where there is an associated deficient intake or increased need for Vitamin B-Complex including folic acid, and Vitamin E.

*Pregnancy may require greater folic acid intake than is provided by Cefol.

Warnings: Folic acid alone is improper therapy in the treatment of pernicious anemia and other megaloblastic anemias where vitamin B_{12} is deficient.

Precautions: Folic acid especially in doses above 1 mg daily may obscure pernicious anemia in that hematologic remission may occur while neurological manifestations remain progressive.

Adverse Reactions: Allergic sensitization has been reported following both oral and parenteral administration of folic acid.

Dosage: Usual adult dose is one tablet daily.

How Supplied: Cefol Filmtab tablets are supplied in bottles of 100 (NDC 0074-6089-13).

Filmtab—Film-sealed tablets, Abbott.

[*Shown in Product Identification Section*]

Ref. 03-0685-4/R5

CLEAR EYES® OTC

Eye Drops

Description: Clear Eyes® is a sterile isotonic buffered solution containing naphazoline hydrochloride 0.012%, boric acid, sodium borate, methylcellulose and water. Disodium edetate 0.1% and benzalkonium chloride 0.01% are added as preservatives.

Indications: Clear Eyes is a decongestant ophthalmic solution specially designed to moisturize as it removes redness from irritated eyes. Clear Eyes contains laboratory tested, and scientifically blended ingredients including an effective vasoconstrictor which narrows swollen blood vessels and rapidly whitens reddened eyes in a moisturizing formulation which produces a refreshing, soothing effect. Clear Eyes is a sterile, isotonic solution compatible with the natural fluids of the eye.

Warning: Clear Eyes should only be used for minor eye irritations. If relief is not obtained within 48 hours, or if irritation persists or increases discontinue use and consult your physician.

Clear Eyes should not be used by individuals with glaucoma and serious eye diseases. In some instances redness or inflammation may be due to serious eye conditions such as acute iritis, acute glaucoma, or corneal trauma. When redness, pain, or blurring persist, a physician should be consulted at once.

Dosage and Administration: One or two drops in eye(s) two or three times daily or as directed by physician. Do not touch bottle tip to

Continued on next page

Abbott—Cont.

any surface, since this may contaminate the solution. Keep container tightly closed. Keep this and all other medicines out of reach of children.

How Supplied: In 0.6 fl. oz. and 1.5 fl. oz. plastic dropper bottle.

CYLERT® ℞ ©
(pemoline)
Tablets

Description: CYLERT (pemoline) is a central nervous system stimulant. Pemoline is structurally dissimilar to the amphetamines and methylphenidate.

It is an oxazolidine compound and is chemically identified as 2-amino-5-phenyl-2-oxazolin-4-one.

Pemoline is a white, tasteless, odorless powder, relatively insoluble (less than 1 mg./ml.) in water, chloroform, ether, acetone, and benzene; its solubility in 95% ethyl alcohol is 2.2 mg./ml.

CYLERT (pemoline) is supplied as tablets for oral administration.

Clinical Pharmacology: CYLERT (pemoline) has a pharmacological activity similar to that of other known central nervous system stimulants; however, it has minimal sympathomimetic effects. Although studies indicate that pemoline may act in animals through dopaminergic mechanisms, the exact mechanism and site of action of the drug in man is not known. There is neither specific evidence which clearly establishes the mechanism whereby CYLERT produces its mental and behavioral effects in children, nor conclusive evidence regarding how these effects relate to the condition of the central nervous system.

The serum half-life of pemoline is approximately 12 hours. Peak serum levels of the drug occur within 2 to 4 hours after ingestion of a single dose. Multiple dose studies in adults at several dose levels indicate that steady state is reached in approximately 2 to 3 days.

Metabolites of pemoline include pemoline conjugate, pemoline dione, mandelic acid, and unidentified polar compounds. CYLERT is excreted primarily by the kidneys; approximately 75% of an oral dose is recovered in the urine within 24 hours. Approximately 43% of pemoline is excreted unchanged.

CYLERT (pemoline) has a gradual onset of action. Using the recommended schedule of dosage titration, significant clinical benefit may not be evident until the third or fourth week of drug administration.

Indications: CYLERT is indicated as an integral part of a total treatment program which typically includes other remedial measures (psychological, educational, social) for a stabilizing effect in children with a behavioral syndrome characterized by the following group of developmentally inappropriate symptoms: moderate to severe distractibility, short attention span, hyperactivity, emotional lability, and impulsivity. The diagnosis of this syndrome should not be made with finality when these symptoms are only of comparatively recent origin. Nonlocalizing (soft) neurological signs, learning disability, and abnormal EEG may or may not be present, and a diagnosis of central nervous system dysfunction may or may not be warranted.

Attention Deficit Disorder and Hyperkinetic Syndrome are among the terms being used to describe the above signs and symptoms. In the past, a variety of terms has been associated with these signs and symptoms, including: Minimal Brain Dysfunction, Hyperkinetic Reaction of Childhood, Hyperkinetic Syndrome, Hyperactive Child Syndrome, Minimal Brain Damage, Minimal Cerebral Dysfunction, and Minor Cerebral Dysfunction.

Contraindications: CYLERT (pemoline) is contraindicated in patients with known hypersensitivity or idiosyncrasy to the drug. (See ADVERSE REACTIONS.)

Warnings: CYLERT is not recommended for children less than 6 years of age since its safety and efficacy in this age group have not been established.

Clinical experience suggests that in psychotic children, administration of CYLERT may exacerbate symptoms of behavior disturbance and thought disorder.

Data are inadequate to determine whether chronic administration of CYLERT may be associated with growth inhibition; therefore, growth should be monitored during treatment.

Precautions: Drug treatment is not indicated in all cases of the behavioral syndrome characterized by moderate to severe distractibility, short attention span, hyperactivity, emotional lability and impulsivity. It should be considered only in light of the complete history and evaluation of the child. The decision to prescribe CYLERT should depend on the physician's assessment of the chronicity and severity of the child's symptoms and their appropriateness for his/her age. Prescription should not depend solely on the presence of one or more of the behavioral characteristics.

When these symptoms are associated with acute stress reactions, treatment with CYLERT is usually not indicated.

Long-term effects of CYLERT in children have not been well established.

Liver function tests should be performed prior to and periodically during therapy with CYLERT. The drug should be discontinued if abnormalities are revealed and confirmed by follow-up tests. (See ADVERSE REACTIONS regarding reports of abnormal liver function tests and jaundice.)

CYLERT should be administered with caution to patients with significantly impaired hepatic or renal function.

The interaction of CYLERT with other drugs has not been studied in humans. Patients who are receiving CYLERT concurrently with other drugs, especially drugs with CNS activity, should be monitored carefully.

CYLERT failed to demonstrate a potential for self-administration in primates. However, the pharmacologic similarity of pemoline to other psychostimulants with known dependence liability suggests that psychological and/or physical dependence might also occur with CYLERT. There have been isolated reports of transient psychotic symptoms occurring in adults following the long-term misuse of excessive oral doses of pemoline. CYLERT should be given with caution to emotionally unstable patients who may increase the dosage on their own initiative.

Usage during Pregnancy and Lactation: The safety of CYLERT (pemoline) for use during pregnancy and lactation has not been established. Studies in rats have shown an increased incidence of stillbirths and cannibalization when pemoline was administered at a dose of 37.5 mg./kg./day. Postnatal survival of offspring was reduced at doses of 18.75 and 37.5 mg./kg./day.

Adverse Reactions: Insomnia is the most frequently reported side effect of CYLERT; it usually occurs early in therapy, prior to an optimum therapeutic response. In the majority of cases it is transient in nature or responds to a reduction in dosage.

Anorexia with weight loss may occur during the first weeks of therapy. In the majority of cases it is transient in nature; weight gain usually resumes within three to six months.

Stomach ache, skin rashes, increased irritability, mild depression, nausea, dizziness, headache, drowsiness, and hallucinations have been reported.

Elevations of SGOT, SGPT, and serum LDH have occurred in patients taking CYLERT, usually after several months of therapy. These effects appear to be reversible upon withdrawal of the drug, and are thought to be manifestations of a delayed hypersensitivity reaction. There have also been a few reports of jaundice occurring in patients taking CYLERT; a causal relationship between the drug and this clinical finding has not been established.

The following CNS effects have been reported with the use of CYLERT: dyskinetic movements of the tongue, lips, face and extremities, nystagmus and nystagmoid eye movements, and convulsive seizures. A definite causal relationship between CYLERT and these reactions has not been established.

Mild adverse reactions appearing early during the course of treatment with CYLERT often remit with continuing therapy. If adverse reactions are of a significant or protracted nature, dosage should be reduced or the drug discontinued.

Overdosage: Signs and symptoms of acute CYLERT overdosage may include agitation, restlessness, hallucinations, dyskinetic movements and tachycardia. The treatment for an acute overdosage of pemoline is essentially the same as that for an overdosage of any CNS stimulant. Management is primarily symptomatic and may include induction of emesis or gastric lavage, sedation, and other appropriate supportive measures.

Results of studies in dogs indicate that extracorporeal hemodialysis may be useful in the management of CYLERT overdosage; forced diuresis and peritoneal dialysis appear to be of little value.

Dosage and Administration: CYLERT (pemoline) is administered as a single oral dose each morning. The recommended starting dose is 37.5 mg./day. This daily dose should be gradually increased by 18.75 mg. at one week intervals until the desired clinical response is obtained. The effective daily dose for most patients will range from 56.25 to 75 mg. The maximum recommended daily dose of pemoline is 112.5 mg.

Clinical improvement with CYLERT is gradual. Using the recommended schedule of dosage titration, significant benefit may not be evident until the third or fourth week of drug administration.

Where possible, drug administration should be interrupted occasionally to determine if there is a recurrence of behavioral symptoms sufficient to require continued therapy.

How Supplied: CYLERT (pemoline) is supplied as monogrammed, grooved tablets in three dosage strengths:

18.75 mg. tablets (white) in bottles of 100 (**NDC** 0074-6025-13)

37.5 mg. tablets (orange-colored) in bottles of 100 (**NDC** 0074-6057-13)

75 mg. tablets (tan-colored) in bottles of 100 (**NDC** 0074-6073-13)

CYLERT Chewable is supplied as monogrammed, grooved tablets in one dosage strength:

37.5 mg. tablets (orange-colored) in bottles of 100 (**NDC** 0074-6088-13)

Ref. No. 03-4196/R3

[Shown in Product Identification Section]

DAYALETS®
Multivitamin Supplement for adults and children 4 or more years of age

DAYALETS® PLUS IRON
Multivitamin Supplement with Iron for adults and children 4 or more years of age

Description: Dayalets provide 100% of the recommended daily allowances of essential vitamins. Dayalets Plus Iron provides 100% of the recommended daily allowances of essential vitamins plus the mineral iron.

Daily dosage (one tablet) provides:

Vitamins			**% U.S. RDA**
Vitamin A	(1.5 mg.)	5000 I.U.	100%
Vitamin D	(10 mcg.)	400 I.U.	100%

Vitamin E	30 I.U.	100%
Vitamin C	60 mg.	100%
Folic Acid	0.4 mg.	100%
Thiamine (Vitamin B_1)	1.5 mg.	100%
Riboflavin (Vitamin B_2)	1.7 mg.	100%
Niacin	20 mg.	100%
Vitamin B_6	2 mg.	100%
Vitamin B_{12}	6 mcg.	100%

Ingredients: Ascorbic acid, cellulose, dl-alpha tocopheryl acetate, niacinamide, pyridoxine hydrochloride, riboflavin, thiamine hydrochloride, vitamin A acetate, folic acid, vitamin A palmitate, ergocalciferol, and cyanocobalamin in a film-coated tablet with vanillin flavoring and artificial coloring added.

Each Dayalets Plus Iron Filmtab® represents all the vitamins in the Dayalets formula in the same concentrations, plus the mineral iron 18 mg. (100% U.S. R.D.A.), as ferrous sulfate. Dayalets Plus Iron contain the same ingredients as Dayalets plus the ingredient povidone.

These products contain no sugar and essentially no calories.

Indications: Dayalets and Dayalets Plus Iron Filmtab tablets are indicated for use as a dietary supplement for adults and children 4 or more years of age.

Administration and Dosage: One Filmtab tablet daily.

How Supplied: In bottles of 100 tablets.

® Filmtab—Film-sealed tablets, Abbott.

[*Shown in Product Identification Section*]

Ref. 02-5322-5/R2, 02-5323-6/R4

DEPAKENE® ℞
Valproic Acid
Capsules and Syrup

Description: DEPAKENE (valproic acid) is a carboxylic acid designated as 2-propylpentanoic acid. It is also known as dipropylacetic acid.

Valproic acid (pKa 4.8) has a molecular weight of 144 and occurs as a colorless liquid with a characteristic odor. It is slightly soluble in water (1.3 mg/ml) and very soluble in organic solvents.

DEPAKENE is supplied as soft elastic capsules and syrup for oral administration.

Clinical Pharmacology: DEPAKENE is an anticonvulsant agent which is chemically unrelated to other drugs used to treat seizure disorders. It has no nitrogen or aromatic moiety characteristic of other anticonvulsant drugs. The mechanism by which DEPAKENE exerts its anticonvulsant effects has not been established. It has been suggested that its activity is related to increased brain levels of gamma-aminobutyric acid (GABA). The effect on the neuronal membrane is unknown.

DEPAKENE is rapidly absorbed after oral administration. Peak serum levels of valproic acid occur approximately one to four hours after a single oral dose of DEPAKENE. The serum half-life ($t_{0.5,\beta}$) of the parent compound is approximately eight to twelve hours. A slight delay in initial absorption occurs when the drug is administered with meals but this does not affect the total absorption.

Valproic acid is rapidly distributed and the drug is strongly bound (90%) to human plasma proteins.

Elimination of DEPAKENE and its metabolites occurs principally in the urine, with minor amounts in the feces and expired air. Very little unmetabolized parent drug is excreted in the urine. The drug is primarily metabolized in the liver and is excreted as the glucuronide conjugate. Other metabolites in the urine are products of beta and omega oxidation (C-3 and C-5 position). The three major oxidative metabolites are 2-propyl-3-keto-pentanoic acid, 2-propyl-5-hydroxypentanoic acid, and 2-propylglutaric acid.

Indications: DEPAKENE (valproic acid) is indicated for use as sole and adjunctive therapy in the treatment of simple and complex absence seizures, including petit mal. DEPAKENE may also be used adjunctively in patients with multiple seizure types which include absence seizures.

In accordance with the International Classification of Seizures, simple absence is defined as very brief clouding of the sensorium or loss of consciousness (lasting usually 2–15 seconds), accompanied by certain generalized epileptic discharges without other detectable clinical signs. Complex absence is the term used when other signs are also present.

Contraindications: DEPAKENE (valproic acid) is contraindicated in patients with known hypersensitivity to the drug.

Warnings: Hepatic failure resulting in fatalities has occurred in patients receiving DEPAKENE. These incidences usually have occurred during the first six months of treatment with DEPAKENE. Liver function tests should be performed prior to therapy and at frequent intervals thereafter. Caution should be observed when administering DEPAKENE to patients with pre-existing hepatic disease.

The drug should be discontinued immediately in the presence of significant hepatic dysfunction, suspected or apparent. The frequency of adverse effects (particularly elevated liver enzymes) may increase with increasing dose. Therefore, the benefit gained by increased seizure control by increasing the dosage must be weighed against the increased incidence of adverse effects sometimes seen at higher dosages.

Usage in Pregnancy: THE EFFECTS OF DEPAKENE IN HUMAN PREGNANCY ARE UNKNOWN. ANIMAL STUDIES HAVE DEMONSTRATED TERATOGENICITY.

Studies in rats demonstrated placental transfer of the drug. Doses greater than 65 mg/kg/day given to pregnant rats and mice produced skeletal abnormalities in the offspring, primarily involving ribs and vertebrae; doses greater than 150 mg/kg/day given to pregnant rabbits produced fetal resorptions and (primarily) soft-tissue abnormalities in the offspring. In rats a dose-related delay in the onset of parturition was noted. Postnatal growth and survival of the progeny were adversely affected, particularly when drug administration spanned the entire gestation and early lactation period.

THERE ARE MULTIPLE REPORTS IN THE CLINICAL LITERATURE WHICH INDICATE THAT THE USE OF ANTICONVULSANT DRUGS DURING PREGNANCY RESULTS IN AN INCREASED INCIDENCE OF BIRTH DEFECTS IN THE OFFSPRING. ALTHOUGH DATA ARE MORE EXTENSIVE WITH RESPECT TO TRIMETHADIONE, PARAMETHADIONE, PHENYTOIN, AND PHENOBARBITAL, REPORTS INDICATE A POSSIBLE SIMILAR ASSOCIATION WITH THE USE OF OTHER ANTICONVULSANT DRUGS. THEREFORE, ANTICONVULSANT DRUGS SHOULD BE ADMINISTERED TO WOMEN OF CHILDBEARING POTENTIAL ONLY IF THEY ARE CLEARLY SHOWN TO BE ESSENTIAL IN THE MANAGEMENT OF THEIR SEIZURES.

Anticonvulsant drugs should not be discontinued in patients in whom the drug is administered to prevent major seizures because of the strong possibility of precipitating status epilepticus with attendant hypoxia and threat to life. In individual cases where the severity and frequency of the seizure disorder are such that the removal of medication does not pose a serious threat to the patient, discontinuation of the drug may be considered prior to and during pregnancy, although it cannot be said with any confidence that even minor seizures do not pose some hazard to the developing embryo or fetus.

The prescribing physician will wish to weigh these considerations in treating or counseling epileptic women of childbearing potential.

Precautions:

Hepatic dysfunction: See WARNINGS.

General: Because of reports of thrombocytopenia and platelet aggregation dysfunction, platelet counts and bleeding time determination are recommended before initiating therapy and at periodic intervals. It is recommended that patients receiving DEPAKENE be monitored for platelet count prior to planned surgery. Clinical evidence of hemorrhage, bruising or a disorder of hemostasis/coagulation is an indication for reduction of DEPAKENE dosage or withdrawal of therapy pending investigation.

Since DEPAKENE (valproic acid) may interact with concurrently administered anticonvulsant drugs, periodic serum level determinations of concomitant anticonvulsant drugs are recommended during the early course of therapy. (See Drug Interactions).

DEPAKENE is partially eliminated in the urine as a keto-metabolite which may lead to a false interpretation of the urine ketone test.

Information For Patients: Since DEPAKENE may produce CNS depression, especially when combined with another CNS depressant (e.g., alcohol), patients should be advised not to engage in hazardous occupations, such as driving an automobile or operating dangerous machinery, until it is known that they do not become drowsy from the drug.

Drug Interactions: DEPAKENE may potentiate the CNS depressant activity of alcohol.

THERE IS EVIDENCE THAT DEPAKENE MAY CAUSE AN INCREASE IN SERUM PHENOBARBITAL LEVELS, ALTHOUGH THE MECHANISM OF THE INTERACTION IS UNKNOWN. ALL PATIENTS RECEIVING CONCOMITANT BARBITURATE THERAPY SHOULD BE CLOSELY MONITORED FOR NEUROLOGICAL TOXICITY, SERUM BARBITURATE DRUG LEVELS OBTAINED, IF POSSIBLE, AND THE BARBITURATE DOSAGE DECREASED, IF APPROPRIATE.

Primidone is metabolized into a barbiturate and, therefore, may also be involved in a similar or identical interaction.

THERE IS CONFLICTING EVIDENCE REGARDING THE INTERACTION OF DEPAKENE WITH PHENYTOIN. IT IS NOT KNOWN IF THERE IS A CHANGE IN UNBOUND (FREE) PHENYTOIN SERUM CONCENTRATIONS. THE DOSAGE OF PHENYTOIN SHOULD BE ADJUSTED AS REQUIRED BY THE CLINICAL SITUATION.

THE CONCOMITANT USE OF VALPROIC ACID AND CLONAZEPAM MAY PRODUCE ABSENCE STATUS.

Caution is recommended when DEPAKENE (valproic acid) is administered with drugs affecting coagulation, e.g., aspirin and warfarin. (See ADVERSE REACTIONS).

Carcinogenesis, Mutagenesis: There has been insufficient study of the drug in animals to determine whether it has carcinogenic potential. Carcinogenicity studies in rats and mice are currently in progress.

Mutagenesis studies on DEPAKENE have been performed using bacterial and mammalian systems. These studies have provided no evidence of a mutagenic potential for DEPAKENE.

Pregnancy: See WARNINGS.

Nursing Mothers: DEPAKENE is excreted in breast milk. It is not known what effect this would have on a nursing infant. As a general rule, nursing should not be undertaken while a patient is receiving DEPAKENE.

Fertility: Chronic toxicity studies in juvenile and adult rats and dogs demonstrated reduced spermatogenesis and testicular atrophy at

Continued on next page

Abbott—Cont.

doses greater than 200 mg/kg/day in rats and greater than 90 mg/kg/day in dogs. Segment I fertility studies in rats have shown doses up to 350 mg/kg/day for 60 days to have no effect on fertility. THE EFFECT OF DEPAKENE (VALPROIC ACID) ON THE DEVELOPMENT OF THE TESTES AND ON SPERM PRODUCTION AND FERTILITY IN HUMANS IS UNKNOWN.

Adverse Reactions: Since DEPAKENE (valproic acid) has usually been used with other anticonvulsant drugs, it is not possible, in most cases, to determine whether the following adverse reactions can be ascribed to DEPAKENE alone, or the combination of drugs.

Gastrointestinal: The most commonly reported side effects at the initiation of therapy are nausea, vomiting and indigestion. These effects are usually transient and rarely require discontinuation of therapy. Diarrhea, abdominal cramps and constipation have been reported. Both anorexia with some weight loss and increased appetite with weight gain have also been reported.

CNS Effects: Sedative effects have been noted in patients receiving valproic acid alone but are found most often in patients receiving combination therapy. Sedation usually disappears upon reduction of other anticonvulsant medication. Ataxia, headache, nystagmus, diplopia, asterixis, "spots before eyes", tremor, dysarthria, dizziness, and incoordination have rarely been noted. Rare cases of coma have been noted in patients also on phenobarbital.

Dermatologic: Transient increases in hair loss have been observed. Skin rash and petechiae have rarely been noted.

Psychiatric: Emotional upset, depression, psychosis, aggression, hyperactivity and behavioral deterioration have been reported.

Musculoskeletal: Weakness has been reported.

Hematopoietic: Thrombocytopenia has been reported. Valproic acid inhibits the secondary phase of platelet aggregation. (See DRUG INTERACTIONS). This may be reflected in altered bleeding time. Bruising, hematoma formation and frank hemorrhage have been reported. Relative lymphocytosis and hypofibrinogenemia have been noted. Leukopenia and eosinophilia have also been reported.

Hepatic: Increases in serum alkaline phosphatase and elevations of serum glutamic oxaloacetic transaminase (SGOT) have been noted. Elevation of SGOT may be dose related. Elevations of SGPT and LDH have been noted less frequently. Isolated cases of severe hepatotoxicity have been reported but do not appear dose related. (See WARNINGS).

Overdosage: A single case of overdosage with valproic acid has been reported. After ingesting 36 grams in combination with phenobarbital and phenytoin, the patient presented in deep coma. An electroencephalogram recorded diffuse slowing, compatible with the state of consciousness. The patient made an uneventful recovery.

Since DEPAKENE is absorbed very rapidly, gastric lavage may be of limited value. General supportive measures should be applied with particular attention being given to the maintenance of adequate urinary output.

Dosage and Administration: DEPAKENE (valproic acid) is administered orally. The recommended initial dose is 15 mg/kg/day, increasing at one week intervals by 5 to 10 mg/kg/day, until seizures are controlled or side effects preclude further increases. The maximum recommended dosage is 60 mg/kg/day. If the total daily dose exceeds 250 mg, it should be given in a divided regimen. The following table is a guide for the initial daily dose of DEPAKENE (valproic acid) (15 mg/kg/day):

[See table below].

Weight (kg)	Weight (lb)	Total Daily Dose (mg)	Number of Capsules or Teaspoonfuls of Syrup: Dose 1	Dose 2	Dose 3
10—24.9	22— 54.9	250	0	0	1
25—39.9	55— 87.9	500	1	0	1
40—59.9	88—131.9	750	1	1	1
60—74.9	132—164.9	1,000	1	1	2
75—89.9	165—197.9	1,250	2	1	2

The frequency of adverse effects (particularly elevated liver enzymes) may increase with increasing dose. Therefore, the benefit gained by increased seizure control by increased dosage must be weighed against the increased incidence of adverse effects sometimes seen at higher doses.

A good correlation has not been established between daily dose, serum level and therapeutic effect, however, therapeutic serum levels for most patients will range from 50 to 100 mcg/ml. Occasional patients may be controlled with serum levels lower or higher than this range.

As the DEPAKENE dosage is titrated upward, blood levels of phenobarbital and/or phenytoin may be affected. (See PRECAUTIONS).

Patients who experience G.I. irritation may benefit from administration of the drug with food or by slowly building up the dose from an initial low level.

THE CAPSULES SHOULD BE SWALLOWED WITHOUT CHEWING TO AVOID LOCAL IRRITATION OF THE MOUTH AND THROAT.

How Supplied: DEPAKENE (valproic acid) is available as orange-colored soft gelatin capsules of 250 mg valproic acid in bottles of 100 capsules (**NDC** 0074-5681-13), and as a red syrup containing the equivalent of 250 mg valproic acid per 5 ml as the sodium salt in bottles of 16 ounces (**NDC** 0074-5682-16).

Ref. No. 01-2036/R2

[Shown in Product Identification Section]

DESOXYN® ℞ Ⓒ

(methamphetamine hydrochloride)
Tablets—Gradument® Tablets

METHAMPHETAMINE HAS A HIGH POTENTIAL FOR ABUSE. IT SHOULD THUS BE TRIED ONLY IN WEIGHT REDUCTION PROGRAMS FOR PATIENTS IN WHOM ALTERNATIVE THERAPY HAS BEEN INEFFECTIVE. ADMINISTRATION OF METHAMPHETAMINE FOR PROLONGED PERIODS OF TIME IN OBESITY MAY LEAD TO DRUG DEPENDENCE AND MUST BE AVOIDED. PARTICULAR ATTENTION SHOULD BE PAID TO THE POSSIBILITY OF SUBJECTS OBTAINING METHAMPHETAMINE FOR NON-THERAPEUTIC USE OR DISTRIBUTION TO OTHERS, AND THE DRUG SHOULD BE PRESCRIBED OR DISPENSED SPARINGLY.

Description: DESOXYN (methamphetamine hydrochloride), previously known as *d*-desoxyephedrine, is a member of the amphetamine group of sympathomimetic amines.

DESOXYN is available as Gradumet tablets and as conventional tablets. The Gradumet is an inert, porous, plastic matrix, which is impregnated with DESOXYN. The drug is leached slowly from the Gradumet as it passes through the gastrointestinal tract. The expended matrix is not absorbed and is excreted in the stool.

Actions: DESOXYN is a sympathomimetic amine with CNS stimulant activity. Peripheral actions include elevation of systolic and diastolic blood pressures and weak bronchodilator and respiratory stimulant action. Drugs of this class used in obesity are commonly known as "anorectics" or "anorexigenics." It has not been established, however, that the action of such drugs in treating obesity is primarily one of appetite suppression. Other central nervous system actions, or metabolic effects, may be involved, for example.

Adult obese subjects instructed in dietary management and treated with "anorectic" drugs, lose more weight on the average than those treated with placebo and diet, as determined in relatively short-term clinical trials. The magnitude of increased weight loss of drug-treated patients over placebo-treated patients is only a fraction of a pound a week. The rate of weight loss is greatest in the first weeks of therapy for both drug and placebo subjects and tends to decrease in succeeding weeks. The origins of the increased weight loss due to the various possible drug effects are not established. The amount of weight loss associated with the use of an "anorectic" drug varies from trial to trial, and the increased weight loss appears to be related in part to variables other than the drug prescribed, such as the physician-investigator, the population treated, and the diet prescribed. Studies do not permit conclusions as to the relative importance of the drug and non-drug factors on weight loss.

The natural history of obesity is measured in years, whereas the studies cited are restricted to a few weeks duration; thus, the total impact of drug-induced weight loss over that of diet alone must be considered clinically limited.

There is neither specific evidence which clearly establishes the mechanism whereby DESOXYN produces its mental and behavioral effects in children, nor conclusive evidence regarding how these effects relate to the condition of the central nervous system.

Indications: *Exogenous Obesity*—as a short-term (i.e., a few weeks) adjunct in a regimen of weight reduction based on caloric restriction, for patients in whom obesity is refractory to alternative therapy, e.g., repeated diets, group programs, and other drugs. The limited usefulness of DESOXYN (see ACTIONS) should be weighed against possible risks inherent in use of the drug, such as those described below.

DESOXYN is indicated as an integral part of a total treatment program which typically includes other remedial measures (psychological, educational, social) for a stabilizing effect in children over 6 years of age with a behavioral syndrome characterized by the following group of developmentally inappropriate symptoms: moderate to severe distractibility, short attention span, hyperactivity, emotional lability, and impulsivity. The diagnosis of this syndrome should not be made with finality when these symptoms are only of comparatively recent origin. Nonlocalizing (soft) neurological signs, learning disability, and abnormal EEG may or may not be present, and a diagnosis of central nervous system dysfunction may or may not be warranted.

Attention Deficit Disorder and Hyperkinetic Syndrome are among the terms being used to describe the above signs and symptoms. In the past, a variety of terms has been associated with these signs and symptoms, including: Minimal Brain Dysfunction, Hyperkinetic Reaction of Childhood, Hyperkinetic Syndrome, Hyperactive Child Syndrome, Minimal Brain Damage, Minimal Cerebral Dysfunction, and Minor Cerebral Dysfunction.

Contraindications: DESOXYN (methamphetamine hydrochloride) is contraindicated during or within 14 days following the administration of monoamine oxidase inhibitors; hypertensive crises may result. It is also contraindicated in patients with glaucoma, advanced arteriosclerosis, symptomatic cardiovascular disease, moderate to severe hypertension, hyperthyroidism or known hypersensitivity or idiosyncrasy to sympathomimetic amines.
Methamphetamine should not be given to patients who are in an agitated state or who have a history of drug abuse.

Warnings: Tolerance to the anorectic effect usually develops within a few weeks. When this occurs, the recommended dose should not be exceeded in an attempt to increase the effect; rather, the drug should be discontinued.
Methamphetamine may impair the ability of the patient to engage in potentially hazardous activities such as operating machinery or driving a motor vehicle; the patient should therefore be cautioned accordingly.

Drug Dependence—DESOXYN has been extensively abused. Tolerance, extreme psychological dependence, and severe social disability have occurred. There are reports of patients who have increased the dosage to many times that recommended. Abrupt cessation following prolonged high dosage administration results in extreme fatigue and mental depression; changes are also noted on the sleep EEG. Manifestations of chronic intoxication with DESOXYN include severe dermatoses, marked insomnia, irritability, hyperactivity, and personality changes. The most severe manifestation of chronic intoxication is psychosis, often clinically indistinguishable from schizophrenia.

Usage in Pregnancy—Safe use in pregnancy has not been established. Reproduction studies in mammals at high multiples of the human dose have suggested both an embryotoxic and a teratogenic potential. Use of methamphetamine by women who are or who may become pregnant, and especially those in the first trimester of pregnancy, requires that the potential benefit be weighed against the possible hazard to mother and infant.

Usage in Children—Methamphetamine is not recommended for use as an anorectic agent in children under 12 years of age.
Clinical experience suggests that in psychotic children, administration of DESOXYN may exacerbate symptoms of behavior disturbance and thought disorder.
Data are inadequate to determine whether chronic administration of DESOXYN may be associated with growth inhibition: therefore, growth should be monitored during treatment.

Precautions: DESOXYN (methamphetamine hydrochloride) should be used with caution in patients with even mild hypertension.
Methamphetamine should not be used to combat fatigue or to replace rest in normal persons.
Insulin requirements in diabetes mellitus may be altered in association with the use of methamphetamine and the concomitant dietary regimen.
Methamphetamine may decrease the hypotensive effect of guanethidine.
Prescribing and dispensing of methamphetamine should be limited to the smallest amount that is feasible at one time in order to minimize the possibility of overdosage.
Drug treatment is not indicated in all cases of the behavioral syndrome characterized by moderate to severe distractibility, short attention span, hyperactivity, emotional lability and impulsivity. It should be considered only in light of the complete history and evaluation of the child. The decision to prescribe DESOXYN should depend on the physician's assessment of the chronicity and severity of the child's symptoms and their appropriateness for his/her age. Prescription should not depend solely on the presence of one or more of the behavioral characteristics.
When these symptoms are associated with acute stress reactions, treatment with DESOXYN is usually not indicated.
Long-term effects of DESOXYN in children have not been well established.

Adverse Reactions: Cardiovascular—Palpitation, tachycardia, elevation of blood pressure.
Central Nervous System—Overstimulation, restlessness, dizziness, insomnia, euphoria, dysphoria, tremor, headache; rarely, psychotic episodes at recommended doses.
Gastrointestinal—Dryness of mouth, unpleasant taste, diarrhea, constipation, and other gastrointestinal disturbances.
Allergic—Urticaria.
Endocrine—Impotence, changes in libido.

Dosage and Administration: DESOXYN (methamphetamine hydrochloride) is given orally.
Methamphetamine should be administered at the lowest effective dosage, and dosage should be individually adjusted. Late evening medication should be avoided because of the resulting insomnia.
For obesity: one Gradumet tablet, 10 or 15 mg. once a day in the morning. When the conventional tablet form is prescribed, one 2.5 or 5 mg tablet should be taken one-half hour before each meal. Treatment should not exceed a few weeks in duration. Methamphetamine is not recommended for use as an anorectic agent in children under 12 years of age.
For treatment of children with a behavioral syndrome characterized by moderate to severe distractibility, short attention span, hyperactivity, emotional lability and impulsivity: an initial dose of 2.5–5 mg DESOXYN (methamphetamine hydrochloride) once or twice a day is recommended. Daily dosage may be raised in increments of 5 mg at weekly intervals until an optimum clinical response is achieved. The usual effective dose is 20–25 mg daily. The total daily dose may be given as conventional tablets in two divided doses daily or once daily using the Gradumet tablet. The Gradumet form should not be utilized for initiation of dosage nor until the conventional titrated daily dosage is equal to or greater than the dosage provided in a Gradumet tablet.
Where possible, drug administration should be interrupted occasionally to determine if there is a recurrence of behavioral symptoms sufficient to require continued therapy.

Overdosage: Manifestations of acute overdosage with methamphetamine include restlessness, tremor, hyperreflexia, rapid respiration, confusion, assaultiveness, hallucinations, and panic states. Fatigue and depression usually follow the central stimulation. Cardiovascular effects include arrhythmias, hypertension or hypotension, and circulatory collapse. Gastrointestinal symptoms include nausea, vomiting, diarrhea, and abdominal cramps. Fatal poisoning usually terminates in convulsions and coma.
Management of acute methamphetamine intoxication is largely symptomatic and includes lavage and sedation with a barbiturate. Experience with hemodialysis or peritoneal dialysis is inadequate to permit recommendations in this regard.
Acidification of urine increases methamphetamine excretion. Intravenous phentolamine (Regitine®) has been suggested for possible acute, severe hypertension, if this complicates methamphetamine overdosage.

How Supplied: DESOXYN (methamphetamine hydrochloride) is supplied as follows:
Gradumet Tablets, 5 mg, white, in bottles of 100 (**NDC** 0074-6941-04); 10 mg, orange, in bottles of 100 (**NDC** 0074-6948-08) and 500 (**NDC** 0074-6948-09); and 15 mg, yellow, in bottles of 100 (**NDC** 0074-6959-07) and 500 (**NDC** 0074-6959-08).
Tablets, 2.5 mg, white, in bottles of 100 (**NDC** 0074-3488-03); and 5 mg, white, in bottles of 100 (**NDC** 0074-3377-04) and 1000 (**NDC** 0074-3377-02).
Ref. No. 01-2010-R7
[*Shown in Product Identification Section*]

DICAL-D®
(Dibasic Calcium Phosphate with Vitamin D)
CAPSULES—WAFERS

Description:
Capsules
Daily dosage (three capsules) provides:
Vitamin D .... 399 IU .... 99% USRDA*
(10 mcg)
Calcium .... 0.35 Gm ... 35% USRDA
Phosphorous ...... 0.27 Gm ... 27% USRDA
Each gelatin capsule contains:
Dibasic Calcium Phosphate, hydrous
(as anhydrous form) .... 500 mg
Vitamin D_2 .... 3.33 mcg (133 IU)
Corn starch added.
Calcium to phosphorous ratio 1.3 to 1.
Wafers
Daily dosage (two wafers) provides:
Vitamin D ...... 400 IU ...... 100% USRDA
(10 mcg)
Calcium :......... 0.464 Gm ..... 46% USRDA
Phosphorous ... 0.36 Gm ...... 36% USRDA
Each wafer contains:
Vitamin D_2................................ 5 mcg (200 IU)
Dibasic Calcium Phosphate, hydrous ... 1 Gm
Added dextrose, sucrose, talc, stearic acid, mineral oil, salt, and natural and artificial flavorings.
Calcium to phosphorous ratio 1.29 to 1.
*% U.S. Recommended Daily Allowance for adults and children 4 or more years of age.

Indications: For those individuals who must restrict their intake of dairy products.

Dosage and Administration: Usual dose for adults and children 4 years and older:
Wafers—Chew 1 wafer twice daily with meals, or as directed by the physician.
Capsules—1 capsule 3 times daily with meals, or as directed by the physician or dentist according to the need of the patient.

How Supplied:
Dical-D Capsules in bottles of 100 (NDC 0074-3594-04) and 500 (NDC 0074-3594-02).
Dical-D Wafers in box of 51 (NDC 0074-3589-01).
Ref. 03-0507-4/R10 & 09-5424-4/R6

DICUMAROL ℞
Tablets, U.S.P.

How Supplied: Dicumarol tablets, U.S.P. are supplied as:
25 mg. tablets,
bottles of 100 (**NDC** 0074-3794-01);
bottles of 1000 (**NDC** 0074-3794-06).
50 mg. tablets,
bottles of 100 (**NDC** 0074-3773-01);
bottles of 1000 (**NDC** 0074-3773-02).
100 mg. tablets,
bottles of 100 (**NDC** 0074-3775-06).
Also available in ABBO-PAC® unit dose packages, of 100 tablets:
25 mg. tablets, (**NDC** 0074-3794-05);
50 mg. tablets, (**NDC** 0074-3773-08);
100 mg. tablets, (**NDC** 0074-3775-05).
[*Shown in Product Identification Section*]

EAR DROPS BY MURINE OTC
See Murine Ear Wax Removal System/Murine Ear Drops

Continued on next page

If desired, additional literature on any Abbott Product will be provided upon request to Abbott Laboratories.

Abbott—Cont.

ENDURON®

℞

(Methyclothiazide Tablets, NF)

Description: ENDURON (methyclothiazide) is a member of the benzothiadiazine (thiazide) family of drugs. It is an analogue of hydrochlorothiazide.

Clinically, ENDURON is an oral diuretic-antihypertensive agent.

Actions: The diuretic and saluretic effects of ENDURON result from a drug-induced inhibition of the renal tubular reabsorption of electrolytes. The excretion of sodium and chloride is greatly enhanced. Potassium excretion is also enhanced to a variable degree, as it is with the other thiazides. Although urinary excretion of bicarbonate is increased slightly, there is usually no significant change in urinary pH. Methyclothiazide has a per mg natriuretic activity approximately 100 times that of the prototype thiazide, chlorothiazide. At maximal therapeutic dosages, all thiazides are approximately equal in their diuretic/natriuretic effects.

There is significant natriuresis and diuresis within two hours after administration of a single dose of methyclothiazide. These effects reach a peak in about six hours and persist for 24 hours following oral administration of a single dose.

Like other benzothiadiazines, ENDURON also has antihypertensive properties, and may be used for this purpose either alone or to enhance the antihypertensive action of other drugs. The mechanism by which the benzothiadiazines, including methyclothiazide, produce a reduction of elevated blood pressure is not known. However, sodium depletion appears to be involved.

ENDURON is readily absorbed from the gastrointestinal tract and is excreted unchanged by the kidneys.

Indications: ENDURON is indicated in the management of hypertension either as the sole therapeutic agent or to enhance the effect of other antihypertensive drugs in the more severe forms of hypertension.

ENDURON (methyclothiazide) is indicated as adjunctive therapy in edema associated with congestive heart failure, hepatic cirrhosis, and corticosteroid and estrogen therapy.

ENDURON has also been found useful in edema due to various forms of renal dysfunction such as the nephrotic syndrome, acute glomerulonephritis, and chronic renal failure.

Usage in Pregnancy: The routine use of diuretics in an otherwise healthy pregnant woman is inappropriate and exposes mother and fetus to unnecessary hazard. Diuretics do not prevent development of toxemia of pregnancy, and there is no satisfactory evidence that they are useful in the treatment of developed toxemia.

Edema during pregnancy may arise from pathological causes or from the physiological and mechanical consequences of pregnancy. Thiazides are indicated in pregnancy when edema is due to pathological causes, just as they are in the absence of pregnancy (however, see Warnings, below). Dependent edema in pregnancy, resulting from restriction of venous return by the expanded uterus, is properly treated through elevation of the lower extremities and use of support hose; use of diuretics to lower intravascular volume in this case is illogical and unnecessary. There is hypervolemia during normal pregnancy which is harmful to neither the fetus nor the mother (in the absence of cardiovascular disease), but which is associated with edema, including generalized edema, in the majority of pregnant women. If this edema produces discomfort, increased recumbency will often provide relief. In rare instances, this edema may cause extreme discomfort which is not relieved by rest. In these cases, a short course of diuretics may provide relief and may be appropriate.

Contraindications: Renal decompensation. Hypersensitivity to this or other sulfonamide-derived drugs.

Warnings: Methyclothiazide shares with other thiazides the propensity to deplete potassium reserves to an unpredictable degree.

Thiazides should be used with caution in patients with renal disease or significant impairment of renal function, since azotemia may be precipitated and cumulative drug effects may occur.

Thiazides should be used with caution in patients with impaired hepatic function or progressive liver disease, since minor alterations of fluid and electrolyte balance may precipitate hepatic coma.

Thiazides may be additive or potentiative of the action of other antihypertensive drugs. Potentiation occurs with ganglionic or peripheral adrenergic blocking drugs.

Sensitivity reactions may occur in patients with a history of allergy or bronchial asthma.

The possibility of exacerbation or activation of systemic lupus erythematosus has been reported.

Usage in Pregnancy: Thiazides cross the placental barrier and appear in cord blood. The use of thiazides in pregnant women requires that the anticipated benefit be weighed against possible hazards to the fetus. These hazards include fetal or neonatal jaundice, thrombocytopenia, and possible other adverse reactions that have occurred in the adult.

Nursing Mothers: Thiazides appear in breast milk. If use of the drug is deemed essential, the patient should stop nursing.

Precautions: Periodic determinations of serum electrolytes should be performed at appropriate intervals for the purpose of detecting possible electrolyte imbalances such as hyponatremia, hypochloremic alkalosis, and hypokalemia. Serum and urine electrolyte determinations are particularly important when a patient is vomiting excessively or receiving parenteral fluids. All patients should be observed for other clinical signs of electrolyte imbalances such as dryness of mouth, thirst, weakness, lethargy, drowsiness, restlessness, muscle pains or cramps, muscular fatigue, hypotension, oliguria, tachycardia, and gastrointestinal disturbances such as nausea and vomiting.

Hypokalemia may develop with thiazides as with any other potent diuretic, especially when brisk diuresis occurs, severe cirrhosis is present, or when corticosteroids or ACTH are given concomitantly. Interference with the adequate oral intake of electrolytes will also contribute to the possible development of hypokalemia. Potassium depletion, even of a mild degree, resulting from thiazide use, may sensitize a patient to the effects of cardiac glycosides such as digitalis.

Any chloride deficit is generally mild and usually does not require specific treatment except under extraordinary circumstances (as in liver disease or renal disease). Dilutional hyponatremia may occur in edematous patients in hot weather; appropriate therapy is water restriction rather than administration of salt, except in rare instances when the hyponatremia is life threatening.

In actual salt depletion, appropriate replacement is the therapy of choice.

Hyperuricemia may occur or frank gout may be precipitated in certain patients receiving thiazide therapy.

Insulin requirements in diabetic patients may be increased, decreased, or unchanged. Latent diabetes mellitus may become manifest during thiazide administration.

Thiazide drugs may increase the responsiveness to tubocurarine.

The antihypertensive effects of the drug may be enhanced in the postsympathectomy patient.

Thiazides may decrease arterial responsiveness to norepinephrine. This diminution is not sufficient to preclude effectiveness of the pressor agent for therapeutic use.

If progressive renal impairment becomes evident as indicated by a rising nonprotein nitrogen or blood urea nitrogen, a careful reappraisal of therapy is necessary with consideration given to withholding or discontinuing diuretic therapy.

Thiazides may decrease serum PBI levels without signs of thyroid disturbance.

Thiazides have been reported, on rare occasions, to have elevated serum calcium to hypercalcemic levels. The serum calcium levels have returned to normal when the medication has been stopped. This phenomenon may be related to the ability of the thiazide diuretics to lower the amount of calcium excreted in the urine.

Adverse Reactions: Gastrointestinal system reactions: Anorexia, gastric irritation, nausea, vomiting, cramping, diarrhea, constipation, jaundice (intrahepatic cholestatic jaundice), pancreatitis.

Central nervous system reactions: Dizziness, vertigo, paresthesias, headache, xanthopsia.

Hematologic reactions: Leukopenia, agranulocytosis, thrombocytopenia, aplastic anemia.

Dermatologic—hypersensitivity reactions: Purpura, photosensitivity, rash, urticaria, necrotizing angiitis (vasculitis) (cutaneous vasculitis).

Cardiovascular reaction: Orthostatic hypotension may occur and may be aggravated by alcohol, barbiturates, or narcotics.

Other: Hyperglycemia, glycosuria, hypercalcemia, hyperuricemia, muscle spasm, weakness, restlessness.

There have been isolated reports that certain nonedematous individuals developed severe fluid and electrolyte derangements after only brief exposure to normal doses of thiazide and non-thiazide diuretics. The condition is usually manifested as severe dilutional hyponatremia, hypokalemia, and hypochloremia. It has been reported to be due to inappropriately increased ADH secretion and appears to be idiosyncratic. Potassium replacement is apparently the most important therapy in the treatment of this syndrome along with removal of the offending drug.

Whenever adverse reactions are severe, treatment should be discontinued.

Dosage and Administration: ENDURON (methyclothiazide) is administered orally. The usual adult dose ranges from 2.5 to 10 mg once daily.

Therapy should be individualized according to patient response. This therapy should be titrated to gain maximal therapeutic response as well as the minimal dose possible to maintain that therapeutic response.

To maintain an edema-free state or as an adjunct in the management of hypertension, 2.5 to 5.0 mg once daily is often adequate.

Maximum effective single dose is 10 mg; larger single doses do not accomplish greater diuresis, and are not recommended.

In the treatment of hypertension methyclothiazide may be either employed alone or concurrently with other antihypertensive drugs. Combined therapy may provide adequate control of hypertension with lower dosage of the component drugs and fewer or less severe side effects. An enhanced response frequently follows its concurrent administration with Harmonyl® (deserpidine) so that dosage of both drugs may be reduced.

For treatment of moderately severe or severe hypertension, supplemental use of other more potent antihypertensive agents such as Eutonyl® (pargyline hydrochloride) may be indicated.

When other antihypertensive agents are to be added to the regimen, this should be accomplished gradually. Ganglionic blocking agents should be given at only half the usual dose since their effect is potentiated by pretreatment with ENDURON.

Overdosage: Symptoms of overdosage include electrolyte imbalance and signs of potassium deficiency such as confusion, dizziness, muscular weakness, and gastrointestinal disturbances. General supportive measures including replacement of fluids and electrolytes may be indicated in treatment of overdosage.

How Supplied: ENDURON (methyclothiazide tablets, NF) is provided in two dosage sizes as monogrammed, grooved, square-shaped tablets:

2.5 mg, orange-colored:
bottles of 100 (**NDC** 0074-6827-01),
bottles of 1000 (**NDC** 0074-6827-02).

5 mg, salmon-colored:
bottles of 100 (**NDC** 0074-6812-01),
bottles of 1000 (**NDC** 0074-6812-02),
bottles of 5000 (**NDC** 0074-6812-03),
Abbo-Pac® unit dose packages of 100 (**NDC** 0074-6812-10).

[*Shown in Product Identification Section*]

Ref. 03-4202-R1

ENDURONYL® ℞

(methyclothiazide and deserpidine)
Tablets

Oral thiazide-rauwolfia therapy for hypertension.

Warning:
This fixed combination drug is not indicated for initial therapy of hypertension. Hypertension requires therapy titrated to the individual patient. If the fixed combination represents the dosage so determined, its use may be more convenient in patient management. The treatment of hypertension is not static, but must be reevaluated as conditions in each patient warrant.

Description: ENDURONYL is an orally-administered combination of Enduron® (methyclothiazide) and Harmonyl® (deserpidine). Methyclothiazide is an oral diuretic-antihypertensive of the benzothiadiazine (thiazide) class. Deserpidine is a purified rauwolfia alkaloid, chemically identified as 11-desmethoxyreserpine, which produces antihypertensive effects.

Actions: The combined antihypertensive actions of methyclothiazide and deserpidine result in a total clinical antihypertensive effect which is greater than can ordinarily be achieved by either drug given individually.

The diuretic and saluretic effects of methyclothiazide result from a drug-induced inhibition of the renal tubular reabsorption of electrolytes. The excretion of sodium and chloride is greatly enhanced. Potassium excretion is also enhanced to a variable degree, as it is with the other thiazides. Although urinary excretion of bicarbonate is increased slightly, there is usually no significant change in urinary pH. Methyclothiazide has a per mg. natriuretic activity approximately 100 times that of the prototype thiazide, chlorothiazide. At maximal therapeutic dosages, all thiazides are approximately equal in their diuretic/natriuretic effects.

There is significant natriuresis and diuresis within two hours after administration of a single dose of methyclothiazide. These effects reach a peak in about six hours and persist for 24 hours following oral administration of a single dose.

Like other benzothiadiazines, methyclothiazide also has antihypertensive properties, and may be used for this purpose either alone or to enhance the antihypertensive action of other drugs. The mechanism by which the benzothiadiazines, including methyclothiazide, produce a reduction of elevated blood pressure is not known. However, sodium depletion appears to be involved.

Methyclothiazide is readily absorbed from the gastrointestinal tract and is excreted unchanged by the kidneys.

The pharmacologic actions of Harmonyl (deserpidine) are essentially the same as those of other active rauwolfia alkaloids. Deserpidine probably produces its antihypertensive effects through depletion of tissue stores of catecholamines (epinephrine and norepinephrine) from peripheral sites. The antihypertensive effect is often accompanied by bradycardia. There is no significant alteration in cardiac output or renal blood flow. The carotid sinus reflex is inhibited, but postural hypotension is rarely seen with the use of conventional doses of Harmonyl alone.

Deserpidine, like other rauwolfia alkaloids, is characterized by slow onset of action and sustained effect which may persist following withdrawal of the drug.

Indications: ENDURONYL (methyclothiazide and deserpidine) is indicated in the treatment of mild to moderately severe hypertension (see boxed warning). In many cases ENDURONYL alone produces an adequate reduction of blood pressure. In resistant or unusually severe cases ENDURONYL also may be supplemented by more potent antihypertensive agents. When administered with ENDURONYL, more potent agents can be given at reduced dosage to minimize undesirable side effects.

Contraindications: Methyclothiazide is contraindicated in patients with renal decompensation and in those who are hypersensitive to this or other sulfonamide-derived drugs.

Deserpidine is contraindicated in patients with known hypersensitivity, mental depression especially with suicidal tendencies, active peptic ulcer, and ulcerative colitis. It is also contraindicated in patients receiving electroconvulsive therapy.

Warnings:

Methyclothiazide

Methyclothiazide shares with other thiazides the propensity to deplete potassium reserves to an unpredictable degree.

Thiazides should be used with caution in patients with renal disease or significant impairment of renal function, since azotemia may be precipitated and cumulative drug effects may occur.

Thiazides should be used with caution in patients with impaired hepatic function or progressive liver disease, since minor alterations of fluid and electrolyte balance may precipitate hepatic coma.

Thiazides may be additive or potentiative of the action of other antihypertensive drugs. Potentiation occurs with ganglionic or peripheral adrenergic blocking drugs.

Sensitivity reactions may occur in patients with a history of allergy or bronchial asthma.

The possibility of exacerbation or activation of systemic lupus erythematosus has been reported.

Deserpidine

Extreme caution should be exercised in treating patients with a history of mental depression. Discontinue the drug at the first sign of despondency, early morning insomnia, loss of appetite, impotence, or self-deprecation. Drug-induced depression may persist for several months after drug withdrawal and may be severe enough to result in suicide.

Usage in Pregnancy and Lactation:

Methyclothiazide

Thiazides cross the placental barrier and appear in cord blood. The use of thiazides in pregnant women requires that the anticipated benefit be weighed against possible hazards to the fetus. These hazards include fetal or neonatal jaundice, thrombocytopenia, and possible other adverse reactions that have occurred in the adult.

Thiazides appear in breast milk. If use of the drug is deemed essential, the patient should stop nursing.

Deserpidine

The safety of deserpidine for use during pregnancy or lactation has not been established; therefore, it should be used in pregnant women or in women of childbearing potential only when in the judgment of the physician its use is deemed essential to the welfare of the patient. Increased respiratory secretions, nasal congestion, cyanosis, and anorexia may occur in infants born to rauwolfia alkaloid-treated mothers, since these preparations are known to cross the placental barrier to enter the fetal circulation and appear in cord blood. They also are secreted by nursing mothers into breast milk.

Studies in rats with deserpidine at multiples of the human therapeutic dose reduced the mating index and neonatal survival indices.

Precautions: Periodic determinations of serum electrolytes should be performed at appropriate intervals for the purpose of detecting possible electrolyte imbalances such as hyponatremia, hypochloremic alkalosis, and hypokalemia. Serum and urine electrolyte determinations are particularly important when a patient is vomiting excessively or receiving parenteral fluids. All patients should be observed for other clinical signs of electrolyte imbalances such as dryness of mouth, thirst, weakness, lethargy, drowsiness, restlessness, muscle pains or cramps, muscular fatigue, hypotension, oliguria, tachycardia, and gastrointestinal disturbances such as nausea and vomiting.

Hypokalemia may develop with thiazides as with any other potent diuretic, especially when brisk diuresis occurs, severe cirrhosis is present, or when corticosteroids or ACTH are given concomitantly. Interference with the adequate oral intake of electrolytes will also contribute to the possible development of hypokalemia. Potassium depletion, even of a mild degree, resulting from thiazide use, may sensitize a patient to the effects of cardiac glycosides such as digitalis.

Any chloride deficit is generally mild and usually does not require specific treatment except under extraordinary circumstances (as in liver disease or renal disease). Dilutional hyponatremia may occur in edematous patients in hot weather; appropriate therapy is water restriction rather than administration of salt, except in rare instances when the hyponatremia is life threatening.

In actual salt depletion, appropriate replacement is the therapy of choice.

Hyperuricemia may occur or frank gout may be precipitated in certain patients receiving thiazide therapy.

Insulin requirements in diabetic patients may be increased, decreased, or unchanged. Latent diabetes mellitus may become manifest during thiazide administration.

Thiazide drugs may increase the responsiveness to tubocurarine.

The antihypertensive effects of the drug may be enhanced in the postsympathectomy patient.

Thiazides may decrease arterial responsiveness to norepinephrine. This diminution is not sufficient to preclude effectiveness of the pressor agent for therapeutic use.

If progressive renal impairment becomes evident as indicated by a rising-nonprotein nitrogen or blood urea nitrogen, a careful reappraisal of therapy is necessary with consideration given to withholding or discontinuing diuretic therapy.

Thiazides may decrease serum PBI levels without signs of thyroid disturbance.

Continued on next page

Abbott—Cont.

Thiazides have been reported, on rare occasions, to have elevated serum calcium to hypercalcemic levels. The serum calcium levels have returned to normal when the medication has been stopped. This phenomenon may be related to the ability of the thiazide diuretics to lower the amount of calcium excreted in the urine.

Because rauwolfia preparations increase gastrointestinal motility and secretion, this drug should be used cautiously in patients with a history of peptic ulcer, ulcerative colitis, or gallstones, where biliary colic may be precipitated.

Caution should be exercised when treating hypertensive patients with renal insufficiency since they adjust poorly to lowered blood pressure levels.

Use deserpidine cautiously with digitalis and quinidine since cardiac arrhythmias have occurred with rauwolfia preparations.

Preoperative withdrawal of deserpidine does not assure that circulatory instability will not occur. It is important that the anesthesiologist be aware of the patient's drug intake and consider this in the overall management, since hypotension has occurred in patients receiving rauwolfia preparations. Anticholinergic and/or adrenergic drugs (metaraminol, norepinephrine) have been employed to treat adverse vagocirculatory effects.

Adverse Reactions:

Methyclothiazide

Gastrointestinal System Reactions: Anorexia, gastric irritation, nausea, vomiting, cramping, diarrhea, constipation, jaundice (intrahepatic cholestatic jaundice), pancreatitis.

Central Nervous System Reactions: Dizziness, vertigo, paresthesias, headache, xanthopsia.

Hematologic Reactions: Leukopenia, agranulocytosis, thrombocytopenia, aplastic anemia.

Dermatologic — Hypersensitivity Reactions: Purpura, photosensitivity, rash, urticaria, necrotizing angiitis (vasculitis) (cutaneous vasculitis).

Cardiovascular Reaction: Orthostatic hypotension may occur and may be aggravated by alcohol, barbiturates, or narcotics.

Other: Hyperglycemia, glycosuria, hypercalcemia, hyperuricemia, muscle spasm, weakness, restlessness.

There have been isolated reports that certain nonedematous individuals developed severe fluid and electrolyte derangements after only brief exposure to normal doses of thiazide and non-thiazide diuretics. The condition is usually manifested as severe dilutional hyponatremia, hypokalemia, and hypochloremia. It has been reported to be due to inappropriately increased ADH secretion and appears to be idiosyncratic. Potassium replacement is apparently the most important therapy in the treatment of this syndrome along with removal of the offending drug.

Whenever adverse reactions are severe, treatment should be discontinued.

Deserpidine

The following adverse reactions have been reported with rauwolfia preparations. These reactions are usually reversible and disappear when the drug is discontinued.

Gastrointestinal: Including hypersecretion, anorexia, diarrhea, nausea, and vomiting.

Cardiovascular: Including angina-like symptoms, arrhythmias (particularly when used concurrently with digitalis or quinidine), and bradycardia.

Central Nervous System: Including drowsiness, depression, nervousness, paradoxical anxiety, nightmares, extrapyramidal tract symptoms, CNS sensitization manifested by dull sensorium, and deafness.

Dermatologic—Hypersensitivity: Including pruritus, rash, and asthma in asthmatic patients.

Ophthalmologic: Including glaucoma, uveitis, optic atrophy, and conjunctival injection.

Hematologic: Thrombocytopenic purpura.

Miscellaneous: Nasal congestion, weight gain, impotence or decreased libido, dysuria, dyspnea, muscular aches, dryness of mouth, dizziness, and headache.

Dosage and Administration: Dosage should be determined by individual titration of ingredients (see boxed warning). Dosage of both components should be carefully adjusted to the needs of the individual patient. Since at least ten days to two weeks may elapse before the full effects of the drugs become manifest, the dosage of the drugs should not be adjusted more frequently.

Two tablet strengths, ENDURONYL (methyclothiazide 5 mg, deserpidine 0.25 mg) and ENDURONYL FORTE (methyclothiazide 5 mg, deserpidine 0.5 mg), each grooved, are provided to permit considerable latitude in meeting the dosage requirements of individual patients.*

The following table will help in determining which dose of ENDURONYL or ENDURONYL FORTE best represents the equivalent of the titrated dose.

Daily Dosage of ENDURONYL	methyclothiazide	deserpidine
½ tablet	2.5 mg	0.125 mg
1 tablet	5.0 mg	0.250 mg
1½ tablet	7.5 mg	0.375 mg
2 tablets	10.0 mg	0.500 mg

Daily Dosage of ENDURONYL FORTE	methyclothiazide	deserpidine
½ tablet	2.5 mg	0.250 mg
1 tablet	5.0 mg	0.500 mg
1½ tablet	7.5 mg	0.750 mg
2 tablets	10.0 mg	1.000 mg

The appropriate dose of ENDURONYL is administered orally, once daily. The usual adult dosage is one lower-strength ENDURONYL tablet daily. There is no contraindication to combining the administration of ENDURONYL with other antihypertensive agents. When other antihypertensive agents are to be added to the regimen, this should be accomplished gradually. Ganglionic blocking agents should be given at only half the usual dose since their effect is potentiated by pretreatment with ENDURONYL.

Overdosage: Symptoms of thiazide overdosage include electrolyte imbalance and signs of potassium deficiency such as confusion, dizziness, muscular weakness, and gastrointestinal disturbances. General supportive measures including replacement of fluids and electrolytes may be indicated in treatment of overdosage.

An overdosage of deserpidine is characterized by flushing of the skin, conjunctival injection, and pupillary constriction. Sedation ranging from drowsiness to coma may occur. Hypotension, hypothermia, central respiratory depression and bradycardia may develop in cases of severe overdosage. Treatment consists of the careful evacuation of stomach contents followed by the usual procedures for the symptomatic management of CNS depressant overdosage. If severe hypotension occurs it should be treated with a direct acting vasopressor such as levarterenol.

How Supplied: ENDURONYL (methyclothiazide and deserpidine) is supplied as monogrammed, grooved, square-shaped tablets in the following dosage sizes and quantities:

ENDURONYL (5 mg of methyclothiazide and 0.25 mg of deserpidine) yellow tablets in bottles of 100 (**NDC** 0074-6838-01) and 1000 (**NDC** 0074-6838-02). Also available in ABBO-PAC® unit dose packages, 100 tablets (**NDC** 0074-6838-06), in strips of 10 tablets.

ENDURONYL FORTE (5 mg of methyclothiazide and 0.5 mg of deserpidine) gray-colored tablets in bottles of 100 (**NDC** 0074-6854-01) and 1000 (**NDC** 0074-6854-02). Also available in ABBO-PAC® unit dose packages, 100 tablets (**NDC** 0074-6854-05), in strips of 10 tablets.

*Each component is separately available as ENDURON (methyclothiazide) and HARMONYL (deserpidine).

[*Shown in Product Identification Section*]
Ref. 03-4200/R4

E.E.S.® ℞
(erythromycin ethylsuccinate)

Description: Erythromycin is produced by a strain of *Streptomyces erythraeus* and belongs to the macrolide group of antibiotics. It is basic and readily forms salts with acids. The base, the stearate salt, and the esters are poorly soluble in water. Erythromycin ethylsuccinate is an ester of erythromycin suitable for oral administration.

The cherry-flavored, chewable tablets are easily ingested and are particularly acceptable for the administration of antibiotic medication to young children who are unable to swallow regular tablets or in whom persuasion of a pleasant taste insures cooperation. Each chewable tablet, providing the equivalent of 200 mg of erythromycin, is conveniently scored for division into half-dose (100 mg) portions.

The granules and drops are intended for reconstitution with water. When reconstituted, they are palatable cherry-flavored suspensions.

The pleasant tasting, fruit-flavored liquids are supplied ready for oral administration.

Granules, drops and ready-made suspensions are intended primarily for pediatric use but can also be used in adults.

The Filmtab® tablets are intended primarily for adults or older children.

Actions: Microbiology: Biochemical tests demonstrate that erythromycin inhibits protein synthesis of the pathogen without directly affecting nucleic acid synthesis. Antagonism has been demonstrated between clindamycin and erythromycin.

NOTE: Many strains of *Hemophilus influenzae* are resistant to erythromycin alone, but are susceptible to erythromycin and sulfonamides together. Staphylococci resistant to erythromycin may emerge during a course of erythromycin therapy. Culture and susceptibility testing should be performed.

Disc Susceptibility Tests

Quantitative methods that require measurement of zone diameters give the most precise estimates of antibiotic susceptibility. One recommended procedure (21 CFR section 460.1) uses erythromycin class discs for testing susceptibility; interpretations correlate zone diameters of this disc test with MIC values for erythromycin. With this procedure, a report from the laboratory of "susceptible" indicates that the infecting organism is likely to respond to therapy. A report of "resistant" indicates that the infective organism is not likely to respond to therapy. A report of "intermediate susceptibility" suggests that the organism would be susceptible if higher doses were used.

Clinical Pharmacology: Erythromycin binds to the 50 S ribosomal subunits of susceptible bacteria and suppresses protein synthesis.

Orally administered erythromycin ethylsuccinate suspensions and Filmtab tablets are readily and reliably absorbed. Erythromycin ethylsuccinate chewable tablets are readily and reliably absorbed when chewed. Comparable serum levels of erythromycin are achieved in the fasting and nonfasting states.

Erythromycin diffuses readily into most body fluids. Only low concentrations are normally achieved in the spinal fluid, but passage of the drug across the blood-brain barrier increases in meningitis. In the presence of normal hepatic function, erythromycin is concentrated in the liver and excreted in the bile; the effect of hepatic dysfunction on excretion of erythromycin by the liver into the bile is not known. Less than 5 percent of the orally administered dose of erythromycin is excreted in active form in the urine.

Erythromycin crosses the placental barrier and is excreted in breast milk.

Indications: *Streptococcus pyogenes* (Group A beta hemolytic streptococcus): Upper and lower respiratory tract, skin, and soft tissue infections of mild to moderate severity.

Injectable benzathine penicillin G is considered by the American Heart Association to be the drug of choice in the treatment and prevention of streptococcal pharyngitis and in long-term prophylaxis of rheumatic fever.

When oral medication is preferred for treatment of the above conditions, penicillin G, V, or erythromycin are alternate drugs of choice. When oral medication is given, the importance of strict adherence by the patient to the prescribed dosage regimen must be stressed. A therapeutic dose should be administered for at least 10 days.

Alpha-hemolytic streptococci (viridans group): Short-term prophylaxis of bacterial endocarditis prior to dental or other operative procedures in patients with a history of rheumatic fever or congenital heart disease who are hypersensitive to penicillin. (Erythromycin is not suitable prior to genitourinary surgery where the organisms likely to lead to bacteremia are gram-negative bacilli or the enterococcus group of streptococci.)

Staphylococcus aureus: Acute infections of skin and soft tissue of mild to moderate severity. Resistant organisms may emerge during treatment.

Streptococcus pneumoniae (Diplococcus pneumoniae): Upper respiratory tract infections (e.g., otitis media, pharyngitis) and lower respiratory tract infections (e.g., pneumonia) of mild to moderate degree.

Mycoplasma pneumoniae (Eaton agent, PPLO): For respiratory infections due to this organism.

Hemophilus influenzae: For upper respiratory tract infections of mild to moderate severity when used concomitantly with adequate doses of sulfonamides. (See sulfonamide labeling for appropriate prescribing information). The concomitant use of the sulfonamides is necessary since not all strains of *Hemophilus influenzae* are susceptible to erythromycin at the concentrations of the antibiotic achieved with usual therapeutic doses.

Treponema pallidum: Erythromycin is an alternate choice of treatment for primary syphilis in patients allergic to the penicillins. In treatment of primary syphilis, spinal fluid examinations should be done before treatment and as part of follow-up after therapy.

Corynebacterium diphtheriae: As an adjunct to antitoxin, to prevent establishment of carriers, and to eradicate the organism in carriers.

Corynebacterium minutissimum: For the treatment of erythrasma.

Entamoeba histolytica: In the treatment of intestinal amebiasis only. Extraenteric amebiasis requires treatment with other agents.

Listeria monocytogenes: Infections due to this organism.

Bordetella pertussis: Erythromycin is effective in eliminating the organism from the nasopharynx of infected individuals, rendering them non-infectious. Some clinical studies suggest that erythromycin may be helpful in the prophylaxis of pertussis in exposed susceptible individuals.

Legionnaires' Disease: Although no controlled clinical efficacy studies have been conducted, *in vitro* and limited preliminary clinical data suggest that erythromycin may be effective in treating Legionnaires' Disease.

Contraindications: Erythromycin is contraindicated in patients with known hypersensitivity to this antibiotic.

Precautions: Erythromycin is principally excreted by the liver. Caution should be exercised in administering the antibiotic to patients with impaired hepatic function. There have been reports of hepatic dysfunction, with or without jaundice occurring in patients receiving oral erythromycin products.

Areas of localized infection may require surgical drainage in addition to antibiotic therapy. Recent data from studies of erythromycin reveal that its use in patients who are receiving high doses of theophylline may be associated with an increase of serum theophylline levels and potential theophylline toxicity. In case of theophylline toxicity and/or elevated serum theophylline levels, the dose of theophylline should be reduced while the patient is receiving concomitant erythromycin therapy.

Usage during pregnancy and lactation: The safety of erythromycin for use during pregnancy has not been established.

Erythromycin crosses the placental barrier. Erythromycin also appears in breast milk.

Adverse Reactions: The most frequent side effects of erythromycin preparations are gastrointestinal, such as abdominal cramping and discomfort, and are dose related. Nausea, vomiting, and diarrhea occur infrequently with usual oral doses.

During prolonged or repeated therapy, there is a possibility of overgrowth of nonsusceptible bacteria or fungi. If such infections occur, the drug should be discontinued and appropriate therapy instituted.

Allergic reactions ranging from urticaria and mild skin eruptions to anaphylaxis have occurred.

Dosage and Administration: Erythromycin ethylsuccinate suspensions, Filmtab tablets and chewable tablets may be administered without regard to meals. For full therapeutic effect, the chewable tablets must be chewed.

Children: Age, weight, and severity of the infection are important factors in determining the proper dosage. In mild to moderate infections the usual dosage of erthromycin ethylsuccinate for children is 30 to 50 mg/kg/day in equally divided doses. For more severe infections this dosage may be doubled.

The following dosage schedule is suggested for mild to moderate infections:

Body Weight	Total Daily Dose
Under 10 lbs	30–50 mg/kg/day 15–25 mg/lb/day
10 to 15 lbs	200 mg
16 to 25 lbs	400 mg
26 to 50 lbs	800 mg
51 to 100 lbs	1200 mg
over 100 lbs	1600 mg

Adults: 400 mg erythromycin ethylsuccinate every 6 hours is the usual dose. Dosage may be increased up to 4 Gm per day according to the severity of the infection.

If twice-a-day dosage is desired in either adults or children, one-half of the total daily dose may be given every 12 hours. Doses may also be given three times daily if desired by administering one-third of the total daily dose every 8 hours.

In the treatment of streptococcal infections, a therapeutic dosage of erythromycin ethylsuccinate should be administered for at least 10 days. In continuous prophylaxis against recurrences of streptococcal infections in persons with a history of rheumatic heart disease, the usual dosage is 400 mg twice a day.

When used prior to surgery to prevent endocarditis (see *Alpha-hemolytic streptococci*), a recommended schedule for adults is 800 mg erythromycin ethylsuccinate before the procedure and 400 mg every 6 hours for 4 doses after the procedure. For small children, 30 to 50 mg/kg/day divided into 3 or 4 evenly spaced doses.

For treatment of primary syphilis: Adults: 48 to 64 Gm given in divided doses over a period of 10 to 15 days.

For intestinal amebiasis: Adults: 400 mg four times daily for 10 to 14 days. Children: 30 to 50 mg/kg/day in divided doses for 10 to 14 days.

For use in pertussis: Although optimal dosage and duration have not been established, doses of erythromycin utilized in reported clinical studies were 40 to 50 mg/kg/day, given in divided doses for 5 to 14 days.

For treatment of Legionnaires' Disease: Although optimal doses have not been established, doses utilized in reported clinical data were those recommended above (1.6 to 4 Gm daily in divided doses.)

How Supplied: E.E.S. 200 LIQUID (erythromycin ethylsuccinate oral suspension) is supplied in 1 pint bottles (**NDC** 0074-6306-16) and in packages of six 100-ml bottles (**NDC** 0074-6306-13). Each 5-ml teaspoonful of fruit-flavored suspension contains activity equivalent to 200 mg of erythromycin.

E.E.S. 400® LIQUID (erythromycin ethylsuccinate oral suspension) is supplied in 1 pint bottles (**NDC** 0074-6373-16) and in packages of six 100-ml bottles (**NDC** 0074-6373-13). Each 5-ml teaspoonful of orange, fruit-flavored suspension contains activity equivalent to 400 mg of erythromycin.

Both liquid products require refrigeration to preserve taste until dispensed. Refrigeration by patient is not required if used within 14 days.

E.E.S. GRANULES (erythromycin ethylsuccinate for oral suspension, USP) is supplied in 60-ml (**NDC** 0074-6369-01), 100-ml (**NDC** 0074-6369-02) and 200-ml (**NDC** 0074-6369-10) size bottles. Each 5-ml teaspoonful of reconstituted cherry-flavored suspension contains activity equivalent to 200 mg of erythromycin. E.E.S. GRANULES is also available in 5-ml bottles (when reconstituted) in the ABBO-PAC® unit dose packages of 100 bottles (**NDC** 0074-6369-05).

E.E.S. DROPS (erythromycin ethylsuccinate for oral suspension, USP) is supplied in 50-ml size bottles (**NDC** 0074-6360-50). Each 2.5-ml dropperful (½ teaspoonful) of reconstituted cherry-flavored suspension contains activity equivalent to 100 mg of erythromycin.

E.E.S. CHEWABLE (erythromycin ethylsuccinate tablets, USP) cherry-flavored wafers containing the equivalent of 200 mg of erythromycin are available in packages of 50 (**NDC** 0074-6371-50). Each wafer is individually sealed in a child-resistant blister package.

E.E.S. 400 Filmtab tablets (erythromycin ethylsuccinate tablets, USP) 400 mg, are available in bottles of 100 (**NDC** 0074-5729-13). Tablets are pink in color.

[*Shown in Product Identification Section*]

ERYTHROCIN® LACTOBIONATE-I.V. ℞

(erythromycin lactobionate for injection, USP)

Description: Erythromycin is produced by a strain of *Streptomyces erythraeus* and belongs to the macrolide group of antibiotics. It is basic and readily forms salts with acids.

ERYTHROCIN LACTOBIONATE (erythromycin lactobionate for injection), is a soluble salt of eryth-

Continued on next page

Abbott—Cont.

romycin suitable for intravenous administration.

Actions

Microbiology: Biochemical tests demonstrate that erythromycin inhibits protein synthesis of the pathogen without directly affecting nucleic acid synthesis. Antagonism has been demonstrated between clindamycin and erythromycin.

NOTE: Many strains of *Hemophilus influenzae* are resistant to erythromycin alone, but are susceptible to erythromycin and sulfonamides together. Staphylococci resistant to erythromycin may emerge during a course of erythromycin therapy. Culture and susceptibility testing should be performed.

Disc Susceptibility Tests: Quantitative methods that require measurement of zone diameters give the most precise estimates of antibiotic susceptibility. One recommended procedure (21 CFR section 460.1) uses erythromycin class discs for testing susceptibility; interpretations correlate zone diameters of this disc test with MIC values for erythromycin. With this procedure, a report from the laboratory of "susceptible" indicates that the infecting organism is likely to respond to therapy. A report of "resistant" indicates, that the infective organism is not likely to respond to therapy. A report of "intermediate susceptibility" suggests that the organism would be susceptible if higher doses were used.

Clinical Pharmacology: Erythromycin binds to the 50 S ribosomal subunits of susceptible bacteria and suppresses protein synthesis.

Intravenous infusion of 500 mg erythromycin lactobionate at a constant rate over 1 hour in fasting adults produced a mean serum erythromycin level of approximately 7 mcg/ml at 20 minutes, 10 mcg/ml at 1 hour, 2.6 mcg/ml at 2.5 hours, and 1 mcg/ml at 6 hours.

Erythromycin diffuses readily into most body fluids. Only low concentrations are normally achieved in the spinal fluid, but passage of the drug across the blood-brain barrier increases in meningitis. In the presence of normal hepatic function, erythromycin is concentrated in the liver and excreted in the bile; the effect of hepatic dysfunction on excretion of erythromycin by the liver into the bile is not known. From 12 to 15 percent of intravenously administered erythromycin is excreted in active form in the urine.

Erythromycin crosses the placental barrier and is excreted in breast milk.

Indications: ERYTHROCIN LACTOBIONATE (erythromycin lactobionate for injection) is indicated in the treatment of patients where oral administration is not possible or where the severity of the infection requires immediate high serum levels of erythromycin. Intravenous therapy should be replaced by oral administration at the appropriate time.

Streptococcus pyogenes (Group A beta hemolytic streptococcus): Upper and lower respiratory tract, skin, and soft tissue infections of mild to moderate severity.

Injectable benzathine penicillin G is considered by the American Heart Association to be the drug of choice in the treatment and prevention of streptococcal pharyngitis and in long-term prophylaxis of rheumatic fever.

When oral medication is preferred for treatment of the above conditions, penicillin G, V, or erythromycin are alternate drugs of choice.

Alpha-hemolytic streptococci (viridans group): Short-term prophylaxis of bacterial endocarditis prior to dental or other operative procedures in patients with a history of rheumatic fever or congenital heart disease who are hypersensitive to penicillin. (Erythromycin is not suitable prior to genitourinary surgery where the organisms likely to lead to bacteremia are gram-negative bacilli or the enterococcus group of streptococci.)

Staphylococcus aureus: Acute infections of skin and soft tissue of mild to moderate severity. Resistant organisms may emerge during treatment.

Streptococcus pneumoniae (Diplococcus pneumoniae): For upper respiratory tract infections (e.g., otitis media, pharyngitis) and lower respiratory tract infections (e.g., pneumonia) of mild to moderate severity.

Mycoplasma pneumoniae (Eaton agent, PPLO): For respiratory infections due to this organism.

Hemophilus influenzae: For upper respiratory tract infections of mild to moderate severity when used concomitantly with adequate doses of sulfonamides. (See sulfonamide labeling for appropriate prescribing information). The concomitant use of the sulfonamides is necessary since not all strains of *Hemophilus influenzae* are susceptible to erythromycin at the concentrations of the antibiotic achieved with usual therapeutic doses.

Corynebacterium diphtheriae: As an adjunct to antitoxin to prevent the establishment of carriers and to eradicate the organism in carriers.

Corynebacterium minutissimum: In the treatment of erythrasma.

Listeria monocytogenes: Infections due to this organism.

Neisseria gonorrhoeae: ERYTHROCIN LACTOBIONATE-I.V. (erythromycin lactobionate for injection) in conjunction with erythromycin stearate or base orally, as an alternative drug in treatment of acute pelvic inflammatory disease caused by *N. gonorrhoeae* in female patients with a history of sensitivity to penicillin. Before treatment of gonorrhea, patients who are suspected of also having syphilis should have a microscopic examination for *T. pallidum* (by immunofluorescence or darkfield) before receiving erythromycin, and monthly serologic tests for a minumum of 4 months.

Legionnaires' Disease: Although no controlled clinical efficacy studies have been conducted, *in vitro* and limited preliminary clinical data suggest that erythromycin may be effective in treating Legionnaires' Disease.

Contraindications: Erythromycin is contraindicated in patients with known hypersensitivity to this antibiotic.

Precautions: Since erythromycin is principally excreted by the liver, caution should be exercised when erythromycin is administered to patients with impaired hepatic function.

Prolonged or repeated use of erythromycin may result in an overgrowth of non-susceptible bacteria or fungi. If superinfection occurs, erythromycin should be discontinued and appropriate therapy instituted.

Areas of localized infection may require surgical drainage in addition to antibiotic therapy.

Recent data from studies of erythromycin reveal that its use in patients who are receiving high doses of theophylline may be associated with an increase of serum theophylline levels and potential theophylline toxicity. In case of theophylline toxicity and/or elevated serum theophylline levels, the dose of theophylline should be reduced while the patient is receiving concomitant erythromycin therapy.

Usage during pregnancy and lactation: The safety of erythromycin for use during pregnancy has not been established.

Erythromycin crosses the placental barrier. Erythromycin also appears in breast milk.

Adverse Reactions: Side effects following the use of intravenous erythromycin are rare. Occasional venous irritation has been encountered, but if the infusion is given slowly, in dilute solution, preferably by continuous intravenous infusion or intermittent infusion in no less than 20 to 60 minutes, pain and vessel trauma are minimized.

Allergic reactions, ranging from urticaria and mild skin eruptions to anaphylaxis, have occurred with intravenously administered erythromycin.

Reversible hearing loss associated with the intravenous infusion of 4 or more grams per day of erythromycin lactobionate has been reported rarely.

Dosage and Administration: Use only Sterile Water for Injection, USP, to dissolve ERYTHROCIN LACTOBIONATE-I.V. (erythromycin lactobionate for injection). Use of other diluents may cause precipitation during reconstitution. Do not use diluents containing preservatives or inorganic salts. After reconstitution, each ml contains 50 mg of erythromycin activity (500 mg in 10 ml or 1,000 mg in 20 ml). The initial solution is stable at refrigerator temperature for 2 weeks, or for 24 hours at room temperature.

Prior to intravenous administration, the initial erythromycin lactobionate solution prepared with Sterile Water for Injection, USP, i.e., without preservatives, is added to Sodium Chloride Injection, USP, or lactated Ringer's, or Normosol®-R solutions. It may also be used with the following solutions to which Neut® (4% sodium bicarbonate, Abbott) is first added to raise the pH. (Add 5 ml of Neut to each 500 or 1,000 ml of solution used. Five ml of Neut contains approximately 2.4 mEq of Na^+ and HCO_3^-.):

Dextrose 5% in water
Dextrose 5% in lactated Ringer's
Dextrose 5% in saline 0.9%
Normosol®-M in D5-W
Normosol®-R in D5-W

The final diluted solution of erythromycin lactobionate should be completely administered within 8 hours since it is not suitable for storage.*

Acidic solutions of erythromycin lactobionate are unstable and lose their potency rapidly. A pH of at least 5.5 is desirable for the final diluted solution of erythromycin lactobionate.

No drug or chemical agent should be added to an erythromycin lactobionate-I.V. fluid admixture unless its effect on the chemical and physical stability of the solution has first been determined.

For the treatment of severe infections in adults and children, the recommended intravenous dose of erythromycin lactobionate is 15 to 20 mg/kg/day. Higher doses, up to 4 Gm/day, may be given for very severe infections.

Continuous infusion of erythromycin lactobionate is preferable; however, intermittent infusion at intervals not greater than every 6 hours is also effective. Intravenous erythromycin should be replaced by oral erythromycin as soon as possible.

For slow continuous infusion: The final diluted solution of erythromycin lactobionate is prepared to give a concentration of 1 Gm per liter.

For intermittent infusion (for administration of one-fourth the total daily dose of erythromycin lactobionate by intravenous infusion in 20 to 60 minutes at intervals not greater than every 6 hours): The final diluted solution of erythromycin lactobionate is prepared to give a concentration of 250 to 500 mg in 100 to 250 ml. Infusion should be sufficiently slow to avoid pain along the vein.

For treatment of acute pelvic inflammatory disease caused by *N. gonorrhoeae*, administer 500 mg erythromycin lactobionate every 6 hours for 3 days, followed by 250 mg erythromycin stearate or base every 6 hours for 7 days.

For treatment of Legionnaires' Disease: Although optimal doses have not been established, doses utilized in reported clinical data were those recommended above (1 to 4 grams daily in divided doses).

How Supplied: ERYTHROCIN LACTOBIONATE-I.V. (erythromycin lactobionate for injection, USP) is supplied as a sterile, lyophilized powder in packages of 5 vials (**NDC** 0074-6342-05), each vial containing the equivalent of 1 Gm of erythromycin with 180 mg benzyl alcohol added as preservative; and in packages of 5

vials (**NDC** 0074-6365-02), each vial containing the equivalent of 500 mg of erythromycin with 90 mg benzyl alcohol added as preservative.
*Contact Abbott Laboratories, Dept. 498 for additional stability data.

ERYTHROCIN® STEARATE ℞
(erythromycin stearate tablets USP)
Filmtab® Tablets

Description: Erythromycin is produced by a strain of *Streptomyces erythraeus* and belongs to the macrolide group of antibiotics. It is basic and readily forms salts with acids. The base, the stearate salt, and the esters are poorly soluble in water, and are suitable for oral administration.
ERYTHROCIN STEARATE (erythromycin stearate) Filmtab tablets contain the stearate salt of the antibiotic in a unique film coating.
Actions: Microbiology: Biochemical tests demonstrate that erythromycin inhibits protein synthesis of the pathogen without directly affecting nucleic acid synthesis. Antagonism has been demonstrated between clindamycin and erythromycin.
NOTE: Many strains of *Hemophilus influenzae* are resistant to erythromycin alone, but are susceptible to erythromycin and sulfonamides together. Staphylococci resistant to erythromycin may emerge during a course of erythromycin therapy. Culture and susceptibility testing should be performed.
Disc Susceptibility Tests
Quantitative methods that require measurement of zone diameters give the most precise estimates of antibiotic susceptibility. One recommended procedure (21 CFR section 460.1) uses erythromycin class discs for testing susceptibility; interpretations correlate zone diameters of this disc test with MIC values for erythromycin. With this procedure, a report from the laboratory of "susceptible" indicates that the infecting organism is likely to respond to therapy. A report of "resistant" indicates that the infective organism is not likely to respond to therapy. A report of "intermediate susceptibility" suggests that the organism would be susceptible if higher doses were used.
Clinical Pharmacology: Erythromycin binds to the 50 S ribosomal subunits of susceptible bacteria and suppresses protein synthesis.
Orally administered ERYTHROCIN STEARATE tablets are readily and reliably absorbed. Optimal serum levels of erythromycin are reached when the drug is taken in the fasting state or immediately before meals.
Erythromycin diffuses readily into most body fluids. Only low concentrations are normally achieved in the spinal fluid, but passage of the drug across the blood-brain barrier increases in meningitis. In the presence of normal hepatic function, erythromycin is concentrated in the liver and excreted in the bile; the effect of hepatic dysfunction on excretion of erythromycin by the liver into the bile is not known. Less than 5 percent of the orally administered dose of erythromycin is excreted in active form in the urine.
Erythromycin crosses the placental barrier and is excreted in breast milk.
Indications: *Streptococcus pyogenes* (Group A beta hemolytic streptococcus): Upper and lower respiratory tract, skin, and soft tissue infections of mild to moderate severity.
Injectable benzathine penicillin G is considered by the American Heart Association to be the drug of choice in the treatment and prevention of streptococcal pharyngitis and in long-term prophylaxis of rheumatic fever.
When oral medication is preferred for treatment of the above conditions, penicillin G, V, or erythromycin are alternate drugs of choice.
When oral medication is given, the importance of strict adherence by the patient to the prescribed dosage regimen must be stressed. A therapeutic dose should be administered for at least 10 days.
Alpha-hemolytic streptococci (viridans group): Short-term prophylaxis of bacterial endocarditis prior to dental or other operative procedures in patients with a history of rheumatic fever or congenital heart disease who are hypersensitive to penicillin. (Erythromycin is not suitable prior to genitourinary surgery where the organisms likely to lead to bacteremia are gram-negative bacilli or the enterococcus group of streptococci.)
Staphylococcus aureus: Acute infections of skin and soft tissue of mild to moderate severity. Resistant organisms may emerge during treatment.
Streptococcus pneumoniae (Diplococcus pneumoniae): Upper respiratory tract infections (e.g., otitis media, pharyngitis) and lower respiratory tract infections (e.g., pneumonia) of mild to moderate degree.
Mycoplasma pneumoniae (Eaton agent, PPLO): For respiratory infections due to this organism.
Hemophilus influenzae: For upper respiratory tract infections of mild to moderate severity when used concomitantly with adequate doses of sulfonamides. (See sulfonamide labeling for appropriate prescribing information). The concomitant use of the sulfonamides is necessary since not all strains of *Hemophilus influenzae* are susceptible to erythromycin at the concentrations of the antibiotic achieved with usual therapeutic doses.
Treponema pallidum: Erythromycin is an alternate choice of treatment for primary syphilis in patients allergic to the penicillins. In treatment of primary syphilis, spinal fluid examinations should be done before treatment and as part of follow-up after therapy.
Corynebacterium diphtheriae: As an adjunct to antitoxin, to prevent establishment of carriers, and to eradicate the organism in carriers.
Corynebacterium minutissimum: For the treatment of erythrasma.
Entamoeba histolytica: In the treatment of intestinal amebiasis only. Extra-enteric amebiasis requires treatment with other agents.
Listeria monocytogenes: Infections due to this organism.
Neisseria gonorrhoeae: Erythrocin Lactobionate-I.V. (erythromycin lactobionate for injection) in conjunction with erythromycin stearate orally, as an alternative drug in treatment of acute pelvic inflammatory disease caused by *N. gonorrhoeae* in female patients with a history of sensitivity to penicillin. Before treatment of gonorrhea, patients who are suspected of also having syphilis should have a microscopic examination for *T. pallidum* (by immunofluorescence or darkfield) before receiving erythromycin, and monthly serologic tests for a minimum of 4 months.
Bordetella pertussis: Erythromycin is effective in eliminating the organism from the nasopharynx of infected individuals, rendering them non-infectious. Some clinical studies suggest that erythromycin may be helpful in the prophylaxis of pertussis in exposed susceptible individuals.
Legionnaires' Disease: Although no controlled clinical efficacy studies have been conducted, *in vitro* and limited preliminary clinical data suggest that erythromycin may be effective in treating Legionnaires' Disease.
Contraindications: Erythromycin is contraindicated in patients with known hypersensitivity to this antibiotic.
Precautions: Erythromycin is principally excreted by the liver. Caution should be exercised in administering the antibiotic to patients with impaired hepatic function. There have been reports of hepatic dysfunction, with or without jaundice occurring in patients receiving oral erythromycin products.
Areas of localized infection may require surgical drainage in addition to antibiotic therapy.
Recent data from studies of erythromycin reveal that its use in patients who are receiving high doses of theophylline may be associated with an increase of serum theophylline levels and potential theophylline toxicity. In case of theophylline toxicity and/or elevated serum theophylline levels, the dose of theophylline should be reduced while the patient is receiving concomitant erythromycin therapy.
Usage during pregnancy and lactation: The safety of erythromycin for use during pregnancy has not been established.
Erythromycin crosses the placental barrier. Erythromycin also appears in breast milk.
Adverse Reactions: The most frequent side effects of oral erythromycin preparations are gastrointestinal, such as abdominal cramping and discomfort, and are dose-related. Nausea, vomiting, and diarrhea occur infrequently with usual oral doses.
During prolonged or repeated therapy, there is a possibility of overgrowth of nonsusceptible bacteria or fungi. If such infections occur, the drug should be discontinued and appropriate therapy instituted.
Allergic reactions ranging from urticaria and mild skin eruptions to anaphylaxis have occurred.
Dosage and Administration: Optimal serum levels of erythromycin are reached when ERYTHROCIN STEARATE (erythromycin stearate) is taken in the fasting state or immediately before meals.
Adults: The usual dosage is 250 mg every 6 hours; or 500 mg every 12 hours, taken in the fasting state or immediately before meals. Up to 4 Gm per day may be administered, depending upon the severity of the infection.
Children: Age, weight, and severity of the infection are important factors in determining the proper dosage. For the treatment of mild to moderate infections the usual dosage is 30 to 50 mg/kg/day in 3 or 4 divided doses. When dosage is desired on a twice-a-day schedule, one-half of the total daily dose may be taken every 12 hours in the fasting state or immediately before meals. For the treatment of more severe infections the total daily dose may be doubled.
In the treatment of streptococcal infections, a therapeutic dosage of erythromycin should be administered for at least 10 days. In continuous prophylaxis of streptococcal infections in persons with a history of rheumatic heart disease, the dose is 250 mg twice a day.
When used prior to surgery to prevent endocarditis (see *Alpha-hemolytic streptococci),* a recommended schedule for adults is: 500 mg before the procedure and 250 mg every 6 hours for 4 doses after the procedure. For small children: 30 to 50 mg/kg/day divided into 3 or 4 evenly spaced doses.
For treatment of primary syphilis: 30 to 40 Gm given in divided doses over a period of 10 to 15 days.
For treatment of acute pelvic inflammatory disease caused by *N. gonorrhoeae:* 500 mg Erythrocin Lactobionate-I.V. (erythromycin lactobionate for injection) every 6 hours for 3 days, followed by 250 mg Erythrocin Stearate every 6 hours for 7 days.
For intestinal amebiasis: Adults: 250 mg four times daily for 10 to 14 days. Children: 30 to 50 mg/kg/day in divided doses for 10 to 14 days.
For use in pertussis: Although optimal dosage and duration have not been established, doses of erythromycin utilized in reported clinical studies were 40 to 50 mg/kg/day, given in divided doses for 5 to 14 days.
For treatment of Legionnaires' Disease: Although optimal doses have not been established, doses utilized in reported clinical data were those recommended above (1 to 4 Gm daily in divided doses).

Continued on next page

If desired, additional literature on any Abbott Product will be provided upon request to Abbott Laboratories.

Abbott—Cont.

How Supplied: ERYTHROCIN STEARATE Filmtab Tablets (erythromycin stearate tablets, USP) are supplied as:

Erythrocin Stearate Filmtab, 125 mg
Bottles of 50 ....(**NDC** 0074-6308-01)

Erythrocin Stearate Filmtab, 250 mg
Bottles of 20 ....(**NDC** 0074-6346-23)
Bottles of 100 ....(**NDC** 0074-6346-20)
Bottles of 500 ....(**NDC** 0074-6346-53)
ABBO-PAC® unit dose strip packages of
100 tablets ....(**NDC** 0074-6346-38)

Erythrocin Stearate Filmtab, 500 mg
Bottles of 100 ....(**NDC** 0074-6316-13)

[*Shown in Product Identification Section*]

ERYTHROMYCIN BASE FILMTAB® ℞
(Erythromycin Tablets, USP)

Description: Erythromycin is produced by a strain of *Streptomyces erythraeus* and belongs to the macrolide group of antibiotics. It is basic and readily forms salts with acids. The base, the stearate salt, and the esters are poorly soluble in water, and are suitable for oral administration.

ERYTHROMYCIN Base Filmtab tablets contain erythromycin, USP, in a unique, nonenteric film coating.

Actions: Microbiology: Biochemical tests demonstrate that erythromycin inhibits protein synthesis of the pathogen without directly affecting nucleic acid synthesis. Antagonism has been demonstrated between clindamycin and erythromycin.

NOTE: Many strains of *Hemophilus influenzae* are resistant to erythromycin alone, but are susceptible to erythromycin and sulfonamides together. Staphylococci resistant to erythromycin may emerge during a course of erythromycin therapy. Culture and susceptibility testing should be performed.

Disc Susceptibility Tests

Quantitative methods that require measurement of zone diameters give the most precise estimates of antibiotic susceptibility. One recommended procedure (21 CFR section 460.1) uses erythromycin class discs for testing susceptibility; interpretations correlate zone diameters of this disc test with MIC values for erythromycin. With this procedure, a report from the laboratory of "susceptible" indicates that the infecting organism is likely to respond to therapy. A report of "resistant" indicates that the infective organism is not likely to respond to therapy. A report of "intermediate susceptibility" suggests that the organism would be susceptible if higher doses were used.

Clinical Pharmacology: Erythromycin binds to the 50 S ribosomal subunits of susceptible bacteria and suppresses protein synthesis.

Orally administered erythromycin is readily absorbed by most patients, especially on an empty stomach, but patient variation is observed. Due to its formulation and nonenteric coating, this erythromycin tablet gives reliable blood levels in the average subject; however, the levels may vary with the individual.

Erythromycin diffuses readily into most body fluids. Only low concentrations are normally achieved in the spinal fluid, but passage of the drug across the blood-brain barrier increases in meningitis. In the presence of normal hepatic function, erythromycin is concentrated in the liver and excreted in the bile; the effect of hepatic dysfunction on excretion of erythromycin by the liver into the bile is not known. Less than 5 percent of the orally administered dose of erythromycin is excreted in active form in the urine.

Erythromycin crosses the placental barrier and is excreted in breast milk.

Indications: *Streptococcus pyogenes* (Group A beta hemolytic streptococcus): Upper and lower respiratory tract, skin, and soft tissue infections of mild to moderate severity.

Injectable benzathine penicillin G is considered by the American Heart Association to be the drug of choice in the treatment and prevention of streptococcal pharyngitis and in long-term prophylaxis of rheumatic fever.

When oral medication is preferred for treatment of the above conditions, penicillin G, V, or erythromycin are alternate drugs of choice.

When oral medication is given, the importance of strict adherence by the patient to the prescribed dosage regimen must be stressed. A therapeutic dose should be administered for at least 10 days.

Alpha-hemolytic streptococci (viridans group): Short-term prophylaxis of bacterial endocarditis prior to dental or other operative procedures in patients with a history of rheumatic fever or congenital heart disease who are hypersensitive to penicillin. (Erythromycin is not suitable prior to genitourinary surgery where the organisms likely to lead to bacteremia are gram-negative bacilli or the enterococcus group of *streptococci.*)

Staphylococcus aureus: Acute infections of skin and soft tissue of mild to moderate severity. Resistant organisms may emerge during treatment.

Streptococcus pneumoniae (Diplococcus pneumoniae): Upper respiratory tract infections (e.g., otitis media, pharyngitis) and lower respiratory tract infections (e.g., pneumonia) of mild to moderate degree.

Mycoplasma pneumoniae (Eaton agent, PPLO): For respiratory infections due to this organism.

Hemophilus influenzae: For upper respiratory tract infections of mild to moderate severity when used concomitantly with adequate doses of sulfonamides. (See sulfonamide labeling for appropriate prescribing information). The concomitant use of the sulfonamides is necessary since not all strains of *Hemophilus influenzae* are susceptible to erythromycin at the concentrations of the antibiotic achieved with usual therapeutic doses.

Treponema pallidum: Erythromycin is an alternate choice of treatment for primary syphilis in patients allergic to the penicillins. In treatment of primary syphilis, spinal fluid examinations should be done before treatment and as part of follow-up after therapy.

Corynebacterium diphtheriae: As an adjunct to antitoxin, to prevent establishment of carriers, and to eradicate the organism in carriers.

Corynebacterium minutissimum: For the treatment of erythrasma.

Entamoeba histolytica: In the treatment of intestinal amebiasis only. Extra-enteric amebiasis requires treatment with other agents.

Listeria monocytogenes: Infections due to this organism.

Neisseria gonorrhoeae: Erythrocin® Lactobionate-I.V. (erythromycin lactobionate for injection) in conjunction with erythromycin base orally, as an alternative drug in treatment of acute pelvic inflammatory disease caused by *N. gonorrhoeae* in female patients with a history of sensitivity to penicillin. Before treatment of gonorrhea, patients who are suspected of also having syphilis should have a microscopic examination for *T. pallidum* (by immunofluorescence or darkfield) before receiving erythromycin, and monthly serologic tests for a minimum of 4 months.

Bordetella pertussis: Erythromycin is effective in eliminating the organism from the nasopharynx of infected individuals, rendering them non-infectious. Some clinical studies suggest that erythromycin may be helpful in the prophylaxis of pertussis in exposed susceptible individuals.

Legionnaires' Disease: Although no controlled clinical efficacy studies have been conducted, *in vitro* and limited preliminary clinical data suggest that erythromycin may be effective in treating Legionnaires' Disease.

Contraindications: Erythromycin is contraindicated in patients with known hypersensitivity to this antibiotic.

Precautions: Erythromycin is principally excreted by the liver. Caution should be exercised in administering the antibiotic to patients with impaired hepatic function. There have been reports of hepatic dysfunction, with or without jaundice occurring in patients receiving oral erythromycin products.

Areas of localized infection may require surgical drainage in addition to antibiotic therapy.

Recent data from studies of erythromycin reveal that its use in patients who are receiving high doses of theophylline may be associated with an increase of serum theophylline levels and potential theophylline toxicity. In case of theophylline toxicity and/or elevated serum theophylline levels, the dose of theophylline should be reduced while the patient is receiving concomitant erythromycin therapy.

Usage during pregnancy and lactation: The safety of erythromycin for use during pregnancy has not been established.

Erythromycin crosses the placental barrier. Erythromycin also appears in breast milk.

Adverse Reactions: The most frequent side effects of oral erythromycin preparations are gastrointestinal, such as abdominal cramping and discomfort, and are dose-related. Nausea, vomiting, and diarrhea occur infrequently with usual oral doses.

During prolonged or repeated therapy, there is a possibility of overgrowth of nonsusceptible bacteria or fungi. If such infections occur, the drug should be discontinued and appropriate therapy instituted.

Allergic reactions ranging from urticaria and mild skin eruptions to anaphylaxis have occurred.

Dosage and Administration: Optimum blood levels are obtained when doses are given on an empty stomach.

Adults: 250 mg every 6 hours is the usual dose; or 500 mg every 12 hours one hour before meals. Dosage may be increased up to 4 Gm per day according to the severity of the infection.

Children: Age, weight, and severity of the infection are important factors in determining the proper dosage. 30 to 50 mg/kg/day, in divided doses, is the usual dose. For more severe infections this dose may be doubled. If dosage is desired on a twice-a-day schedule, one-half of the total daily dose may be given every 12 hours, one hour before meals.

For the treatment of streptococcal infections: a therapeutic dosage should be administered for at least 10 days. In continuous prophylaxis of streptococcal infections in persons with rheumatic heart disease history, the dose is 250 mg twice a day.

To prevent endocarditis prior to surgery (see *Alpha-hemolytic streptococci*), a recommended schedule for adults is: 500 mg before the procedure and 250 mg every 6 hours for 4 doses after the procedure. For small children: 30 to 50 mg/kg/day divided into three or four evenly spaced doses.

For treatment of primary syphilis: 30 to 40 Gm given in divided doses over a period of 10 to 15 days.

For treatment of acute pelvic inflammatory disease caused by *N. gonorrhoeae:* 500 mg Erythrocin Lactobionate-I.V. (erythromycin lactobionate for injection) every 6 hours for 3 days, followed by 250 mg erythromycin base every 6 hours for 7 days.

For intestinal amebiasis: Adults: 250 mg four times daily for 10 to 14 days. Children: 30 to 50 mg/kg/day in divided doses for 10 to 14 days.

For use in pertussis: Although optimal dosage and duration have not been established, doses of erythromycin utilized in reported clinical studies were 40 to 50 mg/kg/day, given in divided doses for 5 to 14 days.

For treatment of Legionnaires' Disease: Although optimal doses have not been established, doses utilized in reported clinical data were those recommended above (1 to 4 Gm daily in divided doses.)

How Supplied: ERYTHROMYCIN Base Filmtab tablets (erythromycin tablets, USP) are supplied as pink capsule-shaped tablets in two dosage strengths:

250 mg tablets:
Bottles of 100 ....(**NDC** 0074-6326-13)
ABBO-PAC® unit dose strip packages of
100 tablets ....(**NDC** 0074-6326-11)
500 mg tablets:
Bottles of 100 ....(**NDC** 0074-6227-13)

FILMTAB—Film-sealed tablets, Abbott.
[*Shown in Product Identification Section*]

EUTONYL® ℞
(pargyline hydrochloride tablets, NF)
FILMTAB®

Description: EUTONYL (pargyline hydrochloride) is a non-hydrazine monoamine oxidase (MAO) inhibitor with hypotensive activity and is chemically identified as N-methyl-N-2-propynylbenzylamine hydrochloride. Clinically, EUTONYL is an effective antihypertensive agent which is primarily useful in the treatment of moderate to severe hypertension.

Actions: EUTONYL (pargyline hydrochloride) is a MAO inhibitor which has a potent antihypertensive action. Its exact mode of action is uncertain. The antihypertensive effect of pargyline is greatest when the patient is in the standing position. In about half of the patients treated, reduction of blood pressure in the sitting and supine positions was nearly as great as in the standing position. An interval of four days to three weeks or more may elapse following initiation of therapy before the full therapeutic effects of a given dosage schedule become manifest. A similar interval may be required for effects to subside after withdrawal of the drug, because the termination of drug effect is dependent on the regeneration of inhibited enzymes.

In rats, about ninety percent of a given dose of pargyline is excreted in the urine within the first twenty-four hours following dosing.

Indications: EUTONYL (pargyline hydrochloride) is indicated in the treatment of moderate to severe hypertension. *It is not recommended for use in patients with mild or labile hypertension.* EUTONYL does not interfere with or obviate the use of diuretic therapy in hypertensive patients who may have an associated edema. EUTONYL may be used alone or concurrently with most other antihypertensive agents. It is often effective at reduced dosage when administered with one of the thiazides and/or rauwolfia alkaloids.

Contraindications:

1. EUTONYL (pargyline hydrochloride) is contraindicated in patients with pheochromocytoma, paranoid schizophrenia, hyperthyroidism, and advanced renal failure.
2. EUTONYL should not be administered to those with malignant hypertension or to children under twelve years of age because significant clinical information concerning the use of the drug in these conditions is not available.
3. In general, the following drugs or agents are contraindicated in patients receiving EUTONYL (pargyline hydrochloride):
   a. Centrally acting sympathomimetic amines such as amphetamine and related compounds (includes most anorectic agents).
   Peripherally acting sympathomimetic drugs such as ephedrine and its derivatives (also found in nasal decongestants, cold remedies, and hay fever preparations).
   b. Aged cheese (e.g., Cheddar, Camembert, and Stilton), processed cheese, beer and wine (especially, Chianti wine), and other foods which require the action of bacteria or molds for their preparation or preservation because of the presence of pressor substances such as tyramine. Other foods which should be avoided during pargyline therapy because of their high pressor amine content include chocolate, yeast extract, avocado, pickled herring, pods of broad beans, ripened bananas, papaya products (including certain meat tenderizers), and chicken livers. Cream cheese, ricotta, and cottage cheese can be allowed in the diet during pargyline therapy since their tyramine content is inconsequential. In some patients receiving pargyline, tyramine may precipitate an abrupt rise in blood pressure accompanied by some or all of the following: severe headache, chest pain, profuse sweating, palpitation, tachycardia or bradycardia, visual disturbances, stertorous breathing, coma, and intracranial bleeding (which could be fatal). Phentolamine may be administered parenterally for treatment of such an acute hypertensive reaction.
   c. Parenteral reserpine or guanethidine. Parenteral use of these drugs in patients receiving monoamine oxidase inhibitors results in a sudden release of accumulated catecholamines which may cause a hypertensive reaction. Reserpine and guanethidine should not be given parenterally during, and for at least one week following, treatment with pargyline.
   d. Imipramine, amitriptyline, desipramine, nortriptyline, protriptyline, doxepin, or their analogues. The use of these drugs with a monoamine oxidase inhibitor has been reported to cause vascular collapse and hyperthermia which may be fatal. A drug-free interval (about two weeks) should separate therapy with EUTONYL (pargyline hydrochloride) and use of these agents.
   e. Other monoamine oxidase inhibitors. These may augment the effects of pargyline.
   f. Methyldopa or dopamine. These drugs may cause hyperexcitability in patients receiving pargyline.
   g. L-dopa. There have been several reports of potentiation of the pressor effects of this drug by various monoamine oxidase inhibitors. At least one month should elapse after the discontinuation of pargyline before L-dopa is given.

Warnings:

A. PATIENTS
1. PATIENTS SHOULD BE WARNED AGAINST THE USE OF ANY OVER-THE-COUNTER PREPARATIONS, PARTICULARLY "COLD PREPARATIONS" AND ANTIHISTAMINES, OR PRESCRIPTION DRUGS WITHOUT THE KNOWLEDGE AND CONSENT OF THE PHYSICIAN.
2. PATIENTS SHOULD BE CAUTIONED ON THE USE OF CHEESE AND OTHER FOODS WITH HIGH TYRAMINE CONTENT (See *Contraindications*) AND ALCOHOLIC BEVERAGES IN ANY FORM.
3. PATIENTS SHOULD BE WARNED ABOUT THE LIKELIHOOD OF THE OCCURRENCE OF ORTHOSTATIC HYPOTENSION.
4. PATIENTS SHOULD BE INSTRUCTED TO REPORT PROMPTLY THE OCCURRENCE OF SEVERE HEADACHE OR OTHER UNUSUAL SYMPTOMS.
5. PATIENTS WITH ANGINA PECTORIS OR CORONARY ARTERY DISEASE SHOULD BE ESPECIALLY WARNED NOT TO INCREASE THEIR PHYSICAL ACTIVITIES IN RESPONSE TO A DIMINUTION IN ANGINAL SYMPTOMS OR AN INCREASE IN WELL-BEING OCCURRING DURING TREATMENT WITH EUTONYL.

B. PHYSICIANS
1. WHEN INDICATED THE FOLLOWING SHOULD BE CAUTIOUSLY PRESCRIBED IN REDUCED DOSAGES:
   a. ANTIHISTAMINES
   b. HYPNOTICS, SEDATIVES, OR TRANQUILIZERS
   c. NARCOTICS (MEPERIDINE SHOULD NOT BE USED)
2. DISCONTINUE EUTONYL AT LEAST TWO WEEKS PRIOR TO ELECTIVE SURGERY.
3. IN EMERGENCY SURGERY THE DOSE OF NARCOTICS OR OTHER PREMEDICATIONS SHOULD BE REDUCED TO ¼ TO ⅕ THE USUAL AMOUNT. CLINICAL EXPERIENCE HAS SHOWN THAT RESPONSE TO ALL ANESTHETIC AGENTS CAN BE EXAGGERATED IN PATIENTS RECEIVING EUTONYL. THEREFORE THE DOSE OF THE ANESTHETIC SHOULD BE CAREFULLY ADJUSTED.
4. EUTONYL MAY INDUCE HYPOGLYCEMIA. THEREFORE, EUTONYL SHOULD BE GIVEN WITH CAUTION TO DIABETICS RECEIVING HYPOGLYCEMIC AGENTS BECAUSE SEVERE HYPOGLYCEMIA MAY OCCUR. IF IT IS NECESSARY TO ADMINISTER EUTONYL TO PATIENTS RECEIVING INSULIN OR OTHER HYPOGLYCEMIC AGENTS, THE DOSE OF THESE AGENTS SHOULD BE REDUCED ACCORDINGLY AND THE PATIENT CAREFULLY MONITORED.
5. CARE SHOULD BE EXERCISED IN USING EUTONYL IN PATIENTS WITH IMPAIRED RENAL FUNCTION.

Use In Pregnancy and Lactation: Safe use of EUTONYL (pargyline hydrochloride) during pregnancy or lactation has not yet been established. Before prescribing EUTONYL in pregnancy, lactation, or in women of childbearing age, the potential benefit of the drug should be weighed against its possible hazard to mother and child.

Precautions: The therapeutic response to a variety of drugs may be changed or exaggerated in patients receiving a monoamine oxidase inhibitor such as pargyline hydrochloride. Caffeine, alcohol, antihistamines, barbiturates, chloral hydrate and other hypnotics, sedatives, tranquilizers, and narcotics (meperidine should not be used) should be used cautiously and at reduced dosage in patients who are taking pargyline.

There have been no substantiated reports of hepatotoxicity associated with pargyline therapy. However, since liver damage has resulted from use of certain other monoamine oxidase inhibitors, and since transient alterations in liver enzyme levels have occasionally occurred with pargyline, it is advisable that patients receiving EUTONYL have periodic liver function tests.

All patients with impaired circulation to vital organs from any cause including those with angina pectoris, coronary artery disease, and cerebral arteriosclerosis should be closely observed for symptoms of orthostatic hypotension. If hypotension develops in these patients, EUTONYL (pargyline hydrochloride) dosage should be reduced or therapy discontinued since severe and/or prolonged hypotension may precipitate cerebral or coronary vessel thrombosis.

Continued on next page

Abbott—Cont.

The hypotensive effect of EUTONYL may be augmented by febrile illnesses. It may be advisable to withdraw the drug during such diseases.

Since pargyline is excreted primarily in the urine, patients with impaired renal function may experience cumulative drug effects. Such patients should also be watched for elevations of blood urea nitrogen and other evidence of progressive renal failure. If such alterations should persist and progress, the drug should be discontinued.

An increased response to central depressants may be manifested by acute hypotension and increased sedative effect. EUTONYL also may augment the hypotensive effects of anesthetic agents, and surgery. For this reason, the drug should be discontinued at least two weeks prior to surgery.

In the event of emergency surgery, ¼ to ⅕ of the usual dose of narcotics, sedatives, analgesics and other premedications should be used. If severe hypotension should occur, this can be controlled by small doses of a vasopressor agent such as levarterenol.

EUTONYL should not be used in individuals with hyperactive or hyperexcitable personalities, as some of these patients show an undesirable increase in motor activity with restlessness, confusion, agitation, and disorientation. Clinical studies have shown that pargyline may unmask severe psychotic symptoms such as hallucinations or paranoid delusions in some patients with pre-existing serious emotional problems. This can usually be controlled by judicious administration of chlorpromazine intramuscularly, or other phenothiazines, the patient remaining supine for one hour after administration.

Pargyline should be used with caution in patients with Parkinsonism, as it may increase symptoms. In addition, great care is required if pargyline is administered in conjunction with anti-parkinsonian agents.

Documented cases of eye changes or optic atrophy have not been reported with the use of pargyline as they have with the use of certain other monoamine oxidase inhibitors. However, since non-specific visual disturbances and aggravation of glaucoma have occurred occasionally, it is advisable that patients receiving EUTONYL be examined for changes in color perception, visual fields, fundi, and visual acuity.

Clinical reports state that certain individuals receiving pargyline for a prolonged period of time are refractory to the nerve-blocking effects of local anesthetics, e.g., lidocaine.

Adverse Reactions: Generally side effects are not severe or serious when the recommended dosages are used and necessary precautions are observed. If side effects are severe or persist the drug should be discontinued. See also *Warnings* and *Precautions*.

The most frequently occurring side effects are those associated with orthostatic hypotension (dizziness, weakness, palpitation, or fainting). These usually respond to a reduction of dosage. Patients should be warned against rising to a standing position too quickly, especially when getting out of bed. Severe and persistent orthostatic hypotension should be avoided by reduction in dosage or discontinuation of therapy.

Mild constipation, fluid retention with or without edema, dry mouth, sweating, increased appetite, arthralgia, nausea and vomiting, blurred vision, headache, insomnia, difficulty in micturition, nightmares, impotence and delayed ejaculation, rash, and purpura have also been encountered. Hyperexcitability, increased neuromuscular activity (muscle twitching), and other extrapyramidal symptoms have been reported. Gain in weight may be due to either edema or increased appetite. Drug fever is extremely rare. In some patients reduction of blood sugar has been noted. Although the significance of this has not been elucidated, the possibility of hypoglycemic effects should be borne in mind. Congestive heart failure has been reported in patients with reduced cardiac reserve.

Dosage and Administration: EUTONYL (pargyline hydrochloride) is orally administered as a single daily dose; there is no known advantage in prescribing the drug more frequently than once daily. Clinical response to the drug is not immediate. Four days to three weeks or more may be required to produce the full effects of a given daily dosage. *For this reason it is generally unwise to increase dosage more frequently than once a week.* Likewise the effects of the drug may persist following reduction of dosage or withdrawal. If therapy must be interrupted because of undesirable side effects, the drug should be withheld until all such effects have disappeared. Therapy is then reinstituted at a lower dosage. Because the drug exerts an orthostatic effect on blood pressure, dosage adjustments should be based upon the blood pressure response *in the standing position.*

The usual adult dosage for initiating therapy in hypertensive patients not receiving other antihypertensive agents is 25 mg once daily. This dosage may be increased once a week by 10 mg increments until the desired response is obtained. The total daily dose of pargyline should not exceed 200 mg if excessive side effects are to be avoided.

Patients over age 65, or those who have undergone sympathectomy may be unusually sensitive to the antihypertensive properties of the drug. In such patients the initial daily dosage should be 10 to 25 mg. When EUTONYL (pargyline hydrochloride) is added to an established antihypertensive regimen, the initial dose should not exceed 25 mg daily (less in sympathectomized or elderly patients).

EUTONYL should not be administered to children under 12 years of age because of limited experience with the drug in this group.

Reduction of blood pressure is often maintained in hypertensive patients with a daily dose of 25 to 50 mg of EUTONYL alone. Larger doses may be tried in resistant cases. In general, dosage should be kept at the minimum level required to maintain a desirable reduction in blood pressure without encountering undue side effects. A few patients may develop a relative tolerance to the antihypertensive effects of the drug. The administration of additional antihypertensive agents may be considered in cases not controlled by EUTONYL alone.

Overdosage: Reported effects of MAOI overdosage include agitation, hallucinations, hyperreflexia, hyperpyrexia, convulsions, and both hypotension and hypertension.

Management must be attempted with great caution because of the potential for interaction with antidotal drugs. Conservative treatment aimed at the maintenance of normal temperature, respiration, blood pressure, and proper fluid and electrolyte balance has generally been successful.

How Supplied: EUTONYL (pargyline hydrochloride, Abbott) is available in Filmtab tablet strengths of 10 mg, 25 mg and 50 mg. The tablets are available in the following packages: 10 mg tablets in bottles of 100 (**NDC** 0074-6876-02); 25 mg tablets in bottles of 100 (**NDC** 0074-6878-01); 50 mg tablets in bottles of 100 (**NDC** 0074-6894-04).

[*Shown in Product Identification Section*]

Ref. 03-4198/R3

EUTRON® ℞
(pargyline hydrochloride and methyclothiazide)
Filmtab®

Warning:
This fixed combination drug is not indicated for initial therapy of hypertension. Hypertension requires therapy titrated to the individual patient. If the fixed combination represents the dosage so determined, its use may be more convenient in patient management. The treatment of hypertension is not static, but must be reevaluated as conditions in each patient warrant.

Description: EUTRON is the Abbott registered trademark for an orally administered tablet combining 25 mg of Eutonyl® (pargyline hydrochloride) and 5 mg of Enduron® (methyclothiazide). Pargyline hydrochloride is a non-hydrazine monoamine oxidase (MAO) inhibitor with hypotensive activity and is chemically identified as N-methyl-N-2-propynylbenzylamine hydrochloride. Methyclothiazide is an oral diuretic-antihypertensive of the benzothiadiazine (thiazide) class.

Actions: Eutonyl (pargyline hydrochloride) is a MAO inhibitor which has a potent antihypertensive action. Its exact mode of action is uncertain. The antihypertensive effect of pargyline is greatest when the patient is in the standing position. In about half of the patients treated, reduction of blood pressure in the sitting and supine positions was nearly as great as in the standing position. An interval of four days to three weeks or more may elapse following initiation of therapy before the full therapeutic effects of a given dosage schedule become manifest. A similar interval may be required for effects to subside after withdrawal of the drug, because the termination of drug effect is dependent on the regeneration of inhibited enzymes.

In rats, about ninety percent of a given dose of pargyline is excreted in the urine within the first twenty-four hours following dosing.

The diuretic and saluretic effects of methyclothiazide result from a drug-induced inhibition of the renal tubular reabsorption of electrolytes. The excretion of sodium and chloride is greatly enhanced. Potassium excretion is also enhanced to a variable degree, as it is with the other thiazides. Although urinary excretion of bicarbonate is increased slightly, there is usually no significant change in urinary pH. Methyclothiazide has a per mg natriuretic activity approximately 100 times that of the prototype thiazide, chlorothiazide. At maximal therapeutic dosages, all thiazides are approximately equal in their diuretic/natriuretic effects.

There is significant natriuresis and diuresis within two hours after administration of a single dose of methyclothiazide. These effects reach a peak in about six hours and persist for 24 hours following oral administration of a single dose.

Like other benzothiadiazines, methyclothiazide also has antihypertensive properties, and may be used for this purpose either alone or to enhance the antihypertensive action of other drugs. The mechanism by which the benzothiadiazines, including methyclothiazide, produce a reduction of elevated blood pressure is not known. However, sodium depletion appears to be involved.

Methyclothiazide is readily absorbed from the gastrointestinal tract and is excreted unchanged by the kidneys.

Indications: EUTRON (pargyline hydrochloride and methyclothiazide) is indicated in the treatment of patients with moderate to severe hypertension, especially those with severe diastolic hypertension. *It is not recommended for use in patients with mild or labile hypertension* (see boxed warning).

Contraindications:

1. Pargyline therapy is contraindicated in patients with pheochromocytoma, paranoid schizophrenia, hyperthyroidism, and advanced renal failure.

2.Pargyline should not be administered to those with malignant hypertension or to children under twelve years of age because significant clinical information concerning the use of the drug in these conditions is not available.

3. In general, the following drugs or agents are contraindicated in patients receiving pargyline hydrochloride:

a. Centrally acting sympathomimetic amines such as amphetamine and its derivatives (also found in anorectic preparations).
Peripherally acting sympathomimetic drugs such as ephedrine and its derivatives (also found in nasal decongestants, hay fever preparations, and cold remedies).

b. Aged cheese (e.g., Cheddar, Camembert, and Stilton), processed cheese, beer and wine (especially, Chianti wine), and other foods which require the action of bacteria or molds for their preparation or preservation because of the presence of pressor substances such as tyramine. Other foods which should be avoided during pargyline therapy because of their high pressor amine content include chocolate, yeast extract, avocado, pickled herring, pods of broad beans, ripened bananas, papaya products (including certain meat tenderizers), and chicken livers. Cream cheese, ricotta, and cottage cheese can be allowed in the diet during pargyline therapy since their tyramine content is inconsequential.
In some patients receiving EUTRON (pargyline hydrochloride and methyclothiazide), tyramine may precipitate an abrupt rise in blood pressure accompanied by some or all of the following: severe headache, chest pain, profuse sweating, palpitation, tachycardia or bradycardia, visual disturbances, stertorous breathing, coma, and intracranial bleeding (which could be fatal). Phentolamine may be administered parenterally for treatment of such an acute hypertensive reaction.

c. Parenteral reserpine or guanethidine. Parenteral use of these drugs in patients receiving monoamine oxidase inhibitors results in a sudden release of accumulated catecholamines which may cause a hypertensive reaction. Reserpine and guanethidine should not be given parenterally during, and for at least one week following, treatment with EUTRON.

d. Imipramine, amitriptyline, desipramine, nortriptyline, protriptyline, doxepin, or their analogues. The use of these drugs with monoamine oxidase inhibitors has been reported to cause vascular collapse and hyperthermia which may be fatal. A drug-free interval (about two weeks) should separate therapy with EUTRON (pargyline hydrochloride and methyclothiazide) and use of these agents.

e. Methyldopa or dopamine. These drugs may cause hyperexcitability in patients receiving pargyline.

f. Other monoamine oxidase inhibitors. These may augment the effects of pargyline.

g. L-dopa. There have been several reports of potentiation of the pressor effects of this drug by various monoamine oxidase inhibitors. At least one month should elapse after the discontinuation of EUTRON before L-dopa is given.

4. Methyclothiazide is contraindicated in patients with renal decompensation and in those who are hypersensitive to this or other sulfonamide-derived drugs.

Warnings:

A. PATIENTS

1. PATIENTS SHOULD BE WARNED AGAINST THE USE OF ANY OVER-THE-COUNTER PREPARATIONS, PARTICULARLY "COLD PREPARATIONS" AND ANTIHISTAMINES, OR PRESCRIPTION DRUGS WITHOUT THE KNOWLEDGE AND CONSENT OF THE PHYSICIAN.
2. PATIENTS SHOULD BE CAUTIONED ON THE USE OF CHEESE AND OTHER FOODS WITH HIGH TYRAMINE CONTENT (SEE CONTRAINDICATIONS) AND ALCOHOLIC BEVERAGES IN ANY FORM.
3. PATIENTS SHOULD BE WARNED ABOUT THE LIKELIHOOD OF THE OCCURRENCE OF ORTHOSTATIC HYPOTENSION.
4. PATIENTS SHOULD BE INSTRUCTED TO REPORT PROMPTLY THE OCCURRENCE OF SEVERE HEADACHE OR OTHER UNUSUAL SYMPTOMS.
5. PATIENTS WITH ANGINA PECTORIS OR CORONARY ARTERY DISEASE SHOULD BE ESPECIALLY WARNED NOT TO INCREASE THEIR PHYSICAL ACTIVITIES IN RESPONSE TO A DIMINUTION IN ANGINAL SYMPTOMS OR AN INCREASE IN WELL-BEING OCCURRING DURING TREATMENT WITH **EUTRON.**

B. PHYSICIANS

1. WHEN INDICATED THE FOLLOWING SHOULD BE CAUTIOUSLY PRESCRIBED IN REDUCED DOSAGES:
   a. ANTIHISTAMINES
   b. HYPNOTICS, SEDATIVES, OR TRANQUILIZERS
   c. NARCOTICS (MEPERIDINE SHOULD NOT BE USED)
2. DISCONTINUE **EUTRON** AT LEAST TWO WEEKS PRIOR TO ELECTIVE SURGERY.
3. IN EMERGENCY SURGERY THE DOSE OF NARCOTICS OR OTHER PREMEDICATIONS SHOULD BE REDUCED TO 1/4 to 1/5 THE USUAL AMOUNT. CLINICAL EXPERIENCE HAS SHOWN THAT RESPONSE TO ALL ANESTHETIC AGENTS CAN BE EXAGGERATED IN PATIENTS RECEIVING **EUTRON.** THEREFORE THE DOSE OF THE ANESTHETIC SHOULD BE CAREFULLY ADJUSTED.
4. PARGYLINE HYDROCHLORIDE MAY INDUCE HYPOGLYCEMIA. THEREFORE, **EUTRON** SHOULD BE GIVEN WITH CAUTION TO DIABETICS RECEIVING HYPOGLYCEMIC AGENTS BECAUSE SEVERE HYPOGLYCEMIA MAY OCCUR. IF IT IS NECESSARY TO ADMINISTER **EUTRON** TO PATIENTS RECEIVING INSULIN OR OTHER HYPOGLYCEMIC AGENTS, THE DOSE OF THESE AGENTS SHOULD BE REDUCED ACCORDINGLY AND THE PATIENT CAREFULLY MONITORED.
5. CARE SHOULD BE EXERCISED IN USING **EUTRON** IN PATIENTS WITH IMPAIRED RENAL FUNCTION.

Methyclothiazide shares with other thiazides the propensity to deplete potassium reserves to an unpredictable degree.

Thiazides should be used with caution in patients with renal disease or significant impairment of renal function, since azotemia may be precipitated and cumulative drug effects may occur.

Thiazides should be used with caution in patients with impaired hepatic function or progressive liver disease, since minor alterations of fluid and electrolyte balance may precipitate hepatic coma.

Thiazides may be additive or potentiative of the action of other antihypertensive drugs. Potentiation occurs with ganglionic or peripheral adrenergic blocking drugs.

Sensitivity reactions may occur in patients with a history of allergy or bronchial asthma. The possibility of exacerbation or activation of systemic lupus erythematosus has been reported.

Use in Pregnancy and Lactation:

Pargyline Hydrochloride

Safe use of pargyline during pregnancy or lactation has not yet been established. Before prescribing pargyline in pregnancy, in lactation, or in women of childbearing age, the potential benefits of the drug should be weighed against its possible hazard to mother and child.

Methyclothiazide

Thiazides cross the placental barrier and appear in cord blood. The use of thiazides in pregnant women requires that the anticipated benefit be weighed against possible hazards to the fetus. These hazards include fetal or neonatal jaundice, thrombocytopenia, and possible other adverse reactions that have occurred in the adult.

Thiazides appear in breast milk. If use of the drug is deemed essential, the patient should stop nursing.

Precautions:

Pargyline Hydrochloride

The therapeutic response to a variety of drugs may be changed or exaggerated in patients receiving a monoamine oxidase inhibitor such as pargyline hydrochloride. Caffeine, alcohol, antihistamines, barbiturates, chloral hydrate and other hypnotics, sedatives, tranquilizers and narcotics (meperidine should not be used) should be used cautiously and at reduced dosage in patients who are taking pargyline.

There have been no substantiated reports of hepatotoxicity associated with pargyline therapy. However, since liver damage has resulted from use of certain other monoamine oxidase inhibitors, and since transient alterations in liver enzyme levels have occasionally occurred with pargyline, it is advisable that patients receiving EUTRON have periodic liver function tests.

All patients with impaired circulation to vital organs from any cause including those with angina pectoris, coronary artery disease, and cerebral arteriosclerosis should be closely observed for symptoms of orthostatic hypotension. If hypotension develops in these patients, EUTRON (pargyline hydrochloride and methyclothiazide) dosage should be reduced or therapy discontinued since severe and/or prolonged hypotension may precipitate cerebral or coronary vessel thrombosis.

The hypotensive effect of pargyline may be augmented by febrile illnesses. It may be advisable to withdraw the drug during such diseases.

Since pargyline is excreted primarily in the urine, patients with impaired renal function may experience cumulative drug effects. Such patients should also be watched for elevations of blood urea nitrogen and other evidence of progressive renal failure. If such alterations should persist and progress, the drug should be discontinued.

An increased response to central depressants may be manifested by acute hypotension and increased sedative effect. Pargyline also may augment the hypotensive effects of anesthetic agents and surgery. For this reason, the drug should be discontinued at least two weeks prior to surgery.

In the event of emergency surgery, smaller than usual doses (1/4 to 1/5) of narcotics, analgesics, sedatives, and other premedications should be used. If severe hypotension should occur, this can be controlled by small doses of a vasopressor agent such as levarterenol.

Continued on next page

Abbott—Cont.

Pargyline therapy should not be used in individuals with hyperactive or hyperexcitable personalities, as some of these patients show an undesirable increase in motor activity with restlessness, confusion, agitation, and disorientation. Clinical studies have shown that pargyline may unmask severe psychotic symptoms such as hallucinations or paranoid delusions in some patients with pre-existing serious emotional problems. This can usually be controlled by judicious administration of chlorpromazine intramuscularly, or other phenothiazines, the patient remaining supine for one hour after administration.
Pargyline should be used with caution in patients with Parkinsonism, as it may increase symptoms. In addition, great care is required if pargyline is administered in conjunction with anti-parkinsonian agents.
Documented cases of eye changes or optic atrophy have not been reported with the use of pargyline as they have with the use of certain other monoamine oxidase inhibitors. However, since non-specific visual disturbances and aggravation of glaucoma have occurred occasionally, it is advisable that patients receiving EUTRON be examined for changes in color perception, visual fields, fundi, and visual acuity.
Clinical reports state that certain individuals receiving pargyline for a prolonged period of time are refractory to the nerve-blocking effects of local anesthetics, e.g., lidocaine.

Methyclothiazide

Periodic determinations of serum electrolytes should be performed at appropriate intervals for the purpose of detecting possible electrolyte imbalances such as hyponatremia, hypochloremic alkalosis, and hypokalemia. Serum and urine electrolyte determinations are particularly important when a patient is vomiting excessively or receiving parenteral fluids. All patients should be observed for other clinical signs of electrolyte imbalances such as dryness of mouth, thirst, weakness, lethargy, drowsiness, restlessness, muscle pains or cramps, muscular fatigue, hypotension, oliguria, tachycardia, and gastrointestinal disturbances such as nausea and vomiting.
Hypokalemia may develop with thiazides as with any other potent diuretic, especially when brisk diuresis occurs, severe cirrhosis is present, or when corticosteroids or ACTH are given concomitantly. Interference with the adequate oral intake of electrolytes will also contribute to the possible development of hypokalemia. Potassium depletion, even of a mild degree, resulting from thiazide use, may sensitize a patient to the effects of cardiac glycosides such as digitalis.
Any chloride deficit is generally mild and usually does not require specific treatment except under extraordinary circumstances (as in liver disease or renal disease). Dilutional hyponatremia may occur in edematous patients in hot weather; appropriate therapy is water restriction rather than administration of salt, except in rare instances when the hyponatremia is life threatening.
In actual salt depletion, appropriate replacement is the therapy of choice.
Hyperuricemia may occur or frank gout may be precipitated in certain patients receiving thiazide therapy.
Insulin requirements in diabetic patients may be increased, decreased, or unchanged. Latent diabetes mellitus may become manifest during thiazide administration.
Thiazide drugs may increase the responsiveness to tubocurarine.
The antihypertensive effects of the drug may be enhanced in the postsympathectomy patient.
Thiazides may decrease arterial responsiveness to norepinephrine. This diminution is not sufficient to preclude effectiveness of the pressor agent for therapeutic use.
If progressive renal impairment becomes evident as indicated by a rising nonprotein nitrogen or blood urea nitrogen, a careful reappraisal of therapy is necessary with consideration given to withholding or discontinuing diuretic therapy.
Thiazides may decrease serum PBI levels without signs of thyroid disturbance.
Thiazides have been reported, on rare occasions, to have elevated serum calcium to hypercalcemic levels. The serum calcium levels have returned to normal when the medication has been stopped. This phenomenon may be related to the ability of the thiazide diuretic to lower the amount of calcium excreted in the urine.

Adverse Reactions: Generally side effects are not severe or serious when the recommended dosages are used and necessary precautions are observed. If side effects are severe or persist the drug should be discontinued. See also *Warnings* and *Precautions.*

Pargyline Hydrochloride

The most frequently occurring side effects are those associated with orthostatic hypotension (dizziness, weakness, palpitation, or fainting). These usually respond to a reduction of dosage. Patients should be warned against rising to a standing position too quickly, especially when getting out of bed. Severe and persistent orthostatic hypotension should be avoided by reduction in dosage or discontinuation of therapy.
Mild constipation, fluid retention with or without edema, dry mouth, sweating, increased appetite, arthralgia, nausea and vomiting, blurred vision, headache, insomnia, difficulty in micturition, nightmares, impotence and delayed ejaculation, rash, and purpura have also been encountered. Hyperexcitability, increased neuromuscular activity (muscle twitching) and other extra-pyramidal symptoms have been reported. Gain in weight may be due either to edema or increased appetite. Drug fever is extremely rare. In some patients reduction of blood sugar has been noted. Although the significance of this has not been elucidated, the possibility of hypoglycemic effects should be borne in mind. Congestive heart failure has been reported in patients with reduced cardiac reserve.

Methyclothiazide

Gastrointestinal system reactions: Anorexia, gastric irritation, nausea, vomiting, cramping, diarrhea, constipation, jaundice (intrahepatic cholestatic jaundice), pancreatitis.
Central nervous system reactions: Dizziness, vertigo, paresthesias, headache, xanthopsia.
Hematologic reactions: Leukopenia, agranulocytosis, thrombocytopenia, aplastic anemia.
Dermatologic — hypersensitivity reactions: Purpura, photosensitivity, rash, urticaria, necrotizing angiitis (vasculitis) (cutaneous vasculitis).
Cardiovascular reaction: Orthostatic hypotension may occur and may be aggravated by alcohol, barbiturates, or narcotics.
Other: Hyperglycemia, glycosuria, hypercalcemia, hyperuricemia, muscle spasm, weakness, restlessness.
There have been isolated reports that certain nonedematous individuals developed severe fluid and electrolyte derangements after only brief exposure to normal doses of thiazide and non-thiazide diuretics. The condition is usually manifested as severe dilutional hyponatremia, hypokalemia, and hypochloremia. It has been reported to be due to inappropriately increased ADH secretion and appears to be idiosyncratic. Potassium replacement is apparently the most important therapy in the treatment of this syndrome along with removal of the offending drug.
Whenever adverse reactions are severe, treatment should be discontinued.

Dosage and Administration: Dosage should be determined by individual titration of ingredients (see boxed warning). Dosage of both components should be carefully adjusted to the needs of the individual patient. Since four days to three weeks or more may be required to produce the full effects of a given daily dosage of pargyline hydrochloride, it is generally unwise to increase the dosage of this drug more frequently than once a week. The maximum recommended dosage of EUTRON (pargyline hydrochloride and methyclothiazide) is two tablets daily. The upper limits of daily dosage of the two components are 10 mg methyclothiazide and 200 mg pargyline hydrochloride. A few patients may develop a relative tolerance to the antihypertensive effects of the drug. In general dosage should be kept at the minimum level required to maintain a desirable reduction in blood pressure without encountering undue side effects.
EUTRON should not be administered to children under 12 years of age because of limited experience with the drug in this group.
EUTRON (25 mg pargyline hydrochloride and 5 mg methyclothiazide) is grooved to permit considerable latitude in meeting the dosage requirements of individual patients.
The table below will help in determining which dose of EUTRON best represents the equivalent of the titrated dose.

Daily Dosage of EUTRON	pargyline hydrochloride	methyclothiazide
½ tablet	12.5 mg	2.5 mg
1 tablet	25.0 mg	5.0 mg
1½ tablets	37.5 mg	7.5 mg
2 tablets	50.0 mg	10.0 mg

The appropriate dose of EUTRON is administered orally, once daily. The usual adult dosage is one tablet daily.

Overdosage:

Pargyline Hydrochloride

Reported effects of MAOI overdosage include agitation, hallucinations, hyperreflexia, hyperpyrexia, convulsions, and both hypotension and hypertension.
Management must be attempted with great caution because of the potential for interaction with antidotal drugs. Conservative treatment aimed at the maintenance of normal temperature, respiration, blood pressure, and proper fluid and electrolyte balance has generally been successful.

Methyclothiazide

Symptoms of overdosage include electrolyte imbalance and signs of potassium deficiency such as confusion, dizziness, muscular weakness, and gastrointestinal disturbances. General supportive measures including replacement of fluids and electrolytes may be indicated in treatment of overdosage.

How Supplied: EUTRON (pargyline hydrochloride, 25 mg and methyclothiazide, 5 mg) is supplied as light purple Filmtab tablets in bottles of 100 (**NDC** 0074-7240-03) and 500 (**NDC** 0074-7240-02).

[*Shown in Product Identification Section*]

03-4190-R6

FERO-FOLIC-500® ℞

(controlled-release Iron with folic acid and vitamin C)
Filmtab® tablets

Description: Fero-Folic-500 contains 525 mg. of ferrous sulfate (equivalent to 105 mg. of elemental iron) in a unique controlled-release vehicle, the Gradumet®. In addition, this product contains 800 mcg. of folic acid and 500 mg. of ascorbic acid present as sodium ascorbate.
Controlled-release of iron from the Gradumet protects against gastric side effects. The Gradumet is an inert, porous, plastic matrix which is impregnated with ferrous sulfate. Iron is leached from the Gradumet as it passes through the gastrointestinal tract, and the expended matrix is excreted harmlessly in the

stool. Controlled-release iron is particularly helpful in patients who have demonstrated intolerance to other oral iron preparations.
Actions: Oral iron is absorbed most efficiently when it is administered between meals. Conventional iron preparations, however, frequently cause gastric irritation when taken on an empty stomach. Studies with iron in the Gradumet have indicated that relatively little of the iron is released in the stomach, gastric intolerance is seldom encountered, and hematologic response ranks with that obtained from plain ferrous sulfate.
Large amounts of ascorbic acid administered orally with ferrous sulfate have been shown to enhance iron absorption. Apparently this is due to the ability of ascorbic acid to prevent the oxidation of ferrous iron to the less effectively absorbed ferric form.
Folic acid and iron are absorbed in the proximal small intestine, particularly the duodenum. Folic acid is absorbed maximally and rapidly at this site, and iron is absorbed in a descending gradient from the duodenum distally.
Except for the folates ingested in liver, yeast, and egg yolk, the percentage of absorption of food folates averages about 10%.
Indications: Fero-Folic-500 is indicated for the treatment of iron deficiency and prevention of concomitant folic acid deficiency in non-pregnant adults. Fero-Folic-500 is also indicated in pregnancy for the prevention and treatment of iron deficiency and to supply a maintenance dosage of folic acid.
Contraindications: Fero-Folic-500 is contraindicated in patients with pernicious anemia.
Warnings: Folic acid alone is improper therapy in the treatment of pernicious anemia and other megaloblastic anemias where vitamin B_{12} is deficient.
Precautions: Where anemia exists, its nature should be established and underlying causes determined.
Fero-Folic-500 contains 800 mcg. of folic acid per tablet. Folic acid especially in doses above 1.0 mg. daily may obscure pernicious anemia, in that hematologic remission may occur while neurological manifestations remain progressive. Accordingly, in older patients and those with conditions tending to lead to vitamin B_{12} depletion, serum B_{12} levels should be regularly assessed during treatment with Fero-Folic-500.
Concomitant parenteral therapy with vitamin B_{12} may be necessary in patients with deficiency of vitamin B_{12}. Pernicious anemia is rare in women of childbearing age, and the likelihood of its occurrence along with pregnancy is reduced by the impairment of fertility associated with vitamin B_{12} deficiency.
Like other oral iron preparations, Fero-Folic-500 should be stored out of the reach of children to guard against accidental iron poisoning (see Overdosage).
Adverse Reactions: The likelihood of gastric intolerance to controlled-release iron is remote. If such should occur, the tablet may be taken after a meal. Allergic sensitization has been reported following both oral and parenteral administration of folic acid.
Dosage and Administration: Fero-Folic-500 is administered orally and may be taken on an empty stomach.
Adults: For treatment of iron deficiency and prevention of folic acid deficiency, the recommended dose is one tablet daily.
Pregnant Adults: For prevention and treatment of iron deficiency and to supply a maintenance dosage of folic acid, the recommended dose is one tablet daily.
Overdosage: Signs of serious toxicity may be delayed because the iron is in a controlled-release dose form. Increased capillary permeability, reduced plasma volume, increased cardiac output, and sudden cardiovascular collapse may occur in acute iron intoxication. In overdosage, efforts should be made to hasten the elimination of the Gradumet tablets ingested. An emetic should be administered as soon as possible, followed by gastric lavage if indicated. Immediately following emesis, a large dose of a saline cathartic should be used to speed passage through the intestinal tract. X-ray examination may then be considered to determine the position and number of Gradumet tablets remaining in the gastrointestinal tract.
How Supplied: FERO-FOLIC-500 is supplied as red Filmtab tablets in bottles of 100 (**NDC** 0074-7079-13) and 500 (**NDC** 0074-7079-53).
[*Shown in Product Identification Section*]
Ref. 01-2772/R3

FERO-GRAD-500®
(Hematinic supplying controlled-release iron with vitamin C)
FERO-GRADUMET®
(Hematinic supplying controlled-release dose of iron)
Filmtab® tablets

Description: Fero-Gradumet and Fero-Grad-500 each contain the equivalent of 105 mg of elemental iron (525 mg of ferrous sulfate) in a unique controlled-release vehicle, the Gradumet®. In addition, Fero-Grad-500 contains 500 mg of vitamin C (as sodium ascorbate) to improve iron absorption.
The Gradumet, an inert, porous, plastic matrix, is impregnated with ferrous sulfate. Iron is leached from the Gradumet as it passes through the gastrointestinal tract, and the expended matrix is excreted harmlessly in the stool. Controlled-release iron is particularly helpful in patients who have demonstrated intolerance to other oral iron preparations.
Indications: Fero-Grad-500: For the treatment of iron deficiency in non-pregnant adults, and for the prevention and treatment of iron deficiency in pregnancy. Fero-Gradumet: For the prevention and treatment of iron deficiency.
Precautions: Where anemia exists, its nature should be established and underlying cause determined.
Like other oral iron preparations Fero-Gradumet and Fero-Grad-500 should be stored out of the reach of children to protect against accidental iron poisoning. (see Overdosage).
Adverse Reactions: The likehood of gastric intolerance to iron in the controlled-release Gradumet vehicle is slight. If it should occur, the tablet may be taken after a meal.
Dosage and Administration: Fero-Gradumet and Fero-Grad-500 are administered orally and may be taken on an empty stomach. The Gradumet controlled-release vehicle reduces the incidence of gastric side effects by delaying the release of almost all the iron until the tablet has passed the stomach.
Fero-Grad-500: Usual adult dose: One tablet daily, or as directed by the physician.
Fero-Gradumet: Usual adult dose: Prevention: One tablet daily; Treatment: One tablet twice daily, or as directed by the physician.
Overdosage: Signs of serious toxicity may be delayed because the iron is in a controlled-release dose form. Increased capillary permeability, reduced plasma volume, increased cardiac output, and sudden cardiovascular collapse may occur in acute iron intoxication. In overdosage, efforts should be made to hasten the elimination of the Gradumet tablets ingested. An emetic should be administered as soon as possible, followed by gastric lavage if indicated. Immediately following emesis, a large dose of a saline cathartic should be used to speed passage through the intestinal tract. X-ray examination may then be considered to determine the position and number of Gradumet tablets remaining in the gastrointestinal tract.
How Supplied: Fero-Gradumet is supplied as red tablets in bottles of 100 (**NDC** 0074-6852-02); Fero-Grad-500 is supplied as red tablets in bottles of 100 (**NDC** 0074-7238-01) and 500 (**NDC** 0074-7238-02). The ingredients of these products are listed in one or more of the Medicare designated compendia.
Ref. 02-5333-6/R22, 02-5307-5/R16

GEMONIL® ℞ Ⓒ
(Metharbital Tablets, NF)

Description: GEMONIL (metharbital) is a synthetic, N-methylated derivative of barbital which is identified chemically as 5,5-diethyl-1-methyl-barbituric acid.
Actions: GEMONIL produces anticonvulsant effects which are similar to those produced by phenobarbital and mephobarbital. In experimental animals the drug has been shown to be unusually effective against pentylenetetrazol-induced convulsions. GEMONIL is less effective against convulsions induced by electroshock. Toxicity studies in mice, rats, cats and dogs indicate that the drug is less toxic and has less sedative effect than phenobarbital.
GEMONIL is adequately absorbed from the gastrointestinal tract following oral administration. It is demethylated in the liver to barbital, and is excreted largely in this form by the kidneys.
Indications: GEMONIL is indicated for the control of grand mal, petit mal, myoclonic and mixed types of seizures.
Contraindications: GEMONIL is contraindicated in patients with known hypersensitivity to barbiturates, and in those with a history of manifest or latent porphyria.
Warnings: Metharbital may be habit forming.
USAGE DURING PREGNANCY AND LACTATION: THERE ARE MULTIPLE REPORTS IN THE CLINICAL LITERATURE WHICH INDICATE THAT THE USE OF ANTICONVULSANT DRUGS DURING PREGNANCY RESULTS IN AN INCREASED INCIDENCE OF BIRTH DEFECTS IN THE OFFSPRING. ALTHOUGH DATA ARE MORE EXTENSIVE WITH RESPECT TO TRIMETHADIONE, PARAMETHADIONE, PHENYTOIN, AND PHENOBARBITAL, REPORTS INDICATE A POSSIBLE SIMILAR ASSOCIATION WITH THE USE OF OTHER ANTICONVULSANT DRUGS. THEREFORE, ANTICONVULSANT DRUGS SHOULD BE ADMINISTERED TO WOMEN OF CHILDBEARING POTENTIAL ONLY IF THEY ARE CLEARLY SHOWN TO BE ESSENTIAL IN THE MANAGEMENT OF THEIR SEIZURES.
ANTICONVULSANT DRUGS SHOULD NOT BE DISCONTINUED IN PATIENTS IN WHOM THE DRUG IS ADMINISTERED TO PREVENT MAJOR SEIZURES BECAUSE OF THE STRONG POSSIBILITY OF PRECIPITATING STATUS EPILEPTICUS WITH ATTENDANT HYPOXIA AND RISK TO BOTH MOTHER AND THE UNBORN CHILD. CONSIDERATION SHOULD, HOWEVER, BE GIVEN TO DISCONTINUATION OF ANTICONVULSANTS PRIOR TO AND DURING PREGNANCY WHEN THE NATURE, FREQUENCY AND SEVERITY OF THE SEIZURES DO NOT POSE A SERIOUS THREAT TO THE PATIENT. IT IS NOT, HOWEVER, KNOWN WHETHER EVEN MINOR SEIZURES CONSTITUTE SOME RISK TO THE DEVELOPING EMBRYO OR FETUS.
REPORTS HAVE SUGGESTED THAT THE MATERNAL INGESTION OF ANTICONVULSANT DRUGS, PARTICULARLY BARBITURATES, IS ASSOCIATED WITH A NEONATAL COAGULATION DEFECT THAT MAY CAUSE BLEEDING DURING THE EARY (USUALLY WITHIN 24 HOURS OF BIRTH) NEONATAL PERIOD. THE POSSIBILITY OF THE OCCURRENCE OF THIS DEFECT WITH THE USE OF GEMONIL

Continued on next page

Abbott—Cont.

SHOULD BE KEPT IN MIND. THE DEFECT IS CHARACTERIZED BY DECREASED LEVELS OF VITAMIN K-DEPENDENT CLOTTING FACTORS, AND PROLONGATION OF EITHER THE PROTHROMBIN TIME OR THE PARTIAL THROMBOPLASTIN TIME, OR BOTH. IT HAS BEEN SUGGESTED THAT VITAMIN K BE GIVEN PROPHYLACTICALLY TO THE MOTHER ONE MONTH PRIOR TO AND DURING DELIVERY, AND TO THE INFANT, INTRAVENOUSLY, IMMEDIATELY AFTER BIRTH.
THE SAFETY OF GEMONIL FOR USE DURING LACTATION HAS NOT BEEN ESTABLISHED.
THE PHYSICIAN SHOULD WEIGH THESE CONSIDERATIONS IN TREATMENT AND COUNSELING OF EPILEPTIC WOMEN OF CHILDBEARING POTENTIAL.

Precautions: There is evidence that some barbiturates stimulate hepatic microsomal enzymes and therefore may increase the rate of metabolism of some drugs including the coumarin anticoagulants. Although metharbital has not been directly associated with such effect, caution is advised in patients receiving such anticoagulants.

Since metharbital is detoxified primarily in the liver, GEMONIL should be used with caution in patients with hepatic impairment.

In patients with convulsive disorders who have been taking regular daily doses, withdrawal of GEMONIL should be gradual since abrupt discontinuation of barbiturates given for the treatment of epilepsy may result in status epilepticus.

Adverse Reactions: GEMONIL (metharbital) has a low toxicity, and side effects are usually infrequent and mild. Gastric distress, dizziness, increased irritability, skin rash and drowsiness (large doses) may occur. If side effects become severe or cannot be controlled by dosage adjustment, the drug should be gradually withdrawn.

Dosage and Administration: GEMONIL is administered orally. As with all antiepileptic therapy, it is particularly important to adjust the dosage for each patient to obtain optimal effect. For adults, the usual starting dose is 100 mg, one to three times daily. The usual initial pediatric dose should be one-half of a 100 mg tablet, one to three times daily, depending on the age and weight of the patient. A dose of 5 to 15 mg/kg per day has been recommended for children. According to the patient's tolerance these dosages may be gradually increased to the level required to control seizures. In some cases very small doses may be effective, whereas in other instances as much as 600 to 800 mg daily are required for adequate control.

GEMONIL may be used alone or in conjunction with other antiepileptic drugs such as Tridione® (trimethadione), Paradione® (paramethadione), Phenurone® (phenacemide), Peganone® (ethotoin), phenytoin sodium, or mephenytoin. Frequently, more effective control of seizures can be achieved by a combination of drugs. When added to an established regimen to replace or supplement other anticonvulsant therapy, the dosage of other medication should be gradually reduced while increasing that of GEMONIL so as to avoid or minimize recurrence of seizures.

Overdosage: Symptoms of overdosage include drowsiness, irritability, dizziness, and gastric distress. Loss of consciousness and coma may occur following very high doses. Treatment is the same as that for barbiturate intoxication.

How Supplied: GEMONIL (metharbital tablets, NF) is supplied as grooved, 100 mg tablets in bottles of 100 (**NDC** 0074-6401-01).

This product is listed in N.F., a Medicare designated compendium.

Ref. 01-2007-R2

HARMONYL® ℞
(deserpidine)
Tablets

Description: Harmonyl (deserpidine) is a purified rauwolfia alkaloid chemically identified as 11-desmethoxyreserpine.

Actions: The pharmacologic actions of HARMONYL (deserpidine) are essentially the same as those of other active rauwolfia alkaloids. Deserpidine probably produces its antihypertensive effects through depletion of tissue stores of catecholamines (epinephrine and norepinephrine) from peripheral sites. By contrast, its sedative and tranquilizing properties are thought to be related to depletion of 5 - hydroxytryptamine from the brain.

The antihypertensive effect is often accompanied by bradycardia. There is no significant alteration in cardiac output or renal blood flow. The carotid sinus reflex is inhibited, but postural hypotension is rarely seen with the use of conventional doses of HARMONYL alone. Deserpidine, like other rauwolfia alkaloids, is characterized by slow onset of action and sustained effect which may persist following withdrawal of the drug.

Indications: HARMONYL (deserpidine) is indicated for the treatment of mild essential hypertension. It is also useful as adjunctive therapy with other antihypertensive agents in the more severe forms of hypertension.

The drug is also indicated for the relief of symptoms in agitated psychotic states, e.g., schizophrenia—primarily in those individuals unable to tolerate phenothiazine derivatives or those who also require antihypertensive medication.

Contraindications: HARMONYL (deserpidine) is contraindicated in patients with known hypersensitivity, mental depression especially with suicidal tendencies, active peptic ulcer, and ulcerative colitis. It is also contraindicated in patients receiving electroconvulsive therapy.

Warnings: Extreme caution should be exercised in treating patients with a history of mental depression. Discontinue the drug at the first sign of despondency, early morning insomnia, loss of appetite, impotence, or self-deprecation. Drug-induced depression may persist for several months after drug withdrawal and may be severe enough to result in suicide.

Usage in Pregnancy and Lactation
The safety of deserpidine for use during pregnancy or lactation has not been established; therefore, it should be used in pregnant women or in women of childbearing potential only when, in the judgment of the physician, its use is deemed essential to the welfare of the patient. Increased respiratory secretions, nasal congestion, cyanosis, and anorexia may occur in infants born to rauwolfia alkaloid-treated mothers since these preparations are known to cross the placental barrier to enter the fetal circulation and appear in cord blood. They also are secreted by nursing mothers into breast milk.

Studies in rats with deserpidine at multiples of the human therapeutic dose reduced the mating index and neonatal survival indices.

Precautions: Because rauwolfia preparations increase gastrointestinal motility and secretion, this drug should be used cautiously in patients with a history of peptic ulcer, ulcerative colitis, or gallstones, where biliary colic may be precipitated.

Caution should be exercised when treating hypertensive patients with renal insufficiency since they adjust poorly to lowered blood pressure levels.

Use HARMONYL (deserpidine) cautiously with digitalis and quinidine since cardiac arrhythmias have occurred with rauwolfia preparations.

Preoperative withdrawal of deserpidine does not assure that circulatory instability will not occur. It is important that the anesthesiologist be aware of the patient's drug intake and consider this in the over-all management, since hypotension has occurred in patients receiving rauwolfia preparations. Anticholinergic and/or adrenergic drugs (metaraminol, norepinephrine) have been employed to treat adverse vagocirculatory effects.

Adverse Reactions: The following adverse reactions have been reported with rauwolfia preparations. These reactions are usually reversible and disappear when the drug is discontinued.

Gastrointestinal: Including hypersecretion, anorexia, diarrhea, nausea, and vomiting.

Cardiovascular: Including angina-like symptoms, arrhythmias (particularly when used concurrently with digitalis or quinidine), and bradycardia.

Central Nervous System: Including drowsiness, depression, nervousness, paradoxical anxiety, nightmares, extrapyramidal tract symptoms, CNS sensitization manifested by dull sensorium, and deafness.

Dermatologic-Hypersensitivity: Including pruritus, rash, and asthma in asthmatic patients.

Ophthalmologic: Including glaucoma, uveitis, optic atrophy, and conjunctival injection.

Hematologic: Thrombocytopenic purpura.

Miscellaneous: Nasal congestion, weight gain, impotence or decreased libido, dysuria, dyspnea, muscular aches, dryness of mouth, dizziness, and headache.

Water retention with edema in patients with hypertensive vascular disease may occur rarely, but the condition generally clears with cessation of therapy or with the administration of a diuretic agent.

Dosage and Administration: HARMONYL (deserpidine) is administered orally. For the management of mild essential hypertension in the average patient not receiving other antihypertensive agents, the usual initial adult dose is 0.75 to 1 mg daily. Because 10 to 14 days are required to produce the full effects of the drug, adjustments in dosage should not be made more frequently. If the therapeutic response is not adequate, it is generally advisable to add another antihypertensive agent to the regimen. For maintenance, dosage should be reduced. A single daily dose of 0.25 mg of deserpidine may suffice for some patients.

Concomitant use of deserpidine with ganglionic blocking agents, guanethidine, veratrum, hydralazine, methyldopa, chlorthalidone, or thiazides necessitates careful titration of dosage with each agent.

For psychiatric disorders: The average initial oral dose is 0.5 mg daily with a range of 0.1 to 1 mg. Adjust dosage upward or downward according to the patient's response.

Overdosage: An overdosage of deserpidine is characterized by flushing of the skin, conjunctival injection, and pupillary constriction. Sedation ranging from drowsiness to coma may occur. Hypotension, hypothermia, central respiratory depression and bradycardia may develop in cases of severe overdosage.

Treatment consists of the careful evacuation of stomach contents followed by the usual procedures for the symptomatic management of CNS depressant overdosage. If severe hypotension occurs, it should be treated with a direct acting vasopressor such as Levophed® (levarterenol).

How Supplied: HARMONYL (deserpidine) Tablets, 0.1 mg, are yellow and supplied in bottles of 100 (**NDC** 0074-6901-01).

HARMONYL (deserpidine) Tablets (grooved), 0.25 mg, are salmon-pink and supplied in bottles of 100 (**NDC** 0074-6906-07) and 1000 (**NDC** 0074-6906-03).

[*Shown in Product Identification Section*]

Ref. No. 01-2019/R5

IBERET®-500
(Hematinic Supplying Controlled-Release Iron, Vitamin C and Vitamin B-Complex.*)
IBERET®
(Hematinic Supplying Controlled-Release Iron, Vitamin C and Vitamin B-Complex.*)
Filmtab® tablets

*Contains no folic acid

Description: Iberet-500 and Iberet Filmtab tablets contain 525 mg. of ferrous sulfate (equivalent to 105 mg. elemental iron) in the Gradumet® controlled-release vehicle. To enhance iron absorption, 500 mg. of vitamin C has been added to each Iberet-500 Filmtab.

The Gradumet is an inert, porous, plastic matrix which is impregnated with ferrous sulfate. Iron is leached from the Gradumet as it passes through the gastrointestinal tract, and the expended matrix is excreted harmlessly in the stool. Controlled-release iron is particularly helpful in patients who have demonstrated intolerance to other oral iron preparations.

Each Iberet-500 Filmtab tablet contains:
Ferrous Sulfate....................................525 mg.
(equivalent to 105 mg. of elemental iron)
Vitamin C (as sodium ascorbate)....................................500 mg.
Niacinamide....................................30 mg.
Calcium Pantothenate....................................10 mg.
Vitamin B_1 (Thiamine Mononitrate)....................................6 mg.
Vitamin B_2 (Riboflavin)....................................6 mg.
Vitamin B_6 (Pyridoxine Hydrochloride)....................................5 mg.
Vitamin B_{12} (Cyanocobalamin)....................................25 mcg.

The formulation of Iberet differs from Iberet-500 only in that it contains a lesser amount of vitamin C, 150 mg. per Filmtab tablet.

Indications: Iberet-500: For conditions in which iron deficiency occurs concomitantly with deficient intake or increased need for the B-complex vitamins.* Iberet: For conditions in which iron deficiency and vitamin C deficiency occur concomitantly with deficient intake or increased need for the B-complex vitamins.*

Precautions: Where anemia exists, its nature should be established and underlying cause determined.

Like other oral iron preparations, Iberet-500 and Iberet should be stored out of the reach of children to protect against accidental iron poisoning (see Overdosage).

Adverse Reactions: The likelihood of gastric intolerance to iron in the controlled-release Gradumet vehicle is slight. If it should occur, the tablet may be taken after a meal.

Dosage and Administration: Iberet-500 and Iberet are administered orally and may be taken on an empty stomach. Iberet-500: Usual Adult Dose: One tablet daily, or as directed by the physician. Iberet: Usual Adult Dose: One tablet daily, or as directed by the physician.

Overdosage: Signs of serious iron toxicity may be delayed because the iron is in a controlled-release dose form. Increased capillary permeability, reduced plasma volume, increased cardiac output, and sudden cardiovascular collapse may occur in acute iron intoxication. In overdosage, efforts should be made to hasten the elimination of the Gradumet tablets. An emetic should be administered as soon as possible, followed by gastric lavage if indicated. Immediately following emesis, a saline cathartic should be administered to hasten passage through the intestinal tract. X-ray examination may then be considered to determine the position and number of Gradumet tablets remaining in the gastrointestinal tract.

How Supplied: Iberet-500 is supplied as red, oval shaped tablets in bottles of 60 (**NDC** 0074-7235-01) and 500 (**NDC** 0074-7235-03); Iberet is supplied as red, round tablets in bottles of 60 (**NDC** 0074-6863-01) and 500 (**NDC** 0074-6863-02).

[*Shown in Product Identification Section*]
Ref. 02-4801-8/R19, 02-5132-6/R15

IBERET-FOLIC-500® ℞
(Controlled-Release Iron with Vitamin C, and B-Complex, including Folic Acid)
Filmtab® Tablets

Description: Iberet-Folic-500 is an Abbott hematinic containing iron in the Gradumet® controlled-release vehicle; vitamin C for enhancement of iron absorption; and the B-Complex vitamins including folic acid.

Each Filmtab tablet provides:
*Ferrous Sulfate....................................525 mg.
(equivalent to 105 mg. of elemental iron)
Ascorbic Acid (present as sodium ascorbate) (C)....................................500 mg.
Niacinamide....................................30 mg.
Calcium Pantothenate....................................10 mg.
Thiamine Mononitrate (B_1)....................................6 mg.
Riboflavin (B_2)....................................6 mg.
Pyridoxine Hydrochloride (B_6)....................................5 mg.
Folic Acid....................................800 mcg.
Cyanocobalamin (Vitamin B_{12})....................................25 mcg.
*In controlled-release form (Gradumet)

The Gradumet is an inert, porous, plastic matrix which is impregnated with ferrous sulfate. Iron is leached from the Gradumet as it passes through the gastrointestinal tract, and the expended matrix is excreted harmlessly in the stool. Controlled-release iron is particularly helpful in patients who have demonstrated intolerance to other oral iron preparations.

Actions: Oral iron is absorbed most efficiently when it is administered between meals. Conventional iron preparations, however, frequently cause gastric irritation when taken on an empty stomach. Studies with iron in the Gradumet have indicated that relatively little of the iron is released in the stomach, gastric intolerance is seldom encountered, and hematologic response ranks with that obtained from plain ferrous sulfate.

Large amounts of ascorbic acid administered orally with ferrous sulfate have been shown to enhance iron absorption. Apparently this is due to the ability of ascorbic acid to prevent the oxidation of ferrous iron to the less effectively absorbed ferric form.

Folic acid and iron are absorbed in the proximal small intestine, particularly the duodenum. Folic acid is absorbed maximally and rapidly at this site, and iron is absorbed in a descending gradient from the duodenum distally.

Except for the folates ingested in liver, yeast, and egg yolk, the percentage of absorption of food folates averages about 10%.

Indications: Iberet-Folic-500 is indicated in non-pregnant adults for the treatment of iron deficiency and prevention of concomitant folic acid deficiency where there is an associated deficient intake or increased need for the B-complex vitamins. Iberet-Folic-500 is also indicated in pregnancy for the prevention and treatment of iron deficiency where there is a concomitant deficient intake or increased need for B-complex vitamins (including folic acid).

Contraindications: Iberet-Folic-500 is contraindicated in patients with pernicious anemia.

Warnings: Folic acid alone is improper therapy in the treatment of pernicious anemia and other megaloblastic anemias where vitamin B_{12} is deficient.

Precautions: Where anemia exists, its nature should be established and underlying causes determined.

Iberet-Folic-500 contains 800 mcg. of folic acid per tablet. Folic acid especially in doses above 1.0 mg. daily may obscure pernicious anemia, in that hematologic remission may occur while neurological manifestations remain progressive. Accordingly, in older patients and those with conditions tending to lead to vitamin B_{12} depletion, serum B_{12} levels should be regularly assessed during treatment with Iberet-Folic-500. Concomitant parenteral therapy with vitamin B_{12} may be necessary in patients with deficiency of vitamin B_{12}. Pernicious anemia is rare in women of childbearing age, and the likelihood of its occurrence along with pregnancy is reduced by the impairment of fertility associated with vitamin B_{12} deficiency.

Like other oral iron preparations, Iberet-Folic-500 should be stored out of the reach of children to guard against accidental iron poisoning (see Overdosage).

Adverse Reactions: The likelihood of gastric intolerance to iron in the controlled release Gradumet vehicle is remote. If such should occur, the tablet may be taken after a meal. Allergic sensitization has been reported following both oral and parenteral administration of folic acid.

Dosage and Administration: Iberet-Folic-500 is administered orally and may be taken on an empty stomach.

Adults: For the treatment of iron deficiency and prevention of concomitant folic acid deficiency where there is an associated deficient intake or increased need for the B-complex vitamins, the recommended dose is one tablet daily.

Pregnant Adults: For the prevention and treatment of iron deficiency where there is a concomitant deficient intake or increased need for the B-complex vitamins including folic acid, the recommended dose is one tablet daily.

Overdosage: Signs of serious toxicity may be delayed because the iron is in a controlled-release dose form. Increased capillary permeability, reduced plasma volume, increased cardiac output, and sudden cardiovascular collapse may occur in acute iron intoxication. In overdosage, efforts should be made to hasten the elimination of the Gradumet tablets ingested. An emetic should be administered as soon as possible, followed by gastric lavage if indicated. Immediately following emesis, a large dose of a saline cathartic should be used to speed passage through the intestinal tract. X-ray examination may then be considered to determine the position and number of Gradumet tablets remaining in the gastrointestinal tract.

How Supplied: Iberet-Folic-500 is supplied as red Filmtab tablets in bottles of 60. (**NDC** 0074-7125-60)

[*Shown in Product Identification Section*]
Ref. 01-2771-R3

IBERET®-500 LIQUID
(Hematinic Supplying Iron, Vitamin C and Vitamin B-Complex*)
IBERET®-LIQUID
(Hematinic Supplying Iron, Vitamin C and Vitamin B-Complex*)

*Contains no folic acid

Description: Iberet-500 Liquid and Iberet-Liquid are hematinic preparations of ferrous sulfate, B-complex vitamins* and ascorbic acid.

Each teaspoonful (5 ml) of Iberet-500 Liquid provides:
Elemental Iron (as ferrous sulfate)....................................26.25 mg
Vitamin C (Ascorbic Acid)....................................125 mg
Niacinamide....................................7.5 mg
Dexpanthenol....................................2.5 mg
Vitamin B_1 (Thiamine Hydrochloride)....................................1.5 mg
Vitamin B_2 (Riboflavin)....................................1.5 mg
Vitamin B_6 (Pyridoxine Hydrochloride)....................................1.25 mg
Vitamin B_{12} (Cyanocobalamin)....................................6.25 mcg

In a citrus-flavored vehicle.

Iberet-Liquid has a raspberry-mint flavored vehicle, alcohol 1%; it has the same formula as Iberet-500 Liquid except for a smaller amount of ascorbic acid: 37.5 mg per teaspoonful.

Continued on next page

If desired, additional literature on any Abbott Product will be provided upon request to Abbott Laboratories.

Abbott—Cont.

Indications: Iberet-500 Liquid: For conditions in which iron deficiency occurs concomitantly with deficient intake or increased need for the B-complex vitamins.* Iberet-Liquid: For conditions in which iron deficiency and vitamin C deficiency occur concomitantly with deficient intake or increased need for the B-complex vitamins.*
Precautions: Where anemia exists, its nature should be established and underlying cause determined. Iberet-500 Liquid and Iberet-Liquid should be stored out of the reach of children because of the possibility of iron intoxication from accidental overdosage.
Adverse Reactions: If gastrointestinal symptoms appear as a sign of iron intolerance, smaller individual doses may be given at more frequent intervals to provide the desired daily amount. Administering Iberet-500 Liquid or Iberet-Liquid after meals may also reduce such effects.
Like other liquid iron preparations, Iberet-500 Liquid or Iberet-Liquid may stain the teeth on continued use. Stains may be prevented to a large extent by taking the dose through a straw, first mixing it with water or fruit juice, and by following the dose with a drink of plain water or juice. Brushing the teeth with sodium bicarbonate or hydrogen peroxide will usually remove existing stains.
Dosage and Administration: Iberet-500 Liquid and Iberet-Liquid are administered orally, preferably after meals. Each has a fruit-flavored vehicle, and is suitable for pediatric patients who are unable to take tablets or capsules, and for patients who prefer or can better tolerate liquid medication. Iberet-500 Liquid and Iberet-Liquid may be administered by spoon or incorporated into infant formulas, water, or fruit juices. Iberet-500 Liquid: Usual dosage: Adults and children 4 years of age and older—2 teaspoonfuls (10 ml) twice daily, after meals; Children 1–3 years of age—1 teaspoonful (5 ml) twice daily, after meals. Otherwise as directed by the physician. Iberet-Liquid: Usual dosage: Adults and children 4 years of age and older—2 teaspoonfuls (10 ml) three times daily, after meals; Children 1–3 years of age—1 teaspoonful (5 ml) three times daily, after meals. Otherwise as directed by the physician.
How Supplied: Iberet-500 Liquid (**NDC** 0074-8422-02) and Iberet-Liquid (**NDC** 0074-7173-01) are supplied in 8 fl oz bottles.
Ref. 02-5560-3/R13, 02-5561-4/R11

JANIMINE® ℞
(imipramine hydrochloride tablets, U.S.P.)
Filmtab® Tablets

How Supplied: JANIMINE (imipramine hydrochloride) is provided in three dosage sizes as monogrammed Filmtab tablets:

10 mg, round-shaped, orange-colored, in bottles of 100 (**NDC** 0074-1897-13) and bottles of 1000 (**NDC** 0074-1897-19).

25 mg. round-shaped, yellow, in bottles of 100 (**NDC** 0074-1898-13) and bottles of 1000 (**NDC** 0074-1898-19).

50 mg, ovaloid-shaped, peach-colored, in bottles of 100 (**NDC** 0074-1899-13) and bottles of 1000 (**NDC** 0074-1899-19).

[*Shown in Product Identification Section*]

K-LOR™ ℞
(Potassium Chloride for Oral Solution, U.S.P.)
Powder

Description: Natural fruit-flavored K-LOR 20 mEq (Potassium Chloride for Oral Solution, USP) and K-LOR 15 mEq (Potassium Chloride for Oral Solution, USP) are for oral use and are offered in individual packets. Each packet of K-LOR 20 mEq contains potassium 20 mEq and chloride 20 mEq provided by potassium chloride 1.5 Gm. Each packet of K-LOR 15 mEq contains potassium 15 mEq and chloride 15 mEq provided by potassium chloride 1.125 Gm.
Indications: K-LOR is indicated in the treatment and prevention of hypokalemia and hypochloremic alkalosis where the severity of the condition does not warrant parenteral therapy. Conditions or factors which may give rise to potassium deficiency include diarrhea and vomiting, decreased potassium intake, increased renal excretion of potassium which may occur in acidosis, diuresis, adrenocortical hyperactivity, or the administration of exogenous adrenocortical steroids, injection of potassium-free fluids, and increased glucose uptake such as occurs in insulin-treated diabetic acidosis.
Potassium chloride may be particularly useful to help prevent the hypokalemia which may be induced by the administration of most diuretic agents.
Contraindications: Potassium chloride is contraindicated in the presence of severe renal impairment with oliguria or azotemia, untreated Addison's disease, adynamia episodica hereditaria, acute dehydration, heat cramps, and hyperkalemia from any cause.
Potassium chloride should not be employed in patients receiving potassium-sparing agents such as aldosterone antagonists and triamterene.
Precautions: With normal kidney function, potassium intoxication from oral administration is not likely to occur, since renal excretion of the ion increases in response to a rise in the concentration of body potassium. Nevertheless, potassium supplements must be administered with caution, since the dietary or daily amount is not accurately known. Frequent checks of the patient's clinical status and periodic ECG and/or serum potassium levels should be done. High serum concentrations of potassium ion may result in death through cardiac depression, arrhythmia, or arrest. The drug should be used with caution in the presence of cardiac disease and systemic acidosis.
Adverse Reactions: Side effects include abdominal discomfort, nausea, vomiting, and diarrhea.
In the presence of renal dysfunction it may be possible to induce hyperkalemia by oral administration of potassium salts. The symptoms and signs of potassium intoxication include paresthesias of the extremities, weakness and heaviness of the legs, flaccid paralysis, listlessness, mental confusion, fall in blood pressure, cardiac arrhythmias, and heart block. Electrocardiographic abnormalities such as disappearance of the P wave, widening and slurring of the QRS complex, changes of the S-T segment and tall peaked T waves may be noted with hyperkalemia.
Dosage and Administration: The dosage depends on the severity of the condition. The usual adult dose is 20 to 80 mEq of potassium per day (1 K-LOR 20 mEq packet 1 to 4 times daily after meals, or 1 K-LOR 15 mEq packet 2 to 5 times daily after meals).
Each 20 mEq (one K-LOR 20 mEq packet) of potassium should be dissolved in at least 4 oz (approximately ½ glassful) cold water or juice. Each 15 mEq (one K-LOR 15 mEq packet) of potassium should be dissolved in at least 3 oz (approximately ½ glassful) cold water or juice. These preparations, like other potassium supplements, must be properly diluted to avoid the possibility of gastrointestinal irritation.
Treatment of Hyperkalemia: Should hyperkalemia occur, treatment measures include the following: (1) elimination of foods or medications containing potassium, (2) the intravenous administration of 300 to 500 ml/hr of dextrose solution (10 or 25%), containing 10 units of insulin/20 Gm dextrose, (3) the use of exchange resins, hemodialysis, or peritoneal dialysis.
In treating hyperkalemia, it should be recalled that in patients who have been stabilized on digitalis, too rapid a lowering of the plasma potassium concentration can produce digitalis toxicity.
How Supplied: K-Lor 20 mEq (Potassium Chloride for Oral Solution, USP) is supplied in cartons of 30 packets (**NDC** 0074-3611-01) and in cartons of 100 packets (**NDC** 0074-3611-02). Each packet contains potassium, 20 mEq and chloride, 20 mEq, provided by potassium chloride, 1.5 Gm.
K-Lor 15 mEq (Potassium Chloride for Oral Solution, USP) is supplied in cartons of 100 packets (**NDC** 0074-3633-11). Each packet contains potassium, 15 mEq, and chloride, 15 mEq, provided by potassium chloride, 1.125 Gm.
[*Shown in Product Identification Section*]
Ref. No. 01-2982/R4

LIDOCAINE HYDROCHLORIDE INJECTION, U.S.P. ℞
Aqueous solutions for acute management of cardiac arrhythmias or for local anesthesia.

Description: Lidocaine hydrochloride is designated chemically as 2-(diethylamino)-2′, 6′-acetoxylidide monohydrochloride and is freely soluble in water. Lidocaine occurs as colorless crystals. The injectable preparation is an aqueous solution of the freely soluble hydrochloride salt. pH adjusted with sodium hydroxide and hydrochloric acid.

FOR CARDIAC ARRHYTHMIAS

Actions: Lidocaine reportedly exerts a cardiac antiarrhythmic effect by increasing the electrical stimulation threshold of the ventricle during diastole. At usual doses, lidocaine produces no change in myocardial contractility, in systemic arterial pressure or in absolute refractory period.
About 90% of an administered dose of the drug is metabolized in the liver. The remaining 10% is excreted unchanged in the urine.
Indications: Lidocaine administered intravenously is specifically indicated in the acute management of (1) ventricular arrhythmias occurring during cardiac manipulation; such as cardiac surgery; and (2) life-threatening arrhythmias, particularly those which are ventricular in origin, such as occur during acute myocardial infarction.
Contraindications: Lidocaine is contraindicated in patients with a known hypersensitivity to local anesthetics of the amide type.
Intravenous injection is contraindicated in patients with Adams-Stokes syndrome or with severe degrees of sinoatrial, atrioventricular or intraventricular heart block.
Warnings: Constant monitoring with an electrocardiograph is essential for proper intravenous administration of lidocaine. Signs of excessive depression of cardiac conductivity, such as prolongation of PR interval and QRS complex and appearance or aggravation of arrhythmias, should be followed by prompt cessation of intravenous injection or infusion of this agent. It is mandatory to have emergency equipment and drugs immediately available to manage possible adverse reactions involving the cardiovascular, respiratory or central nervous systems. Evidence for proper use in children is limited.
Precautions: Caution should be exercised with repeated use of lidocaine in patients with severe liver or renal disease because accumulation may lead to toxic phenomena, since the drug is metabolized mainly in the liver and partially excreted unchanged by the kidney. The drug also should be used with caution in patients with hypovolemia and shock, and all forms of heart block (see CONTRAINDICATIONS and WARNINGS).
In patients with sinus bradycardia the intravenous administration of lidocaine for the elimination of ventricular ectopic beats without prior acceleration in heart rate (e.g., by isopro-

terenol or by electric pacing) may provoke more frequent and serious ventricular arrhythmias.

Adverse Reactions: Systemic reactions of the following types have been reported:

1. Central Nervous System: Light-headedness; drowsiness; dizziness; apprehension; euphoria; tinnitus; blurred or double vision; vomiting; sensation of heat, cold or numbness; twitching; tremors; convulsions; unconsciousness and respiratory depression and arrest.
2. Cardiovascular System: Hypotension; cardiovascular collapse and bradycardia which may lead to cardiac arrest.

There have been no reports of cross sensitivity between lidocaine and procainamide or between lidocaine and quinidine.

Management of Adverse Reactions:

1. In case of severe reaction, discontinue use of the drug.
2. Institute the emergency resuscitative procedures and administer the emergency drugs necessary to manage the severe reaction.
3. For severe convulsions, small doses of an ultrashort-acting barbiturate or a short-acting muscle relaxant (if the patient is under anesthesia) may be used.

Dosage and Administration: For direct intravenous injection, the usual adult dose is 50 to 100 mg. administered at an approximate rate of 25 to 50 mg./minute. Sufficient time should be allowed to enable a slow circulation to carry the drug to the site of action. If the initial injection of 50 to 100 mg. does not produce the desired response, a second dose may be repeated after five minutes.

NO MORE THAN 200 TO 300 MG. OF LIDOCAINE SHOULD BE ADMINISTERED DURING A ONE-HOUR PERIOD.

Patients with reduced hepatic function or diminished hepatic blood flow (as in heart failure and after cardiac surgery), or those over 70 years of age, should receive half the usual loading dose and also receive lower maintenance doses of intravenous lidocaine.

In children, experience with the drug is limited.

For continuous intravenous infusion in patients whose arrhythmia tends to recur following a temporary response to a single or once repeated direct injection, and who are incapable of receiving oral antiarrhythmic therapy, lidocaine hydrochloride may be infused continuously in a concentration of 0.1% (1 mg./ml.) at a rate of 1 to 4 ml./minute (20 to 50 micrograms/kg./minute in the average 70 kg. adult). A 0.2% solution (2 mg./ml.) can be given at a rate of 0.5 to 2 ml./minute. I.V. infusion of the drug must be administered under constant ECG monitoring to avoid potential overdosage and toxicity. I.V. infusion should be terminated as soon as the patient's basic cardiac rhythm appears to be stable or at the earliest signs of toxicity. As soon as possible, and when indicated, patients should be changed to an oral antiarrhythmic agent for maintenance therapy.

When administering lidocaine hydrochloride (or any potent medication) by continuous intravenous infusion, it is advisable to use a precision volume control I.V. set.

A 0.1% solution (1 mg./ml.) for I.V. infusion may be prepared by the addition of one gram of lidocaine hydrochloride injected through the rubber stopper of a 1000 ml bottle of 5% Dextrose Injection (preferred diluent). Infusion of such solution at a rate of 1 to 4 ml./minute will provide approximately 1 to 4 mg./minute.

A 0.2% solution can be prepared by adding two grams of lidocaine hydrochloride to 1000 ml of 5% Dextrose Injection. The rate of administration sufficient to provide 1 to 4 mg./minute is 0.5 to 2 ml./minute.

FOR LOCAL ANESTHESIA

Actions: Lidocaine stabilizes the neuronal membrane and prevents the initiation and transmission of nerve impulses, thereby effecting local anesthetic action.

The onset of action is rapid and the blockade may last from one to one and one-half hours.

Lidocaine, because of its non-ester structure, is not detoxified by the circulating plasma esterases. The liver is the chief site of biotransformation of the drug, and both free and conjugated forms of the drug are excreted in the urine.

Lidocaine does not ordinarily produce irritation or tissue damage following parenteral administration.

Anesthesia may be extended and absorption retarded by the addition of a dilute concentration of epinephrine or other appropriate vasoconstrictor drug.

Indications: Lidocaine hydrochloride injection USP is indicated for production of local anesthesia by nerve block, infiltration injection, caudal or other epidural blocks.

Contraindications: Lidocaine is contraindicated in patients with a known hypersensitivity to local anesthetics of the amide type.

Local anesthetic agents should not be used in patients with severe shock or heart block. Local anesthetic procedures should not be used when there is inflammation in the region of the proposed injection.

Warnings: RESUSCITATIVE EQUIPMENT AND DRUGS SHOULD BE IMMEDIATELY AVAILABLE WHEN ANY LOCAL ANESTHETIC IS USED.

Solutions which contain a vasoconstrictor should be used with extreme caution in patients whose medical history and physical evaluation suggest the existence of hypertension, arteriosclerotic heart disease, cerebral vascular insufficiency, heart block, thyrotoxicosis and diabetes, etc.

Solutions mixed with epinephrine or other vasopressor agents should be used with extreme caution in patients receiving drugs known to produce blood pressure alterations (i.e., MAO inhibitors, tricyclic antidepressants, phenothiazines, etc.) as either severe and sustained hypotension or hypertension may occur.

Usage in Pregnancy: Safe use of lidocaine has not been established with respect to possible adverse effects upon fetal development. Therefore, lidocaine should not be used in women of childbearing potential and particularly during early pregnancy unless, in the judgment of the clinician the potential benefits outweigh the unknown hazards.

This does not exclude use of the drug at term for obstetrical analgesia. Lidocaine has been used effectively for obstetrical analgesia. Adverse effects on the fetus, course of labor or delivery are rare when proper dosage and technique are used. For paracervical block during labor or pudendal block during delivery, the use of local anesthesia without epinephrine is recommended.

In obstetrics, if vasopressor drugs are used either to correct hypotension or added to the local anesthetic solution, it should be noted that some oxytocic drugs may cause severe persistent hypertension and even rupture of a cerebral blood vessel may occur during the postpartum period.

Precautions: The safety and effectiveness of lidocaine depends upon proper dosage, correct technique, adequate precautions and readiness for emergencies.

The lowest dosage that results in effective anesthesia should be used to avoid high plasma levels and serious undesirable systemic side effects.

Injection of repeated doses of lidocaine may cause significant increases in blood levels with each repeated dose due to slow accumulation of the drug or its metabolites or due to slow metabolic degradation. Tolerance varies with the status of the patient. Debilitated, elderly patients, acutely ill patients and children should be given doses commensurate with their age and physical status.

Injection should always be made slowly after aspiration to avoid or reduce the possibility of inadvertent intravascular injection. Intravascular injection may result in serious adverse reactions as well as anesthetic failure.

Lidocaine should be used cautiously in patients with known drug allergies or sensitivities. Patients allergic to a para-aminobenzoic acid ester type of local anesthetic (e.g., procaine, tetracaine, etc.) have not shown cross sensitivity to lidocaine.

Caudal or other epidural block anesthesia should be used with extreme caution in patients with existing neurological disease, spinal deformities, septicemia or severe hypertension and in very young patients.

Solutions admixed with epinephrine or other vasopressor agents should be used with caution in the presence of diseases which may adversely affect the patient's cardiovascular system.

Solutions containing a vasoconstrictor should be used cautiously and in carefully circumscribed quantities in areas of the body supplied by end arteries or having otherwise compromised blood supply (e.g., digits, nose, external ear, penis, etc.).

The decision whether or not to use local anesthesia in the following conditions depends on the physician's appraisal of the advantages as opposed to the risk:

1. Paracervical block when fetal distress is anticipated or when predisposing factors causative of fetal distress are present (i.e., toxemia, prematurity, diabetes, etc.). Fetal bradycardia frequently follows paracervical block and may be associated with fetal acidosis. Fetal heart rate should always be monitored during paracervical anesthesia. When the recommended dose is exceeded the incidence of fetal bradycardia increases.
2. Serious cardiac arrhythmias may occur if preparations containing a vasoconstrictor are employed in patients following the administration of chloroform, trichloroethylene, halothane, etc.

Adverse Reactions: Adverse reactions result from high plasma levels due to rapid absorption, inadvertent intravascular injection, or excessive dosage. Other causes of reactions are hypersensitivity, idiosyncrasy or diminished tolerance.

Reactions due to overdosage (high plasma levels) are systemic and involve the central nervous system and the cardiovascular system.

Reactions involving the central nervous system are characterized by excitation and/or depression. Nervousness, dizziness, blurred vision or tremors may occur followed by drowsiness, convulsions, unconsciousness and possible respiratory arrest. Excitement may be transient or absent, and the first manifestations may be drowsiness merging into unconsciousness and respiratory arrest.

Reactions involving the cardiovascular system include depression of the myocardium, hypotension, bradycardia, and even cardiac arrest.

Allergic reactions are characterized by cutaneous lesions of delayed onset, or urticaria, edema and other manifestations of allergy. The detection of sensitivity by skin testing is of doubtful value.

Treatment of a patient with toxic manifestations consists of maintaining an airway, and supporting ventilation using oxygen and assisted or controlled respiration is required. Supportive treatment of the cardiovascular system consists of using vasopressors, preferably those that stimulate the myocardium (e.g., epinephrine, metaraminol, etc.) and intravenous fluids and, when necessary, external cardiac massage. Convulsions may be con-

If desired, additional literature on any Abbott Product will be provided upon request to Abbott Laboratories.

Continued on next page

Abbott—Cont.

trolled by the intravenous administration of small increments of an anticonvulsive agent such as benzodiazepine (e.g., diazepem) or an ultrashort-acting barbiturate (i.e., thiopental, thiamylal) or a short-acting barbiturate (secobarbital, pentobarbital) or, if these are not available, a short-acting muscle relaxant (succinylcholine), together with oxygen. Muscle relaxants and intravenous barbiturates should only be used by those familiar with their use.

Dosage and Administration: The dosage varies and depends upon the area to be anesthetized, vascularity of the tissues, number of neuronal segments to be blocked, individual tolerance and the technique of anesthesia. The lowest dosage needed to provide effective anesthesia should be administered. For specific techniques and procedures refer to standard textbooks.

THE USUAL INITIAL ADULT DOSE OF LIDOCAINE HYDROCHLORIDE WITHOUT EPINEPHRINE SHOULD NOT EXCEED 2 MG PER POUND.

THE USUAL INITIAL ADULT DOSE WITH EPINEPHRINE SHOULD NOT EXCEED 3 MG PER POUND.

Use of 0.5 or 1% concentrations of lidocaine is recommended in children to minimize the possibility of toxic reactions and the total dose should be reduced in proportion to body weight or surface area.

FOR EPIDURAL OR SPINAL ANESTHESIA, USE ONLY SOLUTIONS WITHOUT PRESERVATIVES

How Supplied: Lidocaine Hydrochloride Injection, U.S.P. is available in a variety of dosage strengths, containers and sizes. Consult Abbott Laboratories for a current listing.

LIDONE® ℞
(molindone hydrochloride)
Capsules

Description: LIDONE (molindone hydrochloride) is a dihydroindolone compound which is not structurally related to the phenothiazines, the butyrophenones or the thioxanthenes.

LIDONE is 3-ethyl-6, 7-dihydro-2-methyl-5-(morpholinomethyl) indol-4(5H)-one hydrochloride. It is a white crystalline powder, freely soluble in water and alcohol and has a molecular weight of 312.67.

Actions: LIDONE has a pharmacological profile in laboratory animals which predominantly resembles that of major tranquilizers causing reduction of spontaneous locomotion and aggressiveness, suppression of a conditioned response and antagonism of the bizarre stereotyped behavior and hyperactivity induced by amphetamines. In addition, LIDONE antagonizes the depression caused by the tranquilizing agent tetrabenazine.

In human clinical studies tranquilization is achieved in the absence of muscle relaxing or incoordinating effects. Based on EEG studies, LIDONE exerts its effect on the ascending reticular activating system.

Human metabolic studies show LIDONE to be rapidly absorbed and metabolized when given orally. Unmetabolized drug reached a peak blood level at 1.5 hours. Pharmacological effect from a single oral dose persists for 24 to 36 hours. There are 36 recognized metabolites with less than 2 to 3% unmetabolized LIDONE being excreted in urine and feces.

Indications: LIDONE is indicated in the management of the manifestations of schizophrenia.

Contraindications: LIDONE is contraindicated in severe central nervous system depression (alcohol, barbiturates, narcotics, etc.) or comatose states, and in patients with known hypersensitivity to the drug.

Warnings:

Usage in Pregnancy: Studies in pregnant patients have not been carried out. Reproduction studies have been performed in the following animals:

Pregnant Rats Oral Dose—
20 mg/kg/day—10 days, no adverse effect
40 mg/kg/day—10 days, no adverse effect

Pregnant Mice Oral Dose—
20 mg/kg/day—10 days, slight increase resorptions
40 mg/kg/day—10 days, slight increase resorptions

Pregnant Rabbits Oral Dose—
5 mg/kg/day—12 days, no adverse effect
10 mg/kg/day—12 days, no adverse effect
20 mg/kg/day—12 days, no adverse effect

Animal reproductive studies have not demonstrated a teratogenic potential. The anticipated benefits must be weighed against the unknown risks to the fetus if used in pregnant patients.

Nursing Mothers: Data are not available on the content of LIDONE in the milk of nursing mothers.

Usage in Children: Use of LIDONE in children below the age of twelve years is not recommended because safe and effective conditions for its usage have not been established.

LIDONE has not been shown effective in the management of behavioral complications in patients with mental retardation.

Precautions: Some patients receiving LIDONE may note drowsiness initially and they should be advised against activities requiring mental alertness until their response to the drug has been established.

Increased activity has been noted in patients receiving LIDONE. Caution should be exercised where increased activity may be harmful.

LIDONE does not lower the seizure threshold in experimental animals to the degree noted with more sedating antipsychotic drugs. However, in humans convulsive seizures have been reported in a few instances.

LIDONE has an antiemetic effect in animals. A similar effect may occur in humans and may obscure signs of intestinal obstruction or brain tumor.

Adverse Reactions:

CNS Effects

The most frequently occurring effect is initial drowsiness that generally subsides with continued usage of the drug or lowering of the dose.

Noted less frequently were depression, hyperactivity and euphoria.

Neurological Extrapyramidal Reactions

Extrapyramidal reactions noted below may occur in susceptible individuals and are usually reversible with appropriate management.

Akathisia: Motor restlessness may occur early.

Parkinson Syndrome: Akinesia, characterized by rigidity, immobility and reduction of voluntary movements and tremor, have been observed. Occurrence is less frequent than akathisia.

Dystonic Syndrome: Prolonged abnormal contractions of muscle groups occur infrequently. These symptoms may be managed by the addition of a synthetic antiparkinson agent (other than L-dopa), small doses of sedative drugs, and/or reduction in dosage.

Autonomic Nervous System

Occasionally blurring of vision, tachycardia, nausea, dry mouth and salivation have been reported. Urinary retention and constipation may occur particularly if anticholinergic drugs are used to treat extrapyramidal symptoms.

Hematological

There have been rare reports of leucopenia and leucocytosis. If such reactions occur, treatment with LIDONE may continue if clinical symptoms are absent. Alterations of blood glucose, liver function tests, B.U.N., and red blood cells have not been considered clinically significant.

Metabolic and Endocrine Effects

Alteration of thyroid function has not been significant. Amenorrhea has been reported infrequently. Resumption of menses in previously amenorrheic women has been reported. Initially heavy menses may occur. Galactorrhea and gynecomastia have been reported infrequently. Increase in libido has been noted in some patients. Impotence has not been reported. Although both weight gain and weight loss have been in the direction of normal or ideal weight, excessive weight gain has not occurred with LIDONE.

Cardiovascular

Rare, transient, non-specific T wave changes have been reported on EKG. Association with a clinical syndrome has not been established. Rarely has significant hypotension been reported.

Ophthalmological

Lens opacities and pigmentary retinopathy have not been reported where patients have received LIDONE (molindone hydrochloride). In some patients, phenothiazine induced lenticular opacities have resolved following discontinuation of the phenothiazine while continuing therapy with LIDONE.

Skin

Early, non-specific skin rash, probably of allergic origin, has occasionally been reported. Skin pigmentation has not been seen with LIDONE usage alone.

LIDONE has certain pharmacological similarities to other antipsychotic agents. Because adverse reactions are often extensions of the pharmacological activity of a drug, all of the known pharmacological effects associated with other antipsychotic drugs should be kept in mind when LIDONE is used. Upon abrupt withdrawal after prolonged high dosage an abstinence syndrome has not been noted.

Tardive Dyskinesia

Although rarely reported with LIDONE, symptoms were reversible upon discontinuation of therapy.

Tardive dyskinesia associated with other agents has appeared in some patients on long-term therapy and has also appeared after drug therapy has been discontinued. The risk appears to be greater in elderly patients on high-dose therapy, especially females. The symptoms are persistent and in some patients appear to be irreversible. The syndrome is characterized by rhythmical involuntary movements of the tongue, face, mouth or jaw (e.g., protrusion of tongue, puffing of cheeks, puckering of mouth, chewing movements). There may be involuntary movements of extremities.

There is no known effective treatment of tardive dyskinesia; antiparkinsonism agents usually do not alleviate the symptoms of this syndrome. It is suggested that all antipsychotic agents be discontinued if these symptoms appear. Should it be necessary to reinstitute treatment or increase the dosage of the agent, or switch to a different agent, the syndrome may be masked. It has been reported that fine vermicular movements of the tongue may be an early sign of the syndrome and if the medication is stopped at that time the syndrome may not develop.

Dosage and Administration: Initial and maintenance doses of LIDONE should be individualized.

Initial Dosage Schedule

The usual starting dosage is 50 to 75 mg/day.

— Increase to 100 mg/day in three or four days.
— Based on severity of symptomatology, dosage may be titrated up or down depending on individual patient response.
— An increase to 225 mg/day may be required in patients with severe symptomatology.

Elderly or debilitated patients should be started on lower dosage.

Maintenance Dosage Schedule

1. Mild — 5 mg to 15 mg three or four times a day.
2. Moderate — 10 mg to 25 mg three or four times a day.
3. Severe — 225 mg/day may be required.

Drug Interactions: Potentiation of drugs administered concurrently with LIDONE has not been reported. Additionally, animal studies

have not shown increased toxicity when LIDONE is given concurrently with representative members of three classes of drugs (i.e., barbiturates, chloral hydrate and antiparkinson drugs).
Management of Overdosage: Symptomatic, supportive therapy should be the rule.
Gastric lavage is indicated for the reduction of absorption of LIDONE which is freely soluble in water.
Since the adsorption of LIDONE by activated charcoal has not been determined, the use of this antidote must be considered of theoretical value.
Emesis in a comatose patient is contraindicated. Additionally, while the emetic effect of apomorphine is blocked by LIDONE in animals, this blocking effect has not been determined in humans.
A significant increase in the rate of removal of unmetabolized LIDONE from the body by forced diuresis, peritoneal or renal dialysis would not be expected. (Only 2% of a single ingested dose of LIDONE is excreted unmetabolized in the urine). However, poor response of the patient may justify use of these procedures.
While the use of laxatives or enemas might be based on general principles, the amount of unmetabolized LIDONE in feces is less than 1%.
Extrapyramidal symptoms have responded to the use of diphenhydramine (Bendadryl*) and the synthetic anticholinergic antiparkinson agents (i.e., Artane*, Cogentin*, Akineton*).
How Supplied: LIDONE (molindone hydrochloride) capsules are supplied in bottles of 100 in the following dosage strengths and colors:
5 mg (**NDC** 0074-5542-13) blue and cream,
10 mg (**NDC** 0074-5543-13) red and cream,
25 mg (**NDC** 0074-5544-13) brown and cream.

U.S. Pat. 3,491,093
*Benadryl—Trademark, Parke Davis and Co.
*Artane—Trademark, Lederle Laboratories
*Cogentin—Trademark, Merck Sharp & Dohme
*Akineton—Trademark, Knoll Pharmaceutical Co.
Ref. 01-2038-R4
[Shown in Product Identification Section]

MURINE EAR WAX REMOVAL SYSTEM/MURINE EAR DROPS — OTC

Description: Carbamide peroxide 6.5% in anhydrous glycerin and a 1.0 fl. oz. soft rubber ear syringe. The MURINE EAR WAX REMOVAL SYSTEM is the only self-treatment method on the market for complete ear wax removal. Application of carbamide peroxide drops followed by warm water irrigation is the only effective, medically recommended way to remove hardened ear wax.
Actions: The carbamide peroxide formula in MURINE EAR DROPS is an aid in the removal of hardened cerumen from the ear canal. Anhydrous glycerin penetrates and softens wax while the release of oxygen from carbamide peroxide provides a mechanical action resulting in the loosening of the softened wax accumulation. It is usually necessary to remove the loosened wax by gentle irrigation with warm water using the soft rubber ear syringe provided.
Indications: The MURINE EAR WAX REMOVAL SYSTEM is indicated as an aid in the removal of hardened or tightly packed cerumen from the ear canal or as an aid in the prevention of ceruminosis.
Caution: If redness, tenderness, pain, dizziness or ear drainage are present or develop, the medication should not be used or continued until a physician is seen. Do not use if ear drum is known to be perforated.
Dosage and Administration: For wax removal, place five drops into affected ear twice daily for three or four days. Tip of bottle should not enter ear canal. Remove softened wax after each application by gently flushing ear with warm (body temperature) water using the soft rubber ear syringe provided. Tip of syringe should be at the edge of the ear canal.
The ear canal can be kept free from accumulated hardened cerumen by regular usage of the MURINE EAR WAX REMOVAL SYSTEM.
How Supplied: The MURINE EAR WAX REMOVAL SYSTEM contains 0.5 fl. oz. drops and a 1.0 fl. oz. soft rubber ear syringe.
Also available in 0.5 fl. oz. drops only, MURINE EAR DROPS

MURINE® — OTC
Eye Drops

Description: Murine® Regular Formula is a sterile isotonic buffered solution containing glycerin, methylcellulose, potassium chloride, sodium chloride, sodium phosphate (monobasic and dibasic), and water. Disodium edetate 0.05% and benzalkonium chloride 0.01% are added as preservatives.
Indications: Murine is non-staining, clear solution formulated to closely match the natural fluid of the eye for gentle, soothing relief from minor eye irritation. Use whenever desired to cleanse or refresh the eyes and to relieve minor irritation due to smog, sun glare, wind, dust, wearing contact lenses and overuse of the eyes in reading, driving, TV and close work.
Warning: Murine Regular Formula should only be used for minor eye irritations. If relief is not obtained within 48 hours, or if irritation persists or increases, discontinue use and consult your physician.
Dosage and Administration: Two or three drops into each eye several times a day or as directed by a physician. Do not touch bottle tip to any surface since this may contaminate solution. Remove contact lenses before using. Keep container tightly closed. Keep this and all medications out of reach of children.
How Supplied: In 0.6 fl. oz. and 1.5 fl. oz. plastic dropper bottle.

MURINE® PLUS — OTC
Eye Drops

Description: Murine® Plus is a sterile isotonic buffered solution containing tetrahydrozoline hydrochloride 0.05%, boric acid, sodium acetate and water. Disodium edetate, 0.1% and benzalkonium chloride 0.01% are added as preservatives.
Indications: Murine Plus is a decongestant ophthalmic solution designed to refresh and soothe as it removes redness from irritated eyes. Murine Plus contains laboratory tested, and scientifically blended ingredients including an effective vasoconstrictor which narrows swollen blood vessels and rapidly whitens reddened eyes in a formulation which produces a refreshing, soothing effect. Murine Plus is a sterile, isotonic solution compatible with the natural fluids of the eye.
Warning: Murine Plus should only be used for minor eye irritations. If relief is not obtained within 48 hours, or if irritation persists or increases, discontinue use and consult your physician.
Murine Plus should not be used by individuals with glaucoma and serious eye diseases. In some instances redness or inflammation may be due to serious eye conditions such as acute iritis, acute glaucoma, or corneal trauma. When redness, pain, or blurring persist, a physician should be consulted at once.
Dosage and Administration: One or two drops in eye(s) two or three times daily or as directed by physician. Do not touch bottle tip to any surface, since this may contaminate the solution. Keep container tightly closed. Keep this and all other medicines out of reach of children.
How Supplied: In 0.6 fl. oz. and 1.5 fl. oz. plastic dropper bottle.

NEMBUTAL® ELIXIR — ℞ Ⓒ
(pentobarbital elixir NF)

WARNING: MAY BE HABIT FORMING
Description: NEMBUTAL (pentobarbital) is a short-acting barbiturate chemically designated as 5-ethyl-5-(1-methylbutyl) barbituric acid. Pentobarbital is a barbituric acid derivative. NEMBUTAL Elixir contains 18.2 mg pentobarbital equivalent to 20 mg pentobarbital sodium per 5-ml teaspoonful. Alcohol, 18%.
Actions: Pentobarbital is a general depressant with the central nervous system being the most sensitive to this effect. In ordinary doses the drug acts as a sedative and hypnotic. The onset of action is from 15 to 30 minutes and the duration of action ranges from 3 to 6 hours. It is detoxified in the liver.
Indications: NEMBUTAL is indicated for use as a sedative or hypnotic. It may be used as a preanesthetic medication.
Contraindications: Pentobarbital is contraindicated in patients with porphyria or in those sensitive to barbiturates. Except in emergencies, it should not be administered to persons with known previous addiction to drugs of the sedative-hypnotic group.
Warnings: This drug may impair the mental and/or physical abilities required for the performance of potentially hazardous tasks such as driving a vehicle or operating machinery. The concomitant use of alcohol or other central nervous system depressants may have an additive effect. Patients should be warned accordingly.
Barbiturates induce liver microsomal enzyme activity. This accelerates the biotransformation of various drugs and is probably part of the mechanism of the tolerance which is seen with barbiturates. Pentobarbital may decrease the potency of the coumarin anticoagulants so that patients receiving such concomitant therapy should have more frequent prothrombin determinations.
Prolonged use of barbiturates, even in therapeutic dosages, may result in psychic dependence. Withdrawal symptoms may occur after chronic use of large doses, resulting in delirium, convulsions, or death.
Usage in Pregnancy: Safe use of pentobarbital has not been established with respect to adverse effects upon fetal development. Therefore, this drug should not be used in women of child-bearing potential and particularly during early pregnancy unless in the judgment of the physician the benefits outweigh the potential hazards.
When administering NEMBUTAL during labor, it must be remembered that barbiturates potentiate the action of narcotic drugs and, when used concomitantly, dosages should be reduced accordingly. Excessive doses to the mother (greater than 200 mg) may result in depression of the newborn. Premature infants are particularly susceptible to the depressant effects of NEMBUTAL and caution should be exercised when delivery of a premature infant is anticipated.
Precautions: Pentobarbital should be used with caution in patients with impaired liver function or in patients with a history of drug dependence or abuse.
Caution is essential when the drug is administered in the presence of any respiratory difficulty. Special care should be taken when pentobarbital is administered to patients in whom the hypnotic effect may be prolonged or intensified, as in those suffering from shock, severe liver disease, uremia, or after recent administration of other respiratory depressants.
Following use of pentobarbital in office procedures, patients should be warned against operating motor vehicles for the remainder of the day.
Adverse Reactions: Possible reactions include respiratory depression, apnea, circulatory collapse, skin rash, allergic reactions, se-

Continued on next page

Abbott—Cont.

vere depression of the central nervous system, drowsiness, lethargy, residual sedation (hangover effect), nausea, vomiting, or paradoxical excitement.
As with other sedative-hypnotic agents, some individuals may develop a psychological dependence on pentobarbital. These persons may increase the dosage without consulting a physician, and may subsequently develop a physical dependence on the drug. In such cases abrupt discontinuance may precipitate typical withdrawal symptoms, including convulsions. Therefore, the drug should be withdrawn *gradually* from any patient known to be taking excessive doses over long periods of time.
Dosage and Administration: Adults: Daytime sedation can ordinarily be provided by one 5-ml teaspoonful of the elixir taken 3 or 4 times per day.
The usual hypnotic dose consists of the equivalent to 100 mg pentobarbital sodium provided by 5 teaspoonfuls NEMBUTAL Elixir.
Children: Daytime sedation can be provided by 8 to 30 mg, depending on age, weight, and the desired degree of sedation.
The proper hypnotic dose for children must be judged on the basis of individual age and weight.
Overdosage: This is manifested by coma, early hypothermia, later fever, sluggish or absent reflexes, respiratory depression, and gradual appearance of circulatory collapse and pulmonary edema. The treatment consists of:
1. Maintain and assist respiration as indicated.
2. Support circulation with vasopressors and intravenous fluids as required.
3. Aspirate stomach contents, taking care to avoid pulmonary aspiration.
4. Use osmotic diuretic and measure intake and output of fluids.
5. Dialysis if indicated.
6. Antibiotics to control pulmonary complications when needed.

How Supplied: NEMBUTAL Elixir (pentobarbital elixir, NF) is supplied in pint and gallon bottles.
Ref. 02-5459-9/R52

NEMBUTAL® SODIUM CAPSULES ℞ ©
(pentobarbital sodium capsules, U.S.P.)

WARNING: MAY BE HABIT FORMING
Description: NEMBUTAL Sodium (pentobarbital sodium, U.S.P.) is a short-acting barbiturate chemically designated as sodium 5-ethyl-5-(1-methylbutyl) barbiturate.
Pentobarbital is a barbituric acid derivative. The sodium salt occurs as a white, slightly bitter powder which is freely soluble in water and alcohol but practically insoluble in benzene and ether.
Actions: Pentobarbital is a general depressant with the central nervous system being the most sensitive to this effect. In ordinary doses the drug acts as a sedative and hypnotic. The onset of action is from 15 to 30 minutes and the duration of action ranges from 3 to 6 hours. It is detoxified in the liver.
Indications: NEMBUTAL Sodium (pentobarbital sodium) is indicated for use as a sedative or hypnotic. It may be used as a pre-anesthetic medication.
Contraindications: NEMBUTAL Sodium (pentobarbital sodium) is contraindicated in patients with porphyria or in those sensitive to barbiturates. Except in emergencies, it should not be administered to persons with known previous addiction to drugs of the sedative-hypnotic group.
Warnings: This drug may impair the mental and/or physical abilities required for the performance of potentially hazardous tasks such as driving a vehicle or operating machinery. The concomitant use of alcohol or other central nervous system depressants may have an additive effect. Patients should be warned accordingly.
Barbiturates induce liver microsomal enzyme activity. This accelerates the biotransformation of various drugs and is probably part of the mechanism of the tolerance which is seen with barbiturates. Pentobarbital may decrease the potency of the coumarin anticoagulants so that patients receiving such concomitant therapy should have more frequent prothrombin determinations.
Prolonged use of barbiturates, even in therapeutic dosages, may result in psychic dependence. Withdrawal symptoms may occur after chronic use of large doses, resulting in delirium, convulsions, or death.
Usage in Pregnancy: Safe use of pentobarbital has not been established with respect to adverse effects upon fetal development. Therefore, this drug should not be used in women of child-bearing potential and particularly during early pregnancy unless in the judgment of the physician the benefits outweigh the potential hazards.
When administering NEMBUTAL (pentobarbital) during labor, it must be remembered that barbiturates potentiate the action of narcotic drugs and, when used concomitantly, dosages should be reduced accordingly. Excessive doses to the mother (greater than 200 mg.) may result in depression of the newborn. Premature infants are particularly susceptible to the depressant effects of NEMBUTAL and caution should be exercised when delivery of a premature infant is anticipated.
Precautions: Pentobarbital should be used with caution in patients with impaired liver function or in patients with a history of drug dependence or abuse.
Caution is essential when the drug is administered in the presence of any respiratory difficulty. Special care should be taken when pentobarbital is administered to patients in whom the hypnotic effect may be prolonged or intensified, as in those suffering from shock, severe liver disease, uremia, or after recent administration of other respiratory depressants.
Following use of pentobarbital in office procedures, patients should be warned against operating motor vehicles for the remainder of the day.
Adverse Reactions: Possible reactions include respiratory depression, apnea, circulatory collapse, skin rash, allergic reactions, severe depression of the central nervous system, drowsiness, lethargy, residual sedation (hangover effect), nausea, vomiting, or paradoxical excitement.
As with other sedative-hypnotic agents, some individuals may develop a psychological dependence on NEMBUTAL Sodium (pentobarbital sodium). These persons may increase the dosage without consulting a physician, and may subsequently develop a physical dependence on the drug. In such cases abrupt discontinuance may precipitate typical withdrawal symptoms, including convulsions. Therefore, the drug should be withdrawn *gradually* from any patient known to be taking excessive doses over long periods of time.
Dosage and Administration: Adults: Daytime sedation can ordinarily be provided by one 30 mg. capsule of NEMBUTAL Sodium (pentobarbital sodium) taken 3 or 4 times per day.
The usual hypnotic dose is 100 mg.
Children: Daytime sedation can be provided by 8 to 30 mg., depending on age, weight, and the desired degree of sedation.
The proper hypnotic dose for children must be judged on the basis of individual age and weight.
Overdosage: This is manifested by coma, early hypothermia, later fever, sluggish or absent reflexes, respiratory depression, and gradual appearance of circulatory collapse and pulmonary edema. The treatment consists of:
1. Maintain and assist respiration as indicated.
2. Support circulation with vasopressors and intravenous fluids as required.
3. Aspirate stomach contents, taking care to avoid pulmonary aspiration.
4. Use osmotic diuretic and measure intake and output of fluids.
5. Dialysis if indicated.
6. Antibiotics to control pulmonary complications when needed.

How Supplied: Nembutal Sodium Capsules (pentobarbital sodium capsules, U.S.P.) are supplied as follows:
30 mg., in bottles of 100 (**NDC** 0074-3120-01);
50 mg., in bottles of 100 (**NDC** 0074-3150-11), 500 (**NDC** 0074-3150-02), and 1000 (**NDC** 0074-3150-03), and in the Abbo-Pac® Unit-of-use Packages of 100 (10 strips of 10 capsules per strip) (**NDC** 0074-3150-13);
100 mg., in bottles of 100 (**NDC** 0074-3114-01), 500 (**NDC** 0074-3114-02), 1000 (**NDC** 0074-3114-03), and 5000 (**NDC** 0074-3114-04), in Strip Packages of 25 (**NDC** 0074-3114-10), and in the Abbo-Pac Unit-of-use Packages of 100 (10 strips of 10 capsules per strip) (**NDC** 0074-3114-21).
[*Shown in Product Identification Section*]
Ref: 03-4156/R1

NEMBUTAL® SODIUM SOLUTION ℞ ©
(pentobarbital sodium injection, USP)
Ampuls—Vials

WARNING: MAY BE HABIT FORMING
DO NOT USE IF MATERIAL HAS PRECIPITATED.
Description: NEMBUTAL Sodium Solution (pentobarbital sodium injection) is a sterile solution for intravenous or intramuscular injection. Each ml contains pentobarbital sodium, 50 mg, in a vehicle of propylene glycol, 40%, alcohol, 10% and water for injection, to volume. The pH is adjusted to approximately 9.5 with hydrochloric acid and/or sodium hydroxide.
NEMBUTAL Sodium is a short-acting barbiturate, chemically designated as sodium 5-ethyl-5-(1-methylbutyl) barbiturate. Pentobarbital is a barbituric acid derivative. The sodium salt occurs as a white, slightly bitter powder which is freely soluble in water and alcohol but practically insoluble in benzene and ether.
Actions: Pentobarbital is a general depressant with the central nervous system being the most sensitive to this effect. In ordinary doses the drug acts as a sedative and hypnotic. It is detoxified in the liver.
Indications: NEMBUTAL Sodium Solution (pentobarbital sodium injection) is indicated for use as a sedative or hypnotic. It may be used as a pre-anesthetic medication. The drug is indicated, in anesthetic doses, for the emergency control of certain acute convulsive conditions; e.g., those associated with tetanus, status epilepticus, and toxic reactions to strychnine and local anesthetics.
Contraindications: NEMBUTAL Sodium Solution (pentobarbital sodium injection) is contraindicated in patients with porphyria or in those sensitive to barbiturates.
Warnings: This drug may impair the mental and/or physical abilities required for the performance of potentially hazardous tasks such as driving a vehicle or operating machinery. The concomitant use of alcohol or other central nervous system depressants may have an additive effect. Patients should be warned accordingly.
Barbiturates induce liver microsomal enzyme activity. This accelerates the biotransformation of various drugs and is probably part of the mechanism of the tolerance which is seen with barbiturates. Pentobarbital may decrease the potency of the coumarin anticoagulants so that patients receiving such concomitant therapy should have more frequent prothrombin determinations.

Prolonged use of barbiturates, even in therapeutic dosages, may result in psychic dependence. Withdrawal symptoms may occur after chronic use of large doses, resulting in delirium, convulsions, or death.

Since NEMBUTAL Sodium Solution (pentobarbital sodium injection) is a potent central depressant, intravenous administration should not be attempted without adequate provisions for supporting respiration and circulation. Too-rapid administration may cause adverse respiratory and circulatory reactions, and should be avoided.

Intramuscular injection should not exceed a volume of 5 ml at any one site because of possible tissue irritation.

Usage in Pregnancy: Safe use of pentobarbital has not been established with respect to adverse effects upon fetal development. Therefore, this drug should not be used in women of childbearing potential and particularly during early pregnancy unless in the judgment of the physician the benefits outweigh the potential hazards.

When administering NEMBUTAL (pentobarbital) during labor, it must be remembered that barbiturates potentiate the action of narcotic drugs and, when used concomitantly, dosages should be reduced accordingly. Excessive doses to the mother (greater than 200 mg) may result in depression of the newborn. Premature infants are particularly susceptible to the depressant effects of NEMBUTAL and caution should be exercised when delivery of a premature infant is anticipated.

Precautions: Pentobarbital should be used with caution in patients with impaired liver function or in patients with a history of drug dependence or abuse.

Caution is essential when the drug is administered in the presence of any respiratory difficulty, *particularly status asthmaticus.* Special care should be taken when pentobarbital is administered to patients in whom the hypnotic effect may be prolonged or intensified, as in those suffering from shock, severe liver disease, uremia, or after recent administration of other respiratory depressants.

Pentobarbital solutions are highly alkaline. Therefore, extreme care should be exercised to avoid perivascular extravasation or intra-arterial injection. Extravascular injection may cause local tissue damage with subsequent necrosis. The consequences of intra-arterial injection may vary from transient pain along the course of the artery to gangrene of the limb. Signs of accidental injection by this route include, in addition to pain, delayed onset of hypnosis, pallor and cyanosis of the extremity, and patchy discoloration of the skin. Any complaint of pain in the limb warrants stopping the injection.

Hypotension may result from intravenous administration of the drug, particularly in patients with hypertension. Slow administration will usually prevent this occurrence.

Aseptic precautions should be observed to avoid contamination of the pentobarbital solution during withdrawal from multiple-dose vials or during transfer from the original container. Solutions which appear cloudy or in which a precipitate has formed should not be used.

Following use of pentobarbital in office procedures, patients should be warned against operating motor vehicles for the remainder of the day.

Adverse Reactions: Possible reactions include respiratory depression, apnea, circulatory collapse, pain, skin rash, allergic reactions, severe depression of the central nervous system, drowsiness, lethargy, residual sedation (hangover effect), nausea, vomiting, or paradoxical excitement.

Coughing, hiccoughing, laryngospasm, and chest-wall spasm have followed the intravenous use of pentobarbital. The occurrence of such effects can be minimized by slow administration of the drug and avoidance of painful stimuli during injection. Bronchospasm may occur, particularly in individuals who are subject to allergic reactions such as bronchial asthma.

Thrombophlebitis, pain at injection site or injury to nerves adjacent to injection site may occur.

Dosage and Administration:

Intravenous Administration

There is no average intravenous dose of NEMBUTAL Sodium Solution (pentobarbital sodium injection) that can be relied on to produce similar effects in different patients. The possibility of overdose and respiratory depression is remote when the drug is injected slowly in fractional doses. The clinical response is the basis for dosage determination, although the patient's weight, age, state of health and temperature may influence the total amount of the drug required. By watching the physical signs closely, the physician can accurately obtain and maintain the desired degree of sedation.

A commonly used initial dose for the 70 kg adult is 100 mg. Proportional reduction in dosage should be made for pediatric or debilitated patients. At least one minute is necessary to determine the full effect of intravenous pentobarbital. If necessary, additional small increments of the drug may be given up to a total of from 200 to 500 mg for normal adults.

In convulsive states, dosage should be kept to a minimum to avoid compounding the depression which may follow convulsions. The injection must be made slowly with due regard to the time required for the drug to penetrate the blood-brain barrier.

Intramuscular Administration

NEMBUTAL Sodium Solution (pentobarbital sodium injection) may be administered intramuscularly if deeply injected into a large muscle mass, preferably the upper outer quadrant of the gluteus maximus.

Dosage should be calculated on the basis of age, weight and the patient's condition. The usual adult dosage is 150 to 200 mg; children's dosage frequently ranges from 25 to 80 mg.

Overdosage: This is manifested by coma, early hypothermia, later fever, sluggish or absent reflexes, respiratory depression, and gradual appearance of circulatory collapse and pulmonary edema. The treatment consists of:

1. Maintain and assist respiration as indicated.
2. Support circulation with vasopressors and intravenous fluids as required.
3. Use osmotic diuretic and measure intake and output of fluids.
4. Dialysis if indicated.
5. Antibiotics to control pulmonary complications when needed.

How Supplied: Each ml contains:

NEMBUTAL Sodium
(Pentobarbital Sodium, derivative of
barbituric acid) .... 50 mg (3/4 gr)
Warning—May be habit forming.
Propylene glycol .... 40% v/v
Alcohol 10%
Water for Injection .... qs
(pH adjusted to approximately 9.5 with hydrochloric acid and/or sodium hydroxide.) Air in container displaced by nitrogen.

NEMBUTAL Sodium Solution (pentobarbital sodium injection) is available in the following sizes:

2-ml ampul, 100 mg (1½ gr), in boxes of 25 (**NDC** 0074-6899-04); 20-ml multiple-dose vial, 1 Gm, in boxes of 5 (**NDC** 0074-3778-04); and 50-ml multiple-dose vial, 2.5 Gm, in boxes of 5 (**NDC** 0074-3778-05).

Ref. 01-2927/R31

NEMBUTAL® SODIUM SUPPOSITORIES ℞ Ⓒ

(pentobarbital sodium suppositories)

WARNING: MAY BE HABIT FORMING

Composition: NEMBUTAL Sodium (pentobarbital sodium, USP) is a short-acting barbiturate chemically designated as sodium 5-ethyl-5-(1-methylbutyl) barbiturate. Pentobarbital is a barbituric acid derivative. The sodium salt occurs as a white, slightly bitter powder which is freely soluble in water and alcohol but practically insoluble in benzene and ether.

Actions: Pentobarbital is a general depressant with the central nervous system being the most sensitive to this effect. In ordinary doses the drug acts as a sedative and hypnotic. It is detoxified in the liver.

Indications: NEMBUTAL Sodium (pentobarbital sodium) is indicated for use as a sedative or hypnotic. It may be used as a pre-anesthetic medication.

NEMBUTAL Sodium Suppositories is a form particularly useful in patients who are unable to accept oral medication, such as nauseated patients or small children. It also provides a convenient means of drug administration during pre-operative fasting.

Contraindications: NEMBUTAL Sodium (pentobarbital sodium) is contraindicated in patients with porphyria or in those sensitive to barbiturates. Except in emergencies, it should not be administered to persons with known previous addiction to drugs of the sedative-hypnotic group.

Warnings: This drug may impair the mental and/or physical abilities required for the performance of potentially hazardous tasks such as driving a vehicle or operating machinery. The concomitant use of alcohol or other central nervous system depressants may have an additive effect. Patients should be warned accordingly.

Barbiturates induce liver microsomal enzyme activity. This accelerates the biotransformation of various drugs and is probably part of the mechanism of the tolerance which is seen with barbiturates. Pentobarbital may decrease the potency of the coumarin anticoagulants so that patients receiving such concomitant therapy should have more frequent prothrombin determinations.

Prolonged use of barbiturates, even in therapeutic dosages, may result in psychic dependence. Withdrawal symptoms may occur after chronic use of large doses, resulting in delirium, convulsions, or death.

Usage in Pregnancy: Safe use of pentobarbital has not been established with respect to adverse effects upon fetal development. Therefore, this drug should not be used in women of child-bearing potential and particularly during early pregnancy unless in the judgment of the physician the benefits outweigh the potential hazards.

When administering NEMBUTAL (pentobarbital) during labor, it must be remembered that barbiturates potentiate the action of narcotic drugs and, when used concomitantly, dosages should be reduced accordingly. Excessive doses to the mother (greater than 200 mg) may result in depression of the newborn. Premature infants are particularly susceptible to the depressant effects of NEMBUTAL and caution should be exercised when delivery of a premature infant is anticipated.

Precautions: Pentobarbital should be used with caution in patients with impaired liver function or in patients with a history of drug dependence or abuse.

Caution is essential when the drug is administered in the presence of any respiratory difficulty. Special care should be taken when pentobarbital is administered to patients in whom the hypnotic effect may be prolonged or inten-

Continued on next page

Abbott—Cont.

sified, as in those suffering from shock, severe liver disease, uremia, or after recent administration of other respiratory depressants.
To assure accuracy of dosage do not administer divided suppositories.
Following use of pentobarbital in office procedures, patients should be warned against operating motor vehicles for the remainder of the day.
Adverse Reactions: Possible reactions include respiratory depression, apnea, circulatory collapse, skin rash, allergic reactions, severe depression of the central nervous system, drowsiness, lethargy, residual sedation (hangover effect), or paradoxical excitement.
As with other sedative-hypnotic agents, some individuals may develop a psychological dependence on NEMBUTAL Sodium (pentobarbital sodium). These persons may increase the dosage without consulting a physician, and may subsequently develop a physical dependence on the drug. In such cases abrupt discontinuance may precipitate typical withdrawal symptoms, including convulsions. Therefore, the drug should be withdrawn gradually from any patient known to be taking excessive doses over long periods of time.
Dosage and Administration: Typical hypnotic doses for adults and children are given below. These are intended only as a guide, and administration should be adjusted to the individual needs of each patient. For sedation, in children 5-14 years and in adults, reduce dose appropriately.
Adults (average to above average weight)—one 120 mg or one 200 mg suppository.
Children—

12-14 years (80-110 lbs)	one 60 mg or one 120 mg suppository
5-12 years (40-80 lbs)	one 60 mg suppository
1-4 years (20-40 lbs)	one 30 mg or one 60 mg suppository
2 months-1 year (10-20 lbs)	one 30 mg suppository

Suppositories should not be divided.
Overdosage: This is manifested by coma, early hypothermia, later fever, sluggish or absent reflexes, respiratory depression, and gradual appearance of circulatory collapse and pulmonary edema. The treatment consists of:

1. Maintain and assist respiration as indicated.
2. Support circulation with vasopressors and intravenous fluids as required.
3. Use osmotic diuretic and measure intake and output of fluids.
4. Dialysis if indicated.
5. Antibiotics to control pulmonary complications when needed.

How Supplied: NEMBUTAL Sodium Suppositories (pentobarbital sodium suppositories) are available as suppositories containing pentobarbital sodium in the amount of 30 mg (**NDC** 0074-3272-01); 60 mg (**NDC** 0074-3148-01); 120 mg (**NDC** 0074-3145-01) and 200 mg (**NDC** 0074-3164-01). Supplied in boxes of 12 suppositories.
Semi-synthetic glycerides provide the base for each suppository.
Ref. No. 01-2979-R6

NORISODRINE® AEROTROL® ℞
(isoproterenol hydrochloride aerosol)
In a Controlled-Dose Nebulizer

Description: Isoproterenol HCl 0.25% w/w (=2.8 mg./ml.) in inert chlorofluorohydrocarbon propellants; alcohol 33%; ascorbic acid 0.1% as preservative; and artificial and natural flavors.
Each depression of the valve delivers approximately 0.12 mg. to the patient.
Actions: Isoproterenol is a short-acting sympathomimetic drug. It produces pharmacologic response in the cardiovascular system and on the smooth muscles of the bronchial tree. The drug will prevent or overcome histamine-induced asthma in both experimental animals and man, and is effective when used prophylactically. It is one of the most potent bronchodilators known and can be used in patients who do not respond to the bronchodilating action of epinephrine. Isoproterenol has a cardio-accelerating effect, but its vasoconstricting action is less pronounced than that of epinephrine. Therapeutic doses may produce a slight increase in systolic blood pressure, but a slight decrease in diastolic. Larger doses may cause peripheral vasodilatation in the renal, mesenteric and femoral beds and some patients respond with a decrease in diastolic, but no change in systolic pressure. Such effects are usually of very short duration.
Indications: Norisodrine is indicated for the treatment of bronchospasm associated with acute and chronic bronchial asthma, pulmonary emphysema, bronchitis, and bronchiectasis.
Contraindications: Use of isoproterenol in patients with pre-existing cardiac arrhythmias associated with tachycardia is contraindicated because the cardiac stimulant effects of the drug may aggravate such disorders.
Warnings: Excessive use of an adrenergic aerosol should be discouraged, as it may lose its effectiveness. Occasional patients have been reported to develop severe paradoxical airway resistance with repeated excessive use of isoproterenol inhalation preparations. The cause of this refractory state is unknown. It is advisable that in such instances the use of this preparation be discontinued immediately and alternative therapy instituted, since in the reported cases the patients did not respond to other forms of therapy until the drug was withdrawn.
Deaths have been reported following excessive use of isoproterenol inhalation preparations and the exact cause is unknown. Cardiac arrest was noted in several instances.
Precautions: Isoproterenol and epinephrine may be used interchangeably if the patient becomes unresponsive to one or the other but should not be used concurrently. If desired, these drugs may be alternated, provided an interval of at least four hours has elapsed.
As with all sympathomimetic drugs, isoproterenol should be used with great caution in the presence of cardiovascular disorders, including coronary insufficiency, hypertension, hyperthyroidism and diabetes, or when there is a sensitivity to sympathomimetic amines.
Although there has been no evidence of teratogenic effects with this drug, use of any drug in pregnancy, lactation, or in women of childbearing age requires that the potential benefit of the drug be weighed against its possible hazard to the mother and child.
Adverse Reactions: Only a small percentage of patients experience any side effects following oral inhalation of aerosolized isoproterenol. Overdosage may produce tachycardia with resultant coronary insufficiency, palpitations, vertigo, nausea, tremors, headache, insomnia, central excitation, and blood pressure changes. These reactions are similar to those produced by other sympathomimetic agents.
Dosage and Administration: The usual dose for the relief of dyspnea in the acute episode is 1 to 2 inhalations. Start with one inhalation. If no relief is evident after 2 to 5 minutes, a second inhalation may be taken. For daily maintenance, use 1 to 2 inhalations 4 to 6 times daily, or as directed by the physician. The physician should be careful to instruct the patient in the proper technique of administration so that the number of inhalations per treatment and the frequency of treatment may be titrated to the patient's response.
No more than two inhalations should be taken at any one time, or more than 6 inhalations in any hour during a 24-hour period, unless advised by the physician.
Directions for Use: Before each use, remove cap and assemble.

1. Breathe out fully. Place mouthpiece well into the mouth, aimed at the back of the throat.
2. As you begin to breathe in deeply, press the vial firmly down into the adapter. This releases one dose. Continue to breathe in until your lungs are completely filled.
3. Remove from mouth. Hold your breath for several seconds, then breathe out slowly.

Warning: Do not exceed the dose prescribed by your physician. If difficulty in breathing persists, contact your physician immediately.
How Supplied: NORISODRINE Aerotrol (isoproterenol hydrochloride aerosol), 0.25% w/w, is supplied in a 15 ml. controlled-dose nebulizer (**NDC** 0074-6869-03).
Ref. No. 01-2822-R2

NORISODRINE® SULFATE ℞
(isoproterenol sulfate)
For Oral Use With The Aerohalor®
To Control Bronchospasm

Description: Isoproterenol sulfate is a white, odorless, crystalline powder which darkens on exposure to air. It is chemically identified as 1,2-Benzenediol,4-[1-hydroxy-2-[(1-methylethyl)amino]ethyl]-, sulfate (2:1) (salt), dihydrate.
Each Aerohalor Cartridge 10% contains 10 mg isoproterenol sulfate and 90 mg lactose as a diluent. Each Aerohalor Cartridge 25% contains 25 mg isoproterenol sulfate and 75 mg lactose as a diluent.
Actions: Isoproterenol is classified as a catecholamine which acts predominantly on beta receptor sites of peripheral inhibitory and cardiac excitatory sympathetic nerves. Therefore, its primary pharmacological actions are to increase both the rate and force of cardiac contraction and to relax the smooth muscle of the bronchi, alimentary tract, and skeletal muscle vasculature. Isoproterenol can prevent or relieve bronchospasm due to drugs, as well as that due to disease. The drug lowers peripheral vascular resistance and reduces the diastolic blood pressure. Systolic pressure is unchanged or slightly increased as a consequence of increased cardiac output.
The calorigenic effects of isoproterenol are similar to those of epinephrine; however, it causes less hyperglycemia than epinephrine. Isoproterenol can also cause central excitation.
Isoproterenol is readily absorbed following inhalation. The duration of action of isoproterenol is the same as that of epinephrine and it is probably metabolized and excreted by the same routes.
Indications: NORISODRINE (isoproterenol) is indicated for the treatment of bronchospasm associated with acute and chronic bronchial asthma, pulmonary emphysema, bronchitis, and bronchiectasis.
Contraindications: NORISODRINE should not be used in those rare instances in which a patient has demonstrated hypersensitivity to isoproterenol or other sympathomimetic amines.
The use of isoproterenol is contraindicated in patients with pre-existing cardiac arrythmias, because the cardiac stimulant effect of the drug may aggravate such disorders.
Warnings: Occasional patients have been reported to develop severe, paradoxical airway resistance of unknown etiology with repeated, excessive use of isoproterenol inhalation preparations. Because of the frequent development of such refractoriness, excessive use of any adrenergic aerosol should be discouraged. Should the refractory state develop, it is advisable to discontinue isoproterenol immediately and institute alternative therapy, since in the reported cases the patients did not respond to

other forms of therapy until isoproterenol was withdrawn.

Deaths have been reported following excessive use of isoproterenol inhalation preparations. The exact cause is unknown. Cardiac arrhythmia or cardiac arrest has been noted.

Bronchial asthma may mask the presence of cardiac asthma (pulmonary edema). A differential diagnosis should be made before instituting therapy.

This product is a powdered formulation which may irritate the oropharynx and tracheobronchial tree. Therefore, its use should be considered secondary to formulations in solution or suspension.

Usage in Pregnancy: Use of isoproterenol in women of childbearing age or during pregnancy or lactation requires that the potential benefit of the drug be weighed against its possible hazards to mother and child.

Precautions: Isoproterenol should be used cautiously in patients with heart disease, hypertension, hyperthyroidism, diabetes, or unstable vasomotor systems.

The concomitant use of NORISODRINE SULFATE (isoproterenol sulfate) AEROHALOR and a parenteral or inhalation form of epinephrine or other adrenergic agent should be avoided since it may result in excessive response and the occurrence of serious cardiovascular symptoms.

Caution should be exercised when NORISODRINE SULFATE AEROHALOR is administered concomitantly with an oral form of adrenergic agent since the effects of these drugs are additive.

In neutral or alkaline solution, isoproterenol may become red on exposure to air. Accordingly, the saliva or sputum may appear pink or red in color after oral inhalation of the drug. This is not harmful but should be explained to patients to allay possible apprehension or confusion with bleeding.

Adverse Reactions: As with other sympathomimetic drugs, NORISODRINE (isoproterenol) may produce undesirable side effects such as nervousness, dizziness, palpitation, nausea, vomiting, headache, tremor, flushing, sweating, weakness, precordial distress and anginal-type pain, and tachycardia. Cardiac arrhythmias may occur, and death from cardiac arrest has been reported with excessive use of isoproterenol.

Swelling of the parotid glands has been reported with the prolonged use of isoproterenol. In such cases the drug should be withdrawn.

Dosage and Administration: NORISODRINE (isoproterenol) SULFATE is administered by oral inhalation. This method is rapidly effective for controlling acute attacks of bronchospasm and is suitable for adults or older children.

Tests done in a mechanical breathing apparatus indicate that one inhalation of the 10% concentration yields about 0.045 mg of isoproterenol sulfate. One inhalation of the 25% concentration yields about 0.11 mg of isoproterenol sulfate.

For the mild or moderate acute attack, 2 to 4 inhalations of normal depth of the 10% concentration, through the Aerohalor, are usually sufficient. The patient should be cautioned not to take a forced, deep inhalation. If the first two to four inhalations do not provide relief within five minutes this dose may be repeated. If relief is still not apparent, a third dose may be taken after an interval of 10 minutes. When therapy has been unsuccessful following three doses the medication should be discontinued as ineffective for that particular attack.

If the 10% concentration does not afford relief and does not induce undesired side effects, the 25% concentration may be used in the same manner.

Symptoms and Treatment of Overdosage: Symptoms may include palpitation, tachycardia, restlessness, tremor, sweating, headache, dizziness, weakness, nausea, and vomiting. Blood pressure may at first be elevated slightly. Later, blood pressure may fall and the general picture of "shock" may develop.

Treatment includes general supportive measures. Sedatives (barbiturates) may be given for restlessness.

How Supplied: NORISODRINE SULFATE (isoproterenol sulfate) 10% (**NDC** 0074-3867-12) and 25% (**NDC** 0074-3882-12) are supplied in bottles containing 12 AEROHALOR cartridges.

Ref. 01-2828-R6

NORISODRINE® WITH CALCIUM IODIDE ℞

(isoproterenol sulfate and calcium iodide) SYRUP

How Supplied: Each teaspoonful of NORISODRINE WITH CALCIUM IODIDE SYRUP contains 3 mg of isoproterenol sulfate, 150 mg of anhydrous calcium iodide and 6% alcohol in a palatable syrup. Norisodrine with Calcium Iodide Syrup is supplied in pint (**NDC** 0074-6953-01) and gallon (**NDC** 0074-6953-02) bottles.

Also available in 5 ml. Abbo-Pac® unit dose packages containing 4 trays of 25 bottles (**NDC** 0074-6953-05).

OGEN® ℞

(piperazine estrone sulfate tablets, N.F.) Tablets

Warning:

1. ESTROGENS HAVE BEEN REPORTED TO INCREASE THE RISK OF ENDOMETRIAL CARCINOMA.

Three independent case control studies have shown an increased risk of endometrial cancer in postmenopausal women exposed to exogenous estrogens for prolonged periods.[1–3] This risk was independent of the other known risk factors for endometrial cancer. These studies are further supported by the finding that incidence rates of endometrial cancer have increased sharply since 1969 in eight different areas of the United States with population-based cancer reporting systems, an increase which may be related to the rapidly expanding use of estrogens during the last decade.[4]

The three case control studies reported that the risk of endometrial cancer in estrogen users was about 4.5 to 13.9 times greater than in nonusers. The risk appears to depend on both duration of treatment[1] and on estrogen dose.[3] In view of these findings, when estrogens are used for the treatment of menopausal symptoms, the lowest dose that will control symptoms should be utilized and medication should be discontinued as soon as possible. When prolonged treatment is medically indicated, the patient should be reassessed on at least a semiannual basis to determine the need for continued therapy. Although the evidence must be considered preliminary, one study suggests that cyclic administration of low doses of estrogen may carry less risk than continuous administration;[3] it therefore appears prudent to utilize such a regimen.

Close clinical surveillance of all women taking estrogens is important. In all cases of undiagnosed persistent or recurring abnormal vaginal bleeding, adequate diagnostic measures should be undertaken to rule out malignancy.

There is no evidence at present that "natural" estrogens are more or less hazardous than "synthetic" estrogens at equiestrogenic doses.

2. OGEN SHOULD NOT BE USED DURING PREGNANCY.

According to some investigators, the use of female sex hormones, both estrogens and progestogens, during early pregnancy may seriously damage the offspring. Studies have reported that females exposed in utero to diethylstilbestrol, a non-steroidal estrogen, have an increased risk of developing in later life a form of vaginal or cervical cancer that is ordinarily extremely rare.[5,6] In one of these studies, this risk was estimated as not greater than 4 per 1000 exposures.[7] Furthermore, there are reports that a high percentage of such exposed women (from 30 to 90 percent) have been found to have vaginal adenosis,[8–12] epithelial changes of the vagina and cervix. Although these reported changes are histologically benign, the investigators have not determined whether they are precursors of adenocarcinoma.

Several reports suggest an association between intrauterine exposure to female sex hormones and congenital anomalies in the offspring, including heart defects and limb reduction defects.[13–16] One case control study[16] estimated a 4.7 fold increased risk of limb reduction defects in infants exposed in utero to sex hormones (oral contraceptives, hormone withdrawal tests for pregnancy, or attempted treatment for threatened abortion). Some of these exposures were very short and involved only a few days of treatment. The data suggest that the risk of limb reduction defects in exposed fetuses is somewhat less than 1 per 1000.

In the past, female sex hormones have been used during pregnancy in an attempt to treat threatened or habitual abortion. OGEN has not been studied for these uses, and therefore should not be used during pregnancy. There is no evidence from well controlled studies that progestogens are effective for these uses.

If OGEN (piperazine estrone sulfate tablets) is used during pregnancy, or if the patient becomes pregnant while taking this drug, she should be apprised of the potential risks to the fetus, and the question of continuation of the pregnancy should be addressed.

Description: OGEN (piperazine estrone sulfate tablets) is an estrogenic substance prepared from purified crystalline estrone, solubilized as the sulfate and stabilized with piperazine. It is appreciably soluble in water and has almost no odor or taste—properties which are ideally suited for oral administration.

The amount of piperazine in OGEN is not sufficient to exert a pharmacological action. Its addition ensures solubility, stability, and uniform potency of the estrone sulfate.

See HOW SUPPLIED section for available dosage forms and ingredient listing.

Clinical Pharmacology: OGEN (piperazine estrone sulfate tablets) owes its therapeutic action to estrone, one of the three principal estrogenic steroid hormones of man: estradiol, estrone, and estriol. Estradiol is rapidly hydrolyzed in the body to estrone, which in turn may be hydrated to the less active estriol. These transformations occur readily, mainly in the liver, where there is also free interconversion between estrone and estradiol.

Gastrointestinal absorption of orally administered estrogens is usually prompt and complete. Inactivation of estrogens in the body occurs mainly in the liver. During cyclic passage through the liver, estrogens are degraded to less active estrogenic compounds and conjugated with sulfuric and glucuronic acids. Estrone is loosely bound to protein as it circulates

Continued on next page

Abbott—Cont.

in the blood, usually as a conjugate with sulfate.

Indications: OGEN (piperazine estrone sulfate tablets) is indicated for the treatment of estrogen deficiency associated with:

1. Moderate to severe *vasomotor* symptoms of menopause. (There is no evidence that estrogens are effective for nervous symptoms or depression which might occur during menopause, and they should not be used to treat these conditions.)
2. Atrophic vaginitis.
3. Kraurosis vulvae.
4. Female hypogonadism.
5. Female castration.
6. Primary ovarian failure.

OGEN (PIPERAZINE ESTRONE SULFATE TABLETS) HAS NOT BEEN TESTED FOR EFFICACY FOR ANY PURPOSE DURING PREGNANCY. SINCE ITS EFFECT UPON THE FETUS IS UNKNOWN, IT CANNOT BE RECOMMENDED FOR ANY CONDITION DURING PREGNANCY (SEE BOXED WARNING).

Contraindications: Ogen should not be used in women with any of the following conditions:

1. Known or suspected cancer of the breast.
2. Known or suspected estrogen-dependent neoplasia.
3. Known or suspected pregnancy (See Boxed Warning).
4. Undiagnosed abnormal genital bleeding.
5. Active thrombophlebitis or thromboembolic disorders.
6. A past history of thrombophlebitis, thrombosis, or thromboembolic disorders associated with previous estrogen use.

Warnings:

1. *Induction of malignant neoplasms.* Long-term continuous administration of natural and synthetic estrogens in certain animal species has been reported by some investigators to increase the frequency of carcinomas of the breast, cervix, vagina, and liver. There is now evidence that estrogens increase the risk of carcinoma of the endometrium in humans. (See Boxed Warning).

At the present time there is no satisfactory evidence that estrogens given to postmenopausal women increase the risk of cancer of the breast,[17] although a recent long-term followup of a single physician's practice has raised this possibility.[18] Therefore, caution should be exercised when administering estrogens to women with a strong family history of breast cancer or who have breast nodules, fibrocystic disease, or abnormal mammograms. Careful breast examinations should be performed periodically.

2. *Gall bladder disease.* A recent study has reported a 2 to 3-fold increase in the risk of surgically confirmed gall bladder disease in women receiving postmenopausal estrogens,[17] similar to the 2-fold increase previously noted in users of oral contraceptives.[19,22] In the case of oral contraceptives, the increased risk appeared after two years of use.[22]

3. *Effects similar to those caused by estrogen-progestogen oral contraceptives.* There are several serious adverse effects of oral contraceptives, most of which have not, up to now, been documented as consequences of postmenopausal estrogen therapy. This may reflect the comparatively low doses of estrogen used in postmenopausal women. It would be expected that the larger doses of estrogen used to treat postpartum breast engorgement would be more likely to result in these adverse effects, and, in fact, it has been shown that there is an increased risk of thrombosis in women receiving estrogens for postpartum breast engorgement.[20,21]

a. *Thromboembolic disease.* It is now well established that users of oral contraceptives have an increased risk of various thromboembolic and thrombotic vascular diseases, such as thrombophlebitis, pulmonary embolism, stroke, and myocardial infarction.[22–29] Cases of retinal thrombosis, mesenteric thrombosis, and optic neuritis have been reported in oral contraceptive users. There is evidence that the risk of several of these adverse reactions is related to the dose of the drug.[30,31] An increased risk of post-surgery thromboembolic complications has also been reported in users of oral contraceptives.[32,33] If feasible, estrogen should be discontinued at least 4 weeks before surgery of the type associated with an increased risk of thromboembolism; it should also be discontinued during periods of prolonged immobilization.

While an increased rate of thromboembolic and thrombotic disease in postmenopausal users of estrogens has not been found[17,34] this does not rule out the possibility that such an increase may be present or that subgroups of women who have underlying risk factors or who are receiving relatively large doses of estrogens may have increased risk. Therefore estrogens should not be used in persons with active thrombophlebitis or thromboembolic disorders, and they should not be used in persons with a history of such disorders in association with estrogen use. They should be used with caution in patients with cerebral vascular or coronary artery disease and only for those in whom estrogens are clearly needed.

Large doses of estrogen (5 mg conjugated estrogens per day), comparable to those used to treat cancer of the prostate and breast, have been shown in a large prospective clinical trial in men[35] to increase the risk of nonfatal myocardial infarction, pulmonary embolism and thrombophlebitis. When estrogen doses of this size are used, any of the thromboembolic and thrombotic adverse effects associated with oral contraceptive use should be considered a clear risk.

b. *Hepatic adenoma.* Benign hepatic adenomas appear to be associated with the use of oral contraceptives.[36–38] Although benign, and rare, these may rupture and cause death through intraabdominal hemorrhage. Such lesions have not yet been reported in association with other estrogen or progestogen preparations but should be considered in estrogen users having abdominal pain and tenderness, abdominal mass, or hypovolemic shock. Hepatocellular carcinoma has also been reported in women taking estrogen-containing oral contraceptives.[37] The relationship of this malignancy to these drugs is not known at this time.

c. *Elevated blood pressure.* Increased blood pressure is not uncommon in women using oral contraceptives. There is now a report that this may occur with use of estrogens in the menopause[39] and blood pressure should be monitored with estrogen use, especially if high doses are used.

d. *Glucose tolerance.* A worsening of glucose tolerance has been observed in a significant percentage of patients on estrogen-containing oral contraceptives. For this reason, diabetic patients should be carefully observed while receiving estrogen.

4. *Hypercalcemia.* Administration of estrogens may lead to severe hypercalcemia in patients with breast cancer and bone metastases.

Precautions:

A. General Precautions.

1. A complete medical and family history should be taken prior to the initiation of any estrogen therapy. The pretreatment and periodic physical examinations should include special reference to blood pressure, breasts, abdomen, and pelvic organs, and should include a Papanicolau smear. As a general rule, estrogen should not be prescribed for longer than one year without another physical examination being performed.
2. Fluid retention—Estrogens may cause some degree of fluid retention. Therefore, patients with conditions such as epilepsy, migraine, and cardiac or renal dysfunction, which might be influenced by this factor, require careful observation.
3. Certain patients may develop undesirable manifestations of excessive estrogenic stimulation, such as abnormal or excessive uterine bleeding, mastodynia, etc.
4. Oral contraceptives appear to be associated with an increased incidence of mental depression.[22] Although it is not clear whether this is due to the estrogenic or progestogenic component of the contraceptive, patients with a history of depression should be carefully observed.
5. Preexisting uterine leiomyomata may increase in size during estrogen use.
6. The pathologist should be advised of the patient's use of estrogen therapy when relevant specimens are submitted.
7. Patients with a past history of jaundice during pregnancy have an increased risk of recurrence of jaundice while receiving estrogen-containing oral contraceptive therapy. If jaundice develops in any patient receiving estrogen, the medication should be discontinued while the cause is investigated.
8. Estrogens may be poorly metabolized in patients with impaired liver function and they should be administered with caution in such patients.
9. Because estrogens influence the metabolism of calcium and phosphorus, they should be used with caution in patients with metabolic bone diseases that are associated with hypercalcemia or in patients with renal insufficiency.
10. Because of the effects of estrogens on epiphyseal closure, they should be used judiciously in young patients in whom bone growth is not complete.
11. Certain endocrine and liver function tests may be affected by estrogen-containing oral contraceptives. The following similar changes may be expected with larger doses of estrogen.
    a. Increased sulfobromophthalein retention.
    b. Increased prothrombin and factors VII, VIII, IX, and X; decreased antithrombin 3; increased norepinephrine-induced platelet aggregability.
    c. Increased thyroid binding globulin (TBG) leading to increased circulating total thyroid hormone, as measured by PBI, T4 by column or T4 by radiommunoassay. Free T3 resin uptake is decreased, reflecting the elevated TBG; free T4 concentration is unaltered.
    d. Impaired glucose tolerance.
    e. Decreased pregnanediol excretion.
    f. Reduced response to metyrapone test.
    g. Reduced serum folate concentration.
    h. Increased serum triglyceride and phospholipid concentration.

B. Information for the patient. See text of Patient Package Insert which appears after PHYSICIAN REFERENCES.

C. OGEN cannot be recommended for use during pregnancy. See Contraindications and Boxed Warning.

D. Nursing Mothers. Estrogens have been reported to be excreted in human breast milk.

Adverse Reactions: (See Warnings regarding reports of possible induction of neoplasia, unknown effects upon the fetus, increased incidence of gall bladder disease, and adverse effects similar to those of oral contraceptives, including thromboembolism.) The following additional adverse reactions have been reported with estrogenic therapy, including oral contraceptives.

1. *Genitourinary system.*

Breakthrough bleeding, spotting, change in menstrual flow.

Dysmenorrhea.

Premenstrual-like syndrome.

Amenorrhea during and after treatment.

Increase in size of uterine fibromyomata.
Vaginal candidiasis.
Change in cervical eversion and in degree of cervical secretion.
Cystitis-like syndrome.

2. *Breast*
Tenderness, enlargement, secretion.

3. *Gastrointestinal*
Nausea, vomiting.
Abdominal cramps, bloating.
Cholestatic jaundice.

4. *Skin*
Chloasma or melasma which may persist when drug is discontinued.
Erythema multiforme.
Erythema nodosum.
Hemorrhagic eruption.
Loss of scalp hair.
Hirsutism.

5. *Eyes*
Steepening of corneal curvature.
Intolerance to contact lenses.

6. *CNS*
Headache, migraine, dizziness.
Mental depression.
Chorea.

7. *Miscellaneous*
Increase or decrease in weight.
Reduced carbohydrate tolerance.
Aggravation of porphyria.
Edema.
Changes in libido.

Acute Overdosage: Numerous reports of ingestion of large doses of estrogen-containing oral contraceptives by young children indicate that serious ill effects do not occur. Overdosage of estrogen may cause nausea and withdrawal bleeding may occur in females.

Dosage and Administration:

1. *Given cyclically for short-term use:*
For treatment of moderate to severe *vasomotor* symptoms, atrophic vaginitis, or kraurosis vulvae associated with the menopause.
The lowest dose that will control symptoms should be chosen and medication should be discontinued as promptly as possible.
Administration should be cyclic (e.g., 3 weeks on and 1 week off).
Attempts to discontinue or taper medication should be made at 3 to 6 month intervals.
The usual dosage range is one OGEN .625 Tablet to one OGEN 5 Tablet per day.

2. *Given cyclically:*
Female hypogonadism. Female castration. Primary ovarian failure. The lowest dose that will control symptoms should be chosen. A daily dose of one OGEN 1.25 Tablet to three OGEN 2.5 Tablets may be given for the first three weeks of a theoretical cycle, followed by a rest period of eight to ten days. The same schedule is repeated if bleeding does not occur by the end of the rest period. The duration of cyclic estrogen therapy necessary to produce withdrawal bleeding will vary according to the responsiveness of the endometrium. If satisfactory withdrawal bleeding does not occur, an oral progestogen may be given in addition to estrogen during the third week of the cycle.
Treated patients with an intact uterus should be monitored closely for signs of endometrial cancer and appropriate diagnostic measures should be taken to rule out malignancy in the event of persistent or recurring abnormal vaginal bleeding.

How Supplied: OGEN (piperazine estrone sulfate tablets) is supplied as OGEN .625 (0.75 mg. piperazine estrone sulfate), yellow tablets, **NDC** 0074-3943-04; OGEN 1.25 (1.5 mg. piperazine estrone sulfate), peach-colored tablets, **NDC** 0074-3946-04; OGEN 2.5 (3 mg. piperazine estrone sulfate), blue tablets, **NDC** 0074-3951-04; and OGEN 5 (6 mg. piperazine estrone sulfate), light green tablets, **NDC** 0074-3958-13. Tablets of all four dosage levels are standardized to provide uniform estrone activity and are grooved (Divide-Tab®) to provide dosage flexibility. All tablet sizes of OGEN are available in bottles of 100.
[*Shown in Product Identification Section*]

Physician References:

[1]Ziel, H. K. and W. D. Finkel, "Increased Risk of Endometrial Carcinoma Among Users of Conjugated Estrogens," *New England Journal of Medicine,* 293:1167-1170, 1975.

[2]Smith, D. C., R. Prentic, D. J. Thompson and W. L. Hermann, "Association of Exogenous Estrogen and Endometrial Carcinoma," *New England Journal of Medicine,* 293:1164-1167, 1975.

[3]Mack, T. M., M. C. Pike, B. E. Henderson, R. I. Pfeffer, V. R. Gerkins, M. Arthur and S. E. Brown, "Estrogens and Endometrial Cancer in a Retirement Community," *New England Journal of Medicine,* 294:1262-1267, 1976.

[4]Weiss, N. S., D. R. Szekely and D. F. Austin, "Increasing Incidence of Endometrial Cancer in the United States," *New England Journal of Medicine,* 294:1259-1262, 1976.

[5]Herbst, A. L., H. Ulfelder and D. C. Poskanzer, "Adenocarcinoma of Vagina," *New England Journal of Medicine,* 284:878-881, 1971.

[6]Greenwald, P., J. Barlow, P. Nasca and W. Burnett, "Vaginal Cancer after Maternal Treatment with Synthetic Estrogens," *New England Journal of Medicine,* 285:390-392, 1971.

[7]Lanier, A., K. Noller, D. Decker, L. Elveback and L. Kurland, "Cancer and Stilbestrol. A Follow-up of 1719 Persons Exposed to Estrogens In Utero and Born 1943-1959," *Mayo Clinic Proceedings,* 48:793-799, 1973.

[8]Herbst, A., R. Kurman and R. Scully, "Vaginal and Cervical Abnormalities After Exposure to Stilbestrol In Utero." *Obstetrics and Gynecology,* 40:287-298, 1972.

[9]Herbst, A., S. Robboy, G. Macdonald and R. Scully, "The Effects of Local Progesterone on Stilbestrol-Associated Vaginal Adenosis," *American Journal of Obstetrics and Gynecology,* 118:607-615, 1974.

[10]Herbst, A., D. Poskanzer, S. Robboy, L. Friedlander and R. Scully, "Prenatal Exposure to Stilbestrol, A Prospective Comparison of Exposed Female Offspring with Unexposed Controls," *New England Journal of Medicine,* 292:334-339, 1975.

[11]Stafl, A., R. Mattingly, D. Foley and W. Fetherston, "Clinical Diagnosis of Vaginal Adenosis," *Obstetrics and Gynecology,* 43:118-128, 1974.

[12]Sherman, A. I., M. Goldrath, A. Berlin, V. Vakhariya, F. Banooni, W. Michaels, P. Goodman and S. Brown, "Cervical-Vaginal Adenosis After *In Utero* Exposure to Synthetic Estrogens," *Obstetrics and Gynecology,* 44:531-545, 1974.

[13]Gal, I., B. Kirman and J. Stern, "Hormone Pregnancy Tests and Congenital Malformation," *Nature,* 216:83, 1967.

[14]Levy, E. P., A. Cohen and F. C. Fraser, "Hormone Treatment During Pregnancy and Congenital Heart Defects." *Lancet,* 1:611, 1973.

[15]Nora, J. and A. Nora, "Birth Defects and Oral Contraceptives," *Lancet,* 1:941-942, 1973.

[16]Janerich, D. T., J. M. Piper and D. M. Glebatis, "Oral Contraceptives and Congenital Limb-Reduction Defects," *New England Journal of Medicine,* 291:697-700, 1974.

[17]Boston Collaborative Drug Surveillance Program "Surgically Confirmed Gall Bladder Disease, Venous Thromboembolism and Breast Tumors in Relation to Post-Menopausal Estrogen Therapy," *New England Journal of Medicine,* 290:15-19, 1974.

[18]Hoover, R., L. A. Gray, Sr., P. Cole and B. MacMahon, "Menopausal Estrogens and Breast Cancer," *New England Journal of Medicine,* 295:401-405, 1976.

[19]Boston Collaborative Drug Surveillance Program, "Oral Contraceptives and Venous Thromboembolic Disease, Surgically Confirmed Gall Bladder Disease and Breast Tumors," *Lancet,* 1:1399-1404, 1973.

[20]Daniel, D. G., H. Campbell and A. C. Turnbull, "Puerperal Thromboembolism and Suppression of Lactation," *Lancet,* 2:287-289, 1967.

[21]Bailar, J. C., "Thromboembolism and Oestrogen Therapy," *Lancet,* 2:560, 1967.

[22]Royal College of General Practitioners, "Oral Contraception and Thromboembolic Disease," *Journal of the Royal College of General Practitioners,* 13:267-279, 1967.

[23]Inman, W. H. W. and M.P. Vessey, "Investigation of Deaths from Pulmonary, Coronary, and Cerebral Thrombosis and Embolism in Women of Child-Bearing Age," *British Medical Journal,* 2:193-199, 1968.

[24]Vessey, M. P. and R. Doll, "Investigation of Relation Between Use of Oral Contraceptives and Thromboembolic Disease. A Further Report," *British Medical Journal,* 2:651-657, 1969.

[25]Sartwell, P. E., A. T. Masi, F. G. Arthes, G. R. Greene and H. E. Smith, "Thromboembolism and Oral Contraceptives: An Epidemiological Case Control Study," *American Journal of Epidemiology,* 90:365-380, 1969.

[26]Collaborative Group for the Study of Stroke in Young Women, "Oral Contraception and Increased Risk of Cerebral Ischemia or Thrombosis," *New England Journal of Medicine,* 288:871-878, 1973.

[27]Collaborative Group for the Study of Stroke in Young Women, "Oral Contraceptives and Stroke in Young Women: Associated Risk Factors," *Journal of the American Medical Association,* 231:718-722, 1975.

[28]Mann, J. I. and W. H. W. Inman, "Oral Contraceptives and Death from Myocardial Infarction," *British Medical Journal* 2:245-248, 1975.

[29]Mann, J. I., M. P. Vessey, M. Thorogood and R. Doll, "Myocardial Infarction in Young Women with Special Reference to Oral Contraceptive Practice," *British Medical Journal,* 2:241-245, 1975.

[30]Inman, W. H. W., V. P. Vessey, B. Westerholm and A. Engelund, "Thromboembolic Disease and the Steroidal Content of Oral Contraceptives," *British Medical Journal,* 2:203-209, 1970.

[31]Stolley, P. D., J. A. Tonascia, M. S. Tockman, P. E. Sartwell, A. H. Rutledge and M. P. Jacobs, "Thrombosis with Low-Estrogen Oral Contraceptives," *American Journal of Epidemiology,* 102:197-208, 1975.

[32]Vessey, M. P., R. Doll, A. S. Fairbairn and G. Glober, "Post-Operative Thromboembolism and the Use of the Oral Contraceptives," *British Medical Journal,* 3:123-126, 1970.

[33]Greene, G. R. and P. E. Sartwell, "Oral Contraceptive Use in Patients with Thromboembolism Following Surgery, Trauma or Infection," *American Journal of Public Health,* 62:680-685, 1972.

[34]Rosenberg, L., M. B. Armstrong and H. Jick, "Myocardial Infarction and Estrogen Therapy in Postmenopausal Women," *New England Journal of Medicine,* 294:1256-1259, 1976.

[35]Coronary Drug Project Research Group, "The Coronary Drug Project: Initial Findings Leading to Modifications of Its Research Protocol, *Journal of the American Medical Association,* 214:1303-1313, 1970.

[36]Baum, J., F. Holtz, J. J. Bookstein and E. W. Klein, "Possible Association Between Benign Hepatomas and Oral Contraceptives," *Lancet,* 2:926-928, 1973.

[37]Mays, E. T., W. M. Christopherson, M. M. Mahr and H. C. Williams, "Hepatic Changes in Young Women Ingesting Contraceptive Steroids, Hepatic Hemorrhage and Primary He-

Continued on next page

Abbott—Cont.

patic Tumors," *Journal of the American Medical Association,*" 235:730-782, 1976.

[38]Edmondson, H. A., B. Henderson and B. Benton, "Liver Cell Adenomas Associated with the Use of Oral Contraceptives," *New England Journal of Medicine,* 294:470-472, 1976.

[39]Pfeffer, R. I. and S. Van Den Noort, "Estrogen Use and Stroke Risk in Postmenopausal Women," *American Journal of Epidemiology,* 103:445-456, 1976.

PATIENT LABELING

WHAT YOU SHOULD KNOW ABOUT ESTROGENS

OGEN®

(Piperazine estrone sulfate)

Estrogens are female hormones produced by the ovaries. The ovaries make several different kinds of estrogens. In addition, scientists have been able to make a variety of synthetic estrogens. As far as we know, all these estrogens have similar properties and therefore much the same usefulness, side effects, and risks. This leaflet is intended to help you understand what estrogens are used for, the risks involved in their use, and how to use them as safely as possible.

This leaflet includes the most important information about estrogens, but not all the information. If you want to know more, you can ask your doctor or pharmacist to let you read the package insert prepared for the doctor.

Uses of Estrogen: Estrogens are prescribed by doctors for a number of purposes, including:

1. To provide estrogen during a period of adjustment when a woman's ovaries no longer produce it, in order to prevent certain uncomfortable symptoms of estrogen deficiency. (All women normally stop producing estrogens, generally between the age of 45 and 55; this is called the menopause.)
2. To prevent symptoms of estrogen deficiency, when a woman's ovaries have been removed surgically before the natural menopause.
3. To prevent pregnancy. (Estrogens are given along with a progestogen, another female hormone; these combinations are called oral contraceptives or birth control pills. Patient labeling is available to women taking oral contraceptives and they will not be discussed in this leaflet.)

THERE IS NO PROPER USE OF OGEN (PIPERAZINE ESTRONE SULFATE) IN A PREGNANT WOMAN.

Estrogens in The Menopause: In the natural course of their lives, all women eventually experience a decrease in estrogen production. This usually occurs between ages 45 and 55 but may occur earlier or later. Sometimes the ovaries may need to be removed before natural menopause by an operation, producing a "surgical menopause."

When the amount of estrogen in the blood begins to decrease, many women may develop typical symptoms: Feelings of warmth in the face, neck, and chest or sudden intense episodes of heat and sweating throughout the body (called "hot flashes" or "hot flushes"). These symptoms are sometimes very uncomfortable. A few women eventually develop changes in the vagina (called "atrophic vaginitis") which cause discomfort, especially during and after intercourse.

Estrogens can be prescribed to treat these symptoms of the menopause. It is estimated that considerably more than half of all women undergoing the menopause have only mild symptoms or no symptoms at all and therefore do not need estrogens. Other women may need estrogens for a few months, while their bodies adjust to lower estrogen levels. Sometimes the need will be for periods longer than six months. In an attempt to avoid over-stimulation of the uterus (womb), estrogens are usually given cyclically during each month of use, that is three weeks of pills followed by one week without pills.

Sometimes women experience nervous symptoms or depression during menopause. There is no evidence that estrogens are effective for such symptoms and they should not be used to treat them, although other treatment may be needed.

You may have heard that taking estrogens for long periods (years) after the menopause will keep your skin soft and supple and keep you feeling young. There is no evidence that this is so, however, and such long-term treatment carries important risks.

The Dangers of Estrogens:

1. *Cancer of the uterus.* If estrogens are used in the postmenopausal period for more than a year, there is an increased risk of *endometrial cancer* (cancer of the uterus). Women taking estrogens have roughly 5 to 10 times as great a chance of getting this cancer as women who take no estrogens. To put this another way, while a postmenopausal woman not taking estrogens has 1 chance in 1,000 each year of getting cancer of the uterus, a women taking estrogens has 5 to 10 chances in 1,000 each year. For this reason *it is important to take estrogens only when you really need them.*

The risk of this cancer is greater the longer estrogens are used and also seems to be greater when larger doses are taken. For this reason *it is important to take the lowest dose of estrogen that will control symptoms and to take it only as long as it is needed.* If estrogens are needed for longer periods of time, your doctor will want to reevaluate your need for estrogens at least every six months.

Women using estrogens should report any irregular vaginal bleeding to their doctors; such bleeding may be of no importance, but it can be an early warning of cancer of the uterus. If you have undiagnosed vaginal bleeding, you should not use estrogens until a diagnosis is made and you are certain there is no cancer of the uterus.

If you have had your uterus completely removed (total hysterectomy), there is no danger of developing cancer of the uterus.

2. *Other possible cancers.* Estrogens can cause development of other tumors in animals, such as tumors of the breast, cervix, vagina, or liver, when given for a long time. At present there is no good evidence that women using estrogen in the menopause have an increased risk of such tumors, but there is no way yet to be sure they do not; and one study raises the possibility that use of estrogens in the menopause may increase the risk of breast cancer many years later. This is a further reason to use estrogens only when clearly needed. While you are taking estrogens, it is important that you go to your doctor at least once a year for a physical examination. Also, if members of your family have had breast cancer or if you have breast nodules or abnormal mammograms (breast x-rays), your doctor may wish to carry out more frequent examinations of your breasts.

3. *Gall bladder disease.* Women who use estrogens after menopause are more likely to develop gall bladder disease needing surgery than women who do not use estrogens. Birth control pills have a similar effect.

4. *Abnormal blood clotting.* Oral contraceptives increase the risk of blood clotting in various parts of the body. This can result in a stroke (if the clot is in the brain), a heart attack (clot in a blood vessel of the heart), or a pulmonary embolus (a clot which forms in the legs or pelvis, then breaks off and travels to the lungs). Any of these can be fatal.

At this time use of estrogens in the menopause is not known to cause such blood clotting, but this has not been fully studied and there could still prove to be such a risk. It is recommended that if you have had clotting in the legs or lungs or a heart attack or stroke while you were using estrogens or birth control pills you should not use estrogens. If you have had a stroke or heart attack or if you have angina pectoris, estrogens should be used with great caution and only if clearly needed (for example, if you have severe symptoms of the menopause).

Special Warning About Pregnancy: You should not receive OGEN (piperazine estrone sulfate) if you are pregnant. Some scientists have reported that, if estrogens are used during pregnancy, there may be a greater than usual chance that the developing baby will be born with a birth defect, although the risk remains small. In addition, other scientists have reported that there is an association between another estrogen-type product (diethylstilbestrol) and appearance of a particular cancer of the vagina or cervix (adenocarcinoma) in young women whose mothers took that drug in pregnancy. Every effort should be made to avoid exposure to OGEN in pregnancy. If exposure occurs, see your doctor.

Other Effects of Estrogens: In addition to the serious known risks of estrogens described above, estrogens have the following side effects and potential risks:

1. *Nausea and vomiting.* The most common side effect of estrogen therapy is nausea. Vomiting is less common.
2. *Effects on breasts.* Estrogens may cause breast tenderness or enlargement and may cause the breasts to secrete a liquid. These effects are not dangerous.
3. *Effects on the uterus.* Estrogens may cause benign fibroid tumors of the uterus to get larger.

Some women will have menstrual bleeding when estrogens are stopped. But if the bleeding occurs on days you are still taking estrogens you should report this to your doctor.

4. *Effects on liver.* Women taking oral contraceptives develop on rare occasions a tumor of the liver which can rupture and bleed into the abdomen. So far, these tumors have not been reported in women using estrogens in the menopause, but you should report any swelling or unusual pain or tenderness in the abdomen to your doctor immediately.

Women with a past history of jaundice (yellowing of the skin and white parts of the eyes) may get jaundice again during estrogen use. If this occurs, stop taking estrogens and see your doctor.

5. *Other effects.* Estrogens may cause excess fluid to be retained in the body. This may make some conditions worse, such as epilepsy, migraine, heart disease, or kidney disease.

Summary: Estrogens have important uses, but they have serious risks as well. You must decide, with your doctor, whether the risks are acceptable to you in view of the benefits of treatment. You should not use OGEN if you have cancer of the breast or uterus, are pregnant, have undiagnosed abnormal vaginal bleeding, clotting in the legs or lungs, or have had a stroke, heart attack or angina, or clotting in the legs or lungs in the past while you were taking estrogens.

You can use estrogens as safely as possible by understanding that your doctor will require regular physical examinations while you are taking them and will try to discontinue the drug as soon as possible and use the smallest dose possible. Be alert for signs of trouble including:

1. Abnormal bleeding from the vagina.
2. Pains in the calves or chest or sudden shortness of breath, or coughing blood (indicating possible clots in the legs, heart or lungs).
3. Severe headache, dizziness, faintness or changes in vision (indicating possible developing clots in the brain or eye).
4. Breast lumps (you should ask your doctor how to examine your own breasts).

5. Jaundice (yellowing of the skin).
6. Mental depression.

Based on his or her assessment of your medical needs, your doctor has prescribed this drug for you. Do not give the drug to anyone else.
Ref. No. 03-4183/R5

OGEN® VAGINAL CREAM ℞
(piperazine estrone sulfate)

Warning:
1. ESTROGENS HAVE BEEN REPORTED TO INCREASE THE RISK OF ENDOMETRIAL CARCINOMA.
Three independent case control studies have shown an increased risk of endometrial cancer in postmenopausal women exposed to exogenous estrogens for prolonged periods.[1–3] This risk was independent of the other known risk factors for endometrial cancer. These studies are further supported by the finding that incidence rates of endometrial cancer have increased sharply since 1969 in eight different areas of the United States with population-based cancer reporting systems, an increase which may be related to the rapidly expanding use of estrogens during the last decade.[4]
The three case control studies reported that the risk of endometrial cancer in estrogen users was about 4.5 to 13.9 times greater than in nonusers. The risk appears to depend on both duration of treatment[1] and on estrogen dose.[3] In view of these findings, when estrogens are used for the treatment of menopausal symptoms, the lowest dose that will control symptoms should be utilized and medication should be discontinued as soon as possible. When prolonged treatment is medically indicated, the patient should be reassessed on at least a semiannual basis to determine the need for continued therapy. Although the evidence must be considered preliminary, one study suggests that cyclic administration of low doses of estrogen may carry less risk than continuous administration;[3] it therefore appears prudent to utilize such a regimen.
Close clinical surveillance of all women taking estrogens is important. In all cases of undiagnosed persistent or recurring abnormal vaginal bleeding, adequate diagnostic measures should be undertaken to rule out malignancy.
There is no evidence at present that "natural" estrogens are more or less hazardous than "synthetic" estrogens at equiestrogenic doses.
2. OGEN VAGINAL CREAM SHOULD NOT BE USED DURING PREGNANCY.
According to some investigators, the use of female sex hormones, both estrogens and progestogens, during early pregnancy may seriously damage the offspring. Studies have reported that females exposed in utero to diethylstilbestrol, a non-steroidal estrogen, have an increased risk of developing in later life a form of vaginal or cervical cancer that is ordinarily extremely rare.[5,6] In one of these studies, this risk was estimated as not greater than 4 per 1000 exposures.[7] Furthermore, there are reports that a high percentage of such exposed women (from 30 to 90 percent) have been found to have vaginal adenosis,[8–12] epithelial changes of the vagina and cervix. Although these reported changes are histologically benign, the investigators have not determined whether they are precursors of adenocarcinoma.
Several reports suggest an association between intrauterine exposure to female sex hormones and congenital anomalies in the offspring, including heart defects and limb reduction defects.[13–16] One case control study[16] estimated a 4.7 fold increased risk of limb reduction defects in infants exposed in utero to sex hormones (oral contraceptives, hormone withdrawal tests for pregnancy, or attempted treatment for threatened abortion). Some of these exposures were very short and involved only a few days of treatment. The data suggest that the risk of limb reduction defects in exposed fetuses is somewhat less than 1 per 1000.
In the past, female sex hormones have been used during pregnancy in an attempt to treat threatened or habitual abortion. OGEN Vaginal Cream is not intended for these uses, nor has it been studied for these uses, and therefore should not be used during pregnancy. There is no evidence from well controlled studies that progestogens are effective for these uses.
If OGEN Vaginal Cream (piperazine estrone sulfate) is used during pregnancy, or if the patient becomes pregnant while taking this drug, she should be apprised of the potential risks to the fetus, and the question of continuation of the pregnancy should be addressed.

Description: OGEN (piperazine estrone sulfate) is a preparation of pure, crystalline estrone, solubilized as the sulfate and stabilized with piperazine. It is appreciably soluble in water and has almost no odor or taste. The amount of piperazine in OGEN is not sufficient to exert a pharmacological action. Its addition ensures solubility, stability, and uniform potency of the estrone sulfate. Each gram of OGEN Vaginal Cream contains 1.5 mg. piperazine estrone sulfate in a base composed of the following ingredients: glycerin, mineral oil, glyceryl monostearate, polyethylene glycol ether complex of higher fatty alcohols, cetyl alcohol, anhydrous lanolin, sodium biphosphate, cis-N-(3-chloroallyl)hexaminium chloride, propylparaben, methylparaben, piperazine hexahydrate, citric acid and water.

Clinical Pharmacology: OGEN (piperazine estrone sulfate) Vaginal Cream owes its therapeutic action to estrone, one of the three principal estrogenic steroid hormones of man; estradiol, estrone, and estriol. These hormones are responsible for the development and maintenance of the female reproductive system and the primary and secondary female sex characteristics. They stimulate endometrial growth, promote the thickening, stratification, and cornification of the vagina, and cause the growth of mammary gland ducts.
A depletion of endogenous estrogens occurs postmenopausally as a result of a decline in ovarian function, and may cause symptomatic vulvovaginal epithelial atrophy. The signs and symptoms of these atrophic changes in the vaginal and vulval epithelia may be alleviated by the topical application of an estrogenic hormone such as OGEN.
OGEN Vaginal Cream may be absorbed transmucosally and may produce systemic estrogenic effects.

Indications: OGEN Vaginal Cream is indicated for the treatment of atrophic vaginitis or kraurosis vulvae.

OGEN VAGINAL CREAM HAS NOT BEEN TESTED FOR EFFICACY FOR ANY PURPOSE DURING PREGNANCY. SINCE ITS EFFECT UPON THE FETUS IS UNKNOWN, IT CANNOT BE RECOMMENDED FOR ANY CONDITION DURING PREGNANCY (SEE BOXED WARNING).

Contraindications: OGEN Vaginal Cream should not be used in women with any of the following conditions:
1. Known or suspected cancer of the breast.
2. Known or suspected estrogen-dependent neoplasia.
3. Known or suspected pregnancy (See Boxed Warning).
4. Undiagnosed abnormal genital bleeding.
5. Active thrombophlebitis or thromboembolic disorders.
6. A past history of thrombophlebitis, thrombosis, or thromboembolic disorders associated with previous estrogen use.

OGEN Vaginal Cream (piperazine estrone sulfate) is contraindicated in patients hypersensitive to its ingredients.

Warnings:
1. *Induction of malignant neoplasms.* Long-term continuous administration of natural and synthetic estrogens in certain animal species has been reported by some investigators to increase the frequency of carcinomas of the breast, cervix, vagina, and liver. There is now evidence that estrogens increase the risk of carcinoma of the endometrium in humans. (See Boxed Warning).
At the present time there is no satisfactory evidence that estrogens given to postmenopausal women increase the risk of cancer of the breast,[17] although a recent long-term followup of a single physician's practice has raised this possibility.[18] Therefore, caution should be exercised when administering estrogens to women with a strong family history of breast cancer or who have breast nodules, fibrocystic disease, or abnormal mammograms. Careful breast examinations should be performed periodically.
2. *Gall bladder disease.* A recent study has reported a 2 to 3-fold increase in the risk of surgically confirmed gall bladder disease in women receiving postmenopausal estrogens,[17] similar to the 2-fold increase previously noted in users of oral contraceptives.[19,22] In the case of oral contraceptives, the increased risk appeared after two years of use.[22]
3. *Effects similar to those caused by estrogen-progestogen oral contraceptives.* There are several serious adverse effects of oral contraceptives, most of which have not, up to now, been documented as consequences of postmenopausal estrogen therapy. This may reflect the comparatively low doses of estrogen used in postmenopausal women. It would be expected that the larger doses of estrogen used to treat postpartum breast engorgement would be more likely to result in these adverse effects, and, in fact, it has been shown that there is an increased risk of thrombosis in women receiving estrogens for postpartum breast engorgement.[20,21]
a. *Thromboembolic disease.* It is now well established that users of oral contraceptives have an increased risk of various thromboembolic and thrombotic vascular diseases, such as thrombophlebitis, pulmonary embolism, stroke, and myocardial infarction.[22–29] Cases of retinal thrombosis, mesenteric thrombosis, and optic neuritis have been reported in oral contraceptive users. There is evidence that the risk of several of these adverse reactions is related to the dose of the drug.[30,31] An increased risk of post-surgery thromboembolic complications has also been reported in users of oral contraceptives.[32,33] If feasible, estrogen should be discontinued at least 4 weeks before surgery of the type associated with an increased risk of thromboembolism; it should also be discontinued during periods of prolonged immobilization.
While an increased rate of thromboembolic and thrombotic disease in postmenopausal users of estrogens has not been found[17,34] this does not rule out the possibility that such an increase may be present or that subgroups of women who have underlying risk factors or who are receiving relatively large doses of es-

Continued on next page

Abbott—Cont.

trogens may have increased risk. Therefore estrogens should not be used in persons with active thrombophlebitis or thromboembolic disorders, and they should not be used in persons with a history of such disorders in association with estrogen use. They should be used with caution in patients with cerebral vascular or coronary artery disease and only for those in whom estrogens are clearly needed.

Large doses of estrogen (5 mg conjugated estrogens per day), comparable to those used to treat cancer of the prostate and breast, have been shown in a large prospective clinical trial in men[35] to increase the risk of nonfatal myocardial infarction, pulmonary embolism and thrombophlebitis. When estrogen doses of this size are used, any of the thromboembolic and thrombotic adverse effects associated with oral contraceptive use should be considered a clear risk.

b. *Hepatic adenoma.* Benign hepatic adenomas appear to be associated with the use of oral contraceptives.[36–38] Although benign, and rare, these may rupture and cause death through intraabdominal hemorrhage. Such lesions have not yet been reported in association with other estrogen or progestogen preparations but should be considered in estrogen users having abdominal pain and tenderness, abdominal mass, or hypovolemic shock. Hepatocellular carcinoma has also been reported in women taking estrogen-containing oral contraceptives.[37] The relationship of this malignancy to these drugs is not known at this time.

c. *Elevated blood pressure.* Increased blood pressure is not uncommon in women using oral contraceptives. There is now a report that this may occur with use of estrogens in the menopause[39] and blood pressure should be monitored with estrogen use, especially if high doses are used.

d. *Glucose tolerance.* A worsening of glucose tolerance has been observed in a significant percentage of patients on estrogen-containing oral contraceptives. For this reason, diabetic patients should be carefully observed while receiving estrogen.

4. *Hypercalcemia.* Administration of estrogens may lead to severe hypercalcemia in patients with breast cancer and bone metastases.

Precautions:

A. General Precautions.

1. A complete medical and family history should be taken prior to the initiation of any estrogen therapy. The pretreatment and periodic physical examinations should include special reference to blood pressure, breasts, abdomen, and pelvic organs, and should include a Papanicolau smear. As a general rule, estrogen should not be prescribed for longer than one year without another physical examination being performed.

2. Diagnostic measures should be taken to rule out gonorrhea or neoplasia before prescribing OGEN Vaginal Cream. Trichomonal, monilial, or bacterial infection should be treated by appropriate anti-microbial therapy.

3. Fluid retention — Estrogens may cause some degree of fluid retention. Therefore, patients with conditions such as epilepsy, migraine, and cardiac or renal dysfunction, which might be influenced by this factor, require careful observation.

4. Certain patients may develop undesirable manifestations of excessive estrogenic stimulation, such as abnormal or excessive uterine bleeding, mastodynia, etc.

5. Oral contraceptives appear to be associated with an increased incidence of mental depression.[22] Although it is not clear whether this is due to the estrogenic or progestogenic component of the contraceptive, patients with a history of depression should be carefully observed.

6. Preexisting uterine leiomyomata may increase in size during estrogen use.

7. The pathologist should be advised of the patient's use of estrogen therapy when relevant specimens are submitted.

8. Patients with a past history of jaundice during pregnancy have an increased risk of recurrence of jaundice while receiving estrogen-containing oral contraceptive therapy. If jaundice develops in any patient receiving estrogen, the medication should be discontinued while the cause is investigated.

9. Estrogens may be poorly metabolized in patients with impaired liver function and they should be administered with caution in such patients.

10. Because estrogens influence the metabolism of calcium and phosphorus, they should be used with caution in patients with metabolic bone diseases that are associated with hypercalcemia or in patients with renal insufficiency.

11. Because of the effects of estrogens on epiphyseal closure, they should be used judiciously in young patients in whom bone growth is not complete.

12. Certain endocrine and liver function tests may be affected by estrogen-containing oral contraceptives. The following similar changes may be expected with larger doses of estrogen:

a. Increased sulfobromophthalein retention.

b. Increased prothrombin and factors VII, VIII, IX, and X; decreased antithrombin 3; increased norepinephrine-induced platelet aggregability.

c. Increased thyroid binding globulin (TBG) leading to increased circulating total thyroid hormone, as measured by PBI, T4 by column, or T4 by radioimmunoassay. Free T3 resin uptake is decreased, reflecting the elevated TBG; free T4 concentration is unaltered.

d. Impaired glucose tolerance.

e. Decreased pregnanediol excretion.

f. Reduced response to metyrapone test.

g. Reduced serum folate concentration.

h. Increased serum triglyceride and phospholipid concentration.

B. Information for the Patient. See text of Patient Package Insert which appears after PHYSICIAN REFERENCES.

C. OGEN Vaginal Cream (piperazine estrone sulfate) cannot be recommended for use during pregnancy. See Contraindications and Boxed Warning.

D. Nursing Mothers. Estrogens have been reported to be excreted in human breast milk.

Adverse Reactions: Hypersensitivity reactions, systemic effects such as breast tenderness, and rarely, withdrawal bleeding have occurred with the use of topical estrogens.

The following additional adverse reactions have been reported with estrogenic therapy, including oral contraceptives (See WARNINGS regarding reports of possible induction of neoplasia, unknown effects upon the fetus, increased incidence of gall bladder disease, and adverse effects similar to those of oral contraceptives, including thromboembolism.):

1. *Genitourinary system.*
Breakthrough bleeding, spotting, change in menstrual flow.
Dysmenorrhea.
Premenstrual-like syndrome.
Amenorrhea during and after treatment.
Increase in size of uterine fibromyomata.
Vaginal candidiasis.
Change in cervical eversion and in degree of cervical secretion.
Cystitis-like syndrome.

2. *Breast.*
Tenderness, enlargement, secretion.

3. *Gastrointestinal.*
Nausea, vomiting.
Abdominal cramps, bloating.
Cholestatic jaundice.

4. *Skin.*
Chloasma or melasma which may persist when drug is discontinued.
Erythema multiforme.
Erythema nodosum.
Hemorrhagic eruption.
Loss of scalp hair.
Hirsutism.

5. *Eyes.*
Steepening of corneal curvature.
Intolerance to contact lenses.

6. *CNS.*
Headache, migraine, dizziness.
Mental depression.
Chorea.

7. *Miscellaneous.*
Increase or decrease in weight.
Reduced carbohydrate tolerance.
Aggravation of porphyria.
Edema.
Changes in libido.

Dosage and Administration: For treatment of atrophic vaginitis or kraurosis vulvae associated with the menopause.

The lowest dose that will control symptoms should be chosen and medication should be discontinued as promptly as possible.

Usual dosage: Intravaginally, 2 to 4 grams of OGEN Vaginal Cream daily, depending upon the severity of the condition.

The following instructions for use are intended for the patient and are printed on the carton label for OGEN Vaginal Cream (piperazine estrone sulfate):

1. Remove cap from tube.
2. Make sure plunger of applicator is all the way into the barrel.
3. Screw nozzle end of applicator onto the tube.
4. Squeeze tube to force sufficient cream into applicator so that number on plunger indicating prescribed dose is level with top of barrel.
5. Unscrew applicator from tube and replace cap on tube.
6. To deliver medication, insert end of applicator into vagina and push plunger all the way down.

Between uses, pull plunger out of barrel and wash applicator in warm, soapy water. DO NOT PUT APPLICATOR IN HOT OR BOILING WATER.

How Supplied: OGEN Vaginal Cream (1.5 mg. piperazine estrone sulfate per gram) is available in packages containing a 1½ oz. (42.5 Gm.) tube with one calibrated plastic applicator. (**NDC** 0074-2467-42).

[*Shown in Product Identification Section*]

Physician References:

[1]Ziel, H. K. and W. D. Finkel, "Increased Risk of Endometrial Carcinoma Among Users of Conjugated Estrogens," *New England Journal of Medicine,* 293:1167–1170, 1975.

[2]Smith, D. C., R. Prentic, D. J. Thompson and W. L. Hermann, "Association of Exogenous Estrogen and Endometrial Carcinoma," *New England Journal of Medicine,* 293:1164–1167, 1975.

[3]Mack, T. M., M. C. Pike, B. E. Henderson, R. I. Pfeffer, V. R. Gerkins, M. Arthur and S. E. Brown, "Estrogens and Endometrial Cancer in a Retirement Community," *New England Journal of Medicine,* 294:1262–1267, 1976.

[4]Weiss, N. S., D. R. Szekely and D. F. Austin, "Increasing Incidence of Endometrial Cancer in the United States," *New England Journal of Medicine,* 294:1259–1262, 1976.

[5]Herbst, A. L., H. Ulfelder and D. C. Poskanzer, "Adenocarcinoma of Vagina," *New England Journal of Medicine,* 284:878–881, 1971.

[6]Greenwald, P., J. Barlow, P. Nasca and W. Burnett, "Vaginal Cancer after Maternal Treatment with Synthetic Estrogens," *New England Journal of Medicine,* 285:390–392, 1971.

[7]Lanier, A., K. Noller, D. Decker, L. Elveback and L. Kurland, "Cancer and Stilbes-

trol. A Follow-up of 1719 Persons Exposed to Estrogens In Utero and Born 1943–1959," *Mayo Clinic Proceedings,* 48:793–799, 1973.

[8]Herbst, A., R. Kurman and R. Scully, "Vaginal and Cervical Abnormalities After Exposure to Stilbestrol In Utero," *Obstetrics and Gynecology,* 40:287–298, 1972.

[9]Herbst, A., S. Robboy, G. Macdonald and R. Scully, "The Effects of Local Progesterone on Stilbestrol-Associated Vaginal Adenosis," *American Journal of Obstetrics and Gynecology,* 118:607–615, 1974.

[10]Herbst, A., D. Poskanzer, S. Robboy, L. Friedlander and R. Scully, "Prenatal Exposure to Stilbestrol, A Prospective Comparison of Exposed Female Offspring with Unexposed Controls," *New England Journal of Medicine,* 292:334–339, 1975.

[11]Stafl, A., R. Mattingly, D. Foley and W. Fetherston, "Clinical Diagnosis of Vaginal Adenosis," *Obstetrics and Gynecology,* 43:118–128, 1974.

[12]Sherman, A. I., M. Goldrath, A. Berlin, V. Vakhariya, F. Banooni, W. Michaels, P. Goodman and S. Brown, "Cervical-Vaginal Adenosis After *In Utero* Exposure to Synthetic Estrogens," *Obstetrics and Gynecology,* 44:531–545, 1974.

[13]Gal, I., B. Kirman and J. Stern, "Hormone Pregnancy Tests and Congenital Malformation," *Nature,* 216:83, 1967.

[14]Levy, E. P., A. Cohen and F. C. Fraser, "Hormone Treatment During Pregnancy and Congenital Heart Defects," *Lancet,* 1:611, 1973.

[15]Nora, J. and A. Nora, "Birth Defects and Oral Contraceptives," *Lancet,* 1:941–942, 1973.

[16]Janerich, D. T., J. M. Piper and D. M. Glebatis, "Oral Contraceptives and Congenital Limb-Reduction Defects," *New England Journal of Medicine,* 291:697–700, 1974.

[17]Boston Collaborative Drug Surveillance Program "Surgically Confirmed Gall Bladder Disease, Venous Thromboembolism and Breast Tumors in Relation to Post-Menopausal Estrogen Therapy," *New England Journal of Medicine,* 290:15–19, 1974.

[18]Hoover, R., L. A. Gray, Sr., P. Cole and B. MacMahon, "Menopausal Estrogens and Breast Cancer," *New England Journal of Medicine,* 295:401–405, 1976.

[19]Boston Collaborative Drug Surveillance Program, "Oral Contraceptives and Venous Thromboembolic Disease, Surgically Confirmed Gall Bladder Disease and Breast Tumors," *Lancet* 1:1399–1404, 1973.

[20]Daniel, D. G., H. Campbell and A. C. Turnbull, "Puerperal Thromboembolism and Suppression of Lactation," *Lancet,* 2:287–289, 1967.

[21]Bailar, J. C., "Thromboembolism and Oestrogen Therapy," *Lancet,* 2:560, 1967.

[22]Royal College of General Practitioners, "Oral Contraception and Thromboembolic Disease," *Journal of the Royal College of General Practitioners,* 13:267–279, 1967.

[23]Inman, W. H. W. and M. P. Vessey, "Investigation of Deaths from Pulmonary, Coronary, and Cerebral Thrombosis and Embolism in Women of Child-Bearing Age," *British Medical Journal,* 2:193–199, 1968.

[24]Vessey, M. P. and R. Doll, "Investigation of Relation Between Use of Oral Contraceptives and Thromboembolic Disease. A Further Report," *British Medical Journal,* 2:651–657, 1969.

[25]Sartwell, P. E., A. T. Masi, F. G. Arthes, G. R. Greene and H. E. Smith, "Thromboembolism and Oral Contraceptives: An Epidemiological Case Control Study," *American Journal of Epidemiology,* 90:365–380, 1969.

[26]Collaborative Group for the Study of Stroke in Young Women, "Oral Contraception and Increased Risk of Cerebral Ischemia or Thrombosis," *New England Journal of Medicine,* 288:871–878, 1973.

[27]Collaborative Group for the Study of Stroke in Young Women, "Oral Contraceptives and Stroke in Young Women: Associated Risk Factors," *Journal of the American Medical Association,* 231:718–722, 1975.

[28]Mann, J. I. and W. H. W. Inman, "Oral Contraceptives and Death from Myocardial Infarction," *British Medical Journal,* 2:245–248, 1975.

[29]Mann, J. I., M. P. Vessey, M. Thorogood and R. Doll, "Myocardial Infarction in Young Women with Special Reference to Oral Contraceptive Practice," *British Medical Journal,* 2:241–245, 1975.

[30]Inman, W. H. W., V. P. Vessey, B. Westerholm and A. Engelund, "Thromboembolic Disease and the Steroidal Content of Oral Contraceptives," *British Medical Journal,* 2:203–209, 1970.

[31]Stolley, P. D., J. A. Tonascia, M. S. Tockman, P. E. Sartwell, A. H. Rutledge and M. P. Jacobs, "Thrombosis with Low-Estrogen Oral Contraceptives," *American Journal of Epidemiology,* 102:197–208, 1975.

[32]Vessey, M. P., R. Doll, A. S. Fairbairn and G. Glober, "Post-Operative Thromboembolism and the Use of the Oral Contraceptives," *British Medical Journal,* 3:123–126, 1970.

[33]Greene, G. R. and P. E. Sartwell, "Oral Contraceptive Use in Patients with Thromboembolism Following Surgery, Trauma or Infection," *American Journal of Public Health,* 62:680–685, 1972.

[34]Rosenberg, L., M. B. Armstrong and H. Jick, "Myocardial Infarction and Estrogen Therapy in Postmenopausal Women," *New England Journal of Medicine,* 294:1256–1259, 1976.

[35]Coronary Drug Project Research Group, "The Coronary Drug Project: Initial Findings Leading to Modifications of Its Research Protocol, *Journal of the American Medical Association,* 214:1303–1313, 1970.

[36]Baum, J., F. Holtz, J. J. Bookstein and E. W. Klein, "Possible Association Between Benign Hepatomas and Oral Contraceptives," *Lancet,* 2:926–928, 1973.

[37]Mays, E. T., W. M. Christopherson, M. M. Mahr and H. C. Williams, "Hepatic Changes in Young Women Ingesting Contraceptive Steroids, Hepatic Hemorrhage and Primary Hepatic Tumors," *Journal of the American Medical Association,* 235:730–782, 1976.

[38]Edmondson, H. A., B. Henderson and B. Benton, "Liver Cell Adenomas Associated with the Use of Oral Contraceptives," *New England Journal of Medicine,* 294:470–472, 1976.

[39]Pfeffer, R. I. and S. Van Den Noort, "Estrogen Use and Stroke Risk in Postmenopausal Women," *American Journal of Epidemiology,* 103:445–456, 1976.

PATIENT LABELING

OGEN® Vaginal Cream

(piperazine estrone sulfate)

You have been given an estrogen cream that is used for the local treatment of certain symptoms of estrogen deficiency: the soreness and itching of the vagina and vulva caused by drying and thinning (atrophy) of these tissues.

The discussion that follows is about estrogens that are taken internally for the treatment of symptoms of estrogen deficiency. Some or all of the information below on the systemic use of estrogens may also apply to the estrogen cream prescribed for you.

What You Should Know About Estrogens: Estrogens are female hormones produced by the ovaries. The ovaries make several different kinds of estrogens. In addition, scientists have been able to make a variety of synthetic estrogens. As far as we know, all these estrogens have similar properties and therefore much the same usefulness, side effects, and risks. This leaflet is intended to help you understand what estrogens are used for, the risks involved in their use, and how to use them as safely as possible.

This leaflet includes the most important information about estrogens, but not all the information. If you want to know more you can ask your doctor or pharmacist to let you read the package insert prepared for the doctor.

Uses of Estrogen: Estrogens are prescribed by doctors for a number of purposes, including:

1. To provide estrogen during a period of adjustment when a woman's ovaries no longer produce it, in order to prevent certain uncomfortable symptoms of estrogen deficiency. (All women normally stop producing estrogens, generally between the ages of 45 and 55; this is called the menopause.)
2. To prevent symptoms of estrogen deficiency when a woman's ovaries have been removed surgically before the natural menopause.
3. To prevent pregnancy. (Estrogens are given along with a progestogen, another female hormone; these combinations are called oral contraceptives or birth control pills. Patient labeling is available to women taking oral contraceptives and they will not be discussed in this leaflet.)

THERE IS NO PROPER USE OF OGEN (PIPERAZINE ESTRONE SULFATE) IN A PREGNANT WOMAN.

Estrogens in the Menopause: In the natural course of their lives, all women eventually experience a decrease in estrogen production. This usually occurs between ages 45 and 55 but may occur earlier or later. Sometimes the ovaries may need to be removed before natural menopause by an operation, producing a "surgical menopause."

When the amount of estrogen in the blood begins to decrease, many women may develop typical symptoms: Feelings of warmth in the face, neck, and chest or sudden intense episodes of heat and sweating throughout the body (called "hot flashes" or "hot flushes"). These symptoms are sometimes very uncomfortable. A few women eventually develop changes in the vagina (called "atrophic vaginitis") which cause discomfort, especially during and after intercourse.

Estrogens can be prescribed to treat these symptoms of the menopause. It is estimated that considerably more than half of all women undergoing the menopause have only mild symptoms or no symptoms at all and therefore do not need estrogens. Other women may need estrogens for a few months, while their bodies adjust to lower estrogen levels. Sometimes the need will be for periods longer than six months. Sometimes women experience nervous symptoms or depression during menopause. There is no evidence that estrogens are effective for such symptoms and they should not be used to treat them, although other treatment may be needed.

You may have heard that taking estrogens for long periods (years) after the menopause will keep your skin soft and supple and keep you feeling young. There is no evidence that this is so, however, and such long-term treatment carries important risks.

The Dangers of Estrogens:

1. *Cancer of the uterus.* If estrogens are used in the postmenopausal period for more than a year, there is an increased risk of *endometrial cancer* (cancer of the uterus). Women taking estrogens have roughly 5 to 10 times as great a chance of getting this cancer as women who take no estrogens. To put this another way, while a postmenopausal woman not taking estrogens has 1 chance in 1,000 each year of getting cancer of the uterus, a woman taking estrogens has 5 to 10 chances in 1,000 each year. For this reason *it is important to take estrogens only when you really need them.*

Continued on next page

Abbott—Cont.

The risk of this cancer is greater the longer estrogens are used and also seems to be greater when larger doses are taken. For this reason *it is important to take the lowest dose of estrogen that will control symptoms and to take it only as long as it is needed.* If estrogens are needed for longer periods of time, your doctor will want to reevaluate your need for estrogens at least every six months.
Women using estrogens should report any irregular vaginal bleeding to their doctors; such bleeding may be of no importance, but it can be an early warning of cancer of the uterus. If you have undiagnosed vaginal bleeding, you should not use estrogens until a diagnosis is made and you are certain there is no cancer of the uterus. If you have had your uterus completely removed (total hysterectomy), there is no danger of developing cancer of the uterus.
2. *Other possible cancers.* Estrogens can cause development of other tumors in animals, such as tumors of the breast, cervix, vagina, or liver, when given for a long time. At present there is no good evidence that women using estrogen in the menopause have an increased risk of such tumors, but there is no way yet to be sure they do not; and one study raises the possibility that use of estrogens in the menopause may increase the risk of breast cancer many years later. This is a further reason to use estrogens only when clearly needed. While you are taking estrogens, it is important that you go to your doctor at least once a year for a physical examination. Also, if members of your family have had breast cancer or if you have breast nodules or abnormal mammograms (breast x-rays), your doctor may wish to carry out more frequent examinations of your breasts.
3. *Gall bladder disease.* Women who use estrogens after menopause are more likely to develop gall bladder disease needing surgery than women who do not use estrogens. Birth control pills have a similar effect.
4. *Abnormal blood clotting.* Oral contraceptives increase the risk of blood clotting in various parts of the body. This can result in a stroke (if the clot is in the brain), a heart attack (clot in a blood vessel of the heart), or a pulmonary embolus (a clot which forms in the legs or pelvis, then breaks off and travels to the lungs). Any of these can be fatal.
At this time use of estrogens in the menopause is not known to cause such blood clotting, but this has not been fully studied and there could still prove to be such a risk. It is recommended that if you have had clotting in the legs or lungs or a heart attack or stroke while you were using estrogens or birth control pills, you should not use estrogens. If you have had a stroke or heart attack or if you have angina pectoris, estrogens should be used with great caution and only if clearly needed (for example, if you have severe symptoms of the menopause).
Special Warning About Pregnancy: You should not receive Ogen (piperazine estrone sulfate) if you are pregnant. Some scientists have reported that, if estrogens are used during pregnancy, there may be a greater than usual chance that the developing baby will be born with a birth defect, although the risk remains small. In addition, other scientists have reported that there is an association between another estrogen-type product (diethylstilbestrol) and appearance of a particular cancer of the vagina or cervix (adenocarcinoma) in young women whose mothers took that drug in pregnancy. Every effort should be made to avoid exposure to Ogen in pregnancy. If exposure occurs, see your doctor.
Other Effects of Estrogens: In addition to the serious known risks of estrogens described above, estrogens have the following side effects and potential risks:
1. *Nausea and vomiting.* The most common side effect of estrogen therapy is nausea. Vomiting is less common.
2. *Effects on breasts.* Estrogens may cause breast tenderness or enlargement and may cause the breasts to secrete a liquid. These effects are not dangerous.
3. *Effects on the uterus.* Estrogens may cause benign fibroid tumors of the uterus to get larger.
Some women will have menstrual bleeding when estrogens are stopped. But if the bleeding occurs on days you are still taking estrogens you should report this to your doctor.
4. *Effects on liver.* Women taking oral contraceptives develop on rare occasions a tumor of the liver which can rupture and bleed into the abdomen. So far, these tumors have not been reported in women using estrogens in the menopause, but you should report any swelling or unusual pain or tenderness in the abdomen to your doctor immediately.
Women with a past history of jaundice (yellowing of the skin and white parts of the eyes) may get jaundice again during estrogen use. If this occurs, stop taking estrogens and see your doctor.
5. *Other effects.* Estrogens may cause excess fluid to be retained in the body. This may make some conditions worse, such as epilepsy, migraine, heart disease, or kidney disease.
Summary: Estrogens have important uses, but they have serious risks as well. You must decide, with your doctor, whether the risks are acceptable to you in view of the benefits of treatment. You should not use OGEN if you have cancer of the breast or uterus, are pregnant, have undiagnosed abnormal vaginal bleeding, clotting in the legs or lungs, or have had a stroke, heart attack or angina, or clotting in the legs or lungs in the past while you were taking estrogens.
You can use estrogens as safely as possible by understanding that your doctor will require regular physical examinations while you are taking them and will try to discontinue the drug as soon as possible and use the smallest dose possible. Be alert for signs of trouble including:
1. Abnormal bleeding from the vagina.
2. Pains in the calves or chest or sudden shortness of breath, or coughing blood (indicating possible clots in the legs, heart or lungs).
3. Severe headache, dizziness, faintness, or changes in vision (indicating possible developing clots in the brain or eye).
4. Breast lumps (you should ask your doctor how to examine your own breasts).
5. Jaundice (yellowing of the skin).
6. Mental depression.

Based on his or her assessment of your medical needs, your doctor has prescribed this drug for you. Do not give the drug to anyone else.
Ref. No. 01-2921/R1

OPTILETS®-500
High potency multivitamin for use in treatment of multivitamin deficiency.*

OPTILETS-M-500®
High potency multivitamin for use in treatment of multivitamin deficiency.* Mineral supplementation added.**

Description: A therapeutic formula of ten important vitamins, with and without minerals, in a small tablet with the Abbott Filmtab® coating. Each Optilets-500 tablet provides:
Vitamin C (as sodium ascorbate)..........500 mg
Niacinamide..........100 mg
Calcium Pantothenate ....20 mg
Vitamin B_1 (thiamine mononitrate).......15 mg
Vitamin B_2 (riboflavin)..........10 mg
Vitamin B_6 (pyridoxine hydrochloride) ...5 mg
Vitamin A (as palmitate 1.5 mg, as acetate 1.5 mg—total 3 mg)..........10,000 IU
Vitamin B_{12} (Cyanocobalamin)..........12 mcg
Vitamin D (ergocalciferol)......(10 mcg) 400 IU
Vitamin E (as dl-alpha tocopheryl acetate)..........30 IU
Each Optilets-M-500 Filmtab contains all the vitamins in the same quantities provided in Optilets-500, plus the following minerals:
Magnesium (as oxide)..........80 mg**
Iron (as dried ferrous sulfate)..........20 mg
Copper (as sulfate)..........2 mg
Zinc (as sulfate)..........1.5 mg**
Manganese (as sulfate)..........1 mg
Iodine (as calcium iodate)..........0.15 mg
* These products contain no folic acid and only dietary supplement levels of vitamins D and E.
** Below USRDA levels.
Dosage and Administration: Usual adult dosage is one Filmtab tablet daily, or as directed by physician.
How Supplied: Optilets-500 tablets are supplied in bottles of 30 (**NDC** 0074-4287-30) and 100 (**NDC** 0074-4287-13). Optilets-M-500 tablets are supplied in bottles of 30 (**NDC** 0074-4286-30) and 100 (**NDC** 0074-4286-13).
[*Shown in Product Identification Section*]
Ref. 02-5548-3/R6, 02-5551-4/R8

ORETIC® ℞
(hydrochlorothiazide tablets, U.S.P.)

Description: ORETIC (hydrochlorothiazide) is a member of the benzothiadiazine (thiazide) family of drugs. It is closely related to chlorothiazide. Clinically, ORETIC is an orally active diuretic-antihypertensive agent.
Actions: The diuretic and saluretic effects of ORETIC result from a drug-induced inhibition of the renal tubular reabsorption of electrolytes. The excretion of sodium and chloride is greatly enhanced. Potassium excretion is also enhanced to a variable degree, as it is with the other thiazides. Although urinary excretion of bicarbonate is increased slightly, there is usually no significant change in urinary pH. Hydrochlorothiazide has a per mg. natriuretic activity approximately 10 times that of the prototype thiazide, chlorothiazide. At maximal therapeutic dosages, all thiazides are approximately equal in their diuretic/natriuretic effects.
There is significant natriuresis and diuresis within two hours after administration of a single oral dose of hydrochlorothiazide. These effects reach a peak in about six hours and persist for about 12 hours following oral administration of a single dose.
Like other benzothiadiazines, ORETIC also has antihypertensive properties, and may be used for this purpose either alone or to enhance the antihypertensive action of other drugs. The mechanism by which the benzothiadiazines, including hydrochlorothiazide, produce a reduction of elevated blood pressure is not known. However, sodium depletion appears to be involved.
ORETIC (hydrochlorothiazide) is readily absorbed from the gastrointestinal tract and is excreted unchanged by the kidneys.
Indications: ORETIC is indicated in the management of hypertension either as the sole therapeutic agent or to enhance the effect of other antihypertensive drugs in the more severe forms of hypertension.
ORETIC is indicated as adjunctive therapy in edema associated with congestive heart failure, hepatic cirrhosis, and corticosteroid and estrogen therapy.
ORETIC has also been found useful in edema due to various forms of renal dysfunction such as the nephrotic syndrome, acute glomerulonephritis and chronic renal failure.
Usage in Pregnancy: The routine use of diuretics in an otherwise healthy pregnant woman is inappropriate and exposes mother and fetus to unnecessary hazard. Diuretics do not prevent development of toxemia of pregnancy, and there is no satisfactory evidence

that they are useful in the treatment of developed toxemia.
Edema during pregnancy may arise from pathological causes or from the physiological and mechanical consequences of pregnancy. Thiazides are indicated in pregnancy when edema is due to pathological causes, just as they are in the absence of pregnancy (however, see Warnings, below). Dependent edema in pregnancy, resulting from restriction of venous return by the expanded uterus, is properly treated through elevation of the lower extremities and use of support hose; use of diuretics to lower intravascular volume in this case is illogical and unnecessary. There is hypervolemia during normal pregnancy which is harmful to neither the fetus nor the mother (in the absence of cardiovascular disease), but which is associated with edema, including generalized edema, in the majority of pregnant women. If this edema produces discomfort, increased recumbency will often provide relief. In rare instances, this edema may cause extreme discomfort which is not relieved by rest. In these cases, a short course of diuretics may provide relief and may be appropriate.
Contraindications: Renal decompensation. Hypersensitivity to this or other sulfonamide-derived drugs.
Warnings: Hydrochlorothiazide shares with other thiazides the propensity to deplete potassium reserves to an unpredictable degree.
Thiazides should be used with caution in patients with renal disease or significant impairment of renal function, since azotemia may be precipitated and cumulative drug effects may occur.
Thiazides should be used with caution in patients with impaired hepatic function or progressive liver disease, since minor alterations of fluid and electrolyte balance may precipitate hepatic coma.
Thiazides may be additive or potentiative of the action of other antihypertensive drugs. Potentiation occurs with ganglionic or peripheral adrenergic blocking drugs.
Sensitivity reactions may occur in patients with a history of allergy or bronchial asthma. The possibility of exacerbation or activation of systemic lupus erythematosus has been reported.
Usage in Pregnancy: Thiazides cross the placental barrier and appear in cord blood. The use of thiazides in pregnant women requires that the anticipated benefit be weighed against possible hazards to the fetus. These hazards include fetal or neonatal jaundice, thrombocytopenia, and possible other adverse reactions that have occurred in the adult.
Nursing Mothers: Thiazides appear in breast milk. If use of the drug is deemed essential, the patient should stop nursing.
Precautions: Periodic determinations of serum electrolytes should be performed at appropriate intervals for the purpose of detecting possible electrolyte imbalances such as hyponatremia, hypochloremic alkalosis, and hypokalemia. Serum and urine electrolyte determinations are particularly important when a patient is vomiting excessively or receiving parenteral fluids. All patients should be observed for other clinical signs of electrolyte imbalances such as dryness of mouth, thirst, weakness, lethargy, drowsiness, restlessness, muscle pains or cramps, muscular fatigue, hypotension, oliguria, tachycardia, and gastrointestinal disturbances such as nausea and vomiting.
Hypokalemia may develop with thiazides as with any other potent diuretic, especially when brisk diuresis occurs, severe cirrhosis is present, or when corticosteroids or ACTH are given concomitantly. Interference with the adequate oral intake of electrolytes will also contribute to the possible development of hypokalemia. Potassium depletion, even of a mild degree, resulting from thiazide use, may sensitize a patient to the effects of cardiac glycosides such as digitalis.
Any chloride deficit is generally mild and usually does not require specific treatment except under extraordinary circumstances (as in liver disease or renal disease). Dilutional hyponatremia may occur in edematous patients in hot weather; appropriate therapy is water restriction rather than administration of salt, except in rare instances when the hyponatremia is life threatening.
In actual salt depletion, appropriate replacement is the therapy of choice.
Hyperuricemia may occur or frank gout may be precipitated in certain patients receiving thiazide therapy.
Insulin requirements in diabetic patients may be increased, decreased, or unchanged. Latent diabetes mellitus may become manifest during thiazide administration.
Thiazide drugs may increase the responsiveness to tubocurarine.
The antihypertensive effects of the drug may be enhanced in the postsympathectomy patient.
Thiazides may decrease arterial responsiveness to norepinephrine. This diminution is not sufficient to preclude effectiveness of the pressor agent for therapeutic use.
If progressive renal impairment becomes evident as indicated by a rising-nonprotein nitrogen or blood urea nitrogen, a careful reappraisal of therapy is necessary with consideration given to withholding or discontinuing diuretic therapy.
Thiazides may decrease serum PBI levels without signs of thyroid disturbance.
Thiazides have been reported, on rare occasions, to have elevated serum calcium to hypercalcemic levels. The serum calcium levels have returned to normal when the medication has been stopped. This phenomenon may be related to the ability of the thiazide diuretics to lower the amount of calcium excreted in the urine.
Adverse Reactions: Gastrointestinal system reactions: Anorexia, gastric irritation, nausea, vomiting, cramping, diarrhea, constipation, jaundice (intrahepatic cholestatic jaundice), pancreatitis.
Central nervous system reactions: Dizziness, vertigo, paresthesias, headache, xanthopsia.
Hematologic reactions: Leukopenia, agranulocytosis, thrombocytopenia, aplastic anemia.
Dermatologic — hypersensitivity reactions: Purpura, photosensitivity, rash, urticaria, necrotizing angiitis (vasculitis) (cutaneous vasculitis).
Cardiovascular reaction: Orthostatic hypotension may occur and may be aggravated by alcohol, barbiturates, or narcotics.
Other: Hyperglycemia, glycosuria, hypercalcemia, hyperuricemia, muscle spasm, weakness, restlessness.
There have been isolated reports that certain nonedematous individuals developed severe fluid and electrolyte derangements after only brief exposure to normal doses of thiazide and non-thiazide diuretics. The condition is usually manifested as severe dilutional hyponatremia, hypokalemia, and hypochloremia. It has been reported to be due to inappropriately increased ADH secretion and appears to be idiosyncratic. Potassium replacement is apparently the most important therapy in the treatment of this syndrome along with removal of the offending drug.
Whenever adverse reactions are severe, treatment should be discontinued.
Dosage and Administration: ORETIC (hydrochlorothiazide) is administered orally. Therapy should be individualized according to patient response. This therapy should be titrated to gain maximal therapeutic response as well as the minimal dose possible to maintain that therapeutic response.
For the management of edema the adult dosage ranges from 25 to 200 mg. daily and may be given in single or divided doses. Usually 75 to 100 mg. will produce the desired diuretic effect.
For the management of hypertension the usual initial adult dosage is 25 to 50 mg. two times daily. The dosage may be increased if necessary to a maximum of 100 mg. twice daily.
When therapy is prolonged or large doses are used, particular attention should be given to the patient's electrolyte status. Supplemental potassium may be required.
In the treatment of hypertension hydrochlorothiazide may be either employed alone or concurrently with other antihypertensive drugs. Combined therapy may provide adequate control of hypertension with lower dosage of the component drugs and fewer or less severe side effects. An enhanced response frequently follows its concurrent administration with Harmonyl® (deserpidine) so that dosage of both drugs may be reduced.
For treatment of moderately severe or severe hypertension, supplemental use of other more potent antihypertensive agents such as Eutonyl® (pargyline hydrochloride) may be indicated.
When other antihypertensive agents are to be added to the regimen, this should be accomplished gradually. Additional potent antihypertensive agents should be given at only half the usual dose since their effect is potentiated by pretreatment with ORETIC.
Overdosage: Symptoms of overdosage include electrolyte imbalance and signs of potassium deficiency such as confusion, dizziness, muscular weakness, and gastrointestinal disturbances. General supportive measures including replacement of fluids and electrolytes may be indicated in treatment of overdosage.
How Supplied: ORETIC (hydrochlorothiazide tablets, U.S.P.) is provided in two dosage sizes as white tablets:
25 mg. tablets:
bottles of 100 (**NDC** 0074-6978-01),
bottles of 1000 (**NDC** 0074-6978-02),
Abbo-Pac® unit dose packages, 100 tablets (**NDC** 0074-6978-05).
50 mg. tablets:
bottles of 100 (**NDC** 0074-6985-01),
bottles of 1000 (**NDC** 0074-6985-02),
Abbo-Pac unit dose packages, 100 tablets (**NDC** 0074-6985-06).
[*Shown in Product Identification Section*]
01-2968-R2

ORETICYL® ℞
(hydrochlorothiazide and deserpidine tablets)

Oral thiazide-rauwolfia therapy for hypertension.

Warning:
This fixed combination drug is not indicated for initial therapy of hypertension. Hypertension requires therapy titrated to the individual patient. If the fixed combination represents the dosage so determined, its use may be more convenient in patient management. The treatment of hypertension is not static, but must be reevaluated as conditions in each patient warrant.

Description: ORETICYL is an orally administered combination of Oretic® (hydrochlorothiazide) and Harmonyl® (deserpidine). Hydrochlorothiazide is a diuretic-antihypertensive agent of the benzothiadiazine (thiazide) class. Deserpidine is a purified rauwolfia alkaloid,

Continued on next page

Abbott—Cont.

chemically identified as 11-desmethoxyreserpine, which produces antihypertensive effects.
Actions: The combined antihypertensive actions of hydrochlorothiazide and deserpidine result in a total clinical antihypertensive effect which is greater than can ordinarily be achieved by either drug given individually.
The diuretic and saluretic effects of hydrochlorothiazide result from a drug-induced inhibition of the renal tubular reabsorption of electrolytes. The excretion of sodium and chloride is greatly enhanced. Potassium excretion is also enhanced to a variable degree, as it is with the other thiazides. Although urinary excretion of bicarbonate is increased slightly, there is usually no significant change in urinary pH.
Hydrochlorothiazide has a per mg natriuretic activity approximately 10 times that of the prototype thiazide, chlorothiazide. At maximal therapeutic dosages, all thiazides are approximately equal in their diuretic/natriuretic effects.
There is significant natriuresis and diuresis within two hours after administration of a single oral dose of hydrochlorothiazide. These effects reach a peak in about six hours and persist for about 12 hours following oral administration of a single dose.
Like other benzothiadiazines, hydrochlorothiazide also has antihypertensive properties, and may be used for this purpose either alone or to enhance the antihypertensive action of other drugs. The mechanism by which the benzothiadiazines, including hydrochlorothiazide, produce a reduction of elevated blood pressure is not known. However, sodium depletion appears to be involved.
Hydrochlorothiazide is readily absorbed from the gastrointestinal tract and is excreted unchanged by the kidneys.
The pharmacologic actions of Harmonyl (deserpidine) are essentially the same as those of other active rauwolfia alkaloids. Deserpidine probably produces its antihypertensive effects through depletion of tissue stores of catecholamines (epinephrine and norepinephrine) from peripheral sites. The antihypertensive effect is often accompanied by bradycardia. There is no significant alteration in cardiac output or renal blood flow. The carotid sinus reflex is inhibited, but postural hypotension is rarely seen with the use of conventional doses of Harmonyl alone.
Deserpidine, like other rauwolfia alkaloids, is characterized by slow onset of action and sustained effect which may persist following withdrawal of the drug.
Indications: ORETICYL (hydrochlorothiazide and deserpidine) is indicated in the treatment of patients with mild to moderately severe hypertension (see boxed warning). It may be used alone for this purpose or added to other antihypertensive agents for the management of more severe hypertension. When administered with ORETICYL, more potent agents can be given at reduced dosage to minimize undesirable side effects.
Contraindications: Hydrochlorothiazide is contraindicated in patients with renal decompensation and in those who are hypersensitive to this or other sulfonamide-derived drugs.
Deserpidine is contraindicated in patients with known hypersensitivity, mental depression especially with suicidal tendencies, active peptic ulcer, and ulcerative colitis. It is also contraindicated in patients receiving electroconvulsive therapy.
Warnings:
Hydrochlorothiazide
Hydrochlorothiazide shares with other thiazides the propensity to deplete potassium reserves to an unpredictable degree.
Thiazides should be used with caution in patients with renal disease or significant impairment of renal function, since azotemia may be precipitated and cumulative drug effects may occur.
Thiazides should be used with caution in patients with impaired hepatic function or progressive liver disease, since minor alterations of fluid and electrolyte balance may precipitate hepatic coma.
Thiazides may be additive or potentiative of the action of other antihypertensive drugs. Potentiation occurs with ganglionic or peripheral adrenergic blocking drugs.
Sensitivity reactions may occur in patients with a history of allergy or bronchial asthma.
The possibility of exacerbation or activation of systemic lupus erythematosus has been reported.
Deserpidine
Extreme caution should be exercised in treating patients with a history of mental depression. Discontinue the drug at the first sign, of despondency, early morning insomnia, loss of appetite, impotence, or self-deprecation. Drug-induced depression may persist for several months after drug withdrawal and may be severe enough to result in suicide.
Usage in Pregnancy and Lactation
Hydrochlorothiazide
Thiazides cross the placental barrier and appear in cord blood. The use of thiazides in pregnant women requires that the anticipated benefit be weighed against possible hazards to the fetus. These hazards include fetal or neonatal jaundice, thrombocytopenia, and possible other adverse reactions that have occurred in the adult.
Thiazides appear in breast milk. If use of the drug is deemed essential, the patient should stop nursing.
Deserpidine
The safety of deserpidine for use during pregnancy or lactation has not been established; therefore, it should be used in pregnant women or in women of childbearing potential only when in the judgment of the physician its use is deemed essential to the welfare of the patient. Increased respiratory secretions, nasal congestion, cyanosis, and anorexia may occur in infants born to rauwolfia alkaloid-treated mothers, since these preparations are known to cross the placental barrier to enter the fetal circulation and appear in cord blood. They also are secreted by nursing mothers into breast milk.
Reproductive and teratology studies in rats reduced the mating index and neonatal survival indices. The no-effect dosage has not been established.
Precautions: Periodic determinations of serum electrolytes should be performed at appropriate intervals for the purpose of detecting possible electrolyte imbalances such as hyponatremia, hypochloremic alkalosis, and hypokalemia. Serum and urine electrolyte determinations are particularly important when a patient is vomiting excessively or receiving parenteral fluids. All patients should be observed for other clinical signs of electrolyte imbalances such as dryness of mouth, thirst, weakness, lethargy, drowsiness, restlessness, muscle pains or cramps, muscular fatigue, hypotension, oliguria, tachycardia, and gastrointestinal disturbances such as nausea and vomiting.
Hypokalemia may develop with thiazides as with any other potent diuretic, especially when brisk diuresis occurs, severe cirrhosis is present, or when corticosteroids or ACTH are given concomitantly. Interference with the adequate oral intake of electrolytes will also contribute to the possible development of hypokalemia. Potassium depletion, even of a mild degree, resulting from thiazide use, may sensitize a patient to the effects of cardiac glycosides such as digitalis.
Any chloride deficit is generally mild and usually does not require specific treatment except under extraordinary circumstances (as in liver disease or renal disease). Dilutional hyponatremia may occur in edematous patients in hot weather; appropriate therapy is water restriction rather than administration of salt, except in rare instances when the hyponatremia is life threatening.
In actual salt depletion, appropriate replacement is the therapy of choice.
Hyperuricemia may occur or frank gout may be precipitated in certain patients receiving thiazide therapy.
Insulin requirements in diabetic patients may be increased, decreased, or unchanged. Latent diabetes mellitus may become manifest during thiazide administration.
Thiazide drugs may increase the responsiveness to tubocurarine.
The antihypertensive effects of the drug may be enhanced in the postsympathectomy patient.
Thiazides may decrease arterial responsiveness to norepinephrine. This diminution is not sufficient to preclude effectiveness of the pressor agent for therapeutic use.
If progressive renal impairment becomes evident as indicated by a rising-nonprotein nitrogen or blood urea nitrogen, a careful reappraisal of therapy is necessary with consideration given to withholding or discontinuing diuretic therapy.
Thiazides may decrease serum PBI levels without signs of thyroid disturbance.
Thiazides have been reported, on rare occasions, to have elevated serum calcium to hypercalcemic levels. The serum calcium levels have returned to normal when the medication has been stopped. This phenomenon may be related to the ability of the thiazide diuretics to lower the amount of calcium excreted in the urine.
Because rauwolfia preparations increase gastrointestinal motility and secretion, this drug should be used cautiously in patients with a history of peptic ulcer, ulcerative colitis, or gallstones, where biliary colic may be precipitated.
Caution should be exercised when treating hypertensive patients with renal insufficiency since they adjust poorly to lowered blood pressure levels.
Use deserpidine cautiously with digitalis and quinidine since cardiac arrhythmias have occurred with rauwolfia preparations.
Preoperative withdrawal of deserpidine does not assure that circulatory instability will not occur. It is important that the anesthesiologist be aware of the patient's drug intake and consider this in the overall management, since hypotension has occurred in patients receiving rauwolfia preparations. Anticholinergic and/or adrenergic drugs (metaraminol, norepinephrine) have been employed to treat adverse vagocirculatory effects.
Adverse Reactions:
Hydrochlorothiazide
Gastrointestinal System Reactions: Anorexia, gastric irritation, nausea, vomiting, cramping, diarrhea, constipation, jaundice (intrahepatic cholestatic jaundice), pancreatitis.
Central Nervous System Reactions: Dizziness, vertigo, paresthesias, headache, xanthopsia.
Hematologic Reactions: Leukopenia, agranulocytosis, thrombocytopenia, aplastic anemia.
Dermatologic — Hypersensitivity Reactions: Purpura, photosensitivity, rash, urticaria, necrotizing angitis (vasculitis) (cutaneous vasculitis).
Cardiovascular Reaction: Orthostatic hypotension may occur and may be aggravated by alcohol, barbiturates, or narcotics.
Other: Hyperglycemia, glycosuria, hypercalcemia, hyperuricemia, muscle spasm, weakness, restlessness.
There have been isolated reports that certain nonedematous individuals developed severe fluid and electrolyte derangements after only brief exposure to normal doses of thiazide and non-thiazide diuretics. The condition is usually

manifested as severe dilutional hyponatremia, hypokalemia, and hypochloremia. It has been reported to be due to inappropriately increased ADH secretion and appears to be idiosyncratic. Potassium replacement is apparently the most important therapy in the treatment of this syndrome along with the removal of the offending drug.

Whenever adverse reactions are severe, treatment should be discontinued.

Deserpidine

The following adverse reactions have been reported with rauwolfia preparations. These reactions are usually reversible and disappear when the drug is discontinued.

Gastrointestinal: Including hypersecretion, anorexia, diarrhea, nausea, and vomiting.

Cardiovascular: Including angina-like symptoms, arrhythmias (particularly when used concurrently with digitalis or quinidine), and bradycardia.

Central Nervous System: Including drowsiness, depression, nervousness, paradoxical anxiety, nightmares, extrapyramidal tract symptoms, CNS sensitization manifested by dull sensorium, and deafness.

Dermatologic—Hypersensitivity: Including pruritus, rash, and asthma in asthmatic patients.

Ophthalmologic: Including glaucoma, uveitis, optic atrophy, and conjunctival injection.

Hematologic: Thrombocytopenic purpura.

Miscellaneous: Nasal congestion, weight gain, impotence or decreased libido, dysuria, dyspnea, muscular aches, dryness of mouth, dizziness and headache.

Dosage and Administration:

Dosage should be determined by individual titration of ingredients (see boxed warning). Dosage of both components should be carefully adjusted to the needs of the individual patient. Since at least ten days to two weeks may elapse before the full effects of the drugs become manifest, the dosage should not be adjusted more frequently.

Three tablet strengths, ORETICYL 25 (hydrochlorothiazide 25 mg, deserpidine 0.125 mg); ORETICYL 50 (hydrochlorothiazide 50 mg, deserpidine 0.125 mg); and ORETICYL FORTE (hydrochlorothiazide 25 mg, deserpidine 0.25 mg), all grooved, are provided to permit considerable latitude in meeting the dosage requirements of individual patients.

The table below will help in determining which dose of ORETICYL 25, ORETICYL 50, or ORETICYL FORTE best represents the equivalent of the titrated dose.

ORETICYL 25	hydro-chlorothiazide	deserpidine
1 tablet bid	25.0 mg bid	0.125 mg bid
1½ tablet bid	37.5 mg bid	0.188 mg bid
2 tablets bid	50.0 mg bid	0.250 mg bid

ORETICYL 50	hydro-chlorothiazide	deserpidine
1 tablet bid	50 mg bid	0.125 mg bid
1½ tablet bid	75 mg bid	0.188 mg bid
2 tablets bid	100 mg bid	0.250 mg bid

ORETICYL FORTE	hydro-chlorothiazide	deserpidine
1 tablet bid	25.0 mg bid	0.250 mg bid
1½ tablet bid	37.5 mg bid	0.375 mg bid
2 tablets bid	50.0 mg bid	0.500 mg bid

The usual adult dosage is one ORETICYL 50 two times daily.

When other antihypertensive agents are to be added to the regimen, this should be accomplished gradually. Ganglionic blocking agents should be given at only half the usual dose since their effect is potentiated by pretreatment with ORETICYL (hydrochlorothiazide and deserpidine).

Overdosage: Symptoms of thiazide overdosage include electrolyte imbalance and signs of potassium deficiency such as confusion, dizziness, muscular weakness, and gastrointestinal disturbances. General supportive measures including replacement of fluids and electrolytes may be indicated in treatment of overdosage.

An overdosage of deserpidine is characterized by flushing of the skin, conjunctival injection, and pupillary constriction. Sedation ranging from drowsiness to coma may occur. Hypotension, hypothermia, central respiratory depression and bradycardia may develop in cases of severe overdosage. Treatment consists of the careful evacuation of stomach contents followed by the usual procedures for the symptomatic management of CNS depressant overdosage. If severe hypotension occurs it should be treated with a direct acting vasopressor such as levarterenol.

How Supplied: ORETICYL is supplied as grooved tablets in the following dosage sizes:

Rose-colored ORETICYL 25, contains hydrochlorothiazide 25 mg, deserpidine 0.125 mg, in bottles of 100 (**NDC** 0074-6922-01) and bottles of 1000 (**NDC** 0074-6922-02).

Rose-colored ORETICYL 50, contains hydrochlorothiazide 50 mg, deserpidine 0.125 mg, in bottles of 100 (**NDC** 0074-6931-01) and bottles of 1000 (**NDC** 0074-6931-02).

Gray-colored ORETICYL FORTE, contains hydrochlorothiazide 25 mg, deserpidine 0.25 mg, in bottles of 100 (**NDC** 0074-6927-01) and bottles of 1000 (**NDC** 0074-6927-02).

[*Shown in Product Identification Section*]

PANHEPRIN® ℞
PANHEPRIN® SDS™
(heparin sodium injection, USP)
PANHEPRIN® LOK™
(heparin lock flush solution, USP)

Description: PANHEPRIN (heparin sodium injection, USP) is derived from porcine intestinal mucosa, standardized for use as an anticoagulant, and supplied in water for injection. The potency is determined by a biological assay using a USP reference standard based upon units of heparin activity per milligram.

Actions: PANHEPRIN (heparin sodium injection, USP) inhibits reactions which lead to the clotting of blood and the formation of fibrin clots both *in vitro* and *in vivo*.

Heparin sodium acts at multiple sites in the normal coagulation system. Small amounts of heparin in combination with antithrombin III (heparin co-factor) can prevent the development of a hypercoagulable state by inactivating activated Factor X, preventing the conversion of prothrombin to thrombin. Once a hypercoagulable state exists, larger amounts of heparin in combination with antithrombin III can inhibit the coagulation process by inactivating thrombin and earlier clotting intermediates, thus preventing the conversion of fibrinogen to fibrin. Heparin also prevents the formation of a stable fibrin clot by inhibiting the activation of the fibrin stabilizing factor.

Bleeding time is usually unaffected by heparin. Clotting time is prolonged by full therapeutic doses of heparin; in most cases it is not measurably affected by low doses of heparin.

Heparin does not have fibrinolytic activity; therefore, it will not lyse existing clots.

Indications: PANHEPRIN injection is indicated for anticoagulant therapy in prophylaxis and treatment of venous thrombosis and its extension; in low-dose regimen for prevention of postoperative deep venous thrombosis and pulmonary embolism in patients undergoing major abdominothoracic surgery who are at risk of developing thromboembolic disease (see DOSAGE AND ADMINISTRATION section); for prophylaxis and treatment of pulmonary embolism; in atrial fibrillation with embolization; for diagnosis and treatment of acute and chronic consumptive coagulopathies (disseminated intravascular coagulation); for prevention of clotting in arterial and cardiac surgery; and for prevention of cerebral thrombosis in evolving stroke.

PANHEPRIN injection is indicated as an adjunct in treatment of coronary occlusion with acute myocardial infarction, and in prophylaxis and treatment of peripheral arterial embolism.

PANHEPRIN injection may also be employed as an anticoagulant in blood transfusions, extracorporeal circulation, dialysis procedures, and in blood samples for laboratory purposes.

PANHEPRIN LOK (heparin lock flush solution, USP) is intended to maintain patency of an indwelling venipuncture device designed for intermittent injection therapy or blood sampling. PANHEPRIN LOK may be used following initial placement of the device in the vein, after each injection of a medication or after withdrawal of blood for laboratory analysis.

PANHEPRIN LOK is not to be used for anticoagulation therapy.

Contraindications: PANHEPRIN injection is contraindicated in patients who are hypersensitive to heparin.

PANHEPRIN injection is contraindicated in any patient for whom suitable blood coagulation tests, such as the whole blood clotting time, partial thromboplastin time, etc., cannot be performed at the required intervals. There is usually no need to monitor the effect of low-dose heparin in patients with normal coagulation parameters.

The drug is also contraindicated during uncontrollable bleeding.

Warnings:

> Heparin sodium should be used with extreme caution in disease states in which there is an increased danger of hemorrhage.

Administration of PANHEPRIN (heparin sodium injection, USP), when used in therapeutic dosage, should be regulated by frequent blood coagulation tests. If these are unduly prolonged or if hemorrhage occurs, heparin sodium should be promptly discontinued. See OVERDOSAGE section.

Some of the conditions in which increased danger of hemorrhage exists are:

Cardiovascular—subacute bacterial endocarditis; arterial sclerosis; increased capillary permeability; during and immediately following a) spinal tap or spinal anesthesia, b) major surgery, especially involving the brain, spinal cord, or eye.

Hematologic—conditions associated with increased bleeding tendencies such as hemophilia, some purpuras, and thrombocytopenia.

Gastrointestinal—inaccessible ulcerative lesions and continuous tube drainage of the stomach or small intestine.

Heparin sodium may prolong the one-stage prothrombin time. Accordingly, when heparin sodium is given with dicumarol or warfarin sodium, a period of at least 5 hours after the last intravenous dose and 24 hours after the last subcutaneous (intrafat) dose of heparin sodium should elapse before blood is drawn, if a valid prothrombin time is to be obtained.

Drugs (such as acetylsalicylic acid, dextran, phenylbutazone, ibuprofen, indomethacin, dipyridamole and hydroxychloroquine) which interfere with platelet aggregation reactions (the main hemostatic defense of heparinized patients) may induce bleeding and should be used with caution in patients on heparin therapy.

While there is experimental evidence that heparin may antagonize the action of ACTH, insu-

Continued on next page

Abbott—Cont.

lin, or corticoids, this effect has not been clearly defined.
There is also evidence in experimental animals that heparin may modify or inhibit allergic reactions. However, the application of these findings to human patients has not been fully defined.
Larger doses of heparin may be necessary in the febrile state.
The use of digitalis, tetracyclines, nicotine, or antihistamines may partially counteract the anticoagulant action of heparin. An increased resistance to heparin is frequently encountered in cases of thrombosis, thrombophlebitis, infections with thrombosing tendency, myocardial infarction, cancer, and in the postoperative patient.
Usage in Pregnancy: Heparin sodium should be used with caution during pregnancy, especially during the last trimester and during the immediate post partum period, because of the risk of maternal hemorrhage.
There is no adequate information as to whether heparin sodium may affect human fertility or have a teratogenic potential or other adverse effects to the fetus.
Heparin sodium does not cross the placental barrier; it is not excreted in human breast milk.
Precautions: Because PANHEPRIN (heparin sodium injection, USP) is derived from animal tissue, it should be used with caution in patients with a history of allergy. Before a therapeutic dose is given to such a patient, a trial dose of 1000 units may be advisable.
Heparin sodium injection should also be used with caution in the presence of hepatic or renal disease, hypertension, during menstruation, or in patients with indwelling catheters.
A higher incidence of bleeding may be seen in women over 60 years of age.
Caution should be exercised when administering ACD-converted blood (i.e. blood collected in heparin sodium and later converted to ACD blood), since the anticoagulant activity of its heparin sodium content persists without loss for 22 days. ACD-converted blood may alter the coagulation system of the recipient, especially if it is given in multiple transfusions.
Adverse Reactions: Hemorrhage is the chief complication that may result from heparin therapy. An overly prolonged clotting time or minor bleeding during therapy can usually be controlled by withdrawing the drug. See OVERDOSAGE section.
The occurrence of significant gastrointestinal or urinary tract bleeding during anticoagulant therapy may indicate the presence of an underlying occult lesion.
Adrenal hemorrhage with resultant acute adrenal insufficiency has occurred during anticoagulant therapy. Anticoagulant therapy should be discontinued in patients who develop signs and symptoms compatible with acute adrenal hemorrhage or insufficiency. Plasma cortisol levels should be measured immediately, and vigorous therapy with intravenous corticosteroids should be instituted promptly. Initiation of therapy should not depend upon laboratory confirmation of the diagnosis, since any delay in an acute situation may result in the patient's death.
Intramuscular injection of heparin sodium frequently causes local irritation, mild pain, or hematoma, and for these reasons should be avoided. These effects are less often seen following deep subcutaneous (intrafat) injection. Histamine-like reactions have also been observed at the site of injection.
Hypersensitivity reactions have been reported with chills, fever and urticaria as the most usual manifestations. Asthma, rhinitis, lacrimation, and anaphylactoid reactions have also been reported. Vasospastic reactions may develop independent of the origin of heparin, 6 to 10 days after the initiation of therapy and last for 4 to 6 hours. The affected limb is painful, ischemic and cyanosed. An artery to this limb may have been recently catheterized. After repeat injections, the reactions may gradually increase, to include generalized vasospasm, with cyanosis, tachypnea, feeling of oppression, and headache. Protamine sulfate treatment has no marked therapeutic effect. Itching and burning, especially on the plantar side of the feet, is possibly based on a similar allergic vasospastic reaction. Chest pain, elevated blood pressure, arthralgias, and/or headache have also been reported in the absence of definite peripheral vasospasm. Anaphylactic shock has been reported rarely following the intravenous administration of heparin sodium. Acute reversible thrombocytopenia following the intravenous administration of heparin sodium has been reported. Osteoporosis, and suppression of renal function following long-term, high-dose administration, suppression of aldosterone synthesis, delayed transient alopecia, priapism, and rebound hyperlipemia following discontinuation of heparin sodium, have also been reported.
Dosage and Administration: PANHEPRIN (heparin sodium injection, USP) is not effective by oral administration and should be given by deep subcutaneous (intrafat, i.e., above iliac crest or into the abdominal fat layer) injection, by intermittent intravenous injection, or intravenous infusion. The intramuscular route of administration should be avoided because of the frequent occurrence of hematoma at the injection site. PANHEPRIN LOK (heparin lock flush solution, USP) is not to be used for anticoagulant therapy.
The dosage of heparin sodium should be adjusted according to the patient's coagulation test results, which, during the first day of treatment, should be determined just prior to each injection. (There is usually no need to monitor the effect of low-dose heparin in patients with normal coagulation parameters.) Dosage is considered adequate when the whole blood clotting time is elevated approximately 2.5 to 3 times the control value.
When heparin sodium is administered by continuous intravenous infusion, coagulation tests should be performed approximately every 4 hours during the early stages of therapy. When it is administered intermittently by intravenous, or deep subcutaneous (intrafat) injection, coagulation tests should be performed before each injection during the early stages of treatment, and daily thereafter.
When an oral anticoagulant of the coumarin, or similar type is administered with heparin sodium, coagulation tests and prothrombin activity should be determined at the start of therapy. For immediate anticoagulant effect, administer heparin sodium in the usual therapeutic dosage. When the results of the initial prothrombin determination are known, administer the first dose of an oral anticoagulant in the usual initial amount. Thereafter, perform a coagulation test and determine the prothrombin activity at appropriate intervals. A period of at least 5 hours after the last intravenous dose and 24 hours after the last subcutaneous (intrafat) dose of heparin sodium should elapse before blood is drawn, if a valid prothrombin time is to be obtained. When the oral anticoagulant shows full effect and prothrombin activity is in the desired therapeutic range, heparin sodium may be discontinued and therapy continued with the oral anticoagulant.

Therapeutic Anticoagulant Effect with Full-Dose Heparin

Although dosage must be adjusted for the individual patient according to the results of suitable laboratory tests, the following dosage schedules may be used as guidelines:
(See table at left)

1. *By deep subcutaneous (intrafat) injection.* After an initial I.V. injection of 5000 units, inject 10,000 to 20,000 units of a concentrated heparin sodium solution subcutaneously, followed by 8000 to 10,000 units of a concentrated solution subcutaneously every 8 hours, or 15,000 to 20,000 units of a concentrated solution subcutaneously every 12 hours. A different site should be used for each injection to prevent the development of a massive hematoma.
2. *By intermittent intravenous injection.* Inject 10,000 units of heparin sodium initially, then 5000 to 10,000 units every 4 to 6 hours. These amounts may be given either undiluted or diluted with 50 to 100 ml of isotonic sodium chloride injection.
3. *By continuous intravenous infusion.* After an initial I.V. injection of 5000 units of heparin sodium, add 20,000 to 40,000 units to 1000 ml of the isotonic sodium chloride solution for infusion. For most patients, the rate of flow should be adjusted to deliver approximately 20,000 to 40,000 units in 24 hours.

Method of Administration	Frequency	Recommended Dose (based on 150 lb (68 kg) patient)
Deep Subcutaneous (Intrafat) Injection	Initial Dose	5,000 units by intravenous injection followed by 10,000–20,000 units of a concentrated solution, subcutaneously
	Every 8 hours	8,000–10,000 units of a concentrated solution
	(or) Every 12 hours	15,000–20,000 units of a concentrated solution
Intermittent Intravenous Injection	Initial Dose	10,000 units, either undiluted or in 50–100 ml isotonic sodium chloride injection
	Every 4 to 6 hours.	5,000–10,000 units, either undiluted or in 50–100 ml isotonic sodium chloride injection
Intravenous Infusion	Initial Dose	5,000 units by intravenous injection
	Continuous	20,000–40,000 units in 1,000 ml of isotonic sodium chloride solution for infusion per day

Surgery of the Heart and Blood Vessels
Patients undergoing total body perfusion for open heart surgery should receive an initial dose of not less than 150 units of heparin sodium per kilogram of body weight. Frequently a dose of 300 units of heparin sodium per kilogram of body weight is used for procedures estimated to last less than 60 minutes; or 400 units per kilogram for those estimated to last longer than 60 minutes.

Low-Dose Prophylaxis of Postoperative Thromboembolism
A number of well-controlled clinical trials have demonstrated that low-dose heparin prophylaxis, given just prior to and after surgery, will reduce the incidence of postoperative deep vein thrombosis in the legs, as measured by the I-125 fibrinogen technique and venography, and of clinical pulmonary embolism. The most widely used dosage has been 5,000 units 2 hours before surgery and 5,000 units every 8 to 12 hours thereafter for 7 days or until the patient is fully ambulatory, whichever is longer. The heparin is given by deep subcutaneous injection in the arm or abdomen with a fine needle (25-26 gauge) to minimize tissue trauma. A concentrated solution of heparin sodium is recommended. Such prophylaxis should be reserved for patients over 40 undergoing major surgery. Patients with bleeding disorders, those having neurosurgery, spinal anesthesia, eye surgery, or potentially sanguinous operations should be excluded, as well as patients receiving oral anticoagulants or platelet-active drugs (see WARNINGS). The value of such prophylaxis in hip surgery has not been established. The possibility of increased bleeding during surgery or postoperatively should be borne in mind. If such bleeding occurs, discontinuance of heparin and neutralization with protamine sulfate is advisable. If clinical evidence of thromboembolism develops despite low-dose prophylaxis, full therapeutic doses of anticoagulants should be given unless contraindicated. All patients should be screened prior to heparinization to rule out bleeding disorders, and monitoring should be performed with appropriate coagulation tests just prior to surgery. Coagulation test values should be normal or only slightly elevated. There is usually no need for daily monitoring of the effect of low-dose heparin in patients with normal coagulation parameters.

Extracorporeal Dialysis Use
Follow equipment manufacturer's operating directions carefully.

Blood Transfusion
Addition of 400 to 600 USP units per 100 ml of whole blood. Usually 7500 USP units of heparin sodium injection are added to 100 ml of Sterile Sodium Chloride Injection (or 75,000 USP units per 1000 ml of Sterile Sodium Chloride Injection) and mixed, and from this sterile solution, 6 ml to 8 ml is added per 100 ml of whole blood. Leukocyte counts should be performed on heparinized blood within two hours after addition of the heparin. Heparinized blood should not be used for isoagglutin, complement, erythrocyte fragility tests, or platelet counts.

Laboratory Samples
Addition of 70 to 150 units of heparin sodium injection per 10 to 20 ml sample of whole blood is usually employed to prevent coagulation of the sample. See comments under "Blood Transfusion".

Heparin Lock
PANHEPRIN LOK (heparin lock flush solution, USP), 100 USP units/ml, is injected as a single dose into the diaphragm injection site of a previously inserted indwelling venipuncture device.

A single dose should be injected following venipuncture when the indwelling unit is not to be used immediately. After each use of the indwelling venipuncture device for injection or infusion of medication, or withdrawal of blood samples, another PANHEPRIN LOK should be injected to restore the effectiveness of the heparin lock. The amount of heparin solution in each single dose is sufficient to maintain anticoagulation within the lumen of indwelling venipuncture devices (usually not holding more than 0.2 to 0.3 ml) for up to four hours. When the indwelling venipuncture device is used to administer a drug which is incompatible with heparin, the entire heparin lock set should be flushed with sterile water or normal saline before and after the medication is administered. Following the second flush, another PANHEPRIN LOK should be injected to restore the effectiveness of the heparin lock.

When the indwelling venipuncture device is used for repeated withdrawal of blood samples for laboratory analyses and the presence of heparin or saline is likely to interfere with or alter results of the desired blood tests, the *in situ* heparin flush solution should be cleared from the device by aspirating and discarding 1 ml of fluid from the device before withdrawing the blood for analysis. After each blood sampling a single PANHEPRIN LOK unit is used to reheparinize the indwelling venipuncture device.

PANHEPRIN LOK is not to be used for anticoagulation therapy.

Overdosage: Protamine sulfate (1% solution) by slow infusion will neutralize heparin. No more than 50 mg should be given very slowly in any 10-minute period. Each mg of protamine sulfate neutralizes approximately 100 USP units of heparin (or 1.0 to 1.5 mg neutralizes approximately 1.0 mg of heparin). Heparins derived from various animal sources require different amounts of protamine sulfate for neutralization. This fact is of most importance during procedures of regional heparinization, including dialysis.

Decreasing amounts of protamine are required as time from the last heparin injection increases. Thirty minutes after a dose of heparin, approximately 0.5 mg of protamine is sufficient to neutralize each 100 units of administered heparin. Blood or plasma transfusions may be necessary; these dilute but do not neutralize heparin.

How Supplied: PANHEPRIN (heparin sodium injection, USP) is supplied in single dose and multiple dose vials. The pH of all PANHEPRIN solutions may have been adjusted with sodium hydroxide and/or hydrochloric acid. In the multiple dose vials, each ml contains 9 mg of benzyl alcohol as preservative. The single dose vials are preservative free:

PANHEPRIN 1000, 10 ml multiple dose vial (**NDC** 0074-3672-02) and 30 ml multiple dose vial (**NDC** 0074-3672-30).
Each milliliter contains 1000 USP units of heparin sodium in an aqueous solution with sufficient sodium chloride to render solution isotonic.

PANHEPRIN 5000, 1 ml single dose vial (**NDC** 0074-6136-01).
Each milliliter contains 5000 USP units of heparin sodium in an aqueous solution with sufficient sodium chloride to render solution isotonic.

PANHEPRIN 5000, 10 ml multiple dose vial (**NDC** 0074-3979-02).
Each milliliter contains 5000 USP units of heparin sodium in an aqueous solution with sufficient sodium chloride to render solution isotonic.

PANHEPRIN 10,000, 1 ml single dose vial (**NDC** 0074-6938-01).
Each milliliter contains 10,000 USP units of heparin sodium in an aqueous solution with sufficient sodium chloride to render solution isotonic.

PANHEPRIN 10,000, 4 ml multiple dose vial (**NDC** 0074-3987-03) and 5 ml multiple dose vial (**NDC** 0074-3987-04).
Each milliliter contains 10,000 USP units of heparin sodium in an aqueous solution with sufficient sodium chloride to render solution isotonic.

PANHEPRIN 20,000, 1 ml single dose vial (**NDC** 0074-6945-01).
Each milliliter contains 20,000 USP units of heparin sodium in an aqueous solution.

PANHEPRIN 20,000, 5 ml multiple dose vial (**NDC** 0074-6957-02).
Each milliliter contains 20,000 USP units of heparin sodium in an aqueous solution.

PANHEPRIN 40,000, 2 ml multiple dose vial (**NDC** 0074-6984-02).
Each milliliter contans 40,000 USP units of heparin sodium in an aqueous solution.

PANHEPRIN SDS (heparin sodium injection, USP) is supplied in 1 ml single dose disposable cartridges. Those cartridges supplied with 1-1/4 inch needles are intended for intravenous use; those with 5/8 inch needles are intended for deep subcutaneous use. The pH in PANHEPRIN SDS cartridges may have been adjusted with sodium hydroxide and/or hydrochloric acid; 9 mg benzyl alcohol is added to each cartridge as preservative:

PANHEPRIN SDS 1000, cartridge with 22 gauge, 1-1/4 inch needle in cartons of 100 (**NDC** 0074-6166-01).
Each milliliter contains 1000 USP units of heparin sodium in an aqueous solution, with sodium chloride sufficient to render solution isotonic.

PANHEPRIN SDS 5000, cartridge with 22 gauge, 1-1/4 inch needle in cartons of 100 (**NDC** 0074-6167-01).
Each milliliter contains 5000 USP units of heparin sodium in an aqueous solution, with sodium chloride sufficient to render solution isotonic.

PANHEPRIN SDS 5000, cartridge with 25 gauge, 5/8 inch needle in cartons of 100 (**NDC** 0074-6168-01).
Each milliliter contains 5000 USP units of heparin sodium in an aqueous solution, with sodium chloride sufficient to render solution isotonic.

PANHEPRIN SDS 10,000, cartridge with 25 gauge, 5/8 inch needle in cartons of 100 (**NDC** 0074-6169-01).
Each milliliter contains 10,000 USP units of heparin sodium in an aqueous solution, with sodium chloride sufficient to render solution isotonic.

PANHEPRIN SDS 20,000, cartridge with 25 gauge, 5/8 inch needle in cartons of 20 (**NDC** 0074-6170-01).
Each milliliter contains 20,000 USP units of heparin sodium in an aqueous solution.

PANHEPRIN LOK (heparin lock flush solution, USP) is supplied in 1 ml disposable cartridges with 25 gauge, 5/8 inch needles in cartons of 100 (**NDC** 0074-5760-01).
Each milliliter contains 100 USP units of heparin sodium and 9 mg of sodium chloride in an aqueous solution. pH may have been adjusted with sodium hydroxide and/or hydrochloric acid.

All PANHEPRIN *solutions should be protected from freezing.*

Ref. 01-2965-R4 and 01-2939-R2

PANWARFIN® ℞
(Warfarin Sodium Tablets, U.S.P.)

How Supplied: PANWARFIN (warfarin sodium tablets, U.S.P.) for oral administration, grooved and bearing dosage strength numerals are available as follows:

2 mg., lavender-colored, in bottles of 100 (**NDC** 0074-6626-03). Also available in ABBO-PAC® unit dose packages of 100 tablets (**NDC** 0074-6626-07).

2½ mg., orange-colored in bottles of 100 (**NDC** 0074-7202-01). Also available in ABBO-PAC

Continued on next page

Abbott—Cont.

unit dose packages of 100 tablets (**NDC** 0074-7202-05).
5 mg., peach-colored, in bottles of 100 (**NDC** 0074-7210-01) and 500 (**NDC** 0074-7210-09). Also available in ABBO-PAC unit dose packages of 100 tablets (**NDC** 0074-7210-05).
7½ mg., yellow, in bottles of 100 (**NDC** 0074-6638-03). Also available in ABBO-PAC unit dose packages of 100 tablets (**NDC** 0074-6638-07).
10 mg., white, in bottles of 100 (**NDC** 0074-7218-01). Also available in ABBO-PAC unit dose packages of 100 tablets (**NDC** 0074-7218-05).
[*Shown in Product Identification Section*]

PARADIONE® ℞
(paramethadione)
Capsules and Oral Solution

BECAUSE OF ITS POTENTIAL TO PRODUCE FETAL MALFORMATIONS AND SERIOUS SIDE EFFECTS, PARADIONE (paramethadione) SHOULD ONLY BE UTILIZED WHEN OTHER LESS TOXIC DRUGS HAVE BEEN FOUND INEFFECTIVE IN CONTROLLING PETIT MAL SEIZURES.

Description: PARADIONE (paramethadione) is an antiepileptic agent. An oxazolidinedione compound, it is chemically identified as 3,5-dimethyl-5-ethyl-oxazolidine-2,4-dione.
PARADIONE is a synthetic, oily, slightly water-soluble liquid. It is supplied in capsular and liquid forms for oral use only.
Clinical Pharmacology: PARADIONE has been shown to prevent pentylenetetrazol-induced and thujone-induced seizures in experimental animals; the drug has a less marked effect on seizures induced by picrotoxin, procaine, cocaine, or strychnine. Unlike the hydantoins and antiepileptic barbiturates, PARADIONE does not modify the maximal seizure pattern in patients undergoing electroconvulsive therapy. PARADIONE has a sedative effect that may increase to the point of ataxia when excessive doses are used. A toxic dose of the drug in animals (approximately 1 Gm/kg) produced sleep, unconsciousness, and respiratory depression.
Paramethadione is rapidly absorbed from the gastrointestinal tract. It is demethylated by liver microsomes to an active N-demethylated metabolite, and is excreted slowly in this form by the kidney; almost no unmetabolized PARADIONE is excreted.
Indications: PARADIONE (paramethadione) is indicated for the control of petit mal seizures that are refractory to treatment with other drugs.
Contraindications: PARADIONE is contraindicated in patients with a known hypersensitivity to the drug.
Warnings: PARADIONE may cause serious side effects. Strict medical supervision of the patient is mandatory, especially during the initial year of therapy.
PARADIONE (paramethadione) should be withdrawn promptly if skin rash appears, because of the grave possibility of the occurrence of exfoliative dermatitis or severe forms of erythema multiforme. Even a minor acneiform or morbilliform rash should be allowed to clear completely before treatment with PARADIONE is resumed; reinstitute therapy cautiously.
A complete blood count should be done prior to initiating therapy with PARADIONE, and at monthly intervals thereafter. A marked depression of the blood count is an indication for withdrawal of the drug. If no abnormality appears within 12 months, the interval between blood counts may be extended. A moderate degree of neutropenia with or without a corresponding drop in the leukocyte count is not uncommon. Therapy need not be withdrawn unless the neutrophil count is 2500 or less; more frequent blood examinations should be done when the count is less than 3,000. Other blood dyscrasias, including leukopenia, eosinophilia, thrombocytopenia, pancytopenia, agranulocytosis, hypoplastic anemia, and fatal aplastic anemia, have occurred with the use of oxazolidinediones.
Patients should be advised to report immediately such signs and symptoms as sore throat, fever, malaise, easy-bruising, petechiae, or epistaxis, or others that may be indicative of an infection or bleeding tendency. PARADIONE should ordinarily not be used in patients with severe blood dyscrasias.
Liver function tests should be done prior to initiating therapy with PARADIONE, and at monthly intervals thereafter. Hepatitis has been associated rarely with the use of oxazolidinediones. Jaundice or other signs of liver dysfunction are an indication for withdrawal of PARADIONE. PARADIONE should ordinarily not be used in patients with severe hepatic impairment.
A urinalysis should be done prior to initiating therapy with PARADIONE and at monthly intervals thereafter. Fatal nephrosis has been reported with the use of oxazolidinediones. Persistent or increasing albuminuria, or the development of any other significant renal abnormality, is an indication for withdrawal of the drug. PARADIONE should ordinarily not be used in patients with severe renal dysfunction.
Hemeralopia has occurred with the use of oxazolidinedione compounds; this appears to be an effect of the drugs on the neural layers of the retina, and usually can be reversed by a reduction in dosage. Scotomata are an indication for withdrawal of the drug. Caution should be observed when treating patients who have diseases of the retina or optic nerve.
Manifestations of systemic lupus erythematosus have been associated with the use of the oxazolidinediones, as they have with the use of certain other anticonvulsants. Lymphadenopathies simulating malignant lymphoma have also occurred. Lupus-like manifestations or lymph node enlargement are indications for withdrawal of PARADIONE. Signs and symptoms may disappear after discontinuation of therapy, and specific treatment may be unnecessary.
A myasthenia gravis-like syndrome has been associated with the chronic use of the oxazolidinediones. Symptoms suggestive of this condition are indications for withdrawal of PARADIONE.
Drugs known to cause toxic effects similar to those of the oxazolidinediones should be avoided or used only with extreme caution during therapy with PARADIONE.
USAGE DURING PREGNANCY AND LACTATION: THERE ARE MULTIPLE REPORTS IN THE CLINICAL LITERATURE WHICH INDICATE THAT THE USE OF ANTICONVULSANT DRUGS DURING PREGNANCY RESULTS IN AN INCREASED INCIDENCE OF BIRTH DEFECTS IN THE OFFSPRING. DATA ARE MORE EXTENSIVE WITH RESPECT TO TRIMETHADIONE, PARAMETHADIONE, PHENYTOIN AND PHENOBARBITAL THAN WITH OTHER ANTICONVULSANT DRUGS.
THEREFORE, ANTICONVULSANT DRUGS SUCH AS PARADIONE (PARAMETHADIONE) SHOULD BE ADMINISTERED TO WOMEN OF CHILD BEARING POTENTIAL ONLY IF THEY ARE CLEARLY SHOWN TO BE ESSENTIAL IN THE MANAGEMENT OF THEIR SEIZURES. EFFECTIVE MEANS OF CONTRACEPTION SHOULD ACCOMPANY THE USE OF PARADIONE IN SUCH PATIENTS. IF A PATIENT BECOMES PREGNANT WHILE TAKING PARADIONE, TERMINATION OF THE PREGNANCY SHOULD BE CONSIDERED. A PATIENT WHO REQUIRES THERAPY WITH PARADIONE AND WHO WISHES TO BECOME PREGNANT SHOULD BE ADVISED OF THE RISKS.
REPORTS HAVE SUGGESTED THAT THE MATERNAL INGESTION OF ANTICONVULSANT DRUGS, PARTICULARLY BARBITURATES, IS ASSOCIATED WITH A NEONATAL COAGULATION DEFECT THAT MAY CAUSE BLEEDING DURING THE EARLY (USUALLY WITHIN 24 HOURS OF BIRTH) NEONATAL PERIOD. THE POSSIBILITY OF THE OCCURRENCE OF THIS DEFECT WITH THE USE OF PARADIONE SHOULD BE KEPT IN MIND. THE DEFECT IS CHARACTERIZED BY DECREASED LEVELS OF VITAMIN K-DEPENDENT CLOTTING FACTORS, AND PROLONGATION OF EITHER THE PROTHROMBIN TIME OR THE PARTIAL THROMBOPLASTIN TIME, OR BOTH. IT HAS BEEN SUGGESTED THAT PROPHYLACTIC VITAMIN K BE GIVEN TO THE MOTHER ONE MONTH PRIOR TO, AND DURING DELIVERY, AND TO THE INFANT, INTRAVENOUSLY, IMMEDIATELY AFTER BIRTH.
THE SAFETY OF PARADIONE FOR USE DURING LACTATION HAS NOT BEEN ESTABLISHED.
Precautions: Abrupt discontinuation of PARADIONE may precipitate petite mal status. PARADIONE (paramethadione) should always be withdrawn gradually unless serious adverse effects dictate otherwise. In the latter case, another anticonvulsant may be substituted to protect the patient.
Usage during Pregnancy and Lactation: See WARNINGS.
Adverse Reactions: The following side effects, some of them serious, have been associated with the use of oxazolidinedione compounds. Although not all of them have been reported with the use of PARADIONE, the possibility of their occurrence should be kept in mind when the drug is prescribed.
Gastrointestinal: nausea, vomiting, abdominal pain, gastric distress.
CNS/Neurologic: drowsiness, fatigue, malaise, insomnia, vertigo, headache, paresthesias, precipitation of grand mal seizures, increased irritability, personality changes.
Drowsiness usually subsides with continued therapy. If it persists, a reduction in dosage is indicated.
Hematologic: bleeding gums, epistaxis, retinal and petechial hemorrhages, vaginal bleeding, neutropenia, leukopenia, eosinophilia, thrombocytopenia, pancytopenia, agranulocytosis, hypoplastic anemia, and fatal aplastic anemia.
Dermatologic: acneiform or morbilliform skin rash that may progress to exfoliative dermatitis or to severe forms of erythema multiforme.
Other: hiccups, anorexia, weight loss, hair loss, changes in blood pressure, albuminuria, hemeralopia, photophobia, diplopia.
Fatal nephrosis has occurred.
Hepatitis has been reported rarely.
Lupus erythematosus, and lymphadenopathies simulating malignant lymphoma, have been reported.
Pruritus associated with lymphadenopathy and hepatosplenomegaly has occurred in hypersensitive individuals.
A myasthenia gravis-like syndrome has been reported.
Overdosage: Symptoms of acute PARADIONE overdosage include drowsiness, nausea, dizziness, ataxia, visual disturbances. Coma may follow massive overdosage.
Gastric evacuation, either by induced emesis, or by lavage, or both, should be done immediately. General supportive care, including frequent monitoring of the vital signs and close observation of the patient, are required.
It has been reported that alkalinization of the urine may be expected to increase the excre-

tion of the N-demethylated metabolite of PARADIONE.
A blood count and a careful evaluation of hepatic and renal function should be done following recovery.
Dosage and Administration: PARADIONE is administered orally.
Because PARADIONE Oral Solution contains alcohol 65%, it may be desirable to dilute the preparation with water before administering it to small children.
Usual Adult Dosage: 0.9–2.4 Gm daily in 3 or 4 equally divided doses (i.e., 300–600 mg. 3 or 4 times daily).
Initially, give 0.9 Gm daily; increase this dose by 300 mg. at weekly intervals until therapeutic results are seen or until toxic symptoms appear.
Maintenance dosage should be the least amount of drug required to maintain control.
Children's Dosage: Usually 0.3–0.9 Gm daily in 3 or 4 equally divided doses.
How Supplied: PARADIONE Capsules (paramethadione capsules, U.S.P.), 150 mg (orange color) (**NDC** 0074-3976-01), and 300 mg (green color) (**NDC** 0074-3838-01) are supplied in bottles of 100.
[*Shown in Product Identification Section*]
PARADIONE Solution (paramethadione oral solution, U.S.P.), 300 mg per ml, is supplied in 50-ml bottles (**NDC** 0074-3860-01). A dropper is provided with each bottle, which is marked to permit easy measurement of 0.5 ml and 1 ml doses.
01-2963/R3

PEGANONE® ℞
(ethotoin tablets)

Description: PEGANONE (ethotoin) is an anticonvulsant of the hydantoin series and is chemically identified as 3 ethyl-5-phenylhydantoin.
Actions: PEGANONE exerts an anticonvulsant effect without causing general central nervous system depression. The mechanism of action is probably very similar to that of phenytoin. The latter drug appears to stabilize rather than to raise the normal seizure threshold, and to prevent the spread of seizure activity rather than to abolish the primary focus of seizure discharges.
In laboratory animals, the drug was found effective against electroshock convulsions, and to a lesser extent, against psychomotor and pentylenetetrazol-induced seizures.
In mice, the duration of anticonvulsant activity was prolonged by hepatic injury but not by bilateral nephrectomy; the drug is apparently biotransformed by the liver.
Indications: PEGANONE is indicated for the control of grand mal and psychomotor seizures.
Contraindications: PEGANONE is contraindicated in patients with hepatic abnormalities or hematologic disorders.
Warnings: USAGE DURING PREGNANCY AND LACTATION—THERE ARE MULTIPLE REPORTS IN THE CLINICAL LITERATURE WHICH INDICATE THAT THE USE OF ANTICONVULSANT DRUGS DURING PREGNANCY RESULTS IN AN INCREASED INCIDENCE OF BIRTH DEFECTS IN THE OFFSPRING. ALTHOUGH DATA ARE MORE EXTENSIVE WITH RESPECT TO TRIMETHADIONE, PARAMETHADIONE, PHENYTOIN, AND PHENOBARBITAL, REPORTS INDICATE A POSSIBLE SIMILAR ASSOCIATION WITH THE USE OF OTHER ANTICONVULSANT DRUGS. THEREFORE, ANTICONVULSANT DRUGS SHOULD BE ADMINISTERED TO WOMEN OF CHILDBEARING POTENTIAL ONLY IF THEY ARE CLEARLY SHOWN TO BE ESSENTIAL IN THE MANAGEMENT OF THEIR SEIZURES.
ANTICONVULSANT DRUGS SHOULD NOT BE DISCONTINUED IN PATIENTS IN WHOM THE DRUG IS ADMINISTERED TO PREVENT MAJOR SEIZURES BECAUSE OF THE STRONG POSSIBILITY OF PRECIPITATING STATUS EPILEPTICUS WITH ATTENDANT HYPOXIA AND RISK TO BOTH MOTHER AND THE UNBORN CHILD. CONSIDERATION SHOULD, HOWEVER, BE GIVEN TO DISCONTINUATION OF ANTICONVULSANTS PRIOR TO AND DURING PREGNANCY WHEN THE NATURE, FREQUENCY AND SEVERITY OF THE SEIZURES DO NOT POSE A SERIOUS THREAT TO THE PATIENT. IT IS NOT, HOWEVER, KNOWN WHETHER EVEN MINOR SEIZURES CONSTITUTE SOME RISK TO THE DEVELOPING EMBRYO OR FETUS.
REPORTS HAVE SUGGESTED THAT THE MATERNAL INGESTION OF ANTICONVULSANT DRUGS, PARTICULARLY BARBITURATES, IS ASSOCIATED WITH A NEONATAL COAGULATION DEFECT THAT MAY CAUSE BLEEDING DURING THE EARLY (USUALLY WITHIN 24 HOURS OF BIRTH) NEONATAL PERIOD. THE POSSIBILITY OF THE OCCURRENCE OF THIS DEFECT WITH THE USE OF PEGANONE SHOULD BE KEPT IN MIND. THE DEFECT IS CHARACTERIZED BY DECREASED LEVELS OF VITAMIN K-DEPENDENT CLOTTING FACTORS, AND PROLONGATION OF EITHER THE PROTHROMBIN TIME OR THE PARTIAL THROMBOPLASTIN TIME, OR BOTH. IT HAS BEEN SUGGESTED THAT VITAMIN K BE GIVEN PROPHYLACTICALLY TO THE MOTHER ONE MONTH PRIOR TO, AND DURING DELIVERY, AND TO THE INFANT, INTRAVENOUSLY, IMMEDIATELY AFTER BIRTH.
THE SAFETY OF PEGANONE FOR USE DURING LACTATION HAS NOT BEEN ESTABLISHED.
THE PHYSICIAN SHOULD WEIGH THESE CONSIDERATIONS IN TREATMENT AND COUNSELING OF EPILEPTIC WOMEN OF CHILDBEARING POTENTIAL.
Precautions: It is recommended that blood counts and urinalyses be performed when therapy is begun and at monthly intervals for several months thereafter. As in patients receiving other hydantoin compounds and other anticonvulsant drugs, blood dyscrasias have been reported in patients receiving PEGANONE (ethotoin). Its use in combination with other drugs known to adversely affect the hematopoietic system should be avoided if possible. Although the etiologic role of PEGANONE has not been definitely established, physicians should be alert for general malaise, sore throat and other symptoms indicative of possible blood dyscrasia. If clinical evidence suggests hepatic dysfunction, liver function tests should be made. Signs of liver damage or marked depression of the blood count are indications for withdrawal of the drug.
There is some evidence suggesting that hydantoin-like compounds may interfere with folic acid metabolism, precipitating a megaloblastic anemia. If this should occur during gestation, folic acid therapy should be considered.
Considerable caution should be exercised if PEGANONE is administered concurrently with Phenurone (phenacemide) since paranoid symptoms have been reported during therapy with this combination.
A two-way interaction between the hydantoin anticonvulsant, phenytoin, and the coumarin anticoagulants has been suggested. Presumably, phenytoin acts as a stimulator of coumarin metabolism and has been reported to cause decreased serum levels of the coumarin anticoagulants and increased prothrombin-proconvertin concentrations. Conversely, the coumarin anticoagulants have been reported to increase the serum levels and prolong the serum half-life of phenytoin by inhibiting its metabolism. Although there is no documentation of such, a similar interaction between ethotoin and the coumarin anticoagulants may occur. Caution is therefore advised when administering PEGANONE to patients receiving coumarin anticoagulants.
Adverse Reactions: Occasionally, nausea or vomiting after ingestion of PEGANONE has been reported, but if the drug is administered after meals, the incidence of gastric distress is reduced. Other side effects have included fatigue, insomnia, dizziness, headache, diplopia, nystagmus, skin rash, numbness, fever, diarrhea and chest pain. Ataxia and gum hypertrophy have occurred only rarely—usually only in patients receiving an additional hydantoin derivative. It is of interest to note that ataxia and gum hypertrophy have subsided in patients receiving other hydantoins when PEGANONE was given as a substitute anticonvulsant. Isolated cases of lymphadenopathy and systemic lupus erythematosus have been reported in patients taking hydantoin compounds and lymphadenopathy has occurred with PEGANONE. Withdrawal of therapy has resulted in remission of the clinical and pathological findings. Therefore, if a lymphoma-like syndrome develops, the drug should be withdrawn and the patient should be closely observed for regression of signs and symptoms before treatment is resumed.
Dosage and Administration: PEGANONE is administered orally in 4 to 6 divided doses daily. The drug should be taken after food, and doses should be spaced as evenly as practicable. Initial dosage should be conservative. For adults, the initial daily dose should be 1 Gm or less, with subsequent gradual dosage increases over a period of several days. The optimum dosage must be determined on the basis of individual response. The usual adult maintenance dose is 2 to 3 Gm daily. Less than 2 Gm daily has been found ineffective in most adults.
Pediatric dosage depends upon the age and weight of the patient. The initial dose should not exceed 750 mg daily. The usual maintenance dose in children ranges from 500 mg to 1 Gm daily, although occasionally 2 or (rarely) 3 Gm daily may be necessary.
If a patient is receiving another anticonvulsant drug, it should not be discontinued when PEGANONE therapy is begun. The dosage of the other drug should be reduced gradually as that of PEGANONE is increased. PEGANONE may eventually replace the other drug or the optimal dosage of both anticonvulsants may be established.
PEGANONE is compatible with all commonly employed anticonvulsant medications with the possible exception of Phenurone® (phenacemide). In grand mal seizures, use of the drug with Gemonil® (metharbital) or phenobarbital may be beneficial. PEGANONE may be used in combination with drugs such as Tridione® (trimethadione) or Paradione® (paramethadione), as an adjunct in those patients with petit mal associated with grand mal.
Overdosage: Symptoms of acute overdosage include drowsiness, visual disturbance, nausea and ataxia. Coma is possible at very high dosage.
Treatment should be begun by inducing emesis; gastric lavage may be considered as an alternative. General supportive measures will be necessary. A careful evaluation of blood-forming organs should be made following recovery.
How Supplied: PEGANONE (ethotoin) Tablets, grooved, 250 mg (NDC 0074-6902-01) are supplied in bottles of 100; 500 mg (NDC 0074-6905-04) are supplied in bottles of 100.
This product is listed in N.D., a Medicare designated compendium.
[*Shown in Product Identification Section*]
Ref. 01-2008-R3

If desired, additional literature on any Abbott Product will be provided upon request to Abbott Laboratories.

Continued on next page

Abbott—Cont.

PENTHRANE® ℞
(methoxyflurane, N.F.)

Description: PENTHRANE (methoxyflurane) is 2,2-dichloro-1, 1-difluoroethyl methyl ether. Certain of the physical constants are:

Molecular weight	164.97
Boiling point at 760 mm. Hg	104.65°C
Partition coefficients at 37°C	
water/gas	4.5
blood/gas (mean range)	10.20 to 14.06*
oil/gas	825
Vapor Pressure 17.7°C	20 mm. Hg
Flash points	
in air	62.8°C
in oxygen (closed system)	32.8°C
in nitrous oxide 50% with 50% oxygen	28.2°C
Lower limits of flammability of vapor concentration	
in air	7.0%
in oxygen	5.4%
in N_2O 50%	4.6%

***As reported by different investigators.**

PENTHRANE (methoxyflurane) is stable and does not decompose in contact with soda lime. It has a mildly pungent odor. An anti-oxidant, butylated hydroxytoluene 0.01% w/w, is added to insure stability on standing. This slowly oxidizes to a yellow pigment that progressively turns to brown, and which may accumulate on the vaporizer wick. The colored matter may be removed by rinsing the wick with diethyl ether. The wick must be dried after cleaning to avoid introducing diethyl ether into the system.

Polyvinyl chloride plastics are extracted by PENTHRANE; therefore, contact should be avoided. PENTHRANE does not extract polyethylene plastics, polypropylene plastics, fluorinated hydrocarbon plastics or nylon. It is very soluble in rubber and soda lime. Disposable conductive plastic circuits should be discarded after a single use to avoid cross contamination and because PENTHRANE may reduce conductivity of such materials below safe limits for subsequent administration of a flammable anesthetic.

The vapor concentration of PENTHRANE is limited by its vapor pressure at room temperature to a maximum of about 3.5% at 23°C. In practice, this concentration is not easily reached due to the cooling effect of vaporization. PENTHRANE is not flammable except at vapor concentrations well above those recommended for its use. Recommended concentrations are nonflammable and nonexplosive in air, oxygen, and nitrous oxide mixtures at ordinary room temperature.

Actions: PENTHRANE provides anesthesia and/or analgesia.

After surgical anesthesia with PENTHRANE, analgesia and drowsiness may persist after consciousness has returned. This may obviate or reduce the need for narcotics in the immediate postoperative period.

When used alone in safe concentration, PENTHRANE (methoxyflurane) will not produce appreciable skeletal muscle relaxation. A muscle relaxing agent, e.g., succinylcholine chloride (Quelicin®) or tubocurarine should be used as an adjunct.

Bronchiolar constriction or laryngeal spasm is not ordinarily provoked by PENTHRANE.

During PENTHRANE anesthesia, the cardiac rhythm is usually regular. The myocardium is only minimally sensitized by PENTHRANE to epinephrine. Some decrease in blood pressure often accompanies light planes of anesthesia. This may be accompanied by bradycardia. The hypotension noted is accompanied by reduced cardiac contractile force and reduced cardiac output.

When used for obstetrical delivery, light planes of PENTHRANE anesthesia have little effect on uterine contractions. There are no known contraindications to the concomitant use of PENTHRANE and oxytocic agents.

Biotransformation of PENTHRANE in man results in the formation of several metabolites which include inorganic fluoride, methoxydifluoroacetic acid, dichloroacetic acid, and, probably, oxalic acid. See WARNINGS.

Indications:

1. PENTHRANE is indicated, usually in combination with oxygen and nitrous oxide, to provide anesthesia for surgical procedures in which the total duration of PENTHRANE administration is anticipated to be 4 hours or less, and in which PENTHRANE is not to be used in concentrations that will provide skeletal muscle relaxation; see WARNINGS regarding time and dose relationships.
2. PENTHRANE (methoxyflurane) may be used alone with hand-held inhalers or in combination with oxygen and nitrous oxide for analgesia in obstetrics and in minor surgical procedures.

Contraindications: See WARNINGS.

Warnings: SEQUENTIAL ANESTHESIA WITH PENTHRANE (METHOXYFLURANE) AND HALOTHANE, OR HALOTHANE AND PENTHRANE, IN EITHER ORDER, HAS BEEN FOLLOWED BY JAUNDICE IN A FEW RARE CASES. WHEN A PREVIOUS EXPOSURE TO PENTHRANE OR HALOTHANE HAS BEEN FOLLOWED BY UNEXPLAINED JAUNDICE, CONSIDERATION SHOULD BE GIVEN TO THE USE OF OTHER AGENTS.

THE NEPHROTOXICITY ASSOCIATED WITH PENTHRANE ADMINISTRATION APPEARS TO BE RELATED TO THE TOTAL DOSE (TIME AND CONCENTRATION). SEE PARAGRAPH 5. THE MANIFESTATIONS RANGE IN SEVERITY FROM REVERSIBLE ALTERATIONS IN LABORATORY FINDINGS TO POLYURIC OR OLIGURIC RENAL FAILURE, SOMETIMES FATAL.

POLYURIC RENAL FAILURE IS CHARACTERIZED BY THE DEVELOPMENT, EARLY IN THE POSTOPERATIVE PERIOD, OF THE FOLLOWING:

WEIGHT LOSS.

URINE: LOW SPECIFIC GRAVITY, LARGE VOLUME EQUAL TO OR IN EXCESS OF FLUID INTAKE, DECREASED OSMOLALITY.

SERUM/BLOOD: ELEVATION OF SODIUM, CHLORIDE, URIC ACID, BUN, CREATININE.

THIS SYNDROME IS BELIEVED TO BE RELATED TO RELEASE OF THE FLUORIDE ION, A METABOLIC PRODUCT OF PENTHRANE AND TO BE RELATED TO THE TOTAL DOSAGE ADMINISTERED. THEREFORE, THE LOWEST EFFECTIVE DOSAGE SHOULD BE ADMINISTERED, ESPECIALLY IN AGED OR OBESE PATIENTS AND IN SURGICAL PROCEDURES OF LONG DURATION, BEARING IN MIND THAT THE TOTAL DOSE DELIVERED TO THE PATIENT IS A FACTOR OF DURATION OF ADMINISTRATION AND CONCENTRATION OF VAPOR.

OXALATE CRYSTALS AND/OR ACUTE TUBULAR NECROSIS HAVE BEEN NOTED AT AUTOPSY.

The guiding principles in minimizing the possibility of renal injury are:

1. AVOID USING PENTHRANE (METHOXYFLURANE) AS THE SOLE OR PRINCIPAL AGENT TO ACHIEVE MUSCULAR RELAXATION.
2. PATIENTS WITH PRE-EXISTING RENAL DISEASE, IMPAIRMENT OF RENAL FUNCTION, TOXEMIA OF PREGNANCY, AND PATIENTS UNDERGOING VASCULAR SURGERY AT OR NEAR THE RENAL VESSELS SHOULD NOT RECEIVE PENTHRANE UNLESS, IN THE JUDGMENT OF THE PHYSICIAN, THE BENEFITS OUTWEIGH THE INCREASED RISK OF NEPHROTOXIC EFFECT.
3. URINARY OUTPUT SHOULD BE MONITORED IN ALL PATIENTS. IF EXCESSIVE URINE OUTPUT OCCURS, APPROPRIATE LABORATORY STUDIES SHOULD BE DONE TO ASSESS RENAL FUNCTION IN HIGH RISK PATIENTS (SEE 2, ABOVE). SERIAL TESTS OF RENAL FUNCTION AND MEASUREMENTS OF FLUID AND ELECTROLYTE BALANCE ARE IMPERATIVE. ALL FLUID AND ELECTROLYTE LOSSES SHOULD BE PROMPTLY REPLACED.
4. THE CONCURRENT USE OF TETRACYCLINE AND PENTHRANE HAS BEEN REPORTED TO RESULT IN FATAL RENAL TOXICITY. THE POSSIBLITY EXISTS THAT PENTHRANE MAY ENHANCE THE ADVERSE RENAL EFFECTS OF OTHER DRUGS INCLUDING CERTAIN ANTIBIOTICS OF KNOWN NEPHROTOXIC POTENTIAL SUCH AS GENTAMICIN, KANAMYCIN, COLISTIN, POLYMYXIN B, CEPHALORIDINE AND AMPHOTERICIN B. THIS SHOULD BE CAREFULLY CONSIDERED WHEN PRESCRIBING SUCH DRUGS DURING THE PREOPERATIVE, OPERATIVE, AND POSTOPERATIVE PERIODS.
5. BECAUSE OF THE DOSE-RELATED NEPHROTOXICITY POTENTIAL OF PENTHRANE (METHOXYFLURANE), IT IS SUGGESTED THAT THE TOTAL DURATION OF LIGHT ANESTHETIC DEPTH WITH PENTHRANE NOT EXCEED APPROXIMATELY 4 HOURS AT A SINGLE ADMINISTRATION.

Usage in Pregnancy: Safe use of PENTHRANE other than for obstetrics has not been established with respect to adverse effects upon fetal development. Therefore, PENTHRANE should not be used in women of childbearing potential and particularly during early pregnancy unless, in the judgment of the physician, the potential benefits outweigh the possible hazards.

Usage in Obstetrics: Attention should be given to the directions for dosage and administration shown below. Fluoride levels in cord blood are usually less than, but may equal those of the mother at delivery. The effect of inorganic fluoride on the infant is not known. However, clinical experience has demonstrated that cases of high output renal failure in either mother or child must be considered unlikely.

Precautions: Diabetic patients may have an increased likelihood of developing nephropathy if they have impaired renal function or polyuria, are obese, or are not optimally controlled.

Caution should be exercised in using PENTHRANE in patients under treatment with enzyme inducing drugs (e.g., barbiturates) as such agents may enhance the metabolism of PENTHRANE, resulting in increased fluoride levels.

Ventilation should be assessed carefully and, if depressed, should be augmented to insure adequate oxygenation and carbon dioxide removal. Parenteral anesthetic adjuncts (ex. barbiturates, narcotics and neuromuscular blocking agents) may also cause depression of respiration requiring assisted or controlled ventilation. A sufficient reduction in respiratory minute volume occurs during deep anesthesia to produce a significant respiratory acidosis if ventilation is not adequately assisted.

PENTHRANE (methoxyflurane) causes a slight metabolic acidosis.

PENTHRANE augments the effect of nondepolarizing muscle relaxants so that their usual dos-

age should be reduced by approximately one-half.
Epinephrine or levarterenol (norepinephrine) should be employed cautiously during PENTHRANE anesthesia.
When PENTHRANE is used under the conditions of dosage and administration shown below, in surgery or obstetrics, inorganic fluoride levels may infrequently reach those at which changes in renal laboratory values have been seen.

Adverse Reactions: Renal dysfunction—see WARNINGS.
Hepatic dysfunction, jaundice, and fatal hepatic necrosis have occurred following PENTHRANE anesthesia. Also, as with other anesthetics, transient alterations in liver function tests may follow PENTHRANE administration. Hepatic complications rarely have involved reported cross reactions between PENTHRANE and Halothane.
Some patients exhibit pallor during recovery after PENTHRANE anesthesia.
Other adverse reactions which have been reported include: cardiac arrest, malignant hyperpyrexia, prolonged postoperative somnolence, respiratory depression, laryngospasm, bronchospasm, nausea, vomiting, postoperative headache, hypotension, and emergence delirium.

Dosage and Administration: THE LOWEST EFFECTIVE DOSAGE OF PENTHRANE (METHOXYFLURANE) SHOULD BE USED IN ORDER TO MINIMIZE THE POSSIBLITY OF NEPHROPATHY AND TO ALLOW FOR OPTIMAL RECOVERY TIME IN CASES OF UNUSUALLY HIGH MAINTENANCE REQUIREMENTS, THE USE OF ANESTHETIC ADJUNCTS OR ANOTHER AGENT MAY BE INDICATED. THE ABSENCE OF HYPOTENSION CANNOT BE RELIED UPON AS EVIDENCE THAT DOSAGE HAS NOT BEEN EXCESSIVE DURING MAINTENANCE.

Analgesia: For analgesia, intermittent inhalation of vapor concentrations in the range of 0.3 to 0.8% are recommended. PENTHRANE may be self-administered by hand-held inhalers (e.g., Analgizer, Cyprane) if the patient is kept under close observation.
For intermittent administration from the hand-held inhaler, dosage for each patient is limited to not more than a single 15 ml. charge of liquid PENTHRANE. Such analgesia in labor should not be instituted before relief becomes necessary. Use of the hand-held inhaler does not preclude transfer of the patient to a conventional anesthesia machine for inhalation anesthesia, but concentrations should be kept at the lowest effective dosage. Total time for anesthesia combined with analgesia should be as short as possible, bearing in mind the recommended duration for continuous anesthesia (four hours).

Anesthesia: A light level of anesthesia should be used. The use of deeper levels to achieve muscle relaxation should be avoided.
Apparatus: PENTHRANE should be vaporized by calibrated, temperature compensated, out-of-circle vaporizers (e.g., Pentec II, Pentomatic) or other methods which provide accurate delivered vapor concentration. Anesthetic up-take by rubber tubing, bags, and soda lime which may prolong induction and recovery time can be reduced by the use of nonabsorptive plastic circuit material (not polyvinyl chloride) and fresh moist Baralyme. The fresh gas inlet should be located downstream of the CO_2 absorber in order to avoid excessive anesthetic absorption, and the rebreathing bag and pop-off valve should be located on the expiratory side.
Premedication: The usual preanesthetic medications may be administered prior to PENTHRANE (methoxyflurane) anesthesia: see PRECAUTIONS.
Induction: Use of a parenteral induction agent (such as an ultra-short acting barbiturate) is recommended unless contraindicated in an individual patient.
Carrier gases: For general surgery, PENTHRANE should usually be administered with a carrier gas flow consisting of oxygen and at least 50% nitrous oxide in order to minimize the total PENTHRANE dose unless nitrous oxide is contraindicated.
Muscle relaxation: PENTHRANE should not be administered at levels required to achieve muscle relaxation. Adequate relaxation should be obtained from adjunctive use of a muscle relaxant, e.g., succinylcholine chloride (Quelicin®) or tubocurarine. The usual dosage of nondepolarizing muscle relaxants should be reduced by approximately one-half.
Vapor concentrations: Initially, PENTHRANE concentrations may be increased as tolerated to the maximum of approximately 2%. This concentration should only be continued for about two to five minutes, or until the patient signs of light anesthesia are evident. The concentration of PENTHRANE should then be reduced by frequent decrements to the lowest possible levels consistent with the maintenance of adequate anesthesia. For example, in a 70 kg. patient, the following sequential reduction in the delivered vapor concentration of PENTHRANE (methoxyflurane) may be appropriate:
[See table above].

Elapsed Minutes	0 to 5	5 to 20	20 to 60	60 to 120	120 to 240
Vapor Conc.*	2.0%	0.6%	0.4%	0.2%	0.1%

*Concentrations are approximate and subject to adjustment according to patient signs of anesthesia. Based on 5 liters per minute gas flow and ventilation rate throughout procedure, 50/50 N_2O and oxygen.

Concentration may be increased or decreased according to the requirements of the individual patient. Four hours of 0.25% delivered methoxyflurane should not be exceeded in normal adult patients unless, in the opinion of the clinician, the anticipated benefits outweigh the increased risk of dose related nephrotoxicity. The product of these two factors (four hours of 0.25% delivered methoxyflurane) may be used to estimate other combinations of time and dose: thus two hours of 0.5%, for example, should not ordinarily be exceeded. In sufficiently long cases, PENTHRANE should be discontinued 30 to 40 minutes before the end of surgery. Rapid flushing will not remove PENTHRANE absorbed by rubber circuit components.
Patient signs and levels: The PENTHRANE level of conscious analgesia is suited for pain relief, as in labor and uncomplicated vaginal deliveries. The level of unconscious analgesia is suitable for many minor surgical procedures. The level of light anesthesia is recommended for general surgical use. Deep anesthesia with PENTHRANE (methoxyflurane) is not recommended.
Appropriate patient signs of PENTHRANE anesthesia should be observed closely as a guide to proper depth. A blood pressure decrease of about 20 mm. Hg may be seen during induction. A greater decrease may occur in hypertensive patients. Blood pressure usually recovers as a level of light anesthesia is reached. The absence of hypotension cannot be relied upon as evidence that dosage has not been excessive during maintenance.

How Supplied: PENTHRANE (methoxyflurane), is supplied in 125 ml. and 15 ml. bottles, List 6864. Butylated hydroxytoluene, 0.01% w/w, is present as an antioxidant.

Caution: Federal (U.S.A.) law prohibits dispensing without prescription.
Ref. No. 06-2556-R24-6/78

PENTOTHAL® Ⓒ

(thiopental sodium for injection, USP)

Description: Pentothal (thiopental sodium for injection, USP) is a thiobarbiturate, the sulfur analogue of sodium pentobarbital. Chemically, Pentothal is sodium 5-ethyl-5-(1-methylbutyl)-2-thiobarbiturate.
All preparations are sterile and as a buffer for stabilization, contain anhydrous sodium carbonate, 60 mg/g of thiopental sodium.

Actions: Pentothal is an ultrashort-acting depressant of the central nervous system which induces hypnosis and anesthesia, but not analgesia. It produces hypnosis within 30 to 40 seconds of intravenous injection. Recovery after a small dose is rapid, with some somnolence and retrograde amnesia. Repeated intravenous doses lead to prolonged anesthesia because fatty tissues act as a reservoir; they accumulate Pentothal in concentrations 6 to 12 times greater than the plasma concentration, and then release the drug slowly to cause prolonged anesthesia.

Indications: Pentothal (thiopental sodium for injection) as indicated (1) as the sole anesthetic agent for brief (15 minute) procedures, (2) for induction of anesthesia prior to administration of other anesthetic agents, (3) to supplement regional anesthesia, (4) to provide hypnosis during balanced anesthesia with other agents for analgesia or muscle relaxation, (5) for the control of convulsive states during or following inhalation anesthesia, local anesthesia, or other causes, (6) in neurosurgical patients with increased intracranial pressure, if adequate ventilation is provided, and (7) for narcoanalysis and narcosynthesis in psychiatric disorders.

Contraindications:
Absolute Contraindications: (1) Absence of suitable veins for intravenous administration, (2) hypersensitivity (allergy) to barbiturates, (3) status asthmaticus, and (4) latent or manifest porphyria.
Relative Contraindications: (1) Severe cardiovascular disease, (2) hypotension or shock, (3) conditions in which the hypnotic effect may be prolonged or potentiated—excessive premedication, Addison's disease, hepatic or renal dysfunction, myxedema, increased blood urea, severe anemia, asthma and myasthenia gravis.

Warning: May be habit forming.
Usage in Pregnancy: Safe use of Pentothal has not been established with respect to adverse effects upon fetal development. Therefore, this drug should not be used in women of childbearing potential and particularly during early pregnancy unless in the judgement of the physician the benefits outweigh the potential hazards.

Precautions: **KEEP RESUSCITATIVE AND ENDOTRACHEAL INTUBATION EQUIPMENT AND OXYGEN READILY AVAILABLE. MAINTAIN PATENCY OF THE AIRWAY AT ALL TIMES.**
This drug should be administered only by persons qualified in the use of intravenous anesthetics.

Continued on next page

Abbott—Cont.

Avoid extravasation or intra-arterial injection.

If used in conditions involving relative contraindications, reduce dosage and administer slowly.

Observe aseptic precautions at all times in preparation and handling of Pentothal (thiopental sodium for injection) solutions. When using 250 ml (List No. 6423) and 500 ml (List No. 6672) Diluent Containers, cleanse external bottle-closure surface with antiseptic before attaching set or adding diluent, and when withdrawing dosage.

Care should be taken in administering the drug to patients with advance cardiac disease, increased intracranial pressure, asthma, myasthenia gravis, and endocrine insufficiency (pituitary, thyroid, adrenal, pancreas).

Adverse Reactions: Adverse reactions include respiratory depression, myocardial depression, cardiac arrhythmias, prolonged somnolence and recovery, sneezing, coughing, bronchospasm, laryngospasm and shivering. Hypersensitivity reactions to barbiturates, including Pentothal, have been reported.

Dosage and Administration: Pentothal (thiopental sodium for injection) is administered by the intravenous route only. Individual response to the drug is so varied that there can be no fixed dosage. The drug should be titrated against patient requirements as governed by age, sex and body weight. Younger patients require relatively larger doses than middle-aged and elderly persons; the latter metabolize the drug more slowly. Pre-puberty requirements are the same for both sexes, but adult females require less than adult males. Dose is usually proportional to body weight, and obese patients require a larger dose than relatively lean persons of the same weight.

Premedication

Premedication usually consists of atropine or scopolamine to suppress vagal reflexes and inhibit secretions. In addition, a barbiturate or an opiate is often given. Sodium pentobarbital injection (Nembutal®) is suggested because it provides a preliminary indication of how the patient will react to barbiturate anesthesia. Ideally, the peak effect of these medications should be reached shortly before the time of induction.

Test Dose

It is advisable to inject a small "test" dose of 25 to 75 mg (1 to 3 ml of a 2.5% solution) of Pentothal (thiopental sodium for injection) to assess tolerance or unusual sensitivity to Pentothal, and pausing to observe patient reaction for at least 60 seconds. If unexpectedly deep anesthesia develops or if respiratory depression occurs, consider these possibilities: (1) the patient may be unusually sensitive to Pentothal, (2) the solution may be more concentrated than had been assumed, or (3) the patient may have received too much premedication.

Use in Anesthesia

Moderately slow induction can usually be accomplished in the "average" adult by injection of 50 to 75 mg (2 to 3 ml of a 2.5% solution) at intervals of 20 to 40 seconds, depending on the reaction of the patient. Once anesthesia is established, additional injections of 25 to 50 mg can be given whenever the patient moves.

Slow injection is recommended to minimize respiratory depression and the possibility of overdosage. The smallest dose consistent with attaining the surgical objective is the desired goal. Momentary apnea following each injection is typical, and progressive decrease in the amplitude of respiration appears with increasing dosage. Pulse remains normal or increases slightly and returns to normal. Blood pressure usually falls slightly but returns toward normal. Muscles usually relax about 30 seconds after unconsciousness is attained, but this may be masked if a skeletal muscle relaxant is used. The tone of jaw muscles is a fairly reliable index. The pupils may dilate but later contract; sensitivity to light is not usually lost until a level of anesthesia deep enough to permit surgery is attained. Nystagmus and divergent strabismus are characteristic during early stages, but at the level of surgical anesthesia, the eyes are central and fixed. Corneal and conjunctival reflexes disappear during surgical anesthesia.

When Pentothal (thiopental sodium for injection) is used for induction in balanced anesthesia with a skeletal muscle relaxant and an inhalation agent, the total dose of Pentothal can be estimated and then injected in two to four fractional doses. With this technique, brief periods of apnea may occur which may require assisted or controlled pulmonary ventilation. As an initial dose, 210 to 280 mg (3 to 4 mg/kg) of Pentothal is usually required for rapid induction in the average adult (70 kg).

When Pentothal (thiopental sodium for injection) is used as the sole anesthetic agent, the desired level of anesthesia can be maintained by injection of small repeated doses as needed or by using a continuous intravenous drip in a 0.2% or 0.4% concentration. (Sterile water should not be used as the diluent in these concentrations, since hemolysis will occur.) With continuous drip, the depth of anesthesia is controlled by adjusting the rate of infusion.

Use in Convulsive States

For the control of convulsive states following anesthesia (inhalation or local) or other causes, 75 to 125 mg (3 to 5 ml of a 2.5% solution) should be given as soon as possible after the convulsion begins. Convulsions following the use of a local anesthetic may require 125 to 250 mg of Pentothal, (thiopental sodium for injection), given over a ten minute period. If the convulsion is caused by a local anesthetic, the required dose of Pentothal will depend upon the amount of local anesthetic given and its convulsant properties.

Use in Neurosurgical Patients with Increased Intracranial Pressure

In neurosurgical patients, intermittent bolus injections of 1.5 to 3.5 mg/kg of body weight may be given to reduce intraoperative elevations of intracranial pressure, if adequate ventilation is provided.

Use in Psychiatric Disorders

For narcoanalysis and narcosynthesis in psychiatric disorders, premedication with an anticholinergic agent may precede administration of Pentothal. After a test dose, Pentothal is injected at a slow rate of 100 mg/min (4 ml/min of a 2.5% solution) with the patient counting backwards from 100. Shortly after counting becomes confused but before actual sleep is produced, the injection is discontinued. Allow the patient to return to a semidrowsy state where conversation is coherent. Alternatively, Pentothal (thiopental sodium for injection) may be administered by rapid I.V. drip using a 0.2% concentration in 5% dextrose and water. At this concentration, the rate of administration should not exceed 50 ml/min.

Management of Some Complications:

Overdosage is to be avoided. In the event of suspected or apparent overdosage the drug should be discontinued, a patent airway established (intubate if necessary) or maintained, and oxygen should be administered, with assisted ventilation if necessary.

Respiratory depression (hypoventilation, apnea), which may result from either unusual responsiveness to Pentothal (thiopental sodium for injection) or overdosage, is managed as stated above. Pentothal should be considered to have the same potential for producing respiratory depression as an inhalation agent, and patency of the airway must be protected at all times.

Laryngospasm may occur with light Pentothal narcosis at intubation, or in the absence of intubation if foreign matter or secretions in the respiratory tract create irritation. Laryngeal and bronchial vagal reflexes can be suppressed, and secretions minimized by giving atropine or scopolamine premedication and a barbiturate or opiate. Use of a skeletal muscle relaxant or positive pressure oxygen will usually relieve laryngospasm. Tracheostomy may be indicated in difficult cases.

Myocardial depression, proportional to the amount of drug in direct contact with the heart, can occur and may cause hypotension, particularly in patients with an unhealthy myocardium. Arrhythmias may appear if PCO_2 is elevated, but they are uncommon with adequate ventilation. Management of myocardial depression is the same as for overdosage. Pentothal (thiopental sodium for injection) does not sensitize the heart to epinephrine or other sympathomimetic animes.

Extravascular infiltration should be avoided. Care should be taken to insure that the needle is within the lumen of the vein before injection of Pentothal. Extravascular injection may cause chemical irritation of the tissues varying from slight tenderness to venospasm, extensive necrosis and sloughing. This is due primarily to the high alkaline pH (10 to 11) of clinical concentrations of the drug. If extravasation occurs, the local irritant effects can be reduced by injection of 1% procaine locally to relieve pain and enhance vasodilatation. Local application of heat also may help to increase local circulation and removal of the infiltrate.

Intra-arterial injection can occur inadvertently, especially if an aberrant superficial artery is present at the medial aspect of the antecubital fossa. The area selected for intravenous injection of the drug should be palpated for detection of an underlying pulsating vessel. Accidental intra-arterial injection can cause arteriospasm and severe pain along the course of the artery, with blanching of the arm and fingers. Appropriate corrective measures should be instituted promptly to avoid possible development of gangrene. Any patient complaint of pain warrants stopping the injection. Methods suggested for dealing with this complication vary with the severity of symptoms. The following have been suggested:

1. Dilute the injected Pentothal (thiopental sodium for injection) by removing the tourniquet and any restrictive garments.
2. Leave the needle in place, if possible.
3. Inject the artery with a dilute solution of papaverine, 40 to 80 mg, or 10 ml of 1% procaine, to inhibit smooth muscle spasm.
4. If necessary, perform sympathetic block of the brachial plexus and/or stellate ganglion to relieve pain and assist in opening collateral circulation. Papaverine can be injected into the subclavian artery, if desired.
5. Unless otherwise contraindicated, institute immediate heparinization to prevent thrombus formation.
6. Consider local infiltration of an alpha-adrenergic blocking agent such as phentolamine into the vasospastic area.
7. Provide additional symptomatic treatment as required.

Shivering after Pentothal anesthesia, manifested by twitching face muscles and occasional progression to tremors of the arms, head, shoulder and body, is a thermal reaction due to increased sensitivity to cold. Shivering appears if the room environment is cold and if a large ventilatory heat loss has been sustained with balanced inhalation anesthesia employing nitrous oxide. Treatment consists of warming the patient with blankets, maintaining room temperature near 22°C (72°F), and administration of chlorpromazine or methylphenidate.

Preparation of Solutions: Pentothal (thiopental sodium for injection,) is supplied as a yellowish, hygroscopic powder in a variety of different containers. Solutions should be prepared aseptically with one of the three following diluents; Sterile Water for Injection, USP,

Sodium Chloride Injection, USP, or 5% Dextrose, Injection, USP. Clinical concentrations used for intermittent intravenous administration vary between 2.0 and 5.0%. A 2.0 or 2.5% solution is most commonly used. A 3.4% concentration in sterile water for injection is isotonic; concentrations less than 2.0% in this diluent are not used because they cause hemolysis. For continuous intravenous drip administration, concentrations of 0.2 or 0.4% are used. Solutions may be prepared by adding Pentothal to 5% Dextrose Injection, USP, Sodium Chloride Injection, USP or Normosol®-R pH 7.4.

Since Pentothal (thiopental sodium for injection) contains no added bacteriostatic agent, extreme care in preparation and handling should be exercised at all times to prevent the introduction of microbial contaminants. Solutions should be freshly prepared and used promptly; when reconstituted for administration to several patients, unused portions should be discarded after 24 hours. Sterilization by heating should not be attempted.

Warning: The 2.5 g and larger sizes contain adequate medication for several patients.

Compatibility: Any solution of Pentothal (thiopental sodium for injection) with a visible precipitate should not be administered. The stability of Pentothal solutions depends upon several factors, including the diluent, temperature of storage, and the amount of carbon dioxide from room air that gains access to the solution. Any factor or condition which tends to lower pH (increase acidity) of Pentothal solutions will increase the likelihood of precipitation of thiopental acid. Such factors include the use of diluents which are too acid and the absorption of carbon dioxide which can combine with water to form carbonic acid.

Solutions of succinylcholine, tubocurarine or other drugs which have an acid pH should not be mixed with Pentothal solutions. The most stable solutions are those reconstituted in water or isotonic saline, kept under refrigeration and tightly stoppered. The presence or absence of a visible precipitate offers a practical guide to the physical compatibility of prepared solutions of Pentothal (thiopental sodium for injection).

CALCULATIONS FOR VARIOUS CONCENTRATIONS

Concentration Desired: Percent	mg/ml	Amounts to Use: Thiopental Sodium g	Diluent ml
0.2	2	1	500
0.4	4	1 2	250 500
2.0	20	5 10	250 500
2.5	25	1 5	40 200
5	50	1 5	20 100

How Supplied: Pentothal (thiopental sodium for injection) is available in a variety of sizes and containers, including combination packages with diluent. Consult Abbott Laboratories for a current listing.

Caution: Federal (USA) law prohibits dispensing without prescription.

Ref. No. 06-2630-R7-2/79

PHENURONE® ℞
(phenacemide tablets, N.F.)

Description: PHENURONE (phenacemide) is a valuable drug for use in selected patients with epilepsy. Since therapy with PHENURONE involves certain risks, *physicians should thoroughly familiarize themselves with the undesirable side effects which may occur and the precautions to be observed.* PHENURONE (phenacemide) is a substituted acetylurea derivative.

Actions: In experimental animals, PHENURONE (phenacemide), in doses well below those causing neurological signs, elevates the threshold for minimal electroshock convulsions and abolishes the tonic phase of maximal electroshock seizures. The drug prevents or modifies seizures induced by pentylenetetrazol or other convulsants. In comparative tests, PHENURONE was found to be equal or more effective than other commonly used anticonvulsants against focal seizures of a psychomotor type which were induced in mice by low frequency stimulation of the cerebral cortex. Studies in mice have shown that PHENURONE exerts a synergistic anticonvulsant effect with mephenytoin, phenobarbital, or trimethadione.

Given orally to laboratory animals, PHENURONE has a low acute toxicity. In mice, slight ataxia appears at 400 mg./kg. and light sleep occurs at 800 mg./kg. In high doses the drug causes marked ataxia and coma, the fatal dose being in the range of 3 to 5 Gm./kg. for mice, rats, and cats.

PHENURONE is well absorbed from the intestine and following a single dose its duration of action is about five hours. It is degraded by the liver with the formation of inactive metabolites which are excreted by the kidney. PHENURONE, as such, does not appear in the urine.

Indications: PHENURONE (phenacemide) is indicated for the control of severe epilepsy, particularly mixed forms of psychomotor seizures, refractory to other drugs.

Warnings: USAGE DURING PREGNANCY AND LACTATION

THERE ARE MULTIPLE REPORTS IN THE CLINICAL LITERATURE WHICH INDICATE THAT THE USE OF ANTICONVULSANT DRUGS DURING PREGNANCY RESULTS IN AN INCREASED INCIDENCE OF BIRTH DEFECTS IN THE OFFSPRING. ALTHOUGH DATA ARE MORE EXTENSIVE WITH RESPECT TO TRIMETHADIONE, PARAMETHADIONE, PHENYTOIN, AND PHENOBARBITAL, REPORTS INDICATE A POSSIBLE SIMILAR ASSOCIATION WITH THE USE OF OTHER ANTICONVULSANT DRUGS. THEREFORE, ANTICONVULSANT DRUGS SHOULD BE ADMINISTERED TO WOMEN OF CHILD BEARING POTENTIAL ONLY IF THEY ARE CLEARLY SHOWN TO BE ESSENTIAL IN THE MANAGEMENT OF THEIR SEIZURES.

ANTICONVULSANT DRUGS SHOULD NOT BE DISCONTINUED IN PATIENTS IN WHOM THE DRUG IS ADMINISTERED TO PREVENT MAJOR SEIZURES BECAUSE OF THE STRONG POSSIBILITY OF PRECIPITATING STATUS EPILEPTICUS WITH ATTENDANT HYPOXIA AND RISK TO BOTH MOTHER AND THE UNBORN CHILD. CONSIDERATION SHOULD, HOWEVER, BE GIVEN TO DISCONTINUATION OF ANTICONVULSANTS PRIOR TO AND DURING PREGNANCY WHEN THE NATURE, FREQUENCY AND SEVERITY OF THE SEIZURES DO NOT POSE A SERIOUS THREAT TO THE PATIENT. IT IS NOT, HOWEVER, KNOWN WHETHER EVEN MINOR SEIZURES CONSTITUTE SOME RISK TO THE DEVELOPING EMBRYO OR FETUS.

REPORTS HAVE SUGGESTED THAT THE MATERNAL INGESTION OF ANTICONVULSANT DRUGS, PARTICULARLY BARBITURATES, IS ASSOCIATED WITH A NEONATAL COAGULATION DEFECT THAT MAY CAUSE BLEEDING DURING THE EARLY (USUALLY WITHIN 24 HOURS OF BIRTH) NEONATAL PERIOD. THE POSSIBILITY OF THE OCCURRENCE OF THIS DEFECT WITH THE USE OF PHENURONE SHOULD BE KEPT IN MIND. THE DEFECT IS CHARACTERIZED BY DECREASED LEVELS OF VITAMIN K-DEPENDENT CLOTTING FACTORS, AND PROLONGATION OF EITHER THE PROTHROMBIN TIME OR THE PARTIAL THROMBOPLASTIN TIME, OR BOTH. IT HAS BEEN SUGGESTED THAT VITAMIN K BE GIVEN PROPHYLACTICALLY TO THE MOTHER ONE MONTH PRIOR TO, AND DURING DELIVERY, AND TO THE INFANT, INTRAVENOUSLY, IMMEDIATELY AFTER BIRTH.

THE SAFETY OF PHENURONE FOR USE DURING LACTATION HAS NOT BEEN ESTABLISHED.

THE PHYSICIAN SHOULD WEIGH THESE CONSIDERATIONS IN TREATMENT AND COUNSELING OF EPILEPTIC WOMEN OF CHILDBEARING POTENTIAL.

Precautions: PHENURONE (phenacemide) can produce serious side effects as well as direct organ toxicity. As a consequence its use entails the assumption of certain risks which must be weighed against the benefit to the patient. *Ordinarily* PHENURONE *should not be administered unless other available anticonvulsants have been found to be ineffective in controlling seizures.*

Extreme caution is essential if PHENURONE is administered with any other anticonvulsant which is known to cause similar toxic effects. Extreme caution must also be exercised in treating patients who previously have shown personality disorders. It may be advisable to hospitalize such patients during the first week of treatment. Personality changes, including attempts at suicide and the occurrence of psychoses requiring hospitalization, have been reported during therapy with PHENURONE (phenacemide). The patient and his family should be aware of these possibilities so that the family can watch for the reported changes in the behavior of the patient such as decreased interest in surroundings, depression, or aggressiveness. Severe or exacerbated personality changes are an indication for withdrawal of the drug. Considerable caution should be exercised if PHENURONE is administered concurrently with PEGANONE (ETHOTOIN) since paranoid symptoms have been reported during therapy with this combination.

Liver function tests should be performed before and during therapy. PHENURONE (phenacemide) should be used with caution in patients with a history of previous liver dysfunction. Death attributable to liver damage during therapy with PHENURONE has been reported. If jaundice or other signs of hepatitis appear, the drug should be discontinued.

Complete blood counts should be made before instituting PHENURONE, and at monthly intervals thereafter. If no abnormality appears within 12 months, the interval between blood counts may be extended. Blood changes have been reported with leukopenia (leukocyte count of 4,000 or less per cubic millimeter of blood) as the most commonly observed effect. However, aplastic anemia has occurred in association with PHENURONE therapy, and death from this condition has been reported. *The total number of each cellular element per cubic millimeter is a better index of possible blood dyscrasia than the percentage of cells.* The patient should be told to report immediately any symptoms indicative of a developing blood dyscrasia such as malaise, sore throat, or fever. Marked depression of the blood count is an indication for withdrawal of the drug.

Similarly, as nephritis has occasionally occurred in patients on PHENURONE, the urine should be examined at regular intervals. Abnormal urinary findings are an indication for discontinuance of therapy.

Continued on next page

Abbott—Cont.

PHENURONE (phenacemide) should be administered with caution to patients with a history of allergy, particularly in association with the administration of other anticonvulsants. The drug should be discontinued at the first sign of a skin rash or other allergic manifestation.
Adverse Reactions: Untoward effects which may occur in association with PHENURONE therapy include gastrointestinal disturbances, anorexia and weight loss, headaches, drowsiness, dizziness, insomnia, paresthesias, psychic changes, hepatitis, blood dyscrasias, skin rash, and nephritis.
Dosage and Administration: PHENURONE (phenacemide) is administered orally.
Since PHENURONE may produce serious toxic effects, it is strongly recommended that the dosage be held to the minimum amount necessary to achieve an adequate therapeutic effect.
For adults the usual starting dose is 1.5 Gm. daily, administered in three divided doses of 500 mg. each. After the first week, if seizures are not controlled and the drug is well tolerated, an additional 500 mg. tablet may be taken upon arising. In the third week, if necessary, the dosage may be further increased by another 500 mg. at bedtime. Satisfactory results have been noted in some patients on an initial dose of 250 mg. three times per day. The effective total daily dose for adults usually ranges from 2 to 3 Gm., although some patients have required as much as 5 Gm. daily.
For the pediatric patient from 5 to 10 years of age, approximately one-half the adult dose is recommended. It should be given at the same intervals as for adults.
PHENURONE may be administered alone or in conjunction with other anticonvulsants. However, extreme caution must be exercised if other anticonvulsants cause toxic effects similar to PHENURONE.
When PHENURONE is to replace other anticonvulsant medication, the latter should be withdrawn gradually as the dosage of PHENURONE is increased to maintain seizure control.
Overdosage: Symptoms of acute overdosage include excitement or mania, followed by drowsiness, ataxia and coma. In one case of acute overdosage, dizziness was followed by coma which lasted nearly 24 hours. Treatment should be started by inducing emesis; gastric lavage may be considered as an alternative or adjunct. General supportive measures will be necessary. A careful evaluation of liver and kidney function, mental state, and the blood-forming organs should be made following recovery.
How Supplied: PHENURONE (Phenacemide Tablets, N.F.), grooved, 500 mg. are supplied in bottles of 100 (**NDC** 0074-3971-05).
Ref. No. 01-2006/R5

PLACIDYL® ℞ Ⓒ
(Ethchlorvynol Capsules, N.F.)
Oral hypnotic

Description: PLACIDYL (ethchlorvynol) is a tertiary carbinol. It is chemically designated as ethyl β-chlorovinyl ethynyl carbinol. It is chemically unrelated to the barbiturates and to nonbarbiturate hypnotics such as chloral hydrate, bromides, paraldehyde or glutethimide.
Actions: The usual hypnotic dose of PLACIDYL induces sleep within 15 minutes to one hour. The duration of the hypnotic effect is about five hours.
PLACIDYL is rapidly absorbed from the gastrointestinal tract. Within the first 24 hours less than 0.1% of the usual dose is excreted in the urine either unchanged or conjugated to glucuronic acid or sulfate. Pharmacokinetic data indicate that ethchlorvynol is highly localized in body lipids.
Indications: PLACIDYL is indicated as short-term hypnotic therapy in the management of insomnia.
Contraindications: PLACIDYL is contraindicated in patients with known hypersensitivity to the drug and in patients with porphyria.
Warnings: PLACIDYL SHOULD BE ADMINISTERED WITH CAUTION TO MENTALLY DEPRESSED PATIENTS WITH OR WITHOUT SUICIDAL TENDENCIES. IT SHOULD ALSO BE ADMINISTERED WITH CAUTION TO THOSE WHO HAVE A PSYCHOLOGICAL POTENTIAL FOR DRUG DEPENDENCE. THE LEAST AMOUNT OF DRUG THAT IS FEASIBLE SHOULD BE PRESCRIBED FOR THESE PATIENTS.
Patients should be advised that, for the duration of the effect of PLACIDYL , mental and/or physical abilities required for the performance of potentially hazardous tasks such as the operation of dangerous machinery including motor vehicles, may be impaired.
Usage During Pregnancy and Lactation: PLACIDYL (ethchlorvynol) is not recommended for use during the first and second trimesters of pregnancy. Also clinical experience has indicated that PLACIDYL when taken during the third trimester of pregnancy may produce CNS depression and transient withdrawal symptoms in the newborn.
Reproductive toxicity testing of PLACIDYL was carried out in rats. A somewhat higher percentage of stillbirths and a lower survival rate of progeny was observed among animals given 40 mg./kg./day.
The safety of use of PLACIDYL during lactation has not been established.
Drug Interactions: Patients should be cautioned that the concomitant use of PLACIDYL and alcohol, barbiturates, other CNS depressants, or MAO inhibitors may produce exaggerated depressant effects.
Ethchlorvynol may cause a decreased prothrombin time response to coumarin anticoagulants; therefore, the dosage of these drugs may require adjustment when therapy with ethchlorvynol is initiated and after it is discontinued.
Transient delirium has been reported with the concomitant use of PLACIDYL and amitriptyline; therefore, PLACIDYL should be administered with caution to patients receiving tricyclic antidepressants.
Usage in Children: PLACIDYL is not recommended for use in children since its safety and effectiveness in the pediatric age group has not been established.
Psychological and Physical Dependence: PROLONGED USE OF PLACIDYL MAY RESULT IN TOLERANCE AND PSYCHOLOGICAL AND PHYSICAL DEPENDENCE. PROLONGED ADMINISTRATION OF THE DRUG IS NOT RECOMMENDED.
Signs and symptoms of intoxication have been reported with the prolonged use of doses as low as 1 Gm/day. Signs and symptoms of chronic intoxication may include incoordination, tremors, ataxia, confusion, slurred speech, hyperreflexia, diplopia, and generalized muscle weakness. Toxic amblyopia, scotoma, nystagmus, and peripheral neuropathy have also been reported with prolonged use of ethchlorvynol; these symptoms are usually reversible.
Pulmonary edema of rapid onset has resulted from the I.V. abuse of PLACIDYL (ethchlorvynol).
Severe withdrawal symptoms similar to those seen during barbiturate and alcohol withdrawal have been reported following abrupt discontinuance of prolonged use of PLACIDYL. These symptoms may appear as late as nine days after sudden withdrawal of the drug. Signs and symptoms of PLACIDYL withdrawal may include convulsions, delirium, schizoid reaction, perceptual distortions, memory loss, ataxia, insomnia, slurring of speech, unusual anxiety, irritability, agitation, and tremors. Other signs and symptoms may include anorexia, nausea, vomiting, weakness, dizziness, sweating, muscle twitching, and weight loss.
Management of a patient who manifests withdrawal symptoms from PLACIDYL involves readministration of the drug to approximately the same level of chronic intoxication that existed before the abrupt discontinuance (Phenobarbital may be substituted for PLACIDYL.) A gradual, stepwise reduction of dosage may then be made over a period of days or weeks. A phenothiazine compound may be used in addition to this regimen for those patients who exhibit psychotic symptoms during the withdrawal period. The patient undergoing withdrawal from PLACIDYL must be hospitalized or closely observed, and given general supportive care as indicated.
Precautions: Elderly or debilitated patients should receive the smallest effective amount of PLACIDYL (ethchlorvynol).
Caution should be exercised when treating patients with impaired hepatic or renal function.
Patients who exhibit unpredictable behavior, or paradoxical restlessness or excitement in response to barbiturates or alcohol may react in this manner to PLACIDYL.
PLACIDYL should not be used for the management of insomnia in the presence of pain unless insomnia persists after pain is controlled with analgesics.
Adverse Reactions: Nausea, vomiting, gastric upset, aftertaste, dizziness, blurred vision, facial numbness, and hypotension have occurred.
Hypersensitivity reactions have included skin rash, urticaria, and occasionally, thrombocytopenia and cholestatic jaundice.
Mild "hangover" has occurred.
The following idiosyncratic responses have been reported occasionally: mild stimulation, marked excitement, hysteria; prolonged hypnosis, profound muscular weakness, syncope without marked hypotension.
Transient giddiness and ataxia have occurred in patients in whom absorption of the drug is especially rapid; these effects can sometimes be controlled by giving PLACIDYL with food.
(See Psychological and Physical Dependence for the signs and symptoms of chronic intoxication.)
Dosage and Administration: The usual adult hypnotic dose of PLACIDYL (ethchlorvynol) is 500 mg. taken orally at bedtime. A dose of 750 mg. may be required for patients whose sleep response to a 500 mg. capsule is inadequate, or for patients being changed from barbiturates or other nonbarbiturate hypnotics. Up to 1000 mg. may be given as a single bedtime dose when insomnia is unusually severe.
A single supplemental dose of 100 to 200 mg. may be given to reinstitute sleep in patients who may awaken after the original bedtime dose of 500 or 750 mg.
For patients whose insomnia is characterized only by untimely awakening during the early morning hours, a single dose of 100 to 200 mg. taken upon awakening may be adequate for relief.
The smallest effective dose of PLACIDYL should be given to elderly or debilitated patients.
PLACIDYL should not be prescribed for prolonged periods. (See Psychological and Physical Dependence.)
Overdosage: Acute intoxication is characterized by prolonged deep coma, severe respiratory depression, hypothermia, hypotension, and relative bradycardia. Nystagmus and pancytopenia resulting from acute PLACIDYL overdose have been reported.
Although death has occurred following the ingestion of 6 Gm. of PLACIDYL, there have been reports of patients who have survived overdoses of 50 Gm. and more with intensive care.
Management of acute PLACIDYL intoxication is similar to that of acute barbiturate intoxication. Gastric evacuation should be performed immediately. (In the unconscious patient, gastric lavage should be preceded by tracheal in-

tubation with a cuffed tube.) Supportive care (assisted ventilation, frequent and careful monitoring of vital signs, control of blood pressure) is essential. Emphasis should be placed on pulmonary care and monitoring of blood gases. Hemodialysis and peritoneal dialysis have each been reported to be of some value in the management of acute PLACIDYL overdose. (Aqueous and oil dialysates have been used.) Forced diuresis with maintenance of a high urinary output has also been reported to be of some value.

(See Psychological and Physical Dependence for the signs and symptoms of chronic intoxication.)

How Supplied: PLACIDYL (ethchlorvynol capsules, N.F.) is supplied as:
100 mg. capsules:
Bottles of 100 ....(**NDC** 0074-6649-04).
200 mg. capsules:
Bottles of 100 ....(**NDC** 0074-6661-08).
500 mg. capsules:
Bottles of 100 ....(**NDC** 0074-6685-15).
Bottles of 500 ....(**NDC** 0074-6685-02).
ABBO-PAC® unit dose strip packages of
100 ....(**NDC** 0074-6685-10).
750 mg. capsules:
Bottles of 100 ....(**NDC** 0074-6630-01).
ABBO-PAC unit dose strip packages of
100 ....(**NDC** 0074-6630-10).
Ref 01-2849/R3
[*Shown in Product Identification Section*]

QUELIDRINE® SYRUP

(non-narcotic, antihistaminic cough suppressant)

Composition: Each teaspoonful (5 ml.) contains:

Dextromethorphan Hydrobromide	10 mg.
Chlorpheniramine maleate	2 mg.
Ephedrine Hydrochloride	5 mg.
Phenylephrine Hydrochloride	5 mg.
Ammonium chloride	40 mg.
Ipecac fluidextract	0.005 ml.
Alcohol	2%

in a palatable, aromatic syrup.

Action and Indications: Quelidrine is designed as an aid in the management of cough associated with acute or subacute simple respiratory infections. Quelidrine provides a wide range of therapeutic action against the cough complex—without the risk of addiction or the production of undue central depression.

Precautions: Quelidrine should be administered with caution to patients with hypertension, serious organic heart disease, angina pectoris, diabetes, thyroid disease, or to persons receiving digitalis. When cough persists or accompanies a high fever, the underlying cause and need for other medication should be reevaluated.

Side Effects: Quelidrine is safe for patients of all ages, but professional supervision of dosage for very young patients is essential. Side effects are infrequent. Drowsiness, nausea, vomiting, nervousness, palpitation, blurred vision and insomnia may occur in susceptible patients. Constipation is seldom a problem. If side effects are encountered, dosage should be reduced or medication withdrawn.

Dosage and Administration: *Adults*—1 teaspoonful, one to four times daily. Children 6 years of age or older, ½ teaspoonful, one to four times daily. Children 2 to 6 years old, ¼ teaspoonful one to four times daily. Under 2, as directed by physician. Quelidrine may be diluted with Syrup, U.S.P., in order to facilitate pediatric administration. Patients should be warned that this medication should be kept from the reach of children.

How Supplied: Quelidrine Syrup is supplied in bottles of 4 fluid ounces (**NDC** 0074-6883-04), 1 pint (**NDC** 0074-6883-02), and 1 gallon (**NDC** 0074-6883-03) with or without a prescription.

SELSUN® ℞

selenium sulfide lotion, U.S.P.

Description: SELSUN (selenium sulfide lotion) is a liquid preparation containing 2.5 percent selenium sulfide suspended in a detergent. The product contains: selenium sulfide 2½%, w/v; bentonite; lauric diethanolamide; ethylene glycol monostearate; titanium dioxide; amphoteric-2; sodium lauryl sulfate; sodium phosphate (monobasic); glyceryl monoricinoleate; citric acid; captan; perfume; and water.

Indications: For the treatment of seborrheic dermatitis of the scalp, including dandruff.

Contraindications: SELSUN (selenium sulfide lotion) should not be used by patients allergic to any of its components.

Warnings: Safety for use on infants has not been established.

Precautions: Cutaneous sensitization of the scalp or adjacent areas has been reported. If sensitivity reactions should occur, the lotion should be discontinued.

Chemical conjunctivitis may result if the preparation enters the eyes.

The product should not be used when acute inflammation or exudation is present as an increase in absorption may occur.

Adverse Reactions: As with other shampoos, oiliness or dryness of the hair and scalp may occur following use and there have been occasional reports of an increase in the amount of normal hair loss. Discoloration of the hair may follow use of the preparation. This can be avoided or minimized by thorough rinsing of the hair after treatment.

Dosage and Administration: For treatment of dandruff or seborrheic dermatitis of the scalp:

1. Massage about 1 or 2 teaspoonfuls of the medicated shampoo into the wet scalp.
2. Allow product to remain on the scalp for 2 to 3 minutes.
3. Rinse the scalp thoroughly.
4. Repeat application and rinse thoroughly.
5. After treatment wash hands.

For the usual case, two applications each week for two weeks will afford control. After this, the lotion may be used at less frequent intervals—weekly, every two weeks, or even every 3 or 4 weeks in some cases. The preparation should not be applied more frequently than required to maintain control.

Accidental Oral Ingestion: There have been no documented reports of serious toxicity in humans resulting from acute ingestion of SELSUN; however, acute toxicity studies in animals suggest that ingestion of large amounts could result in potential human toxicity. For this reason, evacuation of the stomach contents should be considered in cases of acute oral ingestion.

How Supplied: SELSUN (selenium sulfide lotion, U.S.P.) is supplied in 4-fluidounce nonbreakable plastic bottles (**NDC** 0074-2660-04). SELSUN is to be dispensed only on the prescription of a physician.
Ref. No. 01-2878/R1

SELSUN BLUE®

(selenium sulfide)
Lotion

Selsun Blue is a non-prescription anti-dandruff shampoo containing a 1% concentration of selenium sulfide in a freshly scented, pH balanced formula to leave hair clean and manageable. Available in formulations for dry, oily or normal hair types.

Clinical testing has shown it to be safe and effective in helping to control dandruff symptoms with regular use.

Directions: Shake lotion well before using. Use just enough to lather, rinse thoroughly, and repeat. Use once or twice weekly for effective dandruff control.

Caution: For external use only. Keep this and all shampoos out of children's reach. Avoid getting shampoo in eyes—if this happens, rinse thoroughly with water. When used before or after bleaching, tinting or permanent waving, rinse for at least five minutes in cool running water. If irritation occurs, discontinue use. Protect from heat.

SURBEX®

(vitamin B-Complex*)

SURBEX® with C

(vitamin B-Complex* with vitamin C)

Description: Each Surbex Filmtab tablet provides:

Niacinamide	30 mg
Calcium Pantothenate	10 mg
Vitamin B_1 (Thiamine Mononitrate)	6 mg
Vitamin B_2 (Riboflavin)	6 mg
Vitamin B_6 (Pyridoxine Hydrochloride)	2.5 mg
Vitamin B_{12} (Cyanocobalamin)	5 mcg

Each Surbex with C Filmtab tablet provides the same ingredients as Surbex plus 250 mg Vitamin C (as Sodium Ascorbate).

Indications: Surbex is indicated for treatment of Vitamin B-Complex* deficiency.

Surbex with C is indicated for use in treatment of Vitamin B-Complex* with Vitamin C deficiency. Neither product is indicated for the treatment of folate deficiency.

Dosage and Administration: Usual adult dosage is one tablet twice daily or as directed by physician.

How Supplied: Surbex is supplied as bright orange-colored tablets in bottles of 100 (NDC 0074-4876-13).

Surbex with C is supplied as yellow-colored tablets in bottles of 100 (NDC 0074-4877-13) and 500 (NDC 0074-4877-53).

*Contains no folic acid.
Ref. 03-0454-2/R2 & 03-0455-2/R2

SURBEX-T®

(High-Potency Vitamin B-Complex* with 500 mg of Vitamin C)

Description: Each Filmtab® tablet provides:

Vitamin C (as sodium ascorbate)	500 mg
Niacinamide	100 mg
Calcium Pantothenate	20 mg
Vitamin B_1 (Thiamine Mononitrate)	15 mg
Vitamin B_2 (Riboflavin)	10 mg
Vitamin B_6 (Pyridoxine Hydrochloride)	5 mg
Vitamin B_{12} (Cyanocobalamin)	10 mcg

Indications: For use in treatment of Vitamin B-Complex* with Vitamin C deficiency. Not for treatment of folate deficiency.

Administration and Dosage: Usual adult dosage is one Filmtab tablet daily, or as directed by physician.

How Supplied: Orange-colored tablets in bottles of 30 (NDC 0074-4878-30), 50 (NDC 0074-4878-50), 100 (NDC 0074-4878-13), and 500 (NDC 0074-4878-53). Also supplied in Abbo-Pac® (Unit dose packages) 100 tablets in strips of 10 tablets per strip (NDC 0074-4878-11). ®Filmtab—Film-sealed Tablets, Abbott.
[*Shown in Product Identification Section*]

*Contains no folic acid
Ref. 03-0659-2/R3

Continued on next page

If desired, additional literature on any Abbott Product will be provided upon request to Abbott Laboratories.

Abbott—Cont.

SURBEX®-750 with IRON
(High potency B-complex with iron, vitamin E and 750 mg vitamin C)

Description: Each Filmtab® tablet provides:

VITAMINS:	
Vitamin C (as sodium ascorbate)	750 mg
Niacinamide	100 mg
Vitamin B_6 (Pyridoxine Hydrochloride)	25 mg
Calcium Pantothenate	20 mg
Vitamin B_1 (Thiamine Mononitrate)	15 mg
Vitamin B_2 (Riboflavin)	15 mg
Vitamin B_{12} (cyanocobalamin)	12 mcg
Folic Acid	400 mcg
Vitamin E (as dl-alpha tocopheryl acetate)	30 IU
MINERAL:	
Elemental Iron (as dried ferrous sulfate)	27 mg
equivalent to 135 mg ferrous sulfate	

Indications: For the treatment of vitamin C and B-complex deficiencies and to supplement the daily intake of iron and vitamin E.
Dosage and Administration: Usual adult dosage is one tablet daily or as directed by physician.
How Supplied: Bottles of 50 tablets (NDC 0074-8029-50)
Ref. 03-0632-2/R1
[*Shown in Product Identification Section*]

SURBEX®-750 with ZINC
(Zinc, vitamin B-complex and vitamins C and E)

Daily dose (one Filmtab® tablet) provides:

VITAMINS		%U.S. R.D.A.*
Vitamin E	30 IU	100%
Vitamin C	750 mg	1250%
Folic Acid	0.4 mg	100%
Thiamine (B_1)	15 mg	1000%
Riboflavin (B_2)	15 mg	882%
Niacin	100 mg	500%
Vitamin B_6	20 mg	1000%
Vitamin B_{12}	12 mcg	200%
Pantothenic Acid	20 mg	200%
MINERAL		
Zinc	22.5 mg	150%

* % U.S. Recommended Daily Allowance for Adults.
Ingredients: Sodium ascorbate, niacinamide, zinc sulfate, dl-alpha tocopheryl acetate, povidone, cellulose, pyridoxine hydrochloride, calcium pantothenate, thiamine mononitrate, riboflavin, cyanocobalamin, magnesium stearate, colloidal silicon dioxide, folic acid, in a film coated tablet with vanillin flavoring and artificial coloring added.
Usual Adult Dose: One tablet daily.
How Supplied: Bottles of 50 tablets (NDC 0074-8152-50).
Ref. 03-0637-2/R1
[*Shown in Product Identification Section*]

TRAL® ℞
(hexocyclium methylsulfate)
Filmtab® Tablets

Description: TRAL (hexocyclium methylsulfate) is a quaternary ammonium salt. Chemically, it is designated as N-(beta-cyclohexyl-beta-hydroxy-beta-phenylethyl)-N′-methylpiperazine methosulfate. Physically, TRAL is a white powder soluble in water or physiological saline yielding a stable solution.
Actions: Clinically, TRAL is an effective anticholinergic agent which inhibits gastric secretion and gastrointestinal motility.
The drug has an antimuscarinic action similar to that of other quaternary ammonium compounds which produce anticholinergic effects. In experimental animals the drug has been shown to decrease gastric secretion, prevent gastric ulceration, decrease gastrointestinal motility, dilate the pupils, inhibit salivation, increase the heart rate, and counteract the peripheral muscarinic effect of choline esters. With massive overdosage the drug also may produce a peripheral curare-like neuromuscular block and ganglionic blockade. In studies with human subjects, TRAL produced a decrease in gastric acidity, and a decrease in the volume of gastric secretion.
TRAL is absorbed from the gastrointestinal tract but the degree of absorption varies. Following oral administration of a single dose of the drug in conventional tablet form, its effects persist for 3 to 4 hours. The metabolic fate and route of excretion are unknown.
Indications: TRAL is indicated as adjunctive therapy in the treatment of peptic ulcer. IT SHOULD BE NOTED AT THIS POINT IN TIME THAT THERE IS A LACK OF CONCURRENCE AS TO THE VALUE OF ANTICHOLINERGICS IN THE TREATMENT OF GASTRIC ULCER. IT HAS NOT BEEN SHOWN WHETHER ANTICHOLINERGIC DRUGS AID IN THE HEALING OF A PEPTIC ULCER, DECREASE THE RATE OF RECURRENCES OR PREVENT COMPLICATION. To be effective the dosage must be titrated to the individual patient's needs.
Contraindications: TRAL is contraindicated in patients with glaucoma; obstructive uropathy (for example, bladder neck obstruction due to prostatic hypertrophy); obstructive disease of the gastrointestinal tract (as in achalasia, paralytic ileus, pyloroduodenal stenosis, etc.); intestinal atony of the elderly or debilitated patient; unstable cardiovascular status; in acute hemorrhage; severe ulcerative colitis; toxic megacolon complicating ulcerative colitis; myasthenia gravis.
Warnings: In the presence of a high environmental temperature, heat prostration can occur with drug use (fever and heat stroke due to decreased sweating).
TRAL may produce drowsiness or blurred vision. In this event, the patient should be warned not to engage in activities requiring mental alertness such as operating a motor vehicle or other machinery, or perform hazardous work while taking this drug.
Usage in Pregnancy and Lactation: The safety of TRAL for use during pregnancy or lactation has not been established.
Studies in pregnant rabbits at daily oral doses of 2.5 to 40 mg/kg/day produced an increased number of resorption sites and abortions.
As with all anticholinergic drugs, an inhibitory effect on lactation may occur.
Precautions: TRAL should be used with caution in patients with:
- Autonomic neuropathy.
- Hepatic or renal disease.
- Ulcerative colitis—large doses may suppress intestinal motility to the point of producing a paralytic ileus and the use of this drug may precipitate or aggravate the serious complication of toxic megacolon.
- Hyperthyroidism, coronary heart disease, congestive heart failure, cardiac arrhythmias, hypertension and non-obstructing prostatic hypertrophy.
- Hiatal hernia associated with reflux esophagitis since anticholinergic drugs may aggravate this condition.

It should be noted that the use of anticholinergic drugs in the treatment of gastric ulcer may produce a delay in gastric emptying time and may complicate such therapy (antral stasis).
Investigate any tachycardia before giving anticholinergic (atropine-like) drugs since they may increase the heart rate.
With overdosage, a curare-like action may occur.
Adverse Reactions: Adverse reactions may include xerostomia, urinary hesitancy and retention, blurred vision, mydriasis, cycloplegia, increased intra-ocular tension, tachycardia, palpitations, headaches, nervousness, drowsiness, weakness, dizziness, insomnia, nausea, vomiting, impotency, dysphagia, altered taste perception, heartburn, bloated feeling, constipation, paralytic ileus, flushing, decreased sweating, urticaria and other dermal manifestations, severe allergic reaction or drug idiosyncrasies, and some degree of mental confusion and/or excitement especially in elderly persons.
When side effects are severe and cannot be controlled by reduction of dosage, the medication should be withdrawn.
Dosage and Administration: TRAL is administered orally. The usual recommended adult dose of TRAL is one 25 mg Filmtab tablet four times daily, taken before meals and at bedtime.
For optimal therapeutic effect, dosage should be adjusted to the patient's response.
TRAL is not for use in children.
Overdosage: The first sign of overdosage may be indicated by an atropine-like flush, particularly in the blush areas. Other manifestations of overdosage are revealed by the appearance or an increase in intensity of dryness of the mouth or other side effects.
With unusually large doses the quaternary ammonium type of anticholinergic agent may produce a curare-like action and ganglionic blockade manifested by respiratory paralysis and circulatory collapse. This is unlikely to occur with therapeutic doses. Neostigmine methylsulfate at a dose of 0.5 to 2 mg given by slow intravenous injection and repeated as required may be administered as an antidote. Only in exceptional cases should the total dose of neostigmine methylsulfate exceed 5 mg. Artificial respiration and other supportive measures should be applied if needed.
How Supplied: TRAL (hexocyclium methylsulfate) Filmtab tablets, 25 mg, green, (**NDC** 0074-6698-02) are supplied in bottles of 100.
Ref. 01-2992-R4

TRAL® ℞
(hexocyclium methylsulfate)
GRADUMET® TABLETS

Description: TRAL (hexocyclium methylsulfate) is a quaternary ammonium salt. Chemically, it is designated as N-(beta-cyclohexyl-beta-hydroxy-beta-phenylethyl)-N′ methylpiperazine methosulfate. Physically, TRAL is a white powder soluble in water or physiological saline yielding a stable solution.
The Gradumet tablet is designed to provide sustained release of TRAL.
Actions: Clinically, TRAL is an effective anticholinergic agent which inhibits gastric secretion and gastrointestinal motility.
The drug has an antimuscarinic action similar to that of other quaternary ammonium compounds which produce anticholinergic effects. In experimental animals the drug has been shown to decrease gastric secretion, prevent gastric ulceration, decrease gastrointestinal motility, dilate the pupils, inhibit salivation, increase the heart rate, and counteract the peripheral muscarinic effect of choline esters. With massive overdosage the drug also may produce a peripheral curare-like neuro-muscular block and ganglionic blockade. In studies with human subjects, TRAL produced a decrease in gastric acidity, and a decrease in the volume of gastric secretion.
TRAL is absorbed from the gastrointestinal tract but the degree of absorption varies. The duration of significant antisecretory action resulting from a single dose of the Gradumet form is approximately 10 hours. The metabolic fate and route of excretion are unknown.
Indications: As adjunctive therapy in the treatment of peptic ulcer, chiefly for the relief of pain when used as part of a total therapeutic program. IT SHOULD BE NOTED AT THIS POINT IN TIME THAT THERE IS A LACK OF CONCURRENCE AS TO THE VALUE OF ANTICHOLINERGICS IN THE TREAT-

MENT OF GASTRIC ULCER. IT HAS NOT BEEN SHOWN CONCLUSIVELY WHETHER ANTICHOLINERGIC DRUGS AID IN THE HEALING OF A PEPTIC ULCER, DECREASE THE RATE OF RECURRENCES OR PREVENT COMPLICATION. To insure maximum benefit, the dosage must be titrated to the individual patient's needs.

Contraindications: TRAL is contraindicated in patients with glaucoma; obstructive uropathy (for example, bladder neck obstruction due to prostatic hypertrophy); obstructive disease of the gastrointestinal tract (as in achalasia, paralytic ileus, pyloroduodenal stenosis, etc.) intestinal atony of the elderly or debilitated patient; unstable cardiovascular status; in acute hemorrhage; severe ulcerative colitis; toxic megacolon complicating ulcerative colitis; myasthenia gravis.

Warnings: In the presence of high environmental temperature, heat prostration can occur with drug use (fever and heat stroke due to decreased sweating).

TRAL (hexocyclium methylsulfate) may produce drowsiness or blurred vision. In this event, the patient should be warned not to engage in activities requiring mental alertness such as operating a motor vehicle or other machinery or perform hazardous work while taking this drug.

Usage in Pregnancy and Lactation: Safe use in pregnancy and lactation has not been established.

No teratogenic effects with TRAL have been found in humans or in laboratory animal experiments. Although the clinical significance is not clear, recent animal experiments with TRAL have shown that daily oral doses of 2.5 to 40 mg/kg/day given to pregnant rabbits produced an increased number of resorption sites and abortions. No significant effects were observed on the progeny of rats. As with all anticholinergic drugs, an inhibitory effect on lactation may occur.

Precautions: TRAL should be used with caution in patients with:

Autonomic neuropathy.

Hepatic or renal disease.

Ulcerative colitis—large doses may suppress intestinal motility to the point of producing a paralytic ileus and the use of this drug may precipitate or aggravate the serious complication of toxic megacolon.

Hyperthyroidism, coronary heart disease, congestive heart failure, cardiac arrhythmias, hypertension and non-obstructing prostatic hypertrophy.

Hiatal hernia associated with reflux esophagitis since anticholinergic drugs may aggravate this condition.

It should be noted that the use of anticholinergic drugs in the treatment of gastric ulcer may produce a delay in gastric emptying time and may complicate such therapy (antral stasis).

Investigate any tachycardia before giving anticholinergic (atropine-like) drugs since they may increase the heart rate.

With overdosage, a curare-like action may occur.

Adverse Reactions: Adverse reactions may include xerostomia, urinary hesitancy and retention, blurred vision, mydriasis, cycloplegia, increased intra-ocular tension, tachycardia, palpitations, headaches, nervousness, drowsiness, weakness, dizziness, insomnia, nausea, vomiting, impotency, dysphagia, altered taste perception, heartburn, bloated feeling, constipation, paralytic ileus, flushing, decreased sweating, urticaria and other dermal manifestations, severe allergic reaction of drug idiosyncrasies, and some degree of mental confusion and/or excitement especially in elderly persons.

When side effects are severe and cannot be controlled by reduction of dosage, the medication should be withdrawn.

Dosage and Administration: TRAL is administered orally. The usual recommended dose of TRAL Gradumet is one tablet twice daily, taken before lunch and at bedtime, or before breakfast and before the evening meal. The morning and evening doses should be adjusted according to the response of each patient.

The duration of significant antisecretory activity resulting from the use of TRAL Gradumet is approximately 10 hours.

Gradumet tablets should not be chewed. The expended inert Gradumet matrix is not absorbed and is excreted in the stool.

TRAL is not for use in children.

Overdosage: The first sign of overdosage may be indicated by an atropine-like flush, particularly in the blush areas. Other manifestations of overdosage are revealed by the appearance or an increase in intensity of dryness of the mouth or other side effects.

With unusually large doses the quaternary ammonium type of anticholinergic agent may produce a curare-like action and ganglionic blockade manifested by respiratory paralysis and circulatory collapse. This is unlikely to occur with therapeutic doses. Neostigmine methylsulfate at a dose of 0.5 to 2 mg. given by slow intravenous injection and repeated as required may be administered as an antidote. Only in exceptional cases should the total dose of neostigmine methylsulfate exceed 5 mg. Artificial respiration and other supportive measures should be applied if needed.

How Supplied: TRAL (hexocyclium methylsulfate) Gradumet, 50 mg, orange-colored tablets (**NDC** 0074-6920-09) are supplied in bottles of 50.

TRANXENE® ℞ ©

(clorazepate dipotassium)
Capsules

TRANXENE®-SD
& TRANXENE-SD HALF STRENGTH

(clorazepate dipotassium)
Tablets

Description: Chemically, Tranxene (clorazepate dipotassium) is a benzodiazepine. The empirical formula is $C_{16}H_{11}ClK_2N_2O_4$; the molecular weight is 408.92.

The compound occurs as a fine, light yellow, practically odorless powder. It is insoluble in the common organic solvents, but very soluble in water. Aqueous solutions are unstable, clear, light yellow, and alkaline.

Actions: Pharmacologically, clorazepate dipotassium has the characteristics of the benzodiazepines. It has depressant effects on the central nervous system. The primary metabolite, nordiazepam, quickly appears in the blood stream. The serum half-life is about 2 days. The drug is metabolized in the liver and excreted primarily in the urine. (See ANIMAL AND CLINICAL PHARMACOLOGY section).

Indications: TRANXENE is indicated for the symptomatic relief of anxiety and tension associated with anxiety disorders, other psychoneurotic disorders, transient situational disturbances and functional or organic disorders.

TRANXENE is indicated for the symptomatic relief of acute alcohol withdrawal.

The effectiveness of TRANXENE in long-term use, that is, more than 4 months, has not been assessed by systematic clinical studies. The physician should reassess periodically the usefulness of the drug for the individual patient.

Contraindications: TRANXENE is contraindicated in patients with a known hypersensitivity to the drug, and in those with acute narrow angle glaucoma.

Warnings: TRANXENE is not recommended for use in depressive neuroses or in psychotic reactions.

Patients on TRANXENE should be cautioned against engaging in hazardous occupations requiring mental alertness, such as operating dangerous machinery including motor vehicles.

Since TRANXENE has a central nervous system depressant effect, patients should be advised against the simultaneous use of other CNS-depressant drugs, and cautioned that the effects of alcohol may be increased.

Because of the lack of sufficient clinical experience, TRANXENE is not recommended for use in patients less than 18 years of age.

Physical and Psychological Dependence: Withdrawal symptoms (similar in character to those noted with barbiturates and alcohol) have occurred following abrupt discontinuance of clorazepate. Symptoms of nervousness, insomnia, irritability, diarrhea, muscle aches and memory impairment have followed abrupt withdrawal after long-term use of high dosage. Withdrawal symptoms have also been reported following abrupt discontinuance of benzodiazepines taken continuously at therapeutic levels for several months. Caution should be observed in patients who are considered to have a psychological potential for drug dependence.

Evidence of drug dependence has been observed in dogs and rabbits which was characterized by convulsive seizures when the drug was abruptly withdrawn or the dose was reduced; the syndrome in dogs could be abolished by administration of clorazepate.

Usage in Pregnancy: **An increased risk of congenital malformations associated with the use of minor tranquilizers (chlordiazepoxide, diazepam, and meprobamate) during the first trimester of pregnancy has been suggested in several studies. TRANXENE, a benzodiazepine derivative, has not been studied adequately to determine whether it, too, may be associated with an increased risk of fetal abnormality. Because use of these drugs is rarely a matter of urgency, their use during this period should almost always be avoided. The possibility that a woman of childbearing potential may be pregnant at the time of institution of therapy should be considered. Patients should be advised that if they become pregnant during therapy or intend to become pregnant they should communicate with their physician about the desirability of discontinuing the drug.**

Usage during Lactation: TRANXENE should not be given to nursing mothers since it has been reported that nordiazepam is excreted in human breast milk.

Precautions: In those patients in which a degree of depression accompanies the anxiety, suicidal tendencies may be present and protective measures may be required. The least amount of drug that is feasible should be available to the patient.

Patients on TRANXENE for prolonged periods should have blood counts and liver function tests periodically. The usual precautions in treating patients with impaired renal or hepatic function should also be observed.

In elderly or debilitated patients, the initial dose should be small, and increments should be made gradually, in accordance with the response of the patient, to preclude ataxia or excessive sedation.

Adverse Reactions: The side effect most frequently reported was drowsiness. Less commonly reported (in descending order of occurrence) were: dizziness, various gastrointestinal complaints, nervousness, blurred vision, dry mouth, headache, and mental confusion. Other side effects included insomnia, transient skin rashes, fatigue, ataxia, genitourinary complaints, irritability, diplopia, depression and slurred speech.

Continued on next page

Abbott—Cont.

There have been reports of abnormal liver and kidney function tests and of decrease in hematocrit.
Decrease in systolic blood pressure has been observed.
Dosage and Administration: *For the symptomatic relief of anxiety:* TRANXENE is administered orally. The capsules may be given in divided doses. The usual daily dose is 30 mg. The dose should be adjusted gradually within the range of 15 to 60 mg daily in accordance with the response of the patient. In elderly or debilitated patients it is advisable to initiate treatment at a daily dose of 7.5 to 15 mg.
TRANXENE capsules may also be administered as a single dose daily at bedtime; the recommended initial dose is 15 mg. After the initial dose, the response of the patient may require adjustment of subsequent dosage. Lower doses may be indicated in the elderly patient. Drowsiness may occur at the initiation of treatment and with dosage increment.
TRANXENE-SD tablets (22.5 mg) may be administered as a single dose every 24 hours. This tablet is intended as an alternate dosage form for the convenience of patients stabilized on a dose of 7.5 mg capsules three times a day. TRANXENE-SD tablets should not be used to initiate therapy.
TRANXENE-SD HALF STRENGTH tablets (11.25 mg) may be administered as a single dose every 24 hours.
For the symptomatic relief of acute alcohol withdrawal:
The following dosage schedule is recommended:

1st 24 hours (Day 1)	30 mg Tranxene, initially; followed by 30 to 60 mg in divided doses
2nd 24 hours (Day 2)	45 to 90 mg in divided doses
3rd 24 hours (Day 3)	22.5 to 45 mg in divided doses
Day 4	15 to 30 mg in divided doses

Thereafter, gradually reduce the daily dose to 7.5 to 15 mg. Discontinue drug therapy as soon as patient's condition is stable.
The maximum recommended total daily dose is 90 mg. Avoid excessive reductions in the total amount of drug administered on successive days.
Drug Interactions: If TRANXENE is to be combined with other drugs acting on the central nervous system, careful consideration should be given to the pharmacology of the agents to be employed. Animal experience indicates that TRANXENE prolongs the sleeping time after hexobarbital or after ethyl alcohol, increases the inhibitory effects of chlorpromazine, but does not exhibit monoamine oxidase inhibition. Clinical studies have shown increased sedation with concurrent hypnotic medications. The actions of the benzodiazepines may be potentiated by barbiturates, narcotics, phenothiazines, monoamine oxidase inhibitors or other antidepressants.
If TRANXENE is used to treat anxiety associated with somatic disease states, careful attention must be paid to possible drug interaction with concomitant medication.
Management of Overdosage: Overdosage is usually manifested by varying degrees of CNS depression ranging from slight sedation to coma. As in the management of overdosage with any drug, it should be borne in mind that multiple agents may have been taken.
There are no specific antidotes for the benzodiazepines. The treatment of overdosage should consist of the general measures employed in the management of overdosage of any CNS depressant. Gastric evacuation either by the induction of emesis, lavage, or both, should be performed immediately. General supportive care, including frequent monitoring of the vital signs and close observation of the patient, is indicated. Hypotension, though rarely reported, may occur with large overdoses. In such cases the use of agents such as Levophed® Bitartrate (levarterenol bitartrate injection, USP) or Aramine® Injection (metaraminol bitartrate injection, USP) should be considered.
While reports indicate that individuals have survived overdoses of TRANXENE as high as 450 to 675 mg, these doses are not necessarily an accurate indication of the amount of drug absorbed since the time interval between ingestion and the institution of treatment was not always known. Sedation in varying degrees was the most common physiological manifestation of TRANXENE overdosage. Deep coma when it occurred was usually associated with the ingestion of other drugs in addition to TRANXENE.
Animal and Clinical Pharmacology: Studies in rats and monkeys have shown a substantial difference between doses producing tranquilizing, sedative and toxic effects. In rats, conditioned avoidance response was inhibited at an oral dose of 10 mg/kg; sedation was induced at 32 mg/kg; the LD_{50} was 1320 mg/kg. In monkeys aggressive behavior was reduced at an oral dose of 0.25 mg/kg; sedation (ataxia) was induced at 7.5 mg/kg; the LD_{50} could not be determined because of the emetic effect of large doses, but the LD_{50} exceeds 1600 mg/kg.
Twenty-four dogs were given TRANXENE orally in a 22-month toxicity study; doses up to 75 mg/kg were given. Drug-related changes occurred in the liver; weight was increased and cholestasis with minimal hepatocellular damage was found, but lobular architecture remained well preserved.
Eighteen rhesus monkeys were given oral doses of TRANXENE from 3 to 36 mg/kg daily for 52 weeks. All treated animals remained similar to control animals. Although total leucocyte count remained within normal limits it tended to fall in the female animals on the highest doses.
Examination of all organs revealed no alterations attributable to TRANXENE. There was no damage to liver function or structure.
Reproduction Studies: Standard fertility, reproduction, and teratology studies were conducted in rats and rabbits. Oral doses in rats up to 150 mg/kg and in rabbits up to 15 mg/kg produced no abnormalities in the fetuses. TRANXENE (clorazepate dipotassium) did not alter the fertility indices or reproductive capacities of adult animals. As expected, the sedative effect of high doses interfered with care of the young by their mothers (see Usage in Pregnancy).
Clinical Pharmacology: Studies in healthy men have shown that TRANXENE has depressant effects on the central nervous system. Prolonged administration of single daily doses as high as 120 mg was without toxic effects. Abrupt cessation of high doses was followed in some patients by nervousness, insomnia, irritability, diarrhea, muscle aches, or memory impairment.
Absorption—Excretion: After oral administration of TRANXENE there is essentially no circulating parent drug. Nordiazepam, its primary metabolite, quickly appears in the blood stream. In 2 volunteers given 15 mg (50 μC) of ^{14}C-Tranxene, about 80% was recovered in the urine and feces within 10 days. Excretion was primarily in the urine with about 1% excreted per day on day 10.
How Supplied: TRANXENE (clorazepate dipotassium) is supplied as:
3.75 mg gray and white capsules:
Bottles of 100 ....(**NDC** 0074-3417-13)
Bottles of 500 ....(**NDC** 0074-3417-53)
ABBO-PAC® unit dose packages:
100 ....(**NDC** 0074-3417-11).
7.5 mg gray and maroon capsules:
Bottles of 30 ....(**NDC** 0074-3418-30)
Bottles of 100 ....(**NDC** 0074-3418-13)
Bottles of 500 ....(**NDC** 0074-3418-53)
ABBO-PAC unit dose packages:
100 ....(**NDC** 0074-3418-11)
4 cartons of 25 ....(**NDC** 0074-3418-25).
15 mg gray capsules:
Bottles of 100 ....(**NDC** 0074-3419-13)
Bottles of 500 ....(**NDC** 0074-3419-53)
ABBO-PAC unit dose packages:
100 ....(**NDC** 0074-3419-11).
TRANXENE-SD 22.5 mg tan-colored, single dose tablets:
Bottles of 100 ....(**NDC** 0074-2997-13).
TRANXENE-SD HALF STRENGTH 11.25 mg blue-colored, single dose tablets:
Bottles of 30 ....(**NDC** 0074-2699-30)
Bottles of 100 ....(**NDC** 0074-2699-13).
[*Shown in Product Identification Section*]
Ref. 03-4171-R5

TRIDIONE® ℞
(trimethadione)
Tablets, Capsules, and Oral Solution

BECAUSE OF ITS POTENTIAL TO PRODUCE FETAL MALFORMATIONS AND SERIOUS SIDE EFFECTS, TRIDIONE (trimethadione) SHOULD ONLY BE UTILIZED WHEN OTHER LESS TOXIC DRUGS HAVE BEEN FOUND INEFFECTIVE IN CONTROLLING PETIT MAL SEIZURES.

Description: TRIDIONE (trimethadione) is an antiepileptic agent. An oxazolidinedione compound, it is chemically identified as 3,5,5-trimethyloxozolidine-2,4-dione.
TRIDIONE is a synthetic, water-soluble, white, crystalline powder. It is supplied in capsular, tablet, and liquid forms for oral use only.
Clinical Pharmacology: TRIDIONE has been shown to prevent pentylenetetrazol-induced and thujone-induced seizures in experimental animals; the drug has a less marked effect on seizures induced by picrotoxin, procaine, cocaine, or strychnine. Unlike the hydantoins and antiepileptic barbiturates, TRIDIONE does not modify the maximal seizure pattern in patients undergoing electroconvulsive therapy.
TRIDIONE has a sedative effect that may increase to the point of ataxia when excessive doses are used. A toxic dose of the drug in animals (approximately 2 Gm/kg) produced sleep, unconsciousness, and respiratory depression.
Trimethadione is rapidly absorbed from the gastrointestinal tract. It is demethylated by liver microsomes to the active metabolite, dimethadione.
Approximately 3% of a daily dose of TRIDIONE is recovered in the urine as unchanged drug. The majority of trimethadione is excreted slowly by the kidney in the form of dimethadione.
Indications: TRIDIONE (trimethadione) is indicated for the control of petit mal seizures that are refractory to treatment with other drugs.
Contraindications: TRIDIONE is contraindicated in patients with a known hypersensitivity to the drug.
Warnings: TRIDIONE may cause serious side effects. Strict medical supervision of the patient is mandatory, especially during the initial year of therapy.
TRIDIONE (trimethadione) should be withdrawn promptly if skin rash appears, because of the grave possibility of the occurrence of exfoliative dermatitis or severe forms of erythema multiforme. Even a minor acneiform or mor-

billiform rash should be allowed to clear completely before treatment with TRIDIONE is resumed; reinstitute therapy cautiously.
A complete blood count should be done prior to intiating therapy with TRIDIONE, and at monthly intervals thereafter. A marked depression of the blood count is an indication for withdrawal of the drug. If no abnormality appears within 12 months, the interval between blood counts may be extended. A moderate degree of neutropenia with or without a corresponding drop in the leukocyte count is not uncommon. Therapy need not be withdrawn unless the neutrophil count is 2500 or less; more frequent blood examinations should be done when the count is less than 3,000. Other blood dyscrasias, including leukopenia, eosinophilia, thrombocytopenia, pancytopenia, agranulocytosis, hypoplastic anemia, and fatal aplastic anemia, have occurred. Patients should be advised to report immediately such signs and symptoms as sore throat, fever, malaise, easy bruising, petechiae, or epistaxis, or others that may be indicative of an infection or bleeding tendency. TRIDIONE should ordinarily not be used in patients with severe blood dyscrasias.
Liver function tests should be done prior to initiating therapy with TRIDIONE, and at monthly intervals thereafter. Hepatitis has been reported rarely. Jaundice or other signs of liver dysfunction are an indication for withdrawal of the drug. TRIDIONE should ordinarily not be used in patients with severe hepatic impairment.
A urinalysis should be done prior to initiating therapy with TRIDIONE and at monthly intervals thereafter. Fatal nephrosis has been reported. Persistent or increasing albuminuria, or the development of any other significant renal abnormality, is an indication for withdrawal of the drug. TRIDIONE should ordinarily not be used in patients with severe renal dysfunction.
Hemeralopia has occurred; this appears to be an effect of TRIDIONE on the neural layers of the retina, and usually can be reversed by a reduction in dosage. Scotomata are an indication for withdrawal of the drug. Caution should be observed when treating patients who have diseases of the retina or optic nerve.
Manifestations of systemic lupus erythematosus have been associated with the use of TRIDIONE, as they have with the use of certain other anticonvulsants. Lymphadenopathies simulating malignant lymphoma have occurred. Lupus-like manifestations or lymph node enlargement are indications for withdrawal of the drug. Signs and symptoms may disappear after discontinuation of therapy, and specific treatment may be unnecessary.
A myasthenia gravis-like syndrome has been associated with the chronic use of trimethadione. Symptoms suggestive of this condition are indications for withdrawal of the drug.
Drugs known to cause toxic effects similar to those of TRIDIONE should be avoided or used only with extreme caution during therapy with TRIDIONE.

USAGE DURING PREGNANCY AND LACTATION:
THERE ARE MULTIPLE REPORTS IN THE CLINICAL LITERATURE WHICH INDICATE THAT THE USE OF ANTICONVULSANT DRUGS DURING PREGNANCY RESULTS IN AN INCREASED INCIDENCE OF BIRTH DEFECTS IN THE OFFSPRING. DATA ARE MORE EXTENSIVE WITH RESPECT TO TRIMETHADIONE, PARAMETHADIONE, PHENYTOIN AND PHENOBARBITAL THAN WITH OTHER ANTICONVULSANT DRUGS.
THEREFORE, ANTICONVULSANT DRUGS SUCH AS TRIDIONE (TRIMETHADIONE) SHOULD BE ADMINISTERED TO WOMEN OF CHILD BEARING POTENTIAL ONLY IF THEY ARE CLEARLY SHOWN TO BE ESSENTIAL IN THE MANAGEMENT OF THEIR SEIZURES. EFFECTIVE MEANS OF CONTRACEPTION SHOULD ACCOMPANY THE USE OF TRIDIONE IN SUCH PATIENTS. IF A PATIENT BECOMES PREGNANT WHILE TAKING TRIDIONE, TERMINATION OF THE PREGNANCY SHOULD BE CONSIDERED. A PATIENT WHO REQUIRES THERAPY WITH TRIDIONE AND WHO WISHES TO BECOME PREGNANT SHOULD BE ADVISED OF THE RISKS.
REPORTS HAVE SUGGESTED THAT THE MATERNAL INGESTION OF ANTICONVULSANT DRUGS, PARTICULARLY BARBITURATES, IS ASSOCIATED WITH A NEONATAL COAGULATION DEFECT THAT MAY CAUSE BLEEDING DURING THE EARLY (USUALLY WITHIN 24 HOURS OF BIRTH) NEONATAL PERIOD. THE POSSIBILITY OF THE OCCURRENCE OF THIS DEFECT WITH THE USE OF TRIDIONE SHOULD BE KEPT IN MIND. THE DEFECT IS CHARACTERIZED BY DECREASED LEVELS OF VITAMIN K-DEPENDENT CLOTTING FACTORS, AND PROLONGATION OF EITHER THE PROTHROMBIN TIME OR THE PARTIAL THROMBOPLASTIN TIME, OR BOTH. IT HAS BEEN SUGGESTED THAT PROPHYLACTIC VITAMIN K BE GIVEN TO THE MOTHER ONE MONTH PRIOR TO, AND DURING DELIVERY, AND TO THE INFANT, INTRAVENOUSLY, IMMEDIATELY AFTER BIRTH.
THE SAFETY OF TRIDIONE FOR USE DURING LACTATION HAS NOT BEEN ESTABLISHED.

Precautions: Abrupt discontinuation of TRIDIONE may precipitate petit mal status. TRIDIONE should always be withdrawn gradually unless serious adverse effects dictate otherwise. In the latter case, another anticonvulsant may be substituted to protect the patient.
Usage during Pregnancy and Lactation:
See WARNINGS.

Adverse Reactions: The following side effects, some of them serious, have been associated with the use of TRIDIONE.
Gastrointestinal: nausea, vomiting, abdominal pain, gastric distress.
CNS/Neurologic: drowsiness, fatigue, malaise, insomnia, vertigo, headache, paresthesias, precipitation of grand mal seizures, increased irritability, personality changes.
Drowsiness usually subsides with continued therapy. If it persists, a reduction in dosage is indicated.
Hematologic: bleeding gums, epistaxis, retinal and petechial hemorrhages, vaginal bleeding; neutropenia, leukopenia, eosinophilia, thrombocytopenia, pancytopenia, agranulocytosis, hypoplastic anemia, and fatal aplastic anemia.
Dermatologic: acneiform or morbilliform skin rash that may progress to exfoliative dermatitis or to severe forms of erythema multiforme.
Other: hiccups, anorexia, weight loss, hair loss, changes in blood pressure, albuminuria, hemeralopia, photophobia, diplopia.
Fatal nephrosis has occurred.
Hepatitis has been reported rarely.
Lupus erythematosus, and lymphadenopathies simulating malignant lymphoma, have been reported.
Pruritus associated with lymphadenopathy and hepatosplenomegaly has occurred in hypersensitive individuals.
A myasthenia gravis-like syndrome has been reported.

Overdosage: Symptoms of acute TRIDIONE overdosage include drowsiness, nausea, dizziness, ataxia, visual disturbances. Coma may follow massive overdosage.
Gastric evacuation, either by induced emesis, or by lavage, or both, should be done immediately. General supportive care, including frequent monitoring of the vital signs and close observation of the patient, are required.
Alkalinization of the urine has been reported to enhance the renal excretion of dimethadione, the active metabolite of TRIDIONE.
A blood count and a careful evaluation of hepatic and renal function should be done following recovery.

Dosage and Administration: TRIDIONE is administered orally.
Usual Adult Dosage: 0.9–2.4 Gm daily in 3 or 4 equally divided doses (i.e. 300–600 mg 3 or 4 times daily).
Initially, give 0.9 Gm daily; increase this dose by 300 mg at weekly intervals until therapeutic results are seen or until toxic symptoms appear.
Maintenance dosage should be the least amount of drug required to maintain control.
Children's Dosage: Usually 0.3–0.9 Gm daily in 3 or 4 equally divided doses.

How Supplied: TRIDIONE Capsules (trimethadione capsules, U.S.P.), 300 mg (white) are supplied in bottles of 100 (**NDC** 0074-3709-01).
TRIDIONE Dulcet® Tablets (trimethadione tablets, U.S.P.), 150 mg (white) chewable tablets are supplied in bottles of 100 (**NDC** 0074-3753-01).
[*Shown in Product Identification Section*]
TRIDIONE Solution (trimethadione oral solution, U.S.P.), 1.2 Gm per fluidounce (40 mg per ml), is supplied in pint bottles (**NDC** 0074-3721-01).

®Dulcet—Sweetened tablets, Abbott.
Ref. 03-4194/R3

TRONOTHANE® HYDROCHLORIDE
(pramoxine hydrochloride)
Cream, Jelly

Description: Tronothane Hydrochloride (pramoxine hydrochloride) is a surface anesthetic agent, chemically unrelated to the benzoate esters of the "caine" type. It is chemically designated as 4-n-butoxyphenyl gammamorpholinopropyl ether hydrochloride.

Indications: Tronothane Hydrochloride is indicated as a surface anesthetic to relieve pain and itching associated with dermatoses, ano-genital pruritis, hemmorhoids, anal fissure and minor burns.

Contraindications: Tronothane Hydrochloride is not suitable for and should not be injected into the tissues. It should not be used in the eye or nose, for bronchoscopy or gastroscopy, or in patients who are hypersensitive to the drug.

Precautions: Tronothane Hydrochloride should not be applied to extensive areas of skin, and is not intended for indefinitely prolonged use. Discontinue use if redness, irritation, swelling or pain occur.

Adverse Reactions: Local skin reactions, e.g. stinging and burning.

Dosage and Administration: Tronothane Hydrochloride 1% Cream and 1% Jelly are applied externally, directly to the area affected every three to four hours as needed. In cases of severe discomfort, the medication may be applied every two hours.

How Supplied: Tronothane Hydrochloride 1% Cream (pramoxine hydrochloride cream, N.F.), pramoxine hydrochloride 1% in a water miscible cream, is supplied in a 1-oz. tube with rectal applicator (**NDC** 0074-6645-01).
Tronothane Hydrochloride 1% Jelly (pramoxine hydrochloride jelly, N.F.), pramoxine hydrochloride 1% in a water soluble jelly, is supplied in a 1-oz. tube with rectal applicator (**NDC** 0074-6650-01).
These products are listed in N.F., a Medicare designated compendium.

If desired, additional literature on any Abbott Product will be provided upon request to Abbott Laboratories.

Adria Laboratories Inc.
5000 POST ROAD
DUBLIN, OHIO 43017

ADRIAMYCIN™ ℞
(doxorubicin hydrochloride) for Injection
FOR INTRAVENOUS USE ONLY

WARNINGS

1. Severe local tissue necrosis will occur if there is extravasation during administration. Adriamycin must not be given by the intramuscular or subcutaneous route.

2. Serious irreversible myocardial toxicity with delayed congestive failure often unresponsive to any cardiac supportive therapy may be encountered as total dosage approaches 550 mg/m^2. This toxicity may occur at lower cumulative doses in patients with prior mediastinal irradiation or on concurrent cyclophosphamide therapy.

3. Dosage should be reduced in patients with impaired hepatic function.

4. Severe myelosuppression may occur.

5. Adriamycin should be administered only under the supervision of a physician who is experienced in the use of cancer chemotherapeutic agents.

Description: Doxorubicin is a cytotoxic anthracycline antibiotic isolated from cultures of *Streptomyces peucetius* var. *caesius*. It is supplied in the hydrochloride form as a freeze-dried powder containing lactose.

Clinical Pharmacology: Though not completely elucidated, the mechanism of action of doxorubicin is related to its ability to bind to DNA and inhibit nucleic acid synthesis. Cell culture studies have demonstrated rapid cell penetration and perinucleolar chromatin binding, rapid inhibition of mitotic activity and nucleic acid synthesis, mutagenesis and chromosomal aberrations. Animal studies have shown activity in a spectrum of experimental tumors, immunosuppression, carcinogenic properties in rodents, induction of a variety of toxic effects, including delayed and progressive cardiac toxicity in rabbits, myelosuppression in all species and atrophy of testes in rats and dogs.
Pharmacokinetic studies show the intravenous administration of normal or radiolabeled Adriamycin (doxorubicin hydrochloride) for Injection is followed by rapid plasma clearance and significant tissue binding. Urinary excretion, as determined by fluorimetric methods, accounts for approximately 4–5% of the administered dose in five days. Biliary excretion represents the major excretion route, 40–50% of the administered dose being recovered in the bile or the feces in seven days. Impairment of liver function results in slower excretion, and, consequently, increased retention and accumulation in plasma and tissues. Adriamycin does not cross the blood brain barrier.

Indications: Adriamycin has been used successfully to produce regression in disseminated neoplastic conditions such as acute lymphoblastic leukemia, acute myeloblastic leukemia, Wilms' tumor, neuroblastoma, soft tissue and bone sarcomas, breast carcinoma, ovarian carcinoma, transitional cell bladder carcinoma, thyroid carcinoma, lymphomas of both Hodgkin and non-Hodgkin types and bronchogenic carcinoma in which the small cell histologic type is the most responsive compared to other cell types. A number of other solid tumors have also shown some responsiveness but in numbers too limited to justify specific recommendation. Studies to date have shown malignant melanoma, kidney carcinoma, large bowel carcinoma, brain tumors and metastases to the Central Nervous System not to be significantly responsive to Adriamycin therapy.
Contraindications: Adriamycin therapy should not be started in patients who have marked myelosuppression induced by previous treatment with other antitumor agents or by radiotherapy. Conclusive data are not available on pre-existing heart disease as a co-factor of increased risk of Adriamycin induced cardiac toxicity. Preliminary data suggest that in such cases cardiac toxicity may occur at doses lower than the recommended cumulative limit. It is therefore not recommended to start Adriamycin in such cases. Adriamycin treatment is contraindicated in patients who received previous treatment with complete cumulative doses of Adriamycin and daunorubicin.
Warnings: Special attention must be given to the cardiac toxicity exhibited by Adriamycin. Although uncommon, acute left ventricular failure has occurred, particularly in patients who have received total dosage of the drug exceeding the currently recommended limit of 550 mg/m^2. This limit appears to be lower (400 mg/m^2) in patients who received radiotherapy to the mediastinal area or concomitant therapy with other potentially cardiotoxic agents such as cyclophosphamide. The total dose of Adriamycin administered to the individual patient should also take into account a previous or concomitant therapy with related compounds such as daunorubicin. Congestive heart failure and/or cardiomyopathy may be encountered several weeks after discontinuation of Adriamycin therapy.
Cardiac failure is often not favorably affected by presently known medical or physical therapy for cardiac support. Early clinical diagnosis of drug induced heart failure appears to be essential for successful treatment with digitalis, diuretics, low salt diet and bed rest. Severe cardiac toxicity may occur precipitously without antecedent EKG changes. Baseline EKG and periodic follow-up EKG during, and immediately after, active drug therapy is an advisable precaution. Transient EKG changes, such as T-wave flattening, S-T depression, and arrhythmias are presently not considered indications for suspension of Adriamycin therapy. A persistent reduction in the voltage of the QRS wave is presently considered more specifically predictive for cardiac toxicity. If this occurs, the benefit of continued therapy must be carefully evaluated against the risk of producing irreversible cardiac damage.
There is a high incidence of bone marrow depression, primarily of leukocytes, requiring careful hematologic monitoring. With the recommended dosage schedule, leukopenia is usually transient, reaching its nadir at 10–14 days after treatment with recovery usually occurring by the 21st day. White blood cell counts as low as 1000/mm^3 are to be expected during treatment with appropriate doses of Adriamycin. Red blood cell and platelet levels should also be monitored since they may also be depressed. Hematologic toxicity may require dose reduction or suspension or delay of Adriamycin therapy. Persistent severe myelosuppression may result in superinfection or hemorrhage.
Adriamycin may potentiate the toxicity of other anticancer therapies. Exacerbation of cyclophosphamide induced hemorrhagic cystitis and enhancement of the hepatotoxicity of 6-mercaptopurine have been reported. Radiation induced toxicity to the myocardium, mucosae, skin and liver have been reported to be increased by the administration of Adriamycin.
Toxicity to recommended doses of Adriamycin is enhanced by hepatic impairment; therefore, prior to the individual dosing, evaluation of hepatic function is recommended using conventional clinical laboratory tests such as SGOT, SGPT, alkaline phosphatase, bilirubin, and BSP. (See Dosage and Administration.)
On intravenous administration of Adriamycin, a stinging or burning sensation signifies a small degree of extravasation and even if blood return from aspiration of the infusion needle is good, the injection or infusion should be immediately terminated and restarted in another vein.
Adriamycin and related compounds have also been shown to have mutagenic and carcinogenic properties when tested in experimental models.
Usage in Pregnancy: Safe use of Adriamycin in pregnancy has not been established. Adriamycin is embryotoxic and teratogenic in rats and embryotoxic and teratogenic in rabbits. Therefore, the benefits to the pregnant patient should be carefully weighed against the potential toxicity to fetus and embryo. The possible adverse effects on fertility in males and females in humans or experimental animals have not been adequately evaluated.
Precautions: Initial treatment with Adriamycin requires close observation of the patient and extensive laboratory monitoring. It is recommended, therefore, that patients be hospitalized at least during the first phase of the treatment.
Like other cytotoxic drugs, Adriamycin may induce hyperuricemia secondary to rapid lysis of neoplastic cells. The clinician should monitor the patient's blood uric acid level and be prepared to use such supportive and pharmacologic measures as might be necessary to control this problem.
Adriamycin imparts a red coloration to the urine for 1–2 days after administration and patients should be advised to expect this during active therapy.
Adriamycin is not an anti-microbial agent.
Adverse Reactions: Dose limiting toxicities of therapy are myelosuppression and cardiotoxicity (see Warnings). Other reactions reported are:
Cutaneous—Reversible complete alopecia occurs in most cases. Hyperpigmentation of nailbeds and dermal creases, primarily in children, have been reported in a few cases. Recall of skin reaction due to prior radiotherapy has occurred with Adriamycin administration.
Gastrointestinal—Acute nausea and vomiting occurs frequently and may be severe. This may be alleviated by antiemetic therapy. Mucositis (stomatitis and esophagitis) may occur 5–10 days after administration. The effect may be severe leading to ulceration and represent a site of origin for severe infections. The dose regimen consisting of administration of Adriamycin on three successive days results in the greater incidence and severity of mucositis. Anorexia and diarrhea have been occasionally reported.
Vascular—Phlebosclerosis has been reported especially when small veins are used or a single vein is used for repeated administration. Facial flushing may occur if the injection is given too rapidly.
Local—Severe cellulitis, vesication and tissue necrosis will occur if Adriamycin is extravasated during administration. Erythematous streaking along the vein proximal to the site of the injection has been reported.
Hypersensitivity—Fever, chills and urticaria have been reported occasionally. Anaphylaxis may occur. A case of apparent cross sensitivity to lincomycin has been reported.
Other—Conjunctivitis and lacrimation occur rarely.

Dosage and Administration: Care in the administration of Adriamycin will reduce the chance of perivenous infiltration. It may also decrease the chance of local reactions such as urticaria and erythematous streaking.

The recommended dose schedule is 60–75 mg/m^2 as a single intravenous injection administered at 21-day intervals. The lower dose should be given to patients with inadequate marrow reserves due to old age, or prior therapy, or neoplastic marrow infiltration. An alternative dose schedule is 30 mg/m^2 on each of three successive days repeated every 4 weeks.

Adriamycin dosage must be reduced if hepatic function is impaired according to the following table:

Serum Bilirubin Levels	BSP Retention	Recommended Dose
1.2 – 3.0 mg %	9–15%	½ normal dose
>3 mg %	>15%	¼ normal dose

Preparation of Solution: Adriamycin 10 mg vials and 50 mg vials should be reconstituted with 5 ml and 25 ml, respectively, of Sodium Chloride Injection U.S.P. to give a final concentration of 2 mg/ml of doxorubicin hydrochloride. An appropriate volume of air should be withdrawn from the vial during reconstitution to avoid excessive pressure build-up.

Skin reactions associated with Adriamycin have been reported. Caution in the handling and preparation of the powder and solution must be exercised and the use of gloves is recommended. If Adriamycin powder or solution contacts the skin or mucosae, immediately wash thoroughly with soap and water.

After adding the diluent, the vial should be shaken and the contents allowed to dissolve. The reconstituted solution is stable for 24 hours at room temperature and 48 hours under refrigeration (4–10°C). It should be protected from exposure to sunlight and any unused solution should be discarded.

It is recommended that Adriamycin be slowly administered into the tubing of a freely running intravenous infusion of Sodium Chloride Injection U.S.P. or 5% Dextrose Injection U.S.P. The tubing should be attached to a Butterfly needle inserted preferably into a large vein. The rate of administration is dependent on the size of the vein and the dosage. However the dose should be administered in not less than 3 to 5 minutes. Local erythematous streaking along the vein as well as facial flushing may be indicative of too rapid an administration. A burning or stinging sensation may be indicative of perivenous infiltration and the infusion should be immediately terminated and restarted in another vein.

Adriamycin should not be mixed with heparin since it has been reported that these drugs are incompatible to the extent that a precipitate may form. Until specific compatibility data are available, it is not recommended that Adriamycin be mixed with other drugs.

Adriamycin has been used in combination with other approved chemotherapeutic agents. Though evidence is available that at least in some types of neoplastic disease combination chemotherapy is superior to single agents, the benefits and risks of such therapy have not yet been fully elucidated.

How Supplied: ADRIAMYCIN™ (doxorubicin hydrochloride) for Injection is available in two sizes:

10 mg—Each vial contains 10 mg of doxorubicin HC1 and 50 mg of lactose U.S.P. as a sterile red-orange lyophilized powder. Packaged and supplied in 10-vial cartons NDC 38242-874-10.

50 mg—Each vial contains 50 mg of doxorubicin HC1 and 250 mg of lactose U.S.P. as a sterile red-orange lyophilized powder. Packaged and supplied in a single vial carton NDC 38242-875-50.

Distributed by: Adria Laboratories Inc., Columbus, Ohio 43215. Manufactured by: Farmitalia Carlo Erba S.p.A., Italy.

[8740102] Revised Jan. 1979

ADRUCIL® ℞
(fluorouracil, USP)
INJECTABLE
FOR INTRAVENOUS USE ONLY

> **WARNINGS**
> Adrucil should be administered only by or under the supervision of a qualified physician who is experienced in cancer chemotherapy and the use of potent antimetabolites. Because severe toxic reactions may occur, it is recommended that patients be hospitalized during the initial course of therapy. Before administering Adrucil, the contents of this insert should be thoroughly reviewed.

Description: Fluorouracil is a fluorinated pyrimidine belonging to the category of antimetabolites. Fluorouracil resembles the natural uracil molecule except it has been fluorinated in the 5 position.

It is sparingly soluble in water (12.2 mg/ml) at pH 7 and has pK's of 8.0 and 13.0.

Adrucil (Fluorouracil, USP) Injectable is supplied as a sterile aqueous solution for intravenous injection. It has pH of 8.6 to 9.0. The ampules are filled with a 5% excess to permit withdrawal and administration of the labeled volume.

A precipitate may form as a result of exposure to low temperatures. Redissolve by heating to 140°F (60°C) with vigorous shaking, and allow to cool to body temperature prior to use.

Actions: The mechanism of action of fluorouracil is mainly related to competitive inhibition of thymidylate synthetase, the enzyme catalyzing the methylation of deoxyuridylic acid to thymidylic acid. The consequent thymidine deficiency results in inhibition of deoxyribonucleic acid (DNA) synthesis, thus inducing cell death. Also, moderate inhibition of ribonucleic acid (RNA) and incorporation of fluorouracil into RNA have been observed, but these effects do not appear to play a significant role in the determination of the antitumor action of fluorouracil.

The effects of DNA and RNA deprivation are most marked on those cells which grow rapidly and which take up fluorouracil at more rapid pace. Inactive degradation products (e.g., CO_2, urea, α-fluoro-β-alanine) result from the extensive catabolic metabolism of fluorouracil. Following intravenous injection, no intact drug can be detected in the plasma after 3 hours and 60 to 80% of the dose is excreted as respiratory Co_2 in 8 to 12 hours. Within 6 hours approximately 15% of the total drug administered is excreted unchanged in the urine with over 90% of this excretion occurring in the first hour.

Indications: Adrucil is effective in the palliative management of carcinoma of the colon, rectum, breast, stomach and pancreas in patients who are considered incurable by surgery or other means.

Contraindications: Adrucil therapy should not be started in patients with a poor nutritional state, depressed bone marrow function, or potentially serious infections.

Warnings: THE DAILY DOSE OF ADRUCIL IS NOT TO EXCEED 800 MG AND IT IS RECOMMENDED THAT PATIENTS BE HOSPITALIZED DURING THEIR FIRST COURSE OF TREATMENT.

Adrucil (Fluorouracil, USP) should be used with extreme caution in poor risk patients with a history of high-dose pelvic irradiation, previous use of alkylating agents, or who have a widespread involvement of bone marrow by metastatic tumors, or impaired hepatic or renal function. The drug is not intended as an adjuvant to surgery. Although severe toxicity and fatalities are more likely to occur in poor risk patients, these effects have occasionally been encountered in patients in relatively good condition. Severe hematologic toxicity, gastrointestinal hemorrhage, and even death may result from use of Adrucil (Fluorouracil, USP) despite meticulous selection of patients and careful adjustment of dosage.

Usage in Pregnancy: Safe use of Adrucil (Fluorouracil, USP) has not been established with respect to adverse effects on fetal development. Therefore, this drug should not be used during pregnancy, particularly in the first trimester, unless in the judgement of the physician the potential benefits to the patient outweigh the hazards.

Because the risk of mutagenesis has not been evaluated, such possible effects on males and females must be considered.

Combination Therapy: Any form of therapy which adds to the stress of the patient, interfers with nutrition or depresses bone marrow function will increase the toxicity of Adrucil (Fluorouracil, USP).

Precautions: Adrucil® (Fluorouracil, USP) is a highly toxic drug with a narrow margin of safety. Special attention must be given to the toxicity exhibited by fluorouracil. Patients should be carefully supervised since it must be recognized that therapeutic response is unlikely to occur without some evidence of toxicity. Patients should be advised of expected toxic effects, especially oral manifestations. White blood counts with differential are recommended before each dose. Knowledge of WBC nadir is necessary for eventual subsequent dosage adjustments.

Administration of Adrucil (Fluorouracil, USP) is to be discontinued promptly when one of the following signs appear:

1. Stomatitis or esophagopharyngitis (at first visible sign)
2. Leukopenia (WBC < 3500 mm^3) or rapidly falling white blood count
3. Vomiting (intractable)
4. Diarrhea (frequent bowel movements or watery stools)
5. Gastrointestinal ulceration and bleeding
6. Thrombocytopenia (platelets < 100,000 mm^3)
7. Hemorrhage (from any site)

Adverse Reactions: Stomatitis and esophagopharyngitis (which may lead to sloughing and ulceration), diarrhea, anorexia, nausea and emesis are common.

Myelosuppression almost uniformly accompanies a course of adequate therapy with fluorouracil. Low WBC counts are usually first observed between the 9th and 14th day after the first course of treatment with nadir occurring during the third week, although at times delayed for as long as 25 days. By the 30th day the count is usually within the normal range. Thrombocytopenia also may occur.

Alopecia and dermatitis are seen in a substantial number of cases and patients should be advised of this consequence of treatment. The alopecia is reported to be reversible. The dermatitis is often a pruritic maculopapular rash generally appearing on the extremities and less frequently on the trunk. It is usually reversible and responsive to symptomatic treatment. Dry skin and fissuring have also been noted.

Photosensitivity, as manifested by erythema or increased pigmentation of the skin, may occasionally occur. Photophobia, lacrimation, epistaxis, euphoria, acute cerebellar syndrome (which may persist following discontinuation of treatment) and nail changes including loss of nails have also been reported.

Continued on next page

Adria—Cont.

Dosage and Administration:
Note:
The recommended route of administration of Adrucil is only by intravenous injection, using care to avoid extravasation. No dilution of Adrucil is required.
It is recommended that all dosages be based on the patient's actual weight. However, if the patient is obese or if there has been a spurious weight gain due to edema, ascites, or other forms of abnormal fluid retention, then the estimated lean body mass (dry weight) should be used.
Prior to treatment, it is recommended that each patient be carefully evaluated to accurately estimate the optimum initial dosage of Adrucil.
Initial Therapy (See Contraindications, Warnings and Precautions before prescribing):
I. A dose of 12 mg/kg is given intravenously once daily for 4 successive days. The daily dose should not be more than 800 mg. If no toxicity is observed at any time during the course of therapy, 6 mg/kg are given on the 6th, 8th, 10th and 12th days. No therapy is given on the 5th, 7th, 9th or 11th days. Therapy is to be discontinued at the end of the 12th day, even if no toxicity has become apparent.
II. In poor risk patients or those who are not in an adequate nutritional state, a dose level of 6 mg/kg/day for 3 days is recommended. If no toxicity is observed at any time during the treatment, 3 mg/kg may be given on the 5th, 7th and 9th days. No therapy is given on the 4th, 6th or 8th days. The daily dose should not exceed 400 mg.
A sequence of injections on either schedule constitutes a "course of therapy."
Therapy should be discontinued promptly when any of the signs of toxicity listed under PRECAUTIONS appears.
Maintenance Therapy: When toxicity has not been a problem, or after the toxic signs from the initial course of therapy have subsided, therapy should be continued using either of the following schedules:
A. Repeat dosage of the first course, beginning 30 days after the last day of the previous course of treatment.
B. Administer a maintenance dosage of 10 to 15 mg/kg/week. Do not exceed 1 gram per week. Reduced doses should be used for poor risk patients.
The dosage of drug to be used should take into account the patient's reaction to the previous course of therapy and be adjusted accordingly. Some patients have received from 9 to 45 courses of treatment during periods which ranged from 12 to 60 months.
Adrucil (Fluorouracil, USP) should not be mixed with IV additives or chemotherapeutic agents.
How Supplied: Adrucil® (Fluorouracil, USP) Injectable is available in 10 ml ampules, as a colorless to faint yellow aqueous solution containing 500 mg of fluorouracil and pH adjusted with sodium hydroxide to 8.6 to 9.0. Packaged and supplied in individual cartons, there are 10 ampules per shelf container NDC 38242-900-50.
NOTE: Although Adrucil ampule solution may discolor slightly during storage, the potency and safety are not adversely affected. Store at room temperature 59–86°F (15–30°C) and protect from light. If a precipitate occurs due to exposure to low temperatures, re-solubilize by heating to 140°F (60°C) with vigorous shaking; allow to cool to body temperature before using.
Distributed by: Adria Laboratories Inc., Columbus, Ohio 43215
Manufactured by: Taylor Pharmacal Co., Decatur, Illinois 62525
9000100
Revised 10/77

Alba Pharmacal Corporation
**POST OFFICE BOX 628
MUNOZ RIVERA 938
PENUELAS, PUERTO RICO 00724**

ALBA-CE® OTC
**(vitamin C)
Liquid**

Composition:
Alba-Ce Liquid—Each 5 cc contains 500 mg. of Ascorbic Acid in a sorbitol base (sugar free).
How Supplied:
Alba-Ce Liquid—4 oz bottle (NDC 10023-110-04).

ALBAFORT® INJECTABLE ℞
(Iron and B Complex)

Composition: Each ml of Albafort (Iron and B Complex) Injection contains: Iron as ferrous gulconate 50 mg; Vit. B_{12} 100 mcg; 20% Liver Extract N.F., (Vit. B_{12} eq. 10 mcq/ml); Thiamine HCl 12.5 mg; Riboflavin 0.5 mg; Pyridoxine HCl 2.0 mg, Panthenol 1.0 mg; Niacinamide 12.5 mg, with phenol 0.5% and Benzyl alcohol 1.5% as preservatives, water for injection q.s.
Actions: Albafort (Iron and B Complex) provides a combination of the hematinic effect of iron and the hematopoietic effect of liver.
Indications: Albafort (Iron and B Complex) is indicated in the treatment of hypochromic and macrocytic anemias, pernicious anemia and sprue that responds to B_{12} therapy. Hypochromic anemias are mostly due to prolonged loss of blood of the gastrointestinal tract, urinary tract and uterus. In addition, iron requirements must be increased at certain times of life such as, infancy and childhood, puberty (especially in females), during pregnancy and menopause. Albafort offers a balanced and stable formula for the treatment of hypochromic anemias.
Advantages: Iron in Albafort does not stain the skin. A Z-track technique need not be used nor deep needle injection in the gluteal area. No soft-tissue sarcomas have developed at site of injection as with iron dextran; no iron bound permanently to muscle and no fibromyositis. Due to the presence of 20% liver (ferritin present in liver) an excellent iron binding capacity occurs so there is more stimulation of the bone marrow to produce more erythrocites and greater levels of hemoglobin are obtained.
Warnings: As with other iron compounds toxic symptoms may occur at injection. The immediate reactions most frequently found are vomiting, nausea, lowering of blood pressure and pallor. These reactions are transitory and not frequent with ferrous gluconate. Some patients are sensitive to liver. Keep in a dark place at low temperature. DO NOT USE IF SEDIMENTATION OR PRECIPITATION SHOWS.
Contraindication: Individuals who have shown hypersensitivity to any of its components.
Dosage: Children—½ to 1 ml once or twice a week. Adults—1 to 2 ml once or twice a week or as the physician thinks necessary. For intramuscular use only.
How Supplied: 10 ml multidose vials (NDC 10023-100-10).

ALBA-LYBE® OTC

Composition: Each 5 cc contains: Lysine Monohydrochloride 275 mg., Vit. B_{12} Crystalline 10 mcq., Thiamine HCl 5 mg., Riboflavin 4 mg., Pyridoxine HCl 1 mg., Niacinamide 35 mg., Calcium Pantothenate 7 mg., Sorbitol q.s. (imitation sherry wine flavor).
Actions: Alba-Lybe provides lysine as an appetite stimulant and sorbitol q.s. to provide greater absorption of B_{12} and lysine.
Indications: As dietetic supplement of all ages, especially in states of anorexia and convalescence.
Advantages: Alba-Lybe can be administered to patients including the diabetic patient since it contains sorbitol. Sorbitol q.s. base has the advantage over the alcohol base since sorbitol is absorbed much more rapidly than alcohol, as well as the fact that the molecules of lysine and B_{12} adhere to sorbitol. This results in greater appetite and fixing of proteins producing weight increase and better anabolic results.
Dosage: Children—½ to 1 teaspoonful three times a day. Adults—1 tablespoonful three times a day.
How Supplied: 6 oz. bottle (NDC #10023-101-06).

ALBA-TEMP® SUPPOSITORIES OTC
(Rectal acetaminophen)

Composition: Each Alba-Temp Suppository contains Acetaminophen USP 120 mg. or 650 mg.
Indications: Alba-Temp is indicated for the temporary relief of fever, minor aches, pains and headaches.
Administration and Dosage: Alba-Temp 120 mg.—Children 3–6: two suppositories every four to six hours. Under 3 years: one suppository, 120 mg., every four to six hours after consulting a physician. No more than six suppositories during a twenty-four hour period.
Alba-Temp 650 mg.—Adults: two suppositories every four to six hours. No more than six suppositories in a twenty-four hour period. Children 6–12 years: one suppository every four to six hours. No more than 4 suppositories in a twenty-four hour period.
How Supplied: Alba-Temp Suppository is supplied in boxes of 12 foil wrapped suppositories in 120 mg. (NDC 10023-168-12) or 650 mg. (NDC 10023-169-12).
Alba-Temp is also supplied as an elixir in a sugar free base, 120 mg./5 cc, 4 oz. bottle (NDC 10023-105-04); tablets—bottles of 100 (NDC 10023-107-90).

ALBA-3® OINTMENT OTC
(bacitracin-neomycin-polymyxin B)

Composition: Each gram contains: Bacitracin 400 units, Polymyxin B Sulfate 5,000 units, Neomycin Sulfate 5 mg. (eq. to 3.5 mg. neomycin base); white petrolatum base qs.
Indications: *Therapeutically,* (as an adjunct to systemic therapy where indicated), for topical infections, primary or secondary, due to susceptible organisms, as in: infected burns, skin grafts, surgical incisions, otitis externa; primary pyodermas (impetigo, ecthyma, sycosis vulgaris, paronychia); secondarily infected dermatoses (eczema, herpes, and seborrheic dermatitis); traumatic lesions, inflamed or suppurating as a result of bacterial infection. *Prophylactically,* the ointment may be used to prevent bacterial contamination in burns, skin grafts, incisions, and other clean lesions. For abrasions, minor cuts and wounds accidentally incurred, its use may prevent the development of infection and permit wound healing.
Dosage and Administration: Apply to the affected area 2 to 5 times daily, depending on the severity of the condition. May be left exposed or covered with a dressing, as indicated.
How Supplied: Alba-3 Ointment is supplied in 15 gm. tube (NDC 10023-120-15).

ALBATUSSIN® OTC
(Antitussive, Expectorant, Sugar Free)

Composition: Each 5 cc contains: Dextromethorphan HBr 10 mg., pyrilamine maleate 8.33 mg., potassium guaiacolsulfonate 75 mg., phenylephrine HBr 5 mg., sodium citrate 215 mg., citric acid 50 mg., alcohol 4% with menthol, thymol and tolu in a sugar free base.
Actions: Albatussin suppresses coughing, helps in nasal decongestion, sneezing and expectoration.
Indications: For coughing relief due to colds or allergy, as well as an expectorant.
Advantages: Albatussin has a nice, pleasing flavor and can be given to diabetic patients and children of all ages as well as adults.
Dosage: Adults and older children—1 or 2 teaspoonfuls; Children six to twelve years—1 teaspoonful; four to six years—½ to 1 teaspoonful; one to four years—½ teaspoonful; under one year—¼ to ½ teaspoonful. These dosages should be given every four hours.
How Supplied: 4 oz bottle (NDC 10023-104-04).

MYOFORTE® TABLETS ℞
(chlorzoxazone and acetaminophen)

Description: Each Pink tablet contains Chlorzoxazone 250 mg. and Acetaminophen 300 mg.
Actions: Skeletal muscle relaxant and analgesic.
Warnings: *Usage in Pregnancy*—Effect of this drug on the fetus has not been established, therefore, it should not be administered to pregnant women.
Dosage and Administration: *Usual Adult Dosage:* Two tablets 4 times daily.
How Supplied: Bottle of 100's (NDC #10023-167-90) and 500's (NDC #10023-167-75).

PASMIN® ℞
(dicyclomine HCl USP)

Composition:
Pasmin Injectable—Each cc contains 10 mg. Dicyclomine HCl.
Pasmin Capsules—Each capsule contains 10 mg. Dicyclomine HCl.
Pasmin Liquid—Each 5 cc contains 10 mg. Dicyclomine HCl.
How Supplied:
Pasmin Injectable—2 cc vial (NDC 10023-114-20) and 10 cc vial (NDC 10023-114-10).
Pasmin Capsules—Bottle of 100's (NDC 10023-113-90).
Pasmin Liquid—4 oz bottle (NDC 10023-112-04).

SEDARIL ℞
(hydroxyzine HCl)

Composition:
Sedaril 25—Each cc. contains 25 mg. Hydroxyzine HCl
Sedaril 50—Each cc. contains 50 mg. Hydroxyzine HCl
How Supplied:
Sedaril 25—10 cc vial (NDC 10023-172-10)
Sedaril 50—10 cc vial (NDC 10023-173-10)
Sedaril 50— 2 cc vial (NDC 10023-173-02)

TIA-DOCE® INJECTABLE UNIVIAL ℞
(B_{12}—B_1)

Composition: Each cc in the univial, after reconstitution, contains: Cyanocobalamin (Vit. B_{12}) 1000 mcq., Thiamine HCl (Vit. B_1) 100 mg. in bacteriostatic water for injection, 0.9% Benzyl Alcohol, NaOH and HCl for pH control.
Actions and Indications: Tia-Doce Univial is intended for the prevention and treatment of a variety of disorders associated with Vitamin B_1 deficiency as well as for the managment of certain sensory neuropathies responding to massive doses of Vit. B_{12}. Specifically Vitamin B_1 is indicated in the prevention and treatment of beriberi and in the correction of anorexia of dietary origin.
Advantages: Tia-Doce is a stable combination of Vit. B_{12} and Vit. B_1. Since they are separated in the univial there is no reaction between them, resulting in less oxidation of the vitamins and no reduction of vitamin potency. Tia-Doce can be administered either intramuscularly, intravenously, or subcutaneously.
Warnings: Allergic and anaphilactic reactions may occur after frequent I.V. dosage. Contraindicated in persons who are hypersensitive to any of its components.
Dosage: Tia-Doce is administered 0.5 to 1 cc intramuscularly or intravenously daily or as needed. Can be used 1 cc/500 ml of dextrose for I.V. difusion.
How Supplied: Tia-Doce is supplied in 10 cc univials containing the freeze dried Vit. B_1 in the lower chamber and Vit. B_{12} in bacteriostatic water in the upper chamber (NDC 10023-126-10).

Allergan Pharmaceuticals, Inc.
2525 DUPONT DRIVE
IRVINE, CALIFORNIA 92713

OPHTHALMIC PRODUCTS

For information on Allergan prescription and OTC ophthalmic products, consult the Physicians' Desk Reference For Ophthalmology. For literature, service items or sample material, contact Allergan directly. See a complete listing of products in the Manufacturers' Index section of this book.

Alto Pharmaceuticals, Inc.
P.O. BOX 15564
TAMPA, FLORIDA 33684

ZINC-220® CAPSULES
(zinc sulfate 220 mg.)

Composition: Each opaque blue and pink capsule contains zinc sulfate 220 mg. delivering 80 mg. of elemental zinc. Zinc-220 Capsules do not contain dextrose or glucose.
Action and Uses: Zinc-220 Capsules are indicated as a dietary supplement. Normal growth and tissue repair are directly dependent upon an adequate supply of zinc in the diet. Zinc functions as an integral part of a number of enzymes important to protein and carbohydrate metabolism. Zinc-220 Capsules are recommended for deficiencies or the prevention of deficiencies of zinc.
Warnings: Zinc-220 if administered in stat dosages of 2 grams (9 capsules) will cause an emetic effect.
Precaution: It is recommended that Zinc-220 Capsules be taken with meals or milk to avoid gastric distress.
Contraindications: None.
Dosage: One capsule daily with milk or meals. One capsule daily provides approximately 5.3 times the recommended adult requirement for zinc.
How Supplied: Bottles of 100 and 1000 capsules and Unit Dose Strips boxes of 100 capsules. (NDC 0731-0401)
Product Identification Mark: Capsules imprinted 401 on one side, ALTO on the other side.
Samples: Yes, on request.
[*Shown in Product Identification Section*]

American Pharmaceutical Company
245 FOURTH STREET
PASSAIC, NEW JERSEY 07055

AFKO™ EAR DROPS

AFKO-LUBE™ CAPSULES
(Dioctyl Sodium Sulfosuccinate USP 100 mg., 250 mg.)

AFKO-LUBE™ LAX CAPSULES
(Afko Lube 100 mg. with Casanthranol)

AMPICILLIN TRIHYDRATE CAPSULES, USP ℞
250 mg., 500 mg.

APHCO™ HEMORRHOIDAL OINTMENT, SUPPOSITORIES

BACITRACIN OINTMENT

BELEXON™ FORTIFIED CAPSULES

BISACODYL TABLETS AND SUPPOSITORIES

BROMPHENIRAMINE ELIXIR, TABLETS ℞

CHLOROTHIAZIDE TABLETS, USP ℞
250 mg., 500 mg.

CHLORPROMAZINE TABLETS, USP ℞
25 mg., 50 mg., 100 mg.

CODANOL® A&D OINTMENT

CODANOL® MALT WITH HEMOGLOBIN

CORTISONE ACETATE TABLETS, USP ℞
25 mg.

CYCLANDELATE CAPSULES ℞
200 mg., 400 mg.

DAILY DOSE 1 VITAMINS
B-Complex Liver & Iron Tablets
Belaxa™ B-Complex & C Capsules
Fe-ritol Tablets
Gerifort™ Plus
Multiple Vitamins with Iron Tablets
Multiple Vitamins with Minerals Tablets
Nutri-Drops
Super Stress-600 Tablets
Super Stress-600 with Iron Tablets
Super Z Stress-600 Tablets
Thera-Amcaps™
Thera-Amcaps™ M
Vitamin E Capsules

DICYCLOMINE HCl CAPSULES ℞
10 mg.

DI-O-GEST® ANTACID TABLETS

DIPHENHYDRAMINE CAPSULES, ELIXIR, EXPECTORANT ℞

DIPHENOXYLATE WITH ATROPINE SULFATE TABLETS ℞

ERYTHROMYCIN STEARATE TABLETS, USP ℞
250 mg.

FENDON® TABLETS, ELIXIR
(Acetaminophen)

FERROUS SULFATE TABLETS, CAPSULES

FERROUS GLUCONATE TABLETS

GELUMINA™ PLUS LIQUID

GELUMINA™ TABLETS

Continued on next page

American Pharmaceutical—Cont.

GERIFORT™ ELIXIR, TABLETS

HYDRALAZINE TABLETS ℞
25 mg., 50 mg.

HYDROCHLOROTHIAZIDE TABLETS ℞
25 mg., 50 mg.

HYROCAIN™ CREAM

ISO-LO™ EYE WASH, DROPS

ISOXSUPRINE HCl TABLETS ℞
10 mg., 20 mg.

KA-PEK™ SUSPENSION

METHENAMINE MANDELATE TABLETS, USP
0.5 mg., 1 gm.

METHOCARBAMOL TABLETS ℞
500 mg., 750 mg.

NEO-MIST™ NASAL SPRAY

NEOMYCIN TABLETS ℞
0.5 mg.

NITE-REST™ CAPSULES

NUTRI-CAPS™ WITH MINERALS

PAPAVERINE CAPSULES, TABLETS ℞

PENICILLIN V POTASSIUM TABS., USP ℞
125 mg. 200 MU, 250 mg. 400 MU

PERTINEX™ CREAM, SPRAY
Athlete's Foot Control

PHENDEX® ELIXIR, TABLETS ℞

PHENYLAZO TABLETS ℞
100 mg.

PREDNISOLONE TABLETS, USP ℞
5 mg.

PREDNISONE TABLETS, USP ℞
5 mg.

PRENACAPS™

PROCAINAMIDE CAPSULES, USP ℞
250 mg., 500 mg.

PROMETHAZINE TABLETS, EXPECTORANT ℞

PROPYLTHIOURACIL TABLETS, USP ℞
50 mg.

QUINIDINE SULFATE TABLETS, USP ℞
3 gr.

QUININE SULFATE CAPSULES, USP ℞
5 gr.

RHUSTICON™ LOTION
Antihistaminic—Antipruritic

ROMEX® DECONGESTANT COUGH, COLD
Preparations: Liquid, Capsules, Troches

SPD® ANALGESIC CREAM, LOTION

SPECTRO-BIOTIC OINTMENT

TETRACYCLINE CAPSULES, USP ℞
250 mg., 500 mg.

TRIPROLIDINE W/PSEUDOEPHEDRINE TABLETS, SYRUP ℞

VERV® ALERTNESS CAPSULES

Arco Pharmaceuticals, Inc.
105 ORVILLE DRIVE
BOHEMIA, NEW YORK 11716

ARCO-LASE®
(broad pH spectrum digestant)

Composition: Each soft, mint flavored tablet contains Trizyme*, 38 mg., and Lipase, 25 mg.
*Contains the following standardized enzymes: amylolytic 30 mg.; proteolytic 6 mg.; cellulolytic 2 mg.
Action and Uses: Indicated for most gastrointestinal disorders due to poor digestion. Flatulence, gas and bloating, dyspepsia, distention, fullness, heartburn, or in any condition where normal digestion is impaired by digestive insufficiencies. Arcolase provides the highest standardized enzymatic activity, plus the protective action of the widest pH range. Thus it is effective throughout the entire G.I. tract. Requiring no enteric coating, there is assurance of a positive breakdown of its factors. This is advantageous, because quite often patients with digestive disorders cannot digest their food properly, let alone hard, or enteric coated capsules or tablets.
Side Effects: None.
Administration and Dosage: One tablet with or immediately following meals. Tablet may be swallowed or chewed.
Supplied: Bottles of 50's. NDC 275-4040.

ARCO-LASE PLUS ℞

Composition: Same as Arco-Lase, plus the addition of Hyoscyamine sulfate 0.10 mg., atropine sulfate 0.02 mg. and phenobarbital 1/8 gr. (Warning: may be habit forming.)
Action and Uses: Gastrointestinal disturbances, such as cramps, bloating, spasms, diarrhea, nausea, vomiting and peptic ulcer. The enzymes correct the digestive insufficiencies. The antispasmodic and phenobarbital contribute to the symptomatic relief of hypermotility and nervous tension, which usually accompanies functional disturbances of the bowel.
Administration and Dosage: One tablet following meals.
Side Effects: May cause rapid pulse, dryness of mouth and blurred vision.
Contraindications: This product is contraindicated in the presence of glaucoma or prostatic hypertrophy.
Supplied: Bottles of 50's. NDC 275-45-45.
Literature Available: Yes.

MEGA-B®
(super potency vitamin B complex, sugar & starch free)

Composition: Each Mega-B Tablet contains the following Mega Vitamins:

B_1 (Thiamine Mononitrate)	100 mg.
B_2 (Riboflavin)	100 mg.
B_6 (Pyridoxine Hydrochloride)	100 mg.
B_{12} (Cyanocobalamin)	100 mcg.
Choline Bitartrate	100 mg.
Inositol	100 mg.
Niacinamide	100 mg.
Folic Acid	100 mcg.
Pantothenic Acid	100 mg.
d-Biotin	100 mcg.
Para-Aminobenzoic Acid (PABA)	100 mg.

In a base of yeast to provide the identified and unidentified B-Complex Factors.
Advantages: Each Mega-B capsule-shaped tablet provides the highest vitamin B complex available in a single dose.
Mega-B was designed for those patients who require truly Mega vitamin potencies with the convenience of minimum dosage.
Indications: Mega-B is indicated in conditions characterized by depletions or increased demand of the water-soluble B-complex vitamins. It may be useful in the nutritional management of patients during prolonged convalescence associated with major surgery. It is also indicated for stress conditions, as an adjunct to antibiotics and diuretic therapy, pre and post operative cases, liver conditions, gastro-intestinal disorders interferring with intake or absorbtion of water-soluble vitamins, prolonged or wasting diseases, diabetes, burns, fractures, severe infections, and some psychological disorders.
Warning: NOT INTENDED FOR TREATMENT OF PERNICIOUS ANEMIA, OR OTHER PRIMARY OR SECONDARY ANEMIAS.
Dosage: Usual dosage is one Mega-B tablet daily, or varied, depending on clinical needs.
Supplied: Yellow capsule shaped tablets in bottles of 30, 100 and 500.

MEGADOSE™
(multiple mega-vitamin formula with minerals, sugar and starch free)

Composition:

Vitamin A	25,000 USP Units
Vitamin D	1,000 USP Units
Vitamin C w/Rose Hips	250 mg.
Vitamin E	100 IU
Folic Acid	400 mcg.
Vitamin B_1	80 mg.
Vitamin B_2	80 mg.
Niacinamide	80 mg.
Vitamin B_6	80 mg.
Vitamin B_{12}	80 mcg.
Bioten	80 mcg.
Pantothenic Acid	80 mg.
Choline Bitartrate	80 mg.
Inositol	80 mg.
Para-Aminobenzoic Acid	80 mg.
Rutin	30 mg.
Citrus Bioflavonoids	30 mg.
Betaine Hydrochloride	30 mg.
Glutamic Acid	30 mg.
Hesperidin Complex	5 mg.
Iodine (from Kelp)	0.15 mg.
Calcium Gluconate*	50 mg.
Zinc Gluconate*	25 mg.
Potassium Gluconate*	10 mg.
Ferrous Gluconate*	10 mg.
Magnesium Gluconate*	7 mg.
Manganese Gluconate*	6 mg.
Copper Gluconate*	0.5 mg.

*Natural mineral chelates in a base containing natural ingredients.
Dosage: One tablet daily.
Supplied: Capsule shaped tablets in bottles of 30, 100 and 250.

Ar-Ex Products Co.
1036 WEST VAN BUREN STREET
CHICAGO, ILLINOIS 60607

AR-EX HYPO-ALLERGENIC COSMETICS

Composition: Formulated so you can prescribe cosmetics as you prescribe medications or other therapeutic regimen in dermatological, respiratory, gastrointestinal and other allergies where usual cosmetics are contraindicated.
Action and Uses: To provide safe beauty aids and eliminate a whole field of potential irritants and sensitizers that may aggravate or precipitate allergic conditions, as: skin irritations and erythema, contact dermatitis, photosensitivity, dry, chapped skin, lipstick cheilitis, eyelid dermatitis, chronic coryza, chronic vasomotor rhinitis, chronic conjunctivitis, asthma, urticaria, colitis and other G-I symptoms, also other conditions where cosmetics may be prime or contributing offenders.
Unscented Cosmetics: Perfumes, natural or synthetic, and essential oils are known to be capable of irritating the skin, causing Berloque dermatitis (photosensitivity), and causing or

aggravating respiratory symptoms simulating asthma and hay fever. For these persons, all AR-EX Cosmetics are available Unscented, and contain absolutely no perfume, natural or synthetic.

A Complete Line: Following is a list of AR-EX Cosmetics, together with a partial list of potential irritants and allergens which they do NOT contain. When these substances are suspected etiological agents, you can rule them out of your diagnoses when you prescribe AR-EX Cosmetics *by brand name.*

Creams and Lotions: Contain no soap, almond oil, oil of orris, coconut oil, bergamot or other citrus oils, lanolin, cocoa butter, karaya gum, gum arabic, tragacanth, rose water or phenol. Unscented.

Deodorants: Cream, Spray and Roll-On. Contain no aluminum chloride, aluminum chlorhydroxide, aluminum acetate, aluminum sulfate, alum, salicylic acid, formaldehyde, alcohol or hexachlorophene.

Eye Makeup: Contain no lanolin, indelible or aniline dyes, perfume, turpentine, bergamot or other photosensitizers, chromium or nickel compounds, or pharaphenylenediamine.

Hair Preparations: Contain no soap, lanolin, sulfonated oil, palm or coconut oil, gum karaya, gum arabic, tragacanth, resin, lacquer, shellac. Unscented.

Powders: Contain no orris root, oil of orris, bergamot or other citrus oils, corn starch, rice starch, wheat starch, powdered gums or lanolin.

Soap: Low in excess alkali, superfatted. Contains no lanolin, perfumes, essential oils.

Foundation Lotion: Liquid makeup. Contains no gum acacia, karaya or tragacanth, lanolin, corn oil or other vegetable oils, oil of orris, perfumes or essential oils.

AR-EX Special Formula Lipstick: Contains no indelible dyes, eosin, mono-di-tri-or-tetra-bromfluorescein compounds, but achieves shades through use of lake pigments. Contains no perfumes or essential oils, lanolin, almond oil or cocoa butter.

Literature Available: For precise prescription of hypo-allergenic cosmetics in indicated conditions, refer to the AR-EX Professional Formulary. Sent on request.

SAFE SUDS

Composition: Hypo-allergenic, all-purpose detergent for patients whose hands or respiratory membranes are irritated by soaps or detergents. For dishes, laundry, floors, rugs, upholstery, etc. Suds in hard or soft water, with pH approximately 6.8. Contains no enzymes, phosphates, lanolin, fillers or bleaches. Biodegradable. NOT scented.

Armour Pharmaceutical Company

6991 EAST CAMELBACK ROAD
SUITE A-210
SCOTTSDALE, ARIZONA 85251

H.P. ACTHAR® GEL* ℞
(repository corticotropin injection)
and
ACTHAR® ℞
(corticotropin for injection)

Description: H.P. ACTHAR® GEL (Repository Corticotropin Injection) is a Highly Purified preparation of CORTICOTROPIN in gelatin which has both rapid onset and prolonged action. Each milliliter contains the labeled activity of Corticotropin U.S.P., 16% Gelatin, 0.5% Phenol, not more than 0.1% Cysteine (added), Sodium Hydroxide and/or Acetic acid to adjust pH, and Water for Injection, q.s.

ACTHAR® (Corticotropin for Injection) is sterile powdered lyophilized ACTH which in the dry form is stable at room temperature. Each vial contains 25 or 40 Units of Corticotropin U.S.P. and approximately 9 and 14 milligrams of hydrolyzed gelatin respectively.

Acthar must be reconstituted at the time of use by dissolving in a convenient volume of Sterile Water for Injection or Sodium Chloride Injection in such a manner that the individual dose will be contained in 1-2 ml. of solution. The reconstituted solution should be refrigerated and used in 24 hours.

Actions: H.P. ACTHAR® (Repository Corticotropin Injection) and ACTHAR® (Corticotropin for Injection) are the Armour Pharmaceutical Company brands of preparations containing the anterior pituitary hormone. This hormone stimulates the functioning adrenal cortex to produce and secrete the adrenocortical hormones.

Indications: ACTHAR® (Corticotropin for Injection) and H.P. ACTHAR® GEL (Repository Corticotropin Injection) are indicated for diagnostic testing of adrenocortical function.

ACTHAR® (Corticotropin for Injection) and H.P. ACTHAR® GEL (Repository Corticotropin Injection) have limited therapeutic value in those conditions responsive to corticosteroid therapy; in such case, corticosteroid therapy is considered to be the treatment of choice. ACTHAR® (Corticotropin for Injection) and H.P. ACTHAR® GEL (Repository Corticotropin Injection) may be employed in the following disorders:

ENDOCRINE DISORDERS: Nonsuppurative thyroiditis; Hypercalcemia associated with cancer.

RHEUMATIC DISORDERS: As adjunctive therapy for short-term administration (to tide the patient over an acute episode or exacerbation) in:
Psoriatic arthritis; Rheumatoid arthritis, including juvenile rheumatoid arthritis (selected cases may require low-dose maintenance therapy); Ankylosing spondylitis; Acute and subacute bursitis; Acute nonspecific tenosynovitis; Acute gouty arthritis; Posttraumatic arthritis; Synovitis of osteoarthritis; Epicondylitis.

COLLAGEN DISEASES: During an exacerbation or as maintenance therapy in selected cases of:
Systemic lupus erythematosus; Systemic dermatomyositis (polymyositis); Acute rheumatic carditis.

DERMATOLOGIC DISEASES: Pemphigus; Bullous dermatitis herpetiformis; Severe erythema multiforme (Stevens-Johnson syndrome); Exfoliative dermatitis; Severe psoriasis; Severe seborrheic dermatitis; Mycosis fungoides.

ALLERGIC STATES: Control of severe or incapacitating allergic conditions intractable to adequate trials of conventional treatment—Seasonal or perennial allergic rhinitis; Bronchial asthma; Contact dermatitis; Atopic dermatitis; Serum sickness.

OPHTHALMIC DISEASES: Severe acute and chronic allergic and inflammatory processes involving the eye and its adnexa such as:
Allergic conjunctivitis; Keratitis; Herpes zoster ophthalmicus; Iritis and iridocyclitis; Diffuse posterior uveitis and choroiditis; Optic neuritis; Sympathetic ophthalmia; Chorioretinitis; Anterior segment inflammation; Allergic corneal marginal ulcers.

RESPIRATORY DISEASES: Symptomatic sarcoidosis; Loeffler's syndrome not manageable by other means; Berylliosis; Fulminating or disseminated pulmonary tuberculosis when used concurrently with antituberculous chemotherapy; Aspiration pneumonitis.

HEMATOLOGIC DISORDERS: Acquired (autoimmune) hemolytic anemia; Idiopathic thrombocytopenic purpura in adults (I.V. only; I.M. administration is contraindicated); Secondary thrombocytopenia in adults; Erythroblastopenia (RBC anemia); Congenital (erythroid) hypoplastic anemia.

NEOPLASTIC DISEASES: For palliative management of:
Leukemias and lymphomas in adults; Acute leukemia of childhood.

EDEMATOUS STATE: To induce a diuresis or a remission of proteinuria in the nephrotic syndrome without uremia of the idiopathic type or that due to lupus erythematosus.

GASTROINTESTINAL DISEASES: To tide the patient over a critical period of the disease in: Ulcerative colitis; Regional enteritis.

MISCELLANEOUS: Tuberculous meningitis with subarachnoid block or impending block when used concurrently with appropriate anti-tuberculous chemotherapy; Trichinosis with neurologic or myocardial involvement.

Contraindications: Corticotropin is contraindicated in patients with scleroderma, osteoporosis, systemic fungal infections, ocular herpes simplex, recent surgery, history of or the presence of a peptic ulcer, congestive heart failure, hypertension, or sensitivity to proteins of porcine origin.

Treatment of conditions listed within the indication section (see above) when they are accompanied by primary adrenocortical insufficiency or adrenocortical hyperfunction.

Intravenous administration of corticotropin is contraindicated for treatment of conditions listed within the indications section.

Warnings: Chronic administration of corticotropin may lead to adverse effects which are not reversible. Corticotropin may only suppress symptoms and signs of chronic disease without altering the natural course of the disease. Neither H.P. ACTHAR® GEL (Repository Corticotropin Injection) nor ACTHAR® (Corticotropin for Injection) should be administered for treatment until adrenal responsiveness has been verified with the route of administration which will be utilized during treatment, intramuscularly or subcutaneously. A rise in urinary and plasma corticosteroid values provides direct evidence of a stimulatory effect. Prolonged administration of corticotropin increases the risk of hypersensitivity reactions. Although the action of corticotropin is similar to that of exogenous adrenocortical steroids the quantity of adrenocorticoid may be variable. In patients who receive prolonged corticotropin therapy the additional use of rapidly acting corticosteroids before, during, and after an unusual stressful situation is indicated.

Prolonged use of corticotropin may produce posterior subcapsular cataracts and glaucoma with possible damage to the optic nerves.

Corticotropin may mask some signs of infection, and new infections including those of the eye due to fungi or viruses may appear during its use. There may be decreased resistance and inability to localize infection when corticotropin is used.

Usage in pregnancy: Since fetal abnormalities have been observed in experimental animals, use of this drug in pregnancy, nursing mothers, or women of child bearing potential requires that the potential benefits of the drug be weighed against the potential hazards to the mother and embryo or fetus. Infants born of mothers who have received substantial doses of corticotropin during pregnancy should be carefully observed for signs of hypoadrenalism.

Corticotropin can cause elevation of blood pressure, salt and water retention, and increased excretion of potassium. Dietary salt restriction and potassium supplementation may be necessary. Corticotropin increases calcium excretion.

While on corticotropin therapy, patients should not be vaccinated against smallpox. Other immunization procedures should be undertaken with caution in patients who are receiving corticotropin, especially when high doses are administered because of the possible

Continued on next page

Armour—Cont.

hazards of neurological complications and lack of antibody response.

Precautions: Patients with latent tuberculosis or tuberculin reactivity who receive corticotropin should be closely observed as reactivation of the disease may occur. During prolonged corticotropin therapy, these patients should receive chemoprophylaxis.

Skin testing should be performed prior to treatment of all patients with suspected sensitivity to porcine proteins. During intravenous or immediately following intramuscular or subcutaneous administration of corticotropin all patients should be observed carefully for sensitivity reactions.

Relative adrenocortical insufficiency induced by prolonged corticotropin therapy may be minimized by gradual reduction of corticotropin dosage. This type of insufficiency may persist for months after discontinuation of therapy; therefore, in any situation of stress during that period, hormone therapy should be reinstituted.

There is an enhanced effect of corticotropin in patients with hypothyroidism and in those with cirrhosis.

The lowest possible dosage of corticotropin should be used to control the condition under treatment, and when reduction in dosage is possible the reduction should be gradual.

Corticotropin should be administered for treatment only when the disease is intractable to more conventional therapy. Corticotropin should be adjunctive and not the sole therapy in the treatment of a disease.

Since maximal corticotropin stimulation of the adrenals may be limited during the first few days of treatment, other drugs should be administered when an immediate therapeutic effect is desirable.

When infection is present appropriate anti-infective therapy should be administered during corticotropin and following discontinuation of corticotropin therapy.

Treatment of acute gouty arthritis should be limited to a few days. Since rebound attacks may occur when corticotropin is discontinued, conventional concomitant therapy should be administered during corticotropin treatment, and for several days after it is stopped.

Psychic derangements may appear when corticotropin is used, ranging from euphoria, insomnia, mood swings, personality changes, and depression, to frank psychotic manifestations. Also, existing emotional instability or psychotic tendencies may be aggravated by corticotropin.

Aspirin should be used cautiously in conjunction with corticotropin in hypoprothrombinemia. Corticotropin should be used with caution in patients with diabetes, abscess, pyogenic infections, diverticulitis, renal insufficiency, and myasthenia gravis.

Growth and development of infants and children on prolonged corticotropin therapy should be carefully observed.

Adverse Reactions:

Fluid and electrolyte disturbances:
Sodium retention; fluid retention; potassium loss; hypokalemic alkalosis; calcium loss.

Musculoskeletal:
Muscle weakness; steroid myopathy; loss of muscle mass; osteoporosis; vertebral compression fractures; aseptic necrosis of femoral and humeral heads; pathologic fracture of long bones.

Gastrointestinal:
Peptic ulcer with possible perforation and hemorrhage; pancreatitis; abdominal distention; ulcerative esophagitis.

Dermatologic:
Impaired wound healing; thin fragile skin; petechiae and ecchymoses; facial erythema; increased sweating; suppression of skin test reactions; acne; hyperpigmentation.

Cardiovascular:
Hypertension, necrotizing angiitis; congestive heart failure.

Neurological:
Convulsions; increased intracranial pressure with papilledema, (pseudo-tumor cerebri) usually after treatment; headache, vertigo.

Endocrine:
Menstrual irregularities; development of Cushingoid state; suppression of growth in children; secondary adrenocortical pituitary unresponsiveness, particularly in times of stress, as in trauma, surgery or illness; decreased carbohydrate tolerance; manifestations of latent diabetes mellitus; increased requirements for insulin or oral hypoglycemic agents in diabetics; hirsutism.

Ophthalmic:
Posterior subcapsular cataracts; increased intraocular pressure; glaucoma with possible damage to optic nerve; exophthalmos.

Metabolic:
Negative nitrogen balance due to protein catabolism.

Allergic reactions:
Especially in patients with allergic responses to proteins manifesting as dizziness, nausea and vomiting, shock, skin reactions.

Miscellaneous:
Abscess: prolonged use of ACTH may result in antibodies to it and resulting loss of stimulatory effect.

Dosage and Administration: Standard tests for verification of adrenal responsiveness to corticotropin may utilize as much as 80 units as a single injection or one or more injections of a lesser dosage. Verification tests should be performed prior to treatment with corticotropins. The test should utilize the route(s) of administration proposed for treatment. Following verification, dosage should be individualized according to the disease under treatment and the general medical condition of each patient. Frequency and dose of the drug should be determined by considering severity of the disease, plasma and urine corticosteroid levels and the initial response of the patient. Only gradual change in dosage schedules should be attempted, after full drug effects have become apparent.

The chronic administration of more than 40 units daily may be associated with uncontrollable adverse effects.

When reduction in dosage is indicated this should be done gradually by either reducing the amount of each injection, or administering injections at longer intervals, or by a combination of both of the above. During reduction of dosage careful consideration should be given to the disease being treated, the general medical conditions of the patient and the duration over which corticotropin was administered.

H.P. ACTHAR® GEL (Repository Corticotropin Injection) and ACTHAR® (Corticotropin for Injection) may be administered intramuscularly or subcutaneously.

H.P. ACTHAR® GEL (Repository Corticotropin Injection) is given intramuscularly or subcutaneously every 24-72 hours in doses of 40-80 units.

The usual intramuscular or subcutaneous dose for ACTHAR® (Corticotropin for Injection) is 20 units four times a day.

For diagnostic purposes, ACTHAR® (Corticotropin for Injection) may be given intravenously in doses of 10-25 units dissolved in 500 ml. of 5% glucose infused over an 8-hour period.

How Supplied: H.P. ACTHAR® GEL (Repository Corticotropin Injection) is supplied in 5 milliliter multiple dose vials in strengths of 40 and 80 U.S.P. Units per milliliter and 1 milliliter vials containing 40 and 80 U.S.P. Units per milliliter.

ACTHAR® (Corticotropin for Injection) is supplied as a lyophilized powder in vials containing 25 and 40 U.S.P. Units per vial.

*U.S. PAT. NO. 2,992,165

BIOZYME® OINTMENT ℞

(neomycin palmitate—trypsin-chymotrypsin concentrate ointment)

Description: BIOZYME® OINTMENT (Neomycin Palmitate — Trypsin-Chymotrypsin Concentrate Ointment) contains per gram:

Neomycin Palmitate
equivalent to ....3.5 mg. of Neomycin
Trypsin-Chymotrypsin
Concentrate ....10,000 Armour Units of Proteolytic Activity

In a water washable base. (Polyethylene Glycol 4000 and 400, Stearyl Alcohol)

Actions: The anti-infective action of BIOZYME® OINTMENT is accomplished by the broad spectrum antibiotic Neomycin Palmitate. It is effective against most of the organisms, including gram-negative and gram-positive bacteria, frequently found in superficial skin infections, wounds, ulcers and burns. Clinical emergence of resistant strains can occur. The primary action of the Trypsin-Chymotrypsin Concentrate is to digest necrotic tissue, pyogenic membranes and crusts—to cleanse wounds and remove foul odors. This action serves to prepare the area or wounds for the maximum anti-infective action of neomycin. The enzymes are a concentrate derived from mammalian pancreas glands. The proteolytic activity is measured as Armour Units. One Armour Unit is that amount of proteolytic enzyme which upon incubation at 25.0 ± 0.1°C. for ten minutes with a suitable preparation of hemoglobin will cause the decomposition of the hemoglobin to such an extent that the amount of hydroxyaryl substances liberated will upon reaction with Folin-Ciocalteau Phenol Reagent result in the formation of a colored solution of equal intensity to that resulting from the reaction of one microgram of tyrosine in the same manner with Folin-Ciocalteau Phenol Reagent.

A specially prepared water washable ointment base is utilized to provide optimal release of medicaments with ease of application. The base is non-irritating, non-toxic and non-allergenic.

Indications

Based on a review of this drug by the National Academy of Sciences—National Research Council and/or other information, FDA has classified the indications as follows:

"Possibly" effective for the treatment of:
- Abscesses and furuncles—open or incised
- Infected burns
- Pyodermas, such as folliculitis and impetigo
- Infected skin ulcers, such as arteriosclerotic, decubitus, diabetic, stasis, traumatic, varicose, etc.

Final classification of the less-than effective indications requires further investigation.

Contraindications: Local application is contraindicated in those individuals who have shown hypersensitivity to any of its components.

Warning: As with any antibiotic preparation, prolonged use may result in overgrowth of nonsusceptible organisms. If superinfection occurs, the product should be discontinued and appropriate therapy instituted. There are articles in the current medical literature which indicate an increase in the prevalence of persons sensitive to neomycin.

Because of the potential hazard of nephrotoxicity and ototoxicity, prolonged use or use of large amounts of this product should be avoided in the treatment of skin infections following extensive burns, trophic ulceration, and other conditions where absorption of neomycin is possible.

Adverse Reactions: BIOZYME® OINTMENT (Neomycin Palmitate—Trypsin-Chymotrypsin Concentrate Ointment) is generally well tolerated; an itching or stinging sensation is sometimes associated with the first or first few applications. Hypersensitivity or allergenic reactions are occasionally seen. The proteolytic action can be halted by removal of the ointment and irrigation with water.

Ototoxicity and nephrotoxicity have been reported from Neomycin.

Administration: Not for ophthalmic use. Apply directly to the lesions one to three times daily and cover with gauze.

Packaging: Available in one-half ounce (15 g.) and one ounce (30 g.) tubes.

CALCIMAR® SOLUTION ℞
(calcitonin-salmon), Armour

Description: Calcitonin is a polypeptide hormone secreted by the parafollicular cells of the thyroid gland in mammals and by the ultimobranchial gland of birds and fish.

CALCIMAR® (calcitonin-salmon) is a synthetic polypeptide of 32 amino acids in the same linear sequence that is found in calcitonin of salmon origin. This is shown by the following graphic formula:

Cys- Ser- Asn- Leu- Ser-Thr- Cys-Val- Leu-Gly-
1 2 3 4 5 6 7 8 9 10
Lys-Leu- Ser- Gln- Glu- Leu-His- Lys-Leu- Gln-
11 12 13 14 15 16 17 18 19 20
Thr-Tyr- Pro- Arg-Thr- Asn-Thr- Gly- Ser- Gly-
21 22 23 24 25 26 27 28 29 30
Thr-Pro-NH_2
31 32

It is provided in sterile solution for subcutaneous or intramuscular injection. Each milliliter contains 200 MRC units of Calcitonin-Salmon, Armour, 5 mg Phenol (as preservative), with Sodium Chloride, Sodium Acetate, Acetic Acid, and Sodium Hydroxide to adjust tonicity and pH.

The activity of CALCIMAR® is stated in MRC (Medical Research Council) units based on bioassay in comparison with the International Reference Preparation of Calcitonin, Salmon for Bioassay, distributed by the National Institute For Biological Standard And Control, Holly Hill, London.

Clinical Pharmacology: Calcitonin acts primarily on bone, but direct renal effects and actions on the gastrointestinal tract are also recognized. Salmon calcitonin appears to have actions essentially identical to calcitonins of mammalian origin, but its potency per mg is greater and it has a longer duration of action. The actions of calcitonin on bone and its role in normal human bone physiology are still incompletely understood.

Bone—Single injections of calcitonin cause a marked transient inhibition of the ongoing bone resorptive process. With prolonged use, there is a persistent, smaller decrease in the rate of bone resorption. Histologically this is associated with a decreased number of osteoclasts and an apparent decrease in their resorptive activity. Decreased osteocytic resorption may also be involved. There is some evidence that initially bone formation may be augmented by calcitonin through increased osteoblastic activity. However, calcitonin will probably not induce a long-term increase in bone formation.

Animal studies indicate that endogenous calcitonin, primarily through its action on bone, participates with parathyroid hormone in the homeostatic regulation of blood calcium. Thus, high blood calcium levels cause increased secretion of calcitonin which, in turn, inhibits bone resorption. This reduces the transfer of calcium from bone to blood and tends to return blood calcium to the normal level. The importance of this process in humans has not been determined. In normal adults, who have a relatively low rate of bone resorption, the administration of exogenous calcitonin results in only a slight decrease in serum calcium. In normal children and in patients with generalized Paget's disease, bone resorption is more rapid and decreases in serum calcium are more pronounced in response to calcitonin.

Paget's Disease of Bone (osteitis deformans)—Paget's disease is a disorder of uncertain etiology characterized by abnormal and accelerated bone formation and resorption in one or more bones. In most patients only small areas of bone are involved and the disease is not symptomatic. In a small fraction of patients, however, the abnormal bone may lead to bone pain and bone deformity, cranial and spinal nerve entrapment, or spinal cord compression. The increased vascularity of the abnormal bone may lead to high output congestive heart failure.

Active Paget's disease involving a large mass of bone may increase the urinary hydroxyproline excretion (reflecting breakdown of collagen-containing bone matrix) and serum alkaline phosphatase (reflecting increased bone formation).

Salmon calcitonin, presumably by an initial blocking effect on bone resorption, causes a decreased rate of bone turnover with a resultant fall in the serum alkaline phosphatase and urinary hydroxyproline excretion in approximately ⅔ of patients treated. These biochemical changes appear to correspond to changes toward more normal bone, as evidenced by a small number of documented examples of: 1) radiologic regression of Pagetic lesions, 2) improvement of impaired auditory nerve and other neurologic function, 3) decreases (measured) in abnormally elevated cardiac output. These improvements occur extremely rarely, if ever, spontaneously. (elevated cardiac output may disappear over a period of years when the disease slowly enters a sclerotic phase; in the cases treated with calcitonin, however, the decreases were seen in less than one year).

Some patients with Paget's disease who have good biochemical and/or symptomatic responses initially, later relapse. Suggested explanations have included the formation of neutralizing antibodies and the development of secondary hyperparathyroidism, but neither suggestion appears to explain adequately the majority of relapses.

Although the parathyroid hormone levels do appear to rise transiently during each hypocalcemic response to calcitonin, most investigators have been unable to demonstrate persistent hypersecretion of parathyroid hormone in patients treated chronically with calcitonin.

Circulating antibodies to calcitonin after 2–18 months' treatment have been reported in about half of the patients with Paget's disease in whom antibody studies were done, but calcitonin treatment remained effective in many of these cases. Occasionally patients with high antibody titers are found. These patients usually will have suffered a biochemical relapse of Paget's disease and are unresponsive to the acute hypocalcemic effects of calcitonin.

Kidney—Calcitonin increases the excretion of filtered phosphate, calcium, and sodium by decreasing their tubular reabsorption. In some patients the inhibition of bone resorption by calcitonin is of such magnitude that the consequent reduction of filtered calcium load more than compensates for the decrease in tubular reabsorption of calcium. The result in these patients is a decrease rather than an increase in urinary calcium.

Transient increases in sodium and water excretion may occur after the initial injection of calcitonin. In most patients these changes return to pre-treatment levels with continued therapy.

Gastrointestinal tract—Increasing evidence indicates that calcitonin has significant actions on the gastrointestinal tract. Short-term administration results in marked transient decreases in the volume and acidity of gastric juice and in the volume and the trypsin and amylase content of pancreatic juice. Whether these effects continue to be elicited after each injection of calcitonin during chronic therapy has not been investigated.

Metabolism—The metabolism of salmon calcitonin has not yet been studied clinically. Information from animal studies with salmon calcitonin and from clinical studies with calcitonins of porcine and human origin suggest that salmon calcitonin is rapidly metabolized by conversion to smaller inactive fragments, primarily in the kidneys, but also in the blood and peripheral tissues. A small amount of unchanged hormone and its inactive metabolites are excreted in the urine.

It appears that salmon calcitonin cannot cross the placental barrier and its passage to the cerebrospinal fluid or to breast milk has not been determined.

Indications and Usage: Calcimar® (Calcitonin-Salmon) is indicated for the treatment of symptomatic Paget's disease of bone.

At the present time effectiveness has been demonstrated principally in patients with moderate to severe disease characterized by polyostotic involvement with elevated serum alkaline phosphatase and urinary hydroxyproline excretion.

In these patients, the biochemical abnormalities were substantially improved (more than 30% reduction) in about ⅔ of patients studied, and bone pain was improved in a similar fraction. A small number of documented instances of reversal of neurologic deficits has occurred, including improvement in the basilar compression syndrome, and improvement of spinal cord and spinal nerve lesions. At present there is too little experience to predict the likelihood of improvement of any given neurologic lesion. Hearing loss, the most common neurologic lesion of Paget's disease is improved infrequently (4 of 29 patients studied audiometrically).

Patients with increased cardiac output due to extensive Paget's disease have had measured decreases in cardiac output while receiving calcitonin. The number of treated patients in this category is still too small to predict how likely such a result will be.

The large majority of patients with localized, especially monostotic disease do not develop symptoms and most patients with mild symptoms can be managed with analgesics. There is no evidence that the prophylactic use of calcitonin is beneficial in asymptomatic patients, although treatment may be considered in exceptional circumstances in which there is extensive involvement of the skull or spinal cord with the possibility of irreversible neurologic damage. In these instances treatment would be based on the demonstrated effect of calcitonin on Pagetic bone, rather than on clinical studies in the patient population in question.

Contraindications: Clinical allergy to synthetic salmon calcitonin.

Warnings:

Allergic Reactions

Because calcitonin is protein in nature, the possibility of a systemic allergic reaction cannot be overlooked. The usual provisions should be made for the emergency treatment of such a reaction should it occur. Patients with a positive skin test to Calcimar® were excluded from clinical trials.

Skin testing should be considered prior to treatment with calcitonin, particularly for patients with suspected sensitivity to calcitonin. The following procedure is suggested: Prepare a dilution at 10 MRC units per ml by with-

Continued on next page

Armour—Cont.

drawing 1/20 ml (0.05 ml) in a tuberculin syringe and filling it to 1.0 ml with Sodium Chloride Injection, U.S.P. Mix well, discard 0.9 ml and inject intracutaneously 0.1 ml (approximately 1 MRC u) on the inner aspect of the forearm. Observe the injection site 15 minutes after injection. The appearance of more than mild erythema or wheal constitutes a positive response.

The incidence of osteogenic sarcoma is known to be increased in Paget's disease. Pagetic lesions, with or without therapy, may appear by x-ray to progress markedly, possibly with some loss of definition or periosteal margins. Such lesions should be evaluated carefully to differentiate these from osteogenic sarcoma.

Precautions:

1. General
The administration of calcitonin possibly could lead to hypocalcemic tetany under special circumstances although no cases have yet been reported. Provisions for parenteral calcium administration should be available during the first several administrations of calcitonin.

2. Laboratory Tests
Periodic examinations of urine sediment of patients on chronic therapy are recommended. Coarse granular casts and casts containing renal tubular epithelial cells were reported in young adult volunteers at bed rest who were given salmon calcitonin to study the effect on immobilization osteoporosis. There was no other evidence of renal abnormality and the urine sediment became normal after calcitonin was stopped. Urine sediment abnormalities have not been reported by other investigators.

3. Instructions for the patient
Careful instruction in sterile injection technique should be given to the patient, and to other persons who may administer CALCIMAR®.

4. Carcinogenesis
No long-term studies have been performed to evaluate carcinogenic potential of salmon calcitonin.

5. Pregnancy
Salmon calcitonin has been shown to cause decrease in fetal birth weights in rabbits when given in doses 14–56 times the dose recommended for human use. Since calcitonin does not cross the placental barrier, this finding may be due to metabolic effects of calcitonin on the pregnant animal. There are no studies in pregnant women. Salmon calcitonin should be used only when clearly needed in women who are or may become pregnant.

6. Nursing Mothers
It is not known whether this drug is excreted in human milk. As a general rule, nursing should not be undertaken while a patient is on drug since many drugs are excreted in human milk. Calcitonin has been shown to inhibit lactation in animals.

7. Pediatric Use
Disorders of bone in children referred to as juvenile Paget's disease have been reported rarely. The relationship of these disorders to adult Paget's disease has not been established and experience with the use of calcitonin in these disorders is very limited. There are no adequate data to support the use of Calcimar® in children.

Adverse Reactions: Nausea with or without vomiting has been noted in about 10% of patients treated with calcitonin. It is most evident when treatment is first initiated and tends to decrease or disappear with continued administration.

Local inflammatory reactions at the site of subcutaneous or intramuscular injection have been reported in about 10% of patients. Flushing of face or hands occurred in about 2 to 5% of patients. Skin rashes have been reported occasionally.

Overdosage: A dose of 1000 MRC units subcutaneously may produce nausea and vomiting as the only adverse effects. Doses of 32 units per kg per day for one or two days demonstrate no other adverse effects.

Data on chronic high dose administration are insufficient to judge toxicity.

Dosage and Administration: The recommended starting dose of calcitonin in Paget's disease is 100 MRC units (0.5 ml) per day administered subcutaneously (preferred for outpatient self-administration) or intramuscularly. Drug effect should be monitored by periodic measurement of serum alkaline phosphatase and 24-hour urinary hydroxyproline (if available) and evaluation of symptoms. A decrease toward normal of the biochemical abnormalities is usually seen, if it is going to occur, within the first few months. Bone pain may also decrease during that time. Improvement of neurologic lesions, when it occurs, requires a longer period of treatment, often more than one year.

In many patients doses of 50 MRC units (0.25 ml) per day or every other day are sufficient to maintain biochemical and clinical improvement. At the present time, however, there are insufficient data to determine whether this reduced dose will have the same effect as the higher dose on forming more normal bone structure. It appears preferable, therefore, to maintain the higher dose in any patient with serious deformity or neurological involvement.

In any patient with a good response initially who later relapses, either clinically or biochemically, the possibility of antibody formation should be explored. Although specialized tests for antibody titer are not widely available, the patients can be tested for high antibody titer as follows:

> After overnight fasting, a sample of the patient's blood is taken for determination of serum calcium and 100 MRC units of CALCIMAR® (calcitonin-salmon) are injected IM. The patient is then permitted to eat his usual breakfast. At 3 and 6 hours post-injection additional blood samples are drawn and the patient is released. The serum calcium values are then compared. A decrease of 0.5 mg% or more from fasting level at 3 and 6 hours is usually seen in the responsive patient. Decreases of 0.3 mg % or less constitute an inadequate response to calcitonin in the patient with active Paget's disease. If the hypocalcemic action of calcitonin is lost, further therapy with CALCIMAR® will not be effective.

Patient compliance should also be assessed in the event of relapse.

In patients who relapse, whether because of antibodies or for unexplained reasons, a dosage increase beyond 100 MRC units per day does not usually appear to elicit an improved response.

How Supplied: CALCIMAR® Solution (Calcitonin-Salmon) is available as a sterile solution in 2 ml vials containing 200 MRC units per ml.

STORE IN REFRIGERATOR—Between 2°–8° C (36°–46° F)

CHYMORAL®-100 ℞
(trypsin-chymotrypsin tablets, Armour)

CHYMORAL® ℞
(trypsin-chymotrypsin tablets, Armour)

Description: CHYMORAL®-100 (Trypsin-Chymotrypsin Tablets, Armour) and CHYMORAL® (Trypsin-Chymotrypsin Tablets, Armour) are enteric coated tablets specifically formulated to promote systemic absorption of proteolytic enzymes after oral administration. CHYMORAL®-100 is available as 100,000 Armour Units of enzymatic activity per tablet. CHYMORAL® is available as 50,000 Armour Units of enzymatic activity per tablet. The enzymatic activity is present in a purified concentrate containing specific trypsin and chymotrypsin activities in a ratio of approximately six to one. CHYMORAL®-100 and CHYMORAL® are carefully standardized in terms of proteolytic activity. The assay used is a modification of the Anson hemoglobin method, standardized in Armour Units. One Armour Unit of proteolytic activity is that amount which, upon incubation with the hemoglobin substrate, as directed in the method of assay will release a quantity of phenolic substances which when reacted with Folin-Ciocalteau Phenol Reagent, will result in the formation of a colored solution of equal intensity to that produced from the reaction of one microgram of tyrosine with the Folin-Ciocalteau Phenol Reagent.

Indications

Based on a review of this drug by the National Academy of Science—National Research Council and/or other information, FDA has classified the indications as follows:

"Possibly" effective for relieving symptomatology related to episiotomy.

"Lacking substantial evidence of effectiveness" in the reduction of moderate to severe inflammatory response to surgical or accidental trauma when used to supplement and augment other methods of therapy such as immobilization, elevation, compresses, and chemotherapy.

Final classification of less-than-effective indications requires further investigation.

Contraindications: Septicemia, severe generalized or localized infection and in the presence of known disorders of blood coagulation CHYMORAL®-100 (Trypsin-Chymotrypsin Tablets, Armour) or CHYMORAL® (Trypsin-Chymotrypsin Tablets, Armour) should not be given to patients with known sensitivity to any of the components of the drug.

Precautions: Although CHYMORAL®-100 and CHYMORAL® have not been reported to cause a spread of an existing focus of infection, it is recommended that an appropriate antibiotic be used concomitantly where infection is present or suspected.

There is no evidence that CHYMORAL®-100 or CHYMORAL®, in the recommended dosage, affects the blood clotting mechanism. However, the usual laboratory tests and precautions should be observed carefully when anticoagulants are used concomitantly.

Safe use in pregnancy has not been established. In patients with a history of sensitivity to drugs, CHYMORAL®-100 or CHYMORAL® should be used with caution.

Adverse Reactions: An occasional patient may experience gastro-intestinal upset when CHYMORAL®-100 or CHYMORAL® is given. Hematuria, mild skin rash, urticaria or itching has been reported in rare instances. Discontinuance of enzyme therapy is recommended in such cases.

Dosage and Administration: Recommended dosage of CHYMORAL®-100 is one tablet four times daily.

Recommended dosage of CHYMORAL® is one or two tablets four times daily.

CHYMORAL®-100 or CHYMORAL® should be given one hour before meals and at bedtime, and treatment should begin as soon as possible after trauma occurs.

How Supplied: CHYMORAL® is available as red tablets of 50,000 Armour Units in bottles of 48 tablets and CHYMORAL®-100 as red-orange tablets identified by Armacode® CC of 100,000 Armour Units in bottles of 48 and 250 tablets.

[*Shown in Product Identification Section*]

LEVOTHROID™ ℞
(sodium levothyroxine tablets, U.S.P.)

Description: LEVOTHROID™ Tablets provide crystalline sodium levothyroxine, a potent thyroid hormone, in seven different strengths to permit easy convenient dosage adjustment and selection of proper potency for the varying degrees of hypothyroidism. The sodium levothyroxine in LEVOTHROID™ is micronized to provide for optimal absorption, thus helping insure metabolic response for the patient.
Action: Levothyroxine and liothyronine are the two active thyroid hormones.
Sodium L-3, 3′, 5, 5′-tetraiodothyronine
L-Thyroxine is readily absorbed from the gastrointestinal tract. It is carried to tissue cells largely bound to plasma proteins. Deiodinization of L-Thyroxine probably takes place at the cell level, converting to liothyronine which produces the physiologic effect at that level.
Indications: LEVOTHROID™ (Sodium Levothyroxine Tablets, U.S.P.) is indicated as replacement or substitution therapy of diminished or absent thyroid function (e.g., cretinism, myxedema, non-toxic goiter or hypothyroidism generally, including the hypothyroid state in children, in pregnancy and in the elderly resulting from functional deficiency, primary atrophy, from partial or complete absence of the gland or from the effects of surgery, radiation or anti-thyroid agents. Therapy must be maintained continuously to control the symptoms of hypothyroidism.
Contraindications: LEVOTHROID™ administration is contraindicated in thyrotoxicosis and in acute myocardial infarction. LEVOTHROID™ is contraindicated in the presence of uncorrected adrenal insufficiency because it increases the tissue demands for adrenocortical hormones and may cause an acute adrenal crisis in such patients. (See Warnings)

WARNINGS:

> Drugs with thyroid hormone activity, alone or together with other therapeutic agents, have been used for the treatment of obesity. In euthyroid patients, doses within the range of daily hormonal requirements are ineffective for weight reduction. Larger doses may produce serious or even life-threatening manifestations of toxicity, particularly when given in association with sympathomimetic amines such as those used for their anorectic effects.

LEVOTHROID™ should be used with caution in patients with cardiovascular disease, including hypertension. The development of chest pain or other aggravation of cardiovascular disease will require a decrease in dosage.
Injection of epinephrine in patients with coronary disease may precipitate an episode of coronary insufficiency. This may be enhanced in patients receiving thyroid preparations. Careful observation is required if catecholamines are administered to patients in this category. Patients with coronary artery disease should be carefully observed during surgery, since the possibility of precipitating cardiac arrhythmias may be greater in those treated with thyroid hormones.
Thyroid replacement may potentiate anticoagulant effects with agents such as warfarin or bishydroxycoumarin and reduction of one-third in anticoagulant dosage should be undertaken upon initiation of LEVOTHROID™ therapy. Subsequent anticoagulant dosage adjustment should be made on the basis of frequent prothrombin determinations.
In patients whose hypothyroidism is secondary to hypopituitarism, adrenal insufficiency will probably also be present. When adrenal insufficiency and hypothyroidism coexist, the adrenal insufficiency should be corrected by corticosteroids before administering thyroid hormones.
Precautions: Patients with hypothyroidism, and especially myxedema, are particularly sensitive to thyroid preparations so that treatment should begin with small doses and increments should be gradual.
In patients with diabetes mellitus, addition of thyroid hormone therapy may cause an increase in the required dosage of insulin or oral hypoglycemic agents. Conversely, decreasing the dose of thyroid hormone may possibly cause hypoglycemic reactions if the dosage of insulin or oral hypoglycemic agents is not adjusted.
Adverse Reactions: Excessive dosage of thyroid medication may result in symptoms of hyperthyroidism. Since, however, the effects do not appear at once, the symptoms may not appear for one to three weeks after the dosage regimen is begun. The most common signs and symptoms of overdosage are weight loss, palpitation, nervousness, diarrhea or abdominal cramps, sweating, tachycardia, cardiac arrhythmias, angina pectoris, tremors, headache, insomnia, intolerance to heat and fever. If symptoms of overdosage appear, discontinue medication for several days and reinstitute treatment at a lower dosage level.
Dosage and Administration: The goal of therapy should be the restoration of euthyroidism as judged by clinical response and confirmed by appropriate laboratory values. In adults with no complicating endocrine or cardiovascular disease, the predicted full maintenance dose may be achieved immediately with adjustments made as indicated by clinical evaluation. The usual maintenance dose of Levothroid is 0.1 mg to 0.2 mg daily.
In patients with known complications or in case of doubt, individual dose titration at 2 to 4 week intervals is recommended. The usual starting dose is 0.05 mg with increases of 0.05 mg at 2 to 4 week intervals until the patient is euthyroid or symptoms ensue which preclude further dose increase.
In adult myxedema or hypothyroid patients with angina, the starting dose should be 0.025 mg with increases at 2 to 4 week intervals of 0.025 to 0.05 mg as determined by clinical response.
In cretinism or severe hypothyroidism in children, the initial dosage should be 0.025 to 0.05 mg with increases of 0.05 to 0.1 mg at 2 week intervals until the child is clinically euthyroid and laboratory values are in the normal range. In growing children, the usual maintenance dose may be as high as 0.3 to 0.4 mg daily. It is essential in children to reach the euthyroid state as rapidly as possible because of the importance of thyroid in growth and maturation.
How Supplied: LEVOTHROID™ (Sodium Levothyroxine Tablets, U.S.P.) is available in bottles of 100 tablets and larger. The 0.05 mg, 0.1 mg, 0.15 mg, 0.175, 0.2 mg, and 0.3 mg potencies are also available in cartons of 100 (10 strips of 10 tablets) packaged in Unit Dose as Armadose®. Each LEVOTHROID™ Tablet is distinctively colored and bears identifying markings.

Strength (mg)	Tablet Color	Markings	Approx. Equivalent in Armour Thyroid
0.025	Orange	¼ LK	¼ gr
0.05	White	½ LL	½ gr
0.1	Yellow	1 LM	1 gr
0.15	Blue	1½ LN	1½ gr
0.175	Turquoise	1¾ LP	1¾ gr
0.2	Pink	2 LR	2 gr
0.3	Green	3 LS	3 gr

[*Shown in Product Identification Section*]

NICOBID® ℞
(niacin, Armour)
Timed Release Nicotinic Acid Tempules®

Description: Each black-and-clear Tempule® (long-acting, timed-release capsule) contains 125 mg. niacin (nicotinic acid); each green-and-clear Tempule® (long-acting, timed-release capsule) contains 250 mg. niacin (nicotinic acid); and each opaque blue and white long-acting, timed-release capsule (Tempules®) contains 500 mg. niacin (nicotinic acid).
Action: Provides the full actions of nicotinic acid. The effects of the drug are both prompt and prolonged. Portions of the pellets are released immediately and initial effects are observed within the hour. The remainder is released over time to provide long acting effects.
Indications: Indicated in all those disease states in which niacin (nicotinic acid) has been used.
NICOBID® (niacin, Armour) has the advantage of a slower release of niacin (nicotinic acid) than the same drug in tablet form. This may permit its use in those patients who cannot tolerate the tablet form.
Contraindications: Those patients with a known idiosyncrasy to niacin (nicotinic acid) or other components of the drug and patients with arterial bleeding.
Warning: Caution is recommended in patients with glaucoma, severe diabetes, impaired liver function and peptic ulcer.
Precaution: As with all therapeutic agents, use with caution in pregnant patients.
Adverse Reactions: Transient flushing and feeling of warmth may be expected. These effects seldom reach undesirable levels so as to necessitate discontinuation of the drug. Transient headache, itching and tingling, gastric disturbances, skin rash and allergies may occur.
Dosage and Administration: Usual adult dose—one capsule (Tempule®), 125 mg., 250 mg. or 500 mg. morning and evening.
How Supplied: NICOBID® 125 mg. (identified by the Armacode® NC) and NICOBID® 250 mg. (identified by the Armacode® ND) in bottles of 100 and 500 capsules. NICOBID® 500 mg. (identified by the Armacode® NH) is available in bottles of 100 capsules.
Distributed by Armour Pharmaceutical Company

[*Shown in Product Identification Section*]

NICOLAR® ℞
(niacin tablets, Armour)

Description: Nicolar® (niacin tablets, Armour) is a scored yellow colored tablet containing 500 mg. of niacin (nicotinic acid).
Actions: Niacin functions in the body as a component of two hydrogen transporting coenzymes; Coenzyme I (Nicotinamide Adenine Dinucleotide [NAD], sometimes called Diphosphopyridine Nucleotide [DPN]) and Coenzyme II (Nicotinamide Adenine Dinucleotide Phosphate [NADP], sometimes called Triphosphopyridine Nucleotide [TPN]). Niacin in addition to its functions as a vitamin, exerts several distinctive pharmacologic effects which vary according to the dosage level employed.
Niacin, in large doses, causes a reduction in serum lipids. The exact mechanism of this action is unknown.
Indications: Nicolar® is indicated as adjunctive therapy in addition to diet and other measures in the treatment of hypercholesterolemia and hyperbetalipoproteinemia.
Notice: It has not been established whether drug-induced lowering of serum cholesterol or other lipid levels has a detrimental, a beneficial or no effect on the morbidity due to atherosclerosis or coronary heart disease. Several years will be required before current investigations can yield an answer to this question.
Contraindications: Niacin is contraindicated in patients with hepatic dysfunction or in patients with active acute peptic ulcer.
Warnings: Use of this drug in pregnancy, lactation or in women of child-bearing age requires that the potential benefits of the drug be weighed against its possible hazards to the

Continued on next page

Armour—Cont.

mother and child. Although fetal abnormalities have not been reported with this drug, its use as an antilipidemic agent requires high dosages, and animal reproduction or teratology studies have not been done. There are insufficient studies done for usage in children.
Precautions: Patients with gall bladder disease, or those with a past history of jaundice, liver disease or peptic ulcer should be observed closely while taking this medication.
Frequent monitoring of liver function tests and blood glucose should be performed in the initial stage of therapy until it is ascertained that the drug has no adverse effects on these organ systems.
Diabetic or potential diabetic patients should be observed closely in the event of decreased tolerance. Adjustment of diet and/or hypoglycemic therapy may be necessary.
Patients receiving antihypertensive drugs of the adrenal-blocking type may have an additive vasodilating effect and produce postural hypotension.
Elevated uric acid levels have occurred; therefore use with caution in patients predisposed to gout.
Adverse Reactions: Severe generalized flushing
Decreased glucose tolerance
Activation of peptic ulcers
Abnormalities of hepatic functional tests
Jaundice
Gastrointestinal disorders
Dryness of the skin
Keratosis nigricans
Pruritus
Hyperuricemia
Toxic amblyopia
Hypotension
Transient headache
Dosage and Administration: Two to four tablets (1–2 grams) daily with or following meals or as directed by physician.
Since flushing, pruritus and gastrointestinal distress appear frequently, begin therapy with small doses and slowly build up dose in gradual increments observing for adverse effects and efficacy. The usual maximum daily dose is 8 grams.
How Supplied: Nicolar® (niacin tablets, Armour) is available in bottles of 100 scored tablets, each containing 500 mg. of nicotinic acid (identified by the Armacode® NE).
Caution: Federal law prohibits dispensing without prescription.

PENTRITOL®—60 mg. ℞
(pentaerythritol tetranitrate)
timed release tempules® Armour

Description:
Empirical Formula: $C_5H_8N_4O_{12}$
Molecular Weight: 316.15
The pentaerythritol tetranitrate is in a special timed-release base (tempule®) designed to give prolonged systemic effect.
Action: The mechanism of action in the relief of angina pectoris is unknown at this time, although the basic pharmacologic action is to relax smooth muscle.

Indication
Based on a review of this drug by the National Academy of Science—National Research Council and/or other information, FDA has classified the indication as follows:
"Possibly" effective for the relief of angina pectoris (pain of coronary artery disease). It is not intended to abort the acute anginal episode, but is widely regarded as useful in the prophylactic treatment of angina pectoris.
Final classification of the less-than-effective indications requires further investigation.

Contraindications: Idiosyncrasy to this drug.
Warning: Data supporting the use of nitrites during the early days of the acute phase of myocardial infarction (the period during which clinical and laboratory findings are unstable) are insufficient to establish safety.
Precautions: Intraocular pressure is increased; therefore, caution is required in administering to patients with glaucoma. Tolerance to this drug, and cross-tolerance to other nitrites and nitrates may occur.
Adverse Reactions: Cutaneous vasodilation with flushing. Headache is common and may be severe and persistent. Transient episodes of dizziness and weakness, as well as other signs of cerebral ischemia associated with postural hypotension, occasionally may develop. This drug can act as a physiological antagonist to norepinephrine, acetylcholine, histamine, and many other agents. An occasional individual exhibits marked sensitivity to the hypotensive effects of nitrite and severe responses (nausea, vomiting, weakness, restlessness, pallor, perspiration, and collapse) can occur, even with the usual therapeutic dose. Alcohol may enhance this effect. Drug rash and/or exfoliative dermatitis may occasionally occur.
Dosage and Administration: One 60 mg. oral tempule® every 12 hours on an empty stomach. (Not recommended for sublingual use).
Although the onset of effect and the duration of effect of this drug are quite variable, the following are the generally reported ranges for these values:
Onset of effect: estimated to be 30 minutes.
Duration of effect: considered to be up to 12 hours.
How Supplied: Pentritol® 60 mg. tempules® identified by Armacode® PE are available in bottles of 60 and 250. Pentritol® 30 mg. identified by Armacode® PC in bottles of 100 and 250 tempules®.
[*Shown in Product Identification Section*]

ARMOUR THYROID (TABLETS) ℞

Description: Armour Thyroid Tablets are prepared by a *special* process from fresh, desiccated animal thyroid glands. Thus, the active thyroid hormones, l-thyroxine (T_4) and l-triiodothyronine (T_3) are available in their natural state and ratio for full therapeutic availability. Armour Thyroid is standardized both by the official U.S.P. method for iodine content and biologically assayed to assure full metabolic potency.
Action: The principal effect of thyroid hormones is to increase the metabolic rate of body tissues. The effect develops slowly but is prolonged. It begins within 48 hours and reaches a maximum in 8 to 10 days although full effects of continued administration may not be evident for several weeks.
The thyroid hormones are also concerned with growth and differentiation of tissues. In deficiency states in the young there is retardation of growth and failure of maturation of the skeletal and other body systems, especially in failure of ossification in the epiphyses and in the growth and development of the brain.
Thyroid administration increases the basal metabolic rate, increases the protein bound iodine (PBI) in the blood and lowers the level of blood cholesterol.
Euthyroid individuals often tolerate large doses of thyroid without an increase in metabolism.
Indications: Armour Thyroid is indicated as replacement or substitution therapy of diminished or absent thyroid function (e.g., cretinism, myxedema, nontoxic goiter or hypothyroidism generally, including the hypothyroid state in children, in pregnancy and in the elderly) resulting from functional deficiency, primary atrophy, from partial or complete absence of the gland or from the effects of surgery, radiation or anti-thyroid agents. Therapy must be maintained continuously to control the symptoms of hypothyroidism.
Contraindications: Armour Thyroid is contraindicated in the presence of thyrotoxicosis and in acute myocardial infarction uncomplicated by hypothyroidism. However, when hypothyroidism is a complicating or causative factor in myocardial infarction, or heart disease, the judicious use of small doses of Armour Thyroid should be considered. Where hypothyroidism and hypoadrenalism (Addison's Disease) coexist, Armour Thyroid is contraindicated unless treatment of hypoadrenalism with adrenocortical steroids precedes the initiation of Armour Thyroid therapy. (See Warnings)
Warnings:

Drugs with thyroid hormone activity, alone or together with other therapeutic agents, have been used for the treatment of obesity. In euthyroid patients, doses within the range of daily hormonal requirements are ineffective for weight reduction. Larger doses may produce serious or even life-threatening manifestations of toxicity, particularly when given in association with sympathomimetic amines such as those used for their anorectic effects.

Armour Thyroid should be used with caution in patients with cardiovascular disease, including hypertension. The development of chest pain or other aggravation of cardiovascular disease will require a decrease in dosage.
Injection of epinephrine in patients with coronary artery disease may precipitate an episode of coronary insufficiency. This may be enhanced in patients receiving thyroid preparations. Careful observation is required if catecholamines are administered to patients in this category. Patients with coronary artery disease should be carefully observed during surgery, since the possibility of precipitating cardiac arrhythmias may be greater in those treated with thyroid hormones.
Thyroid replacement may potentiate anticoagulant effects with agents such as warfarin or bishydroxy coumarin and reduction of one-third in anticoagulant dosage should be undertaken upon initiation of thyroid therapy. Subsequent anticoagulant dosage adjustment should be made on the basis of frequent prothrombin determinations.
In patients whose hypothyroidism is secondary to hypopituitarism, adrenal insufficiency will probably also be present. When adrenal insufficiency and hypothyroidism co-exist, the adrenal insufficiency should be corrected by corticosteroids before administering thyroid hormones.
Precautions: Patients with hypothyroidism, and especially myxedema, are particularly sensitive to thyroid preparations so that treatment should begin with small doses and increments should be gradual.
In patients with diabetes mellitus, addition of thyroid hormone therapy may cause an increase in the required dosage of insulin or oral hypoglycemic agents. Conversely, decreasing the dose of thyroid hormone may possibly cause hypoglycemic reactions if the dosage of insulin or oral hypoglycemic agents is not adjusted.
Adverse Reactions: Effects of overdosage include palpitation, tachycardia, cardiac arrhythmias, weight loss, angina pectoris, tremors, headache, diarrhea, nervousness, insomnia, sweating, and intolerance to heat and fever. If symptoms of excessive dosage appear, discontinue medication for several days and reinstitute treatment at a lower dosage level.

Dosage and Administration: As with any type of thyroid administration the dosage of Armour Thyroid must be individualized to approximate the deficit in the patient's thyroid secretion. The response of the patient is determined by clinical judgment in conjunction with laboratory findings. Generally, thyroid therapy is instituted at relatively low dosage levels and increased in small increments at intervals until the desired response is obtained. Armour thyroid is given as a single, daily dose, preferably before breakfast. [See table on next page].

In the normal individual PBI values range from 4-8 mcg./100 ml. Values below 4 mcg./100 ml. suggest hypothyroidism and the need for thyroid therapy. When clinical euthyroidism results from the use of Armour Thyroid, PBI values usually fall within the normal range.

In thyroid replacement therapy, observation of the patient is important and the clinical findings are paramount in achieving optimal results. In addition to PBI determinations other useful laboratory procedures include the T_3 Resin Uptake, blood cholesterol, the tendon reflex time and the free thyroxine determination.

Adult Myxedema. In adult myxedema with PBI values of 2.5 mcg./100 ml. or less, give ¼ gr. of Armour Thyroid a day. Usually after two weeks the dosage is increased to one ½ gr. tablet a day and two weeks later increased to one 1 gr. tablet daily. It is suggested that the patient be carefully assessed after one month of treatment with the 1 gr. dose and again after an additional month's treatment.

If necessary, daily dosage may then be increased to 2 gr. per day for two months and the examination repeated. If the values of the laboratory test used are low or if the clinical response is inadequate, dosage may be increased to 3 gr. Further increases, when necessary, may be made in increments of ½ or 1 gr. a day. The usual maintenance dose is from 1 gr. to 3 gr. per day, but it may vary, in individual patients from ½ to 10 gr.

Adult hypothyroidism without myxedema. When the PBI value ranges from 2.5 to 4.5 mcg./100 ml. the initial dose is usually one 1 gr. Armour Thyroid Tablet per day, increasing by 1 gr. every 30 days until the desired result is obtained. Clinical examination at monthly intervals and PBI values every three months are desirable. Maintenance doses are as above.

Children's Dosage. In cretinism or severe hypothyroidism in children the dosage regimen is as for adults with myxedema, with, however, each dosage increment made at intervals of two weeks. The final maintenance dose may be greater in the growing child than in the adult. The sleeping pulse and the basal morning temperature are simple, useful guides to treatment.

How Supplied: Bottles of 100, and larger and ½, 1 and 2 gr. in unit dose boxes of 100.

Armacode®

Potency	Code Marking
¼ gr.	TC
½ gr.	TD
1 gr.	TE
1½ gr.	TJ
2 gr.	TF
3 gr. (scored)	TG
4 gr.	TH
5 gr. (scored)	TI

[Shown in Product Identification Section]

THYROLAR® ℞

(liotrix, Armour)

Description: Thyrolar® tablets provide a combination of the synthetic active thyroid hormones, sodium levothyroxine and sodium liothyronine in a ratio of 4:1 by weight. Thyrolar® is available in six potencies approximately equivalent in therapeutic effect to ¼ gr., ½ gr., 1 gr., 2 gr. and 3 gr. of desiccated thyroid. In Thyrolar® 1 tablets a combination of 50 mcg. of sodium levothyroxine and 12.5 mcg. of sodium liothyronine represent the approximate activity of 1 gr. of desiccated thyroid. The other available potencies are proportional in strength.

Action: Thyrolar® is an effective agent for correcting the hypothyroid state and inducing clinical euthyroidism. The ratio of active hormones present closely simulates the clinical biochemical effects of desiccated thyroid and of the natural endogenous thyroid secretion. Thus, the various thyroid function parameters respond to Thyrolar® as they do to the administration of desiccated thyroid.

The principal effect of thyroid hormones is to increase the metabolic rate of body tissues. Sodium liothyronine is more readily absorbed from the gastrointestinal tract than is sodium levothyroxine. Excretion is rapid so that the action is dissipated more readily than is that of levothyroxine (T_4).

The effects of sodium levothyroxine develop slowly but are more prolonged.

With Thyrolar® the most widely used parameters of thyroid function may be used to aid in the assessment of the response since, when the euthyroid state is achieved, the values may ordinarily be expected to fall within the normal range. This is not true with sodium liothyronine administration alone where subnormal values are present or with sodium levothyroxine alone where abnormally high values are associated with clinical euthyroidism.

Indications: Thyrolar® is indicated in the treatment of hypothyroidism as a source of exogenous thyroid hormone in diminished or absent thyroid function. This may be due to the use of antithyroid agents, radiation therapy, primary atrophy, partial or complete surgical removal of the gland or it may be functional in nature.

Thyrolar® is efficacious in the treatment of hypothyroidism regardless of the etiology. The use of Thyrolar® for suppression therapy in simple (non-toxic) goiter gives prompt results in reducing the size of the gland.

Contraindications: Thyrolar® administration is contraindicated in thyrotoxicosis and in acute myocardial infarction.

Thyrolar® is contraindicated in the presence of uncorrected adrenal insufficiency because it increases the tissue demands for adrenocortical hormones and may cause an acute adrenal crisis in such patients (See Warnings).

Warnings:

> Drugs with thyroid hormone activity, alone or together with other therapeutic agents, have been used for the treatment of obesity. In euthyroid patients, doses within the range of daily hormonal requirements are ineffective for weight reduction. Larger doses may produce serious or even life-threatening manifestations of toxicity, particularly when given in association with sympathomimetic amines such as those used for their anorectic effects.

Thyrolar® should be used with caution in patients with cardiovascular disease, including hypertension. The development of chest pain or other aggravation of cardiovascular disease will require a decrease in dosage.

Injection of epinephrine in patients with coronary artery disease may precipitate an episode of coronary insufficiency. This may be enhanced in patients receiving thyroid preparations. Careful observation is required if catecholamines are administered to patients in this category. Thyrolar® treated patients with concomitant coronary artery disease should be carefully observed during surgery since the possibility of precipitating cardiac arrhythmias may be greater in patients treated with thyroid hormones.

The institution of thyroid replacement therapy may potentiate anticoagulant effects with agents such as warfarin or bishydroxycoumarin and reduction of one-third in anticoagulant dosage should be undertaken upon initiation of Thyrolar® therapy. Subsequent anticoagulant dosage adjustment should be made on the basis of frequent prothrombin determinations.

In patients whose hypothyroidism is secondary to hypopituitarism, adrenal insufficiency will probably also be present. When the adrenal insufficiency and hypothyroidism coexist, the adrenal insufficiency should be corrected by corticosteroids before administering thyroid hormones.

Precautions: Patients with hypothyroidism and especially myxedema are particularly sensitive to thyroid preparations so that treatment should begin with small doses and increments should be gradual. In patients with diabetes mellitus addition of thyroid hormone therapy may cause an increase in the required dosage of insulin or oral hypoglycemic agents. Conversely, decreasing the dose of thyroid hormone may possibly cause hypoglycemic reactions if the dosage of insulin or oral agents is not adjusted.

Adverse Reactions: Excessive dosage of thyroid medication may result in symptoms of hyperthyroidism. Since, however, the effects do not appear at once, the symptoms may not appear for 1 to 3 weeks after the dosage regimen is begun. The most common signs and symptoms of overdosage are weight loss, palpitation, nervousness, diarrhea or abdominal cramps, sweating, tachycardia, cardiac arrhythmias, angina pectoris, tremors, headache, insomnia, intolerance to heat, fever. If symptoms of overdosage appear, discontinue medication for several days and reinstitute treatment at a lower dosage level.

In some individuals who are euthyroid on Thyrolar® headache may appear. Dosage should be decreased. If headache persists or the patient develops signs of hypothyroidism on the lower dosage, another thyroid preparation should be substituted.

Dosage and Administration: As with all thyroid preparations, the dosage of Thyrolar® must be individualized to approximate the deficit in the patient's thyroid secretion. The response of the patient is determined by clinical judgment in conjunction with laboratory findings.

For newly diagnosed or untreated hypothyroidism, therapy may be initiated with one tablet of Thyrolar® ¼ or Thyrolar® ½ daily depending on the patient's status and increased gradually every one or two weeks. In children, increments in dosage should be made every two weeks. For unstabilized hypothyroid patients receiving some form of thyroid therapy direct substitution of Thyrolar® for the current dose of the other product can be made, with gradual increase in dose every one to two weeks.

In patients previously rendered euthyroid with desiccated thyroid, sodium levothyroxine or sodium liothyronine, each Thyrolar®-1 tablet will usually replace 1 grain of desiccated thyroid, 0.1 mg. sodium levothyroxine or 25 mcg. sodium liothyronine. Dosage adjustments, other than those routinely necessary with any thyroid therapy, are seldom necessary.

Thyrolar® is usually given as a single daily dose preferably before breakfast in the morning.

In the normal euthyroid individual, PBI values range from 4 to 8 micrograms/100 ml. and with Thyrolar® values in this range usually correspond to the clinical euthyroid state. Other useful tests include the T_3-resin uptake tests, T_4 by Column and Free thyroxine. In patients rendered euthyroid with Thyrolar®, these

Continued on next page

Armour—Cont.

tests usually give values within the normal range.

How Supplied: Thyrolar® is available in six potencies, coded as follows:
(See table below)
Supplied in bottles of 100, two-layered compressed tablets. Thyrolar®-½, Thyrolar®-1, Thyrolar®-2, and Thyrolar®-3 are also supplied in bottles of 1000.
[*Shown in Product Identification Section*]

THYTROPAR® ℞
(thyrotropin for injection)
U.S. PAT. No. 2,871,159

Description:
THYTROPAR® (Thyrotropin for Injection) is a highly purified and lyophilized thyrotropic or thyroid stimulating hormone (TSH) isolated from bovine anterior pituitary. The potency of THYTROPAR® is designated in terms of International Thyrotropin units and is free of significant amounts of adrenocorticotropic, gonadotropic, somatotropic and posterior pituitary hormones. It is soluble throughout a wide pH range and is stable at room temperature when kept in the dry state. It dissolves readily in physiologic saline and will retain its potency when in solution for at least two weeks if refrigerated.
Thytropar® Diluent (Sodium Chloride Injection) contains in each ml 9 mg. of Sodium Chloride, Water for Injection, q.s.

Action:
The action of the thyrotropic hormone may be briefly described as fourfold, the degree of action depending upon the amount of the hormone acting upon the thyroid:
1. Increases iodine uptake by the thyroid.
2. Increases formation of thyroid hormone.
3. Increases secretion or release of thyroid hormone.
4. Causes a hyperplasia of thyroid cells.

When given exogenously as THYTROPAR® the fourth effect is not significant clinically in doses recommended except as it results in the other three desirable effects. The process is rapidly reversible following a given dose or series of doses.
THYTROPAR® offers a safe and useful tool for both diagnosis and treatment of certain types of thyroid disease. The increase in the thyroid gland's uptake of tracer doses of radioactive iodine and of the serum protein-bound iodine following a single injection of THYTROPAR® has enabled its use in diagnostic tests which are sufficiently simple to be practical for routine clinical application. Through its use the ability of the human thyroid gland to respond to stimulation can now be determined, and this property has certain unique diagnostic advantages. Furthermore, THYTROPAR® has been helpful in the treatment of certain disorders of the thyroid gland.

Indications:
A. Diagnostic applications of Thytropar (Thyrotropin for Injection)
   1. To determine subclinical hypothyroidism or low thyroid reserve.
   2. To differentiate between primary and secondary hypothyroidism.
   3. To differentiate between primary hypothyroidism and euthyroidism in patients whose thyroid function has been suppressed by the administration of thyroid replacement therapy.
   4. To aid in detection of remnants and metastases of thyroid carcinoma.
B. Therapeutic application of Thytropar (Thyrotropin for Injection)
   1. As an adjunct in the management of certain types of functioning thyroid carcinoma and resulting metastases.

Contraindications:
1. Hypersensitivity to thyrotropin.
2. Coronary thrombosis.
3. Untreated Addison's disease.

Precautions:
1. Use THYTROPAR® with caution in the presence of angina pectoris or cardiac failure.
2. Use with care in the presence of hypopituitarism since varying degrees of adrenal cortical atrophy are generally present with this condition. Adrenal cortical suppression as may be seen with corticosteroid therapy should not be overlooked.

Adverse Reactions:
Menstrual irregularities, nausea, vomiting, urticaria, transitory hypotension, tachycardia, auricular fibrillation, fever, headache, thyroid swelling, post injection flare, and anaphylactic reactions have been reported. The hypotension appears to be part of an allergic type reaction whereas the thyroid swelling is related to larger doses (10–20 units) which some workers have employed. The swelling is self-limited when the hormone is discontinued.

Dosage and Administration:
Thytropar (Thyrotropin for Injection) is administered intramuscularly or subcutaneously after dissolving the material in sterile physiologic saline solution. Ten International Units of Thytropar per 2 ml. of diluent is a satisfactory ratio of dilution for injection.
1. Use of Thytropar in PBI or I^{131} uptake determinations in the differential diagnosis of subclinical hypothyroidism or low thyroid reserve: 10 International Units.
2. To determine thyroid status in a patient receiving thyroid medication: 10 International Units for 1–3 days.*
3. In the differential diagnosis of primary and secondary hypothyroidism: 10 International Units for 1–3 days.*
4. Diagnosis of thyroid cancer remnant with I^{131} after surgery: 10 International Units for 3–7 days.
5. Therapy of thyroid carcinoma (local tumor or metastases) with I^{131}: 10 International Units for 3–8 days.

Overdosage:
SYMPTOMS—Headache, irritability, nervousness, sweating, tachycardia, increased bowel motility, menstrual irregularities. Angina pectoris or congestive heart failure may be induced or aggravated. Shock may also develop. Excessive doses may result in symptoms resembling thyroid storm. Chronic excessive dosage will produce the signs and symptoms of hyperthyroidism.
TREATMENT—in shock, supportive measures and treatment of unrecognized adrenal insufficiency should be considered. Thyrotropin is discontinued.

How Supplied:
THYTROPAR® is supplied as a sterile lyophilized powder containing 10 International Units of Thyrotropic activity according to the chick thyroid iodine depletion assay method of Piotrowski (Walaszek) Steelman and Koch (Endocrinology 52: 489, 1953) when compared to the International Reference Standard. Each package contains one vial of THYTROPAR® (Thyrotropin for injection) and one vial of Thytropar® Diluent (Sodium Chloride Injection).

*The 3-day schedule may be indicated in those who have received thyroid medication for prolonged periods or in those with long-standing pituitary myxedema.

Name	Composition (T_4/T_3 per Tablet)	Color	Armacode®	Desiccated Thyroid—Approximate Equivalence
Thyrolar®—¼	12.5 mcg./3.1 mcg.	Violet/White	YC	¼ gr.
Thyrolar®—½	25 mcg./6.25 mcg.	Peach/White	YD	½ gr.
Thyrolar®—1	50 mcg./12.5 mcg.	Pink/White	YE	1 gr.
Thyrolar®—2	100 mcg./25 mcg.	Green/White	YF	2 gr.
Thyrolar®—3	150 mcg./37.5 mcg.	Yellow/White	YH	3 gr.

TUSSAR® DM
Cough Syrup
Non-narcotic, Alcohol Free
Antitussive/Decongestant/Antihistaminic

Each 5 ml (one teaspoonful) contains:
Dextromethorphan
  Hydrobromide, N.F. ....15 mg
Chlorpheniramine Maleate, U.S.P. ....2 mg
Phenylephrine Hydrochloride, U.S.P. ....5 mg
Methylparaben, U.S.P. 0.1%

Indications: For relief of cough due to common cold and minor throat and bronchial irritations. TUSSAR DM provides relief of nasal congestion, running nose and watery eyes as may occur in allergic rhinitis (such as hay fever).

Directions For Use: ADULTS—One or two teaspoonfuls (5 or 10 ml) every six to eight hours, not to exceed eight teaspoonfuls in any 24-hour period.
CHILDREN 6–12 YEARS—One teaspoonful (5 ml) every six to eight hours, not to exceed four teaspoonfuls in any 24-hour period.
CHILDREN UNDER 6 YEARS—Not to be administered unless directed by a physician.

Warnings: Do not take this product for persistent cough which may indicate a serious condition except under the supervision of a physician. Do not take this product if you have high blood pressure, heart disease or thyroid disease unless directed by a physician. Do not exceed recommended dosage.

Cautions: If symptoms persist for more than 7 days or are accompanied by a high fever, rash or persistent headache, consult a physician. If drowsiness occurs, do not drive a car or operate machinery.

TUSSAR®-2 Ⓒ
(exempt narcotic cough syrup)

Each 5 ml (one teaspoonful) contains:
Codeine Phosphate, U.S.P. ....10 mg
(Warning—may be habit-forming)
Carbetapentane Citrate, N.F. ....7.5 mg
Chlorpheniramine Maleate, U.S.P. ....2.0 mg
Glyceryl Guaiacolate, N.F. ....50 mg
Sodium Citrate, U.S.P. ....130 mg
Citric Acid, U.S.P. ....20 mg
Methylparaben, U.S.P. 0.1%
Alcohol 5%

Indications: For relief of severe coughs due to respiratory conditions caused by common cold, bronchitis, and influenza.

Dosage: One teaspoonful 3 to 4 times a day as needed for cough, but no more than 8 teaspoonfuls in any 24-hour period.

Cautions: Persistent cough may indicate the presence of a serious condition. Secure medical advice if there is a high fever or if relief does not occur within 3 days. Persons with a high fever or persistent cough should use only on advice of a physician. Not to be administered to infants or children unless directed by a physician. If drowsiness occurs, do not drive a car or operate machinery.

TUSSAR SF (Sugar Free) ℭ
(exempt narcotic cough syrup)

Formulation identical to Tussar-2, except Tussar SF contains saccharine-sorbitol base for patients who must limit sugar intake. Alcohol content 12 percent instead of 5 percent.

THERAPEUTIC BLOOD DERIVATIVE PRODUCTS

ANTIHEMOPHILIC FACTOR (HUMAN) DRIED FACTORATE® ℞

Antihemophilic Factor (Human)—FACTORATE® is supplied in single dose vials (AHF activity is stated on label of each vial) with sterile diluent and needles for reconstitution and withdrawal.

IMMUNE SERUM GLOBULIN (HUMAN) U.S.P. GAMMAR® ℞

Immune Serum Globulin (Human) U.S.P. is supplied in 2 ml. and 10 ml. vials.

NORMAL SERUM ALBUMIN (HUMAN) U.S.P. 5% ALBUMINAR®-5 ℞

Normal Serum Albumin (Human) ALBUMINAR®-5 is supplied as a 5% solution in:
250 ml. bottles containing 12.5 grams of albumin
500 ml. bottles containing 25.0 grams of albumin
For use with intravenous administration set. See directions on set supplied.

NORMAL SERUM ALBUMIN (HUMAN) U.S.P. 25% ALBUMINAR®-25 ℞

Normal Serum Albumin (Human), ALBUMINAR®-25 is supplied as a 25% solution in:
20 ml. vials containing 5.0 grams of albumin
50 ml. vials containing 12.5 grams of albumin
100 ml. vials containing 25.0 grams of albumin
For use with intravenous administration set. See directions on set supplied.

Arnar-Stone Laboratories, Inc.
McGAW PARK, IL 60085

AMERICAINE® AEROSOL

(See PDR For Nonprescription Drugs)

AMERICAINE® HEMORRHOIDAL OINTMENT

(See PDR For Nonprescription Drugs)

AMERICAINE®-OTIC ℞

Description: Americaine-Otic is a pale yellow, non-aqueous liquid containing 20% benzocaine in a water-soluble base of 1% (w/w) glycerin and polyethylene glycol-300 with benzethonium chloride as a preservative.
Indications: For relief of pain and pruritus in acute congestive and serous otitis media, acute swimmer's ear and otitis externa.
Caution: For external use only. Do not use in infants under one year of age. Discontinue if sensitivity occurs.
Warning: Indiscriminate use of anesthetic ear drops may mask symptoms of fulminating infection of the middle ear.
Administration: Lay patient on side with affected ear up. Clean ear with Americaine-Otic saturated swab. Instill 4–5 drops warm Americaine-Otic along side of auditory canal to prevent air pocket. Insert cotton pledget in meatus. Patient should remain on side for several minutes.
Caution: Federal law prohibits dispensing without prescription.
Supplied: ½ oz. plastic dropper-top bottle.

BRETYLOL® ℞
(bretylium tosylate)
INJECTION
For Intramuscular or Intravenous Use

Description: BRETYLOL (bretylium tosylate) is o-Bromobenzyl ethyl-dimethylammonium p-toluene sulfonate.
BRETYLOL is a white, crystalline powder with an extremely bitter taste. It is freely soluble in water and alcohol. Each ml of sterile, non-pyrogenic solution contains 50 mg bretylium tosylate in Water for Injection, USP. The pH is adjusted, when necessary, with dilute hydrochloric acid or sodium hydroxide. BRETYLOL contains no preservative.
Clinical Pharmacology: BRETYLOL (bretylium tosylate) is a bromobenzyl quaternary ammonium compound which selectively accumulates in sympathetic ganglia and their postganglionic adrenergic neurons where it inhibits norepinephrine release by depressing adrenergic nerve terminal excitability.
BRETYLOL also suppresses ventricular fibrillation and ventricular arrhythmias. The mechanisms of the antifibrillatory and antiarrhythmic actions of BRETYLOL are not established. In efforts to define these mechanisms, the following electrophysiologic actions of BRETYLOL have been demonstrated in animal experiments:
1. Increase in ventricular fibrillation threshold.
2. Increase in action potential duration and effective refractory period without changes in heart rate.
3. Little effect on the rate of rise or amplitude of the cardiac action potential (Phase 0) or in resting membrane potential (Phase 4) in normal myocardium. However, when cell injury slows the rate of rise, decreases amplitude, and lowers resting membrane potential, BRETYLOL restores these parameters toward normal.
4. Increase in impulse formation and spontaneous firing rate of pacemaker tissue as well as increased ventricular induction velocity.

The restoration of injured myocardial cell electrophysiology toward normal, as well as the increase of the action potential duration and effective refractory period without changing their ratio to each other, may be important factors in suppressing re-entry of aberrant impulses and decreasing induced dispersion of local excitable states.
BRETYLOL induces a chemical sympathectomy-like state which resembles a surgical sympathectomy. Catecholamine stores are not depleted by BRETYLOL, but catecholamine effects on the myocardium and on peripheral vascular resistance are often seen shortly after administration because BRETYLOL causes an early release of norepinephrine from the adrenergic postganglionic nerve terminals. Subsequently, BRETYLOL blocks the release of norepinephrine in response to neuron stimulation. Peripheral adrenergic blockade regularly causes orthostatic hypotension but has less effect on supine blood pressure. The relationship of adrenergic blockade to the antifibrillatory and antiarrhythmic actions of BRETYLOL is not clear. In a study in patients with frequent ventricular premature beats, peak plasma concentration of BRETYLOL and peak hypotensive effects were seen within one hour of intramuscular administration, presumably reflecting adrenergic neuronal blockade. However, suppression of premature ventricular beats was not maximal until 6-9 hours after dosing, when mean plasma concentration had declined to less than one-half of peak level. This suggests a slower mechanism, other than neuronal blockade, was involved in suppression of the arrhythmia. On the other hand, antifibrillatory effects can be seen within minutes of an intravenous injection, suggesting that the effect on the myocardium may occur quite rapidly.
BRETYLOL has a positive inotropic effect on the myocardium, but it is not yet certain whether this effect is direct or is mediated by catecholamine release.
BRETYLOL is eliminated intact by the kidneys. No metabolites have been identified following administration of BRETYLOL in man and laboratory animals. In man, approximately 70 to 80% of a ^{14}C-labelled intramuscular dose is excreted in the urine during the first 24 hours, with an additional 10% excreted over the next three days.
In various studies of BRETYLOL excretion, estimates of the terminal half-life have varied from about 5 to about 10 hours, with an even wider range in individual subjects (4 to 17 hours). Whether this represents true intrapatient variability or limitations of methodology remains to be determined.
Effect on Heart Rate: There is sometimes an initial small increase in heart rate when BRETYLOL is administered, but this is an inconsistent and transient occurrence.
Hemodynamic Effects: Following intravenous administration of 5 mg/kg of BRETYLOL to patients with acute myocardial infarction, there was a mild increase in arterial pressure, followed by a modest decrease, remaining within normal limits throughout. Pulmonary artery pressures, pulmonary capillary wedge pressure, right atrial pressure, cardiac index, stroke volume index, and stroke work index were not significantly changed. These hemodynamic effects were not correlated with antiarrhythmic activity.
Onset of Action: Suppression of ventricular fibrillation is rapid, usually occurring within minutes following intravenous administration. Suppression of ventricular tachycardia and other ventricular arrhythmias develops more slowly, usually 20 minutes to 2 hours after parenteral administration.
Indications: BRETYLOL is indicated in the treatment of life-threatening ventricular arrhythmias, principally ventricular fibrillation and ventricular tachycardia, that have failed to respond to adequate doses of a first-line antiarrhythmic agent, such as lidocaine or procainamide. At this time, BRETYLOL should not be considered a first-line antiarrhythmic agent.
Use of BRETYLOL should be limited to intensive care units, coronary care units or other facilities where equipment and personnel for constant monitoring of cardiac arrhythmias and blood pressure are available.
Following injection of BRETYLOL there may be a delay of 20 minutes to 2 hours in the onset of antiarrhythmic action, although it appears to act within minutes in ventricular fibrillation. The delay in effect appears to be longer after intramuscular than after intravenous injection.
Contraindications: There are no contraindications to use in treatment of ventricular fibrillation or life-threatening refractory ventricular arrhythmias.
Warnings:
1. Hypotension
Administration of BRETYLOL regularly results in postural hypotension, subjectively recognized by dizziness, light-headedness, vertigo or faintness. Some degree of hypotension is present in about 50% of patients while they are supine. Hypotension may occur at doses lower than those needed to suppress arrhythmias.

Patients should be kept in the supine position until tolerance to the hypotensive effect of BRETYLOL develops. Tolerance

Continued on next page

Arnar-Stone—Cont.

occurs unpredictably but may be present after several days.

Hypotension with supine systolic pressure greater than 75 mm Hg need not be treated unless there are associated symptoms. If supine systolic pressure falls below 75 mm Hg, an infusion of dopamine or norepinephrine may be used to raise blood pressure. When catecholamines are administered, a dilute solution should be employed and blood pressure monitored closely because the pressor effects of the catecholamines are enhanced by BRETYLOL. Volume expansion with blood or plasma and correction of dehydration should be carried out where appropriate.

2. Transient Hypertension and Increased Frequency of Arrhythmias
Due to the initial release of norepinephrine from adrenergic postganglionic nerve terminals by BRETYLOL, transient hypertension or increased frequency of premature ventricular contractions and other arrhythmias may occur in some patients.

3. Caution During Use with Digitalis Glycosides
The initial release of norepinephrine caused by BRETYLOL may aggravate digitalis toxicity. When a life-threatening cardiac arrhythmia occurs in a digitalized patient, BRETYLOL should be used only if the etiology of the arrhythmia does not appear to be digitalis toxicity and other antiarrhythmic drugs are not effective. Simultaneous initiation of therapy with digitalis glycosides and BRETYLOL should be avoided.

4. Patients with Fixed Cardiac Output
In patients with fixed cardiac output (i.e., severe aortic stenosis or severe pulmonary hypertension), BRETYLOL should be avoided since severe hypotension may result from a fall in peripheral resistance without a compensatory increase in cardiac output. If survival is threatened by the arrhythmia, BRETYLOL may be used but vasoconstrictive catecholamines should be given promptly if severe hypotension occurs.

Use in Pregnancy: The safety of BRETYLOL in human pregnancy has not been established. However, as the drug is intended for use only in life-threatening situations, it may be used in pregnant women when its benefits outweigh the potential risk to the fetus.

Use in Children: The safety and efficacy of this drug in children has not been established. BRETYLOL has been administered to a limited number of pediatric patients, but such use has been inadequate to define fully proper dosage and limitations for use.

Precautions:

1. Dilution for Intravenous Use
BRETYLOL should be diluted (one part BRETYLOL with four parts of Dextrose Injection, USP or Sodium Chloride Injection, USP) prior to intravenous use. Rapid intravenous administration may cause severe nausea and vomiting. Therefore, the diluted solution should be infused over a period greater than 8 minutes. In treating existing ventricular fibrillation BRETYLOL should be given as rapidly as possible and may be given without dilution.

2. Use Various Sites for Intramuscular Injection
When injected intramuscularly, not more than 5 ml should be given in a site, and injection sites should be varied since repeated intramuscular injection into the same site may cause atrophy and necrosis of muscle tissue, fibrosis, vascular degeneration and inflammatory changes.

3. Reduce Dosage in Impaired Renal Function
Since BRETYLOL is excreted principally via the kidney, dosage should be reduced in patients with impaired renal function.

Adverse Reactions: Hypotension and postural hypotension have been the most frequently reported adverse reactions (see Warnings section). Nausea and vomiting occurred in about three percent of patients, primarily when BRETYLOL was administered rapidly by the intravenous route (See Precautions section). Vertigo, dizziness, light-headedness and syncope, which sometimes accompanied postural hypotension, were reported in about 7 patients in 1000.
Bradycardia, increased frequency of premature ventricular contractions, transitory hypertension, initial increase in arrhythmias (see Warnings section), precipitation of anginal attacks, and sensation of substernal pressure have also been reported in a small number of patients, i.e., approximately 1-2 patients in 1000.
Renal dysfunction, diarrhea, abdominal pain, hiccups, erythematous macular rash, flushing, hyperthermia, confusion, paranoid psychosis, emotional lability, lethargy, generalized tenderness, anxiety, shortness of breath, diaphoresis, nasal stuffiness and mild conjunctivitis have been reported in about 1 patient in 1000. The relationship of BRETYLOL administration to these reactions has not been clearly established.

Dosage and Administration: BRETYLOL is to be used clinically only for treatment of life-threatening ventricular arrhythmias under constant electrocardiographic monitoring. Since there is a delay in onset of its antiarrhythmic action, BRETYLOL is not to be considered or used as a replacement for rapidly-acting antiarrhythmic agents currently in use. The clinical use of BRETYLOL is for short-term use only. Patients should either be kept supine during the course of BRETYLOL therapy or be closely observed for postural hypotension. The optimal dose schedule for parenteral administration of BRETYLOL has not been determined. There is comparatively little experience with dosages greater than 30 mg/kg/day, although such doses have been used without apparent adverse effects. The following schedule is suggested:

A. For Immediately Life-threatening Ventricular Arrhythmia, as in Ventricular Fibrillation: Administer undiluted BRETYLOL at a dosage of 5 mg/kg of body weight by rapid intravenous injection. Other usual cardiopulmonary resuscitative procedures, including electrical cardioversion, should be employed prior to and following the injection in accordance with good medical practice. If ventricular fibrillation persists, the dosage may be increased to 10 mg/kg and repeated at 15 to 30 minute intervals until a total dose of not more than 30 mg/kg of body weight has been given. For maintenance dosage, see below.

B. Other Ventricular Arrhythmias:

1. Intravenous Use: **BRETYLOL must be diluted as follows before intravenous administration:** Using aseptic technique, dilute contents of one BRETYLOL ampul (10 ml containing 500 mg bretylium tosylate) to a minimum of 50 ml with Dextrose injection, USP or Sodium Chloride Injection, USP.
   Administer the diluted solution at a dosage of 5 to 10 mg BRETYLOL per kg of body weight by intravenous infusion over a period greater than 8 minutes. More rapid infusion may cause nausea and vomiting. A second dose may be given in 1 to 2 hours if the arrhythmia persists.
2. For Intramuscular Injection: (**Do not dilute BRETYLOL prior to intramuscular injection.**) Inject 5 to 10 mg BRETYLOL per kg of body weight. Dosage may be repeated in 1 to 2 hours if the arrhythmia persists. Thereafter maintain with same dosage every 6 to 8 hours.
   Intramuscular injection should not be made directly into or near a major nerve, and the site of injection should be varied on repeated injection.

C. Maintenance Dosage: The diluted BRETYLOL solution may be administered by intermittent bolus infusion or by constant infusion.

1. Intermittent Infusion: Infuse the diluted solution at a dosage of 5 to 10 mg BRETYLOL per kg body weight, over a period greater than 8 minutes, every 6 hours. More rapid infusion may cause nausea and vomiting.
2. Constant Infusion: Infuse the diluted solution at a dosage of 1 to 2 mg BRETYLOL per minute.

Dosage of BRETYLOL should be reduced and discontinued in 3 to 5 days under electrocardiographic monitoring. Other appropriate antiarrhythmic agents should be substituted, if indicated.

How Supplied: NDC 0094-0012-10: 10 ml ampul containing 500 mg bretylium tosylate in Water for Injection, USP. pH adjusted, when necessary, with dilute hydrochloric acid or sodium hydroxide. Sterile, non-pyrogenic.
Re. Pat. No. 29618

INTROPIN® ℞
(dopamine HCl)
5 ml AMPUL and 5 ml RAP-ADD® Syringe

Description: INTROPIN (dopamine HCl) is 3,4-dihydroxyphenethylamine hydrochloride, a naturally-occurring biochemical catecholamine precursor of norepinephrine.
Dopamine hydrochloride is a white, odorless crystalline powder, freely soluble in water and soluble in alcohol. It is sensitive to light, alkalis, iron salts and oxidizing agents.

5 ml AMPUL AND ADDITIVE SYRINGE: Each ml of sterile, non-pyrogenic INTROPIN Injection contains 40 mg of dopamine hydrochloride (equivalent to 32.3 mg of dopamine base) in Water for Injection, USP, containing 1% sodium bisulfite as a preservative.

Actions: INTROPIN exerts an inotropic effect on the myocardium resulting in an increased cardiac output. INTROPIN produces less increase in myocardial oxygen consumption than isoproterenol and its use is usually not associated with a tachyarrhythmia. Clinical studies indicate that INTROPIN usually increases systolic and pulse pressure with either no effect or a slight increase in diastolic pressure. Total peripheral resistance at low and intermediate therapeutic doses is usually unchanged. Blood flow to peripheral vascular beds may decrease while mesenteric flow increases. INTROPIN has also been reported to dilate the renal vasculature presumptively by activation of a "dopaminergic" receptor. This action is accompanied by increases in glomerular filtration rate, renal blood flow, and sodium excretion. An increase in urinary output produced by dopamine is usually not associated with a decrease in osmolality of the urine.

Indications: INTROPIN is indicated for the correction of hemodynamic imbalances present in the shock syndrome due to myocardial infarctions, trauma, endotoxic septicemia, open heart surgery, renal failure, and chronic cardiac decompensation as in congestive failure.
Where appropriate, restoration of blood volume with a suitable plasma expander or whole blood should be instituted or completed prior to administration of INTROPIN.
Patients most likely to respond adequately to INTROPIN are those in whom physiological parameters, such as urine flow, myocardial function, and blood pressure, have not undergone profound deterioration. Multiclinic trials indicate that the shorter the time interval be-

tween onset of signs and symptoms and initiation of therapy with volume correction and INTROPIN, the better the prognosis.

Poor Perfusion of Vital Organs—Urine flow appears to be one of the better diagnostic signs by which adequacy of vital organ perfusion can be monitored. Nevertheless, the physician should also observe the patient for signs of reversal of confusion or comatose condition. Loss of pallor, increase in toe temperature, and/or adequacy of nail bed capillary filling may also be used as indices of adequate dosage. Clinical studies have shown that when INTROPIN is administered before urine flow has diminished to levels approximately 0.3 ml./minute, prognosis is more favorable. Nevertheless, in a number of oliguric or anuric patients, administration of INTROPIN has resulted in an increase in urine flow which in some cases reached normal levels. INTROPIN may also increase urine flow in patients whose output is within normal limits and thus may be of value in reducing the degree of pre-existing fluid accumulation. It should be noted that at doses above those optimal for the individual patient, urine flow may decrease, necessitating reduction of dosage. Concurrent administration of INTROPIN and diuretic agents may produce an additive or potentiating effect.

Low Cardiac Output—Increased cardiac output is related to INTROPIN's direct inotropic effect on the myocardium. Increased cardiac output at low or moderate doses appears to be related to a favorable prognosis. Increase in cardiac output has been associated with either static or decreased systemic vascular resistance (SVR). Static or decreased SVR associated with low or moderate increments in cardiac output is believed to be a reflection of differential effects on specific vascular beds with increased resistance in peripheral beds (e.g. femoral) and concomitant decreases in mesenteric and renal vascular beds. Redistribution of blood flow parallels these changes so that an increase in cardiac output is accompanied by an increase in mesenteric and renal blood flow. In many instances the renal fraction of the total cardiac output has been found to increase. Increase in cardiac output produced by INTROPIN is not associated with substantial decreases in systemic vascular resistance as may occur with isoproterenol.

Hypotension—Hypotension due to inadequate cardiac output can be managed by administration of low to moderate doses of INTROPIN, which have little effect on SVR. At high therapeutic doses, INTROPIN's alpha adrenergic activity becomes more prominent and thus may correct hypotension due to diminished SVR. As in the case of other circulatory decompensation states, prognosis is better in patients whose blood pressure and urine flow have not undergone profound deterioration. Therefore, it is suggested that the physician administer INTROPIN as soon as a definite trend toward decreased systolic and diastolic pressure becomes evident.

Contraindications: INTROPIN should not be used in patients with pheochromocytoma.

Warnings: INTROPIN should not be administered in the presence of uncorrected tachyarrhythmias or ventricular fibrillation.

Do **NOT** add INTROPIN to any alkaline diluent solution, since the drug is inactivated in alkaline solution.

Patients who have been treated with monamine oxidase (MAO) inhibitors prior to the administration of INTROPIN will require substantially reduced dosage. Dopamine is metabolized by MAO, and inhibition of this enzyme prolongs and potentiates the effect of INTROPIN. The starting dose in such patients should be reduced to at least one-tenth ($^1/_{10}$) of the usual dose.

Usage in Pregnancy—Animal studies have revealed no evidence of teratogenic effects from INTROPIN. In one study, administration of INTROPIN to pregnant rats resulted in a decreased survival rate of the newborn and a potential for cataract formation in the survivors. The drug may be used in pregnant women when, in the judgment of the physician, the expected benefits outweigh the potential risk to the fetus.

Usage in Children—The safety and efficacy of this drug in children has not been established. INTROPIN has been used in a limited number of pediatric patients, but such use has been inadequate to fully define proper dosage and limitations for use. Further studies are in progress.

Precautions: Avoid Hypovolemia—Prior to treatment with INTROPIN, hypovolemia should be fully corrected, if possible, with either whole blood or plasma as indicated.

Decreased Pulse Pressure—If a disproportionate rise in the diastolic pressure (i.e., a marked decrease in the pulse pressure) is observed in patients receiving INTROPIN, the infusion rate should be decreased and the patient observed carefully for further evidence of predominant vasoconstrictor activity, unless such an effect is desired.

Extravasation—INTROPIN should be infused into a large vein whenever possible to prevent the possibility of extravasation into tissue adjacent to the infusion site. Extravasation may cause necrosis and sloughing of surrounding tissue. Large veins of the antecubital fossa are preferred to veins in the dorsum of the hand or ankle. Less suitable infusion sites should be used only if the patient's condition requires immediate attention. The physician should switch to more suitable sites as rapidly as possible. The infusion site should be continuously monitored for free flow.

Occlusive Vascular Disease—Patients with a history of occlusive vascular disease (for example, atherosclerosis, arterial embolism, Raynaud's disease, cold injury, diabetic endarteritis, and Buerger's disease) should be closely monitored for any changes in color or temperature of the skin in the extremities. If a change in skin color or temperature occurs and is thought to be the result of compromised circulation to the extremities, the benefits of continued INTROPIN infusion should be weighed against the risk of possible necrosis. This condition may be reversed by either decreasing or discontinuing the rate of infusion.

IMPORTANT—Antidote for Peripheral Ischemia: To prevent sloughing and necrosis in ischemic areas, the area should be infiltrated as soon as possible with 10 to 15 ml. of Saline solution containing from 5 to 10 mg. of Regitine® (brand of phentolamine), an adrenergic blocking agent. A syringe with a fine hypodermic needle should be used, and the solution liberally infiltrated throughout the ischemic area. Sympathetic blockade with phentolamine causes immediate and conspicuous local hyperemic changes if the area is infiltrated within 12 hours. Therefore, phentolamine should be given as soon as possible after the extravasation is noted.

Avoid Cyclopropane or Halogenated Hydrocarbon Anesthetics—Cyclopropane or halogenated hydrocarbon anesthetics increase cardiac autonomic irritability and therefore may sensitize the myocardium to the action of certain intravenously administered catecholamines. This interaction appears to be related both to pressor activity and to beta adrenergic stimulating properties of these catecholamines. Therefore, as with certain other catecholamines, and because of the theoretical arrhythmogenic potential, INTROPIN should be used with EXTREME CAUTION in patients inhaling cyclopropane or halogenated hydrocarbon anesthetics.

Careful Monitoring Required—Close monitoring of the following indices—urine flow, cardiac output and blood pressure—during INTROPIN infusion is necessary as in the case of any adrenergic agent.

Adverse Reactions: The most frequent adverse reactions observed in clinical evaluation of INTROPIN included ectopic beats, nausea, vomiting, tachycardia, anginal pain, palpitation, dyspnea, headache, hypotension, and vasoconstriction. Other adverse reactions which have been reported infrequently were aberrant conduction, bradycardia, piloerection, widened QRS complex, azotemia, and elevated blood pressure.

Dosage and Administration:

WARNING: This is a potent drug: It must be diluted before administration to patient.

Suggested Dilution—Transfer contents of one or more ampuls or additive syringes (5 ml. containing 200 mg. INTROPIN) by aseptic technique to either a 250 ml. or 500 ml. bottle of one of the following sterile intravenous solutions:

1) Sodium Chloride Injection, USP
2) Dextrose 5% Injection, USP
3) Dextrose (5%) and Sodium Chloride (0.9%) Injection, USP
4) 5% Dextrose in 0.45% Sodium Chloride Solution
5) Dextrose (5%) in Lactated Ringer's Solution
6) Sodium Lactate ($^1/_6$ Molar) Injection, USP
7) Lactated Ringer's Injection, USP

INTROPIN has been found to be stable for a minimum of 24 hours after dilution in the sterile intravenous solutions listed above. However, as with all intravenous admixtures, dilution should be made just prior to administration.

Do **NOT** add INTROPIN Injection to 5% Sodium Bicarbonate or other alkaline intravenous solutions, since the drug is inactivated in alkaline solution.

Rate of Administration—INTROPIN, after dilution, is administered intravenously through a suitable intravenous catheter or needle. An i.v. drip chamber or other suitable metering device is essential for controlling the rate of flow in drops/minute. Each patient must be individually titrated to the desired hemodynamic and/or renal response with INTROPIN. In titrating to the desired increase in systolic blood pressure, the optimum dosage rate for renal response may be exceeded, thus necessitating a reduction in rate after the hemodynamic condition is stablized.

Administration at rates greater than 50 mcg./kg./min. have safely been used in advanced circulatory decompensation states. If unnecessary fluid expansion is of concern, adjustment of drug concentration may be preferred over increasing the flow rate of a less concentrated dilution.

Suggested Regimen:

1. When appropriate, increase blood volume with whole blood or plasma until central venous pressure is 10 to 15 cm. H_2O or pulmonary wedge pressure is 14–18 mm Hg.
2. Begin administration of diluted solution at doses of 2–5 mcg./kg./minute INTROPIN in patients who are likely to respond to modest increments of heart force and renal perfusion. In more seriously ill patients, begin administration of diluted solution at doses of 5 mcg./kg./minute INTROPIN and increase gradually using 5 to 10 mcg./kg./minute increments up to 20 to 50 mcg./kg./minute as needed. If doses of INTROPIN in excess of 50 mcg./kg./minute are required, it is suggested that urine output be checked frequently. Should urine flow begin to decrease in the absence of hypotension, reduction of INTROPIN dosage should be considered. Multiclinic trials have shown that more than 50% of the patients were satisfactorily maintained on doses of INTROPIN less than 20 mcg./kg./minute. In patients who do not respond to these doses

Continued on next page

Arnar-Stone—Cont.

with adequate arterial pressures or urine flow, additional increments of INTROPIN may be employed in an effort to produce an appropriate arterial pressure and central perfusion.

3. Treatment of all patients requires constant evaluation of therapy in terms of the blood volume, augmentation of myocardial contractility, and distribution of peripheral perfusion. Dosage of INTROPIN should be adjusted according to the patient's response, with particular attention to diminution of established urine flow rate, increasing tachycardia or development of new dysrhythmias as indices for decreasing or temporarily suspending the dosage.

4. As with all potent intravenously administered drugs, care should be taken to control the rate of administration so as to avoid inadvertent administration of a bolus of drug.

Overdosage: In case of accidental overdosage, as evidenced by excessive blood pressure elevation, reduce rate of administration or temporarily discontinue INTROPIN until patient's condition stabilizes. Since INTROPIN's duration of action is quite short, no additional remedial measures are usually necessary. If these measures fail to stabilize the patient's condition, use of the short-acting alpha adrenergic blocking agent, phentolamine should be considered.

How Supplied: NDC 0094-0040-05: 5 ml. ampul containing 40 mg. dopamine HCl per ml. NDC 0094-0040-07: 5 ml. additive syringe containing 40 mg. dopamine HCl per ml.

ISOCLOR® EXPECTORANT Ⓒ ℞

Description: Each 5 ml (tsp.) Expectorant contains 10 mg. codeine phosphate (Warning: may be habit forming), 30 mg. pseudoephedrine HCl, 100 mg. guaifenesin and 5% alcohol.

Indications: For temporary relief of troublesome, unproductive coughing associated with runny nose, nasal and sinus congestion.

Contraindications: Severe hypertension or severe cardiac disease. Hypersensitivity to any of the components. Do not use in children under one year of age.

Precautions: Use with caution in patients with hyperthyroidism. Patients susceptible to the soporific effects of codeine should be warned against driving a motor vehicle or operating machinery which requires complete mental alertness.

Dosage: *Adults* — 2 teaspoonsful every 4 hours.

Children: 6–12 yrs. — ½ to 1 teaspoonful every 4 hours; 2–6 yrs. — ¼ to ½ teaspoonful every 4 hours; 1–2 yrs. — ⅛ teaspoonful every 4 hours.

Supplied: Pint and Gallon

DEA Registration Number Required

ISOCLOR® Tablets, Liquid, Timesule® Capsules ℞

Description: Each tablet contains 4 mg. chlorpheniramine maleate and 60 mg. pseudoephedrine HCl. Each 5 ml (tsp.) liquid contains 2 mg. chlorpheniramine maleate and 25 mg. pseudoephedrine HCl. Each sustained-action Timesule capsule contains 8 mg. chlorpheniramine maleate and 120 mg. pseudoephedrine HCl in a special form providing a prolonged therapeutic effect.

Indications: For temporary relief of upper respiratory and nasal congestion associated with the common cold, hay fever and allergies, sinusitis, and vasomotor and allergic rhinitis.

Contraindications: Severe hypertension or severe cardiac disease. Sensitivity to antihistamines or sympathomimetic agents.

Precautions: Use with caution in patients with hyperthyroidism. Patients susceptible to the soporific effects of chlorpheniramine should be warned against driving or operating machinery which requires complete mental alertness.

Dosage: Tablets: *Adults* - 1 tablet every 4 hours.

Liquid: Children: 6–12 yrs., 1 tsp. every 4 hours. Smaller children, as follows, every 4 hours: 40–50 lbs. ¾–1 tsp.; 30–40 lbs. ½–¾ tsp.; 20–30 lbs. ¼–½ tsp.; 15–20 lbs. ⅛–¼ tsp. *Adults* - 2 tsp. every 4 hrs. Timesule Capsules: *Adults* - 1 Timesule Capsule every 12 hrs.

Supplied: Tablets: Bottle of 100. Liquid: Pint or Gallon.

Timesule capsules: Bottles of 100 and 500.

SOPOR™ Ⓒ ℞
(methaqualone tablets - not NF)
150 and 300 mg Tablets

(Note: This product differs from the official NF Methaqualone Tablets in that it meets a different dissolution specification.)

Description: Sopor (methaqualone) is chemically 2-methyl-3-(2-methylphenyl)-4(3H)-quinazolinone. Methaqualone occurs as a white, crystalline powder with a bitter taste and is very slightly soluble in water and freely soluble in alcohol. The drug is highly lipid soluble.

Clinical Pharmacology: Methaqualone is rapidly absorbed from the G.I. tract. The onset of action of the drug is rapid; sleep is usually induced within 30 minutes and lasts 5 to 8 hrs. following usual hypnotic doses.

The decline in serum levels of methaqualone is biphasic. The half-life for the first (distribution) phase is 1 to 4 hrs, and the half-life for the second (elimination) phase has been reported to be 19 to 40 hrs. There is extensive tissue localization of the drug, particularly in adipose tissue. Steady state equilibrium is achieved in less than one week.

Although the metabolic fate of methaqualone has not been completely elucidated, there is considerable evidence that therapeutic doses of methaqualone are almost completely metabolized in the liver by hydroxylation. In doses of up to 300 mg in man, very little unchanged drug is found in the urine.

Indication: Sopor is a hypnotic for the treatment of simple insomnia. The prolonged administration of Sopor is not recommended since it has not been shown to be effective for more than 14 days. Attempts should be made to find alternative non-drug therapy in chronic insomnia.

Contraindications: Sopor is contraindicated in patients with known hypersensitivity to methaqualone and in women who are or may become pregnant. Reproduction studies in the rat revealed minor but clear-cut skeletal abnormalities in the young.

Warnings: The hypnotic dose should be taken only at bedtime, immediately before the patient retires, since methaqualone may produce drowsiness within 10 to 20 minutes.

The patient on Sopor must be warned against driving a car or operating dangerous machinery while on the drug, since methaqualone may impair the ability to perform hazardous activities requiring mental alertness or physical coordination.

The patient should be warned about the possible additive effects when methaqualone is taken concomitantly with other central nervous system depressants such as alcohol or barbiturates.

Usage in Children: Methaqualone is not recommended for use in children, since its safety and effectiveness in the pediatric age group have not been established.

Physical and Psychological Dependence: Psychological and physical dependence with methaqualone have been reported. Excessive use of the drug or abuse of the drug for non-therapeutic purposes may lead to severe psychological or physical dependence.

Since methaqualone is known to have value on the illicit drug market, caution must be exercised in prescribing methaqualone to individuals whose history suggests they may increase the dosage on their own initiative. Ordinarily, an amount adequate for one week is sufficient. The patient should be reevaluated before re-prescribing.

Precautions: The possibility of the use of hypnotic drugs in suicide attempts should be kept in mind and the drugs prescribed in small quantities.

Since methaqualone is metabolized in the liver, it should be given in reduced doses, if at all, to those with impaired hepatic function.

Sopor Tablets—150 & 300 mg contain FD&C yellow #5 (Tartrazine) which may cause allergic-type reactions (including bronchial asthma) in certain susceptible individuals. Although the overall incidence of FD&C yellow #5 (Tartrazine) sensitivity in the general population is low, it is frequently seen in patients who also have aspirin hypersensitivity.

Adverse Reactions:

NEUROPSYCHIATRIC: headache, hangover, fatigue, dizziness, torpor, transient paresthesia of the extremities. Peripheral neuropathy has been reported. Restlessness or anxiety occurs occasionally.

HEMATOLOGIC: Aplastic anemia possibly related to methaqualone has been reported.

GASTROINTESTINAL: dry mouth, anorexia, nausea, emesis, epigastric discomfort, diarrhea.

DERMATOLOGIC: diaphoresis, bromhidrosis, exanthema. Urticaria has been particularly well documented.

Dosage and Administration:

Usual Adult Dosage—The usual adult hypnotic dose of Sopor is 150 to 300 mg at bedtime.

Geriatric Dosage— Dosage for aged, debilitated, or highly agitated patients should be individualized in accordance with the judgment of the physician. The principle to be followed is to observe the response to small doses and determine the desirability of adjusting the dose.

Overdosage: Acute overdosage may result in delirium and coma, with restlessness and hypertonia, progressing to convulsions. Pupillary dilatation, tachycardia, and hyperreflexia may also occur. Spontaneous vomiting and increased secretions are common and may lead to aspiration pneumonitis or respiratory obstruction. Large overdoses have been accompanied by cutaneous edema, pulmonary edema, hepatic damage, renal insufficiency, and bleeding. Shock and respiratory arrest may occasionally occur. Coma has occurred with acute overdoses averaging 2.4 gm. Death has occurred following ingestion of 8 gms of methaqualone.

Recommended management includes prompt evacuation of gastric contents, maintenance of adequate ventilation, support of blood pressure if necessary, and the usual supportive measures for the unconscious patient. Dialysis may be helpful. Analeptics are contraindicated.

Sudden discontinuation of methaqualone in physically dependent patients may produce severe withdrawal symptoms including nausea, vomiting, nervousness, tremulousness, headache, anxiety, confusion, weakness, abdominal cramps, insomnia, nightmares, hallucinations and convulsions. Treatment of methaqualone physical dependence consists of cautious and gradual withdrawal of the drug. Patients being withdrawn from methaqualone should be closely monitored, preferably hospitalized, and general supportive therapy given as needed.

How Supplied:

Sopor—150 mg: Yellow, scored tablets containing 150 mg methaqualone.

Sopor—300 mg: Orange, scored tablets containing 300 mg methaqualone.

Store at room temperature.

Ascher & Company, Inc., B.F.

5100 E. 59TH ST.
KANSAS CITY, MO 64130

ANASPAZ® TABLETS ℞
l-Hyoscyamine Sulfate 0.125 mg
ANASPAZ PB® TABLETS ℞
l-Hyoscyamine Sulfate 0.125 mg
Phenobarbital 15.0 mg
(WARNING: May be habit forming)

For the hyperactive GI tract.
ANTISPASMODIC-ANTISECRETORY

Description: Anaspaz tablets are light yellow in color and Anaspaz PB tablets are raspberry-pink. Both contain chemically pure l-Hyoscyamine Sulfate 0.125 mg, one of the principle parasympatholytic (anticholinergic) alkaloids of belladonna. Anaspaz PB also contains Phenobarbital 15.0 mg.
WARNING: May be habit-forming.
Clinical Pharmacology: ANASPAZ (l-Hyoscyamine Sulfate) acts directly at the effector site to block the action of acetylcholine. ANASPAZ PB (l-Hyoscyamine Sulfate with Phenobarbital) includes the CNS sedative, phenobarbital, to overcome the tension due to spasm.
Indications and Usage: In GI tract disorders due to spasm, hypermotility, hypersecretion, such as peptic ulcer (with diet and antacids), gastritis, pylorospasm, spastic colitis, mild dysenteries; also useful in overcoming spasm of cystitis, dysmenorrhea, renal and biliary colics (with narcotics), and in counteracting hypersecretion of acute rhinitis.
Contraindications: Glaucoma, prostatic hypertrophy, and some cases of cardiac disease.
Adverse Reactions: Side effects are minimal. In high doses, dry mouth, dry nose, urinary difficulty may occur. Vision may blur from pupil dilation; or the heart rate may be speeded, with tachycardia resulting. Decrease of dose usually leads to cessation of discomfort.
Dosage and Administration: One tablet 3 or 4 times a day. Tablets scored to allow individualization of dosage. ANASPAZ (plain) tablets may also be given sublingually. Children, in proportion to age and weight.
How Supplied: ANASPAZ (l-Hyoscyamine Sulfate) and ANASPAZ PB (l-Hyoscyamine Sulfate with Phenobarbital) in bottles of 100, and 500 tablets.
Caution: Federal law prohibits dispensing without prescription.

ETHAQUIN® Tablets ℞
(Ethaverine Hydrochloride)

Description: Each compressed ETHAQUIN Tablet contains Ethaverine Hydrochloride 100 mg.
Clinical Pharmacology: ETHAQUIN (Ethaverine Hydrochloride) acts directly on the smooth muscle cells, without involving the autonomic nervous system or its receptors. It produces smooth muscle relaxation, particularly where spasm exists, affecting the larger blood vessels, especially systemic, peripheral and pulmonary vessels, smooth muscle of the intestines, biliary tree, and ureters.
Indications and Usage: In peripheral and cerebral vascular insufficiency associated with arterial spasm; also useful as a smooth muscle spasmolytic in spastic conditions of the gastrointestinal and genitourinary tracts.
Contraindications: The use of ETHAQUIN (Ethaverine Hydrochloride) is contraindicated in the presence of complete atrioventricular dissociation.
Precautions: As with all vasodilators, ETHAQUIN (Ethaverine Hydrochloride) should be administered with caution to patients with glaucoma.
The safety of Ethaverine Hydrochloride during pregnancy or lactation has not been established; therefore it should not be used in pregnant women or in women of childbearing age unless, in the judgment of the physician, its use is deemed essential to the welfare of the patient.
Adverse Reactions: Even though the incidence of side effects as reported in the literature is very low, it is possible for a patient to évidence nausea, anorexia, abdominal distress, dryness of the throat, hypotension, malaise, lassitude, drowsiness, flushing, sweating, vertigo, respiratory depression, cardiac depression, cardiac arrhythmia and headache. If these side effects occur, reduce dosage or discontinue medication.
Dosage and Administration: In mild or moderate disease, the usual dose for adults is one tablet three times a day: morning, mid-afternoon, evening. In more difficult cases, dosage may be increased to two tablets three times a day. It is most effective given early in the course of the vascular disorder. Because of the chronic nature of the disease, long-term therapy is required.
How Supplied: ETHAQUIN (Ethaverine Hydrochloride) Tablets in bottles of 100, 500, 1000, 2500 and 5000.
Caution: Federal law prohibits dispensing without prescription.
Keep out of reach of children.

MOBIDIN® ℞
(Magnesium Salicylate)

Description: Each compressed tablet contains 600 mg. magnesium salicylate. The yellow tablets are capsule-shaped and scored to permit part dosage.
Clinical Pharmacology: MOBIDIN is thought to act by a number of pathways. MOBIDIN acts to inhibit the synthesis of prostaglandin, one of the chemical mediators of the inflammatory reaction. In addition, salicylates relieve certain types of pain through an effect on the central nervous system.
Indications and Usage: As an analgesic, anti-inflammatory in the daily management of mild to moderately advanced rheumatoid arthritis, osteoarthritis, and related diseases.
Contraindications: To guard against hypermagnesemia, MOBIDIN is contraindicated in patients with advanced chronic renal insufficiency.
Precautions: Since salicylates may exacerbate gastric hemorrhage, MOBIDIN should be given with caution in patients with erosive gastritis or peptic ulcer. It should be used with caution, if at all, in those taking coumarin or indandione anticoagulants, or heparin. The risk of GI ulceration is increased when salicylates are given with steroids, the butazones, or alcohol. Salicylates antagonize the uric acid excretion effect of probenecid and sulfinpyrazone.
Experience with MOBIDIN in children is limited; it is therefore not recommended in the patient under 12 years of age.
Adverse Reactions: On MOBIDIN therapy in usual doses, side effects are rare. Occasionally, epigastric discomfort, nausea, anorexia, occult blood loss may occur. In large doses, and/or prolonged therapy of any salicylate, salicylate intoxication may occur, manifested by tinnitus, headache, dizziness, confusion, fever, sweating, thirst, drowsiness, dimness of vision, impaired hearing, hyperventilation, increased pulse rate, or diarrhea.
Dosage and Administration: The usual dose of MOBIDIN is one tablet 3 or 4 times a day. The number of doses may be increased, if required, to 6 to 8 tablets daily, at intervals of 3 to 6 hours. In rheumatic fever, as many as 16 tablets daily, throughout the 24 hours, may be required to overcome joint pains, especially during the early stage of the disease.
Caution: Federal law prohibits dispensing without prescription.
Supplied: MOBIDIN™ (Magnesium Salicylate 600 mg.) is supplied in bottles of 100 and 500.

MOBISYL® Creme
(Triethanolamine Salicylate)

Description: MOBISYL, a greaseless, odorless, non-staining analgesic creme, is contained in a 3.5 oz. (100 gm) tube and in an 8 oz. (226.8 gm) jar.
Indications: Mobisyl is recommended for relief of pain in arthritis, muscular aches, neuralgia and like-conditions.
Warning: For external use only.
Caution: As with all medications, MOBISYL should be kept out of reach of children. Discontinue use of the medication if excessive irritation of the skin should develop. Avoid contact with the eyes or mucous membranes. If pain persists longer than 10 days, or if redness due to sensitivity to the medication persists, consult your physician without delay.
Directions For Use: A liberal amount of MOBISYL is to be rubbed into the affected area three or four times a day, and before retiring.

Astra Pharmaceutical Products, Inc.

7 NEPONSET ST.
WORCESTER, MA 01606

BRICANYL® (terbutaline sulfate) ℞
SUBCUTANEOUS INJECTION

Description: Bricanyl, α-[(*tert*-butylamino)-methyl]-3,5-dihydroxybenzyl alcohol, sulfate is a synthetic sympathomimetic amine.
Bricanyl, brand of terbutaline sulfate, is a water soluble colorless crystalline solid. Solutions are sensitive to excessive heat and light and ampules should therefore be stored at controlled room temperature with protection from light by storage in their original carton until dispensed. Solutions should not be used if discolored.
Each milliliter of sterile isotonic solution contains 1.0 mg of terbutaline sulfate (equivalent to 0.82 mg of the free base), 8.9 mg of sodium chloride, and hydrochloric acid to adjust the pH to 3.0–5.0.
Actions: Bricanyl, brand of terbutaline sulfate, is a β-adrenergic receptor agonist which has been shown by *in vitro* and *in vivo* pharmacological studies in animals to exert a preferential effect on β_2 adrenergic receptors such as those located in bronchial smooth muscle. Controlled clinical studies in patients who were administered the drug orally have revealed proportionally greater changes in pulmonary function parameters than in heart rate or blood pressure. While this suggests a relative preference for the β_2 receptor in man, the usual cardiovascular effects commonly associated with sympathomimetic agents were also observed with terbutaline sulfate.
Bricanyl (terbutaline sulfate) Subcutaneous Injection has been shown in controlled clinical studies to relieve acute bronchospasm in acute and chronic obstructive pulmonary disease, resulting in a clinically significant increase in pulmonary flow rates, e.g., an increase of 15% or greater in FEV_1. Following administration of 0.25 mg of subcutaneous Bricanyl, a measurable change in flow rate is usually observed within five minutes, and a clinically significant increase in FEV_1 occurs by 15 minutes following the injection. The maximum effect usually occurs within 30–60 minutes and clinically significant bronchodilator activity has been observed to persist for 90 minutes to four

Continued on next page

Astra—Cont.

hours. The duration of clinically significant improvement is comparable to that found with equimilligram doses of epinephrine.

Indications: Bricanyl (terbutaline sulfate) Subcutaneous Injection is indicated as a bronchodilator for bronchial asthma and for reversible bronchospasm which may occur in association with bronchitis and emphysema.

Contraindications: Bricanyl (terbutaline sulfate) Subcutaneous Injection is contraindicated when there is known hypersensitivity to sympathomimetic amines.

Warnings: *Usage in Pregnancy:* Animal reproductive studies have been negative with respect to adverse effects on fetal development. The safe use of Bricanyl Subcutaneous Injection has not, however, been established in human pregnancy. As with any medication, the use of the drug in pregnancy, lactation, or women of childbearing potential requires that the expected therapeutic benefit of the drug be weighed against its possible hazards to the mother or child.

Usage in Pediatrics: Bricanyl Subcutaneous Injection is not presently recommended for children below the age of twelve years due to insufficient clinical data in this pediatric group.

Precautions: Bricanyl (terbutaline sulfate) Subcutaneous Injection should be used with caution in patients with diabetes, hypertension, hyperthyroidism, and history of seizures. As with other sympathomimetic bronchodilator agents, Bricanyl (terbutaline sulfate) Subcutaneous Injection should be administered cautiously to cardiac patients, especially those with associated arrhythmias.

The concomitant use of Bricanyl (terbutaline sulfate) Subcutaneous Injection with other sympathomimetic agents is not recommended, since their combined effect on the cardiovascular system may be deleterious to the patient.

Adverse Reactions: Commonly observed side effects include increases in heart rate, nervousness, tremor, palpitations and dizziness. These occur more frequently at doses in excess of 0.25 mg. Other reported reactions include headache, nausea, vomiting, anxiety and muscle cramps. These reactions are transient in nature and usually do not require treatment. In general, all side effects are characteristic of those commonly seen with sympathomimetic amines such as epinephrine.

Dosage and Administration: The usual subcutaneous dose of Bricanyl, brand of terbutaline sulfate, is 0.25 mg injected into the lateral deltoid area. If significant clinical improvement does not occur by 15–30 minutes, a second dose of 0.25 mg may be administered. A total dose of 0.5 mg should not be exceeded within a four hour period. If a patient fails to respond to a second 0.25 mg dose of Bricanyl Subcutaneous Injection within 15–30 minutes, other therapeutic measures should be considered.

Overdosage: Overdosage experience is limited. Excessive β-adrenergic receptor stimulation may augment the signs or symptoms listed under Adverse Reactions and they may be accompanied by other adrenergic effects. In the case of terbutaline overdosage, the patient should be treated symptomatically for the sympathomimetic overdosage with careful consideration to the appropriateness of any chosen therapy and possible effect on the patient's underlying disease state.

How Supplied: Bricanyl Subcutaneous Injection is supplied in packages of ten 2 ml size ampules each containing one ml of solution [1.0 mg of Bricanyl (terbutaline sulfate)]. Thus, 0.25 ml of solution will provide the usual clinical dose of 0.25 mg. Ampules are expiration dated.

BRICANYL® (terbutaline sulfate) TABLETS ℞

Description: Bricanyl®, brand of terbutaline sulfate, a synthetic sympathomimetic amine, may be chemically described as α-[(tert-butyl-amino)methyl]-3, 5-dihydroxybenzyl alcohol sulfate.

Bricanyl, brand of terbutaline sulfate, is a water soluble, colorless, crystalline solid. Bricanyl Tablets should be stored at controlled room temperature.

Tablets containing 2.5 mg (equivalent to 2.05 mg of free base) and 5 mg (equivalent to 4.1 mg of free base) are white in color, and carry a numerical inscription (i.e., "725" or "750", derived from the NDC # for Bricanyl Tablets).

Actions: Bricanyl, brand of terbutaline sulfate, is a β-adrenergic receptor agonist which has been shown by *in vitro* and *in vivo* pharmacological studies in animals to exert a preferential effect on β_2 adrenergic receptors such as those located in bronchial smooth muscle. Controlled clinical studies in patients who were administered the drug orally have revealed proportionally greater changes in pulmonary function parameters than in heart rate or blood pressure. While this *suggests* a relative preference for the β_2 receptor in man, the usual cardiovascular effects commonly associated with sympathomimetic agents were also observed with Bricanyl Tablets.

Bricanyl Tablets have been shown in controlled clinical studies to relieve bronchospasm in chronic obstructive pulmonary disease. This action is manifested by a clinically significant increase in pulmonary function as demonstrated by an increase of 15% or more in FEV_1 and $FEF_{25\text{-}75}\%$. Following administration of Bricanyl tablets, a measurable change in flow rate is usually observed in 30 minutes, and a clinically significant improvement in pulmonary function occurs at 60–120 minutes. The maximum effect usually occurs within 120–180 minutes. Bricanyl Tablets also produce a clinically significant decrease in airway and pulmonary resistance which persists for at least 4 hours or longer. Significant bronchodilator action, as measured by various pulmonary function determinations (airway resistance, MMEFR, PEFR) has been demonstrated in some studies for periods up to 8 hours.

Clinical studies were conducted in which the effectiveness of Bricanyl Tablets was evaluated in comparison with ephedrine over periods up to 3 months. Both drugs continued to produce significant improvement in pulmonary function throughout this period of treatment.

Indications: Bricanyl (terbutaline sulfate) Tablets are indicated as a bronchodilator for bronchial asthma and for reversible bronchospasm which may occur in association with bronchitis and emphysema.

Contraindications: Bricanyl (terbutaline sulfate) Tablets are contraindicated when there is known hypersensitivity to sympathomimetic amines.

Warnings: *Usage in Pregnancy:* Animal reproductive studies have been negative with respect to adverse effects on fetal development. The safe use of Bricanyl Tablets has not, however, been established in human pregnancy. As with any medication, the use of the drug in pregnancy, lactation, or women of childbearing potential requires that the expected therapeutic benefit of the drug be weighed against its possible hazards to the mother or child.

Usage in Pediatrics: Bricanyl Tablets are not presently recommended for children below the age of twelve years due to insufficient clinical data in this pediatric group.

Precautions: Bricanyl (terbutaline sulfate) Tablets should be used with caution in patients with diabetes, hypertension, and hyperthyroidism.

As with other sympathomimetic bronchodilator agents, Bricanyl Tablets should be administered cautiously to cardiac patients, especially those with associated arrhythmias.

The concomitant use of Bricanyl Tablets with other sympathomimetic agents is not recommended, since their combined effect on the cardiovascular system may be deleterious to the patient. However, this does not preclude the use of an aerosol bronchodilator of the adrenergic stimulant type for the relief of an acute bronchospasm in patients receiving chronic oral therapy with Bricanyl Tablets.

Adverse Reactions: Commonly observed side effects include nervousness and tremor. Other reported reactions include headache, increased heart rate, palpitations, drowsiness, nausea, vomiting, and sweating. These reactions are generally transient in nature and usually do not require treatment. The frequency of these side effects appears to diminish with continued therapy. In general, all the side effects observed are characteristic of those commonly seen with sympathomimetic amines.

Dosage and Administration: The usual oral dose of Bricanyl, brand of terbutaline sulfate, for adults is 5 mg administered at approximately six hour intervals three times daily, during the hours the patient is usually awake. If side effects are particularly disturbing, the dose may be reduced to 2.5 mg three times daily and still provide a clinically significant improvement in pulmonary function. A dose of 2.5 mg three times daily also is recommended for children in the 12–15 year group. Bricanyl Tablets is not recommended at present for use in children below the age of twelve years. In adults, a total dose of 15 mg should not be exceeded in a 24-hour period. In children, a total dose of 7.5 mg should not be exceeded in a 24-hour period.

How Supplied: Both 2.5 mg and 5 mg Bricanyl® (terbutaline sulfate) Tablets are supplied in bottles of 100, 500, and 1,000 and in hospital (unit dose) packs of 100 individually packaged tablets.

CITANEST® (prilocaine HCl) SOLUTIONS ℞

Local anesthetic for infiltration and nerve block

Description: Citanest (prilocaine) is a local anesthetic, chemically designated as 2-propylamino-o-propionotoluidide.

Aqueous solutions of Citanest hydrochloride may be autoclaved repeatedly, if necessary.

Please refer to Table 1 for the exact composition of Citanest hydrochloride solutions.

[See table on next page].

Actions: Citanest stabilizes the neuronal membrane and prevents the initiation and transmission of nerve impulses, thereby effecting local anesthetic action.

Citanest is metabolized in both the liver and the kidney and excreted via the kidney. It is not metabolized by plasma esterases. One of the metabolites of Citanest appears to be o-toluidine. This substance has been found to produce methemoglobin both *in vitro* and *in vivo* (see ADVERSE REACTIONS).

When used for infiltration anesthesia in obstetrical patients, the time of onset of Citanest averages 1–2 minutes with an approximate duration of 60 minutes or longer. For major nerve blocks (e.g. epidural block), the onset of analgesia is approximately two minutes longer for Citanest than for lidocaine, whereas the duration of action is, at least, 30–60 minutes longer for Citanest than for lidocaine.

Indications: Citanest (prilocaine) is indicated for the production of local anesthesia in infiltration procedures, peripheral nerve blocks, and epidural or caudal blocks.

Since Citanest hydrochloride solutions contain no epinephrine, they are particularly useful for patients in whom vasopressor agents may be contraindicated, e.g., patients with hypertension, diabetes, thyrotoxicosis, or other cardiovascular disorders.

Contraindications: Citanest is contraindicated in patients with a known history of hypersensitivity to local anesthetics of the amide type. This agent should not be used in patients with congenital or idiopathic methemoglobinemia.

Local anesthetic agents should not be used in patients with severe shock or heart block. Local anesthetic procedures should not be used when there is inflammation and/or sepsis in the region of the proposed injection.

Warnings:

(1) RESUSCITATIVE EQUIPMENT AND DRUGS SHOULD BE IMMEDIATELY AVAILABLE WHEN ANY LOCAL ANESTHETIC IS USED.

(2) Usage in Pregnancy: The safe use of Citanest (prilocaine) has not been established with respect to adverse effects upon fetal development. Careful consideration should be given to this fact before administering this drug to women of childbearing potential, particularly during early pregnancy. (See ANIMAL STUDIES)

This does not exclude the use of the drug at term for obstetrical analgesia. Adverse effects on the fetus, course of labor, or delivery have rarely been observed when proper dosage and proper technique have been employed.

Precautions: The safety and effectiveness of Citanest depend upon proper dosage, correct technique, adequate precautions, and readiness for emergencies.

The lowest dosage that results in effective anesthesia should be used to avoid high plasma levels and serious adverse effects. Injection of repeated doses of Citanest may cause significant increases in blood levels with each repeated dose due to slow accumulation of the drug or its metabolites. Tolerance varies with the status of the patient. Debilitated, elderly patients, acutely ill patients and children should be given reduced doses commensurate with their age and physical status.

INJECTIONS SHOULD ALWAYS BE MADE SLOWLY AND WITH FREQUENT ASPIRATIONS. Aspiration is advisable since it reduces the possibility of intravascular injection, thereby keeping the incidence of side effects and anesthetic failures at a minimum.

Consult standard textbooks for specific techniques and precautions for various local anesthetic procedures.

Epidural anesthesia and caudal anesthesia should be used with extreme caution in persons with the following conditions: existing neurological disease, spinal deformities, septicemia, severe hypertension, and extreme youth.

The drug should be used with caution in persons with known drug sensitivities.

Local anesthetics react with certain metals and cause the release of their respective ions which, if injected, may cause severe local irritation. Adequate precaution should be taken to avoid this type of interaction.

Adverse Reactions: Adverse reactions may result from high plasma levels due to excessive dosage, rapid absorption or inadvertent intravascular injection, or may result from a hypersensitivity, idiosyncrasy or diminished tolerance on the part of the patient. Such reactions are systemic in nature and involve the central nervous system and/or the cardiovascular system.

CNS reactions are excitatory and/or depressant, and may be characterized by nervousness, dizziness, blurred vision and tremors, followed by drowsiness, convulsions, unconsciousness and possibly respiratory arrest. The excitatory reactions may be very brief or may not occur at all, in which case the first manifestations of toxicity may be drowsiness, merging into unconsciousness and respiratory arrest.

TABLE I COMPOSITION OF AVAILABLE SOLUTIONS

PRODUCT IDENTIFICATION	FORMULA					
	MULTIPLE DOSE VIALS			AMPULES		
Citanest (prilocaine) Hydrochloride (percent)	Prilocaine Hydrochloride (mg per ml)	Sodium Chloride (mg per ml)	Methylparaben (mg per ml)	Prilocaine Hydrochloride (mg per ml)	Sodium Chloride (mg per ml)
1%	10.0	6.0	1.0	10.0	6.0
2%	20.0	6.0	1.0	20.0	6.0
3%	N.S.	N.S.	N.S.	30.0	6.0

NOTE: All solutions are adjusted to a pH of 6.0–7.0 with sodium hydroxide.
N.S. Not supplied.

Cardiovascular reactions are depressant, and may be characterized by hypotension, myocardial depression, bradycardia and possibly cardiac arrest.

Treatment of a patient with toxic manifestations consists of assuring and maintaining a patent airway and supporting ventilation using oxygen and assisted or controlled respiration as required. This usually will be sufficient in the management of most reactions. Should circulatory depression occur, vasopressors, such as ephedrine or metaraminol, and intravenous fluids may be used. Should a convulsion persist despite oxygen therapy, small increments of an ultra-short acting barbiturate (thiopental or thiamylal) or a short acting barbiturate (pentobarbital or secobarbital) may be given intravenously.

Allergic reactions are characterized by cutaneous lesions, urticaria, edema or anaphylactoid reactions. The detection of sensitivity by skin testing is of doubtful value.

Swelling and paresthesia of the lips and oral tissues has been reported following injection of 4% solutions of Citanest into the oral cavity. Such reactions have not been reported with 1%, 2%, or 3% solutions.

Methemoglobinemia

In vivo o-toluidine apparently is formed from the metabolic degradation of Citanest (prilocaine) with the resultant formation of methemoglobinemia. A dose-response relationship appears to exist between the amount of Citanest administered as a single injection and the incidence and degree of methemoglobin formation.

In studies conducted in man to date, the formation of methemoglobin at a dose of 400 mg Citanest has not been statistically significant. Cases of cyanosis at doses between 400 and 600 mg are extremely rare. At a dose of 600 mg, which is the maximum recommended dose for any anesthetic procedure, methemoglobin formation occurred at levels which were less than 15% of the total hemoglobin content in all patients. At no time was the methemoglobinemia associated with any adverse respiratory, cardiovascular, or CNS symptoms. However, cyanosis has been reported at this dosage level. In addition, blood at the time of surgery has appeared somewhat darker than usual in some cases. Cyanosis is reported to be prevalent when 900 or more mg are administered as a single dose. It should be emphasized that this dose exceeds the recommended single dose.

Methemoglobin levels of less than 20 percent of total hemoglobin content are usually not associated with any clinical symptoms of hypoxia. At levels of 20 to 50 percent, fatigue, weakness, dyspnea, tachycardia, headaches, and dizziness may occur. Only one case exhibiting clinical symptoms of lightheadedness and dizziness, which may have been related to a methemoglobin value in excess of 20%, has been reported. The patient received a single injection of 900 mg. The intravenous use of methylene blue alleviated these symptoms within fifteen minutes.

Methemoglobinemia is rapidly and easily treated by 1–2 mg/kg of a 1% solution of methylene blue administered intravenously over a five-minute period. In most patients in whom the maximum recommended dose of Citanest is not exceeded, the appearance of clinical signs and symptoms of hypoxia is probably related to improper ventilation and should be treated with oxygen. If signs and symptoms of hypoxia persist following adequate alveolar ventilation with oxygen, then methemoglobinemia should be suspected and methylene blue treatment initiated. In patients with anemia or cardiac failure in whom the availability of oxygen has already been decreased, the potential disadvantages of a further hypoxic embarrassment due to the use of large doses of this agent must be carefully considered.

Dosage and Administration:

Infiltration Anesthesia—Citanest may be employed for infiltration anesthesia in any of the cases for which this technique is indicated. Selection of appropriate volumes and concentrations is dependent on the nature and extent of the surgical procedure. For most surgical procedures, 20–30 ml of Citanest hydrochloride 1% or 2% will usually provide adequate operative analgesia. The lowest concentration and smallest volume that will produce the desired results should be given. These suggested doses are for adults. Smaller amounts and weaker concentrations should be used for children depending on their age and weight.

Peripheral Nerve Blocks—For therapeutic nerve blocks (e.g. intercostal or paravertebral blocks), 3–5 ml of Citanest hydrochloride will usually be adequate for the management of pain. Selection of the appropriate concentration depends on the degree and duration of the analgesia required. Both parameters increase proportionally as the volume and concentration of drug is increased.

For blocks such as brachial plexus or sciatic-femoral, 20–30 ml of Citanest hydrochloride 2% or 15–20 ml of Citanest hydrochloride 3% will usually provide adequate operative analgesia for most routine surgical procedures involving the upper or lower extremities.

Central Neural Blocks—Citanest may be employed in epidural anesthesia for any of the surgical procedures for which this anesthetic technique is indicated. Volumes of 20–30 ml of Citanest hydrochloride 2% or 15–20 ml of Citanest hydrochloride 3% will usually provide adequate operative analgesia for both minor and major surgical procedures performed under epidural anesthesia.

Caudal anesthesia is useful for obstetrical analgesia and certain pelvic operative procedures such as hysterectomy, transurethral resection, etc. Citanest hydrochloride 1% in volumes of 20–30 ml will usually provide adequate obstetrical analgesia for most routine vaginal deliveries. For surgical procedures requiring more extensive anesthesia, 20–30 ml of Citanest hydrochloride 2% or 15–20 ml of Citanest hydrochloride 3% are recommended.

IMPORTANT: A test dose of 2–5 ml should be administered at least five minutes prior to injecting the total required volume for central neu-

Continued on next page

Astra—Cont.

ral blocks (epidural or caudal anesthesia). It is important that a single dose container be employed for epidural anesthesia.

Table II summarizes the recommended volumes and concentrations of Citanest hydrochloride for various types of anesthetic procedures. These recommended doses serve only as a guide to the amount of anesthetic required for most routine procedures. The actual volume and concentrations to be used depend on a number of factors, such as type and extent of surgical procedure, degree of muscular relaxation required, duration of anesthesia required, the physical state of the patient, etc. In all cases the smallest dose that will produce the desired result should be given.

The onset of anesthesia, the duration of anesthesia and the degree of muscular relaxation are proportional to the volume and concentration of local anesthetic used. Thus, an increase in volume and concentration of Citanest will decrease the onset of anesthesia, prolong the duration of anesthesia, provide a greater degree of muscular relaxation and increase the segmental spread of anesthesia. However, increasing the volume and concentration of Citanest may result in a more profound fall in blood pressure when used in epidural anesthesia. Although the incidence of side effects with Citanest is quite low, caution should be exercised particularly when employing large volumes and concentrations of Citanest since the incidence of side effects is directly proportional to the total dose of local anesthetic agent injected.

Maximum Recommended Dosages

Dosages in excess of those listed in Table II have been administered without serious side effects. However, caution should be exercised in the use of larger dosages, and in general, the amount given at any one time should not exceed that recommended in Table II.

[See table below].

Normal Healthy Adults: No more than 600 mg of Citanest hydrochloride should ever be administered as a single injection, i.e. no more than 8 mg/kg or 4 mg/lb should be given as a single injection. For continuous epidural or caudal anesthesia the maximum recommended dosage should not be administered at intervals of less than two hours.

Children: Experience in children under the age of ten is limited. It is difficult to recommend a maximum dose of any drug for children since this varies as a function of age and weight. With respect to Citanest hydrochloride, 400 mg have been used without toxic effects in children of 10–15 years. However, for children of less than 10 years who have a normal lean body mass and normal body development, the use of one of the standard pediatric drug formulas (e.g. Clark's rule or Young's rule) to determine the maximum dose is recommended. For example, in a child of five years weighing 50 lbs, the dose of Citanest hydrochloride should not exceed 150–200 mg when calculated according to Clark's rule or Young's rule. In order to minimize the possibility of toxic reactions in children the use of a 1% concentration of Citanest hydrochloride is recommended.

Patients with Liver Disease and Debilitated Patients: The use of any local anesthetic agent is undesirable in patients with liver disease or severely debilitated patients. However, for emergency or definitive surgical procedures where a local anesthetic is required, care should be taken to use the lowest dose and concentration of Citanest hydrochloride necessary to provide adequate anesthesia. The maximum safe dose of any drug for such patients depends on the degree of liver damage and degree of debilitation. For most anesthetic procedures, it is advisable to use the 1% concentration of Citanest hydrochloride in order to obtain the minimum dose that will provide adequate anesthesia and avoid possible toxic reactions in these patients. In such patients it is not advisable to exceed a maximum dose of 400 mg.

How Supplied:

Multiple dose vials: 30 ml Citanest hydrochloride 1% and 2%.

Ampules: 30 ml Citanest hydrochloride 1% and 2%; 20 ml Citanest hydrochloride 3%.

All solutions contain sodium chloride 6 mg per ml and are adjusted to a pH of 6.0 to 7.0 with sodium hydroxide. Multiple dose vials contain methylparaben, 1 mg per ml.

Animal Studies: Two studies of the effects of Citanest on reproduction and fetal development have been carried out in animals. In one study, doses of Citanest of 10 and 30 mg/kg (1 to 3 times the maximum human dose) were injected subcutaneously each day for 8 months into male and female rats. During these 8 months the rats were mated three times and the resultant litters were examined. The study revealed no teratogenic effects of Citanest and no adverse effects on the number of litters produced, on the average weight of pups at birth, on the average weight of pups surviving to weaning age, and on the distribution of sex. In the third littering, the average number of pups per litter at birth was lower in the group treated with the high dose of Citanest than in the control group. In all three litterings, the survival of pups in some of the treated groups was less than in their corresponding control groups. Adjustments in the experimental procedure indicated that these differences in survival were at least partially due to experimental artifacts.

In the other study, the effects of Citanest on organogenesis and fetal development was investigated in the rat. Doses ranging from 100 to 300 mg/kg (10 to 30 times the maximum human dose) were injected intramuscularly into pregnant rats from day 7 to day 13 post coitum. On the twenty-first gestational day the fetuses were examined. No external or skeletal malformations were observed and no significant differences were observed in the number of living and dead fetuses among the treated and control groups. The mean fetal weights in the treated groups were, however, less than that of the control group. In addition, hydronephrosis was observed in approximately 1% of the fetuses derived from treated mothers, but in none of the fetuses of the control group. This latter observation was not statistically significant.

TABLE II RECOMMENDED DOSES OF CITANEST (PRILOCAINE) HYDROCHLORIDE FOR VARIOUS ANESTHETIC PROCEDURES IN NORMAL HEALTHY ADULTS

Anesthetic Procedure	Citanest hydrochloride Conc. (%)	Volume (ml)	Total Dose (mg)
Infiltration	1 or 2	20–30	200–600
Peripheral Nerve Blocks			
(a) Therapeutic Nerve Blocks (e.g. intercostal or paravertebral)	1 or 2	3–5	30–100
(b) For blocks such as Brachial Plexus or Sciatic-femoral	2	20–30	400–600
	3	15–20	450–600
Central Neural Blocks			
(a) Epidural	1	20–30	200–300
	2	20–30	400–600
	3	15–20	450–600
(b) Caudal			
(1) Obstetrical Analgesia	1	20–30	200–300
(2) Surgical Anesthesia	2	20–30	400–600
	3	15–20	450–600

Table 1. COMPOSITION OF AVAILABLE SOLUTIONS

Product Identification: Duranest (etidocaine) HCl Concentration	Epinephrine Dilution	Formula: Multiple Dose Vials: Sodium chloride (mg/ml)	Methylparaben (mg/ml)	Sodium metabisulfite (mg/ml)	Ampules and Single Dose Vials: Sodium chloride (mg/ml)	Sodium metabisulfite (mg/ml)	pH
0.5	None	—	—	—	8.07	None	4.0–5.0
0.5	1:200,000	8.07	1.0	0.5	8.07	0.5	3.0–4.5
1.0	None	—	—	—	7.1	None	4.0–5.0
1.0	1:200,000	—	—	—	7.1	0.5	3.0–4.5
1.5	1:200,000	—	—	—	6.2	0.5	3.0–4.5

NOTE: pH of all solutions adjusted with sodium hydroxide or hydrochloric acid

DURANEST® (etidocaine HCl) ℞
STERILE AQUEOUS SOLUTION
Local anesthetic for infiltration and nerve block

Description: Duranest is a local anesthetic of the amide type, chemically related to lidocaine. Its chemical name is (±)-2-(N-ethylpropylamino)-2′,6′-butyroxylidide.

The pKa of Duranest (7.74) is similar to that of lidocaine (7.86). However, Duranest possesses a greater degree of lipid solubility (partition coefficient of 141 in heptane/7.4 phosphate buffer system) and protein binding capacity (94%) as compared to lidocaine (partition coefficient = 3.6, protein binding = 55%).

Duranest HCl solutions are sterile and except for the 1.5% concentration, are available with or without epinephrine 1:200,000. Single dose containers of Duranest without epinephrine may be reautoclaved if necessary.

Please refer to Table 1 for the composition of available solutions.

[See table above].

Actions: Duranest (etidocaine) stabilizes the neuronal membrane and prevents the initiation and conduction of nerve impulses, thereby effecting local anesthetic action. *In vivo* animal studies have shown that Duranest has a rapid onset (3–5 minutes) and a prolonged duration of action (5–10 hours). Based on comparative clinical studies of lidocaine and Duranest, the anesthetic properties of Duranest in man may be characterized as follows: Initial onset of sensory analgesia and motor blockade is rapid (usually 3–5 minutes) and similar to that produced by lidocaine. Duration of sensory analgesia is 1.5 to 2 times longer than that of lidocaine, by the peridural route. The difference in analgesic duration between Duranest and lidocaine may be even greater following peripheral nerve blockade than following central neural block. Duration of analgesia in excess of 9 hours is not infrequent when Duranest is used for peripheral nerve blocks such as brachial plexus blockade. Duranest produces a profound degree of motor blockade and abdominal muscle relaxation when used for peridural analgesia.

Following absorption from the site of injection, Duranest redistributes rapidly and demonstrates a larger volume of distribution than that seen with comparable local anesthetic drugs due to its high tissue solubility.

The rate of metabolism is similar to that of lidocaine. Duranest is metabolized in the liver and its metabolites are excreted via the kidneys. Little unchanged drug is recovered in the urine. Animal studies to date indicate that no single metabolite will account for more than 10% of the administered dose.

Clinical trials to date demonstrate that Duranest HCl does not produce methemoglobinemia or tissue irritation.

Indications: Duranest (etidocaine) HCl is indicated for percutaneous infiltration anesthesia, peripheral nerve blocks, and central neural blocks, i.e., caudal or epidural blocks.

Contraindications: Duranest (etidocaine) HCl is contraindicated in patients with a known history of hypersensitivity to local anesthetic agents of the amide type.

Warnings:

1. RESUSCITATIVE EQUIPMENT AND DRUGS SHOULD BE IMMEDIATELY AVAILABLE WHEN ANY LOCAL ANESTHETIC AGENT IS USED.
2. Use in Pregnancy: Reproductive studies have been performed in rats and rabbits without evidence of harm to the animal fetus. However, the safe use of Duranest (etidocaine) HCl in humans has not been established with respect to adverse effects upon fetal development. Careful consideration should be given to this fact before administering this drug to women of childbearing potential, particularly during early pregnancy. This does not exclude the use of the drug at term for obstetrical analgesia. Duranest HCl has been used for obstetrical analgesia by the peridural route without evidence of adverse effects on the fetus. Fetal effects of Duranest by the paracervical route have *not* been investigated.
3. Local anesthetic procedures should be used with caution when there is inflammation and/or sepsis in the region of the proposed injection.
4. Solutions which contain epinephrine or other vasoconstrictor agents should be used with extreme caution in patients receiving drugs known to produce blood pressure alterations (i.e., MAO inhibitors, tricyclic antidepressants, phenothiazines, etc.) as either severe sustained hypertension or hypotension may occur.
5. Vasopressor agents (administered for the treatment of hypotension related to caudal or other epidural blocks) should be used with extreme caution in the presence of oxytocic drugs as they are known to interact and may produce severe persistent hypertension and/or rupture of cerebral blood vessels.
6. The use of Duranest has not been investigated in children under 14 years of age.

Precautions: The safety and effectiveness of Duranest (etidocaine) HCl depend on proper dosage, correct technique, adequate precautions, and readiness for emergencies. Consult standard textbooks for specific techniques and precautions for various regional anesthetic procedures.

The lowest dosage that results in effective anesthesia should be used to avoid high plasma levels and possible adverse effects. Tolerance varies with the status of the patient. For example, debilitated, elderly or acutely ill patients should be given reduced doses commensurate with their physical status. Duranest HCl should also be used with caution in patients with severe shock or heart block.

INJECTIONS SHOULD ALWAYS BE MADE SLOWLY AND WITH FREQUENT ASPIRATIONS TO AVOID INADVERTENT RAPID INTRAVASCULAR ADMINISTRATION WHICH CAN PRODUCE SYSTEMIC TOXICITY.

Occasionally, duration of motor block may appear to exceed that of sensory block (see ACTIONS). Consideration should be given to the profound motor block and its effect on the need for voluntary expulsive muscles when using Duranest for epidural block in obstetrics.

Epidural anesthesia and caudal anesthesia should be used with extreme caution in persons with the following conditions: existing neurological disease, septicemia, severe hypertension, or spinal deformities which may affect the quality of the block.

Solutions which contain a vasoconstrictor agent should be used with caution in the presence of diseases which may adversely affect the patient's cardiovascular system. Serious cardiac arrhythmias may occur if preparations containing a vasoconstrictor drug are employed in patients during or following the administration of chloroform, halothane, cyclopropane, trichlorethylene, or other related agents. Solutions containing epinephrine should be used cautiously in areas with limited blood supply.

Duranest HCl should be used with caution in persons with known drug sensitivities. Patients allergic to paraaminobenzoic acid derivatives (procaine, tetracaine, benzocaine, etc.) have not shown cross sensitivity to agents of the amide type such as Duranest. Since Duranest is metabolized in the liver and excreted via the kidneys, it should be used cautiously in patients with liver and renal disease.

Consideration should be given to the long duration of peripheral nerve block (8–10 hours) when using this drug for ambulatory patients.

Adverse Reactions: Reactions to Duranest (etidocaine) HCl are similar in character to those observed with other local anesthetic agents such as lidocaine. Adverse reactions may result from high plasma levels due to excessive dosage, rapid absorption or inadvertent intravascular injection. Such reactions are systemic in nature and involve the central nervous system and/or the cardiovascular system. A small number of reactions may result from hypersensitivity, idiosyncrasy or diminished tolerance on the part of the patient.

CNS reactions are excitatory and/or depressant, and are usually characterized by nervousness, dizziness, blurred vision and tremors, followed by drowsiness, convulsions, unconsciousness and possibly respiratory arrest. Excitatory CNS effects commonly represent the initial signs of local anesthetic systemic toxicity. However, these reactions may be very brief or absent in some patients in which case the first manifestations of toxicity may be drowsiness, merging into unconsciousness and respiratory arrest.

Hypotension and bradycardia may occur as normal physiological phenomena following sympathetic block with central neural blocks. Toxic cardiovascular reactions to local anesthetics are usually depressant in nature and are characterized by peripheral vasodilation, hypotension, myocardial depression, bradycardia, and possibly cardiac arrest. However, direct cardiovascular depressant effects have not been seen with Duranest in the absence of central nervous system toxicity.

Treatment of a patient wth toxic manifestations consists of assuring and maintaining a patent airway and supporting ventilation with oxygen and assisted or controlled respiration as required. This usually will be sufficient in the management of most reactions. Should a convulsion persist despite ventilatory therapy, small increments of anticonvulsive agents may be given intravenously such as a benzodiazepine (e.g., diazepam), an ultra-short acting barbiturate (e.g., thiopental or thiamylal) or a short-acting barbiturate (e.g., pentobarbital or secobarbital). Cardiovascular depression may require circulatory assistance with intravenous fluids and/or vasopressor agents as dictated by the clinical situation. Allergic reactions may occur as a result of sensitivity to the local anesthetic or methylparaben used as a preservative and are characterized by cutaneous lesions, urticaria, edema or anaphylactoid type symtomatology. True allergic reactions should be managed by conventional means. The detection of potential sensitivity by skin testing is of limited value.

Dosage and Administration: As with all local anesthetic agents the dose of Duranest (etidocaine) HCl to be employed will depend on the area to be anesthetized, the vascularity of the tissues, the number of neuronal segments to be blocked, the type of regional anesthetic technique and the status and tolerance of the individual patient. The maximum dose of Duranest HCl to be employed as a single injection should be determined on the basis of the status of the patient and the type of regional anesthetic technique to be performed. Although single injections of 450 mg have been employed for regional anesthesia without adverse effects, at present it is strongly recommended that the maximal dose of Duranest HCl as a single injection should not exceed 400 mg (approximately 5.5 mg/kg or 2.7 mg/lb) with epinephrine 1:200,000 and 300 mg (approximately 4 mg/kg or 2 mg/lb) without epinephrine. Because Duranest has been shown to disappear quite rapidly from blood, toxicity is influenced by rapidity of administration, and therefore slow injection in vascular areas is highly recommended. Incremental doses of Duranest HCl may be repeated at 2–3 hour intervals.

The following dosage recommendations are intended as guides for the use of Duranest HCl in the average adult patient. As indicated previously, the dosage should be reduced for elderly or debilitated patients or patients with severe renal disease.

[See table on next page].

No information is available on appropriate pediatric doses.

XYLOCAINE® (lidocaine HCl) STERILE AQUEOUS SOLUTIONS ℞

Local anesthetic for infiltration and nerve block

Description: Xylocaine (lidocaine) is a local anesthetic chemically designated as diethylaminoacet-2,6-xylidide.

Aqueous solutions of Xylocaine hydrochloride (without epinephrine) may be autoclaved repeatedly, if necessary.

Please refer to Table I for the exact composition of available Xylocaine hydrochloride solutions.

(See table bottom left next page)

Actions: Xylocaine (lidocaine) stabilizes the neuronal membrane and prevents the initia-

Continued on next page

Astra—Cont.

TABLE 2. Dosage Recommendations

PROCEDURE	Duranest HCl with epinephrine 1:200,000		
	Conc. (%)	Vol. (ml)	Total Dose (mg)
Percutaneous Infiltration	0.5	1–80	5–400
	0.5	5–80	25–400
Peripheral Nerve Block	or		
	1.0	5–40	50–400
Central Neural Block			
Lumbar Peridural			
Intraabdominal or Pelvic Surgery	1.0	10–30	100–300
Lower Limb Surgery	or		
Caesarean Section	1.5	10–20	150–300
	0.5	10–30	50–150
Vaginal Obstetrical and	or		
Gynecologic Procedures	1.0	5–20	50–200
	0.5	10–30	50–150
Caudal	or		
	1.0	10–30	100–300

How Supplied:

Dosage Form and Volume	Duranest HCl Concentration	Epinephrine Dilution
Multiple Dose Vials		
50 ml	0.5%	1:200,000
Single Dose Vials		
30 ml	0.5%	None
	0.5%	1:200,000
	1.0%	None
	1.0%	1:200,000
Ampules		
30 ml	1.0%	None
	1.0%	1:200,000
20 ml	1.5%	1:200,000

tion and transmission of nerve impulses, thereby effecting local anesthetic action.
Xylocaine is metabolized mainly in the liver and excreted via the kidneys. Approximately 90% of Xylocaine administered is excreted in the form of various metabolites, while less than 10% is excreted unchanged.

Indications: Xylocaine (lidocaine) hydrochloride is indicated for production of local or regional anesthesia by infiltration techniques including percutaneous injection and intravenous regional anesthesia, by peripheral nerve block techniques such as brachial plexus and intercostal blocks, and by central neural techniques including epidural and caudal blocks, when the accepted procedures for these techniques as described in standard textbooks are observed.

Contraindications: Xylocaine hydrochloride is containdicated in patients with a known history of hypersensitivity to local anesthetics of the amide type.
Local anesthetic procedures should not be used in cases in which there is inflammation and/or sepsis in the region of the proposed injection. However, the existence of a region of inflammation or sepsis in a limb does not contraindicate the use of intravenous regional anesthesia if the local anesthetic solution is injected into a vein remote from the region of inflammation or sepsis.

Warnings:

(1) RESUSCITATIVE EQUIPMENT AND DRUGS SHOULD BE IMMEDIATELY AVAILABLE WHEN ANY LOCAL ANESTHETIC IS USED.

(2) *Usage in Pregnancy:* The safe use of Xylocaine (lidocaine) has not been established with respect to adverse effects upon fetal development. Careful consideration should be given to this fact before administering this drug to women of childbearing potential, particularly during early pregnancy.
This does not exclude the use of the drug at term for obstetrical analgesia. Xylocaine has been used effectively for obstetrical analgesia. Adverse effects on the fetus, course of labor, or delivery have rarely been observed when proper dosage and proper technique have been employed.

(3) Solutions which contain a vasoconstrictor should be used with extreme caution in patients receiving drugs known to produce blood pressure alterations (i.e. MAO inhibitors, tricyclic antidepressants, phenothiazines, etc.) as either severe and sustained hypotension or hypertension may occur.

(4) Vasopressor agents (administered for the treatment of hypotension related to caudal or other epidural blocks) should not be used in the presence of oxytocic drugs, as a severe persistent hypertension and even rupture of cerebral blood vessels may occur.

Precautions: The safety and effectiveness of Xylocaine (lidocaine) hydrochloride depends on proper dosage, correct technique, adequate precautions, and readiness for emergencies.
The lowest dosage that results in effective anesthesia should be used to avoid high plasma levels and serious adverse effects. Injection of repeated doses of Xylocaine may cause significant increases in blood levels with each repeated dose due to slow accumulation of the drug or its metabolites. Tolerance varies with the status of the patient. Debilitated, elderly patients, acutely ill patients, and children should be given reduced doses commensurate with their age and physical status. Xylocaine should also be used with caution in patients with severe shock or heart block.
In using Xylocaine for infiltration or regional block anesthesia, injection should always be made slowly and with frequent aspirations.
Epidural anesthesia and caudal anesthesia should be used with extreme caution in persons with the following conditions: existing neurological disease, spinal deformities, septicemia, severe hypertension, and extreme youth.
Fetal bradycardia frequently follows paracervical block and may be associated with fetal acidosis. Fetal heart rate should always be monitored during paracervical anesthesia. Added risk appears to be present in prematurity, toxemia of pregnancy, and fetal distress. The physician should weigh the possible advantages against dangers when considering paracervical block in these conditions. When the recommended dose is exceeded the incidence of fetal bradycardia increases.
Solutions containing a vasoconstrictor should be used cautiously and in carefully circumscribed quantities in areas of the body supplied by end arteries or having otherwise compromised blood supply. Patients with peripheral vascular disease and those with hypertensive vascular disease may exhibit exaggerated vasoconstrictor response. Serious cardiac arrhythmias may occur if preparations containing a vasoconstrictor are employed in patients during or following the administration of chloroform, halothane, cyclopropane, trichlorethylene, or other related agents.
Proper tourniquet technique is essential in the performance of intravenous regional anesthesia. Solutions containing epinephrine or other

TABLE I
COMPOSITION OF AVAILABLE SOLUTIONS

Product Identification		Formula				
		Multiple Dose Vials			Ampules and Single Dose Vials	
Xylocaine (lidocaine) Hydrochloride (percent)	Epinephrine (dilution)	Sodium chloride (mg per ml)	Methylparaben (mg per ml)	Sodium metabisulfite (mg per ml)	Sodium chloride (mg per ml)	Sodium metabisulfite (mg per ml)
0.5	None	8.0	1.0	None	8.0	None
0.5	1:200,000	8.0	1.0	0.5	N.S.	N.S.
1.0	None	7.0	1.0	None	7.0	None
1.0	1:200,000	N.S.	N.S.	N.S.	7.0	0.5
1.0	1:100,000	7.0	1.0	0.5	N.S.	N.S.
1.5	None	N.S.	N.S.	N.S.	6.5	None
1.5	1:200,000	N.S.	N.S.	N.S.	6.5	0.5
2.0	None	6.0	1.0	None	6.0	None
2.0	1:200,000	N.S.	N.S.	N.S.	6.0	0.5
2.0	1:100,000	6.0	1.0	0.5	6.0	0.5

N.S.: Not supplied.
NOTE: pH of all solutions adjusted to U.S.P. limits with sodium hydroxide.

vasoconstrictors should not be used for this technique.

Xylocaine should be used with caution in persons with known drug sensitivities. Patients allergic to para-aminobenzoic acid derivatives (procaine, tetracaine, benzocaine, etc.) have not shown cross sensitivity to Xylocaine.

Local anesthetics react with certain metals and cause the release of their respective ions which, if injected, may cause severe local irritation. Adequate precaution should be taken to avoid this type of interaction.

Adverse Reactions: Adverse reactions may result from high plasma levels due to excessive dosage, rapid absorption or inadvertent intravascular injection, or may result from a hypersensitivity, idiosyncrasy or diminished tolerance on the part of the patient. Such reactions are systemic in nature and involve the central nervous system and/or the cardiovascular system.

CNS reactions are excitatory and/or depressant, and may be characterized by nervousness, dizziness, blurred vision and tremors, followed by drowsiness, convulsions, unconsciousness and possibly respiratory arrest. The excitatory reactions may be very brief or may not occur at all, in which case the first manifestations of toxicity may be drowsiness, merging into unconsciousness and respiratory arrest.

Cardiovascular reactions are depressant, and may be characterized by hypotension, myocardial depression, bradycardia and possibly cardiac arrest.

Treatment of a patient with toxic manifestations consists of assuring and maintaining a patent airway and supporting ventilation using oxygen and assisted or controlled respiration as required. This usually will be sufficient in the management of most reactions. Should circulatory depression occur, vasopressors, such as ephedrine or metaraminol, and intravenous fluids may be used. Should a convulsion persist despite oxygen therapy, small increments of an ultra-short acting barbiturate (thiopental or thiamylal) or a short acting barbiturate (pentobarbital or secobarbital) may be given intravenously.

Allergic reactions are characterized by cutaneous lesions, urticaria, edema or anaphylactoid reactions. The detection of sensitivity by skin testing is of doubtful value.

Dosage and Administration: Table II (Recommended Dosages) summarizes the recommended volumes and concentrations of Xylocaine (lidocaine) hydrochloride for various types of anesthetic procedures. The dosages suggested in this table are for normal healthy adults and refer to the use of epinephrine-free solutions. When larger volumes are required, only solutions containing epinephrine should be used, except in those cases where vasopressor drugs may be contraindicated.

[See table above].

TABLE II (Recommended Dosages)

PROCEDURE	Xylocaine (lidocaine) Hydrochloride (without epinephrine)		
	Conc. (%)	Vol. (ml)	Total Dose (mg)
Infiltration			
Percutaneous	0.5 or 1.0	1–60	5–300
Intravenous regional	0.5	10–60	50–300
Peripheral Nerve Blocks, e.g.			
Brachial	1.5	15–20	225–300
Dental	2.0	1–5	20–100
Intercostal	1.0	3	30
Paravertebral	1.0	3–5	30–50
Pudendal (each side)	1.0	10	100
Paracervical			
Obstetrical analgesia (each side)	1.0	10	100
Sympathetic Nerve Blocks, e.g.			
Cervical (stellate ganglion)	1.0	5	50
Lumbar	1.0	5–10	50–100
Central Neural Blocks			
Epidural*			
Thoracic	1.0	20–30	200–300
Lumbar			
Analgesia	1.0	25–30	250–300
Anesthesia	1.5	15–20	225–300
	2.0	10–15	200–300
Caudal			
Obstetrical analgesia	1.0	20–30	200–300
Surgical anesthesia	1.5	15–20	225–300

*Dose determined by number of dermatomes to be anesthetized (2–3 ml/dermatome).

THE ABOVE SUGGESTED CONCENTRATIONS AND VOLUMES SERVE ONLY AS A GUIDE. OTHER VOLUMES AND CONCENTRATIONS MAY BE USED, PROVIDED THE TOTAL MAXIMUM RECOMMENDED DOSE IS NOT EXCEEDED.

These recommended doses serve only as a guide to the amount of anesthetic required for most routine procedures. The actual volume and concentrations to be used depend on a number of factors, such as type and extent of surgical procedure, degree of muscular relaxation required, duration of anesthesia required, the physical state of the patient, etc. In all cases the lowest concentration and smallest dose that will produce the desired result should be given. Dosages should be reduced for children and for elderly and debilitated patients.

The onset of anesthesia, the duration of anesthesia and the degree of muscular relaxation are proportional to the volume and concentration of local anesthetic used. Thus, an increase in volume and concentration of Xylocaine hydrochloride will decrease the onset of anesthesia, prolong the duration of anesthesia, provide a greater degree of muscular relaxation and increase the segmental spread of anesthesia. However, increasing the volume and concentration of Xylocaine hydrochloride may result in a more profound fall in blood pressure when used in epidural anesthesia. Although the incidence of side effects with Xylocaine hydrochloride is quite low, caution should be exercised particularly when employing large volumes and concentrations of Xylocaine hydrochloride since the incidence of side effects is directly proportional to the total dose of local anesthetic agent injected.

It is important that a single dose container be employed for epidural anesthesia and major peripheral nerve block. For intravenous regional anesthesia, only the single dose containers designated for intravenous regional anesthesia should be used.

Epidural Anesthesia

For epidural anesthesia, only the following dosage forms of Xylocaine hydrochloride are recommended:

1% without epinephrine .... 30 ml ampules
30 ml single dose vials

1% with epinephrine
1:200,000 .... 30 ml ampules

1.5% without epinephrine .... 20 ml ampules
20 ml single dose vials

1.5% with epinephrine
1:200,000 .... 30 ml ampules
30 ml single dose vials

2% without epinephrine .... 10 ml ampules

2% with epinephrine
1:200,000 .... 20 ml ampules
20 ml single dose vials

Although these solutions are intended specifically for epidural anesthesia, they may also be used for infiltration and peripheral nerve block, provided they are employed as single dose units. These solutions contain no bacteriostatic agent.

In epidural anesthesia, the dosage varies with the number of dermatomes to be anesthetized (generally 2-3 ml of the indicated concentration per dermatome).

IMPORTANT: *A test dose of 2-5 ml should be administered at least 5 minutes prior to injecting the total required volume for central neural blocks (epidural or caudal anesthesia).*

Maximum Recommended Dosages

For normal healthy adults, the individual dose of Xylocaine (lidocaine) hydrochloride with epinephrine should be kept below 500 mg and in any case should not exceed 7 mg/kg (3.5 mg/lb) of body weight. When used without epinephrine, the amount of Xylocaine hydrochloride administered should be kept below 300 mg and in any case should not exceed 4.5 mg/kg (2 mg per lb) of body weight. For continuous epidural or caudal anesthesia, the maximum recommended dosage should not be administered at intervals of less than 90 minutes. When continuous epidural or caudal anesthesia is used for non-obstetrical procedures, more drug may be administered if required to produce adequate anesthesia. For paracervical block for obstetrical analgesia, tne maximum recommended dosage (200 mg) should not be administered at intervals of less than 90 minutes. When paracervical block is used for non-obstetrical procedures, more drug may be administered if required to obtain adequate anesthesia. For intravenous regional anesthesia, the dose administered should not exceed 4 mg/kg in adults.

Children:

It is difficult to recommend a maximum dose of any drug for children since this varies as a function of age and weight. For children of less than ten years who have a normal lean body mass and normal body development, the maximum dose may be determined by the application of one of the standard pediatric drug formulas (e.g., Clark's rule or Young's rule). For example, in a child of five years weighing 50 lbs., the dose of Xylocaine hydrochloride should not exceed 75–100 mg when calculated according to Clark's rule or Young's rule. Body surface area may also be used as a guide in determining drug dosage in pediatric patients. In order to minimize the possibility of toxic reactions, the use of 0.5% or 1.0% concentrations of Xylocaine hydrochloride is recommended for most anesthetic procedures involving pediatric patients. The use of even more dilute solutions (i.e., 0.25–0.5%) and total dosages not to exceed

Continued on next page

Astra—Cont.

3 mg/kg are recommended for induction of intravenous regional anesthesia in children.
How Supplied:
[See table below].

Dosage Form	Xylocaine (lidocaine) Hydrochloride concentration	epinephrine (dilution)
Multiple Dose Vials		
50ml	2%	None
	2%	1:100,000
	1%	None
	1%	1:100,000
	0.5%	None
	0.5%	1:200,000
20ml	2%	None
	2%	1:100,000
	1%	None
	1%	1:100,000
Single Dose Vials		
50ml	0.5%	None
30ml	1.5%	1:200,000
	1%	None
20ml	2%	1:200,000
	1.5%	None

Dosage Form	Xylocaine (lidocaine) Hydrochloride concentration	epinephrine (dilution)
Single Dose Ampules		
30ml	1.5%	1:200,000
	1%	None
	1%	1:200,000
20ml	2%	1:200,000
	1.5%	None
10ml	2%	None
5ml	1%	None
2ml	2%	None
	2%	1:100,000
	1%	None
Prefilled Syringe		
5 ml	1%	None

XYLOCAINE® (lidocaine HCl) ℞
INTRAMUSCULAR INJECTION FOR CARDIAC ARRHYTHMIAS

Description: Xylocaine, diethylaminoacet-2,6-xylidide, is a stable colorless crystalline solid. The hydrochloride salt is readily soluble in water. Each ml of the sterile solution for intramuscular injection contains 100 mg of Xylocaine hydrochloride, and sodium hydroxide to adjust pH. This solution is for intramuscular use only.

Actions: Xylocaine (lidocaine) is reported to increase the electrical stimulation threshold of the ventricle during diastole and, thereby, exert an antiarrhythmic effect. In the dosage recommended, Xylocaine produces no change in systolic arterial blood pressure, absolute refractory period, or myocardial contractility.
When an appropriate dose of Xylocaine is administered by the intramuscular (deltoid) route, effective antiarrhythmic blood levels are usually attained within 5–15 minutes and usually persist for 60–90 minutes. Clinical studies in which cardiac arrhythmias were monitored indicated that the onset and duration of antiarrhythmic activity of intramuscular Xylocaine are correlated with the attained blood levels of Xylocaine. As with intravenous Xylocaine, the intramuscular use of this agent has been found to exert beneficial antiarrhythmic activity in approximately 80% of treated patients.
Approximately 90% of an administered dose of Xylocaine is metabolized in the liver. Less than 10% of the drug is excreted unchanged via the kidneys.

Indications: Xylocaine is indicated in the management of cardiac arrhythmias, particularly those of ventricular origin such as occur with acute myocardial infarction.
Intramuscular administration (single dose) is justified in the following exceptional circumstances:
1. by a physician when ECG equipment is not available to verify the diagnosis but in whose opinion the potential benefits outweigh the possible risks.
2. by a physician when facilities for intravenous administration are not readily available.
3. by paramedical personnel in a mobile coronary care unit on direction by a physician viewing the transmitted ECG.

Contraindications: Xylocaine (lidocaine) is contraindicated (1) in patients with a known history of hypersensitivity to local anesthetics of the amide type; and (2) in patients with Adams-Stokes syndrome or with severe degrees of sinoatrial, atrioventricular or intraventricular block.

Warnings: INJECTIONS SHOULD BE MADE WITH FREQUENT ASPIRATIONS TO AVOID POSSIBLE INADVERTENT INTRAVASCULAR ADMINISTRATION.
Monitoring with an electrocardiograph is recommended when Xylocaine is administered by the intramuscular route. In emergency situations when a ventricular rhythm disorder is suspected and electrocardiographic equipment is not available, a single dose may be administered when the physician in attendance has determined that the potential benefits outweigh the possible risks. If possible, emergency resuscitative equipment and drugs should be immediately available to manage potential adverse reactions involving the cardiovascular, respiratory or central nervous systems.
The intramuscular use of Xylocaine may result in an increase in creatine phosphokinase levels. Thus, the use of this enzyme determination, without isoenzyme separation, as a diagnostic test for the presence of acute myocardial infarction may be compromised by the use of intramuscular Xylocaine.
Intramuscular Xylocaine is not recommended for pediatric usage, since evidence concerning proper use in children is not available.

Precautions: Xylocaine (lidocaine) is metabolized mainly in the liver and excreted by the kidney. Therefore, caution should be employed in the repeated or prolonged use of Xylocaine in patients with severe liver or renal disease due to the possible accumulation of Xylocaine or its metabolites which may lead to toxic phenomena. The drug should also be used with caution in patients with hypovolemia and shock, and all forms of heart block.

Adverse Reactions: Serious adverse reactions have been rare following the use of intramuscular Xylocaine. However, systemic reactions of the following types previously have been reported following Xylocaine administration, usually with excessive doses:
(1) Central Nervous System: lightheadedness; drowsiness; dizziness; apprehension; euphoria; tinnitus; blurred or double vision; vomiting; sensations of heat, cold or numbness; twitching; tremors; convulsions; unconsciousness; and respiratory depression and arrest.
(2) Cardiovascular System: hypotension; cardiovascular collapse; and bradycardia which may lead to cardiac arrest.
There have been no reports of cross sensitivity between Xylocaine and procainamide or between Xylocaine and quinidine.
Soreness at the injection site following intramuscular injections has occasionally been reported.

Management of Adverse Reactions:
1. In the case of severe reaction discontinue the use of the drug.
2. Institute the emergency resuscitative procedures, including maintenance of patent airway and assisted respiration, if necessary. Administer the emergency drugs necessary to manage the severe reaction.
3. For severe convulsions, parenteral administration of a rapidly acting anticonvulsant may be used.

Dosage and Administration: The recommended dose of Xylocaine (lidocaine) by the intramuscular route in the average 70 kg or 150 lb man is 300 mg (approximately 4.3 mg/kg or 2.0 mg/lb). The deltoid muscle is recommended as the preferred site of injection, since therapeutic blood levels of Xylocaine occur faster and the peak blood level is significantly higher following deltoid administration as compared to injections into the lateral thigh or gluteus. Injections should be made with frequent aspirations to avoid possible inadvertent intravascular injection.
As soon as possible, and when indicated, patients should be changed to an intravenous infusion of Xylocaine, or to an oral antiarrhythmic preparation for maintenance therapy. However, if necessary, an additional intramuscular injection may be made after an interval of 60–90 minutes.

How Supplied: Xylocaine for intramuscular use is supplied in 5 ml ampules, packed 10 to a carton. Each ml of the sterile solution contains 100 mg of Xylocaine HCl. Thus, 3 ml of solution will provide the recommended dose.

XYLOCAINE® ℞
(lidocaine HCl injection USP)
INTRAVENOUS INJECTION FOR CARDIAC ARRHYTHMIAS

Description: Xylocaine brand of lidocaine HCl is chemically designated as acetamide, 2-(diethylamino)-N-(2.6dimethylphenyl) monohydrochloride. Xylocaine Intravenous Injection for Cardiac Arrhythmias is a sterile solution prepared from lidocaine with the aid of hydrochloric acid in water for injection.
[See Table I].
[See table on next page].

Actions: Xylocaine brand of lidocaine HCl has been reported to exert an antiarrhythmic effect by increasing the electrical stimulation threshold of the ventricle during disatole. In usual therapeutic doses Xylocaine brand of lidocaine HCl produces no changes in myocardial contractility, in systemic arterial pressure, or in absolute refractory period.
Approximately 90% of an administered dose of Xylocaine brand of lidocaine HCl is metabolized in the liver. The remaining 10% is excreted unchanged via the kidneys.

Indications: Xylocaine brand of lidocaine HCl administered intravenously is specifically indicated in the acute management of (1) ventricular arrhythmias occurring during cardiac manipulation such as cardiac surgery, and (2) life-threatening arrhythmias which are ventricular in origin, such as occur during acute myocardial infarction.

Contraindications: Xylocaine brand of lidocaine HCl is contraindicated in patients with a known history of hypersensitivity to local anesthetics of the amide type. Xylocaine brand of lidocaine HCl should not be used in patients with STOKES-ADAMS syndrome, Wolff-Parkinson-White syndrome, or with severe degrees of sinoatrial, atrioventricular, or intraventricular block.

Warnings: Constant monitoring with an electrocardiograph is essential to the proper administration of Xylocaine brand of lidocaine HCl intravenously. Signs of excessive depression of cardiac conductivity, such as prolongation of PR interval and QRS complex and the appearance or aggravation of arrhythmias, should be followed by prompt cessation of the intravenous infusion of this agent. It is mandatory to have emergency resuscitative equipment and drugs immediately available to manage possible adverse reactions involving cardiovascular, respiratory, or central nervous systems.

Occasional acceleration of ventricular rate may occur when Xylocaine brand of lidocaine HCl is administered to patients with atrial fibrillation. Evidence for proper usage in children is limited.

Usage in pregnancy: It is not known whether Xylocaine brand of lidocaine HCl may have adverse effects upon fetal development. The benefits of the drug to the mother should be weighed against possible risk to the fetus.

Precautions: Caution should be employed in the repeated use of Xylocaine brand of lidocaine HCl in patients with severe liver or kidney disease because accumulation may occur and lead to toxic phenomena, since Xylocaine brand of lidocaine HCl is metabolized mainly in the liver and excreted by the kidneys. The drug should also be used with caution in patients with hypovolemia and shock, and in all forms of heart block (see CONTRAINDICATIONS and WARNINGS).

In patients with sinus bradycardia or incomplete heart block, the administration of Xylocaine brand of lidocaine HCl intravenously or the elimination of ventricular ectopic beats without prior acceleration in heart rate (e.g. by isoproterenol or by electric pacing) may promote more frequent and serious ventricular arrhythmias or complete heart block (see CONTRAINDICATIONS).

Adverse Reactions: Systemic reactions of the following types have been reported:

1. Central Nervous System:
   Light-headedness; drowsiness; dizziness; apprehension; euphoria; tinnitus; blurred vision or double vision; vomiting; sensations of heat, cold or numbness; twitching; tremors; convulsions; unconsciousness; respiratory depression and arrest.
2. Cardiovascular System:
   Hypotension; cardiovascular collapse; and bradycardia which may lead to cardiac arrest.
3. Allergic reactions may occur but are infrequent. There have been no reports of cross-sensitivity between Xylocaine brand of lidocaine HCl and procainamide or between Xylocaine brand of lidocaine HCl and quinidine.

Management of Adverse Reactions:

1. In the case of severe reaction, discontinue the use of Xylocaine brand of lidocaine HCl.
2. Institute emergency resuscitative procedures and administer the emergency drugs necessary to manage the severe reaction. For severe convulsions, small increments of diazepam or an ultra-short acting barbiturate (thiopental or thiamylal); or if those are not available a short-acting barbiturate (pentobarbital or secobarbital); or if the patient is under anesthesia, a short-acting muscle relaxant (succinylcholine) may be given intravenously. Muscle relaxants and intravenous medications should only be used by those familiar with their use. Patency of the airway and adequacy of ventilation must be assured.
3. Should circulatory depression occur, vasopressors, such as ephedrine, or metaraminol may be used.

TABLE I Composition of available solutions

	Dosage Form	Composition* Lidocaine HCl (mg per ml)	Sodium Chloride (mg per ml)
For Direct Injection	5 ml (100 mg) prefilled syringe	20	6
	5 ml (100 mg) ampule	20	6
For Preparation of Infusion Solutions	25 ml (One Gram) single use vial	40	None
	50 ml (Two Grams) single use vial	40	None
	5 ml (One Gram) additive syringe	200	None
	10 ml (Two Grams) additive syringe	200	None

*pH of all solutions adjusted with sodium hydroxide
All containers are for single use: solutions do not contain preservatives.

Dosage and Administration:

Single Injection

Only the 5 ml, 100 mg dosage size should be used for direct injection. The usual dose is 50 to 100 mg administered intravenously under ECG monitoring. This dose may be administered at the rate of approximately 20 to 50 mg/min. Sufficient time should be allowed to enable a slow circulation to carry the drug to the site of action. If the initial injection of 50 to 100 mg does not produce a desired response, a second dose may be repeated after 5 minutes. Activate syringe only when prepared to administer injection. See illustrated instructions for use.

NO MORE THAN 200 TO 300 MG OF XYLOCAINE BRAND OF LIDOCAINE HCl SHOULD BE ADMINISTERED DURING A ONE HOUR PERIOD.

Evidence for proper usage in children is limited.

Continuous Infusion

Following a single injection, using a 5 ml, 100 mg dosage size, in those patients in whom the arrhythmia tends to recur and who are incapable of receiving oral antiarrhythmic therapy, intravenous infusions of Xylocaine brand of lidocaine HCl may be administered at the rate of 1 to 4 mg/min. (20 to 50 μg/kg/min. in the average 70 kg man). Intravenous infusions of Xylocaine brand of lidocaine HCl must be administered under constant ECG monitoring to avoid potential overdosage and toxicity. Intravenous infusion should be terminated as soon as the patient's basic cardiac rhythm appears to be stable or at the earliest signs of toxicity. It should rarely be necessary to continue intravenous infusions beyond 24 hours. As soon as possible, and when indicated, patients should be changed to an oral antiarrhythmic agent for maintenance therapy.

Solutions for intravenous infusion may be prepared by the addition of one gram or two grams of Xylocaine brand of lidocaine HCl to one liter of 5% dextrose in water, the preferred diluent using aseptic technique. Approximately a 0.1% to 0.2% solution will result from this procedure, that is, each ml will contain approximately 1 to 2 mg of Xylocaine brand of lidocaine HCl. Thus, 1 to 4 ml/min. will provide 1 to 4 mg of Xylocaine brand of lidocaine HCl/min.

In those cases in which fluid restriction is medically desirable, a more concentrated solution may be prepared.

Xylocaine brand of lidocaine HCl has been found to be chemically stable for a minimum of 24 hours after dilution in the sterile intravenous solution recommended above. However, as with all intravenous admixtures, dilution should be made just prior to administration.

NOTE: Solutions containing 40 mg or 200 mg of Xylocaine brand of lidocaine HCl per ml, without sodium chloride or preservatives, are recommended for the preparation of intravenous infusion solutions.

CAUTION: The flow rate of all intravenous infusion solutions must be closely monitored. Xylocaine brand of lidocaine HCl should not be added to blood transfusion assemblies.

How Supplied: For direct injection Xylocaine brand of lidocaine HCl without preservatives is supplied in 5 ml, 100 mg ampules and in 5 ml, 100 mg prefilled syringes.

For preparing intravenous infusion solutions, Xylocaine brand of lidocaine HCl without sodium chloride or preservatives is supplied in one and two gram additive syringes and in one and two gram single use vials. Each vial is packed with a pre-sterilized transfer unit manufactured by the West Company.

XYLOCAINE® (lidocaine) HYDROCHLORIDE 4% SOLUTION ℞

For transtracheal use, retrobulbar injection, and for topical application

Description: Xylocaine is a local anesthetic chemically designated as diethylaminoacet-2,6-xylidide.

Xylocaine hydrochloride 4% (without epinephrine) in 5 ml ampules may be autoclaved repeatedly, if necessary. The 50 ml screw-cap bottle should not be autoclaved because the closure employed cannot withstand autoclaving temperatures and pressures.

Composition of Xylocaine Hydrochloride 4%

5 ml ampule:
Each ml contains:
diethylaminoacet-2,6-xylidide
(lidocaine) hydrochloride........................40 mg
sodium hydroxide ....to adjust pH to 6.0-7.0
A sterile, aqueous solution.

50 ml screw-cap bottle:
Each ml contains:
diethylaminoacet-2,6-xylidide
(lidocaine) hydrochloride........................40 mg
methylparaben..1 mg
sodium hydroxide ....to adjust pH to 6.0-7.0
An aqueous solution. NOT FOR INJECTION.

Actions: Xylocaine (lidocaine) stabilizes the neuronal membrane and prevents the initiation and transmission of nerve impulses, thereby effecting local anesthetic action.

Xylocaine is metabolized mainly in the liver and excreted via the kidneys. Approximately 90% of Xylocaine administered is excreted in the form of various metabolites, while less than 10% is excreted unchanged.

The onset of action is rapid. For retrobulbar injection, 4 ml of Xylocaine Hydrochloride 4% provides an average duration of action of 1 to 1½ hours. This duration may be extended for ophthalmic surgery by the addition of epinephrine, the usual recommended dilution being 1:50,000 to 1:100,000.

Indications: Xylocaine Hydrochloride 4% sterile solution for parenteral use is indicated for the production of local anesthesia of the mucous membranes of the respiratory tract or the genito-urinary tract. It may be injected

Continued on next page

Astra—Cont.

trans-tracheally to anesthetize the larynx and trachea. It may be administered by retrobulbar injection to provide anesthesia for ophthalmic surgery.

Xylocaine Hydrochloride 4% (50 ml screw-cap bottle) is indicated only for the production of *topical* anesthesia of accessible mucous membranes of the oral and nasal cavities and proximal portions of the digestive tract.

Contraindications: Xylocaine (lidocaine) hydrochloride is contraindicated in patients with a known history of hypersensitivity to local anesthetics of the amide type.

Local anesthetic agents should not be used in patients with severe shock or heart block. Local anesthetic procedures should not be used when there is inflammation in the region of the proposed injection.

The solution from the 50 ml screw-cap bottle should not be used to anesthetize mucous membranes of the tracheobronchial tree and urinary tract, nor should it be used for ophthalmologic procedures.

Warnings:

(1) RESUSCITATIVE EQUIPMENT AND DRUGS SHOULD BE IMMEDIATELY AVAILABLE WHEN ANY LOCAL ANESTHETIC IS USED.

(2) *Usage in Pregnancy:* The safe use of Xylocaine (lidocaine) has not been established with respect to adverse effects upon fetal development. Careful consideration should be given to this fact before administering this drug to women of childbearing potential, particularly during early pregnancy.

(3) If a vasoconstrictor is added to Xylocaine Hydrochloride 4%, the solution should be used with extreme caution in patients receiving drugs known to produce blood pressure alterations (i.e. MAO inhibitors, tricyclic antidepressants, phenothiazines, etc.) as either severe and sustained hypotension or hypertension may occur.

Precautions: The safety and effectiveness of Xylocaine (lidocaine) hydrochloride depends on proper dosage, correct technique, adequate precautions, and readiness for emergencies.

The lowest dosage that results in effective anesthesia should be used to avoid high plasma levels and serious adverse effects. Injection of repeated doses of Xylocaine may cause significant increases in blood levels with each repeated dose due to slow accumulation of the drug or its metabolites. Tolerance varies with the status of the patient. Debilitated, elderly patients, acutely ill patients, and children should be given reduced doses commensurate with their age and physical status.

INJECTIONS (OTHER THAN TRANSTRACHEAL) SHOULD ALWAYS BE MADE SLOWLY AND WITH FREQUENT ASPIRATIONS. Consult standard textbooks for specific techniques and precautions for various local anesthetic procedures.

Xylocaine Hydrochloride 4% should be used with caution in patients with severely traumatized mucosa and sepsis in the region of the proposed application.

If a vasoconstrictor is added to Xylocaine Hydrochloride 4%, the solution should be used with caution in the presence of diseases which may adversely affect the patient's cardiovascular system. Serious cardiac arrhythmias may occur if preparations containing a vasoconstrictor are employed in patients during or following the administration of chloroform, halothane, cyclopropane, trichlorethylene, or other related agents.

Xylocaine should be used with caution in persons with known drug sensitivities. Patients allergic to para-aminobenzoic acid derivatives (procaine, tetracaine, benzocaine, etc.) have not shown cross sensitivity to Xylocaine.

Local anesthetics react with certain metals and cause the release of their respective ions which, if injected, may cause severe local irritation. Adequate precaution should be taken to avoid this type of interaction.

Adverse Reactions: Adverse reactions may result from high plasma levels due to excessive dosage, rapid absorption or inadvertent intravascular injection, or may result from a hypersensitivity, idiosyncrasy or diminished tolerance on the part of the patient. Such reactions are systemic in nature and involve the central nervous system and/or the cardiovascular system.

CNS reactions are excitatory and/or depressant, and may be characterized by nervousness, dizziness, blurred vision and tremors, followed by drowsiness, convulsions, unconsciousness and possibly respiratory arrest. The excitatory reactions may be very brief or may not occur at all, in which case the first manifestations of toxicity may be drowsiness, merging into unconsciousness and respiratory arrest.

Cardiovascular reactions are depressant, and may be characterized by hypotension, myocardial depression, bradycardia and possibly cardiac arrest.

Treatment of a patient with toxic manifestations consists of assuring and maintaining a patent airway and supporting ventilation using oxygen and assisted or controlled respiration as required. This usually will be sufficient in the management of most reactions. Should circulatory depression occur, vasopressors, such as ephedrine or metaraminol, and intravenous fluids may be used. Should a convulsion persist despite oxygen therapy, small increments of an ultra-short acting barbiturate (thiopental or thiamylal) or a short acting barbiturate (pentobarbital or secobarbital) may be given intravenously.

Allergic reactions are characterized by cutaneous lesions, urticaria, edema or anaphylactoid reactions. The detection of sensitivity by skin testing is of doubtful value.

Dosage and Administration: The dosage varies and depends upon the area to be anesthetized, vascularity of the tissues, individual tolerance and the technique of anesthesia. The lowest dosage needed to provide effective anesthesia should be administered. Dosages should be reduced for children and for elderly and debilitated patients. Although the incidence of adverse effects with Xylocaine (lidocaine) hydrochloride is quite low, caution should be exercised particularly when employing large volumes and concentrations of Xylocaine hydrochloride since the incidence of adverse effects is directly proportional to the total dose of local anesthetic agent administered.

For specific techniques and procedures refer to standard textbooks.

The dosages recommended below are for normal, healthy adults:

5 ml ampule

RETROBULBAR INJECTION: The suggested dose for a 70 kg person is 3-5 ml (120-200 mg), i.e. 1.7-3 mg/kg or 0.9-1.5 mg/lb body weight. A portion of this is injected retrobulbarly and the rest may be used to block the facial nerve.

TRANSTRACHEAL INJECTION: For local anesthesia by the transtracheal route 2-3 ml should be injected through a large enough needle so that the injection can be made rapidly. By injecting during inspiration some of the drug will be carried into the bronchi and the resulting cough will distribute the rest of the drug over the vocal cords and the epiglottis. Occasionally it may be necessary to spray the pharynx by oropharyngeal spray to achieve complete analgesia. For the combination of the injection and spray, it should rarely be necessary to utilize more than 5 ml (200 mg), i.e. 3 mg/kg or 1.5 mg/lb body weight.

TOPICAL APPLICATION: For laryngoscopy, bronchoscopy and endotracheal intubation, the pharynx and larynx may be sprayed with 1 ml-5 ml (40 mg-200 mg), i.e. 0.6-3 mg/kg or 0.3-1.5 mg/lb body weight.

50 ml screw-cap bottle

When used as a spray, or when applied by means of cotton applicators or packs, as well as when instilled into a cavity, the suggested dosage of Xylocaine Hydrochloride 4% is 1 ml-5 ml (40 mg-200 mg), i.e. 0.6-3.0 mg/kg or 0.3-1.5 mg/lb body weight.

NOTE: The solution may be applied from a sterile swab which should be discarded after use and never reused under any circumstances. When spraying, transfer the solution from the original container to an atomizer.

Maximum Recommended Dosages:

Normal healthy adults:

The maximum recommended dose of Xylocaine (lidocaine) hydrochloride without epinephrine is 300 mg and in any case should not exceed 4.5 mg/kg (2 mg/lb) body weight.

Children:

It is difficult to recommend a maximum dose of any drug for children since this varies as a function of age and weight. For children of less than ten years who have a normal lean body mass and normal body development, the maximum dose may be determined by the application of one of the standard pediatric drug formulas (e.g. Clark's rule or Young's rule). For example, in a child of five years weighing 50 lbs., the dose of Xylocaine hydrochloride should not exceed 75-100 mg when calculated according to Clark's rule or Young's rule.

How Supplied: Xylocaine (lidocaine) Hydrochloride 4%, Sterile Aqueous Solution: 5 ml ampule, package of 10.

Xylocaine (lidocaine) Hydrochloride 4%, an Aqueous Solution: 50 ml screw-cap bottle, cartoned. NOT FOR INJECTION.

XYLOCAINE® (lidocaine) HYDROCHLORIDE 1.5% WITH DEXTROSE 7.5% ℞

Sterile Aqueous Solution Only for Spinal Anesthesia in Obstetrics

Description: Xylocaine Hydrochloride 1.5% solution with Dextrose 7.5% is a hyperbaric solution for use only for spinal anesthesia in obstetrics. Xylocaine is a local anesthetic chemically designated as diethylaminoacet-2,6-xylidide.

Xylocaine Hydrochloride 1.5% with Dextrose 7.5% may be autoclaved at 15 lbs. pressure at 121°C (250°F) for 15 minutes (USP Standard). Since this preparation contains glucose, caramelization may occur under prolonged heating and in some instances prolonged storage. Therefore, this preparation should be resterilized no more than once and should not be permitted to remain in the sterilizer any longer than necessary. The solution should not be used if a precipitate is present.

Composition of Xylocaine Hydrochloride 1.5% with Dextrose 7.5%

Each ml contains:

Diethylaminoacet-2,6-xylidide (lidocaine) hydrochloride ....15 mg
Dextrose (d-glucose) ....75 mg
Sodium Hydroxide....to adjust pH to ...6.0–6.7
Specific gravity, 1.028–1.034

Actions: Xylocaine (lidocaine) stabilizes the neuronal membrane and prevents the initiation and transmission of nerve impulses, thereby effecting local anesthetic action.

Xylocaine is metabolized mainly in the liver and excreted via the kidneys. Approximately 90% of Xylocaine administered is excreted in the form of various metabolites, while less than 10% is excreted unchanged.

The onset of action is rapid, usually within 30 to 60 seconds of administration. The duration of sensory anesthesia obtained is usually adequate for completion of routine, uncomplicated vaginal delivery while motor anesthesia is limited to the levator and perineal muscles.

Indications: Xylocaine (lidocaine) Hydrochloride 1.5% with Dextrose 7.5% is indicated only for low spinal or "saddle block" anesthesia in vaginal delivery when selective sensory anesthesia is desired.

Contraindications: The following conditions preclude the use of spinal anesthesia:

1. Severe hemorrhage, shock, or heart block.
2. Local infection at the site of proposed puncture.
3. Septicemia.
4. Known sensitivity to the anesthetic agent.

The use of this preparation for spinal anesthesia in obstetrics is contraindicated in the presence of pre-existing neurological disease, and disease of the subarachnoid region.

Warnings:

1. RESUSCITATIVE EQUIPMENT AND DRUGS SHOULD BE IMMEDIATELY AVAILABLE WHEN ANY LOCAL ANESTHETIC IS USED.
2. Vasopressor agents should not be used in the presence of oxytocic drugs, as a severe persistent hypertension and even rupture of cerebral blood vessels may occur.

Precautions: The safety and effectiveness of Xylocaine (lidocaine) hydrochloride depends on proper dosage, correct technique, adequate precautions, and readiness for emergencies.

The lowest dosage that results in effective anesthesia should be used to avoid serious adverse effects.

CONSULT STANDARD TEXTBOOKS FOR SPECIFIC TECHNIQUES AND PRECAUTIONS FOR SPINAL ANESTHETIC PROCEDURES.

Xylocaine should be used with caution in persons with known drug sensitivities. Patients allergic to paraaminobenzoic acid derivatives (procaine, tetracaine, benzocaine, etc.) have not shown cross sensitivity to Xylocaine.

Local anesthetics react with certain metals and cause the release of their respective ions which, if injected, may cause severe local irritation. Adequate precaution should be taken to avoid this type of interaction.

Adverse Reactions: Adverse reactions may result from inadvertent intravascular injection, or may result from a hypersensitivity, idiosyncrasy or diminished tolerance on the part of the patient. However, most adverse reactions seen with spinal anesthesia are related to the technique rather than the drug employed. In addition, use of inappropriate doses or techniques (e.g., improper positioning of patient) may result in extensive spinal blockade leading to occurrences such as profound hypotension, respiratory arrest, etc. Adverse effects on the fetus, course of labor, or delivery have rarely been observed when proper dosage and proper techniques have been employed.

Sympathetic block accompanying spinal anesthesia may result in depression of blood pressure and accentuate supine hypotension which is produced by the gravid uterus compressing the inferior vena cava. High levels or total spinal anesthesia may result in respiratory depression and depressed myocardial contractility. Management consists of uterine displacement, fluid replacement with respiratory support and vasoconstrictors when necessary.

CNS reactions are excitatory and/or depressant, and may be characterized by nervousness, dizziness, blurred vision and tremors, followed by drowsiness, convulsions, unconsciousness, and possibly respiratory arrest. The excitatory reactions may be very brief or may not occur at all, in which case the first manifestations of toxicity may be drowsiness, merging into unconsciousness and respiratory arrest.

Cardiovascular reactions are depressant, and may be characterized by hypotension, myocardial depression, bradycardia and possibly cardiac arrest.

Treatment of a patient with toxic manifestations consists of assuring and maintaining a patent airway and supporting ventilation using oxygen and assisted or controlled respiration as required. This usually will be sufficient in the management of most reactions. Should circulatory depression occur, vasopressors, such as ephedrine or metaraminol, and intravenous fluids may be used. Should a convulsion persist despite oxygen therapy, small increments of an ultra-short acting barbiturate (thiopental or thiamylal) or a short acting barbiturate (pentobarbital or secobarbital) may be given intravenously.

UNDER NO CIRCUMSTANCES SHOULD THE PATIENT BE MOVED OR PLACED IN TRENDELENBERG (HEAD DOWN) POSITION IN AN ATTEMPT TO IMPROVE VENOUS RETURN.

Allergic reactions are characterized by cutaneous lesions, urticaria, edema or anaphylactoid reactions. The detection of sensitivity by skin testing is of doubtful value.

Dosage and Administration: Spinal anesthesia with Xylocaine (lidocaine) Hydrochloride 1.5% with Dextrose 7.5% may be induced in the right or left lateral recumbent or the sitting position. Since this is a hyperbaric solution, the anesthetic will tend to move in the direction in which the table is tilted. After the desired level of anesthesia is obtained and the anesthetic has become fixed, usually in 5–10 minutes with Xylocaine, the patient may be positioned according to the requirement of the surgeon or obstetrician.

INJECTIONS SHOULD BE MADE SLOWLY. Barbotage is not recommended. Consult standard textbooks for specific techniques for spinal anesthetic procedures.

Recommended dosage

The following recommended dosage is for normal healthy adults and serves only as a guide to the amount of anesthetic required for most routine vaginal deliveries. In all cases, the smallest dose that will produce the desired result should be given.

Obstetrical low spinal or "saddle block" anesthesia: The dosage recommended for normal vaginal delivery is approximately 0.6 to 1.0 ml (9–15 mg).

How Supplied: Xylocaine® (lidocaine) Hydrochloride 1.5% solution with Dextrose 7.5% is supplied in 2 ml ampules.

XYLOCAINE® (lidocaine) HYDROCHLORIDE 5% WITH GLUCOSE 7.5% ℞

Sterile Aqueous Solution for Spinal Anesthesia

Description: Xylocaine Hydrochloride 5% solution with Glucose 7.5% is a hyperbaric solution for use in spinal anesthesia. Xylocaine is a local anesthetic chemically designated as diethylaminoacet-2,6-xylidide.

Xylocaine Hydrochloride 5% with Glucose 7.5% may be autoclaved at 15 lbs. pressure at 121°C (250°F) for 15 minutes (USP Standard). Since this preparation contains glucose, caramelization may occur under prolonged heating and in some instances prolonged storage. Therefore, this preparation should be resterilized no more than once or twice and should not be permitted to remain in the sterilizer any longer than necessary. The solution should not be used if a precipitate is present.

Composition of Xylocaine Hydrochloride 5% with Glucose 7.5%

Each ml contains:

Diethylaminoacet-2,6-xylidide (lidocaine) hydrochloride	50 mg
Dextrose (d-glucose)	75 mg
Sodium hydroxide to adjust pH to	6.3-6.7

Specific gravity, 1.030-1.035

Actions: Xylocaine (lidocaine) stabilizes the neuronal membrane and prevents the initiation and transmission of nerve impulses, thereby effecting local anesthetic action.

Xylocaine is metabolized mainly in the liver and excreted via the kidneys. Approximately 90% of Xylocaine administered is excreted in the form of various metabolites, while less than 10% is excreted unchanged.

The onset of action is rapid. The duration of perineal anesthesia provided with 1 ml (50 mg) Xylocaine Hydrochloride 5% with Glucose 7.5% averages 100 minutes with analgesia continuing for an additional 40 minutes. The duration of surgical anesthesia provided with 1.5 to 2 ml (75-100 mg) of this agent is approximately two hours. The duration of anesthesia may be extended by the addition of epinephrine or other appropriate vasoconstrictor agents.

Indications: Xylocaine (lidocaine) Hydrochloride 5% with Glucose 7.5% is indicated for the production of spinal anesthesia.

Contraindications: The following conditions preclude the use of spinal anesthesia:

(1) Severe hemorrhage, shock, or heart block.
(2) Local infection at the site of proposed puncture.
(3) Septicemia.
(4) Known sensitivity to the anesthetic agent.

Warnings:

(1) RESUSCITATIVE EQUIPMENT AND DRUGS SHOULD BE IMMEDIATELY AVAILABLE WHEN ANY LOCAL ANESTHETIC IS USED.
(2) *Usage in Pregnancy:* The safe use of Xylocaine (lidocaine) has not been established with respect to adverse effects upon fetal development. Careful consideration should be given to this fact before administering this drug to women of childbearing potential, particularly during early pregnancy.
This does not exclude the use of the drug at term for obstetrical analgesia. Xylocaine has been used effectively for obstetrical analgesia. Adverse effects on the fetus, course of labor, or delivery have rarely been observed when proper dosage and proper techniques have been employed.
(3) Vasopressor agents should not be used in the presence of oxytocic drugs, as a severe persistent hypertension and even rupture of cerebral blood vessels may occur.

Precautions: The safety and effectiveness of Xylocaine (lidocaine) hydrochloride depends on proper dosage, correct technique, adequate precautions, and readiness for emergencies.

The lowest dosage that results in effective anesthesia should be used to avoid serious adverse effects.

The following conditions may preclude the use of spinal anesthesia, depending upon the physician's ability to deal with the complications which may occur:

(1) Pre-existing neurological disease such as poliomyelitis, pernicious anemia, paralysis from nerve injuries and syphilis.
(2) Disturbance in blood morphology and/or anticoagulant therapy: In these conditions trauma to a blood vessel during needle puncture may result in uncontrollable hemorrhage into the epidural or subarachnoid space. Also profuse hemorrhage into the soft tissue may occur.
(3) Extremes of age.
(4) Chronic backache and preoperative headache.
(5) Hypotension and hypertension.
(6) Arthritis or spinal deformity.
(7) Technical problems (persistent paresthesias, persistent bloody tap).
(8) Psychotic or uncooperative patients.

CONSULT STANDARD TEXTBOOKS FOR SPECIFIC TECHNIQUES AND PRECAUTIONS FOR SPINAL ANESTHETIC PROCEDURES.

Xylocaine should be used with caution in persons with known drug sensitivities. Patients allergic to para-aminobenzoic acid derivatives (procaine, tetracaine, benzocaine, etc.) have not shown cross sensitivity to Xylocaine.

Continued on next page

Astra—Cont.

Local anesthetics react with certain metals and cause the release of their respective ions which, if injected, may cause severe local irritation. Adequate precaution should be taken to avoid this type of interaction.

Adverse Reactions: Adverse reactions may result from inadvertent intravascular injection, or may result from a hypersensitivity, idiosyncrasy or diminished tolerance on the part of the patient. In addition, use of inappropriate doses or techniques (e.g. improper positioning of patient) may result in extensive spinal blockade leading to occurrences such as profound hypotension, respiratory arrest, etc.

CNS reactions are excitatory and/or depressant, and may be characterized by nervousness, dizziness, blurred vision and tremors, followed by drowsiness, convulsions, unconsciousness and possibly respiratory arrest.

The excitatory reactions may be very brief or may not occur at all, in which case the first manifestations of toxicity may be drowsiness, merging into unconsciousness and respiratory arrest.

Cardiovascular reactions are depressant, and may be characterized by hypotension, myocardial depression, bradycardia and possibly cardiac arrest.

Treatment of a patient with toxic manifestations consists of assuring and maintaining a patent airway and supporting ventilation using oxygen and assisted or controlled respiration as required. This usually will be sufficient in the management of most reactions. Should circulatory depression occur, vasopressors, such as ephedrine or metaraminol, and intravenous fluids may be used. Should a convulsion persist despite oxygen therapy, small increments of an ultra-short acting barbiturate (thiopental or thiamylal) or a short acting barbiturate (pentobarbital or secobarbital) may be given intravenously.

Allergic reactions are characterized by cutaneous lesions, urticaria, edema or anaphylactoid reactions. The detection of sensitivity by skin testing is of doubtful value.

Dosage and Administration: Spinal anesthesia with Xylocaine (lidocaine) Hydrochloride 5% with Glucose 7.5% may be induced in the right or left lateral recumbent or the sitting position. Since this is a hyperbaric solution, the anesthetic will tend to move in the direction in which the table is tilted. After the desired level of anesthesia is obtained and the anesthetic has become fixed, usually in 5-10 minutes with Xylocaine, the patient may be positioned according to the requirement of the surgeon or obstetrician.

INJECTIONS SHOULD BE MADE SLOWLY.

Barbotage is not recommended. Consult standard textbooks for specific techniques for spinal anesthetic procedures.

Recommended dosages

The following recommended dosages are for normal healthy adults and serve only as a guide to the amount of anesthetic required for most routine procedures. In all cases, the smallest dose that will produce the desired result should be given.

If the technique is properly performed, and the needle is properly placed in the subarachnoid space, it should not be necessary to administer more than one ampule (100 mg).

Obstetrical low spinal or "saddle block" anesthesia:

The dosage recommended for normal vaginal delivery is approximately 1.0 ml (50 mg). For Cesarean section and those deliveries requiring intrauterine manipulations, 1.5 ml (75 mg) is usually adequate.

Surgical anesthesia:

The dosage recommended for abdominal surgical anesthesia is 1.5-2 ml (75-100 mg).

How Supplied: Xylocaine (lidocaine) Hydrochloride 5% solution with Glucose 7.5% is supplied in 2 ml ampules in packages of 10 and 100.

XYLOCAINE® 2% (lidocaine) HCl JELLY ℞

A Topical Anesthetic for Urological Procedures

Description: Xylocaine is a local anesthetic, chemically designated as diethylaminoacet-2,6-xylidide. Xylocaine Jelly is a sterile, aqueous solution thickened to a suitable viscosity by the addition of carboxymethylcellulose.

Composition of Xylocaine Jelly

Each ml contains:

Diethylaminoacet-2,6-xylidide (lidocaine) hydrochloride	20mg
Methyl-p-hydroxybenzoate	0.7mg
Propyl-p-hydroxybenzoate	0.3mg
Sodium hydroxide	to adjust pH

Sodium carboxymethylcellulose, to adjust to a suitable consistency.

Actions: Xylocaine (lidocaine) stabilizes the neuronal membrane and prevents the initiation and transmission of nerve impulses, thereby effecting local anesthetic action. Xylocaine HCl Jelly contains carboxymethylcellulose, added to an aqueous solution of Xylocaine hydrochloride. The resultant mixture maximizes contact with the urethral mucosa, and provides lubrication for instrumentation.

Indications: Xylocaine (lidocaine) HCl Jelly is indicated for prevention and control of pain in procedures involving the male and female urethra and for topical treatment of painful urethritis.

Contraindications: Xylocaine is contraindicated in patients with a known history of hypersensitivity to local anesthetics of the amide type.

Warnings: RESUSCITATIVE EQUIPMENT AND DRUGS SHOULD BE IMMEDIATELY AVAILABLE WHEN ANY LOCAL ANESTHETIC IS USED.

Precautions: Xylocaine (lidocaine) HCl Jelly should be used with caution in patients with severely traumatized mucosa and sepsis in the region of the proposed application.

As with any local anesthetic, reactions and complications are best averted by employing the minimal effective dosage. Debilitated, elderly patients, and children should be given dosages commensurate with their age and physical condition.

Xylocaine, or any other local anesthetic, should be employed cautiously in persons with known drug sensitivities. Patients with allergic sensitivity to para-aminobenzoic acid derivatives (procaine, tetracaine, benzocaine, etc.) have not shown cross sensitivity to Xylocaine.

Adverse Reactions: Adverse reactions may result from high plasma levels due to excessive dosage, or rapid absorption, or may result from a hypersensitivity, idiosyncrasy or diminished tolerance on the part of the patient. Such reactions are systemic in nature and involve the central nervous system and/or the cardiovascular system.

CNS reactions are excitatory and/or depressant, and may be characterized by nervousness, dizziness, blurred vision and tremors, followed by drowsiness, convulsions, unconsciousness and possibly respiratory arrest. The excitatory reactions may be very brief or may not occur at all, in which case the first manifestations of toxicity may be drowsiness, merging into unconsciousness and respiratory arrest.

Cardiovascular reactions are depressant, and may be characterized by hypotension, myocardial depression, bradycardia and possibly cardiac arrest.

Treatment of a patient with toxic manifestations consists of assuring and maintaining a patent airway and supporting ventilation using oxygen and assisted or controlled respiration as required. This usually will be sufficient in the management of most reactions. Should circulatory depression occur, vasopressors, such as ephedrine or metaraminol, and intravenous fluids may be used. Should a convulsion persist despite oxygen therapy, small increments of an ultra-short acting barbiturate (thiopental or thiamylal) or a short acting barbiturate (pentobarbital or secobarbital) may be given intravenously.

Allergic reactions are characterized by cutaneous lesions, urticaria, edema or anaphylactoid reactions. The detection of sensitivity by skin testing is of doubtful value.

Dosage and Administration:

For surface anesthesia of the male urethra: The outer orifice is washed and cleansed with a disinfectant. The plastic cone is sterilized for 5 minutes in boiling water, cooled, and attached to the tube. The cone may be gas sterilized or cold sterilized, if preferred. The tube key is attached. The jelly is instilled slowly into the urethra by turning the tube key until the patient has a feeling of tension or until almost half the tube (15 ml; 300 mg) is emptied. A penile clamp is then applied for several minutes at the corona and then the remaining contents of the tube are instilled.

Prior to sounding or cystoscopy, a penile clamp should be applied for 5 to 10 minutes to obtain adequate anesthesia. The contents of one tube (30 ml; 600 mg) are usually required to fill and dilate the male urethra.

Prior to catheterization, smaller volumes (5-10 ml; 100-200 mg) are usually adequate.

For surface anesthesia of the female urethra: The outer orifice is washed and cleansed with a disinfectant. The plastic cone is sterilized for 5 minutes in boiling water, cooled, and attached to the tube. The cone may be gas sterilized or cold sterilized, if preferred. The tube key is attached. Three to five ml of the jelly is instilled slowly into the urethra by turning the tube key (approximately 1½ - 2 full turns). If desired, some jelly may be deposited on a cotton swab and introduced into the urethra. In order to obtain adequate anesthesia, several minutes should be allowed prior to performing urological procedures.

Maximum Dosage: No more than one tube should be given in any 12 hour period.

How Supplied: Collapsible tubes which deliver 30 ml. A detachable applicator cone and a key for expressing contents are included in each package.

XYLOCAINE® (lidocaine) 5% OINTMENT ℞

A Water-Soluble Topical Anesthetic Ointment

Description: Xylocaine is a local anesthetic chemically designated as diethylaminoacet-2,6-xylidide.

Composition of Xylocaine 5% Ointment: diethylaminoacet-2,6-xylidide (lidocaine) 5% in a water miscible ointment vehicle consisting of polyethylene glycols and propylene glycol.

Actions: Xylocaine (lidocaine) Ointment 5% effects local topical anesthesia. The onset of action is 3-5 minutes. It is ineffective when applied to intact skin.

Indications: Xylocaine Ointment 5% is indicated for production of anesthesia of accessible mucous membranes of the oropharynx.

It is also useful as an anesthetic lubricant for endotracheal intubation.

> Based on a review of this drug by the National Academy of Sciences - National Research Council and/or other information, FDA has classified the other indications as follows:
> "Possibly" effective: Xylocaine Ointment 5% is indicated for the temporary relief of pain associated with minor abrasions of the skin.

Final classification of the less-than-effective indications requires further investigation.

Contraindications: Xylocaine Ointment 5% is contraindicated in patients with a known history of hypersensitivity to local anesthetics of the amide type.

Precautions: Xylocaine (lidocaine) Ointment 5% should be used with caution in patients with severely traumatized mucosa and sepsis in the region of the proposed application.

Xylocaine, or any other local anesthetic, should be employed cautiously in persons with known drug sensitivities. Patients with allergic sensitivity to para-aminobenzoic acid derivatives (procaine, tetracaine, benzocaine, etc.) have not shown cross sensitivity to Xylocaine.

Usage in Pregnancy: The safe use of Xylocaine has not been established with respect to adverse effects upon fetal development. Careful consideration should be given to this fact before administering or prescribing this drug to women of childbearing potential, particularly during early pregnancy.

Adverse Reactions: Systemic adverse reactions have not been reported with Xylocaine (lidocaine) Ointment. However, as with any local anesthetic, adverse reactions may result from high plasma levels due to excessive dosage or rapid absorption. Hypersensitivity, idiosyncrasy or diminished tolerance may also be a cause of reactions. Systemic reactions due to overdosage (high plasma levels) involve the central nervous system and/or the cardiovascular system.

CNS reactions are excitatory and/or depressant, and may be characterized by nervousness, dizziness, blurred vision and tremors, followed by drowsiness, convulsions, unconsciousness and possibly respiratory arrest. The excitatory reactions may be very brief or may not occur at all, in which case the first manifestations of toxicity may be drowsiness, merging into unconsciousness and respiratory arrest.

Cardiovascular reactions are depressant, and may be characterized by hypotension, myocardial depression, bradycardia and possibly cardiac arrest.

Treatment of a patient with toxic manifestations consists of assuring and maintaining a patent airway and supporting ventilation using oxygen and assisted or controlled respiration as required. This usually will be sufficient in the management of most reactions. Should circulatory depression occur, vasopressors, such as ephedrine or metaraminol, and intravenous fluids may be used. Should a convulsion persist despite oxygen therapy, small increments of an ultra-short acting barbiturate (thiopental or thiamylal) or a short acting barbiturate (pentobarbital or secobarbital) may be given intravenously.

Allergic reactions are characterized by cutaneous lesions, urticaria, edema or anaphylactoid reactions. The detection of sensitivity by skin testing is of doubtful value.

Dosage and Administration: Apply topically for adequate control of symptoms. The use of a sterile gauze pad is suggested for application to broken skin tissue. Apply to the catheter prior to endotracheal intubation.

In dentistry, apply to previously dried oral mucosa. Subsequent removal of excess saliva with cotton rolls or saliva ejector minimizes dilution of the ointment and permits maximum penetration. Avoid cross-contamination between patients by aseptically transferring from its container to a separate plate or small dish the estimated amount of ointment required for each patient. Discard any unused portion. For use in connection with the insertion of new dentures, apply to all denture surfaces contacting mucosa.

IMPORTANT: Patient should consult dentist at intervals not exceeding 36 hours throughout the fitting period.

NOTE: No more than 35 grams should be administered in any one day.

How Supplied: Xylocaine (lidocaine) 5% Ointment is available in 35 gram tubes.

Xylocaine Ointment 5% Flavored, for application within the oral cavity, is dispensed in 3.5 gram tubes, 10 tubes per carton, and in 35 gram jars.

KEEP CONTAINER TIGHTLY CAPPED AT ALL TIMES WHEN NOT IN USE.

XYLOCAINE® (lidocaine) 2.5% OINTMENT

Composition: Diethylaminoacet-2,6-xylidide 2.5% in a water miscible ointment vehicle consisting of polyethylene glycols and propylene glycol.

Action and Uses: A topical anesthetic ointment for fast, temporary relief of pain, burning and itching due to minor burns, sunburn, nonpoisonous insect bites, minor skin irritations and hemorrhoids. The ointment can be easily removed with water. It is ineffective when applied to intact skin.

Administration and Dosage: Apply topically in liberal amounts for adequate control of symptoms. When the anesthetic effect wears off additional ointment may be applied as needed.

Important Warning: *In persistent, severe or extensive skin disorders or bleeding hemorrhoids, advise patient to use only as directed. In case of rectal bleeding, advise patient to consult physician promptly. Keep out of the reach of children.*

Caution: *Do not use in the eyes. Not for prolonged use. If the condition for which this preparation is used persists or if a rash or irritation develops, advise patient to discontinue use and consult a physician.*

How Supplied: Available in tube of 35 grams (approximately 1.25 ounces).

XYLOCAINE® (lidocaine) SUPPOSITORIES ℞

For surface anesthesia of rectal mucous membranes

Description: The base used in these suppositories melts readily at body temperature, leaving no residue, and assuring even and thorough distribution of the active ingredients. Rectal application is facilitated since the base maintains the form of the suppository until after insertion.

Composition:

Each Xylocaine Suppository contains:

Diethylaminoacet-2,6-xylidide (lidocaine)	100 mg (3.8%)
Bismuth subgallate	115 mg
Zinc oxide	375 mg
Aluminum subacetate	75 mg
Peruvian balsam	100 mg
Neutral glycerides of saturated vegetable fatty acids q.s.—ad	2.6 Gm

Actions: These suppositories provide the well-established surface anesthetic effect of Xylocaine which is quick in onset, profound and sustained. They are non-irritating and do not inhibit normal healing processes. Xylocaine Suppositories possess astringent properties which are characteristic of bismuth subgallate, zinc oxide and aluminum subacetate. The effect of Xylocaine Suppositories is usually apparent within 10-15 minutes and lasts, in most cases, for 2-5 hours.

Indications: Xylocaine Suppositories provide temporary relief of pain and discomfort associated with inoperative, irritative or inflammatory anorectal conditions such as hemorrhoids and postoperative edema. They may also be employed pre- and post-operatively in hemorrhoidectomy and sclerosing therapy, and in conjunction with proctoscopic and sigmoidoscopic examinations.

Contraindications: Xylocaine Suppositories are contraindicated in patients with a known history of hypersensitivity to local anesthetics of the amide type or to any of the other components of these suppositories. These suppositories are contraindicated in patients 12 years of age or under.

Warnings: Not for prolonged use. The recommended dose of no more than 5 suppositories in 24 hours should not be exceeded.

KEEP OUT OF THE REACH OF CHILDREN.

Precautions: In case of rectal bleeding, or if a rash, irritation, or other signs of sensitivity develop, discontinue use. Although Xylocaine has been shown to be relatively free from allergic and sensitizing properties, these possibilities should not be overlooked, and appropriate precautions should be observed. Xylocaine, or any other local anesthetic, should be employed cautiously in persons with known drug sensitivities. Patients with allergic sensitivity to para-aminobenzoic acid derivatives (procaine, tetracaine, benzocaine, etc.) have not shown similar sensitivity to Xylocaine.

Adverse Reactions: Systemic adverse reactions have not been reported with Xylocaine Suppositories. However, as with any local anesthetic, adverse reactions may result from high plasma levels due to excessive dosage or rapid absorption. Hypersensitivity, idiosyncrasy or diminished tolerance may also be a cause of reactions. Systemic reactions due to overdosage (high plasma levels) involve the central nervous system and/or the cardiovascular system.

CNS reactions are excitatory and/or depressant, and may be characterized by nervousness, dizziness, blurred vision and tremors, followed by drowsiness, convulsions, unconsciousness and possibly respiratory arrest. The excitatory reactions may be very brief or may not occur at all, in which case the first manifestations of toxicity may be drowsiness, merging into unconsciousness and respiratory arrest.

Cardiovascular reactions are depressant, and may be characterized by hypotension, myocardial depression, bradycardia and possibly cardiac arrest.

Treatment of a patient with toxic manifestations consists of assuring and maintaining a patent airway and supporting ventilation using oxygen and assisted or controlled respiration as required. This usually will be sufficient in the management of most reactions. Should circulatory depression occur, vasopressors, such as ephedrine or metaraminol, and intravenous fluids may be used. Should a convulsion persist despite oxygen therapy, small increments of an ultra-short acting barbiturate (thiopental or thiamylal) or a short acting barbiturate (pentobarbital or secobarbital) may be given intravenously.

Allergic reactions are characterized by cutaneous lesions, urticaria, edema or anaphylactoid reactions. The detection of sensitivity by skin testing is of doubtful value.

Dosage and Administration: Remove from plastic wrapper. Insert one suppository rectally after each bowel movement and before retiring, or as required for control of symptoms; not exceeding five suppositories in 24 hours. This preparation is not recommended for patients 12 years of age or under.

How Supplied: Boxes of 5 and 100 rectal suppositories.

TO BE STORED IN A COOL PLACE

Continued on next page

Astra—Cont.

XYLOCAINE® 2% (lidocaine HCl) VISCOUS ℞

A Topical Anesthetic for the Mucous Membranes of the Mouth and Pharynx

Description: Xylocaine is a local anesthetic, chemically designated as diethylaminoacet-2,6-xylidide.

Composition of Xylocaine 2% Viscous Solution: lidocaine hydrochloride 2% in an aqueous solution adjusted to suitable consistency with sodium carboxymethylcellulose, and pleasantly flavored.

Actions: Xylocaine (lidocaine) stabilizes the neuronal membrane and prevents the initiation and transmission of nerve impulses, thereby effecting local anesthetic action. Xylocaine HCl Viscous contains carboxymethylcellulose, added to an aqueous solution of Xylocaine hydrochloride, creating a solution with high viscosity and low surface tension. As a result of this combination, Xylocaine HCl Viscous spreads well and yet adheres to mucous membranes.

Indications: Xylocaine (lidocaine) HCl Viscous is indicated for the production of topical anesthesia of irritated or inflamed mucous membranes of the mouth and pharynx.

Contraindications: Xylocaine is contraindicated in patients with a known history of hypersensitivity to local anesthetics of the amide type.

Precautions: Xylocaine (lidocaine) HCl Viscous should be used with caution in patients with severely traumatized mucosa and sepsis in the region of the proposed application.

As with any local anesthetic, reactions and complications are best averted by employing the minimal effective dosage. Debilitated, elderly patients, and children should be given dosages commensurate with their age and physical condition.

Although Xylocaine has been shown to be relatively free of allergic and sensitizing properties, these possibilities should not be overlooked and appropriate precautions should be observed.

Xylocaine, or any other local anesthetic, should be employed cautiously in persons with known drug sensitivities. Patients with allergic sensitivity to para-aminobenzoic acid derivatives (procaine, tetracaine, benzocaine, etc.) have not shown cross sensitivity to Xylocaine.

The use of oral topical anesthetic agents may interfere with the second stage (pharyngeal stage) of swallowing. Thus, care should be exercised, particularly in children, when food is ingested within 60 minutes following the use of oral topical anesthetics to prevent the possible aspiration of food.

Adverse Reactions: Systemic adverse reactions are extremely rare with Xylocaine (lidocaine) HCl Viscous 2%. However, as with any local anesthetic, adverse reactions may result from high plasma levels due to excessive dosage, or rapid absorption, or may result from a hypersensitivity, idiosyncrasy or diminished tolerance on the part of the patient. Such reactions are systemic in nature and involve the central nervous system and/or the cardiovascular system.

CNS reactions are excitatory and/or depressant, and may be characterized by nervousness, dizziness, blurred vision and tremors, followed by drowsiness, convulsions, unconsciousness and possibly respiratory arrest. The excitatory reactions may be very brief or may not occur at all, in which case the first manifestations of toxicity may be drowsiness, merging into unconsciousness and respiratory arrest.

Cardiovascular reactions are depressant, and may be characterized by hypotension, myocardial depression, bradycardia and possibly cardiac arrest.

Treatment of a patient with toxic manifestations consists of assuring and maintaining a patent airway and supporting ventilation using oxygen and assisted or controlled respiration as required. This usuually will be sufficient in the management of most reactions. Should circulatory depression occur, vasopressors, such as ephedrine or metaraminol, and intravenous fluids may be used. Should a convulsion persist despite oxygen therapy, small increments of an ultra-short acting barbiturate (thiopental or thiamylal) or a short acting barbiturate (pentobarbital or secobarbital) may be given intravenously.

Allergic reactions are characterized by cutaneous lesions, urticaria, edema or anaphylactoid reactions. The detection of sensitivity by skin testing is of doubtful value.

Dosage and Administration: For symptomatic treatment of irritated or inflamed mucous membranes of the mouth and pharynx, one tablespoonful (15 ml; 300 mg), i.e. 4.5 mg/kg or 2 mg/lb body weight, undiluted is recommended. The solution should be swished around in the mouth and can be swallowed without water. It should rarely be necessary to administer this dose at intervals of less than three hours.

NOTE: No more than 120 ml (approximately 8 tablespoonsful) should be administered in a 24 hour period.

SHAKE WELL BEFORE USING.

How Supplied: 100 ml and 450 ml polyethylene squeeze bottles, cartoned.

Avicon, Inc.
6201 SOUTH FREEWAY
FORT WORTH, TEXAS 76134

AVITENE® ℞
(microfibrillar collagen hemostat)

Description: Avitene is an absorbable topical hemostatic agent prepared as a dry, sterile, fibrous, water insoluble partial hydrochloric acid salt of purified bovine corium collagen. In its manufacture, swelling of the native collagen fibrils is controlled by ethyl alcohol to permit noncovalent attachment of hydrochloric acid to amine groups on the collagen molecule and preservation of the essential morphology of native collagen molecules. Dry heat sterilization causes some crosslinking which is evidenced by reduction of hydrating properties, and a decrease of molecular weight which implies some degradation of collagen molecules. However, the characteristics of collagen which are essential to its effect on the blood coagulation mechanisms are preserved.

Actions: Avitene, in contact with a bleeding surface, attracts platelets which adhere to the fibrils and undergo the release phenomenon to trigger aggregation of platelets into thrombi in the interstices of the fibrous mass. The effect on platelet adhesion and aggregation is not inhibited by heparin in vitro. It has been found effective in heparinized dogs and in eight of nine fully heparinized human subjects. Platelets of patients with clinical thrombasthenia do not adhere to Avitene in vitro. However, in clinical trials it was effective in 50 of 68 patients receiving aspirin. Avitene cannot control bleeding due to systemic coagulation disorders. Appropriate therapy to correct the underlying coagulopathy should be instituted prior to use of the product. Avitene is tenaciously adherent to surfaces wet with blood but excess material not involved in the hemostatic clot may be removed by teasing or irrigation, usually without restarting bleeding. In animal and human studies, it has been shown to stimulate a mild, chronic cellular inflammatory response. When implanted in animal tissues, it is absorbed in less than 84 days. In human studies of hemostasis in osteotomy cuts, it has been shown not to interfere with bone regeneration or healing. In animal studies, it has been demonstrated that Avitene does not predispose to stenosis at vascular anastomotic sites. These findings have not been confirmed in human use. Studies have been performed using Avitene in experimental wounds contaminated with hemolytic Staphylococcus aureus. The presence of Avitene does not enhance or initiate staphylococcus wound infections to a greater or lesser extent than control agents employed for the same purpose. The effects of Avitene on experimental wounds contaminated with a gram-negative aerobic rod and an anaerobic nonspore forming bacteria are currently under investigation.

Indications: Avitene is used in surgical procedures as an adjunct to hemostasis when control of bleeding by ligature or conventional procedures is ineffective or impractical.

Contraindications: Avitene should not be used in the closure of skin incisions as it may interfere with the healing of the skin edges. This is due to simple mechanical interposition of dry collagen and not to any intrinsic interference with wound healing. By filling porosities of cancellous bone, Avitene may significantly reduce the bond strength of methylmethacrylate adhesives. Avitene should not, therefore, be employed on bone surfaces to which prosthetic materials are to be attached with methylmethacrylate adhesives.

Warnings: Avitene is inactivated by autoclaving. Ethylene oxide reacts with bound hydrochloric acid to form ethylene chlorohydrin. This product should not be resterilized. It is not for injection. Moistening Avitene or wetting with saline or thrombin impairs its hemostatic efficacy. It should be used **dry**. Discard any unused portion. As with any foreign substance, use in contaminated wounds may enhance infection.

Precautions: Only that amount of Avitene necessary to produce hemostasis should be used. After several minutes, excess material should be removed; this is usually possible without the re-initiation of active bleeding. Failure to remove excess Avitene may result in bowel adhesion or mechanical pressure sufficient to compromise the ureter. In otolaryngological surgery, precautions against aspiration should include removal of all excess dry material and thorough irrigation of the pharynx. Avitene contains a low, but detectable, level of intercalated bovine serum protein which reacts immunologically as does beef serum albumin. Increases in anti-BSA titer have been observed following treatment with Avitene. About two-thirds of individuals exhibit antibody titers because of ingestion of food products of bovine origin. Intradermal skin tests have occasionally shown a weak positive reaction to BSA or Avitene but these have not been correlated with IgG titers to BSA. Tests have failed to demonstrate clinically significant elicitation of antibodies of the IgE class against BSA following Avitene therapy.

Care should be exercised to avoid spillage on nonbleeding surfaces, particularly in abdominal or thoracic viscera. Teratology studies in rats and rabbits have revealed no harm to the animal fetus. There are no well-controlled studies in pregnant women; therefore, Avitene should be used in pregnant women only when clearly needed.

Adverse Reactions: The most serious adverse reactions reported which may be related to the use of Avitene are potentiation of infection including abscess formation, hematoma, wound dihescence, and mediastinitis. Other reported adverse reactions possibly related are adhesion formation, allergic reaction, foreign body reaction, and subgaleal seroma (report of a single case).

The use of Avitene in dental extraction sockets has been reported to increase the incidence of alveolalgia. Transient laryngospasm due to aspiration of dry materials has been reported following use of Avitene in tonsillectomy.

Dosage and Administration: Avitene must be applied directly to the source of bleeding. Because of its adhesiveness, it may seal over the exit site of deeper hemorrhage and conceal an underlying hematoma as in penetrating liver wounds. Surfaces to be treated should be compressed with dry sponges immediately prior to application of the **dry** Avitene. It is then necessary to apply pressure over the Avitene with a dry sponge for a period of time which varies with the force and severity of bleeding. A minute may suffice for capillary bleeding (e.g., skin graft donor sites, dermatologic curettage) but three to five or more minutes may be required for brisk bleeding (e.g., splenic tears) or high pressure leaks in major artery suture holes. For control of oozing from cancellous bone, it should be firmly packed into the spongy bone surface. After five to ten minutes, excess Avitene should be teased away (see **Precautions**); this can usually be accomplished with blunt forceps and is facilitated by wetting with sterile 0.9% saline solution and irrigation. If break-through bleeding occurs in areas of thin application, additional Avitene may be applied. The amount required depends, again, on the severity of bleeding. In capillary bleeding, one gram will usually be sufficient for a 50 cm^2 area. Thicker coverage will be required for more brisk bleeding. Avitene will adhere to wet gloves, instruments, or tissue surfaces. To facilitate handling, **dry** smooth forceps should be used. Gloved fingers should not be used to apply pressure.

How Supplied: In 1 g and 5 g sterile jars of sterile microfibrillar collagen hemostat all contained in a sealed can. Sterility of the jar exterior cannot be guaranteed if can seal is broken. Content of jar is sterile until opened.

Caution: Federal law prohibits dispensing without prescription.

Ayerst Laboratories

Division of American Home Products Corporation
685 THIRD AVE.
NEW YORK, NY 10017

ANTABUSE® ℞

Brand of disulfiram
In Alcoholism

Indication: ANTABUSE is an aid in the management of selected chronic alcoholic patients who want to remain in a state of enforced sobriety so that supportive and psychotherapeutic treatment may be applied to best advantage. (Used alone, without proper motivation and without supportive therapy, ANTABUSE is not a cure for alcoholism, and it is unlikely that it will have more than a brief effect on the drinking pattern of the chronic alcoholic).

Contraindications: Patients who are receiving or have recently received metronidazole, paraldehyde, alcohol, or alcohol-containing preparations, *e.g.* cough syrups, tonics and the like, should not be given ANTABUSE.

ANTABUSE is contraindicated in the presence of severe myocardial disease or coronary occlusion, psychoses, and hypersensitivity to disulfiram or to other thiuram derivatives used in pesticides and rubber vulcanization.

Warnings

> ANTABUSE should never be administered to a patient when he is in a state of alcohol intoxication or without his full knowledge.
> The physician should instruct relatives accordingly.

The patient must be fully informed of the ANTABUSE-alcohol reaction. He must be strongly cautioned against surreptitious drinking while taking the drug and he must be fully aware of possible consequences. He should be warned to avoid alcohol in disguised form, *i.e.* in sauces, vinegars, cough mixtures, and even aftershave lotions and back rubs. He should also be warned that reactions may occur with alcohol up to 14 days after ingesting ANTABUSE.

The ANTABUSE-ALCOHOL REACTION: ANTABUSE plus alcohol, even small amounts, produces flushing, throbbing in head and neck, throbbing headache, respiratory difficulty, nausea, copious vomiting, sweating, thirst, chest pain, palpitation, dyspnea, hyperventilation, tachycardia, hypotension, syncope, marked uneasiness, weakness, vertigo, blurred vision, and confusion. In severe reactions there may be respiratory depression, cardiovascular collapse, arrhythmias, myocardial infarction, acute congestive heart failure, unconsciousness, convulsions, and death.

The intensity of the reaction varies with each individual, but is generally proportional to the amounts of ANTABUSE and alcohol ingested. Mild reactions may occur in the sensitive individual when the blood alcohol concentration is increased to as little as 5 to 10 mg per 100 ml. Symptoms are fully developed at 50 mg per 100 ml and unconsciousness usually results when the blood alcohol level reaches 125 to 150 mg.

The duration of the reaction varies from 30 to 60 minutes to several hours in the more severe cases, or as long as there is alcohol in the blood.

DRUG INTERACTIONS: Disulfiram appears to decrease the rate at which certain drugs are metabolized and so may increase the blood levels and the possibility of clinical toxicity of drugs given concomitantly.

DISULFIRAM SHOULD BE USED WITH CAUTION IN THOSE PATIENTS RECEIVING PHENYTOIN AND ITS CONGENERS, SINCE THE CONCOMITANT ADMINISTRATION OF THESE TWO DRUGS CAN LEAD TO PHENYTOIN INTOXICATION. PRIOR TO ADMINISTERING DISULFIRAM TO A PATIENT ON PHENYTOIN THERAPY, A BASELINE PHENYTOIN SERUM LEVEL SHOULD BE OBTAINED. SUBSEQUENT TO INITIATION OF DISULFIRAM THERAPY, SERUM LEVELS ON PHENYTOIN SHOULD BE DETERMINED ON DIFFERENT DAYS FOR EVIDENCE OF AN INCREASE OR FOR A CONTINUING RISE IN LEVELS. INCREASED PHENYTOIN LEVELS SHOULD BE TREATED WITH APPROPRIATE DOSAGE ADJUSTMENT.

It may be necessary to adjust the dosage of oral anticoagulants upon beginning or stopping disulfiram, since disulfiram may prolong prothrombin time.

Patients taking isoniazid when disulfiram is given should be observed for the appearance of unsteady gait or marked changes in mental status and the disulfiram discontinued if such signs appear.

In rats, simultaneous ingestion of disulfiram and nitrite in the diet for 78 weeks has been reported to cause tumors, and it has been suggested that disulfiram may react with nitrites in the rat stomach to form a nitrosamine which is tumorigenic. Disulfiram alone in the diet of rats did not lead to such tumors. The relevance of this finding to humans is not known at this time.

CONCOMITANT CONDITIONS: Because of the possibility of an accidental ANTABUSE-alcohol reaction, ANTABUSE should be used with extreme caution in patients with any of the following conditions: diabetes mellitus, hypothyroidism, epilepsy, cerebral damage, chronic and acute nephritis, hepatic cirrhosis or insufficiency.

USAGE IN PREGNANCY: The safe use of this drug in pregnancy has not been established. Therefore, ANTABUSE should be used during pregnancy only when in the judgment of the physician, the probable benefits outweigh the possible risks.

Precautions: Patients with a history of rubber contact dermatitis should be evaluated for hypersensitivity to thiuram derivatives before receiving ANTABUSE (See Contraindications).

It is suggested that every patient under treatment carry an Identification Card, stating that he is receiving ANTABUSE and describing the symptoms most likely to occur as a result of the ANTABUSE-alcohol reaction. In addition, this card should indicate the physician or institution to be contacted in emergency. (Cards may be obtained from Ayerst Laboratories upon request.)

Alcoholism may accompany or be followed by dependence on narcotics or sedatives. Barbiturates have been administered concurrently with ANTABUSE without untoward effects, but the possibility of initiating a new abuse should be considered.

Baseline and follow-up transaminase tests (10–14 days) are suggested to detect any hepatic dysfunction that may result with ANTABUSE therapy. In addition, a complete blood count and a sequential multiple analysis-12 (SMA-12) test should be made every six months.

Patients taking ANTABUSE Tablets should not be exposed to ethylene dibromide or its vapors. This precaution is based on preliminary results of animal research currently in progress which suggests a toxic interaction between inhaled ethylene dibromide and ingested disulfiram resulting in a higher incidence of tumors and mortality in rats. Correlation of this finding to humans, however, has not been demonstrated.

Adverse Reactions: (See Contraindications, Warnings, and Precautions.)

OPTIC NEURITIS, PERIPHERAL NEURITIS AND POLYNEURITIS MAY OCCUR FOLLOWING ADMINISTRATION OF ANTABUSE.

Occasional skin eruptions are, as a rule, readily controlled by concomitant administration of an antihistaminic drug.

In a small number of patients, a transient mild drowsiness, fatigability, impotence, headache, acneform eruptions, allergic dermatitis, or a metallic or garlic-like aftertaste may be experienced during the first two weeks of therapy. These complaints usually disappear spontaneously with the continuation of therapy or with reduced dosage.

Psychotic reactions have been noted, attributable in most cases to high dosage, combined toxicity (with metronidazole or isoniazid), or to the unmasking of underlying psychoses in patients stressed by the withdrawal of alcohol.

One case of cholestatic hepatitis has been reported, but its relationship to ANTABUSE has not been unequivocally established.

Dosage and Administration: ANTABUSE should never be administered until the patient has abstained from alcohol for at least 12 hours.

INITIAL DOSAGE SCHEDULE: In the first phase of treatment, a maximum of 500 mg daily is given in a single dose for one to two weeks. Although usually taken in the morning, ANTABUSE may be taken on retiring by patients who experience a sedative effect. Alternatively, to minimize, or eliminate, the sedative effect, dosage may be adjusted downward.

MAINTENANCE REGIMEN: The average maintenance dose is 250 mg daily (range, 125 to 500 mg); it should not exceed 500 mg daily.

NOTE: Occasional patients, while seemingly on adequate maintenance doses of ANTA-

Continued on next page

Ayerst—Cont.

BUSE, report that they are able to drink alcoholic beverages with impunity and without any symptomatology. All appearances to the contrary, such patients must be presumed to be disposing of their tablets in some manner without actually taking them. Until such patients have been observed reliably taking their daily ANTABUSE tablets (preferably crushed and well mixed with liquid), it cannot be concluded that ANTABUSE is ineffective.
DURATION OF THERAPY: The daily, uninterrupted administration of ANTABUSE must be continued until the patient is fully recovered socially and a basis for permanent self-control is established. Depending on the individual patient, maintenance therapy may be required for months or even years.
TRIAL WITH ALCOHOL: During early experience with ANTABUSE, it was thought advisable for each patient to have at least one supervised alcohol-drug reaction. More recently, the test reaction has been largely abandoned. Furthermore, such a test reaction should never be administered to a patient over 50 years of age. A clear, detailed and convincing description of the reaction is felt to be sufficient in most cases.
However, where a test reaction is deemed necessary, the suggested procedure is as follows:

After the first one to two weeks' therapy with 500 mg daily, a drink of 15 ml (½ oz) of 100 proof whiskey or equivalent is taken slowly. This test dose of alcoholic beverage may be repeated once only so that the total dose does not exceed 30 ml (1 oz) of whiskey. Once a reaction develops, no more alcohol should be consumed. Such tests should be carried out only when the patient is hospitalized, or comparable supervision and facilities, including oxygen, are available.
MANAGEMENT OF ANTABUSE-ALCOHOL REACTION: In severe reactions, whether caused by an excessive test dose or by the patient's unsupervised ingestion of alcohol, supportive measures to restore blood pressure and treat shock should be instituted. Other recommendations include: oxygen, carbogen (95 per cent oxygen and 5 per cent carbon dioxide), vitamin C intravenously in massive doses (1 g), and ephedrine sulfate. Antihistamines have also been used intravenously. Potassium levels should be monitored particularly in patients on digitalis since hypokalemia has been reported.
How Supplied: ANTABUSE—Each tablet (scored) contains 250 mg disulfiram, in bottles of 100 (NDC 0046-0809-81)—Each tablet (scored) contains 500 mg disulfiram, in bottles of 50 (NDC 0046-0810-50) and 1,000 (NDC 0046-0810-91).

[*Shown in Product Identification Section*]

A.P.L.® ℞

Brand of chorionic gonadotropin for injection, U.S.P.
For Intramuscular Injection Only

Description: Human chorionic gonadotropin (HCG), a polypeptide hormone produced by the human placenta, is composed of an alpha and a beta subunit. The alpha subunit is essentially identical to the alpha subunits of the human pituitary gonadotropins, luteinizing hormone (LH) and follicle-stimulating hormone (FSH), as well as to the alpha subunit of human thyroid stimulating hormone (TSH). The beta subunits of these hormones differ in amino acid sequence.
A.P.L. (chorionic gonadotropin for injection, U.S.P.) is a gonad-stimulating principle obtained from the urine of pregnant women. It is an amorphous powder prepared by cryodesiccation, and is freely soluble in water.
Actions: The action of HCG is virtually identical to that of pituitary LH, although HCG appears to have a small degree of FSH activity as well. It stimulates production of gonadal steroid hormones by stimulating the interstitial cells (Leydig cells) of the testis to produce androgens and the corpus luteum of the ovary to produce progesterone. Androgen stimulation in the male leads to the development of secondary sex characteristics and may stimulate testicular descent when no anatomical impediment to descent is present. This descent is usually reversible when HCG is discontinued. During the normal menstrual cycle, LH participates with FSH in the development and maturation of the normal ovarian follicle, and the midcycle LH surge triggers ovulation. HCG can substitute for LH in this function.
During a normal pregnancy, HCG secreted by the placenta maintains the corpus luteum after LH secretion decreases, supporting continued secretion of estrogen and progesterone, and preventing menstruation. HCG HAS NO KNOWN EFFECT ON FAT MOBILIZATION, APPETITE OR SENSE OF HUNGER, OR BODY FAT DISTRIBUTION.
Indications: HCG HAS NOT BEEN DEMONSTRATED TO BE EFFECTIVE ADJUNCTIVE THERAPY IN THE TREATMENT OF OBESITY. THERE IS NO SUBSTANTIAL EVIDENCE THAT IT INCREASES WEIGHT LOSS BEYOND THAT RESULTING FROM CALORIC RESTRICTION, THAT IT CAUSES A MORE ATTRACTIVE OR "NORMAL" DISTRIBUTION OF FAT, OR THAT IT DECREASES THE HUNGER AND DISCOMFORT ASSOCIATED WITH CALORIE RESTRICTED DIETS.

1. Cryptorchidism not due to anatomic obstruction. In general, A.P.L. is thought to induce testicular descent in situations when descent would have occurred at puberty. A.P.L. thus may help to predict whether or not orchiopexy will be needed in the future. Although, in some cases, descent following A.P.L. administration is permanent, in most cases the response is temporary. Therapy is usually instituted between the ages of 4 and 9.
2. Selected cases of male hypogonadism secondary to pituitary failure.
3. Induction of ovulation and pregnancy in the anovulatory, infertile woman in whom the cause of anovulation is secondary and not due to ovarian failure, and who has been appropriately pretreated with human menotropins.

Contraindications: Precocious puberty, prostatic carcinoma or other androgen-dependent neoplasia, prior allergic reaction to chorionic gonadotropin.
Warnings: HCG should be used in conjunction with human menopausal gonadotropins only by physicians experienced with infertility problems who are familiar with the criteria for patient selection, contraindications, warnings, precautions, and adverse reactions described in the package insert for menotropins. The principal serious adverse reactions during this use are: (1) ovarian enlargement, ascites with or without pain, and/or pleural effusion, (2) rupture of ovarian cysts with resultant hemoperitoneum, (3) multiple births, and (4) arterial thromboembolism.
Precautions: Induction of androgen secretion by chorionic gonadotropin may induce precocious puberty in patients treated for cryptorchidism. If signs of precocious puberty occur, therapy should be discontinued.
Since androgens may cause fluid retention, chorionic gonadotropin should be used with caution in patients with epilepsy, migraine, asthma, cardiac or renal disease.
Adverse Reactions:
Headache
Irritability
Restlessness
Depression
Tiredness
Edema
Precocious puberty
Gynecomastia
Pain at site of injection
Dosage and Administration: There is a marked variance of opinion concerning the dosage regimens to be used. Therefore the regimen employed in any particular case will depend upon the indication for use, the age and weight of the patient, and the physician's preference. The following regimens have been advocated by various authorities.
Cryptorchidism: (Therapy is usually instituted between the ages of 4 and 9.)
(1) 4,000 U.S.P. Units three times weekly for three weeks.
(2) 5,000 U.S.P. Units every second day for four injections.
(3) 15 injections of 500 to 1,000 U.S.P. Units over a period of six weeks.
(4) 500 U.S.P. Units three times weekly for four to six weeks. If this course of treatment is not successful, another is begun one month later, giving 1,000 U.S.P. Units per injection.
Selected cases of male hypogonadism secondary to pituitary failure:
(1) 500 to 1,000 U.S.P. Units three times a week for three weeks, followed by the same dose twice a week for three weeks.
(2) 1,000 to 2,000 U.S.P. Units three times weekly.
(3) 4,000 U.S.P. Units three times weekly for six to nine months, following which the dosage may be reduced to 2,000 U.S.P. Units three times weekly for an additional three months.
Induction of ovulation and pregnancy in the anovulatory, infertile woman in whom the cause of anovulation is secondary:
5,000 to 10,000 U.S.P. Units one day following the last dose of menotropins.
How Supplied: A.P.L. (chorionic gonadotropin for injection, U.S.P.)
NDC 0046-0970-10 — Each package provides:
(1) One vial containing 5,000 U.S.P. Units chorionic gonadotropin in dry form, and
(2) One 10 ml ampul sterile diluent.
NDC 0046-0971-10 — Each package provides:
(1) One vial containing 10,000 U.S.P. Units chorionic gonadotropin in dry form, and
(2) One 10 ml ampul sterile diluent.
NDC 0046-0972-10 — Each package provides:
(1) One vial containing 20,000 U.S.P. Units chorionic gonadotropin in dry form, and
(2) One 10 ml ampul sterile diluent.
When reconstituted with 10 ml of accompanying sterile diluent, the resulting solutions also contain 2.0% benzyl alcohol, not more than 0.2% phenol, and the following concentrations of lactose: No. 970, 0.9%; No. 971, 1.8%; No. 972, 3.6%. The pH is adjusted with sodium hydroxide or hydrochloric acid.
MAY BE STORED FOR 90 DAYS IN A REFRIGERATOR AFTER RECONSTITUTION.

ATROMID-S® ℞

Brand of clofibrate
Antilipidemic agent for reduction of elevated serum lipids

Actions: ATROMID-S is an antilipidemic agent. It acts to lower elevated serum lipids by reducing the very low density lipoprotein fraction (S_f20–400) rich in triglycerides. Serum cholesterol, especially the low density lipoprotein fraction (S_f0–20), is also decreased, particularly in those whose cholesterol levels are elevated at the outset.
The mechanism of action has not been established definitively. In man, clofibrate reduces cholesterol formation early in the biosynthetic chain. In addition, clofibrate has been shown to cause increased excretion of neutral sterols.
Animal studies suggest that clofibrate interrupts cholesterol biosynthesis prior to mevalonate formation.

Indications: This is not an innocuous drug. Strict attention should be paid to the Indications, Contraindications, and Warnings.

Treatment of primary hyperlipidemia should begin with a diet specific for the type of hyperlipidemia.[1] Diet, weight reduction, exercise, and good control of diabetes mellitus lead to improved lipid levels and may obviate the need for antilipidemic drugs.

ATROMID-S may be utilized as adjunctive therapy in patients with significant hyperlipidemia and a high risk of coronary artery disease who do not respond adequately to diet and weight loss. Before using ATROMID-S in a patient, consideration should be given to whether other antilipidemic drugs are more appropriate in view of the serious adverse findings with ATROMID-S reported in two large clinical trials (see WARNINGS). In addition, assessment of risk of coronary artery disease should include consideration of such factors, in addition to lipid levels, as strong family history of coronary heart disease, low serum levels of high density lipoprotein, marked obesity, continued smoking, use of oral contraception, and hypertension that is not satisfactorily controlled with medication. Drug therapy should be more strongly considered in younger patients and in those with a history of pancreatitis or abdominal pain associated with markedly elevated triglyceride levels.

ATROMID-S is a drug of first choice for primary dysbetalipoproteinemia (Type III hyperlipidemia), but in other types of hyperlipidemia certain other antilipidemic drugs may prove more effective in individual patients particularly where cholesterol is the lipid of greatest concern.

Clofibrate is not indicated for community-wide prevention of ischemic heart disease, but may be useful in patients individually selected for recognized disorders of fat metabolism which may predispose them to an increased risk of heart disease.

Response to ATROMID-S is variable, and it is not always possible to predict from the lipoprotein type or other factors which patients will obtain favorable results. It is essential that lipid levels be assessed and that the drug be discontinued in any patient in whom lipids are not effectively altered. ATROMID-S usually lowers elevated serum triglycerides to a greater extent than elevated serum cholesterol.

Contraindications: Clofibrate is contraindicated in pregnant women. While teratogenic studies have not demonstrated any effect attributable to clofibrate, it is known that serum of the rabbit fetus accumulates a higher concentration of clofibrate than that found in maternal serum, and it is possible that the fetus may not have developed the enzyme system required for the excretion of clofibrate.

It is contraindicated in lactating women since it is not known if clofibrate is secreted in the milk.

It is contraindicated in patients with clinically significant hepatic or renal dysfunction.

It is contraindicated in patients with primary biliary cirrhosis since it may raise the already elevated cholesterol in these cases.

Warnings

In a large prospective study involving 5,000 patients in a clofibrate-treated group and 5,000 in a placebo-treated group followed for an average of five years on drug or placebo and one year beyond (the WHO study), there was a statistically significant 36% higher mortality due to noncardiovascular causes in the clofibrate-treated group than in a comparable placebo group. Half of this difference was due to malignancy; other causes of death included postcholecystectomy complications and pancreatitis.[2] In another prospective study involving 1,000 clofibrate- and 3,000 placebo-treated patients followed for an average of six years on drug or placebo (the Coronary Drug Project study), the noncardiovascular mortality rate, including that of malignancy, was not significantly different in the clofibrate- and placebo-treated groups.[3] This should not be interpreted to mean that clofibrate is not associated with an increased risk of noncardiovascular death because the patients in the Coronary Drug Project were much older than those in the WHO study and they all had had a previous myocardial infarction so that the deaths in the Coronary Drug Project were overwhelmingly due to cardiovascular causes and it would have been very difficult to discern a clofibrate-associated risk of death due to noncardiovascular causes if it existed. Both studies demonstrated that clofibrate users have twice the risk of developing cholelithiasis and cholecystitis requiring surgery as do nonusers.

A potential benefit of clofibrate was, however, reported in the WHO study which involved patients with hypercholesterolemia and no history of myocardial infarction or angina pectoris. In this study, there was noted a statistically significant 25% decrease in subsequent nonfatal myocardial infarctions in the clofibrate-treated group when compared with the placebo group. There was no difference in incidence of fatal myocardial infarction in the two groups. If the study had been continued longer, had included diet, had been restricted to patients who had both hyperlipidemia and increased risk factors *and* who obtained significant clofibrate-induced reduction in serum lipids, it is possible that it may have shown a decrease in fatal myocardial infarctions. In the Coronary Drug Project study, which involved patients with or without hypercholesterolemia and/or hypertriglyceridemia and with a history of previous myocardial infarction, there was no significant difference in incidence of either nonfatal or fatal myocardial infarction between the clofibrate- and placebo-treated groups.[2]

As a result of these and other studies, the following can be stated:

1. Clofibrate, in general, causes a relatively modest reduction of serum cholesterol and a somewhat greater reduction of serum triglycerides. In Type III hyperlipidemia, however, substantial reductions of both cholesterol and triglycerides can occur with use of clofibrate.
2. No study to date has shown a convincing reduction in incidence of *fatal* myocardial infarction.
3. A significantly increased incidence of cholelithiasis has been demonstrated consistently in clofibrate-treated groups, and an increase in morbidity from this complication and mortality from cholecystectomy must be anticipated during clofibrate treatment.
4. Several types of other undesirable events have been associated in a statistically significant way with clofibrate administration in the WHO or the Coronary Drug Project studies. There was an increase in incidence of noncardiovascular deaths reported in the WHO study. There was an increase in cardiac arrhythmias and intermittent claudication and in definite or suspected thromboembolic events and angina reported in the Coronary Drug Project, which was not, however, reported in the WHO study.
5. Administration of clofibrate to mice and rats in long-term studies at eight times the human dose, and to rats at five times the human dose, resulted in a higher incidence of benign and malignant liver tumors than in controls. Lower doses were not included in these studies.

BECAUSE OF THE HEPATIC TUMORIGENICITY OF CLOFIBRATE IN RODENTS AND THE POSSIBLE INCREASED RISK OF MALIGNANCY ASSOCIATED WITH CLOFIBRATE IN THE HUMAN, AS WELL AS THE INCREASED RISK OF CHOLELITHIASIS, AND BECAUSE THERE IS NOT, TO DATE, SUBSTANTIAL EVIDENCE OF A BENEFICIAL EFFECT ON CARDIOVASCULAR MORTALITY FROM CLOFIBRATE, THIS DRUG SHOULD BE UTILIZED ONLY FOR THOSE PATIENTS DESCRIBED IN THE INDICATIONS SECTION, AND SHOULD BE DISCONTINUED IF SIGNIFICANT LIPID RESPONSE IS NOT OBTAINED.

Concomitant Anticoagulants

CAUTION SHOULD BE EXERCISED WHEN ANTICOAGULANTS ARE GIVEN IN CONJUNCTION WITH ATROMID-S. THE DOSAGE OF THE ANTICOAGULANT SHOULD BE REDUCED USUALLY BY ONE-HALF (DEPENDING ON THE INDIVIDUAL CASE) TO MAINTAIN THE PROTHROMBIN TIME AT THE DESIRED LEVEL TO PREVENT BLEEDING COMPLICATIONS. FREQUENT PROTHROMBIN DETERMINATIONS ARE ADVISABLE UNTIL IT HAS BEEN DEFINITELY DETERMINED THAT THE PROTHROMBIN LEVEL HAS BEEN STABILIZED.

Avoidance of Pregnancy

Strict birth control procedures must be exercised by women of childbearing potential. In patients who plan to become pregnant, clofibrate should be withdrawn several months before conception. Because of the possibility of pregnancy occurring despite birth control precautions in patients taking clofibrate, the possible benefits of the drug to the patient must be weighed against possible hazards to the fetus.

Precautions: Before instituting therapy with clofibrate, attempts should be made to control serum lipids with appropriate dietary regimens, weight loss in obese patients, control of diabetes mellitus, etc.

Because of the long-term administration of a drug of this nature, adequate baseline studies should be performed to determine that the patient has significantly elevated serum lipid levels. Frequent determinations of serum lipids should be obtained during the first few months of ATROMID-S administration, and periodic determinations thereafter. The drug should be withdrawn after three months if response is inadequate. However, in the case of xanthoma tuberosum, the drug should be employed for longer periods (even up to one year) provided that there is a reduction in the size and/or number of the xanthomata.

Subsequent serum lipid determinations should be done to detect a paradoxical rise in serum cholesterol or triglyceride levels. Clofibrate will not alter the seasonal variations of serum cholesterol peak elevations in midwinter and late summer and decreases in fall and spring. If the drug is discontinued, the patient should be continued on an appropriate hypolipidemic diet, and his serum lipids should be monitored until stabilized, as a rise in these values to or above the original baseline may occur.

During clofibrate therapy, frequent serum transaminase determinations and other liver function tests should be performed since the drug may produce abnormalities in these parameters. These effects are usually reversible when the drug is discontinued. Hepatic biopsies are usually within normal limits. If the hepatic function tests steadily rise or show excessive abnormalities, the drug should be with-

Continued on next page

Ayerst—Cont.

drawn. Therefore use with caution in those patients with a past history of jaundice or hepatic disease.
Since cholelithiasis is a possible side effect of clofibrate therapy, appropriate diagnostic procedures should be performed if signs and symptoms related to disease of the biliary system should occur.
Clofibrate may produce "flu like" symptoms (muscular aching, soreness, cramping). The physician should differentiate this from actual viral and/or bacterial disease.
Use with caution in patients with peptic ulcer since reactivation has been reported. Whether this is drug-related is unknown.
Complete blood counts should be done periodically since anemia, and more frequently, leukopenia have been reported in patients who have been taking clofibrate.
Various cardiac arrhythmias have been reported with the use of clofibrate.
Several investigators have observed in their studies that clofibrate may produce a decrease in cholesterol linoleate but an increase in palmitoleate and oleate, the latter being considered atherogenic in experimental animals. The significance of this finding is unknown at this time.
Adverse Reactions: Of the pertinent reactions, the most common is nausea. Less frequently encountered gastrointestinal reactions are vomiting, loose stools, dyspepsia, flatulence, and abdominal distress. Reactions reported less often than gastrointestinal ones are headache, dizziness, and fatigue; muscle cramping, aching, and weakness; skin rash, urticaria, and pruritus; dry brittle hair, and alopecia.
The following reported adverse reactions are listed alphabetically by systems:
Cardiovascular
- Increased or decreased angina
- Cardiac arrhythmias
- Both swelling and phlebitis at site of xanthomas

Dermatologic
- Skin rash
- Alopecia
- Allergic reaction including urticaria
- Dry skin and dry brittle hair
- Puritus

Gastrointestinal
- Nausea
- Diarrhea
- Gastrointestinal upset (bloating, flatulence, abdominal distress)
- Hepatomegaly (not associated with hepatotoxicity)
- Gallstones
- Vomiting
- Stomatitis and gastritis

Genitourinary
- Impotence and decreased libido
- Findings consistent with renal dysfunction as evidenced by dysuria, hematuria, proteinuria, decreased urine output. One patient's renal biopsy suggested "allergic reaction."

Hematologic
- Leukopenia
- Potentiation of anticoagulant effect
- Anemia
- Eosinophilia

Musculoskeletal
- Myalgia (muscle cramping, aching, weakness)
- "Flu like" symptoms
- Arthralgia

Neurologic
- Fatigue, weakness, drowsiness
- Dizziness
- Headache

Miscellaneous
- Weight gain
- Polyphagia

Laboratory Findings
- Abnormal liver function tests as evidenced by increased transaminase (SGOT and SGPT), BSP retention, and increased thymol turbidity
- Proteinuria
- Increased creatine phosphokinase

Reported adverse reactions whose direct relationship with the drug has not been established: peptic ulcer, gastrointestinal hemorrhage, rheumatoid arthritis, tremors, increased perspiration, systemic lupus erythematosus, blurred vision, gynecomastia, thrombocytopenic purpura.
Dosage and Administration:
Initial: The recommended dosage for adults is 2 g daily in divided doses. Some patients may respond to a lower dosage.
Maintenance: Same as for initial dosage.
Note: In children, insufficient studies have been done to show safety and efficacy.
Drug Interactions: Caution should be exercised when anticoagulants are given in conjunction with ATROMID-S. The dosage of the anticoagulant should be reduced usually by one-half (depending on the individual case) to maintain the prothrombin time at the desired level to prevent bleeding complications. Frequent prothrombin determinations are advisable until it has been definitely determined that the prothrombin level has been stabilized.
Management of Overdosage: While there has been no reported case of overdosage, should it occur, symptomatic supportive measures should be taken.
How Supplied: ATROMID-S—Each capsule contains 500 mg clofibrate, in bottles of 100 (NDC 0046-0243-81).
References:
1. Coronary Risk Handbook (1973), American Heart Association.
2. Report from the Committee of Principal Investigators: A cooperative trial in the primary prevention of ischaemic heart disease using clofibrate, Br. Heart J. *40:*1069, 1078.
3. The Coronary Drug Project Research Group: Clofibrate and niacin in coronary heart disease, J.A.M.A. *231:*360, 1975.
[*Shown in Product Identification Section*]

AURALGAN® Otic Solution ℞

Each ml contains:

Antipyrine	54.0 mg
Benzocaine	14.0 mg
Glycerin dehydrated q.s. to	1.0 ml

(contains not more than 1.0% moisture)
(also contains oxyquinoline sulfate)
TOPICAL DECONGESTANT AND ANALGESIC
Description: AURALGAN is an otic solution containing antipyrine, benzocaine, and dehydrated glycerin. The solution congeals at 0° C (32° F), but returns to normal consistency, unchanged, at room temperature.
Actions: AURALGAN combines the hygroscopic property of dehydrated glycerin with the analgesic action of antipyrine and benzocaine to relieve pressure, reduce inflammation and congestion, and alleviate pain and discomfort in acute otitis media.
AURALGAN does not blanch the tympanic membrane or mask the landmarks and, therefore, does not distort the otoscopic picture.
Indications:
Acute otitis media of various etiologies
—prompt relief of pain and reduction of inflammation in the congestive and serous stages
—adjuvant therapy during systemic antibiotic administration for resolution of the infection
Because of the close anatomical relationship of the eustachian tube to the nasal cavity, otitis media is a frequent problem, especially in children in whom the tube is shorter, wider, and more horizontal than in adults.
Removal of cerumen
—facilitates the removal of excessive or impacted cerumen
Contraindications: Hypersensitivity to any of the components or substances related to them. In the presence of spontaneous perforation or discharge.
Dosage and Administration: *Acute otitis media:* Instill AURALGAN, permitting the solution to run along the wall of the canal until it is filled. Avoid touching the ear with dropper. Then moisten a cotton pledget with AURALGAN and insert into meatus. Repeat every one to two hours until pain and congestion are relieved.
Removal of cerumen
Before: Instill AURALGAN three times daily for two or three days to help detach cerumen from wall of canal and facilitate removal.
After: AURALGAN is useful for drying out the canal or relieving discomfort.
Before and after removal of cerumen, a cotton pledget moistened with AURALGAN should be inserted into the meatus following instillation.
NOTE: Do not rinse dropper after use. Replace in bottle and screw cap tightly.
How Supplied: AURALGAN® Otic Solution, in package containing 15 ml (½ fl oz) bottle with separate dropper-screw cap attachment (NDC 0046-1000-15).

BEMINAL®-500
Therapeutic vitamin B complex tablets with 500 mg vitamin C

Each tablet contains:

Thiamine mononitrate (Vit. B_1)	25.0 mg
Riboflavin (Vit. B_2)	12.5 mg
Niacinamide	100.0 mg
Pyridoxine hydrochloride (Vit. B_6)	10.0 mg
Calcium pantothenate	20.0 mg
Ascorbic acid (Vit. C) as sodium ascorbate	500.0 mg
Cyanocobalamin (Vit. B_{12})	5.0 mcg

Does not contain saccharin or other sweeteners.
Indications: Whenever the administration of high potency B complex vitamins with vitamin C is needed—in pre- and postoperative care; in acute infection, long term illness, or debilitating disease; in chronic alcoholism, and whenever nutrition is impaired by digestive problems; to supplement restricted diets prescribed in obesity and other conditions; in geriatrics to help provide nutritional support.
Dosage: Adults—1 tablet daily, or as directed by physician.
How Supplied: BEMINAL-500 Tablets, in bottles of 100 (NDC 0046-0832-81).
[*Shown in Product Identification Section*]

BEMINAL® FORTE with VITAMIN C
Therapeutic vitamin B complex capsules with vitamin C

Each capsule contains:

Thiamine mononitrate (Vit. B_1)	25.0 mg
Riboflavin (Vit. B_2)	12.5 mg
Niacinamide	50.0 mg
Pyridoxine HCl (Vit. B_6)	3.0 mg
Calcium pantothenate	10.0 mg
Ascorbic acid (Vit. C)	250.0 mg
Cyanocobalamin (Vit. B_{12})	2.5 mcg

Indications: Whenever the administration of high potency B complex with vitamin C is needed—pre- and postoperatively; during treatment with sulfonamides and antibiotics; etc.
Dosage: Adults—1 capsule daily, or as directed by physician.

How Supplied: BEMINAL Forte with Vitamin C Capsules, in bottles of 100 (NDC 0046-0817-81).
[*Shown in Product Identification Section*]

CLUSIVOL® SYRUP
Therapeutic vitamin-mineral syrup for children and adults

Each 5 ml (1 teaspoonful) contains:

Vitamin A (as palmitate)	2,500 U.S.P. Units
Cholecalciferol (Vit. D_3)	400 U.S.P. Units
Ascorbic acid (Vit. C)	15.0 mg
Cyanocobalamin (Vit. B_{12})	2.0 mcg
Thiamine HCl (Vit. B_1)	1.0 mg
Riboflavin (Vit. B_2)	1.0 mg
Niacinamide	5.0 mg
d-Panthenol	3.0 mg
Pyridoxine HCl (Vit. B_6)	0.6 mg
Manganese†	0.5 mg
Zinc†	0.5 mg
Magnesium†	3.0 mg

†Supplied as the gluconates of manganese and magnesium, and zinc lactate.

Contains 3.8 mg saccharin, as sodium saccharin, per teaspoonful.

A comprehensive nutritional formula incorporating essential fat- and water-soluble vitamins together with important minerals. Presented in a candy-flavored syrup base; particularly appealing to children, but also enjoyed by older individuals who prefer a liquid preparation.

Action and Uses: A potent nutritional safeguard for better health for the entire family.

Dosage: *Children and Adults:* One teaspoonful (5 ml) daily, or as prescribed by the physician.

How Supplied: CLUSIVOL Syrup, in bottles of 8 fl oz (½ pint) (NDC 0046-0944-08), 16 fl oz (1 pint) (NDC 0046-0944-16), and 32 fl oz (1 quart) (NDC 0046-0944-32).

CLUSIVOL® Tablet/Capsule

CLUSIVOL® 130
Therapeutic vitamin-mineral tablets for adults

Each tablet contains:

Vitamin A (as palmitate)	10,000 U.S.P. Units
Ergocalciferol (Vit. D_2)	400 U.S.P. Units
Ascorbic acid (Vit. C) (as sodium ascorbate)	150.0 mg
Thiamine mononitrate (Vit. B_1)	10.0 mg
Riboflavin (Vit. B_2)	5.0 mg
Pyridoxine HCl (Vit. B_6)	0.5 mg
d-Panthenol	1.0 mg
Cyanocobalamin (Vit. B_{12})	2.5 mcg
Niacinamide	50.0 mg
Vitamin E†	0.5 I.U.
Iron†	15.0 mg
Calcium†	120.0 mg
Manganese†	0.5 mg
Zinc†	0.6 mg
Magnesium†	3.0 mg

†Supplied as *dl-α*-tocopheryl acetate, ferrous fumarate, calcium carbonate, manganese gluconate, zinc oxide, and magnesium oxide.

CLUSIVOL® Capsules
Therapeutic vitamin-mineral capsules for adults

Each capsule contains:

Vitamin A (as palmitate)	10,000 U.S.P. Units
Ergocalciferol (Vit. D_2)	400 U.S.P. Units
Ascorbic acid (Vit. C) (as sodium ascorbate)	150.0 mg
Thiamine mononitrate (Vit. B_1)	10.0 mg
Riboflavin (Vit. B_2)	5.0 mg
Pyridoxine HCl (Vit. B_6)	0.5 mg
d-Panthenol	1.0 mg
Cyanocobalamin (Vit. B_{12})	2.5 mcg
Niacinamide	50.0 mg
Vitamin E†	0.5 I.U.
Iron†	15.0 mg
Calcium†	120.0 mg
Manganese†	0.5 mg
Zinc†	0.6 mg
Magnesium†	3.0 mg

†Supplied as *d-α*-tocopheryl acetate concentrate, ferrous sulfate, calcium carbonate, manganous sulfate, zinc sulfate, and magnesium sulfate.

Indications: For use in vitamin deficiencies, especially for patients with generally inadequate or broadly restricted diets.

Dosage and Administration: One tablet (capsule) daily, or as directed by the physician.

How Supplied: CLUSIVOL 130, bottle of 130 tablets (NDC 0046-0270-81). CLUSIVOL Capsules, bottle of 100 (NDC 0046-0293-81).

DERMOPLAST® Aerosol Spray

Contains (exclusive of propellants) 20% benzocaine and 0.5% menthol in a water-dispersible base of TWEEN® 85 and polyethylene glycol 400 monolaurate with methylparaben as a preservative.

A topical anesthetic and antipruritic spray providing soothing, temporary relief of skin pain, itching, and discomfort due to episiotomy, pruritus vulvae, postpartum hemorrhoids, abrasions, sunburn, minor wounds, burns, and insect bites. May be applied without touching sensitive affected areas.

Warnings: Avoid spraying in eyes. Contents under pressure. Do not puncture or incinerate. Do not expose to heat or temperatures above 120° F. Do not use near open flame. Use only as directed. Intentional misuse by deliberately concentrating and inhaling the contents can be harmful or fatal.

Do not take orally. Not for prolonged use. If the condition for which this preparation is used persists or if a rash or irritation develops, discontinue use and consult physician.

Directions for Use: Hold can in a convenient position at least twelve inches away from affected area. Point spray nozzle and press button. May be administered two or three times daily, or as directed by physician.

How Supplied: DERMOPLAST Aerosol Spray, in Net Wt 3 oz (85 g)—NDC 0046-1008-03; and in Net Wt 6 oz (170 g)—NDC 0046-1008-06.

DIUCARDIN® ℞
Brand of hydroflumethiazide
A diuretic-antihypertensive agent

Actions: DIUCARDIN is a thiazide diuretic and antihypertensive. DIUCARDIN affects the renal tubular mechanism of electrolyte reabsorption. At maximal therapeutic dosage all thiazides are approximately equal in their diuretic potency.

DIUCARDIN increases excretion of sodium and chloride in approximately equivalent amounts. Natriuresis causes a secondary loss of potassium and bicarbonate.

The mechanism of the antihypertensive effect of DIUCARDIN is unknown. DIUCARDIN does not affect normal blood pressure.

Onset of action of DIUCARDIN occurs in two hours and the peak effect at about four hours. Its action persists for approximately 6 to 12 hours. Thiazides are eliminated rapidly by the kidney.

Indications: DIUCARDIN is indicated as adjunctive therapy in edema associated with congestive heart failure, hepatic cirrhosis and corticosteroid and estrogen therapy.

DIUCARDIN has also been found useful in edema due to various forms of renal dysfunction as: nephrotic syndrome; acute glomerulonephritis; and chronic renal failure.

DIUCARDIN is indicated in the management of hypertension either as the sole therapeutic agent or to enhance the effect of other antihypertensive drugs in the more severe forms of hypertension.

Usage in Pregnancy: The routine use of diuretics in an otherwise healthy woman is inappropriate and exposes mother and fetus to unnecessary hazard. Diuretics do not prevent development of toxemia of pregnancy, and there is no satisfactory evidence that they are useful in the treatment of developed toxemia.

Edema during pregnancy may arise from pathological causes or from the physiologic and mechanical consequences of pregnancy. Thiazides are indicated in pregnancy when edema is due to pathologic causes just as they are in the absence of pregnancy (however, see Warnings, below). Dependent edema in pregnancy, resulting from restriction of venous return by the expanded uterus, is properly treated through elevation of the lower extremities and use of support hose. Use of diuretics to lower intravascular volume in this case is illogical and unnecessary. There is hypervolemia during normal pregnancy which is harmful to neither the fetus nor the mother (in absence of cardiovascular disease), but which is associated with edema, including generalized edema, in the majority of pregnant women. If this edema produces discomfort, increased recumbency will often provide relief. In rare instances, this edema may cause extreme discomfort which is not relieved by rest. In these cases, a short course of diuretics may provide relief and may be appropriate.

Contraindications: Anuria.

Hypersensitivity to this or other sulfonamide-derived drugs.

Warnings: Thiazides should be used with caution in severe renal disease. In patients with renal disease, thiazides may precipitate azotemia. Cumulative effects of the drug may develop in patients with impaired renal function.

Thiazides should be used with caution in patients with impaired hepatic function or progressive liver disease, since minor alterations of fluid and electrolyte balance may precipitate hepatic coma.

Thiazides may add to or potentiate the action of other antihypertensive drugs. Potentiation occurs with ganglionic or peripheral adrenergic blocking drugs.

Sensitivity reactions may occur in patients with or without a history of allergy or bronchial asthma.

The possibility of exacerbation or activation of systemic lupus erythematosus has been reported.

Usage in Pregnancy: Thiazides cross the placental barrier and appear in cord blood. The use of thiazides in pregnant women requires that the anticipated benefit be weighed against possible hazards to the fetus. These hazards include fetal or neonatal jaundice, thrombocytopenia, and possibly other adverse reactions which have occurred in the adult.

Nursing Mothers: Thiazides appear in breast milk. If use of the drug is deemed essential, the patient should stop nursing.

Precautions: Periodic determination of serum electrolytes to detect possible electrolyte imbalance should be performed at appropriate intervals.

All patients receiving thiazide therapy should be observed for clinical signs of fluid or electrolyte imbalance: namely, hyponatremia, hypochloremic alkalosis, and hypokalemia. Serum and urine electrolyte determinations are particularly important when the patient is vomiting excessively or receiving parenteral fluids. Medication such as digitalis may also influence serum electrolytes. Warning signs, irrespective of cause are: dryness of mouth, thirst, weakness, lethargy, drowsiness, restlessness, muscle pains or cramps, muscular fatigue, hypotension, oliguria, tachycardia, and gastrointestinal disturbances such as nausea and vomiting.

Hypokalemia may develop, especially with brisk diuresis, when severe cirrhosis is present, or during concomitant use of corticosteroids or ACTH.

Interference with adequate oral electrolyte intake will also contribute to hypokalemia. Hypokalemia can sensitize or exaggerate the

Continued on next page

Ayerst—Cont.

response of the heart to the toxic effects of digitalis (*e.g.,* increased ventricular irritability). Hypokalemia may be avoided or treated by use of potassium supplements such as foods with a high potassium content.
Any chloride deficit is generally mild and usually does not require specific treatment except under extraordinary circumstances (as in liver disease or renal disease). Dilutional hyponatremia may occur in edematous patients in hot weather; appropriate therapy is water restriction, rather than administration of salt, except in rare instances when the hyponatremia is life-threatening. In actual salt depletion, appropriate replacement is the therapy of choice.

Hyperuricemia may occur or frank gout may be precipitated in certain patients receiving thiazide therapy.
Insulin requirements in diabetic patients may be increased, decreased, or unchanged. Diabetes mellitus which has been latent may become manifest during thiazide administration.
Thiazide drugs may increase the responsiveness to tubocurarine.
The antihypertensive effects of the drug may be enhanced in the postsympathectomy patient. Thiazides may decrease arterial responsiveness to norepinephrine. This diminution is not sufficient to preclude effectiveness of the pressor agent for therapeutic use.
If progressive renal impairment becomes evident, consider withholding or discontinuing diuretic therapy.
Thiazides may decrease serum PBI levels without signs of thyroid disturbance.
Calcium excretion is decreased by thiazides. Pathological changes in the parathyroid gland with hypercalcemia and hypophosphatemia have been observed in a few patients on prolonged thiazide therapy. The common complications of hyperparathyroidism such as renal lithiasis, bone resorption, and peptic ulceration have not been seen. Thazides should be discontinued before carrying out tests for parathyroid function.
Adverse Reactions: *Gastrointestinal System:* anorexia, gastric irritation, nausea, vomiting, cramping, diarrhea, constipation, jaundice (intrahepatic cholestatic jaundice), pancreatitis, sialadenitis
Central Nervous System: dizziness, vertigo, paresthesias, headache, xanthopsia
Hematologic: leukopenia, agranulocytosis, thrombocytopenia, aplastic anemia
Cardiovascular: orthostatic hypotension (may be aggravated by alcohol, barbiturates, or narcotics)
Hypersensitivity: purpura, photosensitivity, rash, urticaria, necrotizing angiitis (vasculitis, cutaneous vasculitis), fever, respiratory distress including pneumonitis, anaphylactic reactions
Other: hyperglycemia, glycosuria, hyperuricemia, muscle spasm, weakness, restlessness, transient blurred vision
Whenever adverse reactions are moderate or severe, thiazide dosage should be reduced or therapy withdrawn.
Dosage and Administration: Therapy should be individualized according to patient response. Use the smallest dosage necessary to maintain the required response.
The usual daily dosages for antihypertensive and diuretic effect are:

Diuretic	Antihypertensive
Adult: 25 to 200 mg	50 to 100 mg

Dosage regimens using 25 mg DIUCARDIN may be adequate in some cases.
Dosage should not exceed 200 mg per day.
For Diuresis in the Adult:
Initial recommended dose is 50 mg once or twice a day. Daily maintenance dose may be as little as 25 mg or as much as 200 mg, depending on patient's response. With dosages in excess of 100 mg daily, it is generally preferable to administer DIUCARDIN in divided doses.
Many patients with edema respond to intermittent therapy, i.e., administration on alternate days or on three to five days each week. With an intermittent schedule, excessive response and the resulting undesirable electrolyte imbalance are less likely to occur.
For Control of Hypertension in the Adult:
Usual starting dose is 50 mg twice daily. Dosage is increased or decreased according to the blood pressure response of the patient. Usual maintenance dose is 50 mg to 100 mg per day. Dosage should not exceed 200 mg per day.
Careful observations for changes in blood pressure must be made when this compound is used with other antihipertensive drugs, especially during initial therapy. The dosage of other agents must be reduced by at least 50 percent as soon as it is added to the regimen to prevent excessive drop in blood pressure. As the blood pressure falls under the potentiating effect of this agent, a further reduction in dosage, or even discontinuation, of other antihypertensive drugs may be necessary.
Overdosage: The following information is provided to serve as guidelines in treating overdosage.
HYDROFLUMETHIAZIDE
Signs and Symptoms:
Diuresis is to be expected; lethargy of varying degree may appear and may progress to coma within a few hours, with minimal depression of respiration and cardiovascular function, and without significant serum electrolyte changes or dehydration. The mechanism of CNS depression with thiazide overdosage is unknown.
G.I. irritation and hypermotility may occur; temporary elevation of BUN has been reported and serum electrolyte changes could occur, especially in patients with impairment of renal function.
Treatment:
Evacuate gastric contents but take care to prevent aspiration, especially in the stuporous or comatose patient. G.I. effects are usually of short duration, but may require symptomatic treatment.
Monitor serum electrolyte levels and renal function; institute supportive measures as required individually to maintain hydration, electrolyte balance, respiration, and cardivascular-renal function.
How Supplied: DIUCARDIN—Each scored tablet contains 50 mg hydroflumethiazide, in bottles of 100 (NDC 0046-0702-81) and 1,000 (NDC 0046-0702-91).
[*Shown in Product Identification Section*]

ENZACTIN® Cream
Brand of triacetin

Action: For prevention and treatment of athlete's foot and other superficial fungus infections. The "self-regulating" action of ENZACTIN (triacetin) releases a constant effective level of *free* fatty acid at the site of infection, in a concentration that is nonirritating.
"*Self-regulating*" *action*—At a neutral or higher pH of infected skin and in the presence of the enzyme esterase (found abundantly in skin, serum, and fungi), glycerol and free fatty acid (acetic) are rapidly liberated from triacetin. At this point, the growth of fungi is inhibited by the free acid.
With an accumulation of free acid, the pH drops and esterase activity decreases. Then, as the acid in the skin diffuses or becomes neutralized, the pH rises and esterase is reactivated, to release more free acid for fungistatic control.
Relieves itching and soreness promptly. Helps prevent spread of infection. Nonirritating. Odorless and stainless.
Indications: Athlete's foot and other superficial fungus infections.
Administration: Thoroughly cleanse affected and adjacent areas with dilute alcohol or a mild soap and warm water. Pat dry. Apply cream liberally twice daily, preferably morning and evening.
Note: Rayon fabrics should not come in contact with ENZACTIN Cream. For protection, cover treated areas with clean cotton cloth or bandage. If infection persists, consult a physician.
How Supplied: ENZACTIN *Cream*—250 mg triacetin per gram (in emollient base), in 1 oz (28.35 g) collapsible tubes (NDC 0046-0201-01).

Ayerst
EPITRATE® ℞
Brand of epinephrine bitartrate ophthalmic solution

For management of chronic simple (open-angle) glaucoma

Description: EPITRATE is a sterile aqueous solution of levorotatory epinephrine bitartrate 2%. It has a low surface tension.
Action: Intraocular pressure is lowered by reducing the rate of aqueous formation. Improvement in outflow facility is also observed in certain cases following prolonged therapy.
Indications: Useful in management of chronic simple (open-angle) glaucoma, either alone or in combination with miotics. In selected cases, it may also be used with carbonic anhydrase inhibitors.
Contraindications: Prior to peripheral iridectomy, an epinephrine preparation is contraindicated in eyes that are capable of angle closure since its relatively weak mydriatic action may, nevertheless, precipitate angle block. Gonioscopy should be carried out on all patients before initiating therapy.
Warnings: Topical use of epinephrine in any form should be interrupted prior to general anesthesia with certain anesthetics such as cyclopropane or halothane which sensitize the myocardium to sympathomimetics.
Precautions: EPITRATE (epinephrine bitartrate ophthalmic solution) should be used with caution in the presence of hypertension, diabetes, hyperthyroidism, heart disease, and cerebral arteriosclerosis because of the possibility of systemic action.
Adverse Reactions: As with other epinephrine solutions, transitory stinging on initial instillation may be expected. Headache or browache frequently occur on beginning EPITRATE therapy, but usually diminish as treatment is continued. Conjunctival allergy occurs occasionally. Pigmentary deposits in the lids, conjunctiva or cornea may occur after prolonged use of epinephrine eyedrops. In rare cases, maculopathy with a central scotoma may result from the use of topical epinephrine in aphakic patients; prompt reversal generally follows discontinuance of the drug. Systemic effects have occasionally been reported, such as: palpitation, tachycardia, extrasystoles, hypertension, trembling, sweating, and pallor.
Dosage and Administration: One drop, with frequency of instillation being individualized, from every two or three days to twice daily. More frequent instillation than one drop four times daily does not usually elicit any further improvement in therapeutic response.
How Supplied: EPITRATE—ophthalmic solution of epinephrine bitartrate 2% (equivalent to 1.1% base). [Also contains chlorobutanol (chloral derivative) 0.5%, sodium bisulfite, sodium chloride, polyoxypropylene-polyoxyethylene-diol, and disodium edetate.] Package containing 7.5 ml bottle with separate dropper-screw cap attachment (NDC 0046-1015-07).

ESTRADURIN® ℞

Brand of polyestradiol phosphate

For Intramuscular Injection Only

Description: ESTRADURIN is a water-soluble, high molecular weight polyester of phosphoric acid and 17β-estradiol. It is provided in a SECULE® containing 40 mg polyestradiol phosphate, 0.02 mg phenylmercuric nitrate, and 5.2 mg sodium phosphate. As solubilizing agents for the active ingredient, 25 mg niacinamide and 4 mg propylene glycol are also present. The pH is adjusted with sodium hydroxide.

One 2 ml ampul of sterile diluent is also provided.

Clinical Pharmacology: Estrogens are important in the development and maintenance of the female reproductive system. In responsive tissues estrogens enter the cell and are transported into the nucleus.

In the male patient with androgenic hormone-dependent conditions such as metastatic carcinoma of the prostate gland, estrogens counter the androgenic influence by competing for the receptor sites. As a result of treatment with estrogens, metastatic lesions in the bone may also show improvement.

Biologically active estradiol units are gradually split off from the large parent molecule, thus providing a continuous level of active estrogen over a prolonged period. The liberated estradiol is metabolized by the body in the same manner as the endogenous hormone. There is no depot effect at the site of injection—90 percent of injected dose leaves the bloodstream within 24 hours. Passive storage occurs in the reticuloendothelial system. As circulating levels of estradiol drop, more returns to the bloodstream from the site of storage for an even, continuous therapeutic effect. Increasing the dose acts to prolong the duration of pharmacologic action rather than to increase blood levels.

Metabolism and inactivation occur primarily in the liver. Some estrogens are excreted into the bile; however they are reabsorbed from the intestine and returned to the liver through the portal venous system. Water-soluble estrogen conjugates are strongly acidic and are ionized in body fluids, which favor excretion through the kidneys since tubular reabsorption is minimal.

Indication: ESTRADURIN (polyestradiol phosphate) is indicated in the treatment of prostatic carcinoma—palliative therapy of advanced disease.

Contraindications: Estrogens should not be used in men with any of the following conditions:

1. Known or suspected cancer of the breast except in appropriately selected patients being treated for metastatic disease.
2. Known or suspected estrogen-dependent neoplasia.
3. Active thrombophlebitis or thromboembolic disorders.

Warnings:

1. *Induction of malignant neoplasms.* Long term continuous administration of natural and synthetic estrogens in certain animal species increases the frequency of carcinomas of the breast, cervix, vagina, and liver.
2. *Gallbladder disease.* A recent study has reported a 2 to 3-fold increase in the risk of surgically confirmed gallbladder disease in women receiving postmenopausal estrogens,[1] similar to the 2-fold increase previously noted in users of oral contraceptives.[2,7a]
3. *Effects similar to those caused by estrogen-progestogen oral contraceptives.* There are several serious adverse effects of oral contraceptives. It has been shown that there is an increased risk of thrombosis in men receiving estrogens for prostatic cancer and women for postpartum breast engorgement.[3–6]

a. *Thromboembolic disease.* It is now well established that users of oral contraceptives have an increased risk of various thromboembolic and thrombotic vascular diseases, such as thrombophlebitis, pulmonary embolism, stroke, and myocardial infarction.[7–14] Cases of retinal thrombosis, mesenteric thrombosis, and optic neuritis have been reported in oral contraceptive users. There is evidence that the risk of several of these adverse reactions is related to the dose of the drug.[15,16] An increased risk of postsurgery thromboembolic complications has also been reported in users of oral contraceptives.[17,18] If feasible, estrogen should be discontinued at least 4 weeks before surgery of the type associated with an increased risk of thromboembolism, or during periods of prolonged immobilization.

Estrogens should not be used in persons with active thrombophlebitis or thromboembolic disorders. They should be used with caution in patients with cerebral vascular or coronary artery disease and only for those in whom estrogens are clearly indicated.

Large doses of estrogen (5 mg conjugated estrogens per day), comparable to those used to treat cancer of the prostate, have been shown in a large prospective clinical trial in men[19] to increase the risk of nonfatal myocardial infarction, pulmonary embolism and thrombophlebitis. When estrogen doses of this size are used, any of the thromboembolic and thrombotic adverse effects associated with oral contraceptive use should be considered a clear risk.

b. *Hepatic adenoma.* Benign hepatic adenomas appear to be associated with the use of oral contraceptives.[20–22] Although benign, and rare, these may rupture and may cause death through intra-abdominal hemorrhage. Such lesions have not yet been reported in association with other estrogen or progestogen preparations but should be considered in estrogen users having abdominal pain and tenderness, abdominal mass, or hypovolemic shock. Hepatocellular carcinoma has also been reported in women taking estrogen-containing oral contraceptives.[21] The relationship of this malignancy to these drugs is not known at this time.

c. *Elevated blood pressure.* Women using oral contraceptives sometimes experience increased blood pressure which, in most cases, returns to normal on discontinuing the drug. There is now a report that this may occur with use of estrogens in the menopause[23] and blood pressure should be monitored with estrogen use, especially if high doses are used.

d. *Glucose tolerance.* A worsening of glucose tolerance has been observed in a significant percentage of patients on estrogen-containing oral contraceptives. For this reason, diabetic patients should be carefully observed while receiving estrogen.

4. *Hypercalcemia.* Administration of estrogens may lead to severe hypercalcemia in patients with breast cancer and bone metastases. If this occurs, the drug should be stopped and appropriate measures taken to reduce the serum calcium level.

Precautions:

1. A complete medical and family history should be taken prior to the initiation of any estrogen therapy. The pretreatment and periodic physical examinations should include special reference to blood pressure, breasts, abdomen, and pelvic organs. As a general rule, estrogen should not be prescribed for longer than one year without another physical examination being performed.
2. Fluid retention—Because estrogens may cause some degree of fluid retention, conditions which might be influenced by this factor such as asthma, epilepsy, migraine, and cardiac or renal dysfunction, require careful observation.
3. Certain patients may develop undesirable manifestations of excessive estrogenic stimulation, such as gynecomastia.
4. Oral contraceptives appear to be associated with an increased incidence of mental depression.[7a] Although it is not clear whether this is due to the estrogenic or progestogenic component of the contraceptive, patients with a history of depression should be carefully observed.
5. The pathologist should be advised of estrogen therapy when relevant specimens are submitted.
6. If jaundice develops in any patient receiving estrogen, the medication should be discontinued while the cause is investigated.
7. Estrogens may be poorly metabolized in patients with impaired liver function and they should be administered with caution in such patients.
8. Because estrogens influence the metabolism of calcium and phosphorus, they should be used with caution in patients with metabolic bone diseases that are associated with hypercalcemia or in patients with renal insufficiency.
9. Because of the effects of estrogens on epiphyseal closure, they should be used judiciously in young patients in whom bone growth is not complete.
10. Certain endocrine and liver function tests may be affected by estrogen-containing oral contraceptives. The following similar changes may be expected with larger doses of estrogen:

a. Increased sulfobromophthalein retention.

b. Increased prothrombin and factors VII, VIII, IX, and X; decreased antithrombin 3; increased norepinephrine-induced platelet aggregability.

c. Increased thyroid binding globulin (TBG) leading to increased circulating total thyroid hormone, as measured by PBI, T4 by column, or T4 by radioimmunoassay. Free T3 resin uptake is decreased, reflecting the elevated TBG; free T4 concentration is unaltered.

d. Impaired glucose tolerance.

e. Reduced response to metyrapone test.

f. Reduced serum folate concentration.

g. Increased serum triglyceride and phospholipid concentration.

Adverse Reactions: (See Warnings regarding induction of neoplasia, increased incidence of gallbladder disease, and adverse effects similar to those of oral contraceptives, including thromboembolism.) The following additional adverse reactions have been reported with estrogenic therapy, including oral contraceptives:

1. *Breasts:* Tenderness, enlargement, secretion.
2. *Gastrointestinal:* Nausea, vomiting; abdominal cramps, bloating; cholestatic jaundice.
3. *Skin:* Chloasma or melasma which may persist when drug is discontinued; erythema multiforme, erythema nodosum; hemorrhagic eruption; loss of scalp hair; hirsutism.
4. *Eyes:* Steepening of corneal curvature; intolerance to contact lenses.
5. *CNS:* Headache, migraine, dizziness; mental depression; chorea.
6. *Miscellaneous:* Increase or decrease in weight; reduced carbohydrate tolerance; aggravation of porphyria; edema; changes in libido.

Acute Overdosage: Numerous reports of ingestion of large doses of estrogen-containing oral contraceptives by young children indicate that acute serious ill effects do not occur. Overdosage of estrogen may cause nausea, and withdrawal bleeding may occur in females.

Dosage and Administration: Inoperable progressing prostatic cancer— 40 mg intramuscularly every two to four weeks or less frequently, depending on clinical response of the patient. If the response is not satisfactory doses up to 80 mg may be used. Experimental evidence indicates that increasing the dose primarily prolongs the duration of action, but the amount of estrogen available at any one time is not significantly increased. The dosage should

Continued on next page

Ayerst—Cont.

be adjusted as indicated by careful observation of the patient.

Deep intramuscular injection only is recommended. (Initially, some patients may experience a burning sensation at site of injection. This is transitory, and it may not recur with subsequent injections, or may be obviated by concomitant administration of a local anesthetic.)

If a response to estrogen therapy is going to occur, it will be apparent within three months of the beginning of therapy. If it does occur, the hormone should be continued until the disease is again progressive. The hormone should then be stopped, and the patient may obtain another period of improvement known as "rebound regression." This occurs in 30% of the patients who show objective improvement on estrogens.

DIRECTIONS FOR USE

Reconstitution for use:

1. Introduce sterile diluent into SECULE, preferably with a 20 gauge needle affixed to a 5 ml syringe.
2. Swirl gently until a solution is effected. (DO NOT AGITATE VIOLENTLY.)

Stability: After reconstitution, if storage is desired, the solution should be kept at room temperature and away from direct light. Under these conditions the solution is stable for about 10 days, so long as cloudiness or evidence of a precipitate has not occurred.

How Supplied: NDC 0046-0451-02—Each package provides:

1. One SECULE® containing 40 mg polyestradiol phosphate, 0.02 mg phenylmercuric nitrate, and 5.2 mg sodium phosphate. As solubilizing agents for the active ingredient, 25 mg niacinamide and 4 mg propylene glycol are also present. The pH is adjusted with sodium hydroxide.
2. One 2 ml ampul of sterile diluent.

ESTRADURIN (polyestradiol phosphate) is prepared by cryodesiccation.

Physician References:

1. Boston Collaborative Drug Surveillance Program: N. Engl. J. Med. *290*:15–19, 1974.
2. Boston Collaborative Drug Surveillance Program: Lancet *1*:1399–1404, 1973.
3. Daniel, D. G., *et al.*: Lancet *2*:287–289, 1967.
4. The Veterans Administration Cooperative Urological Research Group: J. Urol. *98*:516–522, 1967.
5. Bailar, J. C.: Lancet *2*:560, 1967.
6. Blackard, C., *et al.*: Cancer *26*:249–256, 1970.
7. Royal College of General Practitioners: J. R. Coll. Gen. Pract. *13*:267–279, 1967.

7a. Royal College of General Practitioners: Oral Contraceptives and Health, New York, Pitman Corp., 1974.

8. Inman, W. H. W., *et al*: Br. Med. J. *2*:193–199, 1968.
9. Vessey, M. P., *et al*: Br. Med. J. *2*:651–657, 1969.
10. Sartwell, P. E., *et al*: Am. J. Epidemiol. *90*:365–380, 1969.
11. Collaborative Group for the Study of Stroke in Young Women: N. Engl. J. Med. *288*:871–878, 1973.
12. Collaborative Group for the Study of Stroke in Young Women: J.A.M.A. *231*:718–722, 1975.
13. Mann, J. I., *et al.*: Br. Med. J. *2*:245–248, 1975.
14. Mann, J. I., *et al*: Br. Med. J. *2*:241–245, 1975.
15. Inman, W. H. W., *et al*: Br. Med. J. *2*:203–209, 1970.
16. Stolley, P. D., *et al*: Am. J. Epidemiol. *102*:197–208, 1975.
17. Vessey, M. P., *et al*: Br. Med. J. *3*:123–126, 1970.
18. Greene, G. R., *et al*: Am. J. Public Health *62*:680–685, 1972.
19. Coronary Drug Project Research Group: J.A.M.A. *214*:1303–1313, 1970.
20. Baum, J., *et al*: Lancet *2*:926–928, 1973.
21. Mays, E. T., *et al*: J.A.M.A. *235*:730–732, 1976.
22. Edmondson, H. A., *et al*: N. Engl. J. Med. *294*:470–472, 1976.
23. Pfeffer, R. I., *et al*: Am. J. Epidemiol. *103*:445–456, 1976.

FLUOTHANE® ℞

Brand of halothane, U.S.P.

Description: FLUOTHANE, brand of halothane, U.S.P., is an inhalation anesthetic. It is 2-bromo-2-chloro-1,1,1-trifluoroethane.

The specific gravity is 1.872-1.877 at 20° C, and the boiling point (range) is 49° C-51° C at 760 mm Hg. The vapor pressure is 243 mm Hg at 20° C. The blood/gas coefficient is 2.5 at 37° C, and the olive oil/water coefficient is 220 at 37° C. Vapor concentrations within anesthetic range are nonirritating and have a pleasant odor. FLUOTHANE is nonflammable, and its vapors mixed with oxygen in proportions from 0.5 to 50 per cent (v/v) are not explosive.

FLUOTHANE does not decompose in contact with warm soda lime. When moisture is present, the vapor attacks aluminum, brass, and lead, but not copper. Rubber, some plastics, and similar materials are soluble in FLUOTHANE; such materials will deteriorate rapidly in contact with FLUOTHANE vapor or liquid. Stability of FLUOTHANE is maintained by the addition of 0.01 per cent thymol (w/w), and storage is in amber colored bottles.

FLUOTHANE should not be kept indefinitely in vaporizer bottles not specifically designed for its use. Thymol does not volatilize along with FLUOTHANE, and therefore accumulates in the vaporizer, and may, in time, impart a yellow color to the remaining liquid or to wicks in vaporizers. The development of such discoloration may be used as an indicator that the vaporizer should be drained and cleaned, and the discolored FLUOTHANE (halothane, U.S.P.) discarded. Accumulation of thymol may be removed by washing with diethyl ether. After cleaning a wick or vaporizer, make certain all the diethyl ether has been removed before reusing the equipment to avoid introducing ether into the system.

Actions: FLUOTHANE is an inhalation anesthetic. Induction and recovery are rapid and depth of anesthesia can be rapidly altered. FLUOTHANE progressively depresses respiration. There may be tachypnea with reduced tidal volume and alveolar ventilation. FLUOTHANE is not an irritant to the respiratory tract, and no increase in salivary or bronchial secretions ordinarily occurs. Pharyngeal and laryngeal reflexes are rapidly obtunded. It causes bronchodilation. Hypoxia, acidosis, or apnea may develop during deep anesthesia.

FLUOTHANE reduces the blood pressure, and frequently decreases the pulse rate. The greater the concentration of the drug, the more evident these changes become. Atropine may reverse the bradycardia. FLUOTHANE does not cause the release of catecholamines from adrenergic stores. FLUOTHANE also causes dilation of the vessels of the skin and skeletal muscles.

Cardiac arrhythmias may occur during FLUOTHANE anesthesia. These include nodal rhythm, AV dissociation, ventricular extrasystoles and asystole. FLUOTHANE sensitizes the myocardial conduction system to the action of epinephrine and norepinephrine, and the combination may cause serious cardiac arrhythmias. FLUOTHANE increases cerebral spinal fluid pressure. FLUOTHANE produces moderate muscular relaxation. Muscle relaxants are used as adjuncts in order to maintain lighter levels of anesthesia. FLUOTHANE augments the action of nondepolarizing relaxants and ganglionic blocking agents. FLUOTHANE is a potent uterine relaxant.

Indications: FLUOTHANE (halothane, U.S.P.) is indicated for the induction and maintenance of general anesthesia.

Contraindications: FLUOTHANE is not recommended for obstetrical anesthesia except when uterine relaxation is required.

Warnings: When previous exposure to FLUOTHANE was followed by unexplained jaundice, consideration should be given to the use of other agents.

FLUOTHANE should be used in vaporizers that permit a reasonable approximation of output, and preferably of the calibrated type. The vaporizer should be placed out of circuit in closed circuit rebreathing systems; otherwise overdosage is difficult to avoid. The patient should be closely observed for signs of overdosage, *i.e.*, depression of blood pressure, pulse rate, and ventilation, particularly during assisted or controlled ventilation.

Usage in Pregnancy. Safe use of FLUOTHANE has not been established with respect to possible adverse effects upon fetal development. Therefore, FLUOTHANE should not be used in women where pregnancy is possible and particularly during early pregnancy, unless, in the judgment of the physician, the potential benefits outweigh the unknown hazards to the fetus.

Precautions: The uterine relaxation obtained with FLUOTHANE unless carefully controlled, may fail to respond to ergot derivatives and oxytocic posterior pituitary extract.

FLUOTHANE increases cerebrospinal fluid pressure. Therefore, in patients with markedly raised intracranial pressure, if FLUOTHANE is indicated, administration should be preceded by measures ordinarily used to reduce cerebrospinal fluid pressure. Ventilation should be carefully assessed, and it may be necessary to assist or control ventilation to insure adequate oxygenation and carbon dioxide removal.

Epinephrine or norepinephrine should be employed cautiously, if at all, during FLUOTHANE (halothane, U.S.P.) anesthesia since their simultaneous use may induce ventricular tachycardia or fibrillation.

Nondepolarizing relaxants and ganglionic blocking agents should be administered cautiously, since their actions are augmented by FLUOTHANE.

Adverse Reactions: The following adverse reactions have been reported: hepatic necrosis, cardiac arrest, hypotension, respiratory arrest, cardiac arrhythmias, hyperpyrexia, shivering, nausea, and emesis.

Dosage and Administration: FLUOTHANE may be administered by the nonrebreathing technic, partial rebreathing, or closed technic. The induction dose varies from patient to patient. The maintenance dose varies from 0.5 per cent to 1.5 per cent.

FLUOTHANE may be administered with either oxygen or a mixture of oxygen and nitrous oxide.

How Supplied: Unit packages of 125 ml (NDC 0046-3125-81) and 250 ml (NDC 0046-3125-82) of halothane, U.S.P. stabilized with 0.01% thymol (w/w).

FORMATRIX® ℞

Each tablet contains:

Premarin®

(Conjugated Estrogens, U.S.P.) ....1.25 mg

Methyltestosterone ....10.0 mg

Ascorbic acid (Vit. C) ....400.0 mg

(as sodium ascorbate)

1. ESTROGENS HAVE BEEN REPORTED TO INCREASE THE RISK OF ENDOMETRIAL CARCINOMA.

Three independent case control studies have reported an increased risk of endometrial cancer in postmenopausal women exposed to exogenous estrogens for more than one year.[1–3] This risk was independent of the other known risk factors for endometrial cancer. These studies are further supported by the finding that incidence rates of endometrial cancer have increased sharply since 1969 in eight different areas of the United States with population-based cancer reporting systems, an increase which may be related to the rapidly expanding use of estrogens during the last decade.[4]

The three case control studies reported that the risk of endometrial cancer in estrogen users was about 4.5 to 13.9 times greater than in nonusers. The risk appears to depend on both duration of treatment[1] and on estrogen dose.[3] In view of these findings, when estrogens are used for the treatment of menopausal symptoms, the lowest dose that will control symptoms should be utilized and medication should be discontinued as soon as possible. When prolonged treatment is medically indicated, the patient should be reassessed on at least a semiannual basis to determine the need for continued therapy. Although the evidence must be considered preliminary, one study suggests that cyclic administration of low doses of estrogen may carry less risk than continuous administration;[3] it therefore appears prudent to utilize such a regimen.

Close clinical surveillance of all women taking estrogens is important. In all cases of undiagnosed persistent or recurring abnormal vaginal bleeding, adequate diagnostic measures should be undertaken to rule out malignancy.

There is no evidence at present that "natural" estrogens are more or less hazardous than "synthetic" estrogens at equiestrogenic doses.

2. ESTROGENS SHOULD NOT BE USED DURING PREGNANCY.

The use of female sex hormones, both estrogens and progestogens, during early pregnancy may seriously damage the offspring. It has been shown that females exposed in utero to diethylstilbestrol, a non-steroidal estrogen, have an increased risk of developing in later life a form of vaginal or cervical cancer that is ordinarily extremely rare.[5,6] This risk has been estimated as not greater than 4 per 1000 exposures.[7] Furthermore, a high percentage of such exposed women (from 30 to 90 percent) have been found to have vaginal adenosis,[8–12] epithelial changes of the vagina and cervix. Although these changes are histologically benign, it is not known whether they are precursors of malignancy. Although similar data are not available with the use of other estrogens, it cannot be presumed they would not induce similar changes.

Several reports suggest an association between intrauterine exposure to female sex hormones and congenital anomalies, including congenital heart defects and limb reduction defects.[13–16] One case control study[16] estimated a 4.7-fold increased risk of limb reduction defects in infants exposed in utero to sex hormones (oral contraceptives, hormone withdrawal tests for pregnancy, or attempted treatment for threatened abortion). Some of these exposures were very short and involved only a few days of treatment. The data suggest that the risk of limb reduction defects in exposed fetuses is somewhat less than 1 per 1000.

In the past, female sex hormones have been used during pregnancy in an attempt to treat threatened or habitual abortion. There is considerable evidence that estrogens are ineffective for these indications, and there is no evidence from well controlled studies that progestogens are effective for these uses.

If FORMATRIX is used during pregnancy, or if the patient becomes pregnant while taking this drug, she should be apprised of the potential risks to the fetus, and the advisability of pregnancy continuation.

Description: FORMATRIX tablets for oral administration contain PREMARIN (Conjugated Estrogens, U.S.P.), methyltestosterone, and ascorbic acid.

PREMARIN (Conjugated Estrogens, U.S.P.) is a mixture of estrogens, obtained exclusively from natural sources, occurring as the sodium salts of water-soluble estrogen sulfates blended to represent the average composition of material derived from pregnant mares' urine. It contains estrone, equilin, and 17 α-dihydroequilin, together with smaller amounts of 17 α-estradiol, equilenin, and 17 α-dihydroequilenin as salts of their sulfate esters.

Methyltestosterone is an androgen. It is a white to light yellow crystalline substance that is virtually insoluble in water but soluble in organic solvents. It is stable in air but decomposes when exposed to light.

Ascorbic acid (vitamin C) is provided as sodium ascorbate which is the monosodium salt of ascorbic acid. It exists as white to faint yellow crystals or a crystalline powder, and is freely soluble in water and relatively stable in air.

Clinical Pharmacology: Estrogens are important in the development and maintenance of the female reproductive system and secondary sex characteristics. They promote growth and development of the vagina, uterus, and fallopian tubes, and enlargement of the breasts. Indirectly, they contribute to the shaping of the skeleton, maintenance of tone and elasticity of urogenital structures, changes in the epiphyses of the long bones that allow for the pubertal growth spurt and its termination, growth of axillary and pubic hair, and pigmentation of the nipples and genitals. Decline of estrogenic activity at the end of the menstrual cycle can bring on menstruation, although the cessation of progesterone secretion is the most important factor in the mature ovulatory cycle. However, in the preovulatory or nonovulatory cycle, estrogen is the primary determinant in the onset of menstruation. Estrogens also affect the release of pituitary gonadotropins.

The pharmacologic effects of conjugated estrogens are similar to those of endogenous estrogens. They are soluble in water and are well absorbed from the gastrointestinal tract.

In responsive tissues (female genital organs, breasts, hypothalamus, pituitary) estrogens enter the cell and are transported into the nucleus. As a result of estrogen action, specific RNA and protein synthesis occurs.

Metabolism and inactivation occur primarily in the liver. Some estrogens are excreted into the bile; however they are reabsorbed from the intestine and returned to the liver through the portal venous system. Water soluble estrogen conjugates are strongly acidic and are ionized in body fluids, which favor excretion through the kidneys since tubular reabsorption is minimal.

Androgens are male sex hormones which mediate the development of the male genital organs and the secondary sex characteristics. Methyltestosterone is also an anabolic agent and promotes the retention of nitrogen, potassium, and phosphate, and increases in protein, skeletal muscle, and body mass. In the female, androgen generally opposes the action of estrogen on the female genital tissues by competing for estrogen-binding receptors.

Methyltestosterone is readily absorbed from the intestine. It is metabolized primarily in the liver and excreted primarily in the urine.

Ascorbic acid deficiency has been associated with pathologic and metabolic abnormalities, the most common of which is scurvy. The exact mechanism of action in relation to disease is not known although the major symptoms arise from lesions in the bones and blood vessels. However, it is not known how ascorbic acid maintains collagen and the intercellular ground substance. Vitamin C is involved in carbohydrate metabolism and occurs in high concentrations in the adrenal cortex and medulla.

Ascorbic acid is readily absorbed from the intestine and is distributed throughout the body. It is excreted primarily by the kidney when plasma levels reach a threshold concentration.

Indications:

1. *Postmenopausal osteoporosis (after a natural or artificial menopause).*
2. *Osteoporosis due to immobilization*—atrophy of disuse—(patient with fracture, bedridden, inactive).
3. *Corticosteroid osteoporosis* following cortisone-like hormone therapy.
4. *Osteoporosis due to malnutrition* (notably protein depletion and ascorbic acid deficiency).

FORMATRIX HAS NOT BEEN SHOWN TO BE EFFECTIVE FOR ANY PURPOSE DURING PREGNANCY AND ITS USE MAY CAUSE SEVERE HARM TO THE FETUS (SEE BOXED WARNING).

Contraindications: Estrogens should not be used in women (or men) with any of the following conditions:

1. Known or suspected cancer of the breast.
2. Known or suspected estrogen-dependent neoplasia.
3. Known or suspected pregnancy (See Boxed Warning).
4. Undiagnosed abnormal genital bleeding.
5. Active thrombophlebitis or thromboembolic disorders.
6. A past history of thrombophlebitis, thrombosis, or thromboembolic disorders associated with previous estrogen use.

Methyltestosterone should not be used in:

1. Persons with known or suspected carcinoma of the prostate and in carcinoma of the male breast.
2. The presence of severe liver damage.
3. Pregnancy and in breast-feeding mothers because of the possibility of masculinization of the female fetus or breast-fed infant.

Warnings:

Associated with Estrogens

1. *Induction of malignant neoplasms.* Long term continuous administration of natural and synthetic estrogens in certain animal species increases the frequency of carcinomas of the breast, cervix, vagina, and liver. There are now reports that estrogens increase the risk of carcinoma of the endometrium in humans. (See Boxed Warning.)

At the present time there is no satisfactory evidence that estrogens given to postmenopausal women increase the risk of cancer of the breast,[17] although a recent long-term followup of a single physician's practice has raised this possibility.[18] Because of the animal data, there is a need for caution in prescribing estrogens for women with a strong family history of breast cancer or who have breast nodules, fibrocystic disease, or abnormal mammograms.

2. *Gallbladder disease.* A recent study has reported a 2 to 3-fold increase in the risk of surgically confirmed gallbladder disease in women receiving postmenopausal estrogens,[17] similar to the 2-fold increase previously noted in users of oral contraceptives.[19,24a]

3. *Effects similar to those caused by estrogen-progestogen oral contraceptives.* There are several serious adverse effects of oral contracep-

Continued on next page

Ayerst—Cont.

tives, most of which have not, up to now, been documented as consequences of postmenopausal estrogen therapy. This may reflect the comparatively low doses of estrogen used in postmenopausal women. It would be expected that the larger doses of estrogen used to treat prostatic or breast cancer or postpartum breast engorgement are more likely to result in these adverse effects, and, in fact, it has been shown that there is an increased risk of thrombosis in men receiving estrogens for prostatic cancer and women for postpartum breast engorgement.[20–23]

a. *Thromboembolic disease.* It is now well established that users of oral contraceptives have an increased risk of various thromboembolic and thrombotic vascular diseases, such as thrombophlebitis, pulmonary embolism, stroke, and myocardial infarction.[24–31] Cases of retinal thrombosis, mesenteric thrombosis, and optic neuritis have been reported in oral contraceptive users. There is evidence that the risk of several of these adverse reactions is related to the dose of the drug.[32,33] An increased risk of postsurgery thromboembolic complications has also been reported in users of oral contraceptives.[34,35] If feasible, estrogen should be discontinued at least 4 weeks before surgery of the type associated with an increased risk of thromboembolism, or during periods of prolonged immobilization.

While an increased rate of thromboembolic and thrombotic disease in postmenopausal users of estrogens has not been found,[17–24,25–36] this does not rule out the possibility that such an increase may be present or that subgroups of women who have underlying risk factors or who are receiving relatively large doses of estrogens may have increased risk. Therefore estrogens should not be used in persons with active thrombophlebitis or thromboembolic disorders, and they should not be used (except in treatment of malignancy) in persons with a history of such disorders in association with estrogen use. They should be used with caution in patients with cerebral vascular or coronary artery disease and only for those in whom estrogens are clearly needed.

Large doses of estrogen (5 mg conjugated estrogens per day), comparable to those used to treat cancer of the prostate and breast, have been shown in a large prospective clinical trial in men[37] to increase the risk of nonfatal myocardial infarction, pulmonary embolism and thrombophlebitis. When estrogen doses of this size are used, any of the thromboembolic and thrombotic adverse effects associated with oral contraceptive use should be considered a clear risk.

b. *Hepatic adenoma.* Benign hepatic adenomas appear to be associated with the use of oral contraceptives.[38–40] Although benign, and rare, these may rupture and may cause death through intra-abdominal hemorrhage. Such lesions have not yet been reported in association with other estrogen or progestogen preparations but should be considered in estrogen users having abdominal pain and tenderness, abdominal mass, or hypovolemic shock. Hepatocellular carcinoma has also been reported in women taking estrogen-containing oral contraceptives.[39] The relationship of this malignancy to these drugs is not known at this time.

c. *Elevated blood pressure.* Women using oral contraceptives sometimes experience increased blood pressure which, in most cases, returns to normal on discontinuing the drug. There is now a report that this may occur with use of estrogens in the menopause[41] and blood pressure should be monitored with estrogen use, especially if high doses are used.

d. *Glucose tolerance.* A worsening of glucose tolerance has been observed in a significant percentage of patients on estrogen-containing oral contraceptives. For this reason, diabetic patients should be carefully observed while receiving estrogen.

4. *Hypercalcemia.* Administration of estrogens may lead to severe hypercalcemia in patients with breast cancer and bone metastases. If this occurs, the drug should be stopped and appropriate measures taken to reduce the serum calcium level.

Associated with Methyltestosterone

1. Female patients should be watched carefully for symptoms or signs of virilization such as hoarseness or deepening of the voice, oily skin, acne, hirsutism, enlarged clitoris, stimulation of libido, and menstrual irregularities. At the dosage necessary to achieve a tumor response, androgens will cause masculinization of a female, but occasionally a sensitive female may exhibit one or more of these signs on small doses. Some of these changes, such as voice changes, may be irreversible even after drug is stopped.
2. Cholestatic hepatitis with jaundice and altered liver function tests, such as increased BSP retention and rises in SGOT levels, have been reported with methyltestosterone. These changes appear to be related to dosage of the drug. Therefore, in the presence of any changes in liver function tests, the drug should be discontinued.

Precautions:

Associated with Estrogens

A. General Precautions.

1. A complete medical and family history should be taken prior to the initiation of any estrogen therapy. The pretreatment and periodic physical examinations should include special reference to blood pressure, breasts, abdomen, and pelvic organs, and should include a Papanicolau smear. As a general rule, estrogen should not be prescribed for longer than one year without another physical examination being performed.
2. Fluid retention—Because estrogens may cause some degree of fluid retention, conditions which might be influenced by this factor such as asthma, epilepsy, migraine, and cardiac or renal dysfunction, require careful observation.
3. Certain patients may develop undesirable manifestations of excessive estrogenic stimulation, such as abnormal or excessive uterine bleeding, mastodynia, etc.
4. Oral contraceptives appear to be associated with an increased incidence of mental depression.[24a] Although it is not clear whether this is due to the estrogenic or progestogenic component of the contraceptive, patients with a history of depression should be carefully observed.
5. Preexisting uterine leiomyomata may increase in size during estrogen use.
6. The pathologist should be advised of estrogen therapy when relevant specimens are submitted.
7. Patients with a past history of jaundice during pregnancy have an increased risk of recurrence of jaundice while receiving estrogen-containing oral contraceptive therapy. If jaundice develops in any patient receiving estrogen, the medication should be discontinued while the cause is investigated.
8. Estrogens may be poorly metabolized in patients with impaired liver function and they should be administered with caution in such patients.
9. Because estrogens influence the metabolism of calcium and phosphorus, they should be used with caution in patients with metabolic bone diseases that are associated with hypercalcemia or in patients with renal insufficiency.
10. Because of the effects of estrogens on epiphyseal closure, they should be used judiciously in young patients in whom bone growth is not complete.
11. Certain endocrine and liver function tests may be affected by estrogen-containing oral contraceptives. The following similar changes may be expected with larger doses of estrogen:

a. Increased sulfobromophthalein retention.
b. Increased prothrombin and factors VII, VIII, IX, and X; decreased antithrombin 3; increased norepinephrine-induced platelet aggregability.
c. Increased thyroid binding globulin (TBG) leading to increased circulating total thyroid hormone, as measured by PBI, T4 by column, or T4 by radioimmunoassay. Free T3 resin uptake is decreased, reflecting the elevated TBG; free T4 concentration is unaltered.
d. Impaired glucose tolerance.
e. Decreased pregnanediol excretion.
f. Reduced response to metyrapone test.
g. Reduced serum folate concentration.
h. Increased serum triglyceride and phospholipid concentration.

B. Information for the Patient. See text which appears after the PHYSICIAN REFERENCES.

C. Pregnancy Category X. See CONTRAINDICATIONS and Boxed Warning.

D. Nursing Mothers. As a general principle, the administration of any drug to nursing mothers should be done only when clearly necessary since many drugs are excreted in human milk.

Associated with Methyltestosterone

A. Prolonged dosage of androgen may result in sodium and fluid retention. This may present a problem, especially in patients with compromised cardiac reserve or renal disease.
B. If priapism or other signs of excessive sexual stimulation develop, discontinue therapy.
C. In the male, prolonged administration or excessive dosage may cause inhibition of testicular function, with resultant oligospermia and decrease in ejaculatory volume. Use cautiously in young boys to avoid possible premature epiphyseal closure or precocious sexual development.
D. Hypersensitivity and gynecomastia may occur rarely.
E. PBI may be decreased in patients taking androgens.
F. Hypercalcemia may occur. If this does occur, the drug should be discontinued.

Adverse Reactions:

Associated with Estrogens

(See Warnings regarding induction of neoplasia, adverse effects on the fetus, increased incidence of gallbladder disease, and adverse effects similar to those of oral contraceptives, including thromboembolism.) The following additional adverse reactions have been reported with estrogenic therapy, including oral contraceptives:

1. *Genitourinary system:* Breakthrough bleeding, spotting, change in menstrual flow; dysmenorrhea; premenstrual-like syndrome; amenorrhea during and after treatment; increase in size of uterine fibromyomata; vaginal candidiasis; change in cervical erosion and in degree of cervical secretion; cystitis-like syndrome.
2. *Breasts:* Tenderness, enlargement, secretion.
3. *Gastrointestinal:* Nausea, vomiting; abdominal cramps, bloating; cholestatic jaundice.
4. *Skin:* Chloasma or melasma which may persist when drug is discontinued; erythema multiforme; erythema nodosum; hemorrhagic eruption; loss of scalp hair; hirsutism.
5. *Eyes:* Steepening of corneal curvature; intolerance to contact lenses.
6. *CNS:* Headache, migraine, dizziness; mental depression; chorea.
7. *Miscellaneous:* Increase or decrease in weight; reduced carbohydrate tolerance; aggravation of porphyria; edema; changes in libido.

Associated with Methyltestosterone
Cholestatic jaundice
Hypercalcemia, particularly in patients with metastatic breast carcinoma. This usually indicates progression of bone metastases.
Sodium and water retention
Priapism
Virilization in female patients
Hypersensitivity

Acute Overdosage: Numerous reports of ingestion of large doses of estrogen-containing oral contraceptives by young children indicate that acute serious ill effects do not occur. Overdosage of estrogen may cause nausea, and withdrawal bleeding may occur in females.

Dosage and Administration:
Usual dose for osteoporosis:
1 tablet daily.

In the female: To avoid continuous stimulation of breast and uterus, administration should be cyclic (e.g., 3 week regimen with 1 week rest period—Withdrawal bleeding may occur during this 1 week rest period).

Treated patients with an intact uterus should be monitored closely for signs of endometrial cancer and appropriate diagnostic measures should be taken to rule out malignancy in the event of persistent or recurring abnormal vaginal bleeding.

In the male: A careful check should be made on the status of the prostate gland when therapy is given for protracted intervals.

Adjunctive measures: A high protein diet is recommended; immobilization should be minimized in order to restore the necessary stress and strain as natural aids to bone repair.

How Supplied: FORMATRIX Tablets, in bottles of 60 (NDC 0046-0883-60) and 500 (NDC 0046-0883-85).

Physician References:

1. Ziel, H. K., *et al.*: N. Engl. J. Med. *293*:1167–1170, 1975.
2. Smith, D. C., *et al.*: N. Engl. J. Med. *293*:1164–1167, 1975.
3. Mack, T. M., *et al.*: N. Engl. J. Med. *294*:1262–1267, 1976.
4. Weiss, N. S., *et al.*: N. Engl. J. Med. *294*:1259–1262, 1976.
5. Herbst, A. L., *et al.*: N. Engl. J. Med. *284*:878–881, 1971.
6. Greenwald, P., *et al.*: N. Engl. J. Med. *285*:390–392, 1971.
7. Lanier, A., *et al.*: Mayo Clin. Proc. *48*:793–799, 1973.
8. Herbst, A., *et al.*: Obstet. Gynecol. *40*:287–298, 1972.
9. Herbst, A., *et al.*: Am. J. Obstet. Gynecol. *118*:607–615, 1974.
10. Herbst, A., *et al.*: N. Engl. J. Med. *292*:334–339, 1975.
11. Stafl, A., *et al.*: Obstet. Gynecol. *43*:118–128, 1974.
12. Sherman A. I., *et al.*: Obstet. Gynecol. *44*:531–545, 1974.
13. Gal, I., *et al.*: Nature *216*:83, 1967.
14. Levy, E. P., *et al.*: Lancet *1*:611, 1973.
15. Nora, J., *et al.*: Lancet *1*:941–942, 1973.
16. Janerich, D. T., *et al.*: N. Engl. J. Med. *291*:697–700, 1974.
17. Boston Collaborative Drug Surveillance Program: N. Engl. J. Med. *290*:15–19, 1974.
18. Hoover, R., *et al.*: N. Engl. J. Med. *295*:401–405, 1976.
19. Boston Collaborative Drug Surveillance Program: Lancet *1*:1399–1404, 1973.
20. Daniel, D. G., *et al.*: Lancet *2*:287–289, 1967.
21. The Veterans Administration Cooperative Urological Research Group: J. Urol. *98*:516–522, 1967.
22. Bailar, J. C.: Lancet *2*:560, 1967.
23. Blackard, C., *et al.*: Cancer *26*:249–256, 1970.
24. Royal College of General Practitioners: J. R. Coll. Gen. Pract. *13*:267–279, 1967.

24a. Royal College of General Practitioners: Oral Contraceptives and Health, New York, Pitman Corp., 1974.
25. Inman, W. H. W., *et al.*: Br. Med. J. *2*:193–199, 1968.
26. Vessey, M. P., *et al.*: Br. Med. J. *2*:651–657, 1969.
27. Sartwell, P. E., *et al.*: Am. J. Epidemiol. *90*:365–380, 1969.
28. Collaborative Group for the Study of Stroke in Young Women: N. Engl. J. Med. *288*:871–878, 1973.
29. Collaborative Group for the Study of Stroke in Young Women: J.A.M.A. *231*:718–722, 1975.
30. Mann, J. I., *et al.*: Br. Med. J. *2*:245–248, 1975.
31. Mann, J. I., *et al.*: Br. Med. J. *2*:241–245, 1975.
32. Inman, W. H. W., *et al.*: Br. Med. J. *2*:203–209, 1970.
33. Stolley, P. D., *et al.*: Am. J. Epidemiol. *102*:197–208, 1975.
34. Vessey, M. P., *et al.*: Br. Med. J. *3*:123–126, 1970.
35. Greene, G. R., *et al.*: Am. J. Public Health *62*:680–685, 1972.
36. Rosenberg, L., *et al.*: N. Engl. J. Med. *294*:1256–1259, 1976.
37. Coronary Drug Project Research Group: J.A.M.A. *214*:1303–1313, 1970.
38. Baum, J., *et al.*: Lancet *2*:926–928, 1973.
39. Mays, E. T., *et al.*: J.A.M.A. *235*:730–732, 1976.
40. Edmondson, H. A., *et al.*: N. Engl. J. Med. *294*:470–472, 1976.
41. Pfeffer, R. I., *et al.*: Am. J. Epidemiol. *103*:445–456, 1976.

INFORMATION FOR THE PATIENT

What You Should Know about Estrogens: Estrogens are female hormones produced by the ovaries. The ovaries make several different kinds of estrogens. In addition, scientists have been able to make a variety of synthetic estrogens. As far as we know, all these estrogens have similar properties and therefore much the same usefulness, side effects, and risks. This leaflet is intended to help you understand what estrogens are used for, the risks involved in their use, and how to use them as safely as possible.

This leaflet includes the most important information about estrogens, but not all the information. If you want to know more, you should ask your doctor for more information or you can ask your doctor or pharmacist to let you read the package insert prepared for the doctor.

Uses of Estrogen: THERE IS NO PROPER USE OF ESTROGENS IN A PREGNANT WOMAN.

Estrogens are prescribed by doctors for a number of purposes, including:

1. To provide estrogen during a period of adjustment when a woman's ovaries stop producing a majority of her estrogens, in order to prevent certain uncomfortable symptoms of estrogen deficiency. (With the menopause, which generally occurs between the ages of 45 and 55, women produce a much smaller amount of estrogens.)
2. To prevent symptoms of estrogen deficiency when a woman's ovaries have been removed surgically before the natural menopause.
3. To prevent pregnancy. (Estrogens are given along with a progestogen, another female hormone; these combinations are called oral contraceptives or birth control pills. Patient labeling is available to women taking oral contraceptives and they will not be discussed in this leaflet.)
4. To treat certain cancers in women and men.
5. To prevent painful swelling of the breasts after pregnancy in women who choose not to nurse their babies.

Estrogens in the Menopause: In the natural course of their lives, all women eventually experience a decrease in estrogen production. This usually occurs between ages 45 and 55 but may occur earlier or later. Sometimes the ovaries may need to be removed before natural menopause by an operation, producing a "surgical menopause."

When the amount of estrogen in the blood begins to decrease, many women may develop typical symptoms: feelings of warmth in the face, neck, and chest or sudden intense episodes of heat and sweating throughout the body (called "hot flashes" or "hot flushes"). These symptoms are sometimes very uncomfortable. Some women may also develop changes in the vagina (called "atrophic vaginitis") which cause discomfort, especially during and after intercourse.

Estrogens can be prescribed to treat these symptoms of the menopause. It is estimated that considerably more than half of all women undergoing the menopause have only mild symptoms or no symptoms at all and therefore do not need estrogens. Other women may need estrogens for a few months, while their bodies adjust to lower estrogen levels. Sometimes the need will be for periods longer than six months. In an attempt to avoid overstimulation of the uterus (womb), estrogens are usually given cyclically during each month of use, such as three weeks of pills followed by one week without pills.

Sometimes women experience nervous symptoms or depression during menopause. There is no evidence that estrogens are effective for such symptoms without associated vasomotor symptoms. In the absence of vasomotor symptoms, estrogens should not be used to treat nervous symptoms, although other treatment may be needed.

You may have heard that taking estrogens for long periods (years) after the menopause will keep your skin soft and supple and keep you feeling young. There is no evidence that this is so, however, and such long-term treatment carries important risks.

Estrogens to Prevent Swelling of the Breasts after Pregnancy: If you do not breast-feed your baby after delivery, your breasts may fill up with milk and become painful and engorged. This usually begins about 3 to 4 days after delivery and may last for a few days to up to a week or more. Sometimes the discomfort is severe, but usually it is not and can be controlled by pain-relieving drugs such as aspirin and by binding the breasts up tightly. Estrogens can be used to try to prevent the breasts from filling up. While this treatment is sometimes successful, in many cases the breasts fill up to some degree in spite of treatment. The dose of estrogens needed to prevent pain and swelling of the breasts is much larger than the dose needed to treat symptoms of the menopause and this may increase your chances of developing blood clots in the legs or lungs (see below). Therefore, it is important that you discuss the benefits and the risks of estrogen use with your doctor if you have decided not to breast-feed your baby.

The Dangers of Estrogens:

1. *Endometrial cancer.* There are reports that if estrogens are used in the postmenopausal period for more than a year, there is an increased risk of *endometrial cancer* (cancer of the lining of the uterus). Women taking estrogens have roughly 5 to 10 times as great a chance of getting this cancer as women who take no estrogens. To put this another way, while a postmenopausal woman not taking estrogens has 1 chance in 1,000 each year of getting endometrial cancer, a woman taking estrogens has 5 to 10 chances in 1,000 each year. For this reason *it is important to take estrogens only when they are really needed.*

Continued on next page

Ayerst—Cont.

The risk of this cancer is greater the longer estrogens are used and when larger doses are taken. Therefore you should not take more estrogen than your doctor prescribes. *It is important to take the lowest dose of estrogen that will control symptoms and to take it only as long as it is needed.* If estrogens are needed for longer periods of time, your doctor will want to reevaluate your need for estrogens at least every six months.
Women using estrogens should report any vaginal bleeding to their doctors; such bleeding may be of no importance, but it can be an early warning of endometrial cancer. If you have undiagnosed vaginal bleeding, you should not use estrogens until a diagnosis is made and you are certain there is no endometrial cancer.
NOTE: If you have had your uterus removed (total hysterectomy), there is no danger of developing endometrial cancer.
2. *Other possible cancers.* Estrogens can cause development of other tumors in animals, such as tumors of the breast, cervix, vagina, or liver, when given for a long time. At present there is no good evidence that women using estrogen in the menopause have an increased risk of such tumors, but there is no way yet to be sure they do not; and one study raises the possibility that use of estrogens in the menopause may increase the risk of breast cancer many years later. This is a further reason to use estrogens only when clearly needed. While you are taking estrogens, it is important that you go to your doctor at least once a year for a physical examination. Also, if members of your family have had breast cancer or if you have breast nodules or abnormal mammograms (breast x-rays), your doctor may wish to carry out more frequent examinations of your breasts.
3. *Gallbladder disease.* Women who use estrogens after menopause are more likely to develop gallbladder disease needng surgery than women who do not use estrogens. Birth control pills have a similar effect.
4. *Abnormal blood clotting.* Oral contraceptives increase the risk of blood clotting in various parts of the body. This can result in a stroke (if the clot is in the brain), a heart attack (clot in a blood vessel of the heart), or a pulmonary embolus (a clot which forms in the legs or pelvis, then breaks off and travels to the lungs). Any of these can be fatal.
At this time use of estrogens in the menopause is not known to cause such blood clotting, but this has not been fully studied and there could still prove to be such a risk. It is recommended that if you have had clotting in the legs or lungs or a heart attack or stroke while you were using estrogens or birth control pills, you should not use estrogens (unless they are being used to treat cancer of the breast or prostate). If you have had a stroke or heart attack or if you have angina pectoris, estrogens should be used with great caution and only if clearly needed (for example, if you have severe symptoms of menopause).
The larger doses of estrogen used to prevent swelling of the breasts after pregnancy have been reported to cause clotting in the legs and lungs.
Special Warning about Pregnancy: You should not receive estrogen if you are pregnant. If this should occur, there is a greater than usual chance that the developing child will be born with a birth defect, although the possibility remains fairly small. A female child may have an increased risk of developing cancer of the vagina or cervix later in life (in the teens or twenties). Every possible effort should be made to avoid exposure to estrogens during pregnancy. If exposure occurs, see your doctor.
Other Effects of Estrogens: In addition to the serious known risks of estrogens decribed above, estrogens have the following side effects and potential risks:
1. *Nausea and vomiting.* The most common side effect of estrogen therapy is nausea. Vomiting is less common.
2. *Effects on breasts.* Estrogens may cause breast tenderness or enlargement and may cause the breasts to secrete a liquid. These effects are not dangerous.
3. *Effects on the uterus.* Estrogens may cause benign fibroid tumors of the uterus to get larger.
4. *Effects on liver.* Women taking oral contraceptives develop on rare occasions a tumor of the liver which can rupture and bleed into the abdomen and may cause death. So far, these tumors have not been reported in women using estrogens in the menopause, but you should report any swelling or unusual pain or tenderness in the abdomen to your doctor immediately.
Women with a past history of jaundice (yellowing of the skin and white parts of the eyes) may get jaundice again during estrogen use. If this occurs, stop taking estrogens and see your doctor.
5. *Other effects.* Estrogens may cause excess fluid to be retained in the body. This may make some conditions worse, such as asthma, epilepsy, migraine, heart disease, or kidney disease.
Summary: Estrogens have important uses, but they have serious risks as well. You must decide, with your doctor, whether the risks are acceptable to you in view of the benefits of treatment. Except where your doctor has prescribed estrogens for use in special cases of cancer of the breast or prostate, you should not use estrogens if you have cancer of the breast or uterus, are pregnant, have undiagnosed abnormal vaginal bleeding, clotting in the legs or lungs, or have had a stroke, heart attack or angina, or clotting in the legs or lungs in the past while you were taking estrogens.
You can use estrogens as safely as possible by understanding that your doctor will require regular physical examinations while you are taking them and will try to discontinue the drug as soon as possible and use the smallest dose possible. Be alert for signs of trouble including:
1. Abnormal bleeding from the vagina.
2. Pains in the calves or chest or sudden shortness of breath, or coughing blood.
3. Severe headache, dizziness, faintness, or changes in vision.
4. Breast lumps (you should ask your doctor how to examine your own breasts).
5. Jaundice (yellowing of the skin).
Your doctor has prescribed this drug for you and you alone. Do not give the drug to anyone else.
How Supplied: FORMATRIX®—tablets for oral administration containing Premarin® (Conjugated Estrogens, U.S.P.), methyltestosterone (an androgen), and ascorbic acid (vitamin C).
MEDIATRIC® —provides estrogen and androgen in small doses, nutritional supplements, and a mild antidepressant. It is supplied as capsules, tablets, and liquid.

[Shown in Product Identification Section]

GRISACTIN® ℞
Brand of griseofulvin (microsize)

Indications: Griseofulvin is indicated for the treatment of ringworm infections of the skin, hair, and nails, namely: *tinea corporis, tinea pedis, tinea cruris, tinea barbae, tinea capitis, tinea unguium* (onychomycosis) when caused by one or more of the following genera of fungi: *Trichophyton rubrum, T. tonsurans, T. mentagrophytes, T. interdigitalis, T. verrucosum, T. megnini, T. gallinae, T. crateriform, T. sulphureum, T. schoenleini, Microsporum audouini, M. canis, M. gypseum, Epidermophyton floccosum.*
NOTE: Prior to therapy, the type of fungi responsible for the infection should be identified.
The use of this drug is not justified in minor or trivial infections which will respond to topical agents alone.
Griseofulvin is *not* effective in the following: Bacterial infections, candidiasis (moniliasis), histoplasmosis, actinomycosis, sporotrichosis, chromoblastomycosis, coccidioidomycosis, North American blastomycosis, cryptococcosis (torulosis), *tinea versicolor,* nocardiosis.
Contraindications: This drug is contraindicated in patients with porphyria, hepatocellular failure, and in individuals with a history of hypersensitivity to griseofulvin.
Warnings: *Prophylactic Usage*—Safety and efficacy of griseofulvin for prophylaxis of fungal infections has not been established.
Animal Toxicology—Chronic feeding of griseofulvin, at levels ranging from 0.5-2.5% of the diet, resulted in the development of liver tumors in several strains of mice, particularly in males. Smaller particle sizes result in an enhanced effect. Lower oral dosage levels have not been tested. Subcutaneous administration of relatively small doses of griseofulvin, once a week, during the first three weeks of life has also been reported to induce hepatomata in mice. Although studies in other animal species have not yielded evidence of tumorigenicity, these studies were not of adequate design to form a basis for conclusions in this regard.
In subacute toxicity studies, orally administered griseofulvin produced hepatocellular necrosis in mice, but this has not been seen in other species. Disturbances in porphyrin metabolism have been reported in griseofulvin-treated laboratory animals. Griseofulvin has been reported to have a colchicine-like effect on mitosis and cocarcinogenicity with methylcholanthrene in cutaneous tumor induction in laboratory animals.
Usage in Pregnancy—The safety of this drug during pregnancy has not been established.
Animal Reproduction Studies—It has been reported in the literature that griseofulvin was found to be embryotoxic and teratogenic on oral administration to pregnant rats. Pups with abnormalities have been reported in the litters of a few bitches treated with griseofulvin. Additional animal reproduction studies are in progress.
Suppression of spermatogenesis has been reported to occur in rats, but investigation in man failed to confirm this.
Precautions: Patients on prolonged therapy with any potent medication should be under close observation. Periodic monitoring of organ system function, including renal, hepatic, and hematopoietic, should be done.
Since griseofulvin is derived from species of Penicillium, the possibility of cross-sensitivity with penicillin exists; however, known penicillin-sensitive patients have been treated without difficulty.
Since a photosensitivity reaction is occasionally associated with griseofulvin therapy, patients should be warned to avoid exposure to intense natural or artificial sunlight. Should a photosensitivity reaction occur, lupus erythematosus may be aggravated.
Griseofulvin decreases the activity of warfarin-type anticoagulants so that patients receiving these drugs concomitantly may require dosage adjustment of the anticoagulant during and after griseofulvin therapy.
Barbiturates usually depress griseofulvin activity and concomitant administration may require a dosage adjustment of the antifungal agent.
Adverse Reactions: When adverse reactions occur, they are most commonly of the hypersensitivity type such as skin rashes, urticaria, and rarely, angioneurotic edema, and may necessitate withdrawal of therapy and appropri-

ate countermeasures. Paresthesias of the hands and feet have been reported rarely after extended therapy. Other side effects reported occasionally are oral thrush, nausea, vomiting, epigastric distress, diarrhea, headache, fatigue, dizziness, insomnia, mental confusion, and impairment of performance of routine activities.

Proteinuria and leukopenia have been reported rarely. Administration of the drug should be discontinued if granulocytopenia occurs.

When rare, serious reactions occur with griseofulvin, they are usually associated with high dosages, long periods of therapy, or both.

Dosage and Administration: Accurate diagnosis of the infecting organism is essential. Identification should be made either by direct microscopic examination of a mounting of infected tissue in a solution of potassium hydroxide or by culture on an appropriate medium.

Medication must be continued until the infecting organism is completely eradicated as indicated by appropriate clinical or laboratory examination. Representative treatment periods are—*tinea capitis*, 4 to 6 weeks; *tinea corporis*, 2 to 4 weeks; *tinea pedis*, 4 to 8 weeks; *tinea unguium*—depending on rate of growth—fingernails, at least 4 months: toenails, at least 6 months.

General measures in regard to hygiene should be observed to control sources of infection or reinfection. Concomitant use of appropriate topical agents is usually required, particularly in treatment of *tinea pedis*. In some forms of athlete's foot, yeasts and bacteria may be involved as well as fungi. Griseofulvin will not eradicate the bacterial or monilial infection.

Adults: 0.5 g daily (125 mg q.i.d., 250 mg b.i.d., or 500 mg/day). Patients with less severe or extensive infections may require less, whereas those with widespread lesions may require a starting dose of 0.75 g to 1.0 g a day. This may be reduced gradually to 0.5 g or less after a response has been noted. In all cases, the dosage should be individualized.

Children: A dosage of 10 mg/kg daily is usually adequate (children from 30 to 50 lb, 125 mg to 250 mg daily; children over 50 lb, 250 mg to 500 mg daily, in divided doses). Dosage should be individualized, as with adults.

Clinical relapse will occur if the medication is not continued until the infecting organism is eradicated.

How Supplied: GRISACTIN [griseofulvin (microsize)]—GRISACTIN 125, each capsule contains 125 mg, in bottles of 100 (NDC 0046-0442-81); GRISACTIN 250, each capsule contains 250 mg, in bottles of 100 (NDC 0046-0443-81) and 500 (NDC 0046-0443-85); and GRISACTIN 500, each tablet (scored) contains 500 mg, in bottles of 60 (NDC 0046-0444-60).

[*Shown in Product Identification Section*]

INDERAL® ℞

Brand of propranolol hydrochloride
A beta-adrenergic blocking agent

BEFORE USING INDERAL (PROPRANOLOL HYDROCHLORIDE), THE PHYSICIAN SHOULD BE THOROUGHLY FAMILIAR WITH THE BASIC CONCEPT OF ADRENERGIC RECEPTORS (ALPHA AND BETA), AND THE PHARMACOLOGY OF THIS DRUG.

Actions: INDERAL is a beta-adrenergic receptor blocking drug, possessing no other autonomic nervous system activity. It specifically competes with beta-adrenergic receptor stimulating agents for available beta receptor sites. When access to beta receptor sites is blocked by INDERAL, the chronotropic, inotropic, and vasodilator responses to beta-adrenergic stimulation are decreased proportionately.

Propranolol is almost completely absorbed from the gastrointestinal tract, but a portion is immediately bound by the liver. Peak effect occurs in one to one and one-half hours. The biologic half-life is approximately two to three hours. Propranolol is not significantly dialyzable. There is no simple correlation between dose or plasma level and therapeutic effect, and the dose-sensitivity range as observed in clinical practice is wide. The principal reason for this is that sympathetic tone varies widely between individuals. Since there is no reliable test to estimate sympathetic tone or to determine whether total beta blockade has been achieved, proper dosage requires titration.

The mechanisms of the antihypertensive and antimigraine effects of INDERAL have not been established. Among the factors that may be involved in the antihypertensive action are (1) decreased cardiac output, (2) inhibition of renin release by the kidneys, and (3) diminution of tonic sympathetic nerve outflow from vasomotor centers in the brain. The antimigraine effect may be due to inhibition of vasodilation or to the fact that beta-adrenergic receptors have been demonstrated in the pial vessels of the brain and that arteriolar spasms over the cortex can be inhibited with INDERAL.

Propranolol hydrochloride decreases heart rate, cardiac output, and blood pressure. Although total peripheral vascular resistance may increase initially, it readjusts to the pretreatment level, or lower, with chronic usage. Earlier studies indicate that plasma volume remains unchanged or may decrease. However, there are certain more recent studies suggesting that in the absence of sodium restriction, plasma volume may increase.

Beta receptor blockade is useful in conditions in which, because of pathologic or functional changes, sympathetic activity is excessive or inappropriate and detrimental to the patient. But there are also situations in which sympathetic stimulation is vital. For example, in patients with severely damaged hearts, adequate ventricular function is maintained by virtue of sympathetic drive which should be preserved. In the presence of AV block, beta blockade may prevent the necessary facilitating effect of sympathetic activity on conduction. Beta blockade results in bronchial constriction by interfering with adrenergic bronchodilator activity which should be preserved in patients subject to bronchospasm.

The proper objective of beta blockade therapy is to decrease adverse sympathetic stimulation but not to the degree that may impair necessary sympathetic support.

Propranolol exerts its antiarrhythmic effects in concentrations associated with beta-adrenergic blockade and this appears to be its principal antiarrhythmic mechanism of action. The membrane effect also plays a role, particularly, some authorities believe, in digitalis-induced arrhythmias. Beta-adrenergic blockade is of unique importance in the management of arrhythmias due to increased levels of circulating catecholamines or enhanced sensitivity of the heart to catecholamines (arrhythmias associated with pheochromocytoma, thyrotoxicosis, exercise).

In dosages greater than required for beta blockade, INDERAL also exerts a quinidine-like or anesthetic-like membrane action which affects the cardiac action potential and depresses cardiac function.

Propranolol may reduce the oxygen requirement of the heart at any given level of effort by blocking catecholamine-induced increases in heart rate, systolic blood pressure, and the velocity and extent of myocardial contraction. On the other hand, propranolol may increase oxygen requirements by increasing left ventricular fiber length, end diastolic pressure, and systolic ejection period.

If the net physiologic effect of beta-adrenergic blockade in angina is advantageous, it would be expected to manifest itself during exercise by delayed onset of pain due to decreased oxygen requirement.

Indications:

Hypertension

INDERAL is indicated in the management of hypertension. It is usually used in combination with other drugs, particularly a thiazide diuretic. INDERAL is not indicated for treatment of hypertensive emergencies.

Angina Pectoris Due to Coronary Atherosclerosis

The initial treatment of angina pectoris involves weight control, rest, cessation of smoking, use of sublingual nitroglycerin, and avoidance of precipitating circumstances. INDERAL is indicated in selected patients with moderate to severe angina pectoris who have not responded to these conventional measures. Propranolol should not be used in patients with angina which occurs only with considerable effort or with infrequent precipitating factors.

INDERAL exerts both favorable and unfavorable effects, the preponderance of which may be beneficial. (See ACTIONS Section.) INDERAL should not be continued unless there is reduced pain or increased work capacity.

Because of the potential for adverse results, treatment should be carefully monitored. The patient should also be reevaluated periodically since the dosage requirement and the need to continue INDERAL may be altered by clinical exacerbations or remissions. (See DOSAGE AND ADMINISTRATION.)

Additional studies of the effects of INDERAL in angina pectoris patients are in progress to better evaluate and define the proper role of INDERAL in this condition.

Cardiac Arrhythmias

1.) Supraventricular arrhythmias
   a) Paroxysmal atrial tachycardias, particularly those arrhythmias induced by catecholamines or digitalis or associated with the Wolff-Parkinson-White syndrome. (See W-P-W under WARNINGS.)
   b) Persistent sinus tachycardia which is noncompensatory and impairs the well-being of the patient.
   c) Tachycardias and arrhythmias due to thyrotoxicosis when causing distress or increased hazard and when immediate effect is necessary as adjunctive, short term (2–4 weeks) therapy. May be used with, but not in place of, specific therapy. (See Thyrotoxicosis under WARNINGS.)
   d) Persistent atrial extrasystoles which impair the well-being of the patient and do not respond to conventional measures.
   e) Atrial flutter and fibrillation when ventricular rate cannot be controlled by digitalis alone, or when digitalis is contraindicated.

2.) Ventricular tachycardias
Ventricular arrhythmias do not respond to propranolol as predictably as do the supraventricular arrhythmias.
   a) Ventricular tachycardias
   With the exception of those induced by catecholamines or digitalis, INDERAL is not the drug of first choice. In critical situations when cardioversion technics or other drugs are not indicated or are not effective, INDERAL may be considered. If, after consideration of the risks involved, INDERAL is used, it should be given intravenously in low dosage and very slowly. (See DOSAGE AND ADMINISTRATION.) *Care in the administration of* INDERAL *with constant electrocardiographic monitoring is essential as the*

Continued on next page

Ayerst—Cont.

failing heart requires some sympathetic drive for maintenance of myocardial tone.

b) Persistent premature ventricular extrasystoles which do not respond to conventional measures and impair the well-being of the patient.

3.) Tachyarrhythmias of digitalis intoxication

If digitalis-induced tachyarrhythmias persist following discontinuance of digitalis and correction of electrolyte abnormalities, they are usually reversible with *oral* INDERAL. Severe bradycardia may occur. (See OVERDOSAGE OR EXAGGERATED RESPONSE.)

Intravenous propranolol hydrochloride is reserved for life-threatening arrhythmias. Temporary maintenance with oral therapy may be indicated. (See DOSAGE AND ADMINISTRATION.)

4.) Resistant tachyarrhythmias due to excessive catecholamine action during anesthesia

Tachyarrhythmias due to excessive catecholamine action during anesthesia may sometimes arise because of release of endogenous catecholamines or administration of catecholamines. When usual measures fail in such arrhythmias, INDERAL may be given intravenously to abolish them. All general inhalation anesthetics produce some degree of myocardial depression. Therefore, when INDERAL is used to treat arrhythmias during anesthesia, it should be used with extreme caution and constant ECG and central venous pressure monitoring. (See WARNINGS.)

Migraine

INDERAL is indicated for the prophylaxis of common migraine headache. The efficacy of INDERAL in the treatment of a migraine attack that has already started has not been established and INDERAL is not indicated for such use.

Vascular headaches of the migraine type are often familial, are recurrent, and vary widely in frequency, duration, and intensity. The attacks are commonly unilateral in onset, and are usually associated with anorexia, and sometimes nausea and vomiting. In females, these headaches often occur premenstrually or early during the menses. Migraine attacks are sometimes preceded by, or associated with, conspicuous sensory, motor, and mood disturbances, but common migraine usually occurs without striking prodromes, and is less often unilateral.

Hypertrophic Subaortic Stenosis

INDERAL is useful in the management of hypertrophic subaortic stenosis, especially for treatment of exertional or other stress-induced angina, palpitations, and syncope. INDERAL also improves exercise performance. The effectiveness of INDERAL in this disease appears to be due to a reduction of the elevated outflow pressure gradient which is exacerbated by beta receptor stimulation. Clinical improvement may be temporary.

Pheochromocytoma

After primary treatment with an alpha-adrenergic blocking agent has been instituted, INDERAL may be useful as *adjunctive* therapy if the control of tachycardia becomes necessary before or during surgery.

It is hazardous to use INDERAL unless alpha-adrenergic blocking drugs are already in use, since this would predispose to serious blood pressure elevation. Blocking only the peripheral dilator (beta) action of epinephrine leaves its constrictor (alpha) action unopposed.

In the event of hemorrhage or shock, there is a disadvantage in having both beta and alpha blockade since the combination prevents the increase in heart rate and peripheral vasoconstriction needed to maintain blood pressure.

With inoperable or metastatic pheochromocytoma, INDERAL may be useful as an adjunct to the management of symptoms due to excessive beta receptor stimulation.

Contraindications: INDERAL is contraindicated in: 1) bronchial asthma; 2) allergic rhinitis during the pollen season; 3) sinus bradycardia and greater than first degree block; 4) cardiogenic shock; 5) right ventricular failure secondary to pulmonary hypertension; 6) congestive heart failure (see WARNINGS) unless the failure is secondary to a tachyarrhythmia treatable with INDERAL; 7) in patients on adrenergic-augmenting psychotropic drugs (including MAO inhibitors), and during the two week withdrawal period from such drugs.

Warnings: CARDIAC FAILURE: Sympathetic stimulation is a vital component supporting circulatory function in congestive heart failure, and inhibition with beta-blockade always carries the potential hazard of further depressing myocardial contractility and precipitating cardiac failure. INDERAL acts selectively without abolishing the inotropic action of digitalis on the heart muscle (*i.e.,* that of supporting the strength of myocardial contractions). In patients already receiving digitalis, the positive inotropic action of digitalis may be reduced by INDERAL's negative inotropic effect. The effects of INDERAL and digitalis are additive in depressing AV conduction.

IN PATIENTS WITHOUT A HISTORY OF CARDIAC FAILURE, continued depression of the myocardium over a period of time can, in some cases, lead to cardiac failure. In rare instances, this has been observed during INDERAL therapy. Therefore, at the first sign or symptom of impending cardiac failure, patients should be fully digitalized and/or given a diuretic, and the response observed closely: a) if cardiac failure continues, despite adequate digitalization and diuretic therapy, INDERAL therapy should be immediately withdrawn; b) if tachyarrhythmia is being controlled, patients should be maintained on combined therapy and the patient closely followed until threat of cardiac failure is over.

> IN PATIENTS WITH ANGINA PECTORIS, there have been reports of exacerbation of angina and, in some cases, myocardial infarction, following *abrupt* discontinuation of INDERAL therapy. Therefore, when discontinuance of INDERAL is planned the dosage should be gradually reduced and the patient carefully monitored. In addition, when INDERAL is prescribed for angina pectoris, the patient should be cautioned against interruption or cessation of therapy without the physician's advice. If INDERAL therapy is interrupted and exacerbation of angina occurs, it usually is advisable to reinstitute INDERAL therapy and take other measures appropriate for the management of unstable angina pectoris. Since coronary artery disease may be unrecognized, it may be prudent to follow the above advice in patients considered at risk of having occult atherosclerotic heart disease, who are given propranolol for other indications.

IN PATIENTS WITH THYROTOXICOSIS, possible deleterious effects from long term use have not been adequately appraised. Special consideration should be given to propranolol's potential for aggravating congestive heart failure. Propranolol may mask the clinical signs of developing or continuing hyperthyroidism or complications and give a false impression of improvement. Therefore, abrupt withdrawal of propranolol may be followed by an exacerbation of symptoms of hyperthyroidism, including thyroid storm. This is another reason for withdrawing propranolol slowly. Propranolol does not distort thyroid function tests.

IN PATIENTS WITH WOLFF-PARKINSON-WHITE SYNDROME, several cases have been reported in which, after propranolol, the tachycardia was replaced by a severe bradycardia requiring a demand pacemaker. In one case this resulted after an initial dose of 5 mg propranolol.

IN PATIENTS DURING ANESTHESIA with agents that require catecholamine release for maintenance of adequate cardiac function, beta blockade will impair the desired inotropic effect. Therefore, INDERAL should be titrated carefully when administered for arrhythmias occurring during anesthesia.

IN PATIENTS UNDERGOING MAJOR SURGERY, beta blockade impairs the ability of the heart to respond to reflex stimuli. For this reason, with the exception of pheochromocytoma, INDERAL should be withdrawn 48 hours prior to surgery, at which time all chemical and physiologic effects are gone according to available evidence. However, in case of emergency surgery, since INDERAL is a competitive inhibitor of beta receptor agonists, its effects can be reversed by administration of such agents, *e.g.,* isoproterenol or levarterenol. However, such patients may be subject to protracted severe hypotension. Difficulty in restarting and maintaining the heart beat has also been reported.

IN PATIENTS PRONE TO NONALLERGIC BRONCHOSPASM (*e.g.,* CHRONIC BRONCHITIS, EMPHYSEMA), INDERAL should be administered with caution since it may block bronchodilation produced by endogenous and exogenous catecholamine stimulation of beta receptors.

DIABETICS AND PATIENTS SUBJECT TO HYPOGLYCEMIA: Because of its beta-adrenergic blocking activity, INDERAL may prevent the appearance of premonitory signs and symptoms (pulse rate and pressure changes) of acute hypoglycemia. This is especially important to keep in mind in patients with labile diabetes. Hypoglycemic attacks may be accompanied by a precipitous elevation of blood pressure.

USE IN PREGNANCY: The safe use of INDERAL in human pregnancy has not been established. Use of any drug in pregnancy or women of childbearing potential requires that the possible risk to mother and/or fetus be weighed against the expected therapeutic benefit. Embryotoxic effects have been seen in animal studies at doses about 10 times the maximum recommended human dose.

Precautions: Patients receiving catecholamine depleting drugs such as reserpine should be closely observed if INDERAL is administered. The added catecholamine blocking action of this drug may then produce an excessive reduction of the resting sympathetic nervous activity. Occasionally, the pharmacologic activity of INDERAL may produce hypotension and/or marked bradycardia resulting in vertigo, syncopal attacks, or orthostatic hypotension.

As with any new drug given over prolonged periods, laboratory parameters should be observed at regular intervals. The drug should be used with caution in patients with impaired renal or hepatic function.

Adverse Reactions:

Cardiovascular: bradycardia; congestive heart failure; intensification of AV block; hypotension; paresthesia of hands; arterial insufficiency, usually of the Raynaud type; thrombocytopenic purpura

Central Nervous System: lightheadedness; mental depression manifested by insomnia, lassitude, weakness, fatigue; reversible mental depression progressing to catatonia; visual disturbances; hallucinations; an acute reversible syndrome characterized by disorientation for time and place, short term memory loss, emotional lability, slightly clouded sensorium,

and decreased performance on neuropsychometrics
Gastrointestinal: nausea, vomiting, epigastric distress, abdominal cramping, diarrhea, constipation, mesenteric arterial thrombosis, ischemic colitis
Allergic: pharyngitis and agranulocytosis, erythematous rash, fever combined with aching and sore throat, laryngospasm and respiratory distress
Respiratory: bronchospasm
Hematologic: agranulocytosis, nonthrombocytopenic purpura, thrombocytopenic purpura
Miscellaneous: reversible alopecia. Oculomucocutaneous reactions involving the skin, serous membranes and conjunctivae reported for a beta blocker (practolol) have not been conclusively associated with propranolol.
Clinical Laboratory Test Findings: Elevated blood urea levels in patients with severe heart disease, elevated serum transaminase, alkaline phosphatase, lactate dehydrogenase

Dosage and Administration:

The dosage range for INDERAL is different for each indication.

ORAL

HYPERTENSION—*Dosage must be individualized.*
The usual initial dosage is 40 mg INDERAL twice daily, whether used alone or added to a diuretic. Dosage may be increased gradually until adequate blood pressure is achieved. The usual dosage is 160 to 480 mg per day. In some instances a dosage of 640 mg may be required. The time needed for full hypertensive response to a given dosage is variable and may range from a few days to several weeks.
While twice-daily dosing is effective and can maintain a reduction in blood pressure throughout the day, some patients, especially when lower doses are used, may experience a modest rise in blood pressure toward the end of the 12 hour dosing interval. This can be evaluated by measuring blood pressure near the end of the dosing interval to determine whether satisfactory control is being maintained throughout the day. If control is not adequate, a larger dose, or 3 times daily therapy may achieve better control.

ANGINA PECTORIS—*Dosage must be individualized.*
Starting with 10–20 mg three or four times daily, before meals and at bedtime, dosage should be gradually increased at three to seven day intervals until optimum response is obtained. Although individual patients may respond at any dosage level, the average optimum dosage appears to be 160 mg per day. In angina pectoris, the value and safety of dosage exceeding 320 mg per day have not been established.
If treatment is to be discontinued, reduce dosage gradually over a period of several weeks. (See WARNINGS.)

ARRHYTHMIAS—10–30 mg three or four times daily before meals and at bedtime.

MIGRAINE—*Dosage must be individualized.*
The initial oral dose is 80 mg INDERAL daily in divided doses. The usual effective dose range is 160–240 mg per day. The dosage may be increased gradually to achieve optimum migraine prophylaxis.
If a satisfactory response is not obtained within four to six weeks after reaching the maximum dose, INDERAL therapy should be discontinued. It may be advisable to withdraw the drug gradually over a period of two weeks.

HYPERTROPHIC SUBAORTIC STENOSIS—20–40 mg three or four times daily, before meals and at bedtime.

PHEOCHROMOCYTOMA—*Preoperatively*—60 mg daily in divided doses for three days prior to surgery, concomitantly with an alpha-adrenergic blocking agent.
—*Management of inoperable tumor*—30 mg daily in divided doses.

PEDIATRIC DOSAGE
At this time the data on the use of the drug in this age group are too limited to permit adequate directions for use.

INTRAVENOUS
Intravenous administration is reserved for life-threatening arrhythmias or those occurring under anesthesia. The usual dose is from 1 to 3 mg administered under careful monitoring, *e.g.* electrocardiographic, central venous pressure. The rate of administration should not exceed 1 mg (1 ml) per minute to diminish the possibility of lowering blood pressure and causing cardiac standstill. Sufficient time should be allowed for the drug to reach the site of action even when a slow circulation is present. If necessary, a second dose may be given after two minutes. Thereafter, additional drug should not be given in less than four hours. Additional INDERAL should not be given when the desired alteration in rate and/or rhythm is achieved.
Transference to oral therapy should be made as soon as possible.
The intravenous administration of INDERAL has not been evaluated adequately in the management of hypertensive emergencies.

Overdosage or Exaggerated Response:
IN THE EVENT OF OVERDOSAGE OR EXAGGERATED RESPONSE, THE FOLLOWING MEASURES SHOULD BE EMPLOYED:

BRADYCARDIA—ADMINISTER ATROPINE (0.25 to 1.0 mg): IF THERE IS NO RESPONSE TO VAGAL BLOCKADE, ADMINISTER ISOPROTERENOL CAUTIOUSLY.

CARDIAC FAILURE—DIGITALIZATION AND DIURETICS

HYPOTENSION—VASOPRESSORS, *e.g.,* LEVARTERENOL OR EPINEPHRINE (THERE IS EVIDENCE THAT EPINEPHRINE IS THE DRUG OF CHOICE.)

BRONCHOSPASM—ADMINISTER ISOPROTERENOL AND AMINOPHYLLINE

How Supplied:

INDERAL
(propranolol hydrochloride)

TABLETS
— Each scored tablet contains 10 mg of propranolol hydrochloride, in bottles of 100 (NDC 0046-0461-81) and 1,000 (NDC 0046-0461-91). Also in unit dose package of 100 (NDC 0046-0461-99).
— Each scored tablet contains 20 mg of propranolol hydrochloride, in bottles of 100 (NDC 0046-0462-81) and 1,000 (NDC 0046-0462-91). Also in unit dose package of 100 (NDC 0046-0462-99).
— Each scored tablet contains 40 mg of propranolol hydrochloride, in bottles of 100 (NDC 0046-0464-81) and 1,000 (NDC 0046-0464-91). Also in unit dose package of 100 (NDC 0046-0464-99).
— Each scored tablet contains 80 mg of propranolol hydrochloride, in bottles of 100 (NDC 0046-0468-81) and 1,000 (NDC 0046-0468-91). Also in unit dose package of 100 (NDC 0046-0468-99).

INJECTABLE
— Each ml contains 1 mg of propranolol hydrochloride in Water for Injection. The pH is adjusted with citric acid. Supplied as: 1 ml ampuls in boxes of 10 (NDC 0046-3265-10).

[*Shown in Product Identification Section*]

INDERIDE® ℞

Brand of propranolol hydrochloride (INDERAL®) and hydrochlorothiazide

No. 474—Each INDERIDE®-40/25 tablet contains:
Propranolol hydrochloride
(INDERAL®) .... 40 mg
Hydrochlorothiazide .... 25 mg

No. 476—Each INDERIDE®-80/25 tablet contains:
Propranolol hydrochloride
(INDERAL®) .... 80 mg
Hydrochlorothiazide .... 25 mg

Warning
This fixed combination drug is not indicated for initial therapy of hypertension. Hypertension requires therapy titrated to the individual patient. If the fixed combination represents the dosage so determined, its use may be more convenient in patient management. The treatment of hypertension is not static, but must be reevaluated as conditions in each patient warrant.

Description: INDERIDE combines two antihypertensive agents: INDERAL (propranolol hydrochloride), a beta-adrenergic blocking agent, and hydrochlorothiazide, a thiazide diuretic-antihypertensive.

Clinical Pharmacology:

Propranolol hydrochloride (INDERAL®):
Propranolol hydrochloride is a beta-adrenergic receptor blocking drug, possessing no other autonomic nervous system activity. It specifically competes with beta-adrenergic receptor stimulating agents for available beta-receptor sites. When access to beta-receptor sites is blocked by propranolol, the chronotropic, inotropic, and vasodilator responses to beta-adrenergic stimulation are decreased proportionately.
Propranolol is almost completely absorbed from the gastrointestinal tract, but a portion is immediately bound by the liver. Peak effect occurs in one to one and one-half hours. The biologic half-life is approximately two to three hours. Propranolol is not significantly dialyzable. There is no simple correlation between dose or plasma level and therapeutic effect and the dose-sensitivity range as observed in clinical practice is wide. The principal reason for this is that sympathetic tone varies widely between individuals. Since there is no reliable test to estimate sympathetic tone or to determine whether total beta blockade has been achieved, proper dosage requires titration.
The mechanism of the antihypertensive effects of propranolol has not been established. Among the factors that may be involved are (1) decreased cardiac output, (2) inhibition of renin release by the kidneys, and (3) diminution of tonic sympathetic nerve outflow from vasomotor centers in the brain.
Propranolol hydrochloride decreases heart rate, cardiac output, and blood pressure. Although total peripheral vascular resistance may increase initially, it readjusts to the pretreatment level or lower with chronic usage. Earlier studies indicate that plasma volume remains unchanged or may decrease. However, there are certain more recent studies suggesting that in the absence of sodium restriction, plasma volume may increase.
Beta-receptor blockade is useful in conditions in which, because of pathologic or functional changes, sympathetic activity is excessive or inappropriate, and detrimental to the patient. But there are also situations in which sympathetic stimulation is vital. For example, in patients with severely damaged hearts, adequate ventricular function is maintained by virtue of sympathetic drive which should be preserved. In the presence of AV block, beta blockade may prevent the necessary facilitating effect of sympathetic activity on conduction. Beta blockade results in bronchial constriction by interfering with adrenergic bronchodilator activity which should be preserved in patients subject to bronchospasm.
The proper objective of beta-blockade therapy is to decrease adverse sympathetic stimulation, but not to the degree that may impair necessary sympathetic support.

Continued on next page

Ayerst—Cont.

Hydrochlorothiazide:
Hydrochlorothiazide is a benzothiadiazine (thiazide) diuretic closely related to chlorothiazide. The mechanism of the antihypertensive effect of the thiazides is unknown. Thiazides do not affect normal blood pressure.
Thiazides affect the renal tubular mechanism of electrolyte reabsorption. At maximal therapeutic dosage, all thiazides are approximately equal in their diuretic potency.
Thiazides increase excretion of sodium and chloride in approximately equivalent amounts. Natriuresis causes a secondary loss of potassium and bicarbonate.
Onset of diuretic action of thiazides occurs in two hours, and the peak effect in about four hours. Its action persists for approximately six to 12 hours. Thiazides are eliminated rapidly by the kidney.
Indication: INDERIDE is indicated in the management of hypertension. (See boxed warning.)
Contraindications:
Propranolol hydrochloride (INDERAL®):
Propranolol hydrochloride is contraindicated in: 1) bronchial asthma; 2) allergic rhinitis during the pollen season; 3) sinus bradycardia and greater than first degree block; 4) cardiogenic shock; 5) right ventricular failure secondary to pulmonary hypertension; 6) congestive heart failure (see WARNINGS) unless the failure is secondary to a tachyarrhythmia treatable with propranolol; 7) in patients on adrenergic-augmenting psychotropic drugs (including MAO inhibitors), and during the two week withdrawal period from such drugs.
Hydrochlorothiazide:
Hydrochlorothiazide is contraindicated in patients with anuria or hypersensitivity to this or other sulfonamide-derived drugs.
Warnings:
Propranolol hydrochloride (INDERAL®):
CARDIAC FAILURE: Sympathetic stimulation is a vital component supporting circulatory function in congestive heart failure, and inhibition with beta blockade always carries the potential hazard of further depressing myocardial contractility and precipitating cardiac failure. Propranolol acts selectively without abolishing the inotropic action of digitalis on the heart muscle (*i.e.* that of supporting the strength of myocardial contractions). In patients already receiving digitalis, the positive inotropic action of digitalis may be reduced by propranolol's negative inotropic effect. The effects of propranolol and digitalis are additive in depressing AV conduction.
IN PATIENTS WITHOUT A HISTORY OF CARDIAC FAILURE, continued depression of the myocardium over a period of time can, in some cases, lead to cardiac failure. In rare instances, this has been observed during propranolol therapy. Therefore, at the first sign or symptom of impending cardiac failure, patients should be fully digitalized and/or given a diuretic, and the response observed closely: a) if cardiac failure continues, despite adequate digitalization and diuretic therapy, propranolol therapy should be immediately withdrawn; b) if tachyarrhythmia is being controlled, patients should be maintained on combined therapy and the patient closely followed until threat of cardiac failure is over.

> IN PATIENTS WITH ANGINA PECTORIS, there have been reports of exacerbation of angina and, in some cases, myocardial infarction, following *abrupt* discontinuation of propranolol therapy. Therefore, when discontinuance of propranolol is planned the dosage should be gradually reduced and the patient carefully monitored. In addition, when propranolol is prescribed for angina pectoris, the patient should be cautioned against interruption or cessation of therapy without the physician's advice. If propranolol therapy is interrupted and exacerbation of angina occurs, it usually is advisable to reinstitute propranolol therapy and take other measures appropriate for the management of unstable angina pectoris. Since coronary artery disease may be unrecognized, it may be prudent to follow the above advice in patients considered at risk of having occult atherosclerotic heart disease, who are given propranolol for other indications.

IN PATIENTS WITH THYROTOXICOSIS, possible deleterious effects from long-term use have not been adequately appraised. Special consideration should be given to propranolol's potential for aggravating congestive heart failure. Propranolol may mask the clinical signs of developing or continuing hyperthyroidism or complications and give a false impression of improvement. Therefore, abrupt withdrawal of propranolol may be followed by an exacerbation of symptoms of hyperthyroidism, including thyroid storm. This is another reason for withdrawing propranolol slowly. Propranolol does not distort thyroid function tests.
IN PATIENTS WITH WOLFF-PARKINSON-WHITE SYNDROME, several cases have been reported in which, after propranolol, the tachycardia was replaced by a severe bradycardia requiring a demand pacemaker. In one case this resulted after an initial dose of 5 mg propranolol.
IN PATIENTS UNDERGOING MAJOR SURGERY, beta blockade impairs the ability of the heart to respond to reflex stimuli. For this reason, with the exception of pheochromocytoma, propranolol should be withdrawn 48 hours prior to surgery, at which time all chemical and physiologic effects are gone according to available evidence. However, in case of emergency surgery, since propranolol is a competitive inhibitor of beta-receptor agonists, its effects can be reversed by administration of such agents, *e.g.,* isoproterenol or levarterenol. However, such patients may be subject to protracted severe hypotension. Difficulty in restarting and maintaining the heart beat has also been reported.
IN PATIENTS PRONE TO NONALLERGIC BRONCHOSPASM (*e.g.,* CHRONIC BRONCHITIS, EMPHYSEMA), propranolol should be administered with caution since it may block bronchodilation produced by endogenous and exogenous catecholamine stimulation of beta receptors.
DIABETICS AND PATIENTS SUBJECT TO HYPOGLYCEMIA: Because of its beta-adrenergic blocking activity, propranolol may prevent the appearance of premonitory signs and symptoms (pulse rate and pressure changes) of acute hypoglycemia. This is especially important to keep in mind in patients with labile diabetes. Hypoglycemic attacks may be accompanied by a precipitous elevation of blood pressure.
Hydrochlorothiazide:
Thiazides should be used with caution in severe renal disease. In patients with renal disease, thiazides may precipitate azotemia. In patients with impaired renal function, cumulative effects of the drug may develop.
Thiazides should also be used with caution in patients with impaired hepatic function or progressive liver disease, since minor alterations of fluid and electrolyte balance may precipitate hepatic coma.
Thiazides may add to or potentiate the action of other antihypertensive drugs. Potentiation occurs with ganglionic or peripheral adrenergic blocking drugs.
Sensitivity reactions may occur in patients with a history of allergy or bronchial asthma.
The possibility of exacerbation or activation of systemic lupus erythematosus has been reported.
USE IN PREGNANCY:
Propranolol hydrochloride (INDERAL®):
The safe use of propranolol in human pregnancy has not been established. Use of any drug in pregnancy or women of childbearing potential requires that the possible risk to mother and/or fetus be weighed against the expected therapeutic benefit. Embryotoxic effects have been seen in animal studies at doses about 10 times the maximum recommended human dose.
Hydrochlorothiazide:
Thiazides cross the placental barrier and appear in cord blood. The use of thiazides in pregnant women requires that the anticipated benefit be weighed against possible hazards to the fetus. These hazards include fetal or neonatal jaundice, thrombocytopenia, and possibly other adverse reactions which have occurred in the adult.
Nursing Mothers: Thiazides appear in breast milk. If the use of the drug is deemed essential, the patient should stop nursing.
Precautions:
Propranolol hydrochloride (INDERAL®):
Patients receiving catecholamine-depleting drugs such as reserpine should be closely observed if propranolol is administered. The added catecholamine blocking action of this drug may then produce an excessive reduction of the resting sympathetic nervous activity.
Occasionally, the pharmacologic activity of propranolol may produce hypotension and/or marked bradycardia resulting in vertigo, syncopal attacks, or orthostatic hypotension.
As with any new drug given over prolonged periods, laboratory parameters should be observed at regular intervals. The drug should be used with caution in patients with impaired renal or hepatic function.
Hydrochlorothiazide:
Periodic determination of serum electrolytes to detect possible electrolyte imbalance should be performed at appropriate intervals.
All patients receiving thiazide therapy should be observed for clinical signs of fluid or electrolyte imbalance, namely: hyponatremia, hypochloremic alkalosis, and hypokalemia. Serum and urine electrolyte determinations are particularly important when the patient is vomiting excessively or receiving parenteral fluids. Medication such as digitalis may also influence serum electrolytes. Warning signs, irrespective of cause are: dryness of mouth, thirst, weakness, lethargy, drowsiness, restlessness, muscle pains or cramps, muscular fatigue, hypotension, oliguria, tachycardia, and gastrointestinal disturbances such as nausea and vomiting.
Hypokalemia may develop, especially with brisk diuresis, when severe cirrhosis is present or during concomitant use of corticosteroids or ACTH.
Interference with adequate oral electrolyte intake will also contribute to hypokalemia. Hypokalemia can sensitize or exaggerate the response of the heart to the toxic effects of digitalis (*e.g.,* increased ventricular irritability). Hypokalemia may be avoided or treated by use of potassium supplements such as foods with a high potassium content.
Any chloride deficit is generally mild, and usually does not require specific treatment except under extraordinary circumstances (as in liver or renal disease). Dilutional hyponatremia may occur in edematous patients in hot weather; appropriate therapy is water restriction, rather than administration of salt, except in rare instances when the hyponatremia is life-threatening. In actual salt depletion, appropriate replacement is the therapy of choice.
Hyperuricemia may occur or frank gout may be precipitated in certain patients receiving thiazide therapy.

Insulin requirements in diabetic patients may be increased, decreased, or unchanged. Diabetes mellitus which has been latent may become manifest during thiazide administration.
Thiazide drugs may increase the responsiveness to tubocurarine.
The antihypertensive effects of the drug may be enhanced in the postsympathectomy patient. Thiazides may decrease arterial responsiveness to norepinephrine. This diminution is not sufficient to preclude effectiveness of the pressor agent for therapeutic use.
If progressive renal impairment becomes evident, consider withholding or discontinuing diuretic therapy.
Thiazides may decrease serum PBI levels without signs of thyroid disturbance.
Calcium excretion is decreased by thiazides. Pathologic changes in the parathyroid gland with hypercalcemia and hypophosphatemia have been observed in a few patients on prolonged thiazide therapy. The common complications of hyperparathyroidism such as renal lithiasis, bone resorption, and peptic ulceration, have not been seen. Thiazides should be discontinued before carrying out tests for parathyroid function.

Adverse Reactions:

Propranolol hydrochloride (INDERAL®):

Cardiovascular: bradycardia; congestive heart failure; intensification of AV block; hypotension; paresthesia of hands; arterial insufficiency, usually of the Raynaud type; thrombocytopenic purpura.
Central Nervous System: lightheadedness; mental depression manifested by insomnia, lassitude, weakness, fatigue; reversible mental depression progressing to catatonia; visual disturbances; hallucinations; an acute reversible syndrome characterized by disorientation for time and place, short term memory loss, emotional lability, slightly clouded sensorium, and decreased performance on neuropsychometrics.
Gastrointestinal: nausea, vomiting, epigastric distress, abdominal cramping, diarrhea, constipation, mesenteric arterial thrombosis, ischemic colitis.
Allergic: pharyngitis and agranulocytosis, erythematous rash, fever combined with aching and sore throat, laryngospasm and respiratory distress.
Respiratory: bronchospasm.
Hematologic: agranulocytosis, nonthrombocytopenic purpura, thrombocytopenic purpura.
Miscellaneous: reversible alopecia. Oculomucocutaneous reactions involving the skin, serous membranes and conjunctivae reported for a beta blocker (practolol) have not been conclusively associated with propranolol.
Clinical Laboratory Test Findings: Elevated blood urea levels in patients with severe heart disease, elevated serum transaminase, alkaline phosphatase, lactate dehydrogenase.

Hydrochlorothiazide:

Gastrointestinal: anorexia, gastric irritation, nausea, vomiting, cramping, diarrhea, constipation, jaundice (intrahepatic cholestatic jaundice), pancreatitis, sialadenitis.
Central Nervous System: dizziness, vertigo, paresthesias, headache, xanthopsia.
Hematologic: leukopenia, agranulocytosis, thrombocytopenia, aplastic anemia.
Cardiovascular: othostatic hypotension (may be aggravated by alcohol, barbiturates, or narcotics).
Hypersensitivity: purpura, photosensitivity, rash, urticaria, necrotizing angiitis (vasculitis, cutaneous vasculitis), fever, respiratory distress including pneumonitis, anaphylactic reactions.
Other: hyperglycemia, glycosuria, hyperuricemia, muscle spasm, weakness, restlessness, transient blurred vision.
Whenever adverse reactions are moderate or severe, thiazide dosage should be reduced or therapy withdrawn.

Dosage and Administration:
The dosage must be determined by individual titration (see boxed warning).
Hydrochlorothiazide is usually given at a dose of 50 to 100 mg per day. The initial dose of propranolol is 40 mg twice daily and it may be increased gradually until optimum blood pressure control is achieved. The usual effective dose is 160 to 480 mg per day.
One to two INDERIDE tablets twice daily can be used to administer up to 320 mg of propranolol and 100 mg of hydrochlorothiazide. For doses of propranolol greater than 320 mg, the combination products are not appropriate because their use would lead to an excessive dose of the thiazide component.
When necessary, another antihypertensive agent may be added gradually beginning with 50 percent of the usual recommended starting dose to avoid an excessive fall in blood pressure.

Overdosage or Exaggerated Response:
The propranolol hydrochloride (INDERAL) component may cause bradycardia, cardiac failure, hypotension, or bronchospasm.
The hydrochlorothiazide component can be expected to cause diuresis. Lethargy of varying degree may appear and may progress to coma within a few hours, with minimal depression of respiration and cardiovascular function, and in the absence of significant serum electrolyte changes or dehydration. The mechanism of central nervous system depression with thiazide overdosage is unknown. Gastrointestinal irritation and hypermotility can occur; temporary elevation of BUN has been reported, and serum electrolyte changes could occur, especially in patients with impairment of renal function.
TREATMENT
The following measures should be employed:
GENERAL—If ingestion is, or may have been, recent, evacuate gastric contents taking care to prevent pulmonary aspiration.
BRADYCARDIA—Administer atropine (0.25 to 1.0 mg). If there is no response to vagal blockade, administer isoproterenol cautiously.
CARDIAC FAILURE—Digitalization and diuretics.
HYPOTENSION—Vasopressors, *e.g.*, levarterenol or epinephrine.
BRONCHOSPASM—Administer isoproterenol and aminophylline.
STUPOR OR COMA—Administer supportive therapy as clinically warranted.
GASTROINTESTINAL EFFECTS—Though usually of short duration, these may require symptomatic treatment.
ABNORMALITIES IN BUN AND/OR SERUM ELECTROLYTES—Monitor serum electrolyte levels and renal function; institute supportive measures as required individually to maintain hydration, electrolyte balance, respiration, and cardiovascular-renal function.

How Supplied:
- Each INDERIDE®-40/25 tablet contains 40 mg propranolol hydrochloride (INDERAL®) and 25 mg hydrochlorothiazide, in bottles of 100 (NDC 0046-0474-81) and 1,000 (NDC 0046-0474-91). Also in unit dose package of 100 (NDC 0046-0474-99).
- Each INDERIDE®-80/25 tablet contains 80 mg propranolol hydrochloride (INDERAL®) and 25 mg hydrochlorothiazide, in bottles of 100 (NDC 0046-0476-81) and 1,000 (NDC 0046-0476-91). Also in unit dose package of 100 (NDC 0046-0476-99).

[*Shown in Product Identification Section*]

KERODEX®

Action and Uses: A specially formulated barrier hand cream to help protect against potentially irritating chemicals, compounds, and solutions in common use. When applied and used as directed, KERODEX provides a barrier film that helps to block contact with skin irritants. KERODEX No. 71 (water repellent) is for use in handling or working with *wet* materials; No. 51 is for *dry* or *oily* work. KERODEX is greaseless and stainless.
Application: 1. Wash hands clean and dry *thoroughly.* 2. Squeeze out ½ inch of cream into palm of one hand. Rub hands together with a washing motion until cream is *lightly* and *evenly* distributed, leaving no excess. Make sure cream reaches under nails, around cuticles, between fingers, across wrists and backs of hands (forearms, if necessary). 3. A second application is recommended. **NOTE:** After applying KERODEX 71, "set" by holding hands under cold running water. Pat dry. After applying KERODEX 51, avoid contact with water. If hands become wet during work, reapply.
How Supplied: KERODEX (water-repellent cream for wet work), in 4 oz (113 g) tubes (NDC 0046-0071-04) and 1 lb. jars (NDC 0046-0071-01). KERODEX (water-miscible cream for dry or oily work), in 4 oz (113 g) tubes (NDC 0046-0051-04) and 1 lb. jars (NDC 0046-0051-01).

LARYLGAN® Throat Spray

An aqueous solution containing:

Antipyrine	0.30%
Pyrilamine maleate	0.05%
Sodium caprylate	0.50%

Also contains menthol, gentian violet, methyl salicylate, methylparaben, propylparaben, peppermint oil, spearmint oil, anise oil, cinnamon oil, isobornyl acetate, benzyl alcohol 0.05%, ethyl alcohol 1.00%, glycerin, sodium saccharin, and other aromatics.
Action: The analgesic-like effect of LARYLGAN helps to allay pain of irritated mucosa. The glycerin dehydrated vehicle provides maximum spreading and penetrating properties to help the medication reach the affected areas. It is non-narcotic.
Indications: A soothing and refreshing spray for dry throat and for minor sore throat due to irritants such as smoking or postnasal drip.
Warning: Severe and persistent sore throat or sore throat accompanied by high fever, headache, nausea, and vomiting may be serious. Consult physician promptly. Do not use more than two days or administer to children under 3 years of age unless directed by physician.
Administration: *Instructions for Use:* Remove cap. Hold close to mouth and spray. Repeat as required. If throat condition persists, consult a physician.
How Supplied: LARYLGAN Throat Spray, in 0.94 fl oz (28 ml) bottles (NDC 0046-1005-01).

MEDIATRIC® Ⓒ℞

Each capsule or tablet contains:

Premarin® (Conjugated Estrogens, U.S.P.)	0.25 mg
Methyltestosterone	2.5 mg
Ascorbic acid (Vit. C)*	100.0 mg
Cyanocobalamin	2.5 mcg
Thiamine mononitrate	10.0 mg
Riboflavin	5.0 mg
Niacinamide	50.0 mg
Pyridoxine HCl	3.0 mg
Calc. pantothenate	20.0 mg
Dried ferrous sulfate	30.0 mg
Methamphetamine HCl	1.0 mg

*For Capsules, provided as ascorbic acid, 70 mg, and as sodium ascorbate, 30 mg.

Also available: MEDIATRIC Liquid
Each 15 ml (3 teaspoonfuls) contains:

Premarin® (Conjugated Estrogens, U.S.P.)	0.25 mg
Methyltestosterone	2.5 mg
Thiamine HCl	5.0 mg
Cyanocobalamin	1.5 mcg
Methamphetamine HCl	1.0 mg

Contains 15% alcohol—some loss unavoidable.

Continued on next page

Ayerst—Cont.

1. ESTROGENS HAVE BEEN REPORTED TO INCREASE THE RISK OF ENDOMETRIAL CARCINOMA.
Three independent case control studies have reported an increased risk of endometrial cancer in postmenopausal women exposed to exogenous estrogens for more than one year.[1–3] This risk was independent of the other known risk factors for endometrial cancer. These studies are further supported by the finding that incidence rates of endometrial cancer have increased sharply since 1969 in eight different areas of the United States with population-based cancer reporting systems, an increase which may be related to the rapidly expanding use of estrogens during the last decade.[4]
The three case control studies reported that the risk of endometrial cancer in estrogen users was about 4.5 to 13.9 times greater than in nonusers. The risk appears to depend on both duration of treatment[1] and on estrogen dose.[3] In view of these findings, when estrogens are used for the treatment of menopausal symptoms, the lowest dose that will control symptoms should be utilized and medication should be discontinued as soon as possible. When prolonged treatment is medically indicated, the patient should be reassessed on at least a semiannual basis to determine the need for continued therapy. Although the evidence must be considered preliminary, one study suggests that cyclic administration of low doses of estrogen may carry less risk than continuous administration;[3] it therefore appears prudent to utilize such a regimen.
Close clinical surveillance of all women taking estrogens is important. In all cases of undiagnosed persistent or recurring abnormal vaginal bleeding, adequate diagnostic measures should be undertaken to rule out malignancy.
There is no evidence at present that "natural" estrogens are more or less hazardous than "synthetic" estrogens at equiestrogenic doses.
2. ESTROGENS SHOULD NOT BE USED DURING PREGNANCY.
The use of female sex hormones, both estrogens and progestogens, during early pregnancy may seriously damage the offspring. It has been shown that females exposed in utero to diethylstilbestrol, a non-steroidal estrogen, have an increased risk of developing in later life a form of vaginal or cervical cancer that is ordinarily extremely rare.[5,6] This risk has been estimated as not greater than 4 per 1000 exposures.[7] Furthermore, a high percentage of such exposed women (from 30 to 90 percent) have been found to have vaginal adenosis,[8–12] epithelial changes of the vagina and cervix. Although these changes are histologically benign, it is not known whether they are precursors of malignancy. Although similar data are not available with the use of other estrogens, it cannot be presumed they would not induce similar changes.
Several reports suggest an association between intrauterine exposure to female sex hormones and congenital anomalies, including congenital heart defects and limb reduction defects.[13–16] One case control study[16] estimated a 4.7-fold increased risk of limb reduction defects in infants exposed in utero to sex hormones (oral contraceptives, hormone withdrawal tests for pregnancy, or attempted treatment for threatened abortion). Some of these exposures were very short and involved only a few days of treatment. The data suggest that the risk of limb reduction defects in exposed fetuses is somewhat less than 1 per 1000.
In the past, female sex hormones have been used during pregnancy in an attempt to treat threatened or habitual abortion. There is considerable evidence that estrogens are ineffective for these indications, and there is no evidence from well controlled studies that progestogens are effective for these uses.
If MEDIATRIC is used during pregnancy, or if the patient becomes pregnant while taking this drug, she should be apprised of the potential risks to the fetus, and the advisability of pregnancy continuation.

Description: MEDIATRIC provides estrogen and androgen in small doses, nutritional supplements, together with a mild antidepressant.
Action: MEDIATRIC provides (1) *steroids* to help counteract declining gonadal hormone secretion, and as important regulators of metabolic processes; (2) *nutritional supplements* specially selected to meet the needs of the aged and aging patient, and to act as necessary catalysts for the maintenance of efficient enzyme systems; and (3) *a mild antidepressant* to impart a gentle emotional uplift.
Indication: For use in aging patients of both sexes.
MEDIATRIC HAS NOT BEEN SHOWN TO BE EFFECTIVE FOR ANY PURPOSE DURING PREGNANCY AND ITS USE MAY CAUSE SEVERE HARM TO THE FETUS (SEE BOXED WARNING).
Contraindications: Estrogens should not be used in women (or men) with any of the following conditions:
1. Known or suspected cancer of the breast except in appropriately selected patients being treated for metastatic disease.
2. Known or suspected estrogen-dependent neoplasia.
3. Known or suspected pregnancy (See Boxed Warning).
4. Undiagnosed abnormal genital bleeding.
5. Active thrombophlebitis or thromboembolic disorders.
6. A past history of thrombophlebitis, thrombosis, or thromboembolic disorders associated with previous estrogen use (except when used in treatment of breast or prostatic malignancy).

Methyltestosterone should not be used in persons with any of the following conditions:
1. Known or suspected carcinoma of the prostate and in carcinoma of the male breast.
2. Severe liver damage.
3. Pregnancy or in breast-feeding mothers because of the possibility of masculinization of the female fetus or breast-fed infant.

Warnings:
Associated with Estrogens
1. *Induction of malignant neoplasms.* Long term continuous administration of natural and synthetic estrogens in certain animal species increases the frequency of carcinomas of the breast, cervix, vagina, and liver. There are now reports that estrogens increase the risk of carcinoma of the endometrium in humans. (See Boxed Warning.)
At the present time there is no satisfactory evidence that estrogens given to postmenopausal women increase the risk of cancer of the breast,[17] although a recent long-term followup of a single physician's practice has raised this possibility.[18] Because of the animal data, there is a need for caution in prescribing estrogens for women with a strong family history of breast cancer or who have breast nodules, fibrocystic disease, or abnormal mammograms.
2. *Gallbladder disease.* A recent study has reported a 2 to 3-fold increase in the risk of surgically confirmed gallbladder disease in women receiving postmenopausal estrogens,[17] similar to the 2-fold increase previously noted in users of oral contraceptives.[19,24a]
3. *Effects similar to those caused by estrogen-progestogen oral contraceptives.* There are several serious adverse effects of oral contraceptives, most of which have not, up to now, been documented as consequences of postmenopausal estrogen therapy. This may reflect the comparatively low doses of estrogen used in postmenopausal women. It would be expected that the larger doses of estrogen used to treat prostatic or breast cancer or postpartum breast engorgement are more likely to result in these adverse effects, and, in fact, it has been shown that there is an increased risk of thrombosis in men receiving estrogens for prostatic cancer and women for postpartum breast engorgement.[20–23]
a. *Thromboembolic disease.* It is now well established that users of oral contraceptives have an increased risk of various thromboembolic and thrombotic vascular diseases, such as thrombophlebitis, pulmonary embolism, stroke, and myocardial infarction.[24–31] Cases of retinal thrombosis, mesenteric thrombosis, and optic neuritis have been reported in oral contraceptive users. There is evidence that the risk of several of these adverse reactions is related to the dose of the drug.[32,33] An increased risk of postsurgery thromboembolic complications has also been reported in users of oral contraceptives.[34,35] If feasible, estrogen should be discontinued at least 4 weeks before surgery of the type associated with an increased risk of thromboembolism, or during periods of prolonged immobilization.
While an increased rate of thromboembolic and thrombotic disease in postmenopausal users of estrogens has not been found,[17–24,25–36] this does not rule out the possibility that such an increase may be present or that subgroups of women who have underlying risk factors or who are receiving relatively large doses of estrogens may have increased risk. Therefore estrogens should not be used in persons with active thrombophlebitis or thromboembolic disorders, and they should not be used (except in treatment of malignancy) in persons with a history of such disorders in association with estrogen use. They should be used with caution in patients with cerebral vascular or coronary artery disease and only for those in whom estrogens are clearly needed.
Large doses of estrogen (5 mg conjugated estrogens per day), comparable to those used to treat cancer of the prostate and breast, have been shown in a large prospective clinical trial in men[37] to increase the risk of nonfatal myocardial infarction, pulmonary embolism and thrombophlebitis. When estrogen doses of this size are used, any of the thromboembolic and thrombotic adverse effects associated with oral contraceptive use should be considered a clear risk.
b. *Hepatic adenoma.* Benign hepatic adenomas appear to be associated with the use of oral contraceptives.[38–40] Although benign, and rare, these may rupture and may cause death through intra-abdominal hemorrhage. Such lesions have not yet been reported in association with other estrogen or progestogen preparations but should be considered in estrogen users having abdominal pain and tenderness, abdominal mass, or hypovolemic shock. Hepatocellular carcinoma has also been reported in women taking estrogen-containing oral contraceptives.[39] The relationship of this malignancy to these drugs is not known at this time.
c. *Elevated blood pressure.* Women using oral contraceptives sometimes experience increased blood pressure which, in most cases, returns to normal on discontinuing the drug. There is now a report that this may occur with use of estrogens in the menopause[41] and blood

pressure should be monitored with estrogen use, especially if high doses are used.
d. *Glucose tolerance.* A worsening of glucose tolerance has been observed in a significant percentage of patients on estrogen-containing oral contraceptives. For this reason, diabetic patients should be carefully observed while receiving estrogen.
4. *Hypercalcemia.* Administration of estrogens may lead to severe hypercalcemia in patients with breast cancer and bone metastases. If this occurs, the drug should be stopped and appropriate measures taken to reduce the serum calcium level.

Associated with Methyltestosterone

1. Female patients should be watched carefully for symptoms or signs of virilization such as hoarseness or deepening of the voice, oily skin, acne, hirsutism, enlarged clitoris, stimulation of libido, and menstrual irregularities. At the dosage necessary to achieve a tumor response, androgens will cause masculinization of a female, but occasionally a sensitive female may exhibit one or more of these signs on smaller doses. Some of these changes, such as voice changes may be irreversible even after drug is stopped.
2. Cholestatic hepatitis with jaundice and altered liver function tests, such as increased BSP retention and rises in SGOT levels, have been reported with methyltestosterone. These changes appear to be related to dosage of the drug. Therefore, in the presence of any changes in liver function tests, the drug should be discontinued.

Precautions:

Associated with Estrogens

A. General Precautions.

1. A complete medical and family history should be taken prior to the initiation of any estrogen therapy. The pretreatment and periodic physical examinations should include special reference to blood pressure, breasts, abdomen, and pelvic organs, and should include a Papanicolau smear. As a general rule, estrogen should not be prescribed for longer than one year without another physical examination being performed.
2. Fluid retention—Because estrogens may cause some degree of fluid retention, conditions which might be influenced by this factor such as asthma, epilepsy, migraine, and cardiac or renal dysfunction, require careful observation.
3. Certain patients may develop undesirable manifestations of excessive estrogenic stimulation, such as abnormal or excessive uterine bleeding, mastodynia, etc.
4. Oral contraceptives appear to be associated with an increased incidence of mental depression.[24a] Although it is not clear whether this is due to the estrogenic or progestogenic component of the contraceptive, patients with a history of depression should be carefully observed.
5. Preexisting uterine leiomyomata may increase in size during estrogen use.
6. The pathologist should be advised of estrogen therapy when relevant specimens are submitted.
7. Patients with a past history of jaundice during pregnancy have an increased risk of recurrence of jaundice while receiving estrogen-containing oral contraceptive therapy. If jaundice develops in any patient receiving estrogen, the medication should be discontinued while the cause is investigated.
8. Estrogens may be poorly metabolized in patients with impaired liver function and they should be administered with caution in such patients.
9. Because estrogens influence the metabolism of calcium and phosphorus, they should be used with caution in patients with metabolic bone diseases that are associated with hypercalcemia or in patients with renal insufficiency.
10. Because of the effects of estrogens on epiphyseal closure, they should be used judiciously in young patients in whom bone growth is not complete.
11. Certain endocrine and liver function tests may be affected by estrogen-containing oral contraceptives. The following similar changes may be expected with larger doses of estrogen:
a. Increased sulfobromophthalein retention.
b. Increased prothrombin and factors VII, VIII, IX, and X; decreased antithrombin 3; increased norepinephrine-induced platelet aggregability.
c. Increased thyroid binding globulin (TBG) leading to increased circulating total thyroid hormone, as measured by PBI, T4 by column, or T4 by radioimmunoassay. Free T3 resin uptake is decreased, reflecting the elevated TBG; free T4 concentration is unaltered.
d. Impaired glucose tolerance.
e. Decreased pregnanediol excretion.
f. Reduced response to metyrapone test.
g. Reduced serum folate concentration.
h. Increased serum triglyceride and phospholipid concentration.

B. Information for the Patient. See text which appears after the PHYSICIAN REFERENCES under FORMATRIX®.

C. Pregnancy Category X. See CONTRAINDICATIONS and Boxed Warning.

D. Nursing Mothers. As a general principle, the administration of any drug to nursing mothers should be done only when clearly necessary since many drugs are excreted in human milk.

Associated with Methyltestosterone

A. Prolonged dosage of androgen may result in sodium and fluid retention. This may present a problem, especially in patients with compromised cardiac reserve or renal disease.
B. If priapism or other signs of excessive sexual stimulation develop, discontinue therapy.
C. In the male, prolonged administration or excessive dosage may cause inhibition of testicular function, with resultant oligospermia and decrease in ejaculatory volume. Use cautiously in young boys to avoid possible premature epiphyseal closure or precocious sexual development.
D. Hypersensitivity and gynecomastia may occur rarely.
E. PBI may be decreased in patients taking androgens.
F. Hypercalcemia may occur. If this does occur, the drug should be discontinued.

Adverse Reactions:

Associated with Estrogens

(See Warnings regarding induction of neoplasia, adverse effects on the fetus, increased incidence of gallbladder disease, and adverse effects similar to those of oral contraceptives, including thromboembolism.) The following additional adverse reactions have been reported with estrogenic therapy, including oral contraceptives:
1. *Genitourinary system:* Breakthrough bleeding, spotting, change in menstrual flow; dysmenorrhea; premenstrual-like syndrome; amenorrhea during and after treatment; increase in size of uterine fibromyomata; vaginal candidiasis; change in cervical erosion and in degree of cervical secretion; cystitis-like syndrome.
2. *Breasts:* Tenderness, enlargement, secretion.
3. *Gastrointestinal:* Nausea, vomiting; abdominal cramps, bloating; cholestatic jaundice.
4. *Skin:* Chloasma or melasma which may persist when drug is discontinued; erythema multiforme; erythema nodosum; hemorrhagic eruption; loss of scalp hair; hirsutism.
5. *Eyes:* Steepening of corneal curvature; intolerance to contact lenses.
6. *CNS:* Headache, migraine, dizziness; mental depression; chorea.
7. *Miscellaneous:* Increase or decrease in weight; reduced carbohydrate tolerance; aggravation of porphyria; edema; changes in libido.

Associated with Methyltestosterone

Cholestatic jaundice
Hypercalcemia, particularly in patients with metastatic breast carcinoma. This usually indicates progression of bone metastases.
Sodium and water retention
Priapism
Virilization in female patients
Hypersensitivity and gynecomastia

Acute Overdosage: Numerous reports of ingestion of large doses of estrogen-containing oral contraceptives by young children indicate that acute serious ill effects do not occur. Overdosage of estrogen may cause nausea, and withdrawal bleeding may occur in females.

Dosage and Administration: *Male and female*—1 MEDIATRIC Capsule or Tablet daily. (MEDIATRIC Liquid, 3 teaspoonfuls daily.)

In the female: To avoid continuous stimulation of breast and uterus, cyclic therapy is recommended (3 week regimen with 1 week rest period—Withdrawal bleeding may occur during this 1 week rest period).

Treated patients with an intact uterus should be monitored closely for signs of endometrial cancer and appropriate diagnostic measures should be taken to rule out malignancy in the event of persistent or recurring abnormal vaginal bleeding.

In the male: A careful check should be made on the status of the prostate gland when therapy is given for protracted intervals.

How Supplied:

MEDIATRIC Capsules, in bottles of 100 (NDC 0046-0252-81).
MEDIATRIC Tablets, in bottles of 100 (NDC 0046-0752-81).
MEDIATRIC Liquid, in bottle of 16 fluidounces (NDC 0046-0910-16).

Physician References:

1. Ziel, H. K., *et al.*: N. Engl. J. Med. *293*:1167–1170, 1975.
2. Smith, D. C., *et al.*: N. Engl. J. Med. *293*:1164–1167, 1975.
3. Mack, T. M., *et al.*: N. Engl. J. Med. *294*:1262–1267, 1976.
4. Weiss, N. S., *et al.*: N. Engl. J. Med. *294*:1259–1262, 1976.
5. Herbst, A. L., *et al.*: N. Engl. J. Med. *284*:878–881, 1971.
6. Greenwald, P., *et al.*: N. Engl. J. Med. *285*:390–392, 1971.
7. Lanier, A., *et al.*: Mayo Clin. Proc. *48*:793–799, 1973.
8. Herbst, A., *et al.*: Obstet. Gynecol. *40*:287–298, 1972.
9. Herbst, A., *et al.*: Am. J. Obstet. Gynecol. *118*:607–615, 1974.
10. Herbst, A., *et al.*: N. Engl. J. Med. *292*:334–339, 1975.
11. Stafl, A., *et al.*: Obstet. Gynecol. *43*:118–128, 1974.
12. Sherman, A. I., *et al.*: Obstet. Gynecol. *44*:531–545, 1974.
13. Gal, I., *et al.*: Nature *216*:83, 1967.
14. Levy, E. P., *et al.*: Lancet *1*:611, 1973.
15. Nora, J., *et al.*: Lancet *1*:941–942, 1973.
16. Janerich, D. T., *et al.*: N. Engl. J. Med. *291*:697–700, 1974.
17. Boston Collaborative Drug Surveillance Program: N. Engl. J. Med. *290*:15–19, 1974.
18. Hoover, R., *et al.*: N. Engl. J. Med. *295*:401–405, 1976.
19. Boston Collaborative Drug Surveillance Program: Lancet *1*:1399–1404, 1973.
20. Daniel, D. G., *et al.*: Lancet *2*:287–289, 1967.
21. The Veterans Administration Cooperative Urological Research Group: J. Urol. *98*:516–522, 1967.

Continued on next page

Ayerst—Cont.

22. Bailar, J. C.: Lancet *2*:560, 1967.
23. Blackard, C., *et al.*: Cancer *26*:249–256, 1970.
24. Royal College of General Practitioners: J. R. Coll. Gen. Pract. *13*:267–279, 1967.
24a. Royal College of General Practitioners: Oral Contraceptives and Health, New York, Pitman Corp., 1974.
25. Inman, W. H. W., *et al.*: Br. Med. J. *2*:193–199, 1968.
26. Vessey, M. P., *et al.*: Br. Med. J. *2*:651–657, 1969.
27. Sartwell, P. E., *et al.*: Am. J. Epidemiol. *90*:365–380, 1969.
28. Collaborative Group for the Study of Stroke in Young Women: N. Engl. J. Med. *288*:871–878, 1973.
29. Collaborative Group for the Study of Stroke in Young Women: J.A.M.A. *231*:718–722, 1975.
30. Mann, J. I., *et al.*: Br. Med. J. *2*:245–248, 1975.
31. Mann, J. I., *et al.*: Br. Med. J. *2*:241–245, 1975.
32. Inman, W. H. W., *et al.*: Br. Med. J. *2*:203–209, 1970.
33. Stolley, P. D., *et al.*: Am. J. Epidemiol. *102*:197–208, 1975.
34. Vessey, M. P., *et al.*: Br. Med. J. *3*:123–126, 1970.
35. Greene, G. R., *et al.*: Am. J. Public Health *62*:680–685, 1972.
36. Rosenberg, L., *et al.*: N. Engl. J. Med. *294*:1256–1259, 1976.
37. Coronary Drug Project Research Group: J.A.M.A. *214*:1303–1313, 1970.
38. Baum, J., *et al.*: Lancet *2*:926–928, 1973.
39. Mays, E. T., *et al.*: J.A.M.A. *235*:730–732, 1976.
40. Edmondson, H. A., *et al.*: N. Engl. J. Med. *294*:470–472, 1976.
41. Pfeffer, R. I., *et al.*: Am. J. Epidemiol. *103*:445–456, 1976.

[*Shown in Product Identification Section*]

MYSOLINE® ℞
Brand of primidone
Anticonvulsant

Actions: MYSOLINE raises electro- or chemoshock seizure thresholds or alters seizure patterns in experimental animals. The mechanism(s) of primidone's antiepileptic action is not known.

Primidone *per se* has anticonvulsant activity as do its two metabolites, phenobarbital and phenylethylmalonamide (PEMA). In addition to its anticonvulsant activity, PEMA potentiates that of phenobarbital in experimental animals.

Indications: MYSOLINE, either alone or used concomitantly with other anticonvulsants, is indicated in the control of grand mal, psychomotor, and focal epileptic seizures. It may control grand mal seizures refractory to other anticonvulsant therapy.

Contraindications: Primidone is contraindicated in: 1) patients with porphyria and 2) patients who are hypersensitive to phenobarbital (see ACTIONS).

Warnings: The abrupt withdrawal of antiepileptic medication may precipitate status epilepticus.

The therapeutic efficacy of a dosage regimen takes several weeks before it can be assessed.

Usage in pregnancy: The effects of MYSOLINE in human pregnancy and nursing infants are unknown.

Recent reports suggest an association between the use of anticonvulsant drugs by women with epilepsy and an elevated incidence of birth defects in children born to these women. Data are more extensive with respect to diphenylhydantoin and phenobarbital, but these are also the most commonly prescribed anticonvulsants; less systematic or anecdotal reports suggest a possible similar association with the use of all known anticonvulsant drugs.

The reports suggesting an elevated incidence of birth defects in children of drug-treated epileptic women cannot be regarded as adequate to prove a definite cause and effect relationship. There are intrinsic methodologic problems in obtaining adequate data on drug teratogenicity in humans; the possibility also exists that other factors, *e.g.*, genetic factors or the epileptic condition itself, may be more important than drug therapy in leading to birth defects. The great majority of mothers on anticonvulsant medication deliver normal infants. It is important to note that anticonvulsant drugs should not be discontinued in patients in whom the drug is administered to prevent major seizures because of the strong possibility of precipitating status epilepticus with attendant hypoxia and threat to life. In individual cases where the severity and frequency of the seizure disorder are such that the removal of medication does not pose a serious threat to the patient, discontinuation of the drug may be considered prior to and during pregnancy, although it cannot be said with any confidence that even minor seizures do not pose some hazard to the developing embryo or fetus.

The prescribing physician will wish to weigh these considerations in treating or counseling epileptic women of childbearing potential.

Neonatal hemorrhage, with a coagulation defect resembling vitamin K deficiency, has been described in newborns whose mothers were taking primidone and other anticonvulsants. Pregnant women under anticonvulsant therapy should receive prophylactic vitamin K_1 therapy for one month prior to, and during, delivery.

Precautions: The total daily dosage should not exceed 2 g. Since MYSOLINE therapy generally extends over prolonged periods, a complete blood count and a sequential multiple analysis-12 (SMA-12) test should be made every six months.

In nursing mothers: There is evidence that in mothers treated with primidone, the drug appears in the milk in substantial quantities. Since tests for the presence of primidone in biological fluids are too complex to be carried out in the average clinical laboratory, it is suggested that the presence of undue somnolence and drowsiness in nursing newborns of MYSOLINE-treated mothers be taken as an indication that nursing should be discontinued.

Adverse Reactions: The most frequently occurring early side effects are ataxia and vertigo. These tend to disappear with continued therapy, or with reduction of initial dosage. Occasionally, the following have been reported: nausea, anorexia, vomiting, fatigue, hyperirritability, emotional disturbances, sexual impotency, diplopia, nystagmus, drowsiness, and morbilliform skin eruptions. Occasionally, persistent or severe side effects may necessitate withdrawal of the drug. Megaloblastic anemia may occur as a rare idiosyncrasy to MYSOLINE and to other anticonvulsants. The anemia responds to folic acid without necessity of discontinuing medication.

Dosage and Administration: The average adult dose is 0.75 to 1.5 g per day. The initial dose is 250 mg. Increments of 250 mg are added, usually at weekly intervals, to tolerance, or therapeutic effectiveness, up to daily doses not exceeding 2.0 g. A typical dosage schedule for the introduction of MYSOLINE is as follows:

Adults and Children Over 8 Years of Age

1st Week	*2nd Week*
250 mg daily at bedtime	250 mg b.i.d.
3rd Week	*4th Week*
250 mg t.i.d.	250 mg q.i.d.

In children under 8 years of age, maintenance levels are established by a similar schedule, but at one-half the adult dosage. It is best to begin with 125 mg, with gradual weekly increases of 125 mg a day, to a daily total usually between 500 mg and 750 mg.

In patients already receiving other anticonvulsants: MYSOLINE should be gradually increased as dosage of the other drug(s) is maintained or gradually decreased. This regimen should be continued until satisfactory dosage level is achieved for combination, or the other medication is completely withdrawn. When therapy with this product alone is the objective, the transition should not be completed in less than two weeks.

MYSOLINE 50 mg Tablet can be used to practical advantage when small fractional adjustments (upward or downward) may be required, as in the following circumstances:

- for initiation of combination therapy
- during "transfer" therapy
- for added protection in periods of stress or stressful situations that are likely to precipitate seizures (menstruation, allergic episodes, holidays, etc.)

How Supplied:
MYSOLINE Tablets
Each tablet contains 250 mg of primidone (scored), in bottles of 100 (NDC 0046-0430-81) and 1,000 (NDC 0046-0430-91).
Also in unit dose package of 100 (NDC 0046-0430-99).
Each tablet contains 50 mg of primidone (scored), in bottles of 100 (NDC 0046-0431-81) and 500 (NDC 0046-0431-85).
MYSOLINE Suspension
Each 5 ml (teaspoonful) contains 250 mg of primidone, in bottles of 8 fluidounces (NDC 0046-3850-08).

[*Shown in Product Identification Section*]

PENBRITIN* ℞
(ampicillin)
Capsules
250 mg and 500 mg

PENBRITIN is an orally active, semisynthetic broad spectrum penicillin. It is inactivated by penicillinase.

Indications: PENBRITIN is indicated in the treatment of infections due to susceptible strains of the following:

GRAM-NEGATIVE organisms: Shigella, Salmonella (including *S. typhosa*), *H. influenzae, E. coli, P. mirabilis, N. gonorrhoeae*, and *N. meningitidis.*

GRAM-POSITIVE organisms: Streptococci, nonpenicillinase-producing staphylococci, and *D. pneumoniae.*

Bacteriologic studies to determine the causative organisms and their sensitivity to ampicillin should be performed. Because PENBRITIN (ampicillin) is a broad spectrum antibiotic, therapy may be instituted prior to the results of sensitivity testing.

Contraindications: PENBRITIN is contraindicated in patients with a history of hypersensitivity to any penicillin.

Warnings: SERIOUS AND OCCASIONALLY FATAL HYPERSENSITIVITY (ANAPHYLACTOID) REACTIONS HAVE BEEN REPORTED IN PATIENTS ON PENICILLIN THERAPY. ALTHOUGH ANAPHYLAXIS IS MORE FREQUENT FOLLOWING PARENTERAL THERAPY, IT HAS OCCURRED IN PATIENTS ON ORAL PENICILLINS. THESE REACTIONS ARE MORE APT TO OCCUR IN INDIVIDUALS WITH A HISTORY OF PENICILLIN HYPERSENSITIVITY AND/OR HYPERSENSITIVITY REACTIONS TO MULTIPLE ALLERGENS.

THERE HAVE BEEN REPORTS OF INDIVIDUALS WITH A HISTORY OF PENICILLIN HYPERSENSITIVITY WHO HAVE EXPERIENCED SEVERE REACTIONS WHEN TREATED WITH CEPHALOSPORINS. BEFORE THERAPY WITH A PENICILLIN, CAREFUL INQUIRY SHOULD BE MADE CONCERNING PREVIOUS HYPERSENSITIVITY REACTIONS TO PENICILLINS, CEPHALOSPORINS, AND OTHER ALLERGENS.

IF AN ALLERGIC REACTION OCCURS, THE DRUG SHOULD BE DISCONTINUED AND THE APPROPRIATE THERAPY INSTITUTED. **SERIOUS ANAPHYLACTOID REACTIONS REQUIRE IMMEDIATE EMERGENCY TREATMENT WITH EPINEPHRINE. OXYGEN, INTRAVENOUS STEROIDS, AND AIRWAY MANAGEMENT, INCLUDING INTUBATION, SHOULD ALSO BE ADMINISTERED AS INDICATED.**

USAGE IN PREGNANCY: Safety for use in pregnancy has not been established.

Precautions: As with any antibiotic preparation, constant observation for signs of overgrowth of nonsusceptible organisms, including fungi, is essential. Should superinfection occur (usually involving Aerobacter, Pseudomonas, or Candida), the drug should be discontinued and/or appropriate therapy instituted.

Periodic assessment of renal, hepatic, and hematopoietic function should be made during prolonged therapy. This is particularly important in prematures, neonates and other infants.

Adverse Reactions: As with other penicillins, it may be expected that untoward reactions will be essentially limited to sensitivity phenomena. These are more likely to occur in individuals with a history of allergy, asthma, hay fever, or urticaria.

The following adverse reactions have been reported as associated with the use of ampicillin:

Gastrointestinal—glossitis, stomatitis, black "hairy" tongue, nausea, vomiting, enterocolitis, pseudomembranous colitis, and diarrhea. (These reactions are usually associated with oral administration.)

Hypersensitivity reactions—erythematous maculopapular rashes have been reported fairly frequently; urticaria, erythema multiforme, and an occasional case of exfoliative dermatitis have been reported. Anaphylaxis is usually associated with parenteral administration.

Note: Urticaria, other skin rashes, and serum sickness-like reactions may be controlled with antihistamines and, if necessary, systemic corticosteroids. Whenever such reactions occur, ampicillin should be discontinued unless, in the opinion of the physician, the condition being treated is life-threatening and amenable only to ampicillin therapy.

Hepatic—A moderate rise in serum glutamic oxaloacetic transaminase (SGOT) has been noted, particularly in infants. The significance of this finding is unknown.

Hemic and lymphatic—anemia, thrombocytopenia, thrombocytopenic purpura, eosinophilia, leukopenia, and agranulocytosis have been reported. These are usually reversible on discontinuation of the drug, and are believed to be hypersensitivity phenomena.

Dosage and Administration:
[See table above].

DURATION OF TREATMENT: Medications should be continued for at least 48 to 72 hours after all symptoms have subsided or cultures have become negative. For any infection caused by hemolytic streptococci, at least 10 days of treatment is recommended to help prevent the occurrence of acute rheumatic fever or glomerulonephritis.

Infection	Usual Dosage* Adults	Usual Dosage* Children†
Respiratory tract	250 mg q 6 h	50 mg/kg/day in equal doses q 6–8 h
Gastrointestinal tract Genitourinary tract	500 mg q 6 h	100 mg/kg/day in equal doses q 6–8 h
Urethritis in Males or Females due to *N. gonorrhoeae*	3.5 g single oral dose administered simultaneously with 1.0 g of probenecid In the treatment of complications of gonorrheal urethritis, such as prostatitis and epididymitis, prolonged and intensive therapy is recommended. Cases of gonorrhea with a suspected primary lesion of syphilis should have dark-field examinations before receiving treatment. In all other cases where concomitant syphilis is suspected, monthly serologic tests should be made for a minimum of four months.	

*Larger than usual dosages may be required for stubborn or severe infections. Smaller doses than those recommended above should not be used.

†The children's dosage is intended for individuals whose weight will not cause a dosage to be calculated greater than that recommended for adults. Children weighing more than 20 kg (44 lb) should be given the adult recommended dosage.

How Supplied:
PENBRITIN (ampicillin) Capsules—
Each capsule contains 250 mg ampicillin as the trihydrate. In bottles of 100 (NDC 0046-0606-81) and 500 (NDC 0046-0606-85).
Each capsule contains 500 mg ampicillin as the trihydrate. In bottles of 50 (NDC 0046-0624-50) and 500 (NDC 0046-0624-85).
*Mfr. lic'd. under ® 705,484
[*Shown in Product Identification Section*]

PENBRITIN* ℞
(ampicillin)
for Oral Suspension
125 mg/5 ml and 250 mg/5 ml

PENBRITIN*
(ampicillin)
PEDIATRIC DROPS
for Oral Suspension
100 mg/ml

PENBRITIN is an orally active, semisynthetic broad spectrum penicillin. It is inactivated by penicillinase.

Indications: PENBRITIN is indicated in the treatment of infections due to susceptible strains of the following:

GRAM-NEGATIVE organisms: Shigella, Salmonella (including *S. typhosa*), *H. influenzae*, *E. coli*, *P. mirabilis*, *N. gonorrhoeae*, and *N. meningitidis*.

GRAM-POSITIVE organisms: Streptococci, nonpenicillinase-producing staphylococci, and *D. pneumoniae*.

Bacteriologic studies to determine the causative organisms and their sensitivity to ampicillin should be performed. Because PENBRITIN is a broad spectrum antibiotic, therapy may be instituted prior to the results of sensitivity testing.

Contraindications: PENBRITIN (ampicillin) is contraindicated in patients with a history of hypersensitivity to any penicillin.

Warnings: SERIOUS AND OCCASIONALLY FATAL HYPERSENSITIVITY (ANAPHYLACTOID) REACTIONS HAVE BEEN REPORTED IN PATIENTS ON PENICILLIN THERAPY. ALTHOUGH ANAPHYLAXIS IS MORE FREQUENT FOLLOWING PARENTERAL THERAPY, IT HAS OCCURRED IN PATIENTS ON ORAL PENICILLINS. THESE REACTIONS ARE MORE APT TO OCCUR IN INDIVIDUALS WITH A HISTORY OF PENICILLIN HYPERSENSITIVITY AND/OR HYPERSENSITIVITY REACTIONS TO MULTIPLE ALLERGENS.

THERE HAVE BEEN REPORTS OF INDIVIDUALS WITH A HISTORY OF PENICILLIN HYPERSENSITIVITY WHO HAVE EXPERIENCED SEVERE REACTIONS WHEN TREATED WITH CEPHALOSPORINS. BEFORE THERAPY WITH A PENICILLIN, CAREFUL INQUIRY SHOULD BE MADE CONCERNING PREVIOUS HYPERSENSITIVITY REACTIONS TO PENICILLINS, CEPHALOSPORINS, AND OTHER ALLERGENS.

IF AN ALLERGIC REACTION OCCURS, THE DRUG SHOULD BE DISCONTINUED AND THE APPROPRIATE THERAPY INSTITUTED. **SERIOUS ANAPHYLACTOID REACTIONS REQUIRE IMMEDIATE EMERGENCY TREATMENT WITH EPINEPHRINE. OXYGEN, INTRAVENOUS STEROIDS, AND AIRWAY MANAGEMENT, INCLUDING INTUBATION, SHOULD ALSO BE ADMINISTERED AS INDICATED.**

USAGE IN PREGNANCY: Safety for use in pregnancy has not been established.

Precautions: As with any antibiotic preparation, constant observation for signs of overgrowth of nonsusceptible organisms, including fungi, is essential. Should superinfection occur (usually involving Aerobacter, Pseudomonas, or Candida), the drug should be discontinued and/or appropriate therapy instituted.

Periodic assessment of renal, hepatic, and hematopoietic function should be made during prolonged therapy. This is particularly important in prematures, neonates and other infants.

Adverse Reactions: As with other penicillins, it may be expected that untoward reactions will be essentially limited to sensitivity phenomena. These are more likely to occur in individuals with a history of allergy, asthma, hay fever, or urticaria.

The following adverse reactions have been reported as associated with the use of ampicillin:

Gastrointestinal—glossitis, stomatitis, black "hairy" tongue, nausea, vomiting, enterocolitis, pseudomembranous colitis, and diarrhea. (These reactions are usually associated with oral administration.)

Hypersensitivity reactions — erythematous maculopapular rashes have been reported

Continued on next page

Ayerst—Cont.

fairly frequently; urticaria, erythema multiforme, and an occasional case of exfoliative dermatitis have been reported. Anaphylaxis is usually associated with parenteral administration.
Note: Urticaria, other skin rashes, and serum sickness-like reactions may be controlled with antihistamines and, if necessary, systemic corticosteroids. Whenever such reactions occur, ampicillin should be discontinued unless, in the opinion of the physician, the condition being treated is life-threatening and amenable only to ampicillin therapy.
Hepatic—A moderate rise in serum glutamic oxaloacetic transaminase (SGOT) has been noted, particularly in infants. The significance of this finding is unknown.
Hemic and lymphatic—anemia, thrombocytopenia, thrombocytopenic purpura, eosinophilia, leukopenia, and agranulocytosis have been reported. These are usually reversible on discontinuation of the drug, and are believed to be hypersensitivity phenomena.

Dosage and Administration:
(See table below)

PEDIATRIC DROPS:
A suggested dosage regimen is:
Under 12 lb—0.6 ml q 6 hours
12–25 lb—1.0 ml q 6 hours
25–44 lb—2.0 ml q 6 hours

DURATION OF TREATMENT: Medications should be continued for at least 48 to 72 hours after all symptoms have subsided or cultures have become negative. For any infection caused by hemolytic streptococci, at least 10 days of treatment is recommended to help prevent the occurrence of acute rheumatic fever or glomerulonephritis.

Directions for Mixing Oral Suspensions: Prepare suspensions at time of dispensing as follows: Tap bottle gently to loosen powder for ease of preparation. Add the required amount of water (see table below) in two portions—shake well after each addition of water. Each teaspoonful (5 ml) of reconstituted Oral Suspension will contain 125 mg or 250 mg ampicillin, depending upon the initial concentration. Each ml of reconstituted Pediatric Drops will contain 100 mg ampicillin.

Bottle Size	Amount of Water Required for Reconstitution
100 ml Oral Suspension	66 ml
200 ml Oral Suspension	132 ml
20 ml Pediatric Drops	11.5 ml

SHAKE WELL BEFORE USING.

Stability: ORAL SUSPENSION: No refrigeration required before mixing. After mixing, suspension may be kept at room temperature [21.1°C (70°F)] for 7 days or in a refrigerator [4.4°C (40°F)] for 14 days without significant loss of potency. KEEP TIGHTLY CLOSED.
PEDIATRIC DROPS: No refrigeration required before mixing. After mixing, suspension may be kept in a refrigerator for 14 days without significant loss of potency. KEEP TIGHTLY CLOSED.

How Supplied:
PENBRITIN (ampicillin) for Oral Suspension—when reconstituted:
Each 5 ml (one teaspoonful) contains 125 mg ampicillin as the trihydrate. Bottles for 100 ml (NDC 0046-0607-86) and 200 ml (NDC 0046-0607-82).
Each 5 ml (one teaspoonful) contains 250 mg ampicillin as the trihydrate. Bottles for 100 ml (NDC 0046-0611-86) and 200 ml (NDC 0046-0611-82).
PENBRITIN (ampicillin) PEDIATRIC DROPS for Oral Suspension—when reconstituted:
Each ml contains 100 mg ampicillin as the trihydrate. Bottles for 20 ml (NDC 0046-0625-20).
*Mfr. lic' d. under ®705,484

PENBRITIN*-S ℞
(sterile ampicillin sodium)
for Injection

Indications: PENBRITIN-S is particularly indicated for the treatment of infections due to susceptible strains of gram-negative bacteria, *e.g.* Shigella, Salmonella (including *S. typhosa*), *Neisseria gonorrhoeae, Neisseria meningitidis, Escherichia coli, Haemophilus influenzae, Proteus mirabilis.* It is also indicated for infections due to susceptible strains of gram-positive bacteria, *e.g.* beta hemolytic streptococcus, nonpenicillinase-producing staphylococci, *Diplococcus pneumoniae,* streptococci.
PENBRITIN-S for Injection, 4 g, is indicated for intravenous use in serious infections when very high levels of antibiotic must reach the site of infection promptly.
Bacteriologic studies to determine the causative organisms and their sensitivity to ampicillin should be performed. (If the Kirby-Bauer method of disc sensitivity is used, a 10 mcg ampicillin disc should be used.) Because PENBRITIN is a broad spectrum antibiotic, therapy may be instituted prior to the results of sensitivity testing.
Indicated surgical procedures should be performed.

Contraindications: PENBRITIN is contraindicated in patients with a history of hypersensitivity to any penicillin.

Warnings: Serious and occasionally fatal hypersensitivity (anaphylactic) reactions have been reported in patients on penicillin therapy. Although anaphylaxis is more frequent following parenteral administration, it has occurred after oral therapy. These reactions are more apt to occur in individuals with a history of sensitivity to multiple allergens.
Cross-sensitivity to penicillin and cephalosporins has been reported. As with any penicillin, before therapy is instituted, careful inquiry should be made concerning previous hypersensitivity reactions to penicillins, cephalosporins, or other allergens. If an allergic reaction occurs, ampicillin should be discontinued, and appropriate therapy instituted (antihistamines, pressor amines, corticosteroids). **Serious anaphylactoid reactions require immediate emergency treatment with epinephrine. Oxygen, intravenous steroids, and airway management, including intubation, should also be administered as indicated.**
Usage in Pregnancy: Safety for use in pregnancy has not been established.

Precautions: As with any potent drug, periodic assessment of renal, hepatic, and hematopoietic function should be made during prolonged therapy. This is particularly important in prematures, neonates, and other infants.
Caution should be used in administering PENBRITIN-S, 2 g–4 g, in instances of complete renal failure.
The possibility of mycotic or bacterial superinfections should be kept in mind during therapy. If they occur, ampicillin should be discontinued and/or appropriate treatment instituted.
Before instituting treatment for gonorrhea in patients with a suspected primary syphilitic lesion, dark-field examinations for *Treponema pallidum* should be made. Serologic tests should be carried out each month for at least four months in all other cases where concomitant syphilis is suspected.

Adverse Reactions: As with other penicillins, it may be expected that untoward reactions will be essentially limited to sensitivity phenomena. These are more likely to occur in individuals with a history of allergy, asthma, hay fever, or urticaria.
The following adverse reactions have been reported as associated with the use of ampicillin:
Gastrointestinal—glossitis, stomatitis, black "hairy" tongue, nausea, vomiting, enterocolitis, pseudomembranous colitis, and diarrhea (These reactions are usually associated with oral administration.)
Hypersensitivity reactions—erythematous maculopapular rashes have been reported fairly frequently; urticaria, erythema multiforme, and an occasional case of exfoliative dermatitis have been reported. Anaphylaxis is usually associated with parenteral administration.
Note: Urticaria, other skin rashes, and serum sickness-like reactions may be controlled with antihistamines and, if necessary, systemic corticosteroids. Whenever such reactions occur, ampicillin should be discontinued unless, in the opinion of the physician, the condition being treated is life-threatening and amenable only to ampicillin therapy.
Hepatic—A moderate rise in serum glutamic oxaloacetic transaminase (SGOT) has been noted, particularly in infants. The significance of this finding is unknown.
Hemic and lymphatic—anemia, thrombocytopenia, thrombocytopenic purpura, eosinophilia, leukopenia, and agranulocytosis have been

Infection	Usual Dosage* Adults	Usual Dosage* Children†
Respiratory tract	250 mg q 6 hours	50 mg/kg/day in equal doses q 6–8 hours
Gastrointestinal tract Genitourinary tract	500 mg q 6 hours	100 mg/kg/day in equal doses q 6–8 hours
Urethritis in Males or Females due to *N. gonorrhoeae*	3.5 g single oral dose administered simultaneously with 1.0 g of probenecid. In the treatment of complications of gonorrheal urethritis, such as prostatitis and epididymitis, prolonged and intensive therapy is recommended. Cases of gonorrhea with a suspected primary lesion of syphilis should have dark-field examinations before receiving treatment. In all other cases where concomitant syphilis is suspected, monthly serologic tests should be made for a minimum of four months.	

*Larger than usual dosages may be required for stubborn or severe infections. Smaller doses than those recommended above should not be used.
†The children's dosage is intended for individuals whose weight will not cause a dosage to be calculated greater than that recommended for adults. Children weighing more than 20 kg (44 lb) should be given the adult recommended dosage.

reported. These are usually reversible on discontinuation of the drug, and are believed to be hypersensitivity phenomena.

Dosage and Administration

PENBRITIN-S (sterile ampicillin sodium) for Injection should be reserved for moderately severe and severe infections and for those patients who, due to poor absorption or difficulty of administration, do not respond adequately to oral dosage forms.
PENBRITIN-S for Injection, 125 mg, is intended primarily for pediatric use. It also serves as a convenient dosage form when small parenteral doses are required.
PENBRITIN-S for Injection, 2 g, and PENBRITIN-S for Injection, 4 g, are recommended for intravenous use in serious infections when very high levels of the antibiotic must reach the site of infection promptly. Such infections which might require high doses include meningitis, subacute bacterial endocarditis, peritonitis, septicemia, and severe infections of other organ systems (e.g., chronic bronchitis, osteomyelitis, pneumonia, and pyelonephritis) due to susceptible organisms.
A change to oral PENBRITIN should be made as soon as appropriate.

Smaller doses than those recommended should not be used. Even higher doses may be required for stubborn or severe infections.
Children weighing more than 20 kg (44 lb) should be given the adult recommended dose.
Usual Dosages: Genitourinary Tract Infections/Gastrointestinal Tract Infections:
ADULTS—500 mg every six hours.
CHILDREN—50 mg/kg/day in equally divided doses every six hours.
Gonorrheal Urethritis:
ADULT MALES—500 mg twice a day. Treatment may be repeated or extended, if required.
ADULT FEMALES—500 mg every six hours. (See **Precautions.**)
Respiratory Tract Infections/Ear Infections/Soft Tissue Infections:
ADULTS—250–500 mg every six hours.
CHILDREN—50 mg/kg/day in equally divided doses every six hours.
Peritonitis, Chronic Bronchitis, Osteomyelitis, Pneumonia, and Pyelonephritis, depending upon the severity of the infection:
ADULTS—2–16 g/day.
CHILDREN—100–200 mg/kg/day.
Bacterial Meningitis, Subacute Bacterial Endocarditis, and Septicemia, depending upon the severity of the infection:
ADULTS—8–16 g/day.
CHILDREN—150–250 mg/kg/day.

NOTE: In order to obtain therapeutic serum levels quickly, an initial direct intravenous injection of approximately 1/6th the calculated daily dose *(but not more than 2 g)* may be given slowly over at least 10–15 minutes. Treatment then should be continued by IV *drip* with the calculated dose every 3–4 hours.
PENBRITIN-S for Injection, 4 g, should be given **only by intravenous drip when more than 2 g are given at one time;** *i.e.* concentrations greater than 2 g should not be given as direct IV injections.
If the patient's veins become inaccessible after three to four days of IV therapy, intramuscular injections may be given in six equally divided doses.

Duration of Treatment: Medications should be continued for at least 48 to 72 hours after all symptoms have subsided or cultures have become negative. For any infection caused by hemolytic streptococci, at least 10 days of treatment is recommended to help prevent the occurrence of acute rheumatic fever or glomerulonephritis. Extended therapy is recommended when treating complications of gonorrheal urethritis, such as prostatitis and epididymitis. In stubborn infections, therapy may be required for several weeks.

For Intramuscular Injection, dissolve contents of a vial with the amount of Sterile Water for Injection, U.S.P., or Bacteriostatic Water for Injection, U.S.P., listed in the table below.

Potency of Product	Recommended Amount of Diluent to Be Added:	Concentration Achieved	Available Volume
125 mg/vial	1.0 ml	125 mg/ml	1.1 ml
250 mg/vial	1.9 ml	125 mg/ml	2.0 ml
500 mg/vial	3.7 ml	125 mg/ml	4.0 ml
1 g/vial*	7.4 ml	125 mg/ml	8.0 ml
250 mg/vial	0.9 ml	250 mg/ml	1.0 ml
500 mg/vial	1.7 ml	250 mg/ml	2.0 ml
1 g/vial*	3.4 ml	250 mg/ml	4.0 ml
2 g/vial*	6.8 ml	250 mg/ml	8.0 ml

*1 g and 2 g potencies may be used for IM injection if the 250 mg or 500 mg concentrations are unavailable. If the desired dosage results in a volume greater than 2 ml, the buttocks should be used for injection; more than 4 ml at any one site is NOT recommended.

For Direct Intravenous Injection, dissolve contents of a vial with the amount of Sterile Water for Injection, U.S.P., or Bacteriostatic Water for Injection, U.S.P. listed in the table below.

Potency of Product	Recommended Amount of Diluent to Be Added:	Time Required for Injection
125 mg/vial	2.0 ml	3–5 min
250 mg/vial	5.0 ml	3–5 min
500 mg/vial	5.0 ml	3–5 min
1 g/vial	7.4 ml	10–15* min
2 g/vial	7.4 ml	10–15* min

*If injected more rapidly, convulsions may ensue.

Directions for Use: *Use only freshly prepared solutions.* Solutions intended for intramuscular or direct intravenous injection should be used as soon as possible because its potency may decrease significantly after one hour.
The potency of intravenous drip solutions can be maintained from four to eight hours, depending upon the concentration of the antibiotic *and* the type of intravenous solution.
[See table above].

For Intravenous Drip, reconstitute the 125 mg through 2 g potencies as for Direct Intravenous Injection prior to diluting with intravenous solution. The 4 g potency should be reconstituted with at least 15 ml of Sterile Water for Injection, U.S.P. or Bacteriostatic Water for Injection, U.S.P.; then added to at least 250 ml of an appropriate intravenous solution. The potency of intravenous drip solutions can be maintained from four to eight hours, depending upon the concentration of the antibiotic and the type of intravenous solution. (See tabulation below.)
Stability studies on ampicillin sodium in various intravenous solutions indicate that the ampicillin sodium will lose less than 10% activity at room temperature (70°F) for the time periods and concentrations stated:
[See table on next page].
How Supplied: PENBRITIN-S (sterile ampicillin sodium) for Injection
Equivalent to 125 mg ampicillin per vial when reconstituted, box of 10 (NDC 0046-0651-10).—Equivalent to 250 mg ampicillin per vial when reconstituted, box of 10 (NDC 0046-0604-10).—Equivalent to 500 mg ampicillin per vial when reconstituted, box of 10 (NDC 0046-0603-10).—Equivalent to 1 g ampicillin per vial when reconstituted, box of 10 (NDC 0046-0623-10).—Equivalent to 2 g ampicillin per vial when reconstituted, box of 10 (NDC 0046-0652-10).—Equivalent to 4 g ampicillin per vial when reconstituted, box of 10 (NDC 0046-0602-10).
*Mfr. lic'd. under ® 705,484

PEPTAVLON® ℞
Brand of pentagastrin
A diagnostic agent for evaluation of gastric acid secretory function.

Actions: PEPTAVLON (pentagastrin) contains the C-terminal tetrapeptide responsible for the actions of the natural gastrins and, therefore, acts as a physiologic gastric acid secretagogue. The recommended dose of 6 mcg/kg subcutaneously produces a peak acid output which is reproducible when used in the same individual.
PEPTAVLON stimulates gastric acid secretion approximately ten minutes after subcutaneous injection, with peak responses occurring in most cases twenty to thirty minutes after administration. Duration of activity is usually between sixty and eighty minutes.
Indications: PEPTAVLON is used as a diagnostic agent to evaluate gastric acid secretory function. It is useful in testing for:
Anacidity:—as a diagnostic aid in patients with suspected pernicious anemia, atrophic gastritis, or gastric carcinoma.
Hypersecretion:—as a diagnostic aid in patients with suspected duodenal ulcer or postoperative stomal ulcer, and for the diagnosis of Zollinger-Ellison tumor.
PEPTAVLON (pentagastrin) is also useful in determining the adequacy of acid-reducing operations for peptic ulcer.
Contraindications: Hypersensitivity or idiosyncrasy to pentagastrin.
Warnings: *Use in Pregnancy*—The use of pentagastrin in pregnancy has NOT been studied, and the benefit of administration of the drug must be weighed against any possible risk to the mother and/or fetus.
Use in Children—There are insufficient data to recommend the use of, or establish a dosage, in children.

Continued on next page

Ayerst—Cont.

****

In amounts in excess of the recommended dose, pentagastrin may cause inhibition of gastric acid secretion.

Precautions: Use with caution in patients with pancreatic, hepatic, or biliary disease. Like gastrin, pentagastrin could, in some cases, have the physiologic effect of stimulating pancreatic enzyme and bicarbonate secretion, as well as biliary flow.

Adverse Reactions: Pentagastrin causes fewer and less severe cardiovascular and other adverse reactions than histamine or betazole. The majority of reactions to pentagastrin are related to the gastrointestinal tract.

The following reactions associated with the use of pentagastrin have been reported.

Gastrointestinal: abdominal pain, desire to defecate, nausea, vomiting, borborygmi, blood-tinged mucus

Cardiovascular: flushing, tachycardia

Central Nervous System: dizziness, faintness or lightheadedness, drowsiness, sinking feeling, transient blurring of vision, tiredness, headache

Allergic and Hypersensitivity Reactions: May occur in some patients.

Miscellaneous: shortness of breath, heavy sensation in arms and legs, tingling in fingers, chills, sweating, generalized burning sensation, warmth, pain at site of injection, bile in collected specimens

Dosage and Administration: *Adults:* 6 mcg/kg subcutaneously. Effect begins in about ten minutes; peak response usually occurs in twenty to thirty minutes. (For discussion of the test and explicit directions, consult Baron, J.H.: Gastric Function Tests, in Wastell, C.: Chronic Duodenal Ulcer, New York, Appleton-Century-Crofts, 1972, pp. 82–114.)

Note: Data are inadequate to recommend the use of, or establish a dosage, in children.

Overdosage: In case of overdosage or idiosyncrasy, symptomatic treatment should be administered as required.

How Supplied: PEPTAVLON—In 2 ml ampuls. Each ml contains 0.25 mg (250 mcg) pentagastrin. Also contains 0.88% sodium chloride, and Water for Injection U.S.P. The pH is adjusted with ammonium hydroxide. Cartons of 10 (NDC 0046-3290-10).

PHOSPHOLINE IODIDE® ℞

(echothiophate iodide for ophthalmic solution)

Description: PHOSPHOLINE IODIDE occurs as a white, crystalline, water-soluble, hygroscopic solid having a slight mercaptan-like odor. When freeze-dried in the presence of potassium acetate, the mixture appears as a white amorphous deposit on the walls of the bottle.

Each package contains materials for dispensing 5 ml of eyedrops: (1) bottle containing PHOSPHOLINE IODIDE in one of four potencies [1.5 mg (0.03%), 3.0 mg (0.06%), 6.25 mg (0.125%), or 12.5 mg (0.25%)] as indicated on the label, with 40 mg potassium acetate in each case. Sodium hydroxide or acetic acid may have been incorporated to adjust pH during manufacturing. (2) a 5 ml bottle of diluent containing chlorobutanol (chloral derivative), 0.5%; mannitol, 1.2%; boric acid, 0.06%; and exsiccated sodium phosphate, 0.026% (3) sterilized dropper.

Actions: PHOSPHOLINE IODIDE is a long-acting cholinesterase inhibitor for topical use which enhances the effect of endogenously liberated acetylcholine in iris, ciliary muscle, and other parasympathetically innervated structures of the eye. It thereby causes miosis, increase in facility of outflow of aqueous humor, fall in intraocular pressure, and potentiation of accommodation.

PHOSPHOLINE IODIDE (echothiophate iodide) will depress both plasma and erythrocyte cholinesterase levels in most patients after a few weeks of eyedrop therapy.

Indications: GLAUCOMA—Chronic open-angle glaucoma. Subacute or chronic angle-closure glaucoma after iridectomy or where surgery is refused or contraindicated. Certain non-uveitic secondary types of glaucoma, especially glaucoma following cataract surgery.

ACCOMMODATIVE ESOTROPIA—Concomitant esotropias with a significant accommodative component.

Contraindications:

1. Active uveal inflammation.
2. Most cases of angle closure glaucoma, due to the possibility of increasing angle block.
3. Hypersensitivity to the active or inactive ingredients.

Warnings:

1. *Use in Pregnancy:* Safe use of anticholinesterase medications during pregnancy has not been established, nor has the absence of adverse effects on the fetus or on the respiration of the neonate.
2. Succinylcholine should be administered only with great caution, if at all, prior to or during general anesthesia to patients receiving anticholinesterase medication because of possible respiratory or cardiovascular collapse.
3. Caution should be observed in treating glaucoma with PHOSPHOLINE IODIDE (echothiophate iodide) in patients who are at the same time undergoing treatment with systemic anticholinesterase medications for myasthenia gravis, because of possible adverse additive effects.

Precautions:

1. Gonioscopy is recommended prior to initiation of therapy.
2. Where there is a quiescent uveitis or a history of this condition, anticholinesterase therapy should be avoided or used cautiously because of the intense and persistent miosis and ciliary muscle contraction that may occur.
3. While systemic effects are infrequent, proper use of the drug requires digital compression of the nasolacrimal ducts for a minute or two following instillation to minimize drainage into the nasal chamber with its extensive absorption area. The hands should be washed immediately following instillation.
4. Temporary discontinuance of medication is necessary if salivation, urinary incontinence, diarrhea, profuse sweating, muscle weakness, respiratory difficulties, or cardiac irregularities occur.
5. Patients receiving PHOSPHOLINE IODIDE who are exposed to carbamate or organophosphate type insecticides and pesticides (professional gardeners, farmers, workers in plants manufacturing or formulating such products, etc.) should be warned of the additive systemic effects possible from absorption of the pesticide through the respiratory tract or skin. During periods of exposure to such pesticides, the wearing of respiratory masks, and frequent washing and clothing changes may be advisable.
6. Anticholinesterase drugs should be used with extreme caution, if at all, in patients with marked vagotonia, bronchial asthma, spastic gastrointestinal disturbances, peptic ulcer, pronounced bradycardia and hypotension, recent myocardial infarction, epilepsy, parkinsonism, and other disorders that may respond adversely to vagotonic effects.
7. Anticholinesterase drugs should be employed prior to ophthalmic surgery only as a considered risk because of the possible occurrence of hyphema.
8. PHOSPHOLINE IODIDE (echothiophate iodide) should be used with great caution, if at all, where there is a prior history of retinal detachment.

Adverse Reactions:

1. Although the relationship, if any, of retinal detachment to the administration of PHOSPHOLINE IODIDE has not been established, retinal detachment has been reported in a few cases during the use of PHOSPHOLINE IODIDE in adult patients without a previous history of this disorder.
2. Stinging, burning, lacrimation, lid muscle twitching, conjunctival and ciliary redness, browache, induced myopia with visual blurring may occur.
3. Activation of latent iritis or uveitis may occur.
4. Iris cysts may form, and if treatment is continued, may enlarge and obscure vision. This occurrence is more frequent in children. The cysts usually shrink upon discontinuance of the medication, reduction in strength of the drops or frequency of instillation. Rarely, they may rupture or break free into the aqueous. Regular examinations are advisable when the drug is being prescribed for the treatment of accommodative esotropia.

Intravenous Solution	Concentration	Stability Period
Sterile Water for Injection	Up to 30 mg/ml	8 hours
Isotonic Sodium Chloride Solution	Up to 30 mg/ml	8 hours
M/6 Sodium Lactate Solution	Up to 30 mg/ml	8 hours
5% Dextrose in water	Up to 2 mg/ml	4 hours
5% Dextrose in Water	10 to 20 mg/ml	2 hours
5% Dextrose in 0.45% Sodium Chloride Solution	Up to 2 mg/ml	4 hours
10% Invert Sugar in Water	Up to 2 mg/ml	4 hours
Lactated Ringer's Solution	Up to 30 mg/ml	8 hours

If the solutions listed below are stored under refrigeration (40° F), they will remain stable for the time periods indicated:

Intravenous Solution	Concentration	Stability Period
Sterile Water for Injection	30 mg/ml	48 hours
Sterile Water for Injection	Up to 20 mg/ml	72 hours
Isotonic Sodium Chloride Solution	30 mg/ml	48 hours
Isotonic Sodium Chloride Solution	Up to 20 mg/ml	72 hours
Lactated Ringer's Solution	Up to 30 mg/ml	24 hours
M/6 Sodium Lactate Solution	Up to 30 mg/ml	8 hours
5% Dextrose in Water	Up to 20 mg/ml	4 hours
5% Dextrose in 0.45% Sodium Chloride Solution	Up to 10 mg/ml	4 hours
10% Invert Sugar in Water	Up to 20 mg/ml	3 hours

5. Prolonged use may cause conjunctival thickening, obstruction of nasolacrimal canals.
6. Lens opacities occurring in patients under treatment for glaucoma with PHOSPHOLINE IODIDE have been reported and similar changes have been produced experimentally in normal monkeys. Routine examinations should accompany clinical use of the drug.
7. Paradoxical increase in intraocular pressure may follow anticholinesterase instillation. This may be alleviated by prescribing a sympathomimetic mydriatic such as phenylephrine.

Dosage and Administration:
GLAUCOMA—
Selection of Therapy: The *medication prescribed* should be that which will control the intraocular pressure around-the-clock with the least risk of side effects or adverse reactions. "Tonometric glaucoma" (ocular hypertension without other evidence of the disease) is frequently not treated with any medication, and PHOSPHOLINE IODIDE (echothiophate iodide) is certainly not recommended for this condition. In early chronic simple glaucoma with field loss or disc changes, pilocarpine is generally used for initial therapy and can be recommended so long as control is thereby maintained over the 24 hours of the day.
When this is not the case, PHOSPHOLINE IODIDE 0.03% may be effective and probably has no greater potential for side effects. If this dosage is inadequate, epinephrine and a carbonic anhydrase inhibitor may be added to the regimen. When still more effective medication is required, the higher strengths of PHOSPHOLINE IODIDE may be prescribed with the recognition that the control of the intraocular pressure should have priority regardless of potential side effects. In secondary glaucoma following cataract surgery, the higher strengths of the drug are frequently needed and are ordinarily very well tolerated.
The *dosage regimen* prescribed should call for the lowest concentration that will control the intraocular pressure around-the-clock. Where tonometry around-the-clock is not feasible, it is suggested that appointments for tension-taking be made at different times of the day so that inadequate control may be more readily detected. Two doses a day are preferred to one in order to maintain as smooth a diurnal tension curve as possible, although a single dose per day or every other day has been used with satisfactory results. Because of the long duration of action of the drug, it is never necessary or desirable to exceed a schedule of twice a day. The daily dose or one of the two daily doses should always be instilled just before retiring to avoid inconvenience due to the miosis.
Early Chronic Simple Glaucoma: PHOSPHOLINE IODIDE (echothiophate iodide) 0.03% instilled twice a day, just before retiring and in the morning, may be prescribed advantageously for cases of early chronic simple glaucoma that are not controlled around-the-clock with pilocarpine. Because of prolonged action, control during the night and early morning hours may then sometimes be obtained. A change in therapy is indicated if, at any time, the tension fails to remain at an acceptable level on this regimen.
Advanced Chronic Simple Glaucoma and Glaucoma Secondary to Cataract Surgery: These cases may respond satisfactorily to PHOSPHOLINE IODIDE 0.03% twice a day as above. When the patient is being transferred to PHOSPHOLINE IODIDE (echothiophate iodide) because of unsatisfactory control with pilocarpine, carbachol, epinephrine, etc., one of the higher strengths, 0.06%, 0.125%, or 0.25% will usually be needed. In this case, a brief trial with the 0.03% eyedrops will be advantageous in that the higher strengths will then be more easily tolerated.
Concomitant Therapy: PHOSPHOLINE IODIDE may be used concomitantly with epinephrine, a carbonic anhydrase inhibitor, or both.
Technic: Good technic in the administration of PHOSPHOLINE IODIDE requires that finger pressure at the inner canthus should be exerted for a minute or two following instillation of the eyedrops, to minimize drainage into the nose and throat. Excess solution around the eye should be removed with tissue and any medication on the hands should be rinsed off.
ACCOMMODATIVE ESOTROPIA—
In Diagnosis: One drop of 0.125% may be instilled once a day in both eyes on retiring, for a period of two or three weeks. If the esotropia is accommodative, a favorable response will usually be noted which may begin within a few hours.
In Treatment: PHOSPHOLINE IODIDE (echothiophate iodide) is prescribed at the lowest concentration and frequency which gives satisfactory results. After the initial period of treatment for diagnostic purposes, the schedule may be reduced to 0.125% every other day or 0.06% every day. These dosages can often be gradually lowered as treatment progresses. The 0.03% strength has proven to be effective in some cases. The maximum usually recommended dosage is 0.125% once a day, although more intensive therapy has been used for short periods.
Technic: See Dosage and Administration, Section on Glaucoma.
Duration of Treatment
In diagnosis, only a short period is required and little time will be lost in instituting other procedures if the esotropia proves to be unresponsive. In therapy, there is no definite limit so long as the drug is well tolerated. However, if the eyedrops, with or without eyeglasses, are gradually withdrawn after about a year or two and deviation recurs, surgery should be considered. As with other miotics, tolerance may occasionally develop after prolonged use. In such cases, a rest period will restore the original activity of the drug.
Overdosage: Antidotes are atropine, 2 mg parenterally; PROTOPAM® CHLORIDE (pralidoxime chloride), 25 mg per kg intravenously; artificial respiration should be given if necessary.

Directions for Preparing Eyedrops
1. Use aseptic technic.
2. Tear off aluminum seals, and remove and discard rubber plugs from both drug and diluent containers.
3. Pour diluent into drug container.
4. Remove dropper assembly from its sterile wrapping. Holding dropper assembly by the screw cap and, WITHOUT COMPRESSING RUBBER BULB, insert into drug container and screw down tightly.
5. Shake for several seconds to ensure mixing.
6. Do not cover nor obliterate instructions to patient regarding storage of eyedrops.

Storage and Stability of Eyedrops
Keep eyedrops in refrigerator to obtain maximum useful life of six months. Room temperature is acceptable if drops will be used up within a month.

How Supplied: Each package contains PHOSPHOLINE IODIDE (echothiophate iodide), diluent, and dropper for dispensing 5 ml eyedrops of the strength indicated on the label. Four potencies are available:
NDC 0046-1062-05 .... 1.5 mg package for 0.03%
NDC 0046-1064-05 .... 3.0 mg package for 0.06%
NDC 0046-1065-05 ....6.25 mg package for 0.125%
NDC 0046-1066-05 ....12.5 mg package for 0.25%

PLEGINE® Tablets ℂ ℞
Brand of phendimetrazine tartrate
Anorexiant

Actions: PLEGINE is a phenylalkylamine sympathomimetic with pharmacologic activity similar to the prototype drugs of this class used in obesity, the amphetamines. Actions include central nervous system stimulation and elevation of blood pressure. Tachyphylaxis and tolerance have been demonstrated with all drugs of this class in which these phenomena have been looked for.
Drugs of this class used in obesity are commonly known as "anorectics" or "anorexigenics." It has not been established, however, that the action of such drugs in treating obesity is primarily one of appetite suppression. Other central nervous system actions, or metabolic effects, may be involved, for example.
Adult obese subjects instructed in dietary management and treated with "anorectic" drugs, lose more weight on the average than those treated with placebo and diet, as determined in relatively short term clinical trials.
The magnitude of increased weight loss of drug-treated patients over placebo-treated patients is only a fraction of a pound a week. The rate of weight loss is greatest in the first weeks of therapy for both drug and placebo subjects and tends to decrease in succeeding weeks. The possible origins of the increased weight loss due to the various drug effects are not established. The amount of weight loss associated with the use of an "anorectic" drug varies from trial to trial, and the increased weight loss appears to be related in part to variables other than the drug prescribed, such as the physician-investigator, the population treated, and the diet prescribed. Studies do not permit conclusions as to the relative importance of the drug and non-drug factors on weight loss.
The natural history of obesity is measured in years, whereas the studies cited are restricted to a few weeks' duration; thus, the total impact of drug-induced weight loss over that of diet alone must be considered clinically limited.
Indications: PLEGINE (phendimetrazine tartrate) is indicated in the management of exogenous obesity as a short term adjunct (a few weeks) in a regimen of weight reduction based on caloric restriction. The limited usefulness of agents of this class should be measured against possible risk factors inherent in their use (see **Actions**).
Contraindications: Known hypersensitivity or idiosyncratic reactions to sympathomimetics.
Advanced arteriosclerosis, symptomatic cardiovascular disease, moderate and severe hypertension, hyperthyroidism
Highly nervous or agitated patients
Patients with a history of drug abuse
Patients taking other CNS stimulants, including monamine oxidase inhibitors
Warnings: DRUG DEPENDENCE: PLEGINE is related chemically and pharmacologically to the amphetamines. Amphetamines and related stimulant drugs have been extensively abused, and the possibility of abuse of PLEGINE should be kept in mind when evaluating the desirability of including a drug as part of a weight reduction program. Abuse of amphetamines and related drugs may be associated with intense psychological dependence and severe social dysfunction. There are reports of patients who have increased the dosage to many times that recommended. Abrupt cessation following prolonged high dosage administration results in extreme fatigue and mental depression; changes are also noted on the sleep EEG. Manifestations of chronic intoxication with anorectic drugs include severe dermatoses, marked insomnia, irritability, hyperactivity, and personality changes. The most severe

Continued on next page

Ayerst—Cont.

manifestation of chronic intoxications is psychosis, often clinically indistinguishable from schizophrenia.

Tolerance to the anorectic effect of PLEGINE develops within a few weeks. When this occurs, its use should be discontinued; the maximum recommended dose should not be exceeded.

Use of PLEGINE (phendimetrazine tartrate) within 14 days following the administration of monamine oxidase inhibitors may result in a hypertensive crisis.

Abrupt cessation of administration following prolonged high dosage results in extreme fatigue and depression. Because of the effect on the central nervous system, PLEGINE may impair the ability of the patient to engage in potentially hazardous activities such as operating machinery or driving a motor vehicle; the patient should therefore be cautioned accordingly.

Usage in Pregnancy: Safe use in pregnancy has not been established. Until more information is available, phendimetrazine tartrate should not be taken by women who are or may become pregnant unless, in the opinion of the physician, the potential benefits outweigh the possible hazards.

Usage in Children: PLEGINE is not recommended for use in children under 12 years of age.

Precautions: PLEGINE should be administered with caution to patients with mild hypertension.

Patients with diabetes mellitus should be followed closely since dosage requirements of antidiabetic drugs may be altered with the use of anorectic agents and concomitant dietary restriction.

Adverse Reactions: *Central Nervous System:* Overstimulation, restlessness, insomnia, agitation, flushing, tremor, sweating, dizziness, headache, psychotic states, blurring of vision

Cardiovascular: Palpitation, tachycardia, elevated blood pressure

Gastrointestinal: Mouth dryness, nausea, diarrhea, constipation, stomach pain

Genitourinary: Urinary frequency, dysuria, changes in libido

Dosage and Administration: *Usual adult dosage:* 1 tablet (35 mg.) b.i.d. or t.i.d., one hour before meals.

Dosage should be individualized to obtain an adequate response with the lowest effective dosage. In some cases, ½ tablet per dose may be adequate; dosage should not exceed 2 tablets t.i.d.

Overdosage: Acute overdosage of phendimetrazine tartrate may manifest itself by the following signs and symptoms: unusual restlessness, confusion, belligerence, hallucinations, and panic states. Fatigue and depression usually follow the central stimulation. Cardiovascular effects include arrhythmias, hypertension, or hypotension and circulatory collapse. Gastrointestinal symptoms include nausea, vomiting, diarrhea, and abdominal cramps. Poisoning may result in convulsions, coma, and death.

The management of overdosage is largely symptomatic. It includes sedation with a barbiturate. If hypertension is marked, the use of a nitrate or rapid-acting alpha receptor-blocking agent should be considered. Experience with hemodialysis or peritoneal dialysis is inadequate to permit recommendations for its use.

How Supplied: PLEGINE—Each scored tablet contains 35 mg. phendimetrazine tartrate, in bottles of 100 (NDC 0046-0755-81) and 1,000 (NDC 0046-0755-91).

[*Shown in Product Identification Section*]

PMB® 200 ℞

Each tablet contains:
Premarin® (Conjugated Estrogens, U.S.P.) ..... 0.45 mg
Meprobamate ..... 200.0 mg

PMB® 400

Each tablet contains:
Premarin® (Conjugated Estrogens, U.S.P.) ..... 0.45 mg
Meprobamate ..... 400.0 mg

1. ESTROGENS HAVE BEEN REPORTED TO INCREASE THE RISK OF ENDOMETRIAL CARCINOMA.

Three independent case control studies have reported an increased risk of endometrial cancer in postmenopausal women exposed to exogenous estrogens for more than one year.[1–3] This risk was independent of the other known risk factors for endometrial cancer. These studies are further supported by the finding that incidence rates of endometrial cancer have increased sharply since 1969 in eight different areas of the United States with population-based cancer reporting systems, an increase which may be related to the rapidly expanding use of estrogens during the last decade.[4]

The three case control studies reported that the risk of endometrial cancer in estrogen users was about 4.5 to 13.9 times greater than in nonusers. The risk appears to depend on both duration of treatment[1] and on estrogen dose.[3] In view of these findings, when estrogens are used for the treatment of menopausal symptoms, the lowest dose that will control symptoms should be utilized and medication should be discontinued as soon as possible. When prolonged treatment is medically indicated, the patient should be reassessed on at least a semiannual basis to determine the need for continued therapy. Although the evidence must be considered preliminary, one study suggests that cyclic administration of low doses of estrogen may carry less risk than continuous administration;[3] it therefore appears prudent to utilize such a regimen.

Close clinical surveillance of all women taking estrogens is important. In all cases of undiagnosed persistent or recurring abnormal vaginal bleeding, adequate diagnostic measures should be undertaken to rule out malignancy.

There is no evidence at present that "natural" estrogens are more or less hazardous than "synthetic" estrogens at equiestrogenic doses.

2. ESTROGENS SHOULD NOT BE USED DURING PREGNANCY.

The use of female sex hormones, both estrogens and progestogens, during early pregnancy may seriously damage the offspring. It has been shown that females exposed in utero to diethylstilbestrol, a non-steroidal estrogen, have an increased risk of developing in later life a form of vaginal or cervical cancer that is ordinarily extremely rare.[5,6] This risk has been estimated as not greater than 4 per 1000 exposures.[7] Furthermore, a high percentage of such exposed women (from 30 to 90 percent) have been found to have vaginal adenosis,[8–12] epithelial changes of the vagina and cervix. Although these changes are histologically benign, it is not known whether they are precursors of malignancy. Although similar data are not available with the use of other estrogens, it cannot be presumed they would not induce similar changes.

Several reports suggest an association between intrauterine exposure to female sex hormones and congenital anomalies, including congenital heart defects and limb reduction defects.[13–16] One case control study[16] estimated a 4.7-fold increased risk of limb reduction defects in infants exposed in utero to sex hormones (oral contraceptives, hormone withdrawal tests for pregnancy, or attempted treatment for threatened abortion). Some of these exposures were very short and involved only a few days of treatment. The data suggest that the risk of limb reduction defects in exposed fetuses is somewhat less than 1 per 1000.

In the past, female sex hormones have been used during pregnancy in an attempt to treat threatened or habitual abortion. There is considerable evidence that estrogens are ineffective for these indications, and there is no evidence from well controlled studies that progestogens are effective for these uses.

If PMB is used during pregnancy, or if the patient becomes pregnant while taking this drug, she should be apprised of the potential risks to the fetus, and the advisability of pregnancy continuation.

3. THIS FIXED COMBINATION DRUG IS NOT INDICATED FOR INITIAL THERAPY.

In cases where estrogen given alone has not alleviated anxiety and tension existing as part of the menopausal symptom complex, therapy may then consist of separate administration of estrogen and meprobamate in order to determine the appropriate dosage of each drug for the patient. If this fixed combination represents the dosage so determined, its use may be more convenient in patient management. The treatment of such patients is not static, but must be reevaluated as conditions in each patient warrant.

Description: PMB is a combination of PREMARIN® (Conjugated Estrogens, U.S.P.) and meprobamate, a tranquilizing agent, in tablet form for oral administration.

PREMARIN (Conjugated Estrogens, U.S.P.) is a mixture of estrogens, obtained exclusively from natural sources, occurring as the sodium salts of water-soluble estrogen sulfates blended to represent the average composition of material derived from pregnant mares' urine. It contains estrone, equilin, and 17α-dihydroequilin, together with smaller amounts of 17α-estradiol, equilenin, and 17 α-dihydroequilenin as salts of their sulfate esters.

Meprobamate is the dicarbamic acid ester of 2-methyl-2-*n*-propyl-1,3-propanediol.

Clinical Pharmacology: Estrogens are important in the development and maintenance of the female reproductive system and secondary sex characteristics. They promote growth and development of the vagina, uterus, and fallopian tubes, and enlargement of the breasts. Indirectly, they contribute to the shaping of the skeleton, maintenance of tone and elasticity of urogenital structures, changes in the epiphyses of the long bones that allow for the pubertal growth spurt and its termination, growth of axillary and pubic hair, and pigmentation of the nipples and genitals. Decline of estrogenic activity at the end of the menstrual cycle can bring on menstruation, although the cessation of progesterone secretion is the most important factor in the mature ovulatory cycle. However, in the preovulatory or nonovulatory cycle, estrogen is the primary determinant in the onset of menstruation. Estrogens also affect the release of pituitary gonadotropins.

The pharmacologic effects of conjugated estrogens are similar to those of endogenous estrogens. They are soluble in water and are well absorbed from the gastrointestinal tract.

In responsive tissues (female genital organs, breasts, hypothalamus, pituitary) estrogens enter the cell and are transported into the nucleus. As a result of estrogen action, specific RNA and protein synthesis occurs.
Metabolism and inactivation occur primarily in the liver. Some estrogens are excreted into the bile; however they are reabsorbed from the intestine and returned to the liver through the portal venous system. Water soluble estrogen conjugates are strongly acidic and are ionized in body fluids, which favor excretion through the kidneys since tubular reabsorption is minimal.
Meprobamate is used clinically for the reduction of anxiety and tension. The precise mechanism(s) of its action is not known. It is well-absorbed from the gastrointestinal tract and has a physiological half-life of about 10 hours. It is excreted in the urine primarily as hydroxymeprobamate and as a glucuronide.

The combination of PREMARIN with meprobamate as provided in PMB relieves the underlying estrogen deficiency and affords tranquilizing activity to ameliorate the anxiety and tension not due to estrogen deficiency.

Indication: For the treatment of moderate to severe vasomotor symptoms of the menopause when anxiety and tension are part of the symptom complex and only in those cases in which the use of estrogens alone has not resulted in alleviation of such symptoms.

PMB HAS NOT BEEN SHOWN TO BE EFFECTIVE FOR ANY PURPOSE DURING PREGNANCY AND ITS USE MAY CAUSE SEVERE HARM TO THE FETUS (SEE BOXED WARNING).

Contraindications: Estrogens should not be used in women with any of the following conditions:
1. Known or suspected cancer of the breast.
2. Known or suspected estrogen-dependent neoplasia.
3. Known or suspected pregnancy (See Boxed Warning).
4. Undiagnosed abnormal genital bleeding.
5. Active thrombophlebitis or thromboembolic disorders.
6. A past history of thrombophlebitis, thrombosis, or thromboembolic disorders associated with previous estrogen use.

Meprobamate should not be used in patients with the following conditions:
1. A history of allergic or idiosyncratic reactions to meprobamate or related compounds such as carisoprodol, mebutamate, tybamate, or carbromal.
2. Acute intermittent porphyria.

Warnings:

USAGE IN PREGNANCY AND LACTATION.

An increased risk of congenital malformations associated with the use of minor tranquilizers (meprobamate, chlordiazepoxide, and diazepam) during the first trimester of pregnancy has been suggested in several studies. Because use of these drugs is rarely a matter of urgency, their use during this period should almost always be avoided. The possibility that a woman of childbearing potential may be pregnant at the time of institution of therapy should be considered. Patients should be advised that if they become pregnant during therapy or intend to become pregnant they should communicate with their physicians about the desirability of discontinuing the drug.

Meprobamate passes the placental barrier. It is present both in umbilical cord blood at or near maternal plasma levels and in breast milk of lactating mothers at concentrations two to four times that of maternal plasma. When use of meprobamate is contemplated in breast-feeding patients, the drug's higher concentrations in breast milk as compared to maternal plasma levels should be considered.

Usage in Children—PMB is not intended for use in children.

Associated with Estrogen Administration:

1. *Induction of malignant neoplasms.* Long term continuous administration of natural and synthetic estrogens in certain animal species increases the frequency of carcinomas of the breast, cervix, vagina, and liver. There are now reports that estrogens increase the risk of carcinoma of the endometrium in humans. (See Boxed Warning.)

At the present time there is no satisfactory evidence that estrogens given to postmenopausal women increase the risk of cancer of the breast,[17] although a recent long-term followup of a single physician's practice has raised this possibility.[18] Because of the animal data, there is a need for caution in prescribing estrogens for women with a strong family history of breast cancer or who have breast nodules, fibrocystic disease, or abnormal mammograms.

2. *Gallbladder disease.* A recent study has reported a 2 to 3-fold increase in the risk of surgically confirmed gallbladder disease in women receiving postmenopausal estrogens,[17] similar to the 2-fold increase previously noted in users of oral contraceptives.[19,24a]

3. *Effects similar to those caused by estrogen-progestogen oral contraceptives.* There are several serious adverse effects of oral contraceptives, most of which have not, up to now, been documented as consequences of postmenopausal estrogen therapy. This may reflect the comparatively low doses of estrogen used in postmenopausal women. It would be expected that the larger doses of estrogen used to treat prostatic or breast cancer or postpartum breast engorgement are more likely to result in these adverse effects, and, in fact, it has been shown that there is an increased risk of thrombosis in men receiving estrogens for prostatic cancer and women for postpartum breast engorgement.[20–23]

a. *Thromboembolic disease.* It is now well established that users of oral contraceptives have an increased risk of various thromboembolic and thrombotic vascular diseases, such as thrombophlebitis, pulmonary embolism, stroke, and myocardial infarction.[24–31] Cases of retinal thrombosis, mesenteric thrombosis, and optic neuritis have been reported in oral contraceptive users. There is evidence that the risk of several of these adverse reactions is related to the dose of the drug.[32,33] An increased risk of postsurgery thromboembolic complications has also been reported in users of oral contraceptives.[34,35] If feasible, estrogen should be discontinued at least 4 weeks before surgery of the type associated with an increased risk of thromboembolism, or during periods of prolonged immobilization.

While an increased rate of thromboembolic and thrombotic disease in postmenopausal users of estrogens has not been found,[17–24,25–36] this does not rule out the possibility that such an increase may be present or that subgroups of women who have underlying risk factors or who are receiving relatively large doses of estrogens may have increased risk. Therefore estrogens should not be used in persons with active thrombophlebitis or thromboembolic disorders, and they should not be used (except in treatment of malignancy) in persons with a history of such disorders in association with estrogen use. They should be used with caution in patients with cerebral vascular or coronary artery disease and only for those in whom estrogens are clearly needed.

Large doses of estrogen (5 mg conjugated estrogens per day), comparable to those used to treat cancer of the prostate and breast, have been shown in a large prospective clinical trial in men[37] to increase the risk of nonfatal myocardial infarction, pulmonary embolism and thrombophlebitis. When estrogen doses of this size are used, any of the thromboembolic and thrombotic adverse effects associated with oral contraceptive use should be considered a clear risk.

b. *Hepatic adenoma.* Benign hepatic adenomas appear to be associated with the use of oral contraceptives.[38–40] Although benign, and rare, these may rupture and may cause death through intra-abdominal hemorrhage. Such lesions have not yet been reported in association with other estrogen or progestogen preparations but should be considered in estrogen users having abdominal pain and tenderness, abdominal mass, or hypovolemic shock. Hepatocellular carcinoma has also been reported in women taking estrogen-containing oral contraceptives.[39] The relationship of this malignancy to these drugs is not known at this time.

c. *Elevated blood pressure.* Women using oral contraceptives sometimes experience increased blood pressure which, in most cases, returns to normal on discontinuing the drug. There is now a report that this may occur with use of estrogens in the menopause[41] and blood pressure should be monitored with estrogen use, especially if high doses are used.

d. *Glucose tolerance.* A worsening of glucose tolerance has been observed in a significant percentage of patients on estrogen-containing oral contraceptives. For this reason, diabetic patients should be carefully observed while receiving estrogen.

4. *Hypercalcemia.* Administration of estrogens may lead to severe hypercalcemia in patients with breast cancer and bone metastases. If this occurs, the drug should be stopped and appropriate measures taken to reduce the serum calcium level.

Associated with Meprobamate Administration:

1. *Drug Dependence*—Physical dependence, psychological dependence, and abuse have occurred. When chronic intoxication from prolonged use occurs, it usually involves ingestion of greater than recommended doses and is manifested by ataxia, slurred speech, and vertigo. Therefore, careful supervision of dose and amounts prescribed is advised, as well as avoidance of prolonged administration, especially for alcoholics and other patients with a known propensity for taking excessive quantities of drugs.

Sudden withdrawal of the drug after prolonged and excessive use may precipitate recurrence of preexisting symptoms, such as anxiety, anorexia, or insomnia, or withdrawal reactions, such as vomiting, ataxia, tremors, muscle twitching, confusional states, hallucinosis, and, rarely, convulsive seizures. Such seizures are more likely to occur in persons with central nervous system damage or preexistent or latent convulsive disorders. Onset of withdrawal symptoms occurs usually within 12 to 48 hours after discontinuation of meprobamate; symptoms usually cease within the next 12 to 48 hours.

When excessive dosage has continued for weeks or months, dosage should be reduced gradually over a period of one or two weeks rather than abruptly stopped. Alternatively, a short-acting barbiturate may be substituted, then gradually withdrawn.

2. *Potentially Hazardous Tasks*—Patients should be warned that this drug may impair the mental and/or physical abilities required for the performance of potentially hazardous tasks such as driving a motor vehicle or operating machinery.

3. *Additive Effects*—Since the effects of meprobamate and alcohol or meprobamate and other CNS depressants or psychotropic drugs may be additive, appropriate caution should be exercised with patients who take more than one of these agents simultaneously.

Precautions:

Associated with Estrogen

A. General Precautions.

1. A complete medical and family history should be taken prior to the initiation of any

Continued on next page

Ayerst—Cont.

estrogen therapy. The pretreatment and periodic physical examinations should include special reference to blood pressure, breasts, abdomen, and pelvic organs, and should include a Papanicolau smear. As a general rule, estrogen should not be prescribed for longer than one year without another physical examination being performed.

2. Fluid retention—Because estrogens may cause some degree of fluid retention, conditions which might be influenced by this factor such as asthma, epilepsy, migraine, and cardiac or renal dysfunction, require careful observation.

3. Certain patients may develop undesirable manifestations of excessive estrogenic stimulation, such as abnormal or excessive uterine bleeding, mastodynia, etc.

4. Oral contraceptives appear to be associated with an increased incidence of mental depression.[24a] Although it is not clear whether this is due to the estrogenic or progestogenic component of the contraceptive, patients with a history of depression should be carefully observed.

5. Preexisting uterine leiomyomata may increase in size during estrogen use.

6. The pathologist should be advised of estrogen therapy when relevant specimens are submitted.

7. Patients with a past history of jaundice during pregnancy have an increased risk of recurrence of jaundice while receiving estrogen-containing oral contraceptive therapy. If jaundice develops in any patient receiving estrogen, the medication should be discontinued while the cause is investigated.

8. Estrogens may be poorly metabolized in patients with impaired liver function and they should be administered with caution in such patients.

9. Because estrogens influence the metabolism of calcium and phosphorus, they should be used with caution in patients with metabolic bone diseases that are associated with hypercalcemia or in patients with renal insufficiency.

10. Because of the effects of estrogens on epiphyseal closure, they should be used judiciously in young patients in whom bone growth is not complete.

11. Certain endocrine and liver function tests may be affected by estrogen-containing oral contraceptives. The following similar changes may be expected with larger doses of estrogen:

a. Increased sulfobromophthalein retention.
b. Increased prothrombin and factors VII, VIII, IX, and X; decreased antithrombin 3; increased norepinephrine-induced platelet aggregability.
c. Increased thyroid binding globulin (TBG) leading to increased circulating total thyroid hormone, as measured by PBI, T4 by column, or T4 by radioimmunoassay. Free T3 resin uptake is decreased, reflecting the elevated TBG; free T4 concentration is unaltered.
d. Impaired glucose tolerance.
e. Decreased pregnanediol excretion.
f. Reduced response to metyrapone test.
g. Reduced serum folate concentration.
h. Increased serum triglyceride and phospholipid concentration.

B. Information for the Patient. See text which appears after the PHYSICIAN REFERENCES under PREMARIN®.

C. Pregnancy Category X. See CONTRAINDICATIONS and Boxed Warning.

D. Nursing Mothers. As a general principle, the administration of any drug to nursing mothers should be done only when clearly necessary since many drugs are excreted in human milk.

Associated with Meprobamate

A. The lowest effective dose should be administered, particularly to debilitated patients, in order to preclude oversedation.

B. The possibility of suicide attempts should be considered and the least amount of drug feasible should be dispensed at any one time.

C. Meprobamate is metabolized in the liver and excreted by the kidney; to avoid its excess accumulation, caution should be exercised in administration to patients with compromised liver or kidney function.

D. Meprobamate occasionally may precipitate seizures in epileptic patients.

Adverse Reactions:

Associated with Estrogen Administration

(See Warnings regarding induction of neoplasia, adverse effects on the fetus, increased incidence of gallbladder disease, and adverse effects similar to those of oral contraceptives, including thromboembolism.) The following additional adverse reactions have been reported with estrogenic therapy, including oral contraceptives:

1. *Genitourinary system:* Breakthrough bleeding, spotting, change in menstrual flow; dysmenorrhea; premenstrual-like syndrome; amenorrhea during and after treatment; increase in size of uterine fibromyomata; vaginal candidiasis; change in cervical erosion and in degree of cervical secretion; cystitis-like syndrome.

2. *Breasts:* Tenderness, enlargement, secretion.

3. *Gastrointestinal:* Nausea, vomiting; abdominal cramps, bloating; cholestatic jaundice.

4. *Skin:* Chloasma or melasma which may persist when drug is discontinued; erythema multiforme; erythema nodosum; hemorrhagic eruption; loss of scalp hair; hirsutism.

5. *Eyes:* Steepening of corneal curvature; intolerance to contact lenses.

6. *CNS:* Headache, migraine, dizziness; mental depression; chorea.

7. *Miscellaneous:* Increase or decrease in weight; reduced carbohydrate tolerance; aggravation of porphyria; edema; changes in libido.

The following have been reported with meprobamate therapy:

1. *Central Nervous System*—Drowsiness, ataxia, dizziness, slurred speech, headache, vertigo, weakness, paresthesias, impairment of visual accommodation, euphoria, overstimulation, paradoxical excitement, fast EEG activity.

2. *Gastrointestinal*—Nausea, vomiting, diarrhea.

3. *Cardiovascular*—Palpitations, tachycardia, various forms of arrhythmia, transient ECG changes, syncope; also, hypotensive crises (including one fatal case).

4. *Allergic or Idiosyncratic*—Allergic or idiosyncratic reactions are usually seen within the period of the first to fourth dose in patients having had no previous contact with the drug. Milder reactions are characterized by an itchy, urticarial, or erythematous maculopapular rash which may be generalized or confined to the groin. Other reactions have included leukopenia, acute nonthrombocytopenic purpura, petechiae, ecchymoses, eosinophilia, peripheral edema, adenopathy, fever, fixed drug eruption with cross reaction to carisoprodol, and cross sensitivity between meprobamate/-mebutamate and meprobamate/carbromal.

More severe hypersensitivity reactions, rarely reported, include hyperpyrexia, chills, angioneurotic edema, bronchospasm, oliguria, and anuria. Also, anaphylaxis, erythema multiforme, exfoliative dermatitis, stomatitis, proctitis, Stevens-Johnson syndrome, and bullous dermatitis, including one fatal case of the latter, following administration of meprobamate in combination with prednisolone.

In case of allergic or idiosyncratic reactions to meprobamate, discontinue the drug and initiate appropriate symptomatic therapy, which may include epinephrine, antihistamines, and in severe cases corticosteroids. In evaluating possible allergic reactions, also consider allergy to excipients (information on excipients is available to physicians on request).

5. *Hematologic* (See also *Allergic or Idiosyncratic.*)—Agranulocytosis and aplastic anemia have been reported, although no causal relationship has been established. These cases rarely were fatal. Rare cases of thrombocytopenic purpura have been reported.

6. *Other*—Exacerbation of porphyric symptoms.

Overdosage:

Acute overdosage (estrogen alone):

Numerous reports of ingestion of large doses of estrogen-containing oral contraceptives by young children indicate that acute serious ill effects do not occur. Overdosage of estrogen may cause nausea, and withdrawal bleeding may occur in females.

Acute simple overdosage (meprobamate alone): Death has been reported with ingestion of as little as 12 grams meprobamate and survival with as much as 40 grams.

Blood levels:

0.5—2.0 mg% represents the usual blood level range of meprobamate after therapeutic doses. The level may occasionally be as high as 3.0 mg%.

3—10 mg% usually corresponds to findings of mild to moderate symptoms of overdosage, such as stupor or light coma.

10—20 mg% usually corresponds to deeper coma, requiring more intensive treatment. Some fatalities occur.

At levels greater than 20 mg%, more fatalities than survivals can be expected.

Acute combined (alcohol or other CNS depressants or psychotropic drugs) **overdosage:** Since effects can be additive, a history of ingestion of a low dose of meprobamate plus any of these compounds (or of a relatively low blood or tissue level) cannot be used as a prognostic indicator.

In cases where excessive doses have been taken, sleep ensues rapidly and blood pressure, pulse, and respiratory rates are reduced to basal levels. Any drug remaining in the stomach should be removed and symptomatic therapy given. Should respiration or blood pressure become compromised, respiratory assistance, central nervous system stimulants, and pressor agents should be administered cautiously as indicated. Meprobamate is metabolized in the liver and excreted by the kidney. Diuresis, osmotic (mannitol) diuresis, peritoneal dialysis, and hemodialysis have been used successfully. Careful monitoring of urinary output is necessary and caution should be taken to avoid overhydration. Relapse and death, after initial recovery, have been attributed to incomplete gastric emptying and delayed absorption. Meprobamate can be measured in biological fluids by two methods: colorimetric[42] and gas chromatographic.[43]

Dosage and Administration:

Given cyclically for short term use only:

For the treatment of moderate to severe vasomotor symptoms of the menopause when anxiety and tension are part of the symptom complex and only in those cases in which the use of estrogens alone has not resulted in alleviation of such symptoms.

The lowest dose that will control symptoms should be chosen and medication should be discontinued as promptly as possible. The usual dosage of conjugated estrogen is 1.25 milligrams daily. The usual dosage of meprobamate is 1,200 to 1,600 milligrams daily.

Administration should be cyclic (e.g., three weeks on and one week off).

Attempts to discontinue or taper medication should be made at three to six month intervals.

PMB® 200 & PMB® 400: The usual dosage is one tablet of either strength three times daily administered cyclically. Use of meprobamate during the rest period should be considered for those patients who may require continuing medication with a tranquilizer. After the first few cycles of therapy, the patient's need for continuing the use of the meprobamate component should be reevaluated.

Daily dosage should be adjusted to individual requirements. The daily dosage should not exceed 6 tablets of PMB 200 per day or 4 tablets of PMB 400 per day.

Treated patients with an intact uterus should be monitored closely for signs of endometrial cancer and appropriate diagnostic measures should be taken to rule out malignancy in the event of persistent or recurring abnormal vaginal bleeding.

How Supplied: PMB® 200, in bottles of 60 (NDC 0046-0880-60).

PMB® 400, in bottles of 60 (NDC 0046-0881-60).

Physician References:

1. Ziel, H. K., *et al.*: N. Engl. J. Med. *293*:1167–1170, 1975.
2. Smith, D. C., *et al.*: N. Engl. J. Med. *293*:1164–1167, 1975.
3. Mack, T. M., *et al.*: N. Engl. J. Med. *294*:1262–1267, 1976.
4. Weiss, N. S., *et al.*: N. Engl. J. Med. *294*:1259–1262, 1976.
5. Herbst, A. L., *et al.*: N. Engl. J. Med. *284*:878–881, 1971.
6. Greenwald, P., *et al.*: N. Engl. J. Med. *285*:390–392, 1971.
7. Lanier, A., *et al.*: Mayo Clin. Proc. *48*:793–799, 1973.
8. Herbst, A., *et al.*: Obstet. Gynecol. *40*:287–298, 1972.
9. Herbst, A., *et al.*: Am. J. Obstet. Gynecol. *118*:607–615, 1974.
10. Herbst, A., *et al.*: N. Engl. J. Med. *292*:334–339, 1975.
11. Stafl, A., *et al.*: Obstet. Gynecol. *43*:118–128, 1974.
12. Sherman, A. I., *et al.*: Obstet. Gynecol. *44*:531–545, 1974.
13. Gal, I., *et al.*: Nature *216*:83, 1967.
14. Levy, E. P., *et al.*: Lancet *1*:611, 1973.
15. Nora, J., *et al.*: Lancet *1*:941–942, 1973.
16. Janerich, D. T., *et al.*: N. Engl. J. Med. *291*:697–700, 1974.
17. Boston Collaborative Drug Surveillance Program: N. Engl. J. Med. *290*:15–19, 1974.
18. Hoover, R., *et al.*: N. Engl. J. Med. *295*:401–405, 1976.
19. Boston Collaborative Drug Surveillance Program: Lancet *1*:1399–1404, 1973.
20. Daniel, D. G., *et al.*: Lancet *2*:287–289, 1967.
21. The Veterans Administration Cooperative Urological Research Group: J. Urol. *98*:516–522, 1967.
22. Bailar, J. C.: Lancet *2*:560, 1967.
23. Blackard, C., *et al.*: Cancer *26*:249–256, 1970.
24. Royal College of General Practitioners: J. R. Coll. Gen. Pract. *13*:267–279, 1967.

24a. Royal College of General Practitioners: Oral Contraceptives and Health New York, Pitman Corp., 1974.

25. Inman, W. H. W., *et al.*: Br. Med. J. *2*:193–199, 1968.
26. Vessey, M. P., *et al.*: Br. Med. J. *2*:651–657, 1969.
27. Sartwell, P. E., *et al.*: Am. J. Epidemiol. *90*:365–380, 1969.
28. Collaborative Group for the Study of Stroke in Young Women: N. Engl. J. Med. *288*:871–878, 1973.
29. Collaborative Group for the Study of Stroke in Young Women: J.A.M.A. *231*:718–722, 1975.
30. Mann, J. I., *et al.*: Br. Med. J. *2*:245–248, 1975.
31. Mann, J. I., *et al.*: Br. Med. J. *2*:241–245, 1975.
32. Inman, W. H. W., *et al.*: Br. Med. J. *2*:203–209, 1970.
33. Stolley, P. D., *et al.*: Am. J. Epidemiol. *102*:197–208, 1975.
34. Vessey, M. P., *et al.*: Br. Med. J. *3*:123–126, 1970.
35. Greene, G. R., *et al.*: Am. J. Public Health *62*:680–685, 1972.
36. Rosenberg, L., *et al.*: N. Engl. J. Med. *294*:1256–1259, 1976.
37. Coronary Drug Project Research Group: J.A.M.A. *214*:1303–1313, 1970.
38. Baum, J., *et al.*: Lancet *2*:926–928, 1973.
39. Mays, E. T., *et al.*: J.A.M.A. *235*:730–732, 1976.
40. Edmondson, H. A., *et al.*: N. Engl. J. Med. *294*:470–472, 1976.
41. Pfeffer, R. I., *et al.*: Am. J. Epidemiol. *103*:445–456, 1976.
42. Hoffman, A. J., *et al.*: J. Am. Pharm. Assoc. *48*:740, 1959.
43. Douglas, J. F., *et al.*: Anal. Chem. *39*:956, 1967.

[*Shown in Product Identification Section*]

PREMARIN® INTRAVENOUS ℞

Brand of Conjugated Estrogens, U.S.P., for Injection

Specially prepared for Intravenous & Intramuscular use

1. ESTROGENS HAVE BEEN REPORTED TO INCREASE THE RISK OF ENDOMETRIAL CARCINOMA.

Three independent case control studies have reported an increased risk of endometrial cancer in postmenopausal women exposed to exogenous estrogens for more than one year.[1–3] This risk was independent of the other known risk factors for endometrial cancer. These studies are further supported by the finding that incidence rates of endometrial cancer have increased sharply since 1969 in eight different areas of the United States with population-based cancer reporting systems, an increase which may be related to the rapidly expanding use of estrogens during the last decade.[4]

The three case control studies reported that the risk of endometrial cancer in estrogen users was about 4.5 to 13.9 times greater than in nonusers. The risk appears to depend on both duration of treatment[1] and on estrogen dose.[3] In view of these findings, when estrogens are used for the treatment of menopausal symptoms, the lowest dose that will control symptoms should be utilized and medication should be discontinued as soon as possible. When prolonged treatment is medically indicated, the patient should be reassessed on at least a semiannual basis to determine the need for continued therapy. Although the evidence must be considered preliminary, one study suggests that cyclic administration of low doses of estrogen may carry less risk than continuous administration;[3] it therefore appears prudent to utilize such a regimen.

Close clinical surveillance of all women taking estrogens is important. In all cases of undiagnosed persistent or recurring abnormal vaginal bleeding, adequate diagnostic measures should be undertaken to rule out malignancy.

There is no evidence at present that "natural" estrogens are more or less hazardous than "synthetic" estrogens at equiestrogenic doses.

2. ESTROGENS SHOULD NOT BE USED DURING PREGNANCY.

The use of female sex hormones, both estrogens and progestogens, during early pregnancy may seriously damage the offspring. It has been shown that females exposed in utero to diethylstilbestrol, a non-steroidal estrogen, have an increased risk of developing in later life a form of vaginal or cervical cancer that is ordinarily extremely rare.[5,6] This risk has been estimated as not greater than 4 per 1000 exposures.[7] Furthermore, a high percentage of such exposed women (from 30 to 90 percent) have been found to have vaginal adenosis,[8–12] epithelial changes of the vagina and cervix. Although these changes are histologically benign, it is not known whether they are precursors of malignancy. Although similar data are not available with the use of other estrogens, it cannot be presumed they would not induce similar changes.

Several reports suggest an association between intrauterine exposure to female sex hormones and congenital anomalies, including congenital heart defects and limb reduction defects.[13–16] One case control study[16] estimated a 4.7-fold increased risk of limb reduction defects in infants exposed in utero to sex hormones (oral contraceptives, hormone withdrawal tests for pregnancy, or attempted treatment for threatened abortion). Some of these exposures were very short and involved only a few days of treatment. The data suggest that the risk of limb reduction defects in exposed fetuses is somewhat less than 1 per 1000.

In the past, female sex hormones have been used during pregnancy in an attempt to treat threatened or habitual abortion. There is considerable evidence that estrogens are ineffective for these indications, and there is no evidence from well controlled studies that progestogens are effective for these uses.

If PREMARIN Intravenous (Conjugated Estrogens, U.S.P., for Injection) is used during pregnancy, or if the patient becomes pregnant while taking this drug, she should be apprised of the potential risks to the fetus, and the advisability of pregnancy continuation.

Description: Each Secule® contains 25 mg of Conjugated Estrogens, U.S.P. in a sterile lyophilized cake which also contains lactose 200 mg, sodium citrate 12.5 mg and simethicone 0.2 mg. The pH is adjusted with sodium hydroxide or hydrochloric acid. A sterile diluent (5 ml) containing 2% benzyl alcohol and Water for Injection, U.S.P. is provided for reconstitution. The reconstituted solution is suitable for intravenous or intramuscular injection.

PREMARIN (Conjugated Estrogens, U.S.P.) is a mixture of estrogens obtained exclusively from natural sources, occurring as the sodium salts of water-soluble estrogen sulfates blended to represent the average composition of material derived from pregnant mares' urine. It contains estrone, equilin, and 17 α-dihydroequilin, together with smaller amounts of 17 α-estradiol, equilenin, and 17 α-dihydroequilenin as salts of their sulfate esters.

Clinical Pharmacology: Estrogens are important in the development and maintenance of the female reproductive system and secondary sex characteristics. They promote growth and development of the vagina, uterus, and fallopian tubes, and enlargement of the breasts. Indirectly, they contribute to the shaping of the skeleton, maintenance of tone and elasticity of urogenital structures, changes in the epiphyses of the long bones that allow for the pubertal growth spurt and its termination, growth of axillary and pubic hair, and pigmentation of the nipples and genitals. Decline of

Continued on next page

Ayerst—Cont.

estrogenic activity at the end of the menstrual cycle can bring on menstruation, although the cessation of progesterone secretion is the most important factor in the mature ovulatory cycle. However, in the preovulatory or nonovulatory cycle, estrogen is the primary determinant in the onset of menstruation. Estrogens also affect the release of pituitary gonadotropins.

The pharmacologic effects of conjugated estrogens are similar to those of endogenous estrogens. They are soluble in water and may be administered by intravenous or intramuscular injection.

In responsive tissues (female genital organs, breasts, hypothalamus, pituitary) estrogens enter the cell and are transported into the nucleus. As a result of estrogen action, specific RNA and protein synthesis occurs.

Metabolism and inactivation occur primarily in the liver. Some estrogens are excreted into the bile; however they are reabsorbed from the intestine and returned to the liver through the portal venous system. Water-soluble estrogen conjugates are strongly acidic and are ionized in body fluids, which favor excretion through the kidneys since tubular reabsorption is minimal.

Indication: PREMARIN Intravenous (Conjugated Estrogens, U.S.P., for Injection) is indicated in the treatment of abnormal uterine bleeding due to hormonal imbalance in the absence of organic pathology.

Contraindications: Estrogens should not be used in women with any of the following conditions:

1. Known or suspected cancer of the breast except in appropriately selected patients being treated for metastatic disease.
2. Known or suspected estrogen-dependent neoplasia.
3. Known or suspected pregnancy (See Boxed Warning).
4. Undiagnosed abnormal genital bleeding.
5. Active thrombophlebitis or thromboembolic disorders.
6. A past history of thrombophlebitis, thrombosis, or thromboembolic disorders associated with previous estrogen use (except when used in treatment of breast malignancy).

Warnings:

1. *Induction of malignant neoplasms.* Long term continuous administration of natural and synthetic estrogens in certain animal species increases the frequency of carcinomas of the breast, cervix, vagina, and liver. There are now reports that estrogens increase the risk of carcinoma of the endometrium in humans. (See Boxed Warning.)

At the present time there is no satisfactory evidence that estrogens given to postmenopausal women increase the risk of cancer of the breast,[17] although a recent long-term followup of a single physician's practice has raised this possibility.[18] Because of the animal data, there is a need for caution in prescribing estrogens for women with a strong family history of breast cancer or who have breast nodules, fibrocystic disease, or abnormal mammograms.

2. *Gallbladder disease.* A recent study has reported a 2 to 3-fold increase in the risk of surgically confirmed gallbladder disease in women receiving postmenopausal estrogens,[17] similar to the 2-fold increase previously noted in users of oral contraceptives.[19,24a]

3. *Effects similar to those caused by estrogen-progestogen oral contraceptives.* There are several serious adverse effects of oral contraceptives, most of which have not, up to now, been documented as consequences of postmenopausal estrogen therapy. This may reflect the comparatively low doses of estrogen used in postmenopausal women. It would be expected that the larger doses of estrogen used to treat prostatic or breast cancer or postpartum breast engorgement are more likely to result in these adverse effects, and, in fact, it has been shown that there is an increased risk of thrombosis in men receiving estrogens for prostatic cancer and women for postpartum breast engorgement.[20–23]

a. *Thromboembolic disease.* It is now well established that users of oral contraceptives have an increased risk of various thromboembolic and thrombotic vascular diseases, such as thrombophlebitis, pulmonary embolism, stroke, and myocardial infarction.[24–31] Cases of retinal thrombosis, mesenteric thrombosis, and optic neuritis have been reported in oral contraceptive users. There is evidence that the risk of several of these adverse reactions is related to the dose of the drug.[32,33] An increased risk of postsurgery thromboembolic complications has also been reported in users of oral contraceptives.[34,35] If feasible, estrogen should be discontinued at least 4 weeks before surgery of the type associated with an increased risk of thromboembolism, or during periods of prolonged immobilization.

While an increased rate of thromboembolic and thrombotic disease in postmenopausal users of estrogens has not been found,[17–24,25–36] this does not rule out the possibility that such an increase may be present or that subgroups of women who have underlying risk factors or who are receiving relatively large doses of estrogens may have increased risk. Therefore estrogens should not be used in persons with active thrombophlebitis or thromboembolic disorders, and they should not be used (except in treatment of malignancy) in persons with a history of such disorders in association with estrogen use. They should be used with caution in patients with cerebral vascular or coronary artery disease and only for those in whom estrogens are clearly needed.

Large doses of estrogen (5 mg conjugated estrogens per day), comparable to those used to treat cancer of the prostate and breast, have been shown in a large prospective clinical trial in men[37] to increase the risk of nonfatal myocardial infarction, pulmonary embolism and thrombophlebitis. When estrogen doses of this size are used, any of the thromboembolic and thrombotic adverse effects associated with oral contraceptive use should be considered a clear risk.

b. *Hepatic adenoma.* Benign hepatic adenomas appear to be associated with the use of oral contraceptives.[38–40] Although benign, and rare, these may rupture and may cause death through intra-abdominal hemorrhage. Such lesions have not yet been reported in association with other estrogen or progestogen preparations but should be considered in estrogen users having abdominal pain and tenderness, abdominal mass, or hypovolemic shock. Hepatocellular carcinoma has also been reported in women taking estrogen-containing oral contraceptives.[39] The relationship of this malignancy to these drugs is not known at this time.

c. *Elevated blood pressure.* Women using oral contraceptives sometimes experience increased blood pressure which, in most cases, returns to normal on discontinuing the drug. There is now a report that this may occur with use of estrogens in the menopause[41] and blood pressure should be monitored with estrogen use, especially if high doses are used.

d. *Glucose tolerance.* A worsening of glucose tolerance has been observed in a significant percentage of patients on estrogen-containing oral contraceptives. For this reason, diabetic patients should be carefully observed while receiving estrogen.

4. *Hypercalcemia.* Administration of estrogens may lead to severe hypercalcemia in patients with breast cancer and bone metastases. If this occurs, the drug should be stopped and appropriate measures taken to reduce the serum calcium level.

Precautions:

A. General Precautions.

1. A complete medical and family history should be taken prior to the initiation of any estrogen therapy. The pretreatment and periodic physical examinations should include special reference to blood pressure, breasts, abdomen, and pelvic organs, and should include a Papanicolau smear. As a general rule, estrogen should not be prescribed for longer than one year without another physical examination being performed.
2. Fluid retention—Because estrogens may cause some degree of fluid retention, conditions which might be influenced by this factor such as asthma, epilepsy, migraine, and cardiac or renal dysfunction, require careful observation.
3. Certain patients may develop undesirable manifestations of excessive estrogenic stimulation, such as abnormal or excessive uterine bleeding, mastodynia, etc.
4. Oral contraceptives appear to be associated with an increased incidence of mental depression.[24a] Although it is not clear whether this is due to the estrogenic or progestogenic component of the contraceptive, patients with a history of depression should be carefully observed.
5. Preexisting uterine leiomyomata may increase in size during estrogen use.
6. The pathologist should be advised of estrogen therapy when relevant specimens are submitted.
7. Patients with a past history of jaundice during pregnancy have an increased risk of recurrence of jaundice while receiving estrogen-containing oral contraceptive therapy. If jaundice develops in any patient receiving estrogen, the medication should be discontinued while the cause is investigated.
8. Estrogens may be poorly metabolized in patients with impaired liver function and they should be administered with caution in such patients.
9. Because estrogens influence the metabolism of calcium and phosphorus, they should be used with caution in patients with metabolic bone diseases that are associated with hypercalcemia or in patients with renal insufficiency.
10. Because of the effects of estrogens on epiphyseal closure, they should be used judiciously in young patients in whom bone growth is not complete.
11. Certain endocrine and liver function tests may be affected by estrogen-containing oral contraceptives. The following similar changes may be expected with larger doses of estrogen:

a. Increased sulfobromophthalein retention.
b. Increased prothrombin and factors VII, VIII, IX, and X; decreased antithrombin 3; increased norepinephrine-induced platelet aggregability.
c. Increased thyroid binding globulin (TBG) leading to increased circulating total thyroid hormone, as measured by PBI, T4 by column, or T4 by radioimmunoassay. Free T3 resin uptake is decreased, reflecting the elevated TBG; free T4 concentration is unaltered.
d. Impaired glucose tolerance.
e. Decreased pregnanediol excretion.
f. Reduced response to metyrapone test.
g. Reduced serum folate concentration.
h. Increased serum triglyceride and phospholipid concentration.

B. Information for the Patient. See text which appears after the PHYSICIAN REFERENCES under PREMARIN®.

C. Pregnancy Category X. See CONTRAINDICATIONS and Boxed Warning.

D. Nursing Mothers. As a general principle, the administration of any drug to nursing mothers should be done only when clearly necessary since many drugs are excreted in human milk.

Adverse Reactions: (See Warnings regarding induction of neoplasia, adverse effects on the fetus, increased incidence of gallbladder disease, and adverse effects similar to those of oral contraceptives, including thromboembolism.) The following additional adverse reactions have been reported with estrogenic therapy, including oral contraceptives:

1. *Genitourinary system:* Breakthrough bleeding, spotting, change in menstrual flow; dysmenorrhea; premenstrual-like syndrome; amenorrhea during and after treatment; increase in size of uterine fibromyomata; vaginal candidiasis; change in cervical erosion and in degree of cervical secretion; cystitis-like syndrome.
2. *Breasts:* Tenderness, enlargement, secretion.
3. *Gastrointestinal:* Nausea, vomiting; abdominal cramps, bloating; cholestatic jaundice.
4. *Skin:* Chloasma or melasma which may persist when drug is discontinued; erythema multiforme; erythema nodosum; hemorrhagic eruption; loss of scalp hair; hirsutism.
5. *Eyes:* Steepening of corneal curvature; intolerance to contact lenses.
6. *CNS:* Headache, migraine, dizziness; mental depression; chorea.
7. *Miscellaneous:* Increase or decrease in weight; reduced carbohydrate tolerance; aggravation of porphyria; edema; changes in libido.

Acute Overdosage: Numerous reports of ingestion of large doses of estrogen-containing oral contraceptives by young children indicate that acute serious ill effects do not occur. Overdosage of estrogen may cause nausea, and withdrawal bleeding may occur in females.

Dosage and Administration:
Abnormal uterine bleeding due to hormonal imbalance: One 25 mg injection, intravenously or intramuscularly. Intravenous use is preferred since more rapid response can be expected from this mode of administration.
Repeat in 6 to 12 hours if necessary. The use of PREMARIN Intravenous (Conjugated Estrogens, U.S.P., for Injection) does not preclude the advisability of other appropriate measures.

The usual precautionary measures governing intravenous administration should be adhered to. Injection should be made SLOWLY to obviate the occurrence of flushes.
Infusion of PREMARIN Intravenous (Conjugated Estrogens, U.S.P., for Injection) with other agents is not generally recommended. In emergencies, however, when an infusion has already been started, it may be expedient to make the injection into the tubing just distal to the infusion needle. If so used, compatibility of solutions must be considered.
Compatibility of solutions: PREMARIN Intravenous is compatible with normal saline, dextrose, and invert sugar solutions. IT IS NOT COMPATIBLE WITH PROTEIN HYDROLYSATE, ASCORBIC ACID, OR ANY SOLUTION WITH AN ACID pH.
Treated patients with an intact uterus should be monitored closely for signs of endometrial cancer and appropriate diagnostic measures should be taken to rule out malignancy in the event of persistent or recurring abnormal vaginal bleeding.

Directions for Storage and Reconstitution:
Storage before reconstitution: Store package in refrigerator, 2–8°C (36–46°F).
To reconstitute: First withdraw air from SECULE so as to facilitate introduction of sterile diluent. Then, flow the sterile diluent slowly against side of SECULE and agitate gently. DO NOT SHAKE VIOLENTLY.
Storage after reconstitution: It is common practice to utilize the reconstituted solution within a few hours. If it is necessary to keep the reconstituted solution for more than a few hours, store the reconstituted solution under refrigeration (2–8°C). Under these conditions, the solution is stable for 60 days, and is suitable for use unless darkening or precipitation occurs.

How Supplied: NDC 0046-0552-05-Each package provides: (1)One SECULE® containing 25 mg of Conjugated Estrogens, U.S.P., for Injection (also lactose 200 mg, sodium citrate 12.5 mg, and simethicone 0.2 mg). The pH is adjusted with sodium hydroxide or hydrochloric acid. (2)One 5 ml ampul sterile diluent with benzyl alcohol 2%, and Water for Injection, U.S.P.
PREMARIN Intravenous (Conjugated Estrogens, U.S.P., for Injection) is prepared by cryodesiccation.

Physician References:

1. Ziel, H. K., *et al.:* N. Engl. J. Med. *293*:1167–1170, 1975.
2. Smith, D. C., *et al.:* N. Engl. J. Med. *293*:1164–1167, 1975.
3. Mack, T. M., *et al.:* N. Engl. J. Med. *294*:1262–1267, 1976.
4. Weiss, N. S., *et al.:* N. Engl. J. Med. *294*:1259–1262, 1976.
5. Herbst, A. L., *et al.:* N. Engl. J. Med. *284*:878–881, 1971.
6. Greenwald, P., *et al.:* N. Engl. J. Med. *285*:390–392, 1971.
7. Lanier, A., *et al.:* Mayo Clin. Proc. *48*:793–799, 1973.
8. Herbst, A., *et al.:* Obstet. Gynecol. *40*:287–298, 1972.
9. Herbst, A., *et al.:* Am. J. Obstet. Gynecol. *118*:607–615, 1974.
10. Herbst, A., *et al.:* N. Engl. J. Med. *292*:334–339, 1975.
11. Stafl, A., *et al.:* Obstet. Gynecol. *43*:118–128, 1974.
12. Sherman, A. I., *et al.:* Obstet. Gynecol. *44*:531–545, 1974.
13. Gal, I., *et al.:* Nature *216*:83, 1967.
14. Levy, E. P., *et al.:* Lancet *1*:611, 1973.
15. Nora, J., *et al.:* Lancet *1*:941–942, 1973.
16. Janerich, D. T., *et al.:* N. Engl. J. Med. *291*:697–700, 1974.
17. Boston Collaborative Drug Surveillance Program: N. Engl. J. Med. *290*:15–19, 1974.
18. Hoover, R., *et al.:* N. Engl. J. Med. *295*:401–405, 1976.
19. Boston Collaborative Drug Surveillance Program: Lancet *1*:1399–1404, 1973.
20. Daniel, D. G., *et al.:* Lancet *2*:287–289, 1967.
21. The Veterans Administration Cooperative Urological Research Group: J. Urol. *98*:516–522, 1967.
22. Bailar, J. C.: Lancet *2*:560, 1967.
23. Blackard, C., *et al.:* Cancer *26*:249–256, 1970.
24. Royal College of General Practitioners: J. R. Coll. Gen. Pract. *13*:267–279, 1967.
24a. Royal College of General Practitioners: Oral Contraceptives and Health, New York, Pitman Corp., 1974.
25. Inman, W. H. W., *et al.:* Br. Med. J. *2*:193–199, 1968.
26. Vessey, M. P., *et al.:* Br. Med. J. *2*:651–657, 1969.
27. Sartwell, P. E., *et al.:* Am. J. Epidemiol. *90*:365–380, 1969.
28. Collaborative Group for the Study of Stroke in Young Women: N. Engl. J. Med. *288*:871–878, 1973.
29. Collaborative Group for the Study of Stroke in Young Women: J.A.M.A. *231*:718–722, 1975.
30. Mann, J. I., *et al.:* Br. Med. J. *2*:245–248, 1975.
31. Mann, J. I., *et al.:* Br. Med. J. *2*:241–245, 1975.
32. Inman, W. H. W., *et al.:* Br. Med. J. *2*:203–209, 1970.
33. Stolley, P. D., *et al.:* Am. J. Epidemiol. *102*:197–208, 1975.
34. Vessey, M. P., *et al.:* Br. Med. J. *3*:123–126, 1970.
35. Greene, G. R., *et al.:* Am. J. Public Health *62*:680–685, 1972.
36. Rosenberg, L., *et al.:* N. Engl. J. Med. *294*:1256–1259, 1976.
37. Coronary Drug Project Research Group: J.A.M.A. *214*:1303–1313, 1970.
38. Baum, J., *et al.:* Lancet *2*:926–928, 1973.
39. Mays, E. T., *et al.:* J.A.M.A. *235*:730–732, 1976.
40. Edmondson, H. A., *et al.:* N. Engl. J. Med. *294*:470–472, 1976.
41. Pfeffer, R. I., *et al.:* Am. J. Epidemiol. *103*:445–456, 1976.

PREMARIN® ℞
Brand of Conjugated Estrogens Tablets, U.S.P.

1. ESTROGENS HAVE BEEN REPORTED TO INCREASE THE RISK OF ENDOMETRIAL CARCINOMA.
Three independent case control studies have reported an increased risk of endometrial cancer in postmenopausal women exposed to exogenous estrogens for more than one year.[1–3] This risk was independent of the other known risk factors for endometrial cancer. These studies are further supported by the finding that incidence rates of endometrial cancer have increased sharply since 1969 in eight different areas of the United States with population-based cancer reporting systems, an increase which may be related to the rapidly expanding use of estrogens during the last decade.[4]
The three case control studies reported that the risk of endometrial cancer in estrogen users was about 4.5 to 13.9 times greater than in nonusers. The risk appears to depend on both duration of treatment[1] and on estrogen dose.[3] In view of these findings, when estrogens are used for the treatment of menopausal symptoms, the lowest dose that will control symptoms should be utilized and medication should be discontinued as soon as possible. When prolonged treatment is medically indicated, the patient should be reassessed on at least a semiannual basis to determine the need for continued therapy. Although the evidence must be considered preliminary, one study suggests that cyclic administration of low doses of estrogen may carry less risk than continuous administration;[3] it therefore appears prudent to utilize such a regimen.
Close clinical surveillance of all women taking estrogens is important. In all cases of undiagnosed persistent or recurring abnormal vaginal bleeding, adequate diagnostic measures should be undertaken to rule out malignancy.
There is no evidence at present that "natural" estrogens are more or less hazardous than "synthetic" estrogens at equiestrogenic doses.

2. ESTROGENS SHOULD NOT BE USED DURING PREGNANCY.
The use of female sex hormones, both estrogens and progestogens, during early pregnancy may seriously damage the offspring. It has been shown that females exposed in utero to diethylstilbestrol, a non-steroidal estrogen, have an increased risk of developing in later life a form of vaginal or cervical cancer that is ordinarily extremely rare.[5,6] This risk has been estimated as not greater than 4 per 1000 exposures.[7] Furthermore, a high percentage of such exposed women (from 30 to 90 percent) have been found to have vaginal adenosis,[8–12] epithelial changes of the vagina and cervix. Although these changes are histologically benign, it is not known whether they are precursors of

Continued on next page

Ayerst—Cont.

malignancy. Although similar data are not available with the use of other estrogens, it cannot be presumed they would not induce similar changes.
Several reports suggest an association between intrauterine exposure to female sex hormones and congenital anomalies, including congenital heart defects and limb reduction defects.[13–16] One case control study[16] estimated a 4.7-fold increased risk of limb reduction defects in infants exposed in utero to sex hormones (oral contraceptives, hormone withdrawal tests for pregnancy, or attempted treatment for threatened abortion). Some of these exposures were very short and involved only a few days of treatment. The data suggest that the risk of limb reduction defects in exposed fetuses is somewhat less than 1 per 1000.
In the past, female sex hormones have been used during pregnancy in an attempt to treat threatened or habitual abortion. There is considerable evidence that estrogens are ineffective for these indications, and there is no evidence from well controlled studies that progestogens are effective for these uses.
If PREMARIN is used during pregnancy, or if the patient becomes pregnant while taking this drug, she should be apprised of the potential risks to the fetus, and the advisability of pregnancy continuation.

Description: PREMARIN (Conjugated Estrogens Tablets, U.S.P.) for oral administration contains a mixture of estrogens, obtained exclusively from natural sources, occurring as the sodium salts of water-soluble estrogen sulfates blended to represent the average composition of material derived from pregnant mares' urine. It contains estrone, equilin, and 17 α-dihydroequilin, together with smaller amounts of 17 α-estradiol, equilenin, and 17 α-dihydroequilenin as salts of their sulfate esters.

Clinical Pharmacology: Estrogens are important in the development and maintenance of the female reproductive system and secondary sex characteristics. They promote growth and development of the vagina, uterus, and fallopian tubes, and enlargement of the breasts. Indirectly, they contribute to the shaping of the skeleton, maintenance of tone and elasticity of urogenital structures, changes in the epiphyses of the long bones that allow for the pubertal growth spurt and its termination, growth of axillary and pubic hair, and pigmentation of the nipples and genitals. Decline of estrogenic activity at the end of the menstrual cycle can bring on menstruation, although the cessation of progesterone secretion is the most important factor in the mature ovulatory cycle. However, in the preovulatory or nonovulatory cycle, estrogen is the primary determinant in the onset of menstruation. Estrogens also affect the release of pituitary gonadotropins.
The pharmacologic effects of conjugated estrogens are similar to those of endogenous estrogens. They are soluble in water and are well absorbed from the gastrointestinal tract.
In responsive tissues (female genital organs, breasts, hypothalamus, pituitary) estrogens enter the cell and are transported into the nucleus. As a result of estrogen action, specific RNA and protein synthesis occurs.
Metabolism and inactivation occur primarily in the liver. Some estrogens are excreted into the bile; however they are reabsorbed from the intestine and returned to the liver through the portal venous system. Water soluble estrogen conjugates are strongly acidic and are ionized in body fluids, which favor excretion through the kidneys since tubular reabsorption is minimal.

Indications: Based on a review of PREMARIN Tablets by the National Academy of Sciences—National Research Council and/or other information, FDA has classified the indications for use as follows:
Effective: 1. Moderate to severe *vasomotor* symptoms associated with the menopause. (There is no evidence that estrogens are effective for nervous symptoms or depression without associated vasomotor symptoms, and they should not be used to treat such conditions.)
2. Atrophic vaginitis.
3. Kraurosis vulvae.
4. Female hypogonadism.
5. Female castration.
6. Primary ovarian failure.
7. Breast cancer (for palliation only) in appropriately selected women and men with metastatic disease.
8. Prostatic carcinoma—palliative therapy of advanced disease.
9. Postpartum breast engorgement—Although estrogens have been widely used for the prevention of postpartum breast engorgement, controlled studies have demonstrated that the incidence of significant painful engorgement in patients not receiving such hormonal therapy is low and usually responsive to appropriate analgesic or other supportive therapy. Consequently, the benefit to be derived from estrogen therapy for this indication must be carefully weighed against the potential increased risk of puerperal thromboembolism associated with the use of large doses of estrogens.[20]
PREMARIN HAS NOT BEEN SHOWN TO BE EFFECTIVE FOR ANY PURPOSE DURING PREGNANCY AND ITS USE MAY CAUSE SEVERE HARM TO THE FETUS (SEE BOXED WARNING).
"Probably" effective: For estrogen deficiency-induced osteoporosis, and only when used in conjunction with other important therapeutic measures such as diet, calcium, physiotherapy, and good general health-promoting measures. Final classification of this indication requires further investigation.

Contraindications: Estrogens should not be used in women (or men) with any of the following conditions:
1. Known or suspected cancer of the breast except in appropriately selected patients being treated for metastatic disease.
2. Known or suspected estrogen-dependent neoplasia.
3. Known or suspected pregnancy (See Boxed Warning).
4. Undiagnosed abnormal genital bleeding.
5. Active thrombophlebitis or thromboembolic disorders.
6. A past history of thrombophlebitis, thrombosis, or thromboembolic disorders associated with previous estrogen use (except when used in treatment of breast or prostatic malignancy).

Warnings:
1. *Induction of malignant neoplasms.* Long term continuous administration of natural and synthetic estrogens in certain animal species increases the frequency of carcinomas of the breast, cervix, vagina, and liver. There are now reports that estrogens increase the risk of carcinoma of the endometrium in humans. (See Boxed Warning.)
At the present time there is no satisfactory evidence that estrogens given to postmenopausal women increase the risk of cancer of the breast,[17] although a recent long-term followup of a single physician's practice has raised this possibility.[18] Because of the animal data, there is a need for caution in prescribing estrogens for women with a strong family history of breast cancer or who have breast nodules, fibrocystic disease, or abnormal mammograms.
2. *Gallbladder disease.* A recent study has reported a 2 to 3-fold increase in the risk of surgically confirmed gallbladder disease in women receiving postmenopausal estrogens,[17] similar to the 2-fold increase previously noted in users of oral contraceptives.[19,24a]
3. *Effects similar to those caused by estrogen-progestogen oral contraceptives.* There are several serious adverse effects of oral contraceptives, most of which have not, up to now, been documented as consequences of postmenopausal estrogen therapy. This may reflect the comparatively low doses of estrogen used in postmenopausal women. It would be expected that the larger doses of estrogen used to treat prostatic or breast cancer or postpartum breast engorgement are more likely to result in these adverse effects, and, in fact, it has been shown that there is an increased risk of thrombosis in men receiving estrogens for prostatic cancer and women for postpartum breast engorgement.[20–23]
a. *Thromboembolic disease.* It is now well established that users of oral contraceptives have an increased risk of various thromboembolic and thrombotic vascular diseases, such as thrombophlebitis, pulmonary embolism, stroke, and myocardial infarction.[24–31] Cases of retinal thrombosis, mesenteric thrombosis, and optic neuritis have been reported in oral contraceptive users. There is evidence that the risk of several of these adverse reactions is related to the dose of the drug.[32,33] An increased risk of postsurgery thromboembolic complications has also been reported in users of oral contraceptives.[34,35] If feasible, estrogen should be discontinued at least 4 weeks before surgery of the type associated with an increased risk of thromboembolism, or during periods of prolonged immobilization.
While an increased rate of thromboembolic and thrombotic disease in postmenopausal users of estrogens has not been found,[17–24,25–36] this does not rule out the possibility that such an increase may be present or that subgroups of women who have underlying risk factors or who are receiving relatively large doses of estrogens may have increased risk. Therefore estrogens should not be used in persons with active thrombophlebitis or thomboembolic disorders, and they should not be used (except in treatment of malignancy) in persons with a history of such disorders in association with estrogen use. They should be used with caution in patients with cerebral vascular or coronary artery disease and only for those in whom estrogens are clearly needed.
Large doses of estrogen (5 mg conjugated estrogens per day), comparable to those used to treat cancer of the prostate and breast, have been shown in a large prospective clinical trial in men[37] to increase the risk of nonfatal myocardial infarction, pulmonary embolism and thrombophlebitis. When estrogen doses of this size are used, any of the thromboembolic and thrombotic adverse effects associated with oral contraceptive use should be considered a clear risk.
b. *Hepatic adenoma.* Benign hepatic adenomas appear to be associated with the use of oral contraceptives.[38–40] Although benign, and rare, these may rupture and may cause death through intra-abdominal hemorrhage. Such lesions have not yet been reported in association with other estrogen or progestogen preparations but should be considered in estrogen users having abdominal pain and tenderness, abdominal mass, or hypovolemic shock. Hepatocellular carcinoma has also been reported in women taking estrogen-containing oral contraceptives.[39] The relationship of this malignancy to these drugs is not known at this time.

c. *Elevated blood pressure.* Women using oral contraceptives sometimes experience increased blood pressure which, in most cases, returns to normal on discontinuing the drug. There is now a report that this may occur with use of estrogens in the menopause[41] and blood pressure should be monitored with estrogen use, especially if high doses are used.
d. *Glucose tolerance.* A worsening of glucose tolerance has been observed in a significant percentage of patients on estrogen-containing oral contraceptives. For this reason, diabetic patients should be carefully observed while receiving estrogen.
4. *Hypercalcemia.* Administration of estrogens may lead to severe hypercalcemia in patients with breast cancer and bone metastases. If this occurs, the drug should be stopped and appropriate measures taken to reduce the serum calcium level.

Precautions:

A. General Precautions.

1. A complete medical and family history should be taken prior to the initiation of any estrogen therapy. The pretreatment and periodic physical examinations should include special reference to blood pressure, breasts, abdomen, and pelvic organs, and should include a Papanicolau smear. As a general rule, estrogen should not be prescribed for longer than one year without another physical examination being performed.
2. Fluid retention—Because estrogens may cause some degree of fluid retention, conditions which might be influenced by this factor such as asthma, epilepsy, migraine, and cardiac or renal dysfunction, require careful observation.
3. Certain patients may develop undesirable manifestations of excessive estrogenic stimulation, such as abnormal or excessive uterine bleeding, mastodynia, etc.
4. Oral contraceptives appear to be associated with an increased incidence of mental depression.[24a] Although it is not clear whether this is due to the estrogenic or progestogenic component of the contraceptive, patients with a history of depression should be carefully observed.
5. Preexisting uterine leiomyomata may increase in size during estrogen use.
6. The pathologist should be advised of estrogen therapy when relevant specimens are submitted.
7. Patients with a past history of jaundice during pregnancy have an increased risk of recurrence of jaundice while receiving estrogen-containing oral contraceptive therapy. If jaundice develops in any patient receiving estrogen, the medication should be discontinued while the cause is investigated.
8. Estrogens may be poorly metabolized in patients with impaired liver function and they should be administered with caution in such patients.
9. Because estrogens influence the metabolism of calcium and phosphorus, they should be used with caution in patients with metabolic bone diseases that are associated with hypercalcemia or in patients with renal insufficiency.
10. Because of the effects of estrogens on epiphyseal closure, they should be used judiciously in young patients in whom bone growth is not complete.
11. Certain endocrine and liver function tests may be affected by estrogen-containing oral contraceptives. The following similar changes may be expected with larger doses of estrogen:
a. Increased sulfobromophthalein retention.
b. Increased prothrombin and factors VII, VIII, IX, and X; decreased antithrombin 3; increased norepinephrine-induced platelet aggregability.
c. Increased thyroid binding globulin (TBG) leading to increased circulating total thyroid hormone, as measured by PBI, T4 by column, or T4 by radioimmunoassay. Free T3 resin uptake is decreased, reflecting the elevated TBG; free T4 concentration is unaltered.
d. Impaired glucose tolerance.
e. Decreased pregnanediol excretion.
f. Reduced response to metyrapone test.
g. Reduced serum folate concentration.
h. Increased serum triglyceride and phospholipid concentration.

B. Information for the Patient. See text which appears after the PHYSICIAN REFERENCES.

C. Pregnancy Category X. See CONTRAINDICATIONS and Boxed Warning.

D. Nursing Mothers. As a general principle, the administration of any drug to nursing mothers should be done only when clearly necessary since many drugs are excreted in human milk.

Adverse Reactions: (See Warnings regarding induction of neoplasia, adverse effects on the fetus, increased incidence of gallbladder disease, and adverse effects similar to those of oral contraceptives, including thromboembolism.) The following additional adverse reactions have been reported with estrogenic therapy, including oral contraceptives:
1. *Genitourinary system:* Breakthrough bleeding, spotting, change in menstrual flow; dysmenorrhea; premenstrual-like syndrome; amenorrhea during and after treatment; increase in size of uterine fibromyomata; vaginal candidiasis; change in cervical erosion and in degree of cervical secretion; cystitis-like syndrome.
2. *Breasts:* Tenderness, enlargement, secretion.
3. *Gastrointestinal:* Nausea, vomiting; abdominal cramps, bloating; cholestatic jaundice.
4. *Skin:* Chloasma or melasma which may persist when drug is discontinued; erythema multiforme; erythema nodosum; hemorrhagic eruption; loss of scalp hair; hirsutism.
5. *Eyes:* Steepening of corneal curvature; intolerance to contact lenses.
6. *CNS:* Headache, migraine, dizziness; mental depression; chorea.
7. *Miscellaneous:* Increase or decrease in weight; reduced carbohydrate tolerance; aggravation of porphyria; edema; changes in libido.

Acute Overdosage: Numerous reports of ingestion of large doses of estrogen-containing oral contraceptives by young children indicate that acute serious ill effects do not occur. Overdosage of estrogen may cause nausea, and withdrawal bleeding may occur in females.

Dosage and Administration:

1. *Given cyclically for short term use only:* For treatment of moderate to severe *vasomotor* symptoms, atrophic vaginitis, or kraurosis vulvae associated with the menopause.
The lowest dose that will control symptoms should be chosen and medication should be discontinued as promptly as possible.
Administration should be cyclic (e.g., three weeks on and one week off).
Attempts to discontinue or taper medication should be made at three to six month intervals.
Usual dosage ranges:
Vasomotor symptoms—1.25 mg daily. If the patient has not menstruated within the last two months or more, cyclic administration is started arbitrarily. If the patient is menstruating, cyclic administration is started on day 5 of bleeding.
Atrophic vaginitis and kraurosis vulvae—0.3 mg to 1.25 mg or more daily, depending upon the tissue response of the individual patient. Administer cyclically.
2. *Given cyclically:* Female hypogonadism; female castration; primary ovarian failure; osteoporosis.
Usual dosage ranges:
Female hypogonadism—2.5 to 7.5 mg daily, in divided doses for 20 days, followed by a rest period of 10 days' duration. If bleeding does not occur by the end of this period, the same dosage schedule is repeated. The number of courses of estrogen therapy necessary to produce bleeding may vary depending on the responsiveness of the endometrium.
If bleeding occurs before the end of the 10 day period, begin a 20 day estrogen-progestin cyclic regimen with PREMARIN, 2.5 to 7.5 mg daily in divided doses, for 20 days. During the last five days of estrogen therapy, give an oral progestin. If bleeding occurs before this regimen is concluded, therapy is discontinued and may be resumed on the fifth day of bleeding.
Female castration and primary ovarian failure—1.25 mg daily, cyclically. Adjust dosage upward or downward according to severity of symptoms and response of the patient. For maintenance, adjust dosage to lowest level that will provide effective control.
Osteoporosis (to retard progression)—1.25 mg daily, cyclically.
3. *Given for a few days:* Prevention of postpartum breast engorgement—3.75 mg every four hours for five doses, or 1.25 mg every four hours for five days.
4. *Given chronically:* Inoperable progessing prostatic cancer—1.25 to 2.5 mg three times daily. The effectiveness of therapy can be judged by phosphatase determinations as well as by symptomatic improvement of the patient.
Inoperable progessing breast cancer in appropriately selected men and postmenopausal women. (See INDICATIONS)—Suggested dosage is 10 mg three times daily for a period of at least three months.
Treated patients with an intact uterus should be monitored closely for signs of endometrial cancer and appropriate diagnostic measures should be taken to rule out malignancy in the event of persistent or recurring abnormal vaginal bleeding.

How Supplied: PREMARIN (Conjugated Estrogens Tablets, U.S.P.)
—Each *purple* tablet contains 2.5 mg, in bottles of 100 (NDC 0046-0865-81) and 1,000 (NDC 0046-0865-91).
—Each *yellow* tablet contains 1.25 mg, in bottles of 100 (NDC 0046-0866-81) and 1,000 (NDC 0046-0866-91). Also in unit dose package of 100 (NDC 0046-0866-99).
—Each *red* tablet contains 0.625 mg, in bottles of 100 (NDC 0046-0867-81) and 1,000 (NDC 0046-0867-91). Also in unit dose package of 100 (NDC 0046-0867-99).
—Each *green* tablet contains 0.3 mg, in bottles of 100 (NDC 0046-0868-81) and 1,000 (NDC 0046-0868-91).

Physician References:

1. Ziel, H. K., *et al.*: N. Engl. J. Med. *293*:1167–1170, 1975.
2. Smith, D. C., *et al.*: N. Engl. J. Med. *293*:1164–1167, 1975.
3. Mack, T. M., *et al.*: N. Engl. J. Med. *294*:1262–1267, 1976.
4. Weiss, N. S., *et al.*: N. Engl. J. Med. *294*:1259–1262, 1976.
5. Herbst, A. L., *et al.*: N. Engl. J. Med. *284*:878–881, 1971.
6. Greenwald, P., *et al.*: N. Engl. J. Med. *285*:390–392, 1971.
7. Lanier, A., *et al.*: Mayo Clin. Proc. *48*: 793–799, 1973.
8. Herbst, A., *et al.*: Obstet. Gynecol. *40*:287–298, 1972.
9. Herbst, A., *et al.*: Am. J. Obstet. Gynecol. *118*:607–615, 1974.
10. Herbst, A., *et al.*: N. Engl. J. Med. *292*: 334–339, 1975.
11. Stafl, A., *et al.*: Obstet. Gynecol. *43*:118–128, 1974.
12. Sherman, A. I., *et al.*: Obstet. Gynecol. *44*:531–545, 1974.
13. Gal, I., *et al.*: Nature *216*:83, 1967.
14. Levy, E. P., *et al.*: Lancet *1*:611, 1973.
15. Nora, J., *et al.*: Lancet *1*:941–942, 1973.

Continued on next page

Ayerst—Cont.

16. Janerich, D. T., *et al.*: N. Engl. J. Med. *291*:697–700, 1974.
17. Boston Collaborative Drug Surveillance Program: N. Engl. J. Med. *290*:15–19, 1974.
18. Hoover, R., *et al.*: N. Engl. J. Med. *295*:401–405, 1976.
19. Boston Collaborative Drug Surveillance Program: Lancet *1*:1399–1404, 1973.
20. Daniel, D. G., *et al.*: Lancet *2*:287–289, 1967.
21. The Veterans Administration Cooperative Urological Research Group: J. Urol. *98*:516–522, 1967.
22. Bailar, J. C.: Lancet *2*:560, 1967.
23. Blackard, C., *et al.*: Cancer *26*:249–256, 1970.
24. Royal College of General Practitioners: J. R. Coll. Gen. Pract. *13*:267–279, 1967.

24a. Royal College of General Practitioners: Oral Contraceptives and Health, New York, Pitman Corp., 1974.

25. Inman, W. H. W., *et al.*: Br. Med. J. *2*:193–199, 1968.
26. Vessey, M. P., *et al.*: Br. Med. J. *2*:651–657, 1969.
27. Sartwell, P. E., *et al.*: Am. J. Epidemiol. *90*:365–380, 1969.
28. Collaborative Group for the Study of Stroke in Young Women: N. Engl. J. Med. *288*:871–878, 1973.
29. Collaborative Group for the Study of Stroke in Young Women: J.A.M.A. *231*:718–722, 1975.
30. Mann, J. I., *et al.*: Br. Med. J. *2*:245–248, 1975.
31. Mann, J. I., *et al.*: Br. Med. J. *2*:241–245, 1975.
32. Inman, W. H. W., *et al.*: Br. Med. J. *2*:203–209, 1970.
33. Stolley, P. D., *et al.*: Am. J. Epidemiol. *102*:197–208, 1975.
34. Vessey, M. P., *et al.*: Br. Med. J. *3*:123–126, 1970.
35. Greene, G. R., *et al.*: Am. J. Public Health *62*:680–685, 1972.
36. Rosenberg, L., *et al.*: N. Engl. J. Med. *294*:1256–1259, 1976.
37. Coronary Drug Project Research Group: J.A.M.A. *214*:1303–1313, 1970.
38. Baum, J., *et al.*: Lancet *2*: 926–928, 1973.
39. Mays, E. T., *et al.*: J.A.M.A. *235*:730–732, 1976.
40. Edmondson, H. A., *et al.*: N. Engl. J. Med. *294*:470–472, 1976.
41. Pfeffer, R. I., *et al.*: Am. J. Epidemiol. *103*:445–456, 1976.

INFORMATION FOR THE PATIENT

What You Should Know about Estrogens: Estrogens are female hormones produced by the ovaries. The ovaries make several different kinds of estrogens. In addition, scientists have been able to make a variety of synthetic estrogens. As far as we know, all these estrogens have similar properties and therefore much the same usefulness, side effects, and risks. This leaflet is intended to help you understand what estrogens are used for, the risks involved in their use, and how to use them as safely as possible.

This leaflet includes the most important information about estrogens, but not all the information. If you want to know more, you should ask your doctor for more information or you can ask your doctor or pharmacist to let you read the package insert prepared for the doctor.

Uses of Estrogen: THERE IS NO PROPER USE OF ESTROGENS IN A PREGNANT WOMAN.

Estrogens are prescribed by doctors for a number of purposes, including:

1. To provide estrogen during a period of adjustment when a woman's ovaries stop producing a majority of her estrogens, in order to prevent certain uncomfortable symptoms of estrogen deficiency. (With the menopause, which generally occurs between the ages of 45 and 55, women produce a much smaller amount of estrogens.)
2. To prevent symptoms of estrogen deficiency when a woman's ovaries have been removed surgically before the natural menopause.
3. To prevent pregnancy. (Estrogens are given along with a progestogen, another female hormone; these combinations are called oral contraceptives or birth control pills. Patient labeling is available to women taking oral contraceptives and they will not be discussed in this leaflet.)
4. To treat certain cancers in women and men.
5. To prevent painful swelling of the breasts after pregnancy in women who choose not to nurse their babies.

Estrogens in the Menopause: In the natural course of their lives, all women eventually experience a decrease in estrogen production. This usually occurs between 45 and 55 but may occur earlier or later. Sometimes the ovaries may need to be removed before natural menopause by an operation, producing a "surgical menopause."

When the amount of estrogen in the blood begins to decrease, many women may develop typical symptoms: feelings of warmth in the face, neck, and chest or sudden intense episodes of heat and sweating throughout the body (called "hot flashes" or "hot flushes"). These symptoms are sometimes very uncomfortable. Some women may also develop changes in the vagina (called "atrophic vaginitis") which cause discomfort, especially during and after intercourse.

Estrogens can be prescribed to treat these symptoms of the menopause. It is estimated that considerably more than half of all women undergoing the menopause have only mild symptoms or no symptoms at all and therefore do not need estrogens. Other women may need estrogens for a few months, while their bodies adjust to lower estrogen levels. Sometimes the need will be for periods longer than six months. In an attempt to avoid overstimulation of the uterus (womb), estrogens are usually given cyclically during each month of use, such as three weeks of pills followed by one week without pills.

Sometimes women experience nervous symptoms or depression during menopause. There is no evidence that estrogens are effective for such symptoms without associated vasomotor symptoms. In the absence of vasomotor symptoms, estrogens should not be used to treat nervous symptoms, although other treatment may be needed.

You may have heard that taking estrogens for long periods (years) after the menopause will keep your skin soft and supple and keep you feeling young. There is no evidence that this is so, however, and such long-term treatment carries important risks.

Estrogens to Prevent Swelling of the Breasts after Pregnancy: If you do not breast-feed your baby after delivery, your breasts may fill up with milk and become painful and engorged. This usually begins about 3 to 4 days after delivery and may last for a few days to up to a week or more. Sometimes the discomfort is severe, but usually it is not and can be controlled by pain-relieving drugs such as aspirin and by binding the breasts up tightly. Estrogens can be used to try to prevent the breasts from filling up. While this treatment is sometimes successful, in many cases the breasts fill up to some degree in spite of treatment. The dose of estrogens needed to prevent pain and swelling of the breasts is much larger than the dose needed to treat symptoms of the menopause and this may increase your chances of developing blood clots in the legs or lungs (see below). Therefore, it is important that you discuss the benefits and the risks of estrogen use with your doctor if you have decided not to breast-feed your baby.

The Dangers of Estrogens:

1. *Endometrial cancer.* There are reports that if estrogens are used in the postmenopausal period for more than a year, there is an increased risk of *endometrial cancer* (cancer of the lining of the uterus). Women taking estrogens have roughly 5 to 10 times as great a chance of getting this cancer as women who take no estrogens. To put this another way, while a postmenopausal woman not taking estrogens has 1 chance in 1,000 each year of getting endometrial cancer, a woman taking estrogens has 5 to 10 chances in 1,000 each year. For this reason *it is important to take estrogens only when they are really needed.*

The risk of this cancer is greater the longer estrogens are used and when larger doses are taken. Therefore you should not take more estrogen than your doctor prescribes. *It is important to take the lowest dose of estrogen that will control symptoms and to take it only as long as it is needed.* If estrogens are needed for longer periods of time, your doctor will want to reevaluate your need for estrogens at least every six months.

Women using estrogens should report any vaginal bleeding to their doctors; such bleeding may be of no importance, but it can be an early warning of endometrial cancer. If you have undiagnosed vaginal bleeding, you should not use estrogens until a diagnosis is made and you are certain there is no endometrial cancer.

NOTE: If you have had your uterus removed (total hysterectomy), there is no danger of developing endometrial cancer.

2. *Other possible cancers.* Estrogens can cause development of other tumors in animals, such as tumors of the breast, cervix, vagina, or liver, when given for a long time. At present there is no good evidence that women using estrogen in the menopause have an increased risk of such tumors, but there is no way yet to be sure they do not; and one study raises the possibility that use of estrogens in the menopause may increase the risk of breast cancer many years later. This is a further reason to use estrogens only when clearly needed. While you are taking estrogens, it is important that you go to your doctor at least once a year for a physical examination. Also, if members of your family have had breast cancer or if you have breast nodules or abnormal mammograms (breast x-rays), your doctor may wish to carry out more frequent examinations of your breasts.
3. *Gallbladder disease.* Women who use estrogens after menopause are more likely to develop gallbladder disease needing surgery than women who do not use estrogens. Birth control pills have a similar effect.
4. *Abnormal blood clotting.* Oral contraceptives increase the risk of blood clotting in various parts of the body. This can result in a stroke (if the clot is in the brain), a heart attack (clot in a blood vessel of the heart), or a pulmonary embolus (a clot which forms in the legs or pelvis, then breaks off and travels to the lungs). Any of these can be fatal.

At this time use of estrogens in the menopause is not known to cause such blood clotting, but this has not been fully studied and there could still prove to be such a risk. It is recommended that if you have had clotting in the legs or lungs or a heart attack or stroke while you were using estrogens or birth control pills, you should not use estrogens (unless they are being used to treat cancer of the breast or prostate). If you have had a stroke or heart attack or if you have angina pectoris, estrogens should be used with great caution and only if clearly needed (for example, if you have severe symptoms of the menopause).

The larger doses of estrogen used to prevent swelling of the breasts after pregnancy have been reported to cause clotting in the legs and lungs.

Special Warning about Pregnancy: You should not receive estrogen if you are pregnant. If this should occur there is a greater than usual chance that the developing child will be born with a birth defect, although the possibility remains fairly small. A female child may have an increased risk of developing cancer of the vagina or cervix later in life (in the teens or twenties). Every possible effort should be made to avoid exposure to estrogens during pregnancy. If exposure occurs, see your doctor.

Other Effects of Estrogens: In addition to the serious known risks of estrogens described above, estrogens have the following side effects and potential risks:

1. *Nausea and vomiting.* The most common side effect of estrogen therapy is nausea. Vomiting is less common.
2. *Effects on breasts.* Estrogens may cause breast tenderness or enlargement and may cause the breasts to secrete a liquid. These effects are not dangerous.
3. *Effects on the uterus.* Estrogens may cause benign fibroid tumors of the uterus to get larger.
4. *Effects on liver.* Women taking oral contraceptives develop on rare occasions a tumor of the liver which can rupture and bleed into the abdomen and may cause death. So far, these tumors have not been reported in women using estrogens in the menopause, but you should report any swelling or unusual pain or tenderness in the abdomen to your doctor immediately.

Women with a past history of jaundice (yellowing of the skin and white parts of the eyes) may get jaundice again during estrogen use. If this occurs, stop taking estrogens and see your doctor.

5. *Other effects.* Estrogens may cause excess fluid to be retained in the body. This may make some conditions worse, such as asthma, epilepsy, migraine, heart disease, or kidney disease.

Summary: Estrogens have important uses, but they have serious risks as well. You must decide, with your doctor, whether the risks are acceptable to you in view of the benefits of treatment. Except where your doctor has prescribed estrogens for use in special cases of cancer of the breast or prostate, you should not use estrogens if you have cancer of the breast or uterus, are pregnant, have undiagnosed abnormal vaginal bleeding, clotting in the legs or lungs, or have had a stroke, heart attack or angina, or clotting in the legs or lungs in the past while you were taking estrogens.

You can use estrogens as safely as possible by understanding that your doctor will require regular physical examinations while you are taking them and will try to discontinue the drug as soon as possible and use the smallest dose possible. Be alert for signs of trouble including:

1. Abnormal bleeding from the vagina.
2. Pains in the calves or chest or sudden shortness of breath, or coughing blood.
3. Severe headache, dizziness, faintness, or changes in vision.
4. Breast lumps (you should ask your doctor how to examine your own breasts).
5. Jaundice (yellowing of the skin).

Your doctor has prescribed this drug for you and you alone. Do not give the drug to anyone else.

How Supplied:

PREMARIN® (Conjugated Estrogens Tablets, U.S.P.)—tablets for oral administration.

PREMARIN® VAGINAL CREAM —PREMARIN® in a nonliquefying base, designed for vaginal use.

PREMARIN® with METHYLTESTOSTERONE —a combination of PREMARIN® and methyltestosterone (an androgen) in tablet form for oral administration.

PMB® 200,400—a combination of PREMARIN® and meprobamate (a tranquilizing agent) in tablet form for oral administration.

PREMARIN® INTRAVENOUS —PREMARIN® specially prepared for intravenous and intramuscular use.

ESTROGENIC SUBSTANCE (Estrone) in Aqueous Suspension—a sterile aqueous suspension of estrone, a short-acting estrogen, for intramuscular injection only.

[*Shown in Product Identification Section*]

PREMARIN® ℞
(Conjugated Estrogens, U.S.P.)
VAGINAL CREAM
in a nonliquefying base

1. ESTROGENS HAVE BEEN REPORTED TO INCREASE THE RISK OF ENDOMETRIAL CARCINOMA.

Three independent case control studies have reported an increased risk of endometrial cancer in postmenopausal women exposed to exogenous estrogens for more than one year.[1–3] This risk was independent of the other known risk factors for endometrial cancer. These studies are further supported by the finding that incidence rates of endometrial cancer have increased sharply since 1969 in eight different areas of the United States with population-based cancer reporting systems, an increase which may be related to the rapidly expanding use of estrogens during the last decade.[4]

The three case control studies reported that the risk of endometrial cancer in estrogen users was about 4.5 to 13.9 times greater than in nonusers. The risk appears to depend on both duration of treatment[1] and on estrogen dose.[3] In view of these findings, when estrogens are used for the treatment of menopausal symptoms, the lowest dose that will control symptoms should be utilized and medication should be discontinued as soon as possible. When prolonged treatment is medically indicated, the patient should be reassessed on at least a semiannual basis to determine the need for continued therapy. Although the evidence must be considered preliminary, one study suggests that cyclic administration of low doses of estrogen may carry less risk than continuous administration;[3] it therefore appears prudent to utilize such a regimen.

Close clinical surveillance of all women taking estrogens is important. In all cases of undiagnosed persistent or recurring abnormal vaginal bleeding, adequate diagnostic measures should be undertaken to rule out malignancy.

There is no evidence at present that "natural" estrogens are more or less hazardous than "synthetic" estrogens at equiestrogenic doses.

2. ESTROGENS SHOULD NOT BE USED DURING PREGNANCY.

The use of female sex hormones, both estrogens and progestogens, during early pregnancy may seriously damage the offspring. It has been shown that females exposed in utero to diethylstilbestrol, a non-steroidal estrogen, have an increased risk of developing in later life a form of vaginal or cervical cancer that is ordinarily extremely rare.[5,6] This risk has been estimated as not greater than 4 per 1000 exposures.[7] Furthermore, a high percentage of such exposed women (from 30 to 90 percent) have been found to have vaginal adenosis,[8–12] epithelial changes of the vagina and cervix. Although these changes are histologically benign, it is not known whether they are precursors of malignancy. Although similar data are not available with the use of other estrogens, it cannot be presumed they would not induce similar changes.

Several reports suggest an association between intrauterine exposure to female sex hormones and congenital anomalies, including congenital heart defects and limb reduction defects.[13–16] One case control study[16] estimated a 4.7-fold increased risk of limb reduction defects in infants exposed in utero to sex hormones (oral contraceptives, hormone withdrawal tests for pregnancy, or attempted treatment for threatened abortion). Some of these exposures were very short and involved only a few days of treatment. The data suggest that the risk of limb reduction defects in exposed fetuses is somewhat less than 1 per 1000.

In the past, female sex hormones have been used during pregnancy in an attempt to treat threatened or habitual abortion. There is considerable evidence that estrogens are ineffective for these indications, and there is no evidence from well controlled studies that progestogens are effective for these uses.

If PREMARIN (Conjugated Estrogens, U.S.P.) Vaginal Cream is used during pregnancy, or if the patient becomes pregnant while taking this drug, she should be apprised of the potential risks to the fetus, and the advisability of pregnancy continuation.

Description: Each gram contains 0.625 mg Conjugated Estrogens, U.S.P., in a nonliquefying base containing cetyl esters wax, cetyl alcohol, white wax, glyceryl monostearate, propylene glycol monostearate, methyl stearate, phenylethyl alcohol, sodium lauryl sulfate, glycerin, and mineral oil.

PREMARIN (Conjugated Estrogens, U.S.P.) is a mixture of estrogens, obtained exclusively from natural sources, occurring as the sodium salts of water-soluble estrogen sulfates blended to represent the average composition of material derived from pregnant mares' urine. It contains estrone, equilin, and 17 α-dihydroequilin, together with smaller amounts of 17 α-estradiol, equilenin, and 17 α-dihydroequilenin as salts of their sulfate esters.

Clinical Pharmacology: Estrogens are important in the development and maintenance of the female reproductive system and secondary sex characteristics. They promote growth and development of the vagina, uterus, and fallopian tubes, and enlargement of the breasts. Indirectly, they contribute to the shaping of the skeleton, maintenance of tone and elasticity of urogenital structures, changes in the epiphyses of the long bones that allow for the pubertal growth spurt and its termination, growth of axillary and pubic hair, and pigmentation of the nipples and genitals. Decline of estrogenic activity at the end of the menstrual cycle can bring on menstruation, although the cessation of progesterone secretion is the most important factor in the mature ovulatory cycle. However, in the preovulatory or nonovulatory cycle, estrogen is the primary determinant in the onset of menstruation. Estrogens also affect the release of pituitary gonadotropins.

The pharmacologic effects of conjugated estrogens are similar to those of endogenous estrogens. They are soluble in water and may be absorbed from mucosal surfaces after local administration.

In responsive tissues (female genital organs, breasts, hypothalamus, pituitary) estrogens enter the cell and are transported into the nucleus. As a result of estrogen action, specific RNA and protein synthesis occurs.

Continued on next page

Ayerst—Cont.

Metabolism and inactivation occur primarily in the liver. Some estrogens are excreted into the bile; however they are reabsorbed from the intestine and returned to the liver through the portal venous system. Water-soluble estrogen conjugates are strongly acidic and are ionized in body fluids, which favor excretion through the kidneys since tubular reabsorption is minimal.

Indications: PREMARIN (Conjugated Estrogens, U.S.P.) Vaginal Cream is indicated in the treatment of atrophic vaginitis and kraurosis vulvae.

PREMARIN Vaginal Cream HAS NOT BEEN SHOWN TO BE EFFECTIVE FOR ANY PURPOSE DURING PREGNANCY AND ITS USE MAY CAUSE SEVERE HARM TO THE FETUS (SEE BOXED WARNING).

Contraindications: Estrogens should not be used in women with any of the following conditions:

1. Known or suspected cancer of the breast except in appropriately selected patients being treated for metastatic disease.
2. Known or suspected estrogen-dependent neoplasia.
3. Known or suspected pregnancy (See Boxed Warning).
4. Undiagnosed abnormal genital bleeding.
5. Active thrombophlebitis or thromboembolic disorders.
6. A past history of thrombophlebitis, thrombosis, or thromboembolic disorders associated with previous estrogen use (except when used in treatment of breast malignancy).

PREMARIN Vaginal Cream should not be used in patients hypersensitive to its ingredients.

Warnings:

1. *Induction of malignant neoplasms.* Long term continuous administration of natural and synthetic estrogens in certain animal species increases the frequency of carcinomas of the breast, cervix, vagina, and liver. There are now reports that estrogens increase the risk of carcinoma of the endometrium in humans. (See Boxed Warning.)

At the present time there is no satisfactory evidence that estrogens given to postmenopausal women increase the risk of cancer of the breast,[17] although a recent long-term followup of a single physician's practice has raised this possibility.[18] Because of the animal data, there is a need for caution in prescribing estrogens for women with a strong family history of breast cancer or who have breast nodules, fibrocystic disease, or abnormal mammograms.

2. *Gallbladder disease.* A recent study has reported a 2 to 3-fold increase in the risk of surgically confirmed gallbladder disease in women receiving postmenopausal estrogens,[17] similar to the 2-fold increase previously noted in users of oral contraceptives.[19,24a]

3. *Effects similar to those caused by estrogen-progestogen oral contraceptives.* There are several serious adverse effects of oral contraceptives, most of which have not, up to now, been documented as consequences of postmenopausal estrogen therapy. This may reflect the comparatively low doses of estrogen used in postmenopausal women. It would be expected that the larger doses of estrogen used to treat breast cancer or postpartum breast engorgement are more likely to result in these adverse effects, and, in fact, it has been shown that there is an increased risk of thrombosis in men receiving estrogens for prostatic cancer and women for postpartum breast engorgement.[20–23]

a. *Thromboembolic disease.* It is now well established that users of oral contraceptives have an increased risk of various thromboembolic and thrombotic vascular diseases, such as thrombophlebitis, pulmonary embolism, stroke, and myocardial infarction.[24–31] Cases of retinal thrombosis, mesenteric thrombosis, and optic neuritis have been reported in oral contraceptive users. There is evidence that the risk of several of these adverse reactions is related to the dose of the drug.[32,33] An increased risk of postsurgery thromboembolic complications has also been reported in users of oral contraceptives.[34,35] If feasible, estrogen should be discontinued at least 4 weeks before surgery of the type associated with an increased risk of thromboembolism, or during periods of prolonged immobilization.

While an increased rate of thromboembolic and thrombotic disease in postmenopausal users of estrogens has not been found,[17–24,25–36] this does not rule out the possibility that such an increase may be present or that subgroups of women who have underlying risk factors or who are receiving relatively large doses of estrogens may have increased risk. Therefore estrogens should not be used in persons with active thrombophlebitis or thromboembolic disorders, and they should not be used (except in treatment of malignancy) in persons with a history of such disorders in association with estrogen use. They should be used with caution in patients with cerebral vascular or coronary artery disease and only for those in whom estrogens are clearly needed.

Large doses of estrogen (5 mg conjugated estrogens per day), comparable to those used to treat cancer of the prostate and breast, have been shown in a large prospective clinical trial in men[37] to increase the risk of nonfatal myocardial infarction, pulmonary embolism and thrombophlebitis. When estrogen doses of this size are used, any of the thromboembolic and thrombotic adverse effects associated with oral contraceptive use should be considered a clear risk.

b. *Hepatic adenoma.* Benign hepatic adenomas appear to be associated with the use of oral contraceptives.[38–40] Although benign, and rare, these may rupture and may cause death through intra-abdominal hemorrhage. Such lesions have not yet been reported in association with other estrogen or progestogen preparations but should be considered in estrogen users having abdominal pain and tenderness, abdominal mass, or hypovolemic shock. Hepatocellular carcinoma has also been reported in women taking estrogen-containing oral contraceptives.[39] The relationship of this malignancy to these drugs is not known at this time.

c. *Elevated blood pressure.* Women using oral contraceptives sometimes experience increased blood pressure which, in most cases, returns to normal on discontinuing the drug. There is now a report that this may occur with use of estrogens in the menopause[41] and blood pressure should be monitored with estrogen use, especially if high doses are used.

d. *Glucose tolerance.* A worsening of glucose tolerance has been observed in a significant percentage of patients on estrogen-containing oral contraceptives. For this reason, diabetic patients should be carefully observed while receiving estrogen.

4. *Hypercalcemia.* Administration of estrogens may lead to severe hypercalcemia in patients with breast cancer and bone metastases. If this occurs, the drug should be stopped and appropriate measures taken to reduce the serum calcium level.

Precautions:

A. General Precautions.

1. A complete medical and family history should be taken prior to the initiation of any estrogen therapy. The pretreatment and periodic physical examinations should include special reference to blood pressure, breasts, abdomen, and pelvic organs, and should include a Papanicolau smear. As a general rule, estrogen should not be prescribed for longer than one year without another physical examination being performed.
2. Fluid retention—Because estrogens may cause some degree of fluid retention, conditions which might be influenced by this factor such as asthma, epilepsy, migraine, and cardiac or renal dysfunction, require careful observation.
3. Certain patients may develop undesirable manifestations of excessive estrogenic stimulation, such as abnormal or excessive uterine bleeding, mastodynia, etc.
4. Oral contraceptives appear to be associated with an increased incidence of mental depression.[24a] Although it is not clear whether this is due to the estrogenic or progestogenic component of the contraceptive, patients with a history of depression should be carefully observed.
5. Preexisting uterine leiomyomata may increase in size during estrogen use.
6. The pathologist should be advised of estrogen therapy when relevant specimens are submitted.
7. Patients with a past history of jaundice during pregnancy have an increased risk of recurrence of jaundice while receiving estrogen-containing oral contraceptive therapy. If jaundice develops in any patient receiving estrogen, the medication should be discontinued while the cause is investigated.
8. Estrogens may be poorly metabolized in patients with impaired liver function and they should be administered with caution in such patients.
9. Because estrogens influence the metabolism of calcium and phosphorus, they should be used with caution in patients with metabolic bone diseases that are associated with hypercalcemia or in patients with renal insufficiency.
10. Because of the effects of estrogens on epiphyseal closure, they should be used judiciously in young patients in whom bone growth is not complete.
11. Certain endocrine and liver function tests may be affected by estrogen-containing oral contraceptives. The following similar changes may be expected with larger doses of estrogen:

a. Increased sulfobromophthalein retention.
b. Increased prothrombin and factors VII, VIII, IX, and X; decreased antithrombin 3; increased norepinephrine-induced platelet aggregability.
c. Increased thyroid binding globulin (TBG) leading to increased circulating total thyroid hormone, as measured by PBI, T4 by column, or T4 by radioimmunoassay. Free T3 resin uptake is decreased, reflecting the elevated TBG; free T4 concentration in unaltered.
d. Impaired glucose tolerance.
e. Decreased pregnanediol excretion.
f. Reduced response to metyrapone test.
g. Reduced serum folate concentration.
h. Increased serum triglyceride and phospholipid concentration.

B. Information for the Patient. See text which appears after the PHYSICIAN REFERENCES.

C. Pregnancy Category X. See CONTRAINDICATIONS and Boxed Warning.

D. Nursing Mothers. As a general principle, the administration of any drug to nursing mothers should be done only when clearly necessary since many drugs are excreted in human milk.

Adverse Reactions: (See Warnings regarding induction of neoplasia, adverse effects on the fetus, increased incidence of gallbladder disease, and adverse effects similar to those of oral contraceptives, including thromboembolism.) The following additional adverse reactions have been reported with estrogenic therapy, including oral contraceptives.

1. *Genitourinary system:* Breakthrough bleeding, spotting, change in menstrual flow; dysmenorrhea; premenstrual-like syndrome; amenorrhea during and after treatment; increase in size of uterine fibromyomata; vaginal candidiasis; change in cervical erosion and in

degree of cervical secretion; cystitis-like syndrome.
2. *Breasts:* Tenderness, enlargement, secretion.
3. *Gastrointestinal:* Nausea, vomiting; abdominal cramps, bloating; cholestatic jaundice.
4. *Skin:* Chloasma or melasma which may persist when drug is discontinued; erythema multiforme; erythema nodosum; hemorrhagic eruption; loss of scalp hair; hirsutism.
5. *Eyes:* Steepening of corneal curvature; intolerance to contact lenses.
6. *CNS:* Headache, migraine, dizziness; mental depression; chorea.
7. *Miscellaneous:* Increase or decrease in weight; reduced carbohydrate tolerance; aggravation of porphyria; edema; changes in libido.

Acute Overdosage: Numerous reports of ingestion of large doses of estrogen-containing oral contraceptives by young children indicate that acute serious ill effects do not occur. Overdosage of estrogen may cause nausea, and withdrawal bleeding may occur in females.

Dosage and Administration:
Given cyclically for short-term use only:
For treatment of atrophic vaginitis, or kraurosis vulvae.
The lowest dose that will control symptoms should be chosen and medication should be discontinued as promptly as possible.
Administration should be cyclic (e.g., three weeks on and one week off).
Attempts to discontinue or taper medication should be made at three to six month intervals.
Usual dosage range: 2 to 4 g daily, intravaginally or topically, depending on the severity of the condition.
Treated patients with an intact uterus should be monitored closely for signs of endometrial cancer and appropriate diagnostic measures should be taken to rule out malignancy in the event of persistent or recurring abnormal vaginal bleeding.

How Supplied: PREMARIN (Conjugated Estrogens, U.S.P.) Vaginal Cream—Each gram contains 0.625 mg Conjugated Estrogens, U.S.P. (Also contains cetyl esters wax, cetyl alcohol, white wax, glyceryl monostearate, propylene glycol monostearate, methyl stearate, phenylethyl alcohol, sodium lauryl sulfate, glycerin, and mineral oil.)
Combination package: Each contains Net Wt. 1½ oz (42.5 g) tube with one calibrated plastic applicator (NDC 0046-0872-93).
Also Available—Refill package: Each contains Net Wt. 1½ oz (42.5 g) tube (NDC 0046-0872-01).

Physician References:

1. Ziel, H. K., *et al.:* N. Engl. J. Med. *293*:1167–1170, 1975.
2. Smith, D. C., *et al.:* N. Engl. J. Med. *293*:1164–1167, 1975.
3. Mack, T. M., *et al.:* N. Engl. J. Med *294*:1262–1267, 1976.
4. Weiss, N. S., *et al.:* N. Engl. J. Med. *294*:1259–1262, 1976.
5. Herbst, A. L., *et al.:* N. Engl. J. Med. *284*:878–881, 1971.
6. Greenwald, P., *et al.:* N. Engl. J. Med. *285*:390–392, 1971.
7. Lanier, A., *et al.:* Mayo Clin. Proc. *48*:793–799, 1973.
8. Herbst, A., *et al.:* Obstet. Gynecol. *40*:287–298, 1972.
9. Herbst, A., *et al.:* Am. J. Obstet. Gynecol. *118*:607–615, 1974.
10. Herbst, A., *et al.:* N. Engl. J. Med. *292*:334–339, 1975.
11. Stafl, A., *et al.:* Obstet. Gynecol. *43*:118–128, 1974.
12. Sherman A. I., *et al.:* Obstet. Gynecol. *44*:531–545, 1974.
13. Gal, I., *et al.:* Nature *216*:83, 1967.
14. Levy, E. P., *et al.:* Lancet *1*:611, 1973.
15. Nora, J., *et al.:*Lancet *1*:941–942, 1973.
16. Janerich, D. T., *et al.:* N. Engl. J. Med. *291*:697–700, 1974.
17. Boston Collaborative Drug Surveillance Program: N. Engl. J. Med. *290*:15–19, 1974.
18. Hoover, R., *et al.:* N. Engl. J. Med. *295*:401–405, 1976.
19. Boston Collaborative Drug Surveillance Program: Lancet *1*:1399–1404, 1973.
20. Daniel, D. G., *et al.:* Lancet *2*:287–289, 1967.
21. The Veterans Administration Cooperative Urological Research Group: J. Urol. *98*:516–522, 1967.
22. Bailar, J. C.: Lancet *2*:560, 1967.
23. Blackard, C., *et al.:* Cancer *26*:249–256, 1970.
24. Royal College of General Practitioners: J. R. Coll. Gen. Pract. *13*:267–279, 1967.
24a. Royal College of General Practitioners: Oral Contraceptives and Health, New York, Pitman Corp., 1974.
25. Inman, W. H. W., *et al.:* Br. Med. J. *2*:193–199, 1968.
26. Vessey, M. P., *et al.:* Br. Med. J. *2*:651–657, 1969.
27. Sartwell, P. E., *et al.:* Am. J. Epidemiol. *90*:365–380, 1969.
28. Collaborative Group for the Study of Stroke in Young Women: N. Engl. J. Med. *288*:871–878, 1973.
29. Collaborative Group for the Study of Stroke in Young Women: J.A.M.A. *231*:718–722, 1975.
30. Mann, J. I., *et al.:* Br. Med. J. *2*:245–248, 1975.
31. Mann. J. I., *et al.:* Br. Med. J. *2*:241–245, 1975.
32. Inman, W. H. W., *et al.:* Br. Med. J. *2*:203–209, 1970.
33. Stolley, P. D., *et al.:* Am. J. Epidemiol. *102*:197–208, 1975.
34. Vessey, M. P., *et al.:* Br. Med. J. *3*:123–126, 1970.
35. Greene, G. R., *et al.:* Am. J. Public Health *62*:680–685, 1972.
36. Rosenberg, L., *et al.:* N. Engl. J. Med. *294*:1256–1259, 1976.
37. Coronary Drug Project Research Group: J.A.M.A. *214*:1303–1313, 1970.
38. Baum, J., *et al.:* Lancet *2*:926–928, 1973.
39. Mays, E. T., *et al.:* J.A.M.A. *235*:730–732, 1976.
40. Edmondson, H. A., *et al.:* N. Engl. J. Med. *294*:470–472, 1976.
41. Pfeffer, R. I., *et al.:* Am. J. Epidemiol. *103*:445–456, 1976.

INFORMATION FOR THE PATIENT

What You Should Know about Estrogens: Estrogens are female hormones produced by the ovaries. The ovaries make several different kinds of estrogens. In addition, scientists have been able to make a variety of synthetic estrogens. As far as we know, all these estrogens have similar properties and therefore much the same usefulness, side effects, and risks.
This leaflet is intended to help you understand what estrogens are used for, the risks involved in their use, and how to use them as safely as possible.
This leaflet includes the most important information about estrogens, but not all the information. If you want to know more, you should ask your doctor for more information or you can ask your doctor or pharmacist to let you read the package insert prepared for the doctor.

Uses of Estrogen: THERE IS NO PROPER USE OF ESTROGENS IN A PREGNANT WOMAN.
Estrogens are prescribed by doctors for a number of purposes, including:
1. To provide estrogen during a period of adjustment when a woman's ovaries stop producing a majority of her estrogens, in order to prevent certain uncomfortable symptoms of estrogen deficiency. (With the menopause, which generally occurs between the ages of 45 and 55, women produce a much smaller amount of estrogens.)
2. To prevent symptoms of estrogen deficiency when a woman's ovaries have been removed surgically before the natural menopause.
3. To prevent pregnancy. (Estrogens are given along with a progestogen, another female hormone; these combinations are called oral contraceptives or birth control pills. Patient labeling is available to women taking oral contraceptives and they will not be discussed in this leaflet.)
4. To treat certain cancers in women and men.
5. To prevent painful swelling of the breasts after pregnancy in women who choose not to nurse their babies.

Estrogens in the Menopause: In the natural course of their lives, all women eventually experience a decrease in estrogen production. This usually occurs between ages 45 and 55 but may occur earlier or later. Sometimes the ovaries may need to be removed before natural menopause by an operation, producing a "surgical menopause."
When the amount of estrogen in the blood begins to decrease, many women may develop typical symptoms: feelings of warmth in the face, neck, and chest or sudden intense episodes of heat and sweating throughout the body (called "hot flashes" or "hot flushes"). These symptoms are sometimes very uncomfortable. Some women may also develop changes in the vagina (called "atrophic vaginitis") which cause discomfort, especially during and after intercourse.
Estrogens can be prescribed to treat these symptoms of the menopause. It is estimated that considerably more than half of all women undergoing the menopause have only mild symptoms or no symptoms at all and therefore do not need estrogens. Other women may need estrogens for a few months, while their bodies adjust to lower estrogen levels. Sometimes the need will be for periods longer than six months. In an attempt to avoid overstimulation of the uterus (womb), estrogens are usually given cyclically during each month of use, such as three weeks of pills followed by one week without pills.
Sometimes women experience nervous symptoms or depression during menopause. There is no evidence that estrogens are effective for such symptoms without associated vasomotor symptoms. In the absence of vasomotor symptoms, estrogens should not be used to treat nervous symptoms, although other treatment may be needed.
You may have heard that taking estrogens for long periods (years) after the menopause will keep your skin soft and supple and keep you feeling young. There is no evidence that this is so, however, and such long-term treatment carries important risks.

Estrogens to Prevent Swelling of the Breasts after Pregnancy: If you do not breast-feed your baby after delivery, your breasts may fill up with milk and become painful and engorged. This usually begins about 3 to 4 days after delivery and may last for a few days to up to a week or more. Sometimes the discomfort is severe, but usually it is not and can be controlled by pain-relieving drugs such as aspirin and by binding the breasts up tightly. Estrogens can be used to try to prevent the breasts from filling up. While this treatment is sometimes successful, in many cases the breasts fill up to some degree in spite of treatment. The dose of estrogens needed to prevent pain and swelliing of the breasts is much larger than the dose needed to treat symptoms of the menopause and this may increase your chances of developing blood clots

Continued on next page

Ayerst—Cont.

in the legs or lungs (see below). Therefore, it is important that you discuss the benefits and the risks of estrogen use with your doctor if you have decided not to breast-feed your baby.

The Dangers of Estrogens:

1. *Endometrial cancer.* There are reports that if estrogens are used in the postmenopausal period for more than a year, there is an increased risk of *endometrial cancer* (cancer of the lining of the uterus). Women taking estrogens have roughly 5 to 10 times as great a chance of getting this cancer as women who take no estrogens. To put this another way, while a postmenopausal woman not taking estrogens has 1 chance in 1,000 each year of getting endometrial cancer, a woman taking estrogens has 5 to 10 chances in 1,000 each year. For this reason *it is important to take estrogens only when they are really needed.*

The risk of this cancer is greater the longer estrogens are used and when larger doses are taken. Therefore you should not take more estrogen than your doctor prescribes. *It is important to take the lowest dose of estrogen that will control symptoms and to take it only as long as it is needed.* If estrogens are needed for longer periods of time, your doctor will want to reevaluate your need for estrogens at least every six months.

Women using estrogens should report any vaginal bleeding to their doctors; such bleeding may be of no importance, but it can be an early warning of endometrial cancer. If you have undiagnosed vaginal bleeding, you should not use estrogens until a diagnosis is made and you are certain there is no endometrial cancer.

NOTE: If you have had your uterus removed (total hysterectomy), there is no danger of developing endometrial cancer.

2. *Other possible cancers.* Estrogens can cause development of other tumors in animals, such as tumors of the breast, cervix, vagina, or liver, when given for a long time. At present there is no good evidence that women using estrogen in the menopause have an increased risk of such tumors, but there is no way yet to be sure they do not; and one study raises the possibility that use of estrogens in the menopause may increase the risk of breast cancer many years later. This is a further reason to use estrogens only when clearly needed. While you are taking estrogens, it is important that you go to your doctor at least once a year for a physical examination. Also, if members of your family have had breast cancer or if you have breast nodules or abnormal mammograms (breast x-rays), your doctor may wish to carry out more frequent examinations of your breasts.

3. *Gallbladder disease.* Women who use estrogens after menopause are more likely to develop gallbladder disease needing surgery than women who do not use estrogens. Birth control pills have a similar effect.

4. *Abnormal blood clotting.* Oral contraceptives increase the risk of blood clotting in various parts of the body. This can result in a stroke (if the clot is in the brain), a heart attack (clot in a blood vessel of the heart), or a pulmonary embolus (a clot which forms in the legs or pelvis, then breaks off and travels to the lungs). Any of these can be fatal.

At this time use of estrogens in the menopause is not known to cause such blood clotting, but this has not been fully studied and there could still prove to be such a risk. It is recommended that if you have had clotting in the legs or lungs or a heart attack or stroke while you were using estrogens or birth control pills, you should not use estrogens (unless they are being used to treat cancer of the breast or prostate). If you have had a stroke or heart attack or if you have angina pectoris, estrogens should be used with great caution and only if clearly needed (for example, if you have severe symptoms of the menopause).

The larger doses of estrogen used to prevent swelling of the breasts after pregnancy have been reported to cause clotting in the legs and lungs.

Special Warning about Pregnancy: You should not receive estrogen if you are pregnant. If this should occur, there is a greater than usual chance that the developing child will be born with a birth defect, although the possibility remains fairly small. A female child may have an increased risk of developing cancer of the vagina or cervix later in life (in the teens or twenties). Every possible effort should be made to avoid exposure to estrogens during pregnancy. If exposure occurs, see your doctor.

Other Effects of Estrogens: In addition to the serious known risks of estrogens described above, estrogens have the following side effects and potential risks:

1. *Nausea and vomiting.* The most common side effect of estrogen therapy is nausea. Vomiting is less common.
2. *Effects on breasts.* Estrogens may cause breast tenderness or enlargement and may cause the breasts to secrete a liquid. These effects are not dangerous.
3. *Effects on the uterus.* Estrogens may cause benign fibroid tumors of the uterus to get larger.
4. *Effects on liver.* Women taking oral contraceptives develop on rare occasions a tumor of the liver which can rupture and bleed into the abdomen and may cause death. So far, these tumors have not been reported in women using estrogens in the menopause, but you should report any swelling or unusual pain or tenderness in the abdomen to your doctor immediately.

Women with a past history of jaundice (yellowing of the skin and white parts of the eyes) may get jaundice again during estrogen use. If this occurs, stop taking estrogens and see your doctor.

5. *Other effects.* Estrogens may cause excess fluid to be retained in the body. This may make some conditions worse, such as asthma, epilepsy, migraine, heart disease, or kidney disease.

Summary: Estrogens have important uses, but they have serious risks as well. You must decide, with your doctor, whether the risks are acceptable to you in view of the benefits of treatment. Except where your doctor has prescribed estrogens for use in special cases of cancer of the breast or prostate, you should not use estrogens if you have cancer of the breast or uterus, are pregnant, have undiagnosed abnormal vaginal bleeding, clotting in the legs or lungs, or have had a stroke, heart attack or angina, or clotting in the legs or lungs in the past while you were taking estrogens.

You can use estrogens as safely as possible by understanding that your doctor will require regular physical examinations while you are taking them and will try to discontinue the drug as soon as possible and use the smallest dose possible. Be alert for signs of trouble including:

1. Abnormal bleeding from the vagina.
2. Pains in the calves or chest or sudden shortness of breath, or coughing blood.
3. Severe headache, dizziness, faintness, or changes in vision.
4. Breast lumps (you should ask your doctor how to examine your own breasts).
5. Jaundice (yellowing of the skin).

Your doctor has prescribed this drug for you and you alone. Do not give the drug to anyone else.

How Supplied:

PREMARIN® (Conjugated Estrogens Tablets, U.S.P.)—tablets for oral administration.

PREMARIN® VAGINAL CREAM—PREMARIN® in a nonliquefying base, designed for vaginal use.

PMB® 200,400—a combination of PREMARIN® and meprobamate (a tranquilizing agent) in tablet form for oral administration.

PREMARIN® INTRAVENOUS—PREMARIN® specially prepared for intravenous and intramuscular use.

ESTROGENIC SUBSTANCE (Estrone) in Aqueous Suspension—a sterile aqueous suspension of estrone, a short-acting estrogen, for intramuscular injection only.

[*Shown in Product Identification Section*]

PREMARIN® ℞
(Conjugated Estrogens, U.S.P.)
with METHYLTESTOSTERONE

No. 879—Each yellow tablet contains:

Premarin® (Conjugated Estrogens, U.S.P.)	1.25 mg
Methyltestosterone	10.0 mg

No. 878—Each red tablet contains:

Premarin® (Conjugated Estrogens, U.S.P.)	0.625 mg
Methyltestosterone	5.0 mg

1. ESTROGENS HAVE BEEN REPORTED TO INCREASE THE RISK OF ENDOMETRIAL CARCINOMA.

Three independent case control studies have reported an increased risk of endometrial cancer in postmenopausal women exposed to exogenous estrogens for more than one year.[1–3] This risk was independent of the other known risk factors for endometrial cancer. These studies are further supported by the finding that incidence rates of endometrial cancer have increased sharply since 1969 in eight different areas of the United States with population-based cancer reporting systems, an increase which may be related to the rapidly expanding use of estrogens during the last decade.[4]

The three case control studies reported that the risk of endometrial cancer in estrogen users was about 4.5 to 13.9 times greater than in nonusers. The risk appears to depend on both duration of treatment[1] and on estrogen dose.[3] In view of these findings, when estrogens are used for the treatment of menopausal symptoms, the lowest dose that will control symptoms should be utilized and medication should be discontinued as soon as possible. When prolonged treatment is medically indicated, the patient should be reassessed on at least a semiannual basis to determine the need for continued therapy. Although the evidence must be considered preliminary, one study suggests that cyclic administration of low doses of estrogen may carry less risk than continuous administration;[3] it therefore appears prudent to utilize such a regimen.

Close clinical surveillance of all women taking estrogens is important. In all cases of undiagnosed persistent or recurring abnormal vaginal bleeding, adequate diagnostic measures should be undertaken to rule out malignancy.

There is no evidence at present that "natural" estrogens are more or less hazardous than "synthetic" estrogens at equiestrogenic doses.

2. ESTROGENS SHOULD NOT BE USED DURING PREGNANCY.

The use of female sex hormones, both estrogens and progestogens, during early pregnancy may seriously damage the offspring. It has been shown that females exposed in utero to diethylstilbestrol, a non-steroidal estrogen, have an increased risk of developing in later life a form of vaginal or cervical cancer that is ordinarily extremely rare.[5,6] This risk has been estimated as not greater than 4 per 1000 exposures.[7] Furthermore, a high percentage of such exposed women (from 30 to 90 percent) have been found to have vaginal adenosis,[8–12] epithelial changes of the vagina and cervix. Although these changes are histologically benign, it is not known whether they are precursors of malignancy. Although similar data are not available with the use of other estrogens, it cannot be presumed they would not induce similar changes.

Several reports suggest an association between intrauterine exposure to female sex hormones and congenital anomalies, including congenital heart defects and limb reduction defects.[13–16] One case control study[16] estimated a 4.7-fold increased risk of limb reduction defects in infants exposed in utero to sex hormones (oral contraceptives, hormone withdrawal tests for pregnancy, or attempted treatment for threatened abortion). Some of these exposures were very short and involved only a few days of treatment. The data suggest that the risk of limb reduction defects in exposed fetuses is somewhat less than 1 per 1000.

In the past, female sex hormones have been used during pregnancy in an attempt to treat threatened or habitual abortion. There is considerable evidence that estrogens are ineffective for these indications, and there is no evidence from well controlled studies that progestogens are effective for these uses.

If PREMARIN with METHYLTESTOSTERONE is used during pregnancy, or if the patient becomes pregnant while taking this drug, she should be apprised of the potential risks to the fetus, and the advisability of pregnancy continuation.

Description: PREMARIN with METHYLTESTOSTERONE is provided in tablets for oral administration.

PREMARIN (Conjugated Estrogens, U.S.P.) is a mixture of estrogens, obtained exclusively from natural sources, occurring as the sodium salts of water-soluble estrogen sulfates blended to represent the average composition of material derived from pregnant mares' urine. It contains estrone, equilin, and 17 α-dihydroequilin, together with smaller amounts of 17 α-estradiol, equilenin, and 17 α-dihydroequilenin as salts of their sulfate esters.

Methyltestosterone is an androgen. It is a white to light yellow crystalline substance that is virtually insoluble in water but soluble in organic solvents. It is stable in air but decomposes in light.

Clinical Pharmacology: Estrogens are important in the development and maintenance of the female reproductive system and secondary sex characteristics. They promote growth and development of the vagina, uterus, and fallopian tubes, and enlargement of the breasts. Indirectly, they contribute to the shaping of the skeleton, maintenance of tone and elasticity of urogenital structures, changes in the epiphyses of the long bones that allow for the pubertal growth spurt and its termination, growth of axillary and pubic hair, and pigmentation of the nipples and genitals. Decline of estrogenic activity at the end of the menstrual cycle can bring on menstruation, although the cessation of progesterone secretion is the most important factor in the mature ovulatory cycle. However, in the preovulatory or nonovulatory cycle, estrogen is the primary determinant in the onset of menstruation. Estrogens also affect the release of pituitary gonadotropins.

The pharmacologic effects of conjugated estrogens are similar to those of endogenous estrogens. They are soluble in water and are well absorbed from the gastrointestinal tract.

In responsive tissues (female genital organs, breasts, hypothalamus, pituitary) estrogens enter the cell and are transported into the nucleus. As a result of estrogen action, specific RNA and protein synthesis occurs.

Metabolism and inactivation occur primarily in the liver. Some estrogens are excreted into the bile; however they are reabsorbed from the intestine and returned to the liver through the portal venous system. Water soluble estrogen conjugates are strongly acidic and are ionized in body fluids, which favor excretion through the kidneys since tubular reabsorption is minimal.

Androgens are male sex hormones which mediate the development of the male genital organs and the secondary sex characteristics. Methyltestosterone is also an anabolic agent and promotes the retention of nitrogen, potassium, and phosphate, and increases in protein, skeletal muscle, and body mass. In the female, androgen generally opposes the action of estrogen on the female genital tissues by competing for estrogen-binding receptors.

Methyltestosterone is readily absorbed from the intestine. It is metabolized primarily in the liver and excreted primarily in the urine.

Indications: PREMARIN (Conjugated Estrogens, U.S.P.) with Methyltestosterone is indicated in the treatment of:

1. Moderate to severe *vasomotor* symptoms associated with the menopause in those patients not improved by estrogens alone. (There is no evidence that estrogens are effective for nervous symptoms or depression without associated vasomotor symptoms, and they should not be used to treat such conditions.)
2. Postpartum breast engorgement—Although estrogens have been widely used for the prevention of postpartum breast engorgement, controlled studies have demonstrated that the incidence of significant painful engorgement in patients not receiving such hormonal therapy is low and usually responsive to appropriate analgesic or other supportive therapy. Consequently, the benefit to be derived from estrogen therapy for this indication must be carefully weighed against the potential increased risk of puerperal thromboembolism associated with the use of large doses of estrogens.[20,22]

PREMARIN with METHYLTESTOSTERONE HAS NOT BEEN SHOWN TO BE EFFECTIVE FOR ANY PURPOSE DURING PREGNANCY AND ITS USE MAY CAUSE SEVERE HARM TO THE FETUS (SEE BOXED WARNING).

Contraindications: Estrogens should not be used in women with any of the following conditions:

1. Known or suspected cancer of the breast except in appropriately selected patients being treated for metastatic disease.
2. Known or suspected estrogen-dependent neoplasia.
3. Known or suspected pregnancy (See Boxed Warning).
4. Undiagnosed abnormal genital bleeding.
5. Active thrombophlebitis or thromboembolic disorders.
6. A past history of thrombophlebitis, thrombosis, or thromboembolic disorders associated with previous estrogen use (except when used in treatment of breast malignancy).

Methyltestosterone should not be used in:

1. The presence of severe liver damage.
2. Pregnancy and in breast-feeding mothers because of the possibility of masculinization of the female fetus or breast-fed infant.

Warnings:

Associated with Estrogens

1. *Induction of malignant neoplasms.* Long term continuous administration of natural and synthetic estrogens in certain animal species increases the frequency of carcinomas of the breast, cervix, vagina, and liver. There are now reports that estrogens increase the risk of carcinoma of the endometrium in humans. (See Boxed Warning.)

At the present time there is no satisfactory evidence that estrogens given to postmenopausal women increase the risk of cancer of the breast,[17] although a recent long-term followup of a single physician's practice has raised this possibility.[18] Because of the animal data, there is a need for caution in prescribing estrogens for women with a strong family history of breast cancer or who have breast nodules, fibrocystic disease, or abnormal mammograms.

2. *Gallbladder disease.* A recent study has reported a 2 to 3-fold increase in the risk of surgically confirmed gallbladder disease in women receiving postmenopausal estrogens,[17] similar to the 2-fold increase previously noted in users of oral contraceptives.[19,24a]

3. *Effects similar to those caused by estrogen-progestogen oral contraceptives.* There are several serious adverse effects of oral contraceptives, most of which have not, up to now, been documented as consequences of postmenopausal estrogen therapy. This may reflect the comparatively low doses of estrogen used in postmenopausal women. It would be expected that the larger doses of estrogen used to treat prostatic or breast cancer or postpartum breast engorgement are more likely to result in these adverse effects, and, in fact, it has been shown that there is an increased risk of thrombosis in men receiving estrogens for prostatic cancer and women for postpartum breast engorgement.[20–23]

a. *Thromboembolic disease.* It is now well established that users of oral contraceptives have an increased risk of various thromboembolic and thrombotic vascular diseases, such as thrombophlebitis, pulmonary embolism, stroke, and myocardial infarction.[24–31] Cases of retinal thrombosis, mesenteric thrombosis, and optic neuritis have been reported in oral contraceptive users. There is evidence that the risk of several of these adverse reactions is related to the dose of the drug.[32,33] An increased risk of postsurgery thromboembolic complications has also been reported in users of oral contraceptives.[34,35] If feasible, estrogen should be discontinued at least 4 weeks before surgery of the type associated with an increased risk of thromboembolism, or during periods of prolonged immobilization.

While an increased rate of thromboembolic and thrombotic disease in postmenopausal users of estrogens has not been found,[17–24,25–36] this does not rule out the possibility that such an increase may be present or that subgroups of women who have underlying risk factors or who are receiving relatively large doses of estrogens may have increased risk. Therefore estrogens should not be used in persons with active thrombophlebitis or thromboembolic disorders, and they should not be used (except in treatment of malignancy) in persons with a history of such disorders in association with estrogen use. They should be used with caution in patients with cerebral vascular or coronary artery disease and only for those in whom estrogens are clearly needed.

Large doses of estrogen (5 mg conjugated estrogens per day), comparable to those used to treat cancer of the prostate and breast, have been shown in a large prospective clinical trial in men[37] to increase the risk of nonfatal myocardial infarction, pulmonary embolism and thrombophlebitis. When estrogen doses of this size are used, any of the thromboembolic and thrombotic adverse effects associated with oral contraceptive use should be considered a clear risk.

b. *Hepatic adenoma.* Benign hepatic adenomas appear to be associated with the use of oral contraceptives.[38–40] Although benign, and rare, these may rupture and may cause death through intra-abdominal hemorrhage. Such lesions have not yet been reported in association with other estrogen or progestogen preparations but should be considered in estrogen users having abdominal pain and tenderness,

Continued on next page

Ayerst—Cont.

abdominal mass, or hypovolemic shock. Hepatocellular carcinoma has also been reported in women taking estrogen-containing oral contraceptives.[39] The relationship of this malignancy to these drugs is not known at this time.

c. *Elevated blood pressure.* Women using oral contraceptives sometimes experience increased blood pressure which, in most cases, returns to normal on discontinuing the drug. There is now a report that this may occur with use of estrogens in the menopause[41] and blood pressure should be monitored with estrogen use, especially if high doses are used.

d. *Glucose tolerance.* A worsening of glucose tolerance has been observed in a significant percentage of patients on estrogen-containing oral contraceptives. For this reason, diabetic patients should be carefully observed while receiving estrogen.

4. *Hypercalcemia.* Administration of estrogens may lead to severe hypercalcemia in patients with breast cancer and bone metastases. If this occurs, the drug should be stopped and appropriate measures taken to reduce the serum calcium level.

Associated with Methyltestosterone

1. Female patients should be watched carefully for symptoms or signs of virilization such as hoarseness or deepening of the voice, oily skin, acne, hirsutism, enlarged clitoris, stimulation of libido, and menstrual irregularities. At the dosage necessary to achieve a tumor response, androgens will cause masculinization of a female, but occasionally a sensitive female may exhibit one or more of these signs on smaller doses. Some of these changes, such as voice changes may be irreversible even after drug is stopped.

2. Cholestatic hepatitis with jaundice and altered liver function tests, such as increased BSP retention and rises in SGOT levels, have been reported with methyltestosterone. These changes appear to be related to dosage of the drug. Therefore, in the presence of any changes in liver function tests, the drug should be discontinued.

Precautions:

Associated with Estrogens

A. General Precautions.

1. A complete medical and family history should be taken prior to the initiation of any estrogen therapy. The pretreatment and periodic physical examinations should include special reference to blood pressure, breasts, abdomen, and pelvic organs, and should include a Papanicolau smear. As a general rule, estrogen should not be prescribed for longer than one year without another physical examination being performed.

2. Fluid retention—Because estrogens may cause some degree of fluid retention, conditions which might be influenced by this factor such as asthma, epilepsy, migraine, and cardiac or renal dysfunction, require careful observation.

3. Certain patients may develop undesirable manifestations of excessive estrogenic stimulation, such as abnormal or excessive uterine bleeding, mastodynia, etc.

4. Oral contraceptives appear to be associated with an increased incidence of mental depression.[24a] Although it is not clear whether this is due to the estrogenic or progestogenic component of the contraceptive, patients with a history of depression should be carefully observed.

5. Preexisting uterine leiomyomata may increase in size during estrogen use.

6. The pathologist should be advised of estrogen therapy when relevant specimens are submitted.

7. Patients with a past history of jaundice during pregnancy have an increased risk of recurrence of jaundice while receiving estrogen-containing oral contraceptive therapy. If jaundice develops in any patient receiving estrogen, the medication should be discontinued while the cause is investigated.

8. Estrogens may be poorly metabolized in patients with impaired liver function and they should be administered with caution in such patients.

9. Because estrogens influence the metabolism of calcium and phosphorus, they should be used with caution in patients with metabolic bone diseases that are associated with hypercalcemia or in patients with renal insufficiency.

10. Because of the effects of estrogens on epiphyseal closure, they should be used judiciously in young patients in whom bone growth is not complete.

11. Certain endocrine and liver function tests may be affected by estrogen-containing oral contraceptives. The following similar changes may be expected with larger doses of estrogen:

a. Increased sulfobromophthalein retention.

b. Increased prothrombin and factors VII, VIII, IX, and X; decreased antithrombin 3; increased norepinephrine-induced platelet aggregability.

c. Increased thyroid binding globulin (TBG) leading to increased circulating total thyroid hormone, as measured by PBI, T4 by column, or T4 by radioimmunoassay. Free T3 resin uptake is decreased, reflecting the elevated TBG; free T4 concentration is unaltered.

d. Impaired glucose tolerance.

e. Decreased pregnanediol excretion.

f. Reduced response to metyrapone test.

g. Reduced serum folate concentration.

h. Increased serum triglyceride and phospholipid concentration.

B. Information for the Patient. See text which appears after the PHYSICIAN REFERENCES under PREMARIN®.

C. Pregnancy Category X. See CONTRAINDICATIONS and Boxed Warning.

D. Nursing Mothers. As a general principle, the administration of any drug to nursing mothers should be done only when clearly necessary since many drugs are excreted in human milk.

Associated with Methyltestosterone

A. Prolonged dosage of androgen may result in sodium and fluid retention. This may present a problem, especially in patients with compromised cardiac reserve or renal disease.

B. Hypersensitivity may occur rarely.

C. PBI may be decreased in patients taking androgens.

D. Hypercalcemia may occur. If this does occur, the drug should be discontinued.

Adverse Reactions:

Associated with Estrogens

(See Warnings regarding induction of neoplasia, adverse effects on the fetus, increased incidence of gallbladder disease and adverse effects similar to those of oral contraceptives, including thromboembolism.) The following additional adverse reactions have been reported with estrogenic therapy, including oral contraceptives:

1. *Genitourinary system:* Breakthrough bleeding, spotting, change in menstrual flow; dysmenorrhea; premenstrual-like syndrome; amenorrhea during and after treatment; increase in size of uterine fibromyomata; vaginal candidiasis; change in cervical erosion and in degree of cervical secretion; cystitis-like syndrome.

2. *Breasts:* Tenderness, enlargement, secretion.

3. *Gastrointestinal:* Nausea, vomiting; abdominal cramps, bloating; cholestatic jaundice.

4. *Skin:* Chloasma or melasma which may persist when drug is discontinued; erythema multiforme; erythema nodosum; hemorrhagic eruption; loss of scalp hair; hirsutism.

5. *Eyes:* Steepening of corneal curvature; intolerance to contact lenses.

6. *CNS:* Headache, migraine, dizziness; mental depression; chorea.

7. *Miscellaneous:* Increase or decrease in weight; reduced carbohydrate tolerance; aggravation of porphyria; edema; changes in libido.

Associated with Methyltestosterone

Cholestatic jaundice

Hypercalcemia, particularly in patients with metastatic breast carcinoma. This usually indicates progression of bone metastases.

Sodium and water retention

Virilization in female patients

Hypersensitivity

Acute Overdosage: Numerous reports of ingestion of large doses of estrogen-containing oral contraceptives by young children indicate that acute serious ill effects do not occur. Overdosage of estrogen may cause nausea, and withdrawal bleeding may occur in females.

Dosage and Administration:

1. *Given cyclically for short-term use only:*

For treatment of moderate to severe *vasomotor* symptoms associated with the menopause in patients not improved by estrogen alone.

The lowest dose that will control symptoms should be chosen and medication should be discontinued as promptly as possible.

Administration should be cyclic (e.g., three weeks on and one week off).

Attempts to discontinue or taper medication should be made at three to six month intervals.

Usual dosage range:

1.25 mg Conjugated Estrogens, U.S.P. and 10.0 mg Methyltestosterone (1 yellow tablet, No. 879, or 2 red tablets, No. 878) daily and cyclically.

2. Given for a few days.

Prevention of postpartum breast engorgement

Usual dosage range:

Using No. 879 (yellow) tablets containing 1.25 mg Conjugated Estrogens, U.S.P. and 10.0 mg Methyltestosterone, either

(a) 3 tablets every four hours for 5 doses, then 2 tablets daily for balance of the week, or

(b) 1 tablet three times each day for the first four days postpartum, then 1 tablet daily for the next 10 days.

Treated patients with an intact uterus should be monitored closely for signs of endometrial cancer and appropriate diagnostic measures should be taken to rule out malignancy in the event of persistent or recurring abnormal vaginal bleeding.

How Supplied: PREMARIN (Conjugated Estrogens, U.S.P.) with Methyltestosterone Tablets

—Each *yellow* tablet contains 1.25 mg PREMARIN and 10.0 mg Methyltestosterone, in bottles of 100 (NDC 0046-0879-81) and 1,000 (NDC 0046-0879-91).

—Each *red* tablet contains 0.625 mg PREMARIN and 5.0 mg Methyltestosterone, in bottles of 100 (NDC 0046-0878-81) and 1,000 (NDC 0046-0878-91).

Physician References:

1. Ziel, H. K., *et al.:* N. Engl. J. Med. *293*:1167–1170, 1975.
2. Smith, D. C., *et al.:* N. Engl. J. Med. *293*:1164–1167, 1975.
3. Mack, T. M., *et al.:* N. Engl. J. Med. *294*:1262–1267, 1976.
4. Weiss, N. S., *et al.:* N. Engl. J. Med. *294*:1259–1262, 1976.
5. Herbst, A. L., *et al.:* N. Engl. J. Med. *284*:878–881, 1971.
6. Greenwald, P., *et al.:* N. Engl. J. Med. *285*:390–392, 1971.
7. Lanier, A., *et al.:* Mayo Clin. Proc. *48*:793–799, 1973.
8. Herbst, A., *et al.:* Obstet. Gynecol. *40*:287–298, 1972.
9. Herbst, A., *et al.:* Am. J. Obstet. Gynecol. *118*:607–615, 1974.
10. Herbst, A., *et al.:* N. Engl. J. Med. *292*:334–339, 1975.
11. Stafl, A., *et al.:* Obstet. Gynecol. *43*:118–128, 1974.

12. Sherman, A. I., *et al.*: Obstet. Gynecol. *44*:531–545, 1974.
13. Gal. I., *et al.*: Nature *216*:83, 1967.
14. Levy, E. P., *et al.*: Lancet *1*:611, 1973.
15. Nora, J., *et al.*: Lancet *1*:941–942, 1973.
16. Janerich, D. T., *et al.*: N. Engl. J. Med. *291*:697–700, 1974.
17. Boston Collaborative Drug Surveillance Program: N. Engl. J. Med. *290*:15–19, 1974.
18. Hoover, R., *et al.*: N. Engl. J. Med. 295 : 401–405, 1976.
19. Boston Collaborative Drug Surveillance Program: Lancet *1*:1399–1404, 1973.
20. Daniel, D. G., *et al.*: Lancet *2*:287–289, 1967.
21. The Veterans Administration Cooperative Urological Research Group: J. Urol. *98*:516–522, 1967.
22. Bailar, J. C.: Lancet *2*:560, 1967.
23. Blackard, C., *et al.*: Cancer *26*:249–256, 1970.
24. Royal College of General Practitioners: J. R. Coll. Gen. Pract. *13*:267–279, 1967.
24a. Royal College of General Practitioners: Oral Contraceptives and Health, New York, Pitman Corp., 1974.
25. Inman, W. H. W., *et al.*: Br. Med. J. *2*:193–199, 1968.
26. Vessey, M. P., *et al.*: Br. Med. J. *2*:651–657, 1969.
27. Sartwell, P. E., *et al.*: Am. J. Epidemiol. *90*:365–380, 1969.
28. Collaborative Group for the Study of Stroke in Young Women: N. Engl. J. Med. *288*:871–878, 1973.
29. Collaborative Group for the Study of Stroke in Young Women: J.A.M.A. *231*: 718–722, 1975.
30. Mann, J. I., *et al.*: Br. Med. J. *2*:245–248, 1975.
31. Mann, J. I., *et al.*: Br. Med. J. *2*:241–245, 1975.
32. Inman, W. H. W., *et al.*: Br. Med. J. *2*:203–209, 1970.
33. Stolley, P. D., *et al.*: Am. J. Epidemiol. *102*:197–208, 1975.
34. Vessey, M. P., *et al.*: Br. Med. J. *3*:123–126, 1970.
35. Greene, G. R., *et al.*: Am. J. Public Health *62*:680–685, 1972.
36. Rosenberg, L., *et al.*: N. Engl. J. Med. *294*: 1256–1259, 1976.
37. Coronary Drug Project Research Group: J.A.M.A. *214*:1303–1313, 1970.
38. Baum, J., *et al.*: Lancet *2*:926–928, 1973.
39. Mays, E. T., *et al.*: J.A.M.A. *235*:730–732, 1976.
40. Edmondson, H. A., *et al.*: N. Engl. J. Med. *294*:470–472, 1976.
41. Pfeffer, R. I., *et al.*: Am. J. Epidemiol. *103*:445–456, 1976.

[Shown in Product Identification Section]

PROTOPAM® CHLORIDE ℞

Brand of pralidoxime chloride

Description: PROTOPAM CHLORIDE is a cholinesterase reactivator.

Chemically, it is 2-formyl-1-methylpyridinium chloride oxime (pyridine-2-aldoxime methochloride), and has the generic name pralidoxime chloride. It has also been referred to as 2-PAM Chloride.

PROTOPAM CHLORIDE occurs as a white, nonhygroscopic, crystalline powder which is soluble in water to the extent of 1 g in less than 1 ml.

The specific activity of the drug resides in the 2-formyl-1-methylpyridinium ion and is independent of the particular salt employed.

Actions: The principal action of PROTOPAM is to reactivate cholinesterase (mainly outside of the central nervous system) which has been inactivated by phosphorylation due to an organophosphate pesticide or related compound. The destruction of accumulated acetylcholine can then proceed and neuromuscular junctions will again function normally. PROTOPAM also slows the process of "aging" of phosphorylated cholinesterase to a non-reactivatable form, and detoxifies certain organophosphates by direct chemical reaction. The drug has its most critical effect in relieving paralysis of the muscles of respiration. Because PROTOPAM is less effective in relieving depression of the respiratory center, atropine is always required concomitantly to block the effect of accumulated acetylcholine at this site. PROTOPAM relieves muscarinic signs and symptoms, salivation, bronchospasm, etc., but this action is relatively unimportant since atropine is adequate for this purpose.

PROTOPAM antagonizes the effects on the neuromuscular junction of the carbamate anticholinesterases, neostigmine, pyridostigmine and ambenonium, used in the treatment of myasthenia gravis. However, it is not nearly as effective as an antidote to these drugs as it is to the organophosphates.

PROTOPAM (pralidoxime) is distributed throughout the extracellular water; it is not bound to plasma protein. The drug is rapidly excreted in the urine partly unchanged, and partly as a metabolite produced by the liver. Consequently. PROTOPAM is relatively short acting and repeated doses may be needed, especially where there is any evidence of continuing absorption of the poison.

Indications: PROTOPAM is indicated as an antidote: (1) in the treatment of poisoning due to those pesticides and chemicals of the organophosphate class which have anticholinesterase activity, and (2) in the control of overdosage by anticholinesterase drugs used in the treatment of myasthenia gravis.

Warnings: Use of PROTOPAM should always be under supervision of the subject's personal physician or of the medical department of his employer.

PROTOPAM is not effective in the treatment of poisoning due to phosphorus, inorganic phosphates or organophosphates not having anticholinesterase activity.

Until further information is available, no recommendation is made as to the use of PROTOPAM in intoxication by pesticides of the carbamate class.

Precautions: PROTOPAM has been very well tolerated in most cases, but it must be remembered that the desperate condition of the organophosphate-poisoned patient will generally mask such minor signs and symptoms as have been noted in normal subjects.

Intravenous administration of PROTOPAM should be carried out slowly and, preferably, by infusion, since certain side effects, such as tachycardia, laryngospasm, and muscle rigidity, have been attributed in a few cases to a too rapid rate of injection. (See Dosage and Administration.)

Because PROTOPAM is excreted in the urine, a decrease in renal function will result in increased blood levels of the drug. Thus, the dosage of PROTOPAM should be reduced in the presence of renal insufficiency.

PROTOPAM should be used with great caution in treating organophosphate overdosage in cases of myasthenia gravis since it may precipitate a myasthenic crisis.

The following precautions should be kept in mind in the treatment of anticholinesterase poisoning, although they do not bear directly on the use of PROTOPAM (pralidoxime): since barbiturates are potentiated by the anticholinesterases, they should be used cautiously in the treatment of convulsions; morphine, theophylline, aminophylline, succinylcholine, reserpine, and phenothiazine-type tranquilizers should be avoided in patients with organophosphate poisoning.

Adverse Reactions: Dizziness, blurred vision, diplopia and impaired accommodation, headache, drowsiness, nausea, tachycardia, hyperventilation, and muscular weakness have been reported after the use of PROTOPAM, but it is very difficult to differentiate the toxic effects produced by atropine or the organophosphate compounds from those of the drug. When atropine and PROTOPAM are used together, the signs of atropinization may occur earlier than might be expected when atropine is used alone. This is especially true if the total dose of atropine has been large and the administration of PROTOPAM has been delayed. Excitement and manic behavior immediately following recovery of consciousness have been reported in several cases. However, similar behavior has occurred in cases of organophosphate poisoning that were not treated with PROTOPAM.

Dosage and Administration:

Organophosphate poisoning

Initial measures should include removal of secretions, maintenance of a patent airway and, if necessary, artificial ventilation.

In the absence of cyanosis, atropine should be given intravenously in doses of 2 to 4 mg; where cyanosis is present, this dose of atropine should be given intramuscularly while simultaneously initiating measures for improving ventilation. Atropine administration should be repeated at 5 to 10 minute intervals until signs of atropine toxicity appear. Some degree of atropinization should be maintained for at least 48 hours.

PROTOPAM administration should be started at the same time as atropine.

In adults, inject an initial dose of 1 to 2 g of PROTOPAM, preferably as an infusion in 100 ml of saline, over a 15 to 30 minute period. If this is not practicable or if pulmonary edema is present, the dose should be given slowly by intravenous injection as a 5 percent solution in water over not less than five minutes. After about an hour, a second dose of 1 to 2 g will be indicated if muscle weakness has not been relieved. Additional doses may be given cautiously if muscle weakness persists. If intravenous administration is not feasible, intramuscular or subcutaneous injection should be used.

In children, the dose should be 20 to 40 mg per kg.

Treatment will be most effective if given within a few hours after poisoning has occurred. Usually, little will be accomplished if the drug is first administered more than 48 hours after exposure, but in severe poisoning, it is, nevertheless, indicated since occasionally patients have responded after such an interval.

In severe cases, especially after ingestion of the poison, it may be desirable to monitor the effect of therapy electrocardiographically because of the possibility of heart block due to the anticholinesterase. Where the poison has been ingested, it is particularly important to take into account the likelihood of continuing absorption from the lower bowel since this constitutes new exposure. In such cases, additional doses of PROTOPAM (pralidoxime) may be needed every three to eight hours. In effect, the patient should be "titrated" with PROTOPAM as long as signs of poisoning recur.

In the absence of severe gastrointestinal symptoms, resulting from the anticholinesterase intoxication, PROTOPAM may be administered orally in doses of 1 to 3 g (2 to 6 tablets) every five hours. As in all cases of organophosphate poisoning, care should be taken to keep the patient under observation for at least 24 hours.

If convulsions interfere with respiration, sodium thiopental (2.5 percent solution) may be given intravenously with care.

Anticholinesterase overdosage

As an antagonist to such anticholinesterases as neostigmine, pyridostigmine, and ambenonium, which are used in the treatment of myasthenia gravis, PROTOPAM may be given in a dosage of 1 to 2 g intravenously followed by increments of 250 mg every five minutes.

Continued on next page

Ayerst—Cont.

Overdosage: Artificial respiration and other supportive therapy should be administered as needed.

How Supplied: NDC 0046-0375-98—*Emergency Kit:* This contains one 20 ml vial of 1 g of sterile PROTOPAM CHLORIDE (pralidoxime chloride) white to off white porous cake*; one 20 ml ampul of Sterile Water for Injection, U.S.P. without preservative to be used as diluent; sterile, disposable 20 ml syringe; needle; alcohol swab. This is a single dose kit for intravenous administration. Intramuscular or subcutaneous injection may be used when intravenous injection is not feasible.
NDC 0046-0374-06—*Hospital Package:* This contains six 20 ml vials of 1 g each of sterile PROTOPAM CHLORIDE (pralidoxime chloride) white to off white porous cake*, without diluent or syringe. Solution may be prepared by adding 20 ml of Sterile Water for Injection, U.S.P. These are single dose vials for intravenous injection or for intravenous infusion after further dilution with physiologic saline. Intramuscular or subcutaneous injection may be used when intravenous injection is not feasible.

*When necessary, sodium hydroxide is added during processing to adjust the pH

PROTOPAM CHLORIDE for Injection is prepared by cryodesiccation.
NDC 0046-0376-81—*Tablets:* Each tablet contains 500 mg of pralidoxime chloride, in bottles of 100.
A FULL DISCUSSION OF THE ACTIONS AND USES OF PROTOPAM (PRALIDOXIME) IS GIVEN IN A PROFESSIONAL BROCHURE WHICH IS AVAILABLE FROM AYERST LABORATORIES ON REQUEST.

Animal Pharmacology and Toxicology: The following table lists chemical and trade or generic names of pesticides, chemicals, and drugs against which PROTOPAM (usually administered in conjunction with atropine) has been found to have antidotal activity on the basis of animal experiments. All compounds listed are organophosphates having anticholinesterase activity. A great many additional substances are in industrial use but have been omitted because of lack of specific information. The use of PROTOPAM should, nevertheless, be considered in any life-threatening situation resulting from poisoning by these compounds, since the limited and arbitrary conditions of pharmacologic screening do not always accurately reflect the usefulness of PROTOPAM in the clinical situation.

AAT—see PARATHION

AFLIX®—see FORMOTHION

ALKRON®—see PARATHION

AMERICAN CYANAMID 3422—see PARATHION

AMITON—diethyl -S- (2-diethyl-aminoethyl) phosphorothiolate

ANTHIO®—see FORMOTHION

APHAMITE—see PARATHION

ARMIN—ethyl-4-nitrophenyl-ethylphosphonate

AZINPHOS-METHYL—dimethyl-S- (4-oxo-1, 2, 3, -benzotriazin-3 (4 H) -ylmethyl) phosphorodithioate

AZODRIN—dimethyl phosphate of 3-hydroxy-N-methyl-cis-crotonamide

BAYER 16259—see ETHYL GUTHION

BAYER 19639—see DISULFOTON

BAYER 25141 — diethyl-4-methyl-sulfinyl-phenylphosphorothionate

BAYER 29493—see FENTHION

BAYER L13/59—see TRICHLOROFON

BAYER E605—see PARATHION

BAYTEX®—see FENTHION

CHIPMAN R6199—see AMITON

COMPOUND 3422—see PARATHION

COMPOUND 4049—see MALATHION

COMPOUND 4072—2-chloro-1-(2,4-dichlorophenyl) vinyl diethyl-phosphate

CO-RAL®—see COUMAPHOS

COROTHION—see PARATHION

COUMAPHOS—3-chloro-4-methyl coumarin-7-yl-diethyl-phosphorothionate

DBD —see AZINPHOS-METHYL

DDVP—see DICHLORVOS

DELNAV—see DIOXATHION

DEMETON—Mixture of SYSTOX® and ISO-SYSTOX®

DEMETON-S—see ISOSYSTOX®

DFP—see ISOFLUROPHATE

DIAZINON—diethyl- (2- isopropyl -4- methyl -6- pyrimidyl) phosphorothionate

DICHLORVOS—dimethyl-2, 2-dichloro vinyl phosphate

DIETHYL-p-NITROPHENYL-PHOSPHOROTHIONATE—see PARATHION

DIETHYL -p- NITROPHENYL - THIONOPHOSPHATE—see PARATHION

DIOXATHION—2, 3-p-dioxanedithio-S, S-bis (0, 0-diethyl phosphorodithioate)

DIPTEREX®—see TRICHLOROFON

DISULFOTON—diethyl -S- (2-ethylthioethyl) phosphorodiothiate

DISYSTON®—see DISULFOTON

DITHIOSYSTOX—see DISULFOTON

DNTP—see PARATHION

DPP—see PARATHION

DSDP—see AMITON

DYFLOS—see DFP

DYLOX®—see TRICHLOROFON

E 600—see PARAOXON

E 601—see METHYL PARATHION

E 605—see PARATHION

E 1059—see SYSTOX

ECHOTHIOPHATE IODIDE—diethoxyphosphinylthio-choline iodide

EKATIN®—see MORPHOTHION

ENDOTHION—2- (dimethoxyphosphinylthiomethyl)-5-methoxy-4-pyrone

ENT 15108—see PARATHION

ENTEX®—see FENTHION

EPN—ethyl -4- nitrophenyl - phenylphosphonothionate

ETHION—0,0,0',0'-tetraethyl-S,S'-methylene-bis-phosphoro dithioate

ETHYL GUSATHION—see ETHYL GUTHION

ETHYL GUTHION®—diethyl-S-(4-oxo-1,2,3,-benzotriazinyl-3-methyl) phosphorodithioate

ETILON—see PARATHION

FENTHION—dimethyl-(4-methylthio-3-tolyl) phosphorothionate

FLOROPRYL®—see DFP

FOLIDOL®—see PARATHION

FORMOTHION—dimethyl -S- (N-formyl -N-methylcarbamyl-methyl) phosphorodithioate

G 24480—see DIAZINON

GB—see SARIN

GENITHION—see PARATHION

GUSATHION®—see AZINPHOSMETHYL

GUTHION®—see AZINPHOSMETHYL

HETP—see TEPP

I-ARMIN—isopropyl -4- nitro-phenyl methylphosphonate

ISOFLUROPHATE—diisopropyl - phosphorofluoridate

ISOSYSTOX®— diethyl-S-(2-ethylmercaptoethyl)-phosphorothiolate

LEBACYD®—see FENTHION

MACKOTHION—see PARATHION

MALATHION—dimethyl -S- (1, 2-dicarbethoxyethyl) -phosphorodithioate

MALATHON—see MALATHION

M-ARMIN—ethyl-4-nitrophenyl methylphosphonate

MECARBAM—0, 0-dimethyl -S- (N-ethoxycarbonyl-N-methyl carbamoylmethyl) phosphorodithioate

METACIDE—see METHYL PARATHION

METASYSTOX®—see METHYL DEMETON

METASYSTOX I®—dimethyl -2- ethyl-mercaptoethylphos-phorothiolate

METASYSTOX R®—see OXYDEMETON-METHYL

METHYL DEMETON—mixture of dimethyl(2-ethylmercapto-ethyl) phosphorothionate and dimethyl-S-(2-ethylmercapto-ethyl) phosphorothiolate

METHYL PARATHION—dimethyl - (4-nitrophenyl) phosphorothionate

MEVINPHOS—1- carbomethoxy-1- propen-2-yl-dimethylphosphate

MINTACOL®—see PARAOXON

ML 97—see PHOSPHAMIDON

MORPHOTHION—dimethyl -S- 2-keto-2- (N-morpholyl ethyl-phosphorodithioate

NEGUVON®—see TRICHLOROFON

NIRAN®—see PARATHION

NITROSTIGMINE—see PARATHION

0, 0-DIETHYL -O- p-NITRO-PHENYL PHOSPHOROTHIOATE—see PARATHION

0, 0-DIETHYL -O- p-NITRO-PHENYLTHIOPHOSPHATE —see PARATHION

OR 1191—see PHOSPHAMIDON

OS 1836—see VINYLPHOS

OXYDEMETONMETHYL—dimethyl -S- 2-(ethylsulfinyl) ethyl phosphorothiolate

PARAOXON—diethyl (4 - nitro - phenyl) phosphate.

PARATHION—diethyl (4-nitro-phenyl) phosphorothionate

PENPHOS—see PARATHION

PHENCAPTON—diethyl -S- (2, 5-dichlorophenylmercaptomethyl) phosphorodithioate

PHOSDRIN®—see MEVINPHOS

PHOS-KIL—see PARATHION

PHOSPHAMIDON—1-chloro -1- diethylcarbamoyl -1- propen -2- yl-dimethylphosphate

PHOSPHOLINE IODIDE®—see echothiophate iodide

PHOSPHOROTHIOIC ACID, 0,0-DIETHYL-0-p-NITRO-PHENYL ESTER—see PARATHION

PLANTHION—see PARATHION

QUELETOX—see FENTHION

RHODIATOX®—see PARATHION

RUELENE®— 4- tert-butyl -2- chlorophenyl-methyl-N-methyl-phosphoroamidate

SARIN— isopropyl - methylphos - phonofluoridate

SHELL OS 1836—see VINYLPHOS

SHELL 2046—see MEVINPHOS

SNP—see PARATHION

SOMAN—pinacolyl - methyl - phosphonofluoridate

SYSTOX®—diethyl - (2-ethyl-mercaptoethyl) phosphorothionate

TEP—see TEPP

TEPP—tetraethylpyro phosphate

THIOPHOS®—see PARATHION

TIGUVON—see FENTHION

TRICHLOROFON—dimethyl -1- hydroxy-2, 2, 2-trichloro ethylphosphonate

VAPONA®—see DICHLORVOS

VAPOPHOS—see PARATHION

VINYLPHOS—diethyl -2- chloro - vinylphosphate

PROTOPAM appears to be ineffective, or marginally effective, against poisoning by:

CIODRIN® (alpha-methylbenzyl-3-[dimethoxyphosphinyloxy]-cis-crotonate)
DIMEFOX (tetramethylphosphorodiamidic fluoride)
DIMETHOATE (dimethyl-S-[N-methylcarbamoylmethyl]phosphorodithioate)
METHYL DIAZINON (dimethyl-[2-isopropyl-4-methylpyrimidyl]-phosphorothionate)
METHYL PHENCAPTON (dimethyl-S- [2, 5-dichlorophenylmercaptomethyl] phosphorodithioate)
PHORATE (diethyl-S-ethylmercaptomethyl-phosphorodithioate)
SCHRADAN (octamethylpyrophosphoramide)
WEPSYN® (5-amino-1-[bis-(dimethylamino)-phosphinyl]-3-phenyl-1,2,4-triazole)

Clinical Studies: The use of PROTOPAM (pralidoxime) has been reported in the treatment of human cases of poisoning by the following substances:

- Azodrin
- Diazinon
- Dichlorvos (DDVP) with chlordane
- Disulfoton
- EPN
- Isoflurophate
- Malathion
- Metasystox I® and Fenthion
- Methyl demeton
- Methyl parathion
- Mevinphos
- Parathion
- Parathion and Mevinphos
- Phosphamidon
- Sarin
- Systox®
- TEPP

Of these cases, over 100 were due to parathion, about a dozen each to malathion, diazinon, and mevinphos, and a few to each of the other compounds.

RIOPAN®
Brand of magaldrate
Antacid

RIOPAN is a chemical entity (not a physical mixture), providing the advantages of a true buffer-antacid (not simply a neutralizing agent): (1) rapid action; (2) uniform buffering action; (3) high acid-consuming capacity; (4) no alkalinization or acid rebound.

Low Sodium Content: Not more than 0.3 mg of sodium—per teaspoonful (5 ml) suspension—per chew tablet—per swallow tablet.

Acid-neutralizing Capacity—13.5 mEq/5 ml or tablet.

Indications: For prompt relief of heartburn, sour stomach, and/or acid indigestion. For symptomatic relief of hyperacidity associated with the diagnosis of peptic ulcer, gastritis, peptic esophagitis, gastric hyperacidity, and hiatal hernia.

Directions: RIOPAN Antacid *Suspension*—Recommended dosage, one or two teaspoonfuls, between meals and at bedtime, or as directed by the physician. RIOPAN Antacid *Chew Tablets*—Recommended dosage, one or two tablets, between meals and at bedtime, or as directed by the physician. Chew before swallowing. RIOPAN Antacid *Swallow Tablets* —Recommended dosage, one or two tablets, between meals and at bedtime, or as directed by the physician. Take with enough water to swallow promptly.

Drug Interaction Precaution: Do not use in patients taking a prescription antibiotic drug containing any form of tetracycline.

Warnings: Patients should not take more than 20 teaspoonfuls (or 20 tablets) in a 24-hour period or use this maximum dosage for more than two weeks and patients with kidney disease should not use in excess of the recommended dosage, except under the advice and supervision of a physician.

How Supplied: RIOPAN Antacid *Suspension* —Each teaspoonful (5 ml) contains 480 mg magaldrate, in 12 fl oz (355 ml) bottles (NDC 0046-0933-12). Individual Cups, 1 fl oz (30 ml) ea., tray of 10—10 trays per packer (NDC 0046-0933-99). RIOPAN Antacid *Chew Tablets*—Each tablet contains 480 mg magaldrate. Packages of 60 (NDC 0046-0928-60) and 100 (NDC 0046-0928-81) in individual film strips (10 x 6 and 10 x 10, respectively). RIOPAN Antacid *Swallow Tablets*—Each tablet contains 480 mg magaldrate. Packages of 60 (NDC 0046-0927-60) and 100 (NDC 0046-0927-81) in individual film strips (6 x 10 and 10 x 10, respectively).

[Shown in Product Identification Section]

RIOPAN PLUS®
magaldrate and SIMETHICONE
Antacid/Anti-Gas

Each teaspoonful (5 ml) of Suspension contains:
Magaldrate .... 480 mg
Simethicone .... 20 mg
Each Chew Tablet contains:
Magaldrate .... 480 mg
Simethicone .... 20 mg

Low Sodium Content: Not more than 0.3 mg per teaspoonful (5 ml) or Chew Tablet.

Acid-neutralizing Capacity—13.5 mEq/5 ml or Chew Tablet.

Indications: For prompt relief of heartburn, sour stomach, and/or acid indigestion, accompanied by the symptoms of gas. For symptomatic relief of hyperacidity associated with the diagnosis of peptic ulcer, gastritis, peptic esophagitis, gastric hyperacidity, and hiatal hernia. For postoperative gas pain or for use in endoscopic examinations.

Directions: RIOPAN PLUS *Suspension*—Recommended dosage, one or two teaspoonfuls between meals and at bedtime, or as directed by the physician.

RIOPAN PLUS *Chew Tablets*—Recommended dosage, one or two tablets, between meals and at bedtime, or as directed by the physician. Chew before swallowing.

Drug Interaction Precaution: Do not use in patients taking a prescription antibiotic drug containing any form of tetracycline.

Warnings: Patients should not take more than 20 teaspoonfuls (or 20 tablets) in a 24-hour period or use this maximum dosage for more than two weeks and patients with kidney disease should not use in excess of the recommended dosage, except under the advice and supervision of a physician.

Continued on next page

Ayerst—Cont.

How Supplied: RIOPAN PLUS *Suspension* —in 12 fl oz (355 ml) plastic bottles (NDC 0046-0937-12). Individual Cups, 1 fl oz (30 ml) ea., tray of 10—10 trays per packer (NDC 0046-0937-99).
RIOPAN PLUS *Chew Tablets*—in packages of 60 (NDC 0046-0930-60).
[*Shown in Product Identification Section*]

THIOSULFIL® ℞
(sulfamethizole)
DUO-PAK®
Package

This package contains 2 products:

Bottle No. 1—24 Tablets (*yellow*)

THIOSULFIL®-A Forte
(sulfamethizole 0.5 g with phenazopyridine HCl)
Each tablet contains:
Sulfamethizole.. 0.5 g
Phenazopyridine HCl .... 50.0 mg

Bottle No. 2—32 Tablets (*white*)

THIOSULFIL® Forte
(sulfamethizole)
Each tablet contains:
Sulfamethizole.. 0.5 g

Indications: THIOSULFIL-A Forte (sulfamethizole 0.5 g with phenazopyridine HCl)—Bottle No. 1.—is indicated for pain, burning, frequency, and urgency due to inflammation associated with urinary tract infection.
THIOSULFIL Forte (sulfamethizole)—Bottle No. 2—is indicated for continuing antibacterial therapy after pain and discomfort have been relieved.
THIOSULFIL is indicated in the treatment of urinary tract infections (primarily pyelonephritis, pyelitis, and cystitis) in the absence of obstructive uropathy or foreign bodies, when these infections are caused by susceptible strains of the following organisms: *Escherichia coli, Klebsiella-Enterobacter, Staphylococcus aureus, Proteus mirabilis,* and *Proteus vulgaris.*

Important note, *In vitro* sulfonamide sensitivity tests are not always reliable. The test must be carefully coordinated with bacteriologic and clinical response. When the patient is already taking sulfonamides, follow-up cultures should have aminobenzoic acid added to the culture media.
Currently, the increasing frequency of resistant organisms is a limitation of the usefulness of antibacterial agents, including the sulfonamides, especially in the treatment of recurrent and complicated urinary tract infections.
Wide variation in blood levels may result with identical doses. Blood levels should be measured in patients receiving sulfonamides for serious infections. Free sulfonamide blood levels of 5–15 mg per 100 ml may be considered therapeutically effective for most infections, with blood levels of 12–15 mg per 100 ml optimal for serious infections; 20 mg per 100 ml should be the maximum total sulfonamide level, as adverse reactions occur more frequently above this level.

Contraindications: Sulfonamides should not be used in patients hypersensitive to sulfa drugs. They should not be used in infants less than two months of age, in pregnancy at term, and during the nursing period because sulfonamides pass the placenta and are excreted in the milk and may cause kernicterus.
Phenazopyridine HCl is contraindicated in renal or hepatic failure, glomerulonephritis, and pyelonephritis of pregnancy with gastrointestinal disturbances.

Warnings: Sulfonamides should not be used to treat group A streptococci infections or their sequelae. The occurrence of sore throat, fever, pallor, purpura, or jaundice during sulfonamide administration may be an early indication of serious blood dyscrasias.
Deaths associated with the administration of sulfonamides have been reported from hypersensitivity reactions, agranulocytosis, aplastic anemia, and other blood dyscrasias.
Frequent blood counts and renal function tests should be carried out during sulfonamide treatment, especially during prolonged administration. Microscopic urinalyses should be done once a week when a patient is treated for longer than two weeks. Urine cultures should be made to confirm eradication of bacteriuria.
Usage in Pregnancy: The safe use of sulfonamides in pregnancy has not been established. The teratogenicity potential of most sulfonamides has not been thoroughly investigated in either animals or humans. However, a significant increase in the incidence of cleft palate and other bony abnormalities of offspring has been observed when certain sulfonamides of the short-, intermediate-, and long-acting types were given to pregnant rats and mice at high oral doses (7 to 25 times the human dose).

Precautions: To allay any possible apprehension, patients should be told that this medication may color the urine orange or red.
The usual precautions used in sulfonamide therapy should be observed, including the maintenance of an adequate fluid intake. Sulfonamides should be used with caution in patients with severe allergy or bronchial asthma, severe impairment of hepatic or renal function, and in patients with glucose-6-phosphate dehydrogenase deficiency since sulfas may cause hemolysis in this latter group.

Adverse Reactions:
Blood dyscrasias. Agranulocytosis, aplastic anemia, thrombocytopenia, leukopenia, hemolytic anemia, purpura, hypoprothrombinemia, and methemoglobinemia.
Allergic reactions. Erythema multiforme (Stevens-Johnson Syndrome), generalized skin eruptions, epidermal necrolysis, urticaria, serum sickness, pruritus, exfoliative dermatitis, anaphylactoid reactions, periorbital edema, conjunctival and scleral injection, photosensitization, arthralgia, and allergic myocarditis.
Gastrointestinal reactions. Nausea, emesis, abdominal pains, hepatitis, diarrhea, anorexia, pancreatitis, and stomatitis.
C.N.S. reactions. Headache, peripheral neuritis, mental depression, convulsions, ataxia, hallucinations, tinnitus, vertigo, and insomnia.
Miscellaneous reactions. Drug fever, chills, and toxic nephrosis with oliguria and anuria. Periarteritis nodosum and L.E. phenomenon have occurred.
The sulfonamides bear certain chemical similarities to some goitrogens, diuretics (acetazolamide and the thiazides), and oral hypoglycemic agents. Goiter production, diuresis, and hypoglycemia have occurred rarely in patients receiving sulfonamides. Cross-sensitivity may exist with these agents.
Rats appear to be especially susceptible to the goitrogenic effects of sulfonamides, and long term administration has produced thyroid malignancies in the species.

Dosage and Administration: *Adult dosage regimen:*
Start—Bottle No. 1 THIOSULFIL-A Forte (sulfamethizole 0.5 g with phenazopyridine HCl)—Two *yellow* tablets (1 g) four times daily for three days.
Continue—Bottle No. 2 THIOSULFIL Forte (sulfamethizole)—Two *white* tablets (1 g) four times daily for four days. Continue medication as recommended by physician.
If pain persists after a course of THIOSULFIL-A Forte, causes for the discomfort other than infection should be investigated.

How Supplied: THIOSULFIL® (sulfamethizole) DUO-PAK®—NDC 0046-0780-98.
Bottle No. 1—THIOSULFIL®-A Forte: 24 tablets (yellow).
Bottle No. 2—THIOSULFIL® Forte: 32 tablets (white).
[*Shown in Product Identification Section*]

THIOSULFIL® FORTE ℞
Brand of sulfamethizole 0.5 g
and
THIOSULFIL®
Brand of sulfamethizole 0.25 g

Bacteriostatic agent for use in Urinary Tract Infection (due to susceptible organisms)

Indications: THIOSULFIL is indicated in the treatment of urinary tract infections (primarily pyelonephritis, pyelitis, and cystitis) in the absence of obstructive uropathy or foreign bodies, when these infections are caused by susceptible strains of the following organisms: *Escherichia coli, Klebsiella-Enterobacter, Staphylococcus aureus, Proteus mirabilis,* and *Proteus vulgaris.*
Important note, *In vitro* sulfonamide sensitivity tests are not always reliable. The test must be carefully coordinated with bacteriologic and clinical reponse. When the patient is already taking sulfonamides, follow-up cultures should have aminobenzoic acid added to the culture media.
Currently, the increasing frequency of resistant organisms is a limitation of the usefulness of antibacterial agents, including the sulfonamides, especially in the treatment of recurrent and complicated urinary tract infections.

Wide variation in blood levels may result with identical doses. Blood levels should be measured in patients receiving sulfonamides for serious infections. Free sulfonamide blood levels of 5–15 mg per 100 ml may be considered therapeutically effective for most infections, with blood levels of 12–15 mg per 100 ml optimal for serious infections; 20 mg per 100 ml should be the maximum total sulfonamide level, as adverse reactions occur more frequently above this level.

Contraindications: Sulfonamides should not be used in patients hypersensitive to sulfa drugs. They should not be used in infants less than two months of age, in pregnancy at term, and during the nursing period because sulfonamides pass the placenta and are excreted in the milk and may cause kernicterus.

Warnings: Sulfonamides should not be used to treat group A streptococci infections or their sequelae. The occurrence of sore throat, fever, pallor, purpura, or jaundice during sulfonamide administration may be an early indication of serious blood dyscrasias.
Deaths associated with the administration of sulfonamides have been reported from hypersensitivity reactions, agranulocytosis, aplastic anemia, and other blood dyscrasias.
Frequent blood counts and renal function tests should be carried out during sulfonamide treatment, especially during prolonged administration. Microscopic urinalyses should be done once a week when a patient is treated for longer than two weeks. Urine cultures should be made to confirm eradication of bacteriuria.

Usage in Pregnancy: The safe use of sulfonamides in pregnancy has not been established. The teratogenicity potential of most sulfonamides has not been thoroughly investigated in either animals or humans. However, a significant increase in the incidence of cleft palate and other bony abnormalities of offspring has been observed when certain sulfonamides of the short-, intermediate-, and long-acting types were given to pregnant rats and mice at high oral doses (7 to 25 times the human dose).

Precautions: The usual precautions used in sulfonamide therapy should be observed, including the maintenance of an adequate fluid intake. Sulfonamides should be used with caution in patients with severe allergy or bronchial asthma, severe impairment of hepatic or renal function, and in patients with glucose-6-phosphate dehydrogenase deficiency since sulfas may cause hemolysis in this latter group.

Adverse Reactions: *Blood dyscrasias.* Agranulocytosis, aplastic anemia, thrombocytopenia, leukopenia, hemolytic anemia, purpura, hypoprothrombinemia, and methemoglobinemia.

Allergic reactions. Erythema multiforme (Stevens-Johnson Syndrome), generalized skin eruptions, epidermal necrolysis, urticaria, serum sickness, pruritus, exfoliative dermatitis, anaphylactoid reactions, periorbital edema, conjunctival and scleral injection, photosensitization, arthralgia, and allergic myocarditis.

Gastrointestinal reactions. Nausea, emesis, abdominal pains, hepatitis, diarrhea, anorexia, pancreatitis, and stomatitis.

C.N.S. reactions. Headache, peripheral neuritis, mental depression, convulsions, ataxia, hallucinations, tinnitus, vertigo, and insomnia.

Miscellaneous reactions. Drug fever, chills, and toxic nephrosis with oliguria and anuria. Periarteritis nodosum and L.E. phenomenon have occurred.

The sulfonamides bear certain chemical similarities to some goitrogens, diuretics (acetazolamide and the thiazides), and oral hypoglycemic agents. Goiter production, diuresis, and hypoglycemia have occurred rarely in patients receiving sulfonamides. Cross-sensitivity may exist with these agents.

Rats appear to be especially susceptible to the goitrogenic effects of sulfonamides, and long term administration has produced thyroid malignancies in the species.

Dosage and Administration: Usual dosage: *Adults:* 0.5 to 1.0 g three or four times daily. *Children and infants* (over 2 months of age): 30 to 45 mg/kg/24 hours, divided into 4 doses.

How Supplied: THIOSULFIL Forte—Each tablet contains sulfamethizole 0.5 g (scored), in bottles of 100 (NDC 0046-0786-81) and 1,000 (NDC 0046-0786-91).

Also in unit dose package of 100 (NDC 0046-0786-99).

THIOSULFIL—Each tablet contains sulfamethizole 0.25 g (scored), in bottles of 100 (NDC 0046-0785-81) and 1,000 (NDC 0046-0785-91).

[*Shown in Product Identification Section*]

THIOSULFIL®-A Forte ℞

(sulfamethizole 0.5 g with phenazopyridine HCl)

Each tablet contains:
Sulfamethizole....................0.5 g
Phenazopyridine HCl....................50.0 mg

and

THIOSULFIL®-A

(sulfamethizole with phenazopyridine HCl)

Each tablet contains:
Sulfamethizole....................0.25 g
Phenazopyridine HCl....................50.0 mg

Where pain is part of the problem in Urinary Tract Infection (due to susceptible organisms)

Indications: Phenazopyridine HCl is indicated for the treatment of pain, burning, frequency, and urgency caused by the inflammation associated with urinary tract infection.

THIOSULFIL is indicated in the treatment of urinary tract infections (primarily pyelonephritis, pyelitis, and cystitis) in the absence of obstructive uropathy or foreign bodies, when these infections are caused by susceptible strains of the following organisms: *Escherichia coli, Klebsiella-Enterobacter, Staphylococcus aureus, Proteus mirabilis,* and *Proteus vulgaris.*

Important note, *In vitro* sulfonamide sensitivity tests are not always reliable. The test must be carefully coordinated with bacteriologic and clinical reponse. When the patient is already taking sulfonamides, follow-up cultures should have aminobenzoic acid added to the culture media.

Currently, the increasing frequency of resistant organisms is a limitation of the usefulness of antibacterial agents, including the sulfonamides, especially in the treatment of recurrent and complicated urinary tract infections.

Wide variation in blood levels may result with identical doses. Blood levels should be measured in patients receiving sulfonamides for serious infections. Free sulfonamide blood levels of 5–15 mg per 100 ml may be considered therapeutically effective for most infections, with blood levels of 12–15 mg per 100 ml optimal for serious infections; 20 mg per 100 ml should be the maximum total sulfonamide level, as adverse reactions occur more frequently above this level.

Contraindications: Sulfonamides should not be used in patients hypersensitive to sulfa drugs. They should not be used in infants less than two months of age, in pregnancy at term, and during the nursing period because sulfonamides pass the placenta and are excreted in the milk and may cause kernicterus.

Phenazopyridine HCl is contraindicated in renal or hepatic failure, glomerulonephritis, and pyelonephritis of pregnancy with gastrointestinal disturbances.

Warnings: Sulfonamides should not be used to treat group A streptococci infections or their sequelae. The occurrence of sore throat, fever, pallor, purpura, or jaundice during sulfonamide administration may be an early indication of serious blood dyscrasias.

Deaths associated with the administration of sulfonamides have been reported from hypersensitivity reactions, agranulocytosis, aplastic anemia, and other blood dyscrasias.

Frequent blood counts and renal function tests should be carried out during sulfonamide treatment, especially during prolonged administration. Microscopic urinalyses should be done once a week when a patient is treated for longer than two weeks. Urine cultures should be made to confirm eradication of bacteriuria.

Usage in Pregnancy: The safe use of sulfonamides in pregnancy has not been established. The teratogenicity potential of most sulfonamides has not been thoroughly investigated in either animals or humans. However, a significant increase in the incidence of cleft palate and other bony abnormalities of offspring has been observed when certain sulfonamides of the short-, intermediate-, and long-acting types were given to pregnant rats and mice at high oral doses (7 to 25 times the human dose).

Precautions: To allay any possible apprehension, patients should be told that this medication may color the urine orange or red.

The usual precautions used in sulfonamide therapy should be observed, including the maintenance of an adequate fluid intake. Sulfonamides should be used with caution in patients with severe allergy or bronchial asthma, severe impairment of hepatic or renal function, and in patients with glucose-6-phosphate dehydrogenase deficiency since sulfas may cause hemolysis in this latter group.

Adverse Reactions:

Blood dyscrasias. Agranulocytosis, aplastic anemia, thrombocytopenia, leukopenia, hemolytic anemia, purpura, hypoprothrombinemia, and methemoglobinemia.

Allergic reactions. Erythema multiforme (Stevens-Johnson Syndrome), generalized skin eruptions, epidermal necrolysis, urticaria, serum sickness, pruritus, exfoliative dermatitis, anaphylactoid reactions, periorbital edema, conjunctival and scleral injection, photosensitization, arthralgia, and allergic myocarditis.

Gastrointestinal reactions. Nausea, emesis, abdominal pains, hepatitis, diarrhea, anorexia, pancreatitis, and stomatitis.

C.N.S. reactions. Headache, peripheral neuritis, mental depression, convulsions, ataxia, hallucinations, tinnitus, vertigo, and insomnia.

Miscellaneous reactions. Drug fever, chills, and toxic nephrosis with oliguria and anuria. Periarteritis nodosum and L.E. phenomenon have occurred.

The sulfonamides bear certain chemical similarities to some goitrogens, diuretics (acetazolamide and the thiazides), and oral hypoglycemic agents. Goiter production, diuresis, and hypoglycemia have occurred rarely in patients receiving sulfonamides. Cross-sensitivity may exist with these agents.

Rats appear to be especially susceptible to the goitrogenic effects of sulfonamides, and long term administration has produced thyroid malignancies in the species.

Dosage and Administration: Usual dosage (based on sulfamethizole content): *Adults:* 0.5 to 1.0 g three or four times daily. *Children and infants* (over 2 months of age): 30 to 45 mg/kg/24 hours, divided into 4 doses.

THIOSULFIL-A Forte and THIOSULFIL-A are recommended for use in the initial phase of urinary tract infection when there is associated pain. After relief of pain has been obtained, treatment of the infection with sulfamethizole alone should be considered. If pain persists, other causes for the discomfort should be investigated.

How Supplied: THIOSULFIL-A Forte Tablets —in bottles of 100 (NDC 0046-0783-81) and 1,000 (NDC 0046-0783-91). THIOSULFIL-A Tablets —in bottles of 100 (NDC 0046-0784-81) and 1,000 (NDC 0046-0784-91).

[*Shown in Product Identification Section*]

VERACILLIN* Capsules ℞

(dicloxacillin sodium)

Description: VERACILLIN (dicloxacillin sodium) is an isoxazolyl penicillin which resists destruction by the enzyme penicillinase (beta lactamase). It is the monohydrate sodium salt of 6-[3-(2, 6-dichlorophenyl)-5-methyl-4-isoxazolecarboxamido] -3, 3-dimethyl-7-oxo-4-thia-1-azabicyclo[3.2.0]heptane-2-carboxylic acid.

Actions:

Pharmacology

VERACILLIN is resistant to destruction by acid and is exceptionally well absorbed from the gastrointestinal tract. Oral administration of VERACILLIN gives blood levels considerably higher than those obtained with equivalent doses of any other presently available oral penicillin.

Microbiology

In vitro, VERACILLIN is active against certain gram-positive cocci including most strains of beta-hemolytic streptococci, pneumococci, penicillin G-sensitive staphylococci and, because of its resistance to penicillinase, penicillin G-resistant staphylococci. Dicloxacillin has less intrinsic antibacterial activity and a narrower spectrum than penicillin G.

Disc Susceptibility Tests

Quantitative methods that require measurement of zone diameters give the most precise estimates of antibiotic susceptibility. One such procedure† has been recommended for use with discs for testing susceptibility to penicillinase-resistant penicillin class antibiotics. Interpretations correlate diameters on the disc test with MIC values for penicillinase-resistant penicillins. With this procedure, a report from the laboratory of "susceptible" indicates that the infecting organism is likely to respond to therapy. A report of "resistant" indicates that the infecting organism is not likely to respond to therapy. A report of "intermediate susceptibility" suggests that the organism would be susceptible if high dosage is used, or if the infection is confined to tissues and fluids (*e.g.,* urine), in which high antibiotic levels are attained.

Continued on next page

Ayerst—Cont.

Indications:
Although the principal indication for VERACILLIN is in the treatment of infections due to penicillinase-producing staphylococci, it may be used to initiate therapy in any patient in whom a staphylococcal infection is suspected. (See Important Note below.)
Bacteriological studies to determine the causative organisms and their sensitivity to dicloxacillin should be performed.
In serious, life-threatening infections, oral preparations of the penicillinase-resistant penicillins should not be relied on for initial therapy.

Important Note

When it is judged necessary that treatment be initiated before definitive culture and sensitivity results are known, the choice of dicloxacillin should take into consideration the fact that it has been shown to be effective only in the treatment of infections caused by pneumococci, Group A beta-hemolytic streptococci, and penicillin G-resistant and penicillin G-sensitive staphylococci. If the bacteriology report later indicates the infection is due to an organism other than a penicllin G-resistant staphylococcus sensitive to dicloxacillin, the physician is advised to continue therapy with a drug other than dicloxacillin or any other penicillinase-resistant penicillin.
Recent studies have shown that the percentage of staphylococcal isolates resistant to penicillin G outside the hospital is increasing, approximating the high percentage of resistant staphylococcal isolates found in the hospital. For this reason, it is recommended that a penicillinase-resistant penicillin be used as initial therapy for any suspected staphylococcal infection until culture and sensitivity results are known.

Dicloxacillin acts through a mechanism similar to that of methicillin against penicillin G-resistant staphylococci. Strains of staphylococci resistant to methicillin have existed in nature and it is known that the number of these strains reported has been increasing. Such strains of staphylococci have been capable of producing serious disease, in some instances resulting in fatality. Because of this, there is concern that widespread use of penicillinase-resistant penicillins may result in the appearance of an increasing number of staphylococcal strains which are resistant to these penicillins.
Methicillin-resistant strains are almost always resistant to all other penicillinase-resistant penicillins (cross resistance with cephalosporin derivatives also occurs frequently). Resistance to any penicillinase-resistant penicillin should be interpreted as evidence of clinical resistance to all in spite of the fact that minor variations in *in vitro* sensitivity may be encountered when more than one penicillinase-resistant penicillin is tested against the same strain of staphylococcus.
Contraindications: A history of a previous hypersensitivity reaction to any of the penicillins is a contraindication.
Warnings: Serious and occasionally fatal hypersensitivity (anaphylactoid) reactions have been reported in patients on penicillin therapy. Although anaphylaxis is more frequent following parenteral therapy, it has occurred in patients on oral penicillins. These reactions are more apt to occur in individuals with a history of sensitivity to multiple allergens.
There have been reports of individuals with a history of penicillin hypersensitivity reactions who experienced severe hypersensitivity reactions when treated with cephalosporins. Before therapy with a penicillin, careful inquiry should be made concerning previous hypersensitivity reactions to penicillins, cephalosporins and other allergens. If an allergic reaction occurs, appropriate therapy should be instituted and discontinuance of dicloxacillin therapy considered. **Serious anaphylactoid reactions require immediate emergency treatment with epinephrine. Oxygen, intravenous steroids, and airway management, including intubation, should also be administered as indicated.**
Precautions: As with any potent drug, periodic assessment of organ system function, including renal, hepatic, and hematopoietic, should be made during prolonged therapy.
The possibility of bacterial and fungal superinfection should be kept in mind during long term therapy. If overgrowth of resistant organisms occurs, appropriate measures should be taken.
This oral preparation should not be relied upon in patients with severe illness or with nausea, vomiting, gastric dilatation, cardiospasm or intestinal hypermotility.
Since experience in neonates is limited, a dose for the newborn is not recommended at this time.
Usage in pregnancy
Safety for use in pregnancy has not been established.
Adverse Reactions: Gastrointestinal disturbances such as nausea, vomiting, epigastric discomfort, flatulence, and loose stools have been noted in some patients receiving dicloxacillin. As with other penicillins, pruritus, urticaria, skin rashes, eosinophilia, anaphylactic reactions, and other allergic symptoms have been occasionally encountered.
Minor changes in the results of liver function tests such as transient elevation of SGOT and changes in cephalin flocculation tests have been reported. The clinical significance of these changes is unknown.
Dosage and Administration: For mild-to-moderate upper respiratory and localized skin and soft tissue infections due to sensitive organisms:
Adults and children weighing 40 kg (88 lb) or more: 125 mg q 6 h.
Children weighing less than 40 kg (88 lb): 12.5 mg/kg/day in equally divided doses q 6 h.
For more severe infections such as those of the lower respiratory tract or disseminated infections:
Adults and children weighing 40 kg (88 lb) or more: 250 mg q 6 h or higher.
Children weighing less than 40 kg (88 lb): 25 mg/kg/day or higher in equally divided doses q 6 h.
Since experience in neonates is limited, a dose for the newborn is not recommended at this time.
Dicloxacillin sodium is best absorbed when taken on an empty stomach, preferably one to two hours before meals.
N.B.: INFECTIONS CAUSED BY GROUP A BETA-HEMOLYTIC STREPTOCOCCI SHOULD BE TREATED FOR AT LEAST 10 DAYS TO HELP PREVENT THE OCCURRENCE OF ACUTE RHEUMATIC FEVER OR ACUTE GLOMERULONEPHRITIS.
How Supplied: VERACILLIN (dicloxacillin sodium) Capsules.
—Each capsule contains dicloxacillin sodium monohydrate equivalent to 250 mg dicloxacillin. In bottles of 100 (NDC 0046-0661-81).
—Each capsule contains dicloxacillin sodium monohydrate equivalent to 500 mg dicloxacillin. In bottles of 50 (NDC 0046-0662-50).
*Mfr. lic'd. under ® 734,467
† Bauer, A. W., Kirby, W. M. M., Sherris, J. C., and Turck, M.: Antibiotic susceptibility testing by a standardized single disk method, Am. J. Clin. Pathol. *45:*493, 1966; Standardized Disc Susceptibility Test, FEDERAL REGISTER *37:*20527-29, 1972.
[*Shown in Product Identification Section*]

Baker/Cummins

Div. Chester A. Baker Laboratories, Inc.
Sub. Key Pharmaceuticals, Inc.
50 N.W. 176TH STREET
MIAMI, FLORIDA 33169

P&S® LIQUID

Composition: P&S Liquid is a specially prepared mixture of liquid paraffin oil, sodium chloride and phenol, less than 1%.
Action and Uses: P&S Liquid provides safe and effective management of scaling conditions of the scalp resulting from psoriasis or seborrhea. It has a relatively high capacity to remove scale from lesions without the disagreeable greasiness, odor, staining and irritation so common to preparations used in psoriasis.
Directions: Shake well before using. Apply P&S Liquid liberally to scalp lesions. Gently massage to loosen scales and crusts, without breaking skin. Use this treatment at night before retiring, and shampoo each morning after treatment. Repeat daily as needed. If other topical agents such as steroid preparations are used during the day, nightly use of P&S Liquid will aid in removing the heavy scale of psoriasis.
Caution: Do not apply to large portions of body surfaces. If irritation should occur during treatment—discontinue use. Keep preparation out of eyes.
How Supplied: P&S Liquid available in 4 and 8 fl oz bottles.

P&S® SHAMPOO
Antiseborrheic Shampoo

Composition: P&S Shampoo contains 2% Salicylic Acid and 0.5% Lactic Acid as active ingredients.
Action and Uses: P&S Shampoo, used regularly, helps control scaling problems of the scalp associated with psoriasis and severe seborrhea. While this unique formulation was designed to complement the action of P&S Liquid treatment, it also effectively controls scaling problems between such treatments while leaving hair clean, fresh and manageable.
Directions: Wet hair thoroughly, apply P&S Shampoo, lather and rinse. Reapply, lather and rinse again. Repeat if necessary, or as directed by physician.
Caution: For external use only. Discontinue use if excessive irritation of the skin develops. Avoid contact with eyes or mucous membranes. Keep out of the reach of children.
How Supplied: P&S Shampoo available in 4 fluid ounce bottles.

PANSCOL®
Lotion and Ointment

Composition: PANSCOL Lotion and Ointment are specially compounded emollients containing 3% salicylic acid, 2% lactic acid and less than 1% phenol.
Action and Uses: PANSCOL Lotion and Ointment provide emollient action for dry, scaly skin and relief of associated itching. PANSCOL Ointment may be preferred for more severe scaling conditions.
Directions: Apply to dry, scaly areas twice daily unless otherwise directed by physician.
Caution: For external use only. Discontinue use if excessive irritation of the skin develops. Avoid contact with eyes or mucous membranes. Keep out of the reach of children.
How Supplied: PANSCOL Lotion available in 4 fl. oz. bottles. PANSCOL Ointment available in 3 oz. jars.

ULTRADERM® MOISTURIZER

Composition: Ultraderm is a lubricating oil-in-water emulsion containing water, propylene glycol, mineral oil, lanolin oil, petrolatum, glyceryl stearate, PEG-50 stearate, proplyene glycol stearate SE, cetyl alcohol, sorbitan laurate, potassium sorbate, phosphoric acid, tetrasodium EDTA, fragrance.
Action & Uses: Ultraderm lubricates and helps hydrate the skin, making it soft and smooth. Indicated for generalized dryness and itching, chapped or chafed skin, sunburn, aging dry skin, detergent hands.
Directions: Apply Ultraderm to dry skin areas several times daily to soothe, moisturize and protect the skin. Use after bathing and exposure to sun, water, soaps and detergents.
Caution: If hypersensitivity develops, discontinue use.
How Supplied: Ultraderm Moisturizer is available in 8-fluid ounce bottles.

XSEB® SHAMPOO

Composition: Contains 4% salicylic acid and a blend of surface active agents to potentiate the keratolytic effect of the salicylic acid.
Action & Uses: Xseb Shampoo helps provide temporary control of scaling associated with dandruff and seborrheic dermatitis.
Directions: Wet hair thoroughly, apply Xseb Shampoo, massaging into scalp for 2–3 minutes. Rinse and reapply. Shampoo once or twice weekly or as directed by physician.
As Oily Skin Cleanser: Massage into moistened skin. Leave on for 2–3 minutes before rinsing off.
Caution: For external use only. Discontinue use if excessive irritation of the skin develops. Avoid contact with eyes or mucous membranes. Keep out of the reach of children.
How Supplied: Xseb Shampoo is available in 4-fluid ounce bottles.

XSEB®-T SHAMPOO

Composition: Contains 10% coal tar solution and 4% salicylic acid in a blend of surface active agents.
Action & Uses: Helps control scaling and itching associated with seborrhea, psoriasis and chronic eczematous conditions of the scalp.
Directions: Wet hair thoroughly. Apply Xseb-T Shampoo, massaging into scalp for 2–3 minutes. Rinse and reapply. Use twice weekly or as directed by physician.
Caution: For external use only. Discontinue use if excessive irritation of the skin develops. Avoid contact with eyes or mucous membranes. Keep out of the reach of children.
How Supplied: Xseb-T Shampoo is available in 4-fluid ounce bottles.

Barnes-Hind Pharmaceuticals, Inc.
895 KIFER ROAD
SUNNYVALE, CA 94086

BARSEB® HC SCALP LOTION ℞
(hydrocortisone)

BARSEB® THERA=SPRAY® ℞
Topical Aerosol

Description: BARSEB® HC contains hydrocortisone 1%, salicylic acid 0.5%, isopropyl alcohol 45%, isopropyl myristate, propylene glycol, ascorbic acid, and citric acid.
BARSEB® THERA=SPRAY—Each 84g bottle contains 360 mg. hydrocortisone, 288 mg. salicylic acid, 14 mg. benzalkonium chloride, propylene glycol, isopropyl myristate, 46 g. alcohol, and butane (propellant). After evaporation of the propellant, the vehicle contains 0.6% hydrocortisone, 0.48% salicylic acid, and 0.024% benzalkonium chloride.

Actions: Primarily effective because of the anti-inflammatory, antipruritic, and vasoconstrictive actions of hydrocortisone, and salicylic acid aids in loosening and removing adherent sebum, crusts, and epithelial debris.

Indications: BARSEB® THERA=SPRAY® and BARSEB® HC are indicated for the relief of the inflammatory manifestations of corticosteroid-responsive dermatoses of the scalp.

Contraindications: Topical steroids are contraindicated in those patients with a history of hypersensitivity to any of the components of the preparations.

Precautions: If irritation develops, discontinue use and institute appropriate therapy.
In the presence of an infection, use of an appropriate antifungal or antibacterial agent should be instituted. If a favorable response does not occur promptly, application of Barseb should be discontinued until the infection has been adequately controlled.
If extensive areas are treated or if the occlusive technique is used, there will be increased systemic absorption of the corticosteroid and suitable precautions should be taken, particularly with children and infants.
Avoid inhalation, ingestion or contact with the eyes or nose. If spray accidentally gets into eyes, flush with copious amounts of water.
Although topical steroids have not been reported to have an adverse effect on human pregnancy, the safety of their use in pregnant women has not absolutely been established. In laboratory animals, increases in incidence of fetal abnormalities have been associated with exposure of gestating females to topical corticosteroids, in some cases at rather low dosage levels. Therefore, drugs of this class should not be used extensively on pregnant patients, in large amounts, or for prolonged periods of time.
These preparations are not for ophthalmic use or use around the eyes.

Adverse Reactions: The following local adverse reactions have been reported with topical corticosteroids, especially under occlusive dressings: burning, itching, irritation, dryness, folliculitis, hypertrichosis, acneform eruptions, hypopigmentation, perioral dermatitis, allergic contact dermatitis, maceration of the skin, secondary infection, skin atrophy, striae, and miliaria.
Transient discomfort may occur when first applied to an inflamed scalp.

Dosage and Administration: BARSEB® THERA=SPRAY should be applied once daily during the acute phase or as directed by a physician. A maintenance schedule may be adjusted to the patient's response to therapy.

Directions For Use: BARSEB® HC Part hair, apply once or twice a day with gentle rubbing. Use BARSEB® HC sparingly. BARSEB® THERA=SPRAY-shake well. Hold the bottle upright (being careful not to spray forehead or eyes); insert applicator tube through hair to scalp at front hairline. Then start spraying and moving applicator tube slowly toward the back of the head. Repeat this procedure until all affected areas of the scalp are treated. Because of the spreading and penetrating properties of BARSEB® THERA=SPRAY it is not necessary to rub or massage medication into the scalp. Assembly directions are provided.

How Supplied: BARSEB® THERA=SPRAY is supplied in 84g aerosol bottles with applicator tube.
BARSEB® HC is supplied in 1¾ fl. oz. (52 ml.) plastic squeeze bottles.

KOMED® Acne Lotion OTC
KOMED® MILD Acne Lotion OTC

	Komed	Komed Mild
Sodium thiosulfate	8%	2%
Salicylic acid	2%	1%
Isopropyl alcohol	25%	25%

The above products also contain menthol, camphor, colloidal alumina, edetate disodium, and purified water.
Indications: Primarily indicated for the treatment of acne associated with oily skin. KOMED MILD Acne Lotion is indicated for topical treatment of acne conditions on delicate skin. KOMED Acne Lotion is indicated in more severe conditions or where stronger keratolytic effect is desired. Komed Lotions feature a thixotropic gel of colloidal alumina. They are greaseless and dry to an almost invisible film, forming a medicated base over which non-oily cosmetics may be applied.
Precautions: Do not use Komed Lotions on or near the eyes.
Dosage and Administration: Wash affected areas thoroughly. Shake lotion well and apply a thin film twice a day.
How Supplied: 1¾ fl. oz. (52.5 ml.) plastic squeeze bottles.

KOMED® HC Lotion ℞
(hydrocortisone)

Description: Contains hydrocortisone acetate 0.5%, sodium thiosulfate 8%, salicylic acid 2%, isopropyl alcohol 25%, menthol, camphor, colloidal alumina, edetate disodium, and purified water.
Indications: KOMED HC Acne Lotion is indicated for topical treatment of acne conditions when accompanied by inflammation. KOMED HC features a thixotropic gel of colloidal alumina. The lotion is greaseless and dries to an almost invisible film, forming a medicated base over which non-oily cosmetics may be applied.
Contraindications: Topical steroids are contraindicated in those patients with a history of hypersensitivity to any of the components of the preparation.
Precautions: If irritation develops, the product should be discontinued and appropriate therapy instituted.
In the presence of an infection, the use of an appropriate antifungal or antibacterial agent should be instituted. If a favorable response does not occur promptly, the corticosteroid should be discontinued until the infection has been adequately controlled.
If extensive areas are treated or if the occlusive technique is used, there will be increased systemic absorption of the corticosteroid and suitable precautions should be taken, particularly in children and infants.
Although topical steroids have not been reported to have an adverse effect on human pregnancy, the safety of their use in pregnant women has not been absolutely established. In laboratory animals, increases in incidence of fetal abnormalities have been associated with exposure of gestating females to topical corticosteroids. Therefore, drugs of this class should not be used extensively on pregnant patients, in large amounts, or for prolonged periods of time.
Not for Ophthalmic Use or Use Around the Eyes.
Adverse Reactions: The following local adverse reactions have been reported with topical corticosteroids especially under occlusive dressings: burning, itching, irritation, dryness, folliculitis, hypertrichosis, acneform eruptions, hypopigmentation, perioral dermatitis, allergic contact dermatitis, maceration of the skin, secondary infection, skin atrophy, striae, and miliaria.
Dosage and Administration: Wash affected areas thoroughly. Shake lotion well and apply a thin film twice a day, or as directed.

Continued on next page

Barnes-Hind—Cont.

How Supplied: 1¾ fl. oz. (52.5 ml.) plastic squeeze bottles.

KOMEX® OTC
(Scrub for Oily Skin and Acne)

Description: KOMEX® is a dissolving cleanser useful as an aid in reducing oily skin conditions associated with acne.
Contents: SCRUBULES, Barnes-Hind brand of dissolving particles (sodium tetraborate decahydrate), in a preserved base containing a unique combination of surface active soapless cleaning agents, and skin conditioners.
Directions: Use Komex in place of your usual soap or cleanser.
Skin Cleansing: Wet the face with warm water. Squeeze Komex onto your fingertips, and gently massage into the face. Continue scrubbing and adding water until Scrubules are completely dissolved (about one minute). Rinse thoroughly and dry. Use once or twice daily.
Caution: Avoid contact with eyes. If granules get into the eyes, flush thoroughly with water and avoid rubbing eyes. If skin irritation or excessive dryness develops, or increases, discontinue use. For external use only. Keep out of reach of children. Not to be used on infants. Do not use on inflamed skin.
How Supplied: 2.65 oz. (75 g.) plastic squeeze tube in unit carton.

TINVER® LOTION ℞

Description: Sodium thiosulfate 25%, salicylic acid 1%, isopropyl alcohol 10%, propylene glycol, menthol, edetate disodium, colloidal alumina, purified water.
Indications: For topical use in treatment of tinea versicolor infections.
Precautions: Discontinue use if irritation or sensitivity develops. Do not use on or about the eyes.
Dosage and Administration: Thoroughly wash, rinse, and dry affected and susceptible areas before application. Apply thin film of TINVER twice a day. Although diagnostic evidence of the disease may disappear in a few days, it is advisable to continue treatment for a much longer period. Clothing should be boiled to prevent reinfection.
How Supplied: 6 fl. oz. (180 ml.) polyethylene squeeze bottles.

Barry Laboratories, Inc.
461 N. E. 27TH STREET
POMPANO BEACH, FL 33064

ALLERGENIC EXTRACTS, DIAGNOSIS AND/OR IMMUNOTHERAPY ℞

Composition: Several hundred fluid allergens are available from the following categories: pollens, foods, dusts, epidermals, insects, fungi (molds & smuts), stinging insects, yeasts, and others.
Action and Uses: For diagnosis and immunotherapy of specific offenders in allergy.
Precautions: Usual precautions used in testing or treating hypersensitive individuals. See product information circulars accompanying each product.
How Supplied: Diagnostic materials are available in liquid form for cutaneous or intracutaneous testing. Autogenous extracts are prepared to order.
Diagnostic Test Sets: The "50 Plus"—includes a comprehensive selection of perennial and seasonal allergens for each of 5 botanical zones. The "60 Plus"—complete food allergen testing set. Regionalized Pollen Test Set—for each of 5 botanical zones.
Immunorex®—Prescription Allergy Treatment Sets—Individualized, four vial treatment sets are prepared from the physician's instructions, based on the patient's skin test reactions and history. Refills of any dilution are available.
Literature Available: Send for free descriptive literature, report and case history forms.

RHUS-ALL® ANTIGEN (Barry) ℞
Poison Ivy, Oak and Sumac Combined

Composition: A triple antigen of the active principles (urushiol) of poison ivy, oak and sumac in an oil vehicle.
Indications: Prophylactic for hyposensitization of Rhus Dermatitis.
Contraindications: Not recommended for treatment of active Rhus Dermatitis.
Administration and Dosage: Usual adult dosage: 1 ml. intramuscular injection a week, for two to three weeks prior to patient's exposure.
How Supplied: 5 ml. multiple dose vial.
Literature Available: Write for free Rhus-All Antigen pamphlet.

STINGING INSECT ANTIGEN ℞
Number 108 (Barry)

Composition: Combined Antigens of Bumble Bee, Honey Bee, Wasp, Hornet and Yellow Jacket.
Action and Uses: For hyposensitization against stinging insect reactions.
Administration and Dosage: Complete suggested administration and dosage recommendations contained in prescription package.
Precautions: Usual precautions observed in vaccine administration.
How Supplied: Three 5 ml. vials, serially diluted. Refills available of any dilution.
Literature Available: Send for free Stinging Insect Antigen No. 108 pamphlet.

Baylor Laboratories, Inc.
P. O. DRAWER 277
HURST, TEXAS 76053

AIRET® TABLETS ℞
AIRET® 400 TABLETS ℞
AIRET® II LIQUID ℞
(dyphylline)

Composition:
Airet® Tablet: Each white monogrammed tablet contains 200 mg. Dyphylline.
Airet® 400 Tablet: Each white monogrammed tablet contains 400 mg. Dyphylline.
Airet® II Liquid: Each 5 ml. (teaspoonful) contains 100 mg. Dyphylline.
Airet® (dyphylline) is the first soluble, stable, neutral derivative of theophylline. Designated chemically as 7-(2,3-Dihydroxypropyl) theophylline, it is a white crystalline compound, freely soluble in water (1 Gm. in 3 ml.). It has a neutral pH in aqueous solution and is soluble over the entire physiologic pH range. Airet® (dyphylline) is a distinct chemical entity, as opposed to the salts or loosely complexed forms of theophylline. Unlike these, it contains no extraneous chemical modifiers.
Action: Airet® (dyphylline) exerts the general pharmacologic actions of theophylline and aminophylline. It acts as a bronchodilator, myocardial stimulant, diuretic, vasodilator (of coronary, pulmonary, and renal vessels), and smooth muscle relaxant. In human therapeutics, its significant action is bronchodilation. By virtue of its high solubility, neutral pH, and stability toward pH changes, Airet® (dyphylline) is readily absorbed and well tolerated upon oral administration, and is uniquely suitable for Intramuscular Injection. This constitutes its basic advantage over theophylline and aminophylline.
Indications: Airet® (dyphylline) is effective for:
1. Relief of acute bronchial asthma
2. Reversible bronchospasm associated with chronic bronchitis and emphysema

Contraindications: Acute myocardial infarction; patients with angina pectoris in whom myocardial stimulation might prove harmful; severe peptic ulcer.
Precautions: Conditions which warrant caution in therapy include hyperthyroidism, severe myocardial damage, renal or hepatic disease and glaucoma.
Despite comparatively low C.N.S. stimulation, the possibility with large doses should be borne in mind. Concomitant therapy with sympathomimetics may occasionally induce restlessness, excitability, insomnia or cardiac arrhythmias. Children have a marked sensitivity to the C.N.S. stimulant action of the theophyllines. Fatalities in children have resulted from a few 100 mg. doses of theophylline and from rectal suppositories of aminophylline. While Airet® (dyphylline) has not been implicated in thse cases, care should be exercised in the treatment of children, the dosage should be titrated carefully, and symptoms of toxicity watched for. Early symptoms of poisoning include anorexia, nausea, occasional vomiting, wakefulness, restlessness, and irritability. Agitated maniacal behaviour and frequent vomiting accompanied by extreme thirst develop later, and lead in fullest severity to delirium, convulsions, hyperthermia, and vasomotor collapse.
Adverse Reactions: Airet® (dyphylline) has a low incidence of gastric irritation. Administration of high doses for long periods of time may cause nausea, vomiting, epigastric or substernal pain, palpitation, dizziness, headache, or nervousness. These side effects can often be controlled by reduction in dosage.
Dosage and Administration: The usual adult dose is 15 mg/kg every 6 hours up to 4 times a day.
For the control of acute attacks of bronchial asthma, the initial dose is 400 to 600 mg., followed in three or four hours by a maintenance dose.
The dosage should be individualized by titration to the condition and response of the patient. Oral bronchodilator therapy for chronic bronchospastic conditions is most effective when administered in individualized doses to accommodate patient-to-patient variations in metabolism. Maintenance therapy may be continued as long as needed, at a dosage level determined by individual requirements and tolerance.
For pediatric use, the usual daily dose is 2 to 3 mg. per pound of body weight administered in divided doses.
Caution: Federal (USA) law prohibits dispensing without prescription.
How Supplied:
Airet® Tablets: Bottles of 100 and 500
Airet® 400 Tablets: Bottles of 100
Airet® II Liquid: Bottles of 1 Pint
NDC Numbers:

Airet® Tablets:	100's	0568-0017-01
	500's	0568-0017-05
Airet® 400 Tablets:	100's	0568-0032-01
Airet® II Liquid:	Pints	0568-0035-22

AIRET® L.A. TABLETS ℞
(dyphylline)

Composition: Each green, scored, long acting tablet contains:
Dyphylline
(Dihydroxypropyl Theophylline)......400 mg.
In a special base which is gradually released over an extended period to provide prolonged therapeutic effect.
Action: Patients with bronchopulmonary insufficiency will achieve prolonged broncho dilation especially during the nocturnal hours. Airet L.A. tablets do not contain ephedrine, as a result night time dosage is less likely to keep

patients awake. The Airet L.A. Tablet is specifically designed for the prophylaxis of allergic and pulmonary diseases and is not effective in the treatment of the acute symptomatic phase.
Indications: For relief of acute bronchial asthma and for reversible bronchospasm associated with chronic bronchitis and emphysema.
Contraindications: In individuals who have shown hypersensitivity to any of its components.
Dyphylline should not be administered concurrently with other xanthine preparations.
Precautions: Use cautiously in cases with severe cardiac disease, renal or hepatic malfunction, glaucoma, hyperthyroidism, peptic ulcer or concurrent use of other xanthine-containing or CNS stimulant drugs.
Adverse Reactions: Dyphylline has a low incidence of gastric irritation. However, administration of high continuous doses may cause nausea, headache, cardiac palpitations and CNS stimulation. Administration after meals may help to avoid gastric discomfort.
Dosage and Administration: Adults, one tablet three times daily every 8 hours, this dosage should be individualized to the condition and response of the patient. Children's dosages have not been established so Airet L.A. is not recommended for children under six. Older children may begin with low doses gradually increased to lowest effective level. This should not exceed 3-4 mg. per pound of body weight daily in divided doses.
Caution: Federal (USA) law prohibits dispensing without prescription.
How Supplied: Bottles of 100 and 500 tablets.

N.D.C. Numbers:	100's 0568-0024-01
	500's 0568-0024-05

COMHIST® TABLET AND LIQUID ℞
COMHIST® L.A. CAPSULE ℞

Description: Comhist® Tablet and Liquid: Each tablet or 5cc (1 teaspoonful) liquid contains Chlorpheniramine Maleate 2 mg., Phenindamine Tartrate 5 mg., Phenylephrine Hydrochloride 10 mg., Hyoscyamine Sulfate 0.1037 mg., Atropine Sulfate 0.0194 mg., Scopolamine Hydrobromide 0.0065 mg.
Comhist® L.A. Capsule: Each long-acting capsule contains Chlorpheniramine Maleate 4 mg., Phenindamine Tartrate 10 mg., Phenylephrine Hydrochloride 20 mg., Hyoscyamine Sulfate 0.1292 mg., Atropine Sulfate 0.0242 mg., Scopolamine Hydrobromide 0.0081 mg.
Action: The belladonna alkaloids complement the drying action of two antihistamines, one of which, Phenindamine Tartrate, is a mild stimulant to many patients. Phenylephrine decongests engorged nasal mucous membranes.
Indications: For the relief of hypersecretion and congestion associated with allergic and vasomotor rhinitis.
Contraindications: Sensitivity to sympathomimetics; glaucoma.
Precautions: Patients should be cautioned against driving or operating mechanical equipment if drowsiness results. Should be used with caution in presence of hypertension, cardiovascular disease, and in patients with incipient glaucoma.
Side Effects: Effects such as blurring of vision, dry mouth and difficult urination may occur infrequently in large doses. An occasional patient may experience mild drowsiness.
Dosage: Comhist® Tablets and Liquid: Adults, 1 or 2 tablets or teaspoonfuls 3 times daily; children 6 to 12 years of age, 1 tablet or teaspoonful 3 times daily; children 3 to 6 years of age, ½ teaspoonful 3 times daily. Tablets are not recommended for children under 6 years of age.
Comhist® L.A. Capsules: Adults and children over 12 years of age, 1 capsule every 8 to 12 hours. Not recommended for children under 12 years of age.
How Supplied:
Comhist® Tablets: Bottles of 100
Comhist® Liquid: Bottles of 1 Pint
Comhist® L.A. Capsules: Bottles of 100 and 500
NDC Numbers:

Comhist® Tablets —	100's:	0568-0015-01
Comhist® Liquid —	Pints:	0568-0016-22
Comhist® L.A. Capsules—		
	100's:	0568-0023-01
	500's:	0568-0023-05

ENTEX® CAPSULES AND LIQUID ℞

Composition: Each monogramed orange and white capsule contains: Phenylephrine HCl 5 mg., Phenylpropanolamine HCl 45 mg., Guaifenesin 200 mg. Each 5cc (one teaspoonful) of Entex Liquid contains: Phenylephrine HCl 5 mg., Phenylpropanolamine HCI 20 mg., Guaifenesin 100 mg., Alcohol 5%.
Indications: Increase of respiratory tract fluids and relief of congestion in the treatment of acute or chronic pulmonary disorders where tenacious mucous plugs and congestion complicate the problem. Such disorders include bronchitis, bronchial asthma, pulmonary emphysema, sinusitis and related conditions.
Contraindications: In individuals with known sensitivity to any of the ingredients, marked hypertension or in patients who are receiving MAO inhibitors.
Caution: Federal (USA) Law prohibits dispensing without prescription.
Precautions: Entex should be used with caution in the presence of hypertension, hyperthyroidism, diabetes, or heart disease, and in those patients who may be sensitive to sympathomimetics.
Adverse Reactions: Central nervous system stimulation may occur with overdosage.
Dosage: Entex Capsule: Adults, orally one capsule four times daily. Entex Liquid: Each of the following is to be prescribed four times daily; Children: 2–4 Years—½ teaspoonful. 4–6 Years—1 teaspoonful. 6–12 Years 1½ teaspoonfuls. Adults:—2 teaspoonfuls.
How Supplied: Entex Capsules 100 and 500, Entex Liquid pints.
N.D.C. Numbers:

Capsules—	100's 0568-0012-01
	500's 0568-0012-05
Liquid——	pints 0568-0014-22

ENTEX® LA ℞

Description: Each blue, scored, capsule-shaped long-acting tablet contains:

Phenylpropanolamine Hydrochloride	75 mg
Guaifenesin	400 mg

In a special base to provide a prolonged therapeutic effect.
Action: Phenylpropanolamine is an effective vasoconstrictor that decongests swollen mucous membranes of the entire respiratory tract. Guaifenesin enhances the flow of respiratory tract fluid, promoting ciliary action and facilitating removal of viscid, inspissated mucus. As a result, sinus and Eustachian tube drainage is improved and dry, unproductive coughs become more productive and less frequent.
Indications: ENTEX® L.A. is indicated in those respiratory conditions where tenacious mucous plugs and congestion complicate the problem. Such problems include sinusitis, pharyngitis, bronchitis, asthma, and, as adjunctive therapy, in serous otitis media. ENTEX® L.A. also may be of value in avoiding secondary middle ear complications of nasopharyngeal congestion accompanying coryza and rhinitis.
Contraindications: ENTEX® L.A. is contraindicated in individuals with known hypersensitivity to sympathomimetics, severe hypertension, or in patients receiving MAO inhibitors.
Precautions: Should be used with caution in presence of hypertension, hyperthyroidism, diabetes, heart disease, and peripheral vascular disease.
Adverse Reactions: Central nervous system stimulation may occur with overdosage. May cause urinary retention in patients with benign prostatic hypertrophy.
Overdosage: Since the effects of ENTEX® L.A. may last up to 12 hours, treatment of overdosage directed toward supporting the patient and reversing the effects of the drug should be continued for at least that length of time. Saline cathartics may be useful in hastening the evacuation of unreleased medication.
Side Effects: Side effects are rare, and seldom, if ever, require discontinuation of therapy. Central nervous system stimulation may occur with overdosage.
Dosage: Adults and children over 12—one tablet twice daily. Not recommended for children under 12 years of age. Tablets may be broken in half for ease of administration without affecting release of medication.
Supplied: Bottles of 100 tablets.
NDC 0568-0036-01
Caution: Federal law prohibits dispensing without prescription.

LĀBID™ 250 mg ℞
(anhydrous theophylline)

Description: LĀBID contains 250 mg anhydrous theophylline in a scored, long-acting dyefree tablet. LĀBID has been specially formulated to provide therapeutic serum levels when administered every 12 hours, and minimizes the peaks and valleys of serum levels commonly found with shorter acting theophylline products.
Indications: For relief and/or prevention of symptoms from asthma and reversible bronchospasm associated with chronic bronchitis and emphysema.
Contraindications: LĀBID is contraindicated in individuals who have shown hypersensitivity to any of its components or to xanthine derivatives.
Warnings: Status asthmaticus is a medical emergency. Optimal therapy frequently requires additional medication including corticosteroids when the patient is not rapidly responsive to bronchodilators.
Since excessive theophylline doses may be associated with toxicity, periodic measurement of serum theophylline levels is recommended to assure maximal benefit without excessive risk. Incidence of toxicity increases at serum levels greater than 20 mcg/ml. Although early signs of theophylline toxicity, such as nausea and restlessness are often seen, in some cases ventricular arrhythmias or seizures may be the first signs of toxicity.
Many patients who have excessive theophylline serum levels exhibit a tachycardia.
Theophylline preparations may worsen preexisting arrhythmias.
Usage in Pregnancy: Safe use in pregnancy has not been established relative to possible adverse effects on fetal development, but neither have adverse effects on fetal development been established. This is, unfortunately, true for most antiasthmatic medications. Therefore, use of theophylline in pregnant women should be balanced against the risk of uncontrolled asthma.
Precautions: Mean half-life in smokers is shorter than non-smokers. Therefore, smokers may require larger doses of theophylline.
Theophylline should not be administered concurrently with other xanthine preparations.
Use with caution in patients with severe cardiac disease, severe hypoxemia, hypertension, hyperthyroidism, acute myocardial injury, cor

Continued on next page

Baylor—Cont.

pulmonale, congestive heart failure, liver disease, and in the elderly (especially males) and in neonates. Great caution should be used in giving theophylline to patients with congestive heart failure. Such patients have shown markedly prolonged theophylline blood levels with theophylline presisting in serum for long periods following discontinuation of the drug.
Use theophylline cautiously in patients with a history of peptic ulcer.
Theophylline may occasionally act as a local gastrointestinal irritant, although G. I. symptoms are more commonly centrally mediated and associated with high serum concentration.
Adverse Reactions: The most consistent adverse reactions are due usually to overdose, and are:
Gastrointestinal: nausea, vomiting, epigastric pain, hematemesis, diarrhea.
Central nervous system: headaches, irritability, restlessness, insomnia, reflex hyperexcitability, muscle twitching, clonic and tonic generalized convulsions.
Cardiovascular: palpitation, tachycardia, extrasystoles, flushing, hypotension, circulatory failure, ventricular arrhythmias.
Respiratory: tachypnea.
Renal: albuminuria, increased excretion of renal tubular cells and red blood cells, potentiation of diuresis.
Others: hyperglycemia and inappropriate ADH syndrome.
Dosage and Administration: THE AVERAGE INITIAL DOSE IS ONE TO TWO LĀBID 250 mg TABLETS EVERY 12 HOURS.
The recommended starting dose of LĀBID for adolescents and adults is 6 mg per kg body weight every 12 hours based upon ideal body weight. If the desired relief is not achieved with this dose and there are no systemic side effects (see Adverse Reactions), the dose may be increased by 1 mg per kg body weight every 2 days. With doses above 8 mg per kg every 12 hours, serum theophylline levels should be monitored.
Doses should be increased until therapeutic responses or side effects occur (higher doses may be necessary and well tolerated).
Occasional patients may require every 8 hours dosing.
THE AVERAGE INITIAL CHILDREN'S DOSE IS ONE-HALF TO ONE LĀBID 250 mg TABLETS EVERY 12 HOURS.
The recommended starting dose for children is 6 mg per kg body weight every 12 hours and this dose can be increased by 1 mg per kg body weight every two days. With doses above 8 mg/kg every 12 hours, serum theophylline levels should be monitored.
How Supplied: LĀBID 250 mg tablets are supplied in bottles of 100.
NDC 0568-0037-01

ORLEX® OTIC ℞

Description: Orlex® Otic Solution is a nonaqueous solution containing 2% Acetic Acid and 0.1% Parachlorometaxylenol in propylene glycol. Buffered with Sodium Acetate 0.015%.
Action: Orlex® Otic Solution is anti-bacterial, antifungal, hydrophilic, has an acid pH and a low surface tension.
Indications: For the treatment of superficial infections of the external auditory canal caused by organisms susceptible to the action of the antimicrobial.
Contraindications: This product is contraindicated in those individuals who have shown hypersensitivity to any of its components. Perforated tympanic membranes are frequently considered a contraindication to the use of external ear canal medications.
Precautions: If sensitization or irritation occurs, medication should be discontinued promptly.
Dosage and Administration: Carefully remove all cerumen and debris to allow Orlex® Otic Solution to contact infected surfaces immediately. To promote continuous contact, insert an Orlex® Otic Solution saturated cotton wick in the ear with instruction to the patient to keep wick moist for the next 24 hours by occasionally adding a few drops on the wick. Remove wick after first 24 hours and continue to instill 5 drops of Orlex® Otic Solution three or four times daily thereafter.
How Supplied: 10ml. dropper tip bottle.
NDC 0568-0300-10

ORLEX® H.C. OTIC ℞

Description: Orlex® H.C. Otic Solution is a nonaqueous solution containing 1% Hydrocortisone, 2% Acetic Acid and 0.1% Parachlorometaxylenol in propylene glycol. Buffered with Sodium Acetate 0.015% and Citric Acid 0.2%.
Action: Orlex® H.C. Otic Solution is antibacterial, anti-fungal, hydrophilic has an acid pH and a low surface tension, and is also antiinflammatory and anti-pruritic.
Indications: For the treatment of superficial infections of the external auditory canal caused by organisms susceptible to the action of the anti-microbial, complicated by inflammation.
Contraindications: This product is contraindicated in those individuals who have shown hypersensitivity to any of its components. It is contraindicated in vaccinia and varicella. Perforated tympanic membranes are frequently considered a contraindication to the use of external ear canal medications.
Precautions: As safety of topical steroids during pregnancy has not been confirmed, they should not be used for an extended period during pregnancy. Systemic side effects may occur with extensive use of steroids. If sensitization or irritation occurs, medication should be discontinued promptly.
Dosage and Administration: Carefully remove all cerumen and debris to allow Orlex® H.C. Otic Solution to contact infected surfaces immediately. To promote continuous contact, insert an Orlex® H.C. Otic Solution saturated cotton wick in the ear with instruction to the patient to keep wick moist for the next 24 hours by occasionally adding a few drops on the wick. Remove wick after first 24 hours and continue to instill 5 drops of Orlex® H.C. Otic Solution three or four times daily thereafter.
How Supplied: 10ml. dropper tip bottle.
NDC 0568-0310-10

Beach Pharmaceuticals

Division of BEACH PRODUCTS, INC.
5220 SOUTH MANHATTAN AVE.
TAMPA, FL 33611

BEELITH Tablets OTC

Description: Each tablet contains: Magnesium oxide 600 mg and pyridoxine hydrochloride (Vitamin B_6) 25 mg equivalent to B_6 20 mg.

K-PHOS® M.F. Tablets ℞
(Modified Formula)*

Description: Each compressed tablet contains potassium acid phosphate 155 mg and sodium acid phosphate, anhydrous 350 mg. Each tablet yields 125.6 mg of phosphorus, 44.5 mg of potassium and 67 mg of sodium.
Actions: K-PHOS **M.F.** (Modified formula) is an effective urinary acidifier that helps keep calcium in solution. This drug also lowers urinary calcium levels and when administered with a low calcium and low Vitamin D diet it effectively reduces the urinary excretion of calcium to quantities unobtainable by any tolerable diet alone.
Indications: Helps Prevent Calcification: K-PHOS **M.F.** (Modified formula) acidifies the urine, lowers urinary calcium levels and increases urinary phosphate and pyrophosphate. These actions help prevent the precipitation of calcium deposits in the urinary tract and in rubber goods placed in the urinary tract. **Helps Control Infection:** By acidifying the urine, this product increases the antibacterial activity of methenamine mandelate, methenamine hippurate and other drugs whose effectiveness is dependent upon an acid pH. **Helps Control Odor-Turbidity:** By acidifying the urine, this product will eliminate odor and turbidity caused by ammoniacal urine.
Precaution: Use with caution if the patient is on a sodium restricted diet.
Contraindications: Renal insufficiency, severe hepatic disease. Addison's disease and hyperkalemia.
Adverse Reactions: Nausea, vomiting, diarrhea and abdominal discomfort may occur.
Dosage and Administration: Two tablets four times daily with a full glass of water.
How Supplied: Bottles of 100, 500 and 5000.

---

* The potassium content has been reduced by use of a sodium salt. This eliminates the required warning concerning gastrointestinal irritation for products containing 100 mg. of potassium. The actions and uses are the same as for the original formula.

[*Shown in Product Identification Section*]

K-PHOS® No. 2 ℞

Description: Each capsule shaped tablet contains potassium acid phosphate 305 mg. & sodium acid phosphate, anhydrous 700 mg.
Actions and Uses: Effectively acidifies the urine and lowers urinary calcium concentration. Increases the antibacterial activity of methenamine and other drugs whose effectiveness is dependent upon acid urine. Helps eliminate odor and turbidity caused by alkaline urine. Increases the urinary calcification inhibitors phosphate and pyrophosphate and lowers urinary calcium; actions which help prevent the precipitation of calcium deposits in the urinary tract and in rubber goods placed in the urinary tract.
Side Effects: Some patients may experience mild laxation which will usually subside by reducing the dosage. If laxation persists, the drug should be discontinued. Hyperacidity and nausea may also occur.
Contraindications: Renal insufficiency, severe hepatic disease, Addison's disease and hyperkalemia.
Precaution: Use with caution if the patient is on a sodium restricted diet.
Dosage and Administration: One tablet four times daily with a full glass of water. When the urine is difficult to acidify administer one tablet every two hours not to exceed eight tablets in a 24 hour period. In all cases Beach's acid ash diet is recommended. Each tablet yields 250 mg. of elemental phosphorus, 88 mg. of potassium or 2.25 mEq. and 134 mg. of sodium or 5.83 mEq.

[*Shown in Product Identification Section*]

K-PHOS® NEUTRAL Tablets OTC

Description: Each tablet contains dibasic sodium phosphate, anhydrous 852 mg; potassium acid phosphate 155 mg and sodium acid phosphate, monohydrate 130 mg. Each tablet yields approximately 250 mg of phosphorus, 298 mg of sodium and 45 mg of potassium.
Actions and Uses: K-PHOS NEUTRAL lowers urinary calcium levels and increases the stone inhibitors, phosphate and pyrophosphate. As a phosphorus supplement, each tablet supplies 25% of the U.S. Recommended Daily Allowance (U.S. RDA) of phosphorus for

adults and children 4 or more years of age and 19% of the U.S. RDA for pregnant or lactating women.
Caution: Consult a physician before using this product if on a sodium restricted diet. Excessive dosage may cause laxation.
Warning: Keep this and all drugs out of the reach of children. In case of accidental overdose, seek professional assistance or contact a Poison Control Center immediately.
Administration and Dosage: One or two tablets four times a day with a full glass of water.
How Supplied: Bottles of 100 and 500 tablets.
[*Shown in Product Identification Section*]

K–PHOS® ORIGINAL (Sodium Free) ℞
(Potassium Acid Phosphate)

Description: Each tablet contains potassium acid phosphate 500 mg. Each tablet yields 114 mg of phosphorus and 144 mg of potassium or 3.67 mEq.
Actions and Uses: Effectively acidifies the urine and lowers urinary calcium concentration.

Helps Control Infection: By acidifying the urine this product increases the antibacterial activity of methenamine mandelate, methenamine hippurate and other drugs whose effectiveness is dependent upon an acid pH.

Helps Control Odor-Turbidity: By acidifying the urine this product will eliminate odor and turbidity caused by ammoniacal urine.

Helps Prevent Calcification: By acidifying the urine, this product lowers urinary calcium levels and increases the calcification inhibitors urinary phosphate and pyrophosphate. These actions help prevent the precipitation of calcium deposits in the urinary tract and in rubber goods placed in the urinary tract.

Side Effects: Some patients may experience mild laxation which will usually subside by reducing the dosage. If laxation persists, the drug should be discontinued. Hyperacidity and nausea may also occur.
Contraindications: Renal insufficiency, severe hepatic disease, Addison's disease and hyperkalemia.
Warning: There have been several reports, published and unpublished, concerning nonspecific small-bowel lesions consisting of stenosis, with or without ulceration, associated with the administration of enteric-coated thiazides with potassium salts. These lesions may occur with enteric-coated potassium tablets alone or when they are used with nonenteric coated thiazides or certain other oral diuretics. These small-bowel lesions have caused obstruction, hemorrhage, and perforation. Surgery was frequently required and deaths have occurred. Based on a large survey of physicians and hospitals, both United States and foreign, the incidence of these lesions is low, and a causal relationship in man has not been definitely established. Available information tends to implicate enteric-coated potassium salts, although lesions of this type also occur spontaneously. Therefore, coated potassium-containing formulations should be administered only when indicated and should be discontinued immediately if abdominal pain, distension, nausea, vomiting or gastrointestinal bleeding occur. Coated potassium tablets should be used only when adequate dietary supplementation is not practicable.
When prescribing this product for patients who are receiving concurrent potassium supplementation (e.g., to replace potassium excreted during thiazide therapy), it should be kept in mind that this product also contains potassium. A decrease in supplemental potassium dosage should be considered in order to help avoid hyperkalemia. Administer with caution in digitalized patients.
Dosage and Administration: Two tablets dissolved in 6–8 oz. of water 4 times daily with meals and at bedtime. For best results let the tablets soak in the water for 2–5 minutes, stir vigorously and swallow.
Caution: Federal law prohibits dispensing without prescription.
[*Shown in Product Identification Section*]

THIACIDE TABLETS ℞
Sodium Free Urinary Acidifer-Antiseptic

Description: Each tablet contains methenamine mandelate 500 mg. and potassium acid phosphate 250 mg.
Actions and Uses: Methenamine mandelate is rapidly absorbed and excreted in the urine. Formaldehyde is released by acid hydrolysis from methenamine with bactericidal levels rapidly reached at pH 5.0. Proportionally less formaldehyde is released as urinary pH approaches 6.0 and insufficient quantities are released above this level for therapeutic response. Since infected urines are frequently above pH 5.0 additional acidification is beneficial. Formaldehyde is 'cidal' against nearly all uropathogens.
Long Term Prophylactic Use: For prevention of reinfection of a sterile urine by converting the urine into an antibacterial medium. Especially useful for long term administration because bacterial resistance will not develop and the components are exceptionally safe.
General Indications: Particularly useful in those infections which are often incurable because of stone or other obstruction, inlying catheter drainage or residual urine in the bladder in neurological disorders. Specifically recommended for the management of chronic urinary tract infections including pyelitis, pyelonephritis, cystitis and infections accompanying neurogenic bladder. Not recommended for acute infections with parenchymal involvement.
Rationale: Methenamine mandelate should not be used unless urinary pH below 6.0 can be maintained. Potassium acid phosphate is a safe, dependable urinary acidifier.
Administration and Dosage: 1 tablet every 2 to 4 hours with a glass of water not to exceed 8 tablets in 24 hours.
Side Effects: A mild laxative effect may be noted in an occasional patient. Methenamine mandelate may cause gastrointestinal upset and/or dysuria.
Precautions: Urine must be kept acid (on the average below 6.0) or therapy should be discontinued as methenamine mandelate is not effective at higher pH. Frequent urine pH tests are essential. This drug is a urine acidifier and can cause metabolic acidosis. Allergic reactions to methenamine mandelate have been reported.
Contraindications: Moderate to severe renal insufficiency with acidosis. Severe hepatic disease.
How Supplied: Bottles of 100 and 500.
Literature Available: Literature and Beach's Low Calcium Acid Ash Diet pads are available on request.
[*Shown in Product Identification Section*]

UROQID–Acid® tablets ℞
UROQID–Acid® No. 2 tablets
Urinary acidifier-Antibacterial

Description: Each UROQID-Acid tablet contains methenamine mandelate 350 mg., sodium acid phosphate, monohydrate 200 mg. Each UROQID-Acid No. 2 tablet contains methenamine mandelate 500 mg., sodium acid phosphate, monohydrate 500 mg.
Actions and Uses: Methenamine mandelate is rapidly absorbed and excreted in the urine. Formaldehyde is released by acid hydrolysis from methenamine with bactericidal levels rapidly reached at pH 5.0. Proportionally less formaldehyde is released as urinary pH approaches 6.0 and insufficient quantities are released above this level for therapeutic response. Since infected urines are frequently above pH 5.0 additional acidification is beneficial. Formaldehyde is 'cidal' against nearly all uropathogens.
Long Term Prophylactic Use: For prevention of reinfection of a sterile urine by converting the urine into an antibacterial medium. Especially useful for long term administration because bacterial resistance will not develop and the components are exceptionally safe.
General Indications: Particularly useful in those infections which are often incurable because of stone or other obstruction, inlying catheter drainage or residual urine in the bladder in neurological disorders. Specifically recommended for the management of chronic urinary tract infections including pyelitis, pyelonephritis, cystitis and infections accompanying neurogenic bladder. Not recommended for acute infections with parenchymal involvement.
Rationale: Methenamine mandelate should not be used unless urinary pH below 6.0 can be maintained. Sodium acid phosphate is a safe, dependable urinary acidifier. The concomitant use of sodium acid phosphate with methenamine mandelate is recommended when the urinary pH is above 6.0. (See U.S. Dispensatory, 1960 Ed., pp 846–847).
Administration and Dosage: UROQID-Acid: initially, 3 tablets 4 times daily. For maintenance, 1 or 2 tablets 4 times daily. UROQID-Acid No. 2: initially, 2 tablets 4 times daily. For maintenance, 2 to 4 tablets daily, in divided doses.
Side Effects: A mild laxative effect may be noted in an occasional patient. Methenamine mandelate may cause gastrointestinal upset and/or dysuria.
Precautions: Urine must be kept acid (on the average below 6.0) or therapy should be discontinued as methenamine mandelate is not effective at higher pH. Frequent urine pH tests are essential. This drug is a urine acidifier and can cause metabolic acidosis. Allergic reactions to methenamine mandelate have been reported.
Use with caution if the patient is on a sodium restricted diet.
Contraindications: Moderate to severe renal insufficiency with acidosis. Severe hepatic disease.
How Supplied: Bottles of 100 and 500.
Literature Available: Literature and Beach's Low Calcium Acid Ash Guide Diet pads are available on request.
[*Shown in Product Identification Section*]

Beecham Products
DIVISION OF BEECHAM INC.
POST OFFICE BOX 1467
PITTSBURGH, PA 15230

MASSENGILL® LIQUID CONCENTRATE
MASSENGILL® POWDER
MASSENGILL® DISPOSABLE DOUCHE

Composition: LIQUID CONCENTRATE—Water, lactic acid, sodium bicarbonate, octoxynol 9, fragrance and color. Alcohol 25%.
POWDER—Boric acid, ammonium alum, fragrance, color.
LIQUID DISPOSABLE DOUCHES:
Vinegar and Water Disposable Douche—water, vinegar, preservative.
Mt. Herbs or Country Flowers Disposable Douche—water, alcohol, lactic acid, sodium lactate, octoxynol 9, cetylpyridinium chloride, fragrance and color.

Continued on next page

Beecham Products—Cont.

Action and Uses: The buffered acid solutions of Massengill Liquid, Disposable Douche, and Powder are valuable adjuncts to specific vaginal therapy, following the prescribed use of vaginal medications or contraceptives and in feminine hygiene.

Directions for Use:
LIQUID CONCENTRATE—Fill cap three quarters full, to measuring line, and pour contents into douche bag containing one quart of warm water. Mix thoroughly.
POWDER—Dissolve two rounded teaspoonfuls in a quart of warm water and mix thoroughly.
LIQUID DISPOSABLE DOUCHE—Twist off cap from bottle containing premixed solution, attach nozzle supplied and use. Unit completely disposable after use.

Warning: Vaginal douches should not be used more than twice weekly except on the advice of a physician. If irritation occurs, discontinue use.

How Supplied: *Liquid,* 4 oz., 8 oz., plastic bottles. Packettes, 12's.
Liquid Disposable Douche, 6 oz.
Powder, 3 oz., 6 oz., 12 oz., 1 lb. Packettes, 12's, 6's.
Is This Product O.T.C.: Yes.

Beecham Laboratories
DIV. OF BEECHAM INC.,
501 FIFTH STREET
BRISTOL, TN 37620

PRODUCT IDENTIFICATION CODES

To provide quick and positive identification of Beecham Laboratories' products, we have imprinted a code number on tablet and capsule products. In order that you may identify a product by its code and number, we have compiled below a numerical list of code numbers with their corresponding product names. The code number as it appears on tablets and capsules bears the letters BMP plus the numerical code.

BMP Code No.	Product
100	ADRENOSEM® SALICYLATE (Carbazochrome Salicylate) Tablets 2.5 mg.
105	ANEXSIA® w/Codeine Tablets
106	ANEXSIA®-D Tablets
107	CONAR®-A Tablets
108	COTROL-D Tablets
109	DASIKON Capsules
112	DASIN® Capsules
119	HYBEPHEN® Tablets
121	LIVITAMIN® Capsules
122	LIVITAMIN® w/INTRINSIC FACTOR Capsules
123	LIVITAMIN® CHEWABLE Tablets
124	LIVITAMIN® PRENATAL Tablets
125	MENEST™ (Esterified Estrogens, U.S.P.) Tablets 0.3 mg.
126	MENEST™ (Esterified Estrogens, U.S.P.) Tablets 0.625 mg.
127	MENEST™ (Esterified Estrogens, U.S.P.) Tablets 1.25 mg.
128	MENEST™ (Esterified Estrogens, U.S.P.) Tablets 2.5 mg.
139	THALFED® Tablets
140	TOTACILLIN® (Ampicillin) Capsules 250 mg.
141	TOTACILLIN® (Ampicillin) Capsules 500 mg.
142	TRISEM Tablets
143	BACTOCILL® (Oxacillin Sodium) Capsules 250 mg.
144	BACTOCILL® (Oxacillin Sodium) Capsules 500 mg.
145	DARICON® (Oxyphencyclimine HCl) Tablets 10 mg.
146	DARICON®-PB (Oxyphencyclimine HCl, 5 mg. and Phenobarbital, 15 mg.) Tablets
147	FASTIN® (Phentermine Hydrochloride) Capsules 30 mg.
148	AMOXIL® (amoxicillin) Capsules 250 mg.
149	AMOXIL® (amoxicillin) Capsules 500 mg.
156	TIGAN® (Trimethobenzamide HCl) Capsules 100 mg.
157	TIGAN® (Trimethobenzamide HCl) Capsules 250 mg.
165	DYCILL® (Dicloxacillin Sodium) Capsules 250 mg.
166	DYCILL® (Dicloxacillin Sodium) Capsules 500 mg.
167	ACTOL EXPECTORANT® Tablets
168	THERALAX® (Bisacodyl, U.S.P.) Tablets 5 mg.
169	CLOXAPEN® (Cloxacillin Sodium) Capsules 250 mg.
170	CLOXAPEN® (Cloxacillin Sodium) Capsules 500 mg.
194	ENARAX®5 (Oxphencyclimine HCl, 5 mg. and Hydroxyzine HCl, 25 mg.) Tablets
195	ENARAX®10 (Oxphencyclimine HCl, 10 mg, and Hydroxyzine HCl, 25 mg.) Tablets

AMOXIL® ℞
(amoxicillin)
CAPSULES and FOR ORAL SUSPENSION

Description: AMOXIL (amoxicillin) is a semisynthetic antibiotic, an analog of ampicillin, with a broad spectrum of bactericidal activity against many Gram-positive and Gram-negative microorganisms. Chemically it is D-(-)-α-amino-p-hydroxybenzyl penicillin trihydrate.

Actions: *PHARMACOLOGY*
Amoxicillin is stable in the presence of gastric acid and may be given without regard to meals. It is rapidly absorbed after oral administration. It diffuses readily into most body tissues and fluids, with the exception of brain and spinal fluid, except when meninges are inflamed. The half-life of amoxicillin is 61.3 minutes. Most of the amoxicillin is excreted unchanged in the urine; its excretion can be delayed by concurrent administration of probenecid. Amoxicillin is not highly protein-bound. In blood serum, amoxicillin is approximately 20% protein-bound as compared to 60% for penicillin-G.
Orally administered doses of 250 mg and 500 mg amoxicillin capsules result in average peak blood levels one to two hours after administration in the range of 3.5 mcg/ml to 5.0 mcg/ml and 5.5 mcg/ml to 7.5 mcg/ml respectively.
Orally administered doses of amoxicillin suspension 125 mg/5 ml and 250 mg/5 ml result in average peak blood levels one to two hours after administration in the range of 1.5 mcg/ml to 3.0 mcg/ml and 3.5 mcg/ml to 5.0 mcg/ml respectively.
Detectable serum levels are observed up to 8 hours after an orally administered dose of amoxicillin. Following a 1 Gm dose and utilizing a special skin window technique to determine levels of the antibiotic, it was noted that therapeutic levels were found in the interstitial fluid. Approximately 60 percent of an orally administered dose of amoxicillin is excreted in the urine within six to eight hours.
MICROBIOLOGY: AMOXIL (amoxicillin) is similar to ampicillin in its bactericidal action against susceptible organisms during the stage of active multiplication. It acts through the inhibition of biosynthesis of cell wall mucopeptide. *In vitro* studies have demonstrated the susceptibility of most strains of the following Gram-positive bacteria: alpha- and beta-hemolytic streptococci, *Diplococcus pneumoniae,* nonpenicillinase-producing staphylococci, and *Streptococcus faecalis.* It is active *in vitro* against many strains of *Haemophilus influenzae, Neisseria gonorrhoeae, Escherichia coli* and *Proteus mirabilis.* Because it does not resist destruction by penicillinase, it is not effective against penicillinase-producing bacteria, particularly resistant staphylococci. All strains of Pseudomonas and most strains of Klebsiella and Enterobacter are resistant.
Disc Susceptibility Tests: Quantitative methods that require measurement of zone diameters give the most precise estimates of antibiotic susceptibility. One such procedure* has been recommended for use with discs for testing susceptibility to ampicillin-class antibiotics. Interpretations correlate diameters of the disc test with MIC values for amoxicillin. With this procedure, a report from the laboratory of "susceptible" indicates that the infecting organism is likely to respond to therapy. A report of "resistant" indicates that the infecting organism is not likely to respond to therapy. A report of "intermediate susceptibility" suggests that the organism would be susceptible if high dosage is used, or if the infection is confined to tissues and fluids (e.g., urine), in which high antibiotic levels are attained.

Indications: AMOXIL (amoxicillin) is indicated in the treatment of infections due to susceptible strains of the following:
Gram-negative organisms—*H. influenzae, E. coli, P. mirabilis* and *N. gonorrhoeae.*
Gram-positive organisms—Streptococci (including *Streptococcus faecalis), D. pneumoniae* and nonpenicillinase-producing staphylococci.
Therapy may be instituted prior to obtaining results from bacteriological and susceptibility studies to determine the causative organisms and their susceptibility to amoxicillin.
Indicated surgical procedures should be performed.

Contraindications: A history of allergic reaction to any of the penicillins is a contraindication.

Warnings: SERIOUS AND OCCASIONALLY FATAL HYPERSENSITIVITY (ANAPHYLACTOID) REACTIONS HAVE BEEN REPORTED IN PATIENTS ON PENICILLIN THERAPY. ALTHOUGH ANAPHYLAXIS IS MORE FREQUENT FOLLOWING PARENTERAL THERAPY, IT HAS OCCURRED IN PATIENTS ON ORAL PENICILLINS. THESE REACTIONS ARE MORE LIKELY TO OCCUR IN INDIVIDUALS WITH A HISTORY OF SENSITIVITY TO MULTIPLE ALLERGENS. THERE HAVE BEEN REPORTS OF INDIVIDUALS WITH A HISTORY OF PENICILLIN HYPERSENSITIVITY WHO HAVE EXPERIENCED SEVERE REACTIONS WHEN TREATED WITH CEPHALOSPORINS. BEFORE THERAPY WITH ANY PENICILLIN, CAREFUL INQUIRY SHOULD BE MADE CONCERNING PREVIOUS HYPER-

SENSITIVITY REACTIONS TO PENICILLINS, CEPHALOSPORINS, OR OTHER ALLERGENS. IF AN ALLERGIC REACTION OCCURS, APPROPRIATE THERAPY SHOULD BE INSTITUTED AND DISCONTINUANCE OF AMOXICILLIN THERAPY CONSIDERED. **SERIOUS ANAPHYLACTOID REACTIONS REQUIRE IMMEDIATE EMERGENCY TREATMENT WITH EPINEPHRINE. OXYGEN, INTRAVENOUS STEROIDS, AND AIRWAY MANAGEMENT, INCLUDING INTUBATION, SHOULD ALSO BE ADMINISTERED AS INDICATED.**

Usage in Pregnancy

Safety for use in pregnancy has not been established.

Precautions: As with any potent drug, periodic assessment of renal, hepatic and hematopoietic function should be made during prolonged therapy.

The possibility of superinfections with mycotic or bacterial pathogens should be kept in mind during therapy. If superinfections occur (usually involving Enterobacter, Pseudomonas or Candida), the drug should be discontinued and/or appropriate therapy instituted.

Adverse Reactions: As with other penicillins, it may be expected that untoward reactions will be essentially limited to sensitivity phenomena. They are more likely to occur in individuals who have previously demonstrated hypersensitivity to penicillins and in those with a history of allergy, asthma, hay fever or urticaria. The following adverse reactions have been reported as associated with the use of the penicillins.

Gastrointestinal: Nausea, vomiting and diarrhea.

Hypersensitivity Reactions: Erythematous maculopapular rashes and urticaria have been reported.

NOTE: Urticaria, other skin rashes and serum sickness-like reactions may be controlled with antihistamines and, if necessary, systemic corticosteroids. Whenever such reactions occur, amoxicillin should be discontinued unless, in the opinion of the physician, the condition being treated is life-threatening and amenable only to amoxicillin therapy.

Liver: A moderate rise in serum glutamic oxaloacetic transaminase (SGOT) has been noted, but the significance of this finding is unknown.

Hemic and Lymphatic Systems: Anemia, thrombocytopenia, thrombocytopenic purpura, eosinophilia, leukopenia and agranulocytosis have been reported during therapy with the penicillins. These reactions are usually reversible on discontinuation of therapy and are believed to be hypersensitivity phenomena.

Dosage and Administration: Infections of the ear, nose and throat due to streptococci, pneumococci, nonpenicillinase-producing staphylococci and *H. influenzae;*

Infections of the genitourinary tract due to *E. coli, Proteus mirabilis* and *Streptococcus faecalis;*

Infections of the skin and soft-tissues due to streptococci, susceptible staphylococci and *E. coli.*

USUAL DOSAGE:

Adults: 250 mg. every 8 hours.

Children: 20 mg./kg./day in divided doses every 8 hours.

Children weighing 20 kg. or more should be dosed according to the adult recommendations.

In severe infections or those caused by less susceptible organisms:

500 mg. every 8 hours for adults, and 40 mg./kg./day in divided doses every 8 hours for children may be needed.

Infections of the lower respiratory tract due to streptococci, pneumococci, nonpenicillinase-producing staphylococci and *H. influenzae:*

USUAL DOSAGE:

Adults: 500 mg. every 8 hours.

Children: 40 mg./kg./day in divided doses every 8 hours.

Children weighing 20 kg. or more should be dosed according to the adult recommendations.

Gonorrhea, acute uncomplicated ano-genital and urethral infections due to *N. gonorrhoeae* (males and females):

3 grams as a single oral dose

Cases of gonorrhea with a suspected lesion of syphilis should have dark-field examinations before receiving amoxicillin, and monthly serological tests for a minimum of four months.

Larger doses may be required for stubborn or severe infections.

The children's dosage is intended for individuals whose weight will not cause a dosage to be calculated greater than that recommended for adults.

It should be recognized that in the treatment of chronic urinary tract infections, frequent bacteriological and clinical appraisals are necessary. Smaller doses than those recommended above should not be used. Even higher doses may be needed at times. In stubborn infections, therapy may be required for several weeks. It may be necessary to continue clinical and/or bacteriological follow-up for several months after cessation of therapy. Except for gonorrhea, treatment should be continued for a minimum of 48 to 72 hours beyond the time that the patient becomes asymptomatic or evidence of bacterial eradication has been obtained. It is recommended that there be at least 10 days' treatment for any infection caused by hemolytic streptococci to prevent the occurrence of acute rheumatic fever or glomerulonephritis.

Dosage and Administration of Pediatric Drops: Usual dosage for all indications except infections of the lower respiratory tract:

Under 6 kg. (13 lbs.): 0.5 ml. every 8 hours

6–8 kg. (13–18 lbs.): 1 ml. every 8 hours

Infections of the lower respiratory tract:

Under 6 kg. (13 lbs.): 1 ml. every 8 hours

6–8 kg. (13–18 lbs.): 2 ml. every 8 hours

Children weighing more than 8 kg. (18 lbs.) should receive the appropriate dose of the Oral Suspension 125 mg. or 250 mg./5 ml.

After reconstitution, the required amount of suspension should be placed directly on the child's tongue for swallowing. Alternate means of administration are to add the required amount of suspension to formula, milk, fruit juice, water, ginger ale or cold drinks. These preparations should then be taken immediately. To be certain the child is receiving full dosage, such preparations should be consumed in entirety.

Directions for Mixing Oral Suspension:

Prepare suspension at time of dispensing as follows: Tap bottle until all powder flows freely. Add approximately ⅓ of the total amount of water for reconstitution (see table below) and shake vigorously to wet powder. Add the remainder of the water and again shake vigorously.

Bottle Size	Amount of Water Required for Reconstitution
80 ml.	53 ml.
100 ml.	66 ml.
150 ml.	100 ml.

Each teaspoonful (5 ml.) will contain 125 mg. or 250 mg. amoxicillin.

125 mg unit dose	5 ml.
250 mg unit dose	5 ml.
3 Gm single dose	40 ml.

Directions for Mixing Pediatric Drops:

Add 11 ml. of water to the bottle and shake vigorously. Each ml. of suspension will contain 50 mg. amoxicillin.

NOTE: SHAKE BOTH ORAL SUSPENSION AND PEDIATRIC DROPS WELL BEFORE USING.

Keep bottle tightly closed. Any unused portion of the reconstituted suspension must be discarded after 14 days. Refrigeration preferable, but not required.

How Supplied: AMOXIL (amoxicillin) Capsules. Each capsule contains 250 mg. or 500 mg. amoxicillin as the trihydrate.

250 mg./Capsule

NDC 0029-6006-24 bottles of 15
NDC 0029-6006-30 bottles of 100
NDC 0029-6006-32 bottles of 500
NDC 0029-6006-31 unit dose cartons of 100

500 mg./Capsule

NDC 0029-6007-24 bottles of 15
NDC 0029-6007-29 bottles of 50
NDC 0029-6007-32 bottles of 500
NDC 0029-6007-31 unit dose cartons of 100

[*Shown in Product Identification Section*]

AMOXIL (amoxicillin) for Oral Suspension.

125 mg./5 ml.

NDC 0029-6008-18 5 ml unit dose bottle
NDC 0029-6008-21 80 ml. bottle
NDC 0029-6008-23 100 ml. bottle
NDC 0029-6008-22 150 ml. bottle

250 mg./5 ml.

NDC 0029-6009-18 5 ml unit dose bottle
NDC 0029-6009-21 80 ml. bottle
NDC 0029-6009-23 100 ml. bottle
NDC 0029-6009-22 150 ml. bottle

Each 5 ml. of reconstituted suspension contains 125 mg. or 250 mg. amoxicillin as the trihydrate.

AMOXIL (amoxicillin) Pediatric Drops for Oral Suspension. Each ml. of reconstituted suspension contains 50 mg. amoxicillin as the trihydrate.

NDC 0029-6035-20 15 ml. bottle

* Bauer, A. W., Kirby, W. M. M., Sherris, J. C., and Turck, M.: Antibiotic Testing by a Standardized Single Disc Method, Am. J. Clin. Pathol., 45: 493, 1966. Standardized Disc Susceptibility Test, FEDERAL REGISTER 37:20527-29, 1972.

BACTOCILL® ℞

(oxacillin sodium)

Capsules and for Injection—Buffered

Description: BACTOCILL (oxacillin sodium) is sodium 5-methyl-3-phenyl-4-isoxazolyl penicillin monohydrate, a penicillinase-resistant, acid-resistant semisynthetic penicillin, derived from the penicillin nucleus, 6-aminopenicillanic acid.

Each gram of BACTOCILL (oxacillin sodium) for Injection is equivalent to 1 Gm. of oxacillin activity, is buffered with 40 mg. dibasic sodium phosphate, preserved with 3.6 mg. methylparaben and 0.4 mg. propylparaben, and contains approximately 3.1 mEq. of sodium.

Actions:

MICROBIOLOGY

Oxacillin sodium displays the ability to resist inactivation by staphylococcal penicillinase. Clinical and laboratory studies show that BACTOCILL demonstrates activity against penicillin G-sensitive staphylococci, penicillin G-resistant staphylococci, pneumococci, and streptococci. In addition, it is more active per μnit weight, *in vitro,* than is methicillin when used against penicillin G-resistant strains of *Staphylococcus aureus.* On an equivalent weight basis, oxacillin sodium is not as active, *in vitro,* as is penicillin G against streptococci, pneumococci, and penicillin G-sensitive staphylococci.

PHARMACOLOGY

Because its resistance to gastric acid is much greater than that of penicillin G, BACTOCILL can be given conveniently by mouth. Oral doses of 500 mg. to 1 gram produce average peak plasma concentrations of 4 to 8 mcg./ml. in one hour (intramuscular doses of 500 mg. to

Continued on next page

Beecham Laboratories—Cont.

1 gram yield a blood concentration of 7 to 13 mcg./ml., but only a negligible amount remains after 4 to 6 hours). Peak serum levels are achieved 30 minutes after intramuscular administration, giving 5.3 mcg./ml. and 10.9 mcg./ml. with a 250 mg. and a 500 mg. dose respectively. Intravenous administration provides peak serum levels approximately 5 minutes after the injection is completed. Slow I.V. administration of 500 mg. gives a peak serum level of 43 mcg./ml. after 5 minutes with a half-life of 20 to 30 minutes. Studies of human distribution have revealed that oxacillin sodium can be detected in bile, pleural and amniotic fluids, cord serum, and milk, but it does not penetrate well into normal cerebrospinal fluid; however, it does appear in cerebrospinal fluid in patients with meningitis. BACTOCILL undergoes rapid excretion by the kidneys. During the 6 hours following an intramuscular dose of 500 mg. to 1 gram, the urinary concentration ranges between 200 mcg./ml. and 2 mg./ml.; 40% of the dose is excreted within this period.

Disc Susceptibility Tests

Quantitative methods that require measurement of zone diameters give the most precise estimates of antibiotic susceptibility. One such procedure* has been recommended for use with discs for testing susceptibility to penicillinase-resistant penicillin-class antibiotics. Interpretations correlate diameters on the disc test with MIC values for penicillinase-resistant penicillins. With this procedure, a report from the laboratory of "susceptible" indicates that the infecting organism is likely to respond to therapy. A report of "resistant" indicates that the infecting organism is not likely to respond to therapy. A report of "intermediate susceptibility" suggests that the organism would be susceptible if high dosage is used, or if the infection is confined to tissues and fluids (e.g., urine), in which high antibiotic levels are attained.

Indications: Although the principal indication for BACTOCILL is in the treatment of infections due to penicillinase-producing staphylococci, it may be used to initiate therapy in any patient in whom a staphylococcal infection is suspected. (See Important Note below.)

Bacteriological studies to determine the causative organisms and their sensitivity to oxacillin sodium should be performed.

In serious, life-threatening infections, oral preparations of the penicillinase-resistant penicillins should not be relied on for initial therapy.

IMPORTANT NOTE

When it is judged necessary that treatment be initiated before definitive culture and sensitivity results are known, the choice of oxacillin sodium should take into consideration the fact that it has been shown to be effective only in the treatment of infections caused by pneumococci, Group A beta-hemolytic streptococci, and penicillin G-resistant and penicillin G-sensitive staphylococci. If the bacteriology report later indicates the infection is due to an organism other than a penicillin G-resistant staphylococcus sensitive to oxacillin sodium, the physician is advised to continue therapy with a drug other than oxacillin sodium or any other penicillinase-resistant semisynthetic penicillin.

Recent studies have reported that the percentage of staphylococcal isolates resistant to penicillin G outside the hospital is increasing, approximating the high percentage of resistant staphylococcal isolates found in the hospital. For this reason, it is recommended that a penicillinase-resistant penicillin be used as initial therapy for any suspected staphylococcal infection until culture and sensitivity results are known.

Oxacillin sodium is a compound that acts through a mechanism similar to that of Methicillin against penicillin G-resistant staphylococci. Strains of staphylococci resistant to methicillin have existed in nature, and it is known that the number of these strains reported has been increasing. Such strains of staphylococci have been capable of producing serious disease, in some instances resulting in fatality. Because of this, there is concern that widespread use of the penicillinase-resistant penicillins may result in the appearance of an increasing number of staphylococcal strains which are resistant to these penicillins.

Methicillin-resistant strains are almost always resistant to all other penicillinase-resistant penicillins. (Cross resistance with cephalosporin derivatives also occurs frequently.) Resistance to any penicillinase-resistant penicillin should be interpreted as evidence of clinical resistance to all, in spite of the fact that minor variations in *in vitro* sensitivity may be encountered when more than one penicillinase-resistant penicillin is tested against the same strain of staphylococcus.

Contraindications: A history of allergic reaction to any of the penicillins is a contraindication.

Warnings: SERIOUS AND OCCASIONALLY FATAL HYPERSENSITIVITY (ANAPHYLACTOID) REACTIONS HAVE BEEN REPORTED IN PATIENTS RECEIVING PENICILLIN. THESE REACTIONS ARE MORE LIKELY TO OCCUR IN PERSONS WITH A HISTORY OF SENSITIVITY TO MULTIPLE ALLERGENS. THERE ARE REPORTS OF PATIENTS WITH A HISTORY OF PENICILLIN HYPERSENSITIVITY REACTIONS WHO EXPERIENCED SEVERE MANIFESTATIONS OF THIS TYPE WHEN TREATED WITH A CEPHALOSPORIN. PRECEDING THERAPY WITH A PENICILLIN, IT IS NECESSARY TO INQUIRE WITH CARE ABOUT PREVIOUS HYPERSENSITIVITY REACTIONS TO PENICILLINS, CEPHALOSPORINS, AND OTHER ALLERGENS. SHOULD SUCH AN UNFAVORABLE RESPONSE OCCUR, THE DRUG MUST BE DISCONTINUED UNLESS, IN THE OPINION OF THE PHYSICIAN, THE CONDITION BEING TREATED THREATENS THE LIFE OF THE PATIENT AND IS AMENABLE ONLY TO THERAPY WITH OXACILLIN SODIUM. **SERIOUS ANAPHYLACTOID REACTIONS REQUIRE IMMEDIATE EMERGENCY TREATMENT WITH EPINEPHRINE. OXYGEN, INTRAVENOUS STEROIDS, AND AIRWAY MANAGEMENT, INCLUDING INTUBATION, SHOULD ALSO BE ADMINISTERED AS INDICATED.**

USAGE DURING PREGNANCY

Safety of BACTOCILL for use during pregnancy has not been established.

Precautions: Penicillin should be used with caution in individuals with histories of significant allergies and/or asthma. The oral route of administration should not be relied upon in patients with severe illness, or with nausea or intestinal hypermotility.

Following the pattern established with other antibiotics, it should be remembered that occurrence of superinfection is a possibility during treatment with oxacillin sodium. Should superinfection appear under these circumstances, it is necessary to institute appropriate measures for its control. As is the case with any potent medication, it is advisable to check periodically for organ system dysfunction during prolonged therapy. Careful monitoring of renal, hepatic, and hematopoietic levels constitutes an important phase of BACTOCILL therapy. Due to the fact that experience with BACTOCILL in premature and newborn infants is limited, caution should be utilized in administering this drug to such patients, and it is recommended that organ system function be frequently evaluated.

Adverse Reactions: This drug has been well tolerated with reactions being infrequent. Included among these are skin rash, urticaria, pruritus, eosinophilia, hairy tongue, fever, gastrointestinal symptoms (such as nausea, vomiting, and diarrhea), and an occasional anaphylactoid response. In a few instances, a moderate elevation of serum glutamic oxaloacetic transaminase (SGOT) has been detected. As with other penicillins, leukopenia, neutropenia, thrombocytopenia, or hemolytic anemia may occur. Transient hematuria, albuminuria, and azotemia have been observed in some newborns and infants who have been administered high doses of oxacillin sodium (150 to 175 mg./kg./day). Although the exact causal relationship of these findings is not clear, such babies should be closely watched for signs of kidney impairment. In addition, small numbers of patients have developed thrombophlebitis following intravenous therapy.

Dosage and Administration: BACTOCILL for Injection is the preferable dosage form for serious infections and for those patients unable to take the drug orally. When parenteral therapy is no longer considered necessary, however, the oral route of administration should be adopted as soon as possible.

Oral:

Usual Adult Dose: For mild-to-moderate infections of the skin, soft tissues or upper respiratory tract: 500 mg. every 4 to 6 hours for a minimum of 5 days.

Oral: Pediatric Dose: Children weighing more than 20 kg. (44 lbs.) should receive adult dosage. Children weighing less than 20 kg. (44 lbs.): For mild to moderately severe infections of the skin, soft tissues or upper respiratory tract: 50 mg./kg./day in equally divided doses at 6-hour intervals for at least 5 days. For follow-up therapy, the dose of oxacillin sodium is 100 mg./kg./day or greater in equally divided doses at 4- to 6-hour intervals. In serious systemic infections, therapy should be continued for at least 1 to 2 weeks after the patient is afebrile and cultures are sterile. Treatment of osteomyelitis may require several months of intensive therapy. The best use for this oral medication is in the prolonged follow-up therapy following successful initial treatment with parenterally administered penicillinase-resistant penicillin. The oral medication is best taken on an empty stomach, preferably 1 to 2 hours before meals.

NOTE: In serious or life-threatening infections, such as staphylococcal septicemia or other deep-seated severe infections, oral preparations of the penicillinase-resistant penicillins should not be relied upon for initial therapy; oral absorption may be unreliable, the patient may vomit the medication or may not actually take it. Parenteral methicillin sodium or parenteral oxacillin sodium is advisable for initial treatment of these conditions if they are due to penicillinase-producing staphylococci. Following initial control of the infections with the parenteral preparations, oral BACTOCILL (oxacillin sodium) may be given for follow-up therapy in a dose of 1 Gm. every 4 to 6 hours.

Parenteral

For mild-to-moderate upper respiratory and localized skin and soft-tissue infections:

Adults: 250 to 500 mg. every 4 to 6 hours.

Children weighing less than 20 kg. (44 lbs.): 50 mg./kg./day (25 mg./lb./day) in equally divided doses every 6 hours.

NOTE: Absorption and excretion data indicate that doses of 25 mg./kg./day (12.5 mg./lb./day) provide adequate therapeutic levels in premature and neonates.

For more severe infections such as those of the lower respiratory tract or disseminated infections:

Adults: 1 Gm. or more every 4 to 6 hours.

Children weighing less than 20 kg. (44 lbs.): 100 mg./kg./day (50 mg./lb./day) or more in equally divided doses every 4 to 6 hours.

Very severe infections may require very high doses and prolonged therapy.
Infections caused by Group A beta-hemolytic streptococci: the use of penicillin G, phenoxymethyl penicillin or phenethicillin is the preferred treatment, because of their greater activity against this agent. Such infections should be treated for at least 10 days to help prevent the occurrence of rheumatic fever or acute glomerulonephritis.

DIRECTIONS FOR USE
INTRAMUSCULAR ADMINISTRATION:
Reconstitution — Use Sterile Water for Injection, U.S.P. or Sodium Chloride Injection, U.S.P. and shake vigorously to reconstitute; withdraw desired volume of solution and inject.

Vial Size	Amount of Diluent to be Added
500 mg	2.8 ml
1 Gm	5.7 ml
2 Gm	11.4 ml
4 Gm	21.8 ml

After reconstitution, each vial will contain 250 mg of Oxacillin per 1.5 ml of solution.
Stability — Discard unused I.M. solutions after 3 days at room temperature or 7 days under refrigeration.
DIRECT INTRAVENOUS ADMINISTRATION:
Reconstitution — Use Sterile Water for Injection,, U.S.P. or Sodium Chloride Injection, U.S.P.

Container Size	Amount of Diluent to be Added
500 mg Vial	5 ml
1 Gm Vial and 1 Gm Piggyback Bottle	10 ml
2 Gm Vial and 2 Gm Piggyback Bottle	20 ml
4 Gm Vial and 4 Gm Bulk Pharmacy Package	40 ml

Shake well until powder is completely dissolved; dilute further as desired, then withdraw contents. Administer as slowly as possible to avoid vein irritation.
Stability — See under Intravenous Drip Infusion.
INTRAVENOUS DRIP INFUSION:
Reconstitution of Standard Vials:
Reconstitute with an appropriate I.V. diluent, shake well until powder is completely dissolved, then further dilute to desired volume.
Reconstitution of 1 Gm, 2 Gm Piggyback Bottles and 4 Gm Bulk Pharmacy Package:

Bottle Size	Amount of Diluent to be Added
1 Gm and 2 Gm Piggyback Bottles	50-100 ml
4 Gm Bulk Pharmacy Package	98 ml

Reconstitute as indicated above with Sterile Water for Injection, U.S.P., Sodium Chloride Injection, U.S.P. or another suitable diluent as indicated below.
Stability
Stability studies on BACTOCILL at concentrations between 10 mg/ml and 100 mg/ml indicate that the resulting solutions will lose less than 10% activity at room temperature (70°F) or under refrigeration (40°F) for the time periods stated below:

Intravenous Solution	Stability Period: Room Temperature	Refrigerated
Sterile Water for Injection	7 days	8 days
Sodium Chloride Injection	7 days	8 days
5% Dextrose in Water	2 days	8 days
Lactated Ringer's Injection	1 day	8 days

After reconstitution, these solutions can be frozen (approx. 0°F) and stored for up to 30 days without loss of potency. The stabilities of the thawed solutions are identical to the unfrozen ones listed above.

BACTOCILL in the followng intravenous solutions at concentrations between 0.5 mg/ml and 40 mg/ml will lose less than 10% activity at room temperature during a 6 hour period:
5% Dextrose in Normal Saline
10% D-Fructose in Water
10% D-Fructose in Normal Saline
Lactated Potassic Saline Injections
10% Invert Sugar in Water
10% Invert Sugar in Normal Saline
10% Invert Sugar plus 0.3% Potassium Chloride in Water
Travert 10% Electrolyte #1
Travert 10% Electrolyte #2
Travert 10% Electrolyte #3
BACTOCILL for intravenous infusion should be reconstituted only in those solutions listed above. The drug concentration and the rate and volume of the infusion should be adjusted so that the total dose of Oxacillin is administered before the drug loses its stability in the diluent.
Unused portions of solutions should be discarded after the time periods mentioned above.
Store dry powder at room temperature or below.

How Supplied:
BACTOCILL (oxacillin sodium) Capsules.
Each capsule contains oxacillin sodium monohydrate equivalent to 250 mg. or 500 mg. oxacillin.
250 mg./Capsule
NDC 0029-6010-30........................bottles of 100
NDC 0029-6010-31....unit dose cartons of 100
500 mg./Capsule
NDC 0029-6015-30........................bottles of 100
NDC 0029-6015-31....unit dose cartons of 100
BACTOCILL (oxacillin sodium) for Injection Buffered.
Each vial contains oxacillin sodium monohydrate equivalent to 500 mg., 1 Gm., 2 Gm., or 4 Gm. oxacillin.
NDC 0029-6020-25 ....500 mg.
NDC 0029-6025-22 ....1 Gm.
NDC 0029-6028-27 ....2 Gm.
NDC 0029-6030-26 ....4 Gm.
NDC 0029-6025-21 .....1 Gm. Piggyback Bottle
NDC 0029-6028-21 .....2 Gm. Piggyback Bottle
NDC 0029-6030-21........4 Gm. Bulk Pharmacy Package

Literature Available: Yes.

*Bauer, A.W., Kirby, W.M.M., Sherris, J.C. and Turck, M.: Antibiotic Testing by a Standardized Single Disc Method, Am.J. Clin. Pathol., 45:493, 1966; Standardized Disc Susceptibility Test, FEDERAL REGISTER 37:20527-29, 1972

CELBENIN® ℞
—(methicillin sodium)
for Injection—Buffered

Description: CELBENIN (Methicillin Sodium) is sodium 2,6-dimethoxyphenyl penicillin monohydrate, a penicillinase-resistant, semisynthetic injectable penicillin, derived from the penicillin nucleus 6-aminopenicillanic acid.
Each 1 Gm. of CELBENIN (methicillin sodium) is equivalent to 900 mg. of 2,6-dimethoxyphenyl penicillin activity, is buffered with 50 mg. of sodium citrate and preserved with 0.9 mg. methylparaben and 0.1 mg. propylparaben. One Gm. of CELBENIN contains approximately 3.1 milliequivalents of sodium.

Actions:
MICROBIOLOGY
CELBENIN is a bactericidal penicillin, highly resistant to staphylococcal penicillinase and equally active against penicillin-sensitive and penicillinase-producing strains of *Staphylococcus aureus.* Although the antimicrobial spectrum of methicillin sodium and penicillin G are qualitatively similar, a higher concentration of the drug is needed for bactericidal activity against streptococci and pneumococci than for penicillin G.
In the presence of staphylococcal penicillinase, the drug is almost completely stable and is not degraded by *B. cereus* penicillinase.
PHARMACOLOGY
Methicillin sodium is not acid resistant and must be administered by intramuscular or intravenous injection. A one-gram dose gives a peak blood level of approximately 10 mcg./ml. which drops off to about 3 mcg./ml. within a 4-hour period. If probenecid is administered concurrently, blood levels of the drug may be improved and prolonged.
Methicillin is excreted unchanged in the urine, about two-thirds of a 1-gram dose being excreted within 4 hours in individuals with normal kidney function. Impairment in kidney function results in elevated blood levels which require downward adjustment of dosage and treatment intervals. Protein binding of methicillin is approximately 40%.
After intramuscular injection in animals, the highest concentrations of the drug are reached in the kidneys, liver, heart, and lung in that order, pointing to an expeditious distribution in the tissues. The spleen and muscles show lower concentrations of the antibiotic. It also diffuses into human pleural, prostatic, pericardial, and synovial fluids. As with all penicillins, higher concentrations of CELBENIN may occur during meningeal inflammation than under normal conditions when absorption is poor. A similar low level of toxicity with CELBENIN and penicillin G has been demonstrated in toxicity studies in animals.
DISC SUSCEPTIBILITY TESTS
Quantitative methods that require measurement of zone diameters give the most precise estimates of antibiotic susceptibility. One such procedure* has been recommended for use with discs for testing susceptibility to penicillinase-resistant penicillin-class antibiotics. Interpretations correlate diameters on the disc test with MIC values for penicillinase-resistant penicillins. With this procedure, a report from the laboratory of "susceptible" indicates that the infecting organism is likely to respond to therapy. A report of "resistant" indicates that the infecting organism is not likely to respond to therapy. A report of "intermediate susceptibility" suggests that the organism would be susceptible if high dosage is used, or if the infection is confined to tissues and fluids (e.g., urine), in which high antibiotic levels are attained.

Indications: Although the principal indication for CELBENIN is in the treatment of infections due to penicillinase-producing staphylococci, it may be used to initiate therapy in any patient in whom a staphylococcal infection is suspected. (See following Important Note.)
Bacteriological studies to determine the causative organisms and their sensitivity to methicillin sodium should be performed.
In serious, life-threatening infections, oral preparations of the penicillinase-resistant penicillins should not be relied on for initial therapy.
Important Note: When it is judged necessary that treatment be initiated before definitive culture and sensitivity results are known, the choice of methicillin sodium should take into consideration the fact that it has been shown to be effective only in the treatment of infections caused by pneumococci, Group A beta-hemolytic streptococci, and penicillin G-resistant and penicillin G-sensitive staphylococci. If the bacteriology report later indicates the infection is due to an organism other than a penicillin G-resistant staphylococcus sensitive to methicillin sodium, the physician is advised to continue therapy with a drug other than methicillin sodium or any other penicillinase-resistant semisynthetic penicillin.

Continued on next page

Beecham Laboratories—Cont.

Recent studies have reported that the percentage of staphylococcal isolates resistant to penicillin G outside the hospital is increasing, approximating the high percentage of resistant staphylococcal isolates found in the hospital. For this reason, it is recommended that a penicillinase-resistant penicillin be used as initial therapy for any suspected staphylococcal infection until culture and sensitivity results are known.

Strains of staphylococci resistant to methicillin have existed in nature and it is known that the number of these strains reported has been increasing. Such strains of staphylococci have been capable of producing serious disease, in some instances resulting in fatality. Because of this, there is concern that widespread use of the penicillinase-resistant penicillins may result in the appearance of an increasing number of staphylococcal strains which are resistant to these penicillins.

Methicillin-resistant strains are almost always resistant to all other penicillinase-resistant penicillins. (Cross resistance with cephalosporin derivatives also occurs frequently.) Resistance to any penicillinase-resistant penicillin should be interpreted as evidence of clinical resistance to all, in spite of the fact that minor variations in *in vitro* sensitivity may be encountered when more than one penicillinase-resistant penicillin is tested against the same strain of staphylococcus.

Contraindications: A history of an allergic reaction to any of the penicillins is a contraindication.

Warning: Serious and occasionally fatal hypersensitivity (anaphylactoid) reactions have been reported in patients on penicillin therapy. Although anaphylaxis is more frequent following parenteral therapy, it has occurred in patients on oral penicillins. These reactions are more apt to occur in individuals with a history of sensitivity to multiple allergens.

There have been reports of individuals with a history of penicillin hypersensitivity reactions who have experienced severe reactions when treated with a cephalosporin. Before therapy with a penicillin, careful inquiry should be made concerning previous hypersensitivity reactions to penicillins, cephalosporins, and other allergens. If an allergic reaction occurs, the drug should be discontinued and the appropriate therapy instituted. **Serious anaphylactoid reactions require immediate emergency treatment with epinephrine. Oxygen, intravenous steroids, and airway management, including intubation, should also be administered as indicated.**

Precautions: Penicillin should be used with caution in individuals with histories of significant allergies and/or asthma.

As with any potent drug, periodic assessment of organ system function, including renal, hepatic, and hematopoietic, should be made during prolonged therapy.

The possibility of bacterial and/or fungal overgrowth should be kept in mind during long-term therapy. If overgrowth of resistant organisms occurs, appropriate measures should be taken.

Safety for use in pregnancy has not been established.

Because of incompletely developed renal function in infants, methicillin may not be completely excreted, with abnormally high blood levels resulting. Frequent blood level measurements are advisable in this age group with dosage adjustments when necessary.

Adverse Reactions: To date, reactions have been infrequent and have included: skin rash, pruritus, urticaria, serum sickness, fever, and oral lesions, such as glossitis and stomatitis. Anaphylactic reactions have also occurred. As with other penicillins, eosinophilia, granulocytopenia, hemolytic anemia, thrombocytopenia, and transient neutropenia with evidence of bone marrow depression have been observed. Occasionally, clinical and laboratory signs of abnormal renal function, including hematuria, casts, azotemia, oliguria, albuminuria, pyuria, and cylindruria have been noted: however, they have disappeared either during therapy or after cessation of the drug. While the causal relationship is not completely evident in all cases, it is recommended that patients under methicillin therapy have periodic blood counts and be observed for signs of progressive renal impairments. Neuropathy and oral and rectal moniliasis have also been noted.

Dosage and Administration:

INTRAMUSCULAR ROUTE:

Adult Dosage: 1 Gm. every 4 to 6 hours.

Infants' and Children's Dosage [Patients weighing less than 20 Kg. (44 lbs.)]: 25 mg./Kg. (12 mg./lb.) every 6 hours.

INTRAVENOUS ROUTE:

Usual Adult Dosage: 1 Gm. every 6 hours.

Infants' and Children's Dosage: Because of an insufficient number of cases, no specific recommendation.

Higher doses should be used in very severe infections.

Therapy should be continued for at least 48 hours (or, in the case of serious systemic infections, for at least 1-2 weeks) after the patient has become afebrile, asymptomatic and cultures are sterile. Treatment of osteomyelitis may require several months of intensive therapy. Oral penicillinase-resistant penicillins may be of special value in follow-up therapy because of the difficulty of maintaining prolonged parenteral treatment.

Note: In the event of a mixed infection or a subsequent superinfection by an organism unsusceptible to methicillin, a supplemental antimicrobial agent may be required. This agent ***should not be physically mixed*** with CELBENIN but should be administered separately, according to its own dosage and administration recommendations.

Directions for Use:

INTRAMUSCULAR ADMINISTRATION:

Reconstitution—Use Sterile Water for Injection, U.S.P. or Sodium Chloride Injection, U.S.P. and shake vigorously to reconstitute; withdraw desired volume of solution and inject.

Vial Size	Amount of Diluent to be Added
1 Gm	At least 1.5 ml
4 Gm	5.7 ml
6 Gm	8.6 ml

After reconstitution each 1 ml of solution contains approximately 500 mg CELBENIN.

Stability—Discard unused I.M. solutions after 24 hours at room temperature or 4 days under refrigeration.

DIRECT INTRAVENOUS ADMINISTRATION:

Standard Vials, 1 Gm, 4 Gm, and 6 Gm:

Reconstitution—Add the following amounts of Sterile Water for Injection, U.S.P. or Sodium Chloride Injection, U.S.P. and shake vigorously until powder is completely dissolved.

Vial Size	Amount of Diluent to be Added
1 Gm	At least 1.5 ml
4 Gm	5.7 ml
6 Gm	8.6 ml

Dilution—Further dilute each 1 ml of solution, reconstituted as directed above, with approximately 20–25 ml of Sterile Water for Injection, U.S.P. or Sodium Chloride Injection, U.S.P. and inject as slowly as possible to avoid vein irritation.

1 Gm, 2 Gm, 4 Gm Piggyback Bottles and 6 Gm Bulk Pharmacy Package:

Reconstitution—*Use Sterile Water for Injection, U.S.P. or Sodium Chloride Injection, U.S.P.*

Bottle Size	Minimum Amount of Diluent to be Added
1 Gm	17 ml
2 Gm	33 ml
4 Gm	65 ml
6 Gm	97 ml

If reconstituted as above, each 17 ml of solution will contain approximately 1 Gm CELBENIN. In order to avoid vein irritation, the solution should be administered as slowly as possible.

Stability—See under Intravenous Drip Infusion

INTRAVENOUS DRIP INFUSION:

Reconstitution of Standard Vials:

Reconstitute with an appropriate I.V. diluent, shake well until powder is completely dissolved, then further dilute to desired volume.

Reconstitution of 1 Gm, 2 Gm, 4 Gm Piggyback Bottles and 6 Gm Bulk Pharmacy Package:

Use Sterile Water for Injection, U.S.P., Sodium Chloride Injection, U.S.P. or another suitable diluent as indicated below.

Bottle Size	Amount of Diluent to be Added
1 Gm	50–100 ml
2 Gm	50–100 ml
4 Gm	At least 65 ml
6 Gm	97 ml

Stability

Stability studies on CELBENIN in various intravenous diluents at concentrations between 10 mg/ml and 60 mg/ml indicate that the resulting solutions will lose less than 10% activity at room temperature (70°F) or under refrigeration (40°F) for the time periods stated below: [See table below].

After reconstitution, these solutions can be frozen (approx. 0°F) and stored for up to 30 days without loss of potency. The stabilities of the thawed solutions are identical to the unfrozen ones listed above.

CELBENIN in the following intravenous solutions at concentrations between 2 mg/ml and 60 mg/ml will lose less than 10% activity at room temperature during an 8 hour period:

5% Dextrose in Normal Saline
10% D-Fructose in Water
10% D-Fructose in Normal Saline
Lactated Potassic Saline Injection
5% Plasma Hydrolysate in Water
10% Invert Sugar in Water
*10% Invert Sugar in Normal Saline
10% Invert Sugar plus 0.3% Potassium Chloride in Water
Travert 10% Electrolyte #1
Travert 10% Electrolyte #2
Travert 10% Electrolyte #3

*At a concentration of 2 mg/ml, Methicillin Sodium is stable for only 4 hours in this solution. Concentrations between 10 mg/ml and 60 mg/ml are stable for 8 hours.

Unused portions of solutions should be discarded after the time periods mentioned above.

Intravenous Solution	Stability Period: Room Temperature	Stability Period: Refrigerated
Sterile Water for Injection	72 hours	14 days
Sodium Chloride Injection	72 hours	14 days
5% Dextrose in Water	72 hours	14 days
M/6 Sodium Lactate Solution	72 hours	14 days
Lactated Ringer's Injection	72 hours	14 days

CELBENIN for intravenous infusion should be reconstituted only in those solutions listed above. The drug concentration and the rate and volume of the infusion should be adjusted so that the total dose of Methicillin is administered before the drug loses its stability in the diluent.
Store dry powder at room temperature or below.
How Supplied: CELBENIN (Methicillin Sodium) for Injection—Buffered. (Contains Methicillin Sodium as the monohydrate.)
NDC 0029-6200-22 ....1 Gm. Vial
NDC 0029-6205-26 ....4 Gm. Vial
NDC 0029-6210-26 ....6 Gm. Vial
NDC 0029-6200-21 .....1 Gm. Piggyback Bottle
NDC 0029-6204-21 .....2 Gm. Piggyback Bottle
NDC 0029-6205-21 .....4 Gm. Piggyback Bottle
NDC 0029-6210-21........6 Gm. Bulk Pharmacy Package
Literature Available: Yes.

*Bauer, A.W., Kirby, W.M.M., Sherris, J.C. and Turck, M.: Antibiotic Testing by a Standardized Single Disc Method, Am. J. Clin. Pathol., 45:493, 1966; Standardized Disc Susceptibility Test, FEDERAL REGISTER 37:20527-29, 1972.

CONAR® EXPECTORANT

Composition: Each 5 ml (teaspoonful) contains: noscapine, 15 mg.; phenylephrine hydrochloride, 10 mg.; guaifenesin, 100 mg.; flavoring.
Action and Uses: For temporary relief of cough and congestion due to the common cold.
Administration and Dosage: 4 times daily (every 3 to 4 hours): *Pediatric dosage:* each dose, 2 to 6 years (27–47 lbs.), 1/4 to 1/2 teaspoonful; 6 to 12 years (over 47 lbs.), 1/2 to 1 teaspoonful; adults and children over 12 years, 1 teaspoonful per dose. Under 2 years of age, only as directed by a physician.
Caution: Use cautiously in individuals with hypertension, cardiovascular diseases, diabetes or hyperthyroidism. Contraindicated in patients receiving MAO inhibitors.
How Supplied: CONAR EXPECTORANT is orange fruit flavored.
NDC 0029-1747-39 ....4 oz., dozen
NDC 0029-1747-35 ....Pint
NDC 0029-1747-35 ....Gallon
Literature Available: Yes.
Is this product O.T.C.: Yes.

CONAR®-A TABLETS

Composition: Each tablet contains: Noscapine, 15 mg.; phenylephrine hydrochloride, 10 mg.; acetaminophen, 300 mg.; guaifenesin, 100 mg.
Action and Uses: A convenient dry expectorant for the temporary relief of cough, congestion, minor aches and pains associated with the common cold.
Administration and Dosage: Adults and children over twelve years of age, 1 tablet four times daily (every 3 or 4 hours) or as directed by physician. Do not exceed recommended dosage.
Caution: Use cautiously in individuals with hypertension, cardiovascular diseases, diabetes or hyperthyroidism. Contraindicated in patients receiving MAO inhibitors.
How Supplied: CONAR-A TABLETS are green, oblong, monogrammed and film-coated
NDC 0029- 1725-39 blister pak of 20
NDC 0029- 1725-30 100
NDC 0029- 1725-33 1000
Literature Available: Yes.
Is This Product O.T.C.: Yes.
[*Shown in Product Identification Section*]
CONAR® Sugarless Syrup
CONAR® A Syrup
For prescribing information write to Beecham Laboratories, Bristol, Tn. 37620, or contact your local Beecham representative.

DARICON® ℞
(oxyphencyclimine HCl)
Tablets

Description: Each Daricon (oxyphencyclimine hydrochloride) tablet contains 10 mg. of oxyphencyclimine HCl. Oxyphencyclimine hydrochloride is (1,4,5,6-tetrahydro-1-methyl-2-pyrimidinyl) methyl- α -phenyl-cyclohexane-glycolate monohydrochloride.
Clinical Pharmacology: The mechanism of action of Daricon is the inhibition of acetylcholine at postganglionic cholinergic sites in structures innervated by postganglionic parasympathetic nerves and on smooth muscle not so innervated but responsive to acetylcholine.
Indications: For use as adjunctive therapy in the treatment of peptic ulcer.
DARICON HAS NOT BEEN SHOWN TO BE EFFECTIVE IN CONTRIBUTING TO THE HEALING OF PEPTIC ULCER, DECREASING THE RATE OF RECURRENCE OR PREVENTING COMPLICATIONS.
Contraindications: Glaucoma; obstructive uropathy (for example, bladder neck obstruction due to prostatic hypertrophy); obstructive disease of the gastrointestinal tract (for example, pyloroduodenal stenosis), paralytic ileus, intestinal atony of the elderly or debilitated patient; unstable cardiovascular status in acute hemorrhage; severe ulcerative colitis; toxic megacolon complicating ulcerative colitis; myasthenia gravis.
Warnings: In the presence of a high environmental temperature, heat prostration (fever and heatstroke due to decreased sweating) can occur with the use of oxyphencyclimine.
Diarrhea may be an early symptom of incomplete intestinal obstruction, especially in patients with ileostomy or colostomy. In this instance treatment with oxyphencyclimine would be inappropriate and possibly harmful.
Daricon may produce drowsiness or blurred vision. The patient should be cautioned regarding activities requiring mental alertness such as operating a motor vehicle or other machinery, or performing hazardous work while taking this drug.
With overdosage, a curare-like action may occur, i.e., neuromuscular blockage leading to muscular weakness and possible paralysis.
Reproduction studies in rats have shown no evidence of impaired fertility or harm to the animal fetus. Information on possible adverse effects in the pregnant human female is limited to uncontrolled data derived from marketing experience. Such experience has revealed no teratogenic effects. No controlled studies to establish the safety of the drug in pregnancy have been performed.
It is not known whether this drug is secreted in human milk. As a general rule, nursing should not be undertaken while a patient is on a drug since many drugs are excreted in human milk.
Since there is no adequate experience in children who have received this drug, safety and efficacy in children have not been established.
Elderly patients may react with excitement, agitation, drowsiness, and other untoward manifestations to even small doses of anticholinergic drugs.
Precautions: Use oxyphencyclimine with caution in the elderly and in all patients with:
Autonomic neuropathy;
Hepatic or renal disease;
Early evidence of ileus as in peritonitis;
Ulcerative colitis—Large doses may suppress intestinal motility to the point of producing a paralytic ileus, and the use of this drug may precipitate or aggravate "toxic megacolon," a serious complication of the disease.
Hyperthroidism, coronary heart disease, congestive heart failure, cardiac tachyarrhythmias, tachycardia, hypertension and prostatic hypertrophy.
Hiatal hernia associated with reflux esophagitis, since anticholinergic drugs may aggravate this condition.
It should be noted that the use of anticholinergic drugs in the treatment of gastric ulcer may produce a delay in gastric emptying time and may complicate such therapy (antral stasis).
Do not rely on the use of the drug in the presence of complication of biliary tract disease.
Investigate any tachycardia before giving anticholinergic (atropine-like) drugs, since they may increase the heart rate.
Adverse Reactions: Anticholinergics produce certain effects which may be physiologic or toxic, depending upon the individual patient's response. The physician must delineate these.
Adverse reactions may include xerostomia, decreased sweating, urinary hesitancy and retention, blurred vision, tachycardia, palpitations, dilatation of the pupil, cycloplegia, increased ocular tension, loss of taste, headaches, nervousness, mental confusion and/or excitement, drowsiness, weakness, dizziness, insomnia, nausea, vomiting, constipation, bloated feeling, impotence, suppression of lactation, severe allergic reactions or drug idiosyncrasies including anaphylaxis, urticaria and other dermal manifestations.
If decreased sweating occurs, it should be noted that adrenergic innervation of the eccrine sweat glands on the palms and soles make complete control of sweating impossible. An end point of complete anhidrosis cannot occur because large doses of the drug would be required, and this would produce severe side effects from parasympathetic paralysis.
Overdosage: The symptoms of overdosage with Daricon progress from an intensification of the usual side effects to CNS disturbances (from restlessness and excitement to psychotic behavior), circulatory changes (flushing, fall in blood pressure, circulatory failure), respiratory failure, paralysis and coma.
Measures to be taken are (1) immediate lavage of the stomach and (2) injection of physostigmine 0.5 to 2 mg intravenously, and repeated as necessary up to a total of 5 mg. Fever may be treated symptomatically (alcohol sponging, ice packs). Excitement of a degree which demands attention may be managed with sodium thiopental 2% solution given slowly intravenously or chloral hydrate (100—200 ml of a 2% solution) by rectal infusion. In the event of progression of the curare-like effect to paralysis of the respiratory muscles, artificial respiration should be instituted and maintained until effective respiratory action returns.
Dosage and Administration: Daricon is administered orally. The usual adult dosage is 10 mg. of Daricon twice daily, preferably in the morning and at night before retiring. Some patients respond well to doses as small as 5 mg. twice daily, while some patients may require a higher dosage on a t.i.d. regimen. Daricon should be administered as long as the physician considers it necessary. Not for use in children under 12 years of age.
It should be noted that the pharmacological effect of the drug is unlikely to be attained without some side effects some of the time.
Drug Interactions: There are no known drug interactions with oxyphencyclimine.
How Supplied: **DARICON**, white, scored tablets containing 10 mg. oxyphencyclimine HCl.
NDC-0029-1930-39 ....bottles of 60
NDC-0029-1930-32 ....bottles of 500
Literature Available: Yes.
[*Shown in Product Identification Section*]

DARICON® PB ℞
(oxyphencyclimine HCl-5 mg. with phenobarbital-15 mg.)
Tablets

Description: Each Daricon PB (oxyphencyclimine hydrochloride with phenobarbital)

Continued on next page

Beecham Laboratories—Cont.

tablet contains 5 mg. of oxyphencyclimine HCl and 15 mg. of phenobarbital. Oxyphencyclimine hydrochloride is (1,4,5,6-tetrahydro-1-methyl-2-pyrimidinyl) methyl-α-phenylcyclohexaneglycolate monohydrochloride.

Clinical Pharmacology: The mechanism of action of Daricon is the inhibition of acetylcholine at postganglionic cholinergic sites in structures innervated by postganglionic parasympathetic nerves and on smooth muscle not so innervated but responsive to acetylcholine. Phenobarbital acts as a central nervous system depressant.

Indications

Based on a review of Daricon PB Tablets by the National Academy of Sciences—National Research Council and/or other information, the FDA has classified the indications as follows:

"Possibly effective":

For use as adjunctive therapy in the treatment of peptic ulcer. DARICON HAS NOT BEEN SHOWN TO BE EFFECTIVE IN CONTRIBUTING TO THE HEALING OF PEPTIC ULCER, DECREASING THE ROLE OF RECURRENCE, OR PREVENTING COMPLICATIONS. May also be useful in the irritable bowel syndrome (irritable colon, spastic colon, mucous colitis, acute enterocolitis, and functional gastrointestinal disorders); and in neurogenic bowel disturbances (including the splenic flexure syndrome and neurogenic colon), WHEN NOT RELIEVED BY SUCH MEASURES AS DIET, SEDATION, REASSURANCE, PHYSICIAN INTEREST AND AMELIORATION OF ENVIRONMENTAL FACTORS. To be effective the dosage must be titrated to the individual patient's needs.

Daricon PB is especially useful when the sedative effects of phenobarbital are desired to allay tension or apprehension which often complicate these disorders.

Final classification of these indications requires further investigation.

Contraindications: Glaucoma; obstructive uropathy (for example, bladder neck obstruction due to prostatic hypertrophy); obstructive disease of the gastrointestinal tract (as in pyloroduodenal stenosis), paralytic ileus, intestinal atony of the elderly or debilitated patient; unstable cardiovascular status in acute hemorrhage; severe ulcerative colitis; toxic megacolon complicating ulcerative colitis; myasthenia gravis.

Phenobarbital is contraindicated in acute intermittent porphyria.

A sensitivity to phenobarbital and/or oxyphencyclimine contraindicates the use of Daricon PB; and in those patients in whom phenobarbital produces restlessness and/or excitement.

Warnings: Phenobarbital in patients taking anticoagulants may decrease the effect of the anticoagulant and thus require larger doses of the anticoagulant for optimal effect. When the phenobarbital is discontinued, the dose of the anticoagulant may have to be decreased. Barbiturates may thus decrease the action of anticoagulant drugs.

Phenobarbital may be habit forming and should not be administered to individuals known to be addiction prone, or to those with a history of physical and/or psychological dependence upon habit forming drugs.

Since barbiturates are metabolized in the liver, use with initial small doses and caution in patients with hepatic dysfunction.

In the presence of a high environmental temperature, heat prostration (fever and heat stroke due to decreased sweating) can occur with use of oxyphencyclimine.

Diarrhea may be an early symptom of incomplete intestinal obstruction, especially in patients with ileostomy or colostomy. In this instance treatment with oxyphencyclimine would be inappropriate and possibly harmful.

Daricon PB may produce drowsiness or blurred vision. The patient should be cautioned regarding activities requiring mental alertness such as operating a motor vehicle or other machinery or performing hazardous work while taking this drug.

With overdosage, a curare-like action may occur, i.e., neuromuscular blockage leading to muscular weakness and possible paralysis.

Reproduction studies in rats have shown no evidence of impaired fertility or harm to the animal fetus. Information of possible adverse effects in the pregnant human female is limited to uncontrolled data derived from marketing experience. Such experience has revealed no teratogenic effects. No controlled studies to establish the safety of the drug in pregnancy have been performed.

It is not known whether this drug is secreted in human milk. As a general rule, nursing should not be undertaken while a patient is on a drug since many drugs are excreted in human milk.

Since there is no adequate experience in children who have received this drug, safety and efficacy in children have not been established.

Elderly patients may react with excitement, agitation, drowsiness, and other untoward manifestations to even small doses of anticholinergic drugs.

Precautions: Use oxyphencyclimine with caution in the elderly and in all patients with:

Autonomic neuropathy;

Hepatic or renal disease;

Early evidence of ileus as in peritonitis;

Ulcerative colitis—Large doses may suppress intestinal motility to the point of producing a paralytic ileus, and the use of this drug may precipitate or aggravate toxic megacolon, a serious complication of the disease.

Hyperthyroidism, coronary heart disease, congestive heart failure, cardiac tachyarrhythmias, tachycardia, hypertension and prostatic hypertrophy.

Hiatal hernia associated with reflux esophagitis, since anticholinergic drugs may aggravate this condition.

It should be noted that the use of anticholinergic drugs in the treatment of gastric ulcer may produce a delay in gastric emptying time and may complicate such therapy (antral stasis).

Do not rely on the use of the drug in the presence of complication of biliary tract disease.

Adverse Reactions: Phenobarbital may produce excitement in some patients rather than a sedative effect. An occasional patient may experience musculoskeletal pain. Some patients may acquire a sensitivity to barbiturates and experience allergic phenomena and/or dermatologic response.

In patients habituated to barbiturates, abrupt withdrawal may produce delirium or convulsions. Anticholinergics produce certain effects which may be physiologic or toxic, depending upon the individual patient's response. The physician must delineate these. Adverse reactions may include xerostomia, decreased sweating, urinary hesitancy and retention, blurred vision, tachycardia, palpitations, dilatation of the pupil, cycloplegia, increased ocular tension, loss of taste, headaches, nervousness, mental confusion and/or excitement, drowsiness, weakness, dizziness, insomnia, nausea, vomiting, constipation, bloated feeling, impotence, suppression of lactation, severe allergic reactions or drug idiosyncrasies including anaphylaxis, urticaria and other dermal manifestations.

If decreased sweating occurs, it should be noted that adrenergic innervation of the eccrine sweat glands on the palms and soles make complete control of sweating impossible. An end point of complete anhidrosis cannot occur because large doses of the drug would be required, and this would produce severe side effects from parasympathetic paralysis.

Overdosage: The symptoms of overdosage with Daricon progress from an intensification of the usual side effects to CNS disturbances (from restlessness and excitement to psychotic behavior), circulatory changes (flushing, fall in blood pressure, circulatory failure), respiratory failure, paralysis and coma.

Measures to be taken are (1) immediate lavage of the stomach and (2) injection of physostigmine 0.5 to 2 mg intravenously, and repeated as necessary up to a total of 5 mg. Fever may be treated symptomatically (alcohol sponging, ice packs). Excitement of a degree which demands attention may be managed with sodium thiopental 2% solution given slowly intravenously or chloral hydrate (100–200 ml of a 2% solution) by rectal infusion. In the event of progression of the curare-like effect to paralysis of the respiratory muscles, artificial respiration should be instituted and maintained until effective respiratory action returns.

Dosage and Administration: Daricon PB is administered orally. Usual initial dosage is 3 tablets daily—in the morning, evening and at bedtime. The usual dosage range is 2 to 4 tablets daily.

Daricon PB should be administered as long as the physician considers it necessary. Not for use in children under 12 years of age.

Drug Interactions: There are no known drug interactions with oxyphencyclimine.

How Supplied: **Daricon PB**, pink, scored tablets containing 5 mg. oxyphencyclimine HCl and 15 mg. phenobarbital.

NDC-0029-1940-30........................bottles of 100

Literature Available: Yes.

[*Shown in Product Identification Section*]

ENARAX® TABLETS ℞

(oxyphencyclimine HCl and hydroxyzine HCl)

Composition:

Each Enarax 5 tablet contains:

oxyphencyclimine HCl ....5 mg.
hydroxyzine HCl N.F. ....25 mg.

Each Enarax 10 tablet contains:

oxyphencyclimine HCl ....10 mg.
hydroxyzine HCl N.F. ....25 mg.

Description: Enarax is a combination of oxyphencyclimine HCl and hydroxyzine HCl. Oxyphencyclimine HCl is a crystalline substance designated chemically as: (1,4,5,6-tetrahydro-1-methyl-2-pyrimidinyl) methyl alpha-phenylcyclohexaneglycolate monohydrochloride.

Hydroxyzine HCl is designated chemically as: 2-[2-[4-(p-chloro-alpha-phenylbenzyl)-1-piperazinyl] ethoxyl] ethanol dihydrochloride.

Actions: Oxyphencyclimine HCl provides long acting suppression of gastric secretion through its anticholinergic action. The mechanism of this action is the inhibition of acetylcholine at postganglionic cholinergic sites in structures innervated by postganglionic parasympathetic nerves and on smooth muscle not so innervated but responsive to acetylcholine.

Hydroxyzine HCl has been shown clinically to be an effective anti-anxiety agent. It induces a calming effect in anxious, tense individuals without impairing mental alertness. It is not a cortical depressant, but its action may be due to a suppression of activity in certain key regions of the subcortical area of the central nervous system.

INDICATIONS

Based on a review of this drug by the National Academy of Sciences-National Research Council and/or other information, FDA has classified the indications as follows:

Possibly Effective: As adjunctive therapy in peptic ulcer; irritable bowel syndrome (irritable colon, spastic colon, mu-

cous colitis, functional gastrointestinal disorders); functional diarrhea; drug induced diarrhea; ulcerative colitis, and urinary bladder spasm and ureteral spasm (i.e. smooth muscle spasm).
Final classification of these less than effective indications requires further investigation.

Contraindications: Because of its anticholinergic activity, Enarax is contraindicated in the presence of glaucoma, obstructive uropathy (i.e. bladder neck obstruction due to prostatic hypertrophy), obstructive disease of the gastrointestinal tract (as in achalasia, pyloroduodenal stenosis, etc.); paralytic ileus; intestinal atony of the elderly or debilitated patient; unstable cardiovascular status in acute hemorrhage; severe ulcerative colitis; toxic megacolon complicating ulcerative colitis; myasthenia gravis.

Warnings: Hydroxyzine, when administered to the pregnant mouse, rat, and rabbit induced fetal abnormalities in the rat at doses substantially above the human therapeutic range.

Clinical data in human beings are inadequate to establish safety in early pregnancy. Until such data are available, hydroxyzine-containing drugs are not advised in early pregnancy.

In the presence of a high environmental temperature, heat prostration can occur with drug use (fever and heatstroke due to decreased sweating).

Diarrhea may be an early symptom of incomplete intestinal obstruction, especially in patients with ileostomy or colostomy. In this instance treatment with this drug would be inappropriate and possibly harmful.

Enarax may produce drowsiness or blurred vision. In this event, the patient should be warned not to engage in activities requiring mental alertness such as operating a motor vehicle or other machinery, or perform hazardous work while taking this drug.

Precautions: Anticholinergics should be used with caution in patients with:
autonomic neuropathy,
hepatic or renal disease,
ulcerative colitis—(Large doses may suppress intestinal motility to the point of producing a paralytic ileus and the use of this drug may precipitate or aggravate the serious complication of toxic megacolon.)
hyperthyroidism, coronary heart disease, congestive heart failure, cardiac arrhythmias, hypertension and nonobstructing prostatic hypertrophy; hiatal hernia associated with reflux esophagitis, since anticholinergic drugs may aggravate this condition.

It should be noted that the use of anticholinergic drugs in the treatment of gastric ulcer may produce a delay in gastric emptying time and may complicate such therapy (antral stasis).

The use of this drug in the presence of complication of biliary tract disease should not be relied upon.

Tachycardia should be thoroughly investigated before giving anticholinergic (atropine-like) drugs since they may increase the heart rate.

With overdosage, a curare-like action may occur.

Adverse Reactions: As with other anticholinergics, oxyphencyclimine HCl produces certain effects which may be physiologic or toxic depending upon the individual patient's response. Th physician must delineate these. Adverse reactions may include xerostomia; urinary hesitancy and retention; blurred vision and tachycardia; palpitations; mydriasis; dilatation of the pupil; cycloplegia, increased ocular tension; loss of taste; headaches; nervousness; drowsiness; weakness; dizziness; insomnia; nausea; vomiting; impotence; suppression of lactation; constipation; bloated feeling; severe allergic reaction or drug idiosyncrasies including anaphylaxis, urticaria and other dermal manifestation; some degree of mental confusion and/or excitement especially in elderly persons.

Decreased sweating is another adverse reaction that may occur. It should be noted that adrenergic innervation of the eccrine sweat glands on the palms and soles make complete control of sweating impossible. An end point of complete anhidrosis cannot occur because large doses of drug would be required, and this would produce severe side effects from parasympathetic paralysis.

Side effects which occasionally occur with hydroxyzine HCl are drowsiness, xerostomia, and at extremely high doses, involuntary motor activity, all of which may be controlled by reduction of the dosage or discontinuation of the medication.

Dosage and Administration: The recommended adult dose is usually one Enarax 5 or one Enarax 10 tablet two times a day or three times a day, depending on individual response. Proper diet and antacids should be used where indicated as concomitant therapy. The safe use of Enarax in children has not been established; therefore, the drug should not be used in children.

Drug Interactions: The potentiating action of hydroxyzine must be considered when the drug is used in combination with central nervous system depressants.

How Supplied: Enarax 5 is available as white scored tablets in bottles of 60.
Enarax 10 is available as black and white scored tablets in bottles of 60.

[*Shown in Product Identification Section*]

FASTIN® CAPSULES ℭ
(phentermine hydrochloride)

Description: Each FASTIN (phentermine hydrochloride) capsule contains phentermine hydrochloride, 30 mg. (equivalent to 24 mg. phentermine).

Phentermine hydrochloride is a white crystalline powder, very soluble in water and alcohol. Chemically, the product is phenyl-tertiary-butylamine hydrochloride.

Actions: FASTIN is a sympathomimetic amine with pharmacologic activity similar to the prototype drugs of this class used in obesity, the amphetamines. Actions include central nervous system stimulation and elevation of blood pressure. Tachyphylaxis and tolerance have been demonstrated with all drugs of this class in which these phenomena have been looked for.

Drugs of this class used in obesity are commonly known as "anorectics" or "anorexigenics." It has not been established, however, that the action of such drugs in treating obesity is primarily one of appetite suppression. Other central nervous system actions, or metabolic effects may be involved, for example.

Adult obese subjects instructed in dietary management and treated with "anorectic" drugs, lose more weight on the average than those treated with placebo and diet, as determined in relatively short-term clinical trials.

The magnitude of increased weight loss of drug-treated patients over placebo-treated patients is only a fraction of a pound a week. The rate of weight loss is greatest in the first weeks of therapy for both drug and placebo subjects and tends to decrease in succeeding weeks. The possible orgins of the increased weight loss due to the various drug effects are not established. The amount of weight loss associated with the use of an "anorectic" drug varies from trial to trial, and the increased weight loss appears to be related in part to variables other than the drugs prescribed, such as the physician-investigator, the population treated, and the diet prescribed. Studies do not permit conclusions as to the relative importance of the drug and non-drug factors on weight loss.

The natural history of obesity is measured in years, whereas the studies cited are restricted to a few weeks duration; thus, the total impact of drug-induced weight loss over that of diet alone must be considered clinically limited.

Indication: FASTIN is indicated in the management of exogenous obesity as a short-term (a few weeks) adjunct in a regimen of weight reduction based on caloric restriction. The limited usefulness of agents of this class (see ACTIONS) should be measured against possible risk factors inherent in their use such as those described below.

Contraindications: Advanced arteriosclerosis, symptomatic cardiovascular disease, moderate-to-severe hypertension, hyperthyroidism, known hypersensitivity, or idiosyncrasy to the sympathomimetic amines, glaucoma.
Agitated states.
Patients with a history of drug abuse.
During or within 14 days following the administration of monoamine oxidase inhibitors (hypertensive crises may result).

Warnings: Tolerance to the anorectic effect usually develops within a few weeks. When this occurs, the recommended dose should not be exceeded in an attempt to increase the effect; rather, the drug should be discontinued.

FASTIN may impair the ability of the patient to engage in potentially hazardous activities such as operating machinery or driving a motor vehicle; the patient should therefore be cautioned accordingly.

Drug Dependence: FASTIN is related chemically and pharmacologically to the amphetamines. Amphetamines and related stimulant drugs have been extensively abused, and the possibility of abuse of FASTIN should be kept in mind when evaluating the desirability of including a drug as part of a weight reduction program. Abuse of amphetamines and related drugs may be associated with intense psychological dependence and severe social dysfunction. There are reports of patients who have increased the dosage to many times that recommended. Abrupt cessation following prolonged high dosage administration results in extreme fatigue and mental depression; changes are also noted on the sleep EEG. Manifestations of chronic intoxication with anorectic drugs include severe dermatoses, marked insomnia, irritability, hyperactivity, and personality changes. The most severe manifestation of chronic intoxications is psychosis, often clinically indistinguishable from schizophrenia.

Usage in Pregnancy: Safe use in pregnancy has not been established. Use of FASTIN by women who are or who may become pregnant, and those in the first trimester of pregnancy, requires that the potential benefit be weighed against the possible hazard to mother and infant.

Usage in Children: FASTIN is not recommended for use in children under 12 years of age.

Precautions: Caution is to be exercised in prescribing FASTIN for patients with even mild hypertension.

Insulin requirements in diabetes mellitus may be altered in association with the use of FASTIN and the concomitant dietary regimen.

FASTIN may decrease the hypotensive effect of guanethidine.

The least amount feasible should be prescribed or dispensed at one time in order to minimize the possibility of overdosage.

Adverse Reactions:
Cardiovascular: Palpitation, tachycardia, elevation of blood pressure.
Central Nervous System: Overstimulation, restlessness, dizziness, insomnia, euphoria, dysphoria, tremor, headache; rarely psychotic episodes at recommended doses.

Continued on next page

Beecham Laboratories—Cont.

Gastrointestinal: Dryness of the mouth, unpleasant taste, diarrhea, constipation, other gastrointestinal disturbances.
Allergic: Urticaria.
Endocrine: Impotence, changes in libido.
Dosage and Administration:
Exogenous Obesity: One capsule at approximately 2 hours after breakfast for appetite control. Late evening medication should be avoided because of the possibility of resulting insomnia.
Administration of one capsule (30 mg.) daily has been found to be adequate in depression of the appetite for twelve to fourteen hours.
FASTIN is not recommended for use in children under 12 years of age.
Overdosage: Manifestations of acute overdosage with phentermine include restlessness, tremor, hyperreflexia, rapid respiration, confusion, assaultiveness, hallucinations, panic states. Fatigue and depression usually follow the central stimulation. Cardiovascular effects include arrhythmias, hypertension or hypotension, and circulatory collapse. Gastrointestinal symptoms include nausea, vomiting, diarrhea, and abdominal cramps. Fatal poisoning usually terminates in convulsions and coma.
Management of acute phentermine intoxication is largely symptomatic and includes lavage and sedation with a barbiturate. Experience with hemodialysis or peritoneal dialysis is inadequate to permit recommendations in this regard. Acidification of the urine increases phentermine excretion. Intravenous phentolamine (REGITINE) has been suggested for possible acute, severe hypertension, if this complicates phentermine overdosage.
Caution: Federal law prohibits dispensing without prescription.
How Supplied: Blue and white capsules containing 30 mg. phentermine hydrochloride (equivalent to 24 mg. Phentermine).
NDC 0029-2205-30........................bottles of 100
Literature Available: Yes.
[*Shown in Product Identification Section*]

MENEST™ ℞
Esterified Estrogens, U.S.P.

Warnings
1. *Estrogens Have Been Reported To Increase The Risk of Endometrial Carcinoma.* Three independent case control studies have shown an increased risk of endometrial cancer in postmenopausal women exposed to exogenous estrogens for prolonged periods.[1–3] This risk was independent of the other known risk factors for endometrial cancer. These studies are further supported by the finding that incidence rates of endometrial cancer have increased sharply since 1969 in eight different areas of the United States with population-based cancer reporting systems, an increase which may be related to the rapidly expanding use of estrogens during the last decade.[4]
The three case control studies reported that the risk of endometrial cancer in estrogen users was about 4.5 to 13.9 times greater than in nonusers. The risk appears to depend on both duration of treatment[1] and on estrogen dose.[3] In view of these findings, when estrogens are used for the treatment of menopausal symptoms, the lowest dose that will control symptoms should be utilized and medication should be discontinued as soon as possible. When prolonged treatment is medically indicated, the patient should be reassessed on at least a semiannual basis to determine the need for continued therapy. Although the evidence must be considered preliminary, one study suggests that cyclic administration of low doses of estrogen may carry less risk than continuous administration;[3] it therefore appears prudent to utilize such a regimen.
Close clinical surveillance of all women taking estrogens is important. In all cases of undiagnosed persistent or recurring abnormal vaginal bleeding, adequate diagnostic measures should be undertaken to rule out malignancy.
There is no evidence at present that "natural" estrogens are more or less hazardous than "synthetic" estrogens at equiestrogenic doses.
2. *Estrogens should not be used during pregnancy.*
The use of female sex hormones, both estrogens and progestagens, during early pregnancy may seriously damage the offspring. It has been shown that females exposed in utero to diethylstilbestrol, a non-steroidal estrogen, have an increased risk of developing in later life a form of vaginal or cervical cancer that is ordinarily extremely rare.[5,6] This risk has been estimated as not greater than 4 per 1000 exposures.[7] Furthermore, a high percentage of such exposed women (from 30 to 90 percent) have been found to have vaginal adenosis,[8–12] epithelial changes of the vagina and cervix. Although these changes are histologically benign, it is not known whether they are precursors of malignancy. Although similar data are not available with the use of other estrogens, it cannot be presumed they would not induce similar changes.
Several reports suggest an association between intrauterine exposure to female sex hormones and congenital anomalies, including congenital heart defects and limb reduction defects.[13–16] One case control study[16] estimated a 4.7 fold increased risk of limb reduction defects in infants exposed in utero to sex hormones (oral contraceptives, hormone withdrawal tests for pregnancy, or attempted treatment for threatened abortion). Some of these exposures were very short and involved only a few days of treatment. The data suggest that the risk of limb reduction defects in exposed fetuses is somewhat less than 1 per 1000.
In the past, female sex hormones have been used during pregnancy in an attempt to treat threatened or habitual abortion. There is considerable evidence that estrogens are ineffective for these indications, and there is no evidence from well controlled studies that progestagens are effective for these uses.
If MENEST (esterified estrogens) is used during pregnancy, or if the patient becomes pregnant while taking this drug, she should be apprised of the potential risks to the fetus, and, the advisability of pregnancy continuation.

Description: Esterified estrogens, U.S.P., is a mixture of the sodium salts of the sulfate esters of the estrogenic substances, principally estrone, that are of the type excreted by pregnant mares. The content of total esterified estrogens is not less than 90 percent and not more than 110 percent of the labeled amount. Esterified estrogens contain not less than 75 percent and not more than 85 percent of sodium estrone sulfate, and not less than 6 percent and not more than 15 percent sodium equilin sulfate, in such proportion that the total of these two components is not less than 90 percent, all percentages being calculated on the basis of the total esterified estrogens content.
The esterified estrogens used in Menest Tablets are standardized by the addition of pure sodium estrone sulfate. Standardization produces a product of more uniform potency to help make dosage adjustment easier and produce a more predictable patient response.
Clinical Pharmacology: Menest (esterified estrogens, U.S.P.) owes its therapeutic action to estrone and equilin. Estrone is one of the three prinicpal human estrogenic steroid hormones... estradiol, estrone and estriol. Estradiol, the major estrogen in the body, is rapidly oxidized to estrone, which in turn may be converted to estriol, the least active of the three compounds. There is free interconversion between estrone and estradiol. Experimental data suggest that the estrogenic activity of equilin is comparable to that of estrone, but details of its metabolism are not known.
While esterified estrogens are rapidly absorbed following oral administration, inactivation occurs in the liver by conversion to less active estrogenic compounds and by conjugation with sulfuric and glucuronic acids. Estrogens circulate in the blood in the free and conjugated forms, both of which are usually bound to certain of the plasma proteins (50–80%). Conjugated estrogens which are more water soluble than free estrogens are well excreted in the urine, the primary route of estrogen elimination.
Indications: MENEST (esterified estrogens) is indicated in the treatment of:
1. Moderate to severe *vasomotor* symptoms associated with the menopause. (There is no evidence that estrogens are effective for nervous symptoms or depression which might occur during menopause, and they should not be used to treat these conditions.)
2. Atrophic vaginitis.
3. Kraurosis vulvae.
4. Female hypogonadism.
5. Female castration.
6. Primary ovarian failure.
7. Breast cancer (for palliation only) in appropriately selected women with metastatic disease.
8. Prostatic carcinoma — palliative therapy of advanced disease.

MENEST (ESTERIFIED ESTROGENS) HAS NOT BEEN SHOWN TO BE EFFECTIVE FOR ANY PURPOSE DURING PREGNANCY AND ITS USE MAY CAUSE SEVERE HARM TO THE FETUS (SEE BOXED WARNING).
Contraindications: Estrogens should not be used in women (or men) with any of the following conditions:
1. Known or suspected cancer of the breast except in appropriately selected patients being treated for metastatic disease.
2. Known or suspected estrogen-dependent neoplasia.
3. Known or suspected pregnancy (See Boxed Warning).
4. Undiagnosed abnormal genital bleeding.
5. Active thrombophlebitis or thromboembolic disorders.
6. A past history of thrombophlebitis, thrombosis, or thromboembolic disorders associated with previous estrogen use (except when used in treatment of breast or prostatic malignancy).
Warnings:
1. *Induction of malignant neoplasms.* Long term continuous administration of natural and synthetic estrogens in certain animal species increases the frequency of carcinomas of the breast, cervix, vagina, and liver. There is now evidence that estrogens increase the risk of carcinoma of the endometrium in humans. (See Boxed Warning).
At the present time there is no satisfactory evidence that estrogens given to postmenopausal women increase the risk of cancer of the breast,[18] although a recent long-term followup of a single physician's practice has raised this possibility.[18a] Because of the animal data, there is a need for caution in prescribing estrogens for women with a strong family history of

breast cancer or who have breast nodules, fibrocystic disease, or abnormal mammograms.

2. *Gall bladder disease.* A recent study has reported a 2 to 3-fold increase in the risk of surgically confirmed gall bladder disease in women receiving postmenopausal estrogens,[18] similar to the 2-fold increase previously noted in users of oral contraceptives.[19] In the case of oral contraceptives the increased risk appeared after two years of use.[24]

3. *Effects similar to those caused by estrogen-progestagen oral contraceptives.* There are several serious adverse effects of oral contraceptives, most of which have not, up to now, been documented as consequences of postmenopausal estrogen therapy. This may reflect the comparatively low doses of estrogen used in postmenopausal women. It would be expected that the larger doses of estrogen used to treat prostatic or breast cancer or postpartum breast engorgement are more likely to result in these adverse effects, and, in fact, it has been shown that there is an increased risk of thrombosis in men receiving estrogens for prostatic cancer and women for postpartum breast engorgement.[20–23]

a. *Thromboembolic disease.* It is now well established that users of oral contraceptives have an increased risk of various thromboembolic and thrombotic vascular diseases, including thrombophlebitis, pulmonary embolism, stroke, and myocardial infarction.[24–31] Cases of retinal thrombosis, mesenteric thrombosis and optic neuritis have been reported in oral contraceptive users. There is evidence that the risk of several of these adverse reactions is related to the dose of the drug.[32/33] An increased risk of postsurgery thromboembolic complications has also been reported in users of oral contraceptives.[34/35] If feasible, estrogen should be discontinued at least 4 weeks before surgery of the type associated with an increased risk of thromboembolism, or during periods of prolonged immobilization.

While an increased rate of thromboembolic and thrombotic disease in postmenopausal users of estrogens has not been found[18/36] this does not rule out the possibility that such an increase may be present or that subgroups of women who have underlying risk factors or who are receiving larger doses of estrogen may have an increased risk. Therefore estrogens should not be used in persons with active thrombophlebitis or thromboembolic disorders, and they should not be used (except in treatment of malignancy) in persons with a history of such disorders in association with estrogen use. They should be used with caution in patients with cerebral vascular or coronary artery disease and only for those in whom estrogens are clearly needed.

Large doses of estrogen (5 mg conjugated estrogens per day), comparable to those used to treat cancer of the prostate and breast, have been shown in a large prospective clinical trial in men[37] to increase the risk of nonfatal myocardial infarction, pulmonary embolism and thrombophlebitis. When estrogen doses of this size are used, any of the thromboembolic and thrombotic adverse effects associated with oral contraceptive use should be considered a clear risk.

b. *Hepatic adenoma.* Benign hepatic adenomas appear to be associated with the use of oral contraceptives.[38–40] Although benign, and rare, these may rupture and may cause death through intraabdominal hemorrhage. Such lesions have not yet been reported in association with other estrogen or progestagen preparations but should be considered in estrogen users having abdominal pain and tenderness, abdominal mass, or hypovolemic shock. Hepatocellular carcinoma has also been reported in women taking estrogen-containing oral contraceptives.[39] The relationship of this malignancy to these drugs is not known at this time.

c. *Elevated blood pressure.* Increased blood pressure is not uncommon in women using oral contraceptives. There is now a report that this may occur with use of estrogens in the menopause[41] and blood pressure should be monitored with estrogen use, especially if high doses are used.

d. *Glucose tolerance.* A worsening of glucose tolerance has been observed in a significant percentage of patients on estrogen-containing oral contraceptives. For this reason, diabetic patients should be carefully observed while receiving estrogen.

4. *Hypercalcemia.* Administration of estrogens may lead to severe hypercalcemia in patients with breast cancer and bone metastases. If this occurs, the drug should be stopped and appropriate measures taken to reduce the serum calcium level.

See footnotes at end of article.

Precautions:

A. General Precautions.

1. A complete medical and family history should be taken prior to the initiation of any estrogen therapy. The pretreatment and periodic physical examinations should include special reference to blood pressure, breasts, abdomen, and pelvic organs, and should include a Papanicolau smear. As a general rule, estrogen should not be prescribed for longer than one year without another physical examination being performed.

2. Fluid retention—Because estrogens may cause some degree of fluid retention, conditions which might be influenced by this factor such as epilepsy, migraine, and cardiac or renal dysfunction, require careful observation.

3. Certain patients may develop undesirable manifestations of excessive estrogenic stimulation, such as abnormal or excessive uterine bleeding, mastodynia, etc.

4. Oral contraceptives appear to be associated with an increased incidence of mental depression.[24] Although it is not clear whether this is due to the estrogenic or progestagenic component of the contraceptive, patients with a history of depression should be carefully observed.

5. Preexisting uterine leiomyomata may increase in size during estrogen use.

6. The pathologist should be advised of estrogen therapy when relevant specimens are submitted.

7. Patients with a past history of jaundice during pregnancy have an increased risk of recurrence of jaundice while receiving estrogen-containing oral contraceptive therapy. If jaundice develops in any patient receiving estrogen, the medication should be discontinued while the cause is investigated.

8. Estrogens may be poorly metabolized in patients with impaired liver function and they should be administered with caution in such patients.

9. Because estrogens influence the metabolism of calcium and phosphorus, they should be used with caution in patients with metabolic bone diseases that are associated with hypercalcemia or in patients with renal insufficiency.

10. Because of the effects of estrogens on epiphyseal closure, they should be used judiciously in young patients in whom bone growth is not complete.

11. Certain endocrine and liver function tests may be affected by estrogen-containing oral contraceptives. The following similar changes may be expected with larger doses of estrogen:

a. Increased sulfobromophthalein retention.

b. Increased prothrombin and factors VII, VIII, IX, and X; decreased antithrombin 3; increased norepinephrine-induced platelet aggregability.

c. Increased thyroid binding globulin (TBG) leading to increased circulating total thyroid hormone, as measured by PBI, T4 by column, or T4 by radioimmunoassay. Free T3 resin uptake is decreased, reflecting the elevated TBG; free T4 concentration is unaltered.

d. Impaired glucose tolerance.

e. Decreased pregnanediol excretion.

f. Reduced response to metyrapone test.

g. Reduced serum folate concentration.

h. Increased serum triglyceride and phospholipid concentration.

B. *Pregnancy Category X*—See Contraindications and Boxed Warning.

C. Nursing Mothers. As a general principle, the administration of any drug to nursing mothers should be done only when clearly necessary since many drugs are excreted in human milk.

Adverse Reactions: (See Warnings regarding induction of neoplasia, adverse effects on the fetus, increased incidence of gall bladder disease, and adverse effects similar to those of oral contraceptives, including thromboembolism.) The following additional adverse reactions have been reported with estrogenic therapy, including oral contraceptives:

1. *Genitourinary system.*

Breakthrough bleeding, spotting, change in menstrual flow.

Dysmenorrhea.

Premenstrual-like syndrome.

Amenorrhea during and after treatment.

Increase in size of uterine fibromyomata.

Vaginal candidiasis.

Change in cervical eversion and in degree of cervical secretion.

Cystitis-like syndrome.

2. *Breast.*

Tenderness, enlargement, secretion.

3. *Gastrointestinal.*

Nausea, vomiting.

Abdominal cramps, bloating.

Cholestatic jaundice.

4. *Skin.*

Chloasma or melasma which may persist when drug is discontinued.

Erythema multiforme.

Erythema nodosum.

Hemorrhagic eruption.

Loss of scalp hair.

Hirsutism.

5. *Eyes.*

Steepening of corneal curvature.

Intolerance to contact lenses.

6. *CNS.*

Headache, migraine, dizziness.

Mental depression.

Chorea.

7. *Miscellaneous.*

Increase or decrease in weight.

Reduced carbohydrate tolerance.

Aggravation of porphyria.

Edema.

Changes in libido.

Overdosage: Numerous reports of ingestion of large doses of estrogen-containing oral contraceptives by young children indicate that serious ill effects do not occur. Overdosage of estrogen may cause nausea, and withdrawal bleeding may occur in females.

Dosage and Administration:

1. *Given cyclically for short term use only:*
   For treatment of moderate-to-severe *vasomotor symptoms, atrophic vaginitis,* or *kraurosis vulvae* associated with the menopause.
   The lowest dose that will control symptoms should be chosen and medication should be discontinued as promptly as possible.
   Administration should be cyclic (e.g., 3 weeks on and 1 week off).
   Attempts to discontinue or taper medication should be made at 3 to 6 month intervals.
   The usual dosage range is 0.3–1.25 mg. daily.
   If the patient has not menstruated within the last two months or more, cyclic admin-

Continued on next page

Beecham Laboratories—Cont.

istration is started arbitrarily. If the patient is menstruating, cyclic administration is started on day 5 of bleeding. If breakthrough bleeding (bleeding or spotting during estrogen therapy) occurs, increase estrogen dosage as needed to stop bleeding. In the following cycle, employ the dosage level used to stop breakthrough bleeding in the previous cycle. In subsequent cycles, the estrogen dosage is gradually reduced to the lowest level which will maintain the patient symptom-free.

2. *Given cyclically:*
   Female Hypogonadism
   In an attempt to bring about sexual and somatic maturation, 2.5 to 7.5 mg. daily, in divided doses for 20 days, followed by a rest period of 10 days' duration. If bleeding does not occur by the end of this period, the same dosage schedule is repeated. The number of courses of estrogen therapy necessary to produce bleeding may vary depending on the responsiveness of the endometrium.
   If bleeding occurs before the end of the 10 day period, begin a 20 day estrogen-progestin cyclic regimen as in primary ovarian failure.
   Female castration; Primary Ovarian failure
   In order to reproduce the hormone pattern of the ovary whereby there is bleeding from a progestational endometrium, begin a 20 day estrogen-progestin cyclic regimen with Menest, 2.5 to 7.5 mg. daily in divided doses, for 20 days. During the last five days of estrogen therapy, give an oral progestin. If bleeding occurs before this regimen is concluded, therapy is discontinued and may be resumed on the fifth day of bleeding.
3. *Given chronically:*
   Inoperable progressing *prostatic cancer* - 1.25 to 2.5 mg. three times daily.
   Inoperable progressing *breast cancer* in appropriately selected men and postmenopausal women. (See indications). 10 mg. three times daily for a period of three months.

Treated patients with an intact uterus should be monitored closely for signs of endometrial cancer and appropriate diagnostic measures should be taken to rule out malignancy in the event of persistent or recurring abnormal vaginal bleeding.

References:

[1]Ziel, H. K. and W. D. Finkel, "Increased Risk of Endometrial Carcinoma Among Users of Conjugated Estrogens," *New England Journal of Medicine,* 293:1167–1170, 1975.
[2]Smith, D. C., R. Prentic, D. J. Thompson, and W. L. Hermann, "Association of Exogenous Estrogen and Endometrial Carcinoma," *New England Journal of Medicine,* 293:1164–1167, 1975.
[3]Mack, T. M., M. C. Pike, B. E. Henderson, R. I. Pfeffer, V. R. Gerkins, M. Arthur, and S. E. Brown, "Estrogens and Endometrical Cancer in a Retirement Community," *New England Journal of Medicine,* 294–1262–1267, 1976.
[4]Weiss, N. S., D. R. Szekely and D. F. Austin, "Increasing Incidence of Endometrial Cancer in the United States," *New England Journal of Medicine,* 294:1259–1262, 1976.
[5]Herbst, A. L., H. Ulfelder and D. C. Poskanzer, "Adenocarcinoma of Vagina," *New England Journal of Medicine,* 284:878–881, 1971.
[6]Greenwald, P., J. Barlow, P. Nasca, and W. Burnett, "Vaginal Cancer after Maternal Treatment with Synthetic Estrogens," *New England Journal of Medicine,* 285:390–392, 1971.
[7]Lanier, A., K. Noller, D. Decker, L. Elveback, and L. Kurland, "Cancer and Stilbestrol. A Follow-up of 1719 Persons Exposed to Estrogens In Utero and Born 1943–1959," *Mayo Clinic Proceedings,* 48:793–799, 1973.
[8]Herbst, A., R. Kurman, and R. Scully, "Vaginal and Cervical Abnormalities After Exposure to Stilbestrol In Utero," *Obstetrics and Gynecology,* 40:287–298, 1972.
[9]Herbst, A., S. Robboy, G. Macdonald, and R. Scully, "The Effects of Local Progesterone on Stilbestrol-Associated Vaginal Adenosis," *American Journal of Obstetrics and Gynecology,* 118:607–615, 1974.
[10]Herbst, A., D. Poskanzer, S. Robboy, L. Friedlander, and R. Scully, "Prenatal Exposure to Stilbestrol, A Prospective Comparison of Exposed Female Offspring with Unexposed Controls," *New England Journal of Medicine,* 292:334–339, 1975.
[11]Stafi, A., R. Mattingly, D. Foley, and W. Fetherston, "Clinical Diagnosis of Vaginal Adenosis," *Obstetrics and Gynecology,* 43:118–128, 1974.
[12]Sherman, A. I., M. Goldrath, A. Berlin, V. Vakhariya, F. Banooni, W. Michaels, P. Goodman, S. Brown, "Cervical-Vaginal Adenosis After *In Utero* Exposure to Synthetic Estrogens," *Obstetrics and Gynecology,* 44:531–545, 1974.
[13]Gal, I., B. Kirman, and J. Stern, "Hormone Pregnancy Tests and Congenital Malformation," *Nature,* 216:83, 1967.
[14]Levy, E. P., A. Cohen, and F. C. Fraser, "Hormone Treatment During Pregnancy and Congenital Heart Defects," *Lancet,* 1:611, 1973.
[15]Nora, J. and A. Nora, "Birth Defects and Oral Contraceptives," *Lancet,* 1:941–942, 1973.
[16]Janerich, D. T., J. M. Piper, and D. M. Glebatis, "Oral Contraceptives and Congenital Limb-Reduction Defects," *New England Journal of Medicine,* 291:697–700, 1974.
[17]"Estrogens for Oral or Parenteral Use," *Federal Register,* 40:8212, 1975.
[18]Boston Collaborative Drug Surveillance Program "Surgically Confirmed Gall Bladder Disease, Venous Thromboembolism and Breast Tumors in Relation to Post-Menopausal Estrogen Therapy," *New England Journal of Medicine,* 290:15–19, 1974.
[18a]Hoover, R., L. A. Gray, Sr., P. Cole, and B. MacMahon, "Menopausal Estrogens and Breast Cancer," *New England Journal of Medicine,* 295:401–405, 1976.
[19]Boston Collaborative Drug Surveillance Program, "Oral Contraceptives and Venous Thromboembolic Disease, Surgically Confirmed Gall Bladder Disease, and Breast Tumors," *Lancet* 1:1399–1404, 1973.
[20]Daniel, D. G., H. Campbell, and A. C. Turnbull, "Puerperal Thromboembolism and Suppression of Lactation," *Lancet,* 2:287–289, 1967.
[21]The Veterans Administration Cooperative Urological Research Group, "Carcinoma of the Prostate: Treatment Comparisons," *Journal of Urology,* 98:516–522, 1967.
[22]Bailar, J. C., "Thromboembolism and Oestrogen Therapy," *Lancet,* 2:560, 1967.
[23]Blackard, C., R. Doe, G. Mellinger, and D. Byar, "Incidence of Cardiovascular Disease and Death in Patients Receivng Diethylstilbestrol for Carcinoma of the Prostate," *Cancer,* 26:249–256, 1970.
[24]Royal College of General Practitioners, "Oral Contraception and Thromboembolic Disease," *Journal of the Royal College of General Practitioners,* 13:267–279, 1967.
[25]Inman, W. H. W. and M. P. Vessey, "Investigation of Deaths from Pulmonary, Coronary, and Cerebral Thrombosis and Embolism in Women of Child-Bearing Age," *British Medical Journal,* 2:193–199, 1968.
[26]Vessey, M. P. and R. Doll, "Investigation of Relation Between Use of Oral Contraceptives and Thromboembolic Disease. A Further Report," *British Medical Journal,* 2:651–657, 1969.
[27]Sartwell, P. E., A. T. Masi, F. G. Arthes, G. R. Greene, and H. E. Smith, "Thromboembolism and Oral Contraceptives: An Epidemiological Case Control Study," *American Journal of Epidemiology,* 90:365–380, 1969.
[28]Collaborative Group for the Study of Stroke in Young Women, "Oral Contraception and Increased Risk of Cerebral Ischemia or Thrombosis," *New England Journal of Medicine,* 288:871–878, 1973.
[29]Collaborative Group for the Study of Stroke in Young Women, "Oral Contraceptives and Stroke in Young Women: Associated Risk Factors," *Journal of the American Medical Association,* 231:718–722, 1975.
[30]Mann, J. I. and W. H. W. Inman, "Oral Contraceptives and Death from Myocardial Infarction," *British Medical Journal,* 2:245–248, 1975.
[31]Mann, J. I., M. P. Vessey, M. Thorogood, and R. Doll, "Myocardial Infarction in Young Women with Special Reference to Oral Contraceptive Practice," *British Medical Journal,* 2:241–245, 1975.
[32]Inman, W. H. W., V. P. Vessey, B. Westerholm, and A. Engelund, "Thromboembolic Disease and the Steroidal Content of Oral Contraceptives," *British Medical Journal,* 2:203–209, 1970.
[33]Stolley, P. D., J. A. Tonascia, M. S. Tockman, P. E. Sartwell, A. H. Rutledge, and M. P. Jacobs, "Thrombosis with Low-Estrogen Oral Contraceptives," *American Journal of Epidemiology,* 102:197–208, 1975.
[34]Vessey, M. P., R. Doll, A. S. Fairbairn, and G. Glober, "Post-Operative Thromboembolism and the Use of the Oral Contraceptives, " *British Medical Journal,* 3:123–126, 1970.
[35]Greene, G. R. and P. E. Sartwell, "Oral Contraceptive Use in Patients with Thromboembolism Following Surgery, Trauma or Infection," *American Journal of Public Health,* 62:680–685, 1972.
[36]Rosenberg, L., M. B. Armstrong and H. Jick, "Myocardial Infarction and Estrogen Therapy in Postmenopausal Women," *New England Journal of Medicine,* 294:1256–1259, 1976.
[37]Coronary Drug Project Research Group, "The Coronary Drug Project: Initial Findings Leading to Modifications of Its Research Protocol," *Journal of the American Medical Association,* 214:1303–1313, 1970.
[38]Baum, J., F. Holtz, J. J. Bookstein, and E. W. Klein, "Possible Association between Benign Hepatomas and Oral Contraceptives," *Lancet,* 2:926–928, 1973.
[39]Mays, E. T., W. M. Christopherson, M. M. Mahr, and H. C. Williams, "Hepatic Changes in Young Women Ingesting Contraceptive Steroids, Hepatic Hemorrhage and Primary Hepatic Tumors, " *Journal of the American Medical Association," 235:730–782, 1976.*
[40]Edmondson, H. A. B. Henderson, and B. Benton, "Liver Cell Adenomas Associated with the Use of Oral Contraceptives," *New England Journal of Medicine,* 294:470–472, 1976.
[41]Pfeffer, R. I. and S. Van Den Noort, "Estrogen Use and Stroke Risk in Postmenopausal Women," *American Journal of Epidemiology,* 103:445–456, 1976.

How Supplied: In order to individualize dosage, MENEST is supplied as film-coated tablets in the following potencies:

0.3 mg./Tablet (Yellow)
NDC 0029-2800-30 100
0.625 mg./Tablet (orange)
NDC 0029-2810-30 100
NDC 0029-2810-33 1000
1.25 mg./Tablet (Green)
NDC 0029-2820-30 100
NDC 0029-2820-33 1000
2.5 mg./Tablet (Pink)
NDC 0029-2830-29 50
NDC 0029-2830-33 1000

Literature Available: Yes.

[*Shown in Product Identification Section*]

NUCOFED® ©

Syrup and Capsules
Antitussive—Decongestant

Description: Each capsule or 5 ml (teaspoonful) contains: Codeine Phosphate, 20 mg (Warning: May Be Habit Forming); Pseudoephedrine HCl, 60 mg.

Actions: NUCOFED® has antitussive and decongestant actions. Codeine, at the recommended dose, causes suppression of the cough reflex by a direct effect on the cough center in the medulla of the brain. Codeine has antitussive, mild analgesic and sedative effects.

Pseudoephedrine Hydrochloride, an orally effective nasal decongestant acts — through vasoconstriction — to promptly reduce edema and congestion of the mucous membranes of the respiratory tract.

Indications: NUCOFED® is indicated for symptomatic relief when both coughing and congestion are associated with upper respiratory infections and related conditions such as common cold, bronchitis, influenza, and sinusitis.

Contraindications: Hypersensitivity to product's active ingredients.

Precautions: Prescribe with caution in patients suffering from hyperthyroidism, hypertension, cardiac disease, diabetes, or chronic pulmonary disease.

Adverse Reactions: Adverse reactions occur infrequently with the usual oral dosage of Nucofed®. However, certain patients may exhibit constipation, nervousness, dizziness or mild stimulation.

Drug Interaction Precaution: Prescribe with caution in patients taking an antihypertensive or an antidepressant drug containing a monoamine oxidase inhibitor.

Dosage and Administration:

Usual Dosage

Adults: 1 teaspoonful or capsule every 4 to 6 hours, not to exceed 6 teaspoonfuls or 6 capsules in 24 hours.

Children: Syrup only

6 to under 12 years: ½ teaspoonful every 4 to 6 hours, not to exceed 3 teaspoonfuls in 24 hours.

2 to under 6 years: ¼ teaspoonful every 4 to 6 hours, not to exceed 1½ teaspoonfuls in 24 hours.

Not recommended for use in children under 2 years of age.

How Supplied: Green, Mint Flavored Liquid

NDC 0029-3135-34 ....Pints

Capsules

NDC 0029-3138-39 ....Bottles of 60's

Caution: Federal law prohibits dispensing without prescription.

PYOPEN® ℞

(sterile carbenicillin disodium)
for Intravenous or Intramuscular Use

Description: PYOPEN (carbenicillin disodium) is a semisynthetic injectable penicillin derived from the penicillin nucleus, 6-aminopenicillanic acid. Chemically, carbenicillin disodium is α-carboxybenzyl-penicillin disodium salt.

Actions:

MICROBIOLOGY:

Carbenicillin is bactericidal and demonstrates activity against both Gram-positive and Gram-negative organisms.

Certain strains of the following organisms are susceptible to carbenicillin *in vitro:*

Staphylococcus aureus
(nonpenicillinase-producing)
Staphylococcus albus
Diplococcus pneumoniae
Beta-hemolytic streptococci
Streptococcus faecalis
Haemophilus influenzae
Neisseria species
Escherichia coli
Salmonella species
Pseudomonas aeruginosa
Proteus mirabilis
Proteus morganii
Proteus rettgeri
Proteus vulgaris
Enterobacter species
Anaerobic bacteria,
including:
Bacteroides species
Peptostreptococcus species
Peptococcus species
Clostridium species
Fusobacterium species

In vitro synergism between carbenicillin and gentamicin sulfate against certain strains of *Pseudomonas aeruginosa* has been demonstrated.

Some strains of such microorganisms as *Mima-Herellea (Acinetobacter), Citrobacter,* and *Serratia* have shown susceptibility. Carbenicillin does not resist destruction by penicillinase-producing staphylococci. *Klebsiella* species are resistant to carbenicillin.

Some strains of *Pseudomonas* have developed resistance fairly rapidly.

PHARMACOLOGY:

Carbenicillin is not absorbed orally; therefore, it must be given intravenously or intramuscularly. Following intramuscular administration, peak blood levels are obtained within 1–2 hours. Somewhat higher and more prolonged serum levels can be achieved with the concurrent administration of probenecid. Although the minimum inhibitory concentrations (MIC) for most *Pseudomonas* and *Bacteroides fragilis* strains is relatively high by usual standards, the low degree of toxicity of carbenicillin permits the use of doses large enough to achieve inhibitory levels for these strains, even in serum or tissues. The successful management of systemic infections and septicemia depends on attainment and maintenance of serum levels at least as high as the MIC. In most *Pseudomonas aeruginosa* and *Bacteroides fragilis* infections, serum levels of 100 mcg./ml. or higher are required, and these can be achieved by intravenous administration. Other susceptible organisms usually require serum levels in the range of 10-25 mcg./ml. Relatively small doses can produce high levels of the antibiotic in the urine of patients with normal renal function. 2,000 to 4,000 mcg./ml. can be obtained in the urine following intramuscular administration of 1 Gm. Lymph levels generally parallel serum levels, and tissue levels are comparable to those obtained with other penicillins.

Indications: PYOPEN is primarily indicated for the treatment of infections due to *Pseudomonas aeruginosa, Proteus* species (particularly indole-positive strains) and certain strains of *Escherichia coli.* PYOPEN has been particularly effective in urinary tract infections caused by one or more of these organisms because of the very high urine levels achieved by intramuscular administration.

Clinical studies have demonstrated the effectiveness of PYOPEN in the following infections caused by these organisms:

1. Severe systemic infections and bacterial septicemia, including meningitis due to *H. influenzae.* Although Carbenicillin possesses *in vitro* activity against many ampicillin-resistant *H. influenzae,* clinical data are insufficient to recommend its use for treatment of meningitis due to ampicillin-resistant strains.
2. Genitourinary tract infections including those due to *Neisseria gonorrhoeae, Enterobacter* and *Streptococcus faecalis* (enterococcus).
3. Acute and chronic respiratory infections. (Though clinical improvement has been shown, bacteriological cures cannot be expected in patients with chronic respiratory disease or cystic fibrosis.)
4. Soft-tissue infections.

Carbenicillin is also indicated in the treatment of the following infections due to susceptible anaerobic bacteria:

1. Bacterial Septicemia.
2. Lower respiratory tract infections such as empyema, anaerobic pneumonitis and lung abscess.
3. Intra-abdominal infections such as peritonitis and intra-abdominal abscess. (Typically resulting from anaerobic organisms resident in the normal gastrointestinal tract.)
4. Infections of the female pelvis and genital tract such as endometritis, pelvic inflammatory disease, pelvic abscess and salpingitis.
5. Skin and soft-tissue infections.

Where there is primary infection due to a Gram-negative organism associated with a Gram-positive organism, the *in vitro* activity of PYOPEN should be considered (see Microbiology above).

In the treatment of infections due to certain susceptible strains of *Pseudomonas aeruginosa,* clinical efficacy may be enhanced by the use of combined therapy with PYOPEN (carbenicillin disodium) and gentamicin sulfate in full therapeutic dosages. For additional prescribing information, see the gentamicin sulfate package insert.

NOTE: Culturing and susceptibility testing should be performed initially and during treatment to monitor the effectiveness of therapy and the antibiotic susceptibility of the bacteria.

Contraindications: A history of allergic reaction to any of the penicillins is a contraindication.

Warnings: Serious and occasionally fatal hypersensitivity (anaphylactoid) reactions have been reported in patients receiving penicillin. These reactions are more likely to occur in persons with a history of sensitivity to multiple allergens.

There have been reports of patients with a history of penicillin hypersensitivity reactions who have experienced severe hypersensitivity reactions when treated with a cephalosporin. Before therapy with a penicillin, careful inquiry should be made about previous hypersensitivity reactions to penicillins, cephalosporins, and other allergens. If a reaction occurs, the drug should be discontinued unless in the opinion of the physician the condition being treated is life-threatening and amenable only to carbenicillin therapy. **Serious anaphylactoid reactions require immediate emergency treatment with epinephrine. Oxygen, intravenous steroids, and airway management, including intubation, should also be administered as indicated.**

Patients with renal impairment should be observed for bleeding manifestations. Such patients should be dosed strictly according to recommendations (see Dosage and Administration). If bleeding manifestations appear, the antibiotic should be discontinued and appropriate therapy instituted.

USAGE DURING PREGNANCY:

Safety for use during pregnancy has not been established.

Precautions: Although PYOPEN exhibits the characteristic low toxicity of the penicillin group of antibiotics, it is advisable to check periodically, as with any other potent agent, for organ system dysfunction (including renal, hepatic, and hematopoietic) during prolonged therapy. Emergence of resistant organisms, such as *Klebsiella* species and *Serratia* species which might cause superinfection, should be kept in mind.

Since the theoretical sodium content is 5.3 milliequivalents (122 mg) per gram of carbenicillin; and the actual vial content can be as high

Continued on next page

Beecham Laboratories—Cont.

as 6.5 mEq/Gm, electrolyte and cardiac status should be monitored carefully.

In a few patients receiving high doses of PYOPEN, hypokalemia has been reported. Periodic serum potassium determinations should be made and corrective measures should be implemented when necessary.

Several uremic patients receiving high doses (24 grams/day) have developed hemorrhagic manifestations associated with abnormalities of coagulation tests such as clotting-time and prothrombin-time. On withdrawal of the antibiotic, the bleeding ceased. The exact relationship of these findings to carbenicillin therapy is not clear.

As with any penicillin preparation, the possibility of an allergic response, including anaphylaxis, exists, particularly in a hypersensitive patient.

Cases of gonorrhea with a suspected lesion of syphilis should have dark-field examinations before treatment. In all other cases where concomitant syphilis is suspected, monthly serological tests should be made for a minimum of 4 months.

Adverse Reactions: Local reactions, such as pain and induration at the site of intramuscu-

PYOPEN DOSAGE and ADMINISTRATION

Indication				
Adults:	*Pseudomonas*	*Proteus and E. coli*	*Enterobacter* and *S. faecalis*	*Anaerobes*
Urinary Tract Infections				
Serious	200 mg/kg/day by I.V. drip.	200 mg/kg/day by I.V. drip.	200 mg/kg/day by I.V. drip.	
Uncomplicated	1–2 grams I.M. or I.V. every 6 hours.	1–2 grams I.M. or I.V. every 6 hours.	1–2 grams I.M. or I.V. every 6 hours.	
Severe Systemic Infections Septicemia Respiratory Infections Soft-Tissue Infections	400–500 mg/kg/day (30–40 grams) I.V. in divided doses or by continuous drip.	250–400 mg/kg/day (15–30 grams) I.V. in divided doses or by continuous drip.		400–500 mg/kg/day (30–40 grams) in divided doses or by continuous drip.
Infections complicated by renal insufficiency (Creatinine clearance less than 5 ml/min).	2 grams I.V. (1) every 8 hours.	2 grams I.V. (1) every 8 hours.		
During peritoneal dialysis	2 grams I.V. every 6 hours.	2 grams I.V. every 6 hours.		
During hemodialysis	2 grams I.V. every 4 hours.	2 grams I.V. every 4 hours.		
Meningitis				*H. influenzae* 400–500 mg/kg/day (30–40 grams) in divided doses or by continuous drip.
Gonorrhea, acute uncomplicated anogenital and urethral infections due to N. gonorrhoeae	MALES and FEMALES Single 4 Gm I.M. injection (divided between 2 sites).			

NOTE: Probenecid in a dosage of 1 gram may be administered orally about 30 minutes prior to the I.M. treatment of acute gonorrhoeal infections. For complete information on probenecid, see manufacturer's product information.

(1) The serum half-life of PYOPEN in patients with severe renal failure is 12.5 hours; therefore, 2 grams of PYOPEN administered intravenously to these patients every 8 hours will give serum levels of PYOPEN of approximately 100 mcg/ml, a level notable free of any untoward effects.

Children:	*Pseudomonas*	*Proteus and E. coli*	*Enterobacter* and *S. faecalis*	*Anaerobes*
Urinary Tract Infections	50–200 mg/kg/day I.M. or I.V. in divided doses every 4 to 6 hours.	50–100 mg/kg/day I.M. or I.V. in divided doses every 4 to 6 hours.	50–200 mg/kg/day I.M. or I.V. in divided doses every 4 to 6 hours.	
Severe Systemic Infections Septicemia Respiratory Infections Soft-Tissue Infections	400–500 mg/kg/day I.V. in divided doses or by continuous drip.	250–400 mg/kg/day I.M. or I.V. in divided doses or by continuous drip.		400–500 mg/kg/day I.V. in divided doses or by continuous drip.
Infections complicated by renal insufficiency (Creatinine clearance less than 5 ml/min)	Clinical data is insufficient to recommend an optimum dose.			
Meningitis				*H. influenzae* 400–500 mg/kg/day I.V. in divided doses or by continuous drip.

Neonates: In the neonate, for severe systemic infections (sepsis) due to susceptible strains of *Pseudomonas, Proteus, E. coli,* and *H. influenzae* the following PYOPEN dosages may be given I.M. or by fifteen (15) minute I.V. infusion:

Infants under 2000 grams body weight:
Initial dose: 100 mg/kg
Subsequent doses during first week:
75 mg/kg/8 hrs (225 mg/kg/day)
After 7 days of age: 100 mg/kg/6 hrs
(400 kg/kg/day)

Infants over 2000 grams body weight:
Initial dose: 100 mg/kg
Subsequent doses during first 3 days:
75 mg/kg/6 hrs (300 mg/kg/day)
After 3 days of age: 100 mg/kg/6 hrs
(400 mg/kg/day)

NOTE: This dosage schedule should give maximum serum levels approximately 150–175 mcg./ml. and minimum levels of approximately 50–75 mcg./ml. of PYOPEN.

lar injection, similar to that noted with other penicillins have been reported. Vein irritation and thrombophlebitis can occur, particularly when undiluted solution is directly injected into the vein.
Allergic reactions, including skin rash, eosinophilia, urticaria, drug fever, and anaphylactic reaction have been reported. Pruritus has also been reported.
Nausea and unpleasant taste have been experienced infrequently during intravenous infusion of large doses.
As with other penicillins, leukopenia, neutropenia, thrombocytopenia, or hemolytic anemia might occur. Hemolytic anemia has been reported in the presence of severe renal impairment and might have been caused by PYOPEN.
Serum glutamic oxaloacetic transaminase (SGOT) and serum glutamic pyruvic transaminase (SGPT) elevations have been observed.
Patients who have impaired renal function may experience convulsions or neuromuscular excitability when large doses are used.
There have been no reports of kidney damage ascribable to the drug.

Dosage and Administration: Clinical experience indicates that in serious urinary tract and systemic infections intravenous therapy in the higher doses should be used. The recommended maximum dose is 40 Gm. per day. Intramuscular injections should not exceed 2 grams per injection.
(See table on preceding page)
Gentamicin may be used concurrently with carbenicillin for initial therapy until results of culture and susceptibility studies are known.
It is recommended that PYOPEN and gentamicin sulfate not be mixed together in the same I.V. solution due to the gradual inactivation of gentamicin sulfate under these circumstances. The therapeutic effect of the two drugs remains unimpaired when administered separately.
Seriously ill patients should receive the higher doses. PYOPEN has proved to be useful in infections in which protective mechanisms are impaired, such as in acute leukemia and during therapy with immunosuppressive or oncolytic drugs.

DIRECTIONS FOR USE

1 Gm., 2 Gm. and 5 Gm. Standard Vials: *Use Sterile Water for Injection, U.S.P.*

Intramuscular Use: Each gram of PYOPEN should be reconstituted with at least 2 ml. of sterile water for injection. In order to facilitate reconstitution, up to 3.6 ml. of sterile water for injection per gram of PYOPEN can be used.

Amount of Diluent to be Added to the 1-Gm. Vial	Volume to be Withdrawn For a 1-Gm. Dose
2.0 ml.	2.5 ml.
2.5 ml.	3.0 ml.
3.6 ml.	4.0 ml.

Amount of Diluent to be Added to the 2-Gm. Vial	Volume to be withdrawn For a 1-Gm. Dose
4.0 ml.	2.5 ml.
5.0 ml.	3.0 ml.
6.6 ml.	4.0 ml.

The 5-Gm. vial should be reconstituted with at least 9.5 ml. of sterile water for injection. In order to facilitate reconstitution, up to 17 ml. of sterile water for injection can be used.

Amount of Diluent to be Added to the 5-Gm. Vial	Volume to be Withdrawn For a 1-Gm. Dose
9.5 ml.	2.5 ml.
12.0 ml.	3.0 ml.
17.0 ml.	4.0 ml.

PYOPEN for intramuscular injection ONLY may also be diluted with one of the following:
1. 0.5% Lidocaine Hydrochloride (without epinephrine).
2. Bacteriostatic Water containing 0.9% Benzyl Alcohol.

Intravenous Solution	Stability Period: Room Temperature	Stability Period: Refrigerated
* Sterile Water for Injection	72 hours	14 days
* Sodium Chloride Injection	72 hours	14 days
* 5% Dextrose in Water	72 hours	14 days
* Ringer's Injection	72 hours	14 days
5% Dextrose in Water with 0.225% Sodium Chloride	24 hours	3 days
5% Dextrose in Water with 0.45% Sodium Chloride	24 hours	3 days
5% Alcohol, 5% Dextrose in Water	24 hours	3 days
5% Alcohol, 5% Dextrose in 0.9% Sodium Chloride Solution	24 hours	3 days
5% Dextrose with Electrolyte No. 48 (Pediatric Maintenance Electrolyte Solution)	24 hours	3 days
Invert Sugar 10% in Water	24 hours	3 days
5% Levugen (Fructose) with Electrolyte No. 75	24 hours	3 days
Lactated Ringer's Injection	24 hours	3 days
Maintenance Electrolyte Solution (Electrolyte No. 75)	24 hours	3 days

*After reconstitution, these solutions can be frozen (approx. 0°F) and stored for up to 30 days without loss of potency. The stabilities of the thawed solutions are identical to the unfrozen ones listed above.
Unused portions of solutions should be discarded after the time periods mentioned above.

For reconstitution of PYOPEN with these diluents, follow the above directions. PYOPEN may be diluted with these solutions and stored for 24 hours at room temperature or for 72 hours under refrigeration. Discard unused solutions stored longer than these time periods. For full product information, refer to the Lidocaine Hydrochloride (without epinephrine) package insert.
As with all intramuscular preparations, PYOPEN (carbenicillin disodium) should be injected well within the body of a relatively large muscle, using usual techniques and precautions.

Intravenous Use: Reconstitute each gram of PYOPEN with at least 4 ml of sterile water for injection; when dissolved, dilute further to desired volume.
Intravenous Injection: In order to avoid vein irritation, administer solution as slowly as possible.
Intravenous Infusion: Reconstitute the required number of vials as described above, using a suitable intravenous solution listed below, then further dilute to the desired volume. Administer by continuous or intermittent intravenous drip. Intermittent infusion should be administered over a 30 minute to 2 hour period in six equally divided doses.
For the stability of PYOPEN in various intravenous solutions see Directions for Use under Piggyback Bottles.

2 Gm, 5 Gm Piggyback Bottles and 10 Gm Bulk Pharmacy Package:
Intravenous Injection:
The 2 gram bottle should be reconstituted with a minimum of 20 ml. Sterile Water for Injection, U.S.P.

Amount of Diluent	Concentration of Solution
100 ml.	1 Gm./50 ml.
50 ml.	1 Gm./25 ml.
20 ml.	1 Gm./10 ml.

The 5 gram bottle should be reconstituted with a minimum of 50 ml. Sterile Water for Injection, U.S.P.

Amount of Diluent	Concentration of Solution
100 ml.	1 Gm./20 ml.
50 ml.	1 Gm./10 ml.

The 10 gram bottle should be reconstituted with a minimum of 95 ml. Sterile Water for Injection, U.S.P.

Amount of Diluent	Concentration of Solution
95 ml.	1 Gm./10 ml.

In order to avoid vein irritation, the solution should be administered as slowly as possible. A dilution of 1 Gm./20 ml. or more, will further reduce the incidence of vein irritation.

Intravenous Infusion:
Stability studies on PYOPEN in various intravenous diluents between 10 mg/ml and 100 mg/ml concentrations indicate that the resulting solutions will lose less than 10% activity at room temperature (70°F) or under refrigeration (40°F) for the time periods stated below:
(See table above)

How Supplied:
PYOPEN (sterile carbenicillin disodium):
Each vial contains carbenicillin disodium equivalent to 1 Gm, 2 Gm, 5 Gm or 10 Gm Carbenicillin.
NDC 0029-6400-22 ....1 Gm Vial
NDC 0029-6402-27 ....2 Gm Vial
NDC 0029-6405-26 ....5 Gm Vial
NDC 0029-6402-21 ......2 Gm Piggyback Bottle
NDC 0029-6405-21 ......5 Gm Piggyback Bottle
NDC 0029-6406-21.......10 Gm Bulk Pharmacy Package

TICAR® ℞
(sterile ticarcillin disodium)
for Intramuscular or Intravenous Use

Description: TICAR (Ticarcillin Disodium) is a semisynthetic injectable penicillin derived from the penicillin nucleus, 6-amino-penicillanic acid. Chemically, it is 6-[(Carboxy-3-thienylacetyl) amino]-3, 3-dimethyl-7-oxo-4-thia-1-azabicyclo [3.2.0] heptane-2-carboxylic acid disodium salt. It is supplied as a white to pale yellow powder or lyophilized cake for reconstitution. The reconstituted solution is clear, colorless or pale yellow, having a pH of 6.0–8.0. Ticarcillin is very soluble in water, its solubility is greater than 600 mg/ml.

Actions:
PHARMACOLOGY
Ticarcillin is not absorbed orally, therefore, it must be given intravenously or intramuscularly. Following intramuscular administration, peak serum concentrations occur within ½–1 hour. Somewhat higher and more prolonged serum levels can be achieved with the concurrent administration of probenecid.
The minimum inhibitory concentrations (MIC) for many strains of *Pseudomonas* are relatively high by usual standards; serum levels of 60 mcg/ml or greater are required. However, the low degree of toxicity of Ticarcillin permits the use of doses large enough to achieve inhibitory levels for these strains in serum or tissues. Other susceptible organisms usually require serum levels in the 10–25 mcg/ml range.
[See table on next page].
As with other penicillins, Ticarcillin is eliminated by glomerular filtration and tubular secretion. It is not highly bound to serum protein (approximately 45%) and is excreted unchanged in high concentrations in the urine.

Continued on next page

Beecham Laboratories—Cont.

After the administration of a 1–2 Gm I.M. dose, a urine concentration of 2000–4000 mcg/ml may be obtained in patients with normal renal function. The serum half-life of Ticarcillin in normal individuals is approximately 70 minutes.

An inverse relationship exists between serum half-life and creatinine clearance, but the dosage of TICAR need only be adjusted in cases of severe renal impairment (see DOSAGE AND ADMINISTRATION). The administered Ticarcillin may be removed from patients undergoing dialysis; the actual amount removed depends on the duration and type of dialysis.

Ticarcillin can be detected in tissues and interstitial fluid following parenteral administration. Penetration into the cerebrospinal fluid, bile and pleural fluid has been demonstrated.

MICROBIOLOGY

Ticarcillin is bactericidal and demonstrates substantial *in vitro* activity against both Gram-positive and Gram-negative organisms. Many strains of the following organisms were found to be susceptible to Ticarcillin *in vitro:*

Pseudomonas aeruginosa (and other species)
Escherichia coli
Proteus mirabilis
Proteus morganii
Proteus rettgeri
Proteus vulgaris
Enterobacter species
Haemophilus influenzae
Neisseria species
Salmonella species
Staphylococcus aureus (non-penicillinase producing)
Staphylococcus albus
Beta-hemolytic streptococci (Group A)
Streptococcus faecalis (Enterococcus)
Streptococcus pneumoniae

Anaerobic bacteria, including:
Bacteroides species, including *B. fragilis*
Fusobacterium species
Veillonella species
Clostridium species
Eubacterium species
Peptococcus species
Peptostreptococcus species

In vitro synergism between Ticarcillin and gentamicin sulfate or tobramycin sulfate against certain strains of *Pseudomonas aeruginosa* has been demonstrated.

Some strains of such microorganisms as *Mima-Herellea (Acinetobacter), Citrobacter* and *Serratia* have shown susceptibility.

Ticarcillin is not stable in the presence of penicillinase.

Some strains of *Pseudomonas* have developed resistance fairly rapidly.

DISC SUSCEPTIBILITY TESTS

Quantitative methods that require measurement of zone diameters give the most precise estimates of antibiotic susceptibility. One such procedure* has been recommended for use with discs for testing susceptibility to carbenicillin-class antibiotics. With this procedure, a report from the laboratory of "susceptible" indicates that the infecting organism is likely to respond to therapy. A report of "resistant" indicates that the infecting organism is not likely to respond to therapy. A report of "intermediate susceptibility" suggests that the organism would be susceptible if high dosage is used, or if the infection is confined to tissues and fluids (e.g., urine), in which high antibiotic levels are attained.

At present, only dilution methods can be recommended for testing antibiotic susceptibility of obligate anaerobes.

Indications: TICAR (Ticarcillin Disodium) is indicated for the treatment of the following infections:

Bacterial septicemia (†)
Skin and soft-tissue infections (†)
Acute and chronic respiratory tract infections (†)(‡);

(†) caused by susceptible strains of *Pseudomonas aeruginosa, Proteus* species (both indole-positive and indole-negative) and *Escherichia coli.*

(‡) (Though clinical improvement has been shown, bacteriological cures cannot be expected in patients with chronic respiratory disease or cystic fibrosis.)

Genitourinary tract infections (complicated and uncomplicated) due to susceptible strains of *Pseudomonas aeruginosa, Proteus* species (both indole-positive and indole-negative), *Escherichia coli, Enterobacter* and *Streptococcus faecalis* (enterococcus).

Ticarcillin is also indicated in the treatment of the following infections due to susceptible anaerobic bacteria:

1. Bacterial septicemia.
2. Lower respiratory tract infections such as empyema, anaerobic pneumonitis and lung abscess.
3. Intra-abdominal infections such as peritonitis and intra-abdominal abscess (typically resulting from anaerobic organisms resident in the normal gastrointestinal tract).
4. Infections of the female pelvis and genital tract such as endometritis, pelvic inflammatory disease, pelvic abscess and salpingitis.
5. Skin and soft-tissue infections.

Although Ticarcillin is primarily indicated in Gram-negative infections, its *in vitro* activity against Gram-positive organisms should be considered in infections caused by both Gram-negative and Gram-positive organisms (see Microbiology).

Based on the *in vitro* synergism between Ticarcillin and gentamicin sulfate or tobramycin sulfate against certain strains of *Pseudomonas aeruginosa,* combined therapy has been successful, using full therapeutic dosages. (For additional prescribing information, see the gentamicin sulfate and tobramycin sulfate package insert.)

NOTE: Culturing and susceptibility testing should be performed initially and during treatment to monitor the effectiveness of therapy and the susceptibility of the bacteria.

Contraindications: A history of allergic reaction to any of the penicillins is a contraindication.

Warnings: Serious and occasionally fatal hypersensitivity (anaphylactoid) reactions have been reported in patients receiving penicillin. These reactions are more likely to occur in persons with a history of sensitivity to multiple allergens.

There are reports of patients with a history of penicillin hypersensitivity reactions who experienced severe hypersensitivity reactions when treated with a cephalosporin. Before therapy with a penicillin, careful inquiry should be made about previous hypersensitivity reactions to penicillins, cephalosporins, and other allergens. If a reaction occurs, the drug should be discontinued unless, in the opinion of the physician, the condition being treated is life-threatening and amenable only to Ticarcillin therapy. **Serious anaphylactoid reactions require immediate emergency treatment with epinephrine. Oxygen, intravenous steroids, airway management, including intubation, should also be administered as indicated.**

Some patients receiving high doses of Ticarcillin may develop hemorrhagic manifestations associated with abnormalities of coagulation tests, such as bleeding time and platelet aggregation. On withdrawal of the drug, the bleeding should cease and the coagulation abnormalities revert to normal. Other causes of abnormal bleeding should also be considered. Patients with renal impairment, in whom excretion of Ticarcillin is delayed, should be observed for bleeding manifestations. Such patients should be dosed strictly according to recommendations (see DOSAGE AND ADMINISTRATION). If bleeding manifestations appear, Ticarcillin treatment should be discontinued and appropriate therapy instituted.

Precautions: Although TICAR (Ticarcillin Disodium) exhibits the characteristic low toxicity of the penicillins, as with any other potent agent, it is advisable to check periodically for organ system dysfunction (including renal, hepatic and hematopoietic) during prolonged treatment. If overgrowth of resistant organisms occurs, the appropriate therapy should be initiated.

Since the theoretical sodium content is 5.2 milliequivalents (120 mg) per gram of Ticarcillin and the actual vial content can be as high as 6.5 mEq/Gm, electrolyte and cardiac status should be monitored carefully.

In a few patients receiving intravenous Ticarcillin, hypokalemia has been reported. Serum potassium should be measured periodically, and, if necessary, corrective therapy should be implemented.

As with any penicillin, the possibility of an allergic response, including anaphylaxis, exists, particularly in hypersensitive patients.

USAGE DURING PREGNANCY

Reproduction studies have been performed in mice and rats and have revealed no evidence of impaired fertility or harm to the fetus due to Ticarcillin. There are no well-controlled studies in pregnant women, but investigational experience does not include any positive evidence of adverse effects on the fetus. Although there is no clearly defined risk, such experience cannot exclude the possibility of infrequent or subtle damage to the fetus. Ticarcillin should be used in pregnant women only when clearly needed.

Adverse Reactions: The following adverse reactions may occur:

Hypersensitivity Reactions: Skin rashes, pruritus, urticaria, drug fever.

TICARILLIN SERUM LEVELS

		mcg/ml						
Dosage	Route	¼ hr.	½ hr.	1 hr.	2 hr.	3 hr.	4 hr.	6 hr.
Adults:								
500 mg	IM	–	7.7	8.6	6.0	4.0	–	2.9
1 Gm	IM	–	31.0	18.7	15.7	9.7	–	3.4
2 Gm	IM	–	63.6	39.7	32.3	18.9	–	3.4
3 Gm	IV	190.0	140.0	107.0	52.2	31.3	13.8	4.2
5 Gm	IV	327.0	280.0	175.0	106.0	63.0	28.5	9.6
3 Gm + 1 Gm Probenecid	IV / Oral	223.0	166.0	123.0	78.0	54.0	35.4	17.1
Neonates:		½ hr.	1 hr.	1½ hr.	2 hr.	4 hr.	8 hr.	
50 mg/kg	IM	64.0	70.7	63.7	60.1	33.2	11.6	

DOSAGE AND ADMINISTRATION

Clinical experience indicates that in serious urinary tract and systemic infections, intravenous therapy in the higher doses should be used. Intramuscular injections should not exceed 2 grams per injection.

Adults:	
Bacterial Septicemia Respiratory Tract Infections Skin and Soft-Tissue Infections Intra-Abdominal Infections Infections of the Female Pelvis and Genital Tract	200-300 mg/kg/day by I.V. infusion in divided doses every 3, 4 or 6 hours. [Usual recommended dosage: 3 grams every 3, 4 or 6 hours, depending on weight and the severity of the infection.]
Urinary Tract Infections	
Complicated:	150-200 mg/kg/day by I.V. infusion in divided doses every 4 or 6 hours. [Usual recommended dosage for average (70 kg) adults: 3 grams q.i.d.]
Uncomplicated:	1 gram I.M. or direct I.V. every 6 hours.
Infections complicated by renal insufficiency: (1)	Initial loading dose of 3 grams I.V. followed by I.V. doses, based on creatinine clearance or type of dialysis, as indicated below:
Creatinine clearance ml/min.:	
over 60	3 grams every 4 hours
30-60	2 grams every 4 hours
10-30	2 grams every 8 hours
less than 10	2 grams every 12 hours (or 1 gram I.M. every 6 hours)
less than 10 with hepatic dysfunction	2 grams every 24 hours (or 1 gram I.M. every 12 hours)
patients on peritoneal dialysis	3 grams every 12 hours
patients on hemodialysis	3 grams after each dialysis

(1)The half-life of Ticarcillin in patients with renal failure is approximately 13 hours.

Children: Under 40 kg (88 lbs)	
The daily dose for children should not exceed the adult dosage.	
Bacterial Septicemia Respiratory Tract Infections Skin and Soft-Tissue Infections Intra-Abdominal Infections Infections of the Female Pelvis and Genital Tract	200-300 mg/kg/day by I.V. infusion in divided doses every 4 or 6 hours.
Urinary Tract Infections	
Complicated:	150-200 mg/kg/day by I.V. infusion in divided doses every 4 or 6 hours.
Uncomplicated	50-100 mg/kg/day I.M. or direct I.V. in divided doses every 6 or 8 hours.
Infections complicated by renal insufficiency:	Clinical data is insufficient to recommend an optimum dose.
Children weighing more than 40 kg (88 lbs) should receive adult dosages.	

Neonates: In the neonate, for severe infections (sepsis) due to susceptible strains of *Pseudomonas, Proteus* and *E. coli*, the following Ticarcillin dosages may be given I.M. or by 10-20 minutes I.V. infusion:

Infants under 2000 grams body weight:	Infants over 2000 grams body weight:
Initial dose: 100 mg/kg	Initial dose: 100 mg/kg
Subsequent doses during first week: 75 mg/kg/8 hours (225 mg/kg/day)	Subsequent doses during first two weeks: 75 mg/kg/4-6 hours (300-450 mg/kg/day)
Over 7 days of age: 100 mg/kg/4 hours (600 mg/kg/day)	Over two weeks of age: 100 mg/kg/4 hours (600 mg/kg/day)

This dosage schedule should provide average maximum Ticarcillin serum levels of approximately 150 mcg/ml and minimum levels of approximately 40-50 mcg/ml.

NOTE: Gentamicin or tobramycin may be used concurrently with Ticarcillin for initial therapy until results of culture and susceptibility studies are known.
Seriously ill patients should receive the higher doses. TICAR has proved to be useful in infections in which protective mechanisms are impaired, such as in acute leukemia and during therapy with immunosuppressive or oncolytic drugs.

Gastrointestinal Disturbances: Nausea and vomiting.
Hemic and Lymphatic Systems: As with other penicillins, anemia, thrombocytopenia, leukopenia, neutropenia and eosinophilia.
Abnormalities of Blood, Hepatic and Renal Laboratory Studies: As with other semisynthetic penicillins, SGOT and SGPT elevations have been reported. To date, clinical manifestations of hepatic or renal disorders have not been observed which could be ascribed solely to Ticarcillin.
CNS: Patients, especially those with impaired renal function, may experience convulsions or neuromuscular excitability when very high doses of the drug are administered.
Other: Local reactions, such as pain (rarely accompanied by induration) at the site of injection have been reported.
Vein irritation and phlebitis can occur, particularly when undiluted solution is directly injected into the vein.
[See table above].

Directions For Use

1 Gm, 3 Gm and 6 Gm Standard Vials:
Intramuscular Use: Each gram of Ticarcillin should be reconstituted with 2 ml of Sterile Water of Injection, U.S.P. or 1% Lidocaine Hydrochloride solution (without epinephrine). Each 2.5 ml of the resulting solution will then contain 1 Gm of Ticarcillin.
[For full product information, refer to manufacturer's package insert for Lidocaine Hydrochloride.]
TICAR may also be diluted with bacteriostatic water containing 0.9% benzyl alcohol.
As with all intramuscular preparations, TICAR (Ticarcillin Disodium) should be injected well within the body of a relatively large muscle, using usual techniques and precautions.
I.M. solutions stored at room temperature must be discarded after 24 hours or after 72 hours if stored under refrigeration.
Intravenous Use: Reconstitute each gram of Ticarcillin with at least 4 ml of Sterile Water for Injection, U.S.P.; when dissolved, dilute further to desired volume.
Direct Intravenous Injection: In order to avoid vein irritation, administer solution as slowly as possible.
Intravenous Infusion: Reconstitute the required number of vials as described above, using a suitable intravenous solution listed below, then further dilute to the desired volume. Administer by continuous or intermittent intravenous drip. Intermittent infusion should be administered over a 30 minute to 2 hour period in six equally divided doses.

Continued on next page

Beecham Laboratories—Cont.

For the stability of TICAR in various intravenous solutions see DIRECTIONS FOR USE under Piggyback Bottles.

3 Gm and 6 Gm Piggyback Bottles:

Direct Intravenous Injection:

The 3 gram bottle should be reconstituted with a minimum of 30 ml Sterile Water for Injection, U.S.P.

Amount of Diluent	Concentration of Solution
100 ml	1 Gm/34 ml
60 ml	1 Gm/20 ml
30 ml	1 Gm/10 ml

The 6 gram bottle should be reconstituted with a minimum of 60 ml Sterile Water for Injection, U.S.P.

Amount of Diluent	Concentration of Solution
100 ml	1 Gm/17 ml
60 ml	1 Gm/10 ml

In order to avoid vein irritation, the solution should be administered as slowly as possible. A dilution of approximately 1 Gm/20 ml or more will further reduce the incidence of vein irritation.

Intravenous Infusion: Stability studies in various intravenous solutions indicate that Ticarcillin Disodium will lose less than 10% activity at room temperature within the stated time periods at concentrations between 10 mg/ml and 50 mg/ml:

Intravenous Solution	Time Period
*Sterile Water for Injection	72 hours
*Sodium Chloride Injection	72 hours
Dextrose 5% in 0.225% Sodium Chloride Solution	72 hours
Dextrose 5% in 0.45% Sodium Chloride Solution	72 hours
*Dextrose Injection 5%	72 hours
5% Alcohol, 5% Dextrose in 0.9% Sodium Chloride Solution	72 hours
*Ringer's Injection	48 hours
*Lactated Ringer's Injection	48 hours
10% Invert Sugar in Water	48 hours
5% Dextrose in Electrolyte #48 Solution	48 hours
5% Dextrose in Electrolyte #75 Solution	48 hours
5% Fructose (Levugen) in Electrolyte #75 Solution	48 hours

The above solutions remain stable for 14 days if stored under refrigeration (4°C); refrigerated solutions stored longer than 72 hours should not be used for multidose purposes.

(*) These solutions remain stable up to 100 mg/ml concentration. After reconstitution, they can be frozen (approx. 0°F) and stored for up to 30 days without loss of potency. The stabilities of the thawed solutions are identical to the unfrozen ones listed above.

Unused solutions should be discarded after the time periods mentioned above.

It is recommended that TICAR and gentamicin sulfate or tobramycin sulfate not be mixed together in the same I.V. solution due to the gradual inactivation of gentamicin sulfate or tobramycin sulfate under these circumstances. The therapeutic effect of TICAR and these aminoglycoside drugs remains unimpaired when administered separately.

How Supplied: TICAR (Sterile Ticarcillin Disodium). Each vial contains Ticarcillin Disodium equivalent to 1 Gm, 3 Gm or 6 Gm Ticarcillin.

NDC 0029-6550-22 ....1 Gm Vial
NDC 0029-6552-26 ....3 Gm Vial
NDC 0029-6555-26 ....6 Gm Vial
NDC 0029-6552-21 .....3 Gm Piggyback Bottle
NDC 0029-6555-21 .....6 Gm Piggyback Bottle

*Bauer, A.W., Kirby, W.M.M., Sherris, J.C. and Turck, M.: Antibiotic Testing by a Standardized Single Disc Method, Am. J. Clin. Pathol., 45:493, 1966. Standardized Disc Susceptibility Test, FEDERAL REGISTER 37:20527-29, 1972.

TIGAN® ℞
(trimethobenzamide HCl)

Description: Tigan is an antiemetic agent. Chemically, trimethobenzamide HCl is N-[*p*-[2-(dimethylamino)-ethoxy] benzyl]-3, 4, 5-trimethoxybenzamide hydrochloride. It has a molecular weight of 424.93.

Capsules; Blue, each containing 250 mg trimethobenzamide hydrochloride; blue and white, each containing 100 mg trimethobenzamide hydrochloride.

Suppositories: (200 mg): Each suppository contains 200 mg trimethobenzamide hydrochloride and 2% benzocaine in a base compounded with polysorbate 80, white beeswax and propylene glycol monostearate.

Suppositories, Pediatric (100 mg): Each suppository contains 100 mg trimethobenzamide hydrochloride and 2% benzocaine in a base compounded with polysorbate 80, white beeswax and propylene glycol monostearate.

Ampuls: Each 2-ml ampul contains 200 mg trimethobenzamide hydrochloride compounded with 0.2% parabens (methyl and propyl) as preservatives, 1 mg sodium citrate and 0.4 mg citric acid as buffers and pH adjusted to approximately 5.0 with sodium hydroxide.

Multiple Dose Vials: Each ml contains 100 mg trimethobenzamide hydrochloride compounded with 0.45% phenol as preservative, 0.5 mg sodium citrate and 0.2 mg citric acid as buffers and pH adjusted to approximately 5.0 with sodium hydroxide.

Thera-Ject™ (Disposable Syringes): Each 2 ml contains 200 mg trimethobenzamide hydrochloride compounded with 0.45% phenol as preservative, 1 mg sodium citrate and 0.4 mg citric acid as buffers, 0.2 mg disodium edetate as stabilizer and pH adjusted to approximately 5.0 with sodium hydroxide.

Actions: The mechanism of action of Tigan as determined in animals is obscure, but may be the chemoreceptor trigger zone (CTZ), an area in the medulla oblongata through which emetic impulses are conveyed to the vomiting center; direct impulses to the vomiting center apparently are not similarly inhibited. In dogs pretreated with trimethobenzamide HCl, the emetic response to apomorphine is inhibited, while little or no protection is afforded against emesis induced by intragastric copper sulfate.

Indications: Tigan is indicated for the control of nausea and vomiting.

Contraindications: The injectable form of Tigan in children, the suppositories in premature or newborn infants, and use in patients with known hypersensitivity to trimethobenzamide are contraindicated. Since the suppositories contain benzocaine they should not be used in patients known to be sensitive to this or similar local anesthetics.

Warnings:

> Caution should be exercised when administering Tigan to children for the treatment of vomiting. Antiemetics are not recommended for treatment of uncomplicated vomiting in children and their use should be limited to prolonged vomiting of known etiology. There are three principal reasons for caution:
>
> 1. There has been some suspicion that centrally acting antimetics may contribute, in combination with viral illnesses (a possible cause of vomiting in children), to development of Reye's syndrome, a potentially fatal acute childhood encephalopathy with visceral fatty degeneration, especially involving the liver. Although there is no confirmation of this suspicion, caution is nevertheless recommended.
>
> 2. The extrapyramidal symptoms which can occur secondary to Tigan may be confused with the cehtral nervous system signs of an undiagnosed primary disease responsible for the vomiting, e.g., Reye's syndrome or other encephalopathy.
>
> 3. It has been suspected that drugs with hepatotoxic potential, such as Tigan, may unfavorably alter the course of Reye's syndrome. Such drugs should therefore be avoided in children whose signs and symptoms (vomiting) could represent Reye's syndrome. It should also be noted that salicylates and acetaminophen are hepatotoxic at large doses. Although it is not known that at usual doses they would represent a hazard in patients with the underlying hepatic disorder of Reye's syndrome, these drugs, too, should be avoided in children whose signs and symptoms could represent Reye's syndrome, unless alternative methods of controlling fever are not successful.

Tigan may produce drowsiness. Patients should not operate motor vehicles or other dangerous machinery until their individual responses have been determined.

Reye's Syndrome has been associated with the use of TIGAN and other drugs, including antiemetics, although their contribution, if any, to the cause and course of the disease hasn't been established. This syndrome is characterized by an abrupt onset shortly following a nonspecific febrile illness, with persistent, severe vomiting, lethargy, irrational behavior, progressive encephalopathy leading to coma, convulsions and death.

Usage in Pregnancy: Trimethobenzamide hydrochloride was studied in reproduction experiments in rats and rabbits and no teratogenicity was suggested. The only effects observed were an increased percentage of embryonic resorptions or stillborn pups in rats administered 20 mg and 100 mg/kg and increased resorptions in rabbits receiving 100 mg/kg. In each study these adverse effects were attributed to one or two dams. The relevance to humans is not known. Since there is no adequate experience in pregnant or lactating women who have received this drug, safety in pregnancy or in nursing mothers has not been established.

Precautions: During the course of acute febrile illness, encephalitides, gastroenteritis, dehydration and electrolyte imbalance, especially in children and the elderly or debilitated, CNS reactions such as opisthotonos, convulsions, coma and extrapyramidal symptoms have been reported with and without use of Tigan or other antiemetic agents. In such disorders caution should be exercised in administering Tigan, particularly to patients who have recently received other CNS-acting agents (phenothiazines, barbiturates, belladonna derivatives). It is recommended that severe emesis should not be treated with an antiemetic drug alone; where possible the cause of vomiting should be established. Primary emphasis should be directed toward the restoration of body fluids and electrolyte balance, the relief of fever and relief of the causative disease process. Overhydration should be avoided since it may result in cerebral edema.

The antiemetic effects of Tigan may render diagnosis more difficult in such conditions as appendicitis and obscure signs of toxicity due to overdosage of other drugs.

Adverse Reactions: There have been reports of hypersensitivity reactions and Parkinson-like symptoms. There have been instances of hypotension reported following parenteral administration to surgical patients. There have been reports of blood dyscrasias, blurring of vision, coma, convulsions, depression of mood, diarrhea, disorientation, dizziness, drowsiness, headache, jaundice, muscle cramps and opisthotonos. If these occur, the administration of the drug should be discontinued. Allergic-type skin reactions have been observed; therefore, the drug should be discontinued at the first sign of sensitization. While these symptoms will usually disappear spontaneously, symptomatic treatment may be indicated in some cases.

Dosage and Administration: (See WARNINGS and PRECAUTIONS.) Dosage should be adjusted according to the indication for therapy, severity of symptoms and the response of the patient.

Capsules, 250 mg and 100 mg

Usual Adult Dosage

One 250-mg capsule t.i.d. or q.i.d.

Usual Children's Dosage

30 to 90 lbs: One or two 100-mg capsules t.i.d. or q.i.d.

Suppositories, 200 mg (Not to be used in premature or newborn infants.)

Usual Adult Dosage

One suppository (200 mg) t.i.d. or q.i.d.

Usual Children's Dosage

Under 30 lbs: One-half suppository (100 mg) t.i.d. or q.i.d.

30 to 90 lbs: One-half to one suppository (100 to 200 mg) t.i.d. or q.i.d.

SUPPOSITORIES, PEDIATRIC, 100 mg (Not to be used in Premature or newborn infants).

Usual Children's Dosage

Under 30 lbs; One suppository (100 mg) t.i.d. or q.i.d.

30 to 90 lbs; One to two suppositories (100 to 200 mg) t.i.d. or q.i.d.

Injectable, 100 mg/ml (Not recommended for use in children.)

Usual Adult Dosage: 2 ml (200 mg) t.i.d. or q.i.d. intramuscularly.

Intramuscular administration may cause pain, stinging, burning, redness and swelling at the site of injection. Such effects may be minimized by deep injection into the upper outer quadrant of the gluteal region, and by avoiding the escape of solution along the route.

Note: The injectable form is intended for intramuscular administration only; it is not recommended for intravenous use.

How Supplied:

Product	Package Sizes	NDC Numbers
Capsules		
100 mg.	100's	NDC-0029-4082-30
250 mg.	100's	NDC-0029-4083-30
	500's	NDC-0029-4083-32
Suppositories		
200 mg.	10's	NDC-0029-4084-38
	50's	NDC-0029-4084-39
Suppositories Pediatric		
100 mg.	10's	NDC-0029-4088-38
Injectable		
Ampuls		
2 ml, 200 mg.	10's	NDC-0029-4085-22
Vials		
20 ml, 100 mg./ml	Each	NDC-0029-4086-22
Thera-Ject® (Disposable Syringe)		
2 ml, 100 mg./ml	25's	NDC-0029-4087-22

[*Shown in Product Identification Section*]

TOTACILLIN®-N ℞

(sterile ampicillin sodium)

Description: TOTACILLIN-N (ampicillin sodium) is derived from the penicillin nucleus, 6-aminopenicillanic acid (6-APA), isolated by Beecham. Chemically, it is D(-)α-aminobenzyl penicillin sodium salt.

Actions:

MICROBIOLOGY:

TOTACILLIN-N (ampicillin sodium) is similar to benzyl penicillin in its bactericidal action against sensitive organisms during the stage of active multiplication. It acts through the inhibition of biosynthesis of cell wall mucopeptide. TOTACILLIN-N (ampicillin sodium) differs in *in vitro* spectrum from benzyl penicillin in the Gram-negative spectrum. It exerts high *in vitro* activity against many strains of *Haemophilus influenzae, Neisseria gonorrhoeae, Neisseria meningitidis, Neisseria catarrhalis, Escherichia coli, Proteus mirabilis, Bacteroides funduliformis, Salmonellae* and *Shigellae.*

In vitro studies have also demonstrated the sensitivity of many strains of the following Gram-positive bacteria: alpha- and beta-hemolytic streptococci, *Diplococcus pneumoniae,* nonpenicillinase-producing staphylococci, *Bacillus anthracis,* and most strains of enterococci and clostridia. Ampicillin generally provides less *in vitro* activity than penicillin-G against Gram-positive bacteria. Because it does not resist destruction by penicillinase, it is not effective against penicillinase-producing bacteria, particularly resistant staphylococci. All strains of Pseudomonas and most strains of Klebsiella and Aerobacter are resistant.

PHARMACOLOGY:

TOTACILLIN-N (ampicillin sodium) diffuses readily into all body tissues and fluids with the exception of brain and spinal fluid except when meninges are inflamed. It produces high and persistent blood levels. Most of the ampicillin is excreted unchanged in the urine and this excretion can be delayed by concurrent administration of probenecid. The active form appears in the bile in higher concentrations than found in the serum. TOTACILLIN-N (ampicillin sodium) is one of the least serum bound of all the penicillins, averaging about 20% compared to approximately 60%-90% for other penicillins.

Indications: TOTACILLIN-N (ampicillin sodium) is indicated in the treatment of infections due to susceptible strains of the following:

Gram-Negative Organisms: *Shigellae, Salmonellae* (including *S. typhosa*), *H. influenzae, E. coli, P. mirabilis, N. gonorrhoeae,* and *N. meningitidis.*

Gram-Positive Organisms: Streptococci, *D. pneumoniae,* and nonpenicillinase-producing staphylococci.

Because of its wide spectrum and bactericidal action, it may be useful in instituting therapy; however, bacteriological studies to determine the causative organisms and their sensitivity to ampicillin should be performed.

Indicated surgical procedures should be performed.

Contraindications: A history of allergic reaction to any of the penicillins is a contraindication.

Warnings: SERIOUS AND OCCASIONALLY FATAL HYPERSENSITIVITY (ANAPHYLACTOID) REACTIONS HAVE BEEN REPORTED IN PATIENTS ON PENICILLIN THERAPY. ALTHOUGH ANAPHYLAXIS IS MORE FREQUENT FOLLOWING PARENTERAL THERAPY, IT HAS OCCURRED IN PATIENTS ON ORAL PENICILLINS. THESE REACTIONS ARE MORE APT TO OCCUR IN INDIVIDUALS WITH A HISTORY OF PENICILLIN HYPERSENSITIVITY AND/OR HYPERSENSITIVITY REACTIONS TO MULTIPLE ALLERGENS. THERE HAVE BEEN REPORTS OF INDIVIDUALS WITH A HISTORY OF PENICILLIN HYPERSENSITIVITY WHO HAVE EXPERIENCED SEVERE REACTIONS WHEN TREATED WITH CEPHALOSPORINS. BEFORE THERAPY WITH A PENICILLIN, CAREFUL INQUIRY SHOULD BE MADE CONCERNING PREVIOUS HYPERSENSITIVITY REACTIONS TO PENICILLINS, CEPHALOSPORINS, AND OTHER ALLERGENS. IF AN ALLERGIC REACTION OCCURS, THE DRUG SHOULD BE DISCONTINUED AND THE APPROPRIATE THERAPY INSTITUTED. **SERIOUS ANAPHYLACTOID REACTIONS REQUIRE IMMEDIATE EMERGENCY TREATMENT WITH EPINEPHRINE. OXYGEN, INTRAVENOUS STEROIDS AND AIRWAY MANAGEMENT, INCLUDING INTUBATION, SHOULD ALSO BE ADMINISTERED AS INDICATED.**

Usage in Pregnancy

Safety for use in pregnancy has not been established.

Precautions: As with any antibiotic preparation, constant observation for signs of overgrowth of nonsusceptible organisms, including fungi, is essential. Should superinfection occur (usually involving Aerobacter, Pseudomonas, or Candida), the drug should be discontinued and/or appropriate therapy instituted.

As with any potent agent, it is advisable to check periodically for organ system dysfunction during prolonged therapy; this includes renal, hepatic, and hematopoietic systems. This is particularly important in prematures, neonates and other infants.

Adverse Reactions: As with other penicillins, it may be expected that untoward reactions will be essentially limited to sensitivity phenomena. They are more likely to occur in individuals who have previously demonstrated hypersensitivity to penicillins and in those with a history of allergy, asthma, hay fever, or urticaria.

The following adverse reactions have been reported as associated with the use of ampicillin:

Gastrointestinal: Glossitis, stomatitis, black "hairy" tongue, nausea, vomiting, and diarrhea. (These reactions are usually associated with oral dosage forms).

Hypersensitivity reactions: An erythematous maculopapular rash has been reported fairly frequently. Urticaria and erythema multiforme have been reported occasionally. A few cases of exfoliative dermatitis have been reported. Anaphylaxis is the most serious reaction experienced and has usually been associated with the parenteral dosage form.

Note: Urticaria, other skin rashes, and serum sickness-like reactions may be controlled with antihistamines and, if necessary, systemic corticosteroids. Whenever such reactions occur, ampicillin should be discontinued unless, in the opinion of the physician, the condition being treated is life-threatening and amenable only to ampicillin therapy.

Liver—A moderate rise in serum glutamic oxaloacetic transaminase (SGOT) has been noted, particularly in infants, but the significance of this finding is unknown.

Hemic and Lymphatic Systems—Anemia, thrombocytopenia, thrombocytopenic purpura, eosinophilia, leukopenia, and agranulocytosis have been reported during therapy with the penicillins. These reactions are usually reversible on discontinuation of therapy and are believed to be sensitivity reactions.

Dosage and Administration: *Infections of the ear, nose, throat, and lower respiratory tract* due to streptococci, pneumococci, and nonpenicillinase-producing staphylococci; and also those infections *of the upper and lower respiratory tract due to H. influenzae:*

ADULTS: 250-500 mg. every 6 hours.

CHILDREN: 12.5 mg./kg. every 6 hours.

Infections of the genitourinary tract caused by sensitive Gram-negative and Gram-positive bacteria:

ADULTS: 500 mg. every 6 hours.

CHILDREN: 12.5 mg./kg. every 6 hours.

Urethritis due to N. gonorrhoeae in adult males: 500 mg. every 12 hours for 1 day. Treatment may be repeated if necessary.

Cases of gonorrhea with a suspected lesion of syphilis should have dark-field examinations before receiving ampicillin, and monthly serological tests for a minimum of 4 months.

Continued on next page

Beecham Laboratories—Cont.

Infections of the gastrointestinal tract:
ADULTS: 500 mg. every 6 hours.
CHILDREN: 12.5 mg./kg. every 6 hours.
Larger doses may be required for stubborn or severe infections. The children's dosage is intended for individuals whose weight will not cause a dosage to be calculated greater than that recommended for adults. Children weighing more than 20 kg. should be dosed according to the adult recommendations.
It should be recognized that in the treatment of chronic urinary tract and intestinal infections, frequent bacteriological and clinical appraisals are necessary. Smaller doses than those recommended above should not be used. Even higher doses may be needed at times. In stubborn infections, therapy may be required for several weeks. It may be necessary to continue clinical and/or bacteriological follow-up for several months after cessation of therapy.
Treatment should be continued for a minimum of 48 to 72 hours beyond the time that the patient becomes asymptomatic or evidence of bacterial eradication has been obtained. It is recommended that there be at least 10 days' treatment for any infection caused by hemolytic streptococci, to help prevent the occurrence of acute rheumatic fever or glomerulonephritis.
Bacterial meningitis:
Children with bacterial meningitis caused by *N. meningitidis* or *H. influenzae* have been successfully treated with doses of 150-200 mg./kg./day. A few adults have been successfully treated for bacterial meningitis with doses ranging from 8 to 14 Gm. daily. Treatment was initiated with intravenous drip therapy for at least 3 days, and continued with frequent (every 3 to 4 hours) intramuscular therapy.
Septicemia:
For adults, a dosage of 8-14 Gm. daily is recommended, starting with I.V. administration for at least 3 days and continuing with the I.M. route every 3 to 4 hours. For children, a dosage of 150-200 mg./kg./day is recommended, starting with I.V. administration for at least 3 days and continuing with the I.M. route every 3 to 4 hours.
[See table below].
Although the 1 Gm and 2 Gm Standard Vials are intended primarily for I.V. use, the desired aliquots from these dosage sizes may be administered intramuscularly when the 125 mg, 250 mg or 500 mg concentrations are unavailable. In such instances, dissolve the 1 Gm in 3.4 ml or the 2 Gm in 6.8 ml Sterile Water for Injection, U.S.P. The resulting solutions will provide a concentration of 250 mg per ml.
Use solutions within one hour after reconstitution, since the potency may decrease significantly after this period.

Intravenous Solution	Concentration	Stability Period
Sterile Water for Injection	up to 30 mg/ml	8 hours
Isotonic Sodium Chloride Solution	up to 30 mg/ml	8 hours
M/6 Sodium Lactate Solution	up to 30 mg/ml	8 hours
5% Dextrose in Water	up to 2 mg/ml	4 hours
5% Dextrose in Water	10 to 20 mg/ml	2 hours
5% Dextrose in 0.45% Sodium Chloride Solution	up to 2 mg/ml	4 hours
10% Invert Sugar in Water	up to 2 mg/ml	4 hours
Lactated Ringer's Solution	up to 30 mg/ml	8 hours

If the solutions listed below are stored under refrigeration (40°F), they will remain stable for the time periods indicated:

Intravenous Solution	Concentration	Stability Period
Sterile Water for Injection	30 mg/ml	48 hours
Sterile Water for Injection	up to 20 mg/ml	72 hours
Isotonic Sodium Chloride Solution	30 mg/ml	48 hours
Isotonic Sodium Chloride Solution	up to 20 mg/ml	72 hours
Lactated Ringer's Solution	up to 30 mg/ml	24 hours
M/6 Sodium Lactate Solution	up to 30 mg/ml	8 hours
5% Dextrose in Water	up to 20 mg/ml	4 hours
5% Dextrose in 0.45% Sodium Choride Solution	up to 10 mg/ml	4 hours
10% Inverted Sugar in Water	up to 20 mg/ml	3 hours

DIRECT INTRAVENOUS ADMINISTRATION:
Dissolve 125 mg., 250 mg. or 500 mg. in 5 ml. of Sterile Water for Injection, U.S.P. Administer every six hours by slow injection (3 to 4 minutes).
Use solutions within one hour after reconstitution, since the potency may decrease significantly after this period.
CONTINUOUS INTRAVENOUS INFUSION:
Reconstitute as directed under INTRAMUSCULAR ADMINISTRATION prior to diluting with intravenous solution.
For the stability of TOTACILLIN-N in various intravenous solutions see **Directions for Use** under Piggyback Bottles.
500 mg, 1 Gm and 2 Gm Piggyback Bottles for Intravenous Drip Use:
Use Sterile Water for Injection, U.S.P. or Sodium Chloride Injection, U.S.P.
500 mg Bottle:
Add a minimum of 50 ml sterile water or saline and shake well. If lower concentrations are desired, the solution could be further diluted with up to a total of 100 ml of diluent.

Amount of Diluent	Concentration of Solution
50 ml	10 mg/ml
100 ml	5 mg/ml

1 Gm. Bottle:
Add a minimum of 49 ml. sterile water or saline and shake well. If lower concentrations are desired, the solution could be further diluted with up to a total of 99 ml. of diluent.

Amount of Diluent	Concentration of Solution
49 ml.	20 mg./ml.
99 ml.	10 mg./ml.

2 Gm. Bottle:
Add 99 ml. sterile water or saline and shake well. The resulting solution will contain 20 mg./ml. ampicillin.
Stability studies on ampicillin sodium in various intravenous solutions indicate that the ampicillin sodium will lose less than 10% activity at room temperature (70°F) for the time periods and concentrations stated:
[See table above].
TOTACILLIN-N (ampicillin sodium) 1 Gm. and 2 Gm. for Intravenous Therapy
Intravenous therapy is recommended in serious infections when prompt, effective levels of the antibiotic must reach the site of the infection. Such infections include meningitis, subacute bacterial endocarditis, peritonitis, septicemia, severe forms of chronic bronchitis, osteomyelitis, pneumonia and pyelonephritis due to susceptible organisms.
The 1 Gm and 2 Gm in the Standard Vials and the Piggyback Bottles may be given by either intravenous drip as indicated above or by direct intravenous injection. For direct intravenous administration, dissolve 1 Gm. or 2 Gm. in at least 7.4 ml. Sterile Water for Injection, U.S.P. and administer slowly over 10 to 15 minutes. **CAUTION:** More rapid administration may result in convulsive seizures.
How Supplied: TOTACILLIN-N (sterile ampicillin sodium). Each vial contains ampicillin sodium equivalent to 125 mg., 250 mg., 500 mg., 1 Gm. or 2 Gm. ampicillin.
NDC 0029-6595-24 ....125 mg. Vial
NDC 0029-6600-24 ....250 mg. Vial
NDC 0029-6605-24 ....500 mg. Vial
NDC 0029-6610-25 .... 1 Gm. Vial
NDC 0029-6612-22 ....2 Gm. Vial
NDC 0029-6605-21 ...500 mg Piggyback Bottle
NDC 0029-6610-21 ....1 Gm. Piggyback Bottles
NDC 0029-6612-21 ....2 Gm. Piggyback Bottles

Directions for TOTACILLIN-N Use
125 mg., 250 mg., 500 mg., 1 Gm. and 2 Gm. Standard Vials:
INTRAMUSCULAR ADMINISTRATION:
Dissolve 125 mg. and 250 mg. in 0.9-1.9 ml. and 500 mg. in 1.7 ml. of Sterile Water for Injection, U.S.P. The entire contents should be withdrawn.

Potency	*Recommended amount of Sterile Water for Injection, U.S.P.*	*Available Volume*	*Concentration mg./ml.*
125 mg.	1.0 ml.	1.0 ml.	125 mg.
250 mg.	0.9 ml.	1.0 ml.	250 mg.
	or 1.9 ml.	2.0 ml.	125 mg.
500 mg.	1.7 ml.	2.0 ml.	250 mg.
1 Gm.	3.4 ml.	4.0 ml.	250 mg.
	or 7.4 ml.	8.0 ml.	125 mg.
2 Gm.	6.8 ml.	8.0 ml.	250 mg.

TOTACILLIN® ℞
(ampicillin)
CAPSULES
250 mg. and 500 mg.
FOR ORAL SUSPENSION
125 mg./5 ml. and 250 mg./5 ml.

Description: TOTACILLIN (ampicillin) is derived from the penicillin nucleus, 6-aminopenicillanic acid (6-APA), isolated by Beecham. Chemically it is D (-) α-aminobenzyl penicillin trihydrate.

Actions:
MICROBIOLOGY:
TOTACILLIN (ampicillin) is similar to benzyl penicillin in its bactericidal action against sensitive organisms during the stage of active multiplication. It acts through the inhibition of biosynthesis of cell wall mucopeptide. TOTACILLIN (ampicillin) differs in *in vitro* spectrum from benzylpenicillin in the Gram-negative spectrum. It exerts high *in vitro* activity against many strains of *Haemophilus influenzae, Neisseria gonorrhoeae, Neisseria meningitidis, Neisseria catarrhalis, Escherichia coli, Proteus mirabilis, Bacteroides funduliformis, Salmonellae* and *Shigellae.*
In vitro studies have also demonstrated the sensitivity of many strains of the following Gram-positive bacteria: alpha- and beta-hemolytic streptococci, *Diplococcus pneumoniae,* nonpenicillinase-producing staphylococci, *Bacillus anthracis,* and most strains of enterococci and clostridia. Ampicillin generally provides less *in vitro* activity than penicillin-G against Gram-positive bacteria. Because it does not resist destruction by penicillinase, it is not effective against penicillinase-producing bacteria, particularly resistant staphylococci. All strains of Pseudomonas and most strains of Klebsiella and Aerobacter are resistant.
PHARMACOLOGY:
TOTACILLIN (ampicillin) is acid stable and, therefore, well absorbed. Food, however, retards absorption. Blood serum levels of approximately 2 mcg./ml. are attained within 1-2 hours following a 250 mg. oral dose given to fasting adults. Detectable amounts persist for about 6 hours. TOTACILLIN (ampicillin) diffuses readily into all body tissues and fluids with the exception of brain and spinal fluid except when meninges are inflamed. Higher serum levels are obtained following I.M. injection. Most of the ampicillin is excreted unchanged in the urine, and this excretion can be delayed by concurrent administration of probenecid. The active form appears in the bile in higher concentrations than found in the serum. TOTACILLIN (ampicillin) is one of the least serum bound of all the penicillins, averaging about 20% compared to approximately 60%-90% for other penicillins.

Indications: TOTACILLIN (ampicillin) is indicated in the treatment of infections due to susceptible strains of the following:
Gram-Negative Organisms: *Shigellae, Salmonellae* (including *S. typhosa*), *H. influenzae, E. coli, P. mirabilis, N. gonorrhoeae,* and *N. meningitidis.*
Gram-Positive Organisms: Streptococci, *D. pneumoniae,* and nonpenicillinase-producing staphylococci.
Because of its wide spectrum and bactericidal action, it may be useful in instituting therapy; however, bacteriological studies to determine the causative organisms and their sensitivity to ampicillin should be performed.
Indicated surgical procedures should be performed.

Contraindications: A history of allergic reaction to any of the penicillins is a contraindication.

Warnings: SERIOUS AND OCCASIONALLY FATAL HYPERSENSITIVITY (ANAPHYLACTOID) REACTIONS HAVE BEEN REPORTED IN PATIENTS ON PENICILLIN THERAPY. ALTHOUGH ANAPHYLAXIS IS MORE FREQUENT FOLLOWING PARENTERAL THERAPY, IT HAS OCCURRED IN PATIENTS ON ORAL PENICILLINS. THESE REACTIONS ARE MORE APT TO OCCUR IN INDIVIDUALS WITH A HISTORY OF PENICILLIN HYPERSENSITIVITY AND/OR HYPERSENSITIVITY REACTIONS TO MULTIPLE ALLERGENS. THERE HAVE BEEN REPORTS OF INDIVIDUALS WITH A HISTORY OF PENICILLIN HYPERSENSITIVITY WHO HAVE EXPERIENCED SEVERE REACTIONS WHEN TREATED WITH CEPHALOSPORINS. BEFORE THERAPY WITH A PENICILLIN, CAREFUL INQUIRY SHOULD BE MADE CONCERNING PREVIOUS HYPERSENSITIVITY REACTIONS TO PENICILLINS, CEPHALOSPORINS, AND OTHER ALLERGENS. IF AN ALLERGIC REACTION OCCURS, THE DRUG SHOULD BE DISCONTINUED AND THE APPROPRIATE THERAPY INSTITUTED. **SERIOUS ANAPHYLACTOID REACTIONS REQUIRE IMMEDIATE EMERGENCY TREATMENT WITH EPINEPHRINE. OXYGEN, INTRAVENOUS STEROIDS AND AIRWAY MANAGEMENT, INCLUDING INTUBATION, SHOULD ALSO BE ADMINISTERED AS INDICATED.**
USAGE IN PREGNANCY:
Safety for use in pregnancy has not been established.

Precautions: As with any antibiotic preparation, constant observation for signs of overgrowth of nonsusceptible organisms, including fungi, is essential. Should superinfection occur (usually involving Aerobacter, Pseudomonas, or Candida), the drug should be discontinued and/or appropriate therapy instituted.
As with any potent agent, it is advisable to check periodically for organ system dysfunction during prolonged therapy; this includes renal, hepatic, and hematopoietic systems. This is particularly important in prematures, neonates and other infants.

Adverse Reactions: As with other penicillins, it may be expected that untoward reactions will be essentially limited to sensitivity phenomena. They are more likely to occur in individuals who have previously demonstrated hypersensitivity to penicillins and in those with a history of allergy, asthma, hay fever, or urticaria.
The following adverse reactions have been reported as associated with the use of ampicillin:
Gastrointestinal—Glossitis, stomatitis, black "hairy" tongue, nausea, vomiting, enterocolitis, pseudomembranous colitis and diarrhea. (These reactions are usually associated with oral dosage forms.)
Hypersensitivity reactions—An erythematous maculopapular rash has been reported fairly frequently. Urticaria and erythema multiforme have been reported occasionally. A few cases of exfoliative dermatitis have been reported. Anaphylaxis is the most serious reaction experienced and has usually been associated with the parenteral dosage form.
Note: Urticaria, other skin rashes, and serum sickness-like reactions may be controlled with antihistamines and, if necessary, systemic corticosteroids. Whenever such reactions occur, ampicillin should be discontinued unless, in the opinion of the physician, the condition being treated is life-threatening and amenable only to ampicillin therapy.
Liver—A moderate rise in serum glutamic oxaloacetic transaminase (SGOT) has been noted, particularly in infants, but the significance of this finding is unknown.
Hemic and Lymphatic Systems—Anemia, thrombocytopenia, thrombocytopenic purpura, eosinophilia, leukopenia, and agranulocytosis have been reported during therapy with the penicillins. These reactions are usually reversible on discontinuation of therapy and are believed to be sensitivity reactions.

Dosage: *Infections of the ear, nose, throat, and lower respiratory tract* due to streptococci, pneumococci, and nonpenicillinase-producing staphylococci, and also those infections of *the upper and lower respiratory tract due to H. influenzae:*
Adults: 250 mg. every 6 hours.
Children: 50 mg./kg./day in divided doses every 6 to 8 hours.
Infections of the genitourinary tract caused by sensitive Gram-negative and Gram-positive bacteria:
Adults: 500 mg. every 6 hours. Larger doses may be required for severe infections.
Children: 100 mg./kg./day in divided doses every 6 hours.
Uncomplicated urethritis due to N. gonorrhoeae. Adult Males and Females—3.5 grams single oral dose administered simultaneously with 1 gram of probenecid.
Cases of gonorrhea with a suspected lesion of syphilis should have dark-field examinations before receiving ampicillin, and monthly serological tests for a minimum of 4 months.
Infections of the gastrointestinal tract:
Adults: 500 mg. every 6 hours.
Children: 100 mg./kg./day in divided doses every 6 hours.
Larger doses may be required for stubborn or severe infections. The children's dosage is intended for individuals whose weight will not cause a dosage to be calculated greater than that recommended for adults. Children weighing more than 20 kg. should be dosed according to the adult recommendations.
It should be recognized that in the treatment of chronic urinary tract and intestinal infections, frequent bacteriological and clinical appraisals are necessary. Smaller doses than those recommended above should not be used. Even higher doses may be needed at times. In stubborn infections, therapy may be required for several weeks. It may be necessary to continue clinical and/or bacteriological follow-up for several months after cessation of therapy.
Treatment should be continued for a minimum of 48 to 72 hours beyond the time that the patient becomes asymptomatic or evidence of bacterial eradication has been obtained. It is recommended that there be at least 10 days' treatment for any infection caused by hemolytic streptococci, to help prevent the occurrence of acute rheumatic fever or glomerulonephritis.

Directions for Mixing Oral Suspension:
Prepare suspension at time of dispensing as follows: Add the required amount of water (see table below) to the bottle. For ease of preparation, add water in two portions. Shake well after each addition of water. Each teaspoonful (5 ml.) will contain 125 mg. or 250 mg. ampicillin.

Bottle size	Amount of Water required for reconstitution
80 ml.	53 ml.
100 ml.	66 ml.
150 ml.	100 ml.
200 ml.	132 ml.

SHAKE WELL BEFORE USING. Keep bottle tightly closed. Any unused portion of the reconstituted suspension must be discarded after 7 days at room temperature or 14 days under refrigeration.

How Supplied: TOTACILLIN (ampicillin) **Capsules.** Each capsule contains 250 mg. or 500 mg. ampicillin as the trihydrate.

250 mg./Capsule
NDC 0029-6615-28............................bottles of 40
NDC 0029-6615-30............................bottles of 100
NDC 0029-6615-32............................bottles of 500
NDC 0029-6615-31............................unit dose cartons of 100

500 mg./Capsule
NDC 0029-6620-28............................bottles of 40
NDC 0029-6620-29............................bottles of 50
NDC 0029-6620-32............................bottles of 500
NDC 0029-6620-31............................unit dose cartons of 100

TOTACILLIN (ampicillin) **for Oral Suspension.** Each 5 ml. of reconstituted suspension contains 125 mg. or 250 mg. ampicillin as the trihydrate.

125 mg./5 ml.
NDC 0029-6625-21.................... 80 ml. bottle
NDC 0029-6625-23.................... 100 ml. bottle
NDC 0029-6625-22.................... 150 ml. bottle
NDC 0029-6625-24.................... 200 ml. bottle

250 mg./5 ml.
NDC 0029-6630-21.................... 80 ml. bottle

Continued on next page

Beecham Laboratories—Cont.

NDC 0029-6630-23 .... 100 ml. bottle
NDC 0029-6630-22 .... 150 ml. bottle
NDC 0029-6630-24 .... 200 ml. bottle

Berlex Laboratories Inc.
CEDAR KNOLLS, NJ 07927

AMINODUR® DURA-TABS® ℞
(aminophylline)

Description: Each tablet contains 300 mg hydrous aminophylline (equivalent to 236 mg anhydrous theophylline) in a tablet matrix specially designed for prolonged release of the drug.
Actions: Aminophylline has the general physiological properties of theophylline. Theophylline, a xanthine derivative, relaxes smooth muscle constrictions of the smaller bronchi, promotes dilation of the small pulmonary arteries, increases cardiac output and is a mild diuretic.
Indications: For relief of acute bronchial asthma and for reversible bronchospasm associated with chronic bronchitis and emphysema.
Contraindications: Sensitivity to any of the ingredients. May be contraindicated in peptic ulcer.
Warning: Xanthine preparations should be used with caution in children.
Precautions: Use cautiously in patients with poor renal function as a decreased rate of excretion may lead to untoward reactions. Use with caution in the presence of cardiovascular diseases, severe hypertension, and with the concurrent use of additional xanthines or sympathomimetic amines from other medications.
Adverse Reactions: Epigastric distress, nausea, vomiting, palpitations, mild CNS stimulation, restlessness and insomnia have been reported.
Dosage and Administration: *Adults:* 1 to 2 tablets every 8 to 12 hours approximately 30 minutes before eating. Not recommended for children under 12 years of age. Patients may develop gastrointestinal disturbances after prolonged use; the simultaneous administration of aluminum hydroxide decreases the incidence of this side effect.
How Supplied: Scored Dura-Tabs in bottles of:
100 ....NDC 50419-131-10
250 ....NDC 50419-131-25
[*Shown in Product Identification Section*]

DECONAMINE® Tablets ℞
DECONAMINE® Elixir ℞
DECONAMINE® SR Capsules ℞
DECONAMINE® Syrup ℞

Description:
Tablets—Each blue color tablet contains:
Chlorpheniramine Maleate ....4 mg
d-Pseudoephedrine Hydrochloride ....60 mg
Elixir—Each 5 ml (teaspoonful) blue color liquid contains:
Chlorpheniramine Maleate ....2 mg
d-Pseudoephedrine Hydrochloride ....30 mg
Alcohol 15%
In a pleasant-tasting aromatic vehicle.
SR Capsules—Each sustained release blue and yellow capsule contains:
Chlorpheniramine Maleate ....8 mg
d-Pseudoephedrine Hydrochloride ....120 mg
The capsules are designed to provide prolonged release of medication.
Syrup—No alcohol. No dye. Each 5 ml (teaspoonful) clear liquid contains
Chlorpheniramine Maleate ....2 mg
d-Pseudoephedrine
Hydrochloride ....30 mg
in a grape-flavored aromatic vehicle.
Actions: Chlorpheniramine maleate antagonizes the physiological action of histamine. d-Pseudoephedrine hydrochloride provides a rapid and sustained decongestant effect on swollen mucosa of the respiratory tract. It does this by vasoconstriction and opens obstructed airways through direct action on the smooth muscle of the bronchi. The vasoconstrictor action of pseudoephedrine is similar to that of ephedrine. In the usual oral dosage, it has minimal vasopressor effects.
Indications: For relief of upper respiratory and bronchial congestion associated with the common cold, hay fever and other allergies, sinusitis, eustachian tube blockage, and vasomotor and allergic rhinitis.
Contraindications: Sensitivity to antihistamines or sympathomimetic agents. It should not be used in patients with severe hypertension or coronary artery disease.
Warnings: Patients should be warned about possible additive effects with alcohol and other central nervous system depressants (hypnotics, sedatives, tranquilizers), and warned against hazardous occupations requiring complete mental alertness such as operating machinery or driving a motor vehicle.
Safety of Deconamine for use during pregnancy has not been established.
Capsules or tablets should not be given to children under 12 years of age.
Precautions: Should be used with caution in the presence of hypertension, coronary artery disease, glaucoma, prostatic hypertrophy, hyperthyroidism and diabetes.
Adverse Reactions: Most patients will have no adverse effects at the usual dosage. However, certain patients may exhibit mild stimulation or mild sedation. Although rare, hypersensitivity to either the antihistamine or decongestant may occur.
Dosage and Administration:
Tablets—Adults and children over 12 years, one tablet three or four times daily. Children under 12 years, Deconomine Elixir or Syrup is recommended.
Elixir or Syrup—Adults and children over 12 years, 1 to 2 teaspoonfuls (5 to 10 ml) 3 or 4 times daily. Children 6 to 12 years, ½ to 1 teaspoonful (2.5 to 5 ml) 3 or 4 times daily. Children 2 to 6 years, ½ teaspoonful (2.5 ml) 3 or 4 times daily, not to exceed 3 teaspoonfuls in 24 hours. Children under 2 years, as directed by physician.
SR Capsules—Adults and children over 12 years, one capsule every 12 hours. Children under 12 years, Deconomine Elixir or Syrup is recommended.
How Supplied: In bottles of:
Tablets:
100 ....NDC 50419-183-10
500 ....NDC 50419-183-50
Elixir:
473 ml ....NDC 50419-182-16
SR Capsules:
100 ....NDC 50419-181-10
500 ....NDC 50419-181-50
Syrup:
473 ml ....NDC 50419-185-16
[*Shown in Product Identification Section*]

ELIXICON® Suspension ℞
(theophylline)

Description: Each 5 ml (teaspoonful) contains 100 mg anhydrous theophylline in an aqueous suspension. Contains no sugar or dye. Preserved with methylparaben and propylparaben.
Indications: For relief of acute bronchial asthma and for reversible bronchospasm as in chronic bronchitis and emphysema.
Contraindications: Sensitivity to any of the ingredients. May be contraindicated in peptic ulcer.
Precautions: Use with caution in the presence of cardiovascular disease and with the concurrent use of additional xanthines or sympathomimetic amines.
Adverse Reactions: Epigastric distress, nausea, vomiting, palpitations, mild CNS stimulation, restlessness and insomnia have been reported.
Dosage and Administration: *Children:* 1 teaspoonful (5 ml) per 55 lbs (25 kg) body weight every 6 hours. Dose should be individualized according to the needs of the patient on a mg/kg basis. *Adults:* 2 teaspoonfuls (10 ml) t.i.d. upon arising, at 3:00 p.m. and at bedtime.
How Supplied: In bottles of:
237 ml ....NDC 50419-112-08

ELIXOPHYLLIN® CAPSULES ℞
100 mg, 200 mg
(theophylline)

ELIXOPHYLLIN® SR CAPSULES ℞
125 mg, 250 mg
(theophylline)

ELIXOPHYLLIN® ELIXIR ℞
(theophylline)

ELIXOPHYLLIN-KI® ELIXIR ℞
(theophylline/potassium iodide)

Elixophyllin product information is consistent with FDA theophylline labeling guidelines. Please see individual products for additional information before prescribing.
Clinical Pharmacology: Theophylline directly relaxes the smooth muscle of the bronchial airways and pulmonary blood vessels, thus acting mainly as a bronchodilator, pulmonary vasodilator and smooth muscle relaxant. The drug also possesses other actions typical of the xanthine derivatives: coronary vasodilator, diuretic, cardiac stimulant, cerebral stimulant and skeletal muscle stimulant. The actions of theophylline may be mediated through inhibition of phosphodiesterase and a resultant increase in intracellular cyclic AMP which could mediate smooth muscle relaxation. At concentrations higher than attained *in vivo*, theophylline also inhibits the release of histamine by mast cells.
In vitro, theophylline has been shown to react synergistically with beta agonists that increase intracellular cyclic AMP through the stimulation of adenyl cyclase (isoproterenol), but synergism has not been demonstrated in patient studies and more data is needed to determine if theophylline and beta agonists have clinically important additive effect *in vivo*.
Apparently, no development of tolerance occurs with chronic use of theophylline.
The half-life is shortened with cigarette smoking. The half-life is prolonged in alcoholism, reduced hepatic or renal function, congestive heart failure, and in patients receiving antibiotics such as TAO (troleandomycin), erythromycin and clindamycin. High fever for prolonged periods may decrease theophylline elimination.

Theophylline Elimination Characteristics

	Theophylline Clearance Rates (mean ± S.D.)	Half-life Average (mean ± S.D.)
Children (over 6 months of age)	1.45 ±0.58 ml/kg/min	3.7 ± 1.1 hours
Adult non-smokers with uncomplicated asthma	0.65 ±0.19 ml/kg/min	8.7 ± 2.2 hours

Newborn infants have extremely slow clearances and half-lives exceeding 24 hours which

approach those seen for older children after about 3–6 months.
Older adults with chronic obstructive pulmonary disease, any patients with cor pulmonale or other causes of heart failure, and patients with liver pathology may have lower clearances with half-lives that may exceed 24 hours.
The half-life of theophylline in smokers (1 to 2 packs/day) averaged 4–5 hours among various studies, much shorter than the half-life in nonsmokers who averaged about 7–9 hours. The increase in theophylline clearance caused by smoking is probably the result of induction of drug-metabolizing enzymes that do not readily normalize after cessation of smoking. It appears that between 3 months and 2 years may be necessary for normalization of the effect of smoking on theophylline pharmacokinetics.

Indications: For relief and/or prevention of symptoms from asthma and reversible bronchospasm associated with chronic bronchitis and emphysema.

Contraindications: In individuals who have shown hypersensitivity to any of its components.

Warnings: Status asthmaticus is a medical emergency. Optimal therapy frequently requires additional medication including corticosteroids when the patient is not rapidly responsive to bronchodilators.
Excessive theophylline doses may be associated with toxicity and serum theophylline levels are recommended to assure maximal benefit without excessive risk. Incidence of toxicity increases at levels greater than 20 mcg/ml. Morphine, curare, and stilbamidine should be used with caution in patients with airflow obstruction since they stimulate histamine release and can induce asthmatic attacks. They may also suppress respiration leading to respiratory failure. Alternative drugs should be chosen whenever possible.
There is an excellent correlation between high blood levels of theophylline resulting from conventional doses and associated clinical manifestations of toxicity in (1) patients with lowered body plasma clearances (due to transient cardiac decomposition), (2) patients with liver dysfunction or chronic obstructive lung disease, (3) patients who are older than 55 years of age, particularly males.
There are often no early signs of less serious theophylline toxicity such as nausea and restlessness, which may appear in up to 50 percent of patients prior to onset of convulsions. Ventricular arrhythmias or seizures may be the first signs of toxicity.
Many patients who have higher theophylline serum levels exhibit a tachycardia.
Theophylline products may worsen pre-existing arrhythmias.

Usage in Pregnancy: Safe use in pregnancy has not been established relative to possible adverse effects on fetal development, but neither have adverse effects on fetal development been established. This is, unfortunately, true for most anti-asthmatic medications. Therefore, use of theophylline in pregnant women should be balanced against the risk of uncontrolled asthma.

Precautions: Mean half-life in smokers is shorter than non-smokers, therefore, smokers may require larger doses of theophylline. Theophylline should not be administered concurrently with other xanthine medications. Use with caution in patients with severe cardiac disease, severe hypoxemia, hypertension, hyperthyroidism, acute myocardial injury, cor pulmonale, congestive heart failure, liver disease, and in the elderly (especially males) and in neonates. Great caution should especially be used in giving theophylline to patients in congestive heart failure. Such patients have shown markedly prolonged theophylline blood level curves with theophylline persisting in serum for long periods following discontinuation of the drug.

Group	Oral Loading Dose (Theophylline)	Maintenance Dose For Next 12 Hours (Theophylline)	Maintenance Dose Beyond 12 Hours (Theophylline)
1. Children 6 months to 9 years	6 mg/kg	4 mg/kg q4hrs	4 mg/kg q6hrs
2. Children age 9–16 and young adult smokers	6 mg/kg	3 mg/kg q4h	3 mg/kg q6h
3. Otherwise healthy nonsmoking adults	6 mg/kg	3 mg/kg q6h	3 mg/kg q8h
4. Older patients and patients with cor pulmonale	6 mg/kg	2 mg/kg q6h	2 mg/kg q8h
5. Patients with congestive heart failure, liver failure	6 mg/kg	2 mg/kg q8h	1–2 mg/kg q12h

Use theophylline cautiously in patients with history of peptic ulcer. Theophylline may occasionally act as a local irritant to G. I. tract although gastrointestinal symptoms are more commonly central and associated with serum concentrations over 20 mcg/ml.

Adverse Reactions: The most consistent adverse reactions are usually due to overdose and are:
Gastrointestinal: nausea, vomiting, epigastric pain, hematemesis, diarrhea.
Central nervous system: headaches, irritability, restlessness, insomnia, reflex hyperexcitability, muscle twitching, clonic and tonic generalized convulsions.
Cardiovascular: palpitation, tachycardia, extra systoles, flushing, hypotension, circulatory failure, life-threatening ventricular arrhythmias.
Respiratory: tachypnea.
Renal: albuminuria, increased excretion of renal tubular cells and red blood cells, potentiation of diuresis.
Others: hyperglycemia and inappropriate ADH syndrome.

Drug Interactions: Toxic synergism with ephedrine has been documented and may occur with some other sympathomimetic bronchodilators.
Recent controlled studies suggest that the addition of ephedrine to adequate dosage regimens of theophylline produces little or no increase in effectiveness over that of theophylline alone, but does produce a synergistic increase in toxic side effects.

Drug	*Effect*
Aminophylline with Lithium Carbonate	Increased excretion of Lithium Carbonate
Aminophylline with Propranolol	Antagonism of Propranolol effect
Theophylline with Furosemide	Increased Diuresis of Furosemide
Theophylline with Hexamethonium	Decreased Hexamethonium-induced chronotropic effect
Theophylline with Reserpine	Reserpine-induced Tachycardia
Theophylline with Chlordiazepoxide	Chlordiazepoxide-induced fatty acid mobilization
Theophylline with Cyclamycin (TAO = Triacetyloleandomycin): erythromycin, lincomycin	Increased Theophylline plasma levels

Overdosage:
Management:
A. If potential oral overdose is established and seizure has not occurred:
 1) Induce vomiting.
 2) Administer a cathartic (this is particularly important if sustained release preparations have been taken).
 3) Administer activated charcoal.
B. If patient is having a seizure:
 1) Establish an airway.
 2) Administer O_2.
 3) Treat the seizure with intravenous diazepam, 0.1 to 0.3 mg/kg up to 10 mg.
 4) Monitor vital signs, maintain blood pressure and provide adequate hydration.
C. Post-Seizure Coma:
 1) Maintain airway and oxygenation.
 2) If a result of oral medication, follow above recommendations to prevent absorption of drug, but intubation and lavage will have to be performed instead of inducing emesis, and the cathartic and charcoal will need to be introduced via a large bore gastric lavage tube.
 3) Continue to provide full supportive care and adequate hydration while waiting for drug to be metabolized. In general, the drug is metabolized sufficiently rapidly so as to not warrant consideration of dialysis.
D. Animal studies suggest that phenobarbital may decrease theophylline toxicity. There is as yet, however, insufficient data to recommend pre-treatment of an overdosage with phenobarbital.

Dosage and Administration: Therapeutic serum levels associated with optimal likelihood for benefit and minimal risk of toxicity are considered to be between 10 mcg/ml and 20 mcg/ml. Levels above 20 mcg/ml may produce toxic effects. There is great variation from patient to patient in dosage needed in order to achieve a therapeutic blood level because of variable rates of elimination. Because of this wide variation from patient to patient, and the relatively narrow therapeutic blood level range, dosage must be individualized and monitoring of theophylline serum levels is highly recommended.
Dosage should be calculated on the basis of lean (ideal) body weight where mg/kg doses are stated. Theophylline does not distribute into fatty tissue.
Giving theophylline with food may prevent the rare case of stomach irritation; and though absorption may be slower, it is still complete. When rapidly absorbed products such as solutions and capsules with rapid dissolution are used, dosing to maintain "around the clock" blood levels generally requires administration every 6 hours to obtain the greatest efficacy for clinical use in children; dosing intervals up to 8 hours may be satisfactory for adults because of their slower elimination. Children, and adults requiring higher than average doses, may benefit from products with slower absorption which may allow longer dosing intervals and/or less fluctuation in serum concentration over a dosing interval during chronic therapy.

Dosage for Patient Population
Acute Symptoms of Asthma Requiring Rapid Theophyllinization:
1. Not currently receiving theophylline products
[See table above].
II. Those currently receiving theophylline products: Determine, where possible, the time, amount, route of administration and form of the patient's last dose.
The loading dose for theophylline will be based on the principle that each 0.5 mg/kg of theo-

Continued on next page

Berlex—Cont.

phylline administered as a loading dose will result in a 1 mcg/ml increase in serum theophylline concentration. Ideally, then, the loading dose should be deferred if a serum theophylline concentration can be rapidly obtained. If this is not possible, the clinician must exercise his judgment in selecting a dose based on the potential for benefit and risk. When there is sufficient respiratory distress to warrant a small risk, 2.5 mg/kg of theophylline is likely to increase the serum concentration when administered as a loading dose in rapidly absorbed form by only about 5 mcg/ml. If the patient is not already experiencing theophylline toxicity, this is unlikely to result in dangerous adverse effects.
Subsequent to the modified decision regarding loading dose in this group of patients, the subsequent maintenance dosage recommendations are the same as those described above.
Comments: To achieve optimal therapeutic theophylline dosage, it is recommended to monitor serum theophylline concentrations. However, it is not always possible or practical to obtain a serum theophylline level.
Patients should be closely monitored for signs of toxicity. The present data suggest that the above dosage recommendations will achieve therapeutic serum concentrations with minimal risk of toxicity for most patients. However, some risk of toxic serum concentrations is still present.
Adverse reactions to theophylline often occur when serum theophylline levels exceed 20 mcg/ml.
Chronic Asthma: Theophyllinization is a treatment of first choice for the management of chronic asthma (to prevent symptoms and maintain patent airways). Slow clinical titration is generally preferred to assure acceptance and safety of the medication.
Initial dose: 16 mg/kg/day or 400 mg/day (whichever is lower) in 3–4 divided doses at 6–8 hour intervals.
Increased dose: The above dosage may be increased in approximately 25 percent increments at 2–3 day intervals so long as no intolerance is observed, until the maximum indicated below is reached.
Maximum dose without measurement of serum concentration:
Not to exceed the following:
(Warning: Do not attempt to maintain any dose that is not tolerated)
- Age <9 years—24 mg/kg/day
- Age 9–12 years—20 mg/kg/day
- Age 12–16 years—18 mg/kg/day
- Age > 16 years—13 mg/kg/day or 900 mg/day ***(whichever is less)***

NOTE: Use ideal body weight for obese patients.
Measurement of serum theophylline concentration during chronic therapy:
If the above maximum doses are to be maintained or exceeded, serum theophylline measurement is recommended. This should be obtained at the approximate time of peak absorption during chronic therapy for the product used (1–2 hours for liquids and capsules that undergo rapid dissolution, 3–5 hours for sustained release preparations). It is important that the patient will have missed *no* doses during the previous 48 hours and that dosing intervals will have been reasonably typical with no added doses during that period of time. ***Dosage adjustment based on serum theophylline measurements when these instructions have not been followed may result in recommendations that present risk of toxicity to the patient.***
Final dosage adjustment:
See Table I. Caution should be exercised for younger children who cannot complain of minor side effects. Older adults, those with cor pulmonale, congestive heart failure, and/or liver disease, may have unusually low dosage requirements and thus may experience toxicity at the maximal dosage recommended above.
It is important that no patient be maintained on any dosage that he is not tolerating. In instructing patients in increase dosage according to the schedule above, they should be instructed to not take a subsequent dose if apparent side effects occur and to resume therapy at a lower dose once adverse effects have disappeared.
[See table below].

Peak Theophylline Level µg/ml	Adjustment in Total Daily Dose	Comment
< 5 5–7.5	100% increase 50% increase	If patient is asymptomatic, consider trial off drug; repeat blood levels after adjustment.
8–10	20% increase	Even if patient is asymptomatic at this level, an increased serum concentration may prevent symptoms during a viral URI, or heavy exposure to an inhalant allergen.
11–13	cautious 10% increase if clinically indicated	If patient is asymptomatic, no increase is necessary. If symptoms present during URI or exercise, increase as indicated.
14–20	None	If "breakthrough" in asthmatic symptoms present at end of dosing interval, change to sustained-release product and repeat blood level.
	Occasional intolerance requires a 10% decrease	If side effects present, decrease total daily dose as indicated.
21–25	10% decrease	Even if side-effects are absent.
26–34	25–33% decrease	Even if side-effects are absent, omit next dose and decrease total daily dose as indicated. Repeat blood levels.
> 35	50% decrease	Omit next two doses, decrease as indicated and repeat blood levels.

Caution: Federal law prohibits dispensing without prescription.

Elixophyllin® (theophylline) *Capsules*

Description:
100 mg capsule—Each off-white (dye-free) soft gelatin Elixophyllin Capsule contains 100 mg theophylline (anhydrous) in a suspension of polyethylene glycol 400.
200 mg capsule—Each red, soft gelatin Elixophyllin Capsule contains 200 mg theophylline (anhydrous) in a suspension of polyethylene glycol 400.
Dosage and Administration:
Maintenance Dosage:*
Adults and children over 12 years of age:
One 200 mg capsule three times daily, upon arising, at 3:00 p.m. and at bedtime.
Children age 6 to 12:
One 100 mg capsule every 6 hours.
Children under 6:
Non-alcoholic Elixicon® (theophylline) Suspension is recommended.
**Dosage should be individualized.*
How Supplied:
100 mg Capsules
Bottles of 100 ....NDC 50419-126-10
200 mg Capsules
Bottles of 100 ....NDC 50419-125-10
Bottles of 500 ....NDC 50419-125-50
Unit Dose Boses of 100 ......NDC 50419-125-11
[Shown in Product Identification Section]

Elixophyllin® SR (theophylline) *Capsules*

Description: Elixophyllin SR (sustained release) Capsules are designed to provide a prolonged therapeutic effect.
125 mg Capsule—Each white, dye-free capsule contains 125 mg anhydrous theophylline.
250 mg Capsule—Each clear, dye-free capsule contains 250 mg anhydrous theophylline.
Dosage and Administration:
Maintenance Dosage:*
Adults and children over 12 years of age:
One 250 mg capsule every 12 hours. In severe cases, one capsule every 8 hours.
Children age 6 to 12:
One 125 mg capsule every 12 hours. In severe cases, one capsule every 8 hours.
Children under 6:
Non-alcoholic Elixicon® (theophylline) Suspension is recommended.
**Dosage should be individualized.*
How Supplied: In bottles of:
250 mg Capsules:
100 capsules ....NDC 50419-123-10
500 capsules ....NDC 50419-123-50
125 mg Capsules:
100 capsules ....NDC 50419-129-10
500 capsules ....NDC 50419-129-50
[Shown in Product Identification Section]

Elixophyllin® (theophylline) *Elixir*

Description: Each 15 ml (tablespoonful) of Elixophyllin® Elixir contains 80 mg anhydrous theophylline and 20% alcohol in a palatable aromatic base.
Dosage and Administration:
See preceding chart: Dosage for Patient Population
How Supplied:
In bottles of:
473 ml ....NDC 50419-121-16
946 ml ....NDC 50419-121-32
3785 ml ....NDC 50419-121-28

Elixophyllin-KI® (theophylline/potassium iodide) *Elixir*

Description: Each 15 ml (tablespoonful) of Elixophyllin-KI Elixer contains 80 mg anhydrous theophylline and 130 mg potassium iodide. Alcohol 10%.

Clinical Pharmacology: Potassium iodide acts as an expectorant by liquifying tenacious bronchial secretions.
Indications: For excessive tenacious mucus in chronic asthma, severe chronic and allergic bronchitis and chronic obstructive pulmonary emphysema.
Precautions: Occasionally, persons are markedly sensitive to iodides; care should be used in administering Elixophyllin-KI for the first time. Caution is recommended in patients sensitive to iodides, and in patients receiving potassium sparing diuretics or potassium supplements.
Usage in Pregnancy: Iodides readily cross the placenta and may cause thyroid enlargement in the fetus. Therefore, Elixophyllin-KI should not be used in pregnant women unless in the judgment of the physician, the potential benefits outweigh the possible hazards.
Since iodides are secreted in human milk, discontinue or decrease during breast feeding.
Adverse Reactions: Thyroid adenoma, goiter and myxedema are possible side effects of potassium iodide.
Hypersensitivity to iodides may be manifested by angioneurotic edema, cutaneous and mucosal hemorrhages, and symptoms resembling serum sickness, such as fever, arthralgia, lymph node enlargement and eosinophilia.
Iodism or chronic iodine poisoning may occur during prolonged treatment. The symptoms of iodism include: a metallic taste, soreness of the mouth, increased salivation, coryza, sneezing and swelling of the eyelids. There may be a severe headache, productive cough, pulmonary edema and tenderness of the salivary glands. Acneform skin lesions are seen in the seborrheic areas. Severe and sometimes fatal skin eruptions may develop. Gastric disturbance and diarrhea are common. If iodism appears, the drug should be withdrawn and the patient given appropriate supportive therapy.
Drug Interactions:

Drug	*Effect*
Potassium iodide with lithium carbonate	Increased hypothyroid and goitrogenic effect

Dosage and Administration: Usual dose in chronic asthma: *Adults:* 30 ml (2 tablespoonfuls) t.i.d. upon arisng, at 3:00 p.m. and at bedtime; *Children:* 0.2 ml per pound of body weight, t.i.d. as above. *Dosage must be individualized.*
How Supplied: Bottles of
237 ml ....NDC 50419-124-08
3785 ml ....NDC 50419-124-28
[*Shown in Product Identification Section*]

KAY CIEL® Elixir ℞
(potassium chloride)

KAY CIEL® Powder ℞
(potassium chloride)
VA NSN 6505-00-133445
DPSC NSN 6505-00-148-6984

Description: Each 15 ml (tablespoonful) of elixir contains:
Potassium Chloride ....1.5 g
(supplying 20 mEq)
Alcohol 4% in a palatable base. Contains no sugar.
Each powder packet contains:
Potassium Chloride ....1.5 g
(supplying 20 mEq) Flavored. Contains no sugar.
Indications: Treatment and prevention of potassium deficiency occurring especially during thiazide diuretic or corticosteroid therapy, digitalis intoxication, low dietary intake of potassium, or as a result of excessive vomiting and diarrhea and for correction of associated hypochloremic alkalosis.
Contraindications: Impaired renal function, untreated Addison's Disease, dehydration, heat cramps and hyperkalemia.
Warnings: Do not use excessively.
Precautions: Administer with caution and adjust to the requirements of the individual patient. The patient should be checked frequently and periodic ECG and/or plasma potassium levels taken. Use with caution in patients with cardiac disease. In hypokalemic states, attention should be directed toward correction of frequently associated hypochloremic alkalosis. ***PATIENTS SHOULD BE CAUTIONED TO ADHERE TO DILUTION INSTRUCTIONS TO ASSURE AGAINST GASTROINTESTINAL INJURY.***
Adverse Reactions: Potassium intoxication indicated by listlessness, mental confusion, paresthesia of the extremities, weakness of the legs, flaccid paralysis, fall in blood pressure, cardiac depression, arrhythmias, arrest and heartblock. Vomiting, nausea, abdominal discomfort and diarrhea may occur.
Dosage and Administration:
Elixir:
One tablespoonful (15 ml supplying 20 mEq) ***diluted*** in 4 ounces of cold water or fruit juice twice daily (preferably after a meal), or as directed by physician.
Powder:
Contents of 1 packet (supplying 20 mEq) dissolved in 4 ounces of cold water or fruit juice twice daily (preferably after a meal), or as directed by physician.
Overdosage: In case of excessive use resulting in hyperkalemia or potassium intoxication, discontinue use of potassium chloride or take other steps to lower serum levels if indicated.
How Supplied:
Elixir: Bottles of:
118 ml..................NDC 50419-145-04
473 ml..................NDC 50419-145-16
3785 ml..................NDC 50419-145-28
Powder: Boxes of:
30 packets.................. NDC 50419-144-30
100 packets..................NDC 50419-144-11
500 packets..................NDC 50419-144-32

PYOCIDIN-OTIC® ℞
(polymyxin-hydrocortisone)
Sterile

Description: Each ml contains:
Polymyxin B Sulfate ....10,000 USP Units
Hydrocortisone ....5 mg
Purified Water ....0.02 ml
In a propylene glycol base.
Actions: Polymyxin B sulfate is effective against the gram-negative *Pseudomonas aeruginosa*, one of the most resistant microorganisms commonly causing otitis externa. The addition of hydrocortisone to the antibiotic affords an anti-inflammatory effect and relief against allergic manifestations and reduces the possibility of sensitivity and tissue reaction.
Indications: For the treatment of superficial bacterial infections of the external auditory canal caused by organisms susceptible to the action of the antibiotic.
Contraindications: This product is contraindicated in those individuals who have shown hypersensitivity to any of its components, and in herpes simplex, vaccinia and varicella.
Warnings: As with other antibiotic preparations, prolonged treatment may result in overgrowth of nonsusceptible organisms and fungi. If the infection is not improved after one week, cultures and susceptibility tests should be repeated to verify the identity of the organism and to determine whether therapy should be changed.
Patients who prefer to warm the medication before using should be cautioned against heating the solution above body temperature, in order to avoid loss of potency.
Precautions: If sensitization or irritation occurs, medication should be discontinued promptly.
Dosage and Administration: The external auditory canal should be thoroughly cleaned and dried with a sterile cotton applicator.
For adults, 4 drops of the solution should be instilled into the affected ear 3 or 4 times daily. For infants and children, 3 drops are suggested because of the smaller capacity of the ear canal.
The patient should lie with the affected ear upward and then the drops should be instilled. This position should be maintained for 5 minutes to facilitate penetration of the drops into the ear canal. Repeat, if necessary, for the opposite ear.
If preferred, a cotton wick may be inserted into the canal and then the cotton may be saturated with the solution. This wick should be kept moist by adding further solution every four hours. The wick should be replaced at least once every 24 hours.
How Supplied: 10 ml bottle with dropper. Refrigerate until dispensed.
NDC 50419-286-10.

QUINAGLUTE® DURA-TABS® ℞
(quinidine gluconate)
100 Tablets: VA NSN 6505-00-728-2010A
250 Tablets: DPSC NSN 6505-00-728-2009

Description: Each tablet contains:
Quinidine Gluconate ....324 mg
in a tablet matrix specially designed for the prolonged (8 to 12 hours) release of the drug in the gastrointestinal tract.
Quinidine gluconate contains 62.3% of the anhydrous quinidine alkaloid, whereas quinidine sulfate contains 82.86%. In prescribing Quinaglute Dura-Tabs, this factor should be considered.
Actions: The antiarrhythmic activity of quinidine consists of two basic actions: (a) prolongation of effective refractory period of the atrial or ventricular muscle which leads to termination of arrhythmia; (b) decrease in excitability of ectopic foci of the heart. The action is not limited to these two properties on the heart. In addition, quinidine (c) blocks vagal innervation and (d) facilitates conduction in the atrioventricular junction. In the treatment of cardiac arrhythmia, quinidine is administered in a dose that will exert actions (a) and (b) with a minimal effect on (c) and (d).
Indications:
Premature atrial and ventricular contractions.
Paroxysmal atrial tachycardia.
Paroxysmal A-V junctional rhythm.
Atrial flutter.
Paroxysmal atrial fibrillation.
Established atrial fibrillation when therapy is appropriate.
Paroxysmal ventricular tachycardia when not associated with complete heart block.
Maintenance therapy after electrical conversion of atrial fibrillation and/or flutter.
NOTE: Depending upon the response desired, the dosage may need to be varied and the blood level and/or electrocardiographic response closely monitored during initial treatment. See Description Section.
Contraindications: Aberrant impulses and abnormal rhythms due to escape mechanisms should not be treated with quinidine.
Partial A-V or complete heart block, or intraventricular conduction defects, especially those exhibiting a marked grade of QRS widening. Renal disease resulting in significant azotemia, or those developing cardiotoxic effects such as conduction defects; ventricular premature beats, ventricular tachycardia or flutter while on the drug.
Marked cardiac enlargement, particularly with congestive failure, poor renal function, and especially renal tubular acidosis.
Idiosyncrasy or hypersensitivity to quinidine.
Warnings: In the treatment of atrial flutter, reversion to sinus rhythm may be preceded by

Continued on next page

Berlex—Cont.

a progressive reduction in the degree of A-V block to a 1:1 ratio resulting in an extremely rapid ventricular rate.

Precautions: The precautions to be observed include all those applicable to quinidine. A preliminary test dose of a single tablet of quinidine sulfate should be administered to determine if the patient has an idiosyncrasy to quinidine. Hypersensitivity to quinidine, although rare, should constantly be considered, especially during the first weeks of therapy.

Quinidine in large doses may reduce the contractile force of the heart, therefore, extreme caution should be exercised in using the drug in patients with severe heart disease, hypotension or digitalis intoxication. The potential disadvantages and benefits must be weighed.

It should be administered cautiously, if at all, to senile patients. Hospitalization for close clinical observations, electrocardiographic monitoring, and possibly plasma quinidine levels, is indicated when large doses are used, or with patients who present an increased risk.

Adverse Reactions: Symptoms of cinchonism, ringing in ears, headache, nausea and/or disturbed vision may appear in sensitive patients after a single dose of the drug.

Cardiovascular: Widening of QRS complex, cardiac asystole, ventricular ectopic beats, ideoventricular rhythms including ventricular tachycardia and fibrillation, paradoxical tachycardia, arterial embolism, hypotension.

Gastrointestinal: Nausea, vomiting, abdominal pain, diarrhea.

Hematologic: Acute hemolytic anemia, hypoprothrombinemia, thrombocytopenic purpura, agranulocytosis.

Central Nervous System: Headache, fever, vertigo, apprehension, excitement, confusion, delirium and syncope, disturbed hearing (tinnitus, decreased auditory acuity), disturbed vision (mydriasis, blurred vision, disturbed color perception, reduced vision field, photophobia, diplopia, night blindness, scotomata), optic neuritis.

Dermatologic: Cutaneous flushing with intense pruritus.

Hypersensitivity Reactions: Angioedema, acute asthmatic episode, vascular collapse, respiratory arrest.

Dosage and Administration: The dosage varies considerably depending upon the general condition and cardiovascular state of the patient. The quantity and frequency of administration of Quinaglute Dura-Tabs which will achieve the desired clinical results, must be determined for each patient.

The ideal dosage is the minimum amount of total dose and frequency of daily administration that will prevent premature contractions, paroxysmal tachycardias, and maintain normal sinus rhythm.

Prevention of premature atrial, nodal or ventricular contractions:

1 to 2 tablets every 8 or 12 hours.

Maintenance of normal sinus rhythm following conversion of atrial fibrillation, tachycardia, or flutter:

2 tablets every 12 hours or 1½ to 2 tablets every 8 hours are usually required.

Some patients may be maintained in normal rhythm on a dosage of 1 tablet every 8 or 12 hours; other patients may require larger doses or more frequent administration (i.e., every 6 hours) than the usually recommended schedule. Such increased dosage should be instituted only after careful clinical and laboratory evaluation of the patient (including serial electrocardiograms and plasma quinidine levels).

Quinaglute Dura-Tabs are well tolerated with few gastrointestinal disturbances which, if they occur, may be minimized by administering the drug with food.

It is frequently desirable to determine if a patient can tolerate maintenance quinidine therapy prior to electrical conversion of atrial fibrillation or flutter. Therefore, maintenance therapy may be initiated 2 to 3 days before electrical conversion is attempted.

Quinaglute Dura-Tabs are well suited for such a program and can be administered at the maintenance dose felt necessary for a given patient as indicated above.

How Supplied: In bottles of:

100 Tablets	NDC 50419-101-10
250 Tablets	NDC 50419-101-25
500 Tablets	NDC 50419-101-50
Unit Dose Boxes of 100	NDC 50419-101-11

[Shown in Product Identification Section]

SUS-PHRINE ℞

(ephinephrine) 1:200

Aqueous Suspension for Subcutaneous Injection

5 ml Vial: DPSC NSN 6505-01-022-2402

Description: Each ml of Sus-Phrine contains 5.0 mg epinephrine in a sterile aqueous vehicle containing Ascorbic Acid 10 mg and Thioglycolic Acid 6.6 mg (as sodium salts), Phenol 5 mg and Glycerin (USP) 325 mg. Sodium hydroxide is added to adjust the pH. Approximately 80% of the total epinephrine is in suspension.

Clinical Pharmacology: Sus-Phrine (epinephrine) acts at both the alpha and beta receptor sites. Beta stimulation provides bronchodilator action by relaxing bronchial muscle. Alpha stimulation increases vital capacity by relieving congestion of the bronchial mucosa and by constricting pulmonary vessels.

Sus-Phrine provides both rapid and sustained epinephrine activity. The rapid action is due to the epinephrine in solution, while the sustained activity is due to the crystalline epinephrine free base in suspension.

Indications: For the symptomatic treatment of bronchial asthma, and reversible bronchospasm associated with chronic bronchitis and emphysema.

Contraindications: Hypersensitivity to any of the components.

Narrow angle glaucoma, shock, cerebral arteriosclerosis and organic heart disease. Epinephrine is also contraindicated during general anesthesia with halogenated hydrocarbons or cyclopropane, and in local anesthesia of certain areas, e.g., fingers, toes, because of the danger of vasoconstriction producing sloughing of tissue, and in labor because the drug may delay the second stage.

Warnings: SUS-PHRINE SHOULD NOT BE EMPLOYED TO CORRECT DRUG INDUCED HYPOTENSION.

Administer with caution to elderly people; those with cardiovascular disease, diabetes, hypertension or hyperthyroidism; in psychoneurotic individuals and in pregnancy. Administer with extreme caution to patients with long-standing bronchial asthma and emphysema who have developed degenerative heart disease.

Cardiac arrhythmias may follow administration of epinephrine.

Anginal pain may be induced when coronary insufficiency is present.

Precautions: DO NOT USE IF PRODUCT IS DISCOLORED. Discoloration indicates the oxidation of epinephrine and possible loss of potency.

Use of Sus-Phrine with digitalis, mercurial diuretics or other drugs that sensitize the heart to arrhythmias is not recommended.

Sus-Phrine should not be administered concomitantly with other sympathomimetic agents, since their combined effects on the cardiovascular system may be deleterious to the patient.

The effects of epinephrine may be potentiated by tricyclic antidepressants; sodium l-thyroxine, and certain antihistamines, e.g., diphenhydramine, tripelennamine or chlorpheniramine.

Adverse Reactions: In some individuals, restlessness, anxiety, headache, tremor, weakness, dizziness, pallor, respiratory difficulties, palpitation, nausea and vomiting may occur. These reactions may be exaggerated in hyperthyroidism. Occlusion of the central retinal artery and shock have also been reported.

Also, urticaria, wheal and hemorrhage at the site of injection may occur. Repeated injections at the same site may result in necrosis from vascular constriction.

Tolerance to epinephrine may occur with prolonged use.

Overdosage: Overdosage or inadvertent intravenous injection may cause cerebrovascular hemorrhage resulting from the sharp rise in blood pressure. Fatalities may also result from pulmonary edema because of peripheral constriction and cardiac stimulation produced. Rapidly acting vasodilators such as nitrites, or alpha blocking agents may counteract the marked pressor effects. Cardiac arrhythmias may be countered by administering rapidly acting antiarrhythmic or beta blocking agents.

Dosage and Administration:

NOTE: INJECT SUBCUTANEOUSLY.

It is suggested that Sus-Phrine be administered with a tuberculin syringe and a 26 gauge, ½ inch needle.

A small initial test dose may be administered subcutaneously as a possible aid in determining patient sensitivity to epinephrine.

Site of injection should be varied to avoid necrosis at the site of injection.

Each time before withdrawing Sus-Phrine into syringe, shake vial or ampul thoroughly to disperse particles and obtain a uniform suspension. Inject promptly subcutaneously to avoid settling of suspension in the syringe.

Adults:

Adult dosage range is 0.1 to 0.3 ml depending on patient response.

Subsequent doses should be administered only when necessary and not more frequently than every six hours.

Infants 1 month to 2 years and Children 2 to 12 years:

Pediatric dose is 0.005 ml/kg (2.2 lb) body weight injected subcutaneously.

FOR CHILDREN 30 kg OR LESS MAXIMUM SINGLE DOSE IS 0.15 ml.

Subsequent doses should be administered only when necessary and not more frequently than every six hours.

Clinical Studies: Controlled studies comparing the effectiveness of Sus-Phrine and an aqueous solution of epinephrine 1:1000 were conducted in both pediatric and adult asthmatics. The studies demonstrated rapid bronchodilator acitivity following administration of either Sus-Phrine or epinephrine 1:1000; however during the 6 hour study period, a greater improvement in FEV_1 and $FEF_{25-75\%}$ was observed 4 to 6 hours subsequent to Sus-Phrine administration. Improvement in WPEF was greater for Sus-Phrine than epinehrine 1:1000 3 to 8 hours following administration (10 hour study duration).

How Supplied:

In boxes of

12 × 0.5 ml ampuls	NDC 50419-127-12
25 × 0.5 ml ampuls	NDC 50419-127-25
5.0 ml multiple dose vial	NDC 50419-128-01

THERAPAV® ℞

(papaverine hydrochloride)

Capsules 75 mg

Capsules 150 mg

Description:

75 mg Capsule: Each aqua, soft gelatin Therapav Capsule contains 75 mg papaverine hydrochloride in a polyethylene glycol suspension.

150 mg Capsule: Each aqua, soft gelatin Therapav Capsule contains 150 mg papaverine hydrochloride in a polyethylene glycol suspension.

Actions: Papaverine exerts its action on cardiac and smooth muscles. It provides a direct antispasmodic effect on muscles that is unrelated to muscle innervation. Papaverine relaxes smooth muscles of the vasculature, especially coronary, systemic peripheral, cerebral and pulmonary arteries. The muscle cell is not paralyzed and continues to respond to drugs and other stimuli causing contraction.

Indications: For the relief of cerebral and peripheral ischemia associated with arterial spasm and myocardial ischemia complicated by arrhythmias.

Contraindications: Hypersensitivity to any of the components.

Precautions: Use with caution in patients with glaucoma. Hepatic hypersensitivity has been reported with gastrointestinal symptoms, jaundice, eosinophilia and altered liver function tests. Discontinue use if these occur.

Adverse Reactions: Although occurring rarely, the reported side effects of papaverine include nausea, abdominal distress, anorexia, constipation, diarrhea, skin rash, malaise, drowsiness, vertigo, sweating, and headache.

Dosage and Administration:

75 mg Capsule: One or two capsules three or four times daily.

150 mg Capsule: One capsule three or four times daily.

How Supplied:

75 mg Capsule: Bottles of
100 Capsules.................NDC 50419-170-10

150 mg Capsule: Bottles of
100 Capsules.................NDC 50419-171-10
500 Capsules.................NDC 50419-171-50

[*Shown in Product Identification Section*]

Information on the Berlex products described above is based on full prescribing information in use November 6, 1979.

Beutlich, Inc.

7006 N. WESTERN AVE.
CHICAGO, IL 60645

CEO-TWO® SUPPOSITORIES

Composition: Each adult rectal suppository contains sodium bicarbonate and potassium bitartrate in a water soluble polyethylene glycol base.

Actions and Uses: The gentle pressure of the released CO_2 in the rectum stimulates peristalsis, and defecation results usually in 10 to 30 minutes. CEO-TWO is used pre and post partum, pre and post operatively, or whenever the last 25 cm of the lower bowel must be emptied.

Administration and Dosage: Moisten CEO-TWO slightly with water before inserting. Patient should retain as long as possible.

Contraindications: As with other enemas or laxatives.

How Supplied: In packages of 10, white opaque suppositories. Keep in cool, dry place.

MEVANIN-C CAPSULES

Composition: Each capsule contains: Ascorbic Acid 200 mg., Hesperidin Complex 30 mg., Calcium Lactate 300 mg., Cyanocobalamin 1 mcg., Ferrous Sulfate 65 mg., Folic Acid 0.1 mg., Vitamin A 3000 USP units, Vitamin D 300 USP units, Thiamine HCl 2 mg., Riboflavin 2 mg., Pyridoxine HCl 0.5 mg., Niacin 5 mg., plus trace amounts of copper, zinc, manganese, magnesium, potassium and iodine.

Administration and Dosage: One capsule daily.

How Supplied: In bottles of 90 and 450 red and white capsules.

PERIDIN-C®

Composition: Each tablet contains Hesperidin Methyl Chalcone 50 mg., Hesperidin Complex 150 mg., Ascorbic Acid 200 mg.

Dosage: 1 tablet daily.

How Supplied: In bottles of 100 and 500 orange tablets.

Bird Corporation

MARK 7
PALM SPRINGS, CALIFORNIA 92263

microNEFRIN®
(racemic epinephrine)

Description: Each 100 ml contains Racemic methylaminoethanol catechol hydrochloride, 2.25 Gm.; Sodium chloride, Sodium bisulfite and Potassium metabisulfite, 0.99 Gm.; Chlorobutanol, 0.50 Gm.; Benzoic acid, 0.05 Gm.; and Propylene glycol, 8.0 ml.

Action: microNEFRIN is a sympathomimetic amine with a dual affinity for Alpha and Beta receptors. Topically within the respiratory tract, it has vasoconstrictor (Alpha receptor stimulating) properties which result in reduction of mucosal and submucosal edema. It has bronchodilator (Beta receptor stimulating) properties which result in reduction of airway smooth muscle spasm. These pharmacologic effects result in enlargement of airways and facilitate the removal of secretions.

Indications: microNEFRIN is indicated in aerosol Topical Pulmonary Chemotherapy (TPC®) employing a medication nebulizer such as the "bird" microNEBULIZER® which delivers its liquid particles 0.5 to 4 microns in size. The medication nebulizer is intended for respiratory care with a respirator delivering controlled flow rates. Utilizing microNEFRIN TPC by controlling flow rates in conjunction with a medication nebulizer designed to deliver particles in the 0.5–4.0 micron range, the following are indications:

1) Croup (postintubation and infectious)—Reduction of upper airway mucosal edema by employing high flow rates to achieve turbulent flow and drug deposition within the area of the larynx and trachea.
2) Chronic Obstructive Lung Disease (COLD), Chronic Bronchitis, Broncheolitis, Bronchial Asthma and other peripheral airway diseases. The reduction of airway edema, the reduction of bronchospasm and resultant facilitation of secretion removal can be accomplished with Topical Pulmonary Chemotherapy employing microNEFRIN.

Contraindications: microNEFRIN should not be administered to patients who are hypersensitive to any of its ingredients.

Warnings: Topical Pulmonary Chemotherapy with microNEFRIN may, in excessive dosages or in conjunction with other sympathomimetics by inhalation, oral or parenteral administration, result in severe and serious tachyarrhythmias. This excessive systemic response may be controlled by elimination of systemic drugs and temporary termination of topical microNEFRIN. If tachycardia again results from topical chemotherapy, total dosage delivered should be reduced by dilution.

Usage in Pregnancy: Although no evidence of teratogenicity has been reported, it is recommended that the utilization and potential benefit be weighed against the possible hazard to mother or child of women during pregnancy or lactation, or women of child bearing potential.

Precautions: Topical Pulmonary Chemotherapy with microNEFRIN must be dosage regulated for all patients. Systemic effect of tachycardia, palpitation, nausea or headache are indications of overdosage. To achieve an appropriate topical response, dosage adjustment with a more dilute solution and/or slower flow rates conducive to a more laminar flow is recommended. The dosage adjustment is most critical in patients with hyperthyroidism, hypertension, acute coronary disease, limited cardiac reserve and in individuals sensitive to sympathomimetics or other constituents.

Adverse Reactions: Utilizing Topical Pulmonary Chemotherapy, an increased heart rate of greater than 20–40 beats per minute may be noted. A temporary treatment cessation and reinstitution employing a more dilute solution is indicated.

Dosage and Administration: The employment of specific chemotherapy to the airways implies topical rather than systemic administration, thus achieving the desired effect at a specific topical site without excessive side effects. Particularly, it does not imply the employment of turbulent flows and/or large particles raining out in the mouth and pharynx that are absorbed at this point and then act in a generalized systemic fashion. The usual dosage is 1/1000. However, a more concentrated form 1/500 may be indicated by a patient's response. This range is achieved with 0.2 to 0.4 ml (approximately 4 to 8 drops) of microNEFRIN diluted with an appropriate diluent; distilled water 4.8 to 4.6 ml (approximately 77 to 74 drops) volume respectively to a volume of 5.0 ml. All dosages should be employed with recognition that each patient responds differently and all may respond differently at varying stages of a disease process. Therefore, adverse reactions can be avoided by tailoring each dose to each patient and monitoring for optimal therapeutic responses with minimal or no adverse reactions. Usually repeat administration need not be employed more often than every three to four hours, but more frequent therapy in the range of every two hours may be required.

How Supplied: microNEFRIN (2.25%) is available for Topical Pulmonary Chemotherapy in 7.5 ml, 15 ml and 30 ml bottles.

Bock Pharmacal Company

5435 HIGHLAND PARK DRIVE
ST. LOUIS, MO 63110

POLY-HISTINE EXPECTORANT WITH CODEINE ℞ Ⓒ

Each 5 ml. cherry flavored red syrup contains:
Codeine Phosphate ....10.0 mg.
(Warning: May be habit forming.)
Phenylpropanolamine HCl ....12.5 mg.
Brompheniramine Maleate ....2.0 mg.
Potassium Guaiacolsulfonate ....100.0 mg.

How Supplied: Bottles of 16 oz. and 1 gallon.

POLY-HISTINE EXPECTORANT PLAIN ℞

Each 5 ml. cherry flavored red syrup contains:
Phenylpropanolamine HCl ....12.5 mg.
Brompheniramine Maleate ....2.0 mg.
Potassium Guaiacolsulfonate ....100.0 mg.

How Supplied: Bottles of 16 oz. and 1 gallon.

POLY-HISTINE-D CAPSULES ℞
Antihistamines + Decongestant

Each red-clear time release capsule imprinted BOCK contains:
Phenylpropanolamine HCl ....50.0 mg.
Phenyltoloxamine Dihydrogen
Citrate ....10.0 mg.
Pyrilamine Maleate ....10.0 mg.
Pheniramine Maleate ....10.0 mg.
Tripelennamine HCl ....10.0 mg.

How Supplied: Bottles of 100 and 1000.

Continued on next page

Bock—Cont.

POLY-HISTINE-D ELIXIR ℞
Antihistamines + Decongestant

Each 5 ml. wild cherry flavored red elixir contains:

Phenylpropanolamine HCl	12.5 mg.
Phenyltoloxamine Dihydrogen Citrate	2.5 mg.
Pyrilamine Maleate	2.5 mg.
Pheniramine Maleate	2.5 mg.
Tripelennamine HCl	2.5 mg.
Alcohol	4%

How Supplied: Bottles of 16 oz. and 1 gallon.

POLY-HISTINE-DX CAPSULES ℞
Antihistamine + Decongestant

Each purple-clear time release capsule imprinted BOCK contains:

Pseudoephedrine HCl	120.0 mg.
Brompheniramine Maleate	12.0 mg.

How Supplied: Bottles of 100 and 1000.

POLY-HISTINE-DX SYRUP ℞
Antihistamine + Decongestant

Each 5 ml. grape flavored purple syrup contains:

Pseudoephedrine HCl	30.0 mg.
Brompheniramine Maleate	4.0 mg.

How Supplied: Bottles of 16 oz. and 1 gallon.

Boehringer Ingelheim Ltd.
90 EAST RIDGE
POST OFFICE BOX 368
RIDGEFIELD, CT 06877

ALUPENT® ℞
brand of metaproterenol sulfate
Bronchodilator

Tablets 10 mg	**BI-CODE 74**
Tablets 20 mg	**BI-CODE 72**
Metered Dose Inhaler 15 ml	**BI-CODE 70**
Syrup 10mg/5ml	**BI-CODE 73**

Description: Chemically, Alupent, brand of metaproterenol sulfate is 1-(3-5-dihydroxyphenyl)-2-isopropylaminoethanol sulfate, a white crystalline, racemic mixture of two optically active isomers. It differs from isoproterenol hydrochloride by having two hydroxyl groups attached at the meta positions on the benzene ring rather than one at the meta and one at the para position.

Actions: Alupent, brand of metaproterenol sulfate, is a potent beta-adrenergic stimulator with the aerosol having a rapid onset of action. It is postulated that beta-adrenergic stimulants produce many of their pharmacological effects by activation of adenyl cyclase, the enzyme which catalyzes the conversion of adenosine triphosphate to cyclic adenosine monophosphate.

Absorption, biotransformation and excretion studies following administration by inhalation have not been performed. Following oral administration in humans, an average of 40% of the drug is absorbed; it is not metabolized by catechol-O-methyltransferase or sulfatase enzymes in the gut, but is excreted primarily as glucuronic acid conjugates.

When administered orally or by inhalation Alupent, brand of metaproterenol sulfate, decreases reversible bronchospasm. Pulmonary function tests performed concomitantly usually show improvement following Alupent, brand of metaproterenol sulfate, administration, e.g., an increase in the one-second forced expiratory volume (FEV_1), an increase in maximum expiratory flow rate, an increase in peak expiratory flow rate, an increase in forced vital capacity, and/or a decrease in airway resistance. The resultant decrease in airway obstruction may relieve the dyspnea associated with bronchospasm.

Controlled single- and multiple-dose studies have been performed with pulmonary function monitoring. The mean duration of effect of a single dose of 20 mg of Alupent tablets or syrup, brand of metaproterenol sulfate, (ie, the period of time during which there is a 15% or greater increase in FEV_1) was up to four hours. Four controlled multiple-dose 60-day studies, comparing the effectiveness of Alupent tablets with ephedrine tablets, have been performed. Because of difficulties in study design, only one study was available which could be analyzed in depth. This study showed a loss of efficacy with time for both Alupent tablets and ephedrine. Therefore, the physician should take this phenomenon into account in evaluating the individual patient's overall management. Further studies are in progress to adequately explain these results.

The duration of effect of a single dose of 2 to 3 inhalations of Alupent MDI, brand of metaproterenol sulfate (ie, the period of time during which there is a 15% or greater increase in mean FEV_1) has varied from 1 to 5 hours. In repetitive-dosing studies (up to q.i.d.) the duration of effect for a similar dose of Alupent MDI, brand of metaproterenol sulfate, has ranged from about one to two-and-one-half hours. Present studies are inadequate to explain the divergence in duration of the FEV_1 effect between single- and repetitive-dosing studies, respectively.

Indications: Alupent, brand of metaproterenol sulfate, is indicated as a bronchodilator for bronchial asthma, and for reversible bronchospasm which may occur in association with bronchitis and emphysema.

Contraindications: Use in patients with cardiac arrhythmias associated with tachycardia is contraindicated.

Warnings: Excessive use of adrenergic aerosols is potentially dangerous. Fatalities have been reported following excessive use of Alupent MDI, brand of metaproterenol sulfate, as with other sympathomimetic inhalation preparations, and the exact cause is unknown. Cardiac arrest was noted in several cases.

Paradoxical bronchoconstriction with repeated excessive administration has been reported with other sympathomimetic agents. Therefore, it is possible that this phenomenon could occur with Alupent MDI, brand of metaproterenol sulfate.

Patients should be advised to contact their physician in the event that they do not respond to their usual dose of a sympathomimetic amine aerosol.

Precautions: Extreme care must be exercised with respect to the administration of additional sympathomimetic agents. A sufficient interval of time should elapse prior to administration of another sympathomimetic agent.

Because Alupent, brand of metaproterenol sulfate, is a sympathomimetic drug, it should be used with great caution in patients with hypertension, coronary artery disease, congestive heart failure, hyperthyroidism and diabetes, or when there is sensitivity to sympathomimetic amines.

Usage in Pregnancy: Safety in pregnancy has not been established. Metaproterenol should not be used except with caution during pregnancy, weighing the drug's benefit to the patient against potential risk to the fetus. Studies of metaproterenol in mice, rats, and rabbits have revealed no significant teratogenic effects at oral doses up to 50 mg/kg (310 times the recommended daily human inhalational dose and 31 times the recommended daily human oral dose). In rabbits, fetal loss and teratogenic effects have been observed at and above oral doses of 50 and 100 mg/kg, respectively.

Adverse Reactions: Adverse reactions such as tachycardia, hypertension, palpitations, nervousness, tremor, nausea, bad taste and vomiting have been reported. These reactions are similar to those noted with other sympathomimetic agents.

Dosage and Administration: ***Tablets:*** *Adults*—The usual dose is 20 mg three or four times a day. *Children*—aged six to nine years or weight under 60 lbs—10 mg three or four times a day. Over nine years or weight over 60 lbs—20 mg three or four times a day. Alupent tablets are not recommended for use in children under six years at this time. (Please refer to the Actions section for further information on clinical experience with this product.)

Syrup: *Children* aged six to nine years or weight under 60 lbs—one teaspoonful three or four times a day. Children over nine years or weight over 60 lbs—two teaspoonfuls three or four times a day. Experience in children under the age of six is limited to seventy-eight children. Of this number, forty were treated with Alupent syrup for at least one month. In this group, daily doses of approximately 1.3 to 2.6 mg/kg were well tolerated.

Adults—two teaspoonfuls three or four times a day.

Metered Dose Inhaler: The usual single dose is two to three inhalations. With repetitive dosing, inhalation should usually not be repeated more often than about every three to four hours. Total dosage per day should not exceed 12 inhalations.

The Metered Dose Inhaler form of Alupent, brand of metaproterenol sulfate, is not recommended for children under 12 years of age because there is not sufficient data on administration of this dosage form in this age group.

If Alupent, brand of metaproterenol sulfate, is administered before or after other sympathomimetic bronchodilators, caution should be exercised with respect to potentiation of adrenergic effects.

Symptoms of Overdosage: The symptoms of overdosage are those of excessive beta-adrenergic stimulation listed under Adverse Reactions.

How Supplied: ***Tablets:*** Alupent, brand of metaproterenol sulfate, is supplied in two dosage strengths as round, white, scored tablets in bottles of 100.

Tablets of 10 mg coded BI/74.
Tablets of 20 mg coded BI/72.

Syrup: Alupent, brand of metaproterenol sulfate, is available as a cherry-flavored syrup, 10 mg per teaspoonful (5 ml), in 16 oz bottles.

Metered Dose Inhaler: Each Alupent Metered Dose Inhaler contains 225 mg of metaproterenol sulfate as a micronized powder in an inert propellant. This is sufficient medication for 300 inhalations. Each metered dose expressed from the inhaler delivers at the mouthpiece approximately 0.65 mg of metaproterenol sulfate. Alupent Metered Dose Inhaler with mouthpiece (15 ml). Alupent Metered Dose Inhaler refill (15 ml).

AL-713R (5/77)

[*Shown in Product Identification Section*]

CATAPRES® ℞
brand of clonidine hydrochloride
Oral Antihypertensive

Tablets, 0.1 mg.	**BI-CODE 06**
Tablets, 0.2 mg.	**BI-CODE 07**
Tablets, 0.3 mg.	**BI-CODE 11**

Description: Catapres, brand of clonidine hydrochloride, an antihypertensive agent, is an imidazoline derivative and exists as a mesomeric compound. Its chemical name is 2-(2,6-dichlorophenylamino)-2-imidazoline hydrochloride.

It is an odorless, bitter, white crystalline substance soluble in water and alcohol, with a molecular weight of 266.57. The 0.1 mg tablet is equivalent to 0.087 mg of the free base.

Actions: Catapres, brand of clonidine hydrochloride, is an antihypertensive agent whose mechanism of action appears to be central alpha-adrenergic stimulation as demonstrated in animal studies. This results in the inhibition

of bulbar sympathetic cardioaccelerator and sympathetic vasoconstrictor centers, thereby causing a decrease in sympathetic outflow from the brain. Initially, Catapres, brand of clonidine hydrochloride, stimulates peripheral alpha-adrenergic receptors producing transient vasoconstriction.
Catapres, brand of clonidine hydrochloride, acts relatively rapidly. The patient's blood pressure declines within 30 to 60 minutes after an oral dose, the maximum decrease occurring within 2 to 4 hours. The antihypertensive effect in humans lasts approximately 6 to 8 hours. The peak plasma level of Catapres, brand of clonidine hydrochloride, occurs in approximately 3 to 5 hours with a plasma half-life of 12 to 16 hours. Catapres, brand of clonidine hydrochloride, and its metabolites are excreted mainly in the urine. When labeled drug was administered, unchanged drug appearing in the urine accounted for about 32 percent of administered radioactivity.
Orthostatic effects are mild and infrequent since supine pressure is reduced to essentially the same extent as standing pressure. Catapres, brand of clonidine hydrochloride, does not alter normal hemodynamic responses to exercise. Acute studies with Catapres, brand of clonidine hydrochloride, in humans have demonstrated a moderate reduction (15 to 20%) of cardiac output in the supine position with no change in the peripheral resistance, while at a 45° tilt there is a smaller reduction in cardiac output and a decrease of peripheral resistance. Renal blood flow and the glomerular filtration rate remain essentially unchanged. During long-term therapy, cardiac output tends to return to control values, while peripheral resistance remains decreased. Slowing of the pulse rate has been observed in most patients given Catapres, brand of clonidine hydrochloride.
Other studies in humans have provided evidence of a reduction in plasma renin activity and in the excretion of aldosterone and catecholamines in patients treated with Catapres, brand of clonidine hydrochloride.
The exact relationship between these pharmacologic actions of Catapres, brand of clonidine hydrochloride, in humans, and its antihypertensive effect in individual patients, has not been fully elucidated at this time.
Catapres, brand of clonidine hydrochloride, has been administered together with hydralazine, guanethidine, methyldopa, reserpine, spironolactone, furosemide, chlorthalidone and thiazide diuretics without drug-to-drug interactions. The concomitant administration of a diuretic has been shown to enhance the antihypertensive efficacy of Catapres, brand of clonidine hydrochloride.
Indication: Catapres, brand of clonidine hydrochloride, is indicated in the treatment of hypertension. As an antihypertensive drug, Catapres, brand of clonidine hydrochloride, is mild to moderate in potency. It may be employed in a general treatment program with a diuretic and/or other antihypertensive agents as needed for proper patient response.
Warnings: Tolerance may develop in some patients, necessitating a reevaluation of therapy.
Use in Pregnancy: Reproduction studies have been performed with Catapres, brand of clonidine hydrochloride, in three animal species. The findings of these studies reflected no teratogenic effect but some embryotoxicity was evident at doses as low as 0.015 mg/kg (one-third the maximum recommended dose). In view of these findings, and since information on possible adverse effects in pregnant women is limited to uncontrolled clinical data, Catapres, brand of clonidine hydrochloride, is not recommended in women who are or may become pregnant unless the potential benefit outweighs the potential risk to mother and infant.
Use in Children: No clinical experience is available with the use of Catapres, brand of clonidine hydrochloride, in children. Studies are being performed to evaluate its use in the treatment of hypertension in children.
Precautions: When discontinuing Catapres, brand of clonidine hydrochloride, therapy the physician should reduce the dose gradually over 2 to 4 days to avoid a possible rapid rise in blood pressure and associated subjective symptoms such as nervousness, agitation, and headache. Patients on Catapres, brand of clonidine hydrochloride, therapy should be instructed not to discontinue therapy without consulting their physician. Rare instances of hypertensive encephalopathy and death have been recorded after abrupt cessation of Catapres, brand of clonidine hydrochloride, therapy. A causal relationship has not been established in these cases. It has been demonstrated that an excessive rise in blood pressure, should it occur, can be reversed by resumption of Catapres, brand of clonidine hydrochloride, therapy or by intravenous phentolamine.
Patients who engage in potentially hazardous activities, such as operating machinery or driving, should be advised of the sedative effect of Catapres, brand of clonidine hydrochloride. This drug may enhance the CNS-depressive effects of alcohol, barbiturates and other sedatives. Like any other antihypertensive agent, Catapres, brand of clonidine hydrochloride, should be used with caution in patients with severe coronary insufficiency, recent myocardial infarction, cerebrovascular disease or chronic renal failure.
As an integral part of their overall long-term care, patients treated with Catapres, brand of clonidine hydrochloride, should receive periodic eye examinations (see Toxicology).
Adverse Reactions: The most common reactions associated with Catapres, brand of clonidine hydrochloride, therapy are dry mouth (about 40%), drowsiness (about 35%), and sedation (about 8%). Constipation, dizziness, headache, and fatigue have been reported. Generally, these effects tend to diminish with continued therapy.
The following reactions have been associated with the drug, some of them rarely. In some instances an exact causal relationship has not been established.
Gastrointestinal: Anorexia, malaise, nausea, vomiting, parotid pain, mild transient abnormalities in liver function tests. There has been one report of possible drug-induced hepatitis without icterus and hyperbilirubinemia in a patient receiving Catapres, brand of clonidine hydrochloride, chlorthalidone and papaverine hydrochloride.
Metabolic: Weight gain, transient elevation of blood glucose or serum creatine phosphokinase, gynecomastia.
Cardiovascular: Congestive heart failure, Raynaud's phenomenon, and electrocardiographic abnormalities manifested as Wenckebach period or ventricular trigeminy.
Central Nervous System: Vivid dreams or nightmares, insomnia, other behavioral changes, nervousness, restlessness, anxiety, mental depression.
Dermatologic: Rash, angioneurotic edema, hives, urticaria, thinning of the hair, pruritus not associated with a rash.
Genitourinary: Impotence, urinary retention.
Other: Increased sensitivity to alcohol, dryness, itching or burning of the eyes, dryness of the nasal mucosa, pallor, or weakly positive Coombs' test.
Dosage and Administration: The dose of Catapres, brand of clonidine hydrochloride, must be adjusted according to the patient's individual blood pressure response. The following is a general guide to its administration.
Initial dose: One 0.1 mg tablet twice daily.
Maintenance dose: Further increments of 0.1 mg or 0.2 mg per day may be made until the desired response is achieved. The therapeutic doses most commonly employed have ranged from 0.2 mg to 0.8 mg per day given in divided doses. Studies have indicated that 2.4 mg is the maximum effective daily dose but doses as high as this have rarely been employed.
Overdosage: Profound hypotension, weakness, somnolence, diminished or absent reflexes and vomiting followed the accidental ingestion of Catapres, brand of clonidine hydrochloride, by several children from 19 months to 5 years of age. Gastric lavage and administration of an analeptic and vasopressor led to complete recovery within 24 hours. Tolazoline in intravenous doses of 10 mg at 30-minute intervals usually abolishes all effects of Catapres, brand of clonidine hydrochloride, overdosage.
Toxicology: In several studies Catapres, brand of clonidine hydrochloride, produced a dose-dependent increase in the incidence and severity of spontaneously occurring retinal degeneration in albino rats treated for six months or longer. Tissue distribution studies in dogs and monkeys revealed that Catapres, brand of clonidine hydrochloride, was concentrated in the choroid of the eye. In view of the retinal degeneration observed in rats, eye examinations were performed in 908 patients prior to the start of Catapres, brand of clonidine hydrochloride, therapy, who were then examined periodically thereafter. In 353 of these 908 patients, examinations were performed for periods of 24 months or longer. Except for some dryness of the eyes, no drug-related abnormal ophthalmologic findings were recorded and Catapres, brand of clonidine hydrochloride, did not alter retinal function as shown by specialized tests such as the electroretinogram and macular dazzle.
How Supplied: Catapres, brand of clonidine hydrochloride, is available as 0.1 mg (tan) and 0.2 mg (orange) oval, single-scored tablets in bottles of 100 and 1,000. Also available as 0.3 mg (peach) oval, single-scored tablets in bottles of 100.

98-146-073-D (9/79)

[*Shown in Product Identification Section*]

COMBIPRES® ℞
Each tablet contains:
Catapres®, brand of
clonidine hydrochloride,
0.1 mg or 0.2 mg,
and chlorthalidone, 15 mg
Oral Antihypertensive
Tablets 0.1 **BI-CODE 08**
Tablets 0.2 **BI-CODE 09**

WARNING
This fixed combination drug is not indicated for initial therapy of hypertension. Hypertension requires therapy titrated to the individual patient. If the fixed combination represents the dosage so determined, its use may be more convenient in patient management. The treatment of hypertension is not static, but must be reevaluated as conditions in each patient warrant.

Description: Combipres is a combination of Catapres®, brand of clonidine hydrochloride, and chlorthalidone. Catapres, an antihypertensive agent, is an imidazoline derivative and exists as a mesomeric compound. The chemical name for clonidine hydrochloride is 2-(2,6-dichlorophenylamino)-2-imidazoline hydrochloride.
It is an odorless, bitter, white crystalline substance soluble in water and alcohol, with a molecular weight of 266.57. The 0.1 mg tablet is equivalent to 0.087 mg of the free base.
Chlorthalidone is 2-chloro-5-(1-hydroxy-3-oxo-1-isoindolinyl) benzenesulfonamide.
Chlorthalidone is an oral diuretic agent indicated for the treatment of edema and hyper-

Continued on next page

Boehringer Ingelheim—Cont.

tension. The drug has a prolonged action. It differs from other sulfonamide diuretics in that a double ring system is incorporated in its chemical structure.

Actions: Combipres:
Combipres produces a more pronounced antihypertensive response than occurs after either clonidine hydrochloride or chlorthalidone alone in equivalent doses.
Catapres (clonidine hydrochloride):
Catapres, brand of clonidine hydrochloride, is an antihypertensive agent whose mechanism of action appears to be central alpha-adrenergic stimulation as demonstrated in animal studies. This results in the inhibition of bulbar sympathetic cardioaccelerator and sympathetic vasoconstrictor centers, thereby causing a decrease in sympathetic outflow from the brain. Initially, Catapres, brand of clonidine hydrochloride, stimulates peripheral alpha-adrenergic receptors producing transient vasoconstriction.
Catapres, brand of clonidine hydrochloride, acts relatively rapidly. The patient's blood pressure declines within 30 to 60 minutes after an oral dose, the maximum decrease occurring within 2 to 4 hours. The antihypertensive effect in humans lasts approximately 6 to 8 hours. The peak plasma level of Catapres, brand of clonidine hydrochloride, occurs in approximately 3 to 5 hours with a plasma half-life of 12 to 16 hours. Catapres, brand of clonidine hydrochloride, and its metabolites are excreted mainly in the urine. When labeled drug was administered, unchanged drug appearing in the urine accounted for about 32 percent of administered radioactivity.
Orthostatic effects are mild and infrequent since supine pressure is reduced to essentially the same extent as standing pressure. Catapres, brand of clonidine hydrochloride, does not alter normal hemodynamic responses to exercise. Acute studies with Catapres, brand of clonidine hydrochloride, in humans have demonstrated a moderate reduction (15 to 20%) of cardiac output in the supine position with no change in the peripheral resistance, while at a 45° tilt there is a smaller reduction in cardiac output and a decrease of peripheral resistance. Renal blood flow and the glomerular filtration rate remain essentially unchanged. During long-term therapy, cardiac output tends to return to control values, while peripheral resistance remains decreased. Slowing of the pulse rate has been observed in most patients given Catapres, brand of clonidine hydrochloride.
Other studies in humans have provided evidence of a reduction in plasma renin activity and in the excretion of aldosterone and catecholamines in patients treated with Catapres, brand of clonidine hydrochloride.
The exact relationship between these pharmacologic actions of Catapres, brand of clonidine hydrochloride, in humans and its antihypertensive effect in individual patients has not been fully elucidated at this time.
Catapres, brand of clonidine hydrochloride, has been administered together with hydralazine, guanethidine, methyldopa, reserpine, spironolactone, furosemide, chlorthalidone and thiazide diuretics without drug-to-drug interactions.
Chlorthalidone:
The diuretic action of chlorthalidone is thought to be due to inhibition of sodium and chloride reabsorption in the proximal tubule. It has been suggested that the initial antihypertensive action of the drug is due to a reduction of plasma volume.

Indication: Combipres is indicated in the treatment of hypertension (see box warning).

Contraindications: Combipres is contraindicated in patients with known hypersensitivity to chlorthalidone and in patients with severe renal or hepatic diseases.

Warnings: Tolerance may develop in some patients treated with Combipres. When this occurs therapy should be reevaluated.
Use in Pregnancy: No teratogenic changes have been observed following concomitant administration of chlorthalidone and Catapres, brand of clonidine hydrochloride, to pregnant rats in doses up to 0.128 mg/kg of Catapres and 32 mg/kg of chlorthalidone. However, when animals were given Catapres, brand of clonidine hydrochloride, alone in doses as low as 0.015 mg/kg (one-third the maximum recommended dose) some embryotoxicity was evident. In view of these findings and since information on possible adverse effects in pregnant women is limited to uncontrolled clinical data, Combipres is not recommended in women who are or may become pregnant unless the potential benefit outweighs the potential risk to mother and infant.
Use in Children: No clinical experience is available with the use of Combipres in children. Studies are being performed with Catapres, brand of clonidine hydrochloride, to evaluate its use in the treatment of hypertension in children.

Precautions: Catapres (clonidine hydrochloride):
When discontinuing Combipres therapy, the physician should reduce the dose gradually over 2 to 4 days to avoid a possible rapid rise in blood pressure and associated subjective symptoms such as nervousness, agitation, and headache. Patients on Combipres therapy should be instructed not to discontinue therapy without consulting their physician. Rare instances of hypertensive encephalopathy and death have been recorded after abrupt cessation of Catapres, brand of clonidine hydrochloride, therapy. A causal relationship has not been established in these cases. It has been demonstrated that an excessive rise in blood pressure, should it occur, can be reversed by resumption of Combipres therapy or by intravenous phentolamine.
Patients who engage in potentially hazardous activities, such as operating machinery or driving, should be advised of the sedative effect of the Catapres component. This drug may enhance the CNS-depressive effects of alcohol, barbiturates and other sedatives. Like any other antihypertensive agent, Combipres should be used with caution in patients with severe coronary insufficiency, recent myocardial infarction, cerebrovascular disease or chronic renal failure.
As an integral part of their overall long-term care, patients treated with Combipres should receive periodic eye examinations (see Toxicology).
Chlorthalidone:
Patients predisposed toward or affected by diabetes should be tested periodically while receiving Combipres, because of the hyperglycemic effect of chlorthalidone.
Because of the possibility of progression of renal failure, periodic determination of the BUN is indicated. If, in the physician's opinion, a rising BUN is significant, the drug should be stopped.
The chlorthalidone component of Combipres may lead to sodium and/or potassium depletion. Muscular weakness, muscle cramps, anorexia, nausea, vomiting, constipation, lethargy or mental confusion may occur. Severe dietary salt restriction is not recommended in patients receiving Combipres.
Periodic determinations of the serum potassium level will aid the physician in the detection of hypokalemia. Extra care should be given to detection of hypokalemia in patients receiving adrenal corticosteroids, ACTH or digitalis. Hypochloremic alkalosis often precedes other evidences of severe potassium deficiency. Frequently, therefore, more sensitive indicators than the potassium serum level are the serum bicarbonate and chloride concentrations. Also indicative of potassium depletion can be electrocardiographic alterations such as changes in conduction time, reduction in amplitude of the T wave, ST segment depression, prominent U wave. These abnormalities may appear with potassium depletion before the serum level of potassium decreases. To lessen the possibility of potassium deficiency, the diet, in addition to meat and vegetables, should include potassium-rich foods such as citrus fruits and bananas. If significant potassium depletion should occur during therapy, oral potassium supplements in the form of potassium chloride (3 to 4.5 g/day), fruit juice and bananas should be given.

Adverse Reactions: Combipres is generally well tolerated. The most common reactions associated with Combipres are dry mouth (about 40%), drowsiness (about 35%), and sedation (about 8%). Constipation, dizziness, headache, and fatigue have been reported. Generally, these effects tend to diminish with continued therapy.
In addition to the reactions listed above, certain adverse reactions associated with the component drugs of Combipres are shown below.
Catapres (clonidine hydrochloride):
Gastrointestinal: Anorexia, malaise, nausea, vomiting, parotid pain, mild transient abnormalities in liver function tests. One case of possible drug-induced hepatitis without icterus or hyperbilirubinemia has been reported in a patient receiving Catapres, brand of clonidine hydrochloride, chlorthalidone and papaverine hydrochloride.
Metabolic: Weight gain, transient elevation of blood glucose or serum creatine phosphokinase, gynecomastia.
Cardiovascular: Congestive heart failure, Raynaud's phenomenon, and electrocardiographic abnormalities manifested as Wenckebach period or ventricular trigeminy.
Central Nervous System: Vivid dreams or nightmares, insomnia, other behavioral changes, nervousness, restlessness, anxiety, mental depression.
Dermatologic: Rash, angioneurotic edema, hives, urticaria, thinning of the hair, pruritus not associated with a rash.
Genitourinary: Impotence, urinary retention.
Other: Increased sensitivity to alcohol, dryness, itching or burning of the eyes, dryness of the nasal mucosa, pallor, or weakly positive Coombs' test.
Chlorthalidone:
Symptoms such as nausea, gastric irritation, anorexia, constipation and cramping, weakness, dizziness, transient myopia and restlessness are occasionally observed. Headache and impotence or dysuria may occur rarely. Orthostatic hypotension has been reported and may be potentiated when chlorthalidone is combined with alcohol, barbiturates or narcotics. Skin rashes, urticaria and purpura have been reported in a few instances.
A decreased glucose tolerance evidenced by hyperglycemia and glycosuria may develop inconsistently. This condition, usually reversible on discontinuation of therapy, responds to control with antidiabetic treatment. Diabetics and those predisposed should be checked regularly.
As with other diuretic agents, hypokalemia may occur (see Precautions). Hyperuricemia may be observed on occasion and acute attacks of gout have been precipitated. In cases where prolonged and significant elevation of blood uric acid concentration is considered potentially deleterious, concomitant use of a uricosuric agent is effective in reversing hyperuricemia without loss of diuretic and/or antihypertensive activity.
Idiosyncratic drug reactions such as aplastic anemia, thrombocytopenia, leukopenia, agranulocytosis and necrotizing angiitis have occurred, but are rare.

The remote possibility of pancreatitis should be considered when epigastric pain or unexplained gastrointestinal symptoms develop after prolonged administration.
Other adverse reactions which have been reported with this general class of compounds include: jaundice, xanthopsia, paresthesia and photosensitization.

Dosage and Administration: *Dosage:* As determined by individual titration of Catapres, brand of clonidine hydrochloride, and chlorthalidone (see box warning).
The following is a general guide to the administration of the individual components of Combipres:
Catapres (clonidine hydrochloride):
Initial dose: One 0.1 mg tablet twice daily.
Maintenance dose: Further increments of 0.1 mg or 0.2 mg per day may be made until the desired response is achieved. The therapeutic doses most commonly employed have ranged from 0.2 to 0.8 mg per day, given in divided doses. Studies have indicated that 2.4 mg is the maximum effective daily dose but doses as high as this have rarely been employed.
Chlorthalidone:
The usual initial dose is 50 mg daily, which may be given in divided doses.
If the individual doses of Catapres, brand of clonidine hydrochloride, and chlorthalidone determined by titration represent the dose contained in Combipres, for convenience the patient may then be given Combipres.

Overdosage: Catapres (clonidine hydrochloride):
Profound hypotension, weakness, somnolence, diminished or absent reflexes and vomiting followed the accidental ingestion of Catapres, brand of clonidine hydrochloride, by several children from 19 months to 5 years of age. Gastric lavage and administration of an analeptic and vasopressor led to complete recovery within 24 hours. Tolazoline in intravenous doses of 10 mg at 30-minute intervals usually abolishes all effects of Catapres, brand of clonidine hydrochloride, overdosage.
Chlorthalidone:
Symptoms of overdosage include nausea, weakness, dizziness, and disturbances of electrolyte balance. There is no specific antidote, but gastric lavage is recommended, followed by supportive treatment. Where necessary, this may include intravenous dextrose and saline with potassium, administered with caution.

Toxicology: In several studies Catapres, brand of clonidine hydrochloride, produced a dose-dependent increase in the incidence and severity of spontaneously occurring retinal degeneration in albino rats treated for 6 months or longer. Tissue distribution studies in dogs and monkeys revealed that Catapres, brand of clonidine hydrochloride, was concentrated in the choroid of the eye. In view of the retinal degeneration observed in rats, eye examinations were performed in 908 patients prior to the start of Catapres, brand of clonidine hydrochloride, therapy, who were then examined periodically thereafter. In 353 of these 908 patients, examinations were performed for periods of 24 months or longer. Except for some dryness of the eyes, no drug-related abnormal ophthalmologic findings were recorded and Catapres, brand of clonidine hydrochloride, did not alter retinal function as shown by specialized tests such as the electroretinogram and macular dazzle.

How Supplied: Combipres® 0.1 (each tablet contains clonidine hydrochloride, 0.1 mg + chlorthalidone, 15 mg). It is available as pink, oval, single-scored compressed tablets in bottles of 100.
Combipres® 0.2 (each tablet contains clonidine hydrochloride, 0.2 mg + chlorthalidone, 15 mg). It is available as blue, oval, single-scored compressed tablets in bottles of 100.
98-146-074-A (7/74)

[*Shown in Product Identification Section*]

DULCOLAX®
brand of bisacodyl USP
Tablets of 5 mg ....BI-CODE 12
Suppositories of 10 mg.............BI-CODE 52
Laxative

Description: Dulcolax is a contact laxative acting directly on the colonic mucosa to produce normal peristalsis throughout the large intestine. Its unique mode of action permits either oral or rectal administration, according to the requirements of the patient. Because of its gentleness and reliability of action without side effects, Dulcolax may be used whenever constipation is a problem. In preparation for surgery, proctoscopy, or radiologic examination, Dulcolax provides satisfactory cleansing of the bowel, obviating the need for an enema. Dulcolax is a colorless, tasteless compound that is practically insoluble in water and alkaline solution. It is designated chemically bis(p-acetoxyphenyl)-2-pyridylmethane.

Actions: Dulcolax differs markedly from other laxatives in its mode of action: it is virtually nontoxic, and its laxative effect occurs on contact with the colonic mucosa, where it stimulates sensory nerve endings to produce parasympathetic reflexes resulting in increased peristaltic contractions of the colon. Administered orally, Dulcolax is absorbed to a variable degree from the small bowel but such absorption is not related to the mode of action of the compound. Dulcolax administered rectally in the form of suppositories is negligibly absorbed. The contact action of the drug is restricted to the colon, and motility of the small intestine is not appreciably influenced. Local axon reflexes, as well as segmental reflexes, are initiated in the region of contact and contribute to the widespread peristaltic activity producing evacuation. For this reason, Dulcolax may often be employed satisfactorily in patients with ganglionic blockage or spinal cord damage (paraplegia, poliomyelitis, etc.).

Indications: *Acute Constipation:* Taken at bedtime, Dulcolax tablets are almost invariably effective the following morning. When taken before breakfast, they usually produce an effect within six hours. For a prompter response and to replace enemas, the suppositories, which are usually effective in 15 minutes to one hour, can be used.
Chronic Constipation and Bowel Retraining: Dulcolax is extremely effective in the management of chronic constipation, particularly in older patients. By gradually lengthening the interval between doses as colonic tone improves, the drug has been found to be effective in redeveloping proper bowel hygiene. There is no tendency to "rebound".
Preparation for Radiography: Dulcolax tablets are excellent in eliminating fecal and gas shadows from x-rays taken of the abdominal area. For barium enemas, no food should be given following the administration of the tablets, to prevent reaccumulation of material in the cecum, and a suppository should be given one to two hours prior to examination.
Preoperative Preparation: Dulcolax tablets have been shown to be an ideal laxative in emptying the G.I. tract prior to abdominal surgery or to other surgery under general anesthesia. They may be supplemented by suppositories to replace the usual enema preparation. Dulcolax will not replace the colonic irrigations usually given patients before intracolonic surgery, but is useful in the preliminary emptying of the colon prior to these procedures.
Postoperative Care: Suppositories can be used to replace enemas, or tablets given as an oral laxative, to restore normal bowel hygiene after surgery.
Antepartum Care: Either tablets or suppositories can be used for constipation in pregnancy without danger of stimulating the uterus.
Preparation for Delivery: Suppositories can be used to replace enemas in the first stage of labor provided that they are given at least two hours before the onset of the second stage.
Postpartum Care: The same indications apply as in postoperative care, with no contraindication in nursing mothers.
Preparation for Sigmoidoscopy or Proctoscopy: For unscheduled office examinations, adequate preparation is usually obtained with a single suppository. For sigmoidoscopy scheduled in advance, however, administration of tablets the night before in addition will result in adequate preparation almost invariably.
Colostomies: Tablets the night before or a suppository inserted into the colostomy opening in the morning will frequently make irrigations unnecessary, and in other cases will expedite the procedure.

Contraindication: There is no contraindication to the use of Dulcolax, other than an acute surgical abdomen.

Precaution: Dulcolax tablets contain FD&C Yellow No. 5 (tartrazine) which may cause allergic-type reactions (including bronchial asthma) in certain susceptible individuals. Although the overall incidence of FD&C Yellow No. 5 (tartrazine) sensitivity in the general population is low, it is frequently seen in patients who also have aspirin hypersensitivity.

Adverse Reactions: As with any laxative, abdominal cramps are occasionally noted, particularly in severely constipated individuals.

Dosage:
Tablets
Tablets must be swallowed whole, not chewed or crushed, and should not be taken within one hour of antacids or milk.
Adults: Two or three (usually two) tablets suffice when an ordinary laxative effect is desired. This usually results in one or two soft, formed stools.
Up to six tablets may be safely given in preparation for special procedures when greater assurance of complete evacuation of the colon is desired. In producing such thorough emptying, these higher doses may result in several loose, unformed stools.
Children: One or two tablets, depending on age and severity of constipation, administered as above. Tablets should not be given to a child too young to swallow them whole.
Suppositories
Adults: One suppository at the time a bowel movement is required. Usually effective in 15 minutes to one hour.
Children: Half a suppository is generally effective for infants and children under two years of age. Above this age, a whole suppository is usually advisable.
Combined
In preparation for surgery, radiography and sigmoidoscopy, a combination of tablets the night before and a suppository in the morning is recommended (see Indications).

How Supplied: Dulcolax, brand of bisacodyl: Yellow, enteric-coated tablets of 5 mg in boxes of 24, bottles of 100, 1000 and unit strip packages of 100; suppositories of 10 mg in boxes of 2, 4, 50 and 500.

Note: Dulcolax suppositories and tablets should be stored at temperatures not above 86°F (30°C).

Also Available: Dulcolax® Bowel Prep Kit. Each kit contains:
1 Dulcolax suppository of 10 mg bisacodyl;
4 Dulcolax tablets of 5 mg bisacodyl;
Complete patient instructions.

Clinical Applications: Dulcolax can be used in virtually any patient in whom a laxative or enema is indicated. It has no effect on the blood picture, erythrocyte sedimentation rate, urinary findings, or hepatic or renal function. It may be safely given to infants and the aged, pregnant or nursing women, debilitated patients, and may be prescribed in the presence

Continued on next page

Boehringer Ingelheim—Cont.

of such conditions as cardiovascular, renal, or hepatic diseases. 026-C (8/79)

[*Shown in Product Identification Section*]

PERSANTINE® ℞

brand of dipyridamole

For Long-Term Therapy of Chronic Angina Pectoris

Tablets of 25 mg..............................BI-CODE 17

Tablets of 50 mg..............................BI-CODE 18

Tablets of 75 mg..............................BI-CODE 19

Description: Persantine, brand of dipyridamole, is classified as a coronary vasodilator. The drug is unrelated chemically to the nitrates or digitalis.

Chemistry: Persantine, brand of dipyridamole, is a homogeneous yellow crystalline powder, odorless but with a bitter taste. It is soluble in dilute acids, methanol, and chloroform. Its basic structure is a double ring of two condensed pyrimidine rings. It is designated chemically as 2,6-bis-(diethanolamino)-4,8-dipiperidino-pyrimido-(5,4-d) pyrimidine.

Actions: *Human:* Persantine, brand of dipyridamole, in therapeutic doses usually produces no significant alteration of systemic blood pressure or of blood flow in peripheral arteries; it increases coronary blood flow primarily by a selective dilation of the coronary arteries. The drug increases coronary sinus oxygen saturation without significantly altering myocardial oxygen consumption. A mild positive inotropic effect has been demonstrated in animals and man.

Animal: Experimental work in dogs subjected to artificial narrowing of one or both branches of the left coronary artery and chronically fed Persantine, brand of dipyridamole, has demonstrated an increase in intercoronary collateral circulation greater than that seen in placebo- or nitrate-treated animals exposed to identical conditions. A similar increase in collateral anastomoses over controls has been shown in healthy animals fed the drug.

In studies with heart preparations, the drug has been shown to protect against disturbances in function and fall in high-energy phosphate levels induced by hypoxia.

In animal (rat) studies using combination therapy with digitalis and dipyridamole, potentiation of digitalis toxicity occurred as measured by an augmentation of phosphorus exchange of the phosphorus-containing fractions of the myocardium. Experiments in cats, on the other hand, have shown that dipyridamole decreases the acute toxicity of digitoxin.

Studies with electron microscopy have demonstrated preservation of the anatomic structure of heart mitochondria (sarcosomes) in animals pretreated with the drug and exposed to hypoxia. Untreated animals showed dissolution of mitochondrial structure under similar conditions.

Indications: Based on a review of this drug by the National Academy of Sciences—National Research Council and/or other information, FDA has classified the indication as follows:

"Possibly" effective: For long-term therapy of chronic angina pectoris. Prolonged therapy may reduce the frequency or eliminate anginal episodes, improve exercise tolerance, and reduce nitroglycerin requirements. The drug is not intended to abort the acute anginal attack.

Final classification of the less-than-effective indications requires further investigation.

Contraindications: No specific contraindications are known.

Precautions: Since excessive doses can produce peripheral vasodilation, the drug should be used cautiously in patients with hypotension.

Persantine tablets, 25 mg, contain FD&C Yellow No. 5 (tartrazine) which may cause allergic-type reactions (including bronchial asthma) in certain susceptible individuals. Although the overall incidence of FD&C Yellow No. 5 (tartrazine) sensitivity in the general population is low, it is frequently seen in patients who also have aspirin hypersensitivity.

Adverse Reactions: Adverse reactions are minimal and transient at recommended dosages.

Instances of headache, dizziness, nausea, flushing, weakness, or syncope, mild gastrointestinal distress and skin rash have been noted during therapy. Rare cases of what appeared to be an aggravation of angina pectoris have been reported, usually at the initiation of therapy. On those uncommon occasions when adverse reactions have been persistent or intolerable to the patient, withdrawal of the medication has been followed promptly by cessation of the undesirable symptoms.

Dosage and Administration: The recommended dosage is 50 mg three times a day, taken at least one hour before meals. In some cases higher doses may be necessary but should be used with the knowledge that a significantly increased incidence of side effects is associated with increased dosage. Clinical response may not be evident before the second or third month of continuous therapy.

How Supplied:

Persantine (dipyridamole): round, orange, sugar-coated tablets of 25 mg, coded 17. Bottles of 100 and 1000. Unit-dose packages of 100.

Persantine-50 (dipyridamole): round, orange, sugar-coated tablets of 50 mg, coded 18. Bottles of 100.

Persantine-75 (dipyridamole): round, orange, sugar-coated tablets of 75 mg, coded 19. Bottles of 100. 98-146-510-H (8/79)

[*Shown in Product Identification Section*]

PRELUDIN® Ⓒ ℞

brand of phenmetrazine hydrochloride

Tablets, 25 mg NF ....BI-CODE 42

Endurets® (prolonged-action tablets), 50 mg..............................BI-CODE 79

Endurets® (prolonged-action tablets), 75 mg..............................BI-CODE 62

Description: Preludin, brand of phenmetrazine hydrochloride, belongs to the oxazine group of compounds and is designated chemically as 2-phenyl-3-methyltetrahydro-1,4-oxazine hydrochloride.

Phenmetrazine hydrochloride is a white, water-soluble, crystalline powder.

Actions: Preludin, brand of phenmetrazine hydrochloride, is a sympathomimetic amine with pharmacologic activity similar to the prototype drugs of this class used in obesity, the amphetamines. Actions include central nervous system stimulation and elevation of blood pressure. Tachyphylaxis and tolerance have been demonstrated with all drugs of this class in which these phenomena have been looked for.

Drugs of this class used in obesity are commonly known as "anorectics" or "anorexigenics". It has not been established, however, that the action of such drugs in treating obesity is primarily one of appetite suppression. Other central nervous system actions, or metabolic effects, may be involved, for example.

Adult obese subjects instructed in dietary management and treated with "anorectic" drugs, lose more weight on the average than those treated with placebo and diet, as determined in relatively short-term clinical trials.

The magnitude of increased weight loss of drug-treated patients over placebo-treated patients is only a fraction of a pound a week. The rate of weight loss is greatest in the first weeks of therapy for both drug and placebo subjects and tends to decrease in succeeding weeks. The possible origins of the increased weight loss due to the various drug effects are not established. The amount of weight loss associated with the use of an "anorectic" drug varies from trial to trial, and the increased weight loss appears to be related in part to variables other than the drug prescribed, such as the physician-investigator, the population treated, and the diet prescribed. Studies do not permit conclusions as to the relative importance of the drug and non-drug factors on weight loss.

The natural history of obesity is measured in years, whereas the studies cited are restricted to a few weeks' duration; thus, the total impact of drug-induced weight loss over that of diet alone must be considered clinically limited.

Preludin Endurets are formulated to release the active drug substance *in vivo* in a more gradual fashion than the standard formulation, as demonstrated by blood levels. The formulation has not been shown superior in effectiveness with respect to weight loss over the same dosage of the standard, noncontrolled-release formulations.

Indication: Preludin, brand of phenmetrazine hydrochloride, is indicated in the management of exogenous obesity as a short-term (a few weeks) adjunct in a regimen of weight reduction based on caloric restriction. The limited usefulness of agents of this class (see Actions) should be measured against possible risk factors inherent in their use such as those described below.

Contraindications: Advanced arteriosclerosis, symptomatic cardiovascular disease, moderate to severe hypertension, hyperthyroidism, known hypersensitivity or idiosyncrasy to sympathomimetic amines, glaucoma. Agitated states. Patients with a history of drug abuse. Concomitant use of CNS stimulants. During or within 14 days following the administration of monoamine oxidase inhibitors (hypertensive crises may result).

Warnings: Tolerance usually develops within a few weeks. When this occurs, the recommended dose should not be exceeded in an attempt to increase anorectic effect; rather, the drug should be discontinued.

Preludin, brand of phenmetrazine hydrochloride, may impair the ability of the patient to engage in potentially hazardous activities such as operating machinery or driving a motor vehicle; the patient should therefore be cautioned accordingly.

Drug Dependence: Preludin, brand of phenmetrazine hydrochloride, is related chemically and pharmacologically to the amphetamines. Amphetamines and related stimulant drugs have been extensively abused, and the possibility of abuse of Preludin, brand of phenmetrazine hydrochloride, should be kept in mind when evaluating the desirability of including a drug as part of a weight reduction program. Abuse of amphetamines and related drugs may be associated with intense psychological dependence and severe social dysfunction. There are reports of patients who have increased the dosage to many times that recommended. Abrupt cessation following prolonged high dosage administration results in extreme fatigue and mental depression; changes are also noted on the sleep EEG. Manifestations of chronic intoxication with anorectic drugs include severe dermatoses, marked insomnia, irritability, hyperactivity, and personality changes. The most severe manifestation of chronic intoxication is psychosis, often clinically indistinguishable from schizophrenia.

Usage in Pregnancy: Safe use in pregnancy has not been established. Animal reproductive studies demonstrated no teratogenic effects. However, the conception rate was adversely affected, as well as survival and body weight of pups at weaning. There have been clinical reports of congenital malformation associated with the use of this compound but a causal re-

lationship has not been proved. Until more information is available, Preludin, brand of phenmetrazine hydrochloride, should not be used by women who are or may become pregnant, particularly in the first trimester, unless in the opinion of the prescribing physician the potential benefits outweigh the possible risks.
Usage in Children: Preludin, brand of phenmetrazine hydrochloride, is not recommended for use in children under 12 years of age.
Precautions: Caution should be exercised in prescribing Preludin, brand of phenmetrazine hydrochloride, for patients with even mild hypertension. Insulin requirements in diabetes mellitus may be altered in association with the use of Preludin, brand of phenmetrazine hydrochloride, and the concomitant dietary regimen. Preludin, brand of phenmetrazine hydrochloride, may decrease the hypotensive effect of guanethidine. The least amount feasible should be prescribed or dispensed at one time in order to minimize the possibility of overdosage.
Preludin Endurets, 75 mg, contain FD&C Yellow No. 5 (tartrazine) which may cause allergic-type reactions (including bronchial asthma) in certain susceptible individuals. Although the overall incidence of FD&C Yellow No. 5 (tartrazine) sensitivity in the general population is low, it is frequently seen in patients who also have aspirin hypersensitivity.
Adverse Reactions: *Cardiovascular:* Palpitation, tachycardia, elevation of blood pressure.
Central Nervous System: Overstimulation, restlessness, dizziness, insomnia, euphoria, dysphoria, tremor, headache; rarely psychotic episodes at recommended doses.
Gastrointestinal: Dryness of the mouth, unpleasant taste, diarrhea, constipation, other gastrointestinal disturbances.
Allergic: Urticaria.
Endocrine: Impotence, changes in libido.
Dosage and Administration: Preludin, brand of phenmetrazine hydrochloride, is not recommended for use in children under 12 years of age.
The maximum adult dosage is 50 to 75 mg administered as one 25-mg tablet two or three times daily, one hour before meals or as one 50-mg or 75-mg Endurets prolonged-action tablet taken daily. The scored 25-mg tablet permits adjustment of dosage to individual needs.
Since an Endurets tablet provides appetite suppression for approximately 12 hours, the time of administration should be determined by the period of the day over which the anorectic effect is desired.
Overdosage: Manifestations of acute overdosage with phenmetrazine hydrochloride include restlessness, tremor, hyperreflexia, rapid respiration, confusion, assaultiveness, hallucinations, panic states. Fatigue and depression usually follow the central stimulation. Cardiovascular effects include arrhythmias, hypertension, or hypotension and circulatory collapse. Gastrointestinal symptoms include nausea, vomiting, diarrhea and abdominal cramps. Poisoning may result in convulsions, coma, and death.
Management of acute phenmetrazine hydrochloride intoxication is largely symptomatic and includes lavage and sedation with a barbiturate. Experience with hemodialysis or peritoneal dialysis is inadequate to permit recommendation in this regard. As with the amphetamines, acidification of the urine should increase phenmetrazine hydrochloride excretion. Intravenous phentolamine has been suggested for possible acute, severe hypertension if this complicates phenmetrazine overdosage.
How Supplied: Preludin, brand of phenmetrazine hydrochloride, is available in three dosage strengths:
White, square, scored tablets of 25 mg, for b.i.d. or t.i.d. administration. Bottles of 100.
White, round Endurets prolonged-action tablets of 50 mg, for once-a-day administration. Bottles of 100.
Pink, round Endurets prolonged-action tablets of 75 mg, for once-a-day administration. Bottles of 100. 98-146-560-N (8/79)
[*Shown in Product Identification Section*]

SERENTIL® ℞

brand of mesoridazine besylate

Tablets, 10 mg .... BI-CODE 20
Tablets, 25 mg .... BI-CODE 21
Tablets, 50 mg .... BI-CODE 22
Tablets, 100 mg .... BI-CODE 23
Concentrate of 25 mg/ml .... BI-CODE 25
Ampuls of 1 ml (25 mg) .... BI-CODE 27

Description: Serentil, brand of mesoridazine, the besylate salt of a metabolite of thioridazine, is a phenothiazine tranquilizer which is effective in the treatment of schizophrenia, organic brain disorders, alcoholism and psychoneuroses.
Serentil, brand of mesoridazine, is 10-[2(1-methyl-2-piperidyl) ethyl]-2-(methyl-sulfinyl)-phenothiazine [as the besylate].
Actions: Based upon animal studies Serentil, brand of mesoridazine, as with other phenothiazines, acts indirectly on reticular formation, whereby neuronal activity into reticular formation is reduced without affecting its intrinsic ability to activate the cerebral cortex. In addition, the phenothiazines exhibit at least part of their activities through depression of hypothalamic centers. Neurochemically, the phenothiazines are thought to exert their effects by a central adrenergic blocking action.
Indications: In clinical studies Serentil, brand of mesoridazine, has been found useful in the following disease states:
Schizophrenia: Serentil is effective in the treatment of schizophrenia. It substantially reduces the severity of emotional withdrawal, conceptual disorganization, anxiety, tension, hallucinatory behavior, suspiciousness and blunted affect in schizophrenic patients. As with other phenothiazines, patients refractory to previous medication may respond to Serentil, brand of mesoridazine.
Behavioral Problems in Mental Deficiency and Chronic Brain Syndrome: The effect of Serentil, brand of mesoridazine, was found to be excellent or good in the management of hyperactivity and uncooperativeness associated with mental deficiency and chronic brain syndrome.
Alcoholism—Acute and Chronic: Serentil, brand of mesoridazine, ameliorates anxiety, tension, depression, nausea and vomiting in both acute and chronic alcoholics without producing hepatic dysfunction or hindering the functional recovery of the impaired liver.
Psychoneurotic Manifestations: Serentil, brand of mesoridazine, reduces the symptoms of anxiety and tension, prevalent symptoms often associated with neurotic components of many disorders, and benefits personality disorders in general.
Contraindications: As with other phenothiazines, Serentil, brand of mesoridazine, is contraindicated in severe central nervous system depression or comatose states from any cause. Serentil, brand of mesoridazine, is contraindicated in individuals who have previously shown hypersensitivity to the drug.
Warnings: Where patients are participating in activities requiring complete mental alertness, (e.g., driving) it is advisable to administer the phenothiazines cautiously and to increase the dosage gradually.
Usage in Pregnancy: The safety of this drug in pregnancy has not been established; hence, it should be given only when the anticipated benefits to be derived from treatment exceed the possible risks to mother and fetus.
Usage in Children: The use of Serentil, brand of mesoridazine, in children under 12 years of age is not recommended, because safe conditions for its use have not been established.
Attention should be paid to the fact that phenothiazines are capable of potentiating central nervous system depressants (e.g., anesthetics, opiates, alcohol, etc.) as well as atropine and phosphorus insecticides.
Precautions: While ocular changes have not to date been related to Serentil, brand of mesoridazine, one should be aware that such changes have been seen with other drugs of this class.
Because of possible hypotensive effects, reserve parenteral administration for bedfast patients or for acute ambulatory cases, and keep patient lying down for at least one-half hour after injection.
Leukopenia and/or agranulocytosis have been attributed to phenothiazine therapy. A single case of transient granulocytopenia has been associated with Serentil, brand of mesoridazine. Since convulsive seizures have been reported, patients receiving anticonvulsant medication should be maintained on that regimen while receiving Serentil, brand of mesoridazine.
Serentil tablets contain FD&C Yellow No. 5 (tartrazine) which may cause allergic-type reactions (including bronchial asthma) in certain susceptible individuals. Although the overall incidence of FD&C Yellow No. 5 (tartrazine) sensitivity in the general population is low, it is frequently seen in patients who also have aspirin hypersensitivity.
Adverse Reactions: Drowsiness and hypotension were the most prevalent side effects encountered. Side effects tended to reach their maximum level of severity early with the exception of a few (rigidity and motoric effects) which occurred later in therapy.
With the exceptions of tremor and rigidity, adverse reactions were generally found among those patients who received relatively high doses early in treatment. Clinical data showed no tendency for the investigators to terminate treatment because of side effects.
Serentil, brand of mesoridazine, has demonstrated a remarkably low incidence of adverse reactions when compared with other phenothiazine compounds.
Central Nervous System: Drowsiness, Parkinson's syndrome, dizziness, weakness, tremor, restlessness, ataxia, dystonia, rigidity, slurring, akathisia, motoric reactions (opisthotonos) have been reported.
Autonomic Nervous System: Dry mouth, nausea and vomiting, fainting, stuffy nose, photophobia, constipation and blurred vision have occurred in some instances.
Genitourinary System: Inhibition of ejaculation, impotence, enuresis, incontinence have been reported.
Skin: Itching, rash, hypertrophic papillae of the tongue and angioneurotic edema have been reported.
Cardiovascular System: Hypotension and tachycardia have been reported. EKG changes have occurred in some instances (see Phenothiazine Derivatives: Cardiovascular Effects).
Phenothiazine Derivatives: It should be noted that efficacy, indications and untoward effects have varied with the different phenothiazines. The physician should be aware that the following have occurred with one or more phenothiazines and should be considered whenever one of these drugs is used:
Autonomic Reactions: Miosis, obstipation, anorexia, paralytic ileus.
Cutaneous Reactions: Erythema, exfoliative dermatitis, contact dermatitis.
Blood Dyscrasias: Agranulocytosis, leukopenia, eosinophilia, thrombocytopenia, anemia, aplastic anemia, pancytopenia.
Allergic Reactions: Fever, laryngeal edema, angioneurotic edema, asthma.
Hepatotoxicity: Jaundice, biliary stasis.
Cardiovascular Effects: Changes in the terminal portion of the electrocardiogram, including prolongation of the Q-T interval, lowering and inversion of the T wave and appearance of a

Continued on next page

Boehringer Ingelheim—Cont.

wave tentatively identified as a bifid T or a U wave have been observed in some patients receiving the phenothiazine tranquilizers, including Serentil, brand of mesoridazine. To date, these appear to be due to altered repolarization and not related to myocardial damage. They appear to be reversible. While there is no evidence at present that these changes are in any way precursors of any significant disturbance of cardiac rhythm, it should be noted that sudden and unexpected deaths apparently due to cardiac arrest have occurred in patients previously showing characteristic electrocardiographic changes while taking the drug. The use of periodic electrocardiograms has been proposed but would appear to be of questionable value as a predictive device.
Hypotension, rarely resulting in cardiac arrest, has been noted.
Extrapyramidal Symptoms: Akathisia, agitation, motor restlessness, dystonic reactions, trismus, torticollis, opisthotonos, oculogyric crises, tremor, muscular rigidity, akinesia.
Persistent Tardive Dyskinesia: As with all antipsychotic agents, tardive dyskinesia may appear in some patients on long-term therapy or may occur after drug therapy has been discontinued. This risk seems to be greater in elderly patients on high-dose therapy, especially females. The symptoms are persistent and in some patients appear to be irreversible. The syndrome is characterized by rhythmical involuntary movements of the tongue, face, mouth or jaw (e.g., protrusion of tongue, puffing of cheeks, puckering of mouth, chewing movements). Sometimes these may be accompanied by involuntary movements of extremities.
There is no known effective treatment for tardive dyskinesia; antiparkinsonism agents usually do not alleviate the symptoms of this syndrome. It is suggested that all antipsychotic agents be discontinued if these symptoms appear.
Should it be necessary to reinstitute treatment, or increase the dosage of the agent, or switch to a different antipsychotic agent, the syndrome may be masked.
It has been reported that fine vermicular movements of the tongue may be an early sign of the syndrome and if the medication is stopped at that time, the syndrome may not develop.
Endocrine Disturbances: Menstrual irregularities, altered libido, gynecomastia, lactation, weight gain, edema. False positive pregnancy tests have been reported.
Urinary Disturbances: Retention, incontinence.
Others: Hyperpyrexia. Behavioral effects suggestive of a paradoxical reaction have been reported. These include excitement, bizarre dreams, aggravation of psychoses and toxic confusional states. More recently, a peculiar skin-eye syndrome has been recognized as a side effect following long-term treatment with phenothiazines. This reaction is marked by progressive pigmentation of areas of the skin or conjunctiva and/or accompanied by discoloration of the exposed sclera and cornea. Opacities of the anterior lens and cornea described as irregular or stellate in shape have also been reported. Systemic lupus erythematosus-like syndrome.

Dosage and Administration: The dosage of Serentil, brand of mesoridazine, as in most medications, should be adjusted to the needs of the individual. The lowest effective dosage should always be used. When maximum response is achieved, dosage may be reduced gradually to a maintenance level.
Schizophrenia: For most patients, regardless of severity, a starting dose of 50 mg. t.i.d. is recommended. The usual optimum total daily dose range is 100-400 mg per day.
Behavioral Problems in Mental Deficiency and Chronic Brain Syndrome: For most patients a starting dose of 25 mg t.i.d. is recommended. The usual optimum total daily dose range is 75-300 mg per day.
Alcoholism: For most patients the usual starting dose is 25 mg b.i.d. The usual optimum total daily dose range is 50-200 mg per day.
Psychoneurotic Manifestations: For most patients the usual starting dose is 10 mg t.i.d. The usual optimum total daily dose range is 30-150 mg per day.
Injectable Form: In those situations in which an intramuscular form of medication is indicated, Serentil, brand of mesoridazine, injectable is available. For most patients a starting dose of 25 mg is recommended. The dose may be repeated in 30 to 60 minutes, if necessary. The usual optimum total daily dose range is 25-200 mg per day.

How Supplied:
Tablets: 10 mg, 25 mg, 50 mg, and 100 mg mesoridazine (as the besylate). Bottles of 100.
Ampuls: 1 ml [25 mg mesoridazine (as the besylate)]. Inactive ingredients: disodium edetate, USP, 0.5 mg; sodium chloride, USP, 7.2 mg; carbon dioxide gas (bone dry) q.s., water for injection, USP, q.s. to 1 ml. Boxes of 20 and 100.
Concentrate: Contains 25 mg mesoridazine (as the besylate) per ml; alcohol, USP, 0.61% by volume. Immediate containers: Amber glass bottles of 4 fl oz (118 ml) packaged in cartons of 12 bottles, with an accompanying dropper graduated to deliver 10 mg, 25 mg and 50 mg of mesoridazine (as the besylate).
Storage: Below 77°F. Protect from light. Dispense in amber glass bottles only.
The concentrate may be diluted with distilled water, acidified tap water, orange juice or grape juice.
Each dose should be so diluted just prior to administration. Preparation and storage of bulk dilutions is not recommended.
Additional information available to physicians.

Pharmacology: Pharmacological studies in laboratory animals have established that Serentil, brand of mesoridazine, has a spectrum of pharmacodynamic actions typical of a major tranquilizer. In common with other tranquilizers it inhibits spontaneous motor activity in mice, prolongs thiopental and hexobarbital sleeping time in mice and produces spindles and block of arousal reaction in the EEG of rabbits. It is effective in blocking spinal reflexes in the cat and antagonizes d-amphetamine excitation and toxicity in grouped mice. It shows a moderate adrenergic blocking activity in vitro and in vivo and antagonizes 5-hydroxytryptamine in vivo. Intravenously administered, it lowers the blood pressure of anesthetized dogs. It has a weak antiacetylcholine effect in vitro.
The most outstanding activity of Serentil, brand of mesoridazine, is seen in tests developed to investigate antiemotive activity of drugs. Such tests are those in which the rat reacts to acute or chronic stress by increased defecation (emotogenic defecation) or tests in which "emotional mydriasis" is elicited in the mouse by an electric shock. In both of these tests Serentil, brand of mesoridazine, is effective in reducing emotive reactions. Its ED_{50} in inhibiting emotogenic defecation in the rat is 0.053 mg/kg (subcutaneous administration). Serentil, brand of mesoridazine, has a potent antiemetic action. The intravenous ED_{50} against apomorphine-induced emesis in the dog is 0.64 mg/kg.
Serentil, brand of mesoridazine, in common with other phenothiazines, demonstrates antiarrhythmic activity in anesthetized dogs. Metabolic studies in the dog and rabbit with tritium labeled mesoridazine demonstrate that the compound is well absorbed from the gastrointestinal tract. The biological half-life of Serentil, brand of mesoridazine, in these studies appears to be somewhere between 24 to 48 hours. Although significant urinary excretion was observed following the administration of Serentil, brand of mesoridazine, these studies also suggest that biliary excretion is an important excretion route for mesoridazine and/or its metabolites.

Toxicity Studies
Acute LD_{50} (mg/kg):
[See table below].

Route	Mouse	Rat	Rabbit	Dog
Oral	560 ± 62.5	644 ± 48	MLD = 800	MLD = 800
I.M.	—	509M 584 F	405	—
I.V.	26 ± 0.08	—	—	—

Chronic toxicity studies were conducted in rats and dogs. Rats were administered Serentil, brand of mesoridazine, orally seven days per week for a period of seventeen months in doses up to 160 mg/kg per day. Dogs were administered Serentil, brand of mesoridazine, orally seven days per week for a period of thirteen months. The daily dosage of the drug was increased during the period of this test such that the "top-dose" group received a daily dose of 120 mg/kg of mesoridazine for the last month of the study. Untoward effects which occurred upon chronic administration of high dose-levels included:
Rats: Reduction of food intake, slowed weight gain, morphological changes in pituitary-supported endocrine organs, and melanin-like pigment deposition in renal tissues.
Dogs: Emesis, muscle tremors, decreased food intake and death associated with aspiration of oral-gastric contents into the respiratory system.
Increased intrauterine resorptions were seen with Serentil, brand of mesoridazine, in rats at 70 mg/kg and in rabbits at 125 mg/kg but not at 60 and 100 mg/kg, respectively. No drug related teratology was suggested by these reproductive studies.
Local irritation from the intramuscular injection of Serentil, brand of mesoridazine, was of the same order of magnitude as with other phenothiazines. SER-Z12 (8/79)

[*Shown in Product Identification Section*]

TORECAN® ℞

brand of thiethylperazine NF
Tablets, 10 mg ....BI-CODE 28
Suppositories, 10 mg ....BI-CODE 29
Injection, 10 mg/2ml ampul ....BI-CODE 30

Description: Torecan, brand of thiethylperazine, is a phenothiazine. Thiethylperazine is characterized by a substituted thioethyl group at position 2 in the phenothiazine nucleus, and a piperazine moiety in the side chain. The chemical designation is: 2-ethyl-mercapto-10-[3′-(1″-methyl-piperazinyl-4″)-propyl-1′] phenothiazine.
Actions: The pharmacodynamic action of Torecan, brand of thiethylperazine, in humans is unknown. However, a direct action of Torecan, brand of thiethylperazine, on both the

CTZ and the vomiting center may be concluded from induced vomiting experiments in animals.

Indications: Based upon the review of this drug by the National Academy of Sciences—National Research Council and/or other information, FDA has classified the indications as follows:
Effective: For the relief of nausea and vomiting.
"Possibly" effective: For the treatment of vertigo.
Final classification of the less-than-effective indication requires further investigation.

Contraindications: Severe central nervous system (CNS) depression and comatose states. In patients who have demonstrated a hypersensitivity reaction (e.g., blood dyscrasias, jaundice) to phenothiazines.
Because severe hypotension has been reported after the intravenous administration of phenothiazines, this route of administration is contraindicated.
Usage in Pregnancy: Torecan, brand of thiethylperazine, is contraindicated in pregnancy.
Warnings: Phenothiazines are capable of potentiating CNS depressants (e.g., anesthetics, opiates, alcohol, etc.) as well as atropine and phosphorous insecticides.
Since Torecan, brand of thiethylperazine, may impair mental and/or physical ability required in the performance of potentially hazardous tasks such as driving a car or operating machinery, it is recommended that patients be warned accordingly.
Postoperative Nausea and Vomiting: With the use of this drug to control postoperative nausea and vomiting occurring in patients undergoing elective surgical procedures, restlessness and postoperative CNS depression during anesthesia recovery may occur. Possible postoperative complications of a severe degree of any of the known reactions of this class of drug must be considered.
Postural hypotension may occur after an initial injection, rarely with the tablet or suppository.
The administration of epinephrine should be avoided in the treatment of drug-induced hypotension in view of the fact that phenothiazines may induce a reversed epinephrine effect on occasion.
Should a vasoconstrictive agent be required, the most suitable are levarterenol and phenylephrine.
The use of this drug has not been studied following intracardiac and intracranial surgery.
Usage in Pediatrics: The safety and efficacy of Torecan, brand of thiethylperazine, in children under 12 years of age has not been established.
Nursing Mothers: Information is not available concerning the secretion of Torecan, brand of thiethylperazine, in the milk of nursing mothers. As a general rule, nursing should not be undertaken while a patient is on a drug, since many drugs are secreted in human milk.
Precautions: Abnormal movements such as extrapyramidal symptoms (EPS) (e.g., dystonia, torticollis, dysphasia, oculogyric crises, akathisia) have occurred. Convulsions have also been reported. The varied symptom complex is more likely to occur in young adults and children. Extrapyramidal effects must be treated by reduction of dosage or cessation of medication.
Torecan tablets contain FD&C Yellow No. 5 (tartrazine) which may cause allergic-type reactions (including bronchial asthma) in certain susceptible individuals. Although the overall incidence of FD&C Yellow No. 5 (tartrazine) sensitivity in the general population is low, it is frequently seen in patients who also have aspirin hypersensitivity.
Postoperative Nausea and Vomiting: When used in the treatment of the nausea and/or vomiting associated with anesthesia and surgery, it is recommended that Torecan, brand of thiethylperazine, should be administered by deep intramuscular injection at or shortly before the termination of anesthesia.
Adverse Reactions: *Central Nervous System:* Serious: Convulsions have been reported. Extrapyramidal symptoms (EPS) may occur, such as dystonia, torticollis, oculogyric crises, akathisia, and gait disturbances. Others: Occasional cases of dizziness, headache, fever and restlessness have been reported.
Drowsiness may occur on occasion, following an initial injection. Generally this effect tends to subside with continued therapy or is usually alleviated by a reduction in dosage.
Autonomic Nervous System: Dryness of the mouth and nose, blurred vision, tinnitus. An occasional case of sialorrhea together with altered gustatory sensation has been observed.
Endocrine System: Peripheral edema of the arms, hands and face.
Hepatotoxicity: An occasional case of cholestatic jaundice has been observed.
Others: An occasional case of cerebral vascular spasm and trigeminal neuralgia has been reported.
Phenothiazine Derivatives: The physician should be aware that the following have occurred with one or more phenothiazines and should be considered whenever one of these drugs is used:
Blood Dyscrasias: Serious: Agranulocytosis, leukopenia, thrombocytopenia, aplastic anemia, pancytopenia. Others: Eosinophilia, leukocytosis.
Autonomic Reactions: Miosis, obstipation, anorexia, paralytic ileus.
Cutaneous Reactions: Serious: Erythema, exfoliative dermatitis, contact dermatitis.
Hepatotoxicity: Serious: Jaundice, biliary stasis.
Cardiovascular Effects: Serious: Hypotension, rarely leading to cardiac arrest; electrocardiographic (ECG) changes.
Extrapyramidal Symptoms: Serious: Akathisia, agitation, motor restlessness, dystonic reactions, trismus, torticollis, opisthotonos, oculogyric crises, tremor, muscular rigidity, akinesia—some of which have persisted for several months or years especially in patients of advanced age with brain damage.
Endocrine Disturbances: Menstrual irregularities, altered libido, gynecomastia, weight gain. False positive pregnancy tests have been reported.
Urinary Disturbances: Retention, incontinence.
Allergic Reactions: Serious: Fever, laryngeal edema, angioneurotic edema, asthma.
Others: Hyperpyrexia. Behavioral effects suggestive of a paradoxical reaction have been reported. These include excitement, bizarre dreams, aggravation of psychoses and toxic confusional states. While there is no evidence at present that ECG changes observed in patients receiving phenothiazines are in any way precursors of any significant disturbance of cardiac rhythm, it should be noted that sudden and unexpected deaths apparently due to cardiac arrest have been reported in a few instances in hospitalized psychotic patients previously showing characteristic ECG changes. A peculiar skin-eye syndrome has also been recognized as a side effect following long-term treatment with certain phenothiazines. This reaction is marked by progressive pigmentation of areas of the skin or conjunctiva and/or accompanied by discoloration of the exposed sclera and cornea. Opacities of the anterior lens and cornea described as irregular or stellate in shape have also been reported.
Drug Interactions: Phenothiazines are capable of potentiating CNS depressants (e.g., anesthetics, opiates, alcohol, etc.) as well as atropine and phosphorous insecticides.
Phenothiazines may induce a reversed epinephrine effect on occasion.
Dosage and Administration:
Adult: Usual daily dose range is 10 mg to 30 mg.
Oral: One tablet, one to three times daily.
Intramuscular: 2 ml IM, one to three times daily. (See Precautions.)
Suppository: Insert one suppository, one to three times daily.
Children: Appropriate dosage of Torecan, brand of thiethylperazine, has not been determined in children.
How Supplied:
Tablets: Each tablet contains 10 mg thiethylperazine maleate, NF, bottles of 100.
Ampuls: Each 2 ml ampul contains in aqueous solution 10 mg thiethylperazine malate, NF; sodium metabisulfite, 0.5 mg; ascorbic acid, USP, 2.0 mg; sorbitol, USP, 40.0 mg; carbon dioxide gas q.s.; water for injection, USP, q.s. Boxes of 20 and 100.
Storage: Below 86° F; light-resistant container. Administer only if clear and colorless.
Suppositories: Each containing 10 mg thiethylperazine maleate, NF and inactive ingredient—cocoa butter, USP; packages of 12.
Storage: Below 77° F; tight container (sealed foil). TOR-Z16 (8/79)
[*Shown in Product Identification Section*]

Boots Pharmaceuticals, Inc.
6540 LINE AVENUE
SHREVEPORT, LOUISIANA 71106

DIACTION ℂ ℞
Anti-diarrheal

Description: Each tablet contains:
Diphenoxylate Hydrochloride................2.5 mg.
(Warning: May be habit forming)
Atropine Sulfate..................................0.025 mg.
Indications: Diaction is effective as adjunctive therapy in the management of diarrhea.
Contraindications: Diaction tablets should not be given to children less than 12 years of age. Diphenoxylate hydrochloride is also contraindicated in patients who are jaundiced or hypersensitive to the ingredients contained in Diaction tablets. The use of this drug is contraindicated in the treatment of diarrhea associated with pseudomembranous colitis occurring during or up to several weeks following treatment with antibiotics such as clindamycin (Cleocin®) or lincomycin (Lincocin®).
Warnings: Do not use Diaction (diphenoxylate with atropine) tablets in children less than 12 years old. Use with extreme caution in patients with cirrhosis and other advanced hepatic disease or abnormal liver function tests, because of possible hepatic coma. Diphenoxylate hydrochloride may potentiate the action of barbiturates, tranquilizers, and alcohol. In theory, concurrent use with monoamine oxidase inhibitors could precipitate hypertensive crisis. In severe dehydration or electrolyte imbalance, withhold Diaction until corrective therapy has been initiated.
Precautions: It is theoretically possible that high doses of diphenoxylate will produce addiction (dependence). Do not exceed recommended doses. Use with caution in patients being treated with addicting drugs or those known to be addiction prone or having a history of drug abuse. The subtherapeutic dose of atropine sulfate is present in Diaction to discourage deliberate overdosing. The warnings, contraindications, and precautions for atropine should be strictly observed. Use with care in patients with actue ulcerative colitis and discontinue use if abdominal distension or other untoward symptoms develop.

Continued on next page

Boots—Cont.

Use in Pregnancy—The potential benefits must be weighed against the possible risks before using during pregnancy or lactation or in women of child bearing age. Diphenoxylate and atropine are both secreted in the milk of lactating mothers.

Adverse Reactions: Reported side effects of Diaction (diphenoxylate with atropine) include nausea, sedation, vomiting, swelling of the gums, abdominal discomfort, numbness of the extremities, headache, dizziness, depression, malaise, respiratory depression, drowsiness, coma, lethargy, anorexia, restlessness, euphoria, pruritus, angioneurotic edema, giant urticaria, paralytic ileus, and toxic megacolon. Atropine effects such as dryness of the skin and mucous membrane, flushing, hyperthermia, tachycardia, and urinary retention may occur.

Overdose: Keep this medication out of reach of children because accidental overdosage can cause severe, even fatal, respiratory depression. Initial signs of overdosage may include dry skin and mucous membranes, flushing, hyperthermia and tachycardia, followed by lethargy or coma, hypotonic reflexes, nystagmus, pinpoint pupils, and respiratory depression. Gastric lavage, establishment of a patent airway and mechanical assistance of respiration when necessary are advised. In severe respiratory depression, a narcotic antagonist such as nalaxone hydrochloride may be used. Continuous observation is necessary until the respiratory depression has passed.

Dosage and Administration: Diaction tablets should not be given to children less than 12 years of age. Adults: The recommended initial dosage is two Diaction tablets four times a day. Most patients will require this dosage until control has been achieved, after which the dosage may be reduced to meet individual requirements.

Diaction (diphenoxylate with atropine) is a Schedule V controlled substance by Federal law. Diphenoxylate is chemically related to meperidine. Overdosage or individual hypersensitivity can result in reactions similar to those produced by overdosage of meperidine or morphine. As in morphine or meperidine poisoning, prolonged and careful monitoring is required. Respiratory depression may recur as long as 30 hours after ingestion and in spite of initial responsiveness to Narcan®, naloxone hydrochloride. DIACTION IS NOT AN INNOCUOUS DRUG. ADHERE STRICTLY TO DOSAGE RECOMMENDATIONS. ESPECIALLY IN CHILDREN. THIS MEDICATION SHOULD BE KEPT OUT OF THE REACH OF CHILDREN.

How Supplied: White tablets containing 2.5 mg. of diphenoxylate hydrochloride and 0.025 mg. of atropine sulfate. Bottles of 100 NDC 0524-0042-01. Bottles of 500 NDC 0524-0043-05.

F-E-P CREME® ℞

Hydrocortisone-Iodochlorhydroxyquin Cream
Antifungal-Antibacterial-
Anti-inflammatory-Anesthetic

Description: Composition contains:

Iodochlorhydroxyquin, NF	3.0%
Pramoxine Hydrochloride, NF	0.5%
Hydrocortisone, USP	1.0%

F-E-P CREME® is water soluble.

F-E-P CREME® also contains as inactive components: Deionized water, Methylparaben, Propylparaben, Glycerin, Octyldodecanol, Cetyl Alcohol, Stearyl Alcohol, and Ethylated Cetyl Stearyl Alcohol.

Indications: Based on a review of this drug by the National Academy of Sciences—National Research Council and/or other information, FDA has classified the indications as follows:

"Possibly" effective: contact or atopic dermatitis; impetiginized eczema; nummular eczema; infantile eczema; endogenous chronic infectious dermatitis; stasis dermatitis; pyoderma; nuchal eczema and chronic eczematoid otitis externa; acne urticata; localized or disseminated neurodermatitis; lichen simplex chronicus; anogenital pruritus (vulvae, scroti, ani); folliculitis; bacterial dermatoses; mycotic dermatoses such as tinea (capitis, cruris, corporis, pedis); moniliasis; intertrigo.

Final classification of the less-than-effective indications requires further investigation.

Pramoxine Hydrochloride promptly relieves pain and itch. This compound may be used safely on the skin of those patients sensitive to the "caine" type local anesthetics.

Contraindications: Hypersensitivity to any of the ingredients, tuberculosis of the skin, viral lesions of the skin (including herpes simplex, varicella and vaccinia).

Precautions: For external application only. If hypersensitivity develops, discontinue use. Not for ophthalmic use. May stain hair.

Adverse Reactions: Rash may occur in the few patients sensitive to topically applied corticosteroids.

Dosage and Administration: Apply a thin layer to the affected parts 3 to 4 times daily.

How Supplied: In ½ ounce tubes. NDC 0524-0026-51.

LOPURIN™ ℞

Allopurinol
100 mg Scored Tablets and
300 mg Scored Tablets

Description: Allopurinol is a xanthine oxidase inhibitor with the chemical name 4-hydroxypyrazolo (3,4-d) pyrimidine (HPP).

Clinical Pharmacology: Lopurin (allopurinol) acts on purine catabolism, without disrupting the biosynthesis of vital purines, thus reducing the production of uric acid by inhibiting the biochemical reactions immediately preceding its formation. Its action differs from that of uricosuric agents, which lower the serum uric acid level by increasing urinary excretion of uric acid. Lopurin reduces both the serum and urinary uric acid levels by inhibiting the formation of uric acid. It thereby avoids the hazard of increased hyperuricosuria in patients with gouty nephropathy or with a predisposition to the formation of uric acid stones.

Lopurin has produced a substantial reduction in serum and urinary uric acid levels in hitherto refractory patients even in the presence of renal damage marked enough to render uricosuric drugs virtually ineffective. Salicylates may be given conjointly for their antirheumatic effect without compromising the action of allopurinol. This is in contrast to the nullifying effect of salicylates on uricosuric drugs.

Lopurin is a structural analogue of the natural purine base, hypoxanthine. It is a potent inhibitor of xanthine oxidase, the enzyme responsible for the conversion of hypoxanthine to xanthine and of xanthine to uric acid, the end product of purine metabolism in man. Lopurin is metabolized to the corresponding xanthine analogue, oxipurinol (alloxanthine), which also is an inhibitor of xanthine oxidase.

Hyperuricemia may be primary, as in gout, or secondary to diseases such as acute and chronic leukemia, polycythemia vera, multiple myeloma, and psoriasis. It may occur with the use of diuretic agents, during renal dialysis, in the presence of renal damage, during starvation or reducing diets and in the treatment of neoplastic disease where rapid resolution of tissue masses may occur.

The major disease manifestations in gout—kidney stones, tophi in soft tissues, and deposits in joints and bones—result from the deposition of urates. If progressive deposition of urates is to be arrested or reversed, it is necessary to reduce the serum uric acid to a level below the saturation point to suppress urate precipitation. Reduction may be achieved by means of uricosuric agents. Uricosurics are less effective in the presence of renal disease, and some patients develop intolerance or sensitivity to these drugs. The use of allopurinol to block the formation of urate avoids the hazard of increased renal excretion of uric acid posed by uricosuric drugs.

The half-life of Lopurin in the body is determined both by renal excretion and by oxidation to 4,6-dihydroxypyrazolo (3,4-d) pyrimidine (oxipurinol). The latter is also an inhibitor of xanthine oxidase, but is somewhat weaker than allopurinol which is bound 15-fold more tightly to the enzyme than is the natural substrate, xanthine. The long half-life of oxipurinol in the plasma (18 to 30 hours), contributes significantly to the enzyme inhibition. Moreover, both allopurinol and oxipurinol tend to inactivate xanthine oxidase, thereby further controlling the level of its activity.

Administration of Lopurin generally results in a fall in both serum and urinary uric acid within two to three days. The magnitude of this decrease can be manipulated almost at will since it is dose-dependent. A week or more of treatment with allopurinol may be required for the full effects of the drug to be manifest; likewise, uric acid may return to pretreatment levels slowly, usually after a period of 7 to 10 days following cessation of therapy. This reflects primarily the accumulation and slow clearance of oxipurinol. In some patients, particularly those with severe tophaceous gout and under-excretors, a dramatic fall in urinary uric acid excretion may not occur. It has been postulated that this may be due to the mobilization of urate from the tissue deposits as the serum uric acid level begins to fall.

The combined increase in hypoxanthine and xanthine excreted in the urine usually, but not always, is considerably less than the accompanying decline in urinary uric acid.

It has been shown that reutilization of both hypoxanthine and xanthine for nucleotide and nucleic acid synthesis is markedly enhanced when their oxidations are inhibited by allopurinol. This reutilization and the normal feedback inhibition which would result from an increase in available purine nucleotides serve to regulate purine biosynthesis and, in essence, the defect of the overproducer of uric acid is thereby compensated.

Innate deficiency of xanthine oxidase, which occurs in congenital xanthuria as an inborn error of metabolism, has been shown to be compatible with normal health. While urinary levels of oxypurines attained with full doses of allopurinol may in exceptional cases equal those (250–600 mg per day) which in xanthinuric subjects have caused formation of urinary calculi, they usually fall in the range of 50–200 mg. Xanthine crystalluria has been reported in a few exceptional cases. Two of these had Lesch-Nyhan syndrome, which is characterized by excessive uric acid production combined with a deficiency in the enzyme, hypoxanthine-guanine phosphoribosyltransferase (HG-PRTase). This enzyme is required for the conversion of hypoxanthine and guanine to their respective nucleotides. The third case was a patient with lymphosarcoma, who produced an extremely large amount of uric acid because of rapid cell lysis during chemotherapy.

The serum concentration of oxypurines in patients receiving allopurinol is usually in the range of 0.3 mg to 0.4 mg percent compared to a normal level of approximately 0.15 mg percent. A maximum of 0.9 mg percent was observed when the serum urate was lowered to less than 2 mg percent by high doses of the drug. In one exceptional case a value of 2.7 mg percent was reached. These are far below the saturation level at which precipitation of xanthine or hypoxanthine would be expected to occur.

The solubilities of uric acid and xanthine in the serum are similar (about 7 mg percent) while hypoxanthine is much more soluble. The finding that the renal clearance of oxypurines is at least 10 times greater than that of uric acid explains the relatively low serum oxypurine concentration at a time when the serum uric acid level has decreased markedly. At serum oxypurine levels of 0.3 mg percent to 0.9 mg percent, oxypurine: inulin clearance ratios were between 0.7 and 1.9. The glomerular filtration rate and urate clearance in patients receiving allopurinol do not differ significantly from those obtained prior to therapy. The rapid renal clearance of oxypurines suggests that allopurinol therapy should be of value in allowing a patient with gout to increase his total purine excretion.

Although the renal clearance of allopurinol is rapid, that of oxipurinol is slow and parallels that of uric acid but is higher by a factor of about three. The clearance of oxipurinol is increased by uricosuric drugs, and as a consequence, the addition of a uricosuric agent may reduce the degree of inhibition of xanthine oxidase by oxipurinol. However, such combined therapy may be useful in achieving minimum serum uric acid levels provided the total urinary uric acid load does not exceed the competence of the patient's renal function. In some patients, where renal function is severely impaired, normal serum urate levels may not be achievable.

The danger of uric acid calculi is diminished as the uric acid excretion is reduced. The amounts of xanthine and hypoxanthine excreted in the urine generally do not exceed the solubilities of these compounds in the urine, particularly if the urine is slightly alkaline. The amounts of allopurinol and oxipurinol excreted are likewise within the limits of their respective solubilities.

Lopurin also inhibits the enzymatic oxidation of mercaptopurine, the sulfur-containing analogue of hypoxanthine, to 6-thiouric acid. This oxidation, which is catalyzed by xanthine oxidase, inactivates mercaptopurine. Hence, the inhibition of such oxidation by allopurinol may result in as much as 75 percent reduction in the therapeutic dose requirement of mercaptopurine when the two compounds are given together.

Indications and Use: THIS IS NOT AN INNOCUOUS DRUG AND STRICT ATTENTION SHOULD BE GIVEN TO THE INDICATIONS FOR ITS USE. PENDING FURTHER INVESTIGATION, ITS USE IN OTHER HYPERURICEMIC STATES IS NOT INDICATED AT THIS TIME.

Lopurin (allopurinol) is intended for:

1. treatment of gout, either primary, or secondary to the hyperuricemia associated with blood dyscrasias and their therapy;
2. treatment of primary or secondary uric acid nephropathy, with or without accompanying symptoms of gout;
3. treatment of patients with recurrent uric acid stone formation;
4. prophylactic treatment to prevent tissue urate deposition, renal calculi, or uric acid nephropathy in patients with leukemias, lymphomas and malignancies who are receiving cancer chemotherapy with its resultant elevating effect on serum uric acid levels.

Allopurinol, by promoting the resolution of tophi and urate crystals in the tissues, has relieved chronic joint pain, increased joint mobility, and permitted urate sinuses to heal. The addition of allopurinol to a uricosuric regimen has reduced the size of tophi which have been refractory to uricosuric agents alone and increased joint mobility.

Lopurin is particularly effective in preventing the occurrence and recurrence of uric acid stones and gravel. Lopurin is useful in therapy and prophylaxis of acute urate nephropathy in patients with neoplastic disease who are particularly susceptible to hyperuricemia and uric acid stone formation, especially after radiation therapy or the use of antineoplastic drugs.

Contraindications: Pending further investigation this drug is contraindicated for use in children with the exception of those with hyperuricemia secondary to malignancy. The drug should not be employed in nursing mothers.

PATIENTS WHO HAVE DEVELOPED A SEVERE REACTION TO LOPURIN SHOULD NOT BE RESTARTED ON THE DRUG.

Warnings: LOPURIN SHOULD BE DISCONTINUED AT THE FIRST APPEARANCE OF SKIN RASH OR ANY SIGN OF ADVERSE REACTION. In some instances a skin rash may be followed by more severe hypersensitivity reactions such as exfoliative, urticarial and purpuric lesions as well as Stevens-Johnson syndrome (erythema multiforme) and very rarely a generalized vasculitis which may lead to irreversible hepatotoxicity and death.

A few cases of reversible clinical hepatotoxicity have been noted in patients taking Lopurin and in some patients asymptomatic rises in serum alkaline phosphate or serum transaminase have been observed. Accordingly, periodic liver function tests should be performed during the early stages of therapy, particularly patients with pre-existing liver disease.

Due to the occasional occurrence of drowsiness, patients should be alerted to the need for due precautions when engaging in activities where alertness is mandatory.

An increase in hepatic iron concentration has been reported in rats given Lopurin. However, laboratory experiments and those of several other investigators have shown no effect of allopurinol on iron metabolism. Nevertheless, iron salts should not be given simultaneously with Lopurin. This drug should not be administered to immediate relatives of patients with idiopathic hemochromatosis.

In patients receiving Purinethol® (mercaptopurine) or Imuran® (azathioprine), the concomitant administration of 300-600 mg of Lopurin per day will require a reduction in dose to approximately one-third to one-fourth of the usual dose of mercaptopurine or azathioprine. Subsequent adjustment of doses of Purinethol or Imuran should be made on the basis of therapeutic response and any toxic effects.

Use in Pregnancy and Women of Childbearing Age: Reproductive studies showed no adverse effect of Lopurin on animal litters. However, since the effect of xanthine oxidase inhibition on the human fetus is still unknown, Lopurin should be used in pregnant women or women of childbearing age only if the potential benefits to the patient are weighed against the possible risk to the fetus.

Precautions: Some investigators have reported an increase in acute attacks of gout during the early stages of allopurinol administration, even when normal or subnormal serum uric acid levels have been attained. Accordingly, maintenance doses of colchicine (0.5 mg twice daily) generally should be given prophylactically when allopurinol is begun. In addition, it is recommended that the patient start with a low dose of allopurinol (100 mg daily) and increase at weekly intervals by 100 mg until a serum uric acid level of 6 mg per 100 ml or less is attained but without exceeding the maximal recommended dose. The use of therapeutic doses of colchicine or anti-inflammatory agents may be required to suppress attacks in some cases. The attacks usually become shorter and less severe after several months of therapy. A possible explanation for these flare-ups may be the mobilization of urates from tissue deposits followed by recrystallization, due to fluctuation in the serum uric acid level. Even with adequate therapy it may require several months to deplete the uric acid pool sufficiently to achieve control of the acute episodes.

The concomitant administration of a uricosuric agent with Lopurin may result in a decrease in urinary excretion of oxypurines as compared to their excretion with allopurinol alone. This may possibly be due to an increased excretion of oxipurinol and a lowering of the degree of inhibition of xanthine oxidase. Such combined therapy is not contraindicated, however, and for many patients, may provide optimum control. A report by Goldfinger, et. al., on a patient treated with sulfinpyrazone and salicylates in addition to allopurinol showed a marked decrease in the excretion of oxypurines which they suggested was due to interference with their clearance at the renal tubular level. However, subsequent laboratory studies have indicated no interference with oxypurine clearance by salicylates. Although clinical evidence to date has not demonstrated renal precipitation of oxypurines in patients either on Lopurin alone or in combination with uricosuric agents, the possibility should be kept in mind. It has been reported that allopurinol prolongs the half-life of the anticoagulant, dicumarol. The clinical significance of this has not been established, but this interaction should be kept in mind when allopurinol is given to patients already on anticoagulant therapy, and the coagulation time should be reassessed.

A fluid intake sufficient to yield a daily urinary output of at least 2 liters and the maintenance of a neutral or, preferably, slightly alkaline urine are desirable to (1) avoid the theoretic possibility of formation of xanthine calculi under the influence of Lopurin therapy and (2) help prevent renal precipitation of urates in patients receiving concomitant uricosuric agents.

A few patients with preexisting renal disease or poor urate clearance have shown a rise in BUN during Lopurin administration although a decrease in BUN has also been observed. Although the relationship of these observations to the drug has not been established, patients with impaired renal function require less drug and should be carefully observed during the early stages of Lopurin administration and the drug withdrawn if increased abnormalities in renal function appear.

In patients with severly impaired renal function, or decreased urate clearance, the half-life of oxipurinol in the plasma is greatly prolonged. Therefore, a dose of 100 mg per day or 300 mg twice a week, or perhaps less, may be sufficient to maintain adequate xanthine oxidase inhibition to reduce serum urate levels. Such patients should be treated with the lowest effective dose, in order to minimize side effects.

Mild reticulocytosis has appeared in some patients, most of whom were receiving other therapeutic agents, so that the significance of this observation is not known.

As with all new agents, periodic determination of liver and kidney function and complete blood counts should be performed especially during the first few months of therapy.

Adverse Reactions:

Dermatologic: Because in some instances skin rash has been followed by severe hypersensitivity reactions, it is recommended that therapy be discontinued at the first sign of rash or other adverse reaction (see WARNINGS).

Skin rash, usually maculopapular, is the adverse reaction most commonly reported.

Exfoliative, urticarial and purpuric lesions, Stevens-Johnson syndrome (erythema multi-

Continued on next page

Boots—Cont.

forme) and toxic epidermal necrolysis have also been reported.
A few cases of alopecia with and without accompanying dermatitis have been reported.
In some patients with a rash, restarting Lopurin therapy at lower doses has been accomplished without untoward incident.
Gastrointestinal: Nausea, vomiting, diarrhea, and intermittent abdominal pain have been reported.
Vascular: There have been rare instances of a generalized hypersensitivity vasculitis or necrotizing angiitis which have led to irreversible hepatotoxicity and death.
Hematopoietic: Agranulocytosis, anemia, aplastic anemia, bone marrow depression, leukopenia, pancytopenia and thrombocytopenia have been reported in patients, most of whom received concomitant drugs with potential for causing these reactions. Lopurin has been neither implicated nor excluded as a cause of these reactions.
Neurologic: There have been a few reports of peripheral neuritis occurring while patients were taking Lopurin. Drowsiness has also been reported in a few patients.
Ophthalmic: There have been a few reports of cataracts found in patients receiving Lopurin. It is not known if the cataracts predated the Lopurin therapy. "Toxic" cataracts were reported in one patient who also received an anti-inflammatory agent; again, the time of onset is unknown. In a group of patients followed by Gutman and Yu for up to five years on Lopurin therapy, no evidence of ophthalmologic effect attributable to Lopurin was reported.
Drug Idiosyncrasy: Symptoms suggestive of drug idiosyncrasy have been reported in a few patients. This was characterized by fever, chills, leukopenia or leukocytosis, eosinophilia, arthralgias, skin rash, pruritus, nausea, and vomiting.
Overdosage: Massive overdosing, or acute poisoning, by Lopurin has not been reported.
Dosage and Administration: The dosage of Lopurin brand Allopurinol to accomplish full control of gout and to lower serum uric acid to normal or near-normal levels varies with the severity of the disease. The average is 200 to 300 mg per day for patients with mild gout and 400 to 600 mg per day for those with moderately severe tophaceous gout. The appropriate dosage may be administered in divided doses or as a single equivalent dose with the 300 mg tablet. Dosage requirements in excess of 300 mg should be supplemented in divided doses. It should also be noted that allopurinol is generally better tolerated if taken following meals. Similar considerations govern the regulation of dosage for maintenance purposes in secondary hyperuricemia. For the prevention of uric acid nephropathy during the vigorous therapy of neoplastic disease, treatment with 600 to 800 mg daily for two to three days is advisable together with a high fluid intake. The minimal effective dosage is 100 to 200 mg daily and the maximal recommended dosage is 800 mg daily. To reduce the possibility of flare-up of acute gouty attacks, it is recommended that the patient start with a low dose of allopurinol (100 mg daily) and increase at weekly intervals by 100 mg until a serum uric acid level of 6 mg per 100 ml or less is attained but without exceeding the maximal recommended dosage.
Normal serum urate levels are achieved in one to three weeks. The upper limit of normal is about 7 mg percent for men and postmenopausal women and 6 mg percent for premenopausal women. Too much reliance should not be placed on a single reading since, for technical reasons, estimation of uric acid may be difficult. By the selection of the appropriate dose, together with the use of uricosuric agents in certain patients, it is possible to reduce the serum uric acid level to normal and, if desired, to hold it as low as 2 to 3 mg percent indefinitely.
A fluid intake sufficient to yield a daily urinary output of at least 2 liters and the maintenance of a neutral or, preferable, slightly alkaline urine are desirable.
Since allopurinol and its metabolites are excreted only by the kidney, accumulation of the drug can occur in renal failure, and the dose of allopurinol should consequently be reduced. With a creatinine clearance of 20 to 10 ml/min, a daily dosage of 200 mg of Lopurin is suitable. When the creatinine clearance is less than 10 ml/min the daily dosage should not exceed 100 mg. With extreme renal impairment (creatinine clearance less than 3 ml/min) the interval between doses may also need to be lengthened. The correct size and frequency of dosage for maintaining the serum uric acid just within the normal range is best determined by using the serum uric acid level as an index.
Children, 6 to 10 years of age, with secondary hyperuricemia associated with malignancies may be given 300 mg allopurinol daily while those under 6 years are generally given 150 mg daily. The response is evaluated after approximately 48 hours of therapy and a dosage adjustment is made if necessary.
In patients who are being treated with cholchicine and/or anti-inflammatory agents, it is wise to continue this therapy while adjusting the dosage of Lopurin until a normal serum uric acid and freedom from acute attacks have been maintained for several months.
In transferring a patient from a uricosuric agent to Lopurin, the dose of the uricosuric agent should be gradually reduced over a period of several weeks and the dose of allopurinol gradually increased to the required dose needed to maintain a normal serum uric acid level.
How Supplied: 100 mg (white) scored tablets, bottles of 100; 300 mg (peach) scored tablets, bottles of 300.
Animal Toxicology: In mice the LD_{50} is 160 mg/kg ip (with death delayed up to five days) and 700 mg/kg po (with deaths delayed up to three days). In rats the acute LD_{50} is 750 mg/kg ip 6000 mg/kg po.
In a 13 week feeding experiment in rats at a drug level of 72 mg/kg per day 2 of 10 rats died and at 225 mg/kg per day 4 of 10 died before the completion of the experiment. Both groups exhibited renal tubular damage due to the deposition of xanthine that was more extensive at the higher dose.
In chronic feeding experiments, rats showed no toxic effects at a level of 14 mg/kg per day after one year. At a level of 24 mg/kg per day for one year the rats showed very slight depression of weight gain and food intake, and 5 out of 10 of the animals showed minor changes in the kidney tubules of the type exhibited by the rats on the higher doses described above.
Dogs survived oral doses of 30 mg/kg per day for one year with nil to minor changes in the kidney and no other significant abnormalities. At 90 mg/kg per day for one year there was some accumulation of xanthine in the kidneys with resultant chronic irritation and slight tubular changes. Occasional hemosiderin-like deposits were seen in the reticuloendothelial system. A higher dose (270 mg/kg per day) resulted in large concretions in the renal pelves, with severe destructive changes in the kidney secondary to xanthine accumulation. The deposition of xanthine appears to be a function both of the metabolic turnover of purines (which is proportionately larger in the smaller animals) and the degree of inhibition of xanthine oxidase.
Reproductive studies in rats and rabbits indicated that Lopurin did not affect litter size, the mean weight of the progeny at birth or at three weeks postpartum, nor did it cause an increase in the number of animals born dead or with malformations.

P-200™ ℞
(papaverine HCl—200 Mg.)
Controlled Dissolution Tablets

Description: Each controlled dissolution tablet contains:
Papaverine hydrochloride ....200 mg.
Clinical Pharmacology: The pharmacological actions of papaverine are most pronounced on cardiac muscle and on smooth muscle. The compound acts directly on heart muscle as does quinidine, that is, conduction rate is depressed and the refractory period is prolonged. Smooth muscle of the large blood vessels is relaxed. This relaxation may be pronounced if spasm exists. Papaverine does not paralyze the muscle, contractions to other drugs and to other stimuli still occur. The antispasmodic effect is a direct one, it is not related to the muscle innervation. The coronary vessels, the cerebral vessels, the pulmonary vessels, and the systemic peripheral vessels are all relaxed by the compound. It is, perhaps, as a result of the direct vasodilation of cerebral blood vessels that papaverine increases cerebral blood flow and decreases cerebrovascular resistance in normal subjects. These effects may explain the reported benefits of papaverine in cerebrovascular encephalopathy.
The direct action of papaverine on cardiac muscle, that is, depression of conduction and prolongation of the refractory period provides the basis for its trial in abrogation of atrial and ventricular premature systoles and ventricular arrhythmias. The coronary vasodilation could be an additional factor of therapeutic value when such rhythms are secondary to insufficiency or occlusion of the coronary arteries. In patients with acute coronary thrombosis the occurrence of ventricular rhythms is serious and requires measures designed to decrease myocardial irritability. Papaverine may have advantages over quinidine, used for a similar purpose, in that it may be given in an emergency by the intravenous route, does not depress myocardial contraction or cause cinchonism, and produces coronary vasodilation.
Indications: For the relief of cerebral and peripheral ischemia associated with arterial spasm and myocardial ischemia complicated by arrhythmias.
Precautions: Use with caution in patients with glaucoma. Hepatic hypersensitivity has been reported with gastrointestinal symptoms, jaundice, eosinophilia, and altered liver function tests. Discontinue treatment with this medication if such responses occur.
Adverse Reactions: Reported side effects of papaverine include nausea, abdominal distress, anorexia, constipation or diarrhea, skin rash, malaise, drowsiness, vertigo, sweating and headache. These effects occur infrequently.
Dosage and Administration: One tablet every 12 hours, or as directed by physician.
How Supplied: P-200™ (papaverine HCl) scored, compressed, controlled dissolution tablets, bottles of 100. NDC 0524-0034-01

RU-TUSS® TABLETS ℞
Decongestant/Antihistaminic

Each Prolonged Action Tablet Contains:
Phenylephrine HCl..25 mg.
Phenylpropanolamine HCl.............................50 mg.
Chlorpheniramine Maleate ....8 mg.
Hyoscyamine Sulfate ....0.1936 mg.
Atropine Sulfate ....0.0362 mg.
Scopolamine HBr...................................0.0121 mg.
Indications and Effects: Vasoconstrictor-antihistaminic combination plus the antisecretory activity of the belladonna alkaloids for prolonged relief of nasal and sinus congestion, watering of the eyes, sneezing, and certain other symptoms common to colds, hay fever, nasal allergies, sinusitis, rhinitis and post nasal drip.

Contraindications: Sensitivity to sympathomimetics, glaucoma, and hypersensitivity to any of the ingredients, or concurrent MAO inhibitor therapy.
Precautions: Hypertension, cardiovascular disease, hyperthyroidism. Due to possible drowsiness, patient should be cautioned against driving or operating mechanical equipment.
Adverse Reactions: May cause drowsiness, xerostomia, anorexia, nausea, vomiting, dizziness, nervousness, insomnia, hypertension, tachycardia, blurring of the vision, and urinary retention. Large overdoses may cause tachypnea, delirium, fever, stupor, coma, and respiratory failure. Since the action of sustained release products may continue for as long as 12 hours, treatment of overdoses directed at reversing the effects of the drug and supporting the patient should be maintained for at least that length of time. Saline cathartics are useful for hastening evacuation of unreleased medication.
Dosage: Adults and children over 12 years of age, 1 tablet morning and evening. Not recommended for children under 12 years of age. Tablets are to be swallowed whole.
How Supplied:
Bottles of 100 tablets (NDC 0524-0058-01).

RU-VERT® ℞
Acute and Chronic Vertigo

Description: Each tablet contains:

Pentylenetetrazol	25 mg.
Pheniramine Maleate	12.5 mg.
Nicotinic Acid	50 mg.

Indications: Ru-Vert® is indicated in the symptomatic management of peripheral vestibular disorders such as idiopathic vertigo as well as that associated with Meniere's syndrome, labyrinthitis and fenestration procedures.
Contraindications: Ru-Vert® should not be used in patients with a known history of sensitivity to any of its ingredients. Because of its vasodilating effect, nicotinic acid is contraindicated in the presence of arterial hypotension.
Precautions and Adverse Reactions: Although there are no absolute contraindications to pentylenetetrazol, it should be used with caution in epileptic patients or those known to have a low convulsive threshold.
Pheniramine maleate, like other antihistamines, may produce sedative side effects in certain patients. This has not been a significant problem with Ru-Vert®.
Transient and mild side effects secondary to the therapeutic vasodilation produced by nicotinic acid, such as flushing and sensations of warmth, may be seen. Gastrointestinal side effects are rare but may occur in some patients.
Dosage & Administration: One or two tablets three times daily.
How Supplied:
Bottles of 100 NDC 0524-0060-01
Bottles of 300 NDC 0524-0061-03

TWIN-K ℞
Potassium Supplement

Description: Each 15 ml (tablespoon) supplies 20 mEq. of elemental potassium as a balanced combination of potassium gluconate (15 mEq.) and potassium citrate (5 mEq.) in a highly palatable base containing D-sorbitol.
Indications: Twin-K® serves as a source of supplemental potassium for use in patients with hypokalemia and as an adjunct in the prevention of potassium depletion.
Because Twin-K® does not contain sucrose, it may be used in patients with diabetes. Sorbitol, the sweetening agent in Twin-K®, is not significantly absorbed in the gastrointestinal tract and will not elevate serum glucose levels.
Contraindications: Hyperkalemia from any cause, renal failure with oliguria or azotemia, untreated Addison's disease, and acute dehydration.
Adverse Reactions: Excessive potassium dosage can result in hyperkalemia as indicated by mental confusion, listlessness, fall in blood pressure, cardiac arrhythmias and heart block. With normal kidney function potassium intoxication from oral administration is not likely to occur since renal excretion of the ion increases in response to an increase in total body potassium.
Dosage and Administration: One tablespoonful of Twin-K® twice daily after meals will supply 40 mEq. of potassium, approximately the normal adult daily requirement. Therapeutic dosage depends upon the requirement of the patient and the severity of the potassium depletion.
How Supplied: Pint bottles. NDC 0524-0021-16

Bowman Pharmaceuticals
Division of Bowman, Inc.
5801 MAYFAIR ROAD, N.W.
NORTH CANTON, OH 44720

GUISTREY FORTIS O.T.C.
Tablets for relief of coughs due to colds.

Description: Each tablet contains: Guaifenesin, 100 mg., Phenylephrine Hydrochloride, 10 mg.; Chlorpheniramine Maleate, 1 mg.
Indications: For the relief of coughs due to colds.
Warning: Persons with a high fever or persistent cough should not use this preparation unless directed by physician.
Caution: Individuals with high blood pressure, heart disease, diabetes, or thyroid disease should use only as directed by physician. This preparation may cause drowsiness. Do not drive or operate machinery while taking this medication. Do not give to children under 6 years of age or exceed the recommended dosage unless directed by physician.
Warning: Keep this and all drugs out of the reach of children. In case of accidental overdose, seek professional assistance or contact a poison control center immediately.
Dosage: ADULT—1 tablet, repeat in 3 hours, if necessary.
How Supplied: Bottles of 100 and 1000 sugar coated oval pink tablets.

Non-Aerosol IVY-CHEX O.T.C.

Description: IVY-CHEX contains: SD Alcohol 40, Polyvinylpyrrolidone-vinylacetate copolymers, Methyl Salicylate, Benzalkonium Cl.
Alcohol content 89.5%. Net Contents 4 fl. oz. SDA-OHIO #1260
Indications: FOR POISON IVY, POISON OAK AND POISON SUMAC—Wash the affected area with soap and water, dry with soft towel. Spray IVY-CHEX, applying only a light coat. Relief from itching and burning is almost instantaneous. Repeat if necessary. IVY-CHEX can be easily removed with soap and water. IVY-CHEX is equally effective in reducing the swelling and itching of insect bites, from chiggers, mosquitoes, bee, wasp, etc.
Directions for Use: Hold in an upright position, approximately 6 inches from the skin, press dispenser with quick short strokes. (If nozzle clogs, pull top off pump, rinse in warm water and replace). Air dry. Warning. Flammable. Do not use near fire or while smoking. Avoid spraying near eyes.
Warning: In case of accidental ingestion seek professional assistance or contact a Poison Control Center immediately. Keep this and all drugs out of reach of children.
How Supplied: 4 oz. Non-Aerosol Spray Bottle.

Boyle & Company
LOS ANGELES, CA 90040

CITRA® CAPSULES

Composition: Each capsule contains: Phenylephrine HCl, 10 mg., Ascorbic Acid, 50 mg., Pheniramine Maleate, 6.25 mg., Chlorpheniramine Maleate, 1 mg., Pyrilamine Maleate, 8.33 mg., Salicylamide, 227 mg., Phenacetin, 120 mg., Caffeine Alkaloid, 30 mg.
Action and Uses: Antihistaminic, Decongestant, analgesic for relief of nasal congestion, muscular aches and pains of the common cold, hay fever, and common pollen allergies.
Administration and Dosage: *Adults*—One capsule every 4 hours. *Children*—(6-12), one half adult dose.
Precautions: Patients should be advised to avoid using machinery or driving until response to antihistamines is established, and not to use longer than 10 days without consulting physician. Use with caution in patients with hypertension, cardiac disease, diabetes or hyperthyroidism.
Warning: If used in large amounts or for long periods of time may damage kidneys.
How Supplied: 100's.

CITRA® FORTE SYRUP Ⓒ ℞
CITRA® FORTE CAPSULES Ⓒ ℞

Composition:	Ea. 5cc	Ea. Cap.
Hydrocodone Bitartrate	5 mg.	5 mg.
(Warning: May be habit forming)		
Ascorbic Acid	30 mg.	50 mg.
Pheniramine Maleate	2.5 mg.	6.25 mg.
Potassium Citrate	150 mg.	
Pyrilamine Maleate	3.33 mg.	8.33 mg.
Chlorpheniramine Maleate		1 mg.
Phenylephrine HCl		10 mg.
Salicylamide		227 mg.
Caffeine Alkaloid		30 mg.
Phenacetin		120 mg.

Syrup in a palatable, alcohol 2% flavored base.
Action and Uses: *CITRA FORTE SYRUP:* Antitussive, Expectorant, Antihistaminic, Analgesic provides effective cough suppressant action, a sodium free expectorant, two antihistamines to help control allergic reactions. *CITRA FORTE CAPSULES:* Antitussive, Antihistaminic, decongestant, analgesic. Also provides cough relief and in addition three antihistamines (each in ⅓ their usual dosage) for fewer side effects and broader control of the patients allergic reaction to the cough/cold process. Decongestant action shrinks mucous membranes.
Administration and Dosage: *CITRA FORTE SYRUP: Usual Adult Dose.*—One or two teaspoonfuls every 3 or 4 hours. *Children* (6-12)—one-half adult dosage. *Children under 6 years*—according to standard method of calculation. *CITRA FORTE CAPSULES: Usual Adult Dose.*—One or two capsules every 3 or 4 hours.
Precautions: Patients should be advised to avoid using machinery or driving until response to antihistamines is established. Use with caution in patients with idiosyncrasies to formula ingredients. CITRA FORTE CAPSULES should be used with caution in patients with hypertension, cardiac disease, diabetes or hyperthyroidism.
How Supplied: CITRA FORTE SYRUP in pints and gallons; CITRA FORTE CAPSULES in bottles of 50 capsules.

Continued on next page

Boyle—Cont.

GLYTINIC®
(For Iron Deficiency Anemia)
Palatable Liquid or Tablets

Composition: Daily adult dose provides:
Iron (ferrous gluconate)........................100 mg.
Aminoacetic acid (Glycine)....................1.3 gm.
Vitamins B_{12} 10 mcg.; B_1 7.5 mg.; B_6 2.25 mg.; niacinamide 45 mg.; d-pantothenyl alcohol 6.5 mg.; liver, 5 gr.
Action and Uses: Ferrous Gluconate, inherently tolerable combined with amino acid, glycine, assures good toleration, assimilation, and utilization. Glycine supplies needed amino nitrogen for rapid, positive hemoglobin and hematocrit response. Patient acceptance is excellent. The liquid is surprisingly free from after-taste making it useful for all ages. Children and elderly patients will like the mild flavor and distinct freedom from gastric irritation and after-taste. Glytinic is particularly useful for patients refractory or intolerant to iron preparations.
Administration and Dosage: Liquid with or between meals: *Adults*—1 tablespoonful b.i.d.; *Children 6 to 12*—1 teaspoonful t.i.d.; 2 to 6, 1 teaspoonful b.i.d. Tablets, with or between meals: *Adults*—2 b.i.d.; *Children 6 to 12*—1 b.i.d.
How Supplied: Liquid—pints; tablets —100's.

TRIVA® COMBINATION ℞
TRIVA® DOUCHE POWDER
TRIVA® JEL ℞

Composition: TRIVA COMBINATION combines therapeutic vaginal douche and jel in a convenient and complete treatment consisting of: TRIVA POWDER containing oxyquinoline sulfate 2%; alkyl aryl sulfonate 35%; disodium edetate 0.33%; sodium sulfate 53%; dispersant (lactose) 9.67% and TRIVA JEL containing per 5 Grams oxyquinoline benzoate 7.5 mg.; alkyl aryl sulfonate 62.5 mg.; disodium edetate 2.5 mg.; aminacrine HCl 10 mg.; copper sulfate .063 mg.; sodium sulfate 6.9 mg.; in an aqueous jel base of tragacanth, Irish moss, modified lanolin, glycerin, sodium bicarbonate preserved with methyl-propyl- and butyl-parahydroxy-benzoate.
Action and Uses: TRIVA COMBINATION effectively treats Monilial and Trichomonal as well as Non-specific Vulvovaginitis. Chronic, stubborn cases as well as Monilia and Trichomonas occurring together can be successfully treated. Organisms are eradicated along with symptoms. Vaginal flora and pH return to normal spontaneously. Fungicidal, trichomonacidal, bactericidal, detergent and chelating agents are provided for a safe, simple, patient-administered 16 day treatment without need for restraints on patient's activities. Flushing and detergent action of the douche combines with the continuous action of the jel to quickly destroy the infection and stop the symptoms. Effectiveness of TRIVA COMBINATION has been demonstrated by clinical tests. Both diagnosis and cure were established by the use of special Papanicolaou smear and Sabouraud culture.
Administration and Dosage: TRIVA COMBINATION, ℞, sig: douche (1 packet in 1 qt water) at night followed immediately by one applicatorfull of JEL, continued for 15 nights followed on 16th morning by douche only. An additional course of treatment may be used if needed. Directions for complete mechanical use of product appear on each package.
TRIVA DOUCHE POWDER (individual packet dissolved in 1 qt water) alone is effective in most cases of Monilial, Trichomonal and Non-specific Vulvovaginitis. It provides rapid relief from symptoms. Particularly useful in pre- and post-operative and post-partum care. May be used adjunctively with oral treatment for Trichomonas.
TRIVA DOUCHE POWDER, sig, douche (1 packet in 1 qt water) morning and night for 12 days.
TRIVA JEL ℞, sig. one or two applicatorsful daily.
IMPORTANT: During menstruation, continue treatment as instructed.
Precautions: Occasionally, irritation occurs at the onset of treatment. In such cases it is recommended that the douche only be prescribed in one-half or less than usual strength for a day or two, then combined therapeutic treatment resumed as directed.
TRIVA COMBINATION, POWDER and JEL are spermicidal.
Side Effects: None.
Contraindications: None.
How Supplied: TRIVA COMBINATION contains 24 individual 3 Gm. packets douche powder, 1 tube 85 Gm. Jel with applicator.
TRIVA DOUCHE POWDER—Available individually, 24 individual 3 Gm. packets.
TRIVA JEL—Available individually, 1 tube 85 Gm. with applicator.

Breon Laboratories Inc.
90 PARK AVE.
NEW YORK, NY 10016

BREOKINASE® ℞
brand of urokinase
FOR INJECTION

BREOKINASE (urokinase for injection) should be used only by physicians with adequate experience in the management of thrombotic disease in hospitals where necessary clinical and laboratory monitoring can be performed (see WARNINGS, PRECAUTIONS and DOSAGE AND ADMINISTRATION).
The physician should carefully assess the overall clinical status and history of the patient before beginning urokinase treatment. Urokinase produces more profound changes in hemostasis and a greater frequency of bleeding than heparin or oral coumarin anticoagulant therapy. Bleeding when it occurs is more severe and more difficult to manage. Such factors as patient's age, physical condition, and underlying bleeding tendency (as described under WARNINGS and PRECAUTIONS) should be taken into consideration when the potential risk of serious hemorrhage is weighed against the potential benefits of urokinase treatment.
Description: BREOKINASE is a sterile preparation of highly purified urokinase isolated from human urine. The urokinase in BREOKINASE is a protein enzyme with a molecular weight predominantly, if not exclusively, in the region of 54,000 daltons (refs. 8–10). It is a potent activator of the endogenous fibrinolytic system.
BREOKINASE is a white cake or powder in lyophilized form intended for intravenous infusion following reconstitution of each vial with 8.0 ml Sterile Water for Injection, USP. Each vial contains 250,000 C.T.A. Units of urokinase activity* and approximately 0.9 millimols of sodium phosphates. Following reconstitution, a clear, practically colorless and isotonic solution of pH 7 is obtained. Each ml of reconstituted BREOKINASE contains 31,250 C.T.A. Units of urokinase activity.
*The C.T.A. (Committee on Thrombolytic Agents) Unit is a standardized measure of the ability of urokinase to cause lysis of a fibrin clot via the plasminogen/plasmin system *in vitro* (see reference 14).
Action: Urokinase activates the endogenous fibrinolytic system by converting plasminogen, an enzyme precursor in blood clots and circulating blood, to the proteolytic enzyme plasmin. Plasmin in turn lyses fibrin in clots as well as fibrinogen and other plasma proteins (ref. 11). Plasmin is rapidly inactivated by a variety of naturally occurring inhibitors in plasma (ref. 1). Since plasminogen is present in thrombi/emboli as well as in the circulating plasma, activation by urokinase occurs both on the surface and within the thrombi/emboli and in the general circulation (refs. 5, 6).

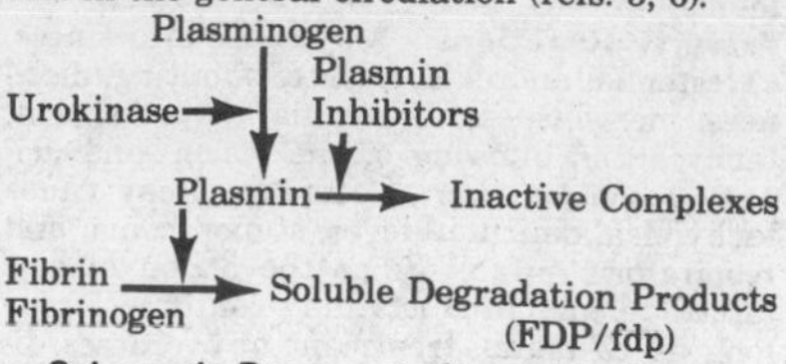

Schematic Representation of Urokinase-Induced Fibrinolysis

Intravenous infusion of BREOKINASE produces a prompt increase in the fibrinolytic activity of the blood which may persist for up to 12 hours after discontinuation of the infusion. This activity is evidenced by a shortening of the whole blood euglobulin clot lysis time, a decrease in plasma levels of fibrinogen and plasminogen, and an increase in plasma levels of fibrinogen-fibrin degradation products (FDP/fdp) (ref. 4).
The efficacy of BREOKINASE in the lysis of pulmonary emboli has been established in controlled clinical studies using angiography, perfusion lung scans, and pulmonary arterial and right heart pressure measurements before and after treatment (refs. 3, 4, 7, 12, 13, 16, 17). In these studies, thrombolysis was accompanied by improved pulmonary capillary perfusion, and by reversal of the cardiopulmonary hemodynamic abnormalities towards normal.
Indications: BREOKINASE is indicated for the thrombolytic treatment of:
—acute massive pulmonary embolism, defined as obstruction or significant filling defects involving two or more lobar pulmonary arteries or an equivalent amount of emboli in other vessels, as seen on pulmonary arteriography;
—pulmonary embolism accompanied by unstable hemodynamics, i.e., inability to maintain blood pressure without supportive measures.
The diagnosis of pulmonary embolism should be confirmed by objective means, preferably pulmonary arteriography.
Urokinase treatment should be started as soon as possible after diagnosis of pulmonary embolism, but no later than five days after onset. Under these circumstances, angiographic and hemodynamic measurements and perfusion lung scans demonstrate a more rapid improvement during the first 24 hours after initiation of therapy than with heparin therapy (Table 1). However, it has not been established that urokinase treatment decreases morbidity or mortality compared to heparin therapy alone. [See table on next page].
Contraindications: thrombolytic therapy increases the risk of bleeding. The risk of hemorrhage in the conditions listed below should be weighed carefully against the anticipated benefits of urokinase therapy in each patient. The benefits and risks associated with urokinase therapy should be compared to the benefits and risks associated with other forms of treatment.

1. Surgical procedures within preceding ten days (including liver or kidney biopsy, lumbar puncture, thoracentesis, paracentesis, extensive or multiple cutdowns).
2. Intraarterial diagnostic procedure within ten days.
3. Ulcerative wound.
4. Recent trauma with possibility of internal injuries.
5. Visceral or intracranial malignancy.
6. Pregnancy and the first ten days post-partum.

7. Actively bleeding lesion of the gastrointestinal or genitourinary tract, or a condition with significant potential for bleeding (including ulcerative colitis, diverticulitis).
8. Severe hypertension.
9. Acute or chronic hepatic or renal insufficiency.
10. Uncontrolled hypocoagulable state (including coagulation factor deficiency, thrombocytopenia, spontaneous fibrinolysis, any purpuric or hemorrhagic disorder).
11. Chronic pulmonary disease with cavitation e.g., tuberculosis.
12. Subacute bacterial endocarditis or rheumatic valvular disease.
13. Recent cerebral embolism, thrombosis or hemorrhage (within at least two months) to avoid risk of bleeding into infarcted cerebral tissue.
14. Any other condition in which bleeding constitutes a significant hazard or would be particularly difficult to locate or control.

Warnings:

Bleeding

Activation of the fibrinolytic system with urokinase causes a more profound change in the hemostatic status of the patient than does anticoagulant therapy with heparin or coumarin agents. The objective of urokinase therapy is the production of sufficient amounts of plasmin to lyse intravascular deposits of fibrin; however, fibrin deposits which provide hemostasis, for example at sites of needle punctures, will also undergo lysis, and bleeding from such sites may occur. The possibility of bruising or hematoma formation, especially with intramuscular injections, is substantial during thrombolytic therapy. Unnecessary clinical or diagnostic procedures should be avoided. It is important that close attention be paid to this section and the CONTRAINDICATIONS section in order to minimize the risk of bleeding.

Intramuscular injections should be avoided during urokinase therapy, as with heparin therapy, because of the high risk of hematoma formation. Bleeding may occur at sites of recent invasive procedures. Therefore, arterial punctures must be avoided before as well as during treatment with urokinase. If arterial puncture is *absolutely* necessary, the radial or brachial artery should be used and the femoral artery must be avoided. Arterial puncture should be performed with great care by an experienced physician and pressure should be applied for at least 15 minutes. This should be followed by the application of a pressure dressing, and the puncture site should be checked frequently for evidence of bleeding. Venipunctures should also be performed as carefully and infrequently as possible. If bleeding from an invasive site occurs during urokinase infusion, but is not severe, treatment may be continued with close clinical observation. Local pressure and other measures should be initiated immediately.

Spontaneous internal bleeding that is not accessible for the application of pressure may also occur. The risk of spontaneous bleeding is greater in patients with preexisting hemostatic abnormalities, including patients whose histories are suggestive of prior bleeding problems whether or not there are demonstrable abnormalities in platelet count, prothrombin time, partial thromboplastin time, or bleeding time. The relative risks and benefits of urokinase treatment must be carefully assessed in such patients before initiating treatment.

Plasmin degrades fibrinogen, Factor V, Factor VIII, and other proteins in addition to fibrin. The products of plasmin degradation of fibrinogen and fibrin (FDP/fdp) possess an anticoagulant effect which may make bleeding difficult to control.

Table 1: Results of National Heart and Lung Institute Study of Urokinase in Pulmonary Embolism†

	Phase I (UPET*)		Phase II (USPET**)	
	Heparin	12-Hours of Urokinase	12-Hours of Urokinase	24-Hours of Urokinase
Change in angiographic severity score based on 4-point system	0.54	1.78	1.66	1.76
Decrease in relative percentage perfusion defect on lung scans	8.3	24.1	20	29.2
Change in pulmonary artery pressure (mmHg)	−1.1	−6.2	−7.28	−7.53
Change in cardiac index (1/min/m^2)	−0.05	+0.02	+0.06	+0.30

* Urokinase pulmonary embolism trial
** Urokinase-streptokinase pulmonary embolism trial
Evaluations were obtained between 18 and 30 hours after the start of therapy.
After several days, there were no differences between the results in the heparin treated patients and those receiving urokinase.
†Adapted from Fratantoni JC, Ness P, Simon TL: Thrombolytic therapy: Current status. *N Eng J Med 293*:1073–1078, 1975.

If serious spontaneous bleeding occurs, the infusion of urokinase should be terminated immediately, and treatment instituted as described under ADVERSE REACTIONS.

Risk of Cerebral Embolism

Urokinase treatment of patients with atrial fibrillation or other conditions which predispose to cerebral embolism may be hazardous because of the risk of bleeding into the infarcted cerebral area.

Use of Anticoagulants

Concurrent use of anticoagulants with urokinase is contraindicated. Before beginning urokinase infusion in patients being treated with heparin, the effects of heparin should be allowed to decrease, as evidenced by a thrombin time of less than twice normal. Similarly, heparin should be withheld following urokinase therapy until the thrombin time is less than twice normal.

Rethrombosis has been observed after completion of urokinase treatment. In order to minimize this risk, administration of intravenous heparin followed by oral anticoagulant therapy is considered a necessary adjunct following urokinase therapy (see DOSAGE AND ADMINISTRATION).

Use in Pregnancy

See CONTRAINDICATIONS.

Use in Children

Safety and effectiveness of urokinase therapy in children have not been established; therefore, treatment of such patients is not recommended.

Precautions:

Drug Interactions

Drugs that may alter platelet function, e.g., aspirin, indomethacin, and phenylbutazone, should be avoided during urokinase treatment. The interaction of BREOKINASE with other drugs has not been studied.

Laboratory Monitoring

In patients who have received heparin, the thrombin time should be measured prior to starting urokinase. (See WARNINGS.) Similarly, the thrombin time should be measured following urokinase therapy prior to instituting heparin. (See DOSAGE AND ADMINISTRATION.) During urokinase administration, the levels of fibrinogen, plasminogen, Factor V, and Factor VIII are usually substantially decreased, and the level of fibrin and fibrinogen degradation products (FDP/fdp) is increased.

Urokinase infusion should be terminated immediately if serious bleeding occurs.

Adverse Reactions: Careful observance of the contraindications, warnings, and precautions to the use of urokinase is essential to minimize the incidence and severity of adverse effects (ref. 7).

Bleeding

Incidence

In controlled clinical trials of streptokinase and urokinase, severe bleeding (requiring a transfusion of greater than two units of blood) was seen in 4% of streptokinase patients and 6% of patients receiving urokinase. Several fatalities due to cerebral hemorrhage have occurred during urokinase therapy.

Spontaneous bleeding of a less severe degree has been observed during urokinase treatment at about twice the frequency as that occurring during heparin therapy. Oozing of blood from sites of skin puncture is frequent; therefore, all invasive procedures, especially arterial punctures and intramuscular injections, should be avoided and intravenous punctures kept to a minimum before and during treatment with urokinase.

A moderate decrease in hematocrit not accompanied by clinically detectable bleeding was observed in about 20% of patients treated with urokinase.

Management of Severe Bleeding

Urokinase therapy must be discontinued if serious bleeding occurs. Packed red cells are indicated for large blood loss. Plasma volume expanders (other than Dextran) may be used to replace blood volume deficit. Whole blood may also be used if it alone is available. The use of aminocaproic acid (ACA, AMICAR®) in humans as an antidote for urokinase has not been documented, but its use may be considered if the hemorrhage is unresponsive to blood replacement (see WARNINGS).

Allergic Reactions: Urokinase is a protein of human origin, and *in vitro* as well as intradermal tests in humans have no evidence of induced antibody formation. However, the possibility of serious allergic reactions (including anaphylaxis) occurring during its use cannot be excluded. There have been rare reports of relatively mild allergic reactions, e.g., bronchospasm and skin rash.

Fever: Febrile episodes occurred in about 2–3% of urokinase-treated patients. A causal relationship to urokinase has not been established. Symptomatic treatment with acetaminophen rather than aspirin is usually sufficient.

Dosage and Administration:

Preparation

Reconstitute each vial of BREOKINASE by aseptically adding 8.0 ml of Sterile Water for Injection, USP (it is important that *only* Sterile Water for Injection, USP, *without* preservatives, be used. Bacteriostatic Water for Injection or other diluents should not be used.) Swirl gently to avoid foaming. (DO NOT SHAKE.)

Continued on next page

Breon—Cont.

Because BREOKINASE contains no preservatives, it should not be reconstituted until immediately before using. Any unused portion of the reconstituted material should be discarded. Each ml of reconstituted BREOKINASE contains 31,250 C.T.A. Units of urokinase activity.

Dosing

BREOKINASE IS INTENDED FOR INTRAVENOUS INFUSION ONLY

Urokinase treatment should be begun as soon as possible after the occurrence of pulmonary embolism, and no later than five days after onset. A priming or loading dose of 2000 C.T.A. Units/lb (4400 C.T.A. Units/kg) of reconstituted BREOKINASE is given over a period of ten minutes. This is followed by a continuous infuson of 2000 C.T.A. Units/lb/hr (4400 C.T.A. Units/kg/hr) for 12 hours (see Table 2). A constant infusion pump independent of all other intravenous systems should be used. Do not expose reconstituted solution to excessive heat, such as high intensity lights, during administration.

[See table below].

Anticoagulation Following BREOKINASE Treatment

At the end of BREOKINASE infusion, treatment with heparin by continuous intravenous infusion followed by oral anticoagulant therapy is recommended to minimize re-thrombosis. Heparin treatment should begin when the thrombin time has returned to less than twice normal. See manufacturer's prescribing information for proper use of heparin.

How Supplied: BREOKINASE is supplied as a sterile lyophilized preparation. Each vial contains 250,000 C.T.A. Units of urokinase activity and approximately 0.9 millimols sodium phosphates. The vials should be stored under refrigeration (2° to 8°C).

Code 1831 BREOKINASE 30 ml Vials
NDC 0057-1000-01

References:

1. Aoki N, Maroi M, Matsuda M, Tachiya K: The behavior of a_2-plasmin inhibitor in fibrinolytic states. *J Clin Invest 60:*361–339, 1977.
2. Bang NU: Physiology and biochemistry of fibrinolysis. In *Thrombosis and Bleeding Disorders* (Bang NU, Beller FK, Deutsch E, Mammen EF, eds). Academic Press, 1971, pp. 292–327.
3. Bell WR: Thrombolytic Therapy: A comparison between urokinase and streptokinase. *Sem Thromb Hemost 2:*1–13, 1975.
4. Bell WR: Streptokinase and urokinase in the treatment of pulmonary thromboemboli. *Thrombos Haemostas 35:*57, 1976.
5. Chesterman CN, Allington MJ, Sharp AA: Relationship of plasminogen activator to fibrin. *Nature (New Biology) 238:*15–17, 1972.
6. Collen D, Wiman B: Fast-acting plasmin inhibitor in human plasma. *Blood 51:*563, 1978.
7. Fratantoni JC, Ness P, Simon TL: Thrombolytic therapy: Current status. *N Engl J Med 293:*1073–1078, 1975.
8. Lesuk A, Terminiello L, Traver JH: Crystalline human urokinase: Some properties. *Science 147:*880, 1965.
9. Lesuk A, Terminiello L, Traver JH: Sephadex gelfiltration of human urokinase preparations. *Fed Proc 25:*194, 1966.
10. Lesuk A, Terminiello L, Traver JH, Groff JL: Biochemical and biophysical studies of human urokinase. *Thrombos Diathes Haemorrh 18:*293, 1967.
11. McNicol GP: The fibrinolytic enzyme system. *Postgrad Med J (Aug Suppl) 49:*10–12, 1973.
12. Sasahara AA, Hyers TM, Cole CM, et al: The urokinase pulmonary embolism trial. *Circulation (Suppl II) 47:*1–108, 1973.
13. Sasahara AA, Bell WR, Simon TL, Stengle JM, and Sherry S: The phase II urokinase-streptokinase pulmonary embolism trial. *Thrombos Diathes Haemorrh* (Stuttg) *33:*464–476, 1975.
14. Sherry S, Alkjaersig N, Fletcher AP: Assay of urokinase preparations with the synthetic substrate acetyl-l-lysine methyl ester. *J Lab Clin Med 64:*145, 1964.
15. Sherry S: Streptokinase, urokinase: Do they really work? *Modern Med:*72–76, Nov. 1, 1976.
16. Urokinase pulmonary embolism trial study group: Urokinase-streptokinase embolism trial. *JAMA 229:*1606–1613, 1974.
17. Urokinase pulmonary embolism trial. *JAMA 214* (12):2163–2172, 1970.

Supplied by:
BREON LABORATORIES INC.
New York, N.Y. 10016
Mfg. by Green Cross Corp.
Osaka, Japan
Revised April 1979 BR 884/0479

Table 2: Dosage and Administration

Patient Weight Lb	Patient Weight Kg	Total Dose C.T.A. Units*	Number Vials BREOKINASE	Total Volume BREOKINASE after Reconstitution (ml)	Loading Dose (ml/10 min)**	12 Hour infusion Rate (ml/hr)
81– 90	36.8– 40.9	2,250,000	9	72	5.5	5.5
91–100	41.4– 45.5	2,500,000	10	80	6.2	6.2
101–110	45.9– 50.0	2,750,000	11	88	6.8	6.8
111–120	50.5– 54.5	3,000,000	12	96	7.4	7.4
121–130	55.0– 59.5	3,250,000	13	104	8.0	8.0
131–140	59.5– 63.6	3,500,000	14	112	8.6	8.6
141–150	64.1– 68.2	3,750,000	15	120	9.2	9.2
151–160	68.6– 72.2	4,000,000	16	128	9.8	9.8
161–170	73.2– 77.3	4,250,000	17	136	10.5	10.5
171–180	77.7– 81.8	4,500,000	18	144	11.1	11.1
181–190	82.3– 86.4	4,750,000	19	152	11.7	11.7
191–200	86.8– 90.9	5,000,000	20	160	12.3	12.3
201–210	91.4– 95.5	5,250,000	21	168	12.9	12.9
211–220	95.9–100.0	5,500,000	22	176	13.5	13.5
221–230	100.5–104.5	5,750,000	23	184	14.2	14.2
231–240	105.0–109.1	6,000,000	24	192	14.8	14.8
241–250	109.5–113.6	6,250,000	25	200	15.4	15.4

*Loading dose plus 12 hour infusion dose
**The loading dose is administered over a ten minute period prior to the 12 hour infusion.

BRONKEPHRINE® ℞

(brand of ethylnorepinephrine hydrochloride)
In Aqueous Solution

Description: Each ml. contains BRONKEPHRINE (ethylnorepinephrine HCl) 2 mg. in a sterile isotonic solution of 0.7% sodium chloride with sodium acetone bisulfite 0.2% as preservative, with pH adjusted to 2.9-4.5 with NaOH or HCl.

Actions: BRONKEPHRINE (ethylnorepinephrine HCl) is a synthetic sympathomimetic amine, largely beta-active in effect. Its bronchodilating properties closely simulate those of epinephrine but without significant pressor effects. It thus may be safer than epinephrine for hypertensive patients and severly ill patients in whom such effects are undesirable. BRONKEPHRINE (ethylnorepinephrine HCl) is particularly adapted for use in children because of its relative lack of adverse effects, especially central nervous system excitation. It also may be of value in diabetic asthmatics due to its lack of glycogenolytic activity.

Indications: BRONKEPHRINE (ethylnorepinephrine HCl) is indicated for the relief of bronchospasm in bronchial asthma.

Contraindications: It is contraindicated in patients with idiosyncrasy to sympathomimetic drugs.

Precautions: BRONKEPHRINE (ethylnorepinephrine HCl) should be used with caution in persons with cardiovascular disease, a history of stroke or coronary artery disease. It is a potent drug and may cause toxic symptoms through idiosyncratic response or overdosage. Care should be taken in anatomical selection of injection sites to avoid inadvertent intraneural or intravascular injection.

Adverse Reactions: BRONKEPHRINE (ethylnorepinephrine HCl) is generally well tolerated. It may, however, produce changes in blood pressure (elevation or depression) or pulse rate (elevation), palpitation, headache, dizziness or nausea.

Dosage and Administration: The usual adult dose by subcutaneous or intramuscular injection is 0.5-1.0 ml. Depending on severity of the asthmatic attack, smaller doses (0.3-0.5 ml.) may suffice. Dosage in children varies according to age and weight; usually 0.1 to 0.5 ml. is sufficient.

How Supplied:
1 ml. sterile single dose ampules, Code No. 1189 (Pkg. of 25) **NDC** 0057-1001-01
Code No. 1188 (Pkg. of 5) **NDC** 0057-1001-05

BRONKODYL® ℞

brand of theophylline, USP (anhydrous)
Capsules
100 mg and 200 mg
ELIXIR
80 mg per 15 ml

Description: Each green and white hard gelatin capsule contains theophylline USP (anhydrous), 200 mg, in a micro-pulverized form. Each brown and white hard gelatin capsule contains 100 mg. The elixir contains 80 mg theophylline per 15 ml in a 20% alcohol elixir (approximately 20 calories, 0.9 gm carbohydrate per tablespoonful). Theophylline, a methylxanthine, is a white, odorless crystalline powder having a bitter taste.

Clinical Pharmacology: Theophylline directly relaxes smooth muscle of bronchi and pulmonary blood vessels, producing bronchodilation and pulmonary vasodilation. Other effects typical of the methylxanthines include coronary vasodilation, diuresis, and cardiac, cerebral and skeletal muscle stimulation. The actions of theophylline may be mediated through inhibition of phosphodiesterase with a resultant increase in intracellular cyclic AMP causing smooth muscle relaxation. At concentrations higher than those usually attained *in vivo,* theophylline also inhibits mast cell release of histamine.

In vitro, theophylline has been shown to act synergistically with beta agonists to increase intracellular cyclic AMP. However, more data are needed to determine whether there are clinically significant additive or synergistic effects *in vivo.*
Tolerance with chronic use of theophylline has not been demonstrated.
Theophylline half-life is prolonged in the presence of alcoholism, reduced hepatic or renal function, congestive heart failure, prolonged periods of high fever, and in patients receiving certain antibiotics such as troleandomycin (TAO), erythromycin and clindamycin. Half-life is shortened in cigarette smokers.

THEOPHYLLINE ELIMINATION

	Clearance (mean ± S.D.)	Half-life (mean ± S.D.)
Adult non-smokers with uncomplicated asthma	0.65 ± 0.19 ml/kg/min	8.7 ± 2.2 hours
Children over six months old	1.45 ± 0.58 ml/kg/min	3.7 ± 1.1 hours

Older adults with chronic obstructive pulmonary disease, patients with cor pulmonale or other heart failure, and patients with liver disease may have much lower clearances with half-life exceeding 24 hours.
Theophylline half-life in smokers of 1–2 packs/day averaged 4–5 hours compared with a half-life of 7–9 hours in nonsmokers. This may be due to induction of drug-metabolizing enzymes and this effect may last months to years after cessation of smoking.
Newborns have extremely slow clearances and half-lives exceeding 24 hours. Theophylline pharmacokinetics approach those in older children after about 3–6 months of life.
Indications: For relief and/or prevention of bronchospasm associated with bronchial asthma, chronic bronchitis and emphysema.
Contraindications: Bronkodyl is contraindicated in persons with hypersensitivity to any of its components.
Warnings: All methylxanthines should be used with caution in children and in others who are currently taking bronchodilator products, especially in rectal dosage form, which may contain theophylline or related drugs.
Status asthmaticus is a medical emergency. Addition of corticosteroids and other medications to bronchodilator therapy may be required.
Because the incidence of toxicity increases at serum theophylline levels greater than 20 mcg/ml, serum theophylline levels should be monitored at appropriate intervals for dosage adjustment. High serum levels of theophylline and resultant toxicity may occur with conventional doses in patients with decreased theophylline clearance as found with cardiac failure, liver disease, chronic obstructive pulmonary disease, and in geriatric patients.
Early signs of theophylline toxicity, such as nausea and restlessness may not occur prior to convulsions or ventricular arrhythmias. Preexisting arrhythmias may be worsened by theophylline.
Usage in Pregnancy: Although theophylline has been used for many years, with no evidence of adverse fetal effect or teratogenicity, its safety in pregnancy has not been established. Therefore, use of Bronkodyl during lactation or in women of childbearing potential requires that possible benefits of the drug be weighed against possible hazards to fetus or child.
Precautions: Smokers may require larger doses of theophylline because of a shorter half-life in these patients.
Theophylline should not be administered concurrently with other xanthines.
Caution should be observed in patients with cardiac disease, severe hypoxemia, hypertension, hyperthyroidism, acute myocardial injury, cor pulmonale, congestive heart failure, liver disease, peptic ulcer, and in the elderly

	ORAL LOADING DOSE	MAINTENANCE DOSE FOR NEXT 12 HOURS	MAINTENANCE DOSE BEYOND 12 HOURS
Children 6 months to 9 years	6 mg/kg	4 mg/kg q4h	4 mg/kg q6h
Children 9-16 years and young adult smokers	6 mg/kg	3 mg/kg q4h	3 mg/kg q6h
Otherwise healthy nonsmoking adults	6 mg/kg	3 mg/kg q6h	3 mg/kg q8h
Older patients and patients with cor pulmonale	6 mg/kg	2 mg/kg q6h	2 mg/kg q8h
Patients with congestive heart failure, liver failure	6 mg/kg	2 mg/kg q8h	1-2 mg/kg q12h

and neonates. Patients with congestive heart failure in particular may have markedly prolonged serum half-lives of theophylline.
Adverse Reactions: Most adverse reactions to theophylline are seen with serum levels exceeding the therapeutic range. *Gastrointestinal:* nausea, vomiting, epigastric pain, hematemesis, diarrhea. *CNS:* headache, irritability, restlessness, insomnia, reflex hyperexcitability, muscle twitching, clonic and tonic generalized convulsions. *Cardiovascular:* palpitations, tachycardia, extrasystoles, flushing, hypotension, circulatory failure, ventricular arrhythmias which may be life-threatening. *Respiratory:* tachypnea. *Renal:* diuresis, albuminuria. *Other:* hyperglycemia, inappropriate ADH secretion.
Drug Interactions: Toxic synergism with ephedrine and other sympathomimetic bronchodilators may occur.

DRUG COMBINATION	EFFECT
Aminophylline with lithium carbonate	Increased excretion of lithium carbonate
Aminophylline with propranolol	Antagonism of propranolol effect
Theophylline with furosemide	Increased diuresis
Theophylline with hexamethonium	Decreased hexamethonium induced chronotropic effect
Theophylline with reserpine	Reserpine-induced tachycardia
Theophylline with chlordiazepoxide	Chlordiazepoxide-induced fatty acid mobilization
Theophylline with TAO (troleandomycin), erythromycin, lincomycin, clindamycin	Increased theophylline plasma levels

Dosage and Administration: Optimum therapeutic serum levels of theophylline are generally considered to lie between 10 and 20 mcg/ml. Levels above 20 mcg/ml may produce toxic effects. Because of great variation of theophylline pharmacokinetics among patients, and in the same patient at different times, dosage must be individualized and serum levels monitored as necessary.
Rapidly absorbed theophylline preparations require administration every 6 hours, especially in children.
When dosage is calculated by body weight, lean or ideal body weight should be used rather than actual weight.
Rapid theophyllinization for Patients with Acute Asthma or Bronchospasm:
For patients not currently receiving theophylline drugs:
[See table above].
For patients currently receiving theophylline drugs, the time, amount, route and form of the last dose should be determined and blood levels measured if possible before beginning treatment.
Patients should be closely monitored for signs of toxicity.
Patients with Chronic Asthma or Bronchospasm:
Slow clinical titration is preferable.
Initial dose: 16 mg/kg/day or 400 mg/day (whichever is lower) in 3 to 4 divided doses at 6 to 8 hour intervals. This may be increased by about 25% at 2 to 3 day intervals if no toxicity occurs until maximum dose is reached (see below).
Maximum dose (dose not to be exceeded in absence of serum determinations):

Under 9 years of age — 24 mg/kg/day
9 to 12 years of age — 20 mg/kg/day
12 to 16 years of age — 18 mg/kg/day
Over 16 years of age — 13 mg/kg/day or 900 mg/day (whichever is lower)

During chronic therapy, periodic serum theophylline levels obtained at the time of peak absorption (1 to 2 hours after a dose of an immediate release preparation) are recommended for dosage adjustments. See Warnings and Precautions for special dosage adjustments in neonates, the elderly, and patients with congestive heart failure, cor pulmonale, liver disease, COPD, etc.
[See table on next page].
Overdosage: See Adverse Reactions for signs and symptoms of theophylline overdosage.
Treatment:
A. If potential oral overdose is established and seizure has not occurred:
1) Induce vomiting.
2) Administer a cathartic.
3) Administer activated charcoal.
B. If patient is having a seizure:
1) Establish an airway.
2) Administer O_2.
3) Treat the seizure with intravenous diazepam, 0.1 to 0.3 mg/kg up to 10 mg.
4) Monitor vital signs, maintain blood pressure and provide adequate hydration.
C. Post-seizure coma:
1) Maintain airway and oxygenation.
2) If a result of oral medication, follow above recommendations to prevent absorption of drug, but intubation and lavage will have to be performed instead of inducing emesis, and the cathartic and charcoal will need to be introduced via a large bore gastric lavage tube.
3) Continue to provide full supportive care and adequate hydration while waiting for drug to be metabolized. In general, the drug is metabolized sufficiently rapidly so as to not warrant consideration of dialysis.
D. Animal studies suggest that phenobarbital may decrease theophylline toxicity. There are as yet, however, insufficient data to recommend pretreatment of an overdosage with phenobarbital.

How Supplied:
Bronkodyl 100 mg,
brown and white capsules in 100's
Code 1831 **NDC** 0057-1030-10
Bronkodyl 200 mg,
green and white capsules in 100's
Code 1833 **NDC** 0057-1031-10
Bronkodyl Elixir,
80 mg per 15 ml, in pints
Code 1835 **NDC** 0057-1032-16
[*shown in Product Identification Section*]

Continued on next page

Breon—Cont.

BRONKOMETER® ℞
(isoetharine mesylate)

***Revised Formula**

Description: BRONKOMETER is a complete pocket nebulizer containing:
Isoetharine mesylate 0.61% (W/W) with saccharin, menthol, alcohol 30% (W/W), and fluorochlorohydrocarbons as gaseous propellants. Preserved with ascorbic acid 0.1% (W/W).
*As originally marketed, BRONKOMETER contained thenyldiamine hydrochloride 0.05% and phenylephrine hydrochloride 0.125%. The present formulation has been revised to delete these ingredients.
Isoetharine is 1-(3,4 dihydroxyphenyl)-2-isopropylamino-1-butanol. The BRONKOMETER unit delivers approximately 20 metered doses per ml. of solution. Each average 56 mg. delivery contains 340 mcg. isoetharine.
Action: Isoetharine is a sympathomimetic amine with preferential affinity for $Beta_2$ adrenergic receptor sites of bronchial and certain arteriolar musculature, and a lower order of affinity for $Beta_1$ adrenergic receptors. Its activity in symptomatic relief of bronchospasm is rapid and of relatively long duration. By relieving bronchospasm, BRONKOMETER helps give prompt relief and significantly increases vital capacity.
Indications: BRONKOMETER is indicated for use as a bronchodilator for bronchial asthma and for reversible bronchospasm that may occur in association with bronchitis and emphysema.
Contraindications: BRONKOMETER should not be administered to patients who are hypersensitive to any of its ingredients.
Warnings: Excessive use of an adrenergic aerosol should be discouraged as it may lose its effectiveness. Occasional patients have been reported to develop severe paradoxical airway resistance with repeated excessive use of an aerosol adrenergic inhalation preparation. The cause of this refractory state is unknown. It is advisable that in such instances the use of the aerosol adrenergic be discontinued immediately and alternative therapy instituted, since in the reported cases the patients did not respond to other forms of therapy until the drug was withdrawn. Cardiac arrest has been noted in several instances.
BRONKOMETER should not be administered along with epinephrine or other sympathomimetic amines, since these drugs are direct cardiac stimulants and may cause excessive tachycardia. They may, however, be alternated if desired.
Usage in Pregnancy: Although there has been no evidence of teratogenic effects with this drug, use of any drug in pregnancy, lactation, or in women of childbearing potential requires that the potential benefit of the drug be weighed against its possible hazard to the mother or child.
Precautions: Dosage must be carefully adjusted in patients with hyperthyroidism, hypertension, acute coronary disease, cardiac asthma, limited cardiac reserve, and in individuals sensitive to sympathomimetic amines, since overdosage may result in tachycardia, palpitation, nausea, headache, or epinephrine-like side effects.
Adverse Reactions: Although BRONKOMETER is relatively free of toxic side effects, too frequent use may cause tachycardia, palpitation, nausea, headache, changes in blood pressure, anxiety, tension, restlessness, insomnia, tremor, weakness, dizziness, and excitement, as in the case with other sympathomimetic amines.
Dosage and Administration: The average adult dose is one or two inhalations. Occasionally, more may be required. It is important, however, to wait one full minute after the initial one or two inhalations in order to be certain whether another is necessary. In most cases, inhalations need not be repeated more often than every four hours, although more frequent administration may be necessary in severe cases.
How Supplied:
BRONKOMETER® 10 ml. Vial with Oral Nebulizer
Code No. 1740 NDC 0057-1040-01
BRONKOMETER® 20 ml. Vial with Oral Nebulizer
Code No. 1742 NDC 0057-1042-02
BRONKOMETER® 10 ml. refill only
Code No. 1743 NDC 0057-1043-01
BRONKOMETER® 20 ml. refill only
Code No. 1741 NDC 0057-1041-02
The bronchodilator isoetharine is also available in a convenient solution for use with conventional nebulizers, by oxygen aerosolization, and in IPPB machines as
BRONKOSOL® (isoetharine HCl) 1.0%
Bottles of 10 ml. Code No. 1771
NDC 0057-1071-10
Bottles of 30 ml. Code No. 1772
NDC 0057-1072-30

Examples of Dosage Adjustments Based on Serum Theophylline Levels:

Peak Theophylline Level mcg/ml	Adjustment in Total Daily Dose	Comment
< 5	100% increase	If patient is asymtomatic, consider trial off drug; repeat blood levels after adjustment.
5–7.5	50% increase	
8–10	20% Increase	Even if patient is asymptomatic at this level, an increased serum concentration may prevent symptoms during a viral URI, or heavy exposure to an inhalant allergen.
11–13	Cautious 10% increase if clinically indicated	If patient is asymptomatic, no increase is necessary. If symptoms are present during URI or exercise, increase as indicated.
14–20	None	If "breakthrough" in asthmatic symptoms occurs at end of dosing interval, change to sustained-release product and repeat blood level.
	Occasional intolerance requires a 10% decrease	If side effects occur, decrease total daily dose as indicated.
21–25	10% decrease	Even if side effects are absent.
26–34	25–33% decrease	Even if side effects are absent, omit next dose and decrease total daily dose as indicated. Repeat blood levels.
> 35	50% decrease	Omit next two doses, decrease as indicated and repeat blood levels.

BRONKOSOL® ℞
(isoetharine HCl)
Bronchodilator Solution For Oral Inhalation
*** Revised Formula**

Description:
Isoetharine HCl . . . 1.0%
in a aqueous-glycerine solution containing sodium chloride, citric acid and sodium hydroxide, with methylparaben, propylparben and acetone sodium bisulfite.
* As originaly marketed, BRONKOSOL contained thenyldiamine hydrochloride 0.10% and phenylephrine hydrochloride 0.25%. The present formulation has been revised to delete those ingredients.
Action: Isoetharine is a sympathomimetic amine with preferential affinity for $Beta_2$adrenergic receptor sites of bronchial and certan arteriolar musculature, and a lower order of affinity for $Beta_1$adrenergic receptors. Its activity in symptomatic relief of bronchospasm is rapid and of relatively long duration. By relieving bronchospasm BRONKOSOL helps give prompt relief and significantly increases vital capacity.
Indications: BRONKOSOL is indicated for use as a bronchodilator for bronchial asthma and for reversible bronchospasm that may occur in associaion with bronchitis and emphysema.
Contraindicaton: BRONKOSOL should not be administered to patients who are hypersensitive to any of its ingredients.
Warnings: Excessive use of an adrenergic aerosol should be discouraged as it may lose its effectiveness. Occasional patients have been reported to develop severe paradoxical airway resistance with repeated excessive use of an aerosol adrenergic inhalation preparation. The cause of this refractory state is unknown. It is advisable that in such instances the use of the aerosol adrenergic be discontinued immediately and alternative therapy instituted, since in the reported cases the patients did not respond to other forms of therapy until the drug was withdrawn. Cardiac arrest has been noted in several instances.
BRONKOSOL should not be administered along with epinephrine or other sympathomimetic amines, since these drugs are direct cardiac stimulants and may cause excessive tachycardia. They may, however, be alternated if desired.
Usage In Pregnancy: Although there has been no evidence of teratogenic effects with this drug, use of any drug in pregnancy, lactation, or in women of childbearing potential requires that the potential benefit of the drug be weighed againt its possible hazard to the mother or child.
Precautions: Dosage must be carefully adjusted in patients with hyperthyroidism, hypertension, acute coronary disease, cardiac asthma, limited cardiac reserve, and in individuals sensitive to sympathomimetic amines, since over-dosage may result in tachycardia, palpitation, nausea, headache, or epinephrine-like side effects.
Adverse Reactions: Although BRONKOSOL is relatively free of toxic side effects, too frequent use may cause tachycardia, palpitation, nausea, headache, changes in blood pressure, anxiety, tension, restlessness, insomnia, tremor, weakness, dizziness, and excitement, as is the case with other sympathomimetic amines.
Dosage and Administration: BRONKOSOL can be administered by hand nebulizer, oxygen aerosolization, or intermittent positive pressure breathing (IPPB). Usually treatment need not be repeated more often than every four hours, although in severe cases more frequent administraton may be necessary.

Method of Administration	Usual Dose	Range	Usual Dilution
Hand	4 inha-	3-7 inha-	

nebulizer	lations	lations	undiluted
Oxygen aerosolization*	½ ml.	¼-½ml.	1:3 with saline or other diluent
IPPB+	½ ml.	¼-1 ml.	1:3 with saline or other diluent

* Administered with oxygen flow adjusted to 4 to 6 liters/minute over a period of 15 to 20 minutes.

+ Usually an inspiratory flow rate of 15 liters/minute at a cycling pressure of 15 cm H_2O is recommended. It may be necessary, according to patient and type of IPPB apparatus, to adjust flow rate to 6 to 30 liters per minute, cycling pressure to 10–15 cm H_2O, and further dilution according to needs of patient.

How Supplied: BRONKOSOL for inhalation-

BRONKOSOL 1% 10 ml.
Code #1771 NDC 0057-1071-10
BRONKOSOL 1% 30 ml.
Code #1772 NDC 0057-1072-30

The bronchodilator isoetharine is also available in convenient, ready-to-use measured dose aerosol containers as:

BRONKOMETER® 10 ml. Vial with Oral Nebulizer
Code #1740 NDC 0057-1041-01
BRONKOMETER® 20 ml. Vial with Oral Nebulizer for desk or bedside.
Code #1742 NDC 0057-1042-02
Bronkometer® 10 ml. Refill only
Code #1743 NDC 0057-1043-01
BRONKOMETER® 20 ml. Refill only
Code #1741 NDC 0057-1041-02
Each contains:
Isoetharine mesylate ....0.61% W/W

BRONKOTABS®

Composition: Each tablet contains ephedrine sulfate 24 mg; guaifenesin 100 mg; theophylline 100 mg; phenobarbital 8 mg (warning: may be habit-forming).

Action and Uses: BRONKOTABS provides bronchodilatation, decongestion,promotes expectoration as well as aids in reducing local bronchial edema, and provides mild sedation—all of which actions are indicated in the treatment of bronchial asthma. For prevention or relief of the symptoms of bronchial asthma, asthmatic bronchitis, chronic bronchitis with emphysema, emphysematous bronchospasm.

Administration and Dosage: *Adults*—Patients will vary in their requirements of BRONKOTABS ; however, a dosage schedule of one tablet administered every three or four hours, four or five times daily, will usually afford symptomatic relief. *Children over six:* One-half the adult dose. *Children under six:* As directed.

Precautions: With BRONKOTABS, sympathomimetic side effects are minimal. Do not exceed the recommended dosage. Frequent or prolonged use may cause nervousness, restlessness, or sleeplessness. Use with caution if hypertension, heart disease, diabetes or hyperthyroidism is present. (Warning: Phenobarbital may be habit-forming.) This preparation may cause drowsiness. Ephedrine may cause urinary retention, especially in the presence of partial obstruction, as in prostatism.

How Supplied: Bottles of 100 and 1000 tablets.

[*Shown in Product Identification Section*]

BRONKOLIXIR®

Composition: Each 5 ml. teaspoonful contains:

Ephedrine sulfate...12 mg.
Guaifenesin ....50 mg.
Theophylline ....15 mg.
Phenobarbital ....4 mg.
(Warning: may be habit forming)

in a cherry-flavored solution containing 19% alcohol (v/v).

Action and Uses: BRONKOLIXIR is a rapidly effective cherry-flavored elixir to aid relief of symptoms of asthma and bronchitis. It promotes removal of tenacious mucus as an expectorant; relieves bronchospasm; reduces bronchial edema; serves as a mild sedative to allay anxiety-tension.

Administration and Dosage: *Adults*—Although individual requirements may vary, 2 teaspoonsful of BRONKOLIXIR every three or four hours, four times daily, usually will provide symptomatic relief. *Children over six:* One-half the adult dose. *Children under six:* As directed by physician.

Precautions: With BRONKOLIXIR, sympathomimetic side effects are minimal. Do not exceed the recommended dosage. Frequent or prolonged use may cause nervousness, restlessness, or sleeplessness. Use with caution if hypertension, heart disease, diabetes, or hyperthyroidism is present. (Warning: Phenobarbital may be habit-forming.) This preparation may cause drowsiness. Ephedrine may cause urinary retention, especially in the presence of partial obstruction, as in prostatism.

How Supplied: Bottles of 16 oz.

CARBOCAINE® Hydrochloride ℞

brand of mepivacaine hydrochloride injection, USP

THESE SOLUTIONS ARE NOT INTENDED FOR SPINAL ANESTHESIA OR DENTAL USE.

Description: Mepivacaine hydrochloride is 1-methyl-2′, 6′-pipecoloxylidide monohydrochloride.

It is a white crystalline, odorless powder, soluble in water, but very resistant to both acid and alkaline hydrolysis. Solutions may be stored for extended periods of time without decomposition and if without vasoconstrictors may be reautoclaved when necessary.

[See table above].

Composition of Available Solutions

Each ml contains	Single-dose 1% vial	Multiple-dose 1% vial	Single dose 1.5% vial	Single-dose 2% vial	Multiple-dose 2% vial
Mepivacaine hydrochloride	10 mg	10 mg	15 mg	20 mg	20 mg
Sodium chloride	6.6 mg	7 mg	5.6 mg	4.6 mg	5 mg
Potassium chloride	0.3 mg	——	0.3 mg	0.3 mg	——
Calcium chloride	0.33 mg	——	0.33 mg	0.33 mg	——
Methylparaben	——	1 mg	——	——	1 mg
Water for injection	30 ml	50 ml	30 ml	20 ml	50 ml

The pH of the solutions is adjusted between 4.5 and 6.8 with sodium hydroxide or hydrochloric acid.

Actions: Mepivacaine stabilizes the neuronal membrane and prevents the initiation and transmission of nerve impulses, thereby effecting local anesthesia.

Onset of anesthesia is rapid, the time of onset for sensory block ranging from about 3 to 20 minutes depending upon such factors as the anesthetic technique, the type of block, the concentration of the solution, and the individual patient. The degree of motor blockade produced is dependent on the concentration of the solution. A 0.5 per cent solution will be effective in small superficial nerve blocks while the 1 per cent concentration will block sensory and sympathetic conduction without loss of motor function. The 1.5 per cent solution will provide extensive and often complete motor block and the 2 per cent concentration of CARBOCAINE will produce complete sensory and motor block of any nerve group.

The duration of anesthesia also varies depending upon the technique and type of block, the concentration, and the individual. Mepivacaine will normally provide anesthesia which is adequate for 2 to 2½ hours of surgery. It has been reported that vasoconstrictors do not significantly prolong anesthesia with mepivacaine but epinephrine (1:200,000) may be added to the mepivacaine solution to promote local hemostasis and to delay systemic absorption of the anesthetic.

Mepivacaine, because of its amide structure, is not detoxified by the circulating plasma esterases. It is rapidly metabolized, with only a small percentage of the anesthetic (5 to 10 per cent) being excreted unchanged in the urine. The liver is the principal site of metabolism, with over 50 per cent of the administered dose being excreted into the bile as metabolites. Most of the metabolized mepivacaine is probably resorbed in the intestine and then excreted into the urine since only a small percentage is found in the feces. The principal route of excretion is via the kidney. Most of the anesthetic and its metabolites are eliminated within 30 hours. It has been shown that hydroxylation and N-demethylation, which are detoxification reactions, play important roles in the metabolism of the anesthetic. Three metabolites of mepivacaine have been identified from adult humans: two phenols, which are excreted almost exclusively as their glucuronide conjugates, and the N-demethylated compound (2′, 6′-pipecoloxylidide).

Mepivacaine does not ordinarily produce irritation or tissue damage.

Indications: CARBOCAINE is indicated for the production of local anesthesia by infiltration injection, peripheral nerve block, and central neural blocks by the lumbar or caudal epidural route.

Contraindications: Mepivacaine is contraindicated in patients with known hypersensitivity to the amide type of local anesthetics or to methylparaben, which is added to the multiple-dose vials.

Warnings: RESUSCITATIVE EQUIPMENT AND DRUGS SHOULD BE IMMEDIATELY AVAILABLE WHENEVER ANY LOCAL ANESTHETIC DRUG IS USED.

Large doses of local anesthetics should not be used in patients with heart block.

Reactions resulting in fatality have occurred on rare occasions with the use of local anesthetics, even in the absence of a history of hypersensitivity.

Solutions which contain a vasoconstrictor should be used with extreme caution in patients receiving drugs known to produce alterations in blood pressure (i.e., monamine oxidase (MAO) inhibitors, tricyclic antidepressants, phenothiazines, etc.) as either severe sustained hypertension or hypotension may occur.

Usage in Children. Great care must be exercised in adhering to safe concentrations and

Continued on next page

Breon—Cont.

dosages for pediatric administration (see Dosage and Administration).
Usage in Pregnancy. Safe use of mepivacaine has not been established with respect to adverse effects on fetal development. Careful consideration should be given to this fact before administering this drug to women of childbearing potential, particularly during early pregnancy. This does not exclude the use of the drug at term for obstetrical analgesia.
Vasopressor agents (administered for the treatment of hypotension related to caudal or other epidural blocks) should be used with extreme caution in the presence of oxytocic drugs as they are known to interact and may produce severe, persistent hypertension and/or rupture of cerebral blood vessels. CARBOCAINE has been used for obstetrical analgesia by the peridural and paracervical routes without evidence of adverse effects on the fetus when no more than the maximum safe dosages are used and strict adherence to technique is followed.
Local anesthetic procedures should be used with caution when there is inflammation and/or sepsis in the region of the proposed injection.
Precautions: Standard textbooks should be consulted for specific techniques and precautions for various regional anesthetic procedures.
The safety and effectiveness of a local anesthetic drug depend upon proper dosage, correct technique, adequate precautions, and readiness for emergencies.
The lowest dosage that results in effective anesthesia should be used to avoid high plasma levels and possible adverse effects. Injection of repeated doses of mepivacaine may cause significant increase in blood levels with each repeated dose due to slow accumulation of the drug or its metabolites or due to slower metabolic degradation than normal.
Tolerance varies with the status of the patient. Debilitated, elderly patients, or acutely ill patients should be given reduced doses commensurate with their weight and physical status.
Mepivacaine should be used with caution in patients with severe disturbances of cardiac rhythm, shock or heart block.
INJECTION SHOULD ALWAYS BE MADE SLOWLY AND WITH FREQUENT ASPIRATIONS TO AVOID INADVERTENT RAPID INTRAVASCULAR ADMINISTRATION WHICH CAN PRODUCE SYSTEMIC TOXICITY.
Fetal bradycardia which frequently follows paracervical block may be indicative of high fetal blood concentrations of CARBOCAINE with resultant fetal acidosis. Fetal heart rate should be monitored prior to and during paracervical block. Added risk appears to be present in prematurity, toxemia of pregnancy, and fetal distress. The physician should weigh the benefits against the risks in considering paracervical block in these conditions. Careful adherence to recommended dosage is of the utmost importance in paracervical block. Failure to achieve adequate analgesia with these doses should arouse suspicion of intravascular or fetal injection.
Case records of maternal convulsions and cardiovascular collapse following use of mepivacaine for paracervical block in early pregnancy (as anesthesia for elective abortion) suggest that systemic absorption under these circumstances may be rapid. Therefore the recommended maximum dose of 100 mg per side should not be exceeded. Injection should be made slowly and with frequent aspiration. Allow a 5-minute interval between sides.
Vasoconstrictors. Solutions containing a vasoconstrictor should be used cautiously. The decision whether or not to use a vasoconstrictor with local anesthesia depends on the physician's appraisal of the benefits as opposed to the risk, e.g., in injection of solutions containing a vasoconstrictor into areas where the blood supply is limited (e.g., ears, nose, digits) or when peripheral vascular disease is present. Furthermore, serious cardiac arrhythmias may occur if preparations containing a vasoconstrictor are employed in patients during or immediately following the administration of halothane, cyclopropane, trichloroethylene, or other related agents.
MEPIVACAINE SHOULD BE USED WITH CAUTION IN PATIENTS WITH KNOWN DRUG ALLERGIES AND SENSITIVITIES. A thorough history of the patient's prior experience with CARBOCAINE or other local anesthetics as well as concomitant or recent drug use should be taken (see Contraindications). Patients allergic to methylparaben or para-aminobenzoic acid derivatives (procaine, tetracaine, benzocaine, etc.) have not shown cross-sensitivity to agents of the amide-type such as mepivacaine. Since mepivacaine is metabolized in the liver and excreted by the kidneys, it should be used cautiously in patients with liver and renal disease.
Adverse Reactions: Systemic adverse reactions involving the central nervous system and the cardiovascular system usually result from high plasma levels due to excessive dosage, rapid absorption, or inadvertent intravascular injection.
A small number of reactions may result from hypersensitivity, idiosyncrasy, or diminished tolerance to normal dosage.
Excitatory CNS effects commonly represent the initial signs of local anesthetic systemic toxicity. However, these reactions may be very brief or absent in some patients in which case the first manifestation of toxicity may be drowsiness merging into unconsciousness and respiratory arrest.
Cardiovascular system reactions include depression of the myocardium, hypotension (or sometimes hypertension), bradycardia, and even cardiac arrest. In obstetrics, cases of fetal bradycardia have occurred (see Precautions).
Allergic reactions are characterized by cutaneous lesions of delayed onset, or urticaria, edema, and other manifestations of allergy. The detection of sensitivity by skin testing is of limited value. As with other local anesthetics, hypersensitivity, idiosyncrasy, and anaphylactoid reactions to CARBOCAINE have occurred rarely. The reaction may be abrupt and severe, and is not usually dose related.
Sensitivity to methylparaben, a preservative added to multiple-dose vials, has been reported. Single dose vials without methylparaben are also available.
Reactions following epidural or caudal anesthesia also may include: high or total spinal block, urinary retention; fecal incontinence; loss of perineal sensation and sexual function; persistent analgesia, paresthesia, and paralysis of the lower extremities; headache and backache; and slowing of labor and consequent increased incidence of forceps delivery.
Treatment of Reactions. Toxic effects of local anesthetics require symptomatic treatment; there is no specific cure. The physician should be prepared to maintain an airway and to support ventilation with oxygen and assisted or controlled respiration as required. Supportive treatment of the cardiovascular system includes intravenous fluids and, when appropriate, vasopressors (preferably those that stimulate the myocardium, such as ephedrine). *Convulsions* may be controlled with oxygen and by the intravenous administration of diazepam or short or ultrashort-acting barbiturates. Intravenous anticonvulsant agents should only be administered by those familiar with their use and only when ventilation and oxygenation are assured. In epidural anesthesia, sympathetic blockade also occurs as a pharmacological reaction, resulting in peripheral vasodilation and often *hypotension.* The extent of the hypotension will usually depend on the number of dermatomes blocked. The blood pressure should therefore be monitored in the early phases of anesthesia. If hypotension occurs, it is readily controlled by vasoconstrictors administered either by the intramuscular or the intravenous route, the dosage of which would depend on the severity of the hypotension and the response to treatment.
Dosage and Administration: As with all local anesthetics, the dose varies and depends upon the area to be anesthetized, the vascularity of the tissues, the number of neuronal segments to be blocked, individual tolerance, and the technique of anesthesia. The lowest dose needed to provide effective anesthesia should be administered. For specific techniques and procedures, refer to standard textbooks.
The recommended single adult dose (or the total of a series of doses given in one procedure) of CARBOCAINE for unsedated, healthy, normal-sized individuals should not usually exceed 400 mg. The recommended dosage is based on requirements for the average adult and should be reduced for elderly or debilitated patients.
While maximum doses of 7 mg/kg (550 mg) have been administered without adverse effect, these are not recommended, except in exceptional circumstances and under no circumstances should the administration be repeated at intervals of less than 1½ hours. The total dose for any 24-hour period should not exceed 1000 mg because of a slow accumulation of the anesthetic or its derivatives or slower than normal metabolic degradation or detoxification with repeat administration (see Actions and Precautions).
Children tolerate the local anesthetic as well as adults. However, the pediatric dose should be carefully measured as a percentage of the total adult dose based on weight, and should not exceed 5 to 6 mg/kg (2.5 to 3 mg/lb) in children, especially those weighing less than 30 lbs. In children under 3 years of age or weighing less than 30 lbs. concentrations less than 2 per cent (e.g., 0.5 to 1.5 per cent) should be employed.
[See table on next page].
How Supplied:
These solutions are not intended for spinal anesthesia or dental use.
Code C-400 1% single-dose vials of 30 ml (NDC 0057-0231-01)
Code C-390 1% multiple-dose vials of 50 ml (NDC 0057-0232-01)
Code C-430 1.5% single-dose vials of 30 ml (NDC 0057-0234-01)
Code C-440 2% single-dose vials of 20 ml (NDC 0057-0236-01)
Code C-410 2% multiple-dose vials of 50 ml (NDC 0057-0237-01)
Supplied by:
BREON LABORATORIES INC., Mfg. by Sterling Drug Inc., New York., N.Y. 10016
Revised March, 1979
BR883/0379

For full prescribing information on the dental use of CARBOCAINE see Cook-Waite laboratories, Inc. product listing in this publication.

DEMEROL® APAP ℂ ℞
(Brand of meperidine hydrochloride, USP with Acetaminophen)

Description: Each round, pink red-mottled tablet contains:
DEMEROL (brand of meperidine) HCl.50 mg.
(Warning: May be habit-forming)
Acetaminophen USP (APAP)..............300 mg.
Actions: Meperidine hydrochloride is a narcotic analgesic with multiple actions qualitatively similar to those of morphine; the most prominent of these involve the central nervous

Recommended Concentrations and Doses of CARBOCAINE

Procedure	Concentration	Total Dose ml	Total Dose mg	Comments
Cervical, brachial, intercostal, pudendal nerve block	1% 2%	5–40 5–20	50–400 100–400	Pudendal block; one half of total dose injected each side.
Transvaginal block (paracervical plus pudendal)	1%	up to 30 (both sides)	up to 300 (both sides)	One half of total dose injected each side. See Precautions.
Paracervical block	1%	up to 20 (both sides)	up to 200 (both sides)	One half of total dose injected each side. This is maximum recommended dose per 90 minute period in obstetrical and non-obstetrical patients. Inject slowly, 5 minutes between sides. See Precautions.
Caudal and Epidural block	1% 1.5% 2%	15–30 10–25 10–20	150–300 150–375 200–400	Use only single dose vials which do not contain a preservative.
Infiltration	1%	up to 40	up to 400	An equivalent amount of a 0.5% solution (prepared by diluting the 1% solution with Sodium Chloride Injection, USP) may be used for large areas.
Therapeutic block	1% 2%	1–5 1–5	10–50 20–50	

Unused portions of solutions not containing preservatives should be discarded.

system and organs composed of smooth muscle. The principal actions of therapeutic value are analgesia and sedation.

There is some evidence which suggests that meperidine may produce less smooth muscle spasm, constipation, and depression of the cough reflex than equianalgesic doses of morphine. Meperidine, in 60- to 80-mg. parenteral doses, is approximately equivalent in analgesic effect to 10 mg. of morphine. The onset of action is slightly more rapid than with morphine, and the duration of action is slightly shorter. Meperidine is significantly less effective by the oral than by the parenteral route, but the exact ratio of oral to parenteral effectiveness is unknown.

Acetaminophen is the active metabolite of acetophenetidin which is responsible for the analgesic and antipyretic actions of the latter.

Indications: For the relief of moderate to severe pain.

Contraindications: Hypersensitivity to meperidine or acetaminophen.

Meperidine is contraindicated in patients who are receiving monoamine oxidase (MAO) inhibitors or those who have received such agents within 14 days.

Therapeutic doses of meperidine have inconsistently precipitated unpredictable, severe, and occasionally fatal reactions in patients who have received such agents within 14 days. The mechanism of these reactions is unclear. Some have been characterized by coma, severe respiratory depression, cyanosis, and hypotension, and have resembled the syndrome of acute narcotic overdose. In other reactions the predominant manifestations have been hyperexcitability, convulsions, tachycardia, hyperpyrexia, and hypertension. Although it is not known that other narcotics are free of the risk of such reactions, virtually all of the reported reactions have occurred with meperidine. If a narcotic is needed in such patients, a sensitivity test should be performed in which repeated, small incremental doses of morphine are administered over the course of several hours while the patient's condition and vital signs are under careful observation.

(Intravenous hydrocortisone or prednisolone have been used to treat severe reactions, with the addition of intravenous chlorpromazine in those cases exhibiting hypertension and hyperpyrexia. The usefulness and safety of narcotic antagonists in the treatment of these reactions is unknown.)

Warnings:

Drug Dependence. Meperidine can produce drug dependence of the morphine type and therefore has the potential for being abused. Psychic dependence, physical dependence, and tolerance may develop upon repeated administration of meperidine, and it should be prescribed and administered with the same degree of caution appropriate to the use of morphine. Like other narcotics, meperidine is subject to the provisions of the Federal narcotic laws.

Interaction with Other Central Nervous System Depressants. Meperidine should be used with great caution and in reduced dosage in patients who are concurrently receiving other narcotic analgesics, general anesthetics, phenothiazines, other tranquilizers, sedative-hypnotics, tricyclic antidepressants, and other CNS depressants (including alcohol). Respiratory depression, hypotension, and profound sedation or coma may result.

Head Injury and Increased Intracranial Pressure. The respiratory depressant effects of meperidine and its capacity to elevate cerebrospinal fluid pressure may be markedly exaggerated in the presence of head injury, other intracranial lesions, or a pre-existing increase in intracranial pressure. Furthermore, narcotics produce adverse reactions which may obscure the clinical course of patients with head injuries. In such patients, meperidine must be used with extreme caution and only if its use is deemed essential.

Asthma and Other Respiratory Conditions. Meperidine should be used with extreme caution in patients having an acute asthmatic attack, patients with chronic obstructive pulmonary disease or cor pulmonale, patients having a substantially decreased respiratory reserve, and patients with pre-existing respiratory depression, hypoxia, or hypercapnia. In such patients, even usual therapeutic doses of narcotics may decrease respiratory drive while simultaneously increasing airway resistance to the point of apnea.

Hypotensive Effect. The administration of meperidine may result in severe hypotension in an individual whose ability to maintain his blood pressure has already been compromised by a depleted blood volume or concurrent administration of drugs such as the phenothiazines or certain anesthetics.

Usage in Ambulatory Patients. Meperidine may impair the mental and/or physical abilities required for the performance of potentially hazardous tasks such as driving a car or operating machinery. The patient should be cautioned accordingly.

Meperidine, like other narcotics, may produce orthostatic hypotension in ambulatory patients.

Usage in Pregnancy and Lactation. Meperidine should not be used in pregnant women prior to the labor period, unless in the judgment of the physician the potential benefits outweigh the possible hazards, because safe use in pregnancy prior to labor has not been established relative to possible adverse effects on fetal development.

When used as an obstetrical analgesic, meperidine crosses the placental barrier and can produce respiratory depression in the newborn; resuscitation may be required (see section on OVERDOSAGE).

Meperidine appears in the milk of nursing mothers receiving the drug.

Precautions:

Supraventricular Tachycardias. Meperidine should be used with caution in patients with atrial flutter and other supraventricular tachycardias because of a possible vagolytic action which may produce a significant increase in the ventricular response rate.

Convulsions. Meperidine may aggravate preexisting convulsions in patients with convulsive disorders. If dosage is escalated substantially above recommended levels because of tolerance development, convulsions may occur in individuals without a history of convulsive disorders.

Acute Abdominal Conditions. The administration of meperidine or other narcotics may obscure the diagnosis or clinical course in patients with acute abdominal conditions.

Special Risk Patients. Meperidine should be given with caution and the initial dose should be reduced in certain patients such as the elderly or debilitated, and those with severe impairment of hepatic or renal function, hypothyroidism, Addison's disease, and prostatic hypertrophy or urethal stricture.

Adverse Reactions: The major hazards of DEMEROL APAP are those of meperidine. As with other narcotic analgesics, these hazards are respiratory depression and to a lesser degree, circulatory depression; respiratory arrest, shock, and cardiac arrest have occurred. The most frequently observed adverse reactions include lightheadedness, dizziness, sedation, nausea, vomiting, and sweating. These effects seem to be more prominent in ambulatory patients and in those who are not experiencing severe pain. In such individuals, lower doses are advisable. Some adverse reactions in ambulatory patients may be alleviated if the patient lies down.

Other adverse reactions include:

Central Nervous System. Euphoria, dysphoria, weakness, headache, agitation, tremor, uncoordinated muscle movements, transient hallucinations and disorientation, visual disturbances.

Continued on next page

Breon—Cont.

Gastrointestinal. Dry mouth, constipation, biliary tract spasm.
Cardiovascular. Flushing of the face, tachycardia, bradycardia, palpitation, faintness, syncope.
Genitourinary. Urinary retention.
Allergic. Pruritus, urticaria, other skin rashes.
Other. Antidiuretic effect.
Dosage and Administration:
For Relief of Pain
Dosage should be adjusted according to the severity of the pain and the response of the patient. Meperidine is less effective orally than on parenteral administration.
The usual adult dose is 1 or 2 tablets, repeated, if necessary, at intervals of three to four hours.
Overdosage:
Symptoms: The major symptoms of overdosage with DEMEROL APAP are those of overdosage with meperidine. Serious overdose with meperidine is characterized by respiratory depression (a decrease in respiratory rate and/or tidal volume, Cheyne-Stokes respiration, cyanosis), extreme somnolence progressing to stupor or coma, skeletal muscle flaccidity, cold and clammy skin, and sometimes bradycardia and hypotension. In severe overdosage, apnea, circulatory collapse, cardiac arrest, and death may occur.
Treatment: Primary attention should be given to the re-establishment of adequate respiratory exchange through provision of a patent airway and institution of assisted or controlled ventilation. The narcotic antagonists, naloxone hydrochloride, nalorphine hydrochloride and levallorphan tartrate, are specific antidotes against respiratory depression which may result from overdosage or unusual sensitivity to narcotics, including meperidine. Therefore, an appropriate dose of one of these antagonists should be administered, preferably by the intravenous route, simultaneously with efforts at respiratory resuscitation.
An antagonist should not be administered in the absence of clinically significant respiratory or cardiovascular depression.
Oxygen, intravenous fluids, vasopressors, and other supportive measures should be employed as indicated.
The stomach should be evacuated by emesis or gastric lavage.
Note: In an individual physically dependent on narcotics, the administration of the usual dose of a narcotic antagonist will precipitate an acute withdrawal syndrome. The severity of this syndrome will depend on the degree of physical dependence and the dose of antagonist administered. The use of narcotic antagonists in such individuals should be avoided if possible. If a narcotic antagonist must be used to treat serious respiratory depression in the physically dependent patient, the antagonist should be administered with extreme care and only one-fifth to one-tenth the usual initial dose administered.
How Supplied: DEMEROL APAP Tablets, bottles of 100. Code 1312 NDC-0057-1022-10
DEA Order Form Required.
Supplied by:
BREON LABORATORIES INC.
New York, N.Y. 10016
Mfg. by Sterling Drug Inc.
New York, N.Y. 10016

Revised July 1977
BR 348/0877
[*Shown in Product Identification Section*]

FERGON®
(Brand of ferrous gluconate)
FERGON ELIXIR

Composition: FERGON (brand of pure ferrous gluconate) is stabilized to maintain a minimum of ferric ions. It contains not less than 11.5 per cent iron. Each FERGON tablet contains 320 mg. FERGON Elixir 6% contains 300 mg per teaspoon.
Action and Uses: FERGON preparations produce rapid hemoglobin regeneration in patients with iron deficiency anemias. FERGON is better utilized and better tolerated than other forms of iron because of its low ionization constant and solubility in the entire pH range of the gastrointestinal tract. It does not precipitate proteins or have the astringency of more ionizable forms of iron, does not interfere with proteolytic or diastatic activities of the digestive system, and will not produce nausea, abdominal cramps, constipation or diarrhea in the great majority of patients.
FERGON preparations are indicated in anemias amenable to iron therapy: (1) hypochromic anemia of infancy and childhood; (2) idiopathic hypochromic anemia; (3) hypochromic anemia of pregnancy; and (4) anemia associated with chronic blood loss.
Administration and Dosage: Adults—one or two FERGON tablets or one or two teaspoons of FERGON Elixir three times daily. Children 6–12 years—one FERGON tablet or one teaspoon of FERGON Elixir one to three times daily, as directed by the physician. Infants—30 drops of FERGON Elixir, gradually increasing to 1 teaspoon daily.
How Supplied: FERGON, tablets of 320 mg (5 grains), bottles of 100, 500 and 1,000. FERGON Elixir 6% (5 grains per teaspoon), bottles of 1 pint.
FERGON registered trademark of Sterling Drug, Inc.
[*Shown in Product Identification Section*]

FERGON® CAPSULES

Composition: Each FERGON Capsule contains 435 mg. of ferrous gluconate, yielding 50 mg. of elemental iron.
Action and Uses: FERGON preparations produce rapid hemoglobin regeneration in patients with iron deficiency anemias. FERGON is better utilized and better tolerated than other forms of iron because of its low ionization constant and solubility in the entire pH range of the gastrointestinal tract. It does not precipitate proteins or have the astringency of more ionizable forms of iron, does not interfere with proteolytic or diastatic activities of the digestive system, and will not produce nausea, abdominal cramps, constipation or diarrhea in the great majority of patients. The pellets of ferrous gluconate contained in FERGON Capsules are coated to permit maximum availability of iron in the upper small bowel, the site of maximum absorption.
FERGON preparations are indicated in anemias amenable to iron therapy: (1) hypochromic anemia of infancy and childhood; (2) idiopathic hypochromic anemia; (3) hypochromic anemia of pregnancy; and (4) anemia associated with chronic blood loss.
Administration and Dosage: 1 FERGON Capsule daily for mild to moderate iron deficiency anemia. For more severe anemia the dosage may be increased.
How Supplied: FERGON Capsules, bottles of 30.
[*Shown in Product Identification Section*]

FERGON® PLUS ℞
FOR IRON DEFICIENCY AND MACROCYTIC ANEMIAS

Description: Each sugar-coated Caplet contains:
FERGON (brand of
ferrous gluconate)............500 mg (5 MDR*)
Vitamin B_{12} With Intrinsic Factor
Concentrate N.F. XI ....½ unit (oral)
Ascorbic acid ....75 mg (2½ MDR*)
*MDR—Adult minimum daily requirement.
Action: Vitamin B_{12} With Intrinsic Factor Concentrate as contained in 2 FERGON Plus Caplets® represents 1 N.F. XI oral unit of anti-anemia activity, that is, the amount of material which, when administered daily by mouth, produces a satisfactory hematologic and symptomatic response in patients in relapse with pernicious anemia.
Vitamin B_{12} is the principal active anti-pernicious anemia factor of liver extract and is believed to be essentially extrinsic factor. Its anti-pernicious anemia activity is approximately the same as that produced by liver extract and, like the latter, it is more effective by injection than by mouth. However, its activity on oral administration is increased by the concomitant ingestion of Intrinsic Factor Concentrate which facilitates absorption of Vitamin B_{12} from the alimentary tract.
Ferrous gluconate is better utilized and better tolerated than other forms of iron and produces rapid hemoglobin regeneration when iron deficiency is present. Vitamin C appears to play a role in the absorption of iron. Its deficiency leads to depression of bone marrow activity.
Indications: *Dietary Supplement*—FERGON Plus is useful as a dietary supplement and as a maintenance source of Vitamin B_{12}, Vitamin C and iron. However, it should be remembered that the development of the classic symptoms of pernicious anemia may in some cases be delayed by oral ingestion of Intrinsic Factor.
Therapy—FERGON Plus is indicated for all anemias amenable to iron therapy including (1) hypochromic anemia of infancy and childhood; (2) idiopathic hypochromic anemia; (3) hypochromic anemia of pregnancy; and (4) anemia associated with chronic blood loss.
FERGON Plus is also indicated for patients with anemias responding to oral Vitamin B_{12} therapy; viz., those in whom the bone marrow is in a state of megaloblastic arrest reflected in the blood stream by macrocytosis, anisocytosis and poikilocytosis, including macrocytic anemia of tropical and nontropical sprue, megaloblastic anemias of pregnancy and infancy, and pernicious anemia amenable to oral B_{12} therapy. Similarly, FERGON Plus may be given orally to patients with pernicious anemia to supplement parenterally administered Vitamin B_{12} therapy.
Note—All patients with pernicious anemia should be given periodic examinations, and laboratory studies should be performed. Some patients may not respond to orally ingested Vitamin B_{12} with Intrinsic Factor Concentrate. There is no known way to predict which patients will respond or which patients may cease to respond.
Dosage: As dietary supplement—1 Caplet daily. Therapeutic dose—1 Caplet twice daily (before the morning and evening meals).
When the condition is severe, the initial dose should be increased to 2 Caplets twice daily for one or two weeks or specific parenteral therapy should be employed.
Caution: Federal law prohibits dispensing without prescription.
How Supplied: Bottles of 100 Caplets. FERGON—registered trade mark of Sterling Drug Inc.

ISUPREL® Hydrochloride ℞
brand of isoproterenol hydrochloride injection, USP
Sterile Injection 1:5000

Description: ISUPREL hydrochloride, brand of isoproterenol hydrochloride, is 3,4-dihydroxy-α-[(isopropylamino) methyl] benzyl alcohol hydrochloride, a synthetic sympathomimetic amine that is structurally related to epinephrine but acts almost exclusively on beta receptors.
Each milliliter of the sterile 1:5000 solution contains 0.2 mg ISUPREL hydrochloride, brand of isoproterenol hydrochloride, 0.12 mg lactic acid, 1.8 mg sodium lactate, 7 mg sodium chloride, and not more than 1 mg sodium bisul-

fite as preservative. The pH is adjusted with hydrochloric acid. The air in the ampuls has been displaced by nitrogen gas.

Action: The primary actions of ISUPREL are on the heart and on smooth muscle of bronchi, skeletal muscle vasculature, and alimentary tract. The positive inotropic and chronotropic actions of the drug increase cardiac output. There is also an increase in venous return to the heart. With usual therapeutic doses, the increase in cardiac output is generally sufficient to maintain or increase systolic blood pressure. ISUPREL also lowers peripheral vascular resistance; the diastolic pressure, therefore, may be expected to fall in normal individuals. Thus, the mean pressure may be reduced. The rate of discharge of cardiac pacemakers is increased with isoproterenol.

ISUPREL relaxes most smooth muscle, the most pronounced effect being on bronchial and gastrointestinal smooth muscle. It produces marked relaxation in the smaller bronchi and may even dilate the trachea and main bronchi past the resting diameter.

The acute toxicity of ISUPREL in animals is much less than that of epinephrine. Excessive doses in animals or man can cause a striking drop in blood pressure, and repeated large doses in animals may result in cardiac enlargement and focal myocarditis.

Indications: Parenteral isoproterenol hydrochloride is indicated as an adjunct in the management of shock (hypoperfusion syndrome) and in the treatment of cardiac standstill or arrest; carotid sinus hypersensitivity; Adams-Stokes syndrome; and ventricular tachycardia and ventricular arrhythmias that require increased inotropic cardiac activity for therapy. It may also be used in the management of bronchospasm during anesthesia.

SHOCK (HYPOPERFUSION SYNDROME)

Shock is a complex clinical syndrome characterized by inadequate tissue perfusion, which results from one or more of the following mechanisms: loss of effective blood volume, cardiac failure, peripheral vascular failure. Rational therapy must be aimed at correcting this perfusion deficit.

Since shock is often, but by no means always, associated with lowered blood pressure, administration of vasoactive drugs that increase blood pressure without increasing blood flow may not be in the best interests of the patient. However, in cases of shock characterized chiefly by peripheral vasodilation and in shock following acute myocardial infarction, according to one group of investigators, a vasopressor such as levarterenol bitartrate injection, USP, may be indicated.[1,2]

In addition to the routine monitoring of systemic blood pressure, heart rate, urine flow, and the use of the electrocardiogram, the shock state and the response to therapy should be monitored by frequent determinations of the central venous pressure, blood pH, and blood pCO_2(or bicarbonate). Determinations of cardiac output and circulation time may also be helpful.

Adequate filling of the intravascular compartment by suitable volume expanders is of primary importance in most cases of shock, and should precede the administration of vasoactive drugs. Determination of central venous pressure is a reliable guide during volume replacement. If evidence of hypoperfusion persists after adequate volume replacement, ISUPREL may be given.

ISUPREL increases cardiac output by increasing the strength of cardiac contraction and, to a limited extent, the rate of contraction. ISUPREL also increases venous return to the heart by mobilizing blood from vascular reservoirs.[3] In addition, the peripheral and coronary vasodilating effects of the drug may aid tissue perfusion. ISUPREL may be given to patients who are fully digitalized;[4,5] in fact, ISUPREL may be particularly useful when cardiac competence cannot be restored by digitalization.

Appropriate measures should be taken to ensure adequate ventilation. Careful attention should be paid to acid-base balance and to the correction of electrolyte disturbance. In cases of shock associated with bacteremia, suitable antimicrobial therapy is, of course, imperative.

In a group of 10 patients with elevated central venous pressures who were in shock from cardiac failure, isoproterenol produced increases in cardiac output of 0.33 to 4.34 liters per minute in nine of the ten.[6] Similarly, in a series of 12 patients with shock due to gram-negative bacteremia, Kardos[7] found isoproterenol to be useful in correcting the hemodynamic alterations.

Although the ultimate effect of ISUPREL on patient survival has not yet been documented, experimental studies in rats have shown that the fatal course of shock caused by transient hemorrhage was reversed by treatment with isoproterenol after replacement of blood volume.[3] In addition, clinical studies[6–15] have indicated that in a majority of patients in shock, administration of ISUPREL tends to correct the hemodynamic abnormalities.

Contraindication: Administration of ISUPREL hydrochloride, brand of isoproterenol hydrochloride, is contraindicated in patients with tachycardia caused by digitalis intoxication.

Warning: ISUPREL infusions may produce an increase in myocardial work and oxygen consumption. These effects may be detrimental to myocardial metabolism and functioning in patients who are in cardiogenic shock secondary to coronary artery occlusion and myocardial infarction.

Precautions: ISUPREL and epinephrine should not be administered simultaneously, since both drugs are direct cardiac stimulants and their combined effects may induce serious arrhythmia. The drugs may, however, be administered alternately provided a proper interval has elapsed between doses.

Dosage of ISUPREL should be carefully adjusted particularly in patients with coronary insufficiency, diabetes, or hyperthyroidism, and in patients sensitive to sympathomimetic amines.

Hypovolemia should be corrected by suitable volume expanders before treatment with ISUPREL. Patients in shock should be closely observed during ISUPREL administration. If the heart rate exceeds 110 beats per minute, it may be advisable to decrease the infusion rate or temporarily discontinue the infusion. Doses of ISUPREL sufficient to increase the heart rate to more than 130 beats per minute may induce ventricular arrhythmia.

There has been no clinical evidence of teratogenic effects attributable to ISUPREL in more than 20 years' use of the drug. However, before administration of any drug to pregnant women or women of childbearing potential, the expected benefit of the drug should be carefully weighed against the possible risk to the mother or child.

Dosage and Administration: ISUPREL hydrochloride Solution 1:5000 should be diluted in 5 per cent Dextrose Injection, USP, before it is administered to patients in shock.

- A convenient dilution is 1 mg ISUPREL (5 ml) in 500 ml diluent (final concentration, 1:500,000).
- Concentrations up to 10 times greater have been used.[6] This may be important in patients in whom limitation of volume is essential.
- Infusion rates of 0.5 to 5 μg per minute (0.25 to 2.5 ml diluted solution 1:500,000) have been recommended.
- Rates over 30 μg per minute have been used in advanced stages of shock.

The speed of infusion should be adjusted on the basis of heart rate, central venous pressure, systemic blood pressure, and urine flow. If the heart rate exceeds 110 beats per minute, it may be advisable to decrease the infusion rate or temporarily discontinue the infusion.

CARDIAC STANDSTILL AND CARDIAC ARRHYTHMIAS

Because it has potent inotropic cardiac stimulant action with little or no pressor activity, ISUPREL hydrochloride, brand of isoproterenol hydrochloride, has been effective for the treatment of the following:

1. Adams-Stokes syndrome—atrioventricular heart block
2. Cardiac standstill (arrest)
3. Carotid sinus hypersensitivity
4. Ventricular arrhythmias, especially certain types of ventricular tachycardia and fibrillation occurring during the course of atrioventricular block.

It should be noted that in symptomatic heart block, electrical pacing is the preferred method of treatment for maintenance of an adequate ventricular rate. Moreover, in ventricular arrhythmias, especially certain types of ventricular tachycardia and fibrillation, electroshock may have to be used, and is usually the treatment of choice.

If, however, therapy with ISUPREL is elected in these conditions, intravenous administration, with constant monitoring, is preferred.

In patients with heart block and episodic ventricular tachycardia or fibrillation, ISUPREL stimulates the higher centers or nodal tissue without exciting the lower ventricular foci. In so doing, the normal idioventricular pacemaker function may take over, thereby abolishing ventricular acceleration. Epinephrine is contraindicated in patients with ventricular fibrillation because it may precipitate or prolong fibrillation by stimulation of multiple higher and lower foci. It also may further embarrass the cardiovascular system by its hypertensive action.

Intravenous administration of ISUPREL has been recommended for the management of patients with complete heart block following closure of ventricular septal defects. A 1:50,000 solution may be administered intravenously in doses ranging from 0.5 to 1.5 ml for infants and from 2 to 3 ml for adults. With such doses the heart rate accelerates and the effect often lasts for 15 or 20 minutes. Sinus rhythm sometimes occurs and persists for a variable period but often relapses again into complete block. In other cases, ISUPREL merely maintains an acceptable heart rate somewhere above 90 to 100 beats per minute. The patient must be monitored constantly by electrocardiography.

Contraindications: Use of isoproterenol in patients with preexisting cardiac arrhythmias associated with tachycardia is generally considered contraindicated because the chronotropic effect of the drug on the heart may aggravate such disorders. Exceptions consist only of those ventricular tachycardias and ventricular arrhythmias which require increased inotropic cardiac activity for therapy.

Administration of ISUPREL is contraindicated in patients with tachycardia caused by digitalis intoxication.

Precautions: ISUPREL and epinephrine should not be administered simultaneously, since both drugs are direct cardiac stimulants and their combined effects may induce serious arrhythmia. The drugs may, however, be administered alternately provided a proper interval has elasped between doses.

Dosage of ISUPREL should be carefully adjusted in patients with coronary insufficiency, diabetes, or hyperthyroidism, and in patients sensitive to sympathomimetic amines.

Continued on next page

Breon—Cont.

If the cardiac rate increases sharply, patients with angina pectoris may experience anginal pain until the cardiac rate decreases.

There has been no clinical evidence of teratogenic effects attributable to ISUPREL in more than 20 years' use of the drug. However, before administration of any drug to pregnant women or women of childbearing potential, the expected benefit of the drug should be carefully weighed against the possible risk to the mother or child.

Adverse Reactions: Serious reactions to ISUPREL are infrequent. The following reactions, however, have been reported: flushing of the face, sweating, mild tremors, nervousness, headache, and tachycardia with palpitation manifested as a sensation of pounding in the chest. These reactions disappear quickly and usually do not require discontinuation of treatment with ISUPREL hydrochloride, brand of isoproterenol hydrochloride. No cumulative effects have been reported. Pulmonary edema has been reported in a patient extremely intolerant to all sympathomimetic drugs.[16]

In a few patients, presumably with organic disease of the A-V node and its branches, ISUPREL has been reported, paradoxically, to precipitate Adams-Stokes seizures during normal sinus rhythm or transient heart block.[16]

Dosage and Administration: In the treatment and prevention of cardiac standstill and cardiac arrhythmias, parenteral ISUPREL may be administered by intravenous injection, infusion, intramuscular and subcutaneous injection, and *in extremis,* by intracardiac injection.

The following table summarizes the dosage regimen suggested for various routes of administration in adults. Children may be given half the initial adult dose. In all patients, subsequent dosage and method of administration depend on the response of the ventricular rate and the rapidity with which the cardiac pacemaker can take over when the drug is gradually withdrawn.

The usual route of administration in emergency treatment of patients threatened with cardiac standstill or arrhythmia is by intravenous injection or infusion. Dosage must be regulated by monitoring of the electrocardiogram. If time is not of utmost importance, initial therapy by intramuscular or subcutaneous injection is preferred.

[See table below, left].
[See table below].

BRONCHOSPASM DURING ANESTHESIA

Parenteral ISUPREL hydrochloride, brand of isoproterenol hydrochloride, has been shown under experimental and clinical conditions to be a potent bronchodilating agent. However, when given in dosages to achieve this effect, it may also have a stimulating effect on the cardiovascular system. Like epinephrine, it may produce arrhythmias in patients anesthetized with cyclopropane, and should be used with caution. ISUPREL can be used for the management of bronchospasm by helping the patient to maintain adequate ventilation and a normally functioning circulatory system.

Precautions and Adverse Reactions: See corresponding sections under "Cardiac Standstill and Cardiac Arrhythmias."

Dosage and Administration: For the management of bronchospasm during anesthesia, 1 ml of ISURPEL Solution 1:5000 is diluted to 10 ml with Sodium Chloride Injection, USP, or 5 per cent Dextrose Injection, USP. An initial dose of 0.01 to 0.02 mg (0.5 to 1 ml of the diluted solution, 1:50,000) is administered intravenously, and may be repeated when necessary.

How Supplied: ISUPREL hydrochloride sterile solution 1:5000 (for parenteral use).

Code I-290 1 ml. ampuls (0.2 mg.)
Box of 5 **NDC-0057-0866-01**
Code I-291 1 ml ampuls (0.2 mg.)
Box of 100 **NDC-0057-0866-06**
Code I-330 5 ml ampuls (1 mg.)
Box of 10 **NDC-0057-0867-02**

Bibliography:

1. Gunnar, R.M., Loeb, H.S., Pietras, R.J., and Tobin, J.R., Jr.: *J.A.M.A. 202*:1124, Dec. 25, 1967.
2. Loeb, H.S., Pietras, R.J., Tobin, J.R., Jr., and Gunnar, R. M.: *Clin. Res. 15*:213, April 1967.
3. Weil, M. H. and Bradley, E.C.: *Bull. N.Y. Acad. Med. 42*:1023, Nov. 1966.
4. Cohn, J. N.: *GP 34*:78, Aug. 1966.
5. du Toit, H. J., du Plessis, J. M. E., Dommisse, J., Rorke, M. J., Theron, M. S., and de Villiers, V. P.: *Lancet 2*:143, July 16, 1966.
6. MacLean, L. D., Duff, J. H., Scott, H. M., and Peretz, D. I.: *Surg. Gynec. Obstet. 120*:1, Jan. 1965.
7. Kardos, G. G.: *New Eng. J. Med. 274*:868, April 21, 1966.
8. Duff, J. H., Scott, H. M., Peretz, D. I., Mulligan, G. W., and MacLean, L. D.: *J. Trauma 6*:145, March 1966.
9. Duff, J. H., McLean, A. P. H., Mulligan, G. W., and MacLean, L. D.: *Acad. Med. New Jersey Bull. 12*:193, Sept. 1966.
10. Duff, J. H., Peretz, D. I., Scott, H. M., Wigmore, R. A., and MacLean, L. D.: *J. Okla. Med. Ass. 59*:437, Aug. 1966.
11. Brown, R. S., Carey, J. S., Mohr, Patricia A., Monson, D. O., and Shoemaker, W. C.: *Circulation 34*:260, Aug. 1966.
12. Brown, R. S., Carey, J. S., Woodward, N. W., Mohr, Patricia A., and Shoemaker, W. C.: *Surg. Gynec. Obstet. 122*:303, Feb. 1966.
13. Wilson, J. N.: *Arch. Surg. 91*:92, July 1965.
14. Loeb, H. S., Stavrakos, C., Pietras, R. J., Tobin, J. R., Jr., and Gunnar, R. M.: *Circulation 34*:III, Oct., Suppl. 3, 1966. (abstr.)
15. Torpey, D. J.: *J.A.M.A. 202*:955, Dec. 4, 1967.
16. Schwartz, S. P. and Schwartz, L. S.: *Amer. Heart J. 57*:849, June 1959.

Dosage of ISUPREL for Cardiac Standstill and Cardiac Arrhythmias in Adults

Route of Administration	Preparation of Dilution	Initial Dose	Subsequent Dose Range
Intravenous	Dilute 1 ml of Solution 1:5000 (0.2 mg) to 10 ml with Sodium Chloride Injection, USP, or 5% Dextrose Injection, USP.	0.02 to 0.06 mg (1 to 3 ml of diluted solution 1:50,000)	0.01 to 0.2 mg (0.5 to 10 ml of diluted solution)
Intravenous infusion	Dilute 10 ml of Solution 1:5000 (2 mg) in 500 ml of 5% Dextrose Injection, USP.	5 μg/min (1.25 ml of diluted solution 1:250,000 per minute)	
Intramuscular	Use Solution 1:5000 undiluted	0.2 mg (1 ml)	0.02 to 1 mg (0.1 to 5 ml)
Subcutaneous	Use Solution 1:5000 undiluted	0.2 mg (1 ml)	0.15 to 0.2 mg (0.75 to 1 ml)
Intracardiac	Use Solution 1:5000 undiluted	0.02 mg (0.1 ml)	

ISUPREL® Hydrochloride ℞

brand of isoproterenol hydrochloride, USP
MISTOMETER®
Potent Bronchodilator

Description: ISUPREL MISTOMETER is a complete nebulizing unit consisting of a plastic-coated vial of aerosol solution, detachable plastic mouthpiece with built-in nebulizer, and protective cap. The vial contains 15 ml of ISUPREL hydrochloride 1:400 or 0.25 per cent w/w (2.8 mg per ml) in inert propellants (dichlorodifluoromethane and dichlorotetrafluorethane) with alcohol 33 per cent (w/w) and ascorbic acid. The contents of the vial permit the delivery of about 300 single oral inhalations. The MISTOMETER unit delivers at the mouthpiece a measured dose of approximately 125 μg of the bronchodilator in a fine, even mist for inhalation.

Action: ISUPREL relaxes bronchial spasm and facilitates expectoration of pulmonary secretions. It is frequently effective when epinephrine and other drugs fail, and it has a wide margin of safety. In dogs the toxic dose is 1000 times the therapeutic dose. Converted to the amount used clinically in man, this would be about 2500 times the therapeutic dose.

Indications: ISUPREL is indicated for the treatment of bronchospasm associated with acute and chronic bronchial asthma, pulmonary emphysema, bronchitis, and bronchiectasis.

Contraindication: Use of isoproterenol in patients with preexisting cardiac arrhythmias associated with tachycardia is generally considered contraindicated because the cardiac stimulant effect of the drug may aggravate such disorders.

Warnings: Excessive use of an adrenergic aerosol should be discouraged as it may lose its effectiveness.

In patients with status asthmaticus and abnormal blood gas tensions, improvement in vital capacity and in blood gas tensions may not accompany apparent relief of bronchospasm. Facilities for administering oxygen mixtures and ventilatory assistance are necessary for such patients.

Occasional patients have been reported to develop severe paradoxical airway resistance with repeated, excessive use of isoproterenol inhalation preparations. The cause of this refractory state is unknown. It is advisable that in such instances the use of the preparation be discontinued immediately and alternative therapy instituted, since in the reported cases the patients did not respond to other forms of therapy until the drug was withdrawn.

Deaths have been reported following excessive use of isoproterenol inhalation preparations and the exact cause is unknown. Cardiac arrest was noted in several instances.

Precautions: Epinephrine should not be administered concomitantly with ISUPREL, as both drugs are direct cardiac stimulants and their combined effects may induce serious ar-

rhythmia. If desired they may, however, be alternated, provided an interval of at least four hours has elapsed.
Isoproterenol should be used with caution in patients with cardiovascular disorders including coronary insufficiency, diabetes, or hyperthyroidism, and in persons sensitive to sympathomimetic amines.
A single treatment with the ISUPREL MISTOMETER unit is usually sufficient for controlling isolated attacks of asthma. Any patient who requires more than three aerosol treatments within a 24-hour period should be under the close supervision of his physician. Further therapy with the bronchodilator aerosol alone is inadvisable when three to five treatments within six to twelve hours produce minimal or no relief.
During the course of over 25 years of use of ISUPREL, isoproterenol, there has been no clinical evidence of teratogenic effects. However, use of any drug in pregnancy, lactation, or in women in childbearing age requires that the potential benefit of the drug be weighed against its possible hazards to the mother or child.
Adverse Reactions: The mist from the ISUPREL MISTOMETER unit contains alcohol but is generally very well tolerated. An occasional patient may experience some transient throat irritation which has been attributed to the alcohol content.
Tachycardia, palpitation, nervousness, nausea, and vomitting may occur from overdosage. Rarely do headache, flushing of the skin, tremor, dizziness, weakness, sweating, precordial distress, or anginal-type pain occur. The inhalation route is usually accompanied by a minimum of side effects. These untoward reactions disappear quickly and do not, as a rule, inconvenience the patient to the extent that the drug must be discontinued. No cumulative effects have been reported.
Dosage and Administration:
Acute Bronchial Asthma: Hold the MISTOMETER unit in an inverted position. Close lips and teeth around open end of mouthpiece. Breathe out, expelling as much air from the lungs as possible; then inhale deeply while pressing down on the bottle to activate spray mechanism. Try to hold breath for a few seconds before exhaling. Wait one full minute in order to determine the effect before considering a second inhalation. A treatment may be repeated up to 5 times daily if necessary. (See Precautions.) If carefully instructed, children quickly learn to keep the stream of mist clear of the teeth and tongue, thereby assuring inhalation into the lungs. Occlusion of the nares of very young children may be advisable to make inhalation certain.
Warm water should be run through the mouthpiece once daily to wash it and prevent clogging.
The mouthpiece may also be sanitized by immersion in alcohol.
Bronchospasm in Chronic Obstructive Lung Disease: The MISTOMETER unit provides a convenient aerosol method for delivering ISUPREL. The treatment described above for Acute Bronchial Asthma may be repeated at not less than 3 to 4 hour intervals as part of a programmed regimen of treatment of obstructive lung disease complicated by a reversible bronchospastic component. One application from the MISTOMETER unit may be regarded as equivalent in effectiveness to 5 to 7 operations of a hand-bulb nebulizer using a 1:100 solution.
Children's Dosage. In general, the technique of ISUPREL hydrochloride, brand of isoproterenol hydrochloride, aerosol solution administration to children is similar to that of adults, since children's smaller ventilatory exchange capacity automatically provides proportionally smaller aerosol intake.
How Supplied: **MISTOMETER** 15 ml (16.8 g)—a complete nebulizing unit and 15 ml (16.8 g) Refill

ISUPREL® Hydrochloride ℞
brand of isoproterenol hydrochloride inhalation, USP
SOLUTION 1:200
SOLUTION 1:100

Potent Bronchodilator

Description: ISUPREL hydrochloride, brand of isoproterenol hydrochloride, is available as:
Solution 1:200 in a buffered aqueous vehicle containing sodium chloride, citric acid, and glycerin with chlorobutanol 0.5 per cent and sodium bisulfite 0.3 per cent as preservatives.
Solution 1:100 in a buffered aqueous vehicle containing sodium chloride, sodium citrate, citric acid, and saccharin with chlorobutanol 0.5 per cent and sodium bisulfite 0.3 per cent as preservatives.
The air in the bottles has been displaced by nitrogen gas.
Do not use the solutions if a precipitate or brownish discoloration is observed. Although ISUPREL solutions left in nebulizers will remain clear and potent for many days, for sanitary reasons it is recommended that they be changed daily.
Action: ISUPREL relaxes bronchial spasm and facilitates expectoration of pulmonary secretions. It is frequently effective when epinephrine and other drugs fail, and it has a wide margin of safety. In dogs the toxic dose is 1000 times the therapeutic dose. Converted to the amount used clinically in man, this would be about 2500 times the therapeutic dose.
Indications: ISUPREL is indicated for the treatment of bronchospasm associated with acute and chronic bronchial asthma, pulmonary emphysema, bronchitis, and bronchiectasis.
Contraindication: Use of isoproterenol in patients with preexisting cardiac arrhythmias associated with tachycardia is generally considered contraindicated because the cardiac stimulant effect of the drug may aggravate such disorders.
Warnings: Excessive use of an adrenergic aerosol should be discouraged as it may lose its effectiveness.
In patients with status asthmaticus and abnormal blood gas tensions, improvement in vital capacity and in blood gas tensions may not accompany apparent relief of bronchospasm. Facilities for administering oxygen mixtures and ventilatory assistance are necessary for such patients.
Occasional patients have been reported to develop severe paradoxical airway resistance with repeated, excessive use of isoproterenol inhalation preparations. The cause of this refractory state is unknown. It is advisable that in such instances the use of this preparation be discontinued immediately and alternative therapy instituted, since in the reported cases the patients did not respond to other forms of therapy until the drug was withdrawn.
Deaths have been reported following excessive use of isoproterenol inhalation preparations and the exact cause is unknown. Cardiac arrest was noted in several instances.
Precautions: Epinephrine should not be administered concomitantly with ISUPREL, as both drugs are direct cardiac stimulants and their combined effects may induce serious arrhythmia. If desired they may, however, be alternated, provided an internal of at least four hours has elapsed.
Isoproterenol should be used with caution in patients with cardiovascular disorders including coronary insufficiency, diabetes, or hyperthyroidism, and in persons sensitive to sympathomimetic amines.
Any patient who requires more than three aerosol treatments within a 24-hour period should be under the close supervision of his physician. Further therapy with the bronchodilator aerosol alone is inadvisable when three to five treatments within six to twelve hours produce minimal or no relief.
During the course of over 25 years of use of ISUPREL, brand of isoproterenol, there has been no clinical evidence of teratogenic effects. However, use of any drug in pregnancy, lactation, or in women of childbearing age requires that the potential benefit of the drug be weighed against its possible hazards to the mother or child.
When compressed oxygen is employed as the aerosol propellant, the percentage of oxygen used should be determined by the patient's individual requirements to avoid depression of respiratory drive.
Adverse Reactions: Tachycardia, palpitation, nervousness, nausea, and vomiting may occur from overdosage. Rarely do headache, flushing of the skin, tremor, dizziness, weakness, sweating, precordial distress, or anginal-type pain occur. The inhalation route is usually accompanied by a minimum of side effects. These untoward reactions disappear quickly and do not, as a rule, inconvenience the patient to the extent that the drug must be discontinued. No cumulative effects have been reported.
Dosage and Administration: ISUPREL hydrochloride solutions can be administered as an aerosol mist by hand-bulb nebulizer, compressed air or oxygen operated nebulizer, or by intermittent positive pressure breathing (IPPB) devices. The method of delivery, and the treatment regimen employed in the management of the reversible bronchospastic element accompanying bronchial asthma, chronic bronchitis, and chronic obstructive lung diseases, will depend on such factors as the severity of the bronchospasm, patient age, tolerance to the medication, complicating cardiopulmonary conditions, and whether therapy is for an intermittent acute attack of bronchospasm or is part of a programmed treatment regimen for constant bronchospasm.
Acute Bronchial Asthma. *Hand-Bulb Nebulizer*—Depending on the frequency of treatment and the type of nebulizer used, a volume of ISUPREL solution, sufficient for not more than one day's treatment, should be placed in the nebulizer using the dropper provided. In time, the patient can learn to adjust the volume required. For adults and children, the 1:200 solution is administered by hand-bulb nebulization in a dosage of 5 to 15 deep inhalations (using an all glass or plastic nebulizer). In adults, the 1:100 solution may be used if a stronger solution seems to be indicated. The dose is 3 to 7 deep inhalations. If after about 5 to 10 minutes inadequate relief is observed, these doses may be repeated one more time. If the acute attack recurs, treatments may be repeated up to 5 times daily if necessary. (See Precautions.)
Bronchospasm in Chronic Obstructive Lung Disease. *Hand-Bulb Nebulizer*—ISUPREL 1:200 or 1:100 solution may be administered daily at not less than 3 to 4 hour intervals for subacute bronchospastic attacks or as part of a programmed treatment regimen in patients with chronic obstructive lung disease with a reversible bronchospastic component. An adequate dose is usually 5 to 15 deep inhalations, using the 1:200 solution. Some patients with severe attacks of bronchospasm may require 3 to 7 deep inhalations using the ISUPREL 1:100 solution.
Nebulization by Compressed Air or Oxygen—A method often used in patients with severe chronic obstructive lung disease is to deliver the ISUPREL, brand of isoproterenol, mist *in more dilute form over a longer period of time.* The purpose is, not so much to increase the dose supplied, as to achieve progressively

Continued on next page

Breon—Cont.

deeped bronchodilatation and thus insure that the mist achieves maximum penetration of the finer bronchioles. In this method, 0.5 ml of an ISUPREL 1:200 solution is diluted to 2 to 2.5 ml with water or isotonic saline to achieve a use concentration of 1:800 to 1:1000. If desired, 0.25 ml of the 1:100 solution may be similarly diluted to achieve the same use concentration. The diluted solution is placed in a nebulizer (e.g., DeVilbiss #640 unit) connected to either a source of compressed air or oxygen. The flow rate is regulated to suit the particular nebulizer so that the diluted ISUPREL solution will be delivered over approximately 10 to 20 minutes. A treatment may be repeated up to 5 times daily if necessary. Although the total delivered dose of ISUPREL is somewhat higher than with the treatment regimen employing the hand-bulb nebulizer, patients usually tolerate it well because of the greater dilution and longer application-time factors.

Intermittent Positive Pressure Breathing (IPPB)—Diluted solutions of ISUPREL 1:200 or 1:100 are used in a programmed regimen for the treatment of reversible bronchospasm in patients with chronic obstructive lung disease who require intermittent positive pressure breathing therapy. These devices generally have a small nebulizer, usually of 3 to 5 ml capacity, on a patient-operated side arm. The effectiveness of IPPB therapy is greatly enhanced by the simultaneous use of aerosolized bronchodilators. As with compressed air or oxygen operated nebulizers, the usual regimen is to place 0.5 ml of ISUPREL 1:200 solution diluted to 2 to 2.5 ml with water or isotonic saline in the nebulizer cup and follow the IPPB manufacturer's operating instructions. IPPB-bronchodilator treatments are usually administered over 15 to 20 minutes, up to 5 times daily if necessary.

Children's Dosage: In general, the technique of ISUPREL hydrochloride solution administration to children is similar to that of adults, since children's smaller ventilatory exchange capacity automatically provides proportionally smaller aerosol intake. However, it is generally recommended that the 1:200 solution (rather than the 1:100) be used for an acute attack of bronchospasm, and no more than 0.25 ml of the 1:200 solution should be used for each 10 to 15 minute programmed treatment in chronic bronchospastic disease.

How Supplied:

Solution 1:100
bottles of 10 ml **NDC** 0057-0873-01
Solution 1:200
bottles of 10 ml **NDC** 0057-0871-01
bottles of 60 ml **NDC** 0057-0871-03

ISUPREL® Hydrochloride ℞
brand of isoproterenol hydrochloride tablets, USP
GLOSSETS®

Description: Isuprel hydrochloride (brand of isoproterenol hydrochloride) is 3,4-dihydroxy-α-[(isopropylamino)methyl]-benzyl alcohol hydrochloride, a synthetic sympathomimetic amine that is structurally related to epinephrine but acts almost exclusively on beta receptors.

Each Isuprel tablet contains 10 or 15 mg isoproterenol hydrochloride in a rapidly disintegrating base consisting of starch, lactose, sodium saccharin, and talcum with sodium bisulfite 2 mg per tablet as antioxidant.

Actions: The primary actions of Isuprel are on the heart and on smooth muscle of bronchi, skeletal muscle vasculature, and alimentary tract. The positive inotropic and chronotropic actions of the drug increase cardiac output. There is also an increase in venous return to the heart. With usual therapeutic doses, the increase in cardiac output is generally sufficient to maintain or increase systolic blood pressure. Isuprel also lowers peripheral vascular resistance; the diastolic pressure, therefore, may be expected to fall in normal individuals. Thus, the mean pressure may be reduced. The rate of discharge of cardiac pacemakers is increased with isoproterenol.

Isuprel relaxes most smooth muscle, the most pronounced effect being on bronchial and gastrointestinal smooth muscle. It produces marked relaxation in the smaller bronchi and may even dilate the trachea and main bronchi past the resting diameter.

The acute toxicity of Isuprel in animals is much less than that of epinephrine. Excessive doses in animals or man can cause a striking drop in blood pressure, and repeated large doses in animals may result in cardiac enlargement and focal myocarditis.

Indications: The sublingual or rectal dosage form of isoproterenol hydrochloride is indicated in the treatment of carotid sinus hypersensitivity, Adams-Stokes syndrome, and atrioventricular heart block. However, the treatment of choice is electrical pacing for heart block and electroshock for emergency conditions involving ventricular arrhythmias. This dosage form of Isuprel may also be used as a bronchodilator in the management of patients with bronchopulmonary disease.

Contraindications: Use of isoproterenol in patients with preexisting cardiac arrhythmias associated with tachycardia is generally considered contraindicated because the chronotropic effect of the drug on the heart may aggravate such disorders.

Administration of Isuprel is also contraindicated in patients with tachycardia caused by digitalis intoxication.

Warnings: In patients with status asthmaticus and abnormal blood gas tensions, improvement in vital capacity and in blood gas tensions may not accompany apparent relief of bronchospasm. Facilities for administering oxygen mixtures and ventilatory assistance are necessary for such patients.

Deaths have been reported following excessive use of isoproterenol inhalation preparations and the exact cause is unknown. Cardiac arrest was noted in several instances.

Precautions: Isuprel and epinephrine should not be administered simultaneously, since both drugs are direct cardiac stimulants and their combined effects may induce serious arrhythmia. The drugs may, however, be administered alternately provided a proper interval has elapsed between doses.

Isoproterenol should be used with caution in patients with cardiovascular disorders including coronary insufficiency, diabetes, or hyperthyroidism, and in persons sensitive to sympathomimetic amines. If precordial distress or anginal-type pain occurs, the drug should be discontinued immediately.

There has been no clinical evidence of teratogenic effects attributable to Isuprel in more than 20 years' use of the drug. However, before administration of any drug to pregnant women or women of childbearing potential, the expected benefit of the drug should be carefully weighed against the possible risk to the mother or child.

Adverse Reactions: Serious reactions to Isuprel are infrequent. The following reactions, however, have been reported: flushing of the face, sweating, mild tremors, nervousness, headache, nausea, vomiting, dizziness, weakness, and tachycardia with palpitation manifested as a sensation of pounding in the chest. These reactions generally disappear quickly and usually do not require discontinuation of treatment with Isuprel. Precordial distress or anginal-type pain occurs rarely. No cumulative effects have been reported. Pulmonary edema has been reported in a patient extremely intolerant to all sympathomimetic drugs.

In a few patients, presumably with organic disease of the A-V node and its branches, Isuprel has been reported, paradoxically, to precipitate Adams-Stokes seizures during normal sinus rhythm or transient heart block.

Dosage and Administration: *For Heart Block and Certain Ventricular Arrhythmias:* The sublingual or rectal administration of Isuprel has proven effective in the control of mild stabilized symptomatic heart block and ventricular arrhythmias. However, it should be noted that in acute symptomatic heart block, particularly in patients with post-cardiac surgery block, electrical pacing is the preferred method of treatment for maintenance of an adequate ventricular rate. Moreover, in ventricular arrhythmias, electroshock may have to be used, and is usually the treatment of choice.

If Isuprel is to be given in acute symptomatic heart block, intravenous administration, with constant monitoring, is preferred. This avoids the irregular absorption which is possible with the sublingual and rectal routes of administration. Rectal administration is more satisfactory for long-term therapy because the effect is produced within 30 minutes and lasts for two to four hours. The patient must be monitored constantly by electrocardiography. Sinus rhythm sometimes occurs and persists for a variable period but often relapses again into complete block. In other cases, Isuprel merely maintains an acceptable heart rate somewhere above 90 to 100 beats per minute.

Carotid sinus hypersensitivity with reflex cardiac standstill, induced either clinically or experimentally, can be abolished successfully by the cardiac stimulative action of Isuprel until normal automaticity returns. From 1 to 2 Isuprel Glossets administered sublingually four to six times daily may prevent heart block in patients with carotid sinus hypersensitivity.

Table 1 summarizes the dosage regimen suggested for adults.

TABLE 1
SUGGESTED DOSAGE FOR HEART BLOCK IN ADULTS

Route of Administration	Initial Dose	Subsequent Dose Range
Sublingual	10 mg	5 to 50 mg
Rectal	5 mg	5 to 15 mg

Children may be given half the initial adult dose. In all patients, subsequent dosage and method of administration depend on the response of the ventricular rate and the rapidity with which the cardiac pacemaker can take over when the drug is gradually withdrawn.

The usual route of administration of Isuprel hydrochloride in emergency treatment of patients with severe heart block is by intravenous injection or infusion. If time is not of utmost importance, initial therapy by intramuscular or subcutaneous injection is preferred. If further maintenance therapy is necessary, Isuprel Glossets may be administered sublingually. Whenever Isuprel is used for these purposes, the electrocardiogram must always be monitored.

The Glossets are particularly useful for prophylaxis and treatment of heart block since patients can administer the medication themselves.

Isuprel Glossets are usually administered sublingually; the Glossets are absorbed directly from the site of administration.

For Pulmonary Conditions with Bronchospasm: The average sublingual dose for adults is 1 tablet of 10 mg. In some cases 1 tablet of 15 mg may be required, or 2 Glossets of 10 mg, depending on the patient's response to sympathomimetic amines. However, a dosage of 15 mg four times daily or 20 mg three times daily (a total of 60 mg in one day) should not be exceeded. For children, the dose is from 5 to 10

mg ($\frac{1}{2}$ to 1 tablet of 10 mg), not exceeding a total of 30 mg in one day.
The Glossets are allowed to disintegrate under the tongue. Until absorption has taken place, patients are instructed not to swallow saliva. Treatment should not be repeated more often than every three or four hours, or more than three times daily.
How Supplied:
Code 1-260 Isuprel Glossets 10 mg bottles of 50
NDC 0057-0875-02
Code 1-270 Isuprel Glossets 15 mg bottles of 50
NDC 0057-0877-02
[*Shown in Product Identification Section*]

ISUPREL® ℞
Compound Elixir

Balanced Expectorant Bronchodilator for the Management of Bronchial Asthma, Allergic Coughs, and Bronchitis

Description: The Elixir has a pleasant vanilla flavor and is mildly sweet. Each tablespoon (15 ml) contains 6 mg of LUMINAL®, brand of phenobarbital, USP, 2.5 mg of ISUPREL hydrochloride, brand of isoproterenol hydrochloride, USP, 12 mg of ephedrine sulfate, USP, 45 mg of theophylline, USP, 150 mg of potassium iodide, USP, and 19 per cent alcohol, USP.
Examine solution before using. Do not use if crystals, precipitaion or cloudiness is observed.
Actions: ISUPREL Hydrochloride is a potent bronchodilator, which produces increased vital capacity.
Ephedrine, when given orally, exerts prolonged bronchodilator and decongestant effects.
Theophylline has a well-established place in the treatment of persons with bronchial asthma because it provides bronchodilating action and a slight stimulating effect on the central nevrous system. When it is combined with ephedrine and LUMINAL, brand of phenobarbital, as in the Elixir, the action obtained provides a valuable preventive effect. The mild sedative property of the barbiturate component offers a twofold benefit to the asthmatic patient who is receiving sympathomimetic drugs: first, it tends to allay the anxiety or tension of the patient, and second, it provides some degree of antagonism to the possible adverse effect of the adrenergic medication.
Potassium iodide, an expectorant, is particularly efffective in relieving the cough associated with the dry type of chronic bronchitis or bronchial asthma.
Indications: The Elixir is indicated for the management of patients with bronchial asthma, allergic coughs, and the chronic bronchitis frequently associated with these respiratory disorders.
Warning: Phenobarbital may be habit forming.
Precautions: The dosage must be carefully adjusted in patients with hyperthyroidism, acute coronary disease, cardiac asthma, hypertension, and limited cardiac reserve and in patients sensitive to sympathomimetic amines, since overdosage may result in tachycardia, palpitation, nausea, headache, or other epinephrine-like side effects. Caution is also recommended in patients with prostatic hypertrophy and glaucoma.
The Elixir should not be given to patients with known sensitivity to iodides. Because of its iodide content, the Elixir may cause elevation of the protein-bound iodine. Large doses of iodides should not be administered during pregnancy since they may cause goiter in the fetus.
Adverse Reactions: Although the Elixir is generally well tolerated, symptoms of adrenergic overstimulation such as tachycardia or nervousness may occur, in which case the preparation should be temporarily discontinued and administered later at a lower dosage. Reactions to iodide include coryza, fever, acneiform eruptions, erythema of the face and chest, and painful swelling of the salivary glands. These side effects quickly subside on discontinuance of medication. Theophylline may cause gastric intolerance (nausea and vomiting).
Dosage and Administration:
For children from 1 to 3 years, 1 or 2 teaspoons (5 to 10 ml); ***from 3 to 6 years,*** 2 or 3 teaspoons (10 to 15 ml); ***from 6 to 12 years,*** 1 or 2 tablespoons (15 to 30 ml). The dose should be administered three times daily as needed to control symptoms.
For adults, 2 tablespoons (30 ml) three or four times daily may be given as needed. Since the severity of the disorder and the response of the patient will vary, the dose should be adjusted to individual needs, the larger doses being reserved for more severe disorders or for patients who do not respond to the smaller doses. Acute or severe attacks of bronchial asthma usually require inhalation and other therapy.
How Supplied:

Bottles of 16 fl oz	NDC 0057-0874-06
Bottles of 1 Gallon	NDC 0057-0874-08

KAYEXALATE® ℞
brand of sodium polystyrene sulfonate, USP

Cation-Exchange Resin

Description: The drug is a light brown to brown, finely ground, powdered form of sodium polystyrene sulfonate, a cation-exchange resin prepared in the sodium phase with an *in vitro* exchange capacity of approximately 3.1 mEq (*in vivo* approximately 1 mEq) of potassium per gram. The sodium content is approximately 100 mg (4.1 mEq) per gram of the drug.
Action: As the resin passes along the intestine or is retained in the colon after administration by enema, the sodium ions are partially released and are replaced by potassium ions. For the most part, this action occurs in the large intestine, which excretes potassium ions to a greater degree than does the small intestine. The efficiency of this process is limited and unpredictably variable. It commonly approximates the order of 33 per cent but the range is so large that definitive indices of electrolyte balance must be clearly monitored.
Indication: KAYEXALATE is indicated for the treatment of hyperkalemia.
Warnings: Since effective lowering of serum potassium with KAYEXALATE may take hours to days, treatment with this drug alone may be insufficient to rapidly correct severe hyperkalemia associated with states of rapid tissue breakdown (e.g., burns and renal failure) or hyperkalemia so marked as to constitute a medical emergency. Therefore, other definitive measures, including dialysis, should always be considered and may be imperative.
Serious potassium efficiency can occur from KAYEXALATE therapy. The effect must be carefully controlled by frequent serum potassium determinations within each 24 hour period. Since intracellular potassium deficiency is not always reflected by serum potassium levels, the level at which treatment with KAYEXALATE should be discontinued must be determined individually for each patient. Important aids in making this determination are the patient's clinical condition and electrocardiogram. Early clinical signs of severe hypokalemia include a pattern of irritable confusion and delayed thought processes. Electrocardiographically, severe hypokalemia is often associated with a lengthened Q-T interval, widening, flattening, or inversion of the T wave, and prominent U waves. Also, cardiac arrhythmias may occur, such as premature atrial, nodal, and ventricular contractions, and supraventricular and ventricular tachycardias. The toxic effects of digitalis are likely to be exaggerated. Marked hypokalemia can also be manifested by severe muscle weakness, at times extending into frank paralysis.
Like all cation-exchange resins, KAYEXALATE is not totally selective (for potassium) in its actions, and small amounts of other cations such as magnesium and calcium can also be lost during treatment. Accordingly, patients receiving KAYEXALATE should be monitored for all applicable electrolyte disturbances. Systemic alkalosis has been reported after cation-exchange resins were administered orally in combination with nonabsorbable cation-donating antacids and laxatives such as magnesium hydroxide and aluminum carbonate. Magnesium hydroxide should not be administered with KAYEXALATE. One case of grand mal seizure has been reported in a patient with chronic hypocalcemia of renal failure who was given KAYEXALATE with magnesium hydroxide as laxative. Also, the simultaneous oral administration of KAYEXALATE with nonabsorbable cation-donating antacids and laxatives may reduce the resin's potassium exchange capability.
Precautions: Caution is advised when KAYEXALATE is administered to patients who cannot tolerate even a small increase in sodium loads (i.e., severe congestive heart failure, severe hypertension, or marked edema). In such instances compensatory restriction of sodium intake from other sources may be indicated.
If constipation occurs, patients should be treated with sorbitol (from 10 to 20 ml of 70 per cent syrup every two hours or as needed to produce one or two watery stools daily), a measure which also reduces any tendency to fecal impaction.
Adverse Reactions: KAYEXALATE may cause some degree of gastric irritation. Anorexia, nausea, vomiting, and constipation may occur especially if high doses are given. Also, hypokalemia, hypocalcemia, and significant sodium retention may occur. Occasionally diarrhea develops. Large doses in elderly individuals may cause fecal impaction (see Precautions). This effect may be obviated through usage of the resin in enemas as described under Dosage and Administration. Intestinal obstruction due to concretions of aluminum hydroxide, when used in combination with KAYEXALATE, has been reported.
Dosage and Administration: Suspensions of this drug should be freshly prepared and not stored beyond 24 hours.
The average daily adult dose of the resin is 15 to 60 g. This is best provided by administering 15 g (approximately 4 *level* teaspoons) of KAYEXALATE, brand of sodium polystyrene sulfonate, one to four times daily. One gram of KAYEXALATE contains 4.1 mEq of sodium; one level teaspoon contains approximately 3.5 g of KAYEXALATE and 15 mEq of sodium. (A heaping teaspoon may contain as much as 10 to 12 g of KAYEXALATE.) Since the *in vivo* efficiency of sodium-potassium exchange resins is approximately 33 per cent, about one third of the resin's actual sodium content is being delivered to the body.
In smaller children and infants lower doses should be employed by using as a guide a rate of 1 mEq of potassium per gram of resin as the basis for calculation.
Each dose should be given as a suspension in a small quantity of water or, for greater palatability, in syrup. The amount of fluid usually ranges from 20 to 100 ml, depending on the dose, or may be simply determined by allowing 3 to 4 ml per gram of resin. Sorbitol may be administered in order to combat constipation. The resin may be introduced into the stomach through a plastic tube and, if desired, mixed with a diet appropriate for a patient in renal failure.

Continued on next page

Breon—Cont.

The resin may also be given, although with less effective results, in a daily enema consisting (for adults) of 30 to 50 g every six hours. Each dose is administered as a warm emulsion (at body temperature) in 100 ml of aqueous vehicle, such as sorbitol. The emulsion should be agitated gently during administration. The enema should be retained as long as possible and followed by a cleansing enema.
After an initial cleansing enema, a soft, large size (French 28) rubber tube is inserted into the rectum for a distance of about 20 cm, with the tip well into the sigmoid colon, and taped in place. The resin is then suspended in the appropriate amount of aqueous vehicle at body temperature and introduced by gravity, while the particles are kept in suspension by stirring. The suspension is flushed with 50 or 100 ml of fluid, following which the tube is clamped and left in place. If back leakage occurs, the hips are elevated on pillows or a knee-chest position is taken temporarily. A somewhat thicker suspension may be used, but care should be taken that no paste is formed, because the latter has a greatly reduced exchange surface and will be particularly ineffective if deposited in the rectal ampulla. The suspension is kept in the sigmoid colon for several hours, if possible. Then, the colon is irrigated with nonsodium containing solution at body temperature in order to remove the resin. Two quarts of flushing solution may be necessary. The returns are drained constantly through a Y tube connection.
The intensity and duration of therapy depend upon the severity and resistance of hyperkalemia.
KAYEXALATE should not be heated for to do so may alter the exchange properties of the resin.
How Supplied: Jars of 1 pound (453.6 g).
Code K-450, **NDC 0057-1075-01**

LEVOPHED® Bitartrate ℞
brand of levarterenol bitartrate injection, USP

Description: Levarterenol (sometimes referred to as *l-arterenol* or *l-norepinephrine*) is a primary amine which differs from epinephrine by the absence of a methyl group on the nitrogen atom.
LEVOPHED is supplied in sterile aqueous solution in the form of the bitartrate. Each 1 ml of LEVOPHED solution contains 1 mg of LEVOPHED base, sodium chloride for isotonicity, and not more than 2 mg of sodium bisulfite as preservative. The air in the ampuls has been displaced by nitrogen gas.
Actions: LEVOPHED functions as a powerful peripheral vasoconstrictor (alpha-adrenergic action) and as a potent inotropic stimulator of the heart and dilator of coronary arteries (beta-adrenergic action). Both of these actions result in an increase in systemic blood pressure and coronary artery blood flow. Cardiac output will vary reflexly in response to systemic hypertension but is usually increased in hypotensive man when the blood pressure is raised to an optimal level. In myocardial infarction accompanied by hypotension, LEVOPHED usually increases aortic blood pressure, coronary artery blood flow, and myocardial oxygenation, thereby helping to limit the area of myocardial ischemia and infarction. Venous return is increased and the heart tends to resume a more normal rate and rhythm than in the hypotensive state.
In hypotension that persists after correction of blood volume deficits, LEVOPHED helps raise the blood pressure to an optimal level and establish a more adequate circulation.
Indications: For the restoration of blood pressure in controlling certain acute hypotensive states (e.g., pheochromocytomectomy, sympathectomy, poliomyelitis, spinal anesthesia, myocardial infarction, septicemia, blood transfusion, and drug reactions).
As an adjunct in the treatment of cardiac arrest and profound hypotension.
Contraindications: LEVOPHED should not be given to patients who are hypotensive from blood volume deficits except as an emergency measure to maintain coronary and cerebral artery perfusion until blood volume replacement therapy can be completed. If LEVOPHED is continuously administered to maintain blood pressure in the absence of blood volume replacement, the following may occur: severe peripheral and visceral vasoconstriction, decreased renal perfusion and urine output, poor systemic blood flow despite "normal" blood pressure, tissue hypoxia, and lactate acidosis.
LEVOPHED should also not be given to patients with mesenteric or peripheral vascular thrombosis (because of the risk of increasing ischemia and extending the area of infarction) unless, in the opinion of the attending physician, the administration of Levophed is necessary as a life-saving procedure.
Cyclopropane and halothane anesthetics increase cardiac autonomic irritability and therefore seem to sensitize the myocardium to the action of intravenously administered epinephrine or levarterenol. Hence, the use of LEVOPHED during cyclopropane and halothane anesthesia is generally considered contraindicated because of the risk of producing ventricular tachycardia or fibrillation. The same type of cardiac arrhythmias may result from the use of LEVOPHED in patients with profound hypoxia or hypercarbia.
Warning: LEVOPHED should be used with extreme caution in patients receiving monoamine oxidase (MAO) inhibitors or antidepressants of the triptyline or imipramine types, because severe, prolonged hypertension may result.
Precautions: *Avoid Hypertension:* Because of the potency of LEVOPHED and because of varying response to pressor substances, the possibility always exists that dangerously high blood pressure may be produced with overdoses of this pressor agent. It is desirable, therefore, to record the blood pressure every two minutes from the time administration is started until the desired blood pressure is obtained, then every five minutes if administration is to be continued. The rate of flow must be watched constantly, and the patient should never be left unattended while receiving LEVOPHED. Headache may be a symptom of hypertension due to overdosage.
Site of Infusion: Whenever possible, LEVOPHED should be given into a large vein, particularly an antecubital vein because, when administered into this vein, the risk of necrosis of the overlying skin from prolonged vasoconstriction is apparently very slight. Some authors have indicated that the femoral vein is also an acceptable route of administration. A catheter tie-in technique should be avoided, if possible, since the obstruction to blood flow around the tubing may cause stasis and increased local concentration of the drug. Occlusive vascular diseases (for example, atherosclerosis, arteriosclerosis, diabetic endarteritis, Buerger's disease) are more likely to occur in the lower than in the upper extremity. Therefore, one should avoid the veins of the leg in elderly patients or in those suffering from such disorders. Gangrene has been reported in a lower extremity when LEVOPHED was given in an ankle vein.
Extravasation: The infusion site should be checked frequently for free flow. Care should be taken to avoid extravasation of LEVOPHED bitartrate, brand of levarterenol bitartrate injection, into the tissues, as local necrosis might ensue due to the vasoconstrictive action of the drug. Blanching along the course of the infused vein, sometimes without obvious extravasation, has been attributed to vasa vasorum constriction with increased permeability of the vein wall, permitting some leakage. This also may progress on rare occasions to superficial slough, particularly during infusion into leg veins in elderly patients or in those suffering from obliterative vascular disease. Hence, if blanching occurs, consideration should be given to the advisability of changing the infusion site at intervals to allow the effects of local vasoconstriction to subside.

IMPORTANT—Antidote for Extravasation Ischemia: To prevent sloughing and necrosis in areas in which extravasation has taken place, the area should be infiltrated as soon as possible with 10 to 15 ml of saline solution containing from 5 to 10 mg of **Regitine® (brand of phentolamine)**, an adrenergic blocking agent. A syringe with a fine hypodermic needle is used, and the solution is infiltrated liberally throughout the area, which is easily identified by its cold, hard, and pallid appearance. Sympathetic blockade with phentolamine causes immediate and conspicuous local hyperemic changes if the area is infiltrated within 12 hours. Therefore, phentolamine should be given as soon as possible after the extravasation is noted.

Some investigators[1] add phentolamine (5 to 10 mg) directly to the infusion flask because it is believed that the drug used in this manner is an effective antidote against sloughing should extravasation occur, whereas the systemic vasopressor activity of the LEVOPHED is not impaired.
Two investigators[2] stated that, in the treatment of patients with severe hypotension following *myocardial infarction*, thrombosis in the infused vein and perivenous reactions and necrosis may usually be prevented if 10 mg of heparin are added to each 500 ml of infusion fluid (5 per cent dextrose) containing LEVOPHED.
Sympathetic nerve block has also been suggested.
Adverse Reactions: When used as directed, LEVOPHED is more certain in action and better tolerated systemically than other pressor amines. Its therapeutic index is four times that of epinephrine. Bradycardia sometimes occurs, probably as a reflex result of a rise in blood pressure. Headache may indicate overdosage and extreme hypertension.
Overdosage with LEVOPHED may also result in severe hypertension, reflex bradycardia, marked increase in peripheral resistance, and decreased cardiac output.
Prolonged administration of any potent vasopressor may result in plasma volume depletion which should be continuously corrected by appropriate fluid and electrolyte replacement therapy. If plasma volumes are not corrected hypotension may recur when LEVOPHED is discontinued, or blood pressure may be maintained at the risk of severe peripheral vasoconstriction with diminution in blood flow and tissue perfusion.
Dosage and Administration:
Restoration of Blood Pressure in Acute Hypotensive States
Blood volume depletion should always be corrected as fully as possible before any vasopressor is administered. When, as an emergency measure, intraaortic pressures must be maintained to prevent cerebral or coronary artery ischemia, LEVOPHED bitartrate, brand of levarterenol bitartrate injection, can be administered before and concurrently with blood volume replacement.
Diluent: LEVOPHED solution should be administered in 5 per cent dextrose solution in distilled water or 5 per cent dextrose in saline solution. These fluids containing dextrose are protection against significant loss of potency

due to oxidation. Administration in saline solution alone is not recommended. Whole blood or plasma, if indicated to increase blood volume, should be administered separately (for example, by use of a Y-tube and individual flasks if given simultaneously).

Average Dosage: Add 4 ml of LEVOPHED solution to 1000 ml of 5 per cent dextrose solution. Each 1 ml of this dilution contains 4 μg of LEVOPHED base. Give this dilution intravenously. Insert a plastic intravenous catheter through a suitable bore needle well advanced centrally into the vein and securely fixed with adhesive tape, avoiding, if possible, a catheter tie-in technique as this promotes stasis. A drip bulb is necessary to permit an accurate estimation of the rate of flow in drops per minute. After observing the response to an initial dose of 2 to 3 ml (from 8 to 12 μg of base) per minute, adjust the rate of flow to establish and maintain a low normal blood pressure (usually 80 to 100 mm Hg systolic) sufficient to maintain the circulation to vital organs. In previously hypertensive patients, it is recommended that the blood pressure should be raised no higher than 40 mm Hg below the preexisting systolic pressure. The average maintenance dose ranges from 0.5 to 1 ml per minute (from 2 to 4 μg of base).

High Dosage: Great individual variation occurs in the dose required to attain and maintain an adequate blood pressure. In all cases, dosage of LEVOPHED should be titrated according to the response of the patient. Occasionally much larger or even enormous daily doses (as high as 68 mg base or 17 ampuls) may be necessary if the patient remains hypotensive, but occult blood volume depletion should always be suspected and corrected when present. Central venous pressure monitoring is usually helpful in detecting and treating this situation.

Fluid Intake: The degree of dilution depends on clinical fluid volume requirements. If large volumes of fluid (dextrose) are needed at a flow rate that would involve an excessive dose of the pressor agent per unit of time, a more dilute solution than 4 μg per ml should be used. On the other hand, when large volumes of fluid are clinically undesirable, a concentration greater than 4 μg per ml may be used.

Duration of Therapy: The infusion should be continued until adequate blood pressure and tissue perfusion are maintained without therapy. LEVOPHED infusion should be reduced gradually, avoiding abrupt withdrawal. In some of the reported cases of vascular collapse due to acute myocardial infarction, treatment was required for up to six days.

Adjunctive Treatment in Cardiac Arrest

LEVOPHED is usually administered intravenously during cardiac resuscitation to restore and maintain an adequate blood pressure after an effective heartbeat and ventilation have been established by other means. [LEVOPHED'S powerful beta-adrenergic stimulating action is also thought to increase the strength and effectiveness of systolic contractions once they occur.]

Average Dosage: To maintain systemic blood pressure during the management of cardiac arrest, LEVOPHED bitartrate, brand of levarterenol bitartrate injection, is used in the same manner as described under Restoration of Blood Pressure in Acute Hypotensive States.

How Supplied: Ampuls of 4 ml containing 4 mg LEVOPHED base, boxes of 10.

Code L-680 **NDC 0057-1123-02**

References:

1. Zucker, G. *et al.: Circulation 22*:935, Nov. 1960.
2. Sampson, J. and Griffith, G.: *Geriatrics 11*:60, Feb. 1956.

Regitine, trademark, CIBA Pharmaceutical Company.

MARCAINE® HYDROCHLORIDE ℞

brand of bupivacaine hydrochloride

Description: Bupivacaine hydrochloride is 1-butyl-2′,6′-pipecoloxylidide hydrochloride, a white crystalline powder that is freely soluble in 95 per cent ethanol, soluble in water, and slightly soluble in chloroform or acetone.

MARCAINE is available in sterile isotonic solutions with and without epinephrine (as bitartrate) 1:200,000. Solutions of MARCAINE may be reautoclaved if they do not contain epinephrine.

MARCAINE is related chemically and pharmacologically to the aminoacyl local anesthetics. It is a homologue of mepivacaine and is chemically related to lidocaine. All three of these anesthetics contain an amide linkage between the aromatic nucleus and the amino or piperidine group. They differ in this respect from the procaine-type local anesthetics, which have an ester linkage.

Actions: Parenteral administration of MARCAINE stabilizes the neuronal membrane and prevents initiation and transmission of nerve impulses, thereby effecting local anesthetic action.

The onset of action is rapid, and anesthesia may last several hours. The duration of anesthesia is significantly longer with MARCAINE than with any other commonly used local anesthetics. Anesthesia may be more prolonged with the addition of a vasoconstrictor such as epinephrine 1:200,000. It has also been noted that there is a period of analgesia that persists after the return of sensation, during which time the need for strong analgesics is reduced.

After injection of MARCAINE for caudal, epidural or peripheral nerve block in man, peak levels of MARCAINE in the blood are reached in 30 to 45 minutes, followed by a decline to insignificant levels during the next three to six hours. Because of its amide structure, MARCAINE is not detoxified by plasma esterases but is detoxified, via conjugation with glucuronic acid, in the liver. When administered in recommended doses and concentrations, MARCAINE does not ordinarily produce irritation or tissue damage, and does not cause methemoglobinemia.

Indications: Peripheral nerve block, infiltration, sympathetic block, caudal, or epidural block.

Contraindication: MARCAINE is contraindicated in patients with known hypersensitivity to it.

Warnings: RESUSCITATIVE EQUIPMENT AND DRUGS SHOULD BE READILY AVAILABLE WHEN ANY LOCAL ANESTHETIC IS USED.

Usage in Pregnancy. Reproduction studies have been performed in rats and rabbits and there is no evidence of harm to the animal fetus. The relevance to the human is not known. Safe use in pregnant women other than those in labor has not been established.

Until further clinical experience is gained, paracervical block with MARCAINE is not recommended. Fetal bradycardia frequently follows paracervical block with some amide-type local anesthetics and may be associated with fetal acidosis. Added risk appears to be present in prematurity, toxemia of pregnancy, and fetal distress.

The obstetrician is warned that severe persistent hypertension may occur after administration of certain oxytocic drugs, if vasopressors have already been used during labor (e.g., in the local anesthetic solution or to correct hypotension).

Solutions containing a vasoconstrictor, particularly epinephrine or norepinephrine, should be used with extreme caution in patients receiving monoamine oxidase (MAO) inhibitors or antidepressants of the triptyline or imipramine types, because severe, prolonged hypertension may result.

Local anesthetics which contain preservatives, i.e., those supplied in multiple-dose vials, should not be used for caudal or epidural anesthesia.

Until further experience is gained in children younger than 12 years, administration of MARCAINE in this age group is not recommended.

Precautions: The safety and effectiveness of local anesthetics depend upon proper dosage, correct technique, adequate precautions, and readiness for emergencies.

The lowest dosage that gives effective anesthesia should be used in order to avoid high plasma levels and serious systemic side effects. Injection of repeated doses of MARCAINE may cause significant increase in blood levels with each additional dose, due to accumulation of the drug or its metabolites or due to slow metabolic degradation. Tolerance varies with the status of the patient. Debilitated, elderly patients and acutely ill patients should be given reduced doses commensurate with age and physical condition.

Solutions containing a vasoconstrictor should be used cautiously in areas with limited blood supply, in the presence of diseases that may adversely affect the patient's cardiovascular system, or in patients with peripheral vascular disease.

MARCAINE hydrochloride, brand of bupivacaine hydrochloride, should be used cautiously in persons with known drugs allergies or sensitivities, particularly to the amide-type local anesthetics.

Serious dose-related cardiac arrhythmias may occur if preparations containing a vasoconstrictor such as epinephrine are employed in patients during or following the administration of chloroform, halothane, cyclopropane, trichloroethylene, or other related agents. In deciding whether to use these products concurrently in the same patient, the combined action of both agents upon the myocardium, the concentration and volume of vasoconstrictor used, and the time since injection, when applicable, should be taken into account.

Caution is advised in administration of repeat doses of MARCAINE to patients with severe liver disease.

Adverse Reactions: Reactions to MARCAINE are characteristic of those associated with other amide-type local anesthetics. A major cause of adverse reactions to this group of drugs is excessive plasma levels, which may be due to overdosage, inadvertent intravascular injection, or slow metabolic degradation.

Excessive plasma levels of the amide-type local anesthetics cause systemic reactions involving the central nervous system and the cardiovascular system. The ***central nervous system effects*** are characterized by excitation or depression. The first manifestation may be nervousness, dizziness, blurred vision, or tremors, followed by drowsiness, convulsions, unconsciousness, and possibly respiratory arrest. Since excitement may be transient or absent, the first manifestation may be drowsiness, sometimes merging into unconsciousness and respiratory arrest. Other central nervous system effects may be nausea, vomiting, chills, constriction of the pupils, or tinnitus. The ***cardiovascular manifestations*** of excessive plasma levels may include depression of the myocardium, blood pressure changes (usually hypotension), and cardiac arrest. In obstetrics, cases of fetal bradycardia have occurred (see Warnings).

Allergic reactions, which may be due to hypersensitivity, idiosyncrasy, or diminished tolerance, are characterized by cutaneous lesions (e.g., urticaria), edema, and other manifestations of allergy. Detection of sensitivity by skin testing is of doubtful value.

Continued on next page

Breon—Cont.

Reactions following epidural or caudal anesthesia also may include: high or total spinal block; urinary retention; fecal incontinence; loss of perineal sensation and sexual function; persistent analgesia, paresthesia, and paralysis of the lower extremities; headache and backache; and slowing of labor and increased incidence of forceps delivery.

Treatment of Reactions. Toxic effects of local anesthetics require symptomatic treatment; there is no specific cure. The physician should be prepared to maintain an airway and to support ventilation with oxygen and assisted or controlled respiration as required. Supportive treatment of the cardiovascular system includes intravenous fluids and, when appropriate, vasopressors (preferably those that stimulate the myocardium). Convulsions may be controlled with oxygen and intravenous administration, in small increments, of a barbiturate, as follows: preferably, an ultrashort-acting barbiturate such as thiopental or thiamylal; if this is not available, a short-acting barbiturate (e.g., secobarbital or pentobarbital) or diazepam. Intravenous barbiturates or anticonvulsant agents should only be administered by those familiar with their use.

Dosage and Administration: As with all local anesthetics, the dosage varies and depends upon the area to be anesthetized, the vascularity of the tissues, the number of neuronal segments to be blocked, individual tolerance, and the technique of anesthesia. The lowest dosage needed to provide effective anesthesia should be administered. For specific techniques and procedures, refer to standard textbooks.

In recommended doses, MARCAINE produces complete sensory block, but the effect on motor function differs among the three concentrations.

0.25%*—when used for caudal, epidural, or peripheral nerve block, produces incomplete motor block. Should be used for operations in which muscle relaxation is not important, or when another means of providing muscle relaxation is used concurrently. Onset of action may be slower than with the 0.5 or 0.75 per cent solutions.

0.5%*—provides motor blockade for caudal, epidural, or nerve block, but muscle relaxation may be inadequate for operations in which complete muscle relaxation is essential.

0.75%—produces complete motor block. Most useful for epidural block in abdominal operations requiring complete muscle relaxation.

The duration of anesthesia with Marcaine is such that for most indications, a single dose is sufficient.

Maximum dosage limit must be individualized in each case after evaluating the size and physical status of the patient, as well as the usual rate of systemic absorption from a particular injection site. Most experience to date is with single doses of MARCAINE up to 225 mg with epinephrine 1:200,000, and 175 mg without epinephrine; more or less drug may be used depending on individualization of each case.

These doses may be repeated up to once every three hours. In clinical studies to date, total daily doses have been up to 400 mg. Until further experience is gained, this dose should not be exceeded in 24 hours. The duration of anesthetic effect may be prolonged by the addition of epinephrine.

The dosages in Table 1 have generally proved satisfactory and are recommended as a guide for use in the average adult. The dosages should be reduced for elderly or debilitated patients. Until further experience is gained, MARCAINE is not recommended for children younger than 12 years.

Unused portions of solutions not containing preservatives., i.e., those supplied in single-dose ampuls, should be discarded following initial use.

*Use only the single dose ampuls for caudal or epidural anesthesia; the multiple dose vials contain a preservative and therefore should not be used for these procedures.

[See table below].

How Supplied:

These solutions are not for spinal anesthesia.

MARCAINE hydrochloride—Sterile isotonic solutions containing sodium chloride. In multiple-dose vials, each 1 ml also contains 1 mg methylparaben as antiseptic preservative. The pH of these solutions is adjusted with sodium hydroxide or hydrochloric acid. Solutions of Marcaine that do not contain epinephrine may be reautoclaved.

0.25%—Contains 2.5 mg. Marcaine hydrochloride per ml.

Single dose ampuls of 50 ml., boxes of 5.
Code M-601, **NDC** 0057-1212-02
Multiple dose vials of 50 ml.
Code M-605 **NDC** 0057-1217-01

0.5%—Contains 5 mg. Marcaine hydrochloride per ml.

Single dose ampuls of 30 ml., boxes of 5.
Code M-611, **NDC** 0057-1213-02
Multiple dose vials of 50 ml.
Code M-615 **NDC** 0057-1218-01

0.75%—Contains 7.5 mg. Marcaine hydrochloride per ml.

Single dose ampuls of 30 ml., boxes of 5.
Code M-621, **NDC** 0057-1214-02

MARCAINE hydrochloride with epinephrine 1:200,000 (as bitartrate)—Sterile isotonic solutions containing sodium chloride. Each 1 ml contains MARCAINE hydrochloride and 0.0091 mg epinephrine bitartrate, USP, with 0.5 mg sodium bisulfite, 0.001 ml thioglycerol, and 2 mg ascorbic acid as antioxidants, 0.0017 ml 60% sodium lactate buffer, and 0.1 mg edetate calcium disodium as stabilizer. In multiple-dose vials, each 1 ml also contains 1 mg methylparaben as antiseptic preservative. The pH of these solutions is adjusted with sodium hydroxide or hydrochloric acid. Solutions of MARCAINE that contain epinephrine should not be autoclaved.

0.25% with epinephrine 1:200,000—Contains 2.5 mg Marcaine hydrochloride per ml

Single dose ampuls of 50 ml, boxes of 5
Code M-631 **NDC** 0057-1222-02
Multiple dose vials of 50 ml, boxes of 10.
Code M-635 **NDC** 0057-1227-01

0.5% with epinephrine 1:200,000—Contains 5 mg Marcaine hydrochloride per ml

Single dose ampuls of 30 ml, boxes of 5.
Code M-641, **NDC** 0057-1223-02
Multiple dose vials of 50 ml, boxes of 10.
Code M-645 **NDC** 0057-1228-01

0.75% with epinephrine 1:200,000—Contains 7.5 mg Marcaine hydrochloride per ml

Single dose ampuls of 30 ml, boxes of 5.
Code M-651, **NDC** 0057-1224-02

The following table presents the solutions and packagings of MARCAINE recommended for each type of block. (An X indicates that the solution may be used for the designated block; an O indicates that it should not be used.)

[See table on next page].

Table 1. Recommended Concentrations and Doses of Marcaine

Type of Block	Conc.	Each Dose (ml)	(mg)	Motor Block[1]
Local infiltration	0.25%	up to max.	up to max.	———
Epidural	0.75%[2]	10–20	75–150	complete
	0.50%	10–20	50–100	moderate to complete
	0.25%	10–20	25–50	partial to moderate
Caudal	0.50%	15–30	75–150	moderate to complete
	0.25%	15–30	37.5–75	moderate
Peripheral nerves	0.50%	5 to max.	25 to max.	moderate to complete
	0.25%	5 to max.	12.5 to max.	moderate to complete
Sympathetic	0.25%	20–50	50–125	———

[1]With continuous (intermittent) techniques, repeat doses increase the degree of motor block. The first repeat dose of 0.5% may produce complete motor block. Intercostal nerve block with 0.25% may also produce complete motor block for intraabdominal surgery.
[2]For single dose use; not for intermittent technique.

MEBARAL® Ⓒ
brand of mephobarbital tablets, NF ℞

Antiepileptic and Sedative

Description: MEBARAL is a white, nearly odorless, and tasteless powder. It is not easily soluble in cold water but more easily soluble in hot water.

Clinical Pharmacology: MEBARAL exerts a strong sedative and anticonvulsive action but has a relatively mild hypnotic effect. It reduces the incidence of epileptic seizures in grand mal and petit mal. MEBARAL usually causes little or no drowsiness or lassitude. Hence, when it is used as a sedative or an anticonvulsant, patients usually become more calm, more cheerful, and better adjusted to their surroundings without clouding of mental faculties.

Indications and Usage: As a sedative, for the relief of anxiety, tension, and apprehension.

As an anticonvulsant, for the treatment of epilepsy in grand and petit mal.

Contraindications: Hypersensitivity to any barbiturate.
Porphyria

Warnings: ***Drug Dependence.*** Tolerance, psychological dependence, and physical dependence may occur with MEBARAL. Special care should be exercised in the treatment of emotionally unstable patients and those with a history of alcoholism or other drug dependence because of the possibility of such patients increasing the dosage on their own initiative. Manifestations of chronic intoxication include ataxia, slurred speech, and vertigo. Abrupt cessation after prolonged ingestion of large doses of MEBARAL may result in withdrawal symptoms which include tremulousness, weakness, insomnia, convulsions, and delirium. Such withdrawal symptoms have also been observed in newborn infants whose mothers required anticonvulsant therapy. (see ***Usage in Pregnancy.***) Appropriate management includes hospitalization and gradual withdrawal over a period of several days. A short-acting barbiturate should be substituted and gradually withdrawn.

Usage in Pregnancy: Safe use of MEBARAL during pregnancy has not been established. Recent reports suggest an association between the use of anticonvulsant medication by women with epilepsy and an increased incidence of birth defects in their children. Therefore, MEBARAL should be administered to women of childbearing potential only when, in the judgment of the physician, the anticipated benefits outweigh the potential risks. Barbiturates readily cross the placental barrier and may have depressant effects on the fetus if administered during labor. They are found in breast milk and may have adverse effects on nursing infants. Also, withdrawal symptoms have been observed in neonates following use of barbiturates during pregnancy.

Usage in Epilepsy. Status epilepticus may result from the abrupt discontinuation of MEBARAL, even when administered in small daily doses in the treatment of epilepsy.

Hazardous Activities. Since MEBARAL may impair the mental and/or physical abilities required for the performance of potentially hazardous tasks, such as driving a motor vehicle or operating machinery, the patient should be warned accordingly.

Drug Interaction. Concomitant use with alcohol and other CNS depressants may result in additive effects including CNS depression. Barbiturates increase the activity of certain drug-metabolizing hepatic enzymes and may thus decrease blood levels and clinical efficacy of drugs given concurrently. It is necessary to monitor closely the dosage of oral anticoagulants when administering or after discontinuing MEBARAL. Administration of MEBARAL may lower the blood levels of coumarin anticoagulants and thus shorten the prothrombin time. Conversely, MEBARAL withdrawal may raise the coumarin blood level, prolong the prothrombin time, and result in hemorrhage. Barbiturates have also been reported to accelerate the metabolism of certain antihistamines, steroids, anticonvulsants, and other drugs. Barbiturates generally have a relatively small and variable effect on the blood level of phenytoin (formerly known as diphenylhydantoin).

Vitamin D Deficiency. MEBARAL may increase vitamin D requirements, possibly by increasing vitamin D metabolism via enzyme induction. Rarely, rickets and osteomalacia have been reported following prolonged usage of barbiturates.

Vitamin K: Bleeding in the early neonatal period due to coagulation defects may follow exposure to anticonvulsant drugs in utero; therefore, vitamin K should be given to the mother before delivery or to the child at birth.

Precautions: Caution and careful adjustment of dosage are required when MEBARAL, brand of mephobarbital tablets, is used in patients with impaired hepatic, renal, cardiac or respiratory function and in patients with myasthenia gravis and myxedema.

Lower doses are also required in elderly and/or debilitated patients in order to preclude oversedation.

The least quantity feasible should be prescribed or dispensed at any one time in order to minimize the possibility of acute or chronic overdosage.

Adverse Reactions: *CNS effects:* dizziness, headache, "hangover", confusion especially in the elderly, paradoxical excitation, exacerbation of preexisting pain. *Gastrointestinal:* nausea, vomiting, epigastric pain. *Cardiovascular:* hypotension. *Allergic:* facial edema, skin rash, bullae and vesicles, purpura, erythema multiforme; and rarely exfoliative dermatitis. Severe allergic reactions may result in degenerative changes in the liver. *Hematologic:* megaloblastic anemia, agranulocytosis, thrombocytopenia.

	INFILTRATION	PERIPHERAL NERVE	CAUDAL	EPIDURAL	SYMPATHETIC
0.25%					
50 ml ampul	X	X	X	X	X
50 ml vial	X	X	O	O	X
0.25% with epinephrine 1:200,000					
50 ml ampul	X	X		X	O
50 ml vial	X	X	O	O	O
0.5%					
30 ml ampul	O	X	X	X	O
50 ml vial	O	X	O	O	O
0.5% with epinephrine 1:200,000					
30 ml ampul	O	X	X	X	O
50 ml vial	O	X	O	O	O
0.75%					
30 ml ampul	O	O	O	X	O
0.75% with epinephrine 1:200,000					
30 ml ampul	O	O	O	X	O

Dosage and Administration:

Epilepsy—Average dose for adults: 400 to 600 mg (6 to 9 grains) daily; children under 5 years, 16 to 32 mg (¼ to ½ grain) three or four times daily; children over 5 years, 32 to 64 mg (½ to 1 grain) three or four times daily. MEBARAL, brand of mephobarbital tablets, is best taken at bedtime if seizures generally occur at night, and during the day if attacks are diurnal.

Treatment should be started with a small dose which is gradually increased over four or five days until the optimum dosage is determined. If the patient has been taking some other antiepileptic drug, it should be tapered off as the doses of MEBARAL are increased, to guard against the temporary marked attacks that may occur when any treatment for epilepsy is changed abruptly. Similarly, when the dose is to be lowered to a maintenance level or to be discontinued, the amount should be reduced gradually over four or five days.

Combination with Other Drugs—MEBARAL may be used in combination with phenobarbital, either in the form of alternating courses or concurrently. When the two drugs are used at the same time, the dose should be about one-half the amount of each used alone. The average daily dose for an adult is from 50 to 100 mg (¾ grain to 1½ grains) of phenobarbital and from 200 to 300 mg (3 to 4½ grains) of MEBARAL.

MEBARAL may also be used with phenytoin sodium; in some cases, combined therapy appears to give better results than either agent used alone, since phenytoin sodium is particularly effective for the psychomotor type of seizure but relatively ineffective for petit mal. When the drugs are employed concurrently, a reduced dose of phenytoin sodium is advisable, but the full dose of MEBARAL may be given. Satisfactory results have been obtained with an average daily dose of 230 mg (3½ grains) of phenytoin sodium plus about 600 mg (9 grains) of MEBARAL, brand of mephobarbital tablets.

As Sedative—Adults: 32 to 100 mg (½ to 1½ grains)—optimum dose, 50 mg (¾ grain)—three or four times daily. In incipient or active delirium tremens, 200 mg (3 grains) three times a day is recommended. Children: 16 to 32 mg (¼ to ½ grain) three or four times daily.

Overdosage: *Manifestations:* Acute overdosage with barbiturates primarily involves the central nervous and cardiovascular systems. Mild overdosage resembles alcohol intoxication. Severe overdose results in shock, coma, and death. Respiratory depression and renal failure may occur.

Treatment: Patent airway must be maintained. Mechanical ventilation and administration of oxygen may be required. Blood pressure must be maintained. If the patient is seen within a few hours of overdosage, gastric lavage may be performed. If the patient cannot protect his own airway during this procedure, endotracheal intubation should be employed. If acute renal failure has not occurred, a forced diuresis and alkalinization of the urine are indicated. Alkalinization increases the concentration of the dissociated form of MEBARAL and, therefore, decreases tubular reabsorption of the drug in the kidney. Drug removal by hemodialysis is very effective, especially in renal failure; peritoneal dialysis is less effective. The use of analeptic agents is controversial.

How Supplied: Tablets

32 mg (½ grain)—bottles of 250 (**NDC** 0057-1231-05) and 1000 (**NDC** 0057-1231-08)

50 mg (¾ grain)—bottles of 250 (**NDC** 0057-1232-05)

100 mg (1½ grains)—bottles of 250 (**NDC** 0057-1233-05)

200 mg (3 grains)—bottles of 250 (**NDC** 0057-1234-05)

[*Shown in Product Identification Section*]

NOVOCAIN® ℞

brand of procaine hydrochloride injection, USP

Local Anesthetic for Major and Minor Surgery

Description: NOVOCAIN occurs as a white crystalline powder that is readily soluble in cold water but less soluble in alcohol. NOVOCAIN is incompatible with caustic alkalis and their carbonates.

Continued on next page

Breon—Cont.

Do not use solutions if crystals, cloudiness, or discoloration is observed. Reautoclaving increases likelihood of crystal formation. Examine solutions carefully before use. Protect solutions from light.

Action: NOVOCAIN is highly efficient and one of the safest local anesthetics. It does not irritate tissues and has a low relative toxicity.

Indications: NOVOCAIN is indicated for production of local anesthesia by infiltration injection, nerve block, caudal, or other epidural blocks.

Precaution: Extreme caution is imperative when any local anesthetic, even in relatively small amounts, is injected into the traumatized urethra or under conditions in which trauma is likely to occur.

Adverse Reactions: The anesthetic can be used with safety in nearly all cases if suitable precautions are observed. However, as with any local anesthetic, idiosyncrasy manifested by the rapid appearance of symptoms, including nausea, vomiting, rapid pulse, talkativeness, syncope, respiratory difficulty, and convulsions, may be encountered. Slow administration and avoidance of accidental intravenous injection are always advisable. If increased sensitivity to the anesthetic is suspected, as in patients with cardiac disease and hyperthyroidism or other endocrine disorders, a small dose may be given first to test tolerance.

Treatment of Reactions—Treatment of reactions hinges on the maintenance of the circulation and respiration and the control of convulsions. Treatment should be prompt.

The use of oxygen by bag and mask at the first sign of a toxic reaction has been recommended in order to prevent the onset of convulsions and circulatory and respiratory collapse.

Convulsions—The immediate administration of oxygen to control convulsions is recommended. If convulsions persist, the slow intravenous infusion of an ultrashort-acting barbiturate, such as thiopental or methohexital, should be considered. An intravenous anticonvulsant such as diazepam may also be administered to control convulsive seizures. Intravenous anticonvulsant agents should be used only by those familiar with their use and only when adequate ventilation and oxygenation are assured.

Respiratory Difficulty—This reaction is due either to central respiratory failure or to spasm of the musculature of the thoracic cage. It is best treated by oxygen inhalation combined, if necessary, with artificial respiration. When facilities are available, endotracheal intubation and administration of oxygen (100 per cent) by intermittent positive pressure are advised. While oxygen is being given, an intravenous infusion (e.g., Dextrose Injection, USP or Sodium Chloride Injection, USP) should be started and maintained, both to support the patient's circulation and to provide ready access to the bloodstream for subsequent intravenous administration of supportive drugs. Unless the infusion is instituted promptly, valuable time may be lost subsequently in accomplishing satisfactory venipuncture after peripheral circulatory collapse has occurred.

Circulatory Collapse—Vasopressor drugs are indicated. Epinephrine should not be given in the presence of anoxia because of the risk of causing ventricular fibrillation.

Dosage and Administration: *For infiltration and extensive field block,* 0.25 or 0.5 per cent solution. From 350 to 600 mg is generally considered to be a single safe total dose. To prepare 60 ml of the 0.5 per cent solution (5 mg/ml), dilute 30 ml of the 1 per cent solution with 30 ml of sterile distilled water. To prepare 60 ml of the 0.25 per cent solution (2.5 mg/ml), dilute 15 ml of the 1 per cent solution with 45 ml of sterile distilled water. From 0.5 to 1 ml of epinephrine solution 1:1000 per 100 ml of anesthetic solution is generally added for its vasoconstrictive effect (= 1:200,000 to 1:100,000).

For conduction anesthesia (nerve block), up to 50 ml of the 1 per cent solution or up to 25 ml of the 2 per cent solution with 0.05 to 0.1 ml (1 to 2 drops) of epinephrine solution 1:1000 in each 10 ml.

How Supplied:

Solution 2 per cent

Vials of 30 ml, made isotonic with sodium chloride and containing not more than 2 mg per ml of acetone sodium bisulfite and chlorobutanol 0.25 per cent as preservatives.

CODE N-190 boxes of 100 **NDC** 0057-1386-01

Solution 1 per cent

Ampuls of 2 ml, made isotonic with sodium chloride and containing not more than 1 mg per ml of acetone sodium bisulfite as preservative.

CODE N-161 boxes of 100 **NDC** 0057-1381-06

Ampuls of 6 ml, made isotonic with sodium chloride and containing not more than 1 mg per ml of acetone sodium bisulfite as preservative.

CODE N-171 boxes of 50 **NDC** 0057-1382-05

Vials of 30 ml, made isotonic with sodium chloride and containing not more than 2 mg per ml of acetone sodium bisulfite and 0.25 per cent chlorobutanol as preservatives.

CODE N-590 boxes of 100 **NDC** 0057-1385-01

The air in all ampuls and vials has been displaced by nitrogen gas.

NOVOCAIN® ℞

brand of procaine hydrochloride injection, USP

10% Solution for Spinal Anesthesia

Description: NOVOCAIN, brand of procaine hydrochloride, is benzoic acid, 4-amino-, 2-(diethylamino) ethyl ester, monohydrochloride, the ester of diethylaminoethanol and para-aminobenzoic acid.

It is a white crystalline, odorless powder that is freely soluble in water, but less soluble in alcohol. Each ml in the ampuls contains 100 mg procaine hydrochloride and 8 mg acetone sodium bisulfite as preservative. DO NOT USE SOLUTIONS IF CRYSTALS, CLOUDINESS, OR DISCOLORATION IS OBSERVED. EXAMINE SOLUTIONS CAREFULLY BEFORE USE. REAUTOCLAVING INCREASES LIKELIHOOD OF CRYSTAL FORMATION.

Clinical Pharmacology: NOVOCAIN stabilizes the neuronal membrane and prevents the initiation and transmission of nerve impulses, thereby effecting local anesthesia. NOVOCAIN lacks surface anesthetic activity. The onset of action is rapid (2 to 5 minutes) and the duration of action is relatively short (average 1 to 1½ hours), depending upon the anesthetic technique, the type of block, the concentration, and the individual patient.

NOVOCAIN is readily absorbed following parenteral administration and is rapidly hydrolyzed by plasma cholinesterase to para-aminobenzoic acid and diethylaminoethanol.

A vasoconstrictor may be added to the NOVOCAIN solution to promote local hemostasis, delay systemic absorption, and increase duration of anesthesia.

Indications and Usage: NOVOCAIN is indicated for spinal anesthesia.

Contraindications: Spinal anesthesia with NOVOCAIN is contraindicated in patients with generalized septicemia; sepsis at the proposed injection site; certain diseases of the cerebrospinal system, e.g., meningitis, syphilis; and a known hypersensitivity to the drug, drugs of a similar chemical configuration, or para-aminobenzoic acid or its derivatives.

The decision as to whether or not spinal anesthesia should be used in an individual case should be made by the physician after weighing the advantages with the risks and possible complications.

Warnings: RESUSCITATIVE EQUIPMENT AND DRUGS SHOULD BE IMMEDIATELY AVAILABLE WHENEVER ANY LOCAL ANESTHETIC DRUG IS USED. Spinal anesthesia should only be administered by those qualified to do so.

Large doses of local anesthetics should not be used in patients with heart block.

Reactions resulting in fatality have occurred on rare occasions with the use of local anesthetics, even in the absence of a history of hypersensitivity.

Usage in Pregnancy. Safe use of NOVOCAIN has not been established with respect to adverse effects on fetal development. Careful consideration should be given to this fact before administering this drug to women of childbearing potential particularly during early pregnancy. This does not exclude the use of the drug at term for obstetrical analgesia.

Vasopressor agents (administered for the treatment of hypotension or added to the anesthetic solution for vasoconstriction) should be used with extreme caution in the presence of oxytocic drugs as they may produce severe, persistent hypertension with possible rupture of a cerebral blood vessel.

Solutions which contain a vasoconstrictor should be used with extreme caution in patients receiving drugs known to produce alterations in blood pressure (i.e., monoamine oxidase (MAO) inhibitors, tricyclic antidepressants, phenothiazines, etc.) as either severe sustained hypertension or hypotension may occur.

Local anesthetic procedures should be used with caution when there is inflammation and/or sepsis in the region of the proposed injection.

Precautions: Standard textbooks should be consulted for specific techniques and precautions for various spinal anesthetic procedures.

The safety and effectiveness of a spinal anesthetic depend upon proper dosage, correct technique, adequate precautions, and readiness for emergencies. The lowest dosage that results in effective anesthesia should be used to avoid high plasma levels and possible adverse effects.

Tolerance varies with the status of the patient. Debilitated, elderly patients, or acutely ill patients should be given reduced doses commensurate with their weight and physical status. Reduced dosages are also indicated for obstetric delivery and patients with increased intraabdominal pressure.

The decision whether or not to use spinal anesthesia in the following disease states depends on the physician's appraisal of the advantages as opposed to the risk: cardiovascular disease (i.e., shock, hypertension, anemia, etc.), pulmonary disease, renal impairment, metabolic or endocrine disorders, gastrointestinal disorders (i.e., intestinal obstruction, peritonitis, etc.), or complicated obstetrical deliveries.

NOVOCAIN SHOULD BE USED WITH CAUTION IN PATIENTS WITH KNOWN DRUG ALLERGIES AND SENSITIVITIES. A thorough history of the patient's prior experience with NOVOCAIN or other local anesthetics as well as concomitant or recent drug use should be taken (see Contraindications). NOVOCAIN should not be used in any condition in which a sulfonamide drug is being employed since para-aminobenzoic acid inhibits the action of sulfonamides.

Solutions containing a vasopressor should be used with caution in the presence of diseases which may adversely affect the cardiovascular system.

NOVOCAIN should be used with caution in patients with severe disturbances of cardiac rhythm, shock or heart block.

Adverse Reactions: Systemic adverse reactions involving the central nervous system and the cardiovascular system usually result from high plasma levels due to excessive dosage, rapid absorption, or inadvertent intravascular injection. In addition, use of inappropriate

doses or techniques may result in extensive spinal blockade leading to hypotension and respiratory arrest.
A small number of reactions may result from hypersensitivity, idiosyncrasy, or diminished tolerance to normal dosage.
Excitatory CNS effect (nervousness, dizziness, blurred vision, tremors) commonly represent the initial signs of local anesthetic systemic toxicity. However, these reactions may be very brief or absent in some patients in which case the first manifestation of toxicity may be drowsiness or convulsions merging into unconsciousness and respiratory arrest.
Cardiovascular system reactions include depression of the myocardium, hypotension (or sometimes hypertension), bradycardia, and even cardic arrest.
Allergic reactions are characterized by cutaneous lesions of delayed onset, or urticaria, edema, and other manifestations of allergy. The detection of sensitivity by skin testing is of limited value. As with other local anesthetics, hypersensitivity, idiosyncrasy and anaphylactoid reactions have occurred rarely. The reaction may be abrupt and severe and is not usually dose related.
The following adverse reactions may occur with spinal anesthesia: *Central Nervous System:* post-spinal headache, meningismus, arachnoiditis, palsies, or spinal nerve paralysis. *Cardiovascular:* hypotension due to vasomotor paralysis and pooling of the blood in the venous bed. *Respiratory:* respiratory impairment or paralysis due to the level of anesthesia extending to the upper thoracic and cervical segments. *Gastrointestinal:* nausea and vomiting.
Treatment of Reactions. Toxic effects of local anesthetics require symptomatic treatment: there is no specific cure. The physician should be prepared to maintain an airway and to support ventilation with oxygen and assisted or controlled respiration as required. Supportive treatment of the cardiovascular system includes intravenous fluids and, when appropriate, vasopressors (preferably those that stimulate the myocardium, such as ephedrine). Convulsions may be controlled with oxygen and by the intravenous administration of diazepam or ultrashort-acting barbiturates or a short-acting muscle relaxant (succinylcholine). Intravenous anticonvulsant agents and muscle relaxants should only be administered by those familiar with their use and only when ventilation and oxygenation are assured. In spinal and epidural anesthesia, sympathetic blockade also occurs as a pharmacological reaction, resulting in peripheral vasodilation and often *hypotension.* The extent of the hypotension will usually depend on the number of dermatomes blocked. The blood pressure should therefore be monitored in the early phases of anesthesia. If hypotension occurs, it is readily controlled by vasoconstrictors administered either by the intramuscular or the intravenous route, the dosage of which would depend on the severity of the hypotension and the response to treatment.
Dosage and Administration: As with all local anesthetics, the dose of NOVOCAIN varies and depends upon the area to be anesthetized, the vascularity of the tissues, the number of neuronal segments to be blocked, individual tolerance, and the technique of anesthesia. The lowest dose needed to provide effective anesthesia should be administered. For specific techniques and procedures, refer to standard textbooks.
[See table above].
THE USUAL INITIAL DOSE SHOULD NOT EXCEED 1000 MG.
The diluent may be sterile normal saline, sterile distilled water, spinal fluid; and for hyperbaric technique, sterile dextrose solution.
The usual rate of injection is 1 ml per 5 seconds. Full anesthesia and fixation usually occur in 5 minutes.

Recommended Dosage
For Spinal Anesthesia

Extent of anesthesia	NOVOCAIN 10% Solution Volume of 10% Solution (ml)	Volume of Diluent (ml)	Total Dose (mg)	Site of Injection (lumbar interspace)
Perineum	0.5	0.5	50	4th
Perineum and lower extremities	1	1	100	3rd or 4th
Up to costal margin	2	1	200	2nd, 3rd or 4th

Sterilization: The drug in intact ampuls is sterile. The preferred method of destroying bacteria on the exterior of ampuls before opening is heat sterilization (autoclaving). Immersion in antiseptic solution is not recommended. **Autoclave at 15-pound pressure, at 121°C (250°F), for 15 minutes.** Dextrose may show some brown discoloration due to caramelization.
How Supplied: NOVOCAIN Solution 10 percent code N-201 ampuls of 2 ml (200 mg) box of 100 **NDC** 0057-1384-06.
Protect solutions from light.
The air in the ampuls has been displaced by nitrogen gas.

Supplied by:
BREON LABORATORIES INC.
Mfg. by Sterling Drug Inc.
New York, N.Y. 10016

Revised April 1979
BR 793/0479

PEDIACOF® Ⓒ ℞

Decongestant and Soothing Cough Syrup for Children

Description:
Each teaspoon (5 ml) contains:
Codeine phosphate, USP ....5.0 mg
(Warning: May be habit forming.)
Neo-Synephrine® hydrochloride ....2.5 mg
(brand of phenylephrine hydrochloride, USP)
Chlorpheniramine maleate, USP ....0.75 mg
Potassium iodide, USP ....75.0 mg
with sodium benzoate 0.2 per cent as preservative and alcohol 5 per cent.
PEDIACOF is a pleasant-tasting, raspberry-flavored cough syrup. It contains four active ingredients in proper proportion for children.
Actions: Codeine phosphate is an antitussive that is well recognized not only because of its efficiency and rapidity of action but also because of its relative safety in clinical use. Thus, irritating, nonproductive cough is suppressed by codeine. The codeine content of PEDIACOF is reduced to the proportion that is most suitable for children. When codeine is combined with the expectorant potassium iodide, which tends to increase bronchial secretion, coughing, although minimized, is more productive when it does occur. The continuous fatiguing effect of useless coughing is thereby avoided. NEO-SYNEPHRINE hydrochloride, brand of phenylephrine hydrochloride, produces effective decongestion of the mucous membranes of the respiratory tract. Chlorpheniramine maleate helps control allergic coughs and mucosal congestion. The mild anticholinergic action of chlorpheniramine maleate may aid in reducing rhinorrhea, and its mild sedative action may also be beneficial to patients whose excessive coughing has caused them to lose sleep. Clinical experience with PEDIACOF has shown it to be a dependable medication for the relief of cough and the reduction of nasal congestion in children.
Indications: Coughs due to colds, as well as coughs and congestive symptoms associated with upper respiratory tract infections such as tracheobronchitis or laryngobronchitis, croup, pharyngitis, allergic bronchitis, and infectious bronchitis, when accompanied by disturbing and fatiguing cough, have been treated successfully with PEDIACOF.
Contraindications: Patients with tuberculosis or those who are known to be sensitive to iodides should not be given PEDIACOF.
Warning: May be habit forming.
Precautions: Caution should be exercised if PEDIACOF is administered to patients with cardiac disorders, hypertension, or hyperthyroidism.
Adverse Reactions: The only significant untoward effects that have occurred are mild anorexia and an occasional tendency to constipation. However, discontinuance of PEDIACOF has seldom been required. Mild drowsiness occurs in some patients but, when cough is relieved, the quieting effect of PEDIACOF is considered beneficial in many instances. Because of its iodide content, PEDIACOF may cause elevation of the protein-bound iodine.
Dosage and Administration: PEDIACOF should be given in accordance with the needs and age of the patient. Frequency of administration may be adjusted as cough is brought under control. The following doses, to be given at 4 to 6 hour intervals, are suggested for patients under 12 years of age: **from 6 months to 1 year,** ¼ teaspoon; **from 1 to 3 years,** ½ to 1 teaspoon; **from 3 to 6 years,** 1 to 2 teaspoons; and **from 6 to 12 years,** 2 teaspoons.
How Supplied:
Bottles of 16 fl oz NDC 0057-1509-06
Gallons NDC 0057-1509-08
Available on prescription only.

PONTOCAINE® Hydrochloride ℞
brand of tetracaine hydrochloride, USP

Prolonged Spinal Anesthesia

Description: PONTOCAINE hydrochloride, brand of tetracaine hydrochloride, is a 2-(dimethylamino)ethyl *p*-(butylamino) benzoate monohydrochloride. It is readily soluble in water and physiologic saline solution. PONTOCAINE hydrochloride in solution is prone to slow hydrolysis and, therefore, crystals may form on aging. The crystals consist of insoluble *p*-butylamino-benzoic acid.
Examine ampuls carefully before use. Do not use solution if crystals, cloudiness, or discoloration is observed. Protect ampuls from light and store under refrigeration.
PONTOCAINE hydrochloride is supplied in two forms for prolonged spinal anesthesia, NIPHANOID® and 1% solution.
NIPHANOID: This sterile and instantly soluble form of the drug consists of a network of extremely fine particles in highly purified form. In appearance the substance resembles snow and hence has been given the designation NIPHANOID, or "snowlike."

Continued on next page

Breon—Cont.

1% Solution: Each 1 ml of this sterile, isotonic, isobaric solution contains 10 mg of PONTOCAINE hydrochloride, 6.7 mg of sodium chloride, and not more than 2 mg of acetone sodium bisulfite. The air in the ampuls has been displaced by nitrogen gas.

Sterilization of Ampuls: The drug in intact ampuls is sterile. The preferred method to destroy bacteria on the exterior of ampuls before opening is heat sterilization (autoclaving). Immersion in antiseptic solution is not recommended.

Autoclave at 15-pound pressure, at 121° C (250° F), for 15 to 20 minutes. The NIPHANOID form also may be autoclaved in the same way but may lose its snowlike appearance and tend to adhere to the sides of the ampul. This effect may slightly decrease the rate at which the drug dissolves but does not interfere with its anesthetic potency.

Autoclaving increases likelihood of crystal formation. Unused autoclaved ampuls should be discarded. In no case should unused autoclaved ampuls be placed back in stock for later use.

Action: PONTOCAINE hydrochloride has been found to possess a number of qualities that make it particularly suitable for spinal anesthesia. When time-consuming surgery is to be performed, adequately prolonged anesthesia of up to two or three hours and even longer can be assured.

Indication: Spinal anesthesia for operations requiring two or three hours.

Contraindications: With the exception of infection in or about the lumbar area and certain serious diseases of the central nervous system or of the lumbar vertebral column, most anesthesiologists consider the following conditions to be only *relative contraindications*. The decision as to whether or not spinal anesthesia should be used for an individual case depends on the physician's appraisal of the advantages as opposed to the risk and on his ability to cope with the complications that may arise.

1. Disease of the cerebrospinal system, such as meningitis, spinal fluid block, cranial or spinal hemorrhage, tumors and syphilis.
2. Suppuration at the site of puncture.
3. Shock. This should be treated before any anesthetic is administered. However, in emergency operations, spinal anesthesia may at times be considered the method of choice.
4. Profound anemia, cachexia, and when death is imminent.
5. Sepsis with positive blood cultures.
6. High blood pressure. Spinal anesthesia is well tolerated if particular care is taken to prevent a sudden or appreciable fall in blood pressure.
7. Low blood pressure. The use of suitable pressor agents and methods of controlling the diffusion of the anesthetic remove the principal objection to spinal anesthesia in patients with low blood pressure.
8. Highly nervous and sensitive persons. Preoperative medication tends to overcome this difficulty.
9. Visceral perforation, bowel strangulation and acute peritonitis. Some surgeons object to contraction of the gastrointestinal musculature; others, however, consider the associated arrest of peristalsis an advantage. With gastrointestinal hemorrhage, spinal anesthesia should be used with caution or may even be contraindicated.
10. Cardiac decompensation, massive pleural effusion, and increased intraabdominal pressure (e.g., full-term pregnancy, massive ascites, large tumor). High spinal anesthesia should not be used in patients with these conditions unless the Trendelenburg position can be omitted or the intraabdominal pressure released slowly. Low spinal (saddle block) anesthesia is satisfactory for normal vaginal delivery.
11. Contraindications to saddle block during delivery include pelvic disproportion, placenta praevia, abruptio placentae, unengaged head, and intrauterine manipulation (e.g., podalic version).
12. Refusal of patient.

Precautions: Whenever a spinal anesthetic is to be administered, oxygen, vasopressors, and equipment for artificial respiration should be immediately available for emergency use. As is the case with all spinal anesthetics, the patient's blood pressure should be monitored during anesthesia.

Spinal anesthesia employing medium or high doses is considered dangerous for vaginal delivery by many anesthesiologists because variations in cerebrospinal fluid pressure during labor contractions may cause undue ascent of the spinal anesthetic. On the other hand, saddle block with small doses (2 to 5 mg), preferably in a hyperbaric (6 per cent) dextrose solution; administered with the patient in a sitting position, has been shown to be satisfactory by many experts.

Hypotension should be corrected promptly, especially if it develops during spinal anesthesia for normal vaginal delivery, since hypoxic fetal bradycardia may occur. If a vasoconstrictor is given to correct hypotension, the obstetrician should be cautioned that if an oxytocic drug of the ergot type is employed, severe persistent hypertension and even rupture of a cerebral blood vessel may occur during the postpartum period.

Adverse Reactions: In isolated instances, one or several of the following complications or side effects may be observed during or after spinal anesthesia:

1. Vasomotor paralysis (due to blocking of the vasomotor fibers by the anesthetic). This complication should not be confused with symptoms of shock due to the operative procedure. The higher the anesthesia, the greater the number of vasoconstrictor fibers blocked and, consequently, the greater the fall in blood pressure. Marked fall in blood pressure is not encountered as commonly as heretofore due to refinements in the technique of injecting the anesthetic agent and to the preoperative administration of a suitable vasopressor. Vomiting, restlessness, pallor, cold sweat, and a weak pulse with shallow respiration accompany a marked decrease in blood pressure. If these signs occur, a parenteral pressor agent should be administered.
2. Respiratory paralysis. This is attributed to diffusion of the anesthetic agent to a high level, producing paralysis of the respiratory center and/or of the motor nerves of respiration. Total spinal anesthesia may occur from *actual overdosage* due to various factors (e.g., increased intraabdominal pressure, decreased size of subarachnoid space, improper technique) or from *relative overdosage* due to improper positioning of patient or such unpredictable factors as failure of or delay in fixation of anesthetic to nerve tissue, increase in cerebrospinal fluid pressure, etc.
3. Meningitis. With the employment of an aseptic technique, septic meningitis is so infrequent as to be practically nonexistent. Some instances of aseptic meningitis, with fever, neck rigidity, and cloudy spinal fluid, have been reported. In such cases, the course is usually rapid and benign, terminating in complete recovery. However, in a few, permanent paralysis (sometimes terminating fatally) and sensory disturbances have been observed. This type of meningitis has also been observed in rare instances following ordinary diagnostic lumbar puncture.
4. Palsies. These are rare and affect either the extraocular muscles or the legs and the anal and vesical sphincters (cauda equina syndrome).
   Paralysis of extraocular muscles and, rarely, of the other cranial nerves usually occurs during the second week after surgery and clears up spontaneously by the third or fourth week. It may be due to stretching of the cranial nerves following changes in cerebrospinal fluid dynamics. Some investigators believe it is caused by low-grade meningitis or meningismus and, therefore, can be eliminated by an absolutely aseptic technique.
   Cauda equina and lumbosacral cord complications (usually consisting of arachnoiditis and demyelinization) result in loss or impairment of motor and sensory function of the saddle area (bladder, rectum) and one or both legs. These complications have occurred after the use of most, if not all, spinal anesthetics. The loss or impairment of motor function may be permanent, or partial recovery may slowly occur. Various explanations for such complications have been advanced, such as hypersensitivity or intolerance to the anesthetic agent with a resultant myelolytic or neurotoxic effect; pooling of relatively high concentrations of anesthetic solution around the cauda equina and spinal cord before diffusion; and accidental injection of irritating antiseptics or detergents (as when syringes are not thoroughly cleaned or when the ampul storage solution enters a cracked ampul). Hence, many anesthesiologists prefer to autoclave ampuls before opening them in order to destory bacteria on the exterior.
   In an article on the hazards of lumbar puncture, Dripps and Vandam (*J.A.M.A.* *147*:1118, Nov. 17, 1951) pointed out that prolonged and occasionally permanent sensory motor abnormalities may result from direct trauma to nerve roots when the puncture is performed. In some of the reported cases of neurologic sequelae it was found that the disturbance was due to preexisting disease of the vertebral column or central nervous system (e.g., cord tumors, malignant metastases, multiple sclerosis).
5. Headache. This may be largely obviated by using the proper needle to prevent spinal fluid leakage and by placing the patient in the horizontal position after operation. Small bore needles (24 or 26 gauge) and needles specially designed to minimize spinal fluid leakage are available.
6. Nausea and vomiting. These may be due to a marked drop in blood pressure, psychic impressions during the course of the operation, undue intraabdominal manipulation, or to preoperative medication (morphine).
7. Systemic side effects. The aforementioned side effects are peculiar to spinal anesthesia and differ from those that may occur when a local anesthetic is applied for surface anesthesia or injected into the tissues for infiltration or conduction anesthesia (nerve block). The latter side effects consist of such symptoms as nausea, vomiting, rapid pulse, talkativeness, syncope, and convulsions and are rarely associated with spinal anesthesia. Avoidance of accidental intravascular injection is imperative.

Treatment of Convulsions. The immediate administration of oxygen to control convulsions is recommended. If convulsions persist, the slow intravenous infusion of an ultrashort-acting barbiturate such as thiopental or methohexital, should be considered. An intravenous anticonvulsant such as diazepam may also be administered to control convulsive seizures. Intravenous anticonvulsant agents should be used only by those familiar with their use and only when adequate ventilation and oxygenation are assured.

Dosage and Administration: Intraspinal use of PONTACAINE hydrochloride is governed by the principles that apply to induction of spinal anesthesia by other agents. The extent and degree of anesthesia depend on a number of well-known factors, the most essential of which include:

1. Dosage
2. Specific gravity of the anesthetic solution.
3. Volume of solution introduced.
4. Force employed in making the injection.
5. Level of puncture.
6. Position of the patient during and immediately after injection.

[See table above].

When spinal fluid is added to either the NIPHANOID or solution, some turbidity results, the degree depending on the pH of the spinal fluid, the temperature of the solution during mixing, as well as the amount of drug and diluent employed. This cloudiness is due to the release of the *base* from the hydrochloride. Liberation of base (which is completed within the spinal canal) is held to be essential for satisfactory results with any spinal anesthetic.

The specific gravity of spinal fluid at 25°/25° C varies under normal conditions from 1.0063 to 1.0075. A solution of the instantly soluble form (NIPHANOID) in spinal fluid has only a slightly greater specific gravity. The 1 per cent concentration in saline solution has a specific gravity of 1.0060 to 1.0074 at 25°/25° C.

A hyperbaric solution may be prepared by mixing equal volumes of the 1 per cent solution and Dextrose Solution 10 per cent (which is available in ampuls of 3 ml).

If the NIPHANOID form is preferred, it is first dissolved in Dextrose Solution 10 per cent in a ratio of 1 ml dextrose to 10 mg of the anesthetic. Further dilution is made with an equal volume of spinal fluid. The resulting solution now contains 5 per cent dextrose with 5 mg of anesthetic agent per milliliter.

A hypobaric solution (for use in Howard Jones or Lund techniques*) may be prepared by dissolving the NIPHANOID in Sterile Water for Injection, USP (1 mg per milliliter). The specific gravity of this solution is essentially the same as that of water, 1.000 at 25°/25° C.

How Supplied: NIPHANOID (instantly soluble): ampuls of 20 mg, boxes of 100.
Code P-841 **NDC** 0057-1577-06
1% isotonic isobaric solution: ampuls of 2 ml., boxes of 25.
Code P-823 **NDC** 0057-1574-04

*For discussion, see Lund, P. C. and Rumball, A. C.: Hypobaric Pontocaine spinal anesthesia; 1640 consecutive cases, *Anesthesiology 8:* 181, March 1947.

SUGGESTED DOSAGE FOR SPINAL ANESTHESIA

	Using NIPHANOID		Using 1 per cent solution		
Extent of anesthesia	Dose of NIPHANOID (mg)	Volume of spinal fluid (ml)	Dose of solution (ml)	Volume of spinal fluid (ml)	Site of injection (lumbar interspace)
Perineum	5*	1	0.5 (=5 mg)*	0.5	4th
Perineum and lower extremities	10	2	1.0 (=10 mg)	1.0	3d or 4th
Up to costal margin	15 to 20†	3	1.5 to 2.0 (=15 to 20 mg)†	1.5 to 2.0	2d, 3d, or 4th

* For vaginal delivery (saddle block), from 2 to 5 mg in dextrose.
† Doses exceeding 15 mg are rarely required and should be used only in exceptional cases.
Inject solution at rate of about 1 ml per 5 seconds.

TRANCOPAL® ℞
brand of chlormezanone
Nonhypnotic Antianxiety Agent

Description: Trancopal (brand of chlormezanone) is [2-(p-chlorophenyl)-tetrahydro-3-methyl-4H-1, 3-thiazin-4-one 1, 1-dioxide], a white, virtually tasteless, crystalline powder with a solubility of less than 0.25 per cent w/v in water.

Clinical Pharmacology: Trancopal improves the emotional state by allaying mild anxiety, usually without impairing clarity of consciousness.

The relief of symptoms is often apparent in fifteen to thirty minutes after administration and may last up to six hours or longer.

Indications and Usage: Trancopal is indicated for the treatment of mild anxiety and tension states.

The effectiveness of chlormezanone in long-term use, that is, more than 4 months, has not been assessed by systematic clinical studies. The physician should periodically reassess the usefulness of the drug for the individual patient.

Contraindication: Contraindicated in patients with a history of a previous hypersensitivity reaction to chlormezanone.

Warnings: Should drowsiness occur, the dose should be reduced. As with other CNS-acting drugs, patients receiving chlormezanone should be warned against performing potentially hazardous tasks which require complete mental alertness, such as operating a motor vehicle or dangerous machinery. Patients should also be warned of the possible additive effects which may occur when the drug is taken with alcohol or other CNS-acting drugs.

Usage in Pregnancy. Safe use of this preparation in pregnancy or lactation has not been established, as no animal reproduction studies have been performed; therefore, use of the drug in pregnancy, lactation, or in women of childbearing age requires that the potential benefit of the drug be weighed against its possible hazards to the mother and fetus.

Adverse Reactions: Adverse effects reported to occur with Trancopal include drowsiness, drug rash, dizziness, flushing, nausea, depression, edema, inability to void, weakness, excitement, tremor, confusion and headache. Medication should be discontinued or modified as the case demands.

Jaundice, apparently of the cholestatic type, has been reported as occurring rarely during the use of chlormezanone, but was reversible on discontinuance of therapy.

Dosage and Administration: The usual adult dosage is 200 mg orally three or four times daily but in some patients 100 mg may suffice. The dosage for children from 5 to 12 years is 50 to 100 mg three or four times daily. Since the effect of CNS-acting drugs varies, treatment, particularly in children, should begin with the lowest dosage which may be increased as needed.

How Supplied:
100 mg (peach colored, scored caplets®)
bottles of 100 NDC=0057-1973-04
200 mg (green colored, scored caplets®)
bottles of 100 NDC=0057-1974-04
bottles of 1000 NDC=0057-1974-08

Supplied by:
BREON LABORATORIES INC.
Mfg. by Sterling Drug Inc.
New York, N.Y. 10016

BR 707/0478 Revised April 1978
[*Shown in Product Identification Section*]

Bristol Laboratories
(Division of Bristol-Myers Co.)
SYRACUSE, NY 13201

AMIKIN™ ℞
(amikacin sulfate)

This is the full text of the latest Official Package Circular dated July 1979 [3015 DIMO-05].

WARNINGS

Patients treated with aminoglycosides should be under close clinical observation because of the potential ototoxicity and nephrotoxicity associated with their use.

Ototoxicity, both auditory and vestibular, can occur in patients treated at higher doses or for periods longer than those recommended. The risk of amikacin-induced ototoxicity is greater in patients with renal damage. High frequency deafness usually occurs first and can be detected only by audiometric testing. Vertigo may occur and may be evidence of vestibular injury.

The ototoxicity potential of amikacin in infants is not known. Until more safety reports become available, amikacin should be used in infants only in those specific circumstances when susceptibility testing indicates that other aminoglycosides cannot be used or are otherwise contraindicated, and when the infant can be observed closely for evidence of toxicity.

Aminoglycosides are potentially nephrotoxic. Renal and eighth-nerve function should be closely monitored in patients with known or suspected renal impairment and also in those whose renal function is initially normal but who develop signs of renal dysfunction during therapy. Such impairment may be characterized by decreased creatinine clearance, the presence of cells or casts, oliguria, proteinuria, decreased urine specific gravity, or evidence of increasing nitrogen retention (increasing BUN or creatinine).

Continued on next page

Bristol—Cont.

Evidence of impairment in renal, vestibular, or auditory function requires discontinuation of the drug or dosage adjustment.
Serum concentrations should be monitored when feasible, and prolonged peak concentrations above 35 mcg./ml. should be avoided. Urine should be examined for increased excretion of protein, the presence of cells and casts, and decreased specific gravity.
Concurrent and/or sequential use of topically or systemically neurotoxic or nephrotoxic antibiotics, particularly kanamycin, gentamicin, tobramycin, neomycin, streptomycin, cephaloridine, paromomycin, viomycin, polymyxin B, colistin, and vancomycin should be avoided.
AMIKIN should not be given concurrently with potent diuretics (ethacrynic acid, furosemide, meralluride sodium, sodium mercaptomerin, or mannitol). Some diuretics themselves cause ototoxicity, and intravenously administered diuretics enhance aminoglycoside toxicity by altering antibiotic concentrations in serum and tissue.

Description: Amikacin sulfate is a semisynthetic aminoglycoside antibiotic derived from kanamycin. It is $C_{22}H_{43}N_5O_{13}$. $2H_2SO_4$. D-Streptamine,0 - 3 -amino- 3 -dioxy- α- D -glucopyranosyl- (1→6) - 0 -[6 -amino- 6 -deoxy-α-D-glycopyranosyl- (1→4)]- N^1- (4 -amino- 2 -hydroxy- l -oxobutyl)- 2 -deoxy-, (S)-,sulfate (1:2) (salt).
The dosage form is supplied as a sterile, colorless to light straw colored solution. The 100 mg. per 2 ml. vial contains, in addition to amikacin sulfate, 0.13% sodium bisulfite and 0.5% sodium citrate with pH adjusted to 4.5 with sulfuric acid. The 500 mg. per 2 ml. vial and the 1.0 Gm. per 4 ml. vial contain 0.66% sodium bisulfite and 2.5% sodium citrate with pH adjusted to 4.5 with sulfuric acid.

Action:

Clinical-Pharmacology

Intramuscular Administration

AMIKIN is rapidly absorbed after intramuscular administration. In normal adult volunteers, average peak serum concentrations of about 12, 16, and 21 mcg/ml are obtained 1 hour after intramuscular administration of 250-mg (3.7 mg/Kg), 375-mg (5 mg/Kg), 500-mg (7.5 mg/Kg), single doses respectively. At 10 hours, serum levels are about 0.3 mcg/ml, 1.2 mcg/ml, and 2.1 mcg/ml, respectively.
Tolerance studies in normal volunteers revealed that amikacin was well tolerated locally following repeated intramuscular dosing and, when given at maximally recommended doses, no ototoxicity or nephrotoxicity was reported. There was no evidence of drug accumulation with repeated dosing for 10 days when administered according to recommended doses.
With normal renal function about 91.9% of an intramuscular dose is excreted unchanged in the urine in the first 8 hours, and 98.2% within 24 hours. Mean urine concentrations for 6 hours are 563 mcg/ml following a 250-mg dose, 697 mcg/ml following a 375-mg dose, and 832 mcg/ml following a 500-mg dose.
Preliminary intramuscular studies in newborns of different weights (less than 1.5 Kg, 1.5 to 2.0 Kg, over 2.0 Kg) at a dose of 7.5 mg/Kg revealed that, like other aminoglycosides, serum half-life values were correlated inversely with post-natal age and renal clearances of amikacin. The volume of distribution indicates that amikacin, like other aminoglycosides, remains primarily in the extracellular fluid space of neonates. Repeated dosing every 12 hours in all the above groups did not demonstrate accumulation after 5 days.

Intravenous Administration

Single doses of 500 mg (7.5 mg/Kg) administered to normal adults as an infusion over a period of 30 minutes produced a mean peak serum concentration of 38 mcg/ml at the end of the infusion, and levels of 24 mcg/ml, 18 mcg/ml, and 0.75 mcg/ml at 30 minutes, 1 hour, and 10 hours post-infusion, respectively. Eighty-four percent of the administered dose was excreted in the urine in 9 hours and about 94% within 24 hours.
Repeat infusions of 7.5 mg/Kg every 12 hours in normal adults were well tolerated and caused no drug accumulation.

General

Pharmacokinetic studies in normal adult subjects reveal the mean serum half-life to be slightly over 2 hours with a mean total apparent volume of distribution of 24 liters (28% of the body weight). By the ultrafiltration technique, reports on serum protein binding range from 0 to 11%. The mean serum clearance rate is about 100 ml/min and the renal clearance rate is 94 ml/min in subjects with normal renal function.
Amikacin is excreted primarily by way of glomerular filtration. Patients with impaired renal function or diminished glomerular filtration pressure excrete the drug much more slowly (effectively prolonging the serum half-life). Therefore, renal function should be monitored carefully and dosage adjusted accordingly (see suggested dosage schedule under "Dosage and Administration").
Amikacin has been found in the cerebrospinal fluid, pleural fluid, and peritoneal cavity following parenteral administration.
Spinal fluid levels in normal infants are approximately 10 to 20% of the serum concentrations and may reach 50% when the meninges are inflamed. AMIKIN has been demonstrated to cross the placental barrier and yield significant concentrations in amniotic fluid. The peak fetal serum concentration is about 16% of the peak maternal serum concentration and maternal and fetal serum half-life values are about 2 and 3.7 hours, respectively.

Microbiology

Gram-negative—Amikacin is active **in vitro** against **Pseudomonas** species, **Escherichia coli, Proteus** species (indole-positive and indole-negative), **Providencia** species, **Klebsiella-Enterobacter-Serratia** species, **Acinetobacter** (formerly **Mima-Herellea**) species and **Citrobacter freundii.**
When strains of the above organisms are found to be resistant to other aminoglycosides, including gentamicin, tobramycin, and kanamycin, many are susceptible to amikacin **in vitro.**
Gram-positive—Amikacin is active **in vitro** against penicillinase and non-penicillinase-producing **Staphylococcus** species including methicillin-resistant strains. However, it has been shown to have a low order of activity against other Gram-positive organisms; viz, **Streptococcus pyogenes,** enterococci, and **Streptococcus pneumoniae** (formerly **Diplococcus pneumoniae**).
Amikacin resists degradation by most aminoglycoside inactivating enzymes known to affect gentamicin, tobramycin, and kanamycin.

Disc Susceptibility Tests

Quantitative methods that require measurement of zone diameters give the most precise estimates of antibiotic susceptibility. One such procedure* has been recommended for use with discs to test susceptibility to amikacin. Interpretation involves correlation of the diameters obtained in the disc test with MIC values for amikacin. When the causative organism is tested by the Kirby-Bauer method of disc susceptibility, a 30-mcg amikacin disc should give a zone of 17 mm or greater to indicate susceptibility. Zone sizes of 14 mm or less indicate resistance. Zone sizes of 15 to 16 mm indicate intermediate susceptibility. With this procedure, a report from the laboratory of "susceptible" indicates that the infecting organism is likely to respond to therapy. A report of "resistant" indicates that the infecting organism is not likely to respond to therapy. A report of "intermediate susceptibility" suggests that the organism would be susceptible if the infection is confined to tissues and fluids (e.g., urine), in which high antibiotic levels are attained.

Indications and Usage: AMIKIN is indicated in the short-term treatment of serious infections due to susceptible strains of Gram-negative bacteria, including **Pseudomonas** species, **Escherichia coli,** species of indole-positive and indole-negative **Proteus, Providencia** species, **Klebsiella-Enterobacter-Serratia** species, and **Acinetobacter (Mima-Herellea)** species.
Clinical studies have shown AMIKIN to be effective in bacteremia and septicemia (including neonatal sepsis); in serious infections of the respiratory tract, bones and joints, central nervous system (including meningitis) and skin and soft tissue; intra-abdominal infections (including pertonitis); and in burns and post-operative infections (including post-vascular surgery). Clinical studies have shown AMIKIN also to be effective in serious complicated and recurrent urinary tract infections due to these organisms. Aminoglycosides, including AMIKIN injectable, are not indicated in uncomplicated initial episodes of urinary tract infections unless the causative organisms are not susceptible to antibiotics having less potential toxicity.
Bacteriologic studies should be performed to identify causative organisms and their susceptibilities to amikacin. AMIKIN may be considered as initial therapy in suspected Gram-negative infections and therapy may be instituted before obtaining the results of susceptibility testing. Clinical trials demonstrated that AMIKIN was effective in infections caused by gentamicin and/or tobramycin resistant strains of Gram-negative organisms, particularly **Proteus rettgeri, Providencia stuartii, Serratia marcescens,** and **Pseudomonas aeruginosa.**
The decision to continue therapy with the drug should be based on results of the susceptibility tests, the severity of the infection, the response of the patient, and the important additional considerations contained in the "Warning" box above.
AMIKIN has also been shown to be effective in staphylococcal infections and may be considered as initial therapy under certain conditions in the treatment of known or suspected staphylococcal disease such as, severe infections where the causative organism may be either a Gram-negative bacterium or a staphylococcus, infections due to susceptible strains of staphylococci in patients allergic to other antibiotics, and in mixed staphylococcal/-Gram-negative infections.
Amikacin may be indicated in the treatment of neonatal sepsis when susceptibility testing indicates that other aminoglycosides cannot be used. In certain severe infections such as neonatal sepsis, concomitant therapy with a penicillin-type drug may be indicated because of the possibility of infections due to Gram-positive organisms such as streptococci or pneumococci.

Contraindications: A history of hypersensitivity to amikacin is a contraindication for its use.

Warning: See "Warning" box above.

Precautions: AMIKIN is potentially nephrotoxic, ototoxic, and neurotoxic. The concurrent or serial use of other ototoxic or nephrotoxic agents should be avoided either systemically or topically because of the potential for additive effects. Such agents include antibacterial drugs such as kanamycin, gentamicin, tobramycin, neomycin, streptomycin, cephaloridine, paromomycin, viomycin, polymyxin B, colistin, and vancomycin as well as certain diuretic agents such as ethacrynic acid or furosemide.

Ototoxicity
See "Warning" box.
Nephrotoxicity
Since AMIKIN is present in high concentrations in the renal excretory system, patients should be well hydrated to minimize chemical irritation of the renal tubules. Kidney function should be assessed by the usual methods prior to starting therapy and daily during the course of treatment.
If signs of renal irritation appear (casts, white or red cells or albumin), hydration should be increased. A reduction in dosage (see "Dosage and Administration") may be desirable if other evidence of renal dysfunction occurs such as decreased creatinine clearance, decreased urine specific gravity, increased BUN, creatinine, or oliguria. If azotemia increases or if a progressive decrease in urinary output occurs, treatment should be stopped.
Note: When patients are well hydrated and kidney function is normal the risk of nephrotoxic reactions with amikacin is low if the dosage recommendations (see "Dosage and Administration") are not exceeded.
Neurotoxicity
Neuromuscular blockade and muscular paralysis have been demonstrated in the cat with high doses of amikacin (188 mg/Kg). The possibility of neuromuscular blockade and respiratory paralysis should be considered when amikacin is administered concomitantly with anesthetic or neuromuscular blocking drugs. If blockade occurs, calcium salts may reverse this phenomenon.
Other
Cross-allergenicity among aminoglycosides has been demonstrated. As with other antibiotics the use of amikacin may result in overgrowth of nonsusceptible organisms. If this occurs, appropriate therapy should be instituted.
Pregnancy
Reproduction studies have been performed in rats and mice and have revealed no evidence of impaired fertility or harm to the fetus due to amikacin. There are no well-controlled studies in pregnant women but investigational experience does not include any positive evidence of adverse effects on the fetus. Although there is no clearly defined risk, such experience cannot exclude the possibility of infrequent or subtle damage to the fetus. AMIKIN should be used in pregnant women only when clearly needed.
It is not known whether this drug is excreted in human milk. As a general rule, nursing should not be undertaken while a patient is on a drug since many drugs are excreted in human milk.
Adverse Reactions:
Ototoxicity
See "Warning" box.
Nephrotoxocity
Albuminuria, presence of red and white cells, casts, azotemia, and oliguria have been reported.
Other
In addition to those described above, other adverse reactions which have been reported on rare occasions are skin rash, drug fever, headache, paresthesia, tremor, nausea and vomiting, eosinophilia, arthralgia, anemia, hypotension.
Overdosage
In the event of overdosage or toxic reaction, peritoneal dialysis or hemodialysis will aid in the removal of amikacin from the blood.
Dosage and Administration: The patient's pretreatment body weight should be obtained for calculation of correct dosage. AMIKIN may be given intramuscularly or intravenously.
Intramuscular Administration for Patients with Normal Renal Function
The recommended dosage for adults, children, and older infants (see Box "Warning") with normal renal function is 15 mg/Kg/day divided into 2 or 3 equal doses administered at equally-divided intervals, i.e., 7.5 mg/Kg q.12h. or 5 mg/Kg q.8h. Treatment of patients in the heavier weight classes shall not exceed 1.5 Gm/day.
When amikacin is indicated in newborns (see Box "Warning"), it is recommended that a loading dose of 10 mg/Kg be administered initially to be followed with 7.5 mg/Kg every 12 hours.
The usual duration of treatment is 7 to 10 days. The total daily dose by all routes of administration should not exceed 15 mg/Kg/day. In the unusual circumstances where treatment beyond 10 days is considered, the use of AMIKIN should be reevaluated and, if continued, renal and auditory functions should be monitored daily.
At the recommended dosage level, uncomplicated infections due to amikacin-sensitive organisms should respond in 24 to 48 hours. If definite clinical response does not occur within 3 to 5 days, therapy should be stopped and the antibiotic sensitivity pattern of the invading organism should be rechecked. Failure of the infection to respond may be due to resistance of the organism or to the presence of septic foci requiring surgical drainage.
When AMIKIN is indicated in uncomplicated urinary tract infections, a dose of 250 mg twice daily may be used.
Intramuscular Administration for Patients with Impaired Renal Function
Whenever possible, serum amikacin concentrations should be monitored by appropriate assay procedures. Doses may be adjusted in patients with impaired renal function either by administering normal doses at prolonged intervals or by administering reduced doses at a fixed interval.
Both methods are based on the patient's creatinine clearance or serum creatinine values since these have been found to correlate with aminoglycoside half-lives in patients with diminished renal function. These dosage schedules must be used in conjunction with careful clinical and laboratory observations of the patient and should be modified as necessary. Neither method should be used when dialysis is being performed.
Normal Dosage at Prolonged Intervals
If the creatinine clearance rate is not available and the patient's condition is stable, a dosage interval in hours for the normal dose can be calculated by multiplying the patient's serum creatinine by nine, e.g., if the serum creatinine concentration is 2 mg/100 ml the recommended single dose (7.5 mg/Kg) should be administered every 18 hours.
Reduced Dosage at Fixed Time Intervals
When renal function is impaired and it is desirable to administer AMIKIN at a fixed time interval, dosage must be reduced. In these patients serum AMIKIN concentrations should be measured to assure accurate administration of AMIKIN and to avoid concentrations above 35 mcg/ml. If serum assay determinations are not available and the patient's condition is stable, serum creatinine and creatinine clearance values are the most readily available indicators of the degree of renal impairment to use as a guide for dosage.
First, initiate therapy by administering a normal dose, 7.5 mg/Kg, as a loading dose. This loading dose is the same as the normally recommended dose which would be calculated for a patient with a normal renal function as described above.
To determine the size of maintenance doses administered every 12 hours, the loading dose should be reduced in proportion to the reduction in the patient's creatinine clearance rate:

$$\text{Maintenance Dose Every 12 Hours} = \frac{\text{observed CC in ml/min}}{\text{normal CC in ml/min}} \times \text{calculated loading dose in mg}$$

(CC—creatinine clearance rate)

An alternate rough guide for determining reduced dosage at twelve-hour intervals (for patients whose steady state serum creatinine values are known) is to divide the normally recommended dose by the patient's serum creatinine.
The above dosage schedules are not intended to be rigid recommendations but are provided as guides to dosage when the measurement of amikacin serum levels is not feasible.
Intravenous Administration
The individual dose, the total daily dose, and the total cumulative dose of AMIKIN are identical to the dose recommended for intramuscular administration. The solution for intravenous use is prepared by adding the contents of a 500-mg vial to 200 ml of sterile diluent such as normal saline or 5% Dextrose in Water or any other compatible solution.
The solution is administered to adults over a 30- to 60-minute period. The total daily dose should not exceed 15 mg/Kg/day and may be divided into either 2 or 3 equally-divided doses at equally-divided intervals.
In pediatric patients the amount of fluid used will depend on the amount ordered for the patient. It should be a sufficient amount to infuse the amikacin over a 30- to 60-minute period. Infants should receive a 1- to 2-hour infusion.
Amikacin should not be physically premixed with other drugs but should be administered separately according to the recommended dose and route.
Supply: AMIKIN is supplied as a colorless solution which requires no refrigeration. It is stable at room temperature for at least two years. At times the solution may become a very pale yellow; this does not indicate a decrease in potency.
AMIKIN (amikacin sulfate injection)
NDC 0015-3015-20—100 mg per 2 ml
NDC 0015-3020-20—500 mg per 2 ml
NDC 0015-3020-21—Disposable Syringe (500 mg per 2 ml)
NDC 0015-3023-20—1.0 gm per 4 ml
For information on package sizes available, refer to the current price schedule.

---

*Bauer, A. W., Kirby, W. M. M., Sherris, J. C., and Turck, M.: Antibiotic Testing by a Standardized Single Disc Method, Am. J. Clin. Pathol., 45:493, 1966; Standardized Disc Susceptibility Test, FEDERAL REGISTER, 37:20527-29, 1972.

AZOTREX® Capsules ℞
(tetracycline phosphate complex with sulfonamide and analgesic)

This is the full text of the latest Official Package Circular dated May 1972 [4325 DIRO-05].
Description: Each capsule contains:
Tetrex® (tetracycline phosphate complex) equivalent to ....125 mg. tetracycline HCl activity
Sulfamethizole ....250 mg.
Phenazopyridine HCl .... 50 mg.
This formula provides comprehensive treatment of common urinary tract infections, since the organisms causing the vast majority of such infections are sensitive to one or more of its antibacterial components.
Tetracycline phosphate complex has the same actions and uses as the parent antibiotic, tetracycline, or its hydrochloride salt. However, the phosphate complex is more rapidly and completely absorbed from the gastrointestinal tract than is the free base or its salts and therefore produces somewhat higher blood levels after oral administration. Tetracycline is excreted primarily by the kidneys.
Laboratory and clinical studies have shown that tetracycline is effective against **D. pneumoniae,** alpha- and beta-hemolytic strepto-

Continued on next page

Bristol—Cont.

cocci, many strains of staphylococci, **N. gonorrhoeae, N. meningitidis, E. coli,** certain clostridia, **H. influenzae, Klebsiella pneumoniae,** Shigella, **Enterobacter aerogenes** and some strains of Salmonella. Tetracycline is also effective against **Entamoeba histolytica,** certain Rickettsia and viruses of the lymphogranuloma-psittacosis-trachoma group.
Sulfamethizole, the sulfonamide component of these capsules, is absorbed rapidly and almost completely from the intestinal tract into the blood stream. It is excreted rapidly by way of the kidneys, with the result that a high concentration is established in the urinary tract 1 to 2 hours after ingestion. The lower degree of acetylation of sulfamethizole assures greater effectiveness with minimum renal toxicity. It may be administered to patients sensitive to other sulfonamides, since there is little cross-sensitization.
Phenazopyridine HCl has a long clinical history of successful use as a urinary analgesic that provides prompt relief of pain and alleviates dysuria, frequency, and urgency.

Indications:
Based on a review of this drug by the National Academy of Sciences—National Research Council and/or other information, FDA has classified the indications as follows:
Lacking substantial evidence of effectiveness for the labeled indications.
Final classification for the less-than-effective indications requires further investigation.
This drug provides systemic and local antibacterial action in acute and chronic urinary tract infections due to organisms sensitive to tetracycline and sulfamethizole. It may be used in mixed infections where the invading organisms are more sensitive to the combination than to either antibacterial agent alone and is not intended for the treatment of infections where complete response to either component might be expected.
It is indicated in the treatment of cystitis, urethritis, pyelonephritis, ureteritis, and prostatitis due to bacterial infection, prior to and following genitourinary surgery and instrumentation, prophylactically in patients with urethrostomies and cord bladders.
In geriatrics this drug is particularly useful when exacerbations of infection occur in such conditions as cystocele, prostatitis, and nonspecific urethritis.
Infections caused by beta-hemolytic streptococci should be treated for at least 10 days to help prevent the occurrence of rheumatic fever or acute glomerulonephritis.

Contraindications: The drug should not be used in patients with a history of sensitivity to one of the components; or in prematures, neonates, pregnant females at term; or in patients with chronic glomerulonephritis, uremia, severe hepatitis, hepatic or renal failure, or severe pyelitis of pregnancy.
Warnings: Certain hypersensitive individuals may develop a photodynamic reaction precipitated by direct exposure to natural or artificial sunlight during the use of tetracycline. This reaction is usually of the photoallergic type which may also be produced by other tetracycline derivatives. Individuals with a history of photosensitivity reactions should be instructed to avoid direct exposure to natural or artificial sunlight while under treatment with this or other tetracycline drugs, and treatment should be discontinued at first evidence of skin discomfort.
n.b. The incidence of photodynamic reactions varies markedly among various drugs of the tetracycline family. Many of these reactions have been reported in the literature from demethylchlortetracycline. Occasional cases from chlortetracycline, a few cases from oxytetracycline, and rare cases from tetracycline, tetracycline hydrochloride, and tetracycline phosphate complex have been reported.
If renal impairment exists, even usual oral or parenteral doses may lead to excessive systemic accumulation of the tetracycline and possible liver toxicity. Under such conditions, lower than usual doses are indicated, and if therapy is prolonged, tetracycline serum level determinations may be advisable.
Severe blood dyscrasias (including granulocytopenia and pancytopenia) have been associated with sulfonamide administration. Deposition of crystals within the kidney can result in oliguria or anuria. Monitoring renal, hepatic, and hematopoietic function is advisable when therapy is prolonged or repetitious.
This drug should be used only after critical appraisal in patients with liver damage, renal damage, urinary obstructions, or blood dyscrasias. Deaths have been reported from hypersensitivity reactions, agranulocytosis, aplastic anemia and other blood dyscrasias associated with sulfonamide administration. When used intermittently or for a prolonged period, blood counts and liver and kidney function tests should be performed.
Precautions: Patients should be informed that the azo dye will impart an orange-red color to the urine.
Prolonged use of these capsules may lead to renal toxicity or to superinfection with resistant organisms (yeasts, Pseudomonas, antibiotic-resistant Staphylococci). If superinfection occurs, appropriate therapy should be instituted.
Infants may occasionally exhibit signs of increased cerebrospinal fluid pressure with bulging fontanels when on full therapeutic doses. Signs and symptoms disappear on cessation of tetracycline therapy.
In the treatment of gonorrhea, patients with a suspected lesion of syphilis should have darkfield examinations before receiving tetracycline and monthly serologic tests for a minimum of four months.
Tetracycline may form a stable calcium complex in any bone-forming tissue with no serious harmful effects reported thus far in humans. However, use of tetracycline during tooth development (last trimester of pregnancy, neonatal period, and early childhood) may cause discoloration of the teeth (yellow-grey-brownish). This effect occurs mostly during long-term use of the drug, but it has also been observed in usual short treatment courses.
Care should be taken to assure adequate fluid intake and urinary output.
This drug should be used with caution in persons having significant allergies and/or asthma.
Adverse Reactions: As in all sulfonamide therapy, the following reactions may occur: nausea, vomiting, diarrhea, hepatitis, pancreatitis, blood dyscrasias, neuropathy, drug fever, skin rash, injection of the conjunctiva and sclera, petechiae, purpura, hematuria and crystalluria. The side effects found with tetracycline therapy, namely glossitis, stomatitis, proctitis and vaginitis may occur. The dosage should be decreased or the drug withdrawn depending upon the severity of the reaction.
Dosage: Adult: One or two capsules 4 times a day. Patients with severe urinary tract infections or those who respond slowly to therapy may require higher doses.
In acute uncomplicated urinary tract infections, therapy should be continued until urine specimens become sterile, i.e., 7 to 14 days.
The medication should be given on an empty stomach. Calcium, in particular, interferes with the absorption of tetracycline.
Supply: AZOTREX Capsules (Tetracycline Phosphate Complex with Sulfonamide and Analgesic).
NDC 0015-4325
For information on package sizes available, refer to the current price schedule.

BETAPEN®-VK ℞

(penicillin V potassium)
Tablets (Film Coated) and Oral Solution

This is the full text of the latest Official Package Circular dated September 1975 [7506 DIRO-06].
Description: Betapen-VK is the potassium salt of penicillin V. The Oral Solutions contain in each 5 ml. (teaspoonful) 125 mg. or 250 mg. of penicillin V activity respectively.
Action and Pharmacology: Penicillin V exerts a bactericidal action against penicillin-sensitive microorganisms during the stage of active multiplication. It acts through the inhibition of biosynthesis of cell wall mucopeptide. It is not active against the penicillinase-producing bacteria, which include many strains of staphylococci. The drug exerts high **in vitro** activity against staphylococci (except penicillinase-producing strains), streptococci (Groups A, C, G, H, L, and M) and pneumococci. Other organisms sensitive **in vitro** to penicillin V are Corynebacterium diphtheriae, Bacillus anthracis, Clostridia, Actinomyces bovis, Streptobacillus moniliformis, Listeria monocytogenes, Leptospira and N. gonorrhoeae. Treponema pallidum is extremely sensitive.
Penicillin V has the distinct advantage over penicillin G in resistance to inactivation by gastric acid. It may be given with meals; however, blood levels are slightly higher when the drug is given on an empty stomach. Average blood levels are two to five times higher than the levels following the same dose of oral penicillin G and also show much less individual variation.
Once absorbed, penicillin V is about 80% bound to serum protein. Tissue levels are highest in the kidney, with lesser amounts in the liver, skin and intestines. Small amounts are found in all other body tissues and the cerebrospinal fluid. The drug is excreted as rapidly as it is absorbed in individuals with normal renal function; however, recovery of the drug from the urine indicates that only about 25% of the dose is absorbed. In neonates, young infants, and individuals with impaired renal function, excretion is considerably delayed.
Indications: Betapen-VK is indicated in the treatment of mild to moderately severe infections due to penicillin G-sensitive microorganisms. Therapy should be guided by bacteriological studies (including sensitivity tests) and by clinical response.
Note: Severe pneumonia, empyema, bacteremia, pericarditis, meningitis, and arthritis should not be treated with oral penicillins during the acute stage.
Indicated surgical procedures should be performed.
The following infections will usually respond to adequate doses of penicillin V: Streptococcal Infections (without bacteremia). Mild to moderate infections of the upper respiratory tract, scarlet fever, and mild erysipelas.
Note: Streptococci in Groups A, C, G, H, L, and M are very sensitive to penicillin. Other groups, including Group D (enterococcus) are resistant.
Pneumococcal Infections—Mild to moderately severe infections of the respiratory tract.
Staphylococcal Infections—penicillin G-sensitive. Mild infections of the skin and soft tissue.
Note: Reports indicate an increasing number of strains of staphylococci resistant to penicillin G, emphasizing the need for culture and sensitivity studies in treating suspected staphylococcal infections.
Fusospirochetosis (Vincent's gingivitis and pharyngitis)—Mild to moderately severe infec-

tions of the oropharynx usually respond to therapy with oral penicillin.
Note: Necessary dental care should be accomplished in infections involving the gum tissue.
Medical conditions in which oral penicillin therapy is indicated as prophylaxis: For the prevention of recurrence following rheumatic fever and/or chorea. Prophylaxis with oral penicillin on a continuing basis has proven effective in preventing recurrence of these conditions.
To prevent bacterial endocarditis in patients with congenital and/or rheumatic heart lesions who undergo dental procedures or minor upper respiratory tract surgery or instrumentation. Prophylaxis should be instituted the day of the procedure and for 2 or more days following. Patients who have a past history of rheumatic fever and are receiving continuous prophylaxis may harbor increased numbers of penicillin-resistant organisms; use of another prophylactic anti-infective agent should be considered. If penicillin is to be used in these patients at surgery, the regular rheumatic fever program should be interrupted 1 week prior to the contemplated surgery. At the time of surgery, penicillin may be reinstituted as a prophylactic measure against the hazards of surgically-induced bacteremia.
Note: Oral penicillin should not be used as adjunctive prophylaxis for genitourinary instrumentation or surgery, lower intestinal tract surgery, sigmoidoscopy and childbirth.
Contraindications: A previous hypersensitivity reaction to any penicillin is a contraindication.
Warning: Serious and occasionally fatal hypersensitivity (anaphylactoid) reactions have been reported in patients on penicillin therapy. Although anaphylaxis is more frequent following parenteral therapy, it has occurred in patients on oral penicillins. These reactions are more apt to occur in individuals with a history of sensitivity to multiple allergens.
There have been well documented reports of individuals with a history of penicillin hypersensitivity reactions who experienced severe hypersensitivity reactions when treated with cephalosporins. Before therapy with a penicillin, careful inquiry should be made concerning previous hypersensitivity reactions to penicillins, cephalosporins, and other allergens. If an allergic reaction occurs, the drug should be discontinued and the patient treated with the usual agents, e.g., antihistamines, pressor amines, corticosteroids.
Precautions: Penicillins should be used with caution in individuals with a history of significant allergies and/or asthma.
The oral route of administration should not be relied upon in patients with severe illness, or with nausea, vomiting, gastric dilatation, cardiospasm or intestinal hypermotility.
Occasional patients will not absorb therapeutic amounts of orally administered penicillin.
In streptococcal infections, therapy must be sufficient to eliminate the organism (10 days minimum); otherwise the sequelae of streptococcal disease may occur. Cultures should be taken following completion of treatment to determine whether streptococci have been eradicated.
Prolonged use of antibiotics may promote the overgrowth of nonsusceptible organisms, including fungi. Should superinfection occur, appropriate measures should be taken.
Adverse Reactions: Although the incidence of reactions to oral penicillins has been reported with much less frequency than following parenteral therapy, it should be remembered that all degrees of hypersensitivity, including fatal anaphylaxis, have been reported with oral penicillin.
The most common reactions to oral penicillin are nausea, vomiting, epigastric distress, diarrhea, and black hairy tongue. The hypersensitivity reactions reported are skin eruptions (maculo-papular to exfoliative dermatitis), urticaria and other serum sickness reactions, laryngeal edema and anaphylaxis. Fever and eosinophilia may frequently be the only reaction observed. Hemolytic anemia, leukopenia, thrombocytopenia, neuropathy, and nephropathy are infrequent reactions and usually associated with high doses of parenteral penicillin.
Administration and Dosage: The dosage of Betapen-VK should be determined according to the sensitivity of the causative organism and the severity of infection, and adjusted to the clinical response of the patient.
The usual dosage recommendations for adults and children 12 years and over are as follows:
Streptococcal Infections—mild to moderately severe—of the upper respiratory tract and including scarlet fever and erysipelas: 125 to 250 mg. (200,000 to 400,000 units) every 6 to 8 hours for 10 days.
Pneumococcal Infections—mild to moderately severe—of the respiratory tract, including otitis media: 250 mg. (400,000 units) every 6 hours until the patient has been afebrile for at least 2 days.
Staphylococcal Infections—mild infections of skin and soft tissue (culture and sensitivity tests should be performed): 250 mg. (400,000 units) every 6 to 8 hours.
Fusospirochetosis (Vincent's Infection) of the oropharynx—mild to moderately severe infections: 250 mg. (400,000 units) every 6 to 8 hours.
For the prevention of recurrence following rheumatic fever and/or chorea: 125 mg. (200,000 units) twice daily on a continuing basis.
To prevent bacterial endocarditis in patients with rheumatic or congenital heart lesions who are to undergo dental or upper respiratory tract surgery or instrumentation: On the day of the procedure prescribe four 250-mg. (400,000 units) doses at 4 to 6 hour intervals plus an extra dose to be taken one hour before the procedure. On each of the two days following the procedure continue to give 250 mg. (400,000 units) four times daily.
Note: Therapy for children under 12 years of age is calculated on the basis of body weight. For infants and small children the suggested dose is 25,000 to 100,000 units/Kg./day (12,500 to 50,000 units/lb./day) in three to six divided doses.
Directions for Dispensing Oral Solutions: Prepare this formulation at the time of dispensing. For ease in preparation, add water to the bottle in two portions and shake well after each addition. Add the total amount of water as directed on the labeling of the package being dispensed. The reconstituted solutions are stable for 14 days under refrigeration.
Supply: BETAPEN-VK (penicillin V potassium) for Oral Solution. Each 5 ml. of reconstituted solution contains penicillin V potassium equivalent to 125 or 250 mg. penicillin V.
NDC 0015-7506—125 mg
125 mg. available in 100 ml. bottles.
NDC 0015-7507—250 mg
250 mg. available in 100, and 200 ml. bottles.
BETAPEN-VK (penicillin V potassium) Tablets (Film Coated). Each tablet contains penicillin V potassium equivalent to 250 or 500 mg. penicillin V.
NDC 0015-7508-250 mg.
NDC 0015-7509-500 mg.
For information on package sizes available, refer to the current price schedule.
[*Shown in Product Identification Section*]

BICNU™ ℞
(carmustine [BCNU])

This is the full text of the latest Official Package Circular dated November 1978 [3012DIMO-05].

WARNING
BiCNU should be administered preferably by individuals experienced in antineoplastic therapy. Since delayed bone marrow toxicity is the major toxicity, complete blood counts should be monitored frequently for at least 6 weeks after a dose. Repeat doses of BiCNU should not be given more frequently than every 6 weeks. The bone marrow toxicity of BiCNU is cumulative, and therefore dosage adjustment must be considered on the basis of nadir blood counts from prior dose (see dosage adjustment table under **Dosage**).
It is recommended that liver function tests also be monitored.

Description: BiCNU (1,3-bis (2-chloroethyl)-1-nitrosourea) is one of the nitrosoureas. It is a white lyophilized powder with a molecular weight of 214.06. It is highly soluble in alcohol and poorly soluble in water. It is also highly soluble in lipids.
Action: BiCNU alkylates DNA and RNA and has also been shown to inhibit several enzymes by carbamoylation of amino acids in proteins.
Intravenously administered BiCNU is rapidly degraded, with no intact drug detectable after 15 minutes. However, in studies with C^{14} labeled drug, prolonged levels of the isotope were observed in the plasma and tissue, probably representing radioactive fragments of the parent compound.
It is thought that the antineoplastic and toxic activities of BiCNU may be due to metabolites.
Approximately 60 to 70% of a total dose is excreted in the urine in 96 hours and about 10% as respiratory CO_2. The fate of the remainder is undetermined.
Because of the high lipid solubility and the relative lack of ionization at a physiological pH, BiCNU crosses the blood brain barrier quite effectively. Levels of radioactivity in the CSF are 50% or greater than those measured concurrently in plasma.
Indications: BiCNU is indicated as palliative therapy as a single agent or in established combination therapy with other approved chemotherapeutic agents in the following:

1. **Brain tumors**—glioblastoma, brainstem glioma, medullablastoma, astrocytoma, ependymoma, and metastatic brain tumors.
2. **Multiple myeloma**—in combination with prednisone.
3. **Hodgkin's Disease**—as secondary therapy in combination with other approved drugs in patients who relapse while being treated with primary therapy, or who fail to respond to primary therapy.
4. **Non-Hodgkin's lymphomas**—as secondary therapy in combination with other approved drugs in patients who relapse while being treated with primary therapy, or who fail to respond to primary therapy.

Contraindications: BiCNU should not be given to individuals who have demonstrated a previous hypersensitivity to it.
BiCNU should not be given to individuals with decreased circulating platelets, leukocytes, or erythrocytes either from previous chemotherapy or other causes.
Warnings: Safe use in pregnancy has not been established. BiCNU is embryotoxic and teratogenic in rats and embryotoxic in rabbits at dose levels equivalent to the human dose. BiCNU also affects fertility in male rats at doses somewhat higher than the human dose. BiCNU is carcinogenic in rats and mice, producing a marked increase in tumor incidence in doses approximating those employed clinically.
Precautions: BiCNU should be administered preferably by individuals experienced in antineoplastic therapy. Since delayed bone marrow toxicity is the major toxicity, complete blood counts should be monitored frequently

Continued on next page

Bristol—Cont.

for at least 6 weeks after a dose. Repeat doses of BiCNU should not be given more frequently than every 6 weeks. The bone marrow toxicity of BiCNU is cumulative, and therefore dosage adjustment must be considered on the basis of nadir blood counts from prior dose (see Dosage Adjustment Table under DOSAGE).

It is recommended that liver function tests also be monitored.

Safe Use in Pregnancy has not been established. Therefore, the benefit to risk of toxicity must be carefully weighed.

Adverse Reactions:

Hematopoietic

The most frequent and most serious toxicity of BiCNU is delayed myelosuppression. It usually occurs 4 to 6 weeks after drug administration and is dose-related. Platelet nadirs occur at 4 to 5 weeks; leukocyte nadirs occur at 5 to 6 weeks post therapy. Thrombocytopenia is generally more severe than leukopenia. However both may be dose limiting toxicities. Anemia also occurs, but is generally less severe.

Gastrointestinal

Nausea and vomiting after IV administration of BiCNU are noted frequently. This toxicity appears within 2 hours of dosing, usually lasting 4 to 6 hours, and is dose-related. Prior administration of antiemetics is effective in diminishing and sometimes preventing this side effect.

Hepatic

When high doses of BiCNU have been employed, a reversible type of hepatic toxicity, manifested by increased transaminase, alkaline phosphatase and bilirubin levels, has been reported in a small percentage of patients.

Local

Burning at the site of injection is common but true thrombosis is rare.

Other

Rapid IV infusion of BiCNU may produce intensive flushing of the skin and suffusion of the conjunctiva within 2 hours, lasting about 4 hours.

Pulmonary toxicity characterized by pulmonary infiltrate and/or fibrosis have been reported in some patients receiving prolonged therapy with BiCNU.

Accidental contact of reconstituted BiCNU with the skin has caused transient hyperpigmentation of the affected areas.

Dosage: The recommended dose of BiCNU as single agent in previously untreated patients, is 200 mg/m^2 intravenously every 6 weeks. This may be given as a single dose or divided into daily injections such as 100 mg/m^2 on 2 successive days.

When BiCNU is used in combination with other myelosuppressive drugs or in patients in whom bone marrow reserve is depleted, the doses should be adjusted accordingly.

A repeat course of BiCNU should not be given until circulating blood elements have returned to acceptable levels (platelets above 100,000/mm^3; leukocytes above 4,000/mm^3), and this is usually in 6 weeks. Blood counts should be monitored frequently and repeat courses should not be given before 6 weeks because of delayed toxicity.

Doses subsequent to the initial dose should be adjusted according to the hematologic response of the patient to the preceding dose. The following schedule is suggested as a guide to dosage adjustment:

Nadir After Prior Dose		Percentage of Prior Dose to be Given
Leukocytes	Platelets	
>4000 -	100,000 -	100%
3000-3999	75,000-99,999	100%
2000-2999	25,000-74,999	70%
<2000 -	<25,000	50%

Preparation of Intravenous Solutions: Dissolve BiCNU with 3 ml of the supplied sterile diluent (absolute ethanol) and then aseptically add 27 ml of Sterile Water for Injection, U.S.P., to the alcohol solution. Each ml of the resulting solution will contain 3.3 mg of BiCNU in 10% ethanol having a pH of 5.6 to 6.0. Accidental contact of reconstituted BiCNU with the skin has caused transient hyperpigmentation of the affected areas.

Reconstitution as recommended results in a clear colorless solution which may be further diluted with Sodium Chloride for Injection, U.S.P., or 5% Dextrose for Injection, U.S.P. The reconstituted solution should be used intravenously only and should be administered by IV drip over a 1 to 2 hour period. Injection of BiCNU over shorter periods of time may produce intense pain and burning at the site of injection.

Important Note: The lyophilized dosage formulation contains no preservatives and is not intended as a multiple dose vial.

Stability: Unopened vials of the dry powder must be stored in a refrigerator (2°C to 8°C). The recommended storage of unopened vials prevents significant decomposition for at least 2 years.

After reconstitution as recommended, decomposition of BiCNU at room temperature is linear with time. After 3 hours, appoximately 6% of the solution has decomposed and after 6 hours, approximately 8%.

Refrigeration (4°C) of the reconstituted BiCNU significantly increases the stability of the solution. After 24 hours, when protected from light, there is only 4% decomposition. Further dilution of the reconstituted solution with 500 ml. of Sodium Chloride for Injection, U.S.P., or 5% Dextrose for Injection, U.S.P., results in a solution which is stable for 48 hours when protected from light and refrigerated.

Important Note: BiCNU has a low melting point (approximately 27°C or 80.6°F). Exposure of the drug to this temperature or above will cause the drug to liquify and appear as an oil film in the bottom of the vials. This is a sign of decomposition and vials should be discarded.

Supply: BiCNU (Carmustine [BCNU]). Each package contains a vial containing 100 mg. carmustine and a vial containing 3 ml. sterile diluent.

NDC 0015-3012

For information on package sizes available, refer to the current price schedule.

BLENOXANE® ℞

(sterile bleomycin sulfate)

This is the full text of the latest Official Package Circular dated October 1978 [3010 DIR-10].

WARNING

It is recommended that Blenoxane be administered under the supervision of a qualified physician experienced in the use of cancer chemotherapeutic agents.

Appropriate management of therapy and complications is possible only when adequate diagnostic and treatment facilities are readily available.

Pulmonary fibrosis is the most severe toxicity associated with Blenoxane. The most frequent presentation is pneumonitis occasionally progressing to pulmonary fibrosis. Its occurrence is higher in elderly patients and in those receiving greater than 400 units total dose, but pulmonary toxicity has been observed in young patients and those treated with low doses.

A severe idiosyncratic reaction consisting of hypotension, mental confusion, fever, chills, and wheezing has been reported in approximately 1% of lymphoma patients treated with Blenoxane.

Description: Blenoxane (sterile bleomycin sulfate) is a mixture of cytotoxic glycopeptide antibiotics isolated from a strain of **Streptomyces verticillus.** It is freely soluble in water.

Note: A unit of bleomycin is equal to the formerly used milligram activity. The term milligram activity is a misnomer and was changed to units to be more precise.

Action: Although the exact mechanism of action of Blenoxane is unknown, available evidence would seem to indicate that the main mode of action is the inhibition of DNA synthesis with some evidence of lesser inhibition of RNA and protein synthesis.

In mice, high concentrations of Blenoxane are found in the skin, lungs, kidneys, peritoneum, and lymphatics. Tumor cells of the skin and lungs have been found to have high concentrations of Blenoxane in contrast to the low concentrations found in hematopoietic tissue. The low concentrations of Blenoxane found in bone marrow may be related to high levels of Blenoxane degradative enzymes found in that tissue.

In patients with a creatinine clearance of >35 ml. per minute, the serum or plasma terminal elimination half-life of bleomycin is approximately 115 minutes. In patients with a creatinine clearance of <35 ml. per minute, the plasma or serum terminal elimination half-life increases exponentially as the creatinine clearance decreases. In humans, 60 to 70% of an administered dose is recovered in the urine as active bleomycin.

Indications: Blenoxane should be considered a palliative treatment. It has been shown to be useful in the management of the following neoplasms either as a single agent or in proven combinations with other approved chemotherapeutic agents:

Squamous Cell Carcinoma—Head and neck including mouth, tongue, tonsil, nasopharynx, oropharynx, sinus, palate, lip, buccal mucosa, gingiva, epiglottis, skin, larynx, penis, cervix, and vulva. The response to Blenoxane is poorer in patients with head and neck cancer previously irradiated.

Lymphomas—Hodgkin's, reticulum cell sarcoma, lymphosarcoma.

Testicular Carcinoma—Embryonal cell, choriocarcinoma, and teratocarcinoma.

Contraindications: Blenoxane is contraindicated in patients who have demonstrated a hypersensitive or an idiosyncratic reaction to it.

Warnings: Patients receiving Blenoxane must be observed carefully and frequently during and after therapy. It should be used with extreme caution in patients with significant impairment of renal function or compromised pulmonary function.

Pulmonary toxicities occur in 10% of treated patients. In approximately 1%, the nonspecific pneumonitis induced by Blenoxane progresses to pulmonary fibrosis, and death. Although this is age and dose related, the toxicity is unpredictable. Frequent roentgenograms are recommended.

Idiosyncratic reactions similar to anaphylaxis have been reported in 1% of lymphoma patients treated with Blenoxane. Since these usually occur after the first or second dose, careful monitoring is essential after these doses.

Renal or hepatic toxicity, beginning as a deterioration in renal or liver function tests, have been reported, infrequently. These toxicities may occur, however, at any time after initiation of therapy.

Usage in Pregnancy: Safe use of Blenoxane in pregnant women has not been established.

Adverse Reactions:

Pulmonary—This is potentially the most serious side effect, occurring in approximately

10% of treated patients. The most frequent presentation is pneumonitis occasionally progressing to pulmonary fibrosis. Approximately 1% of patients treated have died of pulmonary fibrosis. Pulmonary toxicity is both dose and age related, being more common in patients over 70 years of age and in those receiving over 400 units total dose. This toxicity, however, is unpredictable and has been seen occasionally in young patients receiving low doses.

Because of lack of specificity of the clinical syndrome, the identification of patients with pulmonary toxicity due to Blenoxane has been extremely difficult. The earliest symptom associated with Blenoxane pulmonary toxicity is dyspnea. The earliest sign is fine rales.

Radiographically, Blenoxane-induced pneumonitis produces nonspecific patchy opacities, usually of the lower lung fields. The most common changes in pulmonary function tests are a decrease in total lung volume and a decrease in vital capacity. However, these changes are not predictive of the development of pulmonary fibrosis.

The microscopic tissue changes due to Blenoxane toxicity include bronchiolar squamous metaplasia, reactive macrophages, atypical alveolar epithelial cells, fibrinous edema, and interstitial fibrosis. The acute stage may involve capillary changes and subsequent fibrinous exudation into alveoli producing a change similar to hyaline membrane formation and progressing to a diffuse interstitial fibrosis resembling the Hamman-Rich syndrome. These microscopic findings are nonspecific, e.g., similar changes are seen in radiation pneumonitis, pneumocystic pneumonitis.

To monitor the onset of pulmonary toxicity, roentgenograms of the chest should be taken every 1 to 2 weeks. If pulmonary changes are noted, treatment should be discontinued until it can be determined if they are drug related.

Recent studies have suggested that sequential measurement of the pulmonary diffusion capacity for carbon monoxide (DL_{co}) during treatment with Blenoxane may be an indicator of subclinical pulmonary toxicity. It is recommended that the DL_{co} be monitored monthly if it is to be employed to detect pulmonary toxicities, and thus the drug should be discontinued when the DL_{co} falls below 30 to 35% of the pretreatment value.

Idiosyncratic Reactions—In approximately 1% of the lymphoma patients treated with Blenoxane an idiosyncratic reaction, similar to anaphylaxis clinically, has been reported. The reaction may be immediate or delayed for several hours, and usually occurs after the first or second dose. It consists of hypotension, mental confusion, fever, chills, and wheezing. Treatment is symptomatic including volume expansion, pressor agents, antihistamines, and corticosteroids.

Integument and Mucus Membranes—These are the most frequent side effects, being reported in approximately 50% of treated patients. These consist of erythema, rash, striae, vesiculation, hyperpigmentation, and tenderness of the skin. Hyperkeratosis, nail changes, alopecia, pruritus, and stomatitis have also been reported. It was necessary to discontinue Blenoxane therapy in 2% of treated patients because of these toxicities.

Skin toxicity is a relatively late manifestation usually developing in the 2nd and 3rd week of treatment after 150 to 200 units of Blenoxane has been administered and appears to be related to the cumulative dose.

Other—Fever, chills, and vomiting were frequently reported side effects. Anorexia and weight loss are common and may persist long after termination of this medication. Pain at tumor site, phlebitis, and other local reactions were reported infrequently.

There are isolated reports of Raynaud's phenomenon occurring in patients with testicular carcinomas treated with a combination of Blenoxane and Velban®. It is currently unknown if the cause for the Raynaud's phenomenon in these cases is the disease, Blenoxane, Velban, or a combination of any or all of these.

Dosage: Because of the possibility of an anaphylactoid reaction, lymphoma patients should be treated with 2 units or less for the first 2 doses. If no acute reaction occurs, then the regular dosage schedule may be followed.

The following dose schedule is recommended:

Squamous cell carcinoma, lymphosarcoma, reticulum cell sarcoma, testicular carcinoma—0.25 to 0.50 units/Kg. (10 to 20 units/M.^{2}) given intravenously, intramuscularly, or subcutaneously weekly or twice weekly.

Hodgkin's Disease—0.25 to 0.50 units/Kg. (10 to 20 units/M.^{2}) given intravenously, intramuscularly, or subcutaneously weekly or twice weekly. After a 50% response, a maintenance dose of 1 unit daily or 5 units weekly intravenously or intramuscularly should be given.

Pulmonary toxicity of Blenoxane appears to be dose-related with a striking increase when the total dose is over 400 units. Total doses over 400 units should be given with great caution.

Note: When Blenoxane is used in combination with other antineoplastic agents, pulmonary toxicities may occur at lower doses.

Improvement of Hodgkin's Disease and testicular tumors is prompt and noted within two weeks. If no improvement is seen by this time, improvement is unlikely. Squamous cell cancers respond more slowly, sometimes requiring as long as three weeks before any improvement is noted.

Administration: Blenoxane may be given by the intramuscular, intravenous, or subcutaneous routes.

Intramuscular or Subcutaneous—Dissolve the contents of a Blenoxane ampule in 1 to 5 ml. of Sterile Water for Injection, U.S.P., Sodium Chloride for Injection, U.S.P., 5% Dextrose Injection, U.S.P., or Bacteriostatic Water for Injection, U.S.P.

Intravenous—Dissolve the contents of the ampule in 5 ml. or more of a solution suitable for injection, e.g., physiologic saline or glucose, and administer slowly over a period of ten minutes.

Stability: The sterile powder is stable for a period of 18 months and should not be used after the expiration date is reached.

Blenoxane is stable for 24 hours at room temperature in Sodium Chloride or 5% Dextrose Solution.

Blenoxane is stable for 24 hours in 5% Dextrose containing heparin 100 units per ml. or 1000 units per ml.

Supply: Each ampule contains 15 units of Blenoxane as sterile bleomycin sulfate.

NDC 0015-3010-31

For information on package sizes available, refer to the current price sheet.

BRISTAMYCIN® ℞

(erythromycin stearate)
Tablets
Film Coated
250 mg.

This is the full text of the latest Official Package Circular dated July 1978 [8367 DIR-05].

Description: Bristamycin (erythromycin stearate) is produced by a strain of **Streptomyces erythraeus** and belongs to the macrolide group of antibiotics. It is basic and readily forms salts with acids. The base, the stearate salt, and the esters are poorly soluble in water and are suitable for oral administration.

Actions: The mode of action of erythromycin is inhibition of protein synthesis without affecting nucleic acid synthesis. Resistance to erythromycin of some strains of **Haemophilus influenzae** and staphylococci has been demonstrated. Culture and susceptibility testing should be done. If the Kirby-Bauer method of disc susceptibility is used, a 15 mcg. erythromycin disc should give a zone diameter of at least 18 mm. when tested against an erythromycin susceptible organism.

A single oral 250-mg. dose of Bristamycin given to a fasting adult produces in 2 hours a serum level of from 0.4 mcg./ml. to 1.3 mcg./ml. The peak serum level rises with repeated administration.

Orally administered Bristamycin is readily absorbed by most patients, especially on an empty stomach, but patient variation is observed.

After absorption, Bristamycin diffuses readily into most body fluids. In the absence of meningeal inflammation, low concentrations are normally achieved in the spinal fluid but passage of the drug across the blood-brain barrier increases in meningitis. In the presence of normal hepatic function, Bristamycin is concentrated in the liver and excreted in the bile; the effect of hepatic dysfunction on excretion of Bristamycin by the liver into the bile is not known. After oral administration, less than 5 percent of the activity of the administered dose can be recovered in the urine.

Bristamycin crosses the placental barrier but fetal plasma levels are low.

Indications: Streptococcus pyogenes: (Group A beta-hemolytic streptococci.)

Upper and lower respiratory tract, skin, and soft tissue infections of mild to moderate severity.

Injectable penicillin G benzathine is considered by the American Heart Association to be the drug of choice in the treatment and prevention of streptococcal pharyngitis and in long-term prophylaxis of rheumatic fever.

When oral medication is preferred for treatment of streptococcal pharyngitis, penicillin G, V, or erythromycin are alternate drugs of choice.

When oral medication is given, the importance of strict adherence by the patient to the prescribed dosage regimen must be stressed.

A therapeutic dose should be administered for at least 10 days.

Alpha-hemolytic streptococci (viridans group): Short-term prophylaxis against bacterial endocarditis prior to dental or other operative procedures in patients with a history of rheumatic fever or congenital heart disease who are hypersensitive to penicillin. (Erythromycin is not suitable prior to genitourinary surgery where the organisms likely to lead to bacteremia are Gram-negative bacilli or the enterococcus group of streptococci.)

Staphylococcus aureus: Acute infections of skin and soft tissue of mild to moderate severity. Resistance may develop during treatment.

Diplococcus pneumoniae: Upper respiratory tract infections (e.g. otitis media, pharyngitis) and lower respiratory tract infections (e.g. pneumonia) of mild to moderate degree.

Mycoplasma pneumoniae (Eaton agent, PPLO): In the treatment of primary atypical pneumonia, when due to this organism.

Hemophilus influenzae: For upper respiratory tract infections of mild to moderate severity when used concomitantly with adequate doses of sulfonamides. Not all strains of this organism are susceptible at the erythromycin concentrations ordinarily achieved (see appropriate sulfonamide labeling for prescribing information).

Treponema pallidum: Bristamycin is an alternate choice of treatment for primary syphilis in patients allergic to the penicillins. In treatment of primary syphilis, spinal fluid examinations should be done before treatment and as part of follow-up after therapy.

Corynebacterium diphtheriae and **Corynebacterium minutissimum:** As an adjunct to antitoxin, to prevent establishment of carriers, and to eradicate the organism in carriers.

Continued on next page

Bristol—Cont.

In the treatment of erythrasma.
Entamoeba histolytica: In the treatment of intestinal amebiasis only. Extra-enteric amebiasis requires treatment with other agents.
Listeria monocytogenes: Infections due to this organism.
Neisseria gonorrhoeae: Erythromycin lactobionate for injection in conjunction with erythromycin stearate or base orally, as an alternative drug in treatment of acute pelvic inflammatory disease caused by **N. gonorrhoeae** in female patients with a history of sensitivity to penicillin. Before treatment of gonorrhea, patients who are suspected of also having syphilis should have a microscopic examination for **T. pallidum** (by immunofluorescence or darkfield) before receiving erythromycin, and monthly serologic tests for a minimum of 4 months.
Legionnaires' Disease: Although no controlled clinical efficacy studies have been conducted, **in vitro** and limited preliminary clinical data suggest that erythromycin may be effective in treating Legionnaires' Disease.
Contraindications: Bristamycin is contraindicated in patients with known hypersensitivity to this antibiotic.
Warnings: *Usage in Pregnancy:* Safety for use in pregnancy has not been established.
Precautions: Erythromycin is principally excreted by the liver. Caution should be exercised in administering the antibiotic to patients with impaired hepatic function. There have been reports of hepatic dysfunction, with or without jaundice, occurring in patients receiving oral erythromycin products.
Recent data from studies of erythromycin reveal that its use in patients who are receiving high doses of theophylline may be associated with an increase of serum theophylline levels and potential theophylline toxicity. In case of theophylline toxicity and/or elevated serum theophylline levels, the dose of theophylline should be reduced while the patient is receiving concomitant erythromycin therapy.
Surgical procedures should be performed when indicated.
Adverse Reactions: The most frequent side effects of erythromycin preparations are gastrointestinal, such as abdominal cramping and discomfort, and are dose-related. Nausea, vomiting, and diarrhea occur infrequently with usual oral doses.
During prolonged or repeated therapy, there is a possibility of overgrowth of nonsusceptible bacteria or fungi. If such infections occur, the drug should be discontinued and appropriate therapy instituted.
Mild allergic reactions such as urticaria and other skin rashes have occurred. Serious allergic reactions, including anaphylaxis, have been reported.
Dosage and Administration: Optimum blood levels are obtained when doses are given on an empty stomach.
Adults: 250 mg. every 6 hours is the usual dose. Dosage may be increased up to 4 or more Grams per day according to the severity of the infection.
Children: Age, weight, and severity of the infection are important factors in determining the proper dosage. 30 to 50 mg./kg./day (15 to 25 mg./lb./day) in divided doses is the usual dose. For more severe infections this dose may be doubled.
If dosage is desired on a twice-a-day schedule in either adults or children, one-half of the total daily dose may be given every 12 hours, 1 hour before meals.
In the treatment of streptococcal infections, a therapeutic dosage of erythromycin should be administered for at least 10 days. In continuous **prophylaxis** of streptococcal infections in persons with a history of rheumatic heart disease, the dose is 250 mg. twice a day.
When used prior to surgery to prevent endocarditis (see Alpha-hemolytic streptococci), a recommended schedule for adults is: 500 mg. before the procedure and 250 mg. every 6 hours for 4 doses after the procedure. For small children: 30 mg./kg./day (15 mg./lb./day) divided into three or four evenly spaced doses.
For treatment of primary syphilis: 30 to 40 Grams given in divided doses over a period of 10 to 15 days.
For dysenteric amebiasis: 250 mg. four times daily for 10 to 14 days, for adults; 30 to 50 mg./kg./day in divided doses for 10 to 14 days, for children.
For treatment of Legionnaires' Disease: Although optimal doses have not been established, doses utilized in reported clinical data were those recommended above (1 to 4 grams erythromycin stearate, daily in divided doses).
Supply: BRISTAMYCIN (erythromycin stearate) Tablets Film Coated. Erythromycin stearate equivalent to 250 mg. erythromycin per tablet.
NDC 0015-8367—250 mg.
For information on package sizes available, refer to the current price sheet.
[Shown in Product Identification Section]

BRISTOJECT®

The following products are available in prefilled, disposable Bristoject® syringes:

NDC-0015	PRODUCT
	ATROPINE SULFATE ℞
9410-87	0.5 mg in 5 ml, 22 ga × 1½"
9411-87	1 mg in 10 ml, 22 ga × 1½"
	CALCIUM CHLORIDE ℞
9422-78	1 gram in 10 ml (10%), 22 ga × 1½"
9422-75	1 gram in 10 ml (10%), 18 ga × 3½"
	DEXTROSE ℞
9424-87	50% (25 grams in 50 ml), 18 ga × 1½"
	EPINEPHRINE ℞
9423-77	1 mg in 10 ml (1:10,000), 22 ga × 1½"
9423-87	1 mg in 10 ml (1:10,000), 18 ga × 3½"
	LIDOCAINE HCl ℞
9149-87	50 mg in 5 ml (1%), 22 ga × 1½"
9151-87	100 mg in 5 ml (2%), 22 ga × 1½"
9161-87	100 mg in 10 ml (1%), 22 ga × 1½"
9139-87	1 gram in 25 ml (4%), Inject-all™ Syringe
9140-87	2 grams in 50 ml (4%), Inject-all™ Syringe
9115-87	(Infant) 5 mEq in 10 ml (4.2%) 22 ga × 1½"
9142-87	1 gram in 5 ml (20%) Inject-all™ Syringe
9143-87	2 grams in 10 ml (20%) Inject-all™ Syringe
	MAGNESIUM SULFATE ℞
9266-87	50% (5 grams in 10 ml), 20 ga × 2½"
	METARAMINOL BITARTRATE ℞
9440-87	100 mg in 10 ml (1%), Inject-all™ Syringe
	SODIUM BICARBONATE ℞
9121-87	44.6 mEq in 50 ml (7.5%), 18 ga × 1½"
9124-87	50 mEq in 50 ml (8.4%), 18 ga × 1½"
9125-87	(Ped) 10 mEq in 10 ml (8.4%), 22 ga × 1½"

CeeNU® ℞
(lomustine [CCNU])

This is the full text of the latest Official Package Circular dated April 1977 [3030DIMO-05].

WARNING
CeeNU should be administered by individuals experienced in the use of antineoplastic therapy.
Since the major toxicity is delayed bone marrow suppression, blood counts should be monitored weekly for at least 6 weeks after a dose. (See "Adverse Reactions.") At the recommended dosage, courses of CeeNU should not be given more frequently than 6 weeks.
Caution should be used in administering CeeNU to patients with decreased circulating platelets, leukocytes, or erythrocytes. (See "Dosage and Administration.")
Liver function should be monitored periodically. (See "Adverse Reactions.")

Description: CeeNU [1-(2-chloroethyl)-3-cyclohexyl-1-nitrosourea] is one of a group of nitrosoureas. It is a yellow powder with the empirical formula of $C_9H_{16}Cl\ N_3O_2$ and a molecular weight of 233.71. CeeNU is soluble in 10% ethanol (0.05 mg. per ml.) and in absolute alcohol (70 mg. per ml.). CeeNU is relatively insoluble in water ($<$0.05 mg. per ml.). It is relatively unionized at physiological pH.
Action: It is generally agreed that CeeNU acts as an alkylating agent but, as with other nitrosoureas, it may also inhibit several key enzymatic processes.
CeeNU may be given orally. Following oral administration of radioactive CeeNU at doses ranging from 30 mg/M^2 to 100 mg/M^2, about half of the radioactivity given was excreted within 24 hours. The serum half-life of the drug and/or metabolites ranges from 16 hours to 2 days. Tissue levels are comparable to plasma levels at 15 minutes after intravenous administration.
Because of the high lipid solubility and the relative lack of ionization at a physiological pH, CeeNU crosses the blood brain barrier quite effectively. Levels of radioactivity in the CSF are 50% or greater than those measured concurrently in plasma.
Indications: CeeNU is indicated as palliative therapy to be employed in addition to other modalities, or in established combination therapy with other approved chemotherapeutic agents in the following:
Brain tumors—both primary and metastatic, in patients who have already received appropriate surgical and/or radiotherapeutic procedures;
Hodgkin's Disease—as a secondary therapy.
Contraindications: CeeNU should not be given to individuals who have demonstrated a previous hypersensitivity to it.
Warnings: Safe use in pregnancy has not been established. CeeNU is embryotoxic and teratogenic in rats and embryotoxic in rabbits at dose levels equivalent to the human dose. CeeNU also affects fertility in male rats at doses somewhat higher than the human dose. CeeNU is carcinogenic in rats and mice, producing a marked increase in tumor incidence in doses approximating those employed clinically.
Precautions: CeeNU should be administered by individuals experienced in the use of antineoplastic therapy.
Since the major toxicity is delayed bone marrow suppression blood counts should be monitored weekly for at least 6 weeks after a dose. (See "Adverse Reactions"). At the recom-

mended dosage, courses of CeeNU should not be given more frequently than every 6 weeks. Caution should be used in administering CeeNU to patients with decreased circulating platelets, leukocytes, or erythrocytes. (See "Dosage and Administration").
Liver function should be monitored periodically. (See "Adverse Reactions").
Adverse Reactions: Nausea and vomiting may occur 3 to 6 hours after an oral dose and usually last less than 24 hours. The frequency and duration may be reduced by the use of antiemetics prior to dosing and by the administration of CeeNU to fasting patients.
Thrombocytopenia occurs at about 4 weeks after a dose of CeeNU and persists for 1 to 2 weeks.
Leukopenia occurs at about 6 weeks after a dose of CeeNU and persists for 1 to 2 weeks. Approximately 65% of patients develop white blood counts below 5000 wbc/mm^3 and 36% develop white blood counts below 3000 wbc/mm^3.
CeeNU may produce cumulative myelosuppression, manifested by more depressed indices or longer duration of suppression after repeated doses.
Other toxicities: Stomatitis, alopecia, anemia, and hepatic toxicity, manifested by transient reversible elevation of liver function tests, have been reported infrequently.
Neurological reactions such as disorientation, lethargy, ataxia, and dysarthria have been noted in some patients receiving CeeNU. However, the relationship to medication in these patients is unclear.
Dosage and Administration: The recommended dose of CeeNU in adults and children is 130 mg/M^2 as a single dose by mouth every 6 weeks.
In individuals with compromised bone marrow function, the dose should be reduced to 100 mg/M^2 every 6 weeks.
A repeat course of CeeNU should not be given until circulating blood elements have returned to acceptable levels (platelets above 100,000/mm^3; leukocytes above 4,000/mm^3). Blood counts should be monitored weekly and repeat courses should not be given before 6 weeks because the hematologic toxicity is delayed and cumulative.
Doses subsequent to the initial dose should be adjusted according to the hematologic response of the patient to the preceding dose. The following schedule is suggested as a guide to dosage adjustment:

Nadir After Prior Dose Leukocytes	Platelets	Percentage of Prior Dose to be Given
> 4000	> 100,000	100%
3000-3999	75,000-99,999	100%
2000-2999	25,000-74,999	70%
< 2000	< 25,000	50%

When CeeNU is used in combination with myelosuppressive drugs, the doses should be adjusted accordingly.
Stability: CeeNU capsules are stable for at least 2 years when stored at room temperature in well closed containers. Avoid excessive heat (over 40°C).
Supply: This dose pack of CeeNU (Lomustine [CCNU]) Capsules contains;
NDC 0015-3032-13—2—100 mg capsules (Green/Green)
NDC 0015-3031-13—2—40 mg capsules (Purple/Green)
NDC 0015-3030-13—2—10 mg capsules (Purple/Purple)
Directions to the Pharmacist
The capsules are to provide enough medication for a single dose. The total dose prescribed by the physician can be obtained (to within 10 mg) by determining the appropriate combination of the enclosed capsule strengths.
The appropriate number of capsules of each size should be placed in a single vial to which the patient information label (gummed label provided) explaining the differences in the appearance of the capsules is affixed.
Example: A patient dose of 240 mg can be obtained by combining two 100 mg capsules and one 40 mg capsule. The remaining capsules (if any) should be discarded.
A patient information sticker, to be placed on dispensing container, is enclosed.
Also Available: Individual bottles of 20 capsules each.
NDC 0015-3032-20—20—100 mg. capsules (Green/Green)
NDC 0015-3031-20—20—40 mg. capsules (Purple/Green)
NDC 0015-3030-20—20—10 mg. capsules (Purple/Purple)

CEFADYL® ℞
(sterile cephapirin sodium)

This is the full text of the latest Official Package Circular dated December 1977. [7628DIRO-15].
Description: Cefadyl (sterile cephapirin sodium) is a cephalosporin antibiotic intended for intramuscular and intravenous administration only. It is supplied as the sodium salt of 7-[α-(4-pyridylthio)-acetamido]-cephalosporanic acid. Each 500 mg. contains 1.18 milliequivalents of sodium.
Actions:
Human Pharmacology
Following intramuscular administration of single 500-mg. and 1-Gm. doses to normal volunteers, average peak serum levels of 9.0 and 16.4 mcg./ml. respectively, were attained at 30 minutes, declining to 0.7 and 1.0 mcg./ml. respectively, at 4 hours and 0.2 and 0.3 mcg./ml. respectively, at 6 hours.
Cefadyl and its metabolites were excreted primarily by the kidneys. Antibiotic activity in the urine was equivalent to 35% of a 500-mg. dose 6 hours after I.M. injection, and to 65% of a 500-mg. dose 12 hours after injection. Following an I.M. dose of 500 mg., peak urine levels averaged 900 mcg./ml. within the first 6 hours.
Following rapid intravenous administration of single 0.5-Gm., 1-Gm., and 2-Gm. doses, peak serum levels of 35, 67, and 129 mcg./ml. respectively, were attained at 5 minutes, declining to 6.7, 14.0, and 31.7 mcg./ml. respectively, at 30 minutes and 0.27, 0.61, and 1.11 mcg./ml. respectively, at 3 hours.
Seventy percent of the administered dose was recovered in the urine within 6 hours. Repetitive intravenous administration of 1-Gm. doses over 6-hour periods produced serum levels between 4.5 and 5.5 mcg./ml.
At therapeutic drug levels, normal human serum binds Cefadyl to the extent of 44 to 50%.
The average serum half-life of Cefadyl in patients with normal renal function is approximately 36 minutes.
The major metabolite of cephapirin is desacetyl cephapirin which has been shown to contribute to antibacterial activity.
Controlled studies in normal adult volunteers revealed that Cefadyl was well tolerated intramuscularly. In controlled studies of volunteers and of patients receiving I.V. Cefadyl, the incidence of venous irritation was low.
Microbiology
In vitro tests demonstrate that the action of cephalosporins results from inhibition of cell-wall synthesis. Cefadyl is active against the following organisms **in vitro:**
Beta-hemolytic streptococci and other streptococci.
(Many strains of enterococci, e.g., **S. faecalis,** are relatively resistant.)
Staphylococci, including coagulase-positive, coagulase-negative, penicillinase, and nonpenicillinase producing strains.
Diplococcus pneumoniae
Haemophilus influenzae
Proteus mirabilis
Escherichia coli
Klebsiella species
Most strains of enterobacter and indole-positive Proteus **(P. vulgaris, P. morganii, P. rettgeri)** are resistant to Cefadyl. Methicillin-resistant staphylococci, Serratia, Pseudomonas, Mima, and Herellea species are almost uniformly resistant to Cefadyl.
Disc Susceptibility Tests—Quantitative methods that require measurement of zone diameters give the most precise estimates of antibiotic susceptibility. One such procedure* has been recommended for use with discs for testing susceptibility to cephalosporin class antibiotics. Interpretations correlate diameters of the disc test with MIC values for Cefadyl. With this procedure, a report from the laboratory of "susceptible" indicates that the infecting organism is likely to respond to therapy. A report of "resistant" indicates that the infecting organism is not likely to respond to therapy. A report of "intermediate susceptibility" suggests that the organism would be susceptible if high dosage is used, or if the infection is confined to tissues and fluid (e.g., urine), in which high antibiotic levels are attained.
Indications: Cefadyl is indicated for the treatment of serious infections caused by susceptible strains of the designated microorganisms in the diseases listed below. Culture and susceptibility studies should be performed. Therapy may be instituted before results of susceptibility studies are obtained.
Respiratory tract infections caused by **S. pneumoniae** (formerly **D. pneumoniae),** Staphylococcus aureus (penicillinase and nonpenicillinase-producing), **Klebsiella species, H. influenzae** and Group A beta-hemolytic streptococci.
Skin and soft-tissue infections caused by Staphylococcus aureus (penicillinase and nonpenicillinase-producing), **E. coli, P. mirabilis, Klebsiella species** and Group A beta-hemolytic streptococci.
Urinary tract infections caused by Staphylococcus aureus (penicillinase and nonpenicillinase-producing), **E. coli, P. mirabilis, and Klebsiella species.**
Septicemia caused by Staphylococcus aureus (penicillinase and nonpenicillinase-producing), **S. viridans, E. coli, Klebsiella species** and Group A beta-hemolytic streptococci.
Endocarditis caused by Streptococcus viridans and staphylococcus aureus (penicillinase and nonpenicillinase-producing).
Osteomyelitis caused by Staphylococcus aureus (penicillinase and nonpenicillinase-producing), **Klebsiella species, P. mirabilis,** and Group A beta-hemolytic streptococci.
Note: If the susceptibility tests show that the causative organism is resistant to Cefadyl, other appropriate therapy should be instituted.
Contraindications: Cefadyl is contraindicated in persons who have shown hypersensitivity to cephalosporin antibiotics.
Warnings: IN PENICILLIN-ALLERGIC PATIENTS, CEPHALOSPORINS SHOULD BE USED WITH GREAT CAUTION. THERE IS CLINICAL AND LABORATORY EVIDENCE OF PARTIAL CROSS-ALLERGENICITY OF THE PENICILLINS AND THE CEPHALOSPORINS, AND THERE ARE INSTANCES OF PATIENTS WHO HAVE HAD REACTIONS TO BOTH DRUGS (INCLUDING FATAL ANAPHYLAXIS AFTER PARENTERAL USE).
Any patient who has demonstrated some form of allergy, particularly to drugs, should receive antibiotics cautiously and then only when absolutely necessary. No exceptions should be made with regard to Cefadyl.
SERIOUS ANAPHYLACTOID REACTIONS REQUIRE IMMEDIATE EMERGENCY TREATMENT WITH EPINEPHRINE. OXYGEN, INTRAVENOUS STEROIDS, AND AIR-

Continued on next page

Bristol—Cont.

WAY MANAGEMENT, INCLUDING INTUBATION, SHOULD ALSO BE ADMINISTERED AS INDICATED.

Usage in Pregnancy—Safety of this product for use during preganancy has not been established.

Precautions: The renal status of the patients should be determined prior to and during Cefadyl therapy, since in patients with impaired renal function, a reduced dose may be appropriate (see Dosage, Adults). When Cefadyl was given to patients with marked reduction in renal function and to renal transplant patients, no adverse effects were reported.

Prolonged use of Cefadyl may result in the overgrowth of nonsusceptible organisms. Careful observation of the patient is essential. If superinfection occurs during therapy, appropriate measures should be taken.

With high urine concentrations of cephapirin, false-positive glucose reactions may occur if Clinitest, Benedict's Solution or Fehling's Solution are used. Therefore, it is recommended that glucose tests based on enzymatic glucose oxidase reactions (such as Clinistix or Tes-Tape) be used.

Adverse Reactions:

Hypersensitivity—Cephalosporins were reported to produce the following reactions: maculopapular rash, urticaria, reactions resembling serum sickness, and anaphylaxis. Eosinaphilia and drug fever have been observed to be associated with other allergic reactions. These reactions are most likely to occur in patients with a history of allergy, particularly to penicillin.

Blood—During large scale clinical trials, rare instances of neutropenia, leukopenia, and anemia were reported. Some individuals, particularly those with azotemia, have developed positive direct Coombs test during therapy with other cephalosporins.

Liver—Elevations in SGPT or SGOT, alkaline phosphatase, and bilirubin have been reported.

Kidney—Rises in BUN have been observed; their frequency increases in patients over 50 years old.

Dosage:

Adults—The usual dose is 500 mg. to 1 Gm. every 4 to 6 hours intramuscularly or intravenously. The lower dose of 500 mg. is adequate for certain infections, such as skin and soft tissue and most urinary tract infections. However, the higher dose is recommended for more serious infections.

Very serious or life-threatening infections may require doses up to 12 Grams daily. The intravenous route is preferable when high doses are indicated.

Depending upon the causative organism and the severity of infection, patients with reduced renal function (moderately severe oliguria or serum creatinine above 5.0 mg./100 ml.) may be treated adequately with a lower dose, 7.5 to 15 mg./Kg. of cephapirin every 12 hours. Patients with severely reduced renal function and who are to be dialyzed should receive the same dose just prior to dialysis and every 12 hours thereafter.

Children—The dosage is in accordance with age, weight, and severity of infection. The recommended total daily dose is 40 to 80 mg./Kg. (20 to 40 mg./lb.) administered in four equally divided doses.

The drug has not been extensively studied in infants; therefore, in the treatment of children under the age of three months, the relative benefit/risk should be considered.

Therapy in beta-hemolytic streptococcal infections should continue for at least 10 days.

Where indicated, surgical procedures should be performed in conjunction with antibiotic therapy.

Administration: Cefadyl may be administered by the intramuscular or the intravenous routes.

Intramuscular Injection

The 1-Gm. vial should be reconstituted with 2 ml. of Sterile Water for Injection, U.S.P., or Bacteriostatic Water for Injection (with parabens or benzyl alcohol). Each 1.2 ml. contains 500 mg. of cephapirin. All injections should be deep in the muscle mass.

Intravenous Injection

The intravenous route may be preferable for patients with bacteremia, septicemia, or other severe or life-threatening infections who may be poor risks because of lowered resistance resulting from such debilitating conditions as malnutrition, trauma, surgery, diabetes, heart failure, or malignancy, particularly if shock is present or impending. If patient has impaired renal function, a reduced dose may be indicated (see Dosage, Adults). In conditions such as septicemia, 6 to 8 Gm. per day may be given intravenously for several days at the beginning of therapy; then, depending on the clinical response and laboratory findings, the dosage may gradually be reduced.

When the injection has been refractory to previous forms of treatment and mutiple sites have been involved, daily doses up to 12 Gm. have been used.

Intermittent Intravenous Injection

The contents of the 1-Gm. or 2 gm. vial should be diluted with 10 ml. or more of the specified diluent and administered slowly over a 3- to 5-minute period or may be given with intravenous infusions.

Intermittent Intravenous Infusion with Y-Tube

Intermittent intravenous infusion with a Y-type administration set can also be accomplished while bulk intravenous solutions are being infused. However, during infusion of the solution containing Cefadyl it is desirable to discontinue the other solution. When this technique is employed, careful attention should be paid to the volume of the solution containing Cefadyl so that the calculated dose will be infused. When a Y-tube hookup is used, the contents of the 4-Gm. vial of cephapirin should be diluted by addition of 40 ml. of Bacteriostatic Water for Injection, U.S.P., Dextrose Injection, U.S.P., or Sodium Chloride Injection, U.S.P.

STABILITY

Utility Time For Cefadyl In Various Diluents At Concentrations Ranging From 20 to 400 mg./ml.

Diluent	Approximate Concentration (mg./ml.)	Utility Time 25°C	4°C
Water for Injection	50 to 400	12 hours	10 days
Bacteriostatic Water For Injection with Benzyl Alcohol or Parabens	250 to 400	48 hours	10 days
Normal Saline	20 to 100	24 hours	10 days
5% Dextrose in Water	20 to 100	24 hours	10 days

All of the above solutions can be frozen immediately after reconstitution and stored at −15°C for 60 days before use. After thawing, at room temperature (25°C), all of the solutions are stable for at least 12 hours at room temperature or 10 days under refrigeration (4°C).

The pH of the resultant solution ranges from 6.5 to 8.5. During these storage conditions, no precipitation occurs. A change in solution color during this storage time does not affect the potency.

Compatibility with the Infusion Solution

Cefadyl is stable and compatible for 24 hours at room temperature at concentrations between 2 mg./ml. and 30 mg./ml. in the following solutions:

- Sodium Chloride Injection, U.S.P.
- 5% W/V Dextrose in Water, U.S.P.
- Sodium Lactate Injection, U.S.P.
- 5% Dextrose in Normal Saline, U.S.P.
- 10% Invert Sugar in Normal Saline
- 10% Invert Sugar in Water
- 5% Dextrose + 0.2% Sodium Chloride Injection, U.S.P.
- Lactated Ringer's Injection, U.S.P.
- Lactated Ringer's with 5% Dextrose
- 5% Dextrose + 0.45% Sodium Chloride Injection, U.S.P.
- Ringer's Injection, U.S.P.
- 10% Dextrose Injection, U.S.P.
- Sterile Water for Injection, U.S.P.
- 20% Dextrose Injection, U.S.P.
- 5% Sodium Chloride in Water
- 5% Dextrose in Ringer's Injection
- Normosol® R
- Normosol® R in 5% Dextrose Injection
- Ionosol® D-CM
- Ionosol® G in 10% Dextrose Injection

In addition, Cefadyl, at a concentration of 4 mg./ml., is stable and compatible for 10 days under refrigeration (4°C) or 14 days in the frozen state (−15°C) followed by 24 hours at room temperature (25°C) in all of the intravenous solutions listed above.

"Piggyback" I.V. Package: This glass vial contains the labeled quantity of Cefadyl and is intended for intravenous administration. The diluent and volume are specified on the label.

Hospital Bulk Package: This glass vial contains 20 Gm. Cefadyl and is designed for use in the pharmacy in preparing I.V. additives. Add 67 ml. of Sodium Chloride Injection, U.S.P. or Dextrose Injection, U.S.P. The resulting solution will contain 250 mg. cephapirin activity per ml.

Following reconstitution in this manner, the solutions are stable for 24 hours at room temperature or 10 days under refrigeration.

Caution: Not to be dispensed as a unit.

Supply: Cefadyl (Sterile Cephapirin Sodium) for I.M. or I.V. Injection. Cephapirin sodium equivalent to 1 Gm., 2 Gm., 4 Gm., or 20 Gm. cephapirin.

NDC 0015-7628—1-Gm. vial.
NDC 0015-7629—2-Gm. vial.
NDC 0015-7628—1 Gm. "piggy back" vial.
NDC 0015-7629—2 Gm. "piggy back" vial.
NDC 0015-7630—4 Gm. "piggy back" vial.
NDC 0015-7613—20 Gm. hospital bulk package.

*Bauer, A. W., Kirby, W. M. M., Sherris, J. C., and Turck, M.: Antibiotic Testing by a Standardized Single Disc Method, Am. J. Clin. Pathol., 45:493, 1966. Standardized Disc Susceptibility Test, FEDERAL REGISTER 37:20527-29, 1972.

DYNAPEN® ℞

(dicloxacillin sodium)
Capsules-125 mg. and 250 mg.
Dicloxacillin sodium
For Oral Suspension
62.5 mg./5 ml.

This is the full text of the latest Official Package Circular dated February 1978 [7856 DIRO-09].

Description: DYNAPEN (dicloxacillin Sodium monohydrate) is an antibacterial agent of the isoxazolyl penicillin series. It is the monohydrate sodium salt of 3-(2, 6-dichlorophenyl)-5-methyl-4-isoxazolyl penicillin. The drug resists destruction by the enzyme penicillinase (beta-lactamase). It has been demonstrated to be especially efficacious in the treatment of penicillinase-producing staphylococcal infections and effective in the treatment of other commonly encountered Gram-positive coccal infections.

Pharmacology: DYNAPEN (dicloxacillin sodium) is resistant to destruction by acid and is exceptionally well absorbed from the gastrointestinal tract. Oral administration of dicloxacillin gives blood levels considerably in excess of those attained with equivalent doses of any other presently available oral penicillin. The levels are comparable to those achieved with intramuscular administration of similar doses of penicillin G. Studies[1] with an oral dose of 125 mg. gave average serum levels at 60 minutes of 4.74 mcg./ml. At four hours, average levels were 0.62 mcg./ml. The 125 mg. dose gave peak blood levels 5 times higher than those of 250 mg. of penicillin G and 2 to 4 times higher than those of 250 mg. of Penicillin V Potassium. Serum levels after oral administration are directly proportional to dosage at unit doses of 125, 250, 500, and 1000 mg.[1,2,3] as measured at the two-hour level.

Actions (Microbiology): DYNAPEN (dicloxacillin sodium) is active against most Gram-positive cocci including beta-hemolytic streptococci, pneumococci, and susceptible staphylococci. Because of its resistance to the enzyme penicillinase, it is active against penicillinase-producing staphylococci.

The average Minimal Inhibitory Concentrations (M.I.C.'s) of DYNAPEN (dicloxacillin sodium) for these organisms are as follows:

	Average M.I.C. (mcg./ml.)
Group A beta-hemolytic streptococcus	0.05
Diplococcus pneumoniae	0.10
Staphylococcus (nonpenicillinase-producing)	0.20
Staphylococcus (penicillinase-producing)	0.30

Disc Susceptibility Tests

Quantitative methods that require measurement of zone diameters give the most precise estimates of antibiotic susceptibility. One such procedure* has been recommended for use with discs for testing susceptibility to methicillin class antibiotics. Interpretations correlate diameters on the disc test with MIC values for methicillin. With this procedure, a report from the laboratory of "susceptible" indicates that the infecting organism is likely to respond to therapy. A report of "resistant" indicates that the infecting organism is not likely to respond to therapy. A report of "intermediate susceptibility" suggests that the organism would be susceptible if high dosage is used, or if the infection is confined to tissues and fluids (e.g., urine), in which high antibiotic levels are attained.

Indications: Although the principal indication for dicloxacillin sodium is in the treatment of infections due to penicillinase-producing staphylococci, it may be used to initiate therapy in such patients in whom a staphylococcal infection is suspected. (See Important Note below.)

Bacteriologic studies to determine the causative organisms and their susceptibility to dicloxacillin sodium should be performed.

In serious, life-threatening infections, oral preparations of the penicillinase-resistant penicillins should not be relied on for initial therapy.

Important Note: When it is judged necessary that treatment be initiated before definitive culture and susceptibility results are known, the choice of dicloxacillin sodium should take into consideration the fact that it has been shown to be effective only in the treatment of infections caused by pneumococci, Group A beta-hemolytic streptococci, and penicillin G-resistant and penicillin G-susceptible staphylococci. If the bacteriology report later indicates the infection is due to an organism other than a penicillin G-resistant staphylococcus susceptible to dicloxacillin sodium, the physician is advised to continue therapy with a drug other than dicloxacillin sodium or any other penicillinase-resistant semi-synthetic penicillin.

Recent studies have reported that the percentage of staphylococcal isolates resistant to penicillin G outside the hospital is increasing, approximating the high percentage of resistant staphylococcal isolates found in the hospital. For this reason, it is recommended that a penicillinase-resistant penicillin be used as initial therapy for any suspected staphylococcal infection until culture and susceptibility results are known.

Dicloxacillin sodium is a compound that acts through a mechanism similar to that of methicillin against penicillin G-resistant staphylococci. Strains of staphylococci resistant to methicillin have existed in nature and it is known that the number of these strains reported has been increasing. Such strains of staphylococci have been capable of producing serious disease, in some instances resulting in fatality. Because of this, there is concern that widespread use of the penicillinase-resistant penicillins may result in the appearance of an increasing number of staphylococcal strains which are resistant to these penicillins.

Methicillin-resistant strains are almost always resistant to all other penicillinase-resistant penicillins (cross resistance with cephalosporin derivatives also occurs frequently). Resistance to any penicillinase-resistant penicillin should be interpreted as evidence of clinical resistance to all, in spite of the fact that minor variations in **in vitro** susceptibility may be encountered when more than one penicillinase-resistant penicillin is tested against the same strain of staphylococcus.

Contraindications: A history of allergic reactions to penicillins or cephalosporins should be considered a contraindication.

Precautions: As with any penicillin, a careful inquiry about sensitivity or allergic reactions to penicillins, cephalosporins, or other allergens should be made before the drug is prescribed. Allergic reactions are more likely to occur in hypersensitive individuals. Should an allergic reaction occur during therapy, the drug should be discontinued and the patient treated with the usual agents (epinephrine, corticosteroids, antihistamines).

As with other agents capable of altering flora, the possibility of superinfection with mycotic organisms or other pathogens exists during the periods of use of this drug. Should superinfection occur, appropriate treatment should be initiated and discontinuation of dicloxacillin therapy should be considered.

As with any potent drug, periodic assessment of organ system function, including renal, hepatic, and hematopoietic systems, is strongly recommended.

Experience in the neonatal period is limited. Therefore, a dose for the newborn is not recommended at this time.

Safety for use in pregnancy has not been established.

Adverse Reactions: Gastrointestinal disturbances such as nausea, vomiting, epigastric discomfort, flatulence, and loose stools have been noted in some patients receiving DYNAPEN (dicloxacillin sodium). Pruritus, urticaria, skin rashes, and allergic symptoms have been occasionally encountered, as with all penicillins. Mildly elevated SGOT levels (less than 100 units) have been reported in a few patients for whom pretherapeutic determinations were not made. Minor changes in the results of cephalin flocculation tests have been noted without other evidence of hepatic dysfunction. Eosinophilia, with or without overt allergic manifestations, has been noted in some patients during therapy.

Dosage: For mild-to-moderate upper respiratory and localized skin and soft tissue infections due to susceptible organisms:

Adults and children weighing 40 Kg. (88 lbs.) or more: 125 mg. q.6h.

Children weighing less than 40 Kg. (88 lbs.): 12.5 mg./Kg./day in equally-divided doses q.6h.

For more severe infections such as those of the lower respiratory tract or disseminated infections:

Adults and children weighing 40 Kg. (88 lbs.) or more: 250 mg. q.6h. or higher.

Children weighing less than 40 Kg. (88 lbs.): 25 mg./Kg./day or higher in equally-divided doses q.6h.

Experience in the neonatal period is limited. Therefore, a dose for the newborn is not recommended at this time.

Studies indicate that this material is best absorbed when taken on an empty stomach, preferably one to two hours before meals.

N.B. INFECTIONS CAUSED BY GROUP A BETA-HEMOLYTIC STREPTOCOCCI SHOULD BE TREATED FOR AT LEAST 10 DAYS TO HELP PREVENT THE OCCURRENCE OF ACUTE RHEUMATIC FEVER OR ACUTE GLOMERULONEPHRITIS.

Directions for Dispensing Oral Suspension: Prepare these formulations at the time of dispensing. For ease in preparation, add water to the bottle in two portions and shake well after each addition. Add the total amount of water as directed on the labeling of the package being dispensed. The reconstituted formulation is stable for 14 days under refrigeration.

References:

1. Data on file at Bristol Laboratories.
2. Bennett, J.V., Gravenkemper, C.F., Brodie, J.L., and Kirby, W.M.M., "Dicloxacillin, a New Antibiotic: Clinical Studies and Laboratory Comparisons with Oxacillin and Cloxacillin." Antimicrobial Agents and Chemotherapy, 1964, pp. 257-262.
3. Naumann, P. and Kempf, E., "Dicloxacillin, a New Acid and Penicillinase Stable Oral Penicillin." Arzneimittel-Forschung, **15**, pp. 139-145, 1965.

Supply: DYNAPEN (dicloxacillin sodium) for Oral Suspension, 62.5 mg per 5 ml.

NDC 0015-7856—80 ml, 100 ml and 200 ml bottles

DYNAPEN (dicloxacillin sodium) Capsules. Each capsule contains dicloxacillin sodium equivalent to 125 or 250 mg dicloxacillin.

NDC 0015-7892-125 mg
NDC 0015-7893-250 mg
NDC 0015-7658-500 mg

For information on package sizes available, refer to the current price sheet.

[*Shown in Product Identification Section*]

*Bauer, A. W., Kirby, W. M. M., Sherris J. C. and Turck, M.: Antibiotic Testing by a Standardized Single Disc Method, Am. J. Clin. Pathol., 45:493, 1966; Standardized Disc Susceptibility Test, FEDERAL REGISTER 37:20527–29, 1972.

KANTREX® CAPSULES ℞

(kanamycin sulfate)
Not for Systemic Use

This is the full text of the latest Official Package Circular dated January 1978 [3506 DIMO-08].

Description: Kanamycin sulfate is a water soluble aminoglycoside antibiotic derived from **Streptomyces kanamyceticus**. It is supplied in oral formulation for topical effect within the gastrointestinal tract, because it is absorbed only very slightly when administered orally, and is excreted unchanged in the feces.

Actions: Kanamycin is poorly absorbed from the normal gastrointestinal tract. The small absorbed fraction is rapidly excreted with normal kidney function. The unabsorbed portion of the drug is eliminated unchanged in the feces.

Most intestinal bacteria are eliminated rapidly following oral administration of kanamycin,

Continued on next page

Bristol—Cont.

with bacterial suppression persisting for 48 to 72 hours.

Indications:

Suppression of Intestinal Bacteria—Kanamycin is indicated when supression of the normal bacterial flora of the bowel is desirable for short-term adjunctive therapy.

Hepatic Coma—Prolonged administration has been shown to be effective adjunctive therapy in **Hepatic Coma** by reduction of the ammonia-forming bacteria in the intestinal tract. The subsequent reduction in blood ammonia has resulted in neurologic improvement.

Contraindications: This drug is contraindicated in the presence of intestinal obstruction and in individuals with a history of hypersensitivity to the drug.

Warnings: Although negligible amounts of kanamycin are absorbed through intact intestinal mucosa (approximately 1 percent), the possibility of increased absorption from ulcerated or denuded areas should be considered. If renal insufficiency develops during treatment, the dosage should be reduced or the antibiotic discontinued. Urine and blood examinations and audiometric tests should be given prior to and during extended therapy in individuals with hepatic and/or renal disease.

Usage in Pregnancy: Safety for use in pregnancy has not been established.

Precautions: Caution should be taken in concurrent use of other ototoxic and/or nephrotoxic antimicrobial drugs while kanamycin is administered orally. These include streptomycin, neomycin, polymyxin B, colistin, viomycin, gentamicin, and cephaloridine.

The concurrent use of potent diuretics (e.g. ethacrynic acid, furosemide, and mannitol, particularly when the diuretics are given intravenously) should be avoided. They may cause cumulative adverse effects of the kanamycin on the kidney and auditory nerve.

Prolonged use of oral kanamycin may result in overgrowth of nonsusceptible organisms, particularly fungi. If this occurs, appropriate therapy should be instituted.

Adverse Reactions: The most common adverse reactions to oral kanamycin are nausea, vomiting, and diarrhea. The "Malabsorption Syndrome" characterized by increased fecal fat, decreased serum carotene, and fall in xylose absorption has been reported with prolonged therapy. Nephrotoxicity and ototoxicity have been reported following prolonged and high dosage therapy in hepatic coma.

Dosage and Administration For Oral Use Only:

Suppression of Intestinal Bacteria:

1. As an adjunct in therapy of Hepatic Coma for extended therapy: 8 to 12 Gm. per day in divided doses.
2. As an adjunct to mechanical cleansing of the large bowel in short term therapy: 1.0 Gm. (2 capsules) every hour for 4 hours followed by 1.0 Gm. (2 capsules) every 6 hours for 36 to 72 hours.

Duration of therapy within this range depends on the condition of the patient, the type and amount of concurrent mechanical cleansing (catharsis and enemas), and the customary medical routine.

Supply: KANTREX (kanamycin sulfate) Capsules. Kanamycin sulfate equivalent to 500 mg kanamycin per capsule.

NDC 0015-3506—500mg

For information on package sizes available, refer to the current price schedule.

[*Shown in Product Identification Section*]

KANTREX® INJECTION ℞
(kanamycin sulfate injection)
500 mg. per 2 ml.; 1.0 Gm. per 3 ml.

KANTREX® PEDIATRIC INJECTION ℞
(kanamycin sulfate injection)
75 mg. per 2 ml.

This is the full text of the latest Official Package Circular dated November 1978 [3502DIR-09].

WARNING

Patients treated with aminoglycosides by any route should be under close clinical observation because of the potential toxicity associated with their use. As with other aminoglycosides, the major toxic effects of kanamycin sulfate are its action on the auditory and vestibular branches of the eighth nerve and the renal tubules. Loss of high frequency perception usually occurs before clinical hearing loss and can be detected by audiometric testing. There may not be clinical symptoms to warn of developing cochlear damage. Vertigo may occur and may be evidence of vestibular injury. Renal impairment may be characterized by decreased creatinine clearance, the presence of cells or casts, oliguria, proteinuria, decreased urine specific gravity, or evidence of increasing nitrogen retention (increasing BUN, NPN or serum creatinine).

In patients with impaired kidney function, the risks of severe ototoxic and nephrotoxic reactions are sharply increased. In such cases, either the total daily dosage should be reduced, or the interval between doses lengthened, or both. Assessment of renal function and audiograms should be obtained before treatment if possible and monitored frequently during the course of therapy (see "Precautions"). If there is evidence of progressive renal dysfunction (increasing NPN, BUN, serum creatinine or oliguria) during therapy, audiometric tests are advised and discontinuation of the drug should be considered.

Elderly patients, patients with preexisting tinnitus or vertigo or known subclinical deafness, those having received prior ototoxic drugs, and patients receiving a total dose of more than 15 g of kanamycin sulfate should be carefully observed for signs of eighth nerve damage. Loss of hearing may occur in such patients even with normal renal function.

Neuromuscular blockade with respiratory paralysis may occur when kanamycin sulfate is administered intraperitoneally concomitantly with anesthesia and muscle-relaxing drugs. Although there have been isolated reports of respiratory depression following intraperitoneal instillation of kanamycin, there is no conclusive proof that this side effect can be produced with recommended doses of the drug.

The concurrent and or sequential systemic or topical use of kanamycin and other potentially ototoxic, nephrotoxic, and or neurotoxic drugs, particularly streptomycin, polymyxin B, colistin, neomycin, gentamicin, cephaloradine, paromomycin, tobramycin, amikacin, vancomycin and viomycin should be avoided because the toxicity may be additive.

Kanamycin sulfate should not be given concurrently with potent diuretics (ethacrynic acid, furosemide, meralluride sodium, sodium mercaptomerin, or mannitol). Some diuretics themselves cause ototoxicity, and intravenously administered diuretics may enhance aminoglycoside toxicity by altering antibiotic concentrations in serum and tissue.

Description: Kanamycin sulfate is an aminoglycoside antibiotic produced by **Streptomyces kanamyceticus.** It is $C_{18}H_{36}N_4O_{11} \cdot 2H_2$- SO_4·D - Streptomine, 0-3-amino-3-deoxy-α-D- glucopyranosyl— (1→6) - 0-[6-amino-6-deoxy- α-D-glucopyranosyl-(1→4)]-2-deoxy, sulfate 1:2 (salt). It consists of two amino sugars glycosidically linked to deoxystreptamine.

Kanamycin sulfate injection, sterile solution for parenteral administration, contains respectively: kanamycin sulfate 75 mg, 500 mg, and 1 g; sodium bisulfite, an antioxidant, 0.099%, 0.66%, and 0.45%, and sodium citrate, 0.33%, 2.2%, and 2.2% with pH of each dosage form adjusted to 4.5 with sulfuric acid.

Action:

Clinical Pharmacology

The drug is rapidly absorbed after intramuscular injection and peak serum levels are generally reached within approximately one hour. Doses of 7.5 mg/Kg give mean peak levels of 22 mcg/ml. At 8 hours following a 7.5 mg/Kg dose, mean serum levels are 3.2 mcg/ml. Intravenous administration of kanamycin over a period of one hour resulted in serum concentrations similar to those obtained by intramuscular administration.

Kanamycin diffuses rapidly into most body fluids including synovial and peritoneal fluids and bile. Significant levels of the drug appear in cord blood and amniotic fluid following intramuscular administration to pregnant patients. Spinal fluid concentrations in normal infants are approximately 10 to 20 percent of serum levels and may reach 50 percent when the meninges are inflamed.

Studies in normal adult patients have shown only trace levels of kanamycin in spinal fluid. No data are available on adults with meningitis.

The drug is excreted almost entirely by glomerular filtration and is not reabsorbed by the renal tubules. Hence, high concentrations are attained in the nephron, and the urine may contain levels 10 to 20 times higher than those in serum. Renal excretion is extremely rapid. In patients with normal renal function, approximately one-half of the administered dose is cleared within 4 hours and excretion is complete within 24 to 48 hours. Patients with impaired renal function or with diminished glomerular filtration pressure excrete kanamycin more slowly. Such patients may build up excessively high blood levels which greatly increase the risk of ototoxic reactions.

Microbiology

Kanamycin sulfate is a bactericidal antibiotic which acts by inhibiting the synthesis of protein in susceptible microorganisms. Kanamycin sulfate is active **in vitro** against many strains of **Staphylococcus aureus** (including penicillinase and nonpenicillinase-producing strains). **Staphylococcus epidermidis, N. gonorrhoeae, H. influenzae, E. coli, Enterobacter aerogenes,** Shigella, Salmonella, **K. pneumoniae, Serratia marcescens, Acinetobacter,** and many strains of both indole-positive and indole-negative **Proteus** that are frequently resistant to other antibiotics. Bacterial resistance to kanamycin develops slowly in most susceptible organisms. **In vitro** studies have demonstrated that an aminoglycoside combined with an antibiotic which interferes with cell wall synthesis (i.e., penicillins or cephalosporins) acts synergistically against some strains of Gram-negative organisms and enterococci (**Streptococcus faecalis**).

Susceptibility testing: The infecting organism should be cultured and its susceptibility demonstrated as a guide to therapy. If the Kirby-Bauer method of disc susceptibility is used, a 30-mcg kanamycin disc should give a zone of inhibition of 17 mm or more when tested against a kanamycin-susceptible bacterial strain. A zone of 16 mm or less indicates that the infecting organism is likely to be resistant. In certain conditions, it may be desirable to do additional susceptibility testing by the tube or

Agar dilution method. Kanamycin reference standard is available for this purpose.

Indications and Usage: Kanamycin is indicated in the treatment of serious infections caused by susceptible strains of microorganisms. Bacteriological studies to identify the causative organisms and to determine their susceptibility to kanamycin should be performed. Therapy may be instituted prior to obtaining the results of susceptibility testing. Kanamycin may be considered as initial therapy in the treatment of infections where one or more of the following are the known or suspected pathogens: **E. coli, Proteus** species (both indole-positive and indole-negative), **Enterobacter aerogenes, Klebsiella pneumoniae, Serratia marcescens, Acinetobacter.** The decision to continue therapy with the drug should be based on results of the susceptibility tests, the response of the infection to therapy, and the important additional concepts contained in the "Warning" box above.

In serious infections when the causative organisms are unknown, Kantrex may be administered as initial therapy in conjunction with a penicillin- or cephalosporin-type drug before obtaining results of susceptibility testing. If anerobic organisms are suspected, consideration should be given to using other suitable antimicrobial therapy in conjunction with kanamycin.

Although kanamycin is not the drug of choice for staphylococcal infections, it may be indicated under certain conditions for the treatment of known or suspected staphylococcal disease. These situations include the initial therapy of severe infections where the organism is thought to be either a Gram-negative bacterium or a staphylococcus, infections due to susceptible strains of staphylococci in patients allergic to other antibiotics, and mixed staphylococcal/Gram-negative infections.

Contraindications: A history of hypersensitivity or toxic reaction to one aminoglycoside may also contraindicate the use of any other aminoglycoside, because of the known cross-sensitivity and cumulative effects of drugs in this category.

THIS DRUG IS NOT INDICATED IN LONG-TERM THERAPY (e.g. Tuberculosis) BECAUSE OF THE TOXIC HAZARD ASSOCIATED WITH EXTENDED ADMINISTRATION.

Warning: See "Warning" box above.

Precautions:

Ototoxicity: In patients with renal dysfunction an audiogram should be obtained before treatment and repeated frequently during therapy. Therapy should be stopped if tinnitus or subjective hearing loss develops, or if follow-up audiograms show loss of high frequency perception.

It should be emphasized that since renal function may alter appreciably during therapy, the serum creatinine should be checked daily or more frequently. Changes in the concentration would, of course, necessitate changes in the dosage frequency.

Nephrotoxicity: Because of the high concentration of kanamycin sulfate in the urinary excretory system, patients should be well-hydrated to prevent chemical irritation of the renal tubules. Kidney function should be assessed by the usual methods, e.g., urinalysis, BUN, serum creatinine, prior to starting therapy and periodically during the course of treatment. If signs of renal irritation appear, such as casts, white or red cells, and albumin, hydration should be increased and a reduction in dosage may be desirable (see "Dosage and Administration"). These signs usually disappear when treatment is completed. However, if azotemia or a progressive decrease in urine output occurs, treatment should be stopped.

The possibility of neuromuscular blockade with respiratory paralysis should be considered if aminoglycosides are administered by any route in patients receiving anesthetics, in patients receiving neuromuscular-blocking agents such as tubocurarine, succinylcholine, decamethonium or in patients receiving massive transfusions of citrate-anticoagulated blood. In all cases, patients should be observed carefully for signs of respiratory depression. If blockade occurs, calcium salts or neostigmine may reverse this phenomenon.

NOTE: The risk of toxic reactions is low in well-hydrated patients with normal kidney function, who receive a total dose of 15 g of kanamycin or less.

Because of the possibility of additive effects of other potentially ototoxic, neurotoxic, and/or nephrotoxic drugs, the concurrent or sequential administration of these drugs with kanamycin sulfate should be avoided (see "Warning" box).

Increased nephrotoxicity has been reported following concomitant parenteral administration of aminoglycoside antibiotics and cephalothin.

Since kanamycin sulfate and methicillin inactivate each other in vitro, they should not be physically mixed together in the same solution intended for parenteral administration. However, this inactivation has not been demonstrated in patients who receive both drugs by different routes of administration. (See "Dosage and Administration.")

Elderly patients may have reduced renal function which may not be evident in the results of routine screening tests, such as BUN or serum creatinine. A creatinine clearance determination may be more helpful. Monitoring of renal function during treatment is particularly important in such patients.

Aminoglycosides should be used with caution in patients with myasthenia gravis since these drugs may aggrevate muscle weakness because of their curare-like effect on the neuromuscular function.

Kanamycin sulfate should not be given concurrently with potent diuretics (see "Warning" box).

Neurotoxic and nephrotoxic antibiotics may be absorbed from body surfaces after local irrigation or application. The potential toxic effect of aminoglycosides administered in this fashion should be considered (see "Warning" box).

Cross-allergenicity among aminoglycosides has been demonstrated.

As with other antibiotics, kanamycin sulfate administration may result in overgrowth of nonsusceptible organisms, including fungi. If superinfection occurs, appropriate therapy should be instituted.

Pregnancy:

Reproduction studies have been performed in rats and rabbits and have revealed no evidence of impaired fertility or teratogenic effects. Dosages of 200 mg/Kg/day in pregnant rats and pregnant guinea pigs led to hearing impairment in the offspring. There are no well-controlled studies in pregnant women but clinical experience does not include any positive evidence of adverse effects on the fetus. Although there is no clearly defined risk, such experience cannot exclude the possibility of infrequent or subtle damage to the fetus. Kantrex should be used in pregnant women only when clearly needed.

Adverse Reactions:

Nephrotoxicity—Albuminuria, presence of red and white cells, and granular casts; azotemia and oliguria have been reported.

Ototoxicity—Tinnitus, vertigo, and partial reversible to irreversible hearing loss have been reported, usually associated with higher than recommended dosage. Rapid development of hearing loss has been reported in patients with poor kidney function treated concurrently with kanamycin and one of the rapid-acting diuretic agents given intravenously. These have included ethacrynic acid, furosemide, and mannitol.

Other—Some local irritation or pain may follow intramuscular injection. Other adverse reactions of the drug reported on rare occasions are skin rash, drug fever, headache, and paresthesia.

Overdosage: In the event of overdosage or toxic reaction, hemodialysis or peritoneal dialysis will aid in the removal of kanamycin from the blood. In the newborn infant, exchange transfusions may also be considered.

Dosage and Administration:

Intramuscular Route: Inject deeply into the upper outer quadrant of the gluteal muscle. The recommended dose for adults or children is 15 mg/Kg/day in two equally divided dosages administered at equally divided intervals, i.e. 7.5 mg/Kg q12h. If continuously high blood levels are desired, the daily dose of 15 mg/Kg may be given in equally divided doses every 6 or 8 hours. Treatment of patients in the heavier weight classes, i.e. >100 Kg, should not exceed 1.5 g/day.

In patients with impaired renal function, it is desirable to follow therapy by appropriate serum assays. If this is not feasible, a suggested method is to reduce the frequency of administration in patients with renal dysfunction. The interval between doses may be calculated with the following formula:

Serum creatinine (mg/100 ml) $\times$ 9 = Dosage Interval (in hours): e.g., if the serum creatinine is 2 mg, the recommended dose (7.5 mg/Kg) should be administered every 18 hours. Changes in creatinine concentration during therapy would, of course, necessitate changes in the dosage frequency.

The usual duration of treatment is 7 to 10 days. The total daily dose by all routes of administration should not exceed 1.5 g/day.

At the recommended dosage level, uncomplicated infections due to kanamycin-susceptible organisms should respond to therapy in 24 to 48 hours. If definite clinical response does not occur within 3 to 5 days, therapy should be stopped and the antibiotic susceptibility pattern of the invading organism should be rechecked. Failure of the infection to respond may be due to resistance of the organism or to the presence of septic foci requiring surgical drainage.

Intravenous Administration: The dose should not exceed 15 mg/Kg per day and must be administered slowly. The solution for intravenous use is prepared by adding the contents of a 500-mg vial to 100 to 200 ml of sterile diluent such as Normal Saline or 5% Dextrose in Water, or the contents of a 1 g vial to 200 to 400 ml of sterile diluent. The appropriate dose is administered over a 30- to 60-minute period. The total daily dose should be divided into two or three equally divided doses.

In pediatric patients the amount of diluent used should be sufficient to infuse the kanamycin sulfate over a 30- to 60-minute period.

Kanamycin sulfate injection should not be physically mixed with other antibacterial agents but each should be administered separately in accordance with its recommended route of administration and dosage schedule.

Intraperitoneal Use: (following exploration for established peritonitis or after peritoneal contamination due to fecal spill during surgery.)

Adults: 500 mg diluted in 20 ml sterile distilled water may be instilled through a polyethylene catheter sutured into the wound at closure. If possible, instillation should be postponed until the patient has fully recovered from the effects of anesthesia and muscle-relaxing drugs (see "Warning" box).

Aerosol Treatment: 250 mg two to four times a day. Withdraw 250 mg (1 ml) from 500-mg vial and dilute it with 3 ml Physiological Saline and nebulize.

Other Routes of Administration: Kantrex Injection in concentrations of 0.25 percent (2.5 mg/ml) has been used as an irrigating solution

Continued on next page

Bristol—Cont.

in abscess cavities, pleural space, peritoneal and ventricular cavities. Possible absorption of Kantrex by such routes must be taken into account and dosage adjustments should be arranged so that a maximum total dose of 1.5 g/day by all routes of administration is not exceeded.

PEDIATRIC DOSAGE GUIDE FOR KANTREX PEDIATRIC INJECTION, 75 mg/2 ml—
AMOUNT PER 24 HOURS
TO BE GIVEN IN DIVIDED DOSES

Weight in Pounds	Weight in Kilograms	Daily Dosage in Milligrams	Daily Dosage in Milliliters
2.2	1.00	15.0	0.4
2.8	1.25	18.8	0.5
3.3	1.50	22.5	0.6
3.9	1.75	26.2	0.7
4.4	2.00	30.0	0.8
5.0	2.25	33.8	0.9
5.5	2.50	37.5	1.0
6.0	2.75	41.2	1.1
6.6	3.00	45.0	1.2
7.7	3.50	52.5	1.4
8.8	4.00	60.0	1.6
9.9	4.50	67.5	1.8
11.0	5.00	75.0	2.0

Stability: Occasionally, some vials may darken during the shelf-life of the product, but this does not indicate a loss of potency.

How Supplied: KANTREX INJECTION (kanamycin sulfate injection)

NDC 0015-3502-20—500 mg per 2 ml
NDC 0015-3502-24—Disposable Syringe (500 mg per 2 ml)
NDC 0015-3503-20—1 g per 3 ml

KANTREX PEDIATRIC INJECTION (kanamycin sulfate injection)

NDC 0015-3512-20—75 mg per 2 ml
(activity assayed as kanamycin base)

KETAJECT® ℞
(ketamine hydrochloride injection)

This is the full text of the latest Official Package Circular dated June 1976 [8340 DIRO-01].

SPECIAL NOTE

EMERGENCE REACTIONS HAVE OCCURRED IN APPROXIMATELY 12 PERCENT OF PATIENTS.

THE PSYCHOLOGICAL MANIFESTATIONS VARY IN SEVERITY BETWEEN PLEASANT DREAM-LIKE STATES, VIVID IMAGERY, HALLUCINATIONS, AND EMERGENCE DELIRIUM. IN SOME CASES THESE STATES HAVE BEEN ACCOMPANIED BY CONFUSION, EXCITEMENT, AND IRRATIONAL BEHAVIOR WHICH A FEW PATIENTS RECALL AS AN UNPLEASANT EXPERIENCE. THE DURATION ORDINARILY LASTS NO MORE THAN A FEW HOURS; IN A FEW CASES, HOWEVER, RECURRENCES HAVE TAKEN PLACE UP TO 24 HOURS POSTOPERATIVELY. NO RESIDUAL PSYCHOLOGICAL EFFECTS ARE KNOWN TO HAVE RESULTED FROM USE OF KETAJECT.

THE INCIDENCE OF THESE EMERGENCE PHENOMENA IS LEAST IN THE YOUNG (15 YEARS OF AGE OR LESS) AND ELDERLY (OVER 65 YEARS OF AGE) PATIENT. ALSO, THEY ARE LESS FREQUENT WHEN THE DRUG IS GIVEN INTRAMUSCULARLY.

THESE REACTIONS MAY BE REDUCED IF VERBAL, TACTILE, AND VISUAL STIMULATION OF THE PATIENT IS MINIMIZED DURING THE RECOVERY PERIOD. THIS DOES NOT PRECLUDE THE MONITORING OF VITAL SIGNS. IN ADDITION, THE USE OF A SMALL HYPNOTIC DOSE OF A SHORT-ACTING OR ULTRASHORT-ACTING BARBITURATE MAY BE REQUIRED TO TERMINATE A SEVERE EMERGENCE REACTION. THE INCIDENCE OF EMERGENCE REACTIONS IS REDUCED AS EXPERIENCE WITH THE DRUG IS GAINED.

WHEN KETAJECT IS USED ON AN OUTPATIENT BASIS, THE PATIENT SHOULD NOT BE RELEASED UNTIL RECOVERY FROM ANESTHESIA IS COMPLETE AND THEN SHOULD BE ACCOMPANIED BY A RESPONSIBLE ADULT.

Description: Ketaject is a nonbarbiturate anesthetic chemically designated *dl* 2-(o-chlorophenyl)-2-(methylamino) cyclohexanone hydrochloride. It is formulated as a slightly acid (pH 3.5 to 5.5) solution for intravenous or intramuscular injection in concentrations containing the equivalent of either 10, 50, or 100 mg. ketamine base per milliliter and contains 0.1 mg./ml. Phemerol® (benzethonium chloride) as a preservative. The 10 mg./ml. solution has been made isotonic with sodium chloride.

Action: Ketaject is a rapid-acting general anesthetic producing an anesthetic state characterized by profound analgesia, normal pharyngeal-laryngeal reflexes, normal or slightly enhanced skeletal muscle tone, cardiovascular and respiratory stimulation; and occasionally a transient and minimal respiratory depression.

A patent airway is maintained partly by virtue of unimpaired pharyngeal and laryngeal reflexes. (See Warnings and Precautions.)

The anesthetic state produced by Ketaject has been termed "dissociative anesthesia" in that it appears to selectively interrupt association pathways of the brain before producing somesthetic sensory blockade. It may selectively depress the thalamoneocortical system before significantly obtunding the more ancient cerebral centers and pathways (reticular-activating and limbic systems).

Elevation of blood pressure begins shortly after injection, reaches a maximum within a few minutes, and usually returns to preanesthetic values within 15 minutes after injection. The median peak rise has ranged from 20 to 25% of preanesthetic values.

Ketamine has a wide margin of safety; several instances of unintentional administration of overdoses of Ketaject (up to ten times that usually required) have been followed by prolonged but complete recovery.

Indications:

Ketaject is recommended:

1. as the sole anesthetic agent for diagnostic and surgical procedures that do not require skeletal muscle relaxation. Ketaject is best suited for short procedures but it can be used, with additional doses, for longer procedures.
2. for the induction of anesthesia prior to the administration of other general anesthetic agents.
3. to supplement low-potency agents, such as nitrous oxide.

Specific areas of application are described in the section Clinical Studies.

Contraindications: Ketamine hydrochloride is contraindicated in those in whom a significant elevation of blood pressure would constitute a serious hazard and in those who have shown hypersensitivity to the drug.

Warnings:

1. Ketaject should be used by or under the direction of physicians experienced in administering general anesthetics and in maintenance of an airway and in the control of respiration.
2. Cardiac function should be continually monitored during the procedure in patients found to have hypertension or cardiac decompensation.
3. Barbiturates and Ketaject, being chemically incompatible because of precipitate formation, should not be injected from the same syringe.
4. Prolonged recovery time may occur if barbiturates and/or narcotics are used concurrently with Ketaject.
5. Postoperative confusional states may occur during the recovery period.
6. Respiratory depression may occur with overdosage or too rapid a rate of administration of Ketaject, in which case supportive ventilation should be employed. Mechanical support of respiration is preferred to administration of analeptics.

Usage in Pregnancy: Since the safe use in pregnancy, including obstetrics (either vaginal or abdominal delivery), has not been established, such use is not recommended (see Animal Reproduction).

Precautions:

1. Because pharyngeal and laryngeal reflexes are usually active, Ketaject should not be used alone in surgery or diagnostic procedures of the pharynx, larynx, or bronchial tree. Mechanical stimulation of the pharynx should be avoided, whenever possible, if Ketaject is used alone. Muscle relaxants, with proper attention to respiration, may be required in both of these instances.
2. Resuscitative equipment should be ready for use.
3. **The incidence of emergence reactions may be reduced** if verbal and tactile stimulation of the patient is minimized during the recovery period. This does not preclude the monitoring of vital signs (see Special Note).
4. The intravenous dose should be administered over a period of 60 seconds. More rapid administration may result in respiratory depression or apnea and enhanced pressor response.
5. In surgical procedures involving visceral pain pathways, Ketaject should be supplemented with an agent which obtunds visceral pain.
6. Use with caution in the chronic alcoholic and the acutely alcohol-intoxicated patients.
7. An increase in cerebrospinal fluid pressure has been reported following administration of ketamine hydrochloride. Use with extreme caution in patients with preanesthetic elevated cerebrospinal fluid pressure.

Adverse Reactions:

Cardiovascular: Blood pressure and pulse rate are frequently elevated following administration of Ketaject. However, hypotension and bradycardia have been observed. Arrhythmia has also occurred.

Respiration: Although respiration is frequently stimulated, severe depression of respiration or apnea may occur following rapid intravenous administration of high doses of Ketaject. Laryngospasms and other forms of airway obstruction have occurred during Ketaject anesthesia.

Eye: Diplopia and nystagmus have been noted following Ketaject administration. It also may cause a slight elevation in intraocular pressure measurement.

Psychological: (See Special Note.)

Neurological: In some patients, enhanced skeletal muscle tone may be manifested by tonic and clonic movements sometimes resembling seizures (see Dosage and Administration).

Gastrointestinal: Anorexia, nausea, and vomiting have been observed; however, this is not usually severe and allows the great majority of patients to take liquids by mouth shortly after regaining consciousness (see Dosage and Administration).

General: Local pain and exanthema at the injection site have infrequently been reported. Transient erythema and/or morbilliform rash have also been reported.

Dosage and Administration:

Preoperative Preparations:

1. While vomiting has been reported following Ketaject administration, airway protection is usually afforded because of active laryngeal-pharyngeal reflexes. However, since these reflexes may also be diminished by supplementary anesthetics or muscle relaxants, the possibility of aspiration must be considered. Ketaject is recommended for use in the patient whose stomach is not empty when, in the judgment of the practitioner, the benefits of the drug outweigh the possible risks.
2. Atropine, scopolamine, or other drying agents should be given at an appropriate interval prior to induction.

Dosage: As with other general anesthetic agents, the individual response to Ketaject is somewhat varied depending on the dose, route of administration, and age of patients, so that dosage recommendation cannot be absolutely fixed. The drug should be titrated against the patient's requirements.

Onset and Duration: Because of rapid induction following the initial intravenous injection, the patient should be in a supported position during administration.

The onset of action of Ketaject is rapid; an intravenous dose of 2 mg./Kg. (1 mg./lb.) of body weight usually produces surgical anesthesia within 30 seconds after injection, with the anesthetic effect usually lasting five to ten minutes. If a longer effect is desired, additional increments can be administered intravenously or intramuscularly to maintain anesthesia without producing significant cumulative effects.

Intramuscular doses, from experience primarily in children, in a range of 9 to 13 mg./Kg. (4 to 6 mg./lb.) usually produce surgical anesthesia within 3 to 4 minutes following injection, with the anesthetic effect usually lasting 12 to 25 minutes.

Induction:

Intravenous Route: The initial dose of Ketaject administered intravenously may range from 1 mg./Kg. to 4.5 mg./Kg. (0.5 to 2 mg./lb.). The average amount required to produce five to ten minutes of surgical anesthesia has been 2 mg./Kg. (1 mg./lb.).

NOTE: The 100 mg./ml. concentration of Ketaject should not be injected intravenously without proper dilution. It is recommended the drug be diluted with an equal volume of either Sterile Water for Injection, U.S.P., Normal Saline, or 5% Dextrose in Water.

Rate of Administration: It is recommended that Ketaject be administered slowly (over a period of 60 seconds). More rapid administration may result in respiratory depression and enhanced pressor response.

Intramuscular Route: The initial dose of Ketaject administered intramuscularly may range from 6.5 to 13 mg./Kg. (3 to 6 mg./lb.). A dose of 10 mg./Kg. (5 mg./lb.) will usually produce 12 to 25 minutes of surgical anesthesia.

Maintenance of Anesthesia: Increments of one-half to the full induction dose may be repeated as needed for maintenance of anesthesia. However, it should be noted that purposeless and tonic-clonic movements of extremities may occur during the course of anesthesia. These movements do not imply a light plane and are not indicative of the need for additional doses of the anesthetic.

It should be recognized that the larger the total dose of Ketaject administered the longer will be the time to complete recovery.

Supplementary Agents: Ketaject is clinically compatible with the commonly used general and local anesthetic agents when an adequate respiratory exchange is maintained.

Animal Pharmacology and Toxicology:

Toxicity: The acute toxicity of Ketaject has been studied in several species. In mature mice and rats, the intraperitoneal LD_{50} values are approximately 100 times the average human intravenous dose and approximately 20 times the average human intramuscular dose. A slightly higher acute toxicity observed in neonatal rats was not sufficiently elevated to suggest an increased hazard when used in children. Daily intravenous injections in rats of five times the average human intravenous dose and intramuscular injections in dogs at four times the average human intramuscular dose demonstrated excellent tolerance for as long as six weeks. Similarly, twice weekly anesthetic sessions of one, three, or six hours duration in monkeys over a four-to-six week period were well tolerated.

Interaction With Other Drugs Commonly Used for Preanesthetic Medication: Large doses (three or more times the equivalent effective human dose) of morphine, meperidine, and atropine increased the depth and prolonged the duration of anesthesia produced by a standard anesthetizing dose of Ketaject in Rhesus monkeys. The prolonged duration was not of sufficient magnitude to contraindicate the use of these drugs for preanesthetic medication in human clinical trials.

Blood Pressure: Blood pressure responses to Ketaject vary with the laboratory species and experimental conditions. Blood pressure is increased in normotensive and renal hypertensive rats with and without adrenalectomy and under pentobarbital anesthesia.

Intravenous Ketaject produces a fall in arterial blood pressure in the Rhesus monkey and a rise in arterial blood pressure in the dog. In this respect the dog mimics the cardiovascular effect observed in man. The pressor response to Ketaject injected into intact, unanesthetized dogs is accompanied by a tachycardia, rise in cardiac output, and a fall in total peripheral resistance. It causes a fall in perfusion pressure following a large dose injected into an artificially perfused vascular bed (dog hindquarters), and it has little or no potentiating effect upon vasoconstriction responses of epinephrine or norepinephrine. The pressor response to Ketaject is reduced or blocked by chlorpromazine (central depressant and peripheral α-adrenergic blockade), by β-adrenergic blockade, and by ganglionic blockade. The tachycardia and increase in myocardial contractile force seen in intact animals does not appear in isolated hearts (Langendorff) at a concentration of 0.1 mg. of Ketaject nor in Starling dog heart-lung preparations at a Ketaject concentration of 50 mg./Kg. of HLP. These observations support the hypothesis that the hypertension produced by Ketaject is due to selective activation of central cardiac stimulating mechanisms leading to an increase in cardiac output. The dog myocardium is not sensitized to epinephrine and Ketaject appears to have a weak antiarrhythmic activity.

Metabolic Disposition: Ketaject is rapidly absorbed following parenteral administration. Animal experiments indicated that Ketaject was rapidly distributed in body tissues, with relatively high concentrations appearing in body fat, liver, lung, and brain; lower concentrations were found in the heart, skeletal muscle, and blood plasma. Placental transfer of the drug was found to occur in pregnant dogs and monkeys. No significant degree of binding to serum albumin was found with Ketaject.

Balance studies in rats, dogs, and monkeys resulted in the recovery of 85 to 95% of the dose in the urine, mainly in the form of degradation products. Small amounts of drug were also excreted in the bile and feces. Balance studies with tritium-labeled Ketaject in human subjects (1 mg./lb. given intravenously) resulted in the mean recovery of 91% of the dose in the urine and 3% in the feces. Peak plasma levels averaged about 0.75 μg./ml., and CSF levels were about 0.2 μg./ml., one hour after dosing.

Ketaject undergoes N-demethylation and hydroxylation of the cyclohexanone ring, with the formation of water-soluble conjugates which are excreted in the urine. Further oxidation also occurs with the formation of a cyclohexenone derivative. The unconjugated N-demethylated metabolite was found to be less than one sixth as potent as Ketaject. The unconjugated demethyl cyclohexenone derivative was found to be less than one tenth as potent as Ketaject. Repeated doses of Ketaject administered to animals did not produce any detectable increase in microsomal enzyme activity.

Reproduction: Male and female rats, when given five times the average human intravenous dose of Ketaject for three consecutive days about one week before mating had a reproductive performance equivalent to that of saline-injected controls. When given to pregnant rats and rabbits intramuscularly at twice the average human intramuscular dose during the respective periods of organogenesis, the litter characteristics were equivalent to those of saline-injected controls. A small group of rabbits was given a single large dose (six times the average human dose) of Ketaject on Day 6 of pregnancy to simulate the effect of an excessive clinical dose around the period of nidation. The outcome of pregnancy was equivalent in control and treated groups.

To determine the effect of Ketaject on the perinatal and postnatal period, pregnant rats were given twice the average human intramuscular dose during Days 18 to 21 of pregnancy. Litter characteristics at birth and through the weaning period were equivalent to those of the control animals. There was a slight increase in incidence of delayed parturition by one day in treated dams of this group. Three groups each of mated beagle bitches were given 2.5 times the average human intramuscular dose twice weekly for the three weeks of the first, second, and third trimesters of pregnancy, respectively, without the development of adverse effects in the pups.

Clinical Studies: Ketaject was initially studied in over 12,000 operative and diagnostic procedures, involving over 10,000 patients from 105 separate studies. During the course of these studies Ketaject was administered as the sole agent, as induction for other general agents, or to supplement low-potency agents. Specific areas of application have included the following:

1. debridement, painful dressings, and skin grafting in burn patients, as well as other superficial surgical procedures.
2. neurodiagnostic procedures such as pneumoencephalograms, ventriculograms, myelograms, and lumbar punctures.
3. diagnostic and operative procedures of the eye, ear, nose, and mouth, including dental extractions.
4. diagnostic and operative procedures of the pharynx, larynx, or bronchial tree. NOTE: Muscle relaxants, with proper attention to respiration, may be required (see Precautions).
5. sigmoidoscopy and minor surgery of the anus and rectum, and circumcision.
6. extraperitoneal procedures used in gynecology such as dilatation and curettage.
7. orthopedic procedures such as closed reductions, manipulations, femoral pinning, amputations, and biopsies.
8. as an anesthetic in poor-risk patients with depression of vital functions.
9. in procedures where the intramuscular route of administration is preferred.
10. in cardiac catherization procedures.

In these studies, the anesthesia was rated either "excellent" or "good" by the anesthesiologist and the surgeon at 90 and 93%, respectively; rated "fair" at 6 and 4%, respectively; and rated "poor" at 4 and 3%, respectively. In a second method of evaluation, the anesthesia

Continued on next page

Bristol—Cont.

was rated "adequate" in at least 90%, and "inadequate" in 10% or less of the procedures.

How Supplied: Ketaject is supplied as the hydrochloride in concentrations equivalent to ketamine base.

NDC 0015-8340-27—Each 50-ml. vial contains 10 mg./ml.

NDC 0015-8341-10—Each 10-ml. vial contains 50 mg./ml.

NDC 0015-8343-05—Each 5-ml. vial contains 100 mg./ml.

LYSODREN™ ℞
(mitotane)

This is the full text of the latest Official Package Circular dated August 1978 [3080DIM-01].

> Treatment should be instituted in the hospital until a stable dosage regimen is achieved. Lysodren should be temporarily discontinued immediately following shock or severe trauma since adrenal suppression is its prime action. Exogenous steroids should also be administered in such circumstances, since the depressed adrenal may not immediately start to secrete steroids.

LYSODREN (mitotane) is an oral chemotherapeutic agent.

Description: LYSODREN (mitotane) is best known by its trivial name, o,p'-DDD, and is chemically, 1.1 dichloro-2 (o-chlorophenyl)-2-(p-chlorophenyl) ethane.

LYSODREN is a white granular solid composed of clear colorless crystals.

LYSODREN is tasteless and has a slight pleasant aromatic odor.

Action: LYSODREN (mitotane) can best be described as an adrenal cytotoxic agent, although it can cause adrenal inhibition, apparently without cellular destruction. Its biochemical mechanism of action is unknown. Data are available to suggest that the drug modifies the peripheral metabolism of steroids as well as directly suppressing the adrenal cortex. The administration of LYSODREN alters the extra-adrenal metabolism of cortisol in man, leading to a reduction in measurable 17-hydroxy corticosteroids, even though plasma levels of corticosteroids do not fall. The drug apparently causes increased formation of 6-β-hydroxy cortisol.

Indications: LYSODREN is indicated only in the treatment of inoperable adrenal cortical carcinoma of both functional and non-functional types.

Contraindications: The only contraindication for LYSODREN is known hypersensitivity to the drug.

Warnings: Lysodren should be temporarily discontinued immediately following shock or severe trauma, since adrenal suppression is its prime action. Exogenous steroids should also be administered in such circumstances, since the depressed adrenal may not immediately start to secrete steroids.

LYSODREN should be administered with care to patients with liver disease other than metastatic lesions from the adrenal cortex, since the metabolism of LYSODREN may be interfered with and the drug may accumulate.

All possible tumor tissue should be surgically removed from large metastatic masses before LYSODREN administration is instituted. This is necessary to minimize the possibility of infarction and hemorrhage in the tumor due to a rapid positive effect of the drug.

Long-term continuous administration of high doses of LYSODREN may lead to brain damage and impairment of function. Behavioral and neurological assessments should be made at regular intervals when continuous LYSODREN treatment exceeds two years.

Uses in Pregnancy and Lactation: The safety of LYSODREN in pregnancy or lactation has not been established. Treatment of women who are, or who may become pregnant, should be undertaken only after consideration of the benefits versus the possibility of harm to mother and child.

Precautions: Adrenal insufficiency may develop in patients treated with LYSODREN, and adrenal steroid replacement should be considered for these patients.

Since sedation, lethargy, vertigo, and other CNS side effects can occur, ambulatory patients should be cautioned about driving, operating machinery, and other hazardous pursuits requiring mental and physical alertness.

Adverse Reactions: A very high percentage of patients treated with LYSODREN have shown at least one type of side effect. The main types of adverse reactions consist of the following:

1. Gastrointestinal disturbances, which consisted of anorexia, nausea or vomiting, and in some cases diarrhea, occurred in about 80% of the patients.
2. Central nervous system side effects occurred in 40% of the patients. These consisted primarily of depression as manifested by lethargy and somnolence (25%), and dizziness or vertigo (15%).
3. Skin toxicity was observed in about 15% of the cases. In some instances, however, this side effect subsided while the patients were maintained on drug.

Infrequently occurring side effects involve the eye (visual blurring, diplopia, lens opacity, toxic retinopathy); the genitourinary system (hematuria, hemorrhagic cystitis, and albuminuria); cardiovascular system (hypertension, orthostatic hypotension, and flushing); and some miscellaneous complaints including generalized aching, hyperpyrexia, and lowered PBI.

Dosage and Administration: The recommended treatment schedule is to start the patient at 9-10 grams of LYSODREN per day in divided doses, either q.i.d. or t.i.d. If severe side effects appear, the dose should be reduced until the maximum tolerated dose is achieved. If the patient can tolerate higher doses and improved clinical response appears possible, the dose should be increased until adverse reactions interfere. Experience has shown that the maximum tolerated dose (MTD) will vary from 2-16 grams per day, but has usually been 8-10 grams per day. The highest doses used in the studies to date were 18-19 grams per day.

Treatment should be instituted in the hospital until a stable dosage regimen is achieved.

Treatment should be continued as long as clinical benefits are observed. Maintenance of clinical status or slowing of growth of metastatic lesions can be considered clinical benefits if they can clearly be shown to have occurred.

If no clinical benefits are observed after three months at the maximum tolerated dose, the case may be considered a clinical failure. However, 10% of the patients who showed a measurable response required more than three months at the MTD. Early diagnosis and prompt institution of treatment improve the probability of a positive clinical response.

How Supplied: LYSODREN is available as a 500 mg. scored tablet in bottles of 100.

Animal Studies: Dogs were used for much of the experimental work with LYSODREN (1). Doses as low as 4 mg/kg/day may produce some effects upon the canine adrenals. However, most of the data suggest that toxicity occurs between 80-200 mg/kg/day, primarily as a result of LYSODREN'S effect upon the adrenals. At doses of 100 mg/kg/day and higher of LYSODREN, deaths occurred in some of the dogs after two to four weeks of administration. The primary action of LYSODREN is upon the adrenal cortex. The toxicity observed in animals appears to result from suppression of the activity of the adrenal cortex. The production of adrenal steroids has been shown to be reduced in most of the studies.

A toxicity study was conducted in rats at doses as high as 300 mg/kg/day for 28 days. There were no deaths nor was there any evidence of organ changes in these animals. In this study even the adrenal cortex showed no evidence of change, indicating that the rodent appears to be highly resistant to LYSODREN.

In both dogs and rats, there was a dose-related rise in alkaline phosphatase. In dogs, there were signs of histological changes in the liver at the high doses (50-100 mg/kg/day).

A dose of 300 mg/kg/day administered to guinea pigs resulted in death in one of three animals and reduction in cortisol levels. Death was probably due to adrenal insufficiency (2).

Metabolic Studies of LYSODREN in Man: One study (3) with adrenal carcinoma patients indicated that about 40% of oral LYSODREN was absorbed, and approximately 10% was recovered in the urine as a water-soluble metabolite. A small amount was excreted in the bile and the balance was apparently stored in the tissues. When administered parenterally, approximately 25% of the dose was found in the urine as a water-soluble metabolite.

Blood levels were determined during and following administration of LYSODREN. Both unchanged drug and metabolite were measured. The levels in patients receiving doses from 5-15 grams per day varied from 7-90 micrograms/ml of unchanged LYSODREN and 29-54 micrograms/ml of the metabolite. These studies indicated no relationship between blood levels and therapeutic and/or toxic effects.

Following discontinuation of the drug, LYSODREN blood levels fell, but persisted for several weeks. In most patients blood levels became undetectable after six to nine weeks. In one patient who had received a total of 1900 grams of LYSODREN, high blood levels were found ten weeks after stopping the drug. Autopsy data have provided evidence that LYSODREN is found in most tissues of the body. Fat tissues were the primary site of storage. In one patient a very large number of tissues were examined and the drug was found in essentially every tissue. LYSODREN appears to be converted, in part, to a water-soluble metabolite. This material has not been characterized, but is only found in the urine and blood of patients receiving LYSODREN. Examination of bile was made and found to contain no unchanged LYSODREN. There was metabolite in the bile, and this would indicate that biliary excretion is a significant route of removal of this metabolite from the body.

Clinical Studies: Hutter and Kayhoe (4) reported on the clinical features and the results of LYSODREN treatment of 138 patients with adrenal cortical carcinoma, and compared their findings with 48 treated patients previously reported in the literature. Subsequent to their report, 115 patients given drug were studied. There is no evidence of a cure as a consequence of the administration of LYSODREN. A number of patients have been treated intermittently, treatment being restarted when severe symptoms reappeared. Patients often do not respond after the third or fourth such course. Experience accumulated to date suggests that continuous treatment with the maximum possible dosage of LYSODREN would be the best approach.

A substantial percentage of the patients treated showed signs of adrenal insufficiency. It therefore appears necessary to watch for and institute steroid replacement in those patients. It has been shown that the metabolism of exogenous steroids is modified and consequently somewhat higher doses than just replacement therapy may be required.

There was significant reduction in tumor mass following LYSODREN administration in about

50%, and a significant reduction in elevated steroid excretion in about 80% of the evaluable patients studied to date (4). Clinical effectiveness can be shown by reduction in tumor mass, reduction in pain, weakness or anorexia, and reduction of steroid symptoms.

Bibliography:

1. a) Nelson, A A, Woodward, G: *Archives of Pathology,* 48:387, 1949.
   b) Nichols, J: Studies on an Adrenal Cortical Inhibitor, in *The Adrenal Cortex,* Scranton, Pa. Harper and Row, 1961, p 83.
2. Kupfer, D, *et al: Life Sciences,* 3:959, 1964.
3. Moy, R H: *J Lab Clin Med,* 58:296, 1961.
4. Hutter, A M, Kahoe, D E: *Am J Med,* 41:572 581, 1966.

Manufactured by Anabolic, Inc.
Irvine, California 92664

MEXATE™ ℞

(methotrexate sodium injection)

This is the full text of the latest Official Package Circular dated October, 1979 [3050DIM-04].

WARNING

METHOTREXATE MUST BE USED ONLY BY PHYSICIANS EXPERIENCED IN ANTIMETABOLITE CHEMOTHERAPY.

BECAUSE OF THE POSSIBILITY OF FATAL OR SEVERE TOXIC REACTIONS THE PATIENT SHOULD BE FULLY INFORMED BY THE PHYSICIAN OF THE RISK INVOLVED AND SHOULD BE UNDER HIS CONSTANT SUPERVISION.

DEATHS HAVE BEEN REPORTED WITH THE USE OF METHOTREXATE IN THE TREATMENT OF PSORIASIS, IN THE TREATMENT OF PSORIASIS METHOTREXATE SHOULD BE RESTRICTED TO SEVERE, RECALCITRANT, DISABLING PSORIASIS WHICH IS NOT ADEQUATELY RESPONSIVE TO OTHER FORMS OF THERAPY, BUT ONLY WHEN THE DIAGNOSIS HAS BEEN ESTABLISHED AS BY BIOPSY AND/OR AFTER DERMATOLOGIC CONSULTATION.

1. Methotrexate may produce marked depression of bone marrow, anemia, leukopenia, thrombocytopenia and bleeding.
2. Methotrexate may be hepatotoxic, particularly at high dosage or with prolonged therapy. Liver atrophy, necrosis, cirrhosis, fatty changes, and periportal fibrosis have been reported. Since changes may occur without previous signs of gastrointestinal or hematologic toxicity, it is imperative that hepatic function be determined prior to initiation of treatment and monitored regularly throughout therapy. Special caution is indicated in the presence of preexisting liver damage or impaired hepatic function. Concomitant use of other drugs with hepatotoxic potential (including alcohol) should be avoided.
3. Methotrexate has caused fetal death and/or congenital anomalies, therefore, it is not recommended in women of childbearing potential unless there is appropriate medical evidence that the benefits can be expected to outweigh the considered risks. Pregnant psoriatic patients should not receive Methotrexate.
4. Impaired renal function is usually a contraindication.
5. Diarrhea and ulcerative stomatitis are frequent toxic effects and require interruption of therapy; otherwise hemorrhagic enteritis and death from intestinal perforation may occur.

"METHOTREXATE HAS BEEN ADMINISTERED IN VERY HIGH DOSAGE FOLLOWED BY LEUCOVORIN RESCUE IN EXPERIMENTAL TREATMENT OF CERTAIN NEOPLASTIC DISEASES. THIS PROCEDURE IS INVESTIGATIONAL AND HAZARDOUS."

Description: Methotrexate is an antimetabolite used in the treatment of certain neoplastic diseases.

Methotrexate Sodium Parenteral is available in 20, 50, and 100 mg strenths, each available as lyophilized powder in vials, containing no preservatives, for single use only.

Each 20 mg vial contains Methotrexate, 20 mg, prepared as the sodium salt; sodium hydroxide to adjust pH to about 8.5.

Each 50 mg vial contains Methotrexate, 50 mg, prepared as the sodium salt; sodium hydroxide to adjust pH to about 8.5.

Each 100 mg vial contains Methotrexate, 100 mg, prepared as the sodium salt; sodium hydroxide to adjust pH to about 8.5.

Action: Methotrexate has as its principle mechanism of action the competitive inhibition of the enzyme folic acid reductase. Folic acid must be reduced to tetrahydrofolic acid by this enzyme in the process of DNA synthesis and cellular replication. Methotrexate inhibits the reduction of folic acid and interferes with tissue-cell reproduction.

Actively proliferating tissues such as malignant cells, bone marrow, fetal cells, dermal epithelium, buccal and intestinal mucosa and cells of the urinary bladder are in general more sensitive to this effect of Methotrexate. Cellular proliferation in malignant tissue is greater than in most normal tissue and thus Methotrexate may impair malignant growth without irreversible damage to normal tissues.

After parenteral injection, peak serum levels are seen in about 30 to 60 minutes. Approximately one half the absorbed Methotrexate is reversibly bound to serum protein, but exchanges with body fluids easily and diffuses into the body tissue cells.

Excretion of single daily doses occurs through the kidneys in amounts from 55% to 88% or higher within 24 hours. Repeated doses daily result in more sustained serum levels and some retention of Methotrexate over each 24-hour period which may result in accumulation of the drug within the tissues. The liver cells appear to retain certain amounts of the drug for prolonged periods even after a single therapeutic dose. Methotrexate is retained in the presence of impaired renal function and may increase rapidly in the serum and in the tissue cells under such conditions. Methotrexate does not penetrate the blood cerebrospinal fluid barrier in therapeutic amounts when given parenterally. High concentrations of the drug when needed may be attained by direct intrathecal administration.

In psoriasis, the rate of production of epithelial cells in the skin is greatly increased over normal skin. This differential in reproductive rates is the basis for use of Methotrexate to control the psoriatic process.

Indications:

Anti-neoplastic Chemotherapy

Methotrexate is indicated for the treatment of gestational choriocarcinoma, and in patients with chorioadenoma destruens and hydatidiform mole.

Methotrexate is indicated for the palliation of acute lymphocytic leukemia. It is also indicated in the treatment and prophylaxis of meningeal leukemia. Greatest effect has been observed in palliation of acute lymphoblastic (stem-cell) leukemias in children. In combination with other anticancer drugs or suitable agents Methotrexate may be used for induction of remission, but it is most commonly used, as described in the literature, in the maintenance of induced remissions.

Methotrexate is also effective in the treatment of the advanced stages (III and IV, Peters Staging System) of lymphosarcoma, particularly in those cases in children, and in advanced cases of mycosis fungoides.

Psoriasis Chemotherapy (See box warnings.)

Because of high risk attending its use. Methotrexate is only indicated in the symptomatic control of severe, recalcitrant, disabling psoriasis which is not adequately responsive to other forms of therapy, **but only when the diagnosis has been established, as by biopsy and/or after dermatologic consultation.**

Contraindications: Pregnant psoriatic patients should not receive Methotrexate. Psoriatic patients with severe renal or hepatic disorders should not receive Methotrexate. Psoriatic patients with preexisting blood dyscrasias, such as bone marrow hypoplasia, leukopenia, thrombocytopenia or anemia, should not receive Methotrexate.

Warnings: See box warnings.

Precautions: Methotrexate has a high potential toxicity, usually dose-related. The physician should be familiar with the various characteristics of the drug and its established clinical usage. Patients undergoing therapy should be subject to appropriate supervision so that signs or symptoms of possible toxic effects or adverse reactions may be detected and evaluated with minimal delay. Pretreatment and periodic hematologic studies are essential to the use of Methotrexate in chemotherapy because of its common effect of hematopoietic suppression. This may occur abruptly and on apparent safe dosage, and any profound drop in blood-cell count indicates immediate stopping of the drug and appropriate therapy. In patients with malignant disease who have preexisting bone marrow aplasia, leukopenia, thrombocytopenia or anemia, the drug should be used with caution, if at all.

Methotrexate is excreted principally by the kidneys. Its use in the presence of impaired renal function may result in accumulation of toxic amounts or even additional renal damage. The patient's renal status should be determined prior to and during Methotrexate therapy and proper caution exercised should significant renal impairment be disclosed. Drug dosage should be reduced or discontinued until renal function is improved or restored.

In general, the following laboratory tests are recommended as part of essential clinical evaluation and appropriate monitoring of patients chosen for or receiving Methotrexate therapy; complete hemogram; hematocrit; urinalysis; renal function tests; and liver function tests. A chest x-ray is also recommended. The purpose is to determine any existing organ dysfunction or system impairment. The tests should be performed prior to therapy, at appropriate periods during therapy and after termination of therapy. It may be useful or important to perform liver biopsy or bone marrow aspiration studies where high dose or long-term therapy is being followed.

Methotrexate is bound in part to serum albumin after absorption and toxicity may be increased because of displacement by certain drugs such as salicylates, sulfonamides, diphenylhydantoin, phenylbutazone, and some antibacterials as tetracycline, chloramphenicol and para-amino-benzoic acid. These drugs, especially salicylates, phenylbutazone, and sulfonamides, whether antibacterial, hypoglycemic or diuretic, should not be given concurrently until the significance of these findings is established.

Vitamin preparations containing folic acid or its derivatives may alter responses to Methotrexate.

Methotrexate should be used with extreme caution in the presence of infection, peptic ulcer, ulcerative colitis, debility and in extreme youth or old age.

If profound leukopenia occurs during therapy, bacterial infection may occur or become a

Continued on next page

Bristol—Cont.

threat. Cessation of the drug and appropriate antibiotic therapy is usually indicated. In severe bone marrow depression, blood or platelet transfusions may be necessary.
Since it is reported that Methotrexate may have an immunosuppressive action, this factor must be taken into consideration in evaluating the use of the drug where immune responses in a patient may be important or essential.
In all instances where the use of Methotrexate is considered for chemotherapy, the physician must evaluate the need and usefulness of the drug against the risks of toxic effects or adverse reaction. Most such adverse reactions are reversible if detected early. When such effects or reactions do occur, the drug should be reduced in dosage or discontinued and appropriate corrective measures should be taken, according to the clinical judgment of the physician. Reinstitution of Methotrexate therapy should be carried out with caution, with adequate consideration of further need for the drug and alertness as to possible recurrence of toxicity.
Adverse Reactions: The most common adverse reactions include ulcerative stomatitis, leukopenia, nausea and abdominal distress. Others reported are malaise, undue fatigue, chills and fever, dizziness and decreased resistance to infection. In general, the incidence and severity of side effects are considered to be dose-related. Adverse reactions as reported for the various systems are as follows:
Skin: erythematous rashes, pruritus, urticaria, photosensitivity, depigmentation, alopecia, ecchymosis, telangiectasia, acne, furunculosis. Lesions of psoriasis may be aggravated by concomitant exposure to ultraviolet radiation.
Blood: bone marrow depression, leukopenia, thrombocytopenia, anemia, hypogammaglobulinemia, hemorrhage from various sites, septicemia.
Alimentary System: gingivitis, pharyngitis, stomatitis, anorexia, vomiting, diarrhea, hematemesis, melena, gastrointestinal ulceration and bleeding, enteritis, hepatic toxicity resulting in acute liver atrophy, necrosis, fatty metamorphosis, periportal fibrosis, or hepatic cirrhosis.
Urogenital System: renal failure, azotemia, cystitis, hematuria; defective oogenesis or spermatogenesis, transient oligospermia, menstrual dysfunction; infertility, abortion, fetal defects, severe nephropathy.
Central Nervous System: headaches, drowsiness, blurred vision. Aphasia, hemiparesis, paresis and convulsions have also occurred following administration of Methrotrexate.
There have been reports of leucoencephalopathy following intravenous administration of Methotrexate to patients who have had craniospinal irradiation.
After the intrathecal use of Methotrexate, the central nervous system toxicity which may occur can be classified as follows: (1) chemical arachnoiditis manifested by such symptoms as headache, back pain, nuchal rigidity, and fever, (2) paresis, usually transient, manifested by paraplegia associated with involvement with one or more spinal nerve roots, (3) leucoencephalopathy manifested by confusion, irritability, somnolence, ataxia, dementia, and occasionally major convulsions.
Other reactions related to or attributed to the use of Methotrexate such as pneumonitis, metabolic changes, precipitating diabetes, osteoporotic effects, abnormal tissue cell changes, and even sudden death have been reported.
Dosage and Administration:
Anti-neoplastic chemotherapy
Methotrexate sodium parenteral may be given by intramuscular, intravenous, intraarterial or intrathecal route. Initial treatment is usually undertaken with the patient under hospital care.
*For conversion of mg/kg b.w. to mg/M^2 of body surface or the reverse, a ratio of 1:30 is given as a guideline. The conversion factor varies between 1:20 and 1:40 depending on age and body build.
Choriocarcinoma and similar trophoblastic diseases: Methotrexate is administered intramuscularly in doses of 15 to 30 mg daily for a 5 day course. Such courses are usually repeated for 3 to 5 times as required, with rest periods of one or more weeks interposed between courses, until any manifesting toxic symptoms subside. The effectiveness of therapy is ordinarily evaluated by 24 hour quantitative analysis of urinary chorionic gonadotropin hormone (CGH), which should return to normal or less than 50 IU/24 hr usually after the 3rd or 4th course and usually be followed by a complete resolution of measurable lesions in 4 to 6 weeks. One to two courses of Methotrexate after normalization of CGH is usually recommended. Before each course of the drug careful clinical assessment is essential. Cyclic combination therapy of Methotrexate with other antitumor drugs has been reported as being useful.
Since hydatidiform mole may precede or be followed by choriocarcinoma, prophylactic chemotherapy with Methotrexate has been recommended. Chorioadenoma destruens is considered to be an invasive form of hydatidiform mole. Methotrexate is administered in these disease states in doses similar to those recommended for choriocarcinoma.
Leukemia: Acute lymphatic (lymphoblastic) leukemia in children and young adolescents is the most responsive to present day chemotherapy. In young adults and older patients, clinical remission is more difficult to obtain and early relapse is more common. In chronic lymphatic leukemia, the prognosis for adequate response is less encouraging.
Methotrexate alone or in combination with steroids was used initially for induction of remission of lymphoblastic leukemias. More recently corticosteroid therapy in combination with other antileukemic drugs or in cyclic combinations with Methotrexate included appear to produce rapid and effective remissions. When used for induction, Methotrexate in doses of 3.3 mg/M^2 in combination with prednisone 60 mg/M^2, given daily, produced remission in 50% of patients treated, usually within a period of 4 to 6 weeks. Methotrexate alone or in combination with other agents appears to be the drug of choice for securing maintenance of drug-induced remissions. When remission is achieved and supportive care has produced general clinical improvement, maintenance therapy is initiated, as follows: Methotrexate is administered 2 times weekly intramuscularly in doses of 30 mg/M^2. It has also been given in doses of 2.5 mg/kg intravenously every 14 days. If and when relapse does occur, reinduction of remission can again usually be obtained by repeating the initial induction regimen.
Various experts have recently introduced a variety of dosage schedules for both induction and maintenance of remission with various combinations of alkylating and antifolic agents. Multiple drug therapy with several agents, including Methotrexate, given concomitantly is gaining increasing support in both the acute and chronic forms of leukemia. The physician should familiarize himself with the new advances in antileukemic therapy.
Acute granulocytic leukemia is rare in children but common in adults. This form of leukemia responds poorly to chemotherapy and remissions are short with relapses common, and resistance to therapy develops rapidly.
Meningeal leukemia: Patients with leukemia are subject to leukemic invasion of the central nervous system. This may manifest characteristic signs or symptoms or may remain silent and be diagnosed only by examination of the cerebrospinal fluid which contains leukemic cells in such cases. Therefore, the CSF should be examined in all leukemic patients. Since passage of Methotrexate from blood serum to the cerebrospinal fluid is minimal, for adequate therapy the drug is administered intrathecally. It is now common practice because of the noted increased frequency of meningeal leukemia to administer Methotrexate intrathecally as prophylaxis in all cases of lymphocytic leukemia.
By intrathecal injection, the sodium salt of Methotrexate is administered in solution in doses of 12 mg per square meter of body surface or in an empirical dose of 15 mg. The solution is made in a strength of 1 mg per ml with an appropriate, sterile, preservative-free medium such as Sodium Chloride Injection, U.S.P.
For the treatment of meningeal leukemia. Methotrexate is given at intervals of 2 to 5 days. Methotrexate is administered until the cell count of the cerebrospinal fluid returns to normal. At this point one additional dose is advisable.
For prophylaxis against meningeal leukemia, the dosage is the same as for treatment except for the intervals of administration. On this subject, it is advisable for the physician to consult the medical literature.
Large doses may cause convulsions. Untoward side effects may occur with any given intrathecal injection and are commonly neurological in character. Methotrexate given by intrathecal route appears significantly in the systemic circulation and may cause systemic Methotrexate toxicity. Therefore systemic antileukemic therapy with the drug should be appropriately adjusted, reduced or discontinued. Focal leukemic involvement of the central nervous system may not respond to intrathecal chemotherapy and is best treated with radiotherapy.
Lymphomas: In Burkitt's Tumor, Stages I–II, Methotrexate has produced prolonged remissions in some cases. In Stage III Methotrexate is commonly given concomitantly with other antitumor agents. Treatment in all stages usually consists of several courses of the drug interposed with 7 to 10 day rest periods. Lymphosarcomas in Stage III may respond to combined drug therapy with Methotrexate given in doses of 0.625 mg to 2.5 mg/kg daily.
Mycosis fungoides: Therapy with Methotrexate appears to produce clinical remissions in about one half of the cases treated. Dosage is usually daily by mouth for weeks or months. Dose levels of drug and adjustment of dose regimen by reduction or cessation of drug are guided by patient response and hematologic monitoring. Methotrexate has also been given intramuscularly in doses of 50 mg once weekly or 25 mg 2 times weekly.
Psoriasis Chemotherapy
The patient should be fully informed of the risks involved and should be under constant supervision of the physician.
Assessment of renal function, liver function, and blood elements should be made by history, physical examination, and laboratory tests (such as CBC, urinalysis, serum creatinine, liver function studies, and liver biopsy if indicated) before beginning Methotrexate, periodically during Methotrexate therapy, and before reinstituting Methotrexate therapy after a rest period. Appropriate steps should be taken to avoid conception during and for at least eight weeks following Methotrexate therapy.
There are three commonly used general types of dosage schedules:

1. weekly oral or parenteral intermittent large doses
2. divided dose intermittent oral schedule over a 36-hour period
3. daily oral with a rest period

All schedules should be continually tailored to the individual patient. Dose schedules cited below pertain to an average 70 Kg adult. An initial test dose one week prior to initiation of therapy is recommended to detect any idiosyncrasy. A suggested dose range is 5 to 10 mg parenterally.

Recommended starting dose schedule:

Weekly single IM or IV dose schedule:

10 to 25 mg per week until adequate response is achieved. With this dosage schedule, 50 mg per week should ordinarily not be exceeded.

Special Note: Available data suggests that schedule 3 (daily oral with a rest period) may carry an increased risk of serious liver pathology.

Dosages may be gradually adjusted to achieve optimal clinical response, but not to exceed the maximum stated in the schedule.

Once optimal clinical response has been achieved, the dosage schedule should be reduced to the lowest possible amount of drug and to the longest possible rest period. The use of Methotrexate may permit the return to conventional topical therapy, which should be encouraged.

Antidote for Overdosage

Leucovorin (citrovorum factor) is a potent agent for neutralizing the immediate toxic effects of Methotrexate on the hematopoietic system. Where large doses or overdoses are given, Calcium Leucovorin may be administered by intravenous infusion in doses up to 75 mg within 12 hours, followed by 12 mg intramuscularly every 6 hours for 4 doses. Where average doses of Methotrexate appear to have an adverse effect, 2 to 4 ml (6 to 12 mg) of Calcium Leucovorin may be given intramuscularly every 6 hours for 4 doses. In general, where overdosage is suspected, the dose of Leucovorin should be equal to or higher than the offending dose of Methotrexate and should best be administered within the first hour. Use of Calcium Leucovorin after an hour delay is much less effective.

Caution:

Pharmacist: Because of its potential to cause severe toxicity, Methotrexate therapy requires close supervision of the patient by the physician. Pharmacists should dispense no more than a seven (7) day supply of the drug at one time. Refill of such prescriptions should be by direct order (written or oral) of the physician only.

Directions for Use: Reconstitute immediately prior to use with 2 to 10 ml. depending on route of administration, of an appropriate preservative-free medium such as Sodium Chloride Injection, U.S.P.

Note: Store dry powder and reconstituted solution at room temperature protected from light.

Supply: Mexate (Methotrexate Sodium) for Injection.

NDC 0015-3050-20—20 mg vial
NDC 0015-3051-20—50 mg vial
NDC 0015-3052-20—100 mg vial

MUTAMYCIN® ℞
(mitomycin for injection)

This is the full text of the latest Official Package Circular dated December 1978 [3001DIR-12].

WARNING

Mutamycin should be administered under the supervision of a qualified physician experienced in the use of cancer chemotherapeutic agents. Appropriate management of therapy and complications is possible only when adequate diagnostic and treatment facilities are readily available. Bone marrow suppression, notably thrombocytopenia and leukopenia, which may contribute to overwhelming infections in an already compromised patient, is the most common and severe of the toxic effects of Mutamycin (see "Warnings" and "Adverse Reactions" sections).

Description: Mutamycin (also known as mitomycin and/or mitomycin-C) is an antibiotic isolated from the broth of **Streptomyces caespitosus** which has been shown to have antitumor activity. The compound is heat stable, has a high melting point, and is freely soluble in organic solvents.

Action: Mutamycin selectively inhibits the synthesis of deoxyribonucleic acid (DNA). The guanine and cytosine content correlates with the degree of Mutamycin-induced cross-linking. At high concentrations of the drug, cellular RNA and protein synthesis are also suppressed.

In humans, Mutamycin is rapidly cleared from the serum after intravenous administration. Time required to reduce the serum concentration by 50% after a 30 mg. bolus injection is 17 minutes. After injection of 30 mg., 20 mg., or 10 mg. I.V., the maximal serum concentrations were 2.4 mcg./ml., 1.7 mcg./ml., and 0.52 mcg./ml., respectively. Clearance is effected primarily by metabolism in the liver, but metabolism occurs in other tissues as well. The rate of clearance is inversely proportional to the maximal serum concentration because, it is thought, of saturation of the degradative pathways.

Approximately 10% of a dose of Mutamycin is excreted unchanged in the urine. Since metabolic pathways are saturated at relatively low doses, the percent of a dose excreted in urine increases with increasing dose. In children, excretion of intravenously administered Mutamycin is similar.

Animal Toxicology—Mutamycin has been found to be carcinogenic in rats and mice. At doses approximating the recommended clinical dose in man, it produces a greater than 100 percent increase in tumor incidence in male Sprague-Dawley rats, and a greater than 50 percent increase in tumor incidence in female Swiss mice.

Indications: Mutamycin is not recommended as single-agent, primary therapy. It has been shown to be useful in the therapy of disseminated adenocarcinoma of the stomach or pancreas in proven combinations with other approved chemotherapeutic agents and as palliative treatment when other modalities have failed. Mutamycin is not recommended to replace appropriate surgery and/or radiotherapy.

Contraindications: Mutamycin is contraindicated in patients who have demonstrated a hypersensitive or idiosyncratic reaction to it in the past.

Mutamycin is contraindicated in patients with thrombocytopenia, coagulation disorder, or an increase in bleeding tendency due to other causes.

Warnings: Patients being treated with Mutamycin must be observed carefully and frequently during and after therapy.

The use of Mutamycin results in a high incidence of bone marrow suppression, particularly thrombocytopenia and leukopenia. Therefore, the following studies should be obtained repeatedly during therapy and for at least 7 weeks following therapy: platelet count, white blood cell count, differential, and hemoglobin. The occurrence of a platelet count below 150,000, or a WBC below 4,000, or a progressive decline in either is an indication for interruption of therapy.

Patients should be advised of the potential toxicity of this drug, particularly bone marrow suppression. Deaths have been reported due to septicemia as a result of leukopenia due to the drug.

Patients receiving Mutamycin should be observed for evidence of renal toxicity. Mutamycin should not be given to patients with a serum creatinine greater than 1.7 mg. percent.

Usage in Pregnancy—Safe use of Mutamycin in pregnant women has not been established. Teratological changes have been noted in animal studies. The effect of Mutamycin on fertility is unknown.

Adverse Reactions: Bone Marrow Toxicity— This was the most common and most serious toxicity, occurring in 605 of 937 patients (64.4%). Thrombocytopenia and/or leukopenia may occur anytime within 8 weeks after onset of therapy with an average time of 4 weeks. Recovery after cessation of therapy was within 10 weeks. About 25% of the leukopenic or thrombocytopenic episodes did not recover. Mutamycin produces cumulative myelosuppression.

Integument and Mucus Membrane Toxicity— This has occurred in approximately 4% of patients treated with Mutamycin. Cellulitis at the injection site has been reported and is occasionally severe. Stomatitis and alopecia also occurred frequently.

Renal Toxicity—2% of 1,281 patients demonstrated a statistically significant rise in creatinine. There appeared to be no correlation between total dose administered or duration of therapy and the degree of renal impairment.

Pulmonary Toxicity—This has occurred infrequently but can be severe. Dyspnea with a nonproductive cough and radiographic evidence of pulmonary infiltrates may be indicative of Mutamycin-induced pulmonary toxicity. If other etiologies are eliminated, Mutamycin therapy should be discontinued. Steroids have been employed as treatment of this toxicity, but the therapeutic value has not been determined.

Acute Side Effects Due to Mutamycin were fever, anorexia, nausea, and vomiting. They occurred in about 14% of 1,281 patients.

Other Undesirable Side Effects that have been reported during Mutamycin therapy have been headache, blurring of vision, confusion, drowsiness, syncope, fatigue, edema, thrombophlebitis, hematemesis, diarrhea, and pain. These did not appear to be dose related and were not unequivocally drug related. They may have been due to the primary or metastatic disease processes.

Dosage and Administration: Mutamycin should be given intravenously only, using care to avoid extravasation of the compound. If extravasation occurs, cellulitis, ulceration, and slough may result.

Each vial contains either mitomycin 5 mg. and mannitol 10 mg. or mitomycin 20 mg. and mannitol 40 mg. To administer, add Sterile Water for Injection, 10 ml. or 40 ml. respectively. Shake to dissolve. If product does not dissolve immediately, allow to stand at room temperature until solution is obtained.

After full hematological recovery (see guide to dosage adjustment) from any previous chemotherapy, either of the following dosage schedules may be used at 6 to 8 week intervals. Because of cumulative myelosuppression, patients should be fully reevaluated after each course of Mutamycin, and the dose reduced if the patient has experienced any toxicities. Doses greater than 20 mg./M.^{2} have not been shown to be more effective, and are more toxic than lower doses.

(1) 20 mg./M.^{2} intravenously as a single dose via a functioning intravenous catheter.

(2) 2 mg./M.^{2}/day intravenously for 5 days. After a drug-free interval of 2 days, 2 mg./M.^{2}/day for 5 days, thus making the total initial dose 20 mg./M.^{2} given over 10 days. The following schedule is suggested as a guide to dosage adjustment:

Nadir After Prior Dose: Leukocytes	Nadir After Prior Dose: Platelets	Percentage of Prior Dose to be Given
> 4000	> 100,000	100%
3000–3999	75,000–99,999	100%
2000–2999	25,000–74,999	70%
< 2000	< 25,000	50%

Continued on next page

Bristol—Cont.

No repeat dosage should be given until leukocyte count has returned to 3000 and platelet count to 75,000.
When Mutamycin is used in combination with other myelosuppressive agents, the doses should be adjusted accordingly. If the disease continues to progress after two courses of Mutamycin, the drug should be stopped since chances of response are minimal.
Stability:
1. **Unreconstituted** Mutamycin is stable for at least 2 years at room temperature. Avoid excessive heat (over 40°C).
2. **Reconstituted** with Sterile Water for Injection to a concentration of 0.5 mg. per ml., Mutamycin is stable for 14 days refrigerated or 7 days at room temperature.
3. **Diluted** in various IV fluids at room temperature to a concentration of 20 to 40 micrograms per ml.

IV Fluid	Stability
5% Dextrose Injection	3 hours
0.9% Sodium Chloride Injection	12 hours
Sodium Lactate Injection	24 hours

4. **The combination** of Mutamycin (5 mg. to 15 mg.) and heparin (1,000 units to 10,000 units) in 30 ml. of 0.9% Sodium Chloride Injection is stable for 48 hours at room temperature.
Supply:
Mutamycin (mitomycin) for Injection.
NDC 0015-3001-20—Each vial contains 5 mg. mitomycin.
NDC 0015-3002-20—Each vial contains 20 mg. mitomycin.

NAFCIL™ ℞
(nafcillin sodium for injection)
For Intramuscular or Intravenous Injection

This is the full text of the latest Official Package Circular dated May 1979 [7224DIR-07].
Description: NAFCIL (nafcillin sodium as the monohydrate) is 6-(2-ethoxy-1-nophthamido)-penicillanic acid, a penicillinase-resistant semisynthetic penicillin.
Microbiology: NAFCIL is a bactericidal penicillin which has shown activity **in vitro** against both penicillin G-susceptible and penicillin G-resistant strains of **Staphylococcus aureus** as well as against pneumococcus, beta-hemolytic streptococcus, and alpha streptococcus (veridans).
In experimental mouse infections induced with pneumococci, beta-hemolytic streptococci, and both penicillin G-susceptible and penicillin G-resistant strains of **Staphylococcus aureus,** nafcillin sodium was compared with methicillin and oxacillin. Regardless of the route of drug administration (intramuscular or oral) nafcillin sodium was consistently and significantly more effective than the other two penicillins.
The fate of a penicillin G-resistant strain of **Staphylococcus aureus** was determined in the kidneys of mice treated with penicillin G, methicillin, and nafcillin sodium. Animals injected with the nafcillin sodium showed negative cultures after the fourteenth day, whereas positive kidney cultures were obtained during the entire 28-day period from mice treated with penicillin G and methicillin.
Disc Susceptibility Tests
Quantitative methods that require measurement of zone diameters give the most precise estimates of antibiotic susceptibility. One such procedure* has been recommended for use with discs for testing susceptibility to methicillin class antibiotics. Interpretations correlate diameters on the disc test with MIC values for methicillin. With this procedure, a report from the laboratory of "susceptible" indicates that the infecting organism is likely to respond to therapy. A report of "resistant" indicates that the infecting organism is not likely to respond to therapy. A report of "intermediate susceptibility" suggests that the organism would be susceptible if high dosage is used, or if the infection is confined to tissues and fluids (e.g., urine), in which high antibiotic levels are attained.
Pharmacology: NAFCIL is relatively nontoxic for animals. The acute LD^{50} of this product by oral administration in rats and mice was greater than 5 g./Kg.; by intramuscular administration in rats 2800 mg./Kg.; by intraperitoneal administration in rats 1240 mg./Kg.; and by intravenous administration in mice 1140 mg./Kg. The intraperitoneal LD^{50} in dogs is 600 mg./Kg. Animal studies indicated that local tissue responses following intramuscular administration of 25% solutions were minimal and resembled those of penicillin G rather than methicillin.
Animal studies indicate that antibacterial amounts are concentrated in the bile, kidney, lung, heart, spleen, and liver. Eighty-four per cent of an intravenously administered dose can be recovered by biliary cannulation and 13 per cent by renal excretion in 24 hours. High and prolonged tissue levels can be demonstrated by both biological activity assays and C^{14} distribution patterns.
At comparable dosage intramuscular absorption of this product is nearly equivalent to that of intramuscular methicillin, and oral absorption to that of oral oxacillin. Blood concentrations may be tripled by the concurrent use of probenecid. Clinical studies with nafcillin sodium in infants under three days of age and prematures have revealed higher blood levels and slower rates of urinary excretion than in older children and adults.
Studies of the effect of this product on reproduction in rats and rabbits have been completed and reveal no fetal or maternal abnormalities. These studies include the observation of the effects of administration of the drug before conception and continuously through weaning (one generation).
Indications: Although the principal indication for nafcillin sodium is in the treatment of infections due to penicillinase-producing staphylococci, it may be used to initiate therapy in such patients in whom a staphylococcal infection is suspected. (See Important Note below.)
Bacteriologic studies to determine the causative organisms and their susceptibility to nafcillin sodium should be performed.
Important Note: When it is judged necessary that treatment be initiated before definitive culture and susceptibility results are known, the choice of nafcillin sodium should take into consideration the fact that it has been shown to be effective only in the treatment of infections caused by pneumococci, Group A beta-hemolytic streptococci and penicillin G-resistant and penicillin G-susceptible staphylococci. If the bacteriology report later indicates the infection is due to an organism other than a penicillin G-resistant staphylococcus susceptible to nafcillin sodium, the physician is advised to continue therapy with a drug other than nafcillin sodium or any other penicillinase-resistant semisynthetic penicillin.
Recent studies have reported that the percentage of staphylococcal isolates resistant to penicillin G outside the hospital is increasing, approximating the high percentage of resistant staphylococcal isolates found in the hospital. For this reason, it is recommended that a penicillinase-resistant penicillin be used as initial therapy for any suspected staphylococcal infection until culture and susceptibility results are known.
Nafcillin sodium is a compound that acts through a mechanism similar to that of methicillin against penicillin G-resistant staphylococci. Strains of staphylococci resistant to methicillin have existed in nature and it is known that the number of these strains reported has been increasing. Such strains of staphylococci have been capable of producing serious disease, in some instances resulting in fatality. Because of this, there is concern that widespread use of the penicllinase-resistant penicillins may result in the appearance of an increasing number of staphylococcal strains which are resistant to these penicillins.
Methicillin-resistant strains are almost always resistant to all other penicillinase-resistant penicillins (cross resistance with cephalosporin derivatives also occurs frequently). Resistance to any penicillinase-resistant penicillin should be interpreted as evidence of clinical resistance to all, in spite of the fact that minor variations in **in vitro** susceptibility may be encountered when more than one penicillinase-resistant penicillin is tested against the same strain of staphylococcus.
Contraindications: A history of allergic reaction to any of the penicillins is a contraindication.
Warnings:
Warning: Serious and occasionally fatal hypersensitivity (anaphylactoid) reactions have been reported in patients on penicillin therapy. Although anaphylaxis is more frequent following parenteral therapy it has occurred in patients on oral penicillins. These reactions are more apt to occur in individuals with a history of sensitivity to multiple allergens.
There have been reports of individuals with a history of penicillin hypersensitivity reactions who have experienced severe hypersensitivity reactions when treated with a cephalosporin. Before therapy with a penicillin, careful inquiry should be made concerning previous hypersensitivity reactions to penicillins, cephalosporins, and other allergens. If an allergic reaction occurs, appropriate therapy should be instituted, and discontinuation of nafcillin therapy considered. The usual agents (antihistamines, pressor amines, corticosteroids) should be readily available.
Precautions: As with any potent drug, periodic assessment of organ system function, including renal, hepatic and hematopoietic, should be made during prolonged therapy.
The possibility of bacterial and fungal overgrowth should be kept in mind during long-term therapy. If overgrowth of resistant organisms occurs, appropriate measures should be taken.
The oral route of administration should not be relied upon in patients with severe illness, or with nausea, vomiting, gastric dilatation, cardiospasm, or intestinal hypermotility.
Safety for use in pregnancy has not been established.
Particular care should be taken with intravenous administration because of the possibility of thrombophlebitis.
Adverse Reactions: Reactions to nafcillin sodium have been infrequent and mild in nature. As with other penicillins, the possibility of an anaphylactic reaction or serum sickness-like reactions should be considered. A careful history should be taken. Patients with histories of hay fever, asthma, urticaria, or previous sensitivity to penicillin are more likely to react adversely.
The few reactions associated with the intramuscular use of nafcillin sodium have been skin rash, pruritus, and possible drug fever. As with other penicillins, reactions from oral use of the drug have included nausea, vomiting, diarrhea, urticaria, and pruritus.
Dosage and Administration: It is recommended that parenteral therapy be used initially in severe infections. The patient should

be placed on oral therapy with this product as soon as the clinical condition warrants.

Intravenous Route: 500 mg. every 4 hours; double the dose if necessary in very severe infections. The required amount of drug should be diluted in 15 to 30 ml. of Sterile Water for Injection, U.S.P. or Sodium Chloride Injection, U.S.P. and injected over a 5 to 10 minute period. This may be accomplished through the tubing of an intravenous infusion if desirable. Stability studies on nafcillin sodium at concentrations of 2 mg./ml. and 30 mg./ml. in the following intravenous solutions indicate the drug will lose less than 10% activity at room temperature (70°F) during the time period stipulated:

Isotonic sodium chloride	24 hours
5% dextrose in water	24 hours
5% dextrose in 0.4% sodium chloride solution	24 hours
Ringer's solution	24 hours
M/6 sodium lactate solution (conc. of 30 mg./ml.)	24 hours

Discard any unused portions of intravenous solutions after 24 hours. Only those solutions listed above should be used for the intravenous infusion of NAFCIL (nafcillin sodium). The concentration of the antibiotic should fall within the range of 2 to 30 mg./ml. The drug concentrate and the rate and volume of the infusion should be adjusted so that the total dose of nafcillin is administered before the drug loses its stability in the solution in use. There is no clinical experience available on the use of this agent in neonates or infants for this route of administration.

This route of administration should be used for relatively short-term therapy (24 to 48 hours) because of the occasional occurrence of thrombophlebitis particularly in elderly patients.

Intramuscular Route: 500 mg. every 6 hours in adults; decrease the interval to 4 hours if necessary in severe infections. In infants and children a dose of 25 mg. per Kg. (about 12 mg. per pound) twice daily is usually adequate.

For neonates 10 mg. per Kg. is recommended twice daily.

Reconstitute with Sterile Water for Injection, U.S.P., 0.9% Sodium Chloride Injection, U.S.P. or Bacteriostatic water for Injection, U.S.P. (with benzyl alcohol or parabens); add 1.8 ml to the 500 mg vial for 2 ml resulting solution; 3.4 ml to the 1 g vial for 4 ml resulting solution; 6.6 ml to the 2 g vial for 8 ml resulting solution. All reconstituted vials have a concentration of 250 mg per ml.

Reconstituted Stability: Reconstitute with the required amount of Sterile Water for Injection, U.S.P., 0.9% Sodium Chloride Injection, U.S.P., or Bacteriostatic Water for Injection, U.S.P. (with benzyl alcohol or parabens). The resulting solutions are stable for 3 days at room temperature or 7 days under refrigeration and frozen.

When the "piggyback" vial is reconstituted with either Sterile water for Injection, U.S.P. or 0.9% sodium chloride Injection, U.S.P. and the resulting solutions are in a concentration of 10 to 200 mg/ml, the solutions are stable for 24 hours at room temperature or 7 days under refrigeration.

The clear solution should be administered by deep intragluteal injection immediately after reconstitution.

INFECTIONS CAUSED BY GROUP A BETA-HEMOLYTIC STREPTOCOCCI SHOULD BE TREATED FOR AT LEAST 10 DAYS TO HELP PREVENT THE OCCURRENCE OF ACUTE RHEUMATIC FEVER OR ACUTE GLOMERULONEPHRITIS.

"Piggyback" I.V. Package: This glass vial contains the labeled quantity of Nafcillin and is intended for intravenous administration. The diluent and volume are specified on the label of each package.

Reconstituted Stability: Reconsitute with the required amount of Sterile Water for Injection, U.S.P., 0.9% Sodium Chloride Injection, U.S.P. or Bacteriostatic Water for Injection. U.S.P. (with benzyl alcohol or parabens). The resulting solutions are stable for 3 days at room temperature or 7 days under refrigeration and frozen.

When the "piggyback" vial is reconstituted with either Sterile Water for Injection, U.S.P. or 0.9% Sodium Chloride Injection, U.S.P. and the resulting solutions are in a concentration of 10 to 200 mg/ml, the solutions are stable for 24 hours at room temperature of 7 days under refrigeration.

Hospital Bulk Package: This glass vial contains 10 grams Nafcil and is designed for use in the pharmacy in preparing I.V. additives. Add 93 ml Sterile Water for Injection. U.S.P. or 0.9% Sodium Chloride Injection, U.S.P. The resulting solution will contain 100 milligrams natcillin activity per ml. Solutions in a concentration of 10 mg to 200 mg per ml are stable for 24 hours at room temperature or seven days under refrigeration. Solutions in a concentration of 250 mg per ml are stable for three days at room temperature or seven days under refrigeration and frozen.

Caution: NOT TO BE DISPENSED AS A UNIT.

Supply: NAFCIL (nafcillin sodium) for injection. Nafcillin sodium equivalent to 500 mg., 1.0 Gm., 2.0 Gm., and 4.0 Gm. nafcillin per vial.

NDC 0015-7224-20—500 mg. vial
NDC 0015-7225-20—1.0-Gm. vial
NDC 0015-7221-20—2.0-Gm. vial
NDC 0015-7225-28—1.0-Gm. "piggyback" vial.
NDC 0015-7226-28—2.0-Gm. "piggyback" vial.
NDC 0015-7101-28—10 gram Hospital Bulk Package
NDC 0015-7227-28—4.0 Gm. "piggyback" vial.

For information on package sizes available, refer to the current price schedule.

*Bauer, A. W., Kirby, W. M. M., Sherris, J. C. and Turck, M.: Antibiotic Testing by a Standardized Single Disc Method, Am. J. Clin. Pathol., 45:493, 1966; Standardized Disc Susceptibility Test, FEDERAL REGISTER 37:20527-29, 1972.

NALDECON® SYRUP ℞
NALDECON® TABLETS
NALDECON® PEDIATRIC DROPS
NALDECON® PEDIATRIC SYRUP
For oral use only

This is the full text of the latest Official Package Circular dated January 1978 [5600DIMO-11].

Description:
[See table above].

Naldecon Composition Table

	For immediate action	For delayed action	Total content
Each sustained action tablet contains:			
Phenylpropanolamine hydrochloride	20.0 mg.	20.0 mg.	40.0 mg.
Phenylephrine hydrochloride	5.0 mg.	5.0 mg.	10.0 mg.
Phenyltoloxamine citrate	7.5 mg.	7.5 mg.	15.0 mg.
Chlorpheniramine maleate	2.5 mg.	2.5 mg.	5.0 mg.
Each teaspoon (5 ml.) of syrup contains:			
Phenylpropanolamine hydrochloride			20.0 mg.
Phenylephrine hydrochloride			5.0 mg.
Phenyltoloxamine citrate			7.5 mg.
Chlorpheniramine maleate			2.5 mg.
Each pediatric formulation contains the following ingredients:	Pediatric Syrup each 5 ml. contains:	Pediatric Drops each 1 ml. dropper contains:	
Phenylpropanolamine hydrochloride	5.0 mg.	5.0 mg.	
Phenylephrine hydrochloride	1.25 mg.	1.25 mg.	
Phenyltoloxamine citrate	2.0 mg.	2.0 mg.	
Chlorpheniramine maleate	0.5 mg.	0.5 mg.	

Actions: Naldecon is useful for the relief of nasal congestion associated with pollen allergy and minor infections of the upper respiratory tract (the common cold, nasopharyngitis, acute and chronic sinusitis). Naldecon Tablets are compounded with half of each ingredient in the outer layer for immediate action and the remainder in the slowly disintegrating core for a sustained effect.

The actions and uses of individual ingredients in the formulation are as follows:

Phenylpropanolamine Hydrochloride

Phenylpropanolamine hydrochloride[1] acts similarly to ephedrine. It is effective orally for the symptomatic control of allergic manifestations, such as perennial hay fever and bronchial asthma. Its action is more prolonged than that of ephedrine, and it is not so apt to produce anxiety complex as is ephedrine.

Phenylephrine Hydrochloride

Phenylephrine hydrochloride[2] is a more powerful vasoconstrictor than synephrine tartrate. When administered orally, it is a vasopressor and relatively nontoxic. The pressor and antiallergic effects of the drug are produced by oral administration. Therefore, this route may be employed in the treatment of orthostatic hypotension and allergic disorders. The comparatively larger doses required for effective oral treatment are only rarely accompanied by mild gastrointestinal symptoms. These may be avoided by administering the drug after meals.

Phenyltoloxamine Citrate

Phenyltoloxamine citrate[3] is a β-dimethylaminoethyl ether of orthobenzylphenol; as such it belongs to the group of antihistaminics exhibiting the aminoalkyl ether structure. The incidence of side effects is low; at recommended doses, soporific effects occur in less than 7% of patients.

Chlorpheniramine Maleate

Chlorpheniramine maleate[4] has good therapeutic efficacy and low incidence of side effects. It is comparable in therapeutic efficacy to other antihistaminics although administered in very low dosage.

Indications: Relief of distressing symptoms of colds and other upper respiratory infections, acute and chronic sinusitis, hay fever, and other pollen allergies:

- Rhinorrhea
- Postnasal drip
- Nasal congestion
- Sinus congestion
- Lacrimation
- Sneezing
- Itching of eyes and nose
- Head stuffiness

Contraindications: Sensitivity to any of the ingredients.

Precautions. This preparation may cause drowsiness. The patient should be cautioned against engaging in operations requiring alertness such as driving an automobile, operating machinery, etc. Do not exceed the recommended dose unless directed by a physician. Individuals with high blood pressure, heart

Continued on next page

Bristol—Cont.

disease, diabetes mellitus, thyroid disease, glaucoma, peripheral vascular disease, or prostatic hypertrophy should use only as directed by a physician.

Dosage:

The chart represents single dosages for the products listed below. Usual dosage schedule for Naldecon Pediatric Drops, Naldecon Pediatric Syrup, and Naldecon Syrup is every 3 to 4 hours, not to exceed four doses in a 24-hour period. For sustained-action Naldecon Tablets, doses should be administered on arising, midafternoon, and at bedtime.

(See table below)

References:

1. New and Nonofficial Remedies 1955.
2. New and Nonofficial Remedies 1954.
3. A.M.A. Council on Drugs Monograph on Phenyltoloxamine, J.A.M.A. 163:357 (2/2/57).
4. New and Nonofficial Drugs 1959.

Supply:

NDC 0015-5600—Naldecon Tablets.
[*Shown in Product Identification Section*]
NDC 0015-5601—Naldecon Syrup.
NDC 0015-5615—Naldecon Pediatric Drops.
NDC 0015-5616—Naldecon Pediatric Syrup.
For information on package sizes available, refer to the current price sheet.

Single Dosage for...	Naldecon Pediatric Drops	Naldecon Pediatric Syrup	Naldecon Syrup	Naldecon Tablets
3 to 6 months	¼ ml			
6 to 12 months	½ ml	½ teaspoonful		
1 to 6 years	1 ml	1 teaspoonful		
6 to 12 years		2 teaspoonfuls	½ teaspoonful	½ tablet
over 12 years			1 teaspoonful	1 tablet

PLATINOL® ℞
(cisplatin for injection)

This is the full text of the latest Official Package Circular dated August 1979 [3070DIM-06].

WARNING

Platinol (cisplatin) should be administered under the supervision of a qualified physician experienced in the use of cancer chemotherapeutic agents. Appropriate management of therapy and complications is possible only when adequate diagnostic and treatment facilities are readily available.
Cumulative renal toxicity associated with Platinol is severe. Other major dose-related toxicities are myelosuppression and nausea and vomiting.
Ototoxicity, which may be more pronounced in children, and is manifested by tinnitus, and/or loss of high frequency hearing and occasionally deafness, is significant.
Anaphylactic-like reactions to Platinol have been reported. Facial edema, bronchoconstriction, tachycardia, and hypotension may occur within minutes of Platinol administration. Epinephrine, corticosteroids, and antihistamines have been effectively employed to alleviate symptoms (see "Warnings" and "Adverse Reactions" sections).

Description: Platinol (cisplatin) (cis-diamminedichloroplatinum) is a heavy metal complex containing a central atom of platinum surrounded by two chloride atoms and two ammonia molecules in the cis position. It is a white lyophylized powder with the molecular formula Pt $Cl_2H_6N_2$, and a molecular weight of 300.1. It is soluble in water or saline at 1 mg/ml and in dimethylformamide at 24 mg/ml. It has a melting point of 207°C.

Action: Platinol has biochemical properties similar to that of bifunctional alkylating agents producing interstrand and intrastrand crosslinks in DNA. It is apparently cell-cycle non-specific. Following a single I.V. dose, Platinol concentrates in liver, kidneys, and large and small intestines in animals and humans. Platinol apparently has poor penetration into the CNS.
Plasma levels of radioactivity decay in a biphasic manner after an I.V. bolus dose of radioactive Platinol to patients. The initial plasma half-life is 25 to 49 minutes, and the post-distribution plasma half-life is 58 to 73 hours. During the post-distribution phase, greater than 90% of the radioactivity in the blood is protein bound. Platinol is excreted primarily in the urine. However, urinary excretion is incomplete with only 27 to 43% of the radioactivity being excreted within the first 5 days post-dose in human beings. There are insufficient data to determine whether biliary or intestinal excretion occurs.

Indications: Platinol is indicated as palliative therapy to be employed as follows:
Metastatic Testicular Tumors—in established combination therapy with other approved chemotherapeutic agents in patients with metastatic testicular tumors who have already received appropriate surgical and/or radiotherapeutic procedures. An established combination therapy consists of Platinol, Blenoxane (Bleomycin Sulfate) and Velban (Vinblastine Sulfate).
Metastatic Ovarian Tumors—in established combination therapy with other approved chemotherapeutic agents in patients with metastatic ovarian tumors who have already received appropriate surgical and/or radiotherapeutic procedures. An established combination consists of Platinol and Adriamycin (Doxorubicin Hydrochloride). Platinol, as a single agent, is indicated as secondary therapy in patients with metastatic ovarian tumors refractory to standard chemotherapy who have not previously received Platinol therapy.

Contraindications: Platinol is contraindicated in patients with preexisting renal impairment. Platinal should not be employed in myelosuppressed patients, or patients with hearing impairment.
Platinol is contraindicated in patients with a history of allergic reactions to Platinol or other platinum-containing compounds.

Warnings: Platinol produces cumulative nephrotoxicity. The serum creatinine, BUN, and creatinine clearance should be measured prior to initiating therapy, and prior to each subsequent course. At the recommended dosage, Platinol should not be given more frequently than once every 3 to 4 weeks (See "Adverse Reactions").
Anaphylactic-like reactions to Platinol have been reported. These reactions have occurred within minutes of administration to patients with prior exposure to Platinol, and have been alleviated by administration of epinephrine, corticosteroids and antihistamines.
Since ototoxicity of Platinol is cumulative, audiometric testing should be performed prior to initiating therapy and prior to each subsequent dose of drug (see "Adverse Reactions").
Safe use in human pregnancy has not been established. Platinol is mutagenic in bacteria and produces chromosome aberrations in animal cells in tissue culture. In mice Platinol is teratogenic and embryotoxic.
Platinol has not been studied for its carcinogenic potential but compounds with similar mechanisms of action and mutagenicity have been reported to be carcinogenic.

Precautions: Peripheral blood counts should be monitored weekly. Liver function should be monitored periodically. Neurologic examination should also be performed regularly (see "Adverse Reactions").

Adverse Reactions:

Nephrotoxicity

Dose-related and cumulative renal insufficiency is the major dose-limiting toxicity of Platinol. Renal toxicity has been noted in 28 to 36% of patients treated with a single dose of 50 mg/M². It is first noted during the second week after a dose and is manifested by elevations in BUN and creatinine, serum uric acid and/or a decrease in creatinine clearance. **Renal toxicity becomes more prolonged and severe with repeated courses of the drug. Renal function must return to normal before another dose of Platinol can be given.**
Impairment of renal function has been associated with renal tubular damage. The administration of Platinol using a 6- to 8-hour infusion with intravenous hydration, and mannitol has been used to reduce nephrotoxicity. However, renal toxicity still can occur after utilization of these procedures.

Ototoxicity

Ototoxicity has been observed in up to 31% of patients treated with a single dose of Platinol 50 mg/M², and is manifested by tinnitus and/or hearing loss in the high frequency range (4,000 to 8,000 Hz). Decreased ability to hear normal conversational tones may occur occasionally. Ototoxic effects may be more severe in children receiving Platinol. Hearing loss can be unilateral or bilateral and tends to become more frequent and severe with repeated doses. It is unclear whether Platinol-induced ototoxicity is reversible. Careful monitoring of audiometry should be performed prior to initiation of therapy and prior to subsequent doses of Platinol.

Hematologic

Myelosuppression occurs in 25 to 30% of patients treated with Platinol. The nadirs in circulating platelets and leukocytes occur between days 18 to 23 (range 7.5 to 45) with most patients recovering by day 39 (range 13 to 62). Leukopenia and thrombocytopenia are more pronounced at higher doses ($>$ 50 mg/M²). Anemia (decrease of $>$ 2 g hemoglobin/100 ml) occurs at approximately the same frequency and with the same timing as leukopenia and thrombocytopenia.

Gastrointestinal

Marked nausea and vomiting occur in almost all patients treated with Platinol, and are occasionally so severe that the drug must be discontinued. Nausea and vomiting usually begin within one to four hours after treatment and last up to 24 hours. Various degrees of nausea and anorexia may persist for up to one week after treatment.

Other Toxicities:

Hyperuricemia

Hyperuricemia has been reported to occur at approximately the same frequency as the increases in BUN and serum creatinine. It is more pronounced after doses greater than 50 mg/M^2, and peak levels of uric acid generally occur between 3 to 5 days after the dose. Allopurinol therapy for hyperuricemia effectively reduces uric acid levels.

Neurotoxicity

Neurotoxicity, usually characterized by peripheral neuropathies, has occurred in some patients. Loss of taste and seizures have also been reported. Neuropathies resulting from Platinol treatment may occur after prolonged therapy (4 to 7 months); however, neurologic symptoms have been reported to occur after a single dose.

Platinol therapy should be discontinued when the symptoms are first observed. Preliminary evidence suggests peripheral neuropathy may be irreversible in some patients.

Anaphylactic-like Reactions

Anaphylactic-like reactions have been occasionally reported in patients previously exposed to Platinol. The reactions consist of facial edema, wheezing, tachycardia and hypotension within a few minutes of drug administration. Reactions may be controlled by intravenous epinephrine, corticosteroids or antihistamines. Patients receiving Platinol should be observed carefully for possible anaphylactic-like reactions and supportive equipment and medication should be available to treat such a complication.

Other toxicities reported to occur infrequently are cardiac abnormalities, anorexia and elevated SGOT.

Dosage and Administration:

Note: Needles or intravenous sets containing aluminum parts that may come in contact with Platinol should not be used for preparation or administration. Aluminum reacts with Platinol, causing precipitate formation and a loss of potency.

Metastatic Testicular Tumors—An effective combination for the treatment of patients with metastatic testicular carcinomas includes Platinol, Blenoxane (Bleomycin Sulfate) and Velban (Vinblastine Sulfate). Remission induction therapy consists of Platinol, Blenoxane (Bleomycin Sulfate) and Velban (Vinblastine Sulfate) in the following doses:

PLATINOL—20 mg/M^2 I.V. daily for 5 days (days 1–5) every three weeks for three courses.

BLENOXANE® (Bleomycin Sulfate)—30 units I.V. weekly (Day 2 of each week) for 12 consecutive doses.

VELBAN® (Vinblastine Sulfate)—0.15 to 0.2 mg/Kg I.V. twice weekly (Days 1 and 2) every three weeks for four courses (a total of eight doses).

Maintenance therapy for patients who respond to the above regimen consists of Velban (Vinblastine Sulfate) 0.3 mg/Kg I.V. every 4 weeks for a total of 2 years.

For directions for the administration of Blenoxane (Bleomycin Sulfate) and Velban (Vinblastine Sulfate), refer to their respective package insert.

Metastatic Ovarian Tumors—An effective combination for the treatment of patients with metastatic ovarian tumors includes Platinol and Adriamycin (Doxorubicin Hydrochloride) in the following doses:

PLATINOL—50 mg/M^2 I.V. once every 3 weeks (Day 1).

ADRIAMYCIN™ (Doxorubicin Hydrochloride)—50 mg/M^2 I.V. once every 3 weeks (Day 1).

For directions for the administration of Adriamycin (Doxorubicin Hydrochloride), refer to the Adriamycin (Doxorubicin Hydrochloride) package insert.

In combination therapy, Platinol and Adriamycin (Doxorubicin Hydrochloride) are administered sequentially.

As a single agent, Platinol should be administered at a dose of 100 mg/M^2 I.V. once every 4 weeks.

Pretreatment hydration with 1 to 2 liters of fluid infused for 8 to 12 hours prior to a Platinol dose is recommended. The drug is then diluted in 2 liters of 5% Dextrose in ½ or ⅓N Saline containing 37.5 g of mannitol, and infused over a 6- to 8-hour period. Adequate hydration and urinary output must be maintained during the following 24 hours.

A repeat course of Platinol should not be given until the serum creatinine is below 1.5 mg/100 ml, and/or the BUN is below 25 mg/100 ml. A repeat course should not be given until circulating blood elements are at an acceptable level (platelets $\geq$100,000/mm^3, WBC $\geq$4,000/mm^3). Subsequent doses of Platinol should not be given until an audiometric analysis indicates that auditory acuity is within normal limits.

Preparation of Intravenous Solutions: The 10 mg and 50 mg vials should be reconstituted with 10 ml or 50 ml of Sterile Water for Injection, U.S.P., respectively. Each ml of the resulting solution will contain 1 mg of Platinol.

Reconstitution as recommended results in a clear, colorless solution.

The reconstituted solution should be used intravenously only and should be administered by I.V. infusion over a 6- to 8-hour period. (See Dosage and Administration).

Stability: Unopened vials of the dry powder must be stored in a refrigerator (2°C to 8°C). The recommended storage of unopened vials provides a stable product for 2 years.

The reconstituted solution is stable for 20 hours at room temperature (27°C).

Important Note: Once reconstituted, the solution should be kept at room temperature (27°C). If the reconstituted solution is refrigerated a precipitate will form.

Supply: PLATINOL (cisplatin) for Injection

NDC 0015-3070-20—Each amber vial contains 10 mg of cisplatin.

NDC 0015-3072-20—Each amber vial contains 50 mg of cisplatin.

POLYCILLIN® ℞

(ampicillin)

CAPSULES

250 mg. and 500 mg.

For Oral Suspension

125 mg. per 5 ml., 250 mg. per 5 ml., 500 mg. per 5 ml.

Pediatric Drops

100 mg. per ml.

POLYCILLIN-N®

(sterile ampicillin sodium)

For Intramuscular or Intravenous Injection

This is the full text of the latest Combined Official Package Circulars dated October 1977 [7988DIRO-16 Polycillin] *and May 1979* [7401DIRO-24 Polycillin-N]. (S 9/78)

Description: Polycillin (ampicillin) is a synthetic penicillin with a broad spectrum of bactericidal activity against both penicillin-susceptible Gram-positive organisms and many common Gram-negative pathogens.

Polycillin-N (sterile ampicillin sodium) contains 2.9 milliequivalents of sodium per 1 gram of drug.

Actions:

Pharmacology

Polycillin is stable in the presence of gastric acid and is well-absorbed from the gastrointestinal tract. It diffuses readily into most body tissues and fluids. However, penetration into the cerebrospinal fluid and brain occurs only when the meninges are inflamed. Ampicillin is excreted largely unchanged in the urine and its excretion can be delayed by concurrent administration of probenecid. The active form appears in the bile in higher concentrations than those found in serum. Ampicillin is the least serum-bound of all the penicillins, averaging about 20% compared to approximately 60 to 90% for other penicillins. Polycillin is well-tolerated by most patients and has been given in doses of 2 grams daily for many weeks without adverse reactions.

Microbiology

The following bacteria have been shown in **in vitro** studies to be susceptible to Polycillin:

GRAM-POSITIVE ORGANISMS: Hemolytic and nonhemolytic streptococci, **D. pneumoniae,** non-penicillinase-producing staphylococci, Clostridia spp., **B. anthracis, Listeria monocytogenes,** and most strains of enterococci.

GRAM-NEGATIVE ORGANISMS: H. influenzae, N. gonorrhoeae, N. meningitidis, Proteus mirabilis, and many strains of Salmonella, Shigella, and **E. coli.**

Polycillin does not resist destruction by penicillinase. Polycillin Susceptibility Test Discs, 10 mcg. should be used to estimate the **in vitro** susceptibility of bacteria to Polycillin.

Indications: Polycillin is indicated for the treatment of infections due to susceptible Gram-positive organisms including streptococci, pneumococci, penicillin G-susceptible staphylococci, and enterococci, and susceptible strains of Gram-negative bacteria including **H. influenzae, E. coli, Proteus mirabilis, N. gonorrhoeae, N. meningitidis,** Shigella, **S. typhosa** and other Salmonella.

Bacteriology studies to determine the causative organisms and their susceptibility to ampicillin should be performed. Therapy may be instituted prior to obtaining results of susceptibility testing.

It is advisable to reserve the parenteral form of this drug for moderately severe and severe infections and for patients who are unable to take the oral forms. A change to oral Polycillin (ampicillin) may be made as soon as appropriate.

Indicated surgical procedures should be performed.

Contraindications: A history of a previous hypersensitivity reaction to any of the penicillins is a contraindication.

Warning: Serious and occasionally fatal hypersensitivity (anaphylactoid) reactions have been reported in patients on penicillin therapy. Although anaphylaxis is more frequent following parenteral therapy, it has occurred in patients on oral penicillins. These reactions are more apt to occur in individuals with a history of sensitivity to multiple allergens.

There have been well-documented reports of individuals with a history of penicillin hypersensitivity reactions who have experienced severe hypersensitivity reactions when treated with a cephalosporin. Before therapy with a penicillin, careful inquiry should be made concerning previous hypersensitivity reactions to penicillins, cephalosporins, and other allergens.

Serious anaphylactoid reactions require immediate emergency treatment with epinephrine. Oxygen, intravenous steroids, and airway management, including intubation, should also be administered as indicated.

USAGE IN PREGNANCY: Safety for use in pregnancy has not been established.

Precautions: The possibility of superinfections with mycotic organisms or bacterial pathogens should be kept in mind during therapy. In such cases, discontinue the drug and substitute appropriate treatment.

As with any potent drug, periodic assessment of organ system function, including renal, hepatic, and hematopoietic, should be made during prolonged therapy.

Continued on next page

Bristol—Cont.

With high urine concentrations of ampicillin, false-positive glucose reactions may occur if Clinitest, Benedict's Solution, or Fehling's Solution are used. Therefore, it is recommended that glucose tests based on enzymatic glucose oxidase reactions (such as Clinistix or Tes-Tape) be used.

Adverse Reactions: As with other penicillins, it may be expected that untoward reactions will be essentially limited to sensitivity phenomena. They are more likely to occur in individuals who have previously demonstrated hypersensitivity to penicillins and in those with a history of allergy, asthma, hay fever, or urticaria.

The following adverse reactions have been reported as associated with the use of ampicillin:

Gastrointestinal—Glossitis, stomatitis, black "hairy" tongue, nausea, vomiting, enterocolitis, pseudomembranous colitis, and diarrhea. (These reactions are usually associated with oral dosage forms.)

Hypersensitivity reactions—Skin rashes and urticaria have been reported frequently. A few cases of exfoliative dermatitis and erythema multiforme have been reported. Anaphylaxis is the most serious reaction experienced and has usually been associated with the parenteral dosage form.

Note: Urticaria, other skin rashes, and serum sickness-like reactions may be controlled with antihistamines and, if necessary, systemic corticosteroids. Whenever such reactions occur, ampicillin should be discontinued, unless, in the opinion of the physician, the condition being treated is life threatening and amenable only to ampicillin therapy. Serious anaphylactic reactions require the immediate use of epinephrine, oxygen, and intravenous steroids.

Liver—A moderate rise in serum glutamic oxaloacetic transaminase (SGOT) has been noted, particularly in infants, but the significance of this finding is unknown. Mild transitory SGOT elevations have been observed in individuals receiving larger (two to four times) than usual and oft-repeated intramuscular injections. Evidence indicates that glutamic oxaloacetic transaminase (GOT) is released at the site of intramuscular injection of ampicillin sodium and that the presence of increased amounts of this enzyme in the blood does not necessarily indicate liver involvement.

Hemic and Lymphatic Systems—Anemia, thrombocytopenia, thrombocytopenic purpura, eosinophilia, leukopenia, and agranulocytosis have been reported during therapy with the penicillins. These reactions are usually reversible on discontinuation of therapy and are believed to be hypersensitivity phenomena.

Other—Since infectious mononucleosis is viral in origin, ampicillin should not be used in the treatment. A high percentage of patients with mononucleosis who received ampicillin developed a skin rash.

Dosage:

Infections of the respiratory tract and soft tissues:

Oral: Patients weighing 20 Kg. (44 lbs.) or more: 250 mg. every 6 hours.

NDC 0015	Label Claim	Recommended Amount of Diluent	Withdrawable Volume	Concentration (in mg/ml)
7401-20	125 mg.	1.2 ml.	1.0 ml.	125 mg.
7402-20	250 mg.	1.0 ml.	1.0 ml.	250 mg.
7403-20	500 mg.	1.8 ml.	2.0 ml.	250 mg.
7404-20	1.0 gram	3.5 ml.	4.0 ml.	250 mg.
7405-20	2.0 gram	6.8 ml.	8.0 ml.	250 mg.

Patients weighing less than 20 Kg. (44 lbs.): 50 mg./Kg./day in equally divided doses at 6-to 8-hour intervals.

Parenteral: Patients weighing 40 Kg. (88 lbs.) or more: 250 to 500 mg. every 6 hours.

Patients weighing less than 40 Kg. (88 lbs.): 25 to 50 mg./Kg./day in equally divided doses at 6-to 8-hour intervals.

Infections of the gastrointestinal and genitourinary tracts:

Oral: Patients weighing 20 Kg. (44 lbs.) or more: 500 mg. every 6 hours.

Patients weighing less than 20 Kg. (44 lbs.): 100 mg./Kg./day in equally divided doses at 6-to 8-hour intervals.

Infections of the gastrointestinal and genitourinary tracts (including those caused by Neisseria gonorrhea in females).

Parenteral: Patients weighing 40 Kg. (88 lbs.) or more: 500 mg. every 6 hours.

Patients weighing less than 40 Kg. (88 lbs.): 50 mg./Kg./day in equally divided doses at 6-to 8-hour intervals.

In the treatment of chronic urinary tract and intestinal infections, frequent bacteriological and clinical appraisal is necessary. Smaller doses than those recommended above should not be used. Higher doses should be used for stubborn or severe infections. In stubborn infections, therapy may be required for several weeks. It may be necessary to continue clinical and/or bacteriological follow-up for several months after cessation of therapy.

Urethritis in males or females due to N. gonorrhoeae:

Oral: 3.5 Grams, with 1.0 Gram probenecid, administered simultaneously.

Urethritis in males due to N. gonorrhoeae:

Parenteral: Adult: Two doses of 500 mg. each at an interval of 8 to 12 hours. Treatment may be repeated if necessary or extended if required.

In the treatment of complications of gonorrheal urethritis, such as prostatitis and epididymitis, prolonged and intensive therapy is recommended. Cases of gonorrhea with a suspected primary lesion of syphilis should have darkfield examinations before receiving treatment. In all other cases where concomitant syphilis is suspected, monthly serological tests should be made for a minimum of four months. The parenteral doses for the preceding infections may be given by either the intramuscular or intravenous route. A change to oral Polycillin (ampicillin) may be made when appropriate.

Bacterial Meningitis

Parenteral ONLY: Adults and Children: 150 to 200 mg./Kg./day in equally divided doses every 3 to 4 hours. (Treatment may be initiated with intravenous drip therapy and continued with intramuscular injections.) The doses for other infections may be given by either the intravenous or intramuscular route.

Weight		Infection	
Kg.	Lb.	Respiratory	GU/GI
Up to 5	Up to 11	62.5 mg. q. 6h. (½ dropperful q. 6h.)	125 mg. q. 6h. (1 dropperful q. 6h.)
5 to 7.5	11 to 16.5	94 mg. q. 6h. (¾ dropperful q. 6h.)	188 mg. q. 6h. (1½ dropperfuls q. 6h.)
7.6 to 10	16.6 to 22	125 mg. q. 6h. (1 dropperful q. 6h.)	250 mg. q. 6h. (2 dropperfuls q. 6h.)

Septicemia

Parenteral ONLY: Adults and Children: 150 to 200 mg./Kg./day. Start with intravenous administration for at least three days and continue with the intramuscular route every 3 to 4 hours.

Treatment of all infections should be continued for a minimum of 48 to 72 hours beyond the time that the patient becomes asymptomatic or evidence of bacterial eradication has been obtained. A minimum of 10-days treatment is recommended for any infection caused by Group A beta-hemolytic streptococci to help prevent the occurrence of acute rheumatic fever or acute glomerulonephritis.

The following Dosage chart may be useful as a guide to therapy with the Pediatric Drops. [See table below].

Note: For ease in administration, the dropper assembly is calibrated at the 62.5-mg. level (½ dropperful), at the 94-mg. level (¾ dropperful), and at the 125-mg. level (1 dropperful). Children over 10 Kg. (22 pounds) would generally be dosed with Polycillin for Oral Suspension.

Directions for Dispensing Oral Suspension and Pediatric Drops: Prepare these formulations at the time of dispensing. For ease in preparation, add water to the bottle in two portions and shake well after each addition. Add the total amount of water as directed on the labeling of the package being dispensed. The reconstituted formulation is stable for 14 days under refrigeration.

Parenteral—Directions For Use: Use only freshly prepared solutions. Intramuscular and intravenous injections should be administered within one hour after preparation, since the potency may decrease significantly after this period.

For Intramuscular Use: Dissolve contents of a vial with the amount of Sterile Water for Injection, U.S.P. or Bacteriostatic Water for Injection, U.S.P., listed in the table above.

While Polycillin-N, 1.0 g. and 2.0 g., are primarily for intravenous use, they may be administered intramuscularly when the 250-mg. or 500-mg. vials are unavailable. In such instances, dissolve in 3.5 or 6.8 ml. Sterile Water for Injection, U.S.P. or Bacteriostatic Water for Injection, U.S.P., respectively. The resulting solution will provide a concentration of 250 mg. per ml.

Polycillin-N, 125 mg., is intended primarily for pediatric use. It also serves as a convenient dosage form when small parenteral doses of the antibiotic are required.

For Direct Intravenous Use: Add 5 ml. Sterile Water for Injection, U.S.P. or Bacteriostatic Water for Injection, U.S.P. to the 125-, 250-, and 500- mg. vials and administer slowly over a 3- to 5- minute period. Polycillin-N, 1.0 Gm. or 2.0 Gm., may also be given by direct intravenous administration. Dissolve in 7.4 or 14.8 ml. Sterile Water for Injection, U.S.P., or Bacteriostatic Water for Injection, U.S.P. respectively, and administer slowly over at least 10 to 15 minutes. CAUTION: More rapid administration may result in convulsive seizures.

For Administration by Intravenous Drip: Reconstitute as directed above (For Direct Intravenous Use) prior to diluting with Intravenous Solution. Stability studies on ampicillin sodium at several concentrations in various intravenous solutions indicate the drug will

lose less than 10% activity at the temperatures noted for the time periods stated:
(See table at right)
Only those solutions listed at right should be used for the intravenous infusion of Polycillin-N. The concentrations should fall within the range specified. The drug concentration and the rate and volume of the infusion should be adjusted so that the total dose of ampicillin is administered before the drug loses its stability in the solution in use.

"Piggyback" I.V. Package: These glass vials contain the labeled quantity of POLYCILLIN-N and are intended for intravenous administration. The diluent and volume are specified on the label of each package.

Hospital Bulk Package: This glass vial contains 10 grams ampicillin and is designed for use in the pharmacy in preparing I.V. additives. Add 94 ml Sterile Water for Injection, U.S.P. The resulting solution will contain 100 milligrams ampicillin activity per ml, and is stable up to one hour at room temperature. Diluting further within one hour to 5 mg to 10 mg per ml, the resulting solution will remain stable for 8 hours at room temperature or 72 hours under refrigeration.

Caution: NOT TO BE DISPENSED AS A UNIT.

Supply: **Polycillin** (ampicillin) for Oral Suspension. Each 5 ml. of reconstituted suspension contains ampicillin trihydrate equivalent to 125, 250, or 500 mg. ampicillin.

NDC 0015-7988—125 mg., 60 ml., 80 ml., 100 ml., 150 ml. and 200 ml. bottles
NDC 0015-7998—250 mg., 80 ml., 100 ml., 150 ml. and 200 ml. bottle
NDC 0015-7884—500 mg., 100 ml. bottle

Polycillin (ampicillin) Capsules. Ampicillin trihydrate equivalent to 250 or 500 mg. ampicillin per capsule.

NDC 0015-7992—250 mg.
NDC 0015-7993—500 mg.
[*Shown in Product Identification Section*]

Polycillin (ampicillin) for oral suspension. Each ml. of reconstituted pediatric drops contains ampicillin trihydrate equivalent to 100 mg. ampicillin.

NDC 0015-7884—100 mg., 20 ml. bottles.

Polycillin-N (sterile ampicillin sodium) for I.M. or I.V. Injection. Ampicillin sodium equivalent to 125, 250, 500 mg., 1 g or 2 g ampicillin per vial.

NDC 0015-7401-20—125-mg. vial.
NDC 0015-7402-20—250-mg. vial.
NDC 0015-7403-20—500-mg. vial.
NDC 0015-7404-20—1.0-Gm. vial.
NDC 0015-7405-20—2.0 Gm. vial.
NDC 0015-7403-31—500 mg. "piggyback" vial.
NDC 0015-7404-36—1.0 gram "piggyback" vial.
NDC 0015-7405-28—2.0 gram "piggyback" vial.
NDC 0015-7100-28—10 gram Hospital Bulk Package

For information on package sizes available, refer to the current price sheets.

Room Temperature (25°C.)

Diluent	Concentrations	Stability Periods
Sterile Water for Injection	up to 30 mg./ml.	8 hours
Isotonic Sodium Chloride	up to 30 mg./ml.	8 hours
M/6 Sodium Lactate Solution	up to 30 mg./ml.	8 hours
5% Dextrose in Water	10 to 20 mg./ml.	2 hours
5% Dextrose in Water	up to 2 mg./ml.	4 hours
5% Dextrose in 0.45% NaCl	up to 2 mg./ml.	4 hours
10% Invert Sugar in Water	up to 2 mg./ml.	4 hours
Lactated Ringer's Solution	up to 30 mg./ml.	8 hours

Refrigerated (4°C.)

Diluent	Concentrations	Stability Periods
Sterile Water for Injection	30 mg./ml.	48 hours
Sterile Water for Injection	up to 20 mg./ml.	72 hours
Isotonic Sodium Chloride	30 mg./ml.	48 hours
Isotonic Sodium Chloride	up to 20 mg./ml.	72 hours
Lactated Ringer's Solution	up to 30 mg./ml.	24 hours
M/6 Sodium Lactate	up to 30 mg./ml.	8 hours
5% Dextrose in Water	up to 20 mg./ml.	4 hours
5% Dextrose in 0.45% NaCl	up to 10 mg./ml.	4 hours
10% Invert Sugar	up to 20 mg./ml.	3 hours

POLYCILLIN-PRB® ℞
(ampicillin-probenecid)
For Oral Suspension
Ampicillin Trihydrate equivalent to 3.5 Grams ampicillin with 1.0 Gram probenecid

This is the full text of the latest Official Package Circular dated October 1977 [7607 DIRO-06].

Description: Polycillin-PRB (ampicillin-probenecid) is a semisynthetic penicillin in combination with probenecid.

Actions:
Pharmacology
Ampicillin is stable in the presence of gastric acid and is well-absorbed from the gastrointestinal tract. It diffuses readily into most body tissues and fluids. However, penetration into the cerebrospinal fluid and brain occurs only when the meninges are inflamed. Ampicillin is excreted largely unchanged in the urine and its excretion can be delayed by concurrent administration of probenecid. The active form appears in the bile in higher concentrations than those found in serum. Ampicillin is the least serum-bound of all the penicillins, averaging about 20% compared to approximately 60 to 90% for other penicillins. Probenecid inhibits the renal tubular secretion of penicillins causing an increased serum level of the antibiotic.

Microbiology
Neisseria gonorrhoeae has been shown in **in vitro** studies to be susceptible to ampicillin.

Indications: Ampicillin-probenecid is indicated for the treatment of uncomplicated infections (urethral, endocervical, or rectal) due to **N. gonorrhoeae** in males and females.
Susceptibility studies should be performed with recurrent infections or when resistant strains are encountered. Therapy may be instituted prior to obtaining results of susceptibility testing.

Contraindications:
Ampicillin
A history of previous hypersensitivity reactions to any of the penicillins is a contraindication.
Probenecid
Polycillin-PRB should not be given to individuals with a known hypersensitivity to probenecid. It is not recommended for patients with known blood dyscrasias, uric acid kidney stones or during an acute attack of gout.

Warnings: Serious and occasionally fatal hypersensitivity reactions have been reported in patients on penicillin therapy. Although anaphylaxis is more frequent following parenteral therapy, it has occurred in patients on oral penicillins. These reactions are more apt to occur in individuals with a history of sensitivity to multiple allergens.
There have been well-documented reports of individuals with a history of penicillin hypersensitivity reactions who have experienced severe hypersensitivity reactions when treated with a cephalosporin. Before therapy with a penicillin, careful inquiry should be made concerning previous hypersensitivity reactions to penicillins, cephalosporins, and other allergens. If an allergic reaction occurs, the patient should be treated with the usual agents, e.g., pressor amines, antihistamines, and corticosteroids. Serious anaphylactoid reactions require emergency treatment with epinephrine. Oxygen, intravenous steroids, and airway management, including intubation, should also be administered as indicated.

USAGE IN PREGNANCY: Safety for use in pregnancy has not been established.

Precautions: Cases of gonococcal infection with a suspected lesion of syphilis should have darkfield examinations ruling out syphilis before receiving ampicillin. Patients who do not have suspected lesions of syphilis and are treated with ampicillin should have a follow-up serologic test for syphilis each month for four months to detect syphilis that may have been masked by treatment for gonorrhea. Patients with gonorrhea who also have syphilis should be given additional appropriate parenteral penicillin treatment.

Adverse Reactions: As with other penicillins, it may be expected that untoward reactions to ampicillin will be essentially limited to sensitivity phenomena. They are more likely to occur in individuals who have previously demonstrated hypersensitivity to penicillins and in those with a history of allergy, asthma, hay fever, or urticaria.
The following adverse reactions have been reported as associated with the use of ampicillin:
Gastrointestinal—Glossitis, stomatitis, black "hairy" tongue, nausea, vomiting, enterocolitis, pseudomembranous colitis, and diarrhea. (These reactions are usually associated with oral dosage forms.)
Hypersensitivity reactions—Skin rashes and urticaria have been reported frequently. A few cases of exfoliative dermatitis and erythema multiforme have been reported. Anaphylaxis is the most serious reaction experienced and has usually been associated with the parenteral form.
Serious acute hypersensitivity reactions may require the use of epinephrine, oxygen, and airway management, which may include endotracheal intubation, intravenous steroids, and repletion of plasma volume.
Liver—A moderate rise in serum glutamic oxaloacetic transaminase (SGOT) has been noted, but the significance of this finding is unknown.
Hemic and Lymphatic Systems—Anemia, thrombocytopenia, thrombocytopenic purpura, eosinophilia, leukopenia, and agranulocytosis have been reported during therapy with the penicillins. These reactions are usually reversible on discontinuation of therapy and are believed to be hypersensitivity phenomena.

Dosage: Acute N. gonorrhoeae infections in adult males and females.
3.5 Grams ampicillin, with 1.0 Gram probenecid, administered simultaneously. One bottle contains enough of each drug for the required single dose.
It is desirable that follow-up cultures be obtained from the original site(s) of infection 7 to 14 days after therapy.
In women, it is also desirable to obtain culture test-of-cure from both the endocervical and anal canal.

Directions For Dispensing Oral Suspension: Prepare this formulation at the time of dispensing. For ease in preparation, add water to the bottle in two portions and shake well after each addition. Add the total amount of water as directed on the labeling of the package being dispensed. The reconstituted formu-

Continued on next page

Bristol—Cont.

lation is stable for 24 hours at room temperature.
Supply: POLYCILLIN-PRB (Ampicillin-Probenecid) for Oral Suspension. Ampicillin Trihydrate equivalent to 3.5 Grams ampicillin with 1.0 Gram probenecid, single-dose bottle.
NDC 0015-7607

POLYMOX® ℞
(amoxicillin)
CAPSULES
250 mg. and 500 mg.
FOR ORAL SUSPENSION
125 mg. per 5 ml., 250 mg. per 5 ml.
PEDIATRIC DROPS
50 mg. per ml.

This is the full text of the latest Official Package Circular dated May 1976 [7276DIRO-07].
Description: Polymox® (amoxicillin) is a semisynthetic penicillin, an analogue of ampicillin, with a broad spectrum of bactericidal activity against Gram-positive organisms and many Gram-negative pathogens.
Actions:
Pharmacology
Polymox® is stable in the presence of gastric acid and is well absorbed from the gastrointestinal tract and may be given with no regard to food. It diffuses readily into most body tissues and fluids, with the exception of brain and spinal fluid, except when meninges are inflamed. The half-life of amoxicillin is 61.3 minutes. Most of the amoxicillin is excreted unchanged in the urine; its excretion can be delayed by concurrent administration of probenecid. Amoxicillin is not highly protein-bound. In blood serum, amoxicillin is approximately 20% protein-bound as compared to 60% for penicillin-G.
Orally administered doses of 250 mg. and 500 mg. amoxicillin capsules result in average peak blood levels one to two hours after administration in the range of 3.5 mcg./ml. to 5.0 mcg./ml. and 5.5 mcg./ml. to 7.5 mcg./ml. respectively.
Orally administered doses of amoxicillin suspension 125 mg./5 ml., and 250 mg./5 ml., result in average peak blood levels one to two hours after administration in the range of 1.5 mcg./ml. to 3.0 mcg./ml. and 3.5 mcg./ml. to 5.0 mcg./ml. respectively.
Detectable serum levels are observed up to 8 hours after an orally administered dose of amoxicillin. Approximately 60 percent of an orally administered dose of amoxicillin is excreted in the urine within six to eight hours.
Microbiology
Polymox® (amoxicillin) is similar to ampicillin in its bactericidal action against susceptible organisms during the stage of active multiplication. It acts through the inhibition of biosynthesis of cell wall mucopeptides. **In vitro** studies have demonstrated the susceptibility of most strains of the following Gram-positive bacteria: alpha- and beta-hemolytic streptococci, **Diplococcus pneumoniae,** nonpenicillinase-producing staphylococci, and **Streptococcus faecalis.** It is active **in vitro** against many strains of **Haemophilus influenzae, Neisseria gonorrhoeae, Escherichia coli** and **Proteus mirabilis.** Because it does not resist destruction by penicillinase, it is **not** effective against penicillinase-producing bacteria, particularly resistant staphylococci. All strains of Pseudomonas and most strains of Klebsiella and Enterobacter are resistant.
Disc Susceptibility Tests
Quantitative methods that require measurement of zone diameters give the most precise estimates of antibiotic susceptibility. One such procedure* has been recommended for use with discs, for testing susceptibility to ampicillin class antibiotics. Interpretations correlate diameters on the disc test with MIC values for amoxicillin. With this procedure, a report from the laboratory of "susceptible" indicates that the infecting organism is likely to respond to therapy. A report of "resistant" indicates that the infecting organism is not likely to respond to therapy. A report of "intermediate susceptibility" suggests that the organism would be susceptible if high dosage is used, or if the infection is confined to tissues and fluids (e.g., urine), in which high antibiotic levels are attained.
Indications: Polymox® (amoxicillin) is indicated in the treatment of infections due to susceptible strains of the following:
GRAM-NEGATIVE ORGANISMS—**H. influenzae, E. coli, P. mirabilis** and **N. gonorrhoeae.**
GRAM-POSITIVE ORGANISMS—Streptococci (including **Streptococcus faecalis**), **D. pneumoniae** and nonpenicillinase-producing staphylococci.
Therapy may be instituted prior to obtaining results from bacteriological and susceptibility studies to determine the causative organisms and their susceptibility to amoxicillin.
Indicated surgical procedures should be performed.
Contraindications: A history of a previous hypersensitivity reaction to any of the penicillins is a contraindication.
Warning: Serious and occasionally fatal hypersensitivity (anaphylactoid) reactions have been reported in patients on penicillin therapy. Although anaphylaxis is more frequent following parenteral therapy, it has occurred in patients on oral penicillins. These reactions are more apt to occur in individuals with a history of sensitivity to multiple allergens.
There have been well-documented reports of individuals with a history of penicillin hypersensitivity reactions who have experienced severe hypersensitivity reactions when treated with a cephalosporin. Before therapy with a penicillin, careful inquiry should be made concerning previous hypersensitivity reactions to penicillins, cephalosporins, and other allergens.
SERIOUS ANAPHYLACTOID REACTIONS REQUIRE IMMEDIATE EMERGENCY TREATMENT WITH EPINEPHRINE. OXYGEN, INTRAVENOUS STEROIDS, AND AIRWAY MANAGEMENT, INCLUDING INTUBATION, SHOULD ALSO BE ADMINISTERED AS INDICATED.
Usage In Pregnancy: Safety for use in pregnancy has not been established.
Precautions: The possibility of superinfections with mycotic organisms or bacterial pathogens should be kept in mind during therapy. In such cases, discontinue the drug and substitute appropriate treatment.
As with any potent drug, periodic assessment of organ system function, including renal, hepatic, and hematopoietic, should be made during prolonged therapy.
Adverse Reactions: As with other penicillins, it may be expected that untoward reactions will be essentially limited to sensitivity phenomena. They are more likely to occur in individuals who have previously demonstrated hypersensitivity to penicillins and in those with a history of allergy, asthma, hay fever, or urticaria.
The following adverse reactions have been reported as associated with the use of penicillin:
Gastrointestinal—Glossitis, stomatitis, black "hairy" tongue, nausea, vomiting, and diarrhea. (These reactions are usually associated with oral dosage forms.)
Hypersensitivity Reactions—Skin rashes and urticaria have been reported frequently. A few cases of exfoliative dermatitis and erythema multiforme have been reported. Anaphylaxis is the most serious reaction experienced and has usually been associated with the parenteral dosage form.
Note: Urticaria, other skin rashes, and serum sickness-like reactions may be controlled with antihistamines and, if necessary, systemic corticosteroids. Whenever such reactions occur, penicillin should be discontinued unless, in the opinion of the physician, the condition being treated is life threatening and amenable only to penicillin therapy. Serious anaphylactic reactions require the immediate use of epinephrine, oxygen, and intravenous steroids.
Liver—A moderate rise in serum glutamic oxaloacetic transaminase (SGOT) has been noted, particularly in infants, but the significance of this finding is unknown.
Hemic and Lymphatic Systems—Anemia, thrombocytopenia, thrombocytopenic purpura, eosinophilia, leukopenia, and agranulocytosis have been reported during therapy with the penicillins. These reactions are usually reversible on discontinuation of therapy and are believed to be hypersensitivity phenomena.
Dosage and Administration: Infections of the ear, nose and throat due to streptococci, pneumococci, nonpenicillinase-producing staphylococci and **H. influenzae;**
Infections of the genitourinary tract due to **E. coli, Proteus mirabilis** and **Streptococcus faecalis;**
Infections of the skin and soft-tissues due to streptococci, susceptible staphylococci and **E. coli:**

Usual Dosage: Adults: 250 mg. every 8 hours.
Children: 20 mg./Kg./day in divided doses every 8 hours.
Children weighing 20 Kg. or more should be dosed according to the adult recommendations.

In severe infections or those caused by less susceptible organisms: 500 mg. every 8 hours for adults, and 40 mg./Kg./day in divided doses every 8 hours for children may be needed.
Infections of the lower respiratory tract, due to streptococci, pneumococci, nonpenicillinase-producing staphylococci and **H. influenzae:**

Usual Dosage: Adults: 500 mg. every 8 hours
Children: 40 mg./Kg./day in divided doses every 8 hours.
Children weighing 20 Kg. or more should be dosed according to the adult recommendations.

Larger doses may be required for stubborn or severe infections.
The children's dosage is intended for individuals whose weight will not cause a dosage to be calculated greater than that recommended for adults.
Gonorrhea, acute uncomplicated ano-genital and urethral infections due to **N. gonorrhoeae:** (males and females) 3 grams as a single oral dose.
Cases of gonorrhea with a suspected lesion of syphilis should have dark-field examinations before receiving amoxicillin, and monthly serological tests for a minimum of four months.
It should be recognized that in the treatment of chronic urinary tract infections, frequent bacteriological and clinical appraisals are necessary. Smaller doses than those recommended above should not be used. Even higher doses may be needed at times. In stubborn infections, therapy may be required for several weeks. It may be necessary to continue clinical and/or bacteriological follow-up for several months after cessation of therapy. Except for gonorrhea, treatment should be continued for a minimum of 48 to 72 hours beyond the time that the patient becomes asymptomatic or evidence of bacterial eradication has been obtained. It is recommended that there be at least 10 days treatment for any infection caused by hemolytic streptococci to prevent the occurrence of acute rheumatic fever or glomerulonephritis.
Dosage and Administration of Pediatric Drops: Usual dosage for all indications except infections of the lower respiratory tract:

Under 6 Kg. (13 lbs.): 0.5 ml. every 8 hours
6-8 Kg. (13 to 18 lbs.): 1 ml. every 8 hours
Infections of the lower respiratory tract:
Under 6 Kg. (13 lbs.): 1 ml. every 8 hours
6-8 Kg. (13 to 18 lbs.): 2 ml. every 8 hours.

Children weighing more than 8 Kg. (18 lbs.) should receive the appropriate dose of the Oral Suspension 125 mg. or 250 mg./5 ml.

After reconstitution, the required amount of suspension should be placed directly on the child's tongue for swallowing. Alternate means of administration are to add the required amount of suspension to formula, milk, fruit juice, water, ginger ale, or cold drinks. These preparations should then be taken immediately. To be certain the child is receiving full dosage, such preparations should be consumed in entirety.

Directions For Dispensing Oral Suspension and Pediatric Drops:

Prepare these formulations at the time of dispensing. For ease in preparation, add water to the bottle in two portions and shake well after each addition. Add the total amount of water as directed on the labeling of the package being dispensed.

The reconstituted formulation is stable for 14 days at either room temperature or refrigeration.

How Supplied:

Polymox (amoxicillin) Capsules. Each capsule contains amoxicillin trihydrate equivalent to 250 or 500 mg. amoxicillin.

NDC 0015-7278—250 mg., bottles of 100 and 500.

NDC 0015-7279—500 mg., bottles of 50 and 100.

[*Shown in Product Identification Section*]

Polymox (amoxicillin) for Oral Suspension. Each 5 ml. of reconstituted suspension contains amoxicillin trihydrate equivalent to 125 or 250 mg. amoxicillin.

NDC 0015-7276—125 mg., 80 ml., 100 ml. and 150 ml. bottles.

NDC 0015-7277—250 mg., 80 ml., 100 ml. and 150 ml. bottles.

Polymox (amoxicillin) Drops for Oral Suspension. Each ml. of reconstituted pediatric drops contains amoxicillin trihydrate equivalent to 50 mg. amoxicillin.

NDC 0015-7277—50 mg., 15 ml. bottles.

For information on package sizes available, refer to the current price sheets.

*Bauer, A.W., Kirby, W.M.M., Sherris, J.C., and Turck, M.: Antibiotic Testing by a Standardized Single Disc Method, Am. J. Clin. Pathol., 45:493, 1966; Standardized Disc Susceptibility Test, FEDERAL REGISTER 37:20527–29, 1972.

PROSTAPHLIN® ℞
(oxacillin sodium)
Capsules, Oral Solution, I.M. or I.V.

This is the full text of the latest Combined Official Package Circulars dated May 1978 [7977DIRO-09 Prostaphlin Capsules and Oral Solution *May 1978*] [7979DIR-21 Prostaphlin Injectable]. May 1979 (15 8/79)

Description: PROSTAPHLIN (oxacillin sodium monohydrate) is sodium 5-methyl-3-phenyl-4-isoxazolyl penicillin, a penicillinase-resistant, acid-resistant, semi-synthetic penicillin. Each gram of PROSTAPHLIN For Injection contains approximately 2.8 mEq. of sodium and is buffered with 40 mg. dibasic sodium phosphate, and preserved with 3.6 mg. methylparaben and 0.4 mg. propylparaben.

Actions and Pharmacology: Prostaphlin is active against staphylococci (both penicillin G-susceptible and resistant), pneumococci, and streptococci.

It is resistant to destruction by acid and is well-absorbed from the gastrointestinal tract. Distribution studies in man indicate that oxacillin can be detected in bile, amniotic fluid, cord serum and human milk and in trace amounts in normal cerebrospinal fluid.

The drug is well tolerated. Oral doses of 500 mg. to 2.0 Gm. every 6 hours for a period of one month produced no side effects in 40 normal adult volunteers. Intramuscular doses of 250 to 1000 mg. 4 times daily for 30 days produced no side effects in 40 normal adult volunteers. Laboratory and physical examinations showed no significant changes from control levels in the test subjects.

A single 250-mg. oral dose gives a 1-hour peak serum level of 1.65 mcg./ml. A 500-mg. dose peaks at about 2.6 mcg./ml. Peak serum levels with the oral solution occur somewhat earlier, about one-half hour after dosing. A single dose of 250-mg. oral solution gives a peak serum level of 1.9 mcg./ml.; of 500-mg., 4.8 mcg./ml. Intramuscular injections give peak serum levels 30 minutes after injection. A 250-mg. dose gives a level of 5.3 mcg./ml. while a 500-mg. dose peaks at 10.9 mcg./ml. Intravenous injection gives a peak about 5 minutes after the injection is completed. Slow I.V. dosing with 500 mg. gives a 5-minute peak of 43 mcg./ml. with a half-life of 20 to 30 minutes.

PROSTAPHLIN is active against most Gram-positive cocci including beta-hemolytic streptococci, pneumococci and nonpenicillinase-producing staphylococci. Because of its resistance to the enzyme penicillinase, it is also active against penicillinase-producing staphylococci.

Disc Susceptibility Tests: Quantitative methods that require measurement of zone diameters give the most precise estimates of antibiotic susceptibility. One such procedure* has been recommended for use with discs for testing susceptibility to methicillin class antibiotics. Interpretations correlate diameters on the disc test with MIC values for methicillin. With this procedure, a report from the laboratory of "susceptible" indicates that the infecting organism is likely to respond to therapy. A report of "resistant" indicates that the infecting organism is not likely to respond to therapy. A report of "intermediate susceptibility" suggests that the organism would be susceptible if high dosage is used, or if the infection is confined to tissues and fluids (e.g., urine), in which high antibiotic levels are attained.

Indications: Although the principal indication for oxacillin sodium is in the treatment of infections due to penicillinase-producing staphylococci, it may be used to initiate therapy in such patients in whom a staphylococcal infection is suspected. (See Important Note below.)

Bacteriologic studies to determine the causative organisms and their susceptibility to oxacillin sodium should be performed.

In serious life-threatening infections, oral preparations of the penicillinase-resistant penicillins should not be relied on for initial therapy.

Important Note: When it is judged necessary that treatment be initiated before definitive culture and susceptibility results are known, the choice of oxacillin sodium should take into consideration the fact that it has been shown to be effective only in the treatment of infections caused by pneumococci, Group A beta-hemolytic streptococci, and penicillin G-resistant and penicillin G-susceptible staphylococci. If the bacteriology report later indicates the infection is due to an organism other than a penicillin G-resistant staphylococcus susceptible to oxacillin sodium, the physician is advised to continue therapy with a drug other than oxacillin sodium or any other penicillinase-resistant semisynthetic penicillin.

Recent studies have reported that the percentage of staphylococcal isolates resistant to penicillin G outside the hospital is increasing, approximating the high percentage of resistant staphylococcal isolates found in the hospital. For this reason, it is recommended that a penicillinase-resistant penicillin be used as initial therapy for any suspected staphylococcal infection until culture and susceptibility results are known.

Oxacillin sodium is a compound that acts through a mechanism similar to that of methicillin against penicillin G-resistant staphylococci. Strains of staphylococci resistant to methicillin have existed in nature and it is known that the number of these strains reported has been increasing. Such strains of staphylococci have been capable of producing serious disease, in some instances resulting in fatality. Because of this, there is concern that widespread use of the penicillinase-resistant penicillins may result in the appearance of an increasing number of staphylococcal strains which are resistant to these penicillins.

Methicillin-resistant strains are almost always resistant to all other penicillinase-resistant penicillins (cross resistance with cephalosporin derivatives also occurs frequently). Resistance to any penicillinase-resistant penicillin should be interpreted as evidence of clinical resistance to all, in spite of the fact that minor variations in **in vitro** susceptibility may be encountered when more than one penicillinase-resistant penicillin is tested against the same strain of staphylococcus.

Contraindications: A previous hypersensitivity reaction to any penicillin is a contraindication.

Warnings: Serious and occasionally fatal hypersensitivity (anaphylactoid) reactions have been reported in patients on penicillin therapy. Although anaphylaxis is more frequent following parenteral therapy, it has occurred in patients on oral penicillins. These reactions are more apt to occur in individuals with a history of sensitivity to multiple allergens.

There have been well documented reports of individuals with a history of penicillin hypersensitivity reactions who have experienced severe hypersensitivity reactions when treated with a cephalosporin. Before therapy with a penicillin, careful inquiry should be made concerning previous hypersensitivity reactions to penicillins, cephalosporins, and other allergens. If an allergic reaction occurs, the drug should be discontinued and the patient treated with the usual agents e.g., pressor amines, antihistamines, and corticosteroids.

Precautions: Penicillin should be used with caution in individuals with histories of significant allergies and/or asthma.

The oral route of administration should not be relied upon in patients with severe illness, or with nausea, vomiting, gastric dilatation, cardiospasm, or intestinal hypermotility.

Occasional patients will not absorb therapeutic amounts of orally administered penicillin.

The possibility of bacterial and/or fungal overgrowth should be kept in mind during long-term therapy. If overgrowth of resistant organisms occurs, appropriate measures should be taken.

As with any potent drug, periodic assessment of organ system function, including renal, hepatic and hematopoietic, should be made during long-term therapy.

Experience in premature and newborn infants is limited. Caution should be exercised in administration of the drug to such patients and frequent evaluation of organ system function is recommended.

Safety for use in pregnancy has not been established.

Adverse Reactions: The hypersensitivity reactions reported are skin rashes, urticaria, serum sickness and anaphylactic reactions. Symptomatic and asymptomatic elevations of S.G.O.T. and S.G.P.T. have been reported following I.V./I.M. and oral use of oxacillin. Hypersensitivity has been considered to be the cause in most instances which are reversible. Pathological study has shown either a cholestatic or nonspecific hepatitis. Oral lesions

Continued on next page

Bristol—Cont.

such as glossitis and stomatitis have been reported. Fever, eosinophilia, oral and rectal moniliasis have also been reported. Hemolytic anemia, transient neutropenia with evidence of granulocytopenia or thrombocytopenia, neuropathy, and nephrotoxicity (oliguria, albuminuria, hematuria, pyuria, and/or cylindruria) are infrequent and usually associated with high doses of parenteral penicillin. Thrombophlebitis has occurred in a small percentage of patients after intravenous therapy.

In some newborns and infants receiving high doses of oxacillin sodium (150 to 175 mg./Kg./day), transient hematuria, albuminuria and azotemia have been encountered. Although the causal relationship is not entirely clear, infants and newborns treated with high doses of the drug should be observed closely for signs of renal impairment.

Administration and Dosage:

ORAL

Usual Adult Dose: For mild to moderate infections of the skin, soft tissue or upper respiratory tract—500 mg. every 4 to 6 hours for a minimum of 5 days.

Pediatric Dose: Children weighing more than 40 Kg. (88 lbs.) should receive adult dosage. Children weighing less than 40 Kg. (88 lbs.): For mild to moderately severe infections of the skin, soft tissue or upper respiratory tract—50 mg./Kg./day (25 mg./lb./day) in equally-divided doses at 6-hour intervals for at least 5 days.

Note: In serious or life-threatening infections, such as staphylococcal septicemia or other deep-seated severe infections, oral preparations of the penicillinase-resistant penicillins should not be relied upon for initial therapy. Oral absorption may be unreliable. PROSTAPHLIN parenteral or parenteral methicillin sodium is advisable for initial treatment of these conditions.

Following initial control of the infections with the parenteral preparations, oral PROSTAPHLIN may be given for follow-up therapy in the following doses:

Adults: 1.0 Gm. every 4 to 6 hours.
Children: 100 mg/Kg./day (50 mg./lb./day) or greater in equally-divided doses at 4 to 6 hours intervals.

In serious systemic infection, therapy should be continued for at least 1 to 2 weeks after the patient is afebrile and cultures are sterile. Treatment of osteomyelitis may require several months of intensive therapy. The best use for this oral medication is in the prolonged follow-up therapy following successful initial treatment with parenterally administered penicillinase-resistant penicillin.

This medication is best taken on an empty stomach, preferably 1 to 2 hours before meals.

Infections caused by Group A beta-hemolytic streptococci: The use of penicillin G, penicillin V, or phenethicillin is the preferred treatment, because of their greater activity against this agent. Such infections should be treated for at least 10 days to help prevent the occurrence of acute rheumatic fever or acute glomerulonephritis.

Directions for Dispensing Oral Solution

Prepare these formulations at the time of dispensing. For ease in preparation, add water to the bottle in two portions and shake well after each addition. Add the total amount of water as directed on the labeling of the package being dispensed. The reconstituted formulation is stable for 3 days at room temperature or 14 days under refrigeration.

PARENTERAL

The parenteral form of this drug should be considered for patients who are unable to take the oral form. The route of administration, however, should be changed to the oral form when parenteral therapy is no longer necessary.

For mild-to-moderate upper respiratory and localized skin and soft tissue infections:

Adults and children weighing 40 Kg. (88 lbs.) or more: 250 mg. to 500 mg. every 4 to 6 hours.
Children weighing less than 40 Kg. (88 lbs.): 50 mg./Kg./day (25 mg./lb./day) in equally-divided doses every 6 hours.

Note: Absorption and excretion data indicate that doses of 25 mg./Kg./day (12.5 mg./lb./day) in prematures and neonates provide adequate therapeutic levels.

For more severe infections such as those of the lower respiratory tract or disseminated infections:

Adults and children weighing 40 Kg. (88 lbs.) or more: 1 Gm. or higher every 4 to 6 hours.
Children weighing less than 40 Kg. (88 lbs.): 100 mg./Kg./day (50 mg./lb./day) or higher in equally-divided doses every 4 to 6 hours.

Very severe infections may require very high doses and prolonged therapy.

INFECTIONS CAUSED BY GROUP A BETA-HEMOLYTIC STREPTOCOCCI SHOULD BE TREATED FOR AT LEAST 10 DAYS TO HELP PREVENT THE OCCURRENCE OF ACUTE RHEUMATIC FEVER OR ACUTE GLOMERULONEPHRITIS.

Directions For Use:

For Intramuscular Use: Use Sterile Water for Injection, U.S.P. Add 1.4 ml. to the 250-mg. vial, 2.7 ml. to the 500-mg. vial, 5.7 ml. to the 1.0-gram vial, 11.5 ml. to the 2.0-Gm. vial and 23 ml. to the 4.0-Gm. vial. Shake well until a clear solution is obtained. After reconstitution, vials will contain 250 mg. of active drug per 1.5 ml. of solution. The reconstituted solution is stable for 3 days at 70°F. or for one week under refrigeration (40°F.).

For Direct Intravenous Use: Use Sterile Water for Injection, U.S.P. or Sodium Chloride Injection, U.S.P. Add 5 ml. to the 250-mg. and 500-mg. vials, 10 ml. to the 1.0-gram vial, 20 ml. to the 2.0-gram vial, and 40 ml. to the 4.0-gram vial. Withdraw the entire contents and administer slowly over a period of approximately 10 minutes.

For Administration by Intravenous Drip: Reconstitute as directed above (For Direct Intravenous Use) prior to diluting with intravenous Solution. Stability studies on oxacillin sodium at concentrations of 0.5 mg./ml. and 2 mg./ml. in the intravenous solutions listed below indicate that the drug will lose less than 10% activity at room temperature (70°F.) during a six-hour period:

I.V. Solution
Normal Saline Solution
5% Dextrose in Water
5% Dextrose in Normal Saline
10% D-Fructose in Water
10% D-Fructose in Normal Saline
Lactated Ringer's Solution
Lactated Potassic Saline Injection
10% Invert Sugar in Water
10% Invert Sugar in Normal Saline
10% Invert Sugar plus 0.3% Potassium Chloride in Water
Travert 10% Electrolyte #1
Travert 10% Electrolyte #2
Travert 10% Electrolyte #3

Only those solutions listed above should be used for the intravenous infusion of PROSTAPHLIN. The concentration of the antibiotic should fall within the range of 0.5 to 2.0 mg./ml. The drug concentration and the rate and volume of the infusion should be adjusted so that the total dose of oxacillin is administered before the drug loses its stability in the solution in use.

"Piggyback" I.V. Package: This glass vial contains the labeled quantity of Prostaphlin and is intended for intravenous administration. The diluent and volume are specified on the label of each package.

Following reconstitution, the solution is stable for 24 hours at room temperature.

Hospital Bulk Package: This glass vial contains 10 grams Prostaphlin and is designed for use in the pharmacy in preparing I.V. additives. Add 93 ml of Sterile Water for Injection, U.S.P. The resulting solution will contain 100 mg oxacillin activity per ml. Following reconstitution in this manner, the solutions are stable for 24 hours at room temperature.

CAUTION. NOT TO BE DISPENSED AS A UNIT.

Supply: PROSTAPHLIN (oxacillin sodium) Capsules. Each capsule contains oxacillin sodium equivalent to 250 or 500 mg. oxacillin.
NDC-0015-7977—250 mg.
NDC-0015-7982—500 mg.
[*Shown in Product Identification Section*]

PROSTAPHLIN (oxacillin sodium) for Oral Solution. Each 5 ml. of reconstituted solution contains oxacillin sodium equivalent to 250 mg. oxacillin.
NDC-0015-7985—250 mg., 100 ml. bottles.

PROSTAPHLIN (oxacillin sodium) for Injection. Oxacillin sodium equivalent to 250, 500 mg., 1, 2, 4 or 10 grams oxacillin per vial.
NDC 0015-7978—250 mg. vial
NDC 0015-7979—500 mg. vial
NDC 0015-7981—1.0 Gm. vial
NDC 0015-7970—2.0 Gm. vial
NDC 0015-7300—4.0 Gm. vial
NDC 0015-7981—1.0-Gm. "Piggyback" vial.
NDC 0015-7970—2.0-Gm. "Piggyback" vial.
NDC 0015-7300—4.0-Gm. "Piggyback" vial.
NDC 0015-7103-28—10 gram—Hospital Bulk Package

For information on package sizes available, refer to the current price sheets.

---

*Bauer, A.W., Kirby, W.M.M., Sherris, J.C. and Turck, M.: Antibiotic Testing by a Standardized Single Disc Method, Am. J. Clin. Pathol., 45:493, 1966; Standardized Disc Susceptibility Test, FEDERAL REGISTER 37:20527–29, 1972.

SALURON® ℞
(hydroflumethiazide)

This is the full text of the latest Official Package Circular dated December 1976 [5410DIRO-10].

Description: Saluron (hydroflumethiazide) is a potent oral diuretic-antihypertensive agent of low toxicity developed by Bristol Laboratories.

Action: The mechanism of action results in an interference with the renal tubular mechanism of electrolyte reabsorption. At maximal therapeutic dosage all thiazides are approximately equal in their diuretic potency. The mechanism whereby thiazides function in the control of hypertension is unknown.

Indications: Saluron is indicated as adjunctive therapy in edema associated with congestive heart failure, hepatic cirrhosis, and corticosteroid and estrogen therapy.

Saluron has also been found useful in edema due to various forms of renal dysfunction such as nephrotic syndrome, acute glomerulonephritis, and chronic renal failure.

Saluron is indicated in the management of hypertension either as the sole therapeutic agent or to enhance the effectiveness of other antihypertensive drugs in the more severe forms of hypertension.

Usage in Pregnancy: The routine use of diuretics in an otherwise healthy woman is inappropriate and exposes mother and fetus to unnecessary hazard. Diuretics do not prevent development of toxemia of pregnancy, and there is no satisfactory evidence that they are useful in the treatment of developed toxemia.

Edema during pregnancy may arise from pathological causes or from the physiologic and mechanical consequences of pregnancy. Thiazides are indicated in pregnancy when edema is due to pathologic causes, just as they are in the absence of pregnancy (however, see Warnings, below). Dependent edema in pregnancy, resulting from restriction of venous return by the expanded uterus, is properly treated through elevation of the lower extremities and use of support hose; use of diuretics to lower intravascular volume in this case is illogical and unnecessary. There is hypervolemia during normal pregnancy which is harmful to neither the fetus nor the mother (in the absence of cardiovascular disease), but which is associated with edema, including generalized edema, in the majority of pregnant women. If this edema produces discomfort, increased recumbency will often provide relief. In rare instances, this edema may cause extreme discomfort which is not relieved by rest. In these cases, a short course of diuretics may provide relief and may be appropriate.

Contraindications: Patients with anuria or hypersensitivity to this or other sulfonamide derived drugs.

Warnings: Saluron should be used with caution in severe renal disease. In patients with renal disease, thiazides may precipitate azotemia. Cumulative effects of the drug may develop in patients with impaired renal function.

Thiazides should be used with caution in patients with impaired hepatic function or progressive liver disease, since minor alterations of fluid and electrolyte balance may precipitate hepatic coma.

Thiazides may be additive or potentiative of the action of other antihypertensive drugs. Potentiation occurs with ganglionic or peripheral adrenergic blocking drugs.

Sensitivity reactions may occur in patients with a history of allergy or bronchial asthma.

The possibility of exacerbation or activation of systemic lupus erythematosus has been reported.

Usage in Pregnancy: Thiazides cross the placental barrier and appear in cord blood. The use of thiazides in pregnant women requires that the anticipated benefit be weighed against possible hazards to the fetus. These hazards include fetal or neonatal jaundice, thrombocytopenia, and possibly other adverse reactions which have occurred in the adult.

Nursing Mothers: Thiazides appear in breast milk. If use of the drug is deemed essential, the patient should stop nursing.

Precautions: Periodic determination of serum electrolytes to detect possible electrolyte imbalance should be performed at appropriate intervals.

All patients receiving thiazide therapy should be observed for clinical signs of fluid or electrolyte imbalance; namely, hyponatremia, hypochloremic alkalosis, and hypokalemia. Serum and urine electrolyte determinations are particularly important when the patient is vomiting excessively or receiving parenteral fluids. Medication such as digitalis may also influence serum electrolytes. Warning signs, irrespective of cause, are: Dryness of mouth, thirst, weakness, lethargy, drowsiness, restlessness, muscle pains or cramps, muscular fatigue, hypotension, oliguria, tachycardia, and gastrointestinal disturbances such as nausea and vomiting.

Hypokalemia may develop with thiazides as with any other potent diuretic, especially with brisk diuresis, when severe cirrhosis is present, or during concomitant use of corticosteroids or ACTH.

Interference with adequate oral electrolyte intake will also contribute to hypokalemia. Digitalis therapy may exaggerate metabolic effects of hypokalemia especially with reference to myocardial activity.

Any chloride deficit is generally mild and usually does not require specific treatment except under extraordinary circumstances (as in liver disease or renal disease). Dilutional hyponatremia may occur in edematous patients in hot weather; appropriate therapy is water restriction, rather than administration of salt except in rare instances when the hyponatremia is life threatening. In actual salt depletion, appropriate replacement is the therapy of choice.

Hyperuricemia may occur or frank gout may be precipitated in certain patients receiving thiazide therapy.

Insulin requirements in diabetic patients may be increased, decreased, or unchanged. Latent diabetes mellitus may become manifested during thiazide administration.

Thiazide drugs may increase the responsiveness to tubocurarine.

The antihypertensive effects of the drug may be enhanced in the postsympathectomy patient.

Thiazides may decrease arterial responsiveness to norepinephrine. This diminution is not sufficient to preclude effectiveness of the pressor agent for therapeutic use.

If progressive renal impairment becomes evident, as indicated by a rising nonprotein nitrogen or blood urea nitrogen, a careful reappraisal of therapy is necessary with consideration given to withholding or discontinuing diuretic therapy.

Thiazides may decrease serum PBI levels without signs of thyroid disturbance.

Adverse Reactions:

A. Gastrointestinal system reactions: Anorexia, gastric irritation, nausea, vomiting, cramping, diarrhea, constipation, jaundice (intrahepatic cholestatic jaundice), pancreatitis.
B. Central nervous system reactions: Dizziness, vertigo, parasthesias, headache, xanthopsia.
C. Hematologic reactions: Leukopenia, agranulocytosis, thrombocytopenia, aplastic anemia.
D. Dermatologic—Hypersensitivity reactions: Purpura, photo-sensitivity, rash, urticaria, necrotizing angiitis (vasculitis) (cutaneous vasculitis).
E. Cardiovascular reaction: Orthostatic hypotension may occur and may be aggravated by alcohol, barbiturates, or narcotics.
F. Other: Hyperglycemia, glycosuria, hyperuricemia, muscle spasm, weakness, restlessness.

Whenever adverse reactions are moderate or severe, thiazide dosage should be reduced or therapy withdrawn.

Dosage and Administration: The average adult diuretic dose is 25 to 200 mg. per day. The average adult antihypertensive dose is 50 to 100 mg. per day.

Therapy should be individualized according to patient response. This therapy should be titrated to gain maximal therapeutic response as well as the minimal dose possible to maintain that therapeutic response.

How Supplied: NDC 0015-5410—Saluron Tablets, scored, 50 mg., bottles of 100.

[*Shown in product identification Section*]

SALUTENSIN® ℞
SALUTENSIN-Demi™
(hydroflumethiazide, reserpine Antihypertensive Formulation)

This is the full text of the latest Official Package Circular dated March 1977 [5436 DIMO-07].

> **WARNING**
> This fixed combination drug is not indicated for initial therapy of hypertension. Hypertension requires therapy titrated to the individual patient. If the fixed combination represents the dosage so determined, its use may be more convenient in patient management. The treatment of hypertension is not static, but must be reevaluated as conditions in each patient warrant.

Description: Salutensin combines two antihypertensive agents: Saluron® (hydroflumethiazide) and reserpine. The chemical name for hydroflumethiazide is 3,4-dihydro-7-sulfamyl-6-trifluoromethyl-2H-1,2,4-benzothiadiazine-1,1-dioxide. Reserpine (3,4,5-trimethoxybenzoyl methyl reserpate) is a crystalline alkaloid derived from Rauwolfia serpentina.

Each Salutensin tablet contains:

Saluron (hydroflumethiazide)....	50 mg
Reserpine	0.125 mg

Each Salutensin-Demi tablet contains:

Saluron (hydroflumethiazide)....	25 mg
Reserpine	0.125 mg

Actions: Hydroflumethiazide is an oral diuretic-antihypertensive agent. It exerts its effect by inhibiting renal tubular reabsorption, inducing increased excretion of sodium and chloride and water with variable concomitant loss of potassium and bicarbonate as well. When used alone as an antihypertensive agent, hydroflumethiazide usually induces a gradual but sustained decrease in abnormally elevated blood pressure—both systolic and diastolic. Hypertensive patients who have been maintained on chlorothiazide or hydrochlorothiazide may also be maintained on hydroflumethiazide.

The component, reserpine, probably produces its antihypertensive effects through depletion of tissue stores of catecholamines (epinephrine and norepinephrine) from peripheral sites. By contrast, its sedative and tranquilizing properties are thought to be related by depletion of 5-hydroxytryptamine from the brain.

Reserpine is characterized by slow onset of action and sustained effect. Both its cardiovascular and central nervous system effects may persist following withdrawal of the drug.

Careful observation for changes in blood pressure must be made when Salutensin is used with other antihypertensive drugs. The dosage of other agents must be reduced by at least 50 percent as soon as Salutensin is added to the regimen to prevent excessive drop in blood pressure. As the blood pressure falls under the potentiating effect of Salutensin, a further reduction in dosage or even discontinuation of other antihypertensive drugs may be necessary.

Hypertension therapy requires therapy titrated to the individual patient. If a fixed combination represents the dosage so determined its use may be more convenient in patient management.

Indications: Hypertension (see box warning).

Contraindications: Salutensin is contraindicated in patients who have previously demonstrated hypersensitivity to its components. Patients with anuria or oliguria should not be given this medication. The presence of an active peptic ulcer, ulcerative colitis, or severe depression contraindicates the use of reserpine. It is also contraindicated in patients receiving electroconvulsive therapy.

Warnings: Azotemia may be precipitated or increased by hydroflumethiazide. Special caution is necessary in patients with impaired renal function to avoid cumulative or toxic effects.

Since in hepatic cirrhosis, minor alterations of fluid and electrolyte balance may precipitate coma, hydroflumethiazide should be given with caution.

The possibility of sensitivity reactions should be considered in patients with a history of allergy or bronchial asthma.

Hydroflumethiazide potentiates the action of other antihypertensive drugs. Therefore, the dosage of these agents, especially the ganglion blockers, must be reduced by at least 50 percent as soon as hydroflumethiazide is added to the regimen.

The possibility of exacerbation or activation of systemic lupus erythematosus has been re-

Continued on next page

Bristol—Cont.

ported for sulfonamide derivatives (including thiazides) and reserpine.
The occurrence of mental depression due to reserpine in doses of 0.25 mg daily or less is unusual. In any event, Salutensin should be discontinued at the first sign of depression.
There have been several reports, published and unpublished, concerning nonspecific small bowel lesions consisting of stenosis with or without ulceration, associated with the administration of enteric coated thiazides with potassium salts. These lesions may occur with enteric coated potassium tablets alone or when they are used with nonenteric coated thiazides, or certain other oral diuretics.
These small bowel lesions have caused obstruction, hemorrhage, and perforation. Surgery was frequently required and deaths have occurred.
Available information tends to implicate enteric coated potassium salts, although lesions of this type also occur spontaneously. CAUTION: Coated potassium-containing formulations should be administered only when indicated, and should be discontinued immediately if abdominal pain, distention, nausea, vomiting, or gastrointestinal bleeding occurs.
Coated potassium tablets should be used only when adequate dietary supplementation is not practical.

Usage in Pregnancy and the Child-Bearing Age
Since thiazides and reserpine appear in breast milk, Salutensin is contraindicated in nursing mothers. If use of the drug is deemed essential, the patient should stop nursing. Reserpine has been demonstrated to cross the placental barrier in guinea pigs with depression of adrenal catecholamine stores in the newborn. There is some evidence that side effects such as nasal congestion, lethargy, depressed Moro reflex, and bradycardia may appear in infants born of reserpine-treated mothers. Thiazides cross the placental barrier and appear in cord blood. When Salutensin is used in women of child-bearing age, the potential benefits of the drug should be weighed against the possible hazards to the fetus. These hazards include fetal or neonatal jaundice, thrombocytopenia, and possibly other adverse reactions which have occurred in the adult.

Precautions:

Hydroflumethiazide
Careful check should be kept for signs of fluid and electrolyte imbalance. Serum and urine electrolyte determinations are particularly important when the patient is vomiting excessively or receiving parenteral fluids. Warning signs, irrespective of cause, are: dryness of mouth, thirst, weakness, lethargy, drowsiness, restlessness, muscle pains or cramps, muscular fatigue, hypotension, oliguria, tachycardia, and gastrointestinal disturbances.
Potassium excretion is usually minimal. However, hypokalemia may develop with hydroflumethiazide as with any other potent diuretic, especially with brisk diuresis, when severe cirrhosis is present, or during concomitant use of steroids or ACTH. Interference with adequate electrolyte intake will contribute to hypokalemia. Digitalis therapy may exaggerate metabolic effects of hypokalemia especially with reference to myocardial activity. If dietary salt is unduly restricted, especially during hot weather, in severely edematous patients with congestive failure or renal disease, a low salt syndrome may complicate therapy with thiazides.
Hypokalemia may be avoided or treated by use of potassium chloride or giving foods with a high potassium content. Any chloride deficit may similarly be corrected by use of ammonium chloride (excepting patients with hepatic disease) and largely prevented by a near normal salt intake.
Thiazide drugs may increase the responsiveness to tubocurarine. The antihypertensive effect of the drug may be enhanced in the post-sympathectomy patient. Hydroflumethiazide decreases arterial responsiveness to norepinephrine, as do the other thiazides, necessitating due care in surgical patients. It is recommended that thiazides be discontinued 48 hours before elective surgery. Orthostatic hypotension may occur and may be potentiated by alcohol, barbiturates, or narcotics.
Pathological changes in the parathyroid glands with hypercalcemia and hypophosphatemia have been observed in a few patients on prolonged thiazide therapy. The common complications of hyperparathyroidism such as renal lithiasis, bone resorption, and peptic ulceration have not been seen. The effect of discontinuance of thiazide therapy on serum calcium and phosphorus levels may be helpful in assessing the need for parathyroid surgery in such patients. Parathyroidectomy has been followed by subjective clinical improvement in most patients, but is without effect on the hypertension. Following surgery, thiazide therapy may be resumed.
Caution is necessary in patients with hyperuricemia or a history of gout, since gout may be precipitated. Insulin requirements in diabetic patients may be increased, decreased, or unchanged. In latent diabetics, hydroflumethiazide, in common with other benzothiadiazines, may cause hyperglycemia and glycosuria.

Reserpine
Since reserpine may increase gastric secretion and motility, it should be used cautiously in patients with a history of peptic ulcer, ulcerative colitis, or other gastrointestinal disorders. This compound may precipitate biliary colic in patients with gallstones, or bronchial asthma in susceptible persons.
Reserpine may cause hypotension including orthostatic hypotension. In hypertensive patients on reserpine therapy significant hypotension and bradycardia may develop during surgical anesthesia. Therefore, the drug should be discontinued two weeks before giving anesthesia. For emergency surgical procedures, it may be necessary to give vagal blocking agents parenterally to prevent or reverse hypotension and/or bradycardia.
Anxiety or depression, as well as psychosis, may develop during reserpine therapy. If depression is present when therapy is begun, it may be aggravated. Mental depression is unusual with reserpine doses of 0.25 mg daily or less. In any case, Salutensin should be discontinued at the first sign of depression. Extreme caution should be used in treating patients with a history of mental depression, and the possibility of suicide should be kept in mind.
As with most antihypertensive therapy, caution should be exercised when treating hypertensive patients with renal insufficiency, since they adjust poorly to lowered blood pressure levels. Use reserpine cautiously with digitalis and quinidine; cardiac arrhythmias have occurred with reserpine preparations. Thiazides may decrease serum P.B.I. levels without signs of thyroid disturbance.

Adverse Reactions:

Hydroflumethiazide

A. Gastrointestinal System Reactions: Anorexia, gastric irritation, nausea, vomiting, cramping, diarrhea, constipation, jaundice (intrahepatic cholestatic jaundice), pancreatitis, hyperglycemia, and glycosuria.
B. Central Nervous System Reactions: dizziness, vertigo, parasthesias, headache, and xanthopsia.
C. Hematologic Reactions: leukopenia, thrombocytopenia, agranulocytosis, and aplastic anemia.
D. Dermatologic—Hypersensitivity Reactions: purpura, photosensitivity, rash, urticaria, and necrotizing angiitis (vasculitis) (cutaneous vasculitis).
E. Cardiovascular Reaction: orthostatic hypotension may occur and may be aggravated by alcohol, barbiturates or narcotics.
F. Miscellaneous: muscle spasm, weakness, and restlessness.

Whenever adverse reactions are moderate or severe, thiazide dosage should be reduced or therapy withdrawn.

Reserpine
Side effects due to reserpine often disappear with continued use and most can be controlled by reducing the dosage. Rarely, it may be necessary to discontinue therapy. The reactions most often reported include: excessive sedation, nightmares, nasal congestion, conjunctival injection, enhanced susceptibility to colds, muscular aches, headache, dizziness, dyspnea, anorexia, nausea, increased intestinal motility, diarrhea, weight gain, dryness of the mouth, blurred vision, flushing of the skin and pruritus. Skin rash, dysuria, syncope, non-puerperal lactation, impotence or decreased libido, increased salivation, vomiting, bradycardia, mental depression, nervousness, paradoxical anxiety, epistaxis, purpura due to thrombocytopenia, angina pectoris and other direct cardiac effects (e.g., premature ventricular contractions, fluid retention, congestive failure), and central nervous system sensitization manifested by dull sensorium, deafness, glaucoma, uveitis, and optic atrophy also have been noted. In some patients reserpine has produced a syndrome similar to Parkinson's disease, though this effect usually is reversible with decreased dosage or discontinuation of therapy. Salutensin should be given with caution to hypertensive patients who also have coronary artery disease to avoid a precipitous drop in blood pressure.

Dosage: As determined by individual titration (see box warning).
The usual adult dose of Salutensin is one tablet once or twice daily. If a smaller amount of thiazide diuretic is desired, Salutensin-Demi, one tablet once or twice daily, can be given. Most patients will respond to this dosage level. In refractory cases, the physician may carefully increase the dose to three or four tablets per day in divided doses providing the proper precautions are observed—careful attention to serum uric acid, fasting blood sugar, BUN or NPN, and serum electrolyte levels. (See section on Precautions and Warnings above.) When the desired blood pressure reduction has been achieved, the dose should be reduced to the minimum effective dose for the individual patient.
Careful observation for changes in blood pressure must be made when Salutensin is used with other antihypertensive drugs. The dosage of other agents must be reduced by at least 50 percent as soon as Salutensin is added to the regimen to prevent excessive drop in blood pressure. As the blood pressure falls under the potentiating effect of Salutensin, a further reduction in dosage or even discontinuation of other antihypertensive drugs may be necessary.

Supply:
Salutensin Tablets—**NDC** 0015-5436
[*Shown in Product Identification Section*]
Salutensin-Demi Tablets—**NDC** 0015-5455
For information on package sizes available, refer to the current price schedule.

STADOL® ℞
(butorphanol tartrate)

This is the full text of the latest Official Package Circular dated July 1978 [5644DIM-02].

Description: Stadol (butorphanol tartrate), sterile, parenteral, narcotic agonistantagonist, analgesic, is a member of the phenanthrene series. The chemical name is levo-N-cyclobutylmethyl-6, 10aβ-dihydroxy-1,2,3,9,10, 10a-hexahydro-(4H)-10, 4a-iminoethanophenanthrene tartrate. It is a white crystalline substance soluble in aqueous solution. The dose is expressed as the salt. One milligram of tartrate salt is equivalent to 0.68 milligram of base. In addition to Stadol (butorphanol tartrate), each ml contains 3.3 mg citric acid, 6.4 mg sodium citrate and 6.4 mg sodium chloride. The molecular weight is 477.56 and the molecular formula is $C_{21}H_{29}NO_2\text{-}C_4H_6O_6$

Clinical Pharmacology: Stadol is a potent analgesic. The duration of analgesia is generally 3 to 4 hours and is approximately equivalent to that of morphine. The onset time for analgesia appears less than 30 minutes after intramuscular administration and very rapidly following intravenous administration. Peak analgesic activity is obtained at 1 hour following intramuscular injection and at least 30 minutes following intravenous injection.

Narcotic Antagonist Activity

Stadol has narcotic antagonist activity which is approximately equivalent to that of nalorphine, 30 times that of pentazocine and 1/40 that of naloxone (Narcan®) as measured by the antagonism of morphine analgesia in the rattail Flick test.

Mechanism of Analgesic Action

The exact mechanism of action of Stadol is unknown. It is felt that the class of narcotic antagonist analgesics exert their analgesic effect via a central nervous system mechanism. Currently, it is believed the site of action of centrally acting analgesics is subcortical, possibly in the limbic system.

Effect on Respiration

At the analgesic dose of 2 mg, Stadol depresses respiration to a degree equal to 10 mg morphine. The magnitude of respiratory depression with Stadol is not appreciably increased at doses of 4 mg. In contrast to the magnitude of respiratory depression, the duration of respiratory depression with Stadol is dose-related. Any respiratory depression produced by Stadol is reversible by naloxone which is a specific antagonist.

Cardiovascular Effects

The hemodynamic changes after the intravenous administration of Stadol are similar to the reported hemodynamic changes after pentzocine. The changes include increased pulmonary artery pressure, pulmonary wedge pressure, left ventricular end-diastolic pressure, systemic arterial pressure, and pulmonary vascular resistance. Although smaller than those following pentazocine, these changes are nevertheless in a direction which increases the work of the heart, especially in the pulmonary circuit.

Indications and Usage: Stadol is recommended for the relief of moderate to severe pain.

Contraindications: Stadol should not be administered to patients who have been shown to be hypersensitive to it.

Warnings:

Patients Physically Dependent on Narcotics

Because of its antagonist properties, Stadol is not recommended for patients physically dependent on narcotics. Detoxification in such patients is required prior to use.

Due to the difficulty in assessing addiction in patients who have recently received substantial amounts of narcotic medication, caution should be used in the administration of Stadol. Detoxification of such patients prior to usage should be carefully considered.

Drug Dependence

Special care should be exercised in administering Stadol to emotionally unstable patients and to those with a history of drug misuse. When long-term therapy is contemplated, such patients should be closely supervised. Even though Stadol has a low physical dependence liability, care should be taken that individuals who may be prone to drug abuse are closely supervised. It is important to avoid increases in dose and frequency of injections by the patient and to prevent the use of the drug in anticipation of pain rather than for the relief of pain.

Head Injury and Increased Intracranial Pressure

Although there is no clinical experience in patients with head injury, it can be assumed that Stadol, like other potent analgesics, elevates cerebrospinal fluid pressure. Therefore the use of Stadol in cases of head injury can produce effects (e.g., miosis) which may obscure the clinical course of patients with head injuries. In such patients Stadol must be used with extreme caution and only if its use is deemed essential.

Cardiovascular Effects

Because Stadol increases the work of the heart, especially the pulmonary circuit, (see Clinical Pharmacology), the use of this drug in acute myocardial infarction or in cardiac patients with ventricular dysfunction or coronary insufficiency should be limited to those who are hypersensitive to morphine sulfate or meperidine.

Precautions:

Certain Respiratory Conditions

Because Stadol causes some respiratory depression, it should be administered only with caution and low dosage to patients with respiratory depression (e.g., from other medication, uremia, or severe infection), severely limited respiratory reserve, bronchial asthma, obstructive respiratory conditions, or cyanosis.

Impaired Renal or Hepatic Function

Although laboratory tests have not indicated that Stadol causes or increases renal or hepatic impairment, the drug should be administered with caution to patients with such impairment. Extensive liver disease may predispose to greater side effects and greater activity from the usual clinical dose, possibly the result of decreased metabolism of the drug by the liver.

Biliary Surgery

Clinical studies have not been done to establish the safety of Stadol administration to patients about to undergo surgery of the biliary tract.

Usage in Pregnancy

The safety of Stadol for use in pregnancy has not been established; therefore, this drug should be used in pregnant patients only when, in the judgment of the physician, its use is deemed essential to the welfare of the patient. Reproduction studies have been performed in rats, mice, and rabbits and have revealed no evidence of impaired fertility or harm to the fetus due to Stadol at about 2.5 to 5 times the human dose.

Usage in Labor and Delivery

Safety to the mother and fetus following administration of Stadol during labor and delivery has not been established.

Usage in Nursing Mothers

The use of Stadol is not recommended in nursing mothers since it is not known whether this drug is excreted in human milk.

Pediatric Use

Safety and efficacy in children below age 18 years have not been established.

Adverse Reactions: The most frequent adverse reactions in 1250 patients treated with Stadol are: sedation (503, 40%), nausea (82, 6%), clammy/sweating (76, 6%).

Less frequent reactions are: headache (35, 3%), vertigo (33, 3%), floating feeling (33, 3%), dizziness (23, 2%) lethargy (19, 2%), confusion (15, 1%), lightheadedness (12, 1%).

Other adverse reactions which may occur (reported incidence of less than 1%) are:

CNS effects: nervousness, unusual dreams, agitation, euphoria, hallucinations

Autonomic effects: flushing and warmth, dry mouth, sensitivity to cold

Cardiovascular: palpitation, increase or decrease of blood pressure

Gastrointestinal: vomiting

Respiratory: slowing of respiration, shallow breathing

Dermatological: rash or hives

Eye: diplopia or blurred vision

Overdosage:

Manifestations

Although there have been no experiences of overdosage with Stadol during clinical trials, this may occur due to accidental or intentional misuse as well as therapeutic use. Based on the pharmacology of Stadol, overdosage could produce some degree of respiratory depression and variable cardiovascular and central nervous sytem effects.

Treatment

The immediate treatment of suspected Stadol overdosage is intravenous naloxone. The respiratory and cardiac status of the patient should be evaluated constantly and appropriate supportive measures instituted, such as oxygen, intravenous fluids, vasopressors, and assisted or controlled respiration.

Dosage and Administration:

Adults:

Intramuscular—The usual recommended single dose is 2 mg. This may be repeated every three to four hours, as necessary. The effective dosage range, depending on the severity of pain, is 1 to 4 mg repeated every three to four hours. At this time, there is insufficient clinical data to recommend single doses beyond 4 mg.

Intravenous—The usual recommended single dose for intravenous administration is 1 mg repeated every three to four hours as necessary. The effective dosage range, depending on the severity of pain, is 0.5 to 2 mg repeated every three to four hours.

Children:

Since there is no clinical experience in children under 18 years, Stadol is not recommended in this age group.

Storage Conditions

When stored at room temperature, the stability of the solution in vials is 2 years.

Supply: Stadol (butorphanol tartrate) Injection for I.M. or I.V. use, 2 mg per ml, 2 ml vial; 1 mg per ml, 1 ml vial; 2 mg per ml, 1 ml vial; 2 mg per ml, 10 ml multi-dose vial.

NDC 0015-5644—2 mg per ml, 2-ml vials
NDC 0015-5645—1 mg per ml, 1-ml vials
NDC 0015-5646—2 mg per ml, 1-ml vials
NDC 0015-5648—2 mg per ml, 10-ml multi-dose vials.

STAPHCILLIN® ℞

(methicillin sodium for Injection)
Buffered
For I.M. Or I.V. Use

This is the full text of the latest Official Package Circular dated May 1979 [7961DIR-15].

Description: Staphcillin (methicillin sodium monohydrate) is a semisynthetic penicillin: 2,6-dimethoxyphenyl penicillin. It is supplied as the sodium salt in a parenteral dosage form. Each Gm. of Staphcillin is equivalent to 900 mg. methicillin activity and is buffered with 50 mg. sodium citrate and preserved with 0.09% methylparaben and 0.01% propylparaben.

Actions and Pharmacology: Staphcillin is a bactericidal penicillin, highly resistant to staphylococcal penicillinase and equally active against penicillin-susceptible and penicillinase-producing strains of Staphylococcus aureus. Methicillin is considerably less active than penicillin G against streptococci and pneumococci. It is not acid-resistant and must be administered by intramuscular or intravenous injection. A 1-Gram intramuscular dose gives a peak blood level of approximately 12 mcg./ml. which drops off to about 1 mcg./ml. within a 4-hour period. Methicillin is rapidly excreted unchanged in the urine in individuals with normal kidney function. Impairment in kidney function results in elevated blood levels which may require adjustment of dosage and treatment intervals. Protein binding of methi-

Continued on next page

Bristol—Cont.

cillin is approximately 40%. The drug penetrates body tissues well, and diffuses readily into pleural, pericardial, and synovial fluids. As with all penicillins, absorption into spinal fluids is poor under normal conditions. However, higher concentrations may be attained in the presence of meningeal inflammation.

Disc Susceptibility Tests
Quantitative methods that require measurement of zone diameters give the most precise estimates of antibiotic susceptibility. One such procedure* has been recommended for use with discs for testing susceptibility to methicillin class antibiotics. Interpretations correlate diameters on the disc test with MIC values for methicillin. With this procedure, a report from the laboratory of "susceptible" indicates that the infecting organism is likely to respond to therapy. A report of "resistant" indicates that the infecting organism is not likely to respond to therapy. A report of "intermediate susceptibility" suggests that the organism would be susceptible if high dosage is used, or if the infection is confined to tissues and fluids (e.g., urine), in which high antibiotic levels are attained.

Indications: Although the principal indication for methicillin sodium is in the treatment of infections due to penicillinase-producing staphylococci, it may be used to initiate therapy in such patients in whom a staphylococcal infection is suspected. (See Important Note below.)
Bacteriologic studies to determine the causative organisms and their susceptibility to methicillin sodium should be performed.

Important Note: When it is judged necessary that treatment be initiated before definitive culture and susceptibility results are known, the choice of methicillin sodium should take into consideration the fact that it has been shown to be effective only in the treatment of infections caused by pneumococci, Group A beta-hemolytic streptococci, and penicillin G-resistant and penicillin G-susceptible staphylococci. If the bacteriology report later indicates the infection is due to an organism other than a penicillin G-resistant staphylococcus susceptible to methicillin sodium, the physician is advised to continue therapy with a drug other than methicillin sodium or any other penicillinase-resistant semisynthetic penicillin.
Recent studies have reported that the percentage of staphylococcal isolates resistant to penicillin G outside the hospital is increasing, approximating the high percentage of resistant staphylococcal isolates found in the hospital. For this reason, it is recommended that a penicillinase-resistant penicillin be used as initial therapy for any suspected staphylococcal infection until culture and susceptibility results are known.
Strains of staphylococci resistant to methicillin have existed in nature and it is known that the number of these strains reported has been increasing. Such strains of staphylococci have been capable of producing serious disease, in some instances resulting in fatality. Because of this, there is concern that widespread use of the penicillinase-resistant penicillins may result in the appearance of an increasing number of staphylococcal strains which are resistant to these penicillins.
Methicillin-resistant strains are almost always resistant to all other penicillinase-resistant penicillins (cross-resistance with cephalosporin derivatives also occurs frequently). Resistance to any penicillinase-resistant penicillin should be interpreted as evidence of clinical resistance to all, in spite of the fact that minor variations in **in vitro** susceptibility may be encountered when more than one penicillinase-resistant penicillin is tested against the same strain of staphylococcus.

Contraindications: A previous hypersensitivity reaction to any penicillin is a contraindication.

Warning: Serious and occasionally fatal hypersensitivity (anaphylactoid) reactions have been reported in patients on penicillin therapy. Although anaphylaxis is more frequent following parenteral therapy, it has occurred in patients on oral penicillins. These reactions are more apt to occur in individuals with a history of sensitivity to multiple allergens.
There have been well documented reports of individuals with a history of penicillin hypersensitivity reactions who have experienced severe hypersensitivity reactions when treated with a cephalosporin. Before therapy with a penicillin, careful inquiry should be made concerning previous hypersensitivity reactions to penicillins, cephalosporins, and other allergens. If an allergic reaction occurs, the drug should be discontinued and the patient treated with the usual agents e.g., pressor amines, antihistamines, and corticosteroids.

Precautions: Penicillin should be used with caution in individuals with histories of significant allergies and/or asthma.
As with any potent drug, periodic assessment of organ system functions, including renal, hepatic, and hematopoietic, should be made during prolonged therapy.
The possibility of bacterial and/or fungal overgrowth should be kept in mind during long-term therapy. If overgrowth of resistant organisms occurs, appropriate measures should be taken.
Safety for use in pregnancy has not been established.
Because of incompletely developed renal function in infants, methicillin may not be completely excreted, with abnormally high blood levels resulting. Frequent blood levels are advisable in this age group with dosage adjustments when necessary.

Adverse Reactions: The hypersensitivity reactions reported are skin rashes, urticaria, serum sickness, and anaphylactic reactions. Oral lesions such as glossitis and stomatitis have been reported. Fever, eosinophilia, oral and rectal moniliasis have also been reported. Hemolytic anemia, transient neutropenia with evidence of granulocytopenia or thrombocytopenia, neuropathy, and nephrotoxicity (oliguria, albuminuria, hematuria, pyuria, and/or cylindruria) are infrequent and usually associated with high doses of parenteral penicillin.

Dosage and Administration: The drug is well tolerated when given by deep intragluteal or intravenous injection. As is the case with other antibiotics, the duration of therapy should be determined by the clinical and bacteriological response of the patient. Therapy should be continued for at least 48 hours after the patient has become afebrile, asymptomatic, and cultures are negative. In serious systemic infection, therapy should be continued for at least 1 to 2 weeks after the patient is afebrile and cultures are sterile.
Treatment of osteomyelitis may require several months of intensive therapy.
Oral penicillinase-resistant penicillins may be of special value in follow-up therapy because of the difficulty of maintaining prolonged parenteral treatment.

Intramuscular Route: The usual adult dose is 1 Gm. every 4 or 6 hours. Infants' and children's dosage is 25 mg./Kg. (approximately 12 mg./lb.) every 6 hours.

Intravenous Route: The usual adult dose is 1 Gm. every 6 hours using 50 ml. of Sodium Chloride Injection, U.S.P. at the rate of 10 ml. per minute.
The number of instances in which the drug was administered intravenously to infants and children is not large enough to permit specific intravenous dosage recommendations.

Directions For Use:

For Intramuscular Use: Use Sterile Water for Injection, U.S.P. or Sodium Chloride Injection U.S.P. Add 1.5 ml. to the 1.0-Gm. vial, 5.7 ml. to the 4.0-Gm. vial, and 8.6 ml. to the 6.0-Gm. vial, and withdraw the entire contents. Each 1.0 ml. will contain approximately 500 mg. of Staphcillin. The solutions are stable for 24 hours at room temperature and 4 days under refrigeration.

For Direct Intravenous Use: Further dilute each 1.0 ml. of solution, reconstituted as above, with 25 ml. of Sodium Chloride Injection, U.S.P. and inject at the rate of 10 ml. per minute.

For Administration by Intravenous Drip: Reconstitute as directed above (For Intramuscular Use) prior to diluting with Intravenous Solution. Stability studies on Staphcillin at concentrations of 2 mg./ml., 10 mg./ml., and 20 mg./ml. in various intravenous solutions indicate the drug will lose less than 10% activity at room temperature (70°F.) during an 8-hour period.

I.V. Solution
Isotonic Sodium Chloride
5% Dextrose in Water
5% Dextrose in Normal Saline
10% D-Fructose in Water
10% D-Fructose in Normal Saline
M/6 Sodium r-Lactate Solution
Lactated Ringer's Injection
Lactated Potassic Saline Injection
5% Plasma Hydrolysate in Water
10% Invert Sugar in Water
*10% Invert Sugar in Normal Saline
10% Invert Sugar plus 0.3% Potassium Chloride in Water
Travert 10% Electrolyte #1
Travert 10% Electrolyte #2
Travert 10% Electrolyte #3

*At a concentration of 2 mg./ml., Staphcillin is stable for only 4 hours in this solution. Concentrations between 10 mg./ml. and 30 mg./ml. are stable for 8 hours.
Only those solutions listed above should be used for the intravenous infusion of Staphcillin. The concentration of the antibiotic should fall within the range specified. The drug concentration and the rate and volume of the infusion should be adjusted so that the total dose of methicillin is administered before the drug loses its stability in the solution in use.
If another agent is used in conjunction with methicillin therapy, **it should not be physically mixed** with methicillin but should be administered separately.

"Piggyback" I.V. Package: This glass vial contains the labeled quantity of Staphcillin and is intended for intravenous administration. The diluent and volume are specified on the label of each package.
Discard solution after 24 hours at room temperature.

Hospital Bulk Package: This glass vial contains 10 grams Staphcillin and is designed for use in the pharmacy in preparing I.V. additives. Add 94 ml Sterile Water for Injection. U.S.P. or Sodium Chloride Injection, U.S.P. The resulting solution will contain 100 mg methicillin sodium per ml, which is equivalent to 90 mg per ml methicillin activity.
Following reconstitution in this manner, the resulting solutions are stable for 24 hours at room temperature.

Caution: NOT TO BE DISPENSED AS A UNIT.

Supply:
STAPHCILLIN (methicillin sodium for Injection) buffered.

---

*Bauer, A. W., Kirby, W. M. M., Sherris, J. C. and Turck, M.: Antibiotic Testing by a Standard Single Disc Method, Am. J. Clin. Pathol., 45:493, 1966; Standardized Disc Susceptibility Test, FEDERAL REGISTER 37:20527-29, 1972.

NDC 0015-7961-20—1.0-gram vial.
NDC 0015-7964-20—4.0-gram vial.
NDC 0015-7965-20—6.0-gram vial.
NDC 0015-7961-28—1.0-gram "piggyback" vial.
NDC 0015-7964-28—4.0-gram "piggyback" vial.
NDC 0015-7012-28—10-gram Hospital Bulk Package.
For information on package sizes available, refer to the current price sheets.

TEGOPEN® ℞
(cloxacillin sodium)
For Oral Solution
Capsules

This is the full text of the latest Official Package Circular dated January 1978 [7935DIRO-10].

Description: Tegopen (cloxacillin sodium monohydrate) is a member of the Bristol family of synthetic penicillins. It has been demonstrated to be especially efficacious in the treatment of penicillinase-producing staphylococcal infections and effective in the treatment of other commonly encountered Gram-positive coccal infections.

Actions:
Pharmacology
Cloxacillin is resistant to destruction by acid and is well-absorbed from the gastrointestinal tract.
Microbiology
Cloxacillin is active against most Gram-positive cocci including beta-hemolytic streptococci, pneumococci, and nonpenicillinase-producing staphylococci. Because of its resistance to the enzyme penicillinase, it is also active against penicillinase-producing staphylococci.
Disc Susceptibility Tests
Quantitative methods that require measurement of zone diameters give the most precise estimates of antibiotic susceptibility. One such procedure* has been recommended for use with discs for testing susceptibility to methicillin class antibiotics. Interpretations correlate diameters on the disc test with MIC values for methicillin. With this procedure, a report from the laboratory of "susceptible" indicates that the infecting organism is likely to respond to therapy. A report of "resistant" indicates that the infecting organism is not likely to respond to therapy. A report of "intermediate susceptibility" suggests that the organism would be susceptible if high dosage is used, or if the infection is confined to tissues and fluids (e.g. urine), in which high antibiotic levels are attained.

Indications: Although the principal indication for cloxacillin sodium is in the treatment of infections due to penicillinase-producing staphylococci, it may be used to initiate therapy in such patients in whom a staphylococcal infection is suspected. (See Important Note below.)
Bacteriologic studies to determine the causative organisms and their susceptibility to cloxacillin sodium should be performed.
In serious, life-threatening infections, oral preparations of the penicillinase-resistant penicillins should not be relied on for initial therapy.

Important Note: When it is judged necessary that treatment be initiated before definitive culture and susceptibility results are known, the choice of cloxacillin sodium should take into consideration the fact that it has been shown to be effective only in the treatment of infections caused by pneumococci, Group A beta-hemolytic streptococci, and penicillin G-resistant and penicillin G-susceptible staphylococci. If the bacteriology report later indicates the infection is due to an organism other than a penicillin G-resistant staphylococcus susceptible to cloxacillin sodium, the physician is advised to continue therapy with a drug other than cloxacillin sodium or any other penicillinase-resistant semi-synthetic penicillin.
Recent studies have reported that the percentage of staphylococcal isolates resistant to penicillin G outside the hospital is increasing, approximating the high percentage of resistant staphylococcal isolates found in the hospital. For this reason, it is recommended that a penicillinase-resistant penicillin be used as initial therapy for any suspected staphylococcal infection until culture and susceptibility results are known.
Cloxacillin sodium is a compound that acts through a mechanism similar to that of methicillin against penicillin G-resistant staphylococci. Strains of staphylococci resistant to methicillin have existed in nature and it is known that the number of these strains reported has been increasing. Such strains of staphylococci have been capable of producing serious disease, in some instances resulting in fatality. Because of this, there is concern that widespread use of the penicillinase-resistant penicillins may result in the appearance of an increasing number of staphylococcal strains which are resistant to these penicillins.
Methicillin-resistant strains are almost always resistant to all other penicillinase-resistant penicillins (cross resistance with cephalosporin derivatives also occurs frequently). Resistance to any penicillinase-resistant penicillin should be interpreted as evidence of clinical resistance to all, in spite of the fact that minor variations in **in vitro** susceptibility may be encountered when more than one penicillinase-resistant penicillin is tested against the same strain of staphylococcus.

Contraindications: A history of a previous hypersensitivity reaction to any of the penicillins is a contraindication.

Warning: Serious and occasionally fatal hypersensitivity (anaphylactoid) reactions have been reported in patients on penicillin therapy. Although anaphylaxis is more frequent following parenteral therapy it has occurred in patients on oral penicillins. These reactions are more apt to occur in individuals with a history of sensitivity to multiple allergens.
There have been well documented reports of individuals with a history of penicillin hypersensitivity reactions who have experienced severe hypersensitivity reactions when treated with a cephalosporin. Before therapy with a penicillin, careful inquiry should be made concerning previous hypersensitivity reactions to penicillins, cephalosporins, and other allergens. If an allergic reaction occurs, the drug should be discontinued and the patient treated with the usual agents e.g., pressor amines, antihistamines, and corticosteroids.
Usage in Pregnancy
Safety for use in pregnancy has not been established.

Precautions: The possibility of the occurrence of superinfections with mycotic organisms or other pathogens should be kept in mind when using this compound, as with other antibiotics. If superinfection occurs during therapy, appropriate measures should be taken.
As with any potent drug, periodic assessment of organ system function, including renal, hepatic, and hematopoietic, should be made during long-term therapy.

Adverse Reactions: Gastrointestinal disturbances, such as nausea, epigastric discomfort, flatulence, and loose stools, have been noted by some patients. Mildly elevated SGOT levels (less than 100 units) have been reported in a few patients for whom pretherapeutic determinations were not made. Skin rashes and allergic symptoms, including wheezing and sneezing, have occasionally been encountered. Eosinophilia, with or without overt allergic manifestations, has been noted in some patients during therapy.

Dosage: For mild-to-moderate upper respiratory and localized skin and soft tissue infections due to susceptible organisms:
- Adults and children weighing 20 Kg. (44 lbs.) or more: 250 mg. q. 6h.
- Children weighing less than 20 Kg. (44 lbs.): 50 mg./Kg./day in equally-divided doses q. 6h.

For more severe infections such as those of the lower respiratory tract or disseminated infections:
- Adults and children weighing 20 Kg. (44 lbs.) or more: 500 mg. or higher q. 6h.
- Children weighing less than 20 Kg. (44 lbs.): 100 mg./Kg./day or higher in equally-divided doses q. 6h.

Studies indicate that this material is best absorbed when taken on an empty stomach, preferably one to two hours before meals.
N.B.: INFECTIONS CAUSED BY GROUP A BETA-HEMOLYTIC STREPTOCOCCI SHOULD BE TREATED FOR AT LEAST 10 DAYS TO HELP PREVENT THE OCCURRENCE OF ACUTE RHEUMATIC FEVER OR ACUTE GLOMERULONEPHRITIS.

Directions For Dispensing Oral Solution: Prepare solution at the time of dispensing. For ease in preparation add the water in two portions, shaking well after each addition. Add the total amount of water as directed on the labeling of the package being dispensed. Refrigerated, the solution is stable for 14 days.

Supply:
TEGOPEN (cloxacillin sodium) Capsules. Each capsule contains cloxacillin sodium equivalent to 250 mg. or 500 mg. cloxacillin.
NDC 0015-7935—250 mg.
NDC 0015-7496—500 mg.
[*Shown in Product Identification Section*]
TEGOPEN (cloxacillin sodium) for Oral Solution. Each 5 ml. of reconstituted solution contains cloxacillin sodium equivalent to 125 mg. cloxacillin.
NDC 0015-7941—125 mg., 100 ml. and 200 ml. bottles
For information on package sizes available, refer to the current price sheet.

*Bauer, A. W., Kirby, W. M. M., Sherris, J. C. and Turck, M.: Antibiotic Testing by a Standardized Single Disc Method, Am. J. Clin. Pathol., 45:493, 1966; Standardized Disc Susceptibility Test, FEDERAL REGISTER 37:20527-29, 1972.

TETREX® ℞
(tetracycline phosphate complex)
Capsules 250 mg.
bidCAPS® 500 mg.

This is the full text of the latest Official Package Circular dated January 1978 [4322DIRO-14].

Description:
Each capsule contains:
Tetrex (tetracycline phosphate complex equivalent to tetracycline HCl activity) .....250 mg.
bidCaps (tetracycline phosphate complex equivalent to tetracycline HCl activity) ...500 mg.

Actions and Pharmacology: The tetracyclines are primarily bacteriostatic and are thought to exert their antimicrobial effect by inhibition of protein synthesis. Tetracyclines are active against a wide range of Gram-negative and Gram-positive organisms.
The drugs in the tetracycline class have closely similar antimicrobial spectra, and cross-resistance among them appears complete. Microorganisms may be considered highly sensitive if the M.I.C. (minimum inhibitory concentration) is not more than 4.0 mcg./ml. and intermediate if the M.I.C. is 4.0 to 12.5 mcg./ml.
Susceptibility plate testing: A tetracycline disc may be used to determine microbial susceptibility to drugs in the tetracycline class. If the Kirby-Bauer method of disc sensitivity is used, a 30-mcg. tetracycline disc should give a zone of

Continued on next page

Bristol—Cont.

over 18 mm. when tested against a tetracycline-sensitive bacterial strain.
Tetracyclines are readily absorbed and are bound to plasma proteins in varying degree. They are concentrated by the liver in the bile and excreted in the urine and feces at high concentrations and in a biologically active form.
Tetrex has the same actions and uses as the parent antibiotic, tetracycline, or its hydrochloride salt. However, the phosphate complex is more rapidly and more completely absorbed from the gastrointestinal tract than is the free base or its salts and therefore produces somewhat higher blood levels after oral administration.

Indications:
Tetracycline is indicated in infections caused by the following microorganisms:

Rickettsiae: Rocky Mountain spotted fever, typhus fever and the typhus group, Q fever, rickettsialpox, tick fevers,
Mycoplasma pneumoniae (PPLO, Eaton agent),
Agents of psittacosis and ornithosis,
Agents of lymphogranuloma venereum and granuloma inguinale,
The spirochetal agent of relapsing fever (**Borrelia recurrentis**).

The following Gram-negative organisms:

Haemophilus ducreyi (chancroid),
Pasteurella pestis and **Pasteurella tularensis,**
Bartonella bacilliformis,
Bacteroides species,
Vibrio comma and **Vibrio fetus,**
Brucella species (in conjunction with streptomycin).

Because many strains of the following groups of microorganisms have been shown to be resistant to tetracyclines, culture and susceptibility testing are recommended.
Tetracycline is indicated for treatment of infections caused by the following Gram-negative microorganisms, when bacteriologic testing indicates appropriate susceptibility to the drug.

Escherichia coli,
Enterobacter aerogenes (formerly **Aerobacter aerogenes),**
Shigella species,
Mima species and **Herellea** species,
Haemophilus influenzae (respiratory infections),
Klebsiella species (respiratory and urinary infections).

The following Gram-positive organisms when bacteriologic testing indicates appropriate susceptibility to the drug:

Streptococcus species:
Up to 44 percent of strains of **Streptococcus pyogenes** and 74 percent of **Streptococcus faecalis** have been found to be resistant to tetracycline drugs. Therefore, tetracycline should not be used for streptococcal disease unless the organism has been demonstrated to be sensitive.
For upper respiratory infections due to Group A beta-hemolytic streptococci, penicillin is the usual drug of choice, including prophylaxis of rheumatic fever.
Diplococcus pneumoniae,
Staphylococcus aureus, skin and soft tissue infections. Tetracyclines are not the drugs of choice in the treatment of any type of staphylococcal infections.

When penicillin is contraindicated, tetracyclines are alternative drugs in the treatment of infections due to:

Neisseria gonorrhoeae,
Treponema pallidum and **Treponema pertenue** (syphilis and yaws),
Listeria monocytogenes,
Clostridium species,
Bacillus anthracis,
Fusobacterium fusiforme (Vincent's infection),
Actinomyces species.

In acute intestinal amebiasis, the tetracyclines may be a useful adjunct to amebicides.
In severe acne, the tetracyclines may be useful adjunctive therapy.
Tetracyclines are indicated in the treatment of trachoma, although the infectious agent is not always eliminated, as judged by immunofluorescence.
Inclusion conjunctivitis may be treated with oral tetracyclines or with a combination of oral and topical agents.

Contraindications: This drug is contraindicated in persons who have shown hypersensitivity to any of the tetracyclines.

Warnings: THE USE OF DRUGS OF THE TETRACYCLINE CLASS DURING TOOTH DEVELOPMENT (LAST HALF OF PREGNANCY, INFANCY, AND CHILDHOOD TO THE AGE OF 8 YEARS) MAY CAUSE PERMANENT DISCOLORATION OF THE TEETH (YELLOW-GRAY-BROWN.)
This adverse reaction is more common during long-term use of the drugs but has been observed following repeated short-term courses. Enamel hypoplasia has also been reported. TETRACYCLINES, THEREFORE, SHOULD NOT BE USED IN THIS AGE GROUP UNLESS OTHER DRUGS ARE NOT LIKELY TO BE EFFECTIVE OR ARE CONTRAINDICATED.
If renal impairment exists, even usual oral or parenteral doses may lead to excessive systemic accumulation of the drug and possible liver toxicity. Under such conditions, lower than the usual doses are indicated and if therapy is prolonged, serum level determinations of the drug may be advisable.
Photosensitivity manifested by exaggerated sunburn reaction has been observed in some individuals taking tetracyclines. Patients apt to be exposed to direct sunlight or ultraviolet light should be advised that this reaction can occur with tetracycline drugs and treatment should be discontinued at the first evidence of skin erythema.
The anti-anabolic action of the tetracyclines may cause an increase in BUN. While this is not a problem in those with normal renal function, in patients with significantly impaired function, higher serum levels of tetracycline may lead to azotemia, hyperphosphatemia, and acidosis.

Usage in Pregnancy: (See above "Warnings" about use during tooth development.)
Results of animal studies indicate that tetracyclines cross the placenta, are found in fetal tissues, and can have toxic effects on the developing fetus (often related to retardation of skeletal development). Evidence of embryotoxicity has also been noted in animals treated early in pregnancy.

Usage in Newborns, Infants, and Children: (See above "Warning" about use during tooth development.)
All tetracyclines form a stable calcium complex in any bone forming tissue. A decrease in the fibula growth rate has been observed in prematures given oral tetracycline in doses of 25 mg./Kg. every 6 hours. This reaction was shown to be reversible when the drug was discontinued.
Tetracyclines are present in the milk of lactating women who are taking a drug in this class.

Precautions: As with other antibiotics, use of this drug may result in overgrowth of nonsusceptible organisms, including fungi. If superinfection occurs, appropriate therapy should be instituted.
When used in the treatment of gonorrhea, a darkfield examination should be made of any lesions suggestive of syphilis before treatment is started and serologic tests for syphilis should be made monthly for at least 4 months afterwards.
Because the tetracyclines have been shown to depress plasma prothrombin activity, patients who are on anticoagulant therapy may require downward adjustment of their anticoagulant dosage.
In long-term therapy, periodic laboratory evaluation of organ systems, including hematopoietic, renal, and hepatic studies should be performed.
INFECTIONS DUE TO GROUP A BETA-HEMOLYTIC STREPTOCOCCI SHOULD BE TREATED FOR A MINIMUM OF 10 DAYS.
Since bacteriostatic drugs may interfere with the bactericidal action of penicillin, it is advisable to avoid giving tetracyclines in conjunction with penicillin.

Adverse Reactions:
Gastrointestinal: Anorexia, nausea, vomiting, diarrhea, glossitis, dysphagia, enterocolitis, and inflammatory lesions (with monilial overgrowth) in the anogenital region. These reactions have been caused by both oral and parenteral administration of tetracyclines.
Skin: Maculopapular and erythematous rashes. Exfoliative dermatitis has been reported but is uncommon. Photosensitivity is discussed above. (See "Warnings".)
Renal Toxicity: Rise in BUN has been reported and is apparently dose related. (See "Warnings".)
Hypersensitivity reactions: Urticaria, angioneurotic edema, anaphylaxis, anaphylactoid purpura, pericarditis, and exacerbation of systemic lupus erythematosus.
Bulging fontanels have been reported in young infants following therapeutic dosage. This sign disappeared rapidly when the drug was discontinued.
Blood: Hemolytic anemia, thrombocytopenia, neutropenia, and eosinophilia have been reported.
When given over prolonged periods, tetracyclines have been reported to produce brown-black microscopic discoloration of thyroid glands. No abnormalities of thyroid function studies are known to occur.

Administration and Dosage:
Capsules
Adults: The usual dose is 1 Gram per day in 4 divided doses of 250 mg. each. Severe infections require higher doses.
For children above eight years of age: The usual dose is 25 mg./Kg./day (12.5 mg./lb./day) in 4 divided doses. Children weighing more than 40 Kg. (88 lbs.) should be given the adult doses.
bidCAPS
Adults: The usual dose is 500 mg. b.i.d. Severe infections require higher doses.
For treatment of brucellosis, 500 mg. tetracycline four times daily for 3 weeks should be accompanied by streptomycin, 1 Gram intramuscularly twice daily the first week and once daily the second week.
For treatment of syphilis, a total of 30 to 40 Grams in equally divided doses over a period of 10 to 15 days should be given. Close follow-up including laboratory tests is recommended.
For treatment of pustular acne, the dosage may be reduced as soon as pustular element is controlled.
Treatment of uncomplicated gonorrhea, when penicillin is contraindicated, tetracycline may be used for the treatment of both males and females in the following divided dosage schedule: 1.5 Grams initially followed by 0.5 Grams q.i.d. for a total of 9.0 Grams.
Concomitant therapy: Iron salts and antacids containing aluminum, calcium, or magnesium impair absorption and should not be given to patients taking oral tetracycline.
Foods and some dairy products also interfere with absorption. Oral forms of tetracycline should be given 1 hour before or 2 hours after meals. Pediatric oral dosage forms should not

be given with milk formulas and should be given at least 1 hour prior to feeding.
Therapy should be continued for at least 24 to 48 hours after symptoms and fever have subsided.
In patients with renal impairment: (See "Warnings".) Total dosage should be decreased by reduction of recommended individual doses and/or by extending time intervals between doses.
In the treatment of streptococcal infections, a therapeutic dose of tetracycline should be administered for at least 10 days.
Supply:
TETREX (tetracycline phosphate complex) Capsules equivalent to 250 mg. tetracycline HCl activity.
NDC 0015-4322—250 mg.
[*Shown in Product Identification Section*]
TETREX bidCaps (tetracycline phosphate complex) Capsules equivalent to 500 mg. tetracycline HCl activity.
NDC 0015-4330—500 mg.
[*Shown in Product Identification Section*]

VERSAPEN®-K CAPSULES
(hetacillin potassium)
VERSAPEN® ℞
(hetacillin)
Oral Suspension, Pediatric Drops

This is the full text of the latest Official Package Circular dated April 1979 [7805DIR-15].
Description: Versapen (hetacillin) is a semisynthetic antibiotic derived from the penicillin nucleus, 6-amino penicillanic acid. **The antibiotic activity of hetacillin is provided by its rapid conversion to ampicillin.**
Actions:
Pharmacology
Oral preparations of hetacillin are acid stable and, therefore, well absorbed. Food retards absorption. In the conversion of hetacillin to ampicillin at a pH of 7.1, the hetacillin half-life is 20 minutes. Oral formulations of hetacillin and hetacillin potassium equivalent to 225 mg. and 450 mg. of ampicillin activity provide peak blood levels in the range of 1.7 to 2.1 mcg./ml. and 2.5 to 2.7 mcg./ml., respectively.
Ampicillin diffuses readily into most body tissues and fluids. However, penetration into the cerebrospinal fluid and brain occurs only when the meninges are inflamed. Ampicillin is excreted largely unchanged in the urine and its excretion can be delayed by concurrent administration of probenecid. The active form appears in the bile in higher concentrations than those found in the serum. Ampicillin is the least serum-bound of all the penicillins, averaging about 20% compared to approximately 60 to 90% for other penicillins.
Microbiology
No antibacterial activity has been demonstrated for the hetacillin moiety itself. Hetacillin, upon conversion to the active drug, ampicillin, is similar to benzyl penicillin in its bactericidal action against sensitive organisms during the stage of active multiplication.
The following bacteria have been shown in **in vitro** studies to be sensitive to ampicillin.
Gram-Positive Organisms—Hemolytic and nonhemolytic streptococci, **D. pneumoniae,** non-penicillinase-producing staphylococci, Clostridia spp., **B. anthracis, Listeria monocytogenes,** and most strains of enterococci.
Gram-Negative Organisms—H. influenzae, N. gonorrhoeae, N. meningitidis, Proteus mirabilis, and many strains of Salmonella, Shigella, and **E. coli.**
The drug does not resist destruction by penicillinase and hence is not effective against penicillin G-resistant staphylococci. Ampicillin Susceptibility Test Discs, 10 micrograms, should be used to estimate the **in vitro** susceptibility of bacteria to hetacillin.
Indications: Versapen is indicated in the treatment of susceptible strains of the following organisms in the diseases listed. Bacteriology studies to determine the causative organisms and their susceptibility should be performed. Therapy may be instituted prior to obtaining results of susceptibility testing.
Group A beta-hemolytic streptococcus: Tonsillitis, pharyngitis, otitis media, skin and soft tissue infections. (Injectable benzathine penicillin is considered to be the drug of choice in treatment and prevention of streptococcal pharyngitis and in long-term prophylaxis of rheumatic fever. Versapen is effective in the eradication of streptococci from the nasopharynx; however, data establishing the efficacy of orally administered Versapen in the subsequent prevention of rheumatic fever are not available at present.)
Diplococcus pneumoniae: Broncho- and lobar pneumonia, otitis media.
Non-penicillinase-producing **Staphylococcus aureus:** Skin and soft tissue infections, otitis media.
Haemophilus influenzae: Bronchitis, bronchopneumonia, otitis media.
Escherichia coli: Cystitis, pyelonephritis, prostatitis/urethritis, skin and soft tissue infections.
Proteus mirabilis: Cystitis, pyelonephritis, skin and soft tissue infections.
Enterococcus (Streptococcus faecalis): Cystitis, pyelonephritis, prostatitis/urethritis.
Shigella species: Shigellosis.
Indicated surgical procedures should be performed.
Contraindications: A history of a previous hypersensitivity reaction to any of the penicillins is a contraindication.
Warnings: Serious and occasionally fatal hypersensitivity (anaphylactic) reactions have been reported in patients on penicillin therapy. Although anaphylaxis is more frequent following parenteral therapy, it has occurred in patients on oral penicillins. These reactions are more apt to occur in individuals with a history of sensitivity to multiple allergens.
There have been reports of individuals with a history of penicillin hypersensitivity reactions who experienced severe hypersensitivity reactions when treated with cephalosporins. Before therapy with a penicillin, careful inquiry should be made concerning previous hypersensitivity reactions to penicillins, cephalosporins, and other allergens.
Serious anaphylactoid reactions require immediate emergency treatment with epinephrine. Oxygen, intravenous steroids, and airway management, including intubation, should also be administered as indicated.
Usage in Pregnancy: Safety for use in pregnancy has not been established.
Precautions: The possibility of superinfection with mycotic or bacterial pathogens should be kept in mind during therapy. In such cases, discontinue the drug and substitute appropriate treatment.
As with any potent drug, periodic assessment of renal, hepatic, and hematopoietic function should be made during prolonged therapy.
This oral preparation should not be relied upon in patients with severe illness or with nausea, vomiting, gastric dilatation, cardiospasm, or intestinal hypermotility.
Adverse Reactions: As with other penicillins, it may be expected that untoward reactions will be essentially limited to sensitivity phenomena. They are more likely to occur in individuals who have previously demonstrated hypersensitivity to penicillins and in those with a history of allergy, asthma, hay fever, or urticaria.
The following adverse reactions have been reported:
Gastrointestinal: Glossitis, stomatitis, black "hairy" tongue, nausea, vomiting, enterocolitis, pseudomembranous colitis, and diarrhea. (These reactions are usually associated with oral dosage forms.)
Hypersensitivity reactions: Skin rashes and urticaria have been reported frequently. A few cases of exfoliative dermatitis and erythema multiforme have been reported. Anaphylaxis is the most serious reaction experienced and has usually been associated with the parenteral dosage form.
Note: Urticaria, other skin rashes, and serum sickness-like reactions may be controlled with antihistamines and, if necessary, systemic corticosteroids. Whenever such reactions occur, the drug should be discontinued, unless, in the opinion of the physician, the condition being treated is life threatening and amenable only to this therapy.
Liver: A moderate rise in serum glutamic oxaloacetic transaminase (SGOT) has been noted, particularly in infants, but the significance of this finding is unknown.
Hemic and Lymphatic Systems: Anemia, thrombocytopenia, thrombocytopenic purpura, eosinophilia, leukopenia, and agranulocytosis have been reported during therapy with the penicillins. These reactions are usually reversible on discontinuation of therapy and are believed to be hypersensitivity phenomena.
Other: Since infectious mononucleosis is viral in origin, hetacillin should not be used in the treatment. A high percentage of patients with mononucleosis who received ampicillin developed a skin rash.
Dosage: Infections of the upper and lower respiratory tracts; those of the skin and soft tissue; and infections of the gastrointestinal and genitourinary tracts due to sensitive organisms:
Patients weighing 88 lbs. (40 Kg.) or more: 225 to 450 mg. q.i.d. depending on the severity of the infection.
Patients weighing less than 88 lbs. (40 Kg.): 22.5 to 45 mg./Kg./day or 10 to 20 mg./lb./day, depending on the severity of the infection.
Urinary and gastrointestinal tract infections may require prolonged and intensive therapy at doses higher than those recommended above. It may be necessary to maintain therapy for several weeks and to continue bacteriologic and/or clinical follow-up for several months after cessation of therapy.
The oral drug should be administered in a fasting state to insure maximum absorption.
For very severe infections in adults or children, treatment should be initiated with parenteral ampicillin.
INFECTIONS DUE TO GROUP A BETA-HEMOLYTIC STREPTOCOCCI SHOULD BE TREATED FOR A MINIMUM OF TEN DAYS.

Directions for Dispensing Oral Suspension and Pediatric Drops

Prepare these formulations at the time of dispensing. For ease in preparation, add water to the bottle in two portions and shake well after each addition. Add the total amount of water as directed on the labeling of the package being dispensed. The reconstituted formulation is stable 14 days under refrigeration.
Supply: VERSAPEN-K (hetacillin potassium) Capsules. Hetacillin potassium equivalent to 225 or 450 mg. ampicillin per capsule.
NDC 0015-7805—225 mg.
NDC 0015-7806—450 mg.
[*Shown in Product Identification Section*]
VERSAPEN (hetacillin) for Oral Suspension. Each 5 ml. of reconstituted oral suspension contains hetacillin equivalent to 112.5 or 225 mg. ampicillin.
NDC 0015-7808—112.5 mg., 100 ml. bottle
NDC 0015-7809—225 mg., 100 ml. bottle
VERSAPEN (hetacillin) Pediatric Drops. Each ml. of reconstituted pediatric drops contains hetacillin equivalent to 112.5 mg. ampicillin.
NDC 0015-7807—112.5 mg., 15 ml. bottles.

Bristol-Myers Products
(Div. of Bristol-Myers Co.)
345 PARK AVENUE
NEW YORK, NEW YORK 10022

ARTHRITIS STRENGTH BUFFERIN®
Analgesic

Composition: Aspirin 7½ gr. (486 mg.) in a formulation buffered with Di-Alminate,® Bristol-Myers' brand of Aluminum Glycinate 1.125 gr. (72.9 mg.) and Magnesium Carbonate 2.25 gr. (145.8 mg.).
Action and Uses: ARTHRITIS STRENGTH BUFFERIN is specially formulated to give temporary relief from the minor aches and pains, stiffness, swelling and inflammation of arthritis and rheumatism. ARTHRITIS STRENGTH BUFFERIN also reduces pain and fever of colds and "flu" and provides fast, effective pain relief for: simple headache, lower back muscular aches from fatigue, sinusitis, neuralgia, neuritis, tooth extraction, muscle strain, athletic soreness, painful distress associated with normal menstrual periods. The leading aspirin substitute acetaminophen cannot provide relief from inflammation.
ARTHRITIS STRENGTH BUFFERIN PROVIDES INGREDIENTS FOR STOMACH PROTECTION JUST LIKE REGULAR BUFFERIN WHICH HELP PREVENT THE STOMACH UPSET ASPIRIN OFTEN CAUSES.
Contraindications: Hypersensitivity to salicylates.
Caution: If pain persists for more than 10 days or redness is present or in Arthritic or Rheumatic conditions affecting children under 12, consult physician immediately. Do not take without consulting physician if under medical care. WARNING: Keep this and all medicines out of children's reach. In case of accidental overdose, contact a physician immediately.
Administration and Dosage: Two tablets with water. Repeat after four hours if necessary. Do not exceed 8 tablets in any 24 hour period. If dizziness, impaired hearing or ringing in ear occurs, discontinue use. Not recommended for children.
Overdose: (Symptoms and Treatment) Typical of aspirin.
How Supplied: Tablets in bottles of 40 and 100. Samples available upon request.
Product Identification: White elongated tablet.
Literature Available: Upon request.

BUFFERIN® Analgesic

Composition: Aspirin 5 gr. (324 mg.) in a formulation buffered with Di-Alminate®, Bristol-Myers's brand of Aluminum Glycinate ¾ gr. (48.6 mg.), and Magnesium Carbonate 1½ gr. (97.2 mg.).
Action and Uses: Bufferin® is for relief of simple headache; and for temporary relief of: minor arthritic pain, the painful discomforts and fever of colds and "flu", menstrual cramps, muscular aches from fatigue and toothache. Bufferin® helps prevent the stomach upset often caused by plain aspirin.
Contraindications: Hypersensitivity to salicylates.
Caution: If pain persists for more than 10 days or redness is present or, in Arthritic or Rheumatic conditions affecting children under 12, consult physician immediately. Do not take without consulting physician if under medical care. Consult a dentist for toothache promptly.
Warning: Keep this and all medicines out of children's reach. In case of accidental overdose, consult a physician immediately.
Dosage: 2 tablets every four hours as needed. Do not exceed 12 tablets in 24 hours, unless directed by a physician. For children 6-12, one-half dose. Under 6, consult physician.
Overdose: (Symptoms and treatment) Typical of aspirin.
How Supplied: Tablets in bottles of 12, 36, 60, 100, 165, 225, and 375. For hospital and clinical use: bottle—1,000; boxed 200x2 tablet foil packets. Samples available on request.
Product Identification Mark: White tablet with letter "B" on one surface.
Literature Available: Upon request.

COMTREX®
Multi-Symptom Cold Reliever

Composition: Each tablet, fluid ounce (30 ml.), and capsule contains:
[See table below].
Action and Uses: COMTREX® contains safe and effective ingredients including a non-aspirin analgesic, a decongestant, an antihistamine and a cough reliever. COMTREX relieves these major cold symptoms: nasal and sinus congestion, runny nose, sneezing, post nasal drip, watery eyes, coughing, fever, minor sore throat pain (systemically), headache, body aches and pain.
Contraindications: Hypersensitivity to acetaminophen or antihistamines.
Caution: Do not take without consulting a physician if under medical care. Do not drive a car or operate machinery while taking this cold remedy as it may cause drowsiness.
Warning: Keep this and all medicine out of children's reach. In case of accidental overdose, consult a physician immediately. Persistent cough may indicate the presence of a serious condition. Persons with a high fever or persistent cough, or with high blood pressure, diabetes, heart or thyroid disease should not use this preparation unless directed by a physician. Do not use for more than 10 days unless directed by a physician.
Administration and Dosage:
Tablets—Adults: 2 tablets every 4 hours as needed not to exceed 12 tablets in 24 hours. Children 6-12 years: ½ the adult dose. Under 6, consult a physician.
Liquid—Adults: 1 fluid ounce (30 ml.) every 4 hours as needed, not to exceed 6 fluid ounces (180 ml.) in 24 hours. Children 6-12 years: ½ the adult dose. Under 6, consult a physician.
Capsules—Adults 2 capsules every 4 hours as needed not to exceed 12 capsules in 24 hours. Children 6–12 years: ½ the adult dose. Under 6, consult a physician.
Overdose: The signs and symptoms observed would be those produced by the acetaminophen, which may cause hepatotoxicity in some patients. Since clinical and laboratory evidence may be delayed up to 1 week, close clinical monitoring and serial hepatic enzyme determinations are recommended.
How Supplied: Tablets in bottles of 24's, 50's, Capsules in bottles of 16's and 36's, 100's. Liquid in 6 oz. and 10 oz. plastic bottles. Samples available on request.
Product Identification Mark: Yellow tablet with letter "C" on one surface. Orange and Yellow capsules with "Bristol-Myers" and "Comtrex" on one side.
Literature Available: Upon request.

	Tablets	Liquid	Capsules
Acetaminophen	325 mg.	650 mg.	325 mg.
Phenylpropanolamine HCl:	12 ½ mg.	25 mg.	12 ½ mg.
Chlorpheniramine Maleate:	1 mg.	2 mg.	1 mg.
Dextromethorphan HBr	10 mg.	20 mg.	10 mg.
Alcohol:	—	20% by Volume	—

CONGESPIRIN®
Chewable Cold Tablets for Children

Composition: Each tablet contains aspirin 81 mg. (1¼ grains) phenylephrine hydrochloride (1¼ mg.).
Action and Uses: For the temporary relief of nasal congestion, fever, aches and pains of the common cold or "flu". Plus an effective nasal decongestant to help relieve stuffiness, runny nose and sneezing from colds.
Dosage and Administration: Children under three years of age-consult physician. Three years-one tablet. Four to six years-2 tablets. Seven to nine years-3 tablets. Ten to fourteen years-4 tablets. Repeat dose in four hours if necessary. Do not give more than four doses per day unless prescribed by your physician.
Caution: If child is under medical care, do not administer without consulting physician. Do not exceed recommended dosage. Consult your physician if symptoms persist or if high fever, high blood pressure, heart disease, diabetes or thyroid disease is present. Do not administer for more than 10 days unless directed by your physician.
Warning: KEEP THIS AND ALL MEDICINES OUT OF CHILDREN'S REACH. IN CASE OF ACCIDENTAL OVERDOSAGE, CONTACT A PHYSICIAN IMMEDIATELY.
How Supplied: Tablets in bottles of 36.
Product Identification Mark: Two layer (orange/white) circular tablet with letter "C" imprinted on the orange side.

CONGESPRIN®
Liquid Cold Medicine

Composition: Each 5 ml. teaspoon contains Acetaminophen 130 mg, Phenylpropanolamine Hydrochloride 6 ¼ mg., Alcohol 10% by volume.
Action and Uses: Reduces fever and relieves aches and pains associated with colds and "flu". Contains an effective decongestant for the temporary relief of nasal congestion due to the common cold, hay fever or other respiratory allergies. Reduces swelling of nasal passages, shrinks swollen membranes, restores freer breathing.
Dosage and Administration:
Children 3–5, 1 teaspoon every 3–4 hours.
Children 6–12, 2 teaspoons every 3–4 hours.
Children under 3 years use only as directed by your physician.
Do not give more than 4 doses a day unless directed by your physician.
Caution: If child is under medical care, do not administer without consulting physician. Do not exceed recommended dosage. Consult your physician if symptoms persist or if high fever, high blood pressure, heart disease, diabetes or thyroid disease is present. Do not administer for more than 10 days unless directed by your physician.
Warning: KEEP THIS AND ALL MEDICINES OUT OF CHILDREN'S REACH. IN CASE OF ACCIDENTAL OVERDOSAGE, CONTACT A PHYSICIAN IMMEDIATELY.
How Supplied: In 3 oz. plastic, unbreakable bottles.

DATRIL® Analgesic

Composition: Each tablet contains acetaminophen 5 gr. (325 mg.)
Actions and Uses: This is an improved **DATRIL** formula that dissolves faster to get its pain reliever into the bloodstream faster than common acetaminophen tablets. The **DATRIL** formula contains a safe, effective, non-aspirin analgesic that relieves pain fast, without causing the gastric bleeding that aspirin tablets can cause. DATRIL is also less likely to cause the nausea and stomach upset that plain aspirin tablets can cause. DATRIL provides relief from the pain of: • Headache • Colds or "flu" • Bursitis • Menstrual discomfort • Sinusitis • Muscular aches due to fatigue or overexer-

tion • Muscular backache • Neuralgia. DATRIL also helps reduce fever of colds or "flu" and provides temporary relief from toothache and minor arthritic or rheumatic aches and pain. For most persons with peptic ulcer DATRIL may be used safely and comfortably when taken as directed for recommended conditions.
Contraindications: There have been rare reports of skin rash or glossitis attributed to acetaminophen. Discontinue use if a sensitivity reaction occurs. However, acetaminophen is usually well tolerated by aspirin-sensitive patients.
Caution: If pain persists for more than 10 days or redness is present or in arthritic or rheumatic conditions affecting children under 12, consult physician immediately. Do not take without consulting a physician if under medical care. Consult a dentist for toothache promptly.
Warning: Keep this and all medicines out of reach of children. In case of accidental overdose contact a physician promptly.
Dosage: 2 tablets every four hours, 1 to 4 times daily as needed, or as directed by a physician. For children 6–12 years of age use half the adult dose. **Warning:** Do not give to children under 6 or use for more than 10 days unless directed by a physician.
Overdose: A massive overdose of acetaminophen may cause hepatotoxicity in some patients. Since clinical and laboratory evidence may be delayed up to 1 week, close clinical monitoring and serial hepatic enzyme determinations are recommended.
How Supplied: Tablets in bottles of 24, 100 and 250. Samples available on request.
Product Identification Mark: White tablet with name "Datril" on one surface.
Literature Available: Upon request.

DATRIL 500™

Composition: Each tablet contains acetaminophen, 7.5 gr. (500 mg.)
Actions and Uses: DATRIL 500 has been specially developed to provide fast, extra-strength pain relief. It contains a non-aspirin ingredient (acetaminophen) which is less likely to irritate the stomach than plain aspirin. DATRIL 500 is fast-acting. It gets its pain reliever into the bloodstream faster than regular strength (325 mg.) acetaminophen tablets or extra strength acetaminophen capsules. DATRIL 500 Extra-Strength tablets are for the temporary relief of minor aches, pains, headaches and fever. For most persons with peptic ulcer DATRIL 500 may be used when taken as directed for recommended conditions.
Contraindictions: There have been rare reports of skin rash or glossitis attributed to acetaminophen. Discontinue use if a sensitivity reaction occurs. However, acetaminophen is usually well tolerated by aspirin-sensitive patients.
Caution: Severe or recurrent pain or high or continued fever may be indicative of serious illness. Under these conditions consult a physician.
Warning: Keep this and all medicines out of reach of children. In case of accidental overdose contact a physician immediately.
Dosage: Adults: Two tablets. May be repeated in 4 hours if needed. Do not exceed 8 tablets in any 24 hour period.
Warning: Do not give to children 12 and under or use for more than 10 days unless directed by a physician.
Overdose: A massive overdose of acetaminophen may cause hepatotoxicity in some patients. Since clinical and laboratory evidence may be delayed up to 1 week, close clinical monitoring and serial hepatic enzyme determinations are recommended.
How Supplied: Tablets in bottles of 24's, 50's and 72's. Samples available on request.
Product Identification Mark: White tablet with DATRIL 500 on one surface.
Literature Available: Upon request.

EXCEDRIN® Analgesic

Composition: Each tablet contains aspirin 3 gr. (194.4 mg.); Acetaminophen 1½ gr. (97.2 mg.); Salicylamide 2 gr. (129.6 mg.); Caffeine 1 gr. (64.8 mg.).
Action and Uses: The Excedrin formula provides fast, effective relief from pain of: headache, sinusitis, colds or 'flu', muscular aches and menstrual discomfort. Also recommended for temporary relief of toothaches and minor arthritic pains.
Contraindications: Hypersensitivity to salicylates or acetaminophen.
Precaution: Do not give to children under 6 or use for more than 10 days unless directed by physician. If sinus or arthritis pain persists (say for a week) or if skin redness is present, or in arthritic conditions affecting children under 12 consult physician immediately. Consult dentist for toothache promptly. Do not take without consulting physician if under medical care.
Warning: Keep this and all medicines out of children's reach. In case of accidental overdose, contact a physician immediately.
Administration and Dosage: Adults, 2 tablets every 4 hours as needed. Do not exceed 8 tablets in 24 hours unless directed by a physician. For children 6-12, one-half adult dose.
How Supplied: Bottles of 12, 36, 60, 100, 165, 225, and 375 tablets. A metal tin of 12 tablets. All sizes packaged in child resistant safety closure except 60's which is a size not recommended for households with young children.
Product Identification Mark: White, circular tablet with letter "E" imprinted on both sides.
Literature Available: Upon request.

EXCEDRIN P.M.® Nighttime Analgesic

Composition: Each tablet contains Acetaminophen 500 mg. and Pyrilamine Maleate 25 mg.
Action and Uses: Excedrin P.M. has a special formula that provides prompt relief of nighttime pain and aids sleep for people with headache, bursitis, colds or "flu", sinusitis, muscle aches and menstrual discomfort. Also recommended for temporary relief of toothaches and minor arthritic pain.
Contraindications: Hypersensitivity to acetaminophen.
Caution: Do not exceed 2 tablets in 24 hours. Do not give to children under 12 or use for more than 10 days unless directed by physician. If sinus or arthritis pain persists (say for a week) or if skin redness is present, or in arthritic conditions affecting children under 12, consult physician immediately. Do not drive a car or operate machinery after use. Consult dentist promptly for toothache. Do not take without consulting physician if under medical care.
Warning: If sleeplessness persists for more than two weeks, consult your physician. Insomnia may be a symptom of serious underlying medical ailments. Take this product with caution if alcohol is being consumed. **Do not take this product if you have asthma, glaucoma or enlargement of the prostate gland except under the advice and supervision of a physician.** Keep this and all medicines out of children's reach. In case of accidental overdose, contact a physician immediately.
Administration and Dosage: Adults take two tablets at bedtime to help relieve pain and aid sleep.
How Supplied: Bottles of 10, 30, 50, and 80 tablets. All sizes packaged in child resistant safety closure except 50's, which is a size not recommended for households with young children.
Product Identification Mark: Blue/green circular tablet with letters "PM" imprinted on one side.

4-WAY® Cold Tablets

Composition: Each tablet contains aspirin 324 mg., phenylpropanolamine HCl 12 ½ mg., and chlorpheniramine maleate 2 mg.
Action and Uses: For temporary relief of minor aches and pains, fever, nasal congestion and runny nose as may occur in the common cold.
Dosage and Administration:
Adults—2 tablets every 4 hours, if needed. Do not exceed 6 tablets in 24 hours. Children 6–12 years—1 tablet every 4 hours. Do not exceed 4 tablets in 24 hours. Under age 6, consult a physician.
Warning: Do not take without consulting a physician if under medical care.
Caution: This preparation may cause drowsiness. Do not drive or operate machinery while taking this medication. Individuals with high blood pressure, heart disease, diabetes, or thyroid disease should use only as directed by physician. Do not exceed recommended dosage. KEEP THIS AND ALL MEDICINES OUT OF CHILDREN'S REACH. IN CASE OF ACCIDENTAL OVERDOSE, CONTACT PHYSICIAN IMMEDIATELY.
How Supplied: Carded 15's and bottles of 36's and 60's.
Product Identification Mark: Pink and White tablet with number "4" on one surface.

4-WAY® Nasal Spray

Composition: Phenylephrine hydrochloride 0.5%, naphazoline hydrochloride 0.05%, pyrilamine maleate 0.2%, in a buffered isotonic aqueous solution with thimerosal 0.005% added as a preservative. Also available in a mentholated formula.
Action and Uses: For relief of nasal congestion, runny nose, sneezing, itching nose, and watery eyes which may be symptoms of the common cold, sinusitis, nasal allergies, or hay fever.
Dosage and Administration: With head in a normal upright position, put atomizer tip into nostril. Squeeze atomizer with firm, quick pressure while inhaling. Adults-spray twice into each nostril. Children 6-12-spray once. Under 6-consult physician. Repeat in three hours, if needed.
Warning: Overdosage in young children may cause marked sedation. Do not exceed recommended dosage. Follow directions carefully. If symptoms persist, consult physician. Keep out of children's reach.
How Supplied: Atomizers of ½ fluid ounce and 1 fluid ounce.

4-WAY® Long Acting Nasal Spray

Composition: Xylometazoline Hydrochloride 0.1% in a buffered isotonic aqueous solution. Thimerosal, 0.005% added as a preservative. Also available in a mentholated formula.
Action and Uses: Provides temporary relief of nasal congestion due to the common cold, sinusitis, hayfever or other upper respiratory allergies.
Dosage and Administration: With head in a normal upright position, put atomizer tip into nostril. Squeeze atomizer with firm, quick pressure while inhaling. Adults: Spray 2 or 3 times in each nostril every 8 to 10 hours. For children under 12, consult physician.
Warning: For adult use only. Do not give this product to children under 12 years except under the advice and supervision of a physician. Do not exceed recommended dosage because symptoms may occur such as burning, stinging, sneezing, or an increase of nasal discharge.

Continued on next page

Bristol-Myers—Cont.

Do not use this product for more than 3 days. If symptoms persist, consult a physician.
KEEP OUT OF CHILDREN'S REACH.
How Supplied: Atomizers of ½ fluid ounce.

MONSTER®
(Brand)
Monster shaped chewable multiple vitamins

Dosage: One tablet daily for children over two years of age. May be chewed or dissolved in the mouth.
[See table on next page].
Made with NATURAL SWEETENERS, artificial coloring and flavoring.
Action and Uses: MONSTER shaped multiple vitamins, especially made for children, are a dietary supplement to assure necessary vitamin intake. MONSTER contains ten important vitamins.
Administration and Dosage: MONSTER may be chewed, dissolved orally, or crushed and added to foods, either liquid or solid.
Daily: one tablet.
Supplied: MONSTER vitamins are supplied in delicious fruit flavors in bottles of 60's and 100's.

MONSTER® (Brand) with Iron
Monster shaped chewable vitamins with iron

Dosage: One tablet daily for children over two years of age. May be chewed or dissolved in the mouth.
[See table above].
Made with NATURAL SWEETENERS, artificial coloring and flavoring.
KEEP OUT OF REACH OF CHILDREN.
Action and Uses: MONSTER with iron is a specially formulated dietary supplement containing needed vitamins plus iron for children. Each tablet provides ten important vitamins plus iron.
Administration and Dosage: MONSTER with iron may be chewed, dissolved orally, or crushed and added to solid or liquid foods. One tablet daily.
Supplied: MONSTER with iron are supplied in delicious fruit flavors in bottles of 60's and 100's.

NO DOZ® TABLETS

Composition: Each tablet contains 100 mg. Caffeine. No Doz is non-habit forming.
Action and Uses: Helps restore mental alertness.
Dosage and Administration:
For Adults: 2 tablets initially, thereafter, 1 tablet every three hours should be sufficient.
Caution: Do not take without consulting physician if under medical care. No stimulant should be substituted for normal sleep in activities requiring physical alertness.
KEEP THIS AND ALL MEDICINES OUT OF THE REACH OF CHILDREN.
How Supplied: Carded 15's and 36's and bottles of 60's.
Product Identification Mark: A white tablet with No Doz on one side.

Each Tablet Supplies:		Percentage of Recommended Dietary Allowances set by the National Academy of Sciences 2–6	6–12
Vitamin A, U.S.P. units	3500	140%	106%
Vitamin D, U.S.P. units	400	100%	100%
Vitamin C (ascorbic acid), mg.	40	100%	100%
Vitamin B_1 (thiamin), mg.	1.1	122%	92%
Vitamin B_2 (riboflavin), mg.	1.2	109%	100%
Vitamin B_6 (pyridoxine), mg.	1.2	133%	100%
Vitamin B_{12}, mcg.	5	333%	250%
Niacin, mg.	15	125%	94%
Folic acid, mcg.	100	50%	33%
Pantothenic acid, mg.	5	*	*
Iron (ferrous fumarate), mg	10	100%	100%

*Recommended Daily Allowance (RDA) has not been established.

PALS® (Brand)
Animal shaped chewable multiple vitamins

[See table on next page].
Actions and Uses: PALS animal shaped multiple vitamins, especially made for children, are a dietary supplement to assure necessary vitamin intake. PALS contain ten important vitamins.
Administration and Dosage: PALS may be chewed, dissolved orally, or crushed and added to foods, either liquid or solid. Daily: one tablet.
Supplied: PALS are supplied in delicious fruit flavors—grape, lemon, orange, lime and cherry—and in five colors. Bottles of 21, 60, 100.

PALS® (Brand) Plus Iron
Multiple vitamins plus iron

[See table on next page].
Action and Uses: PALS Plus iron is a specially formulated dietary supplement containing needed vitamins plus iron for growing children. Each tablet provides ten important vitamins plus iron.
Administration and Dosage: PALS Plus iron may be chewed, dissolved orally, or crushed and added to solid or liquid foods. One tablet daily.
Supplied: PALS Plus iron are supplied in delicious fruit flavors—grape, lemon, orange, lime and cherry—and in five colors. Bottles of 60 and 100.

Each Tablet Supplies:		Percentage of Recommended Dietary Allowances set by the National Academy of Sciences 2–6	6–12
Vitamin A, U.S.P. units	3500	140%	106%
Vitamin D, U.S.P. units	400	100%	100%
Vitamin C (ascorbic acid), mg.	40	100%	100%
Vitamin B_1 (thiamin), mg.	1.1	122%	92%
Vitamin B_2 (riboflavin), mg.	1.2	109%	100%
Vitamin B_6 (pyridoxine), mg.	1.2	133%	100%
Vitamin B_{12}, mcg.	5	333%	250%
Niacin, mg.	15	125%	94%
Folic acid, mcg.	100	50%	33%
Pantothenic acid, mg.	5	*	*

*Recommended Daily Allowance (RDA) has not been established.

PAZO® HEMORRHOID OINTMENT/SUPPOSITORIES

Composition: Triolyte®, Bristol-Myers brand of the combination of benzocaine (0.8%) and ephedrine sulphate (0.2%); zinc oxide (4.0%); camphor (2.18%) eucalyptus oil (0.25%), in an emollient base.
Action and Uses: Pazo helps shrink swelling of inflamed hemorrhoid tissue. Provides prompt, temporary relief of burning itch and pain in many cases.
Administration:
Ointment—Apply stainless Pazo well up in rectum night and morning, and after each bowel movement. Repeat as often during the day as may be necessary to maintain comfort. Continue for one week after symptoms subside. When applicator is used, lubricate applicator first with Pazo. Insert slowly, then simply press tube.
Suppositories—Remove foil and insert one Pazo suppository night and morning, and after each bowel movement. Repeat as often during the day as may be necessary to maintain comfort. Continue for one week after symptoms subside.
Warning: If the underlying condition persists or recurs frequently, despite treatment, or if any bleeding or hard irreducible swelling is present, consult your physician.
Keep out of children's reach. Keep in a cool place.
How Supplied:
Ointment—1-ounce and 2-ounce tubes with plastic applicator.
Suppositories—Boxes of 12 and 24 wrapped in silver foil.
Literature Available: Yes.

Products are cross-indexed by

generic and chemical names

in the

YELLOW SECTION

TABLE I

Daily Dose: 1 PALS® Vitamin Tablet.

Each tablet contains:		Percentages of Recommended Dietary Allowances set by the National Research Council: 2–6*	6–10*
Vitamin A	3500 USP Units	140%	106%
Vitamin D	400 USP Units	100%	100%
Vitamin C	60 mg.	150%	150%
Vitamin B_1 (thiamine)	0.8 mg.	100%	73%
Vitamin B_2 (riboflavin)	1.3 mg.	145%	108%
Vitamin B_6 (pyridoxine)	1 mg.	111%	83%
Vitamin B_{12} (cyanocobalamin)	2.5 mcg.	62%	50%
Niacin	14 mg.	127%	93%
Folic Acid	50 mcg.	100%	66%
Pantothenic Acid	5 mg.	**	**

*Figures based on values for 6 and 10 year olds respectively. **RDA not established. Made with NATURAL SWEETENERS, artificial colors & flavors.

Brown Pharmaceutical Company, Inc., The

2500 WEST SIXTH STREET
LOS ANGELES, CALIFORNIA 90057

ANDROID®-5 ℞
Methyltestosterone U.S.P. 5 mg.
(Buccal Tablets)

ANDROID®-10 ℞
Methyltestosterone U.S.P. 10 mg.

ANDROID®-25 ℞
Methyltestosterone U.S.P. 25 mg.

Description: Methyltestosterone is an androgenic steroid which occurs as white or creamy white crystals or crystalline powder.

Action: The actions of anabolic steroids are similar to those of male sex hormones.

As methyltestosterone is a 17-methylated steroid it is protected to a certain extent from the liver. Consequently, oral administration does not result in rapid destruction of the preparation by its passage through the hepatic system.

Indications:

In the Male:

1. Eunuchoidism and eunuchism.
2. Climacteric symptoms when these are secondary to androgen deficiency.
3. Impotence due to androgen deficiency.
4. Postpuberal cryptorchidism with evidence of hypogonadism.

In the Female:

1. Prevention of postpartum breast pain and engorgement. There is no satisfactory evidence that this drug prevents or suppresses lactation.
2. Palliation of androgen-responsive, advancing, inoperable mammary cancer in women who are more than 1 year, but less than 5 years postmenopausal or who have been proven to have a hormone-dependent tumor as shown by previous beneficial response to castration.

Contraindications: Carcinoma of the male breast; known or suspected carcinoma of the prostate; cardiac, hepatic, or renal decompensation; hypercalcemia; impaired liver function; prepuberal males; patients easily stimulated; pregnancy; and breast feeding.

Warnings: Hypercalcemia may occur in immobilized patients and in breast cancer patients. In patients with cancer, hypercalcemia may indicate progression of bony metastasis, in which case the drug should be discontinued. Watch female patients closely for signs of virilization. Some effects such as voice changes may not be reversible even when the drug is stopped.

Discontinue the drug if cholestatic hepatitis with jaundice appears or liver function tests become abnormal.

Precautions: Patients with cardiac, renal or hepatic derangement may retain sodium and water with resulting edema formation.

Males, especially the elderly, may become overly stimulated.

Priapism or excessive sexual stimulation may develop.

Oligospermia and reduced ejaculatory volume may occur after prolonged administration or excessive dosage.

Hypersensitivity and gynecomastia may occur.

Alterations in liver function tests (e.g. increased BSP retention and SGOT levels) and rarely jaundice have been reported and appear to be directly related to the dose of the drug. When any of these effects appear, the androgen should be stopped; if restarted, a lower dosage should be utilized.

Use cautiously in young boys to avoid possible premature epiphyseal closure or precocious sexual development.

The PBI may decrease during androgen therapy without clinical significance.

Adverse Reactions: Hypersensitivity, including skin manifestations and anaphylactoid reactions; acne; decreased ejaculatory volume; oligospermia; gynecomastia; edema; priapism; hypercalcemia; especially in immobile patients and those with metastatic breast carcinoma; virilization in females; cholestatic jaundice. There have been rare reports of hepatocellular neoplasms and peliosis hepatis in patients who have received androgenic-anabolic steroids, usually over prolonged periods of time.

Dosage and Administration: Dosage must be strictly individualized. Daily requirements are best administered in divided doses. The following chart is suggested as an average daily dosage guide. Duration of therapy will depend upon the response of the condition being treated and the appearance of adverse reactions.

Note: Buccal tablets have approximately twice the potency of the orally ingested hormone.

Indications:

	Average Daily Dosage Buccal	Tablet
In the Male:		
Eunuchism and eunuchoidism	5 to 20 mg.	10 to 40 mg.
Male climacteric and male impotency	5 to 20 mg.	10 to 40 mg.
Cryptorchidism-postpuberal	15 mg.	30 mg.
In the female:		
Postpartum breast pain & engorgement (3 to 5 days)	40 mg.	80 mg.
Breast cancer	100 mg.	200 mg.

Administration of Buccal Tablets: Buccal tablets should not be swallowed since the hormone is meant to be absorbed through the mucous membranes. Place buccal tablet in the upper or lower buccal pouch between the gum and cheek. Avoid eating, drinking, chewing, or smoking while the buccal tablet is in place. Proper oral hygienic measures are particularly important after the use of buccal tablets.

How Supplied: Tablets of 10 mg. and 25 mg. concentrations and buccal tablets of 5 mg. concentration.

[*Shown in Product Identification Section*]

TABLE II

Daily Dose: 1 PALS® Vitamin Tablet.

Each tablet contains:		Percentages of Recommended Dietary Allowances set by the National Research Council: 2–6*	6–10*
Vitamin A	3500 U.S.P. Units	140%	106%
Vitamin D	400 USP Units	100%	100%
Vitamin C	60 mg.	150%	150%
Vitamin B_1 (thiamine)	0.8 mg.	100%	73%
Vitamin B_2 (riboflavin)	1.3 mg.	145%	108%
Vitamin B_6 (pyridoxine)	1 mg.	111%	83%
Vitamin B_{12} (cyanocobalamin)	2.5 mcg.	62%	50%
Niacin	14 mg.	127%	93%
Folic Acid	50 mcg.	100%	66%
Pantothenic Acid	5 mg.	**	**
Iron (ferrous fumarate)	12 mg.	120%	120%

*Figures based on values for 6 and 10 year olds respectively. **RDA not established. Made with NATURAL SWEETENERS, artificial colors & flavors. KEEP OUT OF REACH OF CHILDREN.

CEREBRO-NICIN® Capsules ℞

Composition: Each capsule:

Pentylenetetrazole	100 mg.
Nicotinic acid	100 mg.
Niacinamide	5 mg.
Vitamin C	100 mg.
Thiamine-HCl	25 mg.
Riboflavin	2 mg.
Pyridoxine	3 mg.
1-Glutamic acid	50 mg.

Action and Uses: A safe and efficient cerebral stimulant and vasodilator for aging patients. Increases cerebral activity, blood flow, nutrition. Pentylenetetrazole is a central nervous system stimulant (analeptic agent), affecting the respiratory, vasomotor and vagal centers of the medulla in the brain. Also affecting the cerebral cortex, the action upon the sympathetic and parasympathetic systems depends upon the status of the organism at the time. The greater the depression of the medullary center, the greater the stimulative effect of the compound. Nicotinic Acid is a vasodilator.

Continued on next page

Brown—Cont.

Administration and Dosage: AVERAGE DOSAGE: One Capsule three times daily.
Precautions: Most persons experience a flushing and tingling sensation after taking a higher potency niacin-containing compound. As a secondary reaction some will complain of nausea and other sensations of discomfort. This reaction is transient and is rarely a cause for discontinuance of the drug if the patient is forewarned to expect the reaction.
Contraindications: Contraindicated in the presence of epilepsy.
How Supplied: AVAILABLE in capsules (bottle of 100).
Literature Available: Samples.

LIPO-NICIN®/100 mg. Tablets ℞
LIPO-NICIN®/250 mg. Tablets
LIPO-NICIN®/300 mg. Timed Caps

Composition:
LIPO-NICIN®/100 mg.
Each blue tablet contains:

Nicotinic Acid	100 mg.
Niacinamide	75 mg.
Ascorbic Acid	150 mg.
Thiamine HCl (B-1)	25 mg.
Riboflavin (B-2)	2 mg.
Pyridoxine HCl (B-6)	10 mg.

LIPO-NICIN /250 mg.
Each yellow tablet contains:

Nicotinic Acid	250 mg.
Niacinamide	75 mg.
Ascorbic Acid	150 mg.
Thiamine HCl (B-1)	25 mg.
Riboflavin (B-2)	2 mg.
Pyridoxine HCl (B-6)	10 mg.

LIPO-NICIN®/300 mg. Timed Caps
Each red capsule contains:

Nicotinic Acid	300 mg.
Vitamin C (Ascorbic Acid)	150 mg.
Vitamin B_1 (Thiamine HCl)	25 mg.
Vitamin B_2 (Riboflavin)	2 mg.
Pyridoxine HCl (B_6)	10 mg.

In a special base so prepared that the active ingredients are released over a period of 6 to 8 hours.
Action and Uses: For use as a vasodilator in the symptoms of cold feet, leg cramps, dizziness, memory loss or tinnitus when associated with impaired peripheral circulation. Also provides concomitant administration of the listed vitamins.
The warm tingling flush which may follow each dose is one of the therapeutic effects that often produce psychologic benefits to the patient.
Side Effects: Flushing with heat and itching, in some cases followed by sweating, nausea and abdominal cramps. This reaction is usually transient. Nausea caused by high acidity can be relieved by nonabsorbable antacid.
Caution: Federal law prohibits dispensing without prescription.
Administration and Dosage:
LIPO-NICIN /100 mg.—1 to 5 tablets daily.
LIPO-NICIN /250 mg.—1 to 3 tablets daily.
LIPO-NICIN® /300 mg Timed— 1 to 2 capsules daily.
Available: Bottles of 100, 500, 1,000.
Literature Available: Samples.

Burroughs Wellcome Co.
3030 CORNWALLIS ROAD
RESEARCH TRIANGLE PARK,
NC 27709

LITERATURE AVAILABLE: Folders, circulars, file cards, films, slides, lecture guides and monographs.

ACTIDIL ℞
brand Triprolidine Hydrochloride
Tablets and Syrup

Description: Actidil brand Triprolidine Hydrochloride is an antihistamine known chemically as *trans*-1-(4-methylphenyl)-1-(2-pyridyl)-3-pyrrolidinoprop-1-ene hydrochloride.
Actions: Actidil brand Triprolidine Hydrochloride is an antihistamine with anticholinergic (drying) and sedative side effects. Antihistamines appear to compete with histamine for cell receptor sites on effector cells.
Indications: For the symptomatic treatment of: perennial and seasonal allergic rhinitis; vasomotor rhinitis; allergic conjunctivitis due to inhalant allergens and foods; mild, uncomplicated allergic skin manifestations of urticaria and angioedema; amelioration of allergic reactions to blood or plasma; dermatographism; as therapy for anaphylactic reactions *adjunctive* to epinephrine and other standard measures after the acute manifestations have been controlled.
Contraindications:
Use in Newborn or Premature Infants: This drug should *not* be used in newborn or premature infants.
Use in Nursing Mothers: Because of the higher risk of antihistamines for infants generally and for newborns and prematures in particular, antihistamine therapy is contraindicated in nursing mothers.
Use in Lower Respiratory Disease: Antihistamines *should NOT* be used to treat lower respiratory tract symptoms including asthma.
Antihistamines are also contraindicated in the following conditions: Hypersensitivity to Actidil® brand Triprolidine Hydrochloride and other antihistamines of similar chemical structure.
Monoamine oxidase inhibitor therapy (see Drug Interaction section).
Warnings: Antihistamines should be used with considerable caution in patients with: narrow angle glaucoma; stenosing peptic ulcer; pyloroduodenal obstruction; symptomatic prostatic hypertrophy and bladder neck obstruction.
Use in Children: In infants and children, especially, antihistamines in *overdosage* may cause hallucinations, convulsions, or death.
As in adults, antihistamines may diminish mental alertness in children. In the young child, particularly, they may produce excitation.
Use in Pregnancy: Experience with this drug in pregnant women is inadequate to determine whether there exists a potential for harm to the developing fetus.
Use With CNS Depressants: Actidil brand Triprolidine has additive effects with alcohol and other CNS depressants (hypnotics, sedatives, tranquilizers, etc.).
Use in Activities Requiring Mental Alertness: Patients should be warned about engaging in activities requiring mental alertness as driving a car or operating appliances, machinery, etc.
Use in The Elderly (approximately 60 years or older): Antihistamines are more likely to cause dizziness, sedation, and hypotension in elderly patients.
Precautions: The anticholinergic or atropine-like effect of Actidil is slight. Nevertheless, as with other antihistamines, this drug should be used with caution in patients with: history of bronchial asthma; increased intraocular pressure; hyperthyroidism; cardiovascular disease and hypertension.
Drug Interactions: MAO inhibitors prolong and intensify the anticholinergic (drying) effects of antihistamines.
Adverse Reactions: The most frequent reactions are underlined:
1. *General:* Urticaria, drug rash, anaphylactic shock, photosensitivity, excessive perspiration, chills, dryness of mouth, nose and throat.
2. *Cardiovascular System:* Hypotension, headache, palpitations, tachycardia, extrasystoles.
3. *Haematologic System:* Hemolytic anemia, thrombocytopenia, agranulocytosis.
4. *Nervous System:* Sedation, sleepiness, dizziness, disturbed coordination, fatigue, confusion, restlessness, excitation, nervousness, tremor, irritability, insomnia, euphoria, paresthesias, blurred vision, diplopia, vertigo, tinnitus, acute labyrinthitis, hysteria, neuritis, convulsions.
5. *G.I. System:* Epigastric distress, anorexia, nausea, vomiting, diarrhea, constipation.
6. *G.U. System:* Urinary frequency, difficult urination, urinary retention, early menses.
7. *Respiratory System:* Thickening of bronchial secretions, tightness of chest and wheezing, nasal stuffiness.

Overdosage: Antihistamine overdosage reactions may vary from central nervous system depression to stimulation. Stimulation is particularly likely in children. Atropine-like signs and symptoms—dry mouth; fixed, dilated pupils; flushing; and gastrointestinal symptoms may also occur.
If vomiting has not occurred spontaneously the patient should be induced to vomit. This is best done by having him drink a glass of water or milk after which he should be made to gag. Precautions against aspiration must be taken, especially in infants and children.
If vomiting is unsuccessful gastric lavage is indicated within 3 hours after ingestion and even later if large amounts of milk or cream were given beforehand. Isotonic and ½ isotonic saline is the lavage solution of choice.
Saline cathartics, as milk of magnesia, by osmosis draw water into the bowel and therefore, are valuable for their action in rapid dilution of bowel content.
Stimulants should *not* be used.
Vasopressors may be used to treat hypotension.
Dosage and Administration:
DOSAGE SHOULD BE INDIVIDUALIZED ACCORDING TO THE NEEDS AND THE RESPONSE OF THE PATIENT.
[See table below].

Usual dose:	Tablets		Syrup teaspoonfuls (5 cc)	
Adults and children 12 years and older	1		2	
Children 6 to 12 years	½	3–4	1	3–4
Children 4 to 6 years	—	times	¾	times
Children 2 to 4 years	—	a day	½	a day
Children 4 months to 2 years	—		¼	

How Supplied: Actidil® brand TRIPROLIDINE HYDROCHLORIDE 2.5 mg Scored Tablets (bottle of 100).
Also Available: Actidil® brand TRIPROLIDINE HYDROCHLORIDE SYRUP 1.25 mg per 5 cc (1 teaspoonful).
Preservatives: sodium benzoate 0.1%, methylparaben 0.1% (bottle of 1 pint).
Tablets bear identification, L2A.
[*Shown in Product Identification Section*]

ACTIFED® Tablets and Syrup ℞

Description: Each scored tablet contains Actidil® (Triprolidine Hydrochloride) 2.5 mg and Sudafed® (Pseudoephedrine Hydrochloride) 60 mg. Each 5 ml teaspoonful of the syrup* contains Actidil (Triprolidine Hydrochloride) 1.25 mg and Sudafed (Pseudoephedrine Hydrochloride) 30 mg.

*Preservatives: sodium benzoate 0.1%, methylparaben 0.1%.

Actidil (Triprolidine Hydrochloride) is *trans*-1-(4-methylphenyl)-1-(2-pyridyl)-3-pyrrolidinoprop-l-ene hydrochloride, a potent antihistamine. It is virtually tasteless and lacking in topical anesthetic effect.

Sudafed (Pseudoephedrine Hydrochloride) is a naturally occurring dextrostereoisomer of ephedrine and is classified as a sympathomimetic amine.

Action: Triprolidine hydrochloride is promptly absorbed and rapidly reaches a therapeutic level which is usually maintained for at least eight hours. It acts as an antagonist of the H1 histamine receptor.

The action of pseudoephedrine hydrochloride is apparently more specific on the blood vessels of the nasal and respiratory tract mucous membrane and less specific for the blood vessels of the systemic circulation. It is absorbed rapidly when administered by mouth. Its decongestant action aids in shrinking swollen mucous membranes of the nasopharynx, sinuses and eustachian tubes.

Actifed Tablets and Syrup appear to provide symptomatic relief by the rapid and sustained decongestant effect of pseudoephedrine hydrochloride together with the antihistaminic activity of triprolidine hydrochloride. In combination these two drugs aid in the symptomatic treatment of seasonal and perennial allergic rhinitis, vasomotor rhinitis and the common cold. In allergic conditions, this combination helps shrink swollen mucous membrane while simultaneously blocking histamine. Many patients who cannot be adequately controlled by antihistamines alone may respond to therapy with Actifed.

Indications: Based on a review of this drug by the National Academy of Sciences—National Research Council and/or other information, FDA has classified the Indications as follows:

"Probably" effective: For the symptomatic treatment of seasonal and perennial allergic rhinitis and vasomotor rhinitis.

"Lacking substantial evidence of effectiveness as a fixed combination": For the prophylaxis and treatment of the symptoms associated with the common cold.

Final classification of the less-than-effective indications requires further investigation.

Contraindications:

Use in Newborn or Premature Infants: This drug should *not* be used in newborn or premature infants.

Use in Nursing Mothers: Because of the higher risk of antihistamines and sympathomimetic amines for infants generally and for newborn and premature in particular, Actifed therapy is contraindicated in nursing mothers.

Use in Lower Respiratory Disease: Actifed is contraindicated for the treatment of lower respiratory symptoms including asthma.

Actifed is also contraindicated in the following conditions:

Hypersensitivity to: 1) Tripolidine Hydrochloride and other antihistamines of similar chemical structure; and/or 2) sympathomimetic amines including pseudoephedrine.

Monoamine oxidase inhibitor therapy (see Drug Interaction Section)

Warnings: Actifed should be used with considerable caution in patients with: increased intraocular pressure (narrow angle glaucoma); stenosing peptic ulcer; pyloroduodenal obstruction; symptomatic prostatic hypertrophy; bladder neck obstruction; hypertension; diabetes mellitus; ischemic heart disease and hyperthyroidism.

Usual Dose:	Tablets		Syrup teaspoonfuls (5 ml)	
Adults and children 12 years and older	1		2	
Children 6 to 12 years	½	3–4	1	3–4
Children 4 to 6 years	—	times	¾	times
Children 2 to 4 years	—	a day	½	a day
Children 4 months to 2 years	—		¼	

Sympathomimetics may produce central nervous stimulation with convulsions or cardiovascular collapse with accompanying hypotension.

Use in Children: As in adults, the combination of an antihistamine and sympathomimetic amine can elicit either mild stimulation or mild sedation in children. In the young child, mild stimulation is the response most frequently seen.

While it is difficult to predict the result of an *overdosage* of a combination of triprolidine and pseudoephedrine, the following is known about the individual components:

In infants and children, especially, antihistamine in overdosage may cause hallucination, convulsion or death. Large doses of pseudoephedrine are known to cause asthenia, lightheadedness, nausea and/or vomiting.

Use in Pregnancy: Experience with this drug in pregnant women is inadequate to determine whether there exists a potential for harm to the developing fetus.

Use with CNS Depressants: Triprolidine has additive effects with alcohol and other CNS depressants (hypnotics, sedatives, tranquilizers, etc.).

Use in Activities Requiring Mental Alertness: Patients should be warned about engaging in activities requiring mental alertness as driving a car or operating appliances, machinery, etc.

Use in the Elderly (approximately 60 years or older): Antihistamines are more likely to cause dizziness, sedation and hypotension in elderly patients. Overdosages of sympathomimetics in this age group may cause hallucinations, convulsions, CNS depression, and death.

Precautions: Actifed should be used with caution in patients with: history of bronchial asthma, increased intraocular pressure, hyperthyroidism, cardiovascular disease and hypertension.

Drug Interactions: MAO inhibitors prolong and intensify the anticholinergic (drying) effects of antihistamines and overall effects of sympathomimetics.

Sympathomimetics may reduce the antihypertension effects of methyldopa, decamylamine, reserpine, and veratrum alkaloids.

Adverse Reactions: The most frequent adverse reactions are underlined:

1. *General:* Urticaria, drug rash, anaphylactic shock, photosensitivity, excessive perspiration, chills, dryness of mouth, nose and throat.
2. *Cardiovascular System:* Hypotension, headache, palpitations, tachycardia, extrasystoles.
3. *Haematologic System:* Hemolytic anemia, thrombocytopenia, agranulocytosis.
4. *Nervous System:* Sedation, sleepiness, dizziness, disturbed coordination, fatigue, confusion, restlessness, excitation, nervousness, tremor, irritability, insomnia, euphoria, paresthesias, blurred vision, diplopia, vertigo, tinnitus, acute labyrinthitis, hysteria, neuritis, convulsions, CNS depression, hallucination.
5. *G.I. System:* Epigastric distress, anorexia, nausea, vomiting, diarrhea, constipation.
6. *G.U. System:* Urinary frequency, difficult urination, urinary retention, early menses.
7. *Respiratory System:* Thickening of bronchial secretions, tightness of chest and wheezing, nasal stuffiness.

Overdosage: Actifed overdosage reactions may vary from central nervous system depression to stimulation. Stimulation is particularly likely in children. Atropine-like signs and symptoms: dry mouth; fixed, dilated pupils; flushing; and gastrointestinal symptoms may also occur.

If vomiting has not occurred spontaneously the patient should be induced to vomit. This is best done by having him drink a glass of water or milk after which he should be made to gag. Precautions against aspiration must be taken, especially in infants and children.

If vomiting is unsuccessful gastric lavage is indicated within 3 hours after ingestion and even later if large amounts of milk or cream were given beforehand. Isotonic and ½ isotonic saline is the lavage solution of choice.

Saline cathartics, as milk of magnesia, draw water by osmosis into the bowel and therefore, are valuable for their action in rapid dilution of bowel content.

Stimulants should *not* be used.

Vasopressors may be used to treat hypotension.

Dosage and Administration:

DOSAGE SHOULD BE INDIVIDUALIZED ACCORDING TO THE NEEDS AND THE RESPONSE OF THE PATIENT.

[See table above].

How Supplied: Actifed® Tablets—Bottles of 100 and 1000; unit dose pack of 100. Actifed® Syrup—Bottles of 1 pint and 1 gallon.

Unit of Use: Tablets—Bottles of 30 and 100 with child-resistant cap. Syrup—4 oz bottle with child-resistant cap.

Tablets bear identification, M2A.

ACTIFED® TABLETS	
30—DoD	**NSN 6505-00-117-8608**
100—DoD	**NSN 6505-00-753-9615**
1000—DoD	**NSN 6505-00-142-9206**
ACTIFED® SYRUP	
4 oz.—DoD	**NSN 6505-00-782-6761**
Pint—DoD	**NSN 6505-00-753-9612**

[*Shown in Product Identification Section*]

ACTIFIED-C® Expectorant ℞ Ⓒ

Description: Each 5 cc (1 teaspoonful) contains: codeine phosphate 10 mg (Warning—may be habit-forming), Actidil® brand Triprolidine Hydrochloride 2 mg, Sudafed® brand Pseudoephedrine Hydrochloride 30 mg, Guaifenesin (glyceryl guaiacolate) 100 mg.

Preservatives: methylparaben 0.1%, sodium benzoate 0.1%.

Action: Actifed-C Expectorant is useful in both "wet" and "dry" coughs, and is effective whether the etiology is infectious or allergic; it is particularly useful in the coughing, wheezing stage of respiratory allergies. In those cases where cough is part of a generalized respiratory tract infection, this expectorant provides the additional benefits of nasal decongestion and prophylaxis against secondary otitis media or sinusitis.

The etiology of cough is such that drug therapy designed to produce relief may be called upon to provide several therapeutic actions simultaneously. The ingredients of Actifed-C Expectorant were selected because they produce the following desirable effects:

Antitussive: For many years codeine has been universally accepted as one of the most consistently effective cough suppressants. As used in Actifed-C brand Expectorant, codeine provides welcome reduction of excessive cough without productive expectoration.

Continued on next page

Burroughs Wellcome—Cont.

Expectorant: Guaifenesin (glyceryl guaiacolate) reduces the viscosity of secretions, thereby increasing the efficiency of the cough reflex and of ciliary action in removing accumulated secretions from the trachea and bronchi. Unlike many other expectorants, guaifenesin (glyceryl guaiacolate) rarely causes gastric irritation.
Decongestant-Bronchodilator: Some degree of mucosal congestion and bronchospasm is usually present along with all coughs. In children and in patients with an asthmatic component, the airway may be narrowed significantly by this congestion and bronchospasm. The bronchodilator and decongestant effect of Sudafed brand Pseudoephedrine Hydrochloride provides gratifying relief to many patients so affected. In cases complicated by upper respiratory congestion, it also helps keep the nasal passages clear and the sinus ostia and eustachian tubes patent.
Antihistaminic: The frequent association of allergy with cough makes antihistaminic action desirable. Whether or not the patient is allergic, the antihistamine will tend to decrease excessive secretions. The potent antihistamine, Actidil brand Triprolidine Hydrochloride, when combined with the sympathomimetic amine, pseudoephedrine hydrochloride, often provides a greater degree of relief from allergy than either drug used alone. This combination has been used successfully in the treatment of asthma, where antihistamines alone may sometimes increase the severity of the condition by thickening the secretions.

Indications: Based on a review of this drug by the National Academy of Sciences—National Research Council and/or other information, FDA has classified the indications as follows:
"Lacking substantial evidence of effectiveness as a fixed combination": For the symptomatic relief of cough in conditions such as: the common cold, acute bronchitis, allergic asthma, bronchiolitis, croup, emphysema, tracheobronchitis.
Final classification of the less-than-effective indications requires further investigation.

Warning: *Use in Pregnancy:* Experience with this drug in pregnant women is inadequate to determine whether there exists a potential for harm to the developing fetus.
Precautions: Although pseudoephedrine hydrochloride causes virtually no pressor effect in normotensive patients, it should be used with caution in patients with hypertension. In addition, even though triprolidine hydrochloride produces only a low incidence of drowsiness, appropriate precautions should be observed.
Side Effects: The great majority of patients will not have any side effects. Only certain patients, sensitive to one or another of the ingredients, may note mild stimulation or mild sedation.
Dosage:
Dosage indicated below may be given 4 times daily.

Adults and children over 12 years of age	2 teaspoonfuls
Children 7 through 12 years of age	1 teaspoonful
Children 2 through 6 years of age	½ teaspoonful

If a more frequent dosage schedule is desired, one-half of the appropriate dose recommended above may be given every 3 hours.
How Supplied: Bottle of 1 pint and 1 gallon.
Subject to DEA Regulations.

AEROSPORIN® ℞
brand Polymyxin B Sulfate
Sterile Powder
Polymyxin B Sulfate for Parenteral and/or Ophthalmic Administration

WARNING
CAUTION: WHEN THIS DRUG IS GIVEN INTRAMUSCULARLY AND/OR INTRATHECALLY, IT SHOULD BE GIVEN ONLY TO HOSPITALIZED PATIENTS, SO AS TO PROVIDE CONSTANT SUPERVISION BY A PHYSICIAN.
RENAL FUNCTION SHOULD BE CAREFULLY DETERMINED AND PATIENTS WITH RENAL DAMAGE AND NITROGEN RETENTION SHOULD HAVE REDUCED DOSAGE. PATIENTS WITH NEPHROTOXICITY DUE TO POLYMYXIN B SULFATE USUALLY SHOW ALBUMINURIA, CELLULAR CASTS, AND AZOTEMIA. DIMINISHING URINE OUTPUT AND A RISING BUN ARE INDICATIONS FOR DISCONTINUING THERAPY WITH THIS DRUG.
NEUROTOXIC REACTIONS MAY BE MANIFESTED BY IRRITABILITY, WEAKNESS, DROWSINESS, ATAXIA, PERIORAL PARESTHESIA, NUMBNESS OF THE EXTREMITIES, AND BLURRING OF VISION. THESE ARE USUALLY ASSOCIATED WITH HIGH SERUM LEVELS FOUND IN PATIENTS WITH IMPAIRED RENAL FUNCTION AND/OR NEPHROTOXICITY. THE CONCURRENT USE OF OTHER NEPHROTOXIC AND NEUROTOXIC DRUGS, PARTICULARLY KANAMYCIN, STREPTOMYCIN, CEPHALORIDINE, PAROMOMYCIN, TOBRAMYCIN, POLYMYXIN E (COLISTIN), NEOMYCIN, GENTAMICIN, AND VIOMYCIN, SHOULD BE AVOIDED.
THE NEUROTOXICITY OF POLYMYXIN B SULFATE CAN RESULT IN RESPIRATORY PARALYSIS FROM NEUROMUSCULAR BLOCKADE, ESPECIALLY WHEN THE DRUG IS GIVEN SOON AFTER ANESTHESIA AND/OR MUSCLE RELAXANTS.
USAGE IN PREGNANCY: THE SAFETY OF THIS DRUG IN HUMAN PREGNANCY HAS NOT BEEN ESTABLISHED.

Description: Polymyxin B sulfate is one of a group of basic polypeptide antibiotics derived from *B polymyxa (B aerosporous).*
Aerosporin brand Sterile Polymyxin B Sulfate is in powder form suitable for preparation of sterile solutions for intramuscular, intravenous drip, intrathecal, or ophthalmic use.
In the medical literature, dosages have frequently been given in terms of equivalent weight of pure polymyxin B base. Each milligram of pure polymyxin B base is equivalent to 10,000 units of polymyxin B and each microgram of pure polymyxin B base is equivalent to 10 units of polymyxin B.
Aqueous solutions of Aerosporin brand Polymyxin B Sulfate may be stored up to 12 months without significant loss of potency if kept under refrigeration. In the interest of safety, solutions for parenteral use should be stored under refrigeration and any unused portion should be discarded after 72 hours. Polymyxin B sulfate should not be stored in alkaline solutions since they are less stable.
Actions: Aerosporin brand Polymyxin B Sulfate has a bactericidal action against almost all gram-negative bacilli except the *Proteus* group. Polymyxins increase the permeability of bacterial cell wall membranes. All gram-positive bacteria, fungi, and the gram-negative cocci, *N gonorrhoeae* and *N meningitidis,* are resistant.
Susceptibility plate testing: If the Kirby-Bauer method of disc susceptibility testing is used, a 300-unit polymyxin B disc should give a zone of over 11 mm when tested against a polymyxin B-susceptible bacterial strain.
Polymyxin B sulfate is not absorbed from the normal alimentary tract. Since the drug loses 50 percent of its activity in the presence of serum, active blood levels are low. Repeated injections may give a cumulative effect. Levels tend to be higher in infants and children. The drug is excreted slowly by the kidneys. Tissue diffusion is poor and the drug does not pass the blood brain barrier into the cerebrospinal fluid. In therapeutic dosage, polymyxin B sulfate causes some nephrotoxicity with tubule damage to a slight degree.
Indications: Acute Infections Caused by Susceptible Strains of *Pseudomonas aeruginosa.*
Polymyxin B sulfate is a drug of choice in the treatment of infections of the urinary tract, meninges, and bloodstream caused by susceptible strains of *Ps aeruginosa.* It may also be used topically and subconjunctivally in the treatment of infections of the eye caused by susceptible strains of *Ps aeruginosa.*
It may be indicated in serious infections caused by susceptible strains of the following organisms, when less potentially toxic drugs are ineffective or contraindicated:
H. influenzae, specifically meningeal infections.
Escherichia coli, specifically urinary tract infections.
Aerobacter aerogenes, specifically bacteremia.
Klebsiella pneumoniae, specifically bacteremia.
Note. In Meningeal Infections, Polymyxin B Sulfate Should Be Administered Only by the Intrathecal Route.
Contraindications: This drug is contraindicated in persons with a prior history of hypersensitivity reactions to the polymyxins.
Precautions: See "Warning" box.
Baseline renal function should be done prior to therapy, with frequent monitoring of renal function and blood levels of the drug during parenteral therapy.
Avoid concurrent use of a curariform muscle relaxant and other neurotoxic drugs (ether, tubocurarine, succinylcholine, gallamine, decamethonium and sodium citrate) which may precipitate respiratory depression. If signs of respiratory paralysis appear, respiration should be assisted as required, and the drug discontinued.
As with other antibiotics, use of this drug may result in overgrowth of nonsusceptible organisms, including fungi. If superinfection occurs, appropriate therapy should be instituted.
Adverse Reactions: See "Warning" box.
Nephrotoxic reactions: Albuminuria, cylinduria, azotemia, and rising blood levels without any increase in dosage.
Neurotoxic reactions: Facial flushing, dizziness progressing to ataxia, drowsiness, peripheral paresthesias (circumoral and stocking-glove), apnea due to concurrent use of curariform muscle relaxants and other neurotoxic drugs or inadvertent overdosage, and signs of meningeal irritation with intrathecal administration, e.g., fever, headache, stiff neck and increased cell count and protein cerebrospinal fluid.
Other reactions occasionally reported: Drug fever, urticarial rash, pain (severe) at intramuscular injection sites, and thrombophlebitis at intravenous injection sites.
Administration and Dosage:
PARENTERAL:
Intravenous. Dissolve 500,000 units polymyxin B sulfate in 300-500 cc of 5 percent dextrose in water for continuous intravenous drip.
Adults and children. 15,000-25,000 units/kg body weight/day in individuals with normal kidney function. This amount should be reduced from 15,000 units/kg downward for individuals with kidney impairment. Infusions may be given every 12 hours; however, the total daily dose must not exceed 25,000 units/kg/day.

Infants. Infants with normal kidney function may receive up to 40,000 units/kg/day without adverse effects.

Intramuscular. Not recommended routinely because of severe pain at injection sites, particularly in infants and children. Dissolve 500,000 units polymyxin B sulfate in 2 cc sterile distilled water (Water for Injection, U.S.P.) or sterile physiologic saline (Sodium Chloride Injection, U.S.P.) or 1 percent procaine hydrochloride solution.

Adults and children. 25,000-30,000 units/kg/day. This should be reduced in the presence of renal impairment. The dosage may be divided and given at either 4- or 6-hour intervals.

Infants. Infants with normal kidney function may receive up to 40,000 units/kg/day without adverse effects.

Note. Doses as high as 45,000 units/kg/day have been used in limited clinical studies in treating prematures and newborn infants for sepsis caused by *Ps aeruginosa.*

Intrathecal. A treatment of choice for *Ps aeruginosa* meningitis. Dissolve 500,000 units polymyxin B sulfate in 10 cc of sterile physiologic saline (Sodium Chloride Injection, U.S.P.) for 50,000 units per ml dosage unit.

Adults and children over 2 years of age. Dosage is 50,000 units once daily intrathecally for 3-4 days, then 50,000 units once every other day for at least 2 weeks after cultures of the cerebrospinal fluid are negative and sugar content has returned to normal.

Children under 2 years of age. 20,000 units once daily, intrathecally for 3-4 days or 25,000 units once every other day. Continue with a dose of 25,000 units once every other day for at least 2 weeks after cultures of the cerebrospinal fluid are negative and sugar content has returned to normal.

IN THE INTEREST OF SAFETY, SOLUTIONS FOR PARENTERAL USE SHOULD BE STORED UNDER REFRIGERATION, AND ANY UNUSED PORTIONS SHOULD BE DISCARDED AFTER 72 HOURS.

TOPICAL:

Ophthalmic. Dissolve 500,000 units polymyxin B sulfate in 20-50 cc sterile distilled water (Water for Injection, U.S.P.) or sterile physiologic saline (Sodium Chloride Injection U.S.P.) for a 10,000-25,000 units per cc concentration.

For the treatment of *Ps aeruginosa* infections of the eye, a concentration of 0.1 percent to 0.25 percent (10,000 units to 25,000 units per cc) is administered 1-3 drops every hour, increasing the intervals as response indicates.

Subconjunctival injection of up to 10,000 units/day may be used for the treatment of *Ps aeruginosa* infections of the cornea and conjunctiva.

Note. Avoid total systemic and ophthalmic instillation over 25,000 units/kg/day.

AVAILABLE DOSAGE FORM

500,000 units.

Rubber-stoppered vial with flip off cap.

Vial—VA NSN 6505-00-913-3124

ALKERAN®

brand Melphalan ℞

Description: Each scored tablet contains 2 mg melphalan, the phenylalanine derivative of nitrogen mustard. Also known as Compound CB 3025 and sometimes referred to as L-Sarcolysin. Chemically, it is *p*-di(2-chloroethyl) amino-L-phenylalanine.

U.S. Pat. Nos. 3,032,584 and 3,032,585.

Action and Uses: Alkeran has the general pharmacologic properties of nitrogen mustard compounds. It is well absorbed when given orally and seems to be equally effective by mouth or intravenously.

Indications: Alkeran brand Melphalan is useful in the treatment of multiple myeloma.

Contraindications: Alkeran brand Melphalan should not be given if other similar chemotherapeutic agents or radiation has been administered in the recent past, or if the neutrophil and/or platelet counts are depressed. The drug should not be administered concurrently with radiation.

Warnings: As with other nitrogen mustard drugs, excessive dosage will produce marked bone marrow depression. Frequent blood counts are essential to determine optimal dosage and to avoid toxicity. The drug should be discontinued or the dosage reduced upon evidence of abnormal depression of the bone marrow.

Usage in Pregnancy: Safe use of melphalan has not been established with respect to adverse effects on fetal development. Therefore, it should be used in women of childbearing potential and particularly during early pregnancy only when, in the judgment of the physician, the potential benefits outweigh the possible hazards.

Precautions: If the leukocyte count falls below 3,000 cells/cu mm, or the platelet count below 100,000/cu mm, the drug should be discontinued until the blood picture has had a chance to recover.

Adverse Reactions: Nausea and vomiting have followed the use of high doses of Alkeran brand Melphalan. Dose related bone marrow depression produces anemia, neutropenia and thrombocytopenia.

Dosage and Administration: The usual oral dose is 6 mg (3 tablets) daily. The entire daily dose may be given at one time. It is adjusted, as required, on the basis of blood counts done at approximately weekly intervals. After 2 to 3 weeks of treatment, the drug should be discontinued for up to 4 weeks during which time the blood count should be followed carefully. When the white blood cell and platelet counts are rising, a maintenance dose of 2 mg daily may be instituted.

Other dosage regimens have been used by various investigators. Osserman has used an initial course of 10 mg/day for 7 to 10 days. He reports that maximal suppression of the leukocyte and platelet counts occurs within 3 to 5 weeks and recovery within 4 to 8 weeks. Continuous maintenance therapy with 2 mg/day is instituted when the white blood cell count is greater than 4000 and the platelet count is greater than 100,000. Dosage is adjusted to between 1 and 3 mg/day depending upon the hematological response. It is desirable to try to maintain a significant degree of bone marrow depression so as to keep the leukocyte count in the range of 3000 to 3500 cells/cu mm.

Hoogstraten has started treatment with 0.15 mg/kg per day for 7 days. This is followed by a rest period of at least 14 days, but it may be as long as 5 to 6 weeks. Maintenance therapy is started when the white blood cell and platelet counts are rising. The maintenance dose is 0.05 mg/kg per day or less and is adjusted according to the blood count.

Available evidence suggests that about one-third to one-half of the patients with multiple myeloma show a favorable response to oral administration of the drug. It is to be emphasized that response may be very gradual over many months; it is important that repeated courses or continuous therapy be given since improvement may continue slowly over many months and the maximum benefit may be missed if treatment is abandoned too soon.

How Supplied: Tablet of 2 mg, scored. Bottle of 50.

Product Identification Marks: Bears Wellcome I.D. code imprint, A2A.

[*Shown in Product Identification Section*]

ANECTINE®

brand Succinylcholine Chloride ℞

THIS DRUG SHOULD BE USED ONLY BY INDIVIDUALS FAMILIAR WITH ITS ACTIONS, CHARACTERISTICS AND HAZARDS.

Description: Anectine brand Succinylcholine Chloride is an ultra short-acting depolarizing type muscle relaxant. Chemically it is a di-quaternary base consisting of the di-chloride salt of the di-choline ester of succinic acid. It is a white, odorless, slightly bitter powder and very soluble in water. The drug is unstable with alkaline solutions, but relatively stable in acid solutions depending upon the concentration of the solution and the storage temperature. While solutions of succinylcholine chloride are sterilized by autoclaving, they should, nevertheless, be stored under refrigeration to preserve their potency.

Actions: Anectine brand Succinylcholine Chloride causes skeletal muscle paralysis by blocking neural transmission at the myoneural junction. It competes with acetylcholine for the cholinergic receptors of the motor end plate. Like acetylcholine, bond with these receptors produces a depolarization followed by an initial transient muscle contraction often visible as fasciculations. Neuromuscular transmission then becomes inhibited and remains so as long as there is an adequate concentration of succinylcholine at the receptor sites. The neuromuscular block so achieved produces a flaccid paralysis of skeletal muscles. Succinylcholine is dissipated through the enzymatic action of pseudocholinesterase at such a rate that the effect of a single paralyzing dose of the drug generally disappears within 8 to 10 minutes. When a single effective dose of the drug is given intravenously, muscular relaxation occurs within a minute, persists for about 2 minutes and returns to normal within 8 to 10 minutes. If a paralyzing dose is given intramuscularly, the onset of action may be delayed for 2 to 3 minutes. When given by intravenous drip, a predetermined degree of muscular relaxation can be closely approximated by adjusting the rate of flow of the infusion.

An important difference between succinylcholine and tubocurarine is that the former is not generally antagonized by anticholinesterases. On the contrary, such drugs as physostigmine, neostigmine and procaine usually prolong the action of succinylcholine. This would support the theory that succinylcholine is hydrolyzed by cholinesterases and that interference with this enzyme action results in persistence of activity of the drug. Succinylcholine is rapidly hydrolyzed by pseudocholinesterase to succinylmonocholine (a weak non-depolarizing type of muscle relaxant), and then more slowly to the normal metabolites succinic acid and choline. However, about 10 percent of the drug is excreted unchanged in the urine. The drug's action may be additionally altered by acetylcholine, dehydration, hypothermia, electrolyte imbalance, certain antibiotics, some carcinomas, procaine-type local anesthetics or the administration of other non-depolarizing or depolarizing muscle relaxants.

The drug has no known effect on consciousness, the pain threshold or cerebration. It should, therefore, be used only during adequate anesthesia.

The paralysis following the administration of succinylcholine is generally initially selective and usually appears in the following muscles consecutively: levator muscles of the eyelids, muscles of mastication, limb muscles, abdominal muscles, muscles of the glottis and finally intercostal muscles and the diaphragm. The drug has no direct effect on the myocardium. Initially a transient bradycardia accompanied by hypotension, arrhythmias and even a sinus arrest may occur during endotracheal intubation due to an increase in vagal tone. This is noted particularly in children and is more apparent with repetitive injections than follow-

Continued on next page

Burroughs Wellcome—Cont.

ing continuous intravenous drip administration. These effects are enhanced by cyclopropane and halothane and are inhibited by thiopental and atropine. Later the drug may cause tachycardia and hypertension as a result of an asphyxial pressor response and mild sympathetic ganglion stimulation.

Succinylcholine causes a slight, transient increase in intraocular pressure. The effect is seen immediately after its injection and during the fasciculation phase. It appears to be the result of brief contraction of the extraocular muscles. This suggests that the drug should not be used when open eye injury is present and should be used with caution, if at all, in intraocular surgery. The opinion is expressed that the effect is probably not sufficient to contraindicate the drug in general surgery or electroshock therapy for patients with glaucoma or in patients undergoing eye surgery under general anesthesia.

Succinylcholine has no direct effect on the uterus or other smooth muscles. The drug is highly ionized and has a low lipid solubility; therefore, it will not cross the placenta readily. Further, the enzymatic destruction of succinylcholine is an important factor in controlling the concentration gradient. Infants are relatively more resistant to depolarizing relaxants than adults.

Tachyphylaxis may occur after repeated doses of succinylcholine.

Note: On rare occasions when succinylcholine is given over a long period of time, the characteristic depolarization block of the myoneural junction changes to a non-depolarizing block resulting in prolonged respiratory depression or apnea similar to the blockade caused by tubocurarine. Under those circumstances small repeated doses of prostigmine may shorten the action of succinylcholine.

Indications: Succinylcholine chloride is indicated as an adjunct to anesthesia to induce skeletal muscle relaxation. It may be employed to reduce the intensity of muscle contractions of pharmacologically or electrically induced convulsions.

Contraindications: Succinylcholine is contraindicated for persons with a known hypersensitivity to the drug.

Warnings:

WARNING: SUCCINYLCHOLINE SHOULD BE USED ONLY BY THOSE SKILLED IN THE MANAGEMENT OF ARTIFICIAL RESPIRATION AND ONLY WHEN FACILITIES ARE INSTANTLY AVAILABLE FOR ENDOTRACHEAL INTUBATION AND FOR PROVIDING ADEQUATE VENTILATION OF THE PATIENT, INCLUDING THE ADMINISTRATION OF OXYGEN UNDER POSITIVE PRESSURE AND THE ELIMINATION OF CARBON DIOXIDE. THE CLINICIAN MUST BE PREPARED TO ASSIST OR TO CONTROL RESPIRATION.

Succinylcholine should not be mixed with short-acting barbiturates in the same syringe, or administered simultaneously during intravenous infusion through the same needle. Solutions of succinylcholine have an acid pH whereas those of barbiturates are alkaline in reaction. Depending upon the resultant pH of a mixture of solutions of these drugs, either free barbituric acid may be precipitated or succinylcholine hydrolyzed.

Usage in Pregnancy: The safe use of succinylcholine has not been established with respect to the possible adverse effects upon fetal development. Therefore, it should not be used in women of childbearing potential and particularly during early pregnancy unless in the judgment of the physician the potential benefits outweigh the unknown hazards.

Precautions: Low levels of, or abnormal variants of plasma cholinesterase may be associated with prolonged respiratory depression or apnea following the use of succinylcholine. Low levels of plasma cholinesterase may occur in patients with severe liver disease or cirrhosis, severe anemia, malnutrition, severe dehydration, changes in body temperature, exposure to neurotoxic insecticides or those receiving antimalarial drugs. Succinylcholine should be administered with extreme care to such patients and dosage should be minimal. If low plasma cholinesterase activity is suspected, a small test dose of from 5 to 10 mg of succinylcholine may be administered, or relaxation may be produced by the cautious administration of a 0.1 percent solution of the drug by intravenous drip. Drugs which either inhibit plasma cholinesterase, such as neostigmine or phospholine iodide, or compete with succinylcholine for the enzyme, as does intravenous procaine, should not be given concurrently with succinylcholine.

Succinylcholine should be administered with great caution to patients with severe burns, those recovering from severe trauma, those suffering from electrolyte imbalance, those receiving quinidine, those who have been digitalized recently or who may have digitalis toxicity as serious cardiac arrhythmias or cardiac arrest may result. Great caution should be observed also in patients with pre-existing hyperkalemia or who are paraplegic, have suffered spinal neuraxis injury, or have degenerative or dystrophic neuromuscular disease, as such patients tend to become severely hyperkalemic when succinylcholine is given.

When succinylcholine is given over a prolonged period of time, the characteristic depolarization block of the myoneural junction may change to a non-depolarizing block which results in prolonged respiratory depression or apnea. Under such circumstances, small repeated doses of neostigmine may possibly act as an antagonist. A peripheral nerve stimulator (e.g. the Wellcome Peripheral Nerve Stimulator) may be used to ascertain the type of neuromuscular blockade. If a depolarization block is present both fast (tetanic) and slow (twitch) rates of nerve stimulation are well sustained, and post-tetanic facilitation is absent. If a non-depolarizing block is present there is post-tetanic facilitation and "fade" of successive stimuli on both fast (tetanic) and slow (twitch) rates of nerve stimulation.

Succinylcholine should be used with caution during ocular surgery and in patients with glaucoma. The drug should be employed with caution in patients with fractures or muscle spasm as the muscle fasciculations may cause additional trauma. Muscle fasciculations and hyperkalemia may be reduced by administering a small dose of a non-depolarizing relaxant. If other relaxants are to be used during the same procedure, the possibility of a synergistic or antagonistic effect should be considered.

During the past few years, reports have called attention to a fulminant syndrome, malignant hyperthermia, observed during anesthesia. Its etiology is not fully understood. Malignant hyperthermia occurs in genetically prone individuals of all ages and both sexes receiving potent anesthetics such as halothane, methoxyflurane, cyclopropane and diethyl ether. It appears to develop irrespective of the concomitant use of a muscle relaxant, but may be triggered by succinylcholine. Because of the seriousness of this syndrome and the need for early effective treatment of the patient; it is suggested that the continuous monitoring of the temperature will serve as an aid to the early recognition of malignant hyperthermia.

Adverse Reactions: Adverse reactions consist primarily of an extension of the drug's pharmacological actions. Profound and prolonged muscle relaxation may occur, resulting in respiratory depression to the point of apnea. Hypersensitivity to the drug may exist in rare instances.

The following adverse reactions have been reported: bradycardia, tachycardia, hypertension, hypotension, arrhythmias, cardiac arrest, prolonged respiratory depression or apnea, hyperthermia, increased intraocular pressure, muscle fasciculation, postoperative muscle pain, myoglobinemia and excessive salivation.

Dosage and Administration: The dosage of succinylcholine is essentially individualized and its administration should always be determined by the clinician after careful assessment of the patient.

To avoid distress to the patient, succinylcholine should be administered only after unconsciousness has been induced.

For Short Surgical Procedures: The average dose for relaxation of short duration is 40 mg (2.0 cc) Anectine brand Succinylcholine Chloride Injection given intravenously. The optimum dose will vary among individuals and may vary from 20 to 80 mg for adults (1.0 to 4.0 cc). Following administration of doses in this range, relaxation develops in about 1 minute; maximum muscular paralysis may persist for about 2 minutes, after which recovery rapidly takes place within 8 to 10 minutes. However, very large doses may result in more prolonged apnea. An initial test dose of 10 mg (0.5 cc) may be used to determine the sensitivity of the patient and the individual recovery time from the drug.

For Long Surgical Procedures: The dosage of succinylcholine chloride administered by infusion depends upon the duration of the surgical procedure and the need for muscle relaxation. The average rate of administration for continuous intravenous infusion is 2.5 mg per minute for adult patients. Solutions containing from 0.1% to 0.2% (1 to 2 mg per cc) succinylcholine chloride have commonly been used for continuous intravenous drip. Solutions of 0.1% or 0.2% may conveniently be prepared by adding 1 g succinylcholine chloride (the contents of one Anectine brand Succinylcholine Chloride Sterile Powder Flo-Pack unit containing 1 g) respectively to 1,000 or 500 cc of sterile solution such as sterile 5% dextrose solution or sterile isotonic saline or lactate solution. The more dilute solution (0.1% or 1 mg per cc) is probably preferable from the standpoint of ease of control of the rate of administration of the drug and, hence, of relaxation. This intravenous drip solution containing 1 mg per cc may be administered at a rate of from 0.5 mg (0.5 cc) to 10 mg (10 cc) per minute to obtain the desired amount of relaxation. The amount required per minute will depend upon the individual response as well as the degree of relaxation required. In the experience of Foldes, the average rate is 2.5 mg per minute. In the series reported by Little, Hampton and Grosskreutz, an average dose of 4.3 mg per minute was used. The 0.2% solution may be especially useful in those cases where it is desired to avoid overburdening the circulation with a large volume of fluid, e.g., cardiac cases. In any case, the rate of administration will be varied from time to time. The degree of relaxation can be regulated to the needs of the surgeon by adjusting the drip. Only freshly prepared solutions of succinylcholine should be used.

Intermittent intravenous injections of succinylcholine may also be used to provide muscular relaxation for long procedures. An initial intravenous injection of 20 to 80 mg may be given initially followed at appropriate intervals by further injections of 3 to 5 mg to maintain the degree of relaxation required.

The intravenous dose of succinylcholine for infants and children is 1.0 to 2.0 mg per kg.

Intramuscular Use: Succinylcholine may be given intramuscularly to infants, older children or adults when a suitable vein is inaccessible. A dose of up to 2.5 mg per kg may be given, but not more than 150 mg total dose should be given.

Management of Adverse Reactions: Apnea or prolonged muscle paralysis should be treated with controlled respiration.

The use of neostigmine to reverse a non-depolarization block is a medical decision which must be made upon the basis of the individual clinical pharmacology and the experience and judgment of the clinician. When neostigmine is used atropine should also be administered.

How Supplied: For immediate injection of single doses for short procedures:

ANECTINE brand SUCCINYLCHOLINE CHLORIDE INJECTION

20 mg in each cc (expressed as anhydrous Succinylcholine Chloride)

Multiple-dose vial of 10 cc—for intravenous injection

ANECTINE Injection is a sterile solution made isotonic with sodium chloride, pH adjusted with hydrochloric acid and preserved with methylparaben 0.1%.

Vial 20 mg/cc × 12 —DoD
NSN 6505-00-133-4309

Flo-Pack 1000 mg × 12 —VA
NSN 6505-00-059-2360

Flo-Pack 1000 mg —DoD
NSN 6505-00-720-9680

Also Available: For preparation of intravenous drip solutions only:

ANECTINE brand SUCCINYLCHOLINE CHLORIDE

(expressed as anhydrous succinylcholine chloride)

FLO-PACK®

500 mg Sterile Powder

For preparation of dilute solutions for intravenous drip only.

HIGH POTENCY ANECTINE brand SUCCINYLCHOLINE CHLORIDE

(expressed as anhydrous succinylcholine chloride)

FLO-PACK®

1000 mg Sterile Powder

For preparation of dilute solutions for intravenous drip only.

ANTEPAR® ℞

brand Piperazine
Syrup/Tablet

Description: (See Table I below).

[See table above].

Piperazine hexahydrate is a white, crystalline substance.

Actions: Clinical investigations in man have demonstrated its activity against the human pinworm, *Enterobius vermicularis,* and against the "common roundworm," *Ascaris lumbricoides.*

Piperazine produces a paralysis of ascaris muscle with resultant expulsion of the worm through intestinal peristalsis.

Systemic absorption of piperazine is variable and the drug is excreted essentially unchanged.

Indications: For the treatment of ascariasis ("common roundworm" infection) and enterobiasis (pinworm infection).

Contraindications: This product is contraindicated in patients with impaired renal or hepatic function, convulsive disorders, or a history of hypersensitivity reactions from piperazine and its salt.

TABLE I

Dosage Form	Contains	Equivalency in Terms of Piperazine Hexahydrate
Syrup	Piperazine Citrate Anhydrous 550 mg per 5 cc (1 teaspoonful)	500 mg per teaspoonful
Scored Tablet	Piperazine Citrate Anhydrous 550 mg per tablet	500 mg per tablet

Warnings: Because of potential neurotoxicity of this drug, especially in children, prolonged or repeated treatment in excess of that recommended should be avoided.

Usage in Pregnancy: Safety of this drug for use during pregnancy has not been established.

Precautions: If CNS, significant gastrointestinal, or hypersensitivity reactions occur, the drug should be discontinued.

In patients with severe malnutrition, or anemia, appropriate caution should be exercised.

Adverse Reactions: The following reactions have been reported, usually due to excessive dosage:

Gastrointestinal—nausea, vomiting, abdominal cramps, and diarrhea.

Central nervous system—headache, vertigo, ataxia, tremors, choreiform movement, muscular weakness, hyporeflexia, paresthesia, blurring of vision, paralytic strabismus, convulsion, EEG abnormalities, sense of detachment, and memory defect.

Hypersensitivity—urticaria, erythema multiforme, purpura, fever, and arthralgia.

Dosage and Administration: *For ascariasis (roundworm infection):*

Adults—a single daily dose of 3.5 g (hexahydrate equivalent) for 2 consecutive days.

Children—a single daily dose of 75 mg (hexahydrate equivalent)/kg of body weight/day for 2 consecutive days, with maximum daily dose of 3.5 g. (See Table II below).

[See table below].

In severe infections, the treatment course may be repeated after a *one* week interval. In circumstances where it is desired to apply mass therapy of ascariasis as a public health measure and where repeated therapy is not practicable, one single dose of 70 mg per pound of body weight, up to a maximum dose of 3 g, may be used, as described by Swartzwelder and Goodwin.* This procedure is successful in removing ascarids in the great majority of cases. However, the maximum cure rate is usually obtained with the multiple-dose regimen.

***References:**

Swartzwelder C, Miller JH, Sappenfield RW: Treatment of ascariasis in children with a single dose of piperazine citrate. Pediatrics 16(1):115, 1955

Goodwin LG, Standen OD: Treatment of roundworm with piperazine citrate (Antepar). Brit MJ 2:1332, 1954

For enterobiasis (pinworm infection): Adults and children—a single daily dose of 65 mg (hexahydrate equivalent)/kg of body weight/day, with a maximum daily dose of 2.5 g, for 7 consecutive days. (See Table III below).

[See table on next page].

In severe infections, the treatment course may be repeated after a *one* week interval.

Use of laxatives or enema and dietary restriction are not necessary.

To prevent reinfection practice of personal and environmental hygiene should be recommended.

How Supplied:

ANTEPAR® brand Piperazine Citrate SYRUP 550 mg per 5 cc (equivalent to 500 mg piperazine hexahydrate). Bottle of 1 pint.

ANTEPAR® brand Piperazine Citrate TABLETS 550 mg scored (equivalent to 500 mg piperazine hexahydrate). Bottles of 100 and 1000. Imprinted Y4A for identification.

[Shown in Product Identification Section]

TABLE II

Patient's Weight	Daily Dose For Two Consecutive Days (For Roundworms)	
15 lbs	1 tablet or teaspoonful	(0.5 g)
30 lbs	2 tablets or teaspoonfuls	(1.0 g)
45 lbs	3 tablets or teaspoonfuls	(1.5 g)
60 lbs	4 tablets or teaspoonfuls	(2.0 g)
75 lbs	5 tablets or teaspoonfuls	(2.5 g)
90 lbs	6 tablets or teaspoonfuls	(3.0 g)
105 lbs or over	7 tablets or teaspoonfuls (maximum daily dose)	(3.5 g)

CARDILATE® ℞

brand Erythrityl Tetranitrate
Oral/Sublingual Tablets (Scored)
5 mg, 10 mg, and 15 mg

CARDILATE® ℞

brand Erythrityl Tetranitrate
Chewable Tablets (Scored) 10 mg

Description: Cardilate brand Erythrityl Tetranitrate is an organic nitrate with empirical formula $C_4H_6(NO_3)_4$.

Riseman noted that the most effective organic nitrates were those which had a molecular configuration similar to that of nitroglycerin with a straight C-atom chain.

The basic action of the nitrates in the body is to relax smooth muscles, especially those of the finer blood vessels; this is independent of innervation. The post-arteriolar vessels—capillaries and venules—are most susceptible, although the larger veins and arteries are also relaxed to some extent.

Pharmacologic Action: The attacks of angina pectoris are believed to be the result of myocardial hypoxia and occur when a discrepancy exists between myocardial demand for oxygen and the supply provided by the coronary circulation. The beneficial effects of nitrates in the treatment of angina pectoris are attributed in part to decreased vascular tone or resistance. Erythrityl tetranitrate has been found to be a potent coronary dilator. Its action is exerted at extremely low blood concentrations.

A second beneficial action of the nitrates is a reduction in cardiac pre-load (ventricular end-diastolic pressure), as the result of pooling of blood in the venous side of the circulation. The reduction in cardiac work through peripheral vasodilation by Cardilate brand Erythrityl Tetranitrate assumes greater significance in light of observations that elevation of blood pressure which follows effort or stress is an important factor in precipitating attacks of angina pectoris by increasing cardiac work. It is felt by Gorlin that "the salutary effect of long-acting nitrites may be due to damping of blood pressure response to effort or anxiety. . . ."

Indications: Cardilate (Erythrityl Tetranitrate) is intended for the prophylaxis and long-term treatment of patients with frequent or

Continued on next page

Burroughs Wellcome—Cont.

recurrent anginal pain and reduced exercise tolerance associated with angina pectoris, rather than for the treatment of the acute attack of angina pectoris, since its onset is somewhat slower than that of nitroglycerin.
Contraindications: Idiosyncrasy to this drug.
Warning: Data supporting the use of nitrates during the early days of the acute phase of myocardial infarction (the period during which clinical and laboratory findings are unstable) are insufficient to establish safety.
Precautions: Intraocular pressure is increased; therefore, caution is required in administering to patients with glaucoma. Tolerance to this drug, and cross-tolerance to other nitrites and nitrates may occur.
Adverse Reactions: Cutaneous vasodilation with flushing. Headache is common and may be severe and persistent. Transient episodes of dizziness and weakness, as well as other signs of cerebral ischemia associated with postural hypotension, may occasionally develop. This drug can act as a physiological antagonist to norepinephrine, acetylcholine, histamine and many other agents. An occasional individual exhibits marked sensitivity to the hypotensive effects of nitrates and severe responses (nausea, vomiting, weakness, restlessness, pallor, perspiration and collapse) can occur even with the usual therapeutic dose. Alcohol may enhance this effect. Drug rash and/or exfoliative dermatitis may occasionally occur.
Dosage and Administration:
Oral/Sublingual Tablets: Cardilate brand Erythrityl Tetranitrate may be administered either sublingually or orally. Therapy may be initiated with 10 mg sublingually prior to each anticipated physical or emotional stress and at bedtime for patients subject to nocturnal attacks. The dose may be increased or decreased as needed.
If oral administration is preferred, therapy may be initiated with 10 mg before each meal, as well as midmorning, midafternoon if needed and at bedtime for patients subject to nocturnal attacks. The dose may be increased or decreased as needed.
Up to 100 mg daily is well tolerated but temporary headache is more apt to occur as with large doses of nitroglycerin. When headache occurs, the dose should be reduced for a few days. If headache is troublesome during adjustment of dosage, it may be effectively relieved with an analgesic.
Administered sublingually, an effect appears within 5 minutes with maximum action developing in 30 to 45 minutes and total duration of effect up to 2 hours against effort-produced angina.
Administered orally, an effect appears in approximately 30 minutes with maximal action developing in about 60 to 90 minutes and with a variable duration of effect.
Chewable: Cardilate brand Erythrityl Tetranitrate Chewable Tablets offer the therapeutic action of erythrityl tetranitrate in a pleasantly flavored (wintergreen) chewable tablet, the action of which parallels that of the sublingual tablets.
One Cardilate brand Erythrityl Tetranitrate 10 mg Chewable Tablet should be chewed prior to each anticipated physical or emotional stress and at bedtime for patients subject to nocturnal attacks. The dose may be increased or decreased as needed.
As many as ten chewable tablets daily are well tolerated but temporary headache is more apt to occur as with large doses of nitroglycerin. When headache occurs, the dose should be reduced for a few days. If headache is troublesome during adjustment of dosage, it may be effectively relieved with an analgesic.
An effect appears within 5 minutes, with maximum action developing in 30 to 45 minutes and total duration of effect up to 2 hours against effort-produced angina. Reduction of left ventricular pre-load has been demonstrated for at least 4 hours.
How Supplied:
CARDILATE brand Erythrityl Tetranitrate TABLETS (Scored) for ORAL or SUBLINGUAL USE 5 mg: Bottles of 100. Bear identification, P2B. 10 mg: Bottles of 100 and 1000. Bear identification, BW & Co. 15 mg: Bottles of 100. Bear identification, R2B.
CHEWABLE TABLETS (Scored) 10 mg: Bottles of 100. Bear identification, X7A.
[Shown in Product Identification Section]

CARDILATE®-P brand ℞
Erythrityl Tetranitrate with Phenobarbital

Description: Each scored tablet contains: erythrityl tetranitrate 10 mg and phenobarbital* 15 mg.
*Warning—may be habit-forming.
For oral use only.
Indications: For the prophylaxis and treatment of patients with frequent or recurrent anginal pain where anxiety and tension may be precipitating factors.
Precautions: As with other effective nitrites, some fall in blood pressure may occur with large doses.
Caution should be observed in administering the drug to patients with a history of recent cerebral hemorrhage, because of the vasodilation which occurs in the area. Although therapy permits more normal activity, the patient should not be allowed to misinterpret freedom from anginal attacks as a signal to drop all restrictions.
Side Effects: As with nitroglycerin or other effective nitrites, temporary vascular headache may occur during the first few days of therapy. This can be controlled by temporary dosage reduction in order to allow adjustment of the cerebral hemodynamics to the initial marked cerebral vasodilation. These headaches usually disappear within one week of continuous therapy but may be minimized by the administration of analgesics.
Mild gastrointestinal disturbances occur occasionally with larger doses and may be controlled by reducing the dose temporarily.
Dosage: For the average patient, one tablet orally before each meal and at bedtime for patients subject to nocturnal attacks. An additional dose may be taken in midmorning and midafternoon if needed.
How Supplied: Bottle of 100 scored tablets. Tablets bear identification, T3B.
[Shown in Product Identification Section]

TABLE III
(For Pinworms)

Patient's Weight	Daily Dose For Seven Consecutive Days	
17 lbs	1 tablet or teaspoonful	(0.5 g)
34 lbs	2 tablets or teaspoonfuls	(1.0 g)
51 lbs	3 tablets or teaspoonfuls	(1.5 g)
68 lbs	4 tablets or teaspoonfuls	(2.0 g)
85 lbs and over	5 tablets or teaspoonfuls (maximum daily dose)	(2.5 g)

CORTISPORIN® CREAM ℞
Polymyxin B—Neomycin—Gramicidin—Hydrocortisone

Description: Each gram contains: Aerosporin® brand Polymyxin B Sulfate 10,000 units; neomycin sulfate 5 mg (equivalent to 3.5 mg neomycin base); gramicidin 0.25 mg; hydrocortisone acetate 5 mg (0.5%).
Preservative: methylparaben 0.25%
The base contains the inactive ingredients liquid petrolatum, white petrolatum, propylene glycol, polyoxyethylene polyoxypropylene compound, emulsifying wax and purified water.
The base is a smooth vanishing cream with a pH of approximately 5.0. The acid pH helps restore normal cutaneous acidity. The cream is cosmetically acceptable and may be easily removed with water. Owing to its excellent spreading and penetrating properties, the cream facilitates treatment of hairy and intertriginous areas. It may also be of value in selective cases where the lesions are moist. The antibiotics diffuse readily from the base into fluids of the skin or tissues.
Action: The cream is useful wherever the anti-inflammatory and antipruritic action of hydrocortisone is indicated in conjunction with the bactericidal action of polymyxin B, neomycin, and gramicidin. For anti-inflammatory action, the acetate salt of the naturally-occurring adrenal corticosteroid hydrocortisone is used. Wide range antibacterial action, approaching the ideal, is provided by the overlapping spectra of polymyxin B, neomycin, and gramicidin. The range of action of this combination includes virtually all pathogenic bacteria found topically, and the three antibacterials are bactericidal, rather than bacteriostatic. The index of allergenicity of this combination has been shown over the years to be low and the rarity of topical irritation has been well demonstrated.
Polymyxin B is one of a group of closely related substances produced by various strains of *Bacillus polymyxa.* Its activity is sharply restricted to gram-negative bacteria, including many strains of *Pseudomonas aeruginosa.*
Neomycin, isolated from *Streptomyces fradiae,* has antibacterial activity *in vitro* against a wide range of gram-negative and gram-positive organisms, with effectiveness against many strains of *Proteus.*
Gramicidin has particular action *in vitro* against certain gram-positive bacteria.

Indications: Based on a review of this drug by the National Academy of Sciences—National Research Council and/or other information, FDA has classified the indications as follows:
"Possibly" effective: General: The cream is indicated in the treatment of topical bacterial infections caused by organisms sensitive to the antibiotic ingredients, and when the anti-inflammatory and/or anti-allergic action of the hydrocortisone is indicated as in burns, wounds, and skin grafts; otitis externa; also following surgical procedures. Dermatologic: Atopic, contact, stasis and infectious eczematoid dermatitis; neurodermatitis; eczema; anogenital pruritus. It may also be useful as an adjunct in certain pyodermas, such as impetigo, during specific systemic antibiotic therapy for these infections.
Final classification of the less-than-effective indications requires further investigation.

Contraindications: Not for use in the eyes or in the external ear canal if the eardrum is perforated. This drug is contraindicated in tuberculous, fungal or viral lesions of the skin (herpes simplex, vaccinia and varicella). This product is contraindicated in those individuals who have shown hypersensitivity to any of its components.

Warning: Because of the potential hazard of nephrotoxicity and ototoxicity due to neomycin, care should be exercised when using this product in treating extensive burns, trophic ulceration and other extensive conditions where absorption of neomycin is possible. In burns where more than 20 percent of the body surface is affected, especially if the patient has impaired renal function or is receiving other aminoglycoside antibiotics concurrently, not more than one application a day is recommended.

When using neomycin-containing products to control secondary infection in the chronic dermatoses, such as chronic otitis externa or stasis dermatitis, it should be borne in mind that the skin in these conditions is more liable than is normal skin to become sensitized to many substances, including neomycin. The manifestation of sensitization to neomycin is usually a low grade reddening with swelling, dry scaling and itching; it may be manifest simply as a failure to heal. During long-term use of neomycin-containing products, periodic examination for such signs is advisable and the patient should be told to discontinue the product if they are observed. These symptoms regress quickly on withdrawing the medication. Neomycin-containing applications should be avoided for that patient thereafter.

Precautions: As with other antibacterial preparations, prolonged use may result in overgrowth of nonsusceptible organisms, including fungi. Appropriate measures should be taken if this occurs. Use of steroids on infected areas should be supervised with care as anti-inflammatory steroids may encourage spread of infection. If this occurs steroid therapy should be stopped and appropriate antibacterial drugs used. Generalized dermatological conditions may require systemic corticosteroid therapy. As the safety of topical steroid preparations during pregnancy has not been fully established, they should not be used unnecessarily, on extended areas, in large amounts, or for prolonged periods of time, in pregnancy.

Adverse Reactions: When steroid preparations are used for long periods of time in intertriginous areas or over extensive body areas, with or without occlusive non-permeable dressings, striae may occur; also there exists the possibility of systemic side effects when steroid preparations are used over larger areas or for a long period of time.

Neomycin is a not uncommon cutaneous sensitizer. Articles in the current literature indicate an increase in the prevalence of persons allergic to neomycin. Ototoxicity and nephrotoxicity have been reported (see Warning section).

Dosage and Administration: A small quantity of the cream should be applied 2 to 4 times daily, as required. The cream should, if conditions permit, be gently rubbed into the affected areas. In chronic conditions, withdrawal of treatment is carried out by decreasing the frequency of application, until the cream finally is applied as infrequently as once a week.

How Supplied: Tube of 7.5 g.

CORTISPORIN® OINTMENT ℞

Polymyxin B-Bacitracin-Neomycin-Hydrocortisone

Description: Each gram contains: Aerosporin® brand Polymyxin B Sulfate 5,000 units; bacitracin zinc 400 units; neomycin sulfate 5 mg (equivalent to 3.5 mg neomycin base); hydrocortisone 10 mg (1%); special white petrolatum qs.

> **Indications:** Based on a review of this drug by the National Academy of Sciences—National Research Council and/or other information, FDA has classified the indications as follows:
>
> "Possibly" effective: General: The ointment is indicated in the treatment of topical bacterial infections caused by organisms sensitive to the antibiotic ingredients, and when the anti-inflammatory and/or anti-allergic action of the hydrocortisone is indicated, e.g., such conditions as burns, wounds, skin grafts; otitis externa; and plastic, proctologic, gynecologic, or general surgical procedures. Dermatologic: Atopic, contact, stasis and infectious eczematoid dermatitis; neurodermatitis; eczema; anogenital pruritus. It may also be useful as an adjunct in certain pyodermas, such as impetigo, during specific systemic antibiotic therapy for these infections.
>
> Final classification of the less-than-effective indications requires further investigation.

Contraindications: This product is contraindicated in those individuals who have shown hypersensitivity to any of its components. Do not use in the external ear canal if the eardrum is perforated.

Warning: Because of the potential hazard of nephrotoxicity and ototoxicity due to neomycin, care should be exercised when using this product in treating extensive burns, trophic ulceration and other extensive conditions where absorption of neomycin is possible. In burns where more than 20 percent of the body surface is affected, especially if the patient has impaired renal function or is receiving other aminoglycoside antibiotics concurrently, not more than one application a day is recommended.

When using neomycin-containing products to control secondary infection in the chronic dermatoses, such as chronic otitis externa or stasis dermatitis, it should be borne in mind that the skin in these conditions is more liable than is normal skin to become sensitized to many substances, including neomycin. The manifestation of sensitization to neomycin is usually a low grade reddening with swelling, dry scaling and itching; it may be manifest simply as a failure to heal. During long-term use of neomycin-containing products, periodic examination for such signs is advisable and the patient should be told to discontinue the product if they are observed. These symptoms regress quickly on withdrawing the medication. Neomycin-containing applications should be avoided for that patient thereafter.

Precautions: As with any antibiotic preparation, prolonged use may result in the overgrowth of nonsusceptible organisms, including fungi. Appropriate measures should be taken if this occurs. Use of steroids on infected areas should be supervised with care as anti-inflammatory steroids may encourage spread of infection. If this occurs steroid therapy should be stopped and appropriate antibacterial drugs used. Generalized dermatological conditions may require systemic corticosteroid therapy. As the safety of topical steroid preparations during pregnancy has not been fully established, they should not be used unnecessarily, on extended areas, in large amounts, or for prolonged periods of time, in pregnancy.

Adverse Reactions: When steroid preparations are used for long periods of time in intertriginous areas or over extensive body areas, with or without occlusive nonpermeable dressings, striae may occur; also there exists the possibility of systemic side effects when steroid preparations are used over larger areas or for a long period of time.

Neomycin is a not uncommon cutaneous sensitizer. Articles in the current literature indicate an increase in the prevalence of persons allergic to neomycin. Ototoxicity and nephrotoxicity have been reported (see Warning section).

Dosage and Administration: A thin film is applied 2 to 4 times daily. In chronic conditions, withdrawal of treatment is carried out by decreasing the frequency of application, until the ointment is applied as infrequently as once a week.

How Supplied: Tube of ½ oz with applicator tip.

CORTISPORIN® OINTMENT ℞

Polymyxin B-Bacitracin-Neomycin-Hydrocortisone

OPHTHALMIC Sterile

Description: Each gram contains: Aerosporin® brand Polymyxin B Sulfate 5,000 units; bacitracin zinc 400 units; neomycin sulfate 5 mg (equivalent to 3.5 mg neomycin base); hydrocortisone 10 mg (1%); special white petrolatum qs.

Action: Hydrocortisone, the naturally occurring adrenal corticosteroid, affords antiallergic, antipruritic and anti-inflammatory activity.

Polymyxin B attacks gram-negative bacilli, including virtually all strains of *Pseudomonas aeruginosa* and *H influenzae* (Koch-Weeks bacillus).

Neomycin provides antibacterial action against many strains of gram-positive and gram-negative organisms, including many strains of *Proteus vulgaris* and *Staphylococcus aureus.*

Bacitracin is highly active against gram-positive bacilli and cocci, and extends the spectrum to include hemolytic streptococci.

In ophthalmology, the ointment is of value in helping to maintain corneal transparency during healing by inhibiting neovascularization and scarring while protecting against bacterial infection.

> **Indications:** Based on a review of this drug by the National Academy of Sciences—National Research Council and/or other information, FDA has classified the indications as follows:
>
> "Possibly" effective: For the treatment of nonpurulent bacterial infections of the eye due to organisms sensitive to the antibiotic ingredients of the drug and when the anti-inflammatory action of the hydrocortisone is indicated as in nonpurulent bacterial, allergic, vernal and phlyctenular conjunctivitis; nonpurulent blepharitis; interstitial, sclerosing, postoperative or acne rosacea keratitis; superficial chemical and thermal burns of the cornea.
>
> Final classification of the less-than-effective indications requires further investigation.

Contraindications: This product is contraindicated in acute purulent conjunctivitis and blepharitis; tuberculous, fungal or viral lesions of the skin or eye, including herpes simplex, dendritic keratitis, vaccinia or varicella; and conditions involving the posterior segment of the eye. It is also contraindicated in those individuals who have shown hypersensitivity to any of its components.

Precautions: Extended ophthalmic use of topical steroid therapy may result in glaucoma with possible damage of the optic nerves, posterior subcapsular cataract formation, or may aid in the establishment of secondary ocular infections from fungi or viruses liberated from ocular tissues. It is advisable that intraocular pressure be checked frequently. In those diseases causing thinning of the cornea, perforation has been known to occur with the use of topical steroids. As with any antibiotic preparation, prolonged use may result in the overgrowth of nonsusceptible organisms, including fungi. Appropriate measures should be taken if this occurs.

Continued on next page

Burroughs Wellcome—Cont.

Adverse Reactions: Articles in the current medical literature indicate an increase in the prevalence of persons allergic to neomycin. The possibility of such a reaction should be borne in mind.
Dosage and Administration: Apply the ointment every 3 or 4 hours, depending on the severity of the infection. In chronic conditions, withdrawal of treatment is carried out by decreasing the frequency of application, until the ointment is applied as infrequently as once a week.
How Supplied: 1/8 oz tube with ophthalmic tip.
1/8 oz.—DoD NSN 6505-00-890-1568

CORTISPORIN® OPHTHALMIC SUSPENSION Sterile ℞
Polymyxin B-Neomycin-Hydrocortisone

Description: Each cc contains: Aerosporin® brand Polymyxin B Sulfate 10,000 units; neomycin sulfate 5 mg (equivalent to 3.5 mg neomycin base); hydrocortisone 10 mg (1%); thimerosal (preservative) 0.001%.
The vehicle contains the inactive ingredients cetyl alcohol, glyceryl monostearate, liquid petrolatum, polyoxyl 40 stearate, propylene glycol and purified water.

Indications:
Based on a review of this drug by the National Academy of Sciences-National Research Council and/or other information, FDA has classified the indications as follows:
"Possibly" effective: For the treatment of nonpurulent bacterial infections of the eye due to organisms sensitive to the antibiotic ingredients of the drug and when the anti-inflammatory action of the hydrocortisone is indicated as in nonpurulent bacterial, allergic, vernal and phlyctenular conjunctivitis; nonpurulent blepharitis; interstitial, sclerosing, postoperative or acne rosacea keratitis; superficial chemical and thermal burns of the cornea.
Final classification of the less-than-effective indications requires further investigation.

Contraindications: This product is contraindicated in acute purulent conjunctivitis and blepharitis; tuberculous, fungal or viral lesions of the skin or eye, including herpes simplex, dendritic keratitis, vaccinia or varicella; and conditions involving the posterior segment of the eye. It is also contraindicated in those individuals who have shown hypersensitivity to any of its components.
Precautions: Extended ophthalmic use of topical steroid therapy may result in glaucoma with possible damage of the optic nerves, posterior subcapsular cataract formation, or may aid in the establishment of secondary ocular infections from fungi or viruses liberated from ocular tissues. It is advisable that intraocular pressure be checked frequently. In those diseases causing thinning of the cornea, perforation has been known to occur with the use of topical steroids. As with any antibiotic preparation, prolonged use may result in the overgrowth of nonsusceptible organisms, including fungi. Appropriate measures should be taken if this occurs.
Adverse Reactions: Articles in the current medical literature indicate an increase in the prevalence of persons allergic to neomycin. The possibility of such a reaction should be borne in mind.
Dosage and Administration: One or two drops in the affected eye every three or four hours, depending on the severity of the condition. The suspension may be used more frequently if necessary. The patient should be instructed to avoid contaminating the dropper with material from the eye, fingers, or other sources. This caution is necessary if the sterility of the suspension is to be preserved. SHAKE WELL BEFORE USING.
How Supplied: Bottle of 5 cc with sterile dropper.
5 cc—DoD NSN 6505-00-764-9042

CORTISPORIN® OTIC SOLUTION Sterile ℞
Polymyxin B-Neomycin-Hydrocortisone

Description: Each cc contains:
Aerosporin® brand Polymyxin B Sulfate ....10,000 Units
Neomycin sulfate ....5 mg
(equivalent to 3.5 mg neomycin base)
Hydrocortisone ....10 mg (1%)
The vehicle contains the inactive ingredients glycerin, hydrochloric acid, propylene glycol, purified water and potassium metabisulfite (preservative) 0.1%.
Action: Hydrocortisone, the naturally occurring adrenal corticosteroid, affords antiallergic, antipruritic and anti-inflammatory activity.
Polymyxin B is one of a group of closely related substances produced by various strains of *Bacillus polymyxa.* Its activity is sharply restricted to gram-negative bacteria, including many strains of *Pseudomonas aeruginosa.*
Neomycin, isolated from *Streptomyces fradiae,* has antibacterial activity *in vitro* against a wide range of gram-negative and gram-positive organisms, with effectiveness against many strains of *Proteus.*
Indications: For the treatment of superficial bacterial infections of the external auditory canal caused by organisms susceptible to the action of the antibiotics.
Contraindications: This product is contraindicated in those individuals who have shown hypersensitivity to any of its components, and in herpes simplex, vaccinia and varicella.
Warnings: As with other antibiotic preparations, prolonged treatment may result in overgrowth of nonsusceptible organisms and fungi. If the infection is not improved after one week, cultures and susceptibility tests should be repeated to verify the identity of the organism and to determine whether therapy should be changed.
When using neomycin-containing products to control secondary infection in the chronic dermatoses, such as chronic otitis externa, it should be borne in mind that the skin in these conditions is more liable than is normal skin to become sensitized to many substances, including neomycin. The manifestation of sensitization to neomycin is usually a low grade reddening with swelling, dry scaling and itching; it may be manifest simply as a failure to heal. During long-term use of neomycin-containing products, periodic examination for such signs is advisable and the patient should be told to discontinue the product if they are observed. These symptoms regress quickly on withdrawing the medication. Neomycin-containing applications should be avoided for that patient thereafter.
Precautions: If sensitization or irritation occurs, medication should be discontinued promptly.
This drug should be used with care when the integrity of the tympanic membrane is in question because of the possibility of ototoxicity caused by neomycin.
Patients who prefer to warm the medication before using should be cautioned against heating the solution above body temperature, in order to avoid loss of potency.
Treatment should not be continued for longer than ten days.
Allergic cross-reactions may occur which could prevent the use of any or all of the following antibiotics for the treatment of future infections: kanamycin, paromomycin, streptomycin, and possibly gentamicin.
Adverse Reactions: Neomycin is a not uncommon cutaneous sensitizer. There are articles in the current literature that indicate an increase in the prevalence of persons sensitive to neomycin.
Stinging and burning have been reported when this drug has gained access to the middle ear.
Dosage and Administration: The external auditory canal should be thoroughly cleansed and dried with a sterile cotton applicator.
For adults, 4 drops of the solution should be instilled into the affected ear 3 or 4 times daily. For infants and children, 3 drops are suggested because of the smaller capacity of the ear canal.
The patient should lie with the affected ear upward and then the drops should be instilled. This position should be maintained for 5 minutes to facilitate penetration of the drops into the ear canal. Repeat, if necessary, for the opposite ear.
If preferred, a cotton wick may be inserted into the canal and then the cotton may be saturated with the solution. This wick should be kept moist by adding further solution every four hours. The wick should be replaced at least once every 24 hours.
The patient should be instructed to avoid contaminating the dropper with material from the ear, fingers, or other source. This caution is necessary if the sterility of the drops is to be preserved.
How Supplied: Bottle of 10 cc with sterile dropper.
10 cc—DoD NSN 6505-01-014-1378
10 cc—VA NSN 6505-01-023-4751

CORTISPORIN® OTIC SUSPENSION Sterile ℞
Polymyxin B-Neomycin-Hydrocortisone

Description: Each cc contains: Aerosporin® brand Polymyxin B Sulfate 10,000 units; neomycin sulfate 5 mg (equivalent to 3.5 mg neomycin base); hydrocortisone 10 mg (1%).
The vehicle contains the inactive ingredients cetyl alcohol, propylene glycol, polysorbate 80, purified water and thimerosal (preservative) 0.01%.
Action: Hydrocortisone, the naturally occurring adrenal corticosteroid, affords antiallergic, antipruritic and anti-inflammatory activity.
Polymyxin B is one of a group of closely related substances produced by various strains of *Bacillus polymyxa.* Its activity is sharply restricted to gram-negative bacteria, including many strains of *Pseudomonas aeruginosa.*
Neomycin, isolated from *Streptomyces fradiae,* has antibacterial activity *in vitro* against a wide range of gram-negative and gram-positive organisms, with effectiveness against many strains of *Proteus.*
Indications: For the treatment of superficial bacterial infections of the external auditory canal caused by organisms susceptible to the action of the antibiotics, and for the treatment of infections of mastoidectomy and fenstration cavities caused by organisms susceptible to the antibiotics.
Contraindications: This product is contraindicated in those individuals who have shown hypersensitivity to any of its components, and in herpes simplex, vaccinia and varicella.
Warnings: As with other antibiotic preparations, prolonged treatment may result in overgrowth of nonsusceptible organisms and fungi. If the infection is not improved after one week, cultures and susceptibility tests should be repeated to verify the identity of the organism and to determine whether therapy should be changed.
When using neomycin-containing products to control secondary infection in the chronic dermatoses, such as chronic otitis externa, it

should be borne in mind that the skin in these conditions is more liable than is normal skin to become sensitized to many substances, including neomycin. The manifestation of sensitization to neomycin is usually a low grade reddening with swelling, dry scaling and itching; it may be manifest simply as a failure to heal. During long-term use of neomycin-containing products, periodic examination for such signs is advisable and the patient should be told to discontinue the product if they are observed. These symptoms regress quickly on withdrawing the medication. Neomycin-containing applications should be avoided for that patient thereafter.

Precautions: If sensitization or irritation occurs, medication should be discontinued promptly.

This drug should be used with care in cases of perforated eardrum and in longstanding cases of chronic otitis media because of the possibility of ototoxicity caused by neomycin.

Patients who prefer to warm the medication before using should be cautioned against heating the solution above body temperature, in order to avoid loss of potency.

Treatment should not be continued for longer than ten days.

Allergic cross-reactions may occur which could prevent the use of any or all of the following antibiotics for the treatment of future infections: kanamycin, paromomycin, streptomycin, and possibly gentamicin.

Adverse Reactions: Neomycin is a not uncommon cutaneous sensitizer. There are articles in the current literature that indicate an increase in the prevalence of persons sensitive to neomycin.

Dosage and Administration: The external auditory canal should be thoroughly cleansed and dried with a sterile cotton applicator.

For adults, 4 drops of the suspension should be instilled into the affected ear 3 or 4 times daily. For infants and children, 3 drops are suggested because of the smaller capacity of the ear canal.

The patient should lie with the affected ear upward and then the drops should be instilled. This position should be maintained for 5 minutes to facilitate penetration of the drops into the ear canal. Repeat, if necessary, for the opposite ear.

If preferred, a cotton wick may be inserted into the canal and then the cotton may be saturated with the suspension. This wick should be kept moist by adding further suspension every four hours. The wick should be replaced at least once every 24 hours.

The patient should be instructed to avoid contaminating the dropper with material from the ear, fingers, or other source. This caution is necessary if the sterility of the drops is to be preserved. SHAKE WELL BEFORE USING.

How Supplied: Bottles of 10 cc with sterile droppers.

10cc DoD **NSN 6505-01-043-0230**
10cc VA **NSN 6505-00-932-3247**

DARAPRIM® ℞
brand Pyrimethamine

Description: Each scored tablet contains 25 mg Daraprim brand Pyrimethamine (2, 4- diamino - 5 - p-chlorophenyl - 6 - ethylpyrimidine), a potent antimalarial drug, discovered by Hitchings, Russell and Falco at the Wellcome Research Laboratories. It is a tasteless and odorless substance.

Actions and Benefits: Daraprim is a folic acid antagonist, and the rationale for its therapeutic action is based on the differential requirement between host and parasite for nucleic acid precursors involved in growth. This activity is highly selective against plasmodia and *Toxoplasma gondii.* Daraprim does not destroy gametocytes, but arrests sporogony in the mosquito.

Indications: Daraprim brand Pyrimethamine is indicated for the chemoprophylaxis of malaria due to susceptible strains of plasmodia. Fast-acting schizonticides (chloroquine, amodiaquin, quinacrine or quinine) are indicated and preferable for the treatment of acute attacks. However, conjoint use of Daraprim will initiate *transmission control* and *suppressive cure.*

Daraprim is also indicated for the treatment of toxoplasmosis. For this purpose the drug should be used conjointly with a sulfonamide since synergism exists with this combination.

Warnings: The dosage of pyrimethamine required for the treatment of toxoplasmosis is 10 to 20 times the recommended antimalarial dosage and approaches the toxic level. If signs of folic or folinic acid deficiency develop (see Adverse Reactions) reduce the dosage or discontinue the drug according to the response of the patient. Folinic acid (leucovorin) may be administered in a dosage of 3 to 9 mg intramuscularly daily for 3 days, or as required to produce a return of depressed platelet or white blood cell counts to safe levels.

Patients should be warned to keep Daraprim out of the reach of children since accidental ingestion has led to fatality.

Use in Pregnancy: Pyrimethamine, like other folic acid antagonists, may, in large doses, produce teratogenic effects in laboratory animals. The large doses required to treat toxoplasmosis should be used only after a definitive diagnosis of acute toxoplasmosis has been made, and the possibility of teratogenic effects from the drug has been carefully weighed against the possible risks of permanent damage to the fetus from the infection.

Concurrent administration of folinic acid is recommended when pyrimethamine is used for treatment of toxoplasmosis during pregnancy.

Precautions: The recommended dosage for malaria suppression should not be exceeded. In patients receiving high dosage, as for the treatment of toxoplasmosis, semi-weekly blood counts, including platelet counts, should be made. In patients with convulsive disorders a small "starting" dose (for toxoplasmosis) is recommended to avoid the potential nervous system toxicity of pyrimethamine.

Adverse Reactions: With large doses, anorexia and vomiting may occur. Vomiting may be minimized by giving the medication with meals; it usually disappears promptly upon reduction of dosage. Also, large doses as used in toxoplasmosis may produce megaloblastic anemia, leukopenia, thrombocytopenia, pancytopenia and atrophic glossitis. Acute intoxication may follow the ingestion of an excessive amount of pyrimethamine; this may involve central nervous system stimulation including convulsions. In such cases a parenteral barbiturate may be indicated followed by folinic acid (leucovorin).

Dosage and Administration:

For Chemoprophylaxis of Malaria: Adults and children over 10 years—25 mg (1 tablet) once weekly.

Children 4 through 10 years—12.5 mg (½ tablet) once weekly.

Infants and children under 4 years—6.25 mg (¼ tablet) once weekly.

Regimens planned to include *suppressive cure* should be extended through any characteristic periods of early recrudescence and late relapse for at least 10 weeks in each case.

For Treatment of Acute Attacks: Daraprim is recommended in areas where only susceptible plasmodia exist. The drug is not recommended alone in the treatment of acute attacks of malaria in non-immune persons. Fast-acting schizonticides (chloroquine, amodiaquin, quinacrine or quinine) are indicated for treatment of acute attacks. However, conjoint Daraprim dosage of 25 mg daily for two days will initiate *transmission control* and *suppressive cure.* Should circumstances arise wherein Daraprim must be used alone in semi-immune persons, the adult dosage for an acute attack is 50 mg daily for 2 days; children 4 through 10 years old may be given 25 mg daily for 2 days. In any event, clinical cure should be followed by the once-weekly regimen described above.

For Toxoplasmosis: The dosage of Daraprim brand Pyrimethamine in the treatment of toxoplasmosis must be carefully adjusted so as to provide maximum therapeutic effect and a minimum of side effects. At the high dosage required, there is a marked variation in the tolerance to the drug. Young patients may tolerate higher doses than older individuals.

The adult *starting* dose is 50 to 75 mg of the drug daily, together with 1 to 4 g daily of a sulfonamide drug of the sulfapyrimidine type, e.g., sulfadiazine, triple-sulfa. This dosage is ordinarily continued for 1 to 3 weeks, depending on the response of the patient and his tolerance of the therapy. The dosage may then be reduced to about one-half that previously given for each drug and continued for an additional 4 or 5 weeks.

The pediatric dosage of Daraprim is 1 mg/kg per day divided into 2 equal daily doses; after 2 to 4 days this dose may be reduced to one-half and continued for approximately one month. The usual pediatric sulfonamide dosage is used in conjunction with Daraprim.

Supplied: Tablets, scored, 25 mg, bottles of 100 and 1000. Tablets bear identification, A3A.

[*Shown in Product Identification Section*]

100—DoD **NSN 6505-00-926-4765**

EMPIRIN
ANALGESIC TABLETS
ASPIRIN—325 mg (5 grs)

For relief of headache, minor muscular aches and pains, toothache, discomfort and fever of colds and flu.

Directions For Adults (5 Grain Tablets): 1 or 2 tablets with a full glass of water. Repeat every 4 hours as needed, up to 12 tablets a day.

Headache: Take 1 or 2 tablets with a full glass of water every 4 hours, as needed, up to 12 tablets a day.

Muscular Aches and Pains: Take 1 or 2 tablets with a full glass of water every 4 hours, as needed, up to 12 tablets a day.

Toothache: Take 1 or 2 tablets with a full glass of water every 4 hours, as needed, up to 12 tablets a day for toothache or for pain following dental procedures.

Colds and Flu: To relieve the pain, discomfort and fever of colds and flu, take 1 or 2 tablets with a full glass of water (or fruit juice) every 4 hours, as needed, up to 12 tablets a day.

Sore Throat Due to Colds and Flu: To relieve the pain and discomfort associated with minor sore throat, take 1 or 2 tablets with a full glass of water every 4 hours, as needed, up to 12 tablets a day.

Neuralgia: For the pain of neuralgia, take 1 or 2 tablets with a glass of water every 4 hours, as needed, up to 12 tablets a day.

Menstrual Pain: For relief of menstrual pain, take 1 or 2 tablets with a full glass of water every 4 hours, as needed, up to 12 tablets a day.

Arthritis and Rheumatism: For the temporary relief of minor aches and pains, take 1 or 2 tablets with a full glass of water every 4 hours, as needed, up to 12 tablets a day. *Caution:* If pain persists for more than 10 days, or redness is present, or in conditions affecting children under 12 years of age, consult a physician immediately.

Bursitis, Lumbago, and Sciatica: For the temporary relief of minor pain, take 1 or 2 tablets with a full glass of water every 4 hours, as needed, up to 12 tablets a day.

Sleeplessness: When sleeplessness is caused by minor pain and discomfort, take 1 or 2 tablets with a full glass of water, every 4 hours, as needed, up to 12 tablets a day.

Continued on next page

Burroughs Wellcome—Cont.

Directions For Children (5 Grain Tablets): To be administered only under adult supervision. For relief of headache, minor muscular aches and pains, toothache, discomfort and fever of colds and flu.

Under 3 years	consult your physician
3 to under 4 years	½ tablet
4 to under 6 years	¾ tablet
6 to under 9 years	1 tablet
9 to under 11 years	1¼ tablets
11 to under 12 years	1½ tablets
12 and over	same as adult

Take with a full glass of water. Indicated dosage may be repeated every 4 hours up to 5 times a day. High or continued fever, severe or persistent sore throat especially when accompanied by high fever, headache, nausea or vomiting, may be serious. Consult your physician.

Warnings: Keep this and all medicines out of children's reach. In case of accidental overdose, contact a physician immediately.

Do not exceed dose unless directed by a physician. Do not take this product if you are allergic to aspirin, have asthma, a gastric ulcer or its symptoms, or are taking a medication that affects the clotting of blood, except under advice of a physician.

How Supplied: Available in bottles of 25, 50, 100 and 250.

Note: Bottle of 250 available without child-resistant cap for people who have no children under 12 in the house and for the elderly or handicapped.

[*Shown in Product Identification Section*]

EMPIRIN® with Codeine ℞ Ⓒ

Description: Each tablet contains aspirin (acetylsalicylic acid) 325 mg plus codeine phosphate in one of the following strengths: No. 2—15 mg, No. 3—30 mg, and No. 4—60 mg. (Warning—may be habit-forming.)

Actions: Aspirin alleviates pain both centrally and peripherally. It also has both antipyretic and anti-inflammatory effects. Codeine is in the category of a narcotic analgesic and antitussive.

Indications: For the relief of mild, moderate, and moderate to severe pain.

Contraindications: Hypersensitivity to aspirin or codeine.

Warnings:

Drug Dependence: Empirin with Codeine can produce drug dependence of the morphine type and, therefore, has the potential for being abused. Psychic dependence, physical dependence, and tolerance may develop upon repeated administration of this drug and it should be prescribed and administered with the same degree of caution appropriate to the use of other oral, narcotic-containing medications. Like other narcotic-containing medications, the drug is subject to the Federal Controlled Substances Act.

Use in ambulatory patients: Empirin with Codeine may impair the mental and/or physical abilities required for the performance of potentially hazardous tasks such as driving a car or operating machinery. The patient using this drug should be cautioned accordingly.

Interaction with other central nervous system (CNS) depressants: Patients receiving other narcotic analgesics, general anesthetics, phenothiazines, other tranquilizers, sedative-hypnotics, or other CNS depressants (including alcohol) concomitantly with Empirin with Codeine may exhibit an additive CNS depression. When such combined therapy is contemplated, the dose of one or both agents should be reduced.

Use in pregnancy: Safe use in pregnancy has not been established relative to possible adverse effects on fetal development. Therefore, Empirin with Codeine should not be used in pregnant women unless, in the judgment of the physician, the potential benefits outweigh the possible hazards.

Precautions:

Head injury and increased intracranial pressure: The respiratory depressant effects of narcotics and their capacity to elevate cerebrospinal fluid pressure may be markedly exaggerated in the presence of head injury, other intracranial lesions or a pre-existing increase in intracranial pressure. Furthermore, narcotics produce adverse reactions which may obscure the clinical course of patients with head injuries.

Acute abdominal conditions: The administration of Empirin with Codeine or other narcotics may obscure the diagnosis or clinical course in patients with acute abdominal conditions.

Allergic: Precautions should be taken in administering salicylates to persons with known allergies: patients with nasal polyps are more likely to be hypersensitive to aspirin.

Special risk patients: Empirin with Codeine should be given with caution to certain patients such as the elderly or debilitated, and those with severe impairment of hepatic or renal function, hypothyroidism, Addison's disease, prostatic hypertrophy or urethral stricture, peptic ulcer, or coagulation disorders.

Adverse Reactions: The most frequently observed adverse reactions to codeine include light-headedness, dizziness, sedation, nausea and vomiting. These effects seem to be more prominent in ambulatory than in nonambulatory patients and some of these adverse reactions may be alleviated if the patient lies down. Other adverse reactions include euphoria, dysphoria, constipation, and pruritus.

The most frequently observed reactions to aspirin include headache, vertigo, ringing in the ears, mental confusion, drowsiness, sweating, thirst, nausea, and vomiting. Occasional patients experience gastric irritation and bleeding with aspirin. Some patients are unable to take salicylates without developing nausea and vomiting. Hypersensitivity may be manifested by a skin rash or even an anaphylactic reaction. With these exceptions, most of the side effects occur after repeated administration of large doses.

Dosage and Administration: Dosage should be adjusted according to the severity of the pain and the response of the patient. It may occasionally be necessary to exceed the usual dosage recommended below in cases of more severe pain or in those patients who have become tolerant to the analgesic effect of narcotics. Empirin with Codeine is given orally. The usual adult dose for Empirin with Codeine No. 2 and No. 3 is one or two tablets every four hours as required. The usual adult dose for Empirin with Codeine No. 4 is one tablet every four hours as required.

Drug Interactions: The CNS depressant effects of Empirin with Codeine may be additive with that of other CNS depressants. See WARNINGS.

Overdosage:

Signs and symptoms: Serious overdose of Empirin with Codeine is characterized by respiratory depression (a decrease in respiratory rate and/or tidal volume, Cheyne-Stokes respiration, cyanosis), extreme somnolence progressing to stupor or coma, skeletal muscle flaccidity, cold and clammy skin and sometimes bradycardia and hypotension. In severe overdose, apnea, circulatory collapse, cardiac arrest and death may occur.

Treatment: Treatment consists primarily of management of codeine intoxication and the correction of the acid-base imbalance due to salicylism. Primary attention should be given to the establishment of adequate respiratory exchange through provision of the patent airway and the institution of assisted or controlled ventilation. The narcotic antagonist naloxone is a specific antidote for respiratory depression which may result from overdose or unusual sensitivity to narcotics. Therefore, an appropriate dose of an antagonist should be administered, preferably by the intravenous route, simultaneously with efforts at respiratory resuscitation. Since the duration of action of Empirin with Codeine may exceed that of the antagonist, the patient should be kept under continued surveillance and repeated doses of the antagonist should be administered as needed to maintain adequate respiration.

An antagonist should not be administered in the absence of clinically significant respiratory or cardiovascular depression.

Oxygen, intravenous fluids, vasopressors and other supportive measures should be employed as indicated.

Gastric emptying may be useful in removing unabsorbed drug.

How Supplied: Empirin with Codeine Nos. 2, 3 and 4, bottles of 100, 500, 1000; Dispenserpak® of 25 tablets.

[*Shown in Product Identification Section*]

EMPRACET® with Codeine Phosphate Nos. 3 and 4 ℞ Ⓒ

Description: Each tablet contains codeine phosphate 30 mg [in No. 3, 60 mg in No. 4] (Warning—may be habit-forming) and acetaminophen 300 mg. Codeine is an alkaloid obtained from opium or prepared from morphine by methylation. Codeine occurs as colorless or white crystals, effloresces slowly in dry air and is affected by light. Acetaminophen is a non-salicylate and occurs as a white, odorless, crystalline powder possessing a slightly bitter taste.

Actions: Acetaminophen is in the category of analgesic and antipyretic, codeine in the category of analgesic and antitussive. Codeine retains at least one-half of its analgesic activity when administered orally.

Indications: For the relief of mild, moderate or severe pain.

Contraindications: Hypersensitivity to acetaminophen or codeine.

Warnings:

Drug dependence: Acetaminophen with codeine can produce drug dependence of the morphine type and, therefore, has the potential for being abused. Psychic dependence, physical dependence and tolerance may develop upon repeated administration of this drug and it should be prescribed and administered with the same degree of caution appropriate to the use of other oral, narcotic-containing medications. Like other narcotic-containing medications, the drug is subject to the Federal Controlled Substances Act.

Use in ambulatory patients: Acetaminophen with codeine may impair the mental and/or physical abilities required for the performance of potentially hazardous tasks such as driving a car or operating machinery. The patient using this drug should be cautioned accordingly.

Interaction with other central nervous system depressants: Patients receiving other narcotic analgesics, general anesthetics, phenothiazines, other tranquilizers, sedative-hypnotics, or other CNS depressants (including alcohol) concomitantly with acetaminophen with codeine may exhibit an additive CNS depression. When such combined therapy is contemplated, the dose of one or both agents should be reduced.

Use in pregnancy: Safe use in pregnancy has not been established relative to possible adverse effects on fetal development. Therefore, acetaminophen with codeine should not be used in pregnant women unless, in the judgment of the physician, the potential benefits outweigh the possible hazards.

Precautions:

Head injury and increased intracranial pressure: The respiratory depressant effects of narcotics and their capacity to elevate cerebrospinal fluid pressure may be markedly exaggerated in the presence of head injury, other

intracranial lesions or a pre-existing increase in intracranial pressure. Furthermore, narcotics produce adverse reactions which may obscure the clinical course of patients with head injuries.
Acute abdominal conditions: The administration of acetaminophen with codeine or other narcotics may obscure the diagnosis or clinical course in patients with acute abdominal conditions.
Special risk patients: Acetaminophen with codeine should be given with caution to certain patients such as the elderly or debilitated, and those with severe impairment of hepatic or renal function, hypothyroidism, Addison's disease, and prostatic hypertrophy or urethral stricture.
Adverse Reactions: The most frequently observed adverse reactions include light-headedness, dizziness, sedation, nausea and vomiting. These effects seem to be more prominent in ambulatory than in nonambulatory patients, and some of these adverse reactions may be alleviated if the patient lies down.
Other adverse reactions include euphoria, dysphoria, constipation and pruritus.
Dosage and Administration: Dosage should be adjusted according to the severity of the pain and the response of the patient. It may occasionally be necessary to exceed the usual dosage recommended below in cases of more severe pain or in those patients who have become tolerant to the analgesic effect of narcotics. Acetaminophen with codeine is given orally. The usual adult dose is one or two tablets every four hours as required.
Drug Interactions: The CNS depressant effects of acetaminophen with codeine may be additive with that of other CNS depressants. See WARNINGS.
Management of Overdose:
Signs and symptoms: Serious overdose of acetaminophen with codeine is characterized by respiratory depression (a decrease in respiratory rate and/or tidal volume, Cheyne-Stokes respiration, cyanosis), extreme somnolence progressing to stupor or coma, skeletal muscle flaccidity, cold and clammy skin and sometimes bradycardia and hypotension. In severe overdose, apnea, circulatory collapse, cardiac arrest and death may occur.
Treatment: Primary attention should be given to the reestablishment of adequate respiratory exchange through provision of a patent airway and the institution of assisted or controlled ventilation. The narcotic antagonists naloxone, nalorphine or levallorphan are specific antidotes against respiratory depression which may result from overdose or unusual sensitivity to narcotics. Therefore, an appropriate dose of one of these antagonists should be administered, preferably by the intravenous route, simultaneously with efforts at respiratory resuscitation. Since the duration of action of acetaminophen with codeine may exceed that of the antagonist, the patient should be kept under continued surveillance and repeated doses of the antagonist should be administered as needed to maintain adequate respiration.
An antagonist should not be administered in the absence of clinically significant respiratory or cardiovascular depression.
Oxygen, intravenous fluids, vasopressors and other supportive measures should be employed as indicated.
Gastric emptying may be useful in removing unabsorbed drug.
How Supplied: Bottles of 100, 500 and Dispenserpak® of 25.
[*Shown in Product Identification Section*]

EMPRAZIL® ℞

Description: Each layered tablet contains Sudafed® brand Pseudoephedrine Hydrochloride 20 mg, phenacetin 150 mg, aspirin 200 mg, caffeine 30 mg.
Indications: Emprazil tablets are a combination of analgesic, antipyretic and decongestant agents for relief of the distressing symptoms of upper respiratory tract infections. Emprazil also gives prophylaxis against secondary otitis media or sinusitis.
Precautions: While pseudoephedrine hydrochloride is virtually without pressor effect in normotensive patients, it should be used with caution in hypertensives.
Side Effects: The great majority of patients will exhibit no side effects. However, certain patients may exhibit mild stimulation—no serious side effects have been noted.
Dosage and Administration: Adults and children over 12 years: 1 or 2 tablets 3 times daily, as required. Children 6 through 12 years: 1 tablet 3 times daily, as required.
How Supplied: Bottles of 100 and 1000 layered tablets.
[*Shown in Product Identification Section*]

EMPRAZIL-C® ℞ Ⓒ

Description: Each tablet contains: codeine phosphate* 15 mg, Sudafed® brand Pseudoephedrine Hydrochloride 20 mg, phenacetin 150 mg, aspirin 200 mg, caffeine 30 mg.
*Warning—May be habit-forming.
Indications: Emprazil-C Tablets provide analgesic, antipyretic, antitussive, and decongestant actions for relief of the distressing symptoms of upper respiratory tract infections. Emprazil-C Tablets provide the additional benefit of prophylaxis against secondary otitis media or sinusitis.
Precautions: While pseudoephedrine hydrochloride is virtually without pressor effect in normotensive patients, it should be used with caution in hypertensives.
Side Effects: The great majority of patients will exhibit no side effects. However, certain patients may exhibit mild stimulation—no serious side effects have been noted.
Dosage and Administration: Adults and children over 12 yrs: 1 or 2 tablets 3 times daily as required. Children 6 through 12 yrs: 1 tablet 3 times daily as required.
Emprazil-C is now classified in Schedule III. Available on oral prescription and may be refilled, if authorized, 5 times within 6 months, unless restricted by state law.
How Supplied: Bottle of 100.
Subject to DEA Regulations.
[*Shown in Product Identification Section*]

FEDRAZIL® TABLETS

Description: Each sugar-coated tablet contains Sudafed® brand Pseudoephedrine Hydrochloride 30 mg and Perazil® brand Chlorcyclizine Hydrochloride 25 mg.
Action and Uses: Decongestant and histamine antagonist in one tablet. Effective orally. Decongests respiratory tract and dilates bronchi. Helps to keep eustachian tubes patent.
For symptomatic relief of acute coryza, allergic and vasomotor rhinitis, acute and subacute sinusitis, and hay fever.
Pregnancy Warning: Do not use if pregnant or likely to become pregnant, unless directed by a physician. This drug may have the potentiality of being injurious to the unborn child.
Precautions: Antihistamines may cause drowsiness. If it occurs, do not drive a car or operate machinery. Should not be used where there is high blood pressure, heart disease, diabetes or thyroid disease unless directed by a physician. Do not exceed recommended dosage. If symptoms persist after three days, see your physician.
Dosage and Administration: Adults and children over 12, one tablet three times daily. Children 12 and under, as directed by a physician.
KEEP THIS AND ALL MEDICINES OUT OF CHILDREN'S REACH
Supplied: Bottles of 100. Vial of 24 tablets.
[*Shown in Product Identification Section*]

IMURAN® ℞

brand
Azathioprine Injection
(as the sodium salt)
equivalent to
100 mg azathioprine
sterile lyophilized material

An adjunct for the prevention of rejection in renal homotransplantation.
Caution: Imuran brand Azathioprine is a potent drug. In view of its hematopoietic toxicity, complete blood counts, including platelets, should be performed frequently. See below under WARNINGS.
Description: Imuran brand Azathioprine is an imidazolyl derivative of mercaptopurine and its action is similar to the latter drug. Chemically azathioprine is 6-[1-methyl-4-nitro imidazol-5-yl)thio]purine. As the Sodium Salt of Imuran brand Azathioprine the drug is sufficiently soluble in water to make a 1.0 percent solution. Such a solution is stable for approximately two weeks when stored at temperatures between 59° and 86° F after which it undergoes increasing hydrolysis to form mercaptopurine. The compound is also split into mercaptopurine by sulfhydryl compounds such as cysteine, glutathione and hydrogen sulfide.
Action:
Metabolism: Following the intravenous administration of therapeutic doses of the Sodium Salt of Imuran to man (equivalent to 150–300 mg per day of azathioprine) the drug quickly leaves the circulation and very little unchanged drug is recovered in the urine. Azathioprine is split extensively to mercaptopurine, which is then subject to catabolic destruction to form a variety of oxidized and methylated derivatives, among which 6-thiouric acid predominates. The latter is formed by the oxidation of mercaptopurine by xanthine oxidase. The proportions of the different metabolites vary from individual to individual depending upon the relative amounts of the catabolic enzymes available. After eight hours there is little or no unchanged drug or mercaptopurine in the urine. A small portion (about 10 percent) of azathioprine is split *in vivo* between the sulfur and the purine ring to give 1-methyl-4-nitro-5-thioimidazole in which the sulfur is derived from the original molecule. Although elimination of azathioprine is mainly by metabolic destruction, small amounts of unchanged drug and mercaptopurine are eliminated by the kidney, and the biological effectiveness and toxicity may, therefore, be increased as much as twofold in the anuric patient. Imuran brand Azathioprine and mercaptopurine show moderate binding (about 30 percent) to serum proteins, but both the unchanged drug and its metabolic products appear to be dialyzable.
Blood levels of Imuran and of the mercaptopurine derived from it are extremely low (below 1 μg/ml) at therapeutic doses, as determined by studies with radio-active material. In any event, blood levels are of little or no predictive value, since the magnitude and duration of the clinical response cannot be predicted from the blood levels. The effects of this drug and its active metabolite, mercaptopurine, may appear long after clearance is complete.
Please see IMURAN® brand Azathioprine Tablets monograph for information on: Immunosuppressive Properties, Human Homotransplantation, Indications, Contraindications, Warnings, Precautions and Adverse Reactions.
Dosage: The intravenous administration of sodium salt of azathioprine has a particular advantage during the first 24–96 hours post-renal homotransplantation, during which time the patient may be unable to receive Imuran

Continued on next page

Burroughs Wellcome—Cont.

orally. As soon as the patient recovers sufficiently from the operation a transfer should be made to oral medication. The dosage of the Sodium Salt of Imuran brand Azathioprine which will be tolerated or will be effective will vary from patient to patient and, therefore, careful management is necessary to obtain the optimum therapeutic effect without incurring toxicity. Caution must be exercised to avoid toxicity, the chief manifestation of which is depression of the bone marrow, resulting most commonly in leukopenia and less often in thrombocytopenia and bleeding. SINCE THIS DRUG MAY HAVE A DELAYED ACTION, IT IS IMPORTANT TO REDUCE DOSAGE OR WITHDRAW THE MEDICATION TEMPORARILY AT THE FIRST SIGN OF AN ABNORMALLY LARGE FALL IN THE LEUKOCYTE COUNT AND/OR OTHER EVIDENCE OF PERSISTENT DEPRESSION OF THE BONE MARROW. The effect of renal failure on tolerance to azathioprine appears to be somewhat variable. Patients with impaired renal function may have slower elimination of the drug and its metabolites, with a consequent cumulative effect; therefore, the dosage may need to be appropriately reduced.

The usual initial post-renal transplantation dose is approximately 3–5 mg/kg per day of azathioprine administered intravenously. Adjunct therapy of various types has generally been used in suppressing rejection of renal homografts and this may add to the toxic potential of the regimen. Dosage must be adjusted to attempt to provide satisfactory maintenance of the homograft without producing toxic effects; it may be possible to reduce maintenance dosage to 1 to 2 mg/kg per day.

Preparation of Solution: Inject into the vial 10 ml sterile water for injection. Swirl the vial until solution results. The resultant solution should be used within 24 hours. It has an approximate pH of 9.6 and is for intravenous use only. For infusion, a further dilution may be made with sterile saline or glucose saline by withdrawing the appropriate dosage from the vial and transferring it aseptically to the infusion solution.

How Supplied: 20 ml vial (contains the equivalent of 100 mg azathioprine). Also available: Imuran® brand Azathioprine Tablets, 50 mg scored.

IMURAN® brand Azathioprine Tablets ℞

Caution: *Imuran® brand Azathioprine is a potent drug. In view of its hematopoietic toxicity, complete blood counts, including platelets, should be performed frequently. See below under WARNINGS.*

Description: Imuran brand Azathioprine is an imidazolyl derivative of mercaptopurine and its action is similar to the latter drug. Chemically it is 6-[(1-methyl-4-nitro-imidazol-5-yl) thio] purine.

Action:

Metabolism: Azathioprine is well absorbed from the gastrointestinal tract when given orally. In man very little unchanged drug is recovered in the urine at the usual therapeutic doses (150-300 mg/day). The drug is split extensively to 6-mercaptopurine, which is then subject to catabolic destruction to form a variety of oxidized and methylated derivatives, among which 6-thiouric acid predominates. The latter is formed by the oxidation of mercaptopurine by xanthine oxidase. The proportions of the different metabolites vary from individual to individual depending upon the relative amounts of the catabolic enzymes available. After eight hours there is little or no unchanged drug or mercaptopurine in the urine. A small portion (about 10%) of azathioprine is split *in vivo* between the sulfur and the purine ring to give 1-methyl-4-nitro-5-thioimidazole in which the sulfur is derived from the original molecule. Although elimination of azathioprine is mainly by metabolic destruction, small amounts of unchanged drug and mercaptopurine are eliminated by the kidney, and the biological effectiveness and toxicity may, therefore, be increased as much as two-fold in the anuric patient. Imuran brand Azathioprine and mercaptopurine show moderate binding (about 30 percent) to serum proteins, but both the unchanged drug and its metabolic products appear to be dialyzable.

Blood levels of Imuran and of the mercaptopurine derived from it are extremely low (below 1 mcg/ml) at therapeutic doses, as determined by studies with radioactive material. In any event, blood levels are of little or no predictive value, since the magnitude and duration of the clinical response cannot be predicted from the blood levels. The effects of this drug and its active metabolite, mercaptopurine, may appear long after clearance is complete.

Immunosuppressive Properties: The rejection of homografts is a complex phenomenon which may involve both circulating antibody and cell-borne immunity of the delayed hypersensitivity type.

Studies by a number of investigators have revealed that the timing of the antigenic stimulus in relation to the administration of mercaptopurine or azathioprine is critical. Maximum effectiveness of the drugs occurred when they were given during the induction period of the antibody response, either starting with the time of antigenic stimulation or within two days thereafter. When the drugs were administered before or after the inductive phase they were relatively ineffective.

In some patients receiving azathioprine, there has been suppression of the delayed hypersensitivity response to keyhole limpet antigen, but not to two contact allergens, DNCB and NDMA. The immunosuppression may thus show specificity against the particular type of antigen or against the type of the response to that antigen.

Although immunosuppression of a varying qualitative and quantitative degree has been demonstrated with mercaptopurine and Imuran, as noted above, anti-kidney antibodies have been detected in the blood of azathioprine-treated patients with successful as well as unsuccessful renal homotransplants. However, the importance of such antibodies in the rejection phenomenon is not known. Infiltration of grafts by small lymphocytes is generally considered as evidence of rejection and has been seen in kidneys which have continued to function. In addition, evaluation of azathioprine-treated patients with kidney transplants of some duration has demonstrated the presence, in many, of other pathologic changes thought to be caused by a low grade immunologic reaction on the part of the host.

Human Homotransplantation: The Fifth Report of the Human Kidney Transplant Registry describes the status of over 1,000 transplants. The following is a summary of the accumulated experiences of centers participating in the Registry.

Approximately one-third of all transplant patients received Imuran brand Azathioprine prior to the transplant operation. Most investigators gave Imuran between one and five days before the operation at a dosage between 1 and 5 mg/kg/day. Imuran treatment almost always started within 24 hours following the transplant whether or not it had been administered preoperatively. The typical postoperative Imuran dosage was in the 1 to 4 mg/kg/day range. During a threatened rejection episode, the Imuran dosage remained relatively stable. Other immunosuppressive therapy was also used in conjunction with Imuran. The most frequently used concomitant agents were the corticosteroids. A variety of other cytotoxic agents was also administered.

During the course of treatment, Imuran therapy was discontinued in some patients, usually because of hematopoietic toxicity. In over half of the cases where Imuran had to be withheld, the transplant either functioned at a reduced level or it was rejected.

In nearly one-third of the transplant cases, toxicity or infection occurred during the first three months of treatment. However, the incidence of complications attributed to Imuran declined the longer the patient survived. For transplants surviving beyond two years, the incidence of complications was approximately three percent. Bone marrow depression—leukopenia, thrombocytopenia, anemia and pancytopenia—was the most frequently occurring complication. Infection and hepatitis were the next most frequent complications observed. Other less frequently occurring complications are described under adverse reactions.

Approximately 80 percent of all transplants in which Imuran was administered were functioning three months after the transplant operation and about 55 percent after two years. Approximately 75 percent of the transplants from siblings were functioning at the end of two years compared to 70 percent for parent, and 35 percent for cadaveric, donors.

Indications: Imuran brand Azathioprine is indicated as an adjunct for the prevention of rejection in renal homotransplantation.

Contraindication: Imuran brand Azathioprine is contraindicated in those patients who have shown hypersensitivity to the drug.

Warnings: Imuran brand Azathioprine is a potent drug which is capable of producing severe and irreversible depression of the bone marrow. Complete blood counts, including platelets, should be performed at least weekly, and more frequently during initiation of treatment and when high doses are used. Persistent decrease or rapid fall in leukocyte count calls for a decrease in dosage or temporary discontinuance of the drug.

In the presence of severe and unremitting rejection, it is probably preferable to allow the kidney transplant to be rejected and removed rather than increase Imuran to very toxic dosage levels in an attempt to prevent rejection. The patient may then be maintained by dialysis until another kidney becomes available.

Infection is always a constant hazard of the therapeutic regimen used for prevention of rejection. There have been reports of fungal, protozoal, viral and uncommon bacterial infections, some of which have been fatal. If intercurrent infection develops, it should be appropriately treated and consideration must be given to the possibility of reducing the dosage of azathioprine, corticosteroids and/or ancillary drugs.

There is a theoretical possibility that prolonged immunological stress and/or immunosuppression may accelerate the rate at which malignant mutations occur or may interfere with their rejection.

Although no causal relationship has been established, there have been a few reports of lymphomas developing in patients receiving immunosuppressive therapy after renal homotransplantation.

Persistent negative nitrogen balance has been observed in some patients on continuous azathioprine and corticosteroid therapy; if this should occur, the dosage should be reduced.

If there is evidence of toxic hepatitis or biliary stasis, consideration should be given to withholding the drug.

Pregnancy Warning: *Drugs of this type have potential teratogenic activity and the benefits and risks must be weighed before use in women of childbearing potential.*

There have been several reports of women who became pregnant while receiving maintenance doses of Imuran and who subsequently gave birth to apparently normal children. Some of these women continued to receive Imuran throughout the pregnancy. Nevertheless, the teratogenic activity of the drug in rabbits and mice suggests the avoidance of its use in pregnancy whenever feasible.

Precautions: *Cadaveric kidneys frequently develop a tubular necrosis with delayed onset of adequate function, and clearance of Imuran brand Azathioprine and its metabolites may be impaired; therefore, the dosage should be appropriately reduced.*

In patients receiving Zyloprim brand Allopurinol, the concomitant administration of Imuran will require a reduction in dose to approximately one-third to one-fourth the usual dose of Imuran.

Adverse Reactions: The chief toxic effect is hematologic manifested by leukopenia, anemia, thrombocytopenia and bleeding. Oral lesions, skin rashes, drug fever, alopecia, pancreatitis, arthralgia and steatorrhea are not generally seen but may occur. Nausea, vomiting, diarrhea and anorexia sometimes occur, especially at higher dosages. Jaundice has been observed in some patients suggesting liver damage or biliary stasis; this has been characterized by extremely high alkaline phosphatase levels with slightly elevated bilirubin.

Dosage: The dosage which will be tolerated or will be effective will vary from patient to patient and, therefore, careful management is necessary to obtain the optimum therapeutic effect without incurring toxicity. Caution must be exercised to avoid toxicity, the chief manifestation of which is depression of the bone marrow, resulting most commonly in leukopenia and less often in thrombocytopenia and bleeding. SINCE THIS DRUG MAY HAVE A DELAYED ACTION, IT IS IMPORTANT TO REDUCE DOSAGE OR WITHDRAW THE MEDICATION TEMPORARILY AT THE FIRST SIGN OF AN ABNORMALLY LARGE FALL IN THE LEUKOCYTE COUNT AND/OR OTHER EVIDENCE OF PERSISTENT DEPRESSION OF THE BONE MARROW. It must be kept in mind that patients with impaired renal function may have slower elimination of the drug with a consequent greater cumulative effect; therefore, the dosage should be appropriately reduced.

The usual initial dose is approximately 3 to 5 mg/kg/day, orally. Adjunct therapy of various types has generally been used in suppressing rejection of renal homografts and this may add to the toxic potential of the regimen. Dosage must be adjusted to attempt to provide satisfactory maintenance of the homograft without producing toxic effects; it may be possible to reduce maintenance dosage to 1 to 2 mg/kg/day.

How Supplied: 50 mg scored tablets, bottle of 100. Tablets bear identification, K7A. Injectable sodium salt is also available in 20 ml vial containing 100 mg.

100—VA & DoD NSN 6505-00-119-9317

[Shown in Product Identification Section]

KEMADRIN® ℞

brand Procyclidine Hydrochloride

Description: 1-cyclohexyl-1-phenyl-3-pyrrolidinopropan-1-ol hydrochloride. Developed in The Wellcome Research Laboratories.

Indications: Kemadrin brand Procyclidine Hydrochloride is indicated for the treatment of parkinsonism including the postencephalitic, arteriosclerotic and idiopathic types. Partial control of the parkinsonism symptoms is the usual therapeutic accomplishment. Procyclidine hydrochloride is usually more efficacious in the relief of rigidity than tremor; but tremor, fatigue, weakness and sluggishness are frequently beneficially influenced. It can be substituted for all previous medications in mild and moderate cases. For the control of more severe cases other drugs may be added to procyclidine therapy as indications warrant.

Clinical reports indicate that procyclidine often successfully relieves the symptoms of extrapyramidal dysfunction (dystonia, dyskinesia, akathisia and parkinsonism) which accompany the therapy of mental disorders with phenothiazine and rauwolfia compounds. In addition to minimizing the symptoms induced by tranquilizing drugs, the drug effectively controls sialorrhea resulting from neuroleptic medication. At the same time freedom from the side effects induced by tranquilizer drugs, as provided by the administration of procyclidine, permits a more sustained treatment of the patient's mental disorder.

Clinical results in the treatment of parkinsonism indicate that most patients experience subjective improvement characterized by a feeling of well-being and increased alertness, together with diminished salivation and a marked improvement in muscular coordination as demonstrated by objective tests of manual dexterity and by increased ability to carry out ordinary self-care activities. While the drug exerts a mild atropine-like action and therefore causes mydriasis, this may be kept minimal by careful adjustment of the daily dosage.

Contraindications: Procyclidine hydrochloride should not be used in angle-closure glaucoma although simple type glaucomas do not appear to be adversely affected.

Warnings:

Use in Children

Safety and efficacy have not been established in the pediatric age group; therefore, the use of procyclidine hydrochloride in this age group requires that the potential benefits be weighed against the possible hazards to the child.

Pregnancy Warning

The safe use of this drug in pregnancy has not been established; therefore, the use of procyclidine hydrochloride in pregnancy, lactation or in women of childbearing age requires that the potential benefits be weighed against the possible hazards to the mother and child.

Precautions: Conditions in which inhibition of the parasympathetic nervous system is undesirable such as tachycardia and urinary retention (such as may occur with marked prostatic hypertrophy) require special care in the administration of the drug. Hypotensive patients who receive the drug should be observed closely. Occasionally, particularly in older patients, mental confusion and disorientation may occur with the development of agitation, hallucinations and psychotic-like symptoms.

Patients with mental disorders occasionally experience a precipitation of a psychotic episode when the dosage of antiparkinsonism drugs is increased to treat the extrapyramidal side effects of phenothiazine and rauwolfia derivatives.

Adverse Reactions: Anticholinergic effects can be produced by therapeutic doses although these can frequently be minimized or eliminated by careful dosage. They include: dryness of the mouth, mydriasis, blurring of vision, giddiness, light headedness and gastrointestinal disturbances such as nausea, vomiting, epigastric distress and constipation. Occasionally an allergic reaction such as a skin rash may be encountered. Feelings of muscular weakness may occur. Acute suppurative parotitis as a complication of dry mouth has been reported.

Dosage and Administration:

For Parkinsonism

The dosage of the drug for the treatment of parkinsonism depends upon the age of the patient, the etiology of the disease, and individual responsiveness. Therefore, the dosage must remain flexible to permit adjustment to the individual tolerance and requirements of each patient. In general, younger and postencephalitic patients require and tolerate a somewhat higher dosage than older patients and those with arteriosclerosis.

For Patients Who Have Received No Other Therapy

The usual dose of procyclidine hydrochloride for initial treatment is 2 to 2.5 mg administered three times daily after meals. If well tolerated, this dose may be gradually increased to 4 to 5 mg three times a day and occasionally 4 to 5 mg given before retiring. In some cases smaller doses may be employed with good therapeutic results.

Occasionally a patient is encountered who cannot tolerate a bedtime dose of the drug. In such cases it may be desirable to adjust dosage so that the bedtime dose is omitted and the total daily requirement is administered in three equal daytime doses. It is best administered during or after meals to minimize the development of side reactions.

To Transfer Patients to Kemadrin brand Procyclidine Hydrochloride from Other Therapy

Patients who have been receiving other drugs may be transferred to procyclidine hydrochloride. This is accomplished gradually by substituting 2 to 2.5 mg three times a day for all or part of the original drug. The dose of procyclidine is then increased as required while that of the other drug is correspondingly omitted or decreased until complete replacement is achieved. The total daily dosage may then be adjusted to the level which produces maximum benefit.

For Drug-Induced Extrapyramidal Symptoms

For treatment of symptoms of extrapyramidal dysfunction induced by tranquilizer drugs during the therapy of mental disorders, the dosage of procyclidine hydrochloride will depend on the severity of side effects associated with tranquilizer administration. In general the larger the dosage of the tranquilizer the more severe will be the associated symptoms, including rigidity and tremors. Accordingly, the drug dosage should be adjusted to suit the needs of the individual patient and to provide maximum relief of the induced symptoms. A convenient method to establish the daily dosage of procyclidine is to begin with the administration of 2 to 2.5 mg three times daily. This may be increased by 2 to 2.5 mg daily increments until the patient obtains relief of symptoms. In most cases excellent results will be obtained with 10 to 20 mg daily.

How Supplied: Scored tablets of 2 mg and 5 mg, bottles of 100 and 1000. 2 mg tablet bears Wellcome I.D. code imprint, F4B.

5 mg 1000—VA NSN 6505-00-687-8469

[Shown in Product Identification Section]

LANOXIN® ℞

brand Digoxin

Description: The cardiac or digitalis glycosides are a closely related group of drugs having specific and powerful effects on the myocardium. These drugs are found in a number of plants. The term "digitalis" is used to designate the whole group. Typically, the glycosides are composed of three portions: a steroid nucleus, a lactone ring, and a sugar (hence "glycosides").

Digoxin, a cardiotonic glycoside obtained from the leaves of *Digitalis lanata*, was discovered and developed in 1930 at the Wellcome Research Laboratories. Lanoxin brand Digoxin has the empirical formula $C_{41}H_{64}O_{14}$, a molecular weight of 780.96, melting and decomposition points above 235°C, and a clearly defined specific optical rotation.

The drug is insoluble in water, chloroform, ether, ethyl acetate or acetone; soluble in dilute (50 percent) alcohol or alcohol-chloroform; and freely soluble in pyridine. It crystallizes from these solutions in characteristic triclinic plates which appear colorless when thin, white when thicker. Digoxin powder is composed of odorless white crystals.

Lanoxin® brand Digoxin Injection is a sterile solution of digoxin for intravenous or intramuscular injection. The vehicle contains 40

Continued on next page

Burroughs Wellcome—Cont.

percent propylene glycol and 10 percent alcohol. The injection is buffered with 0.3 percent sodium phosphate and 0.08 percent anhydrous citric acid. Each 2 cc ampul contains 0.5 mg digoxin (0.25 mg in each cc). Dilution is not required.

Lanoxin® brand Digoxin Injection Pediatric is a sterile solution of digoxin for intravenous or intramuscular injection. The vehicle contains 40 percent propylene glycol and 10 percent alcohol. The injection is buffered with 0.3 percent sodium phosphate and 0.08 percent anhydrous citric acid. Each 1 cc ampul contains 0.1 mg digoxin. Dilution is not required.

Lanoxin® brand Digoxin Tablets are supplied in three strengths: yellow, scored tablets of 0.125 mg bearing ID code Y3B; white, scored tablets of 0.25 mg bearing ID code X3A; and green, scored tablets of 0.5 mg bearing ID code T9A.

Lanoxin® brand Digoxin Elixir Pediatric is a stable solution of digoxin specially formulated for oral use in infants and children. Each cc contains 0.05 mg digoxin. The lime-flavored elixir contains 10 percent alcohol and is preserved with 0.1 percent methylparaben. Each package is supplied with a specially calibrated dropper to facilitate the administration of accurate dosage even in premature infants. Starting with 0.2 cc, this 1 cc dropper is marked in divisions of 0.1 cc, each corresponding to 5 mcg (0.005 mg) digoxin.

Action: The digitalis glycosides have qualitatively the same therapeutic effect on the heart. They (1) increase the force of myocardial contraction, (2) increase the refractory period of the atrioventricular (A-V) node, and (3) to a lesser degree, affect the sinoatrial (S-A) node and conduction system via the parasympathetic and sympathetic nervous systems.

The intravenous administration of Lanoxin brand Digoxin Injection or Injection Pediatric usually produces an initial effect within five to ten minutes, the action becoming maximal in one or two hours. With intramuscular injection the onset of effect occurs within 30 minutes, the action becoming maximal in four to six hours. In cases of atrial fibrillation, dramatic slowing of the ventricular rate may occur. When the rhythm is normal, there may be no substantial change in the cardiac rate; it has been observed, however, that in either case a rapid fall in venous pressure may take place, followed by diuresis (and consequent loss of body weight) and symptomatic relief.

Gastrointestinal absorption of Lanoxin brand Digoxin from the elixir is 65 to 85 percent, and absorption of Lanoxin® brand Digoxin from tablets is 50 to 75 percent.

Digoxin is only 20 to 25 percent bound to plasma proteins and is predominantly excreted by the kidneys unmetabolized unless there is significant renal failure. Renal excretion of digoxin is proportional to glomerular filtration rate and is largely independent of urine flow. Digoxin is not effectively removed from the body by dialysis, exchange transfusions or during cardiopulmonary bypass, presumably because of tissue binding. In subjects with normal renal function, digoxin is excreted exponentially with an average half-life of 36 hours resulting in the loss of 35 to 40 percent of the body stores daily.

Serum levels and pharmacokinetics are essentially unchanged by massive weight loss, suggesting that lean body mass should be used in dosage calculations. The peak blood level from oral dosing with tablets or the elixir occurs one to three hours after administration. The onset of therapeutic action of digoxin after oral tablets is one to two hours (one hour with elixir) with the peak effect occurring six to eight hours after dosing.

Indications:

1. **Congestive heart failure.** Congestive failure of all degrees is the primary indication. The increased cardiac output produced by the drug results in diuresis and general amelioration of the disturbances characteristic of right (venous congestion, edema) and left (dyspnea, orthopnea, cardiac asthma) heart failure.

Digoxin, generally, is most effective in "low output" failure and less effective in "high output" (bronchopulmonary insufficiency, infection, hyperthyroidism) heart failure.

Digitalis should be continued after failure is abolished unless some known precipitating factor has been corrected.

2. **Atrial fibrillation:** Atrial fibrillation, especially when the ventricular rate is elevated. Digoxin rapidly reduces ventricular rates and eliminates the pulse deficit. Palpitation, precordial distress or weakness are relieved and any concomitant congestive failure ameliorated. Digoxin should be continued in doses necessary to maintain the desired ventricular rate and other clinical effects.

3. **Atrial flutter:** Digoxin slows the heart and regular sinus rhythm may appear. Frequently the flutter is converted to atrial fibrillation with a slow ventricular rate. Stopping digoxin at this point may be followed by restoration of sinus rhythm, especially if the flutter was of the paroxysmal type. It is preferable, however, to continue digoxin if failure ensues or if atrial flutter is a frequent occurrence.

4. **Paroxysmal atrial tachycardia:** Oral digoxin may be used, especially if the condition is resistant to lesser measures. Depending on the urgency, a more rapid acting parenteral preparation may be preferable to initiate digitalization, although if heart failure has ensued or paroxysms recur frequently, digoxin should be maintained by oral administration.

Digoxin is not indicated in sinus tachycardia unless due to heart failure.

5. **Cardiogenic shock:** The drug is often employed, especially when the condition is accompanied by pulmonary edema. Digoxin seems to affect adversely shock due to septicemia from gram-negative bacteria.

Contraindications: The presence of toxic effects (see "Overdose") induced by any digitalis preparation is a contraindication to all of the cardiac glycosides.

Allergy, though rare, does occur. It may not extend to all preparations and another may be tried.

Ventricular fibrillation.

Warnings:

> Digitalis alone or with other drugs has been promoted for use in the treatment of obesity. This use of digoxin or other digitalis glycosides is unwarranted. Moreover, since they may cause potentially fatal arrhythmias or other adverse effects, the use of these drugs in the treatment of obesity is dangerous.

Many of the arrhythmias for which digoxin is advised closely resemble those reflecting digoxin intoxication. If the possibility of digoxin intoxication cannot be excluded, cardiac glycosides should be temporarily withheld if permitted by the clinical situation.

The patient with congestive heart failure may complain of nausea and vomiting. These symptoms may also be indications of digoxin intoxication. A clinical determination of the cause of these symptoms must be attempted before further drug administration.

Patients with renal insufficiency require smaller than usual doses of digoxin. See ACTION section for mechanism. Newborn infants display considerable variability in their tolerance to digoxin, depending on their degree of maturity.

Premature and immature infants are particularly sensitive, and dosage must be reduced and digitalization should be even more individualized and cautiously approached than in more mature infants. Impaired renal function must also be carefully taken into consideration.

Congestive heart failure accompanying acute glomerulonephritis requires extreme care in digitalization. A relatively low total dose administered in divided doses and concomitant use of antihypertensive drugs has been recommended. ECG monitoring is essential. Digoxin should be discontinued as soon as possible.

Patients with idiopathic hypertrophic subaortic stenosis must be managed extremely carefully. Unless cardiac failure is severe, it is doubtful whether digoxin should be employed.

Patients with rheumatic carditis, especially when severe, are unusually sensitive to digoxin and prone to disturbances of rhythm. If heart failure develops, digitalization may be initiated with relatively low doses; then it can be cautiously increased until a beneficial effect is obtained. If a therapeutic trial does not result in improvement, the drug should be considered ineffective and be discontinued.

Note: Digitalis glycosides are an important cause of accidental poisoning in children.

Precautions: Atrial arrhythmias associated with hypermetabolic states are particularly resistant to digoxin treatment. Care must be taken to avoid digoxin toxicity if digoxin is used to help the arrhythmia.

Digoxin is not indicated for the treatment of ventricular tachycardia unless congestive heart failure supervenes after a protracted episode not itself due to digoxin.

Potassium depletion sensitizes the myocardium to digoxin and toxicity may develop even with usual dosage. Hypokalemia may also alter the rate of onset and intensity of the positive inotropic effect of digoxin. Therefore, it is desirable to maintain normal serum potassium levels in patients being treated with digoxin. Potassium wastage may result from diuretic or corticosteroid therapy, hemodialysis, and from suction of gastrointestinal secretions. It may accompany malnutrition, diarrhea, prolonged vomiting, old age, and long-standing congestive heart failure. In general, rapid changes in serum potassium or other electrolytes are to be avoided, and intravenous treatment with potassium should be reserved only for special circumstances as described below (see TREATMENT OF ARRHYTHMIAS PRODUCED BY OVERDOSAGES section).

Patients with acute myocardial infarction, severe pulmonary disease, or far advanced heart failure may be more sensitive to digoxin and more prone to disturbances of rhythm.

Calcium affects contractility and excitability of the heart in a manner similar to that of digoxin. Calcium may produce serious arrhythmias in digitalized patients.

In myxedema, the digoxin requirements are less because excretion rate is decreased and blood levels are significantly higher.

In incomplete A-V block, especially in patients subject to Stokes-Adams attacks, advanced or complete heart block may develop if digoxin is given. Heart failure in these patients can usually be controlled by other measures and by increasing the heart rate.

Patients with chronic constrictive pericarditis may to respond unfavorably to digoxin.

Patients with idiopathic hypertrophic subaortic stenosis must be managed extremely carefully. Unless cardiac failure is severe it is doubtful whether digoxin should be employed.

Renal insufficiency delays the excretion of digoxin and dosage must be adjusted accordingly in patients with renal disease. Note: This applies also to potassium administration, should it become necessary.

Electrical conversion of arrhythmias may require adjustment of digoxin dosage.

Dosage must be carefully titrated and differences in the bioavailability of parenteral preparations, elixirs, and tablets should be taken into account when switching patients from one preparation to another.

Electrocardiographic monitoring may be necessary to avoid intoxication.

Premonitory signs of toxicity in the newborn are undue slowing of the sinus rate, sinoatrial arrest, and prolongation of PR interval.

Adverse Reactions:

Gynecomastia: Uncommon

Overdose or toxic effects in adults:

Gastrointestinal: Anorexia, nausea, vomiting, diarrhea are the most common early symptoms of overdosages in the adult (but rarely conspicuous in infants). Uncontrolled heart failure may also produce such symptoms.

Central nervous system: Visual disturbances (blurred vision, yellow vision), headache, weakness, apathy.

Cardiac disturbances (arrhythmias): Ventricular premature beats are the most common, except in infants and young children. Paroxysmal and nonparoxysmal nodal rhythms, atrioventricular (interference) dissociation and paroxysmal atrial tachycardia (PAT) with block are also common arrhythmias due to digoxin overdosage.

Conduction disturbances: Excessive slowing of the pulse is a clinical sign of digoxin overdosage. Atrioventricular block of increasing degree may proceed to complete heart block.

Note: The electrocardiogram is fundamental in determining the presence and nature of these cardiac toxic disturbances. Digoxin may also induce other changes, (as of the ST segment), but these provide no measure of the degree of digitalization.

Overdose or toxic effects in children:

Toxic signs differ from the adult in a number of respects. Cardiac arrhythmias are the more reliable and frequent signs of toxicity.

Vomiting and diarrhea, neurologic and visual disturbances are rare as initial signs.

Premature ventricular systoles are rarely seen; nodal and atrial systoles are more frequent.

Atrial arrhythmias, atrial ectopic rhythms, and paroxysmal atrial tachycardia with A-V block particularly are more common manifestations of toxicity in children.

Ventricular arrhythmias are rare.

Treatment of Toxic Effects Produced by Overdosage: Digoxin should be discontinued until all signs of toxicity are abolished. Discontinuation may be all that is necessary if toxic manifestations are not severe and appear after the time for peak effect of the drug.

Potassium salts are commonly used. Potassium chloride in divided oral doses totaling 4-6 grams for adults (see PEDIATRIC INFORMATION section for pediatric dosage) may be given provided renal function is adequate.

When correction of the arrhythmia is urgent and the serum potassium level is low or normal, potassium should be administered intravenously in a solution of 5 percent dextrose in water. A total of 40-100 milliequivalents (30 milliequivalents per 500 milliliters) is given at the rate of 20 milliequivalents per hour unless limited by pain due to local irritation.

Additional amounts may be given if the arrhythmia is uncontrolled and the potassium well tolerated.

Continuous electrocardiographic monitoring should be performed to watch for any evidence of potassium toxicity, e.g., peaking of T waves, and to observe the effect on the arrhythmia so that the infusion may be promptly stopped when the desired effect is achieved.

Caution: Potassium should not be used and may be dangerous for severe or complete heart block due to digitalis and not related to any tachycardia. A continuous electrocardiogram should be observed so that the infusion may be promptly stopped when the desired effect is achieved.

Other agents which have been used in the treatment of digitalis intoxication include lidocaine, quinidine, procainamide, and beta adrenergic blocking agents. The latter three agents should be used with caution when AV block is a component of digitalis intoxication as they may exaggerate this arrhythmic property.

Pediatric Information: (See adult section for other recommendations for the treatment of arrhythmias produced by overdosages and for additional recommendations and cautions regarding the use of potassium.) Potassium preparations may be given orally in divided doses totaling 1-1.5 milliequivalents/kilogram (1 gram K contains 13.4 milliequivalents). When correction of the arrhythmia is urgent, approximately 0.5 milliequivalents/kilogram of potassium per hour may be given, with careful electrocardiographic monitoring, as a solution of 20 milliequivalents or less for 500 milliliters in 5 percent dextrose in water. The total dose should generally not exceed 2 milliequivalents of potassium/kilogram.

Dosage and Administration: Digoxin is administered slowly or rapidly as required until the desired therapeutic effect is obtained without symptoms of overdose. The amount can be predicted approximately from the lean body mass of the patient with allowances made for excretion during the time taken to induce digitalization. Parenteral administration should be used only when the drug cannot be taken orally, or when rapid digitalization is very urgent.

Subsequent maintenance dosage is also determined tentatively by the amount necessary to sustain the desired therapeutic effect.

Recommended doses are practical average figures that may require considerable modification as dictated by individual sensitivity or associated conditions. Diminished renal function is the most important factor which requires modification of recommended or average doses. (See WARNINGS and PRECAUTIONS section.) Clearance of digoxin from the serum is proportional to the glomerular filtration rate as estimated by renal creatinine clearance. The excretion of digoxin thus varies directly with creatinine clearance, and the ratio of the two clearances is near unity. As a result, an estimate of creatinine clearance gives a reasonable value for digoxin clearance and a dose of digoxin may be reduced in proportion to the observed creatinine clearance (see "Warnings", "Precautions").

The following recommended doses can merely serve as guidelines and should be adjusted according to the circumstances. For example, the lower end of the range should be selected for the very elderly, those with severe heart failure and those with severe renal impairment. On the other hand, patients with fulminating pulmonary edema and rapid heart rate in excess of 130 per minute or atrial fibrillation may require the upper end of the recommended range. It cannot be overemphasized that the values given are averages and substantial individual variation can be expected.

Injection and Injection Pediatric:

Adults and Children 10 Years of Age and Over. The average digitalizing dose (i.e., amount accumulated) with parenteral digoxin is 0.5 to 1.0 mg. The usual initial intravenous or intramuscular dose is 0.25 to 0.50 mg. If required, additional injections of 0.25 mg may be given at four to six hour intervals. Full digitalization may require a total of 1.0 mg. When administered intravenously, it should be injected slowly; when administered intramuscularly, it should be injected deep into the muscle followed by massage. No more than 0.5 mg should be injected into a single site in order to reduce the incidence of discomfort. Because of the local discomfort that occurs with intramuscular administration, this route should be selected only when both intravenous and oral administration are not feasible.

After digitalization has been achieved, the patient may usually be maintained with 0.125 to 0.50 mg Lanoxin brand Digoxin daily (average 0.25 mg) given as a single or divided dose according to the patient's response. Ordinarily, the oral route will be used for maintenance using Lanoxin brand Digoxin Tablets; in special circumstances maintenance by the parenteral route may be preferred, as in patients who cannot tolerate oral medication, or who have lesions of the gastrointestinal tract, making absorption uncertain.

Infants and Children up to 10 Years of Age. Digitalization must be individualized. Generally, premature and immature infants are particularly sensitive requiring reduced dosage which must be determined by careful titration. TOTAL parenteral digitalizing dose (to be given in divided doses): Children from 2 to 10 years: 25 to 40 μg per kg of body weight. Infants from 2 weeks to 2 years: 35 to 50 μg per kg of body weight. Premature and newborn infants (under 2 weeks): 25 to 40 μg per kg of body weight.

Initially, give one-fourth to one-half the calculated total digitalizing dose, followed by one-fourth the total dose at six hour intervals until digitalization is completed. Recommended dosage may be varied in accordance with the requirements of the individual case, but the patient should be followed with careful clinical and electrocardiographic evaluation. The total daily maintenance dose is 20 to 30 percent of the total digitalizing dose. It may be given as one dose or in divided dosage, as indicated.

Long-term use of digitalis is indicated in almost all infants who have been digitalized for acute congestive failure unless the cause is transient. Many favor maintaining digitalis until at least two years of age in all infants with paroxysmal atrial tachycardia or who show either definite or latent failure.

Many children with severe inoperable congenital defects need digitalis throughout childhood and often for life.

ORAL (TABLETS and ELIXIR)

Adults and Children 10 Years of Age and Over. The average digitalizing dose (i.e., amount accumulated) with oral digoxin is 1.0 to 1.5 mg. Digitalization may be accomplished by any of several approaches that vary in dosage and frequency of administration but reach the same end point in terms of total amount accumulated. In previously undigitalized patients, a single loading dose of 0.5 to 0.75 mg orally usually produces a detectable effect in one or two hours that becomes maximal in six to eight hours. Additional doses of 0.25 to 0.50 mg may be given cautiously at six to eight hour intervals to full digitalization.

In previously undigitalized patients, institution of daily maintenance therapy (0.125-0.5 milligram, see next paragraph) without a loading dose results in development of steady-state plateau concentrations in about 7 days in patients with normal renal function.

The average daily oral maintenance dose is 0.125-0.5 milligram, usually 0.25 milligram. In the elderly patient, 0.125-0.25 milligram should be considered the average maintenance dose.

In patients with renal impairment, digoxin excretion is impaired and serum half-life is prolonged (see ACTION section). Digitalizing and maintenance doses are lower than those recommended for patients with normal renal functions. Signs of digoxin toxicity develop sooner in patients with renal impairment, and it takes longer for toxic signs and symptoms to disappear. Because of the prolonged half-life, a longer period of time is required to achieve an initial or new steady-state plateau in patients with renal impairment than in patients with normal renal function.

It cannot be overemphasized that the values given are averages and substantial individual variation can be expected.

Continued on next page

Burroughs Wellcome—Cont.

ORAL (ELIXIR)
Infants and Children.
Digitalization must be individualized. Generally, premature and immature infants are particularly sensitive, requiring reduced dosage which must be determined by careful titration. Beyond the immediate newborn period, children require proportionally greater doses than adults on the basis of body weight or surface area.
Oral Dosage. The following digitalization doses are recommended for children with normal renal function.
Newborns (normal), up to 1 month, require 40 to 60 μg per kg.
Infants, 1 month to 2 years, require approximately 60 to 80 μg per kg.
Children, 2 years to 10 years, require 40 to 60 μg per kg.
Children 10 years of age and over require adult dosages in proportion to their body weight.
Maintenance therapy is 20 to 30 percent of the digitalizing dose administered each day.
Long-term use of digoxin is indicated in almost all infants who have been digitalized for acute congestive failure unless the cause is transient. Many favor maintaining digoxin until at least 2 years of age in all infants with paroxysmal atrial tachycardia or in those who show either definite or latent failure.
Many children with severe inoperable congenital defects need digitalis throughout childhood and often for life.
How Supplied: Oral: Lanoxin brand Digoxin Tablet of 0.125 mg, scored (yellow); bottles of 30, 100 and 1000; unit dose pack of 1000. Tablet of 0.25 mg, scored (white); bottles of 30, 100, 500, 1000 and 5000; and Unit Dose Pack, strips of 10 tablets, 10 boxes of 100 tablets (1000). Tablet of 0.5 mg, scored (green); bottles of 100 and 1000. Lanoxin brand Digoxin Elixir Pediatric, 0.05 mg in each cc. Bottle of 2 fl. oz. with calibrated dropper.
Intramuscular or Intravenous: Lanoxin brand Digoxin Injection, 2 cc ampuls each containing 0.5 mg (0.25 mg per cc) in a vehicle of 40% propylene glycol and 10% alcohol and containing sodium phosphate 0.3% and anhydrous citric acid 0.08%. This injection does not require dilution. Boxes of 12 and 100.
Injection Pediatric also available, 0.1 mg in 1 cc ampuls, box of 50.
Lanoxin 0.125 mg tablets bear identification, Y3B. 0.25 mg tablets are marked X3A. 0.5 mg tablets, T9A. All tablets are also imprinted with the name, LANOXIN.

El. Ped. 60 cc—DoD
NSN 6505-00-890-1726
Inj. 0.5 mg/2 cc Amps × 12—DoD
NSN 6505-00-531-7761
Inj. 0.5 mg/2 cc Amps × 100—VA
NSN 6505-00-147-4974
Tabs. 0.25 mg 30 —VA
NSN 6505-01-035-2104
100 —DoD
NSN 6505-00-116-7750
1000 —VA
NSN 6505-00-616-7898
UDP 100 —DoD
NSN 6505-00-117-5689
Tabs. 0.125 mg 30 —VA
NSN 6505-01-049-6807

[*Shown in Product Identification Section*]

LEUKERAN® ℞
brand Chlorambucil

Description: *p*-(di-2-chlorethyl) aminophenylbutyric acid; a derivative of nitrogen mustard. U.S. Pat. No. 2,944,079.
Caution: Leukeran brand Chlorambucil, a derivative of nitrogen mustard, is a potent drug. Blood counts should be taken once or twice weekly. Discontinue or reduce the dosage upon evidence of abnormal depression of the bone marrow.
Indications: Chlorambucil is indicated in the treatment of chronic lymphocytic leukemia, malignant lymphomas including lymphosarcoma, giant follicular lymphoma and Hodgkin's disease. It is not curative but produces remissions, some of which may be striking, in a substantial proportion of patients. Chlorambucil has been found to be easier to handle than nitrogen mustard and some other related drugs because it produces fewer side effects and is not damaging to the hemopoietic system in therapeutic doses. As with other drugs of this type, excessive or prolonged dosage will produce severe bone marrow depression.
Precautions and Contraindications: Patients must be followed carefully to avoid irreversible damage to the bone marrow during treatment. Weekly examination of the blood should be made to determine hemoglobin levels, and total and differential leukocyte counts. Also, during the first 3 to 6 weeks of therapy, it is recommended that white blood cell counts be made 3 to 4 days after each of the weekly complete blood counts. Galton et al have suggested that in following patients it is helpful to plot the blood counts on a chart at the same time that body weight, temperature, spleen size, etc. are recorded. It is considered dangerous to allow a patient to go more than two weeks without hematological and clinical examination during treatment.
Many patients develop a slowly progressive lymphopenia during treatment. The lymphocyte count usually rapidly returns to normal levels upon completion of drug therapy. Most patients have some neutropenia after the third week of treatment and this may continue for up to ten days after the last dose. Subsequently, the neutrophil count usually rapidly returns to normal. Severe neutropenia appears to be related to dosage and usually occurs only in patients who have received a total dosage of 6.5 mg/kg (about 450 mg) or more in one course. About one-quarter of all patients receiving this dosage, and one-third of those receiving this dosage in eight weeks or less may be expected to develop severe neutropenia.
While it is not necessary to discontinue chlorambucil at the first evidence of a fall in neutrophil count, it must be remembered that the fall may continue for ten days after the last dose and that as the total dose approaches 6.5 mg/kg there is real risk of causing irreversible bone marrow damage. Galton et al. reported that most patients who received benefit from chlorambucil required smaller dosage than this amount.
Chlorambucil should not be given before four weeks after a full course of radiation therapy or chemotherapy because of the vulnerability of the bone marrow to damage under these conditions. Also, the drug should not be given in full dosage when the bone marrow is infiltrated with lymphomatous tissue or is hypoplastic as a result of long-standing and extensively treated disease.
Persistently low neutrophil and platelet counts or peripheral lymphocytosis suggest bone marrow infiltration. If confirmed by bone marrow examination, the dosage of chlorambucil should not exceed 0.1 mg/kg. Chlorambucil appears to be relatively free from gastrointestinal side effects or other evidence of toxicity apart from the bone marrow depressant action.
Pregnancy Warning: Whenever possible avoid use during first trimester of pregnancy.
Dosage and Administration: The usual oral dosage is 0.1 to 0.2 mg/kg body weight daily for three to six weeks as required. This usually amounts to 4 to 10 mg a day for the average patient. The entire daily dose may be given at one time. These dosages are for initiation of therapy or for short courses of treatment. The dosage must be carefully adjusted according to the response of the patient and must be reduced as soon as there is an abrupt fall in the white blood cell count. Patients with Hodgkin's disease usually require 0.2 mg/kg daily whereas patients with other lymphomas or chronic lymphocytic leukemia usually require only 0.1 mg/kg daily. When lymphocytic infiltration of the bone marrow is present, or when the bone marrow is hypoplastic, the daily dose should not exceed 0.1 mg/kg (about 6 mg for the average patient).
Radiation and cytotoxic drugs render the bone marrow more vulnerable to damage and, therefore, chlorambucil should not be used within four weeks of a full course of radiation therapy or chemotherapy. However, small doses of palliative radiation over isolated foci remote from the bone marrow will not usually depress the neutrophil and platelet count. In these cases chlorambucil may be given.
It is presently felt that short courses of treatment are safer than continuous maintenance therapy although both methods have been effective. It must be recognized that continuous therapy may give the appearance of "maintenance" in patients who are actually in remission and have no immediate need for further drug. It may, therefore, be desirable to withdraw the drug for a period in such patients to determine whether maintenance therapy is necessary. If maintenance dosage is used, it should not exceed 0.1 mg/kg daily and may well be as low as 0.03 mg/kg daily. Ordinarily, it is 2 mg to 4 mg daily, or less, depending on the response of the patient.
How Supplied: Tablet of 2 mg, sugar-coated. Bottle of 50.

[*Shown in Product Identification Section*]

LIDOSPORIN® ℞
OTIC SOLUTION, Sterile
Polymyxin B—Lidocaine—Propylene Glycol

Description: Each cc contains Aerosporin brand Polymyxin B Sulfate 10,000 units; lidocaine hydrochloride 50 mg (5%); purified water 0.02 cc; propylene glycol qs.
Action: Polymyxin B attacks most gram-negative bacilli including virtually all strains of *Ps aeruginosa* and *H influenzae* (Koch-Weeks bacillus). Propylene glycol tends to absorb moisture and thus counteract "sogginess", and, *in vitro,* is a potent antimicrobial agent. Lidocaine acts quickly to relieve the pain and itching so often associated with otitis externa.

Indications: Based on a review of this drug by the National Academy of Sciences—National Research Council and/or other information, FDA has classified the indications as follows:
"Possibly" effective: For the prevention of exacerbations and for the treatment of infection, pain and itching associated with otitis and furunculosis.
Final classification of the less-than-effective indications requires further investigation.

Contraindications: This product is contraindicated in those individuals who have shown hypersensitivity to any of its components.
Precautions: Patients who prefer to warm the medication before using should be cautioned to avoid heating it above body temperature to prevent loss of antibiotic potency. While Lidosporin® Otic Solution Sterile (Polymyxin B-Lidocaine-Propylene Glycol) is generally safe for repeated or prolonged use without interruption, as with other antibiotic products, prolonged use may result in overgrowth of nonsusceptible organisms. Appropriate measures should be taken if this occurs.
Dosage and Administration: After preliminary cleansing and thorough but gentle drying, 3 or 4 drops are instilled into the infected ear, 3 or 4 times daily. For infants and children, 2 or 3 drops are suggested because of the

smaller capacity of the ear canal. The drops should be instilled while the affected ear is turned upwards; this position should be maintained for a few minutes to facilitate penetration. In the presence of a perforated eardrum the solution may be induced to flow into the middle ear by gentle intermittent pressure on the tragus. Solution may be applied by saturating a gauze or cotton wick which may be left in the canal for 24 to 48 hours, keeping the wick moist by adding a few drops of solution as required. In the treatment of middle ear infections where sterile technique is indicated, the dropper or other applicator should be sterilized before each use and care should be taken to prevent contamination of the dropper or the solution.

How Supplied: Bottle of 10 cc with sterile dropper.

MANTADIL® CREAM ℞

Description: Each tube contains: chlorcyclizine hydrochloride 2%, hydrocortisone acetate 0.5% in a vehicle containing the inactive ingredients liquid petrolatum, white petrolatum, purified water, emulsifying wax and 0.25% methylparaben as preservative.

Action: Both hydrocortisone and chlorcyclizine are antagonists of the allergic reaction, pruritus and inflammation. Because the two drugs act in entirely different ways, their use in combination enhances and supplements the effectiveness of each, thus providing a dual attack upon the abnormal skin condition.

Indications: Mantadil Cream is indicated for the treatment of itching skin eruptions and a variety of dermatoses, such as: contact dermatitis including poison ivy, oak and sumac; eczema (allergic, nuchal and nummular); dermatitis (atopic, lichenoid and seborrheic); localized neurodermatitis; insect bites; sunburn; intertrigo; anogenital pruritus.

Contraindications: As with other topical products containing hydrocortisone, the cream should not be used in: bacterial infections of the skin unless antibacterial therapy is concomitant; tuberculosis of the skin; viral infections including varicella, dendritic keratitis of the eye, and herpes simplex of the adjacent skin. Not for ophthalmic use.

Dosage and Administration: Apply 2 to 5 times daily. If the skin condition permits, the cream should be rubbed in well.

How Supplied: Tube of 15 g.

MAREZINE® ℞
brand Cyclizine Lactate Injection
50 mg in 1 cc

Description: Chemically, cyclizine is N-benzhydryl-N′ methylpiperazine, and has a molecular weight of 266.4.

It is a white crystalline solid having a bitter taste, and is soluble in water and isotonic saline.

Marezine brand Cyclizine Lactate Injection is a sterile solution for INTRAMUSCULAR INJECTION ONLY.

Action: Marezine brand Cyclizine has antiemetic, anticholinergic and antihistaminic properties. It also reduces the sensitivity of the labyrinthine apparatus. The exact mechanism of action is unknown. In dogs the drug prevents emesis from intravenous threshold doses of apomorphine, but it is much less effective in blocking emesis from orally administered copper sulfate. These data suggest that the action is mediated through the chemoreceptive trigger zone.

Indications: For the treatment of nausea and vomiting of motion sickness when the oral route cannot be used.

Contraindications: Marezine is contraindicated in individuals who have shown a previous hypersensitivity to the drug.

Compatibility Table
Marezine brand Cyclizine Lactate Injection

Forms a clear solution with: (i.e., can be mixed with)	Is not compatible with: (requires separate injection)
Atropine sulfate	Oxytetracycline hydrochloride
Meperidine hydrochloride (Demerol)	Chlortetracycline hydrochloride
Morphine sulfate	Penicillin
Tetracycline hydrochloride	Any solution with pH of 6.8 or higher (this includes Pentothal sodium and other soluble barbiturates)
Streptomycin sulfate	
Pyridoxine hydrochloride*	
Codeine phosphate and sulfate	
Alphaprodine HCl (Nisentil)	
Scopolamine hydrobromide*	
Pantopon (Hydrochlorides of opium alkaloids)*	
Hydromorphone (Dilaudid)*	*Administer within 4–10 minutes

Warnings: Patients may become drowsy while taking Marezine and should be cautioned against engaging in activities requiring mental alertness, e.g., driving a car or operating heavy machinery or appliances.

Use in Children: Clinical studies establishing safety and efficacy in children have not been done; therefore, usage in this age group and nursing mothers cannot be recommended.

Use with CNS Depressants: May have additive effects with alcohol and other CNS depressants (hypnotics, sedatives, tranquilizers, antianxiety agents, etc.).

Precautions: Because of its anticholinergic action, Marezine should be used with caution and appropriate monitoring in patients with glaucoma, obstructive disease of the gastrointestinal or genitourinary tract, and in elderly males with possible prostatic hypertrophy. Incipient glaucoma may be precipitated by anticholinergic drugs such as Marezine. The drug may have a hypotensive action. This may be confusing or dangerous in postoperative patients and should influence the decision on using the drug postoperatively.

Adverse Reactions: Urticaria, drug rash, dryness of mouth, nose and throat, drowsiness, restlessness, excitation, nervousness, insomnia, euphoria, anorexia, nausea, vomiting, diarrhea, constipation, hypotension, blurred vision, diplopia, vertigo, tinnitus, palpitation, tachycardia, urinary frequency, difficult urination, urinary retention, auditory and visual hallucinations have been reported, particularly when dosage recommendations are exceeded. Cholestatic jaundice has occurred in association with the use of Marezine.

Dosage and Administration: Marezine brand Cyclizine Lactate Injection is administered INTRAMUSCULARLY. The usual dose is 1 cc (50 mg) every 4 to 6 hours as necessary.

Overdosage:

Symptoms of Overdosage: Moderate overdosage may cause hyperexcitability alternating with drowsiness. Massive overdosage may cause convulsions; hallucinations; respiratory paralysis.

Treatment: Appropriate supportive and symptomatic treatment. Consider dialysis.

Caution: Do not use morphine or other respiratory depressants.

[See table above].

How Supplied:
MAREZINE® brand CYCLIZINE LACTATE INJECTION
50 mg in 1 cc
Boxes of 100 ampuls
The injection should be stored in a cold place. It may develop a slight yellow tint if stored at room temperature for several months; however, it retains full potency.

Also Available:
MAREZINE® brand CYCLIZINE HYDROCHLORIDE
50 mg Scored TABLETS
Boxes of 12
Bottles of 100 and 1000
[Shown in Product Identification Section]

MIGRAL® TABLETS ℞

Description: Each sugar-coated tablet contains ergotamine tartrate 1 mg, Marezine® brand Cyclizine Hydrochloride 25 mg, caffeine 50 mg.

Action: Ergotamine tartrate is a powerful vasoconstrictor, which is the basis for its therapeutic effectiveness in the treatment of vascular headache, especially migraine. It also depresses the central vasomotor centers and acts as a peripheral adrenergic blocker. Marezine brand Cyclizine Hydrochloride is an antihistamine of the piperazine class noted for its antinauseant and antiemetic effects. Caffeine is employed in the combination because of its direct vasoconstrictor effect on the cerebral blood vessels.

Indications: Based on a review of this drug by the National Academy of Sciences—National Research Council and/or other information, FDA has classified the indications as follows:
"Possibly" effective: For the treatment of vascular headache, that is, migraine, histaminic cephalalgia and related conditions where distention of cranial vessels appears to be the cause.
Final classification of the less-than-effective indications requires further investigation.

Contraindications: The drug is contraindicated in patients with peripheral vascular disease, marked arteriosclerosis, coronary heart disease, hypertension, Buerger's Disease, Raynaud's Disease, thrombophlebitis, thyrotoxicosis, anemia, impaired liver or kidney function, sepsis, and during **pregnancy.** It should be used with caution in the elderly and the undernourished.

Warnings: Undesirable reactions to ergotamine tartrate preparations may best be prevented by avoidance of excessive dosage and careful supervision of the patient so that he will not use the drug in larger dosage, more frequently, or for a longer time than prescribed by the physician. If Migral is used in the correct dosage and in the absence of the above contraindications, few serious complications will ensue.

Chronic ergotism. Because of the possible cumulative effects of ergotamine tartrate it is essential that the dosage of Migral be limited to usually not more than six tablets during one attack and, as a rule, not more than ten tablets in one week. Patients should be cautioned to use the minimal effective dose to control their

Continued on next page

Burroughs Wellcome—Cont.

symptoms. Symptoms of chronic ergotism include cold, pale and numb extremities, muscle pains both with and without activity, decreased or even obliterated peripheral pulses and gangrene of the fingers and toes. Other symptoms of ergotism may occur including anginal pain, tachycardia, bradycardia, changes in blood pressure in either direction, headache, nausea, vomiting, diarrhea, itching, formication, anal burning, weakness, miosis, confusion, depression, drowsiness, increase in muscle tone with pain and trismus and, rarely, convulsions and hemiplegia.

The central nervous system depressant and the atropine-like effects common to all antihistamines may be seen with cyclizine hydrochloride. The patient should be warned that if drowsiness occurs, operation of motor vehicles or other machinery may be potentially hazardous.

Precautions: In rare instances, patients, particularly those who have used the medication indiscriminately over long periods of time, will display withdrawal symptoms consisting primarily of headache upon discontinuation of the drug.

Adverse Reactions: The following reactions have been reported after therapeutic doses of ergotamine tartrate: nausea, vomiting, diarrhea, polydipsia, tingling of the hands and feet, muscle pains and cramps, thrombophlebitis, vascular spasm, rare cases of gangrene, sleepiness, exhaustion, EKG changes, precordial pain, angina and myocardial infarction.

Dosage and Administration: Migral is most effective when taken in the prodromal stage of an attack. This is the period of vasoconstriction during which visual and other sensory disturbances may be experienced. This stage may last for 15 to 30 minutes and, if uncontrolled, it is followed by vasodilation which results in an intense, throbbing headache, usually unilateral, and frequently accompanied by nausea and vomiting. Finally, the cranial blood vessels may become edematous and give rise to a steady, dull headache persisting for hours or days. This may be accompanied by nausea, vomiting, sweating and chilliness.

The lowest effective dosage should be employed but must be determined on an individual basis. It is important that treatment be initiated at the first sign of an attack, preferably prior to the onset of actual headache. If the pathophysiological progression to the vasodilatational stage can be prevented, headaches may actually be eliminated. In the first course of treatment it is suggested that one Migral tablet be taken at the earliest sign of an attack. If symptoms are not relieved, repeated doses at one-half or one hour intervals may be administered. If this proves unsuccessful higher initial doses up to 3 or 4 tablets may be taken at the onset of subsequent attacks with repeated doses at one-half or one hour intervals but **ordinarily no more than six tablets should be administered for each attack, and as a rule not more than ten tablets in one week.**

How Supplied: Bottle of 100 tablets.

[*Shown in Product Identification Section*]

MYLERAN®
brand Busulfan ℞

Caution: Myleran brand Busulfan is a potent cytotoxic drug. Blood counts should be taken at frequent intervals and not less than weekly. Therapy should be discontinued or the dosage reduced at the first signs of abnormal depression of bone marrow.

Description: A sulfonic ester, 1, 4-dimethanesulfonoxybutane.

Indications: Administered orally in therapeutic doses, busulfan has proved to be of value in the treatment of chronic myelocytic leukemia. It is not curative, but affords effective control of symptoms with the expectancy of prolonging life. The drug has been found useful both in patients with prior therapy of radiation or P^{32} and in those untreated by any other means.

Contraindications: Busulfan should not be given if other similar chemotherapeutic agents or radiation has been administered in the recent past, or if neutrophil or platelet counts are depressed.

Warnings:

Use in Pregnancy: Alkylating agents used in treating human cancer are known to produce fetal malformations in certain experimental animals when given in sufficient dosage at the proper time. Also, cases of harmful effects on human conceptus such as fetal death and congenital malformations (early in pregnancy), and intrauterine growth retardation and bone marrow depression (late in gestation), as well as damage to the developing gonads, have been reported with alkylating agents. Although scattered reports of the successful conclusion of pregnancy and of the birth of normal infants to women receiving busulfan have appeared in the literature, nonetheless it is advisable to avoid the use of the drug during the first gestational trimester unless maternal survival will be jeopardized. The possible benefits of the use of busulfan later in pregnancy should be weighed against the considered risks. The safety of its use in lactation has not been established.

Precautions: Use of the drug should be restricted to patients where facilities for complete blood counts at weekly, or more frequent, intervals and other laboratory studies which may seem indicated, are available. The most careful clinical and hematological supervision is essential for early detection and prompt management of the toxic effects.

Adverse Reactions: The chief toxic effect is a dosage related myelosuppression which may cause thrombocytopenia (hemorrhage) and eventually lead to pancytopenia. Rapid destruction of granulocytes may be accompanied by hyperuricemia and uric acid nephropathy. This complication may now be avoided by using allopurinol. Other complications of therapy include instances of nausea, vomiting, diarrhea, cheilosis, glossitis, impotence, sterility, amenorrhea, gynecomastia, generalized skin pigmentation, anhidrosis, alopecia and interstitial pulmonary fibrosis. The melanoderma accompanied at times with digestive troubles, fatigue, muscular weakness and weight loss may simulate adrenocortical insufficiency.

Dosage and Administration: Busulfan is issued as a scored tablet containing 2 mg of the drug for oral administration. Usual dosage is 4 to 8 mg daily depending on the total leukocyte count and the severity of the disease. Therapy is continued until the leukocyte count falls below 10,000/cu mm. During remission the patient is examined at monthly intervals and the treatment is resumed when the white cell count reaches 50,000/cu mm. When remission is shorter than three months, maintenance therapy of 1 to 3 mg daily may be advisable in order to keep the hematological status under control and prevent rapid relapse.

How Supplied: Tablet of 2 mg, scored. Bottles of 25. Bears Wellcome I.D. Code imprint K2A.

[*Shown in Product Identification Section*]

NEOSPORIN® AEROSOL ℞
Polymyxin B—Bacitracin—Neomycin Powder For Topical Use Only (Not Sterile)

Description: Each aerosol spray packing of 90 g contains: Aerosporin® brand Polymyxin B Sulfate 100,000 units; bacitracin zinc 8,000 units; neomycin sulfate 100 mg (equivalent to 70 mg neomycin base).

Inert propellant: dichlorodifluoromethane and trichloromonofluoromethane.

Approximate spraying time of the container is 100 seconds.

Action: The combination of Aerosporin brand Polymyxin B Sulfate with neomycin and bacitracin was selected because it most nearly meets the criteria for an ideal topical antibacterial preparation. The spectrum of action encompasses most pathogenic bacteria found topically, and the three antibiotics are bactericidal rather than bacteriostatic. When used topically, polymyxin B, neomycin and bacitracin are rarely irritating, and absorption from skin or mucous membrane is insignificant. The index of allergenicity of this combination has been shown over the years to be low. And finally, since these antibiotics are seldom used systemically, the patient is spared sensitization to those antibiotics which might later be required systemically.

Polymyxin B is one of a group of closely related substances produced by various strains of *Bacillus polymyxa.* Its activity is sharply restricted to gram-negative bacteria, including many strains of *Pseudomonas aeruginosa.*

Neomycin, isolated from *Streptomyces fradiae,* has antibacterial activity *in vitro* against a wide range of gram-negative and gram-positive organisms, with effectiveness against many strains of *Proteus.*

Bacitracin, an antibiotic substance derived from cultures of *Bacillus subtilis* (Tracy), exerts antibacterial action *in vitro* against a variety of gram-positive and a few gram-negative organisms.

Indications: Based on a review of this drug by the National Academy of Sciences-National Research Council and/or other information, FDA has classified the indications as follows:

"Possibly" effective: For topical administration for the treatment of the listed localized infections or for suppressive therapy in such conditions:

Biopsy sites	Abrasions
Vascular ulcers	Cuts
Decubitus ulcers	Lacerations
Burns	Infected eczemas
Dermabrasion	Infected dermatoses
	Skin grafts and donor sites

Final classification of the less-than-effective indications requires further investigation.

Contraindications: This product is contraindicated in those individuals who have shown hypersensitivity to any of its components.

Warning: Because of the potential hazard of nephrotoxicity and ototoxicity due to neomycin, care should be exercised when using this product in treating extensive burns, trophic ulceration and other extensive conditions where absorption of neomycin is possible. In burns where more than 20 percent of the body surface is affected, especially if the patient has impaired renal function or is receiving other aminoglycoside antibiotics concurrently, not more than one application a day is recommended.

When using neomycin-containing products to control secondary infection in the chronic dermatoses, such as chronic otitis externa or stasis dermatitis, it should be borne in mind that the skin in these conditions is more liable than is normal skin to become sensitized to many substances, including neomycin. The manifestation of sensitization to neomycin is usually a low grade reddening with swelling, dry scaling and itching; it may be manifest simply as failure to heal. During long-term use of neomycin-containing products, periodic examination for such signs is advisable and the patient should be told to discontinue the product if they are observed. These symptoms regress quickly on withdrawing the medication. Neomycin-containing applications should be avoided for that patient thereafter.

Precautions: As with other antibiotic preparations, prolonged use may result in overgrowth of nonsusceptible organisms including fungi. Appropriate measures should be taken if this occurs. Do not spray in the eyes. Contents are under pressure, but are not flammable. Do not puncture or incinerate container.
Adverse Reactions: Neomycin is a not uncommon cutaneous sensitizer. Articles in the current literature indicate an increase in the prevalence of persons allergic to neomycin. Ototoxicity and nephrotoxicity have been reported (see Warning section).
Dosage and Administration: SHAKE WELL before each spraying. Remove cap, twist off tamper-proof seal and press button to spray affected area. Container will operate in either upright or inverted position. Use one-second intermittent sprays from a distance of about 8 inches. Prolonged spraying is unnecessary and wastes medication.
How Supplied: Aerosol spray can of 90 g.

NEOSPORIN®-G CREAM ℞
Polymyxin B—Neomycin—Gramicidin

Description: Each gram contains:
Aerosporin® brand Polymyxin B Sulfate 10,000 units; neomycin sulfate 5 mg (equivalent to 3.5 mg neomycin base); gramicidin 0.25 mg.
Inactive ingredients: liquid petrolatum, white petrolatum, purified water, propylene glycol, polyoxyethylene polyoxypropylene compound, emulsifying wax, and 0.25% methylparaben as preservative.

Indications: Based on a review of this drug by the National Academy of Sciences—National Research Council and/or other information, FDA has classified the indications as follows:
"Possibly" effective: For topical administration for the treatment of the listed localized infections or for suppressive therapy in such conditions: primary pyodermas (impetigo, ecthyma, sycosis vulgaris, paronychia); secondary infected dermatoses (eczema, herpes and seborrheic dermatitis); traumatic lesions (inflamed or suppurating as a result of bacterial infection).
Final classification of the less-than-effective indications requires further investigation.

Contraindications: Not for use in the eyes or in the external ear canal if the eardrum is perforated. This product is contraindicated in those individuals who have shown hypersensitivity to any of its components.
Warning: Because of the potential hazard of nephrotoxicity and ototoxicity due to neomycin, care should be exercised when using this product in treating extensive burns, trophic ulceration and other extensive conditions where absorption of neomycin is possible. In burns where more than 20 percent of the body surface is affected, especially if the patient has impaired renal function or is receiving other aminoglycoside antibiotics concurrently, not more than one application a day is recommended.
When using neomycin-containing products to control secondary infection in the chronic dermatoses, such as chronic otitis externa or stasis dermatitis, it should be borne in mind that the skin in these conditions is more liable than is normal skin to become sensitized to many substances, including neomycin. The manifestation of sensitization to neomycin is usually a low grade reddening with swelling, dry scaling and itching; it may be manifest simply as a failure to heal. During long-term use of neomycin-containing products, periodic examination for such signs is advisable and the patient should be told to discontinue the product if they are observed. These symptoms regress quickly on withdrawing the medication. Neomycin-containing applications should be avoided for that patient thereafter.
Precautions: As with other antibacterial preparations, prolonged use may result in overgrowth of nonsusceptible organisms, including fungi. Appropriate measures should be taken if this occurs.
Adverse Reactions: Neomycin is a not uncommon cutaneous sensitizer. Articles in the current literature indicate an increase in the prevalence of persons allergic to neomycin. Ototoxicity and nephrotoxicity have been reported (see Warning section).
Dosage and Administration: A small quantity of the cream should be applied 2 to 5 times daily, as required. The cream should, if conditions permit, be gently rubbed into the affected areas.
How Supplied: Tube of 15 g.
15 g—DoD & VA NSN 6505-00-926-2159

NEOSPORIN® G.U. IRRIGANT ℞
brand Neomycin Sulfate—Polymyxin B Sulfate G.U. Irrigant, Sterile. A Concentrated Antibiotic Solution To Be Diluted For Urinary Bladder Irrigation. NOT FOR INJECTION.

Description: Each cc contains neomycin sulfate equivalent to neomycin base 40 mg, polymyxin B sulfate 200,000 units, pyrogen-free distilled water qs. Multiple-dose vial contains methylparaben 1 mg (0.1%) as preservative.
Action: Polymyxin B sulfate is bactericidal to most gram-negative bacilli, including clinically isolated strains of *Pseudomonas aeruginosa (B pyocyaneus).* This organism is conspicuously absent from the spectra of most other antibiotic agents, but it is highly susceptible to polymyxin B sulfate, which is acknowledged to be an effective agent for the treatment and prophylaxis of *Pseudomonas* infections.
Neomycin sulfate is bactericidal against a wide range of gram-negative and gram-positive organisms. It is particularly effective against many strains of *Proteus.*
When used topically, polymyxin B sulfate and neomycin are rarely irritating. Since these antibiotics are seldom used systemically, the patient is spared sensitization to those antibiotics which might later be required systemically.
Indications: To be used as a continuous irrigant or rinse for short-term use *(up to 10 days)* in the urinary bladder of abacteriuric patients to help prevent bacteriuria and gram-negative rod bacteremia, associated with the use of indwelling catheters.
Contraindications: This product is contraindicated in those individuals who have shown hypersensitivity to any of its components.
Precautions: As with other antibiotic preparations, prolonged use may result in overgrowth of nonsusceptible organisms, including fungi. Appropriate measures should be taken if this occurs. The safety and effectiveness of this preparation for use in the care of patients with recent lower urinary tract surgery have not been established.
Neomycin toxicity: Neomycin is nephrotoxic and ototoxic, particularly when given parenterally in higher than recommended doses. Cases of nephrotoxicity and/or ototoxicity have been reported following its use in treatment of extensive burns and irrigation of wounds. Although the possibility of these reactions is remote with the use of the minimal amount in bladder irrigations, such may occur if irrigations are continued over the recommended time of "under 10 days"; caution should be observed.
Adverse Reactions: Hypersensitivity reactions: According to current medical literature there has been an increase in the prevalence of neomycin hypersensitivity, however, topical application to mucous membrane rarely result in local or systemic reactions.
Dosage and Administration: This preparation is specifically designed for use with "three-way" catheters or with other catheter systems permitting *continuous* irrigation of the urinary bladder.
Using sterile precautions, one (1) cc of Neosporin G.U. Irrigant should be added to a 1,000 cc container of isotonic saline solution. This container should then be connected to the inflow lumen of the "three-way" catheter which has been inserted with full aseptic precautions; use of a sterile lubricant is recommended during insertion of the catheter. The outflow lumen should be connected, via a sterile disposable plastic tube, to a disposable plastic collection bag.
Inflow rate, for most patients, of the 1,000 cc saline solution of neomycin and polymyxin B, should be adjusted to a slow drip to deliver about 1,000 cc every twenty-four hours. If the patient's urine output exceeds 2 liters per day it is recommended that the inflow rate should be adjusted to deliver 2,000 cc of the solution in a twenty-four hour period.
It is important that the rinse of the bladder be *continuous:* the inflow or rinse solution should not be interrupted for more than a few minutes.
Clinical Background: Extremely high rates of infection of the urinary tract following indwelling catheterization have been reported. The serious sequelae of urinary tract infections, such as hypertension, pregnancy toxemia, premature labor, perinatal mortality, azotemia and renal failure have been substantiated. Recently the seriousness and increasing incidence of gram-negative rod bacteremia have been appreciated—and clear recognition of its close association with indwelling catheterization noted.
Clinical and experimental evidence has demonstrated that organisms gain entrance to the bladder by way of, through, and around the catheter. Significant bacteriuria is then induced by bacterial multiplication in the bladder urine, in the mucoid film often present between catheter and urethra and in other sites. Although recently acquired bacteriuria may or may not have clinical significance, Kass has demonstrated that the hallmark of urinary tract infection is the repeated presence in the urine of large numbers of pathogenic bacteria, usually over 100,000 organisms/ml.
Evidence has been presented that the use of closed systems with indwelling catheters reduces the risk of infection. Such systems, however, demand rigid techniques and probably are appropriate only under ideal conditions.
The effectiveness of a three-way catheter and a continuous neomycin-polymyxin B bladder rinse in preventing bacteriuria after indwelling catheterization was first reported by Martin and Bookrajian: "The selection of neomycin and polymyxin as the active components of a continuous bladder rinse solution was based on the evidence that both compounds are bactericidal in low concentration, that few potential urinary tract pathogens are resistant to both, and that the use of 2 drugs against a pathogen sensitive to both will reduce the probability of acquisition of resistance to either."
In a controlled study of the efficacy of the three-way catheter system with constant neomycin-polymyxin B bladder rinse, Meyers et al demonstrated that the cumulative rates of acquisition of bacteriuria were only 4, 6 and 10 percent after 5, 10 and 15 days of catheterization, respectively.
Elimination of the standard indwelling catheter and institution of routine hospitalwide use of the three-way catheter with continuous neomycin-polymyxin B bladder rinse has been reported to cause a marked reduction in the incidence of both fatal and nonfatal gram-negative rod bacteremia.

Continued on next page

Burroughs Wellcome—Cont.

Supplied: Ampul of 1 cc, boxes of 12 and 100 ampuls. 20 cc multiple-dose vials.

NEOSPORIN® OINTMENT
Polymyxin B-Bacitracin-Neomycin

Description: Each gram contains: Aerosporin® brand Polymyxin B Sulfate 5,000 units; bacitracin zinc 400 units; neomycin sulfate 5 mg (equivalent to 3.5 mg neomycin base); special white petrolatum qs.
Action: The overlapping spectra of the antibiotics provide effective antibacterial action against most commonly occurring bacteria known to be topical invaders. The range of antibacterial activity encompasses many bacteria which are, or have become, resistant to other antibiotics or chemicals—notably *Pseudomonas* and *Staphylococcus.* In susceptible organisms, resistance rarely develops, even on repeated or prolonged use.
Indications: *Therapeutically,* (as an adjunct to systemic therapy when indicated), for topical infections, primary or secondary, due to susceptible organisms, as in: infected burns, skin grafts, surgical incisions, otitis externa; primary pyodermas (impetigo, ecthyma, sycosis vulgaris, paronychia); secondarily infected dermatoses (eczema, herpes, and seborrheic dermatitis); traumatic lesions, inflamed or suppurating as a result of bacterial infection. *Prophylactically,* the ointment may be used to prevent bacterial contamination in burns, skin grafts, incisions, and other clean lesions. For abrasions, minor cuts and wounds accidentally incurred, its use may prevent the development of infection and permit wound healing.
Contraindications: Not for use in the eyes or external ear canal if the eardrum is perforated. This product is contraindicated in those individuals who have shown hypersensitivity to any of its components.
Warning: Because of the potential hazard of nephrotoxicity and ototoxicity due to neomycin, care should be exercised when using this product in treating extensive burns, trophic ulceration and other extensive conditions where absorption of neomycin is possible. In burns where more than 20 percent of the body surface is affected, especially if the patient has impaired renal function or is receiving other aminoglycoside antibiotics concurrently, not more than one application a day is recommended.
When using neomycin-containing products to control secondary infection in the chronic dermatoses, such as chronic otitis externa or stasis dermatitis, it should be borne in mind that the skin in these conditions is more liable than is normal skin to become sensitized to many substances, including neomycin. The manifestation of sensitization to neomycin is usually a low grade reddening with swelling, dry scaling and itching; it may be manifest simply as a failure to heal. During long term use of neomycin-containing products, periodic examination for such signs is advisable and the patient should be told to discontinue the product if they are observed. These symptoms regress quickly on withdrawing the medication. Neomycin-containing applications should be avoided for that patient thereafter.
Precautions: As with other antibiotic products, prolonged use may result in overgrowth of nonsusceptible organisms, including fungi. Appropriate measures should be taken if this occurs.
Adverse Reactions: Neomycin is a not uncommon cutaneous sensitizer. Articles in the current literature indicate an increase in the prevalence of persons allergic to neomycin. Ototoxicity and nephrotoxicity have been reported (see Warning section).
Dosage and Administration: Apply to the affected area 2 to 5 times daily, depending on the severity of the condition. May be left exposed or covered with a dressing, as indicated.
How Supplied: Tubes of 1 oz and ½ oz and foil packet of 1/32 oz (approx.) in box of 144 for topical use only.

NEOSPORIN® OINTMENT ℞
Polymyxin B-Bacitracin-Neomycin
OPHTHALMIC
Sterile

Description: Each gram contains: Aerosporin® brand Polymyxin B Sulfate 5,000 units; bacitracin zinc 400 units; neomycin sulfate 5 mg (equivalent to 3.5 mg. neomycin base); special white petrolatum qs.
Actions: Polymyxin B is one of a group of closely related substances produced by various strains of *Bacillus polymyxa.* Its activity is sharply restricted to gram-negative bacteria, including many strains of *Pseudomonas aeruginosa.*
Neomycin, isolated from *Streptomyces fradiae,* has antibacterial activity *in vitro* against a wide range of gram-negative and gram-positive organisms, with effectiveness against many strains of *Proteus.*
Bacitracin, an antibiotic substance derived from cultures of *Bacillus subtilis* (Tracy), exerts antibacterial action *in vitro* against a variety of gram-positive and a few gram-negative organisms.
Indications: This product is indicated in the short-term treatment of superficial external ocular infections caused by organisms susceptible to one or more of the antibiotics contained therein.
Contraindications: This product is contraindicated in those persons who have shown sensitivity to any of its components.
Warnings: Prolonged use may result in overgrowth of nonsusceptible organisms. Ophthalmic ointment may retard corneal healing.
Precautions: Culture and susceptibility testing should be performed during treatment.
Allergic cross-reactions may occur which could prevent the use of any or all of the following antibiotics for the treatment of future infections: kanamycin, paromomycin, streptomycin, and possibly gentamicin.
Adverse Reactions: Neomycin is a not uncommon cutaneous sensitizer. Articles in the current literature indicate an increase in the prevalence of persons allergic to neomycin.
Dosage and Administration: Apply the ointment every 3 or 4 hours, depending on the severity of the infection.
How Supplied: Tube of ⅛ oz with ophthalmic tip.
⅛ oz. × 12—DoD NSN 6505-00-530-6469

NEOSPORIN® OPHTHALMIC SOLUTION Sterile ℞
Polymyxin B-Neomycin-Gramicidin

Description: Each cc contains: Aerosporin® brand Polymyxin B Sulfate 5,000 units; neomycin sulfate 2.5 mg (equivalent to 1.75 mg neomycin base); gramicidin 0.025 mg. Vehicle contains alcohol 0.5%, thimerosal (preservative) 0.001% and the inactive ingredients propylene glycol, polyoxyethylene polyoxypropylene compound, sodium chloride and purified water.
Indications: This product is indicated in the short-term treatment of superficial external ocular infections caused by organisms susceptible to one or more of the antibiotics contained therein.
Contraindications: This product is contraindicated in those persons who have shown sensitivity to any of its components.
Warnings: Prolonged use may result in overgrowth of nonsusceptible organisms.
Precautions: Culture and susceptibility testing should be performed during treatment.
Allergic cross-reactions may occur which could prevent the use of any or all of the following antibiotics for the treatment of future infections: kanamycin, paromomycin, streptomycin, and possibly gentamicin.
Adverse Reactions: Neomycin is a not uncommon cutaneous sensitizer. Articles in the current literature indicate an increase in the prevalence of persons allergic to neomycin.
Dosage and Administration: The suggested dosage is one or two drops in the affected eye, two to four times daily, or more frequently, as required. In acute infections initiate therapy with one or two drops every 15 to 30 minutes, reducing the frequency of instillation gradually as the infection is controlled.
The patient should be instructed to avoid contaminating the applicator tip with material from an infected eye or other source. This is best done by preventing the tip from touching the eyelid or surrounding areas. This caution is necessary in order to keep the sterile solution as free from contaminating organisms as possible.
How Supplied: 10 cc Drop Dose® (plastic dispenser bottle).
10 cc—DoD NSN 6505-00-890-1299
10 cc—VA NSN 6505-01-012-2906

NEOSPORIN® POWDER ℞
Polymyxin B—Bacitracin—Neomycin
For Topical Use Only (Not Sterile)

Description: Each gram contains: Aerosporin® brand Polymyxin B Sulfate 5,000 units; bacitracin zinc 400 units; neomycin sulfate 5 mg (equivalent to 3.5 mg neomycin base); in a special lactose base.

> **Indications:** Based on a review of this drug by the National Academy of Sciences—National Research Council and/or other information, FDA has classified the indications as follows:
> "Possibly" effective: For topical administration for the treatment of the listed localized infections or for suppressive therapy in such conditions:
> Prophylactic:
> Postoperative and traumatic surface wounds
> Biopsy sites
> Skin grafts and donor sites
> Dermabrasion
> Therapeutic (when infected by susceptible organisms):
> Vascular ulcers
> Decubitus ulcers
> Pyodermas
> Infected eczemas
> Infected dermatoses
> Final classification of the less-than-effective indications requires further investigation.

Contraindications: This product is contraindicated in those individuals who have shown hypersensitivity to any of its components.
Warning: Because of the potential hazard of nephrotoxicity and ototoxicity due to neomycin, care should be exercised when using this product in treating extensive burns, trophic ulceration and other extensive conditions where absorption of neomycin is possible. In burns where more than 20 percent of the body surface is affected, especially if the patient has impaired renal function or is receiving other aminoglycoside antibiotics concurrently, not more than one application a day is recommended.
When using neomycin-containing products to control secondary infection in the chronic dermatoses, such as chronic otitis externa or stasis dermatitis, it should be borne in mind that the skin in these conditions is more liable than is normal skin to become sensitized to many substances, including neomycin. The manifesta-

tion of sensitization to neomycin is usually a low grade reddening with swelling, dry scaling and itching; it may be manifest simply as a failure to heal. During long term use of neomycin-containing products, periodic examination for such signs is advisable and the patient should be told to discontinue the product if they are observed. These symptoms regress quickly on withdrawing the medication. Neomycin-containing applications should be avoided for that patient thereafter.
Precautions: As with other antibiotic preparations, prolonged use may result in overgrowth of nonsusceptible organisms, including fungi. Appropriate measures should be taken if this occurs. It is to be noted that the powder is not intended for sterile use in surgical procedures such as those involving abdominal or thoracic body cavities.
Adverse Reactions: Neomycin is a not uncommon cutaneous sensitizer. Articles in the current literature indicate an increase in the prevalence of persons allergic to neomycin. Ototoxicity and nephrotoxicity have been reported (see Warning section).
Dosage and Administration: Apply lightly to the area to be treated as often as needed; treated area may be covered with a dressing or left exposed, as desired. In biopsy sites, dermabraded areas, etc., the powder may be mixed with a little powdered gelatin foam to provide concurrent hemostasis.
How Supplied: Shaker-top vial of 10 g.

POLYSPORIN® OINTMENT
Polymyxin B-Bacitracin

Description: Each gram contains: Aerosporin brand Polymyxin B Sulfate 10,000 units; bacitracin zinc 500 units in a special petrolatum base.
Action: Combined antibiotic action against gram-negative and gram-positive organisms.
Indications: *Therapeutically,* (as an adjunct to systemic therapy when indicated), for topical infections, primary or secondary, due to susceptible organisms, as in: infected burns, skin grafts, surgical incisions, otitis externa; primary pyodermas (impetigo, ecthyma, sycosis vulgaris, paronychia); secondarily infected dermatoses (eczema, herpes, and seborrheic dermatitis); traumatic lesions, inflamed or suppurating as a result of bacterial infection. *Prophylactically,* the ointment may be used to prevent bacterial contamination in burns, skin grafts, incisions, and other clean lesions. For abrasions, minor cuts and wounds accidentally incurred, its use may prevent the development of infection and permit wound healing.
Contraindication: This product is contraindicated in those individuals who have shown hypersensitivity to any of its components.
Precaution: As with other antibiotic products, prolonged use may result in overgrowth of nonsusceptible organisms including fungi. Appropriate measures should be taken if this occurs.
Dosage and Administration: Apply 2 to 5 times daily, depending on the severity of the infection.
How Supplied: Tubes of ½ oz, 1 oz and ¹⁄₃₂ oz (approx.) foil packet in box of 144.
1 oz.—VA NSN 6505-00-579-9110

POLYSPORIN® OINTMENT ℞
Polymyxin B—Bacitracin
OPHTHALMIC
Sterile

Description: Each gram contains: Aerosporin® brand Polymyxin B Sulfate 10,000 units; bacitracin zinc 500 units; special white petrolatum qs.
Action: Polymyxin B attacks gram-negative bacilli, including virtually all strains of *Pseudomonas aeruginosa* and *H influenzae* species. Bacitracin is active against most gram-positive bacilli and cocci, including hemolytic streptococci.
Indications: For the treatment of superficial ocular infections involving the conjunctiva and/or cornea caused by organisms susceptible to polymyxin B sulfate and bacitracin zinc.
Contraindications: This product is contraindicated in those individuals who have shown hypersensitivity to any of its components.
Warnings: Ophthalmic ointments may retard corneal healing.
Precautions: As with other antibiotic preparations, prolonged use may result in overgrowth of nonsusceptible organisms, including fungi. Appropriate measures should be taken if this occurs.
Dosage and Administration: Apply the ointment every 3 or 4 hours, depending on the severity of the infection.
How Supplied: Tube of ⅛ oz with ophthalmic tip.

PURINETHOL® ℞
brand Mercaptopurine

Caution: Purinethol brand Mercaptopurine is a potent drug. Blood counts should be taken weekly. Discontinue or reduce the dosage immediately at the first sign of abnormal depression of bone marrow.
Description: Mercaptopurine, synthesized and studied at the Wellcome Research Laboratories, is an analogue of the nucleic acid constituent adenine and the purine base hypoxanthine, to both of which it is a metabolic antagonist.
Action: Believed to interfere with nucleic acid biosynthesis.
Indications: This drug is indicated primarily for the treatment of acute leukemia. In general, it appears that a higher proportion of children than adults responds favorably to the drug.
A few patients with chronic myelocytic leukemia have obtained temporary remission after administration of the drug.
It is not indicated in the treatment of chronic lymphatic leukemia, Hodgkin's disease or solid tumors.
Toxicity: Toxicity, studied by Philips et al and by Clarke et al, with mercaptopurine in dogs, cats, rats and mice at doses of the order of 25 mg/kg included anorexia, weight loss, reticulopenia, leukopenia and diarrhea; microscopic lesions included hypoplasia of bone marrow and degenerative changes in the intestinal epithelium and liver. The effects were delayed even when lethal doses were given.
Adverse Reactions:
Hematological effects: The chief toxic effect is hematologic, with leukopenia, and, with excessive dosage, thrombocytopenia and bleeding. In acute leukemia, however, treatment may be given in the presence of thrombocytopenia and bleeding and, in some cases, the bleeding has stopped and the platelet count has risen during treatment.
Dosage must be given cautiously, since the maximum effect on the blood count may be delayed, and the formed elements in the peripheral blood may fall for several days after treatment is stopped. *It is, therefore, important to discontinue the drug temporarily at the first evidence of an abnormally large fall in the white cell count or of abnormal depression of the bone marrow.*
In many patients with severe depression of the formed elements of the blood due to mercaptopurine, the bone marrow appears hypoplastic on aspiration, whereas in other cases it seems normal. The qualitative changes in the erythroid elements towards the megaloblastic series, characteristically seen with the folic acid antagonists, are not seen with this drug.
Oral lesions: Oral lesions are rarely seen, and when they occur they resemble thrush rather than antifolic ulcerations.
Gastrointestinal symptoms: Nausea, vomiting and anorexia are uncommon during administration, but they may occur during toxicity. Mild diarrhea and sprue-like symptoms have been noted occasionally, but it is difficult at present to attribute these to the medication.
Other symptoms: Jaundice has been observed in some instances, suggesting possible liver damage or biliary stasis. In patients with high white cell counts at the onset of treatment or with massive disease, breakdown of tissue may cause hyperuricemia and consequent impairment of renal function, with oliguria. The metabolism of the drug has not been elucidated, thus far, and *it is probably advisable to start with smaller doses in the presence of impaired liver or renal function.* Drug fever has been observed on occasion.
Reversibility: In animals nothing has been found, thus far, including citrovorum factor (folinic acid), xanthine, hypoxanthine, guanine, and adenine, which will prevent or counteract the toxic effects of mercaptopurine.
Precautions: The dosage which will be tolerated or will be effective will vary from patient to patient and, therefore, careful management is necessary to obtain the optimum therapeutic effect without incurring toxicity. Caution must be exercised to avoid toxicity, the chief manifestation of which is depression of the bone marrow, resulting in leukopenia and eventually thrombocytopenia and bleeding. *Since this drug may have a delayed action, it is important to withdraw the medication temporarily at the first sign of an abnormally large fall in the white cell count or of abnormal depression of the bone marrow.* It is probably advisable to start with smaller doses in patients with impaired renal function since the latter might result in slower elimination of the drug and a greater cumulative effect. Jaundice has been observed in a few instances, suggesting possible liver damage or biliary stasis. It is recommended that mercaptopurine be withheld if there is evidence of toxic hepatitis or biliary stasis, as the jaundice may disappear. In some instances jaundice appears and subsequently disappears while the drug is being given; in other cases it may persist even after stopping the drug.
The section on Toxicity should be carefully considered before using the drug. Thus far there is no known antagonist to mercaptopurine and, therefore, the drug should be discontinued when toxicity develops.
Pregnancy Warning: Whenever possible, it seems best to defer use of cancer chemotherapeutic agents during pregnancy until after the first trimester.
Dosage and Administration: The dosage of Purinethol brand Mercaptopurine which will be tolerated or will be effective will vary from patient to patient and, therefore, careful management is necessary to obtain the optimum therapeutic effect without incurring toxicity.
The usual initial dose is approximately 2.5 mg/kg (1 mg per pound) body weight per day, orally (100 to 200 mg in the average adult and 50 mg in an average 5 year old child). Children with acute leukemia have tolerated this dose without difficulty in most cases; it may be continued daily for several weeks or more in some patients. If after four weeks on this dosage there is no clinical improvement and no definite evidence of leukocyte depression, the dosage may be increased up to 5 mg/kg daily.
A dosage of 2.5 mg/kg per day may result in a rapid fall in leukocyte count within 1 to 2 weeks in some adults with acute leukemia and high total leukocyte counts, as well as in certain adults with chronic myelocytic leukemia. Therefore, it is imperative to observe such patients carefully.
A total daily dosage may be given at one time. It is calculated to the closest multiple of 25 mg. The dosage of mercaptopurine should be reduced to ⅓ to ¼ of the usual dose if Zyloprim brand Allopurinol is given concurrently in a dosage of 300 to 600 mg daily to reduce or pre-

Continued on next page

Burroughs Wellcome—Cont.

vent hyperuricemia or to retard the metabolism of mercaptopurine. (Full information on allopurinol is available on request.)
The leukocyte count should be closely followed and since the drug may have a delayed action, it should be discontinued at the first sign of an abnormally large fall in the leukocyte count. If subsequently the leukocyte count remains constant for 2 or 3 days, or rises, treatment should be resumed. It is essential that a suitable maintenance dose be established if early relapse is to be avoided.
How Supplied: Tablet of 50 mg, scored. Bottles of 25 and 250. Tablet bears Wellcome ID Code 04A.
[*Shown in Product Identification Section*]

SEPTRA® TABLETS and SUSPENSION ℞
SEPTRA ® DS TABLETS Double Strength

Description: Septra is a synthetic antibacterial combination product, available in scored pink tablets, each containing 80 mg trimethoprim* and 400 mg sulfamethoxazole and in double strength, pink, scored tablets, each containing 160 mg trimethoprim and 800 mg sulfamethoxazole.
*Mfd. under Pat. 3,956,327
Also available as a pink, cherry flavored oral suspension, each teaspoonful (5 ml) containing the equivalent of 40 mg trimethoprim and 200 mg sulfamethoxazole compounded with 0.26% alcohol.
Trimethoprim is 2,4-diamino-5-(3,4,5-trimethoxybenzl) pyrimidine. It is a white to light yellow, odorless, bitter compound with a molecular weight of 290.3.
Sulfamethoxazole is N^1-(5-methyl-3-isoxazolyl) sulfanilamide. It is an almost white in color, odorless, tasteless compound with a molecular weight of 253.28.
Actions:
Microbiology: Sulfamethoxazole inhibits bacterial synthesis of dihydrofolic acid by competing with *para*-aminobenzoic acid. Trimethoprim blocks the production of tetrahydrofolic acid from dihydrofolic acid by binding to and reversibly inhibiting the required enzyme, dihydrofolate reductase. Thus, Septra blocks two consecutive steps in the biosynthesis of nucleic acids and proteins essential to many bacteria.
In vitro studies have shown that bacterial resistance develops more slowly with Septra than with trimethoprim or sulfamethoxazole alone.
In vitro serial dilution tests have shown that the spectrum of antibacterial activity of Septra includes the common urinary tract pathogens with the exception of *Pseudomonas aeruginosa*. The following organisms are usually susceptible: *Escherichia coli, Klebsiella-Enterobacter, Proteus mirabilis* and indole-positive *Proteus* species.
In addition, the usual spectrum of antimicrobial activity of Septra includes the following bacterial pathogens isolated from middle ear exudate and bronchial secretions: *Haemophilus influenzae,* including ampicillin resistant strains, and *Streptococcus pneumoniae. Shigella flexneri* and *Shigella sonnei* are also usually susceptible.
[See table below].
The recommended quantitative disc susceptibility method (Federal Register *37*:20527–29, 1972; Bauer AW, Kirby WMM, Sherris JC, Turck M: Antibiotic susceptibility testing by a standarized single disk method, Am J Clin Path *45*:493, 1966) may be used for estimating the susceptibility of bacteria to Septra. With this procedure, report from the laboratory of "Susceptible to trimethoprim-sulfamethoxazole" indicates that the infection is likely to respond to therapy with Septra. If the infection is confined to the urine, a report of "Intermediate susceptibility to trimethoprim-sulfamethoxazole" also indicates that the infection is likely to respond. A report of "Resistant to trimethoprim-sulfamethoxazole" indicates that the infection is unlikely to respond to therapy with Septra.
Human Pharmacology: Septra is rapidly absorbed following oral administration. The blood levels of trimethoprim and sulfamethoxazole are similar to those achieved when each component is given alone. Peak blood levels for the individual components occur one to four hours after oral administration. The half-lives of sulfamethoxazole and trimethoprim, 10 and 16 hours respectively, are relatively the same regardless of whether these compounds are administered as individual components or as Septra. Detectable amounts of trimethoprim and sulfamethoxazole are present in the blood 24 hours after drug administration. Free sulfamethoxazole and trimethoprim blood levels are proportionately dose dependent. On repeated administration, the steady-state ratio of trimethoprim to sulfamethoxazole levels in the blood is about 1:20.

REPRESENTATIVE MINIMUM INHIBITORY CONCENTRATION VALUES FOR SEPTRA SUSCEPTIBLE ORGANISMS (MIC-mcg/ml)

Bacteria	TMP Alone	SMX Alone	TMP/SMX (1:19) TMP	SMX
Escherichia coli	0.05–1.5	1.0 –245	0.05 –0.5	0.95 – 9.5
Proteus species (indole positive)	0.5 –5.0	7.35 –300	0.05 –1.5	0.95 –28.5
Proteus mirabilis	0.5 –1.5	7.35 – 30	0.05 –0.15	0.95 – 2.85
Klebsiella-Enterobacter	0.15–5.0	2.45 –245	0.05 –1.5	0.95 –28.5
Haemophilus influenzae	0.15–1.5	2.85 – 95	0.015 –0.15	0.285 – 2.85
Streptococcus pneumoniae	0.15–1.5	7.35 – 24.5	0.05 –0.15	0.95 – 2.85
Shigella flexneri†	<0.01–0.04	<0.16 –>320	<0.002 –0.03	0.04 –0.625
Shigella sonnei†	0.02–0.08	0.625 –>320	0.004 –0.06	0.08 –1.25

TMP = Trimethoprim SMX = Sulfamethoxazole
†Rudoy, R.C., Nelson, J.D., Haltalin, K.C. *Antimicrobial Agents and Chemotherapy 5:*439–43, 1974.

Sulfamethoxazole exists in the blood as free, conjugated and protein-bound forms; trimethoprim is present as free, protein-bound and metabolized forms. The free forms are considered to be the therapeutically active forms. Approximately 44 percent of trimethoprim and 70 percent of sulfamethoxazole are protein-bound in the blood. The presence of 10 mg percent sulfamethoxazole in plasma decreases the protein binding of trimethoprim to an insignificant degree; trimethoprim does not influence the protein binding of sulfamethoxazole.
Excretion of Septra is chiefly by the kidneys through both glomerular filtration and tubular secretion. Urine concentrations of both sulfamethoxazole and trimethoprim are considerably higher than are the concentrations in the blood. When administered together as in Septra, neither sulfamethoxazole nor trimethoprim affects the urinary exretion pattern of the other.
Indications and Usage:
URINARY TRACT INFECTIONS: **For the treatment of urinary tract infections due to susceptible strains of the following organisms:** *Escherichia coli, Klebsiella-Enterobacter, Proteus mirabilis, Proteus vulgaris, Proteus morganii.* **It is recommended that initial episodes of uncomplicated urinary tract infections be treated with a single effective antibacterial agent rather than the combination.**
Note: Currently, the increasing frequency of resistant organisms is a limitation of the usefulness of all antibacterial agents, especially in the treatment of these urinary tract infections.
ACUTE OTITIS MEDIA: **For the treatment of acute otitis media in children due to susceptible strains of** *Haemophilus influenzae* **or** *Streptococcus pneumoniae* **when in the judgment of the physician Septra offers some advantage over the use of other antimicrobial agents. Limited clinical information is presently available on the effectiveness of treatment of otitis media with Septra when the infection is due to** *Haemophilus influenzae* **resistant to ampicillin. To date, there are limited data on the safety of repeated use of Septra in children under two years of age. Septra is not indicated for prophylactic or prolonged administration in otitis media at any age.**
ACUTE EXACERBATIONS OF CHRONIC BRONCHITIS IN ADULTS: **For the treatment of acute exacerbations of chronic bronchitis due to susceptible strains of** *Haemophilus influenzae* **and** *Streptococcus pneumoniae,* **when in the judgment of the physician, Septra offers some advantage over the use of a single antimicrobial agent.**
SHIGELLOSIS: **For the treatment of enteritis caused by susceptible strains of** *Shigella flexneri* **and** *Shigella sonnei* **when antibacterial therapy is indicated.**
PNEUMOCYSTIS CARINII **PNEUMONITIS: Septra is also indicated in the treatment of documented** *Pneumocystis carinii* **pneumonitis. To date, this drug has been tested only in patients 9 months to 16 years of age who were immunosuppressed by cancer therapy.**
Contraindications: Hypersensitivity to trimethoprim or sulfonamides. Pregnancy and during the nursing period (see "Reproduction Studies"). Infants less than two months of age.
Warnings: SEPTRA SHOULD NOT BE USED IN THE TREATMENT OF STREPTOCOCCAL PHARYNGITIS. Clinical studies have documented that patients with Group A β-hemolytic streptococcal tonsillopharyngitis have a greater incidence of bacteriologic failure when treated with Septra than do those patients treated with penicillin as evidenced by failure to eradicate this organism from the tonsillopharyngeal area.
Deaths associated with the administration of sulfonamides have been reported from hypersensitivity reactions, agranulocytosis, aplastic

anemia and other blood dyscrasias. Experience with trimethoprim alone is much more limited, but it has been reported to interfere with hematopoiesis in occasional patients. In elderly patients concurrently receiving certain diuretics, primarily thiazides, an increased incidence of thrombopenia with purpura has been reported.

The presence of clinical signs such as sore throat, fever, pallor, purpura or jaundice may be early indications of serious blood disorders. Complete blood counts should be done frequently in patients receiving Septra. If a significant reduction in the count of any formed blood element is noted, Septra should be discontinued.

Precautions: Septra should be given with caution to patients with impaired renal or hepatic function, to those with possible folate deficiency and to those with severe allergy or bronchial asthma. In glucose-6-phosphate dehydrogenase-deficient individuals, hemolysis may occur. This reaction is frequently dose-related. Adequate fluid intake must be maintained in order to prevent crystalluria and stone formation. Urinalyses with careful microscopic examination and renal function tests should be performed during therapy, particularly for those patients with impaired renal function.

It has been reported that Septra may prolong the prothrombin time of patients who are receiving the anticoagulant warfarin. This interaction should be kept in mind when Septra is given to patients already on anticoagulant therapy, and the coagulation time should be reassessed.

Adverse Reactions: For completeness, all major reactions to sulfonamides and to trimethoprim are included below even though they may not have been with Septra.

Blood Dyscrasias: Agranulocytosis, aplastic anemia, megaloblastic anemia, thrombopenia, leukopenia, hemolytic anemia, purpura, hypoprothrombinemia and methemoglobinemia.

Allergic Reactions: Erythema multiforme, Stevens-Johnson syndrome, generalized skin eruptions, epidermal necrolysis, urticaria, serum sickness, pruritus, exfoliative dermatitis, anaphylactoid reactions, periorbital edema, conjuctival and scleral injection, photosensitization, arthralgia and allergic myocarditis.

Gastrointestinal Reactions: Glossitis, stomatitis, nausea, emesis, abdominal pains, hepatitis, diarrhea and pancreatitis.

C.N.S. Reactions: Headache, peripheral neuritis, mental depression, convulsions, ataxia, hallucinations, tinnitus, vertigo, insomnia, apathy, fatigue, muscle weakness and nervousness.

Miscellaneous Reactions: Drug, chills, and toxic nephrosis with oliguria and anuria. Periarteritis nodosa and L.E. phenomenon have occurred.

The sulfonamides bear certain chemical similarities to some goitrogens, diuretics (acetazolamide and the thiazides) and oral hypoglycemic agents. Goiter production, diuresis and hypoglycemia have occurred rarely in patients receiving sulfonamides. Cross-sensitivity may exist with these agents. Rats appear to be especially susceptible to the goitrogenic effects of sulfonamides, and long-term administration has produced thyroid malignancies in the species.

Dosage and Administration: Not recommended for use in infants less than two months of age.

URINARY TRACT INFECTIONS AND SHIGELLOSIS IN ADULTS AND CHILDREN, ACUTE OTITIS MEDIA IN CHILDREN AND ACUTE EXACERBATIONS OF CHRONIC BRONCHITIS IN ADULTS.

Adults: The usual adult dosage for the treatment of urinary tract infections and acute exacerbations of chronic bronchitis is one Septra DS Tablet every 12 hours for 10 to 14 days. An identical daily dosage is used for 5 days in the treatment of shigellosis.

Children: The recommended dose for children with urinary tract infections or acute otitis media is 8 mg/kg trimethoprim and 40 mg/kg sulfamethoxazole per 24 hours, given in two divided doses every 12 hours for 10 days. An identical daily dosage is used for 5 days in the treatment of shigellosis. The following table is a guideline for the attainment of this dosage using Septra Tablets or Suspension.

Children: Two months of age or older

Weight lb	Weight kg	Dose—every 12 hours Teaspoonfuls	Dose—every 12 hours Tablets
22	10	1 (5 ml)	½
44	20	2 (10 ml)	1
66	30	3 (15 ml)	1 ½
88	40	4 (20 ml)	2 (or 1 DS Tablet)

For patients with renal impairment:

Creatinine Clearance (ml/min)	Recommended Dosage Regimen
Above 30	Usual Standard Regimen
15–30	Half of the usual dosage regimen
Below 15	Use Not Recommended

PNEUMOCYSTIS CARINII **PNEUMONITIS:**
The recommended dosage for patients with documented *Pneumocystis carinii* pneumonitis is 20 mg/kg trimethoprim and 100 mg/kg sulfamethoxazole per 24 hours given in equally divided doses every 6 hours for 14 days. The following table is a guideline for the attainment of this dosage in children.

Weight lb	Weight kg	Dose—every 6 hours Teaspoonfuls	Dose—every 6 hours Tablets
18	8	1 (5 ml)	½
35	16	2 (10 ml)	1
53	24	3 (15 ml)	1 ½
70	32	4 (20 ml)	2 (or 1 DS Tablet)

How Supplied: TABLETS, containing 80 mg trimethoprim and 400 mg sulfamethoxazole—bottles of 40, 100, 500 and 1000 tablets; unit dose pack of 100. Regular strength tablets bear identification, SEPTRA Y2B.

ORAL SUSPENSION, containing the equivalent of 40 mg trimethoprim and 200 mg sulfamethoxazole in each teaspoonful (5 ml), cherry flavored—bottles of 100 ml and 450 ml. Also available in double strength, oval-shaped, pink, scored tablets containing 160 mg trimethoprim and 800 mg sulfamethoxazole—Compliance™ Pak of 20, bottles of 100 and unit dose pack of 100. Double strength tablets bear identification, SEPTRA DS O2C.

Reproduction Studies: In rats, doses of 533 mg/kg sulfamethoxazole or 200 mg/kg trimethoprim produced teratological effects, manifested mainly as cleft palate. The highest dose which did not cause cleft palates in rats was 512 mg/kg sulfamethoxazole or 192 mg/kg trimethoprim when administered separately. In two studies in rats, no teratology was observed when 512 mg/kg of sulfamethoxazole was used in combination with 128 mg/kg of trimethoprim. In one study, however, cleft palates were observed in one litter out of 9 when 355 mg/kg of sulfamethoxazole was used in combination with 88 mg/kg of trimethoprim. In rabbits, trimethoprim administered by intubation from days 8 to 16 of pregnancy at dosages up to 500 mg/kg resulted in higher incidences of dead and resorbed fetuses, particularly at 500 mg/kg. However, there were no significant drug-related teratological effects.

[Shown in Product Identification Section]

SUDAFED®
brand Pseudoephedrine Hydrochloride

Description: Pseudoephedrine hydrochloride. 1 - phenyl - 2 - methylamine - propanol - 1 hydrochloride, a physiologically active stereoisomer of ephedrine; white, crystalline powder, freely soluble in water.

Action: Sudafed brand Pseudoephedrine Hydrochloride is an orally effective nasal decongestant, bronchodilator which takes effect in 15 to 30 minutes after administration. Full effect occurs within 30 to 60 minutes. The mucous membrane of the respiratory tract is gently but promptly decongested through action on the sympathetic nerves.

Indications: For use in acute coryza, vasomotor rhinitis, acute eustachian salpingitis, aerotitis (barotitis) media, serous otitis media with eustachian tube congestion.

In the following conditions, adjunctive therapy with analgesics, antihistaminics, antibiotics, expectorants and other measures may be employed with Sudafed for optimum results: allergic rhinitis, croup, acute and subacute sinusitis, asthma, acute otitis media, acute tracheobronchitis.

Precautions: Although pseudoephedrine is virtually without pressor effect in normotensive patients, it should be used with caution in hypertensives.

Side Effects: While the majority of patients will experience no side effects, those particularly sensitive to sympathomimetic drugs may note mild stimulation.

Dosage and Administration: Dosage indicated below may be given 3-4 times daily.

Syrup (30 mg per 5 cc): Older children and adults—2 tsp; children 4 months through 6 years of age—1 tsp; infants up to 4 months of age—½ tsp.

Tablets (60 mg, scored ℞): Older children and adults—1 tablet; children 4 months through 6 years of age—½ tablet.

Tablets (30 mg, sugar-coated): Older children and adults—2 tablets; children 4 months through 6 years of age—1 tablet.

Sudafed brand Pseudoephedrine Hydrochloride Syrup and 30 mg Tablets may be sold without prescription for the symptomatic relief of nasal and sinus congestion and allergic conditions associated with colds, hay fever; and for minor attacks of bronchial asthma.

O-T-C Caution: Do not exceed recommended dosage unless directed by a physician. If symptoms persist for 5 days or are accompanied by high fever, consult your physician before continuing use. Reduce dosage if nervousness, dizziness, sleeplessness, nausea or headache occur. Individuals with high blood pressure, heart disease, diabetes, urinary retention, glaucoma or thyroid disease should use only as directed by a physician. Consult your physician if pregnant or nursing, or taking other medication.

Recommended O-T-C dosage of 30 mg tablets: Adults and children over 12 years of age, 2 tablets every 4 hours. Children 6–12 years, 1 tablet every 4 hours. For children 2–5 years, use Sudafed® Syrup, ½ teaspoonful every 4 hours. Do not exceed 4 doses in 24 hours. For children under 2 years of age, give only as directed by a physician. **Recommended O-T-C dosage of syrup:** Adults and children over 12 years of age, 2 teaspoonfuls every 4 hours. Children 6–12 years, 1 teaspoonful every 4 hours. Children 2–5 years, ½ teaspoonful every 4 hours. Do not exceed 4 doses in 24 hours. For children under 2 years of age, give only as directed by a physician.

How Supplied: Tablets of 30 mg, sugar-coated (red). Box of 24, bottles of 100 and 1000. Tablets

Continued on next page

Burroughs Wellcome—Cont.

of 60 mg ℞, scored (white) with Wellcome I.D. code imprint S7A. Bottles of 100 and 1000. Syrup, 30 mg per 5 cc tsp. Bottles of 4 fl. oz and 1 pt.

Syrup 4 oz. —DoD
NSN 6505-00-133-4948
Pint —DoD
NSN 6505-00-065-4206

[*Shown in Product Identification Section*]

SUDAFED® PLUS SYRUP/TABLETS

Description: Each scored tablet contains pseudoephedrine HCl 60 mg, chlorpheniramine maleate 4 mg
Each 5 ml of syrup contains pseudoephedrine HCl 30 mg, chlorpheniramine maleate 2 mg
Directions: For the temporary relief of nasal/sinus congestion associated with the common cold; also sneezing; watery, itchy eyes; runny nose and other hay fever/upper respiratory allergy symptons.
Dosage:
Tablets—Adults and children over 12 years of age, 1 tablet every 4 hours.
Children 6–12 years, ½ tablet every 4 hours.
Syrup—Adults and children over 12 years of age, 2 teaspoonfuls every 4 hours.
Children 6–12 years, 1 teaspoonful every 4 hours. For children under 6 years of age, ½ teaspoonful every 4 hours.
Do not exceed 4 doses in 24 hours. However, this dosage may be modified at the discretion of the physician.
Warnings: May cause excitability especially in children. May cause drowsiness. Do not exceed recommended dosage because at higher doses nervousness, dizziness, or sleeplessness may occur. If symptoms do not improve within 7 days, or are accompanied by a high fever, consult a physician before continuing use. Do not take this product if you have high blood pressure, heart disease, diabetes, thyroid disease, asthma, glaucoma, difficulty in urination due to enlargement of the prostate gland or are presently taking a prescription antihypertensive or antidepressant drug containing a monoamine oxidase inhibitor except under the advice and supervision of a physician. Consult your physician if pregnant or nursing, or taking other medication.
Caution: Avoid driving a motor vehicle or operating heavy machinery while taking this product.
Store at 15°–30°C (59°–86°F) and protect from light.
KEEP THIS AND ALL MEDICINES OUT OF CHILDREN'S REACH
How Supplied: Tablets in boxes of 24, syrup in bottles of 4 oz. Tablets bear identification, Wellcome S3C.

SUDAFED® S.A. CAPSULES ℞
SUSTAINED ACTION
(Pseudoephedrine Hydrochloride)

Description: Each Sudafed S.A. Capsule contains 120 mg of pseudoephedrine hydrochloride, the salt of a pharmacologically active stereoisomer of ephedrine (1-phenyl-2-methylaminopropanol). The specially formulated pellets in each Sudafed S.A. Capsule are designed to provide continuous therapeutic effect for 12 hours. About one half of the active ingredient is released soon after administration and the remainder of the ingredient is released slowly over the remaining time period.
Actions: Pseudoephedrine hydrochloride is an orally effective nasal decongestant. Pseudoephedrine is a sympathomimetic amine with peripheral effects similar to epinephrine and central effects similar to, but less intense than, amphetamines. Therefore, it has the potential for excitatory side effects. Pseudoephedrine at the recommended oral dosage has little or no pressor effect in normotensive adults. Patients taking pseudoephedrine orally have not been reported to experience the rebound congestion sometimes experienced with frequent, repeated use of topical decongestants. Pseudoephedrine is not known to produce drowsiness.
Indications: Sudafed S.A. Capsules are indicated for the relief of nasal congestion or eustachian tube congestion. Sudafed S.A. Capsules may be given concurrently, when indicated, with analgesics, antihistamines, expectorants and antibiotics.
Contraindications: Sympathomimetic amines are contraindicated in patients with severe hypertension, severe coronary artery disease, and in patients on MAO inhibitor therapy. Patient idiosyncrasy to adrenergic agents may be manifested by insomnia, dizziness, weakness, tremor or arrhythmias.
Children under 12: Sudafed S.A. Capsules should not be used in children less than 12 years of age.
Nursing mothers: Pseudoephedrine is contraindicated in nursing mothers because of the higher than usual risk for infants from sympathomimetic amines.
Hypersensitivity: This drug is contraindicated in patients with hypersensitivity or idiosyncrasy to sympathomimetic amines.
Warnings: Sympathomimetic amines should be used judiciously and sparingly in patients with hypertension, diabetes mellitus, ischemic heart disease, increased intraocular pressure, hyperthyroidism, and prostatic hypertrophy. Sympathomimetics may produce central nervous stimulation with convulsions or cardiovascular collapse with accompanying hypotension.
Do not exceed recommended dosage.
Use in Pregnancy: The safety of pseudoephedrine for use during pregnancy has not been established.
Use in Elderly: The elderly (60 years and over) are more likely to have adverse reactions to sympathomimetics. Overdosage of sympathomimetics in this age group may cause hallucinations, convulsions, CNS depression, and death. Therefore, safe use of a short-acting sympathomimetic should be demonstrated in the individual elderly patient before considering the use of a sustained-action formulation.
Precautions: Pseudoephedrine should be used with caution in patients with diabetes, hypertension, cardiovascular disease and hyper-reactivity to ephedrine.
Adverse Reactions: Hyper-reactive individuals may display ephedrine-like reactions such as tachycardia, palpitations, headache, dizziness or nausea. Sympathomimetic drugs have been associated with certain untoward reactions including fear, anxiety, tenseness, restlessness, tremor, weakness, pallor, respiratory difficulty, dysuria, insomnia, hallucinations, convulsions, CNS depression, arrhythmias, and cardiovascular collapse with hypotension.
Drug Interactions: MAO inhibitors and beta adrenergic blockers increase the effects of pseudoephedrine (sympathomimetics).
Sympathomimetics may reduce the antihypertensive effects of methyldopa, mecamylamine, reserpine and veratrum alkaloids.
Dosage and Administration: One capsule every 12 hours. Do not give to children under 12 years of age.
How Supplied: Sudafed S.A. is available in capsules of 120 mg (clear red top and clear body) with Wellcome code H9B, bottle of 100. Sudafed is also available in forms other than sustained action: tablets of 30 mg sugar-coated (red), box of 24, bottles of 100 and 1000; tablets of 60 mg scored (white) with Wellcome I.D. code imprint S7A, bottles of 100 and 1000; syrup 30 mg per 5 cc, bottles of 4 fl. oz and 1 pt.
Unit of Use: Tablets of 60 mg—Bottle of 100 with child-resistant cap.

[*Shown in Product Identification Section*]

TABLOID® brand A.P.C. with Codeine ℞ Ⓒ

Description: Each tablet contains aspirin 227 mg (acetylsalicylic acid), phenacetin 162 mg, and caffeine 32 mg; plus codeine phosphate in one of the following strengths: No. 2—15 mg, No. 3—30 mg and No. 4—60 mg.
(Warning—may be habit-forming.)
Actions: Aspirin alleviates pain both centrally and peripherally. It also has both antipyretic and anti-inflammatory effects . Phenacetin's action is similar to aspirin in the relief of pain and as an antipyretic. Caffeine is thought to potentiate the anti-inflammatory effect of aspirin. Codeine is in the category of a narcotic analgesic and antitussive.
Indications: For the relief of mild, moderate, and moderate to severe pain.
Contraindications: Hypersensitivity to aspirin, phenacetin, caffeine, or codeine.
Warnings:
Drug dependence: Tabloid brand A.P.C. with Codeine can produce drug dependence of the morphine type and, therefore, has the potential for being abused. Psychic dependence, physical dependence, and tolerance may develop upon repeated administration of this drug and it should be prescribed and administered with the same degree of caution appropriate to the use of other oral, narcotic-containing medications. Like other narcotic-containing medications, the drug is subject to the Federal Controlled Substances Act.
Use in ambulatory patients: Tabloid brand A.P.C. with Codeine may impair the mental and/or physical abilities required for the performance of potentially hazardous tasks such as driving a car or operating machinery. The patient using this drug should be cautioned accordingly.
Interaction with other central nervous system (CNS) depressants: Patients receiving other narcotic analgesics, general anesthetics, phenothiazines, other tranquilizers, sedative-hypnotics, or other CNS depressants (including alcohol) concomitantly with Tabloid brand A.P.C. with Codeine may exhibit an additive CNS depression. When such combined therapy is contemplated, the dose of one or both agents should be reduced.
Use in pregnancy: Safe use in pregnancy has not been established relative to possible adverse effects on fetal development. Therefore, Tabloid brand A.P.C. with Codeine should not be used in pregnant women unless, in the judgment of the physician, the potential benefits outweigh the possible hazards.
Precautions:
Head injury and increased intracranial pressure: The respiratory depressant effects of narcotics and their capacity to elevate cerebrospinal fluid pressure may be markedly exaggerated in the presence of head injury, other intracranial lesions or a pre-existing increase in intracranial pressure. Furthermore, narcotics produce adverse reactions which may obscure the clinical course of patients with head injuries.
Acute abdominal conditions: The administration of Tabloid brand A.P.C. with Codeine or other narcotics may obscure the diagnosis or clinical course in patients with acute abdominal conditions.
Allergic: Precautions should be taken in administering salicylates to persons with known allergies; patients with nasal polyps are more likely to be hypersensitive to aspirin.
Special risk patients: Tabloid brand A.P.C. with Codeine should be given with caution to certain patients such as the elderly or debilitated, and those with severe impairment of hepatic or renal function, hypothyroidism, Addison's disease, prostatic hypertrophy or urethral stricture, peptic ulcer, or coagulation disorders.
Adverse Reactions: The most frequently observed adverse reactions to codeine include

light-headedness, dizziness, sedation, nausea and vomiting. These effects seem to be more prominent in ambulatory than in nonambulatory patients and some of these adverse reactions may be alleviated if the patient lies down. Other adverse reactions include euphoria, dysphoria, constipation, and pruritus.
The most frequently observed adverse reactions to aspirin include headache, vertigo, ringing in the ears, mental confusion, drowsiness, sweating, thirst, nausea, and vomiting. Occasional patients experience gastric irritation and bleeding with aspirin. Some patients are unable to take salicylates without developing nausea and vomiting. Hypersensitivity may be manifested by a skin rash or even an anaphylactic reaction. With these exceptions, most of the side effects occur after repeated administration of large doses.
Side effects from phenacetin are usually the result of an overdosage. Cyanosis, acute hemolytic anemia, skin lesions, and fever may appear with toxic doses. Abuse of phenacetin-containing analgesic mixtures may lead to renal damage.
Side effects produced by caffeine are almost always the result of overdosage and include insomnia, restlessness, excitement, tense muscles, and diuresis. Tachycardia and extrasystoles may be observed.
Dosage and Administration: Dosage should be adjusted according to the severity of the pain and the response of the patient. It may occasionally be necessary to exceed the usual dosage recommended below in cases of more severe pain or in those patients who have become tolerant to the analgesic effect of narcotics. Tabloid brand A.P.C. with Codeine is given orally. The usual adult dose for Tabloid brand A.P.C. with Codeine No. 2 and No. 3 is one or two tablets every four hours as required. The usual adult dose for Tabloid brand A.P.C. with Codeine No. 4 is one tablet every four hours as required.
Drug Interactions: The CNS depressant effects of Tabloid brand A.P.C. with Codeine may be additive with that of other CNS depressants. See WARNINGS.
Overdosage:
Signs and Symptoms: The primary signs and symptoms of serious overdosage with Tabloid brand A.P.C. with Codeine are mainly due to codeine intoxication and acid-base imbalance due to salicylism. Toxic effects of phenacetin may occur. Since caffeine toxicity usually occurs only at high dosages, the possibility of significant caffeine toxicity from Tabloid brand A.P.C. with Codeine is unlikely. Symptoms resulting from serious overdosage may be the result of one or more of the active ingredients. Therefore, the following signs and symptoms may occur: drowsiness, confusion, tinnitus, restlessness, chills, vomiting, hyperpnea, abdominal pain, respiratory depression (a decrease in respiratory rate and/or tidal volume, Cheyne-Stokes respiration, cyanosis), extreme somnolence progressing to stupor or coma, skeletal muscle flaccidity, cold and clammy skin and sometimes bradycardia and hypotension. Additionally, acid-base distrubances, hypoprothrombinemia, methemoglobinemia, shock, convulsions and coma could occur.
Treatment: Treatment consists primarily of management of codeine intoxication and the correction of the acid-base imbalance due to salicylism. Primary attention should be given to the establishment of adequate respiratory exchange through provision of a patent airway and the institution of assisted or controlled ventilation. The narcotic antagonist, naloxone, is a specific antidote for respiratory depression which may result from overdose or unusual sensitivity to narcotics. Therefore, an appropriate dose of an antagonist should be administered, preferably by the intravenous route, simultaneously with efforts at respiratory resuscitation. Since the duration of action of Tabloid brand A.P.C. with Codeine may exceed that of the antagonist, the patient should be kept under continued surveillance and repeated doses of the antagonist should be administered as needed to maintain adequate respiration.
An antagonist should not be administered in the absence of clinically significant respiratory or cardiovascular depression.
Oxygen, intravenous fluids, vasopressors and other supportive measures should be employed as indicated. Severe methemoglobinemia may be treated with methylene blue administered slowly intravenously.
Gastric emptying may be useful in removing unabsorbed drug.
How Supplied: Nos. 2, 3 and 4, bottles of 100, 500 and 1000.

TABLOID® BRAND THIOGUANINE ℞
40 mg Scored Tablets

CAUTION: Tabloid® brand thioguanine is a potent drug. It should not be used unless a diagnosis of acute leukemia or chronic myelogenous leukemia has been adequately established and the responsible physician is knowledgeable in assessing response to chemotherapy.

Description: Tabloid brand thioguanine (6-thioguanine; 2-amino-6-thiopurine; 2-amino-6-mercaptopurine) was synthesized and developed by Hitchings, Elion, and associates at the Wellcome Research Laboratories. It is one of a large series of purine analogues which interfere with nucleic acid biosynthesis.[1]
Thioguanine is an analogue of the nucleic acid constituent guanine, and is closely related structurally and functionally to Purinethol® brand mercaptopurine (6-mercaptopurine).

1. Thioguanine competes with hypoxanthine and guanine for the enzyme hypoxanthine-guanine phosphoribosyltransferase (HGPRTase) and is itself converted to 6-thioguanylic acid (TGMP). This nucleotide reaches high intracellular concentrations at therapeutic doses. TGMP interferes at several points with the synthesis of guanine nucleotides. It inhibits *de novo* purine biosynthesis by pseudo-feedback inhibition of glutamine-5-phosphoribosylpyrophosphate amidotransferase—the first enzyme unique to the *de novo* pathway for purine ribonucleotide synthesis. TGMP also inhibits the conversion of inosinic acid (IMP) to xanthylic acid (XMP) by competition for the enzyme inosinic acid (IMP) dehydrogenase. At one time TGMP was felt to be a significant inhibitor of ATP:GMP phosphotransferase (guanylate kinase)[2], but recent results have shown this not to be so.[3]
2. Thioguanylic acid is further converted to the di- and tri-phosphates, thioguanosine diphosphate (TGDP) and thioguanosine triphosphate (TGTP) (as well as their 2′-deoxyribosyl analogues), by the same enzymes which metabolize guanine nucleotides.[4] Thioguanine nucleotides are incorporated into both the RNA and the DNA by phosphodiester linkages[5] and it has been argued that incorporation of such fradulent bases contributes to the cytotoxicity of thioguanine.
3. Thus, thioguanine has multiple metabolic effects and, at present, it is not possible to designate one major site of action. Its tumor inhibitory properties may be due to one or more of its effects on (a) feedback inhibition of *de novo* purine synthesis; (b) inhibition of purine nucleotide interconversions; or (c) incorporation into the DNA and the RNA. The net consequence of its actions is a sequential blockade of the synthesis and utilization of the purine nucleotides.[2,4,6]
4. The catabolism of thioguanine and its metabolites is complex and shows significant differences between man and the mouse.[5,7] In both humans and mice, after oral administration of ^{35}S-6-thioguanine, urine contains virtually no detectable intact thioguanine. While deamination and subsequent oxidation to thiouric acid occurs only to a small extent in man, it is the main pathway in mice. The product of deamination by guanase, 6-thioxanthine, is inactive, having negligible antitumor activity. This pathway of thioguanine inactivation is not dependent on the action of xanthine oxidase and an inhibitor of that enzyme (such as Zyloprim® brand allopurinol) will not block the detoxification of thioguanine even though the inactive 6-thioxanthine is normally further oxidized by xanthine oxidase to thiouric acid before it is eliminated. In man, methylation of thioguanine is much more extensive than in the mouse. The product of methylation, 2-amino-6-methylthiopurine, is also substantially less active and less toxic than thioguanine and its formation is likewise unaffected by the presence of allopurinol. Appreciable amounts of inorganic sulfate are also found in both murine and human urine, presumably arising from further metabolism of the methylated derivatives.
5. In some animal tumors, resistance to the effect of thioguanine correlates with the loss of HGPRTase activity and the resulting inability to convert thioguanine to thioguanylic acid. However, other resistance mechanisms, such as increased catabolism of TGMP by a nonspecific phosphatase, may be operative. Although not invariable, it is usual to find cross-resistance between thioguanine and its close analogue, mercaptopurine.

Clinical Pharmacology:

1. Clinical studies have shown that the absorption of an oral dose of thioguanine in man is incomplete and variable, averaging approximately 30% of the administered dose (range: 14–46%).[5,7] Following oral administration of ^{35}S-6-thioguanine, total plasma radioactivity reached a maximum at eight hours and declined slowly thereafter. Parent drug represented only a very small fraction of the total plasma radioactivity at any time, being virtually undetectable throughout the period of measurements.
2. The oral administration of radiolabeled thioguanine revealed only trace quantities of parent drug in the urine. However, a methylated metabolite, 2-amino-6-methylthiopurine (MTG), appeared very early, rose to a maximum six to eight hours after drug administration, and was still being excreted after 12 to 22 hours. Radiolabeled sulfate appeared somewhat later than MTG but was the principal metabolite after eight hours. Thiouric acid and some unidentified products were found in the urine in small amounts.[7]
3. Intravenous administration of ^{35}S-6-thioguanine disclosed a median plasma half-disappearance time of 80 minutes (range: 25–240 minutes) when the compound was given in single doses of 65 to 300 mg/m^2. Although initial plasma levels of thioguanine did correlate with the dose level, there was no correlation between the plasma half-disappearance time and the dose.[5]
4. Thioguanine is incorporated into the DNA and the RNA of human bone marrow cells. Studies with intravenous ^{35}S-6-thioguanine have shown that the amount of thioguanine incorporated into nucleic acids is more than 100 times higher after five daily doses than after a single dose. With the 5-dose schedule, from one-half to virtually all of the guanine in the residual DNA was replaced by thioguanine.[5]
5. Tissue distribution studies of ^{35}S-6-thioguanine in mice showed only traces of

Continued on next page

Burroughs Wellcome—Cont.

radioactivity in brain after oral administration. No measurements have been made of thioguanine concentrations in human cerebrospinal fluid, but observations on tissue distribution in animals, together with the lack of CNS penetration by the closely related compound, mercaptopurine, suggests that thioguanine does not reach therapeutic concentrations in the CSF.

6. Monitoring of plasma levels of thioguanine during therapy is of questionable value.[7] There is technical difficulty in determining plasma concentrations which are seldom greater than 1 to 2 micrograms per ml after a therapeutic oral dose. More significantly, thioguanine enters rapidly into the anabolic acid and catabolic pathways for purines and the active intracellular metabolites have appreciably longer half-lifes than the parent drug. The biochemical effects of a single dose of thioguanine are evident long after the parent drug has disappeared from plasma. Because of this rapid metabolism of thioguanine to active intracellular derivatives, hemodialysis would not be expected to appreciably reduce toxicity of the drug.

Indications:

The Acute Leukemias: Tabloid brand thioguanine is indicated for remission induction, remission consolidation, and maintenance therapy of the acute leukemias. The response to this agent depends upon the particular subclassification of the acute leukemia (lymphatic, myelogenous, undifferentiated, etc.), the age of the patient (child or adult), and whether or not thioguanine is used in previously treated or previously untreated patients. Thioguanine induces complete remissions in approximately 50% of previously untreated children with acute leukemia when the drug is used as a single agent. These results can be improved upon considerably, however, by using multiple carefully selected agents in combination. Reliance upon thioguanine alone is seldom justified for initial remission induction in children with acute leukemia. The duration of complete remission induced in children with acute leukemia is so brief without the use of maintenance therapy that some form of drug therapy is essential following successful remission induction.

In adults, thioguanine has been most frequently employed in combination with other agents (particularly with cytosine arabinoside) for the treatment of acute myelogenous (granulocytic) leukemia and acute lymphatic (lymphocytic, lymphoblastic) leukemia. The incidence of complete remission induction has varied widely, depending upon the particular combination of agents used, the classification of the leukemia (lymphatic, in general, responding better than myelogenous), the age of the patient (younger patients faring better than older), and whether the results are reported by a single institution or a large cooperative group.

Because of the brief duration of "unmaintained" complete remissions following successful remission induction, most therapy for adult acute leukemia currently employs some form of maintenance chemotherapy.

Thioguanine is not effective for prophylaxis or treatment of central nervous system leukemia.

Chronic Myelogenous (Granulocytic) Leukemia: Thioguanine is one of several agents with demonstrated efficacy in the treatment of chronic myelogenous leukemia. Approximately 50% of patients with chronic myelogenous leukemia have an objective response to thioguanine. This is less than the 90% objective responses with busulfan and, of these two agents, Myleran® brand busulfan is usually regarded as the preferred drug for initial therapy.

Other Neoplasms: Tabloid brand thioguanine is not effective in chronic lymphatic leukemia, the lymphomas (including Hodgkin's Disease), multiple myeloma, or solid tumors.

Contraindications: Thioguanine should not be used in patients whose disease has demonstrated prior resistance to this drug. In animals and man, there is usually complete cross-resistance between Purinethol brand mercaptopurine and Tabloid brand thioguanine.

Warnings: While thioguanine may be used in patients with anemia, thrombocytopenia, and granulocytopenia secondary to leukemia, these same abnormalities may be produced as a result of a direct, myelotoxic effect of the drug.

The safe and effective use of thioguanine demands a thorough knowledge of the natural history of the condition being treated. For example, remission induction of acute leukemia in adults virtually always necessitates the production of moderate to severe bone marrow hypoplasia. The degree of myelosuppression acceptable in this disease would not be desirable in the management of chronic granulocytic leukemia. After selection of an initial dosage schedule, therapy will frequently need to be modified depending upon the patient's response and manifestations of toxicity.

Evaluation of response to thioguanine therapy requires frequent examination of the peripheral blood for changes in the formed elements. Bone marrow examination (aspiration and/or biopsy) may be helpful in distinguishing between resistance to therapy, progression of leukemia, and marrow hypoplasia induced by therapy.

The most consistent, dose-related toxicity is bone marrow suppression. This may be manifest by anemia, leukopenia, thrombocytopenia, or any combination of these. Any one of these findings may also reflect progression of the underlying disease. It is imperative that patients be instructed to report promptly the development of fever, sore throat, signs of local infection, bleeding from any site, or symptoms suggestive of anemia. Since thioguanine may have a delayed effect, it is important to withdraw the medication temporarily at the first sign of an abnormally large fall in any of the formed elements of the blood.

It is recommended that evaluation of the hemoglobin concentration or hematocrit, total white blood cell count and differential count, and quantitative platelet count be obtained weekly while the patient is on thioguanine therapy. In cases where the cause of fluctuations in the formed elements in the peripheral blood is obscure, bone marrow examination may be useful for the evaluation of marrow status. The decision to increase, decrease, continue or discontinue a given dosage of thioguanine must be based not only on the absolute hematologic values, but also upon the rapidity with which changes are occurring. In many instances, particularly during the induction phase of acute leukemia, complete blood counts will need to be done more frequently than once weekly in order to evaluate the effect of the therapy. The dosage of thioguanine may need to be reduced when this agent is combined with other drugs whose primary toxicity is myelosuppression.

Although the effect usually occurs slowly over a period of two to four weeks, occasionally there may be a rapid fall in leukocyte count within one to two weeks. This may occur in some adults with acute leukemia and high total leukocyte counts as well as in certain adults with chronic granulocytic leukemia. For this reason, it is important to observe such patients carefully. Since the drug may have a delayed action, it should be discontinued at the first sign of an abnormally large fall in the leukocyte or platelet count. If, subsequently, the leukocyte or platelet count remains constant for two or three days, or rises, treatment may be resumed.

Myelosuppression is often unavoidable during the induction phase of adult acute leukemia if remission induction is to be successful. Whether or not this demands modification or cessation of dosage depends both upon the response of the underlying disease and a careful consideration of supportive facilities (granulocyte and platelet transfusions) which may be available. Life-threatening infections and bleeding have been observed as a consequence of thioguanine induced granulocytopenia and thrombocytopenia.

If it is not the intent to intentionally induce bone marrow hypoplasia, it is important to discontinue the drug temporarily at the first evidence of abnormally large, or excessively rapid, fall in white blood cell count, platelet count, or hemoglobin concentration. In many patients with severe depression of the formed elements of the blood due to thioguanine, the bone marrow appears hypoplastic on aspiration or biopsy, whereas in other cases it may appear normocellular. The qualitative changes in the erythroid elements toward the megaloblastic series, characteristically seen with the folic acid antagonist and some other antimetabolites, are not seen with this drug. Carcinogenic potential exists in man, but the extent of the risk is unknown.

The effect of thioguanine on the immunocompetence of patients is unknown.

Drugs such as thioguanine are potential mutagens and teratogens. Because of the possibility of fetal damage, thioguanine should be used during pregnancy only if the benefit clearly justifies the potential risk to the fetus; whenever possible, use of the drug should be deferred until after the first trimester of pregnancy. The effects of thioguanine upon fertility, both in males and females, together with potential hazards to the fetus are unknown when the drug is employed either as a single agent or is used in combination chemotherapeutic regimens.

Two cases have been reported in which fathers have sired children with congenital abnormalities after chemotherapy with multiple antineoplastic agents (including thioguanine) was stopped.[8]

Precautions: A few cases of jaundice have been reported in patients with leukemia receiving thioguanine. It has been reported that two adult male patients and four children, all with acute myelogenous leukemia, developed veno-occlusive hepatic disease while receiving chemotherapy for their leukemia.[9] All six patients had received cytosine arabinoside prior to treatment with thioguanine and some were receiving other chemotherapy in addition to thioguanine when they became symptomatic. While veno-occlusive hepatic disease has not been reported in patients treated with thioguanine alone, it is recommended that thioguanine be withheld if there is evidence of toxic hepatitis or biliary stasis, and that appropriate clinical and laboratory investigations be initiated to establish the etiology of the hepatic dysfunction.

It is advisable to monitor liver function tests (serum transaminases, alkaline phosphatase, bilirubin) at weekly intervals when first beginning therapy and at monthly intervals thereafter. Liver function tests may be advisable more frequently in patients who are receiving thioguanine with known pre-existing liver disease or with other hepatotoxic drugs. Patients should be instructed to discontinue thioguanine immediately if clinical jaundice is detected.

Deterioration in liver function studies while receiving thioguanine should prompt discontinuation of treatment and a search for an explanation of the hepatotoxicity.

See **WARNINGS** section for information on immunosuppression, carcinogenesis, mutagenesis, and impairment of fertility.

Adverse Reactions:
Gastrointestinal Symptoms: Nausea, vomiting, anorexia, and stomatitis may occur, particularly with overdosage. While no significant clinical differences between thioguanine and mercaptopurine have been noted with respect to action or side effects, it has been observed that occasional patients may experience better gastrointestinal tolerance to one or the other drug. The onset of clinical jaundice, hepatomegaly, or anorexia with tenderness in the right hypochondrium are immediate indications for withholding thioguanine until the exact etiology can be identified.
Other: Hyperuricemia frequently occurs in patients receiving thioguanine as a consequence of rapid cell lysis accompanying the antineoplastic effect. Adverse effects can be minimized by increased hydration, urine alkalinization, and the prophylactic administration of a xanthine oxidase inhibitor such as Zyloprim brand allopurinol. Unlike Purinethol brand mercaptopurine and Imuran® brand azathioprine, thioguanine may be continued in the usual dosage when allopurinol is used conjointly to inhibit uric acid formation.
Overdosage: There is no known pharmacologic antagonist of thioguanine. The drug should be discontinued immediately if unintended toxicity occurs during treatment. Severe hematologic toxicity may require supportive therapy with platelet transfusions for bleeding, and granulocyte transfusions and antibiotics if sepsis is documented. If a patient is seen immediately following an accidental overdosage of the drug, induced emesis may be useful. Hemodialysis is thought to be of marginal use due to the rapid intracellular incorporation of thioguanine into active metabolites with long persistence.
Dosage and Administration: Tabloid brand thioguanine is administered orally. The dosage which will be tolerated or which will be effective varies from patient-to-patient and careful dose titration is necessary to obtain the optimum therapeutic effect without incurring excessive, unintended toxicity. The usual initial dosage for children and adults is approximately 2 mg/kg of body weight per day. If, after four weeks on this dosage, there is no clinical improvement and no leukocyte or platelet depression, the dosage may be cautiously increased to 3 mg/kg per day. The total daily dose may be given at one time. It is usually calculated to the closest multiple of 20 mg.
The dosage of thioguanine used does not depend on whether or not the patient is receiving Zyloprim brand allopurinol; *this is in contradistinction to the dosage reduction which is mandatory when mercaptopurine or azathioprine is used simultaneously with allopurinol.*
If a complete hematologic remission is obtained with thioguanine, either alone or in combination with other agents, maintenance therapy should be instituted. If remission is achieved, maintenance doses and schedules incorporating thioguanine will vary from patient-to-patient depending upon the regimen being used.
How Supplied: Greenish-yellow, scored tablets containing 40 mg thioguanine, imprinted with "WELLCOME" and "U3B" on each tablet; in bottle of 25.
References:
1. Hitchings, G.H., and Elion, G.B: The Chemistry and Biochemistry of Purine Analogs. Ann. N.Y. Acad. Sci. *60:*195–199, 1954.
2. Miech, R.P., Parks, R.E., Jr., Anderson, J.H., Jr., and Sartorelli, A.C.: An Hypothesis on the Mechanism of Action of 6-Thioguanine. Biochem. Pharmacol. *16:*2222–2227, 1967.
3. Miller, R.L., Adamczyk, D.L., and Spector, T.: Reassessment of the Interactions of Guanylate Kinase and 6-Thioguanosine 5'-Phosphate. Proc. Am. Assoc. Cancer Res. *18:*6, 1977. *Abstract.*
4. Paterson, A.R.P., and Tidd, D.N.: 6-Thiopurines. In: *Antineoplastic and Immunosuppressive Agents,* Part II. (Edited by A.C. Sartorelli and D.G. Johns.) Berlin, Springer-Verlag, 384–403, 1975.
5. LePage, G.A., and Whitecar, J.P., Jr.: Pharmacology of 6-Thioguanine in Man. Cancer Res. *31:*1627–1631, 1971.
6. Nelson, J.A., Carpenter, J.W., Rose, L.N., and Adamson, D.J.: Mechanisms of Action of 6-Thioguanine, 6-Mercaptopurine, and 8-Azaguanine. Cancer Res. *35:*2872–2878, 1975.
7. Elion, G.B.: Biochemistry and Pharmacology of Purine Analogues. Fed. Proc. *26:*898–904, 1967.
8. Russell, J.A., Powle, R.L., and Oliver, R.T.D.: Conception and Congenital Abnormalities After Chemotherapy of Acute Myelogenous Leukaemia in Two Men. Brit. Med. J. *1:*1508, 1976.
9. Griner, P.F., Elbadawi, A., and Packman, C.H.: Veno-Occlusive Disease of the Liver After Chemotherapy of Acute Leukemia. Ann. Inter. Med. *85:*578–582, 1976.

VASOXYL® brand ℞
Methoxamine Hydrochloride INJECTION 20 mg in 1 cc
Methoxamine Hydrochloride INJECTION 10 mg in each cc

Description: INJECTION 20 mg in 1 cc: A sterile solution for intramuscular or intravenous injection, made isotonic with sodium chloride, containing citric acid anhydrous 0.3% and sodium citrate 0.3%, and preserved with potassium metabisulfite 0.1%. 1 cc ampuls.
INJECTION 10 mg in each cc: A sterile solution for intramuscular or intravenous injection, made isotonic with sodium chloride, containing disodium edetate 0.025% and calcium chloride 0.01%, and preserved with methylparaben 0.1%. Multi-dose vials of 10 cc.
Methoxamine is a sympathomimetic amine. Chemically, methoxamine is β-hydroxy-β-(2,5-dimethoxyphenyl) isopropylamine. It is available as the hydrochloride in sterile aqueous solution for parenteral use.
Actions: Vasoxyl brand Methoxamine Hydrochloride Injection is a vasopressor agent which produces a prompt and prolonged rise in blood pressure following parenteral administration. It is especially useful for maintaining blood pressure during operations under spinal anesthesia; it may also safely be used during general anesthesia.
The outstanding characteristic is potent, prolonged pressor action following parenteral administration. Unlike most pressor amines, there is no increase in cardiac rate but rather on occasions a decrease in rate develops as the blood pressure increases. This bradycardia is apparently caused by a carotid sinus reflex mediated over the vagus nerve. It is abolished by atropine.
The pressor action appears to be due primarily to peripheral vasoconstriction. Dripps has pointed out that evidence for direct action on blood vessels is provided by the observation of intense constriction along the course of a vein into which methoxamine has been injected. Taube and Fassett have shown that methoxamine increases central venous pressure. Methoxamine hydrochloride has the distinct advantage of being free of central stimulating action. This has been demonstrated by de Beer in laboratory studies as well as by Fassett in electroencephalogram tracings of patients receiving the drug. Pressor action without central stimulation may be especially desirable in patients undergoing surgery under spinal anesthesia.
Of special significance is the conclusion of Stutzman, Pettinga and Fruggiero that "Methoxamine does not increase the irritability of the cyclopropane-sensitized heart. It is a safe pressor agent for use during cyclopropane anesthesia." It has already been noted that it tends to slow the ventricular rate; large doses may produce bradycardia, but do not cause ventricular tachycardia, fibrillation, or an increased sinoauricular rate.
Finally, tachyphylaxis does not appear to be a factor clinically; Dripps states that he has never observed true tachyphylaxis to methoxamine.
Indications: For supporting, restoring or maintaining blood pressure during anesthesia (including cyclopropane anesthesia).
For terminating some episodes of paroxysmal supraventricular tachycardia.
Contraindications: Methoxamine is contraindicated as a combination with local anesthetics to prolong their action at local sites.
Precautions: The use of Vasoxyl brand Methoxamine Hydrochloride Injection is not a substitute for the replacement of blood, plasma, fluids and electrolytes which should promptly be restored when loss has occurred. Caution should be observed when used closely following the parenteral injection of ergot alkaloids, to prevent an excessive rise in blood pressure. Caution should be exercised to avoid overdosage so that undesirably high blood pressure or excessive bradycardia will not occur. (Bradycardia may be abolished with atropine.) While 20 mg Vasoxyl brand Methoxamine Hydrochloride Injection intramuscularly has been used by some anesthesiologists, with favorable results, most studies indicate that 10 to 15 mg intramuscularly is adequate to give a satisfactory pressor response. A second dose should not be given until the previous one has had time to act (about 15 minutes). The intravenous route should be reserved for emergencies where a strong immediate pressor response is imperative, in which case not more than 5 mg may be given slowly.
Vasoxyl brand Methoxamine Hydrochloride Injection, like other vasopressor agents, should be used with care in patients with hyperthyroidism or severe hypertension. It is to be noted, however, that patients with hypertension may suffer greater or more serious fall in blood pressure than those with normal blood pressure when under spinal anesthesia, hence a pressor drug may be especially valuable properly used under these circumstances.
The possibility exists that the increase in peripheral resistance produced by methoxamine may produce or exacerbate heart failure associated with a diseased myocardium, due to the production of an increased workload.
Adverse Reactions: Methoxamine may on occasion produce sustained excessive blood pressure elevations with severe headache, pilomotor response, a desire to void and projectile vomiting, particularly with high dosage.
Dosage: Vasoxyl brand Methoxamine Hydrochloride Injection is administered by either intramuscular or intravenous administration. The usual intravenous dose of methoxamine for emergencies is 3 to 5 mg, injected slowly. Intravenous injection may be supplemented by intramuscular injections to provide a more prolonged effect. The usual intramuscular dose is 10 to 15 mg. This may be given shortly before or at the time of administering spinal anesthesia to prevent a fall in blood pressure. The tendency for the blood pressure to fall is greater with higher levels of spinal anesthesia, hence the dosage may be adjusted accordingly; 10 mg may be adequate at lower spinal levels while 15 to 20 mg may be required at high levels of spinal anesthesia. Repeated doses may be given if necessary but time should be allowed for the previous dose to act (see Precautions). For purposes of correcting a fall in blood pressure an intramuscular injection of 10 to 15 mg methoxamine hydrochloride may be given depending upon the degree of fall. In cases where

Continued on next page

Burroughs Wellcome—Cont.

the systolic pressure falls to 60 mm or less, or whenever an emergency exists, an intravenous injection of 3 to 5 mg Vasoxyl brand Methoxamine Hydrochloride Injection is indicated. This may be accompanied by 10 to 15 mg intramuscularly to provide more prolonged effect. For preoperative and postoperative use in cases of only moderate hypotension 5 to 10 mg intramuscularly may be adequate. In paroxysmal supraventricular tachycardia the average dose is 10 mg intravenously injected slowly.

How Supplied: 20 mg in 1 cc, 1 cc ampul, box of 100.

10 mg in each cc, multi-dose vial of 10 cc, box of 12 vials.

ZYLOPRIM ® ℞

brand Allopurinol*
100 mg Scored Tablets and
300 mg Scored Tablets

Description: Allopurinol is a xanthine oxidase inhibitor with the chemical name 4-hydroxypyrazolo (3,4-d) pyrimidine (HPP).

Clinical Pharmacology: Zyloprim brand Allopurinol acts on purine catabolism, without disrupting the biosynthesis of vital purines, thus reducing the production of uric acid by inhibiting the biochemical reactions immediately preceding its formation. Its action differs from that of uricosuric agents, which lower the serum uric acid level by increasing urinary excretion of uric acid. Zyloprim reduces both the serum and urinary uric acid levels by inhibiting the formation of uric acid. It thereby avoids the hazard of increased hyperuricosuria in patients with gouty nephropathy or with a predisposition to the formation of uric acid stones.

Zyloprim has produced a substantial reduction in serum and urinary uric acid levels in hitherto refractory patients even in the presence of renal damage marked enough to render uricosuric drugs virtually ineffective. Salicylates may be given conjointly for their antirheumatic effect without compromising the action of allopurinol. This is in contrast to the nullifying effect of salicylates on uricosuric drugs.

Zyloprim is a structural analogue of the natural purine base, hypoxanthine. It is a potent inhibitor of xanthine oxidase, the enzyme responsible for the conversion of hypoxanthine to xanthine and of xanthine to uric acid, the end product of purine metabolism in man. Zyloprim is metabolized to the corresponding xanthine analogue, oxipurinol (alloxanthine), which also is an inhibitor of xanthine oxidase.

Hyperuricemia may be primary, as in gout, or secondary to diseases such as acute and chronic leukemia, polycythemia vera, multiple myeloma, and psoriasis. It may occur with the use of diuretic agents, during renal dialysis, in the presence of renal damage, during starvation or reducing diets and in the treatment of neoplastic disease where rapid resolution of tissue masses may occur.

The major disease manifestations in gout—kidney stones, tophi in soft tissues, and deposits in joints and bones—result from the deposition of urates. If progressive deposition of urates is to be arrested or reversed, it is necessary to reduce the serum uric acid to a level below the saturation point to suppress urate precipitation. Reduction may be achieved by means of uricosuric agents. Uricosurics are less effective in the presence of renal disease, and some patients develop intolerance or sensitivity to these drugs. The use of allopurinol to block the formation of urate avoids the hazard of increased renal excretion of uric acid posed by uricosuric drugs.

The half-life of Zyloprim in the body is determined both by renal excretion and by oxidation to 4,6-dihydroxypyrazolo (3,4-d) pyrimidine (oxipurinol). The latter is also an inhibitor of xanthine oxidase, but is somewhat weaker than allopurinol which is bound 15-fold more tightly to the enzyme than is the natural substrate, xanthine. The long half-life of oxipurinol in the plasma (18 to 30 hours), contributes significantly to the enzyme inhibition. Moreover, both allopurinol and oxipurinol tend to inactivate xanthine oxidase, thereby further controlling the level of its activity.

Administration of Zyloprim generally results in a fall in both serum and urinary uric acid within two to three days. The magnitude of this decrease can be manipulated almost at will since it is dose-dependent. A week or more of treatment with allopurinol may be required for the full effects of the drug to be manifest; likewise, uric acid may return to pretreatment levels slowly, usually after a period of seven to 10 days following cessation of therapy. This reflects primarily the accumulation and slow clearance of oxipurinol. In some patients, particularly those with severe tophaceous gout and underexcretors, a dramatic fall in urinary uric acid excretion may not occur. It has been postulated that this may be due to the mobilization of urate from the tissue deposits as the serum uric acid level begins to fall.

The combined increase in hypoxanthine and xanthine excreted in the urine usually, but not always, is considerably less than the accompanying decline in urinary uric acid.

It has been shown that reutilization of both hypoxanthine and xanthine for nucleotide and nucleic acid synthesis is markedly enhanced when their oxidations are inhibited by allopurinol. This reutilization and the normal feedback inhibition which would result from an increase in available purine nucleotides serve to regulate purine biosynthesis and, in essence, the defect of the overproducer of uric acid is thereby compensated.

Innate deficiency of xanthine oxidase, which occurs in congenital xanthinuria as an inborn error of metabolism, has been shown to be compatible with normal health. While urinary levels of oxypurines attained with full doses of allopurinol may in exceptional cases equal those (250–600 mg per day) which in xanthinuric subjects have caused formation of urinary calculi, they usually fall in the range of 50–200 mg. Xanthine crystalluria has been reported in a few exceptional cases. Two of these had Lesch-Nyhan syndrome, which is characterized by excessive uric acid production combined with a deficiency in the enzyme, hypoxanthine-guanine phosphoribosyltransferase (HG-PRTase). This enzyme is required for the conversion of hypoxanthine and guanine to their respective nucleotides. The third case was a patient with lymphosarcoma, who produced an extremely large amount of uric acid because of rapid cell lysis during chemotherapy.

The serum concentration of oxypurines in patients receiving allopurinol is usually in the range of 0.3 mg to 0.4 mg percent compared to a normal level of approximately 0.15 mg percent. A maximum of 0.9 mg percent was observed when the serum urate was lowered to less than 2 mg percent by high doses of the drug. In one exceptional case a value of 2.7 mg percent was reached. These are far below the saturation level at which precipitation of xanthine or hypoxanthine would be expected to occur.

The solubilities of uric acid and xanthine in the serum are similar (about 7 mg percent) while hypoxanthine is much more soluble. The finding that the renal clearance of oxypurines is at least 10 times greater than that of uric acid explains the relatively low serum oxypurine concentration at a time when the serum uric acid level has decreased markedly. At serum oxypurine levels of 0.3 mg to 0.9 mg percent, oxypurine: inulin clearance ratios were between 0.7 and 1.9. The glomerular filtration rate and urate clearance in patients receiving allopurinol do not differ significantly from those obtained prior to therapy. The rapid renal clearance of oxypurines suggests that allopurinol therapy should be of value in allowing a patient with gout to increase his total purine excretion.

Although the renal clearance of allopurinol is rapid, that of oxipurinol is slow and parallels that of uric acid but is higher by a factor of about three. The clearance of oxipurinol is increased by uricosuric drugs, and as a consequence, the addition of a uricosuric agent may reduce the degree of inhibition of xanthine oxidase by oxipurinol. However, such combined therapy may be useful in achieving minimum serum uric acid levels provided the total urinary uric acid load does not exceed the competence of the patient's renal function. In some patients, where renal function is severely impaired, normal serum urate levels may not be achievable.

The danger of uric acid calculi is diminished as the uric acid excretion is reduced. The amounts of xanthine and hypoxanthine excreted in the urine generally do not exceed the solubilities of these compounds in the urine, particularly if the urine is slightly alkaline. The amounts of allopurinol and oxipurinol excreted are likewise within the limits of their respective solubilities.

Zyloprim also inhibits the enzymatic oxidation of mercaptopurine, the sulfur-containing analogue of hypoxanthine, to 6-thiouric acid. This oxidation, which is catalyzed by xanthine oxidase, inactivates mercaptopurine. Hence, the inhibition of such oxidation by allopurinol may result in as much as 75 percent reduction in the therapeutic dose requirement of mercaptopurine when the two compounds are given together.

Indications and Use: This is not an innocuous drug and strict attention should be given to the indications for its use. Pending further investigation, its use in other hyperuricemic states is not indicated at this time.

Zyloprim® (allopurinol) is intended for:

1. treatment of gout, either primary, or secondary to the hyperuricemia associated with blood dyscrasias and their therapy;
2. treatment of primary or secondary uric acid nephropathy, with or without accompanying symptoms of gout;
3. treatment of patients with recurrent uric acid stone formation;
4. prophylactic treatment to prevent tissue urate deposition, renal calculi, or uric acid nephropathy in patients with leukemias, lymphomas and malignancies who are receiving cancer chemotherapy with its resultant elevating effect on serum uric acid levels.

Allopurinol, by promoting the resolution of tophi and urate crystals in the tissues, has relieved chronic joint pain, increased joint mobility and permitted urate sinuses to heal. The addition of allopurinol to a uricosuric regimen has reduced the size of tophi which have been refractory to uricosuric agents alone and increased joint mobility.

Zyloprim is particularly effective in preventing the occurrence and recurrence of uric acid stones and gravel. Zyloprim is useful in therapy and prophylaxis of acute urate nephropathy in patients with neoplastic disease who are particularly susceptible to hyperuricemia and uric acid stone formation, especially after radiation therapy or the use of antineoplastic drugs.

Contraindications: Pending further investigation this drug is contraindicated for use in children with the exception of those with hyperuricemia secondary to malignancy. The drug should not be employed in nursing mothers.

Patients who have developed a severe reaction to Zyloprim should not be restarted on the drug.

Warnings: ZYLOPRIM SHOULD BE DISCONTINUED AT THE FIRST APPEARANCE

OF SKIN RASH OR ANY SIGN OF ADVERSE REACTION. In some instances a skin rash may be followed by more severe hypersensitivity reactions such as exfoliative, urticarial and purpuric lesions as well as Stevens-Johnson syndrome (erythema multiforme) and very rarely a generalized vasculitis which may lead to irreversible hepatotoxicity and death.

A few cases of reversible clinical hepatotoxicity have been noted in patients taking Zyloprim and in some patients asymptomatic rises in serum alkaline phosphatase or serum transaminase have been observed. Accordingly, periodic liver function tests should be performed during the early stages of therapy, particularly in patients with pre-existing liver disease.

Due to the occasional occurrence of drowsiness, patients should be alerted to the need for due precautions when engaging in activities where alertness is mandatory.

An increase in hepatic iron concentration has been reported in rats given Zyloprim. However, experiments in our laboratory and those of several other investigators show no effect of allopurinol on iron metabolism. Nevertheless, iron salts should not be given simultaneously with Zyloprim. This drug should not be administered to immediate relatives of patients with idiopathic hemochromatosis.

In patients receiving Purinethol® (mercaptopurine) or Imuran® (azathioprine), the concomitant administration of 300–600 mg of Zyloprim per day will require a reduction in dose to approximately one-third to one-fourth of the usual dose of mercaptopurine or azathioprine. Subsequent adjustment of doses of Purinethol or Imuran should be made on the basis of therapeutic response and any toxic effects.

Usage in Pregnancy and Women of Childbearing Age: Reproductive studies showed no adverse effect of Zyloprim on animal litters. However, since the effect of xanthine oxidase inhibition on the human fetus is still unknown, Zyloprim should be used in pregnant women or women of childbearing age only if the potential benefits to the patient are weighed against the possible risk to the fetus.

Precautions: Some investigators have reported an increase in acute attacks of gout during the early stages of allopurinol administration, even when normal or subnormal serum uric acid levels have been attained. Accordingly, maintenance doses of colchicine (0.5 mg twice daily) generally should be given prophylactically when allopurinol is begun. In addition, it is recommended that the patient start with a low dose of allopurinol (100 mg daily) and increase at weekly intervals by 100 mg until a serum uric acid level of 6 mg per 100 ml or less is attained but without exceeding the maximal recommended dose. The use of therapeutic doses of colchicine or anti-inflammatory agents may be required to suppress attacks in some cases. The attacks usually become shorter and less severe after several months of therapy. A possible explanation for these flare-ups may be the mobilization of urates from tissue deposits followed by recrystallization, due to fluctuation in the serum uric acid level. Even with adequate therapy it may require several months to deplete the uric acid pool sufficiently to achieve control of the acute episodes.

The concomitant administration of a uricosuric agent with Zyloprim may result in a decrease in urinary excretion of oxypurines as compared to their excretion with allopurinol alone. This may possibly be due to an increased excretion of oxipurinol and a lowering of the degree of inhibition of xanthine oxidase. Such combined therapy is not contraindicated, however, and for many patients, may provide optimum control. A report by Goldfinger, et al on a patient treated with sulfinpyrazone and salicylates in addition to allopurinol showed a marked decrease in the excretion of oxypurines which they suggested was due to interference with their clearance at the renal tubular level. However, subsequent studies in our laboratories have indicated no interference with oxypurine clearance by salicylates. Although clinical evidence to date has not demonstrated renal precipitation of oxypurines in patients either on Zyloprim alone or in combination with uricosuric agents, the possiblity should be kept in mind.

It has been reported that allopurinol prolongs the half-life of the anticoagulant, dicumarol. The clinical significance of this has not been established, but this interaction should be kept in mind when allopurinol is given to patients already on anticoagulant therapy, and the coagulation time should be reassessed.

A fluid intake sufficient to yield a daily urinary output of at least 2 liters and the maintenance of a neutral or, preferably, slightly alkaline urine are desirable to (1) avoid the theoretic possibility of formation of xanthine calculi under the influence of Zyloprim therapy and (2) help prevent renal precipitation of urates in patients receiving concomitant uricosuric agents.

A few patients with preexisting renal disease or poor urate clearance have shown a rise in BUN during Zyloprim administration although a decrease in BUN has also been observed. Although the relationship of these observations to the drug has not been established, patients with impaired renal function require less drug and should be carefully observed during the early stages of Zyloprim administration and the drug withdrawn if increased abnormalities in renal function appear.

In patients with severely impaired renal function, or decreased urate clearance, the half-life of oxipurinol in the plasma is greatly prolonged. Therefore, a dose of 100 mg per day or 300 mg twice a week, or perhaps less, may be sufficient to maintain adequate xanthine oxidase inhibition to reduce serum urate levels. Such patients should be treated with the lowest effective dose, in order to minimize side effects.

Mild reticulocytosis has appeared in some patients, most of whom were receiving other therapeutic agents, so that the significance of this observation is not known.

As with all new agents, periodic determination of liver and kidney function and complete blood counts should be performed especially during the first few months of therapy.

Adverse Reactions:

Dermatologic: Because in some instances skin rash has been followed by severe hypersensitivity reactions, it is recommended that therapy be discontinued at the first sign of rash or other adverse reaction (see WARNINGS). Skin rash, usually maculopapular, is the adverse reaction most commonly reported. Exfoliative, urticarial and purpuric lesions, Stevens-Johnson syndrome (erythema multiforme) and toxic epidermal necrolysis have also been reported.

A few cases of alopecia with and without accompanying dermatitis have been reported. In some patients with a rash, restarting Zyloprim therapy at lower doses has been accomplished without untoward incident.

Gastrointestinal: Nausea, vomiting, diarrhea, and intermittent abdominal pain have been reported.

Vascular: There have been rare instances of a generalized hypersensitivity vasculitis or necrotizing angiitis which have led to irreversible hepatotoxicity and death.

Hematopoietic: Agranulocytosis, anemia, aplastic anemia, bone marrow depression, leukopenia, pancytopenia and thrombocytopenia have been reported in patients, most of whom received concomitant drugs with potential for causing these reactions. Zyloprim has been neither implicated nor excluded as a cause of these reactions.

Neurologic: There have been a few reports of peripheral neuritis occurring while patients were taking Zyloprim.

Drowsiness has also been reported in a few patients.

Ophthalmic: There have been a few reports of cataracts found in patients receiving Zyloprim. It is not known if the cataracts predated the Zyloprim therapy. "Toxic" cataracts were reported in one patient who also received an anti-inflammatory agent; again, the time of onset is unknown. In a group of patients followed by Gutman and Yu for up to five years on Zyloprim therapy, no evidence of ophthalmologic effect attributable to Zyloprim was reported.

Drug Idiosyncrasy: Symptoms suggestive of drug idiosyncrasy have been reported in a few patients. This was characterized by fever, chills, leukopenia or leukocytosis, eosinophilia, arthralgias, skin rash, pruritus, nausea and vomiting.

Overdosage: Massive overdosing, or acute poisoning, by Zyloprim has not been reported.

Dosage and Administration: The dosage of Zyloprim brand Allopurinol to accomplish full control of gout and to lower serum uric acid to normal or near-normal levels varies with the severity of the disease. The average is 200 to 300 mg per day for patients with mild gout and 400 to 600 mg per day for those with moderately severe tophaceous gout. The appropriate dosage may be administered in divided doses or as a single equivalent dose with the 300 mg tablet. Dosage requirements in excess of 300 mg should be supplemented in divided doses. It should also be noted that allopurinol is generally better tolerated if taken following meals. Similar considerations govern the regulation of dosage for maintenance purposes in secondary hyperuricemia. For the prevention of uric acid nephropathy during the vigorous therapy of neoplastic disease, treatment with 600 to 800 mg daily for two or three days is advisable together with a high fluid intake. The minimal effective dosage is 100 to 200 mg daily and the maximal recommended dosage is 800 mg daily. To reduce the possiblity of flare-up of acute gouty attacks, it is recommended that the patient start with a low dose of allopurinol (100 mg daily) and increase at weekly intervals by 100 mg until a serum uric acid level of 6 mg per 100 ml or less is attained but without exceeding the maximal recommended dosage.

Normal serum urate levels are achieved in one to three weeks. The upper limit of normal is about 7 mg percent for men and postmenopausal women and 6 mg percent for premenopausal women. Too much reliance should not be placed on a single reading since, for technical reasons, estimation of uric acid may be difficult. By the selection of the appropriate dose, together with the use of uricosuric agents in certain patients, it is possible to reduce the serum uric acid level to normal and, if desired, to hold it as low as 2 to 3 mg percent indefinitely.

A fluid intake sufficient to yield a daily urinary output of at least 2 liters and the maintenance of a neutral or, preferably, slightly alkaline urine are desirable.

Since allopurinol and its metabolites are excreted only by the kidney, accumulation of the drug can occur in renal failure, and the dose of allopurinol should consequently be reduced. With a creatinine clearance of 20 to 10 ml/min, a daily dosage of 200 mg of Zyloprim is suitable. When the creatinine clearance is less than 10 ml/min the daily dosage should not exceed 100 mg. With extreme renal impairment (creatinine clearance less than 3 ml/min) the interval between doses may also need to be lengthened.

The correct size and frequency of dosage for maintaining the serum uric acid just within

Continued on next page

Burroughs Wellcome—Cont.

the normal range is best determined by using the serum uric acid level as an index.
Children, 6 to 10 years of age, with secondary hyperuricemia associated with malignancies may be given 300 mg allopurinol daily while those under 6 years are generally given 150 mg daily. The response is evaluated after approximately 48 hours of therapy and a dosage adjustment is made if necessary.
In patients who are being treated with colchicine and/or anti-inflammatory agents, it is wise to continue this therapy while adjusting the dosage of Zyloprim, until a normal serum uric acid and freedom from acute attacks have been maintained for several months.
In transferring a patient from a uricosuric agent to Zyloprim, the dose of the uricosuric agent should be gradually reduced over a period of several weeks and the dose of allopurinol gradually increased to the required dose needed to maintain a normal serum uric acid level.
How Supplied: 100 mg (white) scored tablets, bottles of 100 and 1000; unit dose pack of 1000. Tablets bear identification, ZYLOPRIM U4A. 300 mg (peach) scored tablets, bottles of 30, 100, 500 and unit dose pack of 1000. Tablets bear identification, ZYLOPRIM C9B.

100 mg × 100—DoD & VA
NSN 6505-00-998-4381
300 mg × 30—VA
NSN 6505-01-006-5974A
300 mg × 100—VA
NSN 6505-01-004-3952A
300 mg × 100—DoD
NSN 6505-00-149-1438

Animal Toxicology: In mice the LD_{50} is 160 mg/kg ip (with deaths delayed up to five days) and 700 mg/kg po (with deaths delayed up to three days). In rats the acute LD_{50} is 750 mg/kg ip > 6000 mg/kg po.
In a 13 week feeding experiment in rats at a drug level of 72 mg/kg per day 2 of 10 rats died and at 225 mg/kg per day 4 of 10 died before the completion of the experiment. Both groups exhibited renal tubular damage due to the deposition of xanthine that was more extensive at the higher dose.
In chronic feeding experiments, rats showed no toxic effects at a level of 14 mg/kg per day after one year. At a level of 24 mg/kg per day for one year the rats showed very slight depression of weight gain and food intake, and 5 out of 10 of the animals showed minor changes in the kidney tubules of the type exhibited by the rats on the higher doses described above.
Dogs survived oral doses of 30 mg/kg per day for one year with nil to minor changes in the kidney and no other significant abnormalities. At 90 mg/kg per day for one year there was some accumulation of xanthine in the kidneys with resultant chronic irritation and slight tubular changes. Occasional hemosiderin-like deposits were seen in the reticuloendothelial system. A higher dose (270 mg/kg per day) resulted in large concretions in the renal pelves, with severe destructive changes in the kidney secondary to xanthine accumulation. The deposition of xanthine appears to be a function both of the metabolic turnover of purines (which is proportionately larger in the smaller animals) and the degree of inhibition of xanthine oxidase.
Reproductive studies in rats and rabbits indicated that Zyloprim did not affect litter size, the mean weight of the progeny at birth or at three weeks postpartum, nor did it cause an increase in the number of animals born dead or with malformations.

*3,624,205 (Use Patent)
[*Shown in Product Identification Section*]

Burton, Parsons & Company, Inc.
120 WESTHAMPTON AVE.
WASHINGTON, D.C. 20027

KONSYL®
Plantago Ovata Coating
Brand of Psyllium Hydrophilic Mucilloid

Composition: Konsyl contains 100% highly refined mucilloid of the blond psyllium seed. It forms moist, smooth bulk which disperses intimately with the contents of the intestine to promote natural elimination.
Action and Uses: Konsyl provides nonirritating bulk for the treatment of chronic constipation, spastic constipation, nonspecific diarrhea, irritable colon, following anorectal surgery, rectal disorders, obesity, and wherever intensive bulk producing therapy is indicated. If reducing the patient's diet is desired, the bulk of Konsyl helps to prevent overeating when taken before meals.
Administration and Dosage: A rounded teaspoonful one to three times each day. In cases of constipation, each dose should be taken with a full glass of fluid. In cases of diarrhea, each dose should be taken in one-third of a glass of fluid. The patient should be instructed to stir Konsyl into a glass of water, fruit juice, or milk, and drink promptly. Dosage and/or its frequency can be reduced as symptoms disappear.
Side Effects: None.
Precautions: None.
Contraindications: Where obstruction of the bowel exists as the result of growths, adhesions or other causes, Konsyl may, by its bulk, cause difficulty.
How Supplied: Powder, containers of 6 and 12 ounces.

L. A. FORMULA®
Plantago Ovata Coating
Brand of Psyllium Hydrophilic Mucilloid

Composition: L. A. Formula contains 50% Plantago Ovata Coating (blond psyllium) dispersed in an equal amount of dextrose. It forms moist, smooth bulk which disperses intimately with the contents of the intestine to provide natural elimination. Each dose contains approximately 22 calories and a negligible amount of sodium.
Action and Uses: L. A. Formula is prepared by an ultra-fine pulverization process which permits quick dispersion, yet delays gel formation. Its high degree of palatability provides good patient acceptance.
L. A. Formula provides nonirritating bulk for the treatment of chronic constipation, spastic constipation, nonspecific diarrhea, irritable colon, following anorectal surgery, rectal disorders, obesity, and wherever intensive bulk producing therapy is indicated. If reducing the patient's diet is desired, the bulk of L. A. Formula helps to prevent overeating when taken before meals.
Administration and Dosage: A rounded teaspoonful one to three times each day. In cases of constipation, each dose should be taken with a full glass of fluid. In cases of diarrhea, each dose should be taken in one-third glass of fluid. If reducing the patient's appetite is desirable, the dose should be prescribed before meals, since the bulk frequently helps to prevent overeating. The patient should be instructed to stir L. A. Formula into a glass of water, fruit juice, or milk, and drink promptly. Dosage and/or its frequency can be reduced as the symptoms disappear.
Side Effects: None.
Precautions: None.
Contraindications: Where obstruction of the bowel exists as the result of growths, adhesions or other causes, L. A. Formula may, by its bulk, cause difficulty.

How Supplied: Powder, containers of 7 and 14 ounces.

Campbell Laboratories, Inc.
145 EAST 52nd STREET (PH No. 1)
P.O. BOX 812, F.D.R. STATION
NEW YORK, NY 10022

HERPECIN-L® Cold Sore Lip Balm OTC

Composition: A soothing, emollient, cosmetically pleasant lip balm incorporating pyridoxine HCl; allantoin; the sunscreen, octyl p-(dimethylamino)-benzoate (Padimate O); and titanium dioxide in a balanced, acidic lipid system. (All ingredients appear on the package. Does not contain any "caines", antibiotics, phenol or camphor.)
Actions and Uses: HERPECIN-L® relieves dryness and chapping by providing a lipid barrier to help restore normal moisture balance to labial tissues. The sunscreen is effective in 2900-3200 AU range while titanium dioxide blocks, scatters and reflects the sun's rays. Pyridoxine is reputed to act as a co-enzyme in the metabolism of amino acids.
Administration: (1) *Recurrent "cold sores, sun and fever blisters":* Simply put, users report the sooner and more often applied, the better the results. Frequent sufferers report that with *prophylactic* use (B.I.D./P.R.N.), their attacks are fewer and less severe. Most recurrent herpes labialis patients are aware of the *prodromal* symptoms: tingling, itching, burning. At this stage, or if the lesion has already developed, HERPECIN-L should be applied liberally as often as convenient—at least *every hour* (qq. hor.). The prodrome will often persist and remind the patient to continue to reapply HERPECIN-L. (2) *Outdoor sun/winter protection:* Apply during and after exposure (and after swimming) and again at bedtime (h.s.). (3) *Dry, chapped lips:* Apply as needed.
Note: HERPECIN-L is for peri-oral use only; not for "canker sores" (aphthous stomatitis). Primary attacks, usually in children and young adults, are normally intra-oral and accompanied by foul breath, pain and fever. Lasting up to six weeks, they are most resistant to treatment. Adjunctive therapy for pain, fever and secondary infection may be indicated. "Mouth breathing" is often causative of excessive chapping. Malocclusion (narrowed bite) may be suspected in angular chelosis.
Adverse Reactions: Discontinue use if allergic reaction or sensitivity develops.
Contraindications: Concurrent oral or topical corticosteroid therapy is normally contraindicated. (Consult steroid literature.)
How Supplied: 2.5 gm. swivel tubes. O.T.C.
Samples Available: Yes.

Carlton Corporation, The
83 N. SUMMIT STREET
TENAFLY, NJ 07670

CALPHOSAN® ℞
(calcium glycerophosphate/calcium lactate)
calcium/phosphorus solution in metabolic disorders involving low calcium

Composition: CALPHOSAN is a specially processed solution containing calcium glycerophosphate and calcium lactate. CALPHOSAN is isotonic, with a pH of about 7 or above. (Other calcium solutions are usually quite acid, with pH values of 4.5 to 5.5) Each 10 ml. CALPHOSAN contains calcium glycerophosphate 50 mg. and calcium lactate 50 mg. in a physiological solution of sodium chloride, with 0.25% phenol as a preservative.
Advantages: Intramuscular injections of CALPHOSAN raise blood serum calcium lev-

els, do not raise the calcium levels above normal.
Usually intramuscular injections of CALPHOSAN are without pain, inflammatory reactions or sloughing.
Indications: Conditions associated with hypocalcemia: tetany, hypoparathyroidism (postoperative and idiopathic).
Administration: One or two 10 ml. injections of CALPHOSAN each week for the first four or five weeks, and on a when-needed basis thereafter, is usually sufficient to raise blood calcium levels.
Contraindications: Hypercalcemia; and in view of the fact that hypercalcemia is associated with sarcoidosis and bone metastasis of neoplastic processes, it should not be used in those conditions. As there is a similarity in the actions of calcium and digitalis on the contractility and excitability of the heart muscle, CALPHOSAN is contraindicated in fully digitalized patients. **Do not use intramuscularly in infants and young children.**
Availability: 10 ml. ampuls in boxes of 10s and 100s; and 60 ml. multiple dose vials.
Also Available: CALPHOSAN B-12: Calphosan plus 300 mcg. vitamin B_{12} per 10 ml.

Carnrick Laboratories, Inc.
65 HORSE HILL ROAD
CEDAR KNOLLS, NJ 07927

AMEN® ℞
(medroxyprogesterone acetate U.S.P. 10 mg)

Caution: Federal Law Prohibits Dispensing Without Prescription

The Use of Progestational Agents During the First Four Months of Pregnancy is not Recommended.
Progestational agents have been used beginning with the first trimester of pregnancy in an attempt to prevent habitual abortion or treat threatened abortion. There is no adequate evidence that such use is effective and there is evidence of potential harm to the fetus when such drugs are given during the first four months of pregnancy. Furthermore, in the vast majority of women, the cause of abortion is a defective ovum, which progestational agents could not be expected to influence. In addition, the use of progestational agents, with their uterine-relaxant properties, in patients with fertilized defective ova may cause a delay in spontaneous abortion. Therefore, the use of such drugs during the first four months of pregnancy is not recommended.
Several reports suggest an association between intrauterine exposure to female sex hormones and congenital anomalies, including congenital heart defects and limb reduction defects (Refs. 1-5). One study (Ref. 4) estimated a 4.7-fold increased risk of limb reduction defects in infants exposed in utero to sex hormones (oral contraceptives, hormone withdrawal test for pregnancy, or attempted treatment for threatened abortion). Some of these exposures were very short and involved only a few days of treatment. The data suggests that the risk of limb reduction defects in exposed fetuses is somewhat less than 1 in 1,000.
If the patient is exposed to Amen during the first four months of pregnancy or if she becomes pregnant while taking this drug, she should be apprised of the potential risks to the fetus.

Description: Amen (medroxyprogesterone acetate U.S.P.) is a derivative of progesterone. It is a white to off-white, odorless crystalline powder, stable in air, melting between 200° and 210° C. It is freely soluble in chloroform, soluble in acetone and in dioxane, sparingly soluble in alcohol and in methanol, slightly soluble in ether, and insoluble in water.
Actions: Amen (medroxyprogesterone acetate), administered orally in the recommended dose to women with adequate endogenous estrogen, transforms proliferative endometrium into secretory endometrium. Androgenic and anabolic effects have been noted, but the drug is apparently devoid of significant estrogenic activity.
Indications: Amen (medroxyprogesterone acetate) is indicated in secondary amenorrhea and abnormal uterine bleeding due to hormonal imbalance in the absence of organic pathology, such as submucous fibroids or uterine cancer.
Contraindications: **1.** Thrombophlebitis, thromboembolic disorders, cerebral apoplexy or patients with a past history of these conditions. **2.** Liver dysfunction or disease. **3.** Known or suspected malignancy of breast or genital organs. **4.** Undiagnosed vaginal bleeding. **5.** Missed abortion. **6.** As a diagnostic test for pregnancy. **7.** Known sensitivity to medroxyprogesterone acetate.
Warnings: **1.** The physician should be alert to the earliest manifestations of thrombotic disorders (thrombophlebitis, cerebrovascular disorders, pulmonary embolism, and retinal thrombosis). Should any of these occur or be suspected, the drug should be discontinued immediately.
2. Beagle dogs treated with medroxyprogesterone acetate developed mammary nodules, some of which were malignant. Although nodules occasionally appeared in control animals, they were intermittent in nature, whereas the nodules in the drug treated animals were larger, more numerous, persistent, and there were some breast malignancies with metastases, their significance with respect to humans has not been established.
3. Discontinue medication pending examination if there is sudden partial or complete loss of vision, or if there is sudden onset of proptosis, diplopia or migraine. If examination reveals papilledema, or retinal vascular lesions, medication should be withdrawn.
Detectable amounts of progestin have been identified in the milk of mothers receiving the drug. The effect of this on the nursing infant has not been determined. Masculinization of the female fetus has occurred when progestins have been used in pregnant women.
4. Retrospective studies of morbidity and mortality in Great Britain and studies of morbidity in the United States have shown a statistically significant association between thrombophlebitis, pulmonary embolism, and cerebral thrombosis and embolism and the use of oral contraceptives. There have been three principal studies in Great Britain[6–8] leading to this conclusion and one[9] in this country. The estimate of the relative risk of thromboembolism in the study by Vessey and Doll[8] was about sevenfold, while Sartwell and Associates[9] in the United States found a relative risk of 4.4, meaning that the users are several times as likely to undergo thromboembolic disease without evident cause as non-users. The American study also indicated that the risk did not persist after discontinuation of administration, and that it was not enhanced by long continued administration. The American study was not designed to evaluate a difference between products.
Precautions: **1.** The pretreatment physical examination should include special reference to breast and pelvic organs, as well as Papanicolaou smear.
2. Because this drug may cause some degree of fluid retention, conditions which might be influenced by this factor, such as epilepsy, migraine, asthma, cardiac or renal dysfunction require careful observation.
3. In cases of breakthrough bleeding, as in all cases of irregular bleeding per vaginum, nonfunctional causes should be borne in mind. In cases of undiagnosed vaginal bleeding adequate diagnostic measures are indicated.
4. Patients who have a history of psychic depression should be carefully observed and the drug discontinued if the depression recurs to a serious degree.
5. Any possible influence of prolonged progestin therapy on pituitary, ovarian, adrenal, hepatic or uterine functions awaits further study.
6. A decrease in glucose tolerance has been observed in a small percentage of patients on estrogen-progestin combination drugs. The mechanism of this decrease is obscure. For this reason, diabetic patients should be carefully observed while receiving progestin therapy.
7. The age of the patient constitutes no absolute limiting factor although treatment with progestins may mask the onset of the climacteric.
8. The pathologist should be advised of progestin therapy when relevant specimens are submitted.
9. Because of the occasional occurence of thrombotic disorders, (thrombophlebitis, pulmonary embolism, retinal thrombosis, and cerebrovascular disorders) in patients taking estrogen-progestin combinations and since the mechanism is obscure, the physician should be alert to the earliest manifestation of these disorders.
10. Information for the patient. See text of Patient Package Insert which is printed below.
Patient Labeling for Amen—Warning for Women
There is an increased risk of birth defects in children whose mothers take this drug during the first four months of pregnancy.
Amen is similar to the progesterone hormones naturally produced by the body. Progesterone and progesterone-like drugs are used to treat menstrual disorders, to test if the body is producing certain hormones, and to treat some forms of cancer in women.
They have been used as a test for pregnancy but such use is no longer considered safe because of possible damage to a developing baby. Also, more rapid methods for testing for pregnancy are now available. These drugs have also been used to prevent miscarriage in the first few months of pregnancy. No adequate evidence is available to show that they are effective for this purpose and there is evidence of an increased risk of birth defects, such as heart or limb defects, if these drugs are taken during the first four months of pregnancy. Furthermore, most cases of early miscarriage are due to causes which could not be helped by these drugs.
The exact risk of taking this drug early in pregnancy and having a baby with a birth defect is not known. However, one study found that babies born to women who had taken sex hormones (such as progesterone-like drugs) during the first three months of pregnancy were 4 to 5 times more likely to have abnormalities of the arms or legs than if their mothers had not taken such drugs. Some of these women had taken these drugs for only a few days. The chance that an infant whose mother had taken this drug will have this type of defect is about 1 in 1,000.
If you take Amen and later find you were pregnant when you took it, be sure to discuss this with your doctor as soon as possible.

Adverse Reactions: The following adverse reactions have been associated with the use of medroxyprogesterone acetate.
Breast: In a few instances, breast tenderness or galactorrhea have occurred.

Continued on next page

Carnrick—Cont.

Pregnancy: A few cases of clitoral hypertrophy have been reported in new born females, whose mothers received medroxyprogesterone acetate during pregnancy. Prolonged postpartum bleeding, postabortal bleeding and missed abortion have been reported.
Psychic: An occasional patient has experienced nervousness, insomnia, somnolence, fatigue or dizziness.
Thromboembolic phenomena: Thromboembolic phenomena including thrombophlebitis and pulmonary embolism have been reported.
Skin and mucous membranes: Sensitivity reactions ranging from pruritus, urticaria, angioneurotic edema to generalized rash and anaphylaxis have occasionally been reported. Acne, alopecia, or hirsutism have been reported in a few cases.
Gastrointestinal: Rarely, nausea has been reported. Jaundice, including neonatal jaundice, has been noted in a few instances.
Miscellaneous: Rare cases of headache and hyperpyrexia have been reported. The following adverse reactions have been observed in women taking progestins including medroxyprogesterone acetate: breakthrough bleeding; spotting; change in menstrual flow; amenorrhea; edema; change in weight (increase or decrease); changes in cervical erosion and cervical secretions; cholestatic jaundice; rash (allergic) with and without pruritus; melasma or chloasma; mental depression.
A statistically significant association has been demonstrated between use of estrogen-progestin combination drugs and the following serious adverse reactions; thrombophlebitis, pulmonary embolism and cerebral thrombosis and embolism. For this reason patients on progestin therapy should be carefully observed.
Although available evidence is suggestive of an association, such a relationship has been neither confirmed nor refuted for the following serious adverse reactions: neuro-ocular lesions, e.g., retinal thrombosis and optic neuritis.
The following adverse reactions have been observed in patients receiving estrogen-progestin combination drugs; rise in blood pressure in susceptible individuals; premenstrual-like syndrome; changes in libido; changes in appetite; cystitis-like syndrome; headache; nervousness; dizziness; fatigue; backache; hirsutism; loss of scalp hair; erythema multiforme; erythema nodosum; hemorraghic eruption; itching.
In view of these observations, patients on progestin therapy should be carefully observed.
Female fetal masculinization has been observed in patients receiving progestins. The following laboratory results may be altered by the use of estrogen-progestin combination drugs: Increased sulfobromophthalein and other hepatic function tests; Coagulation tests: increase in prothrombin factors VII, VIII, IX and X; Metyrapone test; Pregnanediol determination.
Dosage and Administration: Secondary Amenorrhea—Amen (medroxyprogesterone acetate) may be employed in doses ranging from 5 to 10 mg. daily depending upon the degree of endometrial stimulation desired. The dose should be given daily for 5 to 10 days beginning on the assumed 16th to 21st day of the cycle. In patients with poorly developed endometria, conventional estrogen therapy should be given in conjunction with Amen. Following therapy with the preceding doses of Amen, withdrawal bleeding usually occurs within three days. **Abnormal uterine bleeding, (due to hormonal imbalance in the absence of organic pathology, such as submucous fibroids or uterine cancers)**—Amen may be given in doses ranging from 5 to 10 mg. for 5 to 10 days beginning on the assumed or calculated 16th to 21st day of the cycle. (Hamblen, E.C. et al, Brook Lodge Symposium on Progesterone, page 201, Brook Lodge Press, Augusta, Michigan, 1961). When bleeding is due to a deficiency of both ovarian hormones, as indicated by a poorly developed proliferative endometrium, estrogens should be used in conjunction with Amen. If bleeding is controlled satisfactorily, two subsequent cycles of treatment should be given.
References: 1. Gal, I., B. Kirman, and J. Stern, "Hormonal Pregnancy Tests and Congenital Malformation," Nature, 216:83, 1967.
2. Levy, E. P., A. Cohen, and F. C. Fraser, "Hormone Treatment During Pregnancy and Congenital Heart Defects," Lancet, 1:611, 1973.
3. Nora, J. and A. Nora, "Birth Defects and Oral Contraceptives," Lancet, 1:941, 1973.
4. Janerich, D. T., J. M. Piper, and D. M. Glebatis, "Oral Contraceptives and Congenital Limb-Reduction Defects," New England Journal of Medicine, 291:697, 1974.
5. Heinonen, O. P., D. Slone, R. R. Monson, E. B. Hook, and S. Shapiro, "Cardiovascular Birth Defects and Antenatal Exposure to Female Sex Hormones," New England Journal of Medicine, 296:67, 1977.
6. Royal College of General Practitioners; Oral Contraception and Thromboembolic Disease. J. Coll. Gen. Prac., 13:267–279, 1967.
7. Inman, W. H. W. and Vessey, M. P.: Investigation of Deaths From Pulmonary Coronary and Cerebral Thrombosis and Embolism in Women in Child-Bearing Age, Brit. Med. J., 2:193–199, 1968.
8. Vessey, M. P. and Doll, R.: Investigation of Relation Between Use of Oral Contraceptives and Thromboembolic Disease. A Further Report, Brit. Med. J., 2:651–657, 1969.
9. Sartwell, P. E., Masi, A. T., Arthes, G. R., Greene, R. R., and Smith, H. E.: Thromboembolism and Oral Contraceptives: An Epidemiological Case-Control Study, Am. J. Epidem., 90: 365–380, (Nov.) 1969.
How Supplied: Scored tablets containing 10 mg. of Amen are available in bottles of 50 (NDC 0086-0049-05) and 1000 (NDC 0086-0049-90).
[*Shown in Product Identification Section*]

BONTRIL PDM ©

(brand of phendimetrazine tartrate 35 mg. tablets)

Description: Bontril PDM (phendimetrazine tartrate) is a sympathomimetic amine designated chemically as (+)3,4dimethyl-2-phenylmorpholine tartrate. Phendimetrazine is a white, odorless, powder with a bitter taste. It is soluble in water, methanol and ethanol. It has a molecular weight of 341.
For clinical use, Bontril PDM (phendimetrazine tartrate) is available as a scored 35 mg. tablet.
Actions: Bontril PDM (phendimetrazine tartrate) is a sympathomimetic amine with pharmacologic activity similar to the prototype drugs of this class used in obesity, the amphetamines. Actions include central nervous system stimulation and elevation of blood pressure. Tachyphylaxis and tolerance have been demonstrated with all drugs of this class in which these phenomena have been looked for. Drugs of this class used in obesity are commonly known as "anorectics" or "anorexigenics". It has not been established, however, that the action of such drugs in treating obesity is primarily one of appetite suppression. Other central nervous system actions or metabolic effects, may be involved, for example:
Adult obese subjects instructed in dietary management and treated with "anorectic" drugs, lose more weight on the average than those treated with placebo and diet, as determined in relatively short-term clinical trials.
The magnitude of increased weight loss of drug-treated patients over placebo-treated patients is only a fraction of a pound a week. The rate of weight loss is greatest in the first weeks of therapy for both drug and placebo subjects and tends to decrease in succeeding weeks. The possible origins of the increased weight loss due to the various drug effects are not established. The amount of weight loss associated with the use of "anorectic" drug varies from trial to trial, and the increased weight loss appears to be related in part to variables other than the drug prescribed, such as the physician-investigator, the population treated, and the diet prescribed. Studies do not permit conclusions as to the relative importance of the drug and non-drug factors on weight loss.
The natural history of obesity is measured in years, whereas the studies cited are restricted to a few weeks duration; thus the total impact of drug-induced weight loss over that of diet alone must be considered clinically limited.
Indications: Bontril PDM (phendimetrazine tartrate) is indicated in the management of exogenous obesity as a short term adjunct (a few weeks) in a regimen of weight reduction based on caloric restriction. The limited usefulness of agents of this class (see ACTIONS) should be measured against possible risk factors inherent in their use such as those described below.
Contraindications: Advanced arteriosclerosis, symptomatic cardiovascular disease, moderate to severe hypertension, hyperthyroidism, known hypersensitivity, or idiosyncrasy to the sympathomimetic amines, glaucoma.
Agitated states.
Patients with a history of drug abuse.
During or within 14 days following the administration of monoamine oxidase inhibitors, (hypertensive crises may result).
Warnings: Tolerance to the anorectic effect usually develops within a few weeks. When this occurs, the recommended dose should not be exceeded in an attempt to increase the effect; rather, the drug should be discontinued.
Bontrol PDM (phendimetrazine tartrate) may impair the ability of the patient to engage in potentially hazardous activities such as operating machinery or driving a motor vehicle; the patient should therefore be cautioned accordingly.
Drug Dependence: Bontril PDM (phendimetrazine tartrate) is related chemically and pharmacologically to the amphetamines. Amphetamines and related stimulant drugs have been extensively abused, and the possibility of abuse of Bontril PDM (phendimetrazine tartrate) should be kept in mind when evaluating the desirability of including a drug as part of a weight reduction program. Abuse of amphetamines and related drugs may be associated with intense psychological dependence and severe social dysfunction. There are reports of patients who have increased the dosage to many times that recommended. Abrupt cessation following prolonged high dosage administration results in extreme fatigue and mental depression; changes are also noted on the sleep EEG. Manifestations of chronic intoxication with anorectic drugs include severe dermatoses, marked insomnia, irritability, hyperactivity, and personality changes. The most severe manifestation of chronic intoxications is psychosis, often clinically indistinguishable from schizophrenia.
Usage in Pregnancy: The safety of Bontril PDM (phendimetrazine tartrate) in pregnancy and lactation has not been established. Therefore, use cautiously in women of child bearing age. The potential benefit must be weighed against the possible hazard to mother and infant.
Usage in Children: Bontril PDM (phendimetrazine tartrate) is not recommended for use in children under 12 years of age.
Precautions: Caution is to be exercised in prescribing Bontril PDM (phendimetrazine tartrate) for patients with even mild hypertension.
Insulin requirements in diabetes mellitus may be altered in association with the use of Bontril PDM (phendimetrazine tartrate) and the con-

comitant dietary regimen. Bontril PDM (phendimetrazine tartrate) may decrease the hypotensive effect of guanethidine. The least amount feasible should be prescribed or dispensed at one time in order to minimize the possibility of overdosage.
Adverse Reactions: Cardiovascular: Palpitation, tachycardia, elevation of blood pressure.
Central Nervous System: Overstimulation, restlessness, dizziness, insomnia, euphoria, dysphoria, tremor, headache; rarely psychotic episodes at recommended dose.
Gastrointestinal: Dryness of the mouth, unpleasant taste; diarrhea, constipation, other gastrointestinal disturbances.
Allergic: Urticaria.
Endocrine: Impotence, changes in libido.
Dosage and Administration: Usual Adult Dosage: Dosage should be individualized to obtain an adequate response with the lowest effective dose. In some cases 17½ mg. per dose may be adequate.
1 tablet (35 mg.) b.i.d. or t.i.d. one hour before meals. Dosage should not exceed 2 tablets t.i.d.
Overdosage: Manifestations of acute overdosage with Bontril PDM (phendimetrazine tartrate) include restlessness, tremor, hyperreflexia, rapid respiration, confusion, assaultiveness, hallucinations, panic states.
Fatigue and depression usually follow the central stimulation.
Cardiovascular effects include arrhythmias, hypertension or hypotension and circulatory collapse. Gastrointestinal symptoms include nausea, vomiting, diarrhea and abdominal cramps. Fatal poisoning usually terminates in convulsions and coma. Management of acute Bontril PDM (phendimetrazine tartrate) intoxication is largely symptomatic and includes lavage and sedation with a barbiturate. Experience with hemodialysis or peritoneal dialysis is inadequate to permit recommendation in this regard. Acidification of the urine increases Bontril PDM (phendimetrazine tartrate) excretion. Intravenous phentolamine (Regitine) has been suggested for possible acute, severe hypertension, if this complicates Bontril PDM (phendimetrazine tartrate) overdosage.
How Supplied: NDC 0086-0048-10; Bottles of 100 3-layer green, white and yellow tablets. NDC 0086-0048-90; Bottles of 1,000
Caution: Federal law prohibits dispensing without a prescription.
[*Shown in Product Identification Section*]

CAPITAL® WITH CODEINE SUSPENSION Ⓒ

(acetaminophen with codeine phosphate)
NON-ALCOHOLIC

Caution: Federal law prohibits dispensing without prescription.
Description: Each 5 ml of pink colored suspension contains acetaminophen 120 mg. and codeine phosphate 12 mg. (WARNING: May be habit forming.) Acetaminophen occurs as a white, odorless crystalline powder, possessing a slightly bitter taste. Codeine is an alkaloid obtained from opium or prepared from morphine by methylation. Codeine occurs as colorless or white crystals, effloresces slowly in dry air and is affected by light. Acetaminophen is a non-salicylate.
Actions: Acetaminophen is an analgesic and antipyretic; codeine is an analgesic and antitussive.
Indications: For the relief of mild to moderate pain.
Contraindications: Hypersensitivity to acetaminophen or codeine.
Warnings: Drug Dependence: Codeine can produce drug dependence of the morphine type, and therefore, has the potential for being abused. Psychic dependence, physical dependence and tolerance may develop upon repeated administration of this drug and it should be prescribed and administered with the same degree of caution appropriate to the use of other oral narcotic-containing medications. Like other narcotic-containing medications, the drug is subject to the Federal Controlled Substances Act.
Usage in ambulatory patients: Codeine may impair the mental and/ or physical abilities required for the performance of potentially hazardous tasks such as driving a car or operating machinery. The patient using this drug should be cautioned accordingly.
Interaction with other central nervous system depressants: Patients receiving other narcotic analgesics, general anesthetics, phenothiazines, other tranquilizers, sedative-hypnotics or other CNS depressants (including alcohol) concomitantly with acetaminophen and codeine may exhibit an additive CNS depression. When such combined therapy is contemplated, the dose of one or both agents should be reduced.
Usage in Pregnancy: Safe use in pregnancy has not been established relative to possible adverse effects on fetal development. Therefore acetaminophen and codeine should not be used in pregnant women unless, in the judgment of the physician, the potential benefits outweigh the possible hazards.
Pediatric Use: Safe dosage of this combination has not been established in children below the age of 3.
Precautions: Head injury and increased intracranial pressure: The respiratory depressant effects of narcotics and their capacity to elevate cerebrospinal fluid pressure may be markedly exaggerated in the presence of head injury, other intracranial lesions or a pre-existing increase in intracranial pressure. Furthermore, narcotics produce adverse reactions which may obscure the clinical course of patients with head injuries.
Acute abdominal conditions: The administration of codeine containing products or other narcotics may obscure the diagnosis or clinical course in patients with acute abdominal conditions.
Special risk patients: Acetaminophen and codeine should be given with caution to certain patients such as the elderly or debilitated, and those with severe impairment of hepatic or renal function, hypothyroidism, Addison's disease, and prostatic hypertrophy or urethral stricture.
Adverse Reactions: The most frequently observed adverse reactions include lightheadedness, dizziness, sedation, nausea and vomiting. These effects seem to be more prominent in ambulatory than in nonambulatory patients, and some of these adverse reactions may be alleviated if the patient lies down. Other adverse reactions include euphoria, dysphoria, constipation and pruritus.
Dosage and Administration: Dosage should be adjusted according to the severity of the pain and the response of the patient. It may occasionally be necessary to exceed the usual dosage recommended below in cases of more severe pain or in those patients who have become tolerant to the analgesic effect of narcotics. Acetaminophen with codine suspension is given orally. Usual Dosage—Adults: One tablespoonful (15 ml) every four hours as needed. Children (7–12 years): Two teaspoonfuls (10 ml) three or four times daily. Children (3–6 years): One teaspoonful (5 ml) three or four times daily. Safe dosage of this combination has not been established in children below the age of 3. By weight basis, use this formula:

$$\text{Dose for child} = \frac{\text{adult dose x wt. of child (in lbs.)}}{\text{150 lbs.}}$$

SHAKE WELL BEFORE USING.
Drug Interactions: The CNS depressant effects of acetaminophen and codeine may be additive with that of other CNS depressants. See WARNINGS.
Management of Overdosage: The literature has reported that some adults who have ingested single acute overdoses of 10 gm. or more of acetaminophen have developed hepatotoxicity. Such patients should be closely monitored for signs of hepatotoxicity during seven days following the overdose.
Signs and Symptoms: Codeine in sufficient overdosage produces narcosis sometimes preceded by a feeling of exhilaration and followed by convulsions. Nausea and vomiting are usually prominent symptoms. The pupils are contracted and the pulse rate is usually increased. Cardiorespiratory depression accompanied by cyanosis occurs, followed by a fall in body temperature, circulatory collapse, coma and death.
Treatment: A patent airway must be maintained through the use of an oropharyngeal airway or endotracheal tube, oxygen should be administered, and respiration should be assisted by artificial respiration. A specific antagonist such as naloxone should be administered immediately. Gastric lavage or induction of emesis should be carried out immediately, followed by administration of activated charcoal. Circulatory collapse and shock may be counteracted by use of dextran, plasma, or concentrated albumin and vasopressor drugs, e.g. norepinephrine. Short-acting barbiturates, e.g., thiopental may be used cautiously to control convulsion. Use of analeptic drugs should be avoided.
How Supplied: A pink, pleasantly flavored suspension. 16 oz. NDC 0086-0046-16, 1 gal. NDC 0086-0046-90.
[*Shown in Product Identification Section*]

CAPITAL® WITH CODEINE Ⓒ

(acetaminophen 325 mg., codeine phosphate 30 mg.)

How Supplied: Pale blue tablet
Bottle of 100 - NDC 0086-0044-10
Bottle of 1,000 - NDC 0086-0044-90
[*Shown in Product Indentification Section*]

HORMONIN® No. 1, HORMONIN® No. 2 ℞

Estrogens Have Been Reported To Increase The Risk of Endometrial Carcinoma.
Three independent case control studies have shown an increased risk of endometrial cancer in postmenopausal women exposed to exogenous estrogens for prolonged periods. This risk was independent of the other known risk factors for endometrial cancer. These studies are further supported by the finding that incidence rates of endometrial cancer have increased sharply since 1969 in eight different areas of the United States with population-based cancer reporting systems, an increase which may be related to the rapidly expanding use of estrogens during the last decade.
The three case control studies reported that the risk of endometrial cancer in estrogen users was about 4.5 to 13.9 times greater than in nonusers. The risk appears to depend on both duration of treatment and on estrogen dose. In view of these findings, when estrogens are used for the treatment of menopausal symptoms, the lowest dose that will control symptoms should be utilized and medication should be discontinued as soon as possible. When prolonged treatment is medically indicated, the patient should be reassessed on at least a semiannual basis to determine the need for continued therapy. Although the evidence must be considered preliminary, one study suggests that cyclic admin-

Continued on next page

Carnrick—Cont.

istration of low doses of estrogen may carry less risk than continuous administration, it therefore appears prudent to utilize such a regimen.

Close clinical surveillance of all women taking estrogens is important. In all cases of undiagnosed persistent or recurring abnormal vaginal bleeding, adequate diagnostic measures should be undertaken to rule out malignancy.

There is no evidence at present that "natural" estrogens are more or less hazardous than "synthetic" estrogens at equiestrogenic doses.

Estrogens should not be used during pregnancy.

The use of female sex hormones, both estrogens and progestogens, during early pregnancy may seriously damage the offspring. It has been shown that females exposed in utero to diethylstilbestrol, a non-steroidal estrogen, have an increased risk of developing in later life a form of vaginal or cervical cancer that is ordinarily extremely rare. This risk has been estimated as not greater than 4 per 1000 exposures. Furthermore, a high percentage of such exposed women (from 30 to 90 percent) have been found to have vaginal adenosis, epithelial changes of the vagina and cervix. Although these changes are histologically benign it is not known whether they are precursors of malignancy. Although similar data are not available with the use of other estrogens, it cannot be presumed they would not induce similar changes.

Several reports suggest an association between intrauterine exposure to female sex hormones and congenital anomalies, including congenital heart defects and limb reduction defects. One case control study estimated a 4.7 fold increased risk of limb reduction defects in infants exposed in utero to sex hormones (oral contraceptives, hormone withdrawal tests for pregnancy, or attempted treatment for threatened abortion). Some of these exposures were very short and involved only a few days of treatment. The data suggests that the risk of limb reduction defects in exposed fetuses is somewhat less than 1 per 1000.

In the past, female sex hormones have been used during pregnancy in an attempt to treat threatened or habitual abortion. There is considerable evidence that estrogens are ineffective for these indications, and there is no evidence from well controlled studies that progestogens are effective for these uses.

If HORMONIN is used during pregnancy, or if the patient becomes pregnant while taking this drug, she should be apprised of the potential risks to the fetus, and the advisability of pregnancy continuation.

Description:
Each HORMONIN NO. 1 tablet contains: Estriol 0.135 mg., Estradiol 0.3 mg., Estrone 0.7 mg.
Each HORMONIN NO. 2 tablet contains: Estriol, 0.27 mg., Estradiol 0.6 mg., Estrone 1.4 mg.

Clinical Pharmacology: The estrogens are largely responsible for the changes that take place at puberty in girls and are responsible for development and maintenance of the female reproductive system and secondary sex characteristics. They cause the growth and development of the vagina, uterus, and fallopian tubes. They cause enlargement of the breast through promotion of ductal growth, stromal development and the accretion of fat. They also contribute indirectly in molding the body contours, shaping the skeleton, softening the skin and bringing about changes in the epiphyses of the long bones. Growth of axillary and pubic hair and regional pigmentation of the skin of the nipples and areolae and the genital region are normal effects of estrogen. Estrogens are also involved in psychological and emotional aspects of human behavior. During the follicular phase of the cycle, there is proliferation of vaginal and uterine mucosae, increased secretion of the glands of the uterine cervix, fullness of the breast and enhanced well being and vigor. Decline in estrogen at the end of the cycle can bring about menstruation and its accompanying phenomena, although, cessation of progesterone secretion is the most important factor in the mature ovulatory cycle. In the pre- or non-ovulatory cycle, estrogen is the primary cause of menstruation. Estrogens do not induce ovulation. The changes that follow the slow decline in the secretion of estrogen at the menopause, and during the years following, illustrate the numerous actions of the hormone in the body. Aside from atrophic changes in the genital tract and breast, the lack of estrogen may contribute to such aging processes as the loss of turgor of the skin, thinning of the bones and sclerosis of blood vessels.

Indications: HORMONIN is indicated in the treatment of:
1. Moderate to severe vasomotor symptoms associated with the menopause. (There is no evidence that estrogens are effective for nervous symptoms or depression which might occur during menopause, and they should not be used to treat these conditions.)
2. Atrophic vaginitis.
3. Kraurosis vulvae.
4. Female castration.
5. Primary ovarian failure.

HORMONIN HAS NOT BEEN SHOWN TO BE EFFECTIVE FOR ANY PURPOSE DURING PREGNANCY AND ITS USE MAY CAUSE SEVERE HARM TO THE FETUS (SEE BOXED WARNING).

Contraindications: Estrogens should not be used in women (or men) with any of the following conditions:
1. Known or suspected cancer of the breast except in appropriately selected patients being treated for metastatic disease.
2. Known or suspected estrogen-dependent neoplasia.
3. Known or suspected pregnancy (See Boxed Warning).
4. Undiagnosed abnormal genital bleeding.
5. Thrombophlebitis or thromboembolic disorders.
6. A past history of thrombophlebitis or thromboembolic disorders associated with previous estrogen use.

Warnings:
1. *Induction of malignant neoplasms.* Long term continuous administration of natural and synthetic estrogens in certain animal species increases the frequency of carcinomas of the breast, cervix, vagina, and liver. There is now evidence that estrogens increase the risk of carcinoma of the endometrium in humans. (See Boxed Warning).

At the present time there is no satisfactory evidence that estrogens given to postmenopausal women increase the risk of cancer of the breast although a recent long-term followup of a single physician's practice has raised this possibility. Because of the animal data, there is a need for caution in prescribing estrogens for women with a strong family history of breast cancer or who have breast nodules, fibrocystic disease, or abnormal mammograms.

2. *Gall bladder disease.* A recent study has reported a 2 to 3-fold increase in the risk of surgically confirmed gall bladder disease in women receiving postmenopausal estrogens similar to the 2-fold increase previously noted in users of oral contraceptives. In the case of oral contraceptives the increased risk appeared after two years of use.

3. *Effects similar to those caused by estrogen-progestogen oral contraceptives.* There are several serious adverse effects of oral contraceptives most of which have not, up to now, been documented as consequences of postmenopausal-estrogen therapy. This may reflect the comparatively low doses of estrogen used in postmenopausal women. It would be expected that the larger doses of estrogen used to treat prostatic or breast cancer or postpartum breast engorgement are more likely to result in these adverse effects and, in fact, it has been shown that there is an increased risk of thrombosis in men receiving estrogens for prostatic cancer and women for postpartum breast engorgement.

a. *Thromboembolic disease.* It is now well-established that users of oral contraceptives have an increased risk of various thromboembolic and thrombotic vascular diseases, such as thrombophlebitis, pulmonary embolism, stroke, and myocardial infarction. Cases of retinal thrombosis, mesenteric thrombosis, and optic neuritis have been reported in oral contraceptive users. There is evidence that the risk of several of these adverse reactions is related to the dose of the drug. An increased risk of post-surgery thromboembolic complications has also been reported in users of oral contraceptives. If feasible, estrogen should be discontinued at least 4 weeks before surgery of the type associated with an increased risk of thromboembolism or during periods of prolonged immobilization.

While an increased rate of thromboembolic and thrombotic disease in postmenopausal users of estrogens has not been found, this does not rule out the possibility that such an increase may be present or that subgroups of women who have underlying risk factors or who are receiving relatively large doses of estrogens may have increased risk. Therefore estrogens should not be used in persons with active thrombophlebitis or thromboembolic disorders, and they should not be used (except in treatment of malignancy) in persons with a history of such disorders in association with estrogen use. They should be used with caution in patients with cerebral vascular or coronary artery disease and only for those in whom estrogens are clearly needed.

Large doses of estrogen (5 mg conjugated estrogens per day), comparable to those used to treat cancer of the prostrate and breast, have been shown in a large prospective clinical trial in men to increase the risk of nonfatal myocardial infarction, pulmonary embolism and thrombophlebitis. When estrogen doses of this size are used, any of the thromboembolic and thrombotic adverse effects associated with oral contraceptive use should be considered a clear risk.

b. *Hepatic adenoma.* Benign hepatic adenomas appear to be associated with the use of oral contraceptives. Although benign, and rare, these may rupture and cause death through intraabdominal hemorrhage. Such lesions have not yet been reported in association with other estrogen or progestogen-preparations but should be considered in estrogen users having abdominal pain and tenderness, abdominal mass, or hypovolemic shock. Hepatocellular carcinoma has also been reported in women taking estrogen-containing oral contraceptives. The relationship of this malignancy to these drugs is not known at this time.

c. *Elevated blood pressure.* Increased blood pressure is not uncommon in women using oral contraceptives. There is now a report that this may occur with use of estrogens in the menopause and blood pressure should be monitored with estrogen use, especially if high doses are used.

d. *Glucose tolerance.* A worsening of glucose tolerance has been observed in a significant percentage of patients on estrogen-containing oral contraceptives. For this reason, diabetic patients should be carefully observed while receiving estrogen.

4. *Hypercalcemia.* Administration of estrogens may lead to severe hypercalcemia in patients with breast cancer and bone metastases. If this occurs, the drug should be stopped and appropriate measures taken to reduce the serum calcium level.

Precautions:

A. General Precautions.

1. A complete medical and family history should be taken prior to the initiation of any estrogen therapy. The pre-treatment and periodic physical examinations should include special reference to blood pressure, breasts, abdomen, and pelvic organs, and should include a Papanicolau smear. As a general rule, estrogen should not be prescribed for longer than one year without another physical examination being performed.

2. Fluid retention—Because estrogens may cause some degree of fluid retention, conditions which might be influenced by this factor such as epilepsy, migraine, and cardiac or renal dysfunction, require careful observation.

3. Certain patients may develop undesirable manifestations of excessive estrogenic stimulation, such as abnormal or excessive uterine bleeding, mastodynia, etc.

4. Oral contraceptives appear to be associated with an increased incidence of mental depression. Although it is not clear whether this is due to the estrogenic or progestogenic component of the contraceptive, patients with a history of depression should be carefully observed.

5. Preexisting uterine leiomyomata may increase in size while using estrogen.

6. The pathologist should be advised of estrogen therapy when relevant specimens are submitted.

7. Patients with a past history of jaundice during pregnancy have an increased risk of recurrence of jaundice while receiving estrogen-containing oral contraceptive therapy. If jaundice develops in any patient receiving estrogen, the medication should be discontinued while the cause is investigated.

8. Estrogens may be poorly metabolized in patients with impaired liver function and they should be administered with caution in such patients.

9. Because estrogens influence the metabolism of calcium and phosphorus, they should be used with caution in patients with metabolic bone diseases that are associated with hypercalcemia or in patients with renal insufficiency.

10. Because of the effects of estrogens on epiphyseal closure, they should be used judiciously in young patients in whom bone-growth is not complete.

11. Certain endocrine and liver function tests may be affected by estrogen-containing oral contraceptives. The following similar changes may be expected with larger doses of estrogen:

a. Increased sulfobromophthalein retention.

b. Increased prothrombin and factors VII, VIII, IX, and X; decreased anti-thrombin 3; increased norepinephrine-induced platelet aggregability.

c. Increased thyroid binding globulin (TBG) leading to increased circulating total thyroid hormone, as measured by PBI, T4 by column, or T4 by radioimmunoassay. Free T3 resin uptake is decreased, reflecting the elevated TBG; free T4 concentration is unaltered.

d. Impaired glucose tolerance.

e. Decreased pregnanediol excretion.

f. Reduced response to metyrapone test.

g. Reduced serum folate concentration.

h. Increased serum triglyceride and phospholipid concentration.

B. Information for the Patient. See text of Patient Package Insert reprinted at end of Physician's Labeling.

C. Pregnancy Category. See Contraindications and Boxed Warning.

D. Nursing Mothers. As a general principle, the administration of any drug to nursing mothers should be done only when clearly necessary since many drugs are excreted in human milk.

Adverse Reactions: (See warnings regarding induction of neoplasia, adverse effects on the fetus, increased incidence of gall bladder disease, and adverse effects similar to those of oral contraceptives, including thromboembolism.) The following additional adverse reactions have been reported with estrogenic therapy, including oral contraceptives:

1. *Genitourinary system.* Breakthrough bleeding, spotting, change in menstrual flow. Dysmenorrhea. Premenstrual-like syndrome. Amenorrhea during and after treatment. Increase in size of uterine fibromyomata. Vaginal candidiasis. Change in cervical eversion and in degree of cervical secretion. Cystitis-like syndrome.

2. *Breast.* Tenderness, enlargement, secretion.

3. *Gastrointestinal.* Nausea, vomiting. Abdominal cramps, bloating. Cholestatic jaundice.

4. *Skin.* Chloasma or melasma which may persist when drug is discontinued. Erythema multiforme. Erythema nodosum, Hemorrhagic eruption. Loss of scalp hair. Hirsutism.

5. *Eyes.* Steepening of corneal curvature. Intolerance to contact lenses.

6. *CNS.* Headache, migraine, dizziness. Mental depression. Chorea.

7. *Miscellaneous.* Increase or decrease in weight. Reduced carbohydrate tolerance. Aggravation of porphyria. Edema. Changes in libido.

Acute Overdosage: Numerous reports of ingestion of large doses of estrogen-containing oral contraceptives by young children indicate that serious ill effects do not occur. Overdosage of estrogen may cause nausea, and withdrawal bleeding may occur in females.

Dosage and Administration:

1. *Given cyclically for short term use only:* For treament of moderate to severe *vasomotor* symptoms, atrophic vaginitis, or kraurosis vulvae associated with the menopause.

The lowest dose that will control symptoms should be chosen and medication should be discontinued as promptly as possible.

Administration should be cyclic (e.g., 3 weeks on and 1 week off).

Attempts to discontinue or taper medication should be made at 3 to 6 month intervals.

Treated patients with an intact uterus should be monitored closely for signs of endometrial cancer and appropriate diagnostic measures should be taken to rule out malignancy in the event of persistent or recurring abnormal vaginal bleeding.

DOSAGE: Orally, for the relief of menopausal symptoms, HORMONIN NO. 1, 1 or 2 tablets daily according to severity of symptoms. HORMONIN NO. 2, 1 tablet daily. In severe cases, initial therapy may be supplemented with parenteral estrogens.

How Supplied: HORMONIN NO. 1: NDC 0086-0100-10 Bottle of 100 pink and white tablets. HORMONIN NO. 2: NDC 0086-0105-10 Bottle of 100 aqua and white tablets.

[*Shown in Product Identification Section*]

PATIENT LABELING

What You Should Know About Estrogens: Estrogens are female hormones produced by the ovaries. The ovaries make several different kinds of estrogens. In addition, scientists have been able to make a variety of synthetic estrogens. As far as we know, all these estrogens have similar properties and therefore much the same usefulness, side effects, and risks. This leaflet is intended to help you understand what estrogens are used for, the risks involved in their use, and how to use them as safely as possible.

This leaflet includes the most important information about estrogens, but not all the information. If you want to know more, you can ask your doctor or pharmacist to let you read the package insert prepared for the doctor.

Uses of Estrogen: Estrogens are prescribed by doctors for a number of purposes, including:

1. To provide estrogen during a period of adjustment when a woman's ovaries no longer produce it, in order to prevent certain uncomfortable symptoms of estrogen deficiency. (All women normally stop producing estrogens, generally between the ages of 45 and 55; this is called the menopause.)

2. To prevent symptoms of estrogen deficiency when a woman's ovaries have been removed surgically before the natural menopause.

3. To prevent pregnancy. (Estrogens are given along with a progestogen, another female hormone; these combinations are called oral contraceptives or birth control pills. Patient labeling is available to women taking oral contraceptives and they will not be discussed in this leaflet.)

4. To treat certain cancers in women and men.

5. To prevent painful swelling of the breasts after pregnancy in women who choose not to nurse their babies.

THERE IS NO PROPER USE OF ESTROGENS IN A PREGNANT WOMAN.

Estrogens in the Menopause: In the natural course of their lives, all women eventually experience a decrease in estrogen production. This usually occurs between ages 45 and 55 but may occur earlier or later. Sometimes the ovaries may need to be removed before natural menopause by an operation producing a "surgical menopause."

When the amount of estrogen in the blood begins to decrease, many women may develop typical symptoms: Feelings of warmth in the face, neck, and chest or sudden intense episodes of heat and sweating throughout the body (called "hot flashes" or "hot flushes"). These symptoms are sometimes very uncomfortable. A few women eventually develop changes in the vagina (called "atrophic vaginitis") which cause discomfort, especially during and after intercourse.

Estrogens can be prescribed to treat these symptoms of the menopause. It is estimated that considerably more than half of all women undergoing the menopause have only mild symptoms or no symptoms at all and therefore do not need estrogens. Other women may need estrogens for a few months, while their bodies adjust to lower estrogen levels. Sometimes the need will be for periods longer than six months. In an attempt to avoid over-stimulation of the uterus (womb), estrogens are usually given cyclically during each month of use, that is three weeks of pills followed by one week without pills.

Sometimes women experience nervous symptoms or depression during menopause. There is no evidence that estrogens are effective for such symptoms and they should not be used to treat them, although other treatment may be needed.

You may have heard that taking estrogens for long periods (years) after the menopause will keep your skin soft and supple and keep you feeling young. There is no evidence that this is so, however, and such long-term treatment carries important risks.

Estrogens to Prevent Swelling of the Breasts After Pregnancy: If you do not breast feed your baby after delivery, your breasts may fill up with milk and become painful and engorged. This usually begins about 3 to 4 days after delivery and may last for a few days to up to a week or more. Sometimes the discomfort is severe, but usually it is not and

Continued on next page

Carnrick—Cont.

can be controlled by pain relieving drugs such as aspirin and by binding the breasts up tightly. Estrogens can be used to try to prevent the breasts from filling up. While this treatment is sometimes successful, in many cases the breasts fill up to some degree in spite of treatment. The dose of estrogens needed to prevent pain and swellng of the breasts is much larger than the dose needed to treat symptoms of the menopause and this may increase your chances of developing blood clots in the legs or lungs (see below). Therefore, it is important that you discuss the benefits and risks of estrogen use with your doctor if you have decided not to breast feed your baby.

The Dangers of Estrogens:

1. *Cancer of the uterus.* If estrogens are used in the postmenopausal period for more than a year, there is an increased risk of *endometrial cancer* (cancer of the uterus). Women taking estrogens have roughly 5 to 10 times as great a chance of getting this cancer as women who take no estrogens. To put this another way, while a postmenopausal woman not taking estrogens has 1 chance in 1,000 each year of getting cancer of the uterus, a woman taking estrogens has 5 to 10 chances in 1,000 each year. For this reason *it is important to take estrogens only when you really need them.*

The risk of this cancer is greater the longer estrogens are used and also seems to be greater when larger doses are taken. For this reason *it is important to take the lowest dose of estrogen that will control symptoms and to take it only as long as it is needed.* If estrogens are needed for longer periods of time, your doctor will want to reevaluate your need for estrogens at least every six months.

Women using estrogens should report any irregular vaginal bleeding to their doctors; such bleeding may be of no importance, but it can be an early warning of cancer of the uterus. If you have undiagnosed vaginal bleeding, you should not use estrogens until a diagnosis is made and you are certain there is no cancer of the uterus. If you have had your uterus completely removed (total hysterectomy), there is no danger of developing cancer of the uterus.

2. *Other possible cancers.* Estrogens can cause development of other tumors in animals, such as tumors of the breast, cervix, vagina, or liver, when given for a long time. At present there is no good evidence that women using estrogens in the menopause have an increased risk of such tumors, but there is no way yet to be sure they do not, and one study raises the possibility that use of estrogens in the menopause may increase the risk of breast cancer many years later. This is a further reason to use estrogens only when clearly needed. While you are taking estrogens, it is important that you go to your doctor at least once a year for a physical examination. Also, if members of your family have had breast cancer or if you have breast nodules or abnormal mammograms (breast x-rays), your doctor may wish to carry out more frequent examinations of your breasts.

3. *Gall bladder disease.* Women who use estrogens after menopause are more likely to develop gall bladder disease needing surgery as women who do not use estrogens. Birth control pills have a similar effect.

4. *Abnormal blood clotting.* Oral contraceptives increase the risk of blood clotting in various parts of the body. This can result in a stroke (if the clot is in the brain), a heart attack (clot in a blood vessel of the heart), or a pulmonary embolus (a clot which forms in the legs or pelvis, then breaks off and travels to the lungs). Any of these can be fatal.

At this time use of estrogens in the menopause is not known to cause such blood clotting, but this has not been fully studied and there could still prove to be such a risk. It is recommended that if you have had clotting in the legs or lungs or a heart attack or stroke while you were using estrogens or birth control pills, you should not use estrogens (unless they are being used to treat cancer of the breast or prostate). If you have had a stroke or heart attack or if you have angina pectoris, estrogens should be used with great caution and only if clearly needed (for example, if you have severe symptoms of the menopause).

The larger doses of estrogen used to prevent swelling of the breasts after pregnancy have been reported to cause clotting in the legs and lungs.

Special Warning About Pregnancy: You should not receive estrogen if you are pregnant. If this should occur, there is a greater than usual chance that the developing child will be born with a birth defect, although the possibility remains fairly small. A female child may have an increased risk of developing cancer of the vagina or cervix later in life (in the teens or twenties). Every possible effort should be made to avoid exposure to estrogens during pregnancy. If exposure occurs, see your doctor.

Other Effects of Estrogens: In addition to the serious known risks of estrogens described above, estrogens have the following side effects and potential risks:

1. *Nausea and vomiting.* The most common side effect of estrogen therapy is nausea. Vomiting is less common.
2. *Effects on breasts.* Estrogens may cause breast tenderness or enlargement and may cause the breasts to secrete a liquid. These effects are not dangerous.
3. *Effects on the uterus.* Estrogens may cause benign fibroid tumors of the uterus to get larger.

Some women will have menstrual bleeding when estrogens are stopped. But if the bleeding occurs on days you are still taking estrogens you should report this to your doctor.

4. *Effects on liver.* Women taking oral contraceptives develop on rare occasions a tumor of the liver which can rupture and bleed into the abdomen. So far, these tumors have not been reported in women using estrogens in the menopause, but you should report any swelling or unusual pain or tenderness in the abdomen to your doctor immediately.

Women with a past history of jaundice (yellowing of the skin and white parts of the eyes) may get jaundice again during estrogen use. If this occurs, stop taking estrogens and see your doctor.

5. *Other effects.* Estrogens may cause excess fluid to be retained in the body. This may make some conditions worse, such as epilepsy, migraine, heart disease, or kidney disease.

Summary: Estrogens have important uses, but they have serious risks as well. You must decide, with your doctor, whether the risks are acceptable to you in view of the benefits of treatment. Except where your doctor has prescribed estrogens for use in special cases of cancer of the breast or prostrate, you should not use estrogens if you have cancer of the breast or uterus, are pregnant, have undiagnosed abnormal vaginal bleeding, clotting in the legs or lungs, or have had a stroke, heart attack or angina, or clotting in the legs or lungs in the past while you were taking estrogens.

You can use estrogens as safely as possible by understanding that your doctor will require regular physical examinations while you are taking them and will try to discontinue the drug as soon as possible and use the smallest dose possible. Be alert for signs of trouble including:

1. Abnormal bleeding from the vagina.
2. Pains in the calves or chest or sudden shortness of breath, or coughing blood (indicating possible clots in the legs, heart, or lungs).
3. Severe headache, dizziness, faintness, or changes in vision (indicating possible developing clots in the brain or eye).
4. Breast lumps (you should ask your doctor how to examine your own breasts).
5. Jaundice (yellowing of the skin).
6. Mental depression.

Based on his or her assessment of your medical needs, your doctor has pescribed this drug for you. Do not give the drug to anyone else.

List of references available upon request.

MIDRIN ℞

Caution: Federal law prohibits dispensing without prescription.

Description: Each red capsule with pink band contains Isometheptene Mucate 65 mg., Dichloralphenazone 100 mg., and Acetaminophen 325 mg.

Isometheptene Mucate is a white crystalline powder having a characteristic aromatic odor and bitter taste. It is an unsaturated aliphatic amine with sympathomimetic properties.

Dichloralphenazone is a white, microcrystalline powder, with slight odor and tastes saline at first, becoming acrid. It is a mild sedative.

Acetaminophen, a non-salycylate, occurs as a white, odorless, crystalline powder possessing a slightly bitter taste.

Actions: Isometheptene Mucate, a sympathomimetic amine, acts by constricting dilated cranial and cerebral arterioles, thus reducing the stimuli that lead to vascular headaches. Dichloralphenazone, a mild sedative, reduces the patient's emotional reaction to the pain of both vascular and tension headaches. Acetaminophen raises the threshold to painful stimuli, thus exerting an analgesic effect against all types of headaches.

Indications: For relief of vascular and tension headaches.

> Based on a review for this drug (isometheptene mucate), The National Academy of Sciences-National Research Council and/or other information, FDA has classified the other indication as "Possibly" effective in the treatment of migraine headache.
> Final classification of the less-than-effective indication requires further investigation.

Contraindications: Midrin is contraindicated in Glaucoma and/or severe cases of renal disease, hypertension, organic heart disease, hepatic disease and in those patients who are on monoamine-oxidase (MAO) inhibitor therapy.

Precautions: Caution should be observed in hypertension, peripheral vascular disease and after recent cardiovascular attacks.

Adverse Reactions: Transient dizziness and skin rash may appear in hypersensitive patients. This can usually be eliminated by reducing the dose.

Dosage and Administration: FOR RELIEF OF MIGRAINE HEADACHE: The usual adult dosage is two capsules at once, followed by one capsule every hour until relieved, up to 5 capsules within a twelve hour period.

FOR RELIEF OF TENSION HEADACHE: The usual adult dose is one or two capsules every four hours up to 8 capsules a day.

How Supplied: Bottle of 50 capsules, NDC 0086-0120-05. Bottle of 100 capsules, NDC 0086-0120-10.

[*Shown in Product Identification Section*]

MINOTAL® ℞

Composition: Acetaminophen 325 mg., Sodium Butabarbital 15 mg. (Warning: May be habit forming.)

Indications: Minotal is indicated for the relief of tension headache and the associated symptoms of tension.

Contraindications: Hypersensitivity to either component.

Precautions: Due to presence of a barbiturate, may be habit forming. Excessive prolonged use should be avoided. Should be used with caution in patients with hepatic disease.
Adverse Reactions: In rare instances, drowsiness, nausea, constipation, dizziness and skin rash may occur.
Usual Adult Dosage: 1 or 2 tablets every 4 hours, not to exceed 8 tablets in 24 hours.
How Supplied:
Bottles of 100 tan tablets.
NDC 0086-0043-10
[*Shown in Product Identification Section*]

NOLAMINE ℞

Composition: Each timed-release tablet (formulated to provide 8 to 10 hours of continuous relief) contains: chlorpheniramine maleate 4 mg., phenindamine tartrate 24 mg., phenylpropanolamine HCl 50 mg.
Indications: As a nasal decongestant associated with the common cold, sinusitis, hayfever and other allergies.
Precautions: Antihistamines may cause drowsiness and should be used with caution in patients who operate motor vehicles or dangerous machinery. Use with caution in patients with hypertension, hyperthyroidism or cardiovascular disease.
Adverse Reactions: Drowsiness, tremors, dizziness and nervousness may occur occasionally.
Usual Adult Dosage: Orally, as a nasal decongestant, one tablet every 8 hours. In mild cases, every 10 to 12 hours.
How Supplied:
Bottle of 50 pink timed-release tablets.
NDC 0086-0204-05
Bottle of 250 pink timed-release tablets.
NDC 0086-0204-25
[*Shown in Product Identification Section*]

PHRENILIN® ℞

Composition: Acetaminophen 325 mg., Sodium Butabarbital 15 mg. (Warning: May be habit forming), Caffeine 40 mg.
Indications: Phrenilin is indicated for the relief of tension headache and the associated symptoms of tension.
Contraindications: Hypersensitivity to any of the components.
Precautions: Due to presence of a barbiturate, may be habit forming. Excessive prolonged use should be avoided. Should be used with caution in patients with hepatic disease.
Adverse Reactions: In rare instances, drowsiness, nausea, constipation, dizziness, and skin rash may occur.
Usual Adult Dosage: 1 or 2 tablets every 4 hours, not to exceed 8 tablets in 24 hours.
How Supplied:
Bottles of 100 pale violet tablets.
NDC 0086-0042-10
[*Shown in Product Identification Section*]

SINULIN

Composition: Each tablet contains: phenylpropanolamine HCl 37.5 mg., chlorpheniramine maleate 2 mg., acetaminophen 325 mg., salicylamide 250 mg., homatropine methylbromide 0.75 mg.
Indications: For relief of sinus congestion and headache.
Precautions: Use with caution in presence of hypertension, diabetes, cardiovascular or thyroid disease, manifest glaucoma.
Adverse Reactions: If drowsiness occurs, instruct patients not to drive or operate machinery. If rapid pulse, dizziness, blurring of vision, dryness of mouth occur, reduce dosage.
Dosage: *Adults*—1 tablet every 4 hours. Not more than 4 tablets daily.
Overdosage: In case of accidental overdose, seek professional assistance or contact a poison control center immediately.

How Supplied:
Bottles of 20 peach color tablets.
NDC 0086-0250-02
Bottles of 100 peach color tablets.
NDC 0086-0250-10
[*Shown in Product Identification Section*]

Central Pharmacal Company, The
SEYMOUR, IN 47274

CENALENE® Elixir/Tablet ℞

Composition: Each teaspoonful (5 ml.) or each coated tablet contains:
Pentylenetetrazol ....100 mg.
Thiamine Hydrochloride (Elixir) or Thiamine Mononitrate (Tablet) ....1.67 mg.
Niacinamide ....7.5 mg.
Cyanocobalamin (Vitamin B_{12}) ....2.5 mcg.
Elixir contains 15% alcohol and is sugar-free.
Indications: In older patients with mental confusion, apathy and memory defects as an analeptic agent.
Cenalene also contains thiamine hydrochloride or mononitrate, niacinamide and Vitamin B_{12} (Cyanocobalamin). These vitamins do not contribute directly to the effectiveness of Cenalene and are not present in therapeutic quantities. Their value in this formulation is limited to an occasional patient who may benefit from their administration as a means of preventing the development of a deficiency. It should be noted that although Cenalene contains Vitamin B_{12}, it is not useful in the treatment of any form of anemia.
Contraindications: There are no known contraindications.
Precautions: Caution should be exercised when treating patients with a low convulsive threshold, or with a focal brain lesion.
Caution should be exercised when administering high doses of pentylenetetrazol to patients suffering from heart disease. Pentylenetetrazol does not act directly on the myocardium; the results are from central vagal stimulation. Bradycardia, splanchnic vasodilation and conduction disturbances may occur with a resultant fall in blood pressure.
TOXICITY: Pentylenetetrazol in high doses has toxic symptoms typical of those produced by the central nervous system stimulants which act on the higher motor centers and the spinal cord. Convulsions result which are spontaneous and not induced by external stimuli. They last for several minutes and are followed by profound depression. Death results from anoxia, medullary depression, and respiratory paralysis. Death has been reported from the ingestion of 10 grams of pentylenetetrazol.
Dosage and Administration: Two teaspoonfuls or two tablets 3 times a day. After one month's therapy, dosage may be reduced to one teaspoonful or one tablet three times daily.
How Supplied: Elixir, pint and gallon bottles. Tablets, bottles of 100 and 1,000.

CODIMAL® DH Ⓒ ℞
CODIMAL® DM
CODIMAL® PH Ⓒ
CODIMAL® EXPECTORANT

Composition: Each teaspoonful (5 ml) of CODIMAL DH contains: Hydrocodone Bitartrate 1.66 mg. (Warning—May be habit forming); Phenylephrine Hydrochloride 5.0 mg.; Pyrilamine Maleate 8.33 mg.; Potassium Guaiacolsulfonate 83.3 mg.
Each teaspoonful (5 ml) of CODIMAL DM contains: Dextromethorphan hydrobromide 10 mg.; Phenylephrine hydrochloride 5 mg.; Pyrilamine maleate 8.33 mg.; Potassium guaiacolsulfonate 83.3 mg.; Alcohol 4%. Sugar-free.
Each teaspoonful (5 ml) of CODIMAL PH contains: Codeine Phosphate 10 mg. (Warning—May be habit forming); Phenylephrine Hydrochloride 5 mg.; Pyrilamine Maleate 8.33 mg.; Potassium Guaiacolsulfonate 83.3 mg.
Each teaspoonful (5 ml) of CODIMAL EXPECTORANT contains: Phenylpropanolamine Hydrochloride 25 mg.; Potassium Guaiacolsulfonate 100 mg.
Indications: For temporary relief of cough due to the common cold or other upper respiratory infection or irritation.
Contraindications: In persons with a known hypersensitivity to any of the ingredients.
Precautions: Should be administered with extreme caution to patients with hypertension, heart disease, diabetes, thyroid disease or vascular disease, or those receiving MAO inhibitors. Codeine and its derivative, Hydrocodone Bitartrate, are narcotic agents and the usual precautions in their use should be observed, particularly in infants and elderly patients.
Side Effects: Occasional drowsiness, blurred vision, palpitation, flushing, nervousness or gastrointestinal upsets.
Warnings: Patients should be instructed not to drive or operate machinery while taking the medication; and not to administer it to patients with a high fever or persistent cough unless so directed by a physician.
Administration and Dosage: Codimal DH: Adults and older children—2 teaspoonfuls every 4 hours until symptoms subside; children 6 to 12 years—1 teaspoonful every 4 hours; children 1 to 6 years—½ teaspoonful every 4 hours.
Codimal DM and Codimal PH: Adults and older children—1 to 2 teaspoonfuls; children 6 to 12—1 teaspoonful; children 2 to 6—½ teaspoonful. These doses may be taken every 4 hours. Children 6 months to 2 years—¼ teaspoonful every 6 hours.
Codimal Expectorant: Adults and older children—1 teaspoonful; children, 6 to 12 years—½ teaspoonful; children, 2 to 6—¼ teaspoonful. This dose may be taken every four hours.
How Supplied: Bottles of 4 ounces, pints and gallons.

CODIMAL®-L.A. CENULES® ℞

Composition: Each Cenule® (Timed Release Capsule) contains:
Chlorpheniramine maleate ....8 mg.
Pseudoephedrine hydrochloride ....120 mg.
In a specially prepared base to provide prolonged action.
Action and Uses: Chlorpheniramine maleate is a potent and effective antihistamine which, because of its relatively low dose, seems to cause less drowsiness than some other antihistamines.
Pseudoephedrine hydrochloride is a reliable nasal decongestant with a rapid and sustained activity.
Indications: For the temporary relief of common cold and sinusitis symptoms.
Contraindications: Sensitivity to any of the ingredients.
Precautions: Since drowsiness may occur with chlorpheniramine maleate, patients should be cautioned against engaging in operations requiring alertness, such as driving an automobile, until their response has been determined. Codimal-L.A. should be used with caution in the presence of hypertension, coronary artery disease, narrow-angle glaucoma, prostatic hypertrophy, hyperthyroidism and diabetes.
Adverse Reactions: Slight drowsiness due to chlorpheniramine maleate or mild stimulation due to pseudoephedrine. Other possible adverse reactions are restlessness, dry mouth, dizziness, weakness, anorexia, nausea, head-

Continued on next page

Central—Cont.

ache, nervousness, polyuria, heartburn, diplopia, sweating, dysuria and very rarely, dermatitis.
Dosage and Administration: Adults and children over twelve years of age—one capsule orally every 12 hours.
How Supplied: Bottles of 100 and 1000 Cenules®.
[*Shown in Product Identification Section*]

CO-XAN® (IMPROVED) Syrup ℞

Each tablespoonful (15 ml.) contains:
Theophylline ....165 Mg.
(as 330 mg. Theophylline sodium Glycinate)
Codeine phosphate ....15 mg.
Warning—May be habit forming.
Ephedrine hydrochloride ....25 mg.
Guaifenesin ....100 mg.
Alcohol 10%
Indications: Co-Xan is recommended for the symptomatic treatment of those sufferers from bronchospastic conditions of asthma with symptoms of wheezing, cough, swollen mucous membranes, adherent bronchial mucus and increased nasal secretions.
Contraindications: Co-Xan is contraindicated in individuals with a known hypersensitivity to any of its ingredients.
Precautions: The patient should be advised not to drive a car or operate dangerous machinery if he feels drowsy. This product should be used with caution in patients with hypertension, heart disease, diabetes or thyrotoxicosis. This product should not be administered more frequently than every 6 hours, or within 12 hours after rectal administration of any preparation containing theophylline or aminophylline. Other formulations containing xanthine derivatives should not be given concurrently with this product.
Adverse Reactions: Mild epigastric distress, palpitation, tremulousness, insomnia, difficulty of micturition, and CNS stimulation have been reported.
These effects are more frequent in cardiac patients or in those with interstitial nephritis. In excessive doses in susceptible individuals, albuminuria, gastric hemorrhage or epileptic spasm may appear. These manifestations, however, are rare.
Dosage And Administration:
Adults ....1 tablespoonful
Children over 12 ....2 to 3 teaspoonfuls
Children-6 to 12 ....1 to 2 teaspoonfuls
Children-3 to 6 ....1 teaspoonful
Children-1 to 3 ....½ teaspoonful
Repeat every 6 hours as necessary
How Supplied: Syrup-pint and gallon bottles.

NEOLAX® TABLETS ℞

Composition: Each NEOLAX Tablet contains: Dehydrocholic Acid 240 mg. and Dioctyl sodium sulfosuccinate 50 mg.
Action and Uses: The actions of NEOLAX are the result of the combination of complementary activities of its ingredients. Dehydrocholic acid, the oxidation product of cholic acid, is a potent hydrocholeretic. It is a mild laxative that has shown very low toxicity in both experimental animals and in clinical use. The mechanism by which dehydrocholic acid increases the frequency of bowel movements is unknown. Dioctyl sodium sulfosuccinate effects the surface tension and increases the water content of the stool, making it softer and, therefore, easier to pass. This softening, combined with the laxative effect of dehydrocholic acid, alleviates both of these symptoms of constipation.
Indications: A mild laxative and fecal softener as an aid in the treatment of chronic functional constipation, particularly in the elderly.
Contraindications: Biliary tract obstruction, acute hepatitis, or sensitivity to any of its ingredients.
Precautions: Patients should be examined periodically to prevent fluid and electrolyte deficiencies due to excessive laxative effects or inadequate intake.
Administration and Dosage: One or two tablets three times daily with meals. This dosage should be reduced as the condition is relieved.
How Supplied: Bottles of 100 and 1000, and unit dose packages of 100.

NIFEREX® Tablets/Elixir
NIFEREX®-150 Capsules
NIFEREX® with Vitamin C Tablets
(polysaccharide-iron complex)

Composition: NIFEREX is a highly water-soluble complex of iron and a low molecular weight polysaccharide. Each NIFEREX-150 Capsule contains 150 mg. elemental iron. Each NIFEREX Film Coated Tablet and each NIFEREX with Vitamin C Chewable Tablet contains 50 mg. elemental iron. In addition, each NIFEREX with Vitamin C tablet contains Ascorbic acid, U.S.P., 100 mg. and Sodium ascorbate, 168.75 mg. Each 5 ml. (teaspoonful) NIFEREX Elixir contains 100 mg. elemental iron, alcohol 10% (sugar free).
Action and Uses: NIFEREX is an easily assimilated source of iron for treatment of uncomplicated iron deficiency anemia. Because NIFEREX is a polysaccharide bound iron complex, it is relatively nontoxic and there are relatively few, if any, of the gastrointestinal side effects associated with iron therapy, thus permitting full therapeutic dosage (150 to 300 mg. elemental iron daily) in a single dose if desirable. There is no staining of teeth and no metallic aftertaste.
Indications: For treatment of uncomplicated iron deficiency anemia.
Contraindications: In patients with hemochromatosis and hemosiderosis, and in those with a known hypersensitivity to any of the ingredients.
Administration and Dosage: ADULTS: One or two NIFEREX-150 Capsules daily, or one or two NIFEREX or NIFEREX with Vitamin C Tablets twice daily, *or* one or two teaspoonfuls NIFEREX Elixir daily. CHILDREN 6 to 12 years of age: One or two NIFEREX *or* one NIFEREX with Vitamin C Tablet daily, or one teaspoonful NIFEREX Elixir daily; Children 2 to 6 years of age: ½ teaspoonful NIFEREX Elixir daily. Children under 2 years: ¼ teaspoonful daily.
How Supplied: NIFEREX-150 Capsules: Bottles of 100 and 1,000. NIFEREX Elixir: Bottles of 8 ounces and one gallon. NIFEREX Tablets: Bottles of 100 and 1,000. NIFEREX with Vitamin C Chewable Tablets: Bottles of 50.
[*Shown in Product Identification Section*]

NIFEREX®-150 FORTE Capsules ℞

Each capsule contains:
Iron (Elemental) ....150 mg.
(as polysaccharide-iron complex)
Folic Acid ....1 mg.
Vitamin B_{12} ....25 mcg.
Indications: Iron deficiency anemia and/or nutritional megaloblastic anemias due to inadequate diet.
Warnings: Folic acid alone is improper therapy in the treatment of pernicious anemia and other megaloblastic anemias where vitamin B_{12} is deficient.
Precaution: Folic acid, especially in doses above 1.0 mg. daily, may obscure pernicious anemia, in that hematologic remission may occur while neurological manifestations remain progressive.
Adverse Reactions: Allergic sensitization has been reported following both oral and parenteral administration of folic acid.
Dosage And Administration: One or two capsules daily.
How Supplied: Bottles of 100 and 1000.
[*Shown in Product Identification Section*]

NIFEREX®-PN Tablet ℞

Composition: Each film-coated tablet contains:
Iron (Elemental) ....60 mg.
(as polysaccharide iron complex)
Folic Acid ....1 mg.
Ascorbic Acid ....50 mg.
(as sodium ascorbate)
Cyanocobalamin (Vitamin B_{12}) ....3 mcg.
Vitamin A ....4000 I.U.
Vitamin D_2 ....400 I.U.
Thiamine Mononitrate ....3 mg.
Riboflavin ....3 mg.
Pyridoxine Hydrochloride ....2 mg.
Niacinamide ....10 mg.
Calcium Carbonate ....312 mg.
Indications: For the prevention and/or treatment of dietary vitamin and mineral deficiencies associated with pregnancy and lactation.
Contraindications: Sensitivity to any of the ingredients.
Precautions: Folic acid may correct blood values in pernicious anemia while neurological manifestations remain progressive.
Dosage: Prophylactic—1 tablet daily.
Therapeutic—2 to 4 tablets daily.
How Supplied: Bottles of 100 and 1000
[*Shown in Product Identification Section*]

SYNOPHYLATE® Tablets/Elixir ℞
(theophylline sodium glycinate)
SYNOPHYLATE®-GG Tablets/Syrup ℞
(theophylline sodium glycinate and guaifenesin)

Composition: An equilibrium mixture containing theophylline sodium and glycine in approximately equimolar proportions buffered with an additional mol of glycine. SYNOPHYLATE (theophylline sodium glycinate) Elixir or tablets contain per tbsp. (15 ml.) or per tablet: theophylline sodium glycinate, 330 mg. (equivalent to 165 mg. theophylline). (Alcohol 20% in the elixir).
SYNOPHYLATE-GG Syrup or Tablets contain per tbsp. (15 ml.) or per tablet: theophylline sodium glycinate, 300 mg. (equivalent to 150 mg. theophylline); guaifenesin 100 mg. (Alcohol 10% in the syrup).
Action and Uses: Theophylline sodium glycinate has the typical action of solubilized forms of theophylline with the advantage that it is less irritating to the gastric mucosa. Thus, it is tolerated in larger oral doses than are possible with other theophylline preparations.
It is highly effective in relaxing the smooth muscle of the bronchioles and it is widely used in the treatment of bronchial asthma.
Guaifenesin is an efficient expectorant which provides a marked increase in respiratory tract fluid.
Indications: For relief and/or prevention of symptoms from asthma and reversible bronchospasm associated with chronic bronchitis and emphysema.
Contraindications: These products are contraindicated in patients with a known hypersensitivity to any of their ingredients.
Precautions: These products should not be administered more frequently than every 6 hours, or within 12 hours after rectal administration of any other theophylline or aminophylline containing preparation.
Adverse Reactions: Theophylline sodium glycinate, like other xanthine derivatives, is relatively nontoxic. Therapeutic dosage may cause nausea and vomiting, burning epigastric or substernal pain, palpitation, dizziness, head-

ache, nervousness or similar minor complaints.
These effects are more frequent in cardiac patients or in those with interstitial nephritis. In excessive doses in susceptible individuals, albuminuria, gastric hemorrhage or epileptic spasm may appear. These manifestations, however, are rare.

Administration and Dosage:
Every 6 to 8 hours, preferably after meals:
Adults..1 or 2 tablets or 1 to 2 tablespoonfuls
Children—6 to 12
1 tablet or 2 to 3 teaspoonfuls
Children—3 to 6..............1 to 1½ teaspoonfuls
Children—1 to 3.................½ to 1 teaspoonful

How Supplied: Elixir or Syrup—pint and gallon bottles.
Tablets—bottles of 100 and 1000.

THEOCLEAR® L.A.-130 CENULES® ℞
THEOCLEAR® L.A.-260 CENULES® ℞
THEOCLEAR®-80 Syrup ℞
THEOCLEAR®-100 TABLETS ℞
THEOCLEAR®-200 TABLETS ℞
(theophylline anhydrous)

Description: THEOCLEAR L.A.-130 and THEOCLEAR L.A.-260: Each Cenule® contains 130 mg. or 260 mg. of theophylline anhydrous in a sustained release bead formulation.
THEOCLEAR-80: Each 15 ml. (1 tablespoonful) contains 80 mg. Anhydrous Theophylline as the active ingredient. Other ingredients are saccharin sodium; tartaric acid; benzoic acid; citric acid; sorbitol; glycerin; propylene glycol; artificial flavor and purified water q.s. This formulation provides an alcohol-free, dye-free, and sugar-free vehicle containing no corn by-products.
THEOCLEAR-100 and THEOCLEAR-200: Each tablet contains 100 mg. or 200 mg. of Theophylline Anhydrous.

Indications: For relief and/or prevention of symptoms from asthma and reversible bronchospasm associated with chronic bronchitis and emphysema.

Contraindications: In individuals who have shown hypersensitivity to any of its components.

Warnings: Status asthmaticus is a medical emergency. Optimal therapy frequently requires additional medication including corticosteroids when the patient is not rapidly responsive to bronchodilators.
Excessive theophylline doses may be associated with toxicity thus serum theophylline levels are recommended to assure maximal benefit without excessive risk. Incidence of toxicity increases at levels greater than 20 mcg/ml. Morphine, curare, and stilbamidine should be used with caution in patients with airflow obstruction since they stimulate histamine release and can induce asthmatic attacks. They may also suppress respiration leading to respiratory failure. Alternative drugs should be chosen whenever possible.
There is an excellent correlation between high blood levels of theophylline resulting from conventional doses and associated clinical manifestations of toxicity in (1) patients with lowered body plasma clearances (due to transient cardiac decomposition), (2) patients with liver dysfunction or chronic obstructive lung disease, (3) patients who are older than 55 years of age, particularly males.
There are often no early signs of less serious theophylline toxicity such as nausea and restlessness, which may appear in up to 50 percent of patients prior to onset of convulsions. Ventricular arrhythmias or seizures may be the first signs of toxicity.
Many patients who have higher theophylline serum levels exhibit a tachycardia.
Theophylline products may worsen pre-existing arrhythmias.

Usage in Pregnancy: Safe use in pregnancy has not been established relative to possible adverse effects on fetal development, but neither have adverse effects on fetal development been established. This is, unfortunately, true for most antiasthmatic medications. Therefore, use of theophylline in pregnant women should be balanced against the risk of uncontrolled asthma.

Precautions: Mean half-life in smokers is shorter than non-smokers, therefore, smokers may require larger doses of theophylline. Theophylline should not be administered concurrently with other xanthine medications. Use with caution in patients with severe cardiac disease, severe hypoxemia, hypertension, hyperthyroidism, acute myocardial injury, cor pulmonale, congestive heart failure, liver disease, and in the elderly (especially males) and in neonates. Great caution should especially be used in giving theophylline to patients in congestive heart failure. Such patients have shown markedly prolonged theophylline blood level curves with theophylline persisting in serum for long periods following discontinuation of the drug.
Use theophylline cautiously in patients with history of peptic ulcer. Theophylline may occasionally act as a local irritant to G.I. tract although gastrointestinal symptoms are more commonly central and associated with serum concentrations over 20 mcg/ml.

Adverse Reactions: The most consistent adverse reactions are usually due to overdose and are:
1. Gastrointestinal: nausea, vomiting, epigastric pain, hematemesis, diarrhea.
2. Central nervous system: headaches, irritability, restlessness, insomnia, reflex hyperexcitability, muscle twitching, clonic and tonic generalized convulsions.
3. Cardiovascular: palpitation, tachycardia, extra systoles, flushing, hypotension, circulatory failure, life threatening ventricular arrhythmias.
4. Respiratory: tachypnea.
5. Renal: albuminuria, increased excretion of renal tubular potentiation or diuresis, and red blood cells.
6. Others: hyperglycemia and inappropriate ADH syndrome.

Dosage and Administration: Therapeutic serum levels associated with optimal likelihood for benefit and minimal risk of toxicity are considered to be between 10 mcg/ml and 20 mcg/ml. Levels above 20 mcg/ml may produce toxic effects. There is great variation from patient to patient in dosage needed in order to achieve a therapeutic blood level because of variable rates of elimination. Because of this wide variation from patient to patient, and the relatively narrow therapeutic blood level range, dosage must be individualized and monitoring of theophylline serum levels is highly recommended.
Dosage should be calculated on the basis of lean (ideal) body weight where mg/kg doses are stated. Theophylline does not distribute into fatty tissue.
Giving theophylline with food may prevent the rare case of stomach irritation; and though absorption may be slower, it is still complete. When rapidly absorbed products such as solutions and uncoated tablets with rapid dissolution are used, dosing to maintain "around the clock" blood levels generally requires administration every 6 hours to obtain the greatest efficacy for clinical use in children; dosing intervals up to 8 hours may be satisfactory for adults because of their slower elimination. Children, and adults requiring higher than average doses, may benefit from products with slower absorption which may allow longer dosing intervals and/or less fluctuation in serum concentration over a dosing interval during chronic therapy.
[See table above].

DOSAGE FOR PATIENT POPULATION

Acute Symptoms of Asthma Requiring Rapid Theophyllinization:

I. Not currently receiving theophylline products

GROUP	ORAL LOADING DOSE (THEOPHYLLINE)	MAINTENANCE DOSE FOR NEXT 12 HOURS (THEOPHYLLINE)	MAINTENANCE DOSE BEYOND 12 HOURS (THEOPHYLLINE)
1. Children 6 months to 9 years	6 mg/kg	4 mg/kg q4h	4 mg/kg q6h
2. Children age 9-16 and smoking young adults	6 mg/kg	3 mg/kg q4h	3 mg/kg q6h
3. Otherwise healthy nonsmoking adults	6 mg/kg	3 mg/kg q6h	3 mg/kg q8h
4. Older adults and patients with cor pulmonale	6 mg/kg	2 mg/kg q6h	2 mg/kg q8h
5. Patients with congestive heart failure, liver failure	6 mg/kg	2 mg/kg q8h	1-2 mg/kg q12h

II. Those currently receiving theophylline products: Determine, where possible, the time, amount, route of administration and form of the patient's last dose.

The loading dose for theophylline will be based on the principle that each .5 mg/kg of theophylline administered as a loading dose will result in a 1 mcg/ml increase in serum theophylline concentration. Ideally, then, the loading dose should be deferred if a serum theophylline concentration can be rapidly obtained. If this is not possible, the clinician must exercise his judgment in selecting a dose based on the potential for benefit and risk. When there is sufficient respiratory distress to warrant a small risk, 2.5 mg/kg of theophylline is likely to increase the serum concentration when administered as a loading dose in rapidly absorbed form by only about 5 mcg/ml. If the patient is not already experiencing theophylline toxicity, this is unlikely to result in dangerous adverse effects.
Subsequent to the modified decision regarding loading dose in this group of patients, the subsequent maintenance dosage recommendations are the same as those described above.

Comments: To achieve optimal therapeutic theophylline dosage, it is recommended to monitor serum theophylline concentrations. However, it is not always possible or practical to obtain a serum theophylline level.
Patients should be closely monitored for signs of toxicity. The present data suggest that the above dosage recommendations will achieve therapeutic serum concentrations with minimal risk of toxicity for most patients. However, some risk of toxic serum concentrations is still present.
Adverse reactions to theophylline often occur when serum theophylline levels exceed 20 mcg/ml.

Chronic Asthma:
Theophyllinization is a treatment of first choice for the management of chronic asthma (to prevent symptoms and maintain patent airways). Slow clinical titration is generally preferred to assure acceptance and safety of the medication.
Initial dose: 16 mg/kg/day or 400 mg/day (whichever is

Continued on next page

Central—Cont.

lower) in 3–4 divided doses at 6–8 hour intervals. (520 mg/day in 1–2 divided doses at 12 hour intervals for sustained release formulations.)

Increased dose: The above dosage may be increased in approximately 25 percent increments at 2–3 day intervals so long as no intolerance is observed, until the maximum indicated below is reached.

Maximum dose without measurement of serum concentrations:

Not to exceed the following: (WARNING: DO NOT ATTEMPT TO MAINTAIN ANY DOSE THAT IS NOT TOLERATED)

Age $<$ 9 years - 24 mg/kg/day
Age 9–12 years - 20 mg/kg/day
Age 12–16 years - 18 mg/kg/day
Age $>$ 16 years - 13 mg/kg/day or 900 mg/day (WHICHEVER IS LESS)

Note: Use ideal body weight for obese patients.

Measurement of serum theophylline concentration during chronic therapy:

If the above maximum doses are to be maintained or exceeded, serum theophylline measurement is recommended. This should be obtained at the approximate time of peak absorption during chronic therapy for the product used (1–2 hours for liquids and plain uncoated tablets that undergo rapid dissolution, 3–5 hours for sustained release preparations). It is important that the patient will have missed no doses during the previous 48 hours and that dosing intervals will have been reasonably typical with no added doses during that period of time. DOSAGE ADJUSTMENT BASED ON SERUM THEOPHYLLINE MEASUREMENTS WHEN THESE INSTRUCTIONS HAVE NOT BEEN FOLLOWED MAY RESULT IN RECOMMENDATIONS THAT PRESENT RISK OF TOXICITY TO THE PATIENT.

How Supplied: Theoclear L.A.-260 Cenules, imprinted with "Central Logo and 260 mg." and Theoclear L.A.-130 Cenules, imprinted with "Central Logo and 130 mg:" Supplied in bottles of 100 and 1000 Cenules.
Theoclear-80 Syrup: Supplied in pints and gallons.
Theoclear-100 Tablets and Theoclear-200 Tablets: Supplied in bottles of 100 and 1000.
[*Shown in Product Identification Section*]

Century Pharmaceuticals, Inc.
4553 ALLISONVILLE ROAD
INDIANAPOLIS, INDIANA 46205

POLYDINE–SOLUTION–SCRUB–OINTMENT OTC
(Povidone–Iodine)

Description: Polydine products contain the organic Iodine complex Povidone-Iodine. The therapeutic index is among the highest of the effective antiseptics. Polydine kills gram-positive, gram-negative bacteria (including tubercle bacillus and antibiotic resistant strains), yeast, molds, fungi, spores, viruses, protozoa and metazoa. Development of organism resistant to Polydine has not been reported. Polydine is effective in the presence of blood, pus, oil, grease and soap. Povidone-Iodine prolongs the application of Iodine therapeutically and shows synergistic effect in many cases resulting in greater antimicrobial activity compared to elemental Iodine.

Indications: Solution: For antiseptic and germicidal applications to degerm skin and mucous membranes prior to injections, aspirations, surgery, urinary catheterization; for treatment of cuts, minor wounds, burns, lacerations, abrasions, and pre-operative use (including oral cavity), dressing applications. Scrub: For cleaning as well as degerming-especially pre-operative. Ointment: For topical application when a water soluble base is desired.

Contraindications: Polydine lowers sensitizing effect and toxicity 10 fold compared to elemental Iodine, but do not administer to persons knows to be sensitive to Iodine. Discontinue if sensitivity occurs.

Warning: DO NOT SWALLOW.

Administration: Solution and Ointment. Apply to affected area, may be bandaged. For Scrub: Use about 5 ml., scrub 5 minutes and rinse under running water. Repeat. For pre-operative use: Shave, apply about 1 ml./25 sq. inches and scrub 5 minutes, rinse with water soaked sterile guaze, paint area with solution and let dry. Polydine will not stain natural fabrics.

How Supplied: Polydine Solution and Scrub, 1 oz. (patient unit size), 4 oz., 8 oz., Qt., Gal.
Ointment: 1 oz., 1 lb.

Cetylite Industries, Inc.
9051 RIVER ROAD
PENNSAUKEN, NJ 08110

CETACAINE® ℞
TOPICAL ANESTHETIC

A BRAND OF

Benzocaine	14.0%
Butyl Aminobenzoate	2.0%
Tetracaine Hydrochloride	2.0%
Benzalkonium Chloride	0.5%
Cetyl Dimethyl Ethyl Ammonium Bromide	0.005%

In a bland water soluble base.

Action: Cetacaine produces anesthesia rapidly in approximately 30 seconds.

Indications: Cetacaine is a topical anesthetic indicated for the production of anesthesia of accessible mucous membrane.
Cetacaine Spray is indicated for use to control pain or gagging. Cetacaine in all forms is indicated for use to control pain.

Dosage and Administration: Cetacaine Spray should be applied for approximately one second or less for normal anesthesia. Only limited quantity of Cetacaine is required for anesthesia and a spray in excess of 2 seconds is contraindicated. Average expulsion rate of residue from spray, at normal temperatures, is 295 mg. per second.
Tissue need not be dried prior to application of Cetacaine.
Cetacaine should be applied directly to the site where pain control is required.
Cetacaine Liquid or Cetacaine Ointment may be applied with a cotton pledget or directly to tissue. Cotton pledget should not be held in position for extended periods of time, since local reactions to benzoate topical anesthetics are related to the length of time of application.

Adverse Reactions: Although systemic reactions to Cetacaine have not been reported, local reactions to benzoate topical anesthetics may be associated with the condition of the mucous membrane treated and the length of time of application. Dehydration of the epithelium or a slight escharotic effect may result from prolonged contact. Allergic reactions are known to occur in some patients with preparations containing benzocaine.
Usage in Pregnancy: Safe use of Cetacaine has not been established with respect to possible adverse effects upon fetal development. Therefore Cetacaine should not be used during early pregnancy, unless in the judgment of a physician the potential benefits outweigh the unknown hazards.
Routine precaution for the use of any topical anesthetic should be observed when Cetacaine is used.

Contraindications:
Cetacaine is not for injection.
Do not use in the eyes.
To avoid excessive systemic absorption, Cetacaine should not be applied to large areas of denuded or inflamed tissue.
Cetacaine should not be administered to patients who are hypersensitive to any of its ingredients.
Individual dosage of tetracaine hydrochloride in excess of 20 mg. is contraindicated. Cetacaine should not be used under dentures or cotton rolls, as retention of the active ingredients under a denture or cotton roll could possibly cause a slight escharotic effect.

Jetco Cannula: The Jetco cannula for Cetacaine Spray is specially designed for accessibility and application of Cetacaine, at the required site of pain control.
The Jetco cannula is supplied in various sizes and shapes.
The Jetco cannula is inserted firmly onto the protruding plastic tubing on each bottle of Cetacaine Spray.
The Jetco cannula may be removed and reinserted as many times as required for cleansing or sterilization.

Packaging Available:
Aerosol Spray 56 gm., including propellant.
Liquid 56 gm. bottle.
Ointment, flavored, 37 gram jar.
Hospital Gel, 29 grams in polyethylene tube.

Caution: Federal law prohibits dispensing Cetacaine without prescription.
Keep out of reach of children.

CETYLCIDE® SOLUTION

Composition:

Cetyl Dimethyl Ethyl Ammonium Bromide	6.5%
Benzalkonium Chloride U.S.P.	6.5%
Isopropyl Alcohol	13.0%
Inert Ingredients	74.0%

Formulation contains Sodium Nitrite

Indications and Uses: Cetylcide is for use in the chemical disinfection of dental and surgical instruments. Cetylcide, when diluted, is a potent germicidal solution combining high bactericidal and bacteriostatic action against most kinds of pathogenic bacteria.
Germicides containing a Quarternary Ammonium derivative should not be relied upon to destroy spore bearing organisms, mycobacterium tuberculosis or the etiologic agent of viral hepatitis. Thus, instruments suspected of such contamination should be sterilized by heat. Needles, hypodermic syringes, corroded instruments or those with deep narrow crevices, as well as hinged or defective plated instruments, should be sterilized by heat. To maintain disinfection they may then be immersed in Cetylcide Solution.

How Supplied: 10 cc ampules, 32 ounce bottles, and 16 ounce bottles.

Over 7,000 products are

listed alphabetically

in the

PINK SECTION.

CIBA Pharmaceutical Company

Division of CIBA-GEIGY Corporation
SUMMIT, NJ 07901

To provide a convenient and accurate means of identifying CIBA solid dosage form products, a code number has been imprinted on all tablets and capsules. To help you quickly identify a CIBA Tablet or Capsule by its code number, a numerical listing of codes (with corresponding product names) and an alphabetical listing of products (with corresponding codes and list numbers) have been compiled below.

CIBA Code # ALPHABETICAL LISTING List Number

Antrenyl® bromide
(oxyphenonium bromide)
15 TABLETS, 5 mg (white, scored)
100s 2410

Anturane®
(sulfinpyrazone USP)
41 TABLETS (white, single-scored) each containing 100 mg sulfinpyrazone USP
100s 1910
168 CAPSULES (green) each containing 200 mg sulfinpyrazone USP
100s 1920

Apresazide®
(hydralazine HCl and hydrochlorothiazide)
139 CAPSULES (light blue and white opaque), each containing 25 mg hydralazine HCl and 25 mg hydrochlorothiazide
100s 3131
149 CAPSULES (pink and white opaque), each containing 50 mg hydralazine HCl and 50 mg hydrochlorothiazide
100s 3132
159 CAPSULES (pink flesh and white opaque), each containing 100 mg hydralazine HCl and 50 mg hydrochlorothiazide
100s 3133

Apresoline® hydrochloride
(hydralazine hydrochloride USP)
37 TABLETS, 10 mg (pale yellow, dry-coated)
100s 2629
1000s 2627
Consumer Pack
100s 2603
39 TABLETS, 25 mg (deep blue, dry-coated)
100s 2611
500s 2613
1000s 2615
Accu-Pak® 100s 2647
Consumer Pack
100s 2606
73 TABLETS, 50 mg (light blue, dry-coated
100s 2619
500s 2621
1000s 2623
Accu-Pak® 100s 2648
Consumer Pack
100s 2643
101 TABLETS, 100 mg (peach, dry-coated)
100s 2638

Apresoline®-Esidrix®
(hydralazine hydrochloride and hydrochlorothiazide)
129 TABLETS (orange, dry-coated), each containing 25 mg hydralazine hydrochloride and 15 mg hydrochlorothiazide
100s 3120

Dialog®
(allobarbital and acetaminophen)
105 TABLETS (white, scored), each containing 15 mg allobarbital and 300 mg acetaminophen
30s 3310

Dianabol®
(methandrostenolone NF)
17 TABLETS, 2.5 mg (pale yellow, scored)
100s 0620
20 TABLETS, 5 mg (blue, scored)
100s 0610
1000s 0612

Esidrix®
(hydrochlorothiazide USP)
22 TABLETS, 25 mg (pink, scored)
100s 4310
1000s 4313
5000s 4314
Accu-Pak®
100s 4312
Consumer Pack
100s 4325
46 TABLETS, 50 mg (yellow, scored)
100s 4315
1000s 4318
5000s 4319
Accu-Pak®
100s 4317
Consumer Pack
30s 4328
60s 4331
100s 4330
192 TABLETS, 100 mg (blue, scored)
100s 4340

Esimil®
47 TABLETS (white, scored), each containing 10 mg guanethidine monosulfate and 25 mg hydrochlorothiazide
100s 4503
Accu-Pak®
100s 4505
Consumer Pack
100s 4512

Forhistal® maleate
(dimethindene maleate NF)
45 LONTABS®, 2.5 mg (orange)
100s 4610

Ismelin® sulfate
(guanethidine sulfate USP)
49 TABLETS, 10 mg (pale yellow, scored)
100s 5010
1000s 5012
Accu-Pak®
100s 5005
Consumer Pack
100s 5003
103 TABLETS, 25 mg (white, scored)
100s 5020
1000s 5022
Accu-Pak®
100s 5028
Consumer Pack
100s 5026

Metandren®
(methyltestosterone USP)
30 TABLETS, 10 mg (white, scored)
100s 1414
32 TABLETS, 25 mg (pale yellow, scored)
100s 1418
51 LINGUETS®, 5 mg (white)
100s 1432
64 LINGUETS®, 10 mg (yellow)
100s 1438

Metopirone®
(metyrapone USP)
130 TABLETS, 250 mg (white, scored)
18s 5403

Regitine® hydrochloride
(phentolamine hydrochloride NF)
152 TABLETS, 50 mg (white, scored)
100s 6814

Rimactane®
(rifampin USP)
154 CAPSULES, 300 mg (opaque scarlet and caramel)
30s 8903
60s 8904
100s 8901

Rimactane®/INH Dual Pack
(rifampin USP) (isoniazid USP)
154 Each Dual Pack contains two Rimactane 300-mg CAPSULES and one INH 300-mg TABLET 8912

Ritalin® hydrochloride Ⓒ
(methylphenidate hydrochloride USP)
07 TABLETS, 5 mg (pale yellow)
100s 7410
500s 7412
1000s 7414
03 TABLETS, 10 mg (pale green, scored)
100s 7416
500s 7418
1000s 7420
Accu-Pak® 100s 7415
34 TABLETS, 20 mg (peach, scored)
100s 7422
1000s 7426

Ser-Ap-Es®
71 TABLETS (light salmon pink, dry-coated), each containing 0.1 mg reserpine, 25 mg hydralazine hydrochloride and 15 mg hydrochlorothiazide
100s 6610
1000s 6612
Accu-Pak® 100s 6605
Consumer Pack
100s 6617

Serpasil®
(reserpine USP)
35 TABLETS, 0.1 mg (white)
100s 7610
1000s 7614
36 TABLETS, 0.25 mg (white, scored)
100s 7616
500s 7618
1000s 7620
5000s 7622
Consumer Pack
100s 7607

Serpasil®-Apresoline®
(reserpine and hydralazine hydrochloride)
40 TABLETS #1 (yellow, dry-coated), each containing 0.1 mg reserpine and 25 mg hydralazine hydrochloride
100s 7721
104 TABLETS #2 (yellow, dry-coated), each containing 0.2 mg reserpine and 50 mg hydralazine hydrochloride
100s 7709

Serpasil®-Esidrix®
(reserpine and hydrochlorothiazide)
13 TABLETS #1 (light orange), each containing 0.1 mg reserpine and 25 mg hydrochlorothiazide
100s 7010
1000s 7012
97 TABLETS #2 (light orange), each containing 0.1 mg reserpine and 50 mg hydrochlorothiazide
100s 7020
1000s 7022

Slow-K®
(potassium chloride)
165 TABLETS (pale orange, sugar-coated), each containing 8 mEq (600 mg) potassium chloride
100s 2807
1000s 2811
Accu-Pak®
100s 2817
Consumer Pack
100s 2815

Continued on next page

CIBA—Cont.

CIBA Code # NUMERICAL LISTING

Ritalin® hydrochloride Ⓒ
(methylphenidate hydrochloride USP)
03 TABLETS, 10 mg (pale green, scored)
07 TABLETS, 5 mg (pale yellow)

Serpasil®-Esidrix®
(reserpine and hydrochlorothiazide)
13 TABLETS #1 (light orange), each containing 0.1 mg reserpine and 25 mg hydrochlorothiazide

Antrenyl® bromide
(oxyphenonium bromide)
15 TABLETS, 5 mg (white, scored)

Dianabol®
(methandrostenolone NF)
17 TABLETS, 2.5 mg (pale yellow, scored)
20 TABLETS, 5 mg (blue, scored)

Esidrix®
(hydrochlorothiazide USP)
22 TABLETS, 25 mg (pink, scored)

Metandren®
(methyltestosterone USP)
30 TABLETS, 10 mg (white, scored)

Metandren®
(methyltestosterone USP)
32 TABLETS, 25 mg (pale yellow, scored)

Ritalin® hydrochloride Ⓒ
(methylphenidate hydrochloride USP)
34 TABLETS, 20 mg (peach, scored)

Serpasil®
(reserpine USP)
35 TABLETS, 0.1 mg (white)
36 TABLETS, 0.25 mg (white, scored)

Apresoline® hydrochloride
(hydralazine hydrochloride USP)
37 TABLETS, 10 mg (pale yellow, dry-coated)
39 TABLETS, 25 mg (deep blue, dry-coated)

Serpasil®-Apresoline®
(reserpine and hydralazine hydrochloride)
40 TABLETS #1 (yellow, dry-coated), each containing 0.1 mg reserpine and 25 mg hydralazine hydrochloride

Anturane®
(sulfinpyrazone USP)
41 TABLETS (white, single-scored) each containing 100 mg sulfinpyrazone USP

Forhistal® maleate
(dimethindene maleate NF)
45 LONTABS®, 2.5 mg (orange)

Esidrix®
(hydrochlorothiazide USP)
46 TABLETS, 50 mg (yellow, scored)

Esimil®
47 TABLETS (white, scored), each containing 10 mg guanethidine monosulfate and 25 mg hydrochlorothiazide

Ismelin® sulfate
(guanethidine sulfate USP)
49 TABLETS, 10 mg (pale yellow, scored)

Metandren®
(methyltestosterone USP)
51 LINGUETS®, 5 mg (white)

Metandren®
(methyltestosterone USP)
64 LINGUETS®, 10 mg (yellow)

Ser-Ap-Es®
71 TABLETS (light salmon pink, dry-coated), each containing 0.1 mg reserpine, 25 mg hydralazine hydrochloride and 15 mg hydrochlorothiazide

Apresoline® hydrochloride
(hydralazine hydrochloride USP)
73 TABLETS, 50 mg (light blue, dry-coated)

Serpasil®-Esidrix®
(reserpine and hydrochlorothiazide)
97 TABLETS #2 (light orange), each containing 0.1 mg reserpine and 50 mg hydrochlorothiazide

Apresoline® hydrochloride
(hydralazine hydrochloride USP)
101 TABLETS, 100 mg (peach, dry-coated)

Ismelin® sulfate
(guanethidine sulfate USP)
103 TABLETS, 25 mg (white, scored)

Serpasil®-Apresoline®
(reserpine and hydralazine hydrochloride)
104 TABLETS #2 (yellow, dry-coated), each containing 0.2 mg reserpine and 50 mg hydralazine hydrochloride

Dialog®
(allobarbital and acetaminophen)
105 TABLETS (white, scored), each containing 15 mg allobarbital and 300 mg acetaminophen

Apresoline®-Esidrix®
(hydralazine hydrochloride and hydrochlorothiazide)
129 TABLETS (orange, dry-coated), each containing 25 mg hydralazine hydrochloride and 15 mg hydrochlorothiazide

Metopirone®
(metyrapone USP)
130 TABLETS, 250 mg (white, scored)

Apresazide®
(hydralazine HCl and hydrochlorothiazide)
139 CAPSULES (light blue and white opaque), each containing 25 mg hydralazine hydrochloride and 25 mg hydrochlorothiazide
149 CAPSULES (pink and white opaque), each containing 50 mg hydralazine hydrochloride and 50 mg hydrochlorothiazide

Regitine® hydrochloride
(phentolamine hydrochloride NF)
152 TABLETS, 50 mg (white, scored)

Rimactane®
(rifampin USP)
154 CAPSULES, 300 mg (opaque scarlet and caramel)

Rimactane®/INH Dual Pack
(rifampin USP) (isoniazid USP)
154 Each Dual Pack contains two Rimactane 300-mg CAPSULES and one INH 300-mg TABLET

Apresazide®
(hydralazine HCl and hydrochlorothiazide)
159 CAPSULES (pink flesh and white opaque), each containing 100 mg hydralazine hydrochloride and 50 mg hydrochlorothiazide

Slow-K®
(potassium chloride)
165 TABLETS (pale orange, sugar-coated), each containing 8 mEq (600 mg) potassium chloride

Anturane®
(sulfinpyrazone USP)
168 CAPSULES (green) each containing 200 mg sulfinpyrazone USP

Esidrix®
(hydrochlorothiazide USP)
192 TABLETS, 100 mg (blue, scored)

ANTRENYL® bromide ℞
(oxyphenonium bromide)

Indications: Peptic Ulcer, as adjunctive therapy.

Contraindications: Glaucoma; obstructive uropathy (for example, bladder neck obstruction due to prostatic hypertrophy); obstructive disease of the gastrointestinal tract (as in achalasia, paralytic ileus, pyloroduodenal stenosis, etc.); intestinal atony of the elderly or debilitated patient; unstable cardiovascular status in acute hemorrhage; severe ulcerative colitis; toxic megacolon complicating ulcerative colitis; myasthenia gravis; hypersensitivity.

Warnings: In the presence of a high environmental temperature, heat prostration can occur with drug use (fever and heat stroke due to decreased sweating).

Diarrhea may be an early symptom of incomplete intestinal obstruction, especially in patients with ileostomy or colostomy. In this instance, treatment with Antrenyl would be inappropriate and possibly harmful.

Anticholinergics may produce drowsiness or blurred vision. Therefore, patients should be warned not to engage in activities requiring mental alertness (such as operating a motor vehicle or other machinery) or perform hazardous work while taking Antrenyl.

Usage in Pregnancy
The safe use of this drug in pregnant women or during lactation has not been established. Therefore, the benefits must be weighed against the potential hazards.

Precautions: Give cautiously to patients with autonomic neuropathy; hepatic or renal disease; early evidence of ileus (as in peritonitis); ulcerative colitis (large doses may suppress intestinal motility to the point of producing a paralytic ileus and the use of anticholinergics may precipitate or aggravate the serious complication of toxic megacolon); hyperthyroidism; coronary heart disease; congestive heart failure; cardiac arrhythmias; hypertension; nonobstructing prostatic hypertrophy; hiatal hernia associated with reflux esophagitis, since anticholinergic drugs may aggravate this condition.

It should be noted that the use of anticholinergic drugs in the treatment of gastric ulcer may produce a delay in gastric emptying time and may complicate such therapy (antral stasis). Do not rely on the use of Antrenyl in the presence of biliary tract disease. Investigate any tachycardia before giving anticholinergic (atropine-like) drugs, since they may increase the heart rate.

With overdosage, a curare-like action may occur.

Use cautiously in debilitated patients with chronic lung disease, because reduction in bronchial secretions can lead to inspissation and formation of bronchial plugs. All anticholinergic agents should be used with caution in patients over 40 years of age because of the increased incidence of glaucoma in this age group.

Adverse Reactions: Anticholinergics produce certain effects which may be physiologic or toxic, depending upon the individual patient's response. The physician must delineate these. Adverse reactions may include xerostomia; urinary hesitancy and retention; blurred vision; tachycardia; palpitations; mydriasis; dilatation of the pupil; cycloplegia; increased ocular tension; loss of taste; headaches; nervousness; drowsiness; weakness; dizziness; insomnia; nausea; vomiting; impotence; suppression of lactation; constipation; bloated feeling; severe allergic reaction or drug idiosyncrasies, including anaphylaxis, urticaria, and other dermal manifestation; some degree of mental confusion and/or excitement, especially in elderly persons.

Decreased sweating is another adverse reaction that may occur. It should be noted that adrenergic innervation of the eccrine sweat glands on the palms and soles make complete control of sweating impossible. An end point of complete anhidrosis cannot occur because large doses of drug would be required, and this

would produce severe side effects from parasympathetic paralysis.
Dosage and Administration: Average adult dosage is 10 mg (2 tablets) 4 times daily for several days. Dosage may then be reduced, depending on patient's response.
Not for use in children.
Overdosage: Treatment is the same as for atropine overdosage. Gastric lavage or, in the absence of coma, an emetic should be given, and activated charcoal slurry instilled into the stomach. If central nervous system excitation occurs, a short-acting barbiturate may be used. Avoid long-acting sedatives; the central depressive action of these agents may coincide with depression produced by oxyphenonium in later stages. Fever may be combated with ice bags, alcohol sponges, and other appropriate measures.
How Supplied: *Tablets,* 5 mg (white, scored); bottles of 100. C77-16 Rev. 3/77
[*Shown in Product Identification Section*]

ANTURANE® ℞
(sulfinpyrazone USP)
Tablets Capsules

Indications: Anturane is indicated for the treatment of:
1. Chronic gouty arthritis
2. Intermittent gouty arthritis

Contraindications: Patients with an active peptic ulcer or symptoms of gastrointestinal inflammation or ulceration should not receive the drug.
The drug is contraindicated in patients with a history or the presence of:
1. Hypersensitivity to phenylbutazone or other pyrazoles
2. Blood dyscrasias

Warnings: Studies on the teratogenicity of pyrazole compounds in animals have yielded inconclusive results. Up to the present time, however, there have been no reported cases of human congenital malformation proved to be due to the use of the drug.
It is suggested that Anturane be used with caution in pregnant women, weighing the potential risks against the possible benefits.
Precautions: As with all pyrazole compounds, patients receiving Anturane should be kept under close medical supervision and periodic blood counts are recommended. It may be administered with care to patients with a history of healed peptic ulcer.
Recent reports have indicated that Anturane potentiates the action of certain sulfonamides, such as sulfadiazine and sulfisoxazole. In addition, other pyrazole compounds (phenylbutazone) have been observed to potentiate the hypoglycemic sulfonylurea agents, as well as insulin. In view of these observations, it is suggested that Anturane be used with caution in conjunction with sulfa drugs, the sulfonylurea hypoglycemic agents and insulin.
Because Anturane is a potent uricosuric agent, it may precipitate urolithiasis and renal colic, especially in the initial stages of therapy. For this reason, an adequate fluid intake and alkalinization of the urine are recommended. In cases with significant renal impairment, periodic assessment of renal function is indicated. Occasional cases of renal failure have been reported; but a cause-and-effect relationship has not always been clearly established.
Salicylates antagonize the uricosuric action of Anturane and for this reason their concomitant use is contraindicated in gouty arthritis.
Anturane may accentuate the action of coumarin-type anticoagulants and further depress prothrombin activity when these medications are employed simultaneously.
The Anturane capsules (200 mg) contain FD&C Yellow No. 5 (tartrazine) which may cause allergic-type reactions (including bronchial asthma) in certain susceptible individuals. Although the overall incidence of FD&C Yellow No. 5 (tartrazine) sensitivity in the general population is low, it is frequently seen in patients who also have aspirin hypersensitivity.
Note: Anturane has minimal anti-inflammatory effect and is not intended for the relief of an acute attack of gout.
In the initial stages of therapy, because of the marked ability of Anturane to mobilize urates, acute attacks of gouty arthritis may be precipitated.
Adverse Reactions: The most frequently reported adverse reactions with Anturane have been upper gastrointestinal disturbances. In these patients it is advisable to administer the drug with food, milk, or antacids. Despite this precaution, Anturane may aggravate or reactivate peptic ulcer.
Rash has been reported. In most instances, this reaction did not necessitate discontinuance of therapy. In general, Anturane has not been observed to affect electrolyte balance.
Blood dyscrasias (anemia, leukopenia, agranulocytosis, thrombocytopenia and aplastic anemia) have rarely been reported. There has also been a published report associating Anturane, administered concomitantly with other drugs including colchicine, with leukemia following long-term treatment of patients with gout. However, the circumstances involved in the two cases reported are such that a cause-and-effect relationship to Anturane has not been clearly established.
Overdosage:
Symptoms: Nausea, vomiting, diarrhea, epigastric pain, ataxia, labored respiration, convulsions, coma. Possible symptoms, seen after overdosage with other pyrazolone derivatives: anemia, jaundice, ulceration.
Treatment: No specific antidote. Induce emesis; gastric lavage; supportive treatment (intravenous glucose infusions, analeptics).
Dosage and Administration:
Initial: 200–400 mg daily in two divided doses, with meals or milk, gradually increasing when necessary to full maintenance dosage in one week.
Maintenance:
400 mg daily, given in two divided doses, as above. This dosage may be increased to 800 mg daily, if necessary, and may sometimes be reduced to as low as 200 mg daily after the blood urate level has been controlled. Treatment should be continued without interruption even in the presence of acute exacerbations, which can be concomitantly treated with phenylbutazone or colchicine. Patients previously controlled with other uricosuric therapy may be transferred to Anturane at full maintenance dosage.
How Supplied: White, single-scored tablets of 100 mg, bottles of 100 (NDC 0083-0041-30). Green capsules of 200 mg, bottles of 100 (NDC 0083-0168-30).
Dispense in tight container (USP).
C80-10 (1/80)
[*Shown in Product Identification Section*]

APRESAZIDE® ℞
(hydralazine HCl and hydrochlorothiazide)
25/25 Capsules
50/50 Capsules
100/50 Capsules

Warning
This fixed combination drug is not indicated for initial therapy of hypertension. Hypertension requires therapy titrated to the individual patient. If the fixed combination represents the dosage so determined, its use may be more convenient in patient management. The treatment of hypertension is not static, but must be reevaluated as conditions in each patient warrant.

Indications
Hypertension. (See box warning.)
Contraindications
Hydralazine
Hypersensitivity to hydralazine; coronary artery disease; and mitral valvular rheumatic heart disease.
Hydrochlorothiazide
Anuria; hypersensitivity to this or other sulfonamide-derived drugs.
Warnings
Hydralazine
Hydralazine may produce in a few patients a clinical picture simulating systemic lupus erythematosus. In such patients hydralazine should be discontinued unless the benefit-to-risk determination requires continued antihypertensive therapy with this drug. Symptoms and signs usually regress when the drug is discontinued but residua have been detected many years later. Long-term treatment with steroids may be necessary.
Complete blood counts, L.E. cell preparations, and antinuclear antibody titer determinations are indicated before and periodically during prolonged therapy with hydralazine even though the patient is asymptomatic. These studies are also indicated if the patient develops arthralgia, fever, chest pain, continued malaise or other unexplained signs or symptoms.
A positive antinuclear antibody titer and/or positive L.E. cell reaction requires that the physician carefully weigh the implications of the test results against the benefits to be derived from antihypertensive therapy with hydralazine.
Use MAO inhibitors with caution in patients receiving hydralazine.
When other potent parenteral antihypertensive drugs, such as diazoxide, are used in combination with hydralazine, patients should be continuously observed for several hours for any excessive fall in blood pressure. Profound hypotensive episodes may occur when diazoxide injection and hydralazine are used concomitantly.
Hydrochlorothiazide
Use with caution in severe renal disease. In patients with renal disease, thiazides may precipitate azotemia. Cumulative effects of the drug may develop in patients with impaired renal function.
Thiazides should be used with caution in patients with impaired hepatic function or progressive liver disease, since minor alterations of fluid and electrolyte imbalance may precipitate hepatic coma.
Thiazides may add to or potentiate the action of other antihypertensive drugs. Potentiation occurs with ganglionic or peripheral adrenergic blocking drugs.
Sensitivity reactions are more likely to occur in patients with a history of allergy or bronchial asthma.
The possibility of exacerbation or activation of systemic lupus erythematosus has been reported.
Usage in Pregnancy
Hydralazine
Animal studies indicate that hydralazine is teratogenic in mice, possibly in rabbits, and not in rats. Teratogenic effects observed were cleft palate and malformations of facial and cranial bones. Although clinical experience does not include any positive evidence of adverse effects on the human fetus, hydralazine should not be used during pregnancy unless the expected benefit clearly justifies the potential risk to the fetus.
Hydrochlorothiazide
Thiazides cross the placental barrier and appear in cord blood. The use of thiazides in pregnant women requires that the anticipated benefit be weighed against possible hazards to the

Continued on next page

CIBA—Cont.

fetus. These hazards include fetal or neonatal jaundice, thrombocytopenia, and possibly other adverse reactions which have occurred in the adult.

Nursing Mothers: Thiazides appear in breast milk. If the use of the drug is deemed essential, the patient should stop nursing.

Precautions

Hydralazine

Myocardial stimulation produced by hydralazine can cause anginal attacks and ECG changes of myocardial ischemia. The drug has been implicated in the production of myocardial infarction. It must, therefore, be used with caution in patients with suspected coronary artery disease.

The "hyperdynamic" circulation caused by hydralazine may accentuate specific cardiovascular inadequacies. An example is that hydralazine may increase pulmonary artery pressure in patients with mitral valvular disease. The drug may reduce the pressor responses to epinephrine. Postural hypotension may result from hydralazine but is less common than with ganglionic blocking agents. Use with caution in patients with cerebral vascular accidents.

In hypertensive patients with normal kidneys who are treated with hydralazine, there is evidence of increased renal blood flow and a maintenance of glomerular filtration rate. In some instances improved renal function has been noted where control values were below normal prior to hydralazine administration. However, as with any antihypertensive agent, hydralazine should be used with caution in patients with advanced renal damage.

Peripheral neuritis, evidenced by paresthesias, numbness, and tingling, has been observed. Published evidence suggests an antipyridoxine effect and the addition of pyridoxine to the regimen if symptoms develop.

Blood dyscrasias, consisting of reduction in hemoglobin and red cell count, leukopenia, agranulocytosis, and purpura, have been reported. If such abnormalities develop, discontinue therapy. Periodic blood counts are advised during prolonged therapy.

Hydrochlorothiazide

Periodic determination of serum electrolytes to detect possible electrolyte imbalance should be performed at appropriate intervals. All patients receiving thaizide therapy should be observed for clinical signs of fluid or electrolyte imbalance; namely, hyponatremia, hypochloremic alkalosis, and hypokalemia. Serum and urine electrolyte determinations are particularly important when the patient is vomiting excessively or receiving parenteral fluids. Medication such as digitalis may also influence serum electrolytes. Warning signs are dryness of mouth, thirst, weakness, lethargy, drowsiness, restlessness, muscle pains or cramps, muscular fatigue, hypotension, oliguria, tachycardia, and gastrointestinal disturbance such as nausea or vomiting.

Hypokalemia may develop, especially with brisk diuresis, when severe cirrhosis is present, or during concomitant use of steroids or ACTH. Interference with adequate oral intake of electrolytes will also contribute to hypokalemia. Hypokalemia can sensitize or exaggerate the response of the heart to the toxic effects of digitalis (*eg,* increased ventricular irritability).

Any chloride deficit is generally mild and usually does not require specific treatment except under extraordinary circumstances (as in liver disease or renal disease). Dilutional hyponatremia may occur in edematous patients in hot weather; appropriate therapy is water restriction rather than administration of salt, except in rare instances when the hyponatremia is life-threatening. In actual salt depletion, appropriate replacement is the therapy of choice.

Hyperuricemia may occur or frank gout may be precipitated in certain patients receiving thiazide therapy.

Insulin requirements in diabetic patients may be increased, decreased, or unchanged. Latent diabetes may become manifest during thiazide administration.

Thiazide drugs may increase the responsiveness to tubocurarine.

The antihypertensive effects of the drug may be enhanced in the postsympathectomy patient. Thiazides may decrease arterial responsiveness to norepinephrine. This diminution is not sufficient to preclude effectiveness of the pressor agent for therapeutic use.

If progressive renal impairment becomes evident, withholding or discontinuing diuretic therapy should be considered.

Thiazides may decrease serum PBI levels without signs of thyroid disturbance.

Calcium excretion is decreased by thiazides. Pathological changes in the parathyroid gland with hypercalcemia and hypophosphatemia have been observed in a few patients on prolonged thiazide therapy. The common complications of hyperparathyroidism such as renal lithiasis, bone resorption, and peptic ulceration have not been seen. Thiazides should be discontinued before carrying out tests for parathyroid function.

The Apresazide capsules (100/50) contain FD&C Yellow No. 5 (tartrazine) which may cause allergic-type reactions (including bronchial asthma) in certain susceptible individuals. Although the overall incidence of FD&C Yellow No. 5 (tartrazine) sensitivity in the general population is low, it is frequently seen in patients who also have aspirin hypersensitivity.

Adverse Reactions

Hydralazine

Adverse reactions with hydralazine are usually reversible when dosage is reduced. However, in some cases it may be necessary to discontinue the drug.

Common: Headache; palpitations; anorexia; nausea; vomiting; diarrhea; tachycardia; angina pectoris.

Less frequent: Nasal congestion; flushing; lacrimation; conjunctivitis; peripheral neuritis, evidenced by paresthesias, numbness, and tingling; edema; dizziness; tremors; muscle cramps; psychotic reactions characterized by depression, disorientation, or anxiety; hypersensitivity (including rash, urticaria, pruritus, fever, chills, arthralgia, eosinophilia, and, rarely, hepatitis); constipation; difficulty in micturition; dyspnea; paralytic ileus; lymphadenopathy; splenomegaly; blood dyscrasias, consisting of reduction in hemoglobin and red cell count, leukopenia, agranulocytosis and purpura; hypotension; paradoxical pressor response.

Hydrochlorothiazide

Gastrointestinal: Anorexia, gastric irritation, nausea, vomiting, cramping, diarrhea, constipation, jaundice (intrahepatic cholestatic), pancreatitis, sialadenitis.

Central Nervous System: Dizziness, vertigo, paresthesias, headache, xanthopsia.

Hematologic: Leukopenia, thrombocytopenia, agranulocytosis, aplastic anemia.

Cardiovascular: Orthostatic hypotension (may be potentiated by alcohol, barbiturates, or narcotics).

Hypersensitivity: Purpura, photosensitivity, rash, urticaria, necrotizing angiitis, Stevens-Johnson syndrome, and other hypersensitivity reactions.

Other: Hyperglycemia, glycosuria, hyperuricemia, muscle spasm, weakness, restlessness.

When adverse reactions are moderate or severe, thiazide dosage should be reduced or therapy withdrawn.

Dosage and Administration: As determined by individual titration (see box warning).

Usual dosage is one Apresazide Capsule twice daily, the strength depending upon individual requirement following titration. For maintenance, adjust dosage to lowest effective level. When necessary, other antihypertensives such as sympathetic inhibitors may be added gradually in reduced dosages; watch effects carefully.

How Supplied: *25/25 Capsules* (light blue and white opaque), each containing 25 mg hydralazine hydrochloride and 25 mg hydrochlorothiazide; bottles of 100.

50/50 Capsules (pink and white opaque), each containing 50 mg hydralazine hydrochloride and 50 mg hydrochlorothiazide; bottles of 100.

100/50 Capsules (pink flesh and white opaque), each containing 100 mg hydralazine hydrochloride and 50 mg hydrochlorothiazide; bottles of 100.

Dispense in tight, light-resistant container (USP).

C80-11 (1/80)

[*Shown in Product Identification Section*]

APRESOLINE® hydrochloride (hydralazine hydrochloride USP) Tablets ℞

Listed in USP, a Medicare designated compendium.

Indications: Essential hypertension, alone or as an adjunct.

Contraindications: Hypersensitivity to hydralazine; coronary artery disease; and mitral valvular rheumatic heart disease.

Warnings: Hydralazine may produce in a few patients a clinical picture simulating systemic lupus erythematosus. In such patients hydralazine should be discontinued unless the benefit to risk determination requires continued antihypertensive therapy with this drug. Symptoms and signs usually regress when the drug is discontinued but residua have been detected many years later. Long-term treatment with steroids may be necessary.

Complete blood counts, L. E. cell preparations, and antinuclear antibody titer determinations are indicated before and periodically during prolonged therapy with hydralazine even though the patient is asymptomatic. These studies are also indicated if the patient develops arthralgia, fever, chest pain, continued malaise or other unexplained signs or symptoms.

A positive antinuclear antibody titer and/or positive L.E. cell reaction requires that the physician carefully weigh the implications of the test results against the benefits to be derived from antihypertensive therapy with hydralazine.

Use MAO inhibitors with caution in patients receiving hydralazine.

When other potent parenteral antihypertensive drugs, such as diazoxide, are used in combination with hydralazine, patients should be continuously observed for several hours for any excessive fall in blood pressure. Profound hypotensive episodes may occur when diazoxide injection and Apresoline (hydralazine hydrochloride) are used concomitantly.

Usage in Pregnancy: Animal studies indicate that hydralazine is teratogenic in mice, possibly in rabbits, and not in rats. Teratogenic effects observed were cleft palate and malformations of facial and cranial bones. Although clinical experience does not include any positive evidence of adverse effects on the human fetus, hydralazine should not be used during pregnancy unless the expected benefit clearly justifies the potential risk to the fetus.

Precautions: Myocardial stimulation produced by Apresoline can cause anginal attacks and ECG changes of myocardial ischemia. The drug has been implicated in the production of myocardial infarction. It must, therefore, be used with caution in patients with suspected coronary artery disease.

The "hyperdynamic" circulation caused by Apresoline may accentuate specific cardiovascular inadequacies. An example is that Apresoline may increase pulmonary artery pressure in patients with mitral valvular disease. The drug may reduce the pressor responses to epinephrine. Postural hypotension may result from Apresoline, but is less common than with ganglionic blocking agents. Use with caution in patients with cerebral vascular accidents.
In hypertensive patients with normal kidneys who are treated with Apresoline, there is evidence of increased renal blood flow and a maintenance of glomerular filtration rate. In some instances improved renal function has been noted where control values were below normal prior to Apresoline administration. However, as with any antihypertensive agent, Apresoline should be used with caution in patients with advanced renal damage.
Peripheral neuritis, evidenced by paresthesias, numbness, and tingling, has been observed. Published evidence suggests an antipyridoxine effect and the addition of pyridoxine to the regimen if symptoms develop.
Blood dyscrasias, consisting of reduction in hemoglobin and red cell count, leukopenia, agranulocytosis, and purpura, have been reported. If such abnormalities develop, discontinue therapy. Periodic blood counts are advised during prolonged therapy.
The Apresoline tablets (10 and 100 mg) contain FD&C Yellow No. 5 (tartrazine) which may cause allergic-type reactions (including bronchial asthma) in certain susceptible individuals. Although the overall incidence of FD&C Yellow No. 5 (tartrazine) sensitivity in the general population is low, it is frequently seen in patients who also have aspirin hypersensitivity.
Adverse Reactions: Adverse reactions with Apresoline are usually reversible when dosage is reduced. However, in some cases it may be necessary to discontinue the drug.
Common: Headache; palpitations; anorexia; nausea; vomiting; diarrhea; tachycardia; angina pectoris.
Less Frequent: Nasal congestion; flushing; lacrimation; conjunctivitis; peripheral neuritis, evidenced by paresthesias, numbness, and tingling; edema; dizziness; tremors; muscle cramps; psychotic reactions characterized by depression, disorientation, or anxiety; hypersensitivity (including rash, urticaria, pruritus, fever, chills, arthralgia, eosinophilia, and, rarely, hepatitis); constipation; difficulty in micturition; dyspnea; paralytic ileus; lymphadenopathy; splenomegaly; blood dyscrasias, consisting of reduction in hemoglobin and red cell count, leukopenia, agranulocytosis, and purpura; hypotension; paradoxical pressor response.

Dosage and Administration

Initiate therapy in gradually increasing dosages; adjust according to individual response. Start with 10 mg 4 times daily for the first 2 to 4 days, increase to 25 mg 4 times daily for balance of first week. For second and subsequent weeks, increase dosage to 50 mg 4 times daily. For maintenance, adjust dosage to lowest effective levels.
The incidence of toxic reactions, particularly the L. E. cell syndrome, is high in the group of patients receiving large doses of Apresoline.
In a few resistant patients, up to 300 mg Apresoline daily may be required for a significant antihypertensive effect. In such cases, a lower dosage of Apresoline combined with a thiazide, reserpine, or both may be considered. However, when combining therapy, individual titration is essential to insure the lowest possible therapeutic dose of each drug.

Overdosage

Signs and Symptoms

Hypotension, tachycardia, headache and generalized skin flushing are to be expected. Myocardial ischemia and cardiac arrhythmia can develop; profound shock can occur in severe overdosage.

Treatment

Evacuate gastric contents, taking adequate precautions against aspiration and for protection of the airway; instill activated charcoal slurry, if general conditions permit. These manipulations may have to be omitted or carried out after cardiovascular status has been stabilized, since they might precipitate cardiac arrhythmias or increase the depth of shock.
Support of the cardiovascular system is of primary importance. Shock should be treated with volume expanders without resorting to use of vasopressors, if possible. If a vasopressor is required, use one that is least likely to precipitate or aggravate cardiac arrhythmia. Digitalization may be necessary. Renal function must be monitored and supported as required.
No experience has been reported with extracorporeal or peritoneal dialysis.
How Supplied: *Tablets,* 10 mg (pale yellow, dry-coated); bottles of 100 and 1000. *Tablets,* 25 mg (deep blue, dry-coated) and 50 mg (light blue, dry-coated); bottles of 100, 500, 1000 and Accu-Pak® blister units of 100. *Tablets,* 100 mg (peach, dry-coated); bottles of 100.
Dispense in tight, light-resistant container (USP).

C80-15 (1/80)

Military—1000's, 25 mg, Stock #6505-00-584-2895.
VA—1000's, 25 mg, Stock #6505-00-584-2895A; 1000's, 50 mg, Stock #6505-00-685-5420A

[*Shown in Product Identification Section*]

APRESOLINE® hydrochloride (hydralazine hydrochloride USP) Parenteral ℞

Listed in USP, a Medicare designated compendium.

Indications

Severe essential hypertension when the drug cannot be given orally or when there is an urgent need to lower blood pressure.
Contraindications: Hypersensitivity to hydralazine; coronary artery disease; and mitral valvular rheumatic heart disease.
Warnings: Hydralazine may produce in a few patients a clinical picture simulating systemic lupus erythematosus. In such patients hydralazine should be discontinued unless the benefit to risk determination requires continued antihypertensive therapy with this drug. Symptoms and signs usually regress when the drug is discontinued but residua have been detected many years later. Long-term treatment with steroids may be necessary.
Complete blood counts, L. E. cell preparations, and antinuclear antibody titer determinations are indicated before and periodically during prolonged therapy with hydralazine even though the patient is asymptomatic. These studies are also indicated if the patient develops arthralgia, fever, chest pain, continued malaise, or other unexplained signs or symptoms.
A positive antinuclear antibody titer and/or positive L.E. cell reaction requires that the physician carefully weigh the implications of the test results against the benefits to be derived from antihypertensive therapy with hydralazine.
Use MAO inhibitors with caution in patients receiving hydralazine.
When other potent parenteral antihypertensive drugs, such as diazoxide, are used in combination with hydralazine, patients should be continuously observed for several hours for any excessive fall in blood pressure. Profound hypotensive episodes may occur when diazoxide injection and Apresoline (hydralazine hydrochloride) are used concomitantly.

Usage in Pregnancy

Animal studies indicate that hydralazine is teratogenic in mice, possibly in rabbits, and not in rats. Teratogenic effects observed were cleft palate and malformations of facial and cranial bones. Although clinical experience does not include any positive evidence of adverse effects on the human fetus, hydralazine should not be used during pregnancy unless the expected benefit clearly justifies the potential risk to the fetus.
Precautions: Myocardial stimulation produced by Apresoline can cause anginal attacks and ECG changes of myocardial ischemia. The drug has been implicated in the production of myocardial infarction. It must, therefore, be used with caution in patients with suspected coronary artery disease.
The "hyperdynamic" circulation caused by Apresoline may accentuate specific cardiovascular inadequacies. An example is that Apresoline may increase pulmonary artery pressure in patients with mitral valvular disease. The drug may reduce the pressor responses to epinephrine. Postural hypotension may result from Apresoline, but is less common than with ganglionic blocking agents. Use with caution in patients with cerebral vascular accidents.
In hypertensive patients with normal kidneys who are treated with Apresoline, there is evidence of increased renal blood flow and a maintenance of glomerular filtration rate. In some instances improved renal function has been noted where control values were below normal prior to Apresoline administration. However, as with any antihypertensive agent, Apresoline should be used with caution in patients with advanced renal damage.
Peripheral neuritis, evidenced by paresthesias, numbness, and tingling, has been observed. Published evidence suggests an antipyridoxine effect and the addition of pyridoxine to the regimen if symptoms develop.
Blood dyscrasias, consisting of reduction in hemoglobin and red cell count, leukopenia, agranulocytosis, and purpura, have been reported. If such abnormalities develop, discontinue therapy. Periodic blood counts are advised during prolonged therapy.
Adverse Reactions: Adverse reactions with Apresoline are usually reversible when dosage is reduced. However, in some cases it may be necessary to discontinue the drug.
Common: Headache; palpitations; anorexia; nausea; vomiting; diarrhea; tachycardia; angina pectoris.
Less Frequent: Nasal congestion; flushing; lacrimation; conjunctivitis; peripheral neuritis, evidenced by paresthesias, numbness, and tingling; edema; dizziness; tremors; muscle cramps; psychotic reactions characterized by depression, disorientation, or anxiety; hypersensitivity (including rash, urticaria, pruritus, fever, chills, arthralgia, eosinophilia, and, rarely, hepatitis); constipation; difficulty in micturition; dyspnea; paralytic ileus; lymphadenopathy; splenomegaly; blood dyscrasias, consisting of reduction in hemoglobin and red cell count, leukopenia, agranulocytosis, and purpura; hypotension; paradoxical pressor response.
Dosage and Administration: When there is urgent need, therapy in the hospitalized patient may be initiated intravenously or intramuscularly. Use parenteral Apresoline only when the drug cannot be given orally. Usual dose is 20 to 40 mg, repeated as necessary. Certain patients (especially those with marked renal damage) may require a lower dose. Check blood pressure frequently. It may begin to fall within a few minutes after injection, with an average maximal decrease occurring in 10 to 80 minutes. In cases where there is a previously existing increased intracranial pressure, lowering the blood pressure may increase cere-

Continued on next page

CIBA—Cont.

bral ischemia. Most patients can be transferred to oral Apresoline within 24 to 48 hours.

Overdosage

Signs and Symptoms

Hypotension, tachycardia, headache and generalized skin flushing are to be expected. Myocardial ischemia and cardiac arrhythmia can develop; profound shock can occur in severe overdosage.

Treatment

Support of the cardiovascular system is of primary importance. Shock should be treated with volume expanders without resorting to use of vasopressors, if possible. If a vasopressor is required, use one that is least likely to precipitate or aggravate cardiac arrhythmia. Digitalization may be necessary. Renal function must be monitored and supported as required. No experience has been reported with extracorporeal or peritoneal dialysis.

How Supplied: *Ampuls,* 1 ml, each ml containing 20 mg hydralazine hydrochloride, 0.1 ml propylene glycol with 0.065% methyl-*p*-hydroxybenzoate and 0.035% propyl-*p*-hydroxybenzoate as preservatives in water; cartons of 5. C78-42 (1/79)

Military—Ampuls 5's, Stock #6505-00-685-5425

VA—Ampuls 5's, Stock #6505-00-685-5425A

APRESOLINE®-ESIDRIX® ℞

(hydralazine hydrochloride and hydrochlorothiazide)

> **Warning**
> This fixed combination drug is not indicated for initial therapy of hypertension. Hypertension requires therapy titrated to the individual patient. If the fixed combination represents the dosage so determined, its use may be more convenient in patient management. The treatment of hypertension is not static, but must be reevaluated as conditions in each patient warrant.

Indications

Hypertension. (See box warning.)

Contraindications

Hydralazine

Hypersensitivity to hydralazine; coronary artery disease; and mitral valvular rheumatic heart disease.

Hydrochlorothiazide

Anuria; hypersensitivity to this or other sulfonamide-derived drugs.

Warnings

Hydralazine

Hydralazine may produce in a few patients a clinical picture simulating systemic lupus erythematosus. In such patients hydralazine should be discontinued unless the benefit-to-risk determination requires continued antihypertensive therapy with this drug. Symptoms and signs usually regress when the drug is discontinued but residua have been detected many years later. Long-term treatment with steroids may be necessary.

Complete blood counts, L. E. cell preparations, and antinuclear antibody titer determinations are indicated before and periodically during prolonged therapy with hydralazine even though the patient is asymptomatic. These studies are also indicated if the patient develops arthralgia, fever, chest pain, continued malaise or other unexplained signs or symptoms.

A positive antinuclear antibody titer and/or positive L. E. cell reaction requires that the physician carefully weigh the implications of the test results against the benefits to be derived from antihypertensive therapy with hydralazine.

Use MAO inhibitors with caution in patients receiving hydralazine.

When other potent parenteral antihypertensive drugs, such as diazoxide, are used in combination with hydralazine, patients should be continuously observed for several hours for any excessive fall in blood pressure. Profound hypotensive episodes may occur when diazoxide injection and Apresoline (hydralazine hydrochloride) are used concomitantly.

Hydrochlorothiazide

Use with caution in severe renal disease. In patients with renal disease, thiazides may precipitate azotemia. Cumulative effects of the drug may develop in patients with impaired renal function.

Thiazides should be used with caution in patients with impaired hepatic function or progressive liver disease, since minor alterations of fluid and electrolyte imbalance may precipitate hepatic coma.

Thiazides may add to or potentiate the action of other antihypertensive drugs. Potentiation occurs with ganglionic or peripheral adrenergic blocking drugs.

Sensitivity reactions are more likely to occur in patients with a history of allergy or bronchial asthma.

The possibility of exacerbation or activation of systemic lupus erythematosus has been reported.

Usage in Pregnancy

Hydralazine

Animal studies indicate that hydralazine is teratogenic in mice, possibly in rabbits, and not in rats. Teratogenic effects observed were cleft palate and malformations of facial and cranial bones. Although clinical experience does not include any positive evidence of adverse effects on the human fetus, hydralazine should not be used during pregnancy unless the expected benefit clearly justifies the potential risk to the fetus.

Hydrochlorothiazide

Thiazides cross the placental barrier and appear in cord blood. The use of thiazides in pregnant women requires that the anticipated benefit be weighed against possible hazards to the fetus. These hazards include fetal or neonatal jaundice, thrombocytopenia, and possibly other adverse reactions which have occurred in the adult.

Nursing Mothers: Thiazides appear in breast milk. If the use of the drug is deemed essential, the patient should stop nursing.

Precautions

Hydralazine

Myocardial stimulation produced by hydralazine can cause anginal attacks and ECG changes of myocardial ischemia. The drug has been implicated in the production of myocardial infarction. It must, therefore, be used with caution in patients with suspected coronary artery disease.

The "hyperdynamic" circulation caused by hydralazine may accentuate specific cardiovascular inadequacies. An example is that hydralazine may increase pulmonary artery pressure in patients with mitral valvular disease. The drug may reduce the pressor responses to epinephrine. Postural hypotension may result from hydralazine but is less common than with ganglionic blocking agents. Use with caution in patients with cerebral vascular accidents.

In hypertensive patients with normal kidneys who are treated with hydralazine, there is evidence of increased renal blood flow and a maintenance of glomerular filtration rate. In some instances improved renal function has been noted where control values were below normal prior to hydralazine administration. However, as with any antihypertensive agent, hydralazine should be used with caution in patients with advanced renal damage.

Peripheral neuritis, evidenced by paresthesias, numbness, and tingling, has been observed. Published evidence suggests an antipyridoxine effect and the addition of pyridoxine to the regimen if symptoms develop.

Blood dyscrasias, consisting of reduction in hemoglobin and red cell count, leukopenia, agranulocytosis, and purpura, have been reported. If such abnormalities develop, discontinue therapy. Periodic blood counts are advised during prolonged therapy.

Hydrochlorothiazide

Periodic determination of serum electrolytes to detect possible electrolyte imbalance should be performed at appropriate intervals. All patients receiving thiazide therapy should be observed for clinical signs of fluid or electrolyte imbalance; namely, hyponatremia, hypochloremic alkalosis, and hypokalemia. Serum and urine electrolyte determinations are particularly important when the patient is vomiting excessively or receiving parenteral fluids. Medication such as digitalis may also influence serum electrolytes. Warning signs are dryness of mouth, thirst, weakness, lethargy, drowsiness, restlessness, muscle pains or cramps, muscular fatigue, hypotension, oliguria, tachycardia, and gastrointestinal disturbance such as nausea or vomiting.

Hypokalemia may develop, especially with brisk diuresis, when severe cirrhosis is present, or during concomitant use of steroids or ACTH. Interference with adequate oral intake of electrolytes will also contribute to hypokalemia. Hypokalemia can sensitize or exaggerate the response of the heart to the toxic effects of digitalis (*eg,* increased ventricular irritability).

Any chloride deficit is generally mild and usually does not require specific treatment except under extraordinary circumstances (as in liver disease or renal disease). Dilutional hyponatremia may occur in edematous patients in hot weather; appropriate therapy is water restriction rather than administration of salt, except in rare instances when the hyponatremia is life-threatening. In actual salt depletion, appropriate replacement is the therapy of choice.

Hyperuricemia may occur or frank gout may be precipitated in certain patients receiving thiazide therapy.

Insulin requirements in diabetic patients may be increased, decreased, or unchanged. Latent diabetes may become manifest during thiazide administration.

Thiazide drugs may increase the responsiveness to tubocurarine.

The antihypertensive effects of the drug may be enhanced in the postsympathectomy patient. Thiazides may decrease arterial responsiveness to norepinephrine. This diminution is not sufficient to preclude effectiveness of the pressor agent for therapeutic use.

If progressive renal impairment becomes evident, withholding or discontinuing diuretic therapy should be considered.

Thiazides may decrease serum PBI levels without signs of thyroid disturbance.

Calcium excretion is decreased by thiazides. Pathological changes in the parathyroid gland with hypercalcemia and hypophosphatemia have been observed in a few patients on prolonged thiazide therapy. The common complications of hyperparathyroidism such as renal lithiasis, bone resorption, and peptic ulceration have not been seen. Thiazides should be discontinued before carrying out tests for parathyroid function.

Adverse Reactions

Hydralazine

Adverse reactions with hydralazine are usually reversible when dosage is reduced. However, in some cases it may be necessary to discontinue the drug.

Common: Headache; palpitations; anorexia; nausea; vomiting; diarrhea; tachycardia; angina pectoris.

Less frequent: Nasal congestion; flushing; lacrimation; conjunctivitis; peripheral neuritis, evidenced by paresthesias, numbness, and tingling; edema; dizziness; tremors; muscle cramps; psychotic reactions characterized by depression, disorientation, or anxiety; hypersensitivity (including rash, urticaria, pruritus, fever, chills, arthralgia, eosinophilia, and, rarely, hepatitis); constipation; difficulty in micturition; dyspnea; paralytic ileus; lymphadenopathy; splenomegaly; blood dyscrasias, consisting of reduction in hemoglobin and red cell count, leukopenia, agranulocytosis and purpura; hypotension; paradoxical pressor response.

Hydrochlorothiazide

Gastrointestinal: Anorexia, gastric irritation, nausea, vomiting, cramping, diarrhea, constipation, jaundice (intrahepatic cholestatic), pancreatitis, sialadenitis.

Central Nervous System: Dizziness, vertigo, paresthesias, headache, xanthopsia.

Hematologic: Leukopenia, thrombocytopenia, agranulocytosis, aplastic anemia.

Cardiovascular: Orthostatic hypotension (may be potentiated by alcohol, barbiturates, or narcotics).

Hypersensitivity: Purpura, photosensitivity, rash, urticaria, necrotizing angiitis, Stevens-Johnson syndrome, and other hypersensitivity reactions.

Other: Hyperglycemia, glycosuria, hyperuricemia, muscle spasm, weakness, restlessness.

When adverse reactions are moderate or severe, thiazide dosage should be reduced or therapy withdrawn.

Dosage and Administration: As determined by individual titration (see box warning).

Usual dosage is 1 tablet t.i.d. (maximal dosage is 2 tablets t.i.d.). For maintenance, adjust dosage to lowest effective level.

When necessary, other antihypertensives may be added gradually in reduced dosages. When the drug is given in conjunction with ganglionic blocking agents, dosage must be reduced by at least 50% and effects should be watched carefully.

Overdosage

Hydralazine

Signs and Symptoms

Hypotension, tachycardia, headache and generalized skin flushing are to be expected. Myocardial ischemia and cardiac arrhythmia can develop; profound shock can occur in severe overdosage.

Treatment

Evacuate gastric contents, taking adequate precautions against aspiration and for protection of the airway; instill activated charcoal slurry, if general conditions permit. These manipulations may have to be omitted cr carried out after cardiovascular status has been stabilized, since they might precipitate cardiac arrhythmias or increase the depth of shock.

Support of the cardiovascular system is of primary importance. Shock should be treated with volume expanders without resorting to use of vasopressors, if possible. If a vasopressor is required, use one that is least likely to precipitate or aggravate cardiac arrhythmia. Digitalization may be necessary. Renal function must be monitored and supported as required.

No experience has been reported with extracorporeal or peritoneal dialysis.

Hydrochlorothiazide

Signs and Symptoms

Diuresis is to be expected; lethargy of varying degree may appear and may progress to coma within a few hours, with minimal depression of respiration and cardiovascular function and without significant serum electrolyte changes or dehydration. The mechanism of CNS depression with thiazide overdosage is unknown. GI irritation and hypermotility may occur; temporary elevation of BUN has been reported and serum electrolyte changes could occur, especially in patients with impairment of renal function.

Treatment

Evacuate gastric contents but take care to prevent aspiration, especially in the stuporous or comatose patient. GI effects are usually of short duration, but may require symptomatic treatment.

Monitor serum electrolyte levels and renal function; institute supportive measures as required individually to maintain hydration, electrolyte balance, respiration and cardiovascular-renal function.

How Supplied: *Tablets* (orange, dry-coated), each containing 25 mg hydralazine hydrochloride and 15 mg hydrochlorothiazide; bottles of 100. C78-52 (1/79)

[*Shown in Product Identification Section*]

CORAMINE® ℞
(nikethamide)

Indications: To overcome central nervous system depression, respiratory depression, and circulatory failure, particularly when due to effects of central depressant drugs.

Combined with electroshock therapy, Coramine helps restore respiration more quickly and may reduce the number of treatments required in cases of psychotic excitement.

Contraindications: Hypersensitivity to nikethamide or related compounds.

Warnings: Do not inject intra-arterially as arterial spasm and thrombosis may result.

Usage in Pregnancy

The safety of Coramine for use in pregnancy has not been established; therefore this drug should be used in pregnant patients only when, in the judgment of the physician, its use is deemed essential to the welfare of the patient.

Adverse Reactions: The difference between the clinically effective dose and that producing side effects varies but is often small. The following side effects which have been reported may, in fact, be the result of overdosage.

The most common side effect is an unpleasant feeling of burning or itching, especially at the back of the nose. Flushing or a subjective feeling of warmth, sneezing, coughing, sweating, nausea, vomiting, generalized restlessness, a feeling of fear, changing depth and frequency of respiration, tachycardia, elevated blood pressure, muscle twitching (especially facial), and convulsions have also been reported occasionally.

Dosage and Administration: Although Coramine is readily absorbed after oral, subcutaneous or intramuscular administration, it is most effective by the intravenous route.

Parenteral

Anesthetic Overdosage. *To shorten narcosis:* 4 ml intravenously or intramuscularly. *To increase amplitude of respiration:* 2 to 5 ml intravenously. *To overcome respiratory depression:* 5 to 10 ml intravenously; repeat as necessary. *To combat respiratory paralysis:* 15 ml intravenously as minimal initial dose; repeat as required. Other methods of resuscitation, including artificial respiration, should also be employed as indicated. If cardiac arrest is also present, 0.5 to 1.0 ml administered intracardially may be of some benefit.

Narcotic, Hypnotic, and Carbon Monoxide Poisoning. *Initial dose:* 5 to 10 ml intravenously, followed by 5 ml every 5 minutes for first hour, depending on response. Thereafter, 5-ml booster doses may be given every hour if needed, or, in more serious cases, as often as every half hour. Artificial respiration, gastric lavage, oxygen, and other means of stimulation should also be employed.

Cardiac Decompensation and Coronary Occlusion. *In emergencies:* 5 to 10 ml intravenously or intramuscularly.

Shock. The primary treatment of shock requires oxygen and adequate solutions, including blood or plasma, for volume replacement. Coramine, in doses of 10 to 15 ml intravenously or intramuscularly initially and repeated as indicated by the response, may be of value in compensating peripheral circulation until blood or plasma is available.

Acute Alcoholism. *Initial dose:* 5 to 20 ml intravenously to overcome central depression. Repeat as necessary.

Electroshock Therapy. Recommended dosage is 5 ml Coramine diluted with an equal volume of sterile distilled water in a 10-ml syringe and injected rapidly into an antecubital vein. The electrical stimulus is applied when the patient's face flushes and the respiratory rate increases noticeably, usually within one minute.

Oral

For Maintenance Therapy. 3 to 5 ml of oral solution every 4 to 6 hours, when indicated.

Overdosage

Signs and Symptoms

Coughing, sneezing, hyperpnea, and muscle tremors can occur. Cardiac rate and blood pressure may increase, although probably not markedly. With severe overdosage, as per injection, generalized muscle spasms and convulsive seizures can occur.

Treatment

Treatment is usually not required, except in severe overdosage. In such cases, a short-acting barbiturate is effective in controlling the generalized muscle spasm and convulsions which may be present.

Since the oral solution is rapidly absorbed, attempts to induce emesis or to perform gastric lavage are of little value and, in the presence of paroxysmal coughing or sneezing, could result in complications from aspiration.

How Supplied: Available as a 25% (by weight) aqueous solution in:

Ampuls, 1.5 ml; cartons of 20.

Oral Solution, bottles of 3 fluidounces.

C79-4 (5/79)

DESFERAL® mesylate ℞
(deferoxamine mesylate USP)

Description: Desferal is available as the mesylate salt of deferoxamine. Its solubility in water is greater than 25%; 500 mg will dissolve in 2 ml distilled water.

Chemically, it is N-[5-[3-[(5-Aminopentyl) hydroxycarbamoyl] propionamido] pentyl]-3-[[5-(N-hydroxyacetamido) pentyl] carbamoyl] propionohydroxamic acid monomethanesulfonate (salt).

Actions: Desferal is a compound with a specific ability to chelate iron, forming a stable complex which prevents the iron from entering into further chemical reactions. This chelate is readily soluble in water and passes easily through the kidney, giving the urine a characteristic reddish color. Some is also excreted in the feces via the bile. Theoretically, 100 parts by weight of Desferal are capable of binding approximately 8.5 parts by weight of ferric iron. In studies thus far in man and animals, Desferal does not cause any demonstrable increase in the excretion of electrolytes and trace metals.

Indications: To facilitate the removal of iron in the treatment of acute iron intoxication and in chronic iron overload due to transfusion-dependent anemias.

ACUTE IRON INTOXICATION

Desferal is an adjunct to, and not a substitute for, standard measures generally used in treating acute iron intoxication which may include the following:

1. Induction of emesis with syrup of ipecac.
2. Gastric lavage.
3. Suction and maintenance of clear airway.
4. Control of shock with intravenous fluids, blood, oxygen, and vasopressors.
5. Correction of acidosis.

CHRONIC IRON OVERLOAD

Desferal can promote iron excretion in patients who have secondary iron overload from multiple transfusions (such as occur in some chronic anemias including thalassemia). One controlled study has found that long-term ther-

Continued on next page

CIBA—Cont.

apy with Desferal slows accumulation of hepatic iron and retards or eliminates progression of hepatic fibrosis.
Iron mobilization by Desferal is relatively poor in patients under the age of three with relatively small degrees of iron overload. The drug should ordinarily be withheld in such patients unless a demonstration of significant iron mobilization (eg, one mg of iron per day or more) can be demonstrated.
Desferal is not indicated for the treatment of primary hemochromatosis, since phlebotomy is the method of choice for removing excess iron in this indication.
Contraindications: Desferal is contraindicated in patients with severe renal disease or anuria, since the drug and the chelate which it forms with iron are excreted primarily by the kidney.
Warnings: Rarely, cataracts have been observed in patients who received the drug over prolonged periods in the treatment of chronic iron storage diseases. Slit-lamp examinations performed in patients treated with Desferal for acute iron intoxication have not revealed cataracts. Slit-lamp examinations are recommended periodically in patients treated for chronic iron overload.
Usage in Pregnancy
Skeletal anomalies were noted in the fetuses of two animal species at doses just above those recommended for humans. Therefore, Desferal should not be administered to women of childbearing potential, particularly during early pregnancy, except when in the judgment of the physician the potential benefits outweigh the possible hazards.
Precautions: Flushing of the skin, urticaria, hypotension, and even shock have occurred in a few patients when Desferal has been administered by rapid intravenous injection. To avoid these reactions, DESFERAL SHOULD BE GIVEN INTRAMUSCULARLY, OR BY SLOW SUBCUTANEOUS OR INTRAVENOUS INFUSION.
Adverse Reactions: Occasionally, pain and induration at the site of injection have been reported. Side effects reported in patients treated for acute iron intoxication include generalized erythema, urticaria, and hypotension, which occurred with rapid intravenous injection. Adverse effects reported in patients receiving long-term therapy for chronic iron storage diseases include allergic-type reactions (cutaneous wheal formation, generalized itching, rash, anaphylactic reaction), blurring of vision, dysuria, abdominal discomfort, diarrhea, leg cramps, tachycardia, and fever. Adverse effects reported in patients receiving subcutaneous therapy include localized pain, pruritus, erythema, skin irritation and swelling. These reactions might also occur in an occasional patient treated for acute iron intoxication.
Dosage and Administration: Since little of the drug is absorbed when administered orally, it is necessary to administer Desferal parenterally to chelate the iron that has been absorbed.

ACUTE IRON INTOXICATION

Intramuscular Administration
Intramuscular administration is preferred and should be used for ALL PATIENTS NOT IN SHOCK.
Dose: One gm should be administered initially. This may be followed by 0.5 gm every four hours for two doses. Depending upon the clinical response, subsequent doses of 0.5 gm may be administered every four to twelve hours. The total amount administered should not exceed 6 gm in twenty-four hours.
Preparation of Solution for Intramuscular Administration: Dissolve the Desferal by adding 2 ml sterile water for injection to each vial. Make sure that the drug is completely dissolved and then withdraw the drug and administer intramuscularly.
Intravenous Administration
This route should be used ONLY FOR PATIENTS IN A STATE OF CARDIOVASCULAR COLLAPSE and then ONLY BY SLOW INFUSION. THE RATE OF INFUSION SHOULD NOT EXCEED 15 mg/kg/hour.
Dose: An initial dose of 1 gm should be administered at a rate NOT TO EXCEED 15 mg/kg/hour. This may be followed by 0.5 gm every four hours for two doses. Depending upon the clinical response, subsequent doses of 0.5 gm may be administered every four to twelve hours. The total amount administered should not exceed 6 gm in twenty-four hours. As soon as the clinical condition of the patient permits, intravenous administration should be discontinued and the drug administered intramuscularly.
Preparation of Solution for Intravenous Administration: Dissolve the Desferal by adding 2 ml sterile water for injection to each vial. Make sure that the drug is completely dissolved and then withdraw the drug and add to physiologic saline, glucose in water, or Ringer's lactate solution and administer at a rate NOT TO EXCEED 15 mg/kg/hour.

CHRONIC IRON OVERLOAD

The more effective of the following two routes of administration must be individualized for each patient.
Intramuscular Administration: 0.5 to 1.0 gm daily administered intramuscularly. In addition, 2.0 gm should be administered intravenously with each unit of blood transfused. However, Desferal should be administered separately from blood. The rate of intravenous infusion must not exceed 15 mg/kg/hour.
Subcutaneous Administration: 1.0 gm to 2.0 gm (20–40 mg/kg/day) administered daily over 8 to 24 hours utilizing a small portable pump capable of providing continuous mini-infusion. The duration of infusion must be individualized. In some patients iron excretion will be as great after a short infusion of 8 to 12 hours as it is if the same dose is given over a 24-hour period.
Preparation of Solution for Subcutaneous Administration: Dissolve the Desferal by adding 2.0 ml sterile water to each vial. Make sure that the drug is completely dissolved and then withdraw the drug in syringe to be used for administration.
Note: Desferal reconstituted with sterile water may be stored under sterile conditions and protected from light at room temperature for not longer than one week.
How Supplied: *Vials,* each containing 500 mg lyophilized deferoxamine mesylate sterile, for INTRAMUSCULAR, SUBCUTANEOUS, OR INTRAVENOUS administration; cartons of 4.

C79-24 (6/79)

DIALOG® ℞

(allobarbital and acetaminophen)

Indications: For relief of pain and discomfort of simple headache; neuralgia, myalgia, and musculoskeletal pain; dysmenorrhea; bursitis; sinusitis; fibrositis. Also indicated to relieve the discomfort and reduce the fever caused by respiratory tract infections, influenza, and other febrile conditions.
Contraindications: Hypersensitivity to allobarbital (or related compounds) or acetaminophen; moderate to severe hepatic disease; personal or familial history of acute intermittent porphyria.
Warnings: May be habit-forming. Dosage of coumarin anticoagulants may require adjustments during and on cessation of therapy.
Usage in Pregnancy: The safe use of this drug in pregnant women or during lactation has not been established. Therefore, the benefits must be weighed against the potential hazards.
Precautions: Periodic blood counts are advised during prolonged therapy.
Adverse Reactions: Nausea, transitory dizziness, leukopenia, anemia, pancytopenia, and rash may occur.
Dosage and Administration
Adults: One or 2 tablets every 4 hours. Not to exceed 8 tablets in 24 hours.
Children 6 to 12: One-half to 1 tablet every 4 hours. Not to exceed 4 tablets in 24 hours.
Overdosage: Allobarbital overdosage produces signs and symptoms typical of the intermediate-acting barbiturates. Acetaminophen overdosage can produce gastrointestinal, renal, hepatic, and myocardial damage, severity being directly related to dosage. Gastric emptying, instillation of activated charcoal, diuresis, and intensive supportive care are recommended. Hemodialysis, recommended for removal of allobarbital in severe cases, is apparently not effective for removal of acetaminophen.
How Supplied: *Tablets* (white, scored), each containing 15 mg allobarbital and 300 mg acetaminophen; units of 3 bottles of 30.

C71-29 Rev. 8/71

[*Shown in Product Identification Section*]

DIANABOL® ℞

(methandrostenolone NF)

Indications
Based on a review of this drug by the National Academy of Sciences-National Research Council and/or other information, FDA has classified the indications as follows:
"Probably" effective
As adjunctive therapy in senile and postmenopausal osteoporosis. Anabolic steroids are without value as primary therapy but may be of value as adjunctive therapy. Equal or greater consideration should be given to diet, calcium balance, physiotherapy, and good general health-promoting measures.
Final classification of the less-than-effective indications requires further investigation.

Contraindications: Hypersensitivity: male patients with carcinoma of the prostate or breast; carcinoma of the breast in some females; pregnancy, because of masculinization of the fetus; nephrosis or the nephrotic phase of nephritis.
Warnings: Anabolic steroids do not enhance athletic ability.
Precautions: Hypercalcemia may develop both spontaneously and as a result of hormonal therapy in women with disseminated breast carcinoma. If it develops while on this agent, the drug should be stopped.
Caution is required in administering these agents to patients with cardiac, renal, or hepatic disease. Edema may occur occasionally. Concomitant administration with adrenal steroids or ACTH may add to the edema.
If amenorrhea or menstrual irregularities develop, the drug should be discontinued until the etiology is determined.
Anabolic steroids may increase sensitivity to anticoagulants. Dosage of the anticoagulant may have to be decreased in order to maintain the prothrombin time at the desired therapeutic level.
Anabolic steroids have been shown to alter glucose tolerance tests. Diabetics should be followed carefully and the insulin or oral hypoglycemic dosage adjusted accordingly.
Since Dianabol contains a 17 alpha alkyl group, liver function should be checked at regular intervals in patients receiving this drug. Anabolic steroids should be used with caution in patients with benign prostatic hypertrophy.

Serum cholesterol may increase during therapy. Therefore, caution is required in administering these agents to patients with a history of myocardial infarction or coronary artery disease. Serial determinations of serum cholesterol should be made and therapy adjusted accordingly.

The Dianabol tablets (5 and 2.5 mg) contain FD&C Yellow No. 5 (tartrazine) which may cause allergic-type reactions (including bronchial asthma) in certain susceptible individuals. Although the overall incidence of FD&C Yellow No. 5 (tartrazine) sensitivity in the general population is low, it is frequently seen in patients who also have aspirin hypersensitivity.

Adverse Reactions:

In Males

Prepubertal: phallic enlargement; increased frequency of erections.

Postpubertal: inhibition of testicular function; oligospermia; gynecomastia.

In Females

Hirsutism; male pattern baldness; deepening of the voice; clitoral enlargement. These changes are usually irreversible even after prompt discontinuance of therapy and are not prevented by concomitant use of estrogens. In addition, the following may occur: menstrual irregularities; masculinization of the fetus.

In Both Sexes

Nausea; fullness; loss of appetite; vomiting; burning of the tongue; increased or decreased libido; acne (especially in females and prepubertal males); inhibition of gonadotropin secretion; bleeding in patients on concomitant anticoagulant therapy; premature closure of epiphyses in children; jaundice. There have been rare reports of hepatocellular neoplasms and peliosis hepatis in association with long-term androgenic-anabolic steroid therapy.

Alterations may occur in the following clinical laboratory tests: metyrapone test; glucose tolerance test; thyroid function tests (decrease in protein bound iodine, thyroxine-binding capacity, and radioactive iodine uptake); electrolytes (retention of sodium, chloride, water, potassium, phosphates, and calcium); hepatic function tests (increased BSP, serum cholesterol, SGOT, serum bilirubin, and alkaline phosphatase); blood coagulation tests (suppression of clotting factors II, V, VII, and X); decreased 17-ketosteroid excretion.

Dosage and Administration: Dianabol therapy is adjunctive to and not a replacement for conventional therapy. Duration of therapy will depend on the response of the condition and the appearance of adverse reactions. Therapy should be intermittent and no longer than necessary for optimal results.

The usual initial adult dosage is 5 mg daily. For maintenance, 2.5 to 5 mg daily is usually sufficient. Intermittent therapy is recommended when Dianabol is administered over long periods. For example, after six weeks of treatment, there should be an interval of two to four weeks before resuming therapy.

Proper diet, particularly adequate protein intake, is required to assure the full anabolic benefits of Dianabol.

Overdosage: Signs and symptoms of overdosage are those associated with the known effects of the drug. See Adverse Reactions section.

Treatment is symptomatic and supportive. Evacuate stomach contents by emesis and, if indicated, lavage, taking care to prevent aspiration.

Monitoring of liver function is advised.

How Supplied: *Tablets,* 5 mg (blue, scored); bottles of 100.

Tablets, 2.5 mg (pale yellow, scored); bottles of 100.

Dispense in tight, light-resistant container (USP).

C80-6 (1/80)

[*Shown in Product Identification Section*]

ESIDRIX® ℞

(hydrochlorothiazide USP)

Listed in USP, a Medicare designated compendium.

Indications:

Hypertension: In the management of hypertension either as the sole therapeutic agent or to enhance the effect of other antihypertensive drugs in the more severe forms of hypertension.

Edema: As adjunctive therapy in edema associated with congestive heart failure, hepatic cirrhosis, and corticosteroid and estrogen therapy.

Esidrix has also been found useful in edema due to various forms of renal dysfunction, such as the nephrotic syndrome, acute glomerulonephritis, and chronic renal failure.

Usage in Pregnancy: The routine use of diuretics in an otherwise healthy woman is inappropriate and exposes mother and fetus to unnecessary hazard. Diuretics do not prevent development of toxemia of pregnancy, and there is no satisfactory evidence that they are useful in the treatment of developed toxemia. Edema during pregnancy may arise from pathological causes or from the physiologic and mechanical consequences of pregnancy. Thiazides are indicated in pregnancy when edema is due to pathologic causes, just as they are in the absence of pregnancy (however, see WARNINGS). Dependent edema in pregnancy, resulting from restriction of venous return by the expanded uterus, is properly treated through elevation of the lower extremities and use of support hose; use of diuretics to lower intravascular volume in this case is illogical and unnecessary. There is hypervolemia during normal pregnancy which is not harmful to either the fetus or the mother (in the absence of cardiovascular disease) but which is associated with edema, including generalized edema, in the majority of pregnant women. If this edema produces discomfort, increased recumbency will often provide relief. In rare instances, this edema may cause extreme discomfort which is not relieved by rest. In these cases, a short course of diuretics may provide relief and may be appropriate.

Contraindications: Anuria; hypersensitivity to this or other sulfonamide-derived drugs.

Warnings: Use with caution in severe renal disease. In patients with renal disease, thiazides may precipitate azotemia. Cumulative effects of the drug may develop in patients with impaired renal function.

Thiazides should be used with caution in patients with impaired hepatic function or progressive liver disease, since minor alterations of fluid and electrolyte imbalance may precipitate hepatic coma.

Thiazides may add to or potentiate the action of other antihypertensive drugs. Potentiation occurs with ganglionic or peripheral adrenergic blocking drugs.

Sensitivity reactions are more likely to occur in patients with a history of allergy or bronchial asthma.

The possibility of exacerbation or activation of systemic lupus erythematosus has been reported.

Usage in Pregnancy

Thiazides cross the placental barrier and appear in cord blood. The use of thiazides in pregnant women requires that the anticipated benefit be weighed against possible hazards to the fetus. These hazards include fetal or neonatal jaundice, thrombocytopenia, and possibly other adverse reactions which have occurred in the adult.

Nursing Mothers: Thiazides appear in breast milk. If the use of the drug is deemed essential, the patient should stop nursing.

Precautions: Periodic determination of serum electrolytes to detect possible electrolyte imbalance should be performed at appropriate intervals. All patients receiving thiazide therapy should be observed for clinical signs of fluid or electrolyte imbalance: namely, hyponatremia, hypochloremic alkalosis, and hypokalemia. Serum and urine electrolyte determinations are particularly important when the patient is vomiting excessively or receiving parenteral fluids. Medication such as digitalis may also influence serum electrolytes. Warning signs are dryness of mouth, thirst, weakness, lethargy, drowsiness, restlessness, muscle pains or cramps, muscular fatigue, hypotension, oliguria, tachycardia, and gastrointestinal disturbance such as nausea or vomiting.

Hypokalemia may develop, especially with brisk diuresis, when severe cirrhosis is present, or during concomitant use of steroids or ACTH. Interference with adequate oral intake of electrolytes will also contribute to hypokalemia. Hypokalemia can sensitize or exaggerate the response of the heart to the toxic effects of digitalis (eg, increased ventricular irritability).

Any chloride deficit is generally mild and usually does not require specific treatment except under extraordinary circumstances (as in liver disease or renal disease). Dilutional hyponatremia may occur in edematous patients in hot weather; appropriate therapy is water restriction, rather than administration of salt except in rare instances when the hyponatremia is life-threatening. In actual salt depletion, appropriate replacement is the therapy of choice.

Hyperuricemia may occur or frank gout may be precipitated in certain patients receiving thiazide therapy.

Insulin requirements in diabetic patients may be increased, decreased, or unchanged. Latent diabetes may become manifest during thiazide administration.

Thiazide drugs may increase the responsiveness to tubocurarine.

The antihypertensive effects of the drug may be enhanced in the postsympathectomy patient. Thiazides may decrease arterial responsiveness to norepinephrine. This diminution is not sufficient to preclude effectiveness of the pressor agent for therapeutic use.

If progressive renal impairment becomes evident, withholding or discontinuing diuretic therapy should be considered.

Thiazides may decrease serum PBI levels without signs of thyroid disturbance.

Calcium excretion is decreased by thiazides. Pathological changes in the parathyroid gland with hypercalcemia and hypophosphatemia have been observed in a few patients on prolonged thiazide therapy. The common complications of hyperparathyroidism such as renal lithiasis, bone resorption, and peptic ulceration have not been seen. Thiazides should be discontinued before carrying out tests for parathyroid function.

Adverse Reactions:

Gastrointestinal: Anorexia, gastric irritation, nausea, vomiting, cramping, diarrhea, constipation, jaundice (intrahepatic cholestatic), pancreatitis, sialadenitis

Central Nervous System: Dizziness, vertigo, paresthesias, headache, xanthopsia

Hematologic: Leukopenia, agranulocytosis, thrombocytopenia, aplastic anemia

Cardiovascular: Orthostatic hypotension (may be potentiated by alcohol, barbiturates, or narcotics)

Hypersensitivity: Purpura, photosensitivity, rash, urticaria, necrotizing angiitis, Stevens-Johnson syndrome, and other hypersensitivity reactions

Other: Hyperglycemia, glycosuria, hyperuricemia, muscle spasm, weakness, restlessness

Whenever adverse reactions are moderate or severe, thiazide dosage should be reduced or therapy withdrawn.

Dosage and Administration: Therapy should be individualized according to patient response. Dosage should be titrated to gain maxi-

Continued on next page

CIBA—Cont.

mal therapeutic response as well as the minimal dose possible to maintain that therapeutic response.

Adults

Hypertension

To Initiate Therapy: Usual dose is 75 mg daily. May be given as a single dose every morning.
Maintenance: After a week dosage may be adjusted downward to as little as 25 mg a day, or upward to as much as 100 mg daily.
Combined Therapy: When necessary, other antihypertensive agents may be added cautiously. Since this drug potentiates the antihypertensive effect of other agents, such additions should be gradual. Dosages of ganglionic blockers in particular should be halved initially.

Edema

To Initiate Diuresis: 25 to 200 mg daily for several days, or until dry weight is attained.
Maintenance: 25 to 100 mg daily or intermittently depending on patient's response. A few refractory patients may require up to 200 mg daily.

Infants and Children

The usual pediatric dosage is administered twice daily.
The total daily dosage for infants up to 2 years of age: 12.5 to 37.5 mg; for children 2 to 12 years of age: 37.5 to 100 mg. Dosage should be based on body weight at the rate of 1 mg per pound, but infants below 6 months of age may require 1.5 mg per pound.

Overdosage

Signs and Symptoms

Diuresis is to be expected; lethargy of varying degree may appear and may progress to coma within a few hours, with minimal depression of respiration and cardiovascular function and without significant serum electrolyte changes or dehydration. The mechanism of CNS depression with thiazide overdosage is unknown. GI irritation and hypermotility may occur; temporary elevation of BUN has been reported and serum electrolyte changes could occur, especially in patients with impairment of renal function.

Treatment

Evacuate gastric contents but take care to prevent aspiration, especially in the stuporous or comatose patient. GI effects are usually of short duration, but may require symptomatic treatment.
Monitor serum electrolyte levels and renal function; institute supportive measures as required individually to maintain hydration, electrolyte balance, respiration and cardiovascular-renal function.

How Supplied: *Tablets,* 100 mg (blue, scored); bottles of 100. *Tablets,* 50 mg (yellow, scored); bottles of 30, 60, 100, 1000, 5000 and Accu-Pak® blister units of 100.
Tablets, 25 mg (pink, scored); bottles of 100, 1000 and 5000. C78-1 Rev. 1/78
VA—1000's, 50 mg, Stock 6505-00-880-7929

[*Shown in Product Identification Section*]

ESIMIL® ℞

guanethidine monosulfate 10 mg
hydrochlorothiazide 25 mg

> **Warning**
> This fixed combination drug is not indicated for initial therapy of hypertension. Hypertension requires therapy titrated to the individual patient. If the fixed combination represents the dosage so determined, its use may be more convenient in patient management. The treatment of hypertension is not static, but must be reevaluated as conditions in each patient warrant.

Indications

Hypertension. (See box warning.)

Contraindications

Guanethidine

Known or suspected pheochromocytoma; hypersensitivity; frank congestive heart failure not due to hypertension; use of MAO inhibitors.

Hydrochlorothiazide

Anuria; hypersensitivity to this or other sulfonamide-derived drugs.

Warnings: Guanethidine and hydrochlorothiazide are potent drugs and their use can lead to disturbing and serious clinical problems. Physicians should be familiar with both drugs and their combination before prescribing, and patients should be warned not to deviate from instructions.

Guanethidine

> Orthostatic hypotension can occur frequently and patients should be properly instructed about this potential hazard. Fainting spells may occur unless the patient is forewarned to sit or lie down with the onset of dizziness or weakness. Postural hypotension is most marked in the morning and is accentuated by hot weather, alcohol, or exercise. Dizziness or weakness may be particularly bothersome during the initial period of dosage adjustment and with postural changes, such as arising in the morning. The potential occurrence of these symptoms may require alteration of previous daily activity. The patient should be cautioned to avoid sudden or prolonged standing or exercise while taking the drug.

Concurrent use of guanethidine and rauwolfia derivatives may cause excessive postural hypotension, bradycardia, and mental depression.
If possible, withdraw therapy two weeks prior to surgery to reduce the possibility of vascular collapse and cardiac arrest during anesthesia. If emergency surgery is indicated, preanesthetic and anesthetic agents should be administered cautiously in reduced dosage. Oxygen, atropine, vasopressors, and adequate solutions for volume replacement should be ready for immediate use to counteract vascular collapse in the surgical patient. Vasopressors should be used only with extreme caution, since guanethidine augments the responsiveness to exogenously administered norepinephrine and vasopressors with respect to blood pressure and their propensity for the production of cardiac arrhythmias.
Dosage requirements may be reduced in the presence of fever.
Exercise special care when treating patients with a history of bronchial asthma; asthmatics are more apt to be hypersensitive to catecholamine depletion and their condition may be aggravated.

Hydrochlorothiazide

Use with caution in severe renal disease. In patients with renal disease, thiazides may precipitate azotemia. Cumulative effects of the drug may develop in patients with impaired renal function.
Thiazides should be used with caution in patients with impaired hepatic function or progressive liver disease, since minor alterations of fluid and electrolyte imbalance may precipitate hepatic coma.
Thiazides may add to or potentiate the action of other antihypertensive drugs. Potentiation occurs with ganglionic or peripheral adrenergic blocking drugs.
Sensitivity reactions are more likely to occur in patients with a history of allergy or bronchial asthma.
The possibility of exacerbation or activation of systemic lupus erythematosus has been reported.

Usage in Pregnancy

Guanethidine

The safety of guanethidine for use in pregnancy has not been established; therefore, this drug should be used in pregnant patients only when, in the judgment of the physician, its use is deemed essential to the welfare of the patient.

Hydrochlorothiazide

Thiazides cross the placental barrier and appear in cord blood. The use of thiazides in pregnant women requires that the anticipated benefit be weighed against possible hazards to the fetus. These hazards include fetal or neonatal jaundice, thrombocytopenia, and possibly other adverse reactions which have occurred in the adult.
Nursing Mothers: Thiazides appear in breast milk. If the use of the drug is deemed essential, the patient should stop nursing.

Precautions

Guanethidine

The effects of guanethidine are cumulative over long periods; initial doses should be small and increased gradually in small increments.
Use very cautiously in hypertensive patients with: renal disease and nitrogen retention or rising BUN levels, since decreased blood pressure may further compromise renal function; coronary disease with insufficiency or recent myocardial infarction; cerebral vascular disease, especially with encephalopathy.
Do not give to patients with severe cardiac failure except with extreme caution since guanethidine may interfere with the compensatory role of the adrenergic system in producing circulatory adjustment in patients with congestive heart failure.
In patients with incipient cardiac decompensation, watch for weight gain or edema, which may be averted by the concomitant administration of a thiazide.
Remember that both digitalis and guanethidine slow the heart rate.
Use cautiously in patients with a history of peptic ulcer or other chronic disorders which may be aggravated by a relative increase in parasympathetic tone.
Amphetamine-like compounds, stimulants (*eg,* ephedrine, methylphenidate), tricyclic antidepressants (*eg,* amitriptyline, imipramine, desipramine) and other psychopharmacologic agents (*eg,* phenothiazines and related compounds), and oral contraceptives may reduce the hypotensive effect of guanethidine.
MAO inhibitors should be discontinued for at least one week before starting therapy with guanethidine.

Hydrochlorothiazide

Periodic determination of serum electrolytes to detect possible electrolyte imbalance should be performed at appropriate intervals. All patients receiving thiazide therapy should be observed for clinical signs of fluid or electrolyte imbalance; namely, hyponatremia, hypochloremic alkalosis, and hypokalemia. Serum and urine electrolyte determinations are particularly important when the patient is vomiting excessively or receiving parenteral fluids. Medication such as digitalis may also influence serum electrolytes. Warning signs are dryness of mouth, thirst, weakness, lethargy, drowsiness, restlessness, muscle pains or cramps, muscular fatigue, hypotension, oliguria, tachycardia, and gastrointestinal disturbance such as nausea or vomiting.
Hypokalemia may develop, especially with brisk diuresis, when severe cirrhosis is present, or during concomitant use of steroids or ACTH. Interference with adequate oral intake of electrolytes will also contribute to hypokalemia. Hypokalemia can sensitize or exaggerate the response of the heart to the toxic effects of digitalis (*eg,* increased ventricular irritability).
Any chloride deficit is generally mild and usually does not require specific treatment except under extraordinary circumstances (as in liver disease or renal disease). Dilutional hyponatre-

mia may occur in edematous patients in hot weather; appropriate therapy is water restriction rather than administration of salt, except in rare instances when the hyponatremia is life-threatening. In actual salt depletion, appropriate replacement is the therapy of choice.
Hyperuricemia may occur or frank gout may be precipitated in certain patients receiving thiazide therapy.
Insulin requirements in diabetic patients may be increased, decreased, or unchanged. Latent diabetes may become manifest during thiazide administration.
Thiazide drugs may increase the responsiveness to tubocurarine.
The antihypertensive effects of the drug may be enhanced in the postsympathectomy patient. Thiazides may decrease arterial responsiveness to norepinephrine. This diminution is not sufficient to preclude effectiveness of the pressor agent for therapeutic use.
If progressive renal impairment becomes evident, withholding or discontinuing diuretic therapy should be considered.
Thiazides may decrease serum PBI levels without signs of thyroid disturbance.
Calcium excretion is decreased by thiazides. Pathological changes in the parathyroid gland with hypercalcemia and hypophosphatemia have been observed in a few patients on prolonged thiazide therapy. The common complications of hyperparathyroidism such as renal lithiasis, bone resorption, and peptic ulceration have not been seen. Thiazides should be discontinued before carrying out tests for parathyroid function.

Adverse Reactions

Guanethidine

Frequent reactions due to sympathetic blockade: dizziness, weakness, lassitude, and syncope resulting from either postural or exertional hypotension.

Frequent reactions due to unopposed parasympathetic activity: bradycardia, increase in bowel movements, and diarrhea. Diarrhea may be severe at times and necessitate discontinuance of the medication.

Other common reactions: inhibition of ejaculation, a tendency toward fluid retention and edema with occasional development of congestive heart failure.

Other less common reactions: dyspnea, fatigue, nausea, vomiting, nocturia, urinary incontinence, dermatitis, scalp hair loss, dry mouth, rise in BUN, ptosis of the lids, blurring of vision, parotid tenderness, myalgia, muscle tremor, mental depression, chest pains (angina), chest paresthesias, nasal congestion, weight gain, and asthma in susceptible individuals. Although a causal relationship has not been established, a few instances of blood dyscrasias (anemia, thrombocytopenia, and leukopenia) and of priapism have been reported.

Hydrochlorothiazide

Gastrointestinal: Anorexia, gastric irritation, nausea, vomiting, cramping, diarrhea, constipation, jaundice (intrahepatic cholestatic), pancreatitis, sialadenitis.

Central Nervous System: Dizziness, vertigo, paresthesias, headache, xanthopsia

Hematologic: Leukopenia, thrombocytopenia, agranulocytosis, aplastic anemia

Cardiovascular: Orthostatic hypotension (may be potentiated by alcohol, barbiturates, or narcotics)

Hypersensitivity: Purpura, photosensitivity, rash, urticaria, necrotizing angiitis, Stevens-Johnson syndrome, and other hypersensitivity reactions

Other: Hyperglycemia, glycosuria, hyperuricemia, muscle spasm, weakness, restlessness

Whenever adverse reactions are moderate or severe, thiazide dosage should be reduced or therapy withdrawn.

Dosage and Administration: As determined by individual titration (see box warning).
Ten mg guanethidine monosulfate present in Esimil is equivalent to 8.4 mg guanethidine sulfate USP. The usual dosage of Esimil is 2 tablets daily. As with any antihypertensive, dosage should be individually titrated for the patient. Depending upon the degree of hypertension, the patient should be started on the lowest possible dose (usually 1 tablet daily) and then gradually increased at weekly intervals until the desired response is obtained. Blood pressure should be recorded with the patient in the supine position and again after 10 minutes of standing. Dosage should be increased only if the standing blood pressure has not been reduced to desired levels. Dosage adjustment should be made at not less than weekly intervals; maximal dosage should not exceed 4 tablets daily. If additional effect is desirable, supplement individually with guanethidine tablets.
Do not give MAO inhibitors with Esimil. Stop ganglionic blockers before instituting therapy with Esimil. Wait at least one week after one drug is discontinued before starting Esimil.
When Esimil is to be substituted for other antihypertensive agents, the change should be made gradually. In general, dosage of the agent to be discontinued should be discontinued by one-half, and Esimil should be started at 1 tablet daily. Follow this schedule for at least one week; then, dosage of the previous therapy may be halved again and dosage of Esimil increased to 2 tablets daily. At the next week interval, the previously used drugs can generally be discontinued. Titrate dosage of Esimil at weekly intervals as mentioned above.
Patients receiving more than 75 mg guanethidine alone may do well on a smaller dose if also given hydrochlorothiazide. Because of the ratio of the combination, they are probably not candidates for Esimil.

Overdosage

Guanethidine

Signs and Symptoms

Postural hypotension [with dizziness, blurring of vision, etc., possibly progressing to syncope when standing] and bradycardia are most likely to occur; diarrhea, possibly severe, also may occur. Unconsciousness is unlikely if adequate blood pressure and cerebral perfusion can be maintained by appropriate positioning [supine] and by other treatment as required.

Treatment

In previously normotensive patients, treatment has consisted essentially of restoring blood pressure and heart rate to normal by keeping patient in supine position. Normal homeostatic control usually returns gradually over a 72-hour period in these patients.
In previously hypertensive patients, particularly those with impaired cardiac reserve or other cardiovascular-renal disease, intensive treatment may be required to support vital functions and/or to control cardiac irregularities that might be present. Supine position must be maintained; if vasopressors are required, it must be remembered that guanethidine may increase responsiveness as to blood pressure rise and occurrence of cardiac arrhythmias.
Diarrhea, if severe or persistent, should be treated symptomatically to reduce intestinal hypermotility, with due attention to maintenance of hydration and electrolyte balance.

Hydrochlorothiazide

Signs and Symptoms

Diuresis is to be expected; lethargy of varying degree may appear and may progress to coma within a few hours, with minimal depression of respiration and cardiovascular function and without significant serum electrolyte changes or dehydration. The mechanism of CNS depression with thiazide overdosage is unknown. GI irritation and hypermotility may occur; temporary elevation of BUN has been reported and serum electrolyte changes could occur, especially in patients with impairment of renal function.

Treatment

Evacuate gastric contents but take care to prevent aspiration, especially in the stuporous or comatose patient. GI effects are usually of short duration, but may require symptomatic treatment.
Monitor serum electrolyte levels and renal function; institute supportive measures as required individually to maintain hydration, electrolyte balance, respiration and cardiovascular-renal function.

How Supplied: *Tablets* (white, scored), each containing 10 mg guanethidine monosulfate (equivalent to 8.4 mg guanethidine sulfate USP) and 25 mg hydrochlorothiazide; bottles of 100, and Accu-Pak® blister units of 100.

C78-24 Rev. 12/78

[*Shown in Product Identification Section*]

FORHISTAL® ℞

(dimethindene maleate NF)

Lontabs®

Listed in NF, a Medicare designated compendium.

Indications

Based on a review of this drug by the National Academy of Sciences-National Research Council and/or other information, FDA has classified the indications as follows:

"Probably" effective: Perennial and seasonal allergic rhinitis; vasomotor rhinitis; allergic conjunctivitis due to inhalant allergens and foods; mild, uncomplicated allergic skin manifestations of urticaria and angioedema; amelioration of allergic reactions to blood or plasma; dermographism; anaphylactic reactions as adjunctive therapy to epinephrine and other standard measures after the acute manifestations have been controlled.

Final classification of the less-than-effective indications requires further investigation.

Contraindications: Forhistal should not be used in premature infants, neonates, or nursing mothers; patients receiving MAO inhibitors; patients with narrow-angle glaucoma, stenosing peptic ulcer, symptomatic prostatic hypertrophy, bladder neck obstruction, pyloroduodenal obstruction, lower respiratory tract symptoms (including asthma), or hypersensitivity to dimethindene or related compounds.

Warnings: Antihistamines often produce drowsiness and may reduce mental alertness in children and adults. Patients should be warned about engaging in activities requiring mental alertness (*eg*, driving a car, operating machinery or hazardous appliances). In elderly patients, approximately 60 years or older, antihistamines are more likely to cause dizziness, sedation and hypotension.
Patients should be warned that the central nervous system effects of Forhistal may be additive with those of alcohol and other CNS depressants (*eg*, hypnotics, sedatives, tranquilizers, antianxiety agents).
Antihistamines may produce excitation, particularly in children.

Usage in Pregnancy

Although no Forhistal-related teratogenic potential or other adverse effects on the fetus have been observed in limited animal reproduction studies, the safe use of this drug in pregnancy or during lactation has not been established. Therefore, the drug should not be used during pregnancy or lactation unless, in the judgment of the physician, the expected benefits outweigh the potential hazards.

Continued on next page

CIBA—Cont.

Usage in Children
In infants and children particularly, antihistamines in overdosage may produce hallucinations, convulsions and/or death.
Precautions: Forhistal, like other antihistamines, has atropine-like, anticholinergic activity and should be used with caution in patients with increased intraocular pressure, hyperthyroidism, cardiovascular disease, hypertension, or history of bronchial asthma.
The Forhistal Lontabs® (2.5 mg) contain FD&C Yellow No. 5 (tartrazine) which may cause allergic-type reactions (including bronchial asthma) in certain susceptible individuals. Although the overall incidence of FD&C Yellow No. 5 (tartrazine) sensitivity in the general population is low, it is frequently seen in patients who also have aspirin hypersensitivity.
Adverse Reactions: The most frequent adverse reactions to antihistamines are sedation or drowsiness; sleepiness; dryness of the mouth, nose, and throat; thickening of bronchial secretions; dizziness; disturbed coordination; epigastric distress.
Other adverse reactions which may occur are: fatigue; chills; confusion; restlessness; excitation; hysteria; nervousness; irritability; insomnia; euphoria; anorexia; nausea; vomiting; diarrhea; constipation; hypotension; tightness in the chest; wheezing; blurred vision; diplopia; vertigo; tinnitus; convulsions; headache; palpitations; tachycardia; extrasystoles; nasal stuffiness; urinary frequency; difficult urination; urinary retention; leukopenia; hemolytic anemia; thrombocytopenia; agranulocytosis; aplastic anemia; allergic or hypersensitivity reactions, including drug rash, urticaria, anaphylactic shock, and photosensitivity. Although the following may have been reported to occur in association with some antihistamines, they have not been known to result from the use of Forhistal: excessive perspiration, tremor, paresthesias, acute labyrinthitis, neuritis and early menses.
Dosage and Administration: Dosage should be individualized.
Adults and Children Over 6 Years of Age: One 2.5-mg Lontab once or twice daily.
Overdosage
Signs and Symptoms
The greatest danger from acute overdosage with antihistamines is their central nervous system effects which produce depression and/or stimulation.
In children, stimulation predominates initially in a syndrome which may include excitement, hallucinations, ataxia, incoordination, athetosis, and convulsions followed by postictal depression. Dry mouth, fixed dilated pupils, flushing of the face, and fever are common and resemble the syndrome of atropine poisoning.
In adults, CNS depression (*ie,* drowsiness, coma) is more common. CNS stimulation is rare; fever and flushing are uncommon.
In both children and adults, there can be a terminal deepening of coma and cardiovascular collapse; death can occur, especially in infants and children.
Treatment
There is no specific therapy for acute overdosage with antihistamines. General symptomatic and supportive measures should be instituted promptly and maintained for as long as necessary.
In the conscious patient, vomiting should be induced even though it may have occurred spontaneously. If vomiting cannot be induced, gastric lavage is indicated. Adequate precautions must be taken to protect against aspiration, especially in infants and children. Charcoal slurry or other suitable agent should be instilled into the stomach after vomiting or lavage. Saline cathartics or milk of magnesia may be of additional benefit.
In the unconscious patient, the airway should be secured with a cuffed endotracheal tube before attempting to evacuate the gastric contents. Intensive supportive and nursing care is indicated, as for any comatose patient.
If breathing is significantly impaired, maintenance of an adequate airway and mechanical support of respiration is the safest and most effective means of providing for adequate oxygenation of tissues to prevent hypoxia (especially brain hypoxia during convulsions).
Hypotension is an early sign of impending cardiovascular collapse and should be treated vigorously. Although general supportive measures are important, specific treatment with intravenous infusion of a vasopressor (*eg,* levarterenol bitartrate) titrated to maintain adequate blood pressure may be necessary.
Do *not* use CNS stimulants.
Convulsions should be controlled by careful titration of a short-acting barbiturate, repeated as necessary.
Ice packs and cooling sponge baths can aid in reducing the fever commonly seen in children.
How Supplied
Lontabs, 2.5 mg (orange); bottles of 100.
LONTABS® (long-acting tablets CIBA)
Dispense in tight, light-resistant container (USP).
C80-16 (1/80)
[Shown in Product Identification Section]

INH (isoniazid USP) Tablets ℞

Warning:
Severe and sometimes fatal hepatitis associated with isoniazid therapy may occur and may develop even after many months of treatment. The risk of developing hepatitis is age related. Approximate case rates by age are: 0 per 1,000 for persons under 20 years of age, 3 per 1,000 for persons in the 20–34 year age group, 12 per 1,000 for persons in the 35–49 year age group, 23 per 1,000 for persons in the 50–64 year age group, and 8 per 1,000 for persons over 65 years of age. The risk of hepatitis is increased with daily consumption of alcohol. Precise data to provide a fatality rate for isoniazid-related hepatitis is not available; however, in a U.S. Public Health Service Surveillance Study of 13,838 persons taking isoniazid, there were 8 deaths among 174 cases of hepatitis.
Therefore, patients given isoniazid should be carefully monitored and interviewed at monthly intervals. Serum transaminase concentration becomes elevated in about 10–20 percent of patients, usually during the first few months of therapy but it can occur at any time. Usually enzyme levels return to normal despite continuance of drug but in some cases progressive liver dysfunction occurs. Patients should be instructed to report immediately any of the prodromal symptoms of hepatitis, such as fatigue, weakness, malaise, anorexia, nausea, or vomiting. If these symptoms appear or if signs suggestive of hepatic damage are detected, isoniazid should be discontinued promptly, since continued use of the drug in these cases has been reported to cause a more severe form of liver damage.
Patients with tuberculosis should be given appropriate treatment with alternative drugs. If isoniazid must be reinstituted, it should be reinstituted only after symptoms and laboratory abnormalities have cleared. The drug should be restarted in very small and gradually increasing doses and should be withdrawn immediately if there is any indication of recurrent liver involvement.
Preventive treatment should be deferred in persons with acute hepatic diseases.

Indications: For all forms of tuberculosis in which organisms are susceptible.
For preventive therapy for the following groups, in order of priority:
1. Household members and other close associates of persons with recently diagnosed tuberculous disease.
2. Positive tuberculin skin test reactors with findings on the chest roentgenogram consistent with nonprogressive tuberculous disease, in whom there are neither positive bacteriologic findings nor a history of adequate chemotherapy.
3. Newly infected persons.
4. Positive tuberculin skin test reactors in the following special clinical situations: prolonged therapy with adrenocorticosteroids; immunosuppressive therapy; some hematologic and reticuloendothelial diseases, such as leukemia or Hodgkin's disease; diabetes mellitus; silicosis; after gastrectomy.
5. Other positive tuberculin reactors under 35 years of age.
The risk of hepatitis must be weighed against the risk of tuberculosis in positive tuberculin reactors over the age of 35. However, the use of isoniazid is recommended for those with the additional risk factors listed above (1–4) and on an individual basis in situations where there is likelihood of serious consequences to contacts who may become infected.
Contraindications: Isoniazid is contraindicated in patients who develop severe hypersensitivity reactions, including drug-induced hepatitis. Previous isoniazid-associated hepatic injury: severe adverse reactions to isoniazid, such as drug fever, chills, and arthritis; acute liver disease of any etiology.
Warnings: See the boxed warning.
Ophthalmologic examinations (including ophthalmoscopy) should be done *before* INH is started and periodically thereafter, even without occurrence of visual symptoms.
Carcinogenesis
Isoniazid has been reported to induce pulmonary tumors in a number of strains of mice.
Usage in Pregnancy and Lactation
It has been reported that in both rats and rabbits, isoniazid may exert an embryocidal effect when administered orally during pregnancy, although no isoniazid-related congenital anomalies have been found in reproduction studies in mammalian species (mice, rats, and rabbits). Isoniazid should be prescribed during pregnancy only when therapeutically necessary. The benefit of preventive therapy should be weighed against a possible risk to the fetus. Preventive treatment generally should be started after delivery because of the increased risk of tuberculosis for new mothers.
Since isoniazid is known to cross the placental barrier and to pass into maternal breast milk, neonates and breast-fed infants of isoniazid treated mothers should be carefully observed for any evidence of adverse effects.
Precautions: Use of isoniazid should be carefully monitored in the following:
1. Patients who are receiving phenytoin concurrently. Isoniazid may decrease the excretion of phenytoin or may enhance its effects. To avoid phenytoin intoxication, appropriate adjustment of the anticonvulsant should be made.
2. Daily users of alcohol. Daily ingestion of alcohol may be associated with a higher incidence of isoniazid hepatitis.
3. Patients with current chronic liver disease or severe renal dysfunction.
Adverse Reactions: The most frequent reactions are those affecting the nervous system and the liver.

Nervous system reactions: Peripheral neuropathy is the most common toxic effect. It is dose-related, occurs most often in the malnourished and in those predisposed to neuritis (*eg,* alcoholics and diabetics), and is usually preceded by paresthesias of the feet and hands. The incidence is higher in "slow inactivators".
Other neurotoxic effects, which are uncommon with conventional doses, are convulsions, toxic encephalopathy, optic neuritis and atrophy, memory impairment, and toxic psychosis.
Gastrointestinal reactions: Nausea, vomiting, epigastric distress.
Hepatic reactions: Elevated serum transaminases (SGOT; SGPT), bilirubinemia, bilirubinuria, jaundice and occasionally severe and sometimes fatal hepatitis. The common prodromal symptoms are anorexia, nausea, vomiting, fatigue, malaise, and weakness. Mild and transient elevation of serum transaminase levels, occurs in 10 to 20 percent of persons taking isoniazid. The abnormality usually occurs in the first 4 to 6 months of treatment but can occur at any time during therapy. In most instances, enzyme levels return to normal with no necessity to discontinue medication. In occasional instances, progressive liver damage occurs, with accompanying symptoms. In these cases, the drug should be discontinued immediately. The frequency of progressive liver damage increases with age. It is rare in persons under 20, but occurs in up to 2.3 percent of those over 50 years of age.
Hematologic reactions: Agranulocytosis; hemolytic, sideroblastic, or aplastic anemia; thrombocytopenia; and eosinophilia.
Hypersensitivity reactions: Fever, skin eruptions (morbilliform, maculopapular, purpuric, or exfoliative), lymphadenopathy and vasculitis.
Metabolic and endocrine reactions: Pyridoxine deficiency, pellagra, hyperglycemia, metabolic acidosis, and gynecomastia
Miscellaneous reactions: Rheumatic syndrome and systemic lupus erythematosus-like syndrome.

Overdosage:

Signs and Symptoms

Isoniazid overdosage produces signs and symptoms within 30 minutes to 3 hours after ingestion. Nausea, vomiting, dizziness, slurring of speech, blurring of vision, and visual hallucinations (including bright colors and strange designs), are among the early manifestations. With marked overdosage, respiratory distress and CNS depression, progressing rapidly from stupor to profound coma, are to be expected, along with severe, intractable seizures. Severe metabolic acidosis, acetonuria, and hyperglycemia are typical laboratory findings.

Treatment

Untreated or inadequately treated cases of gross isoniazid overdosage can terminate fatally, but good response has been reported in most patients brought under adequate treatment within the first few hours after drug ingestion.
Secure the airway and establish adequate respiratory exchange. Gastric lavage within the first 2 to 3 hours is advised, but should not be attempted until convulsions are under control. To control convulsions administer I.V. short-acting barbiturates and I.V. pyridoxine (usually 1 mg/1mg isoniazid ingested).
Obtain blood samples for immediate determination of gases, electrolytes, BUN, glucose, etc.; type and crossmatch blood in preparation for possible hemodialysis.
Rapid control of metabolic acidosis is fundamental to management. Give I.V. sodium bicarbonate at once and repeat as needed, adjusting subsequent dosage on the basis of laboratory findings (*ie,* serum sodium, pH, etc.).
Forced osmotic diuresis must be started early and should be continued for some hours after clinical improvement to hasten renal clearance of drug and help prevent relapse; monitor fluid intake and output.
Hemodialysis is advised for severe cases; if this is not available, peritoneal dialysis can be used along with forced diuresis.
Along with measures based on initial and repeated determination of blood gases and other laboratory tests as needed, utilize meticulous respiratory and other intensive care to protect against hypoxia, hypotension, aspiration pneumonitis, etc.

Dosage and Administration (See also indications):
NOTE—For preventive therapy of tuberculous infection it is recommended that physicians be familiar with the joint recommendations of the American Thoracic Society, American Lung Association, and the Center for Disease Control, as published in the American Review of Respiratory Diseases Vol. 110, No. 3, September 1974, or CDC's Morbidity and Mortality Weekly Report, Vol. 24, No. 8, February 22, 1975.

For treatment of active tuberculosis: Isoniazid is used in conjunction with other effective antituberculous agents.
If the bacilli become resistant, therapy must be changed to agents to which the bacilli are susceptible.

Usual oral dosage

Adults: 5 mg/kg up to 300 mg daily in a single dose.
Infants and children: 10–20 mg/kg depending on severity of infection, (up to 300–500 mg daily) in a single dose.

For preventive therapy

Adults: 300 mg/day in a single dose.
Infants and children: 10 mg/kg (up to 300 mg daily) in a single dose.
Continuous administration of isoniazid for a sufficient period is an essential part of the regimen because relapse rates are higher if chemotherapy is stopped prematurely. In the treatment of tuberculosis, resistant organisms may multiply and the emergence of resistant organisms during the treatment may necessitate a change in the regimen.
Concomitant administration of pyridoxine (B_6) is recommended in the malnourished and in those predisposed to neuropathy (*eg,* alcoholics and diabetics).

How Supplied: *Tablets,* 300 mg (white, scored); available as Rimactane® (rifampin USP)/INH Dual Pack containing 30 INH Tablets and 60 Rimactane 300-mg Capsules.
C78-15 Rev. 3/78

ISMELIN® sulfate ℞
(guanethidine sulfate USP)

Listed in USP, a Medicare designated compendium.

Indications: *Moderate and severe hypertension* either alone or as an adjunct.
Renal hypertension, including that secondary to pyelonephritis, renal amyloidosis, and renal artery stenosis.

Contraindications: Known or suspected pheochromocytoma; hypersensitivity; frank congestive heart failure not due to hypertension; use of MAO inhibitors.

Warnings: Ismelin is a potent drug and can lead to disturbing and serious clinical problems. Before prescribing, physicians should familiarize themselves with the details of its use and warn patients not to deviate from instructions.

> Orthostatic hypotension can occur frequently and patients should be properly instructed about this potential hazard. Fainting spells may occur unless the patient is forewarned to sit or lie down with the onset of dizziness or weakness. Postural hypotension is most marked in the morning and is accentuated by hot weather, alcohol, or exercise. Dizziness or weakness may be particularly bothersome during the initial period of dosage adjustment and with postural changes, such as arising in the morning. The potential occurrence of these symptoms may require alteration of previous daily activity. The patient should be cautioned to avoid sudden or prolonged standing or exercise while taking the drug.

Concurrent use of Ismelin and rauwolfia derivatives may cause excessive postural hypotension, bradycardia, and mental depression.
If possible, withdraw therapy two weeks prior to surgery to reduce the possibility of vascular collapse and cardiac arrest during anesthesia. If emergency surgery is indicated, preanesthetic and anesthetic agents should be administered cautiously in reduced dosage. Oxygen, atropine, vasopressors, and adequte solutions for volume replacement should be ready for immediate use to counteract vascular collapse in the surgical patient. Vasopressors should be used only with extreme caution, since Ismelin augments the responsiveness to exogenously administered norepinephrine and vasopressors with respect to blood pressure and their propensity for the production of cardiac arrhythmias.
Dosage requirements may be reduced in the presence of fever.
Exercise special care when treating patients with a history of bronchial asthma; asthmatics are more apt to be hypersensitive to catecholamine depletion and their condition may be aggravated.

Usage in Pregnancy

The safety of Ismelin for use in pregnancy has not been established; therefore this drug should be used in pregnant patients only when, in the judgment of the physician, its use is deemed essential to the welfare of the patient.

Precautions: The effects of guanethidine are cumulative over long periods; initial doses should be small and increased gradually in small increments.
Use very cautiously in hypertensive patients with: renal disease and nitrogen retention or rising BUN levels, since decreased blood pressure may further compromise renal function; coronary disease with insufficiency or recent myocardial infarction; cerebral vascular disease, especially with encephalopathy.
Do not give to patients with severe cardiac failure except with extreme caution since Ismelin may interfere with the compensatory role of the adrenergic system in producing circulatory adjustment in patients with congestive heart failure.
In patients with incipient cardiac decompensation, watch for weight gain or edema, which may be averted by the concomitant administration of a thiazide.
Remember that both digitalis and Ismelin slow the heart rate.
Use cautiously in patients with a history of peptic ulcer or other chronic disorders which may be aggravated by a relative increase in parasympathetic tone.
Amphetamine-like compounds, stimulants (*eg,* ephedrine, methylphenidate), tricyclic antidepressants (*eg,* amitriptyline, imipramine, desipramine) and other psychopharmacologic agents (*eg,* phenothiazines and related compounds), and oral contraceptives may reduce the hypotensive effect of guanethidine.
MAO inhibitors should be discontinued for at least one week before starting therapy with Ismelin.
The Ismelin tablets (10 mg) contain FD&C Yellow No. 5 (tartrazine) which may cause allergic-type reactions (including bronchial asthma) in certain susceptible individuals. Although the overall incidence of FD&C Yellow No. 5 (tartrazine) sensitivity in the general population is low, it is frequently seen in patients who also have aspirin hypersensitivity.

Continued on next page

CIBA—Cont.

Adverse Reactions:
Frequent reactions due to sympathetic blockade: dizziness, weakness, lassitude, and syncope resulting from either postural or exertional hypotension.
Frequent reactions due to unopposed parasympathetic activity: bradycardia, increase in bowel movements, and diarrhea. Diarrhea may be severe at times and necessitate discontinuance of the medication.
Other common reactions: inhibition of ejaculation, a tendency toward fluid retention and edema with occasional development of congestive heart failure.
Other less common reactions: dyspnea, fatigue, nausea, vomiting, nocturia, urinary incontinence, dermatitis, scalp hair loss, dry mouth, rise in BUN, ptosis of the lids, blurring of vision, parotid tenderness, myalgia, muscle tremor, mental depression, chest pains (angina), chest paresthesias, nasal congestion, weight gain, and asthma in susceptible individuals. Although a causal relationship has not been established, a few instances of blood dyscrasias (anemia, thrombocytopenia, and leukopenia) and of priapism have been reported.
Dosage and Administration: Better control may be obtained, especially in the initial phases of treatment, if the patient can have his blood pressure recorded regularly at home.
Ambulatory Patients. Begin treatment with small doses (10 mg). Increase gradually, depending upon the patient's response. Ismelin has a long duration of action; therefore, dosage increases should not be made more often than every 5 to 7 days, unless the patient is hospitalized.
Take blood pressure in the supine position, after standing for ten minutes, and immediately after exercise if feasible. Increase dosage only if there has been *no* decrease in standing blood pressure from the previous levels. The average daily dose is 25 to 50 mg; only 1 dose a day is usually required.

Dosage Chart for Ambulatory Patients

Visits at Intervals of 5 to 7 Days	*Daily Dose*
Visit No. 1 (Start with 10-mg tablets)	10 mg
Visit No. 2	20 mg
Visit No. 3 (Patient can be changed to 25-mg tablets whenever convenient)	30 mg (three 10-mg tablets) or 37.5 mg (one and one-half 25-mg tablets)
Visit No. 4	50 mg

Visit No. 5 (and subsequent). Dosage may be increased by 12.5 mg or 25 mg if necessary.
Reduce dosage in any of the following 3 situations:
1. *Normal supine pressure*
2. *Excessive orthostatic fall in pressure*
3. *Severe diarrhea*

Hospitalized Patients. Initial oral dose is 25 to 50 mg, increased by 25 or 50 mg daily or every other day as indicated. This higher dosage is possible because hospitalized patients can be watched carefully. Unless absolutely impossible, take the standing blood pressure regularly. Patients should not be discharged from the hospital until the effect of the drug on the standing blood pressure is known. *Patients should be told about the possibility of orthostatic hypotension and warned not to get out of bed without help during the period of dosage adjustment.*
Combination Therapy. Ismelin may be added gradually to thiazides and/or hydralazine. Thiazide diuretics enhance the effectiveness of Ismelin and may reduce the incidence of edema. When thiazide diuretics are added to the regimen in patients on Ismelin, it is usually necessary to reduce the dosage of Ismelin. After control is established, reduce dosage of all drugs to the lowest effective level.
When replacing MAO inhibitors, at least one week should elapse before commencing treatment with Ismelin.
In many cases ganglionic blockers will have been stopped before Ismelin is started. It may be advisable, however, to withdraw the blocker gradually to prevent a spiking blood pressure response during the transfer period.

Overdosage

Signs and Symptoms
Postural hypotension [with dizziness, blurring of vision, etc., possibly progressing to syncope when standing] and bradycardia are most likely to occur; diarrhea, possibly severe, also may occur. Unconsciousness is unlikely if adequate blood pressure and cerebral perfusion can be maintained by appropriate positioning [supine] and by other treatment as required.

Treatment
In previously normotensive patients, treatment has consisted essentially of restoring blood pressure and heart rate to normal by keeping patient in supine position. Normal homeostatic control usually returns gradually over a 72-hour period in these patients.
In previously hypertensive patients, particularly those with impaired cardiac reserve or other cardiovascular-renal disease, intensive treatment may be required to support vital functions and/or to control cardiac irregularities that might be present. Supine position must be maintained; if vasopressors are required, it must be remembered that Ismelin may increase responsiveness as to blood pressure rise and occurrence of cardiac arrhythmias.
Diarrhea, if severe or persistent, should be treated symptomatically to reduce intestinal hypermotility, with due attention to maintenance of hydration and electrolyte balance.
How Supplied: *Tablets,* 10 mg (pale yellow, scored) and 25 mg (white, scored); bottles of 100, 1000 and Accu-Pak® blister units of 100.
Dispense in tight container (USP).
C80-17 (1/80)
Military—100's, 10 mg, Stock 6505-00-854-2242; 100's, 25 mg, Stock 6505-00-062-4829; 1000's, 25 mg, Stock 6505-00-964-1551.
VA—100's, 10 mg, Stock 6505-00-854-2242A; 1000's, 10 mg, Stock 6505-00-964-1552A; 100's, 25 mg, Stock 6505-00-062-4829A; 1000's, 25 mg, Stock 6505-00-964-1551A.
[*Shown in Product Identification Section*]

LOCORTEN® ℞
(flumethasone pivalate NF)
anti-inflammatory antipruritic

Listed in NF, a Medicare designated compendium.

Indications: For relief of the inflammatory manifestations of corticosteroid-responsive dermatoses.
Contraindications: Topical steroids are contraindicated in vaccinia and varicella. Topical steroids are also contraindicated in those patients with a history of hypersensitivity to any of the components of the preparation.
Precautions: If irritation develops, the product should be discontinued and appropriate therapy instituted.
In the presence of an infection the use of an appropriate antifungal or antibacterial agent should be instituted. If a favorable response does not occur promptly the corticosteroid should be discontinued until the infection has been adequately controlled.
If extensive areas are treated or if the occlusive technique is used, there will be increased systemic absorption of the corticosteroid and suitable precautions should be taken, particularly in children and infants.
Although topical steroids have not been reported to have an adverse effect on pregnancy, the safety of their use in pregnant women has not been absolutely established. In laboratory animals, increases in incidence of fetal abnormalities have been associated with exposure of gestating females to topical corticosteroids, in some cases at rather low dosage levels. Therefore, drugs of this class should not be used extensively on pregnant patients, in large amounts, or for prolonged periods of time.
The product is not for ophthalmic use.
Adverse Reactions: The following local adverse reactions have been reported with topical corticosteroids, especially under occlusive dressings: burning; itching; irritation; dryness; folliculitis; hypertrichosis; acneiform eruptions; hypopigmentation; perioral dermatitis; allergic contact dermatitis; maceration of the skin; secondary infection; skin atrophy; striae; miliaria.
Dosage and Administration: Apply to affected areas 3 or 4 times daily. Gently rub in the cream until it disappears. Continue treatment for a few days after clearing of the lesions.
Occlusive Dressings: Occlusive dressings may be used for the management of psoriasis or recalcitrant conditions, such as chronic neurodermatitis, lichen planus, or lichen simplex chronicus.
Gently rub in Locorten Cream until it disappears. Then apply an additional thin coating of cream and cover the entire area with a pliable plastic film. If the lesions are dry, make the dressing airtight and watertight. Moist lesions need not be completely sealed. Determine dressing changes on an individual basis. This may be as frequent as once or twice daily or every three or four days. Reapplication of Locorten Cream is required at each dressing change. Usually, the longer the patient is treated by the occlusive technique the more rapid the rate of response.
Note: Sensitivity to occlusive dressings or adhesive may occur. In these cases, substitute hypoallergenic materials. Some plastic films may be flammable; exercise care in their use. Infection may develop when using the occlusive dressing technique; inspect lesions carefully between dressings.
How Supplied: *Cream* (water-washable base); tubes of 15 g and 60 g.
C78-18 Rev. 4/78

METANDREN® ℞
(methyltestosterone USP)
Linguets® and Tablets

Listed in USP, a Medicare designated compendium.

Indications
In the Male
1. Eunuchoidism and eunuchism.
2. Climacteric symptoms when these are secondary to androgen deficiency.
3. Impotence due to androgen deficiency.
4. Postpuberal cryptorchidism with evidence of hypogonadism.

In the Female
1. Prevention of postpartum breast pain and engorgement. There is no satisfactory evidence that this drug prevents or suppresses lactation.
2. Palliation of androgen-responsive, advancing, inoperable mammary cancer, in women who are more than 1 year, but less than 5 years postmenopausal or who have been proven to have a hormone-dependent tumor as shown by previous beneficial response to castration.

Contraindications: Carcinoma of the male breast; known or suspected carcinoma of the prostate; cardiac, hepatic, or renal decompensation; hypercalcemia; impaired liver function; prepuberal males; patients easily stimulated; pregnancy; and breast feeding.
Warnings: Hypercalcemia may occur in immobilized patients and in breast cancer patients. In patients with cancer hypercalcemia

may indicate progression of bony metastasis, in which case the drug should be discontinued. Watch female patients closely for signs of virilization. Some effects such as voice changes may not be reversible even when the drug is stopped.
Discontinue the drug if cholestatic hepatitis with jaundice appears or liver function tests become abnormal.
Precautions: Patients with cardiac, renal, or hepatic derangement may retain sodium and water with resulting edema formation.
Males, especially the elderly, may become overly stimulated.
Priapism or excessive sexual stimulation may develop.
Oligospermia and reduced ejaculatory volume may occur after prolonged administration or excessive dosage.
Hypersensitivity and gynecomastia may occur.
Alterations in liver function tests (*eg,* increased BSP retention and SGOT levels) and rarely jaundice have been reported and appear to be directly related to the dose of the drug. When any of these effects appear, the androgen should be stopped; if restarted, a lower dosage should be utilized.
Use cautiously in young boys to avoid possible premature epiphyseal closure or precocious sexual development.
The PBI may decrease during androgen therapy without clinical significance.
The Metandren Linguets® (10 mg) and tablets (25 mg) contain FD&C Yellow No. 5 (tartrazine) which may cause allergic-type reactions (including bronchial asthma) in certain susceptible individuals. Although the overall incidence of FD&C Yellow No. 5 (tartrazine) sensitivity in the general population is low, it is frequently seen in patients who also have aspirin hypersensitivity.
Adverse Reactions: Hypersensitivity, including skin manifestations and anaphylactoid reactions; acne; decreased ejaculatory volume; oligospermia; gynecomastia; edema; priapism; hypercalcemia, especially in immobile patients and those with metastatic breast carcinoma; virilization in females; cholestatic jaundice. There have been rare reports of hepatocellular neoplasms and peliosis hepatis in association with long-term androgenic-anabolic steroid therapy.
Dosage and Administration: Dosage must be strictly individualized. Daily requirements are best administered in divided doses. The following chart is suggested as an average daily dosage guide. Duration of therapy will depend upon the response of the condition being treated and the appearance of adverse reactions.
NOTE: Linguets have approximately twice the potency of the orally ingested hormone.

INDICATIONS	AVERAGE DAILY DOSAGE *Linguets*	*Tablets*
In the Male		
Eunuchism and eunuchoidism	5 to 20 mg	10 to 40 mg
Male climacteric and male impotence	5 to 20 mg	10 to 40 mg
Cryptorchidism—postpuberal	15 mg	30 mg
In the Female		
Postpartum breast pain and engorgement (3 to 5 days)	40 mg	80 mg
Breast cancer	100 mg	200 mg

Administration of Linguets
Linguets should not be swallowed since the hormone is meant to be absorbed through the mucous membranes. Place Linguet in the upper or lower buccal pouch between the gum and cheek. Avoid eating, drinking, chewing, or smoking while the Linguet is in place. Proper oral hygienic measures are particularly important after the use of Linguets.

How Supplied: *Linguets,* 5 mg (white); bottles of 100. *Linguets,* 10 mg (yellow); bottles of 100. *Tablets,* 10 mg (white, scored) and 25 mg (pale yellow, scored); bottles of 100.
LINGUETS® (tablets for mucosal absorption CIBA)
Dispense in tight, light-resistant container (USP).

C80-18 (1/80)

[*Shown in Product Identification Section*]

METOPIRONE® ℞

(metyrapone USP)
Tablets
Diagnostic Test of Pituitary Function

Description: A synthetic compound prepared in the CIBA Research Laboratories, Metopirone is 2-Methyl-1,2-di-3-pyridyl-1-propanone (USP).
Actions: Immediate effect of reducing cortisol production by inhibition of adrenal 11-β-hydroxylation. In the normal person, a compensatory increase in ACTH release follows and the secretion of 11-desoxycortisol and 11-desoxycorticosterone, "17-hydroxycorticoids," are markedly accelerated.
Indications: A diagnostic test drug for hypothalamico-pituitary function.
Contraindications: Adrenal cortical insufficiency, hypersensitivity.
Warnings: Usage in Pregnancy: The safety of metyrapone in pregnant women has not been established.
Precautions: All corticosteroid therapy must be discontinued prior to and during metyrapone testing.
Ability of adrenals to respond to exogenous ACTH should be demonstrated before metyrapone is employed as a test.
Drug may induce acute adrenal insufficiency in patients with reduced adrenal secretory capacity.
Erroneous results in pituitary function as determined by the metyrapone test may occur in patients taking diphenylhydantoin for as long as two weeks following cessation of therapy. A subnormal response may also occur in pregnant women and in patients on estrogen therapy.
Adverse Reactions: Nausea, abdominal discomfort, dizziness, headache, sedation, and allergic rash have been reported.
Dosage and Administration:
Day 1: Control period—Collect 24-hour urine with measurement of 17-hydroxycorticosteroids (17-OHCS) or 17-ketogenic steroids (17-KGS).
Day 2: ACTH test—Standard ACTH test such as administering 50 units ACTH by infusion over 8 hours and measurement of 24 hours urinary steroids.
Days 3-4: Rest period.
Day 5: Metyrapone administration:
Adults—750 mg orally, every 4 hours for 6 doses. A single dose is approximately equivalent to 15 mg/kg.
Children—15 mg/kg orally, every 4 hours for 6 doses. A minimal single dose of 250 mg is recommended.
Day 6: Post-oral metyrapone measurement—24-hour steroid determination for effect.
Interpretation
ACTH
The normal 24-hour urinary excretion of 17-OHCS ranges from 3 to 12 mg. Following continuous intravenous infusion of 50 units ACTH over a period of 8 hours, the 17-OHCS excretion is increased to 15 to 45 mg per 24 hours.
Metyrapone

a. **Normal response:** In patients with a normally functioning pituitary, the administration of metyrapone is followed by a two- to four-fold increase of 17-OHCS excretion or doubling of 17-KGS excretion.
b. **Subnormal response:** Subnormal response in patients without adrenal insufficiency is indicative of some degree of impairment of pituitary function, either panhypopituitarism or partial hypopituitarism (limited pituitary reserve).
   1. *Panhypopituitarism* is readily diagnosed by the classical clinical and chemical evidences of hypogonadism, hypothyroidism, and hypoadrenocorticism. These patients usually have subnormal basal urinary steroid levels. Depending upon the duration of the disease and degree of adrenal atrophy, they may fail to respond to exogenous ACTH in the normal manner. Metyrapone administration is not essential in the diagnosis, but if given, it will not induce an appreciable increase in urinary steroids.
   2. *Partial hypopituitarism* or limited pituitary reserve is the more difficult diagnosis as these patients do not present the classical signs and symptoms of hypopituitarism. Measurements of target organ functions often are normal under basal conditions. The response to exogenous ACTH is usually normal, producing the expected rise of urinary steroids (17-OHCS or 17-KGS). The response, however, to metyrapone is *subnormal;* that is, no significant increase in 17-OHCS or 17-KGS excretion occurs.
   This failure to respond to metyrapone may be interpreted as evidence of impaired pituitary-adrenal reserve. In view of the normal response to exogenous ACTH, the failure to respond to metyrapone is inferred to be related to a defect in the CNS-pituitary mechanisms which normally regulate ACTH secretions. Presumably the ACTH secreting mechanisms of these individuals are already working at their maximal rates to meet everyday conditions and possess limited "reserve" capacities to secrete additional ACTH either in response to stress or to decreased cortisol levels occurring as a result of metyrapone administration.
c. **Excessive response:** An excessive excretion of 17-OHCS or 17-KGS above the normal range after metyrapone administration is suggestive of Cushing's syndrome associated with adrenal hyperplasia. These patients have an elevated excretion of urinary corticosteroids under basal conditions and will often, but not invariably, show a "supernormal" response to ACTH and also to metyrapone, excreting more than 35 mg per 24 hours of either 17-OHCS or 17-KGS.

How Supplied: *Tablets,* 250 mg (white, scored); bottles of 18.
Dispense in tight, light-resistant container (USP).

C79-3 (7/79)

[*Shown in Product Identification Section*]

NUPERCAINAL®

Anesthetic Ointment
Suppositories
Pain-Relief Cream

CAUTION:
Nupercainal products are not for prolonged or extensive use and should never be applied in or near the eyes.
Consult labels before using.
Keep this and all medications out of reach of children.
NUPERCAINAL SHOULD NOT BE SWALLOWED. SWALLOWING OR USE OF A LARGE QUANTITY IS HAZARDOUS, PARTICULARLY TO CHILDREN.

Continued on next page

CIBA—Cont.

CONSULT A PHYSICIAN OR POISON CONTROL CENTER IMMEDIATELY.

Nupercainal is a fast-acting, long-lasting pain reliever that you can use for a number of painful skin conditions. It comes in 3 different forms: (1) **Nupercainal Anesthetic Ointment** is for hemorrhoids and for general use; (2) **Nupercainal Suppositories** are for hemorrhoids only; (3) **Nupercainal Pain-Relief Cream** is for general use only. The **Cream** is half as strong as the **Ointment.**

How to use Nupercainal Anesthetic Ointment (for general use). This soothing Ointment helps lubricate dry, inflamed skin and gives fast, temporary relief of pain and itching. It is recommended for sunburn, nonpoisonous insect bites, minor burns, cuts, and scratches. **DO NOT USE THIS PRODUCT IN OR NEAR YOUR EYES.**

Apply to affected areas gently. If necessary, cover with a light dressing for protection. Do not use more than 1 ounce of Ointment in a 24-hour period for an adult; do not use more than one-quarter of an ounce in a 24-hour period for a child. If irritation develops, discontinue use and consult your doctor.

How to use Nupercainal Anesthetic Ointment for fast, temporary relief pain and itching due to hemorrhoids (also known as piles).

Remove cap from tube and set it aside. Attach the white plastic applicator to the tube. Squeeze the tube until you see the Ointment begin to come through the little holes in the applicator. Using your finger, lubricate the applicator with the Ointment. Now insert the entire applicator gently into the rectum. Give the tube a good squeeze to get enough Ointment into the rectum for comfort and lubrication. Remove applicator from rectum and wipe it clean. Apply additional Ointment to anal tissues to help relieve pain, burning, and itching. For best results use Ointment morning and night and after each bowel movement. After each use detach applicator, and wash it off with soap and water. Put cap back on tube before storing. In case of rectal bleeding, discontinue use and consult your doctor.

How to use Suppositories for hemorrhoids (also known as piles).

Tear off one suppository along the perforated line. Remove foil wrapper. Insert the suppository, rounded end first, well into the anus until you can feel it moving into your rectum. For best results, use one suppository after each bowel movement. Each suppository is sealed in its own foil packet to reduce danger of leakage when carried in pocket or purse. **To prevent melting, do not store above 86°F (30°C).**

Pain-Relief Cream for general use. This Cream is particularly effective for fast, temporary relief of pain and itching associated with sunburn, cuts, scratches, minor burns and nonpoisonous insect bites. **DO NOT USE THIS PRODUCT IN OR NEAR YOUR EYES.** Apply liberally to affected area and rub in gently. This Cream is water-washable, so be sure to reapply after bathing, swimming or sweating. If irritation develops, discontinue use and consult your doctor.

Nupercainal Anesthetic Ointment contains 1% (one percent) dibucaine NF in a lubricant base. Available in tubes of 1 and 2 ounces.

Nupercainal Suppositories contain 2.5 mg dibucaine NF. Available in boxes of 12 and 24.

Nupercainal Pain-Relief Cream contains 0.5% (one-half of one percent) dibucaine NF in a water-soluble base. Available in 1½ ounce tubes.

Dibucaine NF is officially classified as a "topical anesthetic" and is one of the strongest and longest lasting of all pain relievers. It is not a narcotic. C79-3 (9/79)

NUPERCAINE® hydrochloride ℞
(dibucaine hydrochloride NF)
1:200 (0.5%)

Listed in NF, a Medicare designated compendium.

Specially Prepared for Isobaric Spinal Anesthesia According to the Method of Keyes and McLellan*

*Keyes, E. L., and McLellan, A. M.: *Amer J Surg 9:*1 (July) 1930. Not to be confused with the method of Howard Jones wherein the technique is somewhat different and the dibucaine hydrochloride solution is much weaker (1:1500) or with the Heavy Solution Nupercaine® hydrochloride (dibucaine hydrochloride).

Principle: A small volume of this concentrated solution of dibucaine hydrochloride is mixed with cerebrospinal fluid and injected in a final concentration of 1:1000.

Solution: Nupercaine hydrochloride 1:200 is an isobaric, isotonic, phosphate-buffered solution.

Specific Gravity
1.0062 (15.5°C) 1.0060 (20.0°C) 1.0059 (37.0°C)

Equipment

Syringe: Luer-Lok all-glass syringe, capacity 10 ml.

Needles: One needle of convenient size to transfer solution from the ampul into the syringe. One spinal needle with an accurately fitted stylet. It is suggested that a needle no larger than No. 22 be used. Larger sizes, permitting loss of spinal fluid, contribute to postinjection headache.

The bevel of the needle is important. It should be short with an angle of no less than 45° to decrease the possibility that part of the dibucaine hydrochloride solution might escape into the extradural space during the injection.

Because dibucaine hydrochloride is precipitated by minute amounts of alkali, syringes and needles should be rinsed with acidified distilled water to remove traces of alkaline salts and small foreign particles.

Ampuls: As part of the meticulous technique for administration of any spinal anesthetic agent, ampuls should be prepared as follows: Autoclave sterilization, considered by several authorities to be the best method. Dibucaine hydrochloride 1:200 solution (method of Keyes and McLellan) is stable as to pH, color and chemical assay when subjected to 3 repeated sterilizations at 121°C for 30 minutes.

Preparation of the Patient: Food and liquid, unless otherwise contraindicated, may be given freely up to the night before surgery. Enemas may be given.

It is recommended that a mild hypnotic be given the night before the operation. One-half to one hour before the patient is brought into the operating room, ¼ grain (15 mg) of morphine sulfate [with 1/200 gr (0.33 mg) of scopolamine hydrobromide as recommended by Keyes and McLellan] is administered. If necessary, ⅙ gr (10 mg) of morphine is given shortly before spinal puncture.

Position of the Patient: The sitting position facilitates injection. If necessary, the lateral position may be employed; care must be taken so that the vertebral column is straight and without lateral curvature.

Insertion of the Spinal Needle: The patient sits bending well forward, and the puncture is made at the L_3-L_4 interspace. (If he is in the lateral position he should be fully flexed.) The D_{12}-L_1 interspace can be the site of injection for upper abdominal operations and L_1-L_2 for gynecological surgery.

When the spinal needle is in the correct position, the stylet is removed and about 2 ml cerebrospinal fluid is allowed to escape. The stylet is replaced. If the tapped fluid is bloody after 2 ml have flowed or if there is radiating pain, there has been incorrect placement of the needle. It should be withdrawn and inserted at another interspace.

Once the needle is correctly inserted, it is very important to avoid displacing it from the subdural space.

Suggested Dosages

Surgical Area	*Dose (mg)*	*Volume (ml)*
Perineum and lower limbs	2.5 to 5	0.5 to 1
Lower abdomen	5 to 7.5	1 to 1.5
Upper abdomen	10	2

The size of the individual, the degree of anesthesia desired and particularly the experience of the physician may modify these recommended dosages.

Note: The maximum dose should never be more than 10 mg (2 ml).

Injection: The desired amount of Nupercaine hydrochloride (dibucaine hydrochloride) 1:200 is drawn up into the syringe by the "transfer" needle. With the stylet removed from the positioned spinal needle, the syringe is attached. If the patient is in the upright position, cerebrospinal fluid pressure usually will force the fluid out into the syringe to mix with the dibucaine hydrochloride 1:200 solution. If fluid does not flow easily, gentle aspiration may be used. The appropriate volume of cerebrospinal fluid (4 times the volume of the dibucaine hydrochloride 1:200 solution) is withdrawn and allowed to mix with the dibucaine hydrochloride. [See table below].

About one-third of the mixture is then injected, after which spinal fluid is again aspirated. Following this, one-half of the remaining contents of the syringe is injected. Another aspiration is then followed by injection of the remainder of the mixture.

The whole injection should be carried out very slowly.

Regulation of Anesthesia: When injection is complete, the needle is removed, the skin swabbed with antiseptic, sterile gauze fixed, and the patient is placed in Trendelenburg position.

Immediately after dibucaine hydrochloride is injected subdurally, it is advisable to inject ¾ to 1½ gr (50 to 100 mg) ephedrine intramuscularly. This usually prevents a fall in blood pressure in case the anesthetic solution ascends higher than desired.

For operations on the abdominal viscera a 20° Trendelenburg position is used; with surgery on the lower abdomen, perineum and lower limbs, the tilt may be decreased to 10° to 15°. The level of anesthesia should be determined after 1 or 2 minutes so that the tilt of the table can be adjusted for the desired level of anesthesia.

With correct technique and dosage, anesthesia with Nupercaine hydrochloride (dibucaine hydrochloride) should be sufficiently devel-

Dilution of Dibucaine Hydrochloride 1:200 by Cerebrospinal Fluid

Ml Dibucaine Hydrochloride 1:200	*Ml Cerebrospinal Fluid*	*Final Concentration Dibucaine Hydrochloride*	*Mg Dibucaine Hydrochloride Per Dose*
0.5	2	1:1000	2.5
1	4	1:1000	5
1.5	6	1:1000	7.5
2	8	1:1000	10

oped after 10 to 15 minutes. Failure of this to occur suggests either:
(1) Separation of dibucaine hydrochloride because of alkalinity of the syringe or needle.
(2) Extradural injection of the anesthetic solution.

Anesthesia lasts, on the average, up to six hours. This is followed by a period of slowly returning sensibility during which the patient is free from postoperative discomfort.

General Contraindications

Absolute

1. Disease of the cerebrospinal system, such as meningitis, cranial hemorrhage, tumors, poliomyelitis.
2. Moribund patients.
3. Blood stream infection.
4. Pernicious anemia with cord symptoms.
5. Arthritis, spondylitis, and other diseases of the spinal column rendering spinal puncture impossible. The presence of tuberculosis or metastatic lesions in the column is also a contraindication.
6. Pyogenic infection of the skin at or adjacent to the site of puncture.

Relative

1. **Hysteria or excessive nervous tension.** This difficulty may frequently be overcome by the preoperative administration of morphine sulfate ⅙ to ¼ gr (10 to 15 mg), scopolamine 1/150 to 1/100 gr (0.43 to 0.65 mg), or a sedative.
2. **Chronic backache.** The patient may blame any exacerbation of symptoms, either immediate or late, on the spinal anesthesia.
3. **Preoperative headache of long duration or history of migraine.** Exacerbation of symptoms may follow spinal injection.
4. **Hypersensitivity to drugs.** This drug may be used frequently in patients who have shown a sensitivity to procaine. However, in all patients in whom drug sensitivity is suspected, a skin test should be performed by injecting intradermally a small amount (0.1 ml) of dibucaine hydrochloride and at the same time injecting intradermally a small amount (0.1 ml) of physiologic salt solution as a control. Reaction may be local (redness), or systemic (dyspnea, agitation). Use of the drug is absolutely contraindicated in the presence of local reaction if there is a history of drug idiosyncrasy.
5. **Possibility of severe hemorrhage during operation.** Judgment in this case must include consideration of the amount of possible hemorrhage, the height of anesthesia to be induced, and the facilities available to control shock.
6. **Shock.** All forms of anesthesia are poorly borne by patients in shock. Systolic blood pressure should be raised to at least 105 mm Hg before operation is contemplated.
7. **Hypotension.** In cases not due to Addison's disease or associated with severe shock, this has become of relatively little importance because of the effectiveness of ephedrine in restoring pressure to normal (see *Complications:* Hypotension).
8. **Hemorrhagic spinal fluid.** Where clear spinal fluid cannot be obtained, the needle should be withdrawn and puncture made at another interspace. This is important in order to avoid the possibility of intravenous injection of the drug.
9. **Cardiac decompensation, massive pleural effusions, and markedly increased intra-abdominal pressure** as in massive ascites and tumors.

Warnings

1. An extremely potent anesthetic agent and therefore is to be used in much smaller concentrations than other local anesthetics.
2. As is true for any spinal anesthetic agent, the anesthetist should remain in constant attendance. Ephedrine and oxygen should be held in readiness in order to effectively combat a sudden fall in blood pressure should such occur. Likewise, a quick-acting barbiturate should be readily available so that any evidence of toxicity, as manifested by excitement, may be treated promptly.
3. Persons with known drug sensitivity should be pretested before using any of the local anesthetic agents.

Cautions: Authorities agree that spinal anesthesia should not be induced unless the anesthetist is: (1) equipped to provide a rigidly aseptic technique; (2) prepared to remain in constant attendance; (3) equipped to deal with complications or side effects that may arise; (4) familiar with the contraindications to spinal anesthesia.

Complications and Side Effects

1. **Respiratory.** Cessation of respiration may occur from spread of the anesthetic into the cervical region. This is absolutely prevented by following the technique described. It may also occur because of medullary anoxia which follows the circulatory collapse incident to severe hypotension.
   Treatment: Intubation to assure an adequate airway; artificial respiration; oxygen; respiratory stimulant repeated as necessary.
2. **Hypotension.** The fall of blood pressure produced by spinal anesthesia is due to a number of factors, most important of which are: (1) sudden vasodilatation incident to paralysis of sympathetic vasomotor fibers and (2) loss of muscle tone with decrease in venous pressure, venous return, and cardiac output. The degree of fall therefore depends upon the number of segments involved, being greatest in high spinal anesthesia and practically nonexistent when the effect is confined to the perineal area alone.
   There have been several reports indicating that Nupercaine hydrochloride (dibucaine hydrochloride) has less effect upon blood pressure than does a comparable degree of anesthesia produced by procaine.
   Treatment: The prophylactic use of 25 mg ephedrine given intramuscularly before the anesthetic is injected is advised by many authorities. It may be omitted in low spinals. An additional dose of 25 mg should be given *intravenously* if a fall below 100 mm Hg occurs. This dose may be repeated; total should not exceed 100 mg. Fluids, plasma, or whole blood should be administered intravenously when severe fall of blood pressure occurs. In *obstetrical patients,* raising the legs to the vertical position is the most effective initial procedure to increase blood pressure.
3. **Postanesthetic Headache.** Since this is usually due to leakage of spinal fluid, incidence will decrease as technique improves.
   Prophylaxis: A needle of small caliber (not over 20 or 22 gauge) should be used. Some authorities recommend special needles, one of 20 gauge to penetrate the skin and fascia and an inner needle of 24 gauge to pierce the dura. It has also been recommended that the needle be introduced with the bevel held laterally so as to cut fewer fibers of the dura. The needle should remain in place for several seconds after injection to allow time for equalization of pressure.
   Treatment: Tight abdominal binder. Hydration of the patient with either oral or intravenous fluids. One ml surgical pituitrin or 100 mg ephedrine. Rapid relief has been reported after intraspinal or caudal injection of 30 ml sterile saline.
4. **Nausea and Vomiting.** These may occur from psychic causes, drop in blood pressure, or intra-abdominal manipulation.
   Treatment: When caused by hypotension, inhalations of 100 percent oxygen in conjunction with a vasopressor may be found effective. Light cyclopropane or an intravenous barbiturate will control that which is due to intra-abdominal manipulation.
5. **Palsies.** Transient nerve palsies, usually involving the abducens, have occasionally been reported. This very uncommon complication generally occurs during the second week and clears up by the third or fourth week. Temporary or permanent transverse myelitis may follow the use of spinal anesthetic agents (see *Warnings*).
6. **Meningitis.** An aseptic technique should practically preclude the occurrence of this complication. Aseptic meningitis or meningismus, usually of rapid and benign course, has occurred after spinal anesthesia as it has also in cases where no spinal puncture has been carried out. Lundy has called attention to the fact that meningitides following spinal anesthesia may occur without relation to the method but due to pathologically proved metastases from distant foci. However, even the remote possibility of this complication reinforces the necessity for an absolutely sterile technique.
7. **Drug Idiosyncrasy.** The use of this drug is exceptionally free of this hazard. Patients giving a history of hypersensitivity to drugs, however, should be skin tested (see *Contraindications*).
   Treatment: The occurrence of motor excitement requires the anticonvulsant action of an intravenous barbiturate.

Supplied: *Ampuls,* for spinal anesthesia, 2 ml, 1:200 (method of Keyes and McLellan), each ampul containing 10 mg dibucaine hydrochloride, 10 mg sodium chloride, 4 mg sodium phosphate monobasic, 0.9 mg sodium phosphate dibasic, and water q.s.; cartons of 10.

C76-66 Rev. 9/76

NUPERCAINE® hydrochloride ℞
(dibucaine hydrochloride NF)
1:1500

Listed in NF, a Medicare designated compendium.

Specially Prepared for Hypobaric Spinal Anesthesia According to the Method of Howard Jones*

*Not to be confused with the method of Keyes and McLellan wherein the technique is completely different and the dibucaine hydrochloride solution is much more concentrated.

Principle: A relatively large volume of this solution of dibucaine hydrochloride with a specific gravity *less* than that of the cerebrospinal fluid (hypobaric) is injected without previous removal of fluid.

Solution: Nupercaine hydrochloride 1:1500 in saline. Specific Gravity: 1.0038 (15.5°C), 1.0036 (37°C).

Equipment

Syringe: Luer-Lok syringe with a capacity of 20 ml, accurately gauged, made of neutral glass.

Needles: Rustless needles, 20 gauge and 3½ inches in length; short bevels.

Large needles inflict unnecessary trauma; their use is apt to be followed by postinjection backache and headache, presumably due to trauma and leakage of spinal fluid. With a needle as slender as 22 gauge or more, longer than 3½ inches, bending is apt to occur when the needle is held by the hub and attempt made to puncture the skin; on the other hand, needles less than 3½ inches long may be too short for

Continued on next page

CIBA—Cont.

obese patients. The bevel of the needle is of importance; if it is less than 45 degrees, the chance of having a portion of the lumen outside the dura is increased, although the tip lies in the subdural space; the result being that a part or all of the anesthetic solution escapes extradurally when the attempt is made to inject it. The spinal puncture needle should be furnished with an accurately fitting stylet. The needle should be carefully examined and tested by bending before sterilization.

Syringes and needles are sterilized, preferably in an autoclave, then rinsed in slightly acidulated distilled water or 95% alcohol (2 to 3 drops of dilute hydrochloric acid to the liter), and covered with a sterile towel. This procedure is of importance, both for removing any small foreign particles and also to neutralize any alkalinity.

Ampuls: As part of the meticulous technique for administration of any spinal anesthetic agent, ampuls should be prepared as follows: Autoclave sterilization, considered by several authorities to be the best method. Dibucaine hydrochloride 1:1500 solution (method of Howard Jones) is stable as to pH, color and chemical assay when subjected to 3 repeated sterilizations at 121°C for 30 minutes.

Preoperative Procedure: The patient's confidence should be gained. Food and liquids, unless contraindicated, may be given freely up to the night preceding surgery; enemas may be given.

A mild hypnotic is indicated in order to provide sleep the night preceding the operation; ¼ gr morphine sulfate is administered ½ to 1 hour before the patient is brought to the operating room. If necessary, ⅙ gr morphine may be given shortly before puncture.

Administration: The patient is placed in the right lateral position, after his back has been painted with tincture of iodine over an area extending a palm's breadth below the scapular angle to the gluteal cleft, washed with 70% alcohol and draped with sterile cloth or towels. It is important to have the patient in a lateral position when making the subdural injection, because the solution with the specific gravity lighter than the one of the spinal fluid (usually 1.005 to 1.007) will ascend rapidly in the canal, with possible involvement of the medullary centers, if the sitting position is adopted.

The lumbar puncture is made between the 2nd and 3rd vertebrae or between the 3rd and 4th, according to the level of the operation. The needle, inserted in the proper interspace, is pushed 1 mm further after the first appearance of cerebrospinal fluid, and a few drops are allowed to escape. The syringe is then attached, care being taken not to displace the needle. The injection is made very slowly and should be discontinued for 3 to 4 seconds when an increasing resistance is encountered. The needle is, under these circumstances, maintained strictly in the position adopted to minimize leakage. No efforts should be made to decrease the resistance by moving the needle, but pauses are made after the injection of each succeeding 2 ml of the solution.

While barbotage is practiced in the administration of the buffered (1:200) solution of Nupercaine hydrochloride (dibucaine hydrochloride), it should *never* be employed with the hypobaric (1:1500) concentration.

Upon the completion of the injection, that is, the selected volume of the solution (see dosage), the needle is allowed to remain in place for 1 or 2 minutes to permit increased subdural pressure to return to normal.

Position Following Injection: The needle withdrawn, the patient is immediately turned flat in the prone position for 5 to 10 minutes to enable the light solution to impregnate the posterior roots. If there is a pronounced degree of dorsal curvature, the table may be tilted, fastened down with the head-piece flexed to bring the head below the level of the dorsal region. The patient is then turned on his back in a slight Trendelenburg position (head 2 inches below feet), which is maintained throughout the operation.

Dosage: For anesthesia of the lower extremities as high as the pelvis, 4 mg (6 ml solution, 1:1500) are usually sufficient. 7.5 to 10 mg (11 to 15 ml) will be required for most abdominal operations.

Usually, dosage above 15 ml is not necessary. The volume of solution to pass the level of D_5 is roughly calculated by subtracting from the number of inches given by the measurement of the distance from the spine C_7 to the interiliac line (4 for males and 6 for females). For caudal block, 6 ml is usually sufficient; 10 ml for the level D_{10}, 12 ml for D_7-D_8. For operations of longer duration on the stomach or duodenum, up to 20 ml may be required (16 ml for a 5-foot woman, 17 ml for a 5-foot man with 1 ml added for every 3 inches over 5 feet—to a maximum of 20 ml). For anesthesia in the lower part of the abdomen, divide 100 by the number of the uppermost thoracic nerve segment which is to be anesthetized. The result is the amount (in ml) of Nupercaine hydrochloride (dibucaine hydrochloride) solution to be used.

Approximate Dosage

Dosage for:	Concentration	Amount
Upper Abdominal	1:1500	15 to 18 ml
Lower Abdominal	1:1500	10 to 15 ml
Simple Caudal Block	1:1500	6 ml

Obstetrical Contraindications To Spinal Anesthesia: (1) Pelvic disproportion, (2) placenta praevia, (3) abruptio placenta, (4) unengaged head, and (5) necessity for intrauterine manipulations such as podalic version.

General Contraindications

Absolute

1. Disease of the cerebrospinal system, such as meningitis, cranial hemorrhage, tumors, poliomyelitis.
2. Moribund patients.
3. Blood stream infection.
4. Pernicious anemia with cord symptoms.
5. Arthritis, spondylitis, and other diseases of the spinal column rendering spinal puncture impossible. The presence of tuberculosis or metastatic lesions in the column is also a contraindication.
6. Pyogenic infection of the skin at or adjacent to the site of puncture.

Relative

1. **Hysteria or excessive nervous tension.** This difficulty may frequently be overcome by the preoperative administration of morphine sulfate ⅙ to ¼ gr (10 to 15 mg), scopolamine 1/150 to 1/100 gr (0.43 to 0.65 mg), or a sedative.
2. **Chronic backache.** The patient may blame any exacerbation of symptoms, either immediate or late, on the spinal anesthesia.
3. **Preoperative headache of long duration or history of migraine.** Exacerbation of symptoms may follow spinal injection.
4. **Hypersensitivity to drugs.** This drug may be used frequently in patients who have shown a sensitivity to procaine. However, in all patients in whom drug sensitivity is suspected, a skin test should be performed by injecting intradermally a small amount (0.1 ml) of dibucaine hydrochloride and at the same time injecting intradermally a small amount (0.1 ml) of physiologic salt solution as a control. Reaction may be local (redness), or systemic (dyspnea, agitation). Use of the drug is absolutely contraindicated in the presence of local reaction if there is a history of drug idiosyncrasy.
5. **Possibility of severe hemorrhage during operation.** Judgment in this case must include consideration of the amount of possible hemorrhage, the height of anesthesia to be induced, and the facilities available to control shock.
6. **Shock.** All forms of anesthesia are poorly borne by patients in shock. Systolic blood pressure should be raised to at least 105 mm Hg before operation is contemplated.
7. **Hypotension.** In cases not due to Addison's disease or associated with severe shock, this has become of relatively little importance because of the effectiveness of ephedrine in restoring pressure to normal (see *Complications:* Hypotension).
8. **Hemorrhagic spinal fluid.** Where clear spinal fluid cannot be obtained, the needle should be withdrawn and puncture made at another interspace. This is important in order to avoid the possibility of intravenous injection of the drug.
9. **Cardiac decompensation, massive pleural effusions, and markedly increased intra-abdominal pressure** as in massive ascites and tumors.

Warnings

1. An extremely potent anesthetic agent and therefore is to be used in much smaller concentrations than other local anesthetics.
2. As is true for any spinal anesthetic agent, the anesthetist should remain in constant attendance. Ephedrine and oxygen should be held in readiness in order to effectively combat a sudden fall in blood pressure should such occur. Likewise, a quick-acting barbiturate should be readily available so that any evidence of toxicity, as manifested by excitement, may be treated promptly.
3. Persons with known drug sensitivity should be pretested before using any of the local anesthetic agents.

Cautions: Authorities agree that spinal anesthesia should not be induced unless the anesthetist is: (1) equipped to provide a rigidly aseptic technique; (2) prepared to remain in constant attendance; (3) equipped to deal with complications or side effects that may arise; (4) familiar with the contraindications to spinal anesthesia.

Complications and Side Effects

1. **Respiratory.** Cessation of respiration may occur from spread of the anesthetic into the cervical region. This is absolutely prevented by following the technique described. It may also occur because of medullary anoxia which follows the circulatory collapse incident to severe hypotension.

   Treatment: Intubation to assure an adequate airway; artificial respiration; oxygen; respiratory stimulant repeated as necessary.
2. **Hypotension.** The fall of blood pressure produced by spinal anesthesia is due to a number of factors, most important of which are: (1) sudden vasodilatation incident to paralysis of sympathetic vasomotor fibers and (2) loss of muscle tone with decrease in venous pressure, venous return, and cardiac output. The degree of fall therefore depends upon the number of segments involved, being greatest in high spinal anesthesia and practically nonexistent when the effect is confined to the perineal area alone.

   There have been several reports indicating that Nupercaine hydrochloride (dibucaine hydrochloride) has less effect upon blood pressure than does a comparable degree of anesthesia produced by procaine.

   Treatment: The prophylactic use of 25 mg ephedrine given intramuscularly before the anesthetic is injected is advised by many authorities. It may be omitted in low spinals. An additional dose of 25 mg should be given *intravenously* if a fall below 100 mm Hg occurs. This dose may be repeated; total should not exceed 100 mg. Fluids, plasma, or whole blood should be administered intravenously when severe fall of blood pressure occurs. In *obstetrical patients,* raising the legs to the vertical position is the most effective initial procedure to increase blood pressure.

3. **Postanesthetic Headache.** Since this is usually due to leakage of spinal fluid, incidence will decrease as technique improves.
Prophylaxis: A needle of small caliber (not over 20 or 22 gauge) should be used. Some authorities recommend special needles, one of 20 gauge to penetrate the skin and fascia and an inner needle of 24 gauge to pierce the dura. It has also been recommended that the needle be introduced with the bevel held laterally so as to cut fewer fibers of the dura. The needle should remain in place for several seconds after injection to allow time for equalization of pressure.
Treatment: Tight abdominal binder. Hydration of the patient with either oral or intravenous fluids. One ml surgical pituitrin or 100 mg ephedrine. Rapid relief has been reported after intraspinal or caudal injection of 30 ml sterile saline.
4. **Nausea and Vomiting.** These may occur from psychic causes, drop in blood pressure, or intra-abdominal manipulation.
Treatment: When caused by hypotension, inhalations of 100 percent oxygen in conjunction with a vasopressor may be found effective. Light cyclopropane or an intravenous barbiturate will control that which is due to intra-abdominal manipulation.
5. **Palsies.** Transient nerve palsies, usually involving the abducens, have occasionally been reported. This very uncommon complication generally occurs during the second week and clears up by the third or fourth week. Temporary or permanent transverse myelitis may follow the use of spinal anesthetic agents (see *Warnings*).
6. **Meningitis.** An aseptic technique should practically preclude the occurrence of this complication. Aseptic meningitis or meningismus, usually of rapid and benign course, has occurred after spinal anesthesia as it has also in cases where no spinal puncture has been carried out. Lundy has called attention to the fact that meningitides following spinal anesthesia may occur without relation to the method but due to pathologically proved metastases from distant foci. However, even the remote possibility of this complication reinforces the necessity for an absolutely sterile technique.
7. **Drug Idiosyncrasy.** The use of this drug is exceptionally free of this hazard. Patients giving a history of hypersensitivity to drugs, however, should be skin tested (see *Contraindications*).
Treatment: The occurrence of motor excitement requires the anticonvulsant action of an intravenous barbiturate.

Supplied: *Ampuls,* for spinal anesthesia, 20 ml, 1:1500 (method of Howard Jones), each ml containing 0.667 mg dibucaine hydrochloride, 5 mg sodium chloride, and water q.s.; cartons of 12. C76-65 Rev. 9/76

HEAVY SOLUTION NUPERCAINE® hydrochloride (dibucaine hydrochloride) with Dextrose 5% For Spinal Anesthesia ℞

Indications: Heavy Solution Nupercaine hydrochloride is indicated for the production of low spinal anesthesia.

Contraindications: Shock, hypovolemia due to hemorrhage, and severe anemia; septicemia; pernicious anemia with evidence of spinal cord involvement; infection of the skin or subcutaneous tissue at or near the puncture site; tuberculosis or metastatic lesions in the lumbar spine; history of hypersensitivity to dibucaine or related compounds; in obstetrics: abruptio placenta, placenta praevia with significant bleeding, and early stages of labor (see Dosage and Administration); diseases, syndromes, or situations causing increased intra-abdominal pressure, such as ascites, tumors, or advanced pregnancy (unless in preparation for vaginal delivery).

Warnings: Nupercaine hydrochloride is a highly potent agent and therefore is to be used in lower concentration and lower total dosage than certain other local anesthetic drugs.
Pooling of a concentrated solution of Nupercaine hydrochloride or any other anesthetic agent in the conus may cause irreversible nerve damage. Therefore, the patient must not be kept in the sitting position for more than one minute following injection of the drug.
Do not inject Nupercaine during uterine contractions since spinal fluid currents may carry the drug further cephalad than desired.
The possibility of severe bleeding during planned surgery and the facilities available to manage the resulting complications must be considered in the selection of anesthesia.
To avoid intravascular injection, do not administer spinal anesthesia in the presence of blood noted in attempting lumbar puncture. If the fluid does not clear after entering the dural space, repeat lumbar puncture is recommended; use of another interspace should be considered.
Low spinal anesthesia of the type provided by Heavy Nupercaine is not recommended for delivery involving abdominal operation, nor does it provide the uterine relaxation necessary for obstetrical manipulations such as internal podalic version.

Precautions: Spinal anesthesia should not be undertaken unless the anesthesiologist is familiar with techniques of and contraindications to spinal anesthesia, equipped to provide a rigidly aseptic technique, prepared to remain in constant attendance, monitoring patient's condition continuously, and equipped to deal with any complications that may arise.
Impairment of respiration may result from spread of the anesthetic above the desired level; this can be minimized by following the administration techniques described. It can also occur because of medullary hypoxia associated with circulatory collapse incident to severe hypotension, requiring intensive supportive treatment.
Hypotension during spinal anesthesia may be related to a number of factors, most important of which are sudden vasodilation incident to paralysis of sympathetic vasomotor fibers and loss of muscle tone with decrease in venous pressure, venous return, and cardiac output. The degree of hypotension relates to the number of vasoconstrictor fibers blocked, being greater in a higher level of spinal anesthesia. If the operative conditions permit, it may be possible to restore blood pressure to an acceptable level without drugs by repositioning the patient and administering intravenous fluids. In obstetrics, lateral displacement of the uterus to the left may raise the blood pressure by improving venous return to the heart. If a vasopressor is necessary, one having both central and peripheral actions (*eg,* ephedrine) should be administered as needed. Plasma expanders or whole blood may also be required; adequate respiratory exchange must be maintained.
The use of spinal anesthesia in patients with cardiac disease depends upon the practitioner's evaluation of the type and severity of the physiological disturbance weighed against the possible pharmacological changes resulting from the anesthesia, and upon his ability to manage any possible complications.
In the presence of neurological disease (*eg,* meningitis, spinal block, hemorrhage, poliomyelitis, migraine, headache of long duration) or conditions involving the back (*eg,* arthritis, spondylitis, chronic backache), the decision to use spinal anesthesia will depend upon the practitioner's evaluation of the disease process and its possible implications. In these circumstances, the patient may ascribe signs and symptoms of previously existing disease or exacerbations of chronic backache to the spinal anesthetic.
Selection of another form of anesthesia should be considered if the patient is uncooperative, hysterical, or excessively nervous or apprehensive. Use of spinal anesthesia in such cases will depend upon the practitioner's ability to evaluate and to manage the individual situation.

Adverse Reactions
Postanesthetic Headache. This can be minimized by use of small caliber needles (24 to 26 gauge) specially designed to prevent spinal fluid leakage and by keeping patient flat on back, without a pillow, for appropriate period after delivery or operation.
Nausea and Vomiting. These may result from psychic causes, fall in blood pressure, intra-abdominal manipulation, or concomitant medication.
Palsies. Nerve palsies, involving extra-ocular muscles, legs, vesical and anal sphincters, have occasionally been reported. These usually are transient and clear completely, but in rare instances a permanent residual has been reported.
Meningitis, Myelitis. Careful selection of patients, use of strictest aseptic techniques, and scrupulous care to avoid injury to meninges and cord during anesthetic drug injection should prevent infectious and traumatic complications almost entirely. Instances of aseptic meningitis or myelitis have occurred, occasionally with permanent residual and fatal termination. Aseptic meningitis or myelitis also have been reported in rare instances following diagnostic lumbar puncture without spinal anesthesia, following various operations for which spinal anesthesia was not used and spinal tap was done, and following pregnancy and delivery without use of spinal anesthesia or spinal tap.
Meningismus also has been reported, evidently without infection, and usually clears promptly.

Dosage and Administration: Heavy Solution Nupercaine hydrochloride has a specific gravity greater than that of spinal fluid. When introduced into the spinal subarachnoid space, it will gravitate toward the lowest point; with the patient in sitting position, it settles toward the conus.
If injection is made with patient recumbent and the Trendelenburg position is immediately assumed, flow of anesthetic will be cephalad. Extent of upward spread will depend upon rate, force and volume of fluid injected, and length of time the Trendelenburg position is maintained. **Level of anesthesia and extent of involvement must be precisely regulated by careful attention to the various techniques described herein.**
Syringe should be filled with required amount of solution prior to lumbar puncture in order to reduce possibility of dislodgment of needle. Injection is made as rapidly as gentle pressure will permit, with needle held firmly to prevent dislodgment. The latter detail is of utmost importance, because failure to obtain anesthesia after an apparently satisfactory lumbar puncture may be due to dislodgment of needle during injection of solution. Needle should be kept in place for a few seconds after injection to permit equalization of pressure.

Continued on next page

CIBA—Cont.

Directions for amount of solution, rapidity of injection, and positioning of patient following injection must be followed precisely to obtain desired level of anesthesia and to minimize complications.

Inasmuch as Nupercaine hydrochloride is readily precipitated by even the slightest amount of alkali, needles and syringes must be thoroughly rinsed in distilled water prior to autoclaving. As part of the meticulous technique for administration of any spinal anesthetic agent, ampuls should be autoclaved to assure sterility of exterior surface. Heavy Solution Nupercaine hydrochloride can be resterilized once at 121° C for 30 minutes; repeated autoclaving produces progressive lowering of pH and darkening of color, probably from caramelization of the dextrose contained. Any ampul showing discoloration after resterilization must be discarded.

Heavy Solution Nupercaine hydrochloride should be used only in accordance with the following techniques:

Obstetric Analgesia Not Involving Abdominal Operation

Dose: 1 ml Heavy Solution Nupercaine hydrochloride is the amount most frequently used. However, greater duration of anesthesia will result from the use of 2 ml.

Time of Injection: Low spinal anesthesia is not intended to relieve the pains of early labor; these can be controlled adequately by other methods. There is general agreement that the injection should not be made until the cervix is well effaced, the head fixed in the pelvis, and the labor progressing satisfactorily. Parmley and Adriani advise injection after the cervix is 5 to 6 cm dilated and 60 to 80 percent effaced. Injection must not be made during uterine contractions, since currents in the spinal fluid may carry solution cephalad.

Position of Patient at Injection: Sitting with legs over side of bed or delivery table, supported by an attendant. Downward pressure on the head to increase flexion should be avoided.

Injection: Draw Heavy Solution Nupercaine into syringe before lumbar puncture. After introduction of needle into subarachnoid space, make injection to count of 1-and-2-and-3 (approximately 2 to 3 seconds). Keep patient sitting for exactly 30 seconds, then place her flat, with head supported by two pillows, or in Fowler's position of 5 degrees.

Under no circumstances is patient allowed to remain in sitting position for more than one minute after injection of the hyperbaric solution, since pooling in the conus can produce irreversible nerve damage.

Saddle Block Anesthesia in Rectal and Urologic Surgery Not Involving Abdominal Surgery

Position of Patient at Injection: *Sitting.* Under no circumstances should the patient be allowed to remain in the sitting position for longer than one minute after injection of the hyperbaric solution since pooling of the anesthetic in the conus can produce irreversible nerve damage.

Dose: For anesthesia of the perineum, rectum, lower scrotum, and penis, inject 1 ml Heavy Solution Nupercaine hydrochloride and allow the patient to sit upright for only 60 seconds. For anesthesia of fundus of the uterus, dome of the bladder, and other pelvic structures, in addition to the areas previously mentioned, inject 2 ml Heavy Solution Nupercaine hydrochloride and allow patient to sit upright for 0 to 5 seconds.

Position Following Injection: Place patient down immediately at expiration of the required number of seconds, with head supported by two pillows and table placed in Fowler's position at an angle of 5 degrees. After allowing at least 10 minutes for fixation of the anesthetic level, determining by sensory testing (as by pin-prick) that the level has ceased to rise, place patient in desired position for operation.

How Supplied: *Ampuls,* 2 ml, each ampul containing 5 mg Nupercaine hydrochloride (0.25%) and 100 mg dextrose in water; cartons of 10. C72-37 Rev. 5/73

OCUSERT® ℞
(pilocarpine)
Pilo-20/Pilo-40 Ocular Therapeutic System

For full prescribing information, including placement and removal instructions, consult the Physicians' Desk Reference for Ophthalmology.

PERCORTEN® acetate ℞
(desoxycorticosterone acetate pellets NF)
Pellets

Listed in NF, a Medicare designated compendium.

Indications: As partial replacement therapy for primary and secondary adrenocortical insufficiency in Addison's disease and for the treatment of salt-losing adrenogenital syndrome.

Contraindications: Hypersensitivity to desoxycorticosterone acetate; hypertension; congestive heart failure.

Warnings: Mineralocorticoids should be accompanied by adequate glucocorticoid therapy in adrenal insufficiency or the salt-losing form of the adrenogenital syndrome.

Usage in Pregnancy

If it is necessary to give steroids during pregnancy, the newborn infant should be watched closely for signs of hypoadrenalism and appropriate therapy instituted if such signs are present.

Precautions: All patients receiving Percorten should be watched for evidence of intercurrent infection. Should infection occur, appropriate anti-infective therapy should be initiated.

If edema occurs, dietary sodium restriction may be required. Frequent blood electrolyte determinations should be performed; potassium supplementation may be necessary.

Adverse Reactions: Generalized edema; frontal or occipital headaches; hypertension and cardiac enlargement, especially if hypertension was present before the onset of adrenal insufficiency; arthralgia and tendon contractures; extreme weakness of extremities with ascending paralysis secondary to low serum potassium; cardiac arrhythmias; hypersensitivity reactions; rarely, irritation at site of pellet implantation.

Dosage and Administration: Mineralocorticoid therapy may not be necessary if the patient can be controlled with an adequate salt intake and glucocorticoid therapy.

If mineralocorticoid therapy is necessary, dosage must be individualized according to the severity of the disease and the response of the patient and should be accompanied by adequate amounts of glucocorticoid.

Percorten pellets should be implanted only after the optimal daily maintenance dose of Percorten acetate in Oil has been carefully determined. Any attempt to implant a number of pellets not exactly calculated on the basis of the optimal daily maintenance dose by injection may lead to irreparable damage.

For the determination of the ultimate optimal maintenance dose, several weeks are required. It is advisable, therefore, in order to eliminate the possibility of overdosage, that the patient be maintained on Percorten acetate in Oil for at least 2 to 3 months prior to pellet implantation.

Calculation of Pellet Requirement

One pellet is implanted for each 0.5 mg of the daily injected maintenance dose of Percorten acetate in Oil. For example, an addisonian patient whose optimal maintenance requirement is 5 mg Percorten acetate in Oil should receive a maximum of 10 pellets.

Technique of Pellet Implantation

Pellets should be implanted only in a fully equipped operating room. Aseptic precautions and careful hemostasis are primary requirements for successful implantation.

The infrascapular region has been selected as the most suitable site for the implantation. Strict asepsis is observed. The operative field is prepared with iodine and alcohol, and the site of incision is anesthetized. A 2- to 4-cm transverse incision is made a few centimeters below the inferior angle of the scapula. A number of small pockets, according to the number of pellets to be implanted, are prepared in the subcutaneous tissue by blunt dissection, radiating from the incision.

The pellets, which have been removed previously from the vial under sterile conditions and kept close at hand on a sterile towel, are placed in the pockets with forceps. The use of a nasal dilator, introduced into the opening of the pocket, has been found helpful, as it permits the placing of the pellet sufficiently far away from the incision. If the pellet is not placed at least 2 cm away from the incision, the chances are greatly increased that it may be extruded later. No pellet should be extruded spontaneously if implanted aseptically, sufficiently far away from the incision, and if careful hemostasis is observed. It is a matter of technique and experience whether each single pellet pocket should be closed with an individual suture, or whether the skin incision only should be closed with subcuticular sutures of fine black silk. It is possible to insert as many as 15 pellets through a single incision by this technique.

Observation After Implantation

On the average, the pellets last for a period of 8 to 12 months. In case of infection, disease, or other stress, supplementary Percorten acetate in Oil injections may be necessary until the patient has returned to the condition established when the pellets were implanted.

In a few instances, it has been necessary to remove pellets, although the maintenance dose was adequately determined prior to implantation. The occurrence of edema, excessive gain in weight, and rise in blood pressure are signs of overdosage.

Reimplantation of Pellets

The effect of the implanted pellets fades after approximately 8 to 12 months. A gradual decrease in *blood pressure* and *weight,* increased fatigue, and loss of appetite are usually the first indications of this decrease in hormonal supply, and the patient must be carefully watched. It may be necessary to resume daily injections of Percorten acetate in Oil with slowly increasing doses. During a period of from 4 to 6 weeks, it is possible to ascertain anew the maintenance requirement of Percorten acetate in Oil; from this dosage the number of new pellets to be implanted can be calculated. Under no circumstances should pellets be arbitrarily implanted on the basis of the initial assay, as the condition of the patient may have undergone a definite change in hormone requirement during the year.

How Supplied: *Pellets,* each containing approximately 125 mg desoxycorticosterone acetate; cartons of 1. C72-27 Rev. 3/73

PERCORTEN® pivalate ℞
(desoxycorticosterone pivalate)
INTRAMUSCULAR REPOSITORY

Not NF, differs in pH range (5.0-8.5)

Indications: As partial replacement therapy for primary and secondary adrenocortical insufficiency in Addison's disease and for treatment of salt-losing adrenogenital syndrome.

Contraindications: Hypersensitivity to Percorten pivalate suspension or any of its ingredients. Patients with hypertension or cardiac disease.

Warnings: Since Percorten pivalate is potent and long-acting, do not administer more frequently than once per month.

Usage in Pregnancy

The safe use of this drug in pregnant women or during lactation has not been established. Therefore, the benefits must be weighed against the potential hazards.

Precautions: Patients with Addison's disease are more sensitive to the action of the hormone and may exhibit side effects in an exaggerated degree.

Since Percorten pivalate is a potent adrenocortical preparation which may produce side effects, patients should be closely watched. Treatment should be stopped in the event of a significant increase in weight or blood pressure, or the development of edema or cardiac enlargement.

Sodium retention and the loss of potassium are accelerated by a high intake of sodium. Hence, it may be necessary to restrict intake of sodium and increase that of potassium.

Only if absolutely necessary should a glucose tolerance test (particularly intravenous) be performed, as addisonian patients with or without desoxycorticosterone therapy have the tendency to react with severe hypoglycemia within 3 hours.

Adverse Reactions: Like other adrenocortical hormones, Percorten pivalate may cause severe side effects if dosage is too high or prolonged. It may cause increased blood volume, edema, elevation of blood pressure, and enlargement of the heart shadow. In patients with essential hypertension or a tendency toward its development, a marked rise in blood pressure may follow administration of this drug.

Headache, arthralgia, weakness, ascending paralysis, low potassium syndrome, and hypersensitivity may occur.

On rare occasions, irritation at the site of injection has been reported.

Dosage and Administration: In treating Addison's disease, Percorten pivalate should be used only in conjunction with other supplemental measures (*eg*, other hormonal agents, electrolytes, control of infection).

First determine the daily requirement for maintenance therapy with Percorten acetate in Oil. For each mg of Percorten acetate, inject through a 20-gauge needle 1 ml (25 mg) Percorten pivalate suspension intramuscularly into the upper outer quadrant of one or both buttocks.

The average dose is 25 to 100 mg every 4 weeks.

How Supplied: *Multiple-dose Vials,* 4 ml, each ml containing 25 mg desoxycorticosterone pivalate, 10.5 mg methylcellulose, 3 mg sodium carboxymethylcellulose, 1 mg polysorbate 80, and 8 mg sodium chloride with 0.002% thimerosal added as preservative in aqueous suspension; cartons of 1. *For intramuscular use only.*

C73-57 Rev. 5/73

PRISCOLINE® hydrochloride ℞
(tolazoline hydrochloride NF)
Parenteral/Intra-Arterial

Listed in NF, a Medicare designated compendium.

Indications

Based on a review of this drug by the National Academy of Sciences-National Research Council and/or other information, FDA has classified the indications as follows:

"Possibly" effective: Spastic peripheral vascular disorders associated with acrocyanosis, acroparesthesia, arteriosclerosis obliterans, Buerger's disease, causalgia, diabetic arteriosclerosis, gangrene, endarteritis, frostbite (sequelae), post-thrombotic conditions (thrombophlebitis), Raynaud's disease, and scleroderma.

Final classification of the less-than-effective indications requires further investigation.

Contraindications: Priscoline is contraindicated following a cerebrovascular accident; known or suspected coronary artery disease; hypersensitivity to tolazoline.

Warnings: Priscoline stimulates gastric secretion and may activate peptic ulcers. Use cautiously in patients with gastritis or known or suspected peptic ulcer.

In patients with mitral stenosis, parenterally administered Priscoline may produce either a fall or a rise in pulmonary artery pressure and total pulmonary resistance, hence must be used with caution in known or suspected mitral stenosis.

Usage in Pregnancy

The safe use of this drug in pregnant women or during lactation has not been established. Therefore, the benefits must be weighed against the potential hazards.

Precautions: Because of the risks involved, intra-arterial administration should be used only by those thoroughly familiar with the procedure and, preferably, only in the hospital or a clinic facility (see Dosage and Administration).

Adverse Reactions: Although side effects are generally mild and may decrease progressively during continued therapy, cardiac arrhythmias, anginal pain, and marked hypertension have been reported. Exacerbations of peptic ulcer have also occurred.

Other side effects include nausea, vomiting, diarrhea, epigastric discomfort, tachycardia, flushing, slight rise or fall in blood pressure, increased pilomotor activity with tingling or chilliness, rash and edema.

Thrombocytopenia, leukopenia, psychiatric reactions characterized by confusion or hallucinations, hepatitis, oliguria and hematuria have been reported rarely.

Intra-arterial administration, in addition to the above, may also produce a feeling of warmth or a "burning sensation" in the injected extremity, transient weakness, transient postural vertigo, palpitations, formication, and apprehension. Rarely, a paradoxical response (further decrease in an already impaired blood supply) may occur in a seriously damaged limb with incipient or established gangrene. This usually disappears with continued treatment and may usually be prevented by prior administration of histamine.

Dosage and Administration: Dosage should be individualized according to the condition being treated and the response of the patient.

Subcutaneous, Intramuscular, or *Intravenous:* 10 to 50 mg 4 times daily. Start with low doses, increasing with patient under close observation until optimal dosage (as determined by appearance of flushing) is established. Keeping patient warm will often increase effectiveness of drug.

Intra-arterial: This approach should not be used except in carefully selected cases and only after it has been determined that maximal benefit has been achieved with oral and/or parenteral administration.

Caution: Because of the risks involved, and because of the special technique and strict aseptic precautions required with intra-arterial injection, this approach should be used only by those thoroughly familiar with the procedure and, preferably, only in the hospital or a clinic facility.

Initially, 25 mg (1 ml) is given slowly as a test dose to determine the response. Subsequently, the average single dose may be 50 to 75 mg (2 to 3 ml) per injection, depending on the observed response.

One or 2 injections daily are usually required initially to achieve maximum response. For maintenance, 2 or 3 injections weekly may be enough to sustain improved circulation, but more may be needed. Oral Priscoline may also be given to help maintain vasodilatation between intra-arterial injections.

Overdosage

Signs and Symptoms: Increased pilomotor activity, peripheral vasodilatation and skin flushing, and, in rare instances, hypotension to shock levels.

Treatment: In treating hypotension, placement of the patient in the head-low position and the administration of intravenous fluids is most important. If a vasopressor is necessary, one having both central and peripheral action (*eg*, ephedrine) may be administered as needed. Do not use epinephrine or norepinephrine, since large doses of Priscoline may cause "epinephrine reversal" (further reduction in blood pressure followed by an exaggerated rebound).

How Supplied: *Multiple-dose Vials,* 10 ml, each ml containing 25 mg tolazoline hydrochloride, 0.65% sodium citrate, 0.65% tartaric acid, and 0.5% chlorobutanol as preservative in water; cartons of 1. C78-21 Rev. 9/78

PRIVINE®
0.05% Nasal Solution
0.05% Nasal Spray

Caution: Do not use Privine if you have glaucoma. Privine is an effective nasal decongestant when you use it in the recommended dosage. If you use too much, too long, or too often, Privine may be harmful to your nasal mucous membranes and cause burning, stinging, sneezing or an increased runny nose.

Do not use Privine by mouth.

Keep this and all medications out of the reach of children. Do not use Privine with children under 6 years of age, except with the advice and supervision of a doctor.

OVERDOSAGE IN YOUNG CHILDREN MAY CAUSE MARKED SEDATION AND IF SEVERE, EMERGENCY TREATMENT MAY BE NECESSARY.

IF NASAL STUFFINESS PERSISTS AFTER 3 DAYS OF TREATMENT, DISCONTINUE USE AND CONSULT A DOCTOR.

Privine is a nasal decongestant that comes in two forms: Nasal Solution (in a bottle with a dropper) and Nasal Spray (in a plastic squeeze bottle). Both are for prompt, and prolonged relief of nasal congestion due to common colds, sinusitis, hay fever, etc.

How to use Nasal Solution: Squeeze rubber bulb to fill dropper with proper amount of medication. For best results, tilt head as far back as possible and put two drops of solution into your right nostril. Then lean head forward, inhaling and turning your head to the left. Refill dropper by squeezing bulb. Now tilt head as far back as possible and put two drops of solution into your left nostril. Then lean head forward, inhaling, and turning your head to the right. Use only 2 drops in each nostril. Do not repeat this dosage more than every 3 hours.

The Privine dropper bottle is designed to make administration of the proper dosage easy and to prevent accidental overdosage. Privine will not cause sleeplessness, so you may use it before going to bed.

Important: After use, be sure to rinse the dropper with very hot water. This helps prevent contamination of the bottle with bacteria from nasal secretions. Use of the dispenser by more than one person may spread infection.

Note: Privine Nasal Solution may be used on contact with glass, plastic, stainless steel and specially treated metals used in atomizers. Do not let the solution come in contact with reactive metals, especially aluminum. If solution becomes discolored, it should be discarded.

How to use Nasal Spray: For best results do not shake the plastic squeeze bottle.

Remove cap. With head held upright, spray twice into each nostril. Squeeze the bottle

Continued on next page

CIBA—Cont.

sharply and firmly while sniffing through the nose.
For best results use every 4 to 6 hours. Do not use more often than every 3 hours.
Avoid overdosage. Follow directions for use carefully.
Privine Nasal Solution contains 0.05% naphazoline hydrochloride USP with benzalkonium chloride as a preservative. Available in bottles of .66 fl. oz. (20 ml) with dropper, and bottles of 16 fl. oz. (473 ml). Privine Nasal Spray contains 0.05% naphazoline hydrochloride USP with benzalkonium chloride as a preservative. Available in plastic squeeze bottles of ½ fl. oz. (15 ml).

C80-5 (1/80)

REGITINE®
(phentolamine) ℞

Listed in USP and *NF, Medicare designated compendia.*

Indications

Oral and Parenteral Regitine
Prevention or control of hypertensive episodes that may occur in a patient with pheochromocytoma as a result of stress or manipulation during preoperative preparation and surgical excision.

Parenteral Regitine
Prevention and treatment of dermal necrosis and sloughing following intravenous administration or extravasation of norepinephrine.
Diagnosis of pheochromocytoma—Regitine blocking test.

Contraindications: Myocardial infarction, history of myocardial infarction, coronary insufficiency, angina or other evidence suggestive of coronary artery disease. Hypersensitivity to phentolamine or related compounds.

Warnings: Myocardial infarction, cerebrovascular spasm, and cerebrovascular occlusion have been reported to occur following the administration of phentolamine, usually in association with marked hypotensive episodes with shock-like states which occasionally follow parenteral administration.
For screening tests in patients with hypertension, the generally available urinary assay of catecholamines or other biochemical assays have largely supplanted the Regitine and other pharmacological tests for reasons of accuracy and safety. None of the chemical or pharmacological tests is infallible in the diagnosis of pheochromocytoma. The Regitine test is not the procedure of choice and should be reserved for cases in which additional confirmatory evidence is necessary, and the relative risks involved in conducting the test have been considered.

Usage in Pregnancy: The safe use of this drug in pregnant women or during lactation has not been established. Therefore, the benefits must be weighed against the potential hazards.

Precautions: Tachycardia and cardiac arrhythmias may occur with the use of Regitine or other alpha adrenergic blocking agents. When possible, defer administration of cardiac glycosides until cardiac rhythm returns to normal.

Adverse Reactions: Acute and prolonged hypotensive episodes, tachycardia, and cardiac arrhythmias have been reported, most frequently after parenteral administration. In addition, weakness, dizziness, flushing, orthostatic hypotension, nasal stuffiness, nausea, vomiting, and diarrhea may occur.

Dosage and Administration

1. Prevention or control of hypertensive episodes in the patient with pheochromocytoma.
To control and prevent paroxysmal attacks prior to surgery, the usual adult dosage is 50 mg (1 tablet) of Regitine hydrochloride orally 4 to 6 times daily. In certain severe cases, higher doses may be required. In children, smaller doses generally suffice; 25 mg (½ tablet) orally 4 to 6 times daily is suggested initially.
For use in preoperative reduction of elevated blood pressure, inject 5 mg of Regitine mesylate (1 mg for children) intravenously or intramuscularly 1 or 2 hours before surgery (and repeat if necessary).
During surgery administer Regitine mesylate (5 mg for adults, 1 mg for children) intravenously as indicated to help prevent or control paroxysms of hypertension, tachycardia, respiratory depression, convulsions, or other effects of epinephrine intoxication. (Postoperatively, norepinephrine may be given to control the hypotension which commonly follows complete removal of a pheochromocytoma.)

2. Prevention and treatment of dermal necrosis and sloughing following intravenous administration or extravasation of norepinephrine.
For prevention, add 10 mg Regitine mesylate to each liter of solution containing norepinephrine. The pressor effect of norepinephrine is not affected.
For treatment, inject Regitine mesylate (5 to 10 mg in 10 ml saline) into the area of extravasation within 12 hours.

3. Diagnosis of pheochromocytoma—Regitine blocking test.

a. **Intravenous**
Preparation.
Review the *Contraindications, Warnings,* and *Precautions.* Withhold sedatives, analgesics, and all other medication not deemed essential (such as digitalis and insulin) for at least 24 hours (preferably 48 to 72 hours) prior to the test. Withhold antihypertensive drugs until blood pressure returns to the untreated, hypertensive level. Do not perform test on a patient who is normotensive.
Procedure.
1. Keep patient at rest in the supine position throughout the test, preferably in a quiet, darkened room. Delay Regitine injection until blood pressure is stabilized, as evidenced by blood pressure readings taken every 10 minutes for at least one-half hour.
2. Dissolve 5 mg Regitine mesylate in 1 ml Sterile Water for Injection. Dose for adults is 5 mg; for children, 1 mg.
3. Insert the syringe needle into vein, delay injection until pressor response to venipuncture has subsided.
4. Inject Regitine rapidly. Record blood pressure immediately after injection, at 30-second intervals for the first 3 minutes, and at 60-second intervals for the next 7 minutes.

Interpreting the Test
Positive response, suggestive of pheochromocytoma, is indicated by a drop in blood pressure of more than 35 mm Hg systolic and 25 mm Hg diastolic pressure. A typical positive response may be a drop of 60 mm Hg systolic and 25 mm Hg diastolic. Maximal depressor pressure effect usually is evident within 2 minutes after injection. Return to pre-injection pressure commonly occurs within 15 to 30 minutes, but may return more rapidly.
If blood pressure falls to a dangerous level, treat patient as outlined under "Overdosage."
A positive response should always be confirmed by other diagnostic procedures, preferably the measurement of urinary catecholamines or their metabolites.
Negative response is indicated when the blood pressure is unchanged, elevated, or is reduced less than 35 mm Hg systolic and 25 mm Hg diastolic after injection of Regitine. A negative response to this test does not exclude the diagnosis of pheochromocytoma, especially in patients with paroxysmal hypertension in whom the incidence of false negative responses is high.

b. **Intramuscular**
If the intramuscular test for pheochromocytoma is preferred, preparation is the same as for the intravenous test. Then dissolve 5 mg Regitine mesylate in 1 ml Sterile Water for Injection. Dose for adults is 5 mg intramuscularly; for children, 3 mg. Record blood pressure every 5 minutes for 30 to 45 minutes following intramuscular injection. Positive response is indicated by a drop in blood pressure of 35 mm Hg systolic and 25 mm Hg diastolic or greater within 20 minutes following injection.

c. **Reliability**
The test is most reliable in detecting pheochromocytoma in patients with sustained hypertension, and least reliable in those with paroxysmal hypertension. False positive tests may occur in patients with hypertension without pheochromocytoma.

Overdosage: In the event of a drop in blood pressure to dangerous level or other evidence of shock-like conditions, treat vigorously and promptly. Include intravenous infusion of norepinephrine, titrated to maintain blood pressure to normotensive level, and all available supportive measures. Do not use epinephrine since it may cause a paradoxical fall in blood pressure.

How Supplied
Vials, each containing 5 mg phentolamine mesylate USP and 25 mg mannitol in lyophilized form and accompanied by ampul containing 1 ml Sterile Water for Injection; cartons of 1.
The reconstituted solution should be used upon preparation and should not be stored.
Tablets (white, scored), each containing 50 mg phentolamine hydrochloride NF; bottles of 100. C76-56 Rev. 1/76

[*Shown in Product Identification Section*]

RIMACTANE®
(rifampin USP) ℞

Indications

Pulmonary Tuberculosis
In the initial treatment and in the re-treatment of pulmonary tuberculosis, Rimactane must be used in conjunction with at least one other antituberculous drug.
Frequently used regimens have been the following:
isoniazid and Rimactane
ethambutol and Rimactane
isoniazid, ethambutol, and Rimactane

Neisseria Meningitidis Carriers
Rimactane is indicated for the treatment of asymptomatic carriers of *N. meningitidis* to eliminate meningococci from the nasopharynx.
Rimactane is not indicated for the treatment of meningococcal infection.
To avoid the indiscriminate use of Rimactane, diagnostic laboratory procedures, including serotyping and susceptibility testing, should be performed to establish the carrier state and the correct treatment. In order to preserve the usefulness of Rimactane in the treatment of asymptomatic meningococcal carriers, it is recommended that the drug be reserved for situations in which the risk of meningococcal meningitis is high.
Both in the treatment of tuberculosis and in the treatment of meningococcal carriers, small numbers of resistant cells, present within large populations of susceptible cells, can rapidly become the predominating type. Since rapid emergence of resistance can occur, culture and susceptibility tests should be performed in the event of persistent positive cultures.

Contraindications: A history of previous hypersensitivity reaction to any of the rifamycins.

Warnings: Rifampin has been shown to produce liver dysfunction. There have been fatalities associated with jaundice in patients with liver disease or receiving rifampin concomi-

tantly with other hepatotoxic agents. Since an increased risk may exist for individuals with liver disease, benefits must be weighed carefully against the risk of further liver damage. Periodic liver function monitoring is mandatory.
The possibility of rapid emergence of resistant meningococci restricts the use of Rimactane to short-term treatment of the asymptomatic carrier state. Rimactane is not to be used for the treatment of meningococcal disease.
Several studies of tumorigenicity potential have been done in rodents. In one strain of mice known to be particularly susceptible to the spontaneous development of hepatomas, rifampin given at a level 2–10 times the maximum dosage used clinically, resulted in a significant increase in the occurrence of hepatomas in female mice of this strain after one year of administration. There was no evidence of tumorigenicity in the males of this strain, in males or females of another mouse strain, or rats.
Usage in Pregnancy: Although rifampin has been reported to cross the placental barrier and appear in cord blood, the effect of Rimactane, alone or in combination with other antituberculous drugs, on the human fetus is not known. An increase in congenital malformations, primarily spina bifida and cleft palate, has been reported in the offspring of rodents given oral doses of 150-250 mg/kg/day of rifampin during pregnancy.
The possible teratogenic potential in women capable of bearing children should be carefully weighed against the benefits of therapy.
Precautions: Rimactane is not recommended for intermittent therapy; the patient should be cautioned against intentional or accidental interruption of the daily dosage regimen since rare renal hypersensitivity reactions have been reported when therapy was resumed in such cases.
Rifampin has been observed to increase the requirements for anticoagulant drugs of the coumarin type. The cause of this phenomenon is unknown. In patients receiving anticoagulants and rifampin concurrently, it is recommended that the prothrombin time be performed daily or as frequently as necessary to establish and maintain the required dose of anticoagulant.
Urine, feces, saliva, sputum, sweat, and tears may be colored red-orange by Rimactane and its metabolites. Individuals to be treated should be made aware of these possibilities in order to prevent undue anxiety.
It has been reported that the reliability of oral contraceptives may be affected in some patients being treated for tuberculosis with rifampin in combination with at least one other antituberculous drug. In such cases, alternative contraceptive measures may need to be considered.
Rifampin has been reported to diminish the effects of concurrently administered methadone, oral hypoglycemics, corticosteroids, dapsone, and digitalis preparations; appropriate dosage adjustments may be necessary if indicated by the patient's clinical condition.
Therapeutic levels of rifampin have been shown to inhibit standard assays for serum folate and vitamin B_{12}. Alternative methods must be considered when determining folate and vitamin B_{12} concentrations in the presence of rifampin.
Since rifampin has been reported to cross the placental barrier and appear in cord blood, neonates of rifampin-treated mothers should be carefully observed for any evidence of adverse effects.
Adverse Reactions: Gastrointestinal disturbances such as heartburn, epigastric distress, anorexia, nausea, vomiting, gas, cramps, and diarrhea have been noted in some patients. Headache, drowsiness, fatigue, ataxia, dizziness, inability to concentrate, mental confusion, visual disturbances, muscular weakness, fever, pains in extremities, generalized numbness, and menstrual disturbances have also been noted.
Hypersensitivity reactions have been reported. Encountered occasionally have been pruritus, urticaria, rash, pemphigoid reaction, eosinophilia, sore mouth, sore tongue, and exudative conjunctivitis. Rarely, hepatitis or a shocklike syndrome with hepatic involvement and abnormal liver function tests have been reported. Transient abnormalities in liver function tests (*eg* elevations in serum bilirubin, BSP, alkaline phosphatase, serum transaminases) have also been observed.
Thrombocytopenia, transient leukopenia, hemolytic anemia, and decreased hemoglobin have been observed. Thrombocytopenia has occurred when rifampin and ethambutol were administered concomitantly according to an intermittent dose schedule twice weekly and in high doses.
Elevations in BUN and serum uric acid have occurred. Rarely, hemolysis, hemoglobinuria, hematuria, renal insufficiency or acute renal failure have been reported and are generally considered to be hypersensitivity reactions. These have usually occurred during intermittent therapy or when treatment was resumed following intentional or accidental interruption of a daily dosage regimen and were reversible when rifampin was discontinued and appropriate therapy instituted.
Although rifampin has been reported to have an immunosuppressive effect in some animal experiments, available human data indicate that this has no clinical significance.
Dosage and Administration: It is recommended that Rimactane be administered once daily, either one hour before or two hours after a meal.
Data is not available for determination of dosage for children under 5.

Pulmonary Tuberculosis
Adults: 600 mg (two 300-mg Capsules) in a single daily administration.
Children: 10 to 20 mg/kg, not to exceed 600 mg/day.
In the treatment of pulmonary tuberculosis, Rimactane must be used in conjunction with at least one other antituberculous agent. In general, therapy should be continued until bacterial conversion and maximal improvement have occurred.

Meningococcal Carriers
It is recommended that Rimactane be administered once daily for four consecutive days in the following doses:
Adults: 600 mg (two 300-mg Capsules) in a single daily administration.
Children: 10 to 20 mg/kg, not to exceed 600 mg/day.

Susceptibility Testing
Pulmonary Tuberculosis: Rifampin susceptibility powders are available for both direct and indirect methods of determining the susceptibility of strains of mycobacteria. The MIC's of susceptible clinical isolates when determined in 7H10 or other non-egg-containing media have ranged from 0.1 to 2 mcg/ml.
Meningococcal Carriers: Susceptibility discs containing 5 mcg rifampin are available for susceptibility testing of *N. meningitidis.*
Quantitative methods that require measurement of zone diameters give the most precise estimates of antibiotic susceptibility. One such procedure[1] has been recommended for use with discs for testing susceptibility to rifampin. Interpretations correlate zone diameters from the disc test with MIC (minimal inhibitory concentration) values for rifampin. A range of MIC's from 0.1 to 1 mcg/ml has been found *in vitro* for susceptible strains of *N. meningitidis.* With this procedure, a report from the laboratory of "resistant" indicates that the organism is not likely to be eradicated from the nasopharynx of asymptomatic carriers.
How Supplied: *Capsules,* 300 mg (opaque scarlet and caramel); bottles of 30, 60, 100, and 500.
Also available, Rimactane®/INH (isoniazid USP) Dual Pack containing 60 Rimactane Capsules and 30 INH 300-mg Tablets.

Reference:
1. Bauer, A. W., Kirby, W. M. M., Sherris, J. C., and Turck, M. Antibiotic susceptibility testing by a standardized single disk method. Am. J. Clin. Path. 45:493-496, 1966.

C78-7 Rev. 3/78

[*Shown in Product Identification Section*]

RITALIN® hydrochloride Ⓒ
(methylphenidate hydrochloride USP)
Tablets

Listed in USP, a Medicare designated compendium.

Indications
Based on a review of this drug by the National Academy of Sciences-National Research Council and/or other information, FDA has classified the indications as follows:
Effective: Attention Deficit Disorders (previously known as Minimal Brain Dysfunction in Children). Other terms being used to describe the behavioral syndrome below include: Hyperkinetic Child Syndrome, Minimal Brain Damage, Minimal Cerebral Dysfunction, Minor Cerebral Dysfunction.
Ritalin is indicated as an integral part of a total treatment program which typically includes other remedial measures (psychological, educational, social) for a stabilizing effect in children with a behavioral syndrome characterized by the following group of developmentally inappropriate symptoms: moderate-to-severe distractibility, short attention span, hyperactivity, emotional lability, and impulsivity. The diagnosis of this syndrome should not be made with finality when these symptoms are only of comparatively recent origin. Nonlocalizing (soft) neurological signs, learning disability, and abnormal EEG may or may not be present, and a diagnosis of central nervous system dysfunction may or may not be warranted.
Special Diagnostic Considerations
Specific etiology of this syndrome is unknown, and there is no single diagnostic test. Adequate diagnosis requires the use not only of medical but of special psychological, educational, and social resources. Characteristics commonly reported include: chronic history of short attention span, distractibility, emotional lability, impulsivity, and moderate to severe hyperactivity; minor neurological signs and abnormal EEG. Learning may or may not be impaired. The diagnosis must be based upon a complete history and evaluation of the child and not solely on the presence of one or more of these characteristics.
Drug treatment is not indicated for all children with this syndrome. Stimulants are not intended for use in the child who exhibits symptoms secondary to environmental factors and/or primary psychiatric disorders, including psychosis. Appropriate educational placement is essential and psychosocial intervention is generally necessary. When remedial measures alone are insufficient, the decision to prescribe stimulant medication will depend upon the physician's assessment of the chronicity and severity of the child's symptoms.
Effective: Narcolepsy
"Possibly" effective: Mild depression; Apathetic or Withdrawn Senile Behavior.

Continued on next page

CIBA—Cont.

> Final classification of the less-than-effective indications requires further investigation.

Contraindications: Marked anxiety, tension, and agitation are contraindications to Ritalin, since the drug may aggravate these symptoms. Ritalin is contraindicated also in patients known to be hypersensitive to the drug and in patients with glaucoma.

Warnings: Ritalin should not be used in children under six years, since safety and efficacy in this age group have not been established.

Sufficient data on safety and efficacy of long-term use of Ritalin in children are not yet available. Although a causal relationship has not been established, suppression of growth (*ie,* weight gain and/or height) has been reported with the long-term use of stimulants in children. Therefore, patients requiring long-term therapy should be carefully monitored.

Ritalin should not be used for severe depression of either exogenous or endogenous origin. Clinical experience suggests that in psychotic children, administration of Ritalin may exacerbate symptoms of behavior disturbance and thought disorder.

Ritalin should not be used for the prevention or treatment of normal fatigue states.

There is some clinical evidence that Ritalin may lower the convulsive threshold in patients with prior history of seizures, with prior EEG abnormalities in absence of seizures, and, very rarely, in absence of history of seizures and no prior EEG evidence of seizures. Safe concomitant use of anticonvulsants and Ritalin has not been established. In the presence of seizures, the drug should be discontinued.

Use cautiously in patients with hypertension. Blood pressure should be monitored at appropriate intervals in all patients taking Ritalin, especially those with hypertension.

Symptoms of visual disturbances have been encountered in rare cases. Difficulties with accommodation and blurring of vision have been reported.

Drug Interactions

Ritalin may decrease the hypotensive effect of guanethidine. Use cautiously with pressor agents and MAO inhibitors.

Human pharmacologic studies have shown that Ritalin may inhibit the metabolism of coumarin anticoagulants, anticonvulsants (phenobarbital, diphenylhydantoin, primidone), phenylbutazone, and tricyclic antidepressants (imipramine, desipramine). Downward dosage adjustments of these drugs may be required when given concomitantly with Ritalin.

Usage in Pregnancy

Adequate animal reproduction studies to establish safe use of Ritalin during pregnancy have not been conducted. Therefore, until more information is available, Ritalin should not be prescribed for women of childbearing age unless, in the opinion of the physician, the potential benefits outweigh the possible risks.

> **Drug Dependence**
> Ritalin should be given cautiously to emotionally unstable patients, such as those with a history of drug dependence or alcoholism, because such patients may increase dosage on their own initiative.
> Chronically abusive use can lead to marked tolerance and psychic dependence with varying degrees of abnormal behavior. Frank psychotic episodes can occur, especially with parenteral abuse. Careful supervision is required during drug withdrawal, since severe depression as well as the effects of chronic overactivity can be unmasked. Long-term follow-up may be required because of the patient's basic personality disturbances.

Precautions: Patients with an element of agitation may react adversely; discontinue therapy if necessary.

Periodic CBC, differential, and platelet counts are advised during prolonged therapy.

Drug treatment is not indicated in all cases of this behavioral syndrome and should be considered only in light of the complete history and evaluation of the child. The decision to prescribe Ritalin should depend on the physician's assessment of the chronicity and severity of the child's symptoms and their appropriateness for his/her age. Prescription should not depend solely on the presence of one or more of the behavioral characteristics.

When these symptoms are associated with acute stress reactions, treatment with Ritalin is usually not indicated.

Long-term effects of Ritalin in children have not been well established.

The Ritalin tablets (5 and 20 mg) contain FD&C Yellow No. 5 (tartrazine) which may cause allergic-type reactions (including bronchial asthma) in certain susceptible individuals. Although the overall incidence of FD&C Yellow No. 5 (tartrazine) sensitivity in the general population is low, it is frequently seen in patients who also have aspirin hypersensitivity.

Adverse Reactions: Nervousness and insomnia are the most common adverse reactions but are usually controlled by reducing dosage and omitting the drug in the afternoon or evening. Other reactions include hypersensitivity (including skin rash, urticaria, fever, arthralgia, exfoliative dermatitis, erythema multiforme with histopathological findings of necrotizing vasculitis, and thrombocytopenic purpura); anorexia; nausea; dizziness; palpitations; headache; dyskinesia; drowsiness; blood pressure and pulse changes, both up and down; tachycardia; angina; cardiac arrhythmia; abdominal pain; weight loss during prolonged therapy. Toxic psychosis has been reported. Although a definite causal relationship has not been established, the following have been reported in patients taking this drug: leukopenia and/or anemia; a few instances of scalp hair loss.

In children, loss of appetite, abdominal pain, weight loss during prolonged therapy, insomnia, and tachycardia may occur more frequently; however, any of the other adverse reactions listed above may also occur.

Dosage and Administration

Adults

Administer orally in divided doses 2 or 3 times daily, preferably 30 to 45 minutes before meals. Dosage will depend upon indication and individual response.

Average dosage is 20 to 30 mg daily. Some patients may require 40 to 60 mg daily. In others, 10 to 15 mg daily will be adequate. Patients who are unable to sleep if medication is taken late in the day should take the last dose before 6 p.m.

Children (6 years and over)

Start with small doses (*eg,* 5 mg before breakfast and lunch) with gradual increments of 5 to 10 mg weekly. Daily dosage above 60 mg is not recommended. If improvement is not observed after appropriate dosage adjustment over a one-month period, the drug should be discontinued.

If paradoxical aggravation of symptoms or other adverse effects occur, reduce dosage, or, if necessary, discontinue the drug.

Where possible, drug administration should be interrupted occasionally to determine if there is a recurrence of behavioral symptoms sufficient to require continued therapy. Improvement may be sustained when the drug is either temporarily or permanently discontinued.

Drug treatment should not and need not be indefinite and usually may be discontinued after puberty.

Overdosage: Signs and symptoms of acute overdosage, resulting principally from overstimulation of the central nervous system and from excessive sympathomimetic effects, may include the following: vomiting, agitation, tremors, hyperreflexia, muscle twitching, convulsions (may be followed by coma), euphoria, confusion, hallucinations, delirium, sweating, flushing, headache, hyperpyrexia, tachycardia, palpitations, cardiac arrhythmias, hypertension, mydriasis, and dryness of mucous membranes.

Treatment consists of appropriate supportive measures. The patient must be protected against self-injury and against external stimuli that would aggravate overstimulation already present. If signs and symptoms are not too severe and the patient is conscious, gastric contents may be evacuated by induction of emesis or gastric lavage. In the presence of severe intoxication, use a carefully titrated dosage of a *short-acting* barbiturate *before* performing gastric lavage.

Intensive care must be provided to maintain adequate circulation and respiratory exchange; external cooling procedures may be required for hyperpyrexia.

Efficacy of peritoneal dialysis or extracorporeal hemodialysis for Ritalin overdosage has not been established.

How Supplied: *Tablets,* 20 mg (peach, scored); bottles of 100 and 1000. *Tablets,* 10 mg (pale green, scored); bottles of 100, 500, 1000 and Accu-Pak® blister units of 100. *Tablets,* 5 mg (pale yellow); bottles of 100, 500 and 1000.

Dispense in tight, light-resistant container.

C80-14 (1/80)

Military—1000's, 10 mg, Stock #6505-00-584-3179.

VA—1000's, 10 mg, Stock #6505-00-584-3179A; 1000's, 20 mg, Stock #6505-00-584-3181A.

[*Shown in Product Identification Section*]

SER-AP-ES® ℞

reserpine 0.1 mg
hydralazine hydrochloride 25 mg
hydrochlorothiazide 15 mg
Combination Tablets

> **Warning**
> This fixed combination drug is not indicated for initial therapy of hypertension. Hypertension requires therapy titrated to the individual patient. If the fixed combination represents the dosage so determined, its use may be more convenient in patient management. The treatment of hypertension is not static, but must be reevaluated as conditions in each patient warrant.

Indications

Hypertension. (See box warning.)

Contraindications

Reserpine

Known hypersensitivity, mental depression (especially with suicidal tendencies), active peptic ulcer, ulcerative colitis, and patients receiving electroconvulsive therapy.

Hydralazine

Hypersensitivity to hydralazine; coronary artery disease; and mitral valvular rheumatic heart disease.

Hydrochlorothiazide

Anuria; hypersensitivity to this or other sulfonamide-derived drugs.

Warnings

Reserpine

Extreme caution should be exercised in treating patients with a history of mental depression. Discontinue the drug at first sign of despondency, early morning insomnia, loss of appetite, impotence, or self-deprecation. Drug-induced depression may persist for several months after drug withdrawal and may be severe enough to result in suicide.

MAO inhibitors should be avoided or used with extreme caution.

Hydralazine

Hydralazine may produce in a few patients a clinical picture simulating systemic lupus erythematosus. In such patients hydralazine should be discontinued unless the benefit-to-risk determination requires continued antihypertensive therapy with this drug. Symptoms and signs usually regress when the drug is discontinued but residua have been detected many years later. Long-term treatment with steroids may be necessary.

Complete blood counts, L. E. cell preparations, and antinuclear antibody titer determinations are indicated before and periodically during prolonged therapy with hydralazine, even though the patient is asymptomatic. These studies are also indicated if the patient develops arthralgia, fever, chest pain, continued malaise or other unexplained signs or symptoms.

A positive antinuclear antibody titer and/or positive L. E. cell reaction requires that the physician carefully weigh the implications of the test results against the benefits to be derived from antihypertensive therapy with hydralazine.

Use MAO inhibitors with caution in patients receiving hydralazine.

When other potent parenteral antihypertensive drugs, such as diazoxide, are used in combination with hydralazine, patients should be continuously observed for several hours for any excessive fall in blood presssure. Profound hypotensive episodes may occur when diazoxide injection and hydralazine are used concomitantly.

Hydrochlorothiazide

Use with caution in severe renal disease. In patients with renal disease, thiazides may precipitate azotemia. Cumulative effects of the drug may develop in patients with impaired renal function.

Thiazides should be used with caution in patients with impaired hepatic function or progressive liver disease, since minor alterations of fluid and electrolyte imbalance may precipitate hepatic coma.

Thiazides may add to or potentiate the action of other antihypertensive drugs. Potentiation occurs with ganglionic or peripheral adrenergic blocking drugs.

Sensitivity reactions are more likely to occur in patients with a history of allergy or bronchial asthma.

The possibility of exacerbation or activation of systemic lupus erythematosus has been reported.

Usage in Pregnancy

Reserpine

The safety of reserpine for use during pregnancy or lactation has not been established; therefore, the drug should be used in pregnant patients or in women of childbearing potential only when, in the judgment of the physician, it is essential to the welfare of the patient. Increased respiratory tract secretions, nasal congestion, cyanosis, and anorexia may occur in neonates and breast-fed infants of reserpine-treated mothers since reserpine crosses the placental barrier and appears in maternal breast milk.

Hydralazine

Animal studies indicate that hydralazine is teratogenic in mice, possibly in rabbits, and not in rats. Teratogenic effects observed were cleft palate and malformations of facial and cranial bones. Although clinical experience does not include any positive evidence of adverse effects on the human fetus, hydralazine should not be used during pregnancy unless the expected benefit clearly justifies the potential risk to the fetus.

Hydrochlorothiazide

Thiazides cross the placental barrier and appear in cord blood. The use of thiazides in pregnant women requires that the anticipated benefit be weighed against possible hazards to the fetus. These hazards include fetal or neonatal jaundice, thrombocytopenia, and possibly other adverse reactions which have occurred in the adult.

Nursing Mothers: Thiazides appear in breast milk. If the use of the drug is deemed essential, the patient should stop nursing.

Precautions

Reserpine

Since reserpine increases gastrointestinal motility and secretion, it should be used cautiously in patients with a history of peptic ulcer, ulcerative colitis, or gallstones (biliary colic may be precipitated).

Caution should be exercised when treating hypertensive patients with renal insufficiency since they adjust poorly to lowered blood pressure levels.

Use reserpine cautiously with digitalis and quinidine, since cardiac arrhythmias have occurred with rauwolfia preparations.

Preoperative withdrawal of reserpine does not assure that circulatory instability will not occur. It is important that the anesthesiologist be aware of the patient's drug intake and consider this in the overall management, since hypotension has occurred in patients receiving rauwolfia preparations. Anticholinergic and/or adrenergic drugs (*eg,* metaraminol, norepinephrine) have been employed to treat adverse vagocirculatory effects.

Hydralazine

Myocardial stimulation produced by hydralazine can cause anginal attacks and ECG changes of myocardial ischemia. The drug has been implicated in the production of myocardial infarction. It must, therefore, be used with caution in patients with suspected coronary artery disease.

The "hyperdynamic" circulation caused by hydralazine may accentuate specific cardiovascular inadequacies. An example is that hydralazine may increase pulmonary artery pressure in patients with mitral valvular disease. The drug may reduce the pressor responses to epinephrine. Postural hypotension may result from hydralazine but is less common than with ganglionic blocking agents. Use with caution in patients with cerebral vascular accidents.

In hypertensive patients with normal kidneys who are treated with hydralazine, there is evidence of increased renal blood flow and a maintenance of glomerular filtration rate. In some instances improved renal function has been noted where control values were below normal prior to hydralazine administration. However, as with any antihypertensive agent, hydralazine should be used with caution in patients with advanced renal damage.

Peripheral neuritis, evidenced by paresthesias, numbness, and tingling, has been observed. Published evidence suggests an antipyridoxine effect and the addition of pyridoxine to the regimen if symptoms develop.

Blood dyscrasias, consisting of reduction in hemoglobin and red cell count, leukopenia, agranulocytosis, and purpura, have been reported. If such abnormalities develop, discontinue therapy. Periodic blood counts are advised during prolonged therapy.

Hydrochlorothiazide

Periodic determination of serum electrolytes to detect possible electrolyte imbalance should be performed at appropriate intervals. All patients receiving thiazide therapy should be observed for clinical signs of fluid or electrolyte imbalance; namely, hyponatremia, hypochloremic alkalosis, and hypokalemia. Serum and urine electrolyte determinations are particularly important when the patient is vomiting excessively or receiving parenteral fluids. Medication such as digitalis may also influence serum electrolytes. Warning signs are dryness of mouth, thirst, weakness, lethargy, drowsiness, restlessness, muscle pains or cramps, muscular fatigue, hypotension, oliguria, tachycardia, and gastrointestinal disturbance such as nausea or vomiting.

Hypokalemia may develop, especially with brisk diuresis, when severe cirrhosis is present, or during concomitant use of steroids or ACTH. Interference with adequate oral intake of electrolytes will also contribute to hypokalemia. Hypokalemia can sensitize or exaggerate the response of the heart to the toxic effects of digitalis (*eg,* increased ventricular irritability).

Any chloride deficit is generally mild and usually does not require specific treatment except under extraordinary circumstances (as in liver disease or renal disease). Dilutional hyponatremia may occur in edematous patients in hot weather; appropriate therapy is water restriction rather than administration of salt, except in rare instances when the hyponatremia is life-threatening. In actual salt depletion, appropriate replacement is the therapy of choice.

Hyperuricemia may occur or frank gout may be precipitated in certain patients receiving thiazide therapy.

Insulin requirements in diabetic patients may be increased, decreased, or unchanged. Latent diabetes may become manifest during thiazide administration.

Thiazide drugs may increase the responsiveness to tubocurarine.

The antihypertensive effects of the drug may be enhanced in the postsympathectomy patient. Thiazides may decrease arterial responsiveness to norepinephrine. This diminution is not sufficient to preclude effectiveness of the pressor agent for therapeutic use.

If progressive renal impairment becomes evident, withholding or discontinuing diuretic therapy should be considered.

Thiazides may decrease serum PBI levels without signs of thyroid disturbance.

Calcium excretion is decreased by thiazides. Pathological changes in the parathyroid gland with hypercalcemia and hypophosphatemia have been observed in a few patients on prolonged thiazide therapy. The common complications of hyperparathyroidism such as renal lithiasis, bone resorption, and peptic ulceration have not been seen. Thiazides should be discontinued before carrying out tests for parathyroid function.

Adverse Reactions

Reserpine

Rauwolfia preparations have caused gastrointestinal reactions including hypersecretion, nausea, vomiting, anorexia, and diarrhea; cardiovascular reactions including angina-like symptoms, arrhythmias (particularly when used concurrently with digitalis or quinidine), and bradycardia; central nervous system reactions including drowsiness, depression, nervousness, paradoxical anxiety, nightmares, rare parkinsonian syndrome and other extrapyramidal tract symptoms, and CNS sensitization manifested by dull sensorium, deafness, glaucoma, uveitis, and optic atrophy. Nasal congestion is a frequent occurrence. Pruritus, rash, dryness of mouth, dizziness, headache, dyspnea, syncope, epistaxis, purpura and other hematologic reactions, impotence or decreased libido, dysuria, muscular aches, conjunctival injection, weight gain, breast engorgement, pseudolactation, and gynecomastia have been reported. These reactions are usually reversible and disappear after the drug is discontinued.

Water retention with edema in patients with hypertensive vascular disease may occur rarely, but the condition generally clears with cessation of therapy or with the administration of a diuretic agent.

Continued on next page

CIBA—Cont.

Hydralazine
Adverse reactions with hydralazine are usually reversible when dosage is reduced. However, in some cases it may be necessary to discontinue the drug.
Common: Headache; palpitations; anorexia; nausea; vomiting; diarrhea; tachycardia; angina pectoris.
Less Frequent: Nasal congestion; flushing; lacrimation; conjunctivitis; peripheral neuritis, evidenced by paresthesias, numbness, and tingling; edema; dizziness; tremors; muscle cramps; psychotic reactions characterized by depression, disorientation, or anxiety; hypersensitivity (including rash, urticaria, pruritus, fever, chills, arthralgia, eosinophilia, and, rarely, hepatitis); constipation; difficulty in micturition; dyspnea; paralytic ileus; lymphadenopathy; splenomegaly; blood dyscrasias, consisting of reduction in hemoglobin and red cell count, leukopenia, agranulocytosis, and purpura; hypotension; paradoxical pressor response.
Hydrochlorothiazide
Gastrointestinal: Anorexia, gastric irritation, nausea, vomiting, cramping, diarrhea, constipation, jaundice (intrahepatic cholestatic), pancreatitis, sialadenitis
Central Nervous System: Dizziness, vertigo, paresthesias, headache, xanthopsia
Hematologic: Leukopenia, thrombocytopenia, agranulocytosis, aplastic anemia
Cardiovascular: Orthostatic hypotension (may be potentiated by alcohol, barbiturates, or narcotics)
Hypersensitivity: Purpura, photosensitivity, rash, urticaria, necrotizing angiitis, Stevens-Johnson syndrome, and other hypersensitivity reactions
Other: Hyperglycemia, glycosuria, hyperuricemia, muscle spasm, weakness, restlessness
Whenever adverse reactions are moderate or severe, thiazide dosage should be reduced or therapy withdrawn.
Dosage and Administration: As determined by individual titration (see box warning). Usual dosage is 1 to 2 tablets t.i.d.
Since the antihypertensive effects of reserpine are not immediately apparent, maximal reduction in blood pressure from a given dosage may not occur for 2 weeks. For maintenance, adjust dosage to lowest patient requirement.
When necessary, more potent antihypertensives may be added gradually in dosages reduced by at least 50 percent. Watch effects carefully.
Overdosage
Reserpine
Signs and Symptoms
Impairment of consciousness may occur and may range from drowsiness to coma, depending upon the severity of overdosage. Flushing of the skin, conjunctival injection, and pupillary constriction are to be expected. Hypotension, hypothermia, central respiratory depression, and bradycardia may develop in cases of severe overdosage. Diarrhea may also occur.
Treatment
Evacuate stomach contents, taking adequate precautions against aspiration and for the protection of the airway; instill activated charcoal slurry.
Treat the effect of reserpine overdosage symptomatically. If hypotension is severe enough to require treatment with a vasopressor, use one having a direct action upon vascular smooth muscle (*eg* phenylephrine, levarterenol, metaraminol). Since reserpine is long-acting, observe the patient carefully for at least 72 hours, administering treatment as required.
Hydralazine
Signs and Symptoms
Hypotension, tachycardia, headache and generalized skin flushing are to be expected. Myocardial ischemia and cardiac arrhythmia can develop; profound shock can occur in severe overdosage.
Treatment
Evacuate gastric contents, taking adequate precautions against aspiration and for protection of the airway; instill activated charcoal slurry, if general conditions permit. These manipulations may have to be omitted or carried out after cardiovascular status has been stabilized, since they might precipitate cardiac arrhythmias or increase the depth of shock.
Support of the cardiovascular system is of primary importance. Shock should be treated with volume expanders without resorting to use of vasopressors, if possible. If a vasopressor is required, use one that is least likely to precipitate or aggravate cardiac arrhythmia. Digitalization may be necessary. Renal function must be monitored and supported as required.
No experience has been reported with extracorporeal or peritoneal dialysis.
Hydrochlorothiazide
Signs and Symptoms
Diuresis is to be expected; lethargy of varying degree may appear and may progress to coma within a few hours, with minimal depression of respiration and cardiovascular function and without significant serum electrolyte changes or dehydration. The mechanism of CNS depression with thiazide overdosage is unknown. GI irritation and hypermotility may occur; temporary elevation of BUN has been reported and serum electrolyte changes could occur, especially in patients with impairment of renal function.
Treatment
Evacuate gastric contents but take care to prevent aspiration, especially in the stuporous or comatose patient. GI effects are usually of short duration, but may require symptomatic treatment.
Monitor serum electrolyte levels and renal function; institute supportive measures as required individually to maintain hydration, electrolyte balance, respiration and cardiovascular-renal function.
How Supplied: *Tablets* (light salmon pink, dry-coated), each containing 0.1 mg reserpine, 25 mg hydralazine hydrochloride, and 15 mg hydrochlorothiazide; bottles of 100, 1000 and Accu-Pak® blister units of 100.
C78-53 (1/79)
VA—1000's, Stock #6505-00-774-5857A.
[*Shown in Product Identification Section*]

SERPASIL® ℞
(reserpine USP)
Tablets Elixir

Listed in USP, a Medicare designated compendium.

Indications
Mild essential hypertension; also useful as adjunctive therapy with other antihypertensive agents in the more severe forms of hypertension; relief of symptoms in agitated psychotic states (*eg*, schizophrenia), primarily in those individuals unable to tolerate phenothiazine derivatives or those who also require antihypertensive medication.
Contraindications: Known hypersensitivity, mental depression (especially with suicidal tendencies), active peptic ulcer, ulcerative colitis, and patients receiving electroconvulsive therapy.
Warnings: Extreme caution should be exercised in treating patients with a history of mental depression. Discontinue the drug at first sign of despondency, early morning insomnia, loss of appetite, impotence, or self-deprecation. Drug-induced depression may persist for several months after drug withdrawal and may be severe enough to result in suicide.
MAO inhibitors should be avoided or used with extreme caution.
Usage in Pregnancy
The safety of reserpine for use during pregnancy or lactation has not been established; therefore, the drug should be used in pregnant patients or in women of childbearing potential only when, in the judgment of the physician, it is essential to the welfare of the patient. Increased respiratory tract secretions, nasal congestion, cyanosis, and anorexia may occur in neonates and breast-fed infants of reserpine-treated mothers since reserpine crosses the placental barrier and also appears in maternal breast milk.
Precautions: Since Serpasil increases gastrointestinal motility and secretion, it should be used cautiously in patients with a history of peptic ulcer, ulcerative colitis, or gallstones (biliary colic may be precipitated).
Caution should be exercised when treating hypertensive patients with renal insufficiency since they adjust poorly to lowered blood pressure levels.
Use Serpasil cautiously with digitalis and quinidine since cardiac arrhythmias have occurred with rauwolfia preparations.
Preoperative withdrawal of reserpine does not assure that circulatory instability will not occur. It is important that the anesthesiologist be aware of the patient's drug intake and consider this in the overall management, since hypotension has occurred in patients receiving rauwolfia preparations. Anticholinergic and/or adrenergic drugs (*eg*, metaraminol, norepinephrine) have been employed to treat adverse vagocirculatory effects.
Adverse Reactions: Rauwolfia preparations have caused gastrointestinal reactions including hypersecretion, nausea, vomiting, anorexia, and diarrhea; cardiovascular reactions including angina-like symptoms, arrhythmias (particularly when used concurrently with digitalis or quinidine), bradycardia; central nervous system reactions including drowsiness, depression, nervousness, paradoxical anxiety, nightmares, rare parkinsonian syndrome and other extrapyramidal tract symptoms, and CNS sensitization manifested by dull sensorium, deafness, glaucoma, uveitis, and optic atrophy. Nasal congestion is a frequent occurrence. Pruritus, rash, dryness of mouth, dizziness, headache, dyspnea, syncope, epistaxis, purpura and other hematologic reactions, impotence or decreased libido, dysuria, muscular aches, conjunctival injection, weight gain, breast engorgement, pseudolactation, and gynecomastia have been reported. These reactions are usually reversible and usually disappear after the drug is discontinued.
Water retention with edema in patients with hypertensive vascular disease may occur rarely, but the condition generally clears with cessation of therapy or with the administration of a diuretic agent.
Dosage and Administration
For Hypertension: In the average patient not receiving other antihypertensive agents, the usual initial dose is 0.5 mg daily for 1 or 2 weeks. For maintenance, reduce to 0.1 mg to 0.25 mg daily. Higher doses should be used cautiously, because serious mental depression and other side effects may be increased considerably.
For Psychiatric Disorders: The usual initial dose is 0.5 mg, with a range of 0.1 mg to 1.0 mg. Adjust dosage upward or downward according to the patient's response.
Concomitant use of Serpasil with ganglionic blocking agents, guanethidine, veratrum, hydralazine, methyldopa, chlorthalidone, or thiazides necessitates careful titration of dosage with each agent.
Overdosage
Signs and Symptoms
Impairment of consciousness may occur and may range from drowsiness to coma, depending upon the severity of overdosage. Flushing of the skin, conjunctival injection, and pupillary constriction are to be expected. Hypoten-

sion, hypothermia, central respiratory depression, and bradycardia may develop in cases of severe overdosage. Diarrhea may also occur.

Treatment

Evacuate stomach contents, taking adequate precautions against aspiration and for the protection of the airway; instill activated charcoal slurry.

Treat the effects of reserpine overdosage symptomatically. If hypotension is severe enough to require treatment with a vasopressor, use one having a direct action upon vascular smooth muscle (*eg*, phenylephrine, levarterenol, metaraminol). Since reserpine is long-acting, observe the patient carefully for at least 72 hours, administering treatment as required.

How Supplied

Tablets, 1 mg (white, scored); bottles of 100.
Tablets, 0.25 mg (white, scored); bottles of 100, 500, 1000 and 5000.
Tablets, 0.1 mg (white); bottles of 100, 500 and 1000.
Elixir (green, lemon-lime flavored), 0.2 mg per 4-ml teaspoon; bottles of 1 pint.

C77-5 Rev. 1/77

[*Shown in Product Identification Section*]

SERPASIL® ℞

(reserpine USP)
Parenteral Solution

Listed in USP, a Medicare designated compendium.

Indications: Hypertensive emergencies, such as acute hypertensive encephalopathy, in which it is desired to reduce blood pressure rapidly; psychiatric conditions only to initiate treatment in those patients unable to accept oral medication or to control symptoms of extreme agitation.

Contraindications: Known hypersensitivity, mental depression (especially with suicidal tendencies), active peptic ulcer, ulcerative colitis, and patients receiving electroconvulsive therapy.

Warnings: Extreme caution should be exercised in treating patients with a history of mental depression. Discontinue the drug at first sign of despondency, early morning insomnia, loss of appetite, impotence, or self-deprecation. Drug-induced depression may persist for several months after drug withdrawal and may be severe enough to result in suicide.

MAO inhibitors should be avoided or used with extreme caution.

Usage in Pregnancy

The safety of reserpine for use during pregnancy or lactation has not been established; therefore, the drug should be used in pregnant patients or in women of childbearing potential only when, in the judgment of the physician, it is essential to the welfare of the patient. Increased respiratory tract secretions, nasal congestion, cyanosis, and anorexia may occur in neonates and breast-fed infants of reserpine-treated mothers since reserpine crosses the placental barrier and also appears in maternal breast milk.

Precautions: Since Serpasil increases gastrointestinal motility and secretion, it should be used cautiously in patients with a history of peptic ulcer, ulcerative colitis, or gallstones (biliary colic may be precipitated).

Caution should be exercised when treating hypertensive patients with renal insufficiency since they adjust poorly to lowered blood pressure levels.

Use Serpasil cautiously with digitalis and quinidine since cardiac arrhythmias have occurred with rauwolfia preparations.

Preoperative withdrawal of reserpine does not assure that circulatory instability will not occur. It is important that the anesthesiologist be aware of the patient's drug intake and consider this in the overall management, since hypotension has occurred in patients receiving rauwolfia preparations. Anticholinergic and/or adrenergic drugs (*eg*, metaraminol, norepinephrine) have been employed to treat adverse vagocirculatory effects.

Adverse Reactions: Rauwolfia preparations have caused gastrointestinal reactions including hypersecretion, nausea, vomiting, anorexia, and diarrhea; cardiovascular reactions including angina-like symptoms, arrhythmias (particularly when used concurrently with digitalis or quinidine), bradycardia; central nervous system reactions including drowsiness, depression, nervousness, paradoxical anxiety, nightmares, rare parkinsonian syndrome and other extrapyramidal tract symptoms, and CNS sensitization manifested by dull sensorium, deafness, glaucoma, uveitis, and optic atrophy. Nasal congestion is a frequent occurrence. Pruritus, rash, dryness of mouth, dizziness, headache, dyspnea, syncope, epistaxis, purpura and other hematologic reactions, impotence or decreased libido, dysuria, muscular aches, conjunctival injection, weight gain, breast engorgement, pseudolactation, and gynecomastia have been reported. These reactions are usually reversible and usually disappear after the drug is discontinued.

Water retention with edema in patients with hypertensive vascular disease may occur rarely, but the condition generally clears with cessation of therapy or with the administration of a diuretic agent.

Dosage and Administration: Serpasil may be administered intramuscularly in the short-term treatment of hypertensive crises. Because of the varying responsiveness, a titration procedure should be used. An initial dose of 0.5 to 1 mg intramuscularly is followed at intervals of 3 hours, if necessary, by doses of 2 and 4 mg until the blood pressure falls to the desired level. If the 4-mg dose is ineffective, other antihypertensive agents should be used. An initial dose larger than 0.5 mg may induce severe hypotension, particularly in patients with cerebral hemorrhage.

Serpasil may be administered intramuscularly in psychiatric emergencies to initiate treatment in those patients unable to accept oral medication or to control extreme agitation. The usual dose is from 2.5 mg to 5.0 mg, following a small initial dose to test patient responsiveness.

Concomitant use of Serpasil with ganglionic blocking agents, guanethidine, veratrum, hydralazine, methyldopa, chlorthalidone, or thiazides necessitates careful titration of dosage with each agent.

Overdosage

Signs and Symptoms

Impairment of consciousness may occur and may range from drowsiness to coma, depending upon the severity of overdosage. Flushing of the skin, conjunctival injection, and pupillary constriction are to be expected. Hypotension, hypothermia, central respiratory depression, and bradycardia may develop in cases of severe overdosage. Diarrhea may also occur.

Treatment

Hypotension is likely to require major therapeutic attention. If a vasopressor is necessary, use one having a direct action upon vascular smooth muscle (*eg*, phenylephrine, levarterenol, metaraminol).

If bradycardia becomes marked, especially with cardiac arrhythmia, consider use of vagal blocking agents along with other appropriate measures.

Treat other effects of reserpine overdosage symptomatically. Since reserpine is long-acting, observe the patient carefully for at least 72 hours, administering treatment as required.

How Supplied

Parenteral Solution: Each ml contains 2.5 mg reserpine, 0.1 ml dimethylacetamide, 10 mg adipic acid, 0.1 mg versene, 0.01 ml benzyl alcohol, 0.05 ml polyethylene glycol, 0.5 mg ascorbic acid, and 0.1 mg sodium sulfite in water.
Ampuls, 2 ml; cartons of 5.

C78-62 (3/79)

SERPASIL®-APRESOLINE® ℞

hydrochloride
(reserpine and hydralazine hydrochloride)
Combination Tablets

> **Warning**
> This fixed combination drug is not indicated for initial therapy of hypertension. Hypertension requires therapy titrated to the individual patient. If the fixed combination represents the dosage so determined, its use may be more convenient in patient management. The treatment of hypertension is not static, but must be reevaluated as conditions in each patient warrant.

Indications

Hypertension. (See box warning.)

Contraindications

Reserpine

Known hypersensitivity, mental depression (especially with suicidal tendencies), active peptic ulcer, ulcerative colitis, and patients receiving electroconvulsive therapy.

Hydralazine

Hypersensitivity to hydralazine; coronary artery disease; and mitral valvular rheumatic heart disease.

Warnings

Reserpine

Extreme caution should be exercised in treating patients with a history of mental depression. Discontinue the drug at first sign of despondency, early morning insomnia, loss of appetite, impotence, or self-deprecation. Drug-induced depression may persist for several months after drug withdrawal and may be severe enough to result in suicide.

MAO inhibitors should be avoided or used with extreme caution.

Hydralazine

Hydralazine may produce in a few patients a clinical picture simulating systemic lupus erythematosus. In such patients hydralazine should be discontinued unless the benefit-to-risk determination requires continued antihypertensive therapy with this drug. Symptoms and signs usually regress when the drug is discontinued but residua have been detected many years later. Long-term treatment with steroids may be necessary.

Complete blood counts, L. E. cell preparations, and antinuclear antibody titer determinations are indicated before and periodically during prolonged therapy with hydralazine, even though the patient is asymptomatic. These studies are also indicated if the patient develops arthralgia, fever, chest pain, continued malaise, or other unexplained signs or symptoms.

A positive antinuclear antibody titer and/or positive L. E. cell reaction requires that the physician carefully weigh the implications of the test results against the benefits to be derived from antihypertensive therapy with hydralazine.

Use MAO inhibitors with caution in patients receiving hydralazine.

When other potent parenteral antihypertensive drugs, such as diazoxide, are used in combination with hydralazine, patients should be continuously observed for several hours for any excessive fall in blood pressure. Profound hypotensive episodes may occur when diazoxide injection and Apresoline (hydralazine hydrochloride) are used concomitantly.

Continued on next page

CIBA—Cont.

Usage in Pregnancy
Reserpine
The safety of reserpine for use during pregnancy or lactation has not been established; therefore, the drug should be used in pregnant patients or in women of childbearing potential only when, in the judgment of the physician, it is essential to the welfare of the patient. Increased respiratory tract secretions, nasal congestion, cyanosis, and anorexia may occur in neonates and breast-fed infants of reserpine-treated mothers since reserpine crosses the placental barrier and appears in maternal breast milk.
Hydralazine
Animal studies indicate that hydralazine is teratogenic in mice, possibly in rabbits, and not in rats. Teratogenic effects observed were cleft palate and malformations of facial and cranial bones. Although clinical experience does not include any positive evidence of adverse effects on the human fetus, hydralazine should not be used during pregnancy unless the expected benefit clearly justifies the potential risk to the fetus.

Precautions
Reserpine
Since reserpine increases gastrointestinal motility and secretion, it should be used cautiously in patients with a history of peptic ulcer, ulcerative colitis, or gallstones (biliary colic may be precipitated).
Caution should be exercised when treating hypertensive patients with renal insufficiency, since they adjust poorly to lowered blood pressure levels.
Use reserpine cautiously with digitalis and quinidine since cardiac arrhythmias have occurred with rauwolfia preparations.
Preoperative withdrawal of reserpine does not assure that circulatory instability will not occur. It is important that the anesthesiologist be aware of the patient's drug intake and consider this in the overall management, since hypotension has occurred in patients receiving rauwolfia preparations. Anticholinergic and/or adrenergic drugs (*eg*, metaraminol, norepinephrine) have been employed to treat adverse vagocirculatory effects.
Hydralazine
Myocardial stimulation produced by hydralazine can cause anginal attacks and ECG changes of myocardial ischemia. The drug has been implicated in the production of myocardial infarction. It must, therefore, be used with caution in patients with suspected coronary artery disease.
The "hyperdynamic" circulation caused by hydralazine may accentuate specific cardiovascular inadequacies. An example is that hydralazine may increase pulmonary artery pressure in patients with mitral valvular disease. The drug may reduce the pressor responses to epinephrine. Postural hypotension may result from hydralazine but is less common than with ganglionic blocking agents. Use with caution in patients with cerebral vascular accidents.
In hypertensive patients with normal kidneys who are treated with hydralazine, there is evidence of increased renal blood flow and a maintenance of glomerular filtration rate. In some instances improved renal function has been noted where control values were below normal prior to hydralazine administration. However, as with any antihypertensive agent, hydralazine should be used with caution in patients with advanced renal damage.
Peripheral neuritis, evidenced by paresthesias, numbness, and tingling, has been observed. Published evidence suggests an antipyridoxine effect and the addition of pyridoxine to the regimen if symptoms develop.
Blood dyscrasias, consisting of reduction in hemoglobin and red cell count, leukopenia, agranulocytosis, and purpura, have been reported. If such abnormalities develop, discontinue therapy. Periodic blood counts are advised during prolonged therapy.
The Serpasil-Apresoline tablets (#1 and #2) contain FD&C Yellow No. 5 (tartrazine) which may cause allergic-type reactions (including bronchial asthma) in certain susceptible individuals. Although the overall incidence of FD&C Yellow No. 5 (tartrazine) sensitivity in the general population is low, it is frequently seen in patients who also have aspirin hypersensitivity.

Adverse Reactions
Reserpine
Rauwolfia preparations have caused gastrointestinal reactions including hypersecretion, nausea, vomiting, anorexia, and diarrhea; cardiovascular reactions including angina-like symptoms, arrhythmias (particularly when used concurrently with digitalis or quinidine), and bradycardia; central nervous system reactions including drowsiness, depression, nervousness, paradoxical anxiety, nightmares, rare parkinsonian syndrome and other extrapyramidal tract symptoms, and CNS sensitization manifested by dull sensorium, deafness, glaucoma, uveitis, and optic atrophy. Nasal congestion is a frequent occurrence. Pruritus, rash, dryness of mouth, dizziness, headache, dyspnea, syncope, epistaxis, purpura and other hematologic reactions, impotence or decreased libido, dysuria, muscular aches, conjunctival injection, weight gain, breast engorgement, pseudolactation, and gynecomastia have been reported. These reactions are usually reversible and disappear after the drug is discontinued.
Water retention with edema in patients with hypertensive vascular disease may occur rarely, but the condition generally clears with cessation of therapy or with the administration of a diuretic agent.
Hydralazine
Adverse reactions with hydralazine are usually reversible when dosage is reduced. However, in some cases it may be necessary to discontinue the drug.
Common: Headache; palpitations; anorexia; nausea; vomiting; diarrhea; tachycardia; angina pectoris.
Less Frequent: Nasal congestion; flushing; lacrimation; conjunctivitis; peripheral neuritis, evidenced by paresthesias, numbness, and tingling; edema; dizziness; tremors; muscle cramps; psychotic reactions characterized by depression, disorientation, or anxiety; hypersensitivity (including rash, urticaria, pruritus, fever, chills, arthralgia, eosinophilia, and, rarely, hepatitis); constipation; difficulty in micturition; dyspnea; paralytic ileus; lymphadenopathy; splenomegaly; blood dyscrasias, consisting of reduction in hemoglobin and red cell count, leukopenia, agranulocytosis, and purpura; hypotension; paradoxical pressor response.

Dosage and Administration: As determined by individual titration (see box warning).

Step 1: a. Start with reserpine alone. Average dosage: 0.5 mg daily.
b. Continue for at least one week. If results prove satisfactory—as they will in many cases—no other medication is required. For maintenance, reduce dosage to 0.25 mg or less daily.

Step 2: a. Should more than the therapeutic action of reserpine be indicated, therapy with *Tablet #2* (reserpine 0.2 mg/hydralazine hydrochloride 50 mg) should be initiated—one tablet 4 times a day.
b. When reduction of dosage is indicated, *Tablet #1* (reserpine 0.1 mg/hydralazine hydrochloride 25 mg) should be used—one tablet 4 times a day.

Side effects associated with hydralazine (headache, tachycardia, palpitation) are seldom encountered when the patient has been "primed" with reserpine before combination therapy is begun. Should side effects appear, however, reduction of dosage to one *Tablet #1* two to four times a day for a few days will usually alleviate them.
In cases where further individualization of dosage is necessary, the adjustment may be made by increasing or decreasing the dosage of reserpine and/or hydralazine.
For maintenance, daily dosage of hydralazine should probably not exceed 200 mg, nor should the dosage of reserpine exceed 1 mg.
For Patients on Hydralazine.
Patients already on this drug may be given a combination tablet as required. With the addition of reserpine, it is usually possible to reduce the dose of hydralazine.

Overdosage
Reserpine
Signs and Symptoms
Impairment of consciousness may occur and may range from drowsiness to coma, depending upon the severity of overdosage. Flushing of the skin, conjunctival injection, and pupillary constriction are to be expected. Hypotension, hypothermia, central respiratory depression, and bradycardia may develop in cases of severe overdosage. Diarrhea may also occur.
Treatment
Evacuate stomach contents, taking adequate precautions against aspiration and for the protection of the airway; instill activated charcoal slurry.
Treat the effects of reserpine overdosage symptomatically. If hypotension is severe enough to require treatment with a vasopressor, use one having a direct action upon vascular smooth muscle (*eg*, phenylephrine, levarterenol, metaraminol). Since reserpine is long-acting, observe the patient carefully for at least 72 hours, administering treatment as required.
Hydralazine
Signs and Symptoms
Hypotension, tachycardia, headache and generalized skin flushing are to be expected. Myocardial ischemia and cardiac arrhythmia can develop; profound shock can occur in severe overdosage.
Treatment
Evacuate gastric contents, taking adequate precautions against aspiration and for protection of the airway; instill activated charcoal slurry, if general conditions permit. These manipulations may have to be omitted or carried out after cardiovascular status has been stabilized, since they might precipitate cardiac arrhythmias or increase the depth of shock.
Support of the cardiovascular system is of primary importance. Shock should be treated with volume expanders without resorting to use of vasopressors, if possible. If a vasopressor is required, use one that is least likely to precipitate or aggravate cardiac arrhythmia. Digitalization may be necessary. Renal function must be monitored and supported as required.
No experience has been reported with extracorporeal or peritoneal dialysis.

How Supplied
Tablets #2 (yellow, dry-coated), each containing 0.2 mg reserpine and 50 mg hydralazine hydrochloride; bottles of 100.
Tablets #1 (yellow, dry-coated), each containing 0.1 mg reserpine and 25 mg hydralazine hydrochloride; bottles of 100.
Dispense in tight, light-resistant container (USP).

C80-19 (1/80)

[*Shown in Product Identification Section*]

SERPASIL®-ESIDRIX® ℞
(reserpine and hydrochlorothiazide)
Combination Tablets

Warning
This fixed combination drug is not indicated for initial therapy of hypertension. Hypertension requires therapy titrated to the individual patient. If the fixed combination represents the dosage so determined, its use may be more convenient in patient management. The treatment of hypertension is not static, but must be reevaluated as conditions in each patient warrant.

Indications
Hypertension. (See box warning.)
Contraindications
Reserpine
Known hypersensitivity, mental depression (especially with suicidal tendencies), active peptic ulcer, ulcerative colitis, and patients receiving electroconvulsive therapy.
Hydrochlorothiazide
Anuria; hypersensitivity to this or other sulfonamide-derived drugs.
Warnings
Reserpine
Extreme caution should be exercised in treating patients with a history of mental depression. Discontinue the drug at first sign of despondency, early morning insomnia, loss of appetite, impotence, or self-deprecation. Drug-induced depression may persist for several months after drug withdrawal and may be severe enough to result in suicide.
MAO inhibitors should be avoided or used with extreme caution.
Hydrochlorothiazide
Use with caution in severe renal disease. In patients with renal disease, thiazides may precipitate azotemia. Cumulative effects of the drug may develop in patients with impaired renal function.
Thiazides should be used with caution in patients with impaired hepatic function or progressive liver disease, since minor alterations of fluid and electrolyte imbalance may precipitate hepatic coma.
Thiazides may add to or potentiate the action of other antihypertensive drugs. Potentiation occurs with ganglionic or peripheral adrenergic blocking drugs.
Sensitivity reactions are more likely to occur in patients with a history of allergy or bronchial asthma.
The possibility of exacerbation or activation of systemic lupus erythematosus has been reported.
Usage in Pregnancy
Reserpine
The safety of reserpine for use during pregnancy or lactation has not been established; therefore, the drug should be used in pregnant patients or in women of childbearing potential only when, in the judgment of the physician, it is essential to the welfare of the patient. Increased respiratory tract secretions, nasal congestion, cyanosis, and anorexia may occur in neonates and breast-fed infants of reserpine-treated mothers, since reserpine crosses the placental barrier and appears in maternal breast milk.
Hydrochlorothiazide
Thiazides cross the placental barrier and appear in cord blood. The use of thiazides in pregnant women requires that the anticipated benefit be weighed against possible hazards to the fetus. These hazards include fetal or neonatal jaundice, thrombocytopenia, and possibly other adverse reactions which have occurred in the adult.
Nursing Mothers: Thiazides appear in breast milk. If the use of the drug is deemed essential, the patient should stop nursing.

Precautions
Reserpine
Since reserpine increases gastrointestinal motility and secretion, it should be used cautiously in patients with a history of peptic ulcer, ulcerative colitis, or gallstones (biliary colic may be precipitated).
Caution should be exercised when treating hypertensive patients with renal insufficiency since they adjust poorly to lowered blood pressure levels.
Use reserpine cautiously with digitalis and quinidine since cardiac arrhythmias have occurred with rauwolfia preparations.
Preoperative withdrawal of reserpine does not assure that circulatory instability will not occur. It is important that the anesthesiologist be aware of the patient's drug intake and consider this in the overall management, since hypotension has occurred in patients receiving rauwolfia preparations. Anticholinergic and/or adrenergic drugs (*eg,* metaraminol, norepinephrine) have been employed to treat adverse vagocirculatory effects.
Hydrochlorothiazide
Periodic determination of serum electrolytes to detect possible electrolyte imbalance should be performed at appropriate intervals. All patients receiving thiazide therapy should be observed for clinical signs of fluid or electrolyte imbalance; namely, hyponatremia, hypochloremic alkalosis, and hypokalemia. Serum and urine electrolyte determinations are particularly important when the patient is vomiting excessively or receiving parenteral fluids. Medication such as digitalis may also influence serum electrolytes. Warning signs are dryness of mouth, thirst, weakness, lethargy, drowsiness, restlessness, muscle pains or cramps, muscular fatigue, hypotension, oliguria, tachycardia, and gastrointestinal disturbance such as nausea or vomiting.
Hypokalemia may develop, especially with brisk diuresis, when severe cirrhosis is present, or during concomitant use of steroids or ACTH. Interference with adequate oral intake of electrolytes will also contribute to hypokalemia. Hypokalemia can sensitize or exaggerate the response of the heart to the toxic effects of digitalis (*eg,* increased ventricular irritability).
Any chloride deficit is generally mild and usually does not require specific treatment except under extraordinary circumstances (as in liver disease or renal disease). Dilutional hyponatremia may occur in edematous patients in hot weather; appropriate therapy is water restriction rather than administration of salt, except in rare instances when the hyponatremia is life-threatening. In actual salt depletion, appropriate replacement is the therapy of choice.
Hyperuricemia may occur or frank gout may be precipitated in certain patients receiving thiazide therapy.
Insulin requirements in diabetic patients may be increased, decreased, or unchanged. Latent diabetes may become manifest during thiazide administration.
Thiazide drugs may increase the responsiveness to tubocurarine.
The antihypertensive effects of the drug may be enhanced in the postsympathectomy patient. Thiazides may decrease arterial responsiveness to norepinephrine. This diminution is not sufficient to preclude effectiveness of the pressor agent for therapeutic use.
If progressive renal impairment becomes evident, withholding or discontinuing diuretic therapy should be considered.
Thiazides may decrease serum PBI levels without signs of thyroid disturbance.
Calcium excretion is decreased by thiazides. Pathological changes in the parathyroid gland with hypercalcemia and hypophosphatemia have been observed in a few patients on prolonged thiazide therapy. The common complications of hyperparathyroidism such as renal lithiasis, bone resorption, and peptic ulceration have not been seen. Thiazides should be discontinued before carrying out tests for parathyroid function.
The Serpasil-Esidrix tablets (#1 and #2) contain FD&C Yellow No. 5 (tartrazine) which may cause allergic-type reactions (including bronchial asthma) in certain susceptible individuals. Although the overall incidence of FD&C Yellow No. 5 (tartrazine) sensitivity in the general population is low, it is frequently seen in patients who also have aspirin hypersensitivity

Adverse Reactions
Reserpine
Rauwolfia preparations have caused gastrointestinal reactions including hypersecretion, nausea, vomiting, anorexia, and diarrhea; cardiovascular reactions including angina-like symptoms, arrhythmias (particularly when used concurrently with digitalis or quinidine), and bradycardia; central nervous system reactions including drowsiness, depression, nervousness, paradoxical anxiety, nightmares, rare parkinsonian syndrome and other extrapyramidal tract symptoms, and CNS sensitization manifested by dull sensorium, deafness, glaucoma, uveitis, and optic atrophy. Nasal congestion is a frequent occurrence. Pruritus, rash, dryness of mouth, dizziness, headache, dyspnea, syncope, epistaxis, purpura and other hematologic reactions, impotence or decreased libido, dysuria, muscular aches, conjunctival injection, weight gain, breast engorgement, pseudolactation, and gynecomastia have been reported. These reactions are usually reversible and disappear after the drug is discontinued.
Water retention with edema in patients with hypertensive vascular disease may occur rarely, but the condition generally clears with cessation of therapy or with the administration of a diuretic agent.
Hydrochlorothiazide
Gastrointestinal: Anorexia, gastric irritation, nausea, vomiting, cramping, diarrhea, constipation, jaundice (intrahepatic cholestatic), pancreatitis, sialadenitis
Central Nervous System: Dizziness, vertigo, paresthesias, headache, xanthopsia
Hematologic: Leukopenia, thrombocytopenia, agranulocytosis, aplastic anemia
Cardiovascular: Orthostatic hypotension (may be potentiated by alcohol, barbiturates, or narcotics)
Hypersensitivity: Purpura, photosensitivity, rash, urticaria, necrotizing angiitis, Stevens-Johnson syndrome, and other hypersensitivity reactions
Other: Hyperglycemia, glycosuria, hyperuricemia, muscle spasm, weakness, restlessness
Whenever adverse reactions are moderate or severe, thiazide dosage should be reduced or therapy withdrawn.
Dosage and Administration: As determined by individual titration (see box warning).
Usual dosage is 2 Tablets #2 daily in single or divided doses. For patients requiring less hydrochlorothiazide, substitute Tablets #1.
Since antihypertensive effects of reserpine are not immediately apparent, maximal reduction in blood pressure from a given dosage may not occur for 2 weeks. For maintenance, reduce dosage to lowest effective level; as little as 1 tablet daily may suffice.
When necessary, more potent antihypertensive agents may be added gradually in reduced dosages. Watch effects carefully.
Overdosage
Reserpine
Signs and Symptoms
Impairment of consciousness may occur and may range from drowsiness to coma, depending upon the severity of overdosage. Flushing of the skin, conjunctival injection, and pupillary constriction are to be expected. Hypotension, hypothermia, central respiratory depres-

Continued on next page

CIBA—Cont.

sion, and bradycardia may develop in cases of severe overdosage. Diarrhea may also occur.

Treatment

Evacuate stomach contents, taking adequate precautions against aspiration and for the protection of the airway; instill activated charcoal slurry.

Treat the effects of reserpine overdosage symptomatically. If hypotension is severe enough to require treatment with a vasopressor, use one having a direct action upon vascular smooth muscle (*eg*, phenylephrine, levarterenol, metaraminol). Since reserpine is long-acting, observe the patient carefully for at least 72 hours, administering treatment as required.

Hydrochlorothiazide

Signs and Symptoms

Diuresis is to be expected; lethargy of varying degree may appear and may progress to coma within a few hours, with minimal depression of respiration and cardiovascular function and without significant serum electrolyte changes or dehydration. The mechanism of CNS depression with thiazide overdosage is unknown. GI irritation and hypermotility may occur; temporary elevation of BUN has been reported and serum electrolyte changes could occur, especially in patients with impairment of renal function.

Treatment

Evacuate gastric contents but take care to prevent aspiration, especially in the stuporous or comatose patient. GI effects are usually of short duration, but may require symptomatic treatment.

Monitor serum electrolyte levels and renal function; institute supportive measures as required individually to maintain hydration, electrolyte balance, respiration and cardiovascular-renal function.

How Supplied: *Tablets #1* (light orange), each containing 0.1 mg reserpine and 25 mg hydrochlorothiazide; bottles of 100 and 1000.

Tablets #2 (light orange), each containing 0.1 mg reserpine and 50 mg hydrochlorothiazide; bottles of 100 and 1000.

Dispense in tight, light-resistant container (USP).

C80-20 (1/80)

[*Shown in Product Identification Section*]

SLOW-K® ℞
(potassium chloride)
slow-release tablets

Description: Slow-K is a sugar-coated (not enteric-coated) tablet containing 600 mg potassium chloride (equivalent to 8 mEq) in a wax matrix. This formulation is intended to provide a controlled release of potassium from the matrix to minimize the likelihood of producing high localized concentrations of potassium within the gastrointestinal tract.

Actions: Potassium ion is the principal intracellular cation of most body tissues. Potassium ions participate in a number of essential physiological processes, including the maintenance of intracellular tonicity, the transmission of nerve impulses, the contraction of cardiac, skeletal, and smooth muscle and the maintenance of normal renal function.

Potassium depletion may occur whenever the rate of potassium loss through renal excretion and/or loss from the gastrointestinal tract exceeds the rate of potassium intake. Such depletion usually develops slowly as a consequence of prolonged therapy with oral diuretics, primary or secondary hyperaldosteronism, diabetic ketoacidosis, severe diarrhea, or inadequate replacement of potassium in patients on prolonged parenteral nutrition. Potassium depletion due to these causes is usually accompanied by a concomitant deficiency of chloride and is manifested by hypokalemia and metabolic alkalosis. Potassium depletion may produce weakness, fatigue, disturbances of cardiac rhythm (primarily ectopic beats), prominent U-waves in the electrocardiogram, and in advanced cases flaccid paralysis and/or impaired ability to concentrate urine.

Potassium depletion associated with metabolic alkalosis is managed by correcting the fundamental causes of the deficiency whenever possible and administering supplemental potassium chloride, in the form of high potassium food or potassium chloride solution or tablets. In rare circumstances (*eg*, patients with renal tubular acidosis) potassium depletion may be associated with metabolic acidosis and hyperchloremia. In such patients potassium replacement should be accomplished with potassium salts other than the chloride, such as potassium bicarbonate, potassium citrate, or potassium acetate.

Indications: BECAUSE OF REPORTS OF INTESTINAL AND GASTRIC ULCERATION AND BLEEDING WITH SLOW-RELEASE POTASSIUM CHLORIDE PREPARATIONS, THESE DRUGS SHOULD BE RESERVED FOR THOSE PATIENTS WHO CANNOT TOLERATE OR REFUSE TO TAKE LIQUID OR EFFERVESCENT POTASSIUM PREPARATIONS OR FOR PATIENTS IN WHOM THERE IS A PROBLEM OF COMPLIANCE WITH THESE PREPARATIONS.

1. For therapeutic use in patients with hypokalemia with or without metabolic alkalosis; in digitalis intoxication and in patients with hypokalemic familial periodic paralysis.
2. For prevention of potassium depletion when the dietary intake of potassium is inadequate in the following conditions: Patients receiving digitalis and diuretics for congestive heart failure; hepatic cirrhosis with ascites; states of aldosterone excess with normal renal function; potassium-losing nephropathy, and certain diarrheal states.
3. The use of potassium salts in patients receiving diuretics for uncomplicated essential hypertension is often unnecessary when such patients have a normal dietary pattern. Serum potassium should be checked periodically, however, and, if hypokalemia occurs, dietary supplementation with potassium-containing foods may be adequate to control milder cases. In more severe cases supplementation with potassium salts may be indicated.

Contraindications: Potassium supplements are contraindicated in patients with hyperkalemia since a further increase in serum potassium concentration in such patients can produce cardiac arrest. Hyperkalemia may complicate any of the following conditions: chronic renal failure, systemic acidosis such as diabetic acidosis, acute dehydration, extensive tissue breakdown as in severe burns, adrenal insufficiency, or the administration of a potassium-sparing diuretic (*eg*, spironolactone, triamterene).

Wax-matrix potassium chloride preparations have produced esophageal ulceration in certain cardiac patients with esophageal compression due to an enlarged left atrium.

All solid dosage forms of potassium supplements are contraindicated in any patient in whom there is cause for arrest or delay in tablet passage through the gastrointestinal tract. In these instances, potassium supplementation should be with a liquid preparation.

Warnings:

Hyperkalemia

In patients with impaired mechanisms for excreting potassium, the administration of potassium salts can produce hyperkalemia and cardiac arrest. This occurs most commonly in patients given potassium by the intravenous route but may also occur in patients given potassium orally. Potentially fatal hyperkalemia can develop rapidly and be asymptomatic.

The use of potassium salts in patients with chronic renal disease, or any other condition which impairs potassium excretion, requires particularly careful monitoring of the serum potassium concentration and appropriate dosage adjustment.

Interaction with Potassium-Sparing Diuretics

Hypokalemia should not be treated by the concomitant administration of potassium salts and a potassium-sparing diuretic (*eg*, spironolactone or triamterene), since the simultaneous administration of these agents can produce severe hyperkalemia.

Gastrointestinal lesions

Potassium chloride tablets have produced stenotic and/or ulcerative lesions of the small bowel and deaths. These lesions are caused by a high localized concentration of potassium ion in the region of a rapidly dissolving tablet, which injures the bowel wall and thereby produces obstruction, hemorrhage, or perforation. Slow-K is a wax-matrix tablet formulated to provide a controlled rate of release of potassium chloride and thus to minimize the possibility of a high local concentration of potassium ion near the bowel wall. While the reported frequency of small-bowel lesions is much less with wax-matrix tablets (less than one per 100,000 patient-years) than with enteric-coated potassium chloride tablets (40–50 per 100,000 patient-years) cases associated with wax-matrix tablets have been reported both in foreign countries and in the United States. In addition, perhaps because the wax-matrix preparations are not enteric-coated and release potassium in the stomach, there have been reports of upper gastrointestinal bleeding associated with these products. The total number of gastrointestinal lesions remains less than one per 100,000 patient-years. Slow-K should be discontinued immediately and the possibility of bowel obstruction or perforation considered if severe vomiting, abdominal pain, distention, or gastrointestinal bleeding occurs.

Metabolic acidosis

Hypokalemia in patients with metabolic *acidosis* should be treated with an alkalinizing potassium salt such as potassium bicarbonate, potassium citrate, or potassium acetate.

Precautions: The diagnosis of potassium depletion is ordinarily made by demonstrating hypokalemia in a patient with a clinical history suggesting some cause for potassium depletion. In interpreting the serum potassium level, the physician should bear in mind that acute alkalosis *per se* can produce hypokalemia in the absence of a deficit in total body potassium, while acute acidosis *per se* can increase the serum potassium concentration into the normal range even in the presence of a reduced total body potassium. The treatment of potassium depletion, particularly in the presence of cardiac disease, renal disease, or acidosis, requires careful attention to acid-base balance and appropriate monitoring of serum electrolytes, the electrocardiogram, and the clinical status of the patient.

Adverse Reactions: The most common adverse reactions to oral potassium salts are nausea, vomiting, abdominal discomfort, and diarrhea. These symptoms are due to irritation of the gastrointestinal tract and are best managed by diluting the preparation further, taking the dose with meals, or reducing the dose. One of the most severe adverse effects is hyperkalemia (see Contraindications, Warnings and Overdosage). There also have been reports of upper and lower gastrointestinal conditions including obstruction, bleeding, ulceration and perforation (see Contraindications and Warnings); other factors known to be associated with such conditions were present in many of these patients.

Skin rash has been reported rarely.

Overdosage: The administration of oral potassium salts to persons with normal excretory mechanisms for potassium rarely causes serious hyperkalemia. However, if excretory mechanisms are impaired or if potassium is administered too rapidly intravenously, potentially fatal hyperkalemia can result (see Con-

traindications and Warnings). It is important to recognize that hyperkalemia is usually asymptomatic and may be manifested only by an increased serum potassium concentration and characteristic electrocardiographic changes (peaking of T-waves, loss of P-wave, depression of S-T segment, and prolongation of the QT interval). Late manifestations include muscle paralysis and cardiovascular collapse from cardiac arrest.
Treatment measures for hyperkalemia include the following: (1) elimination of foods and medications containing potassium and of potassium-sparing diuretics; (2) intravenous administration of 300 to 500 ml/hr of 10% dextrose solution containing 10–20 units of insulin per 1,000 ml; (3) correction of acidosis, if present, with intravenous sodium bicarbonate; (4) use of exchange resins, hemodialysis, or peritoneal dialysis.
In treating hyperkalemia, it should be recalled that in patients who have been stabilized on digitalis, too rapid a lowering of the serum potassium concentration can produce digitalis toxicity.
Dosage and Administration: The usual dietary intake of potassium by the average adult is 40 to 80 mEq per day. Potassium depletion sufficient to cause hypokalemia usually requires the loss of 200 or more mEq of potassium from the total body store. Dosage must be adjusted to the individual needs of each patient but is typically in the range of 20 mEq per day for the prevention of hypokalemia to 40–100 mEq per day or more for the treatment of potassium depletion.
Note: Slow-K slow-release tablets must be swallowed whole and never crushed or chewed.
How Supplied: *Tablets* (pale orange, sugar-coated), each containing 600 mg potassium chloride (equivalent to 8 mEq); bottles of 100, 1000 and Accu-Pak® blister units of 100.
C78-23 Rev. 4/78
[*Shown in Product Identification Section*]

VIOFORM®
(iodochlorhydroxyquin NF)

Listed in NF, a Medicare designated compendium.

Indications and Directions For Use:
A soothing antifungal and antibacterial preparation for the treatment of inflamed conditions of the skin, such as eczema, athlete's foot and other fungal infections.
Apply to the affected area 2 or 3 times a day or use as directed by physician.
Caution: May prove irritating to sensitized skin in rare cases. If this should occur, discontinue treatment and consult physician. May stain.
KEEP OUT OF REACH OF CHILDREN.
How Supplied:
Ointment, 3% iodochlorhydroxyquin in a petrolatum base; tubes of 1 ounce.
Cream, 3% iodochlorhydroxyquin in a water-washable base; tubes of 1 ounce.
Rev. 1/76

VIOFORM®-HYDROCORTISONE ℞
(iodochlorhydroxyquin and hydrocortisone)

Indications
Based on a review of this drug by the National Academy of Sciences-National Research Council and/or other information, FDA has classified the indications as follows:
"Possibly" effective: Contact or atopic dermatitis; impetiginized eczema; nummular eczema; infantile eczema; endogenous chronic infectious dermatitis; stasis dermatitis; pyoderma; nuchal eczema and chronic eczematoid otitis externa; acne urticata; localized or disseminated neurodermatitis; lichen simplex chronicus; anogenital pruritus (vulvae, scroti, ani); folliculitis; bacterial dermatoses; mycotic dermatoses such as tinea (capitis, cruris, corporis, pedis); moniliasis; intertrigo.
Final classification of the less-than-effective indications requires further investigation.

Contraindications: Hypersensitivity to Vioform-Hydrocortisone, or any of its ingredients or related compounds; lesions of the eye; tuberculosis of the skin; most viral skin lesions (including herpes simplex, vaccinia, and varicella).
Warnings: *This product is not for ophthalmic use.*
In the presence of systemic infections, appropriate systemic antibiotics should be used.
Usage in Pregnancy: Although topical steroids have not been reported to have an adverse effect on pregnancy, the safety of their use in pregnant women has not been absolutely established. In laboratory animals, increases in incidence of fetal abnormalities have been associated with exposure of gestating females to topical corticosteroids, in some cases at rather low dosage levels. Therefore, drugs of this class should not be used extensively on pregnant patients in large amounts or for prolonged periods of time.
Precautions: May prove irritating to sensitized skin in rare cases. If irritation occurs, discontinue therapy. Staining of skin and fabrics may occur. Additionally, there are rare reports of discoloration of hair and nails.
Signs and symptoms of systemic toxicity, electrolyte imbalance, or adrenal suppression have not been reported with Vioform-Hydrocortisone. Nevertheless, the possibility of suppression of the pituitary-adrenal axis during therapy should be kept in mind, especially when the drug is used under occlusive dressings, for a prolonged period, or for treating extensive cutaneous areas since significant absorption of corticosteroid may occur under these conditions, particularly in children and infants.
Vioform may be absorbed through the skin and interfere with thyroid function tests. If such tests are contemplated, wait at least one month between discontinuation of therapy and performance of these tests. The ferric chloride test for phenylketonuria (PKU) can yield a false-positive result if Vioform is present in the diaper or urine.
Prolonged use may result in overgrowth of nonsusceptible organisms requiring appropriate therapy.
Adverse Reactions: There have been a few reports of rash and hypersensitivity.
The following local adverse reactions have been reported with topical corticosteroids, especially under occlusive dressings: burning; itching; irritation; dryness; folliculitis; hypertrichosis; acneiform eruptions; hypopigmentation; perioral dermatitis; allergic contact dermatitis; maceration of the skin; secondary infection; skin atrophy; striae; miliaria. Discontinue therapy if any untoward reaction occurs.
Dosage and Administration: Apply a thin layer to the affected parts 3 or 4 times daily. The *Cream,* because of its slight drying effect, is primarily useful for moist, weeping lesions; the *Lotion* is particularly suitable for application behind the ears and in intertriginous areas of the body; the *Ointment* is best used for dry lesions accompanied by thickening and scaling of the skin.
The *Mild Cream* and *Mild Ointment* should be used when treating lesions involving extensive body areas or less severe dermatoses.
How Supplied: *Cream,* 3% iodochlorhydroxyquin and 1% hydrocortisone in a water-washable base containing stearyl alcohol, cetyl alcohol, stearic acid, petrolatum, sodium lauryl sulfate, and glycerin in water; tubes of 5 and 20 Gm.
Ointment, 3% iodochlorhydroxyquin and 1% hydrocortisone in a petrolatum base; tubes of 20 Gm.
Lotion, 3% iodochlorhydroxyquin and 1% hydrocortisone in a water-washable base containing stearic acid, cetyl alcohol, lanolin, propylene glycol, sorbitan trioleate, polysorbate 60, triethanolamine, methylparaben, propylparaben, and perfume Flora in water; plastic squeeze bottles of 15 ml.
Mild Cream, 3% iodochlorhydroxyquin and 0.5% hydrocortisone in a water-washable base containing stearyl alcohol, cetyl alcohol, stearic acid, petrolatum, sodium lauryl sulfate, and glycerin in water; tubes of ½ and 1 ounce.
Mild Ointment, 3% iodochlorohydroxyquin and 0.5% hydrocortisone in a petrolatum base; tubes of 1 ounce. C79-1 (5/79)

Circle Pharmaceuticals, Inc.
4553 ALLISONVILLE ROAD
INDIANAPOLIS, IN 46205

AROMATIC ELIXIR, USP OTC
Pleasantly flavored vehicle containing 22% alcohol.
How Supplied: Gallon

TUSQUELIN ℞
Composition: Each teaspoonful (5 ml.) contains: Dextromethorphan HBr, 15 mg.; Chlorpheniramine Maleate, 2 mg.; Phenylpropanolamine HCl, 5 mg.; Phenylephrine HCl, 5 mg.; Fluidextract Ipecac, 0.17 min.; Potassium Guaiacolsulfonate, 44 mg.; Alcohol, 5%.
Action and Uses: Tusquelin is a very palatable antitussive with expectorant, antihistamine, bronchodilating, and nasal decongestant action, suitable for all ages.
Administration and Dosage: *Adults*—One or two teaspoonfuls four times a day, or more, as indicated. *Children*—½ to 1 teaspoonful three or four times a day, as indicated.
Side Effects: If side effects are encountered, dosage should be reduced or medication withdrawn. Professional care in supervising dosage for the very young is essential.
Precautions: This preparation may cause drowsiness. Do not drive or operate machinery while taking this medication. Do not give to children under six years of age or exceed the recommended dosage unless directed by physician. Individuals with high blood pressure, heart disease, diabetes or thyroid disease should use only as directed by physician.
Contraindications: Sensitivity to any of the components.
How Supplied: Syrup, pints. (In a pleasant vanilla-citrus syrup base.)
Literature Available: Yes.

Comatic Laboratories, Inc.
P. O. BOX 42300
HOUSTON, TEXAS 77042

NDC 0552	Product	
5000-32	GUAIFENESIN SYRUP Guaifenesin 100mg/5ml	OTC
5005-16	PSEUDOEPHEDRINE SYRUP Pseudoephedrine HCl 30mg/5 ml	OTC
5010-16	ACETAMINOPHEN WITH CODEINE ELIXIR Acetaminophen 120mg/5ml Codeine Phosphate 12mg/5ml	℞ Ⓒ
5030-12	BISACODYL SUPPOSITORIES Bisacodyl 10mg each	OTC
5035-31	DIBUCAINE OINTMENT Dibucaine 1%	OTC
5045-16	GUAIFENESIN-DEXTROMETHORPHAN SYRUP Guaifenesin 100mg/5ml Dextromethorphan HBr 15 mg/5 ml	OTC
5055-50	ASPIRIN SUPPOSITORIES Aspirin 2, 5, and 10 grains	OTC
5040-16	PHENOBARBITAL ELIXIR Phenobarbital 20mg/5ml	℞ Ⓒ

ANUPHEN® Suppositories (Rectal Acetaminophen) OTC

(See PDR For Nonprescription Drugs)

HEPAHYDRIN TABLETS

(See PDR For Nonprescription Drugs)

MATROPINAL™ AND MATROPINAL FORTE ℞

Composition: *Matropinal Inserts*—Homatropine Methylbromide 10 mg., Pentobarbital 15 mg. each; *Matropinal Forte Inserts*—Homatropine Methylbromide 10 mg., Pentobarbital 90 mg. each; *Matropinal Tablets*—Homatropine Methylbromide 10 mg., Phenobarbital 15 mg. each; *Matropinal Elixir* (per 5 ml.)—Homatropine Methylbromide 10 mg., Phenobarbital 15 mg., Alcohol 15%. WARNING: Phenobarbital & Pentobarbital may be habit forming.
Indications: Matropinal dosage forms are indicated for their anticholinergic and sedative actions in nausea and vomiting.
Contraindications: Patients sensitive to individual ingredients; patients with porphyria or familial tendency severe hepatitis or severe renal disease.
Precautions: Use cautiously in patients with liver disease. Use only under direct physician supervision in the presence of narrow angle glaucoma and prostatic hypertrophy.
Drug Interaction Precaution: No barbiturate therapy should be started or stopped on patients taking anticoagulants without the careful adjustment of the anticoagulant dosage.
Adverse Reactions: In susceptible individuals, dry mouth, blurred vision or drowsiness may occur. Observe caution in operating machinery to avoid injury due to possible impairment of alertness and coordination.
Dosage: Matropinal Inserts: Children and Adults 1 or 2 rectally or vaginally Q3-4 h.
Matropinal Elixir: Children and Adults 1-2 tsp. q.i.d.

Matropinal™ Pediatric Dosage

Weight	Matropinal™ Inserts	Matropinal™ Elixir
11 lbs.	1 Q. 6h	½ tsp Q. 6h
24 lbs.	2 stat. 1 Q. 4h	1 tsp Q. 6h
40 lbs. +	2 Q. 4h	1½ tsp Q. 6h

Individualize Dosage
NOTE: LD_{50} studies have shown that toxicity of the Matropinal combination is almost identical to the toxicity of the barbiturate content alone. Consequently, rectal dosage by weight may be calculated on the basis of 12 mg./kg. of the barbiturate content *per 24 hours.* Oral dosage may be calculated using 6 mg./kg. per 24 hours.
Matropinal Tablets: 1–2 tabs. q.i.d.; children 1 tab. q.i.d.
Matropinal Forte Inserts: Adults 1-2 rectally or vaginally Q4-6 h.
INDIVIDUALIZE ALL DOSAGES TO PATIENT.
How Supplied: *Matropinal Inserts*—NDC 0552-0311-12, Package of 12; *Matropinal Forte Inserts*—NDC 0552-0411-12, Package of 12; *Matropinal Tablets*—NDC 0552-0312-01, Bottle of 100; *Matropinal Elixir*—NDC 0552-0313-16, Pint.
NOTE: MATROPINAL PRODUCTS DO NOT CONTAIN ARTIFICIAL COLORS.
Storage Requirements: Inserts—Store below 95°F.
Tablets and Elixir—Store at room temperature in a tight, light resistant container.
Caution: Federal law prohibits dispensing without a prescription.

ORAPHEN-PD™ (Additive Free) OTC

(See PDR For Nonprescription Drugs)

RHINOSYN® CAPSULES ℞

Composition:
Chlorpheniramine Maleate ....10 mg.
Pseudoephedrine Hydrochloride ....120 mg.
Description: Each sustained release capsule contains chlorpheniramine maleate 10 mg., pseudoephedrine hydrochloride 120 mg. Chlorpheniramine maleate is a synthetic compound that antagonizes many of the characteristic effects of histamine. It has a wide margin of safety, high potency and low frequency of undesirable side effects. Chlorpheniramine maleate controls rhinorrhea, sneezing, and lacrimation in allergic and infectious disorders of the respiratory tract. A physiologically active stereoisomer of ephedrine, pseudoephedrine hydrochloride has a pronounced decongestant effect on nasopharynx and paranasal sinuses as well as on the eustachian tubes. Its action appears to be more specific on blood vessels of the nasal and respiratory tract mucous membranes and less specific on blood vessels of the systemic circulation. The decongestant action takes effect in 15 to 30 minutes, with full effect occurring within 30 to 60 minutes.
Indications: For the relief of congestion, edema, and hypersecretion associated with allergies and infections of the upper respiratory tract, including sinusitis, pharyngitis, the common cold, influenza, vasomotor rhinitis, allergic rhinitis and hay fever, acute eustachian salpingitis and otitis media with eustachian tube congestion.
Contraindications: Sensitivity to the individual ingredients.
Precautions: Although pseudoephedrine is virtually without pressor effect in normotensive patients, it should be used with caution in hypertensives.
Caution: Use with caution in patients with hyperthyroidism, diabetes mellitus, organic heart disease, asthma, difficulty in urination due to prostatic hypertrophy, glaucoma, cardiovascular disease, hypertension, or in patients receiving MAO inhibitors. If drowsiness develops, reduce dosage or discontinue. Persons experiencing drowsiness should not drive or operate machinery. Avoid consuming alcoholic beverages while taking this medication.
Adverse Reactions: While the majority of patients will experience no side effects, those particularly sensitive to sympathomimetic drugs may note mild stimulation. Slight to moderate drowsiness occurs relatively infrequently with chlorpheniramine maleate. Should side effects develop, reduce dosage or discontinue.
Dosage and Administration: Usual adult dosage is one capsule every 12 hours. Individualize dosage.
Storage Requirements: Store at room temperature in a tight, light resistant container.
Supply: NDC 0552-0904-01 bottles of 100 capsules.
Caution: Federal law prohibits dispensing without a prescription.

RHINOSYN® SYRUP (Additive Free) OTC
RHINOSYN®-PD (Additive Free)
RHINOSYN®-DM (Additive Free)
RHINOSYN®-DMX (Additive Free)
RHINOSYN®-X (Additive Free)

(See PDR For Nonprescription Drugs)

Comer Pharmaceuticals, Inc.
POST OFFICE BOX 5471
HAMDEN, CT 06518

NDC-48652	Product	
64280	AMOXICILLIN (Amoxicillin Trihydrate) CAPSULES 250 mg., 100s ea. 500 mg., 50s ea. ORAL SUSPENSION 125 mg./5 cc., 80 cc. ea. 125 mg./5 cc., 100 cc. ea. 125 mg./5 cc., 150 cc. ea. 250 mg./5 cc., 80 cc. ea. 250 mg./5 cc., 100 cc. ea. 250 mg./5 cc., 150 cc. ea.	℞
64290	AMPICILLIN CAPSULES (Maroon & Gray) 250 mg., 100s ea. 250 mg., 500s ea. 500 mg., 100s ea. POWDER (Cherry Flavor) 125 mg., 100 cc. ea. 125 mg., 200 cc. ea. 250 mg., 100 cc. ea. 250 mg., 200 cc. ea.	℞
64300	ERYTHROMYCIN STEARATE FILM TABS., (Pink) 250 mg., 100s ea.	℞
64310	PENICILLIN G POTASSIUM TABLETS (White Scored) 400,000 U. 100s ea.	℞
64320	PENICILLIN VK POWDER (Cherry Flavor) 125 mg., 100 cc. ea. 125 mg., 200 cc. ea. 250 mg., 100 cc. ea. 250 mg., 200 cc. ea. TABLETS (White Scored) 250 mg., 100s (oval) 250 mg., 1000s (oval) 500 mg., 100s (round)	℞
64330	PREDNISONE TABLETS (White Scored) 5 mg., 1000s	℞
64340	TETRACYCLINE HCl CAPSULES (Orange & Yellow) 250 mg., 100s 250 mg., 1000s CAPSULES (Black & Yellow) 500 mg., 100s	℞

Connaught Laboratories, Inc.

SWIFTWATER, PA 18370

Distributed in the Continental U.S.A. by:
Elkins-Sinn, Inc.
2 Esterbrook Lane
Cherry Hill, NJ 08034

The following is a product listing only. Full product and prescribing information is contained in the package insert.

DIPHTHERIA ANTITOXIN, USP ℞
(Purified, Concentrated Globulin, EQUINE)

Expiration Dating—60 Months
How Supplied: 20,000 unit vial.

DIPHTHERIA AND TETANUS TOXOIDS AND PERTUSSIS VACCINE, ADSORBED, USP ℞
(For Pediatric Use)

Expiration Dating—18 Months
How Supplied: 7.5 ml vial.

FLUZONE® ℞
(Influenza Virus Vaccine, USP)
(Formula consistent with current USPHS recommendations)

Expiration Dating—18 Months
How Supplied: 0.5 ml unit dose syringe, package of 5; 5 ml vial (10 doses, 0.5 ml each).

MENOMUNE®- A/C ℞
(Meningococcal Polysaccharide Vaccine, Groups A and C Combined)

Expiration Dating—18 Months
How Supplied: 10 dose vial with 6 ml diluent (needle and syringe administration); 50 dose vial with 27.5 ml diluent (jet injector administration only).
Also available as single-entity vaccines, Group A or Group C. Contact Elkins-Sinn for information.

TETANUS AND DIPHTHERIA TOXOIDS ADSORBED, USP ℞
(For Adult Use)

Expiration Dating—24 Months
How Supplied: 0.5 ml unit dose syringe, package of 5; 5 ml vial.

TETANUS TOXOID ADSORBED, USP ℞

Expiration Dating—24 Months
How Supplied: 0.5 ml unit dose syringe, package of 5; 5 ml vial.

TETANUS TOXOID, USP ℞

Expiration Dating—24 Months
How Supplied: 0.5 ml unit dose syringe, package of 5; 7.5 ml vial

YELLOW FEVER VACCINE, USP ℞

Expiration Dating—12 Months
How Supplied: 5 dose vial with 3 ml diluent; 20 dose vial with 12 ml diluent.

Products are cross-indexed

by product classifications

in the

BLUE SECTION

Connaught Laboratories, Ltd.

1755 STEELES AVENUE WEST
WILLOWDALE, ONTARIO M2N5T8, CANADA

Distributed in the Continental U.S.A. by:
Elkins-Sinn, Inc.
2 Esterbrook Lane
Cherry Hill, NJ 08034

The following is a product listing only. Full product and prescribing information is contained in the package insert.

ALBUCONN™ ℞
(Normal Serum Albumin [Human], USP)

Expiration Dating—36 Months
How Supplied: 5% Concentration 250 ml bottle (12.5g); 500 ml bottle (25g). 25% Concentration 50 ml bottle (12.5g).

POLIOMYELITIS VACCINE (PURIFIED) ℞
(For the prevention of Poliomyelitis [Inactivated, Salk Type])

Expiration Dating—12 Months
How Supplied: 1 ml ampul, package of 5; 10 ml vial.

TET–CONN–G™ ℞
(Tetanus Immune Globulin [Human], USP)

Expiration Dating—24 Months
How Supplied: 250 unit disposable syringe, package of 10; 250 unit vial, package of 10.

TUBERSOL® ℞
Tuberculin Purified Protein Derivative (Mantoux)

Expiration Dating—18 Months
How Supplied: 1 U.S. Unit (TU) per test dose (0.1 ml), package of 10 vials; 5 U.S. Units (TU) per test dose (0.1 ml), package of 10 vials and 50 vials; 250 U.S. Units (TU) per test dose (0.1 ml), package of 10 vials.

TUBERCULIN PURIFIED PROTEIN DERIVATIVE ℞
(Concentrated Solution in 50% Glycerine for Sterneedle® [Heaf] Multiple Puncture Test)

Expiration Dating—24 Months
How Supplied: 1 ml vial.

Important Notice

Before prescribing or administering

any product described in

PHYSICIANS' DESK REFERENCE

always consult the PDR Supplement for

possible new or revised information.

Products are cross-indexed by

generic and chemical names

in the

YELLOW SECTION

Consolidated Chemical, Inc.

3224 SOUTH KINGSHIGHWAY BLVD.
ST. LOUIS, MISSOURI 63139

FORMULA MAGIC® OTC
Antibacterial Body Powder

Composition: Talc, Mineral Oil, Magnesium Carbonate, Fragrance, Triclosan 0.19%. NDC 46706-202.
Action: Talc based body powder and nursing lubricant. Prevents excoriation and friction chafing. Reduces harmful bacteria. Reduces odor.
Precautions: Non-skin irritating. Practically non-toxic (MLD 20,000 mg/kg). Slight eye irritant-in case of eye contact flush with water.
Dosage and Administration: Apply liberally to patients body and bedding. Provides protective film against chafing.
How Supplied: 4 oz., 12 oz.

SATIN™ OTC
Antibacterial Skin Cleanser

Composition: Water, Ammonium Laureth Sulfate, Cocamide DEA, PEG-8, Glycol Stearate, Sodium Cocoyl Sarcosinate, PEG-85 Lanolin, Citric Acid, Fragrance, Triclosan 1:400. NDC 46706-101.
Action: Skin cleanser and shampoo for daily use. Reduces harmful bacteria. Reduces odor.
Precautions: Non-skin irritating. Practically non-toxic (LD_{50} 22,500 mg/kg). Moderate eye irritant-in case of eye contact flush with water.
Dosage and Administration: Apply to dampened washcloth. Wash in the normal manner. Rinse thoroughly.
How Supplied: 8 oz., 16 oz., 1 gallon.

SKIN MAGIC™ OTC
Antibacterial Skin Lotion

Composition: Water, Stearic Acid, Mineral Oil, Propylene Glycol, Isostearyl Alcohol, Glycol Stearate, Stearamide DEA, Triethanolamine, Cetyl Alcohol, Myristyl Propionate, PEG-40 Lanolin, Fragrance, Methylparaben, Carbomer 934, Sodium Borate. Triclosan 0.12%. NDC 46706-201.
Action: Emollient body rub and skin lotion. Soothes and moisturizes dry chapped skin. Reduces harmful bacteria. Reduces odor.
Precautions: Non-skin irritating. Practically non-toxic. (MLD 25,100 mg/kg). Slight eye irritant-in case of eye contact flush with water.
Dosage and Administration: Apply liberally, massage into skin.
How Supplied: 4 oz., 8 oz., 1 gallon.

IDENTIFICATION PROBLEM?

Consult PDR's

Product Identification Section

where you'll find over 900

products pictured actual size

and in full color.

Cook-Waite Laboratories, Inc.

90 PARK AVENUE
NEW YORK, NEW YORK 10016

CARBOCAINE® ℞
hydrochloride 3% Injection
(brand of mepivacaine hydrochloride injection, USP)
CARBOCAINE® ℞
hydrochloride 2%
with NEO-COBEFRIN®
1:20,000 Injection
(brand of mepivacaine hydrochloride and levonordefrin injection, NF)

THESE SOLUTIONS ARE INTENDED FOR DENTAL USE ONLY.

Description: Mepivacaine hydrochloride is 1-methyl-2′, 6′-pipecoloxylidide monohydrochloride.

It is a white, crystalline, odorless powder soluble in water, but very resistant to both acid and alkaline hydrolysis.

Levonordefrin is (−)-α-(1-Aminoethyl)-3, 4-dihydroxybenzyl alcohol.

It is a white or buff-colored crystalline solid, freely soluble in aqueous solutions of mineral acids, but practically insoluble in water.

DENTAL CARTRIDGES MAY NOT BE AUTOCLAVED.

COMPOSITION	CARTRIDGE	
Each ml contains:	2%	3%
mepivacaine hydrochloride	20.0 mg	30.0 mg
levonordefrin	0.05 mg	—
sodium chloride	4.0 mg	3.0 mg
acetone sodium bisulfite not more than	2.0 mg	—
water for injection qs ad	1.0 ml	1.0 ml

The pH of the 2% cartridge solution is adjusted between 3.3 and 5.5 with NaOH or HCl.

The pH of the 3% cartridge solution is adjusted between 4.5 and 6.8 with NaOH or HCl.

Clinical Pharmacology: Carbocaine stabilizes the neuronal membrane and prevents the initiation and transmission of nerve impulses, thereby effecting local anesthesia.

CARBOCAINE is rapidly metabolized, with only a small percentage of the anesthetic (5 to 10 per cent) being excreted unchanged in the urine. CARBOCAINE, because of its amide structure, is not detoxified by the circulating plasma esterases. The liver is the principal site of metabolism, with over 50 per cent of the administered dose being excreted into the bile as metabolites. Most of the metabolized mepivacaine is probably resorbed in the intestine and then excreted into the urine since only a small percentage is found in the feces. The principal route of excretion is via the kidney. Most of the anesthetic and its metabolites are eliminated within 30 hours. It has been shown that hydroxylation and N-demethylation, which are detoxification reactions, play important roles in the metabolism of the anesthetic. Three metabolites of mepivacaine have been identified from adult humans: two phenols, which are excreted almost exclusively as their glucuronide conjugates, and the N-demethylated compound (2′,6′-pipecoloxylidide).

The onset of action is rapid (30 to 120 seconds in the upper jaw; 1 to 4 minutes in the lower jaw) and CARBOCAINE Hydrochloride 3% without vasoconstrictor will ordinarily provide operating anesthesia of 20 minutes in the upper jaw and 40 minutes in the lower jaw.

Carbocaine hydrochloride 2% with Neo-Cobefrin 1:20,000 (brand of mepivacaine hydrochloride and levonordefrin injection) provides anesthesia of longer duration for more prolonged procedures, 1 hour to 2.5 hours in the upper jaw and 2.5 hours to 5.5 hours in the lower jaw. Carbocaine does not ordinarily produce irritation or tissue damage.

Neo-Cobefrin (brand of levonordefrin) is a sympathomimetic amine used as a vasoconstrictor in local anesthetic solutions. It has pharmacologic activity similar to that of epinephrine but it is more stable than epinephrine. In equal concentrations, Neo-Cobefrin is less potent than epinephrine in raising blood pressure, and as a vasoconstrictor.

Indications: Carbocaine is indicated for the production of local anesthesia for dental procedures by infiltration injection or nerve block.

Contraindications: Mepivacaine is contraindicated in patients with a known hypersensitivity to amide type local anesthetics.

Warnings: RESUSCITATIVE EQUIPMENT AND DRUGS SHOULD BE IMMEDIATELY AVAILABLE. (See Adverse Reactions).

Reactions resulting in fatality have occurred on rare occasions with the use of local anesthetics, even in the absence of a history of hypersensitivity.

The solution which contains a vasoconstrictor should be used with extreme caution for patients whose medical history and physical evaluation suggest the existence of hypertension, arteriosclerotic heart disease, cerebral vascular insufficiency, heart block, thyrotoxicosis and diabetes, etc. The solution which contains a vasoconstrictor, should also be used with extreme caution in patients receiving drugs known to produce blood pressure alterations (i.e., MAO inhibitors, tricyclic anti-depressants, phenothiazines, etc.) as either sustained hypotension or hypertension may occur.

Usage in Children. Great care must be exercised in adhering to safe concentrations and dosages for pedodontic administration (see Dosage and Administration).

Usage in Pregnancy. Safe use of mepivacaine has not been established with respect to adverse effects on fetal development. Careful consideration should be given to this fact before administration during pregnancy.

Local anesthetic procedures should be used with caution when there is inflammation and/or sepsis in the region of the proposed injection.

Precautions: The safety and effectiveness of mepivacaine depend upon proper dosage, correct technique, adequate precautions, and readiness for emergencies.

The lowest dose that results in effective anesthesia should be used to avoid high plasma levels and possible adverse effects. Injection of repeated doses of mepivacaine may cause significant increase in blood levels with each repeated dose due to slow accumulation of the drug or its metabolites, or due to slower metabolic degradation than normal.

Tolerance varies with the status of the patient. Debilitated, elderly patients, acutely ill patients, and children should be given reduced doses commensurate with their weight and physical status.

Mepivacaine should be used with caution in patients with a history of severe disturbances of cardiac rhythm or heart block.

INJECTIONS SHOULD ALWAYS BE MADE SLOWLY WITH ASPIRATION TO AVOID INTRAVASCULAR INJECTION AND THEREFORE SYSTEMIC REACTION TO BOTH LOCAL ANESTHETIC AND VASCONSTRICTOR.

If sedatives are employed to reduce patient apprehension, use reduced doses, since local anesthetic agents, like sedatives, are central nervous system depressants which in combination may have an additive effect. Young children should be given minimal doses of each agent.

Changes in sensorium such as excitation, disorientation, drowsiness, may be early indications of a high blood level of the drug and may occur following inadvertent intravascular administration or rapid absorption of mepivacaine.

Solutions containing a vasoconstrictor should be used cautiously in the presence of diseases which may adversely affect the patient's cardiovascular system. Serious cardiac arrhythmias may occur if preparations containing a vasoconstrictor are employed in patients during or following the administration of chloroform, halothane, cyclopropane, trichloroethylene, or other related agents.

Mepivacaine SHOULD BE USED WITH CAUTION IN PATIENTS WITH KNOWN DRUG ALLERGIES AND SENSITIVITIES. A thorough history of the patient's prior experience with mepivacaine or other local anesthetics as well as concomitant or recent drug use should be taken (see Contraindications). Patients allergic to methylparaben or para-aminobenzoic acid derivatives (procaine, tetracaine, benzocaine, etc.) have not shown cross-sensitivity to agents of the amide type such as mepivacaine.

Since mepivacaine is metabolized in the liver and excreted by the kidneys, it should be used cautiously in patients with liver and renal disease.

Adverse Reactions: Systemic adverse reactions involving the central nervous system and the cardiovascular system usually result from high plasma levels due to excessive dosage, rapid absorption, or inadvertent intravascular injection.

A small number of reactions may result from hypersensitivity, idiosyncrasy or diminished tolerance to normal dosage on the part of the patient.

Reactions involving the *central nervous system* are characterized by excitation and/or depression. Nervousness, dizziness, blurred vision, or tremors may occur followed by drowsiness, convulsions, unconsciousness, and possibly respiratory arrest. Since excitement may be transient or absent, the first manifestations may be drowsiness merging into unconsciousness and respiratory arrest.

Reactions involving the *cardiovascular system* include depression of the myocardium, hypotension, bradycardia, and even cardiac arrest.

Allergic reactions are rare and may occur as a result of sensitivity to the local anesthetic and are characterized by cutaneous lesions of delayed onset or urticaria, edema and other manifestations of allergy. The detection of sensitivity by skin testing is of limited value. As with other local anesthetics, anaphylactoid reactions to CARBOCAINE have occurred rarely. The reaction may be abrupt and severe and is not usually dose related.

Treatment of a patient with toxic manifestations consists of assuring and maintaining a patent airway and supporting ventilation (respiration) as required. This usually will be sufficient in the management of most reactions. Should a convulsion persist despite ventilatory therapy, small increments of anticonvulsive agents may be given intravenously, such as benzodiazepine (e.g., diazepam) or ultra-short acting barbiturates (e.g., thiopental or thiamylal) or short-acting barbiturate (e.g., pentobarbital or secobarbital). Cardiovascular depression may require circulatory assistance with intravenous fluids and/or vasopressor (e.g., ephedrine) as dictated by the clinical situation.

Allergic reactions should be managed by conventional means.

Dosage and Administration: As with all local anesthetics, the dose varies and depends upon the area to be anesthetized, the vascularity of the tissues, individual tolerance and the technique of anesthesia. The lowest dose needed to provide effective anesthesia should be administered. For specific techniques and procedures refer to standard dental manuals and textbooks.

For infiltration and block injections in the upper or lower jaw, the average dose of 1 cartridge will usually suffice.

Each cartridge contains 1.8 ml. (36 mg. of 2% or 54 mg. of 3%).

Five cartridges (180 mg. of the 2% solution or 270 mg. of the 3% solution) are usually adequate to effect anesthesia of the entire oral cavity. Whenever a larger dose seems to be necessary for an extensive procedure, the maximum dose should be calculated according to that patient's weight. A dose of up to 3 mg. per pound of body weight may be administered. At any single dental sitting the total dose for all injected sites should not exceed 400 mg.

When using CARBOCAINE for infiltration or regional block anesthesia, injection should always be made slowly and with frequent aspiration.

Any usused portion of a cartridge should be discarded.

Disinfection of Cartridges: As in the case of any cartridge, the diaphragm should be disinfected before needle puncture. The diaphragm should be thoroughly swabbed with either pure 91% isopropyl alcohol or 70% ethyl alcohol, USP just prior to use. Many commercially available alcohol solutions contain ingredients which are injurious to container components, and therefore, should not be used. Cartridges should not be immersed in any solution.

How Supplied: Both formulas are available in 1.8 ml. cartridges, cans of 50, to fit the Carpule® Aspirator.

Carbocaine and Neo-Cobefrin
are the registered trademarks
of Sterling Drug Inc.
Revised September 1979 CO A142A (799)

For full prescribing information on the medical use of Carbocaine, see Breon Laboratories product listing in this publication.

Cooper Laboratories, Inc.

INTERNAL MEDICINE DIVISION
(See Berlex Laboratories Inc.)

Cutter Biological

DIV. CUTTER LABORATORIES, INC.
4TH & PARKER STS.
BERKELEY, CA 94710

GAMASTAN® ℞
(Immune Serum Globulin—Human U.S.P.)
2 ml., 10 ml. vials

HYPERAB® ℞
(Rabies Immune Globulin—Human)
2 ml. (300 IU) pediatric vial
10 ml. (1500 IU) adult vial

HYPERHEP™ ℞
(Hepatitis B Immune Globulin—Human)
1 ml., 4 ml., 5 ml. vials

HYPER-TET® ℞
(Tetanus Immune Globulin—Human U.S.P.)
250 units vial or prefilled disposable syringe

HYPERTUSSIS® ℞
(Pertussis Immune Globulin—Human, U.S.P.)
1.25 ml. vial

HypRho®-D ℞
(Rh$_0$D Immune Globulin—Human)
Unit dose vial with crossmatch reagent and forms.

KOĀTE® ℞
(Antihemophilic Factor—Human—Factor VIII, AHF, AHG)
250 AHF units, approx., with 10 ml. Sterile Water for Injection, U.S.P., and sterile filter needle.
500 AHF units, approx., with 20 ml. Sterile Water for Injection, U.S.P., and sterile filter needle.
1000 AHF units, approx., with 40 ml. Sterile Water for Injection, U.S.P., and sterile filter needle.

KONŸNE® ℞
(Factor IX Complex—Human—Factors II, VII, IX and X)
500 unit vial

PLAGUE VACCINE, U.S.P. ℞
2 ml., 20 ml. vials

Dalin Pharmaceuticals, Inc.

1750 NEW HIGHWAY
FARMINGDALE, NY 11735

DALIDYNE
Lotion
Effective Treatment for the Oral Cavity

Composition: Methylbenzethonium Chloride, Benzocaine, Tannic Acid, Camphor, Chlorothymol, Menthol, Benzyl Alcohol in a Specially Prepared Aromatized Base. Alcohol 61%.

Action and Uses: A cooling, soothing, quick-drying lotion possessing germicidal, fungicidal, anesthetic, astringent and healing properties used in the treatment of: Aphthous Stomatitis • Teething Pains • Herpes Simplex • Denture Irritations • Trench Mouth • Cheilosis, Avitaminosis • Thrush • Gingivitis • Throat Irritations (as mouth wash or gargle).

Administration and Dosage: Topical Application: Dry area and apply several times a day with cotton applicator. As Gargle or Mouth Wash: ½ teaspoonful in ½ glass of warm water several times a day.

How Supplied: 1 Fl. Oz.

SORBUTUSS®
Sugar Free for the Diabetic Cough Patient

Composition: Each teaspoonful (5 cc.) contains d-methorphan hydrobromide 10 mg., glycerol guaiacolate 100 mg., ipecac fluid extract 0.05 min., potassium citrate 85 mg., citric acid 35 mg., in a palatable, mint-flavored, glycerin-sorbitol vehicle.

Action and Uses: Effective sugar-free antitussive and expectorant with demulcent properties for relief of coughs and coughs due to colds.

	• Sugar	• Decongestants
No	• Sodium	• Alcohol
	• Antihistamines	

Recommended for all patients including diabetic, cardiac, hypertensive and geriatric. Soothing for coughs due to smoking.

Administration and Dosage: *Adults*—1 to 2 teaspoonfuls every 3 to 4 hours. *Children*—in proportion.

How Supplied: Pints and gallons.

Remarks: SUGAR-FREE and SODIUM-FREE, NON-NARCOTIC and NON-ALCOHOLIC.

Daywell Laboratories Corporation

78 UNQUOWA PLACE
FAIRFIELD, CT 06430

VERGO®

Composition: Vergo contains Pancin®, a special formulation of calcium pantothenate, ascorbic acid and starch.

Action and Uses: It is believed that warts are caused by a virus, and that the widespread occurrence of warts among children is due to the infectious nature of the wart virus. The child with warts is three times more likely to develop new warts as a child who has not been infected previously. For this reason the early treatment of warts is recommended. Above all, treatment should be conservative and should not affect or injure the surrounding tissues. Vergo gives the same relief and results in the treatment of warts of the adult. Vergo is a conservative, painless and safe treatment of warts. It is convenient, easy to apply, and will not burn, blister or leave scars. The ingredients are essential to the soundness of tissues and skin and will relieve the pain of warts and promote healing. Vergo is not irritating and there are no contraindications to its use. The average treatment time is from 2 to 8 weeks depending on the size of the wart and the response of the patient. It is important that the directions be carefully followed and that treatment be continued without interruption as long as necessary. Mosaic-type warts are more resistant and usually require longer treatment for relief.

Administration and Dosage: Cleanse area with soap and water; rinse thoroughly. Apply Vergo liberally to wart or corn. Do not massage or rub in. Cover with plain Band-Aid® or gauze and adhesive tape. Change dressing and apply Vergo twice a day, morning and evening.

Side Effects: None known.

How Supplied: In one-half ounce tubes.

Product Identification Mark: Vergo®.

Literature Available: Yes.

Delco Chemical Co., Inc.

SELLERSVILLE, PA 18960

DELCOBESE CII ℞
(A SINGLE ENTITY AMPHETAMINE PREPARATION)

Amphetamines have a high potential for abuse. They should thus be tried only in weight reduction programs for patients in whom alternative therapy has been ineffective. Administration of amphetamines for prolonged period of time in obesity may lead to drug dependence and must be avoided. Particular attention should be paid to the possibility of subjects obtaining amphetamines for non-therapeutic use or distribution to others, and the drugs should be prescribed or dispensed sparingly.

Description: DELCOBESE is a single entity amphetamine preparation containing the dextro and dextrolaevo isomers of Amphetamine Adipate and Amphetamine Sulfate.

Actions: Amphetamines are sympathomimetic amines with CNS stimulant activity. Peripheral actions include elevation of systolic and diastolic blood pressures and weak bronchodilator and respiratory stimulant action. Drugs of this class used in obesity are commonly known as "anorectics" or "anorexigenics". It has not been established, however, that the action of such drugs in treating obesity is

Continued on next page

Delco—Cont.

primarily one of appetite suppression. Other central nervous system actions, or metabolic effects, may be involved, for example.
Adult obese subjects instructed in dietary management and treated with "anorectic" drugs, lose more weight on the average than those treated with placebo and diet, as determined in relatively short-term clinical trials.
The magnitude of increased weight loss of drug-treated patients over placebo-treated patients is only a fraction of a pound a week. The rate of weight loss is greatest in the first weeks of therapy for both drug and placebo subjects and tends to decrease in succeeding weeks. The origins of the increased weight loss due to the various possible drug effects are not established. The amount of weight loss associated with the use of an "anorectic" drug varies from trial to trial, and the increased weight loss appears to be related in part to variables other than the drug prescribed, such as the physician-investigator, the population treated, and the diet prescribed. Studies do not permit conclusions as to the relative importance of the drug and non-drug factors on weight loss.
The natural history of obesity is measured in years, whereas the studies cited are restricted to a few weeks duration; thus, the total impact of drug-induced weight loss over that of diet alone must be considered clinically limited.
In the treatment of children with a behavioral syndrome characterized by hyperactivity, distractibility and impulsiveness, there is neither specific evidence which clearly establishes the mechanism whereby DELCOBESE produces its mental and behavioral effects in children, nor conclusive evidence regarding how these effects relate to the condition of the central nervous system.

Indications:
Narcolepsy
Behavioral Syndrome Characterized by Hyperactivity, Distractibility and Impulsiveness in Children:
DELCOBESE Is indicated as an integral part of a total treatment program which typically includes other remedial measures (psychological, educational, social) for a stabilizing effect in children with a behavioral syndrome characterized by the following group of developmentally inappropriate symptoms: moderate to severe distractibility, short attention span, hyperactivity, emotional lability, and impulsivity. The diagnosis of this syndrome should not be made with finality when these symptoms are only of comparatively recent origin. Nonlocalizing (soft) neurological signs, learning disability, and abnormal EEG may or may not be present, and a diagnosis of central nervous system dysfunction may or may not be warranted.
Exogenous obesity: As a short-term (a few weeks) adjunct in a regimen of weight reduction based on caloric restriction, for patients refractory to alternative therapy, e.g., repeated diets, group programs, and other drugs. The limited usefulness of amphetamines (see ACTIONS) should be weighed against possible risks inherent in use of the drug, such as those described below.
Contraindications: Advanced arteriosclerosis, symptomatic cardiovascular disease, moderate to severe hypertension, hyperthyroidism, known hypersensitivity or idiosyncrasy to the sympathomimetic amines, glaucoma.
Agitated states.
Patients with a history of drug abuse.
During or within 14 days following the administration of monoamine oxidase inhibitors (hypertensive crises may result).
Warnings: When tolerance to the "anorectic" effect develops, the recommended dose should not be exceeded in an attempt to increase the effect; rather, the drug should be discontinued.
Amphetamines may impair the ability of the patient to engage in potentially hazardous activities such as operating machinery or driving a motor vehicle; the patient should therefore be cautioned accordingly.
Clinical experience suggests that in psychotic children, administration of DELCOBESE may exacerbate symptoms of behavior disturbance and thought disorder.
Data are inadequate to determine whether chronic administration of DELCOBESE may be associated with growth inhibition; therefore, growth should be monitored during treatment.
Drug Dependence: Amphetamines have been extensively abused. Tolerance, extreme psychological dependence, and severe social disability have occurred. There are reports of patients who have increased the dosage to many times that recommended. Abrupt cessation following prolonged high dosage administration results in extreme fatigue and mental depression; changes are also noted on the sleep EEG. Manifestations of chronic intoxication with amphetamines include severe dermatoses, marked insomnia, irritability, hyperactivity, and personality changes. The most severe manifestation of chronic intoxication is psychosis, often clinically indistinguishable from schizophrenia.
Usage in Pregnancy: Safe use in pregnancy has not been established. Reproduction studies in mammals at high multiples of the human dose have suggested both an embryotoxic and a teratogenic potential. Use of amphetamines by women who are or who may become pregnant, and especially those in the first trimester of pregnancy, requires that the potential benefit be weighed against the possible hazard to mother and infant.
Usage in children: Amphetamines are not recommended for use as anorectic agents in children under 12 years of age.
Precautions: Caution is to be exercised in prescribing amphetamines for patients with even mild hypertension.
Insulin requirements in diabetes mellitus may be altered in association with the use of amphetamines and the concomitant dietary regimen.
Amphetamines may decrease the hypotensive effect of guanethidine.
The least amount feasible should be prescribed or dispensed at one time in order to minimize the possibility of overdosage.
Drug treatment is not indicated in all cases of the behavioral syndrome in children and should be considered only in light of the complete history and evaluation of the child. The decision to prescribe DELCOBESE should depend on the physician's assessment of the chronicity and severity of the child's symptoms and their appropriateness for his/her age. Prescription should not depend solely on the presence of one or more of the behavioral characteristics.
When these symptoms are associated with acute stress reactions, treatment with DELCOBESE is usually not indicated.
Long-term effects of DELCOBESE in children have not been well-established.
Adverse Reactions:
Cardiovascular: Palpitation, tachycardia, elevation of blood pressure.
Central nervous system: Overstimulation, restlessness, dizziness, insomnia, euphoria, dysphoria, tremor, headache; rarely, psychotic episodes at recommended doses.
Gastrointestinal: Dryness of the mouth, unpleasant taste, diarrhea, constipation, other gastrointestinal disturbances. Anorexia and weight loss may occur as undesirable effects when amphetamines are used for other than the anorectic effect.
Allergic: Urticaria.
Endocrine: Impotence, changes in libido.
Dosage and Administration: Regardless of indication, amphetamines should be administered at the lowest effective dosage and dosage should be individually adjusted. Late evening medication should be avoided because of the resulting insomnia.

1. **Narcolepsy:** Usual dose 5 to 60 milligrams per day in divided doses.
2. **Behavioral Syndrome Characterized by Hyperactivity, Distractibility and Impulsiveness in Children:**
   a. Not recommended for children under 3 years of age.
   b. Children from 3 to 5 years of age: 2.5 milligrams daily, raised in increments of 2.5 milligrams at weekly intervals until optimal response is obtained.
   c. Children 6 years of age and older: 5 milligrams once or twice daily, increased in increments of 5 milligrams at weekly intervals. Only in rare cases will it be necessary to exceed a total of 40 milligrams per day.

Where possible, drug administration should be interrupted occasionally to determine if there is a recurrence of behavioral symptoms sufficient to require continued therapy.

3. **Obesity:** Usual adult dose 5 to 30 milligrams per day in divided doses.

Overdosage: Manifestations of acute overdosage with amphetamines include restlessness, tremor, hyperreflexia, rapid respiration, confusion, assaultiveness, hallucinations, panic states.
Fatigue and depression usually follow the central stimulation.
Cardiovascular effects include arrhythmias, hypertension or hypotension and circulatory collapse. Gastrointestinal symptoms include nausea, vomiting, diarrhea, and abdominal cramps. Fatal poisoning usually terminates in convulsions and coma.
Management of acute amphetamine intoxication is largely symptomatic and includes lavage and sedation with a barbiturate. Experience with hemodialysis or peritoneal dialysis is inadequate to permit recommendation in this regard. Acidification of the urine increases amphetamine excretion. Intravenous phentolamine (Regitine) has been suggested for possible acute, severe hypertension, if this complicates amphetamine overdosage.
Dosage: Adults: Tablets or Capsules: One tablet or capsule three times a day ½ hour before meals. Third dose should be taken at 4 P.M. to avoid insomnia.
Time Release Capsules: One sustained release capsule daily; (provides for a prolonged therapeutic effect for approximately 6 to 8 hours).
How Supplied: Available in tablets and capsules for immediate release.
[See table on next page].
Caution: Federal Law Prohibits Dispensing without Prescription.

Important Notice

Before prescribing or administering any product described in PHYSICIANS' DESK REFERENCE always consult the PDR Supplement for possible new or revised information.

DELCOBESE

Each tablet or capsule contains:	5 mg.	10 mg.	15 mg.	20 mg.
Dextroamphetamine sulfate	1.25 mg.	2.5 mg.	3.75 mg.	5 mg.
Dextroamphetamine adipate	1.25 mg.	2.5 mg.	3.75 mg.	5 mg.
Amphetamine adipate	1.25 mg.	2.5 mg.	3.75 mg.	5 mg.
Amphetamine sulfate	1.25 mg.	2.5 mg.	3.75 mg.	5 mg.

In bottles of 1000's

Caution: Federal Law Prohibits Dispensing without Prescription.

Each T. R. Capsule contains:	10 mg.	15 mg.	20 mg.
Dextroamphetamine sulfate	2.5 mg.	3.75 mg.	5 mg.
Dextroamphetamine adipate	2.5 mg.	3.75 mg.	5 mg.
Amphetamine adipate	2.5 mg.	3.75 mg.	5 mg.
Amphetamine sulfate	2.5 mg.	3.75 mg.	5 mg.

In bottles of 1000's

Dermik Laboratories, Inc.
FORT WASHINGTON, PA 19034

ANTHRA-DERM® OINTMENT ℞
(anthralin)

Description: 0.1%, 0.25%, 0.5% or 1% anthralin in a white petrolatum and unsaturated fatty acid ester base.
Action: Skin irritant.
Indication: Psoriasis.
Contraindications: Patients with renal damage. Not to be used on or near the eyes. Use only on quiescent or chronic patches and not in either acute eruptions or where inflammation is present.
Precautions: Anthralin may be absorbed through the skin and excreted partly as chrysophanic acid which is easily formed by its oxidation, especially in alkaline solution. The urine is therefore colored red by alkalies. A part is excreted unchanged and can cause renal irritation, casts and aluminuria. Weekly examination of the urine for evidence of renal irritation should be made by physician. Erythema occurring on normal skin adjacent to lesions is criterion of dosage form concentration. When redness is observed on adjacent normal skin, reduce frequency of application. For external use only. Keep away from eyes. Occular irritant—if accidentally applied, may result in severe conjunctivitis, keratitis and corneal opacity. Anthralin should not be applied to face, genitalia, or intertriginous skin areas. Avoid excessive application as this may produce harmful irritation. Wash thoroughly and carefully after using. (Keep out of the reach of children.)
Adverse Reactions: Occasionally, certain individuals may be sensitive to one or more of the components of this product. If any reaction indicating either sensitivity, pustular folliculitis or renal irritation is observed, discontinue use and consult physician.
Directions: Apply in a thin layer to affected areas once or twice daily as directed by physician.
How Supplied: 1½ oz. tubes.
Caution: Federal law prohibits dispensing without prescription.

MICROGEL™ FORMULA 10-BENZAGEL® (Acne Gel) AND 5-BENZAGEL® (Acne Gel) ℞

Description: 5% or 10% benzoyl peroxide, purified water, carbomer 940, 14% alcohol, sodium hydroxide, dioctyl sodium sulfosuccinate, alkyl polyglycol ether, fragrance.
Action: Provides drying, desquamative and antiseptic activity.
Indication: An aid in the treatment of acne.
Dosage and Administration: Wash and dry affected areas prior to application. Apply sparingly one or more times daily, or as directed by physician.
Contraindications: Should not be used by patients having known sensitivity to benzoyl peroxide or any of the components of this preparation.
Precautions: For External Use Only. Not for ophthalmic use. Keep away from eyes and mucosae. Very fair individuals should begin with a single application at bedtime allowing overnight medication. May bleach colored fabrics. Keep this and all other medications out of the reach of children.
Caution: Federal law prohibits dispensing without prescription.
How Supplied: Plastic tubes, 1½ oz. and 3 oz.

FOMAC® FOAM
(medicated foam cleanser)

Description: Salicylic acid 2% in a soap-free, mild detergent system. (Patent applied for.)
Indications: Acne and oily skin.
Directions: DO NOT SHAKE. Invert container and squeeze a puff of Fomac Foam into palm of hand and massage, gently but thoroughly, into affected area until foam disappears. For best results, do not wet skin. Leave on skin 3 - 5 minutes, then rinse well with lukewarm water and pat dry. Use once or twice daily, or as recommended by physician. Discontinue use of all soaps or other skin cleansers.
Precautions: If redness or irritation occurs or increases, reduce frequency of applications. If irritation persists, discontinue use and consult your physician.
Keep away from eyes.
For external use only.
Keep out of the reach of children.
Keep tightly closed.
Store at room temperature.
How Supplied: 3 fl. oz. non-aerosol bottle.

HYTONE® CREAM ℞
(hydrocortisone)

Description: Hydrocortisone ½%, 1% or 2½% in a water-washable cream containing purified water, propylene glycol, glyceryl monostearate, cholesterol and related sterols, isopropyl myristate, polysorbate 60, cetyl alcohol, sorbitan monostearate, polyoxyl 40 stearate and sorbic acid.
Action: Topical steroids are primarily effective because of their anti-inflammatory, antipruritic and vasoconstrictive actions.
Indications: For relief of the inflammatory manifestations of corticosteroid-responsive dermatoses.
Contraindications: Topical steroids are contraindicated in those patients with a history of hypersensitivity to any of the components of the preparation.
Precautions: If irritation develops, the product should be discontinued and appropriate therapy instituted.
In the presence of an infection the use of an appropriate antifungal or antibacterial agent should be instituted. If a favorable response does not occur promptly, the corticosteroid should be discontinued until the infection has been adequately controlled.
If extensive areas are treated or if the occlusive technique is used there will be increased systemic absorption of the corticosteroid and suitable precautions should be taken, particularly in children and infants.
Although topical steroids have not been reported to have an adverse effect on human pregnancy, the safety of their use in pregnant women has not absolutely been established. In laboratory animals, increases in incidence of fetal abnormalities have been associated with exposure of gestating females to topical corticosteroids, in some cases at rather low dosage levels. Therefore, drugs of this class should not be used extensively on pregnant patients, in large amounts, or for prolonged periods of time.
The product is not for ophthalmic use.
Adverse Reactions: The following local adverse reactions have been reported with topical corticosteroids, especially under occlusive dressings: burning, itching, irritation, dryness, folliculitis, hypertrichosis, acneform eruptions, hypopigmentation, perioral dermatitis, allergic contact dermatitis, maceration of the skin, secondary infection, skin atrophy, striae, miliaria.
Dosage and Administration: Apply to affected areas 3 or 4 times daily.
How Supplied: 2½%—Tube 1 oz. and 2 oz., 1% and ½%—Tube 1 oz. and Jar 4 oz.
Caution: Federal law prohibits dispensing without prescription.

HYTONE® OINTMENT ℞
(hydrocortisone)

Description: Hydrocortisone ½% or 1% in an emollient ointment containing mineral oil, U.S.P., white petrolatum U.S.P. and sorbitan sesquioleate.
Action: Topical steroids are primarily effective because of their anti-inflammatory, antipruritic and vasoconstrictive actions.
Indications: For relief of the inflammatory manifestations of corticosteroid-responsive dermatoses.
Contraindications: Topical steroids are contraindicated in those patients with a history of hypersensitivity to any of the components of the preparation.
Precautions: If irritation develops, the product should be discontinued and appropriate therapy instituted.
In the presence of an infection the use of an appropriate antifungal or antibacterial agent should be instituted. If a favorable response does not occur promptly, the corticosteroid should be discontinued until the infection has been adequately controlled.
If extensive areas are treated or if the occlusive technique is used there will be increased systemic absorption of the corticosteroid and suitable precautions should be taken, particularly in children and infants.
Although topical steroids have not been reported to have an adverse effect on human pregnancy, the safety of their use in pregnant women has not absolutely been established. In laboratory animals, increases in incidence of fetal abnormalities have been associated with exposure of gestating females to topical corticosteroids, in some cases at rather low dosage levels. Therefore, drugs of this class should not be used extensively on pregnant patients, in large amounts, or for prolonged periods of time.
The product is not for ophthalmic use.
Adverse Reactions: The following local adverse reactions have been reported with topical corticosteroids, especially under occlusive dressings: burning, itching, irritation, dryness, folliculitis, hypertrichosis, acneform eruptions, hypopigmentation, perioral dermatitis, allergic contact dermatitis, maceration of the skin, secondary infection, skin atrophy, striae, miliaria.
Dosage and Administration: Apply to affected areas 3 or 4 times daily.

Continued on next page

Dermik—Cont.

How Supplied: Tube 1 oz. and Jar 4 oz.
Caution: Federal law prohibits dispensing without prescription.

KLARON® ACNE LOTION
(Dries on Clear)

Description: Klaron® Acne Lotion contains salicylic acid 2% and colloidal sulfur 5% in an astringent, hydroalcoholic lotion of colloidal magnesium-aluminum silicate, alkyl-aryl sulfonic acid salts, propylene glycol, silicone emulsion, cellulose gum, tetrasodium EDTA, 2 bromo-2-nitropropane-1,3-diol, lauric myristic diethanolamide, butylparaben, fragrance and purified water (alcohol 13.1%).
Actions: Provides keratolytic, peeling, drying and antiseborrheic actions.
Indications: An aid in the treatment of acne vulgaris, acne rosacea and seborrheic dermatitis.
Contraindications: This product is contraindicated for use by patients having known hypersensitivity to salicylic acid, sulfur or any other component of this preparation.
Precautions: For external use only. Keep away from eyes. If irritation develops, discontinue use and consult a physician.
Occasionally certain individuals may be sensitive to one or more components of this product. The object of this therapy is to achieve desquamation without irritation, but salicylic acid and sulfur can cause reddening and scaling of the epidermis. These side effects are not unusual in the treatment of acne and invariably disappear on continued use. Keep out of the reach of children.
Directions: Shake well before using. Apply a small quantity to affected areas with light massaging 1 or 2 times daily or in accordance with the physician's directions.
How Supplied: Plastic squeeze bottles, 2 oz.

LOROXIDE® ACNE LOTION (Flesh Tinted)

Description: Loroxide® Lotion contains (as dispensed) benzoyl peroxide 5.5%, and chlorhydroxyquinoline 0.25% incorporated in a flesh-tinted lotion of propylene glycol, cetyl alcohol, hydroxyethylcellulose, kaolin, caramel, talc, cholesterol and related sterols, propylene glycol stearate, polysorbate 20, lanolin alcohol, propylparaben, methylparaben, tetrasodium EDTA, pH buffers, antioxidants, silicone emulsion, silica, decyl oleate, vegetable oil, purcelline oil syn., titanium dioxide, cyclohexanediamine tetraacetic acid, calcium phosphate, and purified water.
Actions: Provides keratolytic, peeling and drying action.
Indications: An aid in the treatment of acne and oily skin.
Contraindications: This product is contraindicated for use by patients having known hypersensitivity to benzoyl peroxide, chlorhydroxyquinoline or any other component of this preparation.
Precautions: For external use only. Keep away from eyes. Do not add any other medicaments or substances to this lotion unless specifically directed by physician to do so. Patients should be observed carefully for possible local irritation or sensitivity during long-term topical therapy. If any irritation or sensitivity is observed, discontinue use and consult physician. Apply with caution on neck and/or other sensitive areas. There may be a slight, transitory stinging or burning sensation on initial application which invariably disappears on continued use. Ultraviolet and cold quartz light should be employed in lesser amounts as this lotion is keratolytic and drying. Harsh, abrasive cleansers should not be used simultaneously with this lotion. Colored or dyed garments may be bleached by the oxidizing action of benzoyl peroxide. Chlorhydroxyquinoline may cause temporary light-yellowish skin staining in rare cases. Occurrence of excessive redness or peeling indicates that the amount and frequency of application should be reduced. Keep out of the reach of children.
Adverse Reactions: The sensitizing potential of benzoyl peroxide and chlorhydroxyquinoline are low; but they can, on occasion, produce allergic reaction.
Directions: Shake well before using. Apply a thin film to affected areas with light massaging to blend in each application 1 or 2 times daily or in accordance with the physician's directions.
How Supplied: Bottles, 25 grams (0.88 oz.) net weight as dispensed. Trade package contains a bottle of lotion base and a "Benzie Pak"™ vial containing a mixture of benzoyl peroxide 35% and calcium phosphate 65%. Net weight of each vial is 3.8 grams. A "Dermik Color Blender" is also provided which enables the patient to alter the basic shade of the lotion to match the skin color.

LOROXIDE-HC® LOTION ℞
(Flesh-Tinted)

Description: Loroxide-HC® Lotion contains (as dispensed) hydrocortisone 0.5%, benzoyl peroxide 5.5% and chlorhydroxyquinoline 0.25% incorporated in a flesh-tinted lotion of propylene glycol, cetyl alcohol, hydroxyethylcellulose, kaolin, caramel, talc, cholesterol and related sterols, propylene glycol stearate, polysorbate 20, lanolin alcohol, propylparaben, methylparaben, tetrasodium EDTA, pH buffers, antioxidants, silicone emulsion, silica, decyl oleate, vegetable oil, purcelline oil syn., titanium dioxide, cyclohexanediamine tetraacetic acid, calcium phosphate, and purified water.
Actions: Provides keratolytic, peeling and drying action.
Indications: An aid in the treatment of acne and oily skin.
Contraindications: This product is contraindicated for use by patients having known hypersensitivity to hydrocortisone, benzoyl peroxide, chlorhydroxyquinoline or any other component of this preparation. Topical steroids are contraindicated in viral diseases of the skin, such as varicella and vaccinia.
Warning: Usage in Pregnancy: Although topical steroids have not been reported to have an adverse effect on the fetus, the safety of their use during pregnancy has not been absolutely established. Therefore, they should not be used extensively, or in large amounts or for prolonged periods of time on pregnant patients.
Precautions: For external use only. Keep away from eyes. If irritation develops, the product should be discontinued and appropriate therapy instituted. In the presence of an infection, the use of appropriate antifungal or antibacterial agents should be instituted. If a favorable response does not occur promptly, the corticosteroid should be discontinued until the infection has been adequately controlled. If extensive areas are treated, or if the occlusive technique is used, the possibility exists of increased systemic absorption of the corticosteroid and suitable precautions should be taken. Do not add any other medicaments or substances to this lotion unless specifically directed by physician to do so. Patients should be observed carefully for possible local irritation or sensitization during long-term topical therapy. Apply with caution on neck and/or other sensitive areas. There may be a slight, transitory stinging or burning sensation on initial application which invariably disappears on continued use. Ultraviolet and cold quartz light should be employed in lesser amounts as this lotion is keratolytic and drying. Harsh, abrasive cleansers should not be used simultaneously with this lotion. Colored or dyed garments may be bleached by the oxidizing action of benzoyl peroxide. Chlorhydroxyquinoline may cause light-yellowish skin staining in rare cases. Keep out of the reach of children.
Adverse Reactions: The following local adverse reactions have been reported with topical corticosteroids: burning sensation, itching, irritation, dryness, folliculitis, secondary infection, skin atrophy, hypertrichosis, acneform eruptions, and hypopigmentation. The sensitizing potential of benzoyl peroxide and chlorhydroxyquinoline are low, but they can, on occasion, produce allergic reaction. Occurrence of excessive redness or peeling indicates that the amount and frequency of application should be reduced.
Directions: Shake well before using. Apply a thin film to affected areas with light massaging to blend in each application 1 to 3 times daily in accordance with the physician's directions.
How Supplied: Bottles, 25 grams (0.88 oz.) net weight as dispensed. Trade package contains a bottle of lotion base and a "Benzie-Pak"™ vial containing a mixture of benzoyl peroxide 35% and calcium phosphate 65%. Net weight of each vial is 3.8 grams. A "Dermik Color Blender" is also provided which enables the patient to alter the basic shade of the lotion to match the skin color.

REZAMID® ACNE LOTION
(Flesh-Tinted)

Description: Rezamid® Lotion contains resorcinol 2%, sulfur 5%, and parachlorometaxylenol 0.5% incorporated in a flesh-tinted, hydroalcoholic lotion, with alcohol 28.5%.
Actions: Provides peeling, drying, and antiseborrheic action.
Indications: An aid in the treatment of acne and oily skin.
Precautions: For external use only. Keep away from eyes. Persons with sensitive skin may experience a mild transitory stinging sensation which usually disappears on continued use. If irritation develops, discontinue use and consult a physician. Keep out of the reach of children. Keep tightly closed.
Directions: Shake well before using. Apply a thin film once or twice daily as necessary or as directed by physician.
For Best Results: Cleanse area thoroughly. Apply a small quantity of lotion from the inside of cap using fingertips. Beginning with a small patch, spread and massage gently until a thin film covers the entire acne area. Conspicuous blemishes should be retouched to obtain the flesh-tint desired. Consult physician for advice regarding diet and other factors in control of acne. Hair and scalp should be washed once or twice weekly with drying shampoos such as REZAMID® SHAMPOO or ZETAR® SHAMPOO (Dermik).
For light complexions it is suggested that the pharmacist triturate 3 to 5 grams of either titanium dioxide or zinc oxide with glycerin or propylene glycol and add gradually to lotion with agitation. Each package contains a "Dermik Color Blender" which enables the user to darken the basic shade of the lotion so that it matches the skin color.
How Supplied: Bottles 2 oz.

SULFACET-R® LOTION ℞

Description: Sulfacet-R® Lotion contains (as dispensed) sodium sulfacetamide 10% and microsize sulfur 5% in a flesh-tinted lotion of purified water, alkyl-aryl sulfonic acid salts, hydroxyethylcellulose, propylene glycol, xanthan gum, lauric myristic diethanolamide, polyoxyethylene laurate, cyclohexanediamine tetraacetic acid, butylparaben, methylparaben, silicone emulsion, talc, zinc oxide, titanium dioxide, attapulgite, iron oxides, pH buffers and 2-bromo-2-nitropropane-1,3-diol.

Actions: Provides keratolytic, peeling, drying and antiseborrheic action.
Indications: An aid in the treatment of acne vulgaris, acne rosacea and seborrheic dermatitis.
Contraindications: This product is contraindicated for use by patients having known hypersensitivity to sulfonamides, sulfur or any other component of this preparation. Not to be used by patients with kidney disease.
Precautions: For external use only. Keep away from eyes. If irritation develops, discontinue use and consult physician. Sensitivity to sodium sulfacetamide may occur. Therefore, caution and careful supervision should be observed when prescribing this drug for patients who may be prone to hypersensitivity to topical sulfonamides. Particular caution should be employed if areas of denuded or abraded skin are involved. Patients should be carefully observed for possible local irritation or sensitization during long term therapy. Occasionally, certain individuals may be sensitive to one or more components of this preparation. The object of this therapy is to achieve desquamation without irritation, but sodium sulfacetamide and sulfur can cause reddening and scaling of the epidermis. These side effects are not unusual in the treatment of acne vulgaris, but patients should be cautioned about the possibility. Keep out of the reach of children.
Adverse Reactions: Previous toxic reactions such as agranulocytosis, acute hemolytic anemia, purpura hemorrhagica, drug fever, jaundice and contact dermatitis indicates hypersensitivity to sulfonamides.
Directions: Shake well before using. Apply a thin film 1 to 3 times daily with light massaging to blend in each application in accordance with the physician's directions. Each package contains a "Dermik Color Blender" which enables the patient to alter the basic shade of the lotion so that it matches the skin color.
How Supplied: Bottle, 1 oz. (as dispensed).

VANOXIDE® ACNE LOTION
(Dries on Clear)

Description: Vanoxide® Acne Lotion contains (as dispensed) benzoyl peroxide 5% and chlorhydroxyquinoline 0.25% incorporated in a water washable, vanishing lotion consisting of purified water, propylene glycol, hydroxyethylcellulose, FD&C color, cholesterol-sterol, cetyl alcohol, propylene glycol stearate, polysorbate 20, lanolin alcohol, propylparaben, decyl oleate, purcelline oil syn., antioxidants, vegetable oil, methylparaben, tetrasodium EDTA, buffers, cyclohexanediamine tetraacetic acid, calcium phosphate, silicone emulsion, and silica.
Actions: Provides keratolytic, peeling and drying action.
Indications: An aid in the treatment of acne and oily skin
Contraindications: This product is contraindicated for use by patients having known hypersensitivity to benzoyl peroxide, chlorhydroxyquinoline or any other component of this preparation.
Precautions: For external use only. Keep away from eyes. Do not add any other medicaments or substances to this lotion unless specifically directed by physician to do so. Patients should be observed carefully for possible local irritation or sensitization during long-term topical therapy. If any irritation or sensitivity is observed, discontinue use and consult physician. Apply with caution on neck and/or other sensitive areas. There may be a slight, transitory stinging or burning sensation on initial application which invariably disappears on continued use. Ultraviolet and cold quartz light should be employed in lesser amounts as this lotion is keratolytic and drying. Harsh, abrasive cleansers should not be used simultaneously with lotion. Colored or dyed garments may be bleached by the oxidizing action of benzoyl peroxide. Chlorhydroxyquinoline may cause temporary light-yellowish skin staining in rare cases. Occurrence of excessive redness or peeling indicates that the amount and frequency of application should be reduced. Keep out of the reach of children.
Adverse Reactions: The sensitizing potential of benzoyl peroxide and chlorhydroxyquinoline are low but they can, on occasion, produce allergic reaction.
Directions: Shake well before using. Apply a small quantity to affected areas with light massaging 1 or 2 times daily or in accordance with the physician's directions.
How Supplied: Bottles, 25 grams (0.88 oz.) as dispensed and 50 grams (1.76 oz.) as dispensed.

VANOXIDE-HC® LOTION ℞
(Dries on Clear)

Description: Vanoxide-HC® Lotion contains (as dispensed) hydrocortisone 0.5%, benzoyl peroxide 5% and chlorhydroxyquinoline 0.25% incorporated in a water washable, vanishing lotion consisting of propylene glycol, hydroxyethylcellulose, FD&C color, cholesterol-sterol, cetyl alcohol, propylene glycol stearate, polysorbate 20, lanolin alcohol, propylparaben, decyl oleate, purcelline oil syn., antioxidants, vegetable oil, methylparaben, tetrasodium EDTA, buffers, cyclohexanediamine tetraacetic acid, calcium phosphate, silicone emulsion, silica and purified water.
Actions: Provides keratolytic, peeling and drying action.
Indications: An aid in the treatment of acne and oily skin.
Contraindications: This product is contraindicated for use by patients having known hypersensitivity to hydrocortisone, benzoyl peroxide, chlorhydroxyquinoline or any other component of this preparation. Topical steroids are contraindicated in viral diseases of the skin, such as varicella and vaccinia.
Warning: USAGE IN PREGNANCY: Although topical steroids have not been reported to have an adverse effect on the fetus, the safety of their use during pregnancy has not been absolutely established. Therefore, they should not be used extensively, or in large amounts, or for prolonged periods of time on pregnant patients.
Precautions: For external use only. Keep away from eyes. If irritation develops, the product should be discontinued and appropriate therapy instituted. In the presence of an infection, the use of appropriate antifungal or antibacterial agents should be instituted. If a favorable response does not occur promptly, the corticosteroid should be discontinued until the infection has been adequately controlled. If extensive areas are treated, or if the occlusive technique is used, the possibility exists of increased systemic absorption of the corticosteroid and suitable precautions should be taken. Do not add any other medicaments or substances to this lotion unless specifically directed by physician to do so. Patients should be observed carefully for possible local irritation or sensitization during long-term topical therapy. Apply with caution on neck and/or other sensitive areas. There may be a slight, transitory stinging or burning sensation on initial application which invariably disappears on continued use. Ultraviolet and cold quartz light should be employed in lesser amounts as this lotion is keratolytic and drying. Harsh, abrasive cleansers should not be used simultaneously with this lotion. Colored or dyed garments may be bleached by the oxidizing action of benzoyl peroxide. Chlorhydroxyquinoline may cause temporary light yellowish skin staining in rare cases. Occurrence of excessive redness or peeling indicates that the amount and frequency of application should be reduced. Keep out of the reach of children.
Adverse Reactions: The following local adverse reactions have been reported with topical corticosteroids: burning sensations, itching, irritation, dryness, folliculitis, secondary infection, skin atrophy, striae, hypertrichosis, acneform eruptions, and hypopigmentation. The sensitizing potential of benzoyl peroxide and chlorhydroxyquinoline are low; but they can, on occasion, produce allergic reaction.
Directions: Shake well before using. Apply a small quantity to affected areas with light massaging 1 to 3 times daily in accordance with the physician's directions.
How Supplied: Bottles, 25 grams (0.88 oz.) as dispensed.

VYTONE® CREAM ℞
(diiodohydroxyquin-hydrocortisone)

Description: Vytone® Cream contains diiodohydroxyquin 1% and hydrocortisone 0.5% or 1% in a greaseless cream of purified water, propylene glycol, glyceryl monostearate, cholesterol and related sterols, isopropyl myristate, polysorbates 20 and 60, cetyl alcohol, sorbitan monostearate, polyoxyl 40 stearate and sorbic acid.
Actions: Combines the antifungal and antibacterial actions of diiodohydroxyquin with the anti-inflammatory and antipruritic effects of hydrocortisone, providing effective therapy for broader control of various acute and chronic dermatological disorders.

Indications: Based on a review of a related drug by the National Research Council and subsequent FDA classification for the drug, the indications are as follows: "Possibly" Effective: Contact or atopic dermatitis; impetiginized eczema; nummular eczema; infantile eczema; endogeneous chronic infectious dermatitis; stasis dermatitis; pyoderma; nuchal eczema and chronic eczematoid otitis externa; acne urticata; localized or disseminated neurodermatitis; lichen simplex chronicus; anogenital pruritis (vulvae, scroti, ani); folliculitis, bacterial dermatoses; mycotic dermatoses such as tinea (capitis, cruris, corporis, pedis); moniliasis, intertrigo. Final classification of the less-than-effective indications requires further investigation.

Contraindications: Topical steroids are contraindicated in viral diseases of the skin such as varicella and vaccinia and in individuals when circulation is markedly impaired. Vytone Cream is contraindicated in those patients with a history of hypersensitivity to any of the components of the preparation.
Warnings: USAGE IN PREGNANCY: Although topical steroids have not been reported to have an adverse effect on the fetus, the safety of their use on pregnant patients has not been absolutely established. Therefore, they should not be used extensively, or in large amounts or for prolonged periods of time on pregnant patients.
Precautions: For external use only. Keep away from eyes. If irritation develops, the product should be discontinued and appropriate therapy instituted. If extensive areas are treated or if the occulsive technique is used, the possibility exists of increased systemic absorption of the corticosteroid and suitable precautions should be taken. May stain skin, hair, or fabrics. Diiodohydroxyquin may be absorbed through the skin and interfere with thyroid function tests. If such tests are contemplated, wait at least one month after discontinuance of therapy to perform these tests. The ferric chloride test for phenylketonuria (PKU) can yield a false positive result if diiodohydroxyquin is present in the diaper or urine.

Continued on next page

Dermik—Cont.

Prolonged use may result in overgrowth of nonsusceptible organisms requiring appropriate therapy. Keep out of the reach of children.
Adverse Reactions: The following adverse reactions have been reported with topical steroids, either with or without occulsive dressings: burning sensations, itching, irritation, dryness, folliculitis, secondary infection, skin atrophy, striae, hypertrichosis, acneform eruption, and hypopigmentation.
Dosage and Administration: Apply to affected areas 3 or 4 times daily in accordance with physician's directions.
How Supplied: Tubes, 1 oz.

ZETAR® EMULSION For The Bath ℞
(Coal Tar)

Description: Water dispersible emulsion of Zetar® (WHOLE Coal Tar) 300 mg./ml. in polysorbates.
Actions: Antipruritic, keratoplastic, antiseptic and photosensitizing.
Indications: An aid in the treatment of generalized, persistent dermatoses, such as psoriasis, eczema, atopic dermatitis and seborrheic dermatitis.
Contraindications: Not to be used on open or infected lesions. Patients who have previously exhibited sensitivity to tars must be under careful and continuous supervision by the physician.
Precautions: For external use only. Keep away from eyes. Use lukewarm water only, hot water must be avoided. Avoid exposure of treated area(s) to direct sunlight for 84 hours unless directed by physician. Prior to exposure to sunlight, completely remove all tar from skin. Sensitization or dermatitis may occur after prolonged use. If irritation develops or increases, discontinue use and consult physician. Keep out of the reach of children.
Adverse Reactions: In rare cases, may cause allergic irritation attributable to coal tar.
Directions: Shake well before using. Add 3 to 5 capfuls to drawn lukewarm bath water, mixing thoroughly. Use in accordance with physician's directions.
Ultraviolet irradiation may be employed in conjunction with this therapy (see below), but ONLY under careful supervision by the physician.
GOECKERMAN TREATMENT—Photosensitizing effect of coal tar is apparently due to acridine compounds in the anthracene oil fraction. The source of ultraviolet irradiation generally recommended is a standard Hanovia hot quartz ultraviolet lamp emitting wavelengths between 2,400A. and 3,660A. units with an axial average output at 30″ of 1,000 microwatts per sq. cm. of skin surface.
Patients should be given a suberythema dose of ultraviolet irradiation at regular intervals of not more than two weeks. The photosensitization reaction will occur as early as fifteen minutes after the application of tar and last as long as seventy-two hours. For best results, the patient should be exposed to ultraviolet irradiation within 24 hours of application of tar. Initial exposure should be less than one-half minute at an exposure distance of 6 to 8 inches.
Ultraviolet irradiation acts by suppressing the overactivity of the Malpighian layer of the epidermis. The reaction is more intense if all traces of the tar is removed from the skin surface; in fact, any residual tar will have a depressing effect and will lessen the photosensitizing effect of the tar and ultraviolet irradiation.
How Supplied: Plastic bottles of 6 fl. oz.

ZETAR® SHAMPOO

Description: WHOLE Coal Tar (as Zetar®) 1.0%, and parachlorometaxylenol 0.5% in a golden foam shampoo which produces soft, fluffy abundant lather.
Actions and Indications: Antiseptic, antibacterial, antiseborrheic. Loosens and softens scales and crusts. Indicated in psoriasis, seborrhea, dandruff, cradle-cap and other oily, itchy conditions of the body and scalp.
Contraindications: Acute inflammation, open or infected lesions.
Precautions: If undue skin irritation develops or increases, discontinue use and consult physician. In rare instances, temporary discoloration of blond, bleached, or tinted hair may occur. Avoid contact with eyes.
Dosage and Administration: Massage into moistened scalp. Rinse. Repeat; leave on 5 minutes. Rinse thoroughly.
How Supplied: 6 oz. Plastic Bottles.

Dista Products Company

Division of Eli Lilly and Company
P. O. BOX 1407
INDIANAPOLIS, IN 46206

LEGEND

Identi-Code®—*Formula Identification Code, Dista*
Identi-Dose®—*Unit Dose Medication, Dista*
Pulvules®—*Filled Gelatin Capsules, Dista*
℞Pak—*Prescription Package, Dista*

IDENTI-CODE® Index

Illustrations of examples of products bearing Identi-Code® appear in the Product Identification Section.

Identi-Code® Product Name

CO3-C22 (Coated Tablets)

CO3 Ilotycin®
Composition (Each Enteric-Coated Tablet): Erythromycin, USP, 250 mg

C19 Mi-Cebrin®
Composition (Each Coated Tablet): Thiamine (vitamin B_1), 10 mg; riboflavin (vitamin B_2), 5 mg; pyridoxine (vitamin B_6), 1.7 mg; pantothenic acid, 10 mg; niacinamide, 30 mg; vitamin B_{12} (activity equivalent), 3 mcg; ascorbic acid (vitamin C), 100 mg; *dl*-alpha tocopheryl acetate (vitamin E), 5.5 IU (5.5 mg); vitamin A, 10,000 IU (3 mg); vitamin D, 400 IU (10 mcg); contains also (approximately): iron (as ferrous sulfate), 15 mg; copper (as the sulfate), 1 mg; iodine (as potassium iodide), 0.15 mg; manganese (as the glycerophosphate), 1 mg; magnesium (as the hydroxide), 5 mg; zinc (as the chloride), 1.5 mg

C20 Mi-Cebrin T®
Composition (Each Coated Tablet): Thiamine mononitrate (vitamin B_1), 15 mg; riboflavin (vitamin B_2), 10 mg; pyridoxine hydrochloride (vitamin B_6), 2 mg; pantothenic acid (as calcium pantothenate), 10 mg; niacinamide, 100 mg; vitamin B_{12} (activity equivalent), 7.5 mcg; ascorbic acid (vitamin C), 150 mg; *dl*-alpha tocopheryl acetate (vitamin E), 5.5 IU (5.5 mg); vitamin A, 10,000 IU (3 mg); vitamin D, 400 IU (10 mcg); contains also (approximately): iron (as ferrous sulfate), 15 mg; copper (as the sulfate), 1 mg; iodine (as potassium iodide), 0.15 mg; manganese (as the glycerophosphate), 1 mg; magnesium (as the hydroxide), 5 mg; zinc (as the chloride), 1.5 mg

C22 Becotin®-T
Composition (Each Coated Tablet): Thiamine mononitrate (vitamin B_1), 15 mg; riboflavin (vitamin B_2), 10 mg; pyridoxine hydrochloride (vitamin B_6), 5 mg; niacinamide, 100 mg; pantothenic acid (as calcium pantothenate), 20 mg; vitamin B_{12} (activity equivalent), 4 mcg; ascorbic acid (vitamin C) (as sodium ascorbate), 300 mg

F01-H77 (Pulvules®)

F01 Trinsicon®
Composition (Each Pulvule®): Special Liver-Stomach Concentrate, Dista (containing intrinsic factor), 240 mg; Cobalamin Concentrate, NF, equivalent to cobalamin, 7.5 mcg (the total vitamin B_{12} activity in the Special Liver-Stomach Concentrate, Dista, and the Cobalamin Concentrate, NF, is 15 mcg); iron, elemental (as ferrous fumarate), 110 mg; ascorbic acid (vitamin C), 75 mg; folic acid, 0.5 mg

F02 Trinsicon® M
Composition (Each Pulvule®): Special Liver-Stomach Concentrate, Dista (containing intrinsic factor), 240 mg; Cobalamin Concentrate, NF, equivalent to cobalamin, 7.5 mcg (the total vitamin B_{12} activity in the Special Liver-Stomach Concentrate, Dista, and the Cobalamin Concentrate, NF, is 15 mcg); iron, elemental (as ferrous fumarate), 110 mg; ascorbic acid (vitamin C), 75 mg

F62 Becotin®
Composition (Each Pulvule®): Thiamine hydrochloride (vitamin B_1), 10 mg; riboflavin (vitamin B_2), 10 mg; pyridoxine (vitamin B_6), 4.1 mg; niacinamide, 50 mg; pantothenic acid, 25 mg; vitamin B_{12} (activity equivalent), 1 mcg

F77 Becotin® with Vitamin C
Composition (Each Pulvule®): Thiamine hydrochloride (vitamin B_1), 10 mg; riboflavin (vitamin B_2), 10 mg; pyridoxine (vitamin B_6), 4.1 mg; niacinamide, 50 mg; pantothenic acid, 25 mg; vitamin B_{12} (activity equivalent), 1 mcg; ascorbic acid (vitamin C), 150 mg

3043 Co-Pyronil®
Composition (Each Pulvule®): pyrrobutamine phosphate, 15 mg; cyclopentamine hydrochloride, 12.5 mg

3042 Co-Pyronil®, Pediatric
Composition (Each Pulvule®): pyrrobutamine phosphate, 7.5 mg; cyclopentamine hydrochloride, 6.25 mg

H07 Ilosone®
Composition (Each Pulvule®): Erythromycin Estolate, NF, 125 mg (equiv. to erythromycin)

H09 Ilosone®
Composition (Each Pulvule®): Erythromycin Estolate, NF, 250 mg (equiv. to erythromycin)

H69 Keflex®
Composition (Each Pulvule®): Cephalexin, USP, 250 mg

H71 Keflex®
Composition (Each Pulvule®): Cephalexin, USP, 500 mg

©H74 Valmid®
Composition (Each Pulvule®): Ethinamate, NF, 500 mg

H77 Nalfon®
Composition (Each Pulvule®): Fenoprofen calcium, 300 mg (equiv. to fenoprofen)

U05-U59 (Compressed Tablets)

U05 Ilosone® Chewable
Composition (Each Compressed Tablet): Erythromycin Estolate, NF, 125 mg (equiv. to erythromycin)
U25 Ilosone® Chewable
Composition (Each Compressed Tablet): Erythromycin Estolate, NF, 250 mg (equiv. to erythromycin)
U26 Ilosone®
Composition (Each Compressed Tablet): Erythromycin Estolate, NF, 500 mg (equiv. to erythromycin)
U59 Nalfon®
Composition (Each Compressed Tablet): Fenoprofen calcium, 600 mg (equiv. to fenoprofen)

W03-W18 (Miscellaneous)

W03 Ilosone®, for Oral Suspension
Composition (When Mixed as Directed): Each 5 ml contain erythromycin estolate equivalent to 125 mg erythromycin (NF).
W14 Cordran® Tape
Composition: Flurandrenolide, USP, 4 mcg per sq cm
W15 Ilosone® Liquid, Oral Suspension
Composition: Each 5 ml contain erythromycin estolate equivalent to 125 mg erythromycin (NF).
W17 Ilosone® Liquid, Oral Suspension
Composition: Each 5 ml contain erythromycin estolate equivalent to 250 mg erythromycin (NF).
W18 Ilosone® Ready-Mixed Drops
Composition: Each ml contains erythromycin estolate equivalent to 100 mg erythromycin (NF).
W21 For Oral Suspension, Keflex®
Composition (When Mixed as Directed): Each 5 ml contain 125 mg cephalexin (NF).
W22 For Pediatric Drops, Keflex®
Composition (When Mixed as Directed): Each ml contains 100 mg cephalexin (NF).
W68 For Oral Suspension, Keflex®
Composition (When Mixed as Directed): Each 5 ml contain 250 mg cephalexin (NF).

UNIT-DOSE PACKAGING

Identi-Dose® (unit dose medication, Dista)
Closed-circuit control of medication from pharmacy to nurse to patient and return. Simplifies counting and dispensing whether in single-unit or prescription-size quantities. Fits into any dispensing system for ready identification and legibility, better inventory control, protection from contamination, easier handling and recording under Medicare, prevention of drug loss through pilferage or spilling, better control of Federal Controlled Substances, and less chance of medication errors.
The following products are available through normal channels of supply:
Identi-Dose®
Pulvules®
No.
2 Trinsicon®
325 Becotin® with Vitamin C
3043 Co-Pyronil®
375 Ilosone®, 250 mg
Tablets
No.
23 Ilotycin®, 250 mg
1790 Mi-Cebrin®
1807 Mi-Cebrin T®
1810 Becotin®-T
1863 Ilosone®, 500 mg

BECOTIN® OTC
(vitamin B complex)

Description: Each Pulvule® contains—
Thiamine Hydrochloride
(Vitamin B_1) .... 10 mg
Riboflavin
(Vitamin B_2) .... 10 mg
Pyridoxine (Vitamin B_6) .... 4.1 mg
Niacinamide .... 50 mg
Pantothenic Acid .... 25 mg
Vitamin B_{12} (Activity Equivalent) .... 1 mcg
Indications: Prophylaxis or treatment of vitamin B complex deficiencies. Acute B complex deficiencies may be precipitated by concurrent diseases or by surgical procedures, particularly of the gastrointestinal tract. The following symptoms of vitamin B complex deficiencies have been described: loss of appetite, nausea, burning tongue, vomiting, headache, general uneasiness or indisposition, nervousness, apprehensive mental depression, hypersensitivity to noise, mental confusion, fatigue, burning sensation of the skin, sore mouth and tongue, and burning and itching of the eyes.
Dosage: *Prophylaxis*—1 Pulvule a day. *Treatment*—2 or 3 Pulvules a day, or as directed by the physician.
How Supplied: *Pulvules No. 300, Becotin® (vitamin B complex, Dista), F62** (No. 0, Dark-Blue), in bottles of 100. [060178]

*Identi-Code® symbol.

BECOTIN®-T OTC
(vitamin B complex with vitamin C, therapeutic)

Description: Becotin-T is an easy-to-swallow, cinnamon-brown tablet which provides therapeutic quantities of vitamin B complex and vitamin C.
Each tablet contains—
Thiamine Mononitrate (Vitamin B_1) ...... 15 mg
Riboflavin (Vitamin B_2) .... 10 mg
Pyridoxine Hydrochloride
(Vitamin B_6) .... 5 mg
Niacinamide .... 100 mg
Pantothenic Acid
(as Calcium Pantothenate) .... 20 mg
Vitamin B_{12} (Activity Equivalent) .... 4 mcg
Ascorbic Acid (Vitamin C)
(as Sodium Ascorbate) .... 300 mg
Becotin-T is especially useful as an adjunct to specific therapy in medical or surgical aftercare. By restoring normal tissue levels of these easily depleted water-soluble vitamins, Becotin-T reduces morbidity—helps shorten convalescence.
Indications: For the prevention or treatment of concurrent vitamin B complex and vitamin C deficiencies.
Dosage: 1 or 2 tablets a day, or as directed by the physician.
How Supplied: *Tablets No. 1810, Becotin®-T (vitamin B complex with vitamin C, therapeutic, Dista), C22,** Coated, Cinnamon Brown, in bottles of 100 and 1000 and in 10 strips of 10 individually labeled blisters each containing 1 tablet (ID100). [060178]
[*Shown in Product Identification Section*]

*Identi-Code® symbol.

BECOTIN® WITH VITAMIN C OTC
(vitamin B complex with vitamin C)

Description: Each Pulvule® contains—
Thiamine Hydrochloride
(Vitamin B_1) .... 10 mg
Riboflavin
(Vitamin B_2) .... 10 mg
Pyridoxine
(Vitamin B_6) .... 4.1 mg
Niacinamide .... 50 mg
Pantothenic Acid .... 25 mg
Vitamin B_{12} (Activity Equivalent) .... 1 mcg
Ascorbic Acid
(Vitamin C) .... 150 mg
Indications: For the prevention or treatment of concurrent vitamin B complex and vitamin C deficiencies. *See also under* Becotin®.
Dosage: *Prophylaxis*—1 Pulvule a day. *Treatment*—2 or 3 Pulvules a day, or as directed by the physician.
How Supplied: *Pulvules No. 325, Becotin® with Vitamin C (vitamin B complex with vitamin C, Dista), F77** (No. 0, Green Body, Dark-Blue Cap), in bottles of 100, 500, and 1000 and in 10 strips of 10 individually labeled blisters each containing 1 Pulvule (ID100). [060178]
[*Shown in Product Identification Section*]

*Identi-Code® symbol.

CO-PYRONIL® ℞
(pyrrobutamine compound)

Description: Each Pulvule® Co-Pyronil® (pyrrobutamine compound, Dista) contains—
Pyronil® (pyrrobutamine phosphate, Dista) .... 15 mg
Clopane® Hydrochloride (cyclopentamine hydrochloride, Dista) .... 12.5 mg
Each Pulvule Co-Pyronil, Pediatric, contains—
Pyronil® (pyrrobutamine phosphate, Dista) .... 7.5 mg
Clopane® Hydrochloride (cyclopentamine hydrochloride, Dista) .... 6.25 mg
Each 5 ml (approximately 1 teaspoonful) of Suspension Co-Pyronil contain—
Pyrrobutamine naphthalene disulfonate .... 6.73 mg
(Equivalent to 7.5 mg Pyronil)
Cyclopentamine hydroxybenzoyl benzoate .... 13.49 mg
(Equivalent to 6.25 mg Clopane Hydrochloride)
Pyronil is an antihistamine. It is soluble in warm water to the extent of 10 percent.
Clopane Hydrochloride is the hydrochloride of 1-cyclopentyl-2-methylaminopropane.
Actions: Pyronil® (pyrrobutamine phosphate, Dista) is an antihistamine. Side effects of antihistamines include sedation and some anticholinergic (drying) effects.
Pyronil is effective for approximately nine to 11 hours.
Clopane® Hydrochloride (cyclopentamine hydrochloride, Dista) is an ephedrine-like drug that is orally effective as a sympathomimetic and is present in the mixture to provide a constricting effect on the dilated blood vessels of the allergic person's swollen mucous membranes. It results in less central-nervous-system stimulation than ephedrine and, therefore, in fewer side effects, such as tension and insomnia. It also has a more prolonged action than ephedrine.
Indications: Co-Pyronil is indicated in seasonal and perennial allergic rhinitis and in vasomotor rhinitis.
Contraindications: *In Newborn or Premature Infants*—Antihistamines should *not* be used in newborns or premature infants.
In Nursing Mothers—Since antihistamines are hazardous for all infants, especially newborns and prematures, they are contraindicated in nursing mothers.
In Lower Respiratory Disease—Antihistamines should not be used to treat lower respiratory tract symptoms, including asthma.
Co-Pyronil should not be used in patients with hypersensitivity to Pyronil® (pyrrobutamine

Continued on next page

Dista—Cont.

phosphate, Dista), to other antihistamines of similar chemical structure, or to Clopane® Hydrochloride (cyclopentamine hydrochloride, Dista).
Pyronil is contraindicated in patients receiving monoamine oxidase (MAO) inhibitors (*see* Drug Interactions) and in those with narrow-angle glaucoma, stenosing peptic ulcer, symptomatic prostatic hypertrophy, bladder neck obstruction, or pyloroduodenal obstruction.
Warnings: *Use in Children*—In infants and children especially, *overdosage* of antihistamines may cause hallucinations, convulsions, and death.
As in adults, antihistamines may diminish mental alertness in children. In the young child particularly, they may produce excitation.
Use in Pregnancy—Adequate reproduction studies have not been performed in animals. There is insufficient information as to whether this drug may reduce fertility in men or women or have teratogenic or other adverse effects on the fetus.
Use with C.N.S. Depressants—Pyronil® (pyrrobutamine phosphate, Dista) may add to the depressant effects of alcohol and other C.N.S. depressants (hypnotics, sedatives, tranquilizers, antianxiety agents, etc.).
Use When Activities Require Mental Alertness—Patients should be warned against engaging in activities requiring mental alertness, such as driving a car or operating appliances, machinery, etc.
Precautions: Like other antihistamines, Pyronil® (pyrrobutamine phosphate, Dista) has some action similar to that of atropine and, therefore, should be used with caution in patients with a history of bronchial asthma, increased intraocular pressure, hyperthyroidism, cardiovascular-renal disease, hypertension, or diabetes.
In the presence of prostatism, the administration of sympathomimetic drugs may cause urinary retention.
Adverse Reactions: *The most frequent adverse reactions to antihistamines:* sedation; sleepiness; dryness of mouth, nose, and throat; thickening of bronchial secretions; dizziness; epigastric distress; and disturbed coordination.
Other adverse reactions that occur with antihistamines: fatigue, confusion, restlessness, excitation, nervousness, insomnia, euphoria, anorexia, nausea, vomiting, diarrhea, constipation, hypotension, tightness of chest and wheezing, urticaria, drug rash, anaphylactic shock, blurred vision, diplopia, vertigo, tinnitus, headache, palpitation, tachycardia, nasal stuffiness, urinary frequency, difficult urination, urinary retention, photosensitivity, hemolytic anemia, leukopenia, and agranulocytosis.
Persons hypersensitive to sympathomimetics may report nervousness and insomnia. Clopane® Hydrochloride (cyclopentamine hydrochloride, Dista) causes less central-nervous-system stimulation than do other sympathomimetic drugs commonly employed.
The side effects of antihistamines and Clopane Hydrochloride tend to be counteracted by the combined administration of these medications. In most instances, Clopane Hydrochloride, a sympathomimetic, will prevent the drowsiness produced by Pyronil® (pyrrobutamine phosphate, Dista).
Administration and Dosage: Dosage of Co-Pyronil should be adjusted to the requirements and response of the patient.
Pulvules and Suspension
Usual Adult Dosage
Mild symptoms—1 Pulvule or 2 teaspoonfuls q 12 h
Moderate symptoms—1 Pulvule or 2 teaspoonfuls q 8 h
Severe symptoms—2 Pulvules or 4 teaspoonfuls q 8 h or 1 Pulvule or 2 teaspoonfuls q 4 h
Pediatric Pulvules and Suspension
Usual Dosage for Children—40 to 60 Pounds
Mild symptoms—1 Pulvule or 1 teaspoonful q 12 h
Moderate symptoms—1 Pulvule or 1 teaspoonful q 8 h
Severe symptoms—2 Pulvules or 2 teaspoonfuls q 8 h
Suspension
Usual Dosage for Children—20 to 40 Pounds
Mild symptoms—½ teaspoonful q 12 h
Moderate symptoms—½ teaspoonful q 8 h
Severe symptoms—½ to 1 teaspoonful q 8 h
The maximum dosages recommended for severe symptoms should not be exceeded. Side effects will increase with larger doses, but there will be no greater clinical efficacy.
Drug Interactions: MAO inhibitors prolong and intensify the anticholinergic (drying) effects of antihistamines.
Management of Overdosage: Reactions from overdosage of antihistamines may range from central-nervous-system depression to stimulation, especially in children. Also, signs and symptoms similar to those from atropine—dry mouth; fixed, dilated pupils; flushing; etc.—as well as gastrointestinal symptoms may appear.
If vomiting has not occurred spontaneously, the patient should be induced to vomit unless an excessive time has elapsed. Precautions must be taken against aspiration, especially in infants and children.
If vomiting is unsuccessful, gastric lavage is indicated within three hours after ingestion and even later if large amounts of milk or cream were taken beforehand. Isotonic or one-half isotonic saline is the solution of choice for lavage.
Saline cathartics, such as milk of magnesia, draw water into the bowel by osmosis and, therefore, are valuable for their action in the rapid dilution of bowel contents.
Stimulants should *not* be used.
Levarterenol Bitartrate, USP, may be used for hypotension—1 ml of a 0.2 percent solution (0.1 percent base) in 250 ml of diluent. Drip at 0.5 ml per minute to give 2 mcg of base per minute or 2 mcg per m^2 per minute intravenously. The dose should be titrated with blood pressure.
CAUTION: Slough results from extravascular leakage. The extravasated area should be treated quickly by infiltrating Phentolamine Mesylate, USP, or Phentolamine Hydrochloride, NF, 5 to 10 mg in 15 ml of saline solution.
How Supplied: (℞) *Pulvules No. 3043, Co-Pyronil® (pyrrobutamine compound, Dista), 3043** (No. 3, Yellow Opaque Body, Green Opaque Cap), in bottles of 100 and 1000 and in 10 strips of 10 individually labeled blisters each containing 1 Pulvule (ID100).
[*Shown in Product Identification Section*]
(℞) *Pulvules, Pediatric, No. 3042, Co-Pyronil® (pyrrobutamine compound, Dista), 3042**(No. 4, Dark-Red), in bottles of 100.
[*Shown in Product Identification Section*]
(℞) *Suspension No. M-5047, Co-Pyronil® (pyrrobutamine compound, Dista),* in 16-fl-oz bottles. *Avoid freezing.*
[061379]

*Identi-Code® symbol.

CORDRAN® and CORDRAN®SP (flurandrenolide) USP ℞

Description: Cordran® (Flurandrenolide, USP, Dista) is a potent corticosteroid intended for topical use. The chemical formula of Cordran is 6α-fluoro-16α-hydroxyhydrocortisone 16,17-acetonide.
Each gm of Cream Cordran® SP (Flurandrenolide Cream, USP, Dista) contains 0.5 mg (0.05 percent) or 0.25 mg (0.025 percent) flurandrenolide in an emulsified base composed of cetyl alcohol, citric acid, mineral oil, polyoxyl 40 stearate, propylene glycol, sodium citrate, stearic acid, and purified water.
Each gm of Ointment Cordran® (Flurandrenolide Ointment, USP, Dista) contains 0.5 mg (0.05 percent) or 0.25 mg (0.025 percent) flurandrenolide in a base composed of white wax, cetyl alcohol, sorbitan sesquioleate, and white petrolatum.
Each ml of Lotion Cordran® (Flurandrenolide Lotion, USP, Dista) contains 0.5 mg (0.05 percent) flurandrenolide in an oil-in-water emulsion base composed of glycerin, cetyl alcohol, stearic acid, glyceryl monostearate, mineral oil, polyoxyl 40 stearate, menthol, benzyl alcohol, and purified water.
Actions: Cordran® (flurandrenolide, Dista) is primarily effective because of its anti-inflammatory, antipruritic, and vasoconstrictive actions. It is available as cream, ointment, or lotion.
Evaporation of water from the vehicle of Lotion Cordran produces a cooling effect which is often desirable in the treatment of acutely inflamed or weeping lesions.
Indications: For relief of the inflammatory manifestations of corticosteroid-responsive dermatoses.
Contraindications: Topical corticosteroids are contraindicated in patients with a history of hypersensitivity to any of the components of these preparations.
Precautions: If irritation develops, the product should be discontinued and appropriate therapy instituted.
In the presence of an infection, an appropriate antifungal or antibacterial agent should be used. If a favorable response does not occur promptly, the corticosteroid should be discontinued until the infection has been adequately controlled.
If extensive areas are treated or if the occlusive technique is used, there will be increased systemic absorption of the corticosteroid, and suitable precautions should be taken, particularly in children and infants.
Although topical corticosteroids have not been reported to have an adverse effect on human pregnancy, the safety of their use on pregnant women has not been absolutely established. In laboratory animals, increases in incidence of fetal abnormalities have been associated with exposure of gestating females to topical corticosteroids, in some cases at rather low dosage levels. Therefore, drugs of this class should not be used extensively, in large amounts, or for prolonged periods of time on pregnant patients.
These products are not for ophthalmic use.
Adverse Reactions: The following local adverse reactions have been reported with topical corticosteroid formulations:
Acneform eruptions
Allergic contact dermatitis
Burning
Dryness
Folliculitis
Hypertrichosis
Hypopigmentation
Irritation
Itching
Perioral dermatitis
The following may occur more frequently with occlusive dressings:
Maceration of the skin
Miliaria
Secondary infection
Skin atrophy
Striae
Administration and Dosage: For moist lesions, a small quantity of the cream or lotion should be rubbed gently into the affected areas two or three times a day. For dry, scaly lesions, the ointment is applied as a thin film to affected areas two or three times daily.

Use with Occlusive Dressings

The technique of occlusive dressings (for management of psoriasis and other persistent dermatoses) is as follows:

1. Remove as much as possible of the superficial scaling before applying Cream Cordran® SP (flurandrenolide, Dista) or Ointment or Lotion Cordran. Soaking in a bath will help soften the scales and permit easier removal by brushing, picking, or rubbing.
2. Rub Cream Cordran SP or Ointment or Lotion Cordran thoroughly into the affected areas.
3. Cover with an occlusive plastic film, such as polyethylene, Saran Wrap™, or Handi-Wrap®. (When Cream Cordran SP or Lotion Cordran is used, added moisture may be provided by placing a slightly dampened cloth or gauze over the lesion before the plastic film is applied.)
4. Seal the edges to adjacent normal skin with tape or hold in place by a gauze wrapping.
5. For convenience, the patient may remove the dressing during the day. The dressing should then be reapplied each night.
6. For daytime therapy, the condition may be treated by rubbing Cream Cordran SP or Ointment or Lotion Cordran sparingly into the affected areas.
7. In more resistant cases, leaving the dressing in place for three to four days at a time may result in a better response.
8. Thin polyethylene gloves are suitable for treatment of the hands and fingers; plastic garment bags may be utilized for treating lesions on the trunk or buttocks. A tight shower cap is useful in treating lesions on the scalp.

Occlusive Dressings Have the Following Advantages—1. Percutaneous penetration of the corticosteroid is enhanced.

2. Medication is concentrated on the areas of skin where it is most needed.

3. This method of administration frequently is more effective in very resistant dermatoses than is the conventional application of Cordran® (flurandrenolide, Dista).

Precautions to Be Observed in Therapy with Occlusive Dressings—Treatment should be continued for at least a few days after clearing of the lesions. If it is stopped too soon, a relapse may occur. Reinstitution of treatment frequently will cause remission.

Because of the increased hazard of secondary infection from resistant strains of staphylococci among hospitalized patients, it is suggested that the use of occlusive plastic films for corticosteroid therapy in such cases be restricted.

Generally, occlusive dressings should not be used on weeping, or exudative, lesions.

When large areas of the body are covered, thermal homeostasis may be impaired. If elevation of body temperature occurs, use of the occlusive dressing should be discontinued.

Rarely, a patient may develop miliaria, folliculitis, or a sensitivity to either the particular dressing material or a combination of Cordran® (flurandrenolide, Dista) and the occlusive dressing. If miliaria or folliculitis occurs, use of the occlusive dressing should be discontinued. Treatment by inunction with a corticosteroid such as Cordran may be continued. If the sensitivity is caused by the particular material of the dressing, substitution of a different material may be tried.

Warnings—Some plastic films are readily flammable. Patients should be cautioned against the use of any such material.

When plastic films are used on infants and children, the persons caring for the patients must be reminded of the danger of suffocation if the plastic material accidentally covers the face.

How Supplied:

(℞) *Cordran® (Flurandrenolide, USP), 0.05%, Lotion No. M-128,* in 15 and 60-ml plastic squeeze bottles. *Avoid freezing.*

(℞) *Cordran® (Flurandrenolide, USP), 0.025%, Ointment No. 79,* in 30 and 60-gm tubes and in 225-gm jars.

(℞) *Cordran® (Flurandrenolide, USP), 0.05%, Ointment No. 85,* in 15, 30, and 60-gm tubes and in 225-gm jars.

(℞) *Cordran® SP (Flurandrenolide, USP), 0.025%, Cream No. 9,* in 30 and 60-gm tubes and in 225-gm jars.

(℞) *Cordran® SP (Flurandrenolide, USP), 0.05%, Cream No. 11,* in 15, 30, and 60-gm tubes and in 225-gm jars.

Cream No. 9, 0.025%—60 gm—6505-00-917-3681(A)

Cream No. 11, 0.05%—15 gm—6505-00-890-1554(A); 60 gm—6505-00-728-2623A; 225 gm—6505-00-728-2624(A)

Lotion No. M-128, 0.05%—15 ml—6505-00-926-9110

Ointment No. 85, 0.05%—15 gm—6505-00-728-2626; 225 gm—6505-00-728-2625A [040579A]

[*Shown in Product Identification Section*]

CORDRAN®-N ℞

(flurandrenolide with neomycin sulfate)

Description: Cordran® (Flurandrenolide, USP, Dista) is a potent corticosteroid intended for topical use. The chemical formula of Cordran is 6α-fluoro-16α-hydroxyhydrocortisone 16, 17-acetonide.

Each gm of Cordran-N cream contains 0.5 mg (0.05 percent) flurandrenolide and 5 mg neomycin sulfate (equivalent to 3.5 mg neomycin base) in a base composed of stearic acid, cetyl alcohol, mineral oil, polyoxyl 40 stearate, ethylparaben, glycerin, and purified water.

Each gm of Cordran-N ointment contains 0.5 mg (0.05 percent) flurandrenolide and 5 mg neomycin sulfate (equivalent to 3.5 mg neomycin base) in a base composed of white wax, cetyl alcohol, sorbitan sesquioleate, and white petrolatum.

Actions: Cordran® (flurandrenolide, Dista) is primarily effective because of its anti-inflammatory, antipruritic, and vasoconstrictive actions.

The addition of neomycin broadens the usefulness of Cordran so that dermatoses complicated by actual skin infections may be treated more effectively and with safety.

Indications: On the basis of a review of this drug by the National Academy of Sciences—National Research Council and/ or other information, FDA has classified the following indications as "possibly" effective.

For relief of the inflammatory manifestations of corticosteroid-responsive dermatoses complicated by bacterial infections.

Final classification of the less-than-effective indications requires further investigation.

Contraindications: Topical corticosteroids are contraindicated in patients with a history of hypersensitivity to any of the components of these preparations.

Warning: Because of the potential hazard of nephrotoxicity and ototoxicity, prolonged use or use of large amounts of this product should be avoided in the treatment of skin infections following extensive burns, trophic ulceration, and other conditions in which absorption of neomycin is possible.

Precautions: If irritation develops, the product should be discontinued and appropriate therapy instituted.

Patients with superficial fungus or yeast infections should be treated with additional appropriate methods and observed frequently.

Prolonged use of neomycin preparations may result in the overgrowth of nonsusceptible organisms. If this occurs, appropriate measures should be taken.

There are articles in the current medical literature that indicate an increase in the prevalence of persons who are sensitive to neomycin.

If extensive areas are treated or if the occlusive technique is used, there will be increased systemic absorption of the corticosteroid, and suitable precautions should be taken, particularly in children and infants.

Although topical corticosteroids have not been reported to have an adverse effect on human pregnancy, the safety of their use on pregnant women has not been absolutely established. In laboratory animals, increases in incidence of fetal abnormalities have been associated with exposure of gestating females to topical corticosteroids, in some cases at rather low dosage levels. Therefore, drugs of this class should not be used extensively, in large amounts, or for prolonged periods of time on pregnant patients.

These products are not for ophthalmic use.

Adverse Reactions: The following local adverse reactions have been reported with topical corticosteroid formulations:

- Acneform eruptions
- Allergic contact dermatitis
- Burning
- Dryness
- Folliculitis
- Hypertrichosis
- Hypopigmentation
- Irritation
- Itching
- Perioral dermatitis

The following may occur more frequently with occlusive dressings:

- Maceration of the skin
- Miliaria
- Secondary infection
- Skin atrophy
- Striae

Topical neomycin has been reported to cause allergic contact dermatitis, ototoxicity, and nephrotoxicity.

Administration and Dosage: For moist lesions, a small quantity of the cream should be rubbed gently into the affected areas two or three times a day. For dry, scaly lesions, the ointment is applied as a thin film to affected areas two or three times daily.

Use with Occlusive Dressings—See under Cordran and Cordran SP.

How Supplied: (℞) *Cordran®-N (flurandrenolide with neomycin sulfate, Dista), Cream No. 12,* in 15, 30, and 60-gm tubes.

(℞) *Cordran®-N (flurandrenolide with neomycin sulfate, Dista), Ointment No. 86,* in 15, 30, and 60-gm tubes.

[101078]

CORDRAN® TAPE ℞

(flurandrenolide tape)
USP

Description: Cordran Tape is a transparent, inconspicuous, plastic surgical tape, impervious to moisture. It contains Cordran® (flurandrenolide, Dista), a potent corticosteroid. Each square centimeter contains 4 mcg of flurandrenolide uniformly distributed in the adhesive layer. The tape is made of a thin, matte-finish polyethylene film which is slightly elastic and highly flexible.

The adhesive is a synthetic copolymer of acrylate ester and acrylic acid which is free from substances of plant origin. The pressure-sensitive adhesive surface is covered with a protective paper liner to permit handling and trimming before application.

Action: Cordran® (flurandrenolide, Dista) is primarily effective because of its anti-inflammatory, antipruritic, and vasoconstrictive actions.

The tape serves as both a vehicle and an occlusive dressing. Retention of insensible perspiration by the tape results in hydration of the stra-

Continued on next page

Dista—Cont.

tum corneum and improved diffusion of the medication. The skin is protected from scratching, rubbing, desiccation, and chemical irritation. The tape acts as a mechanical splint to fissured skin. Since it prevents removal of the medication by washing or the rubbing action of clothing, the tape formulation provides a sustained action.

Indications: For relief of the inflammatory manifestations of corticosteroid-responsive dermatoses, particularly dry, scaling localized lesions.

Contraindications: Topical corticosteroids are contraindicated in patients with a history of hypersensitivity to any of the components of this preparation.

Use of Cordran® Tape (flurandrenolide tape, Dista) is not recommended for lesions exuding serum or in intertriginous areas.

Precautions: If irritation develops, the product should be discontinued and appropriate therapy instituted.

In the presence of an infection, an appropriate antifungal or antibacterial agent should be used. If a favorable response does not occur promptly, the corticosteroid should be discontinued until the infection has been adequately controlled.

If extensive areas are treated, there will be increased systemic absorption of the corticosteroid, and suitable precautions should be taken, particularly in children and infants.

Although topical corticosteroids have not been reported to have an adverse effect on human pregnancy, the safety of their use on pregnant women has not been absolutely established. In laboratory animals, increases in incidence of fetal abnormalities have been associated with exposure of gestating females to topical corticosteroids, in some cases at rather low dosage levels. Therefore, drugs of this class should not be used extensively, in large amounts, or for prolonged periods of time on pregnant patients.

Adverse Reactions: The following local adverse reactions have been reported with topical corticosteroid formulations:

Acneform eruptions
Allergic contact dermatitis
Burning
Dryness
Folliculitis
Hypertrichosis
Hypopigmentation
Irritation
Itching
Perioral dermatitis

The following may occur more frequently with occlusive dressings (such as Cordran® Tape [flurandrenolide tape, Dista]):

Maceration of the skin
Miliaria
Secondary infection
Skin atrophy
Striae

In addition, the tape vehicle may cause purpura and stripping of the epidermis.

Administration and Dosage: Replacement of the tape every 12 hours produces the lowest incidence of adverse reactions, but it may be left in place for 24 hours if it is well tolerated and adheres satisfactorily. When necessary, the tape may be used at nighttime only and removed during the day.

If ends of the tape loosen prematurely, they may be trimmed off and replaced with fresh tape.

The directions given below are included on a separate package insert for the patient to follow unless otherwise instructed by the physician.

Application of Medicated Transparent Tape

IMPORTANT: Skin should be clean and dry before tape is applied. Tape should always be cut, never torn.

DIRECTIONS FOR USE:

1. Prepare skin as directed by your physician or as follows: Gently clean the area to be covered to remove scales, crusts, dried exudates, and any previously used ointments or creams. A germicidal soap or cleanser should be used to prevent the development of odor under the tape. Shave or clip the hair in the treatment area to allow good contact with the skin and comfortable removal. If shower or tub baths are to be taken, they should be completed before the tape is applied. The skin should be dry before application of the tape.
2. Remove tape from package and cut a piece slightly larger than area to be covered. Round off corners.
3. Pull white paper from transparent tape. Be careful that tape does not stick to itself.
4. Apply tape, keeping skin smooth; press tape into place.

REPLACEMENT OF TAPE:

Unless instructed otherwise by your physician, replace tape after 12 hours. Cleanse skin and allow it to dry for one hour before applying new tape.

IF IRRITATION OR INFECTION DEVELOPS, REMOVE TAPE AND CONSULT PHYSICIAN.

How Supplied: (℞) *Cordran® Tape (Flurandrenolide Tape, USP), M-170, W14,** 4 mcg flurandrenolide per sq cm, in Small Rolls 24 inches long and 3 inches wide (60 cm x 7.5 cm) and in Large Rolls 80 inches long and 3 inches wide (200 cm x 7.5 cm), in single packages.

Directions for the patient are included in each package. [062878]

Cordran Tape is processed for Dista Products Company by Minnesota Mining and Mfg. Co., St. Paul, Minnesota 55101.

M-170—Large Roll—6505-00-168-6813

[*Shown in Product Identification Section*]

*Identi-Code® symbol.

ILOSONE® ℞
(erythromycin estolate)
NF
ORAL PREPARATIONS

WARNING

Hepatic dysfunction with or without jaundice has occurred, chiefly in adults, in association with erythromycin estolate administration. It may be accompanied by malaise, nausea, vomiting, abdominal colic, and fever. In some instances, severe abdominal pain may simulate an abdominal surgical emergency.

If the above findings occur, discontinue Ilosone® (erythromycin estolate, Dista) promptly.

Ilosone is contraindicated for patients with a known history of sensitivity to this drug and for those with preexisting liver disease.

Description: Erythromycin is produced by a strain of *Streptomyces erythraeus* and belongs to the macrolide group of antibiotics. It is basic and readily forms salts with acids. The base, the stearate salt, and the esters are poorly soluble in water and are suitable for oral administration.

Ilosone® (erythromycin estolate, Dista) is the lauryl sulfate salt of the propionyl ester of erythromycin.

Actions: Erythromycin inhibits protein synthesis without affecting nucleic acid synthesis. Some strains of *Haemophilus influenzae* and staphylococci have demonstrated resistance to erythromycin. Culture and susceptibility testing should be done. If the Bauer-Kirby method of disc susceptibility testing is used, a 15-mcg erythromycin disc should give a zone diameter of at least 18 mm when tested against an erythromycin-susceptible organism.

Orally administered erythromycin estolate is readily and reliably absorbed. Because of acid stability, serum levels are comparable whether the estolate is taken in the fasting state or after food. After a single 250-mg dose, blood concentrations average 0.29, 1.2, and 1.2 mcg per ml respectively at two, four, and six hours. Following a 500-mg dose, blood concentrations average 3, 1.9, and 0.7 mcg per ml respectively at two, six, and 12 hours.

After oral administration, serum antibiotic levels consist of erythromycin base and propionyl erythromycin ester. The propionyl ester continuously hydrolyzes to the base form of erythromycin to maintain an equilibrium ratio of approximately 20 percent base and 80 percent ester in the serum. Further, the propionyl ester contributes to the activity of the drug through additional hydrolysis to the base at the bacterial cellular level.

After absorption, erythromycin diffuses readily into most body fluids. In the absence of meningeal inflammation, low concentrations are normally achieved in the spinal fluid, but passage of the drug across the blood-brain barrier increases in meningitis. In the presence of normal hepatic function, erythromycin is concentrated in the liver and excreted in the bile; the effect of hepatic dysfunction on excretion of erythromycin by the liver into the bile is not known. After oral administration, less than 5 percent of the administered dose can be recovered as the active form in the urine.

Erythromycin crosses the placental barrier, but fetal plasma levels are low.

Indications: *Streptococcus pyogenes* (Group A Beta-Hemolytic)—Upper and lower respiratory tract, skin, and soft-tissue infections of mild to moderate severity.

Injectable penicillin G benzathine is considered by the American Heart Association to be the drug of choice in the treatment and prevention of streptococcal pharyngitis and in long-term prophylaxis of rheumatic fever.

When oral medication is preferred for treating the above-mentioned conditions, penicillin G or V or erythromycin is the alternate drug of choice.

The importance of the patient's strict adherence to the prescribed dosage regimen must be stressed when oral medication is given. A therapeutic dose should be administered for at least ten days.

Alpha-Hemolytic Streptococci (Viridans Group)—Short-term prophylaxis against bacterial endocarditis prior to dental or other operative procedures in patients with a history of rheumatic fever or congenital heart disease who are hypersensitive to penicillin. (Erythromycin is not suitable prior to genitourinary surgery when the organisms likely to lead to bacteremia are gram-negative bacilli or belong to the enterococcus group of streptococci.)

Staphylococcus aureus—Acute infections of skin and soft tissue which are mild to moderately severe. Resistance may develop during treatment.

S. (Diplococcus) pneumoniae—Infections of the upper respiratory tract (e.g., otitis media, pharyngitis) and lower respiratory tract (e.g., pneumonia) of mild to moderate severity.

Mycoplasma pneumoniae (Eaton Agent, PPLO)—In the treatment of respiratory tract infections due to this organism.

H. influenzae—May be used concomitantly with adequate doses of sulfonamides in treating upper respiratory tract infections of mild to moderate severity. Not all strains of this organism are susceptible at the erythromycin concentrations ordinarily achieved (see appropriate sulfonamide labeling for prescribing information).

Treponema pallidum—Erythromycin is an alternate choice of treatment for primary syphilis in penicillin-allergic patients. In primary syphilis, spinal-fluid examinations should be done before treatment and as part of follow-up after therapy.

Corynebacterium diphtheriae—As an adjunct to antitoxin, to prevent establishment of carriers, and to eradicate the organism in carriers.

C. minutissimum—In the treatment of erythrasma.

Entamoeba histolytica—In the treatment of intestinal amebiasis only. Extraenteric amebiasis requires treatment with other agents.

Listeria monocytogenes—Infections due to this organism.

Legionnaires' Disease—Although no controlled clinical efficacy studies have been conducted, in vitro and limited preliminary clinical data suggest that erythromycin may be effective in treating Legionnaires' disease.

Contraindication: Erythromycin is contraindicated in patients with known hypersensitivity to this antibiotic.

Warnings: (*See* Warning box above.) The administration of erythromycin estolate has been associated with the infrequent occurrence of cholestatic hepatitis. Laboratory findings have been characterized by abnormal hepatic function test values, peripheral eosinophilia, and leukocytosis. Symptoms may include malaise, nausea, vomiting, abdominal cramps, and fever. Jaundice may or may not be present. In some instances, severe abdominal pain may simulate the pain of biliary colic, pancreatitis, perforated ulcer, or an acute abdominal surgical problem. In other instances, clinical symptoms and results of liver function tests have resembled findings in extrahepatic obstructive jaundice.

Initial symptoms have developed in some cases after a few days of treatment but generally have followed one or two weeks of continuous therapy. Symptoms reappear promptly, usually within 48 hours after the drug is readministered to sensitive patients. The syndrome seems to result from a form of sensitization, occurs chiefly in adults, and has been reversible when medication is discontinued.

Usage in Pregnancy—Safety of this drug for use during pregnancy has not been established.

Precautions: Since erythromycin is excreted principally by the liver, caution should be exercised in administering the antibiotic to patients with impaired hepatic function.

Recent data from studies of erythromycin reveal that its use in patients who are receiving high doses of theophylline may be associated with an increase in serum theophylline levels and potential theophylline toxicity. In case of theophylline toxicity and/or elevated serum theophylline levels, the dose of theophylline should be reduced while the patient is receiving concomitant erythromycin therapy.

Surgical procedures should be performed when indicated.

Adverse Reactions: The most frequent side effects of erythromycin preparations are gastrointestinal (e.g., abdominal cramping and discomfort) and are dose related. Nausea, vomiting, and diarrhea occur infrequently with usual oral doses.

During prolonged or repeated therapy, there is a possibility of overgrowth of nonsusceptible bacteria or fungi. If such infections arise, the drug should be discontinued and appropriate therapy instituted.

Mild allergic reactions, such as urticaria and other skin rashes, have occurred. Serious allergic reactions, including anaphylaxis, have been reported.

Administration and Dosage: *Adults*—The usual dosage is 250 mg every six hours. This may be increased up to 4 gm or more per day according to the severity of the infection.

Children—Age, weight, and severity of the infection are important factors in determining the proper dosage. The usual regimen is 30 to 50 mg per kg per day in divided doses. For more severe infections, this dosage may be doubled. If administration is desired on a twice-a-day schedule in either adults or children, one-half of the total daily dose may be given every 12 hours.

Streptococcal Infections—For the treatment of streptococcal pharyngitis and tonsillitis, the usual dosage range is 20 to 50 mg per kg per day in divided doses.

Body Weight	Total Daily Dose
10 kg or less (less than 25 lb)	250 mg
11–18 kg (25–40 lb)	375 mg
18–25 kg (40–55 lb)	500 mg
25–36 kg (55–80 lb)	750 mg
36 kg or more (more than 80 lb)	1000 mg (adult dose)

In the treatment of group A beta-hemolytic streptococcal infections, a therapeutic dosage of erythromycin should be administered for at least ten days. In continuous prophylaxis of streptococcal infections in persons with a history of rheumatic heart disease, the dosage is 250 mg twice a day.

When Ilosone® (erythromycin estolate, Dista) is used prior to surgery to prevent endocarditis caused by alpha-hemolytic streptococci (viridans group), a recommended schedule for adults is 500 mg before the procedure and 250 mg every eight hours for four doses afterward; for children, 30 to 50 mg per kg per day divided into three or four evenly spaced doses.

Primary Syphilis—A regimen of 20 gm of erythromycin estolate in divided doses over a period of ten days has been shown to be effective in the treatment of primary syphilis.

Dysenteric Amebiasis—Dosage for adults is 250 mg four times daily for 10 to 14 days; for children, 30 to 50 mg per kg per day in divided doses for 10 to 14 days.

Legionnaires' Disease—Although optimum doses have not been established, doses utilized in reported clinical data were those recommended above (1 to 4 gm erythromycin estolate daily in divided doses).

How Supplied: (℞) *Pulvules® Ilosone® (Erythromycin Estolate Capsules, NF): No. 374, H07,** 125 mg (equivalent to erythromycin) (No. 2, Ivory Opaque Body, Red Opaque Cap), in bottles of 24 and 100; *No. 375, H09,** 250 mg (equivalent to erythromycin) (No. 0, Ivory Opaque Body, Red Opaque Cap), in bottles of 24 and 100 and in 10 strips of 10 individually labeled blisters each containing 1 Pulvule (ID100).

(℞) *Tablets Ilosone® (Erythromycin Estolate Tablets, NF), No. 1863, U26,** 500 mg (equivalent to erythromycin), Specially Coated, Light-Pink (capsule-shaped, scored), in bottles of 50 and in 10 strips of 10 individually labeled blisters each containing 1 tablet (ID100).

(℞) *Tablets Ilosone® Chewable (Erythromycin Estolate Tablets, NF), No. 1834, U05,** 125 mg (equivalent to erythromycin), Light-Pink, and *No. 1865, U25,** 250 mg (equivalent to erythromycin), Light-Pink, in bottles of 50.

[*Shown in Product Identification Section*]

(℞) *Ilosone® Liquid (Erythromycin Estolate Oral Suspension, NF), M-148, W15,** in 100-ml and 16-fl-oz bottles.

Each 5 ml contain erythromycin estolate equivalent to 125 mg erythromycin in an orange-flavored vehicle. *Shake well before using. Refrigerate to maintain optimum taste.*

(℞) *Ilosone® Liquid (Erythromycin Estolate Oral Suspension, NF), M-153, W17,** in 100-ml and 16-fl-oz bottles.

Each 5 ml contain erythromycin estolate equivalent to 250 mg erythromycin in a cherry-flavored vehicle. *Shake well before using. Refrigerate to maintain optimum taste.*

(℞) *Ilosone® (Erythromycin Estolate for Oral Suspension, NF), M-104, W03,** in 60 and 150-ml-size packages.

Each 60-ml-size package consists of a bottle containing erythromycin estolate equivalent to 1.5 gm erythromycin. At the time of dispensing, 48 ml of water are added to provide 60 ml of an oral suspension.

Each 150-ml-size package consists of a bottle containing erythromycin estolate equivalent to 3.75 gm erythromycin. At the time of dispensing, 120 ml of water are added to provide 150 ml of an oral suspension.

When mixed as directed, each 5 ml (approximately 1 teaspoonful) will contain erythromycin estolate equivalent to 125 mg erythromycin. After being mixed, the suspension may be kept at room temperature for 14 days without significant loss of potency. *Shake well before using. Keep tightly closed.*

(℞) *Ilosone® Ready-Mixed Drops (Erythromycin Estolate Oral Suspension, NF), M-159, W18,** in 10-ml bottles.

Each package consists of a bottle containing erythromycin estolate equivalent to 1 gm erythromycin in a pleasantly flavored vehicle and a special dropper calibrated at approximately 25 mg and 50 mg.

Each ml contains erythromycin estolate equivalent to 100 mg erythromycin. *Shake well before using. Refrigerate to maintain optimum taste.* [110678]

Pulvules No. 375, 250 mg—100's—6505-00-890-1388A

*Identi-Code® symbol.

ILOTYCIN® ℞
(erythromycin)
Ointment, USP

Description: Ilotycin® (erythromycin, Dista) is a wide-range antibiotic discovered in the research laboratories of Eli Lilly and Company and produced from a strain of *Streptomyces erythraeus.*

Indications: On the basis of a review of this drug by the National Academy of Sciences—National Research Council and/or other information, FDA has classified the following indications as "possibly" effective.

Ilotycin® (erythromycin, Dista) ointment is possibly effective in the treatment of superficial topical infections due to organisms sensitive to its action. The therapeutic spectrum of Ilotycin includes streptococci, staphylococci, pneumococci, and other gram-positive bacteria. In addition, Ilotycin is effective against some gram-negative organisms, *Neisseria, Haemophilus,* corynebacteria, clostridia, and certain parasitic (e.g., *Entamoeba histolytica*), rickettsial, and large-virus infections.

Final classification of the less-than-effective indications requires further investigation.

Contraindication: This drug is contraindicated in patients with a history of sensitivity to erythromycin.

Precautions and Adverse Reactions: The use of antimicrobial agents may be associated with the overgrowth of antibiotic-resistant organisms; in such a case, antibiotic administration should be stopped and appropriate measures taken.

As with any other medicament intended for topical use, there is always the possibility that sensitivity reactions will occur in certain individuals.

Continued on next page

Dista—Cont.

Administration: Ointment Ilotycin® (erythromycin, Dista) should be applied to the affected areas three or four times daily.

How Supplied: (℞) *Ointment No. 90, Ilotycin® (Erythromycin Ointment, USP),* 10 mg per gm, in ½-oz and 1-oz tubes and in 16-oz jars. Contains mineral oil and white petrolatum. *Store at controlled room temperature, 15° to 30°C (59° to 86°F).*

[020678]

ILOTYCIN® ℞
(erythromycin)
Ophthalmic Ointment, USP

Description: Ilotycin® (erythromycin, Dista) is a highly effective wide-range antibiotic discovered in the research laboratories of Eli Lilly and Company and produced from a strain of *Streptomyces erythraeus.* The special sterile ophthalmic ointment base, containing mineral oil and white petrolatum, flows freely over the entire conjunctiva.

Indications: For the treatment of superficial ocular infections involving the conjunctiva and/or cornea caused by organisms susceptible to Ilotycin® (erythromycin, Dista).

Contraindication: This drug is contraindicated in patients with a history of hypersensitivity to erythromycin.

Precautions and Adverse Reactions: As with any other medicament intended for topical use, there is always the possibility that sensitivity reactions will occur in certain individuals.

Administration: In the treatment of external ocular infections, Ophthalmic Ointment Ilotycin® (erythromycin, Dista) should be applied directly to the infected structure one or more times daily, depending on the severity of the infection.

How Supplied: (℞) *Sterile Ophthalmic Ointment No. 52, Ilotycin® (Erythromycin Ophthalmic Ointment, USP),* 5 mg per gm, in ⅛-oz tamperproof tubes. Contains mineral oil and white petrolatum. *Store at controlled room temperature, 15° to 30°C (59° to 86°F).*

[062679]

ILOTYCIN® ℞
(erythromycin)
Tablets, USP
(Enteric-Coated)

Description: Erythromycin is produced by a strain of *Streptomyces erythraeus* and belongs to the macrolide group of antibiotics. It is basic and readily forms salts with acids. The base, the stearate salt, and the esters are poorly soluble in water and are suitable for oral administration.

Actions: Erythromycin inhibits protein synthesis without affecting nucleic acid synthesis. Some strains of *Haemophilus influenzae* and staphylococci have demonstrated resistance to erythromycin. Culture and susceptibility testing should be done. If the Bauer-Kirby method of disc susceptibility testing is used, a 15-mcg erythromycin disc should give a zone diameter of at least 18 mm when tested against an erythromycin-susceptible organism.

Orally administered erythromycin is readily absorbed by most patients, especially on an empty stomach, but patient variation has been observed.

After absorption, erythromycin diffuses readily into most body fluids. In the absence of meningeal inflammation, low concentrations are normally achieved in the spinal fluid, but passage of the drug across the blood-brain barrier increases in meningitis. In the presence of normal hepatic function, erythromycin is concentrated in the liver and excreted in the bile; the effect of hepatic dysfunction on excretion of erythromycin by the liver into the bile is not known. After oral administration, less than 5 percent of the administered dose can be recovered as the active form in the urine.

Erythromycin crosses the placental barrier, but fetal plasma levels are low.

Indications: *Streptococcus pyogenes* (Group A Beta-Hemolytic)—Upper and lower respiratory tract, skin, and soft-tissue infections of mild to moderate severity.

Injectable penicillin G benzathine is considered by the American Heart Association to be the drug of choice in the treatment and prevention of streptococcal pharyngitis and in long-term prophylaxis of rheumatic fever.

When oral medication is preferred for treating the above-mentioned conditions, penicillin G or V or erythromycin is the alternate drug of choice.

The importance of the patient's strict adherence to the prescribed dosage regimen must be stressed when oral medication is given. A therapeutic dose should be administered for at least ten days.

Alpha-Hemolytic Streptococci (Viridans Group)—Short-term prophylaxis against bacterial endocarditis prior to dental or other operative procedures in patients with a history of rheumatic fever or congenital heart disease who are hypersensitive to penicillin. (Erythromycin is not suitable prior to genitourinary surgery when the organisms likely to lead to bacteremia are gram-negative bacilli or belong to the enterococcus group of streptococci.)

Staphylococcus aureus—Acute infections of skin and soft tissue which are mild to moderately severe. Resistance may develop during treatment.

S. (Diplococcus) pneumoniae—Infections of the upper respiratory tract (e.g., otitis media, pharyngitis) and lower respiratory tract (e.g., pneumonia) of mild to moderate severity.

Mycoplasma pneumoniae (Eaton Agent, PPLO)—In the treatment of respiratory tract infections due to this organism.

H. influenzae—May be used concomitantly with adequate doses of sulfonamides in treating upper respiratory tract infections of mild to moderate severity. Not all strains of this organism are susceptible at the erythromycin concentrations ordinarily achieved (see appropriate sulfonamide labeling for prescribing information).

Treponema pallidum—Erythromycin is an alternate choice of treatment for primary syphilis in penicillin-allergic patients. In primary syphilis, spinal-fluid examinations should be done before treatment and as part of follow-up after therapy.

Corynebacterium diphtheriae—As an adjunct to antitoxin, to prevent establishment of carriers, and to eradicate the organism in carriers.

C. minutissimum—In the treatment of erythrasma.

Entamoeba histolytica—In the treatment of intestinal amebiasis only. Extraenteric amebiasis requires treatment with other agents.

Listeria monocytogenes—Infections due to this organism.

Neisseria gonorrhoeae—In female patients with a history of sensitivity to penicillin, a parenteral erythromycin (such as the gluceptate) may be administered in conjunction with an oral erythromycin as alternate therapy in acute pelvic inflammatory disease caused by *N. gonorrhoeae.* In the treatment of gonorrhea, patients suspected of having concomitant syphilis should have microscopic examinations (by immunofluorescence or darkfield) before receiving erythromycin and monthly serologic tests for a minimum of four months.

Legionnaires' Disease—Although no controlled clinical efficacy studies have been conducted, in vitro and limited preliminary clinical data suggest that erythromycin may be effective in treating Legionnaires' disease.

Contraindication: Erythromycin is contraindicated in patients with known hypersensitivity to this antibiotic.

Warning: *Usage in Pregnancy*—Safety of this drug for use during pregnancy has not been established.

Precautions: Since erythromycin is excreted principally by the liver, caution should be exercised in administering the antibiotic to patients with impaired hepatic function. There have been reports of hepatic dysfunction, with or without jaundice, occurring in patients taking oral erythromycin products.

Recent data from studies of erythromycin reveal that its use in patients who are receiving high doses of theophylline may be associated with an increase in serum theophylline levels and potential theophylline toxicity. In case of theophylline toxicity and/or elevated serum theophylline levels, the dose of theophylline should be reduced while the patient is receiving concomitant erythromycin therapy.

Surgical procedures should be performed when indicated.

Adverse Reactions: The most frequent side effects of erythromycin preparations are gastrointestinal (e.g., abdominal cramping and discomfort) and are dose related. Nausea, vomiting, and diarrhea occur infrequently with usual oral doses.

During prolonged or repeated therapy, there is a possibility of overgrowth of nonsusceptible bacteria or fungi. If such infections arise, the drug should be discontinued and appropriate therapy instituted.

Mild allergic reactions, such as urticaria and other skin rashes, have occurred. Serious allergic reactions, including anaphylaxis, have been reported.

Administration and Dosage: Optimum blood levels are obtained when doses are given on an empty stomach.

Adults—The usual dosage is 250 mg every six hours. This may be increased up to 4 gm or more per day according to the severity of the infection.

Children—Age, weight, and severity of the infection are important factors in determining the proper dosage. The usual regimen is 30 to 50 mg per kg per day in divided doses. For more severe infections, this dosage may be doubled. If administration is desired on a twice-a-day schedule in either adults or children, one-half of the total daily dose may be given every 12 hours, one hour before meals.

Streptococcal Infections—In the treatment of group A beta-hemolytic streptococcal infections, a therapeutic dosage of erythromycin should be administered for at least ten days. In continuous prophylaxis of streptococcal infections in persons with a history of rheumatic heart disease, the dosage is 250 mg twice a day. When Ilotycin® (erythromycin, Dista) is used prior to surgery to prevent endocarditis caused by alpha-hemolytic streptococci (viridans group), a recommended schedule for adults is 500 mg before the procedure and 250 mg every six hours for four doses afterward; for children, 30 to 50 mg per kg per day divided into three or four evenly spaced doses.

Primary Syphilis—30 to 40 gm given in divided doses over a period of 10 to 15 days.

Acute Pelvic Inflammatory Disease Caused by N. gonorrhoeae—Ilotycin® Gluceptate (Sterile Erythromycin Gluceptate, USP, Dista), 500 mg intravenously every six hours for at least three days, followed by Ilotycin, 250 mg every six hours for seven days.

Dysenteric Amebiasis—250 mg four times daily for 10 to 14 days for adults; 30 to 50 mg per kg per day in divided doses for 10 to 14 days for children.

Legionnaires' Disease—Although optimum doses have not been established, doses utilized in reported clinical data were those recommended above (1 to 4 gm erythromycin base daily in divided doses).

How Supplied: (℞) *Tablets No. 23, Ilotycin® (Erythromycin Tablets, USP) (Enteric-Coated), C03,** 250 mg, Orange, in bottles of 24, 100, and

500 and in 20 strips of 5 individually labeled blisters each containing 1 tablet (ID100).
[020179]
[*Shown in Product Identification Section*]

*Identi-Code® symbol.

ILOTYCIN® GLUCEPTATE ℞
(erythromycin gluceptate)
Sterile, USP
IntraVenous

Description: Erythromycin is produced by a strain of *Streptomyces erythraeus* and belongs to the macrolide group of antibiotics. It is basic and readily forms salts with acids.

Actions: Erythromycin inhibits protein synthesis without affecting nucleic acid synthesis. Some strains of *Haemophilus influenzae* and staphylococci have demonstrated resistance to erythromycin. Culture and susceptibility testing should be done. If the Bauer-Kirby method of disc susceptibility testing is used, a 15-mcg erythromycin disc should give a zone diameter of at least 18 mm when tested against an erythromycin-susceptible organism.

Intravenous injection of 200 mg of erythromycin produces peak serum levels of 3 to 4 mcg per ml at one hour and 0.5 mcg per ml at six hours.

Erythromycin diffuses readily into the body fluids. Only low concentrations are normally achieved in the spinal fluid, but passage of the drug across the blood-brain barrier increases in meningitis. In the presence of normal hepatic function, erythromycin is concentrated in the liver and excreted in the bile; the effect of hepatic dysfunction on excretion of erythromycin by the liver into the bile is not known. From 12 to 15 percent of intravenously administered erythromycin is excreted in active form in the urine.

Erythromycin crosses the placental barrier, but fetal plasma levels are low.

Indications: *Streptococcus pyogenes* (Group A Beta-Hemolytic)—Upper and lower respiratory tract, skin, and soft-tissue infections of mild to moderate severity.

Injectable penicillin G benzathine is considered by the American Heart Association to be the drug of choice in the treatment and prevention of streptococcal pharyngitis and in long-term prophylaxis of rheumatic fever.

Alpha-Hemolytic Streptococci (Viridans Group)—Short-term prophylaxis against bacterial endocarditis prior to dental or other operative procedures in patients with a history of rheumatic fever or congenital heart disease who are hypersensitive to penicillin. (Erythromycin is not suitable prior to genitourinary surgery when the organisms likely to lead to bacteremia are gram-negative bacilli or belong to the enterococcus group of streptococci.)

Staphylococcus aureus—Acute infections of skin and soft tissue which are mild to moderately severe. Resistance may develop during treatment.

S. (Diplococcus) pneumoniae—Infections of the upper respiratory tract (e.g., otitis media, pharyngitis) and lower respiratory tract (e.g., pneumonia) of mild to moderate severity.

Mycoplasma pneumoniae (Eaton Agent, PPLO)—In the treatment of respiratory tract infections due to this organism.

H. influenzae—May be used concomitantly with adequate doses of sulfonamides in treating upper respiratory tract infections of mild to moderate severity. Not all strains of this organism are susceptible at the erythromycin concentrations ordinarily achieved (see appropriate sulfonamide labeling for prescribing information).

Corynebacterium diphtheriae—As an adjunct to antitoxin.

Listeria monocytogenes—Infections due to this organism.

Neisseria gonorrhoeae—In female patients with a history of sensitivity to penicillin, a parenteral erythromycin (such as the gluceptate) may be administered in conjunction with an oral erythromycin as alternate therapy in acute pelvic inflammatory disease caused by *N. gonorrhoeae*. In the treatment of gonorrhea, patients suspected of having concomitant syphilis should have microscopic examinations (by immunofluorescence or darkfield) before receiving erythromycin and monthly serologic tests for a minimum of four months.

Legionnaires' Disease—Although no controlled clinical efficacy studies have been conducted, in vitro and limited preliminary clinical data suggest that erythromycin may be effective in treating Legionnaires' disease.

Contraindication: Intravenous erythromycin is contraindicated in patients with known hypersensitivity to this antibiotic.

Warning: *Usage in Pregnancy*—Safety of this drug for use during pregnancy has not been established.

Precautions: Side effects following the use of intravenous erythromycin are rare. Occasional venous irritation has been encountered, but if the injection is given slowly, in dilute solution, preferably by continuous intravenous infusion over 20 to 60 minutes, pain and vessel trauma are minimized.

Since erythromycin is excreted principally by the liver, caution should be exercised in administering the antibiotic to patients with impaired hepatic function.

Recent data from studies of erythromycin reveal that its use in patients who are receiving high doses of theophylline may be associated with an increase in serum theophylline levels and potential theophylline toxicity. In case of theophylline toxicity and/or elevated serum theophylline levels, the dose of theophylline should be reduced while the patient is receiving concomitant erythromycin therapy.

Surgical procedures should be performed when indicated.

Adverse Reactions: Allergic reactions, ranging from urticaria and mild skin eruptions to anaphylaxis, have occurred with intravenously administered erythromycin.

During prolonged or repeated therapy, there is a possibility of overgrowth of nonsusceptible bacteria or fungi. If such infections arise, the drug should be discontinued and appropriate therapy instituted.

Variations in liver function have been observed following daily doses at high levels or after prolonged therapy. Hepatic function tests should be performed when such therapy is given.

Reversible hearing loss associated with the intravenous infusion of 4 gm or more per day of erythromycin has been reported rarely.

Administration and Dosage: Prepare the initial solution of Ilotycin® Gluceptate (erythromycin gluceptate, Dista) by (1) adding at least 10 ml of Sterile Water for Injection to the 250 or 500-mg vial or at least 20 ml of Sterile Water for Injection to the 1-gm vial of Ilotycin Gluceptate and (2) shaking the vial until all of the drug is dissolved.

It is important that the product be diluted only *with Sterile Water for Injection without preservatives.*

After reconstitution, the sterile solutions should be stored in a refrigerator and used within seven days.

When all of the drug is dissolved, the solution may then be added to 0.9% Sodium Chloride Injection or to 5% Dextrose in Water to give 1 gm per liter for slow, continuous infusion. I.V. fluid admixtures with a *p*H below 5.5 tend to lose potency rapidly. Therefore, such solutions should be administered completely within four hours after dilution.

If the period of administration is prolonged, the *p*H of the infusion fluid should be buffered to neutrality with a sterile agent such as Neut® (Sodium Bicarbonate 4% Additive Solution, Abbott) or Buff™ (Phosphate-Carbonate Buffer, Travenol). For administration of the antibiotic in 500 or 1000 ml of 5% Dextrose in Water, add one ampoule full-strength Buff or 5 ml of Neut; for administration of the antibiotic in the same volumes of 0.9% Sodium Chloride Injection, add one ampoule half-strength Buff or 5 ml of Neut. These solutions should be completely administered within 24 hours after dilution.

If the medication is to be given in 100 to 250 ml of fluid by a volume control set such as Metriset® (McGaw), Volu-Trole® "B" (Cutter), Soluset® (Abbott), or Buretrol® (Baxter-Travenol), the I.V. fluid should be buffered in its primary container before being added to the volumetric administration set.

If the medication is to be given by intermittent injection, one-fourth of the total daily dose can be given in 20 to 60 minutes by slow intravenous injection of 250 to 500 mg in 100 to 250 ml of 0.9% Sodium Chloride Injection or 5% Dextrose in Water. Injection should be sufficiently slow to avoid pain along the vein.

The recommended I.V. dosage for severe infections in adults and children is 15 to 20 mg per kg of body weight per day. Higher doses (up to 4 gm per day) may be given in very severe infections. Continuous infusion is preferable, but administration in divided doses at intervals of no more than every six hours is also effective.

For treatment of acute pelvic inflammatory disease caused by *N. gonorrhoeae*, administer 500 mg Ilotycin Gluceptate intravenously every six hours for at least three days, followed by 250 mg Ilotycin® (Erythromycin Tablets, USP, Dista) every six hours for seven days.

Patients receiving intravenous erythromycin should be changed to the oral dosage form as soon as possible.

For Treatment of Legionnaires' Disease—Although optimum doses have not been established, doses utilized in reported clinical data were those recommended above (1 to 4 gm daily in divided doses).

How Supplied: (℞) *Ampoules (Vials) Ilotycin® Gluceptate (Sterile Erythromycin Gluceptate, USP), I.V.*, rubber-stoppered (Dry Powder): *No. 524*, 250 mg (equivalent to erythromycin), 20-ml size; *No. 538*, 500 mg (equivalent to erythromycin), 30-ml size; and *No. 646*, 1 gm (equivalent to erythromycin); 50-ml size, in singles (10 per carton).
[021979]

MI-CEBRIN® OTC
(vitamins-minerals)

Description: Each tablet contains—

Thiamine (Vitamin B_1)	10 mg
Riboflavin (Vitamin B_2)	5 mg
Pyridoxine (Vitamin B_6)	1.7 mg
Pantothenic Acid	10 mg
Niacinamide	30 mg
Vitamin B_{12} (Activity Equivalent)	3 mcg
Ascorbic Acid (Vitamin C)	100 mg
dl-Alpha Tocopheryl Acetate (Vitamin E)	5.5 IU (5.5 mg)
Vitamin A	10,000 IU (3 mg)
Vitamin D	400 IU (10 mcg)
Contains also—	approximately
Iron (as Ferrous Sulfate)	15 mg
Copper (as the Sulfate)	1 mg
Iodine (as Potassium Iodide)	0.15 mg
Manganese (as the Glycerophosphate)	1 mg
Magnesium (as the Hydroxide)	5 mg
Zinc (as the Chloride)	1.5 mg

Mi-Cebrin offers a comprehensive vitamin-mineral formula in a yellow tablet of convenient size. The use of synthetic vitamins A and D eliminates any unpleasant fish-liver-oil odor or taste.

Indications: For the prevention or treatment of multiple vitamin and mineral deficien-

Continued on next page

Dista—Cont.

cies and in states of subnutrition. Both vitamins and minerals are essential components of vital physiologic mechanisms, including many enzyme systems. Although trace elements are known constituents of foodstuffs, their exact role in nutrition has not been defined. Studies have shown that foodstuffs may be lacking in these elements when grown in soil notably deprived of its normal constituents.
Dosage: 1 tablet a day, or as directed by the physician.
How Supplied: *Tablets No. 1790, Mi-Cebrin® (vitamins-minerals, Dista), C19,* *Coated, Yellow, in bottles of 60, 100, and 1000 and in 10 strips of 10 individually labeled blisters each containing 1 tablet (ID100). [060178]
[*Shown in Product Identification Section*]

*Identi-Code® symbol.

MI-CEBRIN T® OTC
(vitamin-minerals therapeutic)

Description: Each tablet contains—

Thiamine Mononitrate (Vitamin B_1)	15 mg
Riboflavin (Vitamin B_2)	10 mg
Pyridoxine Hydrochloride (Vitamin B_6)	2 mg
Pantothenic Acid (as Calcium Pantothenate)	10 mg
Niacinamide	100 mg
Vitamin B_{12} (Activity Equivalent)	7.5 mcg
Ascorbic Acid (Vitamin C)	150 mg
dl-Alpha Tocopheryl Acetate (Vitamin E)	5.5 IU (5.5 mg)
Vitamin A	10,000 IU (3 mg)
Vitamin D	400 IU (10 mcg)
Contains also—	approximately
Iron (as Ferrous Sulfate)	15 mg
Copper (as the Sulfate)	1 mg
Iodine (as Potassium Iodide)	0.15 mg
Manganese (as the Glycerophosphate)	1 mg
Magnesium (as the Hydroxide)	5 mg
Zinc (as the Chloride)	1.5 mg

Mi-Cebrin T is an extended-range therapeutic vitamin-mineral tablet formulated to aid patient recovery. Each tablet contains ten vitamins and six minerals and is specially coated to protect the full potency of the ingredients.
Indications: For the therapeutic management of surgical patients and patients with burns or injuries, febrile diseases, or poor dietary intake.
Precaution: Rarely, vitamins A and D in large doses daily for several months or longer cause toxicity.
Dosage: 1 tablet a day, or as directed by the physician.
How Supplied: *Tablets No. 1807, Mi-Cebrin T® (vitamin-minerals therapeutic, Dista), C20,** Coated, Orange, in bottles of 30, 100, and 1000 and in 10 strips of 10 individually labeled blisters each containing 1 tablet (ID100). [060178]
[*Shown in Product Identification Section*]

*Identi-Code® symbol.

NALFON® ℞
(fenoprofen calcium)

Description: Pulvules® Nalfon® (fenoprofen calcium, Dista) for oral administration contain fenoprofen calcium as the dihydrate in an amount equivalent to 300 mg of fenoprofen. Tablets Nalfon contain fenoprofen calcium as the dihydrate in an amount equivalent to 600 mg of fenoprofen. Nalfon is a nonsteroidal, anti-inflammatory, antiarthritic drug. Chemically, it is a propionic acid derivative. The formula is benzeneacetic acid, α-methyl-3-phenoxy-, calcium salt (2:1).-(±)-, dihydrate.
Nalfon is a white crystalline powder, soluble in alcohol (95 percent) to the extent of approximately 15 mg/ml at 25°C, slightly soluble in water, and insoluble in benzene.
The pK_a of Nalfon is 4.5 at 25°C.
Clinical Pharmacology: Nalfon® (fenoprofen calcium, Dista) is a nonsteroidal, anti-inflammatory, antiarthritic compound. In animal systems, it also shows analgesic and antipyretic activity. Its mode of action is unknown.
In patients with rheumatoid arthritis, the anti-inflammatory action of Nalfon has been shown by a reduction in joint swelling, a reduction in pain, a reduction in the duration of morning stiffness, a reduction in disease activity as assessed by both the investigator and the patient, and increased mobility as demonstrated by a reduction in the number of joints with limited motion. In patients with osteoarthritis, the anti-inflammatory and analgesic action of Nalfon in involved joints has been shown by reduction of tenderness with pressure, reduction of pain with motion and at rest, reduction of night pain, stiffness, and swelling, and reduction in overall disease activity as assessed by both patient and investigator and by an increase in range of motion of the knee. Its action is not mediated through the adrenal gland. There is no evidence that Nalfon alters the progressive course of the underlying disease.
To demonstrate further the anti-inflammatory activity of Nalfon in humans, the emergence and degree of erythemic response were measured in adult male volunteers exposed to ultraviolet irradiation. The effects of Nalfon, aspirin, and indomethacin were compared separately with those of placebo. All three drugs demonstrated antierythemic activity. The results in humans confirmed the anti-inflammatory, analgesic activity found in animals.
Nalfon has been shown to inhibit prostaglandin synthetase isolated from bovine seminal vesicles. Reproduction studies in rats have shown Nalfon to be associated with prolonged labor and difficult parturition when given during late pregnancy. Evidence suggested that this may be due to decreased uterine contractility resulting from the inhibition of prostaglandin synthesis.
Under fasting conditions, Nalfon is rapidly absorbed, and peak plasma levels of 50 mcg per ml are achieved within two hours after oral administration of 600-mg doses. Good dose proportionality was observed between 200 mg and 600 mg in fasting male volunteers. The plasma half-life is approximately three hours. Approximately 90 percent of a single oral dose is eliminated within 24 hours as fenoprofen glucuronide and 4′-hydroxyfenoprofen glucuronide, the major urinary metabolites of fenoprofen. Fenoprofen is highly bound (99 percent) to albumin.
The coadministration of aspirin decreases the biologic half-life of fenoprofen because of an increase in metabolic clearance that results in a greater amount of hydroxylated fenoprofen in the urine. Although the mechanism of interaction between fenoprofen and aspirin is not totally known, enzyme induction and displacement of fenoprofen from plasma albumin binding sites are possibilities. Chronic administration of phenobarbital, a known enzyme inducer, may be associated with a decrease in plasma half-life of fenoprofen. The clinical significance of these interactions is not known.
The concomitant administration of antacid (aluminum and magnesium hydroxide) does not interfere with absorption of Nalfon. Food ingestion decreases the rate and extent of absorption.
With single doses of Nalfon® (fenoprofen calcium, Dista), there is less suppression of collagen-induced platelet aggregation than with aspirin.
Fenoprofen shows anti-inflammatory effects in rodents by inhibiting the development of redness and edema in acute inflammatory conditions and by reducing soft-tissue swelling and bone damage associated with chronic inflammation. It exhibits analgesic activity in rodents by inhibiting the writhing response in mice caused by the introduction of an irritant into the peritoneal cavity and by elevating pain thresholds to pressure in edematous hindpaws of rats. In rats made febrile by the subcutaneous administration of brewer's yeast, fenoprofen produces antipyretic action. These effects are characteristic of nonsteroidal, anti-inflammatory, antipyretic, analgesic drugs.
Indications and Usage: Nalfon® (fenoprofen calcium, Dista) is indicated for relief of the signs and symptoms of rheumatoid arthritis and osteoarthritis. It is indicated in the treatment of acute flares and exacerbations and in the long-term management of these diseases. The safety and effectiveness of Nalfon have not been established in those rheumatoid arthritis patients who are designated by the American Rheumatism Association as Functional Class IV (largely or wholly incapacitated with patient bedridden or confined to wheelchair, permitting little or no self-care). Improvement in patients treated with Nalfon for rheumatoid arthritis has been demonstrated by a reduction in joint swelling, a reduction in pain, a reduction in the duration of morning stiffness, a reduction in disease activity as assessed by both the investigator and the patient, and increased mobility as demonstrated by a reduction in the number of joints with limited motion.
Improvement in patients treated with Nalfon for osteoarthritis has been demonstrated in involved joints by reduction of tenderness with pressure, reduction of pain with motion and at rest, reduction of night pain, stiffness, and swelling, and reduction of overall disease activity as assessed by both patient and investigator and by an increase in range of motion of the knee.
In clinical studies in patients with rheumatoid arthritis and osteoarthritis, Nalfon has been shown to be comparable to aspirin in controlling the aforementioned measures of disease activity, but the frequency of the milder gastrointestinal adverse effects (nausea, dyspepsia) and tinnitus was less than in aspirin-treated patients. It is not known whether Nalfon causes less peptic ulceration than aspirin.
In some patients with rheumatoid arthritis, Nalfon has been used in combination with gold salts or corticosteroids. Studies have been inadequate to demonstrate whether or not Nalfon adds any improvement in patients maintained on gold salts or corticosteroids. Whether or not Nalfon could be used in conjunction with partially effective doses of corticosteroid for a "steroid-sparing" effect has not been adequately studied. The use of Nalfon in combination with salicylates is not recommended, because there is no evidence to demonstrate that Nalfon would produce any additional effect beyond that produced by aspirin alone. Furthermore, there is evidence that aspirin increases the rate of excretion of Nalfon.
There have been no studies in children; therefore, the safety and effectiveness of Nalfon in children are unknown.
Contraindications: Nalfon® (fenoprofen calcium, Dista) is contraindicated in patients who have shown hypersensitivity to it.
Because the potential exists for cross-sensitivity to aspirin and other nonsteroidal, anti-inflammatory drugs, Nalfon should not be given to patients in whom aspirin and other nonsteroidal, anti-inflammatory drugs induce the symptoms of asthma, rhinitis, or urticaria.
Warnings: Nalfon® (fenoprofen calcium, Dista) should be given under close supervision to patients with a history of upper gastrointestinal tract disease and only after the section on Adverse Reactions has been consulted. Gastrointestinal bleeding, sometimes severe, has been reported in patients receiving Nalfon.

In patients with active rheumatoid arthritis or osteoarthritis who also have an active peptic ulcer, attempts should be made to treat the arthritis with nonulcerogenic drugs. If Nalfon must be given, the patient should be under close supervision for signs of ulcer perforation or severe gastrointestinal bleeding.

In subacute and chronic studies in rats, Nalfon caused interstitial nephritis, glomerulonephritis, and renal papillary necrosis. These abnormalities were dose related and began to appear at doses approximating the human dose. In chronic studies in monkeys, interstitial nephritis also occurred following administration of Nalfon. Although this was seen at doses considerably above the human dose, lower doses were not studied in this species. During the course of the clinical trials, one patient developed bilateral suppurative pyelonephritis, underwent laparotomy, went on to renal failure, and died with a diagnosis of septicemia and renal papillary necrosis. It is not known whether these events were drug related. A few patients developed mild elevations of BUN during therapy with Nalfon. Since Nalfon is eliminated primarily by the kidney, the drug should not be administered to patients with significantly impaired renal function. It is desirable to perform periodic renal function tests in all patients receiving Nalfon.

Precautions: In chronic studies in rats, high doses of Nalfon® (fenoprofen calcium, Dista) caused elevation of serum transaminase and hepatocellular hypertrophy. In clinical trials, some patients developed elevation of serum transaminase, LDH, and alkaline phosphatase that persisted for some months and usually, but not always, declined despite continuation of the drug. The significance of this is unknown. It is recommended that periodic liver function tests be performed in patients receiving Nalfon and that the drug be discontinued if abnormalities occur.

The safety of this drug in pregnancy and lactation has not been established, and its use during these events is, therefore, not recommended. Reproduction studies have been performed in rats and rabbits. When fenoprofen was given to rats during pregnancy and continued to the time of labor, parturition was prolonged. Similar results have been found with other nonsteroidal, anti-inflammatory drugs that inhibit prostaglandin synthetase.

In vitro studies have shown that fenoprofen, because of its affinity for albumin, may displace from their binding sites other drugs which are also albumin bound, and this may lead to drug interaction. Theoretically, fenoprofen, as well as other nonsteroidal, anti-inflammatory agents, could likewise be displaced. Patients receiving hydantoin, sulfonamides, or sulfonylureas should be observed for signs of toxicity to these drugs. In patients receiving coumarin-type anticoagulants, the addition of Nalfon to therapy could prolong the prothrombin time. Patients receiving both drugs should be under careful observation.

In patients receiving Nalfon and steroid concomitantly, any reduction in steroid dosage should be gradual to avoid the possible complications of sudden steroid withdrawal.

Patients with initial low hemoglobin values who are receiving long-term therapy with Nalfon should have a hemoglobin determination at reasonable intervals.

Peripheral edema has been observed in some patients taking Nalfon; therefore, Nalfon should be used with caution in patients with compromised cardiac function.

Studies to date have not shown changes in the eye attributed to administration of Nalfon. However, because of adverse eye findings in animal studies with some other nonsteroidal, anti-inflammatory drugs, it is recommended that ophthalmologic studies be carried out within a reasonable period of time after chronic therapy with Nalfon has been started and at periodic intervals thereafter.

Since food decreases the blood levels of Nalfon, the drug should be given 30 minutes before or two hours after meals during the daytime.

When phenobarbital, which may enhance the metabolism of Nalfon, is added or withdrawn, dosage adjustment of Nalfon may be required.

Caution should be exercised by patients whose activities require alertness if they experience central-nervous-system side effects from Nalfon.

Since the safety of Nalfon® (fenoprofen calcium, Dista) in patients with impaired hearing has not been established, these patients should have periodic tests of auditory function during chronic therapy with Nalfon.

Nalfon decreases platelet aggregation and may prolong bleeding time. Patients who may be adversely affected by prolongation of the bleeding time should be carefully observed when Nalfon is administered.

Adverse Reactions:

Digestive System—The most common type of adverse reaction concerned the gastrointestinal system. Dyspepsia occurred most frequently, being observed in about one out of seven patients. Other adverse reactions, in descending order of frequency, were constipation, nausea, vomiting, abdominal pain, anorexia, occult blood in the stool, diarrhea, flatulence, and dry mouth.

Three instances of peptic ulceration and/or gastrointestinal hemorrhage that may have been due to the drug and four instances in which drug relationship was questionable were observed in 3391 individuals to whom the drug was administered for periods of time ranging up to 165 weeks.

In less than 2 percent of patients, the drug was discontinued because of adverse gastrointestinal reactions.

Skin and Appendages—The most common adverse effect was pruritus, which was seen in about one out of ten patients. Other adverse reactions were rash, increased sweating, and urticaria.

In about 1 percent of patients, Nalfon® (fenoprofen calcium, Dista) was discontinued because of an adverse effect related to the skin.

Nervous System—The most frequent adverse reaction observed was somnolence, which occurred in about one out of seven patients. Other adverse effects, which occurred less frequently, were dizziness, tremor, confusion, and insomnia.

Nalfon was discontinued in less than 0.2 percent of patients because of these side effects.

Special Senses—The most common adverse reaction was tinnitus, which was seen in about one out of ten patients. Other reactions observed, in descending order of frequency, were blurred vision and decreased hearing.

In about 0.2 percent of patients, Nalfon was discontinued owing to adverse effects related to the special senses.

Cardiovascular—The most frequent adverse effect observed was palpitations. This was noted in about one out of 25 patients. Tachycardia was observed less frequently.

In less than 0.5 percent of patients, Nalfon was discontinued because of adverse cardiovascular reactions.

Laboratory—Anemia was noted in about one out of 500 patients. One patient required discontinuation of therapy with Nalfon because of anemia. Increase in alkaline phosphatase, LDH, and SGOT was observed (*see* Precautions).

Miscellaneous—Headache was seen in about one out of seven patients. Less frequently observed, in descending order of frequency, were nervousness, asthenia, dyspnea, peripheral edema, fatigue, malaise, and dysuria.

Overdosage: No specific information is available on the treatment of overdosage with Nalfon® (fenoprofen calcium, Dista). If it should occur, standard procedures to evacuate gastric contents and to support vital functions should be employed. Since Nalfon is acidic and is excreted in the urine, it may be beneficial to administer alkali and induce diuresis. Furosemide did not lower blood levels.

Administration and Dosage: For the initial treatment of rheumatoid arthritis, the recommended oral dose is 600 mg four times a day. For osteoarthritis, the recommended initial dose is 300 to 600 mg four times a day. Although improvement may be seen in a few days in many patients, an additional two to three weeks may be required to gauge the full benefits of therapy. The dosage should be adjusted in accordance with the patient's age, condition, and changes in disease activity. Daily dosage larger than 3200 mg is not recommended. Nalfon® (fenoprofen calcium, Dista) should be administered 30 minutes before or at least two hours after meals. If gastrointestinal complaints occur, administer Nalfon with meals or with milk.

There have been no studies in children; therefore, the safety and effectiveness of Nalfon in children are unknown.

How Supplied: (℞) *Pulvules No. 416, Nalfon® (fenoprofen calcium, Dista), H77,** 300 mg (equivalent to fenoprofen) (No. 0, Yellow Opaque Body, Ocher Opaque Cap), in an ℞Pak (prescription package, Dista) of 100 and in bottles of 500. All ℞Paks have safety closures.

(℞) *Tablets No. 1900, Nalfon® (fenoprofen calcium, Dista), U59,** 600 mg (equivalent to fenoprofen), Yellow (capsule-shaped, scored), in an ℞Pak of 100 and in bottles of 500. All ℞Paks have safety closures. The tablets are imprinted with DISTA on one side and NALFON on the other.

[101978]

[*Shown in Product Identification Section*]

*Identi-Code® symbol.

TRINSICON® ℞

(hematinic concentrate with intrinsic factor)

Description: Each Pulvule® contains—

Special Liver-Stomach Concentrate, Dista (containing Intrinsic Factor)	240 mg
Cobalamin Concentrate, NF, equivalent to Cobalamin	7.5 mcg

(The total vitamin B_{12} activity in the Special Liver-Stomach Concentrate, Dista, and the Cobalamin Concentrate, NF, is 15 micrograms.)

Iron, Elemental (as Ferrous Fumarate)	110 mg
Ascorbic Acid (Vitamin C)	75 mg
Folic Acid	0.5 mg

Indications: Trinsicon is a multifactor preparation effective in the treatment of anemias that respond to oral hematinics, including pernicious anemia and other megaloblastic anemias and also iron-deficiency anemia. Therapeutic quantities of hematopoietic factors that are known to be important are present in the recommended daily dose.

Vitamin B_{12} with Intrinsic Factor—When secretion of intrinsic factor in gastric juice is inadequate or absent (e.g., in Addisonian pernicious anemia or after gastrectomy), vitamin B_{12} in physiologic doses is absorbed poorly, if at all. The resulting deficiency of vitamin B_{12} leads to the clinical manifestations of pernicious anemia. Similar megaloblastic anemias may develop in fish tapeworm (*Diphyllobothrium latum*) infection or after a surgically created small-bowel blind loop; in these situations, treatment requires freeing the host of the parasites or bacteria which appear to compete for the available vitamin B_{12}. Strict vegetarianism and malabsorption syndromes may also lead to vitamin B_{12} deficiency. In the latter case, parenteral therapy, or oral therapy with

Continued on next page

Dista—Cont.

so-called massive doses of vitamin B_{12}, may be necessary for adequate treatment of the patient.

Potency of intrinsic factor concentrates is determined physiologically, i.e., by their use in patients with pernicious anemia. The liver-stomach concentrate with intrinsic factor and the vitamin B_{12} contained in two Pulvules Trinsicon provide 1½ times the minimum amount of therapeutic agent which, when given daily in an uncomplicated case of pernicious anemia, will produce a satisfactory reticulocyte response and relief of anemia and symptoms.

Concentrates of intrinsic factor derived from hog gastric, pyloric, and duodenal mucosa have been used successfully in patients who lack intrinsic factor. For example, Fouts *et al.* maintained patients with pernicious anemia in clinical remission with oral therapy (liver extracts or intrinsic factor concentrate with vitamin B_{12}) for as long as 29 years.

After total gastrectomy, Ficarra found multifactor preparations taken orally to be "just as effective in maintaining blood levels as any medication that has to be administered parenterally." His study was based on 24 patients who had survived for five years after total gastrectomy for cancer and who had been taking two Pulvules Trinsicon daily.

Folic Acid—Folic acid deficiency is the immediate cause of most, if not all, cases of nutritional megaloblastic anemia and of the megaloblastic anemias of pregnancy and infancy; usually, it is also at least partially responsible for the megaloblastic anemias of malabsorption syndromes, e.g., tropical and nontropical sprue.

It is apparent that in vitamin B_{12} deficiency (e.g., pernicious anemia), lack of this vitamin results in impaired utilization of folic acid. There are other evidences of the close folic acid-vitamin B_{12} interrelationship: (1) B_{12} influences the storage, absorption, and utilization of folic acid, and (2), as a deficiency of B_{12} progresses, the requirement for folic acid increases. However, folic acid does not change the requirement for vitamin B_{12}.

Iron—A very common anemia is that due to iron deficiency. In most cases, the response to iron salts is prompt, safe, and predictable. Within limits, the response is quicker and more certain to large doses of iron than to small doses.

Each Pulvule Trinsicon furnishes 110 mg of elemental iron (as ferrous fumarate) to provide a maximum response.

Ascorbic Acid—Vitamin C plays a role in anemia therapy. It augments the conversion of folic acid to its active form, folinic acid. In addition, ascorbic acid promotes the reduction of ferric iron in food to the more readily absorbed ferrous form. Severe and prolonged vitamin C deficiency is associated with an anemia which is usually hypochromic but occasionally megaloblastic in type.

Contraindications and Precautions: Anemia is a manifestation that requires appropriate investigation to determine its cause or causes.

Folic acid *alone* is unwarranted in the treatment of pure vitamin-B_{12}-deficiency states, such as pernicious anemia. Indeed, the use of folic acid in large doses in pernicious anemia without adequate vitamin B_{12} may result in hematologic remission but neurologic progression.

As with all preparations containing intrinsic factor, resistance may develop in some cases of pernicious anemia to the potentiation of absorption of physiologic doses of vitamin B_{12}. If resistance occurs, parenteral therapy, or oral therapy with so-called massive doses of vitamin B_{12}, may be necessary for adequate treatment of the patient. No single regimen fits all cases, and the status of the patient observed in follow-up is the final criterion for adequacy of therapy. Periodic clinical and laboratory studies are considered essential and are recommended.

Hemochromatosis and hemosiderosis are contraindications to iron therapy.

Adverse Reactions: Rarely, iron in therapeutic doses produces gastrointestinal reactions, such as diarrhea or constipation. Reducing the dose and administering it with meals will minimize these effects in the iron-sensitive patient. In extremely rare instances, skin rash suggesting allergy has been noted following the oral administration of liver-stomach material. Allergic sensitization has been reported following both oral and parenteral administration of folic acid.

Dosage: One Pulvule twice a day. (Two Pulvules daily produce a standard response in the average uncomplicated case of pernicious anemia.)

Overdosage: *Symptoms*—Those of iron intoxication, which may include pallor and cyanosis, vomiting, hematemesis, diarrhea, melena, shock, drowsiness, and coma. *Treatment*—For specific therapy, exchange transfusion and chelating agents. For general management, gastric and rectal lavage with sodium bicarbonate solution or milk, administration of intravenous fluids and electrolytes, and use of oxygen.

How Supplied: (℞) *Pulvules No. 2, Trinsicon® (hematinic concentrate with intrinsic factor, Dista), F01** (No. 0, Dark-Pink Opaque Body, Dark-Red Cap), in an ℞Pak (prescription package, Dista) of 60, in bottles of 500, and in 10 strips of 10 individually labeled blisters each containing 1 Pulvule (ID100). All ℞Paks have safety closures. [042878]

Pulvules No. 2—500's—6505-00-584-4218A; ID100's—6505-00-201-2824A

[*Shown in Product Identification Section*]

*Identi-Code® symbol.

TRINSICON® M ℞
(hematinic concentrate modified)
(Without Folic Acid)

Description: Trinsicon M is a comprehensive hematinic formulation similar to Trinsicon® (hematinic concentrate with intrinsic factor, Dista) but does not contain folic acid.

Each Pulvule® contains—

Special Liver-Stomach Concentrate, Dista (containing Intrinsic Factor) .... 240 mg

Cobalamin Concentrate, NF, equivalent to Cobalamin .... 7.5 mcg

(The total vitamin B_{12} activity in the Special Liver-Stomach Concentrate, Dista, and the Cobalamin Concentrate, NF, is 15 micrograms.)

Iron, Elemental (as Ferrous Fumarate) .... 110 mg

Ascorbic Acid (Vitamin C) .... 75 mg

Indications: Trinsicon M is a multifactor preparation effective in the treatment of pernicious anemia as well as in the hypochromic anemias due to iron deficiency. *See also under* Trinsicon.

Contraindications, Precautions, and Adverse Reactions: *See under* Trinsicon.

Dosage: One Pulvule twice a day. (Two Pulvules daily produce a standard response in the average uncomplicated case of pernicious anemia.)

Overdosage: *See under* Trinsicon.

How Supplied: (℞) *Pulvules No. 3, Trinsicon® M (hematinic concentrate modified, Dista), F02** (No. 0, Pink Opaque Body, Dark-Red Cap), in an ℞Pak (prescription package, Dista) of 60. All ℞Paks have safety closures. [060178]

*Identi-Code® symbol.

VALMID® Ⓒ
(ethinamate)
Capsules, NF

Description: Valmid® (ethinamate, Dista), a nonbarbiturate, is 1-ethinyl-cyclohexyl-carbamate. It is a nonirritating, colorless, faintly bitter, stable crystalline powder with a melting point of 96°-98° C. Valmid is relatively insoluble in water but quite soluble in many alcohols and oils.

Action: Valmid® (ethinamate, Dista) is a hypnotic agent; its site and mechanism of action are unknown.

Clinical Pharmacology: Valmid® (ethinamate, Dista) is rapidly absorbed after oral administration. Following a single oral dose of 1 gm, peak plasma levels are reached in approximately 36 minutes and decline to negligible values over the next eight hours. Approximately 36 percent of the administered dose appears in the urine within 24 hours. The effect of multiple doses and prolonged administration on pharmacodynamics and pharmacokinetics is not known.

Indication: Valmid® (ethinamate, Dista) is a short-acting hypnotic. It has not been sufficiently well studied with currently available sleep laboratory techniques to delimit its value in specific types of insomnia. Valmid is best used for limited periods. Should insomnia persist, drug-free intervals of one week or more should elapse before re-treatment is considered. Attempts should be made to find alternative nondrug therapy for chronic insomnia. The prolonged administration of Valmid is not recommended, since it has not been shown to be effective for a period of more than seven days.

Contraindication: Valmid® (ethinamate, Dista) is contraindicated in patients with known hypersensitivity to the drug.

Warnings: Patients receiving Valmid® (ethinamate, Dista) should be cautioned about possible additive effects when it is taken in combination with alcohol or other C.N.S. depressants. Patients should be cautioned against becoming involved in hazardous occupations requiring complete mental alertness, such as operating machines or driving a motor vehicle, shortly after ingestion of the drug.

Usage in Pregnancy—The absence of adverse effects of this drug on fetal development has not been established. Therefore, the use of Valmid during pregnancy is not recommended.

Usage in Children—The effectiveness and safety of Valmid have not been established in persons under 15 years of age; therefore, its use in such individuals is not currently recommended.

Physical and Psychologic Dependence—Drug dependence characterized by both a psychologic and a physical dependence has occurred when Valmid has been taken at higher than recommended doses for prolonged intervals. It is, therefore, desirable to exercise caution in administering Valmid to individuals who are addiction-prone and to those whose history suggests that they may increase dosage on their own initiative. It is advisable to limit repeated prescriptions without adequate medical supervision.

In the event that an individual has established dependence on Valmid, withdrawal must be accomplished with extreme care. Abrupt withdrawal may cause a typical abstinence syndrome accompanied by convulsions. Withdrawal may be accomplished by hospitalizing the patient and reducing the addictive daily dose at a rate of 500 to 1000 mg every two or three days. Psychiatric follow-up is indicated.

Precautions: Since the risk of oversedation, dizziness, confusion, and/or ataxia substantially increases with the administration of large doses of sedatives in the elderly and de-

bilitated, it is recommended that a single 500-mg Pulvule® be the dose given to such individuals. Should this dose prove to be ineffective, clinical judgment must weigh the risk of increasing the dosage against the potential hazards mentioned above.
If Valmid® (ethinamate, Dista) is to be administered in combination with other drugs known to have a hypnotic or C.N.S.-depressant effect, consideration should be given to the potential additive effects. The usual precautions are indicated for severely depressed patients or those in whom there is any evidence of latent depression, particularly when it is recognized that suicidal tendencies may be present and that protective measures may be necessary.
Adverse Reactions: Rare cases of thrombocytopenic purpura and drug idiosyncrasy with fever have been reported. Paradoxical excitement in children, mild gastrointestinal symptoms, and skin rashes have occurred after the use of Valmid® (ethinamate, Dista).
Dosage and Administration: For insomnia, 1 or 2 Pulvules of Valmid® (ethinamate, Dista) should be taken 20 minutes before retiring.
Overdosage: In suicidal overdosage, C.N.S. and respiratory depression should be treated in the same manner as barbiturate intoxication. Valmid® (ethinamate, Dista) is dialyzable.
How Supplied: (Ⓒ) *Pulvules No. 399, Valmid® (Ethinamate Capsules, NF), H74,** 500 mg (No. 0, Light-Blue Opaque Body, Blue Opaque Cap), in bottles of 100. [021679]
[*Shown in Product Identification Section*]

*Identi-Code® symbol.

Doak Pharmacal Co., Inc.
700 SHAMES DRIVE
WESTBURY, L.I., NY 11590

FORMULA 405 CREAM

Composition: Water, Coconut Oil, Beeswax, PEG-40 Stearate, Petrolatum, Mineral Oil, Lanolin Alcohol, Isopropyl Palmitate, Sweet Almond Oil, Ceresin, Stearyl Alcohol, Acetylated Lanolin, Pregnenolone Succinate, Vitamin E Acetate, Triethanolamine, Imidazolidinyl Urea, Methylparaben, BHA, Propylparaben, Sodium Borate, Fragrance, D & C Red No. 19.
Actions and Uses: For the care of dry, premature aging skin due to epidermal dehydration.
Administration and Dosage: Apply approximately ½" on the face and neck and rub in gently. Should be applied nightly.
Precautions: None.
Contraindications: None.
How Supplied: 2 oz. tubes.

TAR DISTILLATE "DOAK" AND DERIVATIVES

Composition: By-products of fractional distillation of coal in which the active agents are retained while the irritating, staining and odorous factors are removed. Each cc. is equivalent to 1 gm. of whole crude coal tar.
Actions and Uses: Exerts antipruritic, antieczematous and keratoplastic actions of whole crude coal tar without imparting its irritancy, staining and offensive odor. Gratifying results are elicited when used alone in the Goeckerman treatment. Excellent for incorporation in creams, lotions, ointments, alcohol and bath oils. Examples of the combinations and uses of such Tar Distillate "Doak" derivatives are as follows:
DOAK OIL AND DOAK OIL FORTE (Tar Distillate "Doak" 2% and 5% respectively): Moisturizing, lubricating and antipruritic bath oils which may be applied directly to wet skin or added to bathtub of warm water for treatment of psoriasis and other chronic skin disorders. Doak Oil one part mixed with two to three parts of cream containing hydrocortisone or a fluorinated steroid markedly enhances the activity due to the skin-softening action of the oils and the synergistic action of the tar. Doak Oil-Steroid Emulsions are of special value in psoriasis of the scalp and body, seborrheic dermatitis, chronic eczematoid dermatitis and atopic dermatitis. LAVATAR—tar bath (Tar Distillate "Doak" 33⅓%): Useful in generalized pruritis and psoriasis, atopic dermatitis when added to bathtub of water. TARPASTE (Tar Distillate "Doak" 5%): Incorporation of the tar in modified Lassar's Paste renders the product of value in chronic eczematoid dermatitis, infantile eczema and psoriasis.
TAR-DOAK LOTION (Tar Distillate "Doak" 5%): May be used alone in the treatment of psoriasis and other chronic dermatoses with itching and scaling. The combination of the nonionic emulsifiers present in the Lotion offers a high "INCLUSION CAPACITY" for agents such as steroids (powder, cream, lotion or solution), salicylic acid, resorcin, sulfur, iodochlorhydroxyquin, etc.
TERSA-TAR (Tar Distillate "Doak" 3%): Antibacterial soapless tar shampoo which produces copious foaming. Helpful in the treatment of dandruff, seborrhea and psoria sis of the scalp.
UNGUENTUM BOSSI (Tar Distillate "Doak" 5%): See below.
Administration and Dosage: Apply as directed.
Contraindications: Do not use on patients sensitive to tar.
Precautions: Tar Distillate "Doak", as is the case with crude coal tar, may cause allergic irritation in rare instances. Tar Distillate "Doak" and derivatives should not be applied to the acute inflamed skin.
How Supplied: Tar Distillate "Doak" and Doak Oil Forte—2 fl. oz. and 16 fl. oz. bottles; Lavatar, Tersa-Tar, Tar-Doak Lotion—4 fl. oz., 16 fl. oz. and 1 gal. bottles; Doak Oil—8 fl. oz. bottle; Tarpaste—1 oz. tube, 4 oz. and 16 oz. jars.

UNGUENTUM BOSSI ℞

Composition: Tar Distillate "Doak" 5%, Ammoniated Mercury 5%, Methanamine Sulfosalicylate 2%, Doak Oil 40%, Unguentum "Doak" 48%.
Action and Uses: In the treatment of psoriasis, psoriasis of the scalp and seborrheic dermatitis.
Administration and Dosage: Once or twice daily.
Precautions: Applicable to the use of tar and mercury.
Contraindications: Do not use on patients sensitive to mercurials and tars.
How Supplied: 2 oz. tube and 16 oz. jar.

Dome Division
Miles Laboratories, Inc.
400 MORGAN LANE
WEST HAVEN, CT 06516

ACNE-DOME®
Creme and Lotion (acid pH)
(colloidal sulfur, resorcinol)

Composition: Colloidal sulfur and resorcinol in a compatible vehicle adjusted to the pH range for normal skin.
Action and Uses: Medicates acne blemishes. As an aid in drying and peeling acne blemishes.
Caution: If excessive drying or skin irritation develops or increases, discontinue use and consult physician. For external use only. Not for ophthalmic use. Store below 86°F. (30°C.), avoid freezing.
Administration and Dosage: Wash affected parts thoroughly, then dry. Apply sparingly twice daily, preferably in the morning and at bedtime. Follow advice of physician as to diet or other treatment. Shake lotion well.
How Supplied:

Creme	*Lotion*
1 oz. tube	2 fl. oz.

ACNE-DOME® Medicated Cleanser
(acid pH)
(colloidal sulfur, salicylic acid)

Composition: Contains effective anti-acne medications: Colloidal sulfur—to dry excess skin oils. Salicylic acid—to peel away dead skin tissue.
Indications: Medicated skin cleanser as an aid in the treatment of acne.
Caution: WARNING: If excessive drying or skin irritation develops or increases, discontinue use and consult physician. For external use only. Keep away from children. Store below 86°F. (30°C.), avoid freezing. Keep away from eyes.
Administration and Dosage: Use twice daily, preferably in the morning and at bedtime. Wet the skin. Apply the cleanser to moist sponge. Work into lather. Massage for five minutes. Rinse.
How Supplied: In the exclusive 4 oz. DISPENSAJAR® with its "Personal Washcloth"—an applicator sponge so fingers never touch the cleanser.

ALLPYRAL® allergenic extracts, ℞
alum-precipitated, for Subcutaneous Injection
Pollens, Molds, Epithelia, House Dust and Other Inhalants, and Stinging Insects.

Composition: Allpyral allergenic extracts are pyridine/aqueous alkaline solution extracted alum-precipitated antigens in saline suspension.
Indications: Allpyral allergenic extracts, alum-precipitated (pollens, molds, epithelia, house dust or other inhalants, and stinging insects) are indicated for hyposensitization of patients who have been shown by clinical history and/or skin testing to be allergic (hypersensitive) to one or more of these allergens and who have manifested signs and/or symptoms related to exposure to the allergen(s). These manifestations may be referable to the respiratory trace, for example rhinitis, asthma or airway obstruction or they may be ophthalmic such as non-infectious conjunctivitis, pruritus or edema of the eyelids.
Caution: Observe the usual precautions in preparing and administering allergenic extracts. Inject subcutaneously. Avoid depositing material intracutaneously or intravenously. Allpyral extracts may be combined with one another in any proportion. However, in mixing extracts, the total PNU injected shall not be more than the recommended dose (in PNU) of that component with the lowest maximum recommended PNU. This assures that the total aluminum injected shall not exceed 0.85mg. It is desirable to keep ALLPYRAL Mixed Stinging Insects separate from other ALLPYRAL antigens. Admixture with aqueous extracts is not recommended. Never attempt to switch a patient from treatment with Allpyral suspensions to aqueous solutions of allergens. If conversion to an aqueous preparation is necessary, start as though patient were coming for first treatment. Allpyral injections should not be administered more frequently than once a week in the early phases of treatment. Beyond the 1000 PNU dosage level, the interval should be increased to 2 weeks or more. The top dose should not be administered more frequently than every 4 weeks nor less frequently than every 8 weeks. Do not use phosphate-buffered

Continued on next page

Dome—Cont.

saline or bicarbonate saline (Coca's solution) as a diluent.
Reactions: Should a local reaction occur, characterized by moderate edema, erythema and pain at the site of injection, the same or lower dose should be given at the next visit and no increase attempted. If the local reaction is marked, antihistamine drugs may be given. Reduce the dose at the next visit to a previous dose which did not elicit a reaction.
In the event that a delayed constitutional or systemic reaction characterized by urticaria, sneezing, itching, edema of the extremities, respiratory wheezing or asthma, or dyspnea occurs, this will generally appear slowly and gradually, and may last for 2 to 4 days due to continued slow release of the antigen. Injection of 0.3 ml to 0.5 ml of 1:1,000 epinephrine hydrochloride near the site of injection may be given. For children under 12 years of age, the dose of epinephrine 1:1000 is 0.1 ml to 0.3 ml. However, such reactions are rarely critical and are usually readily controlled with antihistamines and steroids. The patient should be supplied with medication and information to prevent undue apprehension and the dose of antigen at the next visit should be reduced.
Acute anaphylactic reactions characterized by difficulty in breathing, cyanosis and shock following Allpyral® therapy are extremely rare but if they do occur, emergency treatment measures must be adopted. Apply a tourniquet above the site of injection and administer 0.3 ml to 0.5 ml of 1:1,000 epinephrine hydrochloride intramuscularly at two sites: (a) at the site of injection and (b) in the opposite arm for systemic effect. In severe anaphylactic reactions, epinephrine may be given intravenously, using a 1:10,000 aqueous solution at a rate not exceeding 0.5 ml per minute and a total no greater than 0.25 mgm. If necessary, this may be repeated in 15 to 20 minutes. Intravenous antihistamine or adrenal corticosteroids should also be considered in severe cases. Oxygen therapy and artificial respiration may be necessary for respiratory failure. If bronchospasm is an important feature of the reaction, intravenous aminophylline may be required and the presence of laryngeal edema or laryngospasm may necessitate tracheotomy. For persistent hypotension an intravenous drip infusion of 5 percent dextrose in water with a vasopressor agent should be administered at a rate sufficient to maintain the blood pressure at reasonably normal levels.
If continuation of Allpyral® therapy is considered necessary in such patients, the dose at the next visit should be greatly reduced and extreme caution exercised.
As with all types of allergenic extracts, Allpyral grass antigens appear to be slightly more reactive than other categories of Allpyral allergens and should be administered on a more conservative basis.
Administration and Dosage: Before administering, see package insert for complete product information.
Literature Available: Upon request.

CANDEX® Creme ℞
(nystatin)

Description: Candex® (nystatin) Creme contains nystatin U.S.P. 100,000 units/g in a base consisting of carboxy vinyl polymer, sodium lauryl sulfate, hexadecyl alcohol, cetyl alcohol, Dowicil® 200, sodium hydroxide, citric acid, sodium citrate, and purified water.
Actions: Nystatin is effective against Candida species (Monilia).
Indications: Candex® (nystatin) Creme is indicated for the treatment of cutaneous or mucocutaneous mycotic infections caused by Candida species (Monilia).
Contraindications: Lesions caused by pathogens not susceptible to nystatin and hypersensitivity to any of the components.
Precautions: If irritation or sensitivity occurs and/or infection persists, discontinue use. If new infections appear, appropriate therapy should be instituted.
Caution: Federal (U.S.A.) law prohibits dispensing without prescription. Store below 86°F. (30°C.), avoid freezing.
For external use only. Not for ophthalmic use.
Dosage and Administration: Apply two or three times daily. Continue use for one week after clinical cure.
How Supplied: Candex® (nystatin) Creme in 15 gram tubes.

CANDEX® Lotion ℞
(nystatin)

Description: Candex® (nystatin) Lotion contains nystatin U.S.P. 100,000 units/ml in a base consisting of carboxy vinyl polymer, sodium lauryl sulfate, hexadecyl alcohol, cetyl alcohol, Dowicil® 200, sodium hydroxide, citric acid, sodium citrate, and purified water.
Actions: Nystatin is effective against Candida species (Monilia).
Indications: Candex® (nystatin) Lotion is indicated for the treatment of cutaneous or mucocutaneous mycotic infections caused by Candida species (Monilia). A lotion is preferred on oozing intertriginous areas.
Contraindications: Lesions caused by pathogens not susceptible to nystatin and hypersensitivity to any of the components.
Precautions: If irritation or sensitivity occurs and/or infection persists, discontinue use. If new infections appear, appropriate therapy should be instituted.
Caution: Federal (U.S.A.) law prohibits dispensing without prescription.
For external use only. Not for ophthalmic use. Store below 86° F. (30° C.), avoid freezing. Shake well.
Dosage and Administration: Apply two or three times daily. Continue use for one week after clinical cure.
How Supplied: Candex® (nystatin) Lotion in 30 ml plastic bottles.

CORT-DOME® 1/8%, 1/4%, 1/2%, and 1% ℞
acid pH Creme
(hydrocortisone)

Description: Cort-Dome® cremes contain microdispersed hydrocortisone (11B, 17, 21-Trihydroxypregn-4-ene-3, 20-dione) in a compatible vehicle buffered to the pH range for normal skin. Each gram of Cort-Dome contains: 1.25 mg/g (1/8%), 2.5 mg/g (1/4%), 5 mg/g (1/2%) and 10 mg/g (1%) of hydrocortisone.
The emollient vehicle for Cort-Dome 1/8% is composed of isopropyl myristate, cholesterol, white petrolatum, synthetic beeswax (B-wax), stearic acid, polyoxyethylene sorbitan monostearate, aluminum sulfate, propylene glycol, calcium acetate, dextrin, perfume and purified water, preserved with methyl and propyl parabens.
The vehicle for Cort-Dome 1/4%, 1/2% and 1% contains glycerin, sodium lauryl sulfate, calcium acetate, cetyl stearyl alcohol, aluminum sulfate, purified water, synthetic beeswax (B-wax), white petrolatum, dextrin, and light mineral oil, preserved with methylparaben.
Actions: Topical steroids are primarily effective because of their anti-inflammatory, antipruritic and vasoconstrictive actions.
Indications: For relief of the inflammatory manifestations of corticosteroid-responsive dermatoses.
Contraindications: Cort-Dome Creme is contraindicated in those patients with a history of hypersensitivity to any of the components.
Precautions: If irritation develops, the product should be discontinued and appropriate therapy instituted. In the presence of an infection the use of an appropriate antifungal or antibacterial agent should be instituted. If a favorable response does not occur promptly, the corticosteroid should be discontinued until the infection has been adequately controlled.
If extensive areas are treated or if the occlusive technique is used there will be increased systemic absorption of the corticosteroid and suitable precautions should be taken, particularly in children and infants.
Although topical steroids have not been reported to have an adverse effect on human pregnancy, the safety of their use in pregnant women has not absolutely been established. In laboratory animals, increases in incidence of fetal abnormalities have been associated with exposure of gestating females to topical corticosteroids, in some cases at rather low dosage levels. Therefore, drugs of this class should not be used extensively on pregnant patients, in large amounts, or for prolonged periods of time.
The product is not for ophthalmic use.
Adverse Reactions: The following local adverse reactions have been reported with topical corticosteroids, especially under occlusive dressings.
1. Burning
2. Itching
3. Irritation
4. Dryness
5. Folliculitis
6. Hypertrichosis
7. Acneiform eruptions
8. Hypopigmentation
9. Perioral dermatitis
10. Allergic Contact Dermatitis
11. Maceration of the skin
12. Secondary infection
13. Skin atrophy
14. Striae
15. Miliaria

Dosage and Administration: Apply to affected areas 3 or 4 times daily.
Caution: Federal (U.S.A.) law prohibits dispensing without prescription.
For external use only. Store at controlled room temperature (59°-86°F.).
How Supplied: Cort-Dome (hydrocortisone) Creme 1/8%-1 oz. tube, 4 oz. DISPENSAJAR®
Cort-Dome 1/4%-1 oz. tube, 4 oz. Dispensajar, 1 lb. jar.
Cort-Dome Creme 1/2%-1/2 oz. tube, 1 oz. tube, 4 oz. and 1 lb. jar.
Cort-Dome Creme 1%-1/2 oz. tube and 1 oz. tube.

CORT-DOME® 1/8%, 1/4%, 1/2%, and 1% ℞
acid pH Lotion
(hydrocortisone)

Description: Contains microdispersed hydrocortisone 1/8%, 1/4%, 1/2% and 1% in a compatible vehicle buffered to the pH range for normal skin. This vehicle is composed of glyceryl monostearate, cetyl alcohol, stearyl alcohol, butyl stearate, aluminum acetate, isopropyl myristate, polyoxyethylene sorbitan monolaurate, glycerin and purified water preserved with methyl and propyl parabens.
Actions: Topical steroids are primarily effective because of their anti-inflammatory antipruritic and vasoconstrictive actions.
Indications: For relief of the inflammatory manifestations of corticosteroid-responsive dermatoses.
Contraindications: Cort-Dome Lotions are contraindicated in those patients with a history of hypersensitivity to any of the components.
Precautions: If irritation develops, the product should be discontinued and appropriate therapy instituted.
In the presence of an infection the use of an appropriate antifungal or antibacterial agent

should be instituted. If a favorable response does not occur promptly, the corticosteroid should be discontinued until the infection has been adequately controlled.
If extensive areas are treated or if the occlusive technique is used there will be increased systemic absorption of the corticosteroid and suitable precautions should be taken, particularly in children and infants.
Although topical steroids have not been reported to have an adverse effect on human pregnancy, the safety of their use in pregnant women has not absolutely been established. In laboratory animals, increases in incidence of fetal abnormalities have been associated with exposure of gestating females to topical corticosteroids, in some cases at rather low dosage levels. Therefore, drugs of this class should not be used extensively on pregnant patients, in large amounts, or for prolonged periods of time.
The product is not for ophthalmic use.
Adverse Reactions: The following local adverse reactions have been reported with topical corticosteroids, especially under occlusive dressings.

1. Burning
2. Itching
3. Irritation
4. Dryness
5. Folliculitis
6. Hypertrichosis
7. Acneiform eruptions
8. Hypopigmentation
9. Perioral dermatitis
10. Allergic Contact Dermatitis
11. Maceration of the skin
12. Secondary infection
13. Skin atrophy
14. Striae
15. Miliaria

Dosage and Administration: Apply to affected areas 3 or 4 times daily.
Caution: Federal (U.S.A.) law prohibits dispensing without prescription.
For external use only. Store at controlled room temperature (59°-86°F.).
How Supplied: Cort-Dome Lotion (hydrocortisone) ⅛%-6 fl. oz. bottle
Cort-Dome Lotion ¼%-4 fl. oz. bottle
Cort-Dome Lotion ½%-½ fl. oz., 1 fl. oz. and 4 fl. oz. bottles
Cort-Dome Lotion 1%-½ fl. oz. and 1 fl. oz. bottles

CORT-DOME® Suppositories ℞
(hydrocortisone acetate)

Composition: Regular: 15 mg. hydrocortisone acetate. High Potency: 25 mg. hydrocortisone acetate. Both are incorporated in a monoglyceride base.
Indications: For use in inflamed hemorrhoids, postirradiation (factitial) proctitis; as an adjunct in the treatment of chronic ulcerative colitis; cryptitis; other inflammatory conditions of anorectum; and pruritus ani.
Contraindications: Cort-Dome Suppositories are contraindicated in those patients with a history of hypersensitivity to any of the components.
Precautions: Do not use unless adequate proctologic examination is made.
If irritation develops, the product should be discontinued and appropriate therapy instituted. In the presence of an infection the use of an appropriate antifungal or antibacterial agent should be instituted. If a favorable response does not occur promptly, the corticosteroid should be discontinued until the infection has been adequately controlled.
Although topical steroids have not been reported to have an adverse effect on human pregnancy, the safety of their use in pregnant women has not absolutely been established. In laboratory animals, increases in incidence of fetal abnormalities have been associated with exposure of gestating females to topical corticosteroids, in some cases at rather low dosage levels. Therefore, drugs of this class should not be used extensively on pregnant patients in large amounts, or for prolonged periods of time.
Adverse Reactions: The following local adverse reactions have been reported with corticosteroids suppositories:

1. Burning
2. Itching
3. Irritation
4. Dryness
5. Folliculitis
6. Hypopigmentation
7. Allergic Contact Dermatitis
8. Secondary Infection

Caution: Federal (U.S.A.) law prohibits dispensing without prescription. Store at controlled room temperature (59°-86°F.).
Dosage and Administration: One suppository inserted in the rectum twice daily, morning and night for two weeks, in nonspecific proctitis. In more severe cases, one suppository three times daily; or, two suppositories twice daily. In factitial proctitis, recommended duration of therapy is six to eight weeks or less, according to response of individual case.
How Supplied: Boxes of 12.

DAXOLIN® ℞
(loxapine succinate)
CAPSULES
For Oral Use

Description: DAXOLIN (loxapine succinate), a dibenzoxazepine compound, represents a new subclass of tricyclic antipsychotic agent, chemically distinct from the thioxanthenes, butyrophenones, and phenothiazines. Chemically, it is 2-chloro-11-(4-methyl-1-piperazinyl) dibenz [b,f] [1,4] oxazepine. It is present in capsules as the succinate salt. Each 1.36 mg of loxapine succinate is equivalent to 1 mg of loxapine.
Actions: Pharmacologically, loxapine is a tranquilizer for which the exact mode of action has not been established. However, changes in the level of excitability of subcortical inhibitory areas have been observed in several animal species in association with such manifestations of tranquilization as calming effects and suppression of aggressive behavior.
In normal human volunteers, signs of sedation were seen within 20 to 30 minutes after administration, were most pronounced within 1½ to 3 hours, and lasted through 12 hours. Similar timing of primary pharmacologic effects was seen in animals.
Absorption of loxapine following oral or parenteral administration is virtually complete. The drug is removed rapidly from the plasma and distributed in tissues. Animal studies suggest an initial preferential distribution in lungs, brain, spleen, heart, and kidney. Loxapine is metabolized extensively and is excreted mainly in the first 24 hours. Metabolites are excreted in the urine in the form of conjugates and in the feces unconjugated.
Indications: DAXOLIN (loxapine succinate) is indicated for the manifestations of schizophrenia.
Contraindications: DAXOLIN is contraindicated in comatose or severe drug-induced depressed states (alcohol, barbiturates, narcotics, etc.).
DAXOLIN is contraindicated in individuals with known hypersensitivity to the drug.
Warnings:
Usage in Pregnancy: Safe use of DAXOLIN (loxapine succinate) during pregnancy or lactation has not been established; therefore, its use in pregnancy, in nursing mothers, or in women of childbearing potential requires that the benefits of treatment be weighed against the possible risks to mother and child. No embryotoxicity or teratology was observed in studies in rats, rabbits or dogs, although with the exception of one rabbit study, the highest dosage was two times the maximum recommended human dose and in some studies they were below this dose. Perinatal studies have shown renal papillary abnormalities in offspring of rats treated from mid-pregnancy with doses of 0.6 and 1.8 mg/kg, doses which approximate the usual human dose but which are considerably below the maximum recommended human dose.
Usage in Children: Studies have not been performed in children; therefore this drug is not recommended for use in children below the age of 16.
DAXOLIN, like other tranquilizers, may impair mental and/or physical abilities, especially during the first few days of therapy. Therefore, ambulatory patients should be warned about activities requiring alertness (eg, operating vehicles or machinery), and about concomitant use of alcohol and other CNS depressants.
DAXOLIN has not been evaluated for the management of behavioral complications in patients with mental retardation, and therefore it cannot be recommended.
Precautions: DAXOLIN should be used with extreme caution in patients with a history of convulsive disorders since it lowers the convulsive threshold. Seizures have been reported in epileptic patients receiving DAXOLIN at antipsychotic dose levels, and may occur even with maintenance of routine anticonvulsant drug therapy.
Loxapine has an antiemetic effect in animals. Since this effect also may occur in man, loxapine may mask signs of overdosage of toxic drugs and obscure conditions such as intestinal obstruction and brain tumor.
DAXOLIN should be used with caution in patients with cardiovascular disease. Increased pulse rates have been reported in the majority of patients receiving antipsychotic doses; and transient hypotension has been reported. In the presence of severe hypotension requiring vasopressor therapy, the preferred drugs may be norepinephrine or angiotensin. Usual doses of epinephrine may be ineffective because of inhibition of its vasopressor effect by loxapine.
The possibility of ocular toxicity from loxapine cannot be excluded at this time. Therefore, careful observation should be made for pigmentary retinopathy and lenticular pigmentation since these have been observed in some patients receiving certain other antipsychotic drugs for prolonged periods.
Because of possible anticholinergic action, the drug should be used cautiously in patients with glaucoma or a tendency to urinary retention, particularly with concomitant administration of anticholinergic-type antiparkinsonian medication.
Adverse Reactions:
CNS Effects: Manifestations of adverse effects on the central nervous system, other than extrapyramidal effects, have been seen infrequently. Drowsiness, usually mild, may occur at the beginning of therapy or when dosage is increased. It usually subsides with continued DAXOLIN (loxapine succinate) therapy. The incidence of sedation has been less than that of certain aliphatic phenothiazines and slightly more than the piperazine phenothiazines. Dizziness, faintness, staggering gait, muscle twitching, weakness, and confusional states have been reported.
Extrapyramidal Reactions—Neuromuscular (extrapyramidal) reactions during the administration of DAXOLIN (loxapine succinate) have been reported frequently, often during the first days of treatment. In most patients, these reactions involved parkinsonism-like symptoms such as tremor, rigidity, excessive salivation, and masked facies. Akathisia (motor restlessness) also has been reported relatively frequently. These symptoms are usually not severe and can be controlled by reduction

Continued on next page

Dome—Cont.

of DAXOLIN dosage or by administration of antiparkinsonian drugs in usual dosage. Dystonic and dyskinetic reactions have occurred less frequently, but may be more severe. Dystonias include spasms of muscles of the neck and face, tongue protrusion, and oculogyric movement. Dyskinetic reaction has been described in the form of choreoathetoid movements. These reactions sometimes require reduction or temporary withdrawal of DAXOLIN dosage in addition to appropriate counteractive drugs.

Persistent Tardive Dyskinesia—As with all antipsychotic agents, tardive dyskinesia may appear in some patients on long-term therapy or may appear after drug therapy has been discontinued. The risk appears to be greater in elderly patients on high-dose therapy, especially females. The symptoms are persistent and in some patients appear to be irreversible. The syndrome is characterized by rhythmical involuntary movement of the tongue, face, mouth, or jaw (eg, protrusion of tongue, puffing of cheeks, puckering of mouth, chewing movements). Sometimes these may be accompanied by involuntary movements of the extremities.

There is no known effective treatment for tardive dyskinesia; antiparkinsonian agents usually do not alleviate the symptoms of this syndrome. It is suggested that all antipsychotic agents be discontinued if these symptoms appear. Should it be necessary to reinstitute treatment, or increase the dosage of the agent, or switch to a different antipsychotic agent, the syndrome may be masked. It has been suggested that fine vermicular movements of the tongue may be an early sign of the syndrome, and if the medication is stopped at that time the syndrome may not develop.

Cardiovascular Effects: Tachycardia, hypotension, hypertension, light-headedness, and syncope have been reported. A few cases of ECG changes similar to those seen with phenothiazines have been reported. It is not known whether these were related to loxapine administration.

Skin Effects: Dermatitis, edema (puffiness of face), pruritus, and seborrhea have been reported with loxapine. The possibility of photosensitivity and/or phototoxicity occurring has not been excluded; skin rashes of uncertain etiology have been observed in a few patients during hot summer months.

Anticholinergic Effects: Dry mouth, nasal congestion, constipation, and blurred vision have occurred; these are more likely to occur with concomitant use of antiparkinsonian agents.

Other Adverse Reactions: Nausea, vomiting, weight gain, weight loss, dyspnea, ptosis, hyperpyrexia, flushed facies, headache, paresthesia, and polydipsia have been reported in some patients. Rarely, galactorrhea and menstrual irregularity of uncertain etiology have been reported.

Dosage and Administration: DAXOLIN (loxapine succinate) is administered orally, usually in divided doses two to four times a day. Daily dosage (in terms of base equivalents) should be adjusted to the individual patient's needs as asessed by the severity of symptoms and previous history of response to antipyschotic drugs. Initial dosage of 10 mg twice daily is recommended, although in severely disturbed patients initial dosage up to a total of 50 mg daily may be desirable. Dosage should then be increased fairly rapidly over the first seven to ten days until there is effective control of psychotic symptoms. The usual therapeutic and maintenance range is 60 mg to 100 mg daily. However, as with other antipsychotic drugs, some patients respond to lower dosage and others require higher dosage for optimal benefit. Daily dosage higher than 250 mg is not recommended. For maintenance therapy, dosage should be reduced to the lowest level compatible with symptom control; many patients have been maintained satisfactorily at dosages in the range of 20 mg to 60 mg daily.

Overdosage: Signs and symptoms of overdosage will depend on the amount ingested and individual patient tolerance. As would be expected from the pharmacologic actions of the drug the clinical findings may range from mild depression of the CNS and cardiovascular systems to profound hypotension, respiratory depression, and unconsciousness. The possibility of occurrence of extrapyramidal symptoms and/or convulsive seizures should be kept in mind.

The treatment of overdosage is essentially symptomatic and supportive. Early gastric lavage and extended dialysis might be expected to be beneficial. Centrally acting emetics may have little effect because of the antiemetic action of loxapine. In addition, emesis should be avoided because of the possibility of aspiration of vomitus. Avoid analeptics, such as pentylenetetrazol, which may cause convulsions. Severe hypotensiion might be expected to respond to the administration of levarterenol or phenylephrine. EPINEPHRINE SHOULD NOT BE USED SINCE ITS USE IN A PATIENT WITH PARTIAL ADRENERGIC BLOCKADE MAY FURTHER LOWER THE BLOOD PRESSURE. Severe extrapyramidal reactions should be treated with anticholinergic antiparkinson agents or diphenhydramine hydrochloride, and anticonvulsant therapy should be initiated as indicated. Additional measures include oxygen and intravenous fluids.

How Supplied: DAXOLIN® (loxapine succinate) is supplied in the following base-equivalent strengths:

CAPSULES Hard Shell Printed "DOME"

10 mg—Light and Dark Blue; bottles of 100, 1000 and Unit Dose 10 × 10's.

25 mg—Blue and White; bottles of 100, 1000 and Unit Dose 10 × 10's.

50 mg—Blue and Maroon; bottles of 100, 1000 and Unit Dose 10 × 10's.

Manufactured for Dome Laboratories by Lederle Laboratories Division, American Cyanamid Company, Pearl River, N.Y.

DAXOLIN® C ℞
(loxapine hydrochloride)
Oral Concentrate
25 mg base/ml*

Description: *Each ml contains the equivalent of 25 mg loxapine base as the hydrochloride (HCl).

DAXOLIN C (loxapine hydrochloride), a dibenzoxazepine compound, represents a new subclass of tricyclic antipsychotic agent, chemically distinct from the thioxanthenes, butyrophenones, and phenothiazines. Chemically, it is 2-chloro-11-(4-methyl-1-piperazinyl) dibenz (b,f) (1,4) oxazepine. It is present in the oral concentrate primarily as the HCl.

Actions: Pharmacologically, loxapine is a tranquilizer for which the exact mode of action has not been established. However, changes in the level of excitability of subcortical inhibitory areas have been observed in several animal species in association with such manifestations of tranquilization as calming effects and suppression of aggressive behavior.

In normal human volunteers, signs of sedation were seen within 20 to 30 minutes after administration. These signs were most pronounced within 1½ to 3 hours after administration and lasted through 12 hours. Similar timing of primary pharmacologic effects was seen in animals.

Absorption of loxapine following oral or parenteral administration is virtually complete. The drug is removed rapidly from the plasma and distributed in tissues. Animal studies suggest an initial preferential distribution in lungs, brain, spleen, heart, and kidney. Loxapine is metabolized extensively and is excreted mainly in the first 24 hours. Metabolites are excreted in the urine in the form of conjugates but are unconjugated in the feces.

Indications: DAXOLIN C Oral Concentrate is indicated for the manifestations of schizophrenia.

DAXOLIN C has not been evaluated for the management of behavioral complications in patients with mental retardation, and therefore it cannot be recommended.

Contraindications: DAXOLIN® C Oral Concentrate is contraindicated in comatose or severe drug induced depressed states (alcohol, barbiturates, narcotics, etc.).

DAXOLIN C is contraindicated in individuals with known hypersensitivity to the drug.

Warnings:

Usage in Pregnancy: Safe use of DAXOLIN C Oral Concentrate during pregnancy or lactation has not been established; therefore, its use in pregnancy, in nursing mothers, or in women of childbearing potential requires that the benefits of treatment be weighed against the possible risks to mother and child. No embryotoxicity or teratogenicity was observed in studies in rats, rabbits or dogs. With the exception of one rabbit study, the highest dosage was two times the maximum recommended human dose and in some studies the dose was lower. Perinatal studies have shown renal papillary abnormalities in offspring of rats treated from mid-pregnancy with doses of 0.6 and 1.8 mg/kg, doses which approximate the usual human dose but which are considerably below the maximum recommended human dose.

Usage in Children: Studies have not been performed in children; therefore this drug is not recommended for use in children below the age of 16.

DAXOLIN C (loxapine hydrochloride) Oral Concentrate, like other tranquilizers, may impair mental and/or physical abilities, especially during the first few days of therapy. Therefore, ambulatory patients should be warned about activities requiring alertness (eg, operating vehicles or machinery), and about concomitant use of alcohol and other CNS depressants.

Precautions: DAXOLIN C should be used with extreme caution in patients with a history of convulsive disorders since it lowers the convulsive threshold. Seizures have been reported in epileptic patients receiving DAXOLIN C at antipsychotic dose levels, and may occur even with maintenance of routine anticonvulsant drug therapy.

DAXOLIN C (loxapine hydrochloride) has an antiemetic effect in animals. Since this effect may also occur in man, loxapine may mask signs of overdosage of toxic drugs and may obscure conditions such as intestinal obstruction and brain tumor.

DAXOLIN C should be used with caution in patients with cardiovascular disease. Increased pulse rates have been reported in the majority of patients receiving antipsychotic doses; and transient hypotension has been reported. In the presence of severe hypotension requiring vasopressor therapy, the preferred drugs may be norepinephrine or angiotensin. Usual doses of epinephrine may be ineffective because of inhibition of its vasopressor effect by loxapine.

The possibility of ocular toxicity from loxapine cannot be excluded at this time. Therefore, careful observation should be made for pigmentary retinopathy and lenticular pigmentation since these have been observed in some patients receiving certain other antipsychotic drugs for prolonged periods.

Because of possible anticholinergic action, the drug should be used cautiously in patients with glaucoma or a tendency to urinary retention, particularly with concomitant administration

of anticholinergic-type antiparkinsonian medication.
Adverse Reactions: *CNS Effects:* Manifestations of adverse effects on the central nervous system, other than extrapyramidal effects, have been seen infrequently. Drowsiness, usually mild, may occur at the beginning of therapy or when dosage is increased. It usually subsides with continued DAXOLIN® C (loxapine hydrochloride) oral concentrate therapy. The incidence of sedation has been less than that of certain aliphatic phenothiazines and slightly more than the piperazine phenothiazines. Dizziness, faintness, staggering gait, muscle twitching, weakness, and confusional states have been reported.
Extrapyramidal Reactions—Neuromuscular (extrapyramidal) reactions during the administration of DAXOLIN C oral concentrate have been reported frequently, often during the first few days of treatment. In most patients, these reactions involved parkinsonism like symptoms such as tremor, rigidity, excessive salivation, and masked facies. Akathisia (motor restlessness) also has been reported relatively frequently. These symptoms are usually not severe and can be controlled by reduction of DAXOLIN C dosage or by administration of antiparkinsonian drugs in usual dosage. Dystonic and dyskinetic reactions have occurred less frequently, but may be more severe. Dystonias include spasms of muscles of the neck and face, tongue protrusion, and oculogyric movement. Dyskinetic reaction has been described in the form of choreoathetoid movements. These reactions sometimes require reduction or temporary withdrawal of DAXOLIN C dosage in addition to appropriate counter-active drugs.
Persistent Tardive Dyskinesia—In keeping with the action of all antipsychotic agents, tardive dyskinesia may appear in some patients on long-term therapy or may appear after drug therapy has been discontinued. The risk appears to be greater in elderly patients (especially females) on high-dose therapy. The symptoms are persistent and, in some patients, appear to be irreversible. The syndrome is characterized by rhythmical involuntary movement of the tongue, face, mouth, or jaw (eg, protrusion of tongue, puffing of cheeks, puckering of mouth, chewing movements). Sometimes these may be accompanied by involuntary movements of extremities.
There is no known effective treatment for tardive dyskinesia; antiparkinsonian agents usually do not alleviate the symptoms of this syndrome. It is suggested that all antipsychotic agents be discontinued if these symptoms appear. Should it be necessary to reinstitute treatment, or increase the dosage of the agent, or switch to a different antipsychotic agent, the syndrome may be masked. It has been suggested that fine vermicular movements of the tongue may be an early sign of the syndrome; if the medication is stopped at that time the syndrome may not develop.
Cardiovascular Effects: Tachycardia, hypotension, hypertension, light-headedness, and syncope have been reported.
A few cases of ECG changes similar to those seen with phenothiazines have been reported. It is not known whether these were related to loxapine administration.
Skin Effects: Dermatitis, edema (puffiness of face), pruritus and seborrhea have been reported with loxapine. The possibility of photosensitivity and/or phototoxicity occurring has not been excluded; skin rashes of uncertain etiology have been observed in a few patients during hot summer months.
Endocrine Effects: No endocrine abnormalities have been reported.
Anticholinergic Effects: Dry mouth, nasal congestion, constipation, and blurred vision have occurred; these are more likely to occur with concomitant use of antiparkinsonian agents.
Other Adverse Reactions: Nausea, vomiting, weight gain, weight loss, dyspnea, ptosis, hyperpyrexia, flushed facies, headache, paresthesia and polydipsia have been reported in some patients. Rarely, galactorrhea and menstrual irregularity of uncertain etiology have been reported.
Dosage and Administration: DAXOLIN® C (loxapine hydrochloride) oral concentrate is administered orally, usually in divided doses, two to four times a day. Daily dosage (in terms of base equivalents) should be adjusted to the individual patient's needs as assessed by the severity of symptoms and previous history of response to antipsychotic drugs. Initial dosage of 10 mg twice daily is recommended although, in severely disturbed patients, initial dosage up to a total of 50 mg daily may be desirable. Dosage should then be increased fairly rapidly over the first seven to ten days until there is effective control of psychotic symptoms. The usual therapeutic and maintenance range is 60 mg to 100 mg daily. However, as with other antipsychotic drugs, some patients respond to lower dosage and others require higher dosage for optimal benefit. Daily dosage higher than 250 mg is not recommended. For maintenance therapy, dosage should be reduced to the lowest level compatible with symptom control; many patients have been maintained satisfactorily at dosages in the range of 20 mg to 60 mg daily.
DAXOLIN C oral concentrate should be mixed with orange or grapefruit juice shortly before administration. A calibrated dropper (10 mg, 15 mg, 25 mg) is enclosed and should be used for dosage.
Overdosage: Signs and symptoms of overdosage will depend on the amount ingested and individual patient tolerance. As would be expected from the pharmacologic actions of the drug, the clinical findings may range from mild depression of the CNS and cardiovascular systems to profound hypotension, respiratory depression, and unconsciousness. The posibility of occurrence of extrapyramidal symptoms and/or convulsive seizures should be kept in mind.
The treatment of overdosage is essentially symptomatic and supportive. Early gastric lavage and extended dialysis might be expected to be beneficial. Centrally acting emetics may have little effect because of the antiemetic action of loxapine. In addition, emesis should be avoided because of the possibility of aspiration of vomitus. Avoid analeptics, such as pentylenetetrazol, which may cause convulsions. Severe hypotension might be expected to respond to the administration of levarterenol or phenylephrine. EPINEPHRINE SHOULD NOT BE USED SINCE ITS USE IN A PATIENT WITH PARTIAL ADRENERGIC BLOCKADE MAY FURTHER LOWER THE BLOOD PRESSURE.
Severe extrapyramidal reactions should be treated with anticholinergic antiparkinsonian agents or diphenhydramine hydrochloride, and anticonvulsant therapy should be initiated as indicated. Additional measures include oxygen and intravenous fluids.
How Supplied: DAXOLIN® C (loxapine hydrochloride) oral concentrate is supplied in 4 fl. oz. bottles (120 ml) with calibrated dropper. Each ml contains the equivalent of 25 mg of loxapine base as the HCl.
Manufactured for Dome Laboratories by Lederle Laboratories Division, American Cyanamid Company, Pearl River, N.Y. 10965

DECHOLIN® Tablets
(dehydrocholic acid)

Composition: Dehydrocholic acid 250 mg. contained in each tablet.
Indications: For the temporary relief of constipation.
Average Adult Dose: One or two tablets, three times daily or as directed by physician.
Warning: Do not use when abdominal pain, nausea or vomiting are present. Frequent use of this preparation may result in dependence on laxatives.
Store at controlled room temperature (59°–86°F.).
KEEP THIS AND ALL MEDICATIONS OUT OF THE REACH OF CHILDREN.
How Supplied: Bottles of 100, 500 and 1000.

DOMEBORO® Powder Packets,
Effervescent Tablets (acid pH)
Astringent Wet Dressing

One packet or tablet dissolved in a pint of water makes a modified Burow's Solution approximately equivalent to a 1:40 dilution, two packets or tablets a 1:20 dilution, and four packets or tablets a 1:10 dilution.
Buffered to an acid pH.
Contains: Aluminum sulfate and calcium acetate.
Indications: A soothing wet dressing for relief of inflammatory conditions of the skin such as insect bites, poison ivy, swellings and bruises or athlete's foot.
Directions: Dissolve one or two packets or tablets in a pint (large glass) of water and stir. When the powder disperses, shake resulting mixture. Do not strain or filter. Bandage the site of application loosely. Pour mixture on bandage every 15 to 30 minutes to keep dressing moist. Continue for 4 to 8 hours unless otherwise directed by physician. Do not use plastic or other impervious material to prevent evaporation without consulting your physician.
Caution: Keep away from eyes. For external use only. Store below 86°F. (30°C.), avoid freezing. Material in diluted form may be stored for 7 days at room temperature.
How Supplied:
Powder Packets: Boxes of 12 and 100. Each packet contains 2.2 gm. Individually foil-wrapped *Tablets:* Boxes of 12, 100 and 1000.

DOME-PASTE® Bandage
3″ and 4″ Bandages
(Medicated Bandage for Leg or Arm, Improved Unna's boot)

Composition: Each medicated bandage is impregnated with zinc oxide, calamine and gelatin. No heating or painting necessary.
Indications: For those conditions of the extremities (e.g. varicose veins and associated ulcers, stasis edema, thrombophlebitis, lymphangitis).
Caution: If skin sensitivity or irritation develops discontinue use and consult a physician.
Administration and Dosage: Detailed instructions for application are supplied on each carton.
How Supplied: 3″ and 4″ cotton bandage by 360″ (10 yd.). Each carton contains one medicated bandage in polyethylene bag.

DOMOL® Bath and Shower Oil
(diisopropyl sebacate, isopropyl myristate)

Composition: Contains sebacate*, a special skin moisturizing agent, refined mineral oil and skin softener.
*Diisopropyl sebacate.
Action and Uses: Effective, pleasant way to lubricate skin and relieve itchy discomfort. It lubricates skin and restores the protective action of skin oils washed away by soaps and detergents. DOMOL helps maintain skin's normal condition by retarding evaporation of skin's moisture.
Directions for Use:
Bath—Add 1 or 2 capfuls to bathtub or water. Soak for 10-20 minutes.
Shower—Pour 1 capful on wet sponge or washcloth. Rub gently over body, rinse under shower.

Continued on next page

Dome—Cont.

Infant's Bath—Add 1 capful to basin or bathinette of water.
Sponge Bath—Add 1 or 2 capfuls to about a pint of water. Sponge body gently with washcloth or cellulose sponge. After bathing the skin should be patted dry rather than rubbed.
How Supplied: 8 fl. oz. unbreakable plastic bottle.

DTIC-Dome® ℞
(dacarbazine)
Sterile

> **Warning:** It is recommended that DTIC-Dome (dacarbazine) be administered under the supervision of a qualified physician experienced in the use of cancer chemotherapeutic agents. Since facilities for necessary laboratory studies must be available, hospitalization of patients is recommended.
> 1. Hemopoietic depression is the most common toxicity with DTIC-Dome (See Warnings).
> 2. Hepatic necrosis has been reported (See Warnings).
> 3. Studies have demonstrated this agent to have a carcinogenic and teratogenic effect when used in animals.
> 4. In treatment of each patient, the physician must weigh carefully the possibility of achieving therapeutic benefit against the risk of toxicity.

Description: DTIC-Dome (dacarbazine) is a colorless to an ivory colored sterile solid which is light sensitive.
Action: Although the exact mechanism of action of DTIC-Dome (dacarbazine) is unknown, three hypotheses have been offered:
1) inhibition of DNA synthesis by acting as a purine analog
2) action as an alkylating agent
3) interaction with SH groups

Pharmacology: The volume of distribution of DTIC-Dome exceeds total body water content, suggesting localization in some body tissue, probably the liver, it is only slightly (approximately 5%) protein-bound. Its plasma half-life after I.V. administration is approximately 35 minutes. In animal study, approximately 46% of a radio-labeled dose was recovered from the urine after six hours. Of this 46%, almost half was unchanged DTIC and a like quantity was AIC (amino imidazole carboxamide) a metabolite. DTIC is subject to renal tubular secretion rather than glomerular filtration.
Indications: DTIC-Dome (dacarbazine) is indicated for the treatment of metastatic malignant melanoma. Combinations of cancer chemotherapeutic agents have often shown an improved response over the use of single agents.
Contraindications: DTIC-Dome (dacarbazine) is contraindicated in patients who have demonstrated a hypersensitivity to it in the past.
Warnings: Hemopoietic depression is the most serious toxicity with DTIC-Dome and involves primarily the leukocytes and platelets, although mild anemia may sometimes occur. Leukopenia and thrombocytopenia may be severe enough to cause death. The possible bone marrow depression requires careful monitoring of white blood cells, red blood cells and platelet levels. Hemopoietic toxicity may warrant temporary suspension or cessation of therapy with DTIC-Dome.
Hepatic toxicity with liver necrosis has been extremely rare and has only been observed in patients in an advanced stage of malignancy when DTIC-Dome has been administered concomitantly with other anti-neoplastic drugs, and when the drug has been used alone in the presence of pre-existing hepatic pathology.
Anaphylaxis can occur following the administration of DTIC-Dome. Safe use of DTIC-Dome in pregnancy has not been established; teratogenic effects have been observed when used in animals.
Precautions: DTIC-Dome (dacarbazine) should be administered preferably to patients who are hospitalized and who can be observed carefully and frequently during and after therapy, with particular reference to the hemopoietic system.
Adverse Reactions: Symptoms of anorexia, nausea, and vomiting are the most frequently noted of all toxic reactions. Over 90% of patients are affected with the initial few doses. The vomiting lasts 1–12 hours and may be completely but unpredictably palliated with phenobarbital and/or prochlorperazine. Rarely intractable nausea and vomiting have necessitated discontinuance therapy with DTIC-Dome (dacarbazine). Rarely, DTIC-Dome (dacarbazine) has caused diarrhea. Some helpful suggestions include restricting the patient's oral intake of food for 4–6 hours prior to treatment. The rapid toleration of these symptoms suggests that a central nervous system mechanism may be involved, and usually these symptoms subside after the first 1 or 2 days.
There are a number of minor toxicities that are infrequently noted. Patients have experienced an influenza-like syndrome of fever to 39°C, myalgias and malaise. These symptoms occur usually after large single doses, may last for several days, and may occur with successive treatments.
Alopecia has been noted as has facial flushing and facial paresthesia. There have been few reports of significant liver or renal function test abnormalities in man. However, these abnormalities have been observed more frequently in animal studies.
Erthematous and urticarial rashes have been observed infrequently after administration of DTIC-Dome. Rarely, photosensitivity reactions may occur.
Dosage and Administration: DTIC-Dome (dacarbazine) 100 mg/vial and 200 mg/vial are reconstituted with 9.9 ml. and 19.7 ml. respectively, of Sterile Water for Injection, USP. The resulting solution contains 10 mg/ml. of dacarbazine having a pH of 3.0 to 4.0.
The recommended dosage is 2 to 4.5 mg/kg/d for 10 days. Treatment may be repeated at 4 week intervals. An alternate recommended dosage is 250 mg./square meter of body surface/day I.V. for five days. Treatment may be repeated every 3 weeks. The calculated dose of the resulting solution is drawn into a syringe and administered *only* intravenously.
The reconstituted solution may be further diluted with 5% dextrose injection, U.S.P. or sodium chloride injection, U.S.P. and administered as an intravenous infusion.
Extravasation of the drug subcutaneously during the intravenous administration may result in tissue damage and severe pain.
After reconstitution and prior to use, the solution in the vial may be stored at 4°C. for up to 72 hours or at normal room conditions (temperature and light) for up to 8 hours. If the reconstituted solution is further diluted in 5% dextrose injection, U.S.P. or sodium chloride injection, U.S.P., the resulting solution may be stored at 4°C. for up to 24 hours or at normal room conditions for up to 8 hours.
Supplied: Vials containing 100 mg or 200 mg of DTIC-Dome as sterile dacarbazine in boxes of 12.

EXZIT® Medicated Cleanser
(acid pH)
(colloidal sulfur, salicylic acid)

Contains: Effective anti-acne medications: colloidal sulfur—to dry excess skin oils; salicylic acid—to peel away dead skin tissue.
Indication: Medicated skin cleanser as an aid in the treatment of acne.
Directions: Use twice daily, preferably in the morning and at bedtime. Wet the skin. Apply the cleanser to moist sponge. Work into lather. Massage for five minutes. Rinse.
Warnings: If excessive drying or skin irritation develops or increases, discontinue use and consult physician. For external use only. Avoid contact with eyes. Keep out of reach of children. Store below 86°F. (30°C.), avoid freezing.
How Supplied: Net weight 4 oz (114 g) in the exclusive **Dome Dispensajar®** with its "personal washcloth"—an applicator sponge so fingers never touch the cleanser. The DISPENSAJAR contains over 4 oz by weight to deliver a full 4 oz through the DISPENSAJAR disc.

EXZIT® Medicated Creme and Lotion
(acid pH)
(colloidal sulfur, resorcinal)

Contains: Colloidal sulfur and resorcinol in a compatible vehicle adjusted to the pH range for normal skin.
Indications: Creme—as an aid in drying and peeling acne blemishes. Lotion—as a colorless aid in drying and peeling blemishes in acne and related skin conditions.
Directions: Wash affected parts thoroughly, then dry. Apply creme or lotion sparingly twice daily, preferably in the morning and at bedtime. Follow advice of physician as to diet or other treatment.
Caution: If excessive drying or skin irritation develops or increases, discontinue use and consult physician. For external use only. Avoid contact with eyes. Keep out of reach of children. Store below 86°F. (30°C.), avoid freezing.
How Supplied: Creme—1 oz tube (28.4 g); Lotion—2 fl oz (60 cc).

LITHANE® ℞
(lithium carbonate)
TABLETS
For Control of Manic Episodes in Manic-Depressive Psychosis

WARNINGS

> Lithium toxicity is closely related to serum lithium levels, and can occur at doses close to therapeutic levels. Facilities for prompt and accurate serum lithium determinations should be available before initiating therapy.

Description: Lithium carbonate is a white, light, alkaline powder with molecular formula Li_2CO_3 and molecular weight 73.89. Lithium is an element of the alkali-metal group with atomic number 3, atomic weight 6.94, and an emission line at 671 mu on the flame photometer.
Actions: Preclinical studies have shown that lithium alters sodium transport in nerve and muscle cells and effects a shift toward intraneuronal metabolism of catecholamines, but the specific biochemical mechanism of lithium action in mania is unknown.
Indications: Lithium carbonate is indicated in the treatment of manic episodes of manic-depressive illness. Maintenance therapy prevents or diminishes the intensity of subsequent episodes in those manic-depressive patients with a history of mania.
Typical symptoms of mania include pressure of speech, motor hyperactivity, reduced need for sleep, flight of ideas, grandiosity, elation, poor judgment, aggressiveness, and possibly hostility. When given to a patient experiencing

a manic episode, lithium may produce a normalization of symptomatology within 1 to 3 weeks.

Warnings: Lithium should generally not be given to patients with significant renal or cardiovascular disease, severe debilitation or dehydration, or sodium depletion, and to patients receiving diuretics, since the risk of lithium toxicity is very high in such patients. If the psychiatric indication is life-threatening, and if such a patient fails to respond to other measures, lithium treatment may be undertaken with extreme caution, including daily serum lithium determinations and adjustment to the usually low doses ordinarily tolerated by these individuals. In such instances, hospitalization is a necessity.

Lithium toxicity is closely related to serum lithium levels, and can occur at doses close to therapeutic levels (see DOSAGE AND ADMINISTRATION).

Outpatients and their families should be warned that the patient must discontinue lithium carbonate therapy and contact his physician if such clinical signs of lithium toxicity as diarrhea, vomiting, tremor, mild ataxia, drowsiness, or muscular weakness occur.

Lithium therapy has been reported in some cases to be associated with morphologic changes in the kidneys. The relationship between such changes and renal function has not been established.

Usage in Pregnancy: Adverse effects on nidation in rats, embryo viability in mice, and metabolism *in vitro* of rat testis and human spermatozoa have been attributed to lithium, as have teratogenicity in submammalian species and cleft palates in mice. Studies in rats, rabbits, and monkeys have shown no evidence of lithium-induced teratology.

There are lithium birth registries in the United States and elsewhere: however there is at the present time insufficient data to determine the effects of lithium carbonate on human fetuses. Therefore, at this point, lithium should not be used in pregnancy, especially the first trimester, unless in the opinion of the physician, the potential benefits outweigh the possible hazards.

Usage in Children: Since information regarding the safety and effectiveness of lithium carbonate in children under 12 years of age is not available, its use in such patients is not recommended at this time.

Combined Use of haloperidol and lithium: An encephalopathic syndrome (characterized by weakness, lethargy, fever, tremulousness and confusion, extrapyramidal symptoms, leucocytosis, elevated serum enzymes, BUN and FBS) followed by irreversible brain damage has occurred in a few patients treated with lithium plus haloperidol. A causal relationship between these events and the concomitant administration of lithium and haloperidol has not been established: however, patients receiving such combined therapy should be monitored closely for early evidence of neurological toxicity and treatment discontinued promptly if such signs appear.

Precautions: The ability to tolerate lithium is greater during the acute manic phase and decreases when manic symptoms subside (see DOSAGE AND ADMINISTRATION).

The distribution space of lithium approximates that of total body water. Lithium is primarily excreted in urine with insignificant excretion in feces. Renal excretion of lithium is proportional to its plasma concentration. The half-elimination time of lithium is approximately 24 hours. Lithium decreases sodium reabsorption by the renal tubules which could lead to sodium depletion. Therefore, it is essential for the patient to maintain a normal diet, including salt, and an adequate fluid intake (2500-3000 ml) at least during the initial stabilization period. Decreased tolerance to lithium has been reported to ensue from protracted sweating or diarrhea, and, if such occur, supplemental fluid and salt should be administered.

In addition to sweating and diarrhea, concomitant infection with elevated temperatures may also necessitate a temporary reduction or cessation of medication.

Untoward reactions to simultaneous use of lithium and other psychoactive drugs have not been reported. However, the possibility of adverse interaction with other anti-psychotic medications remains.

Adverse Reactions: Adverse reactions are seldom encountered at serum lithium levels below 1.5 mEq./1., except in the occasional patient sensitive to lithium. Mild to moderate toxic reactions may occur at levels from 1.5-2.5 mEq./1., and moderate to severe reactions may be seen at levels from 2.0-2.5 mEq./1., depending upon individual response to the drug.

Fine hand tremor, polyuria, and mild thirst may occur during initial therapy for the acute manic phase, and may persist throughout treatment. Transient and mild nausea and general discomfort may also appear during the first few days of lithium administration.

These side effects are an inconvenience rather than a disabling condition, and usually subside with continued treatment or a temporary reduction or cessation of dosage. If persistent, a cessation of dosage is indicated.

Diarrhea, vomiting, drowsiness, muscular weakness, and lack of coordination may be early signs of lithium intoxication, and can occur at lithium levels below 2.0 mEq./1. At higher levels, giddiness, ataxia, blurred vision, tinnitus, and a large output of dilute urine may be seen. Serum lithium levels above 3.0 mEq./1. may produce a complex clinical picture involving multiple organs and organ systems. Serum lithium levels should not be permitted to exceed 2.0 mEq./1. during the acute treatment phase.

The following toxic reactions have been reported and appear to be related to serum lithium levels:

Neuromuscular: tremor, muscle hyperirritability (fasciculations, twitching, clonic movements of whole limbs), ataxia, choreo-athetotic movements, hyperactive deep tendon reflexes.

Central Nervous System: blackout spells, epileptiform seizures, slurred speech, dizziness, vertigo, incontinence of urine or feces, somnolence, psychomotor retardation, restlessness, confusion, stupor, coma.

Cardiovascular: cardiac arrhythmia, hypotension, peripheral circulatory collapse.

Gastrointestinal: anorexia, nausea, vomiting, diarrhea.

Genitourinary: albuminuria, oliguria, polyuria, glycosuria.

Dematologic: drying and thinning of hair, anesthesia of skin, chronic folliculitis, xerosis cutis.

Autonomic Nervous System: blurred vision, dry mouth.

Miscellaneous: fatigue, lethargy, tendency to sleep, dehydration, weight loss, transient scotomata.

Thyroid Abnormalities: Euthyroid goiter and/ or hypothyroidism (including myxedema) accompanied by lower T_3 and T_4. I_{131} iodine uptake may be elevated. Underlying thyroid disorders do not constitute a contraindication to lithium treatment; careful monitoring of thyroid function during lithium stabilization and maintenance allows for correction of changing thyroid parameters, if any. They can be treated by prescribing thyroid in these cases.

EEG. Changes: diffuse slowing, widening of frequency spectrum, potentiation and disorganization of background rhythm.

EKG. Changes: reversible flattening, isoelectricity or inversion of T-waves.

Miscellaneous reactions unrelated to dosage are: transient electroencephalographic and electrocardiographic changes, leucocytosis, headache, diffuse, nontoxic goiter with or without hypothyroidism, transient hyperglycemia, generalized pruritus with or without rash, cutaneous ulcers, albuminuria, worsening of organic brain syndromes, excessive weight gain, edematous swelling of ankles or wrists, and thirst or polyuria, sometimes resembling diabetes insipidus. A single report has been received of the development of painful discoloration of fingers and toes and coldness of the extremities within one day of the starting of treatment of lithium. The mechanism through which these symptoms (resembling Raynaud's Syndrome) developed is not known. Recovery followed discontinuance.

Dosage and Administration:

Acute Mania: Optimal patient response to lithium carbonate usually can be established and maintained with 600 mg t.i.d. Such doses will normally produce an effective serum lithium level ranging between 1.0 and 1.5 mEq./1. Dosage must be individualized according to serum levels and clinical response. Regular monitoring of the patient's clinical state and of serum lithium levels is necessary. Serum levels should be determined twice per week during the acute phase, and until the serum level and clinical condition of the patient have been stabilized.

Long term Control: The desirable lithium levels are 0.6 to 1.2 mEq./1. Dosage will vary from one individual to another, but usually 300 mg t.i.d. or q.i.d. will maintain this level. Serum lithium levels in uncomplicated cases receiving maintenance therapy during remission should be monitored at least every two months.

Patients abnormally sensitive to lithium may exhibit toxic signs at serum levels of 1.0 to 1.5 mEq./1. Elderly patients often respond to reduced dosage, and may exhibit signs of toxicity at serum levels ordinarily tolerated by other patients.

N. B.: Blood samples for serum lithium determinations are drawn 8-12 hours after the previous dose when lithium concentrations are relatively stable. Total reliance must not be placed on serum levels alone. Accurate patient evaluation requires both clinical and laboratory analysis.

Overdosage: The toxic levels for lithium are close to the therapeutic levels. It is therefore important that patients and their families be cautioned to watch for early toxic symptoms and to discontinue the drug and inform the physician should they occur. Toxic symptoms are listed in detail under ADVERSE REACTIONS.

Treatment: No specific antidote for lithium poisoning is known. Early symptoms of lithium toxicity can usually be treated by reduction or cessation of dosage of the drug and resumption of the treatment at a lower dose after 24 to 48 hours. In severe cases of lithium poisoning, the first and foremost goal of treatment consists of elimination of this ion from the organism.

Treatment is essentially the same as that used in barbiturate poisoning: 1) lavage, 2) correction of fluid and electrolyte imbalance, and 3) regulation of kidney functioning. Urea, mannitol, and aminophylline all produce significant increases in lithium excretion. Infection prophylaxis, regular chest X-rays, and preservation of adequate respiration are essential.

How Supplied: Lithane (lithium carbonate) is available as scored tablets containing 300 mg of lithium carbonate in bottles of 100 and 1000.

Manufactured for
Dome Division Miles Laboratories Inc.
West Haven Connecticut 06516
by Pfizer Laboratories, New York, N.Y. 10017

Continued on next page

Dome—Cont.

MITHRACIN® ℞
(mithramycin)
FOR INTRAVENOUS USE

Warning: IT IS RECOMMENDED THAT MITHRACIN (mithramycin) BE ADMINISTERED ONLY TO HOSPITALIZED PATIENTS BY OR UNDER THE SUPERVISION OF A QUALIFIED PHYSICIAN WHO IS EXPERIENCED IN THE USE OF CANCER CHEMOTHERAPEUTIC AGENTS, BECAUSE OF THE POSSIBILITY OF SEVERE REACTIONS. FACILITIES FOR THE DETERMINATION OF NECESSARY LABORATORY STUDIES MUST BE AVAILABLE.

SEVERE THROMBOCYTOPENIA, A HEMORRHAGIC TENDENCY AND EVEN DEATH MAY RESULT FROM THE USE OF MITHRACIN. ALTHOUGH SEVERE TOXICITY IS MORE APT TO OCCUR IN PATIENTS WHO HAVE FAR-ADVANCED DISEASE OR ARE OTHERWISE CONSIDERED POOR RISKS FOR THERAPY, SERIOUS TOXICITY MAY ALSO OCCASIONALLY OCCUR EVEN IN PATIENTS WHO ARE IN RELATIVELY GOOD CONDITION.

IN THE TREATMENT OF EACH PATIENT, THE PHYSICIAN MUST WEIGH CAREFULLY THE POSSIBILITY OF ACHIEVING THERAPEUTIC BENEFIT VERSUS THE RISK OF TOXICITY WHICH MAY OCCUR WITH MITHRACIN THERAPY. THE FOLLOWING DATA CONCERNING THE USE OF MITHRACIN IN THE TREATMENT OF TESTICULAR TUMORS, HYPERCALCEMIC AND/OR HYPERCALCIURIC CONDITIONS ASSOCIATED WITH VARIOUS ADVANCED MALIGNANCIES, SHOULD BE THOROUGHLY REVIEWED BEFORE ADMINISTERING THIS COMPOUND.

Description: Mithracin is a yellow crystalline compound which is produced by a microorganism, *Streptomyces plicatus.* It has an empirical formula of $C_{52}H_{75}O_{24}$.

Actions: Although the exact mechanism by which Mithracin causes tumor inhibition is not yet known, studies have indicated that this compound forms a complex with deoxyribonucleic acid (DNA) and inhibits cellular ribonucleic acid (RNA) and enzymic RNA synthesis. The binding of Mithracin to DNA in the presence of Mg^{11} (or other divalent cations) is responsible for the inhibition of DNA-dependent or DNA-directed RNA synthesis. This action presumably accounts for the biological properties of Mithracin.

Mithracin shows potent cytotoxicity against malignant cells of human origin (Hela cells) growing in tissue culture. Mithracin is lethal to Hela cells in 48 hours at concentrations as low as 0.5 micrograms per milliliter of tissue culture medium. Mithracin has shown significant anti-tumor activity against experimental leukemia in mice when administered intraperitoneally.

Indications: Mithracin is a potent antineoplastic agent which has been shown to be useful in the treatment of carefully selected hospitalized patients with malignant tumors of the testis in whom successful treatment by surgery and/or radiation is impossible. Also, on the basis of limited clinical experience to date, it may be considered in the treatment of certain symptomatic patients with hypercalcemia and hypercalciuria associated with a variety of advanced neoplasms.

The use of Mithracin in other types of neoplastic disease is not recommended at the present time.

Contraindications: Mithracin (mithramycin) is contraindicated in patients with thrombocytopenia, thrombocytopathy, coagulation disorder or an increased susceptibility to bleeding due to other causes. Mithracin should not be administered to any patient with impairment of bone marrow function.

Mithracin should not be used in the treatment of patients who are not hospitalized and who cannot be observed carefully and frequently during and after therapy, or whenever appropriate laboratory facilities are unavailable.

Precautions: Mithracin should be administered only to patients who are hospitalized and who can be observed carefully and frequently during and after therapy.

Severe thrombocytopenia, a hemorrhagic tendency and even death may result from the use of Mithracin. Although severe toxicity is more apt to occur in patients who have far-advanced disease or are otherwise considered poor risks for therapy, serious toxicity may also occasionally occur even in patients who are in relatively good condition.

Electrolyte imbalance, especially hypocalcemia, hypokalemia, and hypophosphatemia, should be corrected with appropriate electrolyte therapy prior to treatment with Mithracin.

Mithracin should be used with extreme caution in patients with significant impairment of renal or hepatic function.

In the treatment of each patient, the physician must weigh carefully the possiblity of achieving therapeutic benefit versus the risk of toxicity which may occur with Mithracin therapy.

The following laboratory studies should be obtained frequently during therapy and for several days following the last dose: platelet count, prothrombin time, bleeding time. The occurrence of thrombocytopenia or a significant prolongation of prothrombin time or bleeding time is an indication for the termination of therapy.

Adverse Reactions: THE MOST IMPORTANT FORM OF TOXICITY ASSOCIATED WITH THE USE OF MITHRACIN CONSISTS OF A BLEEDING SYNDROME WHICH USUALLY BEGINS WITH AN EPISODE OF EPISTAXIS. This bleeding tendency may only consist of a single or several episodes of epistaxis and progress no further. However, in some cases, this hemorrhagic syndrome can start with an episode of hematemesis which may progress to more wide-spread hemorrhage in the gastrointestinal tract or to a more generalized bleeding tendency. This hemorrhagic diathesis is most likely due to abnormalities in multiple clotting factors.

A detailed analysis of the clinical data in 1,160 patients treated with Mithracin indicates that the hemorrhagic syndrome is dose related. With doses of 30 mcg/kg/day or less for 10 or fewer doses, the incidence of bleeding episodes has been 5.4% with an associated drug-related mortality rate of 1.6%. With doses greater than 30 mcg/kg/day and/or for more than 10 doses, a significantly larger number of bleeding episodes occurred (11.9%) and the associated drug-related mortality rate was also significantly higher (5.7%).

The most common side effects reported with the use of Mithracin consist of gastrointestinal symptoms: anorexia, nausea, vomiting, diarrhea, and stomatitis. Other less frequently reported side effects include fever, drowsiness, weakness, lethargy, malaise, headache, depression, phlebitis, facial flushing, and skin rash.

The following laboratory abnormalities have been reported during therapy with Mithracin (mithramycin) and in most instances were reversible following cessation of treatment:

Hematologic Abnormalities: Depression of platelet count, white count, hemoglobin and prothrombin content; elevation of clotting time and bleeding time; abnormal clot retraction.

Thrombocytopenia may be rapid in onset and may occur at any time during therapy or within several days following the last dose. With the occurrence of severe thrombocytopenia, the infusion of platelet concentrates of platelet-rich plasma may be helpful in elevating the platelet count.

The occurrence of leukopenia with the use of Mithracin is relatively uncommon, occurring only in approximately 6% of patients.

It has been uncommon for abnormalities in clotting time or clot retraction to be demonstrated prior to the onset of an overt bleeding episode noted in some patients treated with Mithracin. Nevertheless, the performance of these tests periodically is recommended because in a few instances, an abnormality in one of these studies may have served as a warning to terminate therapy because of impeding serious toxicity.

Abnormal Liver Function Tests: Increased levels of serum glutamic oxalacetic transaminase, serum glutamic pyruvic transaminase, lactic dehydrogenase, alkaline phosphatase, serum bilirubin, ornithine carbamyl transferase, isocitric dehydrogenase, and increased retention of bromsulphalein.

Abnormal Renal Function Tests: Increased blood urea nitrogen and serum creatinine; proteinuria.

Abnormalities in Electrolyte Concentrations: Depression of serum calcium, phosphorus, and potassium.

Dosage: The daily dose of Mithracin is based on the patient's body weight. If a patient has abnormal fluid retention such as edema, hydrothorax or ascites, the patient's ideal weight rather than actual body weight should be used to calculate the dose.

Treatment of Testicular Tumors: In the treatment of patients with testicular tumors the recommended daily dose of Mithracin (mithramycin) is 25 to 30 micrograms per kilogram of body weight. Therapy should be continued for a period of 8 to 10 days unless significant side effects or toxicity occur during therapy. A course of therapy consisting of more than 10 daily doses is not recommended. Individual daily doses should not exceed 30 micrograms per kilogram of body weight.

In those patients with responsive tumors, some degree of tumor regression is usually evident within 3 or 4 weeks following the initial course of therapy. If tumor masses remain unchanged following an initial course of therapy, additional courses of therapy at monthly intervals are warranted.

When a significant tumor regression is obtained, it is suggested that additional courses of therapy be given at monthly intervals until a complete regression of tumor masses is achieved or until definite tumor progression or new tumor masses occur in spite of continued courses of therapy.

Treatment of Hypercalcemia and Hypercalciuria: Reversal of hypercalcemia and hypercalciuria can usually be achieved with Mithracin at doses considerably lower than those recommended for use in the treatment of testicular tumors.

In hypercalcemia and hypercalciuria associated with advanced malignancy the recommended course of treatment with Mithracin is 25 micrograms per kilogram of body weight per day for 3 or 4 days.

If the desired degree of reversal of hypercalcemia or hypercalciuria is not achieved with the initial course of therapy, additional courses of therapy may then be administered at intervals of one week or more to achieve the desired result or to maintain serum calcium and urinary calcium excretion at normal levels. It may be possible to maintain normal calcium balance with single, weekly doses or with a schedule of 2 or 3 doses per week.

NOTE: BECAUSE OF THE DRUG'S TOXICITY AND THE LIMITED CLINICAL EXPERIENCE TO DATE IN THESE INDICATIONS, THE FOLLOWING RECOMMENDATIONS SHOULD BE KEPT IN MIND BY THE PHYSICIAN.

1. CONSIDER CASES OF HYPERCALCEMIA AND HYPERCALCIURIA

NOT RESPONSIVE TO CONVENTIONAL TREATMENT.

2. APPLY SAME CONTRAINDICATIONS AND PRECAUTIONARY MEASURES AS IN ANTITUMOR TREATMENT.
3. RENAL FUNCTION SHOULD BE CAREFULLY MONITORED BEFORE, DURING, AND AFTER TREATMENT.
4. BENEFITS OF USE DURING PREGNANCY OR IN WOMEN OF CHILD-BEARING AGE SHOULD BE WEIGHED AGAINST POTENTIAL TOXICITY TO EMBRYO OR FETUS.

Administration: By IV administration only. The appropriate daily dose of Mithracin should be diluted in one liter of 5% Dextrose Injection, USP or Sodium Chloride Injection, USP and administered by slow intravenous infusion over a period of 4 to 6 hours. Rapid direct intravenous injection of Mithracin should be avoided as it may be associated with a higher incidence and greater severity of gastrointestinal side effects. Extravasation of solutions of Mithracin may cause local irritation and cellulitis at injection sites. Should thrombophlebitis or perivascular cellulitis occur, the infusion should be terminated and reinstituted at another site. The application of moderate heat to the site of extravasation may help to disperse the compound and minimize discomfort and local tissue irritation. The use of antiemetic compounds prior to and during treatment with Mithracin may be helpful in relieving nausea and vomiting.

How Supplied: Mithracin is available in vials as a freeze-dried preparation for intravenous administration. Each vial contains 2500 mcg of Mithracin with 100 mg of mannitol and sufficient disodium phosphate to adjust to pH 7. These vials should be stored at refrigerator temperatures between 2°C. to 8°C. (36°F. to 46°F.).

To reconstitute, add aseptically 4.9 ml of Sterile Water for Injection to the contents of the vial and shake to dissolve. Each ml of the resulting solution will then contain 500 mcg of Mithracin. AFTER REMOVAL OF THE APPROPRIATE DOSE, THE REMAINING UNUSED SOLUTION MUST BE DISCARDED, FRESH SOLUTIONS MUST BE PREPARED IN THE ABOVE MANNER EACH DAY OF THERAPY.

Pharmacology and Toxicology: In mice the average intravenous LD_{50} of Mithracin is 2,000 mcg/kg of body weight. When administered orally, it is not toxic to mice even at doses 100 times greater than the intravenous LD_{50}. In rats the average intravenous LD_{50} of Mithracin is 1,700 mcg/kg of body weight. It is not toxic to rats when administered orally at doses 17 times greater than the intravenous LD_{50}. In dogs and monkeys Mithracin is essentially non-toxic when administered intravenously for 24 days at daily doses as high as 50 and 24 mcg/kg of body weight, respectively. However, at higher doses of 100 mcg/kg/day intravenously it is lethal to dogs and monkeys. Signs of toxicity in dogs and monkeys included anorexia, vomiting, listlessness, melena, anemia, lymphopenia, elevated alkaline phosphatase, serum glutamic oxalacetic transaminase, serum glutamic pyruvic transaminase values, hypochloremia, and azotemia. Dogs also showed marked thrombocytopenia, hyponatremia, hypokalemia, hypocalcemia, and decreased prothrombin consumption. Necropsy findings consisted of necrosis of lymphoid tissue and multiple generalized hemorrhages. Mithracin (mithramycin) was only mildly irritating when injected intramuscularly in rabbits and subcutaneously in guinea pigs. Histologic evidence of inhibition of spermatogenesis was observed in a substantial number of male rats receiving doses of 0.6 mg/kg/day and above. This preclinical finding of selective drug effect constituted the scientific rationale for clinical trials in testicular tumors.

RESULTS IN 305 TESTICULAR TUMOR CASES BY TUMOR TYPE

TYPE OF TESTICULAR TUMOR	TOTAL	COMPLETE RESPONSE	PARTIAL RESPONSE	NO RESPONSE
EMBRYONAL CELL	173	26	42	105
TERATOMA	5	0	1	4
TERATOCARCINOMA	23	0	5	18
SEMINOMA	18	0	7	11
CHORIOCARCINOMA	13	1	6	6
MIXED TUMOR	73	6	19	48
TOTALS	305	33	80	192

Clinical Reports:

Treatment of Patients with Inoperable Testicular Tumors: In a combined series of 305 patients with inoperable testicular tumors treated with Mithracin, 33 patients (10.8%) showed a complete disappearance of tumor masses and an additional 80 patients (26.2%) responded with significant partial regression of tumor masses. The longest duration of a continuing complete response is now over 8½ years. The therapeutic responses in this series of patients have been summarized by type of testicular tumor in the accompanying table. [See table above].

Mithracin may be useful in the treatment of patients with testicular tumors which are resistant to other chemotherapeutic agents. Prior radiation therapy or prior chemotherapy did not alter the response rate with Mithracin. This suggests that there is no significant cross resistance between Mithracin (mithramycin) and other chemotherapeutic agents.

Treatment of Patients with Hypercalcemia and Hypercalciuria: A limited number of patients with hypercalcemia (range: 12.0–25.8 mg%) and patients with hypercalciuria (range 215–492 mg/day) associated with malignant disease were treated with Mithracin. Hypercalcemia and hypercalciuria were promptly reversed in all patients. In some patients, the primary malignancy was of non-testicular origin.

Manufactured for
Dome Division Miles Laboratories Inc.
West Haven Connecticut 06516
by Pfizer laboratories, New York, N.Y. 10017

MYCELEX® 1% ℞
(clotrimazole) Cream

For dematologic use only

Description: Mycelex is clotrimazole [1-(o-chloro-α,α-diphenylbenzyl) imidazole] a synthetic antifungal agent having the chemical formula, $C_{22}H_{17}ClN_2$.

Each gram of Mycelex Cream contains 10 mg. clotrimazole in a vanishing cream base of sorbitan monostearate, polysorbate 60, cetyl esters wax, cetostearyl alcohol, 2-octyldodecanol purified water and, as preservative, benzyl alcohol (1%).

Actions: Clotrimazole is a broad-spectrum antifungal agent that inhibits the growth of pathogenic dermatophytes yeasts and Malassezia furfur. Clotrimazole exhibits fungicidal activity in vitro against isolates of Trichophyton rubrum, Trichophyton mentagrophytes, Epidermophyton floccosum, Microsporum canis, and Candida albicans.

No single-step or multiple-step resistance to clotrimazole has developed during successive passages of Candida albicans and Trichophylon mentagrophytes.

Indications: Mycelex Cream is indicated for the topical treatment of the following dermal infections: tinea pedis, tinea cruris, and tinea corporis due to Trichophyton rubrum, Trichopyton mentagrophytes, Epidermophyton floccosum, and Microsporum canis; candidiasis due to Candida albicans; and tinea versicolor due to Malassezia furfur.

Contraindications: Mycelex Cream is contraindicated in individuals who have shown hypersensitivity to any of its components.

Warnings: Mycelex Cream is not for ophthalmic use.

Precautions: In the first trimester of pregnancy. Mycelex Cream should be used only when considered essential to the welfare of the patient.

If irritation or sensitivity develops with the use of Mycelex, treatment should be discontinued and appropriate therapy instituted.

Adverse Reactions: The following adverse reactions have been reported on connection with the use of this product: erythema, stinging, blistering, peeling, edema, pruritus, urticaria, and general irritation of the skin.

Dosage and Administration: Gently massage sufficient Mycelex Cream into the affected and surrounding skin areas twice a day in the morning and evening.

Clinical improvement, with relief of pruritus, usually occurs within the first week of treatment. If a patient shows no clinical improvement after four weeks of treatment with Mycelex, the diagnosis should be reviewed.

How Supplied: Mycelex Cream 1% is suppled in 15- and 30-gram tubes.

Store between 35 and 86 F.

U.S. Patents No. 3,660,577 and 3,705,172.

Manufactured by Schering Corp., Kenilworth, N.J. 07033 for
Dome Division Miles Laboratories Inc
West Haven Connecticut 06516 USA

MYCELEX® 1% ℞
(clotrimazole) Solution

For dermatologic use only

Description: Mycelex is clotrimazole [1-(o-chloro-α,α-diphenylbenzyl) imidazole] a synthetic antifungal agent having the chemical formula $C_{22}H_{17}C1N_2$.

Each ml. of Mycelex Solution contains 10 mg. clotrimazole in a nonaqueous vehicle of polyethylene glycol 400.

Actions: Clotrimazole is a broad spectrum antifungal agent that inhibits the growth of pathogenic dermatophytes, yeasts, and Malassezia furfur. Clotrimazole exhibits fungicidal activity in vitro against isolates of Trichophyton rubrum, Trichophyton mentagrophytes, Epidermophyton floccosum, Microsporum canis, and Candida albicans.

No single-step or multiple-step resistance to clotrimazole has developed during successive

Continued on next page

Dome—Cont.

passages of Candida albicans and Trichophyton mentagrophytes.
Indications: Mycelex Solution is indicated for the topical treatment of the following dermal infections: tinea pedis, tinea cruris, and tinea corporis due to Trichophyton rubrum, Trichophyton mentagrophytes, Epidermophyton floccosum, and Microsporum canis; candidiasis due to Candida albicans; and tinea versicolor due to Malassezia furfur.
Contraindications: Mycelex Solution is contraindicated in individuals who have shown hypersensitivity to any of its components.
Warnings: Mycelex Solution is not for ophthalmic use.
Precautions: In the first trimester of pregnancy, Mycelex Solution should be used only when considered essential to the welfare of the patient.
If irritation or sensitivity develops with the use of Mycelex, treatment should be discontinued and appropriate therapy instituted.
Adverse Reactions: The following adverse reactions have been reported in connection with the use of this product: erythema, stinging, blistering, peeling, edema, pruritus, urticaria, and general irritation of the skin.
Dosage and Administration: Gently massage sufficient Mycelex Solution into the affected and surrounding skin areas twice a day in the morning and evening.
Clinical improvement, with relief of pruritus, usually occurs within the first week of treatment. If a patient shows no clinical improvement after four weeks of treatment with Mycelex, the diagnosis should be reviewed.
How Supplied: Mycelex Solution 1% is supplied in 10 ml and 30 ml plastic bottles.
Store between 35 and 86 F.
U.S. Patents No. 3,660,577 and 3,705,172

Manufactured by Schering Corp., Kenilworth, N.J. 07033 for
Dome Division Miles Laboratories Inc
West Haven Connecticut 06516 USA

MYCELEX®–G 1% ℞
(clotrimazole) Vaginal Cream

Description: Mycelex-G is clotrimazole [1-(o-Chloro-α,α-diphenylbenzyl) imidazole], a synthetic antifungal agent having the chemical formula, $C_{22}H_{17}ClN_2$.
Each applicatorful of Mycelex-G Vaginal Cream contains approximately 50 mg. clotrimazole dispersed in sorbitan monostearate, polysorbate 60, cetyl esters wax, cetostearyl alcohol, 2-octyldodecanol, purified water, and as a preservative, benzyl alcohol (1%).
Actions: Clotrimazole is a broad spectrum antifungal agent that inhibits the growth of pathogenic yeasts. Clotrimazole exhibits fungicidal activity in vitro against Candida albicans and other species of the genus Candida.
No single-step or multiple-step resistance to clotrimazole has developed during successive passages of Candida albicans.
Indications: Mycelex-G Vaginal Cream is indicated for the local treatment of patients with vulvovaginal candidiasis (moniliasis). As Mycelex-G Vaginal Cream has been shown to be effective only for candidal vulvovaginitis, the diagnosis should be confirmed by KOH smears and/or cultures. Other pathogens commonly associated with vulvovaginitis (Trichomonas and Hemophilus vaginalis) should be ruled out by appropriate laboratory methods.
Studies have shown that women taking oral contraceptives had a cure rate similar to those not taking oral contraceptives.
Contraindications: Mycelex-G Vaginal Cream is contraindicated in women who have shown hypersensitivity to any of the components of the preparation.
Precautions: Laboratory Tests: If there is a lack of response to Mycelex-G Vaginal Cream, appropriate microbiological studies should be repeated to confirm the diagnosis and rule out other pathogens before instituting another course of antimycotic therapy.
Usage in Pregnancy: While Mycelex-G Vaginal Cream has not been studied in the first trimester of pregnancy, use in the second and third trimesters has not been associated with ill effects.
Application of ^{14}C labeled clotrimazole has shown negligible absorption (peak serum level of 0.01 mcg/ml 24 hours after insertion of vaginal cream containing 50 mg. of active drug) from both normal and inflamed human vaginal mucosa.
Adverse Reactions: Three (0.5%) of the 653 patients treated with Mycelex-G Vaginal Cream reported complaints during therapy that were possibly drug related. Vaginal burning occurred in one patient; erythema, irritation and burning in another; intercurrent cystitis was reported in the third.
Dosage and Administration: Mycelex-G Vaginal Cream has been found to be effective when used from seven to fourteen days; studies have shown that patients treated for fourteen days had a significantly higher cure rate. The recommended dose is one applicatorful a day for seven to fourteen consecutive days; using the applicator supplied, insert one applicatorful of cream (approximately 5 grams) intravaginally preferably at bedtime.
How Supplied: Mycelex-G Vaginal Cream 1% is supplied in 45-gram tubes with a measured-dose applicator; box of one for seven-day treatment; box of two for fourteen-day treatment.
Store between 35° and 86° F (2° and 30° C).

Manufactured by Schering Corp., Kenilworth, N.J. 07033 for
Dome Division Miles Laboratories Inc
West Haven Connecticut 06516 USA

MYCELEX–G 100 mg ℞
(clotrimazole) Vaginal Tablets

Description: Mycelex-G is clotrimazole [1-(o-Chloro-α,α-diphenylbenzyl) imidazole]a synthetic antifungal agent having the chemical formula $C_{22}H_{17}ClN_2$.
Each Myclex-G Vaginal Tablet contains 100 mg. clotrimazole dispersed in lactose, povidone, corn starch and magnesium stearate.
Actions: Clotrimazole is a broad-spectrum antifungal agent that inhibits the growth of pathogenic yeasts. Clotrimazole exhibits fungicidal activity *in vitro* against *Candida albicans* and other species of the genus *Candida.*
No single-step or multiple-step resistance to clotrimazole has developed during successive passages of *Candida albicans.*
Indications: Mycelex-G Vaginal Tablets are indicated for the local treatment of vulvovaginal candidasis. The diagnosis should be confirmed by KOH smears and/or cultures.
In randomized double-blind trials where Mycelex-G Vaginal Tablets were compared to Nystatin Vaginal Tablets, cure rates were similar.
Contraindications: Mycelex-G Vaginal Tablets are contraindicated in women who have shown hypersensitivity to this drug.
Precautions: Laboratory Tests: If there is a lack of response to Mycelex-G appropriate microbiological studies should be repeated to confirm the diagnosis and rule out other pathogens.
Usage in Pregnancy: While Mycelex-G Vaginal Tablets have not been studied in the first trimester of pregnancy, use in the second and third trimesters has not been associated with ill effects. Follow-up reports now available on 41 neonates of 107 pregnant patients reveal no adverse effects or complications attributable to Mycelex-G therapy.
Application of ^{14}C-labeled clotrimazole has shown negligible absorption peak of 0.03 mcg/ml of serum 24 hours after insertion of a 100 mg Tablet) from both normal and inflamed human vaginal mucosa.
Adverse Reactions: Eleven (1.6%) of the 689 patients treated with Mycelex-G reported complaints during therapy that were possibly drug-related. Mild burning occurred in four patients while other complaints, such as skin rash, lower abdominal cramps, slight urinary frequency, and burning or irritation in the sexual partner, occurred rarely. In no case was it necessary to discontinue treatment with Mycelex-G.
Dosage and Administration: The recommended dose is one tablet a day for seven consecutive days using the applicator supplied. Insert one tablet intravaginally preferably at bedtime. In the event of treatment failure, other pathogens commonly responsible for vaginitis should be ruled out before instituting another course of antimycotic therapy. There are no studies to show whether a second course of clotrimazole would be effective in patients who fail to respond to the initial course.
How Supplied: Mycelex-G Vaginal Tablets, 100 mg., white, tear-drop-shaped, uncoated tablets, supplied in strip of seven tablets with plastic applicator and patient leaflet of instructions.
Do not store above 35°C (95°F).
U.S. Patents No. 3,660,577 and 3,705,172.
Manufactured by Schering Corporation, Kenilworth, N.J. 07033 for
Dome Division Miles Labortories Inc
West Haven Connecticut 06516 USA

NYSTAFORM® Ointment ℞
(nystatin-iodochlorhydroxyquin ointment)

Description: NYSTAFORM Ointment contains nystatin U.S.P. 100,000 units/Gm and iodochlorhydroxyquin 1% in a water-dispersible, white petrolatum base containing octylphenoxyethanol and paraffin wax.
Actions: Nystatin acts against Candida species (Monilia). Iodochlorhydroxyquin has antibacterial action against bacteria sensitive to this chemotherapeutic agent.
Indications: NYSTAFORM Ointment is indicated for the treatment of cutaneous or mucocutaneous mycotic infections caused by Candida species (Monilia) complicated by iodochlorhydroxyquin-sensitive bacteria.
Contraindications: Lesions caused by pathogens not susceptible to nystatin and iodochlorhydroxyquin and hypersensitivity to any of the components.
Precautions: If irritation or sensitivity occurs and/or infection persists, discontinue use. If new infections appear, appropriate therapy should be instituted. Trace amounts of iodochlorhydroxyquin present in the diaper or urine can yield a false positive test for phenylketonuria (PKU). Percutaneous absorption of iodochlorhydroxyquin may interfere with thyroid function tests. Therapy should be discontinued for one month before these tests are conducted.
Caution: Federal (U.S.A.) law prohibits dispensing without prescription. For external use only. Not for ophthalmic use. Store at controlled room temperature (59°–86°F.). May stain clothing and hair.
Dosage and Administration: Apply two or three times daily. Continue use for one week after clinical cure.
How Supplied: NYSTAFORM Ointment ½ oz. tube

Otic DOMEBORO® Solution (acid pH) ℞
(acetic acid 2%)
(sterile)

Composition: Acetic acid 2% in aluminum acetate (modified Burow's) solution.
Indications: For the treatment of superficial infections of the external auditory canal caused by organisms susceptible to the action of the antimicrobial.
Precautions: If undue irritation or sensitivity develops, discontinue treatment.
Caution: Federal (U.S.A.) law prohibits dispensing without prescription.
For external use only. Not for ophthalmic use. Store at controlled room temperature (59°–86°F).
Administration and Dosage: 4 to 6 drops every 2 to 3 hours.
How Supplied: Packaged under sterile conditions in 2 fl. oz. (60 cc.) plastic squeeze bottle with otic tip.

OTIC NEO-CORT-DOME® ℞
Suspension 1% Sterile
(neomycin sulfate-hydrocortisone-acetic acid suspension)
ACID pH

Description: OTIC NEO-CORT-DOME Suspension contains neomycin sulfate (equivalent to 0.35% neomycin base), microdispersed hydrocortisone 1% and acetic acid 2% with emulsifiers, lubricants and preservatives in a compatible vehicle composed of glyceryl monostearate, stearic acid, propylene glycol, potassium sorbate, methyl and propyl parabens, sodium acetate, and purified water, buffered to the pH range for the normal ear.
Actions: Neomycin sulfate is active against a wide variety of gram-positive and gram-negative pathogens. Hydrocortisone has anti-inflammatory, anti-pruritic and anti-allergic properties.
Indications: For the treatment of superficial bacterial infections of the external auditory canal caused by organisms susceptible to the action of the antibacterials, and for the treatment of infections of mastoidectomy and fenestration cavities by organisms susceptible to the action of the antibacterials.
Contraindications: Tuberculous or fungal lesions of the skin or ear, acute herpes simplex, vaccinia or varicella and hypersensitivity to any of the components of the preparation. Perforated tympanic membranes are frequently considered a contra-indication to the use of external ear canal medication.
Precautions: Use with care in cases of chronic otitis media because of the possibility of ototoxicity. If sensitivity occurs and/or infection persists, discontinue use. If new infections appear, appropriate therapy should be instituted. Articles in the current medical literature indicate an increase in the prevalence of persons sensitive to neomycin.
Caution: Federal (U.S.A.) law prohibits dispensing without prescription. For external use only. Not for ophthalmic use. Store at controlled room temperature (59°–86°F.).
Usual Dosage: Patient should lie on his side with affected ear uppermost. Gently cleanse and dry the infected ear. Instill 3 to 4 drops into the ear; maintain this position for five minutes. Repeat procedure 3 to 4 times daily. To obtain a uniform dispersion of the suspension, the bottle should be shaken before withdrawing each dose. If preferred, a gauze or cotton wick saturated with Otic Neo-Cort-Dome may be inserted in the ear canal and allowed to remain in situ. It should be kept moist by further addition of the suspension, when required.
Supplied: OTIC NEO-CORT-DOME Suspension 10 cc bottle with dropper.

STILPHOSTROL® ℞
(diethylstilbestrol diphosphate)

Actions: Although the mode of action is not known, diethylstilbestrol diphosphate acts in a similar fashion as estrogens and synthetic estrogens in the treatment of prostatic carcinoma.
Important Notes: An increased risk of thromboembolic disease associated with the use of estrogens has now been conclusively established. Retrospective studies have shown a statistically significant association between thrombophlebitis, pulmonary embolism, and cerebral thrombosis and embolism and the use of these drugs. There have been three principal studies in Great Britain[1-3] and one in the United States[4] leading to this conclusion. As a result of these studies, it has been estimated that users of estrogens are 4 to 7 times more likely than nonusers to develop thromboembolic disease without evident cause. The American study also indicated that the increased risk did not persist after discontinuance nor was it enhanced by long-continued administration.
In a more recent analysis of data derived from several national adverse reaction reporting system(s), British investigators concluded that the risk of thromboembolism, including coronary thrombosis, is directly related to the dose of estrogen. Their analysis did suggest, however, that the quantity of estrogen may not be the sole factor involved. Nevertheless, in view of this study, as well as others that have demonstrated a positive relationship between estrogens and thromboembolism, it would seem prudent and in keeping with basic therapeutic principles, to utilize, whenever feasible, the smallest effective dose of estrogen in treating patients.
Risks associated with certain other known adverse reactions, such as elevated blood pressure, liver dysfunction, and reduced tolerance to carbohydrate, have not as yet been quantitated.
Long-term administration of both natural and synthetic estrogens in subprimate animal species in multiples of the human dose increases the frequency for some animal carcinomas. These data cannot be transposed directly to man. The possible carcinogenicity due to the estrogens can neither be confirmed nor refuted at this time. Close clinical surveillance of all persons taking estrogens must be continued.
Indications: STILPHOSTROL (diethylstilbestrol diphosphate) is indicated for the treatment of inoperable progressing prostatic cancer (for palliation only when castration is not feasible or when castration failures or delayed escape following a response to castration have occurred).
Contraindications: 1. Patients with markedly impaired liver function.
2. Patients with thrombophlebitis, thromboembolic disorders, cerebral apoplexy or with a past history of these conditions.
Warning: 1. The physician should be alert to the earliest manifestations of thrombotic disorders (thrombophlebitis, cerebrovascular disorders, pulmonary embolism and retinal thrombosis). If these occur or are suspected the drugs should be discontinued immediately.
2. Discontinue medication pending examination if there is sudden onset of proptosis, diplopia or migraine. If examination reveals papilledema or retinal vascular lesions, medication should be withdrawn.
Precautions: 1. Because of estrogen-induced salt and water retention, these drugs should be used with caution in patients with epilepsy, migraine, asthma, cardiac or renal disease.
2. Patients with a history of psychic depression should be carefully observed and the drug discontinued if the depression recurs to a serious degree.
3. Because of a possible decrease in glucose tolerance, diabetic patients should be followed closely.
4. Because estrogens influence the metabolism of calcium and phosphorus, they should be used with caution in patients with certain metabolic bone diseases that are associated with hypercalcemia or in patients with renal insufficiency.
5. The pathologist should be advised of estrogen therapy when relevant specimens are submitted.
6. Certain endocrine and liver function tests may be affected by treatment with estrogens. If such tests are abnormal in a patient taking these drugs it is recommended that they be repeated after the drug has been withdrawn for two months.
Adverse Reactions: A statistically significant association has been demonstrated between use of estrogen-containing drugs and the following serious reactions: thrombophlebitis, pulmonary embolism and cerebral thrombosis. Although available evidence is suggestive of an association, such a relationship has been neither confirmed nor refuted for the following serious reactions: coronary thrombosis and neuro-ocular lesions (e.g., retinal thrombosis and optic neuritis). The following adverse reactions are known to occur in patients receiving estrogens: nausea, vomiting, anorexia, gastrointestinal symptoms (such as abdominal cramps or bloating), edema, breast tenderness and enlargement, change in body weight (increase or decrease), headache, allergic rash, loss of libido and gynecomastia in the male, sterile abscess (injectable forms only), pain at the site of injection (injectable forms only), post-injection flare (injectable forms only), aggravation of migraine headaches, hepatic cutaneous porphyria becoming manifest, cholestatic jaundice, rise in blood pressure in susceptible individuals, mental depression, cystitis-like syndrome, loss of scalp hair, erythema nodosum, hemorrhagic eruption, changes in libido, changes in appetite, nervousness, dizziness, fatigue, backache, erythema multiforme, itching, irritability, malaise.
Dosage and Administration: TABLETS 50 mg: Start with one tablet t.i.d. and increase this dose level to four or more tablets t.i.d. depending on the tolerance of the patient. Alternatively, if relief is not obtained with high oral dosages, STILPHOSTROL (diethylstilbestrol diphosphate) may be administered intravenously. STILPHOSTROL (diethylstilbestrol diphosphate) solution must be diluted before intravenous infusion.
AMPULS 0.25 g: It is recommended that 0.5 g (2 ampuls) dissolved in 300 ml of saline or 5% dextrose be given intravenously the first day, and that each day thereafter 1 g (4 ampuls) be similarly administered in 300 ml of saline or dextrose. The infusion should be administered slowly (20–30 drops per minute) during the first 10–15 minutes and then the rate of flow adjusted so that the entire amount is given in a period of one hour. This procedure should be followed for five days or more depending on the response of the patient. Following the first intensive course of therapy, 0.25–0.5 g (1 or 2 ampuls) may be administered in a similar manner once or twice weekly or maintenance obtained with STILPHOSTROL (diethylstilbestrol diphosphate) Tablets.
How Supplied: STILPHOSTROL Tablets—Bottles of 50 tablets. Each mottled gray/white tablet contains diethylstilbestrol diphosphate 50 mg.
STILPHOSTROL Ampuls—Boxes of 20 ampuls. Each 5 ml ampul contains diethylstilbestrol diphosphate 0.25 g as a solution of its sodium salts.
References:
1. Royal College of General Practitioners: Oral contraception and throm-

Continued on next page

Dome—Cont.

boembolic disease. *J Coll Gen Pract* 13:267-279, 1967. 2. Inman WHW, Vessey MP: Investigation of deaths from pulmonary, coronary and cerebral thrombosis and embolism in women in childbearing age. *Brit Med J* 2:193-199, 1968. 3. Vessey MP, Doll R: Investigation of relation between use of oral contraceptives and thromboembolic disease. A further report. *Brit Med J* 2:651-657, 1969. 4. Sartwell PE, et al: Thromboembolism and oral contraceptives: An epidemiological case-control study. *Am J Epidemiol* 90:365-380, 1969. 5. Inman, WHW, et al: Thromboembolic disease and the steroidal content of oral contraceptives. *Brit Med J* 2:203-209, 1970. 6. Herbst AL, Ulfelder H, Poskanzer DR: Adenocarcinoma of the vagina. *N Engl J Med* 284:878-881, 1971.

SUNGARD® LOTION
Sunscreen for Sunsensitive Skin

Contains: Sunscreening agents, Padimate-O (a PABA derivative) and dioxybenzone, in a moisturizing emollient base containing 55% ethyl alcohol.
Actions and Uses: SUNGARD Lotion offers protection from the rays of the sun which cause sunburn and are considered harmful to the skin. SUNGARD allows gradual, even tanning while its emollient base helps to prevent drying.
SUNGARD Lotion may help prevent harmful effects of the sun, such as skin cancer and premature aging of the skin, when used regularly as directed.
SUNGARD Lotion's adherent characteristics offer durable protection. Reapplication is usually not required at less than 4-hour intervals, except after swimming and during periods of heavy perspiration.
Directions: Apply evenly to exposed areas of the skin preferably 1 hour prior to exposure. Reapply after swimming or excessive perspiration to continue maximum protection.
Caution: If irritation develops, discontinue use and consult a physician. For external use only. May stain. Avoid the eyes. Keep out of reach of children. Combustible—avoid open flame.
How Supplied: Lotion: 2 oz. net weight and 4 oz. net weight plastic bottles.

TRIDESILON® Creme 0.05% ℞
(desonide)

Description: Tridesilon® (desonide) Creme 0.05% contains a non-fluorinated corticosteroid (16α-hydroxyprednisolone-16, 17-acetonide).
Each gram of Tridesilon (desonide) Creme contains 0.5 milligram of desonide microdispersed in a compatible vehicle buffered to the pH range of normal skin. It contains glycerin, sodium lauryl sulfate, aluminum acetate, purified water, cetyl stearyl alcohol, synthetic beeswax, (B-wax), white petrolatum, and light mineral oil. Preserved with methylparaben.
Action: Tridesilon (desonide) Creme 0.05% is effective because of its anti-inflammatory, anti-pruritic and vasoconstrictive actions.
Indications: Tridesilon (desonide) Creme 0.05% is indicated for the relief of inflammatory manifestations of corticosteroid responsive dermatoses.
Contraindications: Tridesilon (desonide) Creme 0.05%, a topical steroid, is contraindicated in those patients with a history of hypersensitivity to any of the components of the preparation.
Precautions: If irritation develops, the product should be discontinued and appropriate therapy instituted.
In the presence of an infection the use of an appropriate antifungal or anti-bacterial agent should be instituted. If a favorable response does not occur promptly, the corticosteroid should be discontinued until the infection has been adequately controlled.
If extensive areas are treated or if the occlusive technique is used, there will be increased systemic absorption of the corticosteroid and suitable precautions should be taken, particularly in children and infants.
Although topical steroids have not been reported to have an adverse effect on human pregnancy, the safety of their use in pregnant women has not absolutely been established. In laboratory animals, increases in incidence of fetal abnormalities have been associated with exposure of gestating females to topical corticosteroids, in some cases at rather low dosage levels. Therefore, drugs of this class should not be used extensively on pregnant patients, in large amounts, or for proloned periods of time.
The product is not for ophthalmic use.
Adverse Reactions: The following local adverse reactions have been reported with topical corticosteroids, especially under occlusive dressings.
1. Burning
2. Itching
3. Irritation
4. Dryness
5. Folliculitis
6. Hypertrichosis
7. Acneform eruptions
8. Hypopigmentation
9. Perioral dermatitis
10. Allergic Contact Dermatitis
11. Maceration of the skin
12. Secondary infection
13. Skin atrophy
14. Striae
15. Miliaria

Dosage and Administration: Apply a thin film of Tridesilon® (desonide) cream to the affected skin and massage lightly. The usual dosage is two to three times daily.
Caution: Federal (U.S.A.) law prohibits dispensing without prescription. For external use only.
How Supplied: Tridesilon (desonide) Creme 0.05% is supplied in 5, 15 and 60 gram tubes and in 5 pound jars.

TRIDESILON® Ointment 0.05% ℞
(desonide)

Description: Tridesilon® (desonide) Ointment 0.05% contains a non fluorinated corticosteroid (16α-hydroxyprednisolone-16, 17-acetonide).
Each gram of Tridesilon (desonide) Ointment contains 0.5 milligram of desonide microdispersed in white petrolatum.
Action: Tridesilon (desonide) Ointment 0.05% is primarily effective because of its anti-inflammatory, anti-pruritic and vasoconstrictive actions.
Indications: Tridesilon (desonide) Ointment 0.05% is indicated for the relief of inflammatory manifestations of corticosteroid responsive dermatoses.
Contraindications: Tridesilon (desonide) Ointment 0.05%, a topical steroid, is contraindicated in those patients with a history of hypersensitivity to any of the components of the preparation.
Precautions: If irritation develops, the product should be discontinued and appropriate therapy instituted.
In the presence of an infection the use of an appropriate antifungal or antibacterial agent should be instituted. If a favorable response does not occur promptly, the corticosteroid should be discontinued until the infection has been adequately controlled.
If extensive areas are treated or if the occlusive technique is used there will be increased systemic absorption of the corticosteroid and suitable precautions should be taken particularly in children and infants.
Although topical steroids have not been reported to have an adverse effect on human pregnancy, the safety of their uses in pregnant women has not absolutely been established. In laboratory animals, increases in incidence of fetal abnormalities have been associated with exposure of gestating females to topical corticosteroids, in some cases at rather low dosage levels. Therefore, drugs of this class should not be used extensively on pregnant patients, in large amounts, or for prolonged periods of time.
The product is not for ophthalmic use.
Adverse Reactions: The following local adverse reactions have been reported with topical corticosteroids especially under occlusive dressings.
1. Burning
2. Itching
3. Irritation
4. Dryness
5. Folliculitis
6. Hypertrichosis
7. Acneform eruptions
8. Hypopigmentation
9. Perioral dermatitis
10. Allergic Contact Dermatitis
11. Maceration of the skin
12. Secondary infection
13. Skin atrophy
14. Striae
15. Miliaria

Dosage and Administration: Apply a thin film of Tridesilon® (desonide) Ointment to the affected skin and massage lightly. The usual dosage is two or three times daily. This formulation may be particularly useful where an occlusive or lubricating effect is desired.
Caution: Federal (U.S.A. law prohibits dispensing without prescription. For external use only.
How Supplied: Tridesilon (desonide) Ointment 0.05% is supplied in 15 and 60 gram tubes.

Otic TRIDESILON® ℞
Solution 0.05%
(desonide 0.05%—acetic acid 2%)

Description: Otic Tridesilon® Solution contains desonide 0.05% a non-fluorinated corticosteroid (16α- hydroxyprednisolone-16, 17-acetonide) and acetic acid 2% in a compatible vehicle composed of purified water, propylene glycol, sodium acetate, and citric acid.
Actions: Desonide is effective because of its anti-inflammatory, antipruritic and vasoconstrictive actions. Acetic acid has antibacterial and antifungal properties.
Indications: Otic Tridesilon Solution is indicated for the treatment of superficial infections of the external auditory canal caused by organisms susceptible to the action of the antimicrobial and accompanied by inflammation.
Contraindications: Otic Tridesilon Solution (desonide 0.05%—acetic acid 2%) is contraindicated in those patients who have shown hypersensitivity to any of the components of the preparation. Perforated tympanic membranes are frequently considered a contraindication to the use of external ear canal medication.
Precautions: If irritation develops, the product should be discontinued and appropriate therapy instituted.
If infection persists or new infection appears, appropriate therapy should be instituted.
If infection persists or new new infection appears, appropriate therapy should be instituted. If a favorable response does not occur promptly, the corticosteroid should be discontinued until the infection has been adequately controled.
Although topical steroids have not been reported to have an adverse effect on human pregnancy, the safety of their use in pregnant women has not absolutely been established. In laboratory animals, increases in incidence of fetal abnormalities have been associated with

exposure of gestating females to topical corticosteroids, in some cases at rather low dosage levels. Therefore, drugs of this class should not be used extensively on pregnant patients, in large amounts, or for prolonged periods of time.
The product is not for ophthalmic use.
Adverse Reactions: The following local adverse reactions have been reported with otic topical corticosteroids:
1. Burning
2. Itching
3. Irritation
4. Dryness
5. Folliculitis
6. Hypertrichosis
7. Hypopigmentation
8. Allergic Contact Dermatitis
9. Maceration of the skin
10. Secondary Infection
11. Skin Atrophy

Administration and Dosage: All ceruminous material and debris should be carefully removed to permit Otic Tridesilon® Solution (desonide 0.05%—acetic acid 2%) to contact the infected surfaces. Instill 3 to 4 drops into the ear 3 to 4 times daily. If preferred, a gauze or cotton wick saturated with the solution may be inserted in the ear canal and allowed to remain in situ. It should be kept moist by further addition of the solution, as required.
Caution: Federal (U.S.A.) law prohibits dispensing without a prescription. For external use only.
Supplied: Otic Tridesilon Solution (desonide 0.05%—acetic acid 2%) is supplied in 10 cc bottles with dropper.

Dooner Laboratories, Inc.
Subsidiary of William H. Rorer, Inc.
500 VIRGINIA DRIVE
FORT WASHINGTON, PA 19034

D–FEDA® GYROCAPS®, SYRUP
(Pseudoephedrine Hydrochloride)

Description:
GYROCAP® (timed release capsule) ℞
Each Gyrocap contains:
Pseudoephedrine HCl (d-isoephedrine HCl) 60 mg. in a special base that provides for a prolonged therapeutic effect.
SYRUP OTC
Each 5 cc. (one teaspoonful) contains:
Pseudoephedrine HCl (d-isoephedrine HCl) 30 mg. in a grape flavored, dye-free syrup.
Product literature and information available on request.
[*Shown in Product Identification Section*]

FEDAHIST® GYROCAPS®, SYRUP, TABLETS, EXPECTORANT

Description:
GYROCAP (timed release capsule) ℞
Each white and yellow gyrocap contains:
Chlorpheniramine Maleate ....10 mg.
Pseudoephedrine HCl
(d-isoephedrine HCl) ....65 mg.
in a special base that provides for a prolonged therapeutic effect.
SYRUP (nonalcoholic) OTC
Each 5 cc. (one teaspoonful) contains:
Chlorpheniramine Maleate ....2 mg.
Pseudoephedrine HCl
(d-isoephedrine HCl) ....30 mg.
in a pleasant tasting, grape flavored syrup.
TABLET (dye-free) OTC
Each white, scored tablet contains:
Chlorpheniramine Maleate ....4 mg.
Pseudoephedrine HCl
(d-isoephedrine HCl) ....60 mg.
EXPECTORANT (nonalcoholic) OTC
Each 5 cc. (teaspoonful) contains:
Chlorpheniramine Maleate ....2 mg.
Pseudoephedrine HCl
(d-isoephedrine HCl) ....30 mg.
*Guaifenesin ....100 mg.
in a pleasant tasting, red cherry flavored syrup.
Actions: Fedahist provides the antihistaminic activity of chlorpheniramine maleate with the vasoconstrictive actions of pseudoephedrine hydrochloride.
Fedahist Expectorant provides the antihistaminic activity of chlorpheniramine maleate with the decongestant pseudoephedrine hydrochloride and the expectorant guaifenesin.
At the recommended oral dosage, pseudoephedrine has little or no pressor effects in normotensive adults, and is not known to produce drowsiness.
Indications: Fedahist is indicated for the symptomatic relief of seasonal and perennial allergic rhinitis, and eustachian tube congestion.
Fedahist Expectorant is indicated for the temporary relief of the runny nose, sneezing, nasal congestion, bronchial secretions, allergic rhinitis (hay fever).
Contraindications: Sensitivity to antihistamines or sympathomimetic agents. Severe hypertension and coronary artery disease.
Warnings: Patients should be cautioned as to the possible additive effects with alcohol and other central nervous system depressants such as tranquilizers, sedatives, and hypnotics. Patients should be warned against hazardous occupations requiring complete mental alertness, such as operating machinery or driving a motor vehicle.
Precautions: Fedahist should be used with caution in patients with hypertension, coronary artery disease or any other cardiovascular disorder, prostatic hypertropy, hyperthyroidism, glaucoma, or diabetes. In addition, Fedahist Expectorant should be used with caution in patients with asthma, persistent cough, such as occurs with smoking, asthma, emphysema, or where cough is accompanied by excessive secretions.
The effect of pseudoephedrine may be potentiated by monoamine oxidase inhibitors. Sympathomimetics may antagonize antihypertensives, such as methyldopa, reserpine, veratrum alkaloids, and mecamylamine.
Adverse Reactions: The following adverse reactions have been associated with antihistamines and sympathomimetics: Abdominal cramps, angina, anorexia, anxiety, blood pressure elevation, CNS stimulation, circulatory collapse, confusion, dizziness, drowsiness, drug rash, dysuria due to vesicle sphincter spasm, gastric distress, headache, insomnia, mydriasis, nausea, palpitation, restlessness, sweating, tachycardia, tension, vertigo, vomiting, weakness. Sympathomimetics may also produce central nervous stimulation with convulsions or cardiovascular collapse with accompanying hypotension.
Use in Pregnancy: The safety of the use of Fedahist and Fedahist Expectorant in pregnancy has not been established.
Dosage and Administration: Gyrocaps: Adults and children 12 years and older: One capsule twice a day. Not recommended for children under 12 years.
Syrup: Adults and children 12 years and older: Two teaspoonfuls every 4 hours.
Children 6 to under 12 years: One teaspoonful every 4 hours.
Children under 6 years:
12.5–25 lbs.: ¼ teaspoonful 4 times a day
25–37.5 lbs.: ½ teaspoonful 4 times a day
37.5–50 lbs.: ¾ teaspoonful 4 times a day
over 50 lbs.: 1 teaspoonful 4 times a day
Tablets: Adults and children 12 years and older: One tablet every 4 hours. Children 6 to under 12 years: One-half tablet every 4 hours.
Expectorant: Adults and children 12 years and older: Two teaspoonfuls every 4 hours. Children 6 to under 12 years: One teaspoonful every 4 hours. Children 2 to under 6 years: One-half teaspoonful every 4 hours.
How Supplied:
Gyrocaps: Bottles of 100 and 500
Syrup: 4 oz., 8 oz., and gallon bottles.
Tablets: strip packs of 24's, bottles of 100, and 1000.
Expectorant: 4 oz., 8 oz., and gallon bottles

*Official USP name for Glyceryl Guaiacolate as of July 1, 1975.
[*Shown in Product Identification Section*]

SLO-PHYLLIN® GYROCAPS® 60 mg., 125 mg., 250 mg. ℞
(theophylline, anhydrous)
SLO-PHYLLIN® TABLETS 100 mg. and 200 mg. (theophylline, anhydrous)
SLO-PHYLLIN® 80 SYRUP (theophylline, anhydrous)

Composition: Slo-Phyllin® Gyrocaps® (timed release capsules) contain Theophylline (anhydrous) in a special base that provides for a prolonged therapeutic effect. Each Slo-Phyllin® 60 (white color, dye-free) Gyrocap® contains 60 mg. of Theophylline (anhydrous). Each Slo-Phyllin® 125 (brown color) Gyrocap® contains 125 mg. of Theophylline (anhydrous). Each Slo-Phyllin 250 (purple color) Gyrocap® contains 250 mg. of Theophylline (anhydrous). Slo-Phyllin® tablets (white, scored, dye-free) contain prompt acting Theophylline in two strengths. Slo-Phyllin® 100 mg. tablet and Slo-Phyllin® 200 mg. tablet.
Slo-Phyllin® 80 Syrup (orange color, non-alcoholic) contains 80 mg. of Theophylline (anhydrous) per 15 ml. (one tablespoonful).
Indications: Slo-Phyllin® is used in the treatment of asthma and other pulmonary disorders in which a reversible bronchoconstrictive element may be present such as chronic bronchitis and emphysema.
Side Effects: Theophylline may cause gastric irritation, nausea, vomiting, and abdominal discomfort, headache, palpitation, fall in blood pressure, central nervous system stimulation, and diuresis. Slo-Phyllin® Gyrocaps® are formulated in a timed release form to minimize these gastric complaints.
Precautions: Slo-Phyllin® should not be used concurrently with other formulas containing xanthine derivatives.
Warning: Safety in human pregnancy has not been established.
Dosage and Administration:
Slo-Phyllin® Gyrocaps® 60mg.—125mg.—250mg.
CHILDREN UNDER 12: The recommended dosage range is 3–5 mg./kg. body weight every 8 hours. An initial dosage of 4 mg./kg. body weight every 8 hours to a maximum of 16 mg./kg./24 hours is recommended.
If the dosage is to be increased, it should be done in small increments up to a maximum of 24 mg./kg./24 hours or 900 mg./24 hours whichever is less. If the patient is to be maintained at a near maximum of the recommended dosage levels, serum theophylline levels should be determined. In children, not more than 8 mg./kg. every 8 hours should ordinarily be given. If side effects should occur, the dosage should be reduced by 1 mg./kg./dose.
ADULTS AND CHILDREN OVER 12: An initial dosage of 4 mg./kg. body weight every 8 hours is recommended.
The recommended median dose is 8 mg./kg. every 8 hours. This dosage can be approached by increasing the initial dose by increments of 60 mg. to 125 mg. at 3 to 4 day intervals as long as adverse effects are not achieved.
Because of the risk of reaching toxic serum theophylline levels (above 20 ug./ml.), serum theophylline concentrations should be obtained if higher doses are to be maintained.

Continued on next page

Dooner—Cont.

The average adult dose is 930 mg./24 hours. However, some individuals may require doses as high as 2000 mg./24 hours.

For greater flexibility and easier titration of dosage, Slo-Phyllin®Gyrocaps® are available in 3 dosages—60 mg., 125 mg., and 250 mg. These dosages may be used interchangeably or complementary to one another in order to achieve the desired dosage level.

Slo-Phyllin® Tablets and Slo-Phyllin® 80 Syrup

Theophyllinize (titrate) each patient using Slo-Phyllin® at the recommended dosage of 3–5 mg./kg. body weight every six hours. Initially the lower dosage should be administered, then the dosage may be increased if optimal bronchodilator effects are not achieved. It is generally advised that a dosage of 5 mg./kg. body weight every six hours not be exceeded unless it is possible to monitor serum theophylline concentrations during therapy since it has been established that significant variations occur among individuals in the rate at which the drug is eliminated from the body.

Recommended Dosage of SLO-PHYLLIN* Tablets for Various Body Weights

Weight		Dose (in mg)			
lbs.	kg	3 mg/kg	4 mg/kg	5 mg/kg	6 mg/kg
22	10	30	40	50	60
33	15	45	60	75	90
44	20	60	80	100	120
55	25	75	100	125	150
66	30	90	120	150	180
88	40	120	160	200	240
110	50	150	200	250	300
132	60	180	240	300	360
154	70	210	280	350	420
176	80	240	320	400	480
198	90	270	360	450	540
220	100	300	400	500	600

Administered every six hours.

Recommended Dosage of SLO-PHYLLIN® 80 Syrup for Various Body Weights

Weight		Dose (in tsp.)		
lbs.	kg	3 mg/kg	4 mg/kg	5 mg/kg
20	9	1 tsp.	1⅓ tsp.	1½ tsp.
40	18	2 tsp.	2½ tsp.	3 tsp.
60	27	3 tsp.	4 tsp.	5 tsp.
79	36	4 tsp.	5 tsp.	6½ tsp.

Administered every six hours.

The therapeutic serum theophylline concentration is considered to be between 10 and 20 ug./ml. This range may best be reached by individualizing the patient's dosage while concomitantly monitoring the serum theophylline concentrations.

Slo-Phyllin® 80 Syrup U.S. Patent #3928609

How Supplied:

Slo-Phyllin® Gyrocaps®—Bottles of 100 and 1000
unit dose pkgs. (125 mg. and 250 mg. only).
Syrup—4 oz., 16 oz. and gallon bottles
unit dose bottles, 5 ml. and 15 ml.
Tablets—Bottles of 100 and 1000
unit dose pkgs.

[*Shown in Product Identification Section*]

SLO-PHYLLIN® GG CAPSULES, SYRUP ℞

(Theophylline, anhydrous with Guaifenesin)

Description:

SYRUP (nonalcoholic, dye-free)

Each 15 ml. (tablespoonful) contains:

Theophylline (anhydrous)	150 mg.
Guaifenesin	90 mg.

in a lemon-vanilla flavored syrup.

CAPSULES (dye-free)

Each white, liquid filled, soft gelatin capsule contains:

Theophylline (anhydrous)	150 mg.
Guaifenesin	90 mg.

Indications: Slo-Phyllin® GG is used in the treatment of asthma and other pulmonary disorders in which a reversible bronchoconstrictive element may be present, such as chronic bronchitis and emphysema.

Contraindicated: In peptic ulcer.

Side Effects: Theophylline may cause gastric irritation, nausea, vomting, and abdominal discomfort, palpitation, headache, fall in blood pressure, central nervous system stimulation, and diuresis.

Precautions: Slo-Phyllin® GG should not be used concurrently with other formulas containing xanthine derivatives.

Dosage and Administration: Theophyllinize (titrate) each patient using Slo-Phyllin® GG at the theophylline dosage of 3–5mg./kg. body weight every six hours. Initially the lower dose should be administered, then the dosage may be increased if optimal bronchodilator effects are not achieved. It is generally advised that the theophylline dosage not exceed 5mg./kg. body weight every six hours, unless it is possible to monitor serum theophylline concentrations during therapy since it has been established that significant variations occur among individuals in the rate at which the drug is eliminated from the body.

Body Weight		Dosage of Slo-Phyllin GG Syrup Calculated at approximately:		
Expressed in Kilos	Lbs.	3 mg. Per Kilo	4 mg. Per Kilo	5 mg. Per Kilo
9	20	½ tsp.	¾ tsp.	1 tsp.
18	40	1 tsp.	1½ tsp.	2 tsp.
27	60	1½ tsp.	2 tsp.	2¾ tsp.
36	79	2 tsp.	3 tsp.	3½ tsp.
45	99	2¾ tsp.	3½ tsp.	4½ tsp.
54	118	3¼ tsp.	4½ tsp.	5½ tsp.

Administered every six (6) hours.

Warning: Safety in human pregnancy has not been established.

How Supplied:

Capsules—Bottles of 100 and 1000
Unit dose packages.
Syrup— Pints and gallons.

[*Shown in Product Identification Section*]

Dorsey Laboratories

Division of Sandoz, Inc.
LINCOLN, NE 68501

ACID MANTLE® CREME AND LOTION

Description: A greaseless, water-miscible preparation containing buffered aluminum acetate.

Indications: Provides relief from mild skin irritation due to exposure to soaps, detergents, chemicals, alkalis. Aids in the treatment of diaper rash, acne, eczema and dry, rough, scaly skin from varied causes.

Application: Apply several times daily, especially after wet work.

Caution: Limited compatibility and stability with Vitamin A, neomycin and water-soluble antibiotics. For external use only. Not for ophthalmic use.

How Supplied: Creme: 1 oz tubes; 4 oz and 1 lb jars. Lotion: 4 oz and 1 pt bottles.

ASBRON G® INLAY-TABS®/ELIXIR ℞

Description: Each Asbron G Inlay-Tab and tablespoonful (15 ml) of Asbron G Elixir contains theophylline sodium glycinate 300 mg (equivalent to 150 mg theophylline), guaifenesin 100 mg. The elixir supplies the active ingredients in a solution containing 15% alcohol.

Asbron G contains a bronchodilator and an expectorant. Theophylline sodium glycinate is a xanthine bronchodilating agent freely soluble in water. The expectorant component is guaifenesin (formerly called glyceryl guaiacolate) which helps loosen and thus clear the bronchial passageways of bothersome, thickened mucus.

Indications: For relief of acute bronchial asthma and for reversible bronchospasm associated with chronic bronchitis and emphysema.

Contraindications: Sensitivity to any of the ingredients. Xanthines may be contraindicated in patients with peptic ulcers.

Warnings: There is great patient to patient variation in the serum half-life of theophylline. Dosage must be individualized. When possible, serum theophylline levels should be measured to assist in titration of dosage.

Adverse Reactions: Large doses may cause nervousness, agitation, headache, palpitations, tachycardia, nausea and vomiting. Cardiac arrhythmias and ventricular ectopic beats have been associated with the use of theophylline.

Precautions: Use with caution in the presence of hyperthyroidism, hypertension or cardiovascular disease. Acidifying agents can inhibit the action of theophylline by enhancing excretion. Alkalinizing agents can potentiate the action of theophylline by decreasing urinary excretion. Other oral xanthine derivatives should not be given concurrently and intravenous aminophylline should be administered with great caution to a patient having received Asbron G.

Usual Dosage: Adults—1 or 2 tablets or tablespoonfuls (15–30 ml), 3 or 4 times daily. Children 6–12—2 or 3 teaspoonfuls (10–15 ml), 3 or 4 times daily. Children 3–6—1 to 1½ teaspoonfuls (5–7.5 ml), 3 or 4 times daily. Children 1–3—½ to 1 teaspoonful (2.5–5 ml), 3 or 4 times daily.

During the first day of treatment, especially in severe attacks, the higher dosage may be indicated. After the first day, dosage should be adjusted on an individual basis. Administration after meals may reduce the infrequent possibility of gastric distress or CNS stimulation.

How Supplied: Asbron G Inlay-Tabs (green with white inlay), in bottles of 100. Asbron G Elixir (green), in pint bottles.

[*Shown in Product Identification Section*]

BELLERGAL® TABLETS ℞
BELLERGAL-S® TABLETS

Composition: Each Bellergal Tablet contains: phenobarbital, USP, central sedative (Warning: May be habit forming), 20.0 mg; Gynergen® (ergotamine tartrate, USP) sympathetic inhibitor, 0.3 mg; Bellafoline® (levorotatory alkaloids of belladonna, as malates) parasympathetic inhibitor, 0.1 mg. Each Bellergal-S Tablet contains: phenobarbital, USP, central sedative (Warning: May be habit forming), 40.0 mg; Gynergen (ergotamine tartrate, USP) sympathetic inhibitor, 0.6 mg; Bellafoline (levorotatory alkaloids of belladonna, as malates) parasympathetic inhibitor, 0.2 mg.

Properties and Therapeutics: Based on the concept that functional disorders frequently involve hyperactivity of both the sympathetic and parasympathetic nervous systems, the ingredients in Bellergal are combined to provide a balanced preparation designed to correct imbalance of the autonomic nervous system. The integrated action of Bellergal is effected through the combined administration of ergotamine and the levorotatory alkaloids of belladonna, specific inhibitors of the sympathetic and parasympathetic respectively, reinforced by the synergistic action of phenobarbital in dampening the cortical centers.

Indications: Bellergal is employed in the management of disorders characterized by nervous tension and exaggerated autonomic response: *Menopausal disorders* with hot flashes, sweats, restlessness and insomnia. *Cardiovascular disorders* with palpitation, tachycardia, chest oppression and vasomotor disturbances. *Gastrointestinal disorders* with hypermotility, hypersecretion, "nervous stomach," and alternately diarrhea and constipation.
Genitourinary—uterine cramps, etc.
Premenstrual tension.
Interval treatment of *recurrent, throbbing headache.*
Contraindications: Peripheral vascular disease, coronary heart disease, hypertension, impaired hepatic or renal function, sepsis, third trimester of pregnancy and glaucoma. Hypersensitivity to any of the components.
Precautions: Even though the ergotamine tartrate content of this product is extremely low and untoward effects have been rare and insignificant, caution should be exercised if large or prolonged dosage is contemplated, and physicians should be alert to possible peripheral vascular complications in patients highly sensitive to ergot. Due to presence of a barbiturate, may be habit forming.
Side Effects: Blurred vision, dry mouth, flushing, drowsiness occur rarely.
Dosage: Bellergal Tablets: Four tablets daily (one in the morning, one at noon and two at bedtime) is the dose usually employed. In more resistant cases begin with six tablets daily, then gradually reduce dosage at weekly intervals according to response. Where required, continue with the smallest effective dose to maintain the improved status of the patient.
Bellergal-S Tablets: One in the morning and one in the evening.
How Supplied: Bellergal Tablets (flesh pink, sugar-coated) in bottles of 100 and 1000. Bellergal-S Tablets (compressed, scored tablets of tricolored pattern: dark green, orange and light lemon yellow) in bottles of 100.
[*Shown in Product Identification Section*]

CAMA® INLAY-TABS®

Description: Each CAMA INLAY-TAB contains: aspirin 600 mg. (10 grains); magnesium hydroxide, N.F., 150 mg.; aluminum hydroxide dried gel 150 mg.
Indications: An analgesic in arthritis and rheumatism.
Contraindications: Hypersensitivity to salicylates.
Warnings: The antipyretic effect of salicylates may mask the diagnostic importance of persistent fever.
Precautions: The occasional occurrence of mild salicylism may require adjustment of dosage.
Adverse Reactions: Overdosage of salicylates will cause tinnitus, nausea, vomiting and gastrointestinal upsets and bleeding.
Dosage and Administration: Adults—one tablet every four hours. Physicians may increase the dosage as required to provide satisfactory relief of symptoms. Usually, a dose of one to two tablets four times daily is adequate.
How Supplied: Cama Inlay-Tabs (white with salmon inlay) in bottles of 100 and 250.
[*Shown in Product Identification Section*]

DORCOL® PEDIATRIC COUGH SYRUP

Description: Each teaspoonful (5 ml) of DORCOL Pediatric Cough Syrup contains: phenylpropanolamine hydrochloride 6.25 mg, guaifenesin 50 mg, dextromethorphan hydrobromide 5 mg, alcohol 5%.
Indications: Provides prompt relief of cough and nasal congestion due to the common cold. The expectorant component helps loosen bronchial secretions. The decongestant, expectorant and antitussive are provided in an antihistamine-free formula.
Contraindications: DORCOL Pediatric Cough Syrup is contraindicated in the presence of hypersensitivity to any of the ingredients. The use of pressor amines such as phenylpropanolamine hydrochloride is contraindicated in those patients taking monoamine oxidase inhibitors for antihypertensive or antidepressant indications.
Precautions: Exercise prescribing caution in patients with persistent or chronic cough such as occurs with chronic bronchitis, bronchial asthma, or emphysema. Use with caution in patients with hypertension, hyperthyroidism cardiovascular disease or diabetes mellitus.
Adverse Reactions: Occasional blurred vision, cardiac palpitations, flushing, gastrointestinal upsets, nervousness, dizziness, or sleeplessness may occur.
Dosage and Administration: Children 6–12 years—2 teaspoonfuls every 4 hours. Children 2–6 years—1 teaspoonful every 4 hours. The suggested dosage in pediatric patients 3 months to 2 years of age is 3 drops per kilogram of body weight administered every four hours. For nighttime cough relief, give the last dose at bedtime.
How Supplied: DORCOL Pediatric Cough Syrup (grape-colored) in 4 fl oz and 8 fl oz bottles.

GLYSENNID® TABLETS
(Sennosides A and B) N.F.

Description: Each tablet contains sennosides A & B (as calcium salts) N.F. 12 mg.
Indications: Simple constipation, sluggish bowels (as in pregnancy).
Usual Dosage: Adults: One or two tablets at bedtime. Dosage may be increased according to need. Children: Over 10 years old: one or two tablets; six to 10 years: one tablet; under 6 years: at discretion of physician. Take Glysennid at bedtime for morning effect.
Precautions: *Warning:* Not to be used when abdominal pain, nausea, vomiting or other symptoms of appendicitis are present. Frequent or continued use of this preparation may lead to dependence on laxatives.
How Supplied: Tablets, bottles of 100 and 1000.

GRIS-PEG® TABLETS ℞
(griseofulvin ultramicrosize)

Description: Griseofulvin is an antibiotic derived from a species of *Penicillium.*
Gris-PEG is an ultramicrocrystalline solid-state dispersion of griseofulvin in polyethylene glycol 6000.
Gris-PEG Tablets differ from griseofulvin (microsize) tablets USP in that each tablet contains 125 mg of ultramicrosize griseofulvin biologically equivalent to 250 mg of microsize griseofulvin.
Action: *Microbiology*—Griseofulvin is fungistatic with *in vitro* activity against various species of *Microsporum, Epidermophyton* and *Trichophyton.* It has no effect on bacteria or other genera of fungi.
Human Pharmacology—The peak plasma level found in fasting adults given 0.25 g of Gris-PEG occurs at about four hours and ranges between 0.37 to 1.6 mcg/ml.
Comparable studies with microsize griseofulvin indicated that the peak plasma level found in fasting adults given 0.5 g occurs at about four hours and ranges between 0.44 to 1.2 mcg/ml.
Thus, the efficiency of gastrointestinal absorption of the ultramicrocrystalline formulation of Gris-PEG is approximately twice that of conventional microsized griseofulvin. This factor permits the oral intake of half as much griseofulvin per tablet but there is no evidence, at this time, that this confers any significant clinical differences in regard to safety and efficacy.
Griseofulvin is deposited in the keratin precursor cells and has a greater affinity for diseased tissue. The drug is tightly bound to the new keratin which becomes highly resistant to fungal invasions.
Indications: Gris-PEG (griseofulvin ultramicrosize) is indicated for the treatment of the following ringworm infections:
Tinea corporis (ringworm of the body)
Tinea pedis (athlete's foot)
Tinea cruris (ringworm of the thigh)
Tinea barbae (barber's itch)
Tinea capitis (ringworm of the scalp)
Tinea unguium (onychomycosis, ringworm of the nails) when caused by one or more of the following genera of fungi:
Trichophyton rubrum
Trichophyton tonsurans
Trichophyton mentagrophytes
Trichophyton interdigitalis
Trichophyton verrucosum
Trichophyton megnini
Trichophyton gallinae
Trichophyton crateriform
Trichophyton sulphureum
Trichophyton schoenleini
Microsporum audouini
Microsporum canis
Microsporum gypseum
Epidermophyton floccosum
NOTE: Prior to therapy, the type of fungi responsible for the infection should be identified.
The use of the drug is not justified in minor or trivial infections which will respond to topical agents alone.
Griseofulvin is *NOT* effective in the following:
Bacterial infections
Candidiasis (Moniliasis)
Histoplasmosis
Actinomycosis
Sporotrichosis
Chromoblastomycosis
Coccidioidomycosis
North American Blastomycosis
Cryptococcosis (Torulosis)
Tinea versicolor
Nocardiosis
Contraindications: This drug is contraindicated in patients with porphyria, hepatocellular failure, and in individuals with a history of sensitivity to griseofulvin.
Warnings: *Prophylactic Usage*—Safety and Efficacy of Griseofulvin for Prophylaxis of Fungal Infections Has Not Been Established.
Animal Toxicology—Chronic feeding of griseofulvin, at levels ranging from 0.5 to 2.5% of the diet, resulted in the development of liver tumors in several strains of mice, particularly in males. Smaller particle sizes result in an enhanced effect. Lower oral dosage levels have not been tested. Subcutaneous administration of relatively small doses of griseofulvin, once a week, during the first three weeks of life has also been reported to induce hepatomata in mice. Although studies in other animal species have not yielded evidence of tumorigenicity, these studies were not of adequate design to form a basis for conclusions in this regard.
In subacute toxicity studies, orally administered griseofulvin produced hepatocellular necrosis in mice, but this has not been seen in other species. Disturbances in porphyrin metabolism have been reported in griseofulvin treated laboratory animals. Griseofulvin has been reported to have a colchicine-like effect on mitosis and cocarcinogenicity with methylcholanthrene in cutaneous tumor induction in laboratory animals.
Usage in Pregnancy—The safety of this drug during pregnancy has not been established.
Animal Reproduction Studies—It has been reported in the literature that griseofulvin was

Continued on next page

Dorsey—Cont.

found to be embryotoxic and teratogenic on oral administration to pregnant rats. Pups with abnormalities have been reported in the litters of a few bitches treated with griseofulvin. Additional animal reproduction studies are in progress.

Suppression of spermatogenesis has been reported to occur in rats, but investigation in man failed to confirm this.

Precautions: Patients on prolonged therapy with any potent medication should be under close observation. Periodic monitoring of organ system function, including renal, hepatic and hematopoietic, should be done.

Since griseofulvin is derived from species of *Penicillium*, the possibility of cross sensitivity with penicillin exists; however, known penicillin-sensitive patients have been treated without difficulty.

Since a photosensitivity reaction is occasionally associated with griseofulvin therapy, patients should be warned to avoid exposure to intense natural or artificial sunlight. Should a photosensitivity reaction occur, lupus erythematosus may be aggravated.

Griseofulvin decreases the activity of warfarin-type anticoagulants so that patients receiving these drugs concomitantly may require dosage adjustment of the anticoagulant during and after griseofulvin therapy.

Barbiturates usually depress griseofulvin activity and concomitant administration may require a dosage adjustment of the antifungal agent.

Adverse Reactions: When adverse reactions occur, they are most commonly of the hypersensitivity type such as skin rashes, urticaria, and rarely, angioneurotic edema, and may necessitate withdrawal of therapy and appropriate countermeasures. Paresthesias of the hands and feet have been reported rarely after extended therapy. Other side effects reported occasionally are oral thrush, nausea, vomiting, epigastric distress, diarrhea, headache, fatigue, dizziness, insomnia, mental confusion, and impairment of performance of routine activities.

Proteinuria and leukopenia have been reported rarely. Administration of the drug should be discontinued if granulocytopenia occurs.

When rare, serious reactions occur with griseofulvin, they are usually associated with high dosages, long periods of therapy, or both.

Dosage and Administration: Accurate diagnosis of the infecting organism is essential. Identification should be made either by direct microscopic examination of a mounting of infected tissue in a solution of potassium hydroxide or by a culture on an appropriate medium. Medication must be continued until the infecting organism is completely eradicated as indicated by appropriate clinical or laboratory examination. Representative treatment periods are—*tinea capitis*, 4 to 6 weeks; *tinea corporis*, 2 to 4 weeks; *tinea pedis*, 4 to 8 weeks; *tinea unguium*—depending on rate of growth—fingernails, at least 4 months; toenails, at least 6 months.

General measures in regard to hygiene should be observed to control sources of infection or reinfection. Concomitant use of appropriate topical agents is usually required particularly in treatment of *tinea pedis*. In some forms of athlete's foot, yeasts and bacteria may be involved as well as fungi. Griseofulvin will not eradicate the bacterial or monilial infection.

An oral dose of 250 mg of Gris-PEG (griseofulvin ultramicrosize) is biologically equivalent to 500 mg of griseofulvin (microsized) USP (see ACTION Human Pharmacology).

Adults: A daily dose of 250 mg will give a satisfactory response in most patients with *tinea corporis, tinea cruris* and *tinea capitis*. One 125 mg tablet twice per day or two 125 mg tablets once per day is the usual dosage. For those fungal infections more difficult to eradicate such as *tinea pedis* and *tinea unguium*, a divided daily dose of 500 mg is recommended. In all cases, the dosage should be individualized.

Children: Approximately 5 mg per kilogram (2.5 mg per pound) of body weight per day is an effective dose for most children. On this basis the following dosage schedule for children is suggested: Children weighing over 25 kilograms (approximately 50 pounds) 125 mg to 250 mg daily; children weighing 15-25 kilograms (approximately 30 to 50 pounds) 62.5 mg to 125 mg daily; children 2 years of age and younger, dosage has not been established.

Dosage should be individualized, as is done for adults. Clinical experience with griseofulvin in children with *tinea capitis* indicates that a single daily dose is effective. Clinical relapse will occur if the medication is not continued until the infecting organism is eradicated.

How Supplied: Gris-PEG (griseofulvin ultramicrosize) Tablets (white) differ from griseofulvin microsized tablets (USP) in that each tablet contains 125 mg of ultramicrosize griseofulvin, biologically equivalent to 250 mg of microsized griseofulvin. Two 125 mg tablets of Gris-PEG are biologically equivalent to 500 mg of microsized griseofulvin. In bottles of 100 and 500 scored, film-coated tablets.

U.S. Patent No. 4,151,273

[*Shown in Product Identification Section*]

KANULASE® TABLETS

Description: Each KANULASE TABLET contains: Dorase® (cellulase) standardized to 9 mg.; pancreatin, N.F., 500 mg.; glutamic acid hydrochloride 200 mg.; ox bile extract 100 mg.; pepsin 150 mg.

Indications: Kanulase is designed to diminish intestinal gas in healthy persons and in those patients having digestive disorders. Cellulase disintegrates the cell walls of plant foods, releasing starch for digestion in the upper intestinal tract, and thus reducing gas formation in the colon. Kanulase further reduces gas formation by aiding in the digestion of fats, proteins and starches.

Precautions: Kanulase contains glutamic acid hydrochloride which is not usually given to patients with peptic ulcer.

Dosage and Administration: Adults—1 or 2 tablets, swallowed whole, at mealtimes. If looseness of stools occurs decrease the dosage.

How Supplied: Kanulase Tablets (pink) in bottles of 50.

[*Shown in Product Identification Section*]

KLORVESS® EFFERVESCENT GRANULES, TABLETS and KLORVESS® (potassium chloride) 10% LIQUID ℞

Description: Klorvess Effervescent Granules: Each packet (2.8 g) contains 20 mEq each of potassium and chloride supplied by potassium chloride 1.125 g, potassium bicarbonate 0.5 g, L-lysine monohydrochloride 0.913 g in a sodium-, sugar- and carbohydrate-free effervescent formulation. Dissolution of the packet contents in water provides the potassium and chloride available for oral ingestion as potassium chloride, potassium bicarbonate, potassium citrate and L-lysine monohydrochloride.

Klorvess Effervescent Tablets: Each dry, sodium- and sugar-free effervescent tablet contains 20 mEq each of potassium and chloride supplied by potassium chloride 1.125 g, potassium bicarbonate 0.5 g, L-lysine mono- hydrochloride 0.913 g. Dissolution of the tablet in water provides the potassium and chloride available for oral ingestion as potassium chloride, potassium bicarbonate, potassium citrate and L-lysine monohydrochloride.

Klorvess (potassium chloride) 10% Liquid: Each tablespoonful (15 ml) contains 20 mEq of potassium chloride (provided by potassium chloride 1.5 g) in a palatable, cherry-with-pit flavored vehicle, alcohol 1%.

Indications: For the prevention and treatment of potassium depletion and hypokalemic-hypochloremic alkalosis. Deficits of body potassium and chloride can occur as a consequence of therapy with potent diuretic agents and adrenal corticosteroids.

Contraindications: Severe renal impairment characterized by azotemia or oliguria, untreated Addison's disease, Familial Periodic Paralysis, acute dehydration, heat cramps, patients receiving aldosterone-inhibiting or potassium-sparing diuretic agents, or hyperkalemia from any cause.

Precautions: In response to a rise in the concentration of body potassium, renal excretion of the ion is increased. In the presence of normal renal function and hydration, it is difficult to produce potassium intoxication by oral potassium salt supplements.

Since the extent of potassium deficiency cannot be accurately determined, it is prudent to proceed cautiously in undertaking potassium replacement. Periodic evaluations of the patient's clinical status, serum electrolytes and the EKG should be carried out when replacement therapy is undertaken. This is particularly important in patients with cardiac disease and those patients receiving digitalis.

High serum concentrations of potassium may cause death through cardiac depression, arrhythmia or cardiac arrest.

To minimize gastrointestinal irritation associated with potassium chloride preparations, patients should dissolve the packet contents of Klorvess Effervescent Granules or each Klorvess Effervescent Tablet in 3 to 4 ounces of water or fruit juice, or dilute each tablespoonful of Klorvess (potassium chloride) 10% Liquid in 3 to 4 ounces of water. Both of these solutions should be ingested slowly with or immediately after meals.

Adverse Reactions: Abdominal discomfort, diarrhea, nausea and vomiting may occur with the use of potassium salts.

The symptoms and signs of potassium intoxication include paresthesias, heaviness, muscle weakness and flaccid paralysis of the extremities. Potassium intoxication can produce listlessness, mental confusion, a fall in blood pressure, shock, cardiac arrhythmias, heart block and cardiac arrest.

The EKG picture of hyperkalemia is characterized by the early appearance of tall, peaked T waves. The R wave is decreased in amplitude and the S wave deepens; the QRS complex widens progressively. The P wave widens and decreases in amplitude until it disappears. Occasionally, an apparent elevation of the RS-T junction and a cove plane RS-T segment and T wave will be noted in AVL.

Dosage and Administration: Klorvess Effervescent Granules and Tablets: Adults—Contents of one packet or one tablet (20 mEq each of potassium and chloride) completely dissolved in 3 to 4 ounces of cold water, fruit juice or other liquid 2 to 4 times daily depending upon the requirements of the patient.

Klorvess (potassium chloride) 10% Liquid: Adults—One tablespoonful (15 ml) of Klorvess Liquid (20 mEq of potassium chloride) completely diluted in 3 to 4 ounces of water 2 to 4 times daily depending upon the requirements of the patient.

Both of these solutions should be ingested slowly with meals or immediately after eating. Deviations from these recommended dosages may be indicated in certain cases of hypokalemia based upon the patient's status. The average total daily dosage must be governed by the patient's response as determined by frequent evaluation of serum electrolytes, EKG and clinical status.

Overdosage: Potassium intoxication may result from overdosage of potassium or from therapeutic dosage in conditions stated under

"Contraindications." Hyperkalemia, when detected, must be treated immediately because lethal levels can be reached in a few hours.

Treatment of Hyperkalemia:

1. Dextrose solution, 10 or 25% containing 10 units of crystalline insulin per 20 g dextrose, given IV in a dose of 300 to 500 ml in an hour.
2. Adsorption and exchange of potassium using sodium or ammonium cycle cation exchange resins, orally and as retention enema. (Caution: Ammonium compounds should not be used in patients with hepatic cirrhosis.)
3. Hemodialysis and peritoneal dialysis.
4. The use of potassium-containing foods or medicaments must be eliminated.

In digitalized patients too rapid a lowering of plasma potassium concentration can cause digitalis toxicity.

How Supplied: Klorvess Effervescent Granules—packages of 30 packets (2.8 g each). Klorvess Effervescent Tablets (white) – 60 tablets (2 ℞ units of 30 effervescent tablets each). Each tablet is individually foil wrapped. Klorvess (potassium chloride) 10% Liquid (dark red) – as a cherry-with-pit flavored liquid in pint and gallon bottles. Klorvess Tablets and Liquid are also available in institutional packaging as follows: Klorvess Tablets – 30 and 1000 tablets; Klorvess Liquid – 36 (3 × 12) × 4 oz Unit-of-Use bottles and 100 (4 × 25) × 15 ml Unit-Dose bottles.

[*Shown in Product Identification Section*]

MSC TRIAMINIC® TABLETS ℞

Description: Each timed-release tablet contains: phenylpropanolamine hydrochloride 50 mg., pheniramine maleate 25 mg., pyrilamine maleate 25 mg, methscopolamine nitrate 4 mg.

Indications: Relief from symptoms of nasal congestion especially when associated with excessive secretion such as profuse nasal discharge or postnasal drip—as frequently occurs in common colds, sinusitis and nasal allergy.

Contraindications: Glaucoma and prostatic hypertrophy.

Precautions: Patients should be advised not to drive a car or operate dangerous machinery if drowsiness occurs. Use with caution in the presence of hypertension, hyperthyroidism, cardiovascular disease or diabetes.

Adverse Reactions: Occasional drowsiness, blurred vision, cardiac palpitations, flushing, dizziness, nervousness, or gastrointestinal upsets.

Dosage and Administration: Adults - 1 tablet, swallowed whole, in the morning, midafternoon and before retiring.

How Supplied: MSC Triaminic Tablets (dark pink) in bottles of 50.

METAPREL® ℞
(metaproterenol sulfate)
METERED DOSE INHALER, SYRUP and TABLETS

Each Metered Dose Inhaler contains: metaproterenol sulfate 225 mg as a micronized powder in an inert propellant. Each teaspoonful (5 ml) of syrup contains: metaproterenol sulfate 10 mg. Tablets contain: metaproterenol sulfate 10 and 20 mg.

Description: Chemically, Metaprel (metaproterenol sulfate) is 1-(3, 5-dihydroxyphenyl)-2-isopropylaminoethanol sulfate, a white, crystalline, racemic mixture of two optically active isomers. It differs from isoproterenol hydrochloride by having two hydroxyl groups attached at the meta positions on the benzene ring rather than one at the meta and one at the para position.

Actions: Metaprel (metaproterenol sulfate) is a potent beta-adrenergic stimulator. It is postulated that beta-adrenergic stimulants produce many of their pharmacological effects by activation of adenyl cyclase, the enzyme which catalyzes the conversion of adenosine triphosphate to cyclic adenosine monophosphate.

Absorption, biotransformation and excretion studies following administration by inhalation have not been performed. Following oral administration in humans, an average of 40 percent of the drug is absorbed; it is not metabolized by catechol-O-methyltransferase or sulfatase enzymes in the gut but is excreted primarily as glucuronic acid conjugates.

Metered Dose Inhaler: When administered by oral inhalation, Metaprel (metaproterenol sulfate) decreases reversible bronchospasm. Pulmonary function tests performed concomitantly usually show improvement following aerosol Metaprel (metaproterenol sulfate) administration, e.g., an increase in the one-second forced expiratory volume (FEV_1), an increase in maximum expiratory flow rate, an increase in forced vital capacity, and/or a decrease in airway resistance. The resultant decrease in airway obstruction may relieve the dyspnea associated with bronchospasm.

Controlled single- and multiple-dose studies have been performed with pulmonary function monitoring. The duration of effect of a *single dose* of two to three inhalations of Metaprel (metaproterenol sulfate) (that is, the period of time during which there is a 20 percent or greater increase in FEV_1) has varied from one to five hours.

In repetitive-dosing studies (up to q.i.d.) the duration of effect for a similar dose of Metaprel (metaproterenol sulfate) has ranged from about one to two-and-one-half hours. Present studies are inadequate to explain the divergence in duration of the FEV_1 effect between single- and repetitive-dosing studies, respectively.

Syrup: When administered orally, Metaprel (metaproterenol sulfate) decreases reversible bronchospasm. Pulmonary function tests performed after the administration of Metaprel (metaproterenol sulfate) usually show improvement, e.g., an increase in the one-second forced expiratory volume (FEV_1), an increase in maximum expiratory flow rate, an increase in peak expiratory flow rate, an increase in forced vital capacity, and/or a decrease in airway resistance. The decrease in airway obstruction may relieve the dyspnea associated with bronchospasm.

Pulmonary function has been monitored in controlled single- and multiple-dose studies. The duration of effect of a single dose of Metaprel (metaproterenol sulfate) Syrup (that is, the period of time during which there is a 15 percent or greater increase in mean FEV_1) was up to four hours.

Tablets: When administered orally, Metaprel (metaproterenol sulfate) decreases reversible bronchospasm. Pulmonary function tests performed concomitantly usually show improvement following Metaprel (metaproterenol sulfate) administration, e.g., an increase in the one-second forced expiratory volume (FEV_1), an increase in maximum expiratory flow rate, an increase in forced vital capacity, and/or a decrease in airway resistance. The resultant decrease in airway obstruction may relieve the dyspnea associated with bronchospasm.

Controlled single- and multiple-dose studies have been performed with pulmonary function monitoring. The mean duration of effect of a single dose of 20 mg of Metaprel (metaproterenol sulfate) (that is, the period of time during which there is a 15 percent or greater increase in FEV_1) was up to four hours. Four controlled multiple-dose 60-day studies, comparing the effectiveness of metaproterenol sulfate tablets with ephedrine tablets, have been performed. Because of difficulties in study design, only one study was available which could be analyzed in depth. This study showed a loss of efficacy with time for both metaproterenol sulfate and ephedrine. Therefore, the physician should take this phenomenon into account in evaluating the individual patient's overall management. Further studies are in progress to adequately explain these results.

Indications: Metaprel (metaproterenol sulfate) is indicated as a bronchodilator for bronchial asthma, and for reversible bronchospasm which may occur in association with bronchitis and emphysema.

Contraindications: Use in patients with cardiac arrhythmias associated with tachycardia is contraindicated.

Warnings: Excessive use of adrenergic aerosols is potentially dangerous. Fatalities have been reported following excessive use of metaproterenol sulfate as with other sympathomimetic inhalation preparations, and the exact cause is unknown. Cardiac arrest was noted in several cases.

Paradoxical bronchoconstriction with repeated excessive administration has been reported with other sympathomimetic agents. Therefore, it is possible that this phenomenon could occur with Metaprel (metaproterenol sulfate).

Patients should be advised to contact their physician in the event that they do not respond to their *usual dose* of a sympathomimetic amine aerosol.

Precautions: Extreme care must be exercised with respect to the administration of additional sympathomimetic agents. A sufficient interval of time should elapse prior to administration of another sympathomimetic agent.

Because metaproterenol sulfate is a sympathomimetic drug, it should be used with great caution in patients with hypertension, coronary artery disease, congestive heart failure, hyperthyroidism and diabetes, or when there is sensitivity to sympathomimetic amines.

Usage in Pregnancy: Safety in pregnancy has not been established. Metaproterenol should not be used except with caution during pregnancy, weighing the drug's benefit to the patient against potential risk to the fetus. Studies of metaproterenol in mice, rats and rabbits have revealed no significant teratogenic effects at oral doses up to 50 mg/kg (310 times the recommended daily human inhalational dose or 31 times the recommended daily human oral dose). In rabbits, fetal loss and teratogenic effects have been observed at and above oral doses of 50 and 100 mg/kg, respectively.

Adverse Reactions: Adverse reactions such as tachycardia, hypertension, palpitations, nervousness, tremor, nausea and vomiting have been reported. These reactions are similar to those noted with other sympathomimetic agents.

Dosage and Administration: Metered Dose Inhaler: The usual single dose is two to three inhalations. With repetitive dosing, inhalation should usually not be repeated more often than about every three to four hours. Total dosage per day should not exceed 12 inhalations.

Metaprel (metaproterenol sulfate) Metered Dose Inhaler is not recommended for children under 12 years of age because there is not sufficient data on administration of the dosage form in this age group.

Syrup: Children aged 6–9 years or weight under 60 lbs—one teaspoonful three or four times a day. Children over 9 years or weight over 60 lbs—two teaspoonfuls three or four times a day. Experience in children under the age of six is limited to seventy-eight children. Of this number, forty were treated with metaproterenol sulfate syrup for at least one month. In this group, daily doses of approximately 1.3 to 2.6 mg/kg were well tolerated. Adults—two teaspoonfuls three or four times a day.

Tablets: The usual adult dose is one 20 mg tablet three or four times a day. Children aged 6–9 years or weight under 60 lbs—10 mg three or four times a day. Over 9 years or weight over 60 lbs—20 mg three or four times a day. Meta-

Continued on next page

Dorsey—Cont.

prel tablets are not recommended for use in children under 6 years at this time. (Please refer to the Actions section for further information on clinical experience with this product.)
If Metaprel (metaproterenol sulfate) is administered before or after other sympathomimetic bronchodilators, caution should be exercised with respect to possible potentiation of adrenergic effects.
Symptoms of Overdosage: The symptoms of overdosage are those of excessive beta-adrenergic stimulation listed under Adverse Reactions.
How Supplied: Metered Dose Inhaler: Each Metaprel (metaproterenol sulfate) Metered Dose Inhaler contains 225 mg of metaproterenol sulfate as a micronized powder in an inert propellant. This is sufficient medication for 300 inhalations. Each metered dose expressed from the inhaler delivers at the mouthpiece approximately 0.65 mg of metaproterenol sulfate.
Metaprel Metered Dose Inhaler with mouthpiece (15 cc)
Metaprel Metered Dose Inhaler refill (15 cc)
Syrup: Metaprel (metaproterenol sulfate) (red) is available as a cherry-flavored syrup, 10 mg per teaspoonful (5 ml), in pint bottles.
Tablets: Round, scored, white 10 and 20 mg tablets in bottles of 100.
[*Tablets Shown in Product Identification Section*]

NEO-CALGLUCON® SYRUP
(glubionate calcium)

Description: Each teaspoonful (5 ml) of Neo-Calglucon (glubionate calcium) Syrup contains: glubionate calcium 1.8 g (calcium content 115 mg—providing the same amount as 1.2 g calcium gluconate), formic acid (as preservative) 19.0 mg, butylparaben (as preservative) 0.6 mg.
Adequate calcium intake is particularly important during periods of bone growth in childhood and adolescence, during pregnancy and lactation. An adequate supply of calcium is considered necessary in adults, especially those over 40, to prevent a negative calcium balance which may contribute to the development of osteoporosis. The following are the US Government Recommended Daily Allowances (US RDA) of calcium.

Age Period	Calcium Requirements
Infants	0.6 g
Children under 4 years	0.8 g
Adults and children over 4	1.0 g
Pregnant and lactating women	1.3 g

Eight ounces of whole milk provide approximately 267 mg of calcium. One tablespoonful (15 ml) of Neo-Calglucon Syrup contains 345 mg of calcium.
Indications:
1. As a *dietary supplement* where calcium intake may be inadequate:
   a. childhood and adolescence
   b. pregnancy
   c. lactation
   d. postmenopausal females and in the aged
2. In the *treatment* of calcium deficiency states which may occur in diseases such as:
   a. tetany of the newborn*
   b. hypoparathyroidism, acute* and chronic
   c. pseudohypoparathyroidism
   d. postmenopausal and senile osteoporosis
   e. rickets and osteomalacia

*As a supplement to parenterally administered calcium.

Contraindications: Patients with renal calculi.

		Grams of Supplemental Calcium Provided Daily	Percentage of US Recommended Daily Allowance (US RDA)
I.	As a Dietary Supplement: Adults and children 4 or more years of age—1 tablespoonful 3 times daily.	1.0 g	104
	Pregnant or lactating women—1 tablespoonful 4 times daily.	1.4 g	106
	Children under 4 years of age—2 teaspoonfuls 3 times daily.	0.7 g	86
	Infants—1 teaspoonful 5 times daily (may be taken undiluted, mixed with infant's formula or fruit juice). (Part of need is supplied by diet)	0.6 g	96

		Grams of Supplemental Calcium Provided Daily
II.	In the treatment of Calcium Deficiency States: *Tetany of the Newborn* (Tetany of the newborn appears to be a transient physiologic hypoparathyroidism related to the maturation of the parathyroid glands. Adequate parathyroid gland function usually occurs within one week after birth.) Serum calcium should be determined before therapy is instituted. Hypocalcemia is defined as a serum calcium below 8 mg/100 ml or 4 mEq/liter. It is advisable to lower the solute and phosphorus loads in the feeding as well as to provide extra calcium. Intravenous administration of calcium solutions may be necessary for prompt relief of symptoms.	
	Dose: Infants with confirmed hypocalcemia may be benefited by the oral administration of calcium salts so as to provide ELEMENTAL CALCIUM in a dosage of 50 to 150 mg/kg/day divided into three or more doses. (Neo-Calglucon contains 115 mg ELEMENTAL CALCIUM per 5 ml teaspoon.) Oral calcium supplements in neonates should not provide in excess of 1.0 g elemental calcium/day and should be divided into three or more doses in order to minimize gastrointestinal problems. The lower dosage range should be employed if calcium is also being provided by the parenteral route. Whole milk formulas which are high in phosphorus should be eliminated in order to increase the calcium/phosphorus ratio. Supplemental oral calcium should be gradually reduced over a period of two or three weeks after the condition has completely stabilized.	Not to exceed 1.0
	Hypoparathyroidism Acute: Intravenous administration of calcium solutions may be necessary for prompt correction of hypocalcemia. Supplementary calcium should be given orally as soon as possible. Dose: 1–3 tablespoonfuls 3 times daily	1.0–3.1
	Chronic: Dose: 1–3 tablespoonfuls daily	0.3–1.0
	Pseudohypoparathyroidism Dose: 1–3 tablespoonfuls daily	0.3–1.0
	Osteoporosis, postmenopausal and senile Dose: 1–2 tablespoonfuls 3 times daily	1.0–2.1

Rickets and Osteomalacia
Treatment of these disorders consists of the administration of Vitamin D orally. The addition of calcium to the therapeutic regimen may be desirable to provide calcium needed for remineralization and to avoid hypocalcemia which occurs not infrequently in the early days of treatment. Dosages should be those recommended above under Dietary Supplement.

Warnings: Certain dietary substances interfere with the absorption of calcium. These include oxalic acid (found in large quantities in rhubarb and spinach), phytic acid (bran and whole cereals) and phosphorus (milk and other dairy products).
Administration of corticosteroids may interfere with calcium absorption.
Precautions: When calcium is administered in therapeutic amounts for prolonged periods, hypercalcemia and hypercalciuria may result. This is most likely to occur in patients with hypoparathyroidism who are receiving high doses of Vitamin D. It can be avoided by frequent checks of plasma and urine calcium levels. Urine calcium levels may rise before plasma calcium levels. The former may be checked by determining 24-hour calcium excretion or by the Sulkowitch test.
Adverse Reactions: Neo-Calglucon (glubionate calcium) Syrup is exceptionally well tolerated. Gastrointestinal disturbances are exceedingly rare. Hypercalcemia and hypercalciuria have not been reported with Neo-Calglucon Syrup. Symptoms of hypercalcemia include anorexia, nausea, vomiting, con-

stipation, abdominal pain, dryness of the mouth, thirst and polyuria.
Dosage and Administration: Neo-Calglucon (glubionate calcium) Syrup should be administered before meals to enhance absorption.
(See table on preceding page)
How Supplied: Neo-Calglucon Syrup (straw yellow) in bottles of one pint.

PABIRIN® BUFFERED TABLETS

Description: Each BUFFERED PABIRIN TABLET contains: aspirin 300 mg., aminobenzoic acid 300 mg., dried aluminum hydroxide gel 100 mg.
Indications: An analgesic for temporary relief from minor aches and pains associated with arthritis and rheumatism.
Contraindications: Sensitivity to salicylates.
Precautions: When administered concurrently, aminobenzoic acid inhibits bacteriostatic action of sulfonamides.
Dosage and Administration: Adults: 2 tablets every four hours, 4 to 6 times daily.
How Supplied: Buffered Pabirin Tablets (dark pink) in bottles of 100 and 500.

SUNBRELLA® SUNSCREEN LOTION (5% PABA)

Description: Contains: p-aminobenzoic acid (5%), alcohol (60%), water, glycerin, choleth-24, hydroxypropyl cellulose.
Action: Overexposure to the sun may lead to premature aging of the skin and skin cancer—liberal and regular use over the years of Sunbrella Sunscreen Lotion may help reduce the incidence of these harmful effects.
Provides a protective film incorporating moisturizers to help prevent drying of the skin. Does not contain allergy causing parabens as preservatives.
Directions: Apply evenly to exposed areas of the skin and allow to dry. For best protection, apply one hour prior to exposure. To maintain protection, reapply after swimming.
Caution: Avoid contact with the eyes. For external use only. Some individuals may be sensitive to the ingredients. If irritation develops or rashes appear, discontinue use. Slight staining of light colored fabrics may occur if contact is made before application is dry. Alcohol may cause a slight tingling sensation. Contents flammable.
How Supplied: Sunbrella (5% PABA) Sunscreen Lotion in plastic 4 fl oz bottles.

TAVIST-1™ (clemastine fumarate) TABLETS 1.34 mg TAVIST® (clemastine fumarate) TABLETS 2.68 mg ℞

Description: TAVIST (clemastine fumarate) belongs to the benzhydryl ether group of antihistaminic compounds. The chemical name is (+)-2-[-2-[(p-chloro-α-methyl-α-phenyl benzyl) oxy]ethyl]-1-methylpyrrolidine* hydrogen fumarate.
*U.S. Patent No. 3,097,212.
Actions: TAVIST is an antihistamine with anticholinergic (drying) and sedative side effects. Antihistamines appear to compete with histamine for cell receptor sites on effector cells. The inherently long duration of antihistaminic effects of TAVIST has been demonstrated in wheal and flare studies. In normal human subjects who received histamine injections over a 24-hour period, the antihistaminic activity of TAVIST reached a peak at 5–7 hours, persisted for 10–12 hours and, in some cases, for as long as 24 hours. Pharmacokinetic studies in man utilizing ^3H and ^{14}C labeled compound demonstrate that: TAVIST (clemastine fumarate) is rapidly and nearly completely absorbed from the gastrointestinal tract, peak plasma concentrations are attained in 2–4 hours, and urinary excretion is the major mode of elimination.
Indications: TAVIST-1 Tablets 1.34 mg are indicated for the relief of symptoms associated with allergic rhinitis such as sneezing, rhinorrhea, pruritus and lacrimation.
TAVIST Tablets 2.68 mg are indicated for the relief of symptoms associated with allergic rhinitis such as sneezing, rhinorrhea, pruritus, and lacrimation. TAVIST Tablets 2.68 mg are also indicated for the relief of mild, uncomplicated allergic skin manifestations of urticaria and angioedema.
It should be noted that TAVIST (clemastine fumarate) is indicated for the dermatologic indications at the 2.68 mg dosage level only.
Contraindications: *Use in Nursing Mothers:* Because of the higher risk of antihistamines for infants generally and for newborns and prematures in particular, antihistamine therapy is contraindicated in nursing mothers.
Use in Lower Respiratory Disease: Antihistamines <u>should</u> <u>not</u> be used to treat lower respiratory tract symptoms including asthma.
Antihistamines are also contraindicated in the following conditions:
Hypersensitivity to TAVIST (clemastine fumarate) or other antihistamines of similar chemical structure.
Monamine oxidase inhibitor therapy (see Drug Interaction Section).
Warnings: Antihistamines should be used with considerable caution in patients with: narrow angle glaucoma, stenosing peptic ulcer, pyloroduodenal obstruction, symptomatic prostatic hypertrophy, and bladder neck obstruction.
Use in Children: Safety and efficacy of TAVIST have not been established in children under the age of 12.
Use in Pregnancy: Experience with this drug in pregnant women is inadequate to determine whether there exists a potential for harm to the developing fetus.
Use with CNS Depressants: TAVIST has additive effects with alcohol and other CNS depressants (hypnotics, sedatives, tranquilizers, etc.)
Use in Activities Requiring Mental Alertness: Patients should be warned about engaging in activities requiring mental alertness such as driving a car or operating appliances, machinery, etc.
Use in the Elderly (approximately 60 years or older): Antihistamines are more likely to cause dizziness, sedation, and hypotension in elderly patients.
Precautions: TAVIST (clemastine fumarate) should be used with caution in patients with: history of bronchial asthma, increased intraocular pressure, hyperthyroidism, cardiovascular disease, and hypertension.
Drug Interactions: MAO inhibitors prolong and intensify the anticholinergic (drying) effects of antihistamines.
Adverse Reactions: Transient drowsiness, the most common adverse reaction associated with TAVIST (clemastine fumarate), occurs relatively frequently and may require discontinuation of therapy in some instances.
Antihistaminic Compounds: It should been noted that the following reactions have occurred with one or more antihistamines and, therefore, should be kept in mind when prescribing drugs belonging to this class, including TAVIST. The most frequent adverse reactions are underlined.

1. *General:* Urticaria, drug rash, anaphylactic shock, photosensitivity, excessive perspiration, chills, dryness of mouth, nose, and throat.
2. *Cardiovascular System:* Hypotension, headache, palpitations, tachycardia, extrasystoles.
3. *Hematologic System:* Hemolytic anemia, thrombocytopenia, agranulocytosis.
4. *Nervous System:* <u>Sedation</u>, <u>sleepiness</u>, <u>dizziness</u>, <u>disturbed coordination</u>, fatigue, confusion, restlessness, excitation, nervousness, tremor, irritability, insomnia, euphoria, paresthesias, blurred vision, diplopia, vertigo, tinnitus, acute labyrinthitis, hysteria, neuritis, convulsions.
5. *GI System:* <u>Epigastric distress</u>, anorexia, nausea, vomiting, diarrhea, constipation.
6. *GU System:* Urinary frequency, difficult urination, urinary retention, early menses.
7. *Respiratory System:* Thickening of bronchial secretions, tightness of chest and wheezing, nasal stuffiness.

Overdosage: Antihistamine overdosage reactions may vary from central nervous system depression to stimulation. Stimulation is particularly likely in children. Atropine-like signs and symptoms: dry mouth; fixed, dilated pupils; flushing; and gastrointestinal symptoms may also occur.
If vomiting has not occurred spontaneously the conscious patient should be induced to vomit. This is best done by having him drink a glass of water or milk after which he should be made to gag. Precautions against aspiration must be taken, especially in infants and children.
If vomiting is unsuccessful gastric lavage is indicated within 3 hours after ingestion and even later if large amounts of milk or cream were given beforehand. Isotonic and ½ isotonic saline is the lavage solution of choice.
Saline cathartics, such as milk of magnesia, by osmosis draw water into the bowel and therefore, are valuable for their action in rapid dilution of bowel content.
Stimulants should *not* be used.
Vasopressors may be used to treat hypotension.
Dosage and Administration: DOSAGE SHOULD BE INDIVIDUALIZED ACCORDING TO THE NEEDS AND RESPONSE OF THE PATIENT.
TAVIST-1 Tablets 1.34 mg: The recommended starting dose is one tablet twice daily. Dosage may be increased as required, but not to exceed six tablets daily.
TAVIST Tablets 2.68 mg: The maximum recommended dosage is one tablet three times daily. Many patients respond favorably to a single dose which may be repeated as required, but not to exceed three tablets daily.
How Supplied: TAVIST-1 Tablets: 1.34 mg clemastine fumarate. White, oval, compressed tablet, embossed "43" over "80" on one side, "TAVIST" on the other. Packages of 100.
TAVIST Tablets: 2.68 mg clemastine fumarate. White, round compressed tablet, embossed "43" over "70" and scored on one side, "TAVIST" on the other. Packages of 100.

TREST® (methixene hydrochloride) TABLETS ℞

Description: Methixene hydrochloride is 1-methyl-3-(thioxanthen-9-ylmethyl) piperidine Hydrochloride Hydrate.*
Each TREST TABLET contains 1 mg. of methixene hydrochloride.
Actions: Trest (methixene hydrochloride) is a parasympatholytic agent. As an atropine-like anticholinergic, it inhibits actions of acetylcholine on structures innervated by postganglionic cholinergic nerves and on smooth muscles that respond to acetylcholine but lack cholinergic innervation.
Methixene hydrochloride has an inhibitory effect on gastrointestinal motor activity with relatively weaker antisecretory effects than those of atropine. Hence, the usual therapeutic doses have less effect on salivary and gastric secretion than comparable doses of atropine.

Continued on next page

Dorsey—Cont.

Indications: Trest (methixene hydrochloride) is indicated as an adjunct in the treatment of conditions in which abnormal motility of the gastrointestinal tract should be corrected by inhibition of spasm or hypermotility. Conditions of this type include:
biliary dyskinesia, duodenal ulcer, duodenitis, epigastric distress, functional bowel distress, gastric ulcer, gastritis, gastroenteritis, irritable bowel, pylorospasm, rapid transit syndrome, spastic colon, ulcer distress.
Contraindications: The drug is contraindicated in patients with glaucoma (particularly narrow-angle); obstructive uropathy as in bladder neck obstruction due to prostatic hypertrophy; obstructive disease of the gastrointestinal tract as in achalasia, paralytic ileus, pyloroduodenal stenosis, etc.; intestinal atony of the elderly or debilitated; unstable cardiovascular status in acute hemorrhage; toxic megacolon complicating ulcerative colitis; myasthenia gravis.
Warnings: Use in Pregnancy: Use of this drug during pregnancy, lactation, or in women of child-bearing age requires the potential benefits of the drug be weighed against its possible hazards to the mother and child.
In the presence of a high environmental temperature, heat prostration can occur with drug use (fever and heat stroke due to decreased sweating).
Diarrhea may be an early symptom of incomplete intestinal obstruction, especially in patients with ileostomy or colostomy. In this instance treatment with this drug would be inappropriate and possibly harmful.
Precautions: With overdosage, a curare-like action may occur. Investigate any tachycardia before giving anticholinergic (atropine-like) drugs, since they may increase heart rate. Use with caution in the patient with hyperthyroidism, coronary heart disease, congestive heart failure, cardiac arrhythmias, hypertension, and nonobstructing prostatic hypertrophy.
Use with caution in patients with hiatal hernia associated with reflux esophagitis and in those with advanced hepatic or renal disease.
Use with caution in patients with gastric ulcer since anticholinergic drugs may produce the complication of delayed gastric emptying (antral stasis). The control of secretion is believed by some to be less important in gastric than in duodenal ulcers. (Use with caution in ulcerative colitis; large doses may suppress intestinal motility to the point of paralytic ileus thus precipitating or aggravating the serious complication of toxic megacolon.)
Use with caution in patients with autonomic neuropathy. Do not rely on the use of the drug in the presence of complicating biliary tract disease.
Adverse Reactions: Anticholinergics produce certain effects which may be physiologic or toxic depending upon individual patient's response. The physician must delineate these.
Adverse reactions may include: xerostomia, urinary hesitancy and retention; blurred vision and tachycardia; palpitations; mydriasis; dilatation of the pupil; cycloplegia; increased ocular tension; loss of taste; headaches; nervousness, drowsiness, weakness; dizziness; insomnia; nausea; vomiting; impotence; suppression of lactation; constipation; bloated feeling; severe allergic reaction or drug idiosyncrasies including anaphylaxis; urticaria and other dermal manifestation; some degree of mental confusion and/or excitement especially in elderly persons.
In the event of drowsiness or blurred vision, the patient should not operate a motor vehicle or other machinery or perform hazardous work.
Decreased sweating is another adverse reaction that may occur. It should be noted that adrenergic innervation of the eccrine sweat glands on the palms and soles make complete control of sweating impossible. An end point of complete anhidrosis cannot occur because large doses of drug would be required and this would produce severe side effects from parasympathetic paralysis.
Dosage and Administration: Usual adult dosage: 1 or 2 tablets three times daily.
Usage in children: Dosage has not been established for children.
How Supplied: Tablets, 1 mg. (white) in bottles of 100.
*U.S. Patent No. 2,905,590
[*Shown in Product Identification Section*]

TRIAMINIC® PREPARATIONS ℞

Description: TRIAMINIC TIMED-RELEASE TABLETS ℞
Each tablet contains: phenylpropanolamine hydrochloride 50 mg., pheniramine maleate 25 mg., pyrilamine maleate 25 mg.
[*Shown in Product Identification Section*]
TRIAMINIC TIMED-RELEASE JUVELETS® ℞
Each Juvelet contains: phenylpropanolamine hydrochloride 25 mg., pheniramine maleate 12.5 mg., pyrilamine maleate 12.5 mg.
[*Shown in Product Identification Section*]
TRIAMINIC ORAL INFANT DROPS ℞
Each ml. contains: phenylpropanolamine hydrochloride 20 mg., pheniramine maleate 10 mg., pyrilamine maleate 10 mg.
Indications: For relief from such symptoms as nasal congestion, profuse nasal discharge, and postnasal drip associated with colds, nasal allergies, sinusitis and rhinitis. Triaminic decongests and normalizes respiratory passages, reduces irritating secretions, combats allergic symptoms and improves sinus drainage with an orally effective sympathomimetic agent and two antihistamines.
Precautions: Patients should be advised not to drive a car or operate dangerous machinery if drowsiness occurs. Use with caution in the presence of hypertension, hyperthyroidism, cardiovascular disease, or diabetes.
Adverse Reactions: Drowsiness, blurred vision, cardiac palpitations, flushing, dizziness, nervousness or gastrointestinal upsets may occur occasionally.
Dosage and Administration: Tablets—Adults—1 tablet, swallowed whole, in the morning, midafternoon and before retiring. Juvelets—Children 6 to 12, 1 tablet, swallowed whole, in the morning, midafternoon and before retiring. Adults, 2 tablets on same dosage schedule. Oral Infant Drops—1 drop per 2 pounds of body weight administered four times daily.
How Supplied: Triaminic Tablets (yellow) in bottles of 100 and 250. Triaminic Juvelets (pink) in bottles of 50. Triaminic Oral Infant Drops in 15 ml. dropper bottles.

TRIAMINIC® EXPECTORANT

Description: Each teaspoonful (5 ml) of TRIAMINIC Expectorant contains: phenylpropanolamine hydrochloride 12.5 mg, guaifenesin 100 mg, alcohol 5%.
Indications: Provides prompt relief of cough and nasal congestion due to the common cold. The expectorant component helps loosen bronchial secretions. The decongestant and expectorant are provided in an antihistamine-free formula.
Contraindications: TRIAMINIC Expectorant is contraindicated in the presence of hypersensitivity to any of the ingredients. The use of pressor amines such as phenylpropanolamine hydrochloride is contraindicated in those patients taking monoamine oxidase inhibitors for antihypertensive or antidepressant indications.
Precautions: Exercise prescribing caution in patients with persistent or chronic cough such as occurs with chronic bronchitis, bronchial asthma, or emphysema. Use with caution in patients with hypertension, hyperthyroidism, cardiovascular disease or diabetes mellitus.
Adverse Reactions: Occasional blurred vision, cardiac palpitations, flushing, gastrointestinal upsets, nervousness, dizziness, or sleeplessness may occur.
Dosage and Administration: Adults—2 teaspoonfuls every 4 hours. Children 6–12 years—1 teaspoonful every 4 hours. Children 2–6—½ teaspoonful every 4 hours. The suggested dosage in pediatric patients 3 months to 2 years of age is 4 to 5 drops per kilogram of body weight administered every four hours.
How Supplied: TRIAMINIC Expectorant (yellow) in 4 fl oz, 8 fl oz and pint bottles.

TRIAMINIC® ©
Expectorant with Codeine

Description: Each teaspoonful (5 ml) of TRIAMINIC Expectorant with Codeine contains: codeine phosphate 10 mg (Warning: May be habit forming), phenylpropanolamine hydrochloride 12.5 mg, guaifenesin 100 mg, alcohol 5%.
Indications: For use in providing temporary relief of coughs and nasal congestion due to the common cold, when the antitussive properties of codeine are desired. The expectorant component helps loosen bronchial secretions. The ingredients are provided in an antihistamine-free formula.
Contraindications: TRIAMINIC Expectorant with Codeine is contraindicated in the presence of hypersensitivity to any of the ingredients. The use of pressor amines such as phenylpropanolamine hydrochloride is contraindicated in those patients taking monoamine oxidase inhibitors for antihypertensive or antidepressant indications. Continuous dosage over an extended period is generally contraindicated since codeine phosphate may cause addiction.
Precautions: Exercise prescribing caution in patients with persistent or chronic cough such as occurs with chronic bronchitis, bronchial asthma, or emphysema. Use with caution in patients with hypertension, hyperthyroidism, cardiovascular disease, diabetes mellitus, chronic pulmonary disease or shortness of breath. Exercise caution in prescribing this product to children taking other drugs.
Adverse Reactions: Occasional blurred vision, cardiac palpitations, flushing, gastrointestinal upsets, nervousness, dizziness, sleeplessness and drowsiness. May cause or aggravate constipation.
Dosage and Administration: Adults—2 teaspoonfuls every 4 hours. Children 6 to 12 years—1 teaspoonful every 4 hours. Children 2 to 6 years—½ teaspoonful every 4 hours. The suggested dosage in pediatric patients 3 months to 2 years of age is 2 drops per kilogram of body weight administered every four hours.
How Supplied: TRIAMINIC Expectorant with Codeine (green) in 4 fl oz and pint bottles. TRIAMINIC Expectorant with Codeine is a Schedule V controlled substance.

TRIAMINIC® EXPECTORANT DH ©

Description: Each teaspoonful (5 ml) of Triaminic Expectorant DH contains: hydrocodone bitartrate (Warning: May be habit forming) 1.67 mg, Triaminic 25 mg (phenylpropanolamine hydrochloride 12.5 mg, pheniramine maleate 6.25 mg, pyrilamine maleate 6.25 mg), guaifenesin 100 mg, alcohol 5%.
Indications: For relief of troublesome cough and nasal congestion associated with colds, nasal allergies, sinusitis, postnasal drip. Also effective for relief of severe, prolonged or refractory cough associated with other respiratory infections.

Precautions: Patients should be advised not to drive a car or operate dangerous machinery if drowsiness occurs. Use with caution in the presence of hypertension, hyperthyroidism, cardiovascular disease or diabetes.
Hydrocodone is a narcotic and may be habit forming.
Adverse Reactions: Occasional drowsiness, blurred vision, cardiac palpitations, flushing, dizziness, nervousness or gastrointestinal upsets.
Dosage and Administration: Adults—2 teaspoonfuls every 4 hours; children 6 to 12—1 teaspoonful every 4 hours; children 1 to 6—½ teaspoonful every 4 hours.
How Supplied: Triaminic Expectorant DH (green) in pint bottles. Triaminic Expectorant DH is a Schedule III controlled substance.
Remarks: On oral ℞ where state laws permit.

TRIAMINIC® SYRUP

Description: Each teaspoonful (5 ml) of TRIAMINIC Syrup contains: phenylpropanolamine hydrochloride 12.5 mg and chlorpheniramine maleate 2 mg in a nonalcoholic vehicle.
Indications: For the temporary relief of nasal congestion, sneezing, and itchy watery eyes that may occur in hay fever or other upper respiratory allergies, the common cold and sinusitis.
Contraindications: TRIAMINIC Syrup is contraindicated in the presence of hypersensitivity to any of the ingredients. The use of pressor amines such as phenylpropanolamine hydrochloride is contraindicated in those patients taking monoamine oxidase inhibitors for antihypertensive or antidepressant indications.
Precautions: Caution should be observed in operating a motor vehicle or performing potentially hazardous tasks requiring mental alertness. Alcoholic beverages and other CNS depressants may potentiate the sedative effects of antihistamines. Caution should be observed in the presence of hypertension, hyperthyroidism, cardiovascular disease or diabetes mellitus. Because of anticholinergic action of antihistamines they should be administered with caution to patients with bronchial asthma, narrow angle glaucoma, stenosing peptic ulcer, pyloroduodenal obstruction, prostatic hypertrophy or other bladder neck obstruction.
Adverse Reactions: Drowsiness, blurred vision, palpitations, flushing, gastrointestinal upsets, nervousness, dizziness, or sleeplessness may occur. May cause excitability especially in children.
Dosage and Administration: Adults—two teaspoonfuls every 4 hours. Children 6–12 years—1 teaspoonful every 4 hours, children 2–6—½ teaspoonful every 4 hours. The suggested dosage in pediatric patients 3 months to 2 years of age is 4 to 5 drops per kilogram of body weight administered every four hours.
How Supplied: TRIAMINIC Syrup (orange), in 4 fl oz, 8 fl oz and pint bottles.

TRIAMINIC-DM™ COUGH FORMULA

Description: Each teaspoonful (5 ml) of TRIAMINIC-DM Cough Formula contains: phenylpropanolamine hydrochloride 12.5 mg and dextromethorphan hydrobromide 10 mg in a nonalcoholic vehicle.
Indications: Provides prompt, temporary relief of cough and nasal congestion due to the common cold. The decongestant and antitussive are provided in an antihistamine free formula.
Contraindications: TRIAMINIC-DM Cough Formula is contraindicated in the presence of hypersensitivity to any of the ingredients. The use of pressor amines such as phenylpropanolamine hydrochloride is contraindicated in those patients taking monoamine oxidase inhibitors for antihypertensive or antidepressant indications.
Precautions: Exercise prescribing caution in patients with persistent or chronic cough such as occurs with chronic bronchitis, bronchial asthma, or emphysema. Use with caution in patients with hypertension, hyperthyroidism, cardiovascular disease or diabetes mellitus.
Adverse Reactions: Occasional blurred vision, cardiac palpitations, flushing, gastrointestinal upsets, nervousness, dizziness, or sleeplessness may occur.
Dosage and Administration: Adults—2 teaspoonfuls every 4 hours. Children 6–12 years—1 teaspoonful every 4 hours. Children 2–6 years—½ teaspoonful every 4 hours. The suggested dosage in pediatric patients 3 months to 2 years of age is 1½ drops per kilogram of body weight administered every 4 hours.
How Supplied: TRIAMINIC-DM Cough Formula (dark red) in 4 fl oz bottles.

TRIAMINICIN® CHEWABLES

(See PDR For Nonprescription Drugs)

TRIAMINICIN® TABLETS

(See PDR For Nonprescription Drugs)

TRIAMINICOL® DECONGESTANT COUGH SYRUP

Description: Each teaspoonful (5 ml.) of TRIAMINICOL COUGH SYRUP contains: phenylpropanolamine hydrochloride 12.5 mg., pheniramine maleate 6.25 mg., pyrilamine maleate 6.25 mg.; dextromethorphan hydrobromide 15 mg.; ammonium chloride 90 mg., in a palatable vehicle.
Indications: For relief of coughs, especially when accompanied by stuffed and runny noses, due to the common cold. It combines the effective, nonnarcotic, antitussive action of dextromethorphan hydrobromide with a proven nasal decongestant.
Precautions: Patients should be advised not to drive a car or operate dangerous machinery if drowsiness occurs. Use with caution in the presence of hypertension, hyperthyroidism, cardiovascular disease or diabetes.
Adverse Reactions: Occasional drowsiness, blurred vision, cardiac palpitations, flushing, dizziness, nervousness or gastrointestinal upsets.
Dosage and Administration: Adults—2 teaspoonfuls every 4 hours; children 6 to 12—1 teaspoonful every 4 hours; children 2 to 6—½ teaspoonful every 4 to 6 hours. For nighttime cough relief, give the last dose at bedtime.
How Supplied: Triaminicol Decongestant Cough Syrup (dark red) in 4 fl. oz., 8 fl. oz. and pint bottles.

TUSSAGESIC® TABLETS/SUSPENSION

(See PDR For Nonprescription Drugs)

TUSSAMINIC® TABLETS ℞

Description: Each TUSSAMINIC TIMED-RELEASE TABLET contains: Triaminic® 100 mg. (phenylpropanolamine hydrochloride 50 mg., pheniramine maleate 25 mg., pyrilamine maleate 25 mg.); Dormethan® (brand of dextromethorphan hydrobromide) 30 mg.; terpin hydrate 300 mg.
Indications: Relief of cough and nasal congestion due to the common cold, nasal allergies, sinusitis and postnasal drip. The timed-release action helps to provide uninterrupted rest for the patient with night cough.
Precautions: The patient should be advised not to drive a car or operate dangerous machinery if drowsiness occurs. Use with caution in the presence of hypertension, hyperthyroidism, cardiovascular disease or diabetes.
Adverse Reactions: Occasional drowsiness, blurred vision, cardiac palpitations, flushing, dizziness, nervousness or gastrointestinal upsets.
Dosage and Administration: Adults—1 tablet, swallowed whole, in morning, midafternoon and before retiring.
How Supplied: Tussaminic Tablets (green) in bottles of 50.

URSINUS® INLAY-TABS®

(See PDR For Nonprescription Drugs)

UVAL® SUNSCREEN LOTION
(sulisobenzone 10%)

Action: Uval absorbs ultraviolet solar radiation in the wavelength range most damaging to human skin. When properly applied, Uval protects the skin from sunburning and aids in the prevention of visible changes in the skin such as wrinkling, drying and freckling due to overexposure to the sun. Uval deposits an almost invisible protective film on the skin.
Directions: Shake well before using. Apply evenly to exposed skin, rub in well and allow to dry. To maintain protection, reapply after swimming or excessive perspiring.
Caution: Avoid getting lotion into eyes. If skin sensitivity develops, discontinue use. For external use only.
How Supplied: In plastic squeeze bottles of 4 oz.

VACUETTS® EVACUANT SUPPOSITORIES

Description: Each VACUETTS SUPPOSITORY contains sodium biphosphate anhydrous, sodium acid pyrophosphate and sodium bicarbonate in a water-soluble base of polyethylene glycols.
Action and Uses: For safe, rapid and effective evacuation of the lower bowel in most common types of constipation and in preparation for surgery and proctoscopy. When a Vacuetts Suppository is inserted into the rectum, the water-soluble base disintegrates and the released salts react to form carbon dioxide. Gentle pressure from the expanding gas stimulates normal peristaltic and defecation reflexes in the lower bowel.
Precaution: Rectal bleeding or failure to respond may indicate a serious condition.
Dosage and Administration: Remove foil wrapper and moisten suppository under tap or in a cup of water for 10-30 seconds. Do not use mineral oil or petroleum jelly as a lubricant. Gently insert one suppository into rectum. Patient should retain 15-20 minutes, if possible. For bowel retraining, insert one suppository daily, after breakfast, for 7 to 10 days.
How Supplied: Vacuetts Suppositories, Adult—Dozens (in dispensing packages of 2's) and 100's.
U.S. Pat. No. 3,121,663

Dow Pharmaceuticals
THE DOW CHEMICAL COMPANY
P. O. BOX 68511
INDIANAPOLIS, IN 46268

ACCURBRON™ ℞
(theophylline)

Description: Each ml contains anhydrous theophylline 10 mg (50 mg per 5 ml teaspoonful) and alcohol 7.5% in a pleasant tasting vehicle.

Actions: Theophylline, 1,3-dimethylxanthine, is a bronchodilator. It is rapidly absorbed when given as an elixir. It acts by inhibiting the enzyme phosphodiesterase which degrades cyclic AMP. Its plasma half-life ($T\frac{1}{2}$) varies widely because of differences in the rate of metabolism.

Theophylline relaxes the smooth muscle of the respiratory tract and relieves bronchospasm. Its bronchodilator effect is minimal in the absence of bronchospasm.

Other actions of theophylline include dilation of pulmonary, coronary and renal arteries and increased cardiac output, and CNS stimulation. Usual doses increase blood pressure only slightly. Theophylline also has a mild diuretic action.

Indications: For the relief of bronchial asthma (acute or chronic) and reversible bronchospasm associated with obstructive pulmonary diseases such as chronic bronchitis and emphysema.

Theophylline relieves the shortness of breath, wheezing and dyspnea associated with asthma and improves pulmonary function (increases flow rates and vital capacity). In doses sufficient to produce therapeutic serum concentrations (10–20 μg/ml), theophylline would also prevent the symptoms of chronic asthma and suppress exercise-induced asthma. It is especially useful for long-term treatment of bronchospasm because tolerance to the bronchodilator effect of theophylline rarely occurs.

Corticosteroids may be given in conjunction with theophylline, if needed.

Contraindications: Patients with peptic ulcers, active gastritis, and hypersensitivity or idiosyncrasy to theophylline and other methylxanthines.

Warnings: Should not be given concomitantly with other xanthine-containing drugs because of the potential for serious toxicity from elevated xanthine serum levels. Also, liquids containing xanthines (tea, coffee, etc.) should be avoided.

Use in Pregnancy: Safety for use during pregnancy has not been established. Theophylline is excreted in the milk. Use during lactation and in women of childbearing potential requires that benefits be weighed against possible hazards to fetus or child.

Precautions: Use with caution in patients with cardiovascular disease, in young children and the elderly, and in patients with liver, kidney and heart disease.

Adverse Reactions: *Gastrointestinal:* loss of appetite, nausea, vomiting, gastric irritation. *CNS:* irritability, especially in children, insomnia, headache, dizziness, convulsions. These side-effects are usually associated with high theophylline serum levels (exceeding 20 μg/ml). *Cardiovascular:* palpitations, sinus tachycardia and increased pulse rate, usually mild and transient.

Other side-effects may include increased irritation with dehydration, muscle twitching and increased SGOT levels.

Drug Interactions: Theophylline increases the excretion of lithium carbonate and may enhance the sensitivity and toxicity of digitalis derivatives and sympathomimetic amines. Doses higher than usual may increase the effect of oral anticoagulants. Concomitant use with erythromycin, clindamycin, lincomycin and troleandomycin may increase theophylline serum levels.

Colorimetric methods for serum uric acid are affected by theophylline. Spectrophotometric methods of theophylline in serum are affected by furosemide, sulfathiazole, phenylbutazone, probenecid and theobromine.

Dosage and Administration: Dosage must be individualized. Accepted therapeutic serum levels of theophylline are 10–20 μg/ml. Its metabolism may vary greatly with age, among individuals and in patients with liver, kidney and heart disease. Metabolism may be stable within the same individual. Careful monitoring for manifestations of toxicity and periodic determinations of theophylline serum levels are necessary, especially for prolonged therapy and with high doses.

Children: The following table may be used with the graduated measuring spoon for Accurbron:

[See table below].

Adults: Recommended starting dose is 100 to 200 mg (10 to 20 ml) every 6 hours. The adequacy of the dose should be determined by clinical response and periodic monitoring of theophylline serum levels.

May be given after meals with water to minimize possible G.I. irritation.

Overdosage: Theophylline has a narrow therapeutic index and toxicity is likely to occur when serum levels exceed 20 μg/ml. Usual signs of overdosage are anorexia, nausea, vomiting, irritability, headache. Gross overdosage, especially in children, may lead to seizures and death without preceding symptoms of toxicity. Treatment is symptomatic (prompt induction of emesis and gastric lavage, supportive therapy, hemodialysis, etc.).

Caution: Federal law prohibits dispensing without prescription.

How Supplied: As a dye-free liquid in pint bottles (NDC 0183-5002-05) with the graduated measuring spoon for Accurbron.

ACCURBRON™ (theophylline) - PEDIATRIC DOSAGE CALCULATION TABLE

Starting dosage[1]: (All ages for first 3 days[2]) — 4 mg/kg body wt every 6 hours not to exceed 100 mg (10 ml Accurbron)

Age	Body Weight lbs	Body Weight kgs	Dose/6 hours 3 mg/kg	4 mg/kg	5 mg/kg	6 mg/kg	7 mg/kg
Under 9 years*	10	4.5	1 ml	2 ml	2 ml	3 ml	3 ml
average dose	20	9	3 ml	4 ml	5 ml	5 ml	6 ml
4–6 mg/kg/6 hrs.[1]	30	14	4 ml	6 ml	7 ml	8 ml	10 ml
	40	18	5 ml	7 ml	9 ml	11 ml	13 ml
	50	23	7 ml	9 ml	12 ml	14 ml	16 ml
	60	27	8 ml	11 ml	14 ml	16 ml	19 ml
	70	32	10 ml	13 ml	16 ml	19 ml	22 ml
9—12 years*	80	36	11 ml	14 ml	18 ml	22 ml	25 ml
average dose	90	41	12 ml	16 ml	20 ml	25 ml	29 ml
4–5 mg/kg/6 hrs.[1]	100	45	14 ml	18 ml	22 ml	27 ml	32 ml

ACCURBRON contains 10 mg theophylline (anhydrous) per ml.

1. Average dosage from: Wyatt R, Weinberger M, Hendeles L: Oral theophylline dosage for the management of chronic asthma. *J Ped 92*:125–130, 1978.
2. Mitenko PA, Ogilvie RI: Rapidly achieved plasma concentration plateaus, with observations on theophylline kinetics. *Clin Pharmacol Therap 13*:329–335, 1972.

*Do not exceed this dosage without careful clinical monitoring or checking theophylline serum level because of the increased risk of side effects when serum levels exceed 20 μg/ml.

LORELCO® ℞
(probucol)

Description: LORELCO (probucol) is an agent for the reduction of elevated serum cholesterol. The chemical name is 4,4′-(isopropylidenedithio) bis (2,6-di-t-butylphenol). Its chemical structure does not resemble that of any other available cholesterol-lowering agent. It is lipophilic.

Clinical Pharmacology: The pharmacological mode of action by which LORELCO lowers serum cholesterol levels is unknown. However, there is no increase in the cyclic precursors of cholesterol, namely desmosterol and 7-dehydrocholesterol. On this basis it is concluded that LORELCO does not affect the later stages of cholesterol biosynthesis.

Absorption of LORELCO from the gastrointestinal tract is limited and variable. When it is administered with food, peak blood levels are higher and less variable. With continuous administration in a dosage of 500 mg b.i.d., the blood levels of an individual gradually increase over the first three to four months and thereafter remain fairly constant.

At the end of 12 months of treatment in eight patients, blood levels averaged 19.0 μg/ml and ranged from 7.3 to 29.8 μg/ml. Six weeks after cessation of therapy, the average had fallen 60 per cent to 7.8 μg/ml (range from 3.2 to 16.3 μg/ml). After six months the average had fallen 80 per cent to 3.6 μg/ml (range from 1.5 to 6.0 μg/ml).

Indications and Usage: Since no drug is innocuous, strict attention should be paid to the indications and contraindications, particularly when selecting drugs for chronic long-term use.

LORELCO is indicated as adjunctive therapy to diet for the reduction of elevated serum cholesterol in patients with primary hypercholesterolemia (elevated low density lipoproteins). LORELCO may be useful to lower elevated cholesterol that occurs in patients with combined hypercholesterolemia and hypertriglyceridemia, but it is not indicated where hypertriglyceridemia is the abnormality of most concern.

It has not been established whether the drug-induced lowering of serum cholesterol or triglyceride levels has a beneficial effect, no effect, or a detrimental effect on the morbidity or mortality due to atherosclerosis including coronary heart disease. Investigations now in progress may yield an answer to this question.

Contraindications (See also precautions): LORELCO is contraindicated in patients who are known to have a hypersensitivity to it.

Precautions: Before instituting therapy with LORELCO a vigorous attempt should be made to control serum cholesterol by appropriate dietary regimens, weight reduction, and the treatment of any underlying disorder which might be the cause of the hypercholesterolemia.

Because LORELCO (probucol) is intended for long-term administration, adequate baseline studies should be performed to determine that the patient has elevated serum cholesterol levels. Serum cholesterol levels should be determined frequently during the first few months of treatment and periodically thereafter. A favorable trend in cholesterol reduction should be evident during the first two months of probucol administration. The regimen should be followed as long as the trend continues. A decision should be made by the sixth month whether adequate reduction is being attained. A baseline for serum triglycerides should also be established and serum triglyceride levels should be determined periodically. If a marked sustained rise in serum triglycerides is observed during probucol therapy, consideration should be given to improved diet compliance, alcohol abstinence, further calorie restriction or adjustment of carbohydrate intake. LORELCO (probucol) should not be continued if hypertriglyceridemia persists.

Neither oral hypoglycemic agents nor oral anticoagulants alter the effect of LORELCO on serum cholesterol. The dosage of these agents is not usually modified when given with LORELCO.

Use in Pregnancy: Reproduction studies have been performed in rats and rabbits and have revealed no evidence of impaired fertility or harm to the fetus due to LORELCO. Because there are no adequate studies in pregnant women, use of this drug in pregnancy is not recommended. Furthermore, if a patient wishes to become pregnant, it is recommended that the drug be withdrawn, and birth control procedures be used for at least six months because of persistence of the drug in the body for prolonged periods. (See Clinical Pharmacology).

Use in Nursing Mothers: It is not known whether this drug is excreted in human milk, but it is likely to be since such excretion has been shown in animals. It is recommended that nursing not be undertaken while a patient is on LORELCO (probucol).

Use in Children: Safety and effectiveness in children have not been established.

Adverse Reactions: The adverse reactions associated with LORELCO are generally mild to moderate and of short duration.

The most commonly affected system is the gastrointestinal tract. Diarrhea occurs in about one in 10 patients. Other adverse gastrointestinal reactions in descending order of frequency are: flatulence, abdominal pain, nausea and vomiting. These reactions are usually transient and seldom require the drug to be discontinued. During the clinical studies, LORELCO was discontinued in about 2 per cent of the patients because of adverse gastrointestinal reactions.

Less frequent adverse reactions are: hyperhidrosis, fetid sweat and angioneurotic edema which were reported in less than one in 500 subjects.

An idiosyncratic reaction characterized by dizziness, palpitations, syncope, nausea, vomiting and chest pain has been reported.

Other events have been reported in patients treated with LORELCO. The relationship between these events and probucol is not well established. In this group are included totally subjective complaints which are attributed to drugs even though many individuals have symptoms of this sort in the absence of drug ingestion. Also included are events which could have been produced by the patient's state or other modes of therapy. The most frequent were headaches, dizziness, paresthesias and eosinophilia observed in about one of each 50 subjects. Consistently low hemoglobin and/or hematocrit values were observed in about one of each 100 patients. Less frequent were: rash, pruritus, impotency, insomnia, conjunctivitis, tearing, blurred vision, tinnitus, diminished sense of taste and smell, enlargement of a multinodular goiter, anorexia, heartburn, indigestion, gastrointestinal bleeding, ecchymoses and petechiae, thrombocytopenia, nocturia, and peripheral neuritis. These were observed in the range of one to six per thousand subjects.

Elevations of the serum transaminases (glutamic-oxalacetic and glutamic-pyruvic), bilirubin, alkaline phosphatase, creatine phosphokinase, uric acid, blood urea nitrogen and blood glucose above the normal range were observed on one or more occasions in various patients treated with LORELCO (probucol). Most often these were transient and/or could have been related to the patient's clinical state or other modes of therapy. Although the basis for the relationship between probucol and these abnormalities is not firm, the possibility that some of these are drug related cannot be excluded. In the controlled trials, the incidence of abnormal laboratory values was no higher in the patients treated with probucol than in the patients who received placebo.

Dosage and Administration: For adult use only. The recommended dose is 500 mg (2 tablets of 250 mg each) twice daily with the morning and evening meals.

Caution: Federal law prohibits dispensing without prescription.

How Supplied: Each film-coated tablet contains 250 mg probucol and is imprinted with the DOW diamond trademark over the code number 51.

Bottles of 120 tablets, a 30-day supply for one patient (NDC 0183-0051-26). Unit dose packages of 112 tablets (NDC 0183-0051-71).

Keep well closed. Store in a dry place, avoid excessive heat and dispense in light-resistant containers.

Animal Pharmacology and Toxicology: From studies in rats, dogs and monkeys it is known that probucol accumulates slowly in adipose tissue. Approximately 90 per cent of probucol administered orally is unabsorbed. For that which is absorbed, the biliary tract is the major pathway for clearance from the body. After a single dose approximately 10 per cent of the absorbed drug was recovered from bile collected from rats over a period of 30 hours. Very little is excreted by way of the kidneys. Following a single intravenous injection in rats, only one per cent of the drug was recovered in the urine over a 24-hour period.

Probucol has shown no identifiable toxicity in mice, rats and monkeys. In mice and rats the LD_{50} (oral) is in excess of five grams per kilogram of body weight. Two-year chronic toxicity studies in rats and a study in monkeys exceeding seven years in duration have shown probucol to be without adverse effect.

During the performance of a two-year chronic study involving 32 probucol-treated dogs (beagles), there were 12 fatalities. The behavior, physical condition, laboratory findings and post-mortem evaluations were considered to be within normal limits.

Subsequent experiments have indicated that probucol sensitizes the canine myocardium to epinephrine resulting in ventricular fibrillation in many dogs.

Among the animal species in which probucol has been studied, the dog is peculiar with respect to the phenomenon of sudden death and the sensitization of the myocardium to epinephrine. In contrast to findings in the dog, injections of epinephrine to probucol-treated monkeys did not induce ventricular fibrillation. In other studies, monkeys were given probucol either before and after, or only after myocardial infarction induced by coronary artery ligation. In these studies there was no difference between probucol and placebo-treated groups with respect to either survival or detailed blind quantitation of myocardial changes (gross and histopathologic).

Myocardial injury was produced in various groups of rats by one of the following procedures: aortic coarctation, coronary ligation, or cobalt or isoproterenol injection. After probucol administration no deleterious effects related to treatment occurred as measured by survival and microscopic examination of myocardial damage.

Probucol was administered to minipigs beginning 10 days before ligation of a coronary artery and continued for 60 days post surgery. Challenge with epinephrine at the end of 60 days failed to induce ventricular fibrillation in any of the coronary-ligated, probucol-treated minipigs.

In summary, probucol is toxic to the dog; the target organ is the heart. This phenomenon appears to be unique to the dog. Toxic effects were not identified in four other species.

[*Shown in Product Identification Section*]

NEO-POLYCIN®

neomycin sulfate, polymyxin B sulfate and bacitracin zinc ointment, N.F.
Topical Antibiotic

Description: Each gram of Neo-Polycin topical antibiotic ointment contains: neomycin sulfate equivalent to 3.5 mg. neomycin; polymyxin B sulfate, 5000 units; bacitracin zinc, 400 units in a unique Fuzene® ointment base. Inert ingredients are polyethylene glycol dilaurate, polyethylene glycol distearate, light liquid petrolatum, white petrolatum and synthetic glyceride wax.

Actions: All three antibiotics in Neo-Polycin meet most criteria for ideal topical agents. They are rarely used systemically and there is apparently minimal risk of systemic toxicity from their topical use because they are not absorbed to an appreciable extent from denuded skin or mucous membranes. They are essentially non-irritating to the tissues. They are active in the presence of blood or pus, and they diffuse readily into tissue exudates.

Neomycin acts against most of the bacteria that cause topical infection and is especially active against species of *Proteus* and *Staphylococcus*. Bacitracin is primarily effective against gram-positive bacteria, and is especially effective against hemolytic streptococci. Polymyxin is primarily effective against gram-negative bacteria, particularly *Pseudomonas aeruginosa*. This combination of antibiotics makes Neo-Polycin effective against practically all pyogenic bacteria that cause topical infections. Because the Fuzene base is miscible with both tissue exudate and the oils and waxes of the skin, Neo-Polycin can be used in weeping exudative lesions.

Indications: Neo-Polycin may be used in the treatment of bacterial infections of the skin and mucous membrane caused by susceptible bacteria. These include such pyogenic conditions as impetigo, folliculitis, paronychia, and sycosis barbae. It is also effective in controlling secondary bacterial infections in skin carcinoma, burns, eczemas, contact dermatitis, fungal infections, acne, psoriasis, varicose ulcers and neurodermatitis. Its broad antibacterial spectrum and special base make Neo-Polycin especially useful for treating chronic lesions, where mixed infections with relatively resistant bacteria may be present and difficult to identify for definitive therapy.

Neo-Polycin is also indicated as a non-irritating, non-staining dressing for the prevention of bacterial infection of traumatic lesions and surgical incisions.

Contraindications: Hypersensitivity to product ingredients. Not for use in the eyes. Do not use in external ear canal if the eardrum is perforated.

Warning: Because of the potential hazard of nephrotoxicity and ototoxicity due to neomycin, care should be exercised when using Neo-Polycin in treating extensive burns, trophic ulceration and other extensive conditions where absorption of neomycin is possible. Not more than one application a day is recommended where widespread body surfaces are affected, especially if the patient has impaired renal function or is receiving other aminoglycoside antibiotics concurrently.

Continued on next page

Information on Dow products is based on labeling in effect in September, 1979.

Dow—Cont.

Precautions: As with any antibacterial preparation, prolonged use may result in overgrowth of nonsusceptible organisms, including fungi. If this occurs, treatment should be discontinued and appropriate therapy instituted.
Adverse Reactions: Sensitivity, especially to the neomycin ingredient, may develop after continuous, chronic therapy. If itching, burning or inflammation follows application, usage should be discontinued. Articles in the current medical literature indicate an increase in the prevalence of persons sensitive to neomycin.
Administration: Spread Neo-Polycin thinly, with or without a dressing. Reapplication 2 or 3 times daily may be desirable. Avoid using excessive amounts of ointment since it is unnecessary and tends to result in the deposition of undesirable residue.
How Supplied: In ½ ounce tubes (NDC 0183-2010-45) and in 1 ounce tubes (NDC 0183-2010-67).

NEO-POLYCIN® OPHTHALMIC ℞
neomycin sulfate-polymyxin B sulfate-zinc bacitracin ointment
Antibiotic

Description: Each gram contains: neomycin sulfate equivalent to 3.5 mg. neomycin; polymyxin B sulfate, 10,000 units; zinc bacitracin, 500 units; chlorobutonol (chloral derivative) (preservative) 5 mg.; white petrolatum; mineral oil. The ointment is sterile.
Actions: Neomycin, isolated from *Streptomyces fradiae,* has antibacterial activity *in vitro* against a wide range of gram-negative and gram-positive organisms, with effectiveness against many strains of *Proteus.*
Polymyxin B is one of a group of closely related substances produced by various strains of *Bacillus polymyxa.* Its activity is sharply restricted to gram-negative bacteria, including many strains of *Pseudomonas aeruginosa.*
Zinc bacitracin, an antibiotic substance derived from cultures of *Bacillus subtilis* (Tracey), exerts antibacterial action *in vitro* against a variety of gram-positive and a few gram-negative organisms.
Indications: This product is indicated in the short term treatment of superficial external ocular infections caused by organisms susceptible to one or more of the antibiotics contained therein.
Contraindications: This product is contraindicated in those persons who have shown sensitivity to any of its components.
Warning: Prolonged use may result in overgrowth of nonsusceptible organisms. Ophthalmic ointments may retard corneal healing.
Precautions: Culture and susceptibility testing should be performed during treatment. Allergic cross-reactions may occur which could prevent the use of any or all of the following antibiotics for the treatment of future infections: kanamycin, paromomycin, streptomycin, and possibly gentamicin.
Adverse Reactions: Neomycin is a not uncommon cutaneous sensitizer. Articles in the current literature indicate an increase in the prevalence of persons allergic to neomycin.
Administration: Apply to the conjunctival sac two or more times daily as indicated.
Caution: Federal law prohibits dispensing without prescription.
How Supplied: In 3.5 gram tubes with applicator tip (NDC 0183-2009-17).

NEO-POLYCIN® OPHTHALMIC SOLUTION ℞
neomycin sulfate, polymyxin B sulfate and gramicidin ophthalmic solution
Antibiotic

Description: Each ml. contains: neomycin sulfate equivalent to 1.75 mg. neomycin; polymyxin B sulfate, 5000 units; gramicidin, 0.025 mg.; alcohol, 0.5%; and thimerosal, (mercury derivative) 0.01 mg. (preservative) in a sterile isotonic solution. Inert ingredients are: polyoxyalkylene diol, hydrochloric acid if necessary to adjust pH, sodium chloride sufficient to render solution isotonic and purified water.
Actions: Neomycin, isolated from *Streptomyces fradiae,* has antibacterial activity *in vitro* against a wide range of gram-negative and gram-positive organisms, with effectiveness against many strains of *Proteus.*
Polymyxin B is one of a group of closely related substances produced by various strains of *Bacillus polymyxa.* Its activity is sharply restricted to gram-negative bacteria, including many strains of *Pseudomonas aeruginosa.*
Gramicidin has particular action *in vitro* against certain gram-positive bacteria.
Indications: This product is indicated in the short term treatment of superficial external ocular infections caused by organisms susceptible to one or more of the antibiotics contained therein.
Contraindications: This product is contraindicated in those persons who have shown sensitivity to any of its components.
Warnings: Prolonged use may result in overgrowth of nonsusceptible organisms.
Precautions: Culture and susceptibility testing should be performed during treatment. Allergic cross-reactions may occur which could prevent the use of any or all of the following antibiotics for the treatment of future infections: kanamycin, paromomycin, streptomycin, and possibly gentamicin.
A mild, stinging sensation lasting for a few seconds or minutes has been reported, especially if the eyes are inflamed.
Adverse Reactions: Neomycin is a not uncommon cutaneous sensitizer. Articles in the current literature indicate an increase in the prevalence of persons allergic to neomycin.
Administration: One or two drops in the conjunctival sac every 3 or 4 hours. In acute infections more frequent application may be advisable, such as every 15 minutes or half hour.
Caution: Federal law prohibits dispensing without prescription.
How Supplied: In 10 ml. bottles with sterile dropper (NDC 0183-2011-37).

NOVAFED® Capsules ℞
pseudoephedrine hydrochloride

Controlled-Release Decongestant

Description: Each capsule contains 120 mg. of pseudoephedrine hydrochloride in specially formulated pellets designed to provide continuous therapeutic effect for 12 hours. About one half of the active ingredient is released soon after administration and the rest slowly over the remaining time period.
Actions: Pseudoephedrine is an orally effective nasal decongestant with peripheral effects similar to epinephrine and central effects similar to, but less intense than, amphetamines. It has the potential for excitatory side effects. At the recommended oral dosage, it has little or no pressor effect in normotensive adults. Patients have not been reported to experience the rebound congestion sometimes experienced with frequent, repeated use of topical decongestants.
Indications: Relief of nasal congestion or eustachian tube congestion. May be given concomitantly with analgesics, antihistamines, expectorants and antibiotics.
Contraindications: Patients with severe hypertension, severe coronary artery disease, and patients on MAO inhibitor therapy. Also contraindicated in patients with hypersensitivity or idiosyncrasy to sympathomimetic amines which may be manifested by insomnia, dizziness, weakness, tremor or arrhythmias.
Children under 12: Should not be used by children under 12 years.
Nursing Mothers: Contraindicated because of the higher than usual risk for infants from sympathomimetic amines.
Warnings: Use judiciously and sparingly in patients with hypertension, diabetes mellitus, ischemic heart disease, increased intraocular pressure, hyperthyroidism or prostatic hypertrophy. See, however, Contraindications. Sympathomimetics may produce central nervous stimulation with convulsions or cardiovascular collapse with accompanying hypotension.
Do not exceed recommended dosage.
Use in Pregnancy: Safety in pregnancy has not been established.
Use in Elderly: The elderly (60 years and older) are more likely to have adverse reactions to sympathomimetics. Overdosage of sympathomimetics in this age group may cause hallucinations, convulsions, CNS depression, and death. Safe use of a short-acting sympathomimetic should be demonstrated in the individual elderly patient before considering the use of a sustained-action formulation.
Precautions: Patients with diabetes, hypertension, cardiovascular disease and hyper-reactivity to ephedrine.
Adverse Reactions: Hyper-reactive individuals may display ephedrine-like reactions such as tachycardia, palpitations, headache, dizziness or nausea. Sympathomimetics have been associated with certain untoward reactions including fear, anxiety, tenseness, restlessness, tremor, weakness, pallor, respiratory difficulty, dysuria, insomnia, hallucinations, convulsions, CNS depression, arrhythmias, and cardiovascular collapse with hypotension.
Drug Interactions: MAO inhibitors and beta adrenergic blockers increase the effects of pseudoephedrine. Sympathomimetics may reduce the antihypertensive effects of methyldopa, mecamylamine, reserpine and veratrum alkaloids.
Dosage and Administration: One capsule every 12 hours. Do not give to children under 12 years of age.
Caution: Federal law prohibits dispensing without prescription.
How Supplied: Brown and orange colored hard gelatin capsules, monogrammed with the Dow diamond followed by the number 104. Bottle of 100 capsules (NDC 0183-0104-02).
[*Shown in Product Identification Section*]

NOVAFED® Liquid
pseudoephedrine hydrochloride
Decongestant

Description: Each 5 ml. teaspoonful of NOVAFED liquid contains 30 mg. of pseudoephedrine hydrochloride, the salt of a pharmacologically active stereoisomer of ephedrine (1-phenyl-2-methylamino propanol). The formulation also contains 7.5% alcohol.
Actions: Pseudoephedrine hydrochloride is an orally effective nasal decongestant. Pseudoephedrine is a sympathomimetic amine with peripheral effects similar to epinephrine and central effects similar to, but less intense than, amphetamines. Therefore, it has the potential for excitatory side effects. At the recommended oral dosage, pseudoephedrine has little or no pressor effect in normotensive adults. Patients taking pseudoephedrine orally have not been reported to experience the rebound congestion sometimes experienced with frequent, repeated use of topical decongestants. Pseudoephedrine is not known to produce drowsiness.
Indications: NOVAFED liquid is indicated for the relief of nasal congestion associated, for example, with the common cold, acute upper respiratory infections, sinusitis, and hay fever or upper respiratory allergies. Decongestants have been used for many years to relieve eustachian tube congestion associated with acute eustachian salpingitis, aerotitis media, acute otitis media and serous otitis media.

NOVAFED liquid may be given concurrently, when indicated, with analgesics, antihistamines, expectorants and antibiotics.
Contraindications: Patients with severe hypertension, severe coronary artery disease and patients on MAO inhibitor therapy. Also contraindicated in patients with hypersensitivity or idiosyncrasy to sympathomimetic amines which may be manifested by insomnia, dizziness, weakness, tremor or arrythmias.
Nursing Mothers: Contraindicated because of the higher than usual risk for infants from sympathomimetic amines.
Warnings: Use judiciously and sparingly in patients with hypertension, diabetes mellitus, ischemic heart disease, increased intraocular pressure, hyperthyroidism, or prostatic hypertrophy. See, however, Contraindications. Sympathomimetics may produce central nervous stimulation with convulsions or cardiovascular collapse with accompanying hypotension.
Do not exceed recommended dosage.
Use in Pregnancy: Safety has not been established.
Use in Elderly: The elderly (60 years and older) are more likely to have adverse reactions to sympathomimetics. Overdosage of sympathomimetics in this age group may cause hallucinations, convulsions, CNS depression, and death.
Precautions: Patients with diabetes, hypertension, cardiovascular disease and hyper-reactivity to ephedrine.
Adverse Reactions: Hyper-reactive individuals may display ephedrine-like reactions such as tachycardia, palpitations, headache, dizziness, or nausea. Sympathomimetics have been associated with certain untoward reactions including fear, anxiety, tenseness, restlessness, tremor, weakness, pallor, respiratory difficulty, dysuria, insomnia, hallucinations, convulsions, CNS depression, arrhythmias, and cardiovascular collapse with hypotension.
Drug Interactions: MAO inhibitors and beta adrenergic blockers increase the effects of pseudoephedrine. Sympathomimetics may reduce the anti-hypertensive effects of methyldopa, mecamylamine, reserpine and veratrum alkaloids.
Dosage and Administration: Adults, and children over 12 years of age, 2 teaspoonfuls; children 6 to 12 years, 1 teaspoonful, and children under 6 years, ½ teaspoonful, every 4 hours, not to exceed 4 doses in a 24-hour period. However, this dosage may be modified at the discretion of the physician.
Note: NOVAFED liquid does not require a prescription. The package label has dosage instructions as follows: Adults, and children over 12 years of age, 2 teaspoonfuls, every four hours. Children 6 to 12 years, 1 teaspoonful, every four hours. Children 2 to 5 years, ½ teaspoonful, every four hours. Do not exceed four doses in a 24-hour period. For children younger than 2 years, consult a physician.
How Supplied: As a lime green liquid in 4 fluid ounce bottles (NDC 0183-1011-58).

NOVAFED® A CAPSULES ℞
Decongestant Plus Antihistamine Controlled Release

Description: Each capsule contains 120 mg. pseudoephedrine hydrochloride and 8 mg. of chlorpheniramine maleate. The specially formulated pellets in each capsule are designed to provide continuous therapeutic effect for 12 hours. About one-half of the active ingredients is released soon after administration and the rest slowly over the remaining time period.
Actions: Combines the actions of an orally effective nasal decongestant, pseudoephedrine, and an antihistamine, chlorpheniramine. The antihistamine also possesses anticholinergic and sedative effects.
Indications: For the relief of nasal congestion and eustachian tube congestion associated with the common cold, sinusitis and acute upper respiratory infections. Also indicated for symptomatic relief of perennial and seasonal allergic rhinitis, vasomotor rhinitis, allergic conjunctivitis due to inhalant allergens and foods and mild, uncomplicated allergic skin manifestations of urticaria and angioedema. Decongestants in combination with antihistamines have been used to relieve eustachian tube congestion associated with acute eustachian salpingitis, aerotitis, otitis and serous otitis media.
May be given concomitantly, when indicated, with analgesics and antibiotics.
Contraindications: Patients with severe hypertension, severe coronary artery disease; patients on MAO inhibitor therapy; patients with narrow-angle glaucoma, urinary retention, peptic ulcer and during an asthmatic attack. Also contraindicated in patients with hypersensitivity or idiosyncrasy to sympathomimetic amines or antihistamines which may be manifested by insomnia, dizziness, weakness, tremor or arrhythmias, dry mouth, drowsiness and vomiting.
Children under 12: Should not be used by children under 12 years.
Nursing Mothers: Contraindicated because of the higher than usual risk for infants from sympathomimetic amines.
Warnings: Sympathomimetic amines should be used judiciously and sparingly in patients with hypertension, diabetes mellitus, ischemic heart disease, increased intraocular pressure, hyperthyroidism or prostatic hypertrophy. See, however, Contraindications. Sympathomimetics may produce central nervous system stimulation with convulsions or cardiovascular collapse with accompanying hypotension.
Antihistamines may impair mental and physical abilities required for the performance of potentially hazardous tasks, such as driving a vehicle or operating machinery, and may impair mental alertness in children. Chlorpheniramine has an atropine-like action and should be used with caution in patients with increased intraocular pressure, cardiovascular disease, hypertension or in patients with a history of bronchial asthma. See, however, Contraindications.
Do not exceed recommended dosage.
Use in Pregnancy: Safety of pseudoephedrine has not been established.
Use in Elderly: The elderly (60 years and older) are more likely to have adverse reactions to sympathomimetics. Overdosage in this age group may cause hallucinations, convulsions, CNS depression, and death. Therefore, safe use of a short-acting sympathomimetic should be demonstrated in the individual elderly patient before considering the use of a sustained-action formulation.
Precautions: Patients with diabetes, hypertension, cardiovascular disease and hyper-reactivity to ephedrine. The antihistaminic may cause drowsiness and ambulatory patients who operate machinery or motor vehicles should be cautioned accordingly.
Adverse Reactions: Hyper-reactive individuals may display ephedrine-like reactions such as tachycardia, palpitations, headache, dizziness, or nausea. Patients sensitive to antihistamines may experience mild sedation.
Sympathomimetics have been associated with certain untoward reactions including fear, anxiety, tenseness, restlessness, tremor, weakness, pallor, respiratory difficulty, dysuria, insomnia, hallucinations, convulsions, CNS depression, arrhythmias, and cardiovascular collapse with hypotension.
Possible side effects of antihistamines are drowsiness, restlessness, dizziness, weakness, dry mouth, anorexia, nausea, vomiting, headache and nervousness, blurring of vision, polyuria, heartburn, dysuria and very rarely, dermatitis.
Drug Interactions: MAO inhibitors and beta adrenergic blockers increase the effect of sympathomimetics. Sympathomimetics may reduce the antihypertensive effects of methyldopa, mecamylamine, reserpine and veratrum alkaloids. Concomitant use of antihistamines with alcohol, tricyclic antidepressants, barbiturates and other CNS depressants may have an additive effect.
Dosage and Administration: One capsule every 12 hours. Do not give to children under 12 years of age.
Caution: Federal law prohibits dispensing without prescription.
How Supplied: In red and orange colored hard gelatin capsules, monogrammed with the Dow diamond followed by the number 109. Bottles of 100 capsules (NDC 0183-0109-02).
[*Shown in Product Identification Section*]

NOVAFED® A
Decongestant Plus Antihistamine Liquid

Description: Each 5 ml. teaspoonful of NOVAFED A liquid contains: pseudoephedrine hydrochloride, 30 mg. and chlorpheniramine maleate, 2 mg. Pseudoephedrine hydrochloride is the salt of a pharmacologically active stereoisomer of ephedrine (1-phenyl-2-methylamino propanol). Chlorpheniramine is an antihistamine drug of the alkylamine type. Other ingredients include alcohol 5%.
Actions: Combines the actions of an orally effective nasal decongestant, pseudoephedrine, and an antihistamine, chlorpheniramine. The antihistamine also possesses anticholinergic and sedative effects.
Indications: NOVAFED A liquid is indicated for the relief of nasal congestion associated, for example, with the common cold, acute upper respiratory infections, sinusitis, and hay fever or upper respiratory allergies. Decongestants in combination with antihistamines have been used for many years to relieve eustachian tube congestion associated with acute eustachian salpingitis, aerotitis media, acute otitis media and serous otitis media. NOVAFED A liquid may be given concurrently, when indicated, with analgesics and antibiotics.
Contraindications: Patients with severe hypertension, severe coronary artery disease; patients on MAO inhibitor therapy; patients with narrow-angle glaucoma, urinary retention, peptic ulcer and during an asthmatic attack. Also contraindicated in patients with hypersensitivity or idiosyncrasy to sympathomimetic amines or antihistamines which may be manifested by insomnia, dizziness, weakness, tremor or arrhythmias, dry mouth, drowsiness and vomiting.
Nursing Mothers: Contraindicated because of the higher than usual risk for infants from sympathomimetic amines.
Warnings: Sympathomimetic amines should be used judiciously and sparingly in patients with hypertension, diabetes mellitus, ischemic heart disease, increased intraocular pressure, hyperthyroidism or prostatic hypertrophy. See, however, Contraindications. Sympathomimetics may produce central nervous system stimulation with convulsions or cardiovascular collapse with accompanying hypotension.
Antihistamines may impair mental and physical abilities required for the performance of potentially hazardous tasks, such as driving a vehicle or operating machinery, and may impair mental alertness in children. Chlorpheniramine has an atropine-like action and should be used with caution in patients with increased intraocular pressure, cardiovascular disease, hypertension or in patients with a history of bronchial asthma. See, however, Contraindications.

Continued on next page

Information on Dow products is based on labeling in effect in September, 1979.

Dow—Cont.

Do not exceed recommended dosage.
Use in Pregnancy: Safety of pseudoephedrine has not been established.
Use in Elderly: The elderly (60 years and older) are more likely to have adverse reactions to sympathomimetics. Overdosage of sympathomimetics in this age group may cause hallucinations, convulsions, CNS depression, and death.
Precautions: Patients with diabetes, hypertension, cardiovascular disease and hyper-reactivity to ephedrine. The antihistamine may cause drowsiness and ambulatory patients who operate machinery or motor vehicles should be cautioned accordingly.
Adverse Reactions: Hyper-reactive individuals may display ephedrine-like reactions such as tachycardia, palpitations, headache, dizziness or nausea. Patients sensitive to antihistamines may experience mild sedation.
Sympathomimetics have been associated with certain untoward reactions including fear, anxiety, tenseness, restlessness, tremor, weakness, pallor, respiratory difficulty, dysuria, insomnia, hallucinations, convulsions, CNS depression, arrhythmias, and cardiovascular collapse with hypotension.
Possible side effects of antihistamines are drowsiness, dry mouth, anorexia, nausea, vomiting, headache and nervousness, blurring of vision, polyuria, heartburn, dysuria and very rarely, dermatitis.
Drug Interactions: MAO inhibitors and beta adrenergic blockers increase the effects of sympathomimetics. Sympathomimetics may reduce the antihypertensive effects of methyldopa, mecamylamine, reserpine and veratrum alkaloids. Concomitant use of antihistamines with alcohol, tricyclic antidepressants, barbiturates and other CNS depressants may have an additive effect.
Dosage: Adults, and children over 12 years of age, 2 teaspoonfuls; children 6 to 12 years, 1 teaspoonful, and children under 6 years, ½ teaspoonful, every four hours, not to exceed 4 doses in a 24-hour period. However, this dosage may be modified at the discretion of the physician.
Note: NOVAFED A liquid does not require a prescription. The package label has dosage instructions as follows: adults, and children over 12 years of age, 2 teaspoonfuls every 4 hours. Children 6 to 12 years, 1 teaspoonful, every 4 hours. For children under 6 years of age, consult a physician. Do not exceed 4 doses in a 24-hour period.
How Supplied: As a green liquid in 4 fluid ounce bottles (NDC 0183-1010-58).

NOVAHISTINE® DH C
Antitussive-Decongestant-Antihistamine

Description: Each 5 ml. teaspoonful contains codeine phosphate, 10 mg. (Warning: May be habit forming), phenylpropanolamine hydrochloride, 18.75 mg., chlorpheniramine maleate, 2 mg., and alcohol, 5%.
Actions: Antitussive, decongestant and antihistaminic actions.
Codeine, at the recommended dose, causes suppression of the cough reflex by a direct effect on the cough center in the medulla of the brain. Codeine has antitussive, mild analgesic and sedative effects.
Phenylpropanolamine is a sympathomimetic amine similar in action to ephedrine but with less central nervous system stimulation.
Chlorpheniramine possesses antihistaminic, mild anticholinergic and sedative effects. It antagonizes many of the pharmacologic actions of histamine. It prevents released histamine from dilating capillaries and causing edema of the respiratory mucosa.
Indications: For the temporary relief of cough associated with minor throat and bronchial irritation or nasal congestion due to the common cold, sinusitis, and hay fever (allergic rhintis).
A minimum dosage of codeine is provided for the symptomatic relief of nonproductive cough. Phenylpropanolamine is one of the most commonly used oral nasal decongestants. Decongestants have been used to relieve eustachian tube congestion associated with acute eustachian salpingitis, aerotitis, otitis and serous otitis media. Chlorpheniramine maleate provides temporary relief from runny nose, sneezing, itching of nose or throat and itchy and watery eyes as may occur in hay fever (allergic rhinitis).
May be used as supportive therapy for acute otitis media and relief of mild otalgia.
May be given concomitantly, when indicated, with analgesics and antibiotics.
Contraindications: Patients with severe hypertension, severe coronary artery disease, narrow-angle glaucoma, urinary retention, peptic ulcer, during an asthmatic attack, and in patients on MAO inhibitor therapy and nursing mothers. Also contraindicated in patients with hypersensitivity or idiosyncrasy to its ingredients.
Warnings: Codeine should be prescribed and administered with the same degree of caution as all oral medications containing a narcotic analgesic. Codeine appears in the milk of nursing mothers.
If sympathomimetic amines are used in patients with hypertension, diabetes mellitus, ischemic heart disease, hyperthyroidism, increased intraocular pressure or prostatic hypertrophy, judicious caution should be exercised. See, however, Contraindications.
The elderly (60 years and older) are more likely to have adverse reactions to sympathomimetics. Safety for use during pregnancy has not been established.
Antihistamines may cause excitablity, especially in children.
Precautions: If cough persists for more than one week, tends to recur or is accompanied by fever, rash or headache, discontinue treatment. Other medications containing a narcotic analgesic, phenothiazines, tranquilizers, sedatives, hypnotics and other CNS depressants, including alcohol, may have an additive CNS depressant effect when used concomitantly. The dose should be reduced when such combined therapy is contemplated.
Caution should be exercised if used in patients with high blood pressure, heart disease, asthma, emphysema, diabetes or thyroid disease.
The antihistamine may cause drowsiness, and ambulatory patients who operate machinery or motor vehicles should be cautioned accordingly.
Adverse Reactions: Nausea, vomiting, constipation, dizziness, sedation, palpitations or pruritus may occur. More frequent or higher than recommended dosage may cause respiratory depression, especially in patients with respiratory disease associated with carbon dioxide retention.
Drugs containing sympathomimetic amines have been associated with certain untoward reactions including fear, anxiety, tenseness, restlessness, tremor, weakness, pallor, respiratory difficulty, dysuria, insomnia, hallucinations, convulsions, CNS depression, arrhythmias and cardiovascular collapse with hypotension.
Phenylpropanolamine is considered safe when taken at recommended dosage and is relatively free of unpleasant side effects. However, there have been isolated reports of individuals experiencing an acute hypertensive episode after taking therapeutic doses of phenylpropanolamine-containing preparations.
Patients sensitive to antihistamine drugs may experience mild sedation. Other side effects from antihistamines may include dry mouth, dizziness, weakness, anorexia, nausea, vomiting, headache, nervousness, polyuria, heartburn, diplopia, dysuria, and, very rarely, dermatitis.
Drug Interactions: Codeine may potentiate the effects of other narcotics, general anesthetics, tranquilizers, sedatives and hypnotics, tricyclic antidepressants, MAO inhibitors, alcohol and other CNS depressants.
Beta adrenergic blockers and MAO inhibitors potentiate the sympathomimetic effects of phenylpropanolamine. Sympathomimetics may reduce the antihypertensive effects of methyldopa, mecamylamine, reserpine and veratrum alkaloids.
Antihistamines have been shown to enhance one or more of the effects of alcohol, tricyclic antidepressants, barbiturates and other CNS depressants.
Dosage: Adults, 2 teaspoonfuls. Children 50–90 lbs., ½ to 1 teaspoonful; 25–50 lbs., ¼ to ½ teaspoonful. May be given to children under 2 at the discretion of the physician at a dosage of 3 drops/kg. body weight every 4 hours. *Do not exceed 4 doses in a 24-hour period.*
Product label dosage is as follows: Adults, 2 teaspoonfuls; children 6 to 12 years, 1 teaspoonful. May be given every 4 hours, but *do not exceed 4 doses in 24 hours.* For children under 6 years, consult a physician.
How Supplied: In 4 fluid ounce bottles (NDC 0183-1024-58), and pints (NDC 0183-1024-05).

NOVAHISTINE® DMX
Antitussive-Decongestant
Liquid

(See PDR For Nonprescription Drugs)

NOVHASTINE® ELIXIR
NOVAHISTINE® TABLETS
Decongestant—Antihistaminic

(See PDR For Nonprescription Drugs)

NOVAHISTINE® EXPECTORANT C
Antitussive-Decongestant-Expectorant

Description: Each 5 ml. teaspoonful contains codeine phosphate, 10 mg. (Warning: may be habit forming), phenylpropanolamine hydrochloride, 18.75 mg., guaifenesin (glyceryl guaiacolate), 100 mg., and alcohol 7.5%.
Actions: Expectorant, antitussive and decongestant actions. Codeine, at the recommended dose, causes suppression of the cough reflex by a direct effect on the cough center in the medulla of the brain. Codeine has antitussive and mild analgesic and sedative effects.
Phenylpropanolamine is a sympathomimetic amine similar in action to ephedrine but with less central nervous system stimulation.
Guaifenesin helps drainage of bronchial tubes by thinning the mucus, and facilitates expectoration by loosening phlegm and bronchial secretions.
Indications: For loosening tenacious pulmonary secretions associated with cough and respiratory congestion.
A minimum dosage of codeine is provided for the symptomatic relief of nonproductive cough. Phenylpropanolamine is one of the most commonly used oral nasal decongestants. Decongestants have been used to relieve eustachian tube congestion associated with acute eustachian salpingitis, aerotitis, otitis and serous otitis media. Guaifenesin helps loosen phlegm (sputum) and bronchial secretions.
May be used as supportive therapy for acute otitis media and relief of mild otalgia.
May be given concomitantly, when indicated, with analgesics and antibiotics.
Contraindications: Patients with severe hypertension, severe coronary artery disease, in patients on MAO inhibitor therapy and in nursing mothers. Also contraindicated in patients with hypersensitivity or idiosyncrasy to its ingredients.

Warnings: Codeine should be prescribed and administered with the same degree of caution as all oral medications containing a narcotic analgesic. Codeine appears in the milk of nursing mothers.
If sympathomimetic amines are used in patients with hypertension, diabetes mellitus, ischemic heart disease, hyperthyroidism, increased intraocular pressure and prostatic hypertrophy, judicious caution should be exercised. See, however, Contraindications.
The elderly (60 years and older) are more likely to have adverse reactions to sympathomimetics. Safety for use during pregnancy has not been established.
Precautions: If cough persists for more than one week, tends to recur or is accompanied by fever, rash or headache, discontinue treatment.
Other medications containing a narcotic analgesic, phenothiazines, tranquilizers, sedatives, hypnotics, and other CNS depressants, including alcohol, may have an additive CNS depressant effect when used concomitantly. The dose should be reduced when such combined therapy is contemplated.
Caution should be exercised if used in patients with high blood pressure, heart disease, asthma, emphysema, diabetes or thyroid disease.
Adverse Reactions: Nausea, vomiting, constipation, dizziness, sedation, palpitations, or pruritus may occur. More frequent or higher than recommended dosage may cause respiratory depression, especially in patients with respiratory disease associated with carbon dioxide retention.
Drugs containing sympathomimetic amines have been associated with certain untoward reactions including fear, anxiety, tenseness, restlessness, tremor, weakness, pallor, respiratory difficulty, dysuria, insomnia, hallucinations, convulsions, CNS depression, arrhythmias and cardiovascular collapse with hypotension.
Phenylpropanolamine is considered safe when taken at recommended dosage and is relatively free of unpleasant side effects. However, there have been isolated reports of individuals experiencing an acute hypertensive episode after taking therapeutic doses of phenylpropanolamine-containing preparations.

Note: Guaifenesin interferes with the colorimetric determination of 5-hydroxyindoleacetic acid (5-HIAA) and vanilmandelic acid (VMA).

Drug Interactions: Codeine may potentiate the effects of other narcotics, general anesthetics, tranquilizers, sedatives and hypnotics, tricyclic antidepressants, MAO inhibitors, alcohol and other CNS depressants.
Beta adrenergic blockers and MAO inhibitors potentiate the sympathomimetic effects of phenylpropanolamine. Sympathomimetics may reduce the antihypertensive effects of methyldopa, mecamylamine, reserpine and veratrum alkaloids.
Dosage: Adults, 2 teaspoonfuls; children 50–90 lbs., ½ to 1 teaspoonful; 25–50 lbs., ¼ to ½ teaspoonful. May be given to children under 2 at the discretion of the physician at a dosage of 3 drops/kg. body weight every 4 hours. **Do not exceed 4 doses in a 24-hour period.**
Product label dosage is as follows: Adults, 2 teaspoonfuls; children 6 to 12 years, 1 teaspoonful; children 2 to 5 years, ½ teaspoonful. May be given every 4 hours but **do not exceed 4 doses in 24 hours.** For children under 2 years, consult a physician.
How Supplied: As a liquid in 4 fluid ounce bottles (NDC 0183-1023-58) and pints (NDC 0183-1023-05).

NOVAHISTINE®
SINUS TABLETS
Analgesic-Decongestant-Antihistamine
(See PDR For Nonprescription Drugs)

QUIDE® ℞
piperacetazine

Description: Quide (piperacetazine) is a piperidine derivative of phenothiazine having the following chemical designation: 10-{3-[4-(2-Hydroxyethyl)-piperidino] propyl}phenothiazin-2-yl methyl ketone.
Actions: The exact mode of action of the phenothiazines is unclear, but drugs of this class produce changes at all levels of the central nervous system, as well as on multiple organ systems.
Indications: Quide is indicated for use in the management of the manifestations of psychotic disorders.
Quide has not been shown effective in the management of behavioral complications in patients with mental retardation.
Contraindications: Quide is contraindicated in patients who are comatose or markedly depressed from any cause and in the presence of preexisting thrombocytopenia and other blood dyscrasias, bone marrow depression and in patients with significant liver disease. Quide is contraindicated in women who are or may become pregnant since animal reproductive studies adequate to establish safety during pregnancy have not been carried out. Quide is contraindicated in patients who have shown hypersensitivity to the drug. Cross sensitivity between phenothiazine derivatives may occur.
Warnings: Like other phenothiazines, Quide may impair the mental and/or physical abilities required for the performance of potentially hazardous tasks such as driving a car or operating machinery, especially during the first few days of therapy. Therefore, patients should be cautioned accordingly. Concomitant use with alcohol should be avoided due to the potential additive effect. Patients with known suicidal tendencies should not be given Quide except under strict medical supervision.
Use in Children: The use of Quide (piperacetazine) in children under 12 years of age is not recommended because safe conditions for its use have not been established.
Precautions: Use with caution in persons who:

1. are receiving barbiturates or narcotics, because of additive effects on central nervous system depression. The dosage of the narcotic or barbiturate should be reduced when given concomitantly with Quide.
2. are receiving atropine or related drugs, because of additive anticholinergic effects.
3. have a history of epilepsy, because this drug may lower the convulsive threshold. Adequate anticonvulsant therapy must be maintained concomitantly.
4. are exposed to extreme heat or phosphorus insecticides.
5. have cardiovascular disease.
6. have respiratory impairment due to acute pulmonary infections or chronic respiratory disorders such as severe asthma or emphysema.

Keep in mind that the antiemetic effect may mask the toxicity of other drugs or obscure the diagnosis of such conditions as intestinal obstruction or brain tumor.
Any sign of blood dyscrasias requires immediate discontinuance of the drug and the institution of appropriate therapy.
The possibility of liver damage, pigmentary retinopathy, lenticular or corneal deposits, and development of irreversible dyskinesias should be kept in mind when patients are on prolonged therapy.
There is sufficient experimental evidence to conclude that chronic administration of antipsychotic drugs which increase prolactin secretion has the potential to induce mammary neoplasms in rodents under the appropriate conditions. There are recognized differences in the physiological role of prolactin between rodents and humans. Since there are, at present, no adequate epidemiological studies, the relevance to human mammary cancer risk from prolonged exposure to piperacetazine and other antipsychotic drugs is not known.
Abrupt Withdrawal: In general, phenothiazines do not produce psychic dependence, but gastritis, nausea and vomiting, dizziness and tremulousness have been reported following abrupt cessation of high-dose therapy. Reports suggest that these symptoms can be reduced if concomitant antiparkinson agents are continued for several weeks after the phenothiazine is withdrawn.
Adverse Reactions: Not all of the following adverse reactions have been reported with Quide (piperacetazine) but pharmacological similarities among various phenothiazine derivatives require that each be considered.
Note: Sudden Death has occasionally been reported in patients who have received phenothiazines. In some cases death was apparently due to cardiac arrest, in others the cause appeared to be asphyxia due to failure of the cough reflex. In some patients the cause could not be determined, nor could it be established that death was due to the phenothiazine.
Drowsiness: May occur particularly during the first or second week, after which it generally disappears. If troublesome, lower the dosage.
Jaundice: Incidence is low. When it occurs (usually between the second and fourth weeks of therapy) it is generally regarded as a sensitivity reaction. The clinical picture resembles infectious hepatitis with laboratory features of obstructive jaundice It is usually reversible although chronic jaundice has been reported with phenothiazine therapy.
Hematological Disorders: Agranulocytosis, eosinophilia, leukopenia, hemolytic anemia, thrombocytopenic purpura, aplastic anemia and pancytopenia.
Agranulocytosis: Most cases have occurred between the fourth and tenth weeks of therapy. Patients should be watched closely during that period for the sudden appearance of sore throat or other signs of infection. If white blood count and differential show significant cellular depression, discontinue the drug and start appropriate therapy. A slightly lowered white count, however, is not in itself an indication to discontinue the drug.
Cardiovascular: Postural hypotension, tachycardia (especially following rapid increase in dosage), bradycardia, cardiac arrest, faintness and dizziness. Occasionally the hypotensive effect may produce a shock-like condition. In the event a vasoconstrictor is required, levarterenol and phenylephrine are the most suitable. Other pressor agents, including epinephrine, should not be used because a paradoxical further lowering of the blood pressure may ensue. EKG changes, nonspecific, usually reversible, have been observed in some patients receiving phenothiazine tranquilizers. Their relationship to myocardial damage has not been confirmed.
CNS Effects: Neuromuscular (extrapyramidal) Reactions: These are usually dose related and take three forms: (1) pseudoparkinsonism; (2) akathisia; and (3) dystonias (dystonias include spasms of the neck muscles, extensor rigidity of back muscles, carpopedal spasm, eyes rolled back, convulsions, trismus and swallowing difficulties). These resemble serious neurological disorders but usually subside within 48 hours. Management of the extrapyramidal symptoms, depending upon the type and severity, includes sedation, injectable diphenhydramine, and the use of antiparkinsonism agents.

Continued on next page

Information on Dow products is based on labeling in effect in September, 1979.

Dow—Cont.

Hyperreflexia has been reported in the newborn when a phenothiazine was used during pregnancy.
Persistent Tardive Dyskinesia: As with all antipsychotic agents, tardive dyskinesia may appear in some patients on long-term therapy or may appear after drug therapy has been discontinued. The risk appears to be greater in elderly patients on high-dose therapy, especially females. The symptoms are persistent and in some patients appear to be irreversible. The syndrome is characterized by rhythmical involuntary movements of the tongue, face, mouth or jaw (e.g., protrusion of tongue, puffing of cheeks, puckering of the mouth, chewing movements). Sometimes these may be accompanied by involuntary movements of extremities.
There is no known effective treatment for tardive dyskinesia; anti-parkinsonism agents usually do not alleviate the symptoms of this syndrome. It is suggested that all antipsychotic agents be discontinued if these symptoms appear. Should it be necessary to reinstitute treatment, or increase the dosage of the agent, or switch to a different antipsychotic agent, the syndrome may be masked.
It has been reported that fine vermicular movements of the tongue may be an early sign of the syndrome and if the medication is stopped at that time the syndrome may not develop.
Other CNS Effects: Cerebral edema. Abnormality of cerebral spinal fluid proteins. Convulsive seizures, particularly in patients with EEG abnormalities or a history of such disorders. Hyperpyrexia.
Adverse Behavioral Effects: Paradoxical exacerbation of psychotic symptoms.
Allergic Reactions: Urticaria, itching, erythema, photosensitivity (avoid undue exposure to the sun), eczema. Severe reactions include: exfoliative dermatitis (rare); contact dermatitis in nursing personnel administering the drug; asthma; laryngeal edema; angioneurotic edema; and anaphylactoid reactions.
Endocrine Disorders: Lactation and moderate breast engorgement in females and gynecomastia in males on large doses; changes in libido; false-positive pregnancy tests; amenorrhea; hyperglycemia, hypoglycemia, glycosuria.
Autonomic Reactions: Dry mouth, nasal congestion, constipation, adynamic ileus, myosis, mydriasis, urinary retention.
Special Considerations in Long-term Therapy: After prolonged administration of phenothiazines, pigmentation of the skin has occurred chiefly in the exposed areas, especially in females on large doses. Ocular changes consisting of deposition of fine particulate matter in the cornea and lens, progressing in more severe cases to star-shaped lenticular opacities; epithelial keratopathies; pigmentary retinopathy.
Other Adverse Reactions: Increases in appetite and weight; peripheral edema; systemic lupus erythematosus-like syndrome.
Dosage and Administration: Dosage should be individualized, not only initially but during the course of therapy, and the minimal effective dose should always be employed.
A starting dosage of 10 mg. two to four times daily is recommended for adults. The dose may be increased up to 160 mg. daily within a three to five day period. Should side effects occur, dosage should be reduced or discontinued as indicated. For maintenance therapy, up to 160 mg. daily in divided doses may be given.
Overdosage with Phenothiazines:
Manifestations: One of three clinical pictures may be seen.

1. Extreme somnolence; patient can usually be roused with prodding, but if permitted, will fall asleep. General condition is usually satisfactory. The skin, though pale, is warm and dry. Slight blood pressure, respiratory and pulse changes may occur but are not problems.
2. Mild to moderate drop in blood pressure (patient may be conscious or unconscious). Skin is markedly gray, but warm and dry. Nail beds are pink. Respiration is slow and regular. Pulse is strong but rate slightly increased.
3. Severe hypotension, possibly accompanied by weakness, cyanosis, perspiration, rapid, thready pulse and respiratory depression.

TREATMENT: Is essentially symptomatic and supportive. Early gastric lavage and intestinal purges may help. Centrally acting emetics may not help because of the possible antiemetic effect of Quide. Give hot tea or coffee. Severe hypotension usually responds to measures described under hypotensive effects (see ADVERSE REACTIONS: Cardiovascular). Additional measures include pressure bandages to lower limbs, oxygen and I.V. fluids.
Avoid stimulants that may cause convulsions (e.g., picrotoxin and pentylenetetrazol).
Limited experience with dialysis indicates that it is not helpful.
Caution: Federal law prohibits dispensing without prescription.
How Supplied:
Quide (piperacetazine) Tablets-10 mg. (orange)-bottles of 100 (NDC 0183-0052-02). Quide (piperacetazine) Tablets-25 mg. (yellow)-bottles of 100 (NDC 0183-0053-02).
Note: Dispense only in light-resistant containers; the coatings on the tablets contain light-sensitive colors.

RIFADIN® ℞
rifampin
Capsules

Description: Rifadin (rifampin) is a semisynthetic antibiotic derivative of rifamycin B. Specifically, rifampin is the hydrazone, 3-(4-methylpiperazinyliminomethyl) rifamycin SV.
Actions: Rifadin inhibits DNA-dependent RNA polymerase activity in susceptible cells. Specifically, it interacts with bacterial RNA polymerase, but does not inhibit the mammalian enzyme. This is the mechanism of action by which rifampin exerts its therapeutic effect. Cross resistance to Rifadin has only been shown with other rifamycins.
Peak blood levels in normal adults vary widely from individual to individual. Peak levels occur between 2 and 4 hours following the oral administration of a 600 mg. dose. The average peak value is 7 mcg./ml.; however, the peak level may vary from 4 to 32 mcg./ml.
In normal subjects the T ½ (biological half-life) of Rifadin in blood is approximately three hours. Elimination occurs mainly through the bile and, to a much lesser extent, the urine.
Indications: Pulmonary tuberculosis. In the initial treatment and in retreatment of patients with pulmonary tuberculosis, Rifadin must be used in conjunction with at least one other antituberculosis drug. Frequently used regimens have been the following:
isoniazid and Rifadin
ethambutol and Rifadin
isoniazid, ethambutol and Rifadin
Neisseria meningitidis carriers. Rifadin (rifampin) is indicated for the treatment of asymptomatic carriers of *N. meningitidis* to eliminate meningococci from the nasopharynx.
Rifadin is not indicated for the treatment of meningococcal infection.
To avoid the indiscriminate use of Rifadin, diagnostic laboratory procedures, including serotyping and susceptibility testing, should be performed to establish the carrier state and the correct treatment. In order to preserve the usefulness of Rifadin in the treatment of asymptomatic meningococcal carriers, it is recommended that the drug be reserved for situations in which the risk of meningococcal meningitis is high.
Both in the treatment of tuberculosis and in the treatment of meningococcal carriers, small numbers of resistant cells, present within large populations of susceptible cells, can rapidly become the predominating type. Since rapid emergence of resistance can occur, culture and susceptibility tests should be performed in the event of persistent positive cultures.
Contraindications: A history of previous hypersensitivity reaction to any of the rifamycins.
Warnings: Rifampin has been shown to produce liver dysfunction. There have been fatalities associated with jaundice in patients with liver disease or receiving rifampin concomitantly with other hepatoxic agents. Since an increased risk may exist for individuals with liver disease, benefits must be weighed carefully against the risk of further liver damage. Periodic liver function monitoring is mandatory.
The possibility of rapid emergence of resistant meningococci restricts the use of Rifadin to short-term treatment of the asymptomatic carrier state. Rifadin is not to be used for the treatment of meningococcal disease.
Several studies of tumorigenicity potential have been done in rodents. In one strain of mice known to be particularly susceptible to the spontaneous development of hepatomas, rifampin given at a level 2-10 times the maximum dosage used clinically, resulted in a significant increase in the occurrence of hepatomas in female mice of this strain after one year of administration. There was no evidence of tumorigenicity in the males of this strain, in males or females of another mouse strain, or in rats.
Usage in Pregnancy: Although rifampin has been reported to cross the placental barrier and appear in cord blood, the effect of Rifadin, alone or in combination with other antituberculosis drugs, on the human fetus is not known. An increase in congenital malformations, primarily spina bifida and cleft palate, has been reported in the offspring of rodents given oral doses of 150–250 mg/kg/day of rifampin during pregnancy.
The possible teratogenic potential in women capable of bearing children should be carefully weighed against the benefits of therapy.
Precautions: Rifadin (rifampin) is not recommended for intermittent therapy; the patient should be cautioned against intentional or accidental interruption of the daily dosage regimen since rare renal hypersensitivity reactions have been reported when therapy was resumed in such cases.
Rifampin has been observed to increase the requirement for anticoagulant drugs of the coumarin type. The cause of this phenomenon is unknown. In patients receiving anticoagulants and rifampin concurrently, it is recommended that the prothrombin time be performed daily or as frequently as necessary to establish and maintain the required dose of anticoagulant.
Urine, feces, saliva, sputum, sweat and tears may be colored red-orange by rifampin and its metabolites. Soft contact lenses may be permanently stained. Individuals to be treated should be made aware of these possibilities.
It has been reported that the reliability of oral contraceptives may be affected in some patients being treated for tuberculosis with rifampin in combination with at least one other antituberculosis drug. In such cases, alternative contraceptive measures may need to be considered.
It has also been reported that rifampin given in combination with other antituberculosis drugs may affect the blood concentration of methadone, oral hypoglycemics, digitalis derivatives, dapsone and corticosteroids. In these cases,

dosage adjustment of the interacting drugs is recommended.
Therapeutic levels of rifampin have been shown to inhibit standard assays for serum folate and vitamin B_{12}. Alternative methods must be considered when determining folate and vitamin B_{12} concentrations in the presence of rifampin.
Since rifampin has been reported to cross the placental barrier and appear in cord blood, neonates of rifampin-treated mothers should be carefully observed for any evidence of adverse effects.

Adverse Reactions: Gastrointestinal disturbances such as heartburn, epigastric distress, anorexia, nausea, vomiting, gas, cramps and diarrhea have been noted in some patients. Headache, drowsiness, fatigue, menstrual disturbances, ataxia, dizziness, inability to concentrate, mental confusion, visual disturbances, muscular weakness, fever, pains in the extremities and generalized numbness have also been noted.
Hypersensitivity reactions have been reported. Encountered occasionally have been pruritus, urticaria, rash, pemphigoid reaction, eosinophilia, sore mouth, sore tongue and exudative conjunctivitis. Rarely, hepatitis or a shock-like syndrome with hepatic involvement and abnormal liver function tests have been reported.
Transient abnormalities in liver function tests (e.g. elevations in serum bilirubin, BSP, alkaline phosphatase, serum transaminases) have also been observed.
Thrombocytopenia, transient leukopenia, hemolytic anemia and decreased hemoglobin have been observed. Thrombocytopenia has occurred when Rifadin (rifampin) and ethambutol were administered concomitantly according to an intermittent dose schedule twice weekly, and in high doses.
Elevations in BUN and serum uric acid have occurred. Rarely, hemolysis, hemoglobinuria, hematuria, renal insufficiency or acute renal failure have been reported and are generally considered to be hypersensitivity reactions. These have usually occurred during intermittent therapy or when treatment was resumed following intentional or accidental interruption of a daily dosage regimen and were reversible when rifampin was discontinued and appropriate therapy instituted.
Although rifampin has been reported to have an immunosuppressive effect in some animal experiments, available human data indicate that this has no clinical significance.

Dosage and Administration: It is recommended that Rifadin (rifampin) be administered once daily, either one hour before, or two hours after a meal.
Data are not available for determination of dosage for children under 5.

Pulmonary tuberculosis:
- Adults: 600 mg. (two 300 mg. capsules) in a single daily administration.
- Children: 10–20 mg./kg. not to exceed 600 mg./day.

In the treatment of pulmonary tuberculosis, Rifadin (rifampin) must be used in conjunction with at least one other antituberculosis agent. In general, therapy should be continued until bacterial conversion and maximal improvement have occurred.

Meningococcal carriers: It is recommended that Rifadin be administered once daily for four consecutive days in the following doses:
- Adults: 600 mg (two 300 mg Capsules) in a single daily administration.
- Children: 10–20 mg/kg not to exceed 600 mg/day.

Susceptibility testing: Pulmonary tuberculosis. Rifampin susceptibility powders are available for both direct and indirect methods of determining the susceptibility of strains of mycobacteria. The MIC's of susceptible clinical isolates when determined in 7H10 or other non-egg-containing media have ranged from 0.1 to 2 mcg./ml.

Meningococcal carriers: Susceptibility discs containing 5 mcg. of rifampin are available for susceptibility testing of *N. meningitidis*.
Quantitative methods that require measurement of zone diameters give the most precise estimates of antibiotic susceptibility. One such procedure* has been recommended for use with discs for testing susceptibility to rifampin. Interpretations correlate zone diameters from the disc test with MIC (minimal inhibitory concentration) values for rifampin. A range of MIC's from 0.1 to 1 mcg./ml. has been found *in vitro* for susceptible strains of *N. meningitidis*. With this procedure, a report from the laboratory of "resistant" indicates that the organism is not likely to be eradicated from the nasopharynx of asymptomatic carriers.

Overdosage:

Signs and Symptoms

Nausea, vomiting, and increasing lethargy will probably occur within a short time after ingestion; actual unconsciousness may occur with severe hepatic involvement. Brownish-red or orange discoloration of the skin, urine, sweat, saliva, tears and feces is proportional to amount ingested.
Liver enlargement, possibly with tenderness, can develop within a few hours after severe overdosage and jaundice may develop rapidly. Hepatic involvement may be more marked in patients with prior impairment of hepatic function. Other physical findings remain essentially normal.
Direct and total bilirubin levels may increase rapidly with severe overdosage: hepatic enzyme levels may be affected, especially with prior impairment of hepatic function. A direct effect upon the hematopoietic system, electrolyte levels, or acid-base balance is unlikely.

Treatment

Since nausea and vomiting are likely to be present, gastric lavage is probably preferable to induction of emesis. Activated charcoal slurry instilled into the stomach following evacuation of gastric contents could help absorb any remaining drug in the G.I. tract. Antiemetic medication may be required to control severe nausea/vomiting.
Active diuresis (with measured intake and output) will help promote excretion of the drug. Bile drainage may be indicated in the presence of serious impairment of hepatic function lasting more than 24–48 hours; under these circumstances, extracorporeal hemodialysis may be required.
In patients with previously adequate hepatic function, reversal of liver enlargement and impaired hepatic excretory function probably will be noted within 72 hours, with rapid return toward normal thereafter.

Caution: Federal law prohibits dispensing without prescription.

How Supplied: In maroon and scarlet capsules equivalent to 300 mg. rifampin. Bottles of 30 (NDC 0183-0508-30), 60 (NDC 0183-0508-60) and 100 (NDC 0183-0508-02).

**Bauer, A.W., Kirby, W. M. M., Sherris, J. C., and Turck, M. Antibiotic susceptibility testing by a standardized single disk method. Am. J. Clin. Path. 45:493-496, 1966.*

[*Shown in Product Identification Section*]

RIFAMATE™ ℞
rifampin-isoniazid Capsules

WARNING

Severe and sometimes fatal hepatitis associated with isoniazid therapy may occur and may develop even after many months of treatment. The risk of developing hepatitis is age related. Approximate case rates by age are: 0 per 1,000 for persons under 20 years of age, 3 per 1,000 for persons in the 20–34 year age group, 12 per 1,000 for persons in the 35–49 year age group, 23 per 1,000 for persons in the 50–64 year age group, and 8 per 1,000 for persons over 65 years of age. The risk of hepatitis is increased with daily consumption of alcohol. Precise data to provide a fatality rate for isoniazid-related hepatitis are not available; however, in a U.S. Public Health Service Surveillance Study of 13,838 persons taking isoniazid, there were 8 deaths among 174 cases of hepatitis.
Therefore, patients given isoniazid should be carefully monitored and interviewed at monthly intervals. Serum transaminase concentration becomes elevated in about 10–20 percent of patients, usually during the first few months of therapy, but it can occur at any time. Usually enzyme levels return to normal despite continuance of drug, but in some cases progressive liver dysfunction occurs. Patients should be instructed to report immediately any of the prodromal symptoms of hepatitis, such as fatigue, weakness, malaise, anorexia, nausea, or vomiting. If these symptoms appear or if signs suggestive of hepatic damage are detected, isoniazid should be discontinued promptly, since continued use of the drug in these cases has been reported to cause a more severe form of liver damage.
Patients with tuberculosis should be given appropriate treatment with alternative drugs. If isoniazid must be reinstituted, it should be reinstituted only after symptoms and laboratory abnormalities have cleared. The drug should be restarted in very small and gradually increasing doses and should be withdrawn immediately if there is any indication of recurrent liver involvement.
Treatment should be deferred in persons with acute hepatic diseases.

Description: Rifamate is a combination capsule contaning 300 mg rifampin and 150 mg isoniazid.
Rifampin is a semisynthetic antibiotic derivative of rifamycin B. Specifically, rifampin is the hydrazone, 3-(4-methylpiperazinyliminomethyl) rifamycin SV.
Isoniazid is the hydrazide of isonicotinic acid. It exists as colorless or white crystals or as a white, crystalline powder that is water soluble, ordorless, and slowly affected by exposure to air and light.

Actions:

Rifampin

Rifampin inhibits DNA-dependent RNA polymerase activity in susceptible cells. Specifically, it interacts with bacterial RNA polymerase but does not inhibit the mammalian enzyme. This is the mechanism of action by which rifampin exerts its therapeutic effect. Rifampin cross resistance has only been shown with other rifamycins.
In a study of 14 normal human adult males, peak blood levels of rifampin occured 1 ½ to 3 hours following oral administration of two Rifamate capsules. The peaks ranged from 6.9 to 14 mcg/ml with an average of 10 mcg/ml.
In normal subjects the $T^{1/2}$ (biological half-life) of rifampin in blood is approximately 3 hours. Elimination occurs mainly through the bile and, to a much lesser extent the urine.

Isoniazid

Isoniazid acts against actively growing tubercle bacilli.
After oral administration isoniazid produces peak blood levels within 1 to 2 hours which decline to 50% or less within 6 hours. It diffuses readily into all body fluids (cerebrospinal,

Continued on next page

Information on Dow products is based on labeling in effect in September, 1979.

Dow—Cont.

pleural, and ascitic fluids), tissues, organs and excreta (saliva, sputum, and feces). The drug also passes through the placental barrier and into milk in concentrations comparable to those in the plasma. From 50 to 70% of a dose of isoniazid is excreted in the urine in 24 hours.
Isoniazid is metabolized primarily by acetylation and dehydrazination. The rate of acetylation is genetically determined. Approximately 50% of Blacks and Caucasians are "slow inactivators"; the majority of Eskimos and Orientals are "rapid inactivators."
The rate of acetylation does not significantly alter the effectiveness of isoniazid. However, slow acetylation may lead to higher blood levels of the drug, and thus an increase in toxic reactions.
Pyridoxine deficiency (B_6) is sometimes observed in adults with high doses of isoniazid and is considered probably due to its competition with pyridoxal phosphate for the enzyme apotryptophanase.

Indications: For pulmonary tuberculosis in which organisms are susceptible, and when the patient has been titrated on the individual components and it has therefore been established that this fixed dosage is therapeutically effective.
This fixed-dosage combination drug is not recommended for initial therapy of tuberculosis or for preventive therapy.
In the treatment of tuberculosis, small numbers of resistant cells, present within large populations of susceptible cells, can rapidly become the predominating type. Since rapid emergence of resistance can occur, culture and susceptibility tests should be performed in the event of persistent positive cultures.
This drug is *not* indicated for the treatment of meningococcal infections or asymptomatic carriers of *N. meningitidis* to eliminate meningococci from the nasopharynx.

Contraindications: Previous isoniazid-associated hepatic injury; severe adverse reactions to isoniazid, such as drug fever, chills, and arthritis; acute liver disease of any etiology.
A history of previous hypersensitivity reaction to any of the rifamycins or to isoniazid, including drug-induced hepatitis.

Warnings: Rifamate (rifampin-isoniazid) is a combination of two drugs, each of which has been associated with liver dysfunction. Liver function tests should be performed prior to therapy with Rifamate and periodically during treatment.

Rifampin
Rifampin has been shown to produce liver dysfunction. There have been fatalities associated with jaundice in patients with liver disease or receiving rifampin concomitantly with other hepatoxic agents. Since an increased risk may exist for individuals with liver disease, benefits must be weighed carefully against the risk of further liver damage.
Several studies of tumorigenicity potential have been done in rodents. In one strain of mice known to be particularly susceptible to the spontaneous development of hepatomas, rifampin given at a level 2–10 times the maximum dosage used clinically, resulted in a significant increase in the occurrence of hepatomas in female mice of this strain after one year of administration. There was no evidence of tumorigenicity in the males of this strain, in males or females of another mouse strain, or in rats.

Isoniazid
See the boxed warning.

Precautions:

Rifampin
Rifampin is not recommended for intermittent therapy; the patient should be cautioned against intentional or accidental interruption of the daily dosage regimen since rare renal hypersensitivity reactions have been reported when therapy was resumed in such cases.
Rifampin has been observed to increase the requirements for anticoagulant drugs of the coumarin type. The cause of the phenomenon is unknown. In patients receiving anticoagulants and rifampin concurrently, it is recommended that the prothrombin time be performed daily or as frequently as necessary to establish and maintain the required dose of anticoagulant.
Urine, feces, saliva, sputum, sweat and tears may be colored red-orange by rifamin and its metabolites. Soft contact lenses may be permanently stained. Individuals to be treated should be made aware of these possibilities.
It has been reported that the reliability of oral contraceptives may be affected in some patients being treated for tuberculosis with rifampin in combination with at least one other antituberculosis drug. In such cases, alternative contraceptive measures may need to be considered.
It has also been reported that rifampin given in combination with other antituberculosis drugs may affect the blood concentration of methadone, oral hypoglycemics, digitalis derivatives, dapsone and corticosteroids. In these cases, dosage adjustment of the interacting drugs is recommended.
Therapeutic levels of rifampin have been shown to inhibit standard assays for serum folate and vitamin B_{12}. Alternative methods must be considered when determining folate and vitamin B_{12} concentrations in the presence of rifampin.
Since rifampin has been reported to cross the placental barrier and appear in cord blood and in maternal milk, neonates and newborns of rifampin-treated mothers should be carefully observed for any evidence of untoward effects.

Isoniazid
All drugs should be stopped and an evaluation of the patient should be made at the first sign of a hypersensitivity reaction.
Use of isoniazid should be carefully monitored in the following:
1. Patients who are receiving phenytoin (diphenylhydantoin) concurrently. Isoniazid may decrease the excretion of phenytoin or may enhance its effects. To avoid phenytoin intoxication, appropriate adjustment of the anticonvulsant dose should be made.
2. Daily users of alcohol. Daily ingestion of alcohol may be associated with a higher incidence of isoniazid hepatitis.
3. Patients with current chronic liver disease or severe renal dysfunction.

Periodic ophthalmoscopic examination during isoniazid therapy is recommended when visual symptoms occur.

Usage in Pregnancy and Lactation

Rifampin
Although rifampin has been reported to cross the placental barrier and appear in cord blood, the effect of rifampin, alone or in combination with other antituberculosis drugs, on the human fetus is not known. An increase in congenital malformations, primarily spina bifida and cleft palate, has been reported in the offspring of rodents given oral doses of 150–250 mg/kg/day of rifampin during pregnancy.
The possible teratogenic potential in women capable of bearing children should be carefully weighed against the benefits of therapy.

Isoniazid
It has been reported that in both rats and rabbits, isoniazid may exert an embryocidal effect when administered orally during pregnancy, although no isoniazid-related congenital anomalies have been found in reproduction studies in mammalian species (mice, rats, and rabbits).
Isoniazid should be prescribed during pregnancy only when therapeutically necessary. The benefit of preventive therapy should be weighed against a possible risk to the fetus. Preventive treatment generally should be started after delivery because of the increased risk of tuberculosis for new mothers.
Since isoniazid is known to cross the placental barrier and to pass into maternal breast milk, neonates and breast-fed infants of isoniazid treated mothers should be carefully observed for any evidence of adverse effects.

Carcinogenesis:
Isoniazid has been reported to induce pulmonary tumors in a number of strains of mice.

Adverse Reactions:

Rifampin
Nervous system reactions: headache, drowsiness, fatigue, ataxia, dizziness, inability to concentrate, mental confusion, visual disturbances, muscular weakness, pain in extremities and generalized numbness.
Gastrointestinal disturbances: in some patients heartburn, epigastric distress, anorexia, nausea, vomiting, gas, cramps, and diarrhea.
Hepatic reactions: transient abnormalities in liver function tests (e.g. elevations in serum bilirubin, BSP, alkaline phosphatase, serum transaminases) have been observed. Rarely, hepatitis or a shocklike syndrome with hepatic involvement and abnormal liver function tests.
Hematologic reactions: thrombocytopenia, transient leukopenia, hemolytic anemia, eosinophilia and decreased hemoglobin have been observed. Thrombocytopenia has occurred when rifampin and ethambutol were administered concomitantly according to an intermittent dose schedule twice weekly and in high doses.
Allergic and immunological reactions: occasionally pruritus, urticaria, rash, pemphigus, acneiform lesions, eosinophilia, sore mouth, sore tongue and exudative conjunctivitis. Rarely, hemolysis, hemoglobinuria, hematuria, renal insufficiency or acute renal failure have been reported which are generally considered to be hypersensitivity reactions. These have usually occurred during intermittent therapy or when treatment was resumed following intentional or accidental interruption of a daily dosage regimen and were reversible when rifampin was discontinued and appropriate therapy instituted.
Although rifampin has been reported to have an immunosuppressive effect in some animal experiments, available human data indicate that this has no clinical significance.
Metabolic reactions: elevations in BUN and serum uric acid have occurred.
Miscellaneous reactions: fever and menstrual distrubances have been noted.

Isoniazid
The most frequent reactions are those affecting the nervous system and the liver.
Nervous system reactions: Peripheral neuropathy is the most common toxic effect. It is dose-related, occurs most often in the malnourished and in those predisposed to neuritis (e.g., alcoholics and diabetics), and is usually preceded by paresthesias of the feet and hands. The incidence is higher in "slow inactivators".
Other neurotoxic effects, which are uncommon with conventional doses, are convulsions, toxic encephalopathy, optic neuritis and atrophy, memory impairment, and toxic psychosis.
Gastrointestinal reactions: Nausea, vomiting, and epigastric distress.
Hepatic reactions: Elevated serum transaminases (SGOT; SGPT), bilirubinemia, bilirubinuria, jaundice, and occasionally severe and sometimes fatal hepatitis. The common prodromal symptoms are anorexia, nausea, vomiting, fatigue, malaise, and weakness. Mild and transient elevation of serum transaminase levels occurs in 10 to 20 percent of persons taking isoniazid. The abnormality usually occurs in the first 4 to 6 months of treatment but can occur at any time during therapy. In most instances, enzyme levels return to normal with no necessity to discontinue medication. In occasional instances, progressive liver damage occurs, with accompanying symptoms. In these cases, the drug should be discontinued immedi-

ately. The frequency of progressive liver damage increases with age. It is rare in persons under 20, but occurs in up to 2.3 percent of those over 50 years of age.

Hematologic reactions: agranulocytosis, hemolytic sideroblastic or aplastic anemia, thrombocytopenia and eosinophilia.

Hypersensitivity reactions: fever, skin eruptions (morbilliform, maculopapular, purpuric, or exfoliative), lymphadenopathy and vasculitis.

Metabolic and endocrine reactions: pyridoxine deficiency, pellagra, hyperglycemia, metabolic acidosis, and gynecomastia.

Miscellaneous reactions: rheumatic syndrome and systemic lupus erythematosus-like syndrome.

Overdosage:

Rifampin

Signs and Symptoms

Nausea, vomiting, and increasing lethargy will probably occur within a short time after ingestion; actual unconsciousness may occur with severe hepatic involvement. Brownish-red or orange discoloration of the skin, urine, sweat, saliva, tears, and feces is proportional to amount ingested.

Liver enlargement, possibly with tenderness, can develop within a few hours after severe overdosage and jaundice may develop rapidly. Hepatic involvement may be more marked in patients with prior impairment of hepatic function. Other physical findings remain essentially normal.

Direct and total bilirubin levels may increase rapidly with severe overdosage; hepatic enzyme levels may be affected, especially with prior impairment of hepatic function. A direct effect upon hemopoietic system, electrolyte levels or acid-base balance is unlikely.

Isoniazid

Signs and Symptoms

Isoniazid overdosage produces signs and symptoms within 30 minutes to 3 hours. Nausea, vomiting, dizziness, slurring of speech, blurring of vision, visual hallucinations (including bright colors and strange designs), are among the early manifestations. With marked overdosage, respiratory distress and CNS depression, progressing rapidly from stupor to profound coma, are to be expected, along with severe, intractable seizures. Severe metabolic acidosis, acetonuria, and hyperglycemia are typical laboratory findings.

Rifamate (rifampin-isoniazid)

Treatment

The airway should be secured and adequate respiratory exchange established. Only then should gastric emptying (lavage-aspiration) be attempted; this may be difficult because of seizures. Since nausea and vomiting are likely to be present, gastric lavage is probably preferable to induction of emesis.

Activated charcoal slurry instilled into the stomach following evacuation of gastric contents can help absorb any remaining drug in the GI tract. Antiemetic medication may be required to control severe nausea and vomiting.

Blood samples should be obtained for immediate determination of gases, electrolytes, BUN, glucose, etc. Blood should be typed and cross-matched in preparation for possible hemodialysis.

Rapid control of metabolic acidosis is fundamental to management. Intravenous sodium bicarbonate should be given at once and repeated as needed, adjusting subsequent dosage on the basis of laboratory findings (i.e. serum sodium, pH, etc.). At the same time, anticonvulsants should be given intravenously (i.e. barbiturates, diphenylhydantoin, diazepam) as required, and large doses of intravenous pyridoxine.

Forced osmotic diuresis must be started early and should be continued for some hours after clinical improvement to hasten renal clearance of drug and help prevent relapse. Fluid intake and output should be monitored.

Bile drainage may be indicated in presence of serious impairment of hepatic function lasting more than 24–48 hours. Under these circumstances, and for severe cases extra-corporeal hemodialysis may be required; if this is not available, peritoneal dialysis can be used along with forced diuresis.

Along with measures based on initial and repeated determination of blood gases and other laboratory tests as needed, meticulous respiratory and other intensive care should be utilized to protect against hypoxia, hypotension, aspiration, pneumonitis, etc.

In patients with previously adequate hepatic function, reversal of liver enlargement and impaired hepatic excretory function probably will be noted within 72 hours, with rapid return toward normal thereafter.

Untreated or inadequately treated cases of gross isoniazid overdosage can terminate fatally, but good response has been reported in most patients brought under adequate treatment within the first few hours after drug ingestion.

Dosage and Administration: In general, therapy should be continued until bacterial conversion and maximal improvement have occured.

Adults: Two Rifamate (rifampin-isoniazid) capsules (600 mg rifampin, 300 mg isoniazid) once daily, administered one hour before or two hours after a meal.

Concomitant administration of pyridoxine (B_6) is recommended in the malnourished, in those predisposed to neuropathy (e.g. diabetics) and in adolescents.

Susceptibility Testing

Rifampin

Rifampin susceptibility powders are available for both direct and indirect methods of determining the susceptibility of strains of mycobacteria. The MIC's of susceptible clinical isolates when determined in 7H10 or other non-egg-containing media have ranged from 0.1 to 2 mcg/ml.

Quantitative methods that require measurement of zone diameters give the most precise estimates of antibiotic susceptibility. One such procedure has been recommended for use with discs for testing susceptibility to rifampin, Interpretations correlate zone diameters from the disc test with MIC (minimal inhibitory concentration) values for rifampin.

Caution: Federal law prohibits dispensing without prescription.

How Supplied: Capsules (opaque red), containing 300 mg rifampin and 150 mg isoniazid; bottles of 60 (NDC 0183-0509-60).

[*Shown in Product Identification Section*]

SINGLET® ℞

Long-Acting Tablets

Decongestant-Antihistamine-Analgesic

Description: Each SINGLET contains phenylephrine hydrochloride, 40 mg., chlorpheniramine maleate, 8 mg., and acetaminophen, 500 mg.

The long-acting, pink, capsule-shaped tablet is monogrammed with the Dow Diamond and 103 for positive identification.

Actions: Combines the actions of an orally effective nasal decongestant, phenylephrine, an antihistamine, chlorpheniramine, and an analgesic-antipyretic, acetaminophen. The antihistamine also possesses antichlolinergic and sedative effects.

Indications: For the relief of multiple symptoms of nasal and eustachian tube congestion, sneezing, runny nose, watery eyes, myalgia, headache and fever associated with colds and other viral infections, sinusitis, influenza, and seasonal and perennial nasal allergies.

May be given concomitantly, when indicated, with antibiotics.

Contraindications: Patients with severe hypertension, severe coronary artery disease, on MAO inhibitor therapy, narrow-angle glaucoma, urinary retention, peptic ulcer, during an asthmatic attack, seriously impaired liver and kidney function, children under 12 years, in nursing mothers and hypersensitivity to its ingredients.

Warnings: Drugs containing sympathomimetics should be used judiciously and sparingly in patients with hypertension, diabetes mellitus, ischemic heart disease, increased intraocular pressure, hyperthyroidism, or prostatic hypertrophy. Sympathomimetics may produce central nervous system stimulation and convulsions or cardiovascular collapse with accompanying hypotension.

Antihistamines may impair mental and physical abilities required for the performance of potentially hazardous tasks, such as driving a vehicle or operating machinery, and mental alertness in children.

Safety in pregnancy has not been established. The elderly (60 years and older) are more likely to have adverse reactions to sympathomimetics and antihistamines.

Precautions: Patients with hypertension, cardiovascular, liver and kidney disease, anemia, hyperreactivity to ephedrine, or a history of bronchial asthma. See, however, Contraindications. Do not exceed recommended dose.

Adverse Reactions: Sympathomimetics have been associated with certain untoward reactions including fear, anxiety, tenseness, restlessness, tremor, weakness, pallor, respiratory difficulty, dysuria, insomnia, hallucinations, convulsions, CNS depression, arrhythmias, and cardiovascular collapse with hypotension.

Possible side effects of antihistamines are drowsiness, restlessness, dizziness, weakness, dry mouth, anorexia, nausea, headache and nervousness, blurring of vision, heartburn, dysuria and very rarely, dermatitis.

Drug Interactions: MAO inhibitors and beta adrenergic blockers increase the effect of sympathomimetics and the anticholinergic (drying) effects of antihistamines. Sympathomimetics may reduce the antihypertensive effects of methyldopa, mecamylamine, reserpine and veratrum alkaloids. Concomitant use of antihistamines with alcohol, tricyclic antidepressants, barbiturates and other central nervous system depressants may have an additive effect.

Dosage and Administration: Adults, one tablet three times daily. In severe cases, a fourth dose may be indicated. The interval between doses should not be less than six hours.

Note: This product is specifically formulated to provide therapeutic effect up to eight hours. Do not break or crush the tablets.

Overdosage: Acetaminophen in massive overdosage has caused liver damage and fatal hepatic necrosis.

Caution: Federal law prohibits dispensing without prescription.

How Supplied: In bottles of 100 tablets (NDC 0183-0103-02).

[*Shown in Product Identification Section*]

TUSSEND® ℞ Ⓒ

Antitussive-Decongestant

Liquid and Tablets

Description Each 5 ml. teaspoonful or tablet contains hydrocodone bitartrate, 5 mg. (Warning: may be habit forming), and pseudoephedrine hydrochloride, 60 mg. The liquid also contains alcohol, 5%.

Actions: Hydrocodone, at the recommended dose, causes suppression of the cough reflex by

Continued on next page

Information on Dow products is based on labeling in effect in September, 1979.

Dow—Cont.

a direct effect on the cough center in the medulla of the brain. Hydrocodone is an active antitussive with antitussive action approximately three times that of codeine on a weight basis.

Pseudoephedrine is an orally effective nasal decongestant with peripheral effects similar to epinephrine and central effects similar to, but less intense than, amphetamines. It has the potential for excitatory side effects. At the recommended oral dosage, it has little or no pressor effect in normotensive adults. Patients have not been reported to experience the rebound congestion sometimes experienced with frequent, repeated use of topical decongestants.

Indications: For exhausting cough spasms accompanying upper respiratory tract congestion associated with the common cold, influenza, bronchitis, and sinusitis.

Contraindications: Patients with severe hypertension, severe coronary artery disease, and in patients on MAO inhibitor therapy. Patient idiosyncrasy to adrenergic agents may be manifested by insomnia, dizziness, weakness, tremor or arrhythmias.

Nursing mothers: Contraindicated because of the higher than usual risk for infants from sympathomimetic amines.

Hypersensitivity: Contraindicated in patients with hypersensitivity or idiosyncrasy to sympathomimetic amines, phenanthrene derivatives, or to any other formula ingredients.

Warnings: Hydrocodone should be prescribed and administered with the same degree of caution as all oral medications containing a narcotic analgesic.

If sympathomimetic amines are used in patients with hypertension, diabetes mellitus, ischemic heart disease, hyperthyroidism, increased intraocular pressure and prostatic hypertrophy, judicious caution should be exercised. See, however, Contraindications.

The elderly (60 years and older) are more likely to have adverse reactions to sympathomimetics. Safety for use during pregnancy has not been established.

Precautions: Other medications containing a narcotic analgesic, phenothiazines, tranquilizers, sedatives, hypnotics, and other CNS depressants, including alcohol, may have an additive CNS depressant effect when used concomitantly. The dose should be reduced when such combined therapy is contemplated.

Hydrocodone may produce drowsiness, and persons who perform hazardous tasks requiring mental alertness or physicial coordination should be cautioned accordingly.

Caution should be exercised if used in patients with diabetes, hypertension, cardiovascular disease and hyperreactivity to ephedrine. See, however, Contraindications.

Adverse Reactions: Gastrointestinal upset, nausea, drowsiness and constipation. A slight elevation in serum transaminase levels has been noted.

Individuals hyperreactive to pseudoephedrine may display ephedrine-like reactions such as tachycardia, palpitations, headache, dizziness, or nausea. Drugs containing sympathomimetic amines have been associated with certain untoward reactions including fear, anxiety, tenseness, restlessness, tremor, weakness, pallor, respiratory difficulty, dysuria, insomnia, hallucinations, convulsions, CNS depression, arrhythmias and cardiovascular collapse with hypotension.

Drug Interactions: Hydrocodone may potentiate the effects of other narcotics, general anesthetics, tranquilizers, sedatives and hypnotics, tricyclic antidepressants, MAO inhibitors, alcohol and other CNS depressants. Beta adrenergic blockers and MAO inhibitors potentiate the sympathomimetic effects of pseudoephedrine. Sympathomimetics may reduce the anti-hypertensive effects of methyldopa, mecamylamine, reserpine and veratrum alkaloids.

Dosage: Adults, and children over 90 lbs., 1 tablet or teaspoonful; children 50 to 90 lbs., ½ teaspoonful; children 25 to 50 lbs., ¼ teaspoonful. May be given four times a day, as needed. May be taken with meals.

Caution: Federal law prohibits dispensing without prescription.

How Supplied: Tussend liquid in pint bottles (NDC 0183-1018-05). Tussend tablets in bottles of 100 (NDC 0183-0041-02).

TUSSEND® EXPECTORANT ℞ Ⓒ

Antitussive-Decongestant
Liquid

Description: Each 5 ml. teaspoonful of Tussend Expectorant contains: hydrocodone bitartrate, 5 mg. (Warning: may be habit-forming), pseudoephedrine hydrochloride 60 mg., and guaifenesin (glyceryl guaiacolate), 200 mg. The formulation also contains alcohol, 12.5%.

Actions: Hydrocodone, at the recommended dose, causes suppression of the cough reflex by a direct effect on the cough center in the medulla of the brain. Hydrocodone is an active antitussive with antitussive action approximately three times that of codeine on a weight basis.

Pseudoephedrine is an orally effective nasal decongestant with peripheral effects similar to epinephrine and central effects similar to, but less intense than, amphetamines. It has the potential for excitatory side effects. At the recommended oral dosage it has little or no pressor effect in normotensive adults. Patients have not been reported to experience the rebound congestion sometimes experienced with frequent, repeated use of topical decongestants.

Guaifenesin helps drainage of bronchial tubes by thinning the mucus and facilitates expectoration by loosening phlegm and bronchial secretions.

Indications: For exhausting, nonproductive cough accompanying respiratory tract congestion associated with the common cold, influenza, sinusitis and bronchitis.

Contraindications: Patients with severe hypertension, severe coronary artery disease, and in patients on MAO inhibitor therapy. Patient idiosyncrasy to adrenergic agents may be manifested by insomnia, dizziness, weakness, tremor or arrhythmias.

Nursing Mothers: Contraindicated because of the higher than usual risk for infants from sympathomimetic amines.

Hypersensitivity: Contraindicated in patients with hypersensitivity or idiosyncrasy to sympathomimetic amines, phenanthrene derivatives, or to any other formula ingredients.

Warnings: Hydrocodone should be prescribed and administered with the same degree of caution as all oral medications containing a narcotic analgesic.

If sympathomimetic amines are used in patients with hypertension, diabetes mellitus, ischemic heart disease, hyperthyroidism, increased intraocular pressure, and prostatic hypertrophy, judicious caution should be exercised. See, however, Contraindications.

The elderly (60 years and older) are more likely to have adverse reactions to sympathomimetics. Safety for use during pregnancy has not been established.

Precautions: Other medications containing a narcotic analgesic, phenothiazines, tranquilizers, sedatives, hypnotics and other CNS depressants, including alcohol, may have an additive CNS depressant effect when used concomitantly. The dose should be reduced when such combined therapy is contemplated.

Hydrocodone may produce drowsiness, and persons who perform hazardous tasks requiring mental alertness or physical coordination should be cautioned accordingly.

Caution should be exercised if used in patients with diabetes, hypertension, cardiovascular disease and hyperreactivity to ephedrine. See, however, Contraindications.

Adverse Reactions: Gastrointestinal upset, nausea, dizziness, drowsiness, and constipation. A slight elevation in serum transaminase levels has been noted.

Individuals hyperreactive to pseudoephedrine may display ephedrine-like reactions such as tachycardia, palpitations, headache, dizziness or nausea. Drugs containing sympathomimetic amines have been associated with certain untoward reactions including fear, anxiety, tenseness, restlessness, tremor, weakness, pallor, respiratory difficulty, dysuria, insomnia, hallucinations, convulsions, CNS depression, arrhythmias and cardiovascular collapse with hypotension.

Note: Guaifenesin interferes with the colorimetric determination of 5-hydroxyindoleacetic acid (5-HIAA) and vanilmandelic acid (VMA).

Drug Interactions: Hydrocodone may potentiate the effects of other narcotics, general anesthetics, tranquilizers, sedatives and hypnotics, tricyclic antidepressants, MAO inhibitors, alcohol and other CNS depressants. Beta adrenergic blockers and MAO inhibitors potentiate the sympathomimetic effects of pseudoephedrine. Sympathomimetics may reduce the anti-hypertensive effects of methyldopa, mecamylamine, reserpine and veratrum alkaloids.

Dosage: Adults, and children over 90 lbs., 1 teaspoonful; children 50 to 90 lbs., ½ teaspoonful; children 25 to 50 lbs., ¼ teaspoonful. May be given four times a day, as needed. May be given with meals.

Caution: Federal law prohibits dispensing without prescription.

How Supplied: In pint bottles (NDC 0183-1016-05).

2/G®

guaifenesin syrup, N.F.
Expectorant

(See PDR For Nonprescriptin Drug)

2/G–DM®

guaifenesin with d-methorphan
Expectorant-Antitussive

(See PDR For Nonprescription Drugs)

Information on Dow products is based on labeling in effect in September, 1979.

Doyle Pharmaceutical Co., The

A Division of The Delmark Company, Inc.
5320 WEST 23rd STREET
MINNEAPOLIS, MN 55416

CITROTEIN®

Powder
Protein-Vitamin-Mineral Food

Composition (Orange Flavor): Sucrose, pasteurized egg white solids, maltodextrin, calcium glycerophosphate, citric acid, natural and artificial flavor, mono and diglycerides, magnesium oxide, ammonium phosphate, partially hydrogenated soybean oil, ascorbic acid, ferrous sulfate, choline bitartrate, artificial color, niacin, zinc sulfate, alpha tocopheryl acetate, calcium pantothenate, manganese sulfate, copper gluconate, pyridoxine hydrochloride, thiamin hydrochloride, vitamin A

palmitate, riboflavin, folic acid, d-biotin, potassium iodide, cyanocobalamin, vitamin D_2.
Action and Uses: Prescribed for supplemental feeding when patients lack appetite or tolerance for enough ordinary food to meet their nutritional requirements. Specifically prescribed as: Supplementary Nourishment in rapid growth periods, pre- and post-operative states, convalescence, chronic illness, geriatrics, pediatrics, anorexia, pregnancy and postpartum; Fortification for Special Diets—lactose free, bland, liquid, sodium restricted, low fat, cholesterol free, low purine, gluten free, low residue.
Administration and Dosage: Supplemental Feeding—3 servings per day, with meals, between meals or at bedtime. Three servings provide more than 50% of the U.S. RDA for protein and all known essential vitamins and minerals. For use only under medical supervision.
How Supplied: In 1.18 oz individual serving packets and 12 oz cans in Orange and Grape Flavors.

COMPLEAT-B®
Meat Base Blenderized Tube Feeding Formula

Composition: Deionized water, beef puree, hydrolyzed cereal solids, green bean puree, pea puree, nonfat dry milk, corn oil, maltodextrin, peach puree, orange juice, mono and diglycerides, sodium phosphate, carrageenan, magnesium oxide, choline bitartrate, ascorbic acid, calcium carbonate, ferric ammonium citrate, potassium chloride, alpha tocopheryl acetate, calcium pantothenate, manganese sulfate, copper gluconate, niacin, zinc sulfate, thiamin hydrochloride, pyridoxine hydrochloride, riboflavin, biotin, folic acid, vitamin A palmitate, vitamin D_3, vitamin B_{12}.
Action and Uses: COMPLEAT-B provides a nutritionally complete, balanced diet of natural foods with normal proportions of meat, vegetables, milk and fruit in a blenderized feeding, uniform in consistency for gravity or syringe feeding. It is a sterilized tube feeding of rigidly controlled quality and proven safety. Precise quality control assures consistent content and analysis of feedings. Excellent tolerance and utilization in conditions requiring total nutrition or supplementation by tube feeding are proven in clinical trials and long term use.
Administration and Dosage: Four cans (1600 ml) or six bottles (1500 ml) provide 1600 Calories and 100% or more of the U.S. RDA for protein and all known essential vitamins and minerals. Feed slowly at room temperature through nasogastric, gastrostomy or jejunostomy tubes. For use only under medical supervision.
How Supplied: 13.6 fl oz (400 ml) cans and 250 ml bottles for use with Ready To Use Disposable DOYLE TUBE FEEDING SETS™.

CONTROLYTE®
High Calorie Dietary Supplement With Restricted Protein and Electrolyte Content

Composition: Polysaccharides obtained by deionization of a partial hydrolysate of corn starch, partially hydrogenated soybean oil with BHA as freshness preserver, hydroxylated lecithin, polyglycerol esters of fatty acids. Approximate analysis of 14 oz can of CONTROLYTE: 2000 Calories, 286 g carbohydrate, 96 g fat, 0.16 g protein, 8 mg phenylalanine, 40 mg sodium (1.7 mEq), 16 mg potassium (0.4 mEq), 16 mg calcium (0.8 mEq), 32 mg phosphorus.
Action and Uses: CONTROLYTE is a concentrated source of well-tolerated calories for caloric fortification of general and restricted diets such as High Calorie Diets (burns, post surgical, acute or chronic diseases), Tube Feedings and Oral Liquid Diets, Protein/Electrolyte Restricted Diets (renal disease, liver disease, disorders of protein metabolism), Sodium-Restricted Diets, Clinical Balance Studies, Diagnostic Test Meals.
Administration and Dosage: Add CONTROLYTE (one can) to 2 to 3 cups (480 to 720 ml) water, depending on fluid allowance and taste. Use CONTROLYTE as needed to meet the caloric requirements of each individual diet. Fortification of Foods—add CONTROLYTE in varying amounts to foods normally included in the diet. Supplementary Nourishment—Prepare CONTROLYTE with fruit juices and other beverages; add CONTROLYTE Powder to nutritional supplements, milk and tube feedings as desired. For use only under medical supervision.
How Supplied: 14 oz cans.

DIETENE®
For Use In Reducing Diets

Composition (Chocolate Malt Flavor): Specially processed nonfat dry milk, sucrose, cocoa, calcium caseinate, magnesium sulfate, carrageenan, artificial flavor, lecithin, polysorbate 80, zinc sulfate, ascorbic acid, malt, alpha tocopheryl acetate, niacin, iron, copper gluconate, calcium pantothenate, vitamin A palmitate, pyridoxine hydrochloride, thiamin hydrochloride, folic acid, biotin, vitamin D_2.
Action and Uses: DIETENE Nourishments are used as part of DIETENE Weight Reduction Diets. The DIETENE 1000 Calorie Diet (including two DIETENE Nourishments) provides 83 g protein, 26 g fat and 110 g carbohydrate and 100% of the U.S. RDA for all vitamins and minerals. NOTE: A free set of professional weight reduction diets available upon request.
Administration and Dosage: Use the DIETENE 1000, 1200 and 1400 Calorie Diets which include DIETENE Nourishments. For use only under medical supervision.
How Supplied: In 1 lb and 4½ lb cans in Vanilla, Chocolate Malt and Strawberry Flavors.

MERITENE® Powder
Protein-Vitamin-Mineral Food

Composition (Plain Flavor): Specially processed nonfat dry milk, corn syrup solids, calcium caseinate, magnesium sulfate, natural and artificial flavors, ascorbic acid, lecithin, ferrous sulfate, zinc sulfate, alpha tocopheryl acetate, niacin, manganese sulfate, copper gluconate, riboflavin, calcium pantothenate, pyridoxine hydrochloride, vitamin A palmitate, thiamin hydrochloride, folic acid, biotin, vitamin D_2.
Action and Uses: Prescribed for total or supplemental feeding when patients lack appetite or tolerance for enough ordinary food to meet their nutritional requirements.
Specifically prescribed as: Supplementary Nourishment in debilitation and stress conditions—pre- and post-operative, convalescence, chronic illnesses, anemias, geriatrics, anorexia, underweight, pregnancy, post-partum and rapid growth periods; Fortification for Special Diets—ulcer, colitis, liver and gallbladder diseases, gastrointestinal disorders and surgery; Total Feeding—Oral or Tube—immediate post-operative care, fractured jaws, plastic surgery, cancer of throat and oral cavity. NOTE: Complimentary Professional Diet Service available upon request.
Administration and Dosage: Supplemental Feeding: 2 or 3 servings per day between meals and at bedtime. Total Feeding—Oral or Tube—Four servings of MERITENE Nourishment provide 1107 Calories and 100% of the U.S. RDA for protein and all known essential vitamins and minerals. Serve chilled for oral feeding and at room temperature for tube feeding. May be fed through nasogastric, gastrostomy or jejunostomy tubes. For use only under medical supervision.
How Supplied: In 1 lb and 4½ lb cans in Vanilla, Plain, Chocolate and Egg Nog Flavors.

MERITENE® Liquid
Protein-Vitamin-Mineral Food

Composition (Vanilla Flavor): Concentrated sweet skim milk, corn syrup solids, corn oil, sodium caseinate, sucrose, artificial flavor, cellulose flour, mono and diglycerides, magnesium sulfate, salt, magnesium oxide, cellulose gum, sodium ascorbate, ferric orthophosphate, choline chloride, carrageenan, alpha tocopheryl acetate, niacinamide, zinc oxide, copper gluconate, manganese sulfate, calcium pantothenate, ascorbic acid, pyridoxine hydrochloride, thiamin hydrochloride, riboflavin phosphate, vitamin A palmitate, folic acid, biotin, potassium iodide, vitamin D_3, vitamin B_{12}.
Action and Uses: Please refer to "MERITENE Powder Action and Uses".
Administration and Dosage: Supplemental Feeding: 2 or 3 servings per day between meals and at bedtime. Total Feeding—Oral or Tube—Five 250 ml cans provide 1200 Calories and 100% of the U.S. RDA for protein and all known essential vitamins and minerals. Serve chilled for oral feeding and at room temperature for tube feeding. May be fed through nasogastric, gastrostomy or jejunostomy tubes. For use only under medical supervision.
How Supplied: In 250 ml "Easy-Open" individual serving cans in Vanilla, Chocolate and Egg Nog Flavors.

PRECISION HIGH NITROGEN DIET®
PRECISION LR DIET®
NUTRITIONALLY COMPLETE LOW-RESIDUE FOODS
For Oral or Tube Feeding

Composition, PRECISION HIGH NITROGEN DIET (Citrus Fruit Flavor): Maltodextrin, pasteurized egg white solids, sucrose, natural and artificial flavor, calcium glycerophosphate, potassium bitartrate, medium chain triglycerides, magnesium sulfate, citric acid, partially hydrogenated soybean oil, ammonium phosphate, choline bitartrate, mono and diglycerides, polysorbate 80, ascorbic acid, ferrous sulfate, artificial color, alpha tocopheryl acetate, zinc sulfate, copper gluconate, d-calcium pantothenate, niacin, manganese sulfate, vitamin A palmitate, pyridoxine hydrochloride, thiamin hydrochloride, riboflavin, d-biotin, potassium iodide, folic acid, phytonadione (vitamin K_1), vitamin D_2, cyanocobalamin.
Composition, PRECISION LR DIET (Fruit Flavors): Maltodextrin, pasteurized egg white solids, sucrose, calcium glycerophosphate, potassium bitartrate, magnesium sulfate, medium chain triglycerides, partially hydrogenated soybean oil, citric acid, natural and artificial flavor, ammonium phosphate, choline bitartrate, mono and diglycerides, polysorbate 80, ascorbic acid, ferrous sulfate, alpha tocopheryl acetate, zinc sulfate, niacin, artificial color, copper gluconate, d-calcium pantothenate, manganese sulfate, vitamin A palmitate, pyridoxine hydrochloride, thiamin hydrochloride, riboflavin, folic acid, d-biotin, potassium iodide, phytonadione (vitamin K_1), vitamin D_2, cyanocobalamin.
Action and Uses: PRECISION HIGH NITROGEN DIET is a nutritionally complete, low-residue food with high nitrogen content. PRECISION LR DIET is a nutritionally complete, low-residue food with a maintenance level of nitrogen. PRECISION HIGH NITROGEN DIET and PRECISION LR DIET are palatable and well-tolerated for total or supplemental feeding—oral or tube, containing no bulk, fiber, lactose, gluten or cholesterol.

Continued on next page

Doyle—Cont.

Administration: PRECISION HIGH NITROGEN DIET, ten servings (10—2.93 oz packets) provide 3000 Calories, 125 g of highest biological value protein (egg albumin) containing 20 g nitrogen and 100% of the U.S. RDA for protein and all known essential vitamins and minerals. PRECISION LR DIET, six servings (6—3 oz packets) provide 1900 Calories, 45 g of the highest biological value protein (egg albumin) containing 7.2 g nitrogen and 100% of the U.S. RDA for all known essential vitamins and minerals.
Oral Feeding, PRECISION HIGH NITROGEN DIET and PRECISION LR DIET: have patient drink slowly within 4 hours.
Tube Feeding, PRECISION HIGH NITROGEN DIET and PRECISION LR DIET: administer at a slow rate within 4 hours. May be fed through nasogastric, gastrostomy or jejunostomy tubes.
Precautions: PRECISION HIGH NITROGEN DIET and PRECISION LR DIET should not be administered parenterally. Provide additional water to meet fluid requirements, especially for patients with limited renal concentrating capacity, fever, dehydration or who are comatose. Postoperative feedings should not be initiated until peristalsis is re-established. The caloric contribution from carbohydrate in PRECISION HIGH NITROGEN DIET and PRECISION LR DIET may produce elevated blood sugar levels and these diets should not be used for patients with impaired ability to utilize carbohydrate. For children under 10, reduce amount fed downward to match recommended dietary allowances for the age group involved. For use only under medical supervision.
How Supplied: PRECISION HIGH NITROGEN DIET is available in cartons of 10—2.93 oz individual serving packets in Citrus Fruit and Vanilla Flavors. PRECISION LR DIET is available in cartons of 6—3 oz individual serving packets in Cherry, Lemon, Lime, Orange and Vanilla Flavors.

PRECISION ISOTONIC DIET®
NUTRITIONALLY BALANCED ISOTONIC FORMULA
For Oral or Tube Feeding

Composition (Vanilla Flavor): Glucose oligosaccharides, pasteurized egg white solids, sucrose, partially hydrogenated soybean oil with BHA, natural and artificial flavor, sodium caseinate, calcium phosphate, potassium phosphate, citric acid, carrageenan, mono and diglycerides, magnesium oxide, choline bitartrate, sodium iron pyrophosphate, ascorbic acid, alpha tocopheryl acetate, zinc sulfate, artificial color, vitamin A palmitate, niacin, copper gluconate, manganese sulfate, d-calcium pantothenate, pyridoxine hydrochloride, thiamin hydrochloride, riboflavin, folic acid, d-biotin, potassium iodide, phytonadione (vitamin K_1), vitamin D_2, cyanocobalamin.
Action and Uses: PRECISION ISOTONIC DIET is a nutritionally balanced formula with an osmolality isotonic to body fluids for excellent tolerance. It is formulated specifically for patients with a potential or actual intolerance to feedings.
Precautions: PRECISION ISOTONIC DIET should not be administered parenterally. Provide additional water to meet fluid requirements, especially for patients with limited renal concentrating capacity, fever, dehydration or who are comatose. Postoperative feedings should not be initiated until peristalsis is reestablished. The use of PRECISION ISOTONIC DIET should be determined on an individual basis for those patients with an impaired ability to utilize carbohydrate. For children under 10, reduce amount fed downward to match recommended dietary allowances for the age group involved. For use only under medical supervision.
Administration and Dosage: Six servings (6—2.06 oz packets) provide 1500 Calories, 45 g of highest biological value protein (egg albumin) containing 7.2 g nitrogen and 100% of the U.S. RDA for all known essential vitamins and minerals. Oral Feeding, have patient drink slowly within 4 hours. Tube Feeding, administer at a slow rate within 4 hours. May be fed through nasogastric, gastrostomy or jejunostomy tubes.
How Supplied: In 6—2.06 oz individual serving packets in Vanilla and Orange Flavors.

Drug Industries Co., Inc.
13700 WOODWARD AVE.
DETROIT, MICHIGAN 48203

AL-VITE ℞
(high potency vitamin formula with intrinsic factor)

Composition: Each capsule shaped tablet contains: Vitamin A Palmitate, 10,000 USP Units, Vitamin D_3 (activ. 7-Dehydrocholesterol), 400 USP Units, Vitamin E (from D-Alpha Tocopheryl Acetate Concentrate), 25 int. Units, Vitamin C (Ascorbic Acid), 200 mg., Vitamin B_1 (Thiamine Mononitrate), 20 mg., Vitamin B_2 (Riboflavin), 10 mg., Vitamin B_6 (pyridoxine Hydrochloride), 6 mg., Calcium Pantothenate, 20 mg., Niacinamide, 100 mg., Vitamin B_{12} with Intrinsic Factor Concentrate, ½ N.F. Unit (oral).
Action and Uses: Provides Vitamins A, D, C and B Complex factors in therapeutic amounts. For use in multiple vitamin deficiencies.
Administration and Dosage: One or two tablets daily or as directed by the physician.
Side Effects: None known when taken as directed.
Caution: This preparation is not a reliable substitute for parenterally administered cyanocobalamin (vitamin B_{12}) in the management of pernicious anemia. Periodic examinations and laboratory studies of pernicious anemia patients are essential.
Contraindications: Idiosyncrasy to any component.
How Supplied: Bottles of 100 and 500 light orange capsule shaped tablets.
[*Shown in Product Identification Section*]

BILAX CAPSULES™ ℞

Composition: Each Bilax Capsule contains:
Dehydrocholic Acid....................50 mg.
Dioctyl Sodium Sulfosuccinate............100 mg.
Action and Uses: The actions of Bilax are the result of the combination of complementary activities of its ingredients. Dioctyl Sodium Sulfosuccinate effects the surface tension and increases the water content of the stool, making it softer and therefore, easier to pass. The softening, combined with the laxative effect of Dehydrocholic Acid, alleviates symptoms of constipation.
Indications: A mild laxative and fecal softener designed as an aid in the treatment of functional constipation, particularly in the elderly.
Contraindications: Biliary tract obstruction, acute hepatitis, or sensitivity to any of its ingredients.
Precautions: Patients should be examined periodically to prevent fluid and electrolyte deficiencies due to excessive laxative effects or inadequate intake.
Administration and Dosage: One or two capsules three times daily with meals. This dosage should be reduced as the condition is relieved.
How Supplied: Bottles of 100.
Bottles of 500.
NDC 261-0157-01
[*Shown in Product Identification Section*]

HEMO-VITE ℞
(hematinic with vitamins and intrinsic factor)

Composition: Each tablet contains: Ferrous Fumarate, 240.0 mg., Copper Sulfate, 1.0 mg., Vitamin C (ascorbic acid) 150.0 mg., Vitamin B_1(Thiamine Hydrochloride) 5.0 mg., Vitamin B_2(Riboflavin), 5.0 mg., Vitamin B_6(Pyridoxine Hydrochloride), 1.0 mg., Calcium Pantothenate, 10.0 mg., Niacinamide, 50.0 mg., Folic Acid, .2 mg., Vitamin B_{12}(Crystalline with Intrinsic Factor Concentrate), ½ N.F. Unit (oral)
Action and Uses: For the treatment and prevention of iron deficiency anemias. Contains the well tolerated effective fumarate salt of iron.
Administration and Dosage: One or two tablets daily after meals or as directed by the physician.
Precautions: If any symptoms of intolerance appear, the medication should be discontinued. Prolonged administration requires closer medical supervision. Folic acid may obscure the symptoms of pernicious anemia while neurological destruction is progressive. Patients with pernicious anemia should be treated with parenteral B_{12}
HEMO-VITE should not be used in cases of serious folic acid deficiency where therapeutic amounts of folic acid are needed.
Side Effects: None known when used as directed.
Contraindications: Idiosyncrasy to any component.
How Supplied: Bottles of 100 and 500. Black capsule shaped tablets
[*Shown in Product Identification Section*]

SINOVAN TIMED™ ℞

Composition: Each black and clear timed capsule contains 8 mg. Chlorpheniramine Maleate, 20 mg. of Phenylephrine Hydrochloride, and 2.5 mg. of Methscopolamine Nitrate in a special base that provides a prolonged therapeutic effect of from about 10 to 12 hours.
Action and Uses: Provides temporary relief of the distressing symptoms accompanying the common cold, hay fever, and similar allergic conditions.
Contraindications: Pyloric obstruction, prostatic hypertrophy, intolerance to anticholinergic or antisecretory drugs, glaucoma, hepatitis, asthma, and toxemia of pregnancy.
Administration and Dosage: One capsule in the morning and at bedtime.
How Supplied: In bottles of 100 and 1000.

TRILAX™ ℞
(laxative, fecal softener, choleretic)

Composition: Each blue and white capsule contains:
Dioctyl Sodium Sulfosuccinate............200 mg.
Yellow Phenolphthalein..........................30 mg.
Dehydrocholic Acid.................................20 mg.
Action and Uses: Provides softening of the feces, homogenization, and laxative action without the discomfort of bowel distention, pain, cramping, or interference of vitamin absorption. For use in geriatric, obstetric, cardiac and surgical patients, and in those with hepatic or biliary disease or other conditions causing biliary stasis without complete mechanical obstruction of the common duct where increase in volume of fluid bile is desired.
Contraindications: TRILAX is contraindicated in patients with biliary tract obstruction and severe acute hepatitis.
Administration and Dosage: One or two capsules at bedtime for 2 or 3 days. Dosage may then be adjusted to meet individual needs.

How Supplied: Bottles of 100.
Bottles of 500.
NDC 261-0103-01
[*Shown in Product Identification Section*]

Eaton Laboratories

See NORWICH-EATON PHARMACEUTICALS
Professional Products Group

Elder, Inc., Thomas C.

P.O. BOX 125
HAMILTON, IN 46742

PHOTOSENSITIZERS

OXSORALEN® CAPSULES ℞

(8-MOP)® Brand of Methoxsalen

Caution: OXSORALEN (Methoxsalen, Elder) IS A POTENT DRUG.
READ ENTIRE BROCHURE BEFORE PRESCRIBING OR DISPENSING THIS MEDICATION.
Description: OXSORALEN Capsules, 10 mg. OXSORALEN (Methoxsalen, Elder) is the pure, crystalline form of the active principle contained in the fruit of *Ammi majus Linn.*

Indications

Based on a review of this drug by the National Academy of Sciences-National Research Council and/or other information, the FDA has classified the indications as follows:
Possibly Effective: Repigmentation of idiopathic vitiligo.
Final classification of the less-than-effective indications requires further investigation.

Actions: PIGMENT FORMATION WITH OXSORALEN (Methoxsalen, Elder). Normal pigmentation of skin is due to melanin produced in the cytoplasm of melanocytes, located in the basal layer of the epidermis at its junction with the dermis. Melanin is formed by the oxidation of tyrosine to DOPA (Dihydroxyphenylalanine), with tyrosinase as a catalyst. This enzymatic reaction can be activated by radiant energy in the form of ultraviolet light, preferably between 290 and 380 nanometers. The exact mechanism of the action of psoralens in the process of melanogenesis is not known. One group of investigators feels that the psoralens have a specific effect on the epidermis or, more specifically, on the melanocytes. Another group feels that the primary response to the psoralens is an inflammatory one, and that the process of melanogenesis is secondary.
Contraindications: Hepatic insufficiency and in those diseases associated with photosensitivity; such as porphyria, acute lupus erythematosis, hydroa, and polymorphic light eruptions. In leukoderma of infectious origin and in albinism, OXSORALEN (Methoxsalen, Elder) has no effect on pigmentation. It does, however, effect an increase in tolerance of the skin to sunlight. Prior clinical and investigative use has not been sufficient to establish safety in children under twelve years of age. No preparation with any photosensitizing capacity, internal or external, should be used concomitantly with OXSORALEN (Methoxsalen, Elder) therapy.
Warning: OXSORALEN is a potent drug. Read entire brochure before prescribing or dispensing this medication.
Precautions: The dosage of this medication should NOT be increased. Overdosage and/or overexposure may result in serious burning and blistering. To prevent harmful effects, the physician should carefully instruct the patient to adhere to the prescribed dosage schedule and procedure. In patients with vitiligo undergoing OXSORALEN (Methoxsalen, Elder) therapy, liver function tests should be performed monthly for the first few months and less frequently thereafter. While liver damage directly due to the drug has not been reported in human subjects, OXSORALEN (Methoxsalen, Elder) should be given in smaller daily doses or discontinued if impairment of liver function is suspected.
Adverse Reactions: Occasionally, there may occur gastric discomfort, nausea, nervousness, insomnia or depressed mood. To minimize gastric effect, the capsules may be taken with milk or a meal. Reduction in dosage will produce the same therapeutic effect but more slowly.
Dosage and Administration: (Adults and Children over 12)
VITILIGO: Two capsules daily in one dose. Taken two to four hours before measured periods of ultraviolet exposure. Start with five minutes. May be gradually increased to thirty minutes.
SUGGESTED SUN EXPOSURE GUIDE
The exposure time to sunlight should be limited according to the following plan:

	Basic Skin Color Light	Medium
Initial Exposure	15 min.	20 min.
Second Exposure	20 min.	25 min.
Third Exposure	25 min.	30 min.
Fourth Exposure	30 min.	35 min.
Subsequent Exposure:	Gradually increase exposure based on erythema and tenderness.	

Sunglasses should be worn during exposure and the lips protected with a light-screening lipstick.
SUN-LAMP EXPOSURE: Should be initiated according to directions of the sun-lamp manufacturer.
Accidental Overdosage: If an overdose of OXSORALEN (Methoxsalen, Elder) or ultraviolet light, has been taken, emesis should be encouraged. The individual should be kept in a darkened room for eight hours or until cutaneous reactions subside. The treatment for severe reactions resulting from overdosage or overexposure should follow accepted procedures for treatment of severe burns.
How Supplied: OXSORALEN Capsules, 10 mg. in bottles of 30 and 100.
Also Available: OXSORALEN Lotion (Methoxsalen 1%) in 1 ounce bottles for topical use.
[*Shown in Product Identification Section*]

TRISORALEN® ℞

(Trioxsalen-Elder)

To facilitate repigmentation in vitiligo, increase tolerance to solar exposure and enhance pigmentation.
Caution: THIS IS A POTENT DRUG.
Caution: Federal (U.S.A.) law prohibits dispensing without prescription.
Description: Trisoralen Tablets 5 mg.
TRISORALEN (TRIOXSALEN) ELDER is the first synthetic psoralen compound made available to the medical profession. It possesses greater activity than Methoxsalen, yet the LD 50 of (TRIOXSALEN) ELDER is six times that of Methoxsalen.
Actions: Pigment formation with TRISORALEN (TRIOXSALEN) ELDER
The normal pigmentation of the skin is due to melanin which is produced in the cytoplasm of the melanocytes located in the basal layers of the epidermis at its junction with the dermis. Melanin is formed by the oxidation of tyrosine to DOPA (Dihydroxyphenylalanine) with tyrosinase as catalyst. This enzymatic reaction, however, must be activated by radiant energy in the form of ultraviolet light, preferably between 2900 and 3800 angstroms (black light). The exact mechanism of the action of psoralens in the process of melanogenesis is not known. One group of investigators feel that the psoralens have a specific effect on the epidermis or, more specifically, on the melanocytes. Another group feels that the primary response to the psoralens is an inflammatory one and that the process of melanogenesis is secondary.
Indications: TRISORALEN (TRIOXSALEN) ELDER, taken approximately two hours before measured periods of exposure to ultraviolet facilitates:
1. Repigmentation of idiopathic vitiligo. Repigmentation, not equally reversible in every patient, will vary in completeness, time of onset, and duration. The rate of completeness of pigmentation with respect to locations of lesions, occurs more rapidly on fleshy regions, such as the face, abdomen, and buttocks, and less rapidly over bony areas such as the dorsum of the hands and feet. Repigmentation may begin after a few weeks; however, significant results may take as long as six to nine months, and repigmentation, at the optimum level, may, in some cases, require maintenance dosage to retain the new pigment. If follicular repigmentation is not apparent after three months of daily treatment, treatment should be discontinued.
2. Increasing tolerance to sunlight. In blond persons and those with fair complexions who suffer painful reactions when exposed to sunlight, TRISORALEN (TRIOXSALEN) ELDER aids in increasing resistance to solar damage. Certain persons who are allergic to sunlight or exhibit sun sensitivity may be benefited by the protective action of TRISORALEN (TRIOXSALEN) ELDER. In albinism, TRISORALEN (TRIOXSALEN) ELDER will increase the tolerance of the skin to sunlight, although no pigment is formed. This protective action seems to be related to the thickening of the horny layer and retention of melanin which produced a thickened melanized stratum corneum and formation of a stratum lucidum.
3. Enhancing pigmentation. The use of TRISORALEN (TRIOXSALEN) ELDER accelerates pigmentation only when the administration of the drug is followed by exposure of the skin to sunlight or ultraviolet irradiation. The increase in pigmentation is not immediate but occurs gradually within a few days of repeated exposure and may become equivalent in a degree to that achieved by a full summer of sun exposure. Since sufficient pigment will have been formed within two weeks of continuous therapy, the use of TRISORALEN (TRIOXSALEN) ELDER should not be continued beyond this period. Pigmentation can be maintained by periodic exposure to sunlight.
Contraindications: In those diseases associated with photosensitivity, such as porphyria, acute lupus erythematosus, or leukoderma of infectious origin. To date, the safety of this drug in young persons (12 and under), has not been established and is, therefore contraindicated. No preparation with any photosensitizing capacity, internal or external should be used concomitantly with TRISORALEN (TRIOXSALEN) ELDER therapy.
Warnings: TRISORALEN IS A POTENT DRUG.
Read entire brochure before prescribing or dispensing this medication. The dosage of this medication should not be increased.
The dosage of TRISORALEN (TRIOXSALEN) ELDER and exposure time should not be increased. Overdosage and/or overexposure may result in serious burning and blistering. When used to increase tolerance to sunlight or accelerate tanning, TRISORALEN (TRIOXSALEN) ELDER total dosage should not exceed 28 tab-

Continued on next page

Elder—Cont.

lets, taken in daily single doses of two tablets on a continuous or interrupted regimen. To prevent harmful effects, the physician should carefully instruct the patient to adhere to the prescribed dosage schedule and procedure.
Precautions: Accidental Overdosage: If an overdose of TRISORALEN (TRIOXSALEN) ELDER or ultraviolet light has been taken, emesis should be encouraged. The individual should be kept in a darkened room for eight hours or until cutaneous reactions subside. The treatment for severe reactions resulting from overdosage or overexposure should follow accepted procedures for treatment of severe burns. There have not been any clinical reports or tests to verify that more severe reactions may result from the concomitant ingestion of furocoumarin-containing food while on TRISORALEN (TRIOXSALEN) ELDER therapy; but the physician should warn the patient that taking limes, figs, parsley, parsnips, mustard, carrots and celery, might be dangerous.
Adverse Reactions and Side Effects: Severe burns can result from excessive sunlight or sun lamp ultraviolet exposure.
Occasionally, there may occur gastric discomfort; to minimize this gastric effect, the tablets may be taken with milk or after a meal. Some patients who are unable to tolerate 10 mg. will tolerate 5 mg. This dosage produces the same therapeutic effect but more slowly.
Dosage: (Adults and children over 12 years of age)
VITILIGO: Two tablets daily, taken two to four hours before measured periods of ultraviolet exposure or fluorescent black light. (See suggested sun exposure guide.)
TO INCREASE TOLERANCE TO SUNLIGHT AND/OR ENHANCE PIGMENTATION: Two tablets daily, taken two hours before measured periods of exposure to sun or ultraviolet irradiation. Not to be continued for longer than 14 days. The dosage should NOT be increased, as severe burning may occur. (See suggested sun exposure guide.)

SUGGESTED SUN EXPOSURE GUIDE
The exposure time to sunlight should be limited according to the following plan:

	Basic Skin Color Light	Medium
Initial Exposure	15 min.	20 min.
Second Exposure	20 min.	25 min.
Third Exposure	25 min.	30 min.
Fourth Exposure	30 min.	35 min.
Subsequent Exposure:	Gradually increase exposure based on erythema and tenderness.	

Sunglasses should be worn during exposure and the lips protected with a light-screening lipstick.

SUN-LAMP EXPOSURE: Should be initiated according to directions of the sun-lamp manufacturer.

How Supplied: TRISORALEN Tablets 5 mg. In Bottles of 28 and 100.
*U.S. Patent 3,201,421
[*Shown in Product Identification Section*]

SKIN BLEACHES

ELDOPAQUE–Forte®
(for use during the day)

Composition: 4% Hydroquinone in a hydrophilic, stabilized, nongreasy base.
Action and Uses: ELDOPAQUE-Forte is indicated in temporary bleaching of hyperpigmented skin blemishes such as freckles, old age spots, cholasma due to oral contraceptives, and other cosmetic liabilities due to melanin. Clinical evidence indicates that hydroquinone bleaching is faster, more dependable and easier if the treated area is protected from ultraviolet light. ELDOPAQUE-Forte is in an opaque base which occludes all light.
ELDOPAQUE-Forte therefore bleaches in full sunlight.
Administration and Dosage: Determine sensitivity before using: spread ELDOPAQUE-Forte to cover the treated area. Do not rub in. Make-up may then be applied over ELDOPAQUE-Forte. At night, remove it with a mild cleansing cream and rub ELDOQUIN-Forte into the skin.
Precautions: For external use only. If rash or irritation develops, discontinue treatment. Do not use on children under 12.
Contraindications: Do not apply to skin which is affected by prickly heat, depilatory application or is otherwise irritated. Do not use near eyes or open cuts.
How Supplied: In ½ ounce and 1 ounce tubes. Patient instruction sheets are also available.
Also Available: ELDOPAQUE® (2% Hydroquinone) in ½ ounce tubes.

ELDOQUIN–Forte™
(for use at night)

Composition: 4% Hydroquinone in a hydrophilic stabilized, nongreasy base.
Action and Uses: ELDOQUIN-Forte is indicated in temporary bleaching of hyperpigmented skin blemishes such as freckles, old age spots, cholasma due to oral contraceptives, and other forms of melanin hyperpigmentation.
Administration and Dosage: Determine sensitivity before using. Apply ELDOQUIN-Forte before bedtime to the affected areas rubbing it into the skin. During the day, use ELDOPAQUE-Forte®.
Precautions: For external use only. If rash or irritation develops, discontinue treatment. Do not use on children under 12.
Contraindications: Do not apply to skin which is affected by prickly heat, depilatory application or is otherwise irritated. Do not use near eyes or open cuts.
How Supplied: In tubes of ½ ounce and 1 ounce. Patient instruction sheets are also available.
Also Available: ELDOQUIN® (2% Hydroquinone) in ½ ounce and 1 ounce tubes; ELDOQUIN lotion (2% Hydroquinone) in ½ ounce bottles.

VITADYE™
(Cosmetic Cover for hypopigmented skin)

Composition: Certified dyes and dihydroxyacetone in a special solvent base.
Use: To cover light colored or white patches of skin. For external use only.
Administration: Apply Vitadye to hypopigmented areas with the applicator provided and let it dry for ten to fifteen minutes. To obtain a darker shade, additional applications may be made. Allow each application to dry before reapplying. After the desired shade is achieved, allow three hours before washing or rubbing the area. The artificial color will normally last two to four days. Use Vitadye to maintain the desired color.
Concomitant Therapy: Vitadye transmits most UVA radiation so it can be used concurrently with psoralens in vitiligo therapy.
Precaution: If rash or irritation of the skin develops, discontinue use and contact a physician.
Caution: Vitadye when wet will stain clothing.
Warning: Keep this and all drugs out of the reach of children. In case of accidental ingestion, seek professional assistance or contact a poison control center immediately. Avoid open flame.
How Supplied: Vitadye is available is a ½ fluid ounce package. NDC 0163-0413-35.

SUN SCREENS

PABANOL®
(Sunburn Preventative)
(5% PABA in Ethanol)

Composition: 5% Para Aminobenzoic Acid, 70% special denatured alcohol. Oil and perfume-free lotion.
Action and Uses: PABANOL combines with the stratum corneum to provide solar protection at 290-320 nanometers, resisting immersion and perspiration. In vitro tests demonstrated that the prolonged effectiveness of PABA in ethyl alcohol was greater than that of many other ultraviolet absorbing compounds tested. PABANOL protection results from the apparent adsorption of PABA onto intact epidermis and partial chemical conjugation of PABA with constituents of the horny layer.
Administration: Apply evenly to exposed areas and allow to dry before contact with clothing. Should staining result, wash with soap and water, not a synthetic detergent.
Caution: Individuals sensitive to PABA should not use PABANOL.
How Supplied: 4 Ounce Plastic Bottle.

RVPaba® LIP STICK
5% ParaAminobenzoic Acid (PABA) + Red Petrolatum (RVP)

Actions and Uses: RVPaba LIP STICK is a topical sunscreen and protectant for lips and small areas of exposed dermis. ParaAminobenzoic Acid (Paba) in Red Petrolatum (RVP) absorbs burning UV in a wide spectrum. RVPaba LIP STICK contains no perfumes or colors.
Dosage and Administration: Apply to lips and other small areas of skin as often as needed.
Caution: Individuals sensitive to Paba should not use RVPaba LIP STICK.
Supply: 1/7 oz. lipstick tubes.

RVP®
(Red Petrolatum-ELDER)

Composition: Red Petrolatum. Paraben and lanolin-free sunscreen. Now improved with 2.5% surfactants for easier application and easier removal with soap and water.
Action and Use: Topical sunscreen. Absorbs erythemal spectrum through 340 nanometers, but allows the tanning rays to pass. RVP gives sun protection and sun tanning when applied before sun exposure in the thinnest possible film.
Resists water and perspiration; safe around the eyes and on the lips.
How Supplied: 2 ounce tube.
Also Available: RVPlus™, 30% RVP emulsion in a base containing Micasorb to reflect light; in 2 ounce tubes.

RVPaque® (Opaque Sunshade)

Composition: Red Petrolatum, Zinc Oxide, and 2-Ethoxyethyl p-Methoxycinnamate in a greaseless, water-resistant base.
Action and Uses: RVPaque (pronounced aree-vee-pake) is NOT A SUNSCREEN, but an opaque sunshade. Unlike chemical light absorbers, RVPaque blocks all actinic rays; a .002 inch film prevents sunburning and tanning and protects the treated area through the visible light range. Tinted to blend with most skin tones.
Indications: RVPaque provides sun protection in any condition in which light is contraindicated; may be used adjunctively with depigmenting and bleaching agents, and for complete ultraviolet shielding of limited areas of denuded skin after dermabrasion, chemosurgery, cryosurgery, electrocoagulation, and in

certain diseases which require the exclusion of light.
To Use: Apply in a uniformly thin film which is visible to areas requiring exclusion of light. Reapply if removed by abrasion.
Contraindications: None reported; discontinue use if reaction develops.
How Supplied: ½ Ounce and 1¼ Ounce Tubes.

OTHER

PSORALITE®

Psoralite® is a portable UV system specifically designed for the photoactivation of photosensitizing drugs (e.g. Oxsoralen® and Trisoralen®) that are activated by radiation in the 320–400 nanometer range.
Precise dosages of UV radiation are delivered using a dual control system. A remote sensor measures the exact power output of the unit and Psoralite is shut off when the prescribed dose has been given. For added safety, a timing mechanism operates concurrently and acts as a back up system.
The unit is well ventilated, opens to a full 180° to allow easy entry and egress, and is mounted on castors to facilitate cleaning of the treatment area and movability from room to room. A 30 amp, 220 volt, single phase grounded circuit is required.
Psoralite is the registered trademark of the Paul B. Elder Company.

Elkins-Sinn, Inc.
A subsidiary of A. H. Robins Company
2 ESTERBROOK LANE
P.O. BOX 5483
CHERRY HILL, NJ 08034

Elkins-Sinn's DOSETTE® line offers a broad spectrum of injectable products in a variety of single-dose containers—DOSETTE vials, DOSETTE ampuls, and DOSETTE syringes. Easily adaptable to any hospital pharmacy set-up, the DOSETTE system combines easily identifiable, clearly printed product labeling with space-conserving packaging. Each DOSETTE single-dose container is characterized by product name and strength in large, bold-faced type, important usage and storage data, lot identification number, and expiration date.
Elkins-Sinn also produces a vast number of multiple dose vials. Listed below are some major ESI products. Additional syringe products are currently being marketed. For a complete catalog and price list, direct inquiries to Customer Service. For specific product information, direct inquiries to Technical Services Department.

DOSETTE SYRINGE

Dexamethasone Sodium Phosphate Injection, USP
 4 mg/ml
Digoxin Injection, USP
 0.25 mg/ml
Diphenhydramine Hydrochloride Injection, USP
 50 mg/ml
Hep-Lock (Heparin Sodium for IV Flush)
 100 USP U/ml
Heparin Sodium Injection, USP
 5000 USP U/ml
 10,000 USP U/ml
Hydroxyzine Hydrochloride Intramuscular Injection
 50 mg/ml

DOSETTE VIAL

Atropine Sulfate Injection, USP
 400 mcg/ml (0.4 mg-1/150 gr)
 1.0 mg/ml
 1.2 mg/ml
Codeine Phosphate Injection, USP
 30 mg/ml
 60 mg/ml
Cyanocobalamin Injection, USP (Vit. B-12)
 1 mg/ml (1000 mcg)
Dexamethasone Sodium Phosphate Injection, USP
 4 mg/ml
Dexpanthenol Injection
 500 mg/2 ml
Dextrose Injection, USP, 50%
Diphenhydramine Hydrochloride Injection, USP
 50 mg/ml
Hep-Lock (Heparin Sodium for IV Flush)
 10 USP U/ml
 100 USP U/ml
Heparin Sodium Injection, USP
 1000 USP U/ml
 5000 USP U/ml
 10,000 USP U/ml
Hydromorphone Hydrochloride Injection, NF
 2 mg/ml
Hydroxyzine Hydrochloride Intramuscular Injection
 50 mg/ml
Lidocaine Hydrochloride Injection, USP
 1% and 2%
Lidocaine Hydrochloride Injection for Intravenous Use in Cardiac Arrhythmias
 50 mg/5 ml
 100 mg/5 ml
 1 gram/25 ml
 2 grams/50 ml
Meperidine Hydrochloride Injection, USP
 25 mg/ml
 50 mg/ml
 75 mg/ml
 100 mg/ml
Mineral Oil, Sterile Light
Morphine Sulfate Injection, USP
 5 mg/ml
 8 mg/ml (⅛ gr)
 10 mg/ml (⅙ gr)
 15 mg/ml (¼ gr)
Pentobarbital Sodium Injection, USP
 100 mg/2 ml
Phenobarbital Sodium, USP (powder)
 65 mg and 130 mg
Phenobarbital Sodium Injection, USP
 65 mg/ml
 130 mg/ml
Phenytoin Sodium Injection
(formerly Sodium Diphenylhydantoin)
 100 mg/2 ml
 250 mg/5 ml
Scopolamine Hydrobromide Injection, USP
 400 mcg/ml (0.4 mg-1/150 gr)
Secobarbital Sodium, USP (powder) 100 mg
Thiamine Hydrochloride Injection, USP
 100 mg/ml
Vials, Sterile Empty
 2 ml

DOSETTE AMPUL

Aminophylline Injection, USP
 250 mg/10 ml
 500 mg/20 ml
Atropine Sulfate Injection, USP
 400 mcg/ml (0.4 mg-1/150 gr)
 400 mcg/0.5 ml (0.4 mg-1/150 gr)
Calcium Chloride Injection, USP, 10%
Calcium Gluconate Injection, USP, 10%
Chlorpromazine Hydrochloride Injection, USP
 25 mg/ml
 50 mg/2 ml
Cyanocobalamin Injection, USP (Vit. B-12)
 1 mg/ml (1000 mcg)
Digoxin Injection, USP
 0.5 mg/2 ml
Epinephrine Injection, USP, 1:1000
Isoproterenol Hydrochloride Injection, USP
 1:5000
Magnesium Sulfate Injection, USP, 50%
Meperidine Hydrochloride Injection, USP
 25 mg/ml
 50 mg/ml
 75 mg/ml
 100 mg/ml
Methylene Blue Injection, USP, 1%
Morphine Sulfate Injection, USP
 8 mg/ml (⅛ gr)
 10 mg/ml (⅙ gr)
 15 mg/ml (¼ gr)
Paraldehyde Sterile, USP
Phenytoin Sodium Injection
(formerly Sodium Diphenylhydantoin)
 100 mg/2 ml
 250 mg/5 ml
Potassium Chloride Injection, USP
 20 mEq/10 ml
 40 mEq/20 ml
Promethazine Hydrochloride Injection, USP
 25 mg/ml
 50 mg/ml
Sodium Chloride Injection, USP
Sotradecol® (Sodium Tetradecyl Sulfate)
 1% and 3%
Water for Injection, USP

MULTIPLE DOSE VIAL

Atropine Sulfate Injection, USP
 400 mcg/ml (0.4 mg-1/150 gr)
Chlorpromazine Hydrochloride Injection, USP
 25 mg/ml
Cyanocobalamin Injection, USP (Vit. B-12)
 1 mg/ml (1000 mcg)
Dexamethasone Sodium Phosphate Injection, USP
 4 mg/ml
Hydroxyzine Hydrochloride Intramuscular Injection
 50 mg/ml
Lidocaine Hydrochloride Injection, USP
 1% and 2%
Lidocaine Hydrochloride Injection, USP and Epinephrine 1:100,000
 1% and 2%
Metaraminol Bitartrate Injection, USP
 10 mg/ml-1%
Neostigmine Methylsulfate Injection, USP
 1:1000
Potassium Chloride Injection, USP
 60 mEq/30 ml, 20 mEq/10 ml, 30 mEq/15 ml, 40 mEq/20 ml
Procaine Hydrochloride Injection, USP
 1% and 2%
Sodium Chloride Injection, USP
Vials, Sterile Empty
 5 ml
 10 ml
 30 ml
Water for Injection, USP

SOTRADECOL® ℞
(Sodium Tetradecyl Sulfate)
For Intravenous Use Only

Description: Sotradecol (sodium tetradecyl sulfate) Injection is a sterile solution containing in each ml sodium tetradecyl sulfate 10 mg (1%) or 30 mg (3%) in Water for Injection with 0.02 ml benzyl alcohol and buffered with dibasic sodium phosphate. pH is adjusted to 7–8.1 with monobasic sodium phosphate or sodium hydroxide.
Actions: The product is a mild sclerosing agent which acts by irritation of the vein intimal endothelium.
Indications: Indicated in the treatment of small uncomplicated varicose veins of the lower extremities.
The benefit-to-risk ratio should be considered in selected patients who are great surgical risks due to conditions such as old age.
Contraindications: Contraindicated in acute superficial thrombophlebitis; underlying arterial disease; varicosities caused by abdominal and pelvic tumors, uncontrolled diabetes mellitus, thyrotoxicosis, tuberculosis, neoplasms, asthma, sepsis, blood dyscrasias, acute respiratory or skin diseases; and any condition which causes the patient to be bedridden. Do not use if precipitated.

Continued on next page

Elkins-Sinn—Cont.

Warnings: Sotradecol (sodium tetradecyl sulfate) should be used in pregnant women only when clearly needed. See Precautions.

Precautions: For varicosities, sclerotherapy should not be undertaken if tests such as the Trendelenberg and Perthes, and angiography show significant valvular or deep venous incompetence. The physician should bear in mind the fact that injection necrosis may result from direct injection of sclerosing agents. The drug should be administered by physicians who are familiar with an acceptable injection technique. Because of the danger of extension of thrombosis into the deep venous system, thorough pre-injection evaluation for valvular competency should be carried out, and slow injections with a small amount (not over 2 ml) of the preparation should be injected into the varicosity. In particular, deep venous patency must be determined by angiography and/or the Perthes test before sclerotherapy is undertaken.

No well controlled studies have been performed on patients taking anti-ovulatory agents. The physician must use judgment and evaluate any patient taking anti-ovulatory drugs prior to initiating treatment with Sotradecol (sodium tetradecyl sulfate). See Adverse Reactions.

Pregnancy category C. Adequate reproduction studies have not been performed in animals to determine whether this drug affects fertility in males or females, has teratogenic potential, or has other adverse effects on the fetus. There are no well-controlled studies in pregnant women, but investigational and marketing experience does not include any positive evidence of adverse effects on the fetus. Although there is no clearly defined risk, such experience cannot exclude the possibility of infrequent or subtle damage to the human fetus.

Adverse Reactions: Post-operative complication of sloughing may occur. A permanent discoloration, usually small and hardly noticeable may occur at the site of injection, and may be objectionable from a cosmetic viewpoint. Allergic reactions have been reported. Therefore, as a precaution against anaphylactic shock, it is recommended that an injection of 0.5 ml of the product into a varicosity be followed by observance of the patient for several hours before a larger injection is administered. The possibility of an anaphylactic reaction should always be kept in mind, and the physician should be prepared to treat it appropriately. In extreme emergencies, 0.25 ml of a 1:1000 solution of epinephrine (0.25 mg) intravenously should be used and side reactions controlled with antihistamines.

One death has been reported in a patient who received Sotradecol (sodium tetradecyl sulfate) and who had been receiving an anti-ovulatory agent. Another death (fatal pulmonary embolism) has been reported in a 36-year-old female treated with sodium tetradecyl acetate and who was not taking oral contraceptives.

Dosage and Administration: For intravenous use only. Do not use if precipitated. The strength of solution required depends on the size and degree of varicosity. In general, the 3% solution will be found most useful, with the 1% solution preferred for small varicosities. The dosage should be kept small, using 0.5 to 2 ml for each injection, and the maximum single treatment should not exceed 10 ml.

Literature describing various current techniques of administration is available upon request from the Technical Services Department.

How Supplied:
1% — 2 ml Dosette® Ampuls, 5's — #341514 (NDC 0641-1514-34)
3% — 2 ml Dosette® Ampuls, 5's — #341516 (NDC 0641-1516-34)

CAUTION: Federal law prohibits dispensing without prescription.

Endo Laboratories, Inc.
Subsidiary of the DuPont Company
1000 STEWART AVENUE
GARDEN CITY, NEW YORK 11530

Endo Inc.
MANATI, PUERTO RICO 00701
Subsidiary of Endo Laboratories, Inc.
Subsidiary of the DuPont Company

Products indicated by a dagger are products of Endo Inc.

PRODUCT IDENTIFICATION CODES

The Endo Logo and a code number is imprinted on all Endo tablets and a code number appears on the following capsules. This identifies each specific Endo product. Below is an alphabetical listing of each Endo product with the corresponding identification number.

PRODUCT	IDENT. NO.
AZENE® clorazepate monopotassium Capsules Ⓒ	
3.25 mg	501
6.5 mg	502
13 mg	503
COUMADIN® crystalline warfarin sodium Tablets	
2 mg	170
2½ mg	171
5 mg	172
7½ mg	173
10 mg	174
ENDECON® (decongestant, analgesic, antipyretic) Tablets	030
HYCODAN® (hydrocodone bitartrate/homatropine methylbromide combination) Tablets Ⓒ	042
HYCOMINE® COMPOUND (hydrocodone bitartrate/chlorpheniramine maleate/phenylephrine hydrochloride/APC combination) Tablets Ⓒ	048
MOBAN® molindone hydrochloride Tablets	
5 mg	072
10 mg	073
25 mg	074
PERCOBARB® (oxycodone/hexobarbital/APC combination) Capsules Ⓒ	570
†**PERCOCET® 5** (oxycodone/APAP combination) Tablets Ⓒ	127
†**PERCODAN®** (oxycodone/APC combination) Tablets Ⓒ	122
†**PERCODAN®-DEMI** (oxycodone/APC combination) Tablets Ⓒ	123
PERCOGESIC® (analgesic) Tablets	132
PERCOGESIC® with CODEINE (analgesic with codeine) Tablets Ⓒ	133
REMSED® promethazine hydrochloride Tablets	
50 mg	051
SYMMETREL® amantadine hydrochloride Capsules	
100 mg	105
VALPIN® 50 anisotropine methylbromide Tablets	
50 mg	161
VALPIN® 50-PB (anisotropine methylbromide with phenobarbital) Tablets	162

AZENE® Capsules Ⓒ
clorazepate monopotassium

Description: Chemically, AZENE® (clorazepate monopotassium) is a benzodiazepine. The empirical formula is $C_{16}H_{10}O_3N_2ClK$; the molecular weight is 352.82.

The compound occurs as a fine, off-white, practically odorless powder. It is insoluble in the common organic solvents, but very soluble in water. Aqueous solutions are unstable, clear, and slightly alkaline.

Actions: Pharmacologically, AZENE® has the characteristics of the benzodiazepines. It has depressant effects on the central nervous system. The primary metabolite, nordiazepam, reaches peak level in the blood stream at approximately 1 hour. The average serum half-life from bioavailability studies is approximately 2 days. The drug is metabolized in the liver and excreted primarily in the urine.

Indications: AZENE® is indicated for the symptomatic relief of anxiety associated with anxiety neurosis, in other psychoneuroses in which anxiety symptoms are prominent features, and as an adjunct in disease states in which anxiety is manifested.

AZENE® is indicated for the symptomatic relief of acute alcohol withdrawal.

The effectiveness of AZENE® in long-term use, that is, more than four months, has not been assessed by systematic clinical studies. The physician should reassess periodically the usefulness of the drug for the individual patient.

Contraindications: AZENE® is contraindicated in patients with a known hypersensitivity to the drug, and in those with acute narrow angle glaucoma.

Warnings: AZENE® is not recommended for use in depressive neuroses or in psychotic reactions.

Patients on AZENE® should be cautioned against engaging in hazardous occupations requiring mental alertness, such as operating dangerous machinery including motor vehicles.

Since AZENE® has a central nervous system depressant effect, patients should be advised against the simultaneous use of other CNS-depressant drugs, and cautioned that the effects of alcohol may be increased.

Because of the lack of sufficient clinical experience, AZENE® is not recommended for use in patients less than 18 years of age.

Physical and Psychological Dependence: Withdrawal symptoms (similar in character to those noted with barbiturates and alcohol) have occurred following abrupt discontinuance of clorazepates. Symptoms of nervousness, insomnia, irritability, diarrhea, muscle aches and memory impairment have followed abrupt withdrawal after long-term use of high dosage. Caution should be observed in patients who are considered to have a psychological potential for drug dependence.

Tolerance developed within 3 to 9 days in dogs. Evidence of drug dependence has been observed in dogs and rabbits which was characterized by convulsive seizures when the drug was abruptly withdrawn or the dose was reduced; the syndrome in dogs could be abolished by administration of clorazepate.

Usage in Pregnancy: **An increased risk of congenital malformations associated with the use of minor tranquilizers (chlordiazepoxide, diazepam, and meprobamate) during the first trimester of pregnancy has been suggested in several studies. AZENE®, a benzodiazepine derivative, has not been studied adequately to determine whether it, too, may be associated with an increased risk of fetal abnormality. Because use of these drugs is rarely a matter of urgency, their use during this period should almost always be avoided. The possibility that a woman of childbearing potential may be pregnant at the time of institution of therapy should be considered. Patients should be advised that if they become pregnant during therapy or intend to become pregnant they should communicate with their physician about the desirability of discontinuing the drug.**

Usage during Lactation: AZENE® should not be given to nursing mothers since it has been reported that nordiazepam is excreted in human breast milk.

Precautions: In those patients in which a degree of depression accompanies the anxiety, suicidal tendencies may be present and protective measures may be required. The least amount of drug that is feasible should be available to the patient.

Periodic blood counts and liver function tests are advisable for patients on AZENE® for prolonged periods. The usual precautions in treating patients with impaired renal or hepatic function should also be observed.

In elderly or debilitated patients, the initial dose should be small, and increments should be made gradually, in accordance with the response of the patient, to preclude ataxia or excessive sedation.

Adverse Reactions: The side effect most frequently reported with the use of benzodiazepines is drowsiness. Less commonly reported side effects are: dizziness, various gastrointestinal complaints, nervousness, blurred vision, dry mouth, headache, and mental confusion. Other side effects include insomnia, transient skin rashes, fatigue, ataxia, genitourinary complaints, irritability, diplopia, depression and slurred speech.

There have been reports of abnormal liver and kidney function tests and of decrease in hematocrit.

Decrease in systolic blood pressure has been observed with clorazepates.

Dosage and Administration: *For the symptomatic relief of anxiety:* AZENE® is administered orally in divided doses. The usual daily dose is 26 mg. The dose should be adjusted gradually within the range of 13 to 52 mg daily in accordance with the response of the patient. Drowsiness may occur at the initiation of treatment and with dosage increments. In elderly or debilitated patients it is advisable to initiate treatment at a daily dose of 6.5 to 13 mg. AZENE® capsules may also be administered as a single dose daily at bedtime; the recommended initial dose is 13 mg. After the initial dose, the response of the patient may require adjustment of subsequent dosage. Lower doses may be indicated in the elderly patient. Drowsiness may occur at the initiation of treatment and with dosage increments.

For the symptomatic relief of acute alcohol withdrawal: The following dosage schedule is recommended:

1st 24 hours (Day 1)	26 mg AZENE®, initially; followed by 26 to 52 mg in divided doses
2nd 24 hours (Day 2)	39 to 78 mg in divided doses
3rd 24 hours (Day 3)	19.5 to 39 mg in divided doses
Day 4	13 to 26 mg in divided doses

Thereafter, gradually reduce the daily dose to 6.5 to 13 mg. Discontinue drug therapy as soon as patient's condition is stable.

The maximum recommended total daily dose is 78 mg. Avoid excessive reductions in the total amount of drug administered on successive days.

Drug Interactions: If AZENE® is to be combined with other drugs acting on the central nervous system, careful consideration should be given to the pharmacology of the agents to be employed. Animal experience indicates that clorazepates prolong the sleeping time after hexobarbital or after ethyl alcohol, increase the inhibitory effects of chlorpromazine, but do not exhibit monoamine oxidase inhibition. Clinical studies have shown increased sedation with concurrent hypnotic medications. The actions of the benzodiazepines may be potentiated by barbiturates, narcotics, phenothiazines, monoamine oxidase inhibitors or other antidepressants.

If AZENE® is used to treat anxiety associated with somatic disease states, careful attention must be paid to possible drug interaction with concomitant medication.

Management of Overdosage: Overdosage is usually manifested by varying degrees of CNS depression ranging from slight sedation to coma. As in the management of overdosage with any drug, it should be borne in mind that multiple agents may have been taken.

There are no specific antidotes for the benzodiazepines. The treatment of overdosage should consist of the general measures employed in the management of overdosage of any CNS depressant. Gastric evacuation either by the induction of emesis, lavage, or both, should be performed immediately. General supportive care, including frequent monitoring of the vital signs and close observation of the patient, is indicated. Hypotension, though rarely reported, may occur with large overdoses. In such cases the use of agents such as Levophed† (levarterenol) or Aramine‡ (metaraminol) should be considered.

How Supplied: AZENE® is supplied as capsules in three dosage strengths: 3.25 mg capsules (light tan-colored) in bottles of 100 and 500. 6.5 mg capsules (orange-colored) in bottles of 100 and 500. 13 mg capsules (blue-colored) in bottles of 100.

6092-3

†Registered Trademark, Winthrop Laboratories

‡Registered Trademark, Merck Sharp & Dohme

AZENE® is an Endo registered U.S. trademark. Manufactured by Abbott Laboratories, North Chicago, IL 60064, for Endo Laboratories, Inc.

[*Shown in Product Identification Section*]

COUMADIN® ℞

crystalline warfarin sodium, U.S.P.
TABLETS
Anticoagulant

Description: COUMADIN® (crystalline warfarin sodium), a prothrombinopenic anticoagulant, is chemically crystalline sodium warfarin isopropanol clathrate. The crystallization of warfarin sodium virtually eliminates trace impurities present in amorphous warfarin sodium, thus achieving a crystalline product of the highest purity. Warfarin* is the coined generic name for 3-(α-Acetonylbenzyl)-4-hydroxycoumarin. On a dose-for-dose basis, COUMADIN® (crystalline warfarin sodium) is therapeutically equivalent to amorphous warfarin sodium.

Actions: COUMADIN® and other coumarin anticoagulants act by depressing synthesis in the liver of several factors which are known to be active in the coagulation mechanisms in a variety of diseases characterized by thromboembolic phenomena. The resultant **in vivo** effect is a sequential depression of Factors VII, IX, X and II. The degree of depression is dependent upon the dosage administered. Anticoagulants have no direct effect on an established thrombus, nor do they reverse ischemic tissue damage. However, once a thrombosis has occurred, anticoagulant treatment aims to prevent further extension of the formed clot and prevents secondary thromboembolic complications which may result in serious and possible fatal sequelae.

After oral administration, absorption is essentially complete, and maximal plasma concentrations are reached in 1 to 9 hours. Approximately 97% is bound to albumin within the plasma. COUMADIN® usually induces hypoprothrombinemia in 36 to 72 hours, and its duration of action may persist for 4 to 5 days, thus producing a smooth, long lasting response curve. Little is known of the metabolic pathways involved in the biotransformation of oral anticoagulants in man. However, their metabolites appear to be eliminated principally in the urine.

Indications: Based on a review of this drug by the National Academy of Sciences—National Research Council and/or other information, FDA has classified the indications as follows:

Effective: COUMADIN® is indicated for the prophylaxis and treatment of venous thrombosis and its extension, the treatment of atrial fibrillation with embolization, the prophylaxis and treatment of pulmonary embolism, and as an adjunct in the treatment of coronary occlusion.

"Possibly" effective: as an adjunct in the treatment of transient cerebral ischemic attacks.

Final classification of the less-than-effective indication requires further investigation.

Contraindications: Anticoagulation is contraindicated in any localized or general physical condition or personal circumstance in which the hazard of hemorrhage might be greater than its potential clinical benefits, such as:

Pregnancy—COUMADIN® is contraindicated in pregnancy because the drug passes through the placental barrier and may cause fatal hemorrhage to the fetus in utero. Furthermore, there have been reports of birth malformations in children born to mothers who have been treated with warfarin during pregnancy. Women of childbearing potential who are candidates for anticoagulant therapy should be carefully evaluated and the indications critically reviewed with the patient. If the patient becomes pregnant while taking this drug, she should be apprised of the potential risks to the fetus, and the possibility of termination of the pregnancy should be discussed in light of those risks.

Hemorrhagic tendencies or blood dyscrasias.

Recent or contemplated surgery of: (1) central nervous system; (2) eye; (3) traumatic surgery resulting in large open surfaces.

Bleeding tendencies associated with active ulceration or overt bleeding of: (1) gastrointestinal, genitourinary or respiratory tracts; (2) cerebrovascular hemorrhage; (3) aneurysms—cerebral, dissecting aorta; (4) pericarditis and pericardial effusions; (5) subacute bacterial endocarditis.

Threatened abortion, eclampsia and preeclampsia.

Inadequate laboratory facilities or unsupervised senility, alcoholism, psychosis; or lack of patient cooperation.

Spinal puncture and other diagnostic or therapeutic procedures with potential for uncontrollable bleeding.

Miscellaneous: major regional, lumbar block anesthesia and malignant hypertension.

Warnings: Warfarin sodium is a potent drug with a half-life of 2½ days; therefore its effects may become more pronounced as daily maintenance doses overlap. It cannot be emphasized too strongly that treatment of each patient is a highly individualized matter. Dosage should be controlled by periodic determinations of prothrombin time or other suitable coagulation tests. Determinations of whole blood clotting and bleeding times are not effective measures for control of therapy. Heparin prolongs the one-stage prothrombin time. Therefore, to obtain a valid prothrombin time when heparin and COUMADIN® are given together, a period of at least 5 hours should elapse after the last intravenous dose and 24 hours after the last subcutaneous dose of heparin, before blood is drawn.

Caution should be observed when warfarin sodium is administered in any situation or

Continued on next page

Endo—Cont.

physical condition where added risk of hemorrhage is present.

Administration of anticoagulants in the following conditions will be based upon clinical judgment in which the risks of anticoagulant therapy are weighed against the risk of thrombosis or embolization in untreated cases. The following may be associated with these increased risks:

Lactation—coumarins may pass into the milk of mothers and cause a prothrombinopenic state in the nursing infant.

Severe to moderate hepatic or renal insufficiency.

Infectious diseases or disturbances of intestinal flora—sprue, antibiotic therapy.

Trauma which may result in internal bleeding.

Surgery or trauma resulting in large exposed raw surfaces.

Indwelling catheters.

Severe to moderate hypertension.

Miscellaneous: polycythemia vera, vasculitis, severe diabetes, severe allergic and anaphylactic disorders.

Patients with congestive heart failure may become more sensitive to COUMADIN®, thereby requiring more frequent laboratory monitoring, and reduced doses of COUMADIN®.

Concurrent use of anticoagulants with streptokinase or urokinase is not recommended and may be hazardous. (Please note recommendations accompanying these preparations.)

Abrupt cessation of anticoagulant therapy is not generally recommended; taper dose gradually over three to four weeks.

Precautions: Periodic determination of prothrombin time or other suitable coagulation test is essential.

Numerous factors, alone or in combination, including travel, changes in diet, environment, physical state and medication may influence response of the patient to anticoagulants. It is generally good practice to monitor the patient's response with additional prothrombin time determinations in the period immediately after discharge from the hospital, and whenever other medications are initiated, discontinued or taken haphazardly. The following factors are listed for your reference; however, other factors may also affect the prothrombin response.

The following factors, alone or in combination, may be responsible for increased prothrombin time response:

ENDOGENOUS FACTORS: Carcinoma; collagen disease; congestive heart failure; diarrhea; elevated temperature; hepatic disorders—infectious hepatitis, jaundice; poor nutritional state; vitamin K deficiency—steatorrhea.

EXOGENOUS FACTORS: Alcohol†; allopurinol; aminosalicylic acid; anabolic steroids; antibiotics; bromelains; chloral hydrate†; chlorpropamide; chymotrypsin; cimetidine; cinchophen; clofibrate; COUMADIN® overdosage; dextran; dextrothyroxine; diazoxide; dietary deficiencies; diuretics†; disulfiram; drugs affecting blood elements; ethacrynic acid; glucagon; hepatotoxic drugs; indomethacin; inhalation anesthetics; mefenamic acid; methyldopa; methylphenidate; metronidazole; monoamine oxidase inhibitors; nalidixic acid; oxolinic acid; oxyphenbutazone; phenylbutazone; phenyramidol; prolonged hot weather; prolonged narcotics; quinidine; quinine; salicylates; sulfinpyrazone; sulfonamides, long acting; thyroid drugs; tolbutamide; triclofos sodium; trimethoprim/sulfamethoxazole; unreliable prothrombin time determinations.

†Increased and decreased prothrombin time responses have been reported.

The following factors, alone or in combination, may be responsible for decreased prothrombin time response:

ENDOGENOUS FACTORS: Diabetes mellitus; edema; hereditary resistance to coumarin therapy; hyperlipemia; hypothyroidism.

EXOGENOUS FACTORS: Adrenocortical steroids; alcohol†; antacids; antihistamines; barbiturates; chloral hydrate†; chlordiazepoxide; cholestyramine; COUMADIN® underdosage; diet high in vitamin K (vegetables, fish, fish oil, onions); diuretics†; ethchlorvynol; glutethimide; griseofulvin; haloperidol; meprobamate; oral contraceptives; paraldehyde; primidone; rifampin; unreliable prothrombin time determinations; vitamin C.

†Increased and decreased prothrombin time responses have been reported.

A patient may be exposed to a combination of the above factors, some of which may increase and some decrease his sensitivity to COUMADIN®. Because the net effect on his prothrombin time response may be unpredictable under these circumstances, more frequent laboratory monitoring is advisable.

Drugs not yet shown to interact or not to interact with coumarins are best regarded with suspicion, and when their administration is started or stopped, the prothrombin time should be determined more often than usual.

Coumarins also affect the action of other drugs. Hypoglycemic agents (chlorpropamide and tolbutamide) and anticonvulsants (diphenylhydantoin and phenobarbital) may accumulate in the body as a result of interference with either their metabolism or excretion.

Adverse Reactions: Potential side effects of COUMADIN® (crystalline warfarin sodium) include:

1. Minor or major hemorrhage from any tissue or organ—which is an extension of the physiologic activity of prothrombinopenia. The signs and symptoms will vary according to the location and degree or extent of the bleeding. Therefore the possibility of hemorrhage should be considered in evaluating the condition of any anticoagulated patient with complaints which do not indicate an obvious diagnosis. Bleeding during anticoagulant therapy does not always correlate with prothrombin activity. (See TREATMENT FOR OVERDOSAGE.) Bleeding which occurs when the prothrombin time is within the therapeutic range warrants diagnostic investigation since it may unmask a previously unsuspected lesion, e.g. tumor, ulcer etc.
2. Side effects other than hemorrhage are infrequent and consist of alopecia, urticaria, dermatitis, fever, nausea, diarrhea, abdominal cramping, a syndrome called "purple toes", hypersensitivity reactions and reaction consisting of hemorrhagic infarction and necrosis of the skin.
3. Priapism has been associated with anticoagulant administration however, a causal relationship has not been established.

Dosage and Laboratory Control: The aim of anticoagulant therapy is to impede the coagulation or clotting mechanism to such an extent that thrombosis will not occur, but at the same time avoiding such extensive impairment as might produce spontaneous bleeding. Effective therapeutic levels with minimal complications can best be achieved in cooperative and well-instructed patients, who keep the doctor informed of their status between visits. COUMADIN® patient aids are available to physicians on request.

The administration and dosage of COUMADIN® must be individualized for each patient according to the particular patient's sensitivity to the drug as indicated by the prothrombin time. The prothrombin time reflects the depression of vitamin K dependent Factors VII, X and II. These factors, in addition to Factor IX, are affected by coumarin anticoagulants. There are several modifications of the Quick one-stage prothrombin time and the physician should become familiar with the specific method used in his laboratory.

Administration of COUMADIN® should be gauged according to prothrombin time determinations by a suitable method. The blood prothrombin time should usually be determined daily after the administration of the initial dose until prothrombin time results stabilize in the therapeutic range. Intervals between subsequent prothrombin time determinations should be based upon the physician's judgment of the patient's reliability and response to warfarin in order to maintain the individual within the therapeutic range. Acceptable intervals for prothrombin time determinations have usually fallen within the range of one to four weeks. Satisfactory levels for maintenance of therapeutic anticoagulation are $1\frac{1}{2}$ to $2\frac{1}{2}$ times the normal prothrombin time (e.g. 18 to 30 seconds, with a control of 12 seconds).

Induction—40 to 60 mg for average adult or 20 to 30 mg for elderly and/or debilitated patients for one dose only administered orally, intravenously or intramuscularly.

Alternatively, the large priming dose may be decreased for all patients to minimize the possibility of excessive increases in prothrombin time. Induction may be initiated with 10 to 15 mg daily and thereafter (usually 2 or 3 days) adjusted according to prothrombin time response. The basis for the no-loading dose regimen is that the depression of Factors II, IX and X are not accelerated by the administration of a loading dose.

Maintenance—Most patients are satisfactorily maintained at a dose of 2 to 10 mg daily. Flexibility of dosage is provided by breaking scored tablets in half. The individual dose and interval should be gauged by the patient's prothrombin response.

Duration of therapy—The duration of therapy in each patient should be individualized. In general, anticoagulant therapy should be continued until the danger of thrombosis and embolism has passed.

Treatment during dentistry and surgery—The management of patients who undergo dental and surgical procedures requires close liaison between attending physicians, surgeons and dentists. Interruption of anticoagulant therapy may precipitate thromboembolism, and conversely, if anticoagulants are maintained at full doses, some patients may hemorrhage excessively. If it is elected to administer anticoagulants prior to, during, or immediately following dental or surgical procedures, it is recommended that the dosage of COUMADIN® be adjusted to maintain the prothrombin time at approximately $1\frac{1}{2}$ to $2\frac{1}{2}$ times the control level. The operative site should be sufficiently limited to permit the effective use of local procedures for hemostasis including absorbable hemostatic agents, sutures, and pressure dressings if necessary. Under these conditions dental and surgical procedures may be performed without undue risk of hemorrhage.

COUMADIN® with Heparin — Since a delay intervenes between the administration of the initial dose and the therapeutic prolongation of prothrombin time, it may be advisable in emergency situations to administer sodium heparin initially along with COUMADIN®. The initial dose of heparin and injectable COUMADIN® may be administered together in the same syringe. It should be noted that heparin may affect the prothrombin time, and therefore, when patients are receiving both heparin and COUMADIN®, the blood sample for prothrombin time determination should be drawn just prior to the next heparin dosage, at least 5 hours after the last intravenous injection or 24 hours after the last subcutaneous injection.

Treatment For Overdosage: Excessive prothrombinopenia, with or without bleeding, is readily controlled by discontinuing COUMADIN® (crystalline warfarin sodium), and if necessary, the oral or parenteral administration of vitamin K_1. The appearance of mi-

croscopic hematuria, excessive menstrual bleeding, melena, petechiae or oozing from nicks made while shaving are early manifestations of hypoprothrombinemia beyond a safe and satisfactory level.
In excessive prothrombinopenia with mild or no bleeding, omission of one or more doses of COUMADIN® may suffice; and if necessary, small doses of vitamin K_1 orally, 2.5 to 10 mg, will usually correct the problem.
If minor bleeding persists, or progresses to frank bleeding, vitamin K_1 in doses of 5 to 25 mg may be given parenterally. (Please note recommendations accompanying vitamin K preparations prior to use.)
Fresh whole blood transfusions should be considered in cases of severe bleeding or prothrombinopenic states unresponsive to vitamin K_1.
Resumption of COUMADIN® administration reverses the effect of vitamin K_1, and a therapeutic hypoprothrombinemia level can again be obtained.
Supplied: Tablets: COUMADIN® (crystalline warfarin sodium). For oral use, single scored, imprinted numerically with potency as follows:
2 mg lavender 5 mg peach 10 mg white
2½ mg orange 7½ mg yellow
In bottles of 100 and 1000.
Also available in Hospital Unit-Dose blister package of 100.
Injection: Available as single injection units of amorphous warfarin sodium lyophilized for intravenous or intramuscular use in a box of 6 units for use immediately after reconstitution.
50 mg: Unit consists of 1 vial, 50 mg; sodium chloride, 10 mg; thimerosal, 0.2 mg. pH is adjusted with sodium hydroxide; accompanied by a 2 ml ampul Sterile Water for Injection.
Sterile Water for Injection contains no antimicrobial or other substance, and it is not suitable for intravascular injection without first having been made approximately isotonic by the addition of a suitable solute. Use only for reconstitution of the lyophilized product.
6037-14

---

*Present as crystalline sodium warfarin isopropanol clathrate.
Licensed by Wisconsin Alumni Research Foundation.
COUMADIN® is an Endo Registered U.S. Trademark; U.S. Pat. No. 3,077,481 (Reissue No. 25,866)
[*Shown in Product Identification Section*]

HYCODAN®
Tablets and Syrup

Description: Each HYCODAN® Tablet or teaspoonful (5 ml) contains:
Hydrocodone bitartrate .... 5 mg
WARNING: May be habit forming
Homatropine methylbromide.............. 1.5 mg
Hydrocodone is 7, 8-dihydrocodeinone, a derivative of codeine.
Actions: Hydrocodone is a centrally acting narcotic antitussive providing cough relief for up to 6 hours.

> **Indications:** Based on a review of this drug by the National Academy of Sciences-National Research Council and/or other information, FDA has classified HYCODAN® Tablets and Syrup as follows:
> "Probably" effective: for the symptomatic relief of cough.
> Final classification of this "probably" effective indication requires further investigation.

Contraindications: HYCODAN® should not be used in patients with glaucoma or hypersensitivity to hydrocodone or homatropine methylbromide.

HYCODAN® DOSAGE AND ADMINISTRATION
Usual Dosage

	TABLETS Initial dose	TABLETS Maximum single dose	SYRUP teaspoonful (5 ml) Initial dose	SYRUP teaspoonful (5 ml) Maximum single dose
Adults	1	3	1 tsp.	3 tsps.
Children				
over 12 years	1	2	1 tsp.	2 tsps.
2 to 12 years	½	1	½ tsp.	1 tsp.
under 2 years	¼	¼	¼ tsp.	¼ tsp.

Warnings: HYCODAN® should be prescribed and administered with the same degree of caution appropriate for the use of other oral narcotic-containing medications since it can produce drug dependence and, therefore, has the potential for abuse. Patients should be warned not to drive a car or operate machinery if they become drowsy or show impaired mental and/or physical abilities while taking HYCODAN®. Patients receiving narcotic analgesics, phenothiazines, other tranquilizers, sedative-hypnotics or other central nervous system depressants (including alcohol) concomitantly with HYCODAN® may exhibit an additive central nervous system depression. When such combined therapy is contemplated, the dose of one or both agents should be reduced.
Precautions: Before prescribing medication to suppress or modify cough, it is important to ascertain that the underlying cause of cough is identified, that modification of cough does not increase the risk of clinical or physiologic complications, and that appropriate therapy for the primary disease is provided.
Adverse Reactions: Adverse reactions when they occur include sedation, nausea, vomiting and constipation.
Dosage and Administration: HYCODAN® should be taken after meals and at bedtime, not less than 4 hours apart. Treatment should be started with the suggested initial dose and subsequent doses adjusted if required.
[See table above].
Drug Interactions: The central nervous system depressant effects of HYCODAN® may be additive with that of other central nervous system depressants. See WARNINGS.
Management of Overdosage:
Signs and Symptoms: Serious overdose with HYCODAN® may be characterized by respiratory depression, extreme somnolence progressing to stupor or coma, skeletal muscle flaccidity, cold and clammy skin, and sometimes bradycardia and hypotension. In severe overdosage, apnea, circulatory collapse, cardiac arrest and death may occur. The ingestion of very large amounts of HYCODAN® may, in addition, result in acute homatropine intoxication.
Treatment: Primary attention should be given to the reestablishment of adequate respiratory exchange through provision of a patent airway and the institution of assisted or controlled ventilation. The narcotic antagonists naloxone, nalorphine or levallorphan are specific antidotes against respiratory depression which may result from overdosage or unusual sensitivity to narcotics, including hydrocodone. An appropriate dose of one of these antagonists should be administered, preferably by the intravenous route, simultaneously with efforts at respiratory resuscitation. Since the duration of action of hydrocodone may exceed that of the antagonist, the patient should be kept under continued surveillance and repeated doses of the antagonist should be administered as needed to maintain adequate respiration. Oxygen, intravenous fluids, vasopressors and other supportive measures should be employed as indicated, including treatment for anticholinergic drug intoxication. Gastric emptying may be useful in removing unabsorbed drug. Activated charcoal may be of benefit.
How Supplied: As white, scored tablets in bottles of 100, 500 and 1000 or as a red-colored, wild cherry flavored syrup in bottles of one pint and one gallon.
Oral prescription where permitted by State law.
HYCODAN® is an Endo registered U.S. trademark.
6014-8

HYCOMINE® PEDIATRIC
Syrup

Description: Each teaspoonful (5 ml) contains:
Hydrocodone bitartrate ....2.5 mg
(WARNING: May be habit forming)
Phenylpropanolamine hydrochloride. .12.5 mg
Actions: Hydrocodone bitartrate is an effective semisynthetic narcotic antitussive. Phenylpropanolamine is a sympathomimetic amine which provides nasal decongestion.
Indications: To control cough and to provide symptomatic relief of congestion in the upper respiratory tract due to the common cold, pharyngitis, tracheitis, and bronchitis.
Contraindications: Hypersensitivity to any component of the drug.
Precautions: Use with caution in diabetes, hyperthyroidism, hypertension and cardiovascular disease. Since drowsiness and dizziness may occur, patients should be cautioned about activities requiring alertness.
Before prescribing antitussive medication to suppress or modify cough, it is important to ascertain that the underlying cause of the cough is identified, that modification of the cough does not increase the risk of clinical or physiologic complications, and that appropriate therapy for the primary disease is provided.
Adverse Reactions: HYCOMINE® Pediatric Syrup is generally well tolerated. Occasional drowsiness, cardiac palpitation, dizziness, nervousness or gastrointestinal upset may occur.
Dosage and Administration: Usual Dosage: (Age 6–12 yrs.) 1 teaspoonful after meals and at bedtime not less than 4 hours apart (not to exceed 6 teaspoonfuls in a 24 hour period).
How Supplied: As a green-colored, fruit-flavored syrup in bottles of one pint and one gallon.
Oral prescription where permitted by State Law.
HYCOMINE® is an Endo registered U.S. trademark.
ODP

HYCOMINE®
Syrup

Description: Each teaspoonful (5 ml) contains:
Hydrocodone bitartrate ....5 mg
(WARNING: May be habit forming)
Phenylpropanolamine hydrochloride ....25 mg
Actions: Hydrocodone bitartrate is an effective semisynthetic narcotic antitussive.

Continued on next page

Endo—Cont.

Phenylpropanolamine is a sympathomimetic amine which provides nasal decongestion.

Indications: To control cough and to provide symptomatic relief of congestion in the upper respiratory tract due to the common cold, pharyngitis, tracheitis, and bronchitis.

Contraindications: Hypersensitivity to any component of the drug. Should not be used in patients receiving monoamine oxidase inhibitors.

Precautions: Use with caution in diabetes, hyperthyroidism, hypertension, cardiovascular disease and in the aged. Since drowsiness and dizziness may occur, patients should be cautioned about driving or operating machinery.

Before prescribing antitussive medication to suppress or modify cough, it is important to ascertain that the underlying cause of the cough is identified, that modification of the cough does not increase the risk of clinical or physiologic complications, and that appropriate therapy for the primary disease is provided.

Adverse Reactions: HYCOMINE® Syrup is generally well tolerated. Occasional drowsiness, cardiac palpitation, dizziness, nervousness, or gastrointestinal upset may occur.

Dosage and Administration: Usual Adult Dose: 1 teaspoonful after meals and at bedtime, not less than 4 hours apart (not to exceed 6 teaspoonfuls in a 24 hour period).

How Supplied: As an orange-colored, fruit-flavored syrup in bottles of one pint and one gallon.

Oral prescription where permitted by State Law.

HYCOMINE® is an Endo registered U.S. trademark.

NA

HYCOTUSS® EXPECTORANT Ⓒ ℞

Description: Each teaspoonful (5 ml) contains:

Hydrocodone bitartrate ....5 mg
WARNING: May be habit forming
Guaifenesin ....100 mg
Alcohol U.S.P. 10% v/v

Hydrocodone is 7, 8-dihydrocodeinone, a derivative of codeine.

Actions: Hydrocodone is a centrally acting narcotic antitussive providing cough relief for up to 6 hours. Guaifenesin exerts its expectorant action by producing a less viscous exudate thereby facilitating its expulsion.

Indications: Indicated for the symptomatic relief of coughs. Especially useful in unproductive coughs associated with upper and lower respiratory tract congestion.

Contraindications: HYCOTUSS Expectorant should not be used in patients with hypersensitivity to hydrocodone or guaifenesin.

Warnings: HYCOTUSS Expectorant should be prescribed and administered with the same degree of caution appropriate for the use of other oral narcotic-containing medications since it can produce drug dependence and, therefore, has the potential for abuse. Patients should be warned not to drive a car or operate machinery if they become drowsy or show impaired mental and/or physical abilities while taking HYCOTUSS Expectorant. Patients receiving narcotic analgesics, phenothiazines, other tranquilizers, sedative-hypnotics or other central nervous system depressants (including alcohol) concomitantly with HYCOTUSS Expectorant may exhibit an additive central nervous system depression. When such combined therapy is contemplated, the dose of one or both agents should be reduced.

Precautions: Before prescribing medication to suppress or modify cough, it is important to ascertain that the underlying cause of cough is identified, that modification of cough does not increase the risk of clinical or physiologic complications, and that appropriate therapy for the primary disease is provided.

Adverse Reactions: Adverse reactions, when they occur, include sedation, nausea, vomiting and constipation.

Dosage and Administration: HYCOTUSS Expectorant should be taken after meals and at bedtime, not less than 4 hours apart. Treatment should be started with the suggested initial dose and subsequent doses adjusted if required.

HYCOTUSS Expectorant Usual Dosage
SYRUP
teaspoonful (5ml)

	Initial dose	Maximum single dose
Adults	1 tsp.	3 tsps.
Children		
over 12 years	1 tsp.	2 tsps.
2 to 12 years	½ tsp.	1 tsp.
under 2 years	Dosage should be calculated as Hydrocodone, 0.3 mg/kg/24 hrs., divided into four equal doses.	

Drug Interactions: The central nervous system depressant effects of HYCOTUSS Expectorant may be additive with that of other central nervous system depressants. See WARNINGS.

Management of Overdosage:

Signs and Symptoms: Serious overdose with HYCOTUSS Expectorant may be characterized by respiratory depression, extreme somnolence progressing to stupor or coma, skeletal muscle flaccidity, cold and clammy skin, and sometimes bradycardia and hypotension. In severe overdosage, apnea, circulatory collapse, cardiac arrest and death may occur.

Treatment: Primary attention should be given to the reestablishment of adequate respiratory exchange through provision of a patent airway and the institution of assisted or controlled ventilation. The narcotic antagonists naloxone, nalorphine or levallorphan are specific antidotes against respiratory depression which may result from overdosage or unusual sensitivity to narcotics, including hydrocodone. An appropriate dose of one of these antagonists should be administered, preferably by the intravenous route, simultaneously with efforts at respiratory resuscitation. Since the duration of action of hydrocodone may exceed that of the antagonist, the patient should be kept under continued surveillance and repeated doses of the antagonist should be administered as needed to maintain adequate respiration. Oxygen, intravenous fluids, vasopressors and other supportive measures should be employed as indicated. Gastric emptying may be useful in removing unabsorbed drug. Activated charcoal may be of benefit.

How Supplied: In bottles of one pint as an orange syrup with butterscotch flavor.

Oral prescription where permitted by State law.

HYCOTUSS is an Endo Registered U.S. Trademark.

6070-3

MOBAN® ℞
molindone hydrochloride
Tablets

Description: MOBAN® (molindone hydrochloride) is a dihydroindolone compound which is not structurally related to the phenothiazines, the butyrophenones or the thioxanthenes.

MOBAN® is 3-ethyl-6, 7-dihydro-2-methyl-5-(morpholinomethyl) indol-4(5H)-one hydrochloride. It is a white crystalline powder, freely soluble in water and alcohol and has a molecular weight of 312.67.

Actions: MOBAN® (molindone hydrochloride) has a pharmacological profile in laboratory animals which predominantly resembles that of major tranquilizers causing reduction of spontaneous locomotion and aggressiveness, suppression of a conditioned response and antagonism of the bizarre stereotyped behavior and hyperactivity induced by amphetamines. In addition, MOBAN® antagonizes the depression caused by the tranquilizing agent tetrabenazine.

In human clinical studies tranquilization is achieved in the absence of muscle relaxing or incoordinating effects. Based on EEG studies, MOBAN® exerts its effect on the ascending reticular activating system.

Human metabolic studies show MOBAN® (molindone hydrochloride) to be rapidly absorbed and metabolized when given orally. Unmetabolized drug reached a peak blood level at 1.5 hours. Pharmacological effect from a single oral dose persists for 24–36 hours. There are 36 recognized metabolites with less than 2–3% unmetabolized MOBAN® being excreted in urine and feces.

Indications: MOBAN® (molindone hydrochloride) is indicated in the management of the manifestations of schizophrenia.

Contraindications: MOBAN® (molindone hydrochloride) is contraindicated in severe central nervous system depression (alcohol, barbiturates, narcotics, etc.) or comatose states, and in patients with known hypersensitivity to the drug.

Warnings:

Usage in Pregnancy: Studies in pregnant patients have not been carried out. Reproduction studies have been performed in the following animals:

Pregnant Rats oral dose—	20 mg/kg/day —10 days
no adverse effect	
	40 mg/kg/day —10 days
no adverse effect	
Pregnant Mice oral dose—	20 mg/kg/day —10 days
slight increase resorptions	
	40 mg/kg/day —10 days
slight increase resorptions	
Pregnant Rabbits oral dose—	5 mg/kg/day —12 days
no adverse effect	
	10 mg/kg/day —12 days
no adverse effect	
	20 mg/kg/day —12 days
no adverse effect	

Animal reproductive studies have not demonstrated a teratogenic potential. The anticipated benefits must be weighed against the unknown risks to the fetus if used in pregnant patients.

Nursing Mothers: Data are not available on the content of MOBAN® (molindone hydrochloride) in the milk of nursing mothers.

Usage in Children: Use of MOBAN® (molindone hydrochloride) in children below the age of twelve years is not recommended because safe and effective conditions for its usage have not been established.

Moban has not been shown effective in the management of behavorial complications in patients with mental retardation.

Precautions: Some patients receiving MOBAN® (molindone hydrochloride) may note drowsiness initially and they should be advised against activities requiring mental alertness until their response to the drug has been established.

Increased activity has been noted in patients receiving MOBAN®. Caution should be exercised where increased activity may be harmful. MOBAN® does not lower the seizure threshold in experimental animals to the degree noted with more sedating antipsychotic drugs. However, in humans convulsive seizures have been reported in a few instances.

The physician should be aware that this tablet preparation contains calcium sulfate as an excipient and that calcium ions may interfere with the absorption of preparations containing phenytoin sodium and tetracyclines.

MOBAN® has an antiemetic effect in animals. A similar effect may occur in humans and may obscure signs of intestinal obstruction or brain tumor.

Adverse Reactions:

CNS Effects

The most frequently occurring effect is initial drowsiness that generally subsides with continued usage of the drug or lowering of the dose.

Noted less frequently were depression, hyperactivity and euphoria.

Neurological

Extrapyramidal Reactions

Extrapyramidal reactions noted below may occur in susceptible individuals and are usually reversible with appropriate management.

Akathisia

Motor restlessness may occur early.

Parkinson Syndrome

Akinesia, characterized by rigidity, immobility and reduction of voluntary movements and tremor, have been observed. Occurrence is less frequent than akathisia.

Dystonic Syndrome

Prolonged abnormal contractions of muscle groups occur infrequently. These symptoms may be managed by the addition of a synthetic antiparkinson agent (other than L-dopa), small doses of sedative drugs, and/or reduction in dosage.

Autonomic Nervous System

Occasionally blurring of vision, tachycardia, nausea, dry mouth and salivation have been reported. Urinary retention and constipation may occur particularly if anticholinergic drugs are used to treat extrapyramidal symptoms.

Hematological

There have been rare reports of leucopenia and leucocytosis. If such reactions occur, treatment with MOBAN® may continue if clinical symptoms are absent. Alterations of blood glucose, liver function tests, B.U.N., and red blood cells have not been considered clinically significant.

Metabolic and Endocrine Effects

Alteration of thyroid function has not been significant. Amenorrhea has been reported infrequently. Resumption of menses in previously amenorrheic women has been reported. Initially heavy menses may occur. Galactorrhea and gynecomastia have been reported infrequently. Increase in libido has been noted in some patients. Impotence has not been reported. Although both weight gain and weight loss have been in the direction of normal or ideal weight, excessive weight gain has not occurred with MOBAN®.

Cardiovascular

Rare, transient, non-specific T wave changes have been reported on E.K.G. Association with a clinical syndrome has not been established. Rarely has significant hypotension been reported.

Ophthalmological

Lens opacities and pigmentary retinopathy have not been reported where patients have received MOBAN® (molindone hydrochloride). In some patients, phenothiazine induced lenticular opacities have resolved following discontinuation of the phenothiazine while continuing therapy with MOBAN®.

Skin

Early, non-specific skin rash, probably of allergic origin, has occasionally been reported. Skin pigmentation has not been seen with MOBAN® usage alone.

MOBAN® (molindone hydrochloride) has certain pharmacological similarities to other antipsychotic agents. Because adverse reactions are often extensions of the pharmacological activity of a drug, all of the known pharmacological effects associated with other antipsychotic drugs should be kept in mind when MOBAN® is used. Upon abrupt withdrawal after prolonged high dosage an abstinence syndrome has not been noted.

Tardive Dyskinesia

Although rarely reported with MOBAN® (molindone hydrochloride) symptoms were reversible upon discontinuation of therapy.

Tardive dyskinesia associated with other agents has appeared in some patients on long-term therapy and has also appeared after drug therapy has been discontinued. The risk appears to be greater in elderly patients on high-dose therapy, especially females. The symptoms are persistent and in some patients appear to be irreversible. The syndrome is characterized by rhythmical involuntary movements of the tongue, face, mouth or jaw (e.g., protrusion of tongue, puffing of cheeks, puckering of mouth, chewing movements). There may be involuntary movements of extremities.

There is no known effective treatment of tardive dyskinesia; antiparkinsonism agents usually do not alleviate the symptoms of this syndrome. It is suggested that all antipsychotic agents be discontinued if these symptoms appear. Should it be necessary to reinstitute treatment, or increase the dosage of the agent, or switch to a different antipsychotic agent, the syndrome may be masked. It has been reported that fine vermicular movements of the tongue may be an early sign of the syndrome and if the medication is stopped at that time the syndrome may not develop.

Dosage and Administration: Initial and maintenance doses of MOBAN® (molindone hydrochloride) should be individualized.

Initial Dosage Schedule: The usual starting dosage is 50–75 mg/day.

—Increase to 100 mg/day in 3 or 4 days.
—Based on severity of symptomatology, dosage may be titrated up or down depending on individual patient response.
—An increase to 225 mg/day may be required in patients with severe symptomatology.

Elderly and debilitated patients should be started on lower dosage.

Maintenance Dosage Schedule:

1. Mild—5 mg–15 mg three or four times a day.
2. Moderate—10 mg–25 mg three or four times a day.
3. Severe—225 mg/day may be required.

Drug Interactions: Potentiation of drugs administered concurrently with MOBAN® (molindone hydrochloride) has not been reported. Additionally, animal studies have not shown increased toxicity when MOBAN® is given concurrently with representative members of three classes of drugs (i.e., barbiturates, chloral hydrate and antiparkinson drugs).

Management of Overdosage: Symptomatic, supportive therapy should be the rule.

Gastric lavage is indicated for the reduction of absorption of MOBAN® (molindone hydrochloride) which is freely soluble in water.

Since the adsorption of MOBAN® (molindone hydrochloride) by activated charcoal has not been determined, the use of this antidote must be considered of theoretical value.

Emesis in a comatose patient is contraindicated. Additionally, while the emetic effect of apomorphine is blocked by MOBAN® in animals, this blocking effect has not been determined in humans.

A significant increase in the rate of removal of unmetabolized MOBAN® from the body by forced diuresis, peritoneal or renal dialysis would not be expected. (Only 2% of a single ingested dose of MOBAN® is excreted unmetabolized in the urine.)

However, poor response of the patient may justify use of these procedures. While the use of laxatives or enemas might be based on general principles, the amount of unmetabolized MOBAN® in feces is less than 1%. Extrapyramidal symptoms have responded to the use of diphenhydramine (Benadryl*) and the synthetic anticholinergic antiparkinson agents (i.e., Artane*, Cogentin*, Akineton*).

How Supplied: As tablets in bottles of 100 and 1000 with potencies and colors as follows:

5 mg orange
10 mg lavender
25 mg light green

*Benadryl—Trademark, Parke Davis and Co.
*Artane—Trademark, Lederle Laboratories
*Cogentin—Trademark, Merck Sharp & Dohme
*Akineton—Trademark, Knoll Pharmaceutical Co.

6069-6

MOBAN® is an Endo Registered U.S. Trademark.

[*Shown in Product Identification Section*]

NARCAN® INJECTION ℞
NARCAN® NEONATAL INJECTION
naloxone hydrochloride

Description: NARCAN (naloxone hydrochloride), a narcotic antagonist, is a synthetic congener of oxymorphone. In structure it differs from oxymorphone in that the methyl group on the nitrogen atom is replaced by an allyl group.

Naloxone hydrochloride occurs as a white to slightly off-white powder, and is soluble in water, in dilute acids, and in strong alkali; slightly soluble in alcohol; practically insoluble in ether and in chloroform.

NARCAN Injection is available in two concentrations, 0.02 mg and 0.4 mg of naloxone hydrochloride per ml. Each ml of either strength contains 8.6 mg of sodium chloride; and 2.0 mg of methylparaben and propylparaben as preservatives in a ratio of 9 to 1. pH is adjusted with hydrochloric acid.

Actions: NARCAN (naloxone hydrochloride) is an essentially pure narcotic antagonist, i.e., it does not possess the "agonistic" or morphine-like properties characteristic of other narcotic antagonists; NARCAN does not produce respiratory depression, psychotomimetic effects or pupillary constriction. In the absence of narcotics or agonistic effects of other narcotic antagonists it exhibits essentially no pharmacologic activity.

In the presence of physical dependence on narcotics NARCAN will produce withdrawal symptoms; it has not been shown to produce tolerance nor to cause physical or psychological dependence.

When NARCAN is administered intravenously the onset of action is generally apparent within two minutes; the onset of action is only slightly less rapid when it is administered subcutaneously or intramuscularly. The duration of action is dependent upon the dose and route of administration of NARCAN. Intramuscular administration produces a more prolonged effect than intravenous administration. The requirement for repeat doses of NARCAN, however, will also be dependent upon the amount, type and route of administration of the narcotic being antagonized.

Indications: NARCAN is indicated for the complete or partial reversal of narcotic depression, including respiratory depression, induced by opioids including natural and synthetic narcotics, propoxyphene and the narcotic-antagonist analgesic pentazocine. NARCAN is also indicated for the diagnosis of suspected acute opioid overdosage.

Contraindications: NARCAN is contraindicated in patients known to be hypersensitive to it.

Warnings: NARCAN should be administered cautiously to persons including newborns of mothers who are known or suspected to be physically dependent on opioids. In such cases an abrupt and complete reversal of narcotic effects may precipitate an acute abstinence syndrome.

Continued on next page

Endo—Cont.

The patient who has satisfactorily responded to NARCAN should be kept under continued surveillance and repeated doses of NARCAN should be administered, as necessary, since the duration of action of some narcotics may exceed that of NARCAN.
NARCAN is not effective against respiratory depression due to non-opioid drugs.
Usage in Pregnancy Safe use of NARCAN during pregnancy (other than labor) has not been established. Animal reproduction studies have not demonstrated teratogenic or other embryotoxic effects (See ANIMAL PHARMACOLOGY AND TOXICOLOGY). However, NARCAN should be administered to pregnant patients only when, in the judgment of the physician, the potential benefits outweigh the possible hazards.
Precautions: In addition to NARCAN, other resuscitative measures such as maintenance of a free airway, artificial ventilation, cardiac massage, and vasopressor agents should be available and employed when necessary to counteract acute narcotic poisoning.
In an isolated report two patients with preexisting ventricular irritability requiring lidocaine, and either isoproterenol or epinephrine for hypotension following cardiopulmonary bypass procedures, developed ventricular tachycardia or fibrillation when given NARCAN I.V. at 9 and 14 hours, respectively, postoperatively for persistent unresponsiveness. Although a direct cause and effect relationship has not been established, NARCAN should be used with caution in patients with cardiac irritability.
In rare cases, very rapid reversal of narcotic anesthesia in cardiac patients has resulted in pulmonary edema.
Adverse Reactions: Abrupt reversal of narcotic depression may result in nausea, vomiting, sweating, tachycardia, increased blood pressure, and tremulousness. In postoperative patients, excessive dosage of NARCAN may result in significant reversal of analgesia, and excitement; in some cardiac patients, the resultant hypertension and tachycardia may result in left ventricular failure and pulmonary edema. In the absence of narcotics naloxone is essentially devoid of side effects.
Dosage and Administration: NARCAN (naloxone hydrochloride) may be administered intravenously, intramuscularly, or subcutaneously. The most rapid onset of action is achieved by intravenous administration and it is recommended in emergency situations.
Since the duration of action of some narcotics may exceed that of NARCAN the patient should be kept under continued surveillance and repeated doses of NARCAN should be administered, as necessary.
Usage in Adults:
Narcotic Overdose—Known or Suspected: The usual initial adult dose is 0.4 mg (1 ml) NARCAN administered I.V., I.M. or S.C. If the desired degree of counteraction and improvement in respiratory function is not obtained immediately following I.V. administration, it may be repeated intravenously at 2 to 3 minute intervals. Failure to obtain significant improvement after 2 or 3 doses suggests that the condition may be due partly or completely to other disease processes or non-opioid drugs.
Postoperative Narcotic Depression: For the partial reversal of narcotic depression following the use of narcotics during surgery, smaller doses of NARCAN are usually sufficient. The dose of NARCAN should be titrated according to the patient's response. For the initial reversal of respiratory depression, NARCAN should be injected in increments of 0.1 to 0.2 mg intravenously at two to three minute intervals to the desired degree of reversal, i.e., adequate ventilation and alertness without significant pain or discomfort. Excessive dosage of NARCAN may result in significant reversal of analgesia and increase in blood pressure. Similarly, too rapid reversal may induce nausea, vomiting, sweating or circulatory stress.
Repeat doses of NARCAN may be required within one to two hour intervals depending upon the amount, type (i.e. short or long acting) and time interval since last administration of narcotic. Supplemental intramuscular doses have been shown to produce a longer lasting effect.
Usage in Children:
Narcotic Overdose—Known or Suspected: The usual initial child dose is 0.01 mg/kg body weight given I.V., I.M. or S.C. This dose may be repeated in accordance with the adult administration guideline. If necessary, NARCAN can be diluted with sterile water for injection.
Usage in Neonates:
Narcotic-induced depression The usual initial dose is 0.01 mg/kg body weight administered I.V., I.M. or S.C. This dose may be repeated in accordance with adult administration guidelines.
How Supplied: 0.4 mg/ml of NARCAN® (naloxone hydrochloride) for intravenous, intramuscular and subcutaneous administration.
Available in 1 ml ampuls in boxes of 10 and 100.
0.02 mg/ml of NARCAN® (naloxone hydrochloride) NEONATAL INJECTION for intravenous, intramuscular and subcutaneous administration.
Available in 2 ml ampuls in boxes of 10 and 100.
Animal Pharmacology and Toxicology: In the mouse and rat the intravenous LD_{50} is 150 ± 5 mg/kg and 109 ± 4 mg/kg respectively. In acute subcutaneous toxicity studies in newborn rats the LD_{50} (95% CL) is 260 (228–296) mg/kg. Subcutaneous injection of 100 mg/kg/day in rats for 3 weeks produced only transient salivation and partial ptosis following injections; no toxic effects were seen at 10 mg/kg/day for 3 weeks.
Reproductive studies including fertility, general reproductive performance, embryotoxicity, teratogenicity, and lactation did not show any abnormality in mice and rats at 10 mg/kg/day.
NARCAN is an Endo registered U.S. trademark.
6077-4

NUBAIN® ℞
(nalbuphine hydrochloride)

Description: NUBAIN (nalbuphine hydrochloride) is a synthetic narcotic agonist-antagonist analgesic of the phenanthrene series. It is chemically related to both the widely used narcotic antagonist, naloxone, and the potent narcotic analgesic, oxymorphone.
Nalbuphine hydrochloride is (-)-17-(cyclobutylmethyl)-4, 5α-epoxy-morphinan-3,6α, 14-triol, hydrochloride.
Each ml of the injectable aqueous solution of NUBAIN contains 10 mg of nalbuphine hydrochloride.
Actions: NUBAIN is a potent analgesic. Its analgesic potency is essentially equivalent to that of morphine on a milligram basis.
Its onset of action occurs within 2 to 3 minutes after intravenous administration, and in less than 15 minutes following subcutaneous or intramuscular injection. The plasma half-life of nalbuphine is 5 hours and in clinical studies the duration of analgesic activity has been reported to range from 3 to 6 hours.
The narcotic antagonist activity of NUBAIN is one-fourth as potent as nalorphine and 10 times that of pentazocine.
Indications: For the relief of moderate to severe pain. NUBAIN can also be used for preoperative analgesia, as a supplement to surgical anesthesia, and for obstetrical analgesia during labor.
Contraindications: NUBAIN should not be administered to patients who are hypersensitive to it.
Warnings:
Drug Dependence NUBAIN has been shown to have a low abuse potential which is approximate to that of pentazocine. When compared with drugs which are not mixed agonist-antagonists, it has been reported that nalbuphine's potential for abuse would be less than that of codeine and propoxyphene. Psychological and physical dependence and tolerance may follow the abuse or misuse of nalbuphine. Therefore, caution should be observed in prescribing it for emotionally unstable patients, or for individuals with a history of narcotic abuse. Such patients should be closely supervised when long-term therapy is contemplated.
Care should be taken to avoid increases in dosage or frequency of administration which in susceptible individuals might result in physical dependence.
Abrupt discontinuation of NUBAIN following prolonged use has been followed by symptoms of narcotic withdrawal, i.e., abdominal cramps, nausea and vomiting, rhinorrhea, lacrimation, restlessness, anxiety, elevated temperature and piloerection.
Use in Ambulatory Patients NUBAIN may impair the mental or physical abilities required for the performance of potentially dangerous tasks such as driving a car or operating machinery. Therefore, NUBAIN should be administered with caution to ambulatory patients who should be warned to avoid such hazards.
Use in Emergency Procedures Maintain patient under observation until recovered from NUBAIN effects that would affect driving or other potentially dangerous tasks.
Use in Children Clinical experience to support administration to patients under 18 years is not available at present.
Use in Pregnancy (other than labor) Safe use of NUBAIN in pregnancy has not been established. Although animal reproductive studies have not revealed teratogenic or embryotoxic effects, nalbuphine should only be administered to pregnant women when, in the judgement of the physician, the potential benefits outweigh the possible hazards.
Use During Labor and Delivery NUBAIN can produce respiratory depression in the neonate. It should be used with caution in women delivering premature infants.
Head Injury and Increased Intracranial Pressure The possible respiratory depressant effects and the potential of potent analgesics to elevate cerebrospinal fluid pressure (resulting from vasodilation following CO_2 retention) may be markedly exaggerated in the presence of head injury, intracranial lesions or a preexisting increase in intracranial pressure. Furthermore, potent analgesics can produce effects which may obscure the clinical course of patients with head injuries. Therefore, NUBAIN should be used in these circumstances only when essential, and then should be administered with extreme caution.
Interaction With Other Central Nervous System Depressants Although NUBAIN possesses narcotic antagonist activity, there is evidence that in nondependent patients it will not antagonize a narcotic analgesic administered just before, concurrently, or just after an injection of NUBAIN. Therefore, patients receiving a narcotic analgesic general anesthetics, phenothiazines, or other tranquilizers, sedatives, hypnotics, or other CNS depressants (including alcohol) concomitantly with NUBAIN may exhibit an additive effect. When such combined therapy is contemplated, the dose of one or both agents should be reduced.
Precautions:
Impaired Respiration At the usual adult dose of 10 mg/70kg, NUBAIN causes some respira-

tory depression approximately equal to that produced by equal doses of morphine. However, in contrast to morphine, respiratory depression is not appreciably increased with higher doses of NUBAIN. Respiratory depression induced by NUBAIN can be reversed by NARCAN® (naloxone hydrochloride) when indicated. NUBAIN should be administered with caution at low doses to patients with impaired respiration (e.g., from other medication, uremia, bronchial asthma, severe infection, cyanosis or respiratory obstructions).

Impaired Renal or Hepatic Function Because NUBAIN is metabolized in the liver and excreted by the kidneys, patients with renal or liver dysfunction may over-react to customary doses. Therefore, in these individuals, NUBAIN should be used with caution and administered in reduced amounts.

Myocardial Infarction As with all potent analgesics, NUBAIN should be used with caution in patients with myocardial infarction who have nausea or vomiting.

Biliary Tract Surgery As with all narcotic analgesics, NUBAIN should be used with caution in patients about to undergo surgery of the biliary tract since it may cause spasm of the sphincter of Oddi.

Adverse Reactions: The most frequent adverse reaction in 1066 patients treated with NUBAIN is sedation 381 (36%).

Less frequent reactions are: sweaty/clammy 99 (9%) nausea/vomiting 68 (6%), dizziness/vertigo 58 (5%), dry mouth 44 (4%), and headache 27 (3%).

Other adverse reactions which may occur (reported incidence of 1% or less) are:

CNS Effects nervousness, depression, restlessness, crying, euphoria, floating, hostility, unusual dreams, confusion, faintness, hallucinations, dysphoria, feeling of heaviness, numbness, tingling, unreality. The incidence of psychotomimetic effects, such as unreality, depersonalization, delusions, dysphoria and hallucinations has been shown to be less than that which occurs with pentazocine.

Cardiovascular Hypertension, hypotension, bradycardia, tachycardia.

Gastrointestinal Cramps, dyspepsia, bitter taste.

Respiration Depression, dyspnea, asthma.

Dermatological Itching, burning, urticaria.

Miscellaneous Speech difficulty, urinary urgency, blurred vision, flushing and warmth.

Dosage and Administration: The usual recommended adult dose is 10 mg for a 70 kg individual, administered subcutaneously, intramuscularly or intravenously; this dose may be repeated every 3 to 6 hours as necessary. Dosage should be adjusted according to the severity of the pain, physical status of the patient, and other medications which the patient may be receiving. (See Interaction with Other Central Nervous System Depressants under WARNINGS). In non-tolerant individuals, the recommended single maximum dose is 20 mg, with a maximum total daily dose of 160 mg.

Patients Dependent on Narcotics Patients who have been taking narcotics chronically may experience withdrawal symptoms upon the administration of NUBAIN. If unduly troublesome, narcotic withdrawal symptoms can be controlled by the slow intravenous administration of small increments of morphine, until relief occurs. If the previous analgesic was morphine, meperidine, codeine, or other narcotic with similar duration of activity, one-fourth of the anticipated dose of NUBAIN can be administered initially and the patient observed for signs of withdrawal, i.e., abdominal cramps, nausea and vomiting, lacrimation, rhinorrhea, anxiety, restlessness, elevation of temperature or piloerection. If untoward symptoms do not occur, progressively larger doses may be tried at appropriate intervals until the desired level of analgesia is obtained with NUBAIN.

Management of Overdosage The immediate intravenous administration of NARCAN® (naloxone hydrochloride) is a specific antidote. Oxygen, intravenous fluids, vasopressors and other supportive measures should be used as indicated.

The administration of single doses of 72 mg of NUBAIN intramuscularly to eight normal subjects has been reported to have resulted primarily in symptoms of sleepiness and mild dysphoria.

How Supplied: NUBAIN® (nalbuphine hydrochloride) injection for intramuscular, subcutaneous, or intravenous use (10 mg/ml) is available in:

NDC #0056-0385 10 mg/ml, 1 ml ampuls (box of 10)
NDC #0056-0384 10 mg/ml, 2 ml ampuls (box of 10)
NDC #0056-0386 10 mg/ml, 10 ml vials

Each ml contains 10 mg nalbuphine hydrochloride, 0.1% sodium chloride, 0.94% sodium citrate, 1.26% citric acid anhydrous, 0.1% sodium metabisulfite, and 0.2% of a 9:1 mixture of methylparaben and propylparaben as preservative; pH is adjusted with hydrochloric acid.

NUBAIN® is an Endo Registered U.S. Trademark
NARCAN® is an Endo Registered U.S. Trademark
6094-2

†PERCOCET®-5 ©

Description:
Each tablet of PERCOCET®-5 contains:
Oxycodone hydrochloride .... 5 mg
WARNING: May be habit forming
Acetaminophen (APAP) .... 325 mg

The oxycodone component is 14-hydroxydihydrocodeinone, a white, odorless crystalline powder which is derived from the opium alkaloid, thebaine.

Actions: The principal analgesic ingredient, oxycodone, is a semisynthetic narcotic with multiple actions qualitatively similar to those of morphine; the most prominent of these involve the central nervous system and organs composed of smooth muscle. The principal actions of therapeutic value of the oxycodone in PERCOCET®-5 are analgesia and sedation.

Oxycodone is similar to codeine and methadone in that it retains at least one half of its analgesic activity when administered orally. PERCOCET®-5 also contains the non-narcotic antipyretic-analgesic acetaminophen.

Indications: For the relief of moderate to moderately severe pain.

Contraindications: Hypersensitivity to oxycodone or acetaminophen.

Warnings:

Drug Dependence: Oxycodone can produce drug dependence of the morphine type and, therefore, has the potential for being abused. Psychic dependence, physical dependence and tolerance may develop upon repeated administration of PERCOCET®-5, and it should be prescribed and administered with the same degree of caution appropriate to the use of other oral narcotic-containing medications. Like other narcotic-containing medications, PERCOCET®-5 is subject to the Federal Controlled Substances Act.

Usage in ambulatory patients: Oxycodone may impair the mental and/or physical abilities required for the performance of potentially hazardous tasks such as driving a car or operating machinery. The patient using PERCOCET®-5 should be cautioned accordingly.

Interaction with other central nervous system depressants: Patients receiving other narcotic analgesics, general anesthetics, phenothiazines, other tranquilizers, sedative-hypnotics or other CNS depressants (including alcohol) concomitantly with PERCOCET®-5 may exhibit an additive CNS depression. When such combined therapy is contemplated, the dose of one or both agents should be reduced.

Usage in pregnancy: Safe use in pregnancy has not been established relative to possible adverse effects on fetal development. Therefore, PERCOCET®-5 should not be used in pregnant women unless, in the judgment of the physician, the potential benefits outweigh the possible hazards.

Usage in children: PERCOCET®-5 should not be administered to children.

Precautions:

Head injury and increased intracranial pressure: The respiratory depressant effects of narcotics and their capacity to elevate cerebrospinal fluid pressure may be markedly exaggerated in the presence of head injury, other intracranial lesions or a pre-existing increase in intracranial pressure. Furthermore, narcotics produce adverse reactions which may obscure the clinical course of patients with head injuries.

Acute abdominal conditions: The administration of PERCOCET®-5 or other narcotics may obscure the diagnosis or clinical course in patients with acute abdominal conditions.

Special risk patients: PERCOCET®-5 should be given with caution to certain patients such as the elderly or debilitated, and those with severe impairment of hepatic or renal function, hypothyroidism, Addison's disease, and prostatic hypertrophy or urethral stricture.

Adverse Reactions: The most frequently observed adverse reactions include light headedness, dizziness, sedation, nausea and vomiting. These effects seem to be more prominent in ambulatory than in nonambulatory patients, and some of these adverse reactions may be alleviated if the patient lies down.

Other adverse reactions include euphoria, dysphoria, constipation, skin rash and pruritus.

Dosage and Administration: Dosage should be adjusted according to the severity of the pain and the response of the patient. It may occasionally be necessary to exceed the usual dosage recommended below in cases of more severe pain or in those patients who have become tolerant to the analgesic effect of narcotics. PERCOCET®-5 is given orally. The usual adult dose is one tablet every 6 hours as needed for pain.

Drug Interactions: The CNS depressant effects of PERCOCET®-5 may be additive with that of other CNS depressants. See WARNINGS.

Management of Overdosage:

Signs and Symptoms: Serious overdose with PERCOCET®-5 is characterized by respiratory depression (a decrease in respiratory rate and/or tidal volume, Cheyne-Stokes respiration, cyanosis), extreme somnolence progressing to stupor or coma, skeletal muscle flaccidity, cold and clammy skin, and sometimes bradycardia and hypotension. In severe overdosage, apnea, circulatory collapse, cardiac arrest and death may occur. The ingestion of very large amounts of PERCOCET®-5 may, in addition, result in acute hepatic toxicity.

Treatment: Primary attention should be given to the reestablishment of adequate respiratory exchange through provision of a patent airway and the institution of assisted or controlled ventilation. The narcotic antagonists naloxone, nalorphine or levallorphan are specific antidotes against respiratory depression which may result from overdosage or unusual sensitivity to narcotics, including oxycodone. Therefore, an appropriate dose of one of these antagonists should be administered, preferably by the intravenous route, simultaneously with efforts at respiratory resuscitation. Since the duration of action of oxycodone may exceed that of the antagonist, the patient should be kept under continued surveillance and repeated doses of the antagonist should be ad-

Continued on next page

Endo—Cont.

ministered as needed to maintain adequate respiration.
An antagonist should not be administered in the absence of clinically significant respiratory or cardiovascular depression.
Oxygen, intravenous fluids, vasopressors and other supportive measures should be employed as indicated.
Gastric emptying may be useful in removing unabsorbed drug.
Acetaminophen in massive overdosage may cause hepatotoxicity in some patients. Clinical and laboratory evidence of hepatotoxicity may be delayed for up to one week. Close clinical monitoring and serial hepatic enzyme determinations are therefore recommended.
Treatment of acute acetaminophen overdosage is purely symptomatic.
How Supplied: White, scored tablets in bottles of 100 and 500; Hospital blister pack of 25 tablets in units of 250 and 1,000 tablets.
DEA Order Form Required
PERCOCET® is a registered Trademark of Endo, Inc.
6090-1
†Product of Endo Inc.
[*Shown in Product Identification Section*]

†PERCODAN® Ⓒ
†PERCODAN®-DEMI
Tablets

Description:
Each yellow, scored tablet of PERCODAN® contains:
Oxycodone hydrochloride ....4.50 mg
WARNING: May be habit forming
Oxycodone terephthalate ....0.38 mg
WARNING: May be habit forming
Aspirin ....224 mg
Phenacetin ....160 mg
Caffeine ....32 mg
Each pink, scored tablet of PERCODAN®-Demi contains:
Oxycodone hydrochloride ....2.25 mg
WARNING: May be habit forming
Oxycodone terephthalate ....0.19 mg
WARNING: May be habit forming
Aspirin ....224 mg
Phenacetin ....160 mg
Caffeine ....32 mg
The oxycodone component is 14-hydroxydihydrocodeinone, a white odorless crystalline powder which is derived from the opium alkaloid, thebaine.
Actions: The principal ingredient, oxycodone, is a semisynthetic narcotic analgesic with multiple actions qualitatively similar to those of morphine; the most prominent of these involve the central nervous system and organs composed of smooth muscle. The principal actions of therapeutic value of the oxycodone in PERCODAN® and PERCODAN®-Demi are analgesia and sedation.
Oxycodone is similar to codeine and methadone in that it retains at least one half of its analgesic activity when administered orally.
PERCODAN® and PERCODAN®-Demi also contain the non-narcotic antipyretic-analgesics, aspirin and phenacetin.
Indications: For the relief of moderate to moderately severe pain.
Contraindications: Hypersensitivity to oxycodone, aspirin, phenacetin or caffeine.
Warnings:
Drug Dependence: Oxycodone can produce drug dependence of the morphine type and, therefore, has the potential for being abused. Psychic dependence, physical dependence and tolerance may develop upon repeated administration of PERCODAN® and PERCODAN®-Demi, and it should be prescribed and administered with the same degree of caution appropriate to the use of other oral narcotic-containing medications. Like other narcotic-containing medications, PERCODAN® and PERCODAN®-Demi are subject to the Federal Controlled Substances Act.
Usage in ambulatory patients: Oxycodone may impair the mental and/or physical abilities required for the performance of potentially hazardous tasks such as driving a car or operating machinery. The patient using PERCODAN® and PERCODAN®-Demi should be cautioned accordingly.
Interaction with other central nervous system depressants: Patients receiving other narcotic analgesics, general anesthetics, phenothiazines, other tranquilizers, sedative-hypnotics or other CNS depressants (including alcohol) concomitantly with PERCODAN® and PERCODAN®-Demi may exhibit an additive CNS depression. When such combined therapy is contemplated, the dose of one or both agents should be reduced.
Usage in pregnancy: Safe use in pregnancy has not been established relative to possible adverse effects on fetal development. Therefore, PERCODAN® and PERCODAN®-Demi should not be used in pregnant women unless, in the judgment of the physician, the potential benefits outweigh the possible hazards.
Usage in children: PERCODAN® should not be administered to children. PERCODAN®-Demi, containing half the amount of oxycodone, can be considered. (See product prescribing information for PERCODAN®-Demi).
Salicylates should be used with caution in the presence of peptic ulcer or coagulation abnormalities.
Precautions:
Head injury and increased intracranial pressure: The respiratory depressant effects of narcotics and their capacity to elevate cerebrospinal fluid pressure may be markedly exaggerated in the presence of head injury, other intracranial lesions or a pre-existing increase in intracranial pressure. Furthermore, narcotics produce adverse reactions which may obscure the clinical course of patients with head injuries.
Acute abdominal conditions: The administration of PERCODAN® and PERCODAN®-Demi or other narcotics may obscure the diagnosis or clinical course in patients with acute abdominal conditions.
Special risk patients: PERCODAN® and PERCODAN®-Demi should be given with caution to certain patients such as the elderly or debilitated, and those with severe impairment of hepatic or renal function, hypothyroidism, Addison's disease, and prostatic hypertrophy or urethral stricture.
Phenacetin has been reported to damage the kidneys when taken in excessive amounts for a long time.
Adverse Reactions: The most frequently observed adverse reactions include light headedness, dizziness, sedation, nausea and vomiting. These effects seem to be more prominent in ambulatory than in nonambulatory patients, and some of these adverse reactions may be alleviated if the patient lies down.
Other adverse reactions include euphoria, dysphoria, constipation and pruritus.
Dosage and Administration: Dosage should be adjusted according to the severity of the pain and the response of the patient. It may occasionally be necessary to exceed the usual dosage recommended below in cases of more severe pain or in those patients who have become tolerant to the analgesic effect of narcotics. PERCODAN® and PERCODAN®-Demi are given orally.
PERCODAN®: The usual adult dose is one tablet every 6 hours as needed for pain.
PERCODAN®-Demi: Adults—One or two tablets every six hours. Children 12 years and older—One-half tablet every six hours. Children 6 to 12 years—One-quarter tablet every six hours. PERCODAN®-Demi is not indicated for children under 6 years of age.
Drug Interactions: The CNS depressant effects of PERCODAN® and PERCODAN®-Demi may be additive with that of other CNS depressants. See WARNINGS.
Aspirin may enhance the effect of anticoagulants and inhibit the uricosuric effects of uricosuric agents.
Management of Overdosage:
Signs and Symptoms: Serious overdose with PERCODAN® or PERCODAN®-Demi is characterized by respiratory depression (a decrease in respiratory rate and/or tidal volume, Cheyne-Stokes respiration, cyanosis), extreme somnolence progressing to stupor or coma, skeletal muscle flaccidity, cold and clammy skin, and sometimes bradycardia and hypotension. In severe overdosage, apnea, circulatory collapse, cardiac arrest and death may occur. The ingestion of very large amounts of PERCODAN® or PERCODAN®-Demi may, in addition, result in acute salicylate intoxication.
Treatment: Primary attention should be given to the reestablishment of adequate respiratory exchange through provision of a patent airway and the institution of assisted or controlled ventilation. The narcotic antagonists naloxone, nalorphine or levallorphan are specific antidotes against respiratory depression which may result from overdosage or unusual sensitivity to narcotics, including oxycodone. Therefore, an appropriate dose of one of these antagonists should be administered, preferably by the intravenous route, simultaneously with efforts at respiratory resuscitation. Since the duration of action of oxycodone may exceed that of the antagonist, the patient should be kept under continued surveillance and repeated doses of the antagonist should be administered as needed to maintain adequate respiration.
An antagonist should not be administered in the absence of clinically significant respiratory or cardiovascular depression.
Oxygen, intravenous fluids, vasopressors and other supportive measures should be employed as indicated.
Gastric emptying may be useful in removing unabsorbed drug.
How Supplied:
PERCODAN®—Yellow, scored tablets in bottles of 100, 500 and 1,000; Hospital blister pack of 25 tablets in units of 250 and 1,000 tablets.
PERCODAN®-Demi—Pink, scored tablets in bottles of 100 and 500.
[*Shown in Product Identification Section*]
DEA Order Form Required.
PERCODAN® is a registered U.S. trademark of Endo Inc.
†Products of Endo Inc.

PERCOGESIC®
Analgesic Tablets

Description: Each tablet contains:
Acetaminophen (APAP)....................325 mg
Phenyltoloxamine citrate .... 30 mg
Uses: For relief of mild to moderate pain and discomfort due to simple headache; for temporary relief of such pain associated with muscle and joint soreness, neuralgia, sinusitis, minor menstrual cramps, the common cold or grippe, toothache, and minor aches and pains of rheumatism and arthritis.
Precautions: If arthritic or rheumatic pain persists for more than 10 days; in the presence of redness or swelling; or in arthritic or rheumatic conditions affecting children under 12 years of age, consult a physician immediately. When used for the temporary symptomatic relief of colds, if relief does not occur within three days, discontinue use and consult physician. This preparation may cause drowsiness. Do not drive or operate machinery while taking this medication. Do not administer to chil-

dren under six years of age or exceed recommended dosage unless directed by physician.

Administration and Dosage: Adults—1 or 2 tablets every 4 hours; maximum daily dose 8 tablets. Children: 6-12 years—one-half adult dose; maximum daily dose 4 tablets. Do not use for more than 10 days unless directed by physician.

How Supplied: PERCOGESIC® tablets are available in blister-strip boxes of 24 and 960 tablets and bottles of 100.

PERCOGESIC® is an Endo registered U.S. trademark.

LK

SYMMETREL® ℞
amantadine hydrochloride

Description: SYMMETREL® is designated generically as amantadine hydrochloride and chemically as 1-adamantanamine hydrochloride.

Amantadine hydrochloride is a stable, white or nearly white crystalline powder, freely soluble in water and soluble in alcohol and in chloroform. It is readily absorbed, is not metabolized, and is excreted unchanged in the urine.

Actions: The mechanism of action of SYMMETREL® in the treatment of Parkinson's disease and drug-induced extrapyramidal reactions is not known. It has been shown to cause an increase in dopamine release in the animal brain. The drug does not possess anticholinergic activity in animal tests at doses similar to those used clinically.

The antiviral activity of SYMMETREL® against the influenza A virus in humans is not completely understood. The mode of action of SYMMETREL® appears to be the prevention of the release of infectious viral nucleic acid into the host cell. SYMMETREL® does not appear to interfere with the immunogenicity of inactivated influenza A virus vaccine.

Indications: Parkinson's Disease/Syndrome and Drug-Induced Extrapyramidal Reactions: SYMMETREL® is indicated in the treatment of idiopathic Parkinson's disease (Paralysis Agitans), postencephalitic parkinsonism, drug-induced extrapyramidal reactions, and symptomatic parkinsonism which may follow injury to the nervous system by carbon monoxide intoxication. It is indicated in those elderly patients believed to develop parkinsonism in association with cerebral arteriosclerosis. In the treatment of Parkinson's disease, SYMMETREL® is less effective than levodopa, (-)-3-(3,4-dihydroxyphenyl)-L-alanine, and its efficacy in comparison with the anticholinergic antiparkinson drugs has not yet been established. Although anticholinergic type side effects have been noted with SYMMETREL® when used in patients with drug-induced extrapyramidal reactions, there is a lower incidence of these side effects than that observed with anticholinergic antiparkinson drugs.

Influenza A Virus Respiratory Tract Illness: SYMMETREL® (amantadine hydrochloride) is indicated in the prevention (prophylaxis) and symptomatic management of respiratory tract illness caused by influenza A virus strains. SYMMETREL® should be considered especially for high risk patients, close household or hospital ward contacts of index cases and patients with severe influenza A virus illness. In the prophylaxis of influenza due to A virus strains, early immunization as periodically recommended by the Public Health Service Advisory Committee on Immunization Practices is the method of choice. When early immunization is not feasible, or when the vaccine is contraindicated or not available, SYMMETREL® can be used for chemoprophylaxis against influenza A virus illness. Because SYMMETREL® does not appear to suppress antibody response, it can be used chemoprophylactically in conjunction with inactivated influenza A virus vaccine until protective antibody responses develop. There is no clinical evidence that this drug has efficacy in the prophylaxis or symptomatic management of viral respiratory tract illnesses other than those caused by influenza A virus strains.

Contraindications: SYMMETREL® is contraindicated in patients with known hypersensitivity to the drug.

Warnings: Patients with a history of epilepsy or other "seizures" should be observed closely for possible increased seizure activity.

Patients with a history of congestive heart failure or peripheral edema should be followed closely as there are patients who developed congestive heart failure while receiving SYMMETREL®.

Patients with Parkinson's disease improving on SYMMETREL® should resume normal activities gradually and cautiously, consistent with other medical considerations, such as the presence of osteoporosis or phlebothrombosis.

Patients receiving SYMMETREL® who note central nervous system effects or blurring of vision should be cautioned against driving or working in situations where alertness is important.

Use in Pregnancy: SYMMETREL® has not been studied in pregnant women. The use of this drug in women of childbearing age should be undertaken only after weighing the possible risks to the fetus against benefit to the patient. SYMMETREL® has been reported to be embryotoxic and teratogenic in rats at 50 mg/kg/day, about 12 times the recommended human dose, but not at 37 mg/kg/day. Embryotoxic and teratogenic effects were not seen in rabbits which received up to 25 times the usual recommended adult human dose.

Nursing Mothers: Since the drug is secreted in the milk, SYMMETREL® should not be administered to nursing mothers.

Precautions: SYMMETREL® (amantadine hydrochloride) should not be discontinued abruptly since a few patients with Parkinson's disease experienced a parkinsonian crisis, i.e., a sudden marked clinical deterioration, when this medication was suddenly stopped. The dose of anticholinergic drugs or of SYMMETREL® should be reduced if atropine-like effects appear when these drugs are used concurrently.

The dose of SYMMETREL® may need careful adjustment in patients with renal impairment, congestive heart failure, peripheral edema, or orthostatic hypotension. Since SYMMETREL® is not metabolized and is mainly excreted in the urine, it may accumulate when renal function is inadequate.

Care should be exercised when administering SYMMETREL® to patients with liver disease, a history of recurrent eczematoid rash, or to patients with psychosis or severe psychoneurosis not controlled by chemotherapeutic agents. Careful observation is required when SYMMETREL® is administered concurrently with central nervous system stimulants.

Adverse Reactions: The most frequently occurring serious adverse reactions are: depression, congestive heart failure, orthostatic hypotensive episodes, psychosis, and urinary retention. Rarely convulsions, leukopenia, and neutropenia have been reported.

Other adverse reactions of a less serious nature which have been observed are the following: hallucinations, confusion, anxiety and irritability; anorexia, nausea, and constipation; ataxia and dizziness (lightheadedness); livedo reticularis and peripheral edema. Adverse reactions observed less frequently are the following: vomiting; dry mouth; headache; dyspnea; fatigue, insomnia, and a sense of weakness. Infrequently, skin rash, slurred speech, and visual disturbances have been observed. Rarely eczematoid dermatitis and oculogyric episodes have been reported.

Overdosage: There is no specific antidote. For acute overdosing, general supportive measures should be employed along with immediate gastric lavage or induction of emesis. Fluids should be forced, and if necessary, given intravenously. The pH of the urine has been reported to influence the excretion rate of SYMMETREL®. Since the excretion rate of SYMMETREL® increases rapidly when the urine is acidic, the administration of urine acidifying fluids may increase the elimination of the drug from the body. The blood pressure, pulse, respiration and temperature should be monitored. The patient should be observed for hyperactivity and convulsions; if required, sedation, and anticonvulsant therapy should be administered. The patient should be observed for the possible development of arrhythmias and hypotension; if required, appropriate antiarrhythmic and antihypotensive therapy should be given. The blood electrolytes, urine pH and urinary output should be monitored. If there is no record of recent voiding, catheterization should be done. The possibility of multiple drug ingestion by the patient should be considered.

Dosage and Administration:

Dosage for Parkinsonism:

Adult: The usual dose of SYMMETREL® (amantadine hydrochloride) is 100 mg twice a day when used alone. SYMMETREL® has an onset of action usually within 48 hours.

The initial dose of SYMMETREL® is 100 mg daily for patients with serious associated medical illnesses or who are receiving high doses of other antiparkinson drugs. After one to several weeks at 100 mg once daily, the dose may be increased to 100 mg twice daily, if necessary. Occasionally, patients whose responses are not optimal with SYMMETREL® at 200 mg daily may benefit from an increase up to 400 mg daily in divided doses. However, such patients should be supervised closely by their physicians.

Patients initially deriving benefit from SYMMETREL® not uncommonly experience a fall-off of effectiveness after a few months. Benefit may be regained by increasing the dose to 300 mg daily. Alternatively, temporary discontinuation of SYMMETREL® for several weeks, followed by reinitiation of the drug, may result in regaining benefit in some patients. A decision to use other antiparkinson drugs may be necessary.

Dosage for Concomitant Therapy

Some patients who do not respond to anticholinergic antiparkinson drugs may respond to SYMMETREL®. When SYMMETREL® or anticholinergic antiparkinson drugs are each used with marginal benefit, concomitant use may produce additional benefit.

When SYMMETREL® and levodopa are initiated concurrently, the patient can exhibit rapid therapeutic benefits. SYMMETREL® should be held constant at 100 mg daily or twice daily while the daily dose of levodopa is gradually increased to optimal benefit.

When SYMMETREL® is added to optimal well-tolerated doses of levodopa, additional benefit may result, including smoothing out the fluctuations in improvement which sometimes occur in patients on levodopa alone. Patients who require a reduction in their usual dose of levodopa because of development of side effects may possibly regain lost benefit with the addition of SYMMETREL®.

Dosage for Drug-Induced Extrapyramidal Reactions:

Adult: The usual dose of SYMMETREL® (amantadine hydrochloride) is 100 mg twice a day. Occasionally, patients whose responses are not optimal with SYMMETREL® at 200 mg daily may benefit from an increase up to 300 mg daily in divided doses.

Dosage for Prophylaxis and Symptomatic Management of Influenza A Virus Respiratory Tract Illness:

Continued on next page

Endo—Cont.

Adult: The adult daily dosage of SYMMETREL® (amantadine hydrochloride) is 200 mg: two 100 mg capsules (or four teaspoonfuls of syrup) as a single daily dose, or the daily dosage may be split into one capsule of 100 mg (or two teaspoonfuls of syrup) twice a day. If central nervous system effects develop on once-a-day dosage, a split dosage schedule may reduce such complaints.
Children: 1 yr.-9 yrs. of age: The total daily dose should be calculated on the basis of 2 mg to 4 mg per pound of body weight per day (but not to exceed 150 mg per day). The daily dose, given as the syrup, should be given in two or three equal portions.
9 yrs.-12 yrs. of age: The total daily dose is 200 mg given as one capsule of 100 mg (or two teaspoonfuls of syrup) twice a day.
Prophylactic dosing should be started in anticipation of contact or as soon as possible after contact with individuals with influenza A virus respiratory illness. SYMMETREL® should be continued daily for at least 10 days following a known exposure. If SYMMETREL® is used chemoprophylactically in conjunction with inactivated influenza A virus vaccine until protective antibody responses develop, then it should be administered for 2 to 3 weeks after the vaccine has been given. When inactivated influenza A virus vaccine is unavailable or contraindicated, SYMMETREL® should be administered for up to 90 days in case of possible repeated and unknown exposures. Symptomatic management of influenza A virus illness should be started as soon as possible after onset of symptoms and should be continued for 24 to 48 hours after the disappearance of symptoms.
How Supplied: SYMMETREL® (amantadine hydrochloride).
Capsules: (bottles of 100 and 500)-each red, soft gelatin capsule contains 100 mg amantadine hydrochloride.
Syrup: (1 pint)-each 5 ml (1 teaspoonful) of syrup contains 50 mg amantadine hydrochloride.
SYMMETREL® is a DuPont
Registered U.S. Trademark
CAPSULES MANUFACTURED BY
R. P. Scherer Corporation
Detroit, Michigan 48213
FOR
Endo Laboratories, Inc.
Subsidiary of the DuPont Company
Garden City, N.Y. 11530
6043-8
[Shown in Product Identification Section]

TESSALON® ℞
(benzonatate NF)

Description: TESSALON®, a nonnarcotic antitussive agent, is 2, 5, 8, 11, 14, 17, 20, 23, 26-nonaoxaoctacosan-28-yl p-(butylamino) benzoate.
Actions: TESSALON® acts peripherally by anesthetizing the stretch receptors located in the respiratory passages, lungs, and pleura by dampening their activity and thereby reducing the cough reflex at its source. It begins to act within 15 to 20 minutes and its effect lasts for 3 to 8 hours. TESSALON® has no inhibitory effect on the respiratory center in recommended dosage.
Indications: Symptomatic relief of cough.
Contraindications: Hypersensitivity to benzonatate or related compounds.
Warnings: Usage in Pregnancy: The safe use of this drug in pregnant women or during lactation has not been established. Therefore, the benefits must be weighed against the potential hazards.
Precautions: Release of TESSALON® from the perle in the mouth can produce a temporary local anesthesia of the oral mucosa. Therefore, the perles should be swallowed without chewing.
Adverse Reactions: Sedation, headache, mild dizziness, pruritus and skin eruptions, nasal congestion, constipation, nausea, gastrointestinal upset, sensation of burning in the eyes, a vague "chilly" sensation, numbness in the chest, and hypersensitivity have been reported.
Dosage and Administration: Adults and Children over 10: Usual dose is one 100 mg perle t.i.d. as required. If necessary, up to 6 perles daily may be given.
Overdosage: No clinically significant cases have been reported, to our knowledge. The drug is chemically related to tetracaine and other topical anesthetics and shares various aspects of their pharmacology and toxicology. Drugs of this type are generally well absorbed after ingestion.
Signs and Symptoms
If perles are chewed or dissolved in the mouth, oropharyngeal anesthesia will develop rapidly. CNS stimulation may cause restlessness and tremors which may proceed to clonic convulsions followed by profound CNS depression.
Treatment
Evacuate gastric contents and administer copious amounts of activated charcoal slurry. Even in the conscious patient, cough and gag reflexes may be so depressed as to necessitate special attention to protection against aspiration of gastric contents and orally administered materials.
Convulsions should be treated with a *short-acting* barbiturate given intravenously and carefully titrated for the smallest effective dosage.
Intensive support of respiration and cardiovascular-renal function is an essential feature of the treatment of severe intoxication from overdosage.
Do not use CNS stimulants.
How Supplied Perles, 100 mg (yellow); bottles of 100.
TESSALON® is an Endo registered U.S. trademark.
6075-3
TESSALON is manufactured by R.P. Scherer Corporation, Detroit, Michigan, 48213, for Endo Laboratories, Inc.
[Shown in Product Identification Section]

VALPIN® 50 ℞
anisotropine methylbromide 50 mg

Description: VALPIN® 50 is anisotropine methylbromide, a quaternary ammonium salt which differs chemically from atropine and most other anticholinergics in the substitution of an aliphatic for an aromatic side chain in the acid moiety of the ester.
Chemically, VALPIN® 50 is 2-propyl pentanoyl tropinium methylbromide. Its stability both to acid and alkaline hydrolysis minimizes inactivation.
Actions: VALPIN® 50 inhibits gastric acid secretion and reduces gastrointestinal motility.
Indications: For use as adjunctive therapy in the treatment of peptic ulcer.
AS WITH ALL ANTICHOLINERGICS, IT SHOULD BE NOTED THAT AT THE PRESENT TIME THERE IS LACK OF CONCURRENCE AS TO THEIR VALUE IN THE TREATMENT OF GASTRIC ULCER. IT HAS NOT BEEN SHOWN CONCLUSIVELY WHETHER ANTICHOLINERGIC DRUGS AID IN THE HEALING OF A PEPTIC ULCER, DECREASE THE RATE OF RECURRENCES OR PREVENT COMPLICATION.
Contraindications: Glaucoma; obstructive uropathy (for example, bladder neck obstruction due to prostatic hypertrophy); obstructive disease of the gastrointestinal tract (as in achalasia, pyloroduodenal stenosis, etc.); paralytic ileus, intestinal atony of the elderly or debilitated patient; unstable cardiovascular status in acute hemorrhage; severe ulcerative colitis; toxic megacolon complicating ulcerative colitis; myasthenia gravis.
Warnings:
Use in Pregnancy Since the safety of these preparations in pregnancy, lactation or in women of child-bearing age has not been established, use of the drugs in such patients requires that the potential benefits of the drug be weighed against possible hazards to the mother and child.
In the presence of a high environmental temperature, heat prostration can occur with drug use (fever and heat stroke due to decreased sweating).
Diarrhea may be an early symptom of incomplete intestinal obstruction, especially in patients with ileostomy or colostomy. In this instance treatment with this drug would be inappropriate and possibly harmful.
VALPIN® 50 may produce drowsiness or blurred vision. In this event, the patient should be warned not to engage in activities requiring mental alertness such as operating a motor vehicle or other machinery or perform hazardous work while taking this drug.
Precautions:
Use with caution in patients with:
—Autonomic neuropathy.
—Hepatic or renal disease.
—Ulcerative colitis—large doses may suppress intestinal motility to the point of producing a paralytic ileus and the use of this drug may precipitate or aggravate the serious complication of toxic megacolon.
—Hyperthyroidism, coronary heart disease, congestive heart failure, cardiac arrhythmias, hypertension and non-obstructing prostatic hypertrophy.
—Hiatal hernia associated with reflux esophagitis since anticholinergic drugs may aggravate this condition.
It should be noted that the use of anticholinergic drugs in the treatment of gastric ulcer may produce a delay in gastric emptying time and may complicate such therapy (antral stasis).
Do not rely on the use of the drug in the presence of complication of biliary tract disease.
Investigate any tachycardia before giving anticholinergic (atropine-like) drugs since they may increase the heart rate.
With overdosage, a curare-like action may occur.
Adverse Reactions: Anticholinergic drugs produce certain effects which may be physiologic or toxic depending upon the individual patient's response. The physician must delineate these.
Adverse reactions may include xerostomia; urinary hesitancy and retention; blurred vision and tachycardia; palpitations; mydriasis; cycloplegia; increased ocular tension; loss of taste; headaches; nervousness; drowsiness; weakness; dizziness; insomnia; nausea; vomiting; impotence; suppression of lactation; constipation; bloated feeling; severe allergic reaction or drug idiosyncrasies including anaphylaxis; urticaria and other dermal manifestations; some degree of mental confusion and/or excitement especially in elderly persons. Decreased sweating is another adverse reaction that may occur.
Dosage and Administration: To be effective dosage must be titrated to individual patient needs. Usual adult dosage—VALPIN® 50 mg tablet; one tablet 3 times daily.
Management of Overdosage: While overdosage intoxication with anisotropine methylbromide has not been reported, theoretically it could occur since anisotropine methylbromide is an anticholinergic drug. When anticholinergic drugs are taken in sufficient overdose to produce severe symptoms, prompt treatment should be instituted. If the drug has been taken orally, gastric lavage and other measures to limit intestinal absorption should be initiated without delay. Physostigmine administered

parenterally may be necessary for treatment of the serious manifestations of intoxication. Additionally, symptomatic therapy, including oxygen, sedatives, and control of hyperthermia may be necessary.

How Supplied: VALPIN® 50: 50 mg anisotropine methylbromide in each scored, beige tablet.

Bottles of 100 and 1000 tablets.

Animal Pharmacology and Toxicology: VALPIN® 50 (anisotropine methylbromide) is a relatively non-toxic drug. In dogs, mice, rats and guinea pigs both acute toxic and chronic toxic dose-levels are at many times in excess of the clinically useful range.

Both **in vitro** and oral **in vivo** data in mice and rats indicate that VALPIN® 50 (anisotropine methylbromide) is at least 2 or 3 times as potent as homatropine methylbromide in antispasmodic action while it is less than two-thirds as active in mydriatic effect. It has less than one-fiftieth of the mydriatic activity of atropine sulfate. In inhibition of salivary flow, VALPIN® 50 (anisotropine methylbromide) is one-fifth as active as homatropine methylbromide and only one-hundredth as active as atropine sulfate. This pharmacologic profile is consistent with relative specificity of action of the gastrointestinal smooth muscle and the lesser tendency to produce side effects.

VALPIN® is an Endo registered U.S. trademark

6083-4

[*Shown in Product Identification Section*]

VALPIN® 50-PB ℞

(anisotropine methylbromide 50 mg with phenobarbital 15 mg)

Description: VALPIN® 50-PB is anisotropine methylbromide with phenobarbital. Anisotropine methylbromide, differs chemically from atropine and most other anticholinergics/ antispasmodics in the substitution of an aliphatic for an aromatic side chain in the acid moiety of the ester.

Chemically, anisotropine methylbromide is 2-propyl pentanoyl tropinium methylbromide. Its stability both to acid and alkaline hydrolysis minimizes inactivation.

Actions: VALPIN® 50-PB (anisotropine methylbromide with phenobarbital), like other anticholinergic/antispasmodic drugs, effectively produces visceral smooth muscle relaxation. Consequently, VALPIN® 50-PB may provide effective control of smooth muscle spasm seen in motility disorders of the gastrointestinal tract, such as spastic colon and functional gastrointestinal disorders.

Indications: AS WITH ALL ANTICHOLINERGICS/ANTISPASMODICS, IT SHOULD BE NOTED THAT AT THE PRESENT TIME THERE IS LACK OF CONCURRENCE AS TO THEIR VALUE IN THE TREATMENT OF GASTRIC ULCER. IT HAS NOT BEEN SHOWN CONCLUSIVELY WHETHER ANTICHOLINERGIC/ANTISPASMODIC DRUGS AID IN THE HEALING OF A PEPTIC ULCER, DECREASE THE RATE OF RECURRENCES OR PREVENT COMPLICATION.

Based on a review of this drug by the National Academy of Sciences—National Research Council and/or other information, FDA has classified the following indications as "possibly" effective.

Indicated for use as adjunctive therapy in the treatment of peptic ulcer; irritable bowel syndrome (irritable colon, spastic colon, mucous colitis, acute enterocolitis, and functional gastrointestinal disorders); and in neurogenic bowel disturbances (including the splenic flexure syndrome and neurogenic colon).

THESE FUNCTIONAL DISORDERS ARE OFTEN RELIEVED BY VARYING COMBINATIONS OF SEDATIVE, REASSURANCE, PHYSICIAN INTEREST, AMELIORATION OF ENVIRONMENTAL FACTORS.

Final classification of the less-than-effective indications requires further investigation.

Contraindications: Glaucoma; obstructive uropathy (for example, bladder neck obstruction due to prostatic hypertrophy); obstructive disease of the gastrointestinal tract (as in achalasia, pyloroduodenal stenosis, etc.); paralytic ileus, intestinal atony of the elderly or debilitated patient; unstable cardiovascular status in acute hemorrhage; severe ulcerative colitis; toxic megacolon complicating ulcerative colitis; myasthenia gravis.

Phenobarbital is contraindicated in acute intermittent porphyria. VALPIN® 50-PB is contraindicated in those patients in whom phenobarbital produces restlessness and/or excitement.

Warnings:

Use in Pregnancy: Since the safety of these preparations in pregnancy, lactation or in women of child-bearing age has not been established, use of the drugs in such patients requires that the potential benefits of the drug be weighed against possible hazards to the mother and child.

In the presence of a high environmental temperature, heat prostration can occur with drug use (fever and heat stroke due to decreased sweating).

Diarrhea may be an early symptom of incomplete intestinal obstruction, especially in patients with ileostomy or colostomy. In this instance treatment with this drug would be inappropriate and possibly harmful.

VALPIN® 50-PB may produce drowsiness or blurred vision. In this event, the patient should be warned not to engage in activities requiring mental alertness such as operating a motor vehicle or other machinery or perform hazardous work while taking this drug.

Phenobarbital: Phenobarbital may decrease the prothrombin time response to oral anticoagulants. More frequent monitoring of prothrombin time responses is indicated whenever phenobarbital is initiated or discontinued, and the dosage of anticoagulants should be adjusted accordingly.

Phenobarbital may be habit forming and should not be administered to individuals known to be addiction prone or to those with a history of physical and/or psychological dependence upon habit forming drugs.

Precautions: Use with caution in patients with:

—Autonomic neuropathy.
—Hepatic or renal disease.
—Ulcerative colitis—large doses may suppress intestinal motility to the point of producing a paralytic ileus and the use of this drug may precipitate or aggravate the serious complication of toxic megacolon.
—Hyperthyroidism, coronary heart disease, congestive heart failure, cardiac arrhythmias, hypertension and non-obstructing prostatic hypertrophy.
—Hiatal hernia associated with reflux esophagitis since anticholinergic/antispasmodic drugs may aggravate this condition.

It should be noted that the use of anticholinergic/antispasmodic drugs in the treatment of gastric ulcer may produce a delay in gastric emptying time and may complicate such therapy (antral stasis).

Do not rely on the use of the drug in the presence of complication of biliary tract disease. Investigate any tachycardia before giving anticholinergic/antispasmodic (atropine-like) drugs since they may increase the heart rate. With overdosage, a curare-like action may occur.

Adverse Reactions: Anticholinergic/antispasmodic drugs produce certain effects which may be physiologic or toxic depending upon the individual patient's response. The physician must delineate these.

Adverse reactions may include xerostomia; urinary hesitancy and retention; blurred vision and tachycardia; palpitations; mydriasis; cycloplegia; increased ocular tension; loss of taste; headaches; nervousness; drowsiness; weakness; dizziness; insomnia; nausea; vomiting; impotence; suppression of lactation; constipation; bloated feeling; severe allergic reaction or drug idiosyncrasies including anaphylaxis; urticaria and other dermal manifestations; some degree of mental confusion and/or excitement especially in elderly persons. Decreased sweating is another adverse reaction that may occur.

Phenobarbital: In some patients phenobarbital may produce excitement rather than a sedative effect, as well as musculoskeletal pain. Some patients may acquire a sensitivity to barbiturates.

Dosage and Administration: To be effective, the dosage must be titrated to the individual patient's needs. Usual adult dosage—VALPIN® 50-PB; one tablet 3 times daily.

Management of Overdosage: While overdosage intoxication with anisotropine methylbromide with phenobarbital has not been reported, theoretically it could occur since anisotropine methylbromide is an anticholinergic/antispasmodic drug. When anticholinergic/antispasmodic drugs are taken in sufficient overdose to produce severe symptoms, prompt treatment should be instituted. If the drug has been taken orally, gastric lavage and other measures to limit intestinal absorption should be initiated without delay. Physostigmine administered parenterally may be necessary for treatment of the serious manifestations of intoxication. Additionally, symptomatic therapy, including oxygen, sedatives, and control of hyperthermia may be necessary.

Acute barbiturate intoxication with VALPIN® 50-PB, while possible, has not been reported. While the usual procedures for handling barbiturate poisoning should be employed, keep in mind the possibility of anticholinergic overdosing effects.

How Supplied: VALPIN® 50-PB: 50 mg anisotropine methylbromide and 15 mg of phenobarbital (*Warning:* May be habit forming) in each scored, white tablet.

Bottles of 100 and 1000 tablets.

Animal Pharmacology and Toxicology: Anisotropine methylbromide is a relatively non-toxic drug. In dogs, mice, rats and guinea pigs both acute toxic and chronic toxic dose-levels are at many times in excess of the clinically useful range.

Both **in vitro** and oral **in vivo** data in mice and rats indicate that anisotropine methylbromide is at least 2 or 3 times as potent as homatropine methylbromide in antispasmodic action while it is less than two-thirds as active in mydriatic effect. It has less than one-fiftieth of the mydriatic activity of atropine sulfate. In inhibition of salivary flow, anisotropine methylbromide is one-fifth as active as homatropine methylbromide and only one-hundredth as active as atropine sulfate. This pharmacologic profile is consistent with relative specificity of action of the gastrointestinal smooth muscle and the lesser tendency to produce side effects.

VALPIN® is an Endo registered U.S. trademark

6084-1

[*Shown in Product Identification Section*]

Everett Laboratories, Inc.
76 FRANKLIN STREET
EAST ORANGE, NEW JERSEY 07017

REPAN ℞

Composition: Each REPAN Tablet contains isobutylallylbarbituric acid (Butalbital, N.F.), (WARNING: May be habit forming.) 50 mg.; caffeine, U.S.P., 40 mg.; phenacetin, U.S.P. 130 mg.; acetaminophen, N.F. 300 mg.

Properties and Therapeutics: Many clinicians report that nervous tension and anxiety underline tension headache. Sustained contraction of head and neck muscles is a major factor in this type of headache. REPAN combines analgesics plus a mild sedative, Butalbital. Acetaminophen may be used safely by most persons sensitive to aspirin. REPAN may be of value in other pain-tension states such as muscle pain, dental pain, menstrual pain, arthritic pain, and bursitis pain.

Indications

Based on a review of this drug by the National Academy of Sciences—National Research Council and/or other information, FDA has classified the indications as follows: "Possibly" effective: For use to relieve pain; in "conditions in which combined sedative and analgesic action is desired, such as, nervous tension and sleeplessness associated with pain, headache, or general malaise"; in nervous and muscular pain accompanied by hyperexcitability and nervousness; and in "all conditions requiring relief of pain or reduction of fever, such as, rheumatic and arthritic conditions, neuralgia, aches and pains, dysmenorrhea, respiratory infections and febrile conditions (common colds and grippe), dental extractions and minor surgical procedures and headaches." Final classification of the less-than-effective indications requires further investigation.

Contraindications: Hypersensitivity to any of the components.

Precautions: Due to presence of a barbiturate, may be habit forming. Excessive or prolonged use should be avoided. Keep out of reach of children. Phenacetin has been reported damaging to the kidneys when taken in large amounts for a long time and should be used with caution in patients with renal disease.

Side Effects: In rare instances drowsiness, nausea, constipation, dizziness, and skin rash may occur. Discontinue if any such reactions occur.

Adult Dosage: One to two tablets, repeated if necessary up to six per day.

Supplied: REPAN Tablets: White compressed tablet, bottle of 100. IMPRINTED EVERETT & Code #62 NDC 0642-0062-10.

Ferndale Laboratories, Inc.
780 W. EIGHT MILE ROAD
FERNDALE, MI 48220

KRONOHIST KRONOCAPS ℞

Composition: Each sustained release capsule contains:

Chlorpheniramine Maleate	4 mg.
Pyrilamine Maleate	25 mg.
Phenylpropanolamine HCl	50 mg.

Action and Uses: Kronohist effectively reduces excessive nasopharyngeal secretions and diminishes inflammatory mucosal edema and congestion in the upper respiratory tract. The antihistaminic action of chlorpheniramine and pyrilamine maleate reduces or abolishes the allergic response of nasal tissue. It is complemented by the mild vasoconstrictor action of phenylpropanolamine hydrochloride, which provides a nasal decongestant effect.

Indications: Kronohist is indicated for symptomatic relief of allergic manifestations of upper respiratory illnesses, such as the common cold, seasonal allergies, sinusitis, rhinitis, conjunctivitis and otitis. In these cases, it quickly reduces inflammatory edema, nasal congestion and excessive upper respiratory secretions, thereby affording relief from nasal stuffiness and postnasal drip.

Precautions: Administer with care to patients with cardiac or peripheral vascular disease or hypertension. Until the patient's response has been determined, he should be cautioned against engaging in operations requiring alertness such as driving an automobile, operating machinery, etc. Patients receiving antihistamines should be warned against possible additive effects with CNS depressants such as alcohol, hypnotics, sedatives, tranquilizers, etc.

Adverse Reactions: In susceptible patients or extreme overdose, drowsiness, nervousness or rapid pulse may occur.

Administration and Dosage: For all patients 12 years and older, one capsule every morning and evening.

How Supplied: Bottles of 30, 100, and 1000 capsules.

Caution: Federal Law prohibits dispensing with out prescription.

Topical ℞
PRAMOSONE CREAM AND LOTION
(Hydrocortisone Acetate)

Description: Pramosone Cream: Contains Hydrocortisone acetate 0.5% or 1% and Pramoxine HCl 1% in a hydrophylic base containing stearic acid, cetyl alcohol, aquaphor, isopropyl palmitate, polyoxyl 40 stearate, propylene glycol, potassium sorbate 0.1%, sorbic acid 0.1%, triethanolamine lauryl sulfate and water.

Pramosone Lotion: Contains Hydrocortisone acetate 0.5%, 1% or 2.5% and Pramoxine HCl 1% in a base containing forlan-L, cetyl alcohol, stearic acid, di-isopropyl adipate, polyoxyl 40 stearate, silicon, triethanolamine glycerine, polyvinylpyrolidone, potassium sorbate 0.1%, sorbic acid 0.1% and water.

Action: Topical steroids are primarily effective because of their anti-inflammatory, antipruritic and vasoconstrictive actions.

Indications: For relief of the inflammatory manifestations of corti-costeroid-responsive dermatoses.

Contraindications: Topical steroids are contraindicated in viral diseases of the skin, such as varicella and vaccinia. Topical steroids are contraindicated in those patients with a history of hypersensitivity to any of the components of the preparation. Topical steroids should not be used when circulation is markedly impaired.

Precautions: If irritation develops, the product should be discontinued and appropriate therapy instituted. In the presence of an infection, the use of appropriate antifungal or antibacterial agents should be instituted. If a favorable response does not occur promptly, the corticosteroid should be discontinued until the infection has been adequately controlled. If extensive areas are treated or if the occlusive technique is used, the possibility exists of increased systemic absorption of the corticosteroid and suitable precautions should be taken. The product is not for opthalmic use.

Warnings: USAGE IN PREGNANCY: Although topical steroids have not been reported to have an adverse effect on the fetus, the safety of their use in pregnant females has not absolutely been established. Therefore, they should not be used extensively on pregnant patients, or in large amounts, or for prolonged periods of time.

Caution: Federal law prohibits despensing without prescription.

Adverse Reactions: The following adverse reactions have been reported with topical corticosteroids, especially under occlusive dressings.

1. Burning
2. Itching
3. Irritation
4. Dryness
5. Folliculitis
6. Hypertrichosis
7. Acneiform eruptions
8. Hypopigmentation
9. Perioral dermatitis
10. Allergic Contact Dermatitis
11. Maceration of the skin
12. Secondary infection
13. Skin atrophy
14. Striae
15. Miliaria

Dosage and Administration: Apply to affected area 3 or 4 times daily.

How Supplied: CREAM: ½% or 1% in 1 oz. tube and lb. jar. LOTION: ½% or 1% in 1¼ fl. oz., 4 fl. oz., and 8 fl. oz., and NEW HIGH POTENCY: 2½% in 2 fl. oz. plastic dispenser bottles.

Ferring Pharmaceuticals, Inc.
475 PARK AVENUE SOUTH
NEW YORK, NY 10016

DDAVP® ℞
(desmopressin acetate)

Description: DDAVP (desmopressin acetate) is a synthetic analogue of 8-argininevasopressin. It is chemically defined as follows: Mol. wt. 1183.2. Empirical formula: $C_{48}H_{74}N_{14}O_{17}S_2$, SCH_2CH_2CO-Tyr-Phe-Gln-Asn-Cys-Pro-D-Arg-Gly-NH_2·$C_2H_4O_2$·$3H_2O$ 1-(3-mercaptopropionic acid)-8-D-argininevasopressin monoacetate (salt) trihydrate.

DDAVP (desmopressin acetate) is provided as a sterile, aqueous solution for intranasal use. Each ml contains:

Desmopressin acetate	0.1 mg
Chlorobutanol	5.0 mg
Sodium Chloride	9.0 mg

Hydrochloric acid to adjust pH to approximately 4

Clinical Pharmacology: DDAVP (desmopressin acetate) contains as active substance 1-(3-mercaptopropionic acid)-8-D-argininevasopressin, which is a synthetic analogue of the natural hormone argininevasopressin. One ml (0.1 mg) of DDAVP (desmopressin acetate) has an antidiuretic activity of about 400 IU as compared with argininevasopressin. Clinical results obtained thus far indicate that DDAVP (desmopressin acetate) is effective in the management of central diabetes insipidus:

1. The biphasic half-lives for DDAVP (desmopressin acetate) were 7.8 and 75.5 minutes for the fast and slow phases, compared with 2.5

and 14.5 minutes for lysinevasopressin, another form of the hormone used in this condition. As a result, DDAVP (desmopressin acetate) provides a prompt onset of antidiuretic action with a long duration after each administration.
2. The change in structure of argininevasopressin to DDAVP (desmopressin acetate) has resulted in a decreased vasopressor action and decreased actions on visceral smooth muscle relative to the enhanced antidiuretic activity, so that clinically effective antidiuretic doses are usually below threshold levels for effects on vascular or visceral smooth muscle.
Indications: Antidiuretic replacement therapy in the management of cranial diabetes insipidus and for the temporary polyuria and polydipsia associated with trauma to, or surgery in, the pituitary region. DDAVP (desmopressin acetate) is ineffective for the treatment of nephrogenic diabetes insipidus.
Contraindications: Hypersensitivity to DDAVP (desmopressin acetate).
Warnings: 1. For intranasal use only.
2. In very young and elderly patients in particular, fluid intake should be adjusted in order to decrease the potential occurrence of water intoxication and hyponatremia.
Precautions: DDAVP (desmopressin acetate) at high dosage has infrequently produced a slight elevation of blood pressure, which disappeared with a reduction in dosage. The drug should be used with caution in patients with coronary artery insufficiency and/or hypertensive cardiovascular disease.
Use in Pregnancy: Reproduction studies performed in rats and rabbits with doses up to 12.5 times the human intranasal dose have revealed no evidence for a harmful action on the fetus from DDAVP (desmopressin acetate). There are no studies in pregnant women.
Adverse Reactions: Infrequently, high dosages have produced transient headache and nausea. Nasal congestion, rhinitis and flushing have been reported occasionally, as well as mild abdominal cramps and vulval pain. These symptoms disappeared with reduction in dosage.
Overdosage: See adverse reactions above. In case of overdosage, the dosage should be reduced, frequency of administration decreased, or the drug withdrawn according to the severity of the condition.
There is no known specific antidote for DDAVP. If considerable fluid retention is causing concern, a saluretic such as furosemide may induce a diuresis.
Dosage and Administration: This drug is administered into the nose through a soft, flexible plastic nasal tube which has three graduation marks on it that measure 0.2, 0.1 and 0.05 ml. However, there is no number designation on the tube next to the 0.05 ml mark. DDAVP (desmopressin acetate) dosage must be determined for each individual patient and adjusted according to the diurnal pattern of response. Response should be estimated by two parameters: adequate duration of sleep and adequate, not excessive, water turnover. Patients with nasal congestion and blockage have often responded well to DDAVP (desmopressin acetate). The usual dosage range in adults is 0.1 to 0.4 ml daily, either as a single dose or divided into two or three doses. Most adults require 0.2 ml daily in two divided doses. The morning and evening doses should be separately adjusted for an adequate diurnal rhythm of water turnover. For children aged 3 months to 12 years, the usual dosage range is 0.05 to 0.3 ml daily, either as a single dose or divided into two doses. About 1/4 to 1/3 of patients can be controlled by a single daily dose.
How Supplied: 2.5 ml per vial, packaged with two applicator tubes per carton. Keep refrigerated at about 4°C.
Issued: January 1978

Distributed by:
Centerchem Products, Inc.
475 Park Avenue South
New York, NY 10016

Fisons Corporation
Pharmaceutical Division
TWO PRESTON COURT
BEDFORD,
MASSACHUSETTS 01730

BACID® CAPSULES — OTC

Composition: A specially cultured human strain of viable Lactobacillus acidophilus in high concentration. Also sodium carboxymethylcellulose 100 mg. per capsule.
Action and Uses: Antidiarrheal. For relief of diarrhea and associated anal discomfort.
Warning: In diarrhea, unless directed by a physician, do not use for more than 2 days or in the presence of high fever or in infants or children under 3 years of age.
Dosage: 2 capsules 2 to 4 times a day, or as directed by a physician. Preferably taken with milk.
How Supplied: Bottles of 50 and 100. Bottles of 100, NSN 6505-00-089-1282, Military Depots.

ERGOMAR® — ℞
(ergotamine tartrate)

Composition: Each sublingual tablet contains specially processed ergotamine tartrate, 2.0 mg.
Actions and Use: Ergomar (ergotamine tartrate) exerts a direct effect on cranial blood vessels, causing vasoconstriction with concomitant decrease in the pulsations probably responsible for migraine and other vascular headache symptoms. It is thus generally considered to be a specific agent for the therapy of this condition.
Indication: Vascular headaches such as migraine, cluster headache (histaminic cephalalgia).
Precautions and Contraindications: Avoid prolonged administration or dosage in excess of that recommended because of the danger of ergotism and gangrene. Contraindicated in sepsis, occlusive vascular disease (thromboangiitis obliterans, luetic arteritis, severe arteriosclerosis, coronary artery disease, thrombophlebitis, Raynaud's disease), hepatic disease, renal disease, severe pruritus, and pregnancy.
Side Effects: No serious complications have been reported from the use of Ergomar (ergotamine tartrate) in the absence of contraindications and in recommended dosages. Unpleasant side effects which may occur include nausea and vomiting, weakness in the legs, muscle pains in the extremities, numbness and tingling of fingers and toes, percordial distress and pain, and transient tachycardia or bradycardia. Localized edema and itching may occur in the rare sensitive patient. Side effects are usually not such as to necessitate interruption of therapy.
Administration and Dosage: All efforts should be made to initiate therapy as soon as possible after the first symptoms of the attack are noted, since success is proportional to rapidity of treatment, and lower dosages will be effective. At the first sign of an attack, or to relieve the symptoms of the full-blown attack, one tablet is placed under the tongue. Another tablet should be taken at half-hourly intervals thereafter, if necessary, but dosage must not exceed three tablets in any 24 hour period. Limit dosage to not more than five tablets (10 mg.) in any one week.
How Supplied: 20 tablets (green), each containing 2.0 mg. ergotamine tartrate, supplied in foil strips in a plastic child proof container.
Caution: Federal law prohibits dispensing without prescription.

INTAL® — ℞
(cromolyn sodium)
20 mg. capsules
For Inhalation Only
For Use With The SPINHALER®
TURBO–INHALER

Description: Chemically, cromolyn sodium is the disodium salt of 1,3-bis (2-carboxychromon-5-yloxy)-2-hydroxypropane.
It is soluble in water. Each capsule contains 20 mg. cromolyn sodium in micronized form together with 20 mg. of lactose powder added to improve the flow properties of the material. The contents of the capsule are intended for inhalation only, with the SPINHALER® turbo-inhaler.
Actions: *In vitro* and *in vivo* animal studies have shown that INTAL® (cromolyn sodium) inhibits the degranulation of sensitized mast cells which occurs after exposure to specific antigens. Cromolyn sodium inhibits the release of histamine and SRS-A (the slow-reacting substance of anaphylaxis). Bronchial asthma induced by the inhalation of specific antigens can be inhibited to varying degrees by pretreatment with INTAL.
Another activity demonstrated *in vitro* is the capacity of cromolyn sodium to inhibit the degranulation of non-sensitized rat mast cells by phospholipase A and the subsequent release of chemical mediators. An additional *in vitro* study showed that cromolyn sodium did not inhibit the enzymic activity of released phospholipase A on its specific substrate.
INTAL has no intrinsic bronchodilator, antihistaminic or anti-inflammatory activity. Because of its prophylactic mechanism of action, INTAL has no role in the treatment of an acute attack of asthma.
INTAL is poorly absorbed from the gastrointestinal tract. After inhalation of the powder, about 8 percent of the total dose administered is deposited in the lung, absorbed, and rapidly excreted unchanged in the bile and urine. The remainder of the dose is either exhaled or deposited in the oropharynx, swallowed and excreted via the alimentary tract.
Indications: INTAL is indicated as an adjunct in the management of patients with severe bronchial asthma in whom the frequency, intensity and predictability of episodes indicate the use of a continuing program of symptomatic medication. Such patients must have a significant bronchodilator-reversible component to their airway obstruction as demonstrated by a generally accepted pulmonary function test of airway mechanics.
If improvement occurs, it will ordinarily occur within the first 4 weeks of administration as manifested by a decrease in the severity of clinical symptoms of asthma, or in the need for concomitant therapy, or both.
A decision to continue the administration of INTAL on a long term basis is justified if introduction of the drug into the patient's regimen:
- produces a significant reduction in the severity of the symptoms of asthma, or
- permits a significant reduction in or elimination of steroids, or
- permits better management of patients who have intolerable side effects to sympathomimetic agents or methylxanthines.

Contraindications: INTAL is contraindicated in those patients who have shown hypersensitivity to it.
Warnings: **INTAL® (cromolyn sodium) has no role in the treatment of an acute attack of asthma, especially status asthmaticus.**
In some animal toxicity studies, a previously unreported proliferative arterial lesion found predominantly in the kidneys occurred in both treated and untreated macaque monkeys. The

Continued on next page

Fisons—Cont.

possibility that the increased incidence of the lesion in the treated monkeys is due to the administration of INTAL can neither be affirmed nor refuted (see Animal Toxicology). The relevance of these data to man is unknown. In considering the long term administration of INTAL to a patient, the physician should take into consideration the possible risk as well as the degree of efficacy achieved in the individual patient.

In view of the biliary and renal routes of excretion for INTAL, consideration should be given to decreasing the dosage or discontinuing the administration of the drug in patients with impaired renal or hepatic function.

If eosinophilic pneumonia (pulmonary infiltrates with eosinophilia) occurs during the course of INTAL therapy, the drug should be discontinued.

Use in Pregnancy: Reproduction studies have been performed in rabbits, rats, and mice. Adverse fetal effects (increased resorptions, decreased fetal weight) were noticed only at very high parenteral doses that produced maternal toxicity. The relevance to the human is not known. Since there is no experience in pregnant women who have received this drug, safety in pregnancy has not been established and its use in pregnancy is not recommended.

Use in Children: Clinical experience in children under 5 years of age is limited due to the necessity for administration by inhalation. Use of INTAL is not recommended for such children. Because of the possibility that adverse effects of the drug could become apparent only after many years, a benefit-risk consideration of the long term use of INTAL is particularly important in pediatric patients.

Precautions: Occasionally patients may experience cough and/or bronchospasm following INTAL inhalation. At times, patients with cromolyn sodium induced bronchospasm may not be able to continue its administration despite prior bronchodilator administration.

Symptoms of asthma may recur if INTAL is reduced below the recommended dosage, or discontinued.

Adverse Reactions: The most frequently reported adverse reactions attributed to INTAL (on the basis of reoccurrence following readministration) involve the respiratory tract and include:

- Bronchospasm
- Cough
- Laryngeal Edema (rare)
- Nasal Congestion
- Pharyngeal Irritation
- Wheezing

Other adverse reactions which have also been attributed to the drug (on the basis of reoccurrence following readministration) are:

- Angioedema
- Dizziness
- Dysuria and Urinary Frequency
- Joint Swelling and Pain
- Lacrimation
- Nausea and Headache
- Rash
- Swollen Parotid Gland
- Urticaria

In addition, the following adverse reactions have been reported as rare events and it is unclear whether these are attributable to the drug:

- Anaphylaxis
- Anemia
- Exfoliative Dermatitis
- Hemoptysis
- Hoarseness
- Myalgia
- Nephrosis
- Periarteritic Vasculitis
- Pericarditis
- Peripheral Neuritis
- Photodermatitis
- Polymyositis
- Pulmonary Infiltrates with Eosinophilia
- Vertigo

The following adverse effects which have occurred are related to the cromolyn sodium delivery system:

- Inhalation of gelatin particles
- Inhalation of mouthpiece or propeller

Dosage and Administration: The usual Starting Dosage for adults and children 5 years of age and over is the contents of one INTAL (cromolyn sodium) capsule inhaled four times daily at regular intervals using a SPINHALER turbo-inhaler. Because INTAL and the Spinhaler represent a different approach to the treatment of asthma, careful explanation and instruction in the use of the Spinhaler should be given to each patient. (Please see the instructions for the use of the Spinhaler included with the device.) **It should be emphasized to the patient that the drug is not absorbed when swallowed and is not effective by this route of administration.** Patients should be advised that the effect of INTAL therapy is dependent upon its administration at regular intervals, as directed. INTAL should be introduced into the patient's therapeutic regimen when the acute episode has been controlled, the airway cleared and the patient is able to inhale adequately. INTAL has no role in the treatment of an acute asthma attack especially status asthmaticus.

Once a patient is stabilized on INTAL, if there is no need for steroids, the frequency of administration may be titrated downward to the least frequent level consistent with the desired effect. The usual decrease is from four to three INTAL capsules per day. It is important that the dosage be reduced slowly, maintaining close supervision of the patient, to avoid exacerbation of asthma. It should be emphasized that in patients who have been titrated to less than four capsules per day, an increase in dosage may be needed if the patient's clinical condition worsens.

Corticosteroid Treatment and its Relation to Intal Use: An attempt to decrease corticosteroid administration and particularly to institute an alternate day regimen should be made in asthmatic patients receiving corticosteroids. Concomitant corticosteroids, as well as bronchodilators, should be continued following the introduction of INTAL. If the patient improves, an attempt to decrease corticosteroids should be made. Even if the steroid-dependent patient fails to improve following INTAL administration, gradual tapering of steroid dosage may nonetheless be attempted. It is important that the dose be reduced slowly, maintaining close supervision of the patient to avoid an exacerbation of asthma. It should be borne in mind that prolonged corticosteroid therapy frequently causes a reduction in the activity and size of the adrenal cortex. Relative adrenocortical insufficiency upon discontinuation of therapy may be avoided by gradual reduction of dosage.

However, a potentially critical degree of insufficiency may persist asymptomatically for some time even after gradual discontinuation of adrenocortical steroids. Therefore, if a patient is subjected to significant stress, such as a severe asthmatic attack, surgery, trauma or severe illness while being treated or within one year (occasionally up to two years) after corticosteroid treatment has been terminated, consideration should be given to reinstituting corticosteroid therapy. When the inhalation of INTAL is impaired, as may occur in severe exacerbation of asthma, a temporary increase in the amount of corticosteroids and/or other medications may be required.

It is particularly important that great care be exercised if for any reason INTAL is withdrawn in cases where it use has permitted a reduction in the maintenance dose of steroids. In such cases, continued close supervision of the patient is essential since there may be sudden reappearance of severe manifestations of asthma which will require immediate therapy and possible reintroduction of corticosteroids.

How Supplied: INTAL capsules, each containing 20 mg. cromolyn sodium in strips of four capsules each, in trade packages of 60, 120 and 300 capsules. SPINHALER turbo-inhalers are supplied separately in individual containers.

Caution: Federal law prohibits dispensing without prescription.

Animal Toxicology: A previously unreported proliferative arterial lesion has been found in some treated and untreated control macaque monkeys in four out of seven toxicity studies with INTAL (cromolyn sodium). In these four studies, the proliferative arterial lesion occurred predominantly in the kidneys, but was also found in other organs. An increased incidence of the lesion in the drug treated group occurred in one of these macaque monkey studies.

Typically, the lesions were multiple, affecting primarily the medium sized arteries of the kidneys. The most characteristic feature was the focal proliferation of cells in the tunica media replacing the normal smooth muscle and causing eccentric thickening of the arterial wall; there was a gap in the elastica interna in areas where the proliferation occurs. There was no thrombosis nor fibrinoid necrosis in the lesion, and there were no secondary effects such as infarction or glomerular or tubular degeneration. None of the animals developed the physical signs or symptoms usually associated with vascular and/or renal disease, e.g., hypertension, elevated blood urea nitrogen, or proteinuria in studies lasting up to 4 months.

In the initial subchronic study of the effect of INTAL in macaque monkeys, the drug was administered by inhalation for a period of four months. An increased incidence of the arterial lesion was found in the treated group (4 of 12) as compared to the control group (1 of 18). A second four month inhalation study was designed to evaluate the earlier findings and the possible effects of cromolyn sodium on renal vasculature. In this study, lesions were found in 1 of 27 treated macaque monkeys and 1 of 18 untreated control macaque monkeys. After examination of tissues from this study, especially the kidneys of monkeys exhibiting the arterial lesions, it was concluded that there were no histopathological or immunohistochemically detectable lesions associated with the administration of INTAL. The results of the first 4 month inhalation study, with respect to the number of lesions and their distribution between the treated and control animals, were therefore not reproduced in the second 4 month inhalation study.

The lesions were also found in one animal in each of 2 other toxicological studies conducted with macaque monkeys. One of these animals received a single intravenous dose of 50 mg/kg and the other received INTAL by inhalation for three months. The lesion was not found in 3 additional studies in macaque monkeys: an acute intravenous study in which the animals received a single dose of up to 1,000 mg/kg, a 6 month study in which animals received up to 100 mg/kg/day intravenously, and a 3 month inhalation study.

The lesion has not been seen in chronic primate studies utilizing baboons or squirrel monkeys treated for 6 months or longer with cromolyn sodium. Neither has the arterial lesion been found in toxicity studies of rodents treated with cromolyn sodium. Parenteral doses greater than 30 mg/kg produced degeneration of the renal tubular epithelium in the macaque monkey and in the various rodent species studied.

The incidence of the renal proliferative arteritis in the 7 studies conducted in macaque monkeys was 7 of 105 cromolyn sodium treated animals and 2 of 67 controls. Examples of this lesion have been found, in low incidence, in tissues obtained on routine pathological examinations of macaque monkeys not exposed to cromolyn sodium from independent primate research centers and in 2 animals from Regional Primate Research Centers. It is inferred that the lesion may reflect a spontaneous disease of macaque monkeys. The possibility that the increased incidence of the lesion in the treated monkeys is due to the administration of INTAL (cromolyn sodium) can neither be affirmed nor refuted.

Clinical Usage: A number of variables must be considered in evaluating the patient response to a drug used in the treatment of bronchial asthma—for example, concomitant treatment with other drugs, the fact that part of the trial may be conducted during the pollen season, the age of the patient, the duration and severity of disease, etc. In most studies of cromolyn sodium the drug has been evaluated as part of the total care program for asthamtic patients, and the role of each of these factors could not be evaluated. It is emphasized that cromolyn sodium is an adjunct to such a total care program and that patients may continue to require sympathomimetic amines, methylxanthines, and corticosteroids and antibiotics when indicated.

Many clinical studies have been performed with cromolyn sodium in patients with bronchial asthma. Controlled evaluations of the drug in comparison with a placebo have usually been of a crossover design with treatment periods lasting 4 to 6 weeks. In most of these studies, the investigator has concluded that cromolyn sodium is efficacious in comparison with the placebo. The proportion of patients responding to cromolyn sodium is usually reported to be in the majority, and an occasional patient is said to have a dramatic response. Significant improvement in pulmonary function tests is rarely reported, with the exception of one study in children in which approximately one-third of the patients showed an increase in Forced Expiratory Volume at 0.75 seconds ($FEV_{0.75}$) after three months therapy with cromolyn sodium.

One collaborative study involving over 250 patients was sufficiently large to permit multivariate statistical analysis of the results. In this study, patients' symptom scores were measured according to the following scale: 0 (no symptoms), 1 (trivial), 2 (mild), 3 (annoying), 4 (moderate), 5 (severe), and 6 (incapacitating). The indices that were measured included day wheezing, night wheezing, day breathlessness, night breathlessness, day cough, night cough, etc. The study was crossover in design and patients were treated with cromolyn sodium and with placebo for a period of four weeks each. The study as a whole included a large number of patients whose mean baseline symptom scores were less than 2. Changes in mean symptom scores as a result of cromolyn sodium treatment were, for the group as a whole, usually less than one unit. Little clinical benefit was manifested in this group with trivial to mild symptoms. In patients who were most symptomatic (i.e., those whose baseline symptom scores ranged from 2 to 6) changes in mean symptom scores due to cromolyn sodium were greater than one unit. Pulmonary function studies in the total group showed no essential changes attributable to cromolyn sodium. It is inferred from this study that a clinically significant response to cromolyn sodium is most likely in patients with severe perennial asthma who are highly symptomatic (see Indications).

Another group of studies has been performed to determine whether the administration of cromolyn sodium has a corticosteroid-sparing effect. These studies have shown that a number of steroid dependent patients who have had several unsuccessful attempts to reduce or omit corticosteroids may do so after the administration of cromolyn sodium (see special section in Dosage and Administration).

Long-term controlled studies relating specifically to the issue of tolerance are not available, but uncontrolled observations have not to this point revealed evidence of resistance or tolerance to the drug. Because the degree of response in an individual patient cannot be predicted, long-term therapy with cromolyn sodium is indicated only in patients who show a significant initial response (see Indications).

KONDREMUL® OTC
KONDREMUL® with Cascara
KONDREMUL® with Phenolphthalein

Composition: Irish Moss as an emulsifier with 55% heavy mineral oil.

Action and Uses: KONDREMUL brand laxative, a pleasantly flavored microemulsion, practically defies breaking down. Contains Irish Moss, a superior emulsifier, for optimal fecal softening and emollient actions. Acts gently without straining or irritation.

Indication: Constipation

Caution: Take only at bedtime. Avoid prolonged use. Do not administer to infants or young children, in pregnancy or to bedridden or aged patients unless directed by physician.

Precautions: Kondremul with Cascara and Kondremul with Phenolphthalein should not be used when abdominal pain (stomach ache), cramps, colic, nausea, vomiting or other symptoms of appendicitis are present. If skin rash appears, discontinue use. Frequent or continued use may result in dependence on laxatives.

Contraindications: See above

Administration and Dosage: Adults—1 tablespoonful at bedtime; Children over six years old—1 to 2 teaspoonfuls at bedtime. All dosages can be administered plain, mixed with a glass of warm or cold water or with the usual dietary beverages such as milk or cocoa.

How Supplied: Kondremul® Plain (White) 8 oz. and 16 oz. and 2 oz. unit dose: Kondremul® with Cascara [660 mg. Cascara extract per 15 cc] (Yellow) - 14 oz.: Kondremul® with Phenolphthalein [147 mg. Phenolphthalein per 15 cc] (White) - 16 oz.

PERSISTIN® OTC

Composition: Each tablet contains
Salicylsalicylic Acid .... 7 ½ gr. (485 mg)
Aspirin .... 2 ½ gr. (160 mg)

Action and Uses: Analgesic, for the temporary day and night relief of minor pains of arthritis and rheumatism.

Warning: Keep this and all medicines out of children's reach. In case of accidental overdose, contact a physician immediately.

Caution: Do not exceed recommended dosage. Overdosage of salicylates may cause temporary hearing or visual disturbances, drowsiness and nausea. If this occurs discontinue use until symptoms disappear. If pains of rheumatism or arthritis persist for more than 10 days, or redness is present, consult physician before continuing with medication.

Administration and Dosage: Adults, one tablet every 4 hours with a maximum of 6 tablets per 24 hour period.

How Supplied: Yellow, scored, uncoated tablets in bottles of 50 and 500.

SOMOPHYLLIN® Oral Liquid ℞
(aminophylline, USP)

Description: Somophyllin Oral Liquid (aminophylline liquid) contains anhydrous aminophyllin (USP) equal to not less than 85.0 percent and not more than 86.5 percent of anhydrous theophylline ($C_7H_8N_4O_2$) and not less than 13.5 percent and not more than 15.0 percent of ethylenediamine ($C_2H_8N_2$) both calculated on the anhydrous basis. Aminophylline is white or slightly yellowish granules, having a slight ammoniacal odor and a bitter taste. Somophyllin Oral Liquid is a red raspberry flavored solution. Each 5 ml (teaspoonful) contains anhydrous aminophylline 105 mg (equivalent to 90 mg anhydrous theophylline) in a palatable, aqueous vehicle.

Each 15 ml (tablespoonful) contains anhydrous aminophylline 315 mg (equivalent to 270 mg anhydrous theophylline).

Theophylline is the active ingredient.

Clinical Pharmacology: Theophylline directly relaxes the smooth muscle of the bronchial airways and pulmonary blood vessels, thus acting mainly as a bronchodilator, pulmonary vasodilator and smooth muscle relaxant. The drug also possesses other actions typical of the xanthine derivatives: coronary vasodilation; diuresis; cardiac, cerebral and skeletal muscle stimulation. The actions of theophylline may be mediated through inhibition of phosphodiesterase and a resultant increase in intracellular cyclic AMP which could mediate smooth muscle relaxation. At concentrations higher than those attained *in vivo,* theophylline also inhibits the release of histamine by mast cells.

In vitro, theophylline has been shown to act synergistically with beta agonists (isoproterenol) that increase intracellular cyclic AMP through the stimulation of adenyl cyclase, but synergism has not been demonstrated in patient studies. More data are needed to determine if theophylline and beta agonists have a clinically important additive effect *in vivo.* Apparently, no development of tolerance occurs with chronic use of theophylline.

The half-life of theophylline is shortened with cigarette smoking. It is prolonged in alcoholism, reduced hepatic or renal function, congestive heart failure, and in patients receiving antibiotics such as TAO (troleandomycin), erythromycin and clindamycin. High fever for prolonged periods may reduce the rate of theophylline elimination.

Theophylline Elimination Characteristics:

	Theophylline Clearance Rates (mean ± S.D.)	Half-life Average (mean ± S.D.)
Children (over 6 months of age)	1.45 ± 0.58 ml/kg/min	3.7 ± 1.1 hrs.
Adult non-smokers with uncomplicated asthma	0.65 ± 0.19 ml/kg/min	8.7 ± 2.2 hrs.

Newborn infants have extremely slow theophylline clearance rates. The theophylline half-life in newborn infants may exceed 24 hours. Not until 3–6 months of age do these rates approach those seen in older children.

Older adults with chronic obstructive pulmonary disease, any patients with cor pulmonale or other causes of heart failure, and patients with liver pathology may have much slower clearance rates with a half-life that may exceed 24 hours.

The half-life of theophylline in smokers (1 to 2 packs/day) averaged 4–5 hours among various studies, much shorter than the half-life in nonsmokers which averaged about 7–9 hours. The increase in theophylline clearance caused by smoking is probably the result of induction of drug-metabolizing enzymes that do not readily normalize after cessation of smoking. It appears that between 3 months and 2 years may be necessary for normalization of the effect of smoking on theophylline pharmacokinetics.

Indications: ***For relief and/or prevention of symptoms from asthma and reversible bronchospasm associated with chronic bronchitis and emphysema.***

Contraindications: This product is contraindicated in individuals who have shown hypersensitivity to its components, including ethylenediamine.

Continued on next page

Fisons—Cont.

Warnings: ***Status asthmaticus is a medical emergency. Optimal therapy frequently requires additional medication including corticosteroids when the patient is not rapidly responsive to bronchodilators.***

Excessive theophylline doses may be associated with toxicity. The determination of serum theophylline levels is recommended to assure maximal benefit without excessive risk. Incidence of toxicity increases at serum theophylline levels greater than 20 mcg/ml. Morphine, curare, and stilbamidine should be used with caution in patients with airflow obstruction because they stimulate histamine release and they can induce asthmatic attacks. These drugs may also suppress respiration leading to respiratory failure. Alternative drugs should be chosen whenever possible.

There is an excellent correlation between high blood levels of theophylline resulting from conventional doses and associated clinical manifestations of toxicity in (1) patients with lowered body plasma clearances (due to transient cardiac decompensation), (2) patients with liver dysfunction or chronic obstructive lung disease, (3) patients who are older than 55 years of age, particularly males.

Less serious signs of theophylline toxicity such as nausea and restlessness may appear in up to 50 percent of patients. However, serious side effects such as ventricular arrhythmias and convulsions may appear without warning as the first signs of toxicity.

Many patients who have higher theophylline serum levels exhibit tachycardia.

Theophylline products may worsen preexisting arrhythmias.

Usage in Pregnancy: Safe use in pregnancy has not been established relative to possible adverse effects on fetal development, but neither have adverse effects on fetal development been established. This is true for most antiasthmatic medications. Use of theophylline in pregnant women should be balanced against the risk of uncontrolled asthma.

Precautions: Mean half-life in smokers is shorter than nonsmokers, therefore smokers may require larger doses of theophylline. Theophylline should not be administered concurrently with other xanthine medications. Use with caution in patients with severe cardiac disease, severe hypoxemia, hypertension, hyperthyroidism, acute myocardial injury, cor pulmonale, congestive heart failure, liver disease, in the elderly (especially males) and in neonates. In particular, great caution should be used in giving theophylline to patients with congestive heart failure. Frequently, such patients have markedly prolonged theophylline serum levels with theophylline persisting in serum for long periods following discontinuation of the drug.

Use theophylline cautiously in patients with history of peptic ulcer. Theophylline may occasionally act as a local irritant to G. I. tract although gastrointestinal symptoms are more commonly centrally medicated and associated with serum drug concentrations over 20 mcg/ml.

Adverse Reactions: The most consistent adverse reactions are usually due to overdose and are:

1. Gastrointestinal: nausea, vomiting, epigastric pain, hematemesis, diarrhea.
2. Central nervous system: headaches, irritability, restlessness, insomnia, reflex hyperexcitability, muscle twitching, clonic and tonic generalized convulsions.
3. Cardiovascular: palpitation, tachycardia, extra systoles, flushing, hypotension, circulatory failure, life threatening ventricular arrhythmias.
4. Respiratory: tachypnea.
5. Renal: albuminuria, increased excretion of renal tubular and red blood cells, potentiates diuresis.
6. Others: hyperglycemia and inappropriate ADH syndrome; rash *(ethylenediamine).*

Drug Interactions:

Toxic synergism with ephedrine has been documented and may occur with some other sympathomimetic bronchodilators.

Drug	**Effect**
Aminophylline with Lithium Carbonate	Increased excretion of Lithium Carbonate
Aminophylline with Propranolol	Antagonism of Propranolol effect
Theophylline with Furosemide	Increased Diuresis of Furosemide
Theophylline with Hexamethonium	Decreased Hexamethonium-induced chronotropic effect
Theophylline with Reserpine	Reserpine-induced Tachycardia
Theophylline with Chlordiazepoxide	Chlordiazepoxide-induced fatty acid mobilization
Theophylline with clindamycin, troleandomycin, erythromycin, lincomycin	Increased Theophylline plasma levels

Overdosage:

Management::

A. If potential oral overdose is established and seizure has not occurred:
   1. Induce vomiting.
   2. Administer a cathartic (this is particularly important if sustained-release preparations have been taken).
   3. Administer activated charcoal.

B. If patient is having a seizure:
   1. Establish an airway.
   2. Administer oxygen.
   3. Treat the seizure with intravenous diazepam, 0.1 to 0.3 mg/kg up to 10 mg.
   4. Monitor vital signs, maintain blood pressure and provide adequate hydration.

C. Post-Seizure Coma:
   1. Maintain airway and oxygenation.
   2. If a result of oral medication, follow above recommendations to prevent absorption of drug, but intubation and lavage will have to be performed instead of inducing emesis, and the cathartic and charcoal will need to be introduced via a large bore gastric lavage tube.
   3. Continue to provide full supportive care and adequate hydration while waiting for drug to be metabolized. In general, the drug is metabolized sufficiently rapid so as not to warrant consideration of dialysis.

D. Animal studies suggest that phenobarbital may decrease theophylline toxicity. There is as yet, however, insufficient data to recommend pretreatment of an overdosage with phenobarbital.

Dosage and Administration: Therapeutic serum levels associated with optimal likelihood for benefit and minimal risk of toxicity are considered to be between 10 mcg/ml and 20 mcg/ml. Levels above 20 mcg/ml may produce toxic effects. There is great variation from patient to patient in dosage needed in order to achieve a therapeutic blood level because of variable rates of elimination. Because of this wide interpatient variation and the relatively narrow therapeutic blood level range, dosage must be individualized. Monitoring of theophylline serum levels is highly recommended. Dosage should be calculated on the basis of lean (ideal) body weight where mg/kg doses are stated. Theophylline does not distribute into fatty tissue.

Giving theophylline with food may prevent the rare case of stomach irritation; and though absorption may be slower, it is still complete. When rapidly absorbed products such as Somophyllin Oral Liquid are used, dosing to maintain "around-the-clock" blood levels generally requires administration every 6 hours to obtain the greatest efficacy for clinical use in children; dosing intervals up to 8 hours may be satisfactory for adults because they eliminate theophylline more slowly. Children, and adults requiring higher than average doses, may benefit from products with slower absorption which may allow longer dosing intervals and/or less fluctuation in serum concentration over a dosing interval during chronic therapy.

Due to the marked variation in theophylline metabolism in infants under 6 months of age, this drug is not recommended for infants under 6 months of age.

Dosage for Patient Population

Acute Symptoms of Asthma Requiring Rapid Theophyllinization:

Anhydrous theophylline indicated in *( )

I. Not currently receiving theophylline products

[See table below].

II. Those currently receiving theophylline products: Determine, where possible, the time, amount, route of administration and form of the patient's last dose.

The loading dose for theophylline will be based on the principle that each 0.5 mg/kg of theophylline administered as a loading dose will result in a 1.0 mcg/ml increased in serum theophylline concentration. Ideally, then, the loading dose should be deferred if a serum theophylline concentration can be obtained rapidly. If this is not possible, the clinician must exercise his judgement in selecting a dose based on the potential for benefit and risk. When there is sufficient respiratory distress to warrant a small risk, 2.5 mg/kg of theophylline is likely to increase the serum concentration when administered as a loading dose in rapidly absorbed form by approximately 5 mcg/ml. If the patient is not experiencing theophylline toxicity, this is unlikely to result in dangerous adverse effects.

Subsequent to the decision regarding modification of the loading dose for this group of patients, the maintenance dosage recommendations are the same as those described above.

Comments: It is recommended that serum theophylline concentrations be monitored in order to obtain optimal therapeutic theophylline dosage. However, it is not always possible

	Oral Loading Dose Aminophylline	Maintenance Dose for Next 12 Hours Aminophylline	Maintenance Dose Beyond 12 Hours Aminophylline
1. Children 6 months to 9 years	7 mg/kg *(6 mg/kg)	4.7 mg/kg q4 hrs *(4 mg/kg q4 hrs)	4.7 mg/kg q6 hrs *(4 mg/kg q6 hrs)
2. Children age 9–16 and young adult smokers	7 mg/kg *(6 mg/kg)	3.5 mg/kg q4 hrs *(3 mg/kg q4 hrs)	3.8 mg/kg q6 hrs *(3 mg/kg q6 hrs)
3. Otherwise healthy nonsmoking adults	7 mg/kg *(6 mg/kg)	3.5 mg/kg q6 hrs *(3 mg/kg q6 hrs)	3.5 mg/kg q8 hrs *(3 mg/kg q8 hrs)
4. Older patients and patients with cor pulmonale	7 mg/kg *(6 mg/kg)	2.4 mg/kg q6 hrs *(2 mg/kg q6 hrs)	2.4 mg/kg q8 hrs *(2 mg/kg q8 hrs)
5. Patients with congestive heart failure, liver failure	7 mg/kg *(6 mg/kg)	2.4 mg/kg q8 hrs *(2 mg/kg q8 hrs)	1.2–2.4 mg/kg q12 hrs *(1–2 mg/kg q12 hrs)

or practical to obtain a serum theophylline level. Therefore, patients should be closely monitored for signs of toxicity. The present data suggest that the above dosage recommendations will achieve therapeutic serum concentrations with minimal risk of toxicity for most patients. However, some risk of toxic serum concentrations is still present.

Adverse reactions to theophylline often occur when serum theophylline levels exceed 20 mcg/ml.

Chronic Asthma: Theophylline administration is a treatment of first choice for the management of chronic asthma (to prevent symptoms and maintain patent airways). Slow clinical titration is generally preferred to assure acceptance and safety of the medications.

Initial Dose: 16 mg/kg/day or 400 mg/day (whichever is lower) in 3–4 divided doses at 6–8 hour intervals.

Increased Dose: The above dosage may be increased in approximately 25 percent increments at 2–3 day intervals so long as no intolerance is observed, until the maximum dose indicated below is reached.

Maximum dose where the serum concentration is not measured:
(Warning: ***Do Not Attempt to Maintain Any Dose That is Not Tolerated)***

Not to exceed the following:

Age <9 years	28.2 mg/kg/day *(24 mg/kg/day)
Age 9–12 years	23.5 mg/kg/day *(20 mg/kg/day)
Age 12–16 years	21.2 mg/kg/day *(18 mg/kg/day)
Age >16 years	15.2 mg/kg/day or 1100 mg/day (WHICHEVER IS LESS) *(13 mg/kg/day or 900 mg/day) (WHICHEVER IS LESS)

NOTE: Use ideal body weight for obese patients.

Anhydrous theophylline indicated in *().

Measurement of serum theophylline concentration during chronic therapy: If the above maximum doses are to be maintained or exceeded, serum theophylline measurement is recommended. This should be obtained at the approximate time of peak absorption (1–2 hours) during chronic therapy. It is important that the patient will have missed *no* doses during the previous 48 hours and that dosing intervals will have been reasonably typical with no added doses during that period of time. *Dosage Adjustment Based on Serum Theophylline Measurements When These Instructions Have Not Been Followed May Result in Recommendations That Present Risk of Toxicity to the Patient.*

Final adjustment of dosage: See Table I.

Caution should be exercised for younger children who cannot complain of minor side effects. Older adults, those with cor pulmonale, congestive heart failure, and/or liver disease, may have unusually low dosage requirements and thus may experience toxicity at the maximal dosage recommended above.

It is important that no patient be maintained on any dosage that is not tolerated. In instructing patients to increase dosage according to the schedule above, they should be instructed not to take a subsequent dose if apparent side effects occur and to resume therapy at a lower dose once adverse effects have disappeared. [See table above].

TABLE I

Peak Theophylline Serum Level mcg/ml	Adjustment in Total Daily Dose	Comment
<5 5–7.5	100% increase 50% increase	If patient is asymptomatic, consider trial off drug; repeat blood levels after adjustment.
8–10	20% increase	Even if patient is asymptomatic at this level, an increased serum concentration may prevent symptoms during a viral URI, or heavy exposure to an inhalant allergen.
11–13	cautious 10% increase if clinically indicated	If patient is asymptomatic, no increase is necessary. If symptoms present during URI or exercise, increase as indicated.
	None	If "breakthrough" in asthmatic symptoms present at end of dosing interval, change to sustained-release product and repeat blood level.
14–20	Occasional intolerance requires a 10% decrease	If side effects present, decrease total daily dose as indicated.
21–25	10% decrease	Even if side effects are absent.
26–34	25–33% decrease	Even if side effects are absent, omit next dose and decrease total daily dose as indicated. Repeat blood levels.
±35	Omit next two doses. 50% decrease	Resume at 50% of previous dose and repeat blood levels.

How Supplied: Bottles of 8 fl. oz.
Dosage cup enclosed.
NDC #0585-2218-80
Bottles of 32 fl. oz.
NDC #0585-2218-82

Caution: Federal law prohibits dispensing without prescription. Keep tightly closed and out of the reach of children.

SOMOPHYLLIN® Rectal Solution ℞
(aminophylline)

Description: Somophyllin® Rectal Solution contains aminophylline as a concentrated aqueous solution for rectal administration, with the Rectal Ject syringe. Each **5 ml** contains aminophylline 300 mg **(equivalent to 255 mg theophylline base)**. Inactive ingredient: ethylenediamine

Actions: The principal pharmacological actions of theophylline and its derivatives are to relax smooth muscle, notably bronchial muscle, stimulate the central nervous system, act on the kidney to produce diuresis and to stimulate cardiac muscle.

Indications: For the symptomatic relief of bronchial asthma, pulmonary emphysema, chronic bronchitis and other pulmonary diseases associated with bronchospasm.

Contraindications: Somophyllin® Rectal Solution is contraindicated in those patients who have shown hypersensitivity to theophylline or theophylline derivatives.

Warnings and Precautions: Use with caution in the presence of severe hypertension, and in infants and young children. Other formulations containing theophylline or its derivatives should not be administered concomitantly. Metabolism of theophylline and its derivatives may be impaired in patients with severe pulmonary, cardiovascular, renal, or hepatic disease.

Adverse Reactions: Toxicity of theophylline and its derivatives may manifest as nausea, vomiting, peripheral vascular collapse, reactivation of peptic ulcers, intestinal bleeding, albuminuria, palpitation, nervousness, insomnia, and, with excessively high dosages, convulsions.

Dosage and Administration: The dose for **adults** is 5 ml (equivalent to 255 mg theophylline base) rectally, one to three times daily. The single dose for **children** is 5 mg/kg not to be given more often than every 6 hours; the total dose administered in a 24 hour period should not exceed 20 mg/kg.

Note: The metabolism of theophylline and its derivatives is a major factor in the observed interpatient serum level variability. Ideally, all individuals should have serum theophylline levels measured and a theophylline half-life calculated which would enable doses and dosing regimens to be tailored to each patient to maintain a serum theophylline level within the recommended therapeutic range (10–20 μg/ml), which insures optimal clinical response and avoidance of toxicity.

How Supplied: Somophyllin® Rectal Solution is available in nonbreakable bottles of 3 oz. solution (and 5 oz. solution for institutional use) with accompanying Rectal Ject syringe, plastic applicator tips and patient instructions.

Caution: Federal law prohibits dispensing without prescription.

SOMOPHYLLIN®-T Capsules ℞
(theophylline, anhydrous)

Description: Dye free, sugar free Somophyllin® Capsules contain theophylline U.S.P., anhydrous, in a non-alcoholic suspension. Somophyllin®-T Capsules are supplied in three strengths, 100mg, 200mg., and 250mg.

Actions: The principal pharmacological actions of theophylline are to relax smooth muscle, notably bronchial muscle, stimulate the central nervous system, act on the kidney to produce diuresis, and to stimulate cardiac muscle.

Indications: For the symptomatic relief of bronchial asthma, pulmonary emphysema, chronic bronchitis and other pulmonary diseases associated with bronchospasm.

Contraindications: Somophyllin®-T Capsules are contraindicated in those patients who have shown hypersensitivity to theophylline or theophylline derivatives.

Warnings and Precautions: Use with caution in the presence of severe hypertension,

Continued on next page

Fisons—Cont.

and in infants and young children. Other formulations containing theophylline or its derivatives should not be administered concomitantly. Metabolism of theophylline may be impaired in patients with severe pulmonary, cardiovascular, renal, or hepatic disease.
Adverse Reactions: Toxicity of theophylline may manifest as nausea, vomiting, peripheral vascular collapse, reactivation of peptic ulcers, intestinal bleeding, albuminuria, palpitation, nervousness, insomnia, and, with excessively high dosages, convulsions.
Dosage and Administration: The dosage and/or frequency of administration should be increased or decreased depending upon the observed clinical response which may vary from patient to patient.
Children: Over four years of age—one 100 mg Somophyllin® Capsule per 40 pounds (18kg) of body weight every six hours.
Children: Under four years of age—dosage at discretion of physician.
Adults: One 200 mg or 250 mg Somophyllin®-T Capsule every six hours.
Note: The metabolism of theophylline is a major factor in the observed interpatient serum level variability. Ideally, all individuals should have serum theophylline levels measured and a theophylline half-life calculated which would enable doses and dosing regimens to be tailored to each patient to maintain a serum theophylline level within the recommended therapeutic range (10–20μg/ml), which insures optimal clinical response and avoidance of toxicity.
Doses should be taken preferably prior to meals with a glass of water.
How Supplied: Somophyllin®-T Capsules, 100 mg, 200 mg, and 250 mg, in white, imprinted, soft gelatin capsules—bottles of 100.
Caution: Federal law prohibits dispensing without prescription.

TUSSCAPINE® OTC
(noscapine)

Composition: Each teaspoonful (5 ml.) or chewable tablet contains 15 mg. of Noscapine, N.F.
Actions and Uses: The superior clinical effectiveness of Tusscapine in the treatment of cough derives from the properties of noscapine, which, like papaverine, is one of the isoquinoline series of alkaloids which are nonnarcotic. Its antitussive potency has been shown in numerous studies to be equivalent to that of codeine but without the side effects of codeine.
Indications: Tusscapine is indicated for temporary relief of cough in the management of conditions such as bronchial asthma, allergies, common colds, bronchitis, laryngitis, pharyngitis, tracheitis, pertussis, influenza, measles, etc.
Administration and Dosage: Syrup: The usual adult dosage is 1 to 2 teaspoonfuls 3 to 4 times a day. Children 2 to 6 years of age, ½ to 1 teaspoonful 3 to 4 times a day (every 4–6 hours). It is not recommended to exceed 4 doses per day.
Tablets: The usual adult dosage is 1 to 2 tablets at 4 to 6 hour intervals not to exceed a total of 8 tablets (120 mg) in 24 hours. Children 6 to 12 years of age, 1 tablet 3 to 4 times per day, not to exceed 4 tablets (60 mg) in 24 hours.
Side Effects: Infrequently, with high dosage, nausea and drowsiness have been reported.
Caution: Keep out of reach of children. Do not administer to children under 2 years of age unless directed by physician. Persistent cough may indicate presence of serious condition. Persons with high fever or persistent cough should not use this preparation unless directed by physician.
Antitussives do not obviate the need for expectorants and mucolytics and the administration of fluids for asthmatics in whom excess mucus production or mucus plugging is suspected.
Contraindications: This preparation is contraindicated in patients who are allergic to noscapine (rare).
How Supplied: Suspension available in 4-ounce bottles; tablets in boxes of 24, and an industrial pack of 600.

VAPONEFRIN® Solution OTC
(racepinephrine)

Description: Vaponefrin Solution is an inhalant solution for use with a conventional nebulizer or with Vaponefrin pocket nebulizer. Vaponefrin Solution contains racemic epinephrine as hydrochloride equivalent to 2.25% epinephrine base, with 0.5% chlorobutanol as preservative.
Administration and Dosage: Instructions for the use of Vaponefrin Solution with the Vaponefrin Pocket Nebulizer:
Hold Nebulizer tip about 2 inches from mouth. Open mouth wide and inhale deeply, while squeezing the rubber bulb very hard. Unless a deep breath is taken at the same time that a very hard squeeze is given the bulb, the vapor will be wasted in clouds about the face.
Take 2 or 3 inhalations, then rest 5 minutes to note effects. Each user differs in dosage requirements and should use enough solution each time to bring relief without producing a feeling of tremor.
If expected relief does not develop within 5 minutes, take 2 or 3 additional inhalations. Use of Nebulizer 4 to 6 times daily is usually sufficient to maintain comfort. Use the smallest amount which will bring relief from wheezing or spasms of bronchial asthma.
Caution: No prescription is required for VAPONEFRIN. Persons using it, however, should be certain that they are suffering from bronchial asthma. Do not use for children under 4 years of age without consulting physician. Rinsing the throat with water after inhalation helps prevent dryness of the throat in those persons to whom this occurs.
Warning: FOR INHALATION ONLY. VAPONEFRIN should not be used without the advice of the physician by persons with high blood pressure, heart disease, diabetes, or thyroid disease. If bronchial irritation, nervousness, restlessness, or sleeplessness occurs, reduce dosage by decreasing the number of inhalations or using less frequently. If prompt relief is not obtained, consult your physician. Do not use epinephrine inhalation if it is brown in color or contains a precipitate.
How Supplied: Vaponefrin Solution is available in bottles of 7.5, 15, and 30 cc.

VITRON-C® OTC

Composition: Each chewable fruit-flavored tablet contains:
Ferrous fumarate....................200 mg.
(66 mg. elemental iron)
Ascorbic Acid (present in part as Sodium Ascorbate)....................125 mg.
Action and Uses: An effective hematinic for iron deficiency anemia. Pleasant to take and well-tolerated. Can be administered between meals when iron absorption is maximal.
Administration and Dosage: Adults —1 or 2 tablets daily or as directed by physician. Tablet is palatable, may be swallowed whole, chewed or sucked like lozenge.
How Supplied: Tablets (light brown): Bottles of 100 and 1000.

VITRON-C-PLUS® ℞

Description: Each maroon coated tablet contains:
Ferrous fumarate....................400 mg.
Ascorbic acid....................250 mg.
Cobalamin Concentrate
(B-12) Activity....................25 mcg.
Folic acid....................1 mg.
Actions: Folic acid (pteroylglutamic acid) and cyanocobalamin (vitamin B-12) are essential for the growth and reproduction of cells and for hematopoiesis. Iron is a necessary element in the biosynthesis of hemoglobin.
Indications: For the prevention and treatment of megaloblastic anemia associated with iron deficiency anemia as may be found in sprue, megaloblastic anemia of pregnancy, and megaloblastic anemia of infants.
For treatment of nutritional megaloblastic anemia associated with vitamin B-12 deficiency and in tropical and non-tropical sprue.
Contraindications: Folic acid (pteroylglutamic acid) is contraindicated in patients with untreated and uncomplicated pernicious anemia and in those with anaphylactic sensitivity to folic acid. Iron therapy is contraindicated in patients with hemochromatosis and patients with iron storage disease or the potential for iron storage disease due to chronic hemolytic anemia (e.g., inherited anomalies of hemoglobin structure or synthesis and/or red cell enzyme deficiences, etc.), pyridoxine responsive anemia, or cirrhosis of the liver.
Cyanocobalamin is contraindicated in patients with sensitivity to cobalt or cyanocobalamin (vitamin B-12).

Warnings: Patients with untreated pernicious anemia may show hematologic improvement with low daily therapeutic doses of folic acid (pteroylglutamic acid); this can occur with therapeutic doses as low as 0.4 mg/day. In such cases, degenerative lesions of the spinal cord may progress irreversibly after 3 months despite the absence of anemia. In patients with suspected pernicious anemia, pernicious anemia must be ruled out prior to folic acid (pteroylglutamic acid) therapy, by means of a Schilling test and a vitamin B-12 level determination.
Resistance to treatment may be due to depressed hematopoiesis, alcoholism, antimetabolic drugs, a deficiency of vitamin E or an increased requirement for vitamin B-6. Iron deficiency anemia may be due to occult blood loss, the cause of which should be determined and treated appropriately.
Prolonged therapeutic use of iron salts may produce iron storage disease.

Precautions: Folic acid (pteroylglutamic acid) and vitamin B-12 microbiologic blood assays are invalidated by the administration of most antibiotics, methotrexate, and pyrimethamine. Folic acid (pteroylglutamic acid) is not effective in reversing the effects of methotrexate. Folinic acid (5-formyl-tetra-hydrofolic acid) must be used in that situation. Black tarry stools may be due either to occult GI bleeding or iron therapy or both.
Adverse Reactions: Allergic sensitivity reactions and gastrointestinal disturbances may occur.
Dosage: Adults and children over 6 years of age: One tablet daily.
Caution: Federal law prohibits dispensing without prescription.
Overdosage: There have been no reports of toxicity due to excessive intake of either folic acid or cyanocobalamin.
The average human lethal dose of iron is about 200–250 mg. iron/kg. body weight.
How Supplied: Bottles of 30, 100 and 500 tablets.

Products are cross-indexed by generic and chemical names in the **YELLOW SECTION**

Fleet Co., Inc., C. B.
4615 MURRAY PL.
LYNCHBURG, VA. 24506

FLEET® BRAND BISACODYL ENEMA
(bisacodyl U.S.P.)

Composition: Each 30 ml (delivered dose) contains 10 mg. of bisacodyl, U.S.P. suspended in an aqueous medium. The FLEET® Bisacodyl Enema unit, with a 2-inch prelubricated Comfortip®, contains 1¼ fl. oz. of enema suspension in a ready-to-use plastic squeeze bottle. Designed for quick, convenient administration by nurse or patient according to instructions. Disposable after single use.
Action and Uses: FLEET® Bisacodyl Enema is a contact laxative acting directly on the colonic mucosa to produce peristalsis. FLEET® Bisacodyl Enema actually produces peristalsis and evacuation of the large intestine by stimulating sensory nerve endings in the colonic mucosa to produce parasympathetic reflexes. FLEET® Bisacodyl Enema is very effective usually producing an evacuation within 15 minutes to one hour. FLEET® Bisacodyl Enema may be used whenever a laxative or enema is indicated. It is useful as a laxative for relief of constipation, in bowel cleansing before X-ray and endoscopic examination.
Warning: Frequent or prolonged use of any laxative may result in dependence. Do not use when nausea, vomiting or abdominal pain is present. If use results in unusual pain or other side effects, contact a physician. Keep this and all medication out of the reach of children. In case of accidental overdose or ingestion, contact the nearest poison control center.
Precautions: Do not administer to children under two years of age.
Dosage and Administration: Adults—one unit or as directed by a physician. This dosage is not recommended for children under two years of age. Administration: Preferred position—Lying on left side with left knee slightly bent and the right leg drawn up, or knee-chest position. Rubber diaphragm at base of tube prevents accidental leakage and assures controlled flow of the enema solution. May be used at room temperature.
How Supplied: FLEET® Bisacodyl Enema is supplied in 1¼ fl. oz. ready-to-use squeeze bottle.
Is this Product OTC: Yes.
Literature Available: Professional literature mailed on request.

FLEET® BRAND ENEMA

Composition: Each 118 ml (delivered dose) contains 19 g. sodium biphosphate and 7 g. sodium phosphate. The FLEET Enema unit, with a 2-inch, prelubricated Comfortip™, contains 4½ fl. oz. of enema solution in a hand-size plastic squeeze bottle. Designed for quick, convenient administration by nurse or patient according to instructions. Disposable after single use.
Action and Uses: FLEET Enema is useful as a laxative in the relief of constipation, and as a bowel evacuant for a variety of diagnostic, surgical, and therapeutic indications. FLEET Enema provides thorough yet safe cleansing action and induces complete emptying of the left colon usually within 2 to 5 minutes without pain or spasm. FLEET Enema may be used for the relief of constipation; as a routine enema; preparation for rectal examination; during pregnancy and pre- and postnatally; preoperative cleansing and general postoperative care; to help relieve fecal or barium impaction.
Contraindications: Do not use when nausea, vomiting, or abdominal pain is present.
Warnings: Frequent or prolonged use of enemas may result in dependence. Do not use in patients with megacolon, as hypernatremic dehydration may occur. Use with caution in patients with impaired renal function as hyperphosphatemia and hypocalcemia may occur.
Precautions: Do not administer to children under two years of age unless directed by a physician.
Administration and Dosage: Preferred position: Lying on left side with left knee slightly bent and the right leg drawn up, or knee-chest position. Dosage: Adults, 4 fl. oz.; Children two years or older, 2 fl. oz., or as directed by physician. Rubber diaphragm at base of tube prevents accidental leakage and assures controlled flow of the enema solution. May be used at room temperature. Each 118 ml. (delivered dose) contains 4.4 g. sodium.
How Supplied: FLEET Enema is supplied in 4½ fl. oz. ready-to-use squeeze bottle. Pediatric size, 2¼ fl. oz.
Is This Product O.T.C.: Yes.
Literature Available: Professional literature mailed on request.

FLEET® BRAND MINERAL OIL ENEMA

Composition: The FLEET Mineral Oil Enema unit, with a 2-inch, prelubricated Comfortip™, contains 4½ fl.oz. (133 ml.) mineral oil USP in a hand-size plastic squeeze bottle.
Action and Uses: Serves to soften and lubricate hard stools, easing their passage without irritating the mucosa. Results approximate a normal bowel movement in that only the rectum, sigmoid, and part or all of the descending colon are evacuated. Indicated for relief of fecal impaction; valuable in relief of constipation when straining must be avoided (in hypertension, coronary occlusion, proctologic procedures, postoperative care); for removal of barium sulfate residues from the colon after barium administration for GI series or outlining the left atrium; to obtain the laxative benefits of mineral oil while avoiding possible untoward effects of oral administration such as (1) interference with intestinal absorption of fatsoluble vitamins A, D, E and K and other nutrients (2) danger of systemic absorption (3) possible risk of lipid pneumonia due to aspiration.
Contraindications: Do not use when nausea, vomiting, or abdominal pain is present.
Warnings: Frequent or prolonged use of enemas may result in dependence. Take only when needed or when prescribed by a physician.
Precautions: Do not administer to children under two years of age unless directed by a physician.
Administration and Dosage: For rectal administration only. Ready-to-use unit permits easy, rapid administration by physician, nurse, or patient; disposable after single use. *Adults,* 4 fl.oz. *Children two years or older,* one quarter to one half the adult dose, or as directed by physician.
How Supplied: FLEET Mineral Oil Enema is supplied in 4½ fl.oz. ready-to-use squeeze bottle.
Is This Product O.T.C.: Yes.
Literature Available: Professional literature and samples available on request.

FLEET® BRAND
Buffered Laxative
PHOSPHO®-SODA

Composition: Each 100 ml. of regular or flavored PHOSPHO-SODA contains 48 g. sodium biphosphate and 18 g. sodium phosphate in a stable, buffered aqueous solution.
Action and Uses: Versatile in action as a gentle laxative or purgative, according to dosage. Usually works within one hour when taken before meals, or overnight when taken at bedtime. Virtually free from likelihood of GI discomfort and irritation, PHOSPHO-SODA is pleasant to take, safe for all age groups. Useful before diagnostic examinations or bowel surgery.
Contraindications: Do not use when nausea, vomiting, or abdominal pain is present.
Warnings: Frequent or prolonged use of this preparation may result in dependence on laxatives. Do not use in patients with megacolon, as hypernatremic dehydration may occur. Use with caution in patients with impaired renal function as hyperphosphatemia and hypocalcemia may occur.
Administration and Dosage: Mix required dose with one-half glass cold water and follow with a full glass of water, preferably on arising or at least 30 minutes before a meal, or at bedtime for overnight action.
As a laxative: 4 teaspoonfuls, diluted as directed.
As a purgative: 8 teaspoonfuls, diluted as directed.
Children: One half the adult dose for children 10 years old or older; one quarter the adult dose for children between 5 and 10 years of age. Each recommended dose (4 teaspoonfuls) contains 96.4 meq. sodium.
How Supplied: Regular or Flavored, in bottles of 2½, 6 and 16 fl. oz.; 1½ fl. oz. size for hospitals.
Is This Product O.T.C.: Yes.
Literature Available: Professional literature and samples on request.

FLEET® BRAND PREP KITS
Bowel Evacuant

Description: FLEET® Prep Kit No. 1 contains:
1. FLEET® Phospho®-Soda—1½ oz. Ingredients: Each teaspoonful (5 ml) contains : Active Ingredients: Sodium Biphosphate 2.4 Gm. and Sodium Phosphate 0.9 Gm.
2. FLEET® Bisacodyl—4 laxative tablets. Ingredients: Each enteric-coated tablet contains Bisacodyl, NF, 5 mg.
3. FLEET® Bisacodyl—1 laxative suppository. Ingredients: Bisacodyl, NF, 10 mg.
4. 1 Patient Instruction Sheet.

FLEET® Prep Kit No. 2 contains:
1. FLEET® Phospho®-Soda—1½ oz.
2. FLEET® Bisacodyl—4 tablets.
3. FLEET® Bagenema—1. Ingredients: Liquid castile soap ⅔ fl. oz.
4. 1 Patient Instruction Sheet.

FLEET® Prep Kit No. 3 contains:
1. FLEET® Phospho®-Soda—1½ oz.
2. FLEET® Bisacodyl—4 tablets.
3. FLEET® Bisacodyl Enema—1 laxative enema. Ingredients: 1–30 ml. dose containing 10 mg. of Bisacodyl.
4. 1 Patient Instruction Sheet.

Actions: Bowel Evacuant.
Indications: Preparation of the colon for radiology (prior to barium enemas or I.V.P.'s), surgery, and many proctologic and colonoscopic procedures.
Warnings: Each recommended dose ((1½ oz.) (45ml)) contains 216.9 milli-equivalents (mEq) of Sodium. Persons on a low salt diet should consult a health professional before use. Do not use in patients with megacolon, as hypernatremic dehydration may occur. Use with caution in patients with impaired renal function as hyperphosphatemia and hypocalcemia may occur.
General Warnings: Do not use when nausea, vomiting, or abdominal pain is present. Frequent or prolonged use may result in a dependence on laxatives.
These Kits should not be used by patients under 6 years of age.
Dosage and Administration: See Patient Instruction Sheet for 12, 18 and 24 hour preparation schedule in each kit.
How Supplied:
FLEET® Prep Kit No. 1 contains:
1. 1½ oz. FLEET® Phospho®-Soda

Continued on next page

Fleet—Cont.

2. 4 tablets—FLEET® Bisacodyl
3. 2 suppositories—FLEET® Bisacodyl
4. 1 Patient Instruction Sheet

FLEET® Prep Kit No. 2 contains:
1. 1½ oz. FLEET® Phospho®-Soda
2. 4 tablets—FLEET® Bisacodyl
3. 1 FLEET® Bagenema
4. 1 Patient Instruction Sheet

FLEET® Prep Kit No. 3 contains:
1. 1½ oz. FLEET® Phospho®-Soda.
2. 4 tablets FLEET® Bisacodyl.
3. 1 FLEET® Bisacodyl Enema.
4. 1 Patient Instruction Sheet.

Shipping Unit: 48 FLEET® Prep Kits per carton.
For full prescribing information on specific products, see individual listings (FLEET® Phospho®-Soda, and FLEET® Bisacodyl Enema).
Is this Product OTC: YES.
Literature Available: YES.

Fleming & Company
**1600 FENPARK DR.
FENTON, MO 63026**

AEROLATE SR & JR & III Capsules ℞
(theophylline, anhydrous T.D.)

AEROLATE LIQUID
(theophylline, anhydrous)

Composition: Contains theophylline 4 grs. (260 mg) as SR, 2 grs (130 mg) as JR, 1 gr. as III (65 mg), in red/clear capsules. Liquid has 160 mg theophyllin/15cc in a non-sugar, non-alcoholic, non-saccharin tangerine flavored base.
Action and Uses: Timed action pellets bypass stomach to prevent gastric upset. Bronchodilation is achieved through bowel absorption only. Liquid is for the acute attack primarily.
Administration and Dosage: One capsule every 12 hours. Every 8 hours in severe attacks. Liquid—adults—40 ml (2.5 tablespoonfuls) for acute attack. Children—0.25 ml/lb. Maintainance therapy—adults—for the first 6 doses, 25 ml (1.5 tablespoonfuls) before breakfast, at 3 p.m., at bedtime. Then 15 ml doses at above times. Children—0.15ml/lb. at these times, then 0.1ml/lb per dose.
Side Effects: Nausea, vomiting, epigastric or substernal pain, palpitation, headache, dizziness may occur.
How Supplied: Capsules in bottles of 100 and 1000.
Liquid in pints and gallons.

EXTENDRYL ℞
Capsules, Syrup and Tablets

Each timed action capsule contains phenylephrine HCl 20 mg; chlorpheniramine maleate 8 mg; methscopolamine nitrate 2.5 mg. Green/red color. Each 5 cc. of root beer flavored syrup & tablet contains: phenylephrine HCl 10 mg; chlorpheniramine maleate 2 mg; methscopolamine nitrate 1.25 mg.
Action and Uses: Antihistaminic-decongestant for relief of respiratory congestion; allergic rhinitis; vasomotor rhinitis; allergic skin reactions of urticaria and angioedema.
Administration and Dosage: Capsules—one every 12 hours; syrup—*Adults*—two teaspoonfuls every 4 hours. *Children*—6-12 yrs. one teaspoonful every 4 hrs.; tablets—*Adults*—two every four hours; *Children* over 6 yrs one tablet every 4 hrs. Do not exceed 4 doses in 24 hrs. *Children* under 6 yrs. as recommended by a physician.
Precautions: Withdraw therapy if drowsiness or nervousness occurs. Patients are cautioned against driving or operating mechanical devices.
Contraindications: Glaucoma, cardiac disease, hyperthyroidism, and hypertension.
How Supplied: Capsules and tablets in bottles of 100 & 1000. Syrup in pints and gallons.

MARBLEN
Suspensions and Tablet

(See PDR Nonprescription Drugs)

NEPHROX SUSPENSION
**(aluminum hydroxide)
Antacid Suspension**

(See PDR For Nonprescription Drugs)

NICOTINEX Elixir
nicotinic acid

(See PDR For Nonprescription Drugs)

OCEAN MIST
(buffered saline)

(See PDR For Nonprescription Drugs)

PIMA Syrup ℞
(potassium iodide)

Composition: Contains KI 5 grs./tsp., in a black raspberry flavored base.
Action and Uses: An expectorant in the symptomatic treatment of chronic pulmonary diseases where tenacious mucus complicates the problem, including bronchial asthma, bronchitis and pulmonary emphysema.
Administration and Dosage: Children—one half to one tsp. and adults one or two tsp. every 4-6 hours.
Side Effects: May include gastrointestinal upset, metallic taste, minor skin eruptions, nausea, vomiting and epigastric pain. Therapy should be withdrawn.
Precautions: In patients sensitive to iodides, in hyperthyroidism, and in rare cases iodine-induced goiter may occur.
How Supplied: Plastic pints and gallons.

RUM-K ℞
(potassium chloride 15% conc.)

Description: Each 10 ml. contains 1.5 Gm. potassium chloride (20 mEq) in a butter/rum synthetic flavored base that is alcohol and sugar free.
Indications: Hypokalemic-hypochloremic alkalosis; digitalis toxicity; hypokalemia prevention secondary to corticosteroid or diuretic administration.
Contraindications: Impaired renal function, untreated Addison's Disease, acute dehydration, heat cramps, hyperkalemia.
Precautions: Do not use in patients with low urinary output or renal decompensation. Potassium replacements vary and should be individualized. Patients should be checked frequently, ECG and plasma K^+ levels should be made. High serum concentrations of K^+ cause death thru cardiac depression, arrhythmias or arrest. Use with caution in cardiac disease.
Adverse Reactions: Vomiting, nausea, abdominal discomfort, diarrhea may occur. Symptoms and signs of potassium overdose include paresthesias of extremities, flaccid paralysis, listlessness, fall in blood pressure, weakness and heaviness of the legs, cardiac arrhythmias and heart block. Hyperkalemia may cause ECG changes as disappearance of the P wave, widening and slurring of QRS complex, changes of the S-T segment, tall peaked T waves.
Dosage and Administration: Adults—two teaspoonsful (10ml) in 4–6 oz water 2 to 4 times daily after meals to supply 40–80 mEq of elemental potassium and chloride. Larger doses may be required and administered under close supervision due to possible potassium intoxication or saline laxative effect.
How Supplied: 2 oz; 4 oz; pints and gallons.

S-P-T ℞
(Pork thyroid "liquid" capsules USP)

Composition: S-P-T is prepared by special process from cleaned, fresh pork thyroid glands, deprived of connective tissue, defatted and suspended in soy bean oil and encapsulated in gelatin for greater oral absorption. The active hormones (T4 and T3) are available in their natural state in a ratio of approximately 2.5:1, as in humans, to insure therapeutic availability. Capsules are standardized by USP method for iodine content and also biologically to insure 100% metabolic potency.
Action: To increase metabolic rate of body tissues. S-P-T is replacement therapy for diminished or absent thyroid function. Effect develops slowly and is fully reached in 10—14 days per grain increase in most instances.
Indications: As replacement therapy in hypothyroidism, cretinism, myxedema, and after surgery following complete thyroidectomy.
Contraindications: In thyrotoxicosis, angina pectoris, myocardial infarction and hypertension unless complicated by hypothyroidism, and uncorrected adrenal insufficiency.
Precaution and Side Effects: Overdosage may cause tachycardia, angina pectoris, diarrhea, nervousness, sweating, headache and increased pulse action. In most cases, reduction of dosage overcomes side effects.
Dosage and Administration: Patients should be titrated starting at lower levels and increasing by 1 gr every 2 weeks until mild thyromimetic effects are noted. Then lower the dose to the level at which the patient felt best, as patients vary widely as to thyroid need.

> **Warnings:** Drugs with thyroid hormone activity, alone or together with other therapeutic agents, have been used for the treatment of obesity. In euthyroid patients, doses within the range of daily hormonal requirements are ineffective for weight reduction. Larger doses may produce serious or even life-threatening manifestations of toxicity, particularly when given in association with sympathomimetic amines such as those used for their anorectic effects.

How Supplied: As 1 gr (green); 2 gr (brown); 3 gr (red); 5 gr (black) gelatin sealed capsules in bottles of 100 and 1000.

Flint Laboratories
**(Division of Travenol Laboratories, Inc.)
DEERFIELD, ILLINOIS 60015**

CHOLOXIN® ℞
(Dextrothyroxine Sodium Tablets, N.F.)

Description: CHOLOXIN (dextrothyroxine sodium) is the sodium salt of the dextrorotatory isomer of thyroxine. It is chemically described as D-3,5,3′,5′-tetraiodothyronine sodium salt.
Actions: The predominant effect of CHOLOXIN (dextrothyroxine sodium) is the reduction of serum cholesterol levels in hyperlipidemic patients. Beta lipoprotein and triglyceride fractions may also be reduced from previously elevated levels.
Most of the available evidence indicates that CHOLOXIN (dextrothyroxine sodium) stimulates the liver to increase catabolism and excretion of cholesterol and its degradation products via the biliary route into the feces. Cholesterol synthesis is not inhibited and abnormal metabolic end-products do not accumulate in the blood.
Indications: This is not an innocuous drug. Strict attention should be paid to the indications and contraindications.
CHOLOXIN (dextrothyroxine sodium) is an antilipidemic agent used as an adjunct to diet

and other measures for the reduction of elevated serum cholesterol (low density lipoproteins) in euthyroid patients with no known evidence of organic heart disease.
The drug is also indicated in the treatment of hypothyroidism in patients with cardiac disease who cannot tolerate other types of thyroid medication. **Before prescribing, note the following: Results from a randomized clinical study have indicated a possible adverse effect when CHOLOXIN (dextrothyroxine sodium) is administered to a patient receiving a digitalis preparation. There may be an additive effect. This additive effect may possibly stimulate the myocardium excessively in patients with significant myocardial impairment. CHOLOXIN (dextrothyroxine sodium) dosage should not exceed 4 mg per day when the patient is receiving a digitalis preparation concomitantly. Careful monitoring of the total effect of both drugs is important.**
It has not been established whether the drug-induced lowering of serum cholesterol or lipid levels has a detrimental, beneficial, or no effect on the morbidity or mortality due to atherosclerosis or coronary heart disease. Several years will be required before current investigations will yield an answer to this question.
Contraindications: The administration of CHOLOXIN (dextrothyroxine sodium) to euthyroid patients with one or more of the following conditions is contraindicated:

1. Known organic heart disease, including angina pectoris; history of myocardial infarction; cardiac arrhythmia or tachycardia, either active or in patients with demonstrated propensity for arrhythmias; rheumatic heart disease; history of congestive heart failure; and decompensated or borderline compensated cardiac status.
2. Hypertensive states (other than mild, labile systolic hypertension).
3. Advanced liver or kidney disease.
4. Pregnancy.
5. Nursing mothers.
6. History of iodism.

Warnings:

> Drugs with thyroid hormone activity, alone or together with other therapeutic agents, have been used for the treatment of obesity. In euthyroid patients, doses within the range of daily hormonal requirements are ineffective for weight reduction. Larger doses may produce serious or even life threatening manifestations of toxicity, particularly when given in association with sympathomimetic amines such as those used for their anorectic effects.

CHOLOXIN (dextrothyroxine sodium) may potentiate the effects of anticoagulants on prothrombin time. Reductions of anticoagulant dosage by as much as 30% have been required in some patients. Consequently, the dosage of anticoagulants should be reduced by one-third upon initiation of CHOLOXIN (dextrothyroxine sodium) therapy and the dosage subsequently readjusted on the basis of prothrombin time. The prothrombin time of patients receiving anticoagulant therapy concomitantly with CHOLOXIN (dextrothyroxine sodium) therapy should be observed as frequently as necessary, but at least weekly, during the first few weeks of treatment.
In the surgical patient, it is wise to consider withdrawal of the drug two weeks prior to surgery if the use of anticoagulants during surgery is contemplated.
When CHOLOXIN (dextrothyroxine sodium) is used as thyroid replacement therapy in hypothyroid patients with concomitant coronary artery disease (especially those with a history of angina pectoris or myocardial infarction) or other cardiac disease, treatment should be initiated with care. Special consideration of the dosage schedule of CHOLOXIN (dextrothyroxine sodium) is required. This drug may increase the oxygen requirements of the myocardium, especially at high dosage levels. Treated subjects with coronary artery disease must be seen at frequent intervals. If aggravation of angina or increased myocardial ischemia, cardiac failure, or clinically significant arrhythmia develops during the treatment of hypothyroid patients, the dosage should be reduced or the drug discontinued.
Special consideration must be given to the dosage of other thyroid medications used concomitantly with CHOLOXIN (dextrothyroxine sodium). As with all thyroactive drugs, hypothyroid patients are more sensitive to a given dose of CHOLOXIN (dextrothyroxine sodium) than euthyroid patients.
Epinephrine injection in patients with coronary artery disease may precipitate an episode of coronary insufficiency. This condition may be enhanced in patients receiving thyroid analogues. These phenomena should be kept in mind when catecholamine injections are required in dextrothyroxine sodium-treated patients with coronary artery disease.
Since the possibility of precipitating cardiac arrhythmias during surgery may be greater in patients treated with thyroid hormones, it may be wise to discontinue CHOLOXIN (dextrothyroxine sodium) in euthyroid patients at least two weeks prior to an elective operation. During emergency surgery in euthyroid patients, and in surgery in hypothyroid patients in whom it may not be advisable or possible to withdraw therapy, the patients should be carefully observed.
There are reports that dextrothyroxine sodium in diabetic patients is capable of increasing blood sugar levels with a resultant increase in requirements of insulin or oral hypoglycemic agents. Special attention should be paid to parameters necessary for good control of the diabetic state in dextrothyroxine sodium-treated subjects and to dosage requirements of insulin or other antidiabetic drugs. If dextrothyroxine sodium is later withdrawn from patients who had required an increase of insulin (or oral hypoglycemic agents) dosage during its administration, the dosage of antidiabetic drugs should be reduced and adjusted to maintain good control of the diabetic state.
When either or both impaired liver or kidney function are present, the advantages of CHOLOXIN (dextrothyroxine sodium) therapy must be weighed against the possibility of deleterious results.
Usage in Women of Childbearing Age: Women of childbearing age with familial hypercholesterolemia or hyperlipemia should not be deprived of the use of this drug; it can be given to those patients exercising strict birth control procedures. Since pregnancy may occur despite the use of birth control procedures, administration of CHOLOXIN (dextrothyroxine sodium) to women of this age group should be undertaken only after weighing the possible risk to the fetus against the possible benefits to the mother. Teratogenic studies in two animal species have resulted in no abnormalities in the offspring.
Precautions: It is expected that patients on dextrothyroxine sodium therapy will show greatly increased serum protein-bound-iodine levels. These increased serum PBI values are evidence of absorption and transport of the drug, and should NOT be interpreted as evidence of hypermetabolism; similarly, they may not be used for titrating the effective dose of CHOLOXIN (dextrothyroxine sodium). PBI values in the range of 10 to 25 mcg% in treated patients are common.
If signs or symptoms of iodism develop during CHOLOXIN (dextrothyroxine sodium) therapy, the drug should be discontinued.
A few children with familial hypercholesterolemia have been treated with CHOLOXIN (dextrothyroxine sodium) for periods of one year or longer with no adverse effects on growth. However, it is recommended that the drug be continued in patients in this age group only if a significant serum cholesterol-lowering effect is observed.
The 2 mg and 6 mg tablets of CHOLOXIN (dextrothyroxine sodium) contain FD&C Yellow No. 5 (tartrazine) which may cause allergic-type reactions (including bronchial asthma) in certain susceptible individuals. Although the overall incidence of FD&C Yellow No. 5 (tartrazine) sensitivity in the general population is low, it is frequently seen in patients who also have aspirin hypersensitivity.
Adverse Reactions: The side effects attributed to dextrothyroxine sodium therapy are, for the most part, due to increased metabolism, and may be minimized by following the recommended dosage schedule. Adverse effects are least commonly seen in euthyroid patients with no signs or symptoms of organic heart disease; the incidence of adverse effects is increased in hypothyroid patients, and is highest in those patients with organic heart disease superimposed on the hypothyroid state.
In the absence of known organic heart disease, some cardiac changes may be precipitated during dextrothyroxine sodium therapy. In addition to angina pectoris, arrhythmia consisting of extrasystoles, ectopic beats, or supraventricular tachycardia, ECG evidence of ischemic myocardial changes and increase in heart size have been observed. Myocardial infarctions, both fatal and non-fatal, have occurred, but these are not unexpected in untreated patients in the age groups studied. It is not known whether any of these infarcts were drug related.
Changes in clinical status that may be related to the metabolic action of the drug include the development of insomnia, nervousness, palpitations, tremors, loss of weight, lid lag, sweating, flushing, hyperthermia, hair loss, diuresis, and menstrual irregularities. Gastrointestinal complaints during therapy have included dyspepsia, nausea and vomiting, constipation, diarrhea, and decrease in appetite.
Other side effects reported to be associated with CHOLOXIN (dextrothyroxine sodium) therapy include the development of headache, changes in libido (increase or decrease), hoarseness, tinnitus, dizziness, peripheral edema, malaise, tiredness, visual disturbances, psychic changes, paresthesia, muscle pain, and various bizarre subjective complaints. Skin rashes, including a few which appeared to be due to iodism, and itching have been attributed to dextrothyroxine sodium by some investigators. Gallstones have been discovered in occasional dextrothyroxine-treated patients and cholestatic jaundice has occurred in one patient, although its relationship to CHOLOXIN (dextrothyroxine sodium) therapy was not established.
In several instances, the previously existing conditions of the patient appeared to continue or progress during the administration of CHOLOXIN (dextrothyroxine sodium); a worsening of peripheral vascular disease, sensorium, exophthalmos, and retinopathy have been reported.
CHOLOXIN (dextrothyroxine sodium) potentiates the effects of anticoagulants, such as warfarin or Dicumarol, on prothrombin time, thus indicating a decrease in the dosage requirements of the anticoagulants. On the other hand, dosage requirements of antidiabetic drugs have been reported to be increased during dextrothyroxine sodium therapy (see WARNINGS section).
Dosage and Administration: For **adult** euthyroid hypercholesterolemic patients, the recommended maintenance dose of CHOLOXIN (dextrothyroxine sodium) is 4 to 8 mg per day. The initial daily dose should be 1 to 2

Continued on next page

Flint—Cont.

mg to be increased in 1 to 2 mg increments at intervals of not less than one month to a maximal level of 4 to 8 mg daily, if that dosage level is indicated to effect the desired lowering of serum cholesterol.

When used as partial or complete substitution therapy for levothyroxine in hypothyroid patients with cardiac disease who cannot tolerate other types of thyroid medication, the initial daily dose should be 1 mg to be increased in 1 mg increments at intervals of not less than one month to a maximal level of 4 to 8 mg daily, preferably the lower dosage. The maximum in patients receiving digitalis therapy is 4 mg.

For **pediatric** hypercholesterolemic patients, the recommended maintenance dose of CHOLOXIN (dextrothyroxine sodium) is approximately 0.1 mg (100 mcg) per kilogram. The initial daily dosage should be approximately 0.05 mg (50 mcg) per kilogram to be increased in up to 0.05 mg (50 mcg) per kilogram increments at monthly intervals. The recommended maximal dose is 4 mg daily, if that dosage is indicated to effect the desired lowering of serum cholesterol.

If new signs or symptoms of cardiac disease develop during the treatment period, the drug should be withdrawn.

How Supplied: CHOLOXIN (dextrothyroxine sodium) is supplied in prescription packages of scored 1, 2, 4, and 6 mg tablets.

Literature Available: Upon request.

[*Shown in Product Identification Section*]

SYNTHROID® ℞

(Levothyroxine Sodium, U.S.P.) Flint

Synthroid Tablets—for oral administration

Synthroid for Injection—for parenteral administration

Description: SYNTHROID (levothyroxine sodium) Tablets and SYNTHROID Injection contain synthetic crystalline levothyroxine sodium (L-thyroxine). L-thyroxine is the principal hormone secreted by the normal thyroid gland.

Actions: SYNTHROID (levothyroxine sodium) Tablets, taken orally, provide hormone that is readily absorbed from the gastrointestinal tract. SYNTHROID Injection is effective by any parenteral route. Following absorption, the synthetic L-thyroxine provided by SYNTHROID (levothyroxine sodium) products cannot be distinguished from L-thyroxine that is endogenously secreted. Each is bound to the same serum proteins and each exhibits a six to seven day circulating half-life in the euthyroid individual.

Both SYNTHROID (levothyroxine sodium) products will provide L- thyroxine as a substrate for physiologic deiodination to L-triiodothyronine. Therefore, patients taking SYNTHROID (levothyroxine sodium) products will demonstrate normal blood levels of L- triiodothyronine even when the thyroid gland has been surgically removed or destroyed by radioiodine. Administration of levothyroxine sodium alone will result in complete physiologic thyroid replacement.

Indications: SYNTHROID (levothyroxine sodium) products serve as specific replacement therapy for reduced or absent thyroid function of any etiology. SYNTHROID (levothyroxine sodium) Injection can be used intravenously whenever a rapid onset of effect is critical, and either intravenously or intramuscularly in hypothyroid patients whenever the oral route is precluded for long periods of time.

Contraindications: There are no absolute contraindications to SYNTHROID (levothyroxine sodium) therapy. Relative contraindications include acute myocardial infarction, uncorrected adrenal insufficiency and thyrotoxicosis (see WARNINGS).

Warnings:

> Drugs with thyroid hormone activity, alone or together with other therapeutic agents, have been used for the treatment of obesity. In euthyroid patients, doses within the range of daily hormonal requirements are ineffective for weight reduction. Larger doses may produce serious or even life threatening manifestations of toxicity, particularly when given in association with sympathomimetic amines such as those used for their anorectic effects.

Patients with cardiovascular diseases warrant particularly close attention during the restoration of normal thyroid function by any thyroid drug. In such cases, low initial dosage increased slowly by small increments is indicated. Occasionally, the cardiovascular capacity of the patient is so compromised that the metabolic demands of the normal thyroid state cannot be met. Clinical judgment will then dictate either a less-than-complete restoration of thyroid status or reduction in thyroid dosage.

Endocrine disorders such as diabetes mellitus, adrenal insufficiency (Addison's disease), hypopituitarism and diabetes insipidus are characterized by signs and symptoms which may be diminished in severity or obscured by hypothyroidism. SYNTHROID (levothyroxine sodium) therapy for such patients may aggravate the intensity of previously obscured symptoms and require appropriate adjustment of therapeutic measures directed at these concomitant disorders.

Thyroid replacement may potentiate the effects of anticoagulants. Patients on anticoagulant therapy should have frequent prothrombin determinations when instituting thyroid replacement to gauge the need to reduce anticoagulant dosage.

Precautions: Overdosage with any thyroid drug may produce the signs and symptoms of thyrotoxicosis, but resistance to such factitious thyrotoxicosis is the general rule. With SYNTHROID (levothyroxine sodium) Tablets, the relatively slow onset of action minimizes the risk of overdose but close observation in the weeks following institution of a dosage regimen is advised. Treatment of thyroid hyperactivity induced by oral medication is confined to interruption of therapy for a week, followed by reinstitution of daily therapy at an appropriately reduced dosage.

The 100 mcg (0.1 mg) and 300 mcg (0.3 mg) tablets of SYNTHROID (levothyroxine sodium) contain FD&C Yellow No. 5 (tartrazine) which may cause allergic-type reactions (including bronchial asthma) in certain susceptible individuals. Although the overall incidence of FD&C Yellow No. 5 (tartrazine) sensitivity in the general population is low, it is frequently seen in patients who also have aspirin hypersensitivity.

Adverse Reactions: Adverse reactions are due to overdose and are those of induced hyperthyroidism.

Dosage and Administration: For most adults, a final dosage of 100 mcg. (0.1 mg.) to 200 mcg. (0.2 mg.) of SYNTHROID (levothyroxine sodium) Tablets daily will restore normal thyroid function and only occasionally will patients require larger doses. Failure to respond adequately to a daily oral intake of 400 mcg. (0.4 mg.) or more is rare and should prompt reconsideration of the diagnosis of hypothyroidism, special investigation of the patient in terms of malabsorption of L-thyroxine from the gastrointestinal tract or poor adherence to therapy.

The concomitant appearance of other diseases, especially cardiovascular diseases, usually dictates a replacement regimen with initial doses smaller than 100 mcg. (0.1 mg.) per day.

In otherwise healthy adults with relatively recent onset of hypothyroidism, full replacement dose of 150 mcg. (0.15 mg.) or 200 mcg. (0.2 mg.) has been instituted immediately without untoward effect and with good therapeutic response. General experience, however, favors a more cautious approach in view of the possible presence of subclinical disorders of the cardiovascular system or endocrinopathies.

The age and general physicial condition of the patient as well as the severity and duration of hypothyroid symptoms determine the starting dosage and the rate of incremental dosage increase leading to a final maintenance dosage.

In the elderly patient with long standing disease, evidence of myxedematous infiltration and symptomatic, functional or electrocardiographic evidence of cardiovascular dysfunction, the starting dose may be as little as 25 mcg. (0.025 mg.) per day. Further incremental increases of 25 mcg. (0.025 mg.) per day may be instituted at three to four week intervals depending on patient response. Conversely, otherwise healthy adults may be started at higher daily dosage and raised to the full replacement dosage in two to three weeks. Clearly it is the physician's judgment of the severity of the disease and close observation of patient response which determine the rate of dosage titration.

Laboratory tests to monitor thyroid replacement therapy are of limited value. Although measurement of normal blood levels of thyroxine in patients on replacement regimens frequently coincides with the clinical impression of normal thyroid status, higher than normal levels on oral replacement of levothyroxine occasionally occur and should not be considered evidence of overdosage per se.

In all cases, clinical impression of the well-being of the patient takes precedence over laboratory determination in determining the appropriate individual dosage.

In infants and children, there is a great urgency to achieve full thyroid replacement because of the critical importance of thyroid hormone in sustaining growth and maturation. Despite the smaller body size, the dosage needed to sustain a full rate of growth, development and general thriving is higher in the child than in the adult, as much as 300 mcg. (0.3 mg.) to 400 mcg. (0.4 mg.) per day.

In myxedema coma or stupor, without concomitant severe heart disease, 200 to 500 mcg. of SYNTHROID (levothyroxine sodium) Injection may be administered intravenously as a solution containing 100 mcg./ml. Although the patient may show evidence of increased responsivity within six to eight hours, full therapeutic effect may not be evident until the following day. An additional 100 to 300 mcg. or more may be given on the second day if evidence of significant and progressive improvement has not occurred. Like the oral dosage form, SYNTHROID (levothyroxine sodium) Injection produces a predictable increase in the circulating level of hormone with a long half-time. This usually precludes the need for multiple injections but continued daily administration of lesser amounts intravenously should be maintained until the patient is fully capable of accepting a daily oral dose.

In the presence of concomitant heart disease, the sudden administration of such large doses of L-thyroxine intravenously is clearly not without its cardiovascular risks. Under such circumstances, intravenous therapy should not be undertaken without weighing the alternative risks of the myxedema coma and the cardiovascular disease. Clinical judgment in this situation may dictate smaller intravenous doses of levothyroxine.

SYNTHROID (levothyroxine sodium) Injection by intravenous or intramuscular routes can be substituted for the oral dosage form when ingestion of SYNTHROID (levothyroxine sodium) Tablets is precluded for long periods of time.

How Supplied: SYNTHROID (levothyroxine sodium) **Tablets** are supplied as scored, color-coded tablets in 6 concentrations: 25 mcg. (0.025 mg.)—orange ... 50 mcg. (0.05 mg.)—white ... 100 mcg. (0.1 mg.)—yellow ... 150 mcg. (0.15 mg.)—blue ... 200 mcg. (0.2 mg.)—pink ... 300 mcg. (0.3 mg.)—green.
SYNTHROID (levothyroxine sodium) **Injection** is supplied in 10 ml. vials containing 500 mcg. of lyophilized active ingredient and 10 mg. of Mannitol, U.S.P.
Directions for Reconstitution: Reconstitute the lyophilized levothyroxine sodium by aseptically adding 5 ml. of 0.9% Sodium Chloride Injection, U.S.P. to the vial. Do not use Bacteriostatic Sodium Chloride Injection, U.S.P. as the bacteriostatic agent may interfere with complete reconstitution. Shake vial to insure complete mixing. **Use immediately** after reconstitution. Discard any unused portion.
Literature Available: Upon request.
[*Shown in Product Identification Section*]

TRAVASE® OINTMENT ℞
(Sutilains Ointment, N.F.)

Description: TRAVASE Ointment (Sutilains Ointment, N.F.) is a sterile preparation of proteolytic enzymes, elaborated by **Bacillus subtilis,** in a hydrophobic ointment base consisting of 95% white petrolatum and 5% polyethylene. One gram of ointment contains approximately 82,000 casein units* of proteolytic activity.
*A casein unit is the amount of enzyme required to produce the same optical density at 275 mμ as that of a solution of 1.5 mcg. tyrosine/ml. after the enzyme has been incubated with 35 mg. of casein at 37° C. for one minute.
Action: TRAVASE Ointment selectively digests necrotic soft tissues by proteolytic action. It dissolves and facilitates the removal of necrotic tissues and purulent exudates that otherwise impair formation of granulation tissue and delay wound healing.
At body temperatures these proteolytic enzymes have optimal activity in the pH range from 6.0 to 6.8.
Indications: For wound debridement—TRAVASE Ointment is indicated as an adjunct to established methods of wound care for biochemical debridement of the following lesions:
Second and third degree burns,
Decubitus ulcers,
Incisional, traumatic, and pyogenic wounds,
Ulcers secondary to peripheral vascular disease.
Contraindications: Application of TRAVASE Ointment is contraindicated in the following conditions:
Wounds communicating with major body cavities,
Wounds containing exposed major nerves or nervous tissue,
Fungating neoplastic ulcers,
Wounds in women of child-bearing potential—because of lack of laboratory evidence of effects of TRAVASE Ointment upon the developing fetus.
Warning: Do not permit TRAVASE Ointment to come into contact with the eyes. In treatment of burns or lesions about the head or neck, should the ointment inadvertently come into contact with the eyes, the eyes should be immediately rinsed with copious amounts of water, preferably sterile.
Precautions: A moist environment is essential to optimal activity of the enzyme. Enzyme activity may also be impaired by certain agents. **In vitro,** several detergents and antiseptics (benzalkonium chloride, hexachlorophene, iodine, and nitrofurazone) may render the substrate indifferent to the action of the enzyme. Compounds such as thimerosal, containing metallic ions interfere directly with enzyme activity to a slight degree, whereas neomycin, sulfamylon, streptomycin, and penicillin do not affect enzyme activity. In cases where adjunctive topical therapy has been used and no dissolution of slough occurs after treatment with TRAVASE Ointment for 24 to 48 hours, further application, because of interference by the adjunctive agents, is unlikely to be rewarding.
In cases where there is existent or threatening invasive infection, appropriate systemic antibiotic therapy should be instituted concurrently.
Although there have been no reports of systemic allergic reaction to TRAVASE Ointment in humans, studies have shown that there may be an antibody response in humans to absorbed enzyme material.
Adverse Reactions: Adverse reactions consist of mild, transient pain, paresthesias, bleeding and transient dermatitis. Pain usually can be controlled by administration of mild analgesics. Side effects severe enough to warrant discontinuation of therapy occasionally have occurred.
If bleeding or dermatitis occurs as a result of the application of TRAVASE Ointment, therapy should be discontinued. No systemic toxicity has been observed as a result of the topical application of TRAVASE Ointment.
Dosage and Administration:
STRICT ADHERENCE TO THE FOLLOWING IS REQUIRED FOR EFFECTIVE RESULTS OF TREATMENT
1. Thoroughly cleanse and irrigate wound area with sodium chloride or water solutions. Wound MUST be cleansed of antiseptics or heavy-metal antibacterials which may denature enzyme or alter substrate characteristics (e.g., hexachlorophene, silver nitrate, benzalkonium chloride, nitrofurazone).
2. Thoroughly moisten wound area either through tubbing, showering, or wet soaks (e.g., sodium chloride or water solutions).
3. Apply TRAVASE Ointment in a thin layer assuring intimate contact with necrotic tissue and complete wound coverage extending to ¼ to ½ inch beyond the area to be debrided.
4. Apply loose wet dressings.
5. Repeat entire procedure 3 to 4 times per day for best results.

How Supplied: TRAVASE Ointment (Sutilains Ointment, N.F.) is supplied sterile in one-half ounce (14.2 g) tubes. Each gram contains 82,000 casein units of proteolytic activity in a hydrophobic ointment base.
The ointment must be stored under refrigeration at 2° to 8° C (35° to 46° F).
[*Shown in Product Identification Section*]

Fluoritab Corporation
P.O. BOX 381
FLINT, MICHIGAN 48501

FLUORITAB® ℞
sodium fluoride (Active Ingredient)

Composition:
Sodium fluoride .... 2.2 mg.
Inert organic filler ....75.8 mg.
Each tablet contains 1 mg. of fluorine (as fluoride ion)
Action and Uses: FLUORITAB dietary fluoride products are straight fluoride and contain no other active ingredients. They are to provide optimum fluoride where water supplies are deficient in fluorine. Dietary fluoride is beneficial in providing teeth that are more resistant to decay. Fluorine combines with calcium to form the apatite molecule of teeth and bone to form fluorapatite crystals.
Administration and Dosage: FLUORITAB dietary fluoride can be given in baby formulas, or in any liquid. They can be swallowed quickly, or permitted to remain in the mouth to dissolve, which may provide surface benefit to tooth enamel. Fluoride must be taken on a continued basis throughout the period of tooth formation to be fully effective.
Dosage should provide the child with ½ mg. per day from birth to 3 years of age and 1 mg. per day from 3 years of age up.
Water supplies with 0.2 parts per million or less require supplementing with ½ mg. and 1 mg. dosage per day for children under and over 3, respectively. Water supplies with 0.2 to 0.6 parts per million require ¼ mg. and ½ mg. dosage per day for children under 3 and over 3 respectively.
Side Effects: Excess fluoride is to be avoided, as it may cause dental fluorosis (mottling of the teeth).
Precautions: Where water with 0.7 P.P.M. of fluoride is used, dietary fluoride ought not be used.
Contraindications: None.
Overdosage: (*Symptoms and Treatment*): The total contents of our safety limited packages can be taken without any effect.
How Supplied: FLUORITAB TABLETS are supplied in bottles of 100, scored, easily divided 1.2 grain tablets, 1 mg. fluorine per tablet. FLUORITAB LIQUID is supplied in 19 cc. (480 drop) (.25 mg. fluorine per drop) polyethelene squeeze type dropper bottles.
Product Identification Mark(s): FLUORITAB products have the "FLUORITAB" name on all packages.
Remarks: FLUORITAB dietary fluoride was the first dietary fluoride product given A.D.A. acceptance (July, 1958). We adhere rigidly to their recommendation of restricting our package size to their safety admonition: *Never* to sell packages containing more than 264 mg. of sodium fluoride.
Literature Available: Yes. Reprints, educational folders, prescription instructions, and a unique multiple label which is attached to each package which automatically identifies the proper label for the age and water supply of the patient. Sent free, on request.

Forest Laboratories, Inc.
919 THIRD AVENUE
NEW YORK, NEW YORK 10022

BROCON® C.R.* Tablets ℞

Description: Each tablet contains:
Brompheniramine Maleate ....12 mg
Phenylephrine Hydrochloride ....15 mg
Phenylpropanolamine Hydrochloride ....15 mg
Actions: Brocon C.R. reduces excessive nasopharyngeal secretion and diminishes inflammatory mucosal edema and congestion in the upper respiratory tract. The antihistaminic action of brompheniramine maleate reduces or abolishes the allergic response of nasal tissue. It is complemented by the mild vasoconstrictor action of phenylephrine hydrochloride and phenylpropanolamine hydrochloride, which provides a nasal decongestant effect.

Indications: Based on a review of this drug by the National Academy of Sciences-National Research Council and/or other information, FDA has classified the indication(s) as follows: "Possibly" effective for the symptomatic treatment of seasonal and perennial allergic rhinitis and vasomotor rhinitis; and for treatment of urticaria and pruritus due to allergens of drugs; and allergic conjunctivitis.
Final classification of the less-than-effective indication requires further investigation.

Contraindications: Hypersensitivity to any of the ingredients. Brompheniramine is con-

Continued on next page

Forest—Cont.

traindicated during pregnancy and in patients who are receiving concurrent MAO inhibitors. Because of its drying and thickening effect on the lower respiratory secretions, it is not recommended in the treatment of bronchial asthma.
Warnings: In infants and children particularly, over-dosage of antihistamines may produce convulsions and death.
Precautions: Administer with caution to patients with cardiac or peripheral vascular disease or hypertension. Until the patient's response has been determined, he should be warned against engaging in operations requiring alertness, such as driving an automobile, operating machinery, etc. Patients receiving antihistamines should be warned against possible additive effects with CNS depressants such as alcohol, hypnotics, sedatives, tranquilizers, etc.
Adverse Reactions: Hypersensitivity reactions such as rash, leukopenia, urticaria, agranulocytosis and thrombocytopenia, drowsiness, lassitude, giddiness, dryness of the mucous membranes, tightness of the chest, thickening of bronchial secretions, palpitation, hypotension/hypertension, urinary frequency and dysuria, headache, faintness, dizziness, tinnitus, incoordination, visual disturbances, mydriasis, CNS-depressant and stimulant effect, anorexia, nausea, vomiting, diarrhea, constipation and epigastric distress.
Dosage and Administration: Adults and children over 12 years of age: One tablet morning and evening. If indicated, one tablet every 8 hours may be given.
How Supplied: Bottles of 100, 500 and 1000.
Caution: Federal law prohibits dispensing without prescription.

*Synchron™ System, a special base to provide a controlled release—U.S. Patent 3,870,790—Other U.S. Patents Pending.

BROCON® Chewable Tablets ℞

Description: Each Chewable Tablet contains:

Brompheniramine Maleate	2.0 mg
Phenylephrine Hydrochloride	2.5 mg
Phenylpropanolamine Hydrochloride	2.5 mg

Actions: Brocon Chewable reduces excessive nasopharyngeal secretion and diminishes inflammatory mucosal edema and congestion in the upper respiratory tract. The antihistaminic action of brompheniramine maleate reduces or abolishes the allergic response of nasal tissue. It is complemented by the mild vasoconstrictor action of phenylephrine hydrochloride and phenylpropanolamine hydrochloride, which provides a nasal decongestant effect.

Indications: Based on a review of this drug by the National Academy of Sciences—National Research Council and/or other information, FDA has classified the following indications as "possibly effective": for the symptomatic treatment of seasonal and perennial allergic rhinitis and vasomotor rhinitis; and "lacking substantial evidence of effectiveness as a fixed combination" for the following indications: The symptomatic relief of upper respiratory infection, acute sinusitis, asthma, nasal congestion, pharyngitis, bronchitis, and otitis. Final classification of the less-than-effective indications requires further investigation.

Contraindications: Hypersensitivity to antihistamines. Not recommended for use during pregnancy.
Precautions: Administer with caution to patients with cardiac or peripheral vascular disease or hypertension. Until the patient's response has been determined, he should be warned against engaging in operations requiring alertness.
Adverse Reactions: Hypersensitivity reactions including skin rashes, urticaria, hypotension and thrombocytopenia have been reported on rare occasions. Drowsiness, lassitude, nausea, giddiness, dryness of the mouth, mydriasis, increased irritability or excitement may be encountered.
Dosage and Administration: Adults 2 to 4 tablets 3 to 4 times daily; Children (1 to 2 years) 1 tablet 3 or 4 times daily; (2 to 4 years) 1½ tablets 3 or 4 times daily; (4 to 12 years) 2 tablets 3 or 4 times daily.

Tablets Must Be Chewed

How Supplied: Pineapple flavored, white, scored, chewable tablets in bottles of 100's.
Caution: Federal law prohibits dispensing without a prescription.

Frye Pharmaceuticals, Inc.
2625 2ND AVENUE, NORTH
P. O. BOX 10163
BIRMINGHAM, ALABAMA 35202

NORCET® Ⓒ ℞

Composition: Each tablet contains:

Acetaminophen	650 mg.
Hydrocodone Bitartrate	7.5 mg.

(WARNING: May be habit forming)
Action and Uses: Analgesic, antitussive. Indicated for the relief of mild-to-moderate pain.
Contraindications: Hypersensitivity to any of the components.
Warnings: NORCET® should be prescribed and administered with the same degree of caution appropriate for the use of other oral narcotic-containing medications since it can produce drug dependence and, therefore, has the potential for abuse. Patients should be warned not to drive a car or operate machinery if they become drowsy or show impared mental and/or physical abilities while taking NORCET®. Patients receiving narcotic analgesics, phenothiazines, other tranquilizers, sedative-hypnotics or other central nervous system depressants (including alcohol) concomitantly with NORCET® may exhibit an additive CNS depression. When such combined therapy is contemplated, the dose of one or both agents should be reduced.
Caution: Federal law prohibits dispensing without prescription. NORCET® has a schedule III classification which permits prescription refill up to six months or five times on doctor specification.
Precautions: The habit-forming potentialities of hydrocodone are less than those of morphine and greater than those of codeine. The usual precautions should be observed as with other opiate analgesics. NORCET® is usually well tolerated by aspirin-sensitive patients.
Adverse Reactions: Adverse reactions when they occur include sedation, nausea, vomiting and constipation.
Dosage and Administration: 1 or 2 tablets as required to relieve pain.
Management of Overdosage:
Signs and Symptoms: Serious overdose with NORCET® may be characterized by respiratory depression, extreme somnolence progressing to stupor or coma, skeletal muscle flaccidity, cold and clammy skin, and sometimes bradycardia and hypotension. In severe overdosage, apnea, circulatory collapse, cardiac arrest and death may occur.
Treatment: Primary attention should be given to the reestablishment of adequate respiratory exchange through provision of a patent airway and the institution of assisted or controlled ventilation. The narcotic antagonists naloxone, nalorphine or levallorphan are specific antidotes against respiratory depression which may result from overdosage or unusual sensitivity to narcotics, including hydrocodone. An appropriate dose of one of these antagonists should be administered, preferably by the intravenous route, simultaneously with effort at respiratory resuscitation. Since the duration of action of hydrocodone may exceed that of the antagonist, the patient should be kept under continued surveillance and repeated doses of the antagonist should be administered as needed to maintain adequate respiration. Oxygen, intravenous fluids, vasopressors and other supportive measures should be employed as indicated. Gastric emptying may be useful in removing unabsorbed drug. Activated charcoal may be of benefit.
How Supplied: White-blue mottled capsule-shaped tablets.
NDC # 12463-216-01, bottle of 100.
Manufactured for Frye
Pharmaceuticals, Inc.,
Birmingham, Ala. 35202.

PSEUDO-BID® ℞
TIME RELEASE CAPSULES

Composition: Each Clear capsule contains:

Pseudoephedrine Hydrochloride	120 mg.
Guaifenesin	250 mg.

The capsules are designed to provide prolonged release of medication.
Action: Decongestant — Pseudoephedrine Hydrochloride provides a rapid and sustained decongestant effect on swollen mucosa of the respiratory tract. It does this by vasoconstriction and opens obstructed airways through direct action on the smooth muscle of the bronchi. The Vasoconstrictor action of pseudoephedrine is similar to that of ephedrine. In the usual oral dosage, it has minimal vasopressor effects.
Guaifenesin enhances the output of lower respiratory tract fluid. The enhanced flow of less viscid secretions promoted ciliary action, and facilitates the removal of inspissated mucus. As a result, dry unproductive coughs become more productive and less frequent.
Indications: For relief of upper respiratory and bronchial congestion.
Contraindications: Sensitivity to sympathomimetic agents. Should not be given to children under 12 years of age. It should not be used in patients with severe hypertension or coronary artery disease.
Warning: Use with caution in patients suffering from hypertension, cardiac disease or hyperthyroidism.
Precautions: Pseudo-Bid should be used with caution in the presence of hypertension, coronary artery disease, narrowangle glaucoma, prostatic hypertrophy, hyperthyroidism, and diabetes. Patients should be cautioned about possible additive effects with alcohol and other central nervous system depressants (hypnotics, sedatives, tranquilizers). If a sensitivity reaction or idiosyncracy should occur, withdraw the drug.
Side Effects: Most patients will have no side effects at the usual dosage. However, certain patients may exhibit mild stimulation or mild sedation. Although rare, hypersensitivity to decongestant may occur.
Usual Adult Dose: One capsule orally every 12 hours.
Caution: Federal law prohibits dispensing without prescription.
How Supplied: Bottles containing 100 capsules. NDC # 12463-130-01.

PSEUDO-HIST® Liquid, Capsules ℞
PSEUDO-Hist® Expectorant ©

Composition: Each tsp (5cc) liquid contains 2 mg chlorpheniramine maleate and 15 mg pseudoephedrine HCl. Each time release capsule contains 10 mg chlorpheniramine maleate and 65 mg pseudophedrine HCl in a special form providing a prolonged therapeutic effect. Each tsp (5cc) Expectorant contains 2.5 mg hydrocodone bitartrate (Warning: May be habit forming.), 2 mg chlorpheniramine maleate, 15 mg. pseudoephedrine HCl and 100 mg glyceryl guaiacolate.
Action and Uses: For relief of upper respiratory and bronchial congestion associated with: the common cold, hay fever and associated allergies, influenza, sinusitis, and rhinitis. Pseudo-Hist capsule provides up to 12 hours relief with a single oral dose.
Contraindications: Severe hypertension or severe cardiac disease, sensitivity to antihistamines or sympathomimetic agents.
Precautions: Use with caution in patients suffering from hyperthyroidism. Patients susceptible to the soporific effect of chlorpheniramine should be warned against driving or operating machinery should drowsiness occur.
Dosage:
Liquid: Children 6–12 yrs 1 tsp. every 3 to 4 hours; smaller children as follows, every 3 to 4 hours: 40–50 lb.—3/4 tsp: 20–30 lbs 1/4–1/2 tsp; 15–20 lbs 1/8–1/4 tsp. Adults: 2 tsp. every 3–4 hours. Adults: 1-Pseudo-Hist capsule every 12 hours or as directed.
Pseudo-Hist Expectorant: Adults: 1 to 2 tsp. every 4 hours. Children 6–12 yrs: 1/2 to 1 tsp. every four hours; 2–6 yrs 1/4 tsp every 4 hours; 1–2 yrs 1/8 tsp. every 4 hours.
Do not use in children under 1 year.
BNDD registry number required for Expectorant.
How Supplied:
Capsules: Bottles of 100. NDC # 12463-140-01
Liquid: Pints and gallons. NDC # 12463-134-16
Expectorant: Pints and gallons. NDC # 12463-133-16

GEIGY Pharmaceuticals
Division of CIBA-GEIGY Corporation
ARDSLEY, NEW YORK 10502

GY-CODE® INDEX

GEIGY Pharmaceuticals has established a Drug Identity Code System entitled GY-CODE. This system affords a convenient and accurate means of uniquely identifying each Geigy solid dosage form on which the GY-CODE number and the name "Geigy" appear. The GY-CODE number also appears as part of the National Drug Code number.

GY-CODE NUMBER	PROD./DESCRIPTION	NATIONAL DRUG CODE
02	**Butazolidin® alka Capsules**	
	Per capsule:	
	phenylbutazone USP 100 mg.	
	dried aluminum hydroxide gel USP 100 mg.	
	magnesium trisilicate USP 150 mg.	
	Orange and white capsules	
	100's	0028-0002-01
	1000's	0028-0002-10
	100's Unit Dose Pkg.	0028-0002-61
	Gy-Pak® 100's	
	One Unit (12 × 100)	0028-0002-01
	Six Units (72 × 100)	0028-0002-01
11	**Tofranil® Tablets**	
	imipramine hydrochloride USP 25 mg.	
	Coral-colored (black Geigy imprint) coated tablets	
	100's	0028-0011-01
	1000's	0028-0011-10
	5000's	0028-0011-51
	100's Unit Dose Pkg.	0028-0011-61
	Gy-Pak® 100's	
	One unit (12 × 100)	0028-0011-01
	Six units (72 × 100)	0028-0011-01
14	**Butazolidin® Tablets**	
	phenylbutazone USP 100 mg.	
	Red, film-coated tablets	
	100's	0028-0014-01
	1000's	0028-0014-10
	100's Unit Dose Pkg.	0028-0014-61
20	**Tofranil-PM® Capsules**	
	imipramine pamoate 75 mg.	
	Coral-colored capsules	
	30's	0028-0020-26
	100's	0028-0020-01
	1000's	0028-0020-10
	100's Unit Dose Pkg.	0028-0020-61
21	**Tofranil® Tablets**	
	imipramine hydrochloride USP 10 mg.	
	Triangular, coral-colored, coated tablets	
	100's	0028-0021-01
	1000's	0028-0021-10
22	**Tofranil-PM® Capsules**	
	imipramine pamoate 150 mg.	
	Coral-colored capsules	
	30's	0028-0022-26
	100's	0028-0022-01
	1000's	0028-0022-10
	100's Unit Dose Pkg.	0028-0022-61
23	**Lioresal® Tablets**	
	baclofen 10 mg.	
	White, oval, scored tablets	
	100's	0028-0023-01
24	**Tandearil® Tablets**	
	oxyphenbutazone NF 100 mg.	
	Tan, coated tablets	
	100's	0028-0024-01
	1000's	0028-0024-10
40	**Tofranil-PM® Capsules**	
	imipramine pamoate 100 mg.	
	Dark yellow/coral-colored capsules	
	30's	0028-0040-26
	100's	0028-0040-01
	1000's	0028-0040-10
43	**PBZ® Tablets**	
	tripelennamine hydrochloride USP 50 mg.	
	Light blue, scored tablets	
	100's	0028-0043-01
	1000's	0028-0043-10
45	**Tofranil-PM® Capsules**	
	imipramine pamoate 125 mg.	
	Light yellow/coral-colored capsules	
	30's	0028-0045-26
	100's	0028-0045-01
	1000's	0028-0045-10
48	**PBZ-SR® Tablets**	
	tripelennamine hydrochloride 100 mg	
	Lavender-colored tablets	
	100's	0028-0048-01
51	**Lopressor® Tablets**	
	metoprolol tartrate 50 mg	
	Light red, capsule-shaped, scored tablets	
	100's	0028-0051-01
	1000's	0028-0051-10
	100's Unit Dose Pkg.	0028-0051-61
54	**Eurax® Cream—10%**	
	crotamiton NF	
	60-gm.	0028-0054-77
56	**Eurax® Lotion**	
	crotamiton	
	2-oz. bottle	0028-0056-56
60	**PBZ® Lontabs® Tablets**	
	tripelennamine hydrochloride 50 mg.	
	Light green Lontabs® tablets	
	100's	0028-0060-01
67	**Tegretol® Tablets**	
	carbamazepine USP 200 mg.	
	White, single-scored tablets	
	100's	0028-0067-01
	1000's	0028-0067-10
	100's Unit Dose Pkg.	0028-0067-61
71	**Lopressor® Tablets**	
	metoprolol tartrate 100 mg	
	Light blue, capsule-shaped, scored tablets	
	100's	0028-0071-01
	1000's	0028-0071-10
	100's Unit Dose Pkg.	0028-0071-61
72	**Brethine® Tablets**	
	terbutaline sulfate 2.5 mg.	
	Oval, white, scored tablets	
	100's	0028-0072-01
	1000's	0028-0072-10
	100's Unit Dose Pkg.	0028-0072-61
74	**Tofranil® Tablets**	
	imipramine hydrochloride USP 50 mg.	
	Coral-colored (white Geigy imprint) coated tablets	
	100's	0028-0074-01
	1000's	0028-0074-10
	5000's	0028-0074-51
	100's Unit Dose Pkg.	0028-0074-61
	Gy-Pak® 100's	
	One unit (12 × 100)	0028-0074-01
	Six units (72 × 100)	0028-0074-01
95	**PBZ® Tablets**	
	tripelennamine hydrochloride USP 25 mg.	
	Green, sugar-coated tablets	
	100's	0028-0095-01
105	**Brethine® Tablets**	
	terbutaline sulfate 5 mg.	
	Round, scored, white tablets	
	100's	0028-0105-01
	1000's	0028-0105-10
	100's Unit Dose Pkg.	0028-0105-61
	Gy-Pak® 100's	
	One unit (12 × 100)	0028-0105-01
	Six units (72 × 100)	0028-0105-01
134	**PBZ® Tablets with Ephedrine**	
	tripelennamine hydrochloride	
	Per Tablet:	
	tripelennamine hydrochloride 25 mg.	
	ephedrine sulfate 12 mg.	
	White, dry-coated tablets	
	100's	0028-0134-01
6114	**Otrivin® Nasal Drops (0.1%)**	
	xylometazoline hydrochloride NF	
	20 ml.	0028-6114-58
6116	**Otrivin® Pediatric (0.05%)**	
	xylometazoline hydrochloride NF	
	20 ml.	0028-6116-58
6118	**Otrivin® Spray (0.1%)**	
	xylometazoline hydrochloride NF	
	15 ml.	0028-6118-57
6925	**PBZ® Elixir**	
	Per 5-ml teaspoon:	
	tripelennamine citrate USP 37.5 mg	
	(equivalent to 25 mg tripelennamine hydrochloride)	
	473 ml	0028-6925-16
6935	**PBZ® Antihistamine Ointment**	
	tripelennamine hydrochloride	
	Ointment 2% (petrolatum base)	
	1 oz.	0028-6935-76
6946	**PBZ® Antihistamine Cream**	
	tripelannamine hydrochloride	
	Cream 2% (water-washable base)	
	1 oz.	0028-6946-76
6965	**PBZ® Expectorant with Ephedrine**	
	Per 4-ml. teaspoon:	
	tripelennamine citrate USP 30 mg. (equivalent to 20 mg. tripelennamine hydrochloride)	
	ephedrine sulfate 10 mg.	
	ammonium chloride 80 mg.	
	473 ml	0028-6965-16

Continued on next page

The full prescribing information for each GEIGY drug is contained herein and is that in effect as of October 1, 1979.

Geigy—Cont.

BRETHINE® ℞
brand of terbutaline sulfate
Tablets of 5 mg. **GY-CODE 105**
Tablets of 2.5 mg. **GY-CODE 72**

Description: Brethine, brand of terbutaline sulfate, a synthetic sympathomimetic amine, may be chemically described as α-[(*tert*-butylamino) methyl]-3,5-dihydroxybenzyl alcohol sulfate.
Brethine, brand of terbutaline sulfate, is a water soluble, colorless, crystalline solid. Tablets containing Brethine, brand of terbutaline sulfate, should be stored at controlled room temperature.
Each scored, white tablet contains 5 mg. (equivalent to 4.1 mg. of free base) or 2.5 mg. (equivalent to 2.05 mg. of free base) of Brethine, brand of terbutaline sulfate.
Actions: Brethine, brand of terbutaline sulfate, is a β-adrenergic receptor agonist which has been shown by *in vitro* and *in vivo* pharmacological studies in animals to exert a preferential effect on β_2 adrenergic receptors such as those located in bronchial smooth muscle. Controlled clinical studies in patients who were administered the drug orally have revealed proportionally greater changes in pulmonary function parameters than in heart rate or blood pressure. While this *suggests* a relative preference for the β_2 receptor in man, the usual cardiovascular effects commonly associated with sympathomimetic agents were also observed with Brethine, brand of terbutaline sulfate.
Brethine, brand of terbutaline sulfate, has been shown in controlled clinical studies to relieve bronchospasm in chronic obstructive pulmonary disease.
This action is manifested by a clinically significant increase in pulmonary function as demonstrated by an increase of 15% or more in FEV_1 and in $FEF_{25\text{-}75\%}$. Following administration of Brethine, brand of terbutaline sulfate, tablets, a measurable change in flow rate is usually observed in 30 minutes, and a clinically significant improvement in pulmonary function occurs at 60–120 minutes. The maximum effect usually occurs within 120-180 minutes. Brethine, brand of terbutaline sulfate, also produces a clinically significant decrease in airway and pulmonary resistance which persists for at least four hours or longer. Significant bronchodilator action, as measured by various pulmonary function determinations (airway resistance, $FEF_{25\text{-}75\%}$, or PEFR), has been demonstrated in some studies for periods up to eight hours.
Clinical studies were conducted in which the effectiveness of Brethine, brand of terbutaline sulfate, was evaluated in comparison with ephedrine over periods up to three months. Both drugs continued to produce significant improvement in pulmonary function throughout this period of treatment.
Indications: Brethine, brand of terbutaline sulfate, is indicated as a bronchodilator for bronchial asthma and for reversible bronchospasm which may occur in association with bronchitis and emphysema.
Contraindications: Brethine, brand of terbutaline sulfate, is contraindicated when there is known hypersensitivity to sympathomimetic amines.
Warnings: *Usage in Pregnancy:* Animal reproductive studies have been negative with respect to adverse effects on fetal development. The safe use of Brethine, brand of terbutaline sulfate, has not, however, been established in human pregnancy. As with any medication, the use of the drug in pregnancy, lactation, or women of childbearing potential requires that the expected therapeutic benefit of the drug be weighed against its possible hazards to the mother or child.
Usage in Pediatrics: Brethine, brand of terbutaline sulfate, tablets are not presently recommended for children below the age of 12 years due to insufficient clinical data in this pediatric group.
Precautions: Brethine, brand of terbutaline sulfate, should be used with caution in patients with diabetes, hypertension, hyperthyroidism, and a history of seizures.
As with other sympathomimetic bronchodilator agents, Brethine, brand of terbutaline sulfate, should be administered cautiously to cardiac patients, especially those with associated arrhythmias.
The concomitant use of Brethine, brand of terbutaline sulfate, with other sympathomimetic agents is not recommended, since their combined effect on the cardiovascular system may be deleterious to the patient. However, this does not preclude the use of an aerosol bronchodilator of the adrenergic stimulant type for the relief of an acute bronchospasm in patients receiving chronic oral Brethine, brand of terbutaline sulfate, therapy.
Adverse Reactions: Commonly observed side effects include nervousness and tremor. Other reported reactions include headache, increased heart rate, palpitations, drowsiness, nausea, vomiting, sweating, and muscle cramps. These reactions are generally transient in nature and usually do not require treatment. The frequency of these side effects appears to diminish with continued therapy. In general, all the side effects observed are characteristic of those commonly seen with sympathomimetic amines.
Dosage and Administration: The usual oral dose of Brethine, brand of terbutaline sulfate, for adults is 5 mg. administered at approximately six-hour intervals, three times daily, during the hours the patient is usually awake. If side effects are particularly disturbing, the dose may be reduced to 2.5 mg., three times daily, and still provide a clinically significant improvement in pulmonary function. A dose of 2.5 mg., three times daily, also is recommended for children in the 12- to 15-year group. Brethine, brand of terbutaline sulfate, is not recommended at present for use in children below the age of 12 years. In adults, a total dose of 15 mg. should not be exceeded in a 24-hour period. In children, a total dose of 7.5 mg. should not be exceeded in a 24-hour period.
Overdosage: Overdosage experience is limited. Excessive beta-adrenergic receptor stimulation may augment the signs or symptoms listed under **Adverse Reactions** and they may be accompanied by other adrenergic effects. Treat the alert patient who has taken excessive oral medication by emptying the stomach by means of induced emesis, followed by gastric lavage. In the unconscious patient, secure the airway with a cuffed endotracheal tube before beginning lavage (do not induce emesis). Instillation of activated charcoal slurry may help reduce absorption of terbutaline sulfate. Maintain adequate respiratory exchange. Provide cardiac and respiratory support as needed. Continue observation until symptom-free.
How Supplied: Brethine, brand of terbutaline sulfate, round, scored, white tablets of 5 mg. are supplied in bottles of 100 and 1,000 and Unit Dose Packages of 100; and oval, scored, white tablets of 2.5 mg. are supplied in bottles of 100 and 1,000 and Unit Dose Packages of 100.
667005 (Rev. 3/78)
C78-9
[*Shown in Product Identification Section*]

BRETHINE® ℞
terbutaline sulfate **GY-CODE 7507**
Ampuls
A sterile aqueous solution
for subcutaneous injection.

Description: Brethine α-[(*tert*-Butylamino) methyl]- 3,5-dihydroxybenzyl alcohol sulfate is a synthetic sympathomimetic amine.
Brethine is a water soluble colorless crystalline solid. Solutions are sensitive to excessive heat and light, and ampuls should therefore be stored at controlled room temperature with protection from light by storage in their original carton until dispensed. Solutions should not be used if discolored.
Each milliliter of sterile isotonic solution contains 1.0 mg of terbutaline sulfate (equivalent to 0.82 mg of free base), 8.9 mg of sodium chloride, and hydrochloric acid to adjust the pH to 3.0–5.0.
Actions: Brethine is a β-adrenergic receptor agonist which has been shown by *in vitro* and *in vivo* pharmacological studies in animals to exert a preferential effect on β_2-adrenergic receptors such as those located in bronchial smooth muscle.
However, controlled clinical studies in patients who were administered the drug subcutaneously have not revealed a preferential β_2 adrenergic effect.
Brethine has been shown in controlled clinical studies to relieve acute bronchospasm in acute and chronic obstructive pulmonary disease, resulting in a clinically significant increase in pulmonary flow rates, e.g., an increase of 15% or greater in FEV_1. Following administration of 0.25 mg of subcutaneous Brethine, a measurable change in flow rate is usually observed within five minutes, and a clinically significant increase in FEV_1 occurs by 15 minutes following the injection. The maximum effect usually occurs within 30–60 minutes and clinically significant bronchodilator activity has been observed to persist for 90 minutes to four hours. The duration of clinically significant improvement is comparable to that found with equimilligram doses of epinephrine.
Indications: Brethine is indicated as a bronchodilator for bronchial asthma and for reversible bronchospasm which may occur in association with bronchitis and emphysema.
Contraindications: Brethine is contraindicated when there is known hypersensitivity to sympathomimetic amines.
Warnings: *Usage in Pregnancy:* Animal reproductive studies have been negative with respect to adverse effects on fetal development. The safe use of Brethine has not, however, been established in human pregnancy. As with any medication, the use of the drug in pregnancy, lactation, or women of childbearing potential requires that the expected therapeutic benefit of the drug be weighed against its possible hazards to the mother or child.
Usage in Pediatrics: Studies are in progress to define the safe and effective dose of Brethine in children. Therefore, until such studies are completed and evaluated, Brethine is not recommended for use in pediatrics.
Precautions: Brethine should be used with caution in patients with diabetes, hypertension, hyperthyroidism, and a history of seizures.
As with other sympathomimetic bronchodilator agents, Brethine should be administered cautiously to cardiac patients, especially those with associated arrhythmias.
The concomitant use of Brethine with other sympathomimetic agents is not recommended, since their combined effect on the cardiovascular system may be deleterious to the patient.
Adverse Reactions: Commonly observed side effects include increases in heart rate, nervousness, tremor, palpitations and dizziness. These occur more frequently at doses in excess of 0.25 mg. Other reported reactions include headache, nausea, vomiting, anxiety, and mus-

cle cramps. These reactions are transient in nature and usually do not require treatment. In general, all side effects are characteristic of those commonly seen with sympathomimetic amines such as epinephrine.

Dosage and Administration: The usual subcutaneous dose of Brethine is 0.25 mg injected into the lateral deltoid area. If significant clinical improvement does not occur by 15–30 minutes, a second dose of 0.25 mg may be administered. A total dose of 0.5 mg should not be exceeded within a four-hour period. If a patient fails to respond to a second 0.25-mg dose of Brethine within 15–30 minutes, other therapeutic measures should be considered.

Overdosage: Overdosage experience is limited. Excessive beta-adrenergic receptor stimulation may augment the signs or symptoms listed under **Adverse Reactions** and they may be accompanied by other adrenergic effects. In the case of subcutaneous injectable terbutaline overdosage, the patient should be treated symptomatically under guidelines for sympathomimetic overdosage.

How Supplied: Brethine is supplied in packages of 10 and 100 2-ml size ampuls each containing one ml of solution (1.0 mg of Brethine). Thus, 0.25 ml of solution will provide the usual clinical dose of 0.25 mg. Ampuls are expiration-dated.

667063 (Rev. 7/79)
C79-18
Distributed by: GEIGY Pharmaceuticals

BUTAZOLIDIN® ℞
phenylbutazone USP **GY-CODE 14**
Tablets
BUTAZOLIDIN® ALKA **GY-CODE 02**
Capsules
Nonhormonal Antiarthritic
Anti-Inflammatory Agent

Each capsule contains: phenylbutazone USP, 100 mg; dried aluminum hydroxide gel USP, 100 mg. magnesium trisilicate USP, 150 mg

Important Note: Butazolidin cannot be considered a simple analgesic and should never be administered casually. Each patient should be carefully evaluated before treatment is started and should remain constantly under the close supervision of the physician. The following cautions should be observed:

1. Therapy should not be initiated until a careful detailed history and complete physical and laboratory examination, including a complete hemogram and urinalysis, etc., of the patient have been made. These examinations should be made at regular, frequent intervals throughout the duration of this drug therapy.
2. Patients should be carefully selected, avoiding those in whom it is contraindicated as well as those who will respond to ordinary therapeutic measures, or those who cannot be observed at frequent intervals.
3. Patients taking this drug should be warned not to exceed the recommended dosage, since this may lead to toxic effects, and should discontinue the drug and report to the physician immediately any sign of:
   1. Fever, sore throat, lesions in the mouth (symptoms of blood dyscrasia).
   b. Dyspepsia, epigastric pain, symptoms of anemia, unusual bleeding, unusual bruising, black or tarry stools or other evidence of intestinal ulceration.
   c. Skin rashes.
   d. Significant weight gain or edema.
4. A trial period of one week of therapy is considered adequate to determine the therapeutic effect of the drug. In the absence of a favorable response, therapy should be discontinued.
   a. In the elderly (sixty years and over) the drug should be restricted to short-term treatment periods only—if possible, *one week* maximum.
5. **Before prescribing Butazolidin for an individual patient, read thoroughly the information contained under each heading which follows:**

Description: Butazolidin should not be considered as a simple analgesic that can be prescribed for indiscriminate use. Butazolidin is closely related chemically and pharmacologically, including toxic effects, to the well-known pyrazolines (pyrazole compounds) amidopyrine and antipyrine.

Butazolidin is 4-Butyl-1,2-diphenyl-3.5-pyrazolidinedione, with a molecular weight of 308.38.

It is very slightly soluble in water; freely soluble in acetone and in ether; soluble in alcohol.

Clinical Pharmacology: Butazolidin is a nonsalicylate, nonsteroidal, anti-inflammatory drug. It has anti-inflammatory, antipyretic, analgesic and mild uricosuric properties that produce symptomatic relief but do not alter the disease process.

The exact mechanism of the anti-inflammatory effects of Butazolidin has not been elucidated, but clinical pharmacology studies have shown that Butazolidin inhibits certain factors believed to be involved in the inflammatory process. These processes are (1) prostaglandin synthesis; (2) leucocyte migration; (3) release and or activity of lysosomal enzymes.

Phenylbutazone is rapidly absorbed after oral administration of Butazolidin. Tests conducted in 18 healthy adult male volunteers indicated that a peak plasma concentration of 43.3 ($\pm$3.1) mg/l was attained within 2.5 ($\pm$1.4) hours after the ingestion of three 100-mg tablets. In these same volunteers, the apparent elimination half-life was 84 ($\pm$23) hours. About 98% of the drug is bound to human serum albumin.

Twenty-one days after oral administration of 14 C-labelled drug, 61% was recovered from the urine and 27% from the feces. However, only about 1% of total urinary radioactivity represents unchanged drug. The sum of non-conjugated urinary metabolites (oxyphenbutazone, γ-hydroxyphenylbutazone, p,γ-dihydroxyphenyl-butazone), and phenylbutazone itself amounted to only about 10%. About 40% of the total urinary radioactivity was excreted as the C(4)-glucuronide of phenylbutazone and an additional 12% was identified as the C(4)-glucuronide of γ-hydroxyphenylbutazone.

The major metabolite of phenylbutazone in human plasma is oxyphenbutazone; steady-state plasma levels about 50% of those of phenylbutazone. Less than 2% of the dose of phenylbutazone appears in the urine as oxyphenbutazone.

Indications: The indications for Butazolidin are:

Acute Gouty Arthritis
Active Rheumatoid Arthritis
Active Ankylosing Spondylitis
Short-term treatment of acute attacks of degenerative joint disease of the hips and knees not responsive to other treatment.
Painful Shoulder (peritendinitis, capsulitis, bursitis, and acute arthritis of that joint)

Contraindications:

1. *Age:* Butazolidin is contraindicated in children 14 years of age or younger since controlled clinical trials in patients of this age group have not been conducted.
2. *Other Medical Conditions.* Butazolidin is contraindicated in patients with incipient cardiac failure, blood dyscrasias, pancreatitis parotitis, stomatitis, polymyalgia rheumatica, temporal arteritis, senility, drug allergy, and in the presence of severe renal, cardiac and hepatic disease, and in patients with a history of peptic ulcer disease, or symptoms of gastrointestinal inflammation or active ulceration because serious adverse reactions or aggravation of existing medical problems can occur.
3. *Concomitant Medications:* Butazolidin should not be used in combination with other drugs which accentuate or share a potential for similar toxicity.

It is also inadvisable to administer Butazolidin in combination with other potent drugs because of the possibility of increased toxic reactions from Butazolidin and other agents. (see also *Drug interactions.*)

Butazolidin is contraindicated in patients with a history or suggestion of prior toxicity, sensitivity, or idiosyncrasy to phenylbutazone or oxyphenbutazone.

Warnings: Based on reports of clinical experience with phenylbutazone and related compounds, the following warnings should be considered by the physician prior to prescribing the drug:

1. *Gastrointestinal:* Upper G.I. diagnostic tests should be performed in patients with persistent or severe dyspepsia. Peptic ulceration, reactivation of latent peptic ulcer, perforation and gastrointestinal bleeding, sometimes severe, have been reported.
2. *Hematologic: Frequent and regular hematologic evaluations should be performed on patients receiving the drug for periods over one week.* Any significant change in the total white count, relative decrease in granulocytes, appearance of immature forms or fall in hematocrit should be a signal for immediate cessation of therapy and a complete hematologic investigation. Serious, sometimes fatal blood dyscrasias, including aplastic anemia have been reported to occur. Hematologic toxicity may occur suddenly or many days or weeks after cessation of treatment as manifest by the appearance of anemia, leukopenia, thrombocytopenia or clinically significant hemorrhagic diathesis. There have been published reports associating phenylbutazone with leukemia. However, the circumstances involved in these reports are such that a cause-and-effect relationship to the drug has not been clearly established.
3. *Pregnancy:* Reproductive studies in animals, although inconclusive, exhibited evidence of possible embryotoxicity. It is, therefore, recommended that this drug should be used with caution during pregnancy. The benefits should be weighed against the potential risk to the fetus.
4. *Nursing Mothers:* Caution is also advised in prescribing Butazolidin in nursing mothers since the drug may appear in cord blood and breast milk.
5. Patients reporting visual disturbances while receiving the drug should discontinue treatment and have an ophthalmologic examination because ophthalmologic adverse reactions have been reported (see **Adverse Reactions:** *Special Senses*)
6. In the aging (forty years and over), there appears to be an increase in the possibility of adverse reactions. Butazolidin should be used with commensurately greater care in the elderly and should be avoided altogether in the senile patient.
7. Like other drugs with prostaglandin synthetase inhibition activity. Butazolidin may precipitate acute episodes of asthmatic attacks in patients with asthma.
8. Butazolidin increases sodium retention. Evidence of fluid retention in patients in whom there is danger of cardiac decompensation is an indication to discontinue the drug.

Precautions: Because of potential serious adverse reactions to Butazolidin, the following precautions should be observed in the use of the drug:

Continued on next page

The full prescribing information for each GEIGY drug is contained herein and is that in effect as of October 1, 1979.

Geigy—Cont.

—A careful diagnostic physical examination and history should be performed on all patients at regular intervals while the patient is receiving the drug.

—Butazolidin is not recommended for chronic use in the elderly.

—Hematologic evaluation should be performed at frequent and regular intervals and additional laboratory examinations performed as indicated.

—Patients should be instructed to report immediately the occurrence of high fever, severe sore throat, stomatitis, salivary gland enlargement, tarry stools, unusual bleeding or bruising, sudden weight gain, or edema.

—The drug reduces iodine uptake by the thyroid and may interfere with laboratory tests of thyroid function (see **Adverse Reactions:** *Endocrine-Metabolic*)

—The patient should be cautioned regarding participation in activities requiring alertness and coordination and that the concomitant ingestion of alcohol with Butazolidin may further impair psychomotor skills.

Drug Interactions: Butazolidin is highly bound to serum proteins. If its affinity for protein binding is higher than other concurrently administered drugs, the actions and toxicity of the other drug may be increased.
Butazolidin accentuates the prothrombin depression produced by coumarin-type anticoagulants. When administered alone, it does not affect prothrombin activity.
The pharmacologic action of insulin, antidiabetic, and sulfonamide drugs may be potentiated by the simultaneous administration of Butazolidin.
Concomitant administration of phenylbutazone and phenytoin may result in increased serum levels of phenytoin which could lead to increased phenytoin toxicity.
The Butazolidin tablets (film-coated 100 mg) and the Butazolidin alka capsules contain FD&C Yellow No. 5 (tartrazine) which may cause allergic-type reactions (including bronchial asthma) in certain susceptible individuals. Although the overall incidence of FD&C Yellow No. 5 (tartrazine) sensitivity in the general population is low, it is frequently seen in patients who also have aspirin hypersensitivity.

Adverse Reactions: Based upon reports of clinical experience with phenylbutazone and related compounds, the following adverse reactions have been reported.
The adverse reactions listed in the following table have been arranged into three groups: (1) incidence greater than 1%. (2) incidence less than 1% and (3) causal relationship unknown. The incidence for group (1) was obtained from sixty-eight (68) clinical trials reported in the literature (5369 patients). The incidence for group (2) was based on reports in clinical trials, in the literature, and on voluntary reports since marketing. The reactions in group (3) have been reported but occurred under circumstances where a causal relationship could not be established. In some patients the reported reactions may have been unrelated to the administration of Butazolidin. However, in these reported events, the possibility cannot be excluded. Therefore these observations are being listed to serve as alerting information to physicians. Before prescribing this drug for an individual patient, the physician should be familiar with the following:

(1) Incidence greater than 1%	**(2) Incidence less than 1%**
*GASTROINTESTINAL (See **Warnings**)*	
nausea dyspepsia/including indigestion and heartburn abdominal discomfort distress*	vomiting abdominal distention with flatulence constipation diarrhea esophagitis gastritis salivary gland enlargement stomatitis, sometimes with ulceration ulceration and perforation of the intestinal tract including acute and reactivated peptic ulcer with perforation, hemorrhage and hematemesis anemia due to gastrointestinal bleeding which may be occult hepatitis, both fatal and nonfatal, sometimes associated with evidence of cholestasis
*HEMATOLOGICAL (See **Warnings**)*	
None	anemia leukopenia thrombocytopenia with associated purpura, petechiae, and hemorrhage pancytopenia aplastic anemia bone marrow depression agranulocytosis and agranulocytic anginal syndrome hemolytic anemia
HYPERSENSITIVITY	
None	urticaria anaphylactic shock arthralgia, drug fever hypersensitivity angiitis (polyarteritis) and vasculitis Lyell's syndrome serum sickness Stevens-Johnson syndrome activation of systemic lupus erythematosus aggravation of temporal arteritis in patients with polymyalgia rheumatica
DERMATOLOGIC	
rash	pruritus erythema nodosum erythema multiforme nonthrombocytopenic purpura
CARDIOVASCULAR, FLUID AND ELECTROLYTE	
edema/water retention*	sodium and chloride retention fluid retention and plasma dilution cardiac decompensation (congestive heart failure) with edema and dyspnea metabolic acidosis respiratory alkalosis hypertension pericarditis interstitial myocarditis with muscle necrosis and perivascular granulomata
RENAL	
None	hematuria proteinuria ureteral obstruction with uric acid crystals anuria glomerulonephritis acute tubular necrosis cortical necrosis renal stones nephrotic syndrome impaired renal function and renal failure associated with azotemia
CENTRAL NERVOUS SYSTEM	
None	headache drowsiness agitation confusional states and lethargy tremors numbness weakness
*ENDOCRINE-METABOLIC (See **Precautions**)*	
None	hyperglycemia
*SPECIAL SENSES (See **Warnings**)*	
Ocular: None	
Otic: None	hearing loss tinnitus

* Reactions occurring in 3% to 9% of patients treated with phenylbutazone (those reactions occurring in less than 3% of the patients are unmarked).

(3) Causal relationship unknown—incidence less than 1%: *Hematological* (see **Warnings**) —Leukemia (There have been reports associating phenylbutazone with leukemia. However, the circumstances involved in these reports are such that a cause-and-effect relationship to the drug has not been clearly established.) *Endocrine—Metabolic* (see **Precautions**)— Thyroid hyperplasia; goiters associated with hyperthyroidism and hypothyroidism; pancreatitis. *Special Senses* (see **Warnings**)—Blurred vision; optic neuritis; toxic amblyopia; scotomata; retinal detachment; retinal hemorrhage; oculomotor palsy.

Overdosage: *Signs and Symptoms:* Include any of the following: nausea, vomiting, epigastric pain, excessive perspiration, euphoria, psychosis, headaches, giddiness, vertigo, hyperventilation, insomnia, tinnitus, difficulty in hearing, edema (sodium retention), hypertension, cyanosis, respiratory depression, agitation, hallucinations, stupor, convulsions, coma, hematuria, and oliguria. Hepatomegaly, jaundice, and ulceration of the buccal or gastrointestinal mucosa have been reported as late manifestations of massive overdosage.
Reported laboratory abnormalities following overdosage include: respiratory or metabolic acidosis, impaired hepatic or renal function, and abnormalities of formed blood elements.
Treatment: In the alert patient, empty the stomach promptly by induced emesis followed by lavage. In the obtunded patient, secure the airway with a cuffed endotracheal tube before beginning lavage (do not induce emesis). Maintain adequate respiratory exchange, do not use respiratory stimulants. Treat shock with appropriate supportive measures. Control seizures with intravenous diazepam or short-acting barbiturates. Dialysis may be helpful if renal function is impaired.

Dosage and Administration: Butazolidin should be used at the smallest effective dosage to afford rapid relief of severe symptoms. It is contraindicated in children under 14 years of age and in senile patients.
If a favorable symptomatic response to treatment is not obtained after one week, the drug should be discontinued. When a favorable therapeutic response has been obtained, the dosage

should be reduced and then discontinued as soon as possible.

In elderly patients (sixty years and over) every effort must be made to discontinue therapy on, or as soon as possible after, the seventh day, because of the exceedingly high risk of severe fatal toxic reactions in this age group.

To minimize gastric upset, the drug should be taken with milk or with meals, or Butazolidin alka capsules may be substituted.

In selecting the appropriate dosage in any specific case, consideration should be given to the patient's age, weight, general health, and any other factors that may influence his response to the drug.

Rheumatoid Arthritis, Ankylosing Spondylitis, Acute Attacks of Degenerative Joint Disease, and Painful Shoulder: Initial Dosage: The initial daily dose in adult patients is 300 to 600 mg as 3 to 4 divided doses. Maximum therapeutic response is usually obtained at a total daily dose of 400 mg. A trial period of one week of therapy is considered adequate to determine the therapeutic effect of the drug. In the absence of a favorable response, therapy should be discontinued.

Maintenance Dosage: When improvement is obtained, dosage should be promptly decreased to the minimum effective level necessary to maintain relief, not exceeding 400 mg daily because of the possibility of cumulative toxicity. A satisfactory clinical response may be obtained with daily doses as low as 100 to 200 mg daily.

Acute Gouty Arthritis: Satisfactory results are obtained after an initial dose of 400 mg followed by 100 mg every 4 hours. The articular inflammation usually subsides within 4 days and treatment should not be continued longer than one week.

How Supplied:

Butazolidin, phenylbutazone USP

Tablets—red, film-coated	100 mg
Bottle of 100	NDC 0028-0014-01
Bottle of 1000	NDC 0028-0014-10
Unit Dose Packages—Blister-Packed	
Box of 100 (strips of 10)	NDC 002-0014-61

Dispense in tight container (USP)

Butazolidin alka
100 mg phenylbutazone USP
100 mg dried aluminum hydroxide gel USP
150 mg magnesium trisilicate USP

Capsules—orange and white	
Bottle of 100	NDC 0028-0002-01
Bottle of 1000	NDC 0028-0002-10
Gy-Pak® 100's One Unit (12 bottles, 100 ea.)	NDC 0028-0002-01
Unit Dose Packages—Blister-Packed	
Box of 100 (strips of 10)	NDC 0028-0002-61

Dispense in tight, light-resistant container (USP).

667153 (1/80) C80-7

[*Shown in Product Identification Section*]

EURAX® ℞
crotamiton NF
Cream (NF) and Lotion
Antipruritic, Scabicide

Description: Eurax provides 10% of the synthetic, N-ethyl-o- crotonotoluide, in a vanishing-cream or emollient-lotion base containing: glyceryl monostearate, lanolin, PEG 6-32, glycerin, polysorbate 80, methylparaben, propylparaben, perfume, and oxyquinoline sulfate. In addition, the cream contains liquid petrolatum and white wax; the lotion, liquid petrolatum and carboxymethylcellulose.

Actions: Eurax has scabicidal and antipruritic actions. The mechanisms of these actions are not known.

Indications: For eradication of scabies *(Sarcoptes scabiei)* and for symptomatic treatment of pruritic skin.

Contraindications: Eurax should not be administered to patients who are allergic to it or who manifest a primary irritation response.

Warnings and Precautions: Eurax should not be applied to acutely inflamed skin, raw, weeping surfaces, or in the eyes or mouth. Its use should be deferred until acute inflammation has subsided.

If severe irritation or sensitization develops, treatment with this product should be discontinued and appropriate therapy instituted.

Adverse Reactions: Allergic sensitivity or primary irritation reactions may occur in some patients.

Dosage and Administration: *In Scabies:* Thoroughly massage into the skin of the whole body from the chin down, paying particular attention to all folds and creases. A second application is advisable 24 hours later. Clothing and bed linen should be changed the next morning. A cleansing bath should be taken 48 hours after the last application.

In Pruritus: Massage gently into affected areas until medication is completely absorbed. Repeat as needed.

How Supplied: Cream: 60-g tubes; Lotion: 2-oz (60 ml) bottles.

Directions for patients with scabies:

1. Take a routine bath or shower. Thoroughly massage Eurax cream or lotion into the skin from the chin to the toes including folds and creases.
2. A second application is advisable 24 hours later.
3. This 60-gram tube or 2-oz (60 ml) bottle is sufficient for two applications.
4. Clothing and bed linen should be changed the next day. Contaminated clothing and bed linen may be dry-cleaned, or washed in the hot cycle of the washing machine.
5. A cleansing bath should be taken 48 hours after the last application.

667500 (Rev. 8/79)
C79-25

LIORESAL® ℞
baclofen
Tablets of 10 mg GY-CODE 23
Muscle Relaxant, Antispastic

Description: Lioresal is 4-amino-3-(*p*-chlorophenyl) butyric acid, a white to off-white crystalline substance.

It is slightly soluble in water and poorly soluble in organic solvents. Molecular weight: 213.67.

Actions: The precise mechanism of action of Lioresal is not fully known. Lioresal is capable of inhibiting both monosynaptic and polysynaptic reflexes at the spinal level, possibly by hyperpolarization of afferent terminals, although actions at supraspinal sites may also occur and contribute to its clinical effect. Although Lioresal is an analog of the putative inhibitory neurotransmitter gamma-aminobutyric acid (GABA), there is no conclusive evidence that actions on GABA systems are involved in the production of its clinical effects. In studies with animals, Lioresal has been shown to have general CNS depressant properties as indicated by the production of sedation with tolerance, somnolence, ataxia, and respiratory and cardiovascular depression. Lioresal is rapidly and extensively absorbed and eliminated. Absorption may be dose-dependent, being reduced with increasing doses. Lioresal is excreted primarily by the kidney in unchanged form and there is relatively large intersubject variation in absorption and/or elimination.

Indications: Lioresal is useful for the alleviation of signs and symptoms of spasticity resulting from multiple sclerosis, particularly for the relief of flexor spasms and concomitant pain, clonus, and muscular rigidity.

Patients should have reversible spasticity so that Lioresal treatment will aid in restoring residual function.

Lioresal may also be of some value in patients with spinal cord injuries and other spinal cord diseases.

Lioresal is not indicated in the treatment of skeletal muscle spasm resulting from rheumatic disorders.

The efficacy of Lioresal in stroke, cerebral palsy, and Parkinson's disease has not been established and, therefore, it is not recommended for these conditions.

Contraindications: Hypersensitivity to baclofen.

Warnings:

a. *Abrupt Drug Withdrawal:* Hallucinations have occurred on abrupt withdrawal of Lioresal. Therefore, except for serious adverse reactions, the dose should be reduced slowly when the drug is discontinued.

b. *Impaired Renal Function:* Because Lioresal is primarily excreted unchanged through the kidneys, it should be given with caution, and it may be necessary to reduce the dosage.

c. *Stroke:* Lioresal has not significantly benefited patients with stroke. These patients have also shown poor tolerability to the drug.

d. *Pregnancy:* Lioresal has been shown to increase the incidence of omphaloceles (ventral hernias) in fetuses of rats given approximately 13 times the maximum dose recommended for human use, at a dose which caused significant reductions in food intake and weight gain in dams. This abnormality was not seen in mice or rabbits. There was also an increased incidence of incomplete sternebral ossification in fetuses of rats given approximately 13 times the maximum recommended human dose, and an increased incidence of unossified phalangeal nuclei of forelimbs and hindlimbs in fetuses of rabbits given approximately 7 times the maximum recommended human dose. In mice, no teratogenic effects were observed, although reductions in mean fetal weight with consequent delays in skeletal ossification were present when dams were given 17 or 34 times the human daily dose. There are no studies in pregnant women. Lioresal should be used during pregnancy only if the benefit clearly justifies the potential risk to the fetus.

Precautions: Safe use of Lioresal in children under age 12 has not been established, and it is, therefore, not recommended for use in children.

Because of the possibility of sedation, patients should be cautioned regarding the operation of automobiles or other dangerous machinery, and activities made hazardous by decreased alertness. Patients should also be cautioned that the central nervous system effects of Lioresal may be additive to those of alcohol and other CNS depressants.

Lioresal should be used with caution where spasticity is utilized to sustain upright posture and balance in locomotion or whenever spasticity is utilized to obtain increased function.

In patients with epilepsy, the clinical state and electroencephalogram should be monitored at regular intervals, since deterioration in seizure control and EEG have been reported occasionally in patients taking Lioresal.

It is not known whether this drug is excreted in human milk. As a general rule, nursing should not be undertaken while a patient is on a drug since many drugs are excreted in human milk.

A dose-related increase in incidence of ovarian cysts and a less marked increase in enlarged and/or hemorrhagic adrenal glands was ob-

Continued on next page

The full prescribing information for each GEIGY drug is contained herein and is that in effect as of October 1, 1979.

Geigy—Cont.

served in female rats treated chronically with Lioresal. The relevance of these findings to humans is not known.

Adverse Reactions: The most common is transient drowsiness (10–63%). In one controlled study of 175 patients, transient drowsiness was observed in 63% of those receiving Lioresal compared to 36% of those in the placebo group. Other common adverse reactions are dizziness (5–15%), weakness (5–15%) and fatigue (2–4%). Others reported:

Neuropsychiatric: Confusion (1–11%), headache (4–8%), insomnia (2–7%); and, rarely, euphoria, excitement, depression, hallucinations, paresthesia, muscle pain, tinnitus, slurred speech, coordination disorder, tremor, rigidity, dystonia, ataxia, blurred vision, nystagmus, strabismus, miosis, mydriasis, diplopia, dysarthria, epileptic seizure.

Cardiovascular: Hypotension (0–9%). Rare instances of dyspnea, palpitation, chest pain, syncope.

Gastrointestinal: Nausea (4–12%), constipation (2–6%); and, rarely, dry mouth, anorexia, taste disorder, abdominal pain, vomiting, diarrhea, and positive test for occult blood in stool.

Genitourinary: Urinary frequency (2–6%); and, rarely, enuresis, urinary retention, dysuria, impotence, inability to ejaculate, nocturia, hematuria.

Other: Instances of rash, pruritus, ankle edema, excessive perspiration, weight gain, nasal congestion.

Some of the CNS and genitourinary symptoms may be related to the underlying disease rather than to drug therapy.

The following laboratory tests have been found to be abnormal in a few patients receiving Lioresal: increased SGOT, elevated alkaline phosphatase, and elevation of blood sugar.

Overdosage: *Signs and Symptoms:* Vomiting, muscular hypotonia, drowsiness, accommodation disorders, coma, respiratory depression, and seizures.

Treatment: In the alert patient, empty the stomach promptly by induced emesis followed by lavage. In the obtunded patient, secure the airway with a cuffed endotracheal tube before beginning lavage (do not induce emesis). Maintain adequate respiratory exchange, do not use respiratory stimulants.

Dosage and Administration: The determination of optimal dosage requires individual titration. Start therapy at a low dosage and increase gradually until optimum effect is achieved (usually between 40–80 mg daily).

The following dosage titration schedule is suggested:

5 mg t.i.d. for 3 days
10 mg t.i.d. for 3 days
15 mg t.i.d. for 3 days
20 mg t.i.d. for 3 days

Thereafter additional increases may be necessary but the total daily dose should not exceed a maximum of 80 mg daily (20 mg q.i.d.).

The lowest dose compatible with an optimal response is recommended. If benefits are not evident after a reasonable trial period, patients should be slowly withdrawn from the drug (see **Warnings** *Abrupt Drug Withdrawal*).

How Supplied: White, oval, single-scored tablets of 10 mg in bottles of 100 and Unit Dose Packages of 100.

C79-27 (Rev. 9/79) 667253

[*Shown in Product Identification Section*]

LOPRESSOR® ℞

metoprolol tartrate

Tablets of 50 mg GY-CODE 51
Tablets of 100 mg GY-CODE 71

An antihypertensive beta-blocking agent

Description: Lopressor a synthetic selective $beta_1$-adrenoreceptor blocking agent, may be chemically described as 1-isopropylamino-3-[p-(2-methoxyethyl)-phenoxy]-2-propanol *dextro*-tartrate.

Lopressor is a water-soluble, white, crystalline solid. It is supplied for oral administration.

Clinical Pharmacology: Lopressor is a beta-adrenergic receptor blocking agent. *In vitro* and *in vivo* animal studies show it has a preferential effect on $beta_1$ adrenoreceptors, chiefly located in cardiac muscle. This preferential effect is not absolute, however, and at higher doses, metoprolol inhibits $beta_2$ adrenoreceptors, chiefly located in the bronchial and vascular musculature.

Clinical pharmacology studies have confirmed the beta-blocking activity as shown by (1) reduction in heart rate and cardiac output at rest and on exercise, (2) reduction of systolic blood pressure on exercise, (3) inhibition of isoproterenol-induced tachycardia, and (4) reduction of reflex orthostatic tachycardia.

$Beta_1$ selectivity has been confirmed: (1) In normal subjects by the inability of Lopressor to reverse the $beta_2$-mediated vasodilating effects of epinephrine. This contrasts with the effect of nonselective ($beta_1$ plus $beta_2$) beta blockers, such as propranolol, which completely reverse the vasodilating effects of epinephrine. (2) In asthmatic patients, Lopressor reduces FEV_1 and FVC significantly less than propranolol in equivalent $beta_1$-receptor blocking doses.

Metoprolol has no intrinsic sympathomimetic activity and only weak membrane-stabilizing activity. Metoprolol crosses the blood brain barrier and has been reported in the CSF in a concentration 78% of the simultaneous plasma concentration. Animal and human experiments indicate that metoprolol slows the sinus rate and decreases AV nodal conduction.

Lopressor has been shown in controlled clinical studies to be an effective antihypertensive agent when used as monotherapy, or as concomitant therapy with thiazide-type diuretics. In hypertension, dosages in the range of 100 to 450 mg daily have been shown to be effective. In controlled, comparative, clinical studies, Lopressor was shown to be as effective an antihypertensive agent as propranolol, methyldopa, and thiazide-type diuretics. It was equally effective in supine and standing positions.

The mechanism of the antihypertensive effects of beta-blocking agents has not been elucidated. However, several possible mechanisms have been proposed and include (1) competitive antagonism of catecholamines at peripheral (especially cardiac) adrenergic neuron sites, leading to decreased cardiac output, (2) a central effect leading to reduced sympathetic outflow to the periphery, and (3) suppression of renin activity.

In man, absorption of Lopressor is rapid and complete. Plasma levels following oral administration, however, approximate 50% of levels following intravenous administration, indicating about 50% first-pass metabolism. Plasma levels achieved are highly variable. Only a small fraction of the drug (about 12 percent) is bound to human serum albumin. Elimination is mainly by biotransformation in the liver and the plasma half-life is three to four hours. Significant beta-blocking effect (as measured by reduction of exercise heart rate) occurs within one hour after oral administration. The duration of pharmacologic effect as measured by reduction of exercise heart rate is dose-related. For example, the time for a 50-percent reduction of the maximum registered effect after single oral doses of 20, 50, and 100 mg was 3.3, 5.0, and 6.4 hours respectively in normal subjects.

Following repeated oral doses of 100 mg twice daily, a significant reduction in exercise systolic blood pressure was evident at 12 hours. Because of variable plasma levels attained with a given dose and the lack of a consistent relationship of antihypertensive activity to dose, selection of proper dosage requires individual titration.

There is a linear relationship between plasma levels and reduction of exercise heart rate. However, antihypertensive activity does not appear to be related to plasma levels.

Indications: Lopressor is indicated in the management of hypertension. It may be used alone or in combination with other antihypertensive agents, especially thiazide-type diuretics.

Contraindications: Lopressor is contraindicated in sinus bradycardia, heart block greater than first degree, cardiogenic shock, and overt cardiac failure (see **Warnings**).

Warnings: ***Cardiac Failure:*** Sympathetic stimulation is a vital component supporting circulatory function in congestive heart failure, and beta blockade carries the potential hazard of further depressing myocardial contractility and precipitating more severe failure. In hypertensive patients who have congestive heart failure controlled by digitalis and diuretics, Lopressor should be administered cautiously. Both digitalis and metoprolol slow AV conduction.

In Patients Without a History of Cardiac Failure continued depression of the myocardium with beta-blocking agents over a period of time can, in some cases, lead to cardiac failure. At the first sign or symptom of impending cardiac failure, patients should be fully digitalized and/or be given a diuretic, and the response observed closely. If cardiac failure continues, despite adequate digitalization and diuretic, Lopressor therapy should be withdrawn.

Ischemic Heart Disease: Following abrupt cessation of therapy with certain beta-blocking agents, exacerbations of angina pectoris and, in some cases, myocardial infarction have been reported. Even in the absence of overt angina pectoris, when discontinuing therapy, Lopressor should not be withdrawn abruptly, and patients should be cautioned against interruption of therapy without the physician's advice.

Bronchospastic Diseases: **PATIENTS WITH BRONCHOSPASTIC DISEASES SHOULD IN GENERAL NOT RECEIVE BETA BLOCKERS. Because of its relative $beta_1$ selectivity, however, Lopressor may be used with caution in patients with bronchospastic disease who do not respond to, or cannot tolerate, other antihypertensive treatment. Since $beta_1$ selectivity is not absolute, a $beta_2$-stimulating agent should be administered concomitantly and the lowest possible dose of metoprolol should be used. It may be prudent initially to administer metoprolol in smaller doses three doses daily, instead of larger doses two times daily, to avoid the higher plasma levels associated with the longer dosing interval. (See Dosage and Administration.)**

Major Surgery: The necessity or desirability of withdrawal of beta-blocking therapy prior to major surgery is controversial. It should be noted, however, that the impaired ability of the heart to respond to reflex adrenergic stimuli may augment the risks of general anesthesia and surgical procedures.

Metoprolol, like other beta blockers is a competitive inhibitor of beta-receptor agonists and its effects can be reversed by administration of such agents, e.g., dobutamine or isoproterenol. However, such patients may be subject to protracted severe hypotension. Difficulty in restarting and maintaining the heart beat has also been reported with beta blockers.

Diabetes Mellitus: Beta-adrenergic blockade may mask symptoms of hypoglycemia (e.g., tachycardia) and may potentiate insulin-induced hypoglycemia. Lopressor should therefore be used with caution in diabetic patients, especially those with labile diabetes.

Thyrotoxicosis: Beta-adrenergic blockade may mask certain clinical signs (e.g., tachycardia) of hyperthyroidism. Patients suspected of developing thyrotoxicosis should be managed carefully to avoid abrupt withdrawal of beta blockade which might precipitate a thyroid storm.

Precautions: ***Impaired Hepatic or Renal Function:*** The drug should be used with caution in patients with impaired hepatic or renal function.

Drug Interactions: Catecholamine-depleting drugs (e.g., reserpine) may have an additive effect when given with beta-blocking agents. Patients treated with Lopressor plus a catecholamine depletor should therefore be closely observed for evidence of hypotension and/or marked bradycardia which may produce vertigo, syncope, or postural hypotension.

Long-Term Animal Studies: Long-term studies in animals have been conducted to evaluate toxic effects and carcinogenic potential. In a one-year study in dogs, there was no evidence of drug-induced toxicity at or below oral doses of 105 mg/kg per day. Two-year studies in rats at three oral dosage levels of up to 800 mg/kg per day did not indicate an increase in the development of spontaneously occurring benign or malignant neoplasms of any type. The only histologic changes which appeared to be drug-related were an increased incidence of generally mild focal accumulation of foamy macrophages in pulmonary alveoli and a slight increase in biliary hyperplasia. Neither finding represents symptoms of a known disease entity in man. In a 21-month study in mice at three oral dose levels of up to 750 mg/kg per day, benign lung tumors (small adenomas) occurred more frequently in female mice receiving the highest dose than in untreated control animals. There was no increase in malignant lung tumors or total (benign plus malignant) lung tumors. The overall incidence of tumors or malignant tumors was also unaffected by metoprolol administration.

Usage in Pregnancy: Reproduction studies in animals did not reveal any evidence of impaired fertility or of teratogenic potential. There was evidence in the rat of increased post-implantation loss and decreased neonatal survival (threshold between 50 and 500 mg/kg). Distribution studies in mice confirm exposure of the fetus when metoprolol is administered to the pregnant animal. There are no well-controlled studies in pregnant women. Lopressor should be used in pregnant women only when clearly needed.

Nursing Mothers: It is not known whether this drug is excreted in human milk. Since most drugs are excreted in human milk, nursing should not be undertaken by mothers receiving metoprolol.

Usage in Children: Safety and effectiveness in children have not been established.

Adverse Reactions: Most adverse effects have been mild and transient.

Central Nervous System: Tiredness and dizziness have occurred in about 10 of 100 patients. Depression was reported in about 5 of 100 patients. Headache, nightmares, and insomnia have also been reported but drug relationship is not clear.

Cardiovascular: Shortness of breath and bradycardia have occurred in approximately 3 of 100 patients. Cold extremities; arterial insufficiency usually of the Raynaud type; palpitations and congestive heart failure have been reported. See **Contraindications, Warnings,** and **Precautions.**

Respiratory: Wheezing (bronchospasm) has been reported in less than 1 of 100 patients. See **Warnings.**

Gastrointestinal: Diarrhea has occurred in about 5 of 100 patients. Nausea, gastric pain, constipation, flatulence, and heartburn have been reported in 1 of 100 or less.

Allergic: Pruritus has occurred in less than 1 of 100 patients.

Miscellaneous: Peyronie's disease has been reported in less than 1 of 100,000 patients.

The oculomucocutaneous syndrome associated with the beta blocker practolol has not been reported with Lopressor during investigational use and foreign marketing experience.

Potential Adverse Effects: In addition, a variety of adverse effects not listed above have been reported with other beta-adrenergic blocking agents, and should be considered potential adverse effects of metoprolol.

Central Nervous System: Reversible mental depression progressing to catatonia; visual disturbances; hallucinations; an acute reversible syndrome characterized by disorientation for time and place, short-term memory loss, emotional lability, slightly clouded sensorium, and decreased performance on neuropsychometrics.

Cardiovascular: Intensification of AV block (See **Contraindications**).

Hematologic: Agranulocytosis, nonthrombocytopenic purpura, thrombocytopenic purpura.

Allergic: Erythematous rash, fever combined with aching and sore throat, laryngospasm and respiratory distress.

Miscellaneous: Reversible alopecia.

Clinical Laboratory Test Findings: Elevated blood urea levels in patients with severe heart disease, elevated serum transaminase, alkaline phosphatase, lactate dehydrogenase.

Overdosage: To date, only one case of extreme overdosage has been reported. A 19-year-old man ingested 200 50-mg tablets (160 mg/kg) and on hospital admission was conscious with peripheral cyanosis, weak heart sounds and an unmeasurable blood pressure. Only the femoral pulse was palpable. EKG showed sinus rhythm 60-70/minute with normal AV conduction, ST segments and T-waves. Blood analysis revealed excess base (−5 mEq/L), pH 7.41 pCO_2 29 mmHg and bicarbonate 20 mEq/L. Treatment consisted of gastric lavage, 2L Ringers solution, metaraminol 10 mg, glucagon 6 mg, 150 mmol sodium bicarbonate. Fluid retention noted during the first 6 hours was treated with furosemide. Two hours after admission, blood levels of Lopressor of 12,200 ng/g of plasma were recorded (normal maximum values after 100 mg orally is about 100/ng/g plasma). Complete recovery occurred within 12 hours without signs of cardiovascular depression.*

No specific information on emergency treatment of overdosage is available. Therefore, on the basis of the pharmacologic actions of Lopressor the following general measures should be employed:

Gastric Lavage.

Bradycardia: Administer atropine. If there is no response to vagal blockade administer isoproterenol cautiously.

Hypotension: Administer vasopressors, e.g., epinephrine or levarterenol.

Bronchospasm: Administer a $beta_2$-stimulating agent and/or a theophylline derivative.

Cardiac Failure: Administer a digitalis glycoside and diuretic. In shock resulting from inadequate cardiac contractility, the administration of dobutamine may be considered.

*Moller, B HS: Massive intoxication with metoprolol. Br Med J *1* (6003):222 (Jan. 24) 1976.

Dosage and Administration: Dosage of Lopressor should be individualized. The usual initial dose is 50 mg twice daily whether used alone or added to a diuretic. The dosage may be increased at weekly (or longer) intervals until optimum blood pressure reduction is achieved. In general, the maximum effect of any given dosage level will be apparent after one week of therapy. Usual maintenance dosage is approximately 100 mg twice a day, with a range of 100 to 450 mg per day. Dosages above 450 mg per day have not been studied. While twice-daily dosing is effective and can maintain a reduction in blood pressure throughout the day, some patients, especially when lower dosages are used, will experience a modest rise in blood pressure toward the end of the 12-hour dosing interval. This can be evaluated by measuring blood pressure near the end of the dosing interval to determine whether satisfactory control is being maintained throughout the day. If control is not adequate, a larger dose, or three times daily therapy, may achieve better control. $Beta_1$ selectivity diminishes as dosage of Lopressor is increased.

This drug should be stored at controlled room temperature and protected from moisture.

How Supplied: Tablets of 50 mg (capsule-shaped, scored, light red, film-coated) and 100 mg (capsule-shaped, scored, light blue, film-coated) are supplied in bottles of 100 and 1,000 and Unit Dose Packages of 100.

Store at controlled room temperature and protect from moisture.

Dispense in tight, light-resistant container (USP).

667292 (8/79) C79-22

[*Shown in Product Identification Section*]

OTRIVIN®

xylometazoline hydrochloride NF
Adult Nasal Spray and Drops 0.1%
Pediatric Nasal Drops 0.05%

Description: Otrivin, xylometazoline HCl, a sympathomimetic amine, is a white, odorless, crystalline powder which is soluble in water and freely soluble in alcohol. Chemically, it is 2- (4-*tert*-butyl-2,6-dimethylbenzyl) -2-imidazoline monohydrochloride.

This preparation is available in 0.1% solution for adults and 0.05% solution for children under 12.

Nasal Spray contains 0.1% and *Nasal Drops* contain 0.1% or 0.05% xylometazoline hydrochloride NF, potassium phosphate monobasic, potassium chloride, sodium phosphate dibasic, sodium chloride, and benzalkonium chloride 1:5,000 as preservative in water.

Actions: Its sympathomimetic (adrenergic) action constricts the smaller arterioles of the nasal passages, effecting a decongesting action. This vasoconstriction results from alpha adrenergic receptor stimulation of vascular smooth muscle.

Indications: For decongestion of the nasal mucosa.

Contraindications: Narrow-angle glaucoma. Concurrent MAO inhibitor therapy. Tricyclic antidepressant therapy. Hypersensitivity to any component of this preparation.

Sensitivity to even small doses of adrenergic substances as manifested by sleeplessness, dizziness, lightheadedness, weakness, tremulousness, or cardiac arrhythmias.

Warnings: Systemic effects from the use of topical decongestants may occur due to rapid absorption through the nasal mucous membrane and from gastrointestinal absorption if given in excess so that the solution is swallowed. Such reactions are most likely to occur in infants and the elderly.

Because of the possibility of generalized vasoconstriction and tachycardia, nose drops (as all sympathomimetic amines) should be used very cautiously in patients with hypertension, heart disease, including angina, hyperthyroidism and advanced arteriosclerotic conditions. Overdosage may produce profound CNS depression in children, possibly requiring intensive supportive treatment.

Usage in Pregnancy: Clinical data are inadequate to establish conditions for safe use of nose drops in pregnancy.

Directions:

Nasal Spray 0.1%—Spray 2 or 3 times into each nostril every 8–10 hours. With head up-

Continued on next page

The full prescribing information for each GEIGY drug is contained herein and is that in effect as of October 1, 1979.

Geigy—Cont.

right, squeeze sharply and firmly while inhaling (sniffing) through the nose.
Nasal Drops 0.1%—For adults and children 12 years and older. Put 2 or 3 drops into each nostril every 8 to 10 hours. Tilt head as far back as possible. Immediately bend head forward toward knees, hold a few seconds, then return to upright position.
Pediatric Nasal Drops 0.05%—For children 2 to 12 years of age. Put 2 or 3 drops into each nostril every 8 to 10 hours. Tilt head as far back as possible. Immediately bend head forward toward knees, hold a few seconds, then return to upright position.
How Supplied: *Otrivin Nasal Spray/Nasal Drops* are available in unbreakable plastic spray packages of ½ fl oz (15 ml) and in plastic dropper bottles of .66 fl oz (20 ml).
Otrivin Pediatric Nasal Drops Available in plastic dropper bottles of .66 fl oz (20 ml).
(8/79)

PBZ-SR® GY-CODE 48 ℞
tripelennaminne HCl
sustained-release tablets
Tablets of 100 mg

Description: PBZ-SR Tablets are available as the hydrochloride salt of tripelennamine, 2-[benzyl[2-(dimethylamino)ethyl]-amino]pyridine, in a wax matrix. This formulation is intended to provide a gradual and prolonged release of tripelennamine from the matrix. Tripelennamine hydrochloride is an antihistamine occurring as a white, crystalline powder that slowly darkens on exposure to light and is freely soluble in water and alcohol.
Actions: Antihistamines are competitive antagonists of histamine, which also produce central nervous system effects (both stimulant and depressant) and peripheral anticholinergic, atropine-like effects (e.g., drying).
Indications: Perennial and seasonal allergic rhinitis; vasomotor rhinitis; allergic conjunctivitis due to inhalant allergens and foods; mild, uncomplicated allergic skin manifestations of urticaria and angioedema; amelioration of allergic reactions to blood or plasma; dermographism; anaphylactic reactions as adjunctive therapy to epinephrine and other standard measures after the acute manifestations have been controlled.
Contraindications: PBZ-SR should not be used in premature infants, neonates, or nursing mothers; patients receiving MAO inhibitors; patients with narrow-angle glaucoma, stenosing peptic ulcer, symptomatic prostatic hypertrophy, bladder neck obstruction, pyloroduodenal obstruction, lower respiratory tract symptoms (including asthma), or hypersensitivity to tripelennamine or related compounds.
Warnings: Antihistamines often produce drowsiness and may reduce mental alertness in children and adults. Patients should be warned about engaging in activities requiring mental alertness (e.g., driving a car, operating machinery or hazardous appliances). In elderly patients, approximately 60 years or older, antihistamines are more likely to cause dizziness, sedation and hypotension.
Patients should be warned that the central nervous system effects of PBZ-SR may be additive with those of alcohol and other CNS depressants (e.g., hypnotics, sedatives, tranquilizers, antianxiety agents).
Antihistamines may produce excitation, particularly in children.
Usage in Pregnancy
Although no tripelennamine-related teratogenic potential or other adverse effects on the fetus have been observed in limited animal reproduction studies, the safe use of this drug in pregnancy or during lactation has not been established. Therefore, the drug should not be used during pregnancy or lactation unless, in the judgment of the physician, the expected benefits outweigh the potential hazards.
Usage in Children
In infants and children particularly, antihistamines in overdosage may produce hallucinations, convulsions and/or death.
Precautions: PBZ-SR, like other antihistamines, has atropine-like, anticholinergic activity and should be used with caution in patients with increased intraocular pressure, hyperthyroidism, cardiovascular disease, hypertension, or history of bronchial asthma.
Adverse Reactions: The most frequent adverse reactions to antihistamines are sedation or drowsiness; sleepiness; dryness of the mouth, nose, and throat; thickening of bronchial secretions; dizziness; disturbed coordination; epigastric distress.
Other adverse reactions which may occur are: fatigue; chills; confusion; restlessness; excitation; hysteria; nervousness; irritability; insomnia; euphoria; anorexia; nausea; vomiting; diarrhea; constipation; hypotension; tightness in the chest; wheezing; blurred vision; diplopia; vertigo; tinnitus; convulsions; headache; palpitations; tachycardia; extrasystoles; nasal stuffiness; urinary frequency; difficult urination; urinary retention; leukopenia; hemolytic anemia; thrombocytopenia; agranulocytosis; aplastic anemia; allergic or hypersensitivity reactions, including drug rash, urticaria, anaphylactic shock, and photosensitivity. Although the following may have been reported to occur in association with some antihistamines, they have not been known to result from the use of PBZ-SR: excessive perspiration, tremor, paresthesias, acute labyrinthitis, neuritis and early menses.
Dosage and Administration: Dosage should be individualized according to the needs and response of the patient.
Adults: One 100-mg PBZ-SR Tablet in the morning and one in the evening is generally adequate. In difficult cases, one 100-mg PBZ-SR Tablet every 8 hours may be required.
Children: PBZ-SR Tablets are not intended for use in children.
Overdosage:
Signs and Symptoms
The greatest danger from acute overdosage with antihistamines is their central nervous system effects which produce depression and/or stimulation.
In children, stimulation predominates initially in a syndrome which may include excitement, hallucinations, ataxia, incoordination, athetosis, and convulsions followed by postictal depression. Dry mouth, fixed dilated pupils, flushing of the face, and fever are common and resemble the syndrome of atropine poisoning.
In adults, CNS depression (i.e., drowsiness, coma) is more common. CNS stimulation is rare; fever and flushing are uncommon.
In both children and adults, there can be a terminal deepening of coma and cardiovascular collapse; death can occur, especially in infants and children.
Treatment
There is no specific therapy for acute overdosage with antihistamines. General symptomatic and supportive measures should be instituted promptly and maintained for as long as necessary.
In the conscious patient, vomiting should be induced even though it may have occurred spontaneously. If vomiting cannot be induced, gastric lavage is indicated. Adequate precautions must be taken to protect against aspiration, especially in infants and children. Charcoal slurry or other suitable agent should be instilled into the stomach after vomiting or lavage. Saline cathartics or milk of magnesia may be of additional benefit.
In the unconscious patient, the airway should be secured with a cuffed endotracheal tube before attempting to evacuate the gastric contents. Intensive supportive and nursing care is indicated, as for any comatose patient.
If breathing is significantly impaired, maintenance of an adequate airway and mechanical support of respiration is the safest and most effective means of providing for adequate oxygenation of tissues to prevent hypoxia (especially brain hypoxia during convulsions).
Hypotension is an early sign of impending cardiovascular collapse and should be treated vigorously. Although general supportive measures are important, specific treatment with intravenous infusion of a vasopressor (e.g., levarterenol bitartrate) titrated to maintain adequate blood pressure is also necessary.
Do *not* use CNS stimulants.
Convulsions should be controlled by careful titration of a short-acting barbiturate, repeated as necessary.
Ice packs and cooling sponge baths can aid in reducing the fever commonly seen in children.
How Supplied: *PBZ-SR Tablets,* 100 mg (lavender), each containing 100 mg tripelennamine hydrochloride; bottles of 100.
Dispense in tight container (USP).
667350 C78-44 (12/78)
[*Shown in Product Identification Section*]

PBZ® ℞
tripelennamine
Tablets GY-CODE 95
Elixir GY-CODE 6925

Listed in USP, a Medicare designated compendium.

Description: PBZ Tablets are available as the hydrochloride salt and PBZ Elixir as the citrate salt of 2-[benzyl[2-(dimethylamino) ethyl]-amino]pyridine. Tripelennamine hydrochloride is an antihistamine occurring as a white, crystalline powder that slowly darkens on exposure to light and is freely soluble in water and alcohol.
Actions: Antihistamines are competitive antagonists of histamine, which also produce central nervous system effects (both stimulant and depressant) and peripheral anticholinergic, atropine-like effects (e.g., drying).
Indications: Perennial and seasonal allergic rhinitis; vasomotor rhinitis; allergic conjunctivitis due to inhalant allergens and foods; mild, uncomplicated allergic skin manifestations of urticaria and angioedema; amelioration of allergic reactions to blood or plasma; dermographism; anaphylactic reactions as adjunctive therapy to epinephrine and other standard measures after the acute manifestations have been controlled.
Contraindications: PBZ should not be used in premature infants, neonates, or nursing mothers; patients receiving MAO inhibitors; patients with narrow-angle glaucoma, stenosing peptic ulcer, symptomatic prostatic hypertrophy, bladder neck obstruction, pyloroduodenal obstruction, lower respiratory tract symptoms (including asthma), or hypersensitivity to tripelennamine or related compounds.
Warnings: Antihistamines often produce drowsiness and may reduce mental alertness in children and adults. Patients should be warned about engaging in activities requiring mental alertness (e.g., driving a car, operating machinery or hazardous appliances). In elderly patients, approximately 60 years or older, antihistamines are more likely to cause dizziness, sedation and hypotension.
Patients should be warned that the central nervous system effects of PBZ may be additive with those of alcohol and other CNS depressants (e.g., hypnotics, sedatives, tranquilizers, antianxiety agents).
Antihistamines may produce excitation, particularly in children.
Usage in Pregnancy
Although no tripelennamine-related teratogenic potential or other adverse effects on the fetus have been observed in limited animal reproduction studies, the safe use of this drug in pregnancy or during lactation has not been

established. Therefore, the drug should not be used during pregnancy or lactation unless, in the judgment of the physician, the expected benefits outweigh the potential hazards.

Usage in Children

In infants and children particularly, antihistamines in overdosage may produce hallucinations, convulsions and/or death.

Precautions: PBZ, like other antihistamines, has atropine-like, anticholinergic activity and should be used with caution in patients with increased intraocular pressure, hyperthyroidism, cardiovascular disease, hypertension, or history of bronchial asthma.

The PBZ tablets (25 mg) contain FD&C Yellow No. 5 (tartrazine) which may cause allergic-type reactions (including bronchial asthma) in certain susceptible individuals. Although the overall incidence of FD&C Yellow No. 5 (tartrazine) sensitivity in the general population is low, it is frequently seen in patients who also have aspirin hypersensitivity.

Adverse Reactions: The most frequent adverse reactions to antihistamines are sedation or drowsiness; sleepiness; dryness of the mouth, nose, and throat; thickening of bronchial secretions; dizziness; disturbed coordination; epigastric distress.

Other adverse reactions which may occur are: fatigue; chills; confusion; restlessness; excitation; hysteria; nervousness; irritability; insomnia; euphoria; anorexia; nausea; vomiting; diarrhea; constipation; hypotension; tightness in the chest; wheezing; blurred vision; diplopia; vertigo; tinnitus; convulsions; headache; palpitations; tachycardia; extrasystoles; nasal stuffiness; urinary frequency; difficult urination; urinary retention; leukopenia; hemolytic anemia; thrombocytopenia; agranulocytosis; aplastic anemia; allergic or hypersensitivity reactions, including drug rash, urticaria, anaphylactic shock, and photosensitivity. Although the following may have been reported to occur in association with some antihistamines, they have not been known to result from the use of PBZ: excessive perspiration, tremor, paresthesias, acute labyrinthitis, neuritis and early menses.

Dosage and Administration: Dosage should be individualized.

Usual Adult Dose: 25 to 50 mg every four to six hours. As little as 25 mg may control symptoms, but as much as 600 mg daily may be given in divided doses, if necessary.

Children and Infants: 5 mg/kg/24 hours or 150 mg/m^2/24 hours divided into four to six doses. Do not exceed maximum total dose of 300 mg/24 hours.

Note: Recommended dosages are based on the hydrochloride salt; each ml of Elixir (tripelennamine citrate) is equivalent to 5 mg tripelennamine hydrochloride.

Overdosage

Signs and Symptoms

The greatest danger from acute overdosage with antihistamines is their central nervous system effects which produce depression and/or stimulation.

In children, stimulation predominates initially in a syndrome which may include excitement, hallucinations, ataxia, incoordination, athetosis, and convulsions followed by postictal depression. Dry mouth, fixed dilated pupils, flushing of the face, and fever are common and resemble the syndrome of atropine poisoning. In adults, CNS depression (i.e., drowsiness, coma) is more common. CNS stimulation is rare; fever and flushing are uncommon.

In both children and adults, there can be a terminal deepening of coma and cardiovascular collapse; death can occur, especially in infants and children.

Treatment

There is no specific therapy for acute overdosage with antihistamines. General symptomatic and supportive measures should be instituted promptly and maintained for as long as necessary.

In the conscious patient, vomiting should be induced even though it may have occurred spontaneously. If vomiting cannot be induced, gastric lavage is indicated. Adequate precautions must be taken to protect against aspiration, especially in infants and children. Charcoal slurry or other suitable agent should be instilled into the stomach after vomiting or lavage. Saline cathartics or milk of magnesia may be of additional benefit.

In the unconscious patient, the airway should be secured with a cuffed endotracheal tube before attempting to evacuate the gastric contents. Intensive supportive and nursing care is indicated, as for any comatose patient.

If breathing is significantly impaired, maintenance of an adequate airway and mechanical support of respiration is the safest and most effective means of providing for adequate oxygenation of tissues to prevent hypoxia (especially brain hypoxia during convulsions).

Hypotension is an early sign of impending cardiovascular collapse and should be treated vigorously. Although general supportive measures are important, specific treatment with intravenous infusion of a vasopressor (e.g., levarterenol bitartrate) titrated to maintain adequate blood pressure may be necessary.

Do *not* use CNS stimulants.

Convulsions should be controlled by careful titration of a short-acting barbiturate, repeated as necessary.

Ice packs and cooling sponge baths can aid in reducing the fever commonly seen in children.

How Supplied:

Tablets (light blue, scored), containing 50 mg PBZ® hydrochloride (tripelennamine hydrochloride USP); bottles of 100 and 1000.

Tablets (green, sugar-coated), containing 25 mg tripelennamine hydrochloride; bottles of 100.

Elixir (green, cinnamon-flavored), containing 37.5 mg PBZ® citrate (tripelennamine citrate USP) per 5 ml (equivalent to 25 mg tripelennamine hydrochloride); bottles of 473 ml (approx. 1 pint).

Dispense in tight, light-resistant container (USP).

667361 C80-12 (1/80)

[*Shown in Product Identification Section*]

PBZ® Lontabs® GY-CODE 60 ℞

tripelennamine

Tablets of 50 mg

Description: PBZ Lontabs (long-acting tablets) are available as the hydrochloride salt of 2-[benzyl[2-(dimethylamino)ethyl]-amino]pyridine. Tripelennamine hydrochloride is an antihistamine occurring as a white, crystalline powder that slowly darkens on exposure to light and is freely soluble in water and alcohol.

Actions: Antihistamines are competitive antagonists of histamine, which also produce central nervous system effects (both stimulant and depressant) and peripheral anticholinergic, atropine-like effects (e.g., drying).

Indications

Based on a review of this drug by the National Academy of Sciences-National Research Council and/or other information, FDA has classified the indications as follows:

"Probably" effective: Perennial and seasonal allergic rhinitis; vasomotor rhinitis; allergic conjunctivitis due to inhalant allergens and foods; mild, uncomplicated allergic skin manifestations of urticaria and angioedema; amelioration of allergic reactions to blood or plasma; dermographism; anaphylactic reactions as adjunctive therapy to epinephrine and other standard measures after the acute manifestations have been controlled.

Final classification of the less-than-effective indications requires further investigation.

Contraindications: PBZ should not be used in premature infants, neonates, or nursing mothers; patients receiving MAO inhibitors; patients with narrow angle glaucoma, stenosing peptic ulcer, symptomatic prostatic hypertrophy, bladder neck obstruction, pyloroduodenal obstruction, lower respiratory tract symptoms (including asthma), or hypersensitivity to tripelennamine or related compounds.

Warnings: Antihistamines often produce drowsiness and may reduce mental alertness in children and adults. Patients should be warned about engaging in activities requiring mental alertness (e.g., driving a car, operating machinery or hazardous appliances). In elderly patients, approximately 60 years or older, antihistamines are more likely to cause dizziness, sedation and hypotension.

Patients should be warned that the central nervous system effects of tripelennamine may be additive with those of alcohol and other CNS depressants (e.g., hypnotics, sedatives, tranquilizers, antianxiety agents).

Antihistamines may produce excitation, particularly in children.

Usage in Pregnancy

Although no tripelennamine-related teratogenic potential or other adverse effects on the fetus have been observed in limited animal reproduction studies, the safe use of this drug in pregnancy or during lactation has not been established. Therefore, the drug should not be used during pregnancy or lactation unless, in the judgment of the physician, the expected benefits outweigh the potential hazards.

Usage in Children

In infants and children particularly, antihistamines in overdosage may produce hallucinations, convulsions and/or death.

Precautions: PBZ, like other antihistamines, has atropine-like, anticholinergic activity and should be used with caution in patients with increased intraocular pressure, hyperthyroidism, cardiovascular disease, hypertension, or history of bronchial asthma.

PBZ Lontab® tablets (50 mg) contain FD&C Yellow No. 5 (tartrazine) which may cause allergic-type reactions (including bronchial asthma) in certain susceptible individuals. Although the overall incidence of FD&C Yellow No. 5 (tartrazine) sensitivity in the general population is low, it is frequently seen in patients who also have aspirin hypersensitivity.

Adverse Reactions: The most frequent adverse reactions to antihistamines are sedation or drowsiness; sleepiness; dryness of the mouth, nose, and throat; thickening of bronchial secretions; dizziness; disturbed coordination; epigastric distress.

Other adverse reactions which may occur are fatigue; chills; confusion; restlessness; excitation; hysteria; nervousness; irritability; insomnia; euphoria; anorexia; nausea; vomiting; diarrhea; constipation; hypotension; tightness in the chest; wheezing; blurred vision; diplopia; vertigo; tinnitus; convulsions; headache; palpitations; tachycardia; extrasystoles; nasal stuffiness; urinary frequency; difficult urination; urinary retention; leukopenia; hemolytic anemia; thrombocytopenia; agranulocytosis; aplastic anemia; allergic or hypersensitivity reactions, including drug rash, urticaria, anaphylactic shock, and photosensitivity. Although the following may have been reported to occur in association with some antihistamines, they have not been known to result

Continued on next page

The full prescribing information for each GEIGY drug is contained herein and is that in effect as of October 1, 1979.

Geigy—Cont.

from the use of PBZ: excessive perspiration, tremor, paresthesias, acute labyrinthitis, neuritis and early menses.

Dosage and Administration: Dosage should be individualized according to the needs and response of the patient.

The effects of PBZ Lontabs begin within 15 to 30 minutes and generally last up to 8 hours.

Adults: 100 mg in the morning and 100 mg in the evening is generally adequate for "around-the-clock" allergic protection. In difficult cases, 100 mg every 8 hours may be required.

Children Over 5: One 50-mg Lontab in the morning and one in the evening is usually sufficient, but some children may require one every 8 hours.

Overdosage:

Signs and Symptoms

The greatest danger from acute overdosage with antihistamines is their central nervous system effects which produce depression and/or stimulation.

In children, stimulation predominates initially in a syndrome which may include excitement, hallucinations, ataxia, incoordination, athetosis, and convulsions followed by postictal depression. Dry mouth, fixed dilated pupils, flushing of the face, and fever are common and resemble the syndrome of atropine poisoning.

In adults, CNS depression (i.e., drowsiness, coma) is more common. CNS stimulation is rare; fever and flushing are uncommon.

In both children and adults, there can be a terminal deepening of coma and cardiovascular collapse; death can occur, especially in infants and children.

Treatment

There is no specific therapy for acute overdosage with antihistamines. General symptomatic and supportive measures should be instituted promptly and maintained for as long as necessary.

In the conscious patient, vomiting should be induced even though it may have occurred spontaneously. If vomiting cannot be induced, gastric lavage is indicated. Adequate precautions must be taken to protect against aspiration, especially in infants and children. Charcoal slurry or other suitable agent should be instilled into the stomach after vomiting or lavage. Saline cathartics or milk of magnesia may be of additional benefit.

In the unconscious patient, the airway should be secured with a cuffed endotracheal tube before attempting to evacuate the gastric contents. Intensive supportive and nursing care is indicated, as for any comatose patient.

If breathing is significantly impaired, maintenance of an adequate airway and mechanical support of respiration is the safest and most effective means of providing for adequate oxygenation of tissues to prevent hypoxia (especially brain hypoxia during convulsions).

Hypotension is an early sign of impending cardiovascular collapse and should be treated vigorously. Although general supportive measures are important, specific treatment with intravenous infusion of a vasopressor (e.g., levarterenol bitartrate) titrated to maintain adequate blood pressure is also necessary.

Do *not* use CNS stimulants.

Convulsions should be controlled by careful titration of a short-acting barbiturate, repeated as necessary.

Ice packs and cooling sponge baths can aid in reducing the fever commonly seen in children.

How Supplied:

Lontabs (light green), containing 50 mg tripelennamine hydrochloride; bottles of 100.

LONTABS® (long-acting tablets)

Dispense in tight, light-resistant container (USP).

667391 C80-8 (1/80)

PBZ® GY-CODE 6965 ℞

tripelennamine

Expectorant with Ephedrine

Description: PBZ Expectorant with Ephedrine contains 30 mg tripelennamine citrate (equivalent to 20 mg tripelennamine hydrochloride), 10 mg ephedrine sulfate, and 80 mg ammonium chloride per 4 ml. Tripelennamine citrate is the salt of 2-[benzyl[2-(dimethylamino)ethyl]-amino] pyridine.

Actions:

Tripelennamine

Antihistamines are competitive antagonists of histamine, which also produce central nervous system effects (both stimulant and depressant) and peripheral anticholinergic, atropine-like effects (e.g., drying).

Ephedrine

Ephedrine differs from epinephrine mainly in its efficacy after oral administration, its much longer duration of action, its more pronounced central actions, and its much lower potency. Bronchial muscle relaxation is less prominent but more sustained with ephedrine than with epinephrine.

Indications:

PBZ Expectorant with Ephedrine often relieves persistent, unproductive cough frequently accompanying bronchitis due to or associated with allergy. Useful in symptomatic treatment of selected cases of asthma.

Before prescribing medication to suppress or modify cough, it is important to ascertain that the underlying cause of cough is identified; that modification of cough does not increase the risk of clinical or physiologic complications; and that appropriate therapy for the primary disease is provided.

Contraindications: PBZ Expectorant with Ephedrine should not be used in premature infants, neonates, or nursing mothers; patients receiving MAO inhibitors; patients with narrow-angle glaucoma, stenosing peptic ulcer, symptomatic prostatic hypertrophy, bladder neck obstruction, pyloroduodenal obstruction, lower respiratory tract symptoms (including asthma), or hypersensitivity to tripelennamine, or related compounds.

Warnings:

Tripelennamine

Antihistamines often produce drowsiness and may reduce mental alertness in children and adults. Patients should be warned about engaging in activities requiring mental alertness (e.g., driving a car, operating machinery or hazardous appliances). In elderly patients, approximately 60 years or older, antihistamines are more likely to cause dizziness, sedation and hypotension.

Patients should be warned that the central nervous system effects of PBZ may be additive with those of alcohol and other CNS depressants (e.g., hypnotics, sedatives, tranquilizers, anti-anxiety agents).

Antihistamines may produce excitation, particularly in children.

Ephedrine

Use cautiously in patients with degenerative heart disease (anginal pain may be induced in patients with angina pectoris) and in hyperthyroid and hypertensive individuals, who are particularly susceptible to the untoward and pressor responses to ephedrine.

Usage in Pregnancy

Although no tripelennamine-related teratogenic potential or other adverse effects on the fetus have been observed in limited animal reproduction studies, the safe use of this drug in pregnancy or during lactation has not been established. Therefore, the drug should not be used during pregnancy or lactation unless, in the judgment of the physician, the expected benefits outweigh the potential hazards.

Usage in Children

In infants and children particularly, antihistamines in overdosage may produce hallucinations, convulsions and/or death.

Precautions: PBZ, like other antihistamines, has atropine-like, anticholinergic activity and should be used with caution in patients with increased intraocular pressure, hyperthyroidism, cardiovascular disease, hypertension, or history of bronchial asthma.

Adverse Reactions:

Tripelennamine

The most frequent adverse reactions to antihistamines are sedation or drowsiness; sleepiness; dryness of the mouth, nose, and throat; thickening of bronchial secretions; dizziness; disturbed coordination; epigastric distress.

Other adverse reactions which may occur are: fatigue; chills; confusion; restlessness; excitation; hysteria; nervousness; irritability; insomnia; euphoria; anorexia; nausea; vomiting; diarrhea; constipation; hypotension; tightness in the chest; wheezing; blurred vision; diplopia; vertigo; tinnitus; convulsions; headache; palpitations; tachycardia; extrasystoles; nasal stuffiness; urinary frequency; difficult urination; urinary retention; leukopenia; hemolytic anemia; thrombocytopenia; agranulocytosis; aplastic anemia; allergic or hypersensitivity reactions, including drug rash, urticaria, anaphylactic shock, and photosensitivity. Although the following may have been reported to occur in association with some antihistamines, they have not been known to result from the use of PBZ: excessive perspiration, tremor, paresthesias, acute labyrinthitis, neuritis and early menses.

Ephedrine

Occasionally peripheral vasoconstriction, irritability, palpitations, tremors, insomnia, in some cases anxiety, or other side effects which may be encountered with the sympathomimetic drugs. Psychotic symptoms with paranoid delusions have been described following chronic overdosage (self-medication).

Dosage and Administration: Dosage should be individualized according to the needs and the response of the patient.

Expectorant with Ephedrine

Adults: 1 or 2 teaspoons every 3 or 4 hours.

Children: ½ or 1 teaspoon every 3 or 4 hours.

Take a full glass of water with each dose.

Overdosage:

Tripelennamine

Signs and Symptoms

The greatest danger from acute overdosage with antihistamines is their central nervous system effects which produce depression and/or stimulation.

In children, stimulation predominates in a syndrome which may include excitement, hallucinations, ataxia, incoordination, athetosis, and convulsions followed by postictal depression. Dry mouth, fixed dilated pupils, flushed face, and fever are common and resemble the syndrome of atropine poisoning.

In adults, CNS depression (i.e., drowsiness, coma) is more common. CNS stimulation is rare; fever and flushing are uncommon.

In both children and adults, there can be a terminal deepening of coma and cardiovascular collapse; death can occur, especially in infants and children.

Treatment

There is no specific therapy for acute overdosage with antihistamines. General symptomatic and supportive measures should be instituted promptly and maintained for as long as necessary.

In the conscious patient, vomiting should be induced even though it may have occurred spontaneously. If vomiting cannot be induced, gastric lavage is indicated. Adequate precautions must be taken to protect against aspiration, especially in infants and children. Charcoal slurry or other suitable agent should be instilled into the stomach after vomiting or lavage. Saline cathartics or milk of magnesia may be of additional benefit.

In the unconscious patient, the airway should be secured with a cuffed endotracheal tube before attempting to evacuate the gastric con-

tents. Intensive supportive and nursing care is indicated, as for any comatose patient.
If breathing is significantly impaired, maintenance of an adequate airway and mechanical support of respiration is the safest and most effective means of providing for adequate oxygenation of tissues to prevent hypoxia (especially brain hypoxia during convulsions).
Hypotension is an early sign of impending cardiovascular collapse and should be treated vigorously. Although general supportive measures are important, specific treatment with intravenous infusion of a vasopressor (e.g., levarterenol bitartrate) titrated to maintain adequate blood pressure is also necessary.
Do *not* use CNS stimulants.
Convulsions should be controlled by careful titration of a short-acting barbiturate, repeated as necessary.
Ice packs and alcohol sponge baths can aid in reducing the fever commonly seen in children.
How Supplied: *Expectorant with Ephedrine* (yellow), containing 30 mg tripelennamine citrate USP (equivalent to 20 mg tripelennamine hydrochloride), 10 mg ephedrine sulfate, and 80 mg ammonium chloride per 4-ml teaspoon; bottles of 473 ml (approx. 1 pint).
Dispense in tight, light-resistant container (USP).
667370 C78-47 (12/78)

PBZ® tripelennamine GY-CODE 134 ℞
Tablets with Ephedrine

Description: PBZ Tablets with Ephedrine contain 25 mg tripelennamine hydrochloride and 12 mg ephedrine sulfate. PBZ hydrochloride is an antihistamine occurring as a white, crystalline powder that darkens slowly on exposure to light and is freely soluble in water and alcohol; chemically, it is 2-[benzyl[2-(dimethylamino)ethyl]-amino]pyridine hydrochloride.
Actions:
Tripelennamine
Antihistamines are competitive antagonists of histamine, which also produce central nervous system effects (both stimulant and depressant) and peripheral anticholinergic, atropine-like effects (e.g., drying).
Ephedrine
Ephedrine differs from epinephrine mainly in its efficacy after oral administration, its much longer duration of action, its more pronounced central actions, and its much lower potency. Bronchial muscle relaxation is less prominent but more sustained with ephedrine than with epinephrine.

Indications
Based on a review of this drug by the National Academy of Sciences-National Research Council and/or other information, FDA has classified the indications as follows:
"Probably" Effective: For the symptomatic treatment of seasonal and perennial allergic rhinitis and vasomotor rhinitis.
Final classification of the less-than-effective indications requires further investigation.

Contraindications: PBZ Tablets with Ephedrine should not be used in premature infants, neonates, or nursing mothers; patients receiving MAO inhibitors; patients with narrow-angle glaucoma, stenosing peptic ulcer, symptomatic prostatic hypertrophy, bladder neck obstruction, pyloroduodenal obstruction, lower respiratory tract symptoms (including asthma), or hypersensitivity to tripelennamine, ephedrine or related compounds.
Warnings:
Tripelennamine
Antihistamines often produce drowsiness and may reduce mental alertness in children and adults. Patients should be warned about engaging in activities requiring mental alertness (e.g., driving a car, operating machinery or hazardous appliances). In elderly patients, approximately 60 years or older, antihistamines are more likely to cause dizziness, sedation and hypotension.
Patients should be warned that the central nervous system effects of PBZ may be additive with those of alcohol and other CNS depressants (e.g., hypnotics, sedatives, tranquilizers, anti-anxiety agents).
Antihistamines may produce excitation, particularly in children.
Ephedrine
Use cautiously in patients with degenerative heart disease (anginal pain may be induced in patients with angina pectoris) and in hyperthyroid and hypertensive individuals, who are particularly susceptible to the untoward and pressor responses to ephedrine.
Usage in Pregnancy
Although no tripelennamine-related teratogenic potential or other adverse effects on the fetus have been observed in limited animal reproduction studies, the safe use of this drug in pregnancy or during lactation has not been established. Therefore, the drug should not be used during pregnancy or lactation unless, in the judgment of the physician, the expected benefits outweigh the potential hazards.
Usage in Children
In infants and children particularly, antihistamines in overdosage may produce hallucinations, convulsions and/or death.
Precautions: PBZ, like other antihistamines, has atropine-like, anticholinergic activity and should be used with caution in patients with increased intraocular pressure, hyperthyroidism, cardiovascular disease, hypertension, or history of bronchial asthma.
Adverse Reactions:
Tripelennamine
The most frequent adverse reactions to antihistamines are sedation or drowsiness; sleepiness; dryness of the mouth, nose, and throat; thickening of bronchial secretions; dizziness; disturbed coordination; epigastric distress.
Other adverse reactions which may occur are: fatigue; chills; confusion; restlessness; excitation; hysteria; nervousness; irritability; insomnia; euphoria; anorexia; nausea; vomiting; diarrhea; constipation; hypotension; tightness in the chest; wheezing; blurred vision; diplopia; vertigo; tinnitus; convulsions; headache; palpitations; tachycardia; extrasystoles; nasal stuffiness; urinary frequency; difficult urination; urinary retention; leukopenia; hemolytic anemia; thrombocytopenia; agranulocytosis; aplastic anemia; allergic or hypersensitivity reactions, including drug rash, urticaria, anaphylactic shock, and photosensitivity. Although the following may have been reported to occur in association with some antihistamines, they have not been known to result from the use of PBZ: excessive perspiration, tremor, paresthesias, acute labyrinthitis, neuritis and early menses.
Ephedrine
Occasionally peripheral vasoconstriction, irritability, palpitations, tremors, insomnia, in some cases anxiety, or other side effects which may be encountered with the sympathomimetic drugs. Psychotic symptoms with paranoid delusions have been described following chronic overdosage (self-medication).
Dosage and Administration: Dosage should be individualized according to the needs and the response of the patient.
Adults: 1 or 2 tablets every 4 hours.
Older Children: 1 tablet 4 times a day.
Overdosage:
Tripelennamine
Signs and Symptoms
The greatest danger from acute overdosage with antihistamines is their central nervous system effects which produce depression and/or stimulation.
In children, stimulation predominates in a syndrome which may include excitement, hallucinations, ataxia, incoordination, athetosis, and convulsions followed by postictal depression. Dry mouth, fixed dilated pupils, flushed face, and fever are common and resemble the syndrome of atropine poisoning.
In adults, CNS depression (i.e., drowsiness, coma) is more common. CNS stimulation is rare; fever and flushing are uncommon.
In both children and adults, there can be a terminal deepening of coma and cardiovascular collapse; death can occur, especially in infants and children.
Treatment
There is no specific therapy for acute overdosage with antihistamines. General symptomatic and supportive measures should be instituted promptly and maintained for as long as necessary.
In the conscious patient, vomiting should be induced even though it may have occurred spontaneously. If vomiting cannot be induced, gastric lavage is indicated. Adequate precautions must be taken to protect against aspiration, especially in infants and children. Charcoal slurry or other suitable agent should be instilled into the stomach after vomiting or lavage. Saline cathartics or milk of magnesia may be of additional benefit.
In the unconscious patient, the airway should be secured with a cuffed endotracheal tube before attempting to evacuate the gastric contents. Intensive supportive and nursing care is indicated, as for any comatose patient.
If breathing is significantly impaired, maintenance of an adequate airway and mechanical support of respiration is the safest and most effective means of providing for adequate oxygenation of tissues to prevent hypoxia (especially brain hypoxia during convulsions).
Hypotension is an early sign of impending cardiovascular collapse and should be treated vigorously. Although general supportive measures are important, specific treatment with intravenous infusion of a vasopressor (e.g., levarterenol bitartrate) titrated to maintain adequate blood pressure is also necessary.
Do *not* use CNS stimulants.
Convulsions should be controlled by careful titration of a short-acting barbiturate, repeated as necessary.
Ice packs and alcohol sponge baths can aid in reducing the fever commonly seen in children.
How Supplied: *Tablets with Ephedrine* (white, dry-coated), each containing 25 mg tripelennamine hydrochloride and 12 mg ephedrine sulfate; bottles of 100.
Dispense in tight container (USP).
667400 C78-46 (12/78)

PBZ® hydrochloride
tripelennamine hydrochloride
Ointment GY-CODE 6935
Cream GY-CODE 6946
Antihistamine

Indications: For the temporary relief of itching due to minor skin disorders, ivy and oak poisoning, hives, sunburn, insect bites (nonpoisonous), and stings.
Directions: Apply gently to the affected area 3 or 4 times daily or according to physician's directions.
Caution: If the condition persists or irritation develops, discontinue use and consult physician. Do not use in eyes.
KEEP OUT OF REACH OF CHILDREN.
How Supplied:
Ointment, 2% tripelennamine hydrochloride in a petrolatum base; tubes of 1 ounce.

Continued on next page

The full prescribing information for each GEIGY drug is contained herein and is that in effect as of October 1, 1979.

Geigy—Cont.

Cream, 2% tripelennamine hydrochloride in a water-washable base; tubes of 1 ounce.

(12/78)

TANDEARIL® ℞
oxyphenbutazone NF
A Potent Anti-Inflammatory Agent
Tablets of 100 mg **GY-CODE 24**

Important Note: Tandearil cannot be considered a simple analgesic and should never be administered casually. Each patient should be carefully evaluated before treatment is started and should remain constantly under the close supervision of the physician. The following cautions should be observed:

1. Therapy should not be initiated until a careful detailed history and complete physical and laboratory examination, including a complete hemogram and urinalysis, etc., of the patient have been made. These examinations should be made at regular, frequent intervals throughout the duration of this drug therapy.
2. Patients should be carefully selected, avoiding those in whom it is contraindicated as well as those who will respond to ordinary therapeutic measures, or those who cannot be observed at frequent intervals.
3. Patients taking this drug should be warned not to exceed the recommended dosage, since this may lead to toxic effects, and should discontinue the drug and report to the physician immediately any sign of:
   a. Fever, sore throat, lesions in the mouth (symptoms of blood dyscrasia).
   b. Dyspepsia, epigastric pain, symptoms of anemia, unusual bleeding, unusual bruising, black or tarry stools or other evidence of intestinal ulceration.
   c. Skin rashes.
   d. Significant weight gain or edema.
4. A trial period of one week of therapy is considered adequate to determine the therapeutic effect of the drug. In the absence of a favorable response, therapy should be discontinued.
   a. In the elderly (sixty years and over) the drug should be restricted to short-term treatment periods only—if possible, *one week* maximum.
5. **Before prescribing Tandearil for an individual patient, read thoroughly the information contained under each heading which follows:**

Description: Tandearil should not be considered as a simple analgesic that can be prescribed for indiscriminate use. Tandearil is closely related chemically and pharmacologically, including toxic effects, to the well-known pyrazolines (pyrazole compounds) amidopyrine and antipyrine.

Chemically, Tandearil is 4-Butyl-1-(p-hydroxyphenyl) 2-phenyl-3,5-pyrazolidinedione monohydrate, the parahydroxy analog of Butazolidin®, brand of phenylbutazone USP.

It has anti-inflammatory and antipyretic action as well as analgesic and mild uricosuric properties resulting in symptomatic relief only. **The disease process itself is unaltered by this drug.**

Clinical Pharmacology: In man, oxyphenbutazone is completely absorbed after oral administration of Tandearil. After ingestion of three 100-mg tablets, peak plasma concentration of oxyphenbutazone has been measured at 34.9 ($\pm$ 5.3) mg/l within six hours. After therapeutic doses, about 98 percent of the drug is bound to human serum albumin. Elimination is mainly by biotransformation in the liver, and the plasma half-life has been measured as 72 ($\pm$ 15 hours). Urinary excretion consists mostly of metabolites.

Indications: The indications for Tandearil are:
Acute Gouty Arthritis
Active Rheumatoid Arthritis
Active Ankylosing Spondylitis
Short-term treatment of acute attacks of degenerative joint disease of the hips and knees not responsive to other treatment.
Painful Shoulder (peritendinitis, capsulitis, bursitis, and acute arthritis of that joint)

Contraindications:

1. *Age:* Tandearil is contraindicated in children 14 years of age or younger since controlled clinical trials in patients of this age group have not been conducted.
2. *Other Medical Conditions:* Tandearil is contraindicated in patients with incipient cardiac failure, blood dyscrasias, pancreatitis, parotitis, stomatitis, polymyalgia rheumatica, temporal arteritis, senility, drug allergy, and in the presence of severe renal, cardiac and hepatic disease, and in patients with a history of peptic ulcer disease, or symptoms of gastrointestinal inflammation or active ulceration because serious adverse reactions or aggravation of existing medical problems can occur.
3. *Concomitant Medications:* Tandearil should not be used in combination with other drugs which accentuate or share a potential for similar toxicity.
   It is also inadvisable to administer Tandearil in combination with other potent drugs because of the possibility of increased toxic reactions from Tandearil and other agents. (See also *Drug Interactions.*)
   Tandearil is contraindicated in patients with a history or suggestion of prior toxicity, sensitivity, or idiosyncrasy to phenylbutazone or oxyphenbutazone.

Warnings: Based on reports of clinical experience with oxyphenbutazone and related compounds, the following warnings should be considered by the physician prior to prescribing the drug:

1. *Gastrointestinal:* Upper G.I. diagnostic tests should be performed in patients with persistent or severe dyspepsia. Peptic ulceration, reactivation of latent peptic ulcer, perforation and gastrointestinal bleeding, sometimes severe, have been reported.
2. *Hematologic: Frequent and regular hematologic evaluations should be performed on patients receiving the drug for periods over one week.* Any significant change in the total white count, relative decrease in granulocytes, appearance of immature forms, or fall in hematocrit should be a signal for immediate cessation of therapy and a complete hematologic investigation. Serious, sometimes fatal blood dyscrasias, including aplastic anemia have been reported to occur. Hematologic toxicity may occur suddenly or many days or weeks after cessation of treatment as manifest by the appearance of anemia, leukopenia, thrombocytopenia or clinically significant hemorrhagic diathesis. There have been published reports associating oxyphenbutazone with leukemia. However, the circumstances involved in these reports are such that a cause-and-effect relationship to the drug has not been clearly established.
3. *Pregnancy:* Reproductive studies in animals, although inconclusive, exhibited evidence of possible embryotoxicity. It is, therefore, recommended that this drug should be used with caution during pregnancy. The benefits should be weighed against the potential risk to the fetus.
4. *Nursing Mothers:* Caution is also advised in prescribing Tandearil in nursing mothers since the drug may appear in cord blood and breast milk.
5. Patients reporting visual disturbances while receiving the drug should discontinue treatment and have an ophthalmologic examination because ophthalmologic adverse reactions have been reported (see **Adverse Reactions:** *Special Senses*).
6. In the aging (forty years and over), there appears to be an increase in the possibility of adverse reactions. Tandearil should be used with commensurately greater care in the elderly and should be avoided altogether in the senile patient.
7. Like other drugs with prostaglandin synthetase inhibition activity. Tandearil may precipitate acute episodes of asthmatic attacks in patients with asthma.
8. Tandearil increases sodium retention. Evidence of fluid retention in patients in whom there is danger of cardiac decompensation is an indication to discontinue the drug.

Precautions: Because of potential serious adverse reactions to Tandearil, the following precautions should be observed in the use of the drug:

—A careful diagnostic physical examination and history should be performed on all patients at regular intervals while the patient is receiving the drug.
—Tandearil is not recommended for chronic use in the elderly.
—Hematologic evaluation should be performed at frequent and regular intervals and additional laboratory examinations performed as indicated.
—Patients should be instructed to report immediately the occurrence of high fever, severe sore throat, stomatitis, salivary gland enlargement, tarry stools, unusual bleeding or bruising, sudden weight gain, or edema.
—The drug reduces iodine uptake by the thyroid and may interfere with laboratory tests of thyroid function (see **Adverse Reactions:** *Endocrine-Metabolic*).
—The patient should be cautioned regarding participation in activities requiring alertness and coordination, and that the concomitant ingestion of alcohol with Tandearil may further impair psychomotor skills.

Drug Interactions: Tandearil is highly bound to serum proteins. If its affinity for protein binding is higher than other concurrently administered drugs, the actions and toxicity of the other drug may be increased.

Tandearil accentuates the prothrombin depression produced by coumarin-type anticoagulants. When administered alone, it does not affect prothrombin activity.

The pharmacologic action of insulin, antidiabetic, and sulfonamide drugs may be potentiated by the simultaneous administration of Tandearil.

Concomitant administration of oxyphenbutazone and phenytoin may result in increased serum levels of phenytoin which could lead to increased phenytoin toxicity.

Adverse Reactions: Based upon reports of clinical experience with oxyphenbutazone and related compounds, the following adverse reactions have been reported.

The adverse reactions listed in the following table have been arranged into three groups: (1) incidence greater than 1%, (2) incidence less than 1% and (3) causal relationship unknown. The incidence for group (1) was obtained from fifty-seven (57) clinical trials reported in the literature (3713 patients). The incidence for group (2) was based on reports in clinical trials, in the literature, and on voluntary reports since marketing. The reactions in group (3) have been reported but occurred under circumstances where a causal relationship could not be established. In some patients the reported reactions may have been unrelated to the administration of Tandearil. However, in these reported events, the possibility cannot be excluded. Therefore these observations are being listed to serve as alerting information to physicians. Before prescribing this drug for an individual patient, the physician should be familiar with the following:

(1) Incidence greater than 1%	(2) Incidence less than 1%
GASTROINTESTINAL (*See* **Warnings**)	
gastrointestinal upset	nausea
	dyspepsia/including indigestion and heartburn
	abdominal and epigastric distress
	vomiting
	abdominal distention with flatulence
	constipation
	diarrhea
	esophagitis
	gastritis
	salivary gland enlargement
	stomatitis, sometimes with ulceration
	ulceration and perforation of the intestinal tract including acute and reactivated peptic ulcer with perforation, hemorrhage and hematemesis
	anemia due to gastrointestinal bleeding which may be occult
	hepatitis, both fatal and nonfatal, sometimes associated with evidence of cholestasis
HEMATOLOGICAL (*See* **Warnings**)	
None	anemia
	leukopenia
	thrombocytopenia with associated purpura, petechiae, and hemorrhage
	pancytopenia
	aplastic anemia
	bone marrow depression
	agranulocytosis and agranulocytic anginal syndrome
	hemolytic anemia
HYPERSENSITIVITY	
None	urticaria
	anaphylactic shock
	arthralgia, drug fever
	hypersensitivity angiitis (polyarteritis) and vasculitis
	Lyell's syndrome
	serum sickness
	Stevens-Johnson syndrome
	activation of systemic lupus erythematosus
	aggravation of temporal arteritis in patients with polymyalgia rheumatica
DERMATOLOGIC	
None	pruritus
	drug rashes
	erythema nodosum
	erythema multiforme
	nonthrombocytopenic purpura
CARDIOVASCULAR, FLUID AND ELECTROLYTE	
None	sodium and chloride retention
	fluid retention and plasma dilution
	cardiac decompensation (congestive heart failure) with edema and dyspnea
	metabolic acidosis
	respiratory alkalosis
	hypertension
	pericarditis
	interstitial myocarditis with muscle necrosis and perivascular granulomata
RENAL	
None	hematuria
	proteinuria
	ureteral obstruction with uric acid crystals
	anuria
	glomerulonephritis
	acute tubular necrosis
	cortical necrosis
	renal stones
	nephrotic syndrome
	impaired renal function and renal failure associated with azotemia
CENTRAL NERVOUS SYSTEM	
None	headache
	drowsiness
	agitation
	confusional states and lethargy
	tremors
	numbness
	weakness
ENDOCRINE-METABOLIC (*See* **Precautions**)	
None	None
SPECIAL SENSES (*See* **Warnings**)	
Ocular:	
None	None
Otic:	
None	hearing loss
	tinnitus

(3) Causal relationship unknown—Incidence less than 1%: *Hematological* (see **Warnings**)—Leukemia (There have been reports associating oxyphenbutazone with leukemia. However, the circumstances involved in these reports are such that a cause-and-effect relationship to the drug has not been clearly established) *Endocrine—Metabolic* (see **Precautions**)— Thyroid hyperplasia; goiters associated with hyperthyroidism and hypothyroidism; pancreatitis; hyperglycemia. *Special Senses* (see **Warnings**)—Blurred vision; optic neuritis; toxic amblyopia; scotomata; retinal detachment; retinal hemorrhage; oculomotor palsy.

Overdosage: *Signs and Symptoms:* Include any of the following: nausea, vomiting, epigastric pain, excessive perspiration, euphoria, psychosis, headaches, giddiness, vertigo, hyperventilation, insomnia, tinnitus, difficulty in hearing, edema (sodium retention), hypertension, cyanosis, respiratory depression, agitation, hallucinations, stupor, convulsions, coma, hematuria, and oliguria. Hepatomegaly, jaundice, and ulceration of the buccal or gastrointestinal mucosa have been reported as late manifestations of massive overdosage.

Reported laboratory abnormalities following overdosage include: respiratory or metabolic acidosis, impaired hepatic or renal function, and abnormalities of formed blood elements.

Treatment: In the alert patient, empty the stomach promptly by induced emesis followed by lavage. In the obtunded patient, secure the airway with a cuffed endotracheal tube before beginning lavage (do not induce emesis). Maintain adequate respiratory exchange, do not use respiratory stimulants. Treat shock with appropriate supportive measures. Control seizures with intravenous diazepam or short-acting barbiturates. Dialysis may be helpful if renal function is impaired.

Dosage and Administration: Tandearil should be used at the smallest effective dosage to afford rapid relief of severe symptoms. It is contraindicated in children under 14 years of age and in senile patients.

If a favorable symptomatic response to treatment is not obtained after one week, the drug should be discontinued. When a favorable therapeutic response has been obtained, the dosage should be reduced and then discontinued as soon as possible.

In elderly patients (sixty years and over) every effort must be made to discontinue therapy on, or as soon as possible after, the seventh day, because of the exceedingly high risk of severe fatal toxic reactions in this age group.

To minimize gastric upset, the drug should be taken with milk or with meals.

In selecting the appropriate dosage in any specific case, consideration should be given to the patient's age, weight, general health, and any other factors that may influence his response to the drug.

Rheumatoid Arthritis, Ankylosing Spondylitis, Acute Attacks of Degenerative Joint Disease, and Painful Shoulder: Initial Dosage: The initial daily dose in adult patients is 300 to 600 mg as 3 to 4 divided doses. Maximum therapeutic response is usually obtained at a total daily dose of 400 mg. A trial period of one week of therapy is considered adequate to determine the therapeutic effect of the drug. In the absence of a favorable response, therapy should be discontinued.

Maintenance Dosage: When improvement is obtained, dosage should be promptly decreased to the minimum effective level necessary to maintain relief, not exceeding 400 mg daily because of the possibility of cumulative toxicity. A satisfactory clinical response may be obtained with daily doses as low as 100 to 200 mg daily.

Acute Gouty Arthritis: Satisfactory results are obtained after an initial dose of 400 mg followed by 100 mg every 4 hours. The articular inflammation usually subsides within 4 days and treatment should not be continued longer than one week.

How Supplied:

Tandearil, oxyphenbutazone NF

Tablets—round, tan, sugar-coated	100 mg
Bottle of 100	NDC 0028-0024-01
Bottle of 1000	NDC 0028-0024-10
Unit Dose Packages—Blister-Packed	
Box of 100	NDC 0028-0024-61

Dispense in tight container (USP).

667142 C79-17(11/79)

[*Shown in Product Identification Section*]

TEGRETOL® ℞

carbamazepine USP

Tablets of 200 mg **GY-CODE 67**

WARNING
SERIOUS AND SOMETIMES FATAL ABNORMALITIES OF BLOOD CELLS (APLASTIC ANEMIA, AGRANULOCYTOSIS, THROMBOCYTOPENIA, AND LEUKOPENIA) HAVE BEEN REPORTED FOLLOWING TREATMENT WITH TEGRETOL, CARBAMAZEPINE. EARLY DETECTION OF HEMATOLOGIC CHANGE IS IMPORTANT SINCE, IN SOME PATIENTS, APLASTIC ANEMIA IS REVERSIBLE.

Continued on next page

The full prescribing information for each GEIGY drug is contained herein and is that in effect as of October 1, 1979.

Geigy—Cont.

COMPLETE PRETREATMENT BLOOD COUNTS, INCLUDING PLATELET AND POSSIBLY RETICULOCYTE AND SERUM IRON, SHOULD BE OBTAINED. ANY SIGNIFICANT ABNORMALITIES SHOULD RULE OUT USE OF THE DRUG. THESE SAME TESTS SHOULD BE REPEATED AT FREQUENT INTERVALS, POSSIBLY WEEKLY DURING THE FIRST THREE MONTHS OF THERAPY AND MONTHLY THEREAFTER FOR AT LEAST TWO TO THREE YEARS. THE DRUG SHOULD BE STOPPED IF ANY EVIDENCE OF BONE MARROW DEPRESSION DEVELOPS. PATIENTS SHOULD BE MADE AWARE OF THE EARLY TOXIC SIGNS AND SYMPTOMS OF A POTENTIAL HEMATOLOGIC PROBLEM, SUCH AS FEVER, SORE THROAT, ULCERS IN THE MOUTH, EASY BRUISING, PETECHIAL OR PURPURIC HEMORRHAGE, AND SHOULD BE ADVISED TO DISCONTINUE THE DRUG AND TO REPORT TO THE PHYSICIAN IMMEDIATELY IF ANY SUCH SIGNS OR SYMPTOMS APPEAR.

This drug is not a simple analgesic and should not be used for the relief of trivial aches or pains. Treatment of epilepsy should be restricted to those classifications listed under "Indications."

Before prescribing Tegretol, the physician should be thoroughly familiar with the details of this prescribing information, particularly regarding use with other drugs, especially those which accentuate toxicity potential.

Description: Tegretol is an iminostilbene derivative, 5H-dibenz [b,f] azepine-5-carboxamide.

It is a white, crystalline substance which is insoluble in water but soluble in propylene glycol. It melts within a range of no more than 3°C between 187°–193°C. Its molecular weight is 236.26.

Actions: Tegretol has demonstrated anticonvulsant properties in rats and mice with convulsions induced by electrical and chemical methods.

Early animal screening tests demonstrated that Tegretol depressed the linguomandibular reflexes in cats. Pain induced by stimulation of the infraorbital nerve of cats and rats was greatly reduced or abolished. Tegretol, brand of carbamazepine, is chemically unrelated to other anticonvulsants or other agents used to control the severe pain of trigeminal neuralgia. Its mechanism of action is obscure.

Monitoring of blood levels has increased the efficacy and safety of anticonvulsants. Plasma levels of Tegretol are variable and may range from 0.5–25 mcg/ml with no apparent relationship to the daily intake of the drug. Therapeutic levels in the adult range should be between 4–12 mcg/ml. Because Tegretol may induce its own metabolism, the half-life is also variable. Initial half-life values have been reported to range from 25–65 hours, with 12–17 hours on repeated doses. Tegretol is metabolized in the liver. In oral studies with ^{14}C-carbamazepine, 72% of the administered radioactivity was found in the urine and 28% in the feces.

Indications: *Epilepsy:* Tegretol is indicated for the following conditions in patients who have not responded satisfactorily to treatment with other agents such as phenytoin, phenobarbital, and/or primidone:

1. Partial seizures with complex symptomatology (psychomotor, temporal lobe). Patients with these seizures appear to show greater improvement than those with other types.
2. Generalized tonic-clonic seizures (grand mal).
3. Mixed seizure patterns which include the above, or other partial or generalized seizures.

Absence seizures (petit mal) do not appear to be controlled by Tegretol.

Because of the necessity for frequent laboratory evaluation for potentially serious side effects, Tegretol is not recommended as the drug of first choice in seizure disorders. It should be reserved for patients whose seizures are difficult to control and/or patients experiencing marked side effects (e.g., excessive sedation).

Trigeminal Neuralgia: Tegretol is indicated in the treatment of the pain associated with true trigeminal neuralgia.

Beneficial results have also been reported in glossopharyngeal neuralgia.

Contraindications: Tegretol should not be used in patients with a history of previous bone marrow depression and/or hypersensitivity to the drug, or in patients with a known sensitivity to any of the tricyclic compounds, such as amitriptyline, desipramine, imipramine, protriptyline, nortriptyline, etc. Likewise, on theoretical grounds its use with monoamine oxidase inhibitors is not recommended. When administering Tegretol to patients receiving MAO inhibitors, the MAO inhibitors should be discontinued and as long a drug-free interval should elapse as the clinical situation permits with a minimum of fourteen days.

Warnings: The drug should be discontinued if evidence of significant bone marrow depression occurs. In general, Tegretol should be discontinued if a patient sustains evidence of marrow suppression as follows:

1) Erythrocytes	less than 4.0 m/cmm
Hematocrit	less than 32%
Hemoglobin	less than 11 gm%
2) Leukocytes	less than 4000/cmm
3) Platelets	less than 100,000/cmm
4) Reticulocytes	less than 0.3% (20,000/cmm)
5) Serum iron	greater than 150 μgm%

Patients with a history of adverse hematologic reaction to any drug may be particularly at risk.

Usage in Pregnancy: The effects of Tegretol in human pregnancy and nursing infants are unknown. Breakthrough bleeding has been reported among patients receiving concomitant oral contraceptives and their reliability may be adversely affected.

Recent reports suggest an association between the use of anticonvulsant drugs by women with epilepsy and an elevated incidence of birth defects in children born to these women. Data are more extensive with respect to diphenylhydantoin and phenobarbital, but these are also the most commonly prescribed anticonvulsants; less systematic or anecdotal reports suggest a possible similar association with the use of all known anticonvulsant drugs.

The reports suggesting an elevated incidence of birth defects in children of drug-treated epileptic women cannot be regarded as adequate to prove a definite cause-and-effect relationship. There are intrinsic methodologic problems in obtaining adequate data on drug teratogenicity in humans; the possibility also exists that other factors, e.g., genetic factors or the epileptic condition itself, may be more important than drug therapy in leading to birth defects. The great majority of mothers on anticonvulsant medication deliver normal infants. It is important to note that anticonvulsant drugs should not be discontinued in patients in whom the drug is administered to prevent major seizures because of the strong possibility of precipitating status epilepticus with attendant hypoxia and threat to life. In individual cases where the severity and frequency of the seizure disorder are such that the removal of medication does not pose a serious threat to the patient, discontinuation of the drug may be considered prior to and during pregnancy, although it cannot be said with any confidence that even minor seizures do not pose some hazard to the developing embryo or fetus.

Adverse effects have been observed in reproduction studies in animals given Tegretol orally. In rat teratology studies, 2 of 135 offspring showed kinked ribs at 250 mg/kg and 4 of 119 offspring at 650 mg/kg showed other anomalies [cleft palate (1), talipes (1), anophthalmos (2)]. In reproduction studies, nursing rats demonstrated a lack of weight gain and an unkempt appearance at a maternal dosage level of 200 mg/kg.

The prescribing physician will wish to weigh these considerations in treating or counseling epileptic women of childbearing potential.

Use of Tegretol in women of childbearing potential should be considered only when the clinical situation warrants the risk. It is inadvisable for mothers taking Tegretol to nurse.

Tegretol has shown mild anticholinergic activity; therefore, patients with increased intraocular pressure should be closely observed during therapy.

Because of the relationship of the drug to other tricyclic compounds, the possibility of activation of a latent psychosis and, in elderly patients, of confusion or agitation should be borne in mind.

Since dizziness and drowsiness may occur, patients should be cautioned about the hazards of operating machinery or automobiles or engaging in other potentially dangerous tasks.

Precautions: Before initiating therapy, the following procedures are recommended:

Detailed history and physical examination.

Therapy should be prescribed only after critical benefit-to-risk appraisal in patients with a history of cardiac, hepatic or renal damage, history of adverse hematologic reaction to other drugs or who have had interrupted courses of therapy with Tegretol.

Complete pretreatment blood counts, including platelet and possibly reticulocyte and serum iron, should be obtained. Any significant abnormalities should rule out use of the drug.

These same tests should be repeated at frequent intervals, possibly weekly, during the first three months of therapy and monthly thereafter for at least two to three years.

Baseline evaluations of liver function, particularly in patients with a history of liver disease. Liver function tests must be performed at regular intervals during treatment with this drug since liver damage may occur. The drug should be discontinued immediately in cases of aggravated liver dysfunction or active liver disease.

Baseline and periodic eye examinations, including slit-lamp, funduscopy and tonometry. These are recommended for patients being treated with this drug since many phenothiazines and related drugs have been shown to cause eye changes.

Baseline and periodic complete urinalysis and BUN determinations. These are recommended for patients treated with this agent because of observed renal dysfunction.

Carcinogenesis and Mutagenesis. Carbamazepine, when administered to Sprague-Dawley rats for two years in the diet at doses of 25, 75, and 250 mg/kg/day, resulted in a dose-related increase in the incidence of hepatocellular tumors in females and in benign interstitial cell adenomas in the testes of males. Carbamazepine must, therefore, be considered to be carcinogenic in Sprague-Dawley rats. Bacterial and mammalian mutagenicity studies using carbamazepine produced negative results. The significance of these findings relative to the use of carbamazepine in humans is, at present, unknown.

Adverse Reactions: If adverse reactions are of such severity that the drug must be discontinued, the physician must be aware that abrupt discontinuation of any anticonvulsant drug in a responsive epileptic patient may lead to seizures or even status epilepticus with its life-threatening hazards.

The adverse reactions most frequently observed, particularly during the initial phases of therapy, are dizziness, drowsiness, unsteadiness, nausea, and vomiting. To minimize the possibility of such reactions, therapy should be initiated at the low dosage recommended.

The following additional adverse reactions have been reported:

Hemopoietic System: Aplastic anemia, leukopenia, agranulocytosis, eosinophilia, leukocytosis, thrombocytopenia, purpura.

Hepatic: Abnormalities in liver function tests and cholestatic and hepatocellular jaundice.

Genitourinary System: Urinary frequency, acute urinary retention, oliguria with elevated blood pressure, renal failure, azotemia and impotence. Albuminuria, glycosuria, elevated BUN and microscopic deposits in the urine have also been reported. Testicular atrophy occurred in rats receiving Tegretol orally from 4 to 52 weeks at dosage levels of 50 to 400 mg/kg/day. In dogs, it produced a brownish discoloration, presumably a metabolite, in the urinary bladder at dosage levels of 50 mg/kg and higher. Relevance of these findings to humans is unknown.

Nervous System: Dizziness, drowsiness, disturbances of coordination, confusion, headache, fatigue, blurred vision, visual hallucinations, transient diplopia and oculomotor disturbances, speech disturbances, and abnormal involuntary movements, peripheral neuritis and paresthesias, depression with agitation, talkativeness, nystagmus, tinnitus, and hyperacusis.

There have been reports of associated paralysis and other symptoms of cerebral arterial insufficiency, but the exact relationship of these reactions to the drug has not been established.

Skin: Pruritic and erythematous rashes, urticaria, Stevens-Johnson syndrome, photosensitivity reactions, alterations in skin pigmentation, exfoliative dermatitis, alopecia, diaphoresis, erythema multiforme and nodosum, and aggravation of disseminated lupus erythematosus. In certain cases, discontinuation of therapy may be necessary.

Digestive System: Nausea, vomiting, gastric distress and abdominal pain, diarrhea, constipation, anorexia, and dryness of the mouth and pharynx, including glossitis and stomatitis.

Cardiovascular System: Congestive heart failure, aggravation of hypertension, hypotension, syncope and collapse, edema, primary thrombophlebitis, recurrence of thrombophlebitis, aggravation of coronary artery disease, and adenopathy or lymphadenopathy.

Some of these cardiovascular complications have resulted in fatalities. Arrhythmias and A-V block have been reported. Myocardial infarction has been associated with other tricyclic compounds.

Eyes: There have been scattered, punctate, cortical lens opacities reported, as well as conjunctivitis. Although a direct causal relationship has not been established, many phenothiazines and related drugs have been shown to cause eye changes.

Musculoskeletal: Aching joints and muscles, and leg cramps.

Metabolic: Fever and chills. Inappropriate antidiuretic hormone syndrome has been reported. Alterations of thyroid function have been reported in combination therapy with other anticonvulsant medications. Thyroid function tests have been reported to have decreased values with Tegretol alone.

Dosage and Administration: Monitoring of blood levels has increased the efficacy and safety of anticonvulsants (see Actions). Dosage should be adjusted to the needs of the individual patient. A low initial daily dosage with a gradual increase is advised. As soon as adequate control is achieved, the dosage may be reduced very gradually to the minimum effective level.

Epilepsy (see **Indications**):

Adults and children over 12 years of age—Initial: One tablet (200 mg) b.i.d. on the first day. Increase gradually by adding up to 200 mg per day using a t.i.d. or q.i.d. regimen until the best response is obtained. Dosage should generally not exceed 1000 mg daily in children 12 to 15 years of age, and 1200 mg daily in patients above 15 years of age. Doses up to 1600 mg daily have been used in adults in rare instances.

Maintenance: Adjust dosage to the minimum effective level, usually 4–6 tablets (800–1200 mg) daily.

Children 6–12 years of age—Initial: One-half tablet (100 mg) b.i.d. on the first day. Increase gradually by adding 100 mg per day using a t.i.d. or q.i.d. regimen until the best response is obtained. Dosage should generally not exceed 1000 mg.

Maintenance: Adjust dosage to the minimum effective level, usually 2–4 tablets (400–800 mg) daily.

Combination Therapy: Tegretol may be used alone or with other anticonvulsants. When added to existing anticonvulsant therapy, the drug should be added gradually while the other anticonvulsants are maintained or gradually decreased.

Trigeminal Neuralgia (see **Indications**):

Initial: One-half tablet (100 mg) b.i.d. on the first day for a total daily dose of 200 mg. This daily dose may be increased by up to 200 mg a day using increments of one-half tablet every 12 hours only as needed to achieve freedom from pain. Do not exceed 1200 mg daily. Tablets should be taken with meals.

Maintenance: Control of pain can be maintained in most patients with 400 mg to 800 mg daily. However, some cases may be maintained on as little as 200 mg daily, while others may require as much as 1200 mg daily. At least once every 3 months throughout the treatment period, attempts should be made to reduce the dose to the minimum effective level or even to discontinue the drug.

Overdosage: *Symptoms and Treatment:* These include dizziness, ataxia, drowsiness, stupor, nausea, vomiting; restlessness, agitation, disorientation, tremor, involuntary movements, opisthotonus, abnormal reflexes (slowed or hyperactive); mydriasis, nystagmus; flushing, cyanosis; urinary retention. Hypotension or hypertension may develop. Coma may ensue.

Laboratory findings in isolated instances of overdosage have included leukocytosis, reduced leukocyte count, glycosuria and acetonuria. EEG may show dysrhythmias.

Treatment: Experience with cases of accidental overdosage is limited. However, since the drug is related to the tricyclic antidepressants, the treatment recommendations suggested for overdosage with Tofranil®, imipramine hydrochloride, may be helpful.

There is no specific antidote. Induced emesis and gastric lavage are recommended. Vital signs should be watched and symptomatic treatment administered. Parenteral barbiturates may be employed to treat hyperirritability. However, barbiturates should not be used if drugs that inhibit monoamine oxidase have also been taken by the patient either in overdosage or in recent therapy (within one week). Barbiturates may induce respiratory depression, particularly in children. It is therefore advisable to have equipment available for artificial ventilation and resuscitation when barbiturates are employed.

Paraldehyde may be used in children to counteract muscular hypertonus without producing respiratory depression.

Shock (circulatory collapse) should be treated with supportive measures such as intravenous fluids, oxygen and corticosteroids.

Because of the relationship of Tegretol to the tricyclic antidepressants, it is recommended that the EKG be monitored, particularly in children, to detect any cardiac arrhythmias or conduction defects.

Treatment of Blood Count Abnormalities: If evidence of bone marrow depression develops, the following recommendations are suggested: (1) stop the drug, (2) perform daily CBC, platelet and reticulocyte counts, (3) do a bone marrow aspiration and trephine biopsy immediately and repeat with sufficient frequency to monitor recovery.

Special periodic studies might be helpful as follows: (1) white cell and platelet antibodies, (2) 59Fe—ferrokinetic studies, (3) peripheral blood cell typing, (4) cytogenetic studies on marrow and peripheral blood, (5) bone marrow culture studies for colony-forming units, (6) hemoglobin electrophoresis for A_2 and F hemoglobin, and (7) serum folic acid and B_{12} levels. A fully developed aplastic anemia will require appropriate, intensive monitoring and therapy, for which specialized consultation should be sought.

How Supplied: Round, white, single-scored tablets of 200 mg in bottles of 100 and 1000, and Unit Dose Packages of 100.

Dispense in tight container (USP).

667104 (7/79) C79-19

[*Shown in Product Identification Section*]

TOFRANIL® ℞

imipramine hydrochloride USP

Tablets of 10 mg GY-CODE 21
Tablets of 25 mg GY-CODE 11
Tablets of 50 mg GY-CODE 74
For oral administration
Ampuls, 2 cc
For intramuscular administration

Each 2 cc ampul contains: imipramine hydrochloride USP, 25 mg; ascorbic acid, 2 mg; sodium bisulfite, 1 mg; sodium sulfite, anhydrous, 1 mg

Description: Tofranil, the original tricyclic antidepressant, is a member of the dibenzazepine group of compounds. It is designated 5-[3-(Dimethylamino)propyl] - 10, 11 - dihydro - 5H-dibenz[b,f]azepine Monohydrochloride. Its molecular weight is 316.9 and its empirical formula is $C_{19}H_{25}N_2Cl$.

Tofranil is a white, crystalline substance that turns yellowish or reddish on long exposure to light. It is easily soluble in water, fairly soluble in acetone or alcohol, but almost insoluble in ether. It melts at 170–174° C.

Clinical Pharmacology: The mechanism of action of Tofranil is not definitely known. However, it does not act primarily by stimulation of the central nervous system. The clinical effect is hypothesized as being due to potentiation of adrenergic synapses by blocking uptake of norepinephrine at nerve endings. The mode of action of the drug in controlling childhood enuresis is thought to be apart from its antidepressant effect.

Indications: *Depression:* For the relief of symptoms of depression. Endogenous depression is more likely to be alleviated than other depressive states. One to three weeks of treatment may be needed before optimal therapeutic effects are evident.

Childhood Enuresis: May be useful as temporary adjunctive therapy in reducing enuresis in children aged 6 years and older, after possible organic causes have been excluded by appropriate tests. In patients having daytime symptoms of frequency and urgency, examination should include voiding cystourethrography and cystoscopy, as necessary. The effectiveness of treatment may decrease with continued drug administration.

Continued on next page

The full prescribing information for each GEIGY drug is contained herein and is that in effect as of October 1, 1979.

Geigy—Cont.

Contraindications: The concomitant use of monoamine oxidase inhibiting compounds is contraindicated. Hyperpyretic crises or severe convulsive seizures may occur in patients receiving such combinations. The potentiation of adverse effects can be serious, or even fatal. When it is desired to substitute Tofranil in patients receiving a monoamine oxidase inhibitor, as long an interval should elapse as the clinical situation will allow, with a minimum of 14 days. Initial dosage should be low and increases should be gradual and cautiously prescribed.
The drug is contraindicated during the acute recovery period after a myocardial infarction. Patients with a known hypersensitivity to this compound should not be given the drug. The possibility of cross-sensitivity to other dibenzazepine compounds should be kept in mind.
Warnings:
Children: A dose of 2.5 mg/kg/day of imipramine hydrochloride should not be exceeded in childhood. ECG changes of unknown significance have been reported in pediatric patients with doses twice this amount.
Extreme caution should be used when this drug is given to:
patients with cardiovascular disease because of the possibility of conduction defects, arrhythmias, congestive heart failure, myocardial infarction, strokes and tachycardia. These patients require cardiac surveillance at all dosage levels of the drug;
patients with increased intraocular pressure, history of urinary retention, or history of narrow-angle glaucoma because of the drug's anticholinergic properties;
hyperthyroid patients or those on thyroid medication because of the possibility of cardiovascular toxicity;
patients with a history of seizure disorder because this drug has been shown to lower the seizure threshold;
patients receiving guanethidine, clonidine, or similar agents, since imipramine hydrochloride may block the pharmacologic effects of these drugs;
patients receiving methylphenidate hydrochloride. Since methylphenidate hydrochloride may inhibit the metabolism of imipramine hydrochloride, downward dosage adjustment of imipramine hydrochloride may be required when given concomitantly with methylphenidate hydrochloride.
Tofranil may enhance the CNS depressant effects of alcohol. Therefore, it should be borne in mind that the dangers inherent in a suicide attempt or accidental overdosage with the drug may be increased for the patient who uses excessive amounts of alcohol. (See **Precautions.**)
Since imipramine hydrochloride may impair the mental and/or physical abilities required for the performance of potentially hazardous tasks, such as operating an automobile or machinery, the patient should be cautioned accordingly.
Precautions: An ECG recording should be taken prior to the initiation of larger-than-usual doses of imipramine hydrochloride and at appropriate intervals thereafter until steady state is achieved. (Patients with any evidence of cardiovascular disease require cardiac surveillance at all dosage levels of the drug. See **Warnings.**) Elderly patients and patients with cardiac disease or a prior history of cardiac disease are at special risk of developing the cardiac abnormalities associated with the use of imipramine hydrochloride.
It should be kept in mind that the possibility of suicide in seriously depressed patients is inherent in the illness and may persist until significant remission occurs. Such patients should be carefully supervised during the early phase of treatment with imipramine hydrochloride, and may require hospitalization. Prescriptions should be written for the smallest amount feasible.
Hypomanic or manic episodes may occur, particularly in patients with cyclic disorders. Such reactions may necessitate discontinuation of the drug. If needed, imipramine hydrochloride may be resumed in lower dosage when these episodes are relieved. Administration of a tranquilizer may be useful in controlling such episodes.
An activation of the psychosis may occasionally be observed in schizophrenic patients and may require reduction of dosage and the addition of a phenothiazine.
Concurrent administration of imipramine hydrochloride with electroshock therapy may increase the hazards; such treatment should be limited to those patients for whom it is essential, since there is limited clinical experience.
Usage During Pregnancy and Lactation:
Animal reproduction studies have yielded inconclusive results. (See also **Animal Pharmacology & Toxicology.**)
There have been no well-controlled studies conducted with pregnant women to determine the effect of imipramine hydrochloride on the fetus. However, there have been clinical reports of congenital malformations associated with the use of the drug. Although a causal relationship between these effects and the drug could not be established, the possibility of fetal risk from the maternal ingestion of imipramine hydrochloride cannot be excluded. Therefore, imipramine hydrochloride should be used in women who are or might become pregnant only if the clinical condition clearly justifies potential risk to the fetus.
Limited data suggest that imipramine hydrochloride is likely to be excreted in human breast milk. As a general rule, a women taking a drug should not nurse since the possibility exists that the drug may be excreted in breast milk and be harmful to the child.
Usage in Children: The effectiveness of the drug in children for conditions other than nocturnal enuresis has not been established.
The safety and effectiveness of the drug as temporary adjunctive therapy for nocturnal enuresis in children less than 6 years of age has not been established.
The safety of the drug for long-term, chronic use as adjunctive therapy for nocturnal enuresis in children 6 years of age or older has not been established; consideration should be given to instituting a drug-free period following an adequate therapeutic trial with a favorable response.
A dose of 2.5 mg/kg/day should not be exceeded in childhood. ECG changes of unknown significance have been reported in pediatric patients with doses twice this amount.
Patients should be warned that imipramine hydrochloride may enhance the CNS depressant effects of alcohol. (See **Warnings.**)
Imipramine hydrochloride should be used with caution in patients with significantly impaired renal or hepatic function.
Patients who develop a fever and a sore throat during therapy with imipramine hydrochloride should have leukocyte and differential blood counts performed. Imipramine hydrochloride should be discontinued if there is evidence of pathological neutrophil depression.
Prior to elective surgery, imipramine hydrochloride should be discontinued for as long as the clinical situation will allow.
In occasional susceptible patients or in those receiving anticholinergic drugs (including antiparkinsonism agents) in addition, the atropine-like effects may become more pronounced (e.g., paralytic ileus). Close supervision and careful adjustment of dosage is required when imipramine hydrochloride is administered concomitantly with anticholinergic drugs.
Avoid the use of preparations, such as decongestants and local anesthetics, which contain any sympathomimetic amine (e.g., epinephrine, norepinephrine), since it has been reported that tricyclic antidepressants can potentiate the effects of catecholamines.
Caution should be exercised when imipramine hydrochloride is used with agents that lower blood pressure.
Imipramine hydrochloride may potentiate the effects of CNS depressant drugs.
Patients taking imipramine hydrochloride should avoid excessive exposure to sunlight since there have been reports of photosensitization.
Both elevation and lowering of blood sugar levels have been reported with imipramine hydrochloride use.
The Tofranil tablets (10, 25, 50 mg) contain FD&C Yellow No. 5 (tartrazine) which may cause allergic-type reactions (including bronchial asthma) in certain susceptible individuals. Although the overall incidence of FD&C Yellow No. 5 (tartrazine) sensitivity in the general population is low, it is frequently seen in patients who also have aspirin hypersensitivity.
Adverse Reactions: Note: Although the listing which follows includes a few adverse reactions which have not been reported with this specific drug, the pharmacological similarities among the tricyclic antidepressant drugs require that each of the reactions be considered when imipramine is administered.
Cardiovascular: Orthostatic hypotension, hypertension, tachycardia, palpitation, myocardial infarction, arrhythmias, heart block, ECG changes, precipitation of congestive heart failure, stroke.
Psychiatric: Confusional states (especially in the elderly) with hallucinations, disorientation, delusions; anxiety, restlessness, agitation; insomnia and nightmares; hypomania; exacerbation of psychosis.
Neurological: Numbness, tingling, paresthesias of extremities; incoordination, ataxia, tremors; peripheral neuropathy; extrapyramidal symptoms; seizures, alterations in EEG patterns; tinnitus.
Anticholinergic: Dry mouth, and, rarely, associated sublingual adenitis; blurred vision, disturbances of accommodation, mydriasis; constipation, paralytic ileus; urinary retention, delayed micturition, dilation of the urinary tract.
Allergic: Skin rash, petechiae, urticaria, itching, photosensitization; edema (general or of face and tongue); drug fever; cross-sensitivity with desipramine.
Hematologic: Bone marrow depression including agranulocytosis; eosinophilia; purpura; thrombocytopenia.
Gastrointestinal: Nausea and vomiting, anorexia, epigastric distress, diarrhea; peculiar taste, stomatitis, abdominal cramps, black tongue.
Endocrine: Gynecomastia in the male; breast enlargement and galactorrhea in the female; increased or decreased libido, impotence; testicular swelling; elevation or depression of blood sugar levels.
Other: Jaundice (simulating obstructive); altered liver function; weight gain or loss; perspiration; flushing; urinary frequency; drowsiness; dizziness, weakness and fatigue; headache; parotid swelling; alopecia; proneness to falling.
Withdrawal Symptoms: Though not indicative of addiction, abrupt cessation of treatment after prolonged therapy may produce nausea, headache and malaise.
Note: In enuretic children treated with Tofranil the most common adverse reactions have been nervousness, sleep disorders, tiredness, and mild gastrointestinal disturbances. These usually disappear during continued drug administration or when dosage is decreased. Other reactions which have been re-

ported include constipation, convulsions, anxiety, emotional instability, syncope, and collapse. All of the adverse effects reported with adult use should be considered.

Dosage and Administration:

Depression: Lower dosages are recommended for elderly patients and adolescents. Lower dosages are also recommended for outpatients as compared to hospitalized patients who will be under close supervision. Dosage should be initiated at a low level and increased gradually, noting carefully the clinical response and any evidence of intolerance. Following remission, maintenance medication may be required for a longer period of time, at the lowest dose that will maintain remission.

Parenteral administration should be used only for starting therapy in patients unable or unwilling to use oral medication. The oral form should supplant the injectable as soon as possible.

Oral:—Usual Adult Dose: Hospitalized patients—Initially, 100 mg/day in divided doses gradually increased to 200 mg/day as required. If no response after two weeks, increase to 250-300 mg/day.

Outpatients—Initially, 75 mg/day increased to 150 mg/day. Dosages over 200 mg/day are not recommended. Maintenance, 50-150 mg/day.

Adolescent and geriatric patients—Initially, 30–40 mg/day; it is generally not necessary to exceed 100 mg/day.

Parenteral: Initially, up to 100 mg/day intramuscularly in divided doses.

Childhood Enuresis: Initially, an oral dose of 25 mg/day should be tried in children aged 6 and older. Medication should be given one hour before bedtime. If a satisfactory response does not occur within one week, increase the dose to 50 mg nightly in children under 12 years; children over 12 may receive up to 75 mg nightly. A daily dose greater than 75 mg does not enhance efficacy and tends to increase side effects. Evidence suggests that in early night bedwetters, the drug is more effective given earlier and in divided amounts, i.e., 25 mg in midafternoon, repeated at bedtime. Consideration should be given to instituting a drug-free period following an adequate therapeutic trial with a favorable response. Dosage should be tapered off gradually rather than abruptly discontinued; this may reduce the tendency to relapse. Children who relapse when the drug is discontinued do not always respond to a subsequent course of treatment.

A dose of 2.5 mg/kg/day should not be exceeded. ECG changes of unknown significance have been reported in pediatric patients with doses twice this amount.

The safety and effectiveness of Tofranil as temporary adjunctive therapy for nocturnal enuresis in children less than 6 years of age has not been established.

Overdosage: Children have been reported to be more sensitive than adults to an acute overdosage of imipramine hydrochloride. An acute overdose of any amount in infants or young children, especially, must be considered serious and potentially fatal.

Signs and Symptoms: These may vary in severity depending upon factors such as the amount of drug absorbed, the age of the patient, and the interval between drug ingestion and the start of treatment. Blood and urine levels of imipramine may not reflect the severity of poisoning; they have chiefly a qualitative rather than quantitative value, and are unreliable indicators in the clinical management of the patient.

CNS abnormalities may include drowsiness, stupor, coma, ataxia, restlessness, agitation, hyperactive reflexes, muscle rigidity, athetoid and choreiform movements, and convulsions. Cardiac abnormalities may include arrhythmia, tachycardia, ECG evidence of impaired conduction, and signs of congestive failure. Respiratory depression, cyanosis, hypotension, shock, vomiting, hyperpyrexia, mydriasis, and diaphoresis may also be present.

Treatment: Because CNS involvement, respiratory depression and cardiac arrhythmia can occur suddenly, hospitalization and close observation are necessary, even when the amount ingested is thought to be small or the initial degree of intoxication appears slight or moderate. All patients with ECG abnormalities should have continuous cardiac monitoring for at least 72 hours and be closely observed until well after cardiac status has returned to normal; relapses may occur after apparent recovery.

The *slow* intravenous administration of physostigmine salicylate has been reported to reverse most of the cardiovascular and CNS effects of overdosage with tricyclic antidepressants. In adults, 1 to 3 mg has been reported to be effective. In children, start with 0.5 mg and repeat at 5-minute intervals to determine the minimum effective dose; do not exceed 2 mg. Because of the short duration of action of physostigmine, repeat the effective dose at 30- to 60-minute intervals, as necessary. Avoid rapid injection to reduce the possibility of physostigmine-induced convulsions.

In the alert patient, empty the stomach promptly by induced emesis followed by lavage. In the obtunded patient, secure the airway with a cuffed endotracheal tube before beginning lavage (do not induce emesis). Continue lavage for 24 hours or longer, depending on the apparent severity of intoxication. Use normal or half-normal saline to avoid water intoxication, especially in children. Instillation of activated charcoal slurry may help reduce absorption of imipramine.

Minimize external stimulation to reduce the tendency to convulsions. If anticonvulsants are necessary, diazepam, short-acting barbiturates, paraldehyde or methocarbamol may be useful. Do not use barbiturates if MAO inhibitors have been taken recently.

Maintain adequate respiratory exchange. Do not use respiratory stimulants.

Shock should be treated with supportive measures, such as intravenous fluids, oxygen and corticosteroids. Digitalis may increase conduction abnormalities and further irritate an already sensitized myocardium. If congestive heart failure necessitates rapid digitalization, particular care must be exercised.

Hyperpyrexia should be controlled by whatever external means are available, including ice packs and cooling sponge baths, if necessary.

Hemodialysis, peritoneal dialysis, exchange transfusions and forced diuresis have been generally reported as ineffective because of the rapid fixation of imipramine in tissues. Blood and urine levels of imipramine may not correlate with the degree of intoxication, and are unreliable indicators in the clinical management of the patient.

How Supplied: Triangular, sugar-coated, coral-colored tablets of 10 mg in bottles of 100 and 1000; round, sugar-coated, coral-colored (black Geigy imprint) tablets of 25 mg in bottles of 100, 1000 and 5000 and unit strip packages of 100; round, sugar-coated, coral-colored (white Geigy imprint) tablets of 50 mg in bottles of 100, 1000 and 5000 and unit strip packages of 100; ampuls for intramuscular administration only, each containing 25 mg in 2 cc of solution (1.25%), in boxes of 10.

Note: On storage, very minute crystals may form in some ampuls. This has no influence on the therapeutic efficacy of the preparation, and the crystals redissolve when the affected ampuls are immersed in hot tap water for one minute.

Animal Pharmacology & Toxicology:

A. *Acute:* Oral LD_{50} ranges are as follows:

Rat	355 to 682 mg/kg
Dog	100 to 215 mg/kg

Depending on the dosage in both species, toxic signs proceeded progressively from depression, irregular respiration and ataxia to convulsions and death.

B. *Reproduction/Teratogenic:* The overall evaluation may be summed up in the following manner:

Oral: Independent studies in three species (rat, mouse and rabbit) revealed that when Tofranil is administered orally in doses up to approximately 2½ times the maximum human dose in the first 2 species and up to 25 times the maximum human dose in the third species, the drug is essentially free from teratogenic potential. In the three species studied, only one instance of fetal abnormality occurred (in the rabbit) and in that study there was likewise an abnormality in the control group. However, evidence does exist from the rat studies that some systemic and embryotoxic potential is demonstrable. This is manifested by reduced litter size, a slight increase in the stillborn rate and a reduction in the mean birth weight.

Parenteral: In contradistinction to the oral data, Tofranil does exhibit a slight but definite teratogenic potential when administered by the subcutaneous route. Drug effects on both the mother and fetus in the rabbit are manifested in higher resorption rates and decrease in mean fetal birth weights, while teratogenic findings occurred at a level of 5 times the maximum human dose. In the mouse, teratogenicity occurred at 1½ and 6½ times the maximum human dose, but no teratogenic effects were seen at levels 3 times the maximum human dose. Thus, in the mouse, the findings are equivocal.

Dispense in tight container (USP).

667223 C80-3 (1/80)

[*Shown in Product Identification Section*]

For full prescribing information on Enuresis, please refer to Tofranil®, imipramine hydrochloride USP, on page 907.

TOFRANIL-PM® ℞

imipramine pamoate

Capsules of 75 mg	**GY-CODE 20**
Capsules of 100 mg	**GY-CODE 40**
Capsules of 125 mg	**GY-CODE 45**
Capsules of 150 mg	**GY-CODE 22**

For oral administration

Each 75-mg capsule contains imipramine pamoate equivalent to 75 mg of imipramine hydrochloride.

Continued on next page

The full prescribing information for each GEIGY drug is contained herein and is that in effect as of October 1, 1979.

Geigy—Cont.

Each 100-mg capsule contains imipramine pamoate equivalent to 100 mg of imipramine hydrochloride.
Each 125-mg capsule contains imipramine pamoate equivalent to 125 mg of imipramine hydrochloride.
Each 150-mg capsule contains imipramine pamoate equivalent to 150 mg of imipramine hydrochloride.

Description: Tofranil-PM is the pamoate salt of imipramine. It is designated bis 5-[3-(Dimethylamino)propyl] - 10, 11 - dihydro - 5H-dibenz[b,f]azepine compound (2:1) with 4,4-methylene-bis- [3-hydroxy-2-naphthoic acid] with the empirical formula $C_{61}H_{64}N_4O_6$.
Tofranil-PM is a fine, yellow, tasteless and odorless powder. It is soluble in ethyl alcohol, acetone, ethyl ether, chloroform and carbon tetrachloride. It is insoluble in water.

Clinical Pharmacology: The mechanism of action of imipramine is not definitely known. However, it does not act primarily by stimulation of the central nervous system. The clinical effect is hypothesized as being due to potentiation of adrenergic synapses by blocking uptake of norepinephrine at nerve endings.

Indications: For the relief of symptoms of depression. Endogenous depression is more likely to be alleviated than other depressive states. One to three weeks of treatment may be needed before optimal therapeutic effects are evident.

Contraindications: The concomitant use of monoamine oxidase inhibiting compounds is contraindicated. Hyperpyretic crises or severe convulsive seizures may occur in patients receiving such combinations. The potentiation of adverse effects can be serious, or even fatal. When it is desired to substitute Tofranil-PM in patients receiving a monoamine oxidase inhibitor, as long an interval should elapse as the clinical situation will allow, with a minimum of 14 days. Initial dosage should be low and increases should be gradual and cautiously prescribed.
The drug is contraindicated during the acute recovery period after a myocardial infarction. Patients with a known hypersensitivity to this compound should not be given the drug. The possibility of cross-sensitivity to other dibenzazepine compounds should be kept in mind.

Warnings: Extreme caution should be used when this drug is given to:
- patients with cardiovascular disease because of the possibility of conduction defects, arrhythmias, congestive heart failure, myocardial infarction, strokes and tachycardia. These patients require cardiac surveillance at all dosage levels of the drug;
- patients with increased intraocular pressure, history of urinary retention, or history of narrow-angle glaucoma because of the drug's anticholinergic properties;
- hyperthyroid patients or those on thyroid medication because of the possibility of cardiovascular toxicity;
- patients with a history of seizure disorder because this drug has been shown to lower the seizure threshold;
- patients receiving guanethidine, clonidine, or similar agents, since imipramine pamoate may block the pharmacologic effects of these drugs;
- patients receiving methylphenidate hydrochloride. Since methylphenidate hydrochloride may inhibit the metabolism of imipramine pamoate, downward dosage adjustment of imipramine pamoate may be required when given concomitantly with methylphenidate hydrochloride.

Since imipramine pamoate may impair the mental and/or physical abilities required for the performance of potentially hazardous tasks, such as operating an automobile or machinery, the patient should be cautioned accordingly.
Tofranil-PM may enhance the CNS depressant effects of alcohol. Therefore, it should be borne in mind that the dangers inherent in a suicide attempt or accidental overdosage with the drug may be increased for the patient who uses excessive amounts of alcohol. (See **Precautions.**)
Usage in Children: Tofrail-PM should not be used in children of any age because of the increased potential for acute overdosage due to the high unit potency (75 mg, 100 mg, 125 mg and 150 mg). Each capsule contains imipramine pamoate equivalent to 75 mg, 100 mg, 125 mg or 150 mg imipramine hydrochloride.

Precautions: An ECG recording should be taken prior to the initiation of larger-than-usual doses of imipramine pamoate and at appropriate intervals thereafter until steady state is achieved. (Patients with any evidence of cardiovascular disease require cardiac surveillance at all dosage levels of the drug. See **Warnings.**) Elderly patients and patients with cardiac disease or a prior history of cardiac disease are at special risk of developing the cardiac abnormalities associated with the use of imipramine pamoate. It should be kept in mind that the possibility of suicide in seriously depressed patients is inherent in the illness and may persist until significant remission occurs. Such patients should be carefully supervised during the early phase of treatment with imipramine pamoate and may require hospitalization. Prescriptions should be written for the smallest amount feasible.
Hypomanic or manic episodes may occur, particularly in patients with cyclic disorders. Such reactions may necessitate discontinuation of the drug. If needed, imipramine pamoate may be resumed in lower dosage when these episodes are relieved. Administration of a tranquilizer may be useful in controlling such episodes.
An activation of the psychosis may occasionally be observed in schizophrenic patients and may require reduction of dosage and the addition of a phenothiazine.
Concurrent administration of imipramine pamoate with electroshock therapy may increase the hazards; such treatment should be limited to those patients for whom it is essential, since there is limited clinical experience.
Usage During Pregnancy and Lactation:
Animal reproduction studies have yielded inconclusive results. (See also **Animal Pharmacology & Toxicology.**)
There have been no well-controlled studies conducted with pregnant women to determine the effect of imipramine on the fetus. However, there have been clinical reports of congenital malformations associated with the use of the drug. Although a causal relationship between these effects and the drug could not be established, the possibility of fetal risk from the maternal ingestion of imipramine cannot be excluded. Therefore, imipramine should be used in women who are or might become pregnant only if the clinical condition clearly justifies potential risk to the fetus.
Limited data suggest that imipramine is likely to be excreted in human breast milk. As a general rule, a woman taking a drug should not nurse since the possibility exists that the drug may be excreted in breast milk and be harmful to the child.
Patients should be warned that imipramine pamoate may enhance the CNS depressant effects of alcohol. (See **Warnings.**)
Imipramine pamoate should be used with caution in patients with significantly impaired renal or hepatic function.
Patients who develop a fever and a sore throat during therapy with imipramine pamoate should have leukocyte and differential blood counts performed. Imipramine pamoate should be discontinued if there is evidence of pathological neutrophil depression.
Prior to elective surgery, imipramine pamoate should be discontinued for as long as the clinical situation will allow.
In occasional susceptible patients or in those receiving anticholinergic drugs (including antiparkinsonism agents) in addition, the atropine-like effects may become more pronounced (e.g., paralytic ileus). Close supervision and careful adjustment of dosage is required when imipramine pamoate is administered concomitantly with anticholinergic drugs.
Avoid the use of preparations, such as decongestants and local anesthetics, which contain any sympathomimetic amine (e.g., epinephrine, norepinephrine), since it has been reported that tricyclic antidepressants can potentiate the effects of catecholamines.
Caution should be exercised when imipramine pamoate is used with agents that lower blood pressure.
Imipramine pamoate may potentiate the effects of CNS depressant drugs.
Patients taking imipramine pamoate should avoid excessive exposure to sunlight since there have been reports of photosensitization.
Both elevation and lowering of blood sugar levels have been reported with imipramine pamoate use.
The Tofranil-PM capsules (100 and 125 mg) contain FD&C Yellow No. 5 (tartrazine) which may cause allergic-type reactions (including bronchial asthma) in certain susceptible individuals. Although the overall incidence of FD&C Yellow No. 5 (tartrazine) sensitivity in the general population is low, it is frequently seen in patients who also have aspirin hypersensitivity.

Adverse Reactions: Note: Although the listing which follows includes a few adverse reactions which have not been reported with this specific drug, the pharmacological similarities among the tricyclic antidepressant drugs require that each of the reactions be considered when imipramine is administered.
Cardiovascular: Orthostatic hypotension, hypertension, tachycardia, palpitation, myocardial infarction, arrhythmias, heart block, ECG changes, precipitation of congestive heart failure, stroke.
Psychiatric: Confusional states (especially in the elderly) with hallucinations, disorientation, delusions; anxiety, restlessness, agitation; insomnia and nightmares; hypomania; exacerbation of psychosis.
Neurological: Numbness, tingling, paresthesias of extremities; incoordination, ataxia, tremors; peripheral neuropathy; extrapyramidal symptoms; seizures, alterations in EEG patterns; tinnitus.
Anticholinergic: Dry mouth, and, rarely, associated sublingual adenitis; blurred vision, disturbances of accommodation, mydriasis; constipation, paralytic ileus; urinary retention, delayed micturition, dilation of the urinary tract.
Allergic: Skin rash, petechiae, urticaria, itching, photosensitization; edema (general or of face and tongue); drug fever; cross-sensitivity with desipramine.
Hematologic: Bone marrow depression including agranulocytosis; eosinophilia; purpura; thrombocytopenia.
Gastrointestinal: Nausea and vomiting, anorexia, epigastric distress, diarrhea; peculiar taste, stomatitis, abdominal cramps, black tongue.
Endocrine: Gynecomastia in the male; breast enlargement and galactorrhea in the female; increased or decreased libido, impotence; tes-

ticular swelling; elevation or depression of blood sugar levels.

Other: Jaundice (simulating obstructive); altered liver function; weight gain or loss; perspiration; flushing; urinary frequency; drowsiness, dizziness, weakness and fatigue; headache; parotid swelling; alopecia; proneness to falling.

Withdrawal Symptoms: Though not indicative of addiction, abrupt cessation of treatment after prolonged therapy may produce nausea, headache and malaise.

Dosage and Administration: The following recommended dosages for Tofranil-PM should be modified as necessary by the clinical response and any evidence of intolerance.

Initial Adult Dosage:

Outpatients—Therapy should be initiated at 75 mg/day. Dosage may be increased to 150 mg/day which is the dose level at which optimum response is usually obtained. If necessary, dosage may be increased to 200 mg/day. Dosage higher than 75 mg/day may also be administered on a once-a-day basis after the optimum dosage and tolerance have been determined. The daily dosage may be given at bedtime. In some patients it may be necessary to employ a divided-dose schedule.

As with all tricyclics, the antidepressant effect of imipramine may not be evident for one to three weeks in some patients.

Hospitalized Patients—Therapy should be initiated at 100–150 mg/day and may be increased to 200 mg/day. If there is no response after two weeks, dosage should be increased to 250–300 mg/day.

Dosage higher than 150 mg/day may also be administered on a once-a-day basis after the optimum dosage and tolerance have been determined. The daily dosage may be given at bedtime. In some patients it may be necessary to employ a divided-dose schedule.

As with all tricyclics, the antidepressant effect of imipramine may not be evident for one to three weeks in some patients.

Adult Maintenance Dosage: Following remission, maintenance medication may be required for a longer period of time at the lowest dose that will maintain remission after which the dosage should gradually be decreased.

The usual maintenance dosage is 75–150 mg/day. The total daily dosage can be administered on a once-a-day basis, preferably at bedtime. In some patients it may be necessary to employ a divided-dose schedule.

In cases of relapse due to premature withdrawal of the drug, the effective dosage of imipramine should be reinstituted.

Adolescent and Geriatric Patients: Therapy in these age groups should be initiated with Tofranil®, brand of imipramine hydrochloride, tablets at a total daily dosage of 25–50 mg, since Tofranil-PM capsules are not available in these strengths. Dosage may be increased according to response and tolerance, but it is generally unnecessary to exceed 100 mg/day in these patients. Tofranil-PM capsules may be used when total daily dosage is established at 75 mg or higher.

The total daily dosage can be administered on a once-a-day basis, preferably at bedtime. In some patients it may be necessary to employ a divided-dose schedule.

As with all tricyclics, the antidepressant effect of imipramine may not be evident for one to three weeks in some patients.

Adolescent and geriatric patients can usually be maintained at lower dosage. Following remission, maintenance medication may be required for a longer period of time at the lowest dose that will maintain remission after which the dosage should gradually be decreased.

The total daily maintenance dosage can be administered on a once-a-day basis, preferably at bedtime. In some patients it may be necessary to employ a divided-dose schedule.

In cases of relapse due to premature withdrawal of the drug, the effective dosage of imipramine should be reinstituted.

Overdosage: Children have been reported to be more sensitive than adults to an acute overdosage of imipramine pamoate. An acute overdose of any amount in infants or young children, especially, must be considered serious and potentially fatal.

Signs and Symptoms: These may vary in severity depending upon factors such as the amount of drug absorbed, the age of the patient, and the interval between drug ingestion and the start of treatment. Blood and urine levels of imipramine may not reflect the severity of poisoning; they have chiefly a qualitative rather than quantitative value, and are unreliable indicators in the clinical management of the patient.

CNS abnormalities may include drowsiness, stupor, coma, ataxia, restlessness, agitation, hyperactive reflexes, muscle rigidity, athetoid and choreiform movements, and convulsions. Cardiac abnormalities may include arrhythmia, tachycardia, ECG evidence of impaired conduction, and signs of congestive failure. Respiratory depression, cyanosis, hypotension, shock, vomiting, hyperpyrexia, mydriasis, and diaphoresis may also be present.

Treatment: Because CNS involvement, respiratory depression and cardiac arrhythmia can occur suddenly, hospitalization and close observation are necessary, even when the amount ingested is thought to be small or the initial degree of intoxication appears slight or moderate. All patients with ECG abnormalities should have continuous cardiac monitoring for at least 72 hours and be closely observed until well after cardiac status has returned to normal; relapses may occur after apparent recovery.

The *slow* intravenous administration of physostigmine salicylate has been reported to reverse most of the cardiovascular and CNS effects of overdosage with tricyclic antidepressants. In adults, 1 to 3 mg has been reported to be effective. In children, start with 0.5 mg and repeat at 5-minute intervals to determine the minimum effective dose; do not exceed 2 mg. Because of the short duration of action of physostigmine, repeat the effective dose at 30- to 60-minute intervals, as necessary. Avoid rapid injection to reduce the possibility of physostigmine-induced convulsions.

In the alert patient, empty the stomach promptly by induced emesis followed by lavage. In the obtunded patient, secure the airway with a cuffed endotracheal tube before beginning lavage (do not induce emesis). Continue lavage for 24 hours or longer, depending on the apparent severity of intoxication. Use normal or half-normal saline to avoid water intoxication, especially in children. Instillation of activated charcoal slurry may help reduce absorption of imipramine.

Minimize external stimulation to reduce the tendency to convulsions. If anticonvulsants are necessary, diazepam, short-acting barbiturates, paraldehyde or methocarbamol may be useful. Do not use barbiturates if MAO inhibitors have been taken recently.

Maintain adequate respiratory exchange. Do not use repiratory stimulants.

Shock should be treated with supportive measures, such as intravenous fluids, oxygen and corticosteroids. Digitalis may increase conduction abnormalities and further irritate an already sensitized myocardium. If congestive heart failure necessitates rapid digitalization, particular care must be exercised.

Hyperpyrexia should be controlled by whatever external means are available, including ice packs and cooling sponge baths, if necessary.

Hemodialysis, peritoneal dialysis, exchange transfusions and forced diuresis have been generally reported as ineffective because of the rapid fixation of imipramine in tissues. Blood and urine levels of imipramine may not correlate with the degree of intoxication, and are unreliable indicators in the clinical management of the patient.

How Supplied: Tofranil-PM is available as follows:

75-mg, coral-colored capsules equivalent to 75 mg imipramine hydrochloride in bottles of 30, 100 and 1,000 capsules, and unit strip packages of 100.

100-mg, dark yellow/coral-colored capsules equivalent to 100 mg imipramine hydrochloride in bottles of 30, 100 and 1,000 capsules.

125-mg, light yellow/coral-colored capsules equivalent to 125 mg imipramine hydrochloride in bottles of 30, 100 and 1,000 capsules.

150-mg, coral-colored capsules equivalent to 150 mg imipramine hydrochloride in bottles of 30, 100 and 1,000 capsules, and unit strip packages of 100.

Animal Pharmacology & Toxicology

A. *Acute:* Oral LD_{50}:

Mouse	2185 mg/kg
Rat (F)	1142 mg/kg
(M)	1807 mg/kg
Rabbit	1016 mg/kg
Dog	693 mg/kg (Emesis ED_{50})

B. *Subacute:*

Two three-month studies in dogs gave evidence of an adverse drug effect on the testes, but only at the highest dose level employed, i.e., 90 mg/kg (10 times the maximum human dose). Depending on the histological section of the testes examined, the findings consisted of a range of degenerative changes up to and including complete atrophy of the seminiferous tubules, with spermatogenesis usually arrested.

Human studies show no definitive effect on sperm count, sperm motility, sperm morphology or volume of ejaculate.

Rat

One three-month study was done in rats at dosage levels comparable to those of the dog studies. No adverse drug effect on the testes was noted in this study, as confirmed by histological examination.

C. *Reproduction/Teratogenic:*

Oral: Imipramine pamoate was fed to male and female albino rats for 28 weeks through two breeding cycles at dose levels of 15 mg/kg/day and 40 mg/kg/day (equivalent to 2½ and 7 times the maximum human dose). No abnormalities which could be related to drug administration were noted in gross inspection. Autopsies performed on pups from the second breeding likewise revealed no pathological changes in organs or tissues; however, a decrease in mean litter size from both matings was noted in the drug-treated groups and significant growth suppression occurred in the nursing pups of both sexes in the high group as well as in the females of the low-level group. Finally, the lactation index (pups weaned divided by number left to nurse) was significantly lower in the second litter of the high-level group.

Dispense in tight container (USP).

667122 C80-9 (1/80)

[*Shown in Product Identification Section*]

Products are cross-indexed by

generic and chemical names

in the

YELLOW SECTION

Gerber Products Company

FREMONT, MI 49412

MBF* (Meat Base Formula) Liquid
Hypoallergenic Infant feeding Formula, Gerber

Composition: Hypoallergenic liquid formula made from water, beef hearts, cane sugar, sesame oil, modified tapioca starch, tricalcium phosphate, calcium citrate, sodium ascorbate, ferrous sulfate, thiamin hydrochloride, tocopheryl acetate, vitamin A palmitate, calcium pantothenate, pyridoxine hydrochloride, vitamin D, cupric sulfate, phytonadione (vitamin K_1) and potassium iodide.
Nutrient Content: 1:1 dilution contains 20 cal/fl.oz., 12.2% solids, 2.7% protein, 3.2% fat and 6.0% carbohydrate with a Ca/P ratio of 1.5. Vitamin and mineral content per 15 fl. oz. can is:

Vitamin A	1600.0	I.U.
Vitamin D	420.0	I.U.
Vitamin E	5.4	I.U.
Vitamin C	54.0	mg
Thiamin	0.54	mg
Riboflavin	0.9	mg
Niacin	6.6	mg
Vitamin B_6	0.78	mg
Vitamin B_{12}	7.8	mcg
Folacin	24.0	mcg
Pantothenic Acid	1.8	mg
Calcium	900.0	mg
Phosphorus	600.0	mg
Iron	12.6	mg
Copper	0.36	mg
Sodium	164.0	mg
Potassium	346.0	mg
Magnesium	36.0	mg
Iodine	30.0	mcg
Zinc	2.5	mg

Action and Uses: A nutritionally adequate formula for infants and children intolerant to cow's and goat's milk whose symptoms may be diarrhea, colic, eczema, upper respiratory, etc. Useful in the management of galactosemia and milk induced steatorrhea.
Administration and Dosage: Provides 20 cal/fl.oz. when diluted 1:1; similar to other milk-based and soy-based infant formulas. Concentrated liquid added to previously boiled (not hot) water is to be divided among prescribed number of bottles, easily fed thru cross-cut nipples.
MBF's content of essential nutrients conforms to the infant formula standard established by the U.S. Food and Drug Administration in 1971.
Side Effects: None.
Precautions: None.
Contraindications: None.
How Supplied: Concentrated Liquid, 15 fl. oz. cans.
Literature Available: Yes.
*Trademark

Geriatric Pharm. Corp.

397 JERICHO TURNPIKE
FLORAL PARK, NY 11001

B-C-BID CAPSULES
B Complex with Vitamin C
SUSTAINED RELEASE
BY MICRODIALYSIS DIFFUSION

Composition: Each capsule contains: Vitamin B-1 15 mg., Vitamin B-2 10 mg., Vitamin B-6 5 mg., Niacinamide 50 mg., Calcium Pantothenate 10 mg., Vitamin C 300 mg., and Vitamin B-12 (Cyanocobalamin) 5 mcg.
Indications: To provide prophylactic and therapeutic nutritional supplementation. Valuable in physiologic stress, pregnancy and lactation, infections, burns, fractures, pre-and post-operatively, peptic ulcer, colitis, diabetes, alcoholism, in special, and weight-reducing diets, and for debilitated patients.
Medication is released at a smooth, continuous, predictable rate dependent only upon the presence of fluid in the G.I. tract, and not dependent on pH and other variables.
On b.i.d. dosage, this smooth, continuous release of B-C-BID's essential vitamins frees your patient from the "peak and valley" effect of ordinary capsules or tablets.
Dosage: For continuous 24 hour therapy, one capsule after breakfast and one after supper.
How Supplied: Bottles of 30, 100, 500.

CEVI-BID Capsules (500 mg. Vitamin C)
SUSTAINED RELEASE
BY MICRO-DIALYSIS DIFFUSION

Composition: Each CEVI-BID capsule contains 500 mg. Vitamin C.
Action and Uses: For treatment of Vitamin C deficiency. CEVI-BID maintains optimal blood levels of Vitamin C around the clock on b.i.d. dosage, and avoids "peak and valley" effects of ordinary Vitamin C tablets. Medication is released at a smooth, continuous, predictable rate dependent only upon the presence of fluid in the G.I. tract and independent of pH or other variables.
Dosage: For continuous 24 hour therapy, one capsule after breakfast and one after supper.
How Supplied: Bottles of 30, 100, 500.

GAYSAL Anti-arthritic, Analgesic Tablets ℞
GAYSAL-S (same formula sine barbiturates)

Composition: Each GAYSAL tablet contains butabarbital sodium* 8 mg (1/8 gr.), phenobarbital* 4 mg. (1/16 gr.) (*Warning: May be habit forming) sodium salicylate 300 mg. (5 gr.), acetaminophen 180 mg. (3 gr.), aluminum hydroxide gel 60 mg. (1 gr.).
Action and Uses: GAYSAL provides analgesia and effective sedation. Indicated in rheumatoid arthritis, osteoarthritis, fibrositis, bursitis, and related conditions.
Also Available: GAYSAL-S (same formula without barbiturates), where barbiturates are contraindicated, or not necessary.
Contraindications: GAYSAL: Salicylate or barbiturate sensitivity.
GAYSAL-S: Salicylate sensitivity.
Dosage: Two or more tablets, as necessary, after meals and before retiring.
How Supplied: Bottles of 100, 1000.

GER-O-FOAM™ Analgesic Anesthetic Foam

Composition: Aerosol foam containing methyl salicylate 30% and benzocaine 3% in a specially-processed oil emulsion.
Action and Uses: For topical application in alleviating minor pains of musculoskeletal conditions such as osteoarthritis, rheumatoid arthritis and low back pain. GER-O-FOAM permits increased range of motion by decreasing pain.
Administration and Dosage: Massage into affected area 2 or 3 times daily.
Precautions: If a rash or irritation occurs, discontinue medication. Avoid application in or near eyes, mucous membranes or open wounds.
How Supplied: 4 oz. Aerosol cans.

GUSTASE® • GUSTASE-PLUS® ℞
Gastrointestinal Enzyme Tablets

Composition: Each GUSTASE tablet contains GERILASE (standardized amylolytic enzyme) 30 mg., GERIPROTASE (standardized proteolytic enzyme) 6 mg., GERICELLULASE (standardized cellulolytic enzyme) 2 mg.
Action and Uses: GUSTASE is indicated in dyspepsia, colitis, flatulence, diverticulitis, abdominal distension, etc. GUSTASE is effective in a broad pH spectrum (3–10), and is not enteric coated.
When spasmolytic and sedative actions are also indicated: GUSTASE-PLUS (℞). containing same enzymes plus homatropine methylbromide 2½ mg., and phenobarbital ⅛ gr. (warning: may be habit forming).
Contraindications: GUSTASE: None known; GUSTASE-PLUS: Glaucoma, renal disease, sensitivity to phenobarbital.
Adverse Reactions: Blurring of vision and dry mouth may occur.
Administration and Dosage: One tablet during or immediately after meals.
How Supplied: Bottles of 42, 100, 500.

ISO-BID CAPSULES 40 mg. ℞
SUSTAINED RELEASE BY
MICRO-DIALYSIS DIFFUSION

Composition: Each ISO-BID SUSTAINED-MEDICATION CAPSULE contains 40 mg. Isosorbide Dinitrate. Medication is released at a smooth, continuous, predictable rate dependent only upon the presence of fluid in the G.I. tract; not dependent on the variable digestive processes.
Mode of Action: The mechanism of action of ISO-BID, like all nitrates, is the relaxation of smooth muscle. The relationship between this and its clinical usefulness is obscure, since the exact cause of anginal pain is presently unknown. ISO-BID is intended to decrease the frequency and severity of anginal attacks, and thus effect a decrease in the need for nitroglycerin. These should be the criteria for the success of ISO-BID therapy, since there is a wide variation in symptomatic response to treatment.

Indications: Based on a review of this drug by the National Academy of Sciences—National Research Council and/or other information, FDA has classified the indications as follows:
"*Possibly*" *effective:* When taken orally ISO-BID SUSTAINED MEDICATION CAPSULES are indicated for the relief of angina pectoris (pain of coronary artery disease). ISO-BID SUSTAINED RELEASE CAPSULES are not intended to abort the acute anginal episode, but are widely regarded as useful in the prophylactic treatment of angina pectoris. Final classification of the less-than-effective indication requires further investigation.

Contraindication: Idiosyncrasy to this drug.
Warnings: Data supporting the use of nitrites during the early days of the acute phase of myocardial infarction (the period during which clinical and laboratory findings are unstable) are insufficient to establish safety.
Precautions: Use with caution in patients with glaucoma. Tolerance to this drug, and cross-tolerance to other nitrites and nitrates may occur.
Patients with gastric hypermotility for any reason, where the duration of passage through the gastrointestinal tract may be less than nor-

mal, should take sublingual nitroglycerin rather than sustained release medications.
Adverse Reactions: Cutaneous vasodilation with flushing. Headache may commonly occur, and may be both severe and persistent. Transient dizziness and weakness, in addition to other signs of cerebral ischemia associated with postural hypotension may occasionally be seen. ISO-BID can act as a physiological antagonist to norepinephrine, histamine, acetylcholine and many other medications. An occasional patient may show marked sensitivity to the hypotensive effects of nitrite; severe responses (nausea, vomiting, weakness, restlessness, pallor, excessive sweating and collapse) can occur, even with the usual therapeutic dosage. Alcohol may enhance this effect. A drug rash and/or exfoliative dermatitis is occasionally seen.
Dosage: ISO-BID SUSTAINED RELEASE CAPSULES: One 40mg. ISO-BID CAPSULE every 12 hours on an empty stomach according to need, for continuous 24-hour therapy. This dosage schedule is particularly convenient in the management of noctural angina. Some patients may require higher dosage levels. In these patients, dosage should be titrated, and may require two ISO-BID CAPSULES b.i.d.
How Supplied: ISO-BID CAPSULES: bottles of 30's, 100's, 500's.

MENIC™ Analeptic, Vasodilator Tablets ℞

Composition: Each MENIC tablet contains pentylenetetrazole 100 mg. (1½ gr.), nicotinic acid 50 mg. (⅚ gr.).
Actions and Uses: To enhance mental and physical activity of elderly patients. Indicated in the treatment of memory defects, mental confusion, deterioration, abnormal behavior, and related symptoms of senility.
Dosage: Two MENIC tablets after each meal.
Side Effects: Occasionally, pruritus associated with niacin administration.
Precautions: Use with caution in patients with low convulsive threshold, focal brain lesions, severely impaired liver function, peptic ulcer, diabetes, and gall bladder or liver diseases. Niacin may potentiate hypotensive drugs, phenothiazine derivatives and inactivate fibrinolysin.
Contraindications: None known.
How Supplied: Bottles of 100, 500.

STIMULAX CAPSULES
Laxative/Stool Softener

Composition: 250 mg. Dioctyl Sodium Sulfosuccinate and 30 mg. Casanthranol.
Action and Uses: STIMULAX produces soft, formed easily evacuated stools, without straining, griping, flatulence, or diarrhea. Indicated to correct chronic functional constipation, particularly in the elderly, the inactive, the cardiac patient, patients with rectal fissures or hemorrhoids, the obstetrical patient, and following surgery.
Warning: Not to be used when abdominal pain, nausea, vomiting are present. Frequent or prolonged use of this preparation may result in dependence on laxatives.
Dosage: One or two capsules on retiring.
How Supplied: Bottles of 30, 100, 500.

Over 7,000 products are

listed alphabetically

in the

PINK SECTION.

Gilbert Laboratories
31 FAIRMOUNT AVENUE
CHESTER, NEW JERSEY 07930

ESGIC® ℞

Composition: Each ESGIC Tablet contains: isobutylallylbarbituric acid (butalbital, N.F.), (WARNING: may be habit forming) 50 mg.; caffeine, U.S.P., 40 mg.; and acetaminophen, N.F., 325 mg.
Properties and Therapeutics: Many clinicians report that nervous tension and anxiety underlie stress or muscle contraction headache. Sustained contraction of head and neck muscles is a major factor in this type of headache. ESGIC was designed to be an effective means of relieving head pain due to these factors by combining the analgesic effect of acetaminophen with the mild sedative effect of isobutylallylbarbituric acid. Acetaminophen may be used safely and comfortably by most persons sensitive to aspirin.

Indications:
Based on a review of this drug by the National Academy of Sciences-National Research Council and/or other information, FDA has classified the indications as folows: "Possibly" effective: For use to relieve pain; in "conditions in which combined sedative and analgesic action is desired, such as, nervous tension and sleeplessness associated with pain, headache, or general malaise"; in nervous and muscular pain accompanied by hyperexcitability and nervousness; and in "all conditions requiring relief of pain or reduction of fever, such as rheumatic and arthritic conditions, neuralgia, aches and pains, dysmenorrhea, respiratory infections and febrile conditions (common colds and grippe), dental extractions and minor surgical procedures and headaches." Final classification of the less-than-effective indications requires further investigation.

Contraindications: Hypersensitivity to any of the components.
Precautions: Due to the presence of a barbiturate, may be habit forming. Excessive or prolonged use should be avoided. Keep out of reach of children.
Side Effects: In rare instances drowsiness, nausea, constipation, dizziness and skin rash may occur. Discontinue use immediately upon occurrence of any such reactions.
Adult Dosage: One to two tablets, repeated if necessary, but not more than 6 per day.
How Supplied: ESGIC Tablets: White (formerly yellow) compressed tablet, bottle of 100. NDC 0535-0011-01
Company's Product Identification Mark: Tablets imprinted with Gilbert trademark on one side and NDC #535-11 on the other.

5/77

[Shown in Product Identification Section]

Important Notice

Before prescribing or administering

any product described in

PHYSICIANS' DESK REFERENCE

always consult the PDR Supplement for

possible new or revised information.

Glaxo Inc.
1900 WEST COMMERCIAL BLVD.
FT. LAUDERDALE, FL 33309

ATHEMOL® Tablets ℞
ATHEMOL®-N Tablets

Composition: ATHEMOL Tablets—Each red sugar coated tablet contains 200 mg. Theobromine Magnesium Oleate.
ATHEMOL-N Tablets—Each light green sugar coated tablet contains 200 mg. Theobromine Magnesium Oleate and 100 mg. Magnesium Nicotinate (equivalent to 75 mg. Nicotinic Acid).
Action and Uses: Athemol and Athemol-N provide a well tolerated treatment for various forms of arteriosclerosis and peripheral vascular circulatory disease resulting from arteriosclerosis. May be of help in the relief of pain and discomfort of angina pectoris and coronary insufficiency as well as leg pains, peripheral vascular circulatory disease and other symptoms of general arteriosclerosis. Athemol and Athemol-N effectively reduce xanthoma in many patients.
Athemol and Athemol-N therefore may be of help in general arteriosclerosis, thromboangiitis obliterans, diabetic endarteritis, and xanthomatosis. In diabetic endarteritis it must be understood that the usual therapeutic measures, in common use for the treatment of diabetes, must be employed.
Side Effects: Gastric upset may occur, although rarely encountered. Administration of Athemol-N may produce flushing (a sensation of warmth) and pruritus, but these reactions are transient and apparently harmless.
Contraindications: Serious kidney disease and obstructive lesions of the urinary tract.
Administration and Dosage: Athemol and Athemol-N are administered orally in doses of 1 or 2 tablets 3 times a day. Prolonged administration is desirable. Initially a 2 tablet dosage t.i.d. can be given and after 6–8 weeks, the dosage may be reduced to 1 tablet t.i.d. A warm tingly flush may follow each dose of Athemol-N. This is one of the therapeutic effects.
How Supplied: Bottles of 100 and 500 tablets.

[Shown in Product Identification Section]

BECLOVENT® INHALER ℞
(beclomethasone dipropionate)
FOR ORAL INHALATION ONLY

Description: Beclomethasone dipropionate, the active component of BECLOVENT® (beclomethasone dipropionate) Inhaler, is an anti-inflammatory steroid having the chemical name 9-Chloro-11B,17,21-trihydroxy-16B-methylpregna-1,4-diene-3,20-dione17,21-dipropionate.
BECLOVENT® Inhaler is a metered-dose aerosol unit containing a microcrystalline suspension of beclomethasone dipropionate-trichloromonofluoromethane clathrate in a mixture of propellants (trichloromonofluoromethane and dichlorodifluoromethane) with oleic acid. Each canister contains beclomethasone dipropionate-trichloromonofluoromethane clathrate having a molecular proportion of beclomethasone dipropionate to trichloromonofluoromethane between 3:1 and 3:2. Each actuation delivers from the mouthpiece a quantity of clathrate equivalent to 42 mcg. of beclomethasone dipropionate. The contents of one canister provide at least 200 oral inhalations.
Clinical Pharmacology: Beclomethasone 17, 21-dipropionate is a diester of beclomethasone, a synthetic corticosteroid which is chemically related to prednisolone. Beclomethasone differs from prednisolone only in having a chlorine at the 9-alpha and a methyl group at the

Continued on next page

Glaxo—Cont.

16-beta position in place of hydrogen. Animal studies showed that beclomethasone dipropionate has potent anti-inflammatory activity. When administered systemically to mice, the anti-inflammatory activity was accompanied by other typical features of glucocorticoid action including thymic involoution, liver glycogen deposition, and pituitary-adrenal suppression. However, after systemic administration to rats, the anti-inflammatory action was associated with little or no effect on other tests of glucocorticoid activity.
Beclomethasone dipropionate is sparingly soluble and is poorly mobilized from subcutaneous or intramuscular injection sites. However, systemic absorption occurs after all routes of administration. When given to animals in the form of an aerosolized suspension of the trichloromonofluoromethane clathrate, the drug is deposited in the mouth and nasal passages, the trachea and principal bronchi, and in the lung; a considerable portion of the drug is also swallowed. Absorption occurs rapidly from all respiratory and gastrointestinal tissues, as indicated by the rapid clearance of radioactively labeled drug from local tissues and appearance of tracer in the circulation. There is no evidence of tissue storage of beclomethasone dipropionate or its metabolites. Lung slices can metabolize beclomethasone dipropionate rapidly to beclomethasone 17-monopropionate and more slowly to free beclomethasone (which has very weak anti-inflammatory activity). However, irrespective of the route of administration (injection, oral, or aerosol), the principal route of excretion of the drug and its metabolites is the feces. Less than 10% of the drug and its metabolites is excreted in the urine. In humans, 12% to 15% of an orally administered dose of beclomethasone dipropionate was excreted in the urine as both conjugated and free metabolites of the drug.
The mechanisms responsible for the anti-inflammatory action of beclomethasone dipropionate are unknown. The precise mechanism of the aerosolized drug's action in the lung is also unknown.
Indications: BECLOVENT® (beclomethasone dipropionate) Inhaler is indicated only for patients who require chronic treatment with corticosteroids for control of the symptoms of bronchial asthma. Such patients would include those already receiving systemic corticosteroids, and selected patients who are inadequately controlled on a non-steroid regimen and in whom steroid therapy has been withheld because of concern over potential adverse effects.
BECLOVENT® Inhaler is NOT indicated:
1. For relief of asthma which can be controlled by bronchodilators and other non-steroid medications.
2. In patients who require systemic corticosteroid treatment infrequently.
3. In the treatment of non-asthmatic bronchitis.
Contraindications: BECLOVENT® Inhaler is contraindicated in the primary treatment of status asthmaticus or other acute episodes of asthma where intensive measures are required.
Hypersensitivity to any of the ingredients of this preparation contraindicates its use.
Warnings:

> Particular care is needed in patients who are transferred from systemically active corticosteroids to BECLOVENT® Inhaler because deaths due to adrenal insufficiency have occurred in asthmatic patients during and after transfer from systemic corticosteroids to aerosol beclomethasone dipropionate. After withdrawal from systemic corticosteroids, a number of months are required for recovery of hypothalamic-pituitary-adrenal (HPA) function. During this period of HPA suppression, patients may exhibit signs and symptoms of adrenal insufficiency when exposed to trauma, surgery or infections, particularly gastroenteritis. Although BECLOVENT® Inhaler may provide control of asthmatic symptoms during these episodes, it does NOT provide the systemic steroid which is necessary for coping with these emergencies.
> During periods of stress or a severe asthmatic attack, patients who have been withdrawn from systemic corticosteroids should be instructed to resume systemic steroids (in large doses) immediately and to contact their physician for further instruction. These patients should also be instructed to carry a warning card indicating that they may need supplementary systemic steroids during periods of stress or a severe asthma attack. To assess the risk of adrenal insufficiency in emergency situations, routine tests of adrenal cortical function, including measurement of early morning resting cortisol levels, should be performed periodically in all patients. An early morning resting cortisol level may be accepted as normal only if it falls at or near the normal mean level.

Localized infections with Candida albicans or Aspergillus niger have occurred frequently in the mouth and pharynx and occasionally in the larynx. Positive cultures for oral Candida may be present in up to 75% of patients. Although the frequency of clinically apparent infection is considerably lower, these infections may require treatment with appropriate antifungal therapy or discontinuance of treatment with BECLOVENT® Inhaler.
BECLOVENT® Inhaler is not to be regarded as a bronchodilator and is not indicated for rapid relief of bronchospasm.
Patients should be instructed to contact their physician immediately when episodes of asthma which are not responsive to bronchodilators occur during the course of treatment with BECLOVENT® (beclomethasone dipropionate). During such episodes, patients may require therapy with systemic corticosteroids.
There is no evidence that control of asthma can be achieved by the administration of BECLOVENT® in amounts greater than the recommended doses.
Transfer of patients from systemic steroid therapy to BECLOVENT® Inhaler may unmask allergic conditions previously suppressed by the systemic steroid therapy, e.g., rhinitis, conjunctivitis, and eczema.
Precautions: During withdrawal from oral steroids, some patients may experience symptoms of systemically active steroid withdrawal, e.g., joint and/or muscular pain, lassitude and depression, despite maintenance or even improvement of respiratory function (See DOSAGE AND ADMINISTRATION for details).
In responsive patients, beclomethasone dipropionate may permit control of asthmatic symptoms without suppression of HPA function, as discussed below (See CLINICAL STUDIES). Since beclomethasone dipropionate is absorbed into the circulation and can be systemically active, the beneficial effects of BECLOVENT® Inhaler in minimizing or preventing HPA dysfunction may be expected only when recommended dosages are not exceeded.
The long-term effects of beclomethasone dipropionate in human subjects are still unknown. In particular, the local effects of the agent on developmental or immunologic processes in the mouth, pharynx, trachea, and lung are unknown. There is also no information about the possible long-term systemic effects of the agent.
In a one-year oral inhalation study in beagle dogs, narrowed or irregular tracheal caliber was observed on postmortem examination of the treated dogs, but not in the control dogs. Further, the possibility of a drug-related interference with sexual maturation or function of female dogs was suggested by this study (See ANIMAL PHARMACOLOGY AND TOXICOLOGY). The relevance to patients of both of these findings following prolonged administration of the drug is not known.
The potential effects of BECLOVENT® on acute, recurrent, or chronic pulmonary infections, including active or quiescent tuberculosis, are not known. Similarly, the potential effects of long-term administration of the drug on lung or other tissues are unknown.
Pulmonary infiltrates with eosinophilia may occur in patients on BECLOVENT® Inhaler therapy. Although it is possible that in some patients this state may become manifest because of systemic steroid withdrawal when inhalational steroids are administered, a causative role for beclomethasone dipropionate and/or it vehicle cannot be ruled out.
Use in Pregnancy: Glucocorticoids are known teratogens in rodent species and beclomethasone dipropionate is no exception.
Teratology studies were done in rats, mice, and rabbits treated with subcutaneous beclomethasone dipropionate. Beclomethasone dipropionate was found to produce fetal resorption, cleft palate, agnathia, microstomia, absence of tongue, delayed ossification and partial agenesis of the thymus. Well-controlled trials relating to fetal risk in humans are not available. Glucocorticoids are secreted in human milk. It is not known whether beclomethasone dipropionate would be secreted in human milk but it is safe to assume that it is likely. The use of beclomethasone dipropionate in pregnancy, nursing mothers, or women of childbearing potential requires that the possible benefits of the drug be weighed against the potential hazards to the mother, embryo, or fetus. Infants born of mothers who have received substantial doses of corticosteroids during pregnancy should be carefully observed for hypoadrenalism.
Adverse Reactions: Deaths due to adrenal insufficiency have occurred in asthmatic patients during and after transfer from systemic corticosteroids to aerosol beclomethasone dipropionate (See WARNINGS).
Suppression of HPA function (reduction of early morning plasma cortisol levels) has been reported in adult patients who received 1600 mcg. daily doses of BECLOVENT® (beclomethasone dipropionate) for one month. A few patients on BECLOVENT® have complained of hoarseness or dry mouth. Bronchospasm and rash have been reported rarely.
Dosage and Administration: Adults: The usual dosage is two inhalations (84 mcg.) given three or four times a day. In patients with severe asthma, it is advisable to start with 12 to 16 inhalations a day and adjust the dosage downward according to the response of the patient. The maximal daily intake should not exceed 20 inhalations, 840 mcg. (0.84 mg.), in adults.
Children 6 to 12 years of age: The usual dosage is one or two inhalations (42 to 84 mcg.) given three or four times a day according to the response of the patient. The maximal daily intake should not exceed ten inhalations, 420 mcg. (0.42 mg.), in children 6 to 12 years of age.
Insufficient clinical data exist with respect to the administration of BECLOVENT® Inhaler in children below the age of 6.
Rinsing the mouth after inhalation is advised. Patients receiving bronchodilators by inhalation should be advised to use the bronchodilator before BECLOVENT® Inhaler in order to enhance penetration of beclomethasone dipropionate into the bronchial tree. After use of an aerosol bronchodilator several minutes should elapse before use of the BECLOVENT® In-

haler to reduce the potential toxicity from the inhaled fluorocarbon propellants in the two aerosols.

Different considerations must be given to the following groups of patients in order to obtain the full therapeutic benefit of BECLOVENT® Inhaler.

Patients not receiving systemic steroids: The use of BECLOVENT® Inhaler is straightforward in patients who are inadequately controlled with non-steroid medications but in whom systemic steroid therapy has been withheld because of concern over potential adverse reactions. In patients who respond to BECLOVENT®, an improvement in pulmonary function is usually apparent within one to four weeks after the start of BECLOVENT® Inhaler.

Patients receiving systemic steroids: In those patients dependent on systemic steroids, transfer to BECLOVENT® and subsequent management may be more difficult because recovery from impaired adrenal function is usually slow. Such suppression has been known to last for up to 12 months. Clinical studies, however, have demonstrated that BECLOVENT® may be effective in the management of these asthmatic patients and may permit replacement or significant reduction in the dosage of systemic corticosteroids.

The patient's asthma should be reasonably stable before treatment with BECLOVENT® Inhaler is started. Initially, the aerosol should be used concurrently with the patient's usual maintenance dose of systemic steroid. After approximately one week, gradual withdrawal of the systemic steroid is started by reducing the daily or alternate daily dose. The next reduction is made after an interval of one or two weeks, depending on the response of the patient. Generally, these decrements should not exceed 2.5 mg of prednisone or its equivalent. A slow rate of withdrawal cannot be overemphasized. During withdrawal, some patients may experience symptoms of systemically active steroid withdrawal, e.g., joint and/or muscular pain, lassitude and depression, despite maintenance or even improvement of respiratory function. Such patients should be encouraged to continue with the Inhaler but should be watched carefully for objective signs of adrenal insufficiency, such as hypotension and weight loss. If evidence of adrenal insufficiency occurs, the systemic steroid dose should be boosted temporarily and thereafter further withdrawal should continue more slowly.

During periods of stress or a severe asthma attack, transfer patients will require supplementary treatment with systemic steroids. Exacerbations of asthma which occur during the course of treatment with BECLOVENT® (beclomethasone dipropionate) Inhaler should be treated with a short course of systemic steroid which is gradually tapered as these symptoms subside. There is no evidence that control of asthma can be achieved by administration of BECLOVENT® in amounts greater than the recommended doses.

Direction for Use: Illustrated patient instructions for proper use accompany each package of BECLOVENT® Inhaler.

CONTENTS UNDER PRESSURE. Do not puncture. Do not use or store near heat or open flame. Exposure to temperatures above 120° F may cause bursting. Never throw container into fire or incinerator. Keep out of reach of children.

How Supplied: BECLOVENT® Inhaler 16.8 g canister; box of one. It is supplied with an oral adapter and patient's instructions; (NDC-0173-0312-88).

Animal Pharmacology and Toxicology: Studies in a number of animal species including rats, rabbits, and dogs have shown no unusual toxicity during acute experiments. However, the effects of beclomethasone dipropionate in producing signs of glucocorticoid excess during chronic administration by various routes were dose related.

Particular note is made of a one-year study in dogs (beagles) which were given beclomethasone dipropionate in the form of the aerosolized suspension of the trichloromonofluoromethane clathrate; some of the animals also received supplementary treatment with oral beclomethasone. The animals which were given the larger treatment doses of beclomethasone dipropionate-trichloromonofluoromethane clathrate, with or without oral beclomethasone dipropionate, developed severe Cushing's syndrome, associated with suppression of pituitary-adrenal function, delayed growth and sexual maturation, obesity, fatty infiltration of the liver, etc. Even in the absence of severe Cushing's syndrome, the following adverse reactions were noted in the young beagles (age 17 weeks at beginning of study): (1) There was a high incidence of convulsions and uncoordinated movements which were attributed to excessive fluorocarbon propellant and/or the possible anoxia caused by the mode of administration of the aerosol. (2) On postmortem examination narrowed or irregular tracheal caliber was noted in the treated, but not in the control groups. (3) In female animals, the possibility of a drug-related interference with sexual maturation or function was suggested by the ovarian and uterine weights which were disproportionately low in relation to body size. It is unknown whether these observations in beagles have any relationship to possible adverse effects of prolonged administration of the drug in man, and additional studies will be carried out to clarify this matter.

Clinical Studies: The effects of beclomethasone dipropionate on hypothalmic-pituitary-adrenal (HPA) function have been evaluated in adult volunteers. There was no suppression of early morning plasma cortisol concentrations when beclomethasone dipropionate was administered in a dose of 1000 mcg./day for one month as an aerosol or for three days by intramuscular injection. However, partial suppression of plasma cortisol concentration was observed when beclomethasone dipropionate was administered in doses of 2000 mcg./day either intramuscularly or by aerosol. Immediate suppression of plasma cortisol concentrations was observed after single doses of 4000 mcg. of beclomethasone dipropionate.

In one study, the effects of beclomethasone dipropionate on HPA function were examined in patients with asthma. There was no change in basal early morning plasma cortisol concentrations or in the cortisol responses to tetracosactrin (ACTH 1:24) stimulation after daily administration of 400, 800 or 1200 mcg. of beclomethasone dipropionate for 28 days. After daily administration of 1600 mcg. each day for 28 days, there was a slight reduction in basal cortisol concentrations and a statistically significant ($P < .01$) reduction in plasma cortisol responses to tetracosactrin stimulation. The effects of a more prolonged period of beclomethasone dipropionate administration on HPA function have not been evaluated. However, a number of investigators have noted that when systemic corticosteroid therapy in asthmatic subjects can be replaced with recommended doses of beclomethasone dipropionate, there is gradual recovery of endogenous cortisol concentrations to the normal range. There is still no documented evidence of recovery from other adverse systemic corticosteroid-induced reactions during prolonged therapy of patients with beclomethasone dipropionate.

Clinical experience has shown that some patients with bronchial asthma who require corticosteroid therapy for control of symptoms can be partially or completely withdrawn from systemic corticosteroid if therapy with beclomethasone dipropionate aerosol is substituted. Beclomethasone dipropionate aerosol is not effective for all patients with bronchial asthma or at all stages of the disease in a given patient.

The early clinical experience has revealed several new problems which may be associated with the use of beclomethasone dipropionate by inhalation for treatment of patients with bronchial asthma.

1. There is a risk of adrenal insufficiency when patients are transferred from systemic corticosteroids to aerosol beclomethasone dipropionate. Although the aerosol may provide adequate control of asthma during the transfer period, it does not provide the systemic steroid which is needed during acute stress situations. Deaths due to adrenal insufficiency have occurred in asthmatic patients during and after transfer from systemic corticosteroids to aerosol beclomethasone dipropionate. (See WARNINGS.)
2. Transfer of patients from systemic steroid therapy to beclomethasone dipropionate aerosol may unmask allergic conditions which were previously controlled by the systemic steroid therapy, e.g., rhinitis, conjunctivitis, and eczema.
3. Localized infections with Candida albicans or Aspergillus niger have occurred frequently in the mouth and pharynx and occasionally in the larynx. It has been reported that up to 75% of the patients who receive prolonged treatment with beclomethasone dipropionate have positive oral cultures for Candida albicans. The incidence of clinically apparent infection is considerably lower but may require therapy with appropriate antifungal agents or discontinuation of treatment with beclomethasone dipropionate aerosol.

The long-term effects of beclomethasone dipropionate in human subjects are still unknown. In particular, the local effects of the agent on developmental or immunologic processes in the mouth, pharynx, trachea and lung are unknown. There is also no information about the possible long-term systemic effects of the agent. The possible relevance of the data in animal studies to results in human subjects cannot be evaluated.

MAY 1979

Manufactured in Ware, England by Glaxo Operations-UK, Ltd. Distributed by Glaxo Inc., Fort Lauderdale, FL 33309

[*Shown in Product Identification Section*]

CORTICAINE® CREAM ℞

Composition: Hydrocortisone 0.5% and Dibucaine 0.5% in a washable, non-greasy, mentholated, cream base composed of mixed saturated fatty esters, stearyl alcohol, glycerin, polysorbate 40 and purified water with methylparaben and propylparaben as preservatives.

Actions: Corticaine contains hydrocortisone and dibucaine in a soothing, lubricant cream base. Hydrocortisone acts to reduce inflammation, swelling and itching. Dibucaine, the other active ingredient, provides relief from pain and itching; it is effective in low concentrations because of its high potency. Since dibucaine differs chemically from procaine and cocaine, it can often be used in patients sensitive to ester-type local anesthetic agents. It is effective on mucous membranes and on abraded and broken skin surfaces.

Uses: Corticaine, when combined with other recognized therapeutic measures, is recommended for the symptomatic relief of itching, pain, irritation and inflammation of certain anorectal and dermatological conditions. On the skin, it offers symptomatic relief in abrasions, itching rash, poison oak, sumac or ivy dermatitis, mild sunburn, minor burns, hives, prickly heat, itching eczema, diaper rash, and intertrigo. When introduced into the rectum, it helps to relieve the itching, pain and inflammation of hemorrhoids, as well as the anorectal discomfort of associated conditions such as

Continued on next page

Glaxo—Cont.

proctitis, papillitis and cyrptitis. When applied perianally, it can provide symptomatic relief from pruritus ani and external hemorrhoids.
Contraindications: Local tuberculous, fungal and viral infection. Not recommended for such diseases as pemphigus and discoid lupus erythematosus.
Precautions: Avoid use in the eyes. Do not apply to extensive areas nor use for prolonged periods. Care should be exercised if the patient is already receiving oral or parenteral corticosteroid therapy. Should not be used rectally without adequate proctologic examination. Any secondary bacterial infection should be controlled by a suitable antibacterial agent, before use of this cream. As with other topical anesthetics, patients should be observed carefully for possible local irritation or sensitization reactions. Not to be used with anorectal fistulas and abscesses.
Administration: FOR RECTAL USE: Cleanse the rectal area and dry thoroughly before use. Attach plastic applicator to tube and squeeze tube lightly to fill applicator with cream. Lubricate applicator with cream, then gently insert into rectum and squeeze tube again lightly to extrude a similar applicator dose of cream into the rectum. Can also be applied topically to irritated anorectal tissues. Use morning and evening and after each bowel movement. Recommended duration of treatment: 2 to 6 days.
FOR TOPICAL USE: Apply to affected areas of the skin 2 to 4 times daily.
Storage: Keep container well-closed and store between 59° and 86°F. (15 and 30°C).
How Supplied: 1 oz. tube with rectal applicator.
[*Shown in Product Identification Section*]

DOCTATE®-P Tablets

Composition: Each orange tablet of Doctate-P contains 60 mg of Dioctyl Sodium Sulfosuccinate and 40 mg of Danthron N.F.
Indications and Usage: Dioctyl sodium sulfosuccinate promotes fecal softening by reducing the surface tension of water in the intestines, allowing dispersion of the water into the feces. Danthron is an anthraquinone derivative which provides gentle peristaltic stimulation by acting mainly in the large bowel. Doctate-P is a safe and reliable agent for use in the management of patients with chronic functional constipation and depressed bowel motility in those who suffer from constipation associated with old age, general debility, pregnancy (and post-partum), cardiac failure and certain neurological disorders. Doctate-P is especially useful as pretreatment prior to anorectal procedure or as an evacuant prior to x-ray examination of the colon in preparing patients for barium enema.
Warnings: Caution: Prolonged or continued use of this product can lead to laxative dependency and loss of normal bowel function. Serious side effects from prolonged use or overdose can occur. This product should be used only occasionally, but in any event no longer than daily for one week, except on the advice of a physician. Do not use this product when abdominal pain, nausea, or vomiting are present. A harmless pink or orange discoloration may appear in alkaline urine. Not for use during breast-feeding.
Administration and Dosage: Adult dose: Two to three tablets before retiring or as directed by a physician.
How Supplied: In bottles of 100 and 1000 tablets. Also available, Doctate-100 and Doctate-300 containing 100 mg and 300 mg respectively of Dioctyl Sodium Sulfosuccinate.

ETHATAB® Tablets ℞
(Ethaverine Hydrochloride)

Description: Each yellow Ethatab tablet contains Ethaverine Hydrochloride 100 mg.
Action: Ethatab acts directly on the smooth muscle cells, without involving the autonomic nervous system or its receptors. It produces smooth muscle relaxation, particularly where spasm exists, affecting the larger blood vessels, especially systemic, peripheral and pulmonary vessels, smooth muscle of the intestines, biliary tree, and ureters.
Indications: In peripheral and cerebral vascular insufficiency associated with arterial spasm; also useful as a smooth muscle spasmolytic in spastic conditions of the gastrointestinal and genitourinary tracts.
Contraindications: The use of Ethatab is contraindicated in the presence of complete atrioventricular dissociation.
Precautions: As with vasodilators, Ethatab should be administered with caution to patients with glaucoma. The safety of ethaverine hydrochloride during pregnancy or lactation has not been established; therefore it should not be used in pregnant women or in women of childbearing age unless, in the judgement of the physician, its use is deemed essential to the welfare of the patient.
Side Effects: Even though the incidence of side effects as reported in the literature is very low, it is possible for a patient to evidence nausea, anorexia, abdominal distress, dryness of the throat, hypotension, malaise, lassitude, drowsiness, flushing, sweating, vertigo, respiratory depression, cardiac depression, cardiac arrhythmia and headache. If these side effects occur, reduce dosage or discontinue medication.
Dosage and Administration: In mild or moderate disease, the usual dose for adults is one tablet three times a day. In more difficult cases, dosage may be increased to two tablets three times a day. It is most effective given early in the course of the vascular disorder. Because of the chronic nature of the disease, long-term therapy is required.
Supplied: Ethatab Tablets. Bottles of 100 and 500 tablets. Also available in unit dose packages of 100's.
[*Shown in Product Identification Section*]

FERROBID® DURACAP®
Timed Action Capsules

Composition: Each brown and clear Ferrobid Duracap capsule contains:
Ferrous fumarate..................................225 mg.
(75 mg. elemental iron)
Ascorbic Acid..100 mg.
Copper Sulfate..8 mg.
The Duracap release of Ferrobid differs from the other Duracap capsules. The pellets are especially coated so that the ingredients of Ferrobid are smoothly released only in the sites of optimal absorption, i.e., the stomach and upper small intestine. This ensures optimal absorption and reduces the possibility of gastric upset since the iron is encased in the Duracap pellet until osmotically released into the G.I. fluids. Controlled release of iron is particularly helpful in patients who have demonstrated intolerance to oral iron preparations.
Indications: For the prevention and treatment of iron deficiency anemias where oral administration of iron is indicated.
Action and Uses: Ferrobid Duracap capsules provide optimal iron absorption due to the Duracap release and the action of ascorbic acid. The Duracap process prevents excessive concentrations of iron at any single site in the GI tract and thereby reduces the possibility of gastric upset. Also, the fumarate form of iron may be better tolerated in some individuals. Copper is a logical component of Ferrobid due to its importance in the normal utilization of iron.
Precaution: Discontinue or reduce dosage if any sign of intolerance develops.
Administration and Dosage: Adults: One Duracap capsule twice a day. In more severe iron deficiencies, one capsule three times daily with meals. Children: As directed by a physician.
How Supplied: Bottles of 60 and 500 capsules.

HISTABID® DURACAP® ℞
Timed Action Capsules

Composition: Each pink and white capsule contains:
Chlorpheniramine Maleate ....8 mg.
Phenylpropanolamine Hydrochloride ..75 mg.
The ingredients are prepared in special DURACAP® form that provides for prolonged therapeutic effect. Does not contain any tartrazine dyes.
Action and Uses: The antihistaminic component of HISTABID®, chlorpheniramine maleate, acts to reduce or abolish the allergic response or nasal tissue and most smooth muscles. This action is complemented by the decongestant actions of phenylpropanolamine hydrochloride and by its ability to produce a physiologic antagonism of the chemical mediators of allergy.
Histabid reduces nasal congestion and secretions, ophthalmic manifestations, and bronchial edema.
Indications: Histabid is indicated in conditions in which nasal decongestion is desired concurrently with the action of an antihistamine. Indicated for the symptomatic relief of upper respiratory allergic reactions (Hay Fever), perennial and seasonal allergic rhinitis or vasomotor rhinitis.
Contraindications: Hypersensitivity to any of the components.
Precautions: Until the patient's response to the medication has been determined, he should be warned against engaging in operations requiring alertness. use with caution in patients with hypertension, cardiac or peripheral vascular disease, glaucoma, enlarged prostate, or hyperthyroidism.
Usage in Pregnancy: Adequate reproduction studies have not been performed in animals to determine whether this drug affects fertility in males or females, has teratogenic potential, or has other adverse effects on the fetus. There are no well controlled studies in pregnant women, but marketing experience does not include any positive evidence of adverse effects in the fetus. Although there is no clearly defined risk, such experience cannot exclude the possibility of infrequent or subtle damage to the human fetus.
Side Effects: Reactions due to hypesensitivity including skin rashes, urticaria, hypotension, and thrombocytopenia have been reported on rare occasions. Drowsiness, lassitude, dryness of the mouth, giddiness, mydriasis, increased irritability, excitement, or nausea may be encountered.
Administration and Dosage: Adults and children over 6 years, one capsule on arising and one capsule 12 hours later.
The DURACAP® form provides prolonged therapeutic effect, providing effect throughout the day, and if taken at bedtime relief is made possible throughout the night.
How Supplied: Bottles of 100 and 500 pink and white capsules.
[*Shown in Product Identification Section*]

THEOBID® & THEOBID® JR. ℞
(Theophylline, Anhydrous)
DURACAP®
Timed Action Capsules

Composition: Two strengths of anhydrous theophylline in timed action capsules are available. Each blue and white THEOBID DURACAP capsule contains:

Theophylline, Anhydrous .... 260 mg.
Each two-toned blue THEOBID JR. DURACAP capsule contains:
Theophylline, Anhydrous .... 130 mg.

Action and Uses: Theobid Duracap capsules are timed action capsules which provide prolonged therapeutic effect. Since theophylline is released slowly from the Duracap pellets, the likelihood of gastric irritation is minimized or eliminated, in most patients.

Theobid Duracap capsules are indicated for patients requiring continuous therapy for the prevention of asthmatic attacks. The bronchodilating action of theophylline helps to relieve bronchospasm. The relaxation of bronchospasm counteracts the entrapment of residual air and the decrease in vital capacity, thus allaying the psychic anxiety of recurrence of asthmatic attacks. By means of the special coating of the pellets, Theobid provides prolonged therapeutic effect, reducing the necessity for night emergency medication. Severe asthamtic attacks may require inhalant and/or other parenteral therapy. THEOBID DURACAP CAPSULES ARE ESPECIALLY INDICATED FOR THOSE PATIENTS WHO CANNOT TOLERATE EPHEDRINE OR OTHER SYMPATHOMIMETIC DRUGS.

Theobid Duracap capsules are useful as a preventive adjunct in the overall management of bronchial asthma.

Indications: Indicated for the symptomatic relief of bronchial asthma, asthmatic bronchitis and related diseases associated with bronchospasm. Theobid Duracap capsules may be used prophylactically.

THEOBID JR. Is designed for administration to adults of small stature, those sensitive to theophylline and those with severe renal, liver or heart disease who cannot tolerate a full adult does of theophylline.

Contraindications: Contraindicated in patients known to be sensitive to any of the ingredients.

Precautions: Adequate reproduction studies have not been performed in animals to determine whether this drug affects fertility in males or females, has teratogenic potential, or has other adverse effects on the fetus. There are no well controlled studies in pregnant women, but marketing experience does not include any positive evidence of adverse effects in the fetus. Although there is no clearly defined risk, such experience cannot exclude the possibility of infrequent or subtle damage to the human fetus.

Adverse Reactions: Side effects are rare. Mild gastric distress, central nervous system stimulation, and palpitation may occur. The risk of adverse reactions increases with theophylline plasma levels over 20 mcg/ml.

Administration and Dosage:

THEOBID

Adults: One capsule on arising and one capsule 12 hours, later. When higher blood levels are required, the dosage is increased as follows: moderate cases—one capsule every 8 hours, severe cases—two capsules every 12 hours the first day, then one capsule every 8 hours.

THEOBID Jr.

Adults: One or two capsules every 8 to 12 hours.

For patients who have difficulty in swallowing the capsule, the contents may be mixed with a vehicle (jam, applesauce, etc.) for oral administration (without chewing).

Note: Dosage of Theobid Duracap Capsules should be adjusted on an individual basis depending on severity of symptoms, body weight and tolerance. When initiating therapy, periodic plasma theophylline determination may be helpful in establishing the optimum dose to maintain plasma concentrations between 10 and 20 mcg/ml.

How Supplied: Bottles of 60 and 500 Capsules. Theobid is also available in unit dose packages of 100.

[Shown in Product Identification Section]

TRI–CONE® Capsules

Composition: Each white and black capsule contains:
Amylase .... 10 mg
Prolase .... 10 mg
Lipase .... 10 mg
Simethicone .... 40 mg

Actions and Uses: Tri-cone is indicated for the symptomatic relief of functional digestive disorders characterized by functional gastric bloating, dyspepsia, and flatulence resulting from failure to chew food properly, inadequate digestive competency due to disease or age, or faulty dietary habits. Tri-Cone is also indicated as a supplement to normal enzyme activity of the body in absorptive and assimilative defects associated with surgery on the stomach, small bowel, or pancreas and associated with chronic pancreatitis and pancreatic insufficiency.

Simethicone acts to relieve or alleviate the pain and other symptoms of gaseousness produced by bacterial fermentation and aerophagia.

The enzymes, particularly the proteolytic enzyme, do not require acid conditions to be activated which may be of special benefit in aiding digestion in geriatric patients with insufficient gastric acidity due to hypochlorhydria.

Contraindications: Known allergy to an ingredient.

Dosage: Two or three capsules after meals as required to relieve the symptoms of gas and aid digestion of fats, starches and proteins.

How Supplied: Bottles of 60 and 500 capsules.

[Shown in Product Identification Section]

TRI–CONE® PLUS Capsules ℞

Composition: Each two-tone green capsule contains:
Amylase .... 10 mg.
Prolase .... 10 mg.
Lipase .... 10 mg.
Simethicone .... 40 mg.
Hyoscyamine Sulfate .... 0.025 mg.

Actions and Uses: Tri-Cone Plus is indicated for the symptomatic relief of functional digestive disorders characterized by functional gastric bloating, dyspepsia, and flatulence resulting from failure to chew food properly, inadequate digestive competency due to disease or age, or faulty dietary habits. Tri-Cone Plus is also indicated as a supplement to normal enzyme activity of the body in absorptive and assimilative defects associated with surgery on the stomach, small bowel, or pancreas and associated with chronic pancreatitis and pancreatic insufficiency. Simethicone acts to relieve or alleviate the pain and other symptoms of gaseousness produced by bacterial fermentation and aerophagia. The enzymes, particularly the proteolytic enzyme, do not require acid conditions to be activated which may be of special benefit in aiding digestion in geriatric patients with insufficient gastric acidity due to hypochlorhydria.

Hyoscyamine is added to Tri-Cone Plus capsules for its spasmolytic effect in the alimentary tract, which aids in the relief of pain due to spasm of the gastrointestinal masculature.

Contraindications: Acute glaucoma, advanced renal or hepatic disease, biliary or gastrointestinal tract obstruction or a hypersensitivity to any ingredient.

Precautions: Administer with caution to patients with incipient glaucoma, prostatic hypertrophy and known sensitivity to pork or enzymes.

Adverse Reactions: Mild dryness of the mouth, blurring of vision and difficult urination may occur at higher dosage levels.

Dosage: Adults—Two or three capsules with or after meals.

How Supplied: Bottles of 60 and 500 capsules.

[Shown in Product Identification Section]

VICON–C® Capsules
(Therapeutic Vitamins and Minerals)

Composition: Each yellow and orange capsule contains:
Ascorbic Acid .... 300 mg.
Niacinamide .... 100 mg.
Thiamine Mononitrate .... 20 mg.
d-Calcium Pantothenate .... 20 mg.
Riboflavin .... 10 mg.
Pyridoxine Hydrochloride .... 5 mg.
Magnesium Sulfate* .... 70 mg.
Zinc sulfate** .... 80 mg.
* As 50 mg. of dried Magnesium Sulfate
** As 50 mg. of dried Zinc Sulfate.

Actions and Uses: VICON-C® is indicated in the treatment of patients with deficiencies of, or increased requirements for Vitamin C, B-Complex vitamins, zinc and/or magnesium. The components of Vicon-C® have important roles in nutrition, tissue growth and repair, and the prevention of hemorrhage. Tissue injury resulting from trauma, burns or surgery may rapidly deplete the body stores of Vitamin C, the B-Complex vitamins and zinc. Patients maintained on parenteral fluids for extended periods or patients with burns, wounds or diarrhea often develop deficiencies of Vitamin C, the B-Complex vitamins and zinc.

VICON-C® is recommended for deficiencies or the prevention of deficiencies of Vitamin C, the B-Complex vitamins, magnesium and/or zinc in conditions such as febrile diseases, chronic or acute infections, burns fractures, surgery, toxic conditions, physiologic stress, alcoholism, pregnancy, lactation, geriatrics, gastritis, peptic ulcer, colitis and in conditions involving special diets and weight-reduction diets. It is also recommended in dentistry for these deficiencies in conditions such as herpetic stomatitis, aphthous stomatitis, cheilosis, herpangina, gingivitis and states involving oral surgery.

Administration and Dosage: One capsule 2 or 3 times daily or as directed by a physician for treatment of deficiencies.

How Supplied: Bottles of 60 and 500 Capsules and Unit Dose Pack of 240 Capsules.

[Shown in Product Identification Section]

VICON®–PLUS Capsules
(Therapeutic Vitamins and Minerals)

Composition: Each red and beige capsule contains:
Vitamin A .... 4,000 I.U.
Vitamin E .... 50 I.U.
Ascorbic Acid .... 150 mg.
Zinc Sulfate* .... 80 mg.
Magnesium Sulfate** .... 70 mg.
Niacinamide .... 25 mg.
Thiamine Mononitrate .... 10 mg.
d-Calcium Pantothenate .... 10 mg.
Riboflavin .... 5 mg.
Manganese Chloride .... 4 mg.
Pyridoxine HCl .... 2 mg.
* As 50 mg. of Dried Zinc Sulfate
** As 50 mg. of Dried Magnesium Sulfate

Vicon-Plus is an extended range vitamin-mineral supplement formulated to aid patient recovery by helping to meet increased nutritional demands.

Indications: For nutritional supplementation of the patient undergoing physiologic stress due to surgery, burns, trauma, febrile illnesses, or poor nutrition.

Dosage: 1 capsule twice daily or as prescribed by a physician for treatment of deficiencies. Dosage should not exceed 8 capsules daily due to the possible toxicity of large dosages of vitamin A.

How Supplied: In bottles of 60 capsules and 500 capsules.

[Shown in Product Identification Section]

Continued on next page

Glaxo—Cont.

VICON FORTE® Capsules ℞
(Therapeutic Vitamins-Minerals)

Description: Each black and orange capsule contains:

Vitamin A	8,000 I.U.
Vitamin E	50 I.U.
Ascorbic Acid	150 mg.
Zinc Sulfate*	80 mg.
Magnesium Sulfate**	70 mg.
Niacinamide	25 mg.
Thiamine Mononitrate	10 mg.
d-Calcium Pantothenate	10 mg.
Riboflavin	5 mg.
Manganese Chloride	4 mg.
Folic Acid	1 mg.
Vitamin B_{12}(Cyanocobalamin)	10 mcg.

* As 50 mg. of dried Zinc Sulfate
** As 50 mg. of dried Magnesium Sulfate

VICON FORTE® contains the cofactors necessary in meeting acute metabolic stress while providing the extended range of vitamin replacement important in convalescence.

Indications: VICON FORTE is indicated for the prophylaxis or treatment of vitamin and mineral deficiencies associated with restricted diets, improper food intake, alcoholism, and decreased absorption or utilization. VICON FORTE is also indicated in patients with increased requirements for vitamins and minerals due to chronic disease, infection, burns and pregnancy. Pre- and post-operative use of VICON FORTE can provide the increased amounts of vitamins and minerals necessary for optimal recovery from the stress of surgery.

Precautions: Folic acid may obscure pernicious anemia in that the peripheral blood picture may revert to normal while neurological manifestations remain progressive.

Dosage: One capsule daily or as directed by the physician.

How Supplied: In bottles of 60 and 500 capsules.

Also Available: Unit dose packages of 100 capsules.

[*Shown in Product Identification Section*]

VICON® with IRON
Multivitamins with Iron and Zinc

Description: Each pink and red Vicon® with Iron capsule for oral administration contains:

Iron (as Fumarate)	30 mg.
Zinc (as Sulfate)*	18.5 mg.
Vitamin C	300 mg.
Vitamin E	30 I.U.
Niacinamide	30 mg.
Pantothenic Acid**	10 mg.
Pyridoxine Hydrochloride	5 mg.
Thaimine Mononitrate	2 mg.
Riboflaviin	2 mg.

*Equivalent to 80 mg, Zinc Sulfate, U.S.P.
**As Calcium Pantothenate

Indications and Usage: Vicon with Iron is specifically formulated for the woman of childbearing age for use in the prevention of deficiencies of vitamin C and E, the B-complex vitamins and the minerals iron and zinc. It provides safe and effective levels of elemental iron (166% of U.S. RDA) in the form of ferrous fumarate. It also provides 123% of the U.S. RDA for zinc, as zinc sulfate, which can help prevent zinc deficiencies that can accompany acute and chronic infections, surgery, alcoholism and drug therapy.

Dosage and Administration: One capsule daily or as directed by physician.

How Supplied: Bottles of 60 and 500 capsules.

VI-ZAC® Capsules
(Therapeutic Vitamin-Mineral)

Composition: Each orange capsule contains:

Vitamin A	5000 I.U.
Ascorbic Acid	500 mg
Vitamin E	50 I.U.
Zinc Sulfate USP*	80 mg

* as 50 mg dried Zinc Sulfate.

Actions and Uses: Vi-ZAC™ is indicated in the treatment of patients with deficiencies of, or increased requirements for, Vitamins A, C and E and zinc. The VI-ZAC formulation is a limited vitamin-mineral formulation designed to meet special needs. It is particularly indicated where there is no requirement for supplemental amounts of the B-Complex vitamins and their attendant appetite stimulation. The formulation is also designed for patients who cannot tolerate magnesium supplements but do need supplemental amounts of zinc.

Precautions: Although rarely encountered, vitamin A in large doses daily for several months or longer may cause toxicity.

Dosage: One or two capsules daily or as directed by the physician for the treatment of deficiencies.

How Supplied: In bottles of 60 and 500 capsules.

[*Shown in Product Identification Section*]

Glenbrook Laboratories
Division of Sterling Drug Inc.
90 PARK AVENUE
NEW YORK, NY 10016

BAYER® ASPIRIN AND BAYER® CHILDREN'S CHEWABLE ASPIRIN
Aspirin (Acetylsalicylic Acid)

Composition: Bayer Aspirin—Aspirin 5 grains. (325 mg.)
Bayer Children's Chewable Aspirin—Aspirin 1¼ grains (81 mg.) per orange flavored chewable tablet.

Action and Uses: Analgesic, antipyretic, anti-inflammatory. For relief of headache; painful discomfort and fever of colds and flu; muscular aches and pains; temporary relief of minor pains of arthritis, rheumatism, bursitis, lumbago, sciatica; toothache, teething pains, and pain following dental procedures; neuralgia and neuritic pain; functional menstrual pain; sleeplessness when caused by minor painful discomforts; painful discomfort and fever accompanying immunizations.

Administration and Dosage: The following dosages are those provided in the packaging, as appropriate for self-medication. Larger or more frequent dosage may be necessary as appropriate to the condition or needs of the patient.

Bayer Aspirin—5 grain (325 mg.) tablets
Adult Dose: One or two tablets with water. May be repeated every four hours as necessary up to 12 tablets a day.
Children's Dose: To be administered only under adult supervision.

Under 2 years	per physician
2 to under 4 years	½ tablet
4 to under 6 years	¾ tablet
6 to under 9 years	1 tablet
9 to under 11 years	1¼ tablets
11 to under 12 years	1½ tablets
Over 12 years	same as adult

Indicated dosage may be repeated every 4 hours, up to but not more than five times a day. Larger dosage may be prescribed per physician.

Bayer Children's Chewable Aspirin—1¼ grain (81 mg.) tablets

Under 2 years	per physician
2 to under 4 years	2 tablets
4 to under 6 years	3 tablets
6 to under 9 years	4 tablets
9 to under 11 years	5 tablets
11 to under 12 years	6 tablets

Indicated dosage may be repeated every 4 hours, up to but not more than five times a day. Larger dosage may be prescribed per physician.

Contraindications: Hypersensitivity to salicylates. To be used with caution in presence of peptic ulcer, asthma, or with anticoagulant therapy.

How Supplied:
Bayer Aspirin 5 grains (325 mg.)—
NDC-12843-101-10, packs of 12 tablets
NDC-12843-101-11, bottles of 24 tablets
NDC-12843-101-17, bottles of 50 tablets
NDC-12843-101-12, bottles of 100 tablets
NDC-12843-101-20, bottles of 200 tablets
NDC-12843-101-13, bottles of 300 tablets
Child-resistant safety closures on 12s, 24s, 50s, 200s, 300s. Bottle of 100s available without safety closure for households without small children.
Bayer Children's Chewable Aspirin 1¼ grains (81 mg.)—
NDC-12843-131-05, bottle of 36 tablets with child-resistant safety closure.
Samples available on request.

BAYER® CHILDREN'S COLD TABLETS

Composition: Each tablet contains phenylpropanolamine HCl 3.125 mg., aspirin 1¼ gr. (81 mg.); the tablets are orange flavored and chewable.

Action and Uses: Bayer Children's Cold Tablets combine two effective ingredients: a gentle decongestant to relieve nasal congestion and ease breathing, and genuine Bayer Aspirin to reduce fever and relieve minor aches and pains of colds and flu.

Administration and Dosage: The following dosage is provided in the packaging, as appropriate for self-medication only under adult supervision.

Under 3 years - consult physician
3 years - 1 tablet
4 to 5 years - 2 tablets
6 to 12 years - 4 tablets

Indicated dosage may be repeated every four hours up to but not more than four times a day. Larger or more frequent dosage may be necessary as appropriate to the condition or needs of the patient.

Contraindications: Side effects at higher doses may include nervousness, dizziness, sleeplessness. To be used with caution in presence of high blood pressure, heart disease, diabetes, asthma, or thyroid disease.

How Supplied: NDC-12843-181-01, bottles of 30 tablets with child-resistant safety closure. Samples available on request.

BAYER® COUGH SYRUP FOR CHILDREN

Composition: Each 5 ml. (1 tsp.) contains phenylpropanolamine HCl 9 mg. and dextromethorphan hydrobromide 7.5 mg., alcohol 5% Cherry flavored.

Action and Uses: Bayer Cough Syrup for Children combines two effective ingredients in a syrup with a very appealing cherry flavor: a gentle nasal decongestant and a cough suppressant.

Administration and Dosage: The following dosage is provided on the packaging, as appropriate for self-medication by an adult:

Under 2 years	per physician
2–5 years:	1 teaspoon every 4 hours, not to exceed 4 teaspoons every 24 hours.
6–12 years:	2 teaspoons every 4 hours, not to exceed 8 teaspoons every 24 hours.

Contraindications and Precautions: Do not give to children under 2, or exceed recommended dosage, unless directed by a physician. Persistent cough may indicate the presence of

a serious condition. Persons with persistent cough, high fever, high blood pressure, heart disease, diabetes or thyroid disease should use only as directed by a physician. Keep out of reach of children.
How Supplied: NDC–12843-401-02, 3.0 oz. bottles. Samples available on request.

BAYER® TIMED-RELEASE ASPIRIN
(aspirin)

Description: Each oblong white scored tablet contains 10 grains (650 mg.) of aspirin in microencapsulation form.
Indications: Bayer Timed-Release Aspirin is indicated for the temporary relief of low grade pain amenable to relief with salicylates, such as in rheumatoid arthritis, osteoarthritis, spondylitis, bursitis and other forms of rheumatism, as well as in many common musculoskeletal disorders. It possesses the same advantages for other types of prolonged aches and pains, such as minor injuries, dental pain and dysmenorrhea. Its long-lasting effectiveness should also make it valuable as an analgesic in simple headache, colds, grippe, flu and other similar conditions in which aspirin is indicated for symptomatic relief, either by itself or as an adjunct to specific therapy.
Dosage: Two Bayer Timed-Release Aspirin tablets q. 8 h. provide effective long-lasting pain relief. This two-tablet (20 grain or 1300 mg.) dose of timed-release aspirin promptly produces salicylate blood levels greater than those achieved by a 10-grain (650 mg.) dose of regular aspirin, and in the second 4 hour period produces a salicylate blood level curve which approximates that of two successive 10-grain (650 mg.) doses of regular aspirin at 4 hour intervals. The 10-grain (650 mg.) scored Bayer Timed-Release Aspirin tablets permit administration of aspirin in multiples of 5 grains (325 mg.), allowing individualization of dosage to meet the specific needs of the patient. For the convenience of patients on a regular aspirin dosage schedule, two 10-grain (650 mg.) Bayer Timed-Release Aspirin tablets may be administered with water every 8 hours. Whenever possible, two tablets (20 grains or 1300 mg.) should be given before retiring to provide effective analgesic and anti-inflammatory action—for relief of pain throughout the night and lessening of stiffness upon arising. Do not exceed 6 tablets in 24 hours. Bayer Timed-Release Aspirin has been made in a special capsule-shaped tablet to permit easy swallowing. However, for patients who do have difficulty, Bayer Timed-Release Aspirin tablets may be gently crumbled in the mouth and swallowed with water without loss of timed-release effect. There is no bitter "aspirin" taste. For children under 12, per physician.
Side Effects: Side effects encountered with regular aspirin may be encountered with Bayer Timed-Release Aspirin. Tinnitus and dizziness are the ones most frequently encountered.
Contraindications and Precautions: Bayer Timed-Release Aspirin is contraindicated in patients with marked aspirin hypersensitivity, and should be given with extreme caution to any patient with a history of adverse reaction to salicylates. It may cautiously be tried in patients intolerant to aspirin because of gastric irritation, but the usual precautions for any form of aspirin should be observed in patients with gastric ulcers, bleeding tendencies, asthma, or hypoprothrombinemia.
Supplied:

Tablets in Bottle of 30's	NDC-12843-191-72
Tablets in Bottle of 72's	NDC-12843-191-74
Tablets in Bottle of 125's	NDC-12843-191-76

All sizes packaged in child-resistant safety closure except 72's which is a size recommended for households without young children.
Samples available upon request.

MIDOL®

Composition: Each Caplet® contains Aspirin 454 mg (7 grains); Cinnamedrine Hydrochloride 14.9 mg; Caffeine 32.4 mg.
Action and Uses: Analgesic, antipyretic, antispasmodic. For fast relief of functional menstrual pain, cramps, irritability; "nervous" headache and the irritability associated with premenstrual tension; headache, neuralgia; low backache due to fatigue, strain or menstruation.
Usage Adult Dosage: Two Caplets with water. Repeat one or two Caplets every four hours as needed, up to eight Caplets per day.
How Supplied: White, capsule-shaped Caplets.
NDC-12843-151-34, strip packs of 12 Caplets
NDC-12843-151-36, bottles of 30 Caplets
NDC-12843-151-38, bottles of 60 Caplets
Child-resistant safety closures on bottles of 30 to 60 Caplets.
Samples Supplied: Available upon request.

PHILLIPS' MILK OF MAGNESIA

Composition: A suspension of magnesium hydroxide, meeting all USP specifications.
Action and Uses: Phillips' Milk of Magnesia is a mild saline laxative and is indicated for the relief of constipation especially in patients with hemorrhoids, obstetric patients, cardiacs, and in geriatric patients where straining at stool is contraindicated. Phillips' also acts as an antacid, and is effective for the relief of symptoms associated with gastric hyperacidity.
Administration and Dosage: As a laxative, adults 2 to 4 tbsp. followed by a glass of water. Children-infants 1 tsp.; over one year ¼ to ½ adult dose, depending on age. As a antacid, 1 to 3 tsps. with a little water, up to four times a day. Children-1 to 12 years: ¼ to ½ adult dose up to four times a day.
Contraindications: Abdominal pain, nausea, vomiting or other symptoms of appendicitis.
How Supplied: Phillips' Milk of Magnesia is available in regular and mint in bottles of:

Regular	
4 fl. oz.	NDC-12843-353-01
12 fl. oz.	NDC-12843-353-02
26 fl. oz.	NDC-12843-353-03
Mint	
4 fl oz.	NDC-12843-363-04
12 fl. oz.	NDC-12843-363-05
26 fl. oz.	NDC-12843-363-06

VANQUISH®

Composition: Each Caplet contains aspirin 227 mg., acetaminophen 194 mg., caffeine 33 mg., dried aluminum hydroxide gel 25 mg.; magnesium hydroxide 50 mg.
Action and Uses: A buffered analgesic, antipyretic for relief of headache; muscular aches and pains; neuralgia and neuritic pain; pain following dental procedures; for painful discomforts and fever of colds and flu; functional menstrual pain, headache and pain due to cramps; temporary relief from minor pains of arthritis, rheumatism, bursitis, lumbago, sciatica.
Usual Adult Dosage: Two caplets with water. May be repeated every four hours if necessary up to 12 tablets per day. Larger or more frequent doses may be prescribed by physician if necessary.
Contraindications: Hypersensitivity to salicylates.
(To be used with caution during anticoagulant therapy or in asthmatic patients.)
How Supplied: White, capsule-shaped Caplets in bottles of:
15 Caplets NDC 12843-17142
30 Caplets NDC 12843-17144
60 Caplets NDC 12843-17146
100 Caplets NDC 12843-17148

Glenwood Laboratories, Inc.
83 N. SUMMIT STREET
TENAFLY, NJ 07670

MYOTONACHOL™ ℞
Bethanechol Chloride—Oral

Description: Bethanechol chloride is an ester of a choline-like compound.
Actions: Bethanechol chloride is a synthetic choline ester with postganglionic parasympathomimetic actions mediated via direct stimulation of cholinergic receptors. Its actions are similar to those of acetylcholine—the natural neurohormonal mediator of postganglionic parasympathetic receptors and of certain sympathetic nerves (sweat glands and some blood vessels)—which usually produce smooth muscle stimulation. However, unlike acetylcholine, bethanechol chloride is not inactivated by cholinesterases and therefore has more prolonged effects. Bethanechol chloride's principal effects are due predominately to its muscarinic action, i.e., stimulating micturition and gastrointestinal peristalsis while its nicotinic action is slight. Its cardiovascular effects when administered orally, are ordinarily inconspicious and constitute a slight transient fall in diastolic pressure with a minor reflex tachycardia. Other effects of bethanechol chloride's parasympathetic stimulating actions include contracted pupils, salivation, constricted bronchi, and dilated splanchnic vessels. The pharmacological actions of bethanechol chloride are more efficaciously produced following subcutaneous than with oral administration.
Indications: Acute postoperative and postpartum nonobstructive (functional) urinary retention, and neurogenic atony of the urinary bladder with retention.
Contraindications: Bethanechol chloride is contraindicated in the presence of mechanical obstruction of the gastrointestinal or urinary tracts and hollow viscera, or in conditions where the integrity of the gastrointestinal or bladder wall is questionable. Also, it is contraindicated in spastic, including peptic ulcer or acute in flammatory conditions of the gastrointestinal tract, or peritonitis.
Other major contraindications to the use of bethanechol chloride are latent or active asthma, hyperthyroidism, and coronary occlusion. Additional contraindications are bradycardia, atrio-ventricular conduction defects, vasomotor instability, hypotention, hypertention, coronary artery disease, epilepsy and parkinsonism.
Precautions: Special care and consideration are required when bethanechol chloride is administered to patients concomitantly being treated with other drugs with which pharmacologic interactions may occur. Examples of drugs with potentials for such interactions are: quinidine and procainamide, which may antagonize cholinergic effects; cholinergic drugs, particularly cholinesterase inhibitors, where additive effects may occur. When administered to patients receiving ganglionic blocking compounds a critical fall in blood pressure may occur which usually is preceeded by severe abdominal symptoms.
Adverse Reactions: Untoward effects are usually due to overdosage but occur infrequently with the oral administration of bethanechol chloride. Abdominal discomfort, salivation, flushing of the skin ("hot feeling"), sweating, nausea and vomiting are early signs of overdosage. Asthmatic attacks, especially in asthmatic individuals may be precipitated. Substernal pressure or pain may occur, however, it is uncertain whether this is due to bronchoconstriction, or spasm of the esophagus. Myocardial hypoxia must be considered if a marked fall in blood pressure occurs.

Continued on next page

Glenwood—Cont.

Transient syncope with cardiac arrest, transient complete heart block, dyspnea, and orthostatic hypotention may be associated with large doses. Patients with hypertention may react to the drug with a precipitious fall in blood pressure. Short periods of atrial fibrillation have been observed in hyperthyroid individuals following the administration of cholinergic drugs. Also, involuntary defecation and urinary urgency may occur after large doses. **Atropine sulfate is a specific antidote.** A dose of 0.5 mg.—1.0 mg. ($\frac{1}{100}$ grain–$\frac{1}{50}$ grain), for intramuscular or intravenous administration, should be readily available to counteract severe toxic cardiovascular or bronchoconstrictor responses to bethanechol chloride.

Dosage and Administration: The usual adult oral dose is administered with 5, 10 or 25 mg. tablets, three or four times daily. The minimum effective dose is determined by giving 5 or 10 mg. initially and repeating in the same amounts at one or two hour intervals, to a maximum of 30 mg., until the desired response is obtained. The drug's effects appear within 60 to 90 minutes and persist for an hour.

How Supplied: Myotonachol.

5 mg. tablets, flat, NDC 0516-0020-01 in bottles of 100s.
10 mg. tablets, flat, NDC 0516-0021-01 in bottles of 100s.
25 mg. tablets, flat, NDC 0516-0022-01 in bottles of 100s.
10 mg. and 25 mg. tablets also available in unit dose packing of 100s.

POTABA® ℞
Potassium p-Aminobenzoate, Glenwood
Systemic ANTIFIBROSIS THERAPY

Formula: POTABA is chemically a pure potassium p-aminobenzoate, KPAB.

> **Indications:** Based on a review of this drug by the National Academy of Sciences-National Research Council and/or other information, FDA has classified the indications as follows:
> "Possibly" effective: Potassium aminobenzoate is possibly effective in the treatment of scleroderma, dermatomyositis, morphea, linear scleroderma, pemphigus, and Peyronie's disease.
> Final classification of the less-than-effective indications requires further investigation.

Advantages: POTABA offers a means of treatment of serious and often chronic entities involving fibrosis and nonsuppurative inflammation.

Pharmacology: P-Aminobenzoate is considered a member of the vitamin B complex. Small amounts are found in cereal, eggs, milk and meats. Detectable amounts are normally present in human blood, spinal fluid, urine, and sweat. PABA is a component of several biologically important systems, and it participates in a number of fundamental biological processes. It has been suggested that the antifibrosis action of POTABA is due to its mediation of increased oxygen uptake at the tissue level. Fibrosis is believed to occur from either too much serotonin or too little monoamine oxidase activity over a period of time. Monoamine oxidase requires an adequate supply of oxygen to function properly. By increasing oxygen supply at the tissue level POTABA may enhance MAO activity and prevent or bring about regression of fibrosis.

Clinical Uses:

PEYRONIE'S DISEASE: 21 patients with Peyronie's disease were placed on POTABA therapy for periods ranging from 3 months to 2 years. Pain disappeared from 16 of 16 cases in which it had been present. There was objective improvement in penile deformity in 10 of 17 patients, and decrease in plaque size in 16 of 21. The authors suggest that this medication offers no hazard of further local injury as may result from other therapy. There were no significant untoward effects encountered on long term POTABA therapy.

SCLERODERMA: Of 135 patients with diffuse systemic sclerosis treated with POTABA every patient but one has shown softening of the involved skin if treatment has been continued for 3 months or longer. The responses have been reported in a number of publications. The treatment program consists of systemic antifibrosis therapy with POTABA, physical therapy, including deep breathing exercises and dynamic traction splints where indicated, and bethanechol chloride (MYOCHOLINE, Glenwood) for relief of dysphagia as well as small doses of reserpine for amelioration of Raynaud's phenomena.

DERMATOMYOSITIS: Five patients with scleroderma and 2 with dermatomyositis were treated with POTABA. There was striking clinical improvement in each patient. Doses of 15-20 grams per day were well tolerated, and patients were easily able to take these doses.

MORPHEA and LINEAR SCLERODERMA: All 14 patients with localized forms of scleroderma placed on long-term Potaba treatment showed softening of the sclerotic component of their disorder. Treatment is particularly indicated in patients where persistent compressive sclerosis may contribute even greater disfigurement or functional embarrassment from secondary pressure atrophy.

Dosage and Administration: The average adult daily dose of POTABA is 12 grams, usually given in four to six divided doses. Tablets and capsules 0.5 gram are given at the rate of 4 tablets or capsules 6 times daily, or 6 given four times daily, usually with meals, and at bedtime with a snack. Tablets must be dissolved in an adequate amount of liquid to prevent gastrointestinal upset.

POTABA Envules contain 2 grams pure drug each, and constitute the individual average dose. 6 Envules are given for a total of 12 grams POTABA daily.

POTABA Powder is used to prepare solutions, which are kept refrigerated, but for no longer than one week. 100 grams POTABA powder make 1 quart of 10% solution when dissolved in potable tap water. Children are given 1 gram POTABA daily in divided doses for each 10 lbs. of body weight.

Side Effects: Anorexia, nausea, fever and rash have occurred infrequently and subside with omission of the drug. Desensitization can be accomplished and treatment resumed.

Precautions: Should anorexia or nausea occur, therapy is interrupted until the patient is eating normally again. This permits prompt subsidence of symptoms and also avoids the possible development of hypoglycemia. Give cautiously to patients with renal disease. If a hypersensitivity reaction should occur, Potaba should be stopped.

Contraindications: POTABA should not be administered to patients taking sulfonamides.

How Supplied: POTABA Capsules 0.5 gm. in 250's and 1,000's; POTABA Envules 2.0 gm. in boxes of 50's; POTABA Powder, pure, in 100 gm. and 1 lb.; POTABA Tablets 0.5 gm. in 100's and 1,000's.

Products are cross-indexed by generic and chemical names in the

YELLOW SECTION

Gray Pharmaceutical Co.
50 WASHINGTON STREET
NORWALK, CT 06856

X-PREP® LIQUID
(standardized extract of senna fruit)

Action and Uses: An easy-to-administer, palatable, highly effective bowel evacuant for the preparation of the intestinal tract prior to G.I. and urological radiography as well as colonoscopy, sigmoidoscopy and other diagnostic bowel procedures. Permits excellent visualization without residual oil droplets. X-PREP Liquid is fully prepared in a single dose container—all the patient has to do is drink the contents of one small bottle (2½ fl. oz.). Good patient cooperation is ensured because of highly pleasant taste. Predictable effectiveness helps reduce or eliminate the need for enemas prior to radiography.

Contraindications: Acute surgical abdomen. X-PREP Liquid is intended solely for bowel evacuation prior to diagnostic examination of the colon.

Caution: In diabetic patients, the physician should be aware of the sugar content of X-PREP Liquid (50 grams per 2½ fl. oz. dose).

Adverse Reactions: As with all potent purgatives, some patients may experience abdominal discomfort and nausea; vomiting is rare.

Administration and Dosage: For adults: X-PREP Liquid: entire contents of bottle should be taken between 2:00 and 4:00 p.m. on the day prior to diagnostic procedure. Patients should be advised to expect a thorough, strong bowel action to begin approximately six hours later. After X-PREP Liquid is taken, diet should be confined to clear fluids.

X-PREP Liquid has proved to be effective following the above regimen. However, at physician's discretion, X-PREP Liquid may be given in divided doses, particularly to elderly or debilitated patients. The following split dosage regimens are equally effective: (1) One-half (½) of the contents of the bottle is taken at bedtime two days prior to diagnostic procedure. On day prior to examination, remaining contents of bottle is taken, also at bedtime. OR (2) On the day prior to examination, one-half (½) contents of bottle is taken at noon and the remaining one-half (½) at 4:00 p.m.

Some physicians prefer the hydration method, with 24-hour liquid diet and consumption of several extra glasses of water during this period, prior to the administration of X-PREP Liquid. Morning enema is optional. X-PREP Liquid may be successfully combined with adjunctive laxative suppositories or citrate of magnesia

How Supplied: 2½ fl. oz. bottles (alcohol 7% by volume), each providing a single, complete adult dose.

Also Available: X-PREP® Powder (standardized senna concentrate), in ¾ oz. containers, each providing a single, complete adult dose.

Now Available—X-PREP™ Bowel Evacuant Kit. Each kit contains: Two SENOKOT® S Tablets (standardized senna concentrate and dioctyl sodium sulfosuccinate), one bottle of X-PREP Liquid 2½ fl. oz., and one RECTOLAX™ Suppository (bisacodyl 10 mg), plus easy-to-follow patient instructions for hydration, clear liquid diet, and the correct time sequence of administering the above laxatives.

Products are cross-indexed

by product classifications

in the

BLUE SECTION

Guardian Chemical Corporation
**230 MARCUS BLVD.
HAUPPAUGE, L.I., NY 11787**

CLORPACTIN® WCS-90
(brand of sodium oxychlorosene)

Composition: Stabilized organic derivative of hypochlorous acid. A white, water soluble powder with a characteristic smell of hypochlorous acid. Active chlorine derived from calcium hypochlorite: 3–4%.
Action and Uses: For use as a topical antiseptic for treating localized infections, particularly when resistant organisms are present. Complete spectrum (bacteria, fungi, viruses, mold, yeast and spores); effective in cases of antibiotic resistance; nontoxic and non-allergenic in use concentrations.
Administration and Dosage: Applied by irrigation, instillations, spray, soaks or wet compresses, preferably thoroughly cleansing with gravity flow irrigation or syringe to provide copious quantities of fresh solution to remove the organic wastes and debris from the site of the involvement. Also for preoperative skin preparation and postoperative protection. Generally applied as the 0.4% solution in water, or isotonic saline, but as the 0.1% to 0.2% in Urology and Ophthalmology.
Contraindications: The use of this product is contraindicated where the site of the infection is not exposed to the direct contact with the solution. Not for systemic use.
How Supplied: In boxes containing 5 x 2 gram bottles.

LUBRASEPTIC® JELLY

Composition: Active ingredients: Aryl phenols, as phenyl phenol 0.1%, Alkyl phenols, as amyl phenol 0.02%, in water miscible form as an acid complex. Phenyl mercuric nitrate 0.007%.
Uses: For urethral instillation, prior to insertion of cystoscopes or sounds; for urethral dilations in the case of strictures. For proctologic use, in cases of hemorrhoids, or for post-hemorrhoidectomies, to provide increased comfort between and during the passage of stools. For endotracheal intubation. For use whenever a sterile water soluble lubricant is required: on cystoscopes and proctoscopes, in urological, rectal, and vaginal examinations or for use as a sterile dressing on burns, abrasions, and decubitus ulcers (bedsores).
Precautions and Side Effects: No serious side effects or contraindications are known. Urethral instillation, in some individuals, may cause a temporary burning or stinging sensation but this usually disappears in several minutes. Excessive pressure should be avoided when instilling where strictures may exist.
How Supplied: In boxes containing 24 sterile packets each with a 10 gram "bellows" shaped tube of jelly and a urethral Disposatip.

pHos-pHaid® ℞
(brand of urinary acidifier)

Composition: Each 0.5 Gm. tablet contains ammonium biphosphate, 190 mg., sodium biphosphate, 200 mg., and sodium acid pyrophosphate, 110 mg. pH: approximately 4.5. Sodium content: less than one grain per tablet.
Action and Uses: pHos-pHaid is a highly effective urinary acidifier which, in conjunction with an acid ash diet, can decrease the urinary pH to a 5–5.5 level. Useful in increasing the solubility of calcium in the urine to assist in preventing formation of calculi in the urinary tract.
Administration and Dosage: In conjunction with an acidifying diet, the recommended dosage is two 0.5 Gm. tablets, followed by a glass of water, t.i.d. Occasionally, higher dosage is required and may be employed when necessary.
Side Effects: Occasional hyperacidity, particularly where gastritis or ulceration exists, and/or occasional nausea have been observed in some patients on a high dosage level. This may be decreased or eliminated by the use of the Enteric-Coated tablets. Excessive doses may also act as a saline cathartic and cause diarrhea. In such cases dosage should be decreased until the symptoms disappear. In cases of severe or extensive renal damage, pHos-pHaid should be administered with caution.
How Supplied: In color-coded tablets, either regular or Enteric- Coated.

Size	*Type*	*Packaged*	*Color*
0.5 Gm.	Reg.	90 & 500	Blue
0.5 Gm.	Ent.-Coat	90 & 500	Orange
0.25 Gm.	Reg.	150	Pink
0.25 Gm.	Ent.-Coat	150	Green

Literature Available: Literature on pHos-pHaid and Acid Ash Diet Sheets are available to physicians on request.

RENACIDIN® ℞

Composition: Active Ingredients (in a 300 gram bottle): Citric acid, anhydrous, 156–171 grams; D-gluconic acid (primarily as the lactone), 21–30 grams. Inert Ingredients: Purified magnesium hydroxycarbonate, 75–87 grams; Magnesium Acid Citrate ($MgHC_6H_5O_7$), 9–15 grams; Calcium (as the carbonate), 2–6 grams; Water, combined and free, 17–21 grams.
Action and Uses: For use in preparing solutions for irrigating indwelling urethral catheters and the urinary bladder in order to dissolve or prevent formation of calcifications.
Administration and Dosage: As a 10% solution (sterile) in distilled water. Irrigation is carried out with 1-2 ounces, b.i.d. or t.i.d. by means of a small, sterile, rubber syringe.
Side Effects: Only occasionally will a patient complain of some temporary pain or burning sensation from this procedure, in which case use of the solution should be discontinued.
Contraindications: It is contraindicated for therapy or preventive therapy above the ureteral-vesical junction; therefore it is contraindicated for ureteral catheters, nephrostomy or pyelostomy tubes or renal lavage for dissolving calculi. Contraindicated for biliary calculi.
How Supplied: In bottles containing 300 grams; also in boxes containing six 25 gram bottles.

Hauck, Inc., W. E.
**P.O. BOX 1065
ROSWELL, GEORGIA 30075**

BESTA CAPSULES® OTC
(Therapeutic Vitamins and Minerals)

Supplied: Bottles of 100.

CANTRI VAGINAL CREAM ℞

Composition: Sulfisoxazole 10%; Aminacrine HCl 0.2%; Allantoin 2.0%.
Supplied: 90 Gm. tube with reusable applicator.

CHLORAFED TIMECELLES* ℞

Composition: Chlorpheniramine Maleate 8 mg.; Pseudoephedrine HCl-120 mg.;
*In special time release beads.
Supplied: Bottles of 100 and 500

ENTUSS TABLETS and LIQUID Ⓒ ℞

Composition: Each tablet and each 5 ml. of liquid contains: Hydrocodone Bitartrate 5 mg.; Guaifenesin 300 mg.
Supplied: Tablets—bottles of 100. Liquid—4 oz. and pints.

G–2 TABLETS ℞
G–3 Capsules Ⓒ ℞

Each oblong light blue tablet contains: Butabarbital 15 mg.; Acetaminophen 325 mg. Supplied in bottles of 100.
Each blue and gray capsule contains: Butabarbital 15 mg.; Acetaminophen 500 mg.; Codeine PO_4 30 mg. Supplied in bottles of 100.

GERAVITE ELIXIR ℞

Each 15 ml. contains: Pentylene tetrazol 100 mg.; Lysine 150 mg.; Thiamine HCl 1 mg.; Riboflavin 1.2 mg.; Niacinamide 10 mg.; Cyanocobalamin 10 mcg.; Alcohol 5%.
Supplied: Pints and gallons.

ISOTRATE ℞
(Isosorbide Dinitrate)

Supplied: Isotrate Chewable 5 mg., orange round tablet; Isotrate Tablet 10 mg., orange oblong scored tablet; Isotrate Timécelles* 40 mg., orange and clear capsule with white beads imprinted HAUCK.
*In special time release beads.
Supplied in bottles of 100.

OTIC–H.C. EAR DROPS ℞

Each ml. contains: Chloroxylenol 1 mg.; Hydrocortisone 10 mg.; Pramoxine 10 mg.; Acetic Acid Glacial 20 mg.; Benzalkonium Chloride 0.2 mg.; non-aqueous Propylene Glycol base qs.
Supplied: 10 ml. dropper tip bottles.

Health Care Industries, Inc.
**4295 S. OHIO STREET
MICHIGAN CITY, IN 46360**

NILCOL® Tablets ℞
NILCOL® Elixir ℞
Oral Decongestants

Description:

	contents in mg Tablet	Elixir-each 15 ml
Phenylpropanolamine HCl	50	25
Chlorpheniramine maleate	4	2
Guaifenesin	200	100
Dextromethorphan HBr	30	15
Alcohol	-	10%

Actions: Each component of Nilcol has been selected to provide symptomatic relief of congestion and cough in upper respiratory disorders. Phenylpropanolamine hydrochloride is a vasoconstrictor which reduces congestion of the nasopharyngeal mucosa. Chlorpheniramine maleate, a widely used antihistamine, helps to control allergic symptoms. The expectorant is guaifenesin which helps to increase the secretion and decrease the viscosity of fluids of the respiratory tract. Dextromethorphan is a well-known, centrally acting antitussive. Nilcol may minimize the need for topical decongestants.
Indications: Nilcol is indicated for nasal and bronchial congestion; coughs and other symptoms of respiratory infections including influenza and the common cold; other respiratory conditions such as sinusitis, allergic rhinitis or hay fever.

Continued on next page

Health—Cont.

Contraindication: Hypersensitivity to any ingredient.
Precautions: Because of the possibility of drowsiness, patients should be cautioned against driving and operating machinery. Administer with caution to patients with hyperthyroidism, hypertensive cardiovascular disease, diabetes mellitus and liver disease. Use in pregnancy is not recommended.
Adverse Reactions: Anxiety, restlessness, tension, insomnia, tremor, weakness, headache, vertigo, sweating, nausea, and vomiting may possibly occur.
Dosage:

	Tablets	Elixir
Adults	one tablet 3 or 4 times a day	two tablespoonsful 3 or 4 times a day
Children		
6–12	one-half tablet 3 or 4 times a day	one tablespoonful 3 or 4 times a day
4–6		two teaspoonsful 3 or 4 times a day
2–4		one teaspoonful 3 or 4 times a day

Caution: Federal law prohibits dispensing without prescription.
How Supplied:
Light pink and violet, scored layered elliptical tablets in bottles of 100
(NDC #11010-004-10)
Deep violet, grape-flavored elixir in bottles of 32 fl. oz. (1 qt.)
(NDC #11010-003-32)
Store between 59°–86° F (15°–30° C)

Manufactured and Distributed by:
HEALTH CARE INDUSTRIES, INC.
4295 South Ohio Street
Michigan City, Indiana 46360

Herbert Laboratories
Dermatology Division of Allergan Pharmaceuticals, Inc.
2525 DUPONT DRIVE
IRVINE, CALIF. 92713

AEROSEB–DEX® ℞
(dexamethasone)
Topical aerosol spray

Description: Dexamethasone is a white to practically white, odorless, crystalline powder. It has a melting point of 250°C with some decomposition. It is practically insoluble in water and sparingly soluble in alcohol.
Chemical Name: 9-Fluoro-11β, 17, 21-trihydroxy-16α-methylpregna-1,4-diene-3,20-dione.
Each aerosol contains:
dexamethasone 0.01%
alcohol 68.5%
with: isopropyl myristate and propellant (butane).
Each 1 second of spray dispenses approximately 0.02 mg of dexamethasone.
Actions: Topical steroids are primarily effective because of their anti-inflammatory, antipruritic and vasoconstrictive actions.
Indications: For relief of the inflammatory manifestations of corticosteroid-responsive dermatoses.
Contraindications: Topical steroids are contraindicated in those patients with a history of hypersensitivity to any of the components of the preparation.
Precautions: If irritation develops, the product should be discontinued and appropriate therapy instituted.
In the presence of an infection, the use of an appropriate antifungal or antibacterial agent should be instituted. If a favorable response does not occur promptly, the corticosteroid should be discontinued until the infection has been adequately controlled.
If extensive areas are treated or if the occlusive technique is used, there will be increased systemic absorption of the corticosteroid and suitable precautions should be taken, particularly in children and infants.
Although topical steroids have not been reported to have an adverse effect on human pregnancy, the safety of their use in pregnant women has not absolutely been established. In laboratory animals, increases in incidence of fetal abnormalities have been associated with exposure of gestating females to topical corticosteroids, in some cases at rather low dosage levels. Therefore, drugs of this class should not be used extensively on pregnant patients, in large amounts, or for prolonged periods of time.
This product is not for ophthalmic use.
When used about the face, the eyes should be covered and inhalation of the spray should be avoided.
This medication contains alcohol. It may produce irritation or burning sensations in open lesions.
Adverse Reactions: The following local adverse reactions have been reported with topical corticosteroids, especially under occlusive dressings.
1. Burning
2. Itching
3. Irritation
4. Dryness
5. Folliculitis
6. Hypertrichosis
7. Acneform eruptions
8. Hypopigmentation
9. Perioral dermatitis
10. Allergic contact dermatitis
11. Maceration of the skin
12. Secondary infection
13. Skin atrophy
14. Striae
15. Miliaria

Dosage and Administration: Apply to affected areas two or three times daily.
For use on the scalp: Apply to dry scalp after shampoo. Shake well before spraying.
1. Hold aerosol upright. Slide applicator tube under hair so that it touches scalp. Spray while moving tube to all affected areas, keeping tube under hair and in contact with scalp throughout treatment. Spraying should take 1 to 2 seconds.
2. If some areas of the scalp are not covered adequately, they may be "spot" sprayed by sliding applicator tube through hair to touch scalp—press and immediately release spray button.
3. It is unnecessary to massage medication into the scalp.
4. Be sure that the tip of the applicator tube stops at the hairline so that forehead and eyes are not sprayed.

For other dermatoses: Remove applicator tube. Shake well before spraying. Hold the can upright, approximately six inches from the area to be treated. Spray each four inch square of affected area for one or two seconds, two or three times a day.
Note: For best results and to avoid wasting medication, it is important to follow the application instructions carefully (application instructions appear on the carton; however, it is preferable that the physician demonstrate the proper application method to the patient).
Caution: Flammable. Do not spray near flame or heated surfaces. If medication accidentally gets in the eyes, wash thoroughly with water and contact physician immediately. Keep out of the reach of children. Contents under pressure. Do not puncture, incinerate, or expose to temperatures above 120°F.
How Supplied: In 58 gm aerosol with applicator tube.* On prescription only.
*U.S. Patent 3,730,182.

AEROSEB–HC® ℞
(hydrocortisone)
Topical aerosol spray

Description: Hydrocortisone is a white to practically white, odorless crystalline powder. It has a melting point of 217 to 220°C with some decomposition. It is very slightly soluble in water and in ether; sparingly soluble in acetone and in alcohol; slightly soluble in chloroform.
Chemical Name:
11β, 17α, 21-trihydroxy-4-pregnene-3, 20-dione
Each aerosol contains:
hydrocortisone 0.5%
alcohol 68%
with: isopropyl myristate and propellant (butane).
Each one second of spray dispenses approximately 1 mg of hydrocortisone.
Actions: Topical steroids are primarily effective because of their anti-inflammatory, antipruritic and vasoconstrictive actions.
Indications: For relief of the inflammatory manifestations of corticosteroid-responsive dermatoses.
Contraindications: Topical steroids are contraindicated in those patients with a history of hypersensitivity to any of the components of the preparation.
Precautions: If irritation develops, the product should be discontinued and appropriate therapy instituted.
In the presence of an infection, the use of an appropriate antifungal or antibacterial agent should be instituted. If a favorable response does not occur promptly, the corticosteroid should be discontinued until the infection has been adequately controlled.
If extensive areas are treated or if the occlusive technique is used, there will be increased systemic absorption of the corticosteroid and suitable precautions should be taken, particularly in children and infants.
Although topical steroids have not been reported to have an adverse effect on human pregnancy, the safety of their use in pregnant women has not absolutely been established. In laboratory animals, increases in incidence of fetal abnormalities have been associated with exposure of gestating females to topical corticosteroids. In some cases at rather low dosage levels. Therefore, drugs of this class should not be used extensively on pregnant patients, in large amounts, or for prolonged periods of time.
This product is not for ophthalmic use.
When used about the face, the eyes should be covered and inhalation of the spray should be avoided.
This medication contains alcohol. It may produce irritation or burning sensations in open lesions.
Adverse Reactions: The following local adverse reactions have been reported with topical corticosteroids, especially under the occlusive dressings.
1. Burning
2. Itching
3. Irritation
4. Dryness
5. Folliculitis
6. Hypertrichosis
7. Acneform eruptions
8. Hypopigmentation
9. Perioral dermatitis
10. Allergic contact dermatitis
11. Maceration of the skin
12. Secondary infection
13. Skin atrophy

14. Striae
15. Miliaria

Dosage and Administration: Apply to affected areas two or three times daily.

For use on the scalp: Apply to dry scalp after shampoo. Shake well before spraying.

1. Hold aerosol upright. Slide applicator tube under hair so that it touches scalp. Spray while moving tube to all affected areas, keeping tube under hair and in contact with scalp throughout treatment. Spraying should take 1 to 2 seconds.
2. If some areas of the scalp are not covered adequately, they may be "spot" sprayed by sliding applicator tube through hair to touch scalp—press and immediately release spray button.
3. It is unnecessary to massage medication into the scalp.
4. Be sure that the tip of the applicator tube stops at the hairline so that forehead and eyes are not sprayed.

For other dermatoses: Remove applicator tube. Shake well before spraying. Hold the can upright, approximately six inches from the area to be treated. Spray each four inch square of affected area for one or two seconds, two or three times a day.

NOTE: For best results and to avoid wasting medication, it is important to follow the application instructions carefully (application instructions appear on the carton; however it is preferable that the physician demonstrate the proper application method to the patient).

Caution: Flammable. Do not spray near flame or heated surfaces. If medication accidentally gets in the eyes, wash thoroughly with water and contact physician immediately. Keep out of the reach of children. Contents under pressure. Do not puncture, incinerate, or expose to temperatures above 120°F.

How Supplied: In 58 gm aerosol with applicator tube.* On prescription only.
*U.S. Patent 3,730,182.

AQUACARE® DRY SKIN CREAM OTC
AQUACARE® DRY SKIN LOTION OTC
(2% urea cream)

(See PDR For Nonprescription Drugs)

AQUACARE®/HP OTC
Dry Skin Lotion
AQUACARE®/HP OTC
Dry Skin Cream
(10% urea cream)

(See PDR For Nonprescription Drugs)

BLUBORO® POWDER ASTRINGENT SOAKING SOLUTION OTC

(See PDR For Nonprescription Drugs)

DANEX® DANDRUFF SHAMPOO OTC

(See PDR For Nonprescription Drugs)

ECLIPSE® AFTER SUN LOTION OTC

(See PDR For Nonprescription Drugs)

ORIGINAL ECLIPSE® OTC
SUNSCREEN GEL
Sun Protection Factor 10
Maximum Protection Against Sunburn for Normal to Oily Skin.

(See PDR For Nonprescription Drugs)

ECLIPSE® SUNSCREEN LIP AND FACE PROTECTANT OTC
Sun Protection Factor 6
Moderate Protection Against Sunburn.

(See PDR For Nonprescription Drugs)

ORIGINAL ECLIPSE® OTC
SUNSCREEN LOTION
Sun Protection Factor 10
Maximum Protection Against Sunburn for Normal to Dry Skin.

(See PDR For Nonprescription Drugs)

TOTAL ECLIPSE® OTC
SUNSCREEN LOTION
Sun Protection Factor 15
Ultra Protection Against Sunburn for Skin that Burns Easily.

(See PDR For Nonprescription Drugs)

PARTIAL ECLIPSE® OTC
SUNTAN LOTION
Sun Protection Factor 5
Moderate Protection Against Sunburn for Normal to Dry Skin.

(See PDR For Nonprescription Drugs)

EXSEL® ℞
(selenium sulfide) 2.5%
Lotion

Description:
Contains:
selenium sulfide 2.5%
with: edetate disodium; bentonite; sodium linear alkylate sulfonate; alphaolefin sulfonate; glyceryl monoricinoleate; silicone; titanium dioxide; citric acid monohydrate; sodium phosphate monobasic, monohydrate; perfume and purified water.

Actions: The mechanism of action of selenium sulfide in seborrheic dermatitis is unknown.

Indications: Selenium sulfide is indicated in the treatment of seborrheic dermatitis of the scalp, including dandruff.

Contraindications: The product should not be used by patients allergic to any of its components.

Warnings: Safety for use in infants has not been established.

Precautions:
1. Chemical conjunctivitis may result if this preparation enters the eyes.
2. The product should be used with caution when acute inflammation or exudation is present as an increase in absorption may occur.

Adverse Reactions:
1. Hair loss has been reported with the use of the product.
2. Discoloration of the hair may follow the use of selenium sulfide. This can be minimized by careful rinsing of the hair after treatment.
3. Oiliness of the hair and scalp may increase following the use of this product.

Dosage and Administration: Shake well before using.
1. Massage about 1 or 2 teaspoonfuls of the medicated shampoo into the wet scalp. Avoid contact with the eyes.
2. Allow product to remain on the scalp for 2 to 3 minutes.
3. Rinse the scalp thoroughly.
4. Repeat application and rinse thoroughly.
5. After treatment, wash hands well.
6. Repeat treatments as directed by physician.

The preparation should not be applied more frequently than required to maintain control of symptoms.

Accidental Oral Ingestion: Selenium sulfide is highly toxic if ingested. Nausea and vomiting usually occur after oral ingestion. Treatment is to induce vomiting or if necessary perform gastric lavage, together with general supportive measures as required. Administer a purgative to hasten elimination.

How Supplied: 4 oz. plastic bottles. On prescription only.

Protect from heat. For external use only. Keep this and all medications out of the reach of children.

FLUONID® ℞
(fluocinolone acetonide)
Ointment 0.025%
Cream 0.01%
Cream 0.025%
Topical Solution 0.01%

Description: Fluonid (fluocinolone acetonide) has the chemical formula 6α,9α–difluoro -16α-hydroxyprednisolone-16,17-acetonide.

Fluonid Ointment 0.025% contains 0.25 mg/g fluocinolone acetonide in white petrolatum.

Fluonid Cream 0.025% and Fluonid Cream 0.01% contain, respectively, 0.25 mg/g and 0.1 mg/g fluocinolone acetonide, in a water-washable aqueous base of stearic acid, propylene glycol, sorbitan monostearate, sorbitan monooleate, polyoxyethylene sorbitan monostearate, purified water and citric acid with methylparaben and propylparaben as preservatives.

Fluonid Topical Solution 0.01% contains 0.1 mg/ml fluocinolone acetonide in a water-washable base of propylene glycol with citric acid.

Actions: Topical steroids are primarily effective because of their anti-inflammatory, antipruritic and vasoconstrictive actions.

Indications: For relief of the inflammatory manifestations of corticosteroid-responsive dermatoses.

Contraindications: Topical steroids are contraindicated in those patients with a history of hypersensitivity to any of the components of the preparation.

Precautions: If irritation develops, the product should be discontinued and appropriate therapy instituted.

In the presence of an infection, the use of appropriate antifungal or antibacterial agents should be instituted. If a favorable response does not occur promptly, the corticosteroid should be discontinued until the infection has been adequately controlled.

If extensive areas are treated or if the occlusive technique is used, there will be increased systemic absorption of the corticosteroid and suitable precautions should be taken, particularly in children and infants.

Although topical steroids have not been reported to have an adverse effect on human pregnancy, the safety of their use in pregnant women has not absolutely been established. In laboratory animals, increases in incidence of fetal abnormalities have been associated with exposure of gestating females to topical corticosteroids, in some cases at rather low dosage levels. Therefore, drugs of this class should not be used extensively on pregnant patients, in large amounts, or for prolonged periods of time.

The product is not for ophthalmic use.

Adverse Reactions: The following local adverse reactions have been reported with topical corticosteroids, especially under occlusive dressings: (1) burning, (2) itching, (3) irritation, (4) dryness, (5) folliculitis, (6) hypertrichosis, (7) acneiform eruptions, (8) hypopigmentation, (9) perioral dermatitis, (10) allergic contact dermatitis, (11) maceration of the skin, (12) secondary infection, (13) skin atrophy, (14) striae and (15) miliaria.

Dosage and Administration: Fluonid (fluocinolone acetonide) preparations should be applied to any affected skin areas two to four times daily as needed.

Fluonid Cream 0.025% and Fluonid Cream 0.01% may be used over long periods of time in specific conditions when deemed necessary. Where an emollient effect is desired, as in atopic dermatitis, the ointment form may be preferred. When large areas are involved, Fluonid Cream 0.01% is recommended. The

Continued on next page

Herbert—Cont.

cream should be massaged gently and thoroughly until it disappears. In occlusive dressing therapy, the cream is sparingly applied to the lesion and gently rubbed in until it disappears. Then the cream is reapplied, leaving a thin coat over the lesion. This area is then completely covered with a pliable nonporous film. Frequency of dressing change is best determined by the physician on an individual basis. It may be changed twice daily, once daily, or left in place for as long as three or four days. Convenience may dictate the use of closed dressings for only part of each day with the use of bland emollients between dressings for dry, fissured lesions. In general, the rate of response of a given lesion is directly related to the total time the lesion is treated with the closed dressing. Reapplication of Fluonid (fluocinolone acetonide) in the method given above is essential at each change of dressing.

For those lesions which are essentially dry, it is important that the dressing be made as airtight and watertight as possible. The edges of the covering film preferably are sealed to adjacent normal skin with an adhesive material, thus preventing evaporation. In some instances it may be advisable to initially increase local water content by briefly soaking the lesion before application, or by covering the lesion with a dampened clean cotton cloth placed between the corticosteroid film and the overlying plastic film.

For those lesions which are essentially moist, especially those of the eczematous dermatitis group, complete sealing of the lesion may not be needed. Here the covering plastic film is useful to keep the medication in place over the lesion and to retain some water, but incomplete sealing of the edges of the film or punctures in the film will allow excess moisture to escape. Patients with eczematous dermatitis may be particularly prone to develop irritation with the use of adhesive materials; hence, it may be preferable to hold the dressings in place with gauze or elastic bandages, stockings, etc.

Fluonid Topical Solution should be applied directly on the lesion, taking note that small quantities are adequate. It should be rubbed in thoroughly but gently at each application, repeating the treatment two or four times daily. In hairy sites the hair should be parted to allow direct contact with the lesion.

In some cases treated with Fluonid Topical Solution, it has been observed that saprophytic or low-grade infections may clear spontaneously as the skin recovers its integrity under the influence of Fluonid Topical Solution alone. This may be partially attributable to the inherent antimicrobial activity of the solution base, propylene glycol.

In indicated lesions, improvement frequently is reported in two to four days. Complete clearing may require one to several weeks, depending upon the nature and chronicity of the dermatitis and the presence or absence of complicating factors. In some indications prone to recurrence, such as seborrheic dermatitis, a program of regular but less frequent use may be needed to maintain the remission.

How Supplied: Fluonid (fluocinolone acetonide)

Cream 0.025%—15 gm. and 60 gm. collapsible tubes and 425 gm. jars.

Cream 0.01%—15 gm. and 60 gm. collapsible tubes and 425 gm. jars.

Ointment 0.025%—15 gm. and 60 gm. collapsible tubes.

Topical Solution 0.01%—20 ml and 60 ml plastic squeeze bottles.

These preparations are available on prescription only.

Manufactured by
Marion Laboratories, Inc.
Kansas City, Missouri 64137
for
Herbert Laboratories
Dermatology Division of
Allergan Pharmaceuticals, Inc.
Irvine, California 92713
U.S. Patent 3,126,375

FLUOROPLEX® ℞
(fluorouracil)
1% Topical Solution
and 1% Topical Cream

Description: Fluoroplex® (fluorouracil) 1% Topical Cream is a stable, standardized cream formulation of fluorouracil in an emulsion base with the following formula:

fluorouracil..1.0%

with: benzyl alcohol (0.5%), ethoxylated stearyl alcohol, mineral oil, isopropyl myristate, sodium hydroxide, purified water.

Fluoroplex® (fluorouracil) 1% Topical Solution is a stable, standardized solution of fluorouracil in a clear propylene glycol base with the following formula:

fluorouracil..1.0%

with: propylene glycol, sodium hydroxide-hydrochloric acid to adjust to pH 9, purified water.

Fluorouracil is a modified pyrimidine similar to uracil and thymine, with whose metabolism it competes. It is a white crystalline substance with a melting point of 283±2° C., an empirical formula of $C_4H_3FN_2O_2$ and a molecular weight of 130.08. It has a characteristic ultraviolet absorption maximum at 266±1 millimicrons in 0.1N HCl.

Actions: There is evidence that fluorouracil (or its biological metabolites) blocks the methylation reaction of deoxyuridylic acid to thymidylic acid. In this fashion fluorouracil interferes with the synthesis of deoxyribonucleic acid (DNA) and to a lesser extent inhibits the formation of ribonucleic acid (RNA).

Indications: Fluoroplex® (fluorouracil) 1% Topical Solution and Fluoroplex® (fluorouracil) 1% Topical Cream are indicated for the topical treatment of multiple actinic (solar) keratoses.

Contraindications: Should not be used in patients with known hypersensitivity to any of the components of the drug.

Warnings:

1. If an occlusive dressing is used there may be an increase in the incidence of inflammatory reactions to the adjacent normal skin.
2. The patient should avoid prolonged exposure to sunlight or other forms of ultraviolet irradiation during treatment with Fluoroplex® as the intensity of the reaction may be increased.

USE IN PREGNANCY: Safety for use in pregnancy has not been established.

Precautions: The medication should be applied with care near the eyes, nose and mouth. Excessive reaction in these areas may occur due to irritation from accumulation of drug. To rule out the presence of a frank neoplasm, a biopsy should be made of those areas failing to respond to treatment or recurring after treatment.

Adverse Reactions: Pain, pruritus, burning, irritation, inflammation, dermatitis and telangiectasia have been reported. Occasionally, hyperpigmentation and scarring have also been reported.

Dosage and Administration: The patient should be instructed to apply sufficient medication to cover the entire face or other affected areas.

Apply medication twice daily with non-metallic applicator or fingertips and wash hands afterwards. A treatment period of 2-6 weeks is usually required.

Increasing frequency of application and a longer period of administration with Fluoroplex® may be required on areas other than the head and neck.

When Fluoroplex® is applied to keratotic skin, a response occurs with the following sequence: erythema, usually followed by scaling, tenderness, erosion, ulceration, necrosis and re-epithelization. When the inflammatory reaction reaches the erosion, necrosis and ulceration stage, the use of the drug should be terminated. Responses may sometimes occur in areas which appear clinically normal. These may be sites of subclinical actinic (solar) keratoses which the medication is affecting.

How Supplied: Fluoroplex® (fluorouracil) 1% Topical Solution is available in 30 ml. plastic dropper bottles. On prescription only. Fluoroplex® (fluorouracil) 1% Topical Cream is available in 30 gm. tubes. On prescription only.

Avoid freezing.

Store at controlled room temperature (59°-86°F).

VANSEB® OTC
Cream Dandruff Shampoo

(See PDR For Nonprescription Drugs)

VANSEB-T® OTC
Cream Tar Shampoo

(See PDR For Nonprescription Drugs)

VANSEB-T® OTC
Lotion Tar Shampoo

(See PDR For Nonprescription Drugs)

Hickam, Inc., Dow B.
5629 GRAPEVINE
HOUSTON, TEXAS 77085

GRANULEX ℞

Composition: Each 0.82 cc. of medication delivered to the wound site contains Trypsin crystallized 0.1 mg., Balsam Peru 72.5 mg., Castor Oil 650.0 mg., and an emulsifier.

Indications: For the treatment of decubitus ulcers, varicose ulcers, debridement of eschar, dehiscent wounds and sunburn.

Action: Trypsin is intended for debridement of eschar and other necrotic tissue. It appears that in many instances removal of wound debris strengthens humoral defense mechanisms sufficiently to retard proliferation of local pathogens. Balsam Peru is an effective capillary bed stimulant used to increase circulation in the wound site area. Also, Balsam Peru has a mildly bactericidal action. Castor Oil is used to improve epithelialization by reducing premature epithelial desiccation and cornification. Also, it can act as a protective covering and aids in the reduction of pain.

Uses: Granulex is in aerosol form which can be important to healing. It must be remembered, healing starts with a thin sheath of epithelium no more than a cell or two thick. Any rough movement or trauma can quickly destroy the healing tissue. Aerosols have the advantage of eliminating all extraneous physical contact with the wound. Granulex is easy to apply and quickly reduces odor frequently accompanying a decubitus ulcer. The wound may be left open or a wet bandage may be applied. As a suggestion; keep in mind wounds heal poorly in the presence of hemoglobin or zinc deficiency.

Dosage: Apply a minimum of twice daily or as often as necessary. Shake well, press the aerosol valve and coat the wound rapidly but not excessively.

Warning: Do not spray on fresh arterial clots. Avoid spraying in eyes. Flammable, do not expose to fire or open flame. Contents under pressure. Do not puncture or incinerate. Do

not store at temperature above 120°F. Keep out of reach of children. Use only as directed. Intentional misuse by deliberately concentrating and inhaling the contents can be harmful or fatal.
How Supplied:
2 oz. Aerosol NDC 0514-0001-01
4 oz. Aerosol NDC 0514-0001-02

High Chemical Co.
Div. Day Frick, Inc.
1760 N. HOWARD ST.
PHILADELPHIA, PA 19122

SARAPIN ℞

Composition: An aqueous distillate of Sarracenia purpurea, pitcher plant, prepared for parenteral administration.
Action and Uses: Local injection therapy for the relief of pain of neuro-muscular or neuralgic origin.
Administration and Dosage: Paravertebral nerve injection—2 to 10 cc. Local neuromuscular infiltration—5 to 10 cc.
Side Effects: None.
Precautions: Non-toxic.
Contraindications: Local inflammation.
How Supplied: One dozen 10 cc. ampuls and 50 cc. multi-dose vials.
Literature Available: Booklet "SARAPIN, Injection Technique in Pain Control."

Hill Dermaceuticals, Inc.
3102 CORRINE DRIVE
ORLANDO, FLORIDA 32803

BURDEO®

Contains: Aluminum Acetate Basic, Boric Acid, and Hexachlorophene in a non-greasy gel base (NDC 28105-0098-08).

DERMA-SMOOTHE® OIL

Contains: Refined peanut oil-mineral oil blend and is a lipophilic, neutral, non-ionic skin cleanser (NDC 28105-0048-08).

FLORIDA FOAM® IMPROVED

Contains: Benzalkonium Chloride, Aluminum Acetate Basic, Boric Acid, Biodegradable Protein and Non-ionic Detergent in a Dermoat (Oat Powder) base (NDC 28105-0065-08).

HILL CORTAC® LOTION ℞

Contains: Hydrocortisone 0.5%, Resorcinol Monoacetate 3%, Sulfur 5%, Zinc Oxide 20%, Isopropyl Alcohol 5% (NDC 28105-0049-02).

HILL-SHADE LOTION

Contains: Para-aminobenzoic Acid 5%, Alcohol 65% (NDC 28105-0160-04).

Hoechst-Roussel Pharmaceuticals Inc.
SOMERVILLE, NJ 08876

DOXIDAN®

Composition: Doxidan is a combination of 60 mg dioctyl calcium sulfosuccinate N.F. and 50 mg danthron N.F. This combination has a highly effective stool softener and a mild peristaltic stimulant that acts mainly in the lower bowel.
Action and Uses: Doxidan is a safe, gentle laxative for the management of chronic functional constipation. Due to the effectiveness of the stool softening component, Doxidan produces soft, formed, easily evacuated stools, with the least possible disturbance of normal body physiology. Doxidan has proved clinically effective in the management of constipation in geriatric or inactive patients, obstetric patients, and following surgery, particularly anorectal procedures. It may be used as a safe and effective evacuant prior to x-ray examination of the colon in preparing patients for barium enema.
Dosages: Adults and children over 12—one or two capsules daily. Children 6 to 12—one capsule daily. Give at bedtime for two or three days or until bowel movements are normal. For children under 6 consult a physician.
Warning: Do not use when abdominal pain, nausea, or vomiting is present. Frequent or prolonged use of this preparation may result in dependence on laxatives. A harmless pink or orange discoloration may appear in alkaline urine. In some patients occasional cramping may occur.
How Supplied: Packs of 10; bottles of 30, 100 (NSN 6505-00-074-3169) and 1000 (NSN 6505-00-890-1247) maroon, soft-gelatin capsules, and Unit Dose 100's (10×10 strips) (NSN 6505-00-118-1700).
[Shown in Product Identification Section]

FESTAL®

Composition: Each enteric-coated tablet contains the following: lipase 10 units,* amylase 10 units,* protease 17 units,* hemicellulase 50 mg, and bile constituents 25 mg.
*Digestive activity expressed as Willstaetter Units, a standardized unit of measurement for enzyme potency.
Action and Uses: Festal provides a high degree of protected digestive activity in a formula of standardized enzyme and bile constituents. Enteric coating of the tablet protects potency from inactivation in the stomach so that high enzymatic potency is delivered to the site in the intestinal tract where digestion normally takes place.
Festal is indicated in any condition where normal digestion is impaired by insufficiency of natural digestive enzymes, or when additional digestive enzymes may be beneficial. These conditions often manifest complaints of discomfort due to excess intestinal gas, such as bloating, cramps and flatulence. The following are conditions or situations where Festal may be helpful: pancreatic insufficiency, enteritis, postgastrectomy syndrome, chronic pancreatitis, pancreatic necrosis, chronic hepatitis, gallbladder disease, surgical patients following cholecystectomy, subtotal gastrectomy, pancreatectomy and other surgery of the upper gastrointestinal tract, removal of gas prior to x-ray examination; and in the healthy individual who may experience temporary digestive deficiency due to over-indulgence in excessively fatty meals.
Dosage: *Adults*—one or two tablets with each meal, or as directed by a physician.
Contraindications: None.
How Supplied: Bottles of 100 and 500 white, enteric-coated tablets for oral use.
Literature Available: Yes.
[Shown in Product Identification Section]

FESTALAN® ℞

Composition: Each tablet contains: In the outer layer: atropine methyl nitrate, 1 mg. In the enteric-coated core: lipase, 10 units;* amylase, 10 units;* protease, 17 units;* hemicellulase, 50 mg; bile constituents, 25 mg.
*Digestive activity expressed as Willstaetter Units, a standardized unit of measurement for enzyme potency.
Action and Uses: Festalan is a combination of a high potency enzyme and bile-salt preparation and atropine methyl nitrate. The standardized enzyme and bile constituents offer a high degree of digestive activity, protected from gastric destruction by enteric coating of the tablet. The specific enzymatic and emulsifying properties promote improved digestion and relief of discomfort due to excess intestinal gas. Atropine methyl nitrate depresses gastrointestinal motility and inhibits gastric secretion. It is, therefore, a useful antispasmodic agent which aids in the relief of pain due to spasm of the gastrointestinal musculature.
Indications: Festalan is indicated in the treatment of intestinal disorders involving an insufficiency of digestive enzymes, hypermotility and nonspecific spasms. It may be helpful in conditions which manifest the complaint of discomfort due to excess intestinal gas, such as malabsorption syndrome due to pancreatic insufficiency, enteritis, chronic pancreatitis, chronic hepatitis, and gallbladder disease. Festalan is often helpful in patients who have undergone pancreatectomy, cholecystectomy, subtotal gastrectomy, and other surgery of the upper gastrointestinal tract. Festalan's spasmolytic action may be of particular value in functional bowel distress, nervous indigestion, irritable bowel syndrome, mucous colitis or spastic colon.
Contraindications: Do not use in patients with glaucoma, known prostatic hypertrophy, or in those who are sensitive to atropine.
Precautions: The occurrence of urinary retention during therapy may indicate the presence of prostatic hypertrophy and may necessitate diminution of dosage or discontinuance of therapy. Festalan should be used with caution in patients with cardiac disease. Overdoses may result in the usual symptoms of atropine toxicity.
Adverse Reactions: Mild dryness of the mouth, blurring of vision, dysuria and constipation may be seen in patients receiving effective doses of atropine, but do not necessitate lowering the dose. Skin rash and flushing may occur in patients sensitive to atropine. The dosage or frequency of administration should be decreased if severe dryness of the mouth, mydriasis, or rapid or irregular pulse occurs.
Usual Adult Dose: One or two tablets with each meal.
How Supplied: Festalan is available in bottles of 100 and 1000 orange tablets.
Literature Available: Yes.
[Shown in Product Identification Section]

LASIX® ℞
(furosemide)
Oral Solution (10 mg/ml)
Tablets/Injection
Diuretic

WARNING: **Lasix (furosemide) is a potent diuretic which, if given in excessive amounts, can lead to a profound diuresis with water and electrolyte depletion. Therefore, careful medical supervision is required, and dose and dose schedule have to be adjusted**

Continued on next page

Hoechst-Roussel—Cont.

to the individual patient's needs. (See under "DOSAGE AND ADMINISTRATION.")

Description: Lasix (furosemide) is an anthranilic acid derivative. Chemically, it is 4-chloro-N-furfuryl-5-sulfamoylanthranilic acid.

Actions: Investigations into the mode of action of Lasix (furosemide) have utilized micropuncture studies in rats, stop flow experiments in dogs, and various clearance studies in both humans and experimental animals.

It has been demonstrated that Lasix (furosemide) inhibits primarily the reabsorption of sodium and chloride not only in the proximal and distal tubules but also in the loop of Henle. The high degree of efficacy is largely due to this unique site of action. The action on the distal tubule is independent of any inhibitory effect on carbonic anhydrase and aldosterone.

The onset of diuresis following oral administration is within 1 hour. The peak effect occurs within the first or second hour. The duration of diuretic effect is 6 to 8 hours.

The onset of diuresis following intravenous administration is within 5 minutes and somewhat later after intramuscular administration. The peak effect occurs within the first half hour. The duration of diuretic effect is approximately 2 hours.

Indications:

Edema—Oral Lasix (furosemide) is indicated for the treatment of edema associated with congestive heart failure, cirrhosis of the liver, and renal disease, including the nephrotic syndrome. Lasix (furosemide) is particularly useful when an agent with greater diuretic potential than that of those commonly employed is desired.

Lasix (furosemide) is indicated as adjunctive therapy in acute pulmonary edema. The intravenous administration of Lasix (furosemide) is indicated when a rapid onset of diuresis is desired, eg, in acute pulmonary edema.

If gastrointestinal absorption is impaired or oral medication is not practical for any reason, Lasix (furosemide) is indicated by the intravenous or intramuscular route. Parenteral use should be replaced with oral Lasix (furosemide) as soon as practical.

Hypertension—Oral Lasix (furosemide) may be used for the treatment of hypertension alone or in combination with other antihypertensive agents. Hypertensive patients who cannot be adequately controlled with thiazides will probably also not be adequately controlled with Lasix (furosemide) alone.

Contraindications: Because animal reproductive studies have shown that Lasix (furosemide) may cause fetal abnormalities, the drug is contraindicated in women of childbearing potential. An exception exists in life-threatening situations where the use of a diuretic such as Lasix (furosemide) by injection is considered of paramount importance over the use of alternative drugs and where the physician has considered the efficacy potential against the risks.

Lasix (furosemide) is contraindicated in anuria. It is contraindicated in patients with a history of hypersensitivity to this compound.

Warnings: Excessive diuresis may result in dehydration and reduction in blood volume with circulatory collapse and with the possibility of vascular thrombosis and embolism, particularly in elderly patients. Excessive loss of potassium in patients receiving digitalis glycosides may precipitate digitalis toxicity. Care should also be exercised in patients receiving potassium-depleting steroids.

Frequent serum electrolyte, CO_2, and BUN determinations should be performed during the first few months of therapy and periodically thereafter, and abnormalities corrected or the drug temporarily withdrawn.

In patients with hepatic cirrhosis and ascites, initiation of therapy with Lasix (furosemide) is best carried out in the hospital. In hepatic coma and in states of electrolyte depletion, therapy should not be instituted until the basic condition is improved. Sudden alterations of fluid and electrolyte balance in patients with cirrhosis may precipitate hepatic coma; therefore, strict observation is necessary during the period of diuresis. Supplemental potassium chloride and, if required, an aldosterone antagonist are helpful in preventing hypokalemia and metabolic alkalosis.

If increasing azotemia and oliguria occur during treatment of severe progressive renal disease, the drug should be discontinued.

As with many other drugs, patients should be observed regularly for the possible occurrence of blood dyscrasias, liver damage, or other idiosyncratic reactions.

Patients with known sulfonamide sensitivity may show allergic reactions to Lasix (furosemide).

Lasix (furosemide) may add to or potentiate the therapeutic effect of other antihypertensive drugs. Potentiation occurs with ganglionic or peripheral adrenergic blocking drugs.

The possibility exists of exacerbation or activation of systemic lupus erythematosus.

Lasix (furosemide) appears in breast milk. If use of the drug is deemed essential, the patient should stop nursing.

Parenterally administered Lasix (furosemide) may increase the ototoxic potential of aminoglycoside antibiotics. Especially in the presence of impaired renal function, the use of parenterally administered Lasix (furosemide) in patients to whom aminoglycoside antibiotics are also being given should be avoided, except in life-threatening situations.

When parenteral use of Lasix (furosemide) precedes its oral use, it should be kept in mind that cases of tinnitus and reversible hearing impairment have been reported. There have also been some reports of cases in which irreversible hearing impairment occurred. Usually, ototoxicity has been reported when Lasix (furosemide) was injected rapidly in patients with severe impairment of renal function at doses exceeding several times the usual recommended dose and in whom other drugs known to be ototoxic were given. If the physician elects to use high dose parenteral therapy in patients with severely impaired renal function, controlled intravenous infusion is advisable [for adults, an infusion rate not exceeding 4 mg Lasix (furosemide) per minute has been used].

Precautions: As with any effective diuretic, electrolyte depletion may occur during therapy with Lasix (furosemide), especially in patients receiving higher doses and a restricted salt intake. Periodic determinations of serum electrolytes to detect possible imbalance should be performed at appropriate intervals.

All patients receiving Lasix (furosemide) therapy should be observed for signs of fluid or electrolyte imbalance, namely, hyponatremia, hypochloremic alkalosis, and hypokalemia. Serum and urine electrolyte determinations are particularly important when the patient is vomiting excessively or receiving parenteral fluids. Medications such as digitalis may also influence serum electrolytes. Warning signs, irrespective of cause, are: dryness of mouth, thirst, weakness, lethargy, drowsiness, restlessness, muscle pains or cramps, muscular fatigue, hypotension, oliguria, tachycardia, arrhythmia, and gastrointestinal disturbances such as nausea and vomiting.

Hypokalemia may develop with Lasix (furosemide) as with any other potent diuretic, especially with brisk diuresis, when cirrhosis is present, or during concomitant use of corticosteroids or ACTH.

Interference with adequate oral electrolyte intake will also contribute to hypokalemia. Digitalis therapy may exaggerate metabolic effects of hypokalemia, especially with reference to myocardial activity.

Asymptomatic hyperuricemia can occur and gout may rarely be precipitated.

Periodic checks on urine and blood glucose should be made in diabetics and even those suspected of latent diabetes when receiving Lasix (furosemide). Increases in blood glucose and alterations in glucose tolerance tests with abnormalities of the fasting and 2-hour postprandial sugar have been observed and rare cases of precipitation of diabetes mellitus have been reported.

Lasix (furosemide) may lower serum calcium levels and rare cases of tetany have been reported. Accordingly, periodic serum calcium levels should be obtained.

Reversible elevations of BUN may be seen. These have been observed in association with dehydration, which should be avoided, particularly in patients with renal insufficiency.

Patients receiving high doses of salicylates, as in rheumatic disease, in conjunction with Lasix (furosemide) may experience salicylate toxicity at lower doses because of competitive renal excretory sites.

Lasix (furosemide) has a tendency to antagonize the skeletal muscle relaxing effect of tubocurarine and may potentiate the action of succinylcholine.

Lithium generally should not be given with diuretics because they reduce its renal clearance and add a high risk of lithium toxicity.

It has been reported in the literature that diuretics such as furosemide may enhance the nephrotoxicity of cephaloridine. Therefore, Lasix (furosemide) and cephaloridine should not be administered simultaneously.

Lasix (furosemide) may decrease arterial responsiveness to norepinephrine. This diminution is not sufficient to preclude effectiveness of the pressor agent for therapeutic use.

It has been reported in the literature that coadministration of indomethacin may reduce the natriuretic and antihypertensive effects of Lasix (furosemide) in some patients. This effect has been attributed to inhibition of prostaglandin synthesis by indomethacin. Indomethacin may also affect plasma renin levels and aldosterone excretion; this should be borne in mind when a renin profile is evaluated in hypertensive patients. Patients receiving both indomethacin and Lasix (furosemide) should be observed closely to determine if the desired diuretic and/or hypertensive effect of Lasix (furosemide) is achieved.

Adverse Reactions:

Gastrointestinal System Reactions

1. anorexia
2. oral and gastric irritation
3. nausea
4. vomiting
5. cramping
6. diarrhea
7. constipation
8. jaundice (intrahepatic cholestatic jaundice)
9. pancreatitis

Central Nervous System Reactions

1. dizziness
2. vertigo
3. paresthesias
4. headache
5. xanthopsia
6. blurred vision
7. tinnitus and hearing loss

Hematologic Reactions

1. anemia
2. leukopenia
3. agranulocytosis (rare)
4. thrombocytopenia
5. aplastic anemia (rare)

Dermatologic—Hypersensitivity Reactions

1. purpura
2. photosensitivity
3. rash
4. urticaria
5. necrotizing angiitis (vasculitis, cutaneous vasculitis)
6. exfoliative dermatitis
7. erythema multiforme
8. pruritus

Cardiovascular Reaction

Orthostatic hypotension may occur and be aggravated by alcohol, barbiturates, or narcotics.

Other

1. hyperglycemia
2. glycosuria
3. hyperuricemia
4. muscle spasm
5. weakness
6. restlessness
7. urinary bladder spasm
8. thrombophlebitis
9. transient pain at the injection site following intramuscular injection

Whenever adverse reactions are moderate or severe, Lasix (furosemide) dosage should be reduced or therapy withdrawn.

Dosage and Administration:

Oral Administration

Edema—Therapy should be individualized according to patient response. This therapy should be titrated to gain maximal therapeutic response as well as the minimal dose possible to maintain that therapeutic response.

ADULTS—The usual initial daily dose of oral Lasix (furosemide) is 20 to 80 mg given as a single dose. Ordinarily a prompt diuresis ensues. Depending on the patient's response, a second dose can be administered 6 to 8 hours later.

If the diuretic response to a single dose of 20 to 80 mg is not satisfactory, increase this dose by increments of 20 or 40 mg not sooner than 6 to 8 hours after the previous dose until the desired diuretic effect has been obtained. This individually determined single dose should then be given once or twice daily (eg, at 8:00 a.m. and 2:00 p.m.). The dose of Lasix (furosemide) may be carefully titrated up to 600 mg/day in those patients with severe clinical edematous states.

The mobilization of edema may be most efficiently and safely accomplished by utilizing an intermittent dosage schedule in which the diuretic is given for 2 to 4 consecutive days each week.

When doses exceeding 80 mg/day are given for prolonged periods, careful clinical and laboratory observations are particularly advisable.

INFANTS AND CHILDREN—The usual initial dose of oral Lasix (furosemide) in infants and children is 2 mg/kg body weight, given as a single dose. If the diuretic response is not satisfactory after the initial dose, dose may be increased by 1 or 2 mg/kg no sooner than 6 to 8 hours after the previous dose. Doses greater than 6 mg/kg body weight are not recommended.

For maintenance therapy in infants and children, the dose should be adjusted to the minimum effective level.

Hypertension—Therapy should be individualized according to the patient's response. This therapy should be titrated to gain maximal therapeutic response as well as the minimal dose possible to maintain that therapeutic response.

ADULTS—The usual initial daily dose of Lasix (furosemide) for antihypertensive therapy is 80 mg, usually divided into 40 mg twice a day. Dosage should then be adjusted according to response. If the patient does not respond, add other antihypertensive agents.

Careful observations for changes in blood pressure must be made when this compound is used with other antihypertensive drugs, especially during initial therapy. The dosage of other agents must be reduced by at least 50 percent as soon as Lasix (furosemide) is added to the regimen, to prevent excessive drop in blood pressure. As the blood pressure falls under the potentiating effect of Lasix (furosemide), a further reduction in dosage or even discontinuation of other antihypertensive drugs may be necessary.

Parenteral Administration

ADULTS—Parenteral therapy should be reserved for patients for whom oral medication is not practical or in emergency situations where prompt diuresis is desired. Parenteral therapy should be replaced by oral therapy as soon as this is practical for continued mobilization of edema.

Edema—The usual initial dose of Lasix (furosemide) is 20 to 40 mg given as a single dose, injected intramuscularly or intravenously. The intravenous injection should be given slowly (1 to 2 minutes). Ordinarily, a prompt diuresis ensues. Depending on the patient's response, a second dose can be administered 2 hours after the first dose or later.

If the diuretic response with a single dose of 20 to 40 mg is not satisfactory, increase this dose by increments of 20 mg not sooner than 2 hours after the previous dose until the desired diuretic effect has been obtained. This individually determined single dose should then be given once or twice daily.

If the physician elects to use high dose parenteral therapy it should be administered as a controlled infusion at a rate not exceeding 4 mg/min. Lasix (furosemide) Injection is a mildly buffered alkaline solution which should not be mixed with acidic solutions of pH below 5.5. To prepare infusion solutions, isotonic saline and lactated Ringer's injection and 5% dextrose injection have been used after pH has been adjusted when necessary.

Therapy should be individualized according to patient response. This therapy should be titrated to gain maximal therapeutic response as well as the minimal dose possible to maintain that therapeutic response. Close medical supervision is necessary.

Acute Pulmonary Edema—The usual initial dose of Lasix (furosemide) is 40 mg injected intravenously. The injection should be given slowly (1 to 2 minutes). If 40 mg Lasix (furosemide) does not produce a satisfactory response within 1 hour the dose may be increased to 80 mg given intravenously (over 1 to 2 minutes). If deemed necessary, additional therapy (eg, digitalis, oxygen) can be administered concomitantly.

INFANTS AND CHILDREN—Parenteral therapy should be reserved for patients for whom oral medication is not practical or in emergency situations where prompt diuresis is desired. Parenteral therapy should be replaced by oral therapy as soon as this is practical for continued mobilization of edema.

The usual initial dose of Lasix (furosemide) Injection (intravenously or intramuscularly) in infants and children is 1 mg/kg body weight and should be given slowly under close medical supervision. If the diuretic response after the initial dose is not satisfactory, dosage may be increased by 1 mg/kg not sooner than 2 hours after the previous dose, until the desired diuretic effect has been obtained. Doses greater than 6 mg/kg body weight are not recommended.

How Supplied: *Lasix (furosemide) Tablets* are supplied as white, round, monogrammed, scored tablets of 40 mg in amber bottles of 100 (NSN 6505-00-062-3336), 500 (NSN 6505-00-254-5546; 5546A), and 1,000, and unit dose 100s (20 strips of 5) (NSN 6505-00-117-5982; 5982A); white, oval monogrammed tablets of 20 mg in amber bottles of 100, 500 and 1000, and unit dose 100s (20 strips of 5); and white, round, monogrammed, facetted-edge tablets of 80 mg in amber bottles of 50 and unit dose 100s (20 strips of 5).

***Note:* Dispense in dark containers. Exposure to light may cause slight discoloration which, however, does not alter potency.**

Lasix (furosemide) Oral Solution is supplied as an orange-flavored liquid containing furosemide 10 mg/ml in bottles of 60 ml (accompanied by graduated dropper) and bottles of 120 ml (accompanied by graduated dispensing spoon).

***Note:* Store in a cold place (refrigerator, 36–46°F). Dispense in light-resistant containers. Protect from freezing.**

Lasix (furosemide) Injection is supplied as a sterile solution in 2 ml amber ampuls, boxes of 5 (NSN 6505-00-435-0377) and 50 (NSN 6505-00-933-8704A); 4 ml amber ampuls, boxes of 5 and 25; 10 ml amber ampuls, boxes of 5 (NSN 6505-00-148-9814) and 25 (NSN 6505-00-516-0515A); 2 ml prefilled syringes in boxes of 5; and 4 ml prefilled syringes in boxes of 5. Each ml contains 10 mg furosemide (with sodium chloride for isotonicity and sodium hydroxide to make the solution slightly alkaline).

***Note:* Store at controlled room temperature. Do not use if solution is yellow. Protect prefilled syringes from light after removing from blister package.**

[*Shown in Product Identification Section*]

STREPTASE® ℞
(streptokinase)

How Supplied: Streptase (streptokinase) is supplied as a lyophilized white powder in 6.5 ml vials (in packages of 10) with color-coded labels corresponding to the amount of purified Streptase (streptokinase) in each vial as follows: yellow—100,000 IU, green—250,000 IU, blue—750,000 IU.

In each vial there is a 20% overfill above that stated on the label. Each vial also contains 25 mg cross-linked gelatin polypeptides and 25 mg sodium L-glutamate as stabilizers.

For hospital use only. Store at controlled room temperature (15–30°C). Use within 24 hours of reconstitution. Unused reconstituted drug should be discarded.

SURFAK®
(dioctyl calcium sulfosuccinate N.F.)

Composition: Surfak is the stool softening agent, dioctyl calcium sulfosuccinate N.F.

Action and Uses: Surfak is indicated in constipation-prone patients where prevention of hard stools is essential to treatment, or in those conditions where laxative therapy is undesirable or contraindicated. Surfak is useful in patients who require only stool softening without propulsive action to accomplish defecation. Surfak does not cause peristaltic stimulation, and because of its safety and lack of systemic drug action, it may be effectively used in patients with heart conditions, anorectal conditions, obstetrical patients, following surgical procedures, ulcerative colitis, diverticulitis and bedridden patients. Surfak provides homogenization and formation of soft, easily evacuated stools without disturbance of body physiology, discomfort of bowel distention, oily leakage or interference with vitamin absorption.

Dosages: Adults—one red 240 mg capsule daily for several days or until bowel movements are normal. Children and adults with minimal needs—one to three orange 50 mg capsules daily.

Side Effects: Surfak is non-habit forming. It has no known side effects or disadvantages, except for the unusual occurrence of mild, transitory cramping pains. Overdosage does not lead to systemic toxicity.

Contraindications: None.

How Supplied: 240 mg red, soft gelatin capsules—bottles of 30 (NSN 6505-00-117-8607), 100 (NSN 6505-00-926-8844), 500 (NSN 6505-00-148-9815) and Unit Dose 100's (10 x 10 strips) (NSN 6505-00-118-1449), 50 mg orange, soft gelatin capsules—bottles of 30 and 100.

Literature Available: Yes.

[*Shown in Product Identification Section*]

TOPICORT® ℞
(desoximetasone)
EMOLLIENT CREAM 0.25%

Description: Topicort (desoximetasone) Emollient Cream 0.25% contains the active syn-

Continued on next page

Hoechst-Roussel—Cont.

thetic corticosteroid desoximetasone. The chemical name of desoximetasone is 9α-fluoro-11β, 21-dihydroxy-16α-methylpregna-1, 4-diene-3, 20-dione.
Each gram of Topicort (desoximetasone) Emollient Cream 0.25% contains 2.5 mg desoximetasone in an emollient cream consisting of isopropyl myristate, cetylstearyl alcohol, white petrolatum, mineral oil, lanolin alcohol and purified water.
Actions: Topical steroids are primarily effective because of their anti-inflammatory, antipruritic and vasoconstrictive actions.
Indications: Topicort (desoximetasone) Emollient Cream is indicated for the relief of inflammatory manifestations of corticosteroid-responsive dermatoses.
Contraindications: Topical steroids are contraindicated in those patients with a history of hypersensitivity to any of the components of the preparation.
Precautions: If irritation or sensitization develops this product should be discontinued and appropriate therapy instituted.
In the presence of an infection the use of an appropriate antifungal or antibacterial agent should be instituted. If a favorable response does not occur promptly, the corticosteroid should be discontinued until the infection has been adequately controlled.
If extensive areas are treated or if the occlusive technique is used there will be increased systemic absorption of the corticosteroid and suitable precautions should be taken, particularly in children and infants.
Although topical steroids have not been reported to have an adverse effect on human pregnancy, the safety of their use in pregnant women has not been absolutely established. In laboratory animals, increases in incidence of fetal abnormalities have been associated with exposure of gestating females to topical corticosteroids, in some cases at rather low dosage levels. Therefore, drugs of this class should not be used extensively on pregnant patients, in large amounts, or for prolonged periods of time.
This product is not for ophthalmic use.
Adverse Reactions: The following local adverse reactions have been reported with topical corticosteroids, especially under occlusive dressings: burning, itching, irritation, dryness, folliculitis, hypertrichosis, acneiform eruptions, hypopigmentation, perioral dermatitis, allergic contact dermatitis, maceration of the skin, secondary infection, skin atrophy, striae, miliaria.
Dosage and Administration: Apply a thin film of Topicort (desoximetasone) Emollient Cream 0.25% to the affected skin areas twice daily. Rub in gently.
How Supplied: Topicort (desoximetasone) Emollient Cream 0.25% is supplied in 5-, 15- and 60-gram tubes.

Holland-Rantos Company, Inc.

P. O. BOX 385
865 CENTENNIAL AVE.
PISCATAWAY, NJ 08854

KORO-FLEX® ℞
ARCING SPRING DIAPHRAGM

Composition: Improved contouring spring; natural latex diaphragm.
Action and Uses: Half-moon shape when compressed, facilitates introduction along vaginal floor beyond cervix for easy, correct placement.
Administration and Dosage: As directed.
How Supplied: Available as a kit containing trial size tubes of KOROMEX^{II} CONTRACEPTIVE JELLY and KOROMEX^{II} CONTRACEPTIVE CREAM (Stock #136). Also available in a set (Plastic Compact Bag) containing regular size KOROMEX^{II} CONTRACEPTIVE JELLY and trial size KOROMEX^{II} CONTRACEPTIVE CREAM. Sizes 60–95 mms.

KOROMEX® COIL SPRING DIAPHRAGM ℞

Action and Uses: The KOROMEX COIL SPRING DIAPHRAGM is made of pure latex rubber. The cadmium plated coil spring is tension-adjusted. The diaphragm is used with KOROMEX^{II} CONTRACEPTIVE JELLY or KOROMEX^{II} CONTRACEPTIVE CREAM for conception control.
How Supplied: Available as a kit containing trial size tubes of KOROMEX^{II} CONTRACEPTIVE JELLY and KOROMEX^{II} CONTRACEPTIVE CREAM (Stock #131). Also available in a set (plastic compact bag) containing an introducer, regular size KOROMEX^{II} CONTRACEPTIVE JELLY, trial size tube KOROMEX^{II} CONTRACEPTIVE CREAM (Stock #541) Sizes 50 mm.–105 mm. at graduations of 5 mm.

KOROMEX® CONTRACEPTIVE FOAM OTC

(See PDR For Nonprescription Drugs)

KOROMEX^{II} CONTRACEPTIVE CREAM OTC

(See PDR For Nonprescription Drugs)

KOROMEX^{II} CONTRACEPTIVE JELLY OTC

(See PDR For Nonprescription Drugs)

KOROMEX^{II}–A CONTRACEPTIVE JELLY OTC

(See PDR For Nonprescription Drugs)

KOROSTATIN® VAGINAL TABLETS ℞
(nystatin vaginal tablets)
Nystatin

Description: KOROSTATIN Nystatin Vaginal Tablets, U.S.P. is an oblong shaped vaginal tablet, each containing 100,000 units Nystatin, U.S.P. Inactive ingredients: starch, lactose, polyvinylpyrrolidone, sorbitol and magnesium stearate.
Actions:
Microbiology
Nystatin is an antifungal antibiotic produced by a strain of Streptomyces noursei. Nystatin is useful in the treatment of infections caused by Candida (Monilia) albicans. Nystatin has no appreciable activity against bacteria.
Human Pharmacology
No detectable blood levels are obtained following topical or vaginal application.
Indications: Nystatin Vaginal Tablets U.S.P. are indicated in the local treatment of vulvo-vaginal candidiasis.
Contraindications: All nystatin preparations are contraindicated in patients with a history of hypersensitivity to nystatin.
Adverse Reactions: Nystatin U.S.P. is virtually nontoxic and nonsensitizing and is well tolerated by all age groups, even on prolonged administration. If irritation during intra-vaginal use should occur, discontinue the medication.
Dosage and Administration: The usual dosage is 1 or 2 vaginal tablets (100,000 or 200,000 units) daily. The tablets should be deposited high in the vagina by means of the applicator supplied with the package. (See "Instructions for the Patient" on permanent panel of package.) In most cases, two weeks of therapy will be sufficient, but more prolonged treatment may be necessary. It is important that therapy be continued during menstruation. Adjunctive measures such as therapeutic douches are unnecessary and sometimes inadvisable. Cleansing douches may be used by nonpregnant women, if desired, for esthetic purposes.
How Supplied: In packages of 15 and 30 individual foil wrapped tablets with applicator. Refrigeration is not required for these tablets. KOROSTATIN Vaginal Tablets should be stored below 30° C. (86° F.).

KORO-SULF™ Vaginal Cream ℞
(sulfisoxazole)

Description: Koro-Sulf (Sulfisoxazole) Vaginal Cream is a non-staining water dispersible, absorptive cream containing 10% Sulfisoxazole in a base of stearic acid, polysorbate 60, sorbitan monostearate, boric acid, glycerin, methyl paraben, propyl paraben and water.
Actions: The 4.5 pH of Koro-Sulf Cream is approximately that of the normal, healthy vaginal tract. The mechanism of action is that of an antibacterial sulfonamide.
Indications: Koro-Sulf Cream is indicated for treatment of *Hemophilus vaginalis* vaginitis. It may also be used as a deodorant for saprophytic infection following radiation therapy.
Contraindications: Koro-Sulf Cream is contraindicated in patients with known hypersensitivity to any of its components.
Warnings: If the patient develops local irritation to the drug, treatment should be discontinued.
Adverse Reactions: In addition to local irritation, the following reactions have been reported rarely: allergic reaction, pruritus, urticaria and vulvitis.
Dosage and Administration: From 2.5 ml to 5 ml (½ to 1 applicatorful) of Koro-Sulf Cream should be introduced into the vagina twice daily, in the morning and upon retiring. Therapy should be continued up to two weeks, and may be repeated if necessary.
How Supplied: Three-ounce (85 grams) tubes, with 5 ml reusable applicator.

NYLMERATE^{II}® Solution Concentrate OTC

(See PDR For Nonprescription Drugs)

Houser Pharmaceuticals, Inc.
6503 WARWICK ROAD
P. O. BOX 25756
RICHMOND, VA 23260

ZYMENOL® OTC
Regular and Chocolate

Composition: An emulsion of Mineral Oil, 50% and Brewer's Yeast Culture (No live cells) 12%. Sugar-Free.
Actions and Uses: ZYMENOL gently softens bowel content and lubricates for easy passage without straining at stool.
Indications: Constipation in all age groups; especially cardiacs, patients with hemorrhoids, following anorectal surgery and for diabetic patients.
Caution: Take only at bedtime. Prolonged use of all laxatives may result in dependence. Do not administer to infants, young children, in pregnancy, and bedridden or aged patients unless directed by physician.
Dosage and Administration: Adults: 1 to 2 tablespoonfuls. Children 6 to 12 years: 1 tablespoonful. Children 3 to 6 years: 1 heaping teaspoonful. Take only at bedtime.
How Supplied: Regular and Chocolate in 14 oz. bottles.

Hoyt Laboratories
Division of Colgate-Palmolive Co.
633 HIGHLAND AVENUE
NEEDHAM, MASSACHUSETTS 02194

LURIDE® Drops ℞
brand of Sodium Fluoride Solution

Description: Each drop from a drop-delivery, tamperproof, plastic bottle provides approximately 0.125 (1/8) mg fluoride ion (from 0.275 mg sodium fluoride). Sugar and saccharin free.
Action and Uses: To aid in the protection against dental caries. Fluoride supplementation should be continued to at least age 12.
Administration and Dosage:

F-Content of Drinking Water	Daily Dosage Birth to Age 2	Age 2-3	Age 3-12
<0.3 ppm	2 drops	4 drops	8 drops
0.3 - 0.7 ppm	One-half above dosage.		
>0.7 ppm	Fluoride supplements contraindicated.		

LURIDE Drops may be administered orally undiluted or mixed with fluids.
Precautions and Contraindications: LURIDE Drops are contraindicated when the fluoride content of drinking water exceeds 0.7 ppm F. Recommended dosage should not be exceeded as prolonged overdosage may result in dental fluorosis.
KEEP BOTTLE OUT OF REACH OF CHILDREN.
How Supplied: Peach-flavored Drops-30 ml drop-delivery plastic bottles.

LURIDE® Lozi-Tabs® Tablets ℞
brand of Sodium Fluoride Tablets

Description: Each LURIDE 1.0 mg Lozi-Tabs pleasantly-flavored (sugar-free) lozenge-type, chewable tablet provides 1.0 mg fluoride ion (from 2.2 mg sodium fluoride).
Each LURIDE-SF 1.0 mg Lozi-Tabs tablet (SF for Special Formula: no artificial color or flavor) provides 1.0 mg fluoride ion (from 2.2 mg sodium fluoride).
Each LURIDE 0.5 mg Lozi-Tabs tablet (half-strength) provides 0.5 mg fluoride ion (from 1.1 mg sodium fluoride).
Each LURIDE 0.25 mg Lozi-Tabs tablet (quarter-strength) provides 0.25 mg fluoride ion (from 0.55 mg sodium fluoride).
Action and Uses: To aid in the protection against dental caries. Fluoride supplementation should be continued to at least age 12.
Administration and Dosage:

F-Content of Drinking Water	Daily Dosage (F ion) Birth to Age 2	Age 2-3	Age 3-12
<0.3 ppm	0.25 mg	0.5 mg	1.0 mg
0.3–0.7 ppm	One-half above dosages.		
>0.7 ppm	Fluoride supplements contraindicated.		

Each LURIDE Lozi-Tabs tablet to be partially dissolved in mouth or chewed before swallowing, preferably at bedtime after brushing teeth.
Precautions and Contraindications: LURIDE and LURIDE-SF tablets are contraindicated when the fluoride content of drinking water is 0.3 ppm F, or more. LURIDE Half-Strength and LURIDE Quarter-Strength tablets are contraindicated when the fluoride content of drinking water exceeds 0.7 ppm F. Recommended dosage should not be exceeded, as prolonged overdosage may result in dental fluorosis. KEEP BOTTLE OUT OF REACH OF CHILDREN.
How Supplied: LURIDE 1.0 mg Lozi-Tabs-bottles of 120; 1000 and 5000 for dispensing only; available in cherry, lemon, lime, orange, and rainbow assortment flavors. LURIDE-SF 1.0 mg Lozi-Tabs-bottles of 120. LURIDE 0.5 mg Lozi-Tabs (Half-Strength) bottles of 120; and 1200 for dispensing only, grape flavored. LURIDE 0.25 mg Lozi-Tabs (Quarter-Strength) bottles of 120, vanilla flavored.

ORABASE® Plain
"The Oral Bandage" ™
(Oral Protective Paste)

Description: Unique preparation designed for the temporary relief and protection of minor irritations of the mouth and gums. It combines gelatin, pectin, and sodium carboxymethylcellulose in a plasticized hydrocarbon gel (a polyethylene and mineral oil gel base). Imitation vanilla flavor.
Action and Uses: Provides a protective soothing covering for minor mouth irritations, and because of its adhesive qualities (it adheres tenaciously to oral mucous membranes), helps protect involved area against further irritation from chewing, swallowing, and other normal mouth activity.
Nonirritating, nontoxic, and harmless if swallowed. It contains no antibiotic, analgesic, nor antiseptic, and is essentially odorless and tasteless.
Indications: Orabase is indicated for minor lesions of the oral mucosa such as abrasions caused by toothbrushing, chewing or facial injuries; irritation from orthodontic appliances; denture irritations; and sensitive post-infection ulcerated sites.
Administration and Dosage: Press small dabs into place until the involved area is coated with a thin film of the paste. Attempting to spread this preparation may result in a granular, gritty sensation, causing it to crumble. After application, however, a smooth slippery film develops.
Use as often as needed for relief-particularly after eating-or as directed by a dentist or a physician.
Precautions and Contraindications: Not intended for use in the presence of infections. If an infection is suspected, or if any mouth irritation does not heal within 7 days, a dentist or physician should be consulted. If irritation is due to dentures that do not fit properly, a dentist should be consulted.
How Supplied: Net Wt. 0.17 oz. (5 gram) tubes and Net Wt. 1/2 oz. (15 gram) tubes.
Also Available: ORABASE® with Benzocaine, analgesic oral protective paste and ORABASE® HCA, oral paste (cortisol acetate 0.5%).

ORABASE® with Benzocaine
"The Oral Bandage" ™
(Analgesic Oral Protective Paste)

Description: Unique preparation designed for the temporary relief of pain and protection of minor irritations of the mouth and gums. It combines benzocaine, gelatin, pectin, and sodium carboxymethylcellulose in a plasticized hydrocarbon gel (a polyethylene and mineral oil gel base). Imitation vanilla flavor.
Action and Uses: Provides temporary relief of pain and a unique, protective covering for minor oral irritations. Because it adheres tenaciously to the oral mucous membranes, it holds pain relief at the site of the lesion to promote healing and prevents further irritation from chewing and other normal mouth activity.
Indications: For minor lesions of the oral mucosa such as denture irritations; abrasions caused by toothbrushing, chewing or facial injuries; irritation from orthodontic appliances; and sensitive post-infection ulcerated sites.
Administration and Dosage: Press small dabs into place until the involved area is coated with a thin film of the paste. Attempting to spread this preparation may result in a granular, gritty sensation, causing it to crumble. After application, however, a smooth slippery film develops.
Use as often as needed for relief-particularly after eating-or as directed by a dentist or a physician.
Precautions and Contraindications: Do not use in the eyes. Not for use in children under six years of age unless under professional direction. Not intended for use in the presence of infections. If an infection is suspected, or if any mouth irritation does not heal within 7 days, a dentist or physician should be consulted. If irritation is due to dentures that do not fit properly, a dentist should be consulted.
Keep this and all medications out of reach of children.
How Supplied: Net Wt. 0.17 oz. (5 gram) tubes and Net Wt. 1/2 oz. (15 gram) tubes.
Also Available: ORABASE® Plain, oral protective paste and ORABASE® HCA, oral paste (cortisol acetate 0.5%).

ORABASE® HCA ℞
(Oral Paste)

Description: Each gram contains cortisol acetate 5 mg (0.5%) in an oral paste vehicle containing pectin, gelatin, sodium carboxymethylcellulose dispersed in a plasticized hydrocarbon gel composed of 5% polyethylene in mineral oil. Imitation vanilla flavor.
Action and Uses: Cortisol acetate is a natural cortico-steroid and possesses properties of an anti-inflammatory, antipruritic and antiallergic nature. The oral paste acts as an adhesive vehicle for applying the active medication to oral tissues. The protective action of the adhesive vehicle may serve to reduce the pain associated with oral irritation.
Indications: Indicated for adjunctive treatment and for the temporary relief of symptoms associated with oral inflammatory lesions and ulcerative lesions resulting from trauma.
Contraindications: Fungal, viral, or bacterial infections of the oral mucosa. Hypersensitivity to any component. This preparation is not for ophthalmic use.
Warning: Although topical steroids have not been reported to have an adverse effect on the fetus, the safety of their use in pregnant females has not absolutely been established. Therefore, they should not be used extensively in pregnant patients, or in large amounts, or for prolonged periods of time.

Continued on next page

Hoyt—Cont.

Precautions: Patients with tuberculosis, peptic ulcer, or diabetes mellitus should not be routinely treated with this steroid preparation.
It should be borne in mind that the normal defensive responses of the oral tissues are depressed in patients receiving topical corticosteroid therapy. Virulent strains of oral microorganisms may multiply without producing the usual warning symptoms of oral infections. If significant regeneration or repair of oral tissues has not occurred in 7 days, additional investigation into the etiology of the oral lesion is advised.
Adverse Reactions: Prolonged administration may elicit the adverse reactions known to occur with systemic steroid preparations; for example, adrenal suppression, alteration of glucose metabolism, protein catabolism, peptic ulcer activations, and others. These are usually reversible and disappear when the hormone is discontinued.
Administration and Dosage: Dab, do not rub, on the lesion until the paste adheres. (Rubbing this preparation on lesion may result in a granular, gritty sensation.) After application, a smooth, slippery film develops. The drug should be applied 2 to 3 times a day following meals and at bedtime. If significant repair or regeneration has not occurred in 7 days, further investigation is advisable.
How Supplied: Net weight 5 gram tubes.
Caution: Federal (U.S.A.) law prohibits dispensing without prescription.
Keep out of the reach of children. Not for ophthalmic use.
Also Available: ORABASE® Plain, oral protective paste and ORABASE® with Benzocaine, analgesic oral protective paste. ℞ not required.

Perio Cal-D™ Tablets
brand of Dibasic Calcium Phosphate

Description: Each tablet contains 600 mg Dibasic Calcium Phosphate and 133 International Units (3.33 mcg) Vitamin D_2. Daily dosage (3 tablets) provides:

Calcium 500 mg	50% USRDA*
Phosphorus 400 mg	40% USRDA
Vitamin D 400 IU.	100% USRDA

Calcium to Phosphorus ratio 1.25 to 1
* U.S. Recommended Daily Allowance for adults and children 4 or more years of age.
Indications: For those individuals with an inadequate intake of dairy products, the major source of dietary calcium.
Administration and Dosage: Usual dosage is one tablet three times a day, or as directed by dentist or physician.
How Supplied: Bottles of 100 film coated, oval-shaped tablets.

PHOS-FLUR® Oral Rinse Supplement ℞
brand of Acidulated Phosphate Fluoride Solution

Description: Each teaspoonful (5 ml) contains 1.0 mg fluoride ion (from 2.2 mg sodium fluoride) in an M/10 phosphate liquid at a pH of approximately 4.0 in cherry, lime or orange flavors. Contains no sugar, saccharin or alcohol.
Action and Uses: PHOS-FLUR is designed to provide both topical and systemic effects of fluoride with daily rinsings of teeth and ingestion of liquid.
Indications: To aid in protection against dental caries.
Administration and Dosage:
AS A DENTAL RINSE—Children age 6 and over—daily, preferably at bedtime after thoroughly brushing teeth, rinse one teaspoonful (5 ml) or two teaspoonfuls (10 ml) vigorously around and between teeth for one minute, then expectorate, DO NOT SWALLOW:
AS A SUPPLEMENT—Children age 3 and over—in areas where drinking water is devoid of fluoride, (less than 0.3 ppm), rinse one teaspoonful (5 ml) daily as above, then swallow. When drinking water contains 0.3 to 0.7 ppm F, inclusive, reduce dose to ½ teaspoonful.
Precautions and Contraindications: Recommended systemic dosage should not be exceeded, as prolonged overdosage may result in dental fluorosis.
DO NOT SWALLOW in areas where the drinking water contains more than 0.7 ppm F or in conjunction with other adequate fluoride supplements.
How Supplied: 250 ml and 500 ml plastic bottles. Choice of cherry, lime and orange flavors.
Caution: Federal (U.S.A.) law prohibits dispensing without prescription.
KEEP OUT OF THE REACH OF CHILDREN.

POINT-TWO® Dental Rinse ℞
(0.2% Neutral Solution of Sodium Fluoride)

Description: 0.2% sodium fluoride in a pleasantly flavored, sugar and saccharin free neutral liquid. Contains 6% alcohol.
Indications: To aid in the protection against dental caries.
Precautions: Limited to topical use in the mouth only. DO NOT SWALLOW. Excessive ingestion may cause nausea and/or dental fluorosis.
Dosage and Administration: Children age 6 and over: Once a week, preferably at bedtime after thoroughly brushing teeth, rinse one or two teaspoonfuls (5-10 ml) around and between teeth for one minute, then expectorate. Do not eat, drink or rinse mouth for at least 15 minutes afterward.
How Supplied: 120 ml bottles.
Caution: Federal (U.S.A.) law prohibits dispensing without prescription.
KEEP OUT OF THE REACH OF CHILDREN.

THERA-FLUR® Topical Gel-Drops ℞
brand of Acidulated Phosphate Fluoride Gel

Description: 0.5% fluoride ion (from 1.1% sodium fluoride), 0.1 molar phosphate, in an aqueous vehicle at pH 4.5 Lime-flavored. Sugar and saccharin free.
Action and Uses: To aid in the protection against dental caries (age 3 to 18). For daily use with applicators supplied by dentist.
Administration and Dosage: Apply 5 to 10 drops, as required, to cover inner surface of each applicator. Spread liquid with tip of bottle. Then place applicators over upper and lower teeth at the same time. Bite down lightly for 6 minutes. Remove applicators. Rinse mouth. Clean applicators with cold water. Repeat treatment every day. . .preferably after brushing teeth in the evening.
Precautions: For application to teeth only. Frequent ingestion below age 12 may result in dental fluorosis.
How Supplied: 24 ml plastic dropper-bottles (approx. one-month supply). Bottle contains only 120 mg F in keeping with A.D.A. recommendations on the safe dispensing of fluoride.
Also Available: THERA-FLUR SELF-TOPICAL KIT: Two preformed thermoplastic trays for use in preparing custom-fitted mouthpiece-applicators for both the upper and lower arch of a patient, plus a 24-ml bottle of THERA-FLUR TOPICAL GEL-DROPS in a plastic case.
Also Available: THERA-FLUR-N Topical Gel-Drops at neutral pH; no artificial flavor or color.

Hynson, Westcott & Dunning

Becton Dickinson Immunodiagnostics
Division of Becton Dickinson and Co.
CHARLES & CHASE STS.
BALTIMORE, MD 21201

BAL IN OIL AMPULES ℞
(Dimercaprol Injection, USP)

Description: Dimercaprol (2,3-dimercapto-1-propanol) is a colorless or almost colorless liquid, having a disagreeable, mercaptan-like odor. Each 1 ml sterile BAL in Oil contains 100 mg Dimercaprol in 200 mg benzyl benzoate and 700 mg peanut oil. The slight sediment which may be noticed in some ampules develops during sterilization. It is not an indication that the solution is deteriorating.
Action: Dimercaprol promotes the excretion of arsenic, gold and mercury in cases of poisoning. It is also used in combination with Edetate Calcium Disodium Injection, USP to promote the excretion of lead.
Indications: BAL in Oil (Dimercaprol Injection, USP) is indicated in the treatment of arsenic, gold and mercury poisoning. It is indicated in acute lead poisoning when used concomitantly with Edetate Calcium Disodium Injection, USP.
Dimercaprol Injection, USP is effective for use in acute poisoning by mercury salts if therapy is begun within one or two hours following ingestion. It is not very effective for chronic mercury poisoning.
Dimercaprol Injection, USP is of questionable value in poisoning caused by other heavy metals such as antimony and bismuth. It should not be used in iron, cadmium, or selenium poisoning because the resulting dimercaprol-metal complexes are more toxic than the metal alone, especially to the kidneys.
Contraindications: BAL in Oil is contraindicated in most instances of hepatic insufficiency with the exception of postarsenical jaundice. The drug should be discontinued or used only with extreme caution if acute renal insufficiency develops during therapy.
Warnings: There may be local pain at the site of the injection. A reaction apparently peculiar to children is fever which may persist during therapy. It occurs in approximately 30% of children. A transient reduction of the percentage of polymorphonuclear leukocytes may also be observed.
Precautions: Because the dimercaprol-metal complex breaks down easily in an acid medium, production of an alkaline urine affords protection to the kidney during therapy. Medicinal iron should not be administered to patients under therapy with BAL. Data is not available regarding the use of dimercaprol during pregnancy and it should not be used unless judged by the physician to be necessary in the treatment of life threatening acute poisoning.
Adverse Reactions: One of the most consistent responses to Dimercaprol Injection, USP is a rise in blood pressure accompanied by tachycardia. This rise is roughly proportional to the dose administered. Doses larger than those recommended may cause other transitory signs and symptoms in approximate order of frequency as follows: (1) nausea and, in some instances, vomiting; (2) headache; (3) a burning sensation in the lips, mouth and throat; (4) a feeling of constriction, even pain, in the throat, chest, or hands; (5) conjunctivitis, lacrimation, blepharal spasm, rhinorrhea, and salivation; (6) tingling of the hands; (7) a burning sensation in the penis; (8) sweating of the forehead, hands and other areas; (9) abdominal pain; and (10) occasional appearance of painful sterile abscesses. Many of the above symptoms are accompanied by a feeling of anxiety, weakness, and unrest and often are relieved by administration of an antihistamine.

Dosage and Administration: By deep intramuscular injection only. For mild arsenic or gold poisoning, 2.5 mg/kg of body weight four times daily for two days, two times on the third day, and once daily thereafter for ten days; for severe arsenic or gold poisoning, 3 mg/kg every four hours for two days, four times on the third day, then twice daily thereafter for ten days. For mercury poisoning, 5 mg/kg initially, followed by 2.5 mg/kg one or two times daily for ten days. For acute lead encephalopathy 4 mg/kg body weight is given alone in the first dose and thereafter at four hour intervals in combination with Edetate Calcium Disodium Injection, USP administered at a separate site. For less severe poisoning the dose can be reduced to 3 mg/kg after the first dose. Treatment is maintained for two to seven days depending on clinical response. Successful treatment depends on beginning injections at the earliest possible moment and on the use of adequate amounts at frequent intervals. Other supportive measures should always be used in conjunction with BAL in Oil therapy.
How Supplied: 3 ml (100 mg/ml, ampules, box of 10, NDC 0011-8341-09).

LACTINEX® TABLETS AND GRANULES
(See PDR For Nonprescription Drugs)

Hyrex Pharmaceuticals
3494 DEMOCRAT RD.
MEMPHIS, TN 38118

GLUKOR INJECTION ℞

Composition: When mixed, each ml contains: Chorionic Gonadotropin 200 U.S.P. units, Thiamine HCl 25 mg, L (+) Glutamic Acid 52.5 ppm, Chlorobutanol 0.5%, Procaine HCl 1.0%, with Mannitol and Sodium Phosphate Dibasic and Monobasic.

HYTINIC CAPSULES AND ELIXIR
(polysaccharide-iron complex)

Composition: HYTINIC is a highly water-soluble complex of iron and a low molecular weight polysaccharide. Each HYTINIC Capsule contains 150 mg. elemental iron. Each 5 ml. (teaspoonful) HYTINIC Elixir contains 100 mg. elemental iron, alcohol 10% (sugar free).
Action and Uses: HYTINIC is an easily assimilated source of iron for treatment of uncomplicated iron deficiency anemia. Because HYTINIC is a polysaccharide bound iron complex, it is relatively nontoxic and there are relatively few, if any, of the gastrointestinal side effects associated with iron therapy, thus permitting full therapeutic dosage (150 to 300 mg. elemental iron daily) in a single dose if desirable. There is no staining of teeth and no metallic aftertaste.
Indications: For treatment of uncomplicated iron deficiency anemia.
Contraindications: In patients with hemochromatosis and hemosiderosis, and in those with a known hypersensitivity to any of the ingredients.
Administration and Dosage: ADULTS: One or two HYTINIC Capsules daily, or one or two teaspoonfuls HYTINIC Elixir daily. CHILDREN 6 to 12 years of age: One teaspoonful HYTINIC Elixir daily; Children 2 to 6 years of age: ½ teaspoonful HYTINIC Elixir daily. For younger children, consult physician.
How Supplied: HYTINIC Capsules: (Green and white) Bottles of 50 and 500. HYTINIC Elixir: Bottles of 8 ounces.
Product Identification Mark: Hyrex.

HYTUSS TABLETS (100 mg)
HYTUSS-2X CAPSULES (200 mg)
Brand of guaifenesin N.F. (formerly called glyceryl guaiacolate)

Composition: Each sugar-free Hytuss Tablet contains guaifenesin 100 mg. Each sugar-free Hytuss-2X Capsule contains guaifenesin 200 mg.
Action and Uses: This preparation utilizes the effective expectorant action of guaifenesin N.F. (formerly called glyceryl guaicolate) which significantly stimulates the secretion of respiratory tract fluid. The increased flow of less viscid fluid favors expectoration and has a demulcent effect on the tracheobronchial mucosa. The primary usefulness of Hytuss Tablets is to promote the change from a dry, unproductive cough to a productive cough. Hytuss is therefore useful in treating coughs due to the common cold, bronchitis, laryngitis, tracheitis, pharyngitis, influenza and the measles. The expectorant action of Hytuss may also provide symptomatic relief in some chronic respiratory disorders when the patient experiences spasms of dry nonproductive coughing.
Precautions: Extremely large amounts may cause nausea and vomiting.
Dosage: HYTUSS TABLETS—*Adults*—1 or 2 tablets four times daily. *Children 6-12 years of age*—½ tablet three or four times daily.
Dosage: HYTUSS-2X CAPSULES—*Adults*—1 capsule four times daily.
How Supplied: 100 mg. Tablet — White, scored, sugar-free, bottles of 100 — 1,000 — 5,000. Also 200 mg. Capsule, red and white, sugar-free, bottles of 100 — 1,000.
Product Identification Mark: Tablet—Hy. Capsule—Hyrex.

NICOZOL CAPSULES & ELIXIR ℞

Composition: Each capsule contains: Pentylenetetrazol 100 mg and Niacin 50 mg. Each 5cc of Elixir contains: Pentylenetetrazol 200 mg and Niacin 100 mg with 5% Alcohol.

TRAC TABS ℞
TRAC TABS 2X

Composition: Each tablet contains: Trac Tabs—Atropine Sulfate 0.03 mg. Hyoscyamine 0.03 mg. Methenamine 40.8 mg. Methylene Blue 5.4 mg. Phenyl Salicylate 18.1 mg. Gelsemium 6.1 mg. Benzoic Acid 4.5 mg. **Trac Tabs 2X is double strength.**
Action and Uses: Trac Tabs is indicated in those urinary tract infections where the invading organisms are susceptible to Methylene Blue and Methenamine, such as E. coli, staphylococcus aureus and albus. The urine must be maintained at an acid pH in order for Trac Tabs to be effective. Prior to urinary tract instrumentation and surgery, Trac Tabs may be prophylactically indicated. The Atropine and Hyoscyamine provide antispasmodic activity to alleviate the smooth muscle spasm often associated with urinary infection. Gelsemium provides analgesic activity.
Contraindications: Glaucoma and myasthenis gravis.
Warning: Gelsemium toxic effects may be delayed for hours. Warning signs are ptosis, double vision, dilated pupils, weakness and depression. Treatment of gelsemium poisoning: Evacuate the stomach. Absolute rest in horizontal position. Administer spinal and arterial stimulants such as Ammonia, Strychnine, and Digitalis.
Precautions: Do not exceed recommended dosage. If dryness of the mouth occurs, decrease dosage. Discontinue use if rapid pulse, dizziness or blurring of vision occurs. Acute urinary retention may result from prostatic hypertrophy.
Dosage: TRAC TABS—*Adults*—Two tablets, 4 times daily, with a full glass of water. *Children*—One-half adult dosage.
Dosage: Trac Tabs 2X—*Adults*—One tablet, 4 times daily, with a full glass of water. Severe infections: Initially take one Trac Tabs 2X every hour for 3 doses, then follow the above recommended daily dose schedule.
Note: Patients should be advised that urine will be blue when taking this medication.
How Supplied: TRAC TABS (purple tablet)—bottles of 100 – 1,000 – 5,000. TRAC TABS 2X (blue-green tablet)—bottles of 100 – 1,000 – 5,000.

ICN Pharmaceuticals, Inc.
222 NORTH VINCENT AVENUE
COVINA, CA 91722

TESTRED® ℞
(brand of Methyltestosterone)

Description: Each capsule contains 10 mg. of Methyltestosterone, a synthetic androgen occurring as white or creamy white crystals or powder.
Actions: The action of methyltestosterone is similar to that of testosterone. However, it is effective when administered orally, this efficacy being attributed to the fact that the molecule is sufficiently stable to escape extensive inactivation in the liver.
The androgenic action of methyltestosterone is responsible for maintenance of secondary sexual characteristics as well as for development of accessory sexual organs in the male.
Indications:
In the male:
1. Eunuchoidism and eunuchism.
2. Male climacteric when symptoms are secondary to androgen deficiency.
3. Impotence resulting from androgen deficiency.
4. Postpubertal cryptorchidism with evidence of hypogonadism.

In the female:
1. Prevention of postpartum breast pain and engorgement in the non-nursing mother. There is no satisfactory evidence that this drug prevents or suppresses lactation per se.
2. Palliation of androgen-responsive, advancing, inoperable breast cancer in women who are more than 1, but less than 5 years postmenopausal or who have been proven to have a hormone-dependent tumor, as shown by previous beneficial response to castration.

Contraindications: Contraindicated in persons with known or suspected carcinoma of the prostate and in carcinoma of the male breast. Contraindicated in the presence of severe liver damage.
Contraindicated during pregnancy and in breast-feeding mothers because of the possibility of masculinization of the female fetus or breast-fed infant.
Warnings: Female patients should be watched carefully for symptoms or signs of virilization such as hoarseness or deepening of the voice, oily skin, acne, hirsutism, enlarged clitoris, stimulation of libido, and menstrual irregularities. At the dosage necessary to achieve a tumor response, androgens will cause masculinization of a female, but occasionally a sensitive female may exhibit one or more of these signs on smaller doses. Some of these changes, such as voice changes, may be irreversible even after drug is stopped.
Cholestatic hepatitis with jaundice and altered liver function tests, such as increased BSP retention and rises in SGOT levels, have been reported after methyltestosterone. These changes appear to be related to dosage of the drug. Therefore, in the presence of any changes in liver function tests, the drug should be discontinued.

Continued on next page

ICN Pharmaceuticals—Cont.

Precautions: Prolonged dosage of androgen may result in sodium and fluid retention. This may present a problem, especially in patients with compromised cardiac reserve or renal disease.
In treating males for symptoms of climacteric, avoid stimulation to the point of increasing the nervous, mental, and physical activities beyond the patient's cardiovascular capacity.
If priapism or other signs of excessive sexual stimulation develop, discontinue therapy.
In the male, prolonged administration or excessive dosage may cause inhibition of testicular function, with resultant oligospermia and decrease in ejaculatory volume. Use cautiously in young boys to avoid possible premature epiphyseal closure or precocious sexual development.
Hypersensitivity and gynecomastia may occur rarely.
PBI may be increased in patients taking androgens.
Hypercalcemia may occur, particularly during therapy for metastatic breast carcinoma. If this occurs, the drug should be discontinued.
Adverse Reactions: Cholestatic jaundice. Oligospermia and decreased ejaculatory volume. Hypercalcemia, particularly in patients with metastatic breast carcinoma. This usually indicates progression of bone metastases. Virilization in female patients. Sodium and water retention. Hypersensitivity and gynecomastia. Priapism.
Dosage and Administration: Dosage must be strictly individualized, as patients vary widely in requirements. Daily requirements are best administered in divided doses. The following chart is suggested as an average daily dosage guide.

Indications	**Average Daily Dosage**
In the male	
Eunuchism and eunuchoidism	10 to 40 mg.
Male climacteric and male impotence	10 to 40 mg.
Cryptorchidism—postpubertal	30 mg.
In the female	
Postpartum breast pain and engorgement (3 to 5 days)	80 mg.
Palliation for women with advancing inoperable breast cancer	*200 mg.

*As long as improvement is maintained. If a response to androgen therapy is going to occur, it will be apparent within 3 months of beginning therapy. When the disease agent becomes progressive, therapy should be stopped and the patient observed for another period of improvement known as "rebound regression".
How Supplied: Bottles of 100, 500 and 1000 capsules.
Caution: Federal law prohibits dispensing without prescription.

Important Notice

Before prescribing or administering any product described in PHYSICIANS' DESK REFERENCE always consult the PDR Supplement for possible new or revised information.

Invenex Laboratories

5885 LAKEHURST DRIVE
ORLANDO, FLORIDA 32809

GENERIC PHARMACEUTICAL INJECTABLE PRODUCTS

AMINOPHYLLIN INJECTION, U.S.P.; VIAL & AMPUL ℞
ASCORBIC ACID INJECTION, U.S.P.; AMPUL ℞
ATROPINE SULFATE INJECTION, U.S.P.; VIAL & AMPUL ℞
CALCIUM CHLORIDE INJECTION, U.S.P.; VIAL ℞
CALCIUM GLUCONATE INJECTION; VIAL & AMPUL ℞
CYANOCOBALAMIN INJECTION, U.S.P.; VIAL & AMPUL ℞
DEXPANTHENOL INJECTION; VIAL ℞
DEXTROSE INJECTION, U.S.P. 10%; AMPUL ℞
DEXTROSE INJECTION, U.S.P. 50%; VIAL ℞
DIGOXIN INJECTION, U.S.P.; AMPUL ℞
DIPHENHYDRAMINE HYDROCHLORIDE INJECTION, U.S.P.; AMPUL ℞
EPHEDRINE SULFATE INJECTION, U.S.P.; AMPUL ℞
ERGONOVINE MALEATE INJECTION, N.F.; AMPUL ℞
HEPARIN LOCK FLUSH SOLUTION, U.S.P.; VIAL ℞
HEPARIN SODIUM INJECTION, U.S.P.; VIAL & AMPUL ℞
ISOPROTERENOL HYDROCHLORIDE INJECTION, U.S.P.; AMPUL ℞
LIDOCAINE HYDROCHLORIDE INJECTION, U.S.P.; VIAL & AMPUL ℞
LIDOCAINE HYDROCHLORIDE INJECTION, U.S.P.; VIAL (FOR CARDIAC ARRHYTHMIAS) ℞
MAGNESIUM SULFATE INJECTION, U.S.P. 50%; VIAL & AMPUL ℞
MANNITOL INJECTION, U.S.P. 25%; VIAL ℞
METARAMINOL BITARTRATE INJECTION, U.S.P.; VIAL ℞
MURI-LUBE (MINERAL OIL), LIGHT/HEAVY; VIAL ℞
OXYTOCIN INJECTION, U.S.P., SYNTHETIC; VIAL & AMPUL ℞
POTASSIUM ACETATE INJECTION, U.S.P.; VIAL ℞
CONCENTRATED POTASSIUM CHLORIDE INJECTION, U.S.P.; VIAL ℞
POTASSIUM CHLORIDE INJECTION, U.S.P.; VIAL & AMPUL ℞
POTASSIUM PHOSPHATE INJECTION; VIAL ℞
PROCAINE HYDROCHLORIDE INJECTION, U.S.P.; VIAL & AMPUL ℞
PYRIDOXINE HYDROCHLORIDE INJECTION, U.S.P.; VIAL ℞
SCOPOLAMINE HYDROBROMIDE INJECTION, U.S.P.; VIAL & AMPUL ℞
SODIUM ACETATE INJECTION; VIAL ℞
SODIUM BICARBONATE INJECTION, U.S.P.; VIAL & AMPUL ℞
CONCENTRATED SODIUM CHLORIDE INJECTION; VIAL ℞
SODIUM CHLORIDE INJECTION, U.S.P.; VIAL & AMPUL ℞
SODIUM CHLORIDE INJECTION, U.S.P.; VIAL (BACTERIOSTATIC) ℞
THIAMINE HYDROCHLORIDE INJECTION, U.S.P.; VIAL & AMPUL ℞
WATER FOR INJECTION, U.S.P.; VIAL & AMPUL ℞
WATER FOR INJECTION, U.S.P.; VIAL (BACTERIOSTATIC) ℞

Ives Laboratories Inc.

685 THIRD AVENUE
NEW YORK, NY 10017

CYCLOSPASMOL® ℞
(cyclandelate)
Capsules-Tablets

Composition: Each *blue* and *red* capsule contains 400 mg. of cyclandelate, and each *blue* capsule contains 200 mg. of cyclandelate. Each *orange* tablet contains 100 mg. cyclandelate.
Actions: CYCLOSPASMOL is an orally acting vasodilator. The activity of this drug, as measured by pharmacological tests against various types of smooth muscle spasm produced by acetylcholine, histamine, and barium chloride, exceeds that of papaverine, particularly in regard to the neurotropic component produced by the acetylcholine. Cyclandelate is musculotropic, acting directly on vascular smooth muscle, and has no significant adrenergic stimulating or blocking actions.
The drug is not intended to substitute for other appropriate medical or surgical programs in the treatment of peripheral or cerebral vascular disease.

Indications
Based on a review of this drug by the National Academy of Sciences—National Research Council and/or other information, FDA has classified the indications as follows:
"Possibly" effective: CYCLOSPASMOL is indicated for adjunctive therapy in intermittent claudication; arteriosclerosis obliterans; thrombophlebitis (to control associated vasospasm and muscular ischemia); nocturnal leg cramps; Raynaud's phenomenon; and for selected cases of ischemic cerebral vascular disease.
Final classification of the less-than-effective indications requires further investigation.

Contraindications: CYCLOSPASMOL is contraindicated in cases of known hypersensitivity to the drug.
Warnings: 1. Cyclandelate should be used with extreme caution in patients with severe obliterative coronary artery or cerebral-vascular disease, since there is a possibility that these diseased areas may be compromised by vasodilatory effects of the drug elsewhere. 2. **Use in Pregnancy:** The safety of cyclandelate for use during pregnancy or lactation has not been established; therefore, it should not be used in pregnant women or in women of childbearing age unless, in the judgment of the physician, its use is deemed absolutely essential to the welfare of the patient. 3. Although no prolongation of bleeding time has been demonstrated in humans in therapeutic dosages, it has been demonstrated in animals at very large doses. Therefore, the hazard of a prolonged bleeding time should be carefully considered when administering cyclandelate to a patient with active bleeding or a bleeding tendency.
Precautions: Since CYCLOSPASMOL (cyclandelate) is a vasodilator, it should be used with caution in patients having glaucoma.
Adverse Reactions: Gastrointestinal distress (pyrosis, pain, and eructation) may occur with CYCLOSPASMOL. These symptoms occur infrequently and are usually mild. Relief can often be obtained by taking the medication with meals or by the concomitant use of antacids.
Mild flush, headache, feeling of weakness, or tachycardia may occur, especially during the first weeks of administration.
Dosage and Administration: It is often advantageous to initiate therapy at higher dosage; e.g.: 1200-1600 mg. per day, given in di-

vided doses before meals and at bedtime. When a clinical response is noted, the dosage can be decreased in 200-mg. decrements until the maintenance dosage is reached. The usual maintenance dosage of CYCLOSPASMOL (cyclandelate) is between 400 and 800 mg. per day given in two to four divided doses.

Although objective signs of therapeutic benefit may be rapid and dramatic, more often, this improvement occurs gradually over weeks of therapy. It is strongly recommended that the patient be educated to the fact that prolonged use may be necessary. Short term use of CYCLOSPASMOL is rarely beneficial, nor is it likely to be of any permanent value.

How Supplied: 400 mg. blue and red capsules in bottles of 100, and 500; 200 mg. blue capsules in bottles of 100, 500, and 1000; 100 mg. orange tablets in bottles of 100 and 500.

Literature Available: Yes.

[Cir. Cl 2958-1 1/26/78]

[*Shown in Product Identification Section*]

ISORDIL® ℞
(isosorbide dinitrate)
(10 Dosage Forms)

Actions: The basic action of ISORDIL is that of all nitrates, the relaxation of smooth muscle. How this relates to its clinical usefulness in the treatment of angina pectoris (pain of coronary artery disease) is not clear, since the exact cause of this pain is also obscure.

The objective of therapy is a decrease in the frequency and severity of attacks of angina pectoris and a decrease in the need to use nitroglycerin. This is the only practical way to judge the effects of therapy, especially since there is a wide variation in symptomatic response to treatment. ISORDIL is widely accepted as a safe and useful therapeutic agent in the treatment of angina pectoris.

Indications

Based on a review of this drug by the National Academy of Sciences—National Research Council and/or other information, FDA has classified the indications as follows:

"Probably" effective: When taken by the sublingual or chewable route ISORDIL SUBLINGUAL and CHEWABLE tablets are indicated for the treatment of acute anginal attacks and for prophylaxis in situations likely to provoke such attacks.

"Possibly" effective: When taken by the oral route, ISORDIL is indicated for the relief of angina pectoris (pain of coronary artery disease). It is not intended to abort the acute anginal episode, but is widely regarded as useful in the prophylactic treatment of angina pectoris.

Final classification of the less-than-effective indications requires further investigation.

Contraindication: Idiosyncrasy to this drug.

Warning: Data supporting the use of nitrites during the early days of the acute phase of myocardial infarction (the period during which clinical and laboratory findings are unstable) are insufficient to establish safety.

Precautions: 1. Tolerance to this drug, and cross-tolerance to other nitrites and nitrates may occur. 2. In patients with functional or organic gastrointestinal hypermotility or malabsorption syndrome, it is suggested that either the ISORDIL 5 mg., 10 mg., 20 mg., or 30 mg. Oral TITRADOSE® tablets, or ISORDIL 2.5 mg. or 5 mg. SUBLINGUAL tablets, or 10 mg. ISORDIL CHEWABLE tablets be the preferred therapy. The reason for this is that a few patients have reported passing partially dissolved ISORDIL TEMBIDS tablets in their stools. This phenomenon is believed to be on the basis of physiologic variability and to reflect rapid gastrointestinal transit of the tablet.

Adverse Reactions: 1. Cutaneous vasodilation with flushing. 2. Headache is common and may be severe and persistent. 3. Transient episodes of dizziness and weakness, as well as other signs of cerebral ischemia associated with postural hypotension, may occasionally develop. 4. This drug can act as a physiological antagonist to norepinephrine, acetylcholine, histamine, and many other agents. 5. An occasional individual exhibits marked sensitivity to the hypotensive effects of nitrite, and severe responses (nausea, vomiting, weakness, restlessness, pallor, perspiration and collapse) can occur even with the usual therapeutic dose. Alcohol may enhance this effect. 6. Drug rash and/or exfoliative dermatitis may occasionally occur.

Dosage and Administration: ISORDIL (isosorbide dinitrate) 2.5 mg. and 5 mg. SUBLINGUAL tablets. The basic dosage is one or two 5 mg. tablets every 2 to 3 hours. The 2.5 mg. tablet facilitates adjustment of dosage in patients who may require it. Both dosage forms are used sublingually for treatment of an angina pectoris attack (including angina decubitus) or prophylactically in situations likely to provoke such attacks.

ISORDIL 10 mg. CHEWABLE tablets. The smallest effective dose should be used. The initial dose should be no more than 5 mg (½ tablet) as an occasional severe hypotensive response may occur. The low dose may be effective in relieving the acute attack, but if no significant hypotension is seen, an increase in dose may permit more effective prevention of attacks. The chewable tablet is scored to permit dosage adjustment. For relief of the acute attack, the medication may be taken p.r.n. For prophylaxis, it may be taken every 2–3 hours.

ISORDIL 5 mg., 10 mg., 20 mg., or 30 mg. ORAL TITRADOSE tablets with E.Z. SPLIT® scoring are administered orally. The dosage range is 5 mg. to 30 mg. q.i.d., with the usual dosage being 10 mg. to 20 mg. q.i.d.

The uniquely-designed and patented **TITRADOSE E.Z. SPLIT** Oral Tablet dosage forms permit clean-cut splitting of the tablet into equal halves to simplify more accurate dosage titration. Thus, the physician may prescribe (or adjust) a dosage regimen to include half-tablet units for optimal relief. To break the tablet into two even halves, the patient has only to place the tablet on a hard, flat surface, scored side up, and then press the scored surface lightly with the index finger or thumb. Isordil Oral 5, 10, 20, and 30 mg. **TITRADOSE** Tablets replace the former, conventionally-scored tablets.

ISORDIL (10 mg.) with PHENOBARBITAL (15 mg.) tablets are indicated when anxiety or emotional disturbances are important factors in the clinical picture and should be administered on a similar dosage regimen to the plain 10 mg. tablets. **(Warning: Phenobarbital may be habit-forming.)**

ISORDIL TEMBIDS *TABLETS* 40 mg. and ISORDIL TEMBIDS *CAPSULES* 40 mg.: These sustained action medications are administered orally every 6 to 12 hours according to need. They are indicated for sustained prophylaxis against angina pectoris attacks including nocturnal angina. Although the latter condition is relatively infrequent, it is nonetheless angina, i.e., pain of coronary artery disease. The drug is gradually released over a 6-hour period to provide 8–10 hours of sustained effect. Although experiencing a reduction in the number of anginal attacks while under TEMBIDS therapy, patients may still have an attack under stressful conditions. In such cases, the therapy should be supplemented with Sublingual ISORDIL Tablets or nitroglycerin. ISORDIL TEMBIDS SHOULD NOT BE CHEWED.

How Supplied: ISORDIL SUBLINGUAL 2.5 mg.: Supplied in bottles of 100 and 500 yellow tablets. ISORDIL SUBLINGUAL 5 mg.: Supplied in bottles of 100, 250, and 500 pink tablets. ISORDIL CHEWABLE 10 mg.: Supplied in bottles of 100 scored, yellow tablets. ISORDIL ORAL TITRADOSE 5 mg.: Supplied in bottles of 100, 500, and 1000 scored, pink tablets. ISORDIL ORAL TITRADOSE 10 mg.: Supplied in bottles of 100, 500, and 1000 scored, white tablets. ISORDIL ORAL TITRADOSE 20 mg.: Supplied in bottles of 100 and 500 scored, green tablets. ISORDIL ORAL TITRADOSE 30 mg.: Supplied in bottles of 100 scored, blue tablets. ISORDIL (10 mg.) WITH PHENOBARBITAL (15 mg.): Supplied in bottles of 100 and 500 scored, orange tablets. ISORDIL TEMBIDS Tablets 40 mg.: Supplied in bottles of 100, 500, and 1000 scored, green, sustained action tablets. ISORDIL TEMBIDS Capsules, 40 mg.: Supplied in bottles of 100 and 500 sustained-action capsules (opaque blue cap and colorless, transparent body).

Clinipak® Unit dose Medication, Boxes of 100 Tablets (20 strips of 5), is available as:
Isordil Sublingual Tablets, 2.5 mg
Isordil Sublingual Tablets, 5 mg
Isordil Chewable Tablets, 10 mg
Isordil Oral Titradose, 5 mg
Isordil Oral Titradose, 10 mg
Isordil Oral Titradose, 20 mg

Clinical Studies: ISORDIL (isosorbide dinitrate) is widely regarded as an effective, long-acting coronary vasodilator for the management of angina pectoris associated with coronary insufficiency. It may significantly reduce the number, duration and severity of angina attacks. Exercise tolerance may be increased in some patients with all forms of ISORDIL. The 5 mg. sublingual tablet, however, provides greater benefit both in regard to the number of patients who respond to it and the amount of exercise tolerated. Clinical improvement has been customarily measured subjectively by reduction in number of angina attacks and by the change in nitroglycerin requirements.

The 5 mg. ISORDIL SUBLINGUAL tablet has been evaluated clinically, and, by employing exercise tolerance tests, it has been found that this dosage has an onset of action within the range of 2 to 5 minutes, which in some instances, is not as rapid as nitroglycerin (but almost equal in magnitude). Duration of action, however, ranges from 1 to 2 hours, which compares with a duration of action of 20 to 30 minutes in the case of nitroglycerin.

Kinetocardiographic clinical studies indicate that the 10 mg. oral tablet and 40 mg. TEMBID tablet are effective for prolonged periods.

In patients subjected to emotional or physical stress, the oral 5 mg., 10 mg., 20 mg., 30 mg., and 40 mg. ISORDIL medications are of limited effectiveness. In situations where the patient may be exposed to unusual stress, it is suggested that the 2.5 mg. and 5 mg. ISORDIL SUBLINGUAL tablets be used supplementally as required.

Cine-coronary arteriographic studies have demonstrated that ISORDIL can produce a marked dilatation of the larger branches of the coronary arteries (larger than 200 microns). Dilatation of these coronary arteries and collateral coronary arteries persists for more than two hours after Sublingual ISORDIL, as demonstrated by cine-coronary arteriography. The correlation of this demonstrated dilation to increased coronary flow or improvement in clinical angina has not been established.

Literature Available: Yes.

TEMBIDS®—Trademark for sustained action dosage forms.

[Cir. 2876-1—Rev. 6/20/79]

[*Shown in Product Identification Section*]

SURMONTIL® ℞
(trimipramine maleate)

Description: SURMONTIL® (trimipramine maleate) is 5-(3-dimethylamino-2-methyl-

Continued on next page

Ives—Cont.

propyl)-10,11-dihydro-5H-dibenz (b,f) azepine acid maleate (racemic form).
Trimipramine maleate is prepared as a racemic mixture which can be resolved into levorotatory and dextrorotatory isomers. Trimipramine maleate is an almost odorless, white or slightly cream-colored crystalline substance melting at 140–144° C. It is virtually insoluble in ether and water; is slightly soluble in ethanol and acetone and freely soluble in chloroform and methanol at 20° C.

Clinical Pharmacology: SURMONTIL® is an antidepressant with an anxiety-reducing, sedative component to its action. The mode of action of SURMONTIL® on the central nervous system is not known. However, unlike amphetamine-type compounds it does not act primarily by stimulation of the central nervous system. It does not act by inhibition of the monoamine oxidase system.

Indications: SURMONTIL® is indicated for the relief of symptoms of depression. Endogenous depression is more likely to be alleviated than other depressive states. In studies with neurotic out-patients, the drug appeared to be equivalent to amitripytyline in the less depressed patients but somewhat less effective than amitriptyline in the more severely depressed patients. In hospitalized depressed patients, trimipramine and imipramine were equally effective in relieving depression.

Contraindications: SURMONTIL® is contraindicated in cases of known hypersensitivity to the drug. The possibility of cross-sensitivity to other dibenzazepine compounds should be kept in mind. SURMONTIL® should not be given in conjunction with drugs of the monoamine oxidase inhibitor class (e.g.: tranylcypromine, isocarboxazid or phenelzine sulfate). The concomitant use of monoamine oxidase inhibitors (MAOI) and tricyclic compounds similar to SURMONTIL® has caused severe hyperpyretic reactions, convulsive crises, and death in some patients. At least two weeks should elapse after cessation of therapy with MAOI before instituting therapy with SURMONTIL®. Initial dosage should be low and increased gradually with caution and careful observation of the patient. The drug is contraindicated during the acute recovery period after a myocardial infarction.

Warnings:

Use in Children—This drug is not recommended for use in children, since safety and effectiveness in the pediatric age group have not been established.

General Consideration for Use—Extreme caution should be used when this drug is given to patients with any evidence of cardiovascular disease because of the possibility of conduction defects, arrhythmias, myocardial infarction, strokes, and tachycardia.

Caution is advised in patients with increased intraocullar pressure, history of urinary retention, or history of narrow-angle glaucoma because of the drug's anticholinergic properties; hyperthyroid patients or those on thyroid medication because of the possibility of cardiovascular toxicity; patients with a history of seizure disorder because this drug has been shown to lower the seizure threshold; patients receiving guanethidine or similar agents since SURMONTIL® may block the pharmacologic effects of these drugs.

Since the drug may impair the mental and/or physical abilities required for the performance of potentially hazardous tasks, such as operating an automobile or machinery, the patient should be cautioned accordingly.

Precautions: The possibility of suicide is inherent in any severely depressed patient, and persists until a significant remission occurs. When a patient with a serious suicidal potential is not hospitalized, the prescription should be for the smallest amount feasible.
In schizophrenic patients activation of the psychosis may occur and require reduction of dosage or the addition of a major tranquilizer to the therapeutic regime.
Manic or hypomanic episodes may occur in some patients, in particular those with cyclic-type disorders. In some cases therapy with SURMONTIL® must be discontinued until the episode is relieved, after which therapy may be reinstituted at lower dosages if still required.
Concurrent administration of SURMONTIL® and electroshock therapy may increase the hazards of therapy. Such treatment should be limited to those patients for whom it is essential. When possible, discontinue the drug for several days prior to elective surgery.
Patients should be warned that the concomitant use of alcoholic beverages may be associated with exaggerated effects.
It has been reported that tricyclic antidepressants can potentiate the effects of catecholamines. Similarly, atropine-like effects may be more pronounced in patients receiving anticholinergic therapy. Therefore, particular care should be exercised when it is necessary to administer tricyclic antidepressants with sympathomimetic amines, local decongestants, local anesthetics containing epinephrine, atropine or drugs with an anticholinergic effect. In resistant cases of depression in adults, a dose of 2.5 mg/kg/day may have to be exceeded. If a higher dose is needed, ECG monitoring should be maintained during the initiation of therapy and at appropriate intervals during stabilization of dose.

Usage in Pregnancy—Pregnancy Category C. SURMONTIL® has shown evidence of embryo-toxicity and/or increased incidence of major anomalies in rats or rabbits at doses 20 times the human dose. There are no adequate and well-controlled studies in pregnant women. SURMONTIL® should be used during pregnancy only if the potential benefit justifies the potential risk to the fetus.
Semen studies in man (four schizophrenics and nine normal volunteers) revealed no significant changes in sperm morphology. It is recognized that drugs having a parasympathetic effect, including tricyclic antidepressants, may alter the ejaculatory response.
Chronic animal studies showed occasional evidence of degeneration of seminiferous tubules at the highest dose of 60 mg/kg/day.
SURMONTIL® should be used with caution in patients with impaired liver function.
Chronic animal studies showed occasional occurrence of hepatic congestion, fatty infiltration, or increased serum liver enzymes at the highest dose of 60 mg/kg/day.
Both elevation and lowering of blood sugar have been reported with tricyclic antidepressants.

Adverse Reactions:
Note: The pharmacological similarities among the tricyclic antidepressants require that each of the reactions be considered when SURMONTIL® is administered. Some of the adverse reactions included in this listing have not in fact been reported with SURMONTIL®.

Cardiovascular—Hypotension, hypertension, tachycardia, palpitation, myocardial infarction, arrhythmias, heart block, stroke.

Psychiatric—Confusional states (especially the elderly) with hallucinations, disorientation, delusions; anxiety, restlessness, agitation; insomnia and nightmares; hypomania; exacerbation of psychosis.

Neurological—Numbness, tingling, paresthesias of extremities; incoordination, ataxia, tremors; peripheral neuropathy; extrapyramidal symptoms; seizures, alterations in EEG patterns; tinnitus.

Anticholinergic—Dry mouth and, rarely, associated sublingual adenitis; blurred vision, disturbances of accommodation, mydriasis, constipation, paralytic ileus; urinary retention, delayed micturition, dilation of the urinary tract.

Allergic—Skin rash, petechiae, urticaria, itching, photo-sensitization, edema of face and tongue.

Hematologic—Bone-marrow depression including agranulocytosis, eosinophilia; purpura; thrombocytopenia. Leukocyte and differential counts should be performed in any patient who develops fever and sore throat during therapy; the drug should be discontinued if there is evidence of pathological neutrophil depression.

Gastrointestinal—Nausea and vomiting, anorexia, epigastric distress, diarrhea, peculiar taste, stomatitis, abdominal cramps, black tongue.

Endocrine—Gynecomastia in the male; breast enlargement and galactorrhea in the female; increased or decreased libido, impotence; testicular swelling; elevation or depression of blood-sugar levels.

Other—Jaundice (simulating obstructive); altered liver function; weight gain or loss; perspiration; flushing; urinary frequency; drowsiness, dizziness, weakness, and fatigue; headache; parotid swelling; alopecia.

Withdrawal Symptoms—Though not indicative of addiction, abrupt cessation of treatment after prolonged therapy may produce nausea, headache, and malaise.

Dosage and Administration: Dosage should be initiated at a low level and increased gradually, noting carefully the clinical response and any evidence of intolerance.
Lower dosages are recommended for elderly patients and adolescents. Lower dosages are also recommended for out-patients as compared to hospitalized patients who will be under close supervision. It is not possible to prescribe a single dosage schedule of SURMONTIL® that will be therapeutically effective in all patients. The physical psychodynamic factors contributing to depressive symptomatology are very complex; spontaneous remissions or exacerbations of depressive symptoms may occur with or without drug therapy. Consequently, the recommended dosage regimens are furnished as a guide which may be modified by factors such as the age of the patient, chronicity and severity of the disease, medical condition of the patient, and degree of psychotherapeutic support.
Most antidepressant drugs have a lag period of ten days to four weeks before a therapeutic response is noted. Increasing the dose will not shorten this period, but rather increase the incidence of adverse reactions.

Usual Adult Dose:

Outpatients and Office Patients—Initially, 75 mg/day in divided doses, increased to 150 mg/day. Dosages over 200 mg/day are not recommended. Maintenance therapy is in the range of 50–150 mg/day. For convenient therapy and to facilitate patient compliance, the total dosage requirement may be given at bedtime.

Hospitalized Patients—Initially, 100 mg/day in divided doses. This may be increased gradually in a few days to 200 mg/day depending upon individual response and tolerance. If improvement does not occur in 2–3 weeks, the dose may be increased to the maximum recommended dose of 250–300 mg/day.

Adolescent and Geriatric Patients—Initially, a dose of 50 mg/day daily is recommended, with gradual increments up to 100 mg/day depending upon patient response and tolerance.

Maintenance—Following remission, maintenance medication may be required for a longer period of time, at the lowest dose that will maintain remission. Maintenance therapy is preferably administered as a single dose at bedtime. To minimize relapse, maintenance therapy should be continued for about three months.

Overdosage:

Signs and Symptoms—The response of the patient to toxic overdosage of tricyclic antidepressants may vary in severity and is conditioned by factors such as age, amount ingested, amount absorbed, interval between ingestion and start of treatment. SURMONTIL® is not recommended for infants or young children. Should accidental ingestion occur in any amount, it should be regarded as serious and potentially fatal.

CNS abnormalities may include drowsiness, stupor, coma, ataxia, restlessness, agitation, hyperactive reflexes, muscle rigidity, athetoid and choreiform movements and convulsions. Cardiac abnormalities may include arrhythmia, tachycardia, ECG evidence of impaired conduction, and signs of congestive failure. Other symptoms may include respiratory depression, cyanosis, hypotension, shock, vomiting, hyperpyrexia, mydriasis, and diaphoresis. Treatment is supportive and symptomatic, as no specific antidote is known. Depending upon need the following measures can be considered:

1. SURMONTIL® is not recommended for use in infants and children. Hospitalization with continuous cardiac monitoring for up to 4 days is recommended for children who have ingested SURMONTIL® in any amount. This is based on the reported greater sensitivity of children to acute overdosage with tricyclic antidepressants.
2. Blood and urine levels may not reflect the severity of the poisoning and are mostly of diagnostic value.
3. CNS involvement, respiratory depression, or cardiac arrhythmia can occur suddenly; hospitalization and close observation are necessary, even when the amount ingested is thought to be small or initial toxicity appears slight. Patients with any alteration of ECG should have continuous cardiac monitoring for at least 72 hours and be observed until well after the cardiac status has returned to normal; relapses may occur after apparent recovery.
4. The slow intravenous administration of physostigmine salicylate has been reported to reverse most of the cardiovascular and CNS effects of overdosage with tricyclic antidepressants. In adults, 1 to 3 mg has been reported to be effective. In children, start with 0.5 mg and repeat at 5-minute intervals to determine the minimum effective dose; do not exceed 2.0 mg. Avoid rapid injection, to reduce the possibility of physostigmine-induced convulsions. Because of the short duration of action of physostigmine, it may be necessary to repeat doses at 30- to 60-minute intervals as necessary.
5. In the alert patient, empty the stomach rapidly by induced emesis, followed by lavage. In the obtunded patient, secure the airway with a cuffed endotracheal tube before beginning lavage (do not induce emesis). Instillation of activated-charcoal slurry may help reduce absorption of trimipramine.
6. Minimize external stimulation to reduce the tendency to convulsions. If anticonvulsants are necessary, diazepam, short-acting barbiturates, paraldehyde, or methocarbamol may be useful. Do not use barbiturates if MAO inhibitors have been taken recently.
7. Maintain adequate respiratory exchange. Do not use respiratory stimulants.
8. Shock should be treated with supportive measures, such as intravenous fluids, oxygen, and corticosteroids. Digitalis may increase conduction abnormalities and further irritate an already sensitized myocardium. If congestive heart failure necessitates rapid digitalization, particular care must be exercised.
9. Hyperpyrexia should be controlled by whatever external means available, including ice packs and cooling sponge baths if necessary.
10. Hemodialysis, peritoneal dialysis, exchange transfusions, and forced diuresis have been generally reported as ineffective in tricyclic poisoning.

How Supplied: SURMONTIL® (trimipramine maleate) Capsules are available as:
25 mg: in bottles of 100 opaque blue and yellow capsules.
50 mg: in bottles of 100 opaque blue and orange capsules.

[*Shown in Product Identification Section*]

SYNALGOS® Capsules ℞

Composition: Each maroon and gray capsule contains:

Promethazine hydrochloride	6.25 mg.
Aspirin	194.4 mg.
Phenacetin	162.0 mg.
Caffeine	30.0 mg.

Actions: Promethazine is a phenothiazine with sedative actions. Synalgos also contains the non-narcotic antipyretic-analgesics, aspirin and phenacetin.

Indications

Based on a review of this drug by the National Academy of Sciences-National Research Council and/or other information, FDA has classified the indications as follows:
"Possibly" effective for the relief of mild to moderate pain in those situations where the physician wishes to add a mild sedative effect.
Final classification of the less-than-effective indications requires further investigation.

Contraindications: Hypersensitivity to aspirin, phenacetin and promethazine.

Warnings: Salicylates should be used with extreme caution in the presence of peptic ulcer or coagulation abnormalities. Promethazine may impair the mental and/or physical abilities required for the performance of potentially hazardous tasks such as driving a car or operating machinery. The patient using Synalgos should be cautioned accordingly.

Use with CNS Depressants: Synalgos may have additive effects with other CNS depressants (hypnotics, sedatives, tranquilizers, antianxiety agents). Patients who have demonstrated a hypersensitivity reaction (e.g. blood dyscrasia, jaundice) with a phenothiazine should not be re-exposed to any phenothiazine, including Synalgos, unless in the judgment of the physician the potential benefits of treatment outweigh the possible hazards.

Usage in Pregnancy: Reproduction studies have not been performed in animals. There is no adequate information on whether this drug may affect fertility in human males or females or has teratogenic potential or other adverse effect on the fetus.

Usage in Children: Since there is no experience in children who have received this drug, safety and efficacy in children have not been established.

Precautions: Phenacetin has been reported to damage the kidneys when taken in large amounts for a long time. Promethazine should be administered cautiously to patients with cardiovascular or liver disease.

Adverse Reactions: Drowsiness, dizziness, light headedness, sedation, skin reactions, nausea, vomiting, constipation, and rarely hypotension.

Dosage and Administration: Dosage should be adjusted according to the severity of the pain and the response of the patient. Synalgos is given orally. The usual adult dose is two capsules every 4 hours as needed for pain.

Drug Interactions: The CNS depressant effects of Synalgos may be additive with that of other CNS depressants. See Warnings. Aspirin may enhance the effects of anti-coagulants and inhibit the uricosuric effects of uricosuric agents.

How Supplied: Synalgos capsules: Supplied in bottles of 100 and 500 capsules.

Literature Available: Yes.

[Cir. 2802—8/20/73]

[*Shown in Product Identification Section*]

SYNALGOS®-DC Capsules Ⓒ ℞

Composition: Each blue and gray capsule contains:

Drocode (dihydrocodeine) bitartrate	16.0 mg.
Warning: May be habit-forming	
Promethazine hydrochloride	6.25 mg.
Aspirin	194.4 mg.
Phenacetin	162.0 mg.
Caffeine	30.0 mg.

Actions: Dihydrocodeine is a semi-synthetic narcotic analgesic, related to codeine, with multiple actions qualitatively similar to those of codeine; the most prominent of these involve the central nervous system and organs with smooth muscle components. The principal actions of therapeutic value are analgesia and sedation.

Promethazine is a phenothiazine with sedative actions.

Synalgos-DC also contains the non-narcotic antipyretic-analgesics, aspirin and phenacetin.

Indications

Based on a review of this drug by the National Academy of Sciences-National Research Council and/or other information, FDA has classified the indications as follows:
"Possibly" effective for the relief of moderate to moderately severe pain in those situations where the physician wishes to add a mild sedative effect.
Final classification of the less-than-effective indications requires further investigation.

Contraindications: Hypersensitivity to dihydrocodeine, promethazine, aspirin, phenacetin.

Warnings: Salicylates should be used with extreme caution in the presence of peptic ulcer or coagulation abnormalities.

Drug Dependence: Dihydrocodeine can produce drug dependence of the codeine type and therefore has the potential of being abused. Psychic dependence, physical dependence and tolerance may develop upon repeated administration of dihydrocodeine and it should be prescribed and administered with the same degree of caution appropriate to the use of other oral narcotic containing medications.

Like other narcotic containing medications, dihydrocodeine is subject to the provisions of the Federal Controlled Substances Act.

Usage in Ambulatory Patients: Dihydrocodeine and promethazine may impair the mental and/or physical abilities required for the performance of potentially hazardous tasks such as driving a car or operating machinery. The patient using Synalgos-DC should be cautioned accordingly.

Interactions with other Central Nervous System Depressants: Patients receiving other narcotic analgesics, general anesthetics, other phenothiazines, tranquilizers, sedative-hypnotics or other CNS depressants (including alcohol) concomitantly with Synalgos-DC may exhibit an additive CNS depression. When such combined therapy is contemplated, the dose of one or both agents should be reduced. Patients who have demonstrated a hypersensitivity reaction (e.g. blood dyscrasia, jaundice) with a phenothiazine should not be re-exposed to any phenothiazine, including Synalgos-DC,

Continued on next page

Ives—Cont.

unless in the judgment of the physician the potential benefits of the treatment outweigh the possible hazards.

Usage in Pregnancy: Reproduction studies have not been performed in animals. There is no adequate information on whether this drug may affect fertility in human males and females or has a teratogenic potential or other adverse effect on the fetus.

Usage in Children: Since there is no experience in children who have received this drug, safety and efficacy in children have not been established.

Precautions: Phenacetin has been reported to damage kidneys when taken in large amounts for a long time.

Promethazine should be administered cautiously to patients with cardiovascular or liver disease. Synalgos-DC should be given with caution to certain patients such as the elderly or debilitated, and those with hypothyroidism, Addison's disease and prostatic hypertrophy and urethral stricture.

Adverse Reactions: The most frequently observed reactions include lightheadedness, dizziness, drowsiness, sedation, nausea, vomiting, constipation, pruritus, skin reactions, and rarely hypotension.

Dosage and Administration: Dosage should be adjusted according to the severity of the pain and the response of the patient. Synalgos-DC is given orally. The usual adult dose is two capsules every 4 hours as needed for pain.

Drug Interactions: The CNS depressant effects of Synalgos-DC may be additive with that of other CNS depressants.

See Warnings.

Aspirin may enhance the effects of anticoagulants and inhibit the uricosuric effects of uricosuric agents.

How Supplied: Synalgos-DC capsules: Supplied in bottles of 100 and 500 capsules (DEA Schedule III).

Literature Available: Yes

[Cir. 2803—8/20/73]

[*Shown in Product Identification Section*]

TRECATOR®-SC ℞
(ethionamide)
Sugar-Coated Tablets

Action: Bacteriostatic against *Mycobacterium tuberculosis.*

Indications: Failure after adequate treatment with primary drugs (i.e. isoniazid, streptomycin, aminosalicylic acid) in any form of active tuberculosis. Ethionamide should only be given with other effective antituberculous agents.

Contraindications:
Severe hypersensitivity.
Severe hepatic damage.

Warning:

Use in Pregnancy: Teratogenic effects have been demonstrated in animals (rabbits, rats) receiving doses in excess of those recommended in humans. Use of the drug should be avoided during pregnancy or in women of childbearing potential, unless the benefits outweigh its possible hazard.

Use in Children: Optimum dosage for children has not been established. This, however, does not preclude use of the drug when its use is crucial to therapy.

Precautions: Pretreatment examinations should include *in vitro* susceptibility tests of recent cultures of *M. tuberculosis* from the patient as measured, against ethionomide and the usual primary antituberculous drugs.

Determinations of serum transaminase (SGOT, SGPT) should be made prior to and every 2 to 4 weeks during therapy.

In patients with diabetes mellitus management may be more difficult and hepatitis occurs more frequently.

Ethionamide may intensify the adverse effects of the other antituberculous drugs administered concomitantly. Convulsions have been reported and special care should be taken particularly when ethionamide is administered with cycloserine.

Adverse Reactions: The most common side effect is gastrointestinal intolerance.

Other adverse effects similar to those seen with isoniazid have been reported: peripheral neuritis, optic neuritis, psychic disturbances (including mental depression), postural hypotension, skin rashes, thrombocytopenia, pellagra-like syndrome, jaundice and/or hepatitis, increased difficulty in management of diabetes mellitus, stomatitis, gynecomastia, and impotence.

Dosage and Administration: Ethionamide should be administered with at least one other effective antituberculous drug.

Average adult dose: 0.5 gram to 1.0 gram/day in divided doses.

Concomitant administration of pyridoxine is recommended.

How Supplied: Trecator-SC (ethionamide) is supplied as 250 mg. *orange,* sugar-coated tablets in bottles of 100 and 500.

Bibliography available upon request

(Cir. 3038-1—8/22/79)

Jacobus Pharmaceutical Co., Inc.
37 CLEVELAND LANE
PRINCETON, NJ 08540

DAPSONE USP ℞
25 mg. & 100 mg.

Dapsone-USP is 4-4′ diaminodiphenylsulfone (DDS), an effective antibacterial drug which has proved satisfactory in the treatment of leprosy. It is issued in tablets of 25 mg. and 100 mg. for oral administration.

Action: By the kinetic method in mice, Dapsone is bactericidal as well as bacteriostatic against M. leprae.

Indication: All forms of leprosy except for cases of proven Dapsone resistance.

Contraindication: Hypersensitivity to Dapsone and/or its derivatives.

Warnings: Deaths associated with the administration of Dapsone have been reported from agranulocytosis, aplastic anemia and other blood dyscrasias. The presence of clinical signs such as sore throat, fever, pallor, purpura or jaundice may be early indications of serious blood disorders.

Complete blood counts should be done frequently in patients receiving Dapsone. If a significant reduction in any formed element is noted, Dapsone should be discontinued and the patient followed intensively.

Dapsone has been found carcinogenic (sarcomagenic) for male rats and female mice causing mesenchymal tumors in the spleen and peritoneum, and thyroid carcinoma in female rats.

Severe anemia should be treated prior to initiation of therapy.

At first sign of hypersensitivity reaction, sulfone therapy must be discontinued at once and appropriate treatment initiated.

Leporsy reactional states are not hypersensitivity reactions to Dapsone and do not require discontinuation. See special section.

Precautions: In glucose-6-phosphate dehydrogenase (G6PD) deficient individuals hemolysis and Heinz body formation may be exaggerated. This reaction is frequently dose-related. Dapsone should be given with caution if the patient is exposed to other agents capable of producing hemolysis in G6PD deficient patients.

Adverse Reactions: In addition to the warnings listed above, the following syndromes and serious reactions have been reported in patients on Dapsone:

Dose-related hemolysis is the most common adverse-effect and is seen in patients with or without G6PD deficiency. Almost all patients demonstrate the interrelated changes of a loss of a 1–2 gms. Hb, have an increase in the reticulocytes (4–12%), a shortened red cell life span and a rise in methemoglobin. G6PD deficient patients have greater responses.

Dermatitis though rare is probably one of the most serious complications of sulfone therapy and is directly due to drug sensitization. If dermatitis occurs, there is danger of exfoliative dermatitis developing along with enlargement of the liver and damage to that structure. Exfoliative dermatitis is not infrequently fatal; therefore, at the first sign of this reaction, sulfone therapy must be discontinued and appropriate therapy instituted.

Peripheral neuropathy is a definite but unusual complication of Dapsone therapy in non-leprosy patients. Motor loss is predominant. If muscle weakness appears, Dapsone should be withdrawn. Recovery on withdrawal is usually substantially complete. The mechanism of recovery is reportedly by axonal regeneration. In leprosy this complication has not been reported and may be difficult to distinguish from a leprosy reactional state.

In addition to the warnings and adverse effects reported above, additional adverse reactions include: nausea, vomiting, abdominal pains, toxic hepatitis, cholestatic jaundice, psychosis, headache, vertigo, blurred vision, tinnitus, insomnia, fever, mobilliform rash, urticaria, phototoxicity, hyperpigmented macules, tachycardia, albuminuria, the nephrotic syndrome, drug-induced Lupus erythematosus and an infectious mononucleosis-like syndrome.

Dosage and Administration: For leprosy: In order to reduce secondary Dapsone resistance the WHO Expert Committee on Leprosy has recommended that Dapsone should be commenced and maintained at full dosage without interruption. The recommended dosage is 6–10 mg/kg of body weight per week. This schedule amounts to 50–100 mg. daily in full-size adults with correspondingly smaller doses for children.

In bacteriologically negative tuberculoid and indeterminate type leprosy patients, an adult dosage of 50 mg. daily is usually sufficient. After all signs of clinical activity are controlled, therapy should be continued a minimum of 3 years for tuberculoid and indeterminate patients.

In lepromatous and border line lepromatous patients, Dapsone therapy in full dosage should be administered for many years, perhaps for life. The WHO Committee recommends administration for at least 10 years after a patient is bacteriologically negative. More than five years of continuous therapy is required to render most patients with lepromatous leprosy bacteriologically negative.

Secondary Dapsone resistance should be suspected whenever a lepromatous or border-line lepromatous patient receiving Dapsone treatment relapses clinically and bacteriologically, solid staining bacilli being found in the smears taken from the new active lesions. If such cases show no response to regular and supervised Dapsone therapy within three to six months, Dapsone resistance should be considered confirmed clinically. Determination of drug sensitivity using the mouse footpad method is recommended and, after prior arrangement, is available without charge from the USPHS at Carville, La. Patients with proven Dapsone resistance should be treated with other drugs.

Complications: Abrupt changes in clinical activity occur in leprosy and are known as reactions. The majority can be classified into two groups.

Erythema nodosum leprosum (ENL) (lepromatous lepra reaction) (Type 2 reaction) occurs mainly in lepromatous patients and small numbers of borderline patients. Approximately 50 percent of treated patients show this reaction in the first year. The principal clinical features are fever and tender erythematous skin nodules sometimes associated with malaise, neuritis, orchitis, albuminuria, joint swelling, iritis, epistaxis or depression. Skin lesions can become pustular and/or ulcerate. Histologically there is a vasculitis with an intense polymorphonuclear infiltrate and elevated circulating immune complexes. If severe, patients should be hospitalized. In general, anti-leprosy treatment is continued. Analgesics, steroids and other agents available from USPHS Carville, La. are used to suppress the reaction.

The "Reversal" reaction (Type 1) may occur in boderline or tuberculoid leprosy patients often soon after chemotherapy is started. The mechanism is presumed to result from a reduction in the antigenic load: the patient is able to mount an enhanced delayed hypersentitivity response to residual infection leading to swelling ("Reversal") of existing skin and nerve lesions. If severe, or if neuritis is present, large doses of steroids should always be used. If severe, the patient should be hospitalized. In general, antileprosy treatment is continued and therapy to suppress the reaction is indicated such as analgesics, steroids, or surgical decompression of swollen nerve trunks. USPHS at Carville, La. should be contacted for advice in management.

Absorption and Excretion: Dapsone, when given orally, is rapidly and almost completely absorbed. About 85 percent of the daily intake is recoverable from the urine mainly in the form of water-soluble metabolities. Excretion of the drug is slow and a constant blood level can be maintained with the usual dosage.

Blood Levels: Detected a few minutes after ingestion, the drug reaches peak concentration in 4–8 hours. Daily administration for at least eight days is necessary to achieve a plateau level. With doses of 200 mg. daily, this level averaged 2.3 μgm/ml with a range of 0.1-7.0 μgm.

In man there are large individual differences in the rate of Dapsone clearance from the body. The half-life in the plasma in different individuals varies from ten hours to fifty hours and averages twenty-eight hours. Repeat tests in the same individual show the clearance rate to be constant. Dapsone acetylation rates have been used to measure the acetylation phenotype. Daily administration (50–100 mg.) in leprosy patients will provide blood levels in excess of the usual minimum inhibitory concentration even for patients with a short Dapsone half-life.

Rifampicin lowers Dapsone levels 7 to 10 fold by accelerating plasma clearance.

Overdosage: Symptoms of nausea, vomiting, hyperexcitability can appear a few minutes up to 24 hours after ingestion of an overdose. Methemoglobin induced depression, convulsions and severe cyanosis require prompt treatment. Methylene blue 1–2 mg/kg of body weight given slowly intravenously is the treatment of choice. The effect is complete in 30 minutes, but may have to be repeated if methemoglobin reaccumulates. For non-emergencies, if treatment is needed, methylene blue may be given orally in doses of 3–5 mg/kg every 4–6 hours.

Properties: Dapsone is a white odorless crystalline powder, practically insoluble in water and insoluble in fixed and vegetable oils. This drug is not self-sterilizing but it may be sterilized by dry heat at 150°C for one hour.

How Supplied: Rx: 25 mg. and 100 mg. tablets in bottles of 100.

Distributed by: Jacobus Pharmaceutical Co., Inc., 37 Cleveland Lane, Princeton, NJ 08540.
Manufactured by: Rowell Laboratories, Inc., Baudette, MN 56623

Jamol Laboratories Inc.
13 ACKERMAN AVENUE
EMERSON, NEW JERSEY 07630

PONARIS
Nasal Mucosal Emollient

Composition: Essential oils of cajeput, eucalyptus, and peppermint in a specially prepared iodized cottonseed oil. (Total Iodine 0.6%) Assimilable hence NON-lipoid potential.

Indications and Uses: Nasal emollient, for relief of nasal congestion due to colds, nasal irritations, atrophic rhinitis, (dry inflamed nasal passages), nasal mucosal encrustations and allergy manifestations.

Also nasal intubations and sterile gauze impregnated for epistaxis packing.

Administration and Dosage: 3 to 4 drops in each nostril 3 to 4 times daily. May be used in a compressed air nebulizer or a DeVilbiss nebulizer No. 33 or 40.

Childrens Dosage: As directed by physician.

How Supplied: One ounce bottle with dropper.

Janssen Pharmaceutica Inc.
501 GEORGE STREET
NEW BRUNSWICK, NEW JERSEY 08903

INAPSINE® (droperidol) Injection ℞

Description:

2 ml. and 5 ml. ampuls
Each ml. contains:
Droperidol ....2.5 mg.
Lactic acid for pH adjustment to 3.4 ± 0.4.

10 ml. vials
Each ml. contains:
Droperidol ....2.5 mg.
With 1.8 mg. methylparaben and 0.2 mg. propylparaben, and lactic acid for pH adjustment to 3.4 ± 0.4.

FOR INTRAVENOUS OR INTRAMUSCULAR USE ONLY

Droperidol is a neuroleptic (tranquilizer) agent.

Actions: INAPSINE (droperidol) produces marked tranquilization and sedation. It also produces an antiemetic effect as evidenced by the antagonism of the emetic effect of apomorphine in dogs. It potentiates other CNS depressants. It also produces mild alpha-adrenergic blockade, peripheral vascular dilatation and reduction of the pressor effect of epinephrine. INAPSINE (droperidol) can produce hypotension and decreased peripheral vascular resistance. It may decrease pulmonary arterial pressure (particularly if it is abnormally high). It may reduce the incidence of epinephrine-induced arrhythmias but it does not prevent other cardiac arrhythmias. The onset of action is from three to ten minutes following intravenous or intramuscular administration. The full effect, however, may not be apparent for 30 minutes. The duration of the sedative and tranquilizing effects of INAPSINE (droperidol) generally is two to four hours. Alteration of consciousness may persist as long as 12 hours.

Indications: INAPSINE (droperidol) is indicated:

to produce tranquilization and to reduce the incidence of nausea and vomiting in surgical and diagnostic procedures; for premedication, induction, and as an adjunct in the maintenance of general and regional anesthesia;

in neuroleptanalgesia in which INAPSINE (droperidol) is given concurrently with a narcotic analgesic, such as *SUBLIMAZE*® (fentanyl) injection, to aid in producing tranquility and decreasing anxiety and pain.

Contraindications: INAPSINE (droperidol) is contraindicated in patients with known intolerance to the drug.

Warnings: FLUIDS AND OTHER COUNTERMEASURES TO MANAGE HYPOTENSION SHOULD BE READILY AVAILABLE. As with other CNS depressant drugs, patients who have received INAPSINE (droperidol) should have appropriate surveillance.

If INAPSINE (droperidol) is administered with a narcotic analgesic such as *SUBLIMAZE* (fentanyl), the user should familiarize himself with the special properties of each drug, particularly the widely differing durations of action. In addition, when such a combination is used, *resuscitative equipment and a narcotic antagonist should be readily available to manage apnea.* See package insert for fentanyl before using.

Narcotic analgesics such as *SUBLIMAZE* (fentanyl) may cause muscle rigidity, particularly involving the muscles of respiration. This effect is related to the speed of injection. Its incidence can be reduced by the use of slow intravenous injection. Once this effect occurs, it is managed by the use of assisted or controlled respiration and, if necessary, by a neuromuscular blocking agent compatible with the patient's condition.

The respiratory depressant effect of narcotics persists longer than their measured analgesic effect. When used with INAPSINE (droperidol), the total dose of all narcotic analgesics administered should be considered by the practitioner before ordering narcotic analgesics during recovery from anesthesia. It is recommended that narcotics, when required, be used initially in reduced doses as low as 1/4 to 1/3 those usually recommended.

Usage in Children—The safety of INAPSINE (droperidol) in children younger than two years of age has not been established.

Usage in Pregnancy—The safe use of INAPSINE (droperidol) has not been established with respect to possible adverse effects upon fetal development. Therefore, it should be used in women of childbearing potential only when, in the judgment of the physician, the potential benefits outweigh the possible hazards. There are insufficient data regarding placental transfer and fetal effects; therefore, safety for the infant in obstetrics has not been established.

Precautions: *The initial dose of INAPSINE (droperidol) should be appropriately reduced in elderly, debilitated and other poor-risk patients. The effect of the initial dose should be considered in determining incremental doses.*

Certain forms of conduction anesthesia, such as spinal anesthesia and some peridural anesthetics, can cause peripheral vasodilatation and hypotension because of sympathetic blockade. Through other mechanisms (see Actions), INAPSINE (droperidol) can also alter circulation. Therefore, when INAPSINE (droperidol) is used to supplement these forms of anesthesia, the anesthetist should be familiar with the physiological alterations involved, and be prepared to manage them in the patients selected for this form of anesthesia.

If hypotension occurs, the possibility of hypovolemia should be considered and managed with appropriate parenteral fluid therapy. Repositioning the patient to improve venous return to the heart should also be considered when operative conditions permit. It should be noted that in spinal and peridural anesthesia, tilting the patient into a head down position may result in a higher level of anesthesia than is desirable, as well as impair venous return to the heart. Care should be exercised in moving and positioning of patients because of the possibility of orthostatic hypotension. If volume expansion with fluids plus other countermeasures do not correct the hypotension, then the administration of pressor agents other than

Continued on next page

Janssen—Cont.

epinephrine should be considered. Epinephrine may paradoxically decrease the blood pressure in patients treated with INAPSINE (droperidol) due to the alpha-adrenergic blocking action of droperidol.
Since INAPSINE (droperidol) may decrease pulmonary arterial pressure, this fact should be considered by those who conduct diagnostic or surgical procedures where interpretation of pulmonary arterial pressure measurements might determine final management of the patient.
Vital signs should be monitored routinely.
Other CNS depressant drugs (e.g. barbiturates, tranquilizers, naroctics, and general anesthetics) have additive or potentiating effects with INAPSINE (droperidol). When patients have received such drugs, the dose of INAPSINE (droperidol) required will be less than usual. Likewise, following the administration of INAPSINE (droperidol), the dose of other CNS depressant drugs should be reduced.
INAPSINE (droperidol) should be administered with caution to patients with liver and kidney dysfunction because of the importance of these organs in the metabolism and excretion of drugs.
When the EEG is used for postoperative monitoring, it may be found that the EEG pattern returns to normal slowly.
Since INAPSINE (droperidol) is frequently used with the narcotic analgesic *SUBLIMAZE* (fentanyl), it should be noted that fentanyl may produce bradycardia, which may be treated with atropine; however, fentanyl should be used with caution in patients with cardiac bradyarrhythmias.
Adverse Reactions: The most common adverse reactions reported to occur with INAPSINE (droperidol) are mild to moderate hypotension and occasionally tachycardia, but these effects usually subside without treatment. If hypotension occurs and is severe or persists, the possibility of hypovolemia should be considered and managed with appropriate parenteral fluid therapy. Postoperative drowsiness is also frequently reported.
Extrapyramidal symptoms (dystonia, akathisia, and oculogyric crisis) have been observed following administration of INAPSINE (droperidol). Restlessness, hyperactivity, and anxiety which can be either the result of inadequate dosage of INAPSINE (droperidol) or a part of the symptom complex of akathisia may occur. When extrapyramidal symptoms occur, they can usually be controlled with anti-parkinson agents.
Other adverse reactions that have been reported are dizziness, chills and/or shivering, laryngospasm, bronchospasm and postoperative hallucinatory episodes (sometimes associated with transient periods of mental depression).
When INAPSINE (droperidol) is used with a narcotic analgesic such as *SUBLIMAZE* (fentanyl), respiratory depression, apnea, and muscular rigidity can occur; if these remain untreated respiratory arrest could occur.
Elevated blood pressure, with or without preexisting hypotension, has been reported following administration of INAPSINE (droperidol) combined with *SUBLIMAZE* (fentanyl) or other parenteral analgesics. This might be due to unexplained alterations in sympathetic activity following large doses; however, it is also frequently attributed to anesthetic or surgical stimulation during light anesthesia.
Dosage and Administration: *Dosage should be individualized.* Some of the factors to be considered in determining the dose are age, body weight, physical status, underlying pathological condition, use of other drugs, type of anesthesia to be used, and the surgical procedure involved.
Vital signs should be monitored routinely.

Usual Adult Dosage

I. *Premedication*—(to be appropriately modified in the elderly, debilitated, and those who have received other depressant drugs) 2.5 to 10 mg. (1 to 4 ml.) may be administered intramuscularly 30 to 60 minutes preoperatively.
II. *Adjunct to General Anesthesia*
Induction–2.5 mg. (1 ml.) per 20 to 25 pounds may be administered (usually intravenously) along with an analgesic and/or general anesthetic. Smaller doses may be adequate. The total amount of INAPSINE (droperidol) administered should be titrated to obtain the desired effect based on the individual patient's response.
Maintenance—1.25 to 2.5 mg. (0.5 to 1 ml.) usually intravenously (see warning regarding use with concomitant narcotic analgesic medication and the possibility of widely differing durations of action).
If *INNOVAR®* injection is administered in addition to INAPSINE (droperidol), the calculation of the recommended dose of INAPSINE (droperidol) should include the droperidol contained in the *INNOVAR* injection. See *INNOVAR* injection Package Insert for full prescribing information.
III. *Use Without A General Anesthetic In Diagnostic Procedures*—Administer the usual I.M. premedication 2.5 to 10 mg. (1 to 4 ml.) 30 to 60 minutes before the procedure. Additional 1.25 to 2.5 mg. (0.5 to 1 ml) amounts of INAPSINE (droperidol) may be administered, usually intravenously (see warning regarding use with concomitant narcotic analgesic medication and the possibility of widely differing durations of action).
Note: When INAPSINE (droperidol) is used in certain procedures, such as bronchoscopy, appropriate topical anesthesia is still necessary.
IV. *Adjunct to Regional Anesthesia*—2.5 to 5 mg. (1 to 2 ml.) may be administered intramuscularly or slowly intravenously when additional sedation is required.

Usual Children's Dosage

For children two to 12 years of age, a reduced dose as low as 1.0 to 1.5 mg. (0.4 to 0.6 ml.) per 20 to 25 pounds is recommended for premedication or for induction of anesthesia.
See Warnings and Precautions for use of INAPSINE (droperidol) with other CNS depressants, and in patients with altered response.

Overdosage:

Manifestations: The manifestations of INAPSINE (droperidol) overdosage are an extension of its pharmacologic actions.
Treatment: In the presence of hypoventilation or apnea, oxygen should be administered and respiration should be assisted or controlled as indicated. A patent airway must be maintained; an oropharyngeal airway or endotracheal tube might be indicated. The patient should be carefully observed for 24 hours; body warmth and adequate fluid intake should be maintained. If hypotension occurs and is severe or persists, the possibility of hypovolemia should be considered and managed with appropriate parenteral fluid therapy.
How Supplied: 2 ml. and 5 ml. ampuls—packages of 10; 10 ml. multiple-dose vials—packages of 10.
U.S. Patent No. 3,161,645

INNOVAR® Injection Ⓒ ℞

FOR INTRAVENOUS OR INTRAMUSCULAR USE ONLY

The two components of INNOVAR injection, fentanyl and droperidol, have different pharmacologic actions. Before administering INNOVAR injection, the user should familiarize himself with the special properties of each drug, particularly the widely differing durations of action.

Description: Each ml. contains (in a 1:50 ratio):
Fentanyl ....0.05 mg.
as the citrate
Warning: May be habit forming
Droperidol ....2.5 mg.
Lactic acid for adjustment of pH to 3.5 ± 0.3
Actions: INNOVAR injection is a combination drug containing a narcotic analgesic, fentanyl, and a neuroleptic (major tranquilizer), droperidol. The combined effect, sometimes referred to as neuroleptanalgesia, is characterized by general quiescence, reduced motor activity, and profound analgesia; complete loss of consciousness usually does not occur from use of INNOVAR injection alone. The incidence of early postoperative pain and emesis may be reduced.
A. Fentanyl is a narcotic analgesic with actions qualitatively similar to those of morphine and meperidine. Fentanyl in a dose of 0.1 mg. (2.0 ml.) is approximately equivalent in analgesic activity to 10 mg. of morphine or 75 mg. of meperidine. The principal actions of therapeutic value are analgesia and sedation. Alterations in respiratory rate and alveolar ventilation, associated with narcotic analgesics, may last longer than the analgesic effect. As the dose of narcotic is increased, the decrease in pulmonary exchange becomes greater. Large doses may produce apnea. Fentanyl appears to have less emetic activity than other narcotic analgesics. Histamine assays, and skin wheal testing in man, as well as *in vivo* testing in dogs indicate that histamine release rarely occurs with fentanyl.
Fentanyl may cause muscle rigidity, particularly involving the muscles of respiration. It may also produce other signs and symptoms characteristic of narcotic analgesics including euphoria, miosis, bradycardia, and bronchoconstriction.
The onset of action of fentanyl is almost immediate when the drug is given intravenously; however, maximal analgesic and respiratory depressant effect may not be noted for several minutes. The usual duration of action of the analgesic effect is 30 to 60 minutes after a single I.V. dose of up to 0.1 mg. Following intramuscular administration, the onset of action is from seven to eight minutes, and the duration of action is from one to two hours.
As with longer-acting narcotic analgesics, the duration of the respiratory depressant effect of *SUBLIMAZE* (fentanyl) may be longer than the analgesic effect. The following observations have been reported concerning altered respiratory response to CO_2 stimulation following administration of fentanyl to man:
1. DIMINISHED SENSITIVITY TO CO_2 STIMULATION MAY PERSIST LONGER THAN DEPRESSION OF RESPIRATORY RATE. Fentanyl frequently slows the respiratory rate but this effect is seldom noted for over 30 minutes regardless of the dose administered.
2. Duration and degree of respiratory depression is dose related.
3. The peak respiratory depressant effect of a single intravenous dose of fentanyl is noted 5 to 15 minutes following injection.
4. Altered sensitivity to CO_2 stimulation has been demonstrated for up to four hours following a single intravenous dose of 0.6 mg. (12 ml.) fentanyl to healthy volunteers.
See also WARNINGS and PRECAUTIONS concerning respiratory depression.
B. Droperidol produces marked tranquilization and sedation. It also produces an antiemetic effect as evidenced by the antago-

nism of apomorphine in dogs. It potentiates other CNS depressants. It also produces mild alpha-adrenergic blockade, peripheral vascular dilatation and reduction of the pressor effect of epinephrine. Droperidol can produce hypotension and decreased peripheral vascular resistance. It may decrease pulmonary arterial pressure (particularly if it is abnormally high). It may reduce the incidence of epinephrine-induced arrhythmias but it does not prevent other cardiac arrhythmias. The onset of action is from three to ten minutes following intravenous or intramuscular administration. The full effect, however, may not be apparent for 30 minutes. The duration of the sedative and tranquilizing effects generally is two to four hours. Alteration of consciousness may persist as long as 12 hours. This is in contrast to the much shorter duration of fentanyl.

Indications: INNOVAR injection is indicated to produce tranquilization and analgesia for surgical and diagnostic procedures. It may be used as an anesthetic premedication, for the induction of anesthesia, and as an adjunct in the maintenance of general and regional anesthesia. If the supplementation of analgesia is necessary, *SUBLIMAZE*® (fentanyl) injection alone rather than the combination drug INNOVAR injection, should usually be used; see Dosage and Administration Section.

Contraindications: INNOVAR injection is contraindicated in patients with known intolerance to either component.

Warnings: AS WITH OTHER CNS DEPRESSANTS, PATIENTS WHO HAVE RECEIVED *INNOVAR* INJECTION SHOULD HAVE APPROPRIATE SURVEILLANCE. RESUSCITATIVE EQUIPMENT AND A NARCOTIC ANTAGONIST SHOULD BE READILY AVAILABLE TO MANAGE APNEA.

See also discussion of narcotic antagonists in PRECAUTIONS and OVERDOSAGE.

FLUIDS AND OTHER COUNTERMEASURES TO MANAGE HYPOTENSION SHOULD ALSO BE AVAILABLE.

The respiratory depressant effect of narcotics persists longer than the measured analgesic effect. When used with INNOVAR *injection, the total dose of all narcotic analgesics administered should be considered by the practitioner before ordering narcotic analgesics during recovery from anestheisa. It is recommended that narcotics, when required, be used in reduced doses initially, as low as ¼ to ⅓ those usually recommended.*

INNOVAR *injection may cause muscle rigidity, particularly involving the muscles of respiration. This effect is due to the fentanyl component and is related to the speed of injection. Its incidence can be reduced by the use of slow intravenous injection. Once the effect occurs, it is managed by the use of assisted or controlled respiration and, if necessary, by a neuromuscular blocking agent compatible with the patient's condition.*

Drug Dependence: *Fentanyl, the narcotic analgesic component, can produce drug dependence of the morphine type and therefore has the potential for being abused.*

Severe and unpredictable potentiation by MAO inhibitors has been reported with narcotic analgesics. Since the safety of fentanyl in this regard has not been established, the use of INNOVAR injection or *SUBLIMAZE* (fentanyl) in patients who have received MAO inhibitors within 14 days is not recommended.

Head injuries and Increased Intracranial Pressure: INNOVAR injection should be used with caution in patients who may be particularly susceptible to respiratory depression such as comatose patients who may have a head injury or brain tumor. In addition, INNOVAR injection may obscure the clinical course of patients with head injury.

Usage in Children: The safety of INNOVAR injection in children younger than two years of age has not been established.

Usage in Pregnancy: The safe use of INNOVAR injection has not been established with respect to possible adverse effects upon fetal development. Therefore, it should be used in women of childbearing potential only when, in the judgment of the physician, the potential benefits outweigh the possible hazards. There are insufficient data regarding placental transfer and fetal effects; therefore, safety for the infant in obstetrics has not been established.

Precautions: *The initial dose of INNOVAR injection should be appropriately reduced in elderly, dibilitated and other poor-risk patients. The effect of the initial dose should be considered in determining incremental doses.*

Certain forms of conduction anesthesia, such as spinal anesthesia and some peridural anesthetics, can alter respiration by blocking intercostal nerves, and can cause peripheral vasodilation and hypotension because of sympathetic blockade. Through other mechanisms (see Actions), fentanyl and droperidol also depress respiration and blood pressure. Therefore, when INNOVAR injection is used to supplement these forms of anesthesia, the anesthetist must be familiar with the physiological alterations involved, and be prepared to manage them in the patients selected for this form of anesthesia.

If hypotension occurs, the possibility of hypovolemia should be considered and managed with appropriate parenteral fluid therapy. Repositioning the patient to improve venous return to the heart should be considered when operative conditions permit. It should be noted that in spinal and peridural anesthesia, tilting the patient into a head down position may result in a higher level of anesthesia than is desirable, as well as impair venous return to the heart. Care should be exercised in the moving and positioning of patients because of a possibility of orthostatic hypotension. If volume expansion with fluids plus these other countermeasures do not correct the hypotension, then the administration of pressor agents other than epinephrine should be considered. Epinephrine may paradoxically decrease the blood pressure in patients treated with INNOVAR injection due to the alpha-adrenergic blocking action of droperidol.

The droperidol component of INNOVAR injection may decrease pulmonary arterial pressure. This fact should be considered by those who conduct diagnostic or surgical procedures where interpretation of pulmonary arterial pressure measurements might determine final management of the patient.

Vital signs should be monitored routinely.

INNOVAR injection, and *SUBLIMAZE* (fentanyl), should be used with caution in patients with chronic obstructive pulmonary disease, patients with decreased respiratory reserve, and others with potentially compromised ventilation. In such patients narcotics may additionally decrease respiratory drive and increase airway resistance. During anesthesia this can be managed by assisted or controlled respiration. Postoperative respiratory depression caused by narcotic analgesics can be reversed by narcotic antagonists. Appropriate surveillance should be maintained because the duration of respiratory depression of doses of fentanyl (as *SUBLIMAZE* (fentanyl) or INNOVAR) employed during anesthesia may be longer than the duration of the narcotic antagonist action. Consult individual prescribing information (levallorphan, nalorphine and naloxone) before employing narcotic antagonists.

Should respiration be compromised by muscle rigidity, assisted or controlled respiration and possibly a neuromuscular blocking agent will be required. The occurrence of muscle rigidity is related to the speed of intravenous injection and the incidence can be reduced by slow intravenous injection.

Other CNS depressant drugs (e.g. barbiturates, tranquilizers, narcotics, and general anesthetics) have additive or potentiating effects with INNOVAR injection. When patients have received such drugs, the dose of INNOVAR injection required will be less than usual. Likewise, following the administration of INNOVAR injection, the dose of other CNS depressant drugs should be reduced.

INNOVAR injection should be administered with caution to patients with liver and kidney dysfunction because of the importance of these organs in the metabolism and excretion of drugs.

The fentanyl component may produce bradycardia, which may be treated with atropine; however, INNOVAR injection should be used with caution in patients with cardiac bradyarrhythmias.

When the EEG is used for postoperative monitoring, it may be found that the EEG patern returns to normal slowly.

Adverse Reactions: The most common serious adverse reactions reported to occur with INNOVAR injection are respiratory depression, apnea, muscular rigidity, and hypotension; if these remain untreated, respiratory arrest, circulatory depression or cardiac arrest could occur.

Extrapyramidal symptoms (dystonia, akathisia, and oculogyric crisis) have been observed following administration of INNOVAR injection. Restlessness, hyperactivity and anxiety which can be either the result of inadequate tranquilization or part of the symptom complex of akathisia may occur. When extrapyramidal symptoms occur, they can usually be controlled with anti-Parkinson agents.

Elevated blood pressure, with and without preexisting hypertension, has been reported following administration of INNOVAR injection. This might be due to unexplained alterations of sympathetic activity following large doses; however, it is also frequently attributed to anesthetic or surgical stimulation during light anesthesia.

Other adverse reactions that have been reported are dizziness, chills and/or shivering, twitching, blurred vision, laryngospasm, bronchospasm, bradycardia, tachycardia, nausea and emesis, diaphoresis, emergence delirium, and postoperative hallucinatory episodes (sometimes associated with transient periods of mental depression).

Postoperative drowsiness is also frequently reported.

Dosage and Administration: *Dosage should be individualized.* Some of the factors to be considered in determining dose are age, body weight, physical status, underlying pathological condition, use of other drugs, the type of anesthesia to be used, and the surgical procedure involved.

Vital signs should be monitored routinely.

Most patients who have received INNOVAR injection do not require narcotic analgesics during the immediate postoperative period. It is recommended that narcotic analgesics, when required, be used initially in reduced doses, as low as ¼ to ⅓ those usually recommended.

Usual Adult Dosage:

I. *Premedication*—(to be appropriately modified in the elderly, debilitated, and those who have received other depressant drugs)—0.5 to 2.0 ml. may be administered *intramuscularly* 45 to 60 minutes prior to surgery with or without atropine.

II. *Adjunct to General Anesthesia*—
Induction—1 ml. per 20 to 25 pounds of body weight may be administered slowly intravenously. Smaller doses may be adequate.
The total amount of INNOVAR injection administered should be carefully titrated to

Continued on next page

Janssen—Cont.

obtain the desired effect based on the individual patient's response.

There are several methods of administration of INNOVAR injection for induction of anesthesia.

A. Intravenous injection—To allow for the variable needs of patients INNOVAR injection may be administered intravenously in fractional parts of the calculated dose. With the onset of somnolence, the general anesthetic may be administered.

B. Intravenous drip—10 ml. of INNOVAR injection are added to 250 ml. of 5% dextrose in water and the drip given rapidly until the onset of somnolence. At that time, the drip may be either slowed or stopped and the general anesthetic administered.

Maintenance—INNOVAR injection is not indicated as the sole agent for the maintenance of surgical anesthesia. It is customarily used in combination with other measures such as nitrous oxide-oxygen, other inhalation anesthetics, and/or topical or regional anesthesia.

To prevent the possibility of excessive accumulation of the relatively long-acting droperidol component, *SULBIMAZE* (fentanyl) alone should be used in increments of 0.025 to 0.05 mg. (0.5 to 1.0 ml.) for the maintenance of analgesia in patients initially given INNOVAR injection as an adjunct to general anesthesia. (See *SUBLIMAZE* (fentanyl) package insert for additional prescribing information.) However, in prolonged operations, additional 0.5 to 1.0 ml. amounts of INNOVAR injection may be administered with caution intravenously if changes in the patient's condition indicate lightening of tranquilization and analgesia.

III. *Use Without a General Anesthetic in Diagnostic Procedures*—Administer the usual I.M. premedication (0.5 to 2.0 ml.) 45 to 60 minutes before the procedure. To prevent the possibility of excessive accumulation of the relatively long-acting droperidol component, *SUBLIMAZE* (fentanyl) alone should be used in increments of 0.025 to 0.05 mg. (0.5 to 1.0 ml.) for the maintenance of analgesia in patients initially given INNOVAR injection. (See *SUBLIMAZE* (fentanyl) package insert for additional information). However, in prolonged operations, additional 0.5 to 1.0 ml. amounts of INNOVAR injection may be administered with caution intravenously if changes in the patient's condition indicate lightening of tranquilization and analgesia.

Note: When INNOVAR injection is used in certain procedures such as bronchoscopy, appropriate topical anesthesia is still necessary.

IV. *Adjunct to Regional Anesthesia*—1 to 2 ml. may be administered intramuscularly or slowly intravenously when additional sedation and analgesia are required.

Usual Children's Dosage:

I. *Premedication*—0.25 ml. per 20 lbs. body weight administered *intramuscularly* 45 to 60 minutes prior to surgery with or without atropine.

II. *Adjunct to General Anesthesia*—The total combined dose for induction and maintenance averages 0.5 ml. per 20 lbs. body weight. Following induction with INNOVAR injection. *SUBLIMAZE* (fentanyl) alone in a dose of 1/4 to 1/3 that recommended in the adult dosage section should usually be used when indicated to avoid the possibility of excessive accumulation of droperidol. However, in prolonged operations, additional increments of INNOVAR injection may be administered with caution when changes in the patient's condition indicate lightening of tranquilization and analgesia.

See Warnings and Precautions for use of INNOVAR injection with other CNS depressants, and in patients with altered response.

Overdosage: ***Manifestations:*** The manifestations of INNOVAR injection overdosage are an extension of its pharmacologic actions.

Treatment: In the presence of hypoventilation or apnea, oxygen should be administered and respiration should be assisted or controlled as indicated. A patent airway must be maintained; an oropharyngeal airway or endotracheal tube might be indicated. If depressed respiration is associated with muscular rigidity, an intravenous neuromuscular blocking agent might be required to facilitate assisted or controlled respiration. The patient should be carefully observed for 24 hours; body warmth and adequate fluid intake should be maintained. If hypotension occurs and is severe or persists, the possibility of hypovolemia should be considered and managed with appropriate parenteral fluid therapy. A specific narcotic antagonist such as nalorphine, levallorphan or naloxone should be available for use as indicated to manage respiratory depression caused by the narcotic component fentanyl. This does not preclude the use of more immediate counter-measures. The duration of respiratory depression following overdose of fentanyl may be longer than the duration of narcotic antagonist action. Consult the package inserts of the individual narcotic antagonists for details about use.

How Supplies: INNOVAR® injection is supplied in 2 ml. and 5 ml. ampuls, in packages of 10.

U.S. Patent No. 3,141,823

MONISTAT i.v.™ ℞

(miconazole for intravenous infusion)

Description: MONISTAT i.v., (miconazole), 1- {2-(2, 4-dichlorophenyl)-2- [(2, 4-dichlorophenyl) methoxyl] ethyl}-1H-imidazole, is a synthetic antifungal supplied as a sterile solution for intravenous infusion. Each ml of this solution contains 10 mg of miconazole with 0.115 ml PEG 40 castor oil, 1.0 mg lactic acid USP, 0.5 mg methylparaben USP, 0.05 mg propylparaben USP in water for injection. Miconazole i.v. is a clear colorless to slightly yellow solution having a pH of 3.7 to 5.7.

Clinical Pharmacology: MONISTAT i.v. is rapidly metabolized in the liver and about 14% to 22% of the administered dose is excreted in the urine, mainly as inactive metabolites. The pharmacokinetic profile fits a three-compartment open model with the following biologic half-life: 0.4, 2.1, and 24.1 hours for each phase respectively. The pharmacokinetic profile of MONISTAT i.v. is unaltered in patients with renal insufficiency, including those patients on hemodialysis. The in-vitro antifungal activity of MONISTAT i.v. is very broad. Clinical efficacy has been demonstrated in patients with the following species of fungi: *Coccidioides immitis, Candida albicans, Cryptoccus neoformans,* and *Paracoccidiodes brasiliensis.*

Recommended doses of MONISTAT i.v. produce serum concentrations of drug which exceed the in-vitro MIC values for the fungal species noted above. Doses above 9 mg/kg of MONISTAT i.v. produce peak blood levels above 1μg/ml in most cases. The drug penetrates into joints.

Indications: MONISTAT i.v. is indicated for the treatment of the following severe systemic fungal infections: coccidioidomycosis, candidiasis, cryptococcosis, paracoccidioidomycosis, and for the treatment of chronic mucocutaneous candidiasis. However, in the treatment of fungal meningitis and urinary bladder infections an intravenous infusion alone is inadequate. It must be supplemented with intrathecal administration and bladder irrigation. Appropriate diagnostic procedures should be followed and MIC's should be determined.

MONISTAT i.v. should not be used to treat common trivial forms of fungal diseases.

Contraindications: MONISTAT i.v. is contraindicated in those patients who have shown hypersensitivity to it.

Warnings: Rapid injection of undiluted MONISTAT i.v. may produce transient tachycardia or arrhythmia.

Precautions: Before a treatment course of MONISTAT i.v. is started, the physician should make sure that the patient is not hypersensitive to the drug product. MONISTAT i.v. should be given by intravenous infusion. The treatment should be started under stringent conditions of hospitalization but subsequently may be given to suitable patients under ambulatory conditions with close clinical monitoring. It is recommended that an initial dose of 200 mg be given with the physician in attendance. It is also recommended that clinical laboratory monitoring including hemoglobin, hematocrit, electrolytes and lipids be performed.

It should be borne in mind that systemic fungal mycoses may be complications of chronic underlying conditions which in themselves may require appropriate measures.

Pregnancy: Reproductive studies with MONISTAT i.v. in rats and rabbits revealed no evidence of impaired fertility or harm to the fetus. There are no data, however, on the use of the drug in pregnant women.

Children: Since the safety of miconazole i.v. in children under one year of age has not been extensively studied, its benefits in this age group must be weighed against the possible risks involved.

Adverse Reactions: Adverse reactions which have been observed with MONISTAT i.v. therapy include phlebitis, pruritus, rash, nausea, vomiting, febrile reactions, drowsiness, diarrhea, anorexia and flushes. In the U.S. studies, 29% of 209 patients studied had phlebitis, 21% pruritus, 18% nausea, 10% fever and chills, 9% rash, and 7% emesis. Transient decreases in hematocrit and serum sodium values have been observed following infusion of MONISTAT i.v. Thrombocytopenia has also been reported. No serious renal or hepatic toxicity has been reported. If pruritus and skin rashes are severe, discontinuation of treatment may be necessary. Nausea and vomiting can be mitigated with antihistaminic or antiemetic drugs given prior to MONISTAT i.v. infusion, or by reducing the dose, slowing the rate of infusion, or avoiding administration at mealtime.

Aggregation of erythroeytes or rouleau formation on blood smears has been reported. Hyperlipemia has occurred in patients and is reported to be due to the vehicle, Cremophor EL (PEG 40 castor oil).

Drug Interactions: Drugs containing cremophor type vehicles are known to cause electrophoretic abnormalities of the lipoprotein. These effects are reversible upon discontinuation of treatment but are usually not an indication that treatment should be discontinued.

Interaction with the coumarin drugs resulting in an enhancement of the anticoagulant effect has also been reported. In cases of simultaneous treatment with MONISTAT i.v. and coumarin drugs, the anticoagulant effect should be carefully titrated since reductions of the anticoagulant doses may be indicated.

Dosage and Administration:

DOSAGE

Adults. The doses may vary with the diagnosis and with the infective agent, from 200 to 1200 mg per infusion. The following daily doses, which may be divided over 3 infusions, are recommended:

[See table on next page].

Children. A total daily dose of about 20 to 40 mg/kg is generally adequate. However, a dose of 15 mg/kg body weight per infusion should not be exceeded.

ADMINISTRATION
MONISTAT i.v. should be diluted in at least 200 ml of fluid. The diluent of choice is 0.9% sodium chloride or alternatively Dextrose 5% injectable solution. The intravenous infusion should be given over a period of 30 to 60 minutes.
Generally, treatment should be continued until all clinical and laboratory tests no longer indicate that active fungal infection is present. Inadequate periods of treatment may yield poor response and lead to early recurrence of clinical symptoms. The dosing intervals and sites and the duration of treatment vary from patient to patient and depend on the causative organism.

Organism	Dosage Range*	Duration of Successful Therapy (weeks)
Coccidioidomycosis:	1800 to 3600 mg per day	3 to > 20
Cryptococcosis:	1200 to 2400 mg per day	3 to > 12
Candidiasis:	600 to 1800 mg per day	1 to > 20
Paracoccidioidomycosis:	200 to 1200 mg per day	2 to > 16

*May be divided over 3 infusions.
Repeated courses may be necessitated by relapse or reinfection.

OTHER MODES OF ADMINISTRATION
Intrathecal. Administration of the undiluted injectable solution of MONISTAT i.v. by the various intrathecal routes (20 mg per dose) is indicated as an adjunct to intravenous treatment in fungal meningitis. Succeeding intrathecal injections may be alternated between lumbar, cervical, and cisternal punctures every 3 to 7 days. Bladder instillation of 200 mg of diluted solution is indicated in the treatment of mycoses of the urinary bladder.
How Supplied: MONISTAT i.v. is supplied in 20 ml ampoules.
MONISTAT i.v. (miconazole) is an original product of Janssen Pharmaceutica, Belgium.

SUBLIMAZE® (fentanyl) injection Ⓒ ℞

Description: Each ml. contains:
Fentanyl ....0.05 mg.
as the citrate
Warning: May be habit forming.
Sodium hydroxide for adjustment of pH to 4.0–7.5.

FOR INTRAVENOUS OR INTRAMUSCULAR USE ONLY

Actions: SUBLIMAZE (fentanyl) is a narcotic analgesic with actions qualitatively similar to those of morphine and meperidine. SUBLIMAZE (fentanyl) in a dose of 0.1 mg. (2.0 ml.) is approximately equivalent in analgesic activity to 10 mg. of morphine or 75 mg. of meperidine. The principal actions of therapeutic value are analgesia and sedation. Alterations in respiratory rate and alveolar ventilation, associated with narcotic analgesics, may last longer than the analgesic effect. As the dose of narcotic is increased, the decrease in pulmonary exchange becomes greater. Large doses may produce apnea. SUBLIMAZE (fentanyl) appears to have less emetic activity than other narcotic analgesics. Histamine assays and skin wheal testing in man, as well as in *in vivo* testing in dogs, indicate that histamine release rarely occurs with SUBLIMAZE (fentanyl).
SUBLIMAZE (fentanyl) may cause muscle rigidity, particularly involving the muscles of respiration. It may also produce other signs and symptoms characteristic of narcotic analgesics including euphoria, miosis, bradycardia, and bronchoconstriction.
The onset of action of SUBLIMAZE (fentanyl) is almost immediate when the drug is given intravenously; however, the maximal analgesic and respiratory depressant effect may not be noted for several minutes. The usual duration of action of the analgesic effect is 30 to 60 minutes after a single I.V. dose of up to 0.1 mg. Following intramuscular administration, the onset of action is from seven to eight minutes, and the duration of action is one to two hours. As with longer acting narcotic analgesics, the duration of the respiratory depressant effect of SUBLIMAZE (fentanyl) may be longer than the analgesic effect. The following observations have been reported concerning altered respiratory response to CO_2 stimulation following administration of fentanyl to man:
1. DIMINISHED SENSITIVITY TO CO_2 STIMULATION MAY PERSIST LONGER THAN DEPRESSION OF RESPIRATORY RATE. Fentanyl frequently slows the respiratory rate, but this effect is seldom noted for over 30 minutes regardless of the dose administered.
2. Duration and degree of respiratory depression is dose related.
3. The peak respiratory depressant effect of a single intravenous dose of fentanyl is noted 5 to 15 minutes following injection.
4. Altered sensitivity to CO_2 stimulation has been demonstrated for up to four hours following a single intravenous dose of 0.6 mg. (12 ml.) fentanyl to healthy volunteers.

See also WARNINGS and PRECAUTIONS concerning respiratory depression.
Indications: SUBLIMAZE (fentanyl) is indicated:
— for analgesic action of short duration during the anesthetic periods, premedication, induction, and maintenance, and in the immediate post-operative period (recovery room) as the need arises.
— for use as a narcotic analgesic supplement in general or regional anesthesia.
— for administration with a neuroleptic such as *INAPSINE®* (droperidol) injection as an anesthetic premedication, for the induction of anesthesia and as an adjunct in the maintenance of general and regional anesthesia.

Contraindications: SUBLIMAZE (fentanyl) is contraindicated in patients with known intolerance to the drug.
Warnings: AS WITH OTHER CNS DEPRESSANTS, PATIENTS WHO HAVE RECEIVED *SUBLIMAZE* (FENTANYL) SHOULD HAVE APPROPRIATE SURVEILLANCE. RESUSCITATIVE EQUIPMENT AND A NARCOTIC ANTAGONIST SHOULD BE READILY AVAILABLE TO MANAGE APNEA.
See also discussion of narcotic antagonists in Precautions and Overdosage.
If SUBLIMAZE (fentanyl) is administered with a tranquilizer such as *INAPSINE* (droperidol), the user should familiarize himself with the special properties of each drug, particularly the widely differing durations of action. In addition, when such a combination is used *fluids and other counter-measures to manage hypotension should be available.*
As with other potent narcotics, the respiratory depressant effect of SUBLIMAZE (fentanyl) persists longer than the measured analgesic effect. The total dose of all narcotic analgesics administered should be considered by the practitioner before ordering narcotic analgesics during recovery from anesthesia. It is recommended that narcotics, when required, should be used in reduced doses initially, as low as ¼ to ⅓ those usually recommended. SUBLIMAZE (fentanyl) may cause muscle rigidity, particularly involving the muscles of respiration. The effect is related to the speed of injection and its incidence can be reduced by the use of slow intravenous injection. Once the effect occurs, it is managed by the use of assisted or controlled respiration and, if necessary, by a neuromuscular blocking agent compatible with the patient's condition.
Drug Dependence—SUBLIMAZE (fentanyl) can produce drug dependence of the morphine type and therefore has the potential for being abused.
Severe and unpredictable potentiation by MAO inhibitors has been reported with narcotic analgesics. Since the safety of fentanyl in this regard has not been established, the use of SUBLIMAZE (fentanyl) in patients who have received MAO inhibitors within 14 days is not recommended.
Head Injuries and Increased Intracranial Pressure—SUBLIMAZE (fentanyl) should be used with caution in patients who may be particularly susceptible to respiratory depression, such as comatose patients who may have a head injury or brain tumor. In addition, SUBLIMAZE (fentanyl) may obscure the clinical course of patients with head injury.
Usage in Children—The safety of SUBLIMAZE (fentanyl) in children younger than two years of age has not been established.
Usage in Pregnancy—The safe use of SUBLIMAZE (fentanyl) has not been established with respect to possible adverse effects upon fetal development. Therefore, it should be used in women of childbearing potential only when, in the judgment of the physician, the potential benefits outweigh the possible hazards. There are insufficient data regarding placental transfer and fetal effects; therefore, safety for the infant in obstetrics has not been established.
Precautions: *The initial dose of SUBLIMAZE (fentanyl) should be appropriately reduced in elderly, debilitated and other poor-risk patients. The effect of the initial dose should be considered in determining incremental doses.*
Certain forms of conduction anesthesia, such as spinal anesthesia and some peridural anesthetics, can alter respiration by blocking intercostal nerves. Through other mechanisms (see Actions) SUBLIMAZE (fentanyl) can also alter respiration. Therefore, when SUBLIMAZE (fentanyl) is used to supplement these forms of anesthesia, the anesthetist should be familiar with the physiological alterations involved, and be prepared to manage them in the patients selected for these forms of anesthesia. When used with a tranquilizer such as *INAPSINE* (droperidol), blood pressure may be altered and hypotension can occur.
Vital signs should be monitored routinely.
SUBLIMAZE (fentanyl) should be used with caution in patients with chronic obstructive pulmonary disease, patients with decreased respiratory reserve, and others with potentially compromised respiration. In such patients, narcotics may additionally decrease respiratory drive and increase airway resistance. During anesthesia, this can be managed by assisted or controlled respiration. Respiratory depression caused by narcotic analgesics can be reversed by narcotic antagonists. Appropriate surveillance should be maintained because the duration of respiratory depression of doses of fentanyl employed during anesthesia may be longer than the duration of the narcotic antagonist action. Consult individual prescribing information (levallorphan, nalorphine and naloxone) before employing narcotic antagonists.
When a tranquilizer such as *INAPSINE* (droperidol) is used with SUBLIMAZE (fentanyl) pulmonary arterial pressure may be decreased. This fact should be considered by those who conduct diagnostic and surgical procedures where interpretation of pulmonary arterial pressure measurements might determine final management of the patient.
Other CNS depressant drugs (e.g. barbiturates, tranquilizers, narcotics, and general anesthetics) will have additive or potentiating effects with SUBLIMAZE (fentanyl). When patients have received such drugs, the dose of SUBLIMAZE (fen-

Continued on next page

Janssen—Cont.

tanyl) required will be less than usual. Likewise, following the administration of SUBLIMAZE (fentanyl), the dose of other CNS depressant drugs should be reduced.
SUBLIMAZE (fentanyl) should be administered with caution to patients with liver and kidney dysfunction because of the importance of these organs in the metabolism and excretion of drugs.
SUBLIMAZE (fentanyl) may produce bradycardia, which may be treated with atropine; however, SUBLIMAZE (fentanyl) should be used with caution in patients with cardiac bradyarrhythmias.
When SUBLIMAZE (fentanyl) is used with a tranquilizer such as *INAPSINE* (droperidol) hypotension can occur. If this occurs, the possibility of hypovolemia should also be considered and managed with appropriate parenteral fluid therapy. Repositioning the patient to improve venous return to the heart should be considered when operative conditions permit. Care should be exercised in moving and positioning of patients because of the possibility of orthostatic hypotension. If volume expansion with fluids plus other countermeasures do not correct hypotension, the administration of pressor agents other than epinephrine should be considered. Because of the alpha-adrenergic blocking action of *INAPSINE* (droperidol), epinephrine may paradoxically decrease the blood pressure in patients treated with *INAPSINE* (droperidol). When *INAPSINE* (droperidol) is used with SUBLIMAZE (fentanyl) and the EEG is used for postoperative monitoring, it may be found that the EEG pattern returns to normal slowly.
Adverse Reactions: As with other narcotic analgesics, the most common serious adverse reactions reported to occur with SUBLIMAZE (fentanyl) are respiratory depression, apnea, muscular rigidity, and bradycardia; if these remain untreated, respiratory arrest, circulatory depression or cardiac arrest could occur. Other adverse reactions that have been reported are hypotension, dizziness, blurred vision, nausea, emesis, laryngospasm, and diaphoresis.
When a tranquilizer such as *INAPSINE* (droperidol) is used with SUBLIMAZE (fentanyl), the following adverse reactions can occur: chills and/or shivering, restlessness, and postoperative hallucinatory episodes (sometimes associated with transient periods of mental depression); extrapyramidal symptoms (dystonia, akathisia, and oculogyric crisis) have been observed up to 24 hours postoperatively. When they occur, extrapyramidal symptoms can usually be controlled with anti-parkinson agents. Postoperative drowsiness is also frequently reported following the use of *INAPSINE* (droperidol).
Elevated blood pressure, with and without preexisting hypertension, has been reported following administration of SUBLIMAZE (fentanyl) combined with INAPSINE (droperidol). This might be due to unexplained alterations in sympathetic activity following large doses; however, it is also frequently attributed to anesthetic and surgical stimulation during light anesthesia.
Dosage and Administration: *Dosage should be individualized.* Some of the factors to be considered in determining the dose are age, body weight, physical status, underlying pathological condition, use of other drugs, type of anesthesia to be used, and the surgical procedure involved.
Vital signs should be monitored routinely.
Usual Adult Dosage:
I. *Premedication* (to be appropriately modified in the elderly, debilitated, and those who have received other depressant drugs)—0.05 to 0.1 mg. (1 to 2 ml.) may be administered *intramuscularly* 30 to 60 minutes prior to surgery.
II. *Adjunct to General Anesthesia*
Induction—0.05 to 0.1 mg. (1 to 2 ml.) may be administered initially intravenously and may be repeated at 2 to 3 minute intervals until desired effect is achieved. A reduced dose as low as 0.025 to 0.05 mg. (0.5 to 1 ml.) is recommended in elderly and poor-risk patients.
Maintenance—0.025 to 0.05 mg. (0.5 to 1 ml.) may be administered intravenously or intramuscularly when movement and/or changes in vital signs indicate surgical stress or lightening of analgesia.
If *INNOVAR* ® injection is administered in addition to SUBLIMAZE (fentanyl), the calculation of the recommended dose of SUBLIMAZE (fentanyl) should include the fentanyl contained in the *INNOVAR* injection. See *INNOVAR* injection Package Insert for full prescribing information.
III. *Adjunct to Regional Anesthesia*—0.05 to 0.1 mg. (1 to 2 ml.) may be administered intramuscularly or slowly intravenously when additional analgesia is required.
IV. *Postoperatively (recovery room)*—0.05 to 0.1 mg. (1 to 2 ml.) may be administered intramuscularly for the control of pain, tachypnea and emergence delirium. The dose may be repeated in one to two hours as needed.
Usual Children's Dosage: For induction and maintenance in children two to 12 years of age, a reduced dose as low as 0.02 to 0.03 mg. (0.4 to 0.6 ml.) per 20 to 25 pounds is recommended. See Warnings and Precautions for use of SUBLIMAZE (fentanyl) with other CNS depressants, and in patients with altered response.
Overdosage: ***Manifestations:*** The manifestations of SUBLIMAZE (fentanyl) overdosage are an extension of its pharmacologic actions.
Treatment: In the presence of hypoventilation or apnea, oxygen should be administered and respiration should be assisted or controlled as indicated. A patent airway must be maintained; an oropharyngeal airway or endotracheal tube might be indicated. If depressed respiration is associated with muscular rigidity, an intravenous neuromuscular blocking agent might be required to facilitate assisted or controlled respiration. The patient should be carefully observed for 24 hours; body warmth and adequate fluid intake should be maintained. If hypotension occurs and is severe or persists, the possibility of hypovolemia should be considered and managed with appropriate parenteral fluid therapy. A specific narcotic antagonist such as nalorphine, levallorphan, or naloxone should be available for use as indicated to manage respiratory depression. This does not preclude the use of more immediate countermeasures. The duration of respiratory depression following overdosage of fentanyl may be longer than the duration of narcotic antagonist action. Consult the package insert of the individual narcotic antagonists for details about use.
How Supplied: 2 ml. and 5 ml. ampuls—packages of 10.
U.S. Patent No. 3,164,600

VERMOX® Chewable Tablets ℞
(mebendazole)

Description: VERMOX (mebendazole) is methyl 5-benzoylbenzimidazole-2-carbamate.
Actions: VERMOX exerts its anthelmintic effect by blocking glucose uptake by the susceptible helminths, thereby depleting the energy level until it becomes inadequate for survival.
In man, approximately 2% of administered mebendazole is excreted in urine as unchanged drug or a primary metabolite. Following administration of 100 mg of mebendazole twice daily for three consecutive days, plasma levels of mebendazole and its primary metabolite, the 2-amine, never exceeded 0.03 μg/ml and 0.09 μg/ml, respectively.
Indications: VERMOX is indicated for the treatment of *Trichuris trichiura* (whipworm), *Enterobius vermicularis* (pinworm), *Ascaris lumbricoides* (roundworm), *Ancylostoma duodenale* (common hookworm), *Necator americanus* (American hookworm) in single or mixed infections.
Efficacy varies as a function of such factors as pre-existing diarrhea and gastrointestinal transit time, degree of infection and helminth strains. Efficacy rates derived from various studies are shown in the table below:
[See table below].
Contraindications: VERMOX is contraindicated in pregnant women (see: Pregnancy Precautions) and in persons who have shown hypersensitivity to the drug.

Precautions:
PREGNANCY:
VERMOX has shown embryotoxic and teratogenic activity in pregnant rats at single oral doses as low as 10 mg/kg. Since VERMOX may have a risk of producing fetal damage if administered during pregnancy, it is contraindicated in pregnant women.
PEDIATRIC USE:
The drug has not been extensively studied in children under two years; therefore, in the treatment of children under two years the relative benefit/risk should be considered.
Adverse Reactions: Transient symptoms of abdominal pain and diarrhea have occurred in cases of massive infection and expulsion of worms.
Dosage and Administration: The same dosage schedule applies to children and adults. The tablet may be chewed, swallowed or crushed and mixed with food. For the control of pinworm (enterobiasis), a single tablet is administered orally, one time. For the control of roundworm (ascariasis), whipworm (trichuriasis), and hookworm infection, one tablet of VERMOX is administered, orally, morning and evening, on three consecutive days.
If the patient is not cured three weeks after treatment, a second course of treatment is advised. No special procedures, such as fasting or purging, are required.
How Supplied: VERMOX is available as chewable tablets, each containing 100 mg of mebendazole, and is supplied in boxes of twelve tablets.
VERMOX (mebendazole) is an original product of Janssen Pharmaceutica, Belgium.
[*Shown in Product Identification Section*]

	Whipworm	Roundworm	Hookworm	Pinworm
cure rates				
mean	68%	98%	96%	95%
(range)	(61–75%)	(91–100%)	—	(90–100%)
egg reduction				
mean	93%	99.7%	99.9%	—
(range)	(70–99%)	(99.5–100%)	—	—

Jayco Pharmaceuticals
890 POPLAR CHURCH DRIVE
SUITE 305
CAMP HILL, PA 17011

HYDRA-LYTE™ OTC
Oral Glucose Electrolyte Drink Mix

Description: A dietary supplement to replace and maintain electrolytes and water lost during mild and moderate diarrhea in children and adults and to provide nutritional support during parenteral therapy.
Formulated to supply electrolytes and water lost through diarrhea, HYDRA-LYTE enhances the absorption of sodium and water through the addition of sugars.
Usage: Intake of HYDRA-LYTE should be adjusted to individual requirements and should be in small frequent amounts. It should be ingested freely, to quench thirst.
All other food intake, except for water, should be discontinued.
HYDRA-LYTE should be used only under medical supervision in conformity with a physician's recommendation.
Ingredients: Dextrose, sucrose, sodium chloride and citrate, potassium citrate, sodium bicarbonate, artificial flavoring and coloring, 0.05% sodium benazoate as preservative.
HYDRA-LYTE provides 84 mEq Sodium, 59 mEq Chloride, 10 mEq Bicarbonate, 10 mEq Potassium, 67 mM Glucose and 35 mM Sucrose.
How Supplied: HYDRA-LYTE is available in convenient foil-lined packets, two packets per box.
References:
1. Sack, R.B., et. al., The current status of oral therapy in the treatment of acute diarrheal illness *American Journal of Clinical Nutrition* 31:2251 1978
2. Pierce, N.F. and Hirschhorn N, Oral fluid—a simple weapon against dehydration in diarrhoea *WHO Chronicle* 31:87 1977
3. Moenginah, P.A., et.al., Oral Sucrose Therapy for diarrhea *Lancet* 1:323 1975

QUIK-PREP OTC
(Saline Lavage)

Description: QUIK-PREP is an artificially flavored and sweetened salt mixture that provides an isotonic solution for saline lavage. QUIK-PREP induces a volumnogenic diarrhea which serves as an irrigating and cleansing mechanism to prepare patients undergoing diagnostic and therapeutic studies upon the large bowel.
QUIK-PREP contains sodium chloride, sodium bicarbonate, potassium citrate, artificial sweetener, flavoring and coloring. When mixed with two liters of water, QUIK-PREP results in a solution of 141 mEq of sodium, 11 mEq of potassium, 111 mEq of chloride, 30 mEq of bicarbonate and 11 mEq of citrate per liter.
Indications: QUIK-PREP is recommended as a means of cleansing the large bowel in preparation for large bowel surgery, barium enema examination and colonoscopy studies which require the large bowel to be free of fecal material.
Warnings: QUIK-PREP is to be used in caution with patients who must restrict their intake of sodium, potassium or water. This includes patients with cardiac or renal insufficiency or who need a sodium restricted diet.
Contraindications: QUIK-PREP is contraindicated for patients with complete obstruction of the gastrointestinal tract.
Dosage and Administration: The patient should restrict all oral nutrients for at least four hours prior to ingesting QUIK-PREP. No other preparation is necessary.
1. Add packet contents to two liters of room temperature water. Mix thoroughly
2. Drink between 1800 to 2000 cc of solution every hour (approximately 8 glasses of solution per hour)
3. The first bowel movement will usually be within 45 minutes. Clear fluid should be passed within two hours after initial ingestion. However, ingestion should be continued for an additional 45 minutes after passing clear fluid to assure complete cleansing.
4. Diagnostic or therapeutic procedures can be started approximately one hour after termination of the irrigation procedure. If the procedure is delayed, up to but not more than 18 hours, a clear liquid diet is permitted. No further preparation is necessary.

The average person will usually require four to six liters of solution for an adequate preparation. The actual volume required is proportional to the patient's weight. Consumption should not exceed ten liters.
How Supplied: Packed in boxes of 4 foil-line packets, each QUIK-PREP packet will make two liters of solution
References:
Hewitt, J., et.al. Whole Gut Irrigation in Preparation for Large Bowel Surgery. *Lancet* 2:337, 1973
Levy, A.G. et. al. Saline Lavage: A Rapid, Effective and Acceptable Method for Cleansing the Gastrointestinal Tract. *Gastroenterology* 70:157 1976
Rhodes, J.B., et.al. Oral Electrolyte Overload to Cleanse the Colon for Colonoscopy. *Gastrointestinal Endoscopy* 24:24 1969
Skucas, J., et.al. Whole Gut Irrigation as a Means of Cleansing the Colon *Radiology* 121:303 1976

Johnson & Johnson Baby Products Company
PROFESSIONAL PRODUCTS DIV.
220 CENTENNIAL AVENUE
PISCATAWAY, NEW JERSEY 08854

PANCREASE® ℞
brand of pancrelipase
(enteric coated microspheres)

Description: PANCREASE™ is a white, dye-free capsule containing enteric coated microspheres of porcine pancreatic enzyme concentrate, predominately steapsin (pancreatic lipase), amylase and protease. Each capsule contains no less than:

Lipase	4,000 N.F. Units
Amylase	20,000 N.F. Units
Protease	25,000 N.F. Units

Actions: PANCREASE™ resists gastric inactivation and delivers predictable, high levels of biologically active enzymes into the duodenum. The enzymes catalyze the hydrolysis of fats into glycerol and fatty acids, protein into proteoses and derived substances, and starch into dextrins and sugars. PANCREASE™ is effective in controlling steatorrhea and its consequences at low daily dosage levels.
Indications: PANCREASE™ is indicated for patients with exocrine pancreatic enzyme deficiency as in:
- cystic fibrosis
- chronic pancreatitis
- post-pancreatectomy
- post-gastrointestinal bypass surgery (e.g., Billroth II gastroenterostomy)
- ductal obstruction from neoplasm (e.g. of the pancreas or common bile duct)

Contraindications: Hypersensitivity to any of the ingredients.
Warnings and Precautions: Pancrelipase should be used with caution in patients known to be hypersensitive to pork protein.
Safe use in pregnancy has not been established. Diethyl phthalate, an enteric coating component, has been shown with high intraperitoneal dosing to be teratogenic in rats.
Adverse Reactions: No adverse reactions have been observed with PANCREASE™. It should be noted, however, that extremely high doses of exogenous pancreatic enzymes have been associated with hyperuricosuria.
Dosage and Administration: Usual dosage: One or two capsules during each meal and one capsule with snacks. Occasionally a third capsule with meals may be required depending upon individual requirements.
In the presence of deficient pancreatic bicarbonate secretion, antacid supplementation may be required for control of steatorrhea.
Where swallowing of capsules is difficult, they may be opened and the microspheres taken with liquids or shaken onto soft foods which do not require chewing.
TO PROTECT ENTERIC COATING, MICROSPHERES SHOULD NOT BE CRUSHED OR CHEWED.
How Supplied: White, dry-free capsules in bottles of:
100 ....NDC 0204-0095-01
250 ....NDC 0204-0095-02
Rev. 4/78
[Shown in Product Identification Section]

Johnson & Johnson Products, Inc.
DERMATOLOGICAL DIVISION
501 GEORGE STREET
NEW BRUNSWICK, N.J. 08903

(See Ortho Pharmaceutical Corporation
Dermatological Division
Raritan, New Jersey 08869
a Johnson & Johnson Company)

Kenwood Laboratories, Inc.
490-A MAIN STREET
NEW ROCHELLE, NY 10801

GLUTOFAC Tablets™

Composition: Each tablet contains: Saccharomyces Siccum (a selected Brewer's Yeast)—390 mg. (contains Glucose Tolerance Factor—Chromium Complex)

		% U.S. RDA
Vitamin C (Ascorbic Acid)	250 mg.	416
Thiamine Hydrochloride (Vitamin B1)	15 mg.	1000
Riboflavin (Vitamin B2)	10 mg.	588
Niacinamide	50 mg.	250
Vitamin B6 (Pyridoxine Hydrochloride)	50 mg.	2500
Calcium Pantothenate	20 mg.	200
Magnesium Sulfate*	70 mg.	17.5
Zinc Sulfate+	80 mg.	533

* AS 50 mg. Dried Magnesiium Sulfate
\+ AS 50 mg. Dried Zinc Sulfate
Indication: For patients with nutritional deficiencies resulting from diabetes mellitus, physiologic stress, alcoholism and for other acute and chronic depletional states.
Dosage: Adults: One (1) tablet three (3) times daily or as directed by a physician.
Supplied: Green (film coated) tablets in bottles of 90 and 500.

I.L.X.® B_{12} Elixir Crystalline

Composition:
Each (15 cc) contain:
Elemental Iron (from Iron Ammonium Citrate, Brown) ....102 mg
Liver Fraction 1 ....98 mg

Continued on next page

Kenwood—Cont.

Thiamine Hydrochloride
(Vitamin B1) .... 5 mg
Riboflavin (Vitamin B2) .... 2 mg
Nicotinamide .... 10 mg
Vitamin B12 Crystalline
(Cyanocobalamin) .... 10 mcg
Alcohol 8% by Volume

Action and Uses: A readily assimilated elixir for oral therapy in the treatment of iron deficiency anemias.

Administration and Dosage: As a hematinic. One teaspoonful 3 times daily or as directed by physician.

How Supplied: 12 ounce bottles.

I.L.X.® B_{12} Tablets

Composition: Each tablet contains:
Ferrous Gluconate .... 5 gr.
Vitamin C .... 60 mg.
Cyanocobalamin (Vit. B_{12}) .... 10 mcg.
Liver Fraction 2 .... 2 gr.
Thiamine Hydrochloride .... 2 mg.
Riboflavin .... 2 mg.
Nicotinamide .... 20 mg.

Indications: A readily assimilated oral hematinic for the treatment of nutritional and iron deficiency anemias such as those commonly seen in older patients, in convalescence from surgical procedures or medical diseases and anemias of pregnancy.

Administration and Dosage: One tablet 3 times a day or as directed by physician.

How Supplied: I.L.X. B_{12}® tablets are supplied in Bottles of 100.

Kessel Laboratories, Inc.
P.O. BOX 6204
SURFSIDE, FLORIDA 33154

SULFADRIN® ℞
Nasal Suspension

Composition: Phenylephrine
Hydrochloride 0.5%
Sulfathiazole 5.0%
In a buffered and preserved aqueous base

Actions: A decongestant antibacterial combination useful in the local treatment of intranasal bacterial infection and resultant post nasal drip.

Indications: For the relief of nasal congestion in a wide variety of allergic and infectious disorders of the upper respiratory tract.

Contraindications: Hypersensitivity to any of the ingredients of Sulfadrin Nasal Suspension.

Warnings: Excessive use of this medication may induce chronic congestion of the nasal mucosa; increase of blood pressure, dizziness, palpitations and in some cases, nervousness. As with all sympathomimetic amines, Sulfadrin should be used with extreme caution in patients receiving MAO inhibitors, since severe hypertensive crises may ensue.

Precautions: Sulfadrin should be administered only to adults and children over 6 years of age. It should be used cautiously in patients with coronary artery disease, hypertension, hyperthyroidism or diabetes mellitus.

Dosage and Administration: For Adults and children 6 years of age and over: 2 or 3 drops in each nostril.
Not To Exceed 4 Times in 24 Hours

How Supplied: Sulfadrin Nasal Suspension 30 cc with dropper.
NDC 12078-493-26

Key Pharmaceuticals, Inc.
50 N.W. 176th ST.
MIAMI, FL 33169

IRCON®-FA ℞

Description: IRCON-FA contains 1.0 mg of folic acid, and 250 mg of ferrous fumarate equivalent to 82 mg of elemental iron.

Actions: IRCON-FA is a prenatal supplemental hematinic agent specifically intended for prophylaxis against two common types of anemia developing as a result of pregnancy. The use of prophylactic iron and prophylactic folic acid during pregnancy is well accepted. Child-bearing (per pregnancy) has an iron "cost" of about 725 mg. It has been shown that 78 mg of elemental iron, taken orally each day during the last half of pregnancy, will protect against iron deficiency anemia; half this dose is insufficient to maintain iron stores. Two hundred fifty mg of ferrous fumarate contain approximately 82 mg of iron. Absorption characteristics of ferrous fumarate are identical to those of ferrous sulfate.

A deficiency of folic acid, typically during pregnancy, has long been known to cause a megaloblastic anemia, similar in some respects to Addisonian pernicious anemia. The vitamin is not storable in the body and the combination of fetal demand during pregnancy and misnourishment can lead to a deficiency, hence anemia. The average daily requirement of folic acid during pregnancy is unknown. It has been found that a dosage of 20 mcg/day is inadequate. In other instances doses of 1000 mcg/day orally have been found to produce a prompt hematological response in megaloblastic anemia of pregnancy.

Daily doses of folic acid greater than 1.0 mg/day have not been shown to be necessary, even in cases of overt folate deficiency anemia. The estimated minimum daily requirement for folic acid in late pregnancy when folate depletion is present is said to be greater than 200 mcg and possibly 400 mcg or more. IRCON-FA contains 1000 mcg. Folic acid is nontoxic and has commonly been given in several times this daily dose. Though folic acid dietary deficiency in the United States is rare, prophylaxis during pregnancy is considered to be justified in view of the possibly serious consequences of its depletion, both for the mother (megaloblastic anemia) and the fetus.

Finally, it has been observed that the rapid production of red blood cells following treatment with iron alone may deplete the body of folate if there is inadequate intake; combining the two substances avoids this complication.

Indications: For maintenance of maternal hematopoiesis during pregnancy, particularly when diet is abnormal or substandard.

Contraindications:
1) Pernicious anemia. Although rare in the population likely to receive IRCON-FA this megaloblastic anemia must be borne in mind. It is due to faulty or blocked absorption of vitamin B_{12}, or extrinsic factor, on either a genetic, immunologic or surgical basis. The particular danger of missing a diagnosis of pernicious anemia—in relation to folic acid therapy—is that folic acid can mask PA by causing a hematologic remission while allowing the neurological complications of the disease to proceed apace. Thus, before IRCON-FA is prescribed for megaloblastic anemia in pregnancy, appropriate diagnostic exclusion of Addisonian pernicious anemia should be carried out.
2) Anemias other than those due to iron deficiency.

Warning: Folic acid alone is improper therapy in the treatment of pernicious anemia and other megaloblastic anemias where vitamin B_{12} is deficient.

Precautions:
1) If, at the time of initial examination, definite anemia is found, a diagnosis of its cause should be made.
2) IRCON-FA is primarily intended to prevent the development of anemia due to a deficiency of either iron or folic acid by reason of the demands of pregnancy. It is not intended for the treatment of these disorders in fully developed form.
3) Blood examinations including hemoglobin and hematocrit should be done at the usual intervals to make certain that therapy is adequate.
4) Use with care in the presence of peptic ulcer, regional enteritis and ulcerative colitis.
5) Folic acid especially in doses above 1.0 mg. daily may obscure pernicious anemia, in that hematologic remission may occur while neurological manifestations remain progressive.

Adverse Reactions:
1) Ferrous fumarate gastric distress, abdominal cramps, diarrhea.
2) Folic acid allergic sensitization has been reported following both oral and parenteral administration of folic acid.

Administration and Dosage: The usual dose in the second and third trimester of pregnancy is one tablet daily, taken in the morning between breakfast and lunch with a glass of water or milk. If hyperemesis gravidarum is a problem, the dose may be taken in mid-afternoon.

How Supplied: IRCON-FA tablets are available in bottles of 100.

Caution: FEDERAL LAW PROHIBITS DISPENSING WITHOUT A PRESCRIPTION.

NICO-SPAN® ℞
(niacin)
Sustained Action Capsules

Description: NICO-SPAN, formulated as sustained action capsules, contains 400 mg of niacin in a specially prepared form to permit prolonged release.

Actions: Niacin functions in the body as a component of two hydrogen transporting coenzymes: Coenzyme I [Nicotinamide Adenine Dinucleotide (NAD), sometimes called Diphosphopyridine Nucleotide (DPN)] and Coenzyme II [Nicotinamide Adenine Dinucleotide Phosphate (NADP), sometimes called Triphosphopyridine Nucleotide (TPN)]. Niacin in addition to its functions as a vitamin, exerts several distinctive pharmacologic effects which vary according to the dosage level employed.

Niacin in large doses, causes a reduction in serum lipids. The exact mechanism of this action is unknown.

Indications: As adjunctive therapy in addition to diet and other measures in the treatment of hypercholesterolemia and hyperbetalipoproteinemia. Because NICO-SPAN has prolonged release, it minimizes flushing, pruritus and gastrointestinal irritation and permits adequate dosage with maximum patient cooperation.

Notice:
It has not been established whether the drug-induced lowering of serum cholesterol or triglyceride levels has a beneficial effect, no effect, or a detrimental effect on the morbidity or mortality due to atherosclerosis including coronary heart disease. Investigations now in progress may yield an answer to this question.

Contraindications: Niacin is contraindicated in patients with hepatic dysfunction or in patients with active acute peptic ulcer.

Warnings: Use of this drug in pregnancy, during lactation, or in women of child-bearing age requires that the potential benefits of the drug should be weighed against its possible hazards to the mother and child. Although fetal abnormalities have not been reported with this drug, its use as an antilipidemic agent requires high dosages, and animal reproduction or teratology studies have not been done. There are insufficient studies done for usage in children.

Precautions: Patients with gall bladder disease, or those with a past history of jaundice, liver disease or peptic ulcer should be observed closely while taking the medication. Frequent monitoring of liver function tests and blood glucose should be performed during therapy to ascertain that the drug has no adverse effects on these organ systems. Diabetic or potential diabetic patients should be observed closely in the event of decreased tolerance. Adjustment of diet and/or hypoglycemic therapy may be necessary. Antihypertensive drugs of the adrenergic-blocking type may have an additive vasodilating effect and produce postural hypotension.

Elevated uric acid levels have occurred; therefore, use with caution in patients predisposed to gout.

Adverse Reactions: Severe flushing, decreased glucose tolerance, activation of peptic ulcer, abnormal liver function tests, jaundice, gastrointestinal disorders, dry skin, keratosis nigricans, pruritus, hyperuricemia, toxic amblyopia, hypotension, transient headache.

Dosage and Administration: The dose and frequency for the administration of NICO-SPAN should be adjusted to the response of the patient. Slow build-up of dosage in gradual increments is recommended to observe efficacy and/or adverse effects. One or two capsules three times a day is the usual dosage. The maximum dosage is 6 g per day.

Caution: FEDERAL LAW PROHIBITS DISPENSING WITHOUT PRESCRIPTION.

How Supplied: NICO-SPAN 400 mg sustained action capsules are available in bottles of 100, and 1000.

[*Shown in Product Identification Section*]

NITROGLYN® ℞

(nitroglycerin)
Sustained Action Tablets

Description: NITROGLYN, formulated as sustained action tablets, contains nitroglycerin (glyceryl trinitrate). NITROGLYN is available in three strengths: 1/50 gr (1.3 mg), 1/25 gr (2.6 mg) and 1/10 gr (6.5 mg).

Actions: The principal action of nitroglycerin is to relax all smooth muscle, most prominently on vascular smooth muscle. The action on small post-capillary vessels dominates the hemodynamic picture. The resulting increase in cardiac output is transient, and followed by a moderate decrease due to reduced venous return, associated with peripheral vasodilation. The mean arterial pressure may not be affected, or may be decreased. The speed and magnitude of response depend on the dose, the rate of release from the tablet, the rate of absorption, and individual susceptibility. Availability of nitroglycerin at 3 dosage levels permits tailoring the required dose to the need of each patient with angina pectoris.

The release of nitroglycerin from NITROGLYN is gradual but the rate of absorption from the gastrointestinal tract in patients with angina pectoris has not been estabished. Dilation of the coronary arteries has been established in some anginal patients following sublingual administration but not in others. More often patients with coronary artery disease show no change or decrease in coronary flow. Nitroglycerin can act as physiological antagonist to norepinephrine, acetylcholine and histamine. While the mechanism of action of nitroglycerin in the treatment of patients with angina pectoris is still to be established, its use has been well documented for more than a century and is considered the drug of choice.

Indications:
Based on a review of this drug by the National Academy of Sciences-National Research Council and/or other information FDA has classified the indications as follows: "Possibly" Effective.
Sustained action tablets of nitroglycerin are possibly effective for indications relating to the management, prophylaxis or treatment of anginal attacks. This possibly effective classification applies also to conventional or extended action oral forms of all other organic nitrate antianginal drugs alone or in combination.

Contraindications: Data supporting the use of organic nitrates during the course of acute myocardial infarction are not sufficient to establish safety. Caution should be used in administration to anginal patients with postural hypotension or with closed-angle glaucoma.

Precautions: Use the smallest dose which proves effective. Tablets must be swallowed whole. FOR ORAL, NOT SUBLINGUAL USE. Store in cool, dry place and keep container tightly capped. Cross tolerance may develop to other organic nitrates. Continued treatment is not recommended unless the patient is benefited.

Adverse Reactions: Some patients exhibit hypersensitivity to the hypotensive effects of nitroglycerin, as shown by nausea, vomiting, restlessness, pallor, perspiration and collapse, from the usual dose. Other patients may develop severe and persistent headaches, cutaneous flushing, dizziness and weakness; occasionally drug rash or exfoliative dermatitis; these responses may disappear with decrease in dosage. Adverse effects are enhanced by ingestion of alcohol, which appears to increase absorption from the gastrointestinal tract.

Dosage and Administration: Administer the smallest effective dose 2 or 3 times daily unless clinical response suggests a different regimen. Discontinue if not effective.

How Supplied: NITROGLYN 1/50 gr (1.3 mg), 1/25 gr (2.6 mg) and 1/10 gr (6.5 mg) sustained action tablets are available in bottles of 100 and 1000.

Caution: FEDERAL LAW PROHIBITS DISPENSING WITHOUT PRESCRIPTION.

[*Shown in Product Identification Section*]

PAVAKEY-300® ℞

(papaverine hydrochloride, 300 mg.)
Sustained Action Capsules

PAVAKEY®

(papaverine hydrochloride, 150 mg.)
Sustained Action Capsules

Description: PAVAKEY, formulated as sustained action capsules, contains papaverine hydrochloride. PAVAKEY is available in two strengths: PAVAKEY contains 150 mg of papaverine hydrochloride and PAVAKEY-300 contains 300 mg of papaverine hydrochloride; both in a specially prepared form to permit sustained action for prolonged activity.

Actions: The main actions of papaverine are exerted on cardiac and smooth muscle. Like quinidine, papaverine acts directly on the heart muscle to depress conduction and prolong the refractory period. Papaverine relaxes various smooth muscles. This relaxation may be prominent if spasm exists. The muscle cell is not paralyzed by papaverine, and still responds to drugs and other stimuli causing contraction. The antispasmodic effect is a direct one, and unrelated to muscle innervation. Papaverine is practically devoid of effects on the central nervous system.

Papaverine relaxes the smooth musculature of the larger blood vessels, especially coronary, systemic, peripheral, and pulmonary arteries. Perhaps by its direct vasodilating action on cerebral blood vessels, papaverine increases cerebral blood flow and decreases cerebral vascular resistance in normal subjects; oxygen consumption is unaltered. These effects may explain the benefit reported from the drug in cerebral vascular encephalopathy.

The direct actions of papaverine on the heart to depress conduction and irritability and to prolong the refractory period of the myocardium provide the basis for its clinical trial in abrogating atrial and ventricular premature systoles and ominous ventricular arrhythmias. The coronary vasodilator action could be an additional factor of therapeutic value when such rhythms are secondary to insufficiency or occlusion of the coronary arteries. In patients with acute coronary thrombosis, the occurence of ventricular rhythms is serious and requires measures designed to decrease myocardial irritability. Papaverine may have advantages over quinidine, used for a similar purpose, in that it may be given in an emergency by the intravenous route, does not depress myocardial contraction or cause cinchonism, and produces coronary vasodilation.

Indications: For the relief of cerebral and peripheral ischemia associated with arterial spasm and myocardial ischemia complicated by arrhythmias.

Precautions: Use with caution in patients with glaucoma. Hepatic hypersensitivity has been reported with gastrointestinal symptoms, jaundice, eosinophilia and altered liver function tests. Discontinue medication if these occur.

Adverse Reactions: Although occurring rarely, the reported side effects of papaverine include nausea, abdominal distress, anorexia, constipation, malaise, drowsiness, vertigo, sweating, headache, diarrhea and skin rash.

Dosage and Administration:
PAVAKEY—One capsule every 12 hours. In difficult cases administration may be increased to one capsule every 8 hours, or two capsules every 12 hours.
PAVAKEY-300—One capsule every twelve hours for difficult cases.

How Supplied: PAVAKEY sustained action capsules are available in bottles of 100 and 1000.
PAVAKEY-300 sustained action capsules are available in bottles of 100.

Caution: FEDERAL LAW PROHIBITS DISPENSING WITHOUT PRESCRIPTION.

PROTERNOL® ℞

(isoproterenol hydrochloride)
Sustained Action Tablets

Description: PROTERNOL, formulated as sustained action tablets, contains isoproterenol hydrochloride. PROTERNOL is available in two strengths, 15mg and 30mg.

Actions: Isoproterenol is a sympathomimetic amine, being two to ten times more effective than epinephrine by action on the beta receptors, thus producing increased peripheral vasodilation, cardioacceleration and bronchial relaxation. Sublingual doses of 5 to 200mg have little effect on blood pressure; larger doses may produce extreme tachycardia, precordial stress, palpitations and ECG changes suggesting coronary insufficiency. The oral administration of plain isoproterenol hydrochloride tablets has not proven satisfactory in many cases, because of inactivation in the gastrointestinal tract, and decreased absorption. Special coatings to delay release after oral administration have decreased such inactivation. Isoproterenol has been found to be safe and effective to increase the ventricular rate in patients with syncopal seizures associated with the Stokes-Adams Syndrome. "The ability of isoproterenol to stimulate the heart, in a manner similar to that of epinephrine, together with an absence of pressor action makes it the

Continued on next page

Key—Cont.

drug of choice in heart block." This clinical use of sustained action isoproterenol was reported originally by Dr. Simon Dack, and Dack and Robbin. Additional investigations have confirmed the effectiveness as well as the safety of such therapy, and that the effective dose must be tailored to the requirements of each patient.

> **Indications:**
> Based on a review of this drug by the National Academy of Sciences—National Research Council and/or other information, FDA has classified the indication as follows:
> "Possibly" effective:
> For heart block and Stokes-Adams Syndrome.
> Final classification of the less-than-effective indication requires further investigation.

Contraindications: Coronary sclerosis, hypertension, central hyperexcitability. NOT TO BE ADMINISTERED WITH EPINEPHRINE.
Precautions: If untoward effects such as tachycardia or palpitations develop, dosage should be reduced to the level at which symptoms disappear. In rare patients, hypersensitivity to very small doses may require discontinuance.
PROTERNOL is not for sublingual use; tablets must be swallowed whole, not broken. Store in cool, dry place in airtight, light-resistant containers, and keep bottle tightly capped after opening.
Adverse Reactions: Hypersensitive patients may develop dizziness, nausea, tremors and excitement; more extensive side effects include flushing, headache, palpitations and precordial aches or anginal pain. Side effects have been observed more frequently after sublingual than after oral administration.
Dosage and Administration: The recommended daily dose of PROTERNOL is 30mg to 180mg. The physician's findings must determine the maintenance dose.
Toxicity: Similar to epinephrine, isoproterenol may cause marked central hyperexcitation.
How Supplied: PROTERNOL 15mg and 30mg sustained action tablets are available in bottles of 100 and 500.
Caution: FEDERAL LAW PROHIBITS DISPENSING WITHOUT A PRESCRIPTION.
[*Shown in Product Identification Section*]

QUINORA® ℞
(quinidine sulfate tablets U.S.P.)

Description: QUINORA tablets contain quinidine sulfate with no color additives in the base. QUINORA is available in two strengths, 200 mg and 300 mg.
Actions: Quinidine is generally regarded as a myocardial depressant drug, because it depresses excitability, conduction velocity, and contractility of the myocardium. Besides these direct effects quinidine exerts some indirect effects on the heart through an anticholinergic action. Large oral doses may reduce the arterial pressure due to peripheral vasodilation. Hypotension of a serious degree is more likely with the parenteral use of the drug.
Quinidine is essentially completely absorbed after oral administration; maximal effects occur within 1 to 3 hours and persist for 6 to 8 or more hours. Blood levels of quinidine can be measured; the average therapeutic range is between 3 and 6 mg per liter of plasma; toxic reactions are almost certain to appear at levels above 8 mg per liter.
Indications: Quinidine sulfate is indicated in the treatment of premature atrial and ventricular contractions, paroxysmal atrial tachycardia, paroxysmal A-V junctional rhythm, atrial flutter, paroxysmal atrial fibrillation, established atrial fibrillation when therapy is appropriate, and paroxysmal ventricular tachycardia when not associated with complete heartblock, and for maintenance therapy after electrical conversion of atrial fibrillation and/or flutter.
Contraindications: Hypersensitivity or idiosyncrasy to the drug. History of thrombocytopenic purpura associated with previous quinidine administration. Digitalis intoxication manifested by A-V conduction disorders. Complete A-V block with an A-V nodal or idioventricular pacemaker. Ectopic impulses and rhythms due to escape mechanisms.
Warnings: In the treatment of atrial flutter, reversion to sinus rhythm may be preceded by a progressive reduction in the degree of A-V block to a 1:1 ratio resulting in extremely rapid ventricular rate. This possible hazard may be decreased by digitalization prior to giving quinidine. Evidence of quinidine cardiotoxicity (50% widening of QRS, frequent ventricular ectopic beats) mandates immediate discontinuation of the drug followed with close observation (ECG-monitoring) of the patient.
Usage in Pregnancy: The use of quinidine in pregnancy should be reserved only for those cases where the benefits outweigh the possible hazards to patient and fetus.
Precautions: Use quinidine with extreme caution in the presence of incomplete A-V block since complete block and asystole may result. Quinidine may cause unpredictable abnormalities of rhythm in digitalized hearts and it should be used with special caution in the presence of digitalis intoxication. **Note:** Quinidine effect is enhanced by potassium and reduced in the presence of hypokalemia.
The depressant actions of quinidine on cardiac contractility and arterial blood pressure limit its use in congestive heart failure and in hypotensive states unless these conditions are due to, or aggravated by, the arrhythmia. The potential disadvantage and benefits must be weighed. Continuous ECG-monitoring and determination of plasma quinidine levels are indicated when large doses, more than 2 g/day, are used.
Adverse Reactions:
Symptoms of cinchonism: (ringing in the ears, headache, nausea, disturbed vision) may appear (in sensitive patients) after a single dose of the drug.
Cardiovascular: widening of QRS-complex, cardiac asystole, ventricular ectopic beats, idioventricular rhythms including ventricular tachycardia and fibrillation, paradoxical tachycardia, arterial embolism.
Gastrointestinal: nausea, vomiting, abdominal pain, diarrhea.
Hematologic: acute hemalytic anemia, hypoprothrombinemia, thrombocytopenic purpura, agranulocytosis.
CNS: headache, fever, vertigo, apprehension, excitement, confusion, delirium and syncope, disturbed hearing (tinnitus, decreased auditory acuity), disturbed vision (mydriasis, blurred vision, disturbed color perception, photophobia, diplopia, night blindness, scotomata), optic neuritis.
Dermatologic: cutaneous flushing with intense pruritus.
Hypersensitivity reactions: Angioedema, acute asthmatic episode, vascular collapse, respiratory arrest.
Dosage and Administration: A preliminary test dose of a single tablet of quinidine sulfate should be administered to determine whether the patient has an idiosyncrasy to it. Continuous ECG-monitoring is recommended in all cases, where quinidine is used in large doses.
Usual Adult Dose: **Premature atrial and ventricular contractions:** 200 to 300 mg three or four times daily.
Paroxysmal supraventricular tachycardias: 400 to 600 mg every 2 or 3 hours until the paroxysm is terminated.
Atrial flutter: Quinidine should be administered after digitalization for this indication. Dosage is to be individualized.
Conversion of atrial fibrillation: Various schedules of quinidine administration have been in clinical use. A widely used technique is the administration of 200 mg of quinidine orally every 2 or 3 hours for 5 to 8 doses, with subsequent daily increase of the individual dose until sinus rhythm is restored or toxic effects occur. The total daily dose should not exceed 3 to 4 g, given by any schedule. Prior to quinidine administration the ventricular rate and congestive failure (if present) should be brought under control by digitalis therapy.
Maintenance therapy: 200 to 300 mg three or four times daily.
Overdose: Cardiotoxic effects of quinidine may be reversed in part by sodium lactate; the hypotension by vasoconstrictors and by catecholamines (since the vasodilation is partly due to α adrenergic blockade).
How Supplied: QUINORA 200 mg and 300 mg tablets are available in bottles of 100 and 1000.
Caution: FEDERAL LAW PROHIBITS DISPENSING WITHOUT A PRESCRIPTION.

THEO-DUR™ ℞
theophylline (anhydrous)
Sustained Action Tablets

Description: THEO-DUR Sustained Action Tablets contain anhydrous theophylline, with no color additives. THEO-DUR is available in three strengths: 100 mg, 200 mg and 300 mg: each tablet is scored for flexibility of dose. Theophylline, a xanthine compound, is a white, odorless crystalline powder, having a bitter taste.
Actions: The pharmacologic actions of theophylline are as a brochodilator, pulmonary vasodilator and smooth muscle relaxant since the drug directly relaxes the smooth muscle of the bronchial airways and pulmonary blood vessels. Theophylline also possesses other actions typical of the xanthine derivatives: coronary vasodilator, diuretic, cardiac stimulant, cerebral stimulant and skeletal muscle stimulant. The actions of theophylline may be mediated through inhibition of phosphodiesterase and a resultant increase in intracellular cyclic AMP which could mediate smooth muscle relaxation.
No development of tolerance appears to occur with chronic use of theophylline.
The half-life is shortened with cigarette smoking and prolonged in alcoholism, reduced hepatic or renal function, congestive heart failure, and in patients receiving certain antibiotics (see DRUG INTERACTIONS). High fever for prolonged periods may decrease theophylline elimination. Children over six months of age have rapid clearances with average half-lives of approximately 3–5 hours. Newborn infants have extremely slow clearances and half-lives exeeding 24 hours. Older adults with chronic obstructive pulmonary disease, any patients with cor pulmonale or other causes of heart failure, and patients with liver pathology may have much lower clearances with half-lives that exceed 24 hours. The half-life of theophylline in smokers (1–2 packs per day) averages 4–5 hours; the half-life in non-smokers averages 7–9 hours.
In single dose studies, THEO-DUR, administered at 8 mg/kg body weight, produced mean peak theophylline blood levels of 7.5 $\pm$ 1.9 mcg/ml at 9.2 $\pm$ 1.9 hours following administration. In the multiple dose, steady-state, 3 and 5 day studies, THEO-DUR achieved remarkably constant intra-subject theophylline levels with an average peak-trough difference of only 4 mcg/ml. This is indicative of smooth

and stable maintenance therapeutic theophylline levels throughout a q12h dosing interval.

Indications: Symptomatic relief and/or prevention of asthma and reversible bronchospasm associated with chronic bronchitis and emphysema.

Contraindications: THEO-DUR is contraindicated in individuals who have shown hypersensitivity to any of its components or xanthine derivatives.

Warnings: Excessive theophylline doses may be associated with toxicity; serum theophylline levels should be monitored to assure maximum benefit with minimum risk. Incidence of toxicity increases at serum levels greater than 20 mcg/ml. High blood levels of theophylline resulting from conventional doses are correlated with clinical manifestations of toxicity in: patients with lowered body plasma clearances; patients with liver dysfunction or chronic obstructive lung disease, and patients who are older than 55 years of age, particularly males. There are often no early signs of less serious theophylline toxicity such as nausea and restlessness, which may appear in up to 50% of patients prior to onset of convulsions. Ventricular arrhythmias or seizures may be the first signs of toxicity. Many patients who have higher theophylline serum levels exhibit a tachycardia. Theophylline products may worsen pre-existing arrhythmias.

Usage in Pregnancy: Safe use in pregnancy has not been established relative to possible adverse effects on fetal development, but neither have adverse effects on fetal development been established. This is, unfortunately, true for most antiasthmatic medications. Therefore, use of theophylline in pregnant women should be balanced against the risk of uncontrolled asthma.

Precautions: THEO-DUR TABLETS SHOULD NOT BE CHEWED OR CRUSHED. Theophyllines should not be administered concurrently with other xanthine medications. It should be used with caution in patients with severe cardiac disease, severe hypoxemia, hypertension, hyperthyroidism, acute myocardial injury, cor pulmonale, congestive heart failure, liver disease and in the elderly, particularly males, and in neonates. Great caution should be used in giving theophylline to patients in congestive heart failure since these patients show markedly prolonged theophylline blood level curves. Use theophylline cautiously in patients with history of peptic ulcer. Theophylline may occasionally act as a local irritant to G.I. tract although gastrointestinal symptoms are more commonly central and associated with high serum concentrations above 20 mcg/ml.

Adverse Reactions: The most consistent adverse reactions are usually due to overdose and are:

Gastrointestinal: Nausea, vomiting, epigastric pain, hematemesis, diarrhea.

Central Nervous System: Headaches, irritability, restlessness, insomnia, reflex hyperexcitability, muscle twitching, clonic and tonic generalized convulsions.

Cardiovascular: Palpitation, tachycardia, extrasystoles, flushing, hypotension, circulatory failure, life threatening ventricular arrhythmias.

Respiratory: Tachypnea.

Renal: Albuminuria, increased excretion of renal tubular cells and red blood cells; potentiation of diuresis.

Others: Hyperglycemia and inappropriate ADH syndrome.

Drug Interactions:

Drug	Effect
Theophylline with Furosemide	Increased Diuresis
Theophylline with Hexamethonium	Decreased Chronotropic Effect
Theophylline with Reserpine	Tachycardia
Theophylline with Cyclamycin (TAO), Erythromycin, or Lincomycin.	Increased Theophylline Blood Levels

Overdosage:

Management:

A. If potential oral overdose is established and seizure has not occurred;
1) Induce vomiting.
2) Administer a cathartic (this is particularly important if sustained release preparations have been taken).
3) Administer activated charcoal.

B. If patient is having a seizure:
1) Establish an airway.
2) Administer O_2.
3) Treat the seizure with intravenous diazepam, 0.1 to 0.3 mg/kg up to 10 mg.
4) Monitor vital signs, maintain blood pressure and provide adequate hydration.

C. Post-Seizure Coma:
1) Maintain airway and oxygenation.
2) If a result of oral medication, follow above recommendations to prevent absorption of drug, but intubation and lavage will have to be performed instead of inducing emesis, and the cathartic and charcoal will need to be introduced via a large bore gastric lavage tube.
3) Continue to provide full supportive care and adequate hydration while waiting for drug to be metabolized. In general, the drug is metabolized sufficiently rapidly so as to not warrant consideration of dialysis.

Dosage and Administration: Therapeutic serum levels associated with optimal likelihood for benefit and minimal risk of toxicity are considered to be between 10 and 20 mcg/ml. There is a great variation from patient to patient in dosage needed in order to achieve a therapeutic blood level due to variable rates of elimination. Because of this wide variation from patient to patient, and the relatively narrow therapeutic range, dosage must be individualized.

THE AVERAGE INITIAL CHILDREN'S (UNDER 9 YEARS OF AGE) DOSE IS ONE THEO-DUR 100 mg TABLET q12h.

THE AVERAGE INITIAL CHILDREN'S (AGES 9–12) DOSE IS ONE-HALF (150 mg) OF A THEO-DUR 300 mg TABLET q12h.

THE AVERAGE INITIAL ADOLESCENT (AGES 12–16) DOSE IS ONE THEO-DUR 200 mg TABLET q12h.

THE AVERAGE INITIAL ADULT DOSE IS ONE THEO-DUR 300 mg TABLET q12h.

If the desired response is not achieved with the above AVERAGE INITIAL DOSAGE recommendations, and there are no adverse reactions, the dose may be safely increased by 2–3 mg/kg body weight per day at 3 day intervals until the following MAXIMUM DOSE WITHOUT MEASUREMENT OF SERUM CONCENTRATION or a maximum of 900 mg in any 24 hour period, whichever is less, is attained:

(See table below)

If higher doses than those contained in the above MAXIMUM DOSE WITHOUT MEASUREMENT OF SERUM CONCENTRATION are necessary, it is recommended that serum theophylline levels be monitored. Check serum theophylline levels between 3 and 8 hours after a dose. It is important that the patient will have missed **no** doses during the previous 72 hours and that dosing intervals will have been reasonably typical with no added doses during that period of time. DOSAGE ADJUSTMENT BASED ON SERUM THEOPHYLLINE MEASUREMENTS WHEN THESE INSTRUCTIONS HAVE NOT BEEN FOLLOWED, MAY RESULT IN RECOMMENDATIONS THAT PRESENT RISK OF TOXICITY TO THE PATIENT.

How Supplied: THEO-DUR 100 mg, 200 mg and 300 mg Sustained Action Tablets are available in bottles of 100 and 1000, and in unit dose packages of 100 (20 × 5's).

Storage Conditions: Keep tightly closed. Store at controlled room temperature 15–30°C (59–86°F).

Caution: Federal law prohibits dispensing without a prescription.

[Shown in Product Identification Section]

MAXIMUM DOSE WITHOUT MEASUREMENT OF SERUM CONCENTRATION

	mg Per kg Body Weight*	Dose Per Interval
Children (under 9)	24 mg per day	12 mg q12h**
Children (9–12)	20 mg per day	10 mg q12h
Adolescents (12–16)	18 mg per day	9 mg q12h
Adults	13 mg per day	6.5 mg q12h

* Use ideal body weight for obese patients.
** Some children under 9 may require 8 mg q8h.

TYZINE® ℞
(tetrahydrozoline hydrochloride)
0.1% NASAL SOLUTION
and
0.05% PEDIATRIC NASAL DROPS

Actions: Tyzine (tetrahydrozoline hydrochloride), a sympathomimetic amine, possesses vasoconstrictor and decongestant actions when applied to the nasal mucosa, resulting in constriction of the smaller arterioles of the nasal passages effecting a decongesting action. Tyzine administered systemically has a central depressant rather than stimulant effect.

Indications: For decongestion of nasal and nasopharyngeal mucosa.

Contraindications: Tyzine is contraindicated for patients who have shown previous hypersensitivity to its components. The 0.1% solution is contraindicated in children under six years of age. Tyzine is not to be used for infants under two years of age. Tyzine Pediatric Solution should be used for children between the ages of 2 and 6 years. (See "Dosage and Administration".) Tyzine should not be used by patients under treatment with MAO inhibitors.

Warnings: Clinical data in human beings are inadequate to establish conditions for safe use in pregnancy. Therefore, Tyzine Nasal Solution should not be used during pregnancy unless, in the judgement of the physician, the expected benefits outweigh the possible hazards.

Overdosage in children may produce profound sedation. This may be accompanied by profuse sweating. (See "Management Of Overdosage".)

Precautions: Avoid doses greater or more frequent than those recommended below. Excessive dosage in children may, on rare occasions, cause severe drowsiness. Profuse sweating may accompany this effect. Overdosage may also cause marked hypotension or even shock.

Use cautiously in patients with cardiovascular disease (e.g., coronary artery disease, hypertension), and metabolic-endocrine disease (e.g., hyperthyroidism, diabetes).

Adverse Reactions: The most frequent adverse reactions are burning, stinging, sneezing,

Continued on next page

Key—Cont.

dryness, headache, drowsiness, weakness, tremors, lightheadedness, insomnia, and palpitations. Prolonged or excessive use may cause rebound congestion.
If adverse reactions occur, discontinue use.
Dosage and Administration:
Adults and Children 6 years and over:
It is recommended that 2 to 4 drops of Tyzine 0.1% Nasal Solution be instilled in each nostril as needed, never more often than every three hours. Less frequent administration is usually sufficient since relief is maintained for four hours or longer in most cases, and often for as long as eight hours. Bedtime instillation usually assures sleep undisturbed by the need for remedication before morning, or by insomnia from central stimulation.
Children 2 to 6 years of age:
It is recommended that 2 to 3 drops of Tyzine 0.05% Pediatric Nasal Drops be instilled in each nostril as needed and never more often than every three hours. Relief usually lasts for several hours so that instillations are usually needed only every four to six hours.
Instillation of nose drops can be most conveniently accomplished with the patient in the lateral head-low position.
Management of Overdosage: The administration or ingestion of overdoses of Tyzine may result in oversedation in young children. Very occasionally in adults with very excessive overdoses, a shock-like syndrome with hypotension and bradycardia may occur. In either case, the treatment of overdosage is usually that of watchful expectancy and general supportive measures. The patient should be kept warm, fluid balance should be maintained orally, if possible, and parenterally, if necessary. If the respiratory rate drops to 10 or below, the patient should be given oxygen, and respiration assisted. Blood pressure should be watched carefully to prevent a hypotensive crisis.
There is no known antidote for Tyzine (tetrahydrozoline hydrochloride). The use of stimulants is contraindicated. To date, we have had no reports of fatalities resulting from overdosages of Tyzine and while the symptoms resulting from Tyzine overdosage may be alarming, they are self-limiting and the patient recovers with no sequelae.
How Supplied:
Tyzine
Nasal Solution (0.1%)
—1 fl. oz. (30 cc.) and 1 pint bottles
—½ fl. oz. (15 cc.) plastic squeeze bottles
Pediatric Nasal Drops (0.05%)—½ fl. oz. (15 cc.) bottles
Caution: FEDERAL LAW PROHIBITS DISPENSING WITHOUT A PRESCRIPTION.

Knoll Pharmaceutical Company
WHIPPANY, NJ 07981

AKINETON® ℞
(biperiden)

Description: Each AKINETON hydrochloride tablet contains 2 mg. biperiden hydrochloride. Each 1 ml. AKINETON lactate ampule contains 5 mg. of biperiden lactate. Biperiden is α-5-Norbornen-2-yl-α-phenyl-1-piperidinepropanol and is available as the hydrochloride and lactate salts. It is a white crystalline, odorless powder, slightly soluble in water and alcohol. It is stable in air at normal temperatures.
Actions: AKINETON hydrochloride and lactate are weak visceral anticholinergic agents which are somewhat more potent than atropine on a dosage basis in terms of their ability to block nicotine-induced extensor spasm and death in mice. Cardiovascular and respiratory studies in the dog and cat using large intravenous doses of AKINETON hydrochloride reveal that the drug has only minor action on these systems. When given subcutaneously, the drying effect of AKINETON hydrochloride on the salivary glands of rabbits and its mydriatic effect on the mouse pupil are relatively weak compared with atropine. Six hours after an oral dose of 250 mg. of AKINETON hydrochloride per kg. in rats, 87% of the drug had been absorbed. AKINETON lactate (10 mg./ml.) was not irritating to the tissue of rabbits when injected intramuscularly (1.0 ml.) into the sacrospinalis muscles and intradermally (0.25 ml.) and subcutaneously (0.5 ml.) into the shaved abdominal skin. For AKINETON hydrochloride, the acute subcutaneous toxicity (LD_{50}) in mice was found to be 195 mg./kg., and the intravenous toxicity (LD_{50}) in mice 72 mg./kg. The acute oral toxicity (LD_{50}) in rats 750 mg./kg. For AKINETON lactate the intraperitoneal toxicity (LD_{50}) in rats was 270 mg./kg. and the intravenous toxicity (LD_{50}) in dogs was 222 mg./kg.
Clinically, AKINETON hydrochloride reduces akinesia and rigidity and, to a lesser extent, tremor. Excessive flow of saliva and oily skin become less marked or are eliminated. AKINETON hydrochloride can elevate the mood. The parenteral form of AKINETON is an effective and reliable agent for the treatment of acute episodes of extrapyramidal disturbances during treatment with reserpine and the phenothiazines. Akathisia, akinesia, dyskinetic tremors, rigor, oculogyric crises, spasmodic torticollis and profuse sweating are markedly reduced or eliminated. With parenteral AKINETON these drug-induced disturbances are rapidly brought under control. Subsequently this effect can usually be maintained with oral doses which may be given with tranquilizer therapy in psychotic and other conditions requiring an uninterrupted program with phenothiazines or reserpine.
Indications: For use as an adjunct in the therapy of all forms of parkinsonism (post-encephalitic, arteriosclerotic, idiopathic). Useful in the control of extrapyramidal disorders due to central nervous system drugs such as reserpine and phenothiazines. Particularly useful when drug-induced extrapyramidal disturbances interfere with indicated therapy.
Contraindications: The only known contraindication is sensitivity to AKINETON (biperiden).
Warnings: Isolated instances of mental confusion, euphoria, agitation and disturbed behavior have been reported in susceptible patients. Safe use in pregnancy has not been established.
Precautions: Caution should be observed in patients with manifest glaucoma, though no prohibitive rise in intraocular pressure has been noted following either oral or parenteral administration. Patients with prostatism or cardiac arrhythmia should be given this drug with caution. Occasionally, drowsiness may occur.
Adverse Reactions: Minimal with either oral or parenteral administration. Primarily dry mouth and blurred vision. These side effects can be decreased or eliminated by reduction of the oral dosage or by slow parenteral administration. If gastric irritation occurs, it can be avoided by administering during or after meals. A decrease in urinary flow has been noted in a few patients, and some may exhibit short periods of euphoria or disorientation. There have been no significant changes in blood pressure levels or pulse rate in patients who have been given parenteral AKINETON (biperiden), although mild transient postural hypotension may occur. No local tissue reaction has been reported following intramuscular injection.
Dosage and Administration: Orally: Doses required to achieve the therapeutic goal are variable and must be individually and gradually adjusted. *Parkinson's disease:* 1 tablet, three to four times daily. *Drug-induced extrapyramidal disorders:* 1 tablet, one to three times daily. **Parenterally:** *Drug-induced extrapyramidal symptoms:* The average adult dose is 2 mg. intramuscularly or intravenously. May be repeated every half-hour until resolution of symptoms is effected, but not more than four consecutive doses should be administered in a 24-hour period.
Treatment of Overdosage: It may be expected that the effects of Akineton overdosage would resemble atropine toxicity. Treatment should be based on observation and particularly on whether CNS depression or CNS stimulation is observed. Emesis induction or gastric lavage may be beneficial in patients who are neither precomatose nor convulsive.
Respiration must be maintained. If respiratory depression is severe, artificial respiration or mechanical assistance to respiration should be employed. If CNS excitation is observed, a short-acting barbiturate may be administered, remembering that CNS excitation may precede a period of CNS depression. Vasopressor agents may be necessary if circulatory collapse should occur.
Hyperthermia control may be sought by tepid bathing. Simple supportive measures will suffice for less serious problems.
How Supplied: Ampules—1 ml. (each ml. contains 5 mg. AKINETON lactate in an aqueous 1.4 per cent sodium lactate solution. No added preservatives). Boxes of 10. Tablets—2 mg. (bisected) AKINETON hydrochloride. Bottles of 100 and 1000.
[*Shown in Product Identification Section*]

DICODID® TABLETS Ⓒ ℞
(hydrocodone bitartrate)

Description: Each tablet of DICODID contains 5 mg of hydrocodone bitartrate (**Warning:** May be habit forming). Hydrocodone is dihydrocodeinone, a hydrogenated ketone of codeine, available as the bitartrate salt.
Clinical Pharmacology: DICODID is a semisynthetic narcotic with multiple actions qualitatively similar to those of codeine. Most of these involve the central nervous system and smooth muscle. DICODID is an analgesic and antitussive.
Indications and Usage: For the relief of moderate to moderately severe pain; for the suppression of cough.
Contraindications: Hypersensitivity to hydrocodone; intracranial lesion associated with increased intracranial pressure; status asthmaticus.
Warnings:
Drug Dependence: May be habit forming. Hydrocodone can produce drug dependence of the morphine type and therefore has the potential for being abused. Psychic dependence, physical dependence and tolerance may develop upon repeated administration of DICODID and it should be prescribed and administered with the same degree of caution appropriate to the use of other oral narcotic drugs.
Head Injury and Increased Intracranial Pressure: The respiratory depressant effects of narcotics and their capacity to elevate cerebrospinal fluid pressure may be markedly exaggerated in the presence of head injury, other intracranial lesions or a pre-existing increase in intracranial pressure. Furthermore, narcotics produce adverse reactions which may obscure the clinical course of patients with head injuries.
Acute Abdominal Conditions: The administration of DICODID or other narcotics may obscure the diagnosis or clinical course of patients with acute abdominal conditions.
Precautions:
Usage in Ambulatory Patients: Hydrocodone, like all narcotics, may impair the mental and/or physical abilities required for the performance of potentially hazardous tasks such as

driving a car or operating machinery; patients should be cautioned accordingly.

Drug Interactions: Patients receiving other narcotic analgesics, general anesthetics, phenothiazines, other tranquilizers, sedative-hypnotics or other CNS depressants (including alcohol) concomitantly with DICODID may exhibit an additive CNS depression. When such combined therapy is contemplated, the dose of one or both agents should be reduced.

Usage in Pregnancy: Safe use in pregnancy has not been established relative to possible adverse effects on fetal development. Therefore, DICODID should not be used in pregnant women unless, in the judgement of the physician, the potential benefits outweigh the possible hazards.

Usage in Children: DICODID should not be administered to children under 12 because adequate dosing information is not available.

Nursing Mothers: As a general rule, nursing should not be undertaken when a patient is receiving DICODID, since it may be present in the milk of nursing mothers.

Special Risk Patients: DICODID should be used with caution in elderly or debilitated patients and those with severe impairment of hepatic or renal function, hypothyroidism, Addison's disease, prostatic hypertrophy or urethral stricture.

Adverse Reactions: The most frequent adverse reactions are light-headedness, dizziness, sedation, nausea and vomiting. These effects seem to be more prominent in ambulatory than in non-ambulatory patients, and some of these adverse reactions may be alleviated if the patient lies down. Other adverse reactions include euphoria, dysphoria, constipation, skin rash and pruritus.

Overdosage:

Signs and Symptoms: Serious overdosage with DICODID is characterized by respiratory depression (a decrease in respiratory rate and/or tidal volume, Cheyne-Stokes respiration, cyanosis), extreme somnolence progressing to stupor or coma, skeletal muscle flaccidity, cold and clammy skin, and sometimes bradycardia and hypotension. In severe overdosage, apnea, circulatory collapse, cardiac arrest and death may occur.

Treatment: Primary attention should be given to the reestablishment of adequate respiratory exchange through provision of a patent airway and the institution of assisted or controlled ventilation. The narcotic antagonists naloxone, nalorphine and levallorphan are specific antidotes against respiratory depression which may result from overdosage or unusual sensitivity to narcotics, including hydrocodone. Therefore, an appropriate dose of one of these antagonists should be administered, preferably by the intravenous route, simultaneously with ventilatory assistance. Since the duration of action of hydrocodone may exceed that of the antagonist, the patient should be kept under continued surveillance; repeated doses of the antagonist may be required to maintain adequate respiration. An antagonist should not be administered in the absence of clinically significant respiratory or cardiovascular depression. Oxygen, intravenous fluids, vasopressors and other supportive measures should be employed as indicated. Gastric lavage or induced emesis may be useful in removing unabsorbed drug from conscious patients.

Dosage and Administration: DICODID is given orally.

Analgesia: The usual adult dose is 5 or 10 mg every 4–6 hours as needed for pain. Dosage should be adjusted according to the severity of the pain and the response of the patient. It may occasionally be necessary to exceed the usual recommended dosage in cases of more severe pain or in those patients who have become tolerant to the analgesic effect of narcotics.

Cough: The usual adult dose is 5 mg every 4–6 hours as needed.

How Supplied: Flat, round, white tablets inscribed with K logo on one side, "5" on the other side.

5 mg tablets—Bottles of 100—NDC #0044-0721-02.

A Schedule Ⓒ Narcotic.

DEA order form required.

[*Shown in Product Identification Section*]

DILAUDID® Ⓒ ℞

(hydromorphone hydrochloride)

Description: DILAUDID (hydromorphone hydrochloride) (WARNING: May be habit forming), a hydrogenated ketone of morphine, is a narcotic analgesic. It is available in ampules (for parenteral administration) containing 1 mg, 2 mg, 3 mg and 4 mg hydromorphone hydrochloride per ml with 0.2% sodium citrate, 0.2% citric acid solution; in multiple dose vials (for parenteral administration) of 10 ml and 20 ml solutions, each ml containing 2 mg hydromorphone hydrochloride and 0.5 mg edetate disodium with 1.8 mg methylparaben and 0.2 mg propylparaben as preservatives and pH adjusted with sodium hydroxide or hydrochloric acid; in color coded tablets (for oral administration) containing 1 mg, 2 mg, 3 mg and 4 mg hydromorphone hydrochloride; in suppositories (for rectal administration) containing 3 mg hydromorphone hydrochloride in cocoa butter base with 1% colloidal silica as an inactive ingredient; and in powder for prescription compounding. DILAUDID ampules and multiple dose vials are sterile.

Clinical Pharmacology: DILAUDID is a narcotic analgesic; its principal therapeutic effect is relief of pain. The precise mechanism of action of DILAUDID and other opiates is not known, although it is believed to relate to the existence of opiate receptors in the central nervous system. In addition to analgesia, narcotics produce drowsiness, changes in mood and mental clouding, although neither sensory modalities nor motor activity are blocked at therapeutic doses. There is no intrinsic limit to the analgesic effect of DILAUDID; like morphine, adequate doses will relieve even the most severe pain. Clinically, however, dosage limitations are imposed by the adverse effects, primarily respiratory depression, nausea, and vomiting, which can result from high doses.

DILAUDID has diverse additional actions. It depresses the respiratory center and the cough center, stimulates the vomiting center, produces pinpoint constriction of the pupil, enhances parasympathetic activity, elevates cerebrospinal fluid pressure, increases biliary pressure, produces transient hyperglycemia.

Generally, the analgesic action of parenterally administered DILAUDID is apparent within 15 minutes and usually remains in effect for more than five hours. The onset of action of oral DILAUDID is somewhat slower, with measurable analgesia occurring within 30 minutes.

Radioimmunoassay techniques have recently been developed for the analysis of DILAUDID in human plasma. However, little is known as yet about the bioavailability or pharmacokinetics of DILAUDID in humans. Previous investigations reported the half-life of hydromorphone to be 4.6 hours and 6.3 hours. In a recent study of 70 patients, the half-life of hydromorphone was reported to range from 1.2 hours to 13.8 hours with the 50 percentile level of distribution being 4.1 hours. These investigations did not involve direct measurements of hydromorphone plasma levels.

Indications and Usage: DILAUDID is indicated for the relief of moderate to severe pain such as that due to:

Surgery
Cancer
Trauma (soft tissue & bone)
Biliary Colic
Myocardial Infarction
Burns
Renal Colic

Contraindications: As is morphine, DILAUDID is contraindicated in patients known to have a hypersensitivity to it; in the presence of an intracranial lesion associated with increased intracranial pressure; and whenever ventilatory function is depressed (chronic obstructive pulmonary disease, cor pulmonale, emphysema, kyphoscoliosis, status asthmaticus).

Warnings

Respiratory Depression: DILAUDID produces dose-related respiratory depression by acting directly on brain stem respiratory centers. DILAUDID also affects centers that control respiratory rhythm, and may produce irregular and periodic breathing. If significant respiratory depression occurs, it may be antagonized by the use of naloxone hydrochloride, 0.005 mg/kg intravenously. Apply other supportive measures when indicated.

Head Injury and Increased Intracranial Pressure: The respiratory depressant effects of narcotics and their capacity to elevate cerebrospinal fluid pressure may be markedly exaggerated in the presence of head injury, other intracranial lesions or a pre-existing increase in intracranial pressure. Furthermore, narcotics produce adverse reactions which may obscure the clinical course of patients with head injuries.

Acute Abdominal Conditions: The administration of narcotics may obscure the diagnosis or clinical course of patients with acute abdominal conditions.

Precautions

Special Risk Patients: DILAUDID should be used with caution in elderly or debilitated patients and those with impaired renal or hepatic function, hypothyroidism, Addison's disease, prostatic hypertrophy or urethral stricture. As with any narcotic analgesic agent, the usual precautions should be observed and the possibility of respiratory depression should be kept in mind.

Usage in Ambulatory Patients: Narcotics may impair the mental and/or physical abilities required for the performance of potentially hazardous tasks such as driving a car or operating machinery; patients should be cautioned accordingly.

Drug Interactions: Patients receiving other narcotic analgesics, general anesthetics, phenothiazines, tranquilizers, sedative-hypnotics, tricyclic antidepressants or other CNS depressants (including alcohol) concomitantly with DILAUDID may exhibit an additive CNS depression. When such combined therapy is contemplated, the dose of one or both agents should be reduced.

Parenteral Administration: The parenteral form of DILAUDID may be given intravenously, but the injection should be given very slowly. Rapid intravenous injection of narcotic analgesics increases the possibility of side effects such as hypotension and respiratory depression.

Usage in Pregnancy: Pregnancy Category C. DILAUDID has been shown to be teratogenic in hamsters when given in doses 600 times the human dose. There are no adequate and well-controlled studies in pregnant women. DILAUDID should be used during pregnancy only if the potential benefit justifies the potential risk to the fetus.

Nonteratogenic effects: Babies born to mothers who have been taking opioids regularly prior to delivery will be physically dependent. The withdrawal signs include irritability and excessive crying, tremors, hyperactive reflexes, increased respiratory rate, increased stools, sneezing, yawning, vomiting, and fever. The intensity of the syndrome does not always correlate with the duration of maternal opioid

Continued on next page

Knoll—Cont.

use or dose. There is no consensus on the best method of managing withdrawal. Chlorpromazine 0.7–1.0 mg/kg q6h, phenobarbital 2 mg/kg q6h, and paregoric 2–4 drops/kg q4h, have been used to treat withdrawal symptoms in infants. The duration of therapy is 4 to 28 days, with the dosages decreased as tolerated.

Labor and Delivery: As with all narcotics, administration of DILAUDID to the mother shortly before delivery may result in some degree of respiratory depression in the newborn, especially if higher doses are used.

Nursing Mothers: It is not known whether this drug is excreted in human milk. Because many drugs are excreted in human milk and because of the potential for serious adverse reactions in nursing infants from DILAUDID, a decision should be made whether to discontinue nursing or to discontinue the drug, taking into account the importance of the drug to the mother.

Pediatric Use: Safety and effectiveness in children have not been established.

FD&C Yellow No. 5: DILAUDID 1 mg, 2 mg and 4 mg color coded tablets contain FD&C Yellow No. 5 (tartrazine) dye which may cause allergic-type reactions (including bronchial asthma) in certain susceptible individuals. Although the overall incidence of FD&C Yellow No. 5 (tartrazine) dye sensitivity in the general population is low, it is frequently seen in patients who also have aspirin hypersensitivity.

Adverse Reactions

Central Nervous System: Sedation, drowsiness, mental clouding, lethargy, impairment of mental and physical performance, anxiety, fear, dysphoria, dizziness, psychic dependence, mood changes.

Gastrointestinal System: Nausea and vomiting occur more frequently in ambulatory than in recumbent patients. The antiemetic phenothiazines are useful in suppressing these effects; however, some phenothiazine derivatives seem to be antianalgesic and to increase the amount of narcotic required to produce pain relief, while other phenothiazines reduce the amount of narcotic required to produce a given level of analgesia. Prolonged administration of DILAUDID may produce constipation.

Cardiovascular System: Circulatory depression, peripheral circulatory collapse and cardiac arrest have occurred after rapid intravenous injection. Orthostatic hypotension and fainting may occur if a patient stands up suddenly after receiving an injection of DILAUDID.

Genitourinary System: Ureteral spasm, spasm of vesical sphincters and urinary retention have been reported.

Respiratory Depression: DILAUDID produces dose-related respiratory depression by acting directly on brain stem respiratory centers. DILAUDID also affects centers that control respiratory rhythm, and may produce irregular and periodic breathing. If significant respiratory depression occurs, it may be antagonized by the use of naloxone hydrochloride, 0.005 mg/kg intravenously. Apply other supportive measures when indicated.

Cough Reflex: DILAUDID suppresses the cough reflex; as with all narcotics, caution should be exercised when DILAUDID is used postoperatively and in patients with pulmonary disease.

Drug Abuse and Dependence: DILAUDID is a Schedule II narcotic. Psychic dependence, physical dependence, and tolerance may develop upon repeated administration of narcotics; therefore, DILAUDID should be prescribed and administered with caution. However, psychic dependence is unlikely to develop when DILAUDID is used for a short time for the treatment of pain. Physical dependence, the condition in which continued administration of the drug is required to prevent the appearance of a withdrawal syndrome, assumes clinically significant proportions only after several weeks of continued narcotic use, although some mild degree of physical dependence may develop after a few days of narcotic therapy. Tolerance, in which increasingly large doses are required in order to produce the same degree of analgesia, is manifested initially by a shortened duration of analgesic effect, and subsequently by decreases in the intensity of analgesia. The rate of development of tolerance varies among patients.

Overdosage

Signs and Symptoms: Serious overdosage with DILAUDID is characterized by respiratory depression (a decrease in respiratory rate and/or tidal volume, Cheyne-Stokes respiration, cyanosis), extreme somnolence progressing to stupor or coma, skeletal muscle flaccidity, cold and clammy skin, and sometimes bradycardia and hypotension. In severe overdosage, particularly by the intravenous route, apnea, circulatory collapse, cardiac arrest, and death may occur.

Treatment: Primary attention should be given to the reestablishment of adequate respiratory exchange through provision of a patent airway and institution of assisted or controlled ventilation. The narcotic antagonist naloxone hydrochloride is a specific antidote against respiratory depression which may result from overdosage or unusual sensitivity to narcotics, including DILAUDID. Therefore, naloxone hydrochloride, 0.005 mg/kg should be administered intravenously simultaneously with ventilatory assistance.

Since the duration of action of DILAUDID may exceed that of the antagonist, the patient should be kept under continued surveillance; repeated doses of the antagonist may be required to maintain adequate respiration. An antagonist should not be administered in the absence of clinically significant respiratory or cardiovascular depression. Oxygen, intravenous fluids, vasopressors, and other supportive measures should be employed as indicated.

In cases of overdosage with oral DILAUDID, gastric lavage or induced emesis may be useful in removing unabsorbed drug from conscious patients.

Dosage and Administration

Parenteral: The usual dose is 2 mg intramuscularly every 4 to 6 hours as necessary. The dose must be individually adjusted according to severity of pain, patient response and patient size. The subcutaneous route of administration may be utilized, if desired. Intravenous or subcutaneous administration is usually not painful. Should intravenous administration be necessary, the injection should be given very slowly (taking at least 2 to 3 minutes to administer). If the pain increases in severity, analgesia is not adequate or tolerance occurs, a gradual increase in dosage may be required. The first sign of beginning tolerance is usually a reduced duration of effect.

Parenteral drug products should be inspected visually for particulate matter and discoloration prior to administration, whenever solution and container permit. A slight yellowish discoloration may develop in DILAUDID ampules and multiple dose vials. No loss of potency has been demonstrated.

Oral: The usual oral dose is 2 mg every 4 to 6 hours as necessary. The dose must be individually adjusted according to severity of pain, patient response and patient size. More severe pain may require 4 mg or more every 4 to 6 hours. If the pain increases in severity, analgesia is not adequate or tolerance occurs, a gradual increase in dosage may be required. If pain is exceedingly severe, or if prompt response is desired, parenteral DILAUDID should be used initially in adequate amounts to control the pain.

Rectal: DILAUDID suppositories (3 mg) may provide longer duration of relief which could obviate additional medication during the sleeping hours.

How Supplied

Ampules: 1 mg, 2 mg, 3 mg, and 4 mg hydromorphone hydrochloride per ml with 0.2% sodium citrate, 0.2% citric acid solution. No added preservative.

1 mg/ml ampules—Boxes of 10—
NDC# 0044-1011-01.
2 mg/ml ampules—Boxes of 10—
NDC# 0044-1012-01.
Boxes of 25—NDC# 0044-1012-09.
3 mg/ml ampules—Boxes of 10—
NDC# 0044-1013-01.
4 mg/ml ampules—Boxes of 10—
NDC# 0044-1014-01.

Multiple Dose Vials: 10 ml and 20 ml sterile solutions, each ml contains 2 mg hydromorphone hydrochloride and 0.5 mg edetate disodium with 1.8 mg methylparaben and 0.2 mg propylparaben as preservatives. pH adjusted with sodium hydroxide or hydrochloric acid.

2 mg/ml—10 ml multiple dose vials—
NDC# 0044-1062-01.
2 mg/ml—20 ml multiple dose vials—
NDC# 0044-1062-05.

Oral Color Coded Tablets: (NOT FOR INJECTION)

1 mg tablet (green)—Bottles of 100—
NDC# 0044-1021-02.
2 mg tablet (orange)—Bottles of 100—
NDC# 0044-1022-02.
Bottles of 500—NDC# 0044-1022-03.
3 mg tablet (pink)—Bottles of 100—
NDC# 0044-1023-02.
4 mg tablet (yellow)—Bottles of 100—
NDC# 0044-1024-02.
Bottles of 500—NDC# 0044-1024-03.

Rectal Suppositories: 3 mg hydromorphone hydrochloride in cocoa butter base with 1% colloidal silica as an inactive ingredient.
Boxes of 6—NDC# 0044-1053-01.

Powder: For prescription compounding.
15 grain vial—NDC# 0044-1040-01.

Storage: All dosage forms of DILAUDID should be stored at 59°–86°F, 15°–30°C.

A Schedule II Narcotic. DEA order form required.

[*Shown in Product Identification Section*]

DILAUDID® COUGH SYRUP ℭ ℞
(hydromorphone hydrochloride)

Description: Each 5 ml (1 teaspoonful) contains 1 mg DILAUDID (hydromorphone hydrochloride) (**WARNING:** May be habit forming) and 100 mg guaifenesin in a peach-flavored syrup containing 5% alcohol. reduces

Clinical Pharmacology: DILAUDID (hydromorphone hydrochloride), a hydrogenated ketone of morphine, is a centrally acting narcotic antitussive which acts directly on the cough reflex center. DILAUDID is also an analgesic. Guaifenesin reduces the viscosity of secretions, thereby increasing the efficiency of the cough reflex and of ciliary action in removing accumulated secretions from the trachea and bronchi. Unlike many other expectorants, guaifenesin rarely causes gastric irritation.

Indications and Usage: DILAUDID Cough Syrup is indicated for the control of persistent, exhausting cough or dry nonproductive cough.

Contraindications: DILAUDID is contraindicated in the presence of intracranial lesion associated with increased intracranial pressure and whenever ventilatory function is depressed (chronic obstructive pulmonary disease, cor pulmonale, emphysema, kyphoscoliosis, status asthmaticus.)

Warnings:

Drug Dependence: May be habit forming. DILAUDID is a narcotic with an addiction liability similar to that of morphine at equianalgesic doses. Psychic dependence, physical dependence and tolerance may develop upon repeated administration of this drug and it should be prescribed and administered with

the same degree of caution appropriate to the use of other oral narcotic drugs.
Head Injury and Increased Intracranial Pressure: The respiratory depressant effects of narcotics and their capacity to elevate cerebrospinal fluid pressure may be markedly exaggerated in the presence of head injury, other intracranial lesions or a pre-existing increase in intracranial pressure. Furthermore, narcotics produce adverse reactions which may obscure the clinical course of patients with head injuries.
Acute Abdominal Conditions: The administration of narcotics may obscure the diagnosis or clinical course of patients with acute abdominal conditions.
Precautions:
Usage in Ambulatory Patients: Narcotics may impair the mental and or physical abilities required for the performance of potentially hazardous tasks such as driving a car or operating machinery; patients should be cautioned accordingly.
Drug Interactions: Patients receiving other narcotics, general anesthetics, phenothiazines, other tranquilizers, sedative-hypnotics or other CNS depressants (including alcohol) concomitantly with DILAUDID Cough Syrup may exhibit an additive CNS depression. When such combined therapy is contemplated, the dose of one or both agents should be reduced.
Usage in Pregnancy: Safe use in pregnancy has not been established relative to possible adverse effects on fetal development. Therefore, DILAUDID Cough Syrup should not be used in pregnant women unless, in the judgement of the physician, the potential benefits outweigh the possible hazards.
Nursing Mothers: As a general rule, nursing should not be undertaken when a patient is receiving DILAUDID, since it may be present in the milk of nursing mothers.
Special Risk Patients: DILAUDID Cough Syrup should be used with caution in elderly or debilitated patients or those with severe impairment of hepatic or renal function, hypothyroidism, Addison's disease, prostatic hypertrophy or urethral stricture.
Adverse Reactions:
Central Nervous System: Sedation, drowsiness, mental clouding, lethargy, impairment of mental and physical performance, anxiety, fear, dysphoria, dizziness, psychic dependence, mood changes.
Gastrointestinal System: Nausea and vomiting occur more frequently in ambulatory than in recumbent patients. The antiemetic phenothiazines are useful in suppressing these effects; however, some phenothiazine derivatives seem to be antianalgesic and to increase the amount of narcotic required to produce pain relief, while other phenothiazines reduce the amount of narcotic required to produce a given level of analgesia. Prolonged administration of DILAUDID may produce constipation.
Genitourinary System: Ureteral spasm, spasm of vesical sphincters and urinary retention have been reported.
Respiratory Depression: DILAUDID produces dose-related respiratory depression by acting directly on brain stem respiratory centers. DILAUDID also affects centers that control respiratory rhythm, and may produce irregular and periodic breathing. If significant respiratory depression occurs, it may be antagonized by the use of naloxone, nalorphine or levallorphan as recommended by the manufacturer. Apply other supportive measures when indicated.
Cough Relex: DILAUDID suppresses the cough reflex; as with all narcotics, caution should be exercised when DILAUDID is used postoperatively and in patients with pulmonary disease.
Overdosage:
Signs and Symptons: Serious overdosage with DILAUDID Cough Syrup is characterized by respiratory depression (a decrease in respiratory rate and/or tidal volume, Cheyne-Stokes respiration, cyanosis) extreme somnolence progressing to stupor or coma, skeletal muscle flaccidity, cold and clammy skin, and sometimes bradycardia and hypotension. In severe overdosage, apnea, circulatory collapse, cardiac arrest and death may occur.
Treatment: Primary attention should be given to the reestablishment of adequate respiratory exchange through provision of a patent airway and the institution of assisted or controlled ventilation. The narcotic antagonists naloxone, nalorphine or levallorphan are specific antidotes against respiratory depression which may result from overdosage or unusual sensitivity to narcotics. Therefore, an appropriate dose of one of these antagonists should be administered, preferably by the intravenous route, simultaneously with ventilatory assistance. Since the duration of action of the narcotic may exceed that of the antagonist, the patient should be kept under continued surveillance and repeated doses of the antagonist should be administered as needed to maintain adequate respiratory function. An antagonist should not be administered in the absence of clinically significant respiratory or cardiovascular depression. Oxygen, intravenous fluids, vasopressors and other supportive measures should be employed as indicated. Gastric lavage or induced emesis may be useful in removing unabsorbed drug from conscious patients.
Dosage and Administration: The usual adult dose of DILAUDID Cough Syrup is one teaspoonful (5 ml) every 3 to 4 hours. For children, the dose is adjusted according to age and body weight.
How Supplied: Bottles of 1 pint (473 ml)—NDC #0044-1080-01.
A Schedule Ⓒ Narcotic.
DEA order form required.

METRAZOL® ℞
(pentylenetetrazol)

Description: Each tablet or 5 ml. (1 teaspoonful) Liquidum contains 100 mg. METRAZOL (original brand of pentylenetetrazol). The wine-flavored elixir contains 15% alcohol. METRAZOL ampules, 1 ml. of a 10% solution. Each ml. contains 100 mg. pentylenetetrazol in aqueous solution with 0.53 mg. disodium phosphate. pH adjusted with phosphoric acid. No added preservative.
Actions: METRAZOL is a central nervous system stimulant.
Indications: METRAZOL is administered orally to enhance mental and physical activity of elderly patients.
Contraindications: There are no known contraindications to METRAZOL.
Warnings: At recommended oral dosage, side effects occur infrequently or not at all.
Precautions: Caution should be exercised when treating patients with a low convulsive threshold, or with a focal brain lesion.
Adverse Reactions: High doses, parenterally, may precipitate clonic convulsions.
Dosage and Administration: *Orally*—1 or 2 tablets or 1 or 2 teaspoonfuls of the Liquidum three times a day.
How Supplied: METRAZOL Tablets, 100 mg.—bottles of 100 and 1000. METRAZOL Liquidum—bottles of 1 pint (473 ml.). METRAZOL Ampules, 1 ml. (100 mg.)—boxes of 10.

NICO-METRAZOL® Elixir and Tablets ℞

Description: Each tablet or 5 ml. (1 teaspoonful) of the Elixir contains METRAZOL® (original brand of pentylenetetrazol) 100 mg. and niacin 50 mg. The wine flavored Elixir contains 15% alcohol.
Actions: METRAZOL is a central nervous system stimulant. Niacin increases peripheral blood flow.
Indications: NICO-METRAZOL is administered to enhance mental and physical activity of elderly patients.
Contraindications: There are no known contraindications to NICO-METRAZOL.
Warnings: At recommended oral dosage, side effects occur infrequently or not at all.
Precautions: Caution should be exercised when treating patients with a low convulsive threshold or with a focal brain lesion, or severely impaired liver function. Use with caution in patients with peptic ulcer, gall bladder or liver diseases. Niacin may potentiate hypotensive drugs, phenothiazine derivatives and inactivate fibrinolysin. Since decreased glucose tolerance and mild diabetes have been reported with average or excessive doses of niacin, diabetic patients should use the drug with caution.
Adverse Reactions: The occasional pruritus associated with niacin administration may occur.
Dosage and Administration: Average dose—1 or 2 tablets or 1 or 2 teaspoonfuls of the Elixir three times a day.
How Supplied: NICO-METRAZOL Elixir—bottles of 1 pint (473 ml.). NICO-METRAZOL Tablets—bottles of 100.

QUADRINAL™ Tablets and Suspension ℞

Description: Each tablet contains ephedrine hydrochloride 24 mg.; phenobarbital 24 mg. [Warning: May be habit forming]; theophylline calcium salicylate 130 mg. (provides 65 mg. anhydrous theophylline); potassium iodide 320 mg. Each 5 ml. (1 teaspoonful) of the fruit-flavored Suspension is equivalent to ½ tablet.
Actions: QUADRINAL contains two bronchodilators, theophylline and ephedrine. Phenobarbital serves as a mild sedative to help counteract central nervous system stimulation which may be caused by ephedrine. Wheezing and coughing are relieved by improved bronchodilation while expectorant action of potassium iodide helps to remove a source of irritation in the bronchial tree. Dyspnea is thus relieved or prevented and acute episodes of bronchospasm are often eliminated with consequent lessening of apprehension and distress.
Indications: For chronic respiratory disease in which tenacious mucus and bronchospasm are dominant symptoms, such as bronchial asthma, chronic bronchitis and pulmonary emphysema.
Contraindications: Avoid using QUADRINAL in combination with other theophylline preparations since this will elevate theophylline blood levels and may produce adverse effects.
Warning: Phenobarbital may be habit forming.
Use in pregnancy: Caution is recommended. Although an extremely rare occurrence, iodide-induced goiter with hypothyroidism in the newborn has been reported.
Precautions: Caution is recommended in patients sensitive to iodides, in patients receiving potassium-sparing diuretics or potassium supplements, in the presence of cardiovascular disease, hyperthyroidism and diabetes. In some patients, prolonged use of iodides can lead to hypothyroidism. Salicylates block the uricosuric action of probenecid and sulfinpyrazone; therefore, QUADRINAL should be used with caution in patients with gout. Particular caution in dose administration must be exercised in patients with peptic ulcers, as this condition may be exacerbated. Theophylline increases the excretion of lithium. Theophylline clearance has been reported to be larger and more variable in smokers than in non-smokers. There have been reports that troleandomycin (TAO) reduced theophylline clearance by one-half, resulting in a doubling of theophylline blood levels. The effect of other macrolide anti-

Continued on next page

Knoll—Cont.

biotics (such as erythromycin) is not known, but may be similar.

Adverse Reactions: QUADRINAL is usually well tolerated. Gastrointestinal irritation is rarely encountered; if it occurs, administration of QUADRINAL with or after meals is recommended.

Dosage and Administration: Adults and children over 12 years—1 tablet or 2 teaspoonfuls Suspension three or four times daily; if needed, an additional 1 tablet or 2 teaspoonfuls upon retiring for nighttime relief. Children 6 to 12 years—½ tablet or 1 teaspoonful Suspension three times a day. Children under 6 years—dose is proportionately less.

How Supplied: Suspension (strawberry-colored, fruit flavored) pint bottles (473 ml.). Tablets (white, scored, embossed triangle on one side) bottles of 100 and 1000.

[*Shown in Product Identification Section*]

SANTYL® Ointment ℞
(collagenase)

Description: SANTYL® OINTMENT is a sterile enzymatic debriding ointment which contains 250 collagenase units per gram of white pertrolatum USP. The enzyme collagenase is derived from the fermentation by *Clostridium histolyticum.* It possesses the unique ability to digest native and denatured collagen in necrotic tissue.

Action: Since collagen accounts for 75% of the dry weight of skin tissue, the ability of collagenase to digest collagen in the physiological pH range and temperature makes it particularly effective in the removal of detritus.[1] Collagenase thus contributes towards the formation of granulation tissue and subsequent epithelization of dermal ulcers and severely burned areas.[2,3,4,5,6] Collagen in healthy tissue or in newly formed granulation tissue is not attacked.[2,3,4,5,6,7,8]

Indications: Santyl Ointment is indicated for debriding chronic dermal ulcers[2,3,4,5,6,8,9,10,11,12,13,14,15,16,17,18] and severely burned areas.[3,4,5,7,16,19,20,21]

Contraindications: Santyl Ointment is contraindicated in patients who have shown local or systemic hypersensitivity to collagenase.

Precautions: The optimal pH range of collagenase is 6 to 8. Higher or lower pH conditions will decrease the enzyme's activity and appropriate precautions should be taken. The enzymatic activity is also adversely affected by detergents, hexachlorophene and heavy metal ions such as mercury and silver which are used in some antiseptics. When it is suspected such materials have been used, the site should be carefully cleansed by repeated washings with normal saline before Santyl Ointment is applied. Soaks containing metal ions or acidic solutions such as Burow's solution should be avoided because of the metal ion and low pH. Cleansing materials such as hydrogen peroxide, Dakin's solution, and sterile saline are compatible with Santyl Ointment.

Debilitated patients should be closely monitored for systemic bacterial infections because of the theoretical possibility that debriding enzymes may increase the risk of bacteremia. A slight transient erythema has been noted occasionally in the surrounding tissue, particularly when Santyl Ointment was not confined to the lesion. Therefore, the ointment should be applied carefully within the area of the lesion.

Adverse Reactions: No allergic sensitivity or toxic reactions have been noted in the recorded clinical investigations. However, one case of systemic manifestations of hypersensitivity to collagenase in a patient treated for more than one year with a combination of collagenase and cortisone has been reported to us.

Dosage and Administration: Santyl Ointment should be applied once daily (or more frequently if the dressing becomes soiled, as from incontinence) in the following manner:

(1) Prior to application the lesion should be cleansed of debris and digested material by gently rubbing with a gauze pad saturated with hydrogen peroxide or Dakin's solution followed by sterile normal saline.
(2) Whenever infection is present it is desirable to use an appropriate topical antibacterial agent. Neomycin-Bacitracin-Polymyxin B (Neosporin) powder has been found to be compatible with Santyl Ointment. The antibiotic should be applied to the lesion prior to the application of Santyl Ointment. Should the infection not respond, therapy with Santyl Ointment should be discontinued until remission of the infection.
(3) Santyl Ointment should be applied directly to deep lesions with a wooden tongue depressor or spatula. For shallow lesions, Santyl Ointment may be applied to a sterile gauze pad which is then applied to the wound and properly secured.
(4) Crosshatching thick eschar with a #10 blade allows collagenase more surface contact with necrotic debris. It is also desirable to remove, with forceps and scissors, as much loosened detritus as can be done readily.
(5) All excess ointment should be removed each time dressing is changed.
(6) Use of Santyl Ointment should be terminated when debridement of necrotic tissue is complete and granulation tissue is well established.

Overdose: Action of the enzyme may be stopped, should this be desired, by the application of Burow's solution USP (pH 3.6-4.4) to the lesion.

How Supplied: Santyl Ointment contains 250 units of collagenase enzyme per gram of white petrolatum USP. The potency assay of collagenase is based on the digestion of undenatured collagen (from bovine Achilles tendon) at pH 7.2 and 37°C for 24 hours. The number of peptide bonds cleaved are measured by reaction with ninhydrin. Amino groups released by a trypsin digestion control are subtracted. One net collagenase unit will solubilize ninhydrin reactive material equivalent to 4 micromoles of leucine.

[*Shown in Product Identification Section*]

References:

1— Mandl, I., Adv. Enzymol. 23:163, 1961.
2— Boxer, A.M., Gottesman, N., Bernstein, H., & Mandl, I., Geriatrics 24:75, 1969.
3— Mazurek, I., Med. Welt 22:150, 1971.
4— Zimmerman, W.E., in "Collagenase," I. Mandl, ed., Gordon & Breach, Science Publishers, New York, 1971, p. 131, p. 185.
5— Vetra, H., & Whittaker, D., Geriatrics 30:53, 1975.
6— Rao, D.B., Sane, P.G., & Georgiev, E.L., J. Am. Geriatrics Soc. 23:22, 1975.
7— Vrabec, R., Moserova, J., Konickova, Z., Behounkova, E., & Blaha, J., J. Hyg. Epidemiol. Microbiol. Immunol. 18:496, 1974.
8— Lippmann, H.I., Arch. Phys. Med. Rehabil. 54:588, 1973.
9— German, F.M., in "Collagenase," I., Mandl, ed. Gordon & Breach, Science Publishers, New York, 1971, p. 165.
10— Haimovici, H. & Strauch, B., in "Collagenase," I. Mandl, ed., Gordon & Breach, Science Publishers, New York, 1971, p. 177.
11— Lee, L.K., & Ambrus, J.L., Geriatrics 30:91, 1975.
12— Locke, R.K., & Heifitz, N.M., J. Am. Pod. Assoc. 65:242, 1975.
13— Varma, A.O., Bugatch, E., & German, F.M., Surg. Gynecol. Obstet. 136:281, 1973.
14— Barrett, D., Jr., & Klibanski, A., Am. J. Nurs. 73:849, 1973.
15— Bardfeld, L.A., J. Pod. Ed. 1:41, 1970.
16— Blum, G., Schweiz. Rundschau Med. Praxis 62:820, 1973. Abstr. in Dermatology Digest, Feb. 1974, p. 36.
17— Zaruba, F., Lettl, A., Brozkova, L., Skrdlantova, H., & Krs, V., J. Hyg. Epidemiol. Microbiol. Immunol. 18:499, 1974.
18— Altman, M.I., Goldstein, L., Horowitz, S., J. Am. Pod. Assoc. 68:11, 1978.
19— Rehn, V.J., Med. Klin. 58:799, 1963.
20— Krauss, H., Koslowski, L., & Zimmermann, W.E., Langenbecks Arch. Klin. Chir. 303:23, 1963.
21— Gruenagel, H.H., Med. Klin. 58:442, 1963.

THEOPHYL® CHEWABLE TABLETS ℞
(anhydrous theophylline USP)

Description: Each scored white tablet contains not less than 94.0 percent and not more than 106.0 percent of 100 mg anhydrous theophylline USP. Theophylline ($C_7H_8N_4O_2$), a xanthine compound, is a white, odorless crystalline powder, having a bitter taste. The scoring of THEOPHYL® Chewable Tablets allows for titration in 25 mg (¼ tablet) increments.

Clinical Pharmacology: Theophylline directly relaxes the smooth muscle of the bronchial airways and pulmonary blood vessels, thus acting mainly as a bronchodilator, pulmonary vasodilator and smooth muscle relaxant. It also possesses other actions typical of the xanthine deriviatives: coronary vasodilator, diuretic, and cardiac, cerebral, and skeletal muscle stimulant. The actions of theophylline may be mediated through inhibition of phosphodiesterase and a resultant increase in intracellular cyclic AMP which could mediate smooth muscle relaxation.

In vitro, theophylline has been shown to react synergistically with beta agonists (such as isoproterenol) that increase intracellular cyclic AMP through the stimulation of adenyl cyclase, but synergism has not been demonstrated in clinical studies and more data are needed to determine if theophylline and beta agonists have clinically important additive effects **in vivo.**

Apparently, tolerance does not develop with chronic use of theophylline.

The half-life is shortened with cigarette smoking. The half-life is prolonged in alcoholism, reduced hepatic or renal function, congestive heart failure, and in patients receiving antibiotics such as troleandomycin (TAO, Cyclamycin), erythromycin, lincomycin and clindamycin. High fever for prolonged periods may decrease theophylline elimination.

Theophylline Elimination Characteristics

	Theophylline Clearance Rates (mean ± S.D.)	Half-Life Average (mean ± S.D.)
Children (over 6 months of age)	1.45 ± .58 ml/kg/min	3.7 ± 1.1 hours
Adult nonsmokers with uncomplicated asthma	.65 ± .19 ml/kg/min	8.7 ± 2.2 hours

Newborn infants have extremely slow clearances with half-lives exceeding 24 hours. These approach those seen for older children after about 3–6 months.

Older adults with chronic obstructive pulmonary disease, patients with cor pulmonale or other causes of heart failure, and patients with liver pathology may have much lower clearances with half-lives that may exceed 24 hours. The half-life is prolonged in alcoholism, reduced hepatic or renal function, congestive heart failure, and in patients receiving certain antibiotics such as troleandomycin (TAO, Cyclamycin), erythromycin, lincomycin and clin-

		LOADING DOSE	MAINTENANCE DOSE FOR NEXT 12 HOURS	MAINTENANCE DOSE BEYOND 12 HOURS
1.	Children 6 months to 9 years	6 mg/kg	4 mg/kg q4h	4 mg/kg q6h
2.	Children age 9–16 and young adult smokers	6 mg/kg	3 mg/kg q4h	3 mg/kg q6h
3.	Otherwise healthy non-smoking adults	6 mg/kg	3 mg/kg q6h	3 mg/kg q8h
4.	Older patients and patients with cor pulmonale	6 mg/kg	2 mg/kg q6h	2 mg/kg q8h
5.	Patients with congestive heart failure, liver failure	6 mg/kg	2 mg/kg q8h	1–2 mg/kg q12h

damycin. High fever for prolonged periods may decrease theophylline elimination.
The half-life of theophylline in smokers (1 to 2 packs/day) averaged 4 to 5 hours in various studies, much shorter than the 7 to 9 hour half-life in nonsmokers. The increase in theophylline clearance caused by smoking is probably the result of induction of drug-metabolizing enzymes that do not readily normalize after cessation of smoking. It appears that between 3 months and 2 years may be necessary for normalization of the effect of smoking on theophylline pharmacokinetics.
THEOPHYL® Chewable Tablets are a rapidly releasing form of theophylline. Bioavailability of these tablets has been shown to be 98% ± 5% when chewed and 101% ± 4% when swallowed whole.
Indications: For relief and/or prevention of symptoms of asthma and reversible bronchospasm associated with chronic bronchitis and emphysema.
Contraindications: Avoid using THEOPHYL® Chewable Tablets in individuals who have shown hyprsensitivity to any of its components.
Warnings: Excessive theophylline doses may be associated with toxicity determination of serum theophylline levels is recommended to assure maximal benefit without excessive risk. Incidence of toxicity increases at serum levels greater than 20 mcg/ml.
Morphine, curare, and stilbamidine should be used with caution in patients with airflow obstruction since they stimulate histamine release and can induce asthmatic attacks. They may also suppress respiration leading to respiratory failue. Alternative drugs should be chosen whenever possible.
There is an excellent correlation between clinical manifestations of toxicity and high blood levels of theophylline resulting from conventional doses in patients with lowered body plasma clearances (due to transient cardiac decompensation), in patients with liver dysfunction or chronic obstructive lung disease, and in patients who are older than 55 years of age, particularly males. In about 50% of patients, nausea and restlessness precede more severe manifestations of toxicity. In other patients, ventricular arrhythmias or seizures may be the first sign of toxicity. These more serious side effects are more likely to occur after intravenous administration of theophylline. Many patients who have high theophylline serum levels exhibit a tachycardia, and theophylline may worsen pre-existing arrhythmias.
Usage in Pregnancy: Safe use in pregnancy has not been established relative to possible adverse effects on fetal development, but neither have adverse effects on fetal development been established. This is, unfortunately, true for most antiasthmatic medications. Therefore, use of theophylline in pregnant women should be balanced against the risk of uncontrolled asthma.
Precautions: Mean half-life in smokers is shorter than in nonsmokers; therefore, smokers may require larger doses of theophylline. THEOPHYL® Chewable Tablets, like all theophylline products, should not be administered concurrently with other xanthine medications. Use with caution in patients with severe cardiac disease, severe hypoxemia, hypertension, hyperthyroidism, acute myocardial injury, cor pulmonale, congestive heart failure, liver disease, peptic ulcer and in the elderly (especially males) and in neonates. Great caution should be used especially in giving theophylline to patients in congestive heart failure; such patients have shown markedly prolonged theophylline blood level curves with theophylline persisting in serum for long periods following discontinuation of the drug.
Theophylline may occasionally act as a local irritant to the G.I. tract although gastrointestinal symptoms are more commonly central in origin and associated with serum concentrations over 20 mcg/ml.
Adverse Reactions: The most frequent adverse reactions to theophylline are usually due to overdose (serum levels in excess of 20 mcg/ml) and are:
1. Gastrointestinal: nausea, vomiting, epigastric pain, hematemesis, diarrhea.
2. Central nervous system: headaches, irritability, restlessness, insomnia, reflex hyperexcitability, muscle twitching, clonic and tonic generalized convulsions.
3. Cardiovascular: palpitations, tachycardia, extra systoles, flushing, hypotension, circulatory failure, ventricular arrhythmias.
4. Respiratory: tachypnea.
5. Renal: albuminuria, increased excretion of renal tubular cells and red blood cells, potentiation of diuresis.
6. Others: hyperglycemia and inappropriate ADH syndrome.
Drug Interactions: Toxic synergism with ephedrine has been documented and may occur with some other sympathomimetic bronchodilators.

Drug	Effect
Aminophylline with lithium carbonate	Increased excretion of lithium carbonate
Aminophylline with propranolol	Antagonism of propranolol effect
Theophylline with furosemide	Increased diuresis
Theophylline with hexamethonium	Decreased hexamethonium-induced chromatropic effect
Theophylline with reserpine	Reserpine-induced tachycardia
Theophylline with chlordiazepoxide	Chlordiazepoxide-induced fatty acid mobilization
Theophylline with troleandomycin (TAO, Cyclamycin), erythromycin, lincomycin, clindamycin	Increased theophylline plasma levels

Management of Overdose:
A. If potential overdose is established and seizure has not occurred:
1) Induce vomiting.
2) Administer a cathartic.
3) Administer activated charcoal.
B. If patient is having a seizure:
1) Establish an airway.
2) Administer O_2.
3) Treat the seizure with intravenous diazepam, 0.1 to 0.3 mg/kg up to 10 mg.
4) Monitor vital signs, maintain blood pressure and provide adequate hydration.
C. Post-seizure coma:
1) Maintain airway and oxygenation.
2) Follow above recommendations to prevent absorption of drug, but intubation and lavage will have to be performed instead of inducing emesis, and introduce the cathartic and charcoal via a large bore gastric lavage tube.
3) Continue to provide full supportive care and adequate hydration while waiting for drug to be metabolized. In general, the drug is metabolized sufficiently rapidly so as not to require dialysis.

Dosage and Administraion:
Therapeutic serum levels associated with optimal likelihood for benefit and minimal risk of toxicity are considered to be between 10 mcg/ml and 20 mcg/ml. Levels above 20 mcg/ml may produce toxic effects. There is great variation from patient to patient in dosage needed to achieve a therapeutic blood level because of variable rates of elimination. Therefore, dosage must be individualized and monitoring of theophylline serum levels is highly recommended. Serum theophylline measurement should be obtained at the time of peak absorption, which has been shown to be 2 ± 0.3 hours for THEOPHYL® Chewable Tablets when chewed and 2.2 ± .03 hours when swallowed whole. Samples for serum theophylline measurement should be taken after a patient has been on a given dose for at least 3 days and has missed no doses during the previous 48 hours. Unless the above instructions with regard to serum theophylline measurement are followed, the results may be misleading and dosage adjustments based on these results may be incorrect, possibly increasing the risk of toxicity.
As theophylline does not distribute into fatty tissue, dosage should be calculated on the basis of lean (ideal) body weight. Giving theophylline with food may prevent the rare case of stomach irritation; though absorption may be slower, it is still complete.
When rapidly absorbed products such as solutions and uncoated tablets with rapid dissolution are used, dosing to maintain "around the clock" blood levels generally requires administration every 6 hours in children; dosing intervals up to 8 hours may be satisfactory for adults because of their slower elimination rate. Once a patient is stabilized on a particular dose of theophylline, his blood levels tend to remain constant with that dose.
Pulmonary function measurements before and after a period of treatment permit an objective assessment of response to THEOPHYL® Chewable Tablets.
I. Dosage of THEOPHYL® Chewable Tablets for Patients Exhibiting Acute Symptoms of Asthma Requiring Rapid Theophyllinization and Not Currently Receiving Theophylline Products.
[See table above].
II. Dosage for Patients Currently Receiving Theophylline Products.
Determine, where possible the time, amount, route of administration and form of the patient's last dose. Ideally, the loading dose should be deferred if a serum theophylline determination can be rapidly obtained. If this is not possible, the clinician must exercise his judgment in selecting a dose based on the potential for benefit and risk. The loading dose of theophylline is based on the principle that each .5 mg/kg of theophylline administered as a loading dose will result in a 1 mcg/ml increase in serum theophylline concentration.

Continued on next page

Knoll—Cont.

When there is sufficient respiratory distress to warrant a small risk 2.5 mg/kg of theophylline is likely to increase the serum concentration by only about 5 mcg/ml when administered as a loading dose. If the patient is not already experiencing theophylline toxicity, this is unlikely to result in dangerous adverse effects. Subsequent maintenance dosage recommendations are the same as those described above.

III. Dosage for Chronic Asthma

Theophyllinization is a treatment of first choice for the management of chronic asthma (to prevent symptoms and maintain patent airways). Slow clinical titration is generally preferred to assure acceptance and safety of the medication.

Initial Dose: 16 mg/kg/day or 400 mg/day (whichever is lower) in 3–4 divided doses at 6–8 hour intervals.

Increased Dose: The above dosage may be increased in approximately 25 percent increments at 2–3 day intervals so long as no intolerance is observed, until a maximum indicated below is reached.

Maximum Dose Without Measurement of Serum Concentration:

Not to exceed the following: **(WARNING: DO NOT ATTEMPT TO MAINTAIN ANY DOSE THAT IS NOT TOLERATED)**

Age Less than 9 years	—24 mg/kg/day
Age 9–12 years	—20 mg/kg/day
Age 12–16 years	—18 mg/kg/day
Age Greater than 16 years	—13 mg/kg/day or 900 mg/day (WHICHEVER IS LESS)

NOTE: Use ideal body weight for obese patients.

How Supplied:

Tablets—white, round, double-bisected one side, inscribed with K logo on other side. Each tablet contains 100 mg of anhydrous theophylline USP.

Bottles of 100—NDC #0044-6521-02.

[Shown in Product Identification Section]

THEOPHYL®-SR CAPSULES ℞
(anhydrous theophylline USP)

Description: Each capsule contains not less than 94.0 percent and not more than 106.0 percent of 125 mg (yellow and clear capsules) or 250 mg (green and clear capsules) anhydrous theophylline USP in a coated bead timed-release formulation. Theophylline ($C_7H_8N_4O_2$), a xanthine compound, is a white, odorless crystalline powder, having a bitter taste.

Clinical Pharmacology: Theophylline directly relaxes the smooth muscle of the bronchial airways and pulmonary blood vessels, thus acting mainly as a bronchodilator, pulmonary vasodilator and smooth muscle relaxant. It also possesses other actions typical of the xanthine derivatives: coronary vasodilator, diuretic, and cardiac, cerebral, and skeletal muscle stimulant. The actions of theophylline may be mediated through inhibition of phosphodiesterase and a resultant increase in intracellular cyclic AMP which could mediate smooth muscle relaxation.

In vitro, theophylline has been shown to react synergistically with beta agonists (such as isoproterenol) that increase intracellular cyclic AMP through the stimulation of adenyl cyclase, but synergism has not been demonstrated in clinical studies and more data are needed to determine if theophylline and beta agonists have clinically important additive effects *in vivo*.

Apparently, tolerance does not develop with chronic use of theophylline.

The half-life is shortened with cigarette smoking. The half-life is prolonged in alcoholism, reduced hepatic or renal function, congestive heart failure, and in patients receiving antibiotics such as troleandomycin (TAO, Cyclamycin), erythromycin, lincomycin and clindamycin. High fever for prolonged periods may decrease theophylline elimination.

Theophylline Elimination Characteristics

	Theophylline Clearance Rates (mean ± S.D.)	Half-Life Average (mean ± S.D.)
Children (over 6 months of age)	1.45 ± .58 ml/kg/min	3.7 ± 1.1 hours
Adult nonsmokers with uncomplicated asthma	.65 ± .19 ml/kg/min	8.7 ± 2.2 hours

Newborn infants have extremely slow clearances with half-lives exceeding 24 hours. These approach those seen for older children after about 3–6 months.

Older adults with chronic obstructive pulmonary disease, patients with cor pulmonale or other causes of heart failure, and patients with liver pathology may have much lower clearances with half-lives that may exceed 24 hours. The half-life is prolonged in alcoholism, reduced hepatic or renal function, congestive heart failure, and in patients receiving certain antibiotics such as TAO (Cyclamycin), erythromycin, lincomycin and clindamycin. High fever for prolonged periods may decrease theophylline elimination.

The half-life of theophylline in smokers (1 to 2 packs/day) averaged 4 to 5 hours in various studies, much shorter than the 7 to 9 hour half-life in nonsmokers. The increase in theophylline clearance caused by smoking is probably the result of induction of drug-metabolizing enzymes that do not readily normalize after cessation of smoking. It appears that between 3 months and 2 years may be necessary for normalization of the effect of smoking on theophylline pharmacokinetics.

Bioavailability of THEOPHYL®-SR Capsules is 99% ± 6%.

Indications: For relief and/or prevention of symptoms of asthma and reversible bronchospasm associated with chronic bronchitis and emphysema, especially in patients requiring chronic therapy.

Contraindications: Avoid using THEOPHYL®-SR Capsules in individuals who have shown hyprsensitivity to any of its components.

Warnings: Excessive theophylline doses may be associated with toxicity; determination of serum theophylline levels is recommended to assure maximal benefit without excessive risk. Incidence of toxicity increases at serum levels greater than 20 mcg/ml.

Morphine, curare, and stilbamidine should be used with caution in patients with airflow obstruction since they stimulate histamine release and can induce asthmatic attacks. They may also suppress respiration leading to respiratory failure. Alternative drugs should be chosen whenever possible.

There is an excellent correlation between clinical manifestations of toxicity and high blood levels of theophylline resulting from conventional doses in patients with lowered body plasma clearances (due to transient cardiac decompensation), patients with liver dysfunction or chronic obstructive lung disease, and patients who are older than 55 years of age, particularly males. In about 50% of patients, nausea and restlessness precede more severe manifestations of toxicity. In other patients, ventricular arrhythmias or seizures may be the first signs of toxicity. These more serious side effects are more likely to occur after intravenous administration of theophylline. Many patients who have high theophylline serum levels exhibit a tachycardia, and theophylline may worsen pre-existing arrhythmias.

Usage in Pregnancy: Safe use in pregnancy has not been established relative to possible adverse effects on fetal development, but neither have adverse effects on fetal development been established. This is, unfortunately, true for most antiasthmatic medications. Therefore, use of theophylline in pregnant women should be balanced against the risk of uncontrolled asthma.

Precautions: Mean half-life in smokers is shorter than in nonsmokers; therefore, smokers may require larger doses of theophylline. THEOPHYL®-SR Capsules, like all theophylline products, should not be administered concurrently with other xanthine medications. Use with caution in patients with severe cardiac disease, severe hypoxemia, hypertension, hyperthyroidism, acute myocardial injury, cor pulmonale, congestive heart failure, liver disease, peptic ulcer and in the elderly (especially males) and in neonates. Great caution should be used especially in giving theophylline to patients in congestive heart failure; such patients have shown markedly prolonged theophylline blood level curves with theophylline persisting in serum for long periods following discontinuation of the drug.

Theophylline may occasionally act as a local irritant to the G.I. tract although gastrointestinal symptoms are more commonly central and associated with serum concentrations over 20 mcg/ml.

Adverse Reactions: The most frequent adverse reactions to theophylline are usually due to overdose (serum levels in excess of 20 mcg/ml) and are:

1. Gastrointestinal: nausea, vomiting, epigastric pain, hematemesis, diarrhea.
2. Central nervous system: headaches, irritability, restlessness, insomnia, reflex hyperexcitability, muscle twitching, clonic and tonic generalized convulsions.
3. Cardiovascular: palpitations, tachycardia, extra systoles, flushing, hypotension, circulatory failure, ventricular arrhythmias.
4. Respiratory: tachypnea.
5. Renal: albuminuria, increased excretion of renal tubular cells and red blood cells, potentiation of diuresis.
6. Others: hyperglycemia and inappropriate ADH syndrome.

Drug Interactions: Toxic synergism with high doses of ephedrine has been documented and may occur with some other sympathomimetic bronchodilators.

Drug	Effect
Aminophylline with lithium carbonate	Increased excretion of lithium carbonate
Aminophylline with propranolol	Antagonism of propranolol effect
Theophylline with furosemide	Increased diuresis
Theophylline with hexamethonium	Decreased hexamethonium—induced chromatropic effect
Theophylline with reserpine	Reserpine-induced tachycardia
Theophylline with chlordiazepoxide	Chlordiazepoxide-induced fatty acid mobilization
Theophylline with troleandomycin (TAO, Cyclamycin), erythromycin, lincomycin, clindamycin	Increased theophylline plasma levels

Management Of Overdose:

A. If potential overdose is established and seizure has not occurred:
   1) Induce vomiting.
   2) Administer a cathartic.
   3) Administer activated charcoal.

B. If patient is having a seizure:
   1) Establish an airway.
   2) Administer O_2.
   3) Treat the seizure with intravenous diazepam, 0.1 to 0.3 mg/kg up to 10 mg.
   4) Monitor vital signs, maintain blood pressure and provide adequate hydration.

C. Post-seizure coma:
1) Maintain airway and oxygenation.
2) Follow above recommendations to prevent absorption of drug, but intubation and lavage will have to be performed instead of inducing emesis, and introduce the cathartic and charcoal via a large bore gastric lavage tube.
3) Continue to provide full supportive care and adequate hydration while waiting for drug to be metabolized. In general, the drug is metabolized sufficiently rapidly so as not to require dialysis.

Dosage and Administration: Therapeutic serum levels associated with optimal likelihood for benefit and minimal risk of toxicity are considered to be between 10 mcg/ml and 20 mcg/ml. Levels above 20 mcg/ml may produce toxic effects. There is great variation from patient to patient in dosage needed to achieve a therapeutic blood level because of variable rates of elimination. Therefore, dosage must be individualized and monitoring of theophylline serum levels is highly recommended. Serum theophylline measurement should be obtained at the time of peak absorption. Average time to peak theophylline plasma concentrations in 14 patient volunteers after taking a dose of THEOPHYL®-SR Capsules was 5.3 ± 0.5 hours (mean ± standard error). Samples for serum theophylline measurement should be taken after a patient has been on a given dose for at least 3 days and has missed no doses during the previous 48 hours. *Unless the above instructions with regard to serum theophylline measurement are followed, the results may be misleading and dosage adjustments based on these results may be incorrect, possibly increasing the risk of toxicity.*

As theophylline does not distribute into fatty tissue, dosage should be calculated on the basis of lean (ideal) body weight. Giving theophylline with food may prevent the rare case of stomach irritation; though absorption may be slower, it is still complete.

When rapidly absorbed products such as solutions and uncoated tablets with rapid dissolution are used, dosing to maintain "around the clock" blood levels generally requires administration every 6 hours in children; dosing intervals up to 8 hours may be satisfactory for adults because of their slower elimination.

Children, and adults requiring higher than average doses, may benefit from products with slower absorption, such as THEOPHYL®-SR Capsules, which may allow longer dosing intervals and/or less fluctuation in serum concentration over a dosing interval during chronic therapy.

Once a patient is stabilized on a particular dose of theophylline, his blood levels tend to remain constant with that dose.

Pulmonary function measurements before and after a period of treatment permit an objective assessment of response to THEOPHYL®-SR Capsules.

I. Dosage of THEOPHYL®-SR for Patients With Chronic Asthma Not Currently Receiving Theophylline Therapy
Patients not currently receiving theophylline therapy should be started on conventional rapidly absorbed theophylline products, such as THEOPHYL®-225 Tablets. Once the patient is stabilized on a particular dose of theophylline, therapy with THEOPHYL®-SR Capsules should be initiated at the same total daily dose, with half the total daily dose administered every 12 hours. If satisfactory control of symptoms is not maintained for the full 12 hour period, or if unacceptable adverse effects occur, one third of the total daily dosage should be administered on an every 8 hour schedule.
If theophylline therapy is initiated with THEOPHYL®-SR Capsules, the recommended starting dose is 250 mg twice daily. If this dosage is not effective after three days, the dosage may be increased to 375 mg every 12 hours or 250 mg every 8 hours.

II. Dosage of THEOPHYL®-SR for Patients with Chronic Asthma Currently Receiving Theophylline Therapy.
Therapy with THEOPHYL®-SR should be initiated at the patient's current total daily dosage, with half the total daily dose administered every 12 hours. If satisfactory control of symptoms is not maintained for the full 12 hours, or if unacceptable adverse effects occur, one third of the total daily dosage should be administered every 8 hours. If this dosage is not effective after three days, the dosage may be increased to 375 mg every 12 hours or 250 mg every 8 hours.

Maximum Dose Without Measurement of Serum Concentration: Not to exceed the following: (WARNING: DO NOT ATTEMPT TO MAINTAIN ANY DOSE THAT IS NOT TOLERATED)
Age Less than 9 years—24 mg/kg/day
Age 9–12 years—20 mg/kg/day
Age 12–16 years—18 mg/kg/day
Age Greater than 16 years—13 mg/kg/day or 900 mg/day (WHICHEVER IS LESS)

Note: Use ideal body weight for obese patients.

How Supplied: THEOPHYL®-SR Capsules are identified with K logo and mg strength.
125 mg—yellow and clear capsules—bottles of 100—NDC #0044-6531-02. Also available in Unit-of-Use package—bottles of 100—NDC #0044-6531-12.
250 mg—green and clear capsules—bottles of 100—NDC #0044-6532-02. Also available in Unit-of-Use package—bottles of 100—NDC #0044-6532-12.
[*Shown in Product Identification Section*]
Distributed by KNOLL PHARMACEUTICAL COMPANY
Whippany, New Jersey 07981
Manufactured by Cord Laboratories, Inc.
Broomfield, Colorado 80020

THEOPHYL®-225 TABLETS AND ELIXIR ℞
(anhydrous theophylline USP)

Description: Each scored white tablet and each 30 ml (2 TABLESPOONfuls) of the banana-mint flavored Elixir contains not less than 94.0 percent and not more than 106.0 percent of 225 mg anhydrous theophylline USP. Each 30 ml of the Elixir contains 225 mg calcium salicylate as a solubilizing agent, with 5% alcohol. Theophylline ($C_7H_8N_4O_2$), a xanthine compound, is a white, odorless crystalline powder, having a bitter taste.

Clinical Pharmacology: Theophylline directly relaxes the smooth muscle of the bronchial airways and pulmonary blood vessels, thus acting mainly as a bronchodilator, pulmonary vasodilator and smooth muscle relaxant. It also possesses other actions typical of the xanthine derivatives: coronary vasodilator, diuretic, and cardiac, cerebral, and skeletal muscle stimulant. The actions of theophylline may be mediated through inhibition of phosphodiesterase and a resultant increase in intracellular cyclic AMP which could mediate smooth muscle relaxation.

In vitro, theophylline has been shown to react synergistically with beta agonists (such as isoproterenol) that increase intracellular cyclic AMP through the stimulation of adenyl cyclase, but synergism has not been demonstrated in clinical studies and more data are needed to determine if theophylline and beta agonists have clinically important additive effects *in vivo*.

Apparently, tolerance does not develop with chronic use of theophylline.

The half-life is shortened with cigarette smoking. The half-life is prolonged in alcoholism, reduced hepatic or renal function, congestive heart failure, and in patients receiving antibiotics such as troleandomycin (TAO, Cyclamycin), erythromycin, lincomycin and clindamycin. High fever for prolonged periods may decrease theophylline elimination.

Theophylline Elimination Characteristics

	Theophylline Clearance Rates (mean ± S.D.)	Half-Life Average (Mean ± S.D.)
Children (over 6 months of age)	1.45 ± .58 ml/kg/min	3.7 ± 1.1 hours
Adult nonsmokers with uncomplicated asthma	.65 ± .19 ml/kg/min	8.7 ± 2.2 hours

Newborn infants have extremely slow clearances with half-lives excedding 24 hours. These approach those seen for older children after about 3–6 months.

Older adults with chronic obstructive pulmonary disease, patients with cor pulmonale or other causes of heart failure, and patients with liver pathology may have much lower clearances with half-lives that may exceed 24 hours. The half-life is prolonged in alcoholism, reduced hepatic or renal function, congestive heart failure, and in patients receiving certain antibiotics such as troleandomycin (TAO, Cyclamycin), erythromycin, lincomycin and clindamycin. High fever for prolonged periods may decrease theophylline elimination.

The half-life of theophylline in smokers (1 to 2 packs/day) averaged 4 to 5 hours in various studies, much shorter than the 7 to 9 hour half-life in nonsmokers. The increase in theophylline clearance caused by smoking is probably the result of induction of drug-metabolizing enzymes that do not readily normalize after cessation of smoking. It appears that between 3 months and 2 years may be necessary for normalization of the effect of smoking on theophylline pharmacokinetics.

THEOPHYL®-225 TABLETS are a rapidly releasing form of theophylline. Bioavailability of these tablets has been shown to be 96% ± 3%.

THEOPHYL®-225 ELIXIR is a rapidly releasing form of theophylline. Bioavailability has been shown to be 99% ± 2%, with 85% ± 5% of the drug absorbed within one hour.

Indications: For relief and/or prevention of symptoms of asthma and reversible bronchospasm associated with chronic bronchitis and emphysema.

Contraindications: Avoid using THEOPHYL®-225 TABLETS and ELIXIR in individuals who have shown hypersensitivity to any of their components.

Warnings: Excessive theophylline doses may be associated with toxicity; determination of serum theophylline levels is recommended to assure maximal benefit without excessive risk. Incidence of toxicity increases at serum levels greater than 20 mcg/ml.

Morphine, curare, and stilbamidine should be used with caution in patients with airflow obstruction since they stimulate histamine release and can induce asthmatic attacks. They may also suppress respiration leading to respiratory failure. Alternative drugs should be chosen whenever possible.

There is an excellent correlation between clinical manifestations of toxicity and high blood levels of theophylline resulting from conventional doses in patients with lowered body plasma clearances (due to transient cardiac decompensation), patients with liver dysfunction or chronic obstructive lung disease, and patients who are older than 55 years of age, particularly males. In about 50% of patients, nausea and restlessness precede more severe manifestations of toxicity. In other patients, ventricular arrhythmias or seizures may be the first signs of toxicity. These more serious side effects are more likely to occur after intravenous administration of theophylline. Many patients who have high theophylline serum levels exhibit a tachycardia, and theophylline may worsen pre-existing arrhythmias.

Continued on next page

Knoll—Cont.

THEOPHYL®-225 ELIXIR contains 37.5 mg of calcium salicylate per 5 cc as a solubilizing agent. Therefore, concomitant use of aspirin should either be avoided (by use of acetaminophin for analgesia and antipyresis) or should be confined to a dose that provides a total (aspirin and calcium salicylate) of no more than 15 mg/kg at intervals of 6 hours or longer.
Intolerance to aspirin is not intolerance to salicylates generally; aspirin-sensitive patients are no more likely to react to other salicylates such as calcium salicylate than to unrelated materials.

Usage in Pregnancy: Safe use in pregnancy has not been established relative to possible adverse effects on fetal development, but neither have adverse effects on fetal development been established. This is, unfortunately, true for most antiasthmatic medications. Therefore, use of theophylline in pregnant women should be balanced against the risk of uncontrolled asthma.

Precautions: Mean half-life in smokers is shorter than in nonsmokers; therefore, smokers may require larger doses of theophylline. THEOPHYL®-225 TABLETS and ELIXIR, like all theophylline products, should not be administered concurrently with other xanthine medications. Use with caution in patients with severe cardiac disease, severe hypoxemia, hypertension, hyperthyroidism, acute myocardial injury, cor pulmonale, congestive heart failure, liver disease, peptic ulcer and in the elderly (especially males) and in neonates. Great caution should be used especially in giving theophylline to patients in congestive heart failure; such patients have shown markedly prolonged theophylline blood level curves with theophylline persisting in serum for long periods following discontinuation of the drug.
Theophylline may occasionally act as a local irritant to the G.I. tract although gastrointestinal symptoms are more commonly central in origin and associated with serum concentrations over 20 mcg/ml.

Adverse Reactions: The most frequent adverse reactions to theophylline are usually due to overdose (serum levels in excess of 20 mcg/ml) and are:

1. Gastrointestinal: nausea, vomiting, epigastric pain, hematemesis, diarrhea.
2. Central nervous system: headaches, irritability, restlessness, insomnia, reflex hyperexcitability, muscle twitching, clonic and tonic generalized convulsions.
3. Cardiovascular: palpitations, tachycardia, extra systoles, flushing, hypotension, circulatory failure, ventricular arrhythmias.
4. Respiratory: tachypnea.
5. Renal: albuminuria, increased excretion of renal tubular cells and red blood cells, potentiation of diuresis.
6. Others: hyperglycemia and inappropriate ADH syndrome.

Drug Interactions: Toxic synergism with ephedrine has been documented and may occur with some other sympathomimetic bronchodilators.

Drug	Effect
Aminophylline with lithium carbonate	Increased excretion of lithium carbonate
Aminophylline with propranolol	Antagonism of propranolol effect
Theophylline with furosemide	Increased diuresis
Theophylline with hexamethonium	Decreased hexamethonium-induced chromatropic effect
Theophylline with reserpine	Reserpine-induced tachycardia
Theophylline with chlordiazepoxide	Chlordiazepoxide-induced fatty acid mobilization
Theophylline with troleandomycin (TAO, Cyclamycin), erythromycin, lincomycin, clindamycin	Increased theophylline plasma levels

Management Of Overdose:

A. If potential overdose is established and seizure has not occurred:
   1) Induce vomiting.
   2) Administer a cathartic.
   3) Administer activated charcoal.

B. If patient is having a seizure:
   1) Establish an airway.
   2) Administer O_2.
   3) Treat the seizure with intravenous diazepam, 0.1 to 0.3 mg/kg up to 10 mg.
   4) Monitor vital signs, maintain blood pressure and provide adequate hydration.

C. Post-seizure coma:
   1) Maintain airway and oxygenation.
   2) Follow above recommendations to prevent absorption of drug, but intubation and lavage will have to be performed instead of inducing emesis, and introduce the cathartic and charcoal via a large bore gastric lavage tube.
   3) Continue to provide full supportive care and adequate hydration while waiting for drug to be metabolized. In general, the drug is metabolized sufficiently rapidly so as not to require dialysis.

Dosage and Administration: Therapeutic serum levels associated with optimal likelihood for benefit and minimal risk of toxicity are considered to be between 10 mcg/ml and 20 mcg/ml. Levels above 20 mcg/ml may produce toxic effects. There is great variation from patient to patient in dosage needed to achieve a therapeutic blood level because of variable rates of elimination. Therefore, dosage must be individualized and monitoring of theophylline serum levels is highly recommended. Serum theophylline measurement should be obtained at the time of peak absorption, which has been shown to be 2 $\pm$ 0.3 hours for THEOPHYL®-225 TABLETS and 1.4 $\pm$ 0.3 hours for THEOPHYL®-225 ELIXIR. Samples for serum theophylline measurement should be taken after a patient has been on a given dose for at least 3 days and has missed no doses during the previous 48 hours. *Unless the above instructions with regard to serum theophylline measurement are followed, the results may be misleading and dosage adjustments based on these results may be incorrect, possibly increasing the risk of toxicity.*

As theophylline does not distribute into fatty tissue, dosage should be calculated on the basis of lean (ideal) body weight. Giving theophylline with food may prevent the rare case of stomach irritation; though absorption may be slower, it is still complete.

When rapidly absorbed products such as solutions and uncoated tablets with rapid dissolution are used, dosing to maintain "around the clock" blood levels generally requires administration every 6 hours in children; dosing intervals up to 8 hours may be satisfactory for adults because of their slower elimination rate. Once a patient is stabilized on a particular dose of theophylline, his blood levels tend to remain constant with that dose.

Pulmonary function measurements before and after a period of treatment permit an objective assessment of response to THEOPHYL®-225 TABLETS and ELIXIR.

I. Dosage of THEOPHYL®-225 TABLETS and ELIXIR for Patients Exhibiting Acute Symptoms of Asthma Requiring Rapid Theophyllinization and Not Currently Receiving Theophylline Products

[See table below].

	LOADING DOSE	MAINTENANCE DOSE FOR NEXT 12 HOURS	MAINTENANCE DOSE BEYOND 12 HOURS
1. Children 6 months to 9 years	6 mg/kg	4 mg/kg q4h	4 mg/kg q6h
2. Children age 9–16 and young adult smokers	6 mg/kg	3 mg/kg q4h	3 mg/kg q6h
3. Otherwise healthy nonsmoking adults	6 mg/kg	3 mg/kg q6h	3 mg/kg q8h
4. Older patients and patients with cor pulmonale	6 mg/kg	2 mg/kg q6h	2 mg/kg q8h
5. Patients with congestive heart failure, liver failure	6 mg/kg	2 mg/kg q8h	1–2 mg/kg q12h

II. Dosage for Patients Currently Receiving Theophylline Products

Determine, where possible, the time, amount, route of administration and form of the patient's last dose. Ideally, the loading dose should be deferred if a serum theophylline determination can be rapidly obtained. If this is not possible, the clinician must exercise his judgment in selecting a dose based on the potential for benefit and risk. The loading dose of theophylline is based on the principle that each .5 mg/kg of theophylline administered as a loading dose will result in a 1 mcg/ml increase in serum theophylline concentration. When there is sufficient respiratory distress to warrant a small risk, 2.5 mg/kg of theophylline is likely to increase the serum concentration by only about 5 mcg/ml when administered as a loading dose. If the patient is not already experiencing theophylline toxicity, this is unlikely to result in dangerous adverse effects. Subsequent maintenance dosage recommendations are the same as those described above.

III. Dosage for Chronic Asthma

Theophyllinization is a treatment of first choice for the management of chronic asthma (to prevent symptoms and maintain patent airways). Slow clinical titration is generally preferred to assure acceptance and safety of the medication.

Initial Dose: 16 mg/kg/day or 450 mg/day (whichever is lower) in 3–4 divided doses at 6–8 hour intervals.

Increased Dose: The above dosage may be increased in approximately 25 percent increments at 2–3 day intervals so long as no intolerance is observed, until a maximum indicated below is reached.

Maximum Dose Without Measurement of Serum Concentration: Not to exceed the following: (WARNING: DO NOT ATTEMPT TO MAINTAIN ANY DOSE THAT IS NOT TOLERATED)

Age Less than 9 years—24 mg/kg/day
Age 9–12 years—20 mg/kg/day
Age 12–16 years—18 mg/kg/day
Age Greater than 16 years—13 mg/kg/day or 900 mg/day (WHICHEVER IS LESS)

Note: Use ideal body weight for obese patients.

How Supplied:
Tablets—white, triangle shaped, bisected one side, inscribed with K logo on other side. Each tablet contains 225 mg of theophylline anhydrous USP.
Bottles of 100—NDC#0044-6502-92.
Each 30 ml (2 TABLESPOONfuls) of the banana-mint flavored, orange-yellow elixir contains 225 mg of anhydrous theophylline, USP.
Available in pint bottles (473 ml)—NDC#0044-6581-01.
[*Shown in Product Identification Section*]

VEREQUAD® Tablets and Suspension

Description: Each tablet contains phenobarbital 8 mg. [Warning: May be habit forming]; theophylline calcium salicylate 130 mg. (provides 65 mg. anhydrous theophylline); ephedrine hydrochloride 24 mg.; Guaifenesin 100 mg. Each 5 ml. (1 teaspoonful) of the root beer flavored Suspension is equivalent to ½ tablet.
Actions: The comprehensive antispasmodic and expectorant action of VEREQUAD helps dilate the bronchioles and helps clear the bronchial tree so that dyspnea is relieved or prevented and wheezing and coughing are brought under control. Phenobarbital serves as a mild sedative to help counteract central nervous system stimulation caused by ephedrine.
Indications: For chronic respiratory disease in which tenacious mucus and bronchospasm are dominant symptoms, such as chronic bronchitis, bronchial asthma and pulmonary emphysema.
Contraindications: Avoid using VEREQUAD in combination with other theophylline preparations since this will elevate theophylline blood levels and may produce adverse effects.
Warning: Phenobarbital may be habit forming.
Precautions: Caution is indicated in the presence of cardiovascular disease, hyperthyroidism, and diabetes. Salicylates block the uricosuric action of probenecid and sulfinpyrazone; therefore, VEREQUAD should be used with caution in patients with gout. Particular caution in dose administration must be exercised in patients with peptic ulcers, as this condition may be exacerbated. Theophylline increases the excretion of lithium. Theophylline clearance has been reported to be larger and more variable in smokers than in non-smokers.
There has been a report indicating that troleandomycin (TAO) reduced theophylline clearance by one-half, resulting in a doubling of blood theophylline levels. The effect of concomitant administration of other macrolide antibiotics (such as erythromycin) is not known, but may be similar.
Usage in Pregnancy: Safe use in pregnancy has not been established relative to possible adverse effects on fetal development. Therefore, theophylline should not be used in pregnant women unless in the judgment of the physician, the potential benefits outweigh the possible hazards.
Adverse Reactions: VEREQUAD is well tolerated. Gastrointestinal irritation is rarely encountered; if it occurs, administration of VEREQUAD with or after meals is recommended.
Dosage and Administration: Adults and children over 12 years—1 tablet or 2 teaspoonfuls of Suspension three or four times daily; if needed, an additional 1 tablet or 2 teaspoonfuls upon retiring for nighttime relief. Children 6 to 12 years—½ tablet or 1 teaspoonful of Suspension three times a day. Children under 6 years—dose is proportionately less.
How Supplied: Suspension (reddish orange, root beer flavored)—bottles of 1 pint (473 ml.). Tablets (salmon-colored, uncoated)—bottles of 100.

VICODIN® Ⓒ ℞

Description: Each tablet of VICODIN contains:
Hydrocodone Bitartrate 5 mg
Warning: May be habit forming
Acetaminophen (APAP) 500 mg
Acetaminophen occurs as a white, odorless crystalline powder, possessing a slightly bitter taste.
The hydrocodone component is dihydrocodeinone, a white, odorless crystalline powder which is derived from the opium alkaloid, thebaine.
Actions: The principal analgesic ingredient, hydrocodone, is a semisynthetic narcotic with multiple actions qualitatively similar to those of morphine; most of these involve the central nervous system and organs composed of smooth muscle. The principal action of therapeutic value of the hydrocodone in this drug is analgesia.
Hydrocodone is similar to codeine and methadone in that it retains at least one half of its analgesic activity when administered orally. This drug also contains the non-narcotic antipyretic-analgesic acetaminophen.
Indications: For the relief of moderate to moderately severe pain.
Contraindications: Hypersensitivity to hydrocodone or acetaminophen.
Warnings:
Drug Dependence: Hydrocodone can produce drug dependence of the morphine type and, therefore, has the potential for being abused. Psychic dependence, physical dependence and tolerance may develop upon repeated administration of this drug and it should be prescribed and administered with the same degree of caution appropriate to the use of other oral narcotic-containing medications. Like other narcotic-containing medications, VICODIN (hydrocodone bitartrate with acetaminophen) is subject to the Federal Controlled Substances Act.
Usage in Ambulatory Patients: Hydrocodone may impair the mental and/or physical abilities required for the performance of potentially hazardous tasks such as driving a car or operating machinery. The patient using this drug should be cautioned accordingly.
Interaction with other central nervous system depressants:
Patients receiving other narcotic analgesics, general anesthetics, phenothiazines, other tranquilizers, sedative-hypnotics or other CNS depressants (including alcohol) concomitantly with hydrocodone and acetaminophen may exhibit an additive CNS depression. When such combined therapy is contemplated, the dose of one or both agents should be reduced.
Usage in Pregnancy: Safe use in pregnancy has not been established relative to possible adverse effects on fetal development. Therefore, VICODIN should not be used in pregnant women unless, in the judgment of the physician, the potential benefits outweigh the possible hazards.
Usage in Children: VICODIN should not be administered to children under 12, because adequate dosing information is not available.
Precautions:
Head injury and increased intracranial pressure: The respiratory depressant effects of narcotics and their capacity to elevate cerebrospinal fluid pressure may be markedly exaggerated in the presence of head injury, other intracranial lesions or a pre-existing increase in intracranial pressure. Furthermore, narcotics produce adverse reactions which may obscure the clinical course of patients with head injuries.
Acute abdominal conditions: The administration of VICODIN or other narcotics may obscure the diagnosis or clinical course in patients with acute abdominal conditions.
Special risk patients: VICODIN should be given with caution to certain patients such as the elderly or debilitated, and those with severe impairment of hepatic or renal function, hypothyroidism, Addison's disease and prostatic hypertrophy or urethral stricture.
Adverse Reactions: The most frequently observed adverse reactions include light-headedness, dizziness, sedation, nausea and vomiting. These effects seem to be more prominent in ambulatory than in nonambulatory patients, and some of these adverse reactions may be alleviated if the patient lies down.
Other adverse reactions include euphoria, dysphoria, constipation, skin rash and pruritus.
Dosage and Administration: The usual adult dose is one tablet every six hours as needed for pain. In cases of more severe pain, two tablets every 6 hours or one tablet more frequently than every 6 hours may be required. VICODIN is given orally.
Drug Interactions: The CNS depressant effects of this drug may be additive with that of other CNS depressants. See **WARNINGS.**
Management of Overdosage:
Signs and Symptoms: Serious overdose with VICODIN (hydrocodone bitartrate with acetaminophen) is characterized by respiratory depression (a decrease in respiratory rate and/or tidal volume, Cheyne-Stokes respiration, cyanosis), extreme somnolence progressing to stupor or coma, skeletal muscle flaccidity, cold and clammy skin, and sometimes bradycardia and hypotension. In severe overdosage, apnea, circulatory collapse, cardiac arrest and death may occur. The ingestion of very large amounts of this drug may, in addition, result in acute hepatic toxicity.
Treatment: Primary attention should be given to the reestablishment of adequate respiratory exchange through provision of a patent airway and the institution of assisted or controlled ventilation. The narcotic antagonists naloxone, nalorphine or levallorphan are specific antidotes against respiratory depression which may result from overdosage or unusual sensitivity to narcotics, including hydrocodone. Therefore, an appropriate dose of one of these antagonists should be administered, preferably by the intravenous route, simultaneously with efforts at respiratory resuscitation. Since the duration of action of hydrocodone may exceed that of the antagonist, the patient should be kept under continued surveillance and repeated doses of the antagonist should be administered as needed to maintain adequate respiration.
An antagonist should not be administered in the absence of clinically significant respiratory or cardiovascular depression.
Oxygen, intravenous fluids, vasopressors and other supportive measures should be employed as indicated.
Gastric emptying may be useful in removing unabsorbed drug. Acetaminophen in massive overdosage may cause hepatotoxicity in some patients. Clinical and laboratory evidence of hepatotoxicity may be delayed for up to one week. Close clinical monitoring and serial hepatic enzyme determinations are therefore recommended.
Treatment of acute acetaminophen overdosage is purely symptomatic.
How Supplied: VICODIN tablets are white, bisected, flat capsule-shaped tablets with a double K logo.
NDC #0044-0727-02—Bottles of 100
NDC #0044-0727-41—Hospital Unit-Dose dispenser 100's (4 × 25 reverse numbered)
[*Shown in Product Identification Section*]

VITA-METRAZOL® Elixir and Tablets ℞

Description: Each 5 ml. of the Elixir contains 100 mg. METRAZOL (pentylenetetrazol), 10 mg. niacinamide, 1 mg. each of thiamine HCl and pyridoxine HCl, 1.4 mg. of riboflavin-5'-phosphate sodium, in a 15% alcoholic solution.

Continued on next page

Knoll—Cont.

Each tablet contains 100 mg. METRAZOL (pentylenetetrazol), 10 mg. niacinamide, 1 mg. each of thiamine mononitrate, pyridoxine HCl and riboflavin, and 25 mg. ascorbic acid.
Actions: METRAZOL is a central nervous system stimulant. VITA-METRAZOL supplies the amounts of the vitamins listed above.
Indications: VITA-METRAZOL is administered to enhance mental and physical activity of elderly patients.
Contraindications: There are no known contraindications to VITA-METRAZOL.
Warnings: At recommended dosage, side effects occur infrequently or not at all.
Precautions: Caution should be exercised when treating patients with a low convulsive threshold or with a focal brain lesion.
Dosage and Administration: Average dose—1 or 2 tablets or 1 or 2 teaspoonfuls of the Elixir three times a day.
How Supplied: Elixir—bottles of 1 pint (473 ml.). Tablets—bottles of 100.

Kremers-Urban Company
BOX 2038
MILWAUKEE, WI 53201

CALCIFEROL™ ℞
(Ergocalciferol, Vitamin D_2)
50,000 USP Unit Tablets

Description: Each tablet contains 1.25 mg. (50,000 USP units) of Ergocalciferol USP (Vit. D_2).
Indications: For use in the treatment of hypoparathyroidism and refractory rickets.
Contraindications and Precautions: Treatment of patients with coronary disease, impaired renal function, and arteriosclerosis, especially in the elderly, should be cautious. Large doses of Vitamin D are potentially dangerous and frequent determinations for calcium in blood and urine are mandatory.
Adverse Reactions: Adult doses of 100,000 units or more per day or 200,000 units per day in children can produce toxic effects. Elevated serum levels of calcium and phosphorus as well as drowsiness, gastrointestinal symptoms, renal failure, metastatic calcification and hypertension are manifestations of Vitamin D toxicity.
Dosage: REFRACTORY RICKETS 50,000 to 1,000,000 units per day. HYPOPARATHYROIDISM - 50,000 to 400,000 units per day. Dosage must be adjusted to the needs of the patient. Blood calcium concentration should be kept between 9 and 10 mg.%. Blood and urine calcium levels should be checked frequently.
How Supplied: 50,000 unit tablets, bottles of 100 (NDC 0091-3150-01).
[Shown in Product Identification Section]

KUDROX® SUSPENSION OTC
(DOUBLE STRENGTH) ANTACID
KUDROX TABLETS

Composition: A pleasantly flavored SUSPENSION containing a concentrated combination of aluminum hydroxide gel and magnesium hydroxide in d-sorbitol.
Each TABLET contains 400 mg. of a special coprecipitate of aluminum hydroxide and magnesium carbonate.
One teaspoonful of KUDROX Liquid contains not more than 0.65 mEq (15 mg.) of sodium. Each tablet contains 0.70 mEq (17 mg.) of sodium.
Action and Uses: A palatable antacid to alleviate acid indigestion, heartburn and/or sour stomach, or whenever antacid therapy is the treatment indicated for symptomatic relief of hyperacidity associated with the diagnosis of peptic ulcer, gastritis, peptic esophagitis, gastric hyperacidity, and hiatal hernia. The ratio of aluminum hydroxide to magnesium hydroxide is such that undesirable bowel effects are minimal. Each 5cc dose of SUSPENSION or 2 tablets will neutralize approximately 25 mEq of HCl. High concentration of the active ingredients produces prompt, long lasting neutralization without the acid rebound associated with calcium carbonate containing antacids.
Dosage: KUDROX SUSPENSION, half that ordinarily employed with other liquid antacids. Usual dose only 1 teaspoonful 30 minutes after meals and at bedtime. May be taken undiluted or mixed with water or milk. In peptic ulcer, 2 to 4 teaspoonfuls after meals and at bedtime. KUDROX TABLETS should be chewed or crushed and swallowed with a little water or milk. A usual dose is one or two tablets 30 minutes after meals and at bedtime.
Warning: Antacids containing magnesium hydroxide or magnesium salts should be administered cautiously in patients with renal insufficiency.
Drug Interaction Precaution: This product should not be taken if the patient is currently taking a prescription drug containing any form of tetracycline.
Supplied: KUDROX SUSPENSION, 12 oz. plastic bottles (NDC 0091-4475-42) and 6 oz. plastic bottles (NDC 0091-4475-06). KUDROX TABLETS in handy strips, boxes of 60 (NDC 0091-3470-60).

KUTRASE® CAPSULES ℞

Composition: Each green and white capsule contains: amylolytic enzyme 30 mg., proteolytic enzyme 6 mg., lipolytic enzyme 75 mg., cellulolytic enzyme 2 mg., phenyltoloxamine citrate 15 mg., Levsin® (l-hyoscyamine sulfate) 0.0625 mg.
Action and Uses: KUTRASE is an enzymatic digestant, calmative, antispasmodic indicated for relief of symptoms of functional indigestion accompanied by reduced digestive enzyme capacity.
Dosage: 1 or 2 capsules *during* mealtime.
Precautions: Not for pediatric use. Maximum daily dosage, 6 capsules. Administer with caution to patients with glaucoma, heart disease and prostatic hypertrophy. Phenyltoloxamine may cause drowsiness. If so, driving and operation of machinery should be avoided. It is possible that a patient could develop allergy to one of the enzymes, though this has not been reported.
Supplied: Bottles of 100 (NDC 0091-3475-01) and bottles of 500 (NDC 0091-3475-05).
[Shown in Product Identification Section]

KU-ZYME® CAPSULES ℞

Composition: Each yellow and white capsule contains: amylolytic enzyme 30 mg., proteolytic enzyme 6 mg., lipolytic enzyme 75 mg., cellulolytic enzyme 2 mg.
Action and Uses: KU-ZYME, enzymatic digestant. Aids patients with reduced digestive enzyme capacities to enjoy a more varied, normal and satisfying diet. Helps them digest proteins, carbohydrates, cellulose and fats. Aids in preventing digestive distress and improving nutritional status.
Dosage: 1 capsule 3 times daily *during* meals. If difficult to swallow, capsule may be opened and contents sprinkled on food or dispersed in liquid. Where enzyme deficiency is marked (e.g. following partial gastrectomy, pancreatitis), dosage may be increased as required.
Side Effects and Precautions: Virtually none. Slight looseness of the stools very occasionally. It is theoretically possible that a patient could develop allergy to one of the enzymes, though this has not been reported.
Supplied: Bottles of 100 (NDC 0091-3522-01), bottles of 500 (NDC 0091-3522-05), and Unit Dose in strips, boxes of 100 (NDC 0091-3522-02).
[Shown in Product Identification Section]

KU-ZYME® HP ℞
(Pancrelipase Capsules N.F.)

Description: KU-ZYME HP (pancrelipase NF) is a standardized concentrate of pancreatic enzymes. Each white capsule contains:

Lipase	8,000 NF units
Protease	30,000 NF units
Amylase	30,000 NF units

Actions: A pancreatic enzyme concentrate, which hydrolyzes fats to glycerol and fatty acids, changes protein into proteoses and derived substances, and converts starch into dextrins and sugars. The administration of pancrelipase reduces the fat and nitrogen content of the stool.
Indications: KU-ZYME HP is effective in patients with deficient exocrine pancreatic secretions. Thus, KU-ZYME HP may be used as enzyme replacement therapy in cystic fibrosis, chronic pancreatitis, post pancreatectomy, in ductal obstructions caused by cancer of the pancreas, pancreatic insufficiency and for steatorrhea of malabsorption syndrome and post gastrectomy (Billroth II and Total). May also be used as a presumptive test for pancreatic function (especially in pancreatic insufficiency due to chronic pancreatitis).
Contraindications: There are no known contraindications for the use of pancrelipase although sensitivity to pork protein may preclude its use.
Warnings and Precautions: Harmful effects of pancrelipase therapy have not been reported. It should be used with caution in patients known to be hypersensitive to pork protein. It is important to maintain a proper balance of fat, protein and starch in the diet as well as a carefully adjusted dosage of KU-ZYME HP to maintain optimum digestion.
Dosage: Proper dosage depends on the conditions being treated and the digestive requirements as related to the diet of the patient. Generally, 1 to 3 capsules with each meal or snack may suffice, but larger doses may be taken.
Caution: Federal law prohibits dispensing without prescription.
Supplied: White capsules, bottles of 100. NDC 0091-3525-01.

LEVSIN® TABLETS ℞
(l-hyoscyamine sulfate tablets, N.F.)
LEVSIN® WITH PHENOBARBITAL TABLETS
LEVSIN® ELIXIR
LEVSIN® WITH PHENOBARBITAL ELIXIR
LEVSIN® DROPS
LEVSIN®-PB DROPS
LEVSIN® INJECTION
LEVSINEX™ TIMECAPS™
LEVSINEX™ WITH PHENOBARBITAL TIMECAPS™

Composition: LEVSIN is chemically pure *levo*-rotatory-hyoscyamine sulfate, one of the principal parasympatholytic (anticholinergic) alkaloids of belladonna.
Action and Uses: Indicated whenever antispasmodic or anticholinergic therapy is required. Use in conjunction with diet and antacids, for the medical management of peptic ulcer. To aid in the control of gastric hypersecretion, intestinal hypermotility and associated abdominal cramps. May be used in functional intestinal disorders to relieve symptoms such as those seen in mild dysenteries and diverticulitis. Along with morphine or other narcotics in symptomatic relief of biliary and renal colic. As a "drying agent" in the relief of symptoms of acute rhinitis. In preanesthesia to control salivation and respiratory tract secretions. In the therapy for Parkinsonism to re-

duce rigidity and tremors and to control associated sialorrhea and hyperhidrosis. May be used to reduce pain and hypersecretion in pancreatitis. May be used in the therapy for poisoning by anticholinesterase agents.
LEVSIN TABLETS are scored to permit adjustments of dosage required for optimal control of symptoms. The ELIXIRS provide not only infinite dosage adjustment, but also are pleasant tasting for patients young and old, who have difficulty swallowing tablets and capsules. The high purity allows effective action at very low dosage, with a minimal incidence of unwanted side reactions.
Dosage: LEVSIN TABLETS, plain or with phenobarbital: 1 to 2 tablets 3 or 4 times daily as needed to suppress hyperparasympathetic activity. Plain tablets may be taken sublingually.
LEVSIN ELIXIR, plain or with phenobarbital: infants up to 2 years, ¼ to ½ tsp. Children, 2 to 10 years, ½ to 1 tsp. Adults, 1 to 2 tsps. Dose may be repeated at 4 hour intervals.
LEVSIN DROPS, plain or with phenobarbital: Infants 5-20 lbs., 0.1-0.25 cc.; Children 1-10 yrs., 0.5-1 cc.; Adults, 1-2 cc.
LEVSIN INJECTION, plain: 1 or 2 cc. subcutaneously, intramuscularly, or intravenously as indicated. As a antisialogog in preanesthesia, usual adult dose, 0.5 mg. Levsin.
LEVSINEX TIMECAPS, plain or with phenobarbital: 1 Timecap every 12 hours. (Each LEVSINEX TIMECAP Capsule contains the equivalent of 3 LEVSIN plain or 3 LEVSIN with phenobarbital tablets, formulated to provide prolonged therapeutic effect).
WARNING: LEVSIN and LEVSINEX products with phenobarbital may be habit forming.
Side Effects: Excessive dryness of the mouth, blurred vision, urinary difficulty and tachycardia may indicate overdosage.
Contraindications: May be contraindicated in glaucoma, prostatic hypertrophy and some cases of cardiac disease.
SUPPLIED:
LEVSIN Tablets (0.125 mg. l-hyoscyamine sulfate tablets, N.F.) white, scored tablets; bottles of 100 (NDC 0091-3531-01), bottles of 500 (NDC 0091-3531-05), and Unit Dose in strips, boxes of 100 (NDC 0091-3531-02).
[*Shown in Product Identification Section*]
LEVSIN with Phenobarbital Tablets (0.125 mg. l-hyoscyamine sulfate and 15 mg. Phenobarbital) pink, scored tablets; bottles of 100 (NDC 0091-3534-01), and 500 (NDC 0091-3534-05).
[*Shown in Product Identification Section*]
LEVSIN Elixir (0.125 mg. l-hyoscyamine sulfate per 5 cc.) orange colored and flavored; pints. (NDC 0091-4532-16).
LEVSIN with Phenobarbital Elixir (0.125 mg. l-hyoscyamine sulfate and 15 mg. Phenobarbital per 5 cc.) red, raspberry flavored; pints. (NDC 0091-4530-16).
LEVSIN DROPS (0.125 mg. l-hyoscyamine sulfate per cc.), orange colored and flavored, 15 cc. (NDC 0091-4538-15)
LEVSIN-PB DROPS (0.125 mg. l-hyoscyamine sulfate and 15 mg. phenobarbital per cc.), red, cherry flavored, 15 cc. (NDC 0091-4536-15)
LEVSIN Injection (0.25 mg. l-hyoscyamine sulfate per cc.) 10 cc multiple dose vials. (NDC 0091-1532-70)
LEVSINEX TIMECAPS (0.375 mg. l-hyoscyamine sulfate) brown and white sustained release beadlets in brown and clear capsules; bottles of 100. (NDC 0091-3537-01).
[*Shown in Product Identification Section*]
LEVSINEX with Phenobarbital TIMECAPS (0.375 mg. l-hyoscyamine sulfate and 45 mg. Phenobarbital) pink and white sustained release beadlets in pink and clear capsules; bottles of 100. (NDC 0091-3539-01).
[*Shown in Product Identification Section*]

MILKINOL® OTC

Composition: MILKINOL is a unique formulation containing liquid petrolatum for lubrication, dioctyl sodium sulfosuccinate to aid in penetration and softening of the fecal mass, and a special emulsifier to make oil and water mix for complete dispersion.
Action and Uses: Pleasant, dependable MILKINOL provides safe, gentle lubrication for the constipation problem. No oily taste, no purgative griping, not habit forming, sugar free.
Dosage: Adults 1 to 2 tablespoonfuls. Children over 6: 1 to 2 teaspoonfuls. Infants, young children, expectant mothers, aged or bedridden patients, use only as directed by physician. Pour MILKINOL in a glass, add ¼ glass fruit juice, soft drink, milk, or even water. Stir and drink.
Precautions: Prolonged usage, without intermission is not advised. Should be given at bedtime ONLY.
Supplied: 12 oz. glass bottles (NDC 0091-7580-42).

NITROL® OINTMENT ℞

Description: Nitrol® Ointment contains 2% nitroglycerin (glyceryl trinitrate) in a special lanolin-petrolatum base. It is a prompt acting vasodilator, effective in the relief and prevention of anginal attacks.
Action: When the ointment is spread on the skin, the active ingredient (nitroglycerin) is continuously absorbed through the skin into the circulation, thus exerting prolonged vasodilator effect. Nitroglycerin ointment is effective in the control of angina pectoris, regardless of the site of application.
Nitroglycerin relaxes smooth muscles, principally in the smaller blood vessels and dilates the arterioles and capillaries, especially in the coronary circulation. In therapeutic doses, this allows increased blood supply to the myocardium, tending to relieve myocardial ischemia which has been suggested as the basis for the pain of angina pectoris. Nitrol Ointment has been found to produce peripheral vasodilation with decreased arteriolar resistance and increased volume. Recent controlled studies suggest that Nitrol Ointment favorably affects peripheral vascular resistance, venous capacitance, preload and after load. It exerts a favorable influence on myocardial oxygen consumption, resulting in increased myocardial efficiency and significant improvement in left ventricular function. Nitrol Ointment also produces sustained, enhanced exercise capacity; attenuation of ischemic EKG changes; concomittant changes in heart rate and blood pressure without evidence of tolerance or toxicity. Nitrol Ointment induces hemodynamic alterations similar to those of sublingual nitroglycerin, but onset (15 minutes) is delayed and the effect (up to 4 hours) is prolonged.
Indications: Nitrol Ointment is indicated for prevention and treatment of angina pectoris associated with or resulting from coronary insufficiency, coronary artery disease, coronary occlusion, or subacute myocardial infarction.
Contraindications: Nitrol Ointment may be contraindicated in patients with marked anemia, increased intraocular pressure or increased intracranial pressure. Nitrol Ointment should not be employed in patients with known idiosyncrasies to nitrites.
Warning: In terminating treatment of anginal patients, both the dosage and frequency of application must be gradually reduced over a period of 4 to 6 weeks to prevent sudden withdrawal reactions, which are characteristic of all vasodilators in the nitroglycerin class.
Precautions: A hypotensive headache is a sign of overdosage. Occasionally elderly patients may have no untoward symptoms while recumbent but may develop postural hypotension with faintness upon suddenly arising.
Dosage and Administration: For angina pectoris the ointment may be applied every 3 to 4 hours as required. The usual dose is 1 to 2 inches, as squeezed from the tube, although some patients may require as much as 4 to 5 inches. The ointment should be spread in a thin uniform layer on the skin. The optimum dosage is determined by starting with an application of ½ inch of ointment and increasing the dose in ½ inch increments each successive application until headache occurs, then decreasing to the largest dose which does not cause headache. Nitrol Ointment can be applied to any convenient skin area but psychologically, many patients prefer the chest. Measurement and application of the ointment is easily accomplished with the aid of the specially designed Appli-Ruler supplied with the ointment. The ointment can be squeezed onto the graduated area of the Appli-Ruler and conveniently spread over the desired skin area. Keep the tube tightly closed and store at controlled room temperatures.
Caution: Federal law prohibits dispensing without prescription.
How Supplied:
30 gram tube (NDC 0091-5617-31)
60 gram tube (NDC 0091-5617-02)
30 gram 6 Pack Unit (NDC 0091-5617-61)
60 gram 6 Pack Unit (NDC 0091-5617-62)
[*Shown in Product Identification Section*]

PRE-PEN® ℞
(Benzylpenicilloyl-polylysine)
Skin Test Antigen

Description: PRE-PEN® is a sterile solution of benzylpenicilloyl-polylysine in a concentration of 6.0×10^{-5}M. (penicilloyl) in 0.01 M phosphate buffer and 0.15 M sodium chloride. The benzylpenicilloyl-polylysine in PRE-PEN® is a derivative of poly-l-lysine, where the epsilon amino groups are substituted with benzylpenicilloyl groups (50-70%) forming benzylpenicilloyl alpha amide. Each single dose ampule contains 0.25 ml of PRE-PEN®.
Action: PRE-PEN® (benzylpenicilloyl-polylysine) reacts specifically with benzylpenicilloyl skin sensitizing antibodies (reagins: IgE class) to initiate release of chemical mediators which produce an immediate wheal and flare reaction at a skin test site. All individuals exhibiting a positive skin test to PRE-PEN® possess reagins against the benzylpenicilloyl group which is a haptene. A haptene is a low molecular weight chemical which, when conjugated to a carrier, e.g., poly-l-lysine, has the properties under appropriate conditions of an antigen with the haptene's specificity.
It is to be noted that individuals who have previously received therapeutic penicillin may have positive skin test reactions to PRE-PEN® as well as to a number of other non-benzylpenicilloyl haptenes. The latter are designated as minor determinants, in that they are present in lesser amounts than the major determinant, benzylpenicilloyl. The minor determinants may nevertheless be associated with examples of significant clinical hypersensitivity.
Virtually everyone who receives penicillin develops specific antibodies to the drug as measured by hemagglutination studies, but (a) positive skin tests to various penicillin and penicillin-derived reagents become positive in less than 10% of patients who have tolerated penicillin in the past and (b) allergic responses are infrequent (less than 1%).
Many individuals reacting positively to PRE-PEN® will not develop a systemic allergic reaction on subsequent exposure to therapeutic penicillin. Thus, the PRE-PEN® skin test facilitates assessing the local allergic skin reactivity of a patient to benzylpenicilloyl.

Continued on next page

Kremers-Urban—Cont.

Indications: PRE-PEN® is useful as an adjunct in assessing the risk of administering penicillin (benzylpenicillin or penicillin G) when it is the preferred drug of choice in adult patients who have previously received penicillin and have a history of clinical penicillin hypersensitivity. In this situation, a negative skin test to PRE-PEN® is associated with an incidence of allergic reactions of less than 5% after the administration of therapeutic penicillin, whereas the incidence may be more than 20% in the presence of a positive skin test to PRE-PEN®.

These allergic reactions are predominantly dermatologic. Because of the extremely low incidence of anaphylactic reactions, there are insufficient data at present to document that a decreased incidence of anaphylactic reactions following the administration of penicillin will occur in patients with a negative skin test to PRE-PEN®. Similarly, when deciding the risk of proposed penicillin treatment, there are not enough data at present to permit relative weighting in individual cases of a history of clinical penicillin hypersensitivity as compared to positive skin tests to PRE-PEN® and/or minor penicillin determinants.

It should be borne in mind that no reagent, test, or combination of tests will completely assure that a reaction to penicillin therapy will not occur.

Contraindications: PRE-PEN® is contraindicated in those patients who have exhibited either a systemic or marked local reaction to its previous administration. Patients known to be extremely hypersensitive to penicillin should not be skin tested.

Warnings: There are insufficient data to assess the potential danger of sensitization to penicillin from repeated skin testing with PRE-PEN®.

Rarely, a systemic allergic reaction (see below) may follow a skin test with PRE-PEN®. This can be avoided by making the first application by scratch test and very carefully following the instructions below in administering the intradermal test, using the intradermal route only if the scratch test has been entirely negative. Skin testing with penicillin and/or other penicillin-derived reagents should not be performed simultaneously.

No controlled studies have been made of the safety of PRE-PEN® skin testing in pregnant women and therefore, the hazard of skin testing of such patients should be weighed against the hazards of penicillin therapy without skin testing.

Precautions: There are insufficient data derived from well-controlled studies to determine the value of the PRE-PEN® skin test as a means of assessing the risk of administering therapeutic penicillin (when penicillin is the preferred drug of choice) in the following situations:

(1) Adult patients who give no history of clinical penicillin hypersensitivity.

(2) Pediatric patients.

In addition, there are no data at present to assess the clinical value of PRE-PEN® where exposure to penicillin is suspected as a cause of a drug reaction and in patients who are undergoing routine allergy evaluation.

Furthermore, there are no data relating the clinical value of PRE-PEN® skin tests to the risk of administering semi-synthetic penicillins (phenoxymethyl penicillin, ampicillin, carbenicillin, dicloxacillin, methicillin, nafcillin, oxacillin, phenethicillin) and cephalosporin-derived antibiotics.

Recognition that the following clinical outcomes are possible makes it imperative for the physician to weigh risk to benefit in every instance where the decision to administer or not to administer penicillin is based in part on a PRE-PEN® skin test.

(1) An allergic reaction to therapeutic penicillin may occur in a patient with a negative skin test to PRE-PEN®.

(2) It is possible for a patient to have an anaphylactic reaction to therapeutic penicillin in the presence of a negative PRE-PEN® skin test and a negative history of clinical penicillin hypersensitivity.

(3) If penicillin is the absolute drug of choice in a life-threatening situation, successful desensitization with therapeutic penicillin may be possible irrespective of a positive skin test and/or a positive history of clinical penicillin hypersensitivity.

Adverse Reactions: Occasionally, patients may develop an intense local inflammatory response at the skin test site. Rarely, patients will develop a systemic allergic reaction, manifested by generalized erythema, pruritus, angioneurotic edema, urticaria, dyspnea, and/or hypotension. The usual methods of treating a skin test antigen induced reaction—the application of a venous occlusion tourniquet proximal to the skin test site and administration of epinephrine (and, at times, an injection of an antihistamine) — are recommended and will usually control the reaction. As a rule, systemic allergic reactions following skin test procedures are of short duration and controllable, but the patient should be kept under observation for several hours.

Skin Testing Dosage and Technique:
SCRATCH TESTING

Skin testing is usually performed on the inner volar aspect of the forearm. The skin test material should **always** be applied first by the scratch technique. After preparing the skin surface, a sterile 20 gauge needle should be used to make a 3–5 mm scratch of the epidermis. Very little pressure is required to break the epidermal continuity. If bleeding occurs, prepare a second site and scratch more lightly with the needle—sufficient to produce a nonbleeding scratched surface. Apply a small drop of PRE-PEN® solution to the scratch and rub gently with an applicator, toothpick, or the side of the needle. Observe for the appearance of a wheal, erythema, and the occurrence of itching at the test site during the succeeding 15 minutes at which time the solution over the scratch is wiped off. A positive reaction is unmistakable and consists of the development within 10 minutes of a pale wheal, usually with pseudopods, surrounding the scratch site and varying in diameter from 5 to 15 mm (or more). This wheal may be surrounded by a variable diameter of erythema, and accompanied by a variable degree of itching. The most sensitive individuals develop itching almost instantly, and the wheal and erythema are prompt in their appearance. As soon as a positive response as defined above is clearly evident, the solution over the scratch should be immediately wiped off. If the scratch test is either negative or equivocally positive (less than 5 mm wheal and little or no erythema, and no itching), an intradermal test may be performed.

THE INTRADERMAL TEST

Using a tuberculin syringe with a 3/8" to 5/8" long, 26 to 30 gauge, short bevel needle, withdraw the contents of the ampule. Prepare a sterile skin test area on the upper, outer arm, sufficiently below the deltoid muscle to permit proximal application of a tourniquet later, if necessary. Be sure to eject all air from the syringe through the needle, then insert the needle, bevel up immediately below the skin surface. Inject an amount of PRE-PEN® sufficient to raise the smallest possible perceptible bleb. This volume will be between 0.01 and 0.02 ml. Using a separate syringe and needle, inject a like amount of saline as a control at least 1½ inches removed from the test site. Most skin reactions will develop within 5–15 minutes and response to the skin test is read as follows:

(—) Negative response—no increase in size of original bleb and/or no greater reaction than the control site.

(±) Ambiguous response—wheal being only slightly larger than initial injection bleb, with or without accompanying erythematous flare and larger than the control site.

(+) Positive response—itching and marked increase in size of original bleb. Wheal may exceed 20 mm in diameter and exhibit pseudopods.

The control site should be completely reactionless. If it exhibits a wheal greater than 2–3 mm, repeat the test, and if the same reaction is observed, a physician experienced with allergy skin testing should be consulted.

How Supplied: PRE-PEN® is supplied in ampules containing 0.25 ml. and packaged in boxes of 5 (NDC 0091-1640-05).

PRE-PEN® is stable only when kept under refrigeration. It is, therefore, recommended that test materials subjected to ambient temperatures for over a day be discarded.

Further information on these and other Kremers-Urban products will be furnished upon request to our Professional Service Department.

Lambda Pharmacal Corporation

Subsidiary of A. J. Bart, Inc.
PLAINVIEW, NY 11803

DEXTROTUSSIN™

(Cough and Cold Syrup)
Alcohol and Sugar Free

Description: Each fluid ounce contains: Dextromethorphan Hydrobromide 60 mg. (10 mg./teaspoonful), Prophenpyridamine 25 mg., Ammonium Chloride 500 mg., Phenylpropanolamine HCl. 25 mg., Ascorbic Acid 30 mg. in a base of sorbitol, purified water and wild cherry flavor.
Indications: For temporary relief of cough due to the common cold.
Advantages: Can be given to alcoholic as well as to diabetic patients since it neither contains sugar or alcohol.
Caution: May cause drowsiness. Patients receiving this preparation should be cautioned against operating machinery.
Dosage and Administration: Adults and children over 12 years—1 to 2 teaspoonfuls; children 8 to 12 years—1 teaspoonful; under 8 years—from ½ to 1 teaspoonful. These doses may be taken every four hours.
How Supplied: In 4 oz. bottles (NDC 49326-118-04).

FERAPLEX™ LIQUID

(Iron and B Complex)
Alcohol and Sugar Free

Description: Each 30 cc contains: Iron Ammonium Citrate 100 mg., Pyridoxine HCl 1 mg., Riboflavin 2 mg., Thiamine HCl 10 mg., Cyanocobalamin 10 mg., in a peach flavored base of sorbitol.
Indications: FERAPLEX LIQUID is for the treatment of B Complex and Iron deficiencies.
Advantages: Can be given to every patient including the diabetic patient since it does not contain sugar; can be given to alcoholic patients since it does not contain alcohol.
Dosage and Administration: ADULTS—1 tablespoonful with meals. CHILDREN—1 to 2 teaspoonfuls with meals.
How Supplied: FERAPLEX LIQUID is supplied in 4 oz. bottles (NDC 49326-120-04).

MIGRALAM™ CAPSULES ℞

Description: Each white MIGRALAM capsule contains: Isometheptene Mucate 65 mg., Caffeine 100 mg., Acetaminophen 325 mg.
Actions: Isometheptene Mucate, a sympathomimetic amine, acts by constricting dilated cranial and cerebral arterioles, thus reducing the stimuli that lead to vascular headaches. It is particularly desirable in patients predisposed to nausea and vomiting and where ergotamines are precluded. Its action is similar to ergotamine but possessed of a low order of toxicity. Caffeine, also a cranial vasoconstrictor, is added to further enhance the vasoconstrictor effect. Acetaminophen, an effective non-narcotic analgesic, reduces the perception of pain impulses originating from dilated cerebral vessels. It is unlikely to produce many of the side effects associated with aspirin.
Indications: For relief of vascular and tension headaches.

Based on a review for this drug (isometheptene mucate), The National Academy of Sciences-National Research Council and/or other information, FDA has classified the other indications as "Possibly" effective in the treatment of migraine headache.
Final classification of the less-than-effective indication requires further investigation.

Contraindications: MIGRALAN is contraindicated in Glaucoma and/or severe cases of renal disease, hypertension, organic heart disease, hepatic disease and in those patients who are on monoamine-oxidase (MAO) inhibitor therapy.
Precautions: Caution should be observed in hypertension, peripheral vascular disease and after recent cardiovascular attacks.
Adverse Reactions: Transient dizziness and skin rash may appear in hypersensitive patients. This can usually be eliminated by reducing the dose.
Dosage and Administration: **FOR RELIEF OF MIGRAINE HEADACHE.** The usual adult dosage is two capsules at once, followed by one capsule every hour until relieved, up to 5 capsules within a twelve hour period.
FOR RELIEF OF TENSION HEADACHE. The usual adult dose is one or two capsules every four hours up to 8 capsules a day.
How Supplied: Bottles of 100 capsules (NDC 49326-116-90) and 500 capsules (NDC 49326-116-75).

NEURO™ B-12 INJECTABLE ℞

(B-12, B-1)

Description: Each cc in NEURO B-12 contains: Cyanocobalamin (Vitamin B-12) 1000 mcg., Thiamine HCl. (Vitamin B-1) 100 mg., Benzyl Alcohol 1.5% and Disodium E.D.T.A. 0.5 mg. in a sterile aqueous solution.
Indications: NEURO B-12 is intended for the prevention and treatment of a variety of disorders associated with vitamin B-1 deficiency as well as for the management of certain sensory neuropathies responding to massive doses of vitamin B-12. Specifically, vitamin B-1 is indicated in the prevention and treatment of beriberi and in the correction of anorexia of dietary origin.
Contraindications: Hypersensitivity to Thiamine HCl.
Precautions: The usual precautions associated with parenteral medication should be observed.
Dosage and Administration: Dosage requirements of NEURO B-12 vary with the individual patient and with the condition being treated. In disorders due to vitamin B-1 deficiency, the suggested average daily dose is 12.5 to 100 mg. of vitamin B-1 (Thiamine) given subcutaneously or intramuscularly. In trigeminal neuralgia, the suggested daily dose may range from 250 to 1000 mcg. of vitamin B-12 administered by subcutaneous or intramuscular injection. Treatment should be continued until relief is obtained. Additional NEURO B-12 therapy may be advisable if paroxysmal pain recurs after the initial course of treatment.
How Supplied: NEURO B-12 Injectable is supplied in a 10 cc multidose vial (NDC 49326-114-10).

NEURO™ B-12 FORTE INJECTABLE ℞

(B-12, B-1, B-6)

Description: Each cc in NEURO B-12 FORTE contains: Cyanocobalamin 1000 mcg., Thiamine HCl 100 mg., Pyridoxine HCl 100 mg., Benzyl Alcohol 1.5% in a physiological salt solution q.s.
How Supplied: NEURO B-12 FORTE Injectable is supplied in 10 cc multidose vials (NDC 49326-115-10).

The Lannett Company, Inc.

9000 STATE ROAD
PHILADELPHIA, PA 19136

ACNEDERM™ LOTION

(See PDR For Nonprescription Drugs)

CODALAN™ Ⓒ ℞

Composition: Each tablet contains: Codeine Phosphate* gr. ⅛ in No. 1; gr. ¼ in No. 2; gr. ½ in No. 3; Acetaminophen 2½ grs.; Salicylamide 3½ grs.; and caffeine ½ gr.
*Warning: May be habit-forming.
Action and Uses: Analgesic, antitussive. Indicated for the relief of pain of all degrees of severity up to that which requires morphine.
Administration and Dosage: One (No. 1, No. 2 or No. 3) as required to relieve pain.
How Supplied: No. 1 orange color, No. 2 white color, No. 3 green color; all strengths in bottles of 100 and 500. No. 2 and No. 3 also available in bottles of 1000.
Literature Available: Complete Data Card.

DISONATE™ Capsules and Liquid

(dioctyl sodium sulfosuccinate)

Composition: Dioctyl sodium sulfosuccinate, an effective stool-softener.
Action and Uses: Disonate keeps stools soft for easy passage. It is not a laxative and does not irritate the intestinal tract. Useful in treating constipation due to hard stools, in painful anorectal conditions, in cardiac and other patients who must avoid straining at stool.
Dosage: Adults and older children 60 to 240 mg. daily. Children 6 to 12 years of age 40 to 120 mg. daily. Higher doses are recommended for initial therapy and the effect on stools is usually apparent one to three days after the initial dose. Divided dosage may be used and dosage should be adjusted to individual response.
How Supplied: Capsules of 60 mg., 100 mg., and 240 mg. Bottles of 100, 500 and 1000 capsules. Solution, 10 mg/cc Pint Bottle. Syrup, 20 mg/5 cc Pint and Gallon Bottle.
Literature Available: Yes.

MAGNATRIL™ SUSPENSION AND TABLETS

(See PDR For Nonprescription Drugs)

Laser, Inc.

2000 N. MAIN ST.
CROWN POINT, IN 46307

DALLERGY® Syrup, Tablets and Sustained-Release Capsules ℞

Composition: Each teaspoonful (5 cc) of purple, grape flavored syrup contains: chlorpheniramine maleate 2 mg., phenylephrine hydrochloride 10 mg., methscopolamine nitrate 0.625 mg. Each white scored tablet contains: chlorpheniramine maleate 4 mg., phenylephrine hydrochloride 10 mg., methscopolamine nitrate 1.25 mg. Each pink and white sustained-release capsule contains: chlorpheniramine maleate 8 mg., phenylephrine hydrochloride 20 mg., methscopolamine nitrate 2.5 mg.

DONATUSSIN™ DROPS ℞

Composition: Each cc. of orange syrup contains: Chlorpheniramine Maleate 1 mg., Phenylephrine hydrochloride 2 mg., Guaifenesin 20 mg.

KIE® SYRUP and TABLETS ℞

Composition: Each teaspoonful (5cc.) of green syrup contains: potassium iodide 150 mg.,

Continued on next page

Laser—Cont.

ephedrine hydrochloride 8 mg. Each green, scored, tablet contains: potassium iodide 400 mg. ephedrine hydrochloride 24 mg.

THEOSPAN® 80 SYRUP ℞
(theophylline anhydrous USP)

THEOSPAN® TABLETS 100 mg. ℞
(theophylline anhydrous USP)

THEOSPAN® TABLETS 200 mg. ℞
(theophylline anhydrous USP)

THEOSPAN® SR CAPSULES 130 mg. ℞
(theophylline anhydrous USP)

THEOSPAN® SR CAPSULES 260 mg. ℞
(theophylline anhydrous USP)

Composition: Each 15 ml. of dye-free Theospan Syrup contains theophylline anhydrous USP 80 mg., alcohol 1%. Each white, dye-free, quad-scored Theospan Tablet, 100 mg. contains theophylline anhydrous USP 100 mg. Each white, dye-free, quad-scored Theospan Tablet, 200 mg. contains theophylline anhydrous USP 200 mg. Each sustained-release Theospan SR Capsule 130 mg. (white and clear capsule with orange and white pellets) contains theophylline anhydrous USP 130 mg. Each sustained-release Theospan SR Capsule 260 mg. (dye-free, white and clear capsule with white pellets) contains theophylline anhydrous USP 260 mg.

TRIMSTAT® TABLETS Ⓒ ℞
(phendimetrazine tartrate)

Composition: Each tan tablet contains: phendimetrazine tartrate 35 mg.

Lederle Laboratories
A Division of American Cyanamid Co.
WAYNE, NEW JERSEY 07470

ACHROMYCIN® V ℞
(tetracycline HCl)
Capsules and Syrup
ACHROMYCIN Intramuscular
ACHROMYCIN Intravenous

Description: ACHROMYCIN *tetracycline HCl* is an antibiotic isolated from *Streptomyces aureofaciens.* Chemically it is the hydrochloride of 4-dimethylamino-1,4,4a,5,5a,6,11, 12a-octahydro-3, 6, 10, 12, 12a-pentahydroxy-6-methyl -1, 11- dioxo - 2 - naphthacenecarbox - amide.

Actions: The tetracyclines are primarily bacteriostatic and are thought to exert their antimicrobial effect by the inhibition of protein synthesis. Tetracyclines are active against a wide range of gram-negative and gram-positive organisms.

The drugs in the tetracycline class have closely similar antimicrobial spectra, and cross-resistance among them is common. Microorganisms may be considered susceptible if the M.I.C. (minimum inhibitory concentration) is not more than 4.0 mcg./ml. and intermediate if the M.I.C. is 4.0 to 12.5 mcg./ml.

Susceptibility plate testing: A tetracycline disc may be used to determine microbial susceptibility to drugs in the tetracycline class. If the Kirby-Bauer method of disc susceptibility testing is used, a 30 mcg. tetracycline HCl disc should give a zone of at least 19 mm. when tested against a tetracycline-susceptible bacterial strain.

Tetracyclines are readily absorbed and are bound to plasma proteins in varying degree. They are concentrated by the liver in the bile and excreted in the urine and feces at high concentrations and in a biologically active form.

Indications: ACHROMYCIN *tetracycline HCl* is indicated in infections caused by the following micro-organisms:

Rickettsiae: (Rocky Mountain spotted fever, typhus fever and the typhus group, Q fever, rickettsialpox, tick fevers.)
Mycoplasma pneumoniae (PPLO, Eaton agent).
Agents of psittacosis and ornithosis.
Agents of lymphogranuloma venereum and granuloma inguinale.
The spirochetal agent of relapsing fever *(Borrelia recurrentis).*
The following gram-negative micro-organisms:
Haemophilus ducreyi (chancroid),
Pasteurella pestis and *Pasteurella tularensis,*
Bartonella bacilliformis,
Bacteroides species,
Vibrio comma and *Vibrio fetus.*
Brucella species (in conjunction with streptomycin).

Because many strains of the following groups of micro-organisms have been shown to be resistant to tetracyclines, culture and susceptibility testing are recommended.

Tetracycline is indicated for treatment of infections caused by the following gram-negative micro-organisms, when bacteriologic testing indicates appropriate susceptibility to the drug:
Escherichia coli,
Enterobacter aerogenes (formerly *Aerobacter aerogenes*),
Shigella species,
Mima species and *Herellea* species,
Haemophilus influenzae (respiratory infections),
Klebsiella species (respiratory and urinary infections).

Tetracycline is indicated for treatment of infections caused by the following gram-positive micro-organisms when bacteriologic testing indicates appropriate susceptibility to the drug:
Streptococcus species:
Up to 44 percent of strains of *Streptococcus pyogenes* and 74 percent of *Streptococcus faecalis* have been found to be resistant to tetracycline drugs. Therefore, tetracyclines should not be used for streptococcal disease unless the organism has been demonstrated to be sensitive.
For upper respiratory infections due to group A beta-hemolytic streptococci, penicillin is the usual drug of choice, including prophylaxis of rheumatic fever.
Diplococcus pneumoniae,
Staphylococcus aureus, skin and soft tissue infections. Tetracyclines are not the drug of choice in the treatment of any type of staphylococcal infection.

When penicillin is contraindicated, tetracyclines are alternative drugs in the treatment of infections due to:
Neisseria gonorrhoeae,
Treponema pallidum and *Treponema pertenue* (syphilis and yaws),
Listeria monocytogenes,
Clostridium species,
Bacillus anthracis,
Fusobacterium fusiforme (Vincent's infection),
Actinomyces species.

In acute intestinal amebiasis, the tetracyclines may be a useful adjunct to amebicides.

In severe acne, the tetracyclines may be useful adjunctive therapy. (This indication is for the Oral Use only. Not for IM or IV.)

ACHROMYCIN *tetracycline HCl* is indicated in the treatment of trachoma, although the infectious agent is not always eliminated, as judged by immunofluorescence.

Inclusion conjunctivitis may be treated with oral tetracyclines or with a combination of oral and topical agents.

Contraindications: This drug is contraindicated in persons who have shown hypersensitivity to any of the tetracyclines.

Warnings: In the presence of renal dysfunction, particularly in pregnancy, intravenous tetracycline therapy in daily doses exceeding 2 grams has been associated with deaths through liver failure.

When the need for intensive treatment outweighs its potential dangers (mostly during pregnancy or in individuals with known or suspected renal or liver impairment), it is advisable to perform renal and liver function tests before and during therapy. Also tetracycline serum concentrations should be followed.

If renal impairment exists, even usual oral or parenteral doses may lead to excessive systemic accumulation of the drug and possible liver toxicity. Under such conditions, lower than usual total doses are indicated, and if therapy is prolonged, serum level determinations of the drug may be advisable. This hazard is of particular importance in the parenteral administration of tetracyclines to pregnant or postpartum patients with pyelonephritis. When used under these circumstances, the blood level should not exceed 15 micrograms/ml. and liver function tests should be made at frequent intervals. Other potentially hepatotoxic drugs should not be prescribed concomitantly.

THE USE OF DRUGS OF THE TETRACYCLINE CLASS DURING TOOTH DEVELOPMENT (LAST HALF OF PREGNANCY, INFANCY, AND CHILDHOOD TO THE AGE OF 8 YEARS) MAY CAUSE PERMANENT DISCOLORATION OF THE TEETH (YELLOW-GRAY-BROWN). This adverse reaction is more common during long-term use of the drugs but has been observed following repeated short-term courses. Enamel hypoplasia has also been reported. TETRACYCLINES, THEREFORE, SHOULD NOT BE USED IN THIS AGE GROUP UNLESS OTHER DRUGS ARE NOT LIKELY TO BE EFFECTIVE OR ARE CONTRAINDICATED.

Photosensitivity manifested by an exaggerated sunburn reaction has been observed in some individuals taking tetracyclines. Patients apt to be exposed to direct sunlight or ultraviolet light should be advised that this reaction can occur with tetracycline drugs, and treatment should be discontinued at the first evidence of skin erythema.

The antianabolic action of the tetracyclines may cause an increase in BUN. While this is not a problem in those with normal renal function, in patients with significantly impaired function, higher serum levels of tetracycline may lead to azotemia, hyperphosphatemia, and acidosis.

Usage in pregnancy: (See above "Warnings" about use during tooth development.)

Results of animal studies indicate that tetracyclines cross the placenta, are found in fetal tissues and can have toxic effects on the developing fetus (often related to retardation of skeletal development). Evidence of embryotoxicity has also been noted in animals treated early in pregnancy.

Usage in newborns, infants, and children: (See above "Warnings" about use during tooth development.)

All tetracyclines form a stable calcium complex in any bone forming tissue. A decrease in the fibula growth rate has been observed in prematures given oral tetracycline in doses of 25 mg./kg. every 6 hours. This reaction was shown to be reversible when the drug was discontinued.

Tetracyclines are present in the milk of lactating women who are taking a drug in this class.

Precautions: As with other antibiotic preparations, use of this drug may result in overgrowth of nonsusceptible organisms, including fungi. If superinfection occurs, the antibiotic should be discontinued and appropriate therapy instituted.

In venereal diseases when coexistent syphilis is suspected, darkfield examination should be done before treatment is started and the blood serology repeated monthly for at least 4 months.

Because the tetracyclines have been shown to depress plasma prothrombin activity, patients who are on anticoagulant therapy may require downward adjustment of their anticoagulant dosage.

In long-term therapy, periodic laboratory evaluation of organ systems, including hematopoietic, renal and hepatic studies should be performed.

All infections due to Group A beta hemolytic streptococci should be treated for at least 10 days.

Since bacteriostatic drugs may interfere with the bactericidal action of penicillin, it is advisable to avoid giving tetracycline in conjunction with penicillin.

Adverse Reactions: Local irritation may be present after intramuscular injection. The injection should be deep, with care taken not to injure the sciatic nerve nor inject intravascularly.

Gastrointestinal: Anorexia, nausea, vomiting, diarrhea, glossitis, dysphagia, enterocolitis, and inflammatory lesions (with monilial overgrowth) in the anogenital region. These reactions have been caused by both the oral and parenteral administration of tetracyclines.

Skin: Maculopapular and erythematous rashes. Exfoliative dermatitis has been reported but is uncommon. Photosensitivity is discussed above. (See "Warnings".)

Renal toxicity: Rise in BUN has been reported and is apparently dose related. (See "Warnings".)

Hypersensitivity reactions: Urticaria, angioneurotic edema, anaphylaxis, anaphylactoid purpura, pericarditis and exacerbation of systemic lupus erythematosus.

Bulging fontanels have been reported in young infants following full therapeutic dosage. This sign disappeared rapidly when the drug was discontinued.

Blood: Hemolytic anemia, thrombocytopenia, neutropenia and eosinophilia have been reported.

When given over prolonged periods, tetracyclines have been reported to produce brown-black microscopic discoloration of thyroid glands. No abnormalities of thyroid function studies are known to occur.

ORAL FORMS:

Dosage and Administration: Therapy should be continued for at least 24-48 hours after symptoms and fever have subsided.

Concomitant therapy: Antacids containing aluminum, calcium, or magnesium impair absorption and should not be given to patients taking oral tetracycline.

Foods and some dairy products also interfere with absorption. Oral forms of tetracycline should be given 1 hour before or 2 hours after meals. Pediatric oral dosage forms should not be given with milk formulas and should be given at least 1 hour prior to feeding.

In patients with renal impairment: (See "Warnings".) Total dosage should be decreased by reduction of recommended individual doses and/or by extending time intervals between doses.

In the treatment of streptococcal infections, a therapeutic dose of tetracycline should be administered for at least 10 days.

Adults: Usual daily dose, 1-2 Grams divided in two or four equal doses, depending on the severity of the infection.

For children above eight years of age: Usual daily dose, 10-20 mg. (25-50 mg./kg.) per pound of body weight divided in two or four equal doses.

For treatment of brucellosis, 500 mg. tetracycline four times daily for 3 weeks should be accompanied by streptomycin, 1 gram intramuscularly twice daily the first week and once daily the second week.

For treatment of syphilis, a total of 30-40 grams in equally divided doses over a period of 10-15 days should be given. Close followup, including laboratory tests, is recommended.

Gonorrhea patients sensitive to penicillin may be treated with tetracycline, administered as an initial oral dose of 1.5 grams followed by 0.5 grams every 6 hours for 4 days to a total dosage of 9 grams.

INTRAMUSCULAR:

Preparation of Solution: Add 2 ml. of Sterile Water for Injection U.S.P. (or Sodium Chloride Injection U.S.P.) to the 100 mg. or 250 mg. vial. The resulting solution may be stored at room temperature and should not be used after 24 hours.

Dosage and Administration:

Intramuscular administration, Adults: The usual daily dose is 250 mg. administered once every 24 hours or 300 mg. given in divided doses at 8-to 12-hour intervals.

For children above eight years of age: 15-25 mg./kg. body weight up to a maximum of 250 mg. per single daily injection. Dosage may be divided and given at 8- to 12-hour intervals.

Gonorrhea patients sensitive to penicillin may be treated with tetracycline administered as an initial oral dose of 1.5 grams followed by 0.5 grams every 6 hours for 4 days, a total dosage of 9 grams. Intramuscular therapy should be reserved for situations in which oral therapy is not feasible.

In patients with renal impairment: (See "Warnings".)

Total dosage should be decreased by reduction of recommended individual doses and/or by extending time intervals between doses.

The intramuscular administration of ACHROMYCIN *sterile tetracycline hydrochloride* produces lower blood levels than oral administration in the recommended dosages. Patients placed on intramuscular tetracyclines should be changed to the oral dosage form as soon as possible. If rapid, high blood levels are needed, ACHROMYCIN should be administered intravenously.

Administration: ACHROMYCIN Intramuscular should be injected deeply into a large muscle mass such as the gluteal region. Inadvertent injection into the subcutaneous or fat layers may cause pain and induration, which can be relieved by applying an ice pack.

INTRAVENOUS:

Preparation of Solution: The vials should be initially reconstituted by adding 5 ml. of Sterile Water for Injection to the 250 mg. vial and 10 ml. of Sterile Water for Injection to the 500 mg. vial, and then further diluted prior to administration to at least 100 ml. (up to 1000 ml.) with any of the following diluents:

Ringer's Injection, U.S.P.
Sodium Chloride Injection, U.S.P.
Dextrose Injection, U.S.P. (5% Dextrose in Sterile Water for Injection, U.S.P.)
Dextrose and Sodium Chloride Injection, U.S.P. (5% in Sodium Chloride Injection U.S.P.)
Lactated Ringer's Injection, U.S.P.
Protein Hydrolysate Injection, Low Sodium, U.S.P. 5%, 5% with Dextrose 5%, 5% with Invert Sugar 10%

The initial reconstituted solutions are stable at room temperature for twelve hours without significant loss of potency. The final dilution for administration should be administered immediately.

Note: The use of solutions containing calcium should be avoided as these tend to form precipitates (especially in neutral to alkaline solution) and, therefore, should not be used unless necessary. However, Ringer's Injection, U.S.P. and Lactated Ringer's Injection, U.S.P. can be used with caution since the calcium ion content in these diluents does not normally precipitate tetracycline in an acid media.

Dosage and Administration:

Note: Rapid administration is to be avoided. Parenteral therapy is indicated only when oral therapy is not adequate or tolerated. Oral therapy should be instituted as soon as possible. If intravenous therapy is given over prolonged periods of time, thrombophlebitis may result.

Adults: The usual adult dose: 250 to 500 mg. every 12 hours and should not exceed 500 mg. every 6 hours. The drug may be dissolved and then diluted in 100-1,000 ml. of Dextrose 5 percent in water, Isotonic Sodium Chloride Solution or Ringer's solution, but not in other solutions containing calcium (a precipitate may form).

For children above eight years of age: The usual dose: 12 mg./kg./day, divided into 2 doses, but from 10 to 20 mg./kg./day may be given, depending on the severity of the infection.

Gonorrhea patients sensitive to penicillin may be treated with tetracycline administered as an initial oral dose of 1.5 grams followed by 0.5 grams every 6 hours for 4 days, a total dosage of 9 grams. Intravenous therapy should be reserved for situations in which oral therapy is not feasible.

In patients with renal impairment: (See "Warnings".)

Total dosage should be decreased by reduction of recommended individual doses and/or by extending time intervals between doses.

How Supplied:

CAPSULES:

500 mg. Tetracycline HCl (hard shell yellow and blue) bottles of 100 and 1000. Unit Dose 10-10's.

250 mg. Tetracycline HCl (hard shell yellow and blue) bottles of 100, 1000, Unit Dose 10 x 10's, Unit of Issue bottles of 20, 28 and 40.

SYRUP:

Tetracycline equivalent to 125 mg. Tetracycline HCl per teaspoonful (5 ml.). Preserved with Methylparaben 0.12% and Propylparaben 0.03%. Cherry-flavored in bottles of 2 fl. oz. and 16 fl. oz.

INTRAMUSCULAR:

Sterile Tetracycline HCl	100 mg./vial	250 mg./vial
Procaine HCl	40 mg./vial	40 mg./vial
Magnesium Chloride	46.84 mg./vial	46.84 mg./vial
Ascorbic Acid	250 mg./vial packages of 1 and 100 vials.	275 mg./vial packages of 1 and 100 vials.

INTRAVENOUS:

Sterile Tetracycline HCl 250 mg. with 625 mg. ascorbic acid/vial.

Sterile Tetracycline HCl 500 mg. with 1250 mg. ascorbic acid/vial.

A.H.F.S. 8:12.24

ACHROMYCIN® V Capsules:
Military Depot: NSN 6505-00-117-8544

[*Capsules shown in Product Identification Section*]

ACHROMYCIN®
(tetracycline)

is also supplied in a number of other dosage forms and combinations for special purposes (for details of indications, dosage, administration and precautions, see circular in package.)

Continued on next page

The information on each product appearing here is based on labelling effective in August, 1979 and is either the entire official brochure or an accurate condensation therefrom. Official brochures are enclosed in product packages. Information concerning all Lederle products may be obtained from the Medical Department, Lederle Laboratories, Pearl River, New York, 10965.

Lederle—Cont.

ACHROMYCIN ℞
(tetracycline HCl)
Ophthalmic Ointment 1% (sterile)
⅛ oz. tube

ACHROMYCIN
(tetracycline HCl)
3% Ointment
(For topical use)—½ and 1 oz. tubes. ℞ not required.

ACHROMYCIN ℞
(tetracycline HCl)
Ophthalmic Suspension 1% (sterile)
4 ml. plastic dropper bottle.

ACHROSTATIN® V ℞
(tetracycline HCl and nystatin)

Each capsule contains:
Tetracycline HCl....................................250 mg.
Nystatin ....250,000 units
How Supplied: CAPSULES: (hard shell, pink)—bottles of 16 and 100.
[*Shown in Product Identification Section*]

AMICAR® ℞
(aminocaproic acid)
Intravenous, Syrup, and Tablets

Description: AMICAR *aminocaproic acid Lederle* is a monaminocarboxylic acid which acts as an effective inhibitor of fibrinolysis.
Actions: The beneficial fibrinolysis-inhibitory effects of AMICAR appear to be principally via inhibition of plasminogen activator substances and, to a lesser degree, through antiplasmin activity. The drug is absorbed rapidly following oral administration. Whether administered by the oral or intravenous route, a major portion of the compound is recovered unmetabolized in the urine. The renal clearance of AMICAR is high (about 75 percent of the creatinine clearance). Thus the drug is excreted rapidly. After prolonged administration, AMICAR distributes throughout both the extravascular and intravascular compartments of the body and readily penetrates human red blood and other tissue cells.
Indications: AMICAR has proved useful, in many instances, in the treatment of excessive bleeding which results from *systemic hyperfibrinolysis and urinary fibrinolysis.* In life-threatening situations, fresh whole blood transfusions, fibrinogen infusions, and other emergency measures may be required.
Systemic hyperfibrinolysis, a pathological condition, may frequently be associated with *surgical complications* following heart surgery (with or without cardiac bypass procedures) and portacaval shunt; *hematological disorders* such as aplastic anemia, *abruptio placentae, hepatic cirrhosis, neoplastic disease* such as carcinoma of the prostate, lung, stomach, and cervix.
Urinary fibrinolysis, usually a normal physiological phenomenon, may frequently be associated with life-threatening complications following severe trauma, anoxia, and shock. Symptomatic of such complications is *surgical hematuria* (following prostatectomy and nephrectomy) or *non-surgical hematuria* (accompanying polycystic or neoplastic diseases of the genitourinary system).
Contraindications: AMICAR should not be used when there is evidence of an active intravascular clotting process.
Warnings: Safe use of AMICAR has not been established with respect to adverse effects upon fetal development. Therefore, it should not be used in women of childbearing potential and particularly during early pregnancy, unless in the judgment of the physician the potential benefits outweigh the possible hazards.
Precautions: AMICAR *aminocaproic acid* has a very specific action in that it inhibits both plasminogen activator substances and, to a lesser degree, plasmin activity. The drug should NOT be administered without a definite diagnosis, and/or laboratory findings indicative of hyperfibrinolysis (hyperplasminemia).*
The use of AMICAR should be accompanied by tests designed to determine the amount of fibrinolysis present. There are presently available (a) general tests, such as those for the determination of the lysis of a clot of blood or plasma and (b) more specific tests for the study of various phases of fibrinolytic mechanisms. These latter tests include both semi-quantitative and quantitative technics for the determination of profibrinolysin, fibrinolysin, and antifibrinolysin.
Animal experiments indicate particular caution should be taken in administering AMICAR to patients with cardiac, hepatic or renal diseases.
Demonstrable animal pathology in some cases have shown endocardial hemorrhages and myocardial fat degeneration. The use of this drug should thus be restricted to patients in whom the benefit hoped for would outweigh the hazard. Physicians are cautioned in the use of this product because of animal data showing rat teratogenicity and kidney concretions.
Rapid intravenous administration of the drug should be avoided since this may induce hypotension, bradycardia and/or arrhythmia.
One case of *cardiac* and *hepatic lesions* observed in man has been reported. The patient received 2 grams of aminocaproic acid every 6 hours for a total dose of 26 grams. Death was due to continued cerebral vascular hemorrhage. Necrotic changes in the heart and liver were noted at autopsy.
If it is accepted that fibrinolysis is a normal process, potentially active at all times to ensure the fluidity of blood, then it must also be accepted that inhibition of fibrinolysis by aminocaproic acid *may* result in clotting or thrombosis. However, there is no definite evidence that administration of aminocaproic acid has been responsible for the few reported cases of *intravascular clotting* which followed this treatment. Rather, it appears that such intravascular clotting was most likely a result of the fibrinolytic disease being treated.
It has been postulated that *extravascular clots* formed *in vivo* with incorporated aminocaproic acid may not undergo spontaneous lysis as do normal clots.
Adverse Reactions: Occasionally nausea, cramps, diarrhea, dizziness, tinnitus, malaise, conjunctival suffusion, nasal stuffiness, headache, and skin rash have been reported as results of the administration of aminocaproic acid. Only rarely has it been necessary to discontinue or reduce medication because of one or more of these effects.
Thrombophlebitis, a possibility with all intravenous therapy, should be guarded against by strict attention to the proper insertion of the needle and the fixing of its position.
Dosage and Administration: Initial Therapy—An initial priming dose of 5 grams of AMICAR administered either orally or intravenously followed by 1 to 1¼ gram doses at hourly intervals thereafter should achieve and sustain plasma levels of 0.130 mg./ml. of the drug. This is the concentration apparently necessary for the inhibition of systemic hyperfibrinolysis. Administration of more than 30 grams in any 24-hour period is not recommended.
Intravenous—AMICAR *aminocaproic acid* Intravenous is administered by infusion, utilizing the usual compatible intravenous vehicles (e.g. Sterile Water for Injection, physiologic saline, 5% dextrose or Ringer's solution). RAPID INJECTION OF AMICAR INTRAVENOUS UNDILUTED INTO A VEIN IS NOT RECOMMENDED.
For the treatment of *acute* bleeding syndromes due to elevated fibrinolytic activity, it is suggested that 16 to 20 ml. (4 to 5 grams) of AMICAR Intravenous be administered by infusion during the first hour of treatment, followed by a continuing infusion at the rate of 4 ml. (1.0 gram) per hour. This method of treatment would ordinarily be continued for about 8 hours or until the bleeding situation has been controlled.
Oral Therapy—If the patient is able to take medication by mouth, an identical dosage regimen may be followed by administering AMICAR Tablets or 25% Syrup as follows: For the treatment of *acute* bleeding syndromes due to elevated fibrinolytic activity, it is suggested that 10 tablets (5 grams) or 4 teaspoonfuls of syrup (5 grams) of AMICAR be administered during the first hour of treatment, followed by a continuing rate of 2 tablets (1 gram) or 1 teaspoonful of syrup (1¼ grams) per hour. This method of treatment would ordinarily be continued for about 8 hours or until the bleeding situation has been controlled.
How Supplied:
AMICAR *Lederle Intravenous*
Each 20 ml vial contains 5.0 Grams of Aminocaproic Acid (250 mg per ml) as an aqueous solution, with 0.9% benzyl alcohol as a preservative. The pH is adjusted to approx. 6.8 with Hydrochloric Acid. 20 cc vials.
Also Available:
AMICAR *Lederle 25% Syrup*
Each ml of raspberry flavored syrup contains 250 mg of Aminocaproic Acid with 0.1% Sodium Benzoate and 0.2% Potassium Sorbate as preservative. 16 Fl. Oz. bottles.
AMICAR *Lederle Tablets*
Each tablet contains 500 mg of Aminocaproic Acid. Bottles of 100.
A.H.F.S. 20:12.16
Intravenous
Military Depot NSN 6505-00-926-1442
V.A. Depot System NSN 6505-00-926-1442A

*Stefanini, M. and Dameshek, W.: The Hemorrhagic Disorders, Ed. 2, New York, Grune and Stratton, pp. 510–514, 1962.

ARISTOCORT® ℞
(triamcinolone)
TABLETS
ARISTOCORT®
(triamcinolone diacetate)
SYRUP

Description: ARISTOCORT *triamcinolone* is a synthetic adrenocorticosteroid. The tablets contain Triamcinolone, 9α-fluoro-16α-hydroxyprednisolone, Syrup contains Triamcinolone Diacetate, 9α-fluoro-16α-hydroxyprednisolone diacetate. It is readily absorbed from the gastrointestinal tract.
Action: ARISTOCORT is primarily glucocorticoid in action and has potent anti-inflammatory, hormonal and metabolic effects common to cortisone-like drugs. It is essentially devoid of mineralocorticoid activity when administered in therapeutic doses, causing little or no sodium retention, with potassium excretion minimal or absent. The body's immune responses to diverse stimuli is also modified by its action.
Indications:
1. Endocrine Disorders:
Primary or secondary adrenocortical insufficiency (hydrocortisone or cortisone is the first choice; synthetic analogs may be used in conjunction with mineralocorticoids where applicable. In infancy mineralocorticoid supplementation is of particular importance).
Congenital adrenal hyperplasia.
Nonsuppurative thyroiditis.
Hypercalcemia associated with cancer.
2. Rheumatic Disorders:
As adjunctive therapy for short-term administration (to tide the patient over an acute episode or exacerbation) in:

Psoriatic arthritis.
Rheumatoid arthritis including juvenile rheumatoid arthritis (selected cases may require low-dose maintenance therapy).
Ankylosing spondylitis.
Acute and subacute bursitis.
Acute nonspecific tenosynovitis.
Acute gouty arthritis.
Post-traumatic osteoarthritis.
Synovitis of osteoarthritis.
Epicondylitis.

3. Collagen Diseases:
During an exacerbation or as maintenance therapy in selected cases of—
Systemic lupus erythematosus.
Acute rheumatic carditis.

4. Dermatologic Diseases:
Pemphigus.
Bullous dermatitis herpetiformis.
Severe erythema multiforme (Stevens-Johnson syndrome).
Exfoliative dermatitis.
Mycosis fungoides.
Severe psoriasis.
Severe seborrheic dermatitis.

5. Allergic States:
Control of severe or incapacitating allergic conditions intractable to adequate trials of conventional treatment:
Seasonal or perennial allergic rhinitis.
Bronchial asthma.
Contact dermatitis.
Atopic dermatitis.
Serum sickness.
Drug hypersensitivity reactions.

6. Ophthalmic Diseases:
Severe acute and chronic allergic and inflammatory processes involving the eye and its adnexa such as—
Allergic conjunctivitis.
Keratitis.
Allergic corneal marginal ulcers.
Herpes zoster ophthalmicus.
Iritis and iridocyclitis.
Chorioretinitis.
Anterior segment inflammation.
Diffuse posterior uveitis and choroiditis.
Optic neuritis.
Sympathetic ophthalmia.

7. Respiratory Diseases:
Symptomatic sarcoidosis.
Loeffler's syndrome not manageable by other means.
Berylliosis.
Fulminating or disseminated pulmonary tuberculosis when used concurrently with appropriate antituberculous chemotherapy.
Aspiration pneumonitis.

8. Hematologic Disorders:
Idiopathic thrombocytopenic purpura in adults.
Secondary thrombocytopenia in adults.
Acquired (autoimmune) hemolytic anemia.
Erythroblastopenia (RBC anemia).
Congenital (erythroid) hypoplastic anemia.

9. Neoplastic Diseases:
For palliative management of:
Leukemias and lymphomas in adults.
Acute leukemia of childhood.

10. Edematous States:
To induce a diuresis or remission of proteinuria in the nephrotic syndrome, without uremia, of the idiopathic type or that due to lupus erythematosus.

11. Gastrointestinal Diseases:
To tide the patient over a critical period of the disease in:
Ulcerative Colitis.
Regional enteritis.

12. Nervous System:
Acute exacerbations of multiple sclerosis.

13. Miscellaneous:
Tuberculous meningitis with subarachnoid block or impending block when used concurrently with appropriate antituberculous chemotherapy.
Trichinosis with neurologic or myocardial involvement.

Contraindications:
Systemic fungal infections.
Sensitivity to the drug or any of its components.

Warnings: In patients on corticosteroid therapy subjected to unusual stress, increased dosage of rapidly acting corticosteroids before, during, and after the stressful situation is indicated.

Corticosteroids may mask some signs of infection, and new infections may appear during their use. There may be decreased resistance and inability to localize infection when corticosteroids are used.

Prolonged use of corticosteroids may produce posterior subcapsular cataracts, glaucoma with possible damage to the optic nerves, and may enhance the establishment of secondary ocular infections due to fungi or viruses.

Usage in pregnancy: Since adequate human reproduction studies have not been done with corticosteroids, the use of these drugs in pregnancy, nursing mothers or women of childbearing potential requires that the possible benefits of the drug be weighed against the potential hazards to the mother and embryo or fetus. Infants born of mothers who have received substantial doses of corticosteroids during pregnancy should be carefully observed for signs of hypoadrenalism.

Average and large doses of hydrocortisone or cortisone can cause elevation of blood pressure, salt and water retention, and increased excretion of potassium. These effects are less likely to occur with ARISTOCORT *triamcinolone* except when used in large doses. Dietary salt restriction and potassium supplementation may be necessary. All corticosteroids increase calcium excretion.

While on Corticosteroid Therapy Patients Should Not Be Vaccinated Against Smallpox. Other Immunization Procedures Should Not Be Undertaken in Patients Who are on Corticosteroids, Especially on High Dose, Because of Possible Hazards of Neurological Complications and a Lack of Antibody Response.

The use of Triamcinolone in active tuberculosis should be restricted to those cases of fulminating or disseminated tuberculosis in which the corticosteroid is used for the management of the disease in conjunction with an appropriate antituberculous regimen.

If corticosteroids are indicated in patients with latent tuberculosis or tuberculin reactivity, close observation is necessary as reactivation of the disease may occur. During prolonged corticosteroid therapy, these patients should receive chemoprophylaxis.

Precautions: Drug-induced secondary adrenocortical insufficiency may be minimized by gradual reduction of dosage. This type of relative insufficiency may persist for months after discontinuation of therapy; therefore, in any situation of stress occurring during that period, hormone therapy should be reinstituted. Since mineralocorticoid secretion may be impaired, salt and/or a mineralocorticoid should be administered concurrently.

There is an enhanced effect of corticosteroids on patients with hypothyroidism and in those with cirrhosis.

Corticosteroids should be used cautiously in patients with ocular herpes simplex because of possible corneal perforation.

The lowest possible dose of corticosteroid should be used to control the condition under treatment, and when reduction in dosage is possible, the reduction should be gradual.

Psychic derangements may appear when corticosteroids are used, ranging from euphoria, insomnia, mood swings, personality changes, and severe depression, to frank psychotic manifestations. Also, existing emotional instability or psychotic tendencies may be aggravated by corticosteroids.

Aspirin should be used cautiously in conjunction with corticosteroids in hypoprothrombinemia.

Steroids should be used with caution in nonspecific ulcerative colitis if there is a probability of impending perforation, abscess or other pyogenic infection; diverticulitis; fresh intestinal anastomoses; active or latent peptic ulcer; renal insufficiency; hypertension; osteoporosis; and myasthenia gravis.

Growth and development of infants and children on prolonged corticosteroid therapy should be carefully observed.

Although controlled clinical trials have shown corticosteroids to be effective in speeding the resolution of acute exacerbations of multiple sclerosis they do not show that they affect the ultimate outcome or natural history of the disease. The studies do show relatively high doses of corticosteroids are necessary to demonstrate a significant effect. (See Dosage and Administration).

Since complications of treatment with glucocorticoid are dependent on the size of the dose and the duration of treatment a risk benefit decision must be made in each individual case as to dose and duration of treatment and as to whether daily or intermittent therapy should be used.

Adverse Reactions:

Fluid and Electrolyte Disturbances.
Sodium retention.
Fluid retention.
Congestive heart failure in susceptible patients.
Potassium loss.
Hypokalemic alkalosis.
Hypertension.

Musculoskeletal.
Muscle weakness.
Steroid myopathy.
Loss of muscle mass.
Osteoporosis.
Vertebral compression fractures.
Aseptic necrosis of femoral and humeral heads.
Pathologic fracture of long bones.

Gastrointestinal.
Peptic ulcer with possible perforation and hemorrhage.
Pancreatitis.
Abdominal distention.
Ulcerative esophagitis.

Dermatologic.
Impaired wound healing.
Thin fragile skin.
Petechiae and ecchymoses.
Facial erythema.
Increased sweating.
May suppress reactions to skin tests.

Neurological.
Convulsions.
Increased intracranial pressure with papilledema (pseudo-tumor cerebri) usually after treatment.
Vertigo.
Headache.

Endocrine.
Menstrual irregularities.
Development of Cushingoid state.
Suppression of growth in children.
Secondary adrenocortical and pituitary unresponsiveness, particularly in times of stress, as in trauma, surgery or illness.

Continued on next page

The information on each product appearing here is based on labelling effective in August, 1979 and is either the entire official brochure or an accurate condensation therefrom. Official brochures are enclosed in product packages. Information concerning all Lederle products may be obtained from the Medical Department, Lederle Laboratories, Pearl River, New York, 10965.

Lederle—Cont.

Decreased carbohydrate tolerance.
Manifestations of latent diabetes mellitus.
Increased requirements for insulin or oral hypoglycemic agents in diabetics.

Ophthalmic.
Posterior subcapsular cataracts.
Increased intraocular pressure.
Glaucoma.
Exophthalmos.

Metabolic.
Negative nitrogen balance due to protein catabolism.

Dosage and Administration:

General Principles:

1. The initial dosage of ARISTOCORT *triamcinolone* may vary from 4 mg. to 48 mg. per day depending on the specific disease entity being treated. In situations of less severity lower doses will generally suffice while in selected patients higher initial doses may be required. The initial dosage should be maintained or adjusted until a satisfactory response is noted. If after a reasonable period of time there is a lack of satisfactory clinical response, the drug should be discontinued and the patient transferred to other appropriate therapy. *IT SHOULD BE EMPHASIZED THAT DOSAGE REQUIREMENTS ARE VARIABLE AND MUST BE INDIVIDUALIZED ON THE BASIS OF THE DISEASE UNDER TREATMENT AND THE RESPONSE OF THE PATIENT.* After a favorable response is noted, the proper maintenance dosage should be determined by decreasing the initial drug dosage in small increments at appropriate time intervals until the lowest dosage which will maintain an adequate clinical response is reached. It should be kept in mind that constant monitoring is needed in regard to drug dosage. Included in the situations which may make dosage adjustments necessary are changes in clinical status secondary to remissions or exacerbations in the disease process, the patient's individual drug responsiveness, and the effect of patient exposure to stressful situations not directly related to the disease entity under treatment; in this latter situation it may be necessary to increase the dosage of ARISTOCORT for a period of time consistent with the patient's condition. If after long-term therapy the drug is to be stopped, it is recommended that it be withdrawn gradually rather than abruptly.
2. Dosage should be individualized according to the severity of the disease and the response of the patient. For infants and children, the recommended dosage should be governed by the same considerations rather than by strict adherence to the ratio indicated by age or body weight.
3. Hormone therapy is an adjunct to, and not a replacement for, conventional therapy.
4. The severity, prognosis and expected duration of the disease and the reaction of the patient to medication are primary factors in determining dosage.
5. If a period of spontaneous remission occurs in a chronic condition, treatment should be discontinued.
6. Blood pressure, body weight, routine laboratory studies, including 2-hour postprandial blood glucose and serum potassium, and a chest X-ray should be obtained at regular intervals during prolonged therapy. Upper GI X-rays are desirable in patients with known or suspected peptic ulcer disease.
7. Suppression of autogenous pituitary function, a common effect of exogenous corticosteroid administration, may be reduced, modified or minimized by revision of dose schedules. The time of maximum corticoid effect is from midnight to 8 a.m. and minimal during the intervening hours. Use of a single daily dose beginning at or after 8 a.m. will be effective in most conditions, will lower corticoid overload and will cause the least interference with the diurnal system of endogenous secretion and hypothalamopituitary-adrenal function; alternate-day dosage in some conditions and intermittent administration in certain severe disorders requiring long-term and/or high dose maintenance levels have proven both clinically effective and less likely to produce adverse reactions. The maximum daily morning dose not associated with lasting adrenocorticoid suppression is 8 mg.
8. *Alternate-Day Therapy.* After the conventional dose has been established, some patients may be maintained on alternate day therapy. It has been shown that the activity of the adrenal cortex varies throughout the day, being greatest from about midnight to 8:00 a.m. Exogenous corticoid suppresses this activity least when given at the time of maximum activity. A 48-hour interval appears to be necessary since shorter intervals are accompanied by adrenal suppression similar to that of conventional daily divided doses. Therefore, with the alternate day dose plan, a total 48-hour requirement is given every other day at 8:00 a.m. As with other regimens, the minimum effective dose level should be sought.
9. *Intermittent-Type Therapy.* An additional modification of corticosteroid usage has been recommended and used for treatment of disorders often requiring long-term administration of medium or high dose range. It is generally recommended that treatment be initiated with a single calculated dose of ARISTOCORT given once daily and continued daily until clinical response is adequate or appropriate. The time of maximum corticoid effect is from midnight to 8 a.m. and minimal during the intervening hours. Therefore, dosage beginning at or after 8 a.m. will offer good effect and lower corticoid overload. Thereafter, the patient is maintained on a calculated single daily dose given each morning for 3-4 consecutive days, followed by a "rest period" of 3 days, during which no corticosteroid is administered. This schedule is continued for as long as therapeutically indicated.

Specific Dosage Recommendations:

1. *Endocrine Disorders:* Wide variation in dosage requirements for the endocrine disorders such as *congenital adrenal hyperplasia, non-suppurative thyroiditis,* and *hypercalcemia associated* with *cancer* precludes specific recommendation except for *adrenocortical insufficiency* where the dose is usually 4-12 mg. daily in addition to mineralocorticoid therapy.
2. *Rheumatic Disorders: Rheumatoid arthritis; acute gouty arthritis; ankylosing spondylitis;* and *selected cases of psoriatic arthritis;* in *acute* and *subacute bursitis;* and in *acute nonspecific tenosynovitis.* The initial suppressive dose of ARISTOCORT in these conditions ranges from 8 mg. to 16 mg. per day, although the occasional patient may require higher doses. Patients may show an early or a delayed effect, characterized by a reduction in the inflammatory reaction and in joint swelling, together with alleviation of pain and stiffness, resulting in an increased range of motion of the affected joints or tissues. Maintenance doses are adjusted to keep symptoms at a level tolerable to the patient. Rapid reduction of the steroid or its abrupt discontinuance may result in recurrence or even exacerbation of signs and symptoms. Short-term administration is desirable as a rule. ARISTOCORT *triamcinolone* is ordinarily administered as a single morning dose daily or on alternate days, depending on the need of the patient. Occasional patients may secure more effective relief on divided daily doses, either 2 to 4 times daily.
3. *Collagen Diseases: Systemic Lupus Erythematosus:* The initial dose is usually 20 mg. to 32 mg. daily continued until the desired response is obtained, when reduced maintenance levels are sought. Patients with more severe symptoms may require higher initial doses, 48 mg. or more daily, and higher maintenance doses. Although some patients with systemic lupus erythematosus appear to have spontaneous remissions or to tolerate the disorder in its milder forms for prolonged periods of time, adjustment of dosage scheduling to reduce adverse suppression of the pituitary-adrenal axis may be useful. Intermittent higher doses may be given daily for 3 or 4 successive days followed by a rest period of several days; this regimen being repeated each week.
Acute Rheumatic Carditis: In severely ill patients with carditis, pericardial effusion and/or congestive heart failure, corticosteroid therapy is effective in the control of the acute and severe inflammatory changes and may be lifesaving. Initial doses of ARISTOCORT may be from 20 mg. to 60 mg. daily, clinical response is usually rapid and the drug can then be reduced. Maintenance therapy should be continued for at least 6 to 8 weeks and is seldom required beyond a period of 3 months. Corticosteroid therapy does not preclude conventional treatment, including antibiotics and salicylization.
4. *Dermatological Disorders: Pemphigus; bullous dermatitis herpetiformis, severe erythema multiforme* (Stevens-Johnson Syndrome); *exfoliative dermatitis;* and *mycosis fungoides.* The initial dose is 8 mg. to 16 mg. daily. In these conditions, as well as in certain allergic dermatoses, *alternate-day* administration has been found effective and apparently less likely to produce adverse side effects.
Severe psoriasis: ARISTOCORT may produce reduction or remission of the disabling skin manifestations following initial doses of 8 mg. to 16 mg. daily. The period of maintenance is dependent on the clinical response. Corticosteroid reduction or discontinuation of therapy should be attempted with caution since relapse may occur and may appear in a more aggravated form, the so-called "rebound phenomenon".
5. *Allergic States:* ARISTOCORT *triamcinolone* is administered in doses of 8 mg. to 12 mg. daily in acute seasonal or perennial *allergic rhinitis.* Intractable cases may require high initial and maintenance doses. In *bronchial asthma,* 8 mg. to 16 mg. daily are usually effective. The usual therapeutic measures for control of bronchial asthma should be carried out in addition to ARISTOCORT therapy. In both allergic rhinitis and bronchial asthma, therapy is directed at alleviation of acute distress and chronic long-term use of corticosteroids is neither desirable nor often essential. In such conditions as *contact dermatitis* and *atopic dermatitis,* topical therapy may be supplemented with short courses of ARISTOCORT by mouth in doses of 8 mg. to 16 mg. daily. In severely ill patients with *serum sickness,* epinephrine may be the drug of choice for immediate therapy, often supplemented by antihistamines. ARISTOCORT is frequently useful as adjunctive treatment in such cases, with the dosage determined by the severity of the disorder, the speed with which therapeutic response is desired and the response of the patient to initial therapy.
6. *Ophthalmological Disease: Allergic conjunctivitis; keratitis; allergic corneal marginal ulcers, iritis* and *iridocyclitis; chorioretinitis; anterior segment inflammation; diffuse posterior uveitis* and *choroiditis; optic neuritis* and *sympathetic ophthalmia.* Initial doses range from 12 mg. to 40 mg. daily depending on the severity of the condition, the nature and degree of involvement of ocular structure, but response is usually rapid and therapy of short-term duration.
7. *Respiratory Diseases: Symptomatic sarcoidosis; Loeffler's Syndrome; berylliosis;* and in certain cases of *fulminating* or *disseminated pulmonary tuberculosis* when concurrently accompanied by appropriate antituberculous chemotherapy. Initial doses are usually in the range of 16 mg. to 48 mg. daily.
8. *Hematologic Disorders: Idiopathic* and *secondary thrombocytopenia* in *adults, acquired*

(autoimmune) hemolytic anemia; erythroblastopenia (RBC anemia); congenital (erythroid) hypoplastic anemia. ARISTOCORT is used to produce a remission of symptoms and may, in some instances, produce an apparent regression of abnormal cellular blood elements to normal states, temporary or permanent. The recommended dose varies between 16 mg. and 60 mg. daily, with reduction after adequate clinical response.

9. *Neoplastic Diseases: Acute leukemia in childhood.* The usual dose of ARISTOCORT is 1 mg. per kilogram of body weight daily, although as much as 2 mg. per kilogram may be necessary. Initial response is usually seen within 6 to 21 days and therapy continued from 4 to 6 weeks.

Acute leukemia and *lymphoma in adults.* The usual dose of ARISTOCORT is 16 mg. to 40 mg. daily, although it may be necessary to give as much as 100 mg. daily in leukemia. ARISTOCORT therapy in these neoplasias is only palliative and not curative. Other therapeutic and supportive measures must be used when appropriate.

10. *Edematous States: Nephrotic Syndrome:* ARISTOCORT may be used to induce a diuresis or remission of proteinuria in the *nephrotic syndrome,* without uremia, of the idiopathic type or that due to *lupus erythematosus.* The average dose is 16 to 20 mg. (up to 48 mg.) daily until diuresis occurs. The diuresis may be massive and usually occurs by the 14th day, but occasionally may be delayed. After diuresis begins it is advisable to continue treatment until maximal or complete chemical and clinical remission occurs, at which time the dosage should be reduced gradually and then discontinued. In less severe cases maintenance dosages of as little as 4 mg. daily may be adequate. Alternatively and when maintenance therapy may be prolonged, ARISTOCORT may be administered on intermittent or alternate-day dose schedules.

11. *Miscellaneous: Tuberculous meningitis:* ARISTOCORT may be useful when accompanied by appropriate antituberculous therapy when there is subarachnoid block or impending block. The average dosage is 32 to 48 mg. daily in either single or divided doses.

[See table above].

	Anti-inflammatory Relative Potency		Frequently Used Tablet Strength (mg)		Tablet × Potency Equivalent Value
Hydrocortisone	1	×	20	=	20
Prednisolone	4	×	5	=	20
ARISTOCORT®					
Triamcinolone	5	×	4	=	20
Dexamethasone	25	×	0.75	=	18.75

How Supplied:
1 mg. Tablets-Scored yellow; bottles of 50.
2 mg. Tablets-Scored pink; bottles of 30, 100.
4 mg. Tablets-Scored white; bottles of 30, 100, 500 and ARISTO-PAK® *triamcinolone* 16's (for 6 days therapy).
8 mg. Tablets-Scored yellow; bottles of 50.
16 mg. Tablets-Scored white; bottles of 30.
Syrup 2 mg./5 ml. triamcinolone diacetate; cherry flavored; bottles of 4 fl. oz. Preservatives: Methylparaben 0.08% and Propylparaben 0.02%.
A.H.F.S. 68:04
[*Tablets, and ARISTO-PAK 4 mg. Shown in Product Identification Section*]

ARISTOCORT® ℞
(triamcinolone acetonide)
Topical Products

[See table below].
ARISTOCORT *triamcinolone acetonide* Topicals contain the highly active steroid, Triamcinolone Acetonide, which is a derivative of triamcinolone.

Actions: Topical steroids are primarily effective because of their anti-inflammatory, antipruritic and vasoconstrictive actions.

Indications: For relief of the inflammatory manifestations of corticosteroid-responsive dermatoses.

Contraindications: Topical steroids are contraindicated in those patients with a history of hypersensitivity to any of the components of the preparation.

Precautions: If irritation develops, the product should be discontinued and appropriate therapy instituted.

In the presence of an infection the use of appropriate antifungal or antibacterial agents should be instituted. If a favorable response does not occur promptly, the corticosteroid should be discontinued until the infection has been adequately controlled.

If extensive areas are treated or if the occlusive technique is used there will be increased systemic absorption of the corticosteroid and suitable precautions should be taken, particularly in children and infants.

Although topical steroids have not been reported to have an adverse effect on human pregnancy, the safety of their uses in pregnant women has not absolutely been established. In laboratory animals, increases in incidence of fetal abnormalities have been associated with exposure of gestating females to topical corticosteroids, in some cases at rather low dosage levels. Therefore, drugs of this class should not be used extensively on pregnant patients, in large amounts, or for prolonged periods of time.

The product is not for ophthalmic use.

Adverse Reactions: The following local adverse reactions have been reported with topical corticosteroids, especially under occlusive dressings.

1. Burning 2. Itching 3. Irritation 4. Dryness 5. Folliculitis 6. Hypertrichosis 7. Acneiform eruptions 8. Hypopigmentation 9. Perioral dermatitis 10. Allergic Contact Dermatitis 11. Maceration of the skin 12. Secondary infection 13. Skin atrophy 14. Striae 15. Miliaria

A.H.F.S. 84:06
[*Shown in Product Identification Section*]

ARISTOCORT® Triamcinolone Acetonide TOPICAL PRODUCTS

	Cream 0.025%	Cream 0.1%	Cream 0.5%	Ointment 0.1%	Ointment 0.5%
Each gram contains Triamcinolone Acetonide	0.25 mg.	1 mg.	5 mg.	1 mg.	5 mg.
Preservatives: Sorbic Acid	0.1%	0.1%	0.1%		
Potassium Sorbate	0.1%	0.1%	0.1%		
Inactive Ingredients:	In a water base: Mono and Diglycerides, Squalane, Polysorbate 80 USP, Cetyl Esters Wax NF, Polysorbate 60, Stearyl Alcohol USP, Tenox II, and Sorbitol Solution USP			white petroleum	
Dosage and Administration	Apply to the affected areas 3 or 4 times daily. The Cream should be rubbed in gently and thoroughly until it disappears.			Apply to the affected areas 3 or 4 times daily.	
How Supplied	15 and 75 gram tubes, 240 gram and 5.25 lb. jars	15 and 75 gram tubes 240 gram and 5.25 lb. jars	15 gram tubes and 240 gram jars	15 and 75 gram tubes, 240 gram and 5 lb. jars	15 gram tubes, 240 gram jars

Suspensions
ARISTOCORT® ℞
(triamcinolone diacetate)
Forte parenteral
Intralesional

NOT FOR INTRAVENOUS USE

FORTE PARENTERAL:

Description: A suspension of 40 mg./ml. of *triamcinolone diacetate* micronized in:

Polysorbate 80 USP	0.20%
Polyethylene Glycol 4000 USP	3%
Sodium Chloride	0.85%
Benzyl Alcohol	0.90%
Water for Injection q.s.	100%

Hydrochloric Acid and Sodium Hydroxide to approx. pH 6

This preparation is a slightly soluble suspension suitable for parenteral administration through a 24-gauge needle (or larger), but NOT suitable for intravenous use. It may be administered by the intramuscular, intra-articular, or intrasynovial routes, depending upon the situation. The response to each glucocorticoid varies considerably with each type of disease indication and each corticosteroid prescribed. Irreversible clumping occurs when product is frozen.

Continued on next page

The information on each product appearing here is based on labelling effective in August, 1979 and is either the entire official brochure or an accurate condensation therefrom. Official brochures are enclosed in product packages. Information concerning all Lederle products may be obtained from the Medical Department, Lederle Laboratories, Pearl River, New York, 10965.

Lederle—Cont.

Chemically Triamcinolone Diacetate NF is Pregna - 1, 4 - diene - 3, 20 - dione, 16, 21-bis-(acetyloxy) - 9 - fluoro-11, 17- dihydroxy-, (11β, 16α) - 9 - Fluoro-11β, 16α, 17,21-tetrahydroxy-pregna-1, 4-diene-3, 20-dione 16, 21-diacetate. Molecular weight is 478.51.

Action: ARISTOCORT is primarily glucocorticoid in action and has potent anti-inflammatory, hormonal and metabolic effects common to cortisone-like drugs. It is essentially devoid of mineralocorticoid activity when administered in therapeutic doses, causing little or no sodium retention, with potassium excretion minimal or absent. The body's immune responses to diverse stimuli is also modified by its action.

Indications: Where oral therapy is not feasible or temporarily desirable in the judgment of the physician, ARISTOCORT *triamcinolone diacetate* FORTE 40 mg./ml. is indicated for intramuscular use as follows:

1. Endocrine disorders.
   Primary or secondary adrenocortical insufficiency (hydrocortisone or cortisone is the drug of choice; synthetic analogs may be used in conjunction with mineralocorticoids where applicable; in infancy, mineralocorticoid supplementation is of particular importance).
   Preoperatively and in the event of serious trauma or illness, in patients with known adrenal insufficiency or when adrenocortical reserve is doubtful.
   Congenital adrenal hyperplasia.
   Nonsuppurative thyroiditis.
   Hypercalcemia associated with cancer.
2. Rheumatic disorders. As adjunctive therapy for short-term administration to tide the patient over an acute episode or exacerbation) in:
   Post-traumatic osteoarthritis.
   Synovitis of osteoarthritis.
   Rheumatoid arthritis including juvenile rheumatoid arthritis (selected cases may require low-dose maintenance therapy).
   Acute and subacute bursitis.
   Epicondylitis.
   Acute nonspecific tenosynovitis.
   Acute gouty arthritis.
   Psoriatic arthritis.
   Ankylosing spondylitis.
3. Collagen diseases. During an exacerbation or as maintenance therapy in selected cases of:
   Systemic lupus erythematosus.
   Acute rheumatic carditis.
4. Dermatologic diseases. Pemphigus.
   Severe erythema multiforme (Stevens-Johnson syndrome).
   Exfoliative dermatitis.
   Bullous dermatitis herpetiformis.
   Severe seborrheic dermatitis.
   Severe psoriasis.
   Mycosis fungoides.
5. Allergic states. Control of severe or incapacitating allergic conditions intractable to adequate trials of conventional treatment in:
   Bronchial asthma.
   Contact dermatitis.
   Seasonal or perennial allergic rhinitis.
   Drug hypersensitivity reactions.
   Urticarial transfusion reactions.
   Atopic dermatitis.
   Serum sickness.
   Acute noninfectious laryngeal edema (epinephrine is the drug of first choice).
6. Ophthalmic diseases. Severe acute and chronic allergic and inflammatory processes involving the eye, such as:
   Herpes zoster ophthalmicus.
   Iritis, iridocyclitis.
   Chorioretinitis.
   Sympathetic ophthalmia.
   Diffuse posterior uveitis and choroiditis.
   Optic neuritis.
   Keratitis.
   Allergic conjunctivitis.
   Allergic corneal marginal ulcers.
7. Gastrointestinal diseases. To tide the patient over a critical period of disease in:
   Ulcerative colitis - (Systemic therapy).
   Regional enteritis - (Systemic therapy).
8. Respiratory diseases.
   Symptomatic sarcoidosis.
   Berylliosis.
   Fulminating or disseminated pulmonary tuberculosis when concurrently accompanied by appropriate antituberculous chemotherapy.
   Aspiration pneumonitis.
   Loeffler's syndrome not manageable by other means.
9. Hematologic disorders.
   Acquired (autoimmune) hemolytic anemia.
   Secondary thrombocytopenia in adults.
   Erythroblastopenia (RBC anemia).
   Congenital (erythroid) hypoplastic anemia.
10. Neoplastic diseases. For palliative management of:
   Leukemias and lymphomas in adults.
   Acute leukemia of childhood.
11. Edematous state. To induce diuresis or remission of proteinuria in the nephrotic syndrome without uremia, of the idiopathic type or that due to lupus erythematosus.
12. Nervous System.
   Acute exacerbations of multiple sclerosis.
13. Miscellaneous. Tuberculosis meningitis with subarachnoid block or impending block when concurrently accompanied by appropriate antituberculous chemotherapy.
   Trichinosis with neurologic or myocardial involvement.

ARISTOCORT *triamcinolone diacetate* FORTE 40 mg./ml. is indicated for intra-articular or soft tissue use as follows:
As adjunctive therapy for short-term administration (to tide the patient over an acute episode or exacerbation) in:
- Synovitis of osteoarthritis.
- Rheumatoid arthritis.
- Acute and subacute bursitis.
- Acute gouty arthritis.
- Epicondylitis.
- Acute nonspecific tenosynovitis.
- Post-traumatic osteoarthritis.

ARISTOCORT FORTE is indicated for intralesional use as follows:
- Keloids
- Localized hypertrophic, infiltrated, inflammatory lesions of: lichen planus, psoriatic plaques, granuloma annulare and lichen simplex chronicus (neurodermatitis).
- Discoid lupus erythematosus.
- Necrobiosis lipoidica diabeticorum.
- Alopecia areata.
- They may also be useful in cystic tumors of an aponeurosis or tendon (ganglia).

INTRALESIONAL:

Description: ARISTOCORT *triamcinolone diacetate,* 9α fluoro 16α hydroxy prednisolone diacetate possesses glucocorticoid properties while being essentially devoid of mineralocorticoid activity thus causing little or no sodium retention.

A suspension of 25 mg./ml. micronized in:

Polysorbate 80 USP	0.20%
Polyethylene Glycol 4000 USP	3%
Sodium Chloride	0.85%
Benzyl Alcohol	0.90%
Water for Injection q.s.	100%

Hydrochloric Acid to approx. pH 6

Chemically triamcinolone diacetate NF is Pregna - 1, 4 - diene - 3, 20 - dione, 16, 21 - bis-(acetyloxy) - 9 - fluoro - 11, 17-dihydroxy-,(11β, 16α)- or 9-Fluoro-11β, 16α, 17, 21-tetrahydroxypregna-1, 4-diene-3,20-dione 16,21-diacetate. Molecular weight is 478.51.

Actions: Naturally occurring glucocorticoids (hydrocortisone), which also have salt-retaining properties, are used as replacement therapy in adrenocortical deficiency states. Their synthetic analogs are primarily used for their potent anti-inflammatory effects in disorders of many organ systems.
Glucocorticoids cause profound and varied metabolic effects. In addition, they modify the body's immune responses to diverse stimuli.

Indications: ARISTOCORT INTRALESIONAL is indicated by the intralesional route for: Keloids
- Localized hypertrophic, infiltrated, inflammatory lesions of:
- lichen planus, psoriatic plaques, granuloma annulare and lichen simplex chronicus (neurodermatitis).
- Discoid lupus erythematosus.
- Necrobiosis lipoidica diabeticorum.
- Alopecia areata.

It may also be useful in cystic tumors of an aponeurosis or tendon (ganglia).
When used intra-articularly it is also indicated for:
Adjunctive therapy for short-term administration (to tide the patient over an acute episode or exacerbation) in:
- Synovitis of osteoarthritis.
- Rheumatoid arthritis.
- Acute and subacute bursitis.
- Acute gouty arthritis.
- Epicondylitis.
- Acute nonspecific tenosynovitis.
- Post-traumatic osteoarthritis.

FORTE AND INTRALESIONAL:

Contraindications: Systemic fungal infections.

Warnings: In patients on corticosteroid therapy subjected to any unusual stress, increased dosage of rapidly acting corticosteroids before, during, and after the stressful situation is indicated.
Corticosteroids may mask some signs of infection, and new infections may appear during their use. There may be decreased resistance and inability to localize infection when corticosteroids are used.
Prolonged use of corticosteroids may produce posterior subcapsular cataracts, glaucoma with possible damage to the optic nerves, and may enhance the establishment of secondary ocular infections due to fungi or viruses.

Usage in pregnancy

Since adequate human reproduction studies have not been done with corticosteroids, the use of these drugs in pregnancy, nursing mothers, or women of childbearing potential requires that the possible benefits of the drug be weighed against the potential hazards to the mother and embryo or fetus. Infants born of mothers who have received substantial doses of corticosteroids during pregnancy should be carefully observed for signs of hypoadrenalism.
Average and large doses of cortisone or hydrocortisone can cause elevation of blood pressure, salt and water retention, and increased excretion of potassium. These effects are less likely to occur with the synthetic derivatives except when used in large doses. Dietary salt restriction and potassium supplementation may be necessary. All corticosteroids increase calcium excretion.
While on Corticosteroid Therapy Patients Should Not Be Vaccinated Against Smallpox. Other Immunization Procedures Should Not Be Undertaken in Patients Who Are on Corticosteroids, Especially in High Doses, Because of Possible Hazards of Neurological Complications and Lack of Antibody Response.
The use of ARISTOCORT *triamcinolone diacetate* in active tuberculosis should be restricted to those cases of fulminating or disseminated tuberculosis in which the corticosteroid is used for the management of the disease in conjunc-

tion with appropriate antituberculous regimen.
If corticosteroids are indicated in patients with latent tuberculosis or tuberculin reactivity, close observation is necessary as reactivation of the disease may occur. During prolonged corticosteroid therapy, these patients should receive chemoprophylaxis.
Because rare instances of anaphylactoid reactions have occurred in patients receiving parenteral corticosteroid therapy, appropriate precautionary measures should be taken prior to administration, especially when the patient has a history of allergy to any drug.
Postinjection flare (following intra-articular) and Charcot-like arthropathy have been associated with parenteral corticosteroid therapy.
Intralesional or Sublesional injection of excessive dosage whether by single or multiple injection into any given area may cause cutaneous or subcutaneous atrophy.

Precautions: Drug-induced secondary adrenocortical insufficiency may be minimized by gradual reduction of dosage. This type of relative insufficiency may persist for months after discontinuation of therapy; therefore, in any situation of stress occurring during that period, hormone therapy should be reinstituted.
Since mineralocorticoid secretion may be impaired, salt and/or a mineralocorticoid should be administered concurrently.
There is an enhanced effect of corticosteroids in patients with hypothyroidism and in those with cirrhosis.
Corticosteroids should be used cautiously in patients with ocular herpes simplex for fear of corneal perforation.
The lowest possible dose of corticosteroid should be used to control the condition under treatment, and when reduction in dosage is possible, the reduction must be gradual.
Psychic derangements may appear when corticosteroids are used, ranging from euphoria, insomnia, mood swings, personality changes, and severe depression to frank psychotic manifestations. Also, existing emotional instability or psychotic tendencies may be aggravated by corticosteroids.
Aspirin should be used cautiously in conjunction with corticosteroids in hypoprothrombinemia.
Steroids should be used with caution in nonspecific ulcerative colitis, if there is a probability of impending perforation, abscess or other pyogenic infection, also in diverticulitis, fresh intestinal anastomoses, active or latent peptic ulcer, renal insufficiency, hypertension, osteoporosis, and myasthenia gravis.
Growth and development of infants and children on prolonged corticosteroid therapy should be carefully followed.
The following additional precautions apply for parenteral corticosteroids. Intra-articular injection of a corticosteroid may produce systemic as well as local effects.
Appropriate examination of any joint fluid present is necessary to exclude a septic process.
A marked increase in pain accompanied by local swelling, further restriction of joint motion, fever, and malaise are suggestive of septic arthritis. If this complication occurs and the diagnosis of sepsis is confirmed, appropriate antimicrobial therapy should be instituted.
Local injection of a steroid into a previously infected joint is to be avoided.
Corticosteroids should not be injected into unstable joints.
The slower rate of absorption by intramuscular administration should be recognized.
Routine laboratory studies, such as urinalysis, two-hour postprandial blood sugar, determination of blood pressure and body weight, and a chest x-ray should be made at regular intervals during prolonged therapy. Upper GI x-rays are desirable in patients with an ulcer history or significant dyspepsia.
Accidental injection into soft tissue during intra-articular administration decreases local effectiveness in the joint and, by increasing rate of absorption, may produce systemic effects.
Although controlled clinical trials have shown corticosteroids to be effective in speeding the resolution of acute exacerbations of multiple sclerosis they do not show that they affect the ultimate outcome or natural history of the disease. The studies do show that relatively high doses of corticosteroids are necessary to demonstrate a significant effect. (See Dosage and Administration).
Since complications of treatment with glucocorticoid are dependent on the size of the dose and the duration of treatment a risk/benefit decision must be made in each individual case as to dose and duration of treatment and as to whether daily or intermittent therapy should be used.

Adverse Reactions:
Fluid and electrolyte disturbances:
- Sodium retention.
- Fluid retention.
- Congestive heart failure in susceptible patients.
- Potassium loss.
- Hypokalemic alkalosis.
- Hypertension.

Musculoskeletal:
- Muscle weakness.
- Steroid myopathy.
- Loss of muscle mass.
- Osteoporosis.
- Vertebral compression fractures.
- Aseptic necrosis of femoral and humeral heads.
- Pathologic fracture of long bones.

Gastrointestinal:
- Peptic ulcer with possible subsequent perforation and hemorrhage.
- Pancreatitis.
- Abdominal distention.
- Ulcerative esophagitis.

Dermatologic:
- Impaired wound healing.
- Thin fragile skin.
- Petechiae and ecchymoses.
- Facial erythema.
- Increased sweating.
- May suppress reactions to skin tests.

Neurological:
- Increased intracranial pressure with papilledema (pseudotumor cerebri) usually after treatment.
- Convulsions.
- Vertigo.
- Headache.

Endocrine:
- Menstrual irregularities.
- Development of Cushingoid state.
- Suppression of growth in children.
- Secondary adrenocortical and pituitary unresponsiveness, particularly in times of stress, as in trauma, surgery, or illness.
- Decreased carbohydrate tolerance.
- Manifestations of latent diabetes mellitus.
- Increased requirements for insulin or oral hypoglycemic agents in diabetics.

Ophthalmic:
- Posterior subcapsular cataracts.
- Increased intraocular pressure.
- Glaucoma.
- Exophthalmos.

Metabolic:
- Negative nitrogen balance due to protein catabolism.

The following additional adverse reactions are related to parenteral and intralesional corticosteroid therapy:
- Rare instances of blindness associated with intralesional therapy around the orbit or intranasally.
- Hyperpigmentation or hypopigmentation.
- Subcutaneous and cutaneous atrophy.
- Sterile abscess.

Dosage and Administration:
General
The initial dosage of ARISTOCORT *triamcinolone diacetate* may vary from 3 to 48 mg. per day depending on the specific disease entity being treated. In situations of less severity, lower doses will generally suffice while in selected patients higher initial doses may be required. Usually the parenteral dosage ranges are one-third to one-half the oral dose given every 12 hours. However, in certain overwhelming, acute, life-threatening situations, administration in dosages exceeding the usual dosages may be justified and may be in multiples of the oral dosages.
The initial dosage should be maintained or adjusted until a satisfactory response is noted. If after a reasonable period of time there is a lack of satisfactory clinical response, ARISTOCORT *triamcinolone diacetate* should be discontinued and the patient transferred to other appropriate therapy. It Should Be Emphasized That Dosage Requirements Are Variable and Must Be Individualized on the Basis of the Disease Under Treatment and the Response of the Patient. After a favorable response is noted, the proper maintenance dosage should be determined by decreasing the initial drug dosage in small increments at appropriate time intervals until the lowest dosage which will maintain an adequate clinical response is reached. It should be kept in mind that constant monitoring is needed in regard to drug dosage. Included in the situations which may make dosage adjustments necessary are changes in clinical status secondary to remissions or exacerbations in the disease process, the patient's individual drug responsiveness, and the effect of patient exposure to stressful situations not directly related to the disease entity under treatment; in this latter situation, it may be necessary to increase the dosage of ARISTOCORT *triamcinolone diacetate* for a period of time consistent with the patient's condition. If after long-term therapy the drug is to be stopped, it is recommended that it be withdrawn gradually rather than abruptly.
For intra-articular, intralesional and soft tissue use, a lesser initial dosage range of Triamcinolone Diacetate may produce the desired effect when the drug is administered to provide a localized concentration. The site of the injection and the volume of the injection should be carefully considered when Triamcinolone Diacetate is administered for this purpose.
Specific
Forte:
ARISTOCORT FORTE Parenteral is a suspension of 40 mg./ml. of *triamcinolone diacetate*. The full-strength suspension may be employed. If preferred, the suspension may be diluted with normal saline or water. The diluent may also be prepared by mixing equal parts of normal saline and 1% procaine hydrochloride or other similar local anesthetic. The use of diluents containing preservatives such as methylparaben, propylparaben, phenol, etc. must be avoided as these preparations tend to cause flocculation of the steroid. These dilutions retain full potency for at least one week. Topical ethyl chloride spray may be used locally prior to injection.
Intramuscular: Although ARISTOCORT FORTE Parenteral may be administered intra-

Continued on next page

The information on each product appearing here is based on labelling effective in August, 1979 and is either the entire official brochure or an accurate condensation therefrom. Official brochures are enclosed in product packages. Information concerning all Lederle products may be obtained from the Medical Department, Lederle Laboratories, Pearl River, New York, 10965.

Lederle—Cont.

muscularly for initial therapy, most physicians prefer to adjust the dose orally until adequate control is attained. Intramuscular administration provides a sustained or depot action which can be used to supplement or replace initial oral therapy. With intramuscular therapy, greater supervision of the amount of steroid used is made possible in the patient who is inconsistent in following an oral dosage schedule. In maintenance therapy, the patient-to-patient response is not uniform and, therefore, the dose must be individualized for optimal control.
Although triamcinolone diacetate may possess greater anti-inflammatory potency than many glucocorticoids, this is only dose-related since side effects, such as osteoporosis, peptic ulcer, etc. related to glucocorticoid activity, have not been diminished.
The average dose is 40 mg. (1 ml.) administered intramuscularly once a week for conditions in which anti-inflammatory action is required.
In general, a single parenteral dose 4 to 7 times the oral daily dose may be expected to control the patient from 4 to 7 days up to 3 to 4 weeks. Dosage should be adjusted to the point where adequate but not necessarily complete relief of symptoms is obtained.
Intra-Articular and Intrasynovial: The usual dose varies from 5 to 40 mg. The average for the knee, for example, is 25 mg. The duration of effect varies from one week to 2 months. However, acutely inflamed joints may require more frequent injections.
A lesser initial dosage range of Triamcinolone Diacetate may produce the desired effect when the drug is administered to provide a localized concentration. The site of the injection and the volume of the injection should be carefully considered when Triamcinolone Diacetate is administered for this purpose.
A specific dose depends largely on the size of the joint.
Strict surgical asepsis is mandatory. The physician should be familiar with anatomical relationships as described in standard text books. ARISTOCORT FORTE Parenteral may be used in any accessible joint except the intervertebrals. In general, intrasynovial therapy is suggested under the following circumstances:

1. When systemic steroid therapy is contraindicated because of side effects such as peptic ulcer.
2. When it is desirable to secure relief in one or two specific joints.
3. When good systemic maintenance fails to control flare-ups in a few joints and it is desirable to secure relief without increasing oral therapy.

Such treatment should not be considered to constitute a cure; although this method will ameliorate the joint symptoms, it does not preclude the need for the conventional measures usually employed.
It is suggested that infiltration of the soft tissue by local anesthetic precede intra-articular injection. A 24-gauge or larger needle on a dry syringe may be inserted into the joint and excess fluid aspirated. For the first few hours following injection, there may be local discomfort in the joint but this is usually followed rapidly by effective relief of pain and improvement in local function.
[See table below].

	Anti-inflammatory Relative Potency		Frequently Used Tablet Strength (mg)		Tablet × Potency Equivalent Value
Hydrocortisone	1	×	20	=	20
Prednisolone	4	×	5	=	20
ARISTOCORT® triamcinolone	5	×	4	=	20
Dexamethasone	25	×	0.75	=	18.75

Intralesional
When ARISTOCORT INTRALESIONAL is administered by injection strict aseptic technique is mandatory. Full strength suspensions may be employed, or if preferred, the suspension may be diluted, either to a 1:1 or 1:10 concentration, thus obtaining a working concentration of 12.5 mg./ml. or approximately 2.5 mg./ml. respectively. Normal (isotonic) saline solution alone or equal parts of normal (isotonic saline solution and 1% procaine or other local anesthetics, may be used as diluents. These dilutions usually retain full potency for at least one week. Topical ethyl chloride spray may be used as a local anesthetic. The use of diluents containing preservatives such as methylparaben, propylparaben, phenol, etc. must be avoided as these preparations tend to cause flocculations of the steroid.
Intralesional or Sublesional: For small lesions, injection is usually well tolerated and a local anesthetic is not necessary. The location and type of lesion will determine the route of injection: intralesional, sublesional, intradermal, subdermal, intracutaneous, or subcutaneous. The size of the lesion will determine: the total amount of drug needed, the concentration used, and the number and pattern of injection sites utilized (e.g. from a total of 5 mg. ARISTOCORT INTRALESIONAL in a 2 ml. volume divided over several locations in small lesions, ranging up to 48 mg. total ARISTOCORT INTRALESIONAL for large psoriatic plaques).
Avoid injecting too superficially. In general, no more than 12.5 mg. per injection site should be used. An average of 25 mg. is the usual limit for any one lesion. Large areas require multiple injections with smaller doses per injection.
For a majority of conditions, sublesional injection directly through the lesion into the deep dermal tissue is suggested. In cases where it is difficult to inject intradermally, the suspension may be introduced subcutaneously, as superficially as possible.
Two or three injections at one to two week intervals may suffice as an average course of treatment for many conditions. Within 5-7 days after initial injection involution of the lesion can usually be seen, with pronounced clearing towards normal tissue after 12-14 days. Multiple injections of small amounts of equal strength may be convenient in alopecia areata and in psoriasis where there are large or confluent lesions. This is best accomplished by a series of fan-like injections ½ to 1 inch apart.
Alopecia areata and totalis require an average dose of 25 mg. to 30 mg. in a concentration of 10 mg./ml. subcutaneously 1 to 2 times a week, to stimulate hair regrowth. Results may be expected in 3 to 6 weeks on this dosage, and hair growth may last 3-6 months after initial injection. No more than 0.5 ml. should be given in any one site, because excessive deposition may produce local skin atrophy. Continued periodic local injections may be necessary to maintain response and continued hair growth. Use of more dilute solutions diminish the incidence and degree of local atrophy in the injection site.
In keloids and similar dense scars, injections are usually made directly into the lesion. Injections may be repeated as required, but probably a total of no more than 75 mg. of ARISTOCORT *triamcinolone* a week should be given to any one patient. The need for repeated injections is best determined by clinical response. Remissions may be expected to last from a few weeks up to eleven months.
Intra-articular or Intrasynovial: Strict surgical asepsis is mandatory. The physician should be familiar with anatomical relationships as described in standard text books. A recent paper details the anatomy and the technical approach in arthrocentesis.
It is usually recommended that infiltration by local anesthetic of the soft tissue precede intra-articular injection. A 22-gauge or larger needle on a dry syringe should be inserted into the joint and excess fluid if present should be aspirated. The specific dose depends primarily on the size of the joint. The usual dose varies from 5 mg. to 40 mg. with the average for the knee being 25 mg. Smaller joints as in the fingers require 2 mg. to 5 mg. The duration of effect varies from one week to two months. However, acutely inflamed joints may require more frequent injections. Accidental injection into soft tissue is usually not harmful but decreases the local effectiveness and, because the drug is more rapidly absorbed, may produce a systemic effect. Injection into subcutaneous lipoid tissue may produce "pseudo-atrophy" with a persistent depression of the overlying dermis, lasting several weeks or months.
Administration and dosage of ARISTOCORT INTRALESIONAL must be individualized according to the nature, severity and chronicity of the disease or disorder treated, and should be undertaken with a view of the patient's entire clinical condition. Corticosteroid therapy is considered an adjunct to and not usually a replacement for conventional therapy. Therapy with ARISTOCORT INTRALESIONAL, as with all steroids, is of the suppressive type, related to its anti-inflammatory effect. The dose should be regulated during therapy according to the degree of therapeutic response, and should be reduced gradually to maintenance levels, whereby the patient obtains adequate or acceptable control of symptoms. When such control occurs, consideration should be given to gradual decrease in dosage and eventual cessation of therapy. Remission of symptoms may be due to therapy or may be spontaneous and a therapeutic test of gradual withdrawal of steroid treatment is usually indicated.

How Supplied:
Intralesional: (25 mg./ml.); 5 ml. Vials.
Forte: (40 mg./ml.); 1 ml. and 5 ml. Vials.
A.H.F.S. 68:04
Forte Parenteral:
Military Depot NSN 6505-00-926-9089

ARISTOCORT® A ℞
Triamcinolone Acetonide
Topical Products

[See table on next page].
Actions: Topical steroids are primarily effective because of their anti-inflammatory, antipruritic and vasoconstrictive actions.
Indications: For relief of the inflammatory manifestations of corticosteroid-responsive dermatoses.
Contraindications: Topical steroids are contraindicated in those patients with a history of hypersensitivity to any of the components of the preparation.
Precautions: If irritation develops, the product should be discontinued and appropriate therapy instituted.
In the presence of an infection the use of an appropriate antifungal or antibacterial agent should be instituted. If a favorable response does not occur promptly, the corticosteroid should be discontinued until the infection has been adequately controlled.
If extensive areas are treated or if the occlusive technique is used there will be increased sys-

temic absorption of the corticosteroid and suitable precautions should be taken, particularly in children and infants.

Although topical steroids have not been reported to have an adverse effect on human pregnancy, the safety of their use in pregnant women has not absolutely been established. In laboratory animals, increases in incidence of fetal abnormalities have been associated with exposure of gestating females to topical corticosteroids, in some cases at rather low dosage levels. Therefore, drugs of this class should not be used extensively on pregnant patients, in large amounts, or for prolonged periods of time.

The product is not for ophthalmic use.

Adverse Reactions: The following local adverse reactions have been reported with topical corticosteroids, especially under occlusive dressings.

1. Burning 2. Itching 3. Irritation 4. Dryness 5. Folliculitis 6. Hypertrichosis 7. Acneiform eruptions 8. Hypopigmentation 9. Perioral dermatitis 10. Allergic Contact Dermatitis 11. Maceration of the skin 12. Secondary infection 13. Skin atrophy 14. Striae 15. Miliaria

Military Depots: 0.1% cream, 75 Gm. tube NSN 6505-01-063-3110

VA Depots: 0.1% cream, 75 Gm. tube NSN 6505-00-604-1617A

[*Shown in Product Identification Section*]

	Cream 0.025%	Cream 0.1%	Cream 0.5%	Ointment 0.1%	Ointment 0.5%
Each gram contains Triamcinolone Acetonide	0.25 mg	1 mg	5 mg	1 mg	5 mg
Base	AQUATAIN™ Hydrophilic Base Emulsifying wax NF, isopropyl palmitate, glycerin USP, sorbitol solution USP, lactic acid, 2% benzyl alcohol, purified water. AQUATAIN is non-staining, water-washable, paraben-free, spermaceti-free and has a light texture and consistency.			Emulsifying wax NF, white petrolatum, propylene glycol, Tenox II, lactic acid.	
Dosage and Administration	Apply to affected areas 3 or 4 times daily. The cream should be rubbed in gently and thoroughly until it disappears.			Apply to affected areas 3 or 4 times daily.	
How Supplied	15 and 75 gram tubes	15 and 75 gram tubes, 240 gram jar	15 gram tube, 240 gram jar	15 and 75 gram tubes	15 gram tube

ARISTOSPAN® ℞

(Sterile Triamcinolone Hexacetonide)
Suspension, USP
For Intralesional Administration
5 mg./ml.—Parenteral
For Intra-articular Administration
20 mg./ml.—Parenteral
NOT FOR INTRAVENOUS USE

Description:

Intralesional:

A sterile suspension containing 5 mg./ml. of micronized triamcinolone hexacetonide in the following inactive ingredients:

Polysorbate 80 USP	0.20% w/v
Sorbitol Solution USP	50.00% v/v
Water for Injection qs ad	100.00% V
Preservative:	
Benzyl Alcohol	0.90% w/v

Intra-articular:

A sterile suspension containing 20 mg./ml. of micronized triamcinolone hexacetonide in the following inactive ingredients:

Polysorbate 80 USP	0.40% w/v
Sorbitol Solution USP	50.00% v/v
Water for Injection qs ad	100.00% V
Preservative:	
Benzyl Alcohol	0.90% w/v

The hexacetonide ester of the potent glucocorticoid triamcinolone is relatively insoluble (0.0002% at 25° C. in water). When injected intralesionally, sublesionally, or intra-articularly, it can be expected to be absorbed slowly from the injection site.

Chemically triamcinolone hexacetonide USP is 9-Fluoro-11β, 16α, 17,21-tetrahydroxypregna-1,4-diene-3,20-dione cyclic 16,17-acetal with acetone 21-(3,3-dimethylbutyrate). Molecular weight 532.65.

Actions: Naturally occurring glucocorticoids (hydrocortisone), which also have salt-retaining properties, are used as replacement therapy in adrenocortical deficiency states. Their synthetic analogs are primarily used for their potent anti-inflammatory effects in disorders of many organ systems.

Glucocorticoids cause profound and varied metabolic effects. In addition, they modify the body's immune responses to diverse stimuli.

Indications:

Intralesional or sublesional ARISTOSPAN *sterile triamcinolone hexacetonide suspension* is indicated for the following:

Keloids.
Localized hypertrophic, infiltrated, inflammatory lesions of: lichen planus, psoriatic plaques, granuloma annulare and lichen simplex chronicus (neurodermatitis).
Discoid lupus erythematosus.
Necrobiosis lipoidica diabeticorum.
Alopecia areata.

They may also be useful in cystic tumors of an aponeurosis or tendon (ganglia).

Indications:

Intra-articular:

As adjunctive therapy for short-term administration (to tide the patient over an acute episode or exacerbation) in:

Synovitis of osteoarthritis
Acute and subacute bursitis
Epicondylitis
Posttraumatic osteoarthritis
Rheumatoid arthritis
Acute gouty arthritis
Acute nonspecific tenosynovitis

Contraindications: Systemic fungal infections.

Warnings: In patients on corticosteroid therapy subjected to any unusual stress, increased dosage of rapidly acting corticosteroids before, during, and after the stressful situation is indicated.

Corticosteroids may mask some signs of infection, and new infections may appear during their use. There may be decreased resistance and inability to localize infection when corticosteroids are used.

Prolonged use of corticosteroids may produce posterior subcapsular cataracts, glaucoma with possible damage to the optic nerves and may enhance the establishment of secondary ocular infections due to fungi or viruses.

Usage in pregnancy

Since adequate human reproduction studies have not been done with corticosteroids, the use of these drugs in pregnancy, nursing mothers, or women of childbearing potential requires that the possible benefits of the drug be weighed against the potential hazards to the mother and embryo or fetus.

Infants born of mothers who have received substantial doses of corticosteroids during pregnancy should be carefully observed for signs of hypoadrenalism.

Average and large doses of cortisone or hydrocortisone can cause elevation of blood pressure, salt and water retention, and increased excretion of potassium. These effects are less likely to occur with the synthetic derivatives except when used in large doses. Dietary salt restriction and potassium supplementation may be necessary. All corticosteroids increase calcium excretion.

While on Corticosteroid Therapy Patients Should Not Be Vaccinated Against Smallpox. Other Immunization Procedures Should Not Be Undertaken in Patients Who Are on Corticosteroids, Especially in High Doses, Because of Possible Hazards of Neurological Complications and Lack of Antibody Response.

The use of ARISTOSPAN *sterile triamcinolone hexacetonide suspension* in active tuberculosis should be restricted to those cases of fulminating or disseminated tuberculosis in which the corticosteroid is used for the management of the disease in conjunction with appropriate antituberculous regimen.

If corticosteroids are indicated in patients with latent tuberculosis or tuberculin reactivity, close observation is necessary as reactivation of the disease may occur. During prolonged corticosteroid therapy, these patients should receive chemoprophylaxis.

Because rare instances of anaphylactoid reactions have occurred in patients receiving parenteral corticosteroid therapy, appropriate precautionary measures should be taken prior to administration, especially when the patient has a history of allergy to any drug.

Intralesional or sublesional injection of excessive dosage whether by single or multiple injection into any given area may cause cutaneous or subcutaneous atrophy.

Precautions: Drug-induced secondary adrenocortical insufficiency may be minimized by gradual reduction of dosage. This type of relative insufficiency may persist for months after discontinuation of therapy; therefore, in any situation of stress occurring during that period, hormone therapy should be reinstituted.

Since mineralocorticoid secretion may be impaired, salt and/or a mineralocorticoid should be administered concurrently.

There is an enhanced effect of corticosteroids in patients with hypothyroidism and in those with cirrhosis.

Continued on next page

The information on each product appearing here is based on labelling effective in August, 1979 and is either the entire official brochure or an accurate condensation therefrom. Official brochures are enclosed in product packages. Information concerning all Lederle products may be obtained from the Medical Department, Lederle Laboratories, Pearl River, New York, 10965.

Lederle—Cont.

Corticosteroids should be used cautiously in patients with ocular herpes simplex for fear of corneal perforation.
The lowest possible dose of corticosteroid should be used to control the condition under treatment, and when reduction in dosage is possible, the reduction must be gradual.
Psychic derangements may appear when corticosteroids are used, ranging from euphoria, insomnia, mood swings, personality changes, and severe depression to frank psychotic manifestations. Also, existing emotional instability or psychotic tendencies may be aggravated by corticosteroids.
Aspirin should be used cautiously in conjunction with corticosteroids in hypoprothrombinemia.
Steroids should be used with caution in nonspecific ulcerative colitis, if there is a probability of impending perforation, abscess or other pyogenic infection, also in diverticulitis, fresh intestinal anastomoses, active or latent peptic ulcer, renal insufficiency, hypertension, osteoporosis, and myasthenia gravis.
Growth and development of infants and children on prolonged corticosteroid therapy should be carefully followed.
The following additional precautions apply for parenteral corticosteroids.
Intra-articular injection of a corticosteroid may produce systemic as well as local effects.
Appropriate examination of any joint fluid present is necessary to exclude a septic process..
A marked increase in pain accompanied by local swelling, further restriction of joint motion, fever, and malaise are suggestive of septic arthritis. If this complication occurs and the diagnosis of sepsis is confirmed, appropriate antimicrobial therapy should be instituted.
Local injection of a steroid into a previously infected joint is to be avoided.
Corticosteroids should not be injected into unstable joints.
The slower rate of absorption by intramuscular administration should be recognized.
Routine laboratory studies, such as urinalysis, two-hour postprandial blood sugar, determination of blood pressure and body weight, and a chest X-ray should be made at regular intervals during prolonged therapy. Upper GI X-rays are desirable in patients with an ulcer history or significant dyspepsia.

Adverse Reactions:

Fluid and electrolyte disturbances:
- Sodium retention.
- Fluid retention.
- Congestive heart failure in susceptible patients.
- Potassium loss.
- Hypokalemic alkalosis.
- Hypertension.

Musculoskeletal:
- Muscle weakness.
- Steroid myopathy.
- Loss of muscle mass.
- Osteoporosis.
- Vertebral compression fractures.
- Aseptic necrosis of femoral and humeral heads.
- Pathologic fracture of long bones.

Gastrointestinal:
- Peptic ulcer with possible subsequent perforation and hemorrhage.
- Pancreatitis.
- Abdominal distention.
- Ulcerative esophagitis.

Dermatologic:
- Impaired wound healing.
- Thin fragile skin.
- Petechiae and ecchymoses.
- Facial erythema.
- Increased sweating.
- May suppress reactions to skin tests.

Neurological:
- Convulsions
- Increased intracranial pressure with papilledema (pseudotumor cerebri) usually after treatment.
- Vertigo.
- Headache.

Endocrine:
- Menstrual irregularities.
- Development of Cushingoid state.
- Suppression of growth in children.
- Secondary adrenocortical and pituitary unresponsiveness, particularly in times of stress, as in trauma, surgery, or illness.
- Decreased carbohydrate tolerance.
- Manifestations of latent diabetes mellitus.
- Increased requirements for insulin or oral hypoglycemic agents in diabetics.

Ophthalmic:
- Posterior subcapsular cataracts.
- Increased intraocular pressure.
- Glaucoma.
- Exophthalmos.

Metabolic:
- Negative nitrogen balance due to protein catabolism.

The following additional adverse reactions are related to parenteral and intralesional corticosteroid therapy:
- Rare instances of blindness associated with intralesional therapy around the face and head.
- Hyperpigmentation or hypopigmentation.
- Sterile abscess.
- Charcot-like arthropathy.

Dosage and Administration:

General

The initial dosage of ARISTOPAN *sterile triamcinolone hexacetonide suspension* may vary from 2 to 48 mg. per day depending on the specific disease entity being treated. In situations of less severity, lower doses will generally suffice while in selected patients higher initial doses may be required. Usually the parenteral dosage ranges are one-third to one-half the oral dose given every 12 hours. However, in certain overwhelming, acute, life-threatening situations, administration in dosages exceeding the usual dosages may be justified and may be in multiples of the oral dosages.
The initial dosage should be maintained or adjusted until a satisfactory response is noted. If after a reasonable period of time there is a lack of satisfactory clinical response, ARISTOSPAN should be discontinued and the patient transferred to other appropriate therapy.
It Should Be Emphasized That Dosage Requirements Are Variable and Must Be Individualized on the Basis of the Disease Under Treatment and the Response of the Patient.
After a favorable response is noted, the proper maintenance dosage should be determined by decreasing the initial drug dosage in small increments at appropriate time intervals until the lowest dosage which will maintain an adequate clinical response is reached. It should be kept in mind that constant monitoring is needed in regard to drug dosage. Included in the situations which may make dosage adjustments necessary are changes in clinical status secondary to remissions or exacerbations in the disease process, the patient's individual drug responsiveness, and the effect of patient exposure to stressful situations not directly related to the disease entity under treatment; in this latter situation it may be necessary to increase the dosage of ARISTOSPAN for a period of time consistent with the patient's condition. If after long-term therapy the drug is to be stopped, it is recommended that it be withdrawn gradually rather than abruptly.

Directions for Use

Strict aseptic administration technique is mandatory. Topical ethyl chloride spray may be used locally before injection.
The syringe should be gently agitated to achieve uniform suspension before use. Since ARISTOSPAN suspension has been designed for ease of administration, a small bore needle (25 or 26 gauge) may be used.

Dilution—Intralesional 5 mg./ml.

ARISTOSPAN suspension may be diluted, if desired, with Dextrose and Sodium Chloride Injection USP, (5% and 10% Dextrose), Sodium Chloride Injection USP, or Sterile Water for Injection USP.
The optimum dilution, i.e., 1:1, 1:2, 1:4, should be determined by the nature of the lesion, its size, the depth of injection, the volume needed, and location of the lesion. In general, more superficial injections should be performed with greater dilution. Certain conditions, such as keloids, require a less dilute suspension such as 5 mg./ml., with variation in dose and dilution as dictated by the condition of the individual patient. Subsequent dosage, dilution, and frequency of injections are best judged by the clinical response.
The suspension may also be mixed with 1% or 2% Lidocaine Hydrochloride, using the formulations which do not contain parabens. Similar local anesthetics may also be used. Diluents containing methylparaben, propylparaben, phenol, etc., should be avoided since these compounds may cause flocculation of the steroid. These dilutions will retain full potency for one week, but care should be exercised to avoid contamination of the vial's contents and the dilutions should be discarded after 7 days.

Intralesional or Sublesional

Average Dose—to 0.5 mg. per square inch of affected skin injected intralesionally or sublesionally. The frequency of subsequent injections is best determined by the clinical response. If desired, the vial may be diluted as indicated under DIRECTIONS FOR USE.
A lesser initial dosage range of ARISTOSPAN may produce the desired effect when the drug is administered to provide a localized concentration. The site of the injection and the volume of the injection should be carefully considered when ARISTOSPAN is administered for this purpose.

Dilution—Intra-articular 20 mg./ml.

ARISTOSPAN suspension may be mixed with 1% or 2% Lidocaine Hydrochloride, using the formulations which do not contain parabens. Similar local anesthetics may also be used. Diluents containing methylparaben, propylparaben, phenol, etc., should be avoided since these compounds may cause flocculation of the steroid. These dilutions will retain full potency for one week, but care should be exercised to avoid contamination.

Intra-articular

Average dose—2 to 20 mg. (0.1 ml. to 1.0 ml.) The dose depends on the size of the joint to be injected, the degree of inflammation, and the amount of fluid present. In general, large joints (such as knee, hip, shoulder) require 10 to 20 mg. For small joints (such as interphalangeal, metacarpophalangeal), 2 to 6 mg, may be employed. When the amount of synovial fluid is increased, aspiration may be performed before administering ARISTOSPAN. Subsequent dosage and frequency of injections can best be judged by clinical response.
The usual frequency of injection into a single joint is every three or four weeks, and injection more frequently than that is generally not advisable. To avoid possible joint destruction from repeated use of intra-articular corticosteroids, injection should be as infrequent as possible, consistent with adequate patient care. Attention should be paid to avoiding deposition of drug along the needle path which might produce atrophy.

How Supplied:

Intralesional, 5 ml. (in a 12.5 ml. vial).
Intra-articular, 1 ml. vial and 5 ml. vial.
A.H.F.S. 68:04

Military Depots: 5 ml vial
NSN-6505-00-148-6985
VA Depots: 5 ml vial
NSN-6505-00-148-6985A

ARTANE® ℞
(trihexyphenidyl HCl)
Tablets, Elixir, and SEQUELS®
Sustained Release Capsules

Description: ARTANE *trihexyphenidyl HCl Lederle* is a synthetic antispasmodic drug available in the following forms:
TABLETS: 2 mg. and 5 mg.; scored, white.
ELIXIR: 2 mg./5 ml. in a clear, lime-mint flavored preparation with 0.08% methylparaben, 0.02% propylparaben, and 5% Alcohol as preservatives.
SEQUELS: The 5 mg. Sustained Release Capsules are soft shelled and blue colored, with visible granules, each capsule is compounded to release approximately 1.25 mg. immediately and the remainder gradually over a period of six to eight hours.
Actions: ARTANE *trihexyphenidyl HCl Lederle* is the substituted piperidine salt, 3-(1-piperidyl)-1-phenyl-cyclohexyl-1-propanol hydrochloride, which exerts a direct inhibitory effect upon the parasympathetic nervous system. It also has a relaxing effect on smooth musculature; exerted both directly upon the muscle tissue itself and indirectly through an inhibitory effect upon the parasympathetic nervous system. Its therapeutic properties are similar to those of atropine, although undesirable side effects are ordinarily less frequent and severe than with the latter.
Indications:
This drug is indicated as an adjunct in the treatment of all forms of parkinsonism (postencephalitic, arteriosclerotic, and idiopathic). It is often useful as adjuvant therapy when treating these forms of parkinsonism with levodopa. Additionally, it is indicated for the control of extrapyramidal disorders caused by central nervous system drugs such as the dibenoxazepines, phenothiazines, thioxanthenes, and butyrophenones.
SEQUELS—For maintenance therapy after patients have been stabilized on trihexyphenidyl hydrochloride in conventional dosage forms (tablets or elixir).
Warning: Patients to be treated with ARTANE should have a gonioscope evaluation and close monitoring of intraocular pressures at regular periodic intervals.
Precautions: Although Trihexyphenidyl HCl is *not* contraindicated for patients with cardiac, liver, or kidney disorders, or with hypertension, such patients should be maintained under close observation.
Since the use of Trihexyphenidyl HCl may, in some cases continue indefinitely and since it has atropine-like properties, patients should be subjected to constant and careful long-term observation to avoid allergic and other untoward reactions. Inasmuch as Trihexyphenidyl HCl possesses some parasympatholytic activity, it should be used with caution in patients with glaucoma, obstructive disease of the gastrointestinal or genitourinary tracts, and in elderly males with possible prostatic hypertrophy. Geriatric patients, particularly over the age of 60, frequently develop increased sensitivity to the actions of drugs of this type, and hence, require strict dosage regulation. Incipient glaucoma may be precipitated by parasympatholytic drugs such as Trihexyphenidyl HCl.
Adverse Reactions: Minor side effects, such as dryness of the mouth, blurring of vision, dizziness, mild nausea or nervousness, will be experienced by 30 to 50 per cent of all patients. These sensations, however, are much less troublesome with ARTANE *trihexyphenidyl HCl* than with belladonna alkaloids and are usually less disturbing than unalleviated Parkinsonism. Such reactions tend to become less pronounced, and even to disappear, as treatment continues. Even before these reactions have remitted spontaneously, they may often be controlled by careful adjustment of dosage form, amount of drug, or interval between doses.
Isolated instances of suppurative parotitis secondary to excessive dryness of the mouth, skin rashes, dilatation of the colon, paralytic ileus, and certain psychiatric manifestations such as delusions and hallucinations, plus one doubtful case of paranoia all of which may occur with any of the atropine-like drugs, have been rarely reported with ARTANE.
Patients with arteriosclerosis or with a history of idiosyncrasy to other drugs may exhibit reactions of mental confusion, agitation, disturbed behavior, or nausea and vomiting. Such patients should be allowed to develop a tolerance through the initial administration of a small dose and gradual increase in dose until an effective level is reached. If a severe reaction should occur, administration of the drug should be discontinued for a few days and then resumed at a lower dosage. Psychiatric disturbances can result from indiscriminate use (leading to overdosage) to sustain continued euphoria.
Potential side effects associated with the use of any atropine-like drugs include constipation, drowsiness, urinary hesitancy or retention, tachycardia, dilation of the pupil, increased intraocular tension, weakness, vomiting, and headache.
The occurrence of angle-closure glaucoma due to long-term treatment with trihexyphenidyl hydrochloride has been reported.
Dosage and Administration: Dosage should be individualized. The initial dose should be low and then increased gradually, especially in patients over 60 years of age. Whether ARTANE *trihexyphenidyl HCl* may best be given before or after meals should be determined by the way the patient reacts. Postencephalitic patients, who are usually more prone to excessive salivation, may prefer to take it after meals and may, in addition, require small amounts of atropine which, under such circumstances, is sometimes an effective adjuvant. If ARTANE tends to dry the mouth excessively, it may be better to take it before meals, unless it causes nausea. If taken after meals, the thirst sometimes induced can be allayed by mint candies, chewing gum or water.
ARTANE Trihexyphenidyl HCl in Idiopathic Parkinsonism
As initial therapy for Parkinsonism, 1 mg of ARTANE in tablet or elixir form may be administered the first day. The dose may then be increased by 2 mg increments at intervals of three to five days, until a total of 6 to 10 mg is given daily. The total daily dose will depend upon what is found to be the optimal level. Many patients derive maximum benefit from this daily total of 6 to 10 mg, but some patients, chiefly those in the postencephalitic group, may require a total daily dose of 12 to 15 mg.
ARTANE Trihexyphenidyl HCl in Drug-Induced Parkinsonism
The size and frequency of dose of ARTANE needed to control extrapyramidal reactions to commonly employed tranquilizers, notably the phenothiazines, thioxanthenes, and butyrophenones, must be determined empirically. The total daily dosage usually ranges between 5 and 15 mg although, in some cases, these reactions have been satisfactorily controlled on as little as 1 mg daily. It may be advisable to commence therapy with a single 1 mg dose. If the extrapyramidal manifestations are not controlled in a few hours, the subsequent doses may be progressively increased until satisfactory control is achieved. Satisfactory control may sometimes be more rapidly achieved by temporarily reducing the dosage of the tranquilizer on instituting ARTANE trihexyphenidyl HCl therapy and then adjusting dosage of both drugs until the desired ataractic effect is retained without onset of extrapyramidal reactions.
It is sometimes possible to maintain the patient on a reduced ARTANE dosage after the reactions have remained under control for several days. Instances have been reported in which these reactions have remained in remission for long periods after ARTANE therapy was discontinued.
Concomitant Use of ARTANE Trihexyphenidyl HCl with Levodopa
When ARTANE is used concomitantly with levodopa, the usual dose of each may need to be reduced. Careful adjustment is necessary, depending on side effects and degree of symptom control. ARTANE dosage of 3 to 6 mg daily, in divided doses, is usually adequate.
Concomitant Use of ARTANE Trihexyphenidyl HCl with Other Parasympathetic Inhibitors
ARTANE *trihexyphenidyl HCl* may be substituted, in whole or in part, for other parasympathetic inhibitors. The usual technique is partial substitution initially, with progressive reduction in the other medication as the dose of trihexyphenidyl HCl is increased.
ARTANE TABLETS and ELIXIR—The total daily intake of ARTANE tablets or elixir is tolerated best if divided into 3 doses and taken at mealtimes. High doses (> 10 mg daily) may be divided into 4 parts, with 3 doses administered at mealtimes and the fourth at bedtime.
ARTANE SEQUELS—Because of the relatively high dosage in each controlled release capsule, this dosage form should not be used for initial therapy. After patients are stabilized on trihexyphenidyl HCl in conventional dosage forms (tablet or elixir), for convenience of administration they may be switched to the controlled release capsules on a milligram per milligram total daily dose basis, as a single dose after breakfast or in two divided doses 12 hours apart. Most patients will be adequately maintained on the controlled release form, but some may develop an exacerbation of parkinsonism and have to be returned to the conventional form.
How Supplied:
TABLETS 2 mg
BOTTLES of 100, 1000 and Unit Dose
10 × 10's
TABLETS 5 mg
BOTTLES of 100, 1000 and Unit Dose
10 × 10's
ELIXIR 2mg/5 ml
BOTTLES of 16 fl. oz.
SEQUELS SUSTAINED RELEASE
CAPSULES 5 mg
BOTTLES of 60 and 500
A.H.F.S. 12:08
ELIXIR:
VA Depots NSN 6505-890-1378A
[*Tablets and SEQUELS Shown in Product Identification Section*]

AUREOMYCIN®
(chlortetracycline HCl)
OINTMENT

Description: Each gram contains:
Chlortetracycline HCl 30 mg. (3%)
in a white petrolatum-anhydrous lanolin base.
AUREOMYCIN *chlortetracycline HCl* is one of the most versatile of the broad spectrum antibiotics and is effective against many Gram-positive and Gram-negative organisms, as well as rickettsial, viral and virus-like infections.
Indications: AUREOMYCIN Ointment, for topical application only, is indicated for the treatment of superficial pyogenic infections of the skin. It is effective against both Gram-positive cocci (streptococci, staphylococci and

Continued on next page

The information on each product appearing here is based on labelling effective in August, 1979 and is either the entire official brochure or an accurate condensation therefrom. Official brochures are enclosed in product packages. Information concerning all Lederle products may be obtained from the Medical Department, Lederle Laboratories, Pearl River, New York, 10965.

Lederle—Cont.

pneumococci) and Gram-negative bacteria (coli-aerogenes group).

Precautions: The use of antibiotics may result in the overgrowth of nonsusceptible organisms. If new infections appear during therapy, appropriate measures should be taken.

If adverse reaction or idiosyncrasy occurs, discontinue medication.

Administration and Dosage: In the treatment of local skin infections, apply the ointment directly to the involved area, preferably on sterile gauze, one or more times daily as the condition warrants. In severe local infection, topical application should be supplemented by oral administration of an appropriate antibiotic.

How Supplied: ½ and 1 oz. tubes. Rx not required.

CENTRUM™
High Potency Multivitamin-Multimineral Formula

Composition: Each tablet contains:

	For Adults, and Children 4 or more years of age.	Percentage of U.S. Recommended Daily Allowance (U.S. RDA)
Vitamin A (as Acetate)	5000 I.U.	(100%)
Vitamin E (as *dl*-Alpha Tocopheryl Acetate)	30 I.U.	(100%)
Vitamin C (as Ascorbic Acid)	90 mg	(150%)
Folic Acid (as Folacin)	400 mcg	(100%)
Vitamin B_1 (as Thiamine Mononitrate)	2.25 mg	(150%)
Vitamin B_2 (as Riboflavin)	2.6 mg	(153%)
Niacinamide	20 mg	(100%)
Vitamin B_6 (as Pyridoxine Hydrochloride)	3 mg	(150%)
Vitamin B_{12} (as Cyanocobalamin)	9 mcg	(150%)
Vitamin D	400 I.U.	(100%)
Biotin	150 mcg	(50%)
Pantothenic Acid (as Calcium Pantothenate)	10 mg	(100%)
Calcium (as Dibasic Calcium Phosphate)	162 mg	(16%)
Phosphorus (as Dibasic Calcium Phosphate)	125 mg	(13%)
Iodine (as Potassium Iodide)	150 mcg	(100%)
Iron (as Ferrous Fumarate)	27 mg	(150%)
Magnesium (as Magnesium Oxide)	100 mg	(25%)
Copper (as Cupric Oxide)	3 mg	(150%)
Manganese (as Manganese Dioxide)	7.5 mg*	
Potassium (as Potassium Sulfate)	7.5 mg*	
Zinc (as Zinc Oxide)	22.5 mg	(150%)

*Recognized as essential in human nutrition, but no U.S. RDA established.

Recommended Intake: Adults, 1 tablet daily.

How Supplied:
Capsule-shaped tablets, light peach, engraved LL
Bottles of 100 tablets
[*Shown in Product Identification Section*]

CHOLERA VACCINE ℞
(India Strains)

How Supplied: 1 ml. vial (1 immunization)
COMPLETE INFORMATION FURNISHED IN THE PACKAGE.

CYCLOCORT® ℞
(amcinonide cream 0.1% with AQUATAIN™ hydrophilic base)

Description: 0.1% topical cream with AQUATAIN™ hydrophilic base:
Each gram of CYCLOCORT topical cream contains 1 mg (0.1%) of the active steroid, amcinonide in AQUATAIN, a specially formulated base composed of emulsifying wax NF, isopropyl palmitate, glycerin USP, sorbitol solution USP, lactic acid, 2% benzyl alcohol and purified water.

Action: Topical steroids are primarily effective because of their anti-inflammatory, antipruritic, and vasoconstrictive actions.

Indications: For relief of the inflammatory manifestations of corticosteroid responsive dermatoses.

Contraindications: Topical steroids are contraindicated in those patients with a history of hypersensitivity to any of the components of the preparation.

Precautions: If irritation develops, the product should be discontinued and appropriate therapy instituted.

In the presence of an infection the use of an appropriate antifungal or antibacterial agent should be instituted. If a favorable response does not occur promptly, the corticosteroid should be discontinued until the infection has been adequately controlled.

If extensive areas are treated or if an occlusive technique is used there will be increased systemic absorption of the corticosteroid and suitable precautions should be taken, particularly in children and infants.

Although topical steroids have not been reported to have an adverse effect on human pregnancy, the safety of their use in pregnant women has not absolutely been established. In laboratory animals, increases in incidence of fetal abnormalities have been associated with exposure of gestating females to topical corticosteroids, in some cases at rather low dosage levels. Therefore, drugs of this class should not be used extensively on pregnant patients, in large amounts, or for prolonged periods of time.

The product is not for ophthalmic use.

Adverse Reactions: The following local adverse reactions have been reported with topical corticosteroids, especially under occlusive dressings: burning, itching, irritation, dryness, folliculitis, hypertrichosis, acneiform eruptions, hypopigmentation, perioral dermatitis, allergic contact dermatitis, maceration of the skin, secondary infection, skin atrophy, striae and miliaria.

Dosage and Administration: Apply a light film to affected areas 2 or 3 times daily. The cream should be rubbed in gently and thoroughly until it disappears.

How Supplied: 0.1% (Product No. 9183) Topical Cream Available in 15 and 60 Gram tubes.

DECLOMYCIN® ℞
(demeclocycline hydrochloride)

Description: DECLOMYCIN *demeclocycline hydrochloride* is an antibiotic isolated from a mutant strain of *Streptomyces aureofaciens.* Chemically it is the hydrochloride of 7-chloro-4-dimethylamino-1, 4, 4a, 5, 5a, 6, 11, 12a-octahydro-3, 6, 10, 12, 12a-pentahydroxy-1, 11-dioxo-2-naphthacenecarboxamide.

Actions: The tetracyclines are primarily bacteriostatic and are thought to exert their antimicrobial effect by the inhibition of protein synthesis. Tetracyclines are active against a wide range of gram-negative and gram-positive organisms.

The drugs in the tetracycline class have closely similar antimicrobial spectra, and cross-resistance among them is common. Micro-organisms may be considered susceptible if the M.I.C. (minimum inhibitory concentration) is not more than 4.0 mcg./ml. and intermediate if the M.I.C. is 4.0 to 12.5 mcg./ml.

Susceptibility plate testing: A tetracycline disc may be used to determine microbial susceptibility to drugs in the tetracycline class. If the Kirby-Bauer method of disc susceptibility testing is used, a 30 mcg. tetracycline disc should give a zone of at least 19 mm. when tested against a tetracycline-susceptible bacterial strain.

Tetracyclines are readily absorbed and are bound to plasma proteins in varying degree. They are concentrated by the liver in the bile and excreted in the urine and feces at high concentrations and in a biologically active form.

Indications: DECLOMYCIN *demeclocycline hydrochloride* is indicated in infections caused by the following micro-organisms:

Rickettsiae: (Rocky Mountain spotted fever, typhus fever and the typhus group, Q fever, rickettsialpox, tick fevers.)
Mycoplasma pneumoniae (PPLO, Eaton agent).
Agents of psittacosis and ornithosis.
Agents of lymphogranuloma venereum and granuloma inguinale.
The spirochetal agent of relapsing fever *(Borrelia recurrentis).*

The following gram-negative micro-organisms:
Haemophilus ducreyi (chancroid),
Pasteurella pestis and *Pasteurella tularensis,*
Bartonella bacilliformis,
Bacteroides species,
Vibrio comma and *Vibrio fetus.*
Brucella species (in conjunction with streptomycin).

Because many strains of the following groups of micro-organisms have been shown to be resistant to tetracyclines, culture and susceptibility testing are recommended.

Demeclocycline is indicated for treatment of infections caused by the following gram-negative micro-organisms, when bacteriologic testing indicates appropriate susceptibility to the drug:
Escherichia coli,
Enterobacter aerogenes (formerly *Aerobacter aerogenes*),
Shigella species,
Mima species and *Herellea* species,
Haemophilus influenzae (respiratory infections),
Klebsiella species (respiratory and urinary infections).

Demeclocycline is indicated for treatment of infections caused by the following gram-positive micro-organisms when bacteriologic testing indicates appropriate susceptibility to the drug:
Streptococcus species:
Up to 44 percent of strains of *Streptococcus pyogenes* and 74 percent of *Streptococcus faecalis* have been found to be resistant to tetracycline drugs. Therefore, tetracyclines should not be used for streptococcal disease unless the organism has been demonstrated to be sensitive.
For upper respiratory infections due to group A beta-hemolytic streptococci, penicillin is the usual drug of choice, including prophyaxis of rheumatic fever.
Diplococcus pneumoniae,
Staphylococcus aureus, skin and soft tissue infections. Tetracyclines are not the drugs of choice in the treatment of any type of staphylococcal infection.

When penicillin is contraindicated, tetracyclines are alternative drugs in the treatment of infections due to:
Neisseria gonorrhoeae,
Treponema pallidum and *Treponema pertenue* (syphilis and yaws),
Listeria monocytogenes,
Clostridium species,
Bacillus anthracis,
Fusobacterium fusiforme (Vincent's infection),
Actinomyces species.

In acute intestinal amebiasis, the tetracyclines may be a useful adjunct to amebicides.
DECLOMYCIN *demeclocycline hydrochloride* is indicated in the treatment of trachoma, although the infectious agent is not always eliminated, as judged by immunofluorescence.
Inclusion conjunctivitis may be treated with oral tetracyclines or with a combination of oral and topical agents.

Contraindications: This drug is contraindicated in persons who have shown hypersensitivity to any of the tetracyclines.
Warnings: THE USE OF DRUGS OF THE TETRACYCLINE CLASS DURING TOOTH DEVELOPMENT (LAST HALF OF PREGNANCY, INFANCY AND CHILDHOOD TO THE AGE OF 8 YEARS) MAY CAUSE PERMANENT DISCOLORATION OF THE TEETH (YELLOW-GRAY-BROWN).
This adverse reaction is more common during long-term use of the drugs but has been observed following repeated short-term courses. Enamel hypoplasia has also been reported. TETRACYCLINE DRUGS, THEREFORE, SHOULD NOT BE USED IN THIS AGE GROUP UNLESS OTHER DRUGS ARE NOT LIKELY TO BE EFFECTIVE OR ARE CONTRAINDICATED.
If renal impairment exists, even usual oral or parenteral doses may lead to excessive systemic accumulation of the drug and possible liver toxicity. Under such conditions, lower than usual total doses are indicated and, if therapy is prolonged, serum level determinations of the drug may be advisable.
Phototoxic reactions can occur in individuals taking demeclocycline, and are characterized by severe burns of exposed surfaces resulting from direct exposure of patients to sunlight during therapy with moderate or large doses of demeclocycline. Patients apt to be exposed to direct sunlight or ultraviolet light should be advised that this reaction can occur, and treatment should be discontinued at the first evidence of skin erythema.
The anti-anabolic action of the tetracyclines may cause an increase in BUN. While this is not a problem in those with normal renal function, in patients with significantly impaired function, higher serum levels of tetracycline may lead to azotemia, hyperphosphatemia, and acidosis.
Administration of demeclocycline has resulted in appearance of the diabetes insipidus syndrome (polyuria, polydipsia and weakness) in some patients on long term therapy. The syndrome has been shown to be nephrogenic, dose-dependent and reversible on discontinuance of therapy.
Usage in pregnancy (See above "Warnings" about use during tooth development.)
Results of animal studies indicate that tetracyclines cross the placenta, are found in fetal tissues and can have toxic effects on the developing fetus (often related to retardation of skeletal development). Evidence of embryotoxicity has also been noted in animals treated early in pregnancy.
Usage in newborns, infants, and children (See above "Warnings" about use during tooth development.)
All tetracyclines form a stable calcium complex in any bone forming tissue. A decrease in the fibula growth rate has been observed in prematures given oral tetracycline in doses of 25 mg./kg. every 6 hours. This reaction was shown to be reversible when the drug was discontinued.
Tetracyclines are present in the milk of lactating women who are taking a drug in this class.
Precautions: As with other antibiotic preparations, use of this drug may result in overgrowth of nonsusceptible organisms, including fungi. If superinfection occurs, the antibiotic should be discontinued and appropriate therapy should be instituted.
In venereal diseases when coexistent syphilis is suspected, darkfield examination should be done before treatment is started and the blood serology repeated monthly for at least 4 months.
Because the tetracyclines have been shown to depress plasma prothrombin activity, patients who are on anticoagulant therapy may require downward adjustment of their anticoagulant dosage.
In long-term therapy, periodic laboratory evaluation of organ systems, including hematopoietic, renal and hepatic studies should be performed.
All infections due to Group A beta-hemolytic streptococci should be treated for at least 10 days.
Since bacteriostatic drugs may interfere with the bactericidal action of penicillin, it is advisable to avoid giving demeclocycline in conjunction with penicillin.
Interpretation of Bacteriologic Studies: Following a course of therapy, persistence for several days in both urine and blood of bacteriosuppressive levels of demeclocycline may interfere with culture studies. These levels should not be considered therapeutic.
Adverse Reactions: Gastrointestinal: Anorexia, nausea, vomiting, diarrhea, glossitis, dysphagia, enterocolitis, and inflammatory lesions (with monilial overgrowth) in the anogenital region. These reactions have been caused by both the oral and parenteral administration of tetracyclines.
Skin: Maculopapular and erythematous rashes. Exfoliative dermatitis has been reported but is uncommon. Photosensitivity is discussed above. (See "Warnings".)
Renal toxicity: Rise in BUN has been reported and is apparently dose related. Nephrogenic diabetes insipidus. (See "Warnings".)
Hypersensitivity reactions: Urticaria, angioneurotic edema, anaphylaxis, anaphylactoid purpura, pericarditis and exacerbation of systemic lupus erythematosus.
Bulging fontanels have been reported in young infants following full therapeutic dosage. This sign disappeared rapidly when the drug was discontinued.
Blood: Hemolytic anemia, thrombocytopenia, neutropenia and eosinophilia have been reported.
When given over prolonged periods, tetracyclines have been reported to produce brown-black microscopic discoloration of thyroid glands. No abnormalities of thyroid function studies are known to occur.
Dosage and Administration: Therapy should be continued for at least 24-48 hours after symptoms and fever have subsided.
Concomitant therapy: Antacids containing aluminum, calcium, or magnesium impair absorption and should not be given to patients taking oral tetracycline.
Foods and some dairy products also interfere with absorption. Oral forms of tetracycline should be given 1 hour before or 2 hours after meals. Pediatric oral dosage forms should not be given with milk formulas and should be given at least 1 hour prior to feeding.
In patients with renal impairment: (See "Warnings.") Total dosage should be decreased by reduction of recommended individual doses and/or by extending time intervals between doses.
In the treatment of streptococcal infections, a therapeutic dose of demeclocycline should be administered for at least 10 days.
Adults: Usual daily dose—Four divided doses of 150 mg. each or two divided doses of 300 mg. each.
For children above eight years of age: Usual daily dose, 3-6 mg. per pound body weight per day, depending upon the severity of the disease, divided into 2 or 4 doses.
Gonorrhea patients sensitive to penicillin may be treated with demeclocycline administered as an initial oral dose of 600 mg. followed by 300 mg. every 12 hours for 4 days to a total of 3 grams.
How Supplied:
CAPSULES: 150 mg. *demeclocycline hydrochloride* (soft shell two tone coral) bottles of 16 and 100.
TABLETS: 75 mg. *demeclocycline hydrochloride* (Film Coated Red) bottles of 25.
150 mg. *demeclocycline hydrochloride* (Film Coated Red) bottles of 16 and 100.
300 mg. *demeclocycline hydrochloride* (Film Coated Red) bottles of 12, 48 and Unit Dose 10 x 10's.
A.H.F.S. 8:12.24
[*Shown in Product Identification Section*]

DECLOSTATIN® ℞
(demeclocycline hydrochloride and nystatin) for Oral Use

Description:
Tablets
Each tablet contains 300 mg. of DECLOMYCIN® *demeclocycline HCl* and 500,000 units of Nystatin.
Capsules
Each capsule contains 150 mg. of DECLOMYCIN *demeclocycline HCl* and 250,000 units of Nystatin.
DECLOMYCIN *demeclocycline hydrochloride* is an antibiotic isolated from a mutant strain of *Streptomyces aureofaciens.* Chemically it is the hydrochloride of 7-chloro-4-dimethylamino-1, 4, 4a, 5, 5a, 6, 11, 12a-octahydro-3, 6, 10, 12, 12a-pentahydroxy-1, 11- dioxo -2-naphthacenecarboxamide.
Nystatin is an antibiotic with antifungal activity produced by a strain of *Streptomyces noursei.*
Actions: The tetracyclines are primarily bacteriostatic and are thought to exert their antimicrobial effect by the inhibition of protein synthesis. Tetracyclines are active against a wide range of gram-negative and gram-positive organisms.
The drugs in the tetracycline class have closely similar antimicrobial spectra, and cross-resistance among them is common. Micro-organisms may be considered susceptible if the M.I.C. (minimum inhibitory concentration) is not more than 4.0 mcg./ml. and intermediate if the M.I.C. is 4.0 to 12.5 mcg./ml.
Susceptibility plate testing: A tetracycline disc may be used to determine microbial susceptibility to drugs in the tetracycline class. If the Kirby-Bauer method of disc susceptibility testing is used, a 30 mcg. tetracycline disc should give a zone of at least 19 mm. when tested against a tetracycline-susceptible bacterial strain.
Tetracyclines are readily absorbed and are bound to plasma proteins in varying degree. They are concentrated by the liver in the bile and excreted in the urine and feces at high concentrations and in a biologically active form.
Nystatin is an antifungal agent against *Candida* (monilia) *albicans.* It is absorbed very sparingly following oral administration, with no detectable blood levels when given in recommended doses. Most of the unabsorbed nystatin is passed unchanged in the stool.

Indications: Based on a review of this drug by the National Academy of Scien-

Continued on next page

The information on each product appearing here is based on labelling effective in August, 1979 and is either the entire official brochure or an accurate condensation therefrom. Official brochures are enclosed in product packages. Information concerning all Lederle products may be obtained from the Medical Department, Lederle Laboratories, Pearl River, New York, 10965.

Lederle—Cont.

ces—National Research Council and/or other information, FDA has classified the indications section as follows:
Ineffective as a fixed combination. DECLOMYCIN *demeclocycline hydrochloride* is indicated in infections caused by the following micro-organisms:
Rickettsiae: (Rocky Mountain spotted fever, typhus fever and the typhus group, Q fever, rickettsialpox, tick fevers.)
Mycoplasma pneumoniae (PPLO, Eaton agent).
Agents of psittacosis and ornithosis.
Agents of lymphogranuloma venereum and granuloma inguinale.
The spirochetal agent of relapsing fever *(Borrelia recurrentis).*
The following gram-negative micro-organisms:
Haemophilus ducreyi (chancroid),
Pasteurella pestis and *Pasteurella tularensis,*
Bartonella bacilliformis,
Bacteroides species,
Vibrio comma and *Vibrio fetus.*
Brucella species (in conjunction with streptomycin).
Because many strains of the following groups of micro-organisms have been shown to be resistant to tetracyclines, culture and susceptibility testing are recommended.
Demeclocycline is indicated for treatment of infections caused by the following gram-negative micro-organisms, when bacteriologic testing indicates appropriate susceptibility to the drug:
Escherichia coli,
Enterobacter aerogenes (formerly *Aerobacter aerogenes*),
Shigella species
Mima species and *Herellea* species,
Haemophilus influenzae (respiratory infections),
Klebsiella species (respiratory and urinary infections).
Demeclocycline is indicated for treatment of infections caused by the following gram-positive micro-organisms when bacteriologic testing indicates appropriate susceptibility to the drug:
Streptococcus species:
Up to 44 percent of strains of *Streptococcus pyogenes* and 74 percent of *Streptococcus faecalis* have been found to be resistant to tetracycline drugs. Therefore, tetracyclines should not be used for streptococcal disease unless the organism has been demonstrated to be sensitive.
For upper respiratory infections due to group A beta-hemolytic streptococci, penicillin is the usual drug of choice, including prophylaxis of rheumatic fever.
Diplococcus pneumoniae,
Staphylococcus aureus, skin and soft tissue infections. Tetracyclines are not the drugs of choice in the treatment of any type of staphylococcal infection.
When penicillin is contraindicated, tetracyclines are alternative drugs in the treatment of infections due to:
Neisseria gonorrhoeae,
Treponema pallidum and *Treponema pertenue* (syphilis and yaws),
Listeria monocytogenes,
Clostridium species,
Bacillus anthracis,
Fusobacterium fusiforme (Vincent's infection),
Actinomyces species.
In acute intestinal amebiasis, the tetracyclines may be a useful adjunct to amebicides.

DECLOMYCIN *demeclocycline hydrochloride* is indicated in the treatment of trachoma, although the infectious agent is not always eliminated, as judged by immunofluorescence.
Inclusion conjunctivitis may be treated with oral tetracyclines or with a combination of oral and topical agents.
Nystatin, the antifungal antibiotic is combined for added protection against monilial superinfection thought to be associated with the use of broad-spectrum antibiotics.

Contraindications: This drug is contraindicated in persons who have shown hypersensitivity to any of the tetracyclines or nystatin.
Warnings: THE USE OF DRUGS OF THE TETRACYCLINE CLASS DURING TOOTH DEVELOPMENT (LAST HALF OF PREGNANCY, INFANCY AND CHILDHOOD TO THE AGE OF 8 YEARS) MAY CAUSE PERMANENT DISCOLORATION OF THE TEETH (YELLOW-GRAY-BROWN). This adverse reaction is more common during long-term use of the drugs but has been observed following repeated short-term courses. Enamel hypoplasia has also been reported. TETRACYCLINE DRUGS, THEREFORE, SHOULD NOT BE USED IN THIS AGE GROUP UNLESS OTHER DRUGS ARE NOT LIKELY TO BE EFFECTIVE OR ARE CONTRAINDICATED.
If renal impairment exists, even usual oral or parenteral doses may lead to excessive systemic accumulation of the drug and possible liver toxicity. Under such conditions, lower than usual total doses are indicated and, if therapy is prolonged, serum level determinations of the drug may be advisable.
Phototoxic reactions can occur in individuals taking demeclocycline, and are characterized by severe burns of exposed surfaces resulting from direct exposure of patients to sunlight during therapy with moderate or large doses of demeclocycline. Patients apt to be exposed to direct sunlight or ultraviolet light should be advised that this reaction can occur, and treatment should be discontinued at the first evidence of skin erythema.
The anti-anabolic action of the tetracyclines may cause an increase in BUN. While this is not a problem in those with normal renal function, in patients with significantly impaired function, higher serum levels of tetracycline may lead to azotemia, hyperphosphatemia, and acidosis.
Usage in pregnancy (See above "Warnings" about use during tooth development.)
Results of animal studies indicate that tetracyclines cross the placenta, are found in fetal tissues and can have toxic effects on the developing fetus (often related to retardation of skeletal development). Evidence of embryotoxicity has also been noted in animals treated early in pregnancy.
Usage in newborns, infants, and children (See above "Warnings" about use during tooth development.)
All tetracyclines form a stable calcium complex in any bone forming tissue. A decrease in the fibula growth rate has been observed in prematures given oral tetracycline in doses of 25 mg./kg. every 6 hours. This reaction was shown to be reversible when the drug was discontinued.
Tetracyclines are present in the milk of lactating women who are taking a drug in this class.
Precautions: As with other antibiotic preparations, use of this drug may result in overgrowth of nonsusceptible organisms, including fungi. If superinfection occurs, the antibiotic should be discontinued and appropriate therapy should be instituted.
In venereal diseases when coexistent syphilis is suspected, darkfield examination should be done before treatment is started and the blood serology repeated monthly for at least 4 months.
Because the tetracyclines have been shown to depress plasma prothrombin activity, patients who are on anticoagulant therapy may require downward adjustment of their anticoagulant dosage.
In long-term therapy, periodic laboratory evaluation of organ systems, including hematopoietic, renal and hepatic studies should be performed.
All infections due to Group A beta-hemolytic streptococci should be treated for at least 10 days.
Since bacteriostatic drugs may interfere with the bactericidal action of penicillin, it is advisable to avoid giving demeclocycline in conjunction with penicillin.
Interpretation of Bacteriologic Studies: Following a course of therapy, persistence for several days in both urine and blood of bacteriosuppressive levels of demeclocycline may interfere with culture studies. These levels should not be considered therapeutic.
Adverse Reactions:
Gastrointestinal: Anorexia, nausea, vomiting, diarrhea, glossitis, dysphagia, enterocolitis, and inflammatory lesions (with monilial overgrowth) in the anogenital region. These reactions have been caused by both the oral and parenteral administration of tetracyclines.
Skin: Maculopapular and erythematous rashes. Exfoliative dermatitis has been reported but is uncommon. Photosensitivity is discussed above. (See "Warnings".)
Renal toxicity: Rise in BUN has been reported and is apparently dose related. (See "Warnings".)
Hypersensitivity reactions: Urticaria, angioneurotic edema, anaphylaxis, anaphylactoid purpura, pericarditis and exacerbation of systemic lupus erythematosus.
Bulging fontanels have been reported in young infants following full therapeutic dosage. This sign disappeared rapidly when the drug was discontinued.
Blood: Hemolytic anemia, thrombocytopenia, neutropenia and eosinophilia have been reported.
When given over prolonged periods, tetracyclines have been reported to produce brown-black microscopic discoloration of thyroid glands. No abnormalities of thyroid function studies are known to occur.
Nystatin has been associated with nausea and vomiting, gastrointestinal distress and diarrhea (occasionally with large doses.)
Dosage and Administration:
Adults: Usual daily dose—Four divided doses of 150 mg. each or two divided doses of 300 mg. each, based on demeclocycline HCl content.
For children above eight years of age: Usual daily dose, 3-6 mg. per pound body weight per day, depending upon the severity of the disease, divided into 2 or 4 doses, based on the demeclocycline HCl content.
Therapy should be continued for at least 24-48 hours after symptoms and fever have subsided.
Concomitant therapy: Antacids containing aluminum, calcium, or magnesium impair absorption and should not be given to patients taking oral tetracycline.
Foods and some dairy products also interfere with absorption. Oral forms of tetracycline should be given 1 hour before or 2 hours after meals. Pediatric oral dosage forms should not be given with milk formulas and should be given at least 1 hour prior to feeding.
In patients with renal impairment: (See "Warnings.") Total dosage should be decreased by reduction of recommended individual doses and/or by extending time intervals between doses.
In the treatment of streptococcal infections, a therapeutic dose of demeclocycline should be administered for at least 10 days.
Gonorrhea patients sensitive to penicillin may be treated with demeclocycline administered

as an initial oral dose of 600 mg. followed by 300 mg. every 12 hours for 4 days to a total of 3 grams.

How Supplied:
Capsules
150 mg. demeclocycline HCl and 250,000 units of nystatin soft shell—coral, Bottles of 16 and 100.
Tablets
300 mg. demeclocycline HCl and 500,000 units of nystatin film coated—pink, Bottles of 12 and 48.
A.H.F.S. 8:12.24

[*Tablets and Capsules shown in Product Identification Section*]

DIAMOX® ℞
(acetazolamide)
TABLETS, PARENTERAL AND SEQUELS®
Sustained Release Capsules

Description:
Tablets: 125 mg. of acetazolamide, one quarter scored, flat, circular, white and engraved tablets. 250 mg. of acetazolamide, one quarter scored, convex, circular, white and engraved tablets.
Parenteral: *Each vial contains acetazolamide 500 mg (as sodium salt) and pH adjusted to aproximately 9.2 with sodium hydroxide and, if necessary, hydrochloric acid.
SEQUELS: DIAMOX *acetazolamide* SEQUELS Lederle are sustained-release capsules each containing 500 mg. of acetazolamide.
Actions: DIAMOX is a potent carbonic anhydrase inhibitor, effective in the control of fluid secretion (e.g. some types of glaucoma), in the treatment of certain convulsive disorders (e.g. epilepsy) and in the promotion of diuresis in instances of abnormal fluid retention (e.g. cardiac edema).
DIAMOX is not a mercurial diuretic. Rather it is a nonbacteriostatic sulfonamide possessing a chemical structure and pharmacological activity distinctly different from the bacteriostatic sulfonamides.
DIAMOX is an enzyme inhibitor which acts specifically on carbonic anhydrase, the enzyme which catalyzes the reversible reaction involving the hydration of carbon dioxide and the dehydration of carbonic acid. In the eye, this inhibitory action of acetazolamide decreases the secretion of aqueous humor and results in a drop in intraocular pressure, a reaction considered desirable in cases of glaucoma and even in certain non-glaucomatous conditions. Evidence seems to indicate that DIAMOX has utility as an adjuvant in the treatment of certain dysfunctions of the central nervous system (e.g. epilepsy). Inhibition of carbonic anhydrase in this area appears to retard abnormal, paroxysmal, excessive discharge from central nervous system neurons. The diuretic effect of DIAMOX *acetazolamide* is due to its action in the kidney on the reversible reaction involving hydration of carbon dioxide and dehydration of carbonic acid. The result is renal loss of HCO_3 ion, which carries out sodium, water, and potassium. Alkalinization of the urine and promotion of diuresis are thus effected.
SEQUELS: DIAMOX Acetazolamide SEQUELS Sustained Release Capsules provide prolonged action to inhibit aqueous humor secretion for 18 to 24 hours after each dose, whereas tablets act for only 8 to 12 hours. The prolonged/continuous effect of SEQUELS permits a reduction in dosage frequency.
Blood level concentrations of acetazolamide peak between 8 to 12 hours after administration of DIAMOX SEQUELS, compared to 2 to 4 hours with tablets.
Indications—Tablets and Parenteral: For adjunctive treatment of: edema due to congestive heart failure; drug-induced edema; centrencephalic epilepsies (petit mal, unlocalized seizures); chronic simple (open angle) glaucoma, secondary glaucoma, and preoperatively in acute angle closure glaucoma where delay of surgery is desired in order to lower intraocular pressure.
Indications—SEQUELS: For adjunctive treatment of: chronic simple (open angle) glaucoma, secondary glaucoma, and preoperatively in acute angle closure glaucoma where delay of surgery is desired in order to lower intraocular pressure.
Contraindications: Acetazolamide therapy is contraindicated in situations in which sodium and/or potassium blood serum levels are depressed, in cases of marked kidney and liver disease or dysfunction, suprarenal gland failure, and hyperchloremic acidosis.
Long-term administration of DIAMOX *acetazolamide* is contraindicated in patients with chronic noncongestive angle closure glaucoma since it may permit organic closure of the angle to occur while the worsening glaucoma is masked by lowered intraocular pressure.
Warning: Studies of acetazolamide in rats and mice have demonstrated teratogenic and embryocidal effects at doses in excess of ten times those recommended in human beings. There is no evidence of these effects in human beings, however acetazolamide should not be used in pregnancy, especially during the first trimester, unless the benefits to be expected outweigh these potential adverse effects.
Precautions: Increasing the dose does not increase the diuresis and may increase the incidence of drowsiness and/or paresthesia. Increasing the dose often results in a decrease in diuresis. Under certain circumstances, however, very large doses have been given in conjunction with other diuretics in order to secure diuresis in complete refractory failure.
Adverse reactions common to all sulfonamide derivatives may occur: fever, rash, crystalluria, renal calculus, bone marrow depression, thrombocytopenic purpura, hemolytic anemia, leukopenia, pancytopenia and agranulocytosis. Precaution is advised for early detection of such reactions and the drug should be discontinued and appropriate therapy instituted.
In patients with pulmonary obstruction or emphysema where alveolar ventilation may be impaired, Diamox acetazolamide which may precipitate or aggravate acidosis, should be used with caution.
Adverse Reactions: Adverse reactions during short-term therapy are minimal. Those effects which have been noted include: paresthesias, particularly a "tingling" feeling in the extremities; some loss of appetite; polyuria and occasional instances of drowsiness and confusion. During long-term therapy, an acidotic state may occasionally supervene. This can usually be corrected by the administration of bicarbonate.
Transient myopia has been reported. This condition invariably subsides upon diminution or discontinuance of the medication.
Other occasional adverse reactions include: urticaria; melena; hematuria; glycosuria; hepatic insufficiency; flaccid paralysis; and convulsions.

Dosage and Administration:
Preparation and Storage of Parenteral Solution:
Each 500 mg. vial containing DIAMOX *sterile acetazolamide sodium* Parenteral should be reconstituted with at least 5 ml. of Sterile Water for Injection prior to use. Reconstituted solutions, stored at room temperature, retain potency for two weeks or, if refrigerated, four weeks. However, since this product contains no preservative, use within 24 hours of reconstitution is strongly recommended. The direct intravenous route of administration is preferred. Intramuscular administration may be employed but is painful, due to the alkaline pH of the solution.
Glaucoma: DIAMOX *acetazolamide* should be used as an adjunct to the usual therapy. The dosage employed in the treatment of *chronic simple (open-angle) glaucoma* ranges from 250 mg. to 1 Gram of DIAMOX per 24 hours, usually in divided doses for amounts over 250 mg. It has usually been found that a dosage in excess of 1 Gram per 24 hours does not produce an increased effect. In all cases, the dosage should be adjusted with careful individual attention both to symptomatology and ocular tension. Continuous supervision by a physician is advisable.
In the treatment of secondary glaucoma and in the preoperative treatment of some cases of *acute congestive (closed-angle) glaucoma,* the preferred dosage is 250 mg. every 4 hours, although some cases have responded to 250 mg. twice daily on short-term therapy. In some acute cases, it may be more satisfactory to administer an initial dose of 500 mg. followed by 125 or 250 mg. every 4 hours depending on the individual case. Intravenous therapy may be used for rapid relief of ocular tension in acute cases. A complementary effect has been noted when DIAMOX has been used in conjunction with miotics or mydriatics as the case demanded.
Epilepsy: It is not clearly known whether the beneficial effects observed in epilepsy are due to direct inhibition of carbonic anhydrase in the central nervous system or whether they are due to the slight degree of acidosis produced by the divided dosage. The best results to date have been seen in petit mal in children. Good results, however, have been seen in patients, both children and adult, in other types of seizures such as grand mal, mixed seizure patterns, myoclonic jerk patterns, etc. The suggested total daily dose is 8 to 30 mg. per Kg. in divided doses. Although some patients respond to a low dose, the optimum range appears to be from 375 to 1000 mg. daily. However, some investigators feel that daily doses in excess of 1 Gram do not produce any better results than a 1 Gram dose. When DIAMOX is given in combination with other anti-convulsants, it is suggested that the starting dose should be 250 mg. once daily in addition to the existing medications. This can be increased to levels as indicated above.
The change from other medication to DIAMOX should be gradual in accordance with usual practice in epilepsy therapy.
Congestive Heart Failure: For diuresis in congestive heart failure, the starting dose is usually 250 to 375 mg. once daily in the morning (5 mg./Kg.). If after an initial response, the patient fails to continue to lose edema fluid, do not increase the dose but allow for kidney recovery by skipping medication for a day. DIAMOX *acetazolamide* yields best diuretic results when given on alternate days, or for 2 days alternating with a day of rest.
Failures in therapy may be due to overdosage or too frequent dosage. The use of DIAMOX does not eliminate the need for other therapy such as digitalis, bed rest, and salt restriction.
Drug-Induced Edema: Recommended dosage is 250 mg. to 375 mg. of DIAMOX once a day for 1 or 2 days, alternating with a day of rest.
Note: The dosage recommendations for glaucoma and epilepsy differ considerably from those for congestive heart failure, since the first two conditions are not dependent upon carbonic anhydrase inhibition in the kidney which requires intermittent dosage if it is to recover from the inhibitory effect of the therapeutic agent.

Continued on next page

The information on each product appearing here is based on labelling effective in August, 1979 and is either the entire official brochure or an accurate condensation therefrom. Official brochures are enclosed in product packages. Information concerning all Lederle products may be obtained from the Medical Department, Lederle Laboratories, Pearl River, New York, 10965.

Lederle—Cont.

SEQUELS: The recommended dose is 1 capsule (500 mg.) 2 times a day. Usually 1 capsule is administered in the morning and 1 capsule in the evening. It may be necessary to adjust the dose but it has usually been found that dosage in excess of 2 capsules (1 Gram) does not produce an increased effect. The dosage should be adjusted with careful individual attention both to symptomatology and intraocular tension. In all cases, continuous supervision by a physician is advisable.
In those unusual instances where adequate control is not obtained by the twice-a-day administration of DIAMOX *acetazolamide* SEQUELS, sustained release capsules, the desired control may be established by means of DIAMOX (Tablets or Parenteral). Use tablets or parenteral in accordance with the more frequent dosage schedules recommended for these items, such as 250 mg. every 4 hours, or an initial dose of 500 mg. followed by 250 mg. or 125 mg. every 4 hours; depending on the case in question.
How Supplied: *Tablets* (white quarter-scored) 125 mg.-bottles of 100; 250 mg.-bottles of 100 and 1,000; unit-dose 10 x 10's. *Parenteral*-vials of 500 mg. *SEQUELS* (soft shell, orange) 500 mg.-bottles of 30 and 100.
A.H.F.S. 40:28
Military Depot: NSN 6505-00-664-0857, 250 mg. Tablets, 100's.
NSN 6505-00-880-4949, 500 mg. SEQUELS, 100's.
V. A. Depot: NSN 6505-00-584-4303A, 250 mg. Tablets, 1000's.
NSN 6505-00-880-4949A, 500 mg. SEQUELS, 100's.
[*250 mg. Tablets and SEQUELS, 500 mg. Shown in Product Identification Section*]

DIPHTHERIA AND TETANUS TOXOIDS, COMBINED PUROGENATED® ℞

How Supplied: 5 ml. vials (5 immunizations). COMPLETE INFORMATION FURNISHED IN THE PACKAGE.

FERRO-SEQUELS®
(sustained release iron)
Capsules

Composition: Each capsule contains 150 mg. of ferrous fumarate equivalent to approximately 50 mg. of elemental iron, so prepared that it is released over a 5 to 6 hour period, and 100 mg. of docusate sodium (DSS) to counteract constipating effect of iron.
Indications: For the treatment of iron deficiency anemias.
Dosage: 1 capsule, once or twice daily or as prescribed by the physician.
Precautions: In case of accidental overdose, seek professional assistance or contact a Poison Control Center immediately.
How Supplied: Capsules (green)—bottles of 30, 100, and 1,000; unit-dose 10 x 10's.
Military Depot NSN-6505-00-149-0103, 30's
NSN 6505-00-074-2981, 1,000's
NSN 6505-00-031-8870, individually sealed 100's
USPHS Depot: NSN 6505-00-149-0103, 30's
NSN 6505-00-074-2981, 1000's
A.H.F.S. 20:04.04
[*Shown in Product Identification Section*]

FILIBON®
(prenatal tablets)

Each tablet contains:

	For Pregnant or Lactating Women Percentage of U.S. Recommended Daily Allowance (U.S. RDA)
Vitamin A (as Acetate)	5000 I.U. (63%)
Vitamin D_2	400 I.U. (100%)
Vitamin E (as *dl*-Alpha Tocopheryl Acetate)	30 I.U. (100%)
Vitamin C (Ascorbic Acid)	60 mg (100%)
Folic Acid (Folacin)	0.4 mg (50%)
Vitamin B_1 (as Thiamine Mononitrate)	1.5 mg (88%)
Vitamin B_2 (as Riboflavin)	1.7 mg (85%)
Niacinamide	20 mg (100%)
Vitamin B_6 (as Pyridoxine Hydrochloride)	2 mg (80%)
Vitamin B_{12} (as Cyanocobalamine)	6 mcg (75%)
Calcium (as Calcium Carbonate)	125 mg (10%)
Iodine (as Potassium Iodide)	150 mcg (100%)
Iron (as Ferrous Fumarate)	18 mg (100%)
Magnesium (as Magnesium Oxide)	100 mg (22%)

A PHOSPHORUS-FREE VITAMIN AND MINERAL DIETARY SUPPLEMENT FOR USE IN PRENATAL CARE AND LACTATION.
Recommended Intake: 1 daily, or as prescribed by the physician.
How Supplied: Capsule-shaped tablets (film-coated, pink) engraved LL—bottles of 100.
[*Shown in Product Identification Section*]

FILIBON® F.A. ℞
(prenatal tablets)

Each tablet contains:

	Percentage of U.S. Recommended Daily Allowance (U.S. RDA)
Vitamin A (as Acetate)	8000 I.U. (100%)
Vitamin D_2	400 I.U. (100%)
Vitamin E (as *dl*-Alpha Tocopheryl Acetate)	30 I.U. (100%)
Vitamin C (as Ascorbic Acid)	60 mg (100%)
Folic Acid (as Folacin)	1 mg (125%)
Vitamin B_1 (as Thiamine Mononitrate)	1.7 mg (100%)
Vitamin B_2 (as Riboflavin)	2 mg (100%)
Niacinamide	20 mg (100%)
Vitamin B_6 (as Pyridoxine Hydrochloride)	4.0 mg (160%)
Vitamin B_{12} (as Cyanocobalamin)	8 mcg (100%)
Calcium (as Calcium Carbonate)	250 mg (19%)
Iodine (as Potassium Iodide)	150 mcg (100%)
Iron (as Ferrous Fumarate)	45 mg (250%)
Magnesium (as Magnesium Oxide)	100 mg (22%)

Precaution: Folic acid may obscure pernicious anemia in that the peripheral blood picture may revert to normal while neurological manifestations remain progressive.
How Supplied: Capsule-shaped tablets (film-coated, pink) engraved LL—bottles of 100.
[*Shown in Product Identification Section*]

FILIBON® FORTE ℞
(prenatal tablets)

Each tablet contains:

	Percentage of U.S. Recommended Daily Allowance (U.S. RDA)
Vitamin A (as Acetate)	8000 I.U. (100%)
Vitamin D_2	400 I.U. (100%)
Vitamin E (as *dl*-Alpha Tocopheryl Acetate)	45 I.U. (150%)
Vitamin C (Ascorbic Acid)	90 mg (150%)
Folic Acid (Folacin)	1 mg (125%)
Vitamin B_1 (as Thiamine Mononitrate)	2 mg (118%)
Vitamin B_2 (as Riboflavin)	2.5 mg (125%)
Niacinamide	30 mg (150%)
Vitamin B_6 (as Pyridoxine Hydrochloride)	3 mg (120%)
Vitamin B_{12} (as Cyanocobalamin)	12 mcg (150%)
Calcium (as Calcium Carbonate)	300 mg (23%)
Iodine (as potassium Iodide)	200 mg (133%)
Iron (as Ferrous Fumarate)	45 mg (250%)
Magnesium (as Magnesium Oxide)	100 mg (22%)

Recommended Intake: 1 tablet daily. This dosage provides 23% and 22% the Recommended Daily Allowance of calcium and magnesium respectively, therefore, supplementation of the diet by milk or other sources of calcium may be advisable.
Precaution: Folic Acid may obscure pernicious anemia in that the peripheral blood picture may revert to normal while neurological manifestations remain progressive.
How Supplied: Tablets—film coated (pink)—bottles of 100.
[*Shown in Product Identification Section*]

FILIBON® OT ℞
(prenatal tablets)

Each tablet contains:

	Percentage of U.S. Recommended Daily Allowance (U.S. RDA)
Vitamin A (as Acetate)	8000 I.U. (100%)
Vitamin D_2	400 I.U. (100%)
Vitamin E (as *dl*-Alpha Tocopheryl Acetate)	30 I.U. (100%)
Vitamin C (as Ascorbic Acid)	60 mg (100%)
Folic Acid (as Folacin)	1 mg (125%)
Vitamin B_1 (as Thiamine Mononitrate)	1.7 mg (100%)
Vitamin B_2 (as Riboflavin)	2 mg (100%)
Niacinamide	20 mg (100%)
Vitamin B_6 (as PyridoxineHydrochloride)	2.5 mg (100%)
Vitamin B_{12} (as Cyanocobalamin)	8 mcgm (100%)
Calcium (as Calcium Carbonate)	250 mg (19%)
Iodine (as Potassium Iodide)	150 mcgm (100%)
Iron (as Ferrous Furmarate)	30 mg (166%)
Magnesium (as Magnesium Oxide)	100 mg (22%)
Docusate Sodium Sulfosuccinate USP (DSS)	100 mg

Precaution: Folic acid may obscure pernicious anemia in that the peripheral blood picture may revert to normal while neurological manifestations remain progressive.
How Supplied: Tablets (film-coated blue)—bottles of 100.
[*Shown in Product Identification Section*]

FOLVITE® ℞
(folic acid)
Tablets—Parenteral Solution

Composition: Each Tablet contains: 0.25 mg. or 1 mg. of folic acid.
Each ml. of Parenteral Solution contains: Sodium folate equivalent to 5 mg. of folic acid. Inactive ingredients: Sequestrene sodium, 0.2%; Water for Injection, q.s. 100%; Sodium hydroxide to approx. pH 9. Preservative: Benzyl alcohol 1.5%.
How Supplied: Tablets (Scored, orange), 1 mg.—bottles of 100 and 1,000; Unit-dose 10 x 10's. **Parenteral Solution,** 5 mg./ml.—10 ml. vials.
A.H.F.S. 88:08

FOLVRON® ℞
(folic acid and iron)
Capsules

Composition: Each Capsule contains:
Folic acid .... 0.33 mg.
Dried ferrous sulfate ....182 mg.
(Elemental iron 57 mg.)

How Supplied: Capsules (soft shell, red)—bottles of 100.

GEVRABON®
(vitamin-mineral supplement)

(See PDR for Nonprescription Drugs)

GEVRAL®
Multivitamin and Multimineral Supplement for Adults and Children 4 or More Years of Age
TABLETS

(See PDR for Nonprescription Drugs)

GEVRAL® T
High Potency
Multivitamin and Multimineral Supplement for Adults and Children 4 or More Years of Age
TABLETS

(See PDR for Nonprescription Drugs)

HETRAZAN® ℞
(diethylcarbamazine citrate)

Tablets, U.S.P. 50 mg. (scored, white)— bottles of 100.

HYDROMOX® ℞
(quinethazone)
Tablets

Description: Chemistry: HYDROMOX is a quinazoline derivative, in which a cyclic carbamyl group replaces the cyclic sulfamyl group present in the thiazide derivatives.
Chemical name: 7 - Chloro - 2 - ethyl - 1, 2, 3, 4-tetrahydro-4-oxo-6-sulfamyl-quinazoline
Tablet Size: 50 mg. scored
Actions: HYDROMOX produces urinary excretion of sodium and chloride in approximately equivalent amounts (saluresis), while potassium is excreted to a much lesser degree. The saluretic effect of HYDROMOX is rapid and relatively prolonged, beginning within 2 hours after administration, reaching a peak at 6 hours, and lasting for 18 to 24 hours. While HYDROMOX is chemically different, it is pharmacologically genetic to the benzothiadiazine group of drugs.
The dominant action of quinethazone is to increase the renal excretion of sodium and chloride and an accompanying volume of water. This results from inhibition of the tubular mechanism of electrolyte reabsorption. The renal effect is virtually independent of alterations in acid-base balance.
Quinethazone, like other drugs in this class, inhibits the proximal reabsorption of sodium and chloride. The excretion of potassium results from increased potassium secretion by the distal tubule where potassium is exchanged for sodium.
Quinethazone may exert its antihypertensive effect by diuresis and sodium loss and/or on vascular function to reduce peripheral resistance.
Indications: HYDROMOX *quinethazone* Lederle, a nonmercurial oral diuretic agent is indicated as adjunctive therapy in edema associated with congestive heart failure, hepatic cirrhosis and corticosteroid and estrogen therapy.
HYDROMOX has also been found useful in edema due to various forms of renal dysfunction such as: nephrotic syndrome; acute glomerulonephritis; and chronic renal failure.
HYDROMOX is indicated in the management of hypertension either as the sole therapeutic agent or to enhance the effectiveness of other antihypertensive drugs in the more severe forms of hypertension.
Usage in Pregnancy: The routine use of diuretics in an otherwise healthy woman is inappropriate and exposes mother and fetus to unnecessary hazard. Diuretics do not prevent development of toxemia of pregnancy, and there is no satisfactory evidence that they are useful in the treatment of developed toxemia.
Edema during pregnancy may arise from pathological causes or from the physiologic and mechanical consequences of pregnancy. Diuretics are indicated in pregnancy when edema is due to pathologic causes, just as they are in the absence of pregnancy (however, see Warnings, below). Dependent edema in pregnancy, resulting from restriction of venous return by the expanded uterus, is properly treated through elevation of the lower extremities and use of support hose; use of diuretics to lower intravascular volume in this case is illogical and unnecessary. There is hypervolemia during normal pregnancy which is harmful to neither the fetus nor the mother (in the absence of cardiovascular disease), but which is associated with edema, including generalized edema, in the majority of pregnant women. If this edema produces discomfort, increased recumbency will often provide relief. In rare instances, this edema may cause extreme discomfort which is not relieved by rest. In these cases, a short course of diuretics may provide relief and may be appropriate.
Contraindications:
A. Anuria
B. Hypersensitivity to this or other sulfonamide derived drugs.
Warnings: Diuretics should be used with caution in severe renal disease. In patients with renal disease, diuretics may precipitate azotemia. Cumulative effects of the drug may develop in patients with impaired renal function.
Diuretics should be used with caution in patients with impaired hepatic function or progressive liver disease, since minor alterations of fluid and electrolyte balance may precipitate hepatic coma.
Quinethazone may add to or potentiate the action of other antihypertensive drugs. Potentiation occurs with ganglionic or peripheral adrenergic blocking drugs.
Sensitivity reactions may occur in patients with a history of allergy or bronchial asthma.
The possibility of exacerbation or activation of systemic lupus erythematosus has been reported.
Usage in Pregnancy: Quinethazone crosses the placental barrier and appears in cord blood. The use of quinethazone in pregnant women requires that the anticipated benefit be weighed against possible hazards to the fetus. These hazards include fetal or neonatal jaundice, thrombocytopenia, and possible other adverse reactions which have occurred in the adult.
Nursing Mothers: Quinethazone appears in breast milk. If use of the drug is deemed essential, the patient should stop nursing.
Precautions: (1) Quinethazone should be used with caution in patients with impaired hepatic function or progressive liver disease, since minor alterations of fluid and electrolyte balance may precipitate hepatic coma. (2) Whereas electrolyte abnormalities are often present in such conditions as heart failure and cirrhosis as a result of underlying disease process, they may also be aggravated or may be produced independently by any potent diuretic affecting electrolyte excretion. Caution is especially important during prolonged or intensive therapy and when salt intake is restricted or during concomitant use of steroids or ACTH. Hypokalemia attributable to HYDROMOX *quinethazone* therapy has been mild and infrequent, and other electrolyte abnormalities have been rare.
The possibility of potassium depletion and its toxic sequelae must be kept in mind, particularly in cirrhotics and patients receiving digitalis. As a preventive measure the use of foods rich in potassium, such as orange juice, or supplements of potassium chloride may be desirable. (3) In patients with impaired renal function, azotemia and/or excessive drug accumulation may develop. (4) As with other potent diuretics, when HYDROMOX is added to a regimen that includes ganglionic-blocking agents, the dosage of these latter preparations should be reduced to avoid a sudden drop in blood pressure. Reduction of dosage is also necessary when one or more of these antihypertensive agents is added to an established HYDROMOX regimen. (5) As with the thiazide diuretics, increases of serum uric acid may occur but precipitation of gout has been rare. (6) A decreased glucose tolerance as evidenced by hyperglycemia and glycosuria thus aggravating or provoking diabetes mellitus has occurred. (7) Quinethazone may decrease arterial responsiveness to norepinephrine and therefore should be withdrawn 48 hours before elective surgery. If emergency surgery is indicated, pre-anesthetic and anesthetic agents should be administered in reduced dosage. Quinethazone may also increase the responsiveness to tubocurarine. The antihypertensive effects of the drug may be enhanced in the post-sympathectomy patient. (8) Sensitivity reactions may be more likely to occur in patients with a history of allergy or bronchial asthma. (9) The possibility of exacerbation or activation of systemic lupus erythematosus has been suggested for sulfonamide derived drugs.
Adverse Reactions: The following adverse reactions have been reported with the diuretic drugs some of which may be expected to occur with quinethazone:
A. *Gastrointestinal System reactions:* 1. anorexia, 2. gastric irritation, 3. nausea, 4. vomiting, 5. cramping, 6. diarrhea, 7. constipation, 8. jaundice (intrahepatic cholestatic jaundice), 9. pancreatitis, 10. hyperglycemia, 11. glycosuria.
B. *Central Nervous System reactions:* 1. dizziness, 2. vertigo, 3. paresthesias, 4. headache, 5. xanthopsia.
C. *Hematologic Reactions:* 1. leukopenia, 2. thrombocytopenia, 3. agranulocytosis, 4. aplastic anemia.
D. *Dermatologic—hypersensitivity reactions:* 1. purpura, 2. photosensitivity, 3. rash, 4. urticaria, 5. necrotizing angiitis (vasculitis) (cutaneous vasculitis).
E. *Cardiovascular Reactions:* 1. orthostatic hypotension may occur and may be potentiated by alcohol, barbiturates or narcotics.
F. *Miscellaneous:* 1. muscle spasm, 2. weakness, 3. restlessness. Whenever adverse reactions are moderate or severe, thiazide dosage should be reduced or therapy withdrawn.
Dosage: Average Adult Dosage: One or two 50 mg. tablets, orally, once a day. Because of its relatively prolonged duration of activity, a single daily dose is generally sufficient. Occasionally, 1 tablet (50 mg.) is administered twice a day. Infrequently, a total daily dose of 3 to 4 tablets (150 to 200 mg.) may be necessary. The dosage employed depends upon the severity of

Continued on next page

The information on each product appearing here is based on labelling effective in August, 1979 and is either the entire official brochure or an accurate condensation therefrom. Official brochures are enclosed in product packages. Information concerning all Lederle products may be obtained from the Medical Department, Lederle Laboratories, Pearl River, New York, 10965.

Lederle—Cont.

the condition being treated and the responsiveness of the patient, and often must be adjusted at the beginning or during the course of therapy. When HYDROMOX *quinethazone* is used in combination with other antihypertensive agents, the dosage of each drug may often be reduced because of potentiation. (see under Precautions concerning the necessity for dosage adjustment when one or more of these drugs is added to an already established therapeutic regimen.)

How Supplied: 50 mg. tablets (scored)—bottles of 100 and 500.

[*Shown in Product Identification Section*]

HYDROMOX® R ℞
(quinethazone with reserpine)
TABLETS

Warnings:

> This fixed combination drug is not indicated for initial therapy of hypertension. Hypertension requires therapy titrated to the individual patient. If the fixed combination represents the dosage so determined, its use may be more convenient in patient management. The treatment of hypertension is not static, but must be reevaluated as conditions in each patient warrant.

Description: HYDROMOX R tablets each contain 50 mg. quinethazone and 0.125 mg. reserpine. *HYDROMOX® quinethazone Lederle is a nonmercurial oral diuretic agent, effective in the treatment of edema and hypertension. It is chemically distinct from the benzothiadiazine series of compounds.* Reserpine, an antihypertensive agent, has been combined with quinethazone in a dosage form designed to be useful in the treatment of hypertension with or without edema.

Chemistry: HYDROMOX is a quinazoline derivative, in which a cyclic carbamyl group replaces the cyclic sulfamyl group present in the thiazide derivatives.

Quinethazone is 7-Chloro-2-ethyl-1, 2, 3, 4- tetrahydro-4-oxo-6-sulfamyl-quinazoline.

Reserpine is 3, 4, 5 trimethoxybenzyl methyl reserpate.

Actions: HYDROMOX produces urinary excretion of sodium and chloride in approximately equivalent amounts (saluresis), while potassium is excreted to a much lesser degree. The saluretic effect of HYDROMOX is rapid and relatively prolonged, beginning within 2 hours after administration, reaching a peak at 6 hours, and lasting for 18 to 24 hours. While HYDROMOX is chemically different, it is pharmacologically genetic to the benzothiadiazine group of drugs.

The dominant action of quinethazone is to increase the renal excretion of sodium and chloride and an accompanying volume of water. This results from inhibition of the tubular mechanism of electrolyte reabsorption. The renal effect is virtually independent of alterations in acid-base balance.

Quinethazone, like other drugs in this class, inhibits the proximal reabsorption of sodium and chloride. The excretion of potassium results from increased potassium secretion by the distal tubule where potassium is exchanged for sodium.

Quinethazone may exert its antihypertensive effect by diuresis and sodium loss and/or on vascular function to reduce peripheral resistance.

Reserpine is an antihypertensive agent which produces a mild type of sedation that is tranquilizing rather than hypnotic. The most prominent actions of reserpine are upon the cardiovascular and central nervous systems. In clinical hypertension, reserpine produces a gradual and moderate fall in both systolic and diastolic blood pressures after oral administration for several days to 2-3 weeks. Its effects persist about 3-4 weeks after medication is withdrawn. With an increase in dose, a prolongation of hypotensive effect, rather than an intensification of blood pressure fall, tends to occur. The doses employed in the therapy of hypertension are smaller than those used in psychiatric disorders.

The dosage form combining Quinethazone with Reserpine is designed to provide effective antihypertensive action upon patients who have failed to show satisfactory response to the use of quinethazone or reserpine alone. This combination of quinethazone and reserpine frequently permits use of a lower dosage of each agent and hence tends to produce the desired antihypertensive effect while eliminating, or at least minimizing, adverse reactions. Blood pressure reductions averaging about –30/–15 have been demonstrated within the first 2 weeks of treatment. Continuation of therapy beyond 2 weeks may be expected to produce further *small* drops in blood pressure. The enhanced reduction in blood pressure produced by quinethazone with reserpine appears to be an additive rather than a potentiating effect.

Indications: HYDROMOX R is indicated in the management of hypertension (see box warnings) either as the sole therapeutic agent or to enhance the effectiveness of other antihypertensive drugs in the more severe forms of hypertension.

Usage in Pregnancy

The routine use of diuretics in an otherwise healthy woman is inappropriate and exposes mother and fetus to unnecessary hazard. Diuretics do not prevent development of toxemia of pregnancy, and there is no satisfactory evidence that they are useful in the treatment of developed toxemia.

Edema during pregnancy may arise from pathological causes or from the physiologic and mechanical consequences of pregnancy. Diuretics are indicated in pregnancy when edema is due to pathologic causes, just as they are in the absence of pregnancy (however, see WARNINGS, below). Dependent edema in pregnancy, resulting from restriction of venous return by the expanded uterus, is properly treated through elevation of the lower extremities and use of support hose; use of diuretics to lower intravascular volume in this case is illogical and unnecessary. There is hypervolemia during normal pregnancy which is harmful to neither the fetus nor the mother (in the absence of cardiovascular disease), but which is associated with edema, including generalized edema, in the majority of pregnant women. If this edema produces discomfort, increased recumbency will often provide relief. In rare instances, this edema may cause extreme discomfort which is not relieved by rest. In these cases, a short course of diuretics may provide relief and may be appropriate.

Contraindications:

A. Anuria
B. Hypersensitivity to this or other sulfonamide derived drugs.
C. Progressively impaired renal function. Since reserpine may increase gastric secretion and motility, its use alone or in combination requires caution and is sometimes contraindicated in patients with a history of peptic or duodenal ulcer or other gastrointestinal disorders.
D. HYDROMOX R should not be administered to patients with severe hepatic dysfunction. The use of the drug should be avoided in patients with a history of mental depression or psychosis. HYDROMOX R should not be used by patients who are known to be hypersensitive to either agent.

Warnings: Diuretics should be used with caution in several renal disease. In patients with renal disease, diuretics may precipitate azotemia. Cumulative effects of the drug may develop in patients with impaired renal function.

Diuretics should be used with caution in patients with impaired hepatic function or progressive liver disease, since minor alterations of fluid and electrolyte balance may precipitate hepatic coma.

HYDROMOX R may add to or potentiate the action of other antihypertensive drugs. Potentiation occurs with ganglionic or peripheral adrenergic blocking drugs.

Sensitivity reactions may occur in patients with a history of allergy or bronchial asthma. The possibility of exacerbation or activation of systemic lupus erythematosus has been reported with sulfonamide-derived drugs.

Usage in Pregnancy

HYDROMOX R crosses the placental barrier and appears in cord blood. The use of HYDROMOX R in pregnant women requires that the anticipated benefit be weighed against possible hazards to the fetus. These hazards include fetal or neonatal jaundice, thrombocytopenia, and possibly other adverse reactions which have occurred in the adult.

Nursing Mothers

HYDROMOX R appears in breast milk. If use of drug is essential, the patient should stop nursing.

Reserpine has been reported to cause central nervous system depression of the newborn infant when given to the mother in the immediate ante partum period.

HYDROMOX R should be discontinued promptly if any symptoms of mental depression occur with the use of the drug.

Precautions:

Quinethazone:

(1) Quinethazone should be used with caution in patients with impaired hepatic function or progressive liver disease, since minor alterations of fluid and electrolyte balance may precipitate hepatic coma.
(2) Whereas electrolyte abnormalities are often present in such conditions as heart failure and cirrhosis as a result of underlying disease process, they may also be aggravated or may be produced independently by any potent diuretic affecting electrolyte excretion. Caution is especially important during prolonged or intensive therapy and when salt intake is restricted or during concomitant use of steroids or ACTH. Hypokalemia attributable to HYDROMOX *quinethazone* therapy has been mild and infrequent, and other electrolyte abnormalities have been rare.
The possibility of potassium depletion and its toxic sequelae must be kept in mind, particularly in cirrhotics and patients receiving digitalis. As a preventive measure the use of foods rich in potassium, such as orange juice, or supplements of potassium chloride may be desirable.
(3) In patients with impaired renal function, azotemia and/or excessive drug accumulation may develop.
(4) As with other potent diuretics, when HYDROMOX is added to a regimen that includes ganglionic-blocking agents, the dosage of these latter preparations should be reduced to avoid a sudden drop in blood pressure. Reduction of dosage is also necessary when one or more of these antihypertensive agents is added to an established HYDROMOX regimen.
(5) As with the thiazide diuretics, increases of serum uric acid may occur but precipitation of gout has been rare.
(6) A decreased glucose tolerance as evidenced by hyperglycemia and glycosuria thus aggravating or provoking diabetes mellitus has occurred.

(7) Quinethazone may decrease arterial responsiveness to norepinephrine and therefore should be withdrawn 48 hours before elective surgery. If emergency surgery is indicated, pre-anesthetic and anesthetic agents should be administered in reduced dosage. Quinethazone may also increase the responsiveness to tubocurarine. The antihypertensive effects of the drug may be enhanced in the post-sympathectomy patient.

(8) Sensitivity reactions may be more likely to occur in patients with a history of allergy or bronchial asthma.

(9) The possibility of exacerbation or activation of systemic lupus erythematosus has been suggested for sulfonamide derived drugs.

Reserpine:
Reserpine may precipitate biliary colic in patients with gallstones, or bronchial asthma in susceptible patients. Reserpine preparations should be used with caution in patients with a history of peptic ulcer, ulcerative colitis and other gastrointestinal disorders. It may cause severe depression and suicidal risk and may produce pseudoparkinsonism (a paralysis agitans-like syndrome). Administration of reserpine should be discontinued 2 weeks or more before electroconvulsant therapy if possible to preclude severe, even fatal, reactions.
Reserpine may cause cardiotoxic effects, e.g. premature ventricular contractions and other arrhythmias, possible sensitization to digitalis (which might be further complicated by any hypokalemic effects of quinethazone), fluid retention, and congestive failure.

Adverse Reactions: The following adverse reactions have been reported with the diuretic drugs some of which may be expected to occur with quinethazone:

A. Gastrointestinal System reactions
1. anorexia 2. gastric irritation 3. nausea 4. vomiting 5. cramping 6. diarrhea 7. constipation 8. jaundice (intrahepatic cholestatic jaundice) 9. pancreatitis 10. hyperglycemia 11. glycosuria

B. Central Nervous System reactions
1. dizziness 2. vertigo 3. paresthesias 4. headache 5. xanthopsia

C. Hematologic reactions
1. leukopenia 2. thrombocytopenia 3. agranulocytosis 4. aplastic anemia

D. Dermatologic-hypersensitivity reactions
1. purpura 2. photosensitivity 3. rash 4. urticaria 5. necrotizing angiitis (vasculitis) (cutaneous vasculitis)

E. Cardiovascular reactions
1. orthostatic hypotension may occur and may be potentiated by alcohol, barbiturates or narcotics.

F. Miscellaneous
1. muscle spasm 2. weakness 3. restlessness

Reserpine:
With reserpine, nasal congestion, weight gain, and diarrhea are the most frequently noted side effects. The drug may reactivate old peptic ulcers because it increases hydrochloric acid secretion by the stomach. More serious reactions are excessive drowsiness, fatigue, weakness, insomnia, nightmares, excitement, irrational behavior, and incipient parkinsonism. Sodium retention edema may occur when reserpine is used.
Whenever adverse reactions are moderate or severe, thiazide dosage should be reduced or therapy withdrawn.

Dosage and Administration:
Dosage: As determined by individual titration (see box warning).
Usual Initial Adult Loading Dosage: If considered necessary, 3 to 4 HYDROMOX R Tablets (150 mg. quinethazone with 0.375 mg. reserpine to 200 mg. quinethazone with 0.5 mg. reserpine) may be administered orally, once a day, for not more than 2 weeks.
Average (or Maintenance) Adult Dosage: 1 to 2 HYDROMOX R Tablets (50 mg. quinethazone with 0.125 mg. reserpine to 100 mg. quinethazone with 0.25 mg. reserpine) administered orally, once a day.
Because of the relatively prolonged effect of HYDROMOX R, a single daily dose is usually sufficient. Occasionally 1 tablet is administered twice a day, but ordinarily medication is administered only in the morning to avoid the inconvenience of nocturia.
With the exception of the initial loading phase, a total dose of 3 to 4 tablets of HYDROMOX R Quinethazone with Reserpine is not recommended since the 0.375 mg. to 0.5 mg. of reserpine thus provided is more than is routinely necessary for a hypotensive effect and serves to increase the risk of adverse reactions. If more than 100 mg. of quinethazone per day is desired, it is recommended that HYDROMOX Quinethazone Tablets be used to supplement HYDROMOX R.
The dosage of HYDROMOX R to be employed depends upon the severity of the condition being treated and the responsiveness of the individual patient and often must be adjusted at the beginning of, or during the course of, therapy. Reduction of dosage is often possible after 2 weeks, when as little as 1 tablet a day may be sufficient for maintenance.
When HYDROMOX R Tablets are used in combination with other antihypertensive drugs, the dosage of each drug may often be reduced because of potentiation. (See under Precautions concerning the necessity for dosage adjustment when one or more of these drugs is added to an already established therapeutic regimen).

How Supplied: Yellow Tablets Scored - Bottles of 100 and 500.
[*Shown in Product Identification Section*]

INCREMIN®
WITH IRON • SYRUP
(vitamins B_1, B_6, B_{12}-lysine-iron)
Dietary Supplement

(See PDR for Nonprescription Drugs)

LEDERCILLIN® VK ℞
(penicillin V potassium)
For Oral Use

How Supplied:
LEDERCILLIN VK—For Oral Solution
125 mg. (200,000 Units) per 5 ml.—100 ml. 150 ml. and 200 ml. bottles (cherry-punch flavor)
250 mg. (400,000 Units) per 5 ml.—100 ml., 150 ml. and 200 ml. bottles (cherry-punch flavor)
LEDERCILLIN VK Tablets—U.S.P.
250 mg. (400,000 Units) bottles of 100 and 1000, Unit-dose 10 x 10's.
500 mg. (800,000 Units) bottles of 100; Unit-dose 10 x 10's.
USPHS Depot: Tablets, 250 mg—40's, NSN 6505-00-282-5271; 28's-NSN 6505-00-926-2188

LEDERPLEX®
Dietary Supplement of B-Complex Vitamins for Adults and Children 4 or More Years of Age
Capsules—Liquid—Tablets

(See PDR For Nonprescription Drugs)

LEUCOVORIN CALCIUM INJECTION ℞

Description: Each 1 ml ampul of LEUCOVORIN CALCIUM *Lederle* contains Leucovorin 3 mg as the calcium salt which is the form preferred for intramuscular injection. Preservatives: Propylparaben 0.02% w/v, Methylparaben 0.08% w/v. The inactive ingredient is Water for Injection q.s. 100% and sodium hydroxide or hydrochloric acid is used to adjust the pH to approximately 7.8.
Each 50 mg vial of Leucovorin Calcium cryodessicated powder when reconstituted with 5 ml of water for injection contains Leucovorin 10 mg per ml as the calcium salt which is the form preferred for intramuscular injection. Preservatives: Methylparaben 0.08% w/v and Propylparaben 0.02% w/v. The inactive ingredients are Sodium Chloride and Sodium Hydroxide q.s. pH approximately 7.8. Reconstituted solutions should be used as soon as possible since precipitation may occur on prolonged standing.

Actions: Leucovorin (folinic acid) is the formyl derivative and active form of folic acid. Leucovorin Calcium is useful clinically in circumventing the action of folate reductase. There is no evidence that intramuscular doses of greater than 1 mg have greater efficacy than those of 1 mg.

Indications: Indicated (a) to diminish the toxicity and counteract the effect of inadvertently administered overdosages of folic acid antagonists. (See warnings). (b) In the treatment of the megaloblastic anemias due to sprue, nutritional deficiency, pregnancy, and infancy when oral therapy is not feasible.

Contraindications: Not to be administered for the treatment of pernicious anemia or other megaloblastic anemias where Vitamin B_{12} is deficient.

Warnings: Leucovorin is improper therapy for pernicious anemia and other megaloblastic anemias secondary to lack of vitamin B_{12}. A hematologic remission may occur while neurologic manifestations remain progressive.
In the treatment of overdosage of folic acid antagonists leucovorin must be administered within 1 hour, if possible, and is usually ineffective if administered after a delay of 4 hours.

Precautions: In the presence of pernicious anemia a hematologic remission may occur while neurologic manifestations remain progressive.

Adverse Reactions: Allergic sensitization has been reported following both oral and parenteral administration of folic acid.

Dosage: Megaloblastic anemia: No more than or up to 1 mg daily. There is no evidence that intramuscular doses greater than 1 mg daily have greater efficacy than those of 1 mg; additionally, loss of folate in the urine becomes roughly logarithmic as the amount administered exceeds 1 mg.
For the treatment of overdosage of folic acid antagonists: To be given in amounts equal to the weight of the antagonist given.

How Supplied:
6 — 1 ml ampuls.
50 mg vials of cryodessicated powder.

LOXITANE® ℞
(loxapine succinate)
Capsules

and LOXITANE® C
(loxapine hydrochloride)
Oral Concentrate
For oral Use

LOXITANE® IM
(loxapine hydrochloride)
For Intramuscular Use Only

Description: LOXITANE *loxapine*, a dibenzoxazepine compound, represents a new sub-

Continued on next page

The information on each product appearing here is based on labelling effective in August, 1979 and is either the entire official brochure or an accurate condensation therefrom. Official brochures are enclosed in product packages. Information concerning all Lederle products may be obtained from the Medical Department, Lederle Laboratories, Pearl River, New York, 10965.

Lederle—Cont.

class of tricyclic antipsychotic agent, chemically distinct from the thioxanthenes, butyrophenones, and phenothiazines. Chemically, it is 2-chloro-11-(4-methyl-1-piperazinyl)dibenz[b,f]-[1,4]oxazepine. It is present in capsules as the succinate salt, and in the concentrate and parenteral primarily as the HCl.

CAPSULES—Each capsule contains loxapine succinate equivalent to 5, 10, 25 or 50 mg of loxapine base.

ORAL CONCENTRATE—Each ml contains loxapine hydrochloride equivalent to 25 mg of loxapine base.

INTRAMUSCULAR—(Sterile)—Not for Intravenous Use—Each ml contains loxapine hydrochloride equivalent to 50 mg of loxapine base. Inactive Ingredients: polysorbate 80 USP 5% w/v; propylene glycol 70% v/v; and water for injection qs ad 100% v. Hydrochloric acid or Sodium hydroxide qs pH approx. 6.0.

Actions: Pharmacologically, loxapine is a tranquilizer for which the exact mode of action has not been established. However, changes in the level of excitability of subcortical inhibitory areas have been observed in several animal species in association with such manifestations of tranquilization as calming effects and suppression of aggressive behavior.

In normal human volunteers, signs of sedation were seen within 20 to 30 minutes after administration, were most pronounced within 1½ to 3 hours, and lasted through 12 hours. Similar timing of primary pharmacologic effects was seen in animals.

Absorption of loxapine following oral or parenteral administration is virtually complete. The drug is removed rapidly from the plasma and distributed in tissues. Animal studies suggest an initial preferential distribution in lungs, brain, spleen, heart, and kidney. Loxapine is metabolized extensively and is excreted mainly in the first 24 hours. Metabolites are excreted in the urine in the form of conjugates and in the feces unconjugated.

Indications: LOXITANE is indicated for the manifestations of schizophrenia.

Contraindications: LOXITANE is contraindicated in comatose or severe drug-induced depressed states (alcohol, barbiturates, narcotics, etc.)

LOXITANE is contraindicated in individuals with known hypersensitivity to the drug.

Warnings:

Usage in Pregnancy: Safe use during pregnancy or lactation has not been established; therefore, its use in pregnancy, in nursing mothers, or in women of childbearing potential requires that the benefits of treatment be weighed against the possible risks to mother and child. No embryotoxicity or teratology was observed in studies in rats, rabbits or dogs, although with the exception of one rabbit study, the highest dosage was only two times the maximum recommended human dose and in some studies they were below this dose. Perinatal studies have shown renal papillary abnormalities in offspring of rats treated from mid-pregnancy with doses of 0.6 and 1.8 mg/kg, doses which approximate the usual human dose but which are considerably below the maximum recommended human dose.

Usage in Children: Studies have not been performed in children; therefore this drug is not recommended for use in children below the age of 16.

LOXITANE, like other tranquilizers, may impair mental and/or physical abilities, especially during the first few days of therapy. Therefore, ambulatory patients should be warned about activities requiring alertness (eg, operating vehicles or machinery), and about concomitant use of alcohol and other CNS depressants.

LOXITANE has not been evaluated for the management of behavioral complications in patients with mental retardation, and therefore it cannot be recommended.

Precautions: LOXITANE should be used with extreme caution in patients with a history of convulsive disorders since it lowers the convulsive threshold. Seizures have been reported in epileptic patients receiving LOXITANE at antipsychotic dose levels, and may occur even with maintenance of routine anticonvulsant drug therapy.

Loxapine has an antiemetic effect in animals. Since this effect may also occur in man, loxapine may mask signs of overdosage of toxic drugs and may obscure conditions such as intestinal obstruction and brain tumor.

LOXITANE should be used with caution in patients with cardiovascular disease. Increased pulse rates have been reported in the majority of patients receiving antipsychotic doses; transient hypotension has been reported. In the presence of severe hypotension requiring vasopressor therapy, the preferred drugs may be norepinephrine or angiotensin. Usual doses of epinephrine may be ineffective because of inhibition of its vasopressor effect by loxapine.

The possibility of ocular toxicity from loxapine cannot be excluded at this time. Therefore, careful observation should be made for pigmentary retinopathy and lenticular pigmentation since these have been observed in some patients receiving certain other antipsychotic drugs for prolonged periods.

Because of possible anticholinergic action, the drug should be used cautiously in patients with glaucoma or a tendency to urinary retention, particularly with concomitant administration of anticholinergic-type anti-parkinson medication.

Experience to date indicates the possibility of a slightly higher incidence of extrapyramidal effects following intramuscular administration than normally anticipated with oral formulations. The increase may be attributable to higher plasma levels following intramuscular injection.

Adverse Reactions:

CNS Effects: Manifestations of adverse effects on the central nervous system, other than extrapyramidal effects, have been seen infrequently. Drowsiness, usually mild, may occur at the beginning of therapy or when dosage is increased.

It usually subsides with continued LOXITANE therapy. The incidence of sedation has been less than that of certain aliphatic phenothiazines and slightly more the piperazine phenothiazines. Dizziness, faintness, staggering gait, muscle twitching, weakness, and confusional states have been reported.

Extrapyramidal Reactions—Neuromuscular (extra-pyramidal) reactions during the administration of LOXITANE have been reported frequently, often during the first few days of treatment. In most patients, these reactions involved Parkinson-like symptoms such as tremor, rigidity, excessive salivation, and masked facies. Akathisia (motor restlessness) also has been reported relatively frequently. These symptoms are usually not severe and can be controlled by reduction of LOXITANE dosage or by administration of antiparkinson drugs in usual dosage. Dystonic and dyskinetic reactions have occurred less frequently, but may be more severe. Dystonias include spasms of muscles of the neck and face, tongue protrusion, and oculogyric movement. Dyskinetic reaction has been described in the form of choreo-athetoid movements. These reactions sometimes require reduction or temporary withdrawal of LOXITANE dosage in addition to appropriate counteractive drugs.

Persistent Tardive Dyskinesia—As with all antipsychotic agents, tardive dyskinesia may appear in some patients on long-term therapy or may appear after drug therapy has been discontinued. The risk appears to be greater in elderly patients on high-dose therapy, especially females. The symptoms are persistent and in some patients appear to be irreversible. The syndrome is characterized by rhythmical involuntary movement of the tongue, face, mouth, or jaw (eg, protrusion of tongue, puffing of cheeks, puckering of mouth, chewing movements). Sometimes these may be accompanied by involuntary movements of extremities.

There is no known effective treatment for tardive dyskinesia; antiparkinson agents usually do not alleviate the symptoms of this syndrome. It is suggested that all antipyschotic agents be discontinued if these symptoms appear. Should it be necessary to reinstitute treatment, or increase the dosage of the agent, or switch to a different antipsychotic agent, the syndrome may be masked. It has been suggested that fine vermicular movements of the tongue may be an early sign of the syndrome, and if the medication is stopped at that time the syndrome may not develop.

Cardiovascular Effects: Tachycardia, hypotension, hypertension, lightheadedness, and syncope have been reported.

A few cases of ECG changes similar to those seen with phenothiazines have been reported. It is not known whether these were related to loxapine administration.

Skin: Dermatitis, edema (puffiness of face), pruritus, and seborrhea have been reported with loxapine. The possibility of photosensitivity and/or phototoxicity occurring has not been excluded; skin rashes of uncertain etiology have been observed in a few patients during hot summer months.

Anticholinergic Effects: Dry mouth, nasal congestion, constipation, and blurred vision have occurred; these are more likely to occur with concomitant use of antiparkinson agents.

Other Adverse Reactions: Nausea, vomiting, weight gain, weight loss, dyspnea, ptosis, hyperpyrexia, flushed facies, headache, paresthesia, and polydipsia have been reported in some patients.

Rarely, galactorrhea and menstrual irregularity of uncertain etiology have been reported.

Dosage and Administration: LOXITANE is administered, usually in divided doses, two or four times a day. Daily dosage (in terms of base equivalents) should be adjusted to the individual patient's needs as assessed by the severity of symptoms and previous history of response to antipsychotic drugs.

Oral Administration

Initial dosage of 10 mg twice daily is recommended, although in severely disturbed patients initial dosage up to a total of 50 mg daily may be desirable. Dosage should then be increased fairly rapidly over the first seven to ten days until there is effective control of psychotic symptoms. The usual therapeutic and maintenance range is 60 mg to 100 mg daily. However, as with other antipsychotic drugs, some patients respond to lower dosage and others require higher dosage for optimal benefit. Daily dosage higher than 250 mg is not recommended.

LOXITANE C Oral Concentrate should be mixed with orange or grapefruit juice shortly before administration. Use only the enclosed calibrated (10 mg, 15 mg, 20 mg, 25 mg) dropper for dosage.

Maintenance Therapy

For maintenance therapy, dosage should be reduced to the lowest level compatible with symptom control; many patients have been maintained satisfactorily at dosages in the range of 20 mg to 60 mg daily.

Intramuscular Administration

LOXITANE IM is utilized for prompt symptomatic control in the acutely agitated patient and in patients whose symptoms render oral medication temporarily impractical. During clinical trial there were no reports of significant local tissue reaction.

LOXITANE IM is administered by intramuscular (not intravenous) injection in doses of 12.5 mg (¼ ml) to 50 mg (1 ml) at intervals of four to six hours or longer, both dose and interval depending on patient response. Many patients have responded satisfactorily to twice-daily dosage. As described above for oral administration, attention is directed to the necessity for dosage adjustment on an individual basis over the early days of loxapine administration.

Once the desired symptomatic control is achieved and the patient is able to take medication orally, loxapine should be administered in capsule or oral concentrate form. Usually this should occur within five days.

Overdosage: Signs and symptoms of overdosage will depend on the amount ingested and individual patient tolerance. As would be expected from the pharmacologic actions of the drug, the clinical findings may range from mild depression of the CNS and cardiovascular systems to profound hypotension, respiratory depression, and unconsciousness. The possibility of occurrence of extrapyramidal symptoms and/or convulsive seizures should be kept in mind.

The treatment of overdosage is essentially symptomatic and supportive. Early gastric lavage and extended dialysis might be expected to be beneficial. Centrally acting emetics may have little effect because of the antiemetic action of loxapine. In addition, emesis should be avoided because of the possibility of aspiration of vomitus. Avoid analeptics, such as pentylenetetrazol, which may cause convulsions. Severe hypotension might be expected to respond to the administration of levarterenol or phenylephrine. EPINEPHRINE SHOULD NOT BE USED SINCE ITS USE IN A PATIENT WITH PARTIAL ADRENERGIC BLOCKADE MAY FURTHER LOWER THE BLOOD PRESSURE. Severe extrapyramidal reactions should be treated with anticholinergic antiparkinson agents or diphenhydramine hydrochloride, and anticonvulsant therapy should be initiated as indicated. Additional measures include oxygen and intravenous fluids.

How Supplied: LOXITANE *loxapine succinate* capsules are supplied in the following base equivalent strengths:

Hard Shell Printed "Lederle"

- 5 mg – Green; Bottles of 100, 1000, and unit dose 10 × 10's
- 10 mg – Green and Yellow; Bottles of 100, 1000, and unit dose 10 × 10's
- 25 mg – Green Two Tone; Bottles of 100, 1000, and unit dose 10 × 10's
- 50 mg – Green and Blue; Bottles of 100, 1000, and unit dose 10 × 10's

LOXITANE C *loxapine hydrochloride* Oral Concentrate (Product Number 5387) is supplied in bottles of 4 FL. Oz. (120 ml) with calibrated dropper. Each ml contains the equivalent of 25 mg loxapine base as the HCl.

LOXITANE IM *loxapine hydrochloride* for Intramuscular use only (Product Number 5385) is supplied in sterile 1 ml ampuls and 10 ml vials. Each ml contains the equivalent of 50 mg loxapine base as the HCl.

Keep package closed to protect from light. Intensification of the straw color to a light amber will not alter potency or therapeutic efficacy; if noticeably discolored, ampul or vial should not be used.

A.H.F.S. 28:16.08

Oral Concentrate

VA Depot

NSN 6505-01-026-0101A.

[*Shown in Product Identification Section*]

MATERNA™ 1•60 ℞

Prenatal Tablets (Film Coated)

Each tablet contains:		For Pregnant or Lactating Women % of U.S. RDA
Vitamin A Acetate	8,000 I.U.	(100%)
Vitamin D	400 I.U.	(100%)
Vitamin E (as *dl*-Alpha Tocopheryl Acetate)	30 I.U.	(100%)
Vitamin C (Ascorbic Acid)	120 mg.	(200%)
Folic Acid (Folacin)	1 mg.	(125%)
Thiamine (as Thiamine Mononitrate Vitamin B_1)	3 mg.	(176%)
Riboflavin (Vitamin B_2)	3.4 mg.	(170%)
Vitamin B_6 (as Pyridoxine Hydrochloride)	4 mg.	(160%)
Niacinamide	20 mg.	(100%)
Vitamin B_{12} (Cyanocobalamin)	12 mcgm.	(150%)
Calcium (as Calcium Carbonate)	350 mg.	(26%)
Iodine (as Potassium Iodide)	0.3 mg.	(200%)
Elemental Iron (as Ferrous Fumarate)	60 mg.	(333%)
Magnesium (as Magnesium Oxide)	100 mg.	(22%)
Copper (as Cupric Oxide)	2 mg.	(100%)
Zinc (as Zinc Oxide)	15 mg.	(100%)
Docusate Sodium USP (DSS) (Stool Softener)	50 mg.	

A phosphorus-free vitamin and mineral dietary supplement with surfactant, for use during pregnancy and lactation. Recommended intake: 1 daily or as prescribed by physician.

Precaution: Folic acid may obscure pernicious anemia in that the peripheral blood picture may revert to normal while neurological manifestations remain progressive.

Allergic sensitization has been reported following both oral and parenteral administration of Folic Acid.

How Supplied: Tablets (film-coated, pink) —bottles of 100.

[*Shown in Product Identification*]

METHOTREXATE ℞

Tablets and Parenteral

WARNING

METHOTREXATE MUST BE USED ONLY BY PHYSICIANS EXPERIENCED IN ANTIMETABOLITE CHEMOTHERAPY.

BECAUSE OF THE POSSIBILITY OF FATAL OR SEVERE TOXIC REACTIONS THE PATIENT SHOULD BE FULLY INFORMED BY THE PHYSICIAN OF THE RISKS INVOLVED AND SHOULD BE UNDER HIS CONSTANT SUPERVISION.

DEATHS HAVE BEEN REPORTED WITH THE USE OF METHOTREXATE IN THE TREATMENT OF PSORIASIS.

IN THE TREATMENT OF PSORIASIS METHOTREXATE SHOULD BE RESTRICTED TO SEVERE, RECALCITRANT, DISABLING, PSORIASIS WHICH IS NOT ADEQUATELY RESPONSIVE TO OTHER FORMS OF THERAPY, BUT ONLY WHEN THE DIAGNOSIS HAS BEEN ESTABLISHED, AS BY BIOPSY AND/OR AFTER DERMATOLOGIC CONSULTATION.

1. Methotrexate may produce marked depression of bone marrow, anemia, leukopenia, thrombocytopenia and bleeding.
2. Methotrexate may be hepatotoxic, particularly at high dosage or with prolonged therapy. Liver atrophy, necrosis, cirrhosis, fatty changes, and periportal fibrosis have been reported. Since changes may occur without previous signs of gastrointestinal or hematologic toxicity, it is imperative that hepatic function be determined prior to initiation of treatment and monitored regularly throughout therapy. Special caution is indicated in the presence of preexisting liver damage or impaired hepatic function. Concomitant use of other drugs with hepatotoxic potential (including alcohol) should be avoided.
3. Methotrexate has caused fetal death and/or congenital anomalies, therefore, it is not recommended in women of childbearing potential unless there is appropriate medical evidence that the benefits can be expected to outweigh the considered risks. Pregnant psoriatic patients should not receive Methotrexate.
4. Impaired renal function is usually a contraindication.
5. Diarrhea and ulcerative stomatitis are frequent toxic effects and require interruption of therapy; otherwise hemorrhagic enteritis and death from intestinal perforation may occur.

METHOTREXATE HAS BEEN ADMINISTERED IN VERY HIGH DOSAGE FOLLOWED BY LEUCOVORIN RESCUE IN EXPERIMENTAL TREATMENT OF CERTAIN NEOPLASTIC DISEASES. THIS PROCEDURE IS INVESTIGATIONAL AND HAZARDOUS.

Description: Methotrexate Lederle (formerly A-methopterin) is an antimetabolite used in the treatment of certain neoplastic diseases.

Methotrexate Tablets contain 2.5 mg of Methotrexate.

Methotrexate Sodium Parenteral is available both in 2.5 mg/ml and 25 mg/ml strengths each available in 2 ml vials.

Each 2.5 mg/ml (5.0 mg) vial contains per 2 ml: Methotrexate Sodium equivalent to 5 mg Methotrexate, 0.90% w/v of benzyl alcohol as a preservative, and the following Inactive Ingredients. Sodium Chloride 0.630% w/v and Water for Injection qs ad 100% V. Sodium Hydroxide to adjust pH to approx. 8.5.

Each 25 mg/ml (50 mg) vial contains per 2 ml: Methotrexate Sodium equivalent to 50 mg Methotrexate, 0.90% w/v of benzyl alcohol as a preservative, and the following Inactive Ingredients: Sodium Chloride 0.260% w/v and Water for Injection qs ad 100% V. Sodium Hydroxide to adjust pH to approx. 8.5.

If desired, the solution may be further diluted with a compatible medium such as Sodium Chloride Injection USP. Storage for 24 hours at a temperature of 21° to 25° C results in a product which is within 90% of label potency.

Each 20 mg vial of sterile cryodesiccated powder, for single use only, contains: Methotrexate Sodium equivalent to 20 mg Methotrexate. Contains no preservative, with Sodium Hydroxide as an inactive ingredient. Contains approximately 0.14 milliequivalents of sodium per vial. Reconstitute immediately prior to use with 20 ml of an appropriate sterile, preservative-free medium such as Sodium Chloride Injection, USP.

Action: Methotrexate has as its principal mechanism of action the competitive inhibi-

Continued on next page

The information on each product appearing here is based on labelling effective in August, 1979 and is either the entire official brochure or an accurate condensation therefrom. Official brochures are enclosed in product packages. Information concerning all Lederle products may be obtained from the Medical Department, Lederle Laboratories, Pearl River, New York, 10965.

Lederle—Cont.

tion of the enzyme folic acid reductase. Folic acid must be reduced to tetrahydrofolic acid by this enzyme in the process of DNA synthesis and cellular replication. Methotrexate inhibits the reduction of folic acid and interferes with tissue-cell reproduction.

Actively proliferating tissues such as malignant cells, bone marrow, fetal cells, dermal epithelium, buccal and intestinal mucosa and cells of the urinary bladder are in general more sensitive to this effect of Methotrexate. Cellular proliferation in malignant tissue is greater than in most normal tissue and thus Methotrexate may impair malignant growth without irreversible damage to normal tissues.

Orally administered Methotrexate is absorbed rapidly in most, but not all patients, and reaches peak serum levels in 1–2 hours. After parenteral injection, peak serum levels are seen in about one-half this period. Approximately one-half the absorbed Methotrexate is reversibly bound to serum protein, but exchanges with body fluids easily and diffuses into the body tissue cells.

Excretion of single daily doses occurs through the kidneys in amounts from 55% to 88% or higher within 24 hours. Repeated doses daily result in more sustained serum levels and some retention of Methotrexate over each 24 hour period which may result in accumulation of the drug within the tissues. The liver cells appear to retain certain amounts of the drug for prolonged periods even after a single therapeutic dose. Methotrexate is retained in the presence of impaired renal function and may increase rapidly in the serum and in the tissue cells under such conditions. Methotrexate does not penetrate the blood cerebrospinal fluid barrier in therapeutic amounts when given orally or parenterally. High concentrations of the drug when needed may be attained by direct intrathecal administration.

In psoriasis, the rate of production of epithelial cells in the skin is greatly increased over normal skin. This differential in reproductive rates is the basis for the use of Methotrexate to control the psoriatic process.

Indications:

Anti-neoplastic Chemotherapy

Methotrexate is indicated for the treatment of gestational choriocarcinoma, and in patients with chorioadenoma destruens and hydatidiform mole.

Methotrexate is indicated for the palliation of acute lymphocytic leukemia. It is also indicated in the treatment and prophylaxis of meningeal leukemia. Greatest effect has been observed in palliation of acute lymphoblastic (stem-cell) leukemias in children. In combination with other anticancer drugs or suitable agents Methotrexate may be used for induction of remission, but it is most commonly used, as described in the literature, in the maintenance of induced remissions.

Methotrexate may be used alone or in combination with other anticancer agents in the management of breast cancer, epidermoid cancers of the head and neck, and lung cancer, particularly squamous cell and small cell types.

Methotrexate is also effective in the treatment of the advanced stages (III and IV, Peters Staging System) of lymphosarcoma, particularly in those cases in children; and in advanced cases of mycosis fungoides.

Psoriasis Chemotherapy **[See box warnings at top of Insert]** Because of high risk attending its use, Methotrexate is only indicated in the symptomatic control of severe, recalcitrant, disabling psoriasis which is not adequately responsive to other forms of therapy, *but only when the diagnosis has been established, as by biopsy and/or after dermatologic consultation.*

Contraindications: Pregnant psoriatic patients should not receive Methotrexate. Psoriatic patients with severe renal or hepatic disorders should not receive Methotrexate.

Psoriatic patients with pre-existing blood dyscrasias, such as bone marrow hypoplasia, leukopenia, thrombocytopenia or anemia, should not receive Methotrexate.

Warnings: See Box Warnings

Precautions: Methotrexate has a high potential toxicity, usually dose-related. The physician should be familiar with the various characteristics of the drug and its established clinical usage. Patients undergoing therapy should be subject to appropriate supervision so that signs or symptoms of possible toxic effects or adverse reactions may be detected and evaluated with minimal delay. Pretreatment and periodic hematologic studies are essential to the use of Methotrexate in chemotherapy because of its common effect of hematopoietic suppression. This may occur abruptly and on apparent safe dosage, and any profound drop in blood-cell count indicates immediate stopping of the drug and appropriate therapy. In patients with malignant disease who have preexising bone marrow aplasia, leukopenia, thrombocytopenia or anemia, the drug should be used with caution, if at all.

Methotrexate is excreted principally by the kidneys. Its use in the presence of impaired renal function may result in accumulation of toxic amounts or even additional renal damage. The patient's renal status should be determined prior to and during Methotrexate therapy and proper caution exercised should significant renal impairment be disclosed. Drug dosage should be reduced or discontinued until renal function is improved or restored.

In general, the following laboratory tests are recommended as part of essential clinical evaluation and appropriate monitoring of patients chosen for or receiving Methotrexate therapy: complete hemogram; hematocrit; urinalysis; renal function tests; and liver function tests. A chest x-ray is also recommended. The purpose is to determine any existing organ dysfunction or system impairment. The tests should be performed prior to therapy, at appropriate periods during therapy and after termination of therapy. It may be useful or important to perform liver biopsy or bone marrow aspiration studies where high dose or long-term therapy is being followed.

Methotrexate is bound in part to serum albumin after absorption and toxicity may be increased because of displacement by certain drugs such as salicylates, sulfonamides, diphenylhydantoin, phenylbutazone, and some antibacterials as tetracycline, chloramphenicol and para-amino-benzoic acid. These drugs, especially salicylates, phenylbutazone, and sulfonamides, whether antibacterial, hypoglycemic or diuretic, should not be given concurrently until the significance of these findings is established.

Vitamin preparations containing folic acid or its derviatives may alter responses to Methotrexate.

Methotrexate should be used with extreme caution in the presence of infection, peptic ulcer, ulcerative colitis, debility, and in extreme youth and old age.

If profound leukopenia occurs during therapy, bacterial infection may occur or become a threat. Cessation of the drug and appropriate antibiotic therapy is usually indicated. In severe bone marrow depression, blood or platelet transfusions may be necessary.

Since it is reported that Methotrexate may have an immunosuppressive action, this factor must be taken into consideration in evaluating the use of the drug where immune responses in a patient may be important or essential.

In all instances where the use of Methotrexate is considered for chemotherapy, the physician must evaluate the need and usefulness of the drug against the risks of toxic effects or adverse reaction. Most such adverse reactions are reversible if detected early. When such effects or reactions do occur, the drug should be reduced in dosage or discontinued and appropirate corrective measures should be taken, according to the clinical judgment of the physician. Reinstitution of Methotrexate therapy should be carried out with caution, with adequate consideration of further need for the drug and alertness as to possible recurrence of toxicity.

Adverse Reactions: The most common adverse reactions include ulcerative stomatitis, leukopenia, nausea and abdominal distress. Others reported are malaise, undue fatigue, chills and fever, dizziness and decreased resistance to infection. In general, the incidence and severity of side effects are considered to be dose-related. Adverse reactions as reported for the various systems are as follows:

Skin: erythematous rashes, pruritus, urticaria, photosensitivity, depigmentation, alopecia, ecchymosis, telangiectasia, acne, furunculosis. Lesions of psoriasis may be aggravated by concomitant exposure to ultraviolet radiation.

Blood: bone marrow depression, leukopenia, thrombocytopenia, anemia, hypogammaglobulinemia, hemorrhage from various sites, septicemia.

Alimentary System: gingivitis, pharyngitis, stomatitis, anorexia, vomiting, diarrhea, hematemesis, melena, gastrointestinal ulceration and bleeding, enteritis, hepatic toxicity resulting in acute liver atrophy, necrosis, fatty metamorphosis, periportal fibrosis, or hepatic cirrhosis.

Urogenital System: renal failure, azotemia, cystitis, hematuria; defective oogenesis or spermatogenesis, transient oligospermia, menstrual dysfunction; infertility, abortion, fetal defects, severe nephropathy.

Pulmonary System: Interstitial Pneumonitis. Deaths have been reported and chronic interstitial obstructive pulmonary disease has occasionally occurred.

Central Nervous System: Headaches, drowsiness, blurred vision. Aphasia, hemiparesis, paresis and convulsions have also occurred following administration of Methotrexate.

There have been reports of leucoencephalopathy following intravenous administration of Methotrexate to patients who have had craniospinal irradiation.

After the intrathecal use of Methotrexate, the central nervous system toxicity which may occur can be classified as follows: (1) chemical arachnoiditis manifested by such symptoms as headache, back pain, nuchal rigidity, and fever; (2) paresis, usually transient, manifested by paraplegia associated with involvement with one or more spinal nerve roots; (3) leucoencephalopathy manifested by confusion, irritability, somnolence, ataxia, dementia, and occasionally major convulsions.

Other reactions related to or attributed to the use of Methotrexate such as metabolic changes, precipitating diabetes; osteoporotic effects, abnormal tissue cell changes, and even sudden death have been reported.

Dosage and Administration:

Anti-neoplastic chemotherapy

Oral administration in tablet form is often preferred since absorption is rapid and effective serum levels are obtained. Methotrexate sodium parenteral may be given by intramuscular, intravenous, intraarterial or intrathecal route. Initial treatment is usually undertaken with the patient under hospital care.

*For conversion of mg/kg b.w. to mg/M^2 of body surface or the reverse, a ratio of 1:30 is given as a guide line. The conversion factor varies between 1:20 and 1:40 depending on age and body build.

Choriocarcinoma and similar trophoblastic diseases: Methotrexate is administered orally or intramuscularly in doses of 15 to 30 mg daily for a 5 day course. Such courses are usually repeated for 3 to 5 times as required, with rest periods of one or more weeks interposed between courses, until any manifesting toxic symptoms subside. The effectiveness of therapy is ordinarily evaluated by 24 hour quantitative analysis of urinary chorionic gonadotropin hormone (CGH), which should return to normal or less than 50 IU/24 hr. usually after the 3rd or 4th course and usually be followed by a complete resolution of measurable lesions in 4 to 6 weeks. One to two courses of Methotrexate after normalization of CGH is usually recommended. Before each course of the drug careful clinical assessment is essential. Cyclic combination therapy of Methotrexate with other antitumor drugs has been reported as being useful. Since hydatidiform mole may precede or be followed by choriocarcinoma, prophylactic chemotherapy with Methotrexate has been recommended. Chorioadenoma destruens is considered to be an invasive form of hydatidiform mole. Methotrexate is administered in these disease states in doses similar to those recommended for choriocarcinoma.

Leukemia: acute lymphatic (lymphoblastic) leukemia in children and young adolescents is the most responsive to present day chemotherapy. In young adults and older patients, clinical remission is more difficult to obtain and early relapse is more common. In chronic lymphatic leukemia, the prognosis for adequate response is less encouraging.

Methotrexate alone or in combination with steroids was used initially for induction of remission of lymphoblastic leukemias. More recently corticosteroid therapy in combination with other antileukemic drugs or in cyclic combinations with Methotrexate included appear to produce rapid and effective remissions. When used for induction. Methotrexate in doses of 3.3 mg/M^2 in combination with prednisone 60 mg/M^2, given daily, produced remission in 50% of patients treated, usually within a period of 4 to 6 weeks. Methotrexate alone or in combination with other agents appears to be the drug of choice for securing maintenance of drug-induced remissions. When remission is achieved and supportive care has produced general clinical improvement, maintenance therapy is initiated, as follows: Methotrexate is administered 2 times weekly either by mouth or intramuscularly in doses of 30 mg/M^2. It has also been given in doses of 2.5 mg/kg intravenously every 14 days. If and when relapse does occur, reinduction of remission can again usually be obtained by repeating the initial induction regimen. Various experts have recently introduced a variety of dosage schedules for both induction and maintenance of remission with various combinations of alkylating and antifolic agents. Multiple drug therapy with several agents, including Methotrexate given concomitantly is gaining increasing support in both the acute and chronic forms of leukemia. The physician should familiarize himself with the new advances in antileukemic therapy.

Acute granulocytic leukemia is rare in children but common in adults. This form of leukemia responds poorly to chemotherapy and remissions are short with relapses common, and resistance to therapy develops rapidly.

Meningeal leukemia: Patients with leukemia are subject to leukemic invasion of the central nervous system. This may manifest characteristic signs or symptoms or may remain silent and be diagnosed only by examination of the cerebrospinal fluid which contains leukemic cells in such cases. Therefore, the CSF should be examined in all leukemic patients. Since passage of Methotrexate from blood serum to the cerebrospinal fluid is minimal, for adequate therapy the drug is administered intrathecally. It is now common practice because of the noted increased frequency of meningeal leukemia to administer Methotrexate intrathecally as prophylaxis in all cases of lymphocytic leukemia.

By intrathecal injection, the sodium salt of Methotrexate is administered in solution in doses of 12 mg per square meter of body surface or in an empirical dose of 15 mg. The solution is made in a strength of 1 mg per ml as stated above with an appropriate, sterile, preservative-free medium such as Sodium Chloride Injection, USP.

For the treatment of meningeal leukemia, Methotrexate is given at intervals of 2 to 5 days. Methotrexate is administered until the cell count of the cerebrospinal fluid returns to normal. At this point one additional dose is advisable.

For prophylaxis against meningeal leukemia, the dosage is the same as for treatment except for the intervals of administration.

On this subject, it is advisable for the physician to consult the medical literature.

Large doses may cause convulsions. Untoward side effects may occur with any given intrathecal injection and are commonly neurological in character. Methotrexate given by intrathecal route appears significantly in the systemic circulation and may cause systemic Methotrexate toxicity. Therefore systemic antileukemic therapy with the drug should be appropriately adjusted, reduced or discontinued. Focal luekemic involvement of the central nervous system may not respond to intrathecal chemotherapy and is best treated with radiotherapy.

Lymphomas: in Burkitt's Tumor, Stages I-II, Methotrexate has produced prolonged remissions in some cases. Recommended dosage is 10 to 25 mg per day orally for 4 to 8 days. In stage III, Methotrexate is commonly given concomitantly with other antitumor agents. Treatment in all stages usually consists of several courses of the drug interposed with 7 to 10 day rest periods. Lymphosarcomas in Stage III may respond to combined drug therapy with Methotrexate given in doses of 0.625 mg to 2.5 mg/kg daily. Hodgkin's Disease responds poorly to Methotrexate and to most types of chemotherapy.

Mycosis fungoides: therapy with Methotrexate appears to produce clinical remissions in one half of the cases treated. Dosage is usually 2.5 to 10 mg daily by mouth for weeks or months. Dose levels of drug and adjustment of dose regimen by reduction or cessation of drug are guided by patient response and hematologic monitoring. Methotrexate has also been given intramuscularly in doses of 50 mg once weekly or 25 mg 2 times weekly.

Psoriasis Chemotherapy

The patient should be fully informed of the risks involved and should be under constant supervision of the physician.

Assessment of renal function, liver function, and blood elements should be made by history, physical examination, and laboratory tests (such as CBC, urinalysis, serum creatinine, liver function studies, and liver biopsy if indicated) before beginning Methotrexate, periodically during Methotrexate therapy, and before reinstituting Methotrexate therapy after a rest period. Appropriate steps should be taken to avoid conception during and for at least eight weeks following Methotrexate therapy.

There are three commonly used general types of dosage schedules:

1) weekly oral or parenteral intermittent large doses
2) divided dose intermittent oral schedule over a 36 hour period
3) daily oral with a rest period

All schedules should be continually tailored to the individual patient. Dose schedules cited below pertain to an average 70 Kg adult. An initial test dose one week prior to initiation of therapy is recommended to detect any idiosyncrasy. A suggested dose range is 5–10 mg parenterally.

Recommended starting dose schedules:

1. Weekly single oral, IM or IV dose schedule: 10–25 mg per week until adequate response is achieved. With this dosage schedule, 50 mg per week should ordinarily not be exceeded.
2. Divided oral dose schedule: 2.5 mg at 12 hour intervals for three doses or at 8 hour intervals for four doses each week. With this dosage schedule, 30 mg per week should not be exceeded.
3. Daily oral dose schedule: 2.5 mg daily for five days followed by at least a two day rest period. With this dosage schedule, 6.25 mg per day should not be exceeded.

SPECIAL NOTE: Available data suggest that schedule 3 may carry an increased risk of serious liver pathology.

Dosages in each schedule may be gradually adjusted to achieve optimal clinical response, but not to exceed the maximum stated for each schedule.

Once optimal clinical response has been achieved, each dosage schedule should be reduced to the lowest possible amount of drug and to the longest possible rest period. The use of Methotrexate may permit the return to conventional topical therapy, which should be encouraged.

Antidote for Overdosage: Leucovorin (citrovorum factor) is a potent agent for neutralizing the immediate toxic effects of Methotrexate on the hematopoietic system. Where large doses or overdoses are given, Calcium Leucovorin may be administered by intravenous infusion in doses up to 75 mg within 12 hours, followed by 12 mg intramuscularly every 6 hours for 4 doses. Where average doses of Methotrexate appear to have an adverse effect, 2 to 4 ml (6 to 12 mg) of Calcium Leucovorin may be given intramuscularly every 6 hours for 4 doses. In general, where overdosage is suspected, the dose of Leucovorin should be equal to or higher than the offending dose of Methotrexate and should best be administered within the first hour. Use of Calcium Leucovorin after an hour delay is much less effective.

CAUTION: Pharmacist: Because of its potential to cause severe toxicity, Methotrexate therapy requires close supervision of the patient by the physician. Pharmacists should dispense no more than a seven (7) day supply of the drug at one time. Refill of such prescriptions should be by direct order (written or oral) of the physician only.

How Supplied:
2.5 mg Tablets—Bottles of 100.
2.5 mg per ml—2 ml Vials.
25 mg per ml—2 ml Vials.
20 mg Vial.

Military Depots
25 mg/ml—2 ml vial
NSN 6505-01-020-2367

MINOCIN® ℞

(minocycline hydrochloride)
Oral and Intravenous

Description: MINOCIN *minocycline hydrochloride* is a semi-synthetic derivative of tetracycline, 7-dimethylamino-6-deoxy-6-demethyltetracycline hydrochloride.

Intravenous: Each vial, dried by cryodesiccation, contains sterile Minocycline Hydrochloride equivalent to 100 mg. Minocycline. When reconstituted with 5 ml. of Sterile Water For Injection the pH ranges from 2.0 to 2.8.

Actions: Microbiology—The tetracyclines are primarily bacteriostatic and are thought to exert their antimicrobial effect by the inhibition of protein synthesis. Minocycline HCl is a

Continued on next page

The information on each product appearing here is based on labelling effective in August, 1979 and is either the entire official brochure or an accurate condensation therefrom. Official brochures are enclosed in product packages. Information concerning all Lederle products may be obtained from the Medical Department, Lederle Laboratories, Pearl River, New York, 10965.

Lederle—Cont.

tetracycline with antibacterial activity comparable to other tetracyclines with activity against a wide range of gram-negative and gram-positive organisms.

Tube dilution testing: Microorganisms may be considered susceptible (likely to respond to minocycline therapy) if the minimum inhibitory concentration (M.I.C.) is not more than 4.0 mcg./ml. Microorganisms may be considered intermediate (harboring partial resistance) if the M.I.C. is 4.0 to 12.5 mcg./ml. and resistant (not likely to respond to minocycline therapy) if the M.I.C. is greater than 12.5 mcg./ml.

Susceptibility plate testing: If the Kirby-Bauer method of susceptibility testing (using a 30 mcg. tetracycline disc) gives a zone of 18 mm. or greater, the bacterial strain is considered to be susceptible to any tetracycline. Minocycline shows moderate *in vitro* activity against certain strains of staphylococci which have been found resistant to other tetracyclines. For such strains, minocycline susceptibility powder may be used for additional susceptibility testing.

Human Pharmacology: Oral—Following a single dose of two 100 mg. of Minocycline HCl capsules administered to ten normal adult volunteers, serum levels ranged from 0.74 to 4.45 mcg./ml. in one hour (average 2.24), after 12 hours they ranged from 0.34 to 2.36 mcg./ml. (average 1.25). The serum half-life following a single 200 mg. dose in 12 essentially normal volunteers ranged from 11 to 17 hours, in 7 patients with hepatic dysfunction ranged from 11 to 16 hours, and in 5 patients with renal dysfunction from 18 to 69 hours. The urinary and fecal recovery of minocycline when administered to 12 normal volunteers is one-half to one-third that of other tetracyclines.

Human Pharmacology: Intravenous—Following a single dose of 200 mg. administered intravenously to 10 healthy male volunteers, serum levels ranged from 2.52 to 6.63 mcg./ml. (average 4.18), after 12 hours they ranged from 0.82 to 2.64 mcg./ml. (average 1.38). In a group of 5 healthy male volunteers, serum levels of 1.4-1.8 mcg./ml. were maintained at 12 and 24 hours with doses of 100 mg. every 12 hours for three days. When given 200 mg. once daily for three days the serum levels had fallen to approximately 1 mcg./ml. at 24 hours. The serum half-life following I.V. doses of 100 mg. every 12 hours or 200 mg. once daily did not differ significantly and ranged from 15 to 23 hours. The serum half-life following a single 200 mg. oral dose in 12 essentially normal volunteers ranged from 11 to 17 hours, in 7 patients with hepatic dysfunction ranged from 11 to 16 hours, and in 5 patients with renal dysfunction from 18 to 69 hours.

Intravenously administered Minocycline appears similar to oral doses in excretion. The urinary and fecal recovery of oral minocycline when administered to 12 normal volunteers is one-half to one-third that of other tetracyclines.

Indications: MINOCIN *minocycline HCl* is indicated in infections caused by the following microorganisms:

Rickettsiae: (Rocky Mountain spotted fever, typhus fever and the typhus group, Q fever, rickettsialpox, tick fevers.)

Mycoplasma pneumoniae (PPLO, Eaton agent).

Agents of psittacosis and ornithosis.

Agents of lymphogranuloma venereum and granuloma inguinale.

The spirochetal agent of relapsing fever *(Borrelia recurrentis).*

The following gram-negative microorganisms:

Hemophilus ducreyi (chancroid),

Pasteurella pestis and *Pasteurella tularensis,*

Bartonella bacilliformis,

Bacteroides species,

Vibrio comma and *Vibrio fetus,*

Brucella species (in conjunction with streptomycin).

Because many strains of the following groups of microorganisms have been shown to be resistant to tetracyclines, culture and susceptibility testing are recommended.

MINOCIN *minocycline hydrochloride* is indicated for treatment of infections caused by the following gram-negative microorganisms, when bacteriologic testing indicates appropriate susceptibility to the drug:

Escherichia coli,

Enterobacter aerogenes (formerly *Aerobacter aerogenes*),

Shigella species,

Mima species and *Herellea* species,

Haemophilus influenzae (respiratory infections).

Klebsiella species (respiratory and urinary infections).

MINOCIN is indicated for treatment of infections caused by the following gram-positive microorganisms when bacteriologic testing indicates appropriate susceptibility to the drug:

Streptococcus species:

Up to 44 percent of strains of *Streptococcus pyogenes* and 74 percent of *Streptococcus faecalis* have been found to be resistant to tetracycline drugs. Therefore, tetracyclines should not be used for streptococcal disease unless the organism has been demonstrated to be sensitive.

For upper respiratory infections due to group A beta-hemolytic streptococci, penicillin is the usual drug of choice, including prophylaxis of rheumatic fever.

Diplococcus pneumoniae,

Staphylococcus aureus, skin and soft tissue infections. Tetracyclines are not the drug of choice in the treatment of any type of staphylococcal infection.

When penicillin is contraindicated, tetracyclines are alternative drugs in the treatment of infections due to:

Neisseria gonorrhoeae, and *Neisseria meningitidis* (I.V. only)

Treponema pallidum and *Treponema pertenue* (syphilis and yaws),

Listeria monocytogenes,

Clostridium species,

Bacillus anthracis,

Fusobacterium fusiforme (Vincent's infection),

Actinomyces species.

In acute intestinal amebiasis, the tetracyclines may be a useful adjunct to amebicides.

MINOCIN is indicated in the treatment of trachoma, although the infectious agent is not always eliminated as judged by immunofluorescence.

Inclusion conjunctivitis may be treated with oral tetracyclines or with a combination of oral and topical agents.

Oral Only: In severe acne, the tetracyclines may be useful adjunctive therapy.

Minocycline is indicated in the treatment of asymptomatic carriers of *N. meningitidis* to eliminate meningococci from the nasopharynx.

In order to preserve the usefulness of MINOCIN *minocycline HCl* in the treatment of asymptomatic meningococcal carriers, diagnostic laboratory procedures, including serotyping and susceptibility testing, should be performed to establish the carrier state and the correct treatment. It is recommended that the drug be reserved for situations in which the risk of meningococcal meningitis is high.

Minocycline by oral administration is not indicated for the treatment of meningococcal infection.

Although no controlled clinical efficacy studies have been conducted, limited clinical data show that oral minocycline hydrochloride has been used successfully in the treatment of infections caused by Mycobacterium marinum.

Contraindications: This drug is contraindicated in persons who have shown hypersensitivity to any of the tetracyclines.

Warnings: In the presence of renal dysfunction, particularly in pregnancy, intravenous tetracycline therapy in daily doses exceeding 2 grams has been associated with deaths through liver failure.

When the need for intensive treatment outweighs its potential dangers (mostly during pregnancy or in individuals with known or suspected renal or liver impairment), it is advisable to perform renal and liver function tests before and during therapy. Also tetracycline serum concentrations should be followed.

If renal impairment exists, even usual oral or parenteral doses may lead to excessive systemic accumulation of the drug and possible liver toxicity. Under such conditions, lower than usual total doses are indicated, and if therapy is prolonged, serum level determinations of the drug may be advisable. This hazard is of particular importance in the parenteral administration of tetracyclines to pregnant or postpartum patients with pyelonephritis. When used under these circumstances, the blood level should not exceed 15 micrograms/ml. and liver function tests should be made at frequent intervals. Other potentially hepatotoxic drugs should not be prescribed concomitantly.

THE USE OF TETRACYCLINES DURING TOOTH DEVELOPMENT (LAST HALF OF PREGNANCY, INFANCY AND CHILDHOOD TO THE AGE OF 8 YEARS) MAY CAUSE PERMANENT DISCOLORATION OF THE TEETH (YELLOW-GRAY-BROWN). This adverse reaction is more common during long-term use of the drugs but has been observed following repeated short-term courses. Enamel hypoplasia has also been reported. TETRACYCLINES, THEREFORE, SHOULD NOT BE USED IN THIS AGE GROUP UNLESS OTHER DRUGS ARE NOT LIKELY TO BE EFFECTIVE OR ARE CONTRAINDICATED.

Photosensitivity manifested by an exaggerated sunburn reaction has been observed in some individuals taking tetracyclines. Patients apt to be exposed to direct sunlight or ultraviolet light should be advised that this reaction can occur with tetracycline drugs, and treatment should be discontinued at the first evidence of skin erythema. Studies to date indicate that photosensitivity is rarely reported with MINOCIN *minocycline HCl.*

The antianabolic action of the tetracyclines may cause an increase in BUN. While this is not a problem in those with normal renal function, in patients with significantly impaired function, higher serum levels of tetracyclines may lead to azotemia, hyperphosphatemia, and acidosis.

CNS side effects including lightheadedness, dizziness or vertigo have been reported. Patients who experience these symptoms should be cautioned about driving vehicles or using hazardous machinery while on minocycline therapy. These symptoms may disappear during therapy and always disappear rapidly when the drug is discontinued.

Usage in Pregnancy—(See above "Warnings" about use during tooth development.) Results of animal studies indicate that tetracyclines cross the placenta, are found in fetal tissues and can have toxic effects on the developing fetus (often related to retardation of skeletal development). Evidence of embryotoxicity has also been noted in animals treated early in pregnancy.

The safety of minocycline HCl for use during pregnancy has not been established.

Usage in newborns, infants, and children—(See above "Warnings" about use during tooth development.)

All tetracyclines form a stable calcium complex in any bone forming tissue. A decrease in the fibula growth rate has been observed in

prematures given oral tetracycline in doses of 25 mg./kg. every 6 hours. This reaction was shown to be reversible when the drug was discontinued.
Tetracyclines are present in the milk of lactating women who are taking a drug in this class.
Precautions: As with other antibiotic preparations, use of this drug may result in overgrowth of nonsusceptible organisms, including fungi. If superinfection occurs, the antibiotic should be discontinued and appropriate therapy should be instituted.
In venereal diseases when coexistent syphilis is suspected, darkfield examination should be done before treatment is started and the blood serology repeated monthly for at least 4 months.
Because tetracyclines have been shown to depress plasma prothrombin activity, patients who are on anticoagulant therapy may require downward adjustment of their anticoagulant dosage.
In long-term therapy, periodic laboratory evaluation of organ systems, including hematopoietic, renal and hepatic studies, should be performed.
All infections due to Group A beta-hemolytic streptococci should be treated for at least 10 days.
Since bacteriostatic drugs may interfere with the bactericidal action of penicillin, it is advisable to avoid giving tetracycline in conjunction with penicillin.
Adverse Reactions: Gastrointestinal: Anorexia, nausea, vomiting, diarrhea, glossitis, dysphagia, enterocolitis, and inflammatory lesions (with monilial overgrowth) in the anogenital region.
These reactions have been caused by both the oral and parenteral administration of tetracyclines.
Skin: Maculopapular and erythematous rashes. Exfoliative dermatitis has been reported but is uncommon. Photosensitivity is discussed above. (See "Warnings".) Pigmentation of skin and mucous membranes has been reported.
Renal toxicity: Rise in BUN has been reported and is apparently dose related. (See "Warnings".)
Hypersensitivity reactions: Urticaria, angioneurotic edema, anaphylaxis, anaphylactoid purpura, pericarditis and exacerbation of systemic lupus erythematosus.
Bulging fontanels have been reported in young infants following full therapeutic dosage. This sign disappeared rapidly when the drug was discontinued.
Blood: Hemolytic anemia, thrombocytopenia, neutropenia and eosinophilia have been reported.
CNS: (See "Warnings".)
When given over prolonged periods, tetracyclines have been reported to produce brown-black microscopic discoloration of thyroid glands. No abnormalities of thyroid function studies are known to occur.
Dosage and Administration: Oral—Therapy should be continued for at least 24-48 hours after symptoms and fever have subsided.
Concomitant therapy: Antacids containing aluminum, calcium, or magnesium impair absorption and should not be given to patients taking oral tetracycline.
Studies to date have indicated that the absorption of MINOCIN is not notably influenced by foods and dairy products.
In patients with renal impairment: (See "Warnings".) Total dosage should be decreased by reduction of recommended individual doses and/or by extending time intervals between doses.
In the treatment of streptococcal infections, a therapeutic dose of tetracycline should be administered for at least 10 days.
Adults: The usual dosage of MINOCIN *minocycline HCl* is 200 mg. initially followed by 100 mg. every 12 hours. Alternatively, if more frequent doses are preferred, two or four 50 mg. capsules may be given initially followed by one 50 mg. capsule four times daily.
For children above eight years of age: The usual dosage of MINOCIN *minocycline HCl* is 4 mg./kg. initially followed by 2 mg./kg. every 12 hours.
For treatment of syphilis, the usual dosage of MINOCIN should be administered over a period of 10-15 days. Close follow-up, including laboratory tests, is recommended.
Gonorrhea patients sensitive to penicillin may be treated with MINOCIN, administered as 200 mg. initially followed by 100 mg. every twelve hours for a minimum of 4 days, with post-therapy cultures within 2-3 days.
In the treatment of meningococcal carrier state recommended dose is 100 mg. every 12 hours for five days. *Mycobacterium Marinum* Infections–Although optimal doses have not been established, 100 mg twice a day for 6–8 weeks have been used successfully in a limited number of cases.
Dosage and Administration: Intravenous
Note: Rapid administration is to be avoided. Parenteral therapy is indicated only when oral therapy is not adequate or tolerated. Oral therapy should be instituted as soon as possible. If intravenous therapy is given over prolonged periods of time thrombophlebitis may result.
Adults: Usual adult dose: 200 mg. followed by 100 mg. every 12 hours and should not exceed 400 mg. in 24 hours. The drug should be initially dissolved and then further diluted to 500-1,000 ml. with either Sodium Chloride Injection USP, Dextrose Injection USP, Dextrose and Sodium Chloride Injection USP, Ringer's Injection USP, or Lactated Ringer's Injection USP but not in other solutions containing calcium (a precipitate may form).
The reconstituted solutions are stable at room temperature for 24 hours without significant loss of potency. Any unused portion must be discarded after that period. The final dilution for administration should be administered immediately.
For children above eight years of age: Usual pediatric dose: 4 mg./kg. followed by a 2 mg./kg. every 12 hours. In patients with renal impairment: (See "Warnings".)
Total dosage should be decreased by reduction of recommended individual doses and/or by extending time intervals between doses.
How Supplied: CAPSULES: Minocycline Hydrochloride equivalent to 100 mg. Minocycline. Hardshell purple and orange. Bottles of 50 and 100; Unit Dose 10 x 10's.
Minocycline Hydrochloride equivalent to 50 mg. Minocycline. Hardshell orange. Bottles of 100 and Unit Dose 10 x 10's.
SYRUP: Minocycline Hydrochloride equivalent to 50 mg. Minocycline per teaspoonful (5 ml.) Preserved with propylparaben 0.10% and butylparaben 0.06% with Alcohol USP 5% v/v. Custard-flavored in bottles of 2 fl. oz.
INTRAVENOUS—100 mg. vials of sterile cryodesiccated powder.
Animal Pharmacology and Toxicology: MINOCIN *minocycline HCl* has been found to produce high blood concentrations following oral dosage to various animal species and to be extensively distributed to all tissues examined in ^{14}C-labeled drug studies in dogs. MINOCIN has been found experimentally to produce discoloration of the thyroid glands. This finding has been observed in rats and dogs. Changes in thyroid function have also been found in these animal species. However, no change in thyroid function has been observed in humans.

[*Shown in Product Identification Section*]

Capsules, 100 mg
Military Depot NSN 6505-00-003-5112, 50's
VA Depot NSN 6505-00-003-5112, 50's
Capsules, 50 mg.
Military Depot NSN 6505-01-015-4147, 100's
Intravenous, 100 mg.
Military Depot NSN 6505-00-149-0574

MYAMBUTOL® ℞
(ethambutol hydrochloride)
Tablets

Description: MYAMBUTOL *ethambutol hydrochloride Lederle* is an oral chemotherapeutic agent which is specifically effective against actively growing microorganisms of the genus *Mycobacterium*, including *M. tuberculosis*.
Action: MYAMBUTOL, following a single oral dose of 25 mg./Kg. of body weight, attains a peak of 2 to 5 micrograms/ml. in serum 2 to 4 hours after administration. When the drug is administered daily for longer periods of time at this dose, serum levels are similar. The serum level of MYAMBUTOL falls to undetectable levels by 24 hours after the last dose except in some patients with abnormal renal function. The intracellular concentrations of erythrocytes reach peak values approximately twice those of plasma and maintain this ratio throughout the 24 hours.
During the 24-hour period following oral administration of MYAMBUTOL, approximately 50 percent of the initial dose is excreted unchanged in the urine, while an additional 8 to 15 percent appears in the form of metabolites. The main path of metabolism appears to be an initial oxidation of the alcohol to an aldehydic intermediate, followed by conversion to a dicarboxylic acid. From 20 to 22 percent of the initial dose is excreted in the feces as unchanged drug. No drug accumulation has been observed with consecutive single daily doses of 25 mg./Kg. in patients with normal kidney function, although marked accumulation has been demonstrated in patients with renal insufficiency.
MYAMBUTOL diffuses into actively growing *mycobacterium* cells such as tubercle bacilli. MYAMBUTOL appears to inhibit the synthesis of one or more metabolites, thus causing impairment of cell metabolism, arrest of multiplication, and cell death. No cross resistance with other available antimycobacterial agents has been demonstrated.
MYAMBUTOL has been shown to be effective against strains of *Mycobacterium tuberculosis* but does not seem to be active against fungi, viruses, or other bacteria.
Mycobacterium tuberculosis strains previously unexposed to MYAMBUTOL have been uniformly sensitive to concentrations of 8 or less micrograms/ml., depending on the nature of the culture media. When MYAMBUTOL has been used alone for treatment of tuberculosis, tubercle bacilli from these patients have developed resistance to MYAMBUTOL by *in vitro* susceptibility tests; the development of resistance has been unpredictable and appears to occur in a step-like manner. No cross resistance between MYAMBUTOL and other antituberculous drugs has been reported. MYAMBUTOL has reduced the incidence of the emergence of mycobacterial resistance to isoniazid when both drugs have been used concurrently.
An agar diffusion microbiologic assay, based upon inhibition of *Mycobacterium smegmatis* (ATCC 607) may be used to determine concentrations of MYAMBUTOL in serum and urine. This technique has not been published, but further information can be obtained upon inquiry to Lederle Laboratories.
Animal Pharmacology: Toxicological studies in dogs on high prolonged doses produced evi-

Continued on next page

The information on each product appearing here is based on labelling effective in August, 1979 and is either the entire official brochure or an accurate condensation therefrom. Official brochures are enclosed in product packages. Information concerning all Lederle products may be obtained from the Medical Department, Lederle Laboratories, Pearl River, New York, 10965.

Lederle—Cont.

dence of myocardial damage and failure, and depigmentation of the tapetum lucidum of the eyes, the significance of which is not known. Degenerative changes in the central nervous system, apparently not dose-related, have also been noted in dogs receiving ethambutol hydrochloride over a prolonged period.
In the rhesus monkey, neurological signs appeared after treatment with high doses given daily over a period of several months. These were correlated with specific serum levels of ethambutol hydrochloride and with definite neuro-anatomical changes in the central nervous system. Focal interstitial carditis was also noted in monkeys which received ethambutol hydrochloride in high doses for a prolonged period.
When pregnant mice or rabbits were treated with high doses of ethambutol hydrochloride, fetal mortality was slightly but not significantly ($P > 0.05$) increased. Female rats treated with ethambutol hydrochloride displayed slight but insignificant ($P > 0.05$) decreases in fertility and litter size.
In fetuses born of mice treated with high doses of ethambutol hydrochloride during pregnancy, a low incidence of cleft palate, exencephaly and abnormality of the vertebral column were observed. Minor abnormalities of the cervical vertebra were seen in the newborn of rats treated with high doses of ethambutol hydrochloride during pregnancy. Rabbits receiving high doses of ethambutol hydrochloride during pregnancy gave birth to two fetuses with monophthalmia, one with a shortened right forearm accompanied by bilateral wrist-joint contracture and one with hare lip and cleft palate.
Indications: MYAMBUTOL *ethambutol hydrochloride* is indicated for the treatment of pulmonary tuberculosis. It should not be used as the sole antituberculous drug, but should be used in conjunction with at least one other antituberculous drug. Selection of the companion drug should be based on clinical experience, considerations of comparative safety and appropriate *in vitro* susceptibility studies.
In patients who have not received previous antituberculous therapy, i.e. initial treatment, the most frequently used regimens have been the following:
MYAMBUTOL plus isoniazid
MYAMBUTOL plus isoniazid plus streptomycin.
In patients who have received previous antituberculous therapy, mycobacterial resistance to other drugs used in initial therapy is frequent. Consequently in such retreatment patients, MYAMBUTOL should be combined with at least one of the second line drugs not previously administered to the patient and to which bacterial susceptibility has been indicated by appropriate *in vitro* studies. Antituberculous drugs used with MYAMBUTOL have included cycloserine, ethionamide, pyrazinamide, viomycin and other drugs. Isoniazid, aminosalicylic acid, and streptomycin have also been used in multiple drug regimens. Alternating drug regimens have also been utilized.
Contraindications: MYAMBUTOL is contraindicated in patients who are known to be hypersensitive to this drug. It is also contraindicated in patients with known optic neuritis unless clinical judgment determines that it may be used.
Precautions: The effects of combinations of ethambutol hydrochloride with other antituberculous drugs on the fetus is not known. While administration of this drug to pregnant human patients has produced no detectable effect upon the fetus, the possible teratogenic potential in women capable of bearing children should be weighed carefully against the benefits of therapy. There are published reports of five women who received the drug during pregnancy without apparent adverse effect upon the fetus.
MYAMBUTOL is not recommended for use in children under thirteen years of age since safe conditions for use have not been established.
Patients with decreased renal function need the dosage reduced as determined by serum levels of MYAMBUTOL, since the main path of excretion of this drug is by the kidneys.
Because this drug may have adverse effects on vision, physical examination should include ophthalmoscopy, finger perimetry and testing of color discrimination. In patients with visual defects such as cataracts, recurrent inflammatory conditions of the eye, optic neuritis, and diabetic retinopathy, the evaluation of changes in visual acuity is more difficult, and care should be taken to be sure the variations in vision are not due to the underlying disease conditions. In such patients, consideration should be given to relationship between benefits expected and possible visual deterioration since evaluation of visual changes is difficult. (For recommended procedures, see next paragraphs under Adverse Reactions.)
As with any potent drug, periodic assessment of organ system functions, including renal, hepatic, and hematopoietic, should be made during long-term therapy.
Adverse Reactions: MYAMBUTOL may produce decreases in visual acuity which appear to be due to optic neuritis and to be related to dose and duration of treatment. The effects are generally reversible when administration of the drug is discontinued promptly.
In rare cases recovery may be delayed for up to one year or more and the effect may possibly be irreversible in these cases.
Patients should be advised to report promptly to their physician any change of visual acuity. The change in visual acuity may be unilateral or bilateral and hence *each eye must be tested separately and both eyes tested together.* Testing of visual acuity should be performed before beginning MYAMBUTOL *ethambutol hydrochloride* therapy and periodically during drug administration, except that it should be done monthly when a patient is on a dosage of more than 15 mg. per Kilogram per day. Snellen eye charts are recommended for testing of visual acuity. Studies have shown that there are definite fluctuations of one or two lines of the Snellen chart in the visual acuity of many tuberculous patients *not* receiving MYAMBUTOL.
The table may be useful in interpreting possible changes in visual acuity attributable to MYAMBUTOL.
[See table below].
In general, changes in visual acuity less than those indicated under "Significant Number of Lines" and "Decreases-Number of Points", may be due to chance variation, limitations of the testing method or physiologic variability. Conversely, changes in visual acuity equaling or exceeding those under "Significant Number of Lines" and "Decreases-Number of Points" indicate need for retesting and careful evaluation of the patient's visual status. If careful evaluation confirms the magnitude of visual change and fails to reveal another cause, MYAMBUTOL should be discontinued and the patient reevaluated at frequent intervals. Progressive decreases in visual acuity during therapy must be considered to be due to MYAMBUTOL.
If corrective glasses are used prior to treatment, these must be worn during visual acuity testing. During 1 to 2 years of therapy, a refractive error may develop which must be corrected in order to obtain accurate test results. Testing the visual acuity through a pinhole eliminates refractive error. Patients developing visual abnormality during MYAMBUTOL treatment may show subjective visual symptoms before, or simultaneously with, the demonstration of decreases in visual acuity, and all patients receiving MYAMBUTOL should be questioned periodically about blurred vision and other subjective eye symptoms.
Recovery of visual acuity generally occurs over a period of weeks to months after the drug has been discontinued. Patients have then received MYAMBUTOL again without recurrence of loss of visual acuity.
Other adverse reactions reported include: anaphylactoid reactions, dermatitis, pruritus and joint pain; anorexia, nausea, vomiting, gastrointestinal upset, abdominal pain; fever, malaise, headache, and dizziness; mental confusion, disorientation and possible hallucinations. Numbness and tingling of the extremities due to peripheral neuritis have been reported infrequently.
Elevated serum uric acid levels occur and precipitation of acute gout has been reported. Transient impairment of liver function as indicated by abnormal liver function tests is not an unusual finding. Since MYAMBUTOL is recommended for therapy in conjunction with one or more other antituberculous drugs, these changes may be related to the concurrent therapy.
Dosage and Administration: MYAMBUTOL should not be used alone, in initial treatment or in retreatment. MYAMBUTOL should be administered on a once every 24-hour basis only. Absorption is not significantly altered by administration with food. Therapy, in general, should be continued until bacteriological conversion has become permanent and maximal clinical improvement has occurred.
MYAMBUTOL is not recommended for use in children under thirteen years of age since safe conditions for use have not been established.
Initial Treatment: In patients who have not received previous antituberculous therapy, administer MYAMBUTOL 15 mg. per Kilogram (7 mg. per pound) of body weight, as a single oral dose once every 24 hours. In the more recent studies, isoniazid has been administered concurrently in a single, daily, oral dose.
Retreatment: In patients who have received previous antituberculous therapy, administer MYAMBUTOL 25 mg. per Kilogram (11 mg. per pound) of body weight, as a single oral dose once every 24 hours. Concurrently administer at least one other antituberculous drug to which the organisms have been demonstrated to be susceptible by appropriate *in vitro* tests. Suitable drugs usually consist of those not previously used in the treatment of the patient. After 60 days of MYAMBUTOL (ethambutol hydrochloride) administration, decrease the dose to 15 mg. per Kilogram (7 mg. per pound) of body weight, and administer as a single oral dose once every 24 hours.
During the period when a patient is on a daily dose of 25 mg./kg., monthly eye examinations are advised.
See Table for easy selection of proper weight-dose tablet(s).

Initial Snellen Reading	Reading Indicating Significant Decrease	Significant Number of Lines	Decreases Number of Points
20/13	20/25	3	12
20/15	20/25	2	10
20/20	20/30	2	10
20/25	20/40	2	15
20/30	20/50	2	20
20/40	20/70	2	30
20/50	20/70	1	20

Weight-Dose Table

15 mg./Kg. (7 mg./lb.) Schedule

Weight Range Pounds	Kilograms	Daily Dose In mg.
Under 85 lbs.	Under 37 Kg	500
85–94.5	37–43	600
95–109.5	43–50	700
110–124.5	50–57	800
125–139.5	57–64	900
140–154.5	64–71	1000
155–169.5	71–79	1100
170–184.5	79–84	1200
185–199.5	84–90	1300
200–214.5	90–97	1400
215 and Over	Over 97	1500
25 mg./Kg. (11 mg./lb.) Schedule		
Under 85 lbs.	Under 38 Kg.	900
85–92.5	38–42	1000
93–101.5	42–45.5	1100
102–109.5	45.5–50	1200
110–118.5	50–54	1300
119–128.5	54–58	1400
129–136.5	58–62	1500
137–146.5	62–67	1600
147–155.5	67–71	1700
156–164.5	71–75	1800
165–173.5	75–79	1900
174–182.5	79–83	2000
183–191.5	83–87	2100
192–199.5	87–91	2200
200–209.5	91–95	2300
210–218.5	95–99	2400
219 and Over	Over 99	2500

How Supplied: Tablets: 100 mg., white—bottles of 100 and 1,000; 400 mg., film-coated, with a bisecting line on each side—bottles of 100 and 1,000, unit dose 10 × 10's.

A.H.F.S. 8:16

100 mg. Tablets
Military Depots:
NSN 6505-00-403-7645, 100's
400 mg. Tablets
NSN 6505-00-812-2579, 100's
VA Depots:
400 mg Tablets
NSN 6505-00-812-2543A

NEOLOID®
(emulsified castor oil)

Composition: NEOLOID Emulsified Castor Oil U.S.P. 36.4% (w/w) with preservative, emulsifying and flavoring agents in water. NEOLOID is an emulsion with an exceptionally bland, pleasant taste.

Indications: For the treatment of isolated bouts of constipation.

Administration and Dosage:

Infants—½ to 1½ teaspoonfuls.

Children—Adjust between infant and adult dose.

Adult— Average dose, 2 to 4 tablespoonfuls.

Precautions: Not to be used when abdominal pain, nausea, vomiting, or other symptoms of appendicitis are present. Frequent or continued use of this preparation may result in dependence on laxatives. Do not use during pregnancy except on competent advice. Keep this and all drugs out of the reach of children. In case of accidental overdosage seek professional assistance or contact a Poison Control Center immediately.

How Supplied: Bottles of 4 fl. oz. (peppermint flavor).

NILSTAT® ℞
Nystatin Oral Suspension

Description: This antifungal agent is obtained from *Streptomyces noursei*. It is a polyene antibiotic of undetermined structural formula.

Nystatin is an antibiotic with antifungal activity produced by a strain of *Streptomyces noursei*. NILSTAT *nystatin* Oral Suspension, Lederle, is a cherry flavored, ready-to-use suspension containing 100,000 units of nystatin per ml.-with methylparaben (0.12%) and propylparaben (0.03%) as preservatives.

Actions: Nystatin probably acts by binding to sterols in the cell membrane of the fungus with a resultant change in membrane permeability allowing leakage of intracellular components. It is absorbed very sparingly following oral administration, with no detectable blood levels when given in the recommended doses.

Indications: For the treatment of infections of the oral cavity caused by *Candida* (Monilia) *albicans*.

Contraindications: Hypersensitivity to the drug.

Adverse Reactions:

Nausea and vomiting, Gastrointestinal distress, Diarrhea.

Dosage and Administration:

Infants: 2 ml. (200,000 units) four times daily (1 ml. in each side of mouth).

Children and adults: 4-6 ml. (400,000 to 600,000 units) four times daily (one-half of dose in each side of mouth).

Note: Limited clinical studies in prematures and low birth weight infants indicate that 1 ml. four times daily is effective.

Local treatment should be continued at least 48 hours after perioral symptoms have disappeared and cultures returned to normal.

It is recommended that the drug be retained in the mouth as long as possible before swallowing.

How Supplied: 16 fl. oz. bottles and 60 ml. bottles with dropper.

NILSTAT® ℞
Nystatin Vaginal Tablets U.S.P.

Description: NILSTAT *nystatin Vaginal Tablets*, USP are oblong shaped vaginal tablets, each containing 100,000 units Nystatin, USP.

Nystatin is a polyene antibiotic of undetermined structural formula that is obtained from *streptomyces noursei*.

Clinical Pharmacology: Nystatin is an antifungal antibiotic which is both fungistatic and fungicidal *in vitro* against a wide variety of yeasts and yeast-like fungi. It probably acts by binding to sterols in the cell membrane of the fungus with a resultant change in membrane permeability allowing leakage of intracellular components. It exhibits no apreciable activity against bacteria or trichomonads.

Indications and Usage: NILSTAT *nystatin Vaginal Tablets*, USP are effective for the local treatment of vulvovaginal candidiasis (moniliasis). The diagnosis should be confirmed, prior to therapy, by KOH smears and/or cultures. Other pathogens commonly associated with vulvovaginitis (Trichomonas and *Haemophilus vaginalis)* do not respond to nystatin and should be ruled out by appropriate laboratory methods.

Contraindications: This preparation is contraindicated in patients with a history of hypersensitivity to any of its components.

Precautions:

General

Discontinue treatment if sensitization or irritation is reported during use.

Laboratory Tests:

If there is a lack of response to NILSTAT *nystatin Vaginal Tablets*, USP, appropriate michrobiological studies should be repeated to confirm the diagnosis and rule out other pathogens, before instituting another course of antimycotic therapy.

Usage in Pregnancy:

No adverse effects or complications have been attributed to nystatin in infants born to women treated with nystatin vaginal tablets.

Adverse Reactions: Nystatin is virtually nontoxic and nonsensitizing and is well tolerated by all age groups, even on prolonged administration. Rarely, irritation or sensitization may occur (see PRECAUTIONS).

Dosage and Administration: The usual dosage is one tablet (100,000 units nystatin) daily for two weeks. The tablets should be deposited high in the vagina by means of the applicator. "Instructions for the Patient" are enclosed in each package.

Even though symptomatic relief may occur within a few days, treatment should be continued for the full course.

It is important that therapy be continued during menstruation. Adjunctive measures such as therapeutic douches are unnecessary and sometimes inadvisable. Cleansing douches may be used by nonpregnant women, if desired, for esthetic purposes.

How Supplied: In packages of 15 and 30 Vaginal Tablets with Applicator.

NILSTAT ℞
(nystatin)
Oral Tablets (film-coated)

500,000 Units per tablet, bottles of 100; unit-dose 10 x 10's.

[*Shown in Product Identification Section*]

NILSTAT ℞
(nystatin)
Topical Cream, 100,000 Units per Gm.
Military Depot NSN 6505-01-063-1141, 240 gm jar

Inactive ingredients in a water base: Emulsifying Wax, NF, Isopropyl Myristate, Glycerin, Lactic Acid and Sodium Hydroxide. Preservative: Sorbic Acid 0.2%.

How Supplied: 15 gm tube, 240 gm jar.

NILSTAT ℞
(nystatin)
Topical Ointment, 100,000 Units per Gm.

Inactive Ingredients: Light Mineral Oil and Plastibase 50 W.

15 Gm. tubes.

ORIMUNE® POLIOVIRUS VACCINE, LIVE, ORAL, TRIVALENT ℞
0.5 ml Dose Contains Sorbitol
SABIN STRAINS TYPES 1, 2 and 3
FOR ORAL ADMINISTRATION—NOT FOR INJECTION

Description: *Manufacture and Composition:* ORIMUNE® TRIVALENT VACCINE is a mixture of three types of attenuated polioviruses which have been propagated in cercopithecus monkey kidney cell culture. The cells are grown in the presence of a nutrient medium consisting of Earle's balanced salt solution containing lactalbumin hydrolysate, antibiotics and calf serum. After cell growth, the medium is removed and replaced with fresh medium containing the inoculating virus but no calf serum. The final vaccine is diluted with a modified cell culture maintenance medium containing sorbitol. Each dose (0.5 ml.) contains less than 25 micrograms of each of the antibiotics, streptomycin, neomycin and nystatin.

The potency is expressed in terms of the amount of virus contained in the recommended dose as tissue culture infective doses ($TCID_{50}$). The human dose of vaccine containing all three virus types shall be constituted to have infectivity titers in the final container material of $10^{5.4}$ to $10^{6.4}$ for Type I, $10^{4.5}$ to $10^{5.5}$ for Type II and $10^{5.2}$ to $10^{6.2}$ for Type III.[1]

Continued on next page

The information on each product appearing here is based on labelling effective in August, 1979 and is either the entire official brochure or an accurate condensation therefrom. Official brochures are enclosed in product packages. Information concerning all Lederle products may be obtained from the Medical Department, Lederle Laboratories, Pearl River, New York, 10965.

Lederle—Cont.

Color Change: This vaccine contains phenol red as a pH indicator. The usual color of the vaccine is pink, although some containers of vaccine shipped or stored in dry ice, may exhibit a yellow coloration due to the very low temperature or possible absorption of carbon dioxide. The color of the vaccine prior to use (red—pink—yellow) has no effect on the virus or efficacy of the vaccine.

Action and Use: The purpose of administering any attenuated, live, virus vaccine is to stimulate the body mechanism to produce an active immunity by simulating the natural infection without producing untoward symptoms of the disease. To accomplish this with live poliovirus vaccine, it is necessary for the virus to multiply in the intestinal tract. A primary series of this vaccine is designed to produce an antibody response to poliovirus Types 1, 2 and 3. This response is comparable to the immunity induced by the natural disease.

The antibodies thus formed help protect the individual against clinical poliomyelitis infection by any of the three types of poliovirus. When used in the prescribed manner for primary immunization, type specific neutralizing antibodies will be induced in 90% or more of susceptibles.

Indications: *This vaccine is indicated for use in the prevention of poliomyelitis caused by Poliovirus Types 1, 2 and 3.*

Infants starting at six to twelve weeks of age, *all unimmunized children* and *adolescents* through age 18 are the usual candidates for routine prophylaxis.

Trivalent oral polio vaccine (TOPV) and inactivated polio vaccine (IPV) are both effective in preventing poliomyelitis. When the benefits and risks for the population as a whole were evaluated in 1977 by a special expert committee of the Institute of Medicine, National Academy of Science, TOPV was the preferred vaccine for primary vaccination of children, and for control of epidemic disease in the United States.[6]

The choice of TOPV as the principal polio vaccine in the United States has also been made by the Committee on Infectious Disease of the American Academy of Pediatrics.[5] This is because TOPV establishes intestinal immunity to reinfection, is simple to administer, is well accepted by patients, does not require periodic booster doses, and has a record of having essentially eliminated disease associated with wild polioviruses in this country.[2]

Past history of clinical poliomyelitis or prior vaccination with IPV in otherwise healthy individuals does not preclude the administration of TOPV when otherwise indicated.

Serologic evidence indicates that measles and rubella vaccines or combinations (measles-mumps-rubella vaccine) given simultaneously with trivalent oral poliovirus vaccine can be expected to give adequate antibody response.[14]

Use in Pregnancy: Pregnancy is neither an indication for vaccination against poliomyelitis nor a contraindication when protection is needed, as during an epidemic.[2] (See Contraindications and Adverse Reactions.)

Routine poliomyelitis immunization for adults residing in the continental United States may not be necessary because of extreme unlikelihood of exposure. However, immunization with either TOPV or IPV is recommended for those unimmunized adults subject to *increased risk* of exposure, as by travel to or contact with epidemic or endemic areas and for those employed in hospitals, medical laboratories, clinics or sanitation facilities. Immunization may be indicated for unimmunized parents and those in other special situations where, in the judgment of the attending physician, protection may be needed. (See Contraindications and Adverse Reactions.)

Contraindications: *Under no circumstances should this vaccine be administered parenterally.*

Administration of the vaccine should be postponed or avoided in those experiencing any acute illness and in those with any advanced debilitated condition or persistent vomiting or diarrhea.

GRIMUNE *must not* be administered to patients with immune deficiency diseases such as combined immunodeficiency, hypogammaglobulinemia and agammaglobulinemia. It would also be prudent to withhold ORIMUNE from siblings of a child known to have an immunodeficiency syndrome. Further, ORIMUNE *must not* be administered to patients with altered immune states such as those occuring in thymic abnormalities, leukemia, lymphoma or generalized malignancy or by lowered resistance from therapy with corticosteroids, alkylating drugs, antimetabolites or radiation. When possible, all persons with altered immune status should avoid close household-type contact with recipients of the vaccine for at least 6–8 weeks. IPV may be preferred for immunizing all persons in this setting.[2,3,4,5,6]

Precautions: Other viruses (including poliovirus and other enterovirus) may interfere with the desired response to this vaccine since their presence in the intestinal tract may interfere with the replication of the attenuated strains of poliovirus in the vaccine.

The vaccine will not be effective in modifying or preventing cases of existing and/or incubating poliomyelitis.

Adverse Reactions: Paralytic disease following the ingestion of live poliovirus vaccines has been, on rare occasion, reported in individuals receiving the vaccine, as well as in persons who were in close contact with vaccinees.[6,7,8,9,10] Most reports of paralytic disease following ingestion of the vaccine or contact with a recent vaccinee are based on epidemiological analysis and temporal association between vaccination or contact and the onset of symptoms. Most authorities believe that a causal relationship exists.[2,11,12]

The Center for Disease Control reports that during the years 1969 through 1976 approximately 193 million doses of TOPV were distributed in the United States. In the same 8 years, 10 "vaccine-associated" and 34 "contact vaccine-associated" paralytic cases were reported. Eleven other "vaccine-associated" cases have been reported in persons (recipients or contacts) with immune deficiency conditions.[2]

The risk is estimated to be one case in a recipient for every 20 million doses of vaccine distributed and one case in a contact for every 6 million doses distributed.[6]

The risk of vaccine-associated paralysis is extremely small for vaccinees, susceptible family members and other close personal contacts. However, the responsible physician should convey or specifically direct personnel acting under his authority to convey the warnings to the vaccinee, parent, guardian or other responsible person of the possibility of vaccine-associated paralysis prior to administration of the vaccine. When the attenuated vaccine strains are to be introduced into a household with adults who have never been vaccinated, some physicians may choose to give these adults at least two doses of IPV a month apart, if not a full primary series, before the children receive ORIMUNE.[2] The benefit of being protected against polio is believed to greatly outweigh any risk from polio vaccine.[13]

Administration: ORIMUNE Is to be administered *orally, under the supervision of a physician. Under no circumstances should this vaccine be administered parenterally.* For convenience, the vaccine is supplied in a disposable pipette containing a single dose of 0.5 ml. The vaccine can be administered directly or mixed with distilled water, tap water free of chlorine, simple syrup USP or milk. Alternatively, it may be adsorbed on any one of a number of foods such as bread, cake or cube sugar.

Community Programs

Poliovirus Vaccine, Live, Oral, Trivalent has been recommended for epidemic control. Within an epidemic area, TOPV should be provided for all persons over 6 weeks of age who have not been completely immunized or whose immunization status is unknown.[2,5]

Dosage:

Dose: Each single dose consists of 0.5 ml of POLIOVIRUS VACCINE, LIVE, ORAL, TRIVALENT ORIMUNE.

Initial Administration (Primary Series)

Infants: The primary series is three doses. The Advisory Committee on Immunization Practices (Public Health Service) recommends that the three dose immunization series be started at 6 to 12 weeks of age, commonly with the first DTP inoculation. The second dose should be given not less than 6 and preferably 8 weeks later. The third dose is an integral part of the primary immunization and should be administered 8 to 12 months after the second dose.[2]

The American Academy of Pediatrics recommends that the vaccine be administered at 2 months, 4 months, and at approximately 18 months.[5]

Administration to the newborn (under 6 weeks) is not generally recommended because of the varying persistence of maternal antibodies. However in certain tropical endemic areas, where poliomyelitis has been increasing in recent years, the physician may wish to administer TOPV to the infant at birth, and complete the basic course during the first six months of life.[5]

Older Children and Adolescents (through age 18): Two doses, given not less than 6 and preferably 8 weeks apart and the third dose 6 to 12 months after the second dose.[2,5]

Adults: See Indications and Adverse Reactions. Where ORIMUNE is given to unimmunized adults, the dosage is as indicated for children and adolescents.

Booster Doses—School Entrance: On entering elementary school, all children who have completed the primary series should be given a single follow-up dose of trivalent oral poliovirus vaccine.[2,5] All others should complete the primary series.

The Public Health Service Advisory Committee does not recommend routine booster doses of vaccine on the basis of current information beyond that given at the time of entering school.[2] Recent data indicates that over 95% of children studied five years after full immunization with oral poliovirus vaccine had protective antibodies to all three types of poliovirus.[15]

Increased risk: If an individual who has completed a primary series is subjected to a substantially increased risk by virtue of contact, travel or occupation, a single dose of TOPV has been suggested.[2]

Storage: To maintain potency it is necessary to store this vaccine at a temperature which will maintain ice continuously in a solid state. This vaccine may remain fluid at temperatures above −14°C (+7°F) because of its sorbitol content. If frozen, the vaccine must be completely thawed prior to use. An *unopened* container of vaccine that has been frozen and then is thawed may be carried through a maximum of 10 freeze-thaw cycles, provided the temperature does not exceed 8°C (46°F) during the periods of thaw and provided the total cumulative duration of thaw does not exceed 24 hours. If the 24-hour period is exceeded, the vaccine then must be used within 30 days, during which time it must be stored at a temperature between 2–8°C (36–46°F).

Disclaimer of Representations and Warranties: This vaccine has been produced and tested in accordance with the regulations of the United States Food and Drug Administration for the production of Poliovirus Vaccine,

Live, Oral, Trivalent. The manufacturer makes no representation or warranty, expressed or implied, with respect to the merchantability or fitness for use of this vaccine other than that the vaccine has been produced in accordance with the standards for its production prescribed by the United States Food and Drug Administration and applicable thereto at the time of its release by the manufacturer. While the use of this preparation and other measures described herein are consistent with accepted standards of medical practice, their use as described cannot be expected necessarily to assure a specific result.

How Supplied:
0.5 ml dose—contains Sorbitol
10 (0.5 ml) Dispettes® Disposable Pipettes
25 (0.5 ml) Dispettes®
U.S.P.H.S. Depot: 10 × 1 dose
NSN 6505-00-762-1056

Also Available:
2 Drop Dose: (contains no Sorbitol)
10 dose vial with dropper

PATHIBAMATE®-200 ℞
(tridihexethyl chloride-meprobamate)
PATHIBAMATE®-400 ℞
(tridihexethyl chloride-meprobamate)
Tablets

Description: PATHILON® *tridihexethyl chloride* is a synthetic quaternary ammonium compound. Meprobamate is 2-methyl-2-propyltrimethylene dicarbamate.

Actions: *PATHIBAMATE tridihexethyl chloride-meprobamate* combines tridihexethyl chloride, an anticholinergic agent with meprobamate, a tranquilizing agent.

Tridihexethyl chloride
Tridihexethyl chloride possesses antimuscarinic actions. Gastrointestinal actions include reduction in both gastric secretion and gastrointestinal motility.

Meprobamate
Meprobamate is a carbamate derivative which has been shown in animal studies to have effects at multiple sites in the central nervous system, including the thalamus and limbic system.

INDICATIONS
Based on a review of this drug by the National Academy of Sciences-National Research Council and/or other information, FDA has classified the indications as follows:
Possibly Effective: as adjunctive therapy in peptic ulcer and in the irritable bowel syndrome (irritable colon, spastic colon, mucous colitis, and functional gastrointestinal disorders), especially when accompanied by anxiety or tension. It should be used as an adjunct to other appropriate measures such as proper diet and antacids.

Contraindications:
Tridihexethyl chloride
Allergic or idiosyncratic reactions to tridihexethyl chloride or related compounds; glaucoma; obstructive uropathy (e.g., bladder neck obstruction due to prostatic hypertrophy); obstructive disease of the gastrointestinal tract (as in achalasia, paralytic ileus, pyloroduodenal stenosis, etc.); intestinal atony of the elderly or debilitated patient; unstable cardiovascular status in acute hemorrhage; severe ulcerative colitis; toxic megacolon complicating ulcerative colitis; myasthenia gravis.

Meprobamate
Acute intermittent porphyria as well as allergic or idiosyncratic reactions to meprobamate or related compounds such as carisoprodol, mebutamate, tybamate, or carbromal.

Warnings:
Tridihexethyl chloride
In the presence of a high environment temperature, heat prostration can occur with drug use (fever and heat stroke due to decreased sweating).
Diarrhea may be an early symptom of incomplete intestinal obstruction, especially in patients with ileostomy or colostomy. In this instance treatment with this drug would be inappropriate and possibly harmful.
This drug may produce drowsiness or blurred vision. In this event, the patient should be warned not to engage in activities requiring mental alertness such as operating a motor vehicle or other machinery or perform hazardous work while taking this drug.

Meprobamate
Drug Dependence—Physical dependence, psychological dependence, and abuse have occurred. When chronic intoxication from prolonged use occurs, it usually involves ingestion of greater than recommended doses and is manifested by ataxia, slurred speech, and vertigo. Therefore, careful supervision of dose and amounts prescribed is advised, as well as avoidance of prolonged administration, especially for alcoholics and other patients with a known propensity for taking excessive quantities of drugs. Sudden withdrawal of the drug after prolonged and excessive use may precipitate recurrence of pre-existing symptoms, such as anxiety, anorexia, or insomnia, or withdrawal reactions, such as vomiting, ataxia, tremors, muscle twitching, confusional states, hallucinosis, and, rarely, convulsive seizures. Such seizures are more likely to occur in persons with central nervous system damage or pre-existent or latent convulsive disorders. Onset of withdrawal symptoms occurs usually within 12 to 48 hours after discontinuation of meprobamate; symptoms usually cease within the next 12 to 48 hours.
When excessive dosage has continued for weeks or months, dosage should be reduced gradually over a period of one or two weeks rather than abruptly stopped. Alternatively, a short-acting barbiturate may be substituted, then gradually withdrawn.
Potentially Hazardous Tasks—Patients should be warned that this drug may impair the mental and/or physical abilities required for the performance of potentially hazardous tasks such as driving a motor vehicle or operating machinery.
Additive Effects—Since the effects of meprobamate and alcohol or meprobamate and other CNS depressants or psychotropic drugs may be additive, appropriate caution should be exercised with patients who take more than one of these agents simultaneously.
***Usage in Pregnancy and Lactation*—An increased risk of congenital malformations associated with the use of minor tranquilizers (meprobamate, chlordiazepoxide, and diazepam) during the first trimester of pregnancy has been suggested in several studies. Because use of these drugs is rarely a matter of urgency, their use during this period should also always be avoided. The possibility that a woman of childbearing potential may be pregnant at the time of institution of therapy should be considered. Patients should be advised that if they become pregnant during therapy or intend to become pregnant, they should communicate with their physicians about the desirability of discontinuing the drug.**
Meprobamate passes the placental barrier. It is present both in umbilical cord blood at or near maternal plasma levels and in breast milk of lactating mothers at concentrations two to four times that of maternal plasma. When use of meprobamate is contemplated in breast-feeding patients, the drug's higher concentrations in breast milk as compared to maternal plasma levels should be considered.

Precautions:
Tridihexethyl chloride
Use with caution in patients with:
Autonomic neuropathy.
Hepatic or renal disease.
Early evidence of ileus as in peritonitis.
Ulcerative colitis-large doses may suppress intestinal motility to the point of producing a paralytic ileus and the use of this drug may precipitate or aggravate the serious complication of toxic megacolon.
Hyperthyroidism, coronary heart disease, congestive heart failure, cardiac arrhythmias, hypertension and non-obstructing prostatic hypertrophy.
Hiatal hernia associated with reflux esophagitis since anticholinergic drugs may aggravate this condition.
It should be noted that the use of anticholinergic drugs in the treatment of gastric ulcer may produce a delay in gastric emptying time and may complicate such therapy (antral stasis).
Do not rely on the use of the drug in the presence of complication of biliary tract disease.
Investigate any tachycardia before giving anticholinergic (atropine-like) drugs since they may increase the heart rate.
With overdosage, a curare-like action may occur.

Meprobamate
The lowest effective dose should be administered, particularly to elderly and/or debilitated patients, in order to preclude oversedation.
The possibility of suicide attempts should be considered and the least amount of drug feasible should be dispensed at any one time.
Meprobamate is metabolized in the liver and excreted by the kidney; to avoid its excess accumulation, caution should be exercised in administration to patients with compromised liver or kidney function.
Meprobamate occasionally may precipitate seizures in epileptic patients.

Adverse Reactions: In evaluating adverse reactions to this combination, consider the possibility of adverse reactions that can occur with either component, as listed below:

Tridihexethyl chloride
Adverse reactions may be physiologic or toxic, depending upon the individual patient's response, and may include xerostomia; urinary hesitancy and retention; tachycardia; palpitations; blurred vision; mydriasis; cycloplegia; increased ocular tension; loss of taste; headaches; nervousness; drowsiness; weakness; dizziness; insomnia; nausea; vomiting; impotence; suppression of lactation; constipation; bloated feeling; severe allergic reaction or drug idiosyncrasies including anaphylaxis; urticaria and other dermal manifestations; decreased sweating; some degree of mental confusion and/or excitement especially in elderly persons.

Meprobamate
Central Nervous System—Drowsiness, ataxia, dizziness, slurred speech, headache, vertigo, weakness, paresthesias, impairment of visual accommodation, euphoria, overstimulation, paradoxical excitement, fast EEG activity.
Gastrointestinal—Nausea, vomiting, diarrhea.
Cardiovascular—Palpitations, tachycardia, various forms of arrhythmia, transient ECG changes, syncope; also, hypotensive crises (including one fatal case).

Continued on next page

The information on each product appearing here is based on labelling effective in August, 1979 and is either the entire official brochure or an accurate condensation therefrom. Official brochures are enclosed in product packages. Information concerning all Lederle products may be obtained from the Medical Department, Lederle Laboratories, Pearl River, New York, 10965.

Lederle—Cont.

Allergic or Idiosyncratic—Allergic or idiosyncratic reactions are usually seen within the period of the first to fourth dose in patients having had no previous contact with the drug. Milder reactions are characterized by an itchy, urticarial, or erythematous maculopapular rash which may be generalized or confined to the groin. Other reactions have included leukopenia, acute nonthrombocytopenic purpura, petechiae, ecchymoses, eosinophilia, peripheral edema, adenopathy, fever, fixed drug eruption with cross reaction to carisoprodol, and cross sensitivity between meprobamate/-mebutamate and meprobamate/carbromal.
More severe hypersensitivity reactions, rarely reported, include hyperpyrexia, chills, angioneurotic edema, bronchospasm, oliguria, and anuria. Also, anaphylaxis, erythema multiforme, exfoliative dermatitis, stomatitis, proctitis, Stevens-Johnson syndrome, and bullous dermatitis, including one fatal case of the latter following administration of meprobamate in combination with prednisolone.
In case of allergic or idiosyncratic reactions to meprobamate, discontinue the drug and initiate appropriate symptomatic therapy, which may include epinephrine, antihistamines, and in severe cases, corticosteroids. In evaluating possible allergic reactions, also consider allergy to excipients (information on excipients is available to physicians on request).
Hematologic (See also *Allergic or Idiosyncratic.*)—Agranulocytosis and aplastic anemia have been reported, although no causal relationship has been established. These cases rarely were fatal. Rare cases of thrombocytopenic purpura have been reported.
Other—Exacerbation of porphyric symptoms.
Dosage and Administration: The usual adult dose of PATHIBAMATE *tridihexethyl chloride-meprobamate*-400 (meprobamate 400 mg. + tridihexethyl chloride 25 mg.) is one tablet three times a day at mealtimes, and two tablets at bedtime. If a greater anticholinergic effect is desired, the usual adult dose is two PATHIBAMATE *tridihexethyl chloride-meprobamate*-200 (meprobamate 200 mg. + tridihexethyl chloride 25 mg.) tablets three times a day at mealtimes, and two tablets at bedtime. Doses of meprobamate above 2400 mg. daily are not recommended.
Not for use in children under age 12.
Overdosage: Overdosage information on this combination is lacking. However, consider the possibility of signs and symptoms that can occur with either component, as listed below:
Tridihexethyl chloride
Acute overdosage of anticholinergic agents can produce dry mouth, difficulty in swallowing, marked thirst; blurred vision, photophobia; flushed, hot, dry skin; rash; hyperthermia; palpitations, tachycardia with weak pulse, elevated blood pressure; urinary urgency with difficulty in micturition; abdominal distention; restlessness, confusion, delirium and other signs suggestive of an acute organic psychosis. Treatment should include removal of remaining drug from stomach after administration of Universal Antidote, and supportive and symptomatic therapy as indicated. Universal Antidote is a mixture of 2 parts activated charcoal, 1 part magnesium oxide, and 1 part tannic acid, given as ½ ounce in a half glass of warm water.
Meprobamate
Suicidal attempts with meprobamate have resulted in drowsiness, lethargy, stupor, ataxia, coma, shock, vasomotor and respiratory collapse. Some suicidal attempts have been fatal.
The following data on meprobamate tablets have been reported in the literature and from other sources. These data are not expected to correlate with each case (considering factors such as individual susceptibility and length of time from ingestion to treatment), but represent the *usual ranges* reported.
Acute simple overdose (meprobamate alone): Death has been reported with ingestion of as little as 12 Grams meprobamate and survival with as much as 40 Grams.
Blood Levels:
0.5-2.0 mg.% represents the usual blood level range of meprobamate after therapeutic doses. The level may occasionally be as high as 3.0 mg.%.
3-10 mg.% usually corresponds to findings of mild to moderate symptoms of overdosage, such as stupor or light coma.
10-20 mg.% usually corresponds to deeper coma, requiring more intensive treatment. Some fatalities occur.
At levels greater than 20 mg.%, more fatalities than survivals can be expected.
Acute combined overdose (meprobamate with alcohol or other CNS depressants or psychotropic drugs): Since effects can be additive, a history of ingestion of a low dose of meprobamate plus any of these compounds (or of a relatively low blood or tissue level) cannot be used as a prognostic indicator.
In cases where excessive doses have been taken, sleep ensues rapidly; and blood pressure, pulse, and respiratory rates are reduced to basal levels. Any drug remaining in the stomach should be removed and symptomatic therapy given. Should respiration or blood pressure become compromised, respiratory assistance, central nervous system stimulants, and pressor agents should be administered cautiously as indicated. Meprobamate is metabolized in the liver and excreted by the kidney. Diuresis, osmotic (mannitol) diuresis, peritoneal dialysis, and hemodialysis have been used successfully. Careful monitoring of urinary output is necessary and caution should be taken to avoid overhydration. Relapse and death, after initial recovery, have been attributed to incomplete gastric emptying and delayed absorption. Meprobamate can be measured in biological fluids by two methods: colorimetric (Hoffman, A.J. and Ludwig, B.J.: *J Amer Pharm Assn 48:*740,1959) and gas chromatographic (Douglas, J.F. et al: *Anal Chem 39:*956, 1967).
How Supplied: PATHIBAMATE *tridihexethyl chloride-meprobamate* is available in two formulations:
PATHIBAMATE-400: Yellow.
Each tablet contains:
meprobamate .... 400 mg.
tridihexethyl chloride......................... 25 mg.
Bottles of 100 and 1000; drum of 5000.
PATHIBAMATE-200: Yellow, coated tablets.
Each tablet contains:
meprobamate .... 200 mg.
tridihexethyl chloride......................... 25 mg.
Bottles of 100 and 1000.
A.H.F.S. 12:08
[*Shown in Product Identification Section*]

PATHILON® ℞
(tridihexethyl chloride)
Products

Description: PATHILON *tridihexethyl chloride* is a synthetic anticholinergic quaternary ammonium compound.
Phenobarbital is 5-Ethyl-5-phenylbarbituric acid.
The following dosage forms are available:
Tablets 25 mg. Tridihexethyl Chloride
SEQUELS Sustained Release Capsules 75 mg. Tridihexethyl Chloride
SEQUELS Sustained Release Capsules 75 mg. Tridihexethyl Chloride with 45 mg. Phenobarbital
Tablets 25 mg. Tridihexethyl Chloride with 15 mg. Phenobarbital
Actions: PATHILON relieves pain by reducing spasm of the gastrointestinal tract. Phenobarbital is a hypnotic acid sedative drug with anticonvulsive properties. WARNING: May be habit forming.

INDICATIONS
Based on a review of these products by the National Academy of Sciences-National Research Council and/or other information, FDA has classified the indications as follows:
Tablets—Effective as adjunctive therapy in the treatment of peptic ulcer. Probably effective as adjunctive therapy in the irritable bowel syndrome (irritable colon, spastic colon, mucous colitis, acute enterocolitis, and functional gastrointestinal disorders).
SEQUELS—Probably effective as adjunctive therapy in the treatment of peptic ulcer. May also be useful in the irritable bowel syndrome (see above) and in neurogenic bowel disturbances (including the splenic flexure syndrome and neurogenic colon).
SEQUELS with phenobarbital and Tablets with phenobarbital—Possibly effective for the indications for SEQUELS (above).
To be effective the dosage must be titrated to the individual patient's needs.

Contraindications: Glaucoma; obstructive uropathy (for example, bladder neck obstruction due to prostatic hypertrophy); obstructive disease of the gastrointestinal tract (as in achalasia, paralytic ileus, pyloroduodenal stenosis, etc.); intestinal atony of the elderly or debilitated patient; unstable cardiovascular status in acute hemorrhage; severe ulcerative colitis; toxic megacolon complicating ulcerative colitis; myasthenia gravis.
Phenobarbital is contraindicated in acute intermittent porphyria. A sensitivity to phenobarbital contraindicates the use of PATHILON *tridihexethyl chloride* with Phenobarbital Sustained Release Capsules or Tablets and in those patients in whom phenobarbital produces restlessness and/or excitement.
Warnings: USE IN PREGNANCY—The use of any drug in pregnancy, lactation, or in women of child-bearing potential, requires that the potential benefit of the drug be weighed against its possible hazards to the mother and child. As with all anticholinergic drugs, an inhibiting effect on lactation may occur.
In the presence of a high environmental temperature, heat prostration can occur with drug use (fever and heat stroke due to decreased sweating). Diarrhea may be an early symptom of incomplete intestinal obstruction, especially in patients with ileostomy or colostomy. In this instance treatment with this drug would be inappropriate and possibly harmful.
PATHILON *tridihexethyl chloride* may produce drowsiness or blurred vision. In this event, the patient should be warned not to engage in activities requiring mental alertness such as operating a motor vehicle or other machinery or perform hazardous work while taking this drug.
Phenobarbital in patients taking anticoagulants may decrease the effect of the anticoagulant and thus require larger doses of the anticoagulant for optimal effect. When the phenobarbital is discontinued, the dose of the anticoagulant may have to be decreased. Barbiturates may thus decrease the action of anticoagulant drugs.
Phenobarbital may be habit forming and should not be administered to individuals known to be addiction prone or to those with a history of physical and/or psychological dependence upon habit forming drugs.
Since barbiturates are metabolized in the liver, use with initial small doses and caution in patients with hepatic dysfunction.

Precautions: Use with caution in patients with:
Autonomic neuropathy.
Hepatic or renal disease.
Early evidence of ileus as in peritonitis.
Ulcerative colitis—large doses may suppress intestinal motility to the point of producing a paralytic ileus and the use of this drug may precipitate or aggravate the serious complication of toxic megacolon.
Hyperthyroidism, coronary heart disease, congestive heart failure, cardiac arrhythmias, hypertension and non-obstructing prostatic hypertrophy.
Hiatal hernia associated with reflux esophagitis since anticholinergic drugs may aggravate this condition.
It should be noted that the use of anticholinergic drugs in the treatment of gastric ulcer may produce a delay in gastric emptying time and may complicate such therapy (antral stasis).
Do not rely on the use of the drug in the presence of complication of biliary tract disease.
Investigate any tachycardia before giving anticholinergic (atropine-like) drugs since they may increase the heart rate.
With overdosage, a curare-like action may occur.
Adverse Reactions: Anticholinergics produce certain effects which may be physiologic or toxic depending upon the individual patient's response. The physician must delineate these. Adverse reactions may include xerostomia; urinary hesitancy and retention; blurred vision and tachycardia; palpitations; mydriasis; dilatation of the pupil; cycloplegia; increased ocular tension; loss of taste; headaches; nervousness; drowsiness; weakness; dizziness; insomnia; nausea; vomiting; impotence; suppression of lactation; constipation; bloated feeling; severe allergic reaction or drug idiosyncrasies including anaphylaxis; urticaria and other dermal manifestation; some degree of mental confusion and/or excitement especially in elderly persons.
Decreased sweating is another adverse reaction that may occur. It should be noted that adrenergic innervation of the eccrine sweat glands on the palms and soles make complete control of sweating impossible. An end point of complete anhidrosis cannot occur because large doses of drug would be required, and this would produce severe side effects from parasympathetic paralysis.
Phenobarbital may produce excitement in some patients rather than a sedative effect. An occasional patient may experience musculoskeletal pain. Some patients may acquire a sensitivity to barbiturates and experience allergic phenomena and/or dermatologic response.
In patients habituated to barbiturates, abrupt withdrawal may produce delirium or convulsions.
Dosage and Administration: For effective therapeutic results, in particular with anticholinergic drugs, it is absolutely necessary to titrate dosage against the patient's individual needs and response.
Tablets:
The average oral adult dose is 25 to 50 mg. of PATHILON *tridihexethyl chloride* (with or without 15 to 30 mg. of Phenobarbital) 3 to 4 times per day. The usual bedtime dose has been 50 mg. A few patients are well controlled on as little as 10 mg. 3 times per day, while some require as much as 75 mg. 4 times per day. The suggested initial dose is 25 mg. 3 times per day before meals and 50 mg. at bedtime.
SEQUELS:
PATHILON *tridihexethyl chloride* and PATHILON with Phenobarbital are available in a sustained release form which allows less frequent dosage administration with comparable clinical effect obtained by the usual dosage form. SEQUELS Sustained Release Capsules are prepared by a unique process whereby the basic drug is coated with an inert waxy material in a controlled manner. It is possible, therefore, to obtain 24-hour drug effects, including the anticholinergic activity, during the entire normal sleeping period. The average dosage is one 75 mg. capsule, with or without Phenobarbital, every 12 hours; however, if more anticholinergic effect is desired, the SEQUELS may be given as frequently as 1 capsule every 6 hours depending on tolerance.
Overdosage:
Tridihexethyl chloride:
Acute overdosage of anticholinergic agents can produce dry mouth, difficulty swallowing, marked thirst; blurred vision, photophobia; flushed, hot, dry skin; rash; hyperthermia; palpitations, tachycardia with weak pulse, elevated blood pressure; urinary urgency with difficulty in micturition; abdominal distention; restlessness, confusion, delirium and other signs suggestive of an acute organic psychosis. Treatment should include removal of remaining drug from stomach after administration of Universal Antidote, and supportive and symptomatic therapy as indicated. Universal Antidote is a mixture of 2 parts activated charcoal, 1 part magnesium oxide, and 1 part tannic acid, given as ½ ounce in a half glass of warm water.
Phenobarbital:
Early symptoms are sleepiness, mental confusion, and unsteadiness. These are followed by coma (which may last as long as 7 days), slow, shallow respiration, flaccid muscles and absent deep reflexes. Death occurs most often from pulmonary involvement. Shock should be treated with appropriate measures. Absorption of ingested drug should be delayed by giving tap water, milk, or "Universal Antidote", and then removing by thorough gastric lavage or emesis followed by catharsis. The probability of removing a significant amount of drug is good if treatment is started within two hours after ingestion. In comatose patients, care must be taken to prevent aspiration during gastric lavage and emesis.
When the Sustained Release SEQUELS have been used, prolonged intestinal absorption and prolonged drug action may necessitate treatment over an extended period of time.
If necessary to maintain adequate airway, mucous secretions should be removed from the trachea by suction with a soft rubber catheter, or an oropharyngeal airway may be used. If laryngeal stridor or laryngeal edema occurs, a laryngeal airway or tracheotomy may be necessary. It is important to maintain adequate oxygen intake and carbon dioxide removal. If respiration is depressed, moistened 40 to 60% oxygen may be administered. Mechanical assistance to respiration may be needed.
Experimental data have indicated that alkalinization reduces the penetration of phenobarbital into cells. Large quantities of hypertonic $NaHCO_3$ intravenously, usually in concentrations of 14% have produced satisfactory results and the average duration of the coma has been substantially reduced. Hemodialysis has been successfully employed in severe barbiturate intoxication.
How Supplied: *SEQUELS* (75 mg., two-tone pink)—bottles of 30; *Tablets* (25 mg., coated pink—bottles of 100 and 1,000; *SEQUELS*, 75 mg. with phenobarbital, 45 mg.(two-tone blue)—bottles of 30; *Tablets*, 25 mg. with phenobarbital, 15 mg. (coated blue)—bottles of 100 and 1,000.
A.H.F.S. 12:08
V.A. Depots—25 mg. Tablets
NSN 6505-00-584-3272A, 1,000's
[*Tablets and SEQUELS Shown in Product Identification Section*]

PERIHEMIN® ℞
(hematinic)
Capsules

Description: PERIHEMIN *hematinic* Capsules for children over 12 and adults.
Each capsule contains: Vitamin B_{12} (as Cyanocobalamin U.S.P.) 5 mcg.; Intrinsic Factor Concentrate 25 mg.; Ferrous Fumarate 168 mg., (Elemental Iron 55 mg.); Folic Acid 0.33 mg.; Ascorbic Acid (C) 50 mg.
Actions: PERIHEMIN *Lederle* products are general hematinics for the oral treatment of the common anemias. They contain the common substances used in the prevention and treatment of anemic conditions produced or aggravated by insufficient food intake.
Indications: PERIHEMIN is primarily indicated in the hypochromic, microcytic anemias due to insufficient iron intake or absorption. It is also useful in the treatment of macrocytic hyperchromic anemias where an increased intake of oral B_{12} or folic acid is desirable.
Warnings: Folic Acid alone is improper therapy in the treatment of pernicious anemia and other megaloblastic anemias where vitamin B_{12} is deficient.
Precautions: Some patients affected with pernicious anemia may not respond to orally administered Vitamin B_{12} with intrinsic factor concentrate and there is no known way to predict which patients will respond or which patients may cease to respond. Periodic examinations and laboratory studies of pernicious anemia patients are essential and recommended.
Folic acid especially in doses above 1.0 mg. daily may obscure pernicious anemia, in that hematologic remission may occur while neurological manifestations remain progressive.
Overdosage or accidental overingestion of iron-containing compounds may lead to gastrointestinal hemorrhage in children. If symptoms of intolerance develop, the drug should be temporarily or permanently discontinued.
PERIHEMIN *hematinic* preparations should not be relied on to correct the serious folic acid deficiency characterizing sprue or the malabsorption syndromes. In these conditions therapeutic amounts of folic acid should be administered.
Adverse Reactions: Allergic sensitization has been reported following both oral and parenteral administration of Folic Acid.
Dosage: PERIHEMIN Capsules for children over 12 and adults.
1 capsule 3 times daily with or after meals.
How Supplied: Capsules—soft shell red—Bottles of 100.

PERITINIC®
(hematinic with vitamins and fecal softener)
Tablets

Composition: Each tablet contains:
Elemental Iron
(as Ferrous Fumarate) ....100 mg.
Docusate Sodium U.S.P.
(DSS) (to counteract the
constipating effect of iron) ....100 mg.
Vitamin B_1
(as Thiamine Mononitrate)................7.5 mg.
(7 ½ MDR)
Vitamin B_2 (Riboflavin)..........................7.5 mg.
(6¼ MDR)

Continued on next page

The information on each product appearing here is based on labelling effective in August, 1979 and is either the entire official brochure or an accurate condensation therefrom. Official brochures are enclosed in product packages. Information concerning all Lederle products may be obtained from the Medical Department, Lederle Laboratories, Pearl River, New York, 10965.

Lederle—Cont.

Vitamin B_6
(Pyridoxine Hydrochloride)................7.5 mg.
Vitamin B_{12} (Cyanocobalamin) ....50 mcgm.
Vitamin C (Ascorbic Acid)....................200 mg.
(6⅔ MDR)
Niacinamide..30 mg.
(3 MDR)
Folic Acid ....0.05 mg.
Pantothenic Acid
(as D-Pantothenyl Alcohol..................15 mg.
MDR—Adult Minimum Daily Requirement

Action and Uses: In the prevention of nutritional anemias, certain vitamin deficiencies, and iron-deficiency anemias.

Administration and Dosage:
Adults: 1 or 2 tablets daily.

How Supplied: Tablets (maroon capsule-shaped, film coated)—bottles of 60.

PNU-IMUNE® ℞
(pneumococcal vaccine, polyvalent)

Description: PNU-IMUNE is a vaccine consisting of a mixture of purified capsular polysaccharides from 14 pneumococcal types:
[See table below].
It is indicated for immunization against infections caused by the 14 most prevalent types of pneumococci responsible for 80 or more percent of serious pneumococcal disease in the United States and the rest of the world.[1–4]
Each of the pneumococcal polysaccharide types is produced separately by Lederle Laboratories to give a high degree of purity. After an individual pneumococcal type is grown, the polysaccharide is separated from the cell and purified by a series of steps including ethanol fractionation. The resultant 14 purified polysaccharides are combined in amounts to give 50 micrograms of each type per dose (0.5 ml) in the final vaccine. Thimerosal at a concentration of 0.01% is added as a preservative.

Actions: Pneumococci are the etiologic agents for a significant number of the pneumonias occurring throughout the world. The emergence of strains of pneumococci with increased resistance to one or more of the common antibiotics[4] and recent isolations of pneumococci with multiple-antibiotic resistance[5] emphasize the importance of vaccine prophylaxis against pneumococcal disease.
Based on projections from limited observations[2] in the United States, it has been estimated that 400,000 to 500,000 cases of pneumococcal pneumonia may occur annually. The overall case fatality rate ranges from 5–10%.[2]
Populations at high risk are the elderly,[6–7] individuals with immune deficiencies, asplenics and patients with splenic deficiencies including sickle cell anemia and other severe hemoglobinopathies, alcoholics and patients with the following diseases: chronic respiratory illness, the nephrotic syndrome, multiple myeloma, Hodgkin's disease and cirrhosis. Antibiotics have only been partially effective in reducing the mortality of pneumococcal pneumonia. As many as 60 percent of all deaths among patients with pneumococcal bacteremia treated with penicillin or tetracycline occur within five days of onset of the illness.[5]
Thus, vaccination offers an effective means for further reducing the mortality and morbidity of this disease. The pneumococcus is also the chief infectious agent in meningitis[8] and otitis media. Other illnesses caused by pneumococci include sinus infection, arthritis and conjunctivitis. The annual incidence of pneumococcal meningitis is approximately 1.5 to 2.5 per 100,000 population. One-half of the cases occur in children in whom the fatality rate is about 40%.[1,7]
The polysaccharide capsules of pneumococci endow these organisms with resistance to the phagocytic action of polymorphonuclear leukocytes and monocytes. The opsonin activity of type-specific antibody facilitates their destruction in the body by complement-mediated activities. The protection induced by the vaccine is of long duration but its extent is not yet known. Elevated antibody levels have been shown to persist for at least 5 years after immunization with other pneumococcal vaccines.[1] Studies with pneumococcal polysaccharide vaccines prepared in the immediate post-World War II era demonstrated persistence of antibody for as long as 5 years.[9] Children under 2 years of age do not respond adequately to some of the important polysaccharide types. There appears to be no increase in serum antibodies after a second injection (no booster effect). Recipients of polyvalent vaccines acquired less nasopharyngeal carriage of pneumococcal types included in the vaccine.[2,10]
In recent clinical studies with PNU-IMUNE, at least 90% of all adults showed a 4-fold or greater increase in geometric mean antibody titer for each vaccine capsular type.[11]
Patients over the age of 2 years with anatomical or functional asplenia and otherwise intact lymphoid function responded to PNU-IMUNE *pneumococcal vaccine, polyvalent* and other comparable pneumococcal vaccines with a serological conversion comparable to that observed in healthy individuals of the same age.[12]
Polyvalent pneumococcal vaccines, from other sources, were shown to be effective in preventing pneumococcal disease. Controlled field trials in South Africa involving 12,000 gold miners have shown polyvalent vaccine to be 78.5% effective in preventing type-specific pneumococcal pneumonia and 82.3% effective in preventing pneumococcal bacteremia with the types in the vaccine.[13] In a preliminary study of an octavalent polysaccharide vaccine in a group consisting of 77 patients with sickle cell disease and 19 asplenic persons, there were no pneumococcal infections in the immunized patients within two years of immunization. There were eight cases of pneumococcal infection in 106 unimmunized, age-matched patients with sickle cell disease. Antibody response of the asplenic patients was comparable to normal controls.[14]
In a study carried out by Austrian et al.[13] with pneumococcal vaccines prepared for the National Institutes of Allergy and Infectious Disease, the reduction in pneumonias caused by the capsular types in the vaccines was 79%. Reduction in type-specific pneumococcal bacteremia was 82%.
In a double-blind study of a 14-valent pneumococcal vaccine carried out in Papua New Guinea, pneumococcal infection was less in the vaccinated group by 84%. Mortality from pneumonia was less by 44%.[15]

Indications: PNU-IMMUNE is indicated for immunization against pneumococcal disease caused by those pneumococcal types included in the vaccine.
Use in Selected Individuals as Follows: persons over 2 years of age as follows: (1) who have anatomical asplenia or who have splenic dysfunction due to sickle cell disease or other causes; (2) persons with chronic illnesses in which there is an increased risk of pneumococcal disease, such as diabetes mellitus, functional impairment of cardiorespiratory, hepatic and renal systems; (3) persons 50 years of age or older.
Use in Communities. Persons over 2 years of age as follows: (1) closed groups such as those in residential schools, nursing homes and other institutions; (2) groups epidemiologically at risk in the community when there is a generalized outbreak in the general population due to a single pneumococcal type included in the vaccine; (3) patients at high risk of influenza complications, particularly pneumonia.[10]

Contraindications:
Pregnancy. Safety, immunogenicity and efficacy of the vaccine in pregnancy has not been established, and vaccination is not recommended during pregnancy.
Children below 2 years of age. Children in this age group respond poorly to the current vaccine, and vaccination of children in this age group *should not be undertaken.*
Hypersensitivity. Known hypersensitivity to any component of the vaccine including hypersensitivity to thimerosal. Remedial measures for anaphylactoid reactions, including epinephrine injection (1:1000), must be available for immediate use. Prior immunization with pneumococcal polysaccharide vaccine appears to induce hypersensitivity to components of the vaccine.
Additional doses. use of more than one dose, booster doses or revaccination has not yet been established as a useful or safe procedure. Administration of vaccine within three years after initial immunization has been found to result in severe local reactions at the site of injection, especially in persons retaining a high antibody level. There appears to be no booster effect with an additional dose.[9]

Warnings: *PNU-IMUNE is not an effective agent for prophylaxis against pneumococcal disease caused by types not present in the vaccine.*
The vaccine may not be effective in patients undergoing treatment causing therapeutic suppression of the immune-response system.
Patients who have received extensive chemotherapy and/or splenectomy for the treatment of Hodgkin's Disease have been shown to have an impaired serum antibody response to pneumococcal vaccine.[16]

Precautions: The vaccine should be injected deeply subcutaneously or intramuscularly. Do not inject intravenously.
In the presence of any febrile respiratory illness or other active infection, the vaccine should not be used.
The parenteral administration of any biological product should be surrounded by every known precaution for the prevention and arrest of allergic and other untoward reactions. When administering this vaccine, a separate heat-sterilized syringe and needle or a new disposable equivalent should be used for each patient to prevent transmission of hepatitis B (homologous serum hepatitis) or other infectious agents.

Adverse Reactions: PNU-IMUNE *pneumococcal vaccine, polyvalent* is associated with a relatively low incidence of adverse reactions as compared with injectable vaccines presently in use. The adverse reactivity observed in clinical studies was not serious and of short duration. In a study of 32 individuals who received PNU-IMUNE, 23 (72%) experienced local reaction characterized by local soreness at the injection site within 3 days after vaccination.
Low grade fever (less than 100° F) occurs occasionally with PNU-IMUNE and is usually confined to the 24-hour period following vaccination.
Although rare, fever over 102° and marked local swelling has been reported with pneumococcal polysaccharide vaccine.
Reactions of greater severity, or extent are unusual. Rarely, anaphylactoid reactions have been reported.

Dosage and Administration: Do not inject intravenously. The immunization schedule consists of a single 0.5 ml dose given subcutaneously or intramuscularly. See CONTRAINDICATIONS for information regarding doses.

Nomenclature	Pneumococcal Types													
Danish	1	2	3	4	6A	7F	8	9N	12F	14	18C	19F	23F	25
U.S.	1	2	3	4	6	51	8	9	12	14	56	19	23	25

Directions for Use of the LEDERJECT® Disposable Syringe

1. Twist the plunger rod clockwise to be sure that rod is secure to rubber plunger base.
2. Hold needle shield in place with index finger and thumb of one hand while with other thumb exert light pressure on plunger rod until the plunger base has been freed and demonstrates slight movement when pressure is applied.
3. Grasp the rubber needle shield at its base; twist and pull to remove.
4. Pull back plunger rod slowly and carefully to insure smooth plunger operation.
5. Expel the air bubble.

Storage and Use: Store syringes and unopened or opened vials at 2–8° C (35.6—46.4° F). The vaccine is used directly as supplied. No dilution or reconstitution is necessary. Thimerosal in 0.01% concentration is present in the vaccine as preservative. Discard unused vials beyond expiration date.

How Supplied: PNU-IMUNE *pneumococcal vaccine, polyvalent* is supplied as follows:
5 Dose Vial. For use with syringe only.
5 × One Dose Vials. For use with syringe only.
5 × One Dose LEDERJECT® Disposable Syringes

References:

1. Austrian, R. "Surveillance of Pneumococcal Infection for Field Trials of Polyvalent Vaccines." Annual Contract Prog. Report to the Nat. Inst. of Allerg. and Inf. Dis. (1975) Updated to Dec. 1977, personal communication.
2. Editors. Pneumococcal Polysaccharide Vaccine. Morb. Mort. Weekly Report 27 (1978) 25.
3. Lund, E. "Distribution of Pneumococcal Types at Different Times and Different Areas" in *Bayer Symposium III. Bacterial Infections.* "Changes in Their Causative Agents, Trends and Possible Basis." M. Finland, W. Marget and K. Bartman (eds.) Berlin, Springer — Verlag (1971) 49.
4. Mufson, M.A., Kruss, D.M., Wasil, R.E. and Metzger, W.I. "Capsular Types and Outcome of Bacteremic Pneumococcal Disease in the Antibiotic Era." Arch. Int. Med., 134 (1974) 505.
5. Editors. Multiple-Antibiotic Resistance of Pneumococci-South Africa. Morb. Mort. Weekly Report 26 (1977) 285.
6. Austrian, R., and Gold, J. "Pneumococcal Bacteremia with Especial Reference to Bacteremic Pneumococcal Pneumonia." Ann. Int. Med., 60 (1964) 759.
7. Valenti, W.M., Jenzer, M. and Bently, W. "Type-Specific Pneumococcal Respiratory Disease in the Elderly and Chronically Ill." Am. Rev. Resp. Dis., 117 (1978) 233.
8. Fraser, D.W., Geil, C.C., and Feldman, R.A. "Meningitis in Bernalillo County, New Mexico. A Comparison with Three Other American Populations." Am. J. Epidemiol., 100 (1974) 29.
9. Heidelberger, M., Dilapi, M.M., Seigel, M. and Walter, A.N. "Persistence of Antibodies in Human Subjects Injected with Pneumococcal Polysaccharides." J. Immunol., 65 (1950) 535.
10. Mufson, M.A. and Krause, H.E. "Role of Antibody in Prevention of Acquisition of Pneumococcal Carriage Among Vaccinees." Clin. Res., 24 (1976) 577A.
11. Data on File, Lederle Laboratories.
12. Sullivan, J.L., Ochs, H.D., Schiffman, G., Hammerschlag, M.R., Miser, J., Vichinsky, E., and Wedgwood, R.J. "Immune Response After Splenectomy." Lancet, (1978) 178.
13. Austrian, R., Douglas, R.M., Schiffman, G., Coetzee, A.M., Koornhof, H.J., Hayden-Smith, S. and Reid, R.D.W. "Prevention of Pneumococcal Pneumonia by Vaccination." Trans Ass. Am. Physicians, 89 (1976) 184.
14. Amman, A.J., Addiego, K., Wara, D.W., Lubin, B., Smith, W.B. and Mentzer, W.C. "Polyvalent Pneumococcal-Polysaccharide Immunization of Patients with Sickle-Cell Anemia and Patients with Splenectomy." New Eng. J. Med., 297 (1977) 897.
15. Riley, I.D., Andrews, M., Howard, R., Tarr, P.I., Pfeiffer, M., Challands, P. and Jennison, G. "Immunization with Polyvalent Pneumococcal Vaccine." Lancet, (1977) 1338.
16. Siber, G.R. Weitzman, S.A., Aisenberg, A.C., Weinstein, H.J., and Schiffman, G. "Impaired Antibody Response to Pneumococcal Vaccine After Treatment for Hodgkin's Disease." New Eng J. Med., 299 (1978) 442.

PRONEMIA® ℞
(hematinic)
Capsules

Composition: Each capsule contains: Vitamin B_{12} (as Cobalamin Concentrate) 15 mcg.; Intrinsic Factor Concentrate 75 mg.; Ferrous Fumarate 350 mg. (Elemental Iron 115 mg.); Ascorbic Acid (Vitamin C) 150 mg. and Folic Acid 1 mg.

Indications: Indicated for treatment and maintenance in common anemias, including iron-deficiency anemia, megaloblastic anemias of pregnancy, and those of nutritional origin. All of the other means that are recognized as suited to the treatment of these anemias should also be employed. If cases prove resistant to this form of therapy, further exploration of the etiology and additional therapeutic measures should be instituted.

Warnings: Folic Acid alone is improper therapy in the treatment of pernicious anemia and other megaloblastic anemias where vitamin B_{12} is deficient.

Precautions: Some patients affected with pernicious anemia may not respond to orally administered Vitamin B_{12} with intrinsic factor concentrate and there is no known way to predict which patients will respond or which patients may cease to respond. Periodic examinations and laboratory studies of pernicious anemia patients are essential and recommended. If any symptoms of intolerance occur, the drug should be temporarily or permanently discontinued.
Folic acid, especially in doses above 1.0 mg. daily, may obscure pernicious anemia, in that hematologic remission may occur while neurological manifestations remain progressive.

Adverse Reactions: Allergic sensitization has been reported following both oral and parenteral administration of Folic Acid.

Administration and Dosage: One capsule daily with or after meals to treat and maintain the average uncomplicated case of anemia.

How Supplied: Capsules (red)—bottles of 30, 100 and 500.

RHULICREAM®
RHULIGEL®
RHULIHIST®
RHULISPRAY®
(analgesic-anesthetic)

(See PDR For Nonprescription Drugs)

STRESSCAPS®
(stress formula B+C vitamins)

(See PDR For Nonprescription Drugs)

STRESSTABS® 600
High Potency
Stress Formula Vitamins

Each tablet contains:

	For Adults-Percentage of U.S. Recommended Daily Allowance (U.S. RDA)
Vitamin E (as *dl*-Alpha Tocopheryl Acetate)	30 Int. Units (100%)
Vitamin C (L-Ascorbic Acid)	600 mg (1000%)
Vitamin B_1 (as Thiamine Mononitrate)	15 mg (1000%)
Vitamin B_2 (as Riboflavin)	15 mg (882%)
Niacinamide	100 mg (500%)
Vitamin B_6 (as Pyridoxine Hydrochloride)	5 mg (250%)
Vitamin B_{12} (as Cyanocobalamin)	12 mcgm (200%)
Pantothenic Acid (as Calcium Pantothenate USP)	20 mg (200%)

Recommended Intake: Adults, 1 tablet daily or as directed by physician.

Supplied: Capsule-shaped tablets (film-coated orange)-bottles of 30, 60 and 500; unit-dose 10 x 10's.

VA Depot: NSN 6505-00-375-4618A

[*Shown in Product Identification Section*]

STRESSTABS® 600 with IRON
High Potency
Stress Formula Vitamins

Each tablet contains:

	For Adults-Percentage of U.S. Recommended Daily Allowance (U.S. RDA)
Vitamin E (as *dl*-Alpha Tocopheryl Acetate)	30 Int. Units (100%)
Vitamin C (L-Ascorbic Acid)	600 mg (1000%)
Folic Acid (as Folacin)	400 mcgm (100%)
Vitamin B_1 (as Thiamine Mononitrate)	15 mg (1000%)
Vitamin B_2 (as Riboflavin)	15 mg (882%)
Niacinamide	100 mg (500%)
Vitamin B_6 (as Pyridoxine Hydrochloride)	25 mg (1250%)
Vitamin B_{12} (as Cyanocobalamin)	12 mcgm (200%)
Pantothenic Acid (as Calcium Pantothenate USP)	20 mg (200%)
Iron (as Ferrous Fumarate)	27 mg (150%)

Recommended Intake: Adults, 1 tablet daily or as directed by physician.

Supplied: Capsule-shaped tablets (film-coated orange-red scored)—bottles of 30 and 60.

[*Shown in Product Identification Section*]

STRESSTABS® 600 with ZINC
High Potency
Stress Formula Vitamins

Composition: Each tablet contains:

		For Adults-Percentage of U.S. Recommended Daily Allowance (U.S. RDA)
Vitamin E (as *dl*-Alpha Tocopheryl Acetate)	45 I.U.	(150%)
Vitamin C (L-Ascorbic Acid)	600 mg.	(1000%)
Folic Acid (as Folacin)	400 mcg.	(100%)
Vitamin B_1 (as Thiamine Mononitrate)	20 mg.	(1333%)
Vitamin B_2 (as Riboflavin)	10 mg.	(588%)
Niacinamide	100 mg.	(500%)
Vitamin B_6 (as Pyridoxine Hydrochloride)	10 mg.	(500%)

Continued on next page

The information on each product appearing here is based on labelling effective in August, 1979 and is either the entire official brochure or an accurate condensation therefrom. Official brochures are enclosed in product packages. Information concerning all Lederle products may be obtained from the Medical Department, Lederle Laboratories, Pearl River, New York, 10965.

Lederle—Cont.

Vitamin B_{12} (as Cyanocobalamin)	25 mcg.	(417%)
Pantothenic Acid (as Calcium Pantothenate USP)	25 mg.	(250%)
Copper (as Cupric Oxide)	3 mg.	(150%)
Zinc (as 105 mg. of Zinc Sulfate)	23.9 mg.	(159%)

Recommended Intake: Adults, 1 tablet daily or as directed by the physician.
Supplied: Capsule-shaped Tablet (film coated peach color)—bottles of 30 and 60.
[*Shown in Product Identification Section*]

TETANUS AND DIPHTHERIA TOXOIDS, ADSORBED PUROGENATED® ℞

How Supplied: 5 ml. vial; 10 x 0.5 ml. LEDERJECT® Disposable Syringe.
COMPLETE INFORMATION FURNISHED IN THE PACKAGE.

TETANUS TOXOID, ADSORBED PUROGENATED® ℞

How Supplied: 5 ml. vial (5 immunizations); 10 x 0.5 ml. and 100 x 0.5 ml. LEDERJECT Disposable Syringe.
COMPLETE INFORMATION FURNISHED IN THE PACKAGE.

TETANUS TOXOID PUROGENATED® ℞
(Tetanus Toxoid fluid)

How Supplied: 7.5 ml. vial (5 immunizations); 10 x 0.5 ml. and 100 x 0.5 ml. LEDERJECT® Disposable Syringe.
COMPLETE INFORMATION FURNISHED IN THE PACKAGE.

THIOTEPA ℞
parenteral
Sterile

THIOTEPA Lederle is a polyfunctional alkylating agent used in the chemotherapy of certain neoplastic diseases.

Description: THIOTEPA is the ethylenimine-type compound N, N′, N″-Triethylenethiophosphoramide and is available in powder form in vials which contain 15 mg. THIOTEPA, 80 mg. NaCl, and 50 mg. $NaHCO_3$. THIOTEPA has also been known as TESPA and TSPA and is not the same as TEPA. Vials containing THIOTEPA should be stored at 2°–8° C. (35°–46° F.). Reconstituted solutions may be kept for 5 days in a refrigerator without substantial loss of potency. THIOTEPA is stable in alkaline medium and unstable in acid medium.

Action: THIOTEPA is a cytotoxic agent of the polyfunctional alkylating type (more than one reactive ethylenimine group) related chemically and pharmacologically to nitrogen mustard. Its radiomimetic action is believed to occur through the release of ethylenimine radicals which, like irradiation, disrupt the bonds of DNA. One of the principal bond disruptions is initiated by alkylation of guanine at the N-7 position, which severs the linkage between the purine base and the sugar and liberates alkylated guanines. On the basis of tissue concentration studies, it is reported that THIOTEPA has no differential affinity for neoplasms. Most of the drug appears to be excreted unchanged in the urine.

Indications: THIOTEPA has been tried with varying results in the palliation of a wide variety of neoplastic diseases. However, the most consistent results have been seen in the following tumors:

1. Adenocarcinoma of the breast.
2. Adenocarcinoma of the ovary.
3. For controlling intracavitary effusions secondary to diffuse or localized neoplastic disease of various serosal cavities.
4. For the treatment of superficial papillary carcinoma of the urinary bladder.

While now largely superseded by other treatments, THIOTEPA has been effective against lymphomas, such as lymphosarcoma and Hodgkin's disease.

Contraindications: Therapy is probably contraindicated in cases of existing hepatic, renal, or bone-marrow damage. However, if the need overweighs the risk in such patients, THIOTEPA may be used in low dosage, and accompanied by hepatic, renal, and hemopoietic function tests.
THIOTEPA is contraindicated in patients with a known hypersensitivity (allergy) to this preparation.

Warnings: The administration of THIOTEPA to pregnant women is not recommended except in cases where the benefit to be gained outweighs the risk of teratogenicity involved.
THIOTEPA is highly toxic to the hematopoietic system. A rapidly falling white blood cell or platelet count indicates the necessity for discontinuing or reducing the dosage of THIOTEPA. Weekly blood and platelet counts are recommended during therapy and for at least three weeks after therapy has been discontinued.
THIOTEPA is a polyfunctional alkylating agent, capable of cross-linking the DNA within a cell and changing its nature. The replication of the cell is, therefore, altered, and THIOTEPA may be described as mutagenic. An *in vitro* study has shown that it causes chromosomal aberrations of the chromatid type and that the frequency of induced aberrations increases with the age of the subject.
Like all alkylating agents, THIOTEPA is carcinogenic. Carcinogenicity is shown most clearly in mouse studies, but there is strong circumstantial evidence of carcinogenicity in man.

Precautions: The serious complication of excessive THIOTEPA therapy, or sensitivity to the effects of THIOTEPA, is bone-marrow depression. If proper precautions are not observed THIOTEPA may cause leukopenia, thrombocytopenia, and anemia. Death from septicemia and hemorrhage has occurred as a direct result of hematopoietic depression by THIOTEPA.
It is not advisable to combine simultaneously or sequentially cancer chemotherapeutic agents or a cancer chemotherapeutic agent and a therapeutic modality having the same mechanism of action. Therefore, THIOTEPA combined with other alkylating agents such as nitrogen mustard or cyclophosphamide or THIOTEPA combined with irradiation would serve to intensify toxicity rather than to enhance therapeutic response. If these agents must follow each other, it is important that recovery from the first agent, as indicated by white blood cell count, be complete before therapy with the second agent is instituted.
The most reliable guide to THIOTEPA toxicity is the white blood cell count. If this falls to 3000 or less, the dose should be discontinued. Another good index of THIOTEPA toxicity is the platelet count; if this falls to 150,000, therapy should be discontinued. Red blood cell count is a less accurate indicator of THIOTEPA toxicity.
Other drugs which are known to produce bone-marrow depression should be avoided.
There is no known antidote for overdosage with THIOTEPA. Transfusions of whole blood or platelets or leukocytes have proved beneficial to the patient in combatting hematopoietic toxicity.

Adverse Reactions: Apart from its effect on the blood-forming elements, THIOTEPA may cause other adverse reactions. These include pain at the site of injection, nausea, vomiting, anorexia, dizziness, headache, amenorrhea, and interference with spermatogenesis.
Febrile reaction and weeping from a subcutaneous lesion may occur as the result of breakdown of tumor tissue.
Allergic reactions are rare, but hives and skin rash have been noted occasionally. One case of alopecia has been reported. In addition, a patient who had received THIOTEPA and other anticancer agents experienced prolonged apnea after succinylcholine administered prior to surgery. It was theorized that this was caused by decrease of pseudocholinesterase activity caused by the anticancer drugs.

Dosage: Parenteral routes of administration are most reliable since absorption of THIOTEPA from the gastrointestinal tract is variable.
Since THIOTEPA is nonvesicant, intravenous doses may be given directly and rapidly without need for slow drip or large volumes of diluent. Some physicians prefer to give THIOTEPA directly into the tumor mass. This may be effected transrectally, transvaginally, or intracerebrally. The technique is discussed in the appropriate section which follows. For the control of malignant effusions, THIOTEPA is instilled directly into the cavity involved.
Dosage must be carefully individualized. A slow response to THIOTEPA may be deceptive and may occasion unwarranted frequency of administration with subsequent signs of toxicity. After maximum benefit is obtained by initial therapy, it is necessary to continue patient on maintenance therapy (1 to 4 week intervals). In order to continue optimal effect, maintenance doses should be no more frequent than weekly in order to preserve correlation between dose and blood counts.
Initial and Maintenance Doses: Initially the higher dose in the given range is commonly administered. The maintenance dose should be adjusted weekly on the basis of pretreatment control blood counts and subsequent blood counts.
Intravenous Administration: THIOTEPA may be given by rapid intravenous administration in doses of 0.3–0.4 mg/kg. Doses should be given at 1–4 week intervals.
For conversion of mg/kg of body weight to mg/M^2 of body surface or the reverse, a ratio of 1:30 is given as a guideline. The conversion factor varies between 1:20 and 1:40 depending on age and body build.
Intratumor Administration: THIOTEPA in initial doses of 0.6–0.8 mg/kg may be injected directly into a tumor by means of a 22-gauge needle. A small amount of local anesthetic is injected first; then the syringe is removed and the THIOTEPA solution is injected through the same needle. The drug is diluted in sterile water, 10 mg per 1 ml. Maintenance doses at one to four week intervals range from 0.07 mg/kg to 0.8 mg/kg depending on the condition of the patient.
Intracavitary Administration: The dosage recommended is 0.6–0.8 mg/kg. Administration is usually effected through the same tubing which is used to remove the fluid from the cavity involved.
Intravesical Administration: Patients with papillary carcinoma of the bladder are dehydrated for 8 to 12 hours prior to treatment. Then 60 mg of THIOTEPA in 30–60 ml of distilled water is instilled into the bladder by catheter. For maximum effect, the solution should be retained for 2 hours. If the patient finds it impossible to retain 60 ml for 2 hours, the dose may be given in a volume of 30 ml. If desired, the patient may be positioned every 15 minutes for maximum area contact. The usual course of treatment is once a week for 4 weeks. The course may be repeated if necessary, but second and third courses must be given with caution since bone-marrow depression may be increased. Deaths have occurred after intravesical administration, caused by bone-mar-

row depression from systemically absorbed drug.

Preparation of Solution: The powder should be reconstituted preferably in Sterile Water for Injection. The amount of diluent most often used is 1.5 ml. resulting in a drug concentration of 5 mg. in each 0.5 ml. of solution. Larger volumes are usually employed for intracavity use, intravenous drip, or perfusion therapy. The 1.5 ml. reconstituted preparation may be added to larger volumes of other diluents: Sodium Chloride Injection USP, Dextrose Injection USP, Dextrose and Sodium Chloride Injection USP, Ringer's Injection USP, or Lactated Ringer's Injection USP. Reconstituted solutions should be clear to slightly opaque but solutions that are grossly opaque or precipitated should not be used.

Since the original powder form contains 15 mg. THIOTEPA, 80 mg. NaCl, 50 mg. $NaHCO_3$, the addition of Sterile Water for Injection produces an isotonic solution. The addition of other diluents may result in hypertonic solutions, which may cause mild to moderate discomfort on injection.

For local use into single or multiple sites, THIOTEPA may be mixed with procaine HCl 2%, epinephrine HCl 1:1000, or both.

Whether in its original powder form or in reconstituted solution, THIOTEPA must be stored in the refrigerator at 2°–8° C. (35–46° F.).

How Supplied: 15 mg. vials, sterile.

A.H.F.S. 10:00

TriHEMIC® 600 ℞
(hematinic)
Tablets

Description:

Each tablet contains:

Vitamin C (Ascorbic Acid) 600 mg.

Vitamin B_{12} (Cyanocobalamin) 25 mcg.

Intrinsic Factor Concentrate 75 mg.

Folic Acid (Folacin) 1 mg.

Vitamin E (*dl*-Alpha Tocopheryl Acid) 30 Int. Units

Elemental Iron (as 350 mg. of Ferrous Fumarate) 115 mg.

Docusate Sodium USP (DSS) 50 mg.

Actions: TriHEMIC 600 *hematinic* is a preparation containing those ingredients essential to normal erythropoiesis, plus a stool softener to counteract the constipating effects of iron.

Indications: TriHEMIC 600 is a multiphasic preparation for use in the treatment of most megaloblastic, macrocytic and iron-deficiency anemias, in the anemias of pregnancy, in those anemias occurring in a variety of malabsorption syndromes, and those of nutritional origin. It is a useful adjuvant in patients in whom erythropoiesis is suppressed due to severe infections, malignancies or to the toxic effects of certain chemotherapeutic agents. A deficiency of Vitamin E may increase the fragility of red blood cells, with resultant enhanced hemolysis. Vitamin C is present to aid in the absorption of iron.

Warnings: Folic Acid alone is improper therapy in the treatment of pernicious anemia and other megaloblastic anemias where Vitamin B_{12} is deficient.

Precautions: Some patients affected with pernicious anemia may not respond to orally administered Vitamin B_{12} with intrinsic factor concentrate and there is no known way to predict which patients will respond or which patients may cease to respond. Periodic examinations and laboratory studies of pernicious anemia patients are essential and recommended. If any symptoms of intolerance occur, the drug should be temporarily or permanently discontinued.

Folic Acid alone, especially in doses above 1.0 mg. daily, may obscure pernicious anemia, in that hematologic remission may occur while neurological manifestations remain progressive.

Adverse Reactions: Gastrointestinal intolerance may develop and be manifest by nausea, vomiting, diarrhea or abdominal pain. Skin rashes of various types may occur. Such reactions may necessitate temporary or permanent changes in dosage or usage.

Allergic sensitization has been reported following both oral and parenteral administration of Folic Acid.

Dosage and Administration: One tablet daily. Adjustment of dosage is dependent on patient response and the physician's clinical judgment.

How Supplied: Bottles of 30 tablets, and 500 tablets.

[*Shown in Product Identification Section*]

TRI-IMMUNOL® ℞
(diphtheria and tetanus toxoids and pertussis vaccine adsorbed)

How Supplied: 7.5 ml. vials. (5 immunizations).

COMPLETE INFORMATION FURNISHED IN THE PACKAGE.

VARIDASE® ℞
(streptokinase-streptodornase)
For Intramuscular Use

Description: STREPTOKINASE-STREPTODORNASE VARIDASE, *Lederle* is an enzyme mixture which activates a fibrinolytic system in human serum. It is prepared from a strain of streptococcus and is cultivated in a medium containing acid hydrolyzed casein fortified with sugar, minerals, vitamins and a reducing substance. This medium is suitably buffered near neutrality.

Refining of the culture filtrate is carried out by a variation of the Cohn five-variable system in which concentrations of protein, alcohol, ionic strength, pH and temperature are carefully controlled. Each vial contains 20,000 units of Streptokinase and at least 5,000 units of Streptodornase with Thimerosal (mercury derivative) 0.2 mg. per vial added as a preservative.

Actions: Streptokinase acts indirectly upon a substrate of fibrin or fibrinogen by activating a fibrinolytic enzyme in human serum. Upon treatment with streptokinase the activation of this fibrinolytic system brings about rapid dissolution of blood clots and the fibrinous portion of exudates. Streptodornase liquefies the viscous nucleoprotein of dead cells or pus, and has no effect on living cells. Thus, the action of the enzymes results in the liquefaction of the two main viscous substances resulting from inflammatory or infectious processes thereby facilitating drainage. They do not lyse living cells.

Indications: *Intramuscular Use.* The administration of VARIDASE intramuscularly, in dosages of 5,000 units of streptokinase twice daily, has been recommended in the treatment of edema associated with infection and trauma. In some stubborn cases 10,000 units twice daily may be indicated. The best results have been with infections which do not produce necrosis of tissue, such as thrombophlebitis, epididymitis and cellulitis. Streptokinase evokes a beneficial effect on the inflammatory reaction and edema within two days after the start of treatment. In all patients, the degree of redness and edema decreased considerably by the end of two days, and in a small number of patients, an effect was observed in a period of hours. An aggravation of the infection was not observed in any of the patients, but a rise in temperature, attributable to streptokinase, was noted in about 10 percent of these patients. No significant change in the white blood cell count or in the differential count was observed. There was no significant prolongation of the prothrombin time. Fibrinolysis, as determined by the whole blood technique, was not observed in periods up to seventy-two hours after the fifth intramuscular injection of 5,000 units of streptokinase on the third day of treatment. Hemorrhage, the formation of hematomas or petechiae were not seen. IN TREATMENT OF CASES OF EDEMA OR INFLAMMATION ACCOMPANYING INFECTION CONSIDERATION SHOULD BE GIVEN TO THE CONCOMITANT USE OF AN ANTIMICROBIAL AGENT. THE USE OF STREPTOKINASE INTRAMUSCULARLY IN PATIENTS WITH ABSCESSES IS HELPFUL IN REDUCING THE ACCOMPANYING CELLULITIS, BUT SHOULD NOT BE SUBSTITUTED FOR SOUND SURGICAL PRINCIPLES. IT SHOULD BE EMPHASIZED THAT VARIDASE SHOULD NOT BE INJECTED INTRAMUSCULARLY WHEN THERE IS EVIDENCE OF A DEFECT IN BLOOD COAGULATION OR WHERE THE LIVER FUNCTION IS DEPRESSED AND BLOOD COAGULATION MAY BE PROLONGED THEREBY.

Contraindications: VARIDASE should not be used in the presence of active hemorrhage and is not intended for and cannot act upon fibrous tissues, mucoproteins or collagens.

Warning: VARIDASE should never be administered intravenously. Allergic reactions are rare, but the physician should take every precaution to prevent or arrest them.

Precautions: Pyrogenic reactions to VARIDASE may be minimized with careful and frequent removal of exudates, especially from closed areas. The action of the enzymes causes a localized leukocytosis and accumulation of tissue fluid in the first 24 hours. This reaction must be considered in providing drainage and aspiration, particularly of closed spaces.

If bronchopleural fistulae have been present, there is danger of reopening, especially with active tuberculosis; but with traumatic fistulae or those of nontuberculous, pyogenic origin, VARIDASE can facilitate healing when used with proper precaution.

Streptokinase and streptodornase are antigenic, and antienzymes develop in patients, particularly following prolonged therapy. They also appear after acute hemolytic streptococcal infections. A high antienzyme titer is not harmful, but dosage may have to be increased to overcome its effects.

A separate heat-sterilized syringe and needle or new disposable equivalent unit should be used for each individual patient to prevent transmission of homologous serum hepatitis and other infectious agents from one person to another.

Adverse Reactions: Allergic reactions occur but are rare. Pyrogenic reactions are the most common to VARIDASE.

Administration and Dosage: All treatment should be on an individual basis. The physician should be thoroughly familiar with the principles of enzyme action, and with the literature found in published reports.

Add 2 cc. of Sterile Water for Injection or sterile physiological saline solution to make a solution containing 5,000 units of streptokinase per 0.5 cc. This will provide 4 doses or treatment for two days; 0.5 cc. of the reconstituted enzymes preparation, containing 5,000 units of streptokinase, is injected intramuscularly, preferably in the gluteal region, twice a day.

Continued on next page

The information on each product appearing here is based on labelling effective in August, 1979 and is either the entire official brochure or an accurate condensation therefrom. Official brochures are enclosed in product packages. Information concerning all Lederle products may be obtained from the Medical Department, Lederle Laboratories, Pearl River, New York, 10965.

Lederle—Cont.

Solutions of VARIDASE are stable for two weeks after reconstitution, if kept in a refrigerator, when not in use, at 2–8° C. (35–46° F.). At room temperatures, preparations will not remain stable for more than 24 hours.
How Supplied: 25,000 Units/Vial.
A.H.F.S. 44:00

VARIDASE® ℞
(streptokinase-streptodornase)
For Local or Topical Use

Description: For the preparation of Streptokinase-Streptodornase, VARIDASE, *Lederle* a strain of streptococcus is cultivated in a medium containing acid hydrolyzed casein fortified with sugar, minerals, vitamins and a reducing substance. This medium is suitably buffered near neutrality. Refining of the culture filtrate is carried out by a variation of the Cohn five-variable system in which concentrations of protein, alcohol, ionic strength, pH and temperature are carefully controlled. Each vial contains 100,000 units of Streptokinase and at least 25,000 units of Streptodornase with Thimerosal (mercury derivative) 2.0 mg. per vial added as preservative.
Actions: Streptokinase acts indirectly upon a substrate of fibrin or fibrinogen by activating a fibrinolytic enzyme in human serum. Upon application of streptokinase *in situ,* the activation of this fibrinolytic system brings about rapid dissolution of blood clots and the fibrinous portion of exudates. Streptodornase liquefies the viscous nucleoprotein of dead cells or pus, and has no effect on living cells. Thus, the action of the enzymes results in the liquefaction of the two main viscous substances resulting from inflammatory or infectious processes thereby facilitating drainage. They do not lyse living cells.
VARIDASE acts rapidly under favorable conditions upon direct application.
Indications: *Local use:* Indicated wherever clotted blood, fibrinous or purulent accumulations are undesirably present following trauma or infectious processes which have led to ulceration or abscess formation. Indicated in the treatment of: suppurative surface tissues, including ulcers, radiation necrosis, infected wounds, burns, and surgical incisions, hemothorax and hematoma (postoperative or traumatic), empyema (postpneumonic, loculated, bacterial or selected types of tuberculosis), purulent nontuberculous meningitis, purulent pericarditis, chronic suppurations (draining sinuses, osteomyelitis, infected wounds or ulcers, suppurative tuberculous adenitis, sinusitis, otitis media, and arthritis), bronchiectasis, arthritis, suppurative joint infections, skin grafting, and following perineal resections. It is also effective in dissolving clots in the urinary bladder, and clots occluding drainage tubes and catheters.
Contraindications: VARIDASE should not be used in the presence of active hemorrhage and is not intended for and cannot act upon fibrous tissues, mucoproteins or collagens.
Precautions: VARIDASE 125,000 units is intended for local use only, in areas where adequate drainage is maintained, or in closed spaces such as the pleural space when adequate drainage or aspiration is possible. Do not employ this 125,000 unit package for intramuscular use.
Pyrogenic reactions to VARIDASE may be minimized with careful and frequent removal of exudates, especially from closed areas. The action of the enzymes causes a localized leucocytosis and accumulation of tissue fluid in the first 24 hours. This reaction is beneficial, but must be considered in providing drainage and aspiration, particularly of closed spaces.
If bronchopleural fistulae have been present, there is danger of reopening, especially with active tuberculosis, but with traumatic fistulae or those of nontuberculous, pyogenic origin, VARIDASE can facilitate healing when used with proper precaution.
Streptokinase and streptodornase are antigenic, and antienzymes develop in patients, particularly following prolonged therapy. They also appear after acute hemolytic streptococcal infections. A high antienzyme titer is not harmful, but dosage may have to be increased to overcome its effects.
A separate heat-sterilized syringe and needle or new disposable equivalent unit should be used for each individual patient to prevent transmission of homologous serum hepatitis and other infectious agents from one person to another.
Adverse Reactions: Allergic reactions occur but are rare. Pyrogenic reactions are the most common to VARIDASE.
Preparation of Solutions: To prepare VARIDASE solutions, add 10 to 20 cc. of Sterile Water for Injection or sterile physiological saline to a 125,000 unit vial. (If the water used in the saline preparation has a high calcium content or contains a preservative such as benzyl alcohol, the solution may become opalescent, but this does not affect the potency of the enzymes). This dilution gives a solution containing approximately 5,000 to 10,000 units of streptokinase and 1,000 to 2,000 units of streptodornase per cc. More dilute solutions of VARIDASE may be effective, but more concentrated solutions are contraindicated, because of the presence of enzyme inhibitors in concentrated solutions. Solutions of VARIDASE and VARIDASE-JELLY mixtures after reconstitution, are stable for 2 weeks, if kept in a refrigerator (35-46°F.) when not in use. At room temperatures, preparations will not remain stable for more than 24 hours.
Preparation of Jelly: To prepare Carboxymethylcellulose Jelly *Lederle* with VARIDASE dissolve a 125,000 unit vial in 5 cc. of Sterile Water for Injection or sterile physiological saline, and thoroughly mix this volume with the accompanying jar of jelly. This gives a concentration of approximately 5,000 units of streptokinase and 1,250 units of streptodornase per cc. or gram, since each jar of jelly contains 15 cc. of material. Certain antibiotics may be added to VARIDASE solutions and the VARIDASE-jelly mixture. VARIDASE is compatible with Tetracycline and other antibiotics, such as penicillin, streptomycin and dihydrostreptomycin.
Administration and Dosage: All treatment should be on an individual basis. The physician should be thoroughly familiar with the principles of enzyme action, and with the literature found in published reports.
For a hemothorax or thoracic empyema, an initial dose of 200,000 units of streptokinase and 50,000 units of streptodornase is suggested, with this amount injected in single or multiple sites, as the case warrants. Instillation of VARIDASE solution through a closed thoracotomy tube is useful, particularly in children. For exudates with small, enclosed spaces in diverse anatomical sites, a general rule is that the size of the dose and amount of fluid injected should be related to the size of the cavity. It must be remembered, in treating hemothorax or empyema in fixed rigid spaces, that the volume may be increased by the liquefying and associated actions of streptokinase and streptodornase. A suitable initial treatment, for example, in maxillary sinus empyema, would be from 10,000 to 15,000 units of streptokinase and 2,500 to 3,750 units of streptodornase in a volume of 2 to 3 cc. Adequate provision must be made for drainage of the liquefied exudate. Aspiration of closed spaces should be done every one-half to 6 hours, depending on the size of the space and amount of exudate. In using VARIDASE for enzymatic debridement of exudate in chronically infected wounds and similar suppurations, the desirable effect will be achieved only when direct contact is maintained between enzymes and substrate. The method of maintaining this contact will vary with the local situation. Rubber dams, gauze and nylon dressings have been used successfully in individual cases. Surface lesions may be treated with the use of VARIDASE mixed with Carboxymethylcellulose Jelly *Lederle.* For application to the hands, the carboxymethylcellulose jelly containing VARIDASE may be placed inside a loose rubber glove, which is fastened at the wrist.
In purulent nontuberculous meningitis, a lumbar or cisternal puncture should be made with removal of 1 to 3 cc. more of spinal fluid than the amount of VARIDASE to be instilled, and 2 to 4 cc. of VARIDASE solution instilled. Exudate must be removed by intrathecal puncture within 8 hours, or sooner, if fever or signs of increased intracranial pressure appear. Treatment should be repeated once or twice a day until improvement is evident.
Purulent pericarditis may be treated by daily instillations of VARIDASE and antibiotics through a pericardiostomy. This should be followed by irrigation. Careful supervision of the patient is essential, and drainage must be instituted immediately if signs of cardiac embarrassment occur.
How Supplied: Vials of 125,000 units. Combination package: 1 vial of VARIDASE (streptokinase-streptodornase) topical, 125,000 units; 1 jar carboxymethylcellulose (CMC) jelly 4.5%, 15 ml.
A.H.F.S. 44:00

VARIDASE® ℞
(streptokinase-streptodornase)
Oral Tablets

Description: VARIDASE Streptokinase-Streptodornase Oral Tablets *Lederle* contain 10,000 units of Streptokinase and at least 2,500 units of Streptodornase with Thimerosal (not more than 20 mcg./tablet) as a preservative. Streptokinase is thought to be the only active ingredient in oral therapy. The manufacture of Streptokinase involves extracellular elaboration by Lancefield Group C strains of streptococci, separation from the producing microorganisms, and subsequent concentration and purification.
Action and Indications: Streptokinase is a "kinase" not a protease, hence it functions indirectly, by activating a normal physiological constituent of the body, plasminogen, transforming it enzymatically into the physiological protease, plasmin. Plasmin, by digesting the fibrinogen or fibrin or both, which can be found in areas of inflammation and in blood clots, has the physiological function of clot lysis and reduction of edema and inflammation.
VARIDASE Streptokinase-Streptodornase is an anti-inflammatory agent and as such may aid in the relief of such symptoms of inflammation as pain, swelling, tenderness, and erythema, and may assist in the resolution of extravasated blood. Thus VARIDASE Streptokinase-Streptodornase may be useful in the management of edema and of localized extravasation of blood associated with infection or trauma in such conditions as abscesses, acute thrombophlebitis, cellulitis, sinusitis, hematomas, contusions, sprains and fractures, and in certain dental conditions such as local surgical trauma and pericoronitis resulting from extractions.
VARIDASE Streptokinase-Streptodornase may be useful in the treatment of acute edema or inflammation complicating chronic conditions, such as chronic thrombophlebitis, bronchiectasis, chronic bronchitis, and varicose and stasis ulcers.
The use of VARIDASE Streptokinase-Streptodornase should be considered as an adjunct to appropriate therapeutic measures, including surgical procedures. In the presence of infec-

tion, simultaneous administration of an appropriate antibiotic is important.
Because VARIDASE Streptokinase-Streptodornase does not act upon fibrous tissues, mucoproteins, or collagen, its use in conditions involving scarring, organized exudate or organized blood clots is not recommended.
VARIDASE Streptokinase-Streptodornase aids in the activation of the physiological plasminogen system and can be expected to be beneficial only when it can act as a further stimulant of such a system and when the normal process has not been inhibited.
Contraindications: VARIDASE Streptokinase-Streptodornase is contraindicated in patients with reduced plasminogen or fibrinogen.
Precautions: Allergic manifestations are rare but proper precautions should be taken.
Antibodies against Streptokinase may be elicited by VARIDASE Streptokinase-Streptodornase treatment, especially if prolonged. The high antibody titer is apparently not harmful, but necessitates higher dosage.
Side Effects: There have been occasional reports of nausea, vomiting, diarrhea, skin rash and urticaria associated with the use of VARIDASE Streptokinase-Streptodornase which rarely required cessation of therapy.
Dosage: The average oral dose is one tablet (10,000 units of Streptokinase) four times daily. In acute situations, higher doses may be advisable. Normally treatment is continued for 4 to 6 days.
How Supplied: Tablets (Peach color, scored) bottles of 24 and 100.
A.H.F.S. 44:00
Military Depots
NSN 6505-00-067-7176L - 100's

ZINCON®
Dandruff Shampoo

(See PDR For Nonprescription Drugs)

Leeming Division
Pfizer, Inc.
100 JEFFERSON ROAD
PARSIPPANY, NJ 07054

DESITIN® OINTMENT

(See PDR For Nonprescription Drugs)

NYTILAX® TABLETS
(sennosides A and B)

Description: Each blue Nytilax Tablet contains 12 mg. of crystalline Sennosides A and B calcium salts, the most highly purified form available for these glycosides, derived from the *Cassia Acutifolia* plant and standardized by chemical rather than biological assay.
Actions and Uses: Indicated for relief of chronic or occasional functional constipation. Recent additional support has been given to the current theory that upon ingestion, the sugar glycosides Sennosides A and B are transported without chemical change through the alimentary canal to the colon, where they are hydrolyzed to their aglycone derivatives by the colonic flora, leading to localized nerve plexus stimulation and peristalsis-induced defecation. The effect is gentle and predictable, with well-formed stools being produced, usually within 8–10 hours. Contrary to a previously published opinion, the clinical evidence now available strongly indicates that the senna glycosides are not excreted into the milk of lactating mothers and, therefore, have no effect on the bowel function of nursing infants. The high chemical purity of the Sennoside A and B calcium salts facilitates individualized dosage regulation and further minimizes the possibility of rare adverse reactions such as loose stools or abdominal discomfort. Sennosides A and B, as contained in Nytilax Tablets, have been found in numerous clinical studies to be highly effective for varieties of functional constipation: chronic, geriatric, antepartum and postpartum, drug-induced, pediatric and surgical-related, and in lower bowel x-ray preparative procedures.
Dosage and Administration:
Adults—1 or 2 tablets at bedtime. If you do not readily respond to laxatives, take 3 tablets at bedtime.
Children—Consult a physician.
Warnings: Do not take any laxative when abdominal pain, nausea or vomiting are present. Frequent or prolonged use of laxatives may result in dependence.
Keep out of the reach of children.
How Supplied: Boxes of 12 or 24 tablets.

RHEABAN® TABLETS and LIQUID
(attapulgite)

Description: Rheaban is a fast acting, highly concentrated diarrhea medication for effective relief of diarrhea and the cramps and pains that accompany it. Rheaban is offered in convenient tablet and liquid forms. **Liquid** (5.5 oz.) a mint flavored liquid with each fluid ounce containing 4.2 gm of colloidal activated attapulgite. **Tablets** (white—package of 12's) containing 600 mg of colloidal activated attapulgite. Rheaban contains no narcotics, opiates or other habit forming drugs.
Actions and Uses: Rheaban is a highly concentrated gastrointestinal absorbent that acts on noxious gases, irritants, toxins and some bacteria and viruses that are common causes of diarrhea.
Dosage and Administration:
Liquid
Adults—2 tablespoons after initial bowel movement, 1 tablespoon after subsequent bowel movements.
Children 6 to 12 years—1 tablespoon after initial bowel movement, 1 tablespoon after subsequent bowel movements.
Children 3 to 6 years—½ tablespoon after initial bowel movement, ½ tablespoon after each subsequent bowel movements.
Infant and Children under 3 years—Only as directed by physician.
Tablets
Adults—2 tablets after initial bowel movement, 2 tablets after each subsequent bowel movement.
Children 6 to 12 years—1 tablet after initial bowel movement, 1 tablet after subsequent bowel movements.
Children 3 to 6 years—use Rheaban liquid.
Warnings: Do not use for more than two days, or in the presence of high fever. Tablets should not be used for children under 6 years of age and liquid should not be used for children under 3 years of age unless directed by a physician. If diarrhea persists consult a physician.

UNISOM® NIGHTTIME SLEEP-AID OTC
(doxylamine succinate)

Description: Pale blue oval scored tablets containing 25 mg. of doxylamine succinate, 2-(α-(2-dimethylaminoethoxy)α-methylbenzyl) pyridine succinate.
Action and Uses: Doxylamine succinate is an antihistamine of the ethanolamine class, which characteristically shows a high incidence of sedation. In a comparative clinical study of over 20 antihistamines on more than 3000 subjects, doxylamine succinate 25 mg. was one of the three most sedating antihistamines, producing a significantly reduced latency to end of wakefulness and comparing favorably with established hypnotic drugs such as secobarbital and pentobarbital in sedation activity. It was chosen as the antihistamine, based on dosage, causing the earliest onset of sleep. In another clinical study, doxylamine succinate 25 mg. scored better than secobarbital 100 mg. as a nighttime hypnotic. Two additional, identical clinical studies involving a total of 121 subjects demonstrated that doxylamine succinate 25 mg. reduced the sleep latency period by a third, compared to placebo. Duration of sleep was 26.6% longer with doxylamine succinate, and the quality of sleep was rated higher with the drug than with placebo. An EEG study on 6 subjects confirmed the results of these studies.
Administration and Dosage: One tablet 30 minutes before retiring. Not for children under 12 years of age.
Side Effects: Occasional anticholinergic effects may be seen.
Precautions: Unisom® should be taken only at bedtime.
Contraindications: Asthma, glaucoma, enlargement of the prostate gland. This product should not be taken by pregnant women, or those who are nursing a baby.
Warnings: Should be taken with caution if alcohol is being consumed. Product should not be taken if patient is concurrently on any other drug, without prior consultation with physician. Should not be taken for longer than two weeks unless approved by physician.
How Supplied: Boxes of 8 or 16 tablets.

VISINE® Eye Drops
(tetrahydrozoline HCl)

Composition: Tetrahydrozoline hydrochloride 0.05%; sodium chloride; boric acid; sodium borate; with benzalkonium chloride 0.01% and disodium ethylene diamine tetraacetate 0.1% added as preservatives.
Uses: For fast, lasting relief from minor irritation of eyes due to Dust-Smoke-Smog-Contact Lens adaptation (after removal of lenses). Plant Allergies such as hay fever and rose fever. Minor eye irritation from or due to night driving, reading, T.V., sewing, swimming, wind and sun glare.
Refreshes, soothes and helps relieve redness caused by minor irritations.
Warning: Use only in the eyes. If relief is not obtained within 48 hours, or if irritation or redness persists or increases, discontinue use and consult your physician. Infection, pus, draining, foreign body in the eye, any mechanical, chemical, heat or other injury to the eye require the immediate attention of your physician. As with other eye medications, Visine should not be used by individuals with glaucoma or other serious eye diseases.
Parents: Keep this and all other medications out of the reach of children. Before using with children, consult your physician.
Directions: Place 1 or 2 drops in each eye two or three times a day as directed by physician. Visine is produced under sterile conditions.

Legere & Co., Inc., R. J.
7326 E. EVANS ROAD
SCOTTSDALE, AZ 85260

Product Number	Product	
1066	ACETACO Tablets	℞ Ⓒ
	Acetaminophen	325 mg.
	Codeine Phosphate	30 mg.
1040	ALLERPHEN 12 Tablets	℞
	Chlorpheniramine	12 mg.
1051	APECTOL Tablets	℞ Ⓒ
	Butalbital	50 mg.
	Aspirin	200 mg.
	Phenacetin	130 mg.
	Caffeine	40 mg.
1053	AZO-SULFISOXAZOLE Tablets	℞
	Sulfisoxazole	500 mg.
	Phenazopyridine	50 mg.
005	B COMPLEX 100 30 ml	℞

Continued on next page

Legere—Cont.

	Thiamine HCl	100 mg.
	Riboflavin	2 mg.
	Pyridoxine HCl	2 mg.
	Panthenol	2 mg.
	Niacinamide	100 mg.
1012	BENZIDE	℞
	Benzthiazide	50 mg.
1112	CAFAMINE T.D. Capsules	OTC
	Caffeine	75 mg.
	Phenylpropanolamine	25 mg.
007	CEE-500 50 ml	℞
	Sodium Ascorbate	500 mg.
1088	CEE-500 T.D. Capsules	OTC
	Ascorbic Acid	500 mg.
055	CINALONE 40 5 ml	℞
	Triamcinolone Diacetate	40 mg.
101	CINONIDE 40 5 ml	℞
	Triamcinolone Acetonide	40 mg.
109	DEKABOLIN 2 ml	℞
	Nandrolone Decanoate	50 mg.
062	DEPO-PREDATE 80 5 ml	℞
	Methylprednisolone Acetate	80 mg.
010	DEXASONE 4 5 ml	℞
	Dexamethasone Phosphate	4 mg.
011	DEXASONE L.A.	℞
	Dexamethasone Acetate	8 mg.
065	DEXTRARON-50 10 ml	℞
	Iron Dextran	50 mg.
1111	DI-ATRO Tablets	℞ Ⓒ
	Diphenoxylate HCl	2.5 mg.
	Atropine Sulfate	0.025 mg.
080	E.D.T.A. 20 ml	℞
	Edetate Disodium	150 mg.
015	E-CYPIONATE 10 ml	℞
	Estradiol Cypionate	5 mg.
1002	HYDROCHLOR 50	℞
	Hydrochlorothiazide	50 mg.
1104	HYSER PLUS Tablets	℞
	Hydralazine	25 mg.
	Hydrochlorothiazide	15 mg.
	Reserpine	0.1 mg.
1047	IMOTEP	℞
	Chlorpheniramine	9 mg.
	Phenylephrine	21 mg.
091	MAG-5 30 ml	℞
	Magnesium Sulfate	500 mg.
016	MENAVAL-10 10 ml	℞
	Estradiol Valerate	10 mg.
106	MYOTROL 2 ml	℞
	Orphenadrine Citrate	30 mg.
1022	PHENAZINE Tablets & Capsules	℞ Ⓒ
	Phendimetrazine	35 mg.
090	PREDATE-100 10 ml	℞
	Prednisolone Acetate	100 mg.
066	PREDATE-L.A.S.A. 10 ml	℞
	Prednisolone Acetate	80 mg.
	Prednisolone Sodium Phosphate	20 mg.
067	PROBACON 10 ml	℞
	Chlorpheniramine Maleate	5 mg.
	Phenylpropanolamine HCl	12.5 mg.
	Atropine Sulfate	0.2 mg.
1023	PROBACON II Capsules	℞
	Chlorpheniramine Maleate	8 mg.
	Phenylpropanolamine	50 mg.
	Isopropamide Iodide	2.5 mg.
1095	SPASGESIC	℞
	Chlorzoxazone	250 mg.
	Acetaminophen	300 mg.
1025	TERAMINE Capsules	℞ Ⓒ
	Phentermine HCl	30 mg.
050	TESTAVAL 90/4 10 ml	℞
	Testosterone Enanthate	90 mg.
	Estradiol Valerate	4 mg.

Lemmon Company
SELLERSVILLE PA 18960

ADIPEX-P® Capsules 30 mg. Ⓒ ℞
(phentermine hydrochloride)

Composition: Each capsule contains:
Phentermine Hydrochloride ....30 mg.
(equivalent to 24 mg. of Phentermine base)

How Supplied: Capsules (#3 blue and white, imprinted Lemmon 95) in bottles of 100 and 1000 (NDC 0093-0095).

Also Available: Pelletized capsules (#2 blue and clear, imprinted 853) in bottles of 100 and 1000 (NDC 0093-0853).

[*Shown in Product Identification Section*]

ADIPEX-P® Tablets Ⓒ ℞
(phentermine hydrochloride)

Description: Each tablet contains:
Phentermine Hydrochloride, 37.5 mg. (equivalent to 30 mg. of Phentermine base)
Phentermine hydrochloride is designated chemically as phenyl-tert-butylamine hydrochloride. It is a white crystalline powder, very soluble in water and alcohol.

Actions: Phentermine hydrochloride is a sympathomimetic amine with pharmacologic activity similar to the prototype drugs of this class used in obesity, the amphetamines. Actions include central nervous system stimulation and elevation of blood pressure. Tachyphylaxis and tolerance have been demonstrated with all drugs of this class in which these phenomena have been looked for.
Drugs of this class used in obesity are commonly known as "anorectics" or "anorexigenics". It has been established, however, that the action of such drugs in treating obesity is primarily one of appetite suppression. Other central nervous system actions, or metabolic effects, may be involved, for example.
Adult obese subjects instructed in dietary management and treated with "anorectic" drugs, lose more weight on the average than those treated with placebo and diet, as determined in relatively short-term clinical trials.
The magnitude of increased weight loss of drug-treated patients over placebo-treated patients is only a fraction of a pound a week. The rate of weight loss is greatest in the first weeks of therapy for both drug and placebo subjects and tends to decrease in succeeding weeks. The possible origins of the increased weight loss due to the various drug effects are not established. The amount of weight loss associated with the use of an "anorectic" drug varies from trial to trial, and the increased weight loss appears to be related in part to variables other than the drug prescribed, such as the physician-investigator, the population treated, and the diet prescribed. Studies do not permit conclusions as to the relative importance of the drug and non-drug factors on weight loss.
The natural history of obesity is measured in years, whereas, the studies cited are restricted to a few weeks duration; thus, the total impact of drug-induced weight loss over that of diet alone must be considered clinically limited.

Indications: Phentermine hydrochloride is indicated in the management of exogenous obesity as a short term adjunct (a few weeks) in a regimen of weight reduction based on caloric restriction.
The limited usefulness of agents of this class (see ACTIONS) should be measured against possible risk factors in their use such as those described below.

Contraindications: Advanced arteriosclerosis, symptomatic cardiovascular disease, moderate to severe hypertension, hyperthyroidism, known hypersensitivity or idiosyncrasy to the sympathomimetic amines, glaucoma.
Agitated states.
Patients with a history of drug abuse.
During or within 14 days following the administration of monoamine oxidase inhibitors (hypertensive crisis may result).

Warnings: Tolerance to the anorectic effect usually develops within a few weeks. When this occurs, the recommended dose should not be exceeded in an attempt to increase the effect; rather, the drug should be discontinued. Phentermine hydrochloride may impair the ability of the patient to engage in potentially hazardous activities such as operating machinery or driving a motor vehicle; the patient should therefore be cautioned accordingly.

Drug Dependence: Phentermine hydrochloride is related chemically and pharmacologically to the amphetamines. Amphetamines and related stimulant drugs have been extensively abused, and the possibility of abuse of phentermine hydrochloride should be kept in mind when evaluating the desirability of including a drug as part of a weight reduction program. Abuse of amphetamines and related drugs may be associated with intense psychological dependence and severe social dysfunction. There are reports of patients who have increased the dosage to many times that recommended. Abrupt cessation following prolonged high dosage administration results in extreme fatigue and mental depression; changes are also noted in the sleep EEG. Manifestations of chronic intoxication with anorectic drugs include severe dermatoses, marked insomnia, irritability, hyperactivity, and personality changes. The most severe manifestation of chronic intoxications is psychosis, often clinically indistinguishable from schizophrenia.

Usage in Pregnancy: No reproduction studies or teratology studies of phentermine hydrochloride, in animals or humans, have been published. Therefore, use of phentermine hydrochloride by women who are or may become pregnant, requires that the potential benefit be weighed against the possible hazard to mother and infant.

Usage In Children: Phentermine hydrochloride is not recommended for use in children under 12 years of age.

Precautions: Caution is to be exercised in prescribing phentermine hydrochloride for patients with even mild hypertension.
Insulin requirements in diabetes mellitus may be altered in association with the use of phentermine hydrochloride and the concomitant dietary regimen.
Phentermine hydrochloride may decrease the hypotensive effect of guanethidine.
The least amount feasible should be prescribed or dispensed at one time in order to minimize the possibility of overdosage.

Adverse Reactions:
Cardiovascular: Palpitation, tachycardia, elevation of blood pressure.
Central Nervous System: Overstimulation, restlessness, dizziness, insomnia, euphoria, dysphoria, tremor, headache; rarely psychotic episodes at recommended doses.
Gastrointestinal: Dryness of the mouth, unpleasant taste, diarrhea, constipation, other gastrointestinal disturbances.
Allergic: Urticaria.
Endocrine: Impotence, changes in libido.

Dosage and Administration: The usual adult dose is one tablet daily, administered approximately 2 hours after breakfast. Dosage may be adjusted to the patient's need.
Phentermine hydrochloride is not recommended for use in children under 12 years of age.

Overdosage: Manifestations of acute overdosage with phentermine hydrochloride include restlessness, tremor, hyperreflexia, rapid respiration, confusion, assaultive behavior hallucinations, panic states.
Fatigue and depression usually follow the central stimulation.

Cardiovascular effects include arrhythmias, hypertension or hypotension and circulatory collapse. Gastrointestinal symptoms include nausea, vomiting, diarrhea, and abdominal cramps. In fatal poisoning, death is usually preceded by convulsions and coma.
Management of acute phentermine hydrochloride intoxication is largely symptomatic and includes lavage and sedation with a barbiturate. Experience with hemodialysis or peritoneal dialysis is inadequate to permit recommendation in this regard. Acidification of the urine increases phentermine hydrochloride excretion. Intravenous phentolamine (Regitine) has been suggested for possible acute, severe hypertension, if this complicates phentermine hydrochloride overdosage.
How Supplied: Tablets (white with blue specks, oblong, $^{13}/_{32}''$ length, scored, engraved Lemmon) in bottles of 100 and 1000 (NDC 0093-0009).

[*Shown in Product Identification Section*]

BUFFADYNE–Lemmon

Composition: Each tablet contains:

Aspirin ....230 mg.
Phenacetin ....150 mg.
Caffeine ....30 mg.

Buffered with Dried Aluminum Hydroxide Gel and Magnesium Hydroxide.
How Supplied: Tablets (white with pink specks, $^7/_{16}''$, raspberry aroma) in bottles of 100 and 1000 (NDC 0093-0357).

DEXAMPEX® Tablets and Capsules Ⓒ ℞
(dextroamphetamine sulfate)

Composition: Each blue tablet contains:
Dextroamphetamine Sulfate....5 mg.
Each pink tablet contains:
Dextroamphetamine Sulfate....10 mg.
Each capsule contains:
Dextroamphetamine Sulfate....15 mg.

How Supplied:
DEXAMPEX® 5 mg. (blue oblong, 13/32" length, engraved Lemmon) in bottles of 100 and 1000 (NDC 0093-0179).
DEXAMPEX® 10 mg. (pink oblong, 13/32" length, engraved Lemmon) in bottles of 100 and 1000 (NDC 0093-0180).
DEXAMPEX® Capsules 15 mg (#5 green and clear, imprinted Lemmon 133) in bottles of 1000 (NDC 0093-0133).

[*Shown in Product Identification Section*]

KEFF® ℞
(potassium and chloride supplement)
20 mEq. effervescent tablet
Sugar Free

Description: Each tablet contains 20 mEq. each of potassium and chloride supplied by 1.118 gm potassium chloride, 0.768 gm betaine hydrochloride, 0.401 gm potassium bicarbonate and 0.069 gm potassium carbonate with saccharin, natural and artificial fruit flavors and artificial colors.
Actions: Potassium and chloride supplement.
Indications: Hypokalemic-hypochloremic alkalosis and for the prevention and treatment of hypokalemia which may occur secondary to diuretic or corticosteroid administration. It may be used in the treatment of cardiac arrhythmias due to digitalis intoxication.
Contraindications: Severe renal impairment with oliguria or azotemia, untreated Addison's disease, adynamia episodica hereditaria, acute dehydration, heat cramps and hyperkalemia from any cause.
Precautions: In response to a rise in the concentration of body potassium, renal excretion of the ion is increased. With normal kidney function, it is difficult, therefore, to produce potassium intoxication by oral administration. However, potassium supplements must be administered with caution, since the amount of the deficiency or daily dosage is not accurately known. Frequent checks of the clinical status of the patient, and periodic ECG and/or serum potassium levels should be made. High serum concentrations of potassium ion may cause death through cardiac depression, arrhythmias or arrest. This drug should be used with caution in the presence of cardiac disease. If the basic disturbance produces metabolic acidosis, as in some renal tubular disorders, an organic salt such as potassium gluconate may be more advantageous.
Adverse Reactions: Nausea, vomiting, diarrhea and abdominal discomfort have been reported. The symptoms and signs of potassium intoxication include paresthesias of the extremities, flaccid paralysis, listlessness, mental confusion, weakness and heaviness of the legs, fall in blood pressure, cardiac arrhythmias and heart block. Hyperkalemia may exhibit the following electrocardiographic abnormalities: disappearance of the P wave, widening and slurring of QRS complex, changes of the S-T segment, tall peaked T waves, etc.
Dosage and Administration: The usual adult dosage is one KEFF tablet dissolved in four fluid ounces (about ½ glass) or more of water 2 to 4 times daily after meals. This preparation like other potassium supplements must be properly diluted to avoid the possibility of gastrointestinal irritation. This supplies 40 to 80 mEq. of elemental potassium and chloride. The approximate minimum adult daily requirement for potassium is 40 mEq. Deviations from this recommendation may be indicated, since no average total daily dose can be defined but must be governed by close observation for clinical effects. Potassium intoxication may result from any therapeutic dosage. See "Overdosage" and "Precautions."
Overdosage: Potassium intoxication may result from overdosage of potassium or from therapeutic dosage in conditions stated under "Contraindications." Hyperkalemia, when detected, must be treated immediately because lethal levels can be reached in a few hours.
Treatment of Hyperkalemia:
1. Dextrose solution, 10 or 25% containing 10 units of crystalline insulin per 20 gm. dextrose, given I.V. in a dose of 300 to 500 ml. in an hour.
2. Adsorption and exchange of potassium using sodium or ammonium cycle cation exchange resin, orally and as retention enema. (Caution: Ammonium compounds should not be used in patients with hepatic cirrhosis.)
3. Hemodialysis and peritoneal dialysis.
4. The use of potassium-containing foods or medicaments must be eliminated. In cases of digitalization too rapid a lowering of plasma potassium concentration can cause digitalis toxicity.

How Supplied: Each dispensing carton of 60 (Dual Pack of 30's) or 240 (8 packs of 30) tablets contain five different flavors, (grape, cherry, lemon, orange, lime). Each tablet individually sealed in foil and color coded to indicate flavor.
NDC 0093-0142-06; 60's
NDC 0093-0142-42; 240's

[*Shown in Product Identification Section*]

MEQUIN™ Ⓒ ℞
(methaqualone)

Composition: Each tablet contains
Methaqualone ....300 mg
How Supplied: Tablets (white, scored, ½", engraved LMN 300) in bottles of 30 and 100 (NDC 0093-0300).
For full disclosure, refer to QUĀĀLUDE® monograph.

NEOTHYLLINE® Tablets ℞
NEOTHYLLINE® Elixir
NEOTHYLLINE® Injection
(dyphylline)

Composition: Tablets contain Dyphylline 200 mg. and 400 mg. Elixir contains Dyphylline 160 mg. in each 15 ml. (tablespoonful) with 18% alcohol. Injection contains Dyphylline 500 mg. in each 2 ml. with water for injection; may contain sodium hydroxide or hydrochloric acid to adjust pH.
Description: Dyphylline [7-(2,3-Dihydroxypropyl) theophylline] [$C_{10}H_{14}N_4O_4$] is a white, extremely bitter, crystalline solid, freely soluble in water and slightly soluble in alcohol. Dyphylline contains the equivalent of about 70 percent of anhydrous theophylline, on a molecular weight basis.
Actions: As a xanthine derivative, dyphylline possesses the peripheral vasodilator and bronchodilator actions characteristic of theophylline. It has diuretic and myocardial stimulant effects, and is effective orally. Dyphylline may show fewer side effects than aminophylline, but its blood levels and possibly its activity are also lower.
Indications: For relief of acute bronchial asthma and for reversible bronchospasm associated with chronic bronchitis and emphysema.
Contraindications: In individuals who have shown hypersensitivity to any of its components.
Dyphylline should not be administered concurrently with other xanthine preparations.
Warnings: Status asthmaticus is a medical emergency. Excessive doses may be expected to be toxic.
Usage in Pregnancy: Safe use in pregnancy has not been established from the standpoint of possible adverse effects on fetal development. Therefore, dyphylline should not be used in pregnant women unless, in the judgment of the physician, the potential benefits outweigh the possible hazards.
In children treated with dyphylline elixir, the alcoholic vehicle of the product poses a significant factor of drug dependence including all three components of tolerance, physical dependence and compulsive abuse.
Precautions: Use with caution in patients with severe cardiac disease, hypertension, hyperthyroidism, or acute myocardial injury. Particular caution in dose administration must be exercised in patients with peptic ulcers, since the condition may be exacerbated. Chronic oral administration in high doses (500 to 1,000 mg.) is usually associated with gastrointestinal irritation.
Great caution should be used in giving dyphylline to patients in congestive heart failure. Such patients have shown markedly prolonged blood level curves which have persisted for long periods following discontinuation of the drug.
Adverse Reactions: Note: Included in the listing which follows are a few adverse reactions which may not have been reported with this specific drug. However, pharmacological similarities among the xanthine drugs require that each of the reactions be considered when dyphylline in administered.
The most consistent adverse reactions are:

1. Gastrointestinal irritation: nausea, vomiting, and epigastric pain, generally preceded by headache, hematemesis, diarrhea.
2. Central nervous system stimulation: irritability, restlessness, insomnia, reflex hyperexcitability, muscle twitching, clonic and tonic generalized convulsions, agitation.
3. Cardiovascular: palpitation, tachycardia, extra systoles, flushing, marked hypotension, and circulatory failure.
4. Respiratory: tachypnea, respiratory arrest.
5. Renal: albuminuria, increased excretion of renal tubule and red blood cells.

Continued on next page

Lemmon—Cont.

6. Other: fever, dehydration.

Overdosage: Symptoms: In infants and small children: agitation, headache, hyperreflexia, fasciculations, and clonic and tonic convulsions. In adults: nervousness, insomnia, nausea, vomiting, tachycardia, and extra systoles.

Therapy: Discontinue drug immediately. No specific treatment. Ipecac syrup for oral ingestion. Avoid sympathomimetics. Supporting treatment for hypotension, seizure, arrhythmias and dehydration. Sedatives such as short acting barbiturates will help control central nervous system stimulation. Restore the acid-base balance with lactate or bicarbonate. Oxygen and antibiotics provide supportive treatment.

Drug Interactions: Toxic synergism with ephedrine and other sympathomimetic bronchodilator drugs may occur.

Recent controlled studies suggest that the addition of ephedrine to adequate dosage regimens of dyphylline produces no increase in effectiveness over that of dyphylline alone, but does produce an increase in toxic effects.

Dosage and Administration: When administered orally dyphylline produces less nausea than aminophylline and other alkaline theophylline compounds. Absorption orally appears to be faster on an empty stomach; preferably the drug is to be given at six hour intervals.

Adults: Usual Dose—15 mg/kg every 6 hours, up to four times a day. The dosage should be individualized by titration to the condition and response of the patient.

Therapeutic blood levels are considered to be between 10 micrograms/ml. and 20 mcg/ml. Levels above 20 mcg/ml. may produce toxic effects. There is great variation from patient to patient in dosage needed in order to achieve a therapeutic blood level. Also, the duration of action of oral theophylline preparations varies widely from one patient to another. Because of this wide variation from patient to patient and the relatively narrow therapeutic blood level range, dosage must be individualized with monitoring of dyphylline blood levels, particularly when prolonged or repeated use is planned.

Pulmonary functional measurements before and after a period of treatment allow an objective assessment of whether or not therapy should be continued in patients with chronic bronchitis and emphysema.

Injection: Intramuscular administration of Neothylline (dyphylline) is indicated when rapid onset of action is desired or oral therapy is not possible.

The usual dose is 2 ml (500 mg) I.M. and may be repeated several times daily if necessary. The dosage should be individualized to the condition and response of the patient.

Intramuscular administration is virtually painless because of the neutral pH of the solution. Neothylline (dyphylline) should be injected very slowly to allow tissue adaptation to the volume of fluid injected. The usual precautions to avoid the intravenous route should be observed.

How Supplied: Neothylline Tablets 200 mg (white, 11/32" scored, engraved Lemmon) in bottles of 100 and 1000. (NDC-0093-0030) Neothylline Tablets 400 mg (white, oblong 17/32" length, scored, engraved Lemmon) in bottles of 100 and 500. (NDC-0093-0037) Neothylline Elixir (colorless) in pints (473 ml) and gallons (3.78 L.). (NDC-0093-0035) Neothylline Injection, 2 ml ampuls in boxes of 10. (NDC-0093-0036)

[*Shown in Product Identification Section*]

NEOTHYLLINE®-GG Tablets ℞
NEOTHYLLINE®-GG Elixir

Each white tablet contains:
NEOTHYLLINE® (dyphylline) ....200 mg.
Guaifenesin ....200 mg.
Each 30 ml. (two tablespoonfuls) of Elixir contains:
NEOTHYLLINE® (dyphylline) ....200 mg.
Guaifenesin ....200 mg.
Alcohol 10%

NEOTHYLLINE® (dyphylline) is designated chemically as 7-(2,3-Dihydroxypropyl) theophylline. It is a white, bitter crystalline solid, freely soluble in water. It has a neutral pH in aqueous solution and is soluble over the entire physiologic pH range.

NEOTHYLLINE® (dyphylline) is a distinct chemical entity, as opposed to the salts or loosely complexed forms of theophylline. Unlike these, it contains no extraneous chemical modifiers.

Guaifenesin, formerly called glyceryl guaiacolate, is the glyceryl ether of guaiacol.

Actions: NEOTHYLLINE® (dyphylline) exerts the general pharmacologic actions of theophylline and aminophylline. It acts as a bronchodilator, myocardial stimulant, diuretic, vasodilator (of coronary, pulmonary, and renal vessels), and smooth muscle relaxant. In human therapeutics, its significant action is bronchodilation.

By virtue of its high solubility, neutral pH, and stability toward pH changes, NEOTHYLLINE® (dyphylline) is readily absorbed and well tolerated upon oral administration. This constitutes its basic advantage over theophylline and aminophylline.

Guaifenesin exerts its expectorant action by increasing respiratory fluid, thereby reducing the viscosity of tenacious secretions.

NEOTHYLLINE®-GG combines the bronchodilating effect of dyphylline with the expectorant action of guaifenesin.

Indications: For the treatment of acute and chronic bronchitis, bronchial asthma, asthmatic bronchitis, emphysema and related conditions—to relieve bronchospasm and its associated dyspnea, non-productive cough, and tracheobronchial irritation.

Contraindications: In individuals who have shown hypersensitivity to any of the components.

Dyphylline should not be administered concurrently with other xanthine preparations.

Warnings: Usage in Pregnancy: Safe use in pregnancy has not been established from the standpoint of possible adverse effects on fetal development. Therefore, this product should not be used in pregnant women unless, in the judgment of the physician, the potential benefits outweigh the possible hazards.

Precautions: Conditions which warrant caution in therapy include hyperthyroidism, severe myocardial damage, renal or hepatic disease and glaucoma.

Despite comparatively low C.N.S. stimulation, the possibility with large doses should be borne in mind. Concomitant therapy with sympathomimetics may occasionally induce restlessness, excitability, insomnia or cardiac arrhythmias. Children have a marked sensitivity to the C.N.S. stimulant action of the thophyllines. Fatalities in children have resulted from a few 100 mg. doses of theophylline and from rectal suppositories of aminophylline. While dyphylline has not been implicated in these cases, care should be excercised in the treatment of children. The dosage should be titrated carefully, and symptoms of toxicity watched for. Early symptoms of poisoning include anorexia, nausea, occasional vomiting, wakefulness, restlessness, and irritability. Agitated maniacal behavior and frequent vomiting accompanied by extreme thirst develop later, and lead in fullest severity to delirium, convulsions, hyperthermia, and vasomotor collapse.

Guaifenesin has been shown to produce a color interference with certain clinical laboratory determinations of 5-hydroxyindoleacetic acid (5-HIAA) and vanilmandelic acid (VMA).

Adverse Reactions: Occasional side effects include headache, nausea, vomiting, burning, epigastric or substernal pain, palpitation, dizziness or nervousness. These can usually be controlled by reduction in dosage. Other side effects as restlessness, excitability, insomnia or cardiac arrhythmias may occur but are usually seen during concomitant therapy with sympathomimetics. Administration after meals may help to avoid gastric discomfort.

Dosage and Administration: Adults: The usual dose is 1 tablet (or 30 ml. of Elixir) four times a day.

Children, 6 years and older: The usual dose is ½ tablet (or 15 ml. of Elixir) per 60 pounds body weight, four times a day.

The dosage should be titrated to the condition and response of the patient. Oral bronchodilator therapy for chronic bronchospastic conditions is most effective when administered in individualized doses to accomodate patient-to-patient variations in metabolism. Maintenance therapy may be continued as long as required and at a dosage level determined by individual requirements.

How Supplied: Tablets (white, 7/16", scored, engraved Lemmon) in bottles of 100 and 1000 (NDC 0093-0128). Elixir (orange) in pints (473 ml.) and gallons (3.78L.) (NDC 0093-0131).

NEUTRALOX Suspension

(See PDR For Nonprescription Drugs)

OTOCORT® Ear Drops ℞

Composition: Each ml. contains:
Neomycin Sulfate, equiv.
to Neomycin ....3.5 mg.
Polymyxin B Sulfate* ....2000 U.
Hydrocortisone 0.1%
Antipyrine 5%
Dibucaine Hydrochloride..........0.25%
With methylparaben, propylparaben, sodium bisulfite and glycerin in purified water.

*Licensed under U.S. Patent No. 2,565,057.

OTOCORT is a clear, colorless solution in a plastic squeeze bottle suitable for application directly to the external auditory canal. OTOCORT has a physiological pH and is virtually non-irritating.

Action: OTOCORT combines the antibacterial action of neomycin and polymyxin, the anti-inflammatory action of hydrocortisone, and the local anesthetic action of antipyrine and dibucaine.

Indications: Based on a review of this drug by the National Academy of Sciences-National Research Council and/or other information, FDA has classified the indications as follows:

"Possibly" effective in the treatment of bacterial infections of the external auditory canal due to organisms sensitive to neomycin and polymyxin and when the anti-inflammatory and/or antiallergic action of hydrocortisone and anesthetic action of dibucaine is indicated.

Final classification of the less-than-effective indications requires further investigation.

Contraindications: Contraindicated in perforated ear drum or tuberculous, fungal and viral conditions of the skin such as herpes simplex, vaccinia and varicella. Contraindicated in individuals with a history of hypersensitivity to any of the components.

Precautions: As with any antibiotic preparation, overgrowth of non-susceptible organisms may result; if this occurs, discontinue use and

institute appropriate therapy. Use with care in the presence of long-standing cases of otitis media due to the possibility of ototoxicity.
Neomycin is a cutaneous sensitizer. Allergic cross-reactions may occur which might prevent the use of any or all of the following antibiotics for the treatment of future infections: kanamycin, paromomycin, streptomycin, and possibly gentamicin. The wide usage of topical neomycin has resulted in the emergence of bacterial strains resistant to neomycin, kanamycin, paromomycin and streptomycin.
Dosage and Administration: Gently cleanse the ear canal and dry. Loosely pack OTO-CORT-soaked gauze wick in external ear canal, or if preferred, instill 3 to 5 drops, 3 or 4 times daily.
How Supplied: 10 ml. plastic drop bottles (NDC 0093-0024).

QUAALUDE®-150 QUAALUDE®-300 Ⓒ ℞
(methaqualone)

Description: Quaalude (methaqualone) is chemically 2 - methyl - 3 - (2 - methylphenyl) -4 [3H]-quinazolinone. Methaqualone occurs as a white crystalline powder with a bitter taste and is slightly soluble in water and freely soluble in alcohol. The drug is highly lipid soluble.
Clinical Pharmacology: Methaqualone is rapidly absorbed from the G.I. tract. The onset of action of the drug is rapid; sleep is usually induced within 30 minutes and lasts 5 to 8 hours following usual hypnotic doses; and patients usually awaken without "hangover", i.e. without post-hypnotic CNS depression.
The decline of serum levels of methaqualone is biphasic. The half-life for the first (distribution phase is 1 to 4 hours. There is extensive tissue distribution of the drug, particularly in adipose tissue.
Although the metabolic fate of methaqualone has not been completely elucidated, there is considerable evidence that therapeutic doses of methaqualone are almost completely metabolized in the liver by hydroxylation. In doses of up to 300 mg in man, very little unchanged drug is found in the urine. Quaalude may be administered in conjunction with oral anticoagulant therapy without significant clinical interaction.
Indications: Quaalude (methaqualone) is a hypnotic agent useful in the treatment of insomnia and in medical situations requiring restful sleep.
Contraindications: Quaalude (methaqualone) is contraindicated in patients with known hypersensitivity to methaqualone, and in women who are or may become pregnant. Reproduction studies in the rat revealed minor but clearcut skeletal abnormalities in the young.
Warnings: The hypnotic dose should be taken only at bedtime, immediately before the patient retires, since Quaalude (methaqualone) may produce drowsiness within 10 to 20 minutes. The patient on Quaalude must be warned against driving a car or operating dangerous machinery while on the drug, since methaqualone may impair the ability to perform hazardous activities requiring mental alertness or physical coordination.
The patient shall be warned about the possible additive effects when methaqualone is taken concomitantly with other central nervous system depressants such as alcohol or barbiturates.
Since insomnia is often transient and intermittent, the prolonged administration of Quaalude (methaqualone) is generally not necessary or recommended.
Usage in Children—Methaqualone is not recommended for use in children, since its safety and effectiveness in the pediatric age group have not been established.
Psychological and Physical Dependence—Illicit use of the drug or abuse of the drug for non-therapeutic purposes may lead to severe psychological dependence. Physical dependence has been reported on occasion. In the presence of dependence, dosage should be reduced gradually. Caution must be exercised in prescribing methaqualone to individuals whose history suggests they may increase dosage on their own initiative. For this reason, care must be taken not to prescribe an excessive amount of the drug. As with all hypnotic agents, good medical practice suggests that the patient should be reevaluated before repeating the prescription.
Precautions: The possibility of the use of sedative/hypnotic drugs in suicide attempts should be kept in mind and the drugs prescribed in small quantities. Since methaqualone is metabolized in the liver, it should be given in reduced doses, if at all, to those with impaired hepatic function.
Adverse Reactions:
Neuropsychiatric: headache, hangover, fatigue, dizziness, torpor, transient paresthesia of the extremities. Restlessness or anxiety occur occasionally. Peripheral neuropathy has been reported.
Hematologic: Aplastic anemia possibly related to methaqualone has been reported.
Gastrointestinal: dry mouth, anorexia, nausea, emesis, epigastric discomfort, diarrhea.
Dermatologic: diaphoresis, bromhidrosis, exanthema. Urticaria has been particularly well documented.
Dosage and Administration:
Usual Adult Dosage: For sleep, the usual adult hypnotic dose of methaqualone is 150 to 300 mg at bedtime.
Geriatric Dosage: Dosage for aged, debilitated or highly agitated patients should be individualized in accordance with the judgment of the physician. The principle to be followed is to observe the response to small doses and determine the desirability of adjusting the dose.
Overdosage: Acute overdosage may result in delirium and coma with restlessness and hypertonia progressing to convulsions. Spontaneous vomiting and increased secretions are common and may lead to aspiration pneumonitis or respiratory obstruction. Large overdoses have been accompanied by cutaneous edema, plumonary edema, hepatic damage, renal insufficiency, and bleeding. Pupillary dilation, tachycardia and hyperreflexia may also occur. Overdoses of methaqualone appear to be less often associated with cardiac or respiratory depression than are overdoses of the oral barbiturates, but shock and respiratory arrest may ocassionally occur. Coma has occurred with acute overdosages averaging 2400 mg. Death has occurred following ingestion of 8000 mg. Recommended management includes prompt evacuation of gastric contents, maintenance of adequate ventilation, support of blood pressure if necessary, and the usual supportive measures of the unconscious patient. Dialysis may be helpful. Analeptics are contraindicated.

[*Shown in Product Identification Section*]

RACET® Cream ℞
RACET®-1% Cream
(clioquinol and cortisol)*

*Note: Clioquinol is the new official title for iodochlorhydroxyquin; cortisol is the new official title for hydrocortisone.
Composition:
RACET Cream contains 3% clioquinol and 0.5% cortisol;
RACET—1% Cream contains 3% clioquinol and 1% cortisol; with stearic acid, cetyl alcohol, petrolatum, polyoxyl 40 stearate, sorbitol, propylene glycol, methylparaben, propylparaben, heather aroma and purified water.
Action: RACET combines the antifungal and antibacterial actions of clioquinol with the anti-inflammatory and anti-pruritic effects of cortisol, providing effective therapy for broader control of various acute and chronic dermatological disorders.

Indications: Based on a review of this drug by the National Academy of Sciences—National Research Council and/or other information, FDA has classified the indications as follows:
"Possibly" effective: for contact or atopic dermatitis, impetiginized eczema; nummular eczema; infantile eczema; endogenous chronic infectious dermatitis; stasis dermatitis; pyoderma; nuchal eczema and chronic eczematoid otitis externa; acne urticata; localized or disseminated neurodermatitis; lichen simplex chronicus; anogenital pruritus (vulvae, scroti, ani); folliculitis; bacterial dermatoses; mycotic dermatoses, such as tinea (capitis, cruris, corporis, pedis); moniliasis; intertrigo, and many similar conditions.
For broader control of various acute and chronic dermatological disorders. Especially useful for eczematous conditions and for control of inflammation and pruritus. Often effective where antibiotics and steroids alone are not.
Final classification of the less-than-effective indications requires further investigation.

Contraindications: Not for use in the eye or in the presence of tuberculosis, vaccinia, varicella or other viral skin conditions.
Precautions: May be irritating to sensitized skin in rare cases; if this occurs, discontinue use. The cream may stain fabric, hair, or skin. The remote possibility of systemic toxicity, electrolyte imbalance or adrenal suppression should be borne in mind, particularly if used under occlusive dressings or for prolonged periods. While topical steroids have not been reported to have an adverse effect on pregnancy, they should not be used extensively during pregnancy in large amounts or for prolonged periods until their absolute safety has been established. Thyroid function tests should not be performed until one month after discontinuation of therapy due to the possible absorption of clioquinol and resultant interference with these tests. The ferric chloride test for phenylketonuria (PKU) can yield a false positive result if RACET is present in the diaper or urine.
Adverse Reactions: Occasionally, local burning, irritation and itching may occur. Prolonged use in intertriginous areas may cause striae in rare cases.
Dosage: Apply 3 or 4 times daily.
How Supplied: Racet, in 15 Gm. and 30 Gm. tubes, 454 Gm. (lb.) jars and 450 × 1 Gm industrial pac (NDC 0093-0043). Racet–1%, in 15 Gm. tubes and 450X1 Gm industrial pac (NDC 0093-0034).

RACET® LCD Cream ℞
(clioquinol, cortisol, and coal tar)*

*Note: Clioquinol is the new official title for iodochlorhydroxyquin; cortisol is the new official title for hydrocortisone.
Composition:

Clioquinol	3%
Cortisol	0.5%
Coal Tar Topical Solution	5%

With stearic acid, cetyl alcohol, petrolatum, polyoxyl 40 stearate, sorbitol, propylene glycol, methylparaben, propylparaben, heather aroma, rose oil, and purified water.
How Supplied: In 30 Gm. tubes and 454 Gm. (1 lb.) jars (NDC 0093-0101).

Continued on next page

Lemmon—Cont.

RHINEX®

Composition: Each tablet contains:

Aspirin	150 mg.
Chlorpheniramine Maleate	1.25 mg.
Phenylephrine Hydrochloride	2.5 mg.

Buffered with Dried Aluminum Hydroxide Gel and Magnesium Hydroxide.

How Supplied: Tablets (pink and white, oval, scored, orange aroma) in bottles of 100 and 1000 (NDC 0093-0022).

RHINEX® D • LAY ℞

Each tablet contains:

Acetaminophen	300 mg.
Salicylamide	300 mg.
Phenylpropanolamine Hydrochloride	60 mg.
Chlorpheniramine Maleate	4 mg.

D•Lay is the Lemmon brand of timed-release medication.

Indications: For symptomatic relief of upper respiratory congestion and postnasal drip due to vasomotor rhinitis, allergic rhinitis and the common cold, especially when pain and fever accompany such conditions.

Precautions: While the occurrence of drowsiness is rare, driving or operation of machinery should be avoided until its absence is determined. Individuals with high blood pressure, heart disease, diabetes or thyroid disease should use only as directed by the physician.

Dosage: The usual adult dose is one tablet twice daily. Where congestion is marked, one tablet every six hours may be required.

How Supplied: Tablets (white, ½" flat bev. scored, engraved Lemmon) in bottles of 100 and 1000 (NDC 0093-0110).

RHINEX® DM SYRUP

Composition: Each teaspoonful (5 ml) contains:

Dextromethorphan Hydrobromide	7.5 mg.
Chlorpheniramine Maleate	1 mg.
Guaifenesin	50 mg.
Phenylpropanolamine Hydrochloride	12.5 mg.
Ammonium Chloride	100 mg.
Alcohol	5%

Indications: For the temporary relief of coughs due to colds, allergies and other minor throat irritations.

Warning: While the occurrence of drowsiness is rare, driving or operation of machinery should be avoided until its absence is determined. Individuals with high blood pressure, heart disease, diabetes or thyroid disease should use only as directed by the physician. Persistent cough or high fever may indicate the presence of a serious condition.

Dosage: The average dose three or four times daily is as follows:

Children 2–4 years	½ tsp.
4–12 years	1–2 tsp.
Adults (over 12 years)	2–4 tsp.

How Supplied: Syrup (pink) in 4 fl. oz. (120 ml.) and gallon bottles (3.78 L.) (NDC 0093-0066).

RHINEX® DM TABLETS

Composition: Each tablet contains:

Dextromethorphan Hydrobromide	10 mg.
Phenylephrine Hydrochloride	5 mg.
Chlorpheniramine Maleate	2 mg.

Indications: For temporary relief of cough, running nose, sneezing and nasal congestion as may be associated with the common cold.

Warning: May cause marked drowsiness. Avoid driving motor vehicle or operating heavy machinery. If you have high blood pressure, heart disease, diabetes, or thyroid disease, do not take except as directed by a physician. Persistent cough may be a sign of a serious condition. If cough persists for more than 1 week, recurs, or is accompanied by high fever, rash, or persistent headaches, consult a physician. Do not give to children under 6 years of age except under the advice and supervision of a physician. Keep this and all medicines out of the reach of children. In case of accidental overdose, seek professional help or contact a poison control center immediately.

Dosage: Adults: 2 tablets; children, 6 to under 12; 1 tablet; for children under 6, consult a physician. Repeat dosage every 4 hours if needed, not to exceed 6 doses daily, or as directed by a physician.

How Supplied: Tablets (white, scored, oval) in bottles of 100 and 1000 (NDC 0093-0166).

RHINSPEC

Composition: Each tablet contains:

Acetaminophen	300 mg
Guaifenesin	100 mg
Phenylephrine Hydrochloride	5 mg

How Supplied: Tablets (pink, oblong, 17/32" length, engraved Lemmon) in bottles of 100 and 1000 (NDC-0093-0005).

RHUS TOX ANTIGEN™ ℞
(poison ivy extract)

Composition: Each ml. of sterile solution contains 40 mg. poison ivy extract in a 35 per cent aqueous-alcoholic menstruum, with 4 per cent benzyl alcohol to reduce pain of injection; pH adjusted with lactic acid.

Indications: For prophylaxis and treatment of rhus dermatitis.

Precautions: Attention is directed to reports that renal complications may follow extensive dermatitis of various types, and that with severe rhus dermatitis there may be an aggravation of symptoms following administration of poison ivy extract.

Dosage and Administration: Specific Treatment of Rhus Dermatitis—1 ml. intramuscularly every 12 to 24 hours until symptoms are controlled. A minimum of four injections is recommended even if symptoms are alleviated within a few hours; the tendency to future attacks will be lessened. Children usually tolerate the same dose as adults.

Prophylactic Treatment—Susceptible persons can usually be protected against attacks of rhus dermatitis for a season or longer by preseasonal injections of RHUS TOX ANTIGEN. Dose: 1 ml. intramuscularly every 4 to 7 days for four or more injections. In very sensitive individuals it may be advisable to start with a smaller dose—0.25 to 0.5 ml.—and increase the dose gradually to 1 ml., giving a total of 4 ml. or more.

Note: The patient usually complains of a burning sensation at site of the injection. This is due to the alcohol and disappears in a few seconds. In some individuals, localized soreness or a dull ache may be noted for 24 to 48 hours.

How Supplied: Boxes of four 1 ml. vials. Refrigeration not required. Full prescribing information is available on request (NDC 0093-0401).

RHUS TOX™ LOTION

Composition: A soothing, water-washable lotion containing:

Aluminum Acetate Solution (Burow's Solution)	10%
Phenol	1%

Indications: For relief of mild cases of poison ivy, oak, and sumac when accompanied by itching and weeping; for relief of itching and burning due to insect bites and other minor skin irritations.

Warnings: When applied to fingers and toes, do not use a bandage. Apply according to directions for use, and in no case to large areas of the body.

Keep this and all medications out of the reach of children. In case of accidental ingestion, seek professional assistance or contact a poison control center immediately.

Directions for Use: Apply locally. Keep away from the eyes. Weeping lesions, apply and cover with gauze; do not rub. Non-weeping lesions; apply and message gently into the affected area.

How Supplied: Lotion (white) in boxes of one dozen 30 Gm. plastic squeeze dispenser bottles. (NDC-0093-0285).

RUHEXATAL® WITH RESERPINE ℞
(mannitol hexanitrate and reserpine)

Composition: Each tablet contains:

Reserpine	0.1 mg.
Mannitol Hexanitrate	30 mg.

How Supplied: Tablets (pink, oblong, 17/32" length, engraved Lemmon) in bottles of 100 and 1000 (NDC 0093-0341).

STATOBEX® Ⓒ ℞
(phendimetrazine tartrate)

Composition: Each green tablet, speckled tablet, or green and white capsule contains:

Phendimetrazine Tartrate	35 mg.

Description: Phendimetrazine tartrate is a sympathomimetic amine designated chemically as *d*-3,4-dimethyl-2-phenylmorpholine tartrate. It is a white, crystalline powder freely soluble in water.

Actions: Phendimetrazine tartrate is a sympathomimetic amine with pharmacologic activity similar to the prototype drugs of this class used in obesity, the amphetamines. Actions include central nervous system stimulation and elevation of blood pressure. Tachyphylaxis and tolerance have been demonstrated with all drugs of this class in which these phenomena have been looked for.

Drugs of this class used in obesity are commonly known as "anorectics" or "anorexigenics". It has not been established, however, that the action of such drugs in treating obesity is primarily one of appetite suppression. Other central nervous system actions, or metabolic effects, may be involved, for example.

Adult obese subjects instructed in dietary management and treated with "anorectic" drugs, lose more weight on the average than those treated with placebo and diet, as determined in relatively short-term clinical trials. The magnitude of increased weight loss of drug-treated patients over placebo-treated patients is only a fraction of a pound a week. The rate of weight loss is greatest in the first weeks of therapy for both drug and placebo subjects and tends to decrease in succeeding weeks. The possible origins of the increased weight loss due to the various drug effects are not established. The amount of weight loss associated with the use of an "anorectic" drug varies from trial to trial, and the increased weight loss appears to be related in part to variables other than the drug prescribed, such as the physician-investigator, the population treated, and the diet prescribed. Studies do not permit conclusions as to the relative importance of the drug and non-drug factors on weight loss.

The natural history of obesity is measured in years, whereas the studies cited are restricted to a few weeks duration; thus, the total impact of drug-induced weight loss over that of diet alone must be considered clinically limited.

Indications: STATOBEX (phendimetrazine tartrate) is indicated in the management of exogenous obesity as a short term adjunct (a few weeks) in a regimen of weight reduction based on caloric restriction.

The limited usefulness of agents of this class (see ACTIONS) should be measured against possible risk factors inherent in their use such as those described below.

Contraindications: Advanced arteriosclerosis, symptomatic cardiovascular disease, moderate to severe hypertension, hyperthyroidism,

known hypersensitivity or idiosyncrasy to the sympathomimetic amines, glaucoma.
Agitated states.
Patients with a history of drug abuse.
During or within 14 days following the administration of monoamine oxidase inhibitors (hypertensive crises may result).
Warnings: Tolerance to the anorectic effect usually develops within a few weeks. When this occurs, the recommended dose should not be exceeded in an attempt to increase the effect; rather, the drug should be discontinued. Phendimetrazine tartrate may impair the ability of the patient to engage in potentially hazardous activities such as operating machinery or driving a motor vehicle; the patient should therefore be cautioned accordingly.
Drug Dependence: Phendimetrazine tartrate is related chemically and pharmacologically to the amphetamines. Amphetamines and related stimulant drugs have been extensively abused, and the possibility of abuse of phendimetrazine tartrate should be kept in mind when evaluating the desirability of including a drug as part of a weight reduction program. Abuse of amphetamines and related drugs may be associated with intense psychological dependence and severe social dysfunction. There are reports of patients who have increased the dosage to many times that recommended. Abrupt cessation following prolonged high dosage administration results in extreme fatigue and mental depression; changes are also noted on the sleep EEG. Manifestations of chronic intoxication with anorectic drugs include severe dermatoses, marked insomnia, irritability, hyperactivity, and personality changes. The most severe manifestation of chronic intoxications is psychosis, often clinically indistinguishable from schizophrenia.
Usage in Pregnancy: No reproduction studies or teratology studies of phendimetrazine tartrate, in animals or humans, have been published. Therefore, use of phendimetrazine tartrate by women who are or may become pregnant requires that the potential benefit be weighed against the possible hazard to mother and infant.
Usage in Children: Phendimetrazine tartrate is not recommended for use in children under 12 years of age.
Precautions: Caution is to be exercised in prescribing phendimetrazine tartrate for patients with even mild hypertension.
Insulin requirements in diabetes mellitus may be altered in association with the use of phendimetrazine tartrate and the concomitant dietary regimen.
Phendimetrazine tartrate may decrease the hypotensive effect of guanethidine.
The least amount feasible should be prescribed or dispensed at one time in order to minimize the possibility of overdosage.
Adverse Reactions:
Cardiovascular: Palpitation, tachycardia, elevation of blood pressure.
Central Nervous System: Overstimulation, restlessness, dizziness, insomnia, euphoria, dysphoria, tremor, headache; rarely psychotic episodes at recommended doses.
Gastrointestinal: Dryness of the mouth, unpleasant taste, diarrhea, constipation, other gastrointestinal disturbances.
Allergic: Urticaria.
Endocrine: Impotence, changes in libido.
Dosage and Administration: TABLETS: The usual adult dosage is 1 tablet 2 or 3 times daily, one hour before meals. Dosage may be adjusted to the patient's need. A dosage range from 17.5 mg. to 70 mg., 2 or 3 times daily may be used. CAPSULES: Dosage should be individualized to obtain an adequate response with the lowest effective dose. In some cases 17.5 mg. per dose may be adequate. One capsule (35 mg.) twice a day or three times a day, one hour before meals. Dosage should not exceed 2 capsules three times daily.
Phendimetrazine tartrate is not recommended for use in children under 12 years of age.
Overdosage: Manifestations of acute overdosage with phendimetrazine tartrate include restlessness, tremor, hyperreflexia, rapid respiration, confusion, assaultive behavior, hallucinations, panic states.
Fatigue and depression usually follow the central stimulation.
Cardiovascular effects include arrhythmias, hypertension or hypotension and circulatory collapse. Gastrointestinal symptoms include nausea, vomiting, diarrhea, and abdominal cramps. In fatal poisoning, death is usually preceded by convulsions and coma.
Management of acute phendimetrazine tartrate intoxication is largely symptomatic and includes lavage and sedation with a barbiturate. Experience with hemodialysis or peritoneal dialysis is inadequate to permit recommendation in this regard. Acidification of the urine increases phendimetrazine tartrate excretion. Intravenous phentolamine (Regitine) has been suggested for possible acute, severe hypertension, if this complicates phendimetrazine tartrate overdosage.
How Supplied: STATOBEX Tablets (white with green specks, oblong, 17/32" length, scored, engraved Lemmon 71) in bottles of 100 and 1000 (NDC 0093-0071).
STATOBEX-G Tablets (green oblong, 13/32" length, scored, engraved Lemmon) in bottles of 100 and 1000 (NDC 0093-0077).
STATOBEX Capsules (#3 green and white, imprinted Lemmon 277) in bottles of 100 and 1000 (NDC 0093-0277).
Also available in patient-packaged sizes.
[*Shown in Product Identification Section*]

VAGILIA® Cream/Suppositories ℞

Composition: Vagilia Cream contains:

Sulfisoxazole	10.0%
Aminacrine hydrochloride	0.2%
Allantoin	2.0%

in a water-miscible base made from stearic acid, mineral oil, polysorbate 60, sorbitan monostearate, sorbitol, methylparaben, propylparaben and purified water.
Each Vagilia Suppository contains:

Sulfisoxazole	600 mg.
Aminacrine hydrochloride	12 mg.
Allantoin	120 mg.

with lactose, in a base made from polyethylene glycol 400, polyethylene glycol 4000, glycerin and polysorbate 80; buffered with lactic acid to an acid pH. The inert covering of the suppositories consists of gelatin, glycerin, water, methylparaben, propylparaben, and coloring. It dissolves promptly in the vagina.
Action: Vagilia is designed to provide in one preparation efficacious treatment for a variety of infections of the vaginal tract. Vagilia does not attack the vaginal tissues but inhibits those organisms which are usually responsible for infection.
Indications: For the treatment of vaginitis and cervicitis caused by trichomonads, monilia (Candida albicans), Hemophilus vaginalis or other organisms susceptible to sulfisoxazole or aminacrine hydrochloride.
Contraindications: Vagilia should not be used in patients known to be sensitive to sulfonamides.
Precautions: Although some absorption of sulfisoxazole may occur through the vaginal mucosa, systemic reactions attributable to this product are infrequent. Local sensitivity reactions such as increased discomfort or a burning sensation are rare. However, the usual sulfonamide precautions apply.
Adverse Reactions: Patients should be observed for manifestations such as skin rash or other evidence of systemic toxicity; if they occur, the medication should be discontinued.
Dosage and Administration: One applicatorful or 1 suppository intravaginally once or twice daily. Improvement will often be apparent within a few days but treatment should be continued until pathogens have been eliminated or a clinical cure or remission is achieved. Adequate control or eradication of monilia and trichomonads usually requires prolonged treatment. Exacerbation may occur during the menses; for such infections it is therefore advisable to continue the applications for a minimum of one month or through one complete menstrual cycle. Vaginal applicators should not be used after seventh month of pregnancy.
If no improvement occurs within a few days, Vagilia should be discontinued and other treatment initiated.
It is recommended that a pad or tampon be used to protect underclothing.
Douching with a suitable solution before insertion may be recommended for hygienic reasons.
How Supplied: Cream (yellow) in 90 Gm. tubes with reusable applicator. Store at room temperature (NDC 0093-0015). Suppositories (orange) in boxes of 16 with inserter. Store at room temperature; avoid excessive heat (NDC 0093-0315).

Lilly and Company, Eli

307 E. McCARTY ST.
INDIANAPOLIS, IN 46225
P.O. BOX 618
INDIANAPOLIS, IN 46206

LEGEND

Aspirol®—*Inhalant in an Ampoule, Lilly*
Diskets®—*Dispersible Tablets, Lilly*
Enseals®—*Enteric-Release Tablets, Lilly*
Gelseals®—*Filled Elastic Capsules, Lilly*
Hyporets®—*Disposable Syringes, Lilly*
Identi-Code®—*Formula Identification Code, Lilly*
Identi-Dose®—*Unit Dose Medication, Lilly*
Pulvules®—*Filled Gelatin Capsules, Lilly*
Redi Vial®—*Dual Compartment Vial, Lilly*
℞Pak—*Prescription Package, Lilly*
Solvets®—*Soluble Tablets, Lilly*
Traypak™—*Multivial Carton, Lilly*

IDENTI-CODE® Index

Illustrations of examples of products bearing Identi-Code® appear in Product Identification Section.

Identi-Code® **Product Name**

A01-A36 (Enseals®)

A01 **Ammonium Chloride**
Composition (Each Enseal®): Ammonium Chloride, NF, 7½ grs (500 mg)
A02 **Ferrous Sulfate**
Composition (Each Enseal®): Ferrous Sulfate, USP, 5 grs (325 mg) (equiv. to 65 mg elemental iron), Red
A04 **Pancreatin**
Composition (Each Enseal®): Pancreatin, NF, Triple Strength, 5 grs (325 mg)
A05 **Potassium Chloride**
Composition (Each Enseal®): Potassium chloride, 300 mg (5 grs)
A06 **Potassium Iodide**
Composition (Each Enseal®): Potassium iodide, 300 mg (5 grs)

*Identi-Code® symbol.

Continued on next page

Lilly—Cont.

A09 Sodium Chloride
Composition (Each Enseal®): Sodium Chloride, USP, 15½ grs (1 gm)

A10 Sodium Salicylate
Composition (Each Enseal®): Sodium Salicylate, NF, 5 grs (325 mg)

A11 Sodium Salicylate
Composition (Each Enseal®): Sodium Salicylate, NF, 10 grs (650 mg)

A12 Ammonium Chloride
Composition (Each Enseal®): Ammonium Chloride, NF, 15 grs (1 gm)

A14 Thyroid
Composition (Each Enseal®): Thyroid, USP, 30 mg (½ gr)

A15 Thyroid
Composition (Each Enseal®): Thyroid, USP, 60 mg (1 gr)

A16 Thyroid
Composition (Each Enseal®): Thyroid, USP, 120 mg (2 grs)

A17 Thyroid
Composition (Each Enseal®): Thyroid, USP, 200 mg (3 grs)

A19 Diethylstilbestrol
Composition (Each Enseal®): Diethylstilbestrol, USP, 0.1 mg

A20 Diethylstilbestrol
Composition (Each Enseal®): Diethylstilbestrol, USP, 0.25 mg

A21 Diethylstilbestrol
Composition (Each Enseal®): Diethylstilbestrol, USP, 0.5 mg

A22 Diethylstilbestrol
Composition (Each Enseal®): Diethylstilbestrol, USP, 1 mg

A24 Seconal® Sodium
Composition (Each Enseal®): Secobarbital sodium, 100 mg (1½ grs)

A25 A.S.A.®
Composition (Each Enseal®): Aspirin, USP, 5 grs (325 mg)

A26 Ox Bile Extract
Composition (Each Enseal®): Ox bile extract, 5 grs (325 mg)

A27 Amesec®
Composition (Each Enseal®): Aminophylline, 130 mg; ephedrine hydrochloride, 25 mg; amobarbital, 25 mg

A30 Aminosalicylic Acid
Composition (Each Enseal®): Aminosalicylic Acid, NF, 500 mg (7½ grs)

A31 Potassium Chloride
Composition (Each Enseal®): Potassium chloride, 1 gm (15 grs)

A32 A.S.A.®
Composition (Each Enseal®): Aspirin, USP, 10 grs (650 mg)

A33 Diethylstilbestrol
Composition (Each Enseal®): Diethylstilbestrol, USP, 5 mg

A34 Diethylstilbestrol
Composition (Each Enseal®): Diethylstilbestrol, USP, 25 mg

A36 Ferrous Sulfate
Composition (Each Enseal®): Ferrous Sulfate, USP, 5 grs (325 mg) (equiv. to 65 mg elemental iron), Green

C06-C71 (Coated Tablets)

C06 Cascara
Composition (Each Coated Tablet): Cascara, NF, 5 grs (325 mg), Chocolate-Colored

C07 Cascara Compound
Composition (Each Coated Tablet): Ext. cascara, 16 mg; aloin, 16 mg.; podophyllum resin, 10 mg; ext. belladonna, 8 mg (total alkaloids, 0.1 mg); oleoresin ginger, 4 mg

C09 Digiglusin®
Composition (Each Coated Tablet): Digitalis glucosides, 1 NF digitalis unit

C11 Rhinitis, Full Strength
Composition (Each Coated Tablet): Camphor, 32.5 mg; quinine sulfate, 32.5 mg; ext. belladonna leaf, 5.8 mg (total alkaloids, 1/960 gr)

C12 Strychnine Sulfate
Composition (Each Coated Tablet): Strychnine sulfate, 1 mg (1/60 gr)

C13 Ferrous Sulfate
Composition (Each Coated Tablet): Ferrous Sulfate, USP, 5 grs (325 mg) (equiv. to 65 mg elemental iron)

C14 Ferro-Betalin®
Composition (Each Coated Tablet): Ferrous sulfate, 325 mg; thiamine hydrochloride (vitamin B_1), 1 mg

C15 Menadione
Composition (Each Coated Tablet): Menadione, NF, 5 mg

C16 Pagitane® Hydrochloride
Composition (Each Coated Tablet): Cycrimine Hydrochloride, NF, 1.25 mg

C17 Pagitane® Hydrochloride
Composition (Each Coated Tablet): Cycrimine Hydrochloride, NF, 2.5 mg

C27 V-Cillin K®
Composition (Each Coated Tablet): Penicillin V Potassium, USP, 125 mg

C29 V-Cillin K®
Composition (Each Coated Tablet): Penicillin V Potassium, USP, 250 mg

C36 Quinine Sulfate
Composition (Each Coated Tablet): Quinine Sulfate, USP, 5 grs (325 mg)

C37 Stero-Darvon® with A.S.A.®
Composition (Each Coated Tablet): Paramethasone acetate, 0.25 mg; propoxyphene hydrochloride, 32 mg; aspirin, 500 mg

C46 V-Cillin K®
Composition (Each Coated Tablet): Penicillin V Potassium, USP, 500 mg

C47 Hepicebrin®
Composition (Each Coated Tablet): Vitamin A acetate, 5000 IU (1.5 mg); vitamin D (as ergocalciferol), 400 IU (10 mcg); ascorbic acid (vitamin C), 75 mg; thiamine mononitrate (vitamin B_1), 2 mg; riboflavin (vitamin B_2), 3 mg; niacinamide, 20 mg; (NF)

C51 Darvocet-N® 50
Composition (Each Coated Tablet): Propoxyphene napsylate, 50 mg; acetaminophen, 325 mg

C53 Darvon-N®
Composition (Each Coated Tablet): Propoxyphene Napsylate, NF, 100 mg

C54 Darvon-N® with A.S.A.®
Composition (Each Coated Tablet): Propoxyphene napsylate, 100 mg; aspirin, 325 mg

C63 Darvocet-N® 100
Composition (Each Coated Tablet): Propoxyphene napsylate, 100 mg; acetaminophen, 650 mg

C71 Multicebrin®
Composition (Each Coated Tablet): Thiamine (vitamin B_1), 3 mg; riboflavin (vitamin B_2), 3 mg; pyridoxine (vitamin B_6), 1.2 mg; pantothenic acid, 5 mg; niacinamide, 25 mg; vitamin B_{12} (activity equivalent), 3 mcg; ascorbic acid (vitamin C), 75 mg; *dl*-alpha tocopheryl acetate (vitamin E), 6.6 IU (6.6 mg); vitamin A, 10,000 IU (3 mg); vitamin D, 400 IU (10 mcg)

F03-H72 (Pulvules®)

F03 Zentinic®
Composition (Each Pulvule®): Iron, elemental (as ferrous fumarate), 100 mg; folic acid, 0.05 mg; thiamine mononitrate (vitamin B_1), 7.5 mg; riboflavin (vitamin B_2), 7.5 mg; pyridoxine hydrochloride (vitamin B_6), 7.5 mg; vitamin B_{12} (activity equivalent), 50 mcg; pantothenic acid (as calcium pantothenate), 15 mg; niacinamide, 30 mg; ascorbic acid (vitamin C), 200 mg

F04 Seromycin®
Composition (Each Pulvule®): Cycloserine, USP, 250 mg

F05 V-Cillin®
Composition (Each Pulvule®): Penicillin V, USP, 125 mg

F06 V-Cillin®
Composition (Each Pulvule®): Penicillin V, USP, 250 mg

F07 Compren®
Composition (Each Pulvule®): Thiamine mononitrate (vitamin B_1), 0.5 mg; riboflavin (vitamin B_2), 1 mg; vitamin B_{12} (activity equivalent), 2.5 mcg; ascorbic acid (vitamin C), 33.3 mg; niacinamide, 5 mg; vitamin A, 2000 IU (0.6 mg); vitamin D, 133 IU (3.3 mcg); iron (as ferrous sulfate), 5 mg; pyridoxine (vitamin B_6), 1.7 mg; pantothenic acid, 2 mg; calcium (as the carbonate), 250 mg

F10 Amytal® and Aspirin
Composition (Each Pulvule®): Amobarbital, 50 mg; aspirin, 325 mg

F11 A.S.A.®
Composition (Each Pulvule®): Aspirin, NF, 5 grs (325 mg), Clear

F12 A.S.A.®
Composition (Each Pulvule®): Aspirin, NF, 5 grs (325 mg), Pink

F13 A.S.A.® Compound
Composition (Each Pulvule®): Aspirin, 227 mg; phenacetin, 160 mg; caffeine, 32.5 mg; White Opaque

F14 Ephedrine and Amytal®
Composition (Each Pulvule®): Ephedrine sulfate, 25 mg; amobarbital, 50 mg

F15 Lextron®
Composition (Each Pulvule®): Liver-stomach concentrate (as intrinsic powder), 50 mg; iron, elemental (as iron and ammonium citrates green), 30 mg; vitamin B_{12} (activity equivalent), 2 mcg; thiamine hydrochloride (vitamin B_1), 1 mg; riboflavin (vitamin B_2), 0.25 mg; with other factors of vitamin B complex present in the liver-stomach concentrate

F16 Lextron® Ferrous
Composition (Each Pulvule®): Liver-stomach concentrate (as intrinsic powder), 50 mg; iron, elemental (as ferrous sulfate), 35 mg; vitamin B_{12} (activity equivalent), 2 mcg; thiamine hydrochloride (vitamin B_1), 1 mg; riboflavin (vitamin B_2), 0.25 mg; with other factors of vitamin B complex present in the liver-stomach concentrate

F19 Extralin®
Composition (Each Pulvule®): Liver-stomach concentrate (as intrinsic powder), 50 mg

F20 Ephedrine and Seconal® Sodium
Composition (Each Pulvule®): Ephedrine sulfate, 25 mg; secobarbital sodium, 50 mg

F21 Extralin® B
Composition (Each Pulvule®): Liver-stomach concentrate (as intrinsic powder), 67 mg; vitamin B_{12} (activity equivalent), 3 mcg; thiamine hydrochloride (vitamin B_1), 1 mg; riboflavin (vitamin B_2), 0.25 mg; with other factors of vitamin B complex present in the liver-stomach concentrate

F22 Lextron® F. G.
Composition (Each Pulvule®): Liver-stomach concentrate (as intrinsic

powder), 50 mg; iron, elemental (as ferrous gluconate), 20 mg; vitamin B_{12} (activity equivalent), 2 mcg; thiamine hydrochloride (vitamin B_1), 1 mg; riboflavin (vitamin B_2), 0.25 mg; with other factors of vitamin B complex present in the liver-stomach concentrate

F23 Amytal® Sodium
Composition (Each Pulvule®): Amobarbital Sodium, USP, 65 mg (1 gr)

F24 Ephedrine Sulfate
Composition (Each Pulvule®): Ephedrine Sulfate, USP, 25 mg (3/8 gr)

F25 Ephedrine Sulfate
Composition (Each Pulvule®): Ephedrine Sulfate, USP, 50 mg (3/4 gr)

F26 Quinine Sulfate
Composition (Each Pulvule®): Quinine Sulfate, USP, 2 grs (130 mg)

F27 Quinine Sulfate
Composition (Each Pulvule®): Quinine Sulfate, USP, 3 grs (200 mg)

F29 Quinine Sulfate
Composition (Each Pulvule®): Quinine Sulfate, USP, 5 grs (325 mg)

F30 A.S.A.® Compound
Composition (Each Pulvule®): Aspirin, 227 mg; phenacetin, 160 mg; caffeine, 32.5 mg; Pink

F31 Acidulin®
Composition (Each Pulvule®): Glutamic acid hydrochloride, 340 mg

F32 Digitalis
Composition (Each Pulvule®): Digitalis, NF, 100 mg (1 ½ grs)

F33 Amytal® Sodium
Composition (Each Pulvule®): Amobarbital Sodium, USP, 200 mg (3 grs)

F34 Carbarsone
Composition (Each Pulvule®): Carbarsone, NF, 250 mg (4 grs)

F36 Copavin®
Composition (Each Pulvule®): Codeine sulfate, 15 mg; papaverine hydrochloride, 15 mg

F39 Quinidine Sulfate
Composition (Each Pulvule®): Quinidine Sulfate, USP, 200 mg (3 grs)

F40 Seconal® Sodium
Composition (Each Pulvule®): Secobarbital Sodium, USP, 100 mg (1½ grs)

F41 Bilron®
Composition (Each Pulvule®): Iron bile salts, 300 mg (5 grs)

F42 Seconal® Sodium
Composition (Each Pulvule®): Secobarbital Sodium, USP, 50 mg (3/4 gr)

F43 Betalin® Compound
Composition (Each Pulvule®): Thiamine (vitamin B_1), 1 mg; riboflavin (vitamin B_2), 2 mg; pyridoxine (vitamin B_6), 0.4 mg; pantothenic acid, 3.333 mg; niacinamide, 10 mg; vitamin B_{12} (activity equivalent), 1 mcg

F44 Ferrous Gluconate
Composition (Each Pulvule®): Ferrous Gluconate, NF, 5 grs (325 mg)

F45 Epragen™
Composition (Each Pulvule®): Ephedrine hydrochloride, 22 mg; aspirin, 130 mg; phenacetin, 227 mg; amobarbital, 50 mg

F46 Aminophylline and Amytal®
Composition (Each Pulvule®): Aminophylline, 100 mg; amobarbital, 32 mg

F47 Amesec®
Composition (Each Pulvule®): Aminophylline, 130 mg; ephedrine hydrochloride, 25 mg; amobarbital, 25 mg

F50 A.S.A.® and Codeine Compound, No. 2
Composition (Each Pulvule®): Codeine phosphate, 15 mg; phenacetin, 150 mg; aspirin, 230 mg; caffeine, 30 mg

F51 A.S.A.® and Codeine Compound, No. 3
Composition (Each Pulvule®): Codeine phosphate, 30 mg; phenacetin, 150 mg; aspirin, 230 mg; caffeine, 30 mg

F52 Dibasic Calcium Phosphate with Vitamin D
Composition (Each Pulvule®): Dibasic calcium phosphate, anhydrous, equivalent to 500 mg of dibasic calcium phosphate dihydrate; vitamin D synthetic, 33 IU (0.825 mcg)

F53 Trisogel®
Composition (Each Pulvule®): Magnesium trisilicate, 4½ grs; aluminum hydroxide gel, desiccated, 1½ grs

F54 Dicumarol
Composition (Each Pulvule®): Dicumarol, USP, 50 mg

F56 Calcium Gluconate with Vitamin D
Composition (Each Pulvule®): Calcium gluconate, 325 mg; vitamin D synthetic, 0.825 mcg

F59 Histadyl®
Composition (Each Pulvule®): Methapyrilene Hydrochloride, NF, 25 mg

F60 Histadyl®
Composition (Each Pulvule®): Methapyrilene Hydrochloride, NF, 50 mg

F61 Bilron®
Composition (Each Pulvule®): Iron bile salts, 150 mg (2 ½ grs)

F63 Dibasic Calcium Phosphate with Vitamin D and Iron
Composition (Each Pulvule®): Dibasic calcium phosphate, anhydrous, equivalent to 500 mg of dibasic calcium phosphate dihydrate; vitamin D, 33 IU (0.825 mcg); iron (as iron pyrophosphate), 10 mg

F64 Tuinal®
Composition (Each Pulvule®): Secobarbital sodium, 25 mg; amobarbital sodium, 25 mg

F65 Tuinal®
Composition (Each Pulvule®): Secobarbital sodium, 50 mg; amobarbital sodium, 50 mg

F66 Tuinal®
Composition (Each Pulvule®): Secobarbital sodium, 100 mg; amobarbital sodium, 100 mg

F67 A.S.A.® and Codeine Compound, No. 4
Composition (Each Pulvule®): Codeine phosphate, 60 mg; phenacetin, 150 mg; aspirin, 230 mg; caffeine, 30 mg

F71 Dicumarol
Composition (Each Pulvule®): Dicumarol, USP, 25 mg

F72 Seconal® Sodium
Composition (Each Pulvule®): Secobarbital Sodium, USP, 30 mg (½ gr)

F74 Tycopan®
Composition: Three Pulvules® contain thiamine mononitrate (vitamin B_1), 10 mg; riboflavin (vitamin B_2), 8 mg; pyridoxine hydrochloride (vitamin B_6), 10 mg; pantothenic acid (as calcium pantothenate, racemic), 60 mg; niacinamide, 60 mg; vitamin B_{12} (activity equivalent), 15 mcg; ascorbic acid (vitamin C), 200 mg; *dl*-alpha tocopherol (vitamin E), 22 IU (20 mg); biotin, 0.16 mg; folic acid, 0.45 mg; aminobenzoic acid, 33 mg; inositol, 160 mg; choline (as choline bitartrate), 160 mg; lipoic acid, 0.3 mg; vitamin A synthetic, 20,000 IU (6 mg); vitamin D synthetic, 1000 IU (25 mcg)

F90 Pentobarbital Sodium
Composition (Each Pulvule®): Pentobarbital Sodium, USP, 100 mg (1 ½ grs)

F92 Extralin® F
Composition (Each Pulvule®): Special Liver-Stomach Concentrate, Lilly (containing intrinsic factor), 390 mg; Cobalamin Concentrate, NF, equivalent to cobalamin, 15 mcg (the total vitamin B_{12} activity in the Special Liver-Stomach Concentrate, Lilly, and the Cobalamin Concentrate, NF, is 30 mcg); folic acid, 1 mg

F96 Reticulex®
Composition (Each Pulvule®): Liver-stomach concentrate (as intrinsic powder), 222 mg; vitamin B_{12} (activity equivalent), 10 mcg; iron, elemental (as ferrous sulfate), 75 mg; ascorbic acid (vitamin C), 50 mg; folic acid, 0.3 mg

---

G01 Alphalin®
Composition (Each Pulvule®): Vitamin A synthetic (palmitate), 10,000 IU (3 mg)

G19 Zentinic®
Composition (Each Pulvule®): Iron, elemental (as ferrous fumarate), 100 mg; folic acid, 0.05 mg; thiamine mononitrate (vitamin B_1), 7.5 mg; riboflavin (vitamin B_2), 7.5 mg; pyridoxine hydrochloride (vitamin B_6), 7.5 mg; vitamin B_{12} (activity equivalent), 50 mcg; pantothenic acid (as calcium pantothenate), 15 mg; niacinamide, 30 mg; ascorbic acid (vitamin C), 200 mg

---

H02 Darvon®
Composition (Each Pulvule®): Propoxyphene Hydrochloride, USP, 32 mg

H03 Darvon®
Composition (Each Pulvule®): Propoxyphene Hydrochloride, USP, 65 mg

H04 Darvon® with A.S.A.®
Composition (Each Pulvule®): Propoxyphene hydrochloride, 65 mg; aspirin, 325 mg

H05 Darvon® Compound
Composition (Each Pulvule®): Propoxyphene hydrochloride, 32 mg; aspirin, 227 mg; phenacetin, 162 mg; caffeine, 32.4 mg

H06 Darvon® Compound-65
Composition (Each Pulvule®): Propoxyphene hydrochloride, 65 mg; aspirin, 227 mg; phenacetin, 162 mg; caffeine, 32.4 mg

H10 En-Cebrin® F
Composition (Each Pulvule®): Vitamin A synthetic, 4000 IU (1.2 mg); thiamine mononitrate (vitamin B_1), 3 mg; riboflavin (vitamin B_2), 2 mg; niacinamide, 10 mg; pyridoxine hydrochloride (vitamin B_6), 2 mg; folic acid, 1 mg; vitamin B_{12} (activity equivalent), 5 mcg; pantothenic acid (as calcium pantothenate, racemic), 5 mg; ascorbic acid (vitamin C), 50 mg; vitamin D synthetic, 400 IU (10 mcg); calcium (as the carbonate), 250 mg; iron (as ferrous fumarate), 30 mg; iodine (as potassium iodide), 0.15 mg; copper (as the sulfate), 1 mg; magnesium (as

Continued on next page

*Identi-Code® symbol.

Lilly—Cont.

the hydroxide), 5 mg; manganese (as the glycerophosphate), 1 mg; zinc (as the chloride), 1.5 mg

H12 En-Cebrin®
Composition (Each Pulvule®): Vitamin A, 4000 IU (1.2 mg); thiamine mononitrate (vitamin B_1), 3 mg; riboflavin (vitamin B_2), 2 mg; niacinamide, 10 mg; pyridoxine (vitamin B_6), 1.7 mg; vitamin B_{12} (activity equivalent), 5 mcg; pantothenic acid, 5 mg; ascorbic acid (vitamin C), 50 mg; vitamin D, 400 IU (10 mcg); calcium (as the carbonate), 250 mg; iron (as ferrous fumarate), 30 mg; iodine (as potassium iodide), 0.15 mg; copper (as the sulfate), 1 mg; magnesium (as the hydroxide), 5 mg; manganese (as the glycerophosphate), 1 mg; zinc (as the chloride), 1.5 mg

H13 Novrad®
Composition (Each Pulvule®): Levopropoxyphene Napsylate, NF, 50 mg (equivalent to levopropoxyphene)

H14 Novrad®
Composition (Each Pulvule®): Levopropoxyphene Napsylate, NF, 100 mg (equivalent to levopropoxyphene)

H17 Aventyl® HCl
Composition (Each Pulvule®): Nortriptyline Hydrochloride, NF, 10 mg (equiv. to base)

H19 Aventyl® HCl
Composition (Each Pulvule®): Nortriptyline Hydrochloride, NF, 25 mg (equiv. to base)

H66 Kafocin®
Composition (Each Pulvule®): Cephaloglycin, NF, 250 mg

H69 Keflex®
Composition (Each Pulvule®): Cephalexin, USP, 250 mg

H71 Keflex®
Composition (Each Pulvule®): Cephalexin, USP, 500 mg

H72 Theracebrin®
Composition (Each Pulvule®): Thiamine (as the mononitrate) (vitamin B_1), 15 mg; riboflavin (vitamin B_2), 10 mg; pyridoxine (as the hydrochloride) (vitamin B_6), 2.5 mg; pantothenic acid (as *d*-calcium pantothenate), 20 mg; niacinamide, 150 mg; vitamin B_{12} (activity equivalent), 10 mcg; ascorbic acid (vitamin C), 150 mg; *dl*-alpha tocopheryl acetate (vitamin E), 18.5 IU (18.5 mg); vitamin A synthetic, 25,000 IU (7.5 mg); vitamin D synthetic, 1500 IU (37.5 mcg)

3061 Ceclor®
Composition (Each Pulvule®): Cefaclor, 250 mg

3062 Ceclor®
Composition (Each Pulvule®): Cefaclor, 500 mg

3074 Hista-Clopane®
Composition (Each Pulvule®): Chlorpheniramine maleate, 4 mg; cyclopentamine hydrochloride, 12.5 mg

3075 Histadyl® and A.S.A.®
Composition (Each Pulvule®): Chlorpheniramine maleate, 4 mg; aspirin, 325 mg

---

J02-J99 (Compressed Tablets)

J02 Atropine Sulfate
Composition (Each Compressed Tablet): Atropine Sulfate, USP, 0.4 mg (1/150 gr)

J03 Belladonna Extract
Composition (Each Compressed Tablet): Belladonna Extract, NF, 15 mg (1/4 gr) (total alkaloids, 0.187 mg)

J04 Bismuth Subcarbonate
Composition (Each Compressed Tablet): Bismuth subcarbonate, 5 grs (325 mg)

J05 Citrated Caffeine
Composition (Each Compressed Tablet): Citrated caffeine, 1 gr (65 mg)

J09 Codeine Sulfate
Composition (Each Compressed Tablet): Codeine Sulfate, NF, 15 mg (1/4 gr)

J10 Codeine Sulfate
Composition (Each Compressed Tablet): Codeine Sulfate, NF, 30 mg (1/2 gr)

J11 Codeine Sulfate
Composition (Each Compressed Tablet): Codeine Sulfate, NF, 60 mg (1 gr)

J13 Colchicine
Composition (Each Compressed Tablet): Colchicine, USP, 0.6 mg (1/100 gr)

J20 Quinidine Sulfate
Composition (Each Compressed Tablet): Quinidine Sulfate, USP, 200 mg (3 grs)

J23 Soda Mint
Composition (Each Compressed Tablet): Sodium bicarbonate, 5 grs; oil peppermint

J24 Sodium Bicarbonate
Composition (Each Compressed Tablet): Sodium Bicarbonate, USP, 5 grs (325 mg)

J25 Thyroid
Composition (Each Compressed Tablet): Thyroid, USP, 60 mg (1 gr)

J26 Thyroid
Composition (Each Compressed Tablet): Thyroid, USP, 120 mg (2 grs)

J29 Thyroid
Composition (Each Compressed Tablet): Thyroid, USP, 30 mg (1/2 gr)

J30 Thyroid
Composition (Each Compressed Tablet): Thyroid, USP, 15 mg (1/4 gr)

J31 Phenobarbital
Composition (Each Compressed Tablet): Phenobarbital, USP, 15 mg (1/4 gr)

J32 Phenobarbital
Composition (Each Compressed Tablet): Phenobarbital, USP, 30 mg (1/2 gr)

J33 Phenobarbital
Composition (Each Compressed Tablet): Phenobarbital, USP, 100 mg (1 1/2 grs)

J34 Copavin®
Composition (Each Compressed Tablet): Codeine sulfate, 15 mg; papaverine hydrochloride, 15 mg

J36 Ergotrate® Maleate
Composition (Each Compressed Tablet): Ergonovine Maleate, NF, 0.2 mg (1/300 gr)

J37 Phenobarbital
Composition (Each Compressed Tablet): Phenobarbital, USP, 60 mg (1 gr)

J41 Niacin
Composition (Each Compressed Tablet): Niacin, NF, 20 mg

J42 Niacin
Composition (Each Compressed Tablet): Niacin, NF, 100 mg

J43 Niacin
Composition (Each Compressed Tablet): Niacin, NF, 50 mg

J45 Hexa-Betalin®
Composition (Each Compressed Tablet): Pyridoxine Hydrochloride, USP, 25 mg

J46 Niacinamide
Composition (Each Compressed Tablet): Niacinamide, USP, 50 mg

J47 Riboflavin
Composition (Each Compressed Tablet): Riboflavin, USP, 5 mg

J49 Diethylstilbestrol
Composition (Each Compressed Tablet): Diethylstilbestrol, USP, 0.1 mg

J50 Diethylstilbestrol
Composition (Each Compressed Tablet): Diethylstilbestrol, USP, 0.25 mg

J51 Diethylstilbestrol
Composition (Each Compressed Tablet): Diethylstilbestrol, USP, 0.5 mg

J52 Diethylstilbestrol
Composition (Each Compressed Tablet): Diethylstilbestrol, USP, 1 mg

J53 Pantholin®
Composition (Each Compressed Tablet): Calcium Pantothenate, USP, 10 mg

J54 Diethylstilbestrol
Composition (Each Compressed Tablet): Diethylstilbestrol, USP, 5 mg

J55 Phenobarbital and Belladonna, No. 1
Composition (Each Compressed Tablet): Phenobarbital, 30 mg; ext. belladonna, 8 mg (total alkaloids, 0.1 mg)

J56 Hexa-Betalin®
Composition (Each Compressed Tablet): Pyridoxine Hydrochloride, USP, 10 mg

J57 Crystodigin®
Composition (Each Compressed Tablet): Digitoxin, USP, 0.2 mg

J59 Phenobarbital and Belladonna, No. 2
Composition (Each Compressed Tablet): Phenobarbital, 15 mg; ext. belladonna, 4 mg (total alkaloids, 0.05 mg)

J60 Crystodigin®
Composition (Each Compressed Tablet): Digitoxin, USP, 0.1 mg

J61 Papaverine Hydrochloride
Composition (Each Compressed Tablet): Papaverine Hydrochloride, NF, 30 mg (1/2 gr)

J62 Papaverine Hydrochloride
Composition (Each Compressed Tablet): Papaverine Hydrochloride, NF, 60 mg (1 gr)

J63 Riboflavin
Composition (Each Compressed Tablet): Riboflavin, USP, 10 mg

J64 Dolophine® Hydrochloride
Composition (Each Compressed Tablet): Methadone Hydrochloride, USP, 5 mg

J69 Propylthiouracil
Composition (Each Compressed Tablet): Propylthiouracil, USP, 50 mg

J70 Phenobarbital and Belladonna, No. 3
Composition (Each Compressed Tablet): Phenobarbital, 15 mg; ext. belladonna, 8 mg (total alkaloids, 0.1 mg)

J72 Dolophine® Hydrochloride
Composition (Each Compressed Tablet): Methadone Hydrochloride, USP, 10 mg

J73 Methyltestosterone
Composition (Each Compressed Tablet): Methyltestosterone, USP, 10 mg

J74 Methyltestosterone
Composition (Each Compressed Tablet): Methyltestosterone, USP, 25 mg

J75 Crystodigin®
Composition (Each Compressed Tablet): Digitoxin, USP, 0.05 mg

J76 Crystodigin®
Composition (Each Compressed Tablet): Digitoxin, USP, 0.15 mg

J94 Tapazole®
Composition (Each Compressed Tablet): Methimazole, USP, 5 mg

J95 Tapazole®
Composition (Each Compressed Tablet): Methimazole, USP, 10 mg

J96 Tylosterone®
Composition (Each Compressed Tablet): Diethylstilbestrol, 0.25 mg; methyltestosterone, 5 mg

J97 Paveril® Phosphate
Composition (Each Compressed Tablet): Dioxyline phosphate, 100 mg (1½ grs)

J99 Sandril®
Composition (Each Compressed Tablet): Reserpine, USP, 0.1 mg

S02-S17 (Suppositories)

S02 Estrone
Composition (Each Suppository): Estrone, 0.2 mg

S03 Metycaine® Hydrochloride and Merthiolate®
Composition (Each Suppository): Piperocaine hydrochloride, 5 percent; thimerosal, 1:5000

S04 Metycaine® Hydrochloride and Zinc Oxide Compound
Composition (Each Suppository): Piperocaine hydrochloride, 125 mg; extract belladonna, 12.5 mg (total alkaloids, 0.15 mg); bismuth subcarbonate, 125 mg; zinc oxide, 250 mg

S05 Seconal® Sodium
Composition (Each Suppository): Secobarbital sodium, 120 mg

S06 Amytal® Sodium
Composition (Each Suppository): Amobarbital sodium, 200 mg

S07 Diethylstilbestrol
Composition (Each Suppository): Diethylstilbestrol, USP, 0.1 mg

S09 Diethylstilbestrol
Composition (Each Suppository): Diethylstilbestrol, USP, 0.5 mg

S11 Seconal® Sodium
Composition (Each Suppository): Secobarbital sodium, 200 mg

S13 Surfacaine®
Composition (Each Suppository): Cyclomethycaine Sulfate, NF, 10 mg

S14 Seconal® Sodium
Composition (Each Suppository): Secobarbital sodium, 60 mg

S15 A.S.A.®
Composition (Each Suppository): Aspirin, USP, 5 grs (325 mg)

S16 A.S.A.®
Composition (Each Suppository): Aspirin, USP, 10 grs (650 mg)

S17 Seconal® Sodium
Composition (Each Suppository): Secobarbital sodium, 30 mg

T01-U60 (Compressed Tablets)

T01 Zentron® Chewable
Composition (Each Compressed Tablet): Iron, elemental (as ferrous fumarate), 20 mg; thiamine mononitrate (vitamin B_1), 1 mg; riboflavin (vitamin B_2), 1 mg; pyridoxine hydrochloride (vitamin B_6), 1 mg; cyanocobalamin (vitamin B_{12} crystalline), 5 mcg; pantothenic acid (as panthenol), 1 mg; niacinamide, 5 mg; ascorbic acid (vitamin C), 100 mg

T02 Novacebrin® Chewable
Composition (Each Compressed Tablet): Vitamin A, 4000 IU (1.2 mg); vitamin D, 400 IU (10 mcg); ascorbic acid (vitamin C), 60 mg; thiamine mononitrate (vitamin B_1), 1.5 mg; riboflavin (vitamin B_2), 2 mg; pyridoxine (vitamin B_6), 0.8 mg; vitamin B_{12} (activity equivalent), 3 mcg; niacinamide, 12 mg; pantothenic acid, 2.5 mg

T03 Novacebrin® c̄ Fluoride Chewable
Composition (Each Compressed Tablet): Fluoride (as sodium fluoride), 1 mg; vitamin A, 4000 IU (1.2 mg); vitamin D, 400 IU (10 mcg); vitamin C (as sodium ascorbate and ascorbic acid), 60 mg; thiamine mononitrate (vitamin B_1), 1.5 mg; riboflavin (vitamin B_2), 2 mg; pyridoxine hydrochloride (vitamin B_6), 1 mg; cyanocobalamin (vitamin B_{12}), 3 mcg; niacinamide, 12 mg; pantothenic acid (as panthenol), 2.5 mg

T04 Antiseptic No. 3, R. St. J. Perry
Composition (Each Compressed Tablet): Mercury cyanide, 0.5 gm; sodium borate, 0.97 gm

T05 A.S.A.®
Composition (Each Compressed Tablet): Aspirin, USP, 5 grs (325 mg)

T06 A.S.A.®
Composition (Each Compressed Tablet): Aspirin, USP, 5 grs (325 mg), Pink

T07 A.S.A.® Compound
Composition (Each Compressed Tablet): Aspirin, 227 mg; phenacetin, 160 mg; caffeine, 32.5 mg

T13 Calcium Lactate
Composition (Each Compressed Tablet): Calcium Lactate, USP, 5 grs (325 mg)

T14 Calcium Lactate
Composition (Each Compressed Tablet): Calcium Lactate, USP, 10 grs (650 mg)

T17 Diamond® Antiseptics
Composition (Each Compressed Tablet): Mercury bichloride, 475 mg

T19 Methenamine
Composition (Each Compressed Tablet): Methenamine, NF, 5 grs (325 mg)

T21 Methenamine and Sodium Biphosphate
Composition (Each Compressed Tablet): Methenamine, 325 mg; sodium biphosphate, 325 mg; (NF)

T23 Sodium Chloride
Composition (Each Compressed Tablet): Sodium Chloride, USP, 2.25 gm

T24 Sodium Chloride
Composition (Each Compressed Tablet): Sodium Chloride, USP, 1 gm

T26 Pancreatin
Composition (Each Compressed Tablet): Pancreatin, NF, Single Strength, 5 grs (325 mg)

T29 Sodium Bicarbonate
Composition (Each Compressed Tablet): Sodium Bicarbonate, USP, 10 grs (650 mg)

T32 Amytal®
Composition (Each Compressed Tablet): Amobarbital, NF, 100 mg (1½ grs)

T35 Calcium Carbonate
Composition (Each Compressed Tablet): Calcium Carbonate, NF, Aromatic, 10 grs (650 mg)

T36 Calcium Gluconate
Composition (Each Compressed Tablet): Calcium Gluconate, USP, 1 gm (15½ grs)

T37 Amytal®
Composition (Each Compressed Tablet): Amobarbital, NF, 50 mg (¾ gr)

T39 Calcium Gluconate
Composition (Each Compressed Tablet): Calcium Gluconate, USP, 7½ grs (500 mg)

T40 Amytal®
Composition (Each Compressed Tablet): Amobarbital, NF, 15 mg (¼ gr)

T42 A.S.A.® and Codeine Compound, No. 2
Composition (Each Compressed Tablet): Codeine phosphate, 15 mg; aspirin, 230 mg; phenacetin, 150 mg; caffeine, 30 mg

T44 Calcium Gluconate with Vitamin D
Composition (Each Compressed Tablet): Calcium gluconate, 1 gm; vitamin D synthetic, 1.65 mcg

T45 Cevalin®
Composition (Each Compressed Tablet): Ascorbic Acid, USP, 100 mg

T46 Sulfapyridine
Composition (Each Compressed Tablet): Sulfapyridine, USP, 0.5 gm (7.72 grs)

T47 Cevalin®
Composition (Each Compressed Tablet): Ascorbic Acid, USP, 50 mg

T49 A.S.A.® and Codeine Compound, No. 3
Composition (Each Compressed Tablet): Codeine phosphate, 30 mg; aspirin, 230 mg; phenacetin, 150 mg; caffeine, 30 mg

T50 A.S.A.® Compound
Composition (Each Compressed Tablet): Aspirin, 227 mg; phenacetin, 160 mg; caffeine, 32.5 mg; Pink

T52 Betalin® S
Composition (Each Compressed Tablet): Thiamine Hydrochloride, USP, 10 mg

T53 Niacinamide
Composition (Each Compressed Tablet): Niacinamide, USP, 100 mg

T54 Sulfadiazine
Composition (Each Compressed Tablet): Sulfadiazine, USP, 0.5 gm (7.72 grs)

T55 Papaverine Hydrochloride
Composition (Each Compressed Tablet): Papaverine Hydrochloride, NF, 100 mg (1½ grs)

T56 Amytal®
Composition (Each Compressed Tablet): Amobarbital, NF, 30 mg (½ gr)

T59 Betalin® S
Composition (Each Compressed Tablet): Thiamine Hydrochloride, USP, 25 mg

T60 Cevalin®
Composition (Each Compressed Tablet): Ascorbic Acid, USP, 250 mg

T61 Dibasic Calcium Phosphate
Composition (Each Compressed Tablet): Dibasic calcium phosphate, anhydrous, equivalent to 7½ grs (500 mg) of dibasic calcium phosphate dihydrate

T62 Betalin® S
Composition (Each Compressed Tablet): Thiamine Hydrochloride, USP, 50 mg

Continued on next page

*Identi-Code® symbol.

Lilly—Cont.

T63 Betalin® S
Composition (Each Compressed Tablet): Thiamine Hydrochloride, USP, 100 mg

T67 Cevalin®
Composition (Each Compressed Tablet): Ascorbic Acid, USP, 500 mg

T70 Diethylstilbestrol
Composition (Each Compressed Tablet): Diethylstilbestrol, USP, 25 mg

T72 Hexa-Betalin®
Composition (Each Compressed Tablet): Pyridoxine Hydrochloride, USP, 50 mg

T73 Papaverine Hydrochloride
Composition (Each Compressed Tablet): Papaverine Hydrochloride, NF, 200 mg (3 grs)

T74 Penicillin G Potassium
Composition (Each Compressed Tablet): Penicillin G Potassium, USP, Buffered, 250,000 units

T75 Neotrizine®
Composition (Each Compressed Tablet): Sulfadiazine, 167 mg; sulfamerazine, 167 mg; sulfamethazine, 167 mg; (USP)

T76 Penicillin G Potassium
Composition (Each Compressed Tablet): Penicillin G Potassium, USP, 200,000 units

T91 Paveril® Phosphate
Composition (Each Compressed Tablet): Dioxyline phosphate, 200 mg (3 grs)

T93 Isoniazid
Composition (Each Compressed Tablet): Isoniazid, USP, 100 mg

T94 Paveril® Phosphate and Amytal®
Composition (Each Compressed Tablet): Amobarbital, 15 mg; dioxyline phosphate, 200 mg

T96 Neomycin Sulfate
Composition (Each Compressed Tablet): Neomycin Sulfate, USP, 500 mg (equiv. to 350 mg base)

T99 Haldrone®
Composition (Each Compressed Tablet): Paramethasone Acetate, NF, 1 mg

---

U01 Haldrone®
Composition (Each Compressed Tablet): Paramethasone Acetate, NF, 2 mg

U02 Sandril®
Composition (Each Compressed Tablet): Reserpine, USP, 1 mg

U03 Dymelor®
Composition (Each Compressed Tablet): Acetohexamide, USP, 250 mg

U07 Dymelor®
Composition (Each Compressed Tablet): Acetohexamide, USP, 500 mg

U09 Anhydron®
Composition (Each Compressed Tablet): Cyclothiazide, NF, 2 mg

U23 Isoniazid
Composition (Each Compressed Tablet): Isoniazid, USP, 300 mg

U29 Sandril®
Composition (Each Compressed Tablet): Reserpine, USP, 0.25 mg

U53 Methadone Hydrochloride
Composition (Each Disket®): Methadone Hydrochloride, USP, 40 mg

U54 Acetaminophen
Composition (Each Compressed Tablet): Acetaminophen, USP, 325 mg (5 grs)

U56 Folic Acid
Composition (Each Compressed Tablet): Folic Acid, USP, 1 mg

U60 Keflex®
Composition (Each Compressed Tablet): Cephalexin, 1 gm

W07-W68 (Miscellaneous)

W07 V-Cillin K®, for Oral Solution
Composition (When Mixed as Directed): Each 5 ml contain penicillin V potassium equivalent to penicillin V, 125 mg (USP).

W10 V-Cillin® Drops
Composition (When Mixed as Directed): Each 0.6 ml contains penicillin V, 125 mg; buffered with citric acid (USP).

W16 V-Cillin K®, for Oral Solution
Composition (When Mixed as Directed): Each 5 ml contain penicillin V potassium equivalent to penicillin V, 250 mg (USP).

W21 For Oral Suspension, Keflex®
Composition (When Mixed as Directed): Each 5 ml contain cephalexin, 125 mg (NF).

W22 For Pediatric Drops, Keflex®
Composition (When Mixed as Directed): Each ml contains cephalexin, 100 mg (NF).

W68 For Oral Suspension, Keflex®
Composition (When Mixed as Directed): Each 5 ml contain cephalexin, 250 mg (NF).

5057 For Oral Suspension, Ceclor®
Composition (When Mixed as Directed): Each 5 ml contain cefaclor, 125 mg.

5058 For Oral Suspension, Ceclor®
Composition (When Mixed as Directed): Each 5 ml contain cefaclor, 250 mg.

UNIT-DOSE PACKAGING

Dispenser Strip
Hyporets® (disposable syringes, Lilly)
Identi-Dose® (unit dose medication, Lilly)
Reverse-Numbered Package
Closed-circuit control of medication from pharmacy to nurse to patient and return. Simplifies counting and dispensing whether in single-unit or prescription-size quantities. Fits into any dispensing system for ready identification and legibility, better inventory control, protection from contamination, easier handling and recording under Medicare, prevention of drug loss through pilferage or spilling, better control of Federal Controlled Substances, and less chance of medication errors.
The following products are available through normal channels of supply:

Dispenser Strip
Pulvules®
No.
© 240 Seconal® Sodium, 100 mg
© 303 Tuinal®, 100 mg

Hyporets®
No.
8 Duracillin® A.S., 300,000 units, 1 ml
9 Duracillin® A.S., 600,000 units, 1.2 ml
10 Duracillin® A.S., 1,200,000 units, 2 ml
42 Nebcin®, Injection, 80 mg per 2 ml, 2 ml
55 Nebcin®, Injection, 60 mg per 1.5 ml, 1.5 ml

Identi-Dose® (ID100)
Pulvules®
No.
© 222 Amytal® Sodium, 200 mg
© 240 Seconal® Sodium, 100 mg
© 243 Seconal® Sodium, 50 mg
© 286 A.S.A.® and Codeine Compound, No. 3
© 303 Tuinal®, 100 mg
© 304 Tuinal®, 200 mg
© 364 Darvon®, 32 mg
© 365 Darvon®, 65 mg
© 366 Darvon® with A.S.A.®
© 368 Darvon® Compound
© 369 Darvon® Compound-65
387 Aventyl® HCl, 10 mg
389 Aventyl® HCl, 25 mg
402 Keflex®, 250 mg
403 Keflex®, 500 mg
3061 Ceclor®, 250 mg
3062 Ceclor®, 500 mg

Tablets
No.
55 Hepicebrin®
100 Multicebrin®
186 A.S.A.®, 5 grs
189 A.S.A.® Compound
© 558 Codeine Sulfate, NF, 30 mg
1125 Quinidine Sulfate, USP, 200 mg
© 1544 Phenobarbital, USP, 15 mg
© 1545 Phenobarbital, USP, 30 mg
© 1546 Phenobarbital, USP, 100 mg
1572 Ergotrate® Maleate, 0.2 mg
© 1574 Phenobarbital, USP, 60 mg
1671 Papaverine Hydrochloride, NF, 100 mg
1685 Diethylstilbestrol, USP, 5 mg
1703 Crystodigin®, 0.1 mg, Pink
1803 Neomycin Sulfate, USP, 500 mg
1830 V-Cillin K®, 125 mg
1831 V-Cillin K®, 250 mg
1832 V-Cillin K®, 500 mg
1842 Dymelor®, 250 mg
1843 Dymelor®, 500 mg, Yellow
© 1883 Darvon-N®, 100 mg
© 1884 Darvon-N® with A.S.A.®
© 1890 Darvocet-N® 50
© 1893 Darvocet-N® 100
1896 Keflex®, 1 gm

Miscellaneous
M-126 V-Cillin K®, for Oral Solution, 125 mg
© M-135 Darvon-N® Suspension, 100 mg
M-142 V-Cillin K®, for Oral Solution, 250 mg
M-201 For Oral Suspension, Keflex®, 125 mg
M-202 For Oral Suspension, Keflex®, 250 mg
M-5057 For Oral Suspension, Ceclor®, 125 mg
M-5058 For Oral Suspension, Ceclor®, 250 mg

Reverse-Numbered Package
Pulvules®
No.
© 365 Darvon®, 65 mg
© 369 Darvon® Compound-65

Tablets
No.
© 1893 Darvocet-N® 100

Single-Cut Identi-Dose® (ID500)
Pulvules®
No.
© 365 Darvon®, 65 mg
© 369 Darvon® Compound-65

Tablets
No.
© 1883 Darvon-N®, 100 mg
© 1884 Darvon-N® with A.S.A.®
© 1890 Darvocet-N® 50
© 1893 Darvocet-N® 100

©, ©, © Federal Controlled Substances.

ACIDULIN® OTC

(glutamic acid hydrochloride)

Description: Each Pulvule® contains 340 mg glutamic acid hydrochloride and is equivalent to about 10 minims of Diluted Hydrochloric Acid, USP, or to about 16.8 ml of 0.1 *N* hydrochloric acid.
Hydrochloric acid deficiency can be corrected easily and safely with Pulvules Acidulin. The Pulvule form, unlike solutions, is tasteless,

cannot injure mucous membranes or teeth, and is safe and convenient for the patient to carry when traveling or dining out.

Indications: Acidulin is administered to counterbalance deficiency of hydrochloric acid in the gastric juice and to destroy or inhibit the growth of putrefactive microorganisms in ingested food. A deficiency of hydrochloric acid is often associated with pernicious anemia, gastric carcinoma, congenital achlorhydria, and allergy.

Contraindications: Should not be used if gastric hyperacidity or peptic ulcers are present.

Dosage: 1 to 3 Pulvules three times daily before meals, or as directed by the physician.

Overdosage: *Symptoms*—Massive overdosage may produce systemic acidosis. *Treatment*—Alkalies, such as sodium bicarbonate or sodium *r*-lactate solution, one molar (to be diluted).

How Supplied: *Pulvules No. 213, Acidulin® (glutamic acid hydrochloride, Lilly), F31,** 340 mg (No. 1, Pink), in bottles of 100 and 1000.

[060178]

AEROLONE® SOLUTION ℞
(isoproterenol hydrochloride inhalation)
(Not USP)

Description: Aerolone® Solution (isoproterenol hydrochloride inhalation, Lilly) is a bronchodilator. Each 100 ml contain isoproterenol hydrochloride, 0.25 gm, with propylene glycol, ascorbic acid, coloring, and purified water, q.s. Sodium hydroxide is added during manufacture to adjust the *p*H.

This product differs from the USP Inhalation in that it contains 80 percent propylene glycol by volume instead of purified water and it is not isotonic.

Actions: Isoproterenol is an adrenergic (sympathomimetic) agent and relieves bronchospasm by relaxing the smooth muscle of the bronchioles.

Indications: Aerolone® Solution (isoproterenol hydrochloride inhalation, Lilly) is indicated for the treatment of bronchospasm associated with acute and chronic bronchial asthma, pulmonary emphysema, bronchitis, and bronchiectasis.

Contraindications: Aerolone® Solution (isoproterenol hydrochloride inhalation, Lilly) is contraindicated in patients with (1) known hypersensitivity to isoproterenol or (2) cardiac arrhythmia associated with tachycardia.

Warnings: Occasional patients have been reported to develop severe paradoxical airway resistance with repeated excessive use of isoproterenol inhalation preparations. The cause of this refractory state is unknown. It is advisable that, in such instances, the use of this preparation be discontinued immediately and alternative therapy instituted, since in the reported cases the patients did not respond to other forms of therapy until the drug was withdrawn.

Deaths have been reported following excessive use of isoproterenol inhalation preparations, and the exact cause is unknown. Cardiac arrest was noted in several instances.

Usage in Pregnancy—Safe use during pregnancy has not been established relative to possible adverse effects on fetal development. Therefore, Aerolone Solution should not be used in pregnant women unless, in the judgment of the physician, the potential benefits outweigh the possible hazards.

Precautions: Aerolone® Solution (isoproterenol hydrochloride inhalation, Lilly) should be used with caution in patients having serious cardiac disease, hypertension, or hyperthyroidism.

Adverse Reactions: Rarely, insomnia, nervousness, vertigo, tachycardia, and palpitation may occur.

Administration and Dosage: For use by aerosol only. The technique is the same as that for administering epinephrine, 1:100. A nebulizer which produces a fine mist is necessary. The mist is inhaled through the mouth, and the breath is held in momentarily. Usually, 6 to 12 inhalations will bring adequate relief. Mild cases may require only one treatment per day; severe cases may need the treatment repeatedly at intervals of 15 minutes. If relief is not noticeable after three such treatments at 15-minute intervals, consult a physician. Ordinarily, the number of such treatments for repeated attacks should not exceed eight per 24 hours.

Physicians prescribing isoproterenol for use in inhalation therapy equipment should bear in mind the fact that different dosages of medication are delivered into the patient's airways depending upon the proficiency of the therapist and the type of inhalator used.

Proficiency in the use of any of these devices can be gained only by firsthand experience. Furthermore, some equipment can deliver 100 percent of the medication deep into the airways, whereas other inhalators may deliver considerably less than the prescribed dose. The number of inhalations per treatment and the frequency of re-treatment should, therefore, be titrated to the patient's response.

Overdosage: *Symptoms*—Insomnia, nervousness, vertigo, tachycardia, and palpitation resulting from C.N.S. stimulation.

Treatment—No specific treatment; general management consists in controlling symptoms of C.N.S. stimulation by the use of sedatives, such as the barbiturates.

How Supplied: (℞) *Solution No. 50, Aerolone® Solution (isoproterenol hydrochloride inhalation, Lilly),* in 1-fl-oz bottles.

[040678]

ALUMINUM HYDROXIDE GEL AND MAGNESIUM TRISILICATE,

see Trisogel® (magnesium trisilicate and aluminum hydroxide gel, Lilly).

AMESEC® ℞
(aminophylline compound)

Description: Amesec combines the sympathomimetic action of ephedrine, which is valuable in treating the bronchospasm of asthma, with the sedative effect of Amytal® (amobarbital, Lilly). Aminophylline is included in the formula because of its efficacy in the treatment of bronchial asthma.

Each Enseal® or Pulvule® contains—
Aminophylline ....130 mg (2 grs)
Ephedrine Hydrochloride............ 25 mg (3/8 gr)
Amytal® (amobarbital, Lilly).....25 mg (3/8 gr)
WARNING—May be habit-forming.

Indications: Amesec is used in the prevention and symptomatic treatment of asthma.

Contraindications: Since Amesec contains aminophylline and ephedrine, it should not be administered in the presence of massive myocardial damage and/or severe cardiac arrhythmias, marked hypertension, or hyperthyroidism. Because of its amobarbital content, Amesec is contraindicated in patients who are sensitive to the barbiturates and in those with a history of porphyria.

Warnings: The central-nervous-system-depressant effect of amobarbital may be additive with that of other C.N.S. depressants, including alcohol.

Usage in Pregnancy—Safety of this product for use during pregnancy has not been established.

Precautions: This product is not recommended for use in severely agitated patients. It should be administered with caution in persons who are overstimulated by ephedrine or other sympathomimetic drugs. Since the liver is the major site of degradation of barbiturates, caution should be observed when compounds containing these drugs are given to patients with impaired liver function, and lower doses should be used initially.

Adverse Reactions: Untoward effects are usually observed with overdosage. Occasionally, a patient who is hypersensitive to the C.N.S. stimulants may become hyperactive and emotionally upset and may complain of insomnia, nervousness, nausea, or vomiting. Tachycardia and extrasystoles may be produced.

Dosage: 1 to 5 Pulvules over a 24-hour period, or 1 Enseal one, two, or three times in each 24-hour period. To prevent nocturnal asthmatic attacks, 1 Pulvule plus 1 Enseal at bedtime.

Overdosage: *Symptoms*—Nervousness, emotional disturbances, insomnia, nausea, vomiting, tachycardia, and extrasystoles.

Treatment —No specific treatment; general management consists in control of C.N.S. stimulation by the administration of sedatives, such as the short-acting barbiturates.

How Supplied: (℞) *Enseals No. 56, Amesec® (aminophylline compound, Lilly), A27,** in bottles of 100.

(℞) *Pulvules No. 266, F47** (No. 3, Orange Body, Dark-Blue Cap), in bottles of 100 and 500.

[081778]

[Shown in Product Identification Section]

AMINOSALICYLIC ACID ℞
Tablets, NF

Description: Aminosalicylic acid is a white crystalline compound, soluble in water up to 0.2 percent. The chemical formula is $C_7H_7NO_3$. Aqueous solutions are very unstable, since decarboxylation with the formation of meta-aminophenol occurs. The same reaction takes place if the crystalline acid is exposed to moisture, air, or heat.

Enseals® (enteric-release tablets, Lilly) Aminosalicylic Acid are intended to reduce the incidence of gastrointestinal irritation.

Actions: Aminosalicylic acid has a bacteriostatic effect on the organism *Mycobacterium tuberculosis* and inhibits the development of bacterial resistance to streptomycin and isoniazid.

Indications: Aminosalicylic acid is effective in the treatment of pulmonary and extrapulmonary tuberculosis when it is administered with streptomycin, isoniazid, or both and when the organisms are susceptible to the effect of these drugs. Aminosalicylic acid should not be used as the sole therapeutic agent in the treatment of tuberculosis.

Contraindication: Severe hypersensitivity to aminosalicylic acid is a contraindication to the continued use of this drug.

Precautions: If symptoms suggestive of hypersensitivity develop, all medications should be stopped. After the drugs have been discontinued and the symptoms have abated, they may be restarted one at a time in very small but gradually increasing doses to determine whether the symptoms were drug induced and, if so, which medication was responsible. Oral hyposensitization to aminosalicylic acid is only occasionally successful.

Approximately 85 percent of aminosalicylic acid is excreted in the urine. Therefore, this drug should be used cautiously in patients with impaired renal function, decreased hepatic function, or gastric ulcer.

Patients who are being treated with anticoagulants may require an adjustment of the anticoagulant dosage.

Crystalluria due to aminosalicylic acid may be prevented by maintaining the urine at a neutral or alkaline *p*H.

Adverse Reactions: The most common side effect is gastrointestinal intolerance manifested by nausea, vomiting, diarrhea, and abdominal pain.

Continued on next page

*Identi-Code® symbol.

Lilly—Cont.

Hypersensitivity Reactions—Fever, skin eruptions of various types, infectious mononucleosis-like syndrome, leukopenia, agranulocytosis, thrombocytopenia, hemolytic anemia, jaundice, hepatitis, encephalopathy, Löffler's syndrome, and vasculitis.
Endocrine Reactions—Goiter with or without myxedema.
Homeostatic Reactions—Hypokalemia, acidosis.
Administration and Dosage: Aminosalicylic acid should be administered as part of a multiple-drug regimen which includes isoniazid, streptomycin, or both of these drugs.
The adult dosage is 10 to 12 gm orally per day in two or three divided doses. The pediatric dosage is 200 to 300 mg per kg orally per day in three or four divided doses.
Caution—Aminosalicylic acid and its salts deteriorate rapidly in contact with water, heat, and sunlight. A brownish or purplish color of the powder or tablets, and especially of a solution made with them, is indicative of such deterioration. If deterioration is evident, the drug should be discarded.
How Supplied: (℞) *Enseals No. 69, Aminosalicylic Acid Tablets, NF (Enteric), A30,** 500 mg (7½ grs), in bottles of 500.

[092975]

AMYL NITRITE ℞
Inhalant, NF

Description: Amyl nitrite, $C_5H_{11}NO_2$, is a clear, yellowish, volatile, and flammable liquid with a peculiar ethereal and fruity odor. As Aspirols® (inhalants in an ampoule, Lilly), it is supplied in fragile glass containers, enclosed in woven absorbent covering, which can be readily crushed between the fingers and held to the nostrils for inhalation.
Action: Amyl nitrite relaxes smooth muscles and is useful as a coronary vasodilator.
Indication: Amyl nitrite is used for relief of angina pectoris. Its effect appears within approximately 30 seconds and lasts for about three to five minutes.
Contraindications: Since it may increase intraocular and intracranial pressures, amyl nitrite is contraindicated, or should be used with great caution, in patients with glaucoma, head trauma, or cerebral hemorrhage.
Warnings: Transient episodes of dizziness, weakness, or syncope or other signs of cerebral ischemia due to postural hypotension may develop following inhalation of amyl nitrite, particularly if the patient is standing immobile. Measures which facilitate venous return, such as head-low posture, deep breathing, and movements of the extremities, may be used to hasten recovery.
Precautions: Tolerance to amyl nitrite may develop with repeated use of the drug for prolonged periods of time. Tolerance may be minimized by starting with the smallest effective dose and by alternating amyl nitrite with other coronary vasodilators.
Adverse Reactions: Mild transitory headache, dizziness, and flushing of the face are common with the use of amyl nitrite. The following adverse reactions may occur in susceptible patients: nausea, vomiting, weakness, restlessness, pallor, cold sweat, involuntary passing of urine and feces, tachycardia, hypotension, syncope, and collapse. Excessively high doses of amyl nitrite may cause methemoglobinemia.
Administration and Dosage: The usual adult dosage of amyl nitrite is 0.18 ml (Aspirol No. 2) or 0.3 ml (Aspirol No. 3) by inhalation as required.
How Supplied: (℞) *Aspirols Amyl Nitrite Inhalant, NF: No. 2,* 3 minims (0.18 ml), and *No. 3,* 5 minims (0.3 ml), in packages of 12. *Protect from light. CAUTION—FLAMMABLE.*

[062078]

AMYTAL® Ⓒ
(amobarbital)

Description: Amytal® (amobarbital, Lilly) is a moderately long-acting barbiturate.
Indications: Amytal® (amobarbital, Lilly) is indicated in any conditions that require degrees of sedation ranging from minimum doses for the relief of anxiety and tension to hypnotic doses for preanesthetic medication.
Contraindications: Amytal® (amobarbital, Lilly) is contraindicated in patients who are sensitive to the barbiturates and in those with a history of porphyria. Barbiturates should not be administered in the presence of uncontrolled pain, because excitement may be produced.
Warnings: May be habit-forming. Prolonged, uninterrupted use of barbiturates (particularly the short-acting drugs), even in therapeutic doses, may result in psychic and physical dependence.
The central-nervous-system depressant effect of amobarbital may be additive with that of other C.N.S. depressants, including alcohol.
Usage in Pregnancy—Safe use of Amytal® (amobarbital, Lilly) has not been established with respect to possible adverse effects on fetal development. Therefore, if this drug is to be given to pregnant women, particularly during early pregnancy, the potential benefits to the mother should be weighed against the possible risks to the fetus.
Usage in Ambulatory Patients—Amytal may impair the mental and/or physical abilities required for the performance of potentially hazardous tasks, such as driving a car or operating machinery. The patient should be cautioned accordingly.
Precaution: Since the liver is the major site of degradation of sedative-hypnotics, caution should be observed when these drugs are given to patients with impaired liver function, and lower doses should be used initially.
Adverse Reactions: Idiosyncrasy, in the form of excitement, hangover, or pain, may appear. Hypersensitivity reactions occur in some patients, especially in those with asthma, urticaria, or angioneurotic edema.
Dosage: Because of the wide variation in individual response to the barbiturates, the dosage range is relatively great, and doses must be individualized for each patient. The adult dosage range for daytime sedation may be from 15 to 120 mg two to four times a day. However, the usual adult dosage for daytime sedation is 30 to 50 mg two or three times a day. Dosage may be adjusted to relieve tension and anxiety without significant loss of mental acuity. The usual adult hypnotic dose is 100 to 200 mg. On occasion, a larger dose may be necessary to produce the desired degree of hypnosis.
Overdosage: C.N.S. depression. *Symptoms*—Respiratory depression, depression of superficial and deep reflexes, constriction of the pupils to a slight degree (though in severe poisoning they may dilate), decreased urine formation, lowered body temperature, and coma. *Treatment*—General management should consist in symptomatic and supportive therapy, including gastric lavage, administration of intravenous fluids, and maintenance of blood pressure, body temperature, and adequate respiratory exchange. Dialysis will increase the rate of removal of barbiturates from the body fluids.
How Supplied: (Ⓒ) *Elixir No. 237, Amytal® (amobarbital, Lilly),* 880 mg per 100 ml (Not NF), in 16-fl-oz bottles. Alcohol, 34 percent. This product differs from the NF elixir in that it contains a greater proportion of alcohol than the NF drug.
(Ⓒ) *Tablets Amytal® (Amobarbital Tablets, NF)* (scored): *No. 1575, T40,** 15 mg, Light-Green, in bottles of 100 and 500; *No. 1678, T56,** 30 mg, Yellow, in bottles of 100 and 1000; *No. 1550, T37,** 50 mg, Orange, and *No. 1462, T32,** 100 mg, Pink, in bottles of 100 and 500.

[102077]

[*Shown in Product Identification Section*]

AMYTAL® SODIUM Ⓒ
(amobarbital sodium)
Sterile, USP
AMPOULES

WARNING: MAY BE HABIT-FORMING
Caution: These products are to be used by the physician or under his direction. The intravenous administration of Amytal Sodium carries with it the potential dangers inherent in the intravenous use of any potent hypnotic.
Description: Amytal Sodium is a white, friable, granular powder that is odorless, has a bitter taste, and is hygroscopic. It is very soluble in water, soluble in alcohol, and practically insoluble in ether and chloroform. Amytal Sodium is sodium-5-ethyl-5-isopentylbarbiturate and has the empirical formula $C_{11}H_{17}N_2NaO_3$. Ampoules Amytal® Sodium (Sterile Amobarbital Sodium, USP, Lilly) are for parenteral administration. The ampoules contain 125 mg, 250 mg, or 0.5 gm sterile amobarbital sodium.
Clinical Pharmacology: Amobarbital sodium, a short-acting barbiturate, is a central-nervous-system depressant. It is a rapid-acting sedative and hypnotic, with a duration of effect ranging from eight to 11 hours. It is detoxified in the liver.
Indications and Usage: Amytal® Sodium (amobarbital sodium, Lilly) may be used intravenously or intramuscularly for the control of convulsive seizures such as may be due to chorea, eclampsia, meningitis, tetanus, procaine or cocaine reactions, or poisoning from such drugs as strychnine or picrotoxin. It may be administered for the management of catatonic and negativistic reactions, manic reactions, and epileptiform seizures. It is also useful in narcoanalysis and narcotherapy and as a diagnostic aid in schizophrenia.
Contraindications: Amytal® Sodium (amobarbital sodium, Lilly) is contraindicated in patients who are hypersensitive to barbiturates. It is also contraindicated in patients with a history of manifest or latent porphyria, marked impairment of liver function, or respiratory disease in which dyspnea or obstruction is evident. It should not be administered to persons with known previous addiction to the sedative/hypnotic group, since ordinary doses may be ineffectual and may contribute to further addiction. Amytal Sodium should not be administered in the presence of acute or chronic pain, because paradoxical excitement may be induced or important symptoms may be masked.
Warnings: The rate of intravenous injection must not exceed 1 ml per minute.
Either too-rapid injection or relative overdosage may cause apnea or hypotension. Respiratory depression is more likely to occur if other central-nervous-system agents have been used concurrently.
The maximum single dose should not exceed 1 gm in adult patients. The maximum intramuscular dose should not exceed 0.5 gm. No greater volume than 5 ml, irrespective of drug concentration, should be injected intramuscularly at any one site.
Several minutes may be required for the drug to dissolve completely, but under no circumstances should a solution be injected if it has not become absolutely clear within five minutes' time. Also, a solution that forms a precipitate after clearing should not be used. Amytal Sodium hydrolyzes in solution or upon exposure to air. Not more than 30 minutes should elapse from the time the ampoule is opened until its contents are injected. Amytal Sodium supplied in capsules should not be used for injection purposes.

Precautions: *General Precautions*—Barbiturates induce liver microsomal enzyme activity. This accelerates the biotransformation of various drugs and is probably part of the mechanism of the tolerance encountered with barbiturates. Amytal Sodium should, therefore, be used with caution in patients with decreased liver function. This drug should also be administered cautiously to patients with a history of drug dependence or abuse (*see* Drug Abuse and Dependence). Amytal Sodium may decrease the potency of coumarin anticoagulants; therefore, patients receiving such concomitant therapy should have more frequent prothrombin determinations.

As with other sedatives and hypnotics, elderly or debilitated patients may react to barbiturates with marked excitement or depression.

The systemic effects of exogenous hydrocortisone and endogenous hydrocortisone (cortisol) may be diminished by Amytal® Sodium (amobarbital sodium, Lilly). Thus, this product should be administered with caution to patients with borderline hypoadrenal function, regardless of whether it is of pituitary or of primary adrenal origin.

Information for Patients—Amytal Sodium may impair the mental and/or physical abilities required for the performance of potentially hazardous tasks, such as driving a car or operating machinery. The patient should be cautioned accordingly.

Drug Interactions—Amytal Sodium in combination with alcohol, tranquilizers, and other central-nervous-system depressants has additive depressant effects, and the patient should be so advised. Patients taking this drug should be warned not to exceed the dosage recommended by their physician. Toxic effects and fatalities have occurred following overdoses of Amytal Sodium alone and in combination with other central-nervous-system depressants. Caution should be exercised in prescribing unnecessarily large amounts of Amytal Sodium for patients who have a history of emotional disturbances or suicidal ideation or who have misused alcohol and other C.N.S. drugs (*see* overdosage).

Usage in Pregnancy—Pregnancy Category B—Reproduction studies have been performed in animals and have revealed no evidence of impaired fertility or harm to the fetus due to Amytal Sodium. There are, however, no adequate and well-controlled studies in pregnant women. Because animal reproduction studies are not always predictive of human response, this drug should be used during pregnancy only if clearly needed.

Labor and Delivery—Depression has been noted in infants born following the use of Amytal Sodium during labor.

Nursing Mothers—Caution should be exercised when Amytal Sodium is administered to a nursing woman.

Usage in Children—Safety and effectiveness have not been established in children below the age of six years.

Adverse Reactions: In the general use of barbiturates by the intravenous route, respiratory depression is the most serious side effect. Idiosyncrasy, in the form of excitement, hangover, or pain, may appear. Hypersensitivity reactions occur in some patients, especially in those with asthma, urticaria, or angioneurotic edema. Laryngospasm may develop during normal induction or as a result of improper dosage. Rapid intravenous administration may also induce vasodilation and some fall in blood pressure.

Nausea and vomiting, postoperative atelectasis, and circulatory disturbances are uncommon. When they occur, they are usually due to overdosage or extraneous factors. Embolism has not been reported following intravenous use of Amytal® Sodium (amobarbital sodium, Lilly).

Quantity of Sterile Water for Injection Required to Dilute the Contents of a Given Ampoule of Amytal Sodium to Obtain the Percentages Listed. Solutions Derived Will Be in Weight/Volume.

AMYTAL® SODIUM (amobarbital sodium, Lilly)

Ampoule Number	Content in Weight	1 Percent	2.5 Percent	5 Percent	10 Percent	20 Percent
362	125 mg	12.5 ml	5 ml	2.5 ml	1.25 ml	0.625 ml
363 and 386	250 mg	25 ml	10 ml	5 ml	2.5 ml	1.25 ml
364 and 387	0.5 gm	50 ml	20 ml	10 ml	5 ml	2.5 ml

Drug Abuse and Dependence: *Controlled Substance*—Amytal® Sodium (amobarbital sodium, Lilly) is a Schedule II drug.

Dependence—Prolonged, uninterrupted use of barbiturates (particularly the short-acting drugs), even in therapeutic doses, may result in psychic and physical dependence. Withdrawal symptoms due to physical dependence following chronic use of large doses of barbiturates may include delirium, convulsions, and death.

Overdosage: *Symptoms*—The manifestations of overdosage are early hypothermia followed by fever, sluggish or absent reflexes, respiratory depression, gradual appearance of circulatory collapse, pulmonary edema, and coma. *Treatment*—General management should consist in symptomatic and supportive therapy, including gastric lavage, administration of intravenous fluids, and maintenance of blood pressure, body temperature, and adequate respiratory exchange. Dialysis will increase the rate of removal of barbiturates from the body fluids. Antibiotics may be required to control pulmonary complications.

Administration and Dosage: Solutions of Amytal® Sodium (amobarbital sodium, Lilly) should be made up aseptically with Sterile Water for Injection. The accompanying table will aid in preparing solutions of various concentrations. Ordinarily, a 10 percent solution is used; the maximum single dose for an adult is 1 gm. After Sterile Water for Injection is added, the ampoule should be rotated to facilitate solution of the powder. **Do not shake the ampoule.**

[See table above].

Intramuscular Use—No more than 5 ml should be injected at any one site. Depositions should be made deeply in large muscles, such as the gluteus maximus. Superficial intramuscular or subcutaneous injections may be painful and may produce sterile abscesses or sloughs.

The average intramuscular dose ranges from 65 mg to 0.5 gm. Twenty percent solutions may be used so that a small volume can contain a large dose.

Intravenous Use—The rate of intravenous injection should not exceed 1 ml per minute. When the 10 percent solution is used, faster rates of administration may precipitate serious respiratory depression. Because of their higher metabolic rate, children tolerate comparatively larger doses. The final dosage is determined to a great extent by the patient's reaction to the slow administration of the drug. Ordinarily, 65 mg to 0.5 gm may be given to a child six to 12 years of age.

How Supplied: (Ⓒ) *Ampoules Amytal® Sodium (Sterile Amobarbital Sodium, USP)* (Dry Powder): *No. 362,* 125 mg, in packages of 6 (NDC 0002-1645-16); *No. 386,* 250 mg, in packages of 6 (NDC 0002-1654-16) and 25 (NDC 0002-1654-25); *No. 363,* 250 mg (NDC 0002-1646-01), in single ampoules (10 per carton); *No. 387,* 0.5 gm, in packages of 6 (NDC 0002-1655-16) and 25 (NDC 0002-1655-25); *No. 364,* 0.5 gm (NDC 0002-1647-01), in single ampoules (10 per carton). Ampoules No. 363 and No. 364 are supplied with accompanying ampoules of Sterile Water for Injection. [102379]

AMYTAL® SODIUM Ⓒ
(amobarbital sodium)
PULVULES®
Capsules, USP

WARNING: MAY BE HABIT-FORMING

Description: Amytal® Sodium (Amobarbital Sodium, USP, Lilly) is a white, friable, granular powder that is odorless, has a bitter taste, and is hygroscopic. It is very soluble in water, soluble in alcohol, and practically insoluble in ether and chloroform. Amytal Sodium is sodium-5-ethyl-5-isopentylbarbiturate and has the empirical formula $C_{11}H_{17}N_2NaO_3$.

Each Pulvule contains 65 or 200 mg of amobarbital sodium for oral administration.

Clinical Pharmacology: Amobarbital sodium, a short-acting barbiturate, is a central-nervous-system depressant. It is a rapid-acting sedative and hypnotic, with a duration of effect ranging from eight to 11 hours. It is detoxified in the liver.

Indications and Usage: Amytal® Sodium (amobarbital sodium, Lilly) is indicated for sedation and relief of anxiety (in minimum doses); for hypnotic effects; as preanesthetic medication; and to control convulsive disorders. The prolonged administration of Amytal Sodium is not recommended, since it has not been shown to be effective for a period of more than 14 days. If insomnia persists, drug-free intervals of one or more weeks should elapse before re-treatment is considered. Attempts should be made to find alternative nondrug therapy for chronic insomnia.

Contraindications: Amytal® Sodium (amobarbital sodium, Lilly) is contraindicated in patients who are hypersensitive to barbiturates. It is also contraindicated in patients with a history of manifest or latent porphyria, marked impairment of liver function, or respiratory disease in which dyspnea or obstruction is evident. It should not be administered to persons with known previous addiction to the sedative/hypnotic group, since ordinary doses may be ineffectual and may contribute to further addiction. Amytal Sodium should not be administered in the presence of acute or chronic pain, because paradoxical excitement may be induced or important symptoms may be masked.

Precautions: *General Precautions*—Barbiturates induce liver microsomal enzyme activity. This accelerates the biotransformation of various drugs and is probably part of the mechanism of the tolerance encountered with barbiturates. Amytal® Sodium (amobarbital sodium, Lilly) should, therefore, be used with caution in patients with decreased liver function. This drug should also be administered cautiously to patients with a history of drug dependence or abuse (*see* Drug Abuse and Dependence). Amytal Sodium may decrease the potency of coumarin anticoagulants; therefore, patients receiving such concomitant therapy should have more frequent prothrombin determinations. *Continued on next page*

*Identi-Code® symbol.

Lilly—Cont.

As with other sedatives and hypnotics, elderly or debilitated patients may react to barbiturates with marked excitement or depression.
The systemic effects of exogenous hydrocortisone and endogenous hydrocortisone (cortisol) may be diminished by Amytal Sodium. Thus, this product should be administered with caution to patients with borderline hypoadrenal function, regardless of whether it is of pituitary or of primary adrenal origin.
Information for Patients—Amytal Sodium may impair the mental and/or physical abilities required for the performance of potentially hazardous tasks, such as driving a car or operating machinery. The patient should be cautioned accordingly.
Drug Interactions—Amytal Sodium in combination with alcohol, tranquilizers, and other central-nervous-system depressants has additive depressant effects, and the patient should be so advised. Patients taking this drug should be warned not to exceed the dosage recommended by their physician. Toxic effects and fatalities have occurred following overdoses of Amytal Sodium alone and in combination with other central-nervous-system depressants. Caution should be exercised in prescribing unnecessarily large amounts of Amytal Sodium for patients who have a history of emotional disturbances or suicidal ideation or who have misused alcohol and other C.N.S. drugs (*see* Overdosage).
Usage in Pregnancy—Pregnancy Category B—Reproduction studies have been performed in animals and have revealed no evidence of impaired fertility or harm to the fetus due to Amytal Sodium. There are, however, no adequate and well-controlled studies in pregnant women. Because animal reproduction studies are not always predictive of human response, this drug should be used during pregnancy only if clearly needed.
Labor and Delivery—Depression has been noted in infants born following the use of Amytal® Sodium (amobarbital sodium, Lilly) during labor.
Nursing Mothers—Caution should be exercised when Amytal Sodium is administered to a nursing woman.
Usage in Children—Safety and effectiveness in children have not been established.
Adverse Reactions: The following adverse reactions have been reported:
C.N.S. Depression—Residual sedation or "hangover," drowsiness, lethargy.
Respiratory/Circulatory—Respiratory depression, apnea, circulatory collapse.
Allergic—Hypersensitivity reactions, especially in individuals with asthma, urticaria, angioneurotic edema, or similar conditions; skin eruptions.
Other—Nausea and vomiting; headache.
Drug Abuse and Dependence: *Controlled Substance*—Amytal® Sodium (amobarbital sodium, Lilly) is a Schedule II drug.
Dependence—Prolonged, uninterrupted use of barbiturates (particularly the short-acting drugs), even in therapeutic doses, may result in psychic and physical dependence. Withdrawal symptoms due to physical dependence following chronic use of large doses of barbiturates may include delirium, convulsions, and death.
Overdosage: *Symptoms* — The manifestations of overdosage are early hypothermia followed by fever, sluggish or absent reflexes, respiratory depression, gradual appearance of circulatory collapse, pulmonary edema, and coma. *Treatment* — General management should consist in symptomatic and supportive therapy, including gastric lavage, administration of intravenous fluids, and maintenance of blood pressure, body temperature, and adequate respiratory exchange. Dialysis will increase the rate of removal of barbiturates from the body fluids. Antibiotics may be required to control pulmonary complications.
Administration and Dosage: Because of the wide variation in individual response to the barbiturates, the dosage range is relatively great.
For insomnia, 65 to 200 mg by mouth at bedtime. For preanesthetic sedation, 200 mg one or two hours before surgery. In labor, the initial dose is 200 to 400 mg, and additional quantities of 200 to 400 mg may be given at one to three-hour intervals for a total dose of not more than 1 gm.
How Supplied: (©) *Pulvules Amytal® Sodium (Amobarbital Sodium Capsules, USP): No. 111, F23,** 65 mg (No. 4, Blue), in bottles of 100 (NDC 0002-0623-02) and 500 (NDC 0002-0623-03); *No. 222, F33,** 200 mg (No. 2, Blue), in bottles of 100 (NDC 0002-0633-02) and 500 (NDC 0002-0633-03) and in 10 strips of 10 individually labeled blisters each containing 1 Pulvule (ID100) (NDC 0002-0633-33).

[101679]

[*Shown in Product Identification Section*]

ANHYDRON® ℞
(cyclothiazide)
Tablets, NF

Description: Anhydron® (cyclothiazide, Lilly) is 6-chloro-3,4-dihydro-3-(5-norbornen-2-yl) - 7 - sulfamoyl - 1,2,4 - benzothiadiazine-1,1-dioxide. Cyclothiazide is a white crystalline solid with a melting point of approximately 220°C. It is moderately soluble in hot ethyl alcohol and hot dilute alcohol, very soluble in cold ethyl acetate (an ethyl acetate solvate is formed), and relatively insoluble in ether, benzene, or chloroform.
Action: The action of Anhydron® (cyclothiazide, Lilly) results in interference with electrolyte reabsorption by the renal tubules. At maximum therapeutic dosage, all thiazides have approximately equal diuretic potency. The mechanism by which thiazides function in the control of hypertension is unknown.
Indications: Anhydron® (cyclothiazide, Lilly) is indicated as adjunctive therapy in edema associated with congestive heart failure, hepatic cirrhosis, and corticosteroid and estrogen therapy.
Anhydron has also been found useful in edema due to various forms of renal dysfunction, such as nephrotic syndrome, acute glomerulonephritis, and chronic renal failure.
Anhydron is indicated in the management of hypertension either as the sole therapeutic agent or to enhance the effectiveness of other antihypertensive drugs in the more severe forms of hypertension.
Usage in Pregnancy—The routine use of diuretics in an otherwise healty woman is inappropriate and exposes mother and fetus to unnecessary hazard. Diuretics do not prevent development of toxemia of pregnancy, and there is no satisfactory evidence that they are useful in the treatment of developed toxemia.
Edema during pregnancy may arise from pathologic causes or from the physiologic and mechanical consequences of pregnancy. Thiazides are indicated in pregnancy when edema is due to pathologic causes, just as they are in the absence of pregnancy (however, see Warnings below). Dependent edema in pregnancy, resulting from restriction of venous return by the expanded uterus, is properly treated through elevation of the lower extremities and use of support hose; use of diuretics to lower intravascular volume in this case is illogical and unnecessary. There is hypervolemia during normal pregnancy which is harmful to neither the fetus nor the mother (in the absence of cardiovascular disease) but which is associated with edema, including generalized edema, in the majority of pregnant women. If this edema produces discomfort, increased recumbency will often provide relief. In rare instances, such edema may cause extreme discomfort that is not relieved by rest. In these cases, a short course of diuretics may provide relief and may be appropriate.
Contraindications: Anhydron® (cyclothiazide, Lilly) is contraindicated in anuria and in patients who are hypersensitive to cyclothiazide or other sulfonamide-derived drugs.
Warnings: Thiazides should be used with caution in severe renal disease. In patients with renal disease, thiazides may precipitate azotemia. Cumulative effects of the drug may develop in patients with impaired renal function.
Thiazides should be used with caution in patients with impaired hepatic function or progressive liver disease, since minor alterations of fluid and electrolyte balance may precipitate hepatic coma.
Thiazides may add to or potentiate the action of other antihypertensive drugs. Potentiation occurs with ganglionic or peripheral adrenergic blocking drugs.
Sensitivity reactions may occur in patients with a history of allergy or bronchial asthma.
The possibility of exacerbation or activation of systemic lupus erythematosus has been reported.
Usage in Pregnancy—Thiazides cross the placental barrier and appear in cord blood. The use of thiazides in pregnant women requires that the anticipated benefit be weighed against possible hazards to the fetus. These hazards include fetal or neonatal jaundice, thrombocytopenia, and possibly other adverse reactions which have occurred in the adult.
Nursing Mothers—Thiazides appear in breast milk. If use of the drug is deemed essential, the patient should stop nursing.
Precautions: Determination of serum electrolytes to detect possible imbalance should be performed at appropriate intervals.
All patients receiving thiazides should be observed for clinical signs of fluid or electrolyte imbalance, e.g., hyponatremia, hypochloremic alkalosis, and hypokalemia. Serum and urine electrolyte determinations are particularly important when the patient is vomiting excessively or receiving parenteral fluids. Medication such as digitalis may also influence serum electrolytes. Warning signs, irrespective of cause, are dryness of mouth, thirst, weakness, lethargy, drowsiness, restlessness, muscle pains or cramps, muscular fatigue, hypotension, oliguria, tachycardia, and gastrointestinal disturbances, such as nausea and vomiting.
Hypokalemia may develop with use of thiazides as with any other potent diuretic, especially with brisk diuresis, in the presence of severe cirrhosis, or during concomitant use of corticosteroids or ACTH. Interference with adequate oral electrolyte intake will also contribute to hypokalemia. Digitalis therapy may exaggerate metabolic effects of hypokalemia, especially in regard to myocardial activity.
Any chloride deficit is generally mild and usually does not require specific treatment except under extraordinary circumstances (as in liver or renal disease). Dilutional hyponatremia may occur in edematous patients in hot weather. Appropriate therapy is water restriction instead of administration of salt (except in rare instances when the hyponatremia is life threatening). In actual salt depletion, appropriate replacement is the therapy of choice.
Hyperuricemia may occur or frank gout may be precipitated in certain patients receiving thiazide therapy.
Insulin requirements in diabetic patients may be increased, decreased, or unchanged. Latent diabetes mellitus may become manifest during thiazide administration.
Thiazide drugs may increase the responsiveness to tubocurarine.
The antihypertensive effects of the drug may be enhanced in postsympathectomy patients.
Thiazides may decrease arterial responsiveness to norepinephrine. This diminution is not sufficient to preclude effectiveness of the pressor agent for therapeutic use.

If progressive renal impairment becomes evident, as indicated by a rising nonprotein nitrogen or blood urea nitrogen, therapy should be carefully reappraised, because it may be necessary to withhold or discontinue diuretic therapy.
Thiazides may decrease serum PBI levels without signs of thyroid disturbance.
Adverse Reactions: *Gastrointestinal* —Anorexia, gastric irritation, nausea, vomiting, cramping, diarrhea, constipation, jaundice (intrahepatic cholestatic jaundice), pancreatitis
Central Nervous System—Dizziness, vertigo, paresthesias, headache, xanthopsia
Hematologic—Leukopenia, agranulocytosis, thrombocytopenia, aplastic anemia
Dermatologic and Hypersensitivity—Purpura, photosensitivity, rash, urticaria, necrotizing angiitis (vasculitis or cutaneous vasculitis)
Cardiovascular—Orthostatic hypotension may occur and may be aggravated by alcohol, barbiturates, or narcotics.
Other—Hyperglycemia, glycosuria, hyperuricemia, muscle spasm, weakness, restlessness
Whenever adverse reactions are moderate or severe, thiazide dosage should be reduced or therapy withdrawn.
Administration and Dosage: Therapy should be individualized according to patient response. This therapy should be titrated to gain maximum therapeutic response as well as the minimum dose possible to maintain that therapeutic response.
For Diuretic Effect—The usual adult dosage of Anhydron® (cyclothiazide, Lilly) is ½ or 1 tablet (1 or 2 mg) once a day, preferably given early in the morning in order to obtain diuresis predominantly during the day and avoid disturbing the patient's rest at night. After the edema is eliminated, the dosage should be reduced according to the patient's need; body weight is usually a very helpful guide. For maintenance therapy, ½ or 1 tablet given on alternate days or two or three times a week frequently may be sufficient. Such an intermittent dosage schedule reduces the possibility of excessive depletion of body sodium and chloride or of potassium deficiency.
For Antihypertensive Effect—The dosage of Anhydron, like that of other thiazides, is often greater than that required for diuresis. The usual dosage of Anhydron is 1 tablet (2 mg) once a day; in some cases, it may be necessary to give 1 tablet two or three times a day.
Since Anhydron augments the action of other antihypertensive drugs, dosage of the latter should be reduced—perhaps to 50 percent of the usually recommended dosage—at the start of treatment and carefully readjusted upward or downward according to the patient's response and need.
How Supplied: (℞) *Tablets No. 1850, Anhydron® (Cyclothiazide Tablets, NF), U09,** 2 mg, Pink (capsule-shaped, scored), in bottles of 100 and 1000. [092478]
[*Shown in Product Identification Section*]

APOMORPHINE HYDROCHLORIDE ℞

Indications: For use as a centrally acting emetic. Results are usually obtained within ten to 15 minutes after parenteral administration.
Contraindications and Precautions: Do not use in impending shock states; in corrosive-poisoning cases; in narcosis due to opiates, barbiturates, alcohol, or other central-nervous-system depressants; or in patients too inebriated to stand unaided. Use with caution in children, debilitated individuals, those with cardiac decompensation, or persons predisposed to nausea and vomiting.
Adverse Reactions: Therapeutic doses may cause central-nervous-system depression; at times, however, euphoria, tachypnea, restlessness, and tremors may be produced. Peripheral vascular collapse has been reported. Dangerous depression, even death, may occur when the drug is used in patients who are in shock (as from corrosive poisons) or in those narcotized from overdoses of opiates, barbiturates, alcohol, or other central-nervous-system depressants. Excessive doses may cause violent emesis, cardiac depression, and death.
Dosage: *Adults*—Emesis, 5 mg subcutaneously (dosage ranges between 2 and 10 mg). *Do not repeat.*
How Supplied: (℞) *Soluble Tablets No. 7, Apomorphine Hydrochloride,* 6 mg, with lactose, q.s., in bottles of 100.
Note—These tablets should be protected from light and kept in tightly closed bottles. This preparation changes with age owing to conditions that are unavoidable, and we cannot be responsible for any discoloration that might occur. [030679]

ATROPINE SULFATE ℞
Injection, USP

Description: Atropine is a white crystalline alkaloid which may be extracted from belladonna root and hyoscyamine or may be produced synthetically. It is used in the form of atropine sulfate because this compound has much greater solubility in water.
Each ml contains 0.4 mg atropine sulfate, with chlorobutanol (chloroform derivative), 0.5 percent, as a preservative.
Actions: Atropine has two actions. The most important therapeutic action is the inhibition of smooth muscle and glands innervated by postganglionic cholinergic nerves. Atropine also has central-nervous-system activity, which may be stimulating or depressing depending upon the dose.
Indications: Atropine is given parenterally as preanesthetic medication in surgical patients to reduce salivation and bronchial secretions.
The antispasmodic action of atropine is useful in pylorospasm and other spastic conditions of the gastrointestinal tract. For ureteral and biliary colic, atropine concomitantly with morphine may be indicated.
In poisoning by the organic phosphate cholinesterase inhibitors found in certain insecticides and by chemical warfare "nerve gases," large doses of atropine relieve the muscarine-like symptoms and some of the central-nervous-system manifestations. Adults suspected of contact with organic phosphorus insecticides of the parathion type should be given atropine sulfate, 0.8 mg, intramuscularly. If an atropine effect is not apparent within 30 minutes or if definite symptoms of the poisoning occur (nausea, vomiting, diarrhea, pupillary constriction, pulmonary edema, fasciculations of eyelids and tongue, jerky ocular movements, and excessive sweating, salivation, and bronchial secretion), atropine sulfate, 2 mg, should be given intramuscularly at hourly intervals until signs of atropinization are observed. Up to two or three times this dose (4 to 6 mg) may be required in severe cases. Removing contaminated clothing, washing the skin, and commencing artificial respiration and supportive therapy are also indicated.
Contraindications: Glaucoma; adhesions (synechiae) between the iris and lens of the eye; asthma.
Precautions: Doses of 0.5 to 1 mg of atropine are mildly stimulating to the central nervous system. Larger doses may produce mental disturbances; still larger doses are depressing. Death from atropine poisoning, though rare, is usually due to paralysis of the medullary centers.
Adverse Reactions: Toxic effects from overdosage of atropine are not uncommon, especially in children. Individual tolerance varies greatly, but these systemic doses are likely to produce the following effects:
0.5 mg—Slight dryness of nose and mouth; bradycardia.
1 mg—Greater dryness of nose and mouth, with thirst; slowing, then acceleration, of heart; slight mydriasis.
2 mg—Very dry mouth; tachycardia, with palpitation, mydriasis, slight blurring of near vision; flushed, dry skin.
5 mg—Increase in above symptoms plus disturbance of speech; difficulty in swallowing; headache; hot, dry skin; restlessness, with asthenia.
10 mg and over—Above symptoms to extreme degree, plus ataxia, excitement, disorientation, hallucinations, delirium, and coma.
65 mg—May be fatal.
A scarlatiniform rash may occur. Atropine may produce fever, particularly in children, through inhibition of heat loss by evaporation. Although large doses of atropine may cause an alarming condition, recovery is usual.
In the treatment of atropine poisoning, respiratory assistance and symptomatic support are indicated. Pilocarpine is sometimes given but is of limited value.
Administration and Dosage: The usual adult dose of atropine is 0.4 to 0.6 mg. Suggested doses for children are as follows:
7-16 pounds—0.1 mg
17-24 pounds—0.15 mg
24-40 pounds—0.2 mg
40-65 pounds—0.3 mg
65-90 pounds—0.4 mg
Over 90 pounds—0.4 to 0.6 mg
As indicated previously, however, these doses may be considerably exceeded in certain cases.
How Supplied: (℞) *Ampoules (Vials) No. 419, Atropine Sulfate Injection, USP,* 0.4 mg per ml, 20 ml, rubber-stoppered, in singles (10 per carton). [020279]

ATROPINE SULFATE ℞
STERILE OPHTHALMIC OINTMENT

Description: Atropine is a white crystalline alkaloid extracted from belladonna root and hyoscyamine or produced synthetically. It is used in the form of atropine sulfate.
Indications: *Diagnostic*—To produce mydriasis and cycloplegia for thorough examination of the retina and optic disk and accurate measurement of refractive errors.
Therapeutic—To produce mydriasis and cycloplegia in the therapy of acute iritis, iridocyclitis, and keratitis. Complete cycloplegia may be necessary in the treatment of iridocyclitis and choroiditis.
Both the mydriasis and cycloplegia produced by a single instillation in healthy eyes may persist for several days, whereas two or three instillations a day may be required to maintain a full effect in the presence of acute inflammation.
Contraindication: Glaucoma.
Precautions: Great care should be exercised in treating patients with any suggestion of increased intraocular pressure. An attack of acute glaucoma may be precipitated, with deleterious effects.
Intraocular pressure of all older patients should be measured before the drug is administered.
Adverse Reactions: Atropine occasionally causes local irritation of the eye and, in susceptible persons, may produce swelling of the eyelids and conjunctivitis. With continued use of the drug, the conjunctivitis may become chronic.
Administration and Dosage: Apply a small amount of ointment into the conjunctival sac and repeat as necessary to produce the desired intensity and duration of effect.
How Supplied: (℞) *Sterile Ophthalmic Ointment No. 6, Atropine Sulfate, 1%,* in 1/8-oz tamperproof tubes. [082878]

Continued on next page

*Identi-Code® symbol.

Lilly—Cont.

ATROPINE SULFATE ℞
Soluble Tablets and Tablets

Description: Atropine is a white crystalline alkaloid which may be extracted from belladonna root and hyoscyamine or may be produced synthetically. It is used in the form of atropine sulfate because this compound has much greater solubility in water.
Each soluble tablet contains 0.3 mg, 0.4 mg, or 0.6 mg atropine sulfate and lactose.
Each tablet contains 0.4 mg atropine sulfate.
Actions: Atropine has two actions. The most important therapeutic action is the inhibition of smooth muscle and glands innervated by postganglionic cholinergic nerves. Atropine also has central-nervous-system activity, which may be stimulating or depressing depending on the dose.
Indications: Atropine is used to reduce salivation and bronchial secretions.
The antispasmodic action of atropine is useful in pylorospasm and other spastic conditions of the gastrointestinal tract. For ureteral and biliary colic, atropine concomitantly with morphine may be indicated.
In poisoning by the organic phosphate cholinesterase inhibitors found in certain insecticides and by chemical warfare "nerve gases," large doses of atropine relieve the muscarine-like symptoms and some of the central-nervous-system manifestations (*see under* Administration and Dosage).
Contraindications: Narrow-angle glaucoma; adhesions (synechiae) between the iris and lens of the eye.
Precautions: Doses of 0.5 to 1 mg of atropine are mildly stimulating to the central nervous system. Larger doses may produce mental disturbances; still larger doses are depressing. Atropine should be used cautiously in asthmatic patients.
Adverse Reactions: Individual tolerance varies greatly, but these systemic doses are likely to produce the following effects:
0.5 mg—Slight dryness of nose and mouth; bradycardia.
1 mg—Greater dryness of nose and mouth, with thirst; slowing, then acceleration, of heart; slight mydriasis.
2 mg—Very dry mouth; tachycardia, with palpitation, mydriasis, slight blurring of near vision; flushed, dry skin.
5 mg—Increase in above symptoms plus disturbance of speech; difficulty in swallowing; headache; hot, dry skin; restlessness, with asthenia.
10 mg and over—Above symptoms to extreme degree, plus ataxia, excitement, disorientation, hallucinations, delirium, and coma.
65 mg—May be fatal.
A scarlatiniform rash may occur. Atropine may produce fever, particularly in children, through inhibition of heat loss by evaporation.
Although large doses of atropine may cause an alarming condition, recovery is usual.
Toxic effects from overdosage of atropine are not uncommon, especially in children. In the treatment of atropine poisoning, respiratory assistance and symptomatic support are indicated. Neostigmine methylsulfate in doses of 0.5 to 1 mg should be given intramuscularly every two to three hours, followed by 15 mg of neostigmine bromide orally when the patient improves.
Death from atropine poisoning, though rare, is usually due to paralysis of the medullary centers.
Administration and Dosage: The usual oral adult dose of atropine is 0.4 to 0.6 mg.
Adults suspected of contact with organic phosphorus insecticides of the parathion type should be given atropine sulfate, 0.8 mg, intramuscularly. If an atropine effect is not apparent within 30 minutes or if definite symptoms of the poisoning occur (nausea, vomiting, diarrhea, pupillary constriction, pulmonary edema, fasciculations of eyelids and tongue, jerky ocular movements, and excessive sweating, salivation, and bronchial secretion), atropine sulfate, 2 mg, should be given intramuscularly at hourly intervals until signs of atropinization are observed. Up to two or three times this dose (4 to 6 mg) may be required in severe cases. Removing contaminated clothing, washing the skin, and commencing artificial respiration and supportive therapy are also indicated.
Suggested doses for children are as follows:
7–16 pounds—0.1 mg
17–24 pounds—0.15 mg
24–40 pounds—0.2 mg
40–65 pounds—0.3 mg
65–90 pounds—0.4 mg
Over 90 pounds—0.4 to 0.6 mg
These doses may be exceeded in certain cases.
How Supplied: (℞) *Tablets No. 205, Atropine Sulfate, USP, J02,* * 0.4 mg, in bottles of 100.
(℞) *Soluble Tablets Atropine Sulfate: No. 14,* 0.3 mg, *No. 15,* 0.4 mg, and *No. 17,* 0.6 mg, in bottles of 100. Contain lactose, q.s. [041279]

AVENTYL® HCL ℞
(nortriptyline hydrochloride) NF

Description: Aventyl® HCl (nortriptyline hydrochloride, Lilly) is 5-(3-methylaminopropylidene)-10,11-dihydro-5H-dibenzo [a,d] cycloheptene hydrochloride. Its molecular weight is 299.8, and its empirical formula is $C_{19}H_{21}N \bullet HCl$.
Actions: The mechanism of mood elevation by tricyclic antidepressants is at present unknown. Aventyl® HCl (nortriptyline hydrochloride, Lilly) is not a monoamine oxidase inhibitor. It inhibits the activity of such diverse agents as histamine, 5-hydroxytryptamine, and acetylcholine. It increases the pressor effect of norepinephrine but blocks the pressor response of phenethylamine. Studies suggest that Aventyl HCl interferes with the transport, release, and storage of catecholamines. Operant conditioning techniques in rats and pigeons suggest that Aventyl HCl has a combination of stimulant and depressant properties.
Indications: Aventyl® HCl (nortriptyline hydrochloride, Lilly) is indicated for the relief of symptoms of depression. Endogenous depressions are more likely to be alleviated than are other depressive states.
Contraindications: The use of Aventyl® HCl (nortriptyline hydrochloride, Lilly) or other tricyclic antidepressants concurrently with a monoamine oxidase (MAO) inhibitor is contraindicated. Hyperpyretic crises, severe convulsions, and fatalities have occurred when similar tricyclic antidepressants were used in such combinations. It is advisable to have discontinued the MAO inhibitor for at least two weeks before treatment with Aventyl HCl is started. Patients hypersensitive to Aventyl HCl should not be given the drug.
Cross-sensitivity between Aventyl HCl and other dibenzazepines is a possibility.
Aventyl HCl is contraindicated during the acute recovery period after myocardial infarction.
Warnings: Patients with cardiovascular disease should be given Aventyl® HCl (nortriptyline hydrochloride, Lilly) only under close supervision because of the tendency of the drug to produce sinus tachycardia and to prolong the conduction time. Myocardial infarction, arrhythmia, and strokes have occurred. The antihypertensive action of guanethidine and similar agents may be blocked. Because of its anticholinergic activity, Aventyl HCl should be used with great caution in patients who have glaucoma or a history of urinary retention. Patients with a history of seizures should be followed closely when Aventyl HCl is administered, inasmuch as this drug is known to lower the convulsive threshold. Great care is required if Aventyl HCl is given to hyperthyroid patients or to those receiving thyroid medication, since cardiac arrhythmias may develop.
Aventyl HCl may impair the mental and/or physical abilities required for the performance of hazardous tasks, such as operating machinery or driving a car; therefore, the patient should be warned accordingly.
Excessive consumption of alcohol in combination with nortriptyline therapy may have a potentiating effect, which may lead to the danger of increased suicidal attempts or overdosage, especially in patients with histories of emotional disturbances or suicidal ideation.
Use in Pregnancy—Safe use of Aventyl HCl during pregnancy and lactation has not been established; therefore, when the drug is administered to pregnant patients, nursing mothers, or women of childbearing potential, the potential benefits must be weighed against the possible hazards. Animal reproduction studies have yielded inconclusive results.
Use in Children—This drug is not recommended for use in children, since safety and effectiveness in the pediatric age group have not been established.
Precautions: The use of Aventyl® HCl (nortriptyline hydrochloride, Lilly) in schizophrenic patients may result in an exacerbation of the psychosis or may activate latent schizophrenic symptoms. If the drug is given to overactive or agitated patients, increased anxiety and agitation may occur. In manic-depressive patients, Aventyl HCl may cause symptoms of the manic phase to emerge.
Administration of reserpine during therapy with a tricyclic antidepressant has been shown to produce a "stimulating" effect in some depressed patients.
Troublesome patient hostility may be aroused by the use of Aventyl HCl. Epileptiform seizures may accompany its administration, as is true of other drugs of its class.
Close supervision and careful adjustment of the dosage are required when Aventyl HCl is used with other anticholinergic drugs and sympathomimetic drugs.
The patient should be informed that the response to alcohol may be exaggerated.
When it is essential, the drug may be administered with electroconvulsive therapy, although the hazards may be increased. Discontinue the drug for several days, if possible, prior to elective surgery.
The possibility of a suicidal attempt by a depressed patient remains after the initiation of treatment; in this regard, it is important that the least possible quantity of drug be dispensed at any given time.
Both elevation and lowering of blood sugar levels have been reported.
Adverse Reactions: Note—Included in the following list are a few adverse reactions that have not been reported with this specific drug. However, the pharmacologic similarities among the tricyclic antidepressant drugs require that each of the reactions be considered when nortriptyline is administered.
Cardiovascular—Hypotension, hypertension, tachycardia, palpitation, myocardial infarction, arrhythmias, heart block, stroke.
Psychiatric—Confusional states (especially in the elderly) with hallucinations, disorientation, delusions; anxiety, restlessness, agitation; insomnia, panic, nightmares; hypomania; exacerbation of psychosis.
Neurologic—Numbness, tingling, paresthesias of extremities; incoordination, ataxia, tremors; peripheral neuropathy; extrapyramidal symptoms; seizures, alteration in EEG patterns; tinnitus.
Anticholinergic—Dry mouth and, rarely, associated sublingual adenitis; blurred vision, disturbance of accommodation, mydriasis; consti-

pation, paralytic ileus; urinary retention, delayed micturition, dilation of the urinary tract.

Allergic—Skin rash, petechiae, urticaria, itching, photosensitization (avoid excessive exposure to sunlight); edema (general or of face and tongue), drug fever, cross-sensitivity with other tricyclic drugs.

Hematologic—Bone marrow depression, including agranulocytosis; eosinophilia; purpura; thrombocytopenia.

Gastrointestinal—Nausea and vomiting, anorexia, epigastric distress, diarrhea; peculiar taste, stomatitis, abdominal cramps, black-tongue.

Endocrine—Gynecomastia in the male; breast enlargement and galactorrhea in the female; increased or decreased libido, impotence; testicular swelling; elevation or depression of blood sugar levels.

Other—Jaundice (simulating obstructive); altered liver function; weight gain or loss; perspiration; flushing; urinary frequency, nocturia; drowsiness, dizziness, weakness, fatigue; headache; parotid swelling; alopecia.

Withdrawal Symptoms—Though these are not indicative of addiction, abrupt cessation of treatment after prolonged therapy may produce nausea, headache, and malaise.

Administration and Dosage: Aventyl® HCl (nortriptyline hydrochloride, Lilly) is not recommended for children.

Aventyl HCl is administered orally in the form of Pulvules® or liquid. Lower than usual dosages are recommended for elderly patients and adolescents. Lower dosages are also recommended for outpatients than for hospitalized patients who will be under close supervision. The physician should initiate dosage at a low level and increase it gradually, noting carefully the clinical response and any evidence of intolerance. Following remission, maintenance medication may be required for a longer period of time at the lowest dose that will maintain remission.

If a patient develops minor side effects, the dosage should be reduced. The drug should be discontinued promptly if adverse effects of a serious nature or allergic manifestations occur.

Usual Adult Dose—25 mg three or four times daily; dosage should begin at a low level and be increased as required. Doses above 100 mg per day are not recommended.

Elderly and Adolescent Patients—30 to 50 mg per day, in divided doses.

Overdosage: Toxic overdosage may result in confusion, restlessness, agitation, vomiting, hyperpyrexia, muscle rigidity, hyperactive reflexes, tachycardia, ECG evidence of impaired conduction, shock, congestive heart failure, stupor, coma, and C.N.S. stimulation with convulsions followed by respiratory depression. Deaths have occurred following overdosage with drugs of this class.

No specific antidote is known. General supportive measures are indicated, with gastric lavage. Respiratory assistance is apparently the most effective measure when indicated. The use of C.N.S. depressants may worsen the prognosis.

The administration of barbiturates for control of convulsions alleviates an increase in the cardiac work load but should be undertaken with caution to avoid potentiation of respiratory depression.

Intramuscular paraldehyde or diazepam provides anticonvulsant activity with less respiratory depression than do the barbiturates; diazepam seems to be preferred.

The use of digitalis and/or physostigmine may be considered in case of serious cardiovascular abnormalities or cardiac failure.

The value of dialysis has not been established.

How Supplied: (℞) *Liquid No. 38, Aventyl® HCl (Nortriptyline Hydrochloride Solution, NF),* 10 mg (equivalent to base) per 5 ml, in 16-fl-oz bottles. Alcohol, 4 percent.

(℞) *Pulvules Aventyl® HCl (Nortriptyline Hydrochloride Capsules, NF): No. 387, H17** (No. 3, White Opaque Body, Yellow Opaque Cap), 10 mg (equivalent to base), and *No. 389, H19** (No. 1, White Opaque Body, Yellow Opaque Cap), 25 mg (equivalent to base), in bottles of 100 and 500 and in 10 strips of 10 individually labeled blisters each containing 1 Pulvule (ID100).

[081678]

[*Shown in Product Identification Section*]

Pulvules No. 389, 25 mg—
100's—6505-00-926-4773

BETALIN® COMPLEX ℞
(vitamin B complex)
AMPOULES and VIALS

Description: Ampoules and Vials Betalin Complex contain a sterile solution of synthetic B complex factors in sterile distilled water for intramuscular or slow intravenous injection.

Each ml of material in both the ampoules and the vials contains—

Thiamine Hydrochloride (Vitamin B_1)	5 mg
Riboflavin (as Riboflavin 5′ Phosphate Sodium) (Vitamin B_2)	2 mg
Niacinamide	75 mg
Pantothenic Acid (as Panthenol)	2.5 mg
Pyridoxine (Vitamin B_6) Hydrochloride	5 mg
Cyanocobalamin (Vitamin B_{12} Crystalline)	2.5 mcg

Phenol, 0.5 percent, as a preservative.

These are "ready-to-use" preparations; no reconstitution is necessary.

Indications: Betalin Complex is indicated in the prevention and treatment of vitamin B complex deficiencies.

Administration of these factors by injection is necessary whenever rapid tissue saturation is desirable and in severe vitamin depletion states in which absorption from the gastrointestinal tract is likely to be impaired.

Parenteral administration of vitamin B complex is required when prolonged intravenous administration of fluids replaces oral feeding, as in burns, before or after surgery, and in severe illnesses and fractures. If extensive resection of the gastrointestinal tract prevents adequate absorption of vitamins, it may be necessary to give them parenterally to maintain normal nutrition.

Contraindication: Betalin Complex is contraindicated in patients who are allergic to thiamine.

Precautions: The products should be refrigerated as indicated on the label. If storage and handling requirements are not observed, a precipitate may develop in the solution. If this occurs, the material should not be used.

The patient should be advised as to proper dietary habits during treatment so that relapses will be less likely to occur with reduction in dosage or cessation of injection therapy.

Adverse Reactions: An occasional individual may develop a sensitivity or intolerance to thiamine, especially after repeated intravenous administration.

Some tenderness and induration may follow intramuscular use.

Administration and Dosage: Intramuscular injection is preferred. When the intravenous route is used, the material may be given slowly undiluted or may be diluted to avoid "speed reactions." For dilution, normal saline or sterile distilled water may be employed.

Administration with intravenous dextrose infusions is facilitated by injection into the rubber tubing after the infusion is flowing or by direct addition to the contents of the flask. With the latter technique, light should be excluded from the flask. If continuous intravenous-drip infusion is used, the material should be injected into the rubber tubing at appropriate intervals to avoid loss of vitamin potency, which may occur after long standing in dilute glucose solution. Aseptic technique is required with either procedure.

The amount to be administered will depend upon an appraisal of the vitamin B content of the diet that the patient can and will employ, his condition, and whether it is prophylaxis or treatment that is required.

Ordinarily, 2 ml at each injection should be adequate, although 5 ml or even more may be given if indicated. Frequency of injection and length of treatment will depend upon the severity of the patient's condition. A suggested amount to use in initiating therapy in adults is 2 ml daily, and this dosage should be decreased or increased as dictated by the patient's difficulties and his response to therapy. Children require proportionately less.

When used with dextrose or other infusions for prophylactic treatment, 2 to 10 ml for each liter of 5 or 10 percent solution are indicated.

How Supplied: (℞) *Betalin® Complex (vitamin B complex, Lilly): Ampoules No. 390,* 2 ml, in packages of 100; *Ampoules (Vials) No. 391,* 10 ml, rubber-stoppered, in singles (10 per carton) and in packages of 25. *Refrigerate.* [010579]

BETALIN® COMPLEX F.C. ℞
(vitamin B complex, fortified, +vitamin C)

Description: Ampoules and Vials Betalin Complex F.C. contain synthetic vitamin B factors and synthetic ascorbic acid in sterile distilled water.

Each ml of material in both the ampoules and vials contains—

Thiamine Hydrochloride	12.5 mg
Riboflavin (as Riboflavin 5′ Phosphate Sodium)	3 mg
Niacinamide	50 mg
Pantothenic Acid (as Panthenol)	2.5 mg
Pyridoxine Hydrochloride	5 mg
Ascorbic Acid	75 mg
Benzyl Alcohol	2 percent

Phenol, 0.25 percent, is employed as a preservative, and sodium hydroxide is added during manufacture to adjust the *p*H.

These are "ready-to-use" preparations; no reconstitution is necessary.

Indications: Betalin Complex F.C. is indicated in the prevention and treatment of vitamin B complex deficiencies.

Administration of these factors by injection is necessary whenever rapid tissue saturation is desirable and in severe vitamin depletion states in which absorption from the gastrointestinal tract is likely to be impaired.

Parenteral administration of vitamin B complex is required when prolonged intravenous administration of fluids replaces oral feeding, as in burns, before or after surgery, and in severe illnesses and fractures. If extensive resection of the gastrointestinal tract prevents adequate absorption of vitamins, it may be necessary to give them parenterally to maintain normal nutrition.

Contraindication: Betalin Complex F.C. is contraindicated in patients who are allergic to thiamine.

Precautions: The products should be refrigerated as indicated on the label. If storage and handling requirements are not observed, a precipitate may develop in the solution. If this occurs, the material should not be used.

The patient should be advised as to proper dietary habits during treatment so that relapses will be less likely to occur with reduction in dosage or cessation of injection therapy.

Adverse Reactions: An occasional individual may develop a sensitivity or intolerance to thiamine, especially after repeated intravenous administration.

Continued on next page

*Identi-Code® symbol.

Lilly—Cont.

Some tenderness and induration may follow intramuscular use.

Administration and Dosage: Intramuscular injection is preferred. When the intravenous route is used, the material may be given slowly undiluted or may be diluted to avoid "speed reactions." For dilution, normal saline or sterile distilled water may be employed.

Administration with intravenous dextrose infusions is facilitated by injection into the rubber tubing after the infusion is flowing or by direct addition to the contents of the flask. With the latter technique, light should be excluded from the flask. If continuous intravenous-drip infusion is used, the material should be injected into the rubber tubing at appropriate intervals to avoid loss of vitamin potency, which may occur after long standing in dilute glucose solution. Aseptic technique is required with either procedure.

The amount to be administered will depend upon an appraisal of the vitamin B and vitamin C content of the diet that the patient can and will employ, his condition, and whether it is prophylaxis or treatment that is required. Ordinarily, 2 ml at each injection should be adequate, although 5 ml or even more may be given if indicated. Frequency of injection and length of treatment will depend upon the severity of the patient's condition. A suggested amount to use in initiating therapy in adults is 2 ml daily, and this dosage should be decreased or increased as dictated by the patient's difficulties and his response to therapy. Children require proportionately less.

When used with dextrose or other infusions for prophylactic treatment, 2 to 10 ml for each liter of 5 or 10 percent solution are indicated.

How Supplied: (℞) *Betalin® Complex F.C. (vitamin B complex, fortified, + vitamin C, Lilly): Ampoules No. 620,* 2 ml, in packages of 100; *Ampoules (Vials) No. 621,* 10 ml, rubber-stoppered, in singles (10 per carton) and in packages of 25. *Refrigerate. Avoid freezing.*

[111478]

BILRON® OTC
(iron bile salts)

Description: Pulvules® Bilron contain those naturally occurring bile salts from the gallbladder bile of cattle which, when combined with iron, are insoluble in an acid medium. Bilron is inactive in the stomach because it is insoluble in an acid medium. When Bilron enters the alkaline medium of the small intestine, the iron moiety separates, and the bile salts become soluble and physiologically active like endogenously produced bile salts. Bile from cattle is used because the bile-salt content (chiefly salts of cholic, deoxycholic, lithocholic, and sterocholic acids conjugated with glycine and taurine) is similar to that of human bile.

Indications: Bilron is indicated as a physiologic laxative in the symptomatic treatment of uncomplicated constipation.

Contraindications: Bilron is nontoxic in therapeutic doses, and no absolute contraindications to its use have been recognized. However, on theoretical grounds, Bilron should be withheld from patients with complete biliary obstruction.

Precautions: In marked hepatic insufficiency (as in viral hepatitis, suppurative cholangitis, and advanced cirrhosis), therapy with Bilron should be avoided except in the presence of malnutrition with steatorrhea and vitamin K deficiency with hypoprothrombinemia.

Adverse Reactions: Excessive doses can cause loose stools and mild cramping, which are indications for a reduction in dosage.

Administration and Dosage: In adults, the usual dose is 150 to 450 mg, with or after meals, until constipation is relieved.

Overdosage: *Symptoms*—Loose stools and gastrointestinal cramping. *Treatment*—For general management, symptomatic therapy should be employed.

How Supplied: *Pulvules Bilron® (iron bile salts, Lilly): No. 298, F61,** 150 mg (2½ grs) (No. 2, Green), in bottles of 100; *No. 241, F41,** 300 mg (5 grs) (No. 0, Green), in bottles of 100 and 500.

[060178]

BREVITAL® SODIUM ℭ
(methohexital sodium)
For Injection, USP
For Intravenous Use

WARNING

This drug should be administered by persons qualified in the use of intravenous anesthetics and with the ready availability of appropriate resuscitative equipment for prevention and treatment of anesthetic emergencies.

Description: Brevital® Sodium (Methohexital Sodium for Injection, USP, Lilly) is sodium α-*dl*-1-methyl-5-allyl-5-(1-methyl-2-pentynyl) barbiturate. It differs chemically from the established barbiturate anesthetics in that it contains no sulfur.

Action: Methohexital sodium is a rapid, ultrashort-acting barbiturate anesthetic agent.

Indications: For induction of anesthesia, for supplementing other anesthetic agents, as intravenous anesthesia for short surgical procedures with minimum painful stimuli, or as an agent for inducing a hypnotic state.

Contraindications: Methohexital sodium is contraindicated when general anesthesia is contraindicated, in patients with latent or manifest porphyria, or in patients with a known hypersensitivity to barbiturates.

Warnings: May be habit-forming.

Repeated or continuous infusion may cause cumulative effects resulting in prolonged somnolence and respiratory and circulatory depression.

Usage in Pregnancy—Safe use of methohexital sodium has not been established with respect to possible adverse effects on human fetal development. Therefore, if methohexital sodium is to be given to women who are pregnant, the benefits to the mother should be weighed against possible risks to the fetus. When administered to pregnant rabbits and rats at four and seven times the human dose respectively, methohexital sodium produced no evidence of teratogenicity and no fetal abnormalities.

Precautions: Respiratory depression, apnea, or hypotension may occur owing to variations in tolerance from individual to individual or to the physical status of the patient. Caution should be exercised in debilitated patients or in those with impaired function of respiratory, circulatory, renal, hepatic, or endocrine systems.

Methohexital sodium should be used with extreme caution in patients in status asthmaticus.

Extravascular injection may cause pain, swelling, ulceration, and necrosis. Intra-arterial injection is dangerous and may produce gangrene of an extremity. The central-nervous-system depressant effect of methohexital sodium may be additive with that of other C.N.S. depressants, including alcohol.

Adverse Reactions: The following reactions have been reported:

- Circulatory depression
- Thrombophlebitis
- Pain at injection site
- Respiratory depression, including apnea
- Laryngospasm
- Bronchospasm
- Salivation
- Hiccups
- Skeletal-muscle hyperactivity (twitching to convulsive-like movements)
- Emergence delirium
- Headache
- Injury to nerves adjacent to injection site
- Nausea
- Emesis

Acute allergic reactions, such as erythema, pruritus, urticaria, rhinitis, dyspnea, hypotension, restlessness, anxiety, abdominal pain, and peripheral vascular collapse, have been reported with the use of Brevital® Sodium (methohexital sodium, Lilly).

Administration and Dosage: Preanesthetic medication is generally advisable. Brevital® Sodium (methohexital sodium, Lilly) may be used with any of the recognized preanesthetic medications, but the phenothiazines are less satisfactory than the combination of an opiate and a belladonna derivative.

Facilities for assisting respirations and administering oxygen are necessary adjuncts for intravenous anesthesia.

[See table below].

For continuous drip anesthesia, prepare a 0.2% solution by adding 500 mg of Brevital Sodium to 250 ml of diluent. For this dilution, we recommend as solvents either 5% glucose solution or isotonic (0.9%) sodium chloride solution instead of distilled water in order to avoid extreme hypotonicity.

Administration—A 1% solution is recommended for induction of anesthesia and for maintenance by intermittent injection. Dosage of all intravenous barbiturates must be individualized according to the patient's response. The usual range for Brevital® Sodium (methohexital sodium, Lilly) is 5 to 12 ml of a 1% solution (50 to 120 mg). This induction dose will provide anesthesia for five to seven minutes. The rate of injection is not fixed, but it is usu-

Preparation of Solution—FOLLOW DILUTING INSTRUCTIONS EXACTLY.

Diluents—DO NOT USE DILUENTS CONTAINING BACTERIOSTATS.

Sterile Water for Injection is the preferred diluent.

Dextrose Injection (5%) or Sodium Chloride Injection (0.9%) may be used.

(Brevital Sodium is not compatible with Lactated Ringer's Injection.)

Dilution Instructions—For a 1% solution (10 mg per ml), contents of vials should be diluted as follows:

Ampoules (Vials) No. 660 (500 mg)—add 50 ml of diluent
Ampoules (Vials) No. 760 (500 mg)—add 50 ml of accompanying diluent
Ampoules (Vials) No. 664 (2.5 gm)—add 250 ml of diluent
Ampoules (Vials) No. 662 (5 gm)—add 500 ml of diluent

Ampoule (Vial) No.	Amount of Diluent to Be Added to the Vial	For 1 Percent Solution Dilute to
663 (2.5 gm)	15 ml	250 ml
659 (5 gm)	30 ml	500 ml

When the first dilution is made with Ampoules (Vials) No. 663 or No. 659, the solution in the vial will be yellow. When further diluted to make a 1% solution, it must be *clear and colorless* or should not be used.

ally found to be about 1 ml of the 1% solution (10 mg) in five seconds. If intermittent injection of a 1% solution is used for maintenance, additional amounts of about 2 to 4 ml (20 to 40 mg) will be required every four to seven minutes.

Some anesthesiologists have preferred the continuous drip method of maintenance with a 0.2% solution. The rate of flow must be individualized for each patient. As a guide, 1 drop per second may be used.

Storage—Brevital Sodium is stable in Sterile Water for Injection at room temperature (25°C or below) for at least *six weeks.* Dextrose Injection (5%) or isotonic (0.9%) sodium chloride injection may be used as diluents, but these solutions are not stable for much more than *24 hours.* Solutions may be stored and used as long as they remain clear and colorless.

Compatibility Information: Solutions of Brevital® Sodium (methohexital sodium, Lilly) should not be mixed with acid solutions such as atropine sulfate, Metubine® Iodide (Metocurine Iodide Injection, NF, Lilly), and succinylcholine chloride. However, because of numerous requests from anesthesiologists for information regarding the chemical compatibility of these mixtures, the following is provided.

The soluble sodium salts of barbiturates are the forms used for intravenous administration. Solubility is maintained only at a relatively high (basic) *p*H. The accompanying chart contains information obtained from compatibility studies in which a 1% solution of Brevital Sodium was mixed with therapeutic amounts of agents whose solutions have a low (acid) *p*H.

Solutions of Brevital Sodium are incompatible with silicone and should not be allowed to come in contact with rubber stoppers or parts of disposable syringes that have been treated with silicone.

[See table below].

Active Ingredient	Potency per ml	Volume Used	Physical Change: Immediate	15 min	30 min	1 hr
BREVITAL® SODIUM (methohexital sodium, Lilly)	10 mg	10 ml		CONTROL		
Atropine sulfate	1/150 gr	1 ml	None	Haze		
Atropine sulfate	1/100 gr	1 ml	None	Ppt.	Ppt.	
Succinylcholine chloride	0.5 mg	4 ml	None	None	Haze	
Succinylcholine chloride	1 mg	4 ml	None	None	Haze	
Metocurine iodide	0.5 mg	4 ml	None	None	Ppt.	
Metocurine iodide	1 mg	4 ml	None	None	Ppt.	
Scopolamine hydrobromide	1/120 gr	1 ml	None	None	None	Haze
Tubocurarine chloride	3 mg	4 ml	None	Haze		

How Supplied: *Ampoules (Vials) Brevital® Sodium (Methohexital Sodium for Injection, USP)* are supplied as follows:

(Ⓒ) *No. 660,* 500 mg, 50-ml size, rubber-stoppered (Dry Powder), in singles (10 per carton) and in packages of 25.

Each vial contains—
Brevital® Sodium (methohexital sodium, Lilly) .... 500 mg
Anhydrous Sodium Carbonate .... 30 mg
Contains no preservative.

(Ⓒ) *No. 760,* 500 mg, 50-ml size, rubber-stoppered (Dry Powder), in singles (10 per carton). Each package contains one 50-ml vial of Sterile Water for Injection.

Each vial contains—
Brevital® Sodium (methohexital sodium, Lilly) .... 500 mg
Anhydrous Sodium Carbonate .... 30 mg
Contains no preservative.

(Ⓒ) *No. 663,* 2.5 gm, rubber-stoppered (Dry Powder), in singles (10 per carton) and in packages of 25.

Each vial contains—
Brevital® Sodium (methohexital sodium, Lilly) .... 2.5 gm
Anhydrous Sodium Carbonate .... 150 mg
Contains no preservative.

(Ⓒ) *No. 664,* 2.5 gm, 250-ml size, rubber-stoppered (Dry Powder), in singles and in packages of 25.

Each vial contains—
Brevital® Sodium (methohexital sodium, Lilly) .... 2.5 gm
Anhydrous Sodium Carbonate .... 150 mg
Contains no preservative.

(Ⓒ) *No. 659,* 5 gm, rubber-stoppered (Dry Powder), in singles (10 per carton).

Each vial contains—
Brevital® Sodium (methohexital sodium, Lilly) .... 5 gm
Anhydrous Sodium Carbonate .... 300 mg
Contains no preservative.

(Ⓒ) *No. 662,* 5 gm, 500-ml size, rubber-stoppered (Dry Powder), in singles and in packages of 25.

Each vial contains—
Brevital® Sodium (methohexital sodium, Lilly) .... 5 gm
Anhydrous Sodium Carbonate .... 300 mg
Contains no preservative. [081578]

CAFFEINE AND SODIUM BENZOATE ℞
Injection, USP

Description: Caffeine and Sodium Benzoate Injection, USP, is a mixture of approximately equal parts of caffeine (1,3,7-trimethylxanthine) and sodium benzoate ($C_7H_5NaO_2$). A white powder with a slightly bitter taste, it is freely soluble in water (1:1.2) and soluble in alcohol (1:30). The free water solubility of the salt makes it preferable to the caffeine base for parenteral administration.

Action: Caffeine and Sodium Benzoate Injection, USP, is similar to caffeine itself in its physiologic effects and therapeutic use in that it is a potent central-nervous-system stimulant.

Indications: Because of its C.N.S. stimulating effect, Caffeine and Sodium Benzoate is useful as a respiratory stimulant, particularly in the treatment of respiratory depression due to poisoning from morphine or alcohol. It has also been used to stimulate respiration in cases of electric shock and to relieve the headache caused by spinal puncture.

Precaution: Because too-vigorous treatment with Caffeine and Sodium Benzoate can produce further depression in the already depressed patient, a single dose should not exceed 1 gm.

Adverse Reactions: Side effects produced by caffeine include nausea, insomnia, restlessness, excitement, tinnitus, scintillating scotoma, muscular tremor, tachycardia, extrasystoles, and diuresis. Short-acting barbiturates, such as pentobarbital sodium, may be used to counteract these effects on the central nervous system.

Administration and Dosage: For central-nervous-system stimulation, the usual dosage is 500 mg in 2 ml of solution, administered intramuscularly as necessary. (It may be given by intravenous injection in emergency situations of respiratory failure.)

How Supplied: (℞) *Ampoules No. 11, Caffeine and Sodium Benzoate Injection, USP,* 500 mg (7½ grains) in 2 ml, in packages of 12. [110876]

CALCIUM GLUCEPTATE ℞
Injection, USP
For Intravenous or Intramuscular Administration of Calcium

Description: Calcium Gluceptate Injection, USP, contains a sterile, aqueous, approximately neutral solution of the calcium salt of *d*-glucoheptonic acid, $[CH_2OH \bullet (CHOH)_5 \bullet COO]_2\ Ca \bullet H_2O$, stabilized with 0.5 percent monothioglycerol. Each 5 ml contain 1.1 gm calcium gluceptate representing 90 mg calcium (4.5 mEq) and are equivalent in calcium content to 10 ml of 10 percent calcium gluconate; the osmolarity is 0.5 mOsm per ml. Sodium hydroxide and/or glucono delta lactone may have been added during manufacture to adjust the *p*H.

Actions: Calcium is the fifth most abundant element in the body, and the major fraction is in the bony structure. Calcium plays important physiologic roles, many of which are poorly understood. It is essential for the functional integrity of the nervous and muscular systems, is necessary for normal cardiac function, and is one of the factors involved in the coagulation of blood.

Indications: The parenteral administration of calcium is indicated in the treatment of hypocalcemia for those conditions requiring a prompt increase in blood plasma calcium levels, such as neonatal tetany and tetany due to parathyroid deficiency, vitamin D deficiency, and alkalosis. It is also indicated for the prevention of hypocalcemia during exchange transfusions.

Precautions: Because of its additive effect, calcium should be administered very cautiously to a patient who is digitalized or who is taking effective doses of digitalis or digitalis-like preparations.

Although calcium gluceptate given intramuscularly appears to be well tolerated, this route of administration should be used for very young patients only in emergencies when technical difficulty makes intravenous injection impossible.

Adverse Reactions: Following intramuscular administration, mild local reactions may occur; severe inflammatory reactions have not been observed.

Rapid intravenous administration may cause the patient to complain of tingling sensations, a calcium taste, a sense of oppression, or "heat waves."

Administration and Dosage: Calcium gluceptate may be given *intramuscularly* in 2 to 5-ml doses. When 5 ml are administered, the dose should be injected in the gluteal region or, in infants, in the lateral thigh.

The usual *intravenous* dose of calcium gluceptate is from 5 to 20 ml. The usual precautions for intravenous therapy should be observed. The solution should be warmed to body temperature and administered slowly (2 ml per minute). The injection should be halted if the patient complains of any discomfort; it may be resumed when symptoms disappear. Following injection, the patient should remain recumbent for a short time. Repeated injections may be required because of the rapid excretion of calcium.

During exchange transfusions in newborns, the usual dose is 0.5 ml after every 100 ml of blood exchanged.

How Supplied: (℞) *Ampoules No. 483, Calcium Gluceptate Injection, USP,* 5 ml, in packages of 25.

[062078]

Continued on next page

*Identi-Code® symbol.

Lilly—Cont.

CAPASTAT® SULFATE ℞
(capreomycin sulfate)
Sterile, USP
Not for Pediatric Use

Warnings

The use of capreomycin in patients with renal insufficiency or preexisting auditory impairment must be undertaken with great caution, and the risk of additional eighth-nerve impairment or renal injury should be weighed against the benefits to be derived from therapy.

Refer to animal pharmacology section for additional information.

Since other parenteral antituberculosis agents (streptomycin, viomycin) also have similar and sometimes irreversible toxic effects, particularly on eighth-cranial-nerve and renal function, simultaneous administration of these agents with capreomycin is not recommended. Use with nonantituberculosis drugs (polymyxin, colistin sulfate, gentamicin, tobramycin, vancomycin, kanamycin, and neomycin) having ototoxic or nephrotoxic potential should be undertaken only with great caution.

Usage in Pregnancy—The safety of the use of capreomycin in *pregnancy* has not been determined.

Pediatric Usage—Safety of the use of capreomycin in infants and children has not been established.

Description: Capastat® Sulfate (capreomycin sulfate, Lilly) is a polypeptide antibiotic isolated from *Streptomyces capreolus.* It is a complex of four microbiologically active components which have been characterized in part; however, complete structural determination of all the components has not been established. Capreomycin is supplied as the disulfate salt and is soluble in water. In complete solution, it is almost colorless.

Actions: *Human Pharmacology*—Capastat® Sulfate (capreomycin sulfate, Lilly) is not absorbed in significant quantities from the gastrointestinal tract and must be administered parenterally. In two studies of ten patients each, peak serum concentrations following 1 gm of capreomycin given intramuscularly were achieved one to two hours after administration, and average peak levels reached were 28 and 32 mcg/ml respectively (range, 20 to 47 mcg/ml). Low serum concentrations were present at 24 hours. However, 1 gm of capreomycin daily for 30 days or more produced no significant accumulation in subjects with normal renal function. Two patients with marked reduction of renal function had high serum concentrations 24 hours after administration of the drug. When a 1-gm dose of capreomycin was given intramuscularly to normal volunteers, 52 percent was excreted in the urine within 12 hours.

Paper chromatographic studies indicated that capreomycin is excreted essentially unaltered. Urine concentrations averaged 1.68 mg/ml (average urine volume, 228 ml) during the six hours following a 1-gm dose.

Microbiology—Capreomycin is active against human strains of *Mycobacterium tuberculosis.* The susceptibility of strains of *M. tuberculosis* in vitro varies with the media and techniques employed. In general, the minimum inhibitory concentrations for *M. tuberculosis* are lowest in liquid media that are free of egg protein (7H10 or Dubos) and range from 1 to 5 mcg/ml when the indirect method is used. Comparable inhibitory concentrations are obtained when 7H10 agar is used for direct susceptibility testing. When indirect susceptibility tests are performed on standard tube slants with 7H10 media, susceptible strains are inhibited by 10 to 25 mcg/ml. Egg-containing media, such as Löwenstein-Jensen or ATS, require concentrations of 25 to 50 mcg/ml to inhibit susceptible strains.

Cross-Resistance—Frequent cross-resistance occurs between capreomycin and viomycin. Varying degrees of cross-resistance between capreomycin and kanamycin and neomycin have been reported. No cross-resistance has been observed between capreomycin and isoniazid, aminosalicylic acid, cycloserine, streptomycin, ethionamide, or ethambutol.

Indications: Capreomycin, which is to be used concomitantly with other appropriate antituberculosis agents, is indicated in pulmonary infections caused by capreomycin-susceptible strains of *M. tuberculosis* when the primary agents (isoniazid, aminosalicylic acid, and streptomycin) have been ineffective or cannot be used because of toxicity or the presence of resistant tubercle bacilli.

Susceptibility studies should be performed to determine the presence of a capreomycin-susceptible strain of *M. tuberculosis.*

Contraindication: Capreomycin is contraindicated in those patients who are hypersensitive to it.

Precautions: Audiometric measurements and assessment of vestibular function should be performed prior to initiation of therapy with capreomycin and at regular intervals during treatment.

Regular tests of renal function should be made throughout the period of treatment, and reduced dosage should be employed in patients with known or suspected renal impairment.

Renal injury, with tubular necrosis, elevation of the blood urea nitrogen (BUN) or nonprotein nitrogen (NPN), and abnormal urinary sediment, has been noted. Renal function studies should be made both before capreomycin therapy is started and on a weekly basis during treatment. Slight elevation of the BUN or NPN has been observed in a significant number of patients receiving prolonged therapy. The appearance of casts, red cells, and white cells in the urine has been noted in a high percentage of these cases. Elevation of the BUN above 30 mg/100 ml or any other evidence of decreasing renal function with or without a rise in BUN levels calls for careful evaluation of the patient, and the dosage should be reduced or the drug completely withdrawn. The clinical significance of abnormal urine sediment and slight elevation in the BUN (or total NPN) observed during long-term capreomycin therapy has not been established.

Since hypokalemia may occur during capreomycin therapy, serum potassium levels should be determined frequently.

The peripheral neuromuscular blocking action that has been attributed to other polypeptide antibiotics (colistin sulfate, polymyxin A sulfate, paromomycin, and viomycin) and aminoglycoside antibiotics (streptomycin, dihydrostreptomycin, neomycin, and kanamycin) has been studied with capreomycin. A partial neuromuscular block was demonstrated after large intravenous doses of capreomycin. This action was enhanced by ether anesthesia (as has been reported for neomycin) and was antagonized by neostigmine.

Caution should be exercised in the administration of antibiotics, including capreomycin, to any patient who has demonstrated some form of allergy, particularly to drugs.

Adverse Reactions: *Nephrotoxicity*—In 36 percent of 722 patients treated with capreomycin, elevation of the BUN above 20 mg/100 ml and of the NPN above 35 mg/100 ml has been observed. In many instances, there was also depression of PSP excretion and abnormal urine sediment. In 10 percent of this series, the BUN elevation exceeded 30 mg/100 ml or the NPN exceeded 50 mg/100 ml.

Toxic nephritis was reported in one patient with tuberculosis and portal cirrhosis who was treated with capreomycin (1 gm) and aminosalicylic acid daily for one month. This patient developed renal insufficiency and oliguria and died. Autopsy showed subsiding acute tubular necrosis.

Ototoxicity—Subclinical auditory loss was noted in approximately 11 percent of patients undergoing treatment with capreomycin. This has been a 5 to 10-decibel loss in the 4000 to 8000-CPS range. Clinically apparent hearing loss occurred in 3 percent of 722 subjects. Some audiometric changes were reversible. Other cases with permanent loss were not progressive following withdrawal of capreomycin. Tinnitus and vertigo have occurred.

Liver—Serial tests of liver function have demonstrated a decrease in BSP excretion without change in SGOT or SGPT in the presence of preexisting liver disease. Abnormal results in liver function tests have occurred in many persons receiving capreomycin in combination with other antituberculosis agents which also are known to cause changes in hepatic function. The role of capreomycin in producing these abnormalities is not clear; however, periodic determinations of liver function are recommended.

Blood—Leukocytosis and leukopenia have been observed. The majority of patients treated have had eosinophilia exceeding 5 percent while receiving daily injections of capreomycin. This has subsided with reduction of the capreomycin dosage to 2 or 3 gm weekly.

Pain and induration at the injection sites have been observed. Excessive bleeding at the injection site has been reported. Sterile abscesses have been noted.

Hypersensitivity—Urticaria and maculopapular skin rashes associated in some cases with febrile reactions have been reported when capreomycin and other antituberculosis drugs were given concomitantly.

Administration and Dosage: Capastat® Sulfate (capreomycin sulfate, Lilly) should be dissolved in 2 ml of 0.9% Sodium Chloride Injection or Sterile Water for Injection. Two to three minutes should be allowed for complete solution. For administration of a 1-gm dose, the entire contents of the vial should be given. For dosages less than 1 gm, the accompanying dilution table may be used.

[See table below].

The solution may acquire a pale straw color and darken with time, but this is not associated with loss of potency or the development of toxicity. After reconstitution, solutions of Capastat Sulfate may be stored for 48 hours at room

DILUTION TABLE

Diluent Added to 1-gm Vial	Volume of Capastat® Sulfate (capreomycin sulfate, Lilly) Solution	Concentration* (Approx.)
2.15 ml	2.85 ml	350 mg per ml
2.63 ml	3.33 ml	300 mg per ml
3.3 ml	4 ml	250 mg per ml
4.3 ml	5 ml	200 mg per ml

*Stated in terms of mg of capreomycin activity.

temperature and up to 14 days under refrigeration.

Capastat Sulfate should be given by deep intramuscular injection into a large muscle mass, since superficial injections may be associated with increased pain and the development of sterile abscesses.

Capreomycin is always administered in combination with at least one other antituberculosis agent to which the patient's strain of tubercle bacilli is susceptible. The usual dose is 1 gm daily (not to exceed 20 mg/kg per day) given intramuscularly for 60 to 120 days, followed by 1 gm intramuscularly two or three times weekly. (*Note*—Therapy for tuberculosis should be maintained for 18 to 24 months. If facilities for administering injectable medication are not available, a change to appropriate oral therapy is indicated upon the patient's release from the hospital.)

Animal Pharmacology: In addition to renal and eighth-cranial-nerve toxicity demonstrated in animal toxicology studies, two dogs have developed cataracts while on doses of 62 mg/kg and 100 mg/kg for prolonged periods.

In teratology studies, a low incidence of "wavy ribs" was noted in litters of female rats treated with daily doses of 50 mg/kg or more of capreomycin.

How Supplied: (℞) *Ampoules (Vials) No. 718, Capastat® Sulfate (Sterile Capreomycin Sulfate, USP),* equivalent to 1 gm capreomycin activity, 5-ml size, rubber-stoppered (Dry Powder), in singles (10 per carton).

[072479]

CARBARSONE ℞

(Arsenic Derivative)
Capsules, NF

Description: Carbarsone is a pentavalent organic arsenical containing approximately 29 percent arsenic. It is a white, crystalline, odorless solid which is stable in air and has a slightly acid taste. It is practically insoluble in water but is soluble in carbonate or bicarbonate solutions.

Indication: Carbarsone is indicated in the treatment of intestinal amebiasis and is effective against the trophozoite form of *Entamoeba histolytica* in the lumen and shallow ulcers of the colon.

Contraindications: Carbarsone should not be used (1) as the initial agent when amebic hepatitis of any degree may be present, (2) when there is any other liver or kidney disease, (3) in the presence of contracted visual or color fields, or (4) when the patient is hypersensitive or intolerant to organic or inorganic arsenic given systemically or applied topically.

Precautions: Since Carbarsone is absorbed readily from the gastrointestinal tract and excreted rather slowly by way of the kidneys, accumulation of the drug may result. Therefore, the following precautions should be observed. If prolonged treatment is indicated or contemplated, it is mandatory that the recommended daily dose not be exceeded, that a course of treatment be no longer than ten days, and that a rest interval of at least ten days be allowed before another treatment period is started. If there is any evidence of intolerance or toxicity (i.e., increase in severity of gastrointestinal symptoms already present; development of nausea, vomiting, abdominal pain or cramps, or diarrhea when these symptoms have not previously been present; urinary symptoms; dermatitis or other skin lesions suggesting sensitivity to arsenic; any central or peripheral nervous-system changes; or any of the signs or symptoms listed below or under Adverse Reactions), the drug should be discontinued at once. Since Carbarsone accumulates in the tissues and is eliminated slowly, the patient should be instructed to report any unusual signs or symptoms for a period of time after treatment has been discontinued.

Epstein found that individuals who are sensitive to trivalent arsenicals may also exhibit positive skin reactions when tested with pentavalent arsenicals. Four of six such patients showed positive patch tests with Carbarsone. This author also reported a fatality which occurred following a course of therapy with Carbarsone, but he stated that, when correctly administered, this drug is less toxic than other related arsenical preparations. Smithies observed sore throat, splenic enlargement, and edema of ankles, knees, and wrists in patients receiving Carbarsone and reported single instances of icterus, dermatitis, and papillitis with retinal edema.

Adverse Reactions: Although Carbarsone is one of the most innocuous of organic arsenicals, toxic manifestations must be watched for. Such signs include sore throat, edema, splenomegaly, icterus, pruritus, skin eruptions, gastrointestinal irritation, hepatitis, neuritis, and visual disturbances. Fatalities from exfoliative dermatitis and liver necrosis and from hemorrhagic encephalitis are on record.

If it is warranted, untoward reactions to Carbarsone may be treated with the specific antiarsenical compound Dimercaprol (BAL).

Administration and Dosage: *Adults*—The usual course of treatment consists in oral administration of 250 mg (4 grains) of Carbarsone two or three times daily for ten days. Additional courses of treatment are given as indicated following a rest period of ten to 14 days.

Children—The individual and total dosage may be reduced in proportion to weight. The average total dose, based on body weight, is about 75 mg per kg.

The following dosage scale will be effective: ages two to four years, a total dose of 2 gm of Carbarsone over a period of ten days, a dose of 66 mg being given three times a day in half a glass of milk or in orange juice; ages five to eight years, a total dose of 3 gm of Carbarsone over a ten-day period in three daily doses; nine to 12 years, a total dose of 4 gm in three daily doses for ten days; and from puberty on to young adulthood, a total dose of 5 gm.

For children, it will be necessary to divide the contents of a Pulvule® and to give the Carbarsone as suggested above or in a small volume of sodium bicarbonate solution (1 percent), in jelly, or in some other food. The taste is not objectionable. If a solution is made of the Pulvule, it is to be remembered that it will not be clear, but the Carbarsone will be in solution. Should toxic manifestations appear, discontinue therapy at once.

Overdosage: *Symptoms*—Nausea, vomiting, abdominal pain, diarrhea, shock, coma, convulsions, ulceration of mucous membranes and skin, and kidney damage. *Treatment*—Specifically, Dimercaprol, 3 to 4 mg per kg (or 0.3 to 0.4 ml per kg), every six hours for the first two days and then twice daily for a total of ten days. General management should be symptomatic and supportive and may include gastric lavage, administration of oxygen and intravenous fluids, and maintenance of body temperature. Unexplained fatalities have been reported with usual doses.

How Supplied: (℞) *Pulvules No. 227, Carbarsone Capsules, NF, F34,* * 250 mg (4 grs) (No. 2, Pink), in bottles of 20.

[121875]

CECLOR® ℞

(cefaclor)

Description: Ceclor® (cefaclor, Lilly) is a semisynthetic cephalosporin antibiotic for oral administration. It is chemically designated as 3-chloro-7-D-(2-phenylglycinamido)-3-cephem-4-carboxylic acid. Ceclor is available in 250-mg and 500-mg Pulvules® and in a powder for oral suspension containing 125 or 250 mg per 5 ml.

Actions: *Clinical Pharmacology*—Ceclor® (cefaclor, Lilly) is well absorbed after oral administration to fasting subjects. Total absorption is the same whether the drug is given with or without food; however, when it is taken with food, the peak concentration achieved is 50 to 75 percent of that observed when the drug is administered to fasting subjects and generally appears from three-fourths to one hour later. Following administration of 250-mg, 500-mg, and 1-gm doses to fasting subjects, average peak serum levels of approximately 7, 13, and 23 mcg per ml respectively were obtained within 30 to 60 minutes. Approximately 60 to 85 percent of the drug is excreted unchanged in the urine within eight hours, the greater portion being excreted within the first two hours. During this eight-hour period, peak urine concentrations following the 250-mg, 500-mg, and 1-gm doses were approximately 600, 900, and 1900 mcg per ml respectively. The serum half-life in normal subjects is 0.6 to 0.9 hour. In patients with reduced renal function, the serum half-life of cefaclor is slightly prolonged. In those with complete absence of renal function, the biologic half-life of the intact molecule is 2.3 to 2.8 hours. Excretion pathways in patients with markedly impaired renal function have not been determined. Hemodialysis shortens the half-life by 25 to 30 percent.

Microbiology—In vitro tests demonstrate that the bactericidal action of the cephalosporins results from inhibition of cell-wall synthesis. Cefaclor is usually active against the following organisms in vitro and in clinical infections:

- Staphylococci, including coagulase-positive, coagulase-negative, and penicillinase-producing strains
- *Streptococcus pyogenes* (group A beta-hemolytic streptococci)
- *S. pneumoniae* (formerly *Diplococcus pneumoniae*)
- *Escherichia coli*
- *Proteus mirabilis*
- *Klebsiella* species
- *Haemophilus influenzae,* including some beta-lactamase-producing ampicillin-resistant strains

Note: Pseudomonas species, *Acinetobacter calcoaceticus* (formerly *Mima* and *Herellea* species), and most strains of enterococci (*S. faecalis,* group D streptococci), *Enterobacter* species, indole-positive *Proteus,* and *Serratia* species are resistant to Ceclor. When tested by in vitro methods, staphylococci exhibit cross-resistance between cefaclor and methicillin-type antibiotics.

Disc Susceptibility Tests—Quantitative methods that require measurement of zone diameters give the most precise estimates of antibiotic susceptibility. One such procedure* has been recommended for use with discs for testing susceptibility to cephalothin. The currently accepted zone diameter interpretative criteria for the cephalothin disc are appropriate for determining bacterial susceptibility to cefaclor. With this procedure, a report from the laboratory of "resistant" indicates that the infecting organism is not likely to respond to therapy. A report of "intermediate susceptibility" suggests that the organism would be susceptible if the infection is confined to tissues and fluids (e.g., urine) in which high antibiotic levels can be obtained or if high dosage is used.

Indications and Usage: Ceclor® (cefaclor, Lilly) is indicated in the treatment of the following infections when caused by susceptible strains of the designated microorganisms:

- Otitis media caused by *S. pneumoniae (D. pneumoniae), H. influenzae,* staphylococci, and *S. pyogenes* (group A beta-hemolytic streptococci)
- Lower respiratory infections, including pneumonia caused by *S. pneumoniae (D.*

Continued on next page

*Identi-Code® symbol.

Lilly—Cont.

pneumoniae), H. influenzae, and *S. pyogenes* (group A beta-hemolytic streptococci)

Upper respiratory infections, including pharyngitis and tonsillitis caused by *S. pyogenes* (group A beta-hemolytic streptococci)

Note: Penicillin is the usual drug of choice in the treatment and prevention of streptococcal infections, including the prophylaxis of rheumatic fever. Cefaclor is generally effective in the eradication of streptococci from the nasopharynx; however, substantial data establishing the efficacy of cefaclor in the subsequent prevention of rheumatic fever are not available at present.

Urinary tract infections, including pyelonephritis and cystitis caused by *E. coli, P. mirabilis, Klebsiella* species, and coagulase-negative staphylococci

Skin and skin-structure infections caused by *Staphylococcus aureus* and *S. pyogenes* (group A beta-hemolytic streptococci)

Appropriate culture and susceptibility studies should be performed to determine susceptibility of the causative organism to Ceclor.

Contraindication: Ceclor® (cefaclor, Lilly) is contraindicated in patients with known allergy to the cephalosporin group of antibiotics.

Warnings: IN PENICILLIN-SENSITIVE PATIENTS, CEPHALOSPORIN ANTIBIOTICS SHOULD BE ADMINISTERED CAUTIOUSLY. THERE IS CLINICAL AND LABORATORY EVIDENCE OF PARTIAL CROSS-ALLERGENICITY OF THE PENICILLINS AND THE CEPHALOSPORINS, AND THERE ARE INSTANCES IN WHICH PATIENTS HAVE HAD REACTIONS TO BOTH DRUG CLASSES (INCLUDING ANAPHYLAXIS AFTER PARENTERAL USE).

Antibiotics, including Ceclor® (cefaclor, Lilly), should be administered cautiously to any patient who has demonstrated some form of allergy, particularly to drugs.

Precautions: If an allergic reaction to cefaclor occurs, the drug should be discontinued, and, if necessary, the patient should be treated with appropriate agents, e.g., pressor amines, antihistamines, or corticosteroids.

Prolonged use of cefaclor may result in the overgrowth of nonsusceptible organisms. Careful observation of the patient is essential. If superinfection occurs during therapy, appropriate measures should be taken.

Positive direct Coombs tests have been reported during treatment with the cephalosporin antibiotics. In hematologic studies or in transfusion cross-matching procedures when antiglobulin tests are performed on the minor side or in Coombs testing of newborns whose mothers have received cephalosporin antibiotics before parturition, it should be recognized that a positive Coombs test may be due to the drug.

Ceclor® (cefaclor, Lilly) should be administered with caution in the presence of markedly impaired renal function. Under such a condition, careful clinical observation and laboratory studies should be made because safe dosage may be lower than that usually recommended.

Usage in Pregnancy—Although no teratogenic or antifertility effects were seen in reproduction studies in mice and rats receiving up to 12 times the maximum human dose or in ferrets given three times the maximum human dose, the safety of this drug for use in human pregnancy has not been established. The benefits of the drug in pregnant women should be weighed against a possible risk to the fetus.

Usage in Infancy—Safety of this product for use in infants less than one month of age has not been established.

Adverse Reactions: In clinical studies in 1493 patients, adverse effects considered related to cefaclor therapy were uncommon and are listed below:

Gastrointestinal symptoms occurred in about 2.5 percent of patients and included diarrhea (1 in 70) and nausea and vomiting (1 in 90).

Hypersensitivity reactions were reported in about 1.5 percent of patients and included morbilliform eruptions (1 in 100). Pruritus, urticaria, and positive Coombs tests each occurred in less than 1 in 200 patients.

Other effects considered related to therapy included eosinophilia (1 in 50 patients) and genital pruritus or vaginitis (less than 1 in 100 patients).

Causal Relationship Uncertain—Transitory abnormalities in clinical laboratory test results have been reported. Although they were of uncertain etiology, they are listed below to serve as alerting information for the physician.

Hepatic—Slight elevations in SGOT, SGPT, or alkaline phosphatase values (1 in 40).

Hematopoietic—Transient fluctuations in leukocyte count, predominantly lymphocytosis occurring in infants and young children (1 in 40).

Renal—Slight elevations in BUN or serum creatinine (less than 1 in 500) or abnormal urinalysis (less than 1 in 200).

Administration and Dosage: Ceclor® (cefaclor, Lilly) is administered orally.

Adults—The usual adult dosage is 250 mg every eight hours. For more severe infections (such as pneumonia) or those caused by less susceptible organisms, doses may be doubled. Doses of 4 gm per day have been administered safely to normal subjects for 28 days, but the total daily dosage should not exceed this amount.

Children—The usual recommended daily dosage for children is 20 mg/kg/day in divided doses every eight hours, as indicated:

	Ceclor Suspension	
Child's Weight	125 mg/5 ml	250 mg/5 ml
9 kg	½ tsp t i d	
18 kg	1 tsp t i d	½ tsp t i d

In more serious infections, otitis media, and infections caused by less susceptible organisms, 40 mg/kg/day are recommended, with a maximum dosage of 1 gm per day.

Ceclor may be administered in the presence of impaired renal function. Under such a condition, the dosage usually is unchanged (*see* Precautions).

In the treatment of beta-hemolytic streptococcal infections, a therapeutic dosage of Ceclor should be administered for at least ten days.

How Supplied: (℞) *Ceclor® (cefaclor, Lilly), for Oral Suspension, M-5057,* 125 mg per 5 ml (strawberry flavor) and *M-5058,* 250 mg per 5 ml (grape flavor), in 75 and 150-ml-size packages.

Directions for mixing are included on the label. After mixing, store in a refrigerator. Shake well before using. Keep tightly closed. The mixture may be kept for 14 days without significant loss of potency. Discard unused portion after 14 days.

(℞) *Pulvules® Ceclor® (cefaclor, Lilly): No. 3061,* 250 mg (White Opaque Body, Purple Opaque Cap), and *No. 3062,* 500 mg (Gray Opaque Body, Purple Opaque Cap), in bottles of 15 and 100 and in 10 strips of 10 individually labeled blisters each containing one Pulvule (ID100).

---

*Bauer, A. W., Kirby, W. M. M., Sherris, J. C., and Turck, M.: Antibiotic Susceptibility Testing by a Standardized Single Disk Method, Am. J. Clin. Pathol, 45:493, 1966; Standardized Disc Susceptibility Test, Federal Register, *39:*19182–19184, 1974.

[042479]

CEFACLOR, *see* Ceclor® (cefaclor, Lilly).

CEFAMANDOLE NAFATE, *see* Mandol® (cefamandole nafate, Lilly).

CEFAZOLIN SODIUM, *see* Kefzol® (cefazolin sodium, Lilly).

CEPHALEXIN, *see* Keflex® (cephalexin, Lilly).

CEPHALOGLYCIN, *see* Kafocin® (cephaloglycin, Lilly).

CEPHALORIDINE, *see* Loridine® (cephaloridine, Lilly).

CEPHALOTHIN SODIUM, *see* Keflin® (cephalothin sodium, Lilly).

COLCHICINE ℞
AMPOULES

Description: A phenanthrene derivative, colchicine is the active alkaloidal principle derived from various species of *Colchicum;* it is a pale-yellow amorphous powder that is soluble in water (1:25) and freely soluble in alcohol.

Ampoules Colchicine Injection provide an aqueous solution of colchicine for intravenous use. Each ampoule contains 1 mg of colchicine in 2 ml of solution. Sodium hydroxide may have been added during manufacture to adjust the *p*H.

Action: The precise pharmacologic activity of colchicine in gout is not known. However, it is thought to decrease lactic acid production by the leukocytes and thereby decrease urate crystal deposition and subsequent inflammatory response.

Indications: Colchicine is indicated for the treatment of gout. It is effective in relieving the pain of acute attacks, especially if therapy is begun early in the attack and in adequate dosage. Many therapists use colchicine as interval therapy to prevent acute attacks of gout. It has no effect on nongouty arthritis or on uric acid metabolism.

The intravenous use of colchicine is advantageous when a rapid response is desired or when gastrointestinal side effects interfere with oral administration of the medication. Occasionally, intravenous colchicine is effective when the oral preparation is not. After the acute attack has subsided, the patient can usually be given colchicine tablets by mouth.

Precautions: Colchicine should be administered with great caution to aged and debilitated patients, especially those with renal, gastrointestinal, or heart disease. Reduction of dosage is indicated if weakness, anorexia, nausea, vomiting, or diarrhea appears. Rarely, thrombophlebitis occurs at the site of injection.

Adverse Reactions: These are usually gastrointestinal in nature and consist of abdominal pain, nausea, vomiting, and diarrhea. The diarrhea may be severe. The gastrointestinal symptoms may occur even though the drug is given intravenously; however, such symptoms are unusual unless the recommended dose is exceeded.

Chronic administration may cause bone-marrow depression, with agranulocytosis, thrombocytopenia, and aplastic anemia. Peripheral neuritis and depilation have also been reported.

Administration and Dosage: Colchicine Injection must be given intravenously. Severe local irritation occurs if it is administered subcutaneously or intramuscularly.

The injection should take two to five minutes for completion. Colchicine Injection should NOT be diluted with or injected into intravenous tubing containing 0.9% Sodium Chloride Injection, 5% Dextrose Injection, or any other fluid which would even slightly change the *p*H of the colchicine solution, since this may cause precipitation. The *p*H of Colchicine Injection

ranges from 6.0 to 7.2. If a lower concentration is required, Sterile Water for Injection may be used for the dilution. Solutions which thereafter become turbid should not be injected.
In the treatment of acute gouty arthritis, the average initial dose of Colchicine Injection is 2 mg (4 ml). This may be followed by 0.5 mg (1 ml) every six hours until a satisfactory response is achieved. In general, the total dosage for a 24-hour period should not exceed 4 mg (8 ml). Some clinicians recommend a single intravenous dose of 3 mg, whereas others recommend not more than 1 mg of colchicine intravenously for the initial dose, followed by 0.5 mg once or twice daily if needed.
If pain recurs, it may be necessary to administer a daily dose of 1 to 2 mg (2 to 4 ml) for several days. Many patients can be transferred to the oral colchicine in a similar dosage to that being given intravenously.
In the prophylactic or maintenance therapy of recurrent or chronic gouty arthritis, a dosage of 0.5 to 1 mg (1 to 2 ml) once or twice daily may be used. However, in these cases, oral administration of colchicine is preferable, usually in conjunction with a uricosuric agent.
Acute Overdosage: There is usually a latent period between overdosage and the onset of symptoms, regardless of the route of administration. Deaths have been reported with as little as 8 mg, although higher doses have been taken without fatal results. The first symptoms to appear are gastrointestinal—nausea, vomiting, abdominal pain, and diarrhea. The diarrhea may be severe and bloody owing to hemorrhagic gastroenteritis. Burning sensations in the throat, stomach, and skin may also occur. Extensive vascular damage may result in shock. The kidney may show evidence of damage by hematuria and oliguria, since it is an excretory site. Muscular weakness is marked, and an ascending paralysis of the central nervous system may develop. The patient usually remains conscious. However, delirium and convulsions may occur. Death usually is the result of respiratory depression.
Recent studies appear to support the use of hemodialysis or peritoneal dialysis as part of the treatment of acute overdosage. Shock must be combated. Atropine and morphine may relieve the abdominal pain. Respiratory assistance may be needed to insure proper oxygenation and ventilation.
How Supplied: (℞) *Ampoules No. 656, Colchicine Injection,* 1 mg, 2 ml, in packages of 6.
[092578]

COLCHICINE ℞
Tablets, USP

Description: A phenanthrene derivative, colchicine is the active alkaloidal principle derived from various species of *Colchicum;* it is a pale-yellow amorphous powder that is soluble in water (1:25) and freely soluble in alcohol.
Action: The precise pharmacologic activity of colchicine in gout is not known. However, it is thought to decrease lactic acid production by the leukocytes and thereby decrease urate crystal deposition and subsequent inflammatory response.
Indications: Colchicine is indicated for the treatment of gout. It is effective in relieving the pain of acute attacks, especially if therapy is begun early in the attack and in adequate dosage. Many therapists use colchicine as interval therapy to prevent acute attacks of gout. It has no effect on nongouty arthritis or on uric acid metabolism.
Precautions: Colchicine should be administered with great caution to aged and debilitated patients, especially those with renal, gastrointestinal, or heart disease. Reduction of dosage is indicated if weakness, anorexia, nausea, vomiting, or diarrhea appears.
Adverse Reactions: In full dosage, colchicine produces nausea, vomiting, or diarrhea. However, it is generally necessary to reach such dose levels for an adequate therapeutic effect. Paregoric may be given either concurrently or when diarrhea develops.
Prolonged administration may cause bone-marrow depression, with agranulocytosis, thrombocytopenia, and aplastic anemia. Peripheral neuritis and depilation have also been reported.
Administration and Dosage: Colchicine should be started at the first warning of an acute attack; a delay of a few hours impairs its effectiveness. The usual adult dose is 1 or 2 tablets initially, followed by 1 tablet every one to two hours until pain is relieved or nausea, vomiting, or diarrhea develops. Some physicians use 2 tablets every two hours. Since the number of doses required may range from six to 16, the total dose is variable. As interval treatment, 1 tablet may be taken one to four times a week for the mild or moderate case, once or twice daily for the severe case.
Acute Overdosage: There is usually a latent period between overdosage and the onset of symptoms, regardless of the route of administration. Deaths have been reported with as little as 8 mg, although higher doses have been taken without fatal results. The first symptoms to appear are gastrointestinal—nausea, vomiting, abdominal pain, and diarrhea. The diarrhea may be severe and bloody owing to hemorrhagic gastroenteritis. Burning sensations in the throat, stomach, and skin may also occur. Extensive vascular damage may result in shock. The kidney may show evidence of damage by hematuria and oliguria, since it is an excretory site. Muscular weakness is marked, and an ascending paralysis of the central nervous system may develop. The patient usually remains conscious. However, delirium and convulsions may occur. Death usually is the result of respiratory depression.
Recent studies would appear to support the use of hemodialysis or peritoneal dialysis as part of the treatment of acute overdosage in addition to gastric lavage. Shock must be combated. Atropine and morphine may relieve the abdominal pain. Respiratory assistance may be needed to insure proper oxygenation and ventilation.
How Supplied: (℞) *Tablets No. 560, Colchicine Tablets, USP, J13,** 0.6 mg, in bottles of 100 and 1000.
[061978]

COPAVIN® ©
(codeine and papaverine)

Description: Each Pulvule® contains—
Codeine Sulfate ....15 mg (1/4 gr)
WARNING—May be habit-forming.
Papaverine Hydrochloride ....15 mg (1/4 gr)
Indications: For the relief of the general malaise and cough of acute respiratory infections.
Contraindications and Precautions: Habituation and tolerance to papaverine have not been reported. However, since Copavin® (codeine and papaverine, Lilly) contains codeine, it should not be prescribed for persons who have been or are addicted to drugs of the analgesic group.
Adverse Reactions: Unpleasant symptoms, such as nausea, dizziness, headache, and fainting, are encountered only infrequently following the administration of Copavin. Constipation is reported in approximately 6 percent of the cases. If necessary, an appropriate laxative may be prescribed.
Dosage: *Adults*—1 Pulvule after each meal and 2 Pulvules at bedtime for a three-day period. Additional doses may be taken occasionally if the symptoms are severe.
Children—Dosage should be adjusted according to weight, with the average child of elementary school age receiving approximately one-half the usual adult dose.
Overdosage: Narcotic antagonists are indicated for the treatment of toxic doses of codeine. These agents should be repeatedly administered as indicated by patient response. Papaverine is comparatively nontoxic, although in gross overdosage it can cause cardiac arrhythmia.
How Supplied: (©) *Pulvules No. 230, F36,** *Copavin® (codeine and papaverine, Lilly)* (No. 3, Clear), in bottles of 100.
[110876]

CRYSTODIGIN® ℞
(digitoxin)
Injection, USP
AMPOULES

Description: The cardiac (or digitalis) glycosides are a closely related group of drugs having in common specific and powerful effects on the myocardium. Typically, the glycosides are composed of three portions—a steroid nucleus, a lactone ring, and a sugar (hence, "glycosides").
Crystodigin® (digitoxin, Lilly) is a crystalline cardiac glycoside obtained from *Digitalis purpurea.* Crystodigin® Injection (Digitoxin Injection, USP, Lilly) is a sterile solution of digitoxin in water for injection and 49 percent (v/v) alcohol. Each ampoule contains 0.2 mg of digitoxin in each ml.
Actions: Qualitatively, digitalis glycosides have the same therapeutic effect on the heart. They increase the force of myocardial contraction, increase the refractory period of the atrioventricular (AV) node, and, to a lesser degree, affect the sinoatrial (SA) node and conduction system via the parasympathetic and sympathetic nervous systems.
Following intravenous injection of Crystodigin® (digitoxin, Lilly), the action starts in 25 minutes to two hours, is maximal in four to 12 hours, regresses in two to three days, and disappears in two to three weeks.
Indications: Crystodigin® (digitoxin, Lilly) Injection is indicated in the following conditions when the patient cannot take medication by mouth.
Congestive Heart Failure (All Degrees)—The increased cardiac output results in diuresis and general amelioration of the disturbances characteristic of right and left heart failure. Digitalis, generally, is most effective in "low-output" failure and less effective in "high-output" (bronchopulmonary insufficiency, infection, hyperthyroidism) heart failure. The drug should be continued after heart failure is abolished unless some known precipitating factor is corrected.
Atrial Fibrillation—Digitalis is especially indicated when the ventricular rate is elevated. It rapidly reduces ventricular rates and thus the pulse deficit. Digitalis is continued in doses necessary to maintain the desired ventricular rate and other clinical effects.
Atrial Flutter—Digitalis usually slows the heart, and regular sinus rhythm may appear. Flutter may be converted to atrial fibrillation with a slow ventricular rate. Stopping digitalis treatment at this point may result in restoration of sinus rhythm, especially if the flutter was of the paroxysmal type. It is preferable, however, to continue digitalis if failure ensues or if atrial flutter is a frequent occurrence.
Paroxysmal Atrial Tachycardia—Digitalis may be used, especially if the tachycardia is resistant to lesser measures. Depending on the urgency, a more rapidly acting parenteral digitalis preparation may be preferable. If failure has ensued or paroxysms recur frequently, the digitalis effect should be maintained by oral administration.
The value of digitalis is not established in cardiogenic shock.
Contraindications: The presence of toxic effects (*see* Overdosage and Toxic Effects) in-

Continued on next page

*Identi-Code® symbol.

Lilly—Cont.

duced by any digitalis preparation is an absolute contraindication to all of the glycosides. Allergy, though rare, does occur.
Ventricular tachycardia is a contraindication. However, if congestive failure supervenes after a protracted episode of tachycardia and the patient has not already received digitalis, the drug may be used.
Warnings: Many of the arrhythmias for which digitalis is advised are identical with those reflecting digitalis intoxication. When the possibility of digitalis intoxication cannot be excluded, cardiac glycosides should be withheld temporarily if the clinical situation permits.
The patient with congestive heart failure may complain of nausea and vomiting. Since these symptoms may also be associated with digitalis intoxication, a clinical determination of their cause must be attempted before further administration of the drug.
Cases of idiopathic hypertrophic subaortic stenosis must be managed with extreme care. Unless cardiac failure is severe, it is doubtful whether digitalis should be employed.
Children—During the first month of life, infants have a sharply defined tolerance to digitalis. Impaired renal function must also be considered. Premature and immature infants are particularly sensitive, and reduction of dosage may be necessary.
The presence of acute glomerulonephritis accompanied by congestive failure requires extreme care in digitalization. A relatively low total dose, administered in divided doses, and concomitant use of reserpine or other antihypertensive agents have been recommended. Constant ECG monitoring is essential. Digitalis should be discontinued as soon as possible.
Patients with rheumatic carditis, especially when severe, are unusually sensitive to digitalis and prone to disturbances of rhythm. If heart failure develops, digitalization may be tried with relatively low doses; these must be cautiously increased until a beneficial effect is obtained. If a therapeutic trial does not result in improvement, the drug should be discontinued.
Note: Digitalis glycosides are an important cause of accidental poisoning in children.
Precautions: Great caution should be exercised when Crystodigin® (digitoxin, Lilly) Injection is given to patients still under the influence of digitalis from previous medication; to patients with hypercalcemia; and in the presence of multiple ventricular extrasystoles, hypersensitivity of the carotid sinus, Adams-Stokes syndrome, or heart block.
Potassium depletion sensitizes the myocardium to digitalis. Toxicity is apt to develop even with usual dosage. Hypokalemia also tends to reduce the positive inotropic effect of digitalis. Potassium wastage may result from diuretic, corticosteroid, hemodialysis, and other therapy and is liable to accompany malnutrition, old age, and long-standing congestive heart failure.
Patients with acute myocardial infarction, severe pulmonary disease, or far-advanced heart failure are likely to be more sensitive to digitalis and may be more prone to disturbances of rhythm.
Calcium may produce serious arrhythmias in digitalized patients and should not be given to them intravenously.
In myxedema, digitalis requirements are reduced because the excretion rate is decreased and blood levels are significantly higher.
Patients with incomplete atrioventricular block, especially those subject to Stokes-Adams attacks, may develop advanced or complete heart block. Heart failure in these patients can usually be controlled by other measures and by increasing the heart rate.
Patients with chronic constrictive pericarditis are likely to respond unfavorably.
Renal insufficiency delays the excretion of digitalis, and dosage must be adjusted accordingly in patients with renal disease.
Note: This applies also to potassium administration, should it become necessary.
Electrical conversion of arrhythmias may require adjustment of digitalis dosage.
Children—Dosage must be carefully titrated. Electrocardiographic monitoring may be necessary to avoid intoxication. Premonitory signs of toxicity in the newborn are undue slowing of the sinus rate, sinoatrial arrest, and prolongation of the P-R interval.
Adverse Reaction: Gynecomastia can occur, but it is uncommon.
Overdosage and Toxic Effects: *Gastrointestinal*—Anorexia, nausea, vomiting, and diarrhea are the most common early symptoms of overdosage in the adult (but are rarely conspicuous in infants). Uncontrolled heart failure may also produce such symptoms.
Central Nervous System—Headache, weakness, apathy, and visual disturbances may be present. Mental depression may be an early symptom; mental confusion, disorientation, and delirium may be seen with more severe intoxication.
Cardiovascular—The most common arrhythmia is ventricular premature beats (except in infants and young children). Paroxysmal and nonparoxysmal nodal rhythms, atrioventricular (interference) dissociation, and paroxysmal atrial tachycardia with block are also common arrhythmias due to digitalis overdosage.
Excessive slowing of the pulse is a clinical sign of digitalis overdosage. Atrioventricular block of increasing degree may proceed to complete heart block. The electrocardiogram is fundamental in determining the presence and nature of these arrhythmias. Other electrocardiographic changes (as of the S-T segment) provide no measure of the degree of digitalization.
Children—Cardiac arrhythmias are the more reliable and frequent signs of toxicity, whereas vomiting, diarrhea, and neurologic and ophthalmologic disturbances are rare as initial signs.
Premature ventricular systoles are rarely seen; nodal and atrial systoles are more frequent. Atrial arrhythmias, atrial ectopic rhythms, and paroxysmal atrial tachycardia (particularly with atrioventricular block) are more common manifestations of toxicity in children. Ventricular arrhythmias are rare.
Treatment of Toxic Arrhythmias: *Adults*—Digitalis should be discontinued until all signs of toxicity are abolished. This may be all that is necessary if toxic manifestations are not severe and appear after the time for peak effect of the drug.
Potassium salts are commonly used, e.g., potassium chloride in divided doses totaling 4 to 6 gm, provided renal function is adequate. When correction of the arrhythmia is urgently needed, potassium may be administered intravenously in a solution of 5% dextrose in water, for a total dosage of 40 to 100 mEq (40 mEq per 500 ml) at the rate of 40 mEq per hour, unless injection is limited because of pain due to local irritation. Additional amounts may be given if the arrhythmia is uncontrolled and the potassium is well tolerated. Electrocardiographic monitoring is indicated to avoid potassium toxicity, e.g., peaking of T waves. However, potassium should not be used and may be dangerous when severe or complete heart block is due to digitalis (and is not related to tachycardia).
Chelating agents to bind calcium may also be used to counteract the arrhythmia caused by digitalis toxicity, hypokalemia, or elevated serum calcium. Four gm (0.8% solution) of the disodium salt of EDTA (ethylenediaminetetraacetic acid) are dissolved in 500 ml of 5% dextrose in water (50 mg per ml) and administered over a period of two hours, unless the arrhythmia is controlled before the infusion is completed. A continuous electrocardiogram should be observed so that the infusion may be stopped promptly when the desired effect is achieved. Other counteracting agents are quinidine, procainamide, and beta-adrenergic blocking agents.
Children—Potassium preparations may be given orally in divided doses totaling 1 to 2 gm daily. When correction of the arrhythmia is urgent, 5 to 10 mEq of potassium per hour may be given; this amount should be dissolved in 100 ml of 5% dextrose in water. Additional amounts of potassium may be administered if necessary and if well tolerated by the child.
A chelating agent may be tried if other measures fail. EDTA has been recommended in an intravenous dose of 15 mg/kg per hour in 5% dextrose in water, with the total not to exceed 60 mg/kg per day. A continuous electrocardiogram should be observed so that the infusion can be stopped promptly when the desired effect is achieved.
Administration and Dosage: Crystodigin® (digitoxin, Lilly) Injection should be given intravenously.
Adults—Intravenous administration of Crystodigin should be used only when the drug cannot be taken orally.
The average digitalizing dose by the intravenous route is 1.2 to 1.6 mg; this is approximately the same as that used when digitoxin is given orally.
In a patient who has not received digitalis or any digitalis-like preparation during the preceding three weeks, digitalization may be accomplished by the slow intravenous injection of an initial dose of 0.6 mg Crystodigin, followed by 0.4 mg four to six hours later and by 0.2 mg every four to six hours thereafter until the full therapeutic effect becomes apparent. This should occur in eight to 12 hours. Daily intravenous or oral administration of 0.05 to 0.3 mg of Crystodigin will be needed as a maintenance dose. It should be emphasized that the dose of Crystodigin must be proportionately reduced for partially digitalized patients.
The administration of the average digitalizing dose in a single injection is not recommended. Patients who have extensive myocardial damage or conduction defects may require a much smaller quantity of digitoxin than those with less abnormal hearts.
Children—Digitalization must be individualized. Generally, premature and immature infants are particularly sensitive and require reduced dosage that must be determined by careful titration. Intravenous doses should be given slowly with continuous electrocardiographic monitoring to avoid toxic doses.
The digitalizing dose for newborn infants under two weeks, premature infants, and those having reduced renal function or myocarditis is 0.022 mg/kg (0.3 to 0.35 mg/m^2).
After the neonatal period, the dose is as follows:

Under one year of age—0.045 mg/kg
One to two years of age—0.04 mg/kg
Over two years of age—0.03 mg/kg
(0.75 mg/m^2)

The total dose should be divided into three, four, or more portions, with six hours or more between doses.
For a maintenance dose, the patient should be given one-tenth of the digitalizing dose.
How Supplied: (℞) *Ampoules No. 426, Crystodigin® (Digitoxin Injection, USP),* 0.2 mg, 1 ml; in packages of 6 and 100. [082378]

CRYSTODIGIN® ℞
(digitoxin)
Tablets, USP

Description: Crystodigin® (digitoxin, Lilly) is a crystalline-pure single cardiac glycoside obtained from *Digitalis purpurea* and is identical in pharmacologic action with whole-leaf digitalis.

Digitoxin is the most slowly excreted of all digitalis compounds (excretion time is 14 to 21 days). It is most useful in patients with impaired renal function, since excretion and metabolism are independent of renal function.
Crystodigin is noted for its uniform potency, complete absorption, and lack of gastrointestinal irritation. It permits accurate dosage adjustments to produce maximum therapeutic effect smoothly and dependably.
Crystodigin, for oral administration, is available in tablets containing 0.05, 0.1, 0.15, or 0.2 mg crystalline digitoxin.
Digitoxin is a cardiotonic glycoside. The chemical name is card-20 (22) - enolide,3-[(*O*-2,6-dideoxy-*β*- D -*ribo* -hexopyranosyl-(1→4)-*O*-2,6-dideoxy-*β*- D -*ribo* -hexopyranosyl - (1→4)-2,6-dideoxy - *β* - D -*ribo* - hexopyranosyl)oxy]-14-hydroxy, (3*β*,5*β*)-. The empirical formula of digitoxin is $C_{41}H_{64}O_{13}$.

Clinical Pharmacology: The cellular basis for the inotropic effects of digitalis is probably enhancement of excitation-contraction coupling, that process by which chemical energy is converted into mechanical energy when triggered by membrane depolarization. Most evidence relates this process to the entry of calcium ions into the cell during depolarization of the membrane and/or to the release of calcium from intracellular binding sites on the sarcoplasmic reticulum. The free calcium ion mediates the interaction of actin and myosin, resulting in contraction.
The amount of glycoside absorbed depends largely on its polarity, which is a function of the net electronic charge on the molecule. The more nonpolar or lipid soluble, the better is the absorption, because of the greater permeability of lipid membrane of the intestinal mucosa for lipid-soluble substances. The nonpolar, lipophilic digitoxin is completely absorbed; the oral dose, therefore, is the same as the intravenous dose. Other glycosides are not as well absorbed.
Nonpolar digitoxin is over 90 percent bound to tissue proteins. The firm binding of digitoxin to protein is responsible for its long half-life (seven to nine days).
Digitoxin differs from other commonly used glycosides not only in its firm binding to protein but also because it is metabolized in the liver, with the only active metabolite being digoxin, which represents only a small fraction of the total metabolites. All other metabolites are inert and are probably excreted as such in the urine. The portion of digitoxin that is not metabolized is excreted in the bile to the intestines and recycled to the liver until it is completely metabolized. The portion of digitoxin that is bound to protein is in equilibrium with free digitoxin in the serum. Thus, as more and more of the free digitoxin is metabolized after a single dose, there is proportionately less bound digitoxin.

Indications and Usage: Crystodigin® (digitoxin, Lilly) is indicated in the treatment of heart failure, atrial flutter, atrial fibrillation, and supraventricular tachycardia. Parenteral administration of Crystodigin is indicated for neonates and immature infants.

Contraindications: If the indications are carefully observed, there are few contraindications to digitalis therapy except toxic response to digitalis or idiosyncrasy, ventricular tachycardia, beriberi heart disease, and some instances of the hypersensitive carotid sinus syndrome.
Patients already taking digitalis preparations must not be given the rapid digitalizing dose of Crystodigin® (digitoxin, Lilly) or parenteral calcium.

Warnings: Many of the arrhythmias for which digitalis is advised are identical with those reflecting digitalis intoxication. When the possibility of digitalis intoxication cannot be excluded, cardiac glycosides should be withheld temporarily if the clinical situation permits.
The patient with congestive heart failure may complain of nausea and vomiting. Since these symptoms may also be associated with digitalis intoxication, a clinical determination of their cause must be attempted before further administration of the drug.
Cases of idiopathic hypertrophic subaortic stenosis must be managed with extreme care. Unless cardiac failure is severe, it is doubtful whether digitalis should be employed.
Children—During the first month of life, infants have a sharply defined tolerance to digitalis. Impaired renal function must also be considered. Premature and immature infants are particularly sensitive, and reduction in dosage may be necessary.
The presence of acute glomerulonephritis accompanied by congestive failure requires extreme care in digitalization. A relatively low total dose, administered in divided doses, and concomitant use of reserpine or other antihypertensive agents have been recommended. Constant ECG monitoring is essential. Digitalis should be discontinued as soon as possible.
Patients with rheumatic carditis, especially when severe, are unusually sensitive to digitalis and prone to disturbances of rhythm. If heart failure develops, digitalization may be tried with relatively low doses; these must be cautiously increased until a beneficial effect is obtained. If a therapeutic trial does not result in improvement, the drug should be discontinued.
NOTE: Digitalis glycosides are an important cause of accidental poisoning in children.

Precautions: *General Precautions*—When the risk of digitalis intoxication is great, the use of a short-acting, rapidly eliminated glycoside, such as digoxin, is advisable. Although intoxication cannot always be prevented by the selection of one glycoside over another, certain glycosides may be preferred in patients who have fixed disabilities (e.g., liver impairment, drug intolerance). However, digitoxin can be used in patients with impaired renal function.
Newborn infants with heart disease, especially prematures, are particularly susceptible to digitalis intoxication, and frequent electrocardiographic monitoring is essential in these patients. Special care must likewise be exercised in elderly patients receiving digitalis because their body mass tends to be small and renal clearance is likely to be reduced. In addition, digitalis must be used cautiously in the presence of active heart disease, such as acute myocardial infarction or acute myocarditis. In patients with acute or unstable chronic atrial fibrillation, digitalis may not normalize the ventricular rate even when the serum concentration exceeds the usual therapeutic level. Although these patients may be less sensitive to the toxic effects of digitalis than are patients with normal sinus rhythm, dosage should not be increased to potentially toxic levels.
Hypokalemia predisposes to digitalis toxicity, and even a moderate decrease in the concentration of serum potassium can precipitate serious arrhythmias.
Impaired liver function may necessitate reduction in dosage of any digitalis preparation, including digitoxin.
Sensitive radioimmunoassay techniques have been developed for measuring serum levels of digitoxin, and these procedures can be instituted in almost any hospital. Serum levels must, however, be evaluated in conjunction with clinical history and the results of the electrocardiogram and other laboratory tests. A therapeutic serum level for one patient may be excessive or inadequate for another patient.
Drug Interactions—The synthesis of microsomal enzymes that metabolize digitoxin in the liver is subject to stimulation by a number of drugs, such as antihistamines, anticonvulsants, barbiturates, oral hypoglycemic agents, and others.
When digitoxin is the glycoside used for digitalis maintenance, drugs that are liver-microsomal enzyme inducers should not be used at the same time. Phenobarbital, phenylbutazone, and diphenylhydantoin will increase the rate of metabolism of digitoxin. In patients receiving 60 mg of phenobarbital three times a day for 12 weeks, the steady-state concentration of digitoxin in plasma fell approximately 50 percent when the drugs were administered concurrently and returned to previous levels when phenobarbital was discontinued.
When drugs that increase the rate of metabolism of digitoxin in the liver are discontinued, toxicity may occur.
Hypokalemia is most frequently encountered in patients receiving concomitant diuretic therapy, because the most widely used and most effective diuretics (i.e., thiazides and furosemide) increase the urinary loss of potassium. Prescribing a potassium-sparing agent (spironolactone or triamterene) together with the potassium-wasting diuretic is a reliable means for maintaining the serum potassium level. Alternatively, potassium chloride supplements may be prescribed.
Mineralocorticoids (e.g., prednisone) and, rarely, certain antibiotics (e.g., amphotericin B) may also cause increased excretion of potassium.
Usage in Pregnancy—Pregnancy Category C—Animal reproduction studies have not been conducted with Crystodigin. It is also not known whether this drug can cause fetal harm when administered to a pregnant woman or can affect reproduction capacity. Crystodigin should be given to a pregnant woman only if clearly needed.
Labor and Delivery—No information is available concerning the use of Crystodigin in labor and delivery.
Nursing Mothers—It is not known whether this drug is excreted in human milk. Because many drugs are excreted in human milk, caution should be exercised when Crystodigin is administered to a nursing woman.

Adverse Reactions Anorexia, nausea, and vomiting have been reported. These effects are central in origin, but following large oral doses, there is also a local emetic action. Abdominal discomfort or pain and diarrhea may also occur.

Overdosage: Overdosage causes side effects, such as mental depression, anorexia, nausea, vomiting, premature beats, complete heart block, AV dissociation, ventricular tachycardia, ventricular fibrillation, restlessness, yellow vision, mental confusion, disorientation, and delirium.
Alterations in cardiac rate and rhythm occurring in digitalis poisoning may simulate almost any known type of arrhythmia seen clinically. Extrasystoles are probably the most frequent effect. An electrocardiogram is necessary in the clinical management of the patient to aid in the differentiation of arrhythmia due to digitalis poisoning from that due to heart disease. Older patients and particularly those with disease of the coronary arteries and impaired myocardial blood supply are more susceptible to these untoward effects. Sinus arrhythmia may occur early as a minor toxic effect. Paroxysmal atrial and ventricular tachycardia call for immediate cessation of the drug. Atrial fibrillation can occur following large doses of digitalis. Ventricular fibrillation is the most common cause of death from digitalis poisoning.
Potassium ion is probably the best agent for prompt suppression of digitalis arrhythmias. It can be administered intravenously in the form of potassium chloride at a rate of 0.5 mEq per minute in sodium chloride (isotonic) or dextrose (5 percent) solution containing 50 to 100 mEq of potassium per liter. Administration of

Continued on next page

Lilly—Cont.

the potassium salt in normal saline is preferred. Constant electrocardiographic monitoring is essential during injection of the solution. Since the action of potassium ion lasts only minutes after infusion is discontinued, oral therapy with potassium chloride may be given for prolonged suppression of arrhythmias. Potassium is contraindicated in the presence of renal failure. Diphenylhydantoin may be used if potassium fails or is contraindicated. If both potassium and diphenylhydantoin fail, procainamide and quinidine can be used. Disodium edetate has been used for terminating digitalis-induced ventricular arrhythmias and abnormalities of atrioventricular conduction.

Administration and Dosage: *Adults: Slow Digitalization*—0.2 mg twice daily for a period of four days, followed by maintenance dosage. *Rapid Digitalization*—Preferably 0.6 mg initially, followed by 0.4 mg and then 0.2 mg at intervals of four to six hours. *Maintenance Dosage*—Ranges from 0.05 to 0.3 mg daily, the most common dose being 0.15 mg daily.

Children: Digitalization must be individualized. Generally, premature and immature infants are particularly sensitive and require reduced parenteral dosage of Crystodigin that must be determined by careful titration.

After the neonatal period, the dose is as follows:

Under one year of age—0.045 mg/kg
One to two years of age—0.04 mg/kg
Over two years of age—0.03 mg/kg (0.75 mg/m^2)

The total dose should be divided into three, four, or more portions, with six hours or more between doses.

For a maintenance dose, the patient should be given one-tenth of the digitalizing dose.

How Supplied: (℞) *Tablets Crystodigin® (Digitoxin Tablets, USP)* (scored): *No. 1736, J75,** 0.05 mg, Orange, in bottles of 100 (NDC 0002-1075-02) and 500 (NDC 0002-1075-03); *No. 1703, J60,** 0.1 mg, Pink, in bottles of 100 (NDC 0002-1060-02), 500 (NDC 0002-1060-03), and 5000 (NDC 0002-1060-31) and in 10 strips of 10 individually labeled blisters each containing 1 tablet (ID100) (NDC 0002-1060-33); *No. 1737, J76,** 0.15 mg, Yellow, and *No. 1694, J57,** 0.2 mg, White, in bottles of 100 (NDC 0002-1076 and 1057-02) and 500 (NDC 0002-1076 and 1057-03).

[101779]

[*Shown in Product Identification Section*]

CYCLOMETHYCAINE SULFATE, *see* Surfacaine® (cyclomethycaine sulfate, Lilly)

CYCLOSERINE, *see* Seromycin® (cycloserine, Lilly).

CYCLOTHIAZIDE, *see* Anhydron® (cyclothiazide, Lilly).

CYTELLIN® ℞
(sitosterols)

Description: Each 15 ml (approximately 1 tablespoonful) contain 3 gm Cytellin® (sitosterols, Lilly), with alcohol, approximately 0.95 percent.

Actions: The exact mechanism of action is unknown. Cytellin (sitosterols) may lower elevated serum cholesterol by interfering with the intestinal absorption of cholesterol.

Indications: Cytellin® (sitosterols, Lilly) is indicated as adjunctive therapy in the treatment of patients with hypercholesterolemia and hyperbetalipoproteinemia who do not respond adequately to diet and other measures.

Note: The effect of Cytellin in lowering serum cholesterol is usually moderate and variable in magnitude.

Proper assessment of the magnitude and variability of changes in serum cholesterol depends on obtaining several (usually three or more) base-line serum cholesterol values while the subject is on a controlled diet over a period of one to three weeks prior to treatment with Cytellin.

Notice: It has not been established whether drug-induced lowering of serum cholesterol or triglyceride levels has a detrimental, a beneficial, or no effect on the morbidity or mortality due to atherosclerosis, including coronary heart disease. Investigations now in progress may yield an answer to this question.

Contraindications: There are no known contraindications to the use of Cytellin® (sitosterols, Lilly).

Warnings: Since the safety of Cytellin® (sitosterols, Lilly) for use during pregnancy has not been established, the potential hazards of the drug must be weighed against the possible benefits.

Precautions: Cytellin® (sitosterols, Lilly) may interfere with the absorption of other substances and drugs besides cholesterol.

Adverse Reactions: Sitosterols are excreted in the feces and may produce bulky light-colored stools. A mild laxative effect (looseness of the stool) may also occur because of the methylcellulose derivative which is used as a dispersing agent in Cytellin® (sitosterols, Lilly).

Administration and Dosage: Cytellin® (sitosterols, Lilly) is given by mouth. It can be mixed with coffee, tea, fruit juices, or milk. This method of administration has been found to increase the palatability of Cytellin. The suggested dosage is 1 tablespoonful (approximately 15 ml) immediately before meals.

The dose may be increased to 1½ or 2 tablespoonfuls when large or high-fat meals are consumed. To obtain optimum therapeutic effect, any additional food taken between meals should be preceded by a whole or fractional dose of Cytellin. The total daily dose should not exceed 8 to 12 tablespoonfuls (24 to 36 gm).

How Supplied: (℞) *Suspension No. M-100, Cytellin® (sitosterols, Lilly),* in 16-fluid-ounce bottles. *Avoid freezing.*

[100678]

DARVOCET-N® 50 and DARVOCET-N® 100 ©
(propoxyphene napsylate with acetaminophen)

DARVON-N®
(propoxyphene napsylate) NF

DARVON-N® WITH A.S.A.®
(propoxyphene napsylate with aspirin)

Description: Propoxyphene napsylate (Darvon-N®) is an odorless white crystalline solid with a bitter taste. It is very slightly soluble in water and soluble in methanol, ethanol, chloroform, and acetone. Chemically, it is α-(+)-4-(Dimethylamino)-3-methyl-1, 2-diphenyl-2-butanol Propionate (ester) 2-Naphthalenesulfonate (salt) Hydrate.

Propoxyphene napsylate differs from propoxyphene hydrochloride in that it allows more stable liquid dosage forms and tablet formulations. Because of differences in molecular weight, a dose of 100 mg of propoxyphene napsylate is required to supply an amount of propoxyphene equivalent to that present in 65 mg of propoxyphene hydrochloride.

Each tablet of Darvocet-N 50 contains 50 mg propoxyphene napsylate and 325 mg acetaminophen.

Each tablet of Darvocet-N 100 contains 100 mg propoxyphene napsylate and 650 mg acetaminophen.

Each 5 ml of Suspension Darvon-N contain 50 mg propoxyphene napsylate.

Each tablet of Darvon-N contains 100 mg propoxyphene napsylate.

Each tablet of Darvon-N with A.S.A. contains 100 mg propoxyphene napsylate and 325 mg aspirin.

Clinical Pharmacology: Propoxyphene is a centrally acting narcotic analgesic agent. Equimolar doses of propoxyphene hydrochloride or napsylate provide similar plasma concentrations. Following administration of 65, 130, or 195 mg of propoxyphene hydrochloride, the bioavailability of propoxyphene is equivalent to that of 100, 200, or 300 mg respectively of propoxyphene napsylate. Peak plasma concentrations of propoxyphene are reached in two to two and one-half hours. After a 100-mg oral dose of propoxyphene napsylate, peak plasma levels of 0.05 to 0.1 mcg/ml are achieved. As shown in Figure 1, the napsylate salt tends to be absorbed more slowly than the hydrochloride. At or near therapeutic doses, this difference is small when compared with that among subjects and among doses.

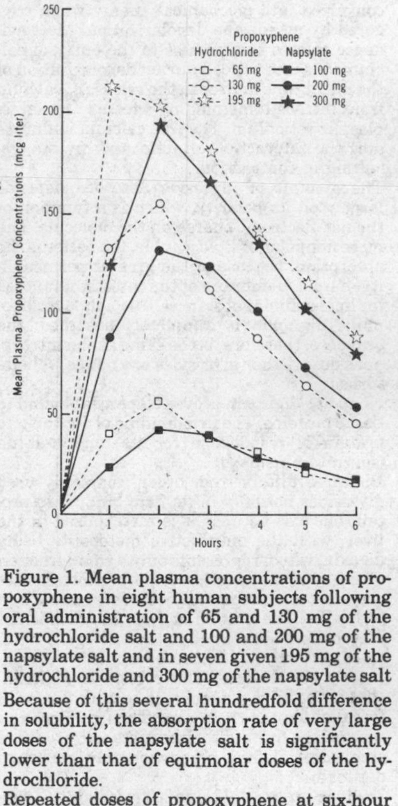

Figure 1. Mean plasma concentrations of propoxyphene in eight human subjects following oral administration of 65 and 130 mg of the hydrochloride salt and 100 and 200 mg of the napsylate salt and in seven given 195 mg of the hydrochloride and 300 mg of the napsylate salt

Because of this several hundredfold difference in solubility, the absorption rate of very large doses of the napsylate salt is significantly lower than that of equimolar doses of the hydrochloride.

Repeated doses of propoxyphene at six-hour intervals lead to increasing plasma concentrations, with a plateau after the ninth dose at 48 hours.

Propoxyphene is metabolized in the liver to yield norpropoxyphene. Propoxyphene has a half-life of six to 12 hours, whereas that of norpropoxyphene is 30 to 36 hours.

Norpropoxyphene has substantially less central-nervous-system-depressant effect than propoxyphene but a greater local anesthetic effect, which is similar to that of amitriptyline and antiarrhythmic agents, such as lidocaine and quinidine.

In animal studies in which propoxyphene and norpropoxyphene were continuously infused in large amounts, intracardiac conduction time (P-R and QRS intervals) was prolonged. Any intracardiac conduction delay attributable to high concentrations of norpropoxyphene may be of relatively long duration.

Actions: Propoxyphene is a mild narcotic analgesic structurally related to methadone.

The potency of propoxyphene napsylate is from two-thirds to equal that of codeine.

Darvocet-N 50 and Darvocet-N 100 provide the analgesic activity of propoxyphene napsylate and the antipyretic-analgesic activity of acetaminophen.

The combination of propoxyphene and acetaminophen produces greater analgesia than that produced by either propoxyphene or acetaminophen administered alone.

The combination of propoxyphene with aspirin produces greater analgesia than that produced by either drug administered alone.

Indications: Darvocet-N 50, Darvocet-N 100, and Darvon-N with A.S.A. are indicated for the relief of mild to moderate pain, either when pain is present alone or when it is accompanied by fever.

Darvon-N® (propoxyphene napsylate, Lilly) is indicated for the relief of mild to moderate pain.

Contraindications: Hypersensitivity to propoxyphene, acetaminophen, or aspirin.

WARNINGS

- **Do not prescribe propoxyphene for patients who are suicidal or addiction-prone.**
- **Prescribe propoxyphene with caution for patients taking tranquilizers or antidepressant drugs and patients who use alcohol in excess.**
- **Tell your patients not to exceed the recommended dose and to limit their intake of alcohol.**

Propoxyphene products in excessive doses, either alone or in combination with other C.N.S. depressants, including alcohol, are a major cause of drug-related deaths. Fatalities within the first hour of overdosage are not uncommon. In a survey of deaths due to overdosage conducted in 1975, in approximately 20 percent of the fatal cases, death occurred within the first hour (5 percent occurred within 15 minutes). Propoxyphene should not be taken in doses higher than those recommended by the physician. The judicious prescribing of propoxyphene is essential to the safe use of this drug. With patients who are depressed or suicidal, consideration should be given to the use of non-narcotic analgesics. Patients should be cautioned about the concomitant use of propoxyphene products and alcohol because of potentially serious C.N.S.-additive effects of these agents. Because of its added depressant effects, propoxyphene should be prescribed with caution for those patients whose medical condition requires the concomitant administration of sedatives, tranquilizers, muscle relaxants, antidepressants, or other C.N.S.-depressant drugs. Patients should be advised of the additive depressant effects of these combinations.

Many of the propoxyphene-related deaths have occurred in patients with previous histories of emotional disturbances or suicidal ideation or attempts as well as histories of misuse of tranquilizers, alcohol, and other C.N.S.-active drugs. Some deaths have occurred as a consequence of the accidental ingestion of excessive quantities of propoxyphene alone or in combination with other drugs. Patients taking propoxyphene should be warned not to exceed the dosage recommended by the physician.

Drug Dependence—Propoxyphene, when taken in higher-than-recommended doses over long periods of time, can produce drug dependence characterized by psychic dependence and, less frequently, physical dependence and tolerance. Propoxyphene will only partially suppress the withdrawal syndrome in individuals physically dependent on morphine or other narcotics. The abuse liability of propoxyphene is qualitatively similar to that of codeine although quantitatively less, and propoxyphene should be prescribed with the same degree of caution appropriate to the use of codeine.

Usage in Ambulatory Patients—Propoxyphene may impair the mental and/or physical abilities required for the performance of potentially hazardous tasks, such as driving a car or operating machinery. The patient should be cautioned accordingly.

Precautions: *General Precautions*— Salicylates should be used with extreme caution in the presence of peptic ulcer or coagulation abnormalities.

Drug Interactions—The C.N.S.-depressant effect of propoxyphene is additive with that of other C.N.S. depressants, including alcohol.

Usage in Pregnancy—Safe use in pregnancy has not been established relative to possible adverse effects on fetal development. Instances of withdrawal symptoms in the neonate have been reported following usage during pregnancy. Therefore, propoxyphene should not be used in pregnant women unless, in the judgment of the physician, the potential benefits outweigh the possible hazards.

Usage in Nursing Mothers—Low levels of propoxyphene have been detected in human milk. In postpartum studies involving nursing mothers who were given propoxyphene, no adverse effects were noted in infants receiving mother's milk.

Usage in Children—Propoxyphene is not recommended for use in children, because documented clinical experience has been insufficient to establish safety and a suitable dosage regimen in the pediatric age group.

A Patient Information Sheet is available for these products. See text following "How Supplied" section below.

Adverse Reactions: In a survey conducted in hospitalized patients, less than 1 percent of patients taking propoxyphene hydrochloride at recommended doses experienced side effects. The most frequently reported have been dizziness, sedation, nausea, and vomiting. Some of these adverse reactions may be alleviated if the patient lies down.

Other adverse reactions include constipation, abdominal pain, skin rashes, lightheadedness, headache, weakness, euphoria, dysphoria, and minor visual disturbances.

Cases of liver dysfunction have been reported.

Administration and Dosage: These products are given orally. The usual dose of Darvocet-N 50 or Darvocet-N 100 is 100 mg propoxyphene napsylate and 650 mg acetaminophen every four hours as needed for pain.

The usual dose of Darvon-N® (propoxyphene napsylate, Lilly) is 100 mg every four hours as needed for pain.

The usual dose of Darvon-N with A.S.A. is 100 mg propoxyphene napsylate and 325 mg aspirin every four hours as needed for pain.

The maximum recommended dose of propoxyphene napsylate is 600 mg per day.

Management of Overdosage: Initial consideration should be given to the management of the C.N.S. effects of propoxyphene overdosage. Resuscitative measures should be initiated promptly.

Symptoms of Propoxyphene Overdosage—The manifestations of acute overdosage with propoxyphene are those of narcotic overdosage. The patient is usually somnolent but may be stuporous or comatose and convulsing. Respiratory depression is characteristic. The ventilatory rate and/or tidal volume is decreased, which results in cyanosis and hypoxia. Pupils, initially pinpoint, may become dilated as hypoxia increases. Cheyne-Stokes respiration and apnea may occur. Blood pressure and heart rate are usually normal initially, but blood pressure falls and cardiac performance deteriorates, which ultimately results in pulmonary edema and circulatory collapse, unless the respiratory depression is corrected and adequate ventilation is restored promptly. Cardiac arrhythmias and conduction delay may be present. A combined respiratory-metabolic acidosis occurs owing to retained CO_2 (hypercapnea) and to lactic acid formed during anaerobic glycolysis. Acidosis may be severe if large amounts of salicylates have also been ingested. Death may occur.

Treatment of Propoxyphene Overdosage — Attention should be directed first to establishing a patent airway and to restoring ventilation. Mechanically assisted ventilation, with or without oxygen, may be required, and positive pressure respiration may be desirable if pulmonary edema is present. The narcotic antagonist naloxone will markedly reduce the degree of respiratory depression and should be administered promptly, preferably intravenously, 0.4 to 0.8 mg, and carefully repeated, as necessary, at 20 to 30-minute intervals. The duration of action of the antagonist may be brief. If no response is observed after 10 mg of naloxone have been administered, the diagnosis of propoxyphene toxicity should be questioned. (Nalorphine and levallorphan may be used if naloxone is not available, but these agents are not as satisfactory as naloxone.)

Blood gases, *p*H, and electrolytes should be monitored in order that acidosis and any electrolyte disturbance present may be corrected promptly. Acidosis, hypoxia, and generalized C.N.S. depression predispose to the development of cardiac arrhythmias. Ventricular fibrillation or cardiac arrest may occur and necessitate the full complement of cardiopulmonary resuscitation (CPR) measures. Respiratory acidosis rapidly subsides as ventilation is restored and hypercapnea eliminated, but lactic acidosis may require intravenous bicarbonate for prompt correction.

Electrocardiographic monitoring is essential. Prompt correction of hypoxia, acidosis, and electrolyte disturbance (when present) will help prevent these cardiac complications and will increase the effectiveness of agents administered to restore normal cardiac function.

In addition to the use of a narcotic antagonist, the patient may require careful titration with an anticonvulsant to control convulsions. Analeptic drugs (for example, caffeine or amphetamine) should not be used because of their tendency to precipitate convulsions.

General supportive measures, in addition to oxygen, include, when necessary, intravenous fluids, vasopressor-inotropic compounds, and, when infection is likely, anti-infective agents. Gastric lavage may be useful, and activated charcoal can adsorb a significant amount of ingested propoxyphene. Dialysis is of little value in poisoning due to propoxyphene. Efforts should be made to determine whether other agents, such as alcohol, barbiturates, tranquilizers, or other C.N.S. depressants, were also ingested, since these increase C.N.S. depression as well as cause specific toxic effects.

Symptoms of Acetaminophen Overdosage—Shortly after oral ingestion of an overdose of acetaminophen and for the next 24 hours, anorexia, nausea, vomiting, and abdominal pain have been noted. The patient may then present no symptoms, but evidence of liver dysfunction may be apparent during the next 24 to 48 hours, with elevated serum transaminase and lactic dehydrogenase levels, an increase in serum bilirubin concentrations, and a prolonged prothrombin time. Death from hepatic failure may result three to seven days after overdosage.

Treatment of Acetaminophen Overdosage—There is no specific antidote currently available for the treatment of acetaminophen intox-

Continued on next page

*Identi-Code® symbol.

Lilly—Cont.

ication. Subject to primary consideration of the C.N.S.-depressant effects of propoxyphene, gastric lavage should be instituted.

Symptoms of Salicylate Overdosage—Such symptoms include central nausea and vomiting, tinnitus and deafness, vertigo and headaches, mental dullness and confusion, diaphoresis, rapid pulse, and increased respiration and respiratory alkalosis.

Treatment of Salicylate Overdosage—When Darvon-N with A.S.A. has been ingested, the clinical picture may be complicated by salicylism.

The treatment of acute salicylate intoxication includes minimizing drug absorption, promoting elimination through the kidneys, and correcting metabolic derangements affecting body temperature, hydration, acid-base balance, and electrolyte balance. The technique to be employed for eliminating salicylate from the bloodstream depends on the degree of drug intoxication.

If the patient is seen within four hours of ingestion, the stomach should be emptied by inducing vomiting or by gastric lavage as soon as possible.

The nomogram of Done is a useful prognostic guide in which the expected severity of salicylate intoxication is based on serum salicylate levels and the time interval between ingestion and taking the blood sample.

Exchange transfusion is most feasible for a small infant. Intermittent peritoneal dialysis is useful for cases of moderate severity in adults. Intravenous fluids alkalinized by the addition of sodium bicarbonate or potassium citrate are helpful. Hemodialysis with the artificial kidney is the most effective means of removing salicylate and is indicated for the very severe cases of salicylate intoxication.

Animal Toxicology: The acute lethal doses of the hydrochloride and napsylate salts of propoxyphene were determined in four species. The results shown in Figure 2 indicate that, on a molar basis, the napsylate salt is less toxic than the hydrochloride. This may be due to the relative insolubility and retarded absorption of propoxyphene napsylate.

Figure 2. Acute oral toxicity of propoxyphene

LD_{50} (mg/kg) ± SE / LD_{50} (mM/kg)

Species	Propoxyphene Hydrochloride	Propoxyphene Napsylate
Mouse	282 ± 39 / 0.75	915 ± 163 / 1.62
Rat	230 ± 44 / 0.61	647 ± 95 / 1.14
Rabbit	ca. 82 / 0.22	> 183 / > 0.32
Dog	ca.100 / 0.27	> 183 / > 0.32

Some indication of the relative insolubility and retarded absorption of propoxyphene napsylate was obtained by measuring plasma propoxyphene levels in two groups of four dogs following oral administration of equimolar doses of the two salts. As shown in Figure 3, the peak plasma concentration observed with propoxyphene hydrochloride was much higher than that obtained after administration of the napsylate salt.

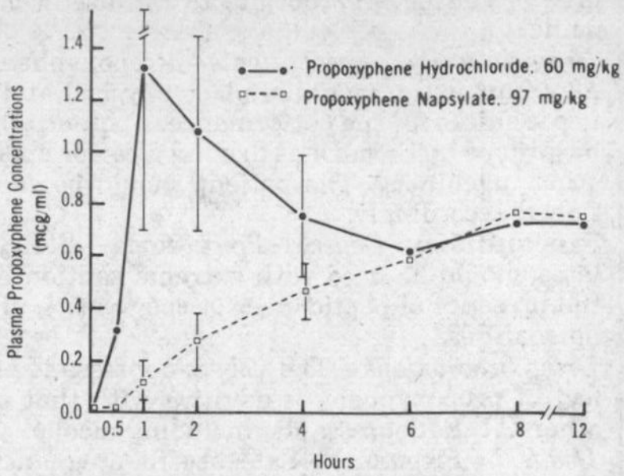

Figure 3. Plasma propoxyphene concentrations in dogs following large doses of the hydrochloride and napsylate salts

Although none of the animals in this experiment died, three of the four dogs given propoxyphene hydrochloride exhibited convulsive seizures during the time interval corresponding to the peak plasma levels. The four animals receiving the napsylate salt were mildly ataxic but not acutely ill.

How Supplied: Ⓔ *Darvocet-N® 50 (propoxyphene napsylate with acetaminophen, Lilly), Tablets No. 1890, C51,* *Specially Coated, Dark-Orange, in bottles of 500, in 10 strips of 10 individually labeled blisters each containing 1 tablet (ID100), in 500 single-cut individually labeled blisters each containing 1 tablet (ID500), and in ℞Paks (prescription packages, Lilly) in bottles of 100 and in 20 packages of 50. All ℞Paks have safety closures.

℞Pak 50—6505-00-135-2156

Ⓔ *Darvocet-N® 100 (propoxyphene napsylate with acetaminophen, Lilly), Tablets No. 1893, C63,* * Specially Coated, Dark-Orange, in bottles of 500, in 10 strips of 10 individually labeled blisters each containing 1 tablet (ID100), in 500 single-cut individually labeled blisters each containing 1 tablet (ID500), in 20 rolls, each consisting of 25 tablets in individual unit-dose packets, reverse-numbered (RN500), and in ℞Paks in bottles of 100, in 25 packages of 30, and in 20 packages of 50. All ℞Paks have safety closures.

℞Pak 30—6505-00-111-8364
ID100—6505-00-111-8373
500's—6505-00-111-8359

Ⓔ *Darvon-N® (Propoxyphene Napsylate Oral Suspension, NF), Suspension No. M-135,* 50 mg per 5 ml, in 16-fl-oz (473-ml) bottles; 100 mg per 10 ml, in unit-dose bottles of 100 (ID100). *Avoid freezing.*

Ⓔ *Darvon-N® (Propoxyphene Napsylate Tablets, NF), Tablets No. 1883, C53,* * 100 mg, Specially Coated, Buff, in bottles of 100 (℞Pak) and 500, in 10 strips of 10 individually labeled blisters each containing 1 tablet (ID100), in 500 single-cut individually labeled blisters each containing 1 tablet (ID500), and in ℞Paks in 25 packages of 30 and 20 packages of 50. All ℞Paks have safety closures.

℞Pak 30—6505-00-083-5750
500's —6505-00-111-8383

Ⓔ *Darvon-N® with A.S.A.® (propoxyphene napsylate with aspirin, Lilly), Tablets No. 1884, C54,* * Specially Coated, Orange, in bottles of 100 (℞Pak) and 500, in 10 strips of 10 individually labeled blisters each containing 1 tablet (ID100), in 500 single-cut individually labeled blisters each containing 1 tablet (ID500), and in ℞Paks in 25 packages of 30 and 20 packages of 50. All ℞Paks have safety closures.

℞Pak 30—6505-00-083-5762

[*Shown in Product Identification Section*]

The following information, including illustrations of dosage forms and the maximum daily dosage of each, is available to patients receiving Darvon products.

Patient Information Sheet

YOUR PRESCRIPTION FOR A DARVON® (PROPOXYPHENE) PRODUCT Ⓔ

Your doctor has chosen to prescribe Darvon®. Darvon is used for the relief of pain.

It is important that you read and understand the information in this leaflet. If you have any questions, ask your doctor or pharmacist.

GENERAL CAUTIONS

Other Drugs: Combinations of excessive doses of Darvon, alcohol, and tranquilizers may be dangerous. Make sure your doctor knows that you are taking tranquilizers, sleep aids, antidepressant drugs, antihistamines, or any other drugs that make you sleepy. The use of these drugs with Darvon increases their sedative effects and may lead to overdosage symptoms, including death (see "Overdosage" below).

Alcohol: Heavy use of alcohol with Darvon is hazardous and may lead to overdosage symptoms (see "Overdosage" below). THEREFORE, LIMIT YOUR INTAKE OF ALCOHOL WHILE TAKING DARVON.

Regular Activities: Darvon may cause drowsiness or impair your mental and/or physical abilities; therefore, use caution when driving a vehicle or operating dangerous machinery. DO NOT perform any hazardous task until you have seen your response to this drug.

Pregnancy: Do not take Darvon or other drugs during pregnancy unless your doctor knows you are pregnant and specifically recommends their use.

Children: Darvon is not recommended for use in children under 12 years of age.

Allergy: Do not take Darvon if you have had an allergic reaction to any dosage form of this drug.

Dependence: Darvon, when taken in higher-than-recommended doses over a long period of time, has produced physical and psychologic dependence (a craving for the drug or an inability to function normally without the drug).

SIDE EFFECTS

When Darvon is taken as directed, side effects are infrequent. Among those reported are drowsiness, dizziness, nausea, and vomiting. If these effects occur, some of them may go away if you lie down.

Less frequently reported side effects include constipation, abdominal pain, skin rashes, lightheadedness, headache, weakness, minor visual disturbances, and feelings of elation or discomfort.

If one of these side effects occurs and becomes severe, contact your physician.

DOSAGE

Your prescription should be taken as directed by your doctor.

Do not exceed the maximum daily dosage shown on the reverse side of this sheet for the product form you are taking. Always follow dosage recommendations carefully—do not increase the dosage without your doctor's approval. If you miss a dose of the drug, do not take twice as much the next time.

OVERDOSAGE

An overdosage of Darvon, alone or in combination with other drugs, including alcohol, may cause weakness, difficulty in breathing, confusion, anxiety, and more severe drowsiness and dizziness. Extreme overdosage may lead to unconsciousness and death.

In any suspected overdosage situation, GET EMERGENCY HELP IMMEDIATELY.

OTHER INFORMATION

This medication was prescribed specifically for you. It should not be given to anyone else even if his/her condition appears to be similar to yours. If you want more information or have any questions about Darvon, ask your doctor or pharmacist. There is a more detailed leaflet available from them. You may need their help in understanding parts of the detailed leaflet. Keep this and all other drugs out of the reach of children.

Prescription Vial Sticker
Tell your doctor if you are taking tranquilizers, antidepressant drugs, or sleep aids. LIMIT alcohol use with Darvon-N® (propoxyphene napsylate) and Darvon® (propoxyphene hydrochloride) products.

[082079]

DARVON® Ⓒ
(propoxyphene hydrochloride)
Capsules, USP

DARVON® COMPOUND and DARVON® COMPOUND-65
(propoxyphene hydrochloride and APC)
Capsules, USP

DARVON® WITH A.S.A®
(propoxyphene hydrochloride and aspirin)

Description: Darvon® (propoxyphene hydrochloride, Lilly) is an odorless white crystalline powder with a bitter taste. It is freely soluble in water. Chemically, it is alpha-(+)-4-(Dimethylamino) - 3 - methyl - 1, 2-diphenyl-2-butanol Propionate Hydrochloride.
Each Pulvule® Darvon contains 32 or 65 mg propoxyphene hydrochloride.

Pulvules No. 368 Darvon® Compound		Pulvules No. 369 Darvon® Compound-65
32 mg	Darvon® (propoxyphene hydrochloride, Lilly)	65 mg
227 mg	A.S.A.® (aspirin, Lilly)	227 mg
162 mg	Phenacetin	162 mg.
32.4 mg	Caffeine	32.4 mg

Each Pulvule Darvon with A.S.A. contains 65 mg propoxyphene hydrochloride and 325 mg aspirin.

Clinical Pharmacology: Propoxyphene is a centrally acting narcotic analgesic agent. Equimolar doses of propoxyphene hydrochloride or napsylate provide similar plasma concentrations. Following administration of 65, 130, or 195 mg of propoxyphene hydrochloride, the bioavailability of propoxyphene is equivalent to that of 100, 200, or 300 mg respectively of propoxyphene napsylate. Peak plasma concentrations of propoxyphene are reached in two to two and one-half hours. After a 65-mg oral dose of propoxyphene hydrochloride, peak plasma levels of 0.05 to 0.1 mcg/ml are achieved.
Repeated doses of propoxyphene at six-hour intervals lead to increasing plasma concentrations, with a plateau after the ninth dose at 48 hours.
Propoxyphene is metabolized in the liver to yield norpropoxyphene. Propoxyphene has a half-life of six to 12 hours, whereas that of norpropoxyphene is 30 to 36 hours.
Norpropoxyphene has substantially less central-nervous-system-depressant effect than propoxyphene but a greater local anesthetic effect, which is similar to that of amitriptyline and antiarrhythmic agents, such as lidocaine and quinidine.
In animal studies in which propoxyphene and norpropoxyphene were continuously infused in large amounts, intracardiac conduction time (P-R and QRS intervals) was prolonged. Any intracardiac conduction delay attributable to high concentrations of norpropoxyphene may be of relatively long duration.

Actions: Propoxyphene is a mild narcotic analgesic structurally related to methadone. The potency of propoxyphene hydrochloride is from two-thirds to equal that of codeine.
The combination of propoxyphene with aspirin or a mixture of aspirin, phenacetin, and caffeine (APC compound) produces greater analgesia than that produced by either propoxyphene or APC compound administered alone.

Indications: Darvon® (propoxyphene hydrochloride, Lilly) is indicated for the relief of mild to moderate pain.
Darvon Compound, Darvon Compound-65, and Darvon with A.S.A. are indicated for the relief of mild to moderate pain, either when pain is present alone or when it is accompanied by fever.

Contraindication: Hypersensitivity to propoxyphene, aspirin, phenacetin, or caffeine.

WARNINGS

- **Do not prescribe propoxyphene for patients who are suicidal or addiction-prone.**
- **Prescribe propoxyphene with caution for patients taking tranquilizers or antidepressant drugs and patients who use alcohol in excess.**
- **Tell your patients not to exceed the recommended dose and to limit their intake of alcohol.**

Propoxyphene products in excessive doses, either alone or in combination with other C.N.S. depressants, including alcohol, are a major cause of drug-related deaths. Fatalities within the first hour of overdosage are not uncommon. In a survey of deaths due to overdosage conducted in 1975, in approximately 20 percent of the fatal cases, death occurred within the first hour (5 percent occurred within 15 minutes). Propoxyphene should not be taken in doses higher than those recommended by the physician. The judicious prescribing of propoxyphene is essential to the safe use of this drug. With patients who are depressed or suicidal, consideration should be given to the use of non-narcotic analgesics. Patients should be cautioned about the concomitant use of propoxyphene products and alcohol because of potentially serious C.N.S.-additive effects of these agents. Because of its added depressant effects, propoxyphene should be prescribed with caution for those patients whose medical condition requires the concomitant administration of sedatives, tranquilizers, muscle relaxants, antidepressants, or other C.N.S.-depressant drugs. Patients should be advised of the additive depressant effects of these combinations.
Many of the propoxyphene-related deaths have occurred in patients with previous histories of emotional disturbances or suicidal ideation or attempts as well as histories of misuse of tranquilizers, alcohol, and other C.N.S.-active drugs. Some deaths have occurred as a consequence of the accidental ingestion of excessive quantities of propoxyphene alone or in combination with other drugs. Patients taking propoxyphene should be warned not to exceed the dosage recommended by the physician.

DARVON COMPOUND AND DARVON COMPOUND-65 CONTAIN PHENACETIN. PHENACETIN, IF TAKEN IN LARGE DOSES FOR LONG PERIODS IN COMBINATION WITH OTHER ANTI-INFLAMMATORY ANALGESICS, IS ASSOCIATED WITH SEVERE KIDNEY DISEASE AND WITH CANCER OF THE KIDNEY.

Drug Dependence—Propoxyphene, when taken in higher-than-recommended doses over long periods of time, can produce drug dependence characterized by psychic dependence and, less frequently, physical dependence and tolerance. Propoxyphene will only partially suppress the withdrawal syndrome in individuals physically dependent on morphine or other narcotics. The abuse liability of propoxyphene is qualitatively similar to that of codeine although quantitatively less, and propoxyphene should be prescribed with the same degree of caution appropriate to the use of codeine.
Usage in Ambulatory Patients—Propoxyphene may impair the mental and/or physical abilities required for the performance of potentially hazardous tasks, such as driving a car or operating machinery. The patient should be cautioned accordingly.

Precautions: *General Precautions*—Kidney disease, often irreversible, has been noted with doses of phenacetin of 1 gm or more per day taken for one to three years and with total ingestion of 2 kg or more. It is not known whether prolonged ingestion of doses of phenacetin lower than 1 gm per day might also result in kidney disease.
Salicylates should be used with extreme caution in the presence of peptic ulcer or coagulation abnormalities.
Drug Interactions—The C.N.S.-depressant effect of propoxyphene is additive with that of other C.N.S. depressants, including alcohol.
Salicylates may enhance the effect of anticoagulants and inhibit the uricosuric effect of uricosuric agents.
Usage in Pregnancy—Safe use in pregnancy has not been established relative to possible adverse effects on fetal development. Instances of withdrawal symptoms in the neonate have been reported following usage during pregnancy. Therefore, propoxyphene should not be used in pregnant women unless, in the judgment of the physician, the potential benefits outweigh the possible hazards.
Usage in Nursing Mothers—Low levels of propoxyphene have been detected in human milk. In postpartum studies involving nursing mothers who were given propoxyphene, no adverse effects were noted in infants receiving mother's milk.
Usage in Children—Propoxyphene is not recommended for use in children, because documented clinical experience has been insufficient to establish safety and a suitable dosage regimen in the pediatric age group.
A Patient Information Sheet is available for these products. See text following "How Supplied" section below.

Adverse Reactions: In a survey conducted in hospitalized patients, less than 1 percent of patients taking propoxyphene hydrochloride at recommended doses experienced side effects. The most frequently reported have been dizziness, sedation, nausea, and vomiting. Some of these adverse reactions may be alleviated if the patient lies down.
Other adverse reactions include constipation, abdominal pain, skin rashes, lightheadedness, headache, weakness, euphoria, dysphoria, and minor visual disturbances.
Cases of liver dysfunction have been reported.

Administration and Dosage: These products are given orally. The usual dosage of Darvon® (propoxyphene hydrochloride, Lilly) is 65 mg every four hours as needed for pain.
The usual dosage of Darvon Compound and Darvon Compound-65 is 32 or 65 mg propoxyphene hydrochloride, 227 mg aspirin, 162 mg phenacetin, and 32.4 mg caffeine every four hours as needed for pain.
The usual dosage of Darvon with A.S.A. is 65 mg propoxyphene hydrochloride and 325 mg aspirin every four hours as needed for pain.
The maximum recommended dose of propoxyphene hydrochloride is 390 mg per day.

Management of Overdosage: Initial consideration should be given to the management of the C.N.S. effects of propoxyphene overdosage. Resuscitative measures should be initiated promptly.
Symptoms of Propoxyphene Overdosage—The manifestations of acute overdosage with pro-

Continued on next page

Ⓒ**Identi-Code® symbol.**

Lilly—Cont.

poxyphene are those of narcotic overdosage. The patient is usually somnolent but may be stuporous or comatose and convulsing. Respiratory depression is characteristic. The ventilatory rate and/or tidal volume is decreased, which results in cyanosis and hypoxia. Pupils, initially pinpoint, may become dilated as hypoxia increases. Cheyne-Stokes respiration and apnea may occur. Blood pressure and heart rate are usually normal initially, but blood pressure falls and cardiac performance deteriorates, which ultimately results in pulmonary edema and circulatory collapse, unless the respiratory depression is corrected and adequate ventilation is restored promptly. Cardiac arrhythmias and conduction delay may be present. A combined respiratory-metabolic acidosis occurs owing to retained CO_2 (hypercapnea) and to lactic acid formed during anaerobic glycolysis. Acidosis may be severe if large amounts of salicylates have also been ingested. Death may occur.

Treatment of Propoxyphene Overdosage — Attention should be directed first to establishing a patent airway and to restoring ventilation. Mechanically assisted ventilation, with or without oxygen, may be required, and positive pressure respiration may be desirable if pulmonary edema is present. The narcotic antagonist naloxone will markedly reduce the degree of respiratory depression and should be administered promptly, preferably intravenously, 0.4 to 0.8 mg, and carefully repeated, as necessary, at 20 to 30-minute intervals. The duration of action of the antagonist may be brief. If no response is observed after 10 mg of naloxone have been administered, the diagnosis of propoxyphene toxicity should be questioned. (Nalorphine and levallorphan may be used if naloxone is not available, but these agents are not as satisfactory as naloxone.)

Blood gases, *p*H, and electrolytes should be monitored in order that acidosis and any electrolyte disturbance present may be corrected promptly. Acidosis, hypoxia, and generalized C.N.S. depression predispose to the development of cardiac arrhythmias. Ventricular fibrillation or cardiac arrest may occur and necessitate the full complement of cardiopulmonary resuscitation (CPR) measures. Respiratory acidosis rapidly subsides as ventilation is restored and hypercapnea eliminated, but lactic acidosis may require intravenous bicarbonate for prompt correction.

Electrocardiographic monitoring is essential. Prompt correction of hypoxia, acidosis, and electrolyte disturbance (when present) will help prevent these cardiac complications and will increase the effectiveness of agents administered to restore normal cardiac function.

In addition to the use of a narcotic antagonist, the patient may require careful titration with an anticonvulsant to control convulsions. Analeptic drugs (for example, caffeine or amphetamine) should not be used because of their tendency to precipitate convulsions.

General supportive measures, in addition to oxygen, include, when necessary, intravenous fluids, vasopressor-inotropic compounds, and, when infection is likely, anti-infective agents. Gastric lavage may be useful, and activated charcoal can adsorb a significant amount of ingested propoxyphene. Dialysis is of little value in poisoning due to propoxyphene. Efforts should be made to determine whether other agents, such as alcohol, barbiturates, tranquilizers, or other C.N.S. depressants, were also ingested, since these increase C.N.S. depression as well as cause specific toxic effects.

Symptoms of Salicylate Overdosage—Such symptoms include central nausea and vomiting, tinnitus and deafness, vertigo and headaches, mental dullness and confusion, diaphoresis, rapid pulse, and increased respiration and respiratory alkalosis.

Treatment of Salicylate Overdosage—When Darvon Compound or Darvon Compound-65 has been ingested, the clinical picture may be complicated by salicylism.

The treatment of acute salicylate intoxication includes minimizing drug absorption, promoting elimination through the kidneys, and correcting metabolic derangements affecting body temperature, hydration, acid-base balance, and electrolyte balance. The technique to be employed for eliminating salicylate from the bloodstream depends on the degree of drug intoxication.

If the patient is seen within four hours of ingestion, the stomach should be emptied by inducing vomiting or by gastric lavage as soon as possible.

The nomogram of Done is a useful prognostic guide in which the expected severity of salicylate intoxication is based on serum salicylate levels and the time interval between ingestion and taking the blood sample.

Exchange transfusion is most feasible for a small infant. Intermittent peritoneal dialysis is useful for cases of moderate severity in adults. Intravenous fluids alkalinized by the addition of sodium bicarbonate or potassium citrate are helpful. Hemodialysis with the artificial kidney is the most effective means of removing salicylate and is indicated for the very severe cases of salicylate intoxication.

How Supplied: Ⓒ *Pulvules Darvon® (Propoxyphene Hydrochloride Capsules, USP): No. 364, HO2,** 32 mg (No. 4, Light-Pink Opaque), in bottles of 100 (℞Pak) and 500 and in 10 strips of 10 individually labeled blisters each containing 1 Pulvule (ID100); *No. 365, HO3,** 65 mg (No. 3, Light-Pink Opaque), in bottles of 100 (℞Pak) and 500, in 10 strips of 10 individually labeled blisters each containing 1 Pulvule (ID100), in 500 single-cut individually labeled blisters each containing 1 Pulvule (ID500), in 20 rolls, each consisting of 25 Pulvules in individual unit-dose packets, reverse-numbered (RN500), and in ℞Paks (prescription packages, Lilly) in 25 packages of 30 and 20 packages of 50. All ℞Paks have safety closures.

65 mg—500's—6505-00-958-2364

Ⓒ *Darvon Compound, Pulvules No. 368, HO5** (No. 0, Light-Pink Opaque Body, Light-Gray Opaque Cap), in bottles of 100 (℞Pak) and 500 and in 10 strips of 10 individually labeled blisters each containing 1 Pulvule (ID100). All ℞Paks have safety closures.

Ⓒ *Darvon Compound-65, Pulvules No. 369, HO6** (No. 0, Red Opaque Body, Light-Gray Opaque Cap), in bottles of 100 (℞Pak) and 500, in 10 strips of 10 individually labeled blisters each containing 1 Pulvule (ID100), in 500 single-cut individually labeled blisters each containing 1 Pulvule (ID500), in 20 rolls, each consisting of 25 Pulvules in individual unit-dose packets, reverse-numbered (RN500), and in ℞Paks in 25 packages of 30 and 20 packages of 50. All ℞Paks have safety closures.

Ⓒ *Darvon with A.S.A., Pulvules No. 366, HO4** (No. 0, Red Opaque Body, Light-Pink Opaque Cap), in bottles of 100 (℞Pak) and 500 and in 10 strips of 10 individually labeled blisters each containing 1 Pulvule (ID100). All ℞Paks have safety closures.

[*Shown in Product Identification Section*]

*Identi-Code® Symbol.

The following information, including illustrations of dosage forms and the maximum daily dosage of each, is available to patients receiving Darvon products.

Patient Information Sheet
YOUR PRESCRIPTION FOR A DARVON® (PROPOXYPHENE) PRODUCT Ⓒ

Your doctor has chosen to prescribe Darvon®. Darvon is used for the relief of pain.

It is important that you read and understand the information in this leaflet. If you have any questions, ask your doctor or pharmacist.

GENERAL CAUTIONS

Other Drugs: Combinations of excessive doses of Darvon, alcohol, and tranquilizers may be dangerous. Make sure your doctor knows that you are taking tranquilizers, sleep aids, antidepressant drugs, antihistamines, or any other drugs that make you sleepy. The use of these drugs with Darvon increases their sedative effects and may lead to overdosage symptoms, including death (see "Overdosage" below).

Alcohol: Heavy use of alcohol with Darvon is hazardous and may lead to overdosage symptoms (see "Overdosage" below). THEREFORE, LIMIT YOUR INTAKE OF ALCOHOL WHILE TAKING DARVON.

Regular Activities: Darvon may cause drowsiness or impair your mental and/or physical abilities; therefore, use caution when driving a vehicle or operating dangerous machinery. DO NOT perform any hazardous task until you have seen your response to this drug.

Pregnancy: Do not take Darvon or other drugs during pregnancy unless your doctor knows you are pregnant and specifically recommends their use.

Children: Darvon is not recommended for use in children under 12 years of age.

Allergy: Do not take Darvon if you have had an allergic reaction to any dosage form of this drug.

Dependence: Darvon, when taken in higher-than-recommended doses over a long period of time, has produced physical and psychologic dependence (a craving for the drug or an inability to function normally without the drug).

SIDE EFFECTS

When Darvon is taken as directed, side effects are infrequent. Among those reported are drowsiness, dizziness, nausea, and vomiting. If these effects occur, some of them may go away if you lie down.

Less frequently reported side effects include constipation, abdominal pain, skin rashes, lightheadedness, headache, weakness, minor visual disturbances, and feelings of elation or discomfort.

If one of these side effects occurs and becomes severe, contact your physician.

DOSAGE

Your prescription should be taken as directed by your doctor. Do not exceed the maximum daily dosage shown on the reverse side of this sheet for the product form you are taking. Always follow dosage recommendations carefully—do not increase the dosage without your doctor's approval. If you miss a dose of the drug, do not take twice as much the next time.

OVERDOSAGE

An overdosage of Darvon, alone or in combination with other drugs, including alcohol, may cause weakness, difficulty in breathing, confusion, anxiety, and more severe drowsiness and dizziness. Extreme overdosage may lead to unconsciousness and death.

In any suspected overdosage situation, GET EMERGENCY HELP IMMEDIATELY.

OTHER INFORMATION

This medication was prescibed specifically for you. It should not be given to anyone else even if his/her condition appears to be similar to yours. If you want more information or have any questions about Darvon, ask your doctor or pharmacist. There is a more detailed leaflet available from them. You may need their help in understanding parts of the detailed leaflet. Keep this and all other drugs out of the reach of children.

Prescription Vial Sticker

Tell your doctor if you are taking tranquilizers, antidepressant drugs, or sleep aids. LIMIT alcohol use with Darvon-N® (propoxyphene napsylate) and Darvon® (propoxyphene hydrochloride) products.

[082079]

DICUMAROL ℞
Capsules, USP

Description: Chemically, dicumarol is bishydroxycoumarin (3,3′-methylenebis [4-hydroxycoumarin]), $C_{19}H_{12}O_6$.
Actions: Dicumarol reduces the concentration of prothrombin in blood and increases the prothrombin time by inhibiting the formation of prothrombin in the liver. Since the drug also interferes with the production of factors VII, IX, and X, their concentration in the blood is lowered during therapy. The inhibition of prothrombin involves interference with the action of vitamin K, and it has been postulated that dicumarol competes with vitamin K for an enzyme essential to prothrombin synthesis.
After oral administration of dicumarol, maximum plasma concentrations are reached in two to eight hours. Greatest effect on prothrombin time is achieved in 36 to 72 hours. Following a single therapeutic dose of the drug, its effect on prothrombin time persists for four to five days.
Indications: Dicumarol is indicated for the prophylaxis and treatment of pulmonary embolism and of venous thrombosis and its extension, for therapy of atrial fibrillation with embolization, and as an adjunct in the treatment of coronary occlusion.
Contraindications: Dicumarol is contraindicated in patients who have active bleeding or subacute bacterial endocarditis.
Dicumarol passes the placental barrier. When pregnant women are treated with the drug, fetal bleeding diathesis may occur and cause fetal death *in utero.* Dicumarol is also secreted in the maternal milk. Therefore, the drug is contraindicated for pregnant patients and for breast-feeding mothers. If anticoagulant therapy is required for such patients, heparin should be considered, because it does not pass through the placenta or into the mother's milk.
Warnings: Dicumarol is a potent drug, and its effects tend to be cumulative and prolonged. Caution should be used when dicumarol is administered in any situation in which the risk of hemorrhage is present. The drug should be withdrawn at the earliest sign of bleeding. It cannot be emphasized too strongly that treatment of each patient is a highly individualized matter. Dosage can be controlled only by periodic determination of prothrombin time. Clotting and bleeding times are not effective measures for control of therapy.
It is important to bear in mind that heparin sodium prolongs the one-stage prothrombin time. Accordingly, when heparin sodium is given with dicumarol, a period of four to five hours after the last intravenous dose and of 12 to 24 hours after the last subcutaneous dose of heparin sodium should elapse before blood is drawn if a valid prothrombin time is to be obtained.
For usage in pregnancy, *see* Contraindications.
Precautions: Several factors may alter the activity of dicumarol (*see also* Factors Influencing Activity of Dicumarol): any change in the intake of vitamin K, fat, or leafy green vegetables; vitamin K deficiency of the newborn; fever; alcoholism; vitamin C deficiency; x-ray therapy; and diarrhea, which causes increased loss in the stool and/or decreased absorption from the gut.
Many drugs can increase or decrease the effect of dicumarol on the prothrombin time. No other agent should be administered with dicumarol unless its potentialities for interacting with an oral anticoagulant are fully appreciated. If a drug is added to or withdrawn from a patient's therapeutic regimen, it is essential that his prothrombin time be carefully monitored. Fatalities have been reported from interactions that affected the metabolism of coumarin anticoagulants or their binding to plasma proteins.
Care in patient selection is desirable to insure cooperation, particularly from alcoholic, emotionally unstable, psychotic, or senile patients. Bleeding during oral anticoagulant therapy may not always correlate with the prothrombin time.
Factors Influencing Activity of Dicumarol: Factors which enhance the anticoagulant effect of dicumarol include decreased dietary intake or absorption of vitamin K, infancy, cachexia, liver impairment, renal insufficiency, fever, scurvy, congestive heart failure, salicylates, sulfas, chloramphenicol, tetracycline, neomycin (and possibly other antibiotics which suppress intestinal bacterial flora), phenylbutazone, oxyphenbutazone, phenyramidol hydrochloride, diphenylhydantoin sodium, pyrazoline drugs, quinine, quinidine, D-thyroxine, clofibrate, anabolic steroids, ACTH, adrenocorticosteroids, alcoholism, methylthiouracil, x-ray, and radioactive compounds.
Factors which reduce the anticoagulant effect of dicumarol include vitamin K, barbiturates, chloral hydrate, glutethimide, meprobamate, griseofulvin, and haloperidol.
Adverse Reactions: Hemorrhage is the principal adverse reaction to overdosage with dicumarol. Hemorrhagic tendency may be manifested by hematuria, petechiae in the skin, hemorrhage into or from a wound or ulcerating lesion, or petechial and purpuric hemorrhages throughout the body. Patients receiving dicumarol should be examined daily for evidence of these complications, and the urine should be tested daily to detect hematuria. When an ulcerative lesion of the gastrointestinal tract is suspected to be present or when dicumarol is administered in the postoperative period to patients who have had an operative procedure upon the gastrointestinal tract, the stools should be examined frequently for evidence of hemorrhage into the bowel.
The occurrence of significant gastrointestinal or urinary tract bleeding during anticoagulant therapy may indicate the presence of an underlying occult lesion.
Paralytic ileus and intestinal obstruction have been reported from submucosal or intramural hemorrhage.
Nonhemorrhagic adverse reactions have been noted. These include dermatitis, urticaria, alopecia, fever, anorexia, nausea, vomiting, cramps, diarrhea, leukopenia, agranulocytosis, mouth ulcers, nephropathy, and red-orange urine.
Administration and Dosage: Dicumarol is given by mouth. The dosage must be individualized and adjusted according to the prothrombin time. Probably the best method of reporting of prothrombin time is to give the patient's prothrombin time together with that of the control, both expressed in seconds. Many laboratories still report prothrombin time in percent of normal, on the basis of a prothrombin dilution curve; if this is done, it is essential for the laboratory to state what type of diluent was used.
There is no general agreement as to the minimum prothrombin time that accomplishes effective anticoagulation. The following schedule serves only as a guide. On the average, the dose for the first day in adults with normal prothrombin activity is 200 to 300 mg. On subsequent days, the dose may range from 25 to 200 mg. When expressed in seconds, the prothrombin time should be maintained, in general, at one and one-half to three times the control value; this ratio varies with the different types of tissue thromboplastin used in performing the prothrombin time test.
Combined Use with Heparin—Because dicumarol has a slow onset of action, heparin should be used when a rapid anticoagulant effect is desired. Both drugs can be given together at the start of therapy, and heparin administration may be continued for 24 to 72 hours or until a satisfactory effect from dicumarol is obtained as determined by prothrombin time studies.
Management of Overdosage: Usually, an overly prolonged prothrombin time or minor hemorrhage will respond satisfactorily to withdrawal of the drug alone, but whole-blood transfusion may also be desirable in some cases.
If prothrombin activity falls below the therapeutic range or if hemorrhage occurs, dicumarol should be temporarily withdrawn.
If warranted by the clinical situation, phytonadione (vitamin K_1) may be administered by slow intravenous injection—1 to 5 mg in cases of mild overdosage and 20 to 40 mg in cases of severe overdosage. Such use of vitamin K_1 complicates subsequent anticoagulant therapy; therefore, caution must be used in determining the need for this vitamin. It has been reported that a hypercoagulable state occurs following the rapid reversal of a prolonged prothrombin time.
How Supplied: (℞) *Pulvules® Dicumarol, Capsules, USP: No. 314, F71,* * 25 mg (No. 4, Clear), and *No. 291, F54,* * 50 mg (No. 3, Clear), in bottles of 100.

[083077]

DICURIN® PROCAINE ℞
(merethoxylline procaine)

Description: Dicurin® Procaine (merethoxylline procaine, Lilly) is an organic mercurial combined with procaine and theophylline (for stabilization of the solution).
Each ml contains—
2-N - (3′-Hydroxy-mercuri-2′-methoxy-ethoxy)-propyl-carbamyl Phenoxyacetic Acid, as the Procaine Salt of the Anhydro Acid..100 mg
(Equivalent to 39.3 mg mercury and 45 mg procaine base)
Theophylline, Anhydrous ....50 mg
Contains 0.5 percent chlorobutanol (chloroform derivative) as a preservative. Sodium hydroxide and/or hydrochloric acid may have been added during manufacture to adjust the *p*H.
Prolonged exposure to direct sunlight should be avoided, since it causes darkening of the solution. Freezing is harmless. Refrigeration storage is recommended.
Actions: Like other mercurial diuretics, Dicurin® Procaine (merethoxylline procaine, Lilly) inhibits the tubular reabsorption of sodium and chloride and, secondarily, water. Mercurial diuretics have a dual action on potassium secretion. Urinary potassium is increased or decreased, depending upon whether the initial secretory rate is low or high. In the treatment of edema, mercurial diuretics usually increase potassium secretion slightly.
Indications: Dicurin® Procaine (merethoxylline procaine, Lilly) is indicated for the treatment of edema secondary to congestive heart failure, the nephrotic syndrome, the nephrotic stage of glomerulonephritis, and hepatic cirrhosis or portal obstruction.
Contraindications: Dicurin® Procaine (merethoxylline procaine, Lilly) is contraindicated for intravenous use.
It should not be given when the patient is hypersensitive to mercury, procaine, or theophylline. In addition, because of the possibility of cross-sensitization, Dicurin Procaine should not be administered to patients who are sensitive to other drugs containing the *p*-aminobenzoic acid group, such as benzocaine, tetracaine, butacaine, etc. It is also contraindicated in patients with acute glomerulonephritis, ulcerative colitis, or gouty diathesis.
Warnings: A few instances of anaphylactic reactions have been reported.

Continued on next page

*Identi-Code® symbol.

Lilly—Cont.

***Use in Pregnancy*—Since the safety of this preparation in pregnancy, during lactation, or in women of childbearing age has not been established, use of the drug in such patients requires that the potential benefits be weighed against the possible hazards to the mother and child.**

Precautions: Diuresis of any kind should be induced with great caution in the presence of benign prostatic hypertrophy; distention of the bladder may precipitate obstruction. If the blood urea nitrogen is more than 60 mg per 100 ml, mercurial diuretics should be used with caution. If definite albuminuria, hematuria, or oliguria appears *after* administration of a mercurial diuretic, the drug should be discontinued.

Lack of the anticipated diuretic response in a patient previously responsive should direct the physician's attention to such possible factors as insufficient restriction of the patient's activity, inadequate dosage of cardiac glycosides, underlying renal disease, or electrolyte imbalance.

Too-frequent or injudicious use of mercurial diuretics may result in excessive loss of body water, sodium, potassium, and chloride, especially if dietary restriction of salt has been too rigid and prolonged.

In edematous patients who are well saturated with digitalis, rapid mobilization of large quantities of edema fluid may be followed by manifestations of digitalis overdosage.

Although Dicurin® Procaine (merethoxylline procaine, Lilly), as a potent mercurial diuretic, is invaluable in the management of edema, it is not a substitute for digitalis or other drugs and therapeutic measures in the treatment of the underlying diseases associated with edema.

Dicurin Procaine should be administered with caution to patients receiving sulfonamide therapy.

Adverse Reactions: As is true of any mercurial diuretic, Dicurin® Procaine (merethoxylline procaine, Lilly) may cause the following:

Hypersensitivity reactions—flushing, pruritus, urticaria, cutaneous rash (which may become exfoliative), and, occasionally, anaphylactic reactions

Gastrointestinal reactions—nausea, vomiting, diarrhea, and abdominal pain

Bone-marrow depression, manifested by neutropenia and agranulocytosis

Mercurialism arising from excessive parenteral therapy or in patients with advanced renal disease (as manifested by stomatitis, marginal gingivitis, metallic taste, diarrhea, and proteinuria)

Local reactions—ecchymoses and induration

Genitourinary reactions—transient azotemia or an increase in preexistent azotemia; acute urinary retention

Rarely, hyperuricemia

Administration and Dosage: Dicurin® Procaine (merethoxylline procaine, Lilly) is not for intravenous use.

Intramuscular Administration—Select a nonedematous area, preferably the upper outer quadrant of the buttocks.

Subcutaneous Administration—Rotate sites of injection and avoid edematous or adipose tissue; local reactions may occur more frequently. Subcutaneous administration should be deep. Superficial deposit of the medication predisposes to local reaction.

Some investigators have recommended that an initial dose of any mercurial should be 0.5 ml or less, to preclude reaction due to mercury idiosyncrasy. The most common dose of an organic mercurial is 2 ml per day. It has been reported that two spaced injections of 1 ml of a mercurial give approximately 20 percent more diuresis than does one injection of 2 ml. During the clinical trial of Dicurin Procaine, a satisfactory diuresis was obtained with 1 ml in many cases, but, in others, 2-ml doses were needed to eliminate edema. A weight record and close clinical observation should be the guides for frequency of administration.

If feasible, mercurial diuretics should be administered early in the morning in order to obtain diuresis predominantly during the day and to avoid disturbance of the patient's rest at night.

The diuretic effect of mercurials is potentiated by (1) ammonium chloride, best given as Enseals® (enteric-release tablets, Lilly), (2) theophylline preparations, and (3) bed rest.

A continued daily loss of body weight of two to four pounds (1 to 2 kg) is preferable to sudden inordinately large diuresis. When edema has disappeared and the body weight reaches a resistant level, the "dry weight" of the patient has been attained.

Pharmacology: The site of action of mercurial diuretics is in the kidneys, where they produce a powerful depression of tubular reabsorption of electrolytes and, secondarily, water. Since the rate of glomerular filtration is unaffected by therapeutic doses, the net result is an increased urinary excretion of water and salts.

When Dicurin® Procaine (merethoxylline procaine, Lilly) was compared with another mercurial in common use, it was found that, with equivalent dosage in terms of mercury content, both drugs produced in dogs an increase of sodium, potassium, and water excretion to about the same degree. Acute toxicity studies with large doses showed that there was no significant difference in the median lethal doses (LD_{50}'s) for the two mercurial compounds.

The excretion of mercury and electrolytes was studied in six patients during three, six, 12, and 24-hour periods following subcutaneous injection of Dicurin Procaine, with another mercurial diuretic used for comparison. There was no significant difference in excretion of mercury, sodium, chloride, or potassium with the two preparations. Following injection of Dicurin Procaine, an average of 73 percent of the administered mercury was excreted in 21 hours.

How Supplied: (℞) *Ampoules (Vials) No. 581, Dicurin® Procaine (merethoxylline procaine, Lilly), Injection,* 10 ml, rubber-stoppered, in singles (10 per carton). *Refrigerate.*

[071073B]

DIETHYLSTILBESTROL USP ℞

1. *PROLONGED USE OF ESTROGENS HAS BEEN REPORTED TO INCREASE THE RISK OF ENDOMETRIAL CARCINOMA*

Three independent case-control studies have reported an increased risk of endometrial cancer in postmenopausal women exposed to exogenous estrogens for prolonged periods. This risk was independent of other known risk factors for endometrial cancer. These studies are further supported by the finding that, since 1969, the incidence rate of endometrial cancer has increased sharply in eight different areas of the United States which have population-based cancer reporting systems.

The three case-control studies reported that the risk of endometrial cancer in estrogen users was about 4.5 to 13.9 times greater than in nonusers. The risk appears to depend on both the duration of treatment and the dose of estrogen. In view of these findings, the lowest dose that will control symptoms should be utilized when estrogens are used for the treatment of menopausal symptoms, and medication should be discontinued as soon as possible. When prolonged treatment is medically indicated, a reassessment should be made on at least a semiannual basis to determine the need for continued therapy. Although the evidence must be considered preliminary, one study suggests that cyclic administration of low doses of estrogen may carry less risk than does continuous administration; it therefore appears prudent to utilize such a regimen.

Close clinical surveillance of all women taking estrogens is important. In all cases of undiagnosed persistent or recurring abnormal vaginal bleeding, adequate diagnostic measures should be undertaken to rule out malignancy.

At present, there is no evidence that "natural" estrogens are more or less hazardous than "synthetic" estrogens at equivalent estrogenic doses.

2. *ESTROGENS SHOULD NOT BE USED DURING PREGNANCY*

The use of female sex hormones, both estrogens and progestogens, during early pregnancy may affect the offspring. It has been reported that females exposed *in utero* to diethylstilbestrol, a nonsteroidal estrogen, may have an increased risk of developing later in life a rare form of vaginal or cervical cancer. This risk has been estimated to be no greater than 4 per 1000 exposures. Furthermore, from 30 to 90 percent of such exposed women have been found to have vaginal adenosis and epithelial changes of the vagina and cervix. Although these changes are histologically benign, it is not known whether they are precursors of malignancy. Even though similar data are not available with the use of other estrogens, it cannot be presumed that they would not induce similar changes.

Several reports suggest that there is an association between intrauterine exposure to female sex hormones and congenital anomalies, including congenital heart defects and limb-reduction defects. One case-control study estimated a 4.7-fold increased risk of limb-reduction defects in infants exposed *in utero* to sex hormones (oral contraceptives, hormone withdrawal tests for pregnancy, or attempted treatment for threatened abortion). Some of these exposures were very short and involved only a few days of treatment. The data suggest that the risk of limb-reduction defects in exposed fetuses is somewhat less than 1 per 1000.

In the past, female sex hormones have been used during pregnancy in an attempt to treat threatened or habitual abortion; however, their efficacy was never conclusively proved or disproved.

If diethylstilbestrol is administered during pregnancy, or if the patient becomes pregnant while taking this drug, she should be apprised of the potential risks to the fetus and of the advisability of pregnancy continuation.

THIS DRUG PRODUCT SHOULD NOT BE USED AS A POSTCOITAL CONTRACEPTIVE

Description: Diethylstilbestrol is a crystalline synthetic estrogenic substance capable of producing all the pharmacologic and therapeutic responses attributed to natural estrogens. Diethylstilbestrol may be administered orally (in the form of Enseals® [enteric-release tablets, Lilly] and tablets) or vaginally (in the form of suppositories). Chemically, diethylstilbestrol is α,α'-diethyl-4,4'-stilbenediol.

Indications: Diethylstilbestrol is indicated in the treatment of:

1. Moderate to severe *vasomotor* symptoms associated with the menopause (There is no evidence that estrogens are effective for nervous symptoms or depression which might occur

during menopause, and they should not be used to treat these conditions.)

2. Atrophic vaginitis
3. Kraurosis vulvae
4. Female hypogonadism
5. Female castration
6. Primary ovarian failure
7. Breast cancer (for palliation only) in appropriately selected women and men with metastatic disease
8. Prostatic carcinoma—palliative therapy of advanced disease

DIETHYLSTILBESTROL SHOULD NOT BE USED FOR ANY PURPOSE DURING PREGNANCY. ITS USE MAY CAUSE SEVERE HARM TO THE FETUS (SEE BOXED WARNING).

Contraindications: Estrogens should not be used in women (or men) with any of the following conditions:

1. Known or suspected cancer of the breast, except in appropriately selected patients being treated for metastatic disease
2. Known or suspected estrogen-dependent neoplasia
3. Known or suspected pregnancy (see boxed warning)
4. Undiagnosed abnormal genital bleeding
5. Active thrombophlebitis or thromboembolic disorders
6. A past history of thrombophlebitis, thrombosis, or thromboembolic disorders associated with previous use of estrogen (except when used in treatment of breast or prostatic malignancy)

Warnings: 1. *Induction of Malignant Neoplasms*—In certain animal species, long-term continuous administration of natural and synthetic estrogens increases the frequency of carcinomas of the breast, cervix, vagina, kidney, and liver. There are now reports that prolonged use of estrogens increases the risk of carcinoma of the endometrium in humans (see boxed warning).

At the present time, there is no satisfactory evidence that administration of estrogens to postmenopausal women increases the risk of cancer of the breast. This possibility, however, has been raised by a recent long-term follow-up of one physician's practice. Because of the animal data, there is a need for caution in prescribing estrogens for women with a family history of breast cancer or for women who have breast nodules, fibrocystic disease, or abnormal mammograms.

2. *Gallbladder Disease*—A recent study reported a two-to-threefold increase in the risk of gallbladder disease occurring in women receiving postmenopausal estrogen therapy, similar to the twofold increased risk previously noted in women using oral contraceptives. In the case of oral contraceptives, this increased risk appeared after two years of use.

3. *Effects Similar to Those Caused by Estrogen-Progestogen Oral Contraceptives*—There are several serious adverse effects associated with the use of oral contraceptives; however, most of these adverse effects have not as yet been documented as consequences of postmenopausal estrogen therapy. This may reflect the comparatively low doses of estrogen used in postmenopausal women. It would be expected that these adverse effects are more likely to occur following administration of the larger doses of estrogen used for treating prostatic or breast cancer. It has, in fact, been shown that there is an increased risk of thrombosis with the administration of estrogens for prostatic cancer in men and for postpartum breast engorgement in women.

a. *Thromboembolic Disease*—It is now well established that women taking oral contraceptives run an increased risk of various thromboembolic and thrombotic vascular diseases, such as thrombophlebitis, pulmonary embolism, stroke, and myocardial infarction. Cases of retinal thrombosis, mesenteric thrombosis, and optic neuritis have been reported in users of oral contraceptives. There is evidence that the risk of several of these adverse reactions is related to the dose of the drug. An increased risk of postsurgical thromboembolic complications has also been reported in users of oral contraceptives. If feasible, estrogen therapy should be discontinued at least four weeks before any surgery that may be associated with an increased risk of thromboembolism or that may require periods of prolonged immobilization.

Although an increased rate of thromboembolic and thrombotic disease has not been noted in postmenopausal users of estrogen, this does not rule out the possiblity that such an increase may be present or that it exists in subgroups of women who have underlying risk factors or who are receiving relatively large doses of estrogens. Therefore, estrogens should not be used in persons with active thrombophlebitis or thromboembolic disorders, nor should they be used (except in treatment of malignancy) in persons with a history of such disorders associated with estrogen therapy. Estrogens should be administered cautiously to patients with cerebral vascular or coronary artery disease and only when such therapy is clearly needed.

In a large prospective clinical trial in men, large doses of estrogen (5 mg of conjugated estrogens per day), comparable to those used to treat cancer of the prostate and breast, have been shown to increase the risk of nonfatal myocardial infarction, pulmonary embolism, and thrombophlebitis. When such large doses of estrogen are used, any of the thromboembolic and thrombotic adverse effects associated with the use of oral contraceptives should be considered a clear risk.

b. *Hepatic Adenoma*—Benign hepatic adenomas appear to be associated with the use of oral contraceptives. Although these adenomas are benign and rare, they may rupture and may cause death by intra-abdominal hemorrhage. Such lesions have not yet been reported in association with the administration of other estrogen or progestogen preparations, but they should be considered when abdominal pain and tenderness, abdominal mass, or hypovolemic shock occurs in persons receiving estrogen therapy. Hepatocellular carcinoma has also been reported in women taking estrogen-containing oral contraceptives. The relationship of this malignancy to such drugs is not known at this time.

c. *Elevated Blood Pressure*—Increased blood pressure is not uncommon in women taking oral contraceptives. There is now one report that this may occur with use of estrogens in the menopause, and blood pressure should be monitored during estrogen therapy, especially if high doses are used.

d. *Glucose Tolerance*—A decrease in glucose tolerance has been observed in a significant percentage of patients on estrogen-containing oral contraceptives. For this reason, diabetic patients should be carefully observed while receiving estrogen.

4. *Hypercalcemia*—Administration of estrogens may lead to severe hypercalcemia in patients with breast cancer and bone metastases. If this occurs, the drug should be stopped and appropriate measures taken to reduce the serum calcium level.

Precautions: A. General Precautions

1. A complete medical and family history should be taken prior to initiation of any estrogen therapy. In the pretreatment and periodic physical examinations, special consideration should be given to blood pressure, breasts, abdomen, and pelvic organs, and a Papanicolaou smear should be performed. As a general rule, estrogen should not be prescribed for over a year without another physical examination.

2. Fluid retention—Because estrogens may cause some degree of fluid retention, conditions which might be influenced by this factor, such as epilepsy, migraine, and cardiac or renal dysfunction, require careful observation.

3. Certain patients may develop undesirable manifestations of excessive estrogenic stimulation, such as abnormal or excessive uterine bleeding, mastodynia, etc.

4. Oral contraceptives appear to be associated with an increased incidence of mental depression. Although it is not clear whether this is due to the estrogenic or progestogenic component of the contraceptive agent, patients with a history of depression should be carefully observed.

5. Preexisting uterine leiomyomata may increase in size with administration of estrogens.

6. The pathologist should be advised of estrogen therapy when relevant specimens are submitted.

7. Patients with a past history of jaundice during pregnancy run an increased risk of recurrence of jaundice while receiving estrogen-containing oral contraceptive therapy. If jaundice develops in any patient receiving estrogen, the medication should be discontinued while the cause is investigated.

8. Estrogens may be poorly metabolized in patients with impaired liver function, and they should therefore be administered with caution in such patients.

9. Because estrogens influence the metabolism of calcium and phosphorus, they should be used with caution in patients with metabolic bone diseases associated with hypercalcemia or in patients with renal insufficiency.

10. Because of the effects of estrogens on epiphyseal closure, they should be used judiciously in young patients in whom bone growth is not complete.

11. Certain endocrine and liver function tests may be affected by estrogen-containing oral contraceptives. The following similar changes may be expected with larger doses of estrogen:

a. Increased sulfobromophthalein retention

b. Increased prothrombin and factors VII, VIII, IX, and X; decreased antithrombin 3; increased norepinephrine-induced platelet aggregability

c. Increased thyroid-binding globulin (TBG) leading to increased circulating total thyroid hormone, as measured by PBI, T^4 by column, or T^4 by radioimmunoassay. Free T^3 resin uptake is decreased, reflecting the elevated TBG; free T^4 concentration is unaltered

d. Impaired glucose tolerance

e. Decreased pregnanediol excretion

f. Reduced response to metyrapone test

g. Reduced serum folate concentration

h. Increased serum triglyceride and phospholipid concentration

B. Information for the Patient. *See* text of Patient Package Insert.

C. Pregnancy Category X. *See* Contraindications and boxed warning.

D. Nursing Mothers. As a general principle, any drug should be administered to nursing mothers only when clearly necessary, since many drugs are excreted in human milk.

Adverse Reactions: (*See* Warnings regarding induction of neoplasia, adverse effects on the fetus, increased incidence of gallbladder disease, and adverse effects similar to those of oral contraceptives, including thromboembolism.) The following additional adverse reactions have been reported with estrogenic therapy, including oral contraceptives:

Continued on next page

•Identi-Code® symbol.

Lilly—Cont.

1. *Genitourinary System*
   Breakthrough bleeding, spotting, change in menstrual flow
   Dysmenorrhea
   Premenstrual-like syndrome
   Amenorrhea during and after treatment
   Increase in size of uterine fibromyomata
   Vaginal candidiasis
   Change in cervical eversion and in degree of cervical secretion
   Cystitis-like syndrome
2. *Breasts*
   Tenderness, enlargement, secretion
3. *Gastrointestinal*
   Nausea, vomiting
   Abdominal cramps, bloating
   Cholestatic jaundice
4. *Skin*
   Chloasma or melasma which may persist when drug is discontinued
   Erythema multiforme
   Erythema nodosum
   Hemorrhagic eruption
   Loss of scalp hair
   Hirsutism
5. *Eyes*
   Steepening of corneal curvature
   Intolerance to contact lenses
6. *C.N.S.*
   Headache, migraine, dizziness
   Mental depression
   Chorea
7. *Miscellaneous*
   Increase or decrease in weight
   Reduced carbohydrate tolerance
   Aggravation of porphyria
   Edema
   Changes in libido

Acute Overdosage: Numerous reports indicate that serious ill effects do not occur when large doses of estrogen-containing oral contraceptives are ingested by young children. Overdosage of estrogen may cause nausea, and withdrawal bleeding may occur in females.

Administration and Dosage: 1. *Given Cyclically for Short-Term Use Only:*
For treatment of moderate to severe *vasomotor* symptoms, atrophic vaginitis, or kraurosis vulvae associated with the menopause.
The lowest dose that will control symptoms should be chosen, and medication should be discontinued as promptly as possible.
Administration should be cyclic (e.g., three weeks on and one week off).
Attempts to discontinue or taper medication should be made at three to six-month intervals.
The usual dosage range is 0.2 to 0.5 mg daily.
Patients with atrophic vaginitis may require up to 2 mg daily, and cyclic administration may be necessary for several years. Patients with atrophic vaginitis may notice relief of symptoms sooner if up to 1 mg of the suppository form is administered daily for ten to 14 days concomitantly with oral diethylstilbestrol. Consideration should also be given to prescribing the suppository form as the only means of estrogenic therapy for patients with atrophic vaginitis or kraurosis vulvae, in which case the dosage may be increased to 5 to 7 mg weekly.

2. *Given Cyclically:*
   Female hypogonadism
   Female castration
   Primary ovarian failure
   0.2 to 0.5 mg daily
3. *Given Chronically:*
   Inoperable progressing prostatic cancer
   1 to 3 mg daily initially, increased in advanced cases; the dosage may later be reduced to an average of 1 mg daily.
   Inoperable progressing breast cancer in appropriately selected men and postmenopausal women (*see* Indications)
   15 mg daily

Patients with an intact uterus should be closely monitored for signs of endometrial cancer, and appropriate diagnostic measures should be taken to rule out malignancy in the event of persistent or recurring abnormal vaginal bleeding.

How Supplied: (℞) *Enseals—Diethylstilbestrol Tablets, USP (Enteric): No. 46, A19,** 0.1 mg, *No. 47, A20,** 0.25 mg, *No. 48, A21,** 0.5 mg, *No. 49, A22,** 1 mg, and *No. 85, A33,** 5 mg, in bottles of 100 and 1000.
(℞) *Diethylstilbestrol Suppositories, USP* (Vaginal): *No. 14, SO7,* *0.1 mg, and *No. 15, SO9,* *0.5 mg, in packages of 6.
(℞) *Tablets—Diethylstilbestrol Tablets, USP: No. 1646, J49,** 0.1 mg, in bottles of 100 and 1000; *No. 1647, J50,** 0.25 mg, in bottles of 100; *No. 1648, J51,** 0.5 mg, and *No. 1649, J52,** 1 mg, in bottles of 100 and 1000; *No. 1685, J54,** 5 mg, in bottles of 100 and 1000 and in 10 strips of 10 individually labeled blisters each containing 1 tablet (ID100). [110278]

DOBUTREX® ℞
(dobutamine hydrochloride)
For Injection

Description: Dobutrex® (dobutamine hydrochloride, Lilly) is (±)-4-[2-[[3-(*p*-hydroxyphenyl)-1-methylpropyl]amino]-ethyl] -pyrocatechol hydrochloride. It is a synthetic catecholamine.
The clinical formulation is supplied in a sterile lyophilized form for intravenous use only. Each vial contains 250 mg of dobutamine and 250 mg of mannitol. Hydrochloric acid is used to adjust the *p*H. The *p*H of the reconstituted solution is between 2.5 and 5.5.

Clinical Pharmacology: Dobutrex® (dobutamine hydrochloride, Lilly) is a direct-acting inotropic agent whose primary activity results from stimulation of the beta receptors of the heart while producing comparatively mild chronotropic, hypertensive, arrhythmogenic, and vasodilative effects. It does not cause the release of endogenous norepinephrine, as does dopamine. In animal studies, dobutamine produces less increase in heart rate and less decrease in peripheral vascular resistance for a given inotropic effect than does isoproterenol.
In patients with depressed cardiac function, both dobutamine and isoproterenol increase the cardiac output to a similar degree. In the case of dobutamine, this increase is usually not accompanied by marked increases in heart rate (although tachycardia is occasionally observed), and the cardiac stroke volume is usually increased. In contrast, isoproterenol increases the cardiac index primarily by increasing the heart rate while stroke volume changes little or declines.
Facilitation of atrioventricular conduction has been observed in human electrophysiologic studies and in patients with atrial fibrillation.
Systemic vascular resistance is usually decreased with administration of dobutamine. Occasionally, minimal vasoconstriction has been observed.
Most clinical experience with dobutamine is short-term—up to several hours in duration. In the limited number of patients who were studied for 24, 48, and 72 hours, a persistent increase in cardiac output occurred in some, whereas the output of others returned toward base-line values.
The onset of action of Dobutrex is within one to two minutes; however, as much as ten minutes may be required to obtain the peak effect of a particular infusion rate.
The plasma half-life of dobutamine in humans is two minutes. The principal routes of metabolism are methylation of the catechol and conjugation. In human urine, the major excretion products are the conjugates of dobutamine and 3-O-methyl dobutamine. The 3-O-methyl derivative of dobutamine is inactive.
Alteration of synaptic concentrations of catecholamines with either reserpine or tricyclic antidepressants does not alter the actions of dobutamine in animals, which indicates that the actions of dobutamine are not dependent on presynaptic mechanisms.

Indications and Usage: Dobutrex® (dobutamine hydrochloride, Lilly) is indicated when parenteral therapy is necessary for inotropic support in the short-term treatment of adults with cardiac decompensation due to depressed contractility resulting either from organic heart disease or from cardiac surgical procedures.
In patients who have atrial fibrillation with rapid ventricular response, a digitalis preparation should be used prior to institution of therapy with Dobutrex.

Contraindication: Dobutrex® (dobutamine hydrochloride, Lilly) is contraindicated in patients with idiopathic hypertrophic subaortic stenosis.

Warnings: 1. *Increase in Heart Rate or Blood Pressure*—Dobutrex® (dobutamine hydrochloride, Lilly) may cause a marked increase in heart rate or blood pressure, especially systolic pressure. Approximately 10 percent of patients in clinical studies have had rate increases of 30 beats/minute or more, and about 7.5 percent have had a 50-mm Hg or greater increase in systolic pressure. Reduction of dosage usually reserves these effects promptly. Because dobutamine facilitates atrioventricular conduction, patients with atrial fibrillation are at risk of developing rapid ventricular response. Patients with preexisting hypertension appear to face an increased risk of developing an exaggerated pressor response.
2. *Ectopic Activity*—Dobutrex may precipitate or exacerbate ventricular ectopic activity, but it rarely has caused ventricular tachycardia.

Precautions: 1. During the administration of Dobutrex® (dobutamine hydrochloride, Lilly), as with any adrenergic agent, ECG and blood pressure should be continuously monitored. In addition, pulmonary wedge pressure and cardiac output should be monitored whenever possible to aid in the safe and effective infusion of Dobutrex.
2. Hypovolemia should be corrected with suitable volume expanders before treatment with Dobutrex is instituted.
3. Animal studies indicate that Dobutrex may be ineffective if the patient has recently received a beta-blocking drug. In such a case, the peripheral vascular resistance may increase.
4. No improvement may be observed in the presence of marked mechanical obstruction, such as severe valvular aortic stenosis.
Usage Following Acute Myocardial Infarction—Clinical experience with Dobutrex following myocardial infarction has been insufficient to establish the safety of the drug for this use. There is concern that any agent which increases contractile force and heart rate may increase the size of an infarction by intensifying ischemia, but it is not known whether dobutamine does so.
Usage in Pregnancy—Reproduction studies performed in rats and rabbits have revealed no evidence of impaired fertility, harm to the fetus, or teratogenic effects due to dobutamine. However, the drug has not been administered to pregnant women and should be used only when the expected benefits clearly outweigh the potential risks to the fetus.
Pediatric Use—The safety and effectiveness of Dobutrex for use in children have not been studied.
Drug Interactions—There was no evidence of drug interactions in clinical studies in which Dobutrex was administered concurrently with other drugs, including digitalis preparations, furosemide, spironolactone, lidocaine, glyceryl trinitrate, isosorbide dinitrate, morphine, atropine, heparin, protamine, potassium chloride, folic acid, and acetaminophen. Preliminary

studies indicate that the concomitant use of dobutamine and nitroprusside results in a higher cardiac output and, usually, a lower pulmonary wedge pressure than when either drug is used alone.

Adverse Reactions: *Increased Heart Rate, Blood Pressure, and Ventricular Ectopic Activity*—A 10 to 20-mm increase in systolic blood pressure and an increase in heart rate of five to 15 beats per minute have been noted in most patients. (*See* Warnings regarding exaggerated chronotropic and pressor effects.) Approximately 5 percent of patients have had increased premature ventricular beats during infusions. These effects are dose related.

Miscellaneous Uncommon Effects—The following adverse effects have been reported in 1 to 3 percent of patients: nausea, headache, anginal pain, nonspecific chest pain, palpitations, and shortness of breath.

No abnormal laboratory values attributable to Dobutrex® (dobutamine hydrochloride, Lilly) have been observed.

Longer-Term Safety—Infusions of up to 72 hours have revealed no adverse effects other than those seen with shorter infusions.

Overdosage: In case of overdosage, as evidenced by excessive alteration of blood pressure or by tachycardia, reduce the rate of administration or temporarily discontinue Dobutrex® (dobutamine hydrochloride, Lilly) until the patient's condition stabilizes. Because the duration of action of Dobutrex is short, usually no additional remedial measures are necessary.

Administration and Dosage: *Reconstitution and Stability*—Dobutrex® (dobutamine hydrochloride, Lilly) is incompatible with alkaline solutions and should not be mixed with products such as 5% Sodium Bicarbonate Injection.

Dobutrex may be reconstituted with Sterile Water for Injection or 5% Dextrose Injection. To reconstitute, add 10 ml of diluent to Vial No. 7051, Dobutrex, 250 mg. If the material is not completely dissolved, add an additional 10 ml of diluent. The reconstituted solution may be stored under refrigeration for 48 hours or at room temperature for six hours.

Reconstituted Dobutrex must be further diluted to at least 50 ml prior to administration in 5% Dextrose Injection, 0.9% Sodium Chloride Injection, or Sodium Lactate Injection. Intravenous solutions should be used within 24 hours.

Solutions containing Dobutrex may exhibit a color that, if present, will increase with time. This color change is due to slight oxidation of the drug, but there is no significant loss of potency during the reconstituted time periods stated above.

Recommended Dosage—The rate of infusion needed to increase cardiac output usually ranges from 2.5 to 10 mcg/kg/min (see table). On rare occasions, infusion rates up to 40 mcg/kg/min have been required to obtain the desired effect.

[See table above].

The rate of administration and the duration of therapy should be adjusted according to the patient's response, as determined by heart rate, presence of ectopic activity, blood pressure, urine flow, and, whenever possible, measurement of central venous or pulmonary wedge pressure and cardiac output.

Concentrations up to 5000 mcg/ml have been administered to humans (250 mg/50 ml). The final volume administered should be determined by the fluid requirements of the patient.

How Supplied: (℞) *Vials No. 7051, Dobutrex® (dobutamine hydrochloride, Lilly), for Injection* (lyophilized), equivalent to 250 mg dobutamine, 20-ml size, rubber-stoppered, in singles (10 per carton). [072178]

[*Shown in Product Identification Section*]

Rates of Infusion for Concentrations of 250, 500, and 1000 mcg/ml

Drug Delivery Rate (mcg/kg/min)	Infusion Delivery Rate 250 mcg/ml* (ml/kg/min)	500 mcg/ml† (ml/kg/min)	1000 mcg/ml‡ (ml/kg/min)
2.5	0.01	0.005	0.0025
5	0.02	0.01	0.005
7.5	0.03	0.015	0.0075
10	0.04	0.02	0.01
12.5	0.05	0.025	0.0125
15	0.06	0.03	0.015

*250 mg per liter of diluent
†500 mg per liter or 250 mg per 500 ml of diluent
‡1000 mg per liter or 250 mg per 250 ml of diluent

DOLOPHINE® HYDROCHLORIDE Ⓒ
(methadone hydrochloride)
Injection, USP

AMPOULES AND VIALS

> CONDITIONS FOR DISTRIBUTION AND USE OF METHADONE PRODUCTS:
> Code of Federal Regulations, Title 21, Sec. 310.505
>
> METHADONE PRODUCTS, WHEN USED FOR THE TREATMENT OF NARCOTIC ADDICTION IN DETOXIFICATION OR MAINTENANCE PROGRAMS, SHALL BE DISPENSED ONLY BY APPROVED HOSPITAL PHARMACIES, APPROVED COMMUNITY PHARMACIES, AND MAINTENANCE PROGRAMS APPROVED BY THE FOOD AND DRUG ADMINISTRATION AND THE DESIGNATED STATE AUTHORITY.
> APPROVED MAINTENANCE PROGRAMS SHALL DISPENSE AND USE METHADONE IN ORAL FORM ONLY AND ACCORDING TO THE TREATMENT REQUIREMENTS STIPULATED IN THE FEDERAL METHADONE REGULATIONS (21 CFR 310.505).
> FAILURE TO ABIDE BY THE REQUIREMENTS IN THESE REGULATIONS MAY RESULT IN CRIMINAL PROSECUTION, SEIZURE OF THE DRUG SUPPLY, REVOCATION OF THE PROGRAM APPROVAL, AND INJUNCTION PRECLUDING OPERATION OF THE PROGRAM.
> A METHADONE PRODUCT, WHEN USED AS AN ANALGESIC, MAY BE DISPENSED IN ANY LICENSED PHARMACY.

Description: Dolophine® Hydrochloride (Methadone Hydrochloride, USP, Lilly) (4,4-diphenyl-6-dimethylamino-heptanone-3 hydrochloride) is a white crystalline material which is water soluble.

Each ml contains methadone hydrochloride, 10 mg, and sodium chloride, 0.9 percent. Sodium hydroxide and/or hydrochloric acid may have been added during manufacture to adjust the *p*H. The 20-ml vials also contain chlorobutanol (chloroform derivative), 0.5 percent, as a preservative.

Actions: Methadone hydrochloride is a synthetic narcotic analgesic with multiple actions quantitatively similar to those of morphine, the most prominent of which involve the central nervous system and organs composed of smooth muscle. The principal actions of therapeutic value are analgesia and sedation and detoxification or temporary maintenance in narcotic addiction. The methadone abstinence syndrome, although qualitatively similar to that of morphine, differs in that the onset is slower, the course is more prolonged, and the symptoms are less severe.

A parenteral dose of 8 to 10 mg of methadone is approximately equivalent in analgesic effect to 10 mg of morphine. With single-dose administration, the onset and duration of analgesic action of the two drugs are similar.

When administered orally, methadone is approximately one-half as potent as when given parenterally. Oral administration results in a delay of the onset, a lowering of the peak, and an increase in the duration of analgesic effect.

Indications: (See Note below.)
For relief of severe pain.
For detoxification treatment of narcotic addiction.
For temporary maintenance treatment of narcotic addiction.

> **NOTE**
>
> If methadone is administered for treatment of heroin dependence for more than three weeks, the procedure passes from treatment of the acute withdrawal syndrome (detoxification) to maintenance therapy. Maintenance treatment is permitted to be undertaken only by approved methadone programs. This does not preclude the maintenance treatment of an addict who is hospitalized for medical conditions other than addiction and who requires temporary maintenance during the critical period of his stay or whose enrollment has been verified in a program which has approval for maintenance treatment with methadone.

Contraindication: Hypersensitivity to methadone.

Warnings: Methadone hydrochloride, a narcotic, is a Schedule II controlled substance under the Federal Controlled Substances Act. Appropriate security measures should be taken to safeguard stocks of methadone against diversion.

DRUG DEPENDENCE—METHADONE CAN PRODUCE DRUG DEPENDENCE OF THE MORPHINE TYPE AND, THEREFORE, HAS THE POTENTIAL FOR BEING ABUSED. PSYCHIC DEPENDENCE, PHYSICAL DEPENDENCE, AND TOLERANCE MAY DEVELOP UPON REPEATED ADMINISTRATION OF METHADONE, AND IT SHOULD BE PRESCRIBED AND ADMINISTERED WITH THE SAME DEGREE OF CAUTION APPROPRIATE TO THE USE OF MORPHINE.

Interaction with Other Central-Nervous-System Depressants—Methadone should be used with caution and in reduced dosage in patients who are concurrently receiving other narcotic analgesics, general anesthetics, phenothiazines, other tranquilizers, sedative-hypnotics, tricy-

Continued on next page

*Identi-Code® symbol.

Lilly—Cont.

clic antidepressants, and other C.N.S. depressants (including alcohol). Respiratory depression, hypotension, and profound sedation or coma may result.

Anxiety—Since methadone, as used by tolerant subjects at a constant maintenance dosage, is not a tranquilizer, patients who are maintained on this drug will react to life problems and stresses with the same symptoms of anxiety as do other individuals. The physician should not confuse such symptoms with those of narcotic abstinence and should not attempt to treat anxiety by increasing the dosage of methadone. The action of methadone in maintenance treatment is limited to the control of narcotic symptoms and is ineffective for relief of general anxiety.

Head Injury and Increased Intracranial Pressure—The respiratory depressant effects of methadone and its capacity to elevate cerebrospinal-fluid pressure may be markedly exaggerated in the presence of increased intracranial pressure. Furthermore, narcotics produce side effects that may obscure the clinical course of patients with head injuries. In such patients, methadone must be used with caution and only if it is deemed essential.

Asthma and Other Respiratory Conditions—Methadone should be used with caution in patients having an acute asthmatic attack, in those with chronic obstructive pulmonary disease or cor pulmonale, and in individuals with a substantially decreased respiratory reserve, preexisting respiratory depression, hypoxia, or hypercapnia. In such patients, even usual therapeutic doses of narcotics may decrease respiratory drive while simultaneously increasing airway resistance to the point of apnea.

Hypotensive Effect—The administration of methadone may result in severe hypotension in an individual whose ability to maintain his blood pressure has already been compromised by a depleted blood volume or concurrent administration of such drugs as the phenothiazines or certain anesthetics.

Use in Ambulatory Patients—Methadone may impair the mental and/or physical abilities required for the performance of potentially hazardous tasks, such as driving a car or operating machinery. The patient should be cautioned accordingly.

Methadone, like other narcotics, may produce orthostatic hypotension in ambulatory patients.

Use in Pregnancy—Safe use in pregnancy has not been established in relation to possible adverse effects on fetal development. Therefore, methadone should not be used in pregnant women unless, in the judgment of the physician, the potential benefits outweigh the possible hazards.

Methadone is not recommended for obstetric analgesia because its long duration of action increases the probability of respiratory depression in the newborn.

Use in Children—Methadone is not recommended for use as an analgesic in children, since documented clinical experience has been insufficient to establish a suitable dosage regimen for the pediatric age group.

Precautions: **Interaction with Pentazocine—Patients who are addicted to heroin or who are on the methadone maintenance program may experience withdrawal symptoms when given pentazocine.**

Interaction with Rifampin—The concurrent administration of rifampin may possibly reduce the blood concentration of methadone to a degree sufficient to produce withdrawal symptoms. The mechanism by which rifampin may decrease blood concentrations of methadone is not fully understood, although enhanced microsomal drug-metabolized enzymes may influence drug disposition.

Acute Abdominal Conditions—The administration of methadone or other narcotics may obscure the diagnosis or clinical course in patients with acute abdominal conditions.

Interaction with Monoamine Oxidase (MAO) Inhibitors—Therapeutic doses of meperidine have precipitated severe reactions in patients concurrently receiving monoamine oxidase inhibitors or those who have received such agents within 14 days. Similar reactions thus far have not been reported with methadone; but if the use of methadone is necessary in such patients, a sensitivity test should be performed in which repeated small incremental doses are administered over the course of several hours while the patient's condition and vital signs are under careful observation.

Special-Risk Patients—Methadone should be given with caution and the initial dose should be reduced in certain patients, such as the elderly or debilitated and those with severe impairment of hepatic or renal function, hypothyroidism, Addison's disease, prostatic hypertrophy, or urethral stricture.

Adverse Reactions: THE MAJOR HAZARDS OF METHADONE, AS OF OTHER NARCOTIC ANALGESICS, ARE RESPIRATORY DEPRESSION AND, TO A LESSER DEGREE, CIRCULATORY DEPRESSION. RESPIRATORY ARREST, SHOCK, AND CARDIAC ARREST HAVE OCCURRED.

The most frequently observed adverse reactions include lightheadedness, dizziness, sedation, nausea, vomiting, and sweating. These effects seem to be more prominent in ambulatory patients and in those who are not suffering severe pain. In such individuals, lower doses are advisable. Some adverse reactions may be alleviated in the ambulatory patient if he lies down.

Other adverse reactions include the following:

Central Nervous System—Euphoria, dysphoria, weakness, headache, insomnia, agitation, disorientation, and visual disturbances.

Gastrointestinal—Dry mouth, anorexia, constipation, and biliary tract spasm.

Cardiovascular—Flushing of the face, bradycardia, palpitation, faintness, and syncope.

Genitourinary—Urinary retention or hesitancy, antidiuretic effect, and reduced libido and/or potency.

Allergic—Pruritus, urticaria, other skin rashes, edema, and, rarely, hemorrhagic urticaria.

In addition, pain at injection site; local tissue irritation and induration following subcutaneous injection, particularly when repeated.

Administration and Dosage: *For Relief of Pain*—Dosage should be adjusted according to the severity of the pain and the response of the patient. Occasionally it may be necessary to exceed the usual dosage recommended in cases of exceptionally severe pain or in those patients who have become tolerant to the analgesic effect of narcotics.

Although subcutaneous administration is suitable for occasional use, intramuscular injection is preferred when repeated doses are required.

The usual adult dosage is 2.5 to 10 mg intramuscularly or subcutaneously every three or four hours as necessary.

For Detoxification Treatment—THE DRUG SHALL BE ADMINISTERED DAILY UNDER CLOSE SUPERVISION AS FOLLOWS:

A detoxification treatment course shall not exceed 21 days and may not be repeated earlier than four weeks after completion of the preceding course.

The oral form of administration is preferred. However, if the patient is unable to ingest oral medication, he may be started on the parenteral form initially.

In detoxification, the patient may receive methadone when there are significant symptoms of withdrawal. The dosage schedules indicated below are recommended but could be varied in accordance with clinical judgment. Initially, a single dose of 15 to 20 mg of methadone will often be sufficient to suppress withdrawal symptoms. Additional methadone may be provided if withdrawal symptoms are not suppressed or if symptoms reappear. When patients are physically dependent on high doses, it may be necessary to exceed these levels. Forty mg per day in single or divided doses will usually constitute an adequate stabilizing dosage level. Stabilization can be continued for two to three days, and then the amount of methadone normally will be gradually decreased. The rate at which methadone is decreased will be determined separately for each patient. The dose of methadone can be decreased on a daily basis or at two-day intervals, but the amount of intake shall always be sufficient to keep withdrawal symptoms at a tolerable level. In hospitalized patients, a daily reduction of 20 percent of the total daily dose may be tolerated and may cause little discomfort. In ambulatory patients, a somewhat slower schedule may be needed. If methadone is administered for more than three weeks, the procedure is considered to have progressed from detoxification or treatment of the acute withdrawal syndrome to maintenance treatment, even though the goal and intent may be eventual total withdrawal.

Overdosage: *Symptoms*—Serious overdosage of methadone is characterized by respiratory depression (a decrease in respiratory rate and/or tidal volume, Cheyne-Stokes respiration, cyanosis), extreme somnolence progressing to stupor or coma, maximally constricted pupils, skeletal-muscle flaccidity, cold and clammy skin, and, sometimes, bradycardia and hypotension. In severe overdosage, particularly by the intravenous route, apnea, circulatory collapse, cardiac arrest, and death may occur.

Treatment—Primary attention should be given to the reestablishment of adequate respiratory exchange through provision of a patent airway and institution of assisted or controlled ventilation. If a nontolerant person, especially a child, takes a large dose of methadone, effective narcotic antagonists are available to counteract the potentially lethal respiratory depression. **The physician must remember, however, that methadone is a long-acting depressant (36 to 48 hours), whereas the antagonists act for much shorter periods (one to three hours).** The patient must, therefore, be monitored continuously for recurrence of respiratory depression and treated repeatedly with the narcotic antagonist as needed. If the diagnosis is correct and respiratory depression is due only to overdosage of methadone, the use of other respiratory stimulants is not indicated.

An antagonist should not be administered in the absence of clinically significant respiratory or cardiovascular depression. Intravenously administered narcotic antagonists (naloxone, nalorphine, and levallorphan) are the drugs of choice to reverse signs of intoxication. These agents should be given repeatedly until the patient's status remains satisfactory. The hazard that the narcotic antagonist will further depress respiration is less likely with the use of naloxone.

Oxygen, intravenous fluids, vasopressors, and other supportive measures should be employed as indicated.

NOTE: IN AN INDIVIDUAL PHYSICALLY DEPENDENT ON NARCOTICS, THE ADMINISTRATION OF THE USUAL DOSE OF A NARCOTIC ANTAGONIST WILL PRECIPITATE AN ACUTE WITHDRAWAL SYNDROME. THE SEVERITY OF THIS SYNDROME WILL DEPEND ON THE DEGREE OF PHYSICAL DEPENDENCE AND THE DOSE OF THE ANTAGONIST ADMINISTERED. THE USE OF A NARCOTIC ANTAGO-

NIST IN SUCH A PERSON SHOULD BE AVOIDED IF POSSIBLE. IF IT MUST BE USED TO TREAT SERIOUS RESPIRATORY DEPRESSION IN THE PHYSICALLY DEPENDENT PATIENT, THE ANTAGONIST SHOULD BE ADMINISTERED WITH EXTREME CARE AND BY TITRATION WITH SMALLER THAN USUAL DOSES OF THE ANTAGONIST.

How Supplied: (Ⓒ) *Dolophine® Hydrochloride (Methadone Hydrochloride Injection, USP): Ampoules No. 456,* 10 mg, 1 ml, in packages of 12 and 100. *Ampoules (Vials) No. 435,* 10 mg per ml, 20 ml, rubber-stoppered, in singles (10 per carton) and in packages of 25.

[022779]

DOLOPHINE® HYDROCHLORIDE Ⓒ
(methadone hydrochloride)
Tablets, USP

CONDITIONS FOR DISTRIBUTION AND USE OF METHADONE PRODUCTS: *See under* Ampoules Dolophine Hydrochloride.

Description, Actions, Indications, and Contraindication: *See under* Ampoules Dolophine Hydrochloride.

Warnings:

Tablets Dolophine® Hydrochloride (methadone hydrochloride, Lilly) are for oral administration only and *must not* be used for injection. It is recommended that Tablets Dolophine Hydrochloride, if dispensed, be packaged in child-resistant containers and kept out of the reach of children to prevent accidental ingestion.

See also under Ampoules Dolophine Hydrochloride.

Precautions and Adverse Reactions: *See under* Ampoules Dolophine Hydrochloride.

Administration and Dosage: *For Relief of Pain*—Dosage should be adjusted according to the severity of the pain and the response of the patient. Occasionally it may be necessary to exceed the usual dosage recommended in cases of exceptionally severe pain or in those patients who have become tolerant to the analgesic effect of narcotics.

The usual adult dosage is 2.5 to 10 mg every three or four hours as necessary.

See also under Ampoules Dolophine Hydrochloride.

If the patient cannot ingest methadone orally, parenteral administration may be substituted.

Overdosage: *See under* Ampoules Dolophine Hydrochloride.

How Supplied: (Ⓒ) *Tablets Dolophine® Hydrochloride (Methadone Hydrochloride Tablets, USP): No. 1712, J64,** 5 mg, in bottles of 100 and 1000; *No. 1730, J72,**10 mg, in bottles of 100.

[041179]

DROLBAN® ℞
(dromostanolone propionate)
Injection, NF

Description: Drolban® (dromostanolone propionate, Lilly) is a synthetic steroid, a variant of testosterone. It is 17β-hydroxy-2α-methyl-5α-androstan-3-one propionate and is also known as 2-α-methyl-dihydrotestosterone propionate.

Indications: Dromostanolone propionate is recommended for use in the palliative treatment of advanced or metastatic carcinoma of the breast in women who are inoperable and are one to five years postmenopausal at the time of diagnosis or who have been proved to have hormone-dependent cancer by previous beneficial response to castration.

Contraindications: Androgens are contraindicated in carcinoma of the male breast and in premenopausal women.

Precautions: In general, the usual precautions pertaining to testosterone propionate should apply to Drolban® (dromostanolone propionate, Lilly), although in the latter the androgenic effects appear to be significantly less marked.

Patients with edema may require diuretics before and during treatment with this steroid.

In patients with bone metastases, the level of the serum calcium should be determined before and at intervals during the course of treatment with Drolban. Hypercalcemia may require other management, such as the use of corticosteroid therapy. Increase in libido appears to be unusual with this steroid; however, if it occurs, the use of sedation may be helpful.

Objective evidence of tumor progression should be evaluated periodically by physical examination, x-rays of known or suspected metastases, and determinations of serum calcium and alkaline phosphatase levels. The latter determination may reflect improvement in osseous lesions if there is a slight to moderate rise after initiation of treatment, or it may be indicative of extensive hepatic metastases if the level is markedly elevated.

Drug-induced jaundice or masculinization of the fetus reported with the use of other anabolic agents has thus far not been seen with Drolban. There are no reports of the use of this agent in carcinoma of the breast during pregnancy or in carcinoma of the breast in males with or without associated carcinoma of the prostate.

Until further information is available, Drolban should be used with caution in the presence of any of the following: liver disease, cardiac decompensation, nephritis, nephrosis, pregnancy, and carcinoma of the prostate.

Adverse Reactions: Side effects are significantly less intense with Drolban® (dromostanolone propionate, Lilly) than with comparable doses of testosterone propionate. The most likely side effects are mild virilism, such as deepening of the voice, acne, facial hair growth, and enlargement of the clitoris. At times, marked virilism will occur after prolonged treatment. Edema occasionally occurs. Hypercalcemia was noted in a few cases but usually accompanied progression of the disease. Libido seldom seems to be affected. Goldenberg reported a single case of "severe C.N.S. side effects, which cleared when the drug was stopped." Local reactions at the site of injection may occur rarely.

Administration and Dosage: It is recommended that 100 mg of Drolban® (dromostanolone propionate, Lilly) be administered by intramuscular injection three times weekly. Treatment probably should be continued as long as satisfactory results are obtained. After treatment has begun, eight to 12 weeks should elapse before any conclusions are drawn as to the efficacy of this steroid. If a significant progression of the disease occurs during the first six to eight weeks of therapy, another form of treatment should be considered.

How Supplied: (℞) *Ampoules (Vials) No. 691, Drolban® (Dromostanolone Propionate Injection, NF),* 50 mg per ml, 10 ml, rubber-stoppered, in singles (10 per carton). Each ml provides 50 mg dromostanolone propionate and sesame oil, q.s., with 0.5 percent phenol as a preservative. *Do not refrigerate.* [120777]

DROMOSTANOLONE PROPIONATE, *see* Drolban® (dromostanolone propionate, Lilly).

DURACILLIN® A.S. ℞
(sterile penicillin G procaine suspension)
USP

Description: Duracillin® A.S. (Sterile Penicillin G Procaine Suspension, USP, Lilly) is a ready-to-use aqueous suspension of Duracillin® (Penicillin G Procaine, USP, Lilly), the original penicillin G procaine, which was developed in the Lilly laboratories to fill a need for a long-acting parenteral penicillin preparation. Penicillin G procaine is a stable crystalline salt which is only slightly soluble in water. When combined with certain dispersing agents and suspended in water, it is slowly absorbed (because of its low solubility in body fluids) from the injection site in the muscle.

Actions and Pharmacology: Penicillin G is bactericidal against penicillin-sensitive microorganisms during the stage of active multiplication. It produces its effect by inhibiting biosynthesis of cell-wall mucopeptide. It is not active against the penicillinase-producing bacteria, which include many strains of staphylococci. Penicillin G exerts high in vitro activity against staphylococci (except penicillinase-producing strains), streptococci (groups A, C, G, H, L, and M), and pneumococci. Other organisms sensitive to penicillin G are *Neisseria gonorrhoeae, Corynebacterium diphtheriae, Bacillus anthracis,* clostridia, *Actinomyces bovis, Streptobacillus moniliformis, Listeria monocytogenes,* and *Leptospira. Treponema pallidum* is extremely sensitive to the bactericidal action of penicillin G.

Disc Susceptibility Tests—Quantitative methods that require measurement of zone diameters give the most precise estimates of antibiotic susceptibility. One such procedure (*Am. J. Clin. Pathol., 45:*493, 1966; *Federal Register, 39:*19182-19184, 1974) has been recommended for use with discs for testing susceptibility to penicillin.

Penicillin G procaine is an equimolecular compound of procaine and penicillin G administered intramuscularly as a suspension. It dissolves slowly at the site of injection and gives a plateau type of blood level at about four hours, which falls slowly over a period of the next 15 to 20 hours.

Approximately 60 percent of penicillin G is bound to serum protein. The drug is distributed throughout the body tissues in widely varying amounts. Highest levels are found in the kidneys, and lesser amounts appear in the liver, skin, and intestines. Small concentrations are found in all other body tissues and the cerebrospinal fluid. With normal kidney function, the drug is excreted rapidly by tubular excretion. In neonates, young infants, and individuals with impaired kidney function, excretion is considerably delayed. Approximately 60 to 90 percent of a dose of parenteral penicillin G is excreted in the urine within 24 to 36 hours.

Indications: Penicillin G procaine is indicated in the treatment of moderately severe infections due to penicillin-G-sensitive microorganisms that are sensitive to the low and persistent serum levels common to this particular dosage form. Therapy should be guided by bacteriologic studies (including susceptibility tests) and by clinical response.

NOTE: When high, sustained serum levels are required, aqueous penicillin G should be used either intramuscularly or intravenously.

The following infections will usually respond to adequate dosages of intramuscular penicillin G procaine:

Streptococcal Infections (Group A) (without Bacteremia)—Moderately severe to severe infections of the upper respiratory tract, skin and soft-tissue infections, scarlet fever, and erysipelas.

NOTE: Streptococci in groups A, C, G, H, L, and M are very sensitive to penicillin G. Other groups, including group D (enterococcus), are resistant. Aqueous penicillin is recommended for streptococcal infections with bacteremia.

Pneumococcal Infections—Moderately severe infections of the respiratory tract.

Continued on next page

*Identi-Code® symbol.

Lilly—Cont.

NOTE: Severe pneumonia, empyema, bacteremia, pericarditis, meningitis, peritonitis, and arthritis of pneumococcal etiology are better treated with aqueous penicillin G during the acute stage.
Staphylococcal Infections Sensitive to Penicillin G—Moderately severe infections of the skin and soft tissues.
NOTE: Reports indicate an increasing number of strains of staphylococci resistant to penicillin G, which emphasizes the need for culture and susceptibility studies in treating suspected staphylococcal infections.
Indicated surgical procedures should be performed.
Fusospirochetosis (Vincent's Gingivitis and Pharyngitis)—Moderately severe infections of the oropharynx respond to therapy with penicillin G procaine.
NOTE: Necessary dental care should be accomplished in infections involving the gum tissue.
Syphilis (T. pallidum)—All stages
Acute and Chronic Gonorrhea (without Bacteremia) (N. gonorrhoeae)
Yaws, Bejel, Pinta
Diphtheria (C. diphtheriae)—Penicillin G procaine as an adjunct to antitoxin for prevention of the carrier stage
Anthrax
Rat-Bite Fever (S. moniliformis and *Spirillum minus)*
Erysipeloid
Subacute Bacterial Endocarditis (Group A Streptococci)—Limited to extremely sensitive infections
Prophylaxis against bacterial endocarditis in patients with congenital and/or rheumatic heart disease when undergoing dental or upper respiratory tract surgery or instrumentation. Prophylaxis should be instituted the day of the procedure and continued for two or more days following.
NOTE: Because patients with a past history of rheumatic fever and receiving continuous prophylaxis may harbor increased numbers of penicillin-resistant organisms, use of another prophylactic anti-infective agent should be considered. If penicillin is to be used in these patients at surgery, the regular rheumatic fever program should be interrupted one week prior to the contemplated surgery. At the time of surgery, penicillin may be reinstituted as a prophylactic measure against the hazards of surgically induced bacteremia.
Contraindication: A previous hypersensitivity reaction to any penicillin is a contraindication.
Warnings: Serious and occasionally fatal hypersensitivity (anaphylactoid) reactions have been reported in patients receiving penicillin therapy. Although anaphylaxis is more frequent following parenteral therapy, it has occurred in patients given oral penicillins. These reactions are more likely in individuals with a history of sensitivity to multiple allergens.
There have been well-documented reports of individuals with a history of penicillin hypersensitivity who have experienced severe reactions when treated with a cephalosporin. Before therapy with a penicillin, careful inquiry should be made concerning previous hypersensitivity reactions to penicillins, cephalosporins, and other allergens. If an allergic reaction occurs, the drug should be discontinued and the patient treated with the usual agents (e.g., epinephrine or other pressor amines, antihistamines, or corticosteroids).
Immediate toxic reactions to procaine may occur in some individuals, particularly when a large single dose is administered in the treatment of gonorrhea (4,800,000 units). These reactions may be manifested by mental disturbances, including anxiety, confusion, agitation, depression, weakness, seizures, hallucinations, combativeness, and expressed "fear of impending death." The reactions noted in carefully controlled studies occurred in approximately one of 500 patients treated for gonorrhea. Reactions are transient and last from 15 to 30 minutes.
Precautions: Penicillin should be used with caution in individuals having histories of significant allergies and/or asthma.
In intramuscular therapy, care should be taken to avoid accidental intravenous administration.
In suspected staphylococcal infections, proper laboratory studies, including susceptibility tests, should be performed.
A small percentage of patients are sensitive to procaine. If there is a history of sensitivity, make the usual test: Inject 0.1 ml. of a 1 to 2 percent procaine solution intradermally. Development of an erythema, wheal, flare, or eruption indicates procaine sensitivity. Sensitivity should be treated by the usual methods, including barbiturates, and penicillin procaine preparations should not be used. Antihistamines appear beneficial in treatment of procaine reactions.
The use of antibiotics may result in overgrowth of nonsusceptible organisms. Constant observation of the patient is essential. If new infections due to bacteria or fungi appear during therapy, the drug should be discontinued and appropriate measures taken. Whenever allergic reactions occur, penicillin should be withdrawn unless, in the opinion of the physician, the condition being treated is life threatening and amenable only to penicillin therapy.
In prolonged therapy with penicillin, and particularly with high dosage schedules, periodic evaluation of the renal and hematopoietic systems is recommended.
When gonococcal infections are treated in which primary or secondary syphilis may be suspected, proper diagnostic procedures, including darkfield examinations, should be performed. In all cases in which concomitant syphilis is suspected, monthly serologic tests should be made for at least four months.
Adverse Reactions: Penicillin is a substance of low toxicity but does have a significant index of sensitization. The following hypersensitivity reactions have been reported: skin rashes ranging from maculopapular eruptions to exfoliative dermatitis; urticaria; and reactions resembling serum sickness, including chills, fever, edema, arthralgia, and prostration. Severe and often fatal anaphylaxis has occurred (*see* Warnings). As with other treatments for syphilis, the Jarisch-Herxheimer reaction has been reported.
Manifestations of procaine toxicity have been reported (*see* Warnings). Procaine hypersensitivity reactions have not been reported with this drug.
Administration and Dosage: Penicillin G procaine (aqueous) is for intramuscular injection only.
Recommended dosage is as follows:
Pneumonia (Pneumococcus)—Moderately severe (uncomplicated): 600,000 to 1,000,000 units daily.
Streptococcal Infections (Group A)—Moderately severe to severe tonsillitis, erysipelas, scarlet fever, and upper respiratory tract, skin, and soft-tissue infections: 600,000 to 1,000,000 units daily for a minimum of ten days.
Staphylococcal Infections—Moderately severe to severe: 600,000 to 1,000,000 units daily.
Bacterial Endocarditis (Group A Streptococci)—Limited to extremely sensitive infections: 600,000 to 1,000,000 units daily.
Prophylaxis against Bacterial Endocarditis—In patients with rheumatic or congenital heart disease when undergoing dental or upper respiratory tract surgery or instrumentation: 600,000 units of aqueous penicillin G procaine the day of the procedure; 600,000 units of aqueous penicillin G one to two hours before surgery; 600,000 units of aqueous penicillin G procaine daily for two days following surgery.
Syphilis—Primary, secondary, and latent with a negative spinal fluid in adults and children over 12 years of age: 600,000 units daily for eight days (total, 4,800,000 units).
Late (tertiary and latent syphilis and neurosyphilis with positive spinal-fluid examination or no spinal-fluid examination): 600,000 units daily for ten to 15 days (total, 6,000,000 to 9,000,000 units).
Congenital syphilis in a patient weighing less than 70 pounds: 10,000 units/kg per day for ten days.
Syphilis in pregnancy: Treatment should correspond to the stage of the disease.
Yaws, Bejel, and Pinta—Same treatment as for syphilis in corresponding stage of disease.
Gonorrheal Infections (Uncomplicated)—Men or women: 4,800,000 units intramuscularly, divided into at least two doses and injected at different sites during one visit, together with 1 gm of oral probenecid, preferably given at least 30 minutes prior to the injection.
NOTE: Gonorrheal endocarditis should be treated intensively with aqueous penicillin G.
Diphtheria—Adjunctive therapy with antitoxin: 300,000 to 600,000 units daily.
Diphtheria Carrier State—300,000 units daily for ten days.
Anthrax (Cutaneous)—600,000 to 1,000,000 units per day.
Vincent's Infection (Fusospirochetosis)—600,000 to 1,000,000 units per day.
Erysipeloid—600,000 to 1,000,000 units per day.
Rat-Bite Fever (S. moniliformis and *S. minus)*—600,000 to 1,000,000 units per day.
How Supplied: (℞) *Ampoules (Vials) No. 554, Duracillin® A.S. (Sterile Penicillin G Procaine Suspension, USP),* 300,000 units per ml, 10 ml, rubber-stoppered, in singles (10 per carton) and in Traypaks™ (multivial cartons, Lilly) of 100. Each vial also contains lecithin, 1 percent; sodium citrate, 4 percent; povidone, 0.1 percent; and 0.015 percent butylparaben as a preservative.
(℞) *Hyporets® Duracillin® A.S. (Sterile Penicillin G Procaine Suspension, USP): No. 8,* 300,000 units, 1 ml, disposable syringe with 22-gauge needle, *No. 9,* 600,000 units, 1.2 ml, disposable syringe with 20-gauge needle, and *No. 10,* 1,200,000 units, 2 ml, disposable syringe with 20-gauge needle, in packages of 10 and 100. Each Hyporet No. 8 also contains sodium citrate, 1 percent; polysorbate 80, 0.15 percent; and 0.015 percent butylparaben as a preservative. Each Hyporet No. 9 and No. 10 also contains sodium citrate, 4 percent; lecithin, 1.5 percent; polysorbate 80, 0.4 percent; and 0.015 percent butylparaben as a preservative.
Refrigerate all preparations of Duracillin A.S. Avoid freezing. [020179]

DYMELOR® ℞
(acetohexamide)
Tablets, USP

Description: Dymelor® (acetohexamide, Lilly) is a sulfonylurea characterized by the presence of an acetyl group in the para position of the phenyl ring and the incorporation of a cyclohexyl group on the urea moiety. Chemically, it is N-(*p*-acetylphenylsulfonyl)-N′-cyclohexylurea.
Action: Dymelor® (acetohexamide, Lilly) is an oral antidiabetic agent which is effective in controlling the blood glucose in properly selected patients with maturity-onset diabetes. The mode of action of Dymelor is stimulation of release of insulin from the beta cells of the pancreas. In addition, a number of extrapancreatic actions of this class of drug have been elucidated; the most important of these is a reduction in glucose output from the liver.
Indications: The principal clinical indication for Dymelor® (acetohexamide, Lilly) is diabetes mellitus of the stable type (without such

complications as ketosis or acidosis), variously described as relatively mild adult, maturity-onset, or nonketotic type.
The use of Dymelor in insulin-dependent patients may reduce the insulin requirements.
Contraindications: Dymelor® (acetohexamide, Lilly) is contraindicated in patients with hyperglycemia and glycosuria which may be associated with primary renal disease. If reduction of the blood sugar becomes essential in these cases, insulin is indicated.
Warnings: *Use in Pregnancy*—Safe use in pregnancy *has not been* established at this time, from the standpoint of either the mother or the fetus. Therefore, the use of Dymelor® (acetohexamide, Lilly) is not recommended for the management of diabetes when complicated by pregnancy. The advisability of administering Dymelor to women of childbearing age should be considered with caution.
Dymelor is of no value in diabetes complicated by acidosis and coma. These conditions require insulin.
In times of stress to the patient, such as fever of any cause, trauma, infection, or surgical procedures, it may be necessary to return the patient to insulin therapy or to use insulin in addition to Dymelor.
Precautions: The principles of management of diabetes mellitus are necessary to insure optimum control with Dymelor® (acetohexamide, Lilly) and are the same as for patients requiring insulin.
In patients with impaired hepatic and/or renal function and in debilitated or malnourished individuals, careful observation of the patient and adjustment of dosage are mandatory to prevent the occurrence of hypoglycemia.
Thiazide-type diuretics may aggravate the diabetic state and alter the dosage of Dymelor required.
Preparations containing phenylbutazone interfere with the excretion of the active metabolite hydroxyhexamide; as a result, increased sulfonylurea levels depress the blood glucose. This may also be true of probenecid and the absorbed antimicrobial sulfas.
Nonsteroidal anti-inflammatory agents have an affinity for albumin and may displace other albumin-bound drugs from their binding sites; this may lead to drug interaction. Patients receiving both Dymelor and nonsteroidal anti-inflammatory agents should be observed for signs of toxicity to these drugs.
Sulfonylurea compounds, like antimicrobial sulfa drugs and barbiturates, may aggravate hepatic porphyria.
Patients receiving sulfonylureas may experience peculiar symptoms, referred to as the "disulfiram reaction," following the ingestion of alcohol.
Secondary failures and the spontaneous tendency of diabetes to fluctuate in severity may occur. Therefore, patients should be seen by their physicians at regular intervals and their diabetes evaluated in order to avoid hyperglycemic and hypoglycemic episodes.
Adverse Reactions: Hypoglycemia may occur in those patients who do not eat regularly or who exercise without caloric supplementation. It is most likely to appear during the period of transition from insulin to Dymelor® (acetohexamide, Lilly) and should be considered in patients who have hepatic or renal disease as well as those who are debilitated or malnourished. Other untoward reactions consist principally in gastrointestinal disturbances (nausea, epigastric fullness, heartburn) and headache, appear to be dose related, and may disappear when dosage is reduced.
Allergic skin manifestations (pruritus, erythema, urticaria, morbilliform or maculopapular eruptions) occur but are usually transient and may disappear with continued dosage. If the skin reactions persist, the drug should be stopped. Photosensitivity reactions may be noted. Jaundice of both the cholestatic and mixed hepatic types has been observed with Dymelor.
As with other sulfonylurea drugs, leukopenia, thrombocytopenia, pancytopenia, agranulocytosis, aplastic anemia, and hemolytic anemia may occur with Dymelor.
Administration and Dosage: Since diabetes may be of various degrees of severity, there can be no fixed dosage of either Dymelor® (acetohexamide, Lilly) or insulin. Daily oral dosage of Dymelor may range between 250 mg and 1.5 gm. No loading dose is required. Patients who do not respond to 1.5 gm daily usually will not respond to a higher dose. For this reason, doses in excess of 1.5 gm daily are not recommended. The majority of patients receiving 1 gm or less per day can be controlled on a convenient once-daily dosage. Patients who need 1.5 gm per day usually benefit from twice-daily dosage, given before the morning and evening meals.
Dymelor may be used in combination with phenformin as well as with insulin.
Various measures have been employed to establish patients on Dymelor, and the following procedures are suggested.
Patients Not Previously Receiving Insulin or Drug Therapy—In mild, stable diabetes (after dietary regulation), therapy may be initiated with 250 mg daily before breakfast; subsequent adjustment of the dosage may be made by increments of 250 to 500 mg every five to seven days as necessary. The 250-mg or the 500-mg tablet (scored and easily broken in half) may be used.
Because of reports of hyperresponsiveness of some elderly diabetics to Dymelor® (acetohexamide, Lilly), patients in this group should be started with a single dose of 250 mg before breakfast, and their blood and urine sugars should be checked during the first 24 hours of therapy. If control appears to be satisfactory, this dose may be continued on a daily basis or, if necessary, gradually increased. If, however, there appears to be a tendency toward hypoglycemia, this dose should be reduced or the drug should be discontinued.
Patients Receiving Other Oral Agents—When transfer is made from tolbutamide, the initial dose of Dymelor® (acetohexamide, Lilly) should be about half the tolbutamide dose (e.g., 250 mg of Dymelor in place of 500 mg of tolbutamide), up to a maximum of 1.5 gm of Dymelor.
When transfer is made from chlorpropamide, the initial dose of Dymelor should be about double the chlorpropamide dose (e.g., 500 mg of Dymelor in place of 250 mg of chlorpropamide). No transition period is required. Subsequent adjustment of dosage should be made according to clinical response. The maximum recommended dose of Dymelor is 1.5 gm.
Clinical reports on the efficacy of once-daily dosage of Dymelor indicate that its effect on the blood sugar is better sustained than that of tolbutamide. However, patients requiring more than 1 gm of Dymelor daily should be treated with divided doses.
Patients Receiving Insulin—In general, patients who were previously maintained on insulin in small dosage (e.g., up to 20 units per day) may be placed on Dymelor® (acetohexamide, Lilly) directly and their insulin administration abruptly discontinued. Patients requiring larger doses of insulin, such as 20 to 40 units or more per day, should have an initial reduction of insulin dosage by 25 or 30 percent daily or every other day and subsequent further reduction depending on the response to Dymelor. An initial dose of 250 mg of Dymelor can be used, with readjustment depending upon response to therapy. Because of the potential hazards of hypoglycemia in the elderly, patients in this age group should be carefully observed during the transition from insulin to Dymelor.
During the period of insulin withdrawal, the patient should test his urine for sugar and acetone at least three times a day and report the results frequently to his physician so that appropriate adjustments of therapy may be made. In some cases, it may be advisable to consider hospitalization during the transition period from insulin to Dymelor.
It should be noted that, as with other sulfonylureas, primary and secondary failures may occur with Dymelor.
Overdosage: Hypoglycemia may appear in those patients who do not eat regularly or who exercise without caloric supplementation. This is treated in the usual manner, by supplying carbohydrate in various forms, dependent upon the clinical status.
In patients with protracted hypoglycemia, treatment with 10 to 50 percent dextrose in water is advisable until the tendency toward hypoglycemia has subsided.
How Supplied: (℞) *Tablets Dymelor® (Acetohexamide Tablets, USP)* (capsule-shaped, scored): *No. 1842, U03,** 250 mg, White, and *No. 1843, U07,** 500 mg, Yellow, in bottles of 50, 200, and 500 and in 10 strips of 10 individually labeled blisters each containing 1 tablet (ID100). [052278]

[*Shown in Product Identification Section*]

Tablets No. 1843, 500 mg—50's—6505-00-765-0589

EN-CEBRIN® OTC
(prenatal vitamin-minerals)

Description: En-Cebrin is a broad and potent vitamin-mineral formulation for use during pregnancy and lactation. Each Pulvule® contains phosphorus-free calcium in the form of calcium carbonate, plus liberal quantities of important vitamins and minerals in well-balanced proportions.

Each Pulvule contains—

Vitamin A	4000 IU (1.2 mg)
Thiamine Mononitrate (Vitamin B_1)	3 mg
Riboflavin (Vitamin B_2)	2 mg
Niacinamide	10 mg
Pyridoxine (Vitamin B_6)	1.7 mg
Vitamin B_{12} (Activity Equivalent)	5 mcg
Pantothenic Acid	5 mg
Ascorbic Acid (Vitamin C)	50 mg
Vitamin D	400 IU (10 mcg)
Calcium (as the Carbonate)	250 mg
Iron (as Ferrous Fumarate)	30 mg
Iodine (as Potassium Iodide)	0.15 mg
Copper (as the Sulfate)	1 mg
Magnesium (as the Hydroxide)	5 mg
Manganese (as the Glycerophosphate)	1 mg
Zinc (as the Chloride)	1.5 mg

Indications: For use during pregnancy and lactation.
Adverse Reactions: Infrequently, nausea and vomiting have been reported after administration.
Dosage: 1 Pulvule a day, or as directed by the physician.
How Supplied: *Pulvules No. 382, En-Cebrin® (prenatal vitamin-minerals, Lilly), H12** (No. 0, Light-Pink Opaque Body, Light-Blue Opaque Cap), in bottles of 100. [060178]

EN-CEBRIN® F ℞
(prenatal vitamin-mineral supplements with folic acid)

Description: Each Pulvule® contains—

Vitamin A Synthetic	4000 IU (1.2 mg)
Thiamine Mononitrate (Vitamin B_1)	3 mg
Riboflavin (Vitamin B_2)	2 mg
Niacinamide	10 mg
Pyridoxine Hydrochloride (Vitamin B_6)	2 mg
Folic Acid	1 mg
Vitamin B_{12} (Activity Equivalent)	5 mcg

Continued on next page

*Identi-Code® symbol.

Lilly—Cont.

Pantothenic Acid (as Calcium Pantothenate, Racemic)	5 mg
Ascorbic Acid (Vitamin C)	50 mg
Vitamin D Synthetic	400 IU (10 mcg)
Calcium (as the Carbonate)	250 mg
Iron (as Ferrous Fumarate)	30 mg
Iodine (as Potassium Iodide)	0.15 mg
Copper (as the Sulfate)	1 mg
Magnesium (as the Hydroxide)	5 mg
Manganese (as the Glycerophosphate)	1 mg
Zinc (as the Chloride)	1.5 mg

Each Pulvule supplies at least the minimum daily requirement of vitamins A and D, thiamine, riboflavin, niacinamide, ascorbic acid, iron, and iodine. In addition, the formula contains pyridoxine to help meet the increased need for this substance in pregnant women.
Calcium (phosphorus-free) is also supplied, as well as other minerals for which the qualitative, but not quantitative, needs seem to be well established.

Indications: En-Cebrin F is indicated whenever a wide-range nutritional supplement is needed during pregnancy.
En-Cebrin F contains 1 mg folic acid per Pulvule. Folic acid deficiency is the cause of most cases of megaloblastic anemia of pregnancy, a condition which may occur in 3 to 4 percent of patients in the temperate zone and in an even higher percentage of patients in the tropics. There is an increased requirement for folic acid during pregnancy, especially in the third trimester. In addition, recent studies suggest that absorption of this substance may be impaired in pregnancy.
A report based on bone-marrow biopsies of pregnant women indicates that megaloblastic erythropoiesis was found in about 4 percent of cases. It is significant that, clinically, many of the women had only a slight anemia.

Contraindications: There are no known contraindications to En-Cebrin F.

Precautions: Although administration of folic acid alone may produce a temporary hematologic remission in Addisonian pernicious anemia, neurologic progression may not be halted. Therefore, vitamin B_{12} in ample doses must be given to patients with this disease. However, true Addisonian pernicious anemia in pregnancy is extremely rare.
In unusual cases of allergy or intolerance to specific ingredients in the formula, the product should be used with caution.

Adverse Reactions: Infrequently, nausea and vomiting have been reported after administration.

Dosage: The usual dosage is 1 Pulvule daily.

How Supplied: (℞) *Pulvules No. 376, En-Cebrin® F (prenatal vitamin-mineral supplements with folic acid, Lilly), H10** (No. 0, Light-Pink Opaque Body, Light-Blue Opaque Cap), in ℞ Paks (prescription packages, Lilly) of 100. ℞Paks have safety closures. [062876]

ERGOTRATE® MALEATE ℞
(ergonovine maleate)
Injection, NF
AMPOULES

Description: Ergonovine is the hydroxyisopropylamide of lysergic acid. It is somewhat soluble in water, and its salts are readily soluble. It is obtained from ergot and has been shown to possess all of the desirable oxytocic activity of ergot itself.
Each ampoule contains 0.2 mg of the active ingredient, ergonovine maleate, with ethyl lactate, 0.1 percent, lactic acid, 0.1 percent, and phenol, 0.25 percent, as a preservative.
The empirical formula of ergonovine maleate is $C_{19}H_{23}N_3O_2 \cdot C_4H_4O_4$. Chemically, it is 9,10-Didehydro- *N*-[(*S*)-2-hydroxy-1-methylethyl]-6-methylergoline-8β-carboxamide maleate (1:1) (salt).

Clinical Pharmacology: Injection Ergotrate® Maleate (Ergonovine Maleate Injection, NF, Lilly) produces a firm contraction of the uterus. Upon the initial tetanic contraction is superimposed a succession of minor relaxations and contractions. The extent of relaxation gradually increases over a period of about one and one-half hours, but vigorous rhythmic contractions continue for a period of three or more hours after injection. The prolonged initial contraction is the type necessary to control uterine hemorrhage.

Indications and Usage: Ergotrate® Maleate (ergonovine maleate, Lilly) is indicated for the prevention and treatment of postpartum and postabortal hemorrhage and of puerperal morbidity.

Contraindications: Ergotrate® Maleate (ergonovine maleate, Lilly) is contraindicated for the induction of labor and in cases of threatened spontaneous abortion. It should not be administered to those patients who have shown allergic or idiosyncratic reactions to it.

Warnings: All oxytocic agents are potentially dangerous. Mothers and infants have been injured, and some have died because of their injudicious use. Hyperstimulation of the uterus during labor may lead to uterine tetany with marked impairment of the uteroplacental blood flow, uterine rupture, cervical and perineal lacerations, amniotic fluid embolism, and trauma to the infant (e.g., hypoxia, intracranial hemorrhage). Because of these hazards which result with overdosage, oxytocic agents must be administered under conditions of meticulous observation.

Precautions: *General Precautions*—Because of the high uterine tone produced, Ergotrate® Maleate (ergonovine maleate, Lilly) is not recommended for routine use prior to the delivery of the placenta unless the operator is versed in the technique described by Davis and others and has adequate facilities and personnel at his disposal.
As is the case with all ergot preparations, prolonged use of Ergotrate Maleate is to be avoided. Discontinue Ergotrate Maleate if symptoms of ergotism appear.
Ergotrate Maleate should be used cautiously in patients with hypertension, heart disease, venoatrial shunts, mitral-valve stenosis, obliterative vascular disease, sepsis, or hepatic or renal impairment.
The character and amount of vaginal bleeding should be observed. Hypocalcemia may affect patient response to the drug. If the patient is not also taking digitalis, cautious administration of calcium gluconate I.V. may produce the desired oxytocic action.
Laboratory Tests—Blood pressure, pulse, and uterine response should be monitored. Sudden changes in vital signs or frequent periods of uterine relaxation should be noted.

Adverse Reactions: Nausea and vomiting may occur, but they are uncommon. Allergic phenomena, including shock, have been reported. Ergotism has also been reported. Elevation of blood pressure (sometimes extreme) may appear in a small percentage of patients, most frequently in association with regional anesthesia (caudal or spinal), previous administration of a vasoconstrictor, and the intravenous route of administration of the oxytocic. The mechanism of such hypertension is obscure, since it may occur in the absence of anesthesia, vasoconstrictors, and oxytocics. These elevations are no more frequent with Ergotrate® Maleate (ergonovine maleate, Lilly) than with other oxytocics. They usually subside promptly following intravenous administration of 15 mg of chlorpromazine.

Overdosage: *Symptoms*—The principal manifestations of serious overdosage are convulsions and gangrene. Symptoms of overdosage include the following: vomiting, diarrhea, dizziness, rise or fall in blood pressure, weak pulse, dyspnea, loss of consciousness, numbness and coldness of the extremities, tingling, pain in the chest, gangrene of the fingers and toes, and hypercoagulability.
Treatment—Treat convulsions. Control hypercoagulability by the administration of heparin, and maintain blood-clotting time at approximately three times the normal. Give a vasodilator such as tolazine as an antidote; the rate of administration may be controlled by monitoring pulse rate and blood pressure. For emergency measures, delay absorption of ingested ergotamine by giving tap water, milk, or activated charcoal and then removing by gastric lavage or emesis followed by catharsis. Gangrene will require surgical amputation.

Administration and Dosage: Ergotrate® Maleate (ergonovine maleate, Lilly) is intended primarily for routine intramuscular injection in obstetric practice. By this route, it usually produces a firm contraction of the uterus within a few minutes.
Intravenous administration leads to a quicker response. However, because of the higher incidence of nausea and other side effects, it is recommended that the intravenous route be confined to emergencies such as excessive uterine bleeding.
The usual intramuscular (or emergency intravenous) dose of Ergotrate Maleate is 0.2 mg, one ampoule. Severe uterine bleeding may call for repeated doses, but injection will rarely be required more often than once in two to four hours.
In some calcium-deficient patients, the uterus may fail to respond to Ergotrate Maleate. In such instances, responsiveness can be immediately restored by the cautious intravenous injection of calcium salts. Calcium should not be given intravenously to patients under the influence of digitalis.
Tablets Ergotrate Maleate are available for oral administration.
Storage—Ampoules Ergotrate Maleate should be stored in a cold place (below 46°F). However, delivery-room stock may be kept at room temperature (although periods of more than 60 days at room temperature prior to use are not recommended).

How Supplied: (℞) *Ampoules No. 302, Ergotrate® Maleate (Ergonovine Maleate Injection, NF),* 0.2 mg, 1 ml, in packages of 6 (NDC 0002-1629-16) and 100 (NDC 0002-1629-02). [101979]

ERGOTRATE® MALEATE ℞
(ergonovine maleate)
Tablets, NF

Description: Ergonovine is the hydroxyisopropylamide of lysergic acid. It is somewhat soluble in water, and its salts are readily soluble. It is obtained from ergot and has been shown to possess all of the desirable oxytocic activity of ergot itself.

Actions: Within six to 15 minutes, Ergotrate® Maleate (ergonovine maleate, Lilly) produces a firm tetanic contraction of the postpartum uterus which, in the course of about 90 minutes, gradually changes to a series of clonic contractions that persist for another 90 minutes or more.

Indications: For prevention and treatment of postpartum and postabortal hemorrhage due to uterine atony.

Contraindications: Ergotrate® Maleate (ergonovine maleate, Lilly) is contraindicated for the induction of labor and in cases of threatened spontaneous abortion. It should not be administered to those patients who have shown allergic or idiosyncratic reactions to it.

Precautions: Because of the high uterine tone produced, Ergotrate® Maleate (ergonovine maleate, Lilly) is not recommended for routine use prior to the delivery of the placenta unless the operator is versed in the technique described by Davis and others and has adequate facilities and personnel at his disposal.
As is the case with all ergot preparations, prolonged use of Ergotrate Maleate is to be

avoided. Discontinue Ergotrate Maleate if symptoms of ergotism appear.
Adverse Reactions: Nausea and vomiting may occur, but they are uncommon. Allergic phenomena, including shock, have been reported. Ergotism has also been reported. Elevations of blood pressure (sometimes extreme) may appear in a small percentage of patients, most frequently in association with regional anesthesia (caudal or spinal), previous administration of a vasoconstrictor, and the intravenous route of administration of the oxytocic. The mechanism of such hypertension is obscure, since it may occur in the absence of anesthesia, vasoconstrictors, and oxytocics. These elevations are no more frequent with Ergotrate® Maleate (ergonovine maleate, Lilly) than with other oxytocics. They usually subside promptly following intravenous administration of 15 mg of chlorpromazine.
Administration and Dosage: The immediate postpartum dose of Ergotrate® Maleate (ergonovine maleate, Lilly) is usually 0.2 mg. It is ordinarily administered parenterally. To minimize late postpartum bleeding, 1 or 2 tablets may be given orally two to four times daily (every six to 12 hours) until the danger of uterine atony has passed—usually 48 hours. Severe cramping is evidence of effectiveness but may justify reduction in dosage. Tablets Ergotrate Maleate may also be administered perlingually.
How Supplied: (℞) *Tablets No. 1572, Ergotrate® Maleate (Ergonovine Maleate Tablets, NF), J36,** 0.2 mg, in bottles of 100 and 1000 and in 10 strips of 10 individually labeled blisters each containing 1 tablet (ID100).[020179]

FOLIC ACID ℞
Tablets, USP

Description: Folic acid is a member of the vitamin B complex.
Action: Folic acid acts on megaloblastic bone marrow to produce a normoblastic marrow.
Indications: It is effective in the treatment of megaloblastic anemias due to a deficiency of folic acid (as may be seen in tropical or nontropical sprue) and in anemias of nutritional origin, pregnancy, infancy, or childhood.
Warning: Administration of folic acid alone is improper therapy for pernicious anemia and other megaloblastic anemias in which vitamin B_{12} is deficient.
Precaution: Folic acid, especially in doses above 1 mg daily, may obscure pernicious anemia; that is, hematologic remission may occur while neurologic manifestations remain progressive.
Adverse Reaction: Allergic sensitization has been reported following both oral and parenteral administration of folic acid.
Administration and Dosage: Folic acid is well absorbed and may be administered orally with satisfactory results except in severe instances of intestinal malabsorption.
The usual therapeutic dosage in adults and children (regardless of age) is up to 1 mg daily. Resistant cases may require larger doses.
When clinical symptoms have subsided and the blood picture has become normal, a daily maintenance level should be used, i.e., 0.1 mg for infants and up to 0.3 mg for children under four years of age, 0.4 mg for adults and children four or more years of age, and 0.8 mg for pregnant and lactating women, but never less than 0.1 mg per day. Patients should be kept under close supervision and adjustment of the maintenance level made if relapse appears imminent.
In the presence of alcoholism, hemolytic anemia, anticonvulsant therapy, or chronic infection, the maintenance level may need to be increased.
How Supplied: (℞) *Tablets No. 1897, Folic Acid, USP, U56,** 1 mg, in bottles of 100.
[102678]

GLUCAGON FOR INJECTION USP ℞

Description: Glucagon is produced in the pancreas (alpha cells of the islands of Langerhans). Purified and crystallized by scientists at the Lilly Research Laboratories, it is used in the treatment of hypoglycemic states and is effective in small doses.
Chemically unrelated to insulin, glucagon is a straight-chain polypeptide containing 29 amino acid residues and having a molecular weight of 3485.
Crystalline glucagon is a white powder containing less than 0.01 percent zinc. It is relatively insoluble in water but is soluble at a *p*H of less than 3 or more than 9.5. Glucagon is stable in lyophilized form at room temperatures. It will remain potent in solution for as long as three months if kept under refrigeration.
Actions: Glucagon causes an increase in blood glucose concentration and is used in the treatment of hypoglycemic states. It is effective in small doses, and no evidence of toxicity has been reported with its use. Glucagon acts only on liver glycogen, converting it to glucose.
Indications: Glucagon is useful in counteracting severe hypoglycemic reactions in diabetic patients or during insulin shock therapy in psychiatric patients. Glucagon is helpful in hypoglycemia only if liver glycogen is available. It is of little or no help in states of starvation, adrenal insufficiency, or chronic hypoglycemia.
The patient with juvenile-type diabetes does not have as great a response in blood glucose levels as does the adult-type stable diabetic. Therefore, supplementary carbohydrate should be given as soon as possible to the juvenile patient especially.
Contraindication: Since glucagon is a protein, hypersensitivity is a possibility.
Precautions: In the treatment of hypoglycemic shock with glucagon, liver glycogen must be available. Glucose by the intravenous route or by gavage should be considered in the hypoglycemic patient.
Adverse Reactions: Glucagon is relatively free of adverse reactions except for occasional nausea and vomiting, which may also occur with hypoglycemia.
Administration and Dosage: The diluent is provided for use only in the preparation of glucagon for *intermittent* parenteral injection and for no other use.
Directions for Use of Glucagon—1. Dissolve the lyophilized glucagon in the accompanying solvent.
2. Give 0.5 to 1 unit of glucagon by subcutaneous, intramuscular, or intravenous injection.
3. The patient will usually awaken in five to 20 minutes. If the response is delayed, there is no contraindication to the administration of one or two additional doses of glucagon; however, in view of the deleterious effects of cerebral hypoglycemia and depending on the duration and depth of coma, the use of parenteral glucose *must* be considered by the physician.
4. Intravenous glucose *must* be given if the patient fails to respond to glucagon.
5. When the patient responds, give supplemental carbohydrate to restore the liver glycogen and prevent secondary hypoglycemia.
General Management of Hypoglycemia—The following are helpful measures in the prevention of hypoglycemic reactions due to insulin:
1. Reasonable uniformity from day to day with regard to diet, insulin, and exercise.
2. Careful adjustment of the insulin program so that the type (or types) of insulin, dose, and time (or times) of administration are suited to the individual patient.
3. Frequent testing of the urine so that a change in insulin requirements can be foreseen.
4. Routine carrying of sugar, candy, or other readily absorbable carbohydrate by the patient so that it may be taken at the first warning of an oncoming reaction.
If the patient is unaware of the symptoms of hypoglycemia, he may lapse into insulin shock; therefore, the physician should instruct the patient in this regard when feasible.
It is important that the patient be aroused as quickly as possible, for prolonged hypoglycemic reactions may result in cortical damage. Glucagon or intravenous glucose will awaken the patient sufficiently so that oral carbohydrates may be taken.
Instructions to the Family—Instructions describing the method of using this preparation are included in the literature which accompanies the patient's package. It is advisable for the patient to become familiar with the technique of preparing glucagon for injection before an emergency arises.
CAUTION—Although glucagon may be used for the treatment of hypoglycemia by the patient during an emergency, the physician must still be notified when hypoglycemic reactions occur so that the dose of insulin may be adjusted more accurately.
Insulin Shock Therapy—Dissolve the lyophilized glucagon in the accompanying solvent.
After one hour of coma, inject 0.5 to 1 unit of glucagon by the subcutaneous, intramuscular, or intravenous route. Larger doses may be employed if desired.
The patient will usually awaken in ten to 25 minutes. If no response occurs within the desired interval, the dose may be repeated. Upon awakening, the patient should be fed orally as soon as possible and the usual dietary regimen followed.
In a very deep state of coma, such as Stage IV or Stage V of Himwich, intravenous glucose should be given in addition to glucagon for a more immediate response. Glucagon and glucose may be used together without decreasing the efficacy of glucose administration.
How Supplied: (℞) *Ampoules (Vials) Glucagon for Injection, USP: No. 666,* 1 unit (1 mg), rubber-stoppered (Dry Powder), with 49 mg of lactose, in single packages (10 per carton). Vial No. 667, Diluting Solution for Glucagon for Injection, USP, 1 ml, included in this package, is not offered separately. It contains glycerin, 1.6 percent, with phenol, 0.2 percent, as a preservative. Sodium hydroxide and/or hydrochloric acid may have been added during manufacture to adjust the *p*H. *No. 668,* 10 units (10 mg), rubber-stoppered (Dry Powder), with 140 mg of lactose, in single packages (10 per carton). Vial No. 669, Diluting Solution for Glucagon for Injection, USP, 10 ml, included in this package, is not offered separately. It contains glycerin, 1.6 percent, with phenol, 0.2 percent, as a preservative. Sodium hydroxide and/or hydrochloric acid may have been added during manufacture to adjust the *p*H. If properly refrigerated, Ampoules (Vials) No. 668 may be used up to three months after reconstitution.
[051276A]

HALDRONE® ℞
(paramethasone acetate)
Tablets, NF

Description: Haldrone® (paramethasone acetate, Lilly) is a synthetic adrenocortical steroid which is readily absorbed from the gastrointestinal tract. It is a white crystalline compound that is soluble in alcohol and acetone and in water. Haldrone has anti-inflammatory activity, and within the usual dose range there is little effect on electrolyte metabolism. Haldrone compares favorably in its met-

Continued on next page

*Identi-Code® symbol.

Lilly—Cont.

abolic actions and side effects with other corticosteroids.

Actions: Naturally occurring glucocorticoids (hydrocortisone and cortisone), which have salt-retaining properties, are used as replacement therapy in adrenocortical deficiency states. Their synthetic analogs are used primarily for their potent anti-inflammatory effects in disorders of many organ systems.

Glucocorticoids cause profound and varied metabolic effects. In addition, they modify the body's immune responses to diverse stimuli.

Indications:

Endocrine Disorders

Primary or secondary adrenocortical insufficiency

(Hydrocortisone or cortisone is the first choice; synthetic analogs may be used in conjunction with mineralocorticoids when applicable; in infancy, mineralocorticoid supplementation is of particular importance.)

Congenital adrenal hyperplasia

Nonsuppurative thyroiditis

Hypercalcemia associated with cancer

Rheumatic Disorders

Psoriatic arthritis—Adjunctive therapy for short-term administration to tide the patient over an acute episode or exacerbation.

Rheumatoid arthritis, including juvenile rheumatoid arthritis—Selected cases may require low-dose maintenance therapy.

Ankylosing spondylitis

Bursitis—Use only in acute and subacute conditions. Not effective in chronic bursitis.

Acute nonspecific tenosynovitis

Acute gouty arthritis

Post-traumatic osteoarthritis

Synovitis of osteoarthritis

Epicondylitis

Collagen Diseases

During an exacerbation or as maintenance therapy in selected cases of the following:

Systemic lupus erythematosus

Acute rheumatic carditis

Dermatologic Diseases

Pemphigus

Bullous dermatitis herpetiformis

Severe erythema multiforme (Stevens-Johnson syndrome)

Exfoliative dermatitis

Mycosis fungoides

Severe psoriasis

Severe seborrheic dermatitis

Allergic States

Control of severe or incapacitating allergic conditions intractable to adequate trials of conventional treatment:

Seasonal or perennial allergic rhinitis

Bronchial asthma

Contact dermatitis

Atopic dermatitis

Serum sickness

Drug hypersensitivity reactions

Ophthalmic Diseases

Severe acute and chronic allergic and inflammatory processes involving the eye and its adnexa, such as:

Allergic conjunctivitis

Keratitis

Allergic corneal marginal ulcers

Herpes zoster ophthalmicus

Iritis and iridocyclitis

Chorioretinitis

Anterior segment inflammation

Diffuse posterior uveitis and choroiditis

Optic neuritis

Sympathetic ophthalmia

Respiratory Diseases

Symptomatic sarcoidosis

Loeffler's syndrome not manageable with other treatment

Pulmonary tuberculosis—Only in fulminating or disseminated disease in conjunction with appropriate and adequate antituberculosis chemotherapy

Berylliosis

Aspiration pneumonitis

Hematologic Disorders

Idiopathic thrombocytopenic purpura in adults

Secondary thrombocytopenia in adults

Acquired (autoimmune) hemolytic anemia

Erythroblastopenia (RBC anemia)

Congenital (erythroid) hypoplastic anemia

Neoplastic Diseases

For the palliative management of leukemias and lymphomas in adults and acute leukemia of childhood

Edematous States

To induce diuresis or a remission of proteinuria in nephrotic syndrome, without uremia, of the idiopathic type or that due to lupus erythematosus

Gastrointestinal Diseases

To tide the patient over a critical period of the disease in ulcerative colitis or regional enteritis

Miscellaneous

Tuberculous meningitis with subarachnoid block or impending block when the patient is receiving appropriate and adequate antituberculosis chemotherapy

Trichinosis with neurologic or myocardial involvement

Contraindications: Therapy with Haldrone® (paramethasone acetate, Lilly) is contraindicated in the presence of systemic fungal infections.

Warnings: In patients on corticosteroid therapy subjected to unusual stress, increased dosage of rapidly acting corticosteroids is indicated before, during, and after the stressful situation.

Corticosteroids may mask some signs of infection, and new infections may appear during their use. There may be decreased resistance and inability to localize infection when corticosteroids are administered.

Prolonged use of corticosteroids may produce posterior subcapsular cataracts, may cause glaucoma with possible damage to the optic nerves, and may increase the possibility of secondary ocular infections due to fungi or viruses.

Usage in Pregnancy—Since adequate human reproduction studies have not been made with corticosteroids, the use of these drugs in pregnancy, nursing mothers, or women of childbearing potential requires that the possible benefits of the drug be weighed against the potential hazards to the mother and embryo or fetus. Infants born of mothers who have received substantial doses of corticosteroids during pregnancy should be carefully observed for signs of hypoadrenalism.

Average and large doses of hydrocortisone or cortisone can cause elevation of blood pressure, salt and water retention, and increased excretion of potassium. These effects are less likely to occur with the synthetic derivatives except when large doses are employed. Dietary salt restriction and potassium supplementation may be necessary. All corticosteroids increase calcium excretion.

PATIENTS ON CORTICOSTEROID THERAPY SHOULD NOT BE VACCINATED AGAINST SMALLPOX. OTHER IMMUNIZATION PROCEDURES SHOULD NOT BE UNDERTAKEN IN PATIENTS WHO ARE RECEIVING CORTICOSTEROIDS, ESPECIALLY WHEN HIGH DOSES ARE BEING GIVEN, BECAUSE OF POSSIBLE HAZARDS OF NEUROLOGIC COMPLICATIONS AND A LACK OF ANTIBODY RESPONSE.

The use of Haldrone® (paramethasone acetate, Lilly) in active tuberculosis should be restricted to cases of fulminating or disseminated disease in which the corticosteroid is used in conjunction with an appropriate antituberculosis regimen.

If corticosteroids are indicated in patients with latent tuberculosis or tuberculin reactivity, close observation is necessary, since reactivation of the disease may occur. During prolonged corticosteroid therapy, such individuals should receive chemoprophylaxis.

Precautions: Drug-induced secondary adrenocortical insufficiency may be minimized by gradual reduction of dosage. This type of relative insufficiency may persist for months after discontinuation of therapy; therefore, in any situation of stress occurring during that period, hormone therapy should be reinstituted. Since mineralocorticoid secretion may be impaired, salt and/or a mineralocorticoid should be administered concurrently.

Corticosteroids have an enhanced effect on patients with hypothyroidism and those with cirrhosis.

Corticosteroids should be used cautiously in patients with ocular herpes simplex because of possible corneal perforation.

The lowest possible dose of corticosteroid should be employed to control the condition under treatment; and when the dose is reduced, it should be done gradually.

Psychic derangements, ranging from euphoria, insomnia, mood swings, personality changes, and severe depression to frank psychotic manifestations, may appear when corticosteroids are given. Also, existing emotional instability or psychotic tendencies may be aggravated by corticosteroids.

Aspirin should be used cautiously in conjunction with corticosteroids in hypoprothrombinemia.

Steroids should be administered with caution in nonspecific ulcerative colitis if there is a probability of impending perforation, abscess, or other pyogenic infection; diverticulitis; fresh intestinal anastomoses; active or latent peptic ulcer; renal insufficiency; hypertension; osteoporosis; and myasthenia gravis.

Growth and development of infants and children on prolonged corticosteroid therapy should be carefully observed.

Adverse Reactions:

Fluid and Electrolyte Disturbances

Sodium retention

Fluid retention

Congestive heart failure in susceptible patients

Potassium loss

Hypokalemic alkalosis

Hypertension

Musculoskeletal

Muscle weakness

Steroid myopathy

Loss of muscle mass

Osteoporosis

Vertebral compression fractures

Aseptic necrosis of femoral and humeral heads

Pathologic fracture of long bones

Gastrointestinal

Peptic ulcer with possible perforation and hemorrhage

Pancreatitis

Abdominal distention

Ulcerative esophagitis

Dermatologic

Impaired wound healing

Thin, fragile skin

Petechiae and ecchymoses

Facial erythema

Increased sweating

Suppression of reactions to skin tests

Neurologic

Convulsions

Increased intracranial pressure with papilledema (pseudotumor cerebri), usually after treatment

Vertigo

Headache

Endocrine

Menstrual irregularities

Development of Cushingoid state

Suppression of growth in children

Secondary adrenocortical and pituitary unresponsiveness, particularly in times of stress, as in trauma, surgery, or illness

Decreased carbohydrate tolerance
Manifestations of latent diabetes mellitus
Increased requirements for insulin or oral hypoglycemic agents in diabetics

Ophthalmic
Posterior subcapsular cataracts
Increased intraocular pressure
Glaucoma
Exophthalmos

Metabolic
Negative nitrogen balance due to protein catabolism

Administration and Dosage: The initial dosage of Haldrone® (paramethasone acetate, Lilly) may vary from 2 to 24 mg per day, depending on the disease entity being treated. In situations of less severity, lower doses will generally suffice, although higher initial quantities may be required in selected patients. The initial regimen should be maintained or adjusted until a satisfactory response is noted. If a satisfactory response does not occur after a reasonable period of time, Haldrone should be discontinued and other appropriate therapy begun. DOSAGE REQUIREMENTS ARE VARIABLE AND MUST BE INDIVIDUALIZED ACCORDING TO THE DISEASE BEING TREATED AND THE RESPONSE OF THE PATIENT.
After a favorable response, the initial dosage should be decreased by small amounts at appropriate intervals until the lowest effective maintenance dosage is reached. Constant monitoring of dosage is needed. Adjustments may be necessary on the basis of clinical changes secondary to remission or exacerbation of the disease, the patient's individual response to the drug, or the effect of stress other than that of the disease under treatment; in the last situation, it may be necessary to increase the dosage for a period of time. If the drug is to be stopped after long-term therapy, it should be withdrawn gradually rather than abruptly.

How Supplied: (℞) *Tablets Haldrone® (Paramethasone Acetate Tablets, NF)* (capsule-shaped, scored): *No. 1818, T99,** 1 mg, Yellow, in bottles of 100; *No. 1819, U01,** 2 mg, Orange, in bottles of 30 and 100. [081578]

HEPARIN SODIUM ℞
Injection, USP

WARNING—This is a potent drug, and serious consequences may result if used other than under constant medical supervision.

Description: Heparin Sodium Injection, USP, is derived from the intestinal mucosa of domestic mammals used for human consumption and is standardized for administration as an anticoagulant. Its potency is determined by a biological assay with a USP reference standard based on units of heparin activity per milligram.
Each vial contains 0.9 percent sodium chloride, with 0.9 percent benzyl alcohol as a preservative. Sodium hydroxide and/or hydrochloric acid may have been added during manufacture to adjust the *p*H.

Actions: Heparin sodium inhibits the clotting of blood and the formation of fibrin clots both in vitro and in vivo. In combination with a cofactor, it inactivates thrombin and thus prevents the conversion of fibrinogen to fibrin. Heparin sodium also prohibits the formation of a stable fibrin clot by delaying the activation of the fibrin stabilizing factor.
Heparin sodium inhibits reactions that lead to clotting but does not significantly alter normal components of the blood. Although clotting time is prolonged by therapeutic doses, bleeding time is usually unaffected. The drug does not have fibrinolytic activity; therefore, it will not lyse existing clots.

Indications: Heparin sodium is indicated for:
Anticoagulant therapy in prophylaxis of venous thrombosis and as treatment to prevent its extension
Low-dose regimen for prevention of postoperative deep venous thrombosis and pulmonary embolism in patients undergoing major abdominothoracic surgery who are at risk of developing thromboembolic disease (*see* Administration and Dosage)
Prophylaxis and treatment of pulmonary embolism
Atrial fibrillation with embolization
Diagnosis and treatment of acute and chronic consumption coagulopathies (disseminated intravascular coagulation)
Prevention of clotting in arterial and heart surgery
Prevention of cerebral thrombosis in evolving stroke
Heparin sodium may be used as an adjunct both in treating coronary occlusion with acute myocardial infarction and in the prophylaxis and treatment of peripheral arterial embolism.
Heparin sodium may also be employed as an anticoagulant in blood transfusions, extracorporeal circulation, and dialysis procedures and in blood samples for laboratory purposes.

Contraindications: Heparin sodium is contraindicated in patients known to be sensitive to the drug.
It is also contraindicated when suitable blood coagulation tests—e.g., the Lee-White whole-blood clotting time, activated partial thromboplastin time (APTT), etc.—cannot be performed at the required intervals.
The drug is contraindicated during any uncontrollable active bleeding state (*see* Warnings).

Warnings:

Heparin sodium should be used with extreme caution in disease states in which there is increased danger of hemorrhage.

When heparin sodium is administered in therapeutic amounts, its dosage should be regulated by frequent blood coagulation tests. If the coagulation test is unduly prolonged or if hemorrhage occurs, heparin sodium should be discontinued promptly (*see* Overdosage).
Some of the conditions in which increased danger of hemorrhage exists are as follows:
Cardiovascular—Subacute bacterial endocarditis; arterial sclerosis; increased capillary permeability; major surgery (during and immediately following), especially of the brain, spinal cord, and, except in low doses, the eye; suspected intracranial hemorrhage; shock; and severe hypertension.
Hematologic—Conditions in which there are increased bleeding tendencies, such as hemophilia, purpuras, jaundice, thrombocytopenia (the exception is bleeding states associated with disseminated intravascular coagulation), postoperative oozing of blood, etc. Prior to therapy with heparin sodium, it is desirable to determine whether the platelet count is adequate.
Gastrointestinal—Inaccessible ulcerative lesions (especially of the gastrointestinal tract) and continuous tube drainage of the stomach or small intestine.
Obstetric—Threatened abortion (unless clearly complicated by disseminated intravascular coagulation).
Heparin sodium may prolong the one-stage prothrombin time. Therefore, when heparin sodium is given with dicumarol or sodium warfarin, a period of at least five hours after the last intravenous dose or 24 hours after the last subcutaneous (intrafat, i.e., above the iliac crest or abdominal fat layer) dose should elapse before blood is drawn if a valid prothrombin time is to be obtained.
Drugs (such as acetylsalicylic acid) that interfere with platelet-aggregation reactions (the main hemostatic defense of heparinized patients) may induce bleeding and should be used with caution in patients receiving heparin sodium.
Although there is experimental evidence that heparin sodium may antagonize the action of ACTH, insulin, or corticoids, this effect has not been clearly defined.
There is also evidence in experimental animals that heparin sodium may modify or inhibit allergic reactions. However, the application of these findings to human patients has not been fully defined.
It may be necessary to increase doses of heparin sodium in the febrile state.
Digitalis, tetracyclines, nicotine, or antihistamines may partially counteract the anticoagulant action of heparin sodium. An increased resistance to the drug is frequently encountered in thrombosis, thrombophlebitis, infections with thrombosing tendencies, myocardial infarction, cancer, and postsurgical patients.
Usage in Pregnancy—Reproduction studies have not been performed in animals. There is inadequate information on whether this drug may affect fertility in human males or females or have a teratogenic potential or other adverse effect on the fetus.

Precautions: Because heparin sodium is derived from animal tissue, it should be used with caution in any patient with a history of allergy. Before a therapeutic dose is given to such a patient, a trial dose of 1000 units may be advisable.
Heparin sodium should be used with caution during pregnancy, especially during the last trimester (even though it does not cross the placental barrier) and in the immediate postpartum period. It should also be used cautiously in the presence of mild hepatic or renal disease, in hypertension, during menstruation, or in patients with indwelling catheters. A higher incidence of bleeding may be seen in women over 60 years of age.

Adverse Reactions: Hemorrhage is the chief complication that may develop as a result of heparin sodium administration. An overly prolonged clotting time or minor bleeding during therapy can usually be controlled by withdrawing the drug (*see* Overdosage).
When administered intramuscularly, heparin sodium may produce local irritation, mild pain, or hematoma at the injection site. These effects are seen less frequently after deep subcutaneous (intrafat) administration. Histamine-like reactions have also been observed at the site of injection.
Hypersensitivity reactions have been reported. The most usual manifestations are chills, fever, and urticaria. However, asthma, rhinitis, lacrimation, and anaphylactoid reactions have also been observed.
Acute reversible thrombocytopenia has occurred following intravenously administered heparin sodium.
Osteoporosis and suppression of renal function after long-term administration of high doses, aldosterone suppression, delayed transient alopecia, priapism, and rebound hyperlipemia upon discontinuation of heparin sodium have also been reported.

Administration and Dosage: Heparin sodium is not effective by oral administration and should be given by intermittent intravenous injection, intravenous infusion, or deep subcutaneous (intrafat) injection. The intramuscular route of administration should be avoided because of the frequent occurrence of hematoma at the injection site.
The dosage of heparin sodium should be adjusted according to the patient's coagulation test results, which, during the first day of treatment, should be determined just prior to each injection. (There is usually no need to monitor the effect of low-dose heparin in patients with normal coagulation parameters.) Dosage is considered adequate when the whole-blood

Continued on next page

*Identi-Code® symbol.

Lilly—Cont.

clotting time is elevated approximately two and one-half to three times the control value. When heparin sodium is given by continuous intravenous infusion, the coagulation time should be determined approximately every four hours in the early stages of treatment.
When the drug is administered intermittently by intravenous or deep subcutaneous (intrafat) injection, coagulation tests should be performed before each injection during the early stages of treatment and daily thereafter.
When an oral anticoagulant of the coumadin or similar type is administered with heparin sodium, coagulation tests and prothrombin activity should be determined at the start of therapy. For an immediate anticoagulant effect, give heparin sodium in the usual therapeutic dosage. When the results of the initial prothrombin tests are known, administer the first dose of an oral anticoagulant in the usual initial amount. Thereafter, determine the clotting time and the prothrombin time at appropriate intervals. A period of at least five hours after the last intravenous dose or 24 hours after the last subcutaneous (intrafat) dose of heparin sodium should elapse before blood is drawn if a valid prothrombin time is to be obtained. When the oral anticoagulant shows its full effect and prothrombin activity is in the desired therapeutic range, heparin sodium may be discontinued and therapy continued with the oral anticoagulant.
Although dosage must be adjusted for the individual patient on the basis of suitable laboratory tests, the following guidelines may be used to achieve a therapeutic anticoagulant effect with full-dose heparin:
1. *Deep Subcutaneous (Intrafat) Injection*—After an initial intravenous injection of 5000 units, inject 10,000 to 20,000 units of a concentrated heparin sodium solution subcutaneously; then, 8000 to 10,000 units every eight hours or 15,000 to 20,000 units every 12 hours. A different site should be used for each injection to prevent the development of a massive hematoma.
2. *Intermittent Intravenous Injection*—Initially, 10,000 units; then, 5000 to 10,000 units every four to six hours. These amounts may be given undiluted or diluted with 50 to 100 ml of isotonic Sodium Chloride Injection.
3. *Continuous Intravenous Infusion*—After an initial intravenous injection of 5000 units, add 20,000 to 40,000 units of heparin sodium to 1000 ml of isotonic Sodium Chloride Solution for infusion. For most patients, the rate of flow should be adjusted to deliver approximately 20,000 to 40,000 units in 24 hours.
[See table below].
Surgery of the Heart and Blood Vessels—Patients undergoing total body perfusion for open-heart surgery should receive an initial dose of not less than 150 units of heparin sodium per kg of body weight. Frequently, a dose of 300 units per kg is used for procedures estimated to last less than 60 minutes or 400 units per kg for those estimated to last longer than 60 minutes. Prior to administration, heparin sodium should be added to the fluids in the pump oxygenator to prevent the patient's blood from clotting in the tube system.
Low-Dose Prophylaxis of Postoperative Thromboembolism—A number of well-controlled clinical trials have demonstrated that low-dose heparin prophylaxis, given just prior to and after surgery, will reduce the incidence of postoperative deep vein thrombosis in the legs (as measured by the I-125 fibrinogen technique and venography) and of clinical pulmonary embolism. The most widely used dosage has been 5000 units two hours before surgery and 5000 units every eight to 12 hours thereafter for seven days or until the patient is fully ambulatory, whichever is longer. The heparin is given by deep subcutaneous (intrafat) injection in the arm or abdomen with a fine (25 to 26-gauge) needle to minimize tissue trauma. A concentrated solution of heparin sodium is recommended. Such prophylaxis should be reserved for patients over the age of 40 who are undergoing major surgery. Patients with bleeding disorders and those having neurosurgery, spinal anesthesia, eye surgery, or potentially sanguineous operations should be excluded, as should patients receiving oral anticoagulants or platelet-active drugs (*see* Warnings). The value of such prophylaxis in hip surgery has not been established. The possibility of increased bleeding during surgery or postoperatively should be borne in mind. If such bleeding occurs, discontinuance of heparin and neutralization with protamine sulfate are advisable. If clinical evidence of thromboembolism develops despite low-dose prophylaxis, full therapeutic doses of anticoagulants should be given unless contraindicated. All patients should be screened prior to heparinization to rule out bleeding disorders, and monitoring with appropriate coagulation tests should be performed just prior to surgery. Coagulation test values should be normal or only slightly elevated. There is usually no need for daily monitoring of the effect of low-dose heparin in patients with normal coagulation parameters.
Extracorporeal Dialysis—Follow equipment manufacturers' operating directions carefully.
Laboratory Samples—Seventy to 150 units of heparin sodium are usually added to 10 to 20 ml of whole blood to prevent coagulation of the sample.
Overdosage: Protamine sulfate (1 percent solution) given by *slow infusion* will neutralize heparin sodium. *No more than 50 mg* should be administered, *very slowly*, in any ten-minute period. Each mg of protamine sulfate neutralizes approximately 100 USP heparin units (or injection of 1 to 1.5 mg neutralizes approximately 1 mg of heparin sodium).
Because heparin sodium disappears rapidly from the circulation, the dose of protamine sulfate required also decreases rapidly as time elapses following intravenous injection. Thirty minutes after a dose of heparin sodium, approximately 0.5 mg of protamine is sufficient to neutralize each 100 units of administered heparin.
In some cases, blood or plasma transfusions may be necessary; these dilute but do not neutralize heparin sodium.
How Supplied: (℞) *Ampoules (Vials) Heparin Sodium Injection, USP: No. 405 (for I.V. use and for addition to blood in the indirect method of transfusion),* 1000 USP units per ml, 10 ml; *No. 520 (for I.V. or deep subcutaneous [intrafat] use),* 10,000 USP units per ml, 5 ml; *No. 622 (for I.V. or deep subcutaneous [intrafat] use),* 20,000 USP units per ml, 1 ml; and *No. 642 (for I.V. or deep subcutaneous [intrafat] use),* 20,000 USP units per ml, 2 ml, rubber-stoppered, in singles (10 per carton).
[102677]

Method of Administration	Frequency	Recommended Dose*
Subcutaneous Injection	Initial dose Every 8 hours or Every 12 hours	10,000-20,000 units† 8000-10,000 units 15,000-20,000 units
Intermittent Intravenous Injection	Initial dose Every 4 to 6 hours	10,000 units 5000-10,000 units
Intravenous Infusion	Continuous	20,000-40,000 units/day in 1000 ml of solution†

*Based on 150-lb (68-kg) patient.
†Immediately preceded by an initial dose of 5000 units intravenously.

HEXA-BETALIN® ℞
(pyridoxine hydrochloride) Injection, USP

Description: Hexa-Betalin® (pyridoxine hydrochloride, Lilly) Injection is a sterile solution of pyridoxine hydrochloride in Water for Injection with a *p*H between 2 and 3.8.
Each vial is preserved with chlorobutanol (chloroform derivative), 0.5 percent. Sodium hydroxide and/or hydrochloric acid may have been added during manufacture to adjust the *p*H.
Pyridoxine hydrochloride is a colorless or white crystal or a white crystalline powder. One gm dissolves in 5 ml of water. It is stable in air and is slowly affected by sunlight.
Its chemical name is 2-methyl-3-hydroxy-4,5-bis(hydroxymethyl) pyridine hydrochloride.
Actions: Natural substances that have vitamin B_6 activity are pyridoxine in plants and pyridoxal or pyridoxamine in animals. All three are converted to pyridoxal phosphate by the enzyme pyridoxal kinase. The physiologically active forms of vitamin B_6 are pyridoxal phosphate (codecarboxylase) and pyridoxamine phosphate. Riboflavin is required for the conversion of pyridoxine phosphate to pyridoxal phosphate.
Vitamin B_6 acts as a coenzyme in the metabolism of protein, carbohydrate, and fat. In protein metabolism, it participates in the decarboxylation of amino acids, conversion of tryptophan to niacin or to serotonin (5-hydroxytryptamine), deamination, and transamination and transulfuration of amino acids. In carbohydrate metabolism, it is responsible for the breakdown of glycogen to glucose-1-phosphate.
The total adult body pool consists of 16 to 25 mg of pyridoxine. Its half-life appears to be 15 to 20 days. Vitamin B_6 is degraded to 4-pyridoxic acid in the liver. This metabolite is excreted in the urine.
The need for pyridoxine increases with the amount of protein in the diet. The tryptophan load test appears to uncover early vitamin B_6 deficiency by detecting xanthinuria. The average adult minimum daily requirement is about 1.25 mg. The "Recommended Dietary Allowance" of the National Academy of Sciences is estimated to be as much as 2 mg for adults and 2.5 mg for pregnant and lactating women. The requirements are more in persons having certain genetic defects or those being treated with isonicotinic acid hydrazide (INH) or oral contraceptives.
Indications: Pyridoxine hydrochloride injection is effective for the treatment of pyridoxine deficiency as seen in the following:
Inadequate dietary intake
Drug-induced deficiency, as from isoniazid (INH) or oral contraceptives
Inborn errors of metabolism, e.g., vitamin-B_6-dependent convulsions or vitamin-B_6-responsive anemia
The parenteral route is indicated when oral administration is not feasible, as in anorexia, nausea and vomiting, and preoperative and

postoperative conditions. It is also indicated when gastrointestinal absorption is impaired.
Contraindication: A history of sensitivity to pyridoxine or to any of the ingredients in Hexa-Betalin® (pyridoxine hydrochloride, Lilly) is a contraindication.
Warning: This product should be protected from exposure to light.
Precautions: Single deficiency, as of pyridoxine alone, is rare. Multiple vitamin deficiency is to be expected in any inadequate diet. Patients treated with levodopa should avoid supplemental vitamins that contain more than 5 mg pyridoxine in the daily dose.
Women taking oral contraceptives may exhibit increased pyridoxine requirements.
Adverse Reactions: Paresthesia, somnolence, and low serum folic acid levels have been reported.
Administration and Dosage: In cases of dietary deficiency, the dosage is 10 to 20 mg daily for three weeks. Follow-up treatment is recommended daily for several weeks with an oral therapeutic multivitamin preparation containing 2 to 5 mg pyridoxine. Poor dietary habits should be corrected, and an adequate, well-balanced diet should be prescribed.
The vitamin-B_6-dependency syndrome may require a therapeutic dosage of as much as 600 mg a day and a daily intake of 30 mg for life.
In deficiencies due to INH, the dosage is 100 mg daily for three weeks followed by a 30-mg maintenance dose daily.
In poisoning caused by ingestion of more than 10 gm of INH, an equal amount of pyridoxine should be given—4 gm intravenously followed by 1 gm intramuscularly every 30 minutes.
Overdosage: Pyridoxine given to animals in amounts of 3 to 4 gm per kg of body weight produces convulsions and death. In man, a dose of 25 mg per kg of body weight is well tolerated.
How Supplied: (℞) *Ampoules (Vials) No. 479, Hexa-Betalin® (Pyridoxine Hydrochloride Injection, USP),* 100 mg per ml, 10 ml, rubber-stoppered, in singles (10 per carton).
Also Available:
*Tablets Hexa-Betalin® (Pyridoxine Hydrochloride Tablets, USP): No. 1691, J56,** 10 mg, *No. 1632, J45,** 25 mg, and *No. 1728, T72,** 50 mg, in bottles of 100.

[041879]

HISTA-CLOPANE® ℞
(chlorpheniramine and cyclopentamine)

Description: Each Pulvule® contains—
Histadyl® (chlorpheniramine maleate, Lilly) .... 4 mg
Clopane® Hydrochloride (cyclopentamine hydrochloride, Lilly) .... 12.5 mg
Histadyl is freely soluble in water, soluble in alcohol and chloroform, and slightly soluble in ether and benzene. Solutions have a *p*H of about 4 and 5.
Clopane Hydrochloride, a sympathomimetic, is the hydrochloride of 1-cyclopentyl-2-methylaminopropane. It is freely soluble in water and in alcohol. In a 1:100 solution, it has a *p*H of 6. Clopane is a white crystalline powder with a characteristic odor and a bitter taste.
Actions: Histadyl® (chlorpheniramine maleate, Lilly) is an antihistamine. Side effects of antihistamines include sedation and some anticholinergic (drying) effects.
Clopane® Hydrochloride (cyclopentamine hydrochloride, Lilly) is an ephedrine-like sympathomimetic drug that is effective orally. Such drugs may cause nervousness and insomnia.

INDICATIONS
On the basis of a review of this drug by the National Academy of Sciences—National Research Council and/or other information, FDA has classified the following indications as "possibly" effective: perennial and seasonal allergic rhinitis, vasomotor rhinitis, allergic conjunctivitis due to inhalant allergens and foods, mild, uncomplicated allergic skin manifestations of urticaria and angioedema, amelioration of allergic reactions to blood or plasma, dermatographism, and as therapy for anaphylactic reactions *adjunctive* to epinephrine and other standard measures after the acute manifestations have been controlled.
Final classification of these less-than-effective indications requires further investigation.

Contraindications: *In Nursing Mothers*—Since antihistamines and sympathomimetic amines are hazardous for all infants, especially newborns and prematures, Hista-Clopane is contraindicated in nursing mothers.
Use in Children under 12—Until its safety has been established in children, it is recommended that the combination of chlorpheniramine maleate and cyclopentamine hydrochloride not be used in children under 12 years of age.
In Lower Respiratory Disease—Antihistamines *should not* be used to treat lower respiratory tract symptoms, including asthma.
Use in Hypersensitivity or Idiosyncrasy—Hista-Clopane should not be used in patients with *hypersensitivity or idiosyncrasy to Histadyl® (chlorpheniramine maleate, Lilly),* to Clopane® Hydrochloride (cyclopentamine hydrochloride, Lilly), or to other antihistamines and sympathomimetic drugs of similar chemical structure.
Hista-Clopane should not be used concomitantly with C.N.S. stimulants. It is contraindicated in patients receiving monoamine oxidase (MAO) inhibitors (*see* Drug Interactions).
Warnings: Antihistamines should be used with considerable caution in patients with:
- Narrow-angle glaucoma
- Stenosing peptic ulcer
- Pyloroduodenal obstruction
- Symptomatic prostatic hypertrophy
- Bladder neck obstruction

Use in Children—Antihistamines in *overdosage* may cause hallucinations, convulsions, or death, especially in infants and children.
As in adults, antihistamines may diminish mental alertness in children. They may produce excitation, particularly in the young child.
Use in Pregnancy—Adequate reproduction studies with this antihistamine and with sympathomimetic amines have not been performed in animals. There is insufficient information as to whether these drugs may reduce fertility or have teratogenic or other adverse effects in the fetus.
Use with C.N.S. Depressants—Histadyl has additive effects with alcohol and other C.N.S. depressants (hypnotics, sedatives, tranquilizers, etc.)
Use When Activities Require Mental Alertness—Patients should be warned about engaging in activities requiring mental alertness, such as driving a car or operating appliances, machinery, etc.
Use in the Elderly (Approximately 60 Years or Older)—Antihistamines are more likely to cause dizziness, sedation, and hypotension in elderly patients.
Precautions: Histadyl® (chlorpheniramine maleate, Lilly) has an atropine-like action and, therefore, should be used with caution in patients with:
- History of bronchial asthma
- Increased intraocular pressure
- Hyperthyroidism
- Cardiovascular disease
- Hypertension

Sympathomimetic drugs such as cyclopentamine hydrochloride should be used with caution in patients with cardiovascular disease, especially ischemic heart disease, hyperthyroidism, diabetes, hypertension, and glaucoma. In the presence of prostatism, the administration of sympathomimetic drugs may cause urinary retention.
Adverse Reactions: The most frequent adverse reactions to antihistamines are italicized:
General—Urticaria, drug rash, anaphylactic shock, photosensitivity, excessive perspiration, chills, dryness of mouth, nose, and throat.
Cardiovascular System—Hypotension, headache, palpitations, tachycardia, extrasystoles.
Hematologic System—Hemolytic anemia, thrombocytopenia, agranulocytosis.
Nervous System—Sedation, sleepiness, dizziness, disturbed coordination, fatigue, confusion, restlessness, excitation, nervousness, tremor, irritability, insomnia, euphoria, paresthesias, blurred vision, diplopia, vertigo, tinnitus, acute labyrinthitis, hysteria, neuritis, convulsions.
Gastrointestinal System—Epigastric distress, anorexia, nausea, vomiting, diarrhea, constipation.
Genitourinary System—Urinary frequency, difficult urination, urinary retention, early menses.
Respiratory System—Thickening of bronchial secretions, tightness of chest and wheezing, nasal stuffiness.
The most frequent adverse reactions to sympathomimetics are:
Nervous System—Nervousness and insomnia. Clopane® Hydrochloride (cyclopentamine hydrochloride, Lilly) causes less central-nervous-system stimulation than other sympathomimetic drugs commonly employed. The sedating side effect of Histadyl® (chlorpheniramine maleate, Lilly) and the excitation side effect of Clopane Hydrochloride *may* be counteracted by their combined administration (there is a great deal of individual variation in this regard).
Cardiovascular System—Increased heart rate and blood pressure.
Administration and Dosage: Dosage of Hista-Clopane should be adjusted according to the needs and response of the patient.
Adults—The usual dosage is 1 or 2 Pulvules four or five times daily. The recommended maximum dosage is 2 Pulvules five times a day.
Children—Until its safety has been established in children, it is recommended that the combination of chlorpheniramine maleate and cyclopentamine hydrochloride not be used in children under 12 years of age.
The maximum dosage should not be exceeded. Side effects will increase with larger doses, but there will be no greater clinical efficacy.
Drug Interactions: MAO inhibitors prolong and intensify the anticholinergic (drying) effects of antihistamines. Sympathomimetic amines may interact with MAO inhibitors or tricyclic antidepressants to cause hypertension or hypertensive crises. Sympathomimetic amines may interact with digitalis and other cardiac glycosides to increase the tendency to cardiac arrhythmias; they may also interact with cyclopropane or halogenated hydrocarbon anesthetics to cause cardiac arrhythmias. Certain antihypertensive drugs, such as methyldopa and reserpine, may have a reduced effect if sympathomimetic amines are administered concurrently.
Management of Overdosage: Antihistamine overdosage reactions may range from central-nervous-system depression to stimulation. Stimulation is particularly likely in children. Atropine-like signs and symptoms—dry mouth; fixed, dilated pupils; flushing—and gastrointestinal symptoms may also occur.

Continued on next page

*Identi-Code® symbol.

Lilly—Cont.

If vomiting has not occurred spontaneously, the patient should be induced to vomit. This is best done by having him drink a glass of water or milk, after which he should be made to gag. Precautions against aspiration must be taken, especially in infants and children.
If vomiting is unsuccessful, gastric lavage is indicated within three hours after ingestion and even later if large amounts of milk or cream were given beforehand. Isotonic or one-half isotonic saline is the lavage solution of choice.
Saline cathartics, such as milk of magnesia, draw water into the bowel by osmosis, and, therefore, are valuable for their action in rapid dilution of bowel contents.
Stimulants should *not* be used.
Vasopressors may be used to treat hypotension.
Information concerning overdosage with Clopane® Hydrochloride (cyclopentamine hydrochloride, Lilly) is limited. Treatment should include that which is appropriate for sympathomimetic drugs. Gastric lavage and avoidance of external stimuli are included. For extreme cases, hypothermic measures (when indicated) as well as peritoneal dialysis may be considered.
How Supplied: (℞) *Pulvules No. 3074, Hista-Clopane® (chlorpheniramine and cyclopentamine, Lilly)*(No. 4, Pink Body, Red Cap), in bottles of 100. [062579]

HISTADYL® E. C. Ⓒ
(chlorpheniramine compound E. C.)

Description: Contains in 30 ml—
Codeine Phosphate ....60 mg (1 gr)
WARNING—May be habit-forming.
Ephedrine Hydrochloride ....30 mg
Chlorpheniramine Maleate ....12 mg
Ammonium Chloride ....660 mg
Menthol ....3.9 mg
Alcohol, 5 percent.
Indications: For the treatment of coughs and colds, especially those of an allergic nature.
Dosage: *Adults*—1 teaspoonful every three hours as needed.
Children Six to 12 Years of Age—½ teaspoonful every three hours as needed. *Children under Six Years of Age*—Only as directed by the physician.
Overdosage: *Symptoms*—Nausea, vomiting, excitement, and signs and symptoms of C.N.S. stimulation ranging in degree from skeletal-muscle fasciculations to true convulsions. These may be followed by coma.
Treatment—No specific antidote. General management consists in symptomatic and supportive therapy. Sedatives such as the short-acting barbiturates may be used judiciously to control C.N.S. stimulation. Treatment may include gastric lavage, oxygen, and intravenous fluids if indicated.
How Supplied: (Ⓒ) *Syrup No. 5125, Histady® E. C. (chlorpheniramine compound E. C., Lilly),* in 4-fl-oz, 16-fl-oz, and gallon bottles. [062179]

ILETIN® (INSULIN, LILLY)— REGULAR AND MODIFIED INSULIN PRODUCTS

All of the insulins listed below are prepared from a mixture of insulin crystals extracted from beef and pork pancreas, except for Regular (Concentrated) Iletin® (insulin injection, Lilly), U-500, which is prepared from pork insulin only. Regular Iletin® (insulin injection, Lilly), Lente® Iletin® (insulin zinc suspension, Lilly), NPH Iletin® (isophane insulin suspension, Lilly), and Protamine, Zinc & Iletin® (protamine zinc insulin suspension, Lilly) made solely from beef or pork source are available on special order in U-100 strength only. When insulin is prepared from a single animal source, the species is indicated on the vial label and on the package.

REGULAR ILETIN®
(insulin injection)
USP

Description: Regular Iletin is an aqueous solution made from the antidiabetic principle of beef pancreas or pork pancreas or both as stated on the label. All Iletin® (insulin, Lilly) is made from zinc-insulin crystals. The potency and stability of each lot of Iletin are carefully determined by approved methods, and the product conforms to established standards. Insulin remains substantially stable if stored in a cold place, preferably a refrigerator.
Insulin, in appropriate doses, enables the diabetic to utilize carbohydrates and fats in a comparatively satisfactory manner; the concentration of sugar in the blood is confined within normal limits; the urine becomes free of sugar and ketone bodies; and diabetic acidosis and coma are prevented. In general, the presence of sugar in the urine is a manifestation of unsuitable insulin dosage or dietary imbalance. Only by frequent estimations of the sugar in the urine or in the blood can a satisfactory adjustment of insulin dosage be made.
Each cubic centimeter (cc) contains approximately 1.6 percent glycerin (w/v) and approximately 0.2 percent phenol (w/v) as a preservative.
Precautions: *Insulin should be used only under the direction of a physician. Each patient requires individual study.*
Diet—It is important that the patient carefully follow a course of diet as prescribed by the physician.
Insulin is usually best administered 15 to 30 minutes before a meal. The time, number, and amount of individual daily doses and the distribution of food among the several meals of the day must be determined by the physician. No change in this regimen should be made unless prescribed by the physician.
Hypoglycemia—The administration of an excessive dose of insulin causes hypoglycemia. This condition may also occur following increased work or exercise; when food is not being absorbed in the usual manner—because of postponement or omission of a meal or in illness with vomiting, diarrhea, or delayed digestion; when insulin is administered too long before a meal; when the patient's requirement of insulin declines; or when large doses of insulin are given at insufficient or irregular intervals. If it becomes necessary to omit a meal because of nausea or vomiting, the physician should be notified, and the urine should be tested every three or four hours.
An early symptom of hypoglycemia may be merely a feeling of fatigue. *Hence it is of utmost importance for the patient to understand clearly that the presence of vague symptoms of fatigue, headache, drowsiness, lassitude, tremulousness, or nausea demands immediate attention.* More marked symptoms of hypoglycemic reactions, such as weakness, sweating, tremor, or nervousness, may also develop, but these are more easily recognized. The occurrence of such symptoms calls for prompt and, if necessary, repeated administration of some form of carbohydrate. (Candy or a lump of sugar is convenient for this purpose and should always be carried by the patient.) If the patient becomes delirious or mentally confused, dilute corn syrup or orange juice with sugar should be administered by mouth. In severe hypoglycemic reactions, it may be desirable for a physician to administer intravenously from 10 to 20 gm of dextrose (D-glucose) in sterile solution. *If symptoms of hypoglycemia occur, the physician should be notified promptly.*

Administration: Regular insulin should not be confused with modified insulins, such as protamine zinc insulin, NPH insulin, or Lente® insulin; and none of these preparations should be used except by direction of a physician.
The patient should be carefully instructed in the administration of insulin and should be cautioned to become familiar with the information in the package insert.
Use of a package of insulin should not be commenced after the expiration date stamped upon it.
IMPORTANT—USE THE CORRECT SYRINGE, NEEDLE
Doses of insulin are measured in UNITS. The number of units in each cc is clearly stated on the package. Three strengths are available for each type of insulin—U-40 (40 units per cc), U-80 (80 units per cc), and U-100 (100 units per cc). For this reason, always use a syringe that correlates with the strength of insulin to be administered. Failure to use the proper syringe can result in an improper dose, with effects ranging from mild abnormalities of the blood glucose to coma or, rarely, death.
Each strength of insulin is identified by the color of the "flip-off" cap. Red identifies U-40; green, U-80; and orange, U-100.
Dosage: The number and size of daily doses and the time of administration, as well as diet and exercise, are problems that require direct and continuous medical supervision. Usually, the most satisfactory time for injection of Iletin is 15 to 30 minutes before a meal.
Important Notes: In general, the presence of sugar in the urine means unsuitable dosage of insulin or dietary imbalance.
Insulin should be stored in a cold place, preferably a refrigerator. Iletin that is not water-clear should not be injected. Discoloration, turbidity, or unusual viscosity indicates deterioration or contamination.
An extra vial of insulin and a spare syringe and needle should always be kept on hand. If a shortage of insulin appears to be inevitable, a temporary reduction of doses may be made, accompanied by limitation of food to two-thirds of its usual quantity and a liberal increase in fluids of little or no food value, such as water, tea, coffee, broths, or clear soups.
If the patient becomes ill from any cause, he should notify the physician at once and drink liberally of water or tea. If delay is experienced in obtaining the advice of a physician, the administration of insulin should be governed by the results of periodic determination of urinary sugar.
How Supplied: *Regular Iletin ® (Insulin Injection, USP)* is supplied in rubber-stoppered vials as follows:
M-240, U-40, forty units per cc, 10 cc (400 units).
M-280, U-80, eighty units per cc, 10 cc (800 units).
M-210, U-100, one hundred units per cc, 10 cc (1000 units).
The above products are supplied 10 per carton.
Refrigerate. Avoid freezing. [060178]
[*Shown in Product Identification Section*]
M-210—6505-00-584-3470

REGULAR (CONCENTRATED) ℞ ILETIN®, U-500
(insulin injection)
USP

WARNING: *Prepared from pork insulin only. The dose of pork insulin for patients with insulin resistance due to antibodies to beef insulin may be only a fraction of that of beef insulin. This insulin preparation contains 500 units of insulin in each milliliter. Extreme caution must be observed in the measurement of dosage because inadvertent overdose may result in irreversible insulin shock. Serious consequences may* *result if it is used other than under constant medical supervision.*

Description: Regular (Concentrated) Iletin® (insulin injection, Lilly), U-500, is an aqueous solution made from the antidiabetic principle of pork pancreas as stated on the label. Each milliliter contains 500 units of regular (unmodified) insulin and approximately 1.6 percent glycerin (w/v), with approximately 0.2 percent phenol (w/v) as a preservative. Sodium hydroxide and hydrochloric acid are added during manufacture to adjust the pH. All preparations of Iletin® (insulin, Lilly) are made from zinc-insulin crystals.

Adequate insulin dosage permits the diabetic patient to utilize carbohydrates and fats in a comparatively satisfactory manner. Regardless of concentration, the action of insulin is basically the same: to enable carbohydrate metabolism to occur and thus to prevent the production of ketone bodies by the liver. Although, under usual circumstances, diabetes can be controlled with doses in the vicinity of 40 to 60 units or less, an occasional patient develops such resistance or becomes so unresponsive to the effect of insulin that daily doses of several hundred, or even several thousand, units are required. Fortunately, there seems to be no condition of absolute resistance; all resistant patients will apparently respond to some dose, if it is large enough.

Occasionally, a cause of the insulin resistance can be found (such as hemochromatosis, cirrhosis of the liver, some complicating disease of the endocrine glands other than the pancreas, allergy, or infection), but in other cases no cause of the high insulin requirement can be determined.

Iletin, U-500, is unmodified by any agent that might prolong its action; however, clinical experience has shown that it frequently has a time action similar to a repository insulin preparation and that a single dose may show activity over a 24-hour period. This effect has been credited to the high concentration of the preparation.

Indications: Iletin® (insulin, Lilly), U-500, is especially useful for the treatment of diabetic patients with marked insulin resistance (daily requirements more than 200 units), since a large dose may be administered subcutaneously in a reasonable volume.

Precautions: Every patient exhibiting insulin resistance who requires Iletin® (insulin, Lilly), U-500, for the control of diabetes should be held under close observation until dosage is established. The response will vary among patients. Some can be controlled with a single dose daily; others may require two or three injections per day. Most patients will show a "tolerance" to insulin, so that minor variations in dosage can occur without the development of untoward symptoms of insulin shock.

Insulin resistance is frequently self-limited; after several weeks or months during which high dosage is required, responsiveness to the pharmacologic effect of insulin may be regained and dosage can be reduced.

Insulin should be kept in a cold place, preferably in a refrigerator. Do not inject insulin that is not water-clear. Discoloration, turbidity, or unusual viscosity indicates deterioration or contamination.

Use of a package of insulin should not be started after the expiration date stamped upon it.

Adverse Reactions: As with other insulin preparations, hypoglycemic reactions may be associated with the administration of Iletin® (insulin, Lilly), U-500. However, deep secondary hypoglycemic reactions may develop 18 to 24 hours after the original injection of Iletin, U-500. Consequently, patients should be carefully observed, and prompt treatment of such reactions should be initiated with glucagon injections and/or with glucose by intravenous injection or gavage.

Administration and Dosage: Iletin® (insulin, Lilly), U-500, can be administered by both the subcutaneous and the intramuscular routes. It is inadvisable to inject Iletin, U-500, intravenously because of the possible development of allergic or anaphylactoid reactions.

It is recommended that a tuberculin type of syringe be utilized for the measurement of dosage. Variations in dosage are frequently possible in the insulin-resistant patient, since the individual is unresponsive to the pharmacologic effect of the insulin. Nevertheless, accuracy of measurement is to be encouraged because of the potential danger of the preparation.

How Supplied: (℞) *M-2500, Regular (Concentrated) Iletin® (Insulin Injection, USP), U-500,* five hundred units per cc, 20 cc, rubber-stoppered vials (10,000 units) (10 per carton). *Refrigerate. Avoid freezing.* [042076]

LENTE® ILETIN®
(insulin zinc suspension)
USP

SEMILENTE® ILETIN®
(prompt insulin zinc suspension)
USP

ULTRALENTE® ILETIN®
(extended insulin zinc suspension)
USP

Note: *The expression "regular insulin," "unmodified insulin," or simply "insulin" is used in referring to aqueous solutions made from the antidiabetic principle of beef pancreas or pork pancreas or both as stated on the label. Lente Iletin, Semilente Iletin, and Ultralente Iletin represent the result of interaction of zinc on insulin under specific chemical conditions so that higher concentrations of the metallic element are made to combine with the insulin present. They are supplied in the form of a suspension of minute particles.*

Description: Semilente Iletin and Ultralente Iletin are stable preparations which have prolonged action without the addition of a modifying protein. Lente Iletin combines approximately 70 percent of the Ultralente and 30 percent of the Semilente insulin.

Semilente Iletin has the smaller particle size and the shorter action, with a total duration of effect of approximately 12 to 16 hours. Ultralente Iletin has the larger particle size and a total duration of effect in excess of 36 hours. (These time activities are based on averages and may vary from patient to patient.) Lente Iletin has a time action which is intermediate between these; its action falls so close to that of NPH insulin that the two can usually be used interchangeably. Patients on NPH insulin may be transferred directly to Lente Iletin on a unit-for-unit basis. However, in some patients, the duration of action may be a little longer than that of NPH insulin.

When these preparations are brought into uniform suspension, each cubic centimeter (cc) contains 40, 80, or 100 USP units of insulin, together with approximately 0.2 mg of zinc per 100 units of insulin. Each cubic centimeter also contains approximately 1 mg of methylparaben as a preservative, approximately 1.6 mg of sodium acetate as buffer, and approximately 7 mg of sodium chloride.

Precautions: *Inasmuch as insulin dosage varies from patient to patient, the Lente insulins should be used only under the direction of a physician.* It is important that the patient carefully follow a course of diet as prescribed by the physician.

Lente Iletin, Semilente Iletin, and Ultralente Iletin are not adapted for use in place of regular (unmodified) insulin in dealing with acidosis and emergencies. They should not under any circumstances be substituted for another insulin preparation except by direction of a physician.

Diet—When the Lente insulins are used, regulation of diet is a factor of fundamental importance. Such regulation should be done under the supervision of—and in close cooperation with—a physician.

Hypoglycemia—The administration of an excessive dose of insulin causes hypoglycemia. This condition may also occur following increased work or exercise; when food is not being absorbed in the usual manner—because of postponement or omission of a meal or in illness with vomiting, diarrhea, or delayed digestion; when insulin is administered too long before a meal; when the patient's requirement of insulin declines; or when large doses of insulin are given at insufficient or irregular intervals. If it becomes necessary to omit a meal because of nausea or vomiting, the physician should be notified, and the urine should be tested every three or four hours.

An early symptom of hypoglycemia may be merely a feeling of fatigue. *Hence it is of utmost importance for the patient to understand clearly that the presence of vague symptoms of fatigue, headache, drowsiness, lassitude, tremulousness, or nausea demands immediate attention.* More marked symptoms of hypoglycemic reactions, such as weakness, sweating, tremor, or nervousness, may also develop, but these are more easily recognized. The occurrence of such symptoms calls for prompt and, if necessary, repeated administration of some form of carbohydrate. (Candy or a lump of sugar is convenient for this purpose and should always be carried by the patient.) If the patient becomes delirious or mentally confused, dilute corn syrup or orange juice with sugar should be administered by mouth. In severe hypoglycemic reactions, it may be desirable for a physician to administer intravenously from 10 to 20 gm of dextrose (D-glucose) in sterile solution. *If symptoms of hypoglycemia occur, the physician should be notified promptly.*

Administration: The patient should be carefully instructed in the administration of the Lente insulins and should be cautioned to become familiar with the information in the package insert.

In Lente Iletin, Semilente Iletin, and Ultralente Iletin, the active material is present in the milky-white precipitate and not in the clear supernatant fluid. *To insure that a constant proportion of this precipitate is present in each dose injected, the vial should be rotated and inverted from end to end several times immediately before the withdrawal of each dose.* Failure to observe this procedure can lead only to marked irregularity in the effects of individual doses. Vigorous shaking, with consequent frothing of the material, should be avoided.

No vial should be used in which the precipitate has become clumped or granular in appearance or has formed a deposit of solid particles on the wall of the vial.

Use of a package of insulin should not be commenced after the expiration date stamped upon it.

IMPORTANT—USE THE CORRECT SYRINGE, NEEDLE

Doses of insulin are measured in UNITS. The number of units in each cc is clearly stated on the package. Three strengths are available for each type of insulin—U-40 (40 units per cc), U-80 (80 units per cc), and U-100 (100 units per cc). For this reason, always use a syringe that correlates with the strength of insulin to be administered. Failure to use the proper syringe can result in an improper dose, with effects ranging from mild abnormalities of the blood glucose to coma or, rarely, death.

Continued on next page

*Identi-Code® symbol.

Lilly—Cont.

Each strength of insulin is identified by the color of the "flip-off" cap. Red identifies U-40; green, U-80; and orange, U-100.

Dosage: The number and size of daily doses and the time of administration, as well as diet and exercise, are problems that require direct and continuous medical supervision. Usually, the most satisfactory time for injection of the Lente insulins is before breakfast.

A mixture of Semilente Iletin and Lente Iletin may be indicated when the control of the blood sugar and glycosuria after meals is inadequate with Lente Iletin alone. Ultralente Iletin may be mixed with Lente Iletin when inadequate control of the blood sugar and glycosuria in the fasting state (before breakfast) is obtained with Lente Iletin alone.

These preparations can be mixed with one another but must not be mixed with other modified insulin preparations.

Important Notes: In general, the presence of sugar in the urine means unsuitable dosage of insulin or dietary imbalance.

Insulin should be stored in a cold place, preferably a refrigerator. *Exposure to either freezing or high temperatures should be avoided.* Vials in use should be kept cold and protected from strong light and their contents used as continuously as practicable. A partially empty vial should be discarded if it has not been used for several weeks' time.

The use of heavily chlorinated water or chemical solutions for sterilizing the syringe prior to injection should be avoided. The use of distilled or clean rainwater rather than hard water is to be preferred if the syringe is to be sterilized by boiling.

In case a meal is unavoidably omitted as a result of fever or nausea and vomiting, the next dose of insulin should not be omitted unless a test of the urine shows that no sugar is present. If no sugar is present, urine tests should be made at intervals not exceeding four hours. Food unavoidably omitted by patients using insulin should be replaced by similar amounts of carbohydrate in the form of orange juice or some other source of available glucose.

If the patient becomes ill from any cause, he should notify the physician immediately, have his urine tested at once, and take plenty of fluids—at least a cupful of hot tea, coffee, milk, broth, or orange juice *every hour.* Coma may be avoided by prompt treatment.

Syringes which have been used for a time may become coated with a precipitate. This opaque layer may be easily removed by a swab of cotton saturated with vinegar, and the syringe should then be thoroughly rinsed in water and sterilized. Very fine needles may become plugged with the precipitate unless cleaned with a wire after use.

How Supplied: *Lente® Iletin® (Insulin Zinc Suspension, USP)* is supplied in rubber-stoppered vials as follows:

M-440, U-40, forty units per cc, 10 cc (400 units).

M-480, U-80, eighty units per cc, 10 cc (800 units).

M-410, U-100, one hundred units per cc, 10 cc (1000 units).

Semilente® Iletin® (Prompt Insulin Zinc Suspension, USP) is supplied in rubber-stoppered vials as follows:

M-540, U-40, forty units per cc, 10 cc (400 units).

M-580, U-80, eighty units per cc, 10 cc (800 units).

M-510, U-100, one hundred units per cc, 10 cc (1000 units).

Ultralente® Iletin® (Extended Insulin Zinc Suspension, USP) is supplied in rubber-stoppered vials as follows:

M-640, U-40, forty units per cc, 10 cc (400 units).

M-680, U-80, eighty units per cc, 10 cc (800 units).

M-610, U-100, one hundred units per cc, 10 cc (1000 units).

The above products are supplied 10 per carton.

Refrigerate. Avoid freezing. [060178]

[*Shown in Product Identification Section*]

Lente Iletin, M-440—6505-00-753-9548
Lente Iletin, M-480—6505-00-754-2580
Lente Iletin, M-410—6505-00-118-1160

NPH ILETIN®
(isophane insulin suspension) USP

Note: *The expression "regular insulin," "unmodified insulin," or simply "insulin" is used in referring to aqueous solutions made from the antidiabetic principle of beef pancreas or pork pancreas or both as stated on the label. NPH Iletin contains an amount of protamine sulfate sufficient to combine chemically with the insulin present to form crystals containing insulin, protamine, and zinc.*

Description: NPH Iletin is supplied in the form of a suspension of minute particles. It has a time action intermediate between those of insulin and protamine zinc insulin. The onset of action of the preparation is usually prompt enough to provide for adequate control of the after-breakfast rise in blood sugar, which formerly called for supplemental doses of regular (unmodified) insulin.

NPH Iletin combines some of the advantages and eliminates some of the disadvantages of both very short and very long-acting preparations.

When this preparation is brought into uniform suspension, each cubic centimeter (cc) of NPH Iletin contains 40, 80, or 100 USP units of insulin, together with protamine in approximately isophane proportions. Each cubic centimeter also contains approximately 1.6 percent glycerin (w/v), approximately 0.2 percent dibasic sodium phosphate (w/v) as buffer, and approximately 0.065 percent phenol (w/v) and approximately 0.16 percent metacresol (w/v) as preservatives.

Precautions, Administration, and Important Notes: *See under* Lente® Iletin®.

Dosage: The number and size of daily doses and the time of administration, as well as diet and exercise, are problems that require direct and continuous medical supervision. Usually, the most satisfactory time for injection of NPH Iletin is before breakfast.

How Supplied: *NPH Iletin® (Isophane Insulin Suspension, USP)* is supplied in rubber-stoppered vials as follows:

M-340, U-40, forty units per cc, 10 cc (400 units).

M-380, U-80, eighty units per cc, 10 cc (800 units).

M-310, U-100, one hundred units per cc, 10 cc (1000 units).

The above products are supplied 10 per carton.

Refrigerate. Avoid freezing. [102478]

[*Shown in Product Identification Section*]

M-310—6505-00-118-1138

PROTAMINE, ZINC & ILETIN®
(protamine zinc insulin suspension) USP

Note: *The expression "regular insulin," "unmodified insulin," or simply "insulin" is used in referring to aqueous solutions made from the antidiabetic principle of beef pancreas or pork pancreas or both as stated on the label. Protamine, Zinc & Iletin represents the modification of preparations of the principle by the addition of protamine and zinc.*

Description: Protamine, Zinc & Iletin is in the form of a suspension of minute particles.

When this preparation is brought into uniform suspension, each cubic centimeter (cc) contains 40, 80, or 100 USP units of insulin, together with approximately 1.25 mg of protamine and approximately 0.2 mg of zinc per 100 units of insulin. Each cubic centimeter also contains approximately 1.6 percent glycerin (w/v), approximately 0.25 percent phenol (w/v) as a preservative, and approximately 0.2 percent dibasic sodium phosphate (w/v) as a buffer.

Precautions: *Inasmuch as insulin dosage varies from patient to patient, Protamine, Zinc & Iletin should be used only under the direction of a physician.* It is important that the patient carefully follow a course of diet as prescribed by the physician.

Protamine, Zinc & Iletin is not adapted for use in place of regular (unmodified) insulin in dealing with acidosis and emergencies.

Protamine, Zinc & Iletin should not under any circumstances be substituted for another insulin preparation except by direction of a physician.

Diet—When Protamine, Zinc & Iletin is used, regulation of diet is a factor of fundamental importance. Each case has to be treated individually, and success in many instances depends upon skillful balancing of diet in relation to prolonged insulin effect rather than upon adjustment of insulin dosage with respect to individual meals, such as is made when regular insulin is being used. Food should not be redistributed, and the dose or time of taking either insulin or Protamine, Zinc & Iletin should not be altered except by direction of a physician.

Hypoglycemia—Fall of blood sugar levels after injections of Protamine, Zinc & Iletin may be so slow that marked hypoglycemia without apparent symptoms is produced. A low blood sugar level may be signified by such symptoms as weakness, nervousness, or sweating or by fatigue, drowsiness, headache, nausea, or tingling sensations in the extremities. If not promptly and adequately treated, hypoglycemia may lead to stupor, unconsciousness, and possibly grave consequences. *If symptoms of hypoglycemia occur, the physician should be notified promptly.*

Hypoglycemia is treated by administration of carbohydrate. With Protamine, Zinc & Iletin, both a soluble and a slowly digestible carbohydrate should be given; for example, corn syrup or honey with bread. It is important for additional carbohydrate to be provided after the lapse of one or two hours. This may be given in the form of a glass of milk and some crackers. In emergencies, from 10 to 20 gm of dextrose (D-glucose) in sterile solution are slowly administered intravenously, followed later by food.

At institution of treatment with Protamine, Zinc & Iletin, a small amount of food may be taken between meals in order to ward off the occurrence of hypoglycemia during periods when a dose of Protamine, Zinc & Iletin may be having its greatest effect. This purpose may be served by two or three crackers between daytime meals and a glass of milk with a small sandwich or some crackers at bedtime.

Administration: *See under* Lente® Iletin®.

Dosage: The number and size of daily doses and the time of administration, as well as diet and exercise, are problems that require direct and continuous medical supervision. Usually, the most satisfactory time for injection of Protamine, Zinc & Iletin is before breakfast. In some severe cases, this is followed or accompanied by a separate small dose of regular insulin.

Several days may elapse before the full therapeutic effect of Protamine, Zinc & Iletin is evident. During this interval, small supplementary doses of regular insulin are often necessary.

Important Notes: *See under* Lente® Iletin®. If both Regular Iletin® and Protamine, Zinc & Iletin are being used, separate injections should be administered unless the physician instructs the patient to mix the preparations.

How Supplied: *Protamine, Zinc & Iletin® (Protamine Zinc Insulin Suspension, USP)* is supplied in rubber-stoppered vials as follows:

M-140, U-40, forty units per cc, 10 cc (400 units).
M-180, U-80, eighty units per cc, 10 cc (800 units).
M-110, U-100, one hundred units per cc, 10 cc (1000 units).
The above products are supplied 10 per carton.
Refrigerate. Avoid freezing. [060178]
[*Shown in Product Identification Section*]

IPECAC ℞
Syrup, USP

Description: Ipecac Syrup contains 7 gm of ipecac per 100 ml (32 grs per fl oz). Contains alcohol, 2 percent.
Indication: It is useful as an emetic (induces vomiting) for emergency use in the treatment of drug overdosage and in certain cases of poisoning.
Contraindication: It should not be given to unconscious patients.
Warnings: Ipecac Syrup may not be effective in those cases in which the ingested substance is an antiemetic.
The drug can exert a cardiotoxic effect if it is not vomited but is absorbed.
Precautions: Emesis is not the proper treatment in all cases of potential poisoning; it should not be induced when such substances as petroleum distillates, strong alkali, acids, or strychnine are ingested.
Note to the Pharmacist:
The Food and Drug Administration has determined that, in the interest of public health, Ipecac Syrup should be available for sale without prescription provided it is packaged in a quantity of 1 fl oz (30 ml) and, in addition to other required labeling, contains the following:
1. A statement, conspicuously boxed and in red letters, to the effect: "For emergency use to cause vomiting in poisoning. Before using, call physician, the Poison Control Center, or hospital emergency room immediately for advice."
2. A warning to the effect: "Warning—Keep out of reach of children. Do not use in unconscious persons. Ordinarily, this drug should not be used if strychnine, corrosives such as alkalies (lye) and strong acids, or petroleum distillates such as kerosene, gasoline, coal oil, fuel oil, paint thinner, or cleaning fluid have been ingested."
3. Usual dosage: 1 tablespoonful (15 ml) in persons over one year of age.
Administration and Dosage: Children less than one year of age, 1 to 2 teaspoonfuls; children over one year of age and adults, 3 teaspoonfuls.
The dosage may be repeated in 20 minutes if vomiting does not occur. Then, if the patient does not vomit, the dosage should be recovered (lavage).
How Supplied: (℞) *Syrup No. 37, Ipecac, USP,* in 16-fl-oz bottles.
[100578]

ISONIAZID ℞
Tablets, USP

WARNING
Severe and sometimes fatal hepatitis associated with isoniazid therapy has been reported and may occur or may develop even after many months of treatment. The risk of developing hepatitis is age related. Approximate case rates by age are 0 per 1000 for persons under 20 years of age, 3 per 1000 for persons in the 20 to 34-year age group, 12 per 1000 for persons in the 35 to 49-year age group, 23 per 1000 for persons in the 50 to 64-year age group, and 8 per 1000 for persons over 65 years of age. The risk of hepatitis is increased with daily consumption of alcohol. Precise data to provide a fatality rate for isoniazid-related hepatitis are not available; however, in a U.S. Public Health Service Surveillance Study of 13,838 persons taking isoniazid, there were eight deaths among 174 cases of hepatitis.
Therefore, patients given isoniazid should be carefully monitored and interviewed at monthly intervals. Serum transaminase concentration becomes elevated in about 10 to 20 percent of patients, usually during the first few months of therapy, but it can occur at any time. Usually, enzyme levels return to normal despite continuance of the drug, but in some cases progressive liver dysfunction occurs. Patients should be instructed to report immediately any of the prodromal symptoms of hepatitis, such as fatigue, weakness, malaise, anorexia, nausea, or vomiting. If these symptoms appear or if signs suggestive of hepatic damage are detected, isoniazid should be discontinued promptly, since continued use of the drug in such cases has been reported to cause a more severe form of liver damage.
Patients with tuberculosis should be given appropriate treatment with alternative drugs. If isoniazid must be reinstituted, it should be done only after symptoms and laboratory abnormalities have cleared. The drug should be restarted in very small and gradually increasing doses and should be withdrawn immediately if there is any indication of recurrent liver involvement. Preventive treatment should be deferred in persons with acute hepatic diseases.

Description: Isoniazid, USP, the hydrazide of isonicotinic acid, is chemically isonicotinyl hydrazine, and the chemical formula is $C_6H_7N_3O$. It exists as colorless or white crystals or as a crystalline powder that is water soluble. It is slowly affected by exposure to air and light.
Actions: Isoniazid acts against actively growing tubercle bacilli.
After oral administraton, isoniazid produces peak blood levels within one or two hours; these decline to 50 percent or less within six hours. It diffuses readily into all body fluids (cerebrospinal, pleural, and ascitic), tissues, organs, and excreta (saliva, sputum, and feces). The drug also passes through the placental barrier and into milk in concentrations comparable to those in the plasma. From 50 to 70 percent of a dose of isoniazid is excreted in the urine within 24 hours.
Isoniazid is metabolized primarily by acetylation and dehydrazination. The rate of acetylation is genetically determined. Approximately 50 percent of blacks and Caucasians are "slow inactivators," and the rest are "rapid inactivators"; the majority of Eskimos and Orientals are "rapid inactivators."
The rate of acetylation does not significantly alter the effectiveness of isoniazid. However, slow acetylation may lead to higher blood levels of the drug and, thus, to an increase in toxic reactions.
Pyridoxine (vitamin B_6) deficiency is sometimes observed in adults taking high doses of isoniazid and is considered probably due to the drug's competition with pyridoxal phosphate for the enzyme apotryptophanase.
Indications: Isoniazid is recommended for all forms of tuberculosis in which organisms are susceptible.
Isoniazid is recommended as preventive therapy for the following individuals, in order of priority:
1. Household members and other close associates of persons with recently diagnosed tuberculous disease.
2. Positive tuberculin skin-test reactors for whom findings on the chest roentgenogram are consistent with nonprogressive tuberculous disease and in whom there are neither positive bacteriologic findings nor a history of adequate chemotherapy.
3. Newly infected persons.
4. Positive tuberculin skin-test reactors in the following special clinical situations:
   a. Prolonged therapy with adrenocorticosteroids
   b. Immunosuppressive therapy
   c. Some hematologic and reticuloendothelial diseases, such as leukemia or Hodgkin's disease
   d. Diabetes mellitus
   e. Silicosis
   f. After gastrectomy
5. Other positive tuberculin reactors who are less than 35 years of age.

The risk of hepatitis must be weighed against the risk of tuberculosis in positive tuberculin reactors over the age of 35. However, the use of isoniazid is recommended for those with the additional risk factors listed above (1–4) and, on an individual basis, in situations in which there is a likelihood of serious consequences to contacts who may become infected.
Contraindications: Isoniazid is contraindicated in patients with previous isoniazid-associated hepatic injury; severe adverse reactions to isoniazid, such as drug fever, chills, and arthritis; or acute liver disease of any etiology.
Warning: See the boxed warning.
Precautions: Use of isoniazid should be carefully monitored in the following:
1. Patients who are receiving phenytoin concurrently. Isoniazid may decrease the excretion of phenytoin or may enhance its effects. To avoid phenytoin intoxication, appropriate dosage adjustment of the anticonvulsant should be made.
2. Daily users of alcohol. Daily ingestion of alcohol may be associated with a higher incidence of isoniazid-related hepatitis.
3. Patients with active chronic liver disease or severe renal dysfunction.

Periodic ophthalmologic examinations during isoniazid therapy are recommended when visual symptoms occur.
Usage in Pregnancy and Lactation: It has been reported that isoniazid may exert an embryocidal effect in both rats and rabbits when administered orally during pregnancy, but no isoniazid-related congenital anomalies have been found in reproduction studies in mammalian species (mice, rats, and rabbits). Isoniazid should be prescribed during pregnancy only when therapeutically necessary. The benefit of preventive therapy should be weighed against a possible risk to the fetus. Preventive treatment generally should be started after delivery because the risk of tuberculosis for new mothers is increased during the postpartum period. Since isoniazid is known to cross the placental barrier and to pass into maternal breast milk, neonates and breast-fed infants of isoniazid-treated mothers should be carefully observed for any evidence of adverse effects.
Carcinogenesis: Isoniazid has been reported to induce pulmonary tumors in a number of strains of mice.
Adverse Reactions: The most frequent reactions are those affecting the nervous system and the liver.
Nervous System Reactions—Peripheral neuropathy is the most common toxic effect. It is dose related, occurs most often in the malnourished and in those predisposed to neuritis (e.g., alcoholics and diabetics), and is usually preceded by paresthesias of the feet and hands. The incidence is higher in "slow inactivators."
Other neurotoxic effects that are uncommon with conventional doses are convulsions, toxic encephalopathy, optic neuritis and atrophy, memory impairment, and toxic psychosis.
Gastrointestinal Reactions—Nausea, vomiting, and epigastric distress.

Continued on next page

*Identi-Code® symbol.

Lilly—Cont.

Hepatic Reactions—Elevated serum transaminase levels (SGOT, SGPT), bilirubinemia, bilirubinuria, jaundice, and occasionally severe and sometimes fatal hepatitis. The common prodromal symptoms are anorexia, nausea, vomiting, fatigue, malaise, and weakness. Mild hepatic dysfunction, evidenced by mild and transient elevation of serum transaminase levels, occurs in 10 to 20 percent of patients taking isoniazid. This abnormality usually appears in the first four to six months of treatment but can develop at any time during therapy. Enzyme levels return to normal in most instances, and there is no necessity to discontinue medication. Occasionally, progressive liver damage with accompanying symptoms may occur. In such cases, the drug should be discontinued immediately. The frequency of progressive liver damage increases with age. It is rare in individuals under 20 but is seen in as many as 2.3 percent of those over 50 years of age.

Hematologic Reactions—Agranulocytosis; hemolytic, sideroblastic, or aplastic anemia; thrombocytopenia; and eosinophilia.

Hypersensitivity Reactions—Fever, skin eruptions (morbilliform, maculopapular, purpuric, or exfoliative), lymphadenopathy, and vasculitis.

Metabolic and Endocrine Reactions—Pyridoxine deficiency, pellagra, hyperglycemia, metabolic acidosis, and gynecomastia.

Miscellaneous Reactions—Rheumatic syndrome and systemic lupus erythematosus-like syndrome.

Overdosage: *Signs and Symptoms*—Isoniazid overdosage produces signs and symptoms within 30 minutes to three hours after ingestion. Nausea, vomiting, dizziness, slurring of speech, blurring of vision, and visual hallucinations (including bright colors and strange designs) are among the early manifestations. With marked overdosage, respiratory distress and C.N.S. depression, progressing rapidly from stupor to profound coma, are to be expected along with severe, intractable seizures. Severe metabolic acidosis, acetonuria, and hyperglycemia are typical laboratory findings.

Treatment — Untreated or inadequately treated cases of gross isoniazid overdosage can terminate fatally, but good response has been reported in most patients brought under adequate therapy within the first few hours after drug ingestion.

Secure the airway and establish adequate respiratory exchange. Gastric lavage is advised within the first two to three hours, but it should not be attempted until convulsions are under control. To control convulsions, administer short-acting barbiturates intravenously, followed by pyridoxine intravenously (usually 1 mg per 1 mg of isoniazid ingested).

Obtain blood samples for immediate determination of gases, electrolytes, BUN, glucose, etc., and type and cross-match blood in preparation for possible hemodialysis.

Rapid control of metabolic acidosis is fundamental to management. Give sodium bicarbonate intravenously at once and repeat as needed, adjusting subsequent dosage on the basis of laboratory findings (i.e., serum sodium, pH, etc.).

Forced osmotic diuresis must be started early and should be continued for some hours after clinical improvement has been noted to hasten renal clearance of the drug and help prevent relapse; monitor fluid intake and output.

Hemodialysis is advised for severe cases; if this is not available, peritoneal dialysis can be used concomitantly with forced diuresis.

In conjunction with measures based on initial and repeated determination of blood gases and other laboratory tests as needed, utilize meticulous respiratory and other intensive care to protect against hypoxia, hypotension, aspiration pneumonitis, etc.

Note: For preventive therapy of tuberculous infection, it is recommended that physicians be familiar with the joint recommendations of the American Thoracic Society, American Lung Association, and the Center for Disease Control, as published in the *American Review of Respiratory Disease, 110:*306, 1974, or CDC's *Morbidity and Mortality Weekly Report, 24:*71, 1975.

Administration and Dosage: *For Treatment of Tuberculosis*—Isoniazid is used in conjunction with other effective antituberculosis agents. If the bacilli become resistant, therapy must be changed to agents to which the bacilli are susceptible.

Usual Oral Dosage

Adults: 5 mg per kg (up to 300 mg) daily in a single dose.

Infants and Children: 10 to 20 mg per kg (up to 300 to 500 mg) daily in a single dose, depending on the severity of the infection.

For Preventive Therapy

Adults: 300 mg daily in a single dose.

Infants and Children: 10 mg per kg (up to 300 mg) daily in a single dose.

Continuous administration of isoniazid for a sufficient period is an essential part of the regimen, because relapse rates are higher if chemotherapy is stopped prematurely. Resistant organisms may multiply in the treatment of tuberculosis, and their emergence during treatment may necessitate a change in the regimen.

Concomitant administration of pyridoxine (B_6) is recommended in the malnourished and in those predisposed to neuropathy (e.g., alcoholics and diabetics).

How Supplied: (℞) *Isoniazid Tablets, USP: No. 1795, T93,** 100 mg (scored), in bottles of 100 and 1000; *No. 1868, U23,** 300 mg, in bottles of 100.

[102578]

Minimum Inhibitory Concentration Values
(MIC—mcg/ml)
with Representative Bacterial Strains

Bacteria	Number of Strains	Cephaloglycin Range	Desacetylcephaloglycin Range
Staphylococcus aureus	15	1–8 (2)*	0.5–4(2)*
Streptococcus sp. (group D)	4	0.25–32	0.5–32
E. coli	27	1–>128 (2)*	4–>128 (8)*
Klebsiella-Enterobacter	6	2–64	8–>128
Proteus sp. (indole-positive)	5	16–>128	32–>128
Proteus mirabilis	6	4–16	8–32

*MIC value for most strains

ISOPROTERENOL HYDROCHLORIDE INHALATION,

see Aerolone® Solution.

KAFOCIN® ℞
(cephaloglycin)
Capsules, NF

Description: Kafocin® (cephaloglycin, Lilly) is a phenylglycine analogue of the antibiotic cephalosporin C. It is the zwitterion form of 7-(D-α-aminophenylacetamido) cephalosporanic acid. It is intended for oral administration.

Actions: *Human Pharmacology*—Cephaloglycin is acid stable and is absorbed after oral administration. Food does not significantly affect the total amount of cephaloglycin absorbed, although the excretion of peak urine levels may be delayed. Urine collected over an eight-hour period shows average concentrations of approximately 200 mcg per ml after administration of 250 mg of the drug and of approximately 350 mcg per ml after administration of 500 mg of the drug. It is excreted almost entirely as the active metabolite desacetylcephaloglycin. Peak urine concentrations may exceed 1300 mcg per ml after the 500-mg dose.

Microbiology—Cephaloglycin and its metabolite desacetylcephaloglycin have an antibacterial spectrum that includes strains of *Escherichia coli, Klebsiella-Enterobacter,* staphylococci, certain of the *Proteus* species, and enterococci. It is ineffective in vivo and in vitro against *Pseudomonas.* The bactericidal activity of the cephalosporins is based on their inhibition of cell-wall synthesis.

Disc Susceptibility Tests—Quantitative methods that require measurement of zone diameters give the most precise estimates of antibiotic susceptibility. Information on disc testing for susceptibility to Kafocin is found in the package literature for "Cephalothin 30-mcg Discs for Testing Susceptibility to Keflin® (Cephalothin Sodium), Loridine® (Cephaloridine), Kefzol® (Cefazolin Sodium), Kafocin® (Cephaloglycin), Keflex® (Cephalexin)." Interpretations correlate zone diameters of the disc test with MIC values for desacetylcephaloglycin.

[See table below].

Indications: Kafocin® (cephaloglycin, Lilly) is indicated for the treatment of acute and chronic infections of the urinary tract, including cystitis, pyelitis, pyelonephritis, and "asymptomatic bacteriuria," when due to susceptible strains of *E. coli, Klebsiella-Enterobacter, Proteus* species, staphylococci, and enterococci.

Note—Culture and susceptibility tests should be initiated prior to and during therapy. Renal function studies should be performed when indicated.

Contraindication: Kafocin® (cephaloglycin, Lilly) is contraindicated in patients with known allergy to the cephalosporin group of antibiotics.

Warnings: IN PENICILLIN-SENSITIVE PATIENTS, CEPHALOSPORIN C DERIVATIVES SHOULD BE USED WITH GREAT CAUTION. THERE IS CLINICAL AND LABORATORY EVIDENCE OF PARTIAL CROSS-ALLERGENICITY OF THE PENICILLINS AND THE CEPHALOSPORINS, AND THERE ARE INSTANCES OF PATIENTS WHO HAVE HAD REACTIONS TO BOTH DRUGS (INCLUDING FATAL ANAPHYLAXIS AFTER PARENTERAL USE).

Any patient who has demonstrated some form of allergy, particularly to drugs, should receive antibiotics cautiously and then only when absolutely necessary. No exception should be made with regard to Kafocin® (cephaloglycin, Lilly).

Usage in Children—Since safety has not been established for use in premature infants and in infants under one year, the administration of Kafocin in this age group is not recommended.

Usage in Pregnancy and Lactation—Safety of this product for use during pregnancy and lactation has not been established.

Precautions: Patients should be followed carefully so that any side effects or unusual manifestations of drug idiosyncrasy may be detected. If an allergic reaction to Kafocin® (cephaloglycin, Lilly) occurs, the drug should be discontinued and the patient treated with the usual agents (e.g., epinephrine or other pressor amines, antihistamines, or corticosteroids).

Prolonged use of Kafocin may result in the overgrowth of nonsusceptible organisms. Careful observation of the patient is essential. If superinfection occurs during therapy, appropriate measures should be taken.

Like other antibacterial agents excreted by the kidney, Kafocin should be administered with caution in the presence of markedly impaired renal function. Under such conditions, careful clinical observation and laboratory studies should be made because safe dosage may be lower than that usually recommended.

Since safety has not been established for use in premature infants and in infants under one year, the administration of Kafocin in this age group is not recommended.

A false-positive reaction for glucose in the urine may occur with Benedict's or Fehling's solution or with Clinitest® tablets but not with Tes-Tape® (Glucose Enzymatic Test Strip, USP, Lilly).

Adverse Reactions: *Gastrointestinal* — Nausea and vomiting have been reported. Diarrhea (ranging from soft stools to frequent bowel movements) is the most frequent adverse reaction noted in clinical studies to date. Diarrhea severe and persistent enough to warrant cessation of therapy has occurred.

Abdominal pain, gastrointestinal bleeding, and severe enterocolitis have been reported during therapy with Kafocin® (cephaloglycin, Lilly). In such cases, Kafocin should be discontinued.

Hypersensitivity—Allergy (in the form of rash, urticaria, angioedema, or exfoliative dermatitis) has occurred.

Other reactions that have been reported are monilial vaginitis, malaise, fever, chills, headache, and dizziness or vertigo. Eosinophilia has been reported.

Administration and Dosage: Kafocin® (cephaloglycin, Lilly) is administered orally. For infections of the urinary tract in the adult, the usual dosage of Kafocin is 250 mg four times daily. For more severe infections, 500 mg four times daily may be required. If larger doses are necessary, initial therapy with the injectable cephalosporins should be considered.

In children with urinary tract infections, the daily dosage is 25 to 50 mg per kg (12 to 25 mg per pound). In infants under one year of age, the administration of Kafocin is not recommended until additional data are available.

Any infection which has not responded to treatment indicates the need for further determination of the antibacterial susceptibility of the infecting organism and/or a thorough study of the urinary tract.

Kafocin can be given without regard to meals.

How Supplied: (℞) *Pulvules® No. 398, Kafocin® (Cephaloglycin Capsules, NF), H66,** 250 mg (No. 0, Light-Turquoise Opaque Body, Dark-Turquoise Opaque Cap), in bottles of 100.

[092975B]

KEFLEX® ℞
(cephalexin)

Description: Keflex® (cephalexin, Lilly) is a semisynthetic cephalosporin antibiotic intended for oral administration. It is 7-(D-α-amino-α-phenylacetamido)-3-methyl-3-cephem-4-carboxylic acid, monohydrate.

Actions: *Human Pharmacology*—Keflex® (cephalexin, Lilly) is acid stable and may be given without regard to meals. It is rapidly absorbed after oral administration. Following doses of 250 mg, 500 mg, and 1 gm, average peak serum levels of approximately 9, 18, and 32 mcg per ml respectively were obtained at one hour. Measurable levels were present six hours after administration. Over 90 percent of the drug was excreted unchanged in the urine within eight hours. During this period, peak urine concentrations following the 250-mg, 500-mg, and 1-gm doses were approximately 1000, 2200, and 5000 mcg per ml respectively.

Microbiology—In vitro tests demonstrate that the cephalosporins are bactericidal because of their inhibition of cell-wall synthesis. Keflex is active against the following organisms in vitro:

- Beta-hemolytic streptococci
- Staphylococci, including coagulase-positive, coagulase-negative, and penicillinase-producing strains
- *Streptococcus (Diplococcus) pneumoniae*
- *Escherichia coli*
- *Proteus mirabilis*
- *Klebsiella* sp.
- *Haemophilus influenzae*
- *Neisseria catarrhalis*

Note—Most strains of enterococci *(S. faecalis)* and a few strains of staphylococci are resistant to Keflex. It is not active against most strains of *Enterobacter* sp., *P. morganii,* and *P. vulgaris.* It has no activity against *Pseudomonas* or *Herellea* species. When tested by in vitro methods, staphylococci exhibit cross-resistance between Keflex and methicillin-type antibiotics.

Disc Susceptibility Tests—Quantitative methods that require measurement of zone diameters give the most precise estimates of antibiotic susceptibility. One such procedure (*Am. J. Clin. Pathol., 45:*493, 1966; *Federal Register, 39:*19182-19184, 1974) has been recommended for use with discs for testing susceptibility to cephalothin. Interpretations correlate zone diameters of the disc test with MIC values for Keflex. With this procedure, a report from the laboratory of "resistant" indicates that the infecting organism is not likely to respond to therapy. A report of "intermediate susceptibility" suggests that the organism would be susceptible if the infection is confined to the urine, in which high antibiotic levels can be obtained, or if high dosage is used in other types of infection.

Indications: Keflex® (cephalexin, Lilly) is indicated for the treatment of the following infections when caused by susceptible strains of the designated microorganisms:

- Respiratory tract infections caused by *S. pneumoniae* and group A beta-hemolytic streptococci (Penicillin is the usual drug of choice in the treatment and prevention of streptococcal infections, including the prophylaxis of rheumatic fever. Keflex is generally effective in the eradication of streptococci from the nasopharynx; however, substantial data establishing the efficacy of Keflex in the subsequent prevention of rheumatic fever are not available at present.)
- Otitis media due to *S. pneumoniae, H. influenzae,* staphylococci, streptococci, and *N. catarrhalis*
- Skin and soft-tissue infections caused by staphylococci and/or streptococci
- Bone infections caused by staphylococci and/or *P. mirabilis*
- Genitourinary tract infections, including acute prostatitis, caused by *E. coli, P. mirabilis,* and *Klebsiella* sp.

Note—Culture and susceptibility tests should be initiated prior to and during therapy. Renal function studies should be performed when indicated.

Contraindication: Keflex® (cephalexin, Lilly) is contraindicated in patients with known allergy to the cephalosporin group of antibiotics.

Warnings: BEFORE CEPHALEXIN THERAPY IS INSTITUTED, CAREFUL INQUIRY SHOULD BE MADE CONCERNING PREVIOUS HYPERSENSITIVITY REACTIONS TO CEPHALOSPORINS AND PENICILLIN. CEPHALOSPORIN C DERIVATIVES SHOULD BE GIVEN CAUTIOUSLY TO PENICILLIN-SENSITIVE PATIENTS.

SERIOUS ACUTE HYPERSENSITIVITY REACTIONS MAY REQUIRE EPINEPHRINE AND OTHER EMERGENCY MEASURES.

There is some clinical and laboratory evidence of partial cross-allergenicity of the penicillins and the cephalosporins. Patients have been reported to have had severe reactions (including anaphylaxis) to both drugs.

Any patient who has demonstrated some form of allergy, particularly to drugs, should receive antibiotics cautiously. No exception should be made with regard to Keflex® (cephalexin, Lilly).

Usage in Pregnancy—Safety of this product for use during pregnancy has not been established.

Precautions: Patients should be followed carefully so that any side effects or unusual manifestations of drug idiosyncrasy may be detected. If an allergic reaction to Keflex® (cephalexin, Lilly) occurs, the drug should be discontinued and the patient treated with the usual agents (e.g., epinephrine or other pressor amines, antihistamines, or corticosteroids).

Prolonged use of Keflex may result in the overgrowth of nonsusceptible organisms. Careful observation of the patient is essential. If superinfection occurs during therapy, appropriate measures should be taken.

Positive direct Coombs tests have been reported during treatment with the cephalosporin antibiotics. In hematologic studies or in transfusion cross-matching procedures when antiglobulin tests are performed on the minor side or in Coombs testing of newborns whose mothers have received cephalosporin antibiotics before parturition, it should be recognized that a positive Coombs test may be due to the drug.

Keflex should be administered with caution in the presence of markedly impaired renal function. Under such conditions, careful clinical observation and laboratory studies should be made because safe dosage may be lower than that usually recommended.

Indicated surgical procedures should be performed in conjunction with antibiotic therapy.

As a result of administration of Keflex, a false-positive reaction for glucose in the urine may occur. This has been observed with Benedict's and Fehling's solutions and also with Clinitest® tablets but not with Tes-Tape® (Glucose Enzymatic Test Strip, USP, Lilly).

Adverse Reactions: *Gastrointestinal*—The most frequent side effect has been diarrhea. It was very rarely severe enough to warrant cessation of therapy. Nausea, vomiting, dyspepsia, and abdominal pain have also occurred.

Hypersensitivity—Allergies (in the form of rash, urticaria, and angioedema) have been observed. These reactions usually subsided upon discontinuation of the drug. Anaphylaxis has also been reported.

Other reactions have included genital and anal pruritus, genital moniliasis, vaginitis and vaginal discharge, dizziness, fatigue, and headache. Eosinophilia, neutropenia, and slight elevations in SGOT and SGPT have been reported.

Administration and Dosage: Keflex® (cephalexin, Lilly) is administered orally.

Adults—The adult dosage ranges from 1 to 4 gm daily in divided doses. The usual adult dose is 250 mg every six hours. For more severe infections or those caused by less susceptible organisms, larger doses may be needed. If daily doses of Keflex greater than 4 gm are required, parenteral cephalosporins, in appropriate doses, should be considered.

Continued on next page

*Identi-Code® symbol.

Lilly—Cont.

Children—The usual recommended daily dosage for children is 25 to 50 mg per kg divided into four doses.
[See table below].
In severe infections, the dosage may be doubled.
In the therapy of otitis media, clinical studies have shown that a dosage of 75 to 100 mg per kg per day in four divided doses is required.
In the treatment of beta-hemolytic streptococcal infections, a therapeutic dosage of Keflex should be administered for at least ten days.
How Supplied: ℞ *For Oral Suspension, Keflex® (Cephalexin for Oral Suspension, NF), M-201, W21,** in 60, 100, and 200-ml-size packages and in unit-dose bottles of 100 (ID100).
Each 60-ml-size package contains 1.5 gm cephalexin in a dry, pleasantly flavored mixture. At the time of dispensing, add 36 ml of water to the dry mixture in the bottle in *two* portions. Shake well after each addition.
Each 100-ml-size package contains 2.5 gm cephalexin in a dry, pleasantly flavored mixture. At the time of dispensing, add 60 ml of water in *two* portions to the dry mixture in the bottle. Shake well after each addition.
Each 200-ml-size package contains 5 gm cephalexin in a dry, pleasantly flavored mixture. At the time of dispensing, add 120 ml of water in *two* portions to the dry mixture in the bottle. Shake well after each addition.
When mixed as directed, each 5 ml (approximately 1 teaspoonful) will contain 125 mg cephalexin. After mixing, store in a refrigerator. The mixture may be kept for 14 days without significant loss of potency. *Shake well before using. Keep tightly closed.*
℞ *For Oral Suspension, Keflex® (Cephalexin for Oral Suspension, NF), M-202, W68,** in 100 and 200-ml-size packages and in unit-dose bottles of 100 (ID100).
Each 100-ml-size package contains 5 gm cephalexin in a dry, pleasantly flavored mixture. At the time of dispensing, add 60 ml of water in *two* portions to the dry mixture in the bottle. Shake well after each addition.
Each 200-ml-size package contains 10 gm cephalexin in a dry, pleasantly flavored mixture. At the time of dispensing, add 124 ml of water in *two* portions to the dry mixture in the bottle. Shake well after each addition.
When mixed as directed, each 5 ml (approximately 1 teaspoonful) will contain 250 mg cephalexin. After mixing, store in a refrigerator. The mixture may be kept for 14 days without significant loss of potency. *Shake well before using. Keep tightly closed.*
℞ *For Pediatric Drops, Keflex® (Cephalexin for Oral Suspension, NF), M-204, W22,** in 10-ml-size packages.
This package contains 1 gm cephalexin in a dry, pleasantly flavored mixture and a special dropper calibrated at approximately 25 and 50 mg.
At the time of dispensing, add 5.5 ml of water to the dry mixture in the bottle. Close with original bottle cap and shake promptly until all of the powder is in suspension. Replace bottle cap with dropper assembly. Remove detachable portion of bottle label but leave white tab affixed.
When mixed as directed, each ml will contain 100 mg cephalexin. After being mixed, the suspension may be kept in a refrigerator for 14 days without significant loss of potency. *Shake well before using. Keep tightly closed.*
℞ *Pulvules® Keflex® (Cephalexin Capsules, USP): No. 402, H69,** 250 mg (No. 0, White Opaque Body, Dark-Green Opaque Cap), and *No. 403, H71,** 500 mg (No. 0, Light-Green Opaque Body, Dark-Green Opaque Cap), in bottles of 20 and 100 and in 10 strips of 10 individually labeled blisters each containing 1 Pulvule (ID100).
℞ *Tablets No. 1896, Keflex® (cephalexin, Lilly), U60,** 1 gm, Green (capsule-shaped), in bottles of 24 and in 10 strips of 10 individually labeled blisters each containing 1 tablet (ID100). [030279]
[*Shown in Product Identification Section*]
Pulvules No. 402, 250 mg—100's—6505-00-165-6545
M-201—For Oral Suspension—100-ml size —6505-00-009-1833

Keflex Suspension

Child's Weight	125 mg/5 ml	250 mg/5 ml
10 kg (22 lb)	½ to 1 tsp q i d	¼ to ½ tsp q i d
20 kg (44 lb)	1 to 2 tsp q i d	½ to 1 tsp q i d
40 kg (88 lb)	2 to 4 tsp q i d	1 to 2 tsp q i d

KEFLIN® ℞
(cephalothin sodium)
For Injection, USP
Neutral

Description: Keflin® (cephalothin sodium, Lilly), Neutral, is a semisynthetic cephalosporin antibiotic for parenteral use. It is the sodium salt of 7-(thiophene-2-acetamido) cephalosporanic acid. Sodium bicarbonate has been added to result in reconstituted solutions having a pH ranging between 6 and 8.5. The total sodium content is approximately 63 mg (2.8 mEq sodium ion) per gm of Keflin.
Actions: *Human Pharmacology*—Keflin® (cephalothin sodium, Lilly) is a broad-spectrum antibiotic for parenteral administration. After administration of a 500-mg dose intramuscularly to normal volunteers, the average peak serum antibiotic level was 10 mcg per ml at one-half hour; with a 1-gm dose, the average was about 20 mcg per ml. Following a single 1-gm intravenous dose of Keflin, blood levels have been about 30 mcg per ml at 15 minutes, have ranged from 3 to 12 mcg at one hour, and have declined to about 1 mcg at four hours. With continuous infusion, at the rate of 500 mg per hour, levels have been from 14 to 20 mcg per ml of serum. Dosages of 2 gm given intravenously over a 30-minute period have produced serum concentrations of 80 to 100 mcg per ml one-half hour after the infusion; levels ranged from 10 to 40 mcg per ml at one hour and from 3 to 6 mcg per ml at two hours and were not assayable after five hours.
Sixty to 70 percent of an intramuscular dose is excreted by the kidneys in the first six hours; this results in high urine levels, e.g., 800 mcg per ml of urine after a 500-mg dose and 2500 mcg per ml following 1 gm. Probenecid slows tubular excretion and almost doubles peak blood levels.
Spinal-fluid levels have ranged from 0.4 to 1.4 mcg per ml in a child and from 0.15 to 5 mcg per ml in adults with meningeal inflammatory states. The antibiotic passes readily into other body fluids, e.g., pleural, joint, and ascitic fluids. Studies of amniotic fluid and cord blood show prompt transfer of Keflin across the placenta. Secondary aqueous-humor levels have averaged 0.5 mcg per ml 30 minutes after a single 1-gm intravenous dose. The antibiotic has been detected in bile.
Microbiology—The in vitro bactericidal action of cephalothin results from inhibition of cell-wall synthesis.
Keflin is usually active against the following organisms in vitro:

- Beta-hemolytic and other streptococci (many strains of enterococci, e.g., *Streptococcus faecalis*, are relatively resistant)
- Staphylococci, including coagulase-positive, coagulase-negative, and penicillinase-producing strains
- *S. (Diplococcus) pneumoniae*
- *Haemophilus influenzae*
- *Escherichia coli* and other coliform bacteria
- *Klebsiella*
- *Proteus mirabilis*
- *Salmonella* sp.
- *Shigella* sp.

Pseudomonas organisms are resistant to Keflin, as are most indole-producing *Proteus* species and motile *Enterobacter* species.
Susceptibility Plate Tests—If the Bauer-Kirby-Sherris-Turck method of disc susceptibility testing is used (*Am. J. Clin. Pathol., 45:*493, 1966; *Federal Register, 39:*19182-19184, 1974), a disc containing 30 mcg cephalothin should give a zone of over 17 mm when tested against a cephalothin-susceptible bacterial strain and a zone of over 14 mm with an organism of intermediate susceptibility.
Indications: Keflin® (cephalothin sodium, Lilly) is indicated for the treatment of serious infections caused by susceptible strains of the designated microorganisms in the diseases listed below. Culture and susceptibility studies should be performed. Therapy may be instituted before results of susceptibility studies are obtained.

- Respiratory tract infections caused by *S. pneumoniae*, staphylococci (penicillinase and non-penicillinase-producing), group A beta-hemolytic streptococci, *Klebsiella*, and *H. influenzae*
- Skin and soft-tissue infections, including peritonitis, caused by staphylococci (penicillinase and non-penicillinase-producing), group A beta-hemolytic streptococci, *E. coli, P. mirabilis*, and *Klebsiella*
- Genitourinary tract infections caused by *E. coli, P. mirabilis*, and *Klebsiella*
- Septicemia, including endocarditis, caused by *S. pneumoniae*, staphylococci (penicillinase and non-penicillinase-producing), group A beta-hemolytic streptococci, *S. viridans, E. coli, P. mirabilis*, and *Klebsiella*
- Gastrointestinal infections caused by *Salmonella* and *Shigella* species
- Meningitis caused by *S. pneumoniae*, group A beta-hemolytic streptococci, and staphylococci (penicillinase and non-penicillinase-producing)

  NOTE: Inasmuch as only low levels of Keflin are found in the cerebrospinal fluid, the drug is not reliable in the treatment of meningitis and cannot be recommended for that purpose. Keflin has, however, proved to be effective in a number of cases of meningitis and may be considered for unusual circumstances in which other, more reliably effective antibiotics cannot be used.
- Bone and joint infections caused by staphylococci (penicillinase and non-penicillinase-producing)

The prophylactic administration of Keflin preoperatively, intraoperatively, and postoperatively may reduce the incidence of certain postoperative infections in patients undergoing surgical procedures (e.g., vaginal hysterectomy) that are classified as contaminated or potentially contaminated.
The perioperative use of Keflin also may be effective in surgical patients in whom infection at the operative site would present a serious risk, e.g., during open-heart surgery and prosthetic arthroplasty.
The prophylactic administration of Keflin should be discontinued within a 24-hour period after the surgical procedure. If there are signs of infection, specimens for culture should be obtained for the identification of the causative organism so that appropriate therapy may be instituted. (*See* Administration and Dosage.)
NOTE: If the susceptibility tests show that the causative organism is resistant to Keflin, other appropriate antibiotic therapy should be instituted.

Contraindication: Keflin® (cephalothin sodium, Lilly) is contraindicated in persons who have shown hypersensitivity to cephalosporin antibiotics.

Warnings: BEFORE CEPHALOTHIN THERAPY IS INSTITUTED, CAREFUL INQUIRY SHOULD BE MADE CONCERNING PREVIOUS HYPERSENSITIVITY REACTIONS TO CEPHALOSPORINS AND PENICILLIN. CEPHALOSPORIN C DERIVATIVES SHOULD BE GIVEN CAUTIOUSLY TO PENICILLIN-SENSITIVE PATIENTS.

SERIOUS ACUTE HYPERSENSITIVITY REACTIONS MAY REQUIRE EPINEPHRINE AND OTHER EMERGENCY MEASURES.

There is some clinical and laboratory evidence of partial cross-allergenicity of the penicillins and the cephalosporins. Patients have been reported to have had severe reactions (including anaphylaxis) to both drugs.

Any patient who has demonstrated some form of allergy, particularly to drugs, should receive antibiotics cautiously and then only when absolutely necessary. No exception should be made with regard to Keflin® (cephalothin sodium, Lilly).

Usage in Pregnancy—Safety of this product for use during pregnancy has not been established.

Precautions: Patients should be followed carefully so that any side effects or unusual manifestations of drug idiosyncrasy may be detected. If an allergic reaction to Keflin® (cephalothin sodium, Lilly) occurs, the drug should be discontinued and the patient treated with the usual agents (e.g., epinephrine or other pressor amines, antihistamines, or corticosteroids).

Although Keflin rarely produces alteration in kidney function, evaluation of renal status is recommended, especially in seriously ill patients receiving maximum doses. Patients with impaired renal function should be placed on the dosage schedule recommended under Administration and Dosage. Usual doses in such individuals may result in excessive serum concentrations.

When intravenous doses of cephalothin larger than 6 gm daily are given by infusion for periods longer than three days, they may be associated with thrombophlebitis, and the veins may have to be alternated. The addition of 10 to 25 mg of hydrocortisone to intravenous solutions containing 4 to 6 gm of cephalothin may reduce the incidence of thrombophlebitis. The use of small I.V. needles in the larger available veins may be preferred.

Prolonged use of Keflin may result in the overgrowth of nonsusceptible organisms. Constant observation of the patient is essential. If superinfection occurs during therapy, appropriate measures should be taken.

A false-positive reaction for glucose in the urine may occur with Benedict's or Fehling's solution or with Clinitest® tablets but not with Tes-Tape® (Glucose Enzymatic Test Strip, USP, Lilly).

Adverse Reactions: *Hypersensitivity*—Maculopapular rash, urticaria, reactions resembling serum sickness, and anaphylaxis have been reported. Eosinophilia and drug fever have been observed to be associated with other allergic reactions. These reactions are most likely to occur in patients with a history of allergy, particularly to penicillin.

Blood—Neutropenia, thrombocytopenia, and hemolytic anemia have been reported. Some individuals, particularly those with azotemia, have developed positive direct Coombs tests during cephalothin therapy.

Liver—Transient rise in SGOT and alkaline phosphatase has been noted.

Kidney—Rise in BUN and decreased creatinine clearance have been reported, particularly in patients with prior renal impairment. The role of Keflin® (cephalothin sodium, Lilly) in renal changes is difficult to assess, because other factors predisposing to prerenal azotemia or to acute renal failure usually have been present.

Local Reactions—Pain, induration, tenderness, and elevation of temperature have been reported following repeated intramuscular injections. Thrombophlebitis has occurred and is usually associated with daily doses of more than 6 gm given by infusion for longer than three days.

Administration and Dosage: *In adults,* the usual dosage range is 500 mg to 1 gm of cephalothin every four to six hours. A dosage of 500 mg every six hours is adequate in uncomplicated pneumonia, furunculosis with cellulitis, and most urinary tract infections. In severe infections, this may be increased by giving the injections every four hours or, when the desired response is not obtained, by raising the dose to 1 gm. In life-threatening infections, doses up to 2 gm every four hours may be required.

For perioperative prophylactic use to prevent postoperative infection in contaminated or potentially contaminated surgery in adults, the following doses are recommended:

(a) 1 to 2 gm administered I.V. just prior to surgery (approximately one-half to one hour before the initial incision);
(b) 1 to 2 gm during surgery (administration modified according to the duration of the operative procedure); and
(c) 1 to 2 gm every six hours postoperatively for 24 hours.

In children, 20 to 30 mg per kg may be given at the times designated above.

Since Keflin has a very short serum half-life (30 to 50 minutes), it is important that (1) the preoperative dose be given just prior to the start of surgery so that adequate antibiotic levels are present in the serum and tissues at the time of initial surgical incision; and (2) Keflin be administered, if necessary, at appropriate intervals during surgery to provide sufficient levels of the antibiotic at the anticipated moments of greatest exposure to infective organisms.

When renal function is reduced, an intravenous loading dose of 1 to 2 gm may be given. Continued dosage schedule should be determined by degree of renal impairment, severity of infection, and susceptibility of the causative organism. The maximum doses administered should be based on the following recommendations.

DOSAGE OF KEFLIN®
(CEPHALOTHIN SODIUM, LILLY)
WHEN RENAL FUNCTION IS IMPAIRED

STATUS OF RENAL FUNCTION	MAXIMUM ADULT DOSAGE (Maintenance)
Mild Impairment (C_{cr}=80–50 ml/min)	2 gm q 6 h
Moderate Impairment (C_{cr}=50–25 ml/min)	1.5 gm q 6 h
Severe Impairment (C_{cr}=25–10 ml/min)	1 gm q 6 h
Marked Impairment (C_{cr}=10–2 ml/min)	0.5 gm q 6 h
Essentially No Function (C_{cr}= <2 ml/min)	0.5 gm q 8 h

In infants and children, the dosage should be proportionately less in accordance with age, weight, and severity of infection. Daily administration of 100 mg per kg (80 to 160 mg per kg or 40 to 80 mg per pound) in divided doses has been found effective for most infections susceptible to Keflin® (cephalothin sodium, Lilly).

Antibiotic therapy in beta-hemolytic streptococcal infections should continue for at least ten days. In staphylococcal infections, surgical procedures, such as incision and drainage, should be carried out in all cases when indicated.

Keflin may be given intravenously or by deep intramuscular injection into a large muscle mass, such as the gluteus or lateral aspect of the thigh, to minimize pain and induration.

Intramuscular—Each gm of cephalothin should be diluted with 4 ml of Sterile Water for Injection. If the vial contents do not completely dissolve, an additional small amount of diluent (e.g., 0.2 to 0.4 ml) may be added and the contents warmed slightly.

Intravenous—The intravenous route may be preferable for patients with bacteremia, septicemia, or other severe or life-threatening infections who may be poor risks because of lowered resistance resulting from such debilitating conditions as malnutrition, trauma, surgery, diabetes, heart failure, or malignancy, particularly if shock is present or impending. For these infections in patients with normal renal function, the intravenous dosage is 4 to 12 gm of cephalothin daily. In conditions such as septicemia, 6 to 8 gm per day may be given intravenously for several days at the beginning of therapy; then, depending on the clinical response and laboratory findings, the dosage may gradually be reduced.

For patients who are to receive cephalothin intravenously, it is convenient to use the 1 or 2-gm 100-ml-size vial (*see* Precautions).

For intermittent intravenous administration, a solution containing 1 gm cephalothin in 10 ml of diluent may be slowly injected directly into the vein over a period of three to five minutes or may be given through the tubing when the patient is receiving parenteral solutions.

Intermittent intravenous infusion with a Y-type administration set can also be accomplished while bulk intravenous solutions are being infused. However, during infusion of the solution containing Keflin® (cephalothin sodium, Lilly), it is desirable to discontinue the other solution. When this technique is employed, careful attention should be paid to the volume of the solution containing Keflin so that the calculated dose will be infused.

For continuous intravenous infusion, 1 or 2 gm of cephalothin, diluted and well mixed with at least 10 ml of Sterile Water for Injection, may be added to an I.V. bottle containing one of the following intravenous solutions: Acetated Ringer's Injection, 5% Dextrose Injection, 5% Dextrose in Lactated Ringer's Injection, Ionosol® B in D5-W, Isolyte® M with 5% Dextrose, Lactated Ringer's Injection, Normosol®-M in D5-W, Plasma-Lyte® Injection, Plasma-Lyte®-M Injection in 5% Dextrose, Ringer's Injection, or 0.9% Sodium Chloride Injection. The choice of solution and the volume to be employed are dictated by fluid and electrolyte management.

Intraperitoneal—In peritoneal dialysis procedures, cephalothin has been added to dialysis fluid in concentrations up to 6 mg per 100 ml and instilled into the peritoneal space throughout an entire dialysis (16 to 30 hours). Careful assay procedures have shown that 44 percent of the administered drug was absorbed into the bloodstream. Serum levels of 10 mcg per ml were reported, with no evidence of accumulation and no untoward local or systemic reactions.

The intraperitoneal administration of solutions containing 0.1 to 4 percent Keflin in saline has been used in treating patients with peritonitis or contaminated peritoneal cavities. (The total daily dosage of Keflin should take into account the amount given by the intraperitoneal route.)

Stability: While stored under *refrigeration,* the solution has a satisfactory potency for 96

Continued on next page

*Identi-Code® symbol.

Lilly—Cont.

hours after reconstitution. Solutions may precipitate; they can be redissolved by being warmed to room temperature with constant agitation. Kept at *room temperature,* solutions for intramuscular injection should be given within 12 hours after being mixed. Intravenous infusions should be started within 12 hours and completed within 24 hours. For prolonged infusions, replace with a freshly prepared solution at least every 24 hours.
The concentrated solution will darken, especially at room temperature. Slight discoloration of the solution is permissible.
Solutions of Keflin® (cephalothin sodium, Lilly) in Sterile Water for Injection, 5% Dextrose Injection, or 0.9% Sodium Chloride Injection that are frozen immediately after reconstitution in the original container are stable for as long as 12 weeks when stored at −20°C. **If the product is warmed, care should be taken to avoid heating it after the thawing is complete. Once thawed, the solution should not be refrozen.**
How Supplied: (℞) *Ampoules (Vials) Keflin® (Cephalothin Sodium for Injection, USP), Neutral,* rubber-stoppered (Dry Powder): *No. 7001,* 1 gm (equivalent to cephalothin), 10-ml size, in singles (10 per carton) and Traypaks™ (multivial cartons, Lilly) of 25; *No. 7000,* 1 gm (equivalent to cephalothin), 100-ml size, *No. 7003,* 2 gm (equivalent to cephalothin), 20-ml size, *No. 7002,* 2 gm (equivalent to cephalothin), 100-ml size, and *No. 7004,* 4 gm (equivalent to cephalothin), 50-ml size, in singles (10 per carton) and Traypaks of 10; *No. 7020,* 20 gm (equivalent to cephalothin), 200-ml size, in Traypaks of 6.

[032879]

KEFZOL® ℞
(cefazolin sodium)
Sterile, USP

Description: Kefzol® (cefazolin sodium, Lilly) is a semisynthetic cephalosporin for parenteral administration. It is the sodium salt of 3-[[(5-methyl-1,3,4-thiadiazol-2-yl) -thio] methyl]-7- [2- (1H-tetrazol-1-yl) acetamido] -3- cephem-4-carboxylic acid. The sodium content is 48.3 mg per gm of cefazolin sodium.
Actions: *Microbiology*—In vitro tests demonstrate that the bactericidal action of cephalosporins results from inhibition of cell-wall synthesis. Kefzol® (cefazolin sodium, Lilly) is active against the following organisms in vitro:
- *Staphylococcus aureus* (penicillin-sensitive and penicillin-resistant)
- Group A beta-hemolytic streptococci and other strains of streptococci (many strains of enterococci are resistant)
- *Streptococcus (Diplococcus) pneumoniae*
- *Escherichia coli*
- *Proteus mirabilis*
- *Klebsiella* species
- *Enterobacter aerogenes*
- *Haemophilus influenzae*

Most strains of *E. cloacae* and indole-positive *Proteus* (*P. vulgaris, P. morganii, P. rettgeri*) are resistant. Methicillin-resistant staphylococci, *Serratia, Pseudomonas, Mima,* and *Herellea* species are almost uniformly resistant to cefazolin.
Human Pharmacology—Table 1 demonstrates the blood levels and duration of cefazolin following intramuscular administration.

TABLE 1. SERUM CONCENTRATIONS AFTER INTRAMUSCULAR ADMINISTRATION

Dose	Serum Concentrations (mcg/ml) ½ hr	1 hr	2 hr	4 hr	6 hr	8 hr
250 mg	15.5	17	13	5.1	2.5	
500 mg	36.2	36.8	37.9	15.5	6.3	3
1 gm*	60.1	63.8	54.3	29.3	13.2	7.1

*Average of two studies

Clinical pharmacology studies in patients hospitalized with infections indicate that cefazolin produces mean peak serum levels approximately equivalent to those seen in normal volunteers.
In a study (using normal volunteers) of constant intravenous infusion with dosages of 3.5 mg/kg for one hour (approximately 250 mg) and 1.5 mg/kg the next two hours (approximately 100 mg), cefazolin produced a steady serum level at the third hour of approximately 28 mcg/ml. Table 2 shows the average serum concentrations after I.V. injection of a single 1-gm dose; average half-life was 1.4 hours.

TABLE 2. SERUM CONCENTRATIONS AFTER 1-GM INTRAVENOUS DOSE

Serum Concentrations (mcg/ml) 5 min	15 min	30 min	1 hr	2 hr	4 hr
188.4	135.8	106.8	73.7	45.6	16.5

Controlled studies on adult normal volunteers receiving 1 gm four times a day for ten days, monitoring CBC, SGOT, SGPT, bilirubin, alkaline phosphatase, BUN, creatinine, and urinalysis, indicated no clinically significant changes attributed to cefazolin.
Cefazolin is excreted unchanged in the urine. Following intramuscular injection of 500 mg, 56 to 89 percent of the administered dose is recovered within six hours and 80 to nearly 100 percent in 24 hours. Cefazolin achieves peak urine concentrations greater than 1000 mcg/ml and 4000 mcg/ml respectively following 500-mg and 1-gm intramuscular doses.
When cefazolin is administered to patients with unobstructed biliary tracts, high concentrations well over serum levels occur in the gallbladder tissue and bile. In the presence of obstruction, however, concentration of the antibiotic is considerably lower in bile than in serum.
Cefazolin readily crosses an inflamed synovial membrane, and the concentration of the antibiotic achieved in the joint space is comparable to levels measured in the serum.
Cefazolin readily crosses the placental barrier into the cord blood and amniotic fluid. It is present in very low concentrations in the milk of nursing mothers.
Disc Susceptibility Tests—Quantitative methods that require measurement of zone diameters give the most precise estimates of antibiotic susceptibility. One such procedure *(Am. J. Clin. Pathol., 45:*493, 1966; *Federal Register, 39:*19182-19184, 1974) has been recommended for use with discs for testing susceptibility to cephalosporin-class antibiotics. Interpretations correlate diameters of the disc test with MIC values for Kefzol® (cefazolin sodium, Lilly). With this procedure, a report from the laboratory of "susceptible" indicates that the infecting organism is likely to respond to therapy. A report of "resistant" indicates that the infecting organism is not likely to respond to therapy. A report of "intermediate susceptibility" suggests that the organism would be susceptible if high dosage is used or if the infection is confined to tissues and fluids (e.g., urine) in which high antibiotic levels are attained.

Indications: Kefzol® (cefazolin sodium, Lilly) is indicated in the treatment of the following serious infections due to susceptible organisms:
Respiratory tract infections due to *S. pneumoniae, Klebsiella* species, *H. influenzae, S. aureus* (penicillin-sensitive and penicillin-resistant), and group A beta-hemolytic streptococci
Injectable penicillin G benzathine is considered to be the drug of choice in the treatment and prevention of streptococcal infections, including the prophylaxis of rheumatic fever.
Kefzol is effective in the eradication of streptococci from the nasopharynx; however, data establishing the efficacy of Kefzol in the subsequent prevention of rheumatic fever are not available at present.
Genitourinary tract infections due to *E. coli, P. mirabilis, Klebsiella* species, and some strains of *Enterobacter* and enterococci
Skin and soft-tissue infections due to *S. aureus* (penicillin-sensitive and penicillin-resistant) and group A beta-hemolytic streptococci and other strains of streptococci
Biliary tract infections due to *E. coli,* various strains of streptococci, *P. mirabilis, Klebsiella* species, and *S. aureus*
Bone and joint infections due to *S. aureus*
Septicemia due to *S. pneumoniae, S. aureus* (penicillin-sensitive and penicillin-resistant), *P. mirabilis, E. coli,* and *Klebsiella* species
Endocarditis due to *S. aureus* (penicillin-sensitive and penicillin-resistant) and group A beta-hemolytic streptococci
Appropriate culture and susceptibility studies should be performed to determine susceptibility of the causative organism to Kefzol.
Contraindication: Kefzol® (cefazolin sodium, Lilly) is contraindicated in patients with known allergy to the cephalosporin group of antibiotics.
Warnings: BEFORE CEFAZOLIN THERAPY IS INSTITUTED, CAREFUL INQUIRY SHOULD BE MADE CONCERNING PREVIOUS HYPERSENSITIVITY REACTIONS TO CEPHALOSPORINS AND PENICILLIN. CEPHALOSPORIN C DERIVATIVES SHOULD BE GIVEN CAUTIOUSLY TO PENICILLIN-SENSITIVE PATIENTS.
SERIOUS ACUTE HYPERSENSITIVITY REACTIONS MAY REQUIRE EPINEPHRINE AND OTHER EMERGENCY MEASURES.
There is some clinical and laboratory evidence of partial cross-allergenicity of the penicillins and the cephalosporins. Patients have been reported to have had severe reactions (including anaphylaxis) to both drugs.
Antibiotics, including Kefzol® (cefazolin sodium, Lilly), should be administered cautiously to any patient who has demonstrated some form of allergy, particularly to drugs.
Usage in Pregnancy—Safety of this product for use during pregnancy has not been established.
Usage in Infants—Safety for use in prematures and infants under one month of age has not been established.
Precautions: If an allergic reaction to Kefzol® (cefazolin sodium, Lilly) occurs, the drug should be discontinued and the patient treated with the usual agents (e.g., epinephrine or other pressor amines, antihistamines, or corticosteroids).
Prolonged use of Kefzol may result in the overgrowth of nonsusceptible organisms. Careful clinical observation of the patient is essential. If superinfection occurs during therapy, appropriate measures should be taken.
When Kefzol is administered to patients with low urinary output because of impaired renal function, lower daily dosage is required (see dosage instructions).
A false-positive reaction for glucose in the urine may occur with Benedict's or Fehling's solution or with Clinitest® tablets but not with Tes-Tape® (Glucose Enzymatic Test Strip, USP, Lilly).
Adverse Reactions: The following reactions have been reported:
Hypersensitivity—Drug fever, skin rash, vulvar pruritus, and eosinophilia have occurred.
Blood—Neutropenia, leukopenia, thrombocythemia, and positive direct and indirect Coombs tests have occurred.
Hepatic and Renal—Transient rise in SGOT, SGPT, BUN, and alkaline phosphatase levels has been observed without clinical evidence of renal or hepatic impairment.

TABLE 3. DILUTION TABLE

Vial Size	Diluent to Be Added	Approximate Available Volume	Approximate Average Concentration
250 mg	2 ml	2 ml	125 mg/ml
500 mg	2 ml	2.2 ml	225 mg/ml
1 gm	2.5 ml	3 ml	330 mg/ml

Gastrointestinal—Nausea, anorexia, vomiting, diarrhea, and oral candidiasis (oral thrush) have been reported.

Other—Pain on intramuscular injection, sometimes with induration, has occurred infrequently. Phlebitis at the site of injection has been noted. Other reactions have included genital and anal pruritus, genital moniliasis, and vaginitis.

Administration and Dosage: Kefzol® (cefazolin sodium, Lilly) may be administered intramuscularly or intravenously after reconstitution.

Intramuscular Administration—Reconstitute with 0.9% Sodium Chloride Injection, Sterile Water for Injection, or Bacteriostatic Water for Injection according to Table 3. Shake well until dissolved. Kefzol should be injected into a large muscle mass. Pain on injection is infrequent with Kefzol.

[See table above].

Intravenous Administration—Kefzol® (cefazolin sodium, Lilly) may be administered by intravenous injection or by continuous or intermittent infusion. Total daily dosages are the same as with intramuscular injection.

Intermittent intravenous infusion: Kefzol can be administered along with primary intravenous fluid management programs in a volume control set or in a separate, secondary I.V. bottle. Reconstituted 500 mg or 1 gm of Kefzol may be diluted in 50 to 100 ml of one of the following intravenous solutions: 0.9% Sodium Chloride Injection, 5% or 10% Dextrose Injection, 5% Dextrose in Lactated Ringer's Injection, 5% Dextrose and 0.9% Sodium Chloride Injection (also may be used with 5% Dextrose and 0.45% or 0.2% Sodium Chloride Injection), Lactated Ringer's Injection, 5% or 10% Invert Sugar in Sterile Water for Injection, Ringer's Injection, Normosol®-M in D5-W, Ionosol® B with Dextrose 5%, or Plasma-Lyte® with 5% Dextrose.

Direct intravenous injection: Dilute the reconstituted 500 mg or 1 gm of Kefzol in a minimum of 10 ml of Sterile Water for Injection. Inject solution slowly over three to five minutes. It may be administered directly into a vein or through the tubing for a patient receiving the above parenteral fluids.

Dosage—The usual adult dosages are given in Table 4.

TABLE 4. USUAL ADULT DOSAGE

Type of Infection	Dose	Frequency
Pneumococcal pneumonia	500 mg	q 12 h
Mild infections caused by susceptible gram-positive cocci	250 to 500 mg	q 8 h
Acute uncomplicated urinary tract infections	1 gm	q 12 h
Moderate to severe infections	500 mg to 1 gm	q 6 to 8 h

Cefazolin has been administered in dosages of 6 to 12 gm per day in life-threatening infections such as endocarditis and septicemia.

In adults with renal impairment, cefazolin is not readily excreted. After a loading dose of 500 mg, the following recommendations for *maintenance dosage* (Table 5) may be used as a guide.

[See table below].

In children, a total daily dosage of 25 to 50 mg/kg (approximately 10 to 20 mg/pound) of body weight, divided into three or four equal doses, is effective for most mild to moderately severe infections (Table 6). Total daily dosage may be increased to 100 mg/kg (45 mg/pound) of body weight for severe infections.

In children with mild to moderate impairment (creatinine clearance of 70 to 40 ml/min), 60 percent of the normal daily dose given in divided doses every 12 hours should be sufficient. In patients with moderate impairment (creatinine clearance of 40 to 20 ml/min), 25 percent of the normal daily dose given in divided doses every 12 hours should be sufficient. In children with severe impairment (creatinine clearance of 20 to 5 ml/min), 10 percent of the normal daily dose given every 24 hours should be adequate. All dosage recommendations apply after an initial loading dose.

TABLE 6. PEDIATRIC DOSAGE GUIDE

Weight		25 mg/kg/Day Divided into 3 Doses		25 mg/kg/Day Divided into 4 Doses	
lb	kg	Approximate Single Dose (mg q 8 h)	Vol. (ml) Needed with Dilution of 125 mg/ml	Approximate Single Dose (mg q 6 h)	Vol. (ml) Needed with Dilution of 125 mg/ml
10	4.5	40 mg	0.35 ml	30 mg	0.25 ml
20	9	75 mg	0.6 ml	55 mg	0.45 ml
30	13.6	115 mg	0.9 ml	85 mg	0.7 ml
40	18.1	150 mg	1.2 ml	115 mg	0.9 ml
50	22.7	190 mg	1.5 ml	140 mg	1.1 ml

Weight		50 mg/kg/Day Divided into 3 Doses		50 mg/kg/Day Divided into 4 Doses	
lb	kg	Approximate Single Dose (mg q 8 h)	Vol. (ml) Needed with Dilution of 225 mg/ml	Approximate Single Dose (mg q 6 h)	Vol. (ml) Needed with Dilution of 255 mg/ml
10	4.5	75 mg	0.35 ml	55 mg	0.25 ml
20	9	150 mg	0.7 ml	110 mg	0.5 ml
30	13.6	225 mg	1 ml	170 mg	0.75 ml
40	18.1	300 mg	1.35 ml	225 mg	1 ml
50	22.7	375 mg	1.7 ml	285 mg	1.25 ml

Since safety for use in premature infants and in infants under one month of age has not been established, the use of Kefzol in these patients is not recommended.

Stability: Reconstituted Kefzol® (cefazolin sodium, Lilly) and dilutions of Kefzol in the recommended intravenous fluids are stable for 24 hours at room temperature and for 96 hours if stored under refrigeration (5°C).

Solutions of Kefzol in Sterile Water for Injection, 5% Dextrose Injection, or 0.9% Sodium Chloride Injection that are frozen immediately after reconstitution in the original container are stable for as long as 12 weeks when stored at −20°C. **If the product is warmed, care should be taken to avoid heating it after the thawing is complete. Once thawed, the solution should not be refrozen.**

How Supplied: (℞) *Ampoules (Vials) Kefzol® (Sterile Cefazolin Sodium, USP),* rubber-stoppered (Dry Powder): *No. 766,* 250 mg (equivalent to cefazolin), 10-ml size, in singles (10 per carton); *No. 767,* 500 mg (equivalent to cefazolin), and *No. 768,* 1 gm (equivalent to cefazolin), 10-ml size, in singles (10 per carton) and in Traypaks™ (multivial cartons, Lilly) of 25; *No. 7018,* 500 mg (equivalent to cefazolin), and *No. 7011,* 1 gm (equivalent to cefazolin), 100-ml size, in singles (10 per carton) and in Traypaks of 10; *No. 7014,* 10 gm (equivalent to cefazolin), 100-ml size, in Traypaks of 6.

(℞) *Redi Vial® (dual compartment vial, Lilly) Kefzol® (cefazolin sodium, Lilly): No. 7082,* 500 mg (equivalent to cefazolin), and *No. 7083,* 1 gm (equivalent to cefazolin), in singles (10 per carton) and in Traypaks of 10. [070579]

LENTE® ILETIN® (insulin zinc suspension, Lilly), *see under* Iletin® (insulin, Lilly).

Continued on next page

TABLE 5. MAINTENANCE DOSAGE OF KEFZOL® (CEFAZOLIN SODIUM) IN ADULTS WITH REDUCED RENAL FUNCTION

Renal Function	BUN* (mg %)	Creatinine Clearance (ml/min)	Dosage: Mild to Moderate Infection	Dosage: Moderate to Severe Infection	Serum Half-Life (Hours)
Mild impairment	20–34	70–40	250 to 500 mg q 12 h	500 mg to 1.25 gm q 12 h	3–5
Moderate impairment	35–49	40–20	125 to 250 mg q 12 h	250 to 600 mg q 12 h	6–12
Severe impairment	50–75	20–5	75 to 150 mg q 24 h	150 to 400 mg q 24 h	15–30
Essentially no function	>75	<5	37.5 to 75 mg q 24 h	75 to 200 mg q 24 h	30–40

*If used to estimate degree of renal impairment, BUN concentrations should reflect a steady state of renal azotemia.

*Identi-Code® symbol.

Lilly—Cont.

LORIDINE® ℞
(cephaloridine)
Sterile, NF

Because of nephrotoxicity (e.g., tubular necrosis) of cephaloridine in dosages above 4 gm daily (*see* Warnings and Adverse Reactions), recommended doses should not be exceeded. Renal status of the patient should be determined prior to initiation of therapy. Patients with known or suspected impairment of renal function should be under close clinical observation for changes in renal function or be hospitalized, and reduced dosage should be employed. If impaired renal function develops during therapy, cephaloridine should be discontinued.

Description: Loridine® (cephaloridine, Lilly) is a semisynthetic cephalosporin antibiotic intended for parenteral administration. It is 7-(thiophene-2-acetamido)-3-(1-pyridylmethyl)-3-cephem-4-carboxylic acid betaine. Loridine is relatively painless when injected intramuscularly. It contains neither inorganic anions nor cations.

Actions: *Human Pharmacology*—Peak blood levels of 7 and 14 mcg per ml respectively were obtained in one-half to one hour following intramuscular doses of 250 and 500 mg in humans. Measurable levels of cephaloridine persisted for longer than 12 hours.

Loridine® (cephaloridine, Lilly) is excreted unchanged largely by glomerular filtration. Doses of 250 and 500 mg produced very high antibacterial concentrations in the urine, in some instances approaching 1000 mcg per ml. Its nucleus and degradation products differ from those of penicillin. However, some patients who are allergic to penicillin or to other cephalosporins may also be allergic to Loridine.

Microbiology—The in vitro bactericidal action of Loridine results from inhibition of cell-wall synthesis. It is not bound significantly to plasma protein.

Loridine is active against the following organisms in vitro:

- Beta-hemolytic and other streptococci (many strains of enterococci, e.g., *Streptococcus faecalis*, are relatively resistant)
- Staphylococci, both coagulase-positive and coagulase-negative (some strains of staphylococci are resistant to cephaloridine)
- Pneumococci
- Gonococci
- *Haemophilus influenzae*
- *Escherichia coli* and other coliform bacteria
- *Klebsiella*
- *Proteus mirabilis*

Loridine® (cephaloridine, Lilly) is active against *Treponema pallidum* in animal studies.

All tested strains of group A streptococci, pneumococci, and penicillin-G-susceptible staphylococci are susceptible to Loridine. However, some strains of penicillinase-producing staphylococci are resistant in vitro to concentrations of Loridine that can be achieved in the serum. The majority of strains of *H. influenzae, P. mirabilis, E. coli,* and *Klebsiella* are also susceptible in vitro.

Pseudomonas organisms are resistant to Loridine, as are most indole-producing *Proteus* species and motile *Enterobacter* species.

Susceptibility Plate Tests—If the Bauer-Kirby-Sherris-Turck method of disc susceptibility testing is used (*Am. J. Clin. Pathol., 45:*493, 1966; *Federal Register, 39:*19182–19184, 1974), a disc containing 30 mcg cephalothin should give a zone of over 17 mm when tested against a bacterial strain susceptible to cephalothin or cephaloridine and a zone of over 14 mm with an organism of intermediate susceptibility.

Indications: Loridine® (cephaloridine, Lilly) is indicated in the treatment of serious infections of the respiratory tract, genitourinary tract, bones and joints, bloodstream, soft tissue, and skin due to susceptible strains of the organisms listed above. It is also indicated for therapy of early syphilis when penicillin may be contraindicated. (*See* Warnings in regard to cross-sensitivity with penicillin.) It is indicated in the treatment of gonorrhea when penicillin is not considered the drug of choice.

Appropriate culture and susceptibility studies should be performed. If the susceptibility tests show that the causative organism is resistant to Loridine, other appropriate antibiotic therapy should be instituted.

Contraindication: Loridine® (cephaloridine, Lilly) is contraindicated in those persons who have shown hypersensitivity to it or other cephalosporins.

Warnings: BEFORE CEPHALORIDINE THERAPY IS INSTITUTED, CAREFUL INQUIRY SHOULD BE MADE CONCERNING PREVIOUS HYPERSENSITIVITY REACTIONS TO CEPHALOSPORINS AND PENICILLIN. CEPHALOSPORIN C DERIVATIVES SHOULD BE GIVEN CAUTIOUSLY TO PENICILLIN-SENSITIVE PATIENTS.

SERIOUS ACUTE HYPERSENSITIVITY REACTIONS MAY REQUIRE EPINEPHRINE AND OTHER EMERGENCY MEASURES.

There is some clinical and laboratory evidence of partial cross-allergenicity of the penicillins and the cephalosporins. Patients have been reported to have had severe reactions (including anaphylaxis) to both drugs.

Antibiotics, including Loridine® (cephaloridine, Lilly), should be administered cautiously to any patient who has demonstrated some form of allergy, particularly to drugs.

Impairment of renal function during treatment may be indicated by the appearance of casts in the urine, proteinuria, falling urinary output, a rising BUN or serum creatinine, or a decreasing creatinine clearance or urine/plasma creatinine ratio.

Cephaloridine should be given cautiously when used with other antibiotics having nephrotoxic potential, e.g., tobramycin, gentamicin, kanamycin, polymyxin B, and colistin.

The results of experimental studies in animals suggest that the concurrent use of potent diuretics, such as furosemide or ethacrynic acid, may increase the risk of renal toxicity.

Usage in Pregnancy—Safety of this product for use during pregnancy has not been established.

DILUTION TABLE

Diluent Added to 1-gm Vial	Volume of Loridine Solution	Concentration (Approx.)
2.5 ml	3.3 ml	300 mg per ml
10 ml	10.8 ml	100 mg per ml

Diluent Added to 500-mg Vial	Volume of Loridine Solution	Concentration (Approx.)
2 ml	2.4 ml	200 mg per ml
5 ml	5.4 ml	100 mg per ml

Precautions: In the case of infections due to beta-hemolytic streptococci, antibiotic therapy should be continued for at least ten days.

In the therapy of gonorrhea, patients in whom there is reason to suspect concomitant syphilis should have darkfield examinations of all suspect lesions before treatment and monthly serologic tests for a minimum of three months.

Indicated surgical procedures should be performed in conjunction with antibiotic therapy.

Superinfections may develop with organisms not in the spectrum of Loridine® (cephaloridine, Lilly), particularly *Pseudomonas*. These can be recognized by clinical observation and by means of appropriate cultures. If they occur, proper therapeutic measures should be taken.

Since safety for use in premature infants and in infants under one month of age has not been established, the use of cephaloridine in these patients is not recommended.

A false-positive reaction for glucose in the urine may occur with Benedict's or Fehling's solution or with Clinitest® tablets but not with Tes-Tape® (Glucose Enzymatic Test Strip, USP, Lilly).

Adverse Reactions: *Hypersensitivity*—Maculopapular and erythematous rashes, urticaria, and anaphylaxis have been reported. Drug fever and eosinophilia also have been noted. Hypersensitivity reactions are more likely to occur in patients with a history of allergy, particularly to penicillin.

Blood—Neutropenia and leukopenia have been reported. Some individuals have developed positive direct Coombs tests during therapy.

Liver—Transient elevations of transaminase and alkaline phosphatase levels have been noted. The significance of these findings is uncertain.

Renal—Severe, acute renal failure, in some cases terminating in death, has occurred in a small number of patients receiving Loridine® (cephaloridine, Lilly). The possibility of this complication seems to be greater in seriously ill patients given more than recommended doses. Acute tubular necrosis has been noted in affected patients coming to autopsy.

Local Reactions—Pain on I.M. injection of Loridine is rare, and phlebitis on I.V. injection occurs infrequently.

Other—Nausea and vomiting have been reported.

Administration and Dosage: Vials should be protected from light. Extemporaneous mixtures of Loridine® (cephaloridine, Lilly) with other antibiotics are not recommended.

Loridine should be dissolved in either 0.9% Sodium Chloride Injection or Sterile Water for Injection. If a diluent containing preservative is to be used, Bacteriostatic Sodium Chloride Injection, USP, containing benzyl alcohol as a preservative, is recommended. Diluents containing parabens may be incompatible with Loridine.

Solution will be facilitated if the vial is warmed (in the hand) to body temperature. The fresh solution may have a pale straw color. If necessary, the solution may be stored 96 hours (four days) under refrigeration. Thereafter, the unused portion should be discarded. Any recrystallization that forms can be dissolved by warming the vial in the hand and shaking the solution.

Dilution—The diluent, previously warmed to body temperature, is added to the contents of the appropriate vial. Shake until dissolved and inject promptly. If recrystallization occurs prior to injection, warm vial in the hand and shake until the crystals are dissolved. For a 1-gm dose, add 2.5 ml to the 1-gm vial. For a 500-mg dose, add 2 ml to the 500-mg vial. (*See* Dilution Table.)

[See table at left].

Intramuscular Injection—Loridine® (cephaloridine, Lilly) is usually injected into a large muscle mass, for example, the gluteal region or the lateral aspect of the thigh.

The usual adult dosage for many infections of moderate severity is 500 mg to 1 gm three times a day at equally spaced intervals. Milder and more susceptible infections have been treated with 250 to 500 mg given two or three times a day. More severe infections may be treated with 500 mg to 1 gm four times a day. A single 2-gm dose is recommended for the treatment of acute gonorrhea.

Early syphilis may be treated with 500 mg to 1 gm daily for ten to 14 days.

Although some clinical experience with high doses for life-threatening conditions has been reported, it has been shown that excessive dosages (above 4 gm daily) may cause serious nephrotoxic reactions. For this reason, Keflin® (cephalothin sodium, Lilly) may be preferred when doses larger than 4 gm daily are considered for life-threatening situations. If more than 2 gm of cephaloridine is injected daily, the patient should be under close clinical observation for changes in renal function or be hospitalized. In addition, reduced dosage should be employed in patients with known or suspected renal impairment.

In adults with renal impairment, the recommendations for *maintenance dosage* after a *loading dose* of 500 mg to 1 gm may be used as an approximate guide (*see* accompanying chart). The serum concentrations achievable with these reduced dosages will approximate those obtainable with 1.5 to 4 gm daily in patients with normal renal function. If possible, serum concentrations should be monitored. Concentrations above 75 mcg per ml should be avoided by appropriate adjustment of dosage. (See table at right)

In children, a daily total of 30 to 50 mg per kg (15 to 25 mg per pound) of body weight, given in divided doses, has been found effective for mild to moderately severe infections. A daily total of 100 mg per kg (50 mg per pound) of body weight (not to exceed recommended adult doses) may be needed for very severe infections. Since safety for use in premature infants and in infants under one month of age has not been established, the use of cephaloridine in these patients is not recommended.

In both adults and children, failures have appeared to be related more closely to insusceptibility of the organism or poor general condition of the patient than to inadequate dosage.

Intravenous Injection—In the presence of extremely serious infections (such as bacteremia) or when any infection seems overwhelming, intravenous administration may be indicated. Total daily dosages are the same as with intramuscular injection. For very susceptible organisms, 500 mg to 1.5 gm per day may suffice; for less susceptible organisms and for serious infections, 2 to 4 gm per day may be needed.

If the physician desires very high intermittent levels of antibiotic, 500 mg or 1 gm of Loridine dissolved respectively in 5 or 10 ml of diluent (*see* Dilution Table) may be injected slowly (over a three or four-minute period three or four times daily) directly into a vein or into the tubing through which the patient is receiving intravenous fluids. Continuous infusion is obtained by adding the total daily dose to the daily volume of fluid being administered intravenously. Loridine is compatible with distilled water, normal saline, or dextrose solutions.

How Supplied: (℞)*Ampoules (Vials) Loridine® (Sterile Cephaloridine, NF)*, rubber-stoppered (Dry Powder): *No. 722*, 500 mg, 10-ml size, and *No. 723*, 1 gm, 10-ml size, in singles (10 per carton). [041779]

APPROXIMATELY EQUIVALENT MAINTENANCE DOSAGES OF CEPHALORIDINE IN RENAL IMPAIRMENT*

Renal Function	Dosage Schedules: Usual Dosage Range			Dosage Schedules: Maximum Dose	Serum Half-Life (Hours)
Normal $C_{cr} > 80$ ml/min BUN < 20 mg% Serum Cr < 1.4 mg%	1.5 gm/day	2 gm/day	3 gm/day	4 gm/day	1.2–1.8
	(For normal schedule, see discussion above)				
Slight Impairment C_{cr} = 80–60 ml/min BUN = 20–24 mg% Serum Cr = 1.4–1.6 mg%	0.4 gm q 8 h	0.5 gm q 8 h	0.75 gm q 8 h	1 gm q 8 h	2–2.5
Mild to Moderate Impairment C_{cr} = 60–40 ml/min BUN = 25–34 mg% Serum Cr = 1.7–2 mg%	0.4 gm q 12 h	0.5 gm q 12 h	0.75 gm q 12 h	1 gm q 12 h	3–4
Moderate Impairment C_{cr} = 40–20 ml/min BUN = 35–49 mg% Serum Cr = 2.1–3.5 mg%	0.25 gm q 12 h	0.3 gm q 12 h	0.5 gm q 12 h	0.6 gm q 12 h	5–8
Marked Impairment C_{cr} = 20–5 ml/min BUN = 50–75 mg% Serum Cr = 3.6–7 mg%	0.25 gm q 24 h	0.3 gm q 24 h	0.5 gm q 24 h	0.6 gm q 24 h	9–14
Essentially No Function $C_{cr} < 5$ ml/min BUN > 75 mg% Serum Cr > 7 mg%	0.25 gm q 48 h†	0.3 gm q 48 h†	0.5 gm q 48 h†	0.6 gm q 48 h†	15–24

*If used to estimate degree of impaired glomerular function, elevated BUN and serum creatinine concentrations should reflect a steady state of renal azotemia.

†When dialysis is not being performed.

MANDOL® ℞

(cefamandole nafate)
For Injection

Description: Mandol® (cefamandole nafate, Lilly) is a semisynthetic broad-spectrum cephalosporin antibiotic for parenteral administration. It is the sodium salt of 7-D-mandelamido-3-[[(1-methyl-1*H*-tetrazol-5-yl)-thio]-methyl]-3-cephem-4-carboxylic acid, formate (ester). Mandol also contains 63 mg sodium carbonate per gm of cefamandole activity. The total sodium content is approximately 77 mg (3.3 mEq sodium ion) per gm of cefamandole activity. After addition of diluent, cefamandole nafate rapidly hydrolyzes to cefamandole, and both compounds have microbiologic activity in vivo. Solutions of Mandol range from light-yellow to amber, depending on concentration and diluent used. The *p*H of freshly reconstituted solutions usually ranges from 6.0 to 8.5.

Actions: *Clinical Pharmacology*—After intramuscular administration of a 500-mg dose of cefamandole to normal volunteers, the mean peak serum concentration was 13 mcg/ml. After a 1-gm dose, the mean peak concentration was 25 mcg/ml. These peaks occurred at 30 to 120 minutes. Following intravenous doses of 1, 2, and 3 gm, serum concentrations were 139, 240, and 533 mcg/ml respectively at ten minutes. These concentrations declined to 0.8, 2.2, and 2.9 mcg/ml at four hours. Intravenous administration of 4-gm doses every six hours produced no evidence of accumulation in the serum. The half-life after an intravenous dose is 32 minutes; after intramuscular administration, the half-life is 60 minutes.

Sixty-five to 85 percent of cefamandole is excreted by the kidneys over an eight-hour period, resulting in high urinary concentrations. Following intramuscular doses of 500 mg and 1 gm, urinary concentrations averaged 254 and 1357 mcg/ml respectively. Intravenous doses of 1 and 2 gm produced urinary levels averaging 750 and 1380 mcg/ml respectively. Probenecid slows tubular excretion and doubles the peak serum level and the duration of measurable serum concentrations.

The antibiotic reaches therapeutic levels in pleural and joint fluids and in bile and bone.

Microbiology—The bactericidal action of cefamandole results from inhibition of cell-wall synthesis. Cephalosporins have in vitro activity against a wide range of gram-positive and gram-negative organisms. Cefamandole is usually active against the following organisms in vitro and in clinical infections:

Gram-positive
- *Staphylococcus aureus,* including penicillinase and non-penicillinase-producing strains
- *S. epidermidis*
- Beta-hemolytic and other streptococci (Most strains of enterococci, e.g., *Streptococcus faecalis,* are resistant.)
- *S. pneumoniae* (formerly *Diplococcus pneumoniae*)

Gram-negative
- *Escherichia coli*
- *Klebsiella* species
- *Enterobacter* species (Initially susceptible organisms occasionally may become resistant during therapy.)
- *Haemophilus influenzae*
- *Proteus mirabilis*
- *P. rettgeri*
- *P. morganii*
- *P. vulgaris* (Some strains of *P. vulgaris* have been shown by in vitro tests to be resistant to cefamandole and other cephalosporins.)

Continued on next page

*Identi-Code® symbol.

Lilly—Cont.

Anaerobic organisms
- Gram-positive and gram-negative cocci (including *Peptococcus* and *Peptostreptococcus* species)
- Gram-positive bacilli (including *Clostridium* species)
- Gram-negative bacilli (including *Bacteroides* and *Fusobacterium* species). Most strains of *Bacteroides fragilis* are resistant.

Pseudomonas, Acinetobacter calcoaceticus (formerly *Mima* and *Herellea* species), and most *Serratia* strains are resistant to cephalosporins. Cefamandole is resistant to degradation by beta-lactamases from certain members of the *Enterobacteriaceae.*

Susceptibility Tests—Quantitative methods that require measurement of zone diameters give the most precise estimates of antibiotic susceptibility. One such procedure[1] has been recommended for use with discs to test susceptibility to cefamandole. Interpretation involves correlation of the diameters obtained in the disc test with minimum inhibitory concentration (MIC) values for cefamandole.

Reports from the laboratory giving results of the standardized single-disc susceptibility test[1] using a 30-mcg cefamandole disc should be interpreted according to the following criteria:
- Susceptible organisms produce zones of 18 mm or greater, indicating that the tested organism is likely to respond to therapy.
- Organisms of intermediate susceptibility produce zones of 15 to 17 mm, indicating that the tested organism would be susceptible if high dosage is used or if the infection is confined to tissues and fluids (e.g., urine), in which high antibiotic levels are attained.
- Resistant organisms produce zones of 14 mm or less, indicating that other therapy should be selected.

For gram-positive isolates, the test may be performed with either the cephalosporin-class disc (30 mcg cephalothin) or the cefamandole disc (30 mcg cefamandole), and a zone of 18 mm is indicative of a cefamandole-susceptible organism.

Gram-negative organisms should be tested with the cefamandole disc (using the above criteria), since cefamandole has been shown by in vitro tests to have activity against certain strains of *Enterobacteriaceae* found resistant when tested with the cephalosporin-class disc. Gram-negative organisms having zones of less than 18 mm around the cephalothin disc are not necessarily of intermediate susceptibility or resistant to cefamandole.

The cefamandole disc should not be used for testing susceptibility to other cephalosporins.

A bacterial isolate may be considered susceptible if the MIC value for cefamandole[2] is not more than 16 mcg/ml. Organisms are considered resistant if the MIC is greater than 32 mcg/ml.

Indications and Usage: Mandol® (cefamandole nafate, Lilly) is indicated for the treatment of serious infections caused by susceptible strains of the designated microorganisms in the diseases listed below:
- Lower respiratory infections, including pneumonia caused by *S. pneumoniae (D. pneumoniae), H. influenzae, Klebsiella* species, *S. aureus* (penicillinase and non-penicillinase-producing), beta-hemolytic streptococci, and *P. mirabilis*
- Urinary tract infections caused by *E. coli, Proteus* species (both indole-negative and indole-positive), *Enterobacter* species, *Klebsiella* species, group D streptococci (*Note:* Most enterococci, e.g., *S. faecalis,* are resistant), and *S. epidermidis*
- Peritonitis caused by *E. coli* and *Enterobacter* species
- Septicemia caused by *E. coli, S. aureus* (penicillinase and non-penicillinase-producing), *S. pneumoniae, S. pyogenes* (group A beta-hemolytic streptococci), *H. influenzae,* and *Klebsiella* species
- Skin and skin-structure infections caused by *S. aureus* (penicillinase and non-penicillinase-producing), *S. pyogenes* (group A beta-hemolytic streptococci), *H. influenzae, E. coli, Enterobacter* species, and *P. mirabilis*
- Bone and joint infections caused by *S. aureus* (penicillinase and non-penicillinase-producing)

Clinical microbiologic studies in nongonococcal pelvic inflammatory disease in females, lower respiratory infections, and skin infections frequently reveal the growth of susceptible strains of both aerobic and anaerobic organisms. Mandol has been used successfully in these infections in which several organisms have been isolated. Most strains of *B. fragilis* are resistant in vitro; however, infections caused by susceptible strains have been treated successfully.

Specimens for bacteriologic cultures should be obtained in order to isolate and identify causative organisms and to determine their susceptibilities to cefamandole. Therapy may be instituted before results of susceptibility studies are known; however, once these results become available, the antibiotic treatment should be adjusted accordingly.

In certain cases of confirmed or suspected gram-positive or gram-negative sepsis or in patients with other serious infections in which the causative organism has not been identified, Mandol may be used concomitantly with an aminoglycoside (*see* Precautions). The recommended doses of both antibiotics may be given, depending on the severity of the infection and the patient's condition. The renal function of the patient should be carefully monitored, especially if higher dosages of the antibiotics are to be administered.

Antibiotic therapy of beta-hemolytic streptococcal infections should continue for at least ten days.

Contraindication: Mandol® (cefamandole nafate, Lilly) is contraindicated in patients with known allergy to the cephalosporin group of antibiotics.

Warnings: BEFORE THERAPY WITH MANDOL® (cefamandole nafate, Lilly) IS INSTITUTED, CAREFUL INQUIRY SHOULD BE MADE TO DETERMINE WHETHER THE PATIENT HAS HAD PREVIOUS HYPERSENSITIVITY REACTIONS TO CEPHALOSPORINS, PENICILLINS, OR OTHER DRUGS. THIS PRODUCT SHOULD BE GIVEN CAUTIOUSLY TO PENICILLIN-SENSITIVE PATIENTS. ANTIBIOTICS SHOULD BE ADMINISTERED WITH CAUTION TO ANY PATIENT WHO HAS DEMONSTRATED SOME FORM OF ALLERGY, PARTICULARLY TO DRUGS. SERIOUS ACUTE HYPERSENSITIVITY REACTIONS MAY REQUIRE EPINEPHRINE AND OTHER EMERGENCY MEASURES.

In newborn infants, accumulation of other cephalosporin-class antibiotics (with resulting prolongation of drug half-life) has been reported.

Precautions: Although Mandol® (cefamandole nafate, Lilly) rarely produces alteration in kidney function, evaluation of renal status is recommended, especially in seriously ill patients receiving maximum doses.

Prolonged use of Mandol may result in the overgrowth of nonsusceptible organisms. Careful observation of the patient is essential. If superinfection occurs during therapy, appropriate measures should be taken.

Nephrotoxicity has been reported following concomitant administration of aminoglycoside antibiotics and cephalosporins.

A false-positive reaction for glucose in the urine may occur with Benedict's or Fehling's solution or with Clinitest® tablets but not with Tes-Tape® (Glucose Enzymatic Test Strip, USP, Lilly). There may be a false-positive test for proteinuria with acid and denaturization-precipitation tests.

As with other broad-spectrum antibiotics, hypoprothrombinemia, with or without bleeding, has been reported rarely, but it has been promptly reversed by administration of vitamin K. Such episodes usually have occurred in elderly, debilitated, or otherwise compromised patients with deficient stores of vitamin K. Treatment of such individuals with antibiotics possessing significant gram-negative and/or anaerobic activity is thought to alter the number and/or type of intestinal bacterial flora, with consequent reduction in synthesis of vitamin K. Prophylactic administration of vitamin K may be indicated in such patients, especially when intestinal sterilization and surgical procedures are performed.

Usage in Pregnancy—Safety of this product for use during pregnancy has not been established.

Usage in Infancy—Mandol has been effectively used in this age group, but all laboratory parameters have not been extensively studied in infants between one and six months of age; safety of this product has not been established in prematures and infants under one month of age. Therefore, if Mandol is administered to infants, the physician should determine whether the potential benefits outweigh the possible risks involved.

Adverse Reactions: *Hypersensitivity*—Maculopapular rash, urticaria, eosinophilia, and drug fever have been reported. These reactions are more likely to occur in patients with a history of allergy, particularly to penicillin.

Blood—Thrombocytopenia has been reported rarely. Neutropenia has been reported, especially in long courses of treatment. Some individuals have developed positive direct Coombs tests during treatment with the cephalosporin antibiotics.

Liver—Transient rise in SGOT, SGPT, and alkaline phosphatase levels has been noted.

Kidney—Decreased creatinine clearance has been reported in patients with prior renal impairment. As with some other cephalosporins, transitory elevations of BUN have occasionally been observed with Mandol® (cefamandole nafate, Lilly); their frequency increases in patients over 50 years of age. In some of these cases, there was also a mild increase in serum creatinine.

Local Reactions—Pain on intramuscular injection is infrequent. Thrombophlebitis occurs rarely.

Administration and Dosage: *Dosage—Adults:* The usual dosage range for cefamandole is 500 mg to 1 gm every four to eight hours. In infections of skin structures and in uncomplicated pneumonia, a dosage of 500 mg every six hours in adequate.

In uncomplicated urinary tract infections, a dosage of 500 mg every eight hours is sufficient. In more serious urinary tract infections, a dosage of 1 gm every eight hours may be needed.

In severe infections, 1-gm doses may be given at four to six-hour intervals.

In life-threatening infections or infections due to less susceptible organisms, doses up to 2 gm every four hours (i.e., 12 gm per day) may be needed.

Infants and Children: Administration of 50 to 100 mg/kg/day in equally divided doses every four to eight hours has been effective for most infections susceptible to Mandol® (cefamandole nafate, Lilly). This may be increased to a total daily dose of 150 mg/kg (not to exceed the maximum adult dose) for severe infections. (*See* Warnings and Precautions for this age group.)

Note: As with antibiotic therapy in general, administration of Mandol should be continued for a minimum of 48 to 72 hours after the patient becomes asymptomatic or after evidence of bacterial eradication has been obtained; a minimum of ten days of treatment is recommended in infections caused by group A beta-hemolytic streptococci in order to guard against the risk of rheumatic fever or glomerulonephritis; frequent bacteriologic and clinical appraisal is necessary during therapy of chronic urinary tract infection and may be required for several months after therapy has been completed; persistent infections may require treatment for several weeks; and doses smaller than those indicated above should not be used.

Impaired Renal Function—When renal function is impaired, a reduced dosage must be employed and the serum levels closely monitored. After an initial dose of 1 to 2 gm (depending on the severity of infection), a maintenance dosage schedule should be followed (see chart). Continued dosage should be determined by degree of renal impairment, severity of infection, and susceptibility of the causative organism.

[See table above].

MAINTENANCE DOSAGE GUIDE FOR PATIENTS WITH RENAL IMPAIRMENT

Creatinine Clearance (ml/min/1.73 m^2)	Renal Function	Life-Threatening Infections—Maximum Dosage	Less Severe Infections
>80	Normal	2 gm q 4 h	1–2 gm q 6 h
80–50	Mild Impairment	1.5 gm q 4 h OR 2 gm q 6 h	0.75–1.5 gm q 6 h
50–25	Moderate Impairment	1.5 gm q 6 h OR 2 gm q 8 h	0.75–1.5 gm q 8 h
25–10	Severe Impairment	1 gm q 6 h OR 1.25 gm q 8 h	0.5–1 gm q 8 h
10–2	Marked Impairment	0.67 gm q 8 h OR 1 gm q 12 h	0.5–0.75 gm q 12 h
<2	None	0.5 gm q 8 h OR 0.75 gm q 12 h	0.25–0.5 gm q 12 h

When only serum creatinine is available, the following formula (based on sex, weight, and age of the patient) may be used to convert this value into creatinine clearance. The serum creatinine should represent a steady state of renal function.

$$\text{Males: } \frac{\text{Weight (kg)} \times (146 - \text{age})}{72 \times \text{serum creatinine}}$$

Females: 0.9 × above value

Modes of Administration—Mandol® (cefamandole nafate, Lilly) may be given intravenously or by deep intramuscular injection into a large muscle mass (such as the gluteus or lateral part of the thigh) to minimize pain.

Intramuscular Administration—Each gm of Mandol should be diluted with 3 ml of one of the following diluents: Sterile Water for Injection, Bacteriostatic Water for Injection, 0.9% Sodium Chloride Injection, or Bacteriostatic Sodium Chloride Injection. Shake well until dissolved.

Intravenous Administration—The intravenous route may be preferable for patients with bacterial septicemia, localized parenchymal abscesses (such as intra-abdominal abscess), peritonitis, or other severe or life-threatening infections when they may be poor risks because of lowered resistance. In those with normal renal function, the intravenous dosage for such infections is 3 to 12 gm of Mandol daily. In conditions such as bacterial septicemia, 6 to 12 gm per day may be given initially by the intravenous route for several days, and dosage may then be gradually reduced according to clinical response and laboratory findings.

If combination therapy with Mandol and an aminoglycoside is indicated, each of these antibiotics should be administered in different sites. *Do not mix an aminoglycoside with Mandol in the same intravenous fluid container.*

A SOLUTION OF 1 GM MANDOL IN 22 ML OF STERILE WATER FOR INJECTION IS ISOTONIC.

The choice of saline, dextrose, or electrolyte solution and the volume to be employed are dictated by fluid and electrolyte management.

For direct intermittent intravenous administration, each gm of cefamandole should be reconstituted with 10 ml of Sterile Water for Injection, 5% Dextrose Injection, or 0.9% Sodium Chloride Injection. Slowly inject the solution into the vein over a period of three to five minutes, or give it through the tubing of an administration set while the patient is also receiving one of the following intravenous fluids:

0.9% Sodium Chloride Injection
5% Dextrose Injection
10% Dextrose Injection
5% Dextrose and 0.9% Sodium Chloride Injection
5% Dextrose and 0.45% Sodium Chloride Injection
5% Dextrose and 0.2% Sodium Chloride Injection
Sodium Lactate Injection (M/6)

Intermittent intravenous infusion with a Y-type administration set or volume control set can also be accomplished while any of the above-mentioned intravenous fluids are being infused. However, during infusion of the solution containing Mandol® (cefamandole nafate, Lilly), it is desirable to discontinue the other solution. When this technique is employed, careful attention should be paid to the volume of the solution containing Mandol so that the calculated dose will be infused. When a Y-tube hookup is used, 100 ml of the appropriate diluent should be added to the 1 or 2-gm piggyback (100-ml) vial. If Sterile Water for Injection is used as the diluent, reconstitute with approximately 20 ml per gm to avoid a hypotonic solution.

For continuous intravenous infusion, each gm of cefamandole should be diluted with 10 ml of Sterile Water for Injection. An appropriate quantity of the resulting solution may be added to an I.V. bottle containing one of the following fluids:

0.9% Sodium Chloride Injection
5% Dextrose Injection
10% Dextrose Injection
5% Dextrose and 0.9% Sodium Chloride Injection
5% Dextrose and 0.45% Sodium Chloride Injection
5% Dextrose and 0.2% Sodium Chloride Injection
Sodium Lactate Injection (M/6)

Stability: Reconstituted Mandol® (cefamandole nafate, Lilly) is stable for 24 hours at room temperature (25°C) and for 96 hours if stored under refrigeration (5°C). *During storage at room temperature, carbon dioxide develops inside the vial after reconstitution. This pressure may be dissipated prior to withdrawal of the vial contents, or it may be used to aid withdrawal if the vial is inverted over the syringe needle and the contents are allowed to flow into the syringe.*

Solutions of Mandol in Sterile Water for Injection, 5% Dextrose Injection, or 0.9% Sodium Chloride Injection that are frozen immediately after reconstitution in the original container are stable for six months when stored at −20°C. If the product is warmed (to a maximum of 37°C), care should be taken to avoid heating it after the thawing is complete. Once thawed, the solution should not be refrozen.

How Supplied: (℞) *Vials Mandol® (cefamandole nafate, Lilly), for Injection,* rubber-stoppered (Dry Powder): *No. 7060,* 500 mg (equivalent to cefamandole activity), and *No. 7061,* 1 gm (equivalent to cefamandole activity), 10-ml size, in singles (10 per carton) and in Traypaks of 25; *No. 7068,* 1 gm (equivalent to cefamandole activity), 100-ml size, in Traypaks of 10; *No. 7064,* 2 gm (equivalent to cefamandole activity), 20-ml size, in singles (10 per carton) and in Traypaks of 10; *No. 7069,* 2 gm (equivalent to cefamandole activity), 100-ml size, in Traypaks of 10. [062679]

1. Bauer, A. W., Kirby, W. M. M., Sherris, J. C., and Turck, M.: Antibiotic Susceptibility Testing by a Standardized Single Disk Method, Am. J. Clin. Pathol., *45*:493, 1966; Standardized Disc Susceptibility Test, Federal Register, *39*:19182-19184, 1974. National Committee for Clinical Laboratory Standards. Approved Standard: ASM-2, Performance Standards for Antimicrobial Disc Susceptibility Tests, July, 1975.
2. Determined by the ICS agar-dilution method (Ericsson, H. M., and Sherris, J. C.: Acta Pathol. Microbiol. Scand. [B], Supplement No. 217, 1971) or any other method that has been shown to give equivalent results.

MERTHIOLATE® OTC
(thimerosal)

Description: Merthiolate is a superior organomercurial antiseptic with long-recognized usefulness in most areas of medicine.

It provides sustained activity against the common pathogens (bacteria and fungi), is relatively nontoxic and nonirritating to body tissues, and maintains activity in high dilution. It is readily soluble in water and is miscible with soap and alcohol. Unlike many other antiseptics, Merthiolate is not inactivated by soaps, cotton materials, or body lipids and proteins.

Continued on next page

Lilly—Cont.

All antiseptics have antagonists that nullify their action. In the case of the mercurial antiseptics, these are the free, active sulfhydryl groups. Their chief source under the artificial conditions of the test tube is thioglycolic acid. In the body, glutathione of the red blood cells has a similar action. Thus, Merthiolate, like other antiseptics, is antagonized by whole blood. However, since the action of Merthiolate, in contrast to that of other antiseptics, is not significantly diminished by plasma, serum, or body fluids in general, it remains effective in the presence of nonsanguineous drainage or discharge.

Merthiolate may also serve as a preservative for serums, antigens, vaccines, arterial grafts, bone, cartilage, antibiotic preparations, and other biological and pharmaceutical products. Merthiolate is supplied in a variety of forms, including cream, glycerite, sterile ophthalmic ointment, powder, aqueous solution, and a specially buffered tincture.

Indications: *Aeropump*—Especially useful in first aid, the treatment of contaminated wounds after appropriate cleansing, antisepsis of intact skin, pustular dermatoses, and dermatomycoses. It is also of value in the presurgical preparation of the skin and in postoperative wound care.

Aeropump Merthiolate may be used whenever external application of Tincture Merthiolate is indicated. Aeropump therapy saves time, eliminates waste, prevents contamination, and obviates direct contact with affected areas.

Cream—For use on the skin when a nonirritating antiseptic preparation easily removed by water is indicated.

Glycerite—For irrigation of open wounds. Particularly suitable for local application to the vagina and cervix.

Sterile Ophthalmic Ointment—For conjunctivitis, corneal ulcer, and prevention of infection following removal of foreign bodies.

Powder—For use as a preservative (see the package literature).

Solution—An aqueous preparation preferred whenever the tincture is contraindicated because of its alcohol-acetone content. When diluted to a 1:5000 solution, Merthiolate may be used in the eye, nose, throat, or genitourinary tract.

Tincture—For antisepsis of the skin prior to surgery and for first-aid treatment of contaminated wounds. Has been used as an antifungal agent in athlete's foot infection.

Contraindications and Precautions: A small group of individuals are hypersensitive to thio or mercuri radicals such as are contained in Merthiolate. The symptoms include erythematous, papular, and vesicular eruptions over the area of application. These persons should avoid contact with Merthiolate.

Prolonged repeated applications of Solution Merthiolate in the mouths of infants should be avoided.

After application, Tincture Merthiolate should be permitted to dry before being covered by bandages or other occlusive dressings. If this is not done, the alcohol and acetone in the solvent may be irritating. Merthiolate is incompatible with strong acids, salts of heavy metals, and iodine and should not be used in combination with or immediately following their application. It may be used with or following soaps or sulfonamides. It should not be used when aluminum may come in contact with treated skin.

Administration and Dosage: Apply locally one to three times a day or as directed by the physician.

Overdosage: The mercury content of Merthiolate is closely bound; apparently it is not split off to an appreciable extent in the gastrointestinal tract or elsewhere in the body.

In over 30 years of widespread use, only rarely have instances of mercury poisoning been reported in relation to products containing Merthiolate. One case involved a three-month-old infant who apparently was exposed to swabbing of the oral mucous membranes with 1:1000 aqueous Merthiolate four to six times daily for five weeks. Symptoms of anorexia and irritability developed after the first three weeks. Lethargy, vomiting, and seizures were manifested during the final two weeks of exposure. Blood and urine mercury levels were found to be abnormally elevated. Another case involved an adult who apparently employed Suppositories Metycaine® Hydrochloride and Merthiolate® (piperocaine hydrochloride and thimerosal, Lilly) rectally each day for approximately five years. Peripheral neuropathy and abnormal urine levels for mercury receded when use of the suppositories was discontinued.

After accidental ingestion of Tincture Merthiolate, account must be taken of the alcohol (50 percent) and acetone (10 percent) content. After accidental ingestion of Solution Merthiolate, account must be taken of the borate content. Solution Merthiolate contains 0.1 percent tetraborate ion ($B_4O_7=$). *Treatment*—Supportive therapy.

How Supplied: *Aeropump™ No. 5100, Merthiolate® (Thimerosal Tincture, NF), 1:1000,* in 6-fl-oz bottles. Contains thimerosal, 0.1 gm, with inert coloring material, in a mixture of alcohol, 52.5 ml; acetone, 10 ml; monoethanolamine, 0.1 gm; ethylenediamine, 0.02 gm; and purified water, q.s. to make 100 ml. Alcohol, 50 percent. *Flammable.*

Cream No. 1, Merthiolate, 1:1000, in 1-oz tubes. Contains thimerosal, 0.1 percent, in a modified vanishing-cream base.

Glycerite No. 10, Merthiolate, 1:1000, in gallon bottles. Each 100 ml contain thimerosal, 100 mg, and monoethanolamine, 100 mg, in Glycerin, USP.

Sterile Ophthalmic Ointment No. 31, Merthiolate, 1:5000, in ⅛-oz tamperproof tubes.

Powder No. 20, Merthiolate® (Thimerosal Powder, NF), in 1-oz bottles.

Solution No. 45, Merthiolate® (Thimerosal Solution, NF), 1:1000, Stainless, in 4-fl-oz, 16-fl-oz, and gallon bottles. *Avoid freezing.*

Tincture No. 99, Merthiolate® (Thimerosal Tincture, NF), 1:1000, in ¾-oz plastic applicator bottles (dozens) and in 4-fl-oz, 16-fl-oz, and gallon bottles. Alcohol, 50 percent. *Flammable.*

[060479]

METHADONE HYDROCHLORIDE Ⓒ
DISKETS® (dispersible tablets, Lilly)
Tablets, USP
(*See also* Dolophine® Hydrochloride)

CONDITIONS FOR DISTRIBUTION AND USE OF METHADONE PRODUCTS:

Code of Federal Regulations,

Title 21, Sec. 310.505

METHADONE PRODUCTS, WHEN USED FOR THE TREATMENT OF NARCOTIC ADDICTION IN DETOXIFICATION OR MAINTENANCE PROGRAMS, SHALL BE DISPENSED ONLY BY APPROVED HOSPITAL PHARMACIES, APPROVED COMMUNITY PHARMACIES, AND MAINTENANCE PROGRAMS APPROVED BY THE FOOD AND DRUG ADMINISTRATION AND THE DESIGNATED STATE AUTHORITY.

APPROVED MAINTENANCE PROGRAMS SHALL DISPENSE AND USE METHADONE IN ORAL FORM ONLY AND ACCORDING TO THE TREATMENT REQUIREMENTS STIPULATED IN THE FEDERAL METHADONE REGULATIONS (21 CFR 310.505).

FAILURE TO ABIDE BY THE REQUIREMENTS IN THESE REGULATIONS MAY RESULT IN CRIMINAL PROSECUTION, SEIZURE OF THE DRUG SUPPLY, REVOCATION OF THE PROGRAM APPROVAL, AND INJUNCTION PRECLUDING OPERATION OF THE PROGRAM.

Description: Methadone Hydrochloride, USP (4, 4- diphenyl -6- dimethylamino - heptanone-3 hydrochloride), is a white crystalline material which is water soluble. However, the Disket preparation of methadone hydrochloride has been specially formulated with insoluble excipients to deter the use of this drug by injection.

Actions: Methadone hydrochloride is a synthetic narcotic analgesic with multiple actions quantitatively similar to those of morphine, the most prominent of which involve the central nervous system and organs composed of smooth muscle. The principal actions of therapeutic value are analgesia and sedation and detoxification or maintenance in narcotic addiction. The methadone abstinence syndrome, although qualitatively similar to that of morphine, differs in that the onset is slower, the course is more prolonged, and the symptoms are less severe.

When administered orally, methadone is approximately one-half as potent as when given parenterally. Oral administration results in a delay of the onset, a lowering of the peak, and an increase in the duration of analgesic effect.

Indications: 1. Detoxification treatment of narcotic addiction (heroin or other morphine-like drugs).

2. Maintenance treatment of narcotic addiction (heroin or other morphine-like drugs), in conjunction with appropriate social and medical services.

NOTE

If methadone is administered for treatment of heroin dependence for more than three weeks, the procedure passes from treatment of the acute withdrawal syndrome (detoxification) to maintenance therapy. Maintenance treatment is permitted to be undertaken only by approved methadone programs. This does not preclude the maintenance treatment of an addict who is hospitalized for medical conditions other than addiction and who requires temporary maintenance during the critical period of his stay or whose enrollment has been verified in a program which has approval for maintenance treatment with methadone.

Contraindication: Hypersensitivity to methadone.

Warnings:

Diskets Methadone Hydrochloride are for oral administration only. This preparation contains insoluble excipients and therefore *must not* be injected. It is recommended that Diskets Methadone Hydrochloride, if dispensed, be packaged in child-resistant containers to prevent accidental ingestion.

Methadone hydrochloride, a narcotic, is a Schedule II controlled substance under the Federal Controlled Substances Act. Appropriate security measures should be taken to safeguard stocks of methadone against diversion.

DRUG DEPENDENCE—METHADONE CAN PRODUCE DRUG DEPENDENCE OF THE MORPHINE TYPE AND, THEREFORE, HAS THE POTENTIAL FOR BEING ABUSED. PSYCHIC DEPENDENCE, PHYSICAL DEPENDENCE, AND TOLERANCE MAY DEVELOP UPON REPEATED ADMINISTRATION OF METHADONE, AND IT SHOULD BE PRESCRIBED

AND ADMINISTERED WITH THE SAME DEGREE OF CAUTION APPROPRIATE TO THE USE OF MORPHINE.

Interaction with Other Central-Nervous-System Depressants—Methadone should be used with caution and in reduced dosage in patients who are concurrently receiving other narcotic analgesics, general anesthetics, phenothiazines, other tranquilizers, sedative-hypnotics, tricyclic antidepressants, and other C.N.S. depressants (including alcohol). Respiratory depression, hypotension, and profound sedation or coma may result.

Anxiety—Since methadone, as used by tolerant subjects at a constant maintenance dosage, is not a tranquilizer, patients who are maintained on this drug will react to life problems and stresses with the same symptoms of anxiety as do other individuals. The physician should not confuse such symptoms with those of narcotic abstinence and should not attempt to treat anxiety by increasing the dosage of methadone. The action of methadone in maintenance treatment is limited to the control of narcotic symptoms and is ineffective for relief of general anxiety.

Head Injury and Increased Intracranial Pressure—The respiratory depressant effects of methadone and its capacity to elevate cerebrospinal-fluid pressure may be markedly exaggerated in the presence of increased intracranial pressure. Furthermore, narcotics produce side effects that may obscure the clinical course of patients with head injuries. In such patients, methadone must be used with caution and only if it is deemed essential.

Asthma and Other Respiratory Conditions—Methadone should be used with caution in patients having an acute asthmatic attack, in those with chronic obstructive pulmonary disease or cor pulmonale, and in individuals with a substantially decreased respiratory reserve, preexisting respiratory depression, hypoxia, or hypercapnia. In such patients, even usual therapeutic doses of narcotics may decrease respiratory drive while simultaneously increasing airway resistance to the point of apnea.

Hypotensive Effect—The administration of methadone may result in severe hypotension in an individual whose ability to maintain his blood pressure has already been compromised by a depleted blood volume or concurrent administration of such drugs as the phenothiazines or certain anesthetics.

Use in Ambulatory Patients—Methadone may impair the mental and/or physical abilities required for the performance of potentially hazardous tasks, such as driving a car or operating machinery. The patient should be cautioned accordingly.

Methadone, like other narcotics, may produce orthostatic hypotension in ambulatory patients.

Use in Pregnancy—Safe use in pregnancy has not been established in relation to possible adverse effects on fetal development. Therefore, methadone should not be used in pregnant women unless, in the judgment of the physician, the potential benefits outweigh the possible hazards.

Precautions: ***Interaction with Pentazocine*—Patients who are addicted to heroin or who are on the methadone maintenance program may experience withdrawal symptoms when given pentazocine.**

Interaction with Rifampin—The concurrent administration of rifampin may possibly reduce the blood concentration of methadone to a degree sufficient to produce withdrawal symptoms. The mechanism by which rifampin may decrease blood concentrations of methadone is not fully understood, although enhanced microsomal drug-metabolized enzymes may influence drug disposition.

Acute Abdominal Conditions—The administration of methadone or other narcotics may obscure the diagnosis or clinical course in patients with acute abdominal conditions.

Interaction with Monoamine Oxidase (MAO) Inhibitors—Therapeutic doses of meperidine have precipitated severe reactions in patients concurrently receiving monoamine oxidase inhibitors or those who have received such agents within 14 days. Similar reactions thus far have not been reported with methadone; but if the use of methadone is necessary in such patients, a sensitivity test should be performed in which repeated small incremental doses are administered over the course of several hours while the patient's condition and vital signs are under careful observation.

Special-Risk Patients—Methadone should be given with caution and the initial dose should be reduced in certain patients, such as the elderly or debilitated and those with severe impairment of hepatic or renal function, hypothyroidism, Addison's disease, prostatic hypertrophy, or urethral stricture.

Adverse Reactions: *Heroin Withdrawal*—During the induction phase of methadone maintenance treatment, patients are being withdrawn from heroin and may therefore show typical withdrawal symptoms, which should be differentiated from methadone-induced side effects. They may exhibit some or all of the following symptoms associated with acute withdrawal from heroin or other opiates: lacrimation, rhinorrhea, sneezing, yawning, excessive perspiration, gooseflesh, fever, chilliness alternating with flushing, restlessness, irritability, "sleepy yen," weakness, anxiety, depression, dilated pupils, tremors, tachycardia, abdominal cramps, body aches, involuntary twitching and kicking movements, anorexia, nausea, vomiting, diarrhea, intestinal spasms, and weight loss.

Initial Administration—Initially, the dosage of methadone should be carefully titrated to the individual. Induction too rapid for the patient's sensitivity is more likely to produce the following effects.

THE MAJOR HAZARDS OF METHADONE, AS OF OTHER NARCOTIC ANALGESICS, ARE RESPIRATORY DEPRESSION AND, TO A LESSER DEGREE, CIRCULATORY DEPRESSION. RESPIRATORY ARREST, SHOCK, AND CARDIAC ARREST HAVE OCCURRED.

The most frequently observed adverse reactions include lightheadedness, dizziness, sedation, nausea, vomiting, and sweating. These effects seem to be more prominent in ambulatory patients and in those who are not suffering severe pain. In such individuals, lower doses are advisable. Some adverse reactions may be alleviated in the ambulatory patient if he lies down.

Other adverse reactions include the following:

Central Nervous System—Euphoria, dysphoria, weakness, headache, insomnia, agitation, disorientation, and visual disturbances.

Gastrointestinal—Dry mouth, anorexia, constipation, and biliary tract spasm.

Cardiovascular—Flushing of the face, bradycardia, palpitation, faintness, and syncope.

Genitourinary—Urinary retention or hesitancy, antidiuretic effect, and reduced libido and/or potency.

Allergic—Pruritus, urticaria, other skin rashes, edema, and, rarely, hemorrhagic urticaria.

Maintenance on a Stabilized Dose—During prolonged administration of methadone, as in a methadone maintenance treatment program, there is a gradual, yet progressive, disappearance of side effects over a period of several weeks. However, constipation and sweating often persist.

Administration and Dosage: *For Detoxification Treatment*—THE DRUG SHALL BE ADMINISTERED DAILY UNDER CLOSE SUPERVISION AS FOLLOWS:

A detoxification treatment course shall not exceed 21 days and may not be repeated earlier than four weeks after completion of the preceding course.

In detoxification, the patient may receive methadone when there are significant symptoms of withdrawal. The dosage schedules indicated below are recommended but could be varied in accordance with clinical judgment. Initially, a single oral dose of 15 to 20 mg of methadone will often be sufficient to suppress withdrawal symptoms. Additional methadone may be provided if withdrawal symptoms are not suppressed or if symptoms reappear. When patients are physically dependent on high doses, it may be necessary to exceed these levels. Forty mg per day in single or divided doses will usually constitute an adequate stabilizing dosage level. Stabilization can be continued for two to three days, and then the amount of methadone normally will be gradually decreased. The rate at which methadone is decreased will be determined separately for each patient. The dose of methadone can be decreased on a daily basis or at two-day intervals, but the amount of intake shall always be sufficient to keep withdrawal symptoms at a tolerable level. In hospitalized patients, a daily reduction of 20 percent of the total daily dose may be tolerated and may cause little discomfort. In ambulatory patients, a somewhat slower schedule may be needed. If methadone is administered for more than three weeks, the procedure is considered to have progressed from detoxification or treatment of the acute withdrawal syndrome to maintenance treatment, even though the goal and intent may be eventual total withdrawal.

For Maintenance Treatment—In maintenance treatment, the initial dosage of methadone should control the abstinence symptoms that follow withdrawal of narcotic drugs but should not be so great as to cause sedation, respiratory depression, or other effects of acute intoxication. It is important that the initial dosage be adjusted on an individual basis to the narcotic tolerance of the new patient. If such a patient has been a heavy user of heroin up to the day of admission, he may be given 20 mg four to eight hours later or 40 mg in a single oral dose. If he enters treatment with little or no narcotic tolerance (e.g., if he has recently been released from jail or other confinement), the initial dosage may be one-half these quantities. When there is any doubt, the smaller dose should be used initially. The patient should then be kept under observation, and, if symptoms of abstinence are distressing, additional 10-mg doses may be administered as needed. Subsequently, the dosage should be adjusted individually, as tolerated and required, up to a level of 120 mg daily. The patient will initially ingest the drug under observation daily, or at least six days a week, for the first three months. After demonstrating satisfactory adherence to the program regulations for at least three months, the patient may be permitted to reduce to three times weekly the occasions when he must ingest the drug under observation. He shall receive no more than a two-day take-home supply. With continuing adherence to the program's requirements for at least two years, he may then be permitted twice-weekly visits to the program for drug ingestion under observation, with a three-day take-home supply. A daily dose of 120 mg or more shall be justified in the medical record. Prior approval from state authority and the Food and Drug Administration is required for any dose above 120 mg administered at the clinic and for any dose above 100 mg to be taken at home. A regular review of dosage level should be made by the responsible physician, with careful consideration given to reduction of dosage as indicated on an individual basis. A new dosage level is only a test level until stability is achieved.

Continued on next page

*Identi-Code® symbol.

Lilly—Cont.

Special Considerations for a Pregnant Patient—Caution shall be taken in the maintenance treatment of pregnant patients. Dosage levels shall be kept as low as possible if continued methadone treatment is deemed necessary. It is the responsibility of the program sponsor to assure that each female patient be fully informed concerning the possible risks to a pregnant woman or her unborn child from the use of methadone.

Special Limitations—
Treatment of Patients under Age 18

1. The safety and effectiveness of methadone for use in the treatment of adolescents have not been proved by adequate clinical study. Special procedures are therefore necessary to assure that patients under age 16 will not be admitted to a program and that patients between 16 and 18 years of age will be admitted to maintenance treatment only under limited conditions.
2. Patients between 16 and 18 years of age who were enrolled and under treatment in approved programs on December 15, 1972, may continue in maintenance treatment. No new patients between 16 and 18 years of age may be admitted to a maintenance treatment program after March 15, 1973, unless a parent, legal guardian, or responsible adult designated by the state authority completes and signs Form FD 2635, "Consent for Methadone Treatment." Methadone treatment of new patients between the ages of 16 and 18 years will be permitted after December 15, 1972, only with a documented history of two or more unsuccessful attempts at detoxification and a documented history of dependence on heroin or other morphine-like drugs beginning two years or more prior to application for treatment. No patient under age 16 may be continued or started on methadone treatment after December 15, 1972, but these patients may be detoxified and retained in the program in a drug-free state for follow-up and aftercare.
3. Patients under age 18 who are not placed on maintenance treatment may be detoxified. Detoxification may not exceed three weeks. A repeat episode of detoxification may not be initiated until four weeks after the completion of the previous detoxification.

Overdosage: *Symptoms*—Serious overdosage of methadone is characterized by respiratory depression (a decrease in respiratory rate and/or tidal volume, Cheyne-Stokes respiration, cyanosis), extreme somnolence progressing to stupor or coma, maximally constricted pupils, skeletal-muscle flaccidity, cold and clammy skin, and, sometimes, bradycardia and hypotension. In severe overdosage, particularly by the intravenous route, apnea, circulatory collapse, cardiac arrest, and death may occur.

Treatment—Primary attention should be given to the reestablishment of adequate respiratory exchange through provision of a patent airway and institution of assisted or controlled ventilation. If a nontolerant person, especially a child, takes a large dose of methadone, effective narcotic antagonists are available to counteract the potentially lethal respiratory depression. **The physician must remember, however, that methadone is a long-acting depressant (36 to 48 hours), whereas the antagonists act for much shorter periods (one to three hours).** The patient must, therefore, be monitored continuously for recurrence of respiratory depression and treated repeatedly with the narcotic antagonist as needed. If the diagnosis is correct and respiratory depression is due only to overdosage of methadone, the use of respiratory stimulants is not indicated.

An antagonist should not be administered in the absence of clinically significant respiratory or cardiovascular depression. Intravenously administered narcotic antagonists (naloxone, nalorphine, and levallorphan) are the drugs of choice to reverse signs of intoxication. These agents should be given repeatedly until the patient's status remains satisfactory. The hazard that the narcotic antagonist will further depress respiration is less likely with the use of naloxone.

Oxygen, intravenous fluids, vasopressors, and other supportive measures should be employed as indicated.

> NOTE: IN AN INDIVIDUAL PHYSICALLY DEPENDENT ON NARCOTICS, THE ADMINISTRATION OF THE USUAL DOSE OF A NARCOTIC ANTAGONIST WILL PRECIPITATE AN ACUTE WITHDRAWAL SYNDROME. THE SEVERITY OF THIS SYNDROME WILL DEPEND ON THE DEGREE OF PHYSICAL DEPENDENCE AND THE DOSE OF THE ANTAGONIST ADMINISTERED. THE USE OF A NARCOTIC ANTAGONIST IN SUCH A PERSON SHOULD BE AVOIDED IF POSSIBLE. IF IT MUST BE USED TO TREAT SERIOUS RESPIRATORY DEPRESSION IN THE PHYSICALLY DEPENDENT PATIENT, THE ANTAGONIST SHOULD BE ADMINISTERED WITH EXTREME CARE AND BY TITRATION WITH SMALLER THAN USUAL DOSES OF THE ANTAGONIST.

How Supplied: (Ⓒ) *Diskets No. 1, Methadone Hydrochloride Tablets, USP, U53,** 40 mg, Peach-Colored (pillow-shaped, cross-scored), in bottles of 100. [121178]

[*Shown in Product Identification Section*]

METUBINE® IODIDE ℞

(metocurine iodide)
Injection, NF

THIS DRUG SHOULD BE ADMINISTERED ONLY BY ADEQUATELY TRAINED INDIVIDUALS WHO ARE FAMILIAR WITH ITS ACTIONS, CHARACTERISTICS, AND HAZARDS.

Description: Metubine® Iodide (Metocurine Iodide Injection, NF, Lilly) is a sterile isotonic solution for intravenous injection.

Each ml contains 2 mg metocurine iodide and sodium chloride, 0.9 percent, with 0.5 percent phenol as a preservative. Sodium carbonate and/or hydrochloric acid may have been added during manufacture to adjust the *p*H.

Actions: Metubine® Iodide (metocurine iodide, Lilly) blocks nerve impulses to skeletal muscles at the myoneural junction. This is a nondepolarizing neuromuscular blockade. When it is administered intravenously (intramuscular injection is unpredictable), the onset of flaccid paralysis occurs within a few minutes.

Muscle paralysis may be expected for periods of 25 to 90 minutes. The use of repeated doses may be accompanied by a cumulative effect. Since Metubine Iodide is excreted by the kidneys, severe renal disease or hypotension may result in a more prolonged action of this drug. Concurrently administered general anesthetics, certain antibiotics, abnormal states (e.g., acidosis), electrolyte imbalance, and neuromuscular disease have been reported to cause a potentiation of this drug's activity.

Rapid intravenous injection may produce increased release of histamine with resultant decreased respiratory capacity due to bronchospasm and paralysis of the respiratory muscles. Hypotension may occur owing to ganglionic blockade, or it may be a complication of positive pressure respiration.

Metubine Iodide does not affect consciousness or cerebration, and it does not relieve pain. A patient in severe pain may not be able to communicate this to the anesthesiologist.

Indications: Metocurine iodide is indicated as an adjunct to anesthesia to induce skeletal-muscle relaxation. It may be employed to reduce the intensity of muscle contractions in pharmacologically or electrically induced convulsions. It may also be employed to facilitate the management of patients undergoing mechanical ventilation.

Contraindications: Metubine® Iodide (metocurine iodide, Lilly) is contraindicated in those persons who have shown an allergic reaction or hypersensitivity to the drug or to its iodide content.

Metubine Iodide is contraindicated in patients in whom histamine release is a definite hazard.

Warnings: METUBINE® IODIDE (METOCURINE IODIDE, LILLY) IS A POTENT DRUG WHICH MAY CAUSE RESPIRATORY DEPRESSION. THEREFORE, IT SHOULD BE USED ONLY BY THOSE EXPERIENCED IN THE TECHNIQUE OF ARTIFICIAL RESPIRATION AND THE ADMINISTRATION OF OXYGEN UNDER POSITIVE PRESSURE. FACILITIES FOR THESE PROCEDURES SHOULD BE IMMEDIATELY AVAILABLE AT ALL TIMES.

Prolonged apnea with its attendant hazards due to hypoxia may result from overdosages of this preparation.

It should be employed with extreme caution in patients with known myasthenia gravis.

Usage in Pregnancy—The safe use of Metubine Iodide has not been established with respect to the possible adverse effects upon child development. Therefore, it should not be administered to women of childbearing potential and especially not during early pregnancy unless, in the judgment of the physician, the potential benefits outweigh the possible hazards.

Precautions: When sufficiently excessive dosage of curare has been administered, there is no antidote. It is again emphasized that dosage should be controlled so that emergency measures need not be instituted.

Metubine® Iodide (metocurine iodide, Lilly) should be used with caution in patients with respiratory depression or with renal, hepatic, or pulmonary diseases.

Hypotension can follow the administration of large doses.

Adverse Reactions: Adverse reactions consist primarily in extension of the drug's pharmacologic actions. Profound and prolonged muscle relaxation may occur, with consequent respiratory depression to the point of apnea. Hypersensitivity to the drug may exist in rare instances.

Idiosyncrasy, interference with physical signs of anesthesia, circulatory depression, ganglionic blockage, and release of histamine are complications that can result from the use of this medication.

Administration and Dosage: Metubine® Iodide (metocurine iodide, Lilly) is administered intravenously as a sustained injection over a period of 30 to 60 seconds. Care must be taken to avoid overdosage.

The type of anesthetic agent to be used will influence the size of the initial dose. With cyclopropane anesthesia, doses of Metubine Iodide range from 2 to 4 mg, the average being 2.68 mg. When the drug is administered as an adjunct to ether anesthesia, doses of 1.5 to 3 mg are given and average 2.1 mg. When Metubine Iodide is used in conjunction with nitrous oxide anesthesia, doses range from 4 to 7 mg, with an average of 4.79 mg. Satisfactory relaxation cannot be obtained with initial doses below 1 mg, irrespective of the type of anesthetic agent used.

Relaxation following the initial dose may be expected to be effective for periods of 25 to 90 minutes, with a mean average of approximately 60 minutes. Supplemental injections of 0.5 to 1 mg may be made as required and indicated by the depth of relaxation.

Metubine Iodide is adjusted to a *p*H sufficiently low to assure full stability for indefinite periods without the need for refrigeration and

dating; therefore, because of the high pH of barbiturate solutions, a precipitate will form when Metubine Iodide is combined with such agents as Brevital® Sodium (Methohexital Sodium for Injection, USP, Lilly) and Thiopental Sodium.
It is recommended that each component be given from a separate syringe to assure more uniform and predictable results with each of the drugs. A single needle and tube attached to a three-way stopcock apparatus can readily be adapted to this method if it is desirable to utilize as few of the patient's veins as possible.
In electroshock therapy, doses required to produce satisfactory relaxation range from 1.75 to 5.5 mg. When the patient is treated for the first time, the drug is administered slowly by the intravenous route as a sustained injection until a head-drop response ensues. After dosage in a given case has been established, subsequent injections are completed in 15 to 30 seconds when the patient is re-treated. Average doses in this series range from 2 to 3 mg.
Management of Adverse Reactions: If hypotension occurs, the etiology should be determined. When it is due to ganglionic blockade, hypotension may be treated with fluid and vasopressors which act at the adrenergic receptors as required. Apnea or prolonged curarization should be treated with controlled respiration. Edrophonium or neostigmine may antagonize the skeletal-muscle-relaxant action of Metubine® Iodide (metocurine iodide, Lilly). Neostigmine injection should be accompanied or preceded by an injection of atropine sulfate or its equivalent. A nerve stimulator may be used to assess the nature and degree of the neuromuscular blockade. The optimum time to administer the antagonist is when the patient is being hyperventilated and the carbon-dioxide level of the blood is low. The effects of neostigmine given intravenously last from 30 to 90 minutes; the effects of edrophonium are usually dissipated within five minutes. The antagonists are merely adjuncts. Before they are used, the package inserts of these drugs should be consulted for prescribing information.
Pharmacology: Metubine® Iodide (metocurine iodide, Lilly) blocks nervous impulses to skeletal muscles at the myoneural junction. The iodide preparation of metocurine is more predictable than is the chloride.
Metubine Iodide is approximately three to nine times more potent than *d*-tubocurarine chloride, and 1 mg may be expected to produce a therapeutic response comparable to that obtained with 3 mg of *d*-tubocurarine chloride.
Renal excretion occurs fairly rapidly; therefore, the physiologic effect is of relatively short duration.
How Supplied: (℞) *Ampoules (Vials) No. 586, Metubine® Iodide (Metocurine Iodide Injection, NF),* 2 mg per ml, 20 ml, rubber-stoppered, in singles (10 per carton).

[121278]

METYCAINE® HYDROCHLORIDE ℞

(piperocaine hydrochloride)
AMPOULES (VIALS) AND POWDER
For Regional, Infiltration, and Topical Anesthesia

Description: Metycaine® Hydrochloride (piperocaine hydrochloride, Lilly) is an odorless, white crystalline powder, easily soluble in water, alcohol, and chloroform but insoluble in ether and in olive oil. Aqueous solutions (1:10) are faintly acid to litmus. Solutions of Metycaine Hydrochloride are stable and retain their potency after sterilization by boiling or autoclaving.
Each 30-ml vial contains Metycaine Hydrochloride, 600 mg; sodium chloride, 260 mg; potassium chloride, 9 mg; calcium chloride, 10 mg; and chlorobutanol (chloroform derivative), 0.5 percent.
Warning—Not for spinal anesthesia.
Note—Since sulfates are incompatible with the calcium in the formula for Vials No. 318, Metycaine Hydrochloride, 2 percent, vasopressor drugs should be added only in the form of the hydrochloride if such solutions are employed as diluents. Vials No. 318 should be protected from light.
Indications: Metycaine® Hydrochloride (piperocaine hydrochloride, Lilly) has been successfully used for all types of tissue infiltration and regional nerve block anesthesia. Anesthesia develops more rapidly than with procaine and is more certain, more intense, and of longer duration. The toxicity of Metycaine Hydrochloride is considerably less than that of cocaine and in clinical use is comparable to that of procaine. When administered by intravenous injection in different species of laboratory animals, Metycaine Hydrochloride has from 1.9 to 2.75 times the toxicity of procaine.
General Uses—For infiltration, solutions of 0.5 to 1 percent are usually employed. For regional nerve block, concentrations of 0.5 to 2 percent are used.
Although the more concentrated solutions have a longer duration of action, the more dilute solutions allow a larger total quantity of drug to be given safely. It is suggested that the most dilute solution possible be used and that the duration of action be increased by the addition of epinephrine, which slows absorption. Woodbridge recommends the addition of 0.2 mg epinephrine (0.2 ml of 1:1000 solution or 0.5 ml of 1:2600) per gm of Metycaine® Hydrochloride (piperocaine hydrochloride, Lilly). Lundy recommends twice this quantity. One gm of Metycaine Hydrochloride is contained in 100 ml of 1 percent, 200 ml of 0.5 percent, or 400 ml of 0.25 percent solution. Epinephrine should be omitted for patients with hypertension, hyperthyroidism, or heart disease and for those who are unusually susceptible to its effects. Epinephrine must also be omitted from solutions infiltrated into or near the digits.
Woodbridge advises that not more than 80 ml of 1 percent solution of Metycaine Hydrochloride or 200 ml of 0.5 percent solution be injected at one time. A pause of ten minutes for signs of toxicity or idiosyncrasy to develop should be allowed before additional quantities of the drug are administered.
Sodium Chloride Injection or Ringer's Injection should be used as diluents for Metycaine Hydrochloride. Since distilled water is hypotonic, it is damaging to tissues and should be avoided.
Animal experiments suggest the possibility that toxic reactions can be minimized by premedication with sedative doses of one of the barbiturates.
Surgery—Metycaine® Hydrochloride (piperocaine hydrochloride, Lilly) is satisfactory in all surgical procedures requiring a local anesthetic of prompt and well-sustained action. The various forms in which Metycaine Hydrochloride is available provide for convenient use of this drug by infiltration, topical application, or regional nerve block. In blocking large nerve trunks such as may be required before dressing sprains or preceding minor operations, 0.5 to 2 percent solution of Metycaine Hydrochloride is suggested. *This preparation is not for spinal anesthesia.*
For instillation into the stomach, urinary bladder, rectum, or other hollow viscus, the concentration of Metycaine Hydrochloride should not exceed 0.25 percent, and no more than 100 ml of such a solution should be used. If solutions of higher concentration are utilized, excesses should be withdrawn after optimum anesthesia is established.
Urology—Metycaine® Hydrochloride (piperocaine hydrochloride, Lilly) may be applied topically to the urethra and bladder before cystoscopy, urethral dilatation, and other procedures. It may be used by infiltration or nerve block for all types of operative procedures.
With regard to urethral application, it is well to note the warning issued by the Council on Pharmacy and Chemistry of the American Medical Association: "The local anesthetics can be used with safety in nearly all cases if suitable precautions are observed; but extreme caution is imperative when any local anesthetic is injected into the traumatized urethra, or under conditions in which trauma is likely to occur."
In the male, 4 to 8 ml of a 2 to 4 percent solution of Metycaine Hydrochloride are injected into the anterior urethra and retained for a few minutes. Then 8 to 16 ml of the solution are injected gently and retained three to ten minutes. In the female, 15 ml of a 2 to 4 percent solution may be deposited in the bladder, and the urethra may be anesthetized by the introduction of a cotton-tipped wooden applicator that has been soaked in the solution of Metycaine Hydrochloride and lubricated with jelly.
If solutions stronger than 0.25 percent are instilled into the bladder, it is important to withdraw the remaining solution after anesthesia is established.
Rhinolaryngology—Metycaine® Hydrochloride (piperocaine hydrochloride, Lilly), 2 percent, applied as a spray, is recommended prior to examination and treatment and also for placing of epinephrine packs, eustachian catheters, etc.
For general use, such as removal of polypi, washing out of antra, and similar procedures, solutions of 5 to 10 percent may be used, according to the experience and technique of the operator.
Ophthalmology—A 2 to 4 percent solution of Metycaine® Hydrochloride (piperocaine hydrochloride, Lilly) applied to the eye by instillation with appropriate technique gives anesthesia in one minute. One application is sufficient for minor procedures which do not cause severe pain. Anesthesia lasts for eight to ten minutes. Greater depth and duration of anesthesia are obtained by repeating instillation at intervals of three minutes. Usually four such instillations will prove sufficient for most purposes. Occasionally, supplementary infiltration with 0.5 to 1 percent Metycaine Hydrochloride may be indicated.
Proctology—Upon topical application in the anal canal, a 5 percent solution of Metycaine® Hydrochloride (piperocaine hydrochloride, Lilly) produces anesthesia in five to 15 minutes, which permits satisfactory dilatation and examination of the rectum.
For certain operative procedures, a 10 to 20 percent solution of Metycaine Hydrochloride may be applied topically. For perirectal infiltration, a concentration of 0.5 percent has been found adequate.
Dentistry—Solutions of Metycaine® Hydrochloride (piperocaine hydrochloride, Lilly) have been used in all phases of dental work requiring local anesthesia. A 1 to 2 percent solution is used most frequently for infiltrative procedures. For topical anesthesia, 5 to 10 percent solutions usually are preferred.
The drug may be used by dentists who have developed an allergy to procaine but who, upon routine skin testing, show no sensitivity to Metycaine Hydrochloride.
Contraindications and Precautions: There seem to be few or no general contraindications to regional anesthesia. Apprehensive patients either should not have it or should receive adequate preliminary sedation. Injection should not be made into or through infected or inflamed tissues.
Except when it is injected intravenously, toxicity is apparently very rare with Metycaine® Hydrochloride (piperocaine hydrochloride,

Continued on next page

*Identi-Code® symbol.

Lilly—Cont.

Lilly). Inadvertent intravenous administration may result in either of two types of reaction: (1) a shocklike reaction, with sharp fall in blood pressure, slow pulse, perhaps unconsciousness, or even death; or (2) nervous symptoms such as pallor, sweating, apprehension, tremors, and, in severe cases, convulsions. The intravenous administration of ordinary doses of any of the barbiturates—for example, Amytal® Sodium (Sterile Amobarbital Sodium, USP, Lilly), 250 mg (4 grains)—is helpful in combating toxicity but is of less value in the shocklike reactions than in those marked by nervous symptoms. Some have recommended oral premedication with barbiturates as a precautionary measure.
How Supplied: (℞) *Ampoules (Vials) No. 318, Metycaine® Hydrochloride (piperocaine hydrochloride, Lilly) Injection, 2%,* 30 ml, rubber-stoppered, in singles (10 per carton).
(℞) *Powder No. 41, Metycaine® Hydrochloride (piperocaine hydrochloride, Lilly),* in 4-oz bottles. For topical and infiltrative use. Solutions intended for injection should be sterilized by boiling or autoclaving.

[062978]

MORRHUATE SODIUM ℞
Injection, NF

Each ampoule contains a sufficient amount to permit withdrawal and administration of the volume specified on the label.
Description: Morrhuate Sodium Injection, NF, is a sterile solution of the sodium salts of the fatty acids of cod liver oil. Each ml contains 50 mg of sodium morrhuate in 3 percent alcohol. Sodium hydroxide and/or morrhuic acid may have been added during manufacture to adjust the *p*H. A 5 percent solution is the accepted strength for injection treatment of varicose veins.
Action: Morrhuate sodium is a mild sclerosing drug that produces its effect by irritation of the intimal endothelium.
Indication: Morrhuate sodium is indicated for the obliteration of varicose veins. The benefit-to-risk ratio should be considered in certain patients who are definite surgical risks because of old age and in patients with small asymptomatic veins when the drug is used for cosmetic reasons.
Contraindications and Precautions: Morrhuate sodium is contraindicated in patients known to be sensitive to it and in those with uncontrolled diabetes and advanced arterial disease of the legs. Cardiac, hyperthyroid, and renal disease may render treatment inadvisable. The drug is also contraindicated in patients with acute superficial thrombophlebitis, varicosities caused by abdominal and pelvic tumors, sepsis, blood dyscrasia, and any condition which causes the patient to be bedridden.
Extensive injection treatment is not advisable in advanced debility and senility. An unusual local reaction at the injection site or any systemic reaction is a contraindication to the continued use of this medication. Persistent occlusion of deep veins definitely contraindicates obliteration of superficial veins. In the opinion of some authorities, veins should not be ligated if infected ulcers are present. Treatment should be delayed if there is any acute local or systemic infection. History of phlebitis or thrombophlebitis may not definitely rule out ligation, but prior to treatment by injection, ligation, or a combination of the two, patency of the deep venous circulation of the leg should be determined.
Great care should be taken when therapy is reinstituted after a period of time has elapsed, because there have been reports of anaphylactoid reactions.
Usage in Pregnancy—Morrhuate sodium may be used in pregnant women only when clearly indicated and after the benefits have been weighed against the risks. Reproduction studies have not been done in animals to determine whether the drug has teratogenic potential or any other adverse effects on the fetus. No well-controlled studies have been done with pregnant women to determine whether the drug has any adverse effects on the fetus, but there has been no positive evidence to date that they may occur. Although there is no clearly defined risk, the possibility of damage to the fetus cannot be excluded.
There have been no well-controlled studies with patients who have been given morrhuate sodium while they were taking antiovulatory drugs. Positive evidence of any adverse effects in such patients is lacking. Although there is no well-defined risk, infrequent adverse reactions cannot be excluded. Therefore, the physician must use his best judgment in giving morrhuate sodium to such patients.
Sclerotherapy should not be undertaken for the treatment of varicosities unless deep-vein patency has been determined. This can be done by the use of such tests as Trendelenburg's and Perthes' and angiography. Because of the danger of extension of thrombosis into the deep veins, a thorough preinjection evaluation for valvular competence should be carried out.
Adverse Reactions: *Expected Results*—The injected vein usually shows a prompt effect. It becomes hard and swollen for two to four inches, depending on the size of the vein and its response. The vein is hard and firm after 24 hours and not very tender to touch (little or no periphlebitis). The skin about the injected vein assumes a light-bronze color. Bronzing usually disappears in a short time. The injection may cause swelling, thickening, tenderness, and redness at the point of injection and for some distance along the vein for a few days. An aching sensation and a feeling of stiffness usually occur and last for approximately 48 hours. A permanent discoloration, usually small and barely noticeable, can occur at the injection site and may be objectionable from the cosmetic viewpoint. Because of this and the side effects noted above, morrhuate sodium is not recommended for the injection of veins for cosmetic purposes.
An occasional individual may have or may develop a sensitivity to morrhuate sodium. Symptoms may include dizziness, weakness, vascular collapse, respiratory depression, gastrointestinal disturbances, and urticaria. Such anaphylactoid reactions are usually noted within a few minutes after the injection and should be treated promptly. When this drug is administered, emergency measures should be readily available. These include epinephrine, oxygen, and pressor drugs for immediate allergic manifestations, as well as antihistamines and corticosteroids for delayed effects. Dermatitis, urticaria, or asthma rarely occurs following injection; pulmonary embolism has proved fatal (J.A.M.A., *118*:1293, 1942).
Morrhuate sodium produces a good thrombus; it rarely causes cramping pain. There is little pain on injection, and severe afterpain is rare. Apply pressure over the puncture in the vein to prevent leakage. If the injection is made outside the vein, a slough will usually result.
Administration and Dosage: The dose necessary to produce sclerosis of the varix is proportional to the size of the vein. In small or medium-size veins, 1 or 2 ml of the 5 percent solution are sufficient; in large veins, 3 to 5 ml are necessary. Morrhuate sodium may be administered in multiple injections at one time or in single doses repeated at intervals; not more than 5 ml should be injected in a single day. Injections may be repeated at intervals of five to seven days and as gauged by the patient's reaction to the drug.
Injection may be made into distended veins or into emptied veins. When injection is made into emptied veins, elevate the limb to empty the vein of some of the blood and apply digital pressure or a tourniquet above the point of injection. Pressure should be maintained for two or three minutes after the injection in order to prevent dilution of the drug by the backflow of blood from above.
When smaller veins are being injected or when the ampoule is cold, it is advisable to immerse the ampoule in hot water. The cold solution should clear entirely upon warming before it is used. Do not use if solution does not clear upon warming.
A large-bore needle should be used to load the syringe, because the solution becomes frothy rather easily; however, a fine needle should be used for injection. Care should be used to prevent extravasation of the solution into the surrounding tissues. If the solution leaks from the veins or is not injected entirely into the veins, necrosis of the tissue surrounding the vein can occur. After the injection, a small piece of sterile gauze is placed over the needle puncture and secured by adhesive tape. Tight bandaging is not necessary. The needle puncture seals rapidly, but the site should be inspected before the patient leaves the office.
How Supplied: (℞) *Ampoules Morrhuate Sodium Injection, NF: No. 296,* 5%, 2 ml, in packages of 12. Two ml contain 100 mg (1½ grs); *No. 279,* 5%, 5 ml, in packages of 6. Five ml contain 250 mg (4 grs).

[030879]

MULTICEBRIN® OTC
(pan-vitamins)

Description: Each tablet contains—

Thiamine (Vitamin B_1)	3 mg
Riboflavin (Vitamin B_2)	3 mg
Pyridoxine (Vitamin B_6)	1.2 mg
Pantothenic Acid	5 mg
Niacinamide	25 mg
Vitamin B_{12} (Activity Equivalent)	3 mcg
Ascorbic Acid (Vitamin C)	75 mg
dl-Alpha Tocopheryl Acetate (Vitamin E)	6.6 IU (6.6 mg)
Vitamin A	10,000 IU (3 mg)
Vitamin D	400 IU (10 mcg)

Indications: One tablet supplies the optimum requirements of six essential vitamins and significant amounts of other important factors for which optimum requirements have not been established. Tablets Multicebrin are indicated in the prophylaxis or treatment of multiple vitamin deficiencies, in patients on restricted diets, in pregnancy, in wasting diseases, and in any situation characterized by improper food intake, utilization, or absorption.
Dosage: 1 tablet a day, or as directed by the physician.
How Supplied: *Tablets No. 100, Multicebrin® (pan-vitamins, Lilly), C71,** Coated, Red, in bottles of 100 and 1000 and in 10 strips of 10 individually labeled blisters each containing 1 tablet (ID100). [073179]

NEBCIN® ℞
(tobramycin sulfate)
Injection, USP

WARNINGS

Patients treated with Nebcin® (tobramycin sulfate, Lilly) should be under close clinical observation, because tobramycin and other aminoglycoside antibiotics have an inherent potential for causing ototoxicity and nephrotoxicity.
Both vestibular and auditory ototoxicity can occur. Eighth-nerve impairment may develop if patients have preexisting renal damage and if Nebcin is administered for longer periods or in higher doses than those recommended.
Tobramycin is potentially nephrotoxic. Renal and eighth-nerve function should be closely monitored in patients with known or suspected renal impairment and also in those whose renal function is initially normal but who develop signs of renal dys-

function during therapy. Such impairment may be characterized by cylindruria, oliguria, proteinuria, or evidence of nitrogen retention (increasing BUN, NPN, or creatinine). Evidence of impairment in renal, vestibular, or auditory function requires discontinuation of the drug or dosage adjustment.
Nebcin should be used with caution in premature and neonatal infants because of their renal immaturity and the resulting prolongation of serum half-life of the drug.
In the case of overdosage or toxic reactions, peritoneal dialysis or hemodialysis will help remove tobramycin from the blood.
Serum concentrations should be monitored when feasible, and prolonged concentrations above 12 mcg/ml should be avoided. Urine should be examined for increased excretion of protein, cells, and casts.
Concurrent and sequential use of other neurotoxic and/or nephrotoxic antibiotics, particularly streptomycin, neomycin, kanamycin, gentamicin, cephaloridine, paromomycin, viomycin, polymyxin B, colistin, and vancomycin, should be avoided.
Nebcin should not be given concurrently with potent diuretics. Some diuretics themselves cause ototoxicity, and intravenously administered diuretics enhance aminoglycoside toxicity by altering antibiotic concentrations in serum and tissue.
Usage in Pregnancy—Safety of this product for use during pregnancy has not been established.

Description: Tobramycin sulfate, a water-soluble antibiotic of the aminoglycoside group, is derived from the actinomycete *Streptomyces tenebrarius.* Nebcin® (tobramycin sulfate, Lilly), Injection, is a clear and colorless sterile aqueous solution for parenteral administration. It is stable and requires no refrigeration. Each ml also contains 5 mg phenol as a preservative, 3.2 mg sodium bisulfite, 0.1 mg edetate disodium, and water for injection, q.s. Sulfuric acid and/or sodium hydroxide may have been added to adjust the *p*H.

Actions: *Clinical Pharmacology*—Peak serum concentrations of tobramycin occur between 30 and 90 minutes after intramuscular administration. Following an intramuscular dose of 1 mg/kg of body weight, maximum serum concentrations reach about 4 mcg/ml, and measurable levels persist for as long as eight hours. When Nebcin® (tobramycin sulfate, Lilly) is administered by intravenous infusion over a one-hour period, the serum concentrations are similar to those obtained by intramuscular administration.
In patients with normal renal function, except neonates, Nebcin administered every eight hours does not accumulate in the serum. However, in those with reduced renal function and in neonates, the serum concentration of the antibiotic is usually higher and can be measured for longer periods of time than in normal adults. Dosage for such patients must, therefore, be adjusted accordingly (*see* Administration and Dosage).
Tobramycin is eliminated almost exclusively by glomerular filtration. Renal clearance is similar to that of endogenous creatinine. Ultrafiltration studies demonstrate that practically no serum protein binding occurs. In patients with normal renal function, up to 84 percent of the dose is recoverable from the urine in eight hours and up to 93 percent in 24 hours. The serum half-life in normal individuals is two hours.
Peak urine concentrations ranging from 75 to 100 mcg/ml have been observed following the intramuscular injection of a single dose of 1 mg/kg. After several days of treatment, the amount of tobramycin excreted in the urine approaches the daily dose administered.
An inverse relationship exists between serum half-life and creatinine clearance, and the dosage schedule should be adjusted according to the degree of renal impairment (see below). In patients undergoing dialysis, 25 to 70 percent of the administered dose may be removed, depending on the duration and type of dialysis.
Tobramycin can be detected in tissues and body fluids after parenteral administration. Concentrations in bile and stools ordinarily have been low, which suggests minimum biliary excretion. Tobramycin has appeared in low concentration in the cerebrospinal fluid following parenteral administration. It has also been found in sputum, peritoneal fluid, and abscess fluids, and it crosses the placental membranes.
Microbiology—In vitro tests demonstrate that tobramycin is bactericidal and that it acts by inhibiting the synthesis of protein in bacterial cells.
Tobramycin is usually active against most strains of the following organisms:
- *Pseudomonas aeruginosa*
- *Proteus* sp. (indole-positive and indole-negative), including *Proteus mirabilis, P. morganii, P. rettgeri,* and *P. vulgaris*
- *Escherichia coli*
- *Klebsiella-Enterobacter-Serratia* group
- *Citrobacter* sp.
- *Providencia* sp.
- Staphylococci, including *Staphylococcus aureus* (coagulase-positive and coagulase-negative)

Although most strains of group D streptococci demonstrate in vitro resistance, some strains in this group are susceptible. In vitro studies have shown that an aminoglycoside combined with an antibiotic which interferes with cell-wall synthesis affects some group D streptococcal strains synergistically. The combination of penicillin G and tobramycin results in a synergistic bactericidal effect in vitro against certain strains of *Streptococcus faecalis.* However, this combination is not synergistic against other closely related organisms, e.g., *S. faecium.* Speciation of group D streptococci alone cannot be used to predict susceptibility. Susceptibility testing and tests for antibiotic synergism are emphasized.
Susceptibility Plate Tests—If the FDA Standardized Disc Test method (formerly the Bauer-Kirby-Sherris-Turck method) of disc susceptibility testing is used, a disc containing 10 mcg tobramycin should give a zone of at least 14 mm when tested against a tobramycin-susceptible bacterial strain, a zone of 12 to 13 mm against strains of intermediate susceptibility, and a zone of 11 mm or less against resistant organisms.

Indications and Usage: Nebcin® (tobramycin sulfate, Lilly) is indicated for the treatment of serious infections caused by susceptible strains of the following microorganisms: *P. aeruginosa, E. coli, Proteus* sp. (indole-positive and indole-negative), *Providencia, Klebsiella-Enterobacter-Serratia* group, *Citrobacter* sp., and staphylococci, including *S. aureus* (coagulase-positive and coagulase-negative).
Nebcin is indicated in the treatment of septicemia; central-nervous-system infections, including meningitis; neonatal sepsis; serious lower respiratory infections; gastrointestinal infections, including peritonitis; and serious skin, bone, and soft-tissue infections, including burns, caused by the susceptible organisms listed above. Clinical studies have shown Nebcin also to be effective in serious complicated and recurrent urinary tract infections due to these organisms. Aminoglycosides, including Nebcin, are not indicated in uncomplicated initial episodes of urinary tract infections unless the causative organisms are not susceptible to antibiotics having less potential toxicity. Nebcin may be considered in serious staphylococcal infections when penicillin or other potentially less toxic drugs are contraindicated and when bacterial susceptibility testing and clinical judgment indicate its use.
Bacterial cultures should be obtained prior to and during treatment to isolate and identify etiologic organisms and to test their susceptibility to tobramycin. If susceptibility tests show that the causative organisms are resistant to tobramycin, other appropriate therapy should be instituted. In patients in whom gram-negative septicemia, neonatal sepsis, or meningitis is suspected, including those in whom concurrent therapy with a penicillin or cephalosporin and an aminoglycoside may be indicated, treatment with Nebcin may be initiated before the results of susceptibility studies are obtained. The decision to continue therapy with Nebcin® (tobramycin sulfate, Lilly) should be based on the results of susceptibility studies, the severity of the infection, and the important additional concepts discussed in the WARNINGS box above.

Contraindication: A history of hypersensitivity to tobramycin is a contraindication to its use.

Warnings: *See* WARNINGS box above.

Precautions: Specimens should be collected during therapy for examination, as recommended in the WARNINGS box.
Neuromuscular blockade and respiratory paralysis have been reported in cats receiving very high doses of tobramycin (40 mg/kg). The possibility that prolonged or secondary apnea may occur should be considered if tobramycin is administered to anesthetized patients who are also receiving neuromuscular blocking agents, such as succinylcholine or tubocurarine.
Cross-allergenicity among aminoglycosides has been demonstrated.
If overgrowth of nonsusceptible organisms occurs, appropriate therapy should be initiated.

Adverse Reactions: *Nephrotoxicity*—Renal function changes, as shown by rising BUN, NPN, and serum creatinine and by oliguria, cylindruria, and increased proteinuria, have been reported, especially in patients with a history of renal impairment who are treated for longer periods or with higher doses than those recommended.
Neurotoxicity—Adverse effects on both the vestibular and auditory branches of the eighth nerve have been noted, especially in patients receiving high doses or prolonged therapy. Symptoms include dizziness, vertigo, tinnitus, roaring in the ears, and hearing loss.
NOTE: The risk of toxic reactions is low in patients with normal renal function who do not receive Nebcin in higher doses or for longer periods of time than those recommended.
Other reported adverse reactions possibly related to Nebcin include increased serum transaminase (SGOT, SGPT) and increased serum bilirubin; anemia, granulocytopenia, and thrombocytopenia; and fever, rash, itching, urticaria, nausea, vomiting, headache, and lethargy.

Administration and Dosage: The patient's pretreatment body weight should be obtained for calculation of correct dosage. Nebcin® (tobramycin sulfate, Lilly) may be given intramuscularly or intravenously.
Intramuscular Administration for Patients with Normal Renal Function—The recommended dosage for adults, children, and older infants with normal renal function who have serious infections is 3 mg/kg/day, administered in three equal doses every eight hours (*see* Table 1).
[See table on next page].
In adults, children, and older infants with life-threatening infections, dosages up to 5 mg/kg/day may be administered in three or

Continued on next page

***Identi-Code® symbol.**

Lilly—Cont.

four equal doses (*see* Table 1). The dosage should be reduced to 3 mg/kg/day as soon as clinically indicated. To prevent increased toxicity due to excessive blood levels, dosage should not exceed 5 mg/kg/day unless serum levels are monitored.

For neonates (one week of age or less), dosages up to 4 mg/kg/day may be administered in two equal doses every 12 hours.

The usual duration of treatment is seven to ten days. A longer course of therapy may be necessary in difficult and complicated infections. In such cases, monitoring of renal, auditory, and vestibular functions is advised, because neurotoxicity is more likely to occur when treatment is extended longer than ten days.

Intramuscular Administration for Patients with Impaired Renal Function—Whenever possible, serum tobramycin concentrations should be determined by bioassay.

Following a loading dose of 1 mg/kg, subsequent dosage in these patients must be adjusted, either with reduced doses administered at eight-hour intervals or with normal doses given at prolonged intervals. Both of these methods are suggested as guides to be used when serum levels of tobramycin cannot be measured directly. They are based on either the creatinine clearance or the serum creatinine of the patient, because these values correlate with the half-life of tobramycin. The dosage schedules derived from either method should be used in conjunction with careful clinical and laboratory observations of the patient and should be modified as necessary. Neither method should be used when dialysis is being performed.

Reduced dosage at eight-hour intervals: When the creatinine clearance rate is 70 ml or less per minute or when the serum creatinine value is known, the amount of the reduced dose can be determined by multiplying the normal dose from Table 1 by the percent of normal dose from the accompanying nomogram.

REDUCED DOSAGE NOMOGRAM*

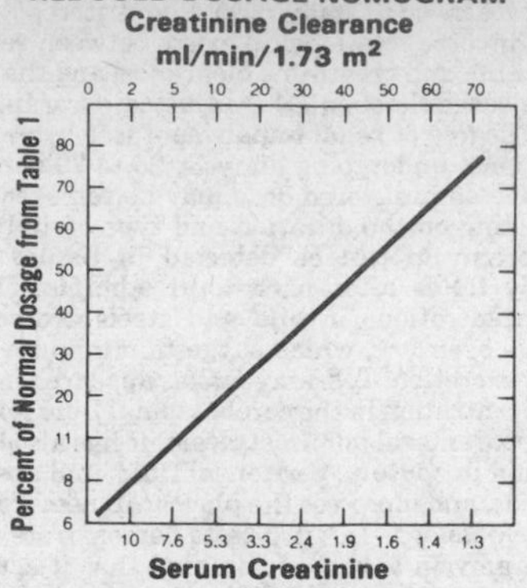

***Scales have been adjusted to facilitate dosage calculations.**

An alternate rough guide for determining reduced dosage at eight-hour intervals (for patients whose steady-state serum creatinine values are known) is to divide the normally recommended dose by the patient's serum creatinine.

Normal dosage at prolonged intervals: If the creatinine clearance rate is not available and the patient's condition is stable, a dosage frequency *in hours* for the dosage given in the table can be determined by multiplying the patient's serum creatinine by six.

Intravenous Administration—The intravenous dose is the same as the intramuscular. For intravenous administration, the usual volume of diluent (0.9% Sodium Chloride Injection or 5% Dextrose Injection) is 50 to 100 ml for adult doses. For children, the volume of diluent should be proportionately less than for adults. The diluted solution usually should be infused over a period of 20 to 60 minutes. Infusion periods of less than 20 minutes are not recommended, because peak serum levels may exceed 12 mcg/ml (*see* WARNINGS box).

Nebcin® (tobramycin sulfate, Lilly) should not be physically premixed with other drugs but should be administered separately according to the recommended dose and route.

How Supplied: (℞) *Ampoules (Vials) No. 781, Nebcin® (Tobramycin Sulfate Injection, USP),* 80 mg (equivalent to tobramycin) per 2 ml, 2 ml, rubber-stoppered, in singles (10 per carton) and in Traypaks™ (multivial cartons, Lilly) of 25.

(℞) *Ampoules (Vials) No. 782, Nebcin® (Tobramycin Sulfate Injection, USP), Pediatric,* 20 mg (equivalent to tobramycin) per 2 ml, 2 ml, rubber-stoppered, in singles (10 per carton).

(℞) *Hyporets® (disposable syringes, Lilly) Nebcin® (Tobramycin Sulfate Injection, USP): No. 55,* 60 mg (equivalent to tobramycin) per 1.5 ml, 1.5 ml, and *No. 42,* 80 mg (equivalent to tobramycin) per 2 ml, 2 ml, in packages of 24. Each Hyporet is scored with a 10-mg (0.25-ml) fractional dose scale. [010279]

TABLE 1. DOSAGE SCHEDULE GUIDE FOR ADULTS WITH NORMAL RENAL FUNCTION
(Dosage at Eight-Hour Intervals)

For Patient Weighing kg	lb	Usual Dose for Serious Infections 1 mg/kg q 8 h (Total, 3 mg/kg/day) mg/dose q 8 h	ml/dose*	Maximum Dose for Life-Threatening Infections (Reduce as soon as possible) 1.66 mg/kg q 8 h (Total, 5 mg/kg/day) mg/dose q 8 h	ml/dose*
120	264	120 mg	3 ml	200 mg	5 ml
115	253	115 mg	2.9 ml	191 mg	4.75 ml
110	242	110 mg	2.75 ml	183 mg	4.5 ml
105	231	105 mg	2.6 ml	175 mg	4.4 ml
100	220	100 mg	2.5 ml	166 mg	4.2 ml
95	209	95 mg	2.4 ml	158 mg	4 ml
90	198	90 mg	2.25 ml	150 mg	3.75 ml
85	187	85 mg	2.1 ml	141 mg	3.5 ml
80	176	80 mg	2 ml	133 mg	3.3 ml
75	165	75 mg	1.9 ml	125 mg	3.1 ml
70	154	70 mg	1.75 ml	116 mg	2.9 ml
65	143	65 mg	1.6 ml	108 mg	2.7 ml
60	132	60 mg	1.5 ml	100 mg	2.5 ml
55	121	55 mg	1.4 ml	91 mg	2.25 ml
50	110	50 mg	1.25 ml	83 mg	2.1 ml
45	99	45 mg	1.1 ml	75 mg	1.9 ml
40	88	40 mg	1 ml	66 mg	1.6 ml

*Applicable to all product forms except Nebcin® (tobramycin sulfate, Lilly), Pediatric, Injection (*see* How Supplied).

NEO-BETALIN® 12 CRYSTALLINE ℞
(hydroxocobalamin)
Injection, NF

Description: Neo-Betalin® 12 Crystalline (Hydroxocobalamin Injection, NF, Lilly) is a form of vitamin B_{12} which differs from cyanocobalamin in that the cyano group is replaced by a hydroxyl group. Vitamin B_{12a}, vitamin B_{12b}, and aquocobalamin are other names that have been used for this form of vitamin B_{12}.

Studies have shown that hydroxocobalamin is as effective as cyanocobalamin in the treatment of patients manifesting vitamin B_{12} deficiency secondary to inadequate secretion of intrinsic factor (pernicious anemia). Studies have also shown that hydroxocobalamin is more slowly absorbed from an injection site and may be taken up by the liver in larger quantities than cyanocobalamin. In addition, it has been demonstrated that there is a more sustained rise in the serum cobalamin level and significantly less urinary excretion of cobalamin after injection of hydroxocobalamin than after injection of the same dose of cyanocobalamin. For these reasons, hydroxocobalamin is believed to have advantages over cyanocobalamin in replenishing vitamin B_{12} stores in the body when deficiency of this vitamin exists.

Indications: Neo-Betalin® 12 Crystalline (hydroxocobalamin, Lilly) may be used in the treatment of all clinical conditions manifesting deficiency of vitamin B_{12}. These include classical pernicious anemia with or without subacute combined degeneration of the spinal cord, malabsorption syndromes, and certain other macrocytic (megaloblastic) anemias which occur in strict vegetarianism, blind-loop syndromes, or fish tapeworm *(Diphyllobothrium latum)* infection. In the last two situations, treatment also requires freeing the host of the bacteria or parasites which appear to compete for the vitamin B_{12} available in the diet.

Although folic acid deficiency is more commonly recognized as the problem in nutritional macrocytic anemias (e.g., of pregnancy, infancy, or chronic liver disease), Neo-Betalin 12 Crystalline may also be used when such anemias likewise involve vitamin B_{12} deficiency.

Patients who show sensitivity to purified liver extracts may be transferred to crystalline vitamin B_{12} without reaction.

Neo-Betalin 12 Crystalline, 1000 micrograms (mcg), is suitable for use as the flushing dose in the Schilling test.

Precautions and Adverse Reactions: Although the possibility of sensitivity-type reactions following administration of any parenteral preparation must always be kept in mind, there is no documented evidence that vitamin B_{12} itself is toxic, even in large doses. Many thousands of injections of a 1000-mcg (1-mg) dose have been administered to humans without toxic or allergic reactions. However, on rare occasions, reactions of an apparently allergic type have been reported following the injection of parenteral preparations of crystalline vitamin B_{12}. It is not known whether these were related to the preservative, the vitamin, or neither. Patients sensitive to parenterally administered purified liver extract or to vitamin B_{12} concentrates obtained from culture filtrates can take crystalline vitamin B_{12} without untoward response.

A few patients may experience mild pain at the injection site after administration of Neo-Betalin® 12 Crystalline (hydroxocobalamin, Lilly).

Administration and Dosage: Neo-Betalin® 12 Crystalline (hydroxocobalamin, Lilly) should be administered by the intramuscular route only.

Treatment with vitamin B_{12} should be sufficient to replenish and, when necessary, to maintain body stores. The human requirement for this vitamin has been estimated to be between 1 and 5 mcg per day; in some exceptional cases, it may be slightly higher.

Although the optimum dosage regimen with any injectable vitamin B_{12} must be individualized for each patient, the indication that 1 mcg of vitamin B_{12} is equivalent to 1 injectable unit of liver extract may be used as a guide for minimum treatment of the individual case of pernicious anemia (vitamin B_{12} deficiency secondary to intrinsic factor deficiency). In such patients, satisfactory responses have been obtained with initial minimum treatment of 15 to 20 mcg of cyanocobalamin daily for two or three days, followed by weekly injections of a minimum of 7 to 15 mcg until the blood picture has returned to normal, followed indefinitely by biweekly or monthly maintenance injections of 15 to 30 mcg.

Since there is a range in individual daily requirements for vitamin B_{12} and since studies suggest that hydroxocobalamin may be given best in larger amounts and at less frequent intervals than cyanocobalamin, it seems reasonable to employ Neo-Betalin 12 Crystalline in doses of at least 100 mcg per injection. Sufficient amounts should be administered to produce a satisfactory reticulocyte response, to effect a return to and maintenance of the red-blood-cell count at normal levels, to cause the disappearance of gastrointestinal symptoms, and to clear neurologic involvement or prevent its further progression. Patients who show extensive neurologic symptoms should be given more than minimum dosage. No single regimen can be expected to apply to all cases. Follow-up of the patient is the final criterion for adequacy of therapy. The optimum maximum interval between maintenance doses can be determined only by empirical means. Follow-up at monthly intervals appears to be reasonable and is often recommended. On the basis of experience with the individual patient, a suitable lifetime maintenance dosage schedule can be determined.

In malabsorption syndromes and in cases of nutritional or other macrocytic anemias, the dose must be individualized according to the response of the patient. Other possible primary or associated deficiencies (e.g., of folic acid or other vitamins) must also be treated as indicated in these situations.

How Supplied: (℞) *Ampoules (Vials) No. 729, Neo-Betalin® 12 Crystalline (Hydroxocobalamin Injection, NF),* 1000 mcg hydroxocobalamin per ml, 10 ml, rubber-stoppered, in singles (10 per carton). Each vial also contains 0.1 percent anhydrous sodium acetate, 0.22 percent acetic acid, and 0.82 percent sodium chloride. Preservatives are methylparaben, 0.15 percent, and propylparaben, 0.02 percent. Sodium hydroxide and/or hydrochloric acid may have been added during manufacture to adjust the *p*H. [061175A]

NEOMYCIN SULFATE ℞
Tablets, USP

Description: Neomycin is an antibiotic obtained from the metabolic products of the actinomycete *Streptomyces fradiae.*

Actions: Neomycin is poorly absorbed from the normal gastrointestinal tract. The small absorbed fraction is rapidly excreted with normal kidney function. The unabsorbed portion of the drug (approximately 97 percent) is eliminated unchanged in the feces.

Growth of most intestinal bacteria is rapidly suppressed following oral administration of neomycin, and the suppression persists for 48 to 72 hours. Nonpathogenic yeasts and, occasionally, resistant strains of *Enterobacter aerogenes* (formerly *Aerobacter aerogenes*) replace the intestinal bacteria.

Indications: *Suppression of Intestinal Bacteria*—Neomycin may be indicated when suppression of the normal bacterial flora of the bowel is desirable for either short-term or long-term adjunctive therapy.

Hepatic Coma—Prolonged administration has been shown to be effective adjunctive therapy in hepatic coma because it reduces the ammonia-forming bacteria in the intestinal tract. The subsequent reduction in blood ammonia has resulted in neurologic improvement.

Diarrhea Due to Enteropathogenic Escherichia coli—Diarrhea caused by enteropathogenic *E. coli* may be effectively treated with neomycin sulfate. When this diarrhea occurs in epidemic form, all patients and carriers should be treated concurrently.

Contraindications: Neomycin sulfate tablets are contraindicated in the presence of intestinal obstruction and in individuals with a history of hypersensitivity to the drug.

Warnings: Patients treated with oral neomycin should be under close clinical observation because of the potential nephrotoxic and ototoxic effects. Patients with renal insufficiency may develop toxic blood levels of the drug unless doses are properly regulated. If renal insufficiency develops during treatment, the dosage should be reduced or the antibiotic discontinued. Urine and blood examinations and audiometric tests should be given prior to and during extended therapy in individuals with hepatic and/or renal disease to avoid nephrotoxicity and eighth-nerve damage from improper dosage.

Usage in Pregnancy—Safety of this product for use during pregnancy has not been established.

Precautions: Caution should be observed in the concurrent use of other ototoxic and/or nephrotoxic antimicrobial drugs while neomycin is being administered orally. These include streptomycin, kanamycin, polymyxin B, colistin, viomycin, gentamicin, cephaloridine, and tobramycin.

The concurrent use of potent diuretics, such as ethacrynic acid, furosemide, urea, and mannitol (particularly when given intravenously), should be avoided. They may cause cumulative adverse effects of the neomycin on the kidney and auditory nerve.

Prolonged oral use of neomycin may result in overgrowth of nonsusceptible organisms, particularly fungi. If this occurs, appropriate therapy should be instituted.

Adverse Reactions: The most common adverse reactions to neomycin given orally are nausea, vomiting, and diarrhea. The "malabsorption syndrome," characterized by increased fecal fat, decreased serum carotene, and fall in xylose absorption, has been reported with prolonged therapy. Nephrotoxicity and ototoxicity have occurred following extended and high-dosage therapy in hepatic coma.

Administration and Dosage: *Adults*—For suppression of intestinal bacteria as an adjunct to mechanical cleansing of the large bowel in short-term therapy prior to bowel surgery, 40 mg per kg every 24 hours in six divided doses may be used. Duration of therapy should not exceed three days.

As adjunctive therapy in the treatment of hepatic coma, the recommended dosage schedule is 100 mg per kg in four divided doses the first 24 hours, followed by 50 mg per kg per day thereafter. The total daily dose should not exceed 3 gm.

Infants and Children—Diarrhea due to enteropathogenic *E. coli* may be treated with 50 mg per kg given in four divided doses daily for two to three days.

How Supplied: (℞) *Tablets No. 1803, Neomycin Sulfate, USP, T96,** 500 mg (equivalent to 350 mg base), in bottles of 20 and 100 and in 10 strips of 10 individually labeled blisters each containing 1 tablet (ID100). [103078]

NOVACEBRIN® c̄ FLUORIDE CHEWABLE ℞
(multiple vitamins with fluoride)

Description: Tablets Novacebrin c̄ Fluoride Chewable are designed to prevent vitamin deficiencies in children and to aid in the prevention of dental caries.

Each tablet contains—

Fluoride (as Sodium Fluoride)	1 mg
Vitamin A	4000 IU (1.2 mg)
Vitamin D	400 IU (10 mcg)
Vitamin C (as Sodium Ascorbate and Ascorbic Acid)	60 mg
Thiamine Mononitrate (Vitamin B_1)	1.5 mg
Riboflavin (Vitamin B_2)	2 mg
Pyridoxine Hydrochloride (Vitamin B_6)	1 mg
Cyanocobalamin (Vitamin B_{12})	3 mcg
Niacinamide	12 mg
Pantothenic Acid (as Panthenol)	2.5 mg

Indications: This fluoride-containing vitamin preparation is intended for use as a dietary supplement in children who consume water containing less than 0.7 part per million (p.p.m.) of fluoride. The vitamin formula is especially indicated for those children who do not eat a well-balanced diet, and it is suitable particularly for children who would rather chew or swallow a tablet than take vitamin drops. The excellent flavor is appreciated by children and helps to assure that the tablets will be taken regularly. Since synthetic vitamins are used, objectionable odors are avoided, and the likelihood of sensitivity to any of the components is decreased.

The inclusion of fluoride in vitamin preparations culminates a long period of medical research. It is now well established that artificial fluoridation of public water supplies is an effective method for the control of dental caries. Apparently, fluoride is incorporated into the chemical complex which makes up tooth enamel. For maximum benefit, fluoride should be available during the entire period of enamel development, i.e., from before birth until eight or ten years of age. With the exception of the third molars, calcification of the teeth is virtually completed by the age of ten. The caries resistance induced by fluoride administration during the developmental period would appear to persist throughout life.

Since not all of the population in the United States has the benefit of either naturally or artificially fluoridated water, the question arises as to whether the daily ingestion of fluoride in other forms might provide the same beneficial effects as fluoridated water. Several studies have now demonstrated that the administration of tablets or liquids containing fluoride is both practical and effective.

The optimum dose of fluoride that will give protection against caries without causing mottling of tooth enamel is not well established. When the source of fluoride is drinking water, one would expect that the amount of fluoride ingested daily by different infants and children might vary quite considerably. Variation in water intake, in fact, might help explain the repeated observation that some children in

Continued on next page

*Identi-Code® symbol.

Lilly—Cont.

fluoridated areas seem to benefit more than others.
In early studies in which sodium fluoride tablets were used, a daily dose of 1 mg of fluoride was given. With this amount, some mottling of the teeth was noted. Subsequently, the dose for the first two years of life was restricted to 0.5 mg daily, and 1 mg per day was given only after the age of two. With this regimen, mottling did not appear, but caries resistance was preserved.
Thus, for the prophylaxis of caries in communities where the water supply contains less than 0.7 p.p.m. of fluoride, it is suggested that a liquid vitamin preparation containing 0.5 mg of fluoride per recommended dose be administered from the time of birth until the age of two or three. At that time, Tablets Novacebrin c̄ Fluoride Chewable may be substituted. These should be continued until the child is at least eight or ten years old. For maximum benefit, it is of utmost importance that the child receive fluoride regularly.
Contraindications and Precautions: In order that dental fluorosis may be avoided, this product should be used only in areas where the drinking water contains less than 0.7 p.p.m. of fluoride. The recommended dose should not be exceeded. When this preparation is being taken, no other medication or vitamin product containing fluoride should be used.
Like all medications, this preparation should be kept out of the reach of children to prevent any possibility of their taking the entire contents of a bottle at one time.
With the passage of time, there is a small gradual decrease in potency of vitamin mixtures. For the protection of the patient, bottles of Novacebrin c̄ Fluoride Chewable are stamped with an expiration date. If the contents are used before the expiration date, the vitamin content will not be less than that stated on the label. To safeguard their potency, vitamin preparations should be protected from direct sunlight.
Adverse Reactions: Ingestion of excessive amounts of fluoride over prolonged periods can result in mottling of the dental enamel. Significant mottling is usually not observed in areas with naturally fluoridated water supplies until the fluoride content reaches approximately 2 p.p.m.
Prolonged use of optimally fluoridated water supplies (1 p.p.m.) has not caused adverse side effects on growth, general health, or well-being or any changes in skeletal density or rate of skeletal maturation. However, it has been reported that patients taking fluoride preparations occasionally developed skin rashes, gastrointestinal upsets, and headache. These complaints disappeared when the drug was discontinued.
Overdosage of fluoride may result in severe illness; a single dose of 230 to 450 mg of fluoride will cause signs of acute toxicity. The lowest recorded human fatal dose is 2 gm. Since the bottle of Novacebrin c̄ Fluoride Chewable contains 100 tablets—a total of 100 mg of fluoride—the possibility of an accidental dangerous overdosage is almost completely obviated.
Administration and Dosage: For children three years of age and older who live in areas where the drinking water contains less than 0.7 p.p.m. of fluoride, 1 tablet daily is recommended. The tablet may be chewed or swallowed with water or other liquid.
How Supplied: (℞) *Tablets No. 52, Novacebrin® c̄ Fluoride Chewable (multiple vitamins with fluoride, Lilly), T03,** Orange, in bottles of 100. [081478]

NOVACEBRIN® c̄ FLUORIDE DROPS ℞
(multiple vitamins with fluoride)

Description: Novacebrin c̄ Fluoride Drops are designed to prevent vitamin deficiencies in infants and young children and to aid in the prevention of dental caries.
Each 0.6 ml contains—
Fluoride (as Sodium Fluoride)............0.5 mg
Vitamin A ....2500 IU (0.75 mg)
Vitamin D............400 IU (10 mcg)
Vitamin C............60 mg
(as Sodium Ascorbate and Ascorbic Acid)
Thiamine Hydrochloride (Vitamin B_1)............1mg
Riboflavin (Vitamin B_2)............1 mg
(as Riboflavin 5′ Phosphate Sodium)
Pyridoxine Hydrochloride (Vitamin B_6)............1 mg
Niacinamide............10 mg
Indications: *See also under* Novacebrin® c̄ Fluoride Chewable.
The vitamin formula is well balanced and is suitable for infants and children from birth until two or three years of age. Multiple vitamins are indicated particularly for infants who do not accept solid foods well and whose intake of certain vitamins may therefore be inadequate.
For the prophylaxis of caries in communities where the water supply contains less than 0.7 p.p.m. of fluoride, it is recommended that Novacebrin c̄ Fluoride Drops be administered from the time of birth until the age of two or three. At that time, Tablets Novacebrin c̄ Fluoride Chewable may be substituted. These should be continued until the child is at least eight or ten years old. For maximum benefit, it is of utmost importance that the child receive fluoride regularly.
Contraindications and Precautions: *See under* Novacebrin c̄ Fluoride Chewable.
Adverse Reactions: *See also under* Novacebrin c̄ Fluoride Chewable.
Overdosage of fluoride may result in severe illness; a single dose of 230 to 450 mg of fluoride will cause signs of acute toxicity. The lowest recorded human fatal dose is 2 gm. An entire bottle of Novacebrin c̄ Fluoride Drops contains 25 mg of fluoride. Thus, the possibility of an accidental dangerous overdosage is completely obviated.
Administration and Dosage: For infants and children under three years of age who live in areas where the drinking water contains less than 0.7 p.p.m. of fluoride, a daily dose of 0.6 ml. Novacebrin c̄ Fluoride Drops is recommended. Fill dropper to mark and dispense contents with one firm squeeze of the bulb. The dropper is designed to compensate for the small amount of solution remaining in the tip. The dose may be dropped directly on the tongue, or it may be mixed with milk, fruit juices, or other foods.
How Supplied: (℞) *Novacebrin® c̄ Fluoride Drops (multiple vitamins with fluoride, Lilly), M-152,* in 30-ml bottles with an accompanying dropper calibrated at 0.6 ml. [081878]

NOVRAD® ℞
(levopropoxyphene napsylate)
NF

Description: Novrad® (levopropoxyphene napsylate, Lilly) is an antitussive which was synthesized by chemists in the Lilly Research Laboratories. When administered orally to humans, it was found to control cough. It is not a cure for any pulmonary disorder, but it is an adjunct to other forms of therapy and will provide symptomatic relief.
Chemistry: Novrad® (α-*l*-4-dimethylamino-1,2-diphenyl-3-methyl-2-propionoxybutane 2-naphthalene sulfonate) is a mildly bitter, white crystalline solid which is very slightly soluble in water.
Indication: Novrad® (levopropoxyphene napsylate, Lilly) is indicated for the symptomatic treatment of cough.
Contraindications: Novrad® (levopropoxyphene napsylate, Lilly) is contraindicated in conditions in which it is inadvisable to decrease the frequency and intensity of cough. Other contraindications include known sensitivity to Novrad.
Precautions: If symptoms of central-nervous-system stimulation or sedation develop, the dosage should be reduced or the medication discontinued.
Levopropoxyphene may impair the mental and/or physical abilities required for the performance of potentially hazardous tasks, such as driving a car or operating machinery. The patient should be cautioned accordingly.
Adverse Reactions: The administration of Novrad® (levopropoxyphene napsylate, Lilly) may be followed by nausea, epigastric burning, skin rash, urticaria, drowsiness, nervousness, and dizziness.
Administration and Dosage: Novrad® (levopropoxyphene napsylate, Lilly) is administered orally.
The usual adult dosage is 100 mg every four hours.
The usual pediatric dosage is approximately 0.5 mg per pound of body weight every four hours. The following dosage table is for convenience in prescribing the suspension.
25 pounds............¼ teaspoonful (12.5 mg)
50 pounds............½ teaspoonful (25 mg)
75–100 pounds............1 teaspoonful (50 mg)
The dose may be varied somewhat, depending on the results produced. The maximum recommended daily dosage of Novrad (in divided doses) is as follows:
Adults—600 mg
Children—25 pounds............75 mg
50 pounds............150 mg
75–100 pounds............200 mg
Overdosage: Symptoms of overdosage include uncontrollable muscle tremor, agitation, and vomiting, followed by sedation. In the event that overdosage with Novrad® (levopropoxyphene napsylate, Lilly) preparations is encountered, gastric lavage along with symptomatic and supportive therapy is recommended. No specific antagonists to Novrad are known. According to animal data, nalorphine is contraindicated in the treatment of overdosage.
How Supplied: (℞) *Pulvules® Novrad® (Levopropoxyphene Napsylate Capsules, NF), No. 384, H14,** 100 mg (equivalent to levopropoxyphene) (No. 1, Ivory Opaque Body, Light-Brown Opaque Cap), in bottles of 50.
(℞) *Suspension No. M-109, Novrad® (Levopropoxyphene Napsylate Oral Suspension, NF),* 50 mg (equivalent to levopropoxyphene) per 5 ml, in 4-fl-oz bottles. Alcohol, 1 percent. *Avoid freezing.* [112178]

ONCOVIN® ℞
(vincristine sulfate)
For Injection, USP

Description: Oncovin® (vincristine sulfate, Lilly) is the salt of an alkaloid obtained from a common flowering herb, the periwinkle plant (*Vinca rosea* Linn.). Originally known as leurocristine, it has also been referred to as LCR and VCR. The empirical formula is $C_{46}H_{56}N_4O_{10} \cdot H_2SO_4$.
The vials contain either 1 mg Oncovin and 10 mg lactose or 5 mg Oncovin and 50 mg lactose. Each size is supplied in a combination package with an accompanying vial of diluting solution (Bacteriostatic Sodium Chloride Injection), 10 ml, containing 90 mg sodium chloride, with 0.9 percent benzyl alcohol as a preservative.
Action: The mode of action of Oncovin® (vincristine sulfate, Lilly) is unknown but is under investigation. Treatment of neoplastic cells in vitro with Oncovin demonstrated that it may

cause an arrest of mitotic division at the stage of metaphase.
Central-nervous-system leukemia has been reported in patients undergoing otherwise successful therapy with Oncovin. This suggests that Oncovin does not penetrate well into the cerebrospinal fluid.
Indications: Oncovin® (vincristine sulfate, Lilly) is indicated in acute leukemia.
It has also been shown to be useful in combination with other oncolytic agents in Hodgkin's disease, lymphosarcoma, reticulum-cell sarcoma, rhabdomyosarcoma, neuroblastoma, and Wilms' tumor.
Contraindications: There are no contraindications to the use of Oncovin® (vincristine sulfate, Lilly), but careful attention should be given to those conditions listed under Warning and Precautions.
Warning: Since reproduction studies have not been performed in animals, there is insufficient information as to whether this drug may affect fertility in men and women or have teratogenic or other adverse effects on the fetus. The physician should weigh the benefits in relation to the risks when using this and other chemotherapeutic agents in populations in which reproduction may be a factor.
Precautions: Acute uric acid nephropathy, which may occur after the administration of oncolytic agents, has also been reported with Oncovin® (vincristine sulfate, Lilly). In the presence of leukopenia or a complicating infection, administration of the next dose of Oncovin warrants careful consideration.
If central-nervous-system leukemia is diagnosed, additional agents and routes of administration may be required, since Oncovin does not appear to cross the blood-brain barrier in adequate amounts.
Particular attention should be given to dosage and neurologic side effects if Oncovin is administered to patients with preexisting neuromuscular disease and also when other drugs with neurotoxic potential are being used.
Adverse Reactions: In general, adverse reactions are reversible and are related to dosage. The most common adverse reaction is hair loss; the most troublesome are neuromuscular in origin.
When single weekly doses of the drug are employed, the adverse reactions of leukopenia, neuritic pain, constipation, and difficulty in walking are usually of short duration (i.e., less than seven days). When the dosage is reduced, these reactions may lessen or disappear. They seem to be increased when the calculated amount of drug is given in divided doses. Other adverse reactions, such as hair loss, sensory loss, paresthesia, slapping gait, loss of deep-tendon reflexes, and muscle wasting, may persist for at least as long as therapy is continued. In most instances, they have disappeared by about the sixth week after discontinuance of treatment, but in some patients the neuromuscular difficulties may persist for prolonged periods.
In addition to constipation (mentioned below), paralytic ileus may occur, particularly in young children. The ileus will reverse itself upon temporary discontinuance of Oncovin and with symptomatic care. It mimics the "surgical abdomen."
Frequently, there is a sequence in the development of neuromuscular side effects. Initially, only sensory impairment and paresthesias may be encountered. With continued treatment, neuritic pain may appear and, later, motor difficulties. No reports have yet been made of any agent that can reverse the neuromuscular manifestations accompanying therapy with Oncovin® (vincristine sulfate, Lilly).
Convulsions, frequently with hypertension, have been reported in a few patients receiving Oncovin.
Rare occurrences of the syndrome attributed to inappropriate antidiuretic hormone secretion have been observed in patients treated with Oncovin. The syndrome has been described in association with several disease states. There is high urinary sodium excretion in the presence of hyponatremia; renal or adrenal disease, hypotension, dehydration, azotemia, and clinical edema are absent. With fluid deprivation, improvement occurs in the hyponatremia and in the renal loss of sodium.
Constipation may take the form of upper-colon impaction, and, on physical examination, the rectum may be found to be empty. Colicky abdominal pain coupled with an empty rectum may mislead the physician. A flat film of the abdomen is useful in demonstrating this condition. All cases have responded to high enemas and laxatives. A routine prophylactic regimen against constipation is recommended for all patients receiving Onocovin.
Other adverse reactions that have been reported are abdominal cramps, ataxia, foot drop, weight loss, fever, cranial nerve manifestations, paresthesia and numbness of the digits, polyuria, dysuria, oral ulceration, headache, vomiting, and diarrhea.
Oncovin does not appear to have any constant or significant effect upon the platelets or the red blood cells. Thrombocytopenia, if present when therapy with Oncovin is begun, may actually improve before the appearance of marrow remission.
Administration and Dosage: Extreme care must be used in calculating and administering the dose of Oncovin® (vincristine sulfate, Lilly), since overdosage may have a very serious or fatal outcome.
The drug is administered intravenously *at weekly intervals.* The usual dose of Oncovin for children is 2 mg/m^2; for adults, 1.4 mg/m^2. Various dosage schedules have been used (see references in package insert).
Oncovin should be mixed with the diluting solution provided (Bacteriostatic Sodium Chloride Injection). The resulting solution of Oncovin may be stored in the refrigerator for 14 days without significant loss of potency.
Oncovin may also be diluted in sterile water or physiological saline to concentrations of 0.01 to 1 mg/ml.
The solution may be injected either directly into a vein or into the tubing of a running intravenous infusion. Injection of the Oncovin may be completed in about one minute.
Caution—It is extremely important that the needle be properly positioned in the vein before any vincristine is injected. If leakage into surrounding tissue should occur during intravenous administration of Oncovin, it may cause considerable irritation. The injection should be discontinued immediately, and any remaining portion of the dose should then be introduced into another vein. Local injection of hyaluronidase and the application of moderate heat to the area of leakage help disperse the drug and are thought to minimize discomfort and the possibility of cellulitis.
How Supplied: (℞) *Ampoules (Vials) Oncovin® (Vincristine Sulfate for Injection, USP)* (Dry Powder): *No. 694,* containing 1 mg Oncovin® (vincristine sulfate, Lilly) and 10 mg lactose, and *No. 695,* containing 5 mg Oncovin® (vincristine sulfate, Lilly) and 50 mg lactose, rubber-stoppered, in singles (10 per carton). *Refrigerate.* [041879]

Ampoules No. 694, 1 mg—
6505-00-904-0024
Ampoules No. 695, 5 mg—
6505-00-903-9990

OUABAIN ℞
Injection, USP

Each ampoule contains a sufficient amount to permit withdrawal and administration of the volume specified on the label.
Description: Ouabain is a crystalline glycoside isolated from the seeds of *Strophanthus gratus.* It is capable of producing the same therapeutic and toxic effects as digitalis and, when given intravenously, acts more rapidly than any other cardiac glycoside now available. Full digitalis effect is obtained within two hours. Ouabain is eliminated more rapidly from the body, and the duration of its effect is shorter than that of the glycosides in either *Digitalis lanata* or *Digitalis purpurea.* Therefore, cumulation is less likely to occur than with other substances possessing a digitalis-like action. Each 2 ml contain Ouabain, USP, 0.5 mg; with sodium chloride, 17 mg; potassium phosphate, monobasic, 2 mg; and sodium phosphate, 6.6 mg; in Sterile Water for Injection, USP, q.s. to make 2 ml.
Indications: Ouabain is primarily indicated to produce rapid digitalization in acute congestive heart failure. It is also recommended in the treatment of atrial or nodal paroxysmal tachycardia and atrial flutter.
Precautions: Since ouabain is a potent and rapidly acting drug, it should be injected slowly. Close observation of the patient is essential. Great care must be exercised if ouabain is given to a patient who has frequent ventricular premature beats or who has received any preparation of digitalis during the preceding three weeks.
Administration and Dosage: The administration of ouabain should be limited to the intravenous route, because it is poorly and irregularly absorbed from the intestinal tract and intramuscular injection is painful. The recommended initial dose is 0.25 mg; but in an emergency in which the full therapeutic effect must be obtained as soon as possible, 0.5 mg can be injected into the vein. After the initial injection, 0.1 mg of the glycoside may be given hourly until the desired result is produced or until a total of 1 mg of the drug has been given within 24 hours. Administration of ouabain should be discontinued if nausea, vomiting, or extreme bradycardia occurs or if cardiac arrhythmia develops in a patient whose heart has been regular. Ouabain is not suitable for maintaining the digitalis effect, and the administration of a cardiac glycoside effective by the oral route should be instituted as soon as the emergency has passed. For example, if one-fourth or one-third of the average digitalizing dose of Crystodigin® (Digitoxin, USP, Lilly) (0.3 to 0.4 mg) is given one hour after the initial injection of ouabain, the transition from the intravenous to oral therapy can be accomplished without loss of the therapeutic effect produced by ouabain.
How Supplied: (℞) *Ampoules No. 112, Ouabain Injection, USP,* 0.5 mg in 2 ml, in packages of 12. [110378]

PAGITANE® HYDROCHLORIDE ℞
(cycrimine hydrochloride)
Tablets, NF

Description: Pagitane® Hydrochloride (cycrimine hydrochloride, Lilly) is α-Cyclopentyl-α-phenyl-1-piperidinepropanol Hydrochloride.
Actions: Pagitane® Hydrochloride (cycrimine hydrochloride, Lilly) has anticholinergic activity. It has been suggested that this action may block the uptake of catecholamines into the corpus striatum.
Indications: Pagitane® Hydrochloride (cycrimine hydrochloride, Lilly) is useful as an adjunct in all three types of Parkinsonism (postencephalitic, arteriosclerotic, or idiopathic).
Contraindication: Pagitane® Hydrochloride (cycrimine hydrochloride, Lilly) is contraindicated in individuals showing hypersensitivity to this drug.
Warning: Caution should be observed in treating patients with glaucoma, because the

Continued on next page

*Identi-Code® symbol.

Lilly—Cont.

possible consequent dilation of the pupil might be harmful.

Usage in Pregnancy—Safety of this product for use during pregnancy has not been established.

Precautions: Use of Pagitane® Hydrochloride (cycrimine hydrochloride, Lilly) should be avoided in those conditions in which inhibition of the parasympathetic nervous system is undesirable.

Great care should be taken in the administration of Pagitane Hydrochloride to patients in the older age groups, particularly those with arteriosclerotic changes, because side effects are likely to be more severe. The drug should be used with caution in patients with tachycardia or any tendency toward urinary retention (such as may be produced by a benign enlargement of the prostate).

Adverse Reactions: Side effects appear to be related to the dosage and to individual sensitivity. Transient nausea associated with anorexia may occur about 30 to 60 minutes after the drug is taken. Some patients may also have blurring of vision and dryness of the mouth, occasionally in conjunction with soreness of the mouth and tongue. These minor side effects often disappear when the drug has been continued for one or two weeks. Epigastric distress can often be overcome if the medication is administered with meals or with a glass of milk. Sucking hard candy at intervals throughout the day usually relieves dryness of the mouth. Lightheadedness, weakness, tachycardia, elevated temperature, flushing, rash, and transitory confusional states have been reported. These side effects quickly disappeared when the drug was discontinued. The more significant side effects were observed in the older age groups, especially in those with arteriosclerotic changes.

Administration and Dosage: Pagitane® Hydrochloride (cycrimine hydrochloride, Lilly) is administered by mouth, preferably with meals. The dosage must be individualized; it is influenced by the type of the disease and by other factors, such as the patient's age. In general, patients with postencephalitic Parkinsonism tolerate larger doses of the drug than do those suffering from the arteriosclerotic or idiopathic types of the disease. Elderly patients, particularly when their disease has an arteriosclerotic basis, do not tolerate large single doses. However, an adequate total daily dosage can often be reached in these patients by frequent administration of very small doses. The following are recommended starting doses.

Type of Parkinsonism	
Postencephalitic	5 mg t i d
Idiopathic	1.25 mg t i d
Arteriosclerotic	1.25 mg t i d

The maximum recommended dose is usually 20 mg daily; however, some postencephalitic patients may require more.

Overdosage: Symptoms of intoxication with Pagitane® Hydrochloride (cycrimine hydrochloride, Lilly) are similar to those of atropine overdosage. They include dryness of the mucous membranes, dilatation of pupils, hot, dry, and flushed skin, hyperpyrexia, tachycardia, nausea and vomiting, restlessness and confusion with coma, circulatory collapse, and respiratory depression. Treatment of overdosage is symptomatic. Gastric lavage should be performed with 4 percent tannic acid or other alkaloidal antidotes. To relieve the peripheral effects, 5 mg of pilocarpine may be given orally at repeated intervals. Artificial respiration and oxygen therapy may be needed for respiratory depression. Urinary retention may require catheterization. The hyperpyrexia is best treated with alcohol sponges. To counteract mydriasis, pilocarpine nitrate, 0.5 percent, may be used. Because of photophobia, the patient may be more comfortable in a darkened room.

How Supplied: (℞) *Tablets Pagitane® Hydrochloride (Cycrimine Hydrochloride Tablets, NF): No. 1783, C16,** 1.25 mg, Sugar-Coated, Orange, and *No. 1784, C17,** 2.5 mg, Sugar-Coated, Brown, in bottles of 100.

[080277]

PAPAVERINE HYDROCHLORIDE ℞
Injection, NF
AMPOULES AND VIALS

Each ampoule or vial contains a sufficient amount to permit withdrawal and administration of the volume specified on the label.

Description: Papaverine hydrochloride is the hydrochloride of an alkaloid obtained from opium or prepared synthetically. It belongs to the benzylisoquinoline group of alkaloids. It does not contain a phenanthrene group as do morphine and codeine.

Indications: Papaverine is recommended in various conditions accompanied by spasm of smooth muscle, such as:

Vascular spasm associated with:
- Acute myocardial infarction (coronary occlusion)
- Angina pectoris
- Peripheral and pulmonary embolism
- Peripheral vascular disease in which there is a vasospastic element
- Certain cerebral angiospastic states

Visceral spasm as in:
- Ureteral colic
- Biliary colic
- Gastrointestinal colic

Contraindications: Intravenous injection of papaverine is contraindicated in the presence of complete atrioventricular heart block. When conduction is depressed, the drug may produce transient ectopic rhythms of ventricular origin, either premature beats or paroxysmal tachycardia.

Precaution: Papaverine Hydrochloride Injection should not be added to Lactated Ringer's Injection, because precipitation would result.

Adverse Reactions: The following side effects have been reported: general discomfort, intensive flushing of the face, perspiration, increase in the depth of respiration, increase in heart rate, a slight rise in blood pressure, and excessive sedation.

Administration and Dosage: Papaverine hydrochloride may be administered intravenously or intramuscularly. The intravenous route is recommended when an immediate effect is desired, but the drug *must* be injected *slowly* over the course of one or two minutes to avoid uncomfortable or alarming side effects. Parenteral administration of papaverine hydrochloride in doses of 1 to 4 ml is repeated every three hours as indicated. In the treatment of cardiac extrasystoles, two doses may be given ten minutes apart.

Pharmacology: The most characteristic effect of papaverine is relaxation of the tonus of all smooth muscle, especially when it has been spasmodically contracted. The action is apparently direct on the muscle itself. This relaxation is noted in the *vascular system* and *bronchial musculature* and in the *gastrointestinal, biliary,* and *urinary tracts.*

No cumulative effects have been noted following the use of papaverine. Its toxicity is low, and neither tolerance nor habituation has been reported after administration.

How Supplied: (℞) *Papaverine Hydrochloride Injection, NF: Ampoules (Vials) No. 423,* 30 mg (½ gr) per ml, 10 ml, rubber-stoppered, in singles (10 per carton) and in packages of 25; *Ampoules No. 396,* 60 mg (1 gr) in 2 ml, in packages of 12 and 100. Each ampoule or vial contains edetate disodium, 0.005 percent. Sodium hydroxide may have been added during manufacture to adjust the *p*H. Ampoules (Vials) No. 423 also contain chlorobutanol (chloroform derivative), 0.5 percent.

[020879]

PAPAVERINE HYDROCHLORIDE ℞
POWDER AND TABLETS
NF

Description and Indications: *See under* Ampoules and Vials Papaverine Hydrochloride.

Contraindication: There is no known contraindication to oral administration of papaverine hydrochloride.

Adverse Reactions: The following side effects have been reported: mild constipation, general discomfort, intensive flushing of the face, perspiration, increase in the depth of respiration, increase in heart rate, a slight rise in blood pressure, and excessive sedation.

Administration and Dosage: The usual adult dosage ranges from 100 to 300 mg three to five times daily.

How Supplied: (℞) *Powder No. 36, Papaverine Hydrochloride, NF,* in 1-oz and 4-oz bottles. (℞) *Tablets Papaverine Hydrochloride, NF: No. 1705, J61,** 30 mg (½ gr), in bottles of 100; *No. 1706, J62,** 60 mg (1 gr), in bottles of 100 and 1000; *No. 1671, T55,** 100 mg (1 ½ grs), in bottles of 100 and 1000 and in 10 strips of 10 individually labeled blisters each containing 1 tablet (ID100); *No. 1733, T73,** 200 mg (3 grs), in bottles of 100.

[020779]

PARATHYROID ℞
Injection, USP

Description: Parathyroid Injection, USP, is prepared from beef glands. One ml possesses a potency of not less than 100 USP parathyroid units and contains glycerin, 1.6 percent, with 0.25 percent phenol as a preservative. Sodium hydroxide and/or hydrochloride acid may have been added during manufacture to adjust the *p*H.

Standard: Parathyroid Injection, USP, is standardized by its capacity to increase the total serum calcium in normal dogs. One USP parathyroid unit is defined as one one-hundredth of the amount required to raise the calcium content of 100 ml of the blood serum of normal dogs 1 mg within 16 to 18 hours after administration. Mature male dogs free from gross evidence of disease and weighing between 10 and 12 kg are used, and the rules of assay as given in the USP are followed.

Physiology: When parathyroid hormone is administered to hypoparathyroid patients or to normal individuals, the following changes occur in this order: (1) hyperphosphaturia, (2) hypophosphatemia, (3) hypercalcemia, and (4) hypercalciuria. There is much evidence that the major effect of parathyroid hormone is an increased renal excretion of phosphorus. On the other hand, there is evidence that this hormone may have a direct action on bone. There is no evidence that calcium absorption from the gastrointestinal tract is increased.

Indications: Parathyroid Injection may be used in the treatment of acute hypoparathyroidism with tetany. Ordinarily, the serum calcium level rises in four hours after each injection. Calcium gluconate administered intravenously is important interim therapy until the effect of parathyroid hormone occurs. Patients soon become refractory to injections of parathyroid hormone; therefore, long-continued use is not recommended. The use of vitamin D_2 (calciferol) plus oral calcium is usually effective in those cases of hypoparathyroidism that need prolonged therapy.

Parathyroid Injection is used in the Ellsworth-Howard test, which is useful in establishing the diagnosis of idiopathic and postoperative hypoparathyroidism. This test also differentiates hypoparathyroidism from pseudohypoparathyroidism. The procedure requires that the patient be in a fasting state. Three urine collections made at hourly intervals are analyzed for phosphorus content. Then 200 units of Parathyroid Injection are administered intravenously. Following this, three to five hourly urine collections are again analyzed for phosphorus content. In order to eliminate the possibility of inactive material, it is generally recommended that this test be performed at the same time with the same parathyroid extract on a normal control patient. Improper refrigeration is the usual cause of inactive extract. Normal patients have a five to sixfold increase in the amount of phosphorus in the urine. Patients with postoperative or idiopathic hypoparathyroidism usually have a tenfold or greater increase in phosphorus excretion. Cases of pseudohypoparathyroidism have a twofold or less increase in phosphorus excretion.

Contraindications and Precautions: Parathyroid Injection should not be given (and, especially, should not be given intravenously) to patients whose blood calcium levels are already above normal. The hormone should be used cautiously in the presence of renal or cardiac disease. Symptoms of overdosage are anorexia, vomiting, diarrhea, and weakness.

The dosage should be so controlled as to maintain the serum calcium level at not more than 12 mg per 100 ml.

Because parathyroid extracts have some of the properties of proteins, caution should be used in their intravenous administration. Preliminary skin tests should be undertaken before intravenous injection, and desensitization should be employed if the tests are positive. Even if sensitivity cannot be demonstrated, intravenous administration should be slow, and a solution of epinephrine should be available in case of reaction. If Parathyroid Injection is to be added to other intravenous solutions, it is recommended that 2.5 to 5 percent dextrose be used. Saline solutions often cause the formation of a precipitate.

Administration and Dosage: Administration may be subcutaneous, intramuscular, or intravenous. The intramuscular route is generally the most satisfactory. Moderate inflammatory reactions are observed at times after subcutaneous injection.

In the acute state of tetany due to hypoparathyroidism, 20 to 40 units of Parathyroid Injection may be administered every 12 hours. Larger doses may be given if needed. The use of intravenous calcium gluconate as well as oral calcium is important. Parathyroid extract ordinarily is continued only for a few days, since patients may soon become refractory to it. If prolonged therapy seems indicated, the use of vitamin D, such as Gelseals® Deltalin® (synthetic oleovitamin D, Lilly), 50,000 IU, is preferred to parathyroid extract.

How Supplied: (℞) *Ampoules (Vials) No. 355, Parathyroid Injection, USP,* 100 USP units per ml, 5 ml, rubber-stoppered, in singles (10 per carton). *To retain full potency, this product should be kept between 2° and 8°C (36° and 46°F). Avoid freezing.*

[062277]

PAVERIL® PHOSPHATE ℞
(dioxyline phosphate)

Description: Paveril® Phosphate (dioxyline phosphate, Lilly) is a synthetic, crystalline, *non-narcotic* compound which has the ability to relax smooth-muscle spasm.

Indications: On the basis of a review of this drug by the National Academy of Sciences — National Research Council and/or other information, FDA has classified the following indications as "possibly" effective.

For the treatment of angina pectoris and conditions in which there is reflex spasm of blood vessels in arms, legs, or lungs. Paveril® Phosphate (dioxyline phosphate, Lilly) also may be tried in other conditions involving spasm of smooth muscle.

Final classification of the less-than-effective indications requires further investigation.

Contraindications: There are no known contraindications to the oral administration of Paveril® Phosphate (dioxyline phosphate, Lilly).

Adverse Reactions: Paveril® Phosphate (dioxyline phosphate, Lilly) given orally in therapeutic doses rarely causes side effects. If they occur, they are mild and include nausea, dizziness, sweating, flushing, sedation, and abdominal cramps.

Dosage: *Adults*—100 to 400 mg three or four times daily as required.

Overdosage: Gastric irritation and vasodilation. *Symptoms*—Nausea, dizziness, sweating, flushing, and abdominal cramping. *Treatment*—General management consists in symptomatic therapy, including gastric lavage immediately following administration of the drug.

How Supplied: (℞) *Tablets Paveril® Phosphate (dioxyline phosphate, Lilly)* (scored): *No. 1781, J97,** 100 mg, White, and *No. 1782, T91,** 200 mg, Pink, in bottles of 100 and 500.

[011279]

PENICILLIN G PROCAINE, *see* Duracillin® A.S. (sterile penicillin G procaine suspension, Lilly).

PENICILLIN G PROCAINE FOR AQUEOUS INJECTION, *see* Duracillin® A.S. (sterile penicillin G procaine suspension, Lilly).

PENICILLIN V POTASSIUM PRODUCTS, *see* V-Cillin K® (penicillin V potassium, Lilly).

POTASSIUM IODIDE ℞

Description: Each Enseal® (enteric-release tablet, Lilly) Potassium Iodide contains 300 mg of the salt in a special coating designed to prevent disintegration in the stomach.

Indications: Potassium iodide is used as an expectorant to liquefy the tenacious bronchial secretions often seen in chronic bronchitis, bronchiectasis, and asthma.

Contraindications: Known sensitivity to iodides is a contraindication to the use of potassium iodide. The drug should not be administered in the presence of acute bronchitis.

Warnings: There have been several reports, published and unpublished, concerning nonspecific small-bowel lesions (consisting of stenosis with or without ulceration) associated with the administration of enteric-coated thiazides with potassium salts. Such lesions may occur when enteric-coated potassium tablets are given alone, with non-enteric-coated thiazides, or with certain other oral diuretics.

These small-bowel lesions have caused obstruction, hemorrhage, and perforation. Surgery has frequently been required, and deaths have occurred.

Available information tends to implicate enteric-coated potassium salts, although lesions of this type also occur spontaneously. Therefore, coated potassium-containing formulations should be administered only when indicated and should be discontinued immediately if abdominal pain, distention, nausea, vomiting, or gastrointestinal bleeding occurs.

Coated potassium tablets should be used only when adequate dietary supplementation is not practical.

Precautions: Occasionally, persons are markedly sensitive to iodides, and care should be used in administering the drug for the first time. Iodides should be given with great caution, if at all, in the presence of tuberculosis. Because of the possible development of fetal goiter, iodide should be administered with caution to pregnant women.

Adverse Reactions: Thyroid adenoma, goiter, and myxedema are possible side effects. Hypersensitivity to iodides may be manifested by angioneurotic edema, cutaneous and mucosal hemorrhages, and symptoms resembling serum sickness, such as fever, arthralgia, lymph node enlargement, and eosinophilia. Iodism or chronic iodine poisoning may occur during prolonged treatment. The symptoms of iodism include a metallic taste, soreness of the mouth, increased salivation, coryza, sneezing, and swelling of the eyelids. There may be a severe headache, productive cough, pulmonary edema, and swelling and tenderness of the salivary glands. Acneform skin lesions are seen in the seborrheic areas. Severe and sometimes fatal skin eruptions may develop. Gastric disturbance and diarrhea are common. If iodism appears, the drug should be withdrawn and the patient given appropriate supportive therapy.

Administration and Dosage: The usual adult daily dose of potassium iodide given to increase secretions is 1 or 2 Enseals three times a day. If symptoms of increased lacrimal and nasal secretions are noted, the dose should be decreased to 1 Enseal three times a day or less. The medication should be used no longer than is necessary to produce the desired effect. However, in chronic conditions, continuous administration may be required.

How Supplied: (℞) *Enseals No. 23, Potassium Iodide, A06,** 300 mg, in bottles of 100 and 1000.

[101178]

POTASSIUM TRIPLEX ℞

Description: Liquid Potassium Triplex, containing potassium acetate, potassium bicarbonate, and potassium citrate (each in 10 percent concentration), supplies approximately 15 mEq of potassium in each 5 ml.

Potassium acetate appears as colorless, monoclinic crystals or white crystalline powder. It is very soluble in water and freely soluble in alcohol. Potassium bicarbonate occurs as white granular powder. It is freely soluble in water but practically insoluble in alcohol. Potassium citrate occurs as transparent crystals or white granular powder. Freely soluble in water, it is almost insoluble in alcohol.

Contains in each 5 ml: Potassium, 15 mEq (approximately), provided by 0.5 gm potassium acetate; 0.5 gm potassium bicarbonate; and 0.5 gm potassium citrate in a sugar-free vehicle containing glycerin, saccharin sodium, water, and aromatics.

Clinical Pharmacology: Potassium, the major intracellular cation, plays a significant part in the control of osmotic pressure and also serves as an essential activator in a number of enzymatic reactions. In addition, the potassium concentration of body fluids has an important influence on the excitability of both skeletal and cardiac muscle and on the structure and function of the kidneys. Disturbances in potassium equilibrium may, therefore, produce a wide range of clinical disorders.

The potassium concentration in extracellular fluid is normally 4 to 5 mEq per liter; that in intracellular fluid is approximately 150 mEq per liter. Since about 20 percent of body weight is extracellular fluid, it can readily be calculated that only a small fraction of the 2500 to 3000 mEq of potassium within the body is contained in the extracellular space. Changes in plasma potassium concentration often mirror those in cellular potassium content; thus, plasma concentration provides a useful clinical

Continued on next page

*Identi-Code® symbol.

Lilly—Cont.

guide to disturbances in potassium balance. By producing large differences in the ratio of intracellular to extracellular potassium, relatively small absolute changes in extracellular concentration may have important effects on neuromuscular activity.

Despite wide variations in dietary intake of potassium (e.g., 40 to 120 mEq per day), plasma potassium concentration is normally stabilized within the narrow range of 4 to 5 mEq per liter by virtue of close renal regulation of potassium balance. Renal potassium excretion is accomplished largely, if not exclusively, by a process of potassium secretion in the distal portion of the nephron; essentially all filtered potassium is reabsorbed in the proximal tubule, and the potassium that appears in the urine is added to the filtrate by a distal process of sodium-cation exchange. Fecal excretion of potassium normally amounts to only a few milliequivalents per day and does not play a significant role in potassium homeostasis.

Indications and Usage: Potassium Triplex is indicated in the treatment of potassium deficiency which may occur in conjunction with (1) long-term diuretic therapy, (2) digitalis intoxication, (3) low dietary intake of potassium, (4) loss of potassium due to vomiting and diarrhea, (5) diabetic acidosis, (6) metabolic alkalosis, (7) corticosteroid therapy, and (8) familial periodic paralysis.

Symptoms and Signs of Potassium Deficiency—These include weakness, drowsiness, anorexia, nausea, chronic ileus with distention, edema, oliguria, shallow and infrequent respirations, dilatation of the heart, low blood pressure, ectopic rhythms, systolic murmurs, hypokalemia, and electrocardiographic changes showing prominent U wave, lengthening of the Q-U (Q-T) interval, depression of the S-T segment, and depression or inversion of the T wave.

Contraindications: Potassium Triplex is contraindicated in severe renal impairment with oliguria, anuria, or azotemia; untreated Addison's disease; adynamia episodica hereditaria; acute dehydration; heat cramps; and hyperkalemia from any cause. Potassium intensifies the symptoms of myotonia congenita.

Warnings: High plasma concentrations of potassium ion may cause death through cardiac depression, arrhythmias, or arrest.

Precautions: *General Precautions*—Potassium Triplex must be administered with caution, since the degree of potassium deficiency or the ideal daily dosage often is not accurately known. Excessive dosage may result in potassium intoxication. The drug should be used with caution in the presence of cardiac disease.

Laboratory Tests—Frequent checks of the clinical status of the patient, ECG, and/or plasma potassium levels should be made.

Usage in Pregnancy—Pregnancy Category C—Animal reproduction studies have not been conducted with Potassium Triplex. It is also not known whether Potassium Triplex can cause fetal harm when administered to a pregnant woman or can affect reproduction capacity. Potassium Triplex should be given to a pregnant woman only if clearly needed.

Nursing Mothers—It is not known whether this drug is excreted in human milk. Because many drugs are excreted in human milk and because of the potential for serious adverse reactions in nursing infants from Potassium Triplex, a decision should be made whether to discontinue nursing or to discontinue the drug, taking into account the importance of the drug to the mother.

Usage in Children—Safety and effectiveness in children have not been established.

Drug Interactions—Mineral acids liberate acetic acid, and, because of the feeble ionization of this acid, acetates act as buffers toward mineral acids, decreasing to some extent the hydrogen-ion concentration.

Aqueous solutions of potassium citrate are slightly alkaline and will react with acidic substances. Alkaloidal salts may be precipitated from their aqueous or hydroalcoholic solutions. Acidification or addition of alcohol will restore the solution. Calcium and strontium salts cause a precipitation of the corresponding citrates.

Potassium bicarbonate is decomposed by acids and salts having an acid reaction with the liberation of carbon dioxide. Acid-reacting vehicles are troublesome in this respect, as are some tinctures, fluid extracts, and solutions. Heating or agitating the aqueous solution partially converts it to the normal carbonate with evolution of carbon dioxide. Potassium bicarbonate intensifies the darkening that occurs in solutions of salicylates. Some alkaloids are precipitated from solutions of their salts.

In powder mixtures, atmospheric moisture or water of crystallization from another ingredient sometimes permits potassium bicarbonate to react with boric acid or a salt such as alum. In liquid mixtures containing bismuth subnitrate, potassium bicarbonate reacts with the acid formed by hydrolysis of the bismuth salt.

Adverse Reactions: Potassium Triplex may cause gastric irritation if taken undiluted and on an empty stomach. Vomiting, diarrhea, nausea, and abdominal discomfort have been reported. The symptoms and signs of potassium intoxication include paresthesia of the extremities, flaccid paralysis, listlessness, mental confusion, weakness and heaviness of the legs, fall in blood pressure, cardiac arrhythmias, heart block, hyperkalemia, and electrocardiographic abnormalities (disappearance of the P wave, depression of the S-T segment, tall and peaked T waves, spreading and slurring of the QRS complex with development of a biphasic curve, and cardiac arrest). Potassium intoxication may result from overdosage of Potassium Triplex or from therapeutic dosage in conditions stated under Contraindications. When detected, hyperkalemia must be treated immediately, because lethal levels can be reached in a few hours.

Overdosage: *Clinical Manifestations*—The clinical manifestations of potassium intoxication are related primarily to the heart and the neuromuscular system. Electrocardiographic abnormalities are the earliest and most frequent sign of disturbed membrane excitability and are characterized by the development of tall, "tent-shaped" T waves, by decreased amplitude of the P waves, and later by atrial asystole. Intraventricular block, with widening of the QRS complex, may lead to the development of a sine wave pattern and ultimately to ventricular standstill. Changes in the electrocardiogram usually appear when the serum potassium concentration reaches 7 to 8 mEq per liter, and cardiac standstill is likely to occur at a concentration of 9 to 10 mEq per liter. Weakness and flaccid paralysis, usually indistinguishable from that seen in hypokalemic paralysis, appear only in association with severe hyperkalemia, and death may occur from cardiac arrest before muscular weakness is evident. For this reason, the electrocardiogram is the single most important guide in appraising the threat posed by the hyperkalemia and in determining how aggressive a therapeutic approach is necessary.

Treatment—The treatment of severe potassium intoxication should be directed toward promoting rapid transfer of potassium into cells in order to lower serum potassium concentration and prevent cardiac arrest. Two approaches to this goal are likely to prove effective. Infusion of glucose and insulin induces the cellular deposition of glycogen and at the same time brings about a shift of potassium to the intracellular space; 1 liter of a 10 percent glucose solution with 50 units of insulin is generally employed for this purpose. A further redistribution of potassium can be achieved in the acidotic patient by the administration of sodium bicarbonate (150 to 300 mEq). In many cases, these measures will induce a striking reduction in plasma potassium concentration and prompt improvement in the electrocardiogram. In some instances, the administration of calcium (as 2 gm of calcium lactate) is also useful because calcium, though it has no effect on the plasma potassium contentration, opposes the cardiotoxic effects of potassium. It should be noted, incidentally, that calcium cannot be given in the same solution with sodium bicarbonate because precipitation of the calcium ion will result.

Because the techniques described above do not remove potassium from the body and may be only temporarily effective, longer-term efforts should be directed toward promoting gastrointestinal losses of potassium. A cation-exchange resin in the sodium cycle, such as Kayexelate, will usually achieve this purpose if administered by mouth in a dose of 20 to 30 gm every six hours. Each gm of resin binds approximately 1 mEq of potassium, and within 24 hours a significant effect on plasma potassium concentration should be achieved. To enhance potassium loss and assure the rapid movement of the resin through the gastrointestinal tract, sorbitol, a nonreabsorbable polyhydric alcohol, should be given in quantities sufficient to induce a soft or semiliquid bowel movement every few hours. The usual dose for this purpose is 20 ml. of a 70 percent solution three or four times a day. If the patient is unable to take medication by mouth, the resin can be administered by rectum as a retention enema of 100 gm in several hundred ml of water.

Hemodialysis is an efficient alternative means of removing the excess potassium but usually will not be required if the program outlined above can be carried out effectively.

Administration and Dosage: Potassium Triplex is given orally after meals and is diluted with a glass of tomato juice, orange juice, or other readily available vehicle. The usual adult dosage is 5 ml (15 mEq) of potassium three or four times a day.

Since no average total daily dose can be defined, deviations from this recommendation may be indicated but must be governed by close observation for clinical effects. However, potassium intoxication may result from any therapeutic dosage. *See under* Precautions *and* Overdosage.

How Supplied: (℞) *Liquid No. 29, Potassium Triplex,* in 16-fl-oz (NDC 0002-2463-05) and gallon bottles (NDC 0002-2463-06).

[102279]

PROPYLTHIOURACIL ℞

Tablets, USP

Description: Propylthiouracil (6-propyl-2-thiouracil) is one of the thiocarbamide compounds. It is a white crystalline substance that has a bitter taste and is very slightly soluble in water.

Actions: Propylthiouracil inhibits the synthesis of thyroid hormones and thus is effective in the treatment of hyperthyroidism. The drug does not inactivate existing thyroxine and triiodothyronine which is stored in colloid or is circulating in the blood, nor does it interfere with the effectiveness of thyroid hormones given by mouth or by injection.

Indications: Propylthiouracil is indicated in the medical treatment of hyperthyroidism. Long-term therapy may lead to remission of the disease. Propylthiouracil may also be used to ameliorate hyperthyroidism in preparation for subtotal thyroidectomy or radioactive iodine therapy.

Contraindication: Propylthiouracil is contraindicated in the presence of hypersensitivity to the drug.

Warnings: *Pregnancy*—Propylthiouracil, used judiciously, is an effective drug in hyperthyroidism complicated by pregnancy. Because the drug readily crosses placental membranes and can induce goiter and even cretinism in the developing fetus, it is important that a sufficient, but not excessive, dose be given. In many pregnant women, the thyroid dysfunction diminishes as the pregnancy proceeds; consequently, a reduction of dosage may be possible. In some instances, propylthiouracil can be withdrawn two or three weeks before delivery. The administration of thyroid during propylthiouracil therapy of the pregnant hyperthyroid woman is also recommended in order to prevent hypothyroidism in the mother and her fetus. Administration should continue throughout the pregnancy and after delivery. Postpartum patients receiving propylthiouracil should not nurse their babies.

Precautions: Patients who receive propylthiouracil should be under close surveillance and should be impressed with the necessity of reporting immediately any evidence of illness, particularly sore throat, skin eruptions, fever, headache, or general malaise. In such cases, white-blood-cell and differential counts should be made to determine whether agranulocytosis has developed. Particular care should be exercised with patients who are receiving additional drugs known to cause agranulocytosis. Because propylthiouracil may cause hypoprothrombinemia and bleeding, prothrombin time should be monitored during therapy with the drug, especially before surgical procedures.

Adverse Reactions: Adverse reactions probably occur in less than 3 percent of patients. Minor adverse reactions include skin rash, urticaria, nausea, vomiting, epigastric distress, arthralgia, paresthesia, loss of taste, abnormal loss of hair, myalgia, headache, pruritus, drowsiness, neuritis, edema, vertigo, skin pigmentation, jaundice, sialadenopathy, and lymphadenopathy.

Major adverse reactions (much less common than the minor adverse reactions) include inhibition of myelopoiesis (agranulocytosis, granulopenia, and thrombocytopenia), drug fever, a lupuslike syndrome, hepatitis, periarteritis, and hypoprothrombinemia and bleeding.

It should be noted that about 10 percent of patients with untreated hyperthyroidism have leukopenia (white-blood-cell count of less than 4000 per cu mm), often with relative granulopenia.

Administration and Dosage: Propylthiouracil is administered orally. The total daily dosage is usually given in three equal doses at approximately eight-hour intervals.

Adult—The initial dosage is 300 mg daily. In patients with severe hyperthyroidism, very large goiters, or both, the beginning dosage usually should be 400 mg daily; an occasional patient will require 600 to 900 mg per day initially. The usual maintenance dosage is 100 to 150 mg daily.

Pediatric—For children six to ten years of age, the initial dosage is 50 to 150 mg daily. For children ten years and over, the initial dosage is 150 to 300 mg daily. The maintenance dosage is determined by the response of the patient.

Overdosage: *See under* Tapazole®.

How Supplied: (℞) *Tablets No. 1723, Propylthiouracil, USP, J69,** 50 mg (scored), in bottles of 100 and 1000. [082878]

PROTAMINE SULFATE ℞
Injection, USP

Description: Protamines are simple proteins of low molecular weight that are rich in arginine and strongly basic. They occur in the sperm of salmon and certain other species of fish.

Each 5-ml ampoule of Protamine Sulfate Injection, USP, contains protamine sulfate equivalent to 50 mg of activity, and each 25-ml vial contains protamine sulfate equivalent to 250 mg of activity. Both products also contain 0.9 percent sodium chloride. Sodium phosphate and/or sulfuric acid may have been added during manufacture to adjust the *p*H. Contain no preservative.

Actions: When administered alone, protamine has an anticoagulant effect. However, when it is given in the presence of heparin (which is strongly acidic), a stable salt is formed which results in the loss of anticoagulant activity of both drugs.

Indication: Protamine sulfate is indicated in the treatment of heparin overdosage.

Warnings: Hyperheparinemia or bleeding has been reported in experimental animals and in some patients 30 minutes to 18 hours after cardiac surgery (under cardiopulmonary bypass) in spite of complete neutralization of heparin by adequate doses of protamine sulfate at the end of the operation.

Therefore, it is important to keep the patient under close observation after cardiac surgery. Additional doses of protamine sulfate should be administered if indicated by coagulation studies, such as the heparin titration test with protamine and the determination of plasma thrombin time.

Protamine sulfate should be given by slow intravenous injection (in one to three minutes) in doses not exceeding 50 mg of protamine sulfate activity in any ten-minute period. Facilities to treat shock should be available.

Usage in Pregnancy—Reproduction studies have not been performed in animals. There is no adequate information as to whether this drug may affect fertility in human males or females or have a teratogenic potential or other adverse effect on the fetus.

Precautions: Because of the anticoagulant effect of protamine, it is unwise to give more than 100 mg over a short period unless there is certain knowledge of a larger requirement.

Patients with a history of allergy to fish may develop hypersensitivity reactions to protamine, although to date no relationship has been established between allergic reactions to protamine and fish allergy. A number of individuals hypersensitive to fish have received protamine sulfate without developing allergic reactions.

Adverse Reactions: Intravenous injections of protamine may cause a sudden fall in blood pressure, bradycardia, dyspnea, or transitory flushing and a feeling of warmth. There have been reports of anaphylaxis that resulted in respiratory embarrassment (*see* Precautions).

Administration and Dosage: Each mg of protamine sulfate neutralizes approximately 90 USP units of heparin activity derived from lung tissue or about 115 USP units of heparin activity derived from intestinal mucosa.

Protamine Sulfate Injection, USP, should be given very slowly (in one to three minutes) by the intravenous route. The dosage should not exceed the equivalent of 50 mg of protamine sulfate activity (5 ml) in any ten-minute period.

Protamine Sulfate is intended for injection without further dilution; however, if further dilution is desired, D5W or normal saline may be used. Diluted solutions should not be stored since they contain no preservative.

Protamine Sulfate should not be mixed with other drugs without knowledge of their compatibility, because Protamine Sulfate has been shown to be incompatible with certain antibiotics, including several of the cephalosporins and penicillins.

Because heparin disappears rapidly from the circulation, the dose of protamine sulfate required also decreases rapidly with the time elapsed following intravenous injection of heparin. For example, if the protamine sulfate is administered 30 minutes after the heparin, one-half the usual dose may be sufficient.

The dosage of protamine sulfate should be guided by blood coagulation studies (*see* Warnings).

How Supplied: (℞) *Protamine Sulfate Injection, USP: Ampoules No. 473,* 5 ml (equivalent to 50 mg of activity), in packages of 6 and 25; *Ampoules (Vials) No. 735,* 25 ml (equivalent to 250 mg of activity), rubber-stoppered, in singles (10 per carton). *Refrigerate. Avoid freezing.* **Both products should be stored in the refrigerator above freezing and below 50°F.**

CAUTION—The total dose of protamine sulfate contained in Vials No. 735 (250 mg of activity in 25 ml) is five times greater than that in Ampoules No. 473 (50 mg of activity in 5 ml). The large-size vials (No. 735) are designed only for antiheparin treatment in certain cases in which large doses of heparin have been given during surgery and are to be neutralized by large doses of protamine sulfate after surgical procedures.

[080779]

QUINIDINE GLUCONATE ℞
Injection, USP

Description: Quinidine gluconate, a white dextrorotatory salt, contains 62.3 percent anhydrous quinidine and 37.7 percent gluconic acid. Quinidine Gluconate Injection, USP, is suitable for parenteral use because of its high efficacy, local tolerance, and stability in solution.

Each vial contains 800 mg of the salt of the alkaloid in 10 ml of Sterile Water for Injection, with 0.005 percent edetate disodium and 0.25 percent phenol. This quantity of quinidine gluconate represents 500 mg of anhydrous quinidine.

Indications: Parenteral administration of quinidine is indicated in the treatment of the following conditions when oral therapy is not feasible or when rapid therapeutic effect is required:

- Premature atrial and ventricular contractions
- Paroxysmal atrial tachycardia
- Paroxysmal atrioventricular junctional rhythm
- Atrial flutter
- Paroxysmal atrial fibrillation
- Established atrial fibrillation when therapy is appropriate
- Paroxysmal ventricular tachycardia when not associated with complete heart block
- Maintenance therapy after electrical conversion of atrial fibrillation and/or flutter

Contraindications: Aberrant impulses and abnormal rhythms due to escape mechanisms should not be treated with quinidine.

The other absolute contraindication to the use of quinidine is the known presence of an idiosyncrasy or hypersensitivity to this alkaloid or to other derivatives of cinchona.

Warnings: In the treatment of atrial flutter, reversion to sinus rhythm may be preceded by a progressive reduction in the degree of atrioventricular block to a 1:1 ratio and a resulting extremely rapid ventricular rate.

The dangers of the parenteral use of quinidine are increased in the presence of atrioventricular heart block or in the absence of atrial activity. The administration of quinidine is more hazardous in patients with extensive myocardial damage than it is in persons with a normal heart who have a cardiac arrhythmia. Occasionally, a cardiac arrhythmia may have been produced by digitalis intoxication, and the use of quinidine in this situation is extremely dangerous because the cardiac glycoside may already have caused serious impairment of the intracardiac conduction system.

Adverse Reactions: As much as 500 mg of quinidine gluconate has been administered into the gluteal muscle without producing irritation.

It was reported that untoward subjective reactions, such as nausea, vomiting, cramps, an urge to defecate or urinate, cold sweat, and

Continued on next page

*Identi-Code® symbol.

Lilly—Cont.

apprehensiveness, occurred in patients who received quinidine lactate by the intravenous route. Such symptoms were unrelated to the dosage and occurred when as little as 130 to 260 mg of this preparation was given. Signs of cinchonism, such as vertigo, tinnitus, headache, fever, and visual disturbances, can be produced by an overdose of quinidine, regardless of the route of administration.

The rate of injection into the vein is all-important. Too-rapid administration of as little as 200 mg of quinidine may cause a fall of 40 to 50 mm Hg in arterial pressure.

Large doses of the alkaloid may have a deleterious effect on the heart and result in heart block or standstill in diastole. Deaths have been reported during the intravenous administration of quinidine, but in every instance the patient was *in extremis* before this treatment was initiated. The undesirable effects are more likely to occur in the presence of a previously damaged myocardium than in the treatment of arrhythmia of a more normal heart.

Administration and Dosage: If the patient's condition is not critical, quinidine gluconate should be given intramuscularly. On the other hand, extreme palpitation, dyspnea, vomiting, and a shocklike state in patients with ventricular tachycardia are signs that the intravenous administration of quinidine may be required as a lifesaving measure.

The patient must be under close clinical observation. Frequent or continuous electrocardiograms are desirable, especially during intravenous injection, to detect any change in rate or rhythm.

Administration of the drug must be stopped when any one of the following occurs: (1) side effects of more than trivial nature, (2) restoration of sinus rhythm, (3) prolongation of QRS complex in excess of 25 percent beyond that observed prior to the injection, (4) disappearance of P waves, and (5) decrease in heart rate to 120 beats per minute.

In the treatment of cardiac arrhythmias with quinidine, therapy should be regulated in such a way that the drug is accumulated in the heart in sufficient quantities to abolish ectopic rhythm without disturbing the normal mechanism of the heartbeat. *The effective dose must be determined for each patient.*

If the patient has not received quinidine before and time permits, an initial dose of 200 mg of quinidine gluconate may be given intramuscularly as a test for idiosyncrasy. The test dose is given intramuscularly, regardless of whether subsequent administration is to be intramuscular or intravenous.

Intramuscular—In the treatment of acute tachycardia, the recommended initial dose is 600 mg. Subsequently, the injection of 400 mg of quinidine gluconate can be repeated as often as every two hours. The amount of each dose must be gauged by the effect of the preceding one.

Intravenous—It has been shown that in about 50 percent of patients who respond successfully to quinidine, the arrhythmia can be terminated by 330 mg or less of quinidine gluconate (or its equivalent in other salts). In some cases, the intravenous administration of as much as 500 to 750 mg may be required.

The quinidine gluconate solution must be injected *slowly*. It is advisable to dilute 10 ml of the preparation to 50 ml, using 5 percent glucose as the diluent. It has been suggested that the diluted quinidine gluconate be given at a rate of 1 ml per minute for maximum safety.

Clinical Reports: Intramuscular administration of quinidine gluconate was found by various investigators to be satisfactory in treating acute arrhythmias. Characteristic quinidine effect was observed as early as 15 minutes after injection, and conversion occurred within two hours. The maximum concentration of quinidine in the blood occurred after one hour, and the peak level was higher with a single dose of quinidine gluconate than with an equivalent intramuscular dose of quinidine sulfate in urea-antipyrine or in propylene glycol.

It has been repeatedly reported that the intravenous use of quinidine was successful in the treatment of urgent cases of tachycardias, particularly ventricular tachycardia. Normal rhythm was restored as quickly as four to six minutes after injection.

How Supplied: (℞) *Ampoules (vials) No. 530, Quinidine Gluconate Injection, USP,* 80 mg per ml, 10 ml, rubber-stoppered, in singles (10 per carton). [041679]
6505-00-864-6298

QUINIDINE SULFATE USP ℞

Description: Quinidine sulfate occurs as minute needlelike white crystals (frequently cohering in masses) or fine white powder. It is odorless, has a very bitter taste, and darkens on exposure to light. It is slightly soluble in water, soluble in alcohol and in chloroform, and insoluble in ether. It contains not less than 99 percent and not more than 101 percent of total alkaloids, calculated as $(C_{20}H_{24}N_2O_2)_2 \bullet H_2SO_4$, on the anhydrous basis.

Actions: Quinidine is generally regarded as a myocardial depressant drug, because it depresses excitability, conduction velocity, and contractility of the myocardium. Besides these direct effects, quinidine exerts some indirect activity on the heart through an anticholinergic action. Large oral doses may reduce the arterial pressure by means of peripheral vasodilation. Hypotension of a serious degree is more likely with the parenteral use of the drug.

Quinidine is essentially completely absorbed after oral administration; maximum effects occur in one to three hours, and activity persists for six to eight or more hours. Blood levels of quinidine can be measured; the average therapeutic range is between 3 and 6 mg per liter of plasma. Toxic reactions are almost certain to appear at levels above 8 mg per liter.

Indications: Quinidine sulfate is indicated in the treatment of:

- Premature atrial and ventricular contractions
- Paroxysmal atrial tachycardia
- Paroxysmal atrioventricular (AV) junctional rhythm
- Atrial flutter
- Paroxysmal atrial fibrillation
- Established atrial fibrillation when therapy is appropriate
- Paroxysmal ventricular tachycardia when not associated with complete heart block
- Maintenance therapy after electrical conversion of atrial fibrillation and/or flutter

Contraindications: Contraindications include hypersensitivity or idiosyncrasy to the drug, history of thrombocytopenic purpura associated with previous quinidine administration, digitalis intoxication manifested by AV conduction disorders, complete AV block with an AV nodal or idioventricular pacemaker, and ectopic impulses and rhythms due to escape mechanisms.

Warnings: In the treatment of atrial flutter, reversion to sinus rhythm may be preceded by a progressive reduction in the degree of AV block to a 1:1 ratio, which results in extremely rapid ventricular rate. This possible hazard may be decreased by digitalization prior to administration of quinidine.

Evidence of quinidine cardiotoxicity (50 percent widening of QRS complex, frequent ventricular ectopic beats) mandates immediate discontinuation of the drug and subsequent close observation (electrocardiographic monitoring) of the patient.

Usage in Pregnancy—The use of quinidine in pregnancy should be reserved only for those cases in which the benefits outweigh the possible hazards to the patient and fetus.

Precautions: Quinidine should be used with extreme caution when there is incomplete AV block, since complete block and asystole may result. The drug may cause unpredictable abnormalities of rhythm in digitalized hearts, and it should be used with special caution in the presence of digitalis intoxication.

Note— The effect of quinidine is enhanced by potassium and reduced if hypokalemia is present.

The depressant actions of quinidine on cardiac contractility and arterial blood pressure limit its use in congestive heart failure and in hypotensive states unless these conditions are due to or aggravated by the arrhythmia. The potential disadvantages and benefits must be weighed.

Continuous electrocardiographic monitoring and determination of plasma quinidine levels are indicated when large doses (more than 2 gm per day) are used.

Adverse Reactions: *Symptoms of Cinchonism* (ringing in the ears, headache, nausea, disturbed vision)—These may appear (in sensitive patients) after a single dose of the drug.

Cardiovascular—Widening of QRS complex, cardiac asystole, ventricular ectopic beats, idioventricular rhythms (including ventricular tachycardia and fibrillation), paradoxical tachycardia, arterial embolism.

Gastrointestinal—Nausea, vomiting, abdominal pain, diarrhea.

Hematologic—Acute hemolytic anemia, hypoprothrombinemia, thrombocytopenic purpura, agranulocytosis.

Central Nervous System—Headache, fever, vertigo, apprehension, excitement, confusion, delirium and syncope, disturbed hearing (tinnitus, decreased auditory acuity), disturbed vision (mydriasis, blurred vision, disturbed color perception, photophobia, diplopia, night blindness, scotomata), optic neuritis.

Dermatologic—Cutaneous flushing with intense pruritus.

Hypersensitivity Reactions — Angioedema, acute asthmatic episode, vascular collapse, respiratory arrest.

Administration and Dosage: A preliminary test dose of a single tablet of quinidine sulfate should be administered to determine whether the patient has an idiosyncrasy to it. Continuous electrocardiographic monitoring is recommended in all cases in which quinidine is used in large doses.

Usual Adult Dose:

Premature Atrial and Ventricular Contractions—0.2 to 0.3 gm three or four times daily.

Paroxysmal Supraventricular Tachycardias—0.4 to 0.6 gm every two or three hours until the paroxysm is terminated.

Atrial Flutter—Quinidine should be administered after digitalization for this indication. Dosage is to be individualized.

Conversion of Atrial Fibrillation—Various schedules of quinidine administration have been in clinical use. A widely used technique is to give 0.2 gm of quinidine orally every two or three hours for five to eight doses, with subsequent daily increase of the individual dose until sinus rhythm is restored or toxic effects occur. The total daily dose should not exceed 3 to 4 gm in any regimen. Prior to quinidine administration, the ventricular rate and congestive failure (if present) should be brought under control by digitalis therapy.

Maintenance Therapy—0.2 to 0.3 gm three or four times daily.

Overdosage: Cardiotoxic effects of quinidine may be reversed in part by molar sodium lactate; the hypotension, by vasoconstrictors and by catecholamines (since the vasodilatation is partly due to α adrenergic blockade).

How Supplied: (℞) *Pulvules No. 239, Capsules, USP, F39,** 200 mg (3 grs) (No. 2, Pink), in bottles of 100.

(℞) *Tablets No. 1125, USP, J20,** 200 mg (3 grs) (scored), in bottles of 100 and 1000 and in 10 strips of 10 individually labeled blisters each containing 1 tablet (ID100).

[052479]

RABIES VACCINE ℞
(DUCK EMBRYO) DRIED KILLED VIRUS USP

Description: Rabies Vaccine, USP (Duck Embryo), Dried Killed Virus, is a suspension of embryonic duck tissue infected with fixed virus, to which beta-propiolactone has been added as a virucidal agent. Beta-propiolactone, as such, does not remain in the final product but hydrolyzes to harmless breakdown materials. The suspending fluid consists of 0.1 percent cysteine hydrochloride, 5 percent lactose, 0.2 percent gelatin, and 0.25 percent dibasic potassium phosphate. The vaccine is preserved with Merthiolate® (thimerosal, Lilly) (sodium ethylmercurithiosalicylate), 1:10,000.

Rabies vaccine of duck-embryo origin was developed by Eli Lilly and Company to circumvent the use of brain tissue, since it has been demonstrated that duck embryos contain little or none of the "paralytic factor" said to be present in brain tissue. Myelin, contained in conventional vaccines of brain origin, has been implicated as the causative factor in rabies treatment paralysis.

The standard requirements of the Food and Drug Administration are adequately met by this vaccine. Of prime importance in rabies immunization is the early development of antibodies. It has been demonstrated that rabies vaccine of duck-embryo origin produces antibodies in most patients by the tenth day and in almost all subjects by the 15th day after the beginning of a course of at least 14 daily doses.

Indications: *Postexposure Immunization*—Indications for and against giving rabies vaccine are difficult to define. In favor of giving it is the fact that, if rabies develops, it will almost certainly have fatal results. Against giving it is the danger of development of severe side effects involving the central nervous system when vaccine contains brain tissue. Experiments have shown that duck-embryo tissue contains little or none of the "paralytic factor," and the incidence of neurologic side effects has been low with the use of duck-embryo vaccine.

The following factors also should be taken into consideration: (1) Approximately 40 percent of persons who are bitten by animals known to be rabid have developed rabies if not treated with rabies vaccine, and (2) rabies rarely occurs unless the individual actually has been bitten by the animal.

The World Health Organization Expert Committee on Rabies has considered various types of exposure to rabies and made the following recommendations:

I. If contact with the rabid animal has been indirect or if there has been only a lick on unabraded skin, no exposure is considered to have occurred and vaccine is not recommended.

II. If the exposure was mild, i.e., a lick on abraded skin or on mucosal surfaces, or for single bites *not* on the head, neck, face, or arm:
   A. If the animal is healthy at the time of exposure, withhold vaccine, but observe the animal for ten days.
   B. If during the ten-day observation period the animal is proved to have rabies or becomes clinically suspicious, start vaccine immediately.
   C. If the animal has signs suspicious of rabies at the time of exposure, start vaccine immediately, but stop injections if the animal is normal on the fifth day after exposure.
   D. If the animal is rabid, if it escapes or is killed, or if it is unknown, give complete course of vaccine. If the biting animal is wild, also give rabies antiserum.

III. If exposure was severe (multiple bites or single bites on the head, neck, face, or arm), the indications for giving vaccine are the same as in mild exposure (*see* II above). In addition, in every category, the administration of rabies antiserum is recommended.

The most recent report of the U.S. Public Health Service Advisory Committee on Immunization Practices recommends the use of passive antibody for treatment of ALL BITES by animals suspected of having rabies and for nonbite exposures inflicted by animals suspected of being rabid. There is evidence that, when antibody is administered concurrently with vaccine, it can interfere with the development of active immunity. If passive antibody is used, this committee recommends supplementary doses of vaccine ten and twenty days after the last usual dose.

When considering the above recommendations, physicians should consult local health officials to obtain information on the presence of rabies in the region.

Preexposure Immunization—Vaccination with duck-embryo rabies vaccine before exposure occurs may be desirable for certain high-risk individuals. These include veterinarians, deliverymen, meter readers, spelunkers, laboratory personnel working with rabies virus, and perhaps others.

Precautions: Caution should be used in administering the vaccine to persons with a history of allergy, especially when the allergy is to chicken or duck eggs or proteins.

Adrenocorticotropin and adrenal corticosteroids may reduce host resistance to certain infectious agents either through suppression of antibody response or through other and as yet poorly understood mechanisms. Therefore, they should not be administered following exposure to infectious agents (such as rabies) for which no satisfactory antimicrobial therapy is available. To do so may alter the host-parasite relationship sufficiently to cause severe or fatal illness in spite of prophylactic administration of a vaccine. Under these circumstances, the occurrence of disease, actually due to the altered pattern of resistance, might be attributed to a vaccine failure.

Usage in Pregnancy—Safety of this product for use during pregnancy has not been established; however, when postexposure rabies immunization is indicated, pregnancy has not been considered to be a contraindication to use of this killed virus vaccine.

Adverse Reactions: Local reactions to the injected material have been observed to be fewer and somewhat less severe than those seen with vaccines of brain origin. Tenderness at the injection site is common. Varying degrees of local erythema and induration have been observed; these reactions tend to appear from the sixth to the tenth day of treatment but may occur after each inoculation. Subsequent injections are likely to cause flare-ups at the sites of previous inoculations. Regional lymphadenopathy may also be encountered.

Since this material is protein and foreign to the human body, systemic sensitivity to the vaccine may be encountered. Urticaria, respiratory distress (including dyspnea and bronchospasm), and gastrointestinal disorders (e.g., abdominal cramps, nausea, vomiting, and diarrhea) have occurred. Anaphylactic reactions have been reported. In one prospective study, anaphylaxis was observed in 0.5 to 0.9 percent of recipients. Epinephrine may be helpful in controlling these situations. Patients with a history of allergy should be tested for hypersensitivity before the vaccine is administered.

Constitutional reactions are difficult to evaluate because of the patient's tendency to be apprehensive about the situation, but the development of fever, malaise, and drowsiness calls for careful observation. Minor neurologic reactions, such as headache, photophobia, paresthesias, listlessness, malaise, and increased fatigability, have been reported. Major neurologic reactions temporally associated with vaccine therapy have been reported rarely. These include transverse myelitis, cranial or peripheral palsy, and encephalitis. If symptoms appear that indicate central-nervous-system involvement, vaccine injections should be discontinued.

Local Treatment: The World Health Organization makes the following recommendations: All bite wounds and scratches that may possibly be contaminated with rabies virus should receive prompt and adequate treatment. This should include adequate cleansing, thorough flushing and scrubbing with 20 percent soap solution, and/or the application of a quaternary ammonium compound or other substance of proved lethal effect on rabies virus. All traces of soap should be removed before quaternary ammonium compounds are applied, because soap neutralizes their activity.

If rabies antiserum is indicated, some of the total dose should be thoroughly infiltrated around the wound. For directions concerning use of rabies antiserum, consult the package literature for the product. When possible, bite wounds should not be immediately sutured. If found to be advisable, tetanus prophylaxis and measures to control bacterial infections should be performed.

Prognosis: Vaccination therapy is known to be highly effective when the incubation period is expected to be more than three or four weeks. In cases of face bites or very severe, extensive bites elsewhere, the incubation period may be as short as 17 days. It is in these latter instances that most of the vaccination failures appear. Such failures may occur even though vaccination is begun immediately; however, since failure is by no means certain, promptness is essential in beginning the course of injections.

Administration and Dosage: *Postexposure Immunization*— A combination of passive and active immunization (vaccine and immune globulin) is considered the best postexposure prophylaxis and is recommended both for treatment of ALL BITES by animals suspected of having rabies and for nonbite exposures inflicted by animals suspected of being rabid. Passive immunization should be used in conjunction with active immunization regardless of the interval between exposure and treatment.

Immunization

Rabies Immune Globulin, Human (RIG), and Duck Embryo Vaccine (DEV): Passive antibody, RIG (Antirabies Serum, Equine [ARS], only if RIG is not available), is administered only once, at the beginning of antirabies therapy. The recommended dose of RIG is 20 IU/kg, or approximately 9 IU/lb body weight. (When ARS must be used, the recommended dose is 40 IU/kg, approximately 18 IU/lb, or one vial of 1000 IU/55 lbs body weight.) Up to one-half the dose of RIG (or ARS) should be thoroughly infiltrated around the wound and the rest administered intramuscularly in the buttocks.

Twenty-three 1-ml doses of DEV should be given, beginning the day that passive antibody is administered.

Vaccine may be given as 21 daily doses or 14 doses in the first seven days (two injections each day) and then seven daily doses. This should be followed by the two "booster" doses, the first booster ten days after the twenty-first

Continued on next page

*Identi-Code® symbol.

Lilly—Cont.

dose and the second booster ten days later. Vaccine should be injected subcutaneously in the abdomen, lower back, or lateral aspect of the thigh; rotation of sites is recommended.
All persons who receive vaccine and RIG (or ARS) should have serum collected for rabies antibody testing at the time of the second booster. Testing for rabies antibody can be arranged by state health department laboratories. If no antibody is detected, additional boosters should be given.
Preexposure Immunization—The two schedules that are currently recommended appear to be equally effective. The first procedure consists of a series of four subcutaneous injections of 1 ml each. The first three injections are given one week apart, and the fourth is given five to six months after the third. The second procedure consists of a series of three subcutaneous injections of 1 ml each. The first two injections are given one month apart, and the third is administered seven months later. Experimental data indicate that, one month after completion of either of the above courses of immunization, over 80 percent of individuals have rabies-neutralizing antibody in their serum and presumably are protected against rabies. It is not known how long immunity lasts, and the frequency with which booster doses are required has not been definitely determined. However, it seems probable that more or less permanent immunity could be maintained by a single 1-ml booster injection every one or two years.
Because the antibody response is not 100 percent, *an antibody titer must be determined* after the course of immunization. Individuals desiring antibody determinations may have them done through their state board of health laboratory by the Rabies Investigations Laboratory, Communicable Disease Center, Atlanta, Georgia. If antibody is not present after the course of immunization, additional booster doses may be given until it is detected.
If mild exposure occurs, individuals in whom rabies antibody has been determined to be present can be given a single 1-ml booster dose of vaccine. If exposure is severe or due to bites of wild animals, the usual postexposure immunization recommended by the WHO Expert Committee on Rabies should be followed (*see* Indications).
Directions for Mixing and Administration—One dose of vaccine is contained in an individual vial accompanied by one ampoule of diluent (Sterile Water for Injection). Withdraw 1.1 ml of the Sterile Water for Injection into a sterile syringe, inject into the vaccine vial, and gently mix with the vaccine. One ml of the reconstituted vaccine is withdrawn into the syringe and then injected subcutaneously. It is recommended that a 23 or 24-gauge needle, approximately ½ to ¾ inch long, be used. Pull back on the syringe plunger after the needle has been inserted into the tissues and before the injection is given to make sure that the end of the needle is not in a blood vessel.
A separate sterile syringe and needle should be used for each patient to prevent transmission of homologous serum hepatitis virus and other infectious agents.
When not in use, the vial should be stored at a uniform temperature between 2° and 8°C (36° and 46°F), preferably at the lower limit.
How Supplied: (℞) *Biologic No. V-1079, Rabies Vaccine, USP (Duck Embryo), Dried Killed Virus.* Contains one single-dose vial of vaccine (Dry Powder) with one ampoule of Sterile Water for Injection as a diluent in each package (7 per carton). [071179]
V-1079—7 per carton—6505-00-754-2727

REGULAR ILETIN® (insulin injection, Lilly), *see under* Iletin® (insulin, Lilly).

SANDRIL® ℞
(reserpine)
Injection, USP
AMPOULES (VIALS)

Description: Sandril® (reserpine, Lilly) is a pure crystalline alkaloid derived from suitable species of *Rauwolfia.* Reserpine alkaloid occurs as an odorless crystalline powder which is white or pale buff to slightly yellowish in color. It darkens slowly on exposure to light but more rapidly when in solution. It is insoluble in water and very slightly soluble in alcohol and in ether. It is slightly soluble in benzene and freely soluble in acetic acid and chloroform.
Actions: Reserpine probably produces its antihypertensive effects through depletion of tissue stores of catecholamines (epinephrine and norepinephrine) from peripheral sites. By contrast, its sedative and tranquilizing properties are thought to be related to depletion of 5-hydroxytryptamine from the brain.
Reserpine is characterized by slow onset of action and sustained effect. Both its cardiovascular and central-nervous-system effects may persist following withdrawal of the drug.
Indications: The parenteral route is indicated in the treatment of hypertensive emergencies, such as acute hypertensive encephalopathy, in which it is desired to reduce the blood pressure promptly.
The parenteral route has been used in psychiatric conditions only to initiate treatment in those patients who are unable to accept oral medication or to control symptoms of extreme agitation.
Contraindications: Do not use in patients with known hypersensitivity to reserpine, mental depression (especially with suicidal tendencies), active peptic ulcer, or ulcerative colitis and in patients receiving electroconvulsive therapy.
Warnings: Sandril® (reserpine, Lilly) Injection is not for intravenous use.
Parenteral reserpine should be used with extreme caution if the patient is under treatment for hypertension with other potent drugs.
Extreme caution should be exercised in treating patients with a history of mental depression. Discontinue the drug at the first sign of despondency, early morning insomnia, loss of appetite, impotence, or self-depreciation. Drug-induced depression may persist for several months after drug withdrawal and may be severe enough to result in suicide.
Usage in Pregnancy—The safety of reserpine for use during pregnancy or lactation has not been established; therefore, the drug should be administered to pregnant patients or to women of childbearing potential only when, in the judgment of the physician, its use is deemed essential to the welfare of the patient. Increased respiratory secretions, nasal congestion, cyanosis, and anorexia may occur in infants born to reserpine-treated mothers, since the preparation is known to cross the placental barrier and to appear in cord blood and breast milk.
The drug should be discontinued for two weeks before electroshock therapy is employed.
Precautions: Because rauwolfia preparations increase gastrointestinal motility and secretion, this drug should be used cautiously in patients with a history of peptic ulcer, ulcerative colitis, or gallstones (a condition in which biliary colic may be precipitated).
Caution should be exercised in the treatment of hypertensive patients with renal insufficiency; they adjust poorly to lowered blood pressure levels.
Cardiac arrhythmias have occurred with rauwolfia preparations; therefore, reserpine should be used cautiously with digitalis and quinidine.
Administration of reserpine during therapy with a tricyclic antidepressant has been shown to produce a "stimulating" effect in some depressed patients.
Preoperative withdrawal of reserpine does not assure that circulatory instability will not take place. It is important that the anesthesiologist be aware of the patient's drug intake and consider this in the overall management, since hypotension has occurred in patients receiving rauwolfia preparations. Anticholinergic and/or adrenergic drugs (metaraminol, norepinephrine) have been employed to treat adverse vagocirculatory effects.
Adverse Reactions: Rauwolfia preparations have caused gastrointestinal reactions, including hypersecretion, ptyalism, nausea and vomiting, anorexia, and diarrhea; cardiovascular reactions, including fall in blood pressure, orthostatic hypotension, syncope, angina-like symptoms, bradycardia, and arrhythmias (particularly when reserpine is used concurrently with digitalis or quinidine); and central-nervous-system reactions, including drowsiness, depression, nervousness, paradoxical anxiety, vivid dreams, nightmares, rare parkinsonian syndrome, and C.N.S. sensitization manifested by dull sensorium, deafness, glaucoma, uveitis, and optic atrophy. Nasal congestion is a frequent complaint, and pruritus, flushing, rash, dryness of mouth, dizziness, headache, dyspnea, purpura, impotence or decreased libido, dysuria, muscular aches, conjunctival injection, and weight gain have been reported. Extrapyramidal tract symptoms have also taken place. These reactions are usually reversible and disappear when the drug is discontinued.
Water retention with edema in patients with hypertensive vascular disease may occur rarely, but the condition generally clears with cessation of therapy or with the administration of a diuretic agent.
Administration and Dosage: Sandril® (reserpine, Lilly) may be administered intramuscularly in the short-term treatment of hypertensive crises. Because of varying responsiveness, a titration procedure should be used. An initial dose of 0.5 to 1 mg intramuscularly is followed by doses of 2 and 4 mg at intervals of three hours, if necessary, until the blood pressure falls to the desired level. If the 4-mg dose is ineffective, other antihypertensive agents should be used. An initial dose larger than 0.5 mg may induce severe hypotension, particularly in patients with cerebral hemorrhage.
In psychiatric emergencies, reserpine may be administered intramuscularly to initiate treatment in those patients who are unable to accept oral medication. The average dose is 2.5 to 5 mg following a small initial dose to test sensitivity.
Concomitant use of reserpine with ganglionic blocking agents, guanethidine, veratrum, hydralazine, methyldopa, chlorthalidone, or thiazides necessitates careful titration of dosage with each agent.
Overdosage: Central depression of vasopressor reflexes and depression of the central nervous system. *Symptoms*—Hypotension and mental depression. *Treatment*—No specific therapy. General management consists in symptomatic and supportive therapy, which may include gastric lavage immediately following oral administration of the drug.
How Supplied: (℞) *Ampoules (Vials) No. 653, Sandril® (Reserpine Injection, USP),* 2.5 mg per ml, 10 ml, rubber-stoppered, in singles (10 per carton). Each vial also contains polyethylene glycol, 30 percent; benzyl alcohol, 2 percent; monothioglycerol, 1 percent; ascorbic acid, 1 percent; and Sterile Water for Injection, q.s. Sodium hydroxide and/or hydrochloric acid may have been added during manufacture to adjust the *p*H.
[120575A]

SANDRIL® ℞
(reserpine)
Tablets, USP

Description and Actions: *See under* Ampoules (Vials) Sandril.
Indications: Sandril® (reserpine, Lilly) is indicated in the treatment of mild essential hypertension. It is useful as adjunctive therapy with other antihypertensive agents in the more severe forms of hypertension.
In addition, Sandril is indicated for the relief of symptoms in agitated psychotic states (e.g., schizophrenia), primarily in those individuals who are unable to tolerate phenothiazine derivatives or those who also require antihypertensive medication.
Contraindications, Warnings, Precautions, and Adverse Reactions: *See under* Ampoules (Vials) Sandril.
Administration and Dosage: *Hypertension*—For the average patient not receiving other antihypertensive agents, the usual initial daily dose is 0.5 mg given orally for one or two weeks. Maintenance dosage is 0.1 to 0.25 mg daily. Higher doses should be used cautiously, because serious mental depression and other side effects may be increased considerably.
Psychiatric Disorders—The average initial dose is 0.5 mg orally, with a range of 0.1 to 1 mg. Dosage should be adjusted upward or downward according to the patient's response.
Concomitant use of reserpine with ganglionic blocking agents, guanethidine, veratrum, hydralazine, methyldopa, chlorthalidone, or thiazides necessitates careful titration of dosage with each agent.
Overdosage: *See under* Ampoules (Vials) Sandril.
How Supplied: (℞) *Tablets Sandril® (Reserpine Tablets, USP): No. 1798, J99,** 0.1 mg, Orange, in bottles of 100; *No. 1805, U29,** 0.25 mg, Green (scored), in bottles of 100 and 1000.
[052576]

SECONAL® Ⓒ
(secobarbital)
Elixir, USP

WARNING: MAY BE HABIT-FORMING
Description: Seconal® (Secobarbital, USP, Lilly) is a barbituric acid derivative for oral administration and occurs as a white, odorless, slightly bitter powder that is soluble in chloroform, freely soluble in alcohol or ether, and very slightly soluble in water. Its saturated solution has a *p*H of about 5.6.
Each 5 ml contain secobarbital, 22 mg; methenamine, 22 mg; glycerin; alcohol, 12 percent; water, and aromatics.
Chemically, it is 5-allyl-5-(1-methylbutyl)barbituric acid, with the empirical formula $C_{12}H_{17}N_2O_3$.
Clinical Pharmacology: Seconal® (secobarbital, Lilly), a short-acting barbiturate, is a central-nervous-system depressant. In ordinary doses, the drug acts as a sedative and hypnotic. Its onset of action is from 15 to 30 minutes, and the duration of action ranges from three to six hours. It is detoxified in the liver.
Indications and Usage: Elixir Seconal® (secobarbital, Lilly) is indicated for intermittent use as a sedative or hypnotic. The prolonged administration of Seconal is not recommended, since it has not been shown to be effective for a period of more than 14 days. If insomnia persists, drug-free intervals of one or more weeks should elapse before re-treatment is considered. Attempts should be made to find alternative nondrug therapy for chronic insomnia.
Contraindications: Seconal® (secobarbital, Lilly) is contraindicated in patients who are hypersensitive to barbiturates. It is also contraindicated in patients with a history of manifest or latent porphyria, marked impairment of liver function, or respiratory disease in which dyspnea or obstruction is evident. It should not be administered to persons with known previous addiction to the sedative/hypnotic group, since ordinary doses may be ineffectual and may contribute to further addiction. Seconal should not be administered in the presence of acute or chronic pain, because paradoxical excitement may be induced or important symptoms may be masked.
Precautions: *General Precautions*—Barbiturates induce liver microsomal enzyme activity. This accelerates the biotransformation of various drugs and is probably part of the mechanism of the tolerance encountered with barbiturates. Seconal® (secobarbital, Lilly) should, therefore, be used with caution in patients with decreased liver function. This drug should also be administered cautiously to patients with a history of drug dependence or abuse (*see* Drug Abuse and Dependence). Seconal may decrease the potency of coumarin anticoagulants; therefore, patients receiving such concomitant therapy should have more frequent prothrombin determinations.
As with other sedatives and hypnotics, elderly or debilitated patients may react to barbiturates with marked excitement or depression.
The systemic effects of exogenous hydrocortisone and endogenous hydrocortisone (cortisol) may be diminished by Seconal. Thus, this product should be administered with caution to patients with borderline hypoadrenal function, regardless of whether it is of pituitary or of primary adrenal origin.
Information for Patients—Seconal may impair the mental and/or physical abilities required for the performance of potentially hazardous tasks, such as driving a car or operating machinery. The patient should be cautioned accordingly.
Drug Interactions—Seconal in combination with alcohol, tranquilizers, and other central-nervous-system depressants has additive depressant effects, and the patient should be so advised. Patients taking this drug should be warned not to exceed the dosage recommended by their physician. Toxic effects and fatalities have occurred following overdoses of Seconal alone and in combination with other central-nervous-system depressants. Caution should be exercised in prescribing unnecessarily large amounts of Seconal for patients who have a history of emotional disturbances or suicidal ideation or who have misused alcohol and other C.N.S. drugs (*see* Overdosage).
Usage in Pregnancy—Pregnancy Category B—Reproduction studies have been performed in animals and have revealed no evidence of impaired fertility or harm to the fetus due to Seconal. There are, however, no adequate and well-controlled studies in pregnant women. Because animal reproduction studies are not always predictive of human response, this drug should be used during pregnancy only if clearly needed.
Nursing Mothers—Caution should be exercised when Seconal is administered to a nursing woman.
Usage in Children—Safety and effectiveness in children have not been established.
Adverse Reactions: The following adverse reactions have been reported:
C.N.S. Depression—Residual sedation or "hangover," drowsiness, lethargy.
Respiratory/Circulatory—Respiratory depression, apnea, circulatory collapse.
Allergic—Hypersensitivity reactions, especially in individuals with asthma, urticaria, angioneurotic edema, or similar conditions; skin eruptions.
Other—Nausea and vomiting; headache.
Drug Abuse and Dependence: *Controlled Substance*—Seconal® (secobarbital, Lilly) is a Schedule II drug.
Dependence—Prolonged, uninterrupted use of barbiturates (particularly the short-acting drugs), even in therapeutic doses, may result in psychic and physical dependence. Withdrawal symptoms due to physical dependence following chronic use of large doses of barbiturates may include delirium, convulsions, and death.
Overdosage: *Symptoms*—The manifestations of overdosage are early hypothermia followed by fever, sluggish or absent reflexes, respiratory depression, gradual appearance of circulatory collapse, pulmonary edema, and coma. *Treatment* — General management should consist in symptomatic and supportive therapy, including gastric lavage, administration of intravenous fluids, and maintenance of blood pressure, body temperature, and adequate respiratory exchange. Dialysis will increase the rate of removal of barbiturates from the body fluids. Antibiotics may be required to control pulmonary complications.
Dosage and Administration: *Adults*—The usual hypnotic dose is 100 mg. For daytime sedation, 20 to 40 mg may be given two or three times per day.
Children—The usual dosage range is 7.5 to 30 mg, depending on age, weight, and the degree of sedation desired.
How Supplied: (Ⓒ) *Elixir No. 247, Seconal® (Secobarbital Elixir, USP),* 440 mg per 100 ml, in 16-fl-oz bottles (NDC 0002-2444-05).
[101579]

SECONAL® SODIUM Ⓒ
(secobarbital sodium)
Injection, USP
AMPOULES (VIALS)

WARNING: This is a potent drug, and serious consequences may result if it is used other than under constant medical supervision. May be habit-forming. Solutions showing evidence of precipitation should not be used.
Description: Each ml contains Seconal® Sodium (Secobarbital Sodium, USP, Lilly), 50 mg, in Sterile Water for Injection, with polyethylene glycol, 50 percent. Phenol, 0.25 percent, is added as a preservative. Sodium hydroxide and/or hydrochloric acid may have been added during manufacture to adjust the *p*H.
Action: Seconal® Sodium (secobarbital sodium, Lilly) Injection is a short-acting barbiturate in a liquid vehicle and acts as a central-nervous-system depressant. Depending upon dosage, the drug will produce responses ranging from mild sedation to profound hypnosis. In large doses, it causes anesthesia; with overdosage, respiratory depression which may be dangerous will result.
Indications: Seconal® Sodium (secobarbital sodium, Lilly) is used as a sedative or hypnotic. It is indicated in anesthetic doses for the emergency control of certain acute convulsive conditions, e.g., those associated with tetanus, status epilepticus, and toxic reactions to strychnine or local anesthetics.
Contraindications: Seconal® Sodium (secobarbital sodium, Lilly) should not be given to patients who are sensitive to barbiturates or to anyone who has a history of porphyria. It should be used with extreme caution in any patient with impaired hepatic function. Respiratory or cardiac disease of more than minimum degree may contraindicate its administration. Although Seconal Sodium itself is not harmful when renal disease exists, the polyethylene glycol vehicle may be irritating to the kidneys.
Use of parenteral Seconal Sodium in obstetric deliveries is contraindicated.
Warnings: Intramuscular injection should be made deeply into a large muscle, and a volume of 5 ml (regardless of dilution) should not be exceeded at one site. After intramuscular injection of large hypnotic doses, the patient

Continued on next page

*Identi-Code® symbol.

Lilly—Cont.

should be observed for 20 to 30 minutes to assure that narcosis will not be excessive.
Intravenous administration of Seconal® Sodium (secobarbital sodium, Lilly) should be undertaken only by those who have familiarized themselves with the work of experienced investigators. The rate of intravenous injection should not exceed 50 mg per 15-second period. Too-rapid administration may cause respiratory depression or apnea, laryngospasm, or vasodilation with fall in blood pressure. Special care is needed when any barbiturate is given to patients who have received analgesics, other sedatives or hypnotics, ether, curare-like drugs, alcohol, or tranquilizers, because an additive respiratory-depressant effect may ensue.
Usage in Pregnancy—Safety of this product for use during pregnancy has not been established in regard to possible harmful effects on the fetus. Therefore, Seconal Sodium should not be used in pregnant women unless, in the judgment of the physician, the benefits outweigh the potential hazards. If the drug is administered to the pregnant patient, the fetal heart should be monitored carefully and oxygen given to the patient by appropriate means in the event that slowing or irregularities occur.
Precautions: After the use of a barbiturate in any office procedure, the patient should be discharged only in the company of another person. The patient should be warned about the possibility of drowsiness if he must operate dangerous machinery or drive a vehicle. The central-nervous-system depressant effect of secobarbital may be additive with that of other C.N.S. depressants, including alcohol.
Secobarbital sodium, like other barbiturates, decreases the response to coumarin anticoagulants, with the result that there is less suppression of prothrombin.
Adverse Reactions: In the general use of barbiturates by the intravenous route, respiratory depression is the most serious side effect. Idiosyncrasy, in the form of excitement, hangover, or pain, may appear. Hypersensitivity reactions occur in some patients, especially in those with asthma, urticaria, or angioneurotic edema. Laryngospasm may develop during normal induction or as a result of improper dosage. Rapid intravenous administration may also induce vasodilation and some fall in blood pressure.
Nausea and vomiting, postoperative atelectasis, and circulatory disturbances are uncommon. When they occur, they are usually due to overdosage or extraneous factors. Embolism has not been reported following intravenous use of Seconal® Sodium (secobarbital sodium, Lilly) Injection.
Administration and Dosage: Doses should be reduced significantly in the elderly or debilitated. Such patients may be unusually sensitive to the recommended doses. No barbiturate should be given parenterally without full knowledge of its particular characteristics, dosage, and recommended rate of administration.
Seconal® Sodium (secobarbital sodium, Lilly) Injection is given intramuscularly, intravenously, or rectally. It may be administered as supplied (in a concentration of 50 mg per ml), or it may be diluted with Sterile Water for Injection, 0.9% Sodium Chloride Injection, or Ringer's Injection.
Following rectal administration of average doses, full hypnotic effects are generally observed in 15 to 20 minutes; following intramuscular injection, after seven to ten minutes; following intravenous injection, after one to three minutes.
Anesthetic Procedures—To provide basal hypnosis for general, spinal, or regional anesthesia or to facilitate intubation procedures, Seconal® Sodium (secobarbital sodium, Lilly) Injection is usually given intravenously. The injection is made at a rate not to exceed 50 mg (1 ml of the undiluted preparation as supplied) per 15-second period. Administration is discontinued as soon as the desired degree of hypnosis is attained. Total dosage in excess of 250 mg is not recommended, even though larger doses have been given without serious side effects. If hypnosis is inadequate after 250 mg, the addition of a small quantity of meperidine is recommended. When Seconal Sodium Injection is employed as an adjunct to spinal or regional anesthesia, usually minimum quantities (50 to 100 mg) are required.
For rectal administration to children prior to ear, nose, and throat procedures, the 5 percent solution as supplied is usually diluted with lukewarm tap water to a concentration of 1 to 1.5 percent. It is administered after a cleansing enema. Children weighing less than 40 kg (88 pounds) may receive 5 mg per kg of body weight (2.3 mg per pound). Some investigators have recommended that larger children should receive only 4 mg per kg of body weight (1.8 mg per pound). Atropine may be administered for its drying effect on respiratory tract secretions. After rectal administration of the barbiturate, hypnosis follows within 15 to 20 minutes. The children should be attended during this period.
Dentistry—As a sedative for apprehensive patients, the usual dose of Seconal® Sodium (secobarbital sodium, Lilly) Injection for adults or children is 1 mg per pound of body weight. Intramuscular rather than intravenous administration is recommended, and the injection should be made 10 to 15 minutes before the procedure is to be started. Sedative effects persist for three to four hours. For light sedation, 0.5 to 0.75 mg per pound will suffice.
In patients who are to receive nerve blocks, 100 to 150 mg may be given intravenously. With this dosage range and this route, the patient can be expected to be awake in 15 minutes and can be discharged in the company of another person after 30 minutes. If nitrous oxide is to be employed, Seconal Sodium Injection should be administered as suggested above (*see* Anesthetic Procedures).
Convulsions in Tetanus—For the control of convulsions in the treatment of tetanus, an initial dose of 2.5 mg per pound of body weight may be employed. This can be repeated every three to four hours as needed.
Overdosage: C.N.S. depression. *Symptoms*—Respiratory depression, depression of superficial and deep reflexes, constriction of the pupils to a slight degree (though in severe poisoning they may dilate), decreased urine formation, lowered body temperature, and coma. *Treatment*—General management should consist in symptomatic and supportive therapy, including gastric lavage, administration of intravenous fluids, and maintenance of blood pressure, body temperature, and adequate respiratory exchange. Dialysis will increase the rate of removal of barbiturates from the body fluids.
How Supplied: (Ⓒ) *Ampoules (Vials) No. 616, Seconal® Sodium (Secobarbital Sodium Injection, USP),* 50 mg per ml, 20 ml, rubber-stoppered, in singles (10 per carton). *Refrigerate. Protect from light. Store in carton until contents have been used.*
[121376]

SECONAL® SODIUM Ⓒ
(secobarbital sodium)
Capsules, USP

WARNING: MAY BE HABIT-FORMING

Description: Seconal® Sodium (Secobarbital Sodium, USP, Lilly) is a barbituric acid derivative and occurs as a white, odorless, bitter powder that is very soluble in water, soluble in alcohol, and practically insoluble in ether.
Each Pulvule contains 50 or 100 mg of secobarbital sodium.
Chemically, the drug is sodium 5-allyl-5-(1-methylbutyl)barbiturate, with the empirical formula $C_{12}H_{17}N_2NaO_3$.
Clinical Pharmacology: *See under* Seconal®.
Indications and Usage: *See under* Seconal.
Contraindications: *See under* Seconal.
Precautions: *See under* Seconal.
Adverse Reactions: *See under* Seconal.
Drug Abuse and Dependence: *See under* Seconal.
Overdosage: *See under* Seconal.
Administration and Dosage: *Adults*—Insomnia, 100 mg. at bedtime. Preoperatively, 200 to 300 mg one to two hours before surgery. *Children*—50 to 100 mg.
How Supplied: (Ⓒ) *Pulvules® Seconal® Sodium (Secobarbital Sodium Capsules, USP): No. 243, F42,**50 mg (No. 4, Orange), in bottles of 100 (NDC 0002-0642-02) and 500 (NDC 0002-0642-03) and in 10 strips of 10 individually labeled blisters each containing 1 Pulvule (ID100) (NDC 0002-0642-33); *No. 240, F40,**100 mg (No. 3, Orange), in bottles of 100 (NDC 0002-0640-02) and 500 (NDC 0002-0640-03), in 10 strips of 10 individually labeled blisters each containing 1 Pulvule (ID100) (NDC 0002-0640-33), and in strip packages of individually sealed Pulvules (DS1000) (NDC 0002-0640-35).
[101779]
[*Shown in Product Identification Section*]

SECONAL® SODIUM Ⓒ
(secobarbital sodium)
SUPPOSITORIES

WARNING: MAY BE HABIT-FORMING

Description: Seconal® Sodium (secobarbital sodium, Lilly) is a barbituric acid derivative and occurs as a white, odorless, bitter powder that is very soluble in water, soluble in alcohol, and practically insoluble in ether. Suppositories Seconal Sodium contain white wax and cocoa butter.
Chemically, the drug is sodium 5-allyl-5-(1-methylbutyl)barbiturate, with the empirical formula $C_{12}H_{17}N_2NaO_3$.
Clinical Pharmacology: *See under* Seconal®.
Indications and Usage: Suppositories Seconal® Sodium (secobarbital sodium, Lilly) are indicated for intermittent use as a sedative or hypnotic whenever rectal administration of the drug is preferred. The prolonged administration of Seconal Sodium is not recommended, since it has not been shown to be effective for a period of more than 14 days. If insomnia persists, drug-free intervals of one or more weeks should elapse before re-treatment is considered. Attempts should be made to find alternative nondrug therapy for chronic insomnia.
Contraindications: *See under* Seconal.
Precautions: *See under* Seconal.
Adverse Reactions: *See under* Seconal.
Drug Abuse and Dependence: *See under* Seconal.
Overdosage: *See under* Seconal.
Administration and Dosage: *Rectal*—Children up to six months of age, 15 to 60 mg; six months to three years, 60 mg; older children, 60 to 120 mg; adults, 120 to 200 mg. These suggested dosages should be considered approximate and should be adjusted according to the patient's general condition, degree of sedation or hypnosis desired, and clinical response.
How Supplied: (Ⓒ) *Suppositories Seconal® Sodium (secobarbital sodium, Lilly)* (Rectal): *No. 46, S17,**30 mg (NDC 0002-1917-12), *No. 25, S14,* *60 mg (NDC 0002-1914-12),*No. 11, S05,** 120 mg (NDC 0002-1905-12), and *No. 17, S11,** 200 mg (NDC 0002-1911-12), in packages of 12. *Refrigerate.*
[101679]

SECONAL® SODIUM (secobarbital sodium, Lilly) and
AMYTAL® SODIUM (amobarbital sodium, Lilly), *see* Tuinal® (secobarbital sodium and amobarbital sodium, Lilly).

SEMILENTE® ILETIN® (prompt insulin zinc suspension, Lilly), *see under* Iletin® (insulin, Lilly).

SEROMYCIN® ℞
(cycloserine)
Capsules, USP

Description: Seromycin® (cycloserine, Lilly), D-4-amino-3-isoxazolidinone, is a broad-spectrum antibiotic which is produced by a strain of *Streptomyces orchidaceus* and has also been synthesized. A white powder that is soluble in water and stable in alkaline solution, it is rapidly destroyed at neutral or acid *p*H.
Actions: Cycloserine inhibits cell-wall synthesis in susceptible strains of gram-positive and gram-negative bacteria and in *Mycobacterium tuberculosis.*
Indications: Seromycin® (cycloserine, Lilly) is indicated in the treatment of active pulmonary and extrapulmonary tuberculosis (including renal disease) when the organisms are susceptible to this drug and after failure of adequate treatment with the primary medications (streptomycin, isoniazid, and ethambutol). Like all antituberculosis drugs, Seromycin should be administered in conjunction with other effective chemotherapy and not as the sole therapeutic agent.
Seromycin may be effective in the treatment of acute urinary tract infections caused by susceptible strains of gram-positive and gram-negative bacteria, especially *Enterobacter* and *Escherichia coli.* It is generally no more and is usually less effective than other antimicrobial agents in the treatment of urinary tract infections caused by bacteria other than mycobacteria. Use of Seromycin in these infections should be considered only when the more conventional therapy has failed and when the organism has been demonstrated to be sensitive to the drug.
Contraindications: Administration is contraindicated in patients with any of the following:
- Hypersensitivity to cycloserine
- Epilepsy
- Depression, severe anxiety, or psychosis
- Severe renal insufficiency
- Excessive concurrent use of alcoholic beverages

Warnings: Administration of Seromycin® (cycloserine, Lilly) should be discontinued or the dosage reduced if the patient develops allergic dermatitis or symptoms of central-nervous-system toxicity, such as convulsions, psychosis, somnolence, depression, confusion, hyperreflexia, headache, tremor, vertigo, paresis, or dysarthria.
The toxicity of Seromycin is closely related to excessive blood levels (above 30 mcg/ml), which are determined by high dosage or inadequate renal clearance. The ratio of toxic dose to effective dose in tuberculosis is small.
The risk of convulsions is increased in chronic alcoholics.
Patients should be monitored by hematologic, renal excretion, blood level, and liver function studies.
Usage in Pregnancy—The safety of the use of Seromycin during pregnancy has not been established.
Usage in Children—Safety and dosage have not been established for pediatric use.
Precautions: Before treatment with Seromycin® (cycloserine, Lilly) is initiated, cultures should be taken and the organism's susceptibility to the drug should be established. In tuberculous infections, its sensitivity to the other antituberculosis agents in the regimen should also be demonstrated.
Blood levels should be determined at least weekly for patients having reduced renal function, for individuals receiving a daily dosage of more than 500 mg, and for those showing signs and symptoms suggestive of toxicity. The dosage should be adjusted to keep the blood level below 30 mcg/ml.
Anticonvulsant drugs or sedatives may be effective in controlling symptoms of central-nervous-system toxicity, such as convulsions, anxiety, and tremor. Patients receiving more than 500 mg of Seromycin daily should be closely observed for such symptoms. The value of pyridoxine in preventing C.N.S. toxicity from cycloserine has not been proved.
Administration of Seromycin and other antituberculosis drugs has been associated in a few instances with vitamin B_{12} and/or folic acid deficiency, megaloblastic anemia, and sideroblastic anemia. If evidence of anemia develops during treatment, appropriate studies and therapy should be instituted.
Adverse Reactions: Most adverse reactions occurring during therapy with Seromycin® (cycloserine, Lilly) involve the nervous system or are manifestations of drug hypersensitivity. The following side effects have been observed in patients receiving Seromycin:
Nervous system symptoms (which appear to be related to higher dosages of drug, i.e., more than 500 mg daily)
- Convulsions
- Drowsiness and somnolence
- Headache
- Tremor
- Dysarthria
- Vertigo
- Confusion and disorientation with loss of memory
- Psychoses, possibly with suicidal tendencies
  - Character changes
  - Hyperirritability
  - Aggression
- Paresis
- Hyperreflexia
- Paresthesias
- Major and minor (localized) clonic seizures
- Coma

Allergic (apparently not related to dosage)
- Skin rash

Miscellaneous
- Elevated serum transaminase, especially in patients with preexisting liver disease

Administration and Dosage: Seromycin® (cycloserine, Lilly) is effective orally and is currently administered only by this route. The usual dosage is 500 mg to 1 gm daily in divided doses monitored by blood levels. The initial adult dosage most frequently given is 250 mg twice daily at 12-hour intervals for the first two weeks. The daily dosage of 1 gm should not be exceeded.
Overdosage: *Symptoms*—C.N.S. depression with accompanying drowsiness, somnolence, dizziness, hyperreflexia, mental confusion, convulsions, and allergic dermatitis. *Treatment*—Pyridoxine (vitamin B_6), 300 mg or more daily, and anticonvulsants may be given to relieve convulsions. General management may include symptomatic and supportive therapy, such as gastric lavage, oxygen, artificial respiration, intravenous fluids, standard measures for management of circulatory shock, and maintenance of body temperature.
How Supplied: (℞) *Pulvules® No. 12, Seromycin® (Cycloserine Capsules, USP), F04,* *250 mg (No. 1, Light-Gray Opaque Body, Red Opaque Cap), in bottles of 40 and 500.

[112278]

[*Shown in Product Identification Section*]

SILVER NITRATE ℞
Ophthalmic Solution, USP
One Percent (Buffered)
Wax Ampoules

For the Prevention of Ophthalmia Neonatorum

This product is to be used by the physician or under his direction.

Administration: Immediately after the child is born, the eyelids should be cleaned with sterile absorbent cotton or gauze and sterile water. A separate pledget should be used for each eye, and the lids, without being opened, should be washed from the nose outward until quite free of all blood, mucus, or meconium.
Next, the lids should be separated, and two drops of 1 percent silver nitrate solution should be dropped into the eye. The lids should be separated and elevated away from the eyeball so that a lake of silver nitrate may lie for a half minute or longer between them, coming in contact with every portion of the conjunctival sac. A mild chemical conjunctivitis should result from a properly performed Credé prophylaxis using silver nitrate.
The American Academy of Pediatrics has endorsed a statement of the Committee on Ophthalmia Neonatorum of the National Society for the Prevention of Blindness which does not recommend irrigation of the eyes following instillation of the silver nitrate.
Method of Use: *See* the package literature for illustrations. Pierce the end of the ampoule with a needle, making sure that its entry into the interior of the ampoule is accomplished.
To express the contents of the ampoule, press between the thumb and first finger.
The ampoule should be kept at controlled room temperature, 59° to 86°F (15° to 30°C). Do not freeze. It should not be used when cold. Protect from light.
How Supplied: (℞) *Wax Ampoules No. 146, Silver Nitrate Ophthalmic Solution, USP, One Percent (Buffered),* in packages of 100. Sodium acetate and acetic acid are contained as buffers.

[083178]

STREPTOMYCIN SULFATE ℞
Sterile, USP

STREPTOMYCIN SULFATE
Injection, USP
For Intramuscular Use Only

Warning

The risk of severe neurotoxic reactions is sharply increased in patients with impaired kidney function or prerenal azotemia. Reactions include disturbances of the auditory and/or optic nerve, peripheral neuritis, arachnoiditis, and encephalopathy. Renal function should be carefully determined, and patients with renal damage and nitrogen retention should have reduced dosage. The peak serum concentration in individuals with kidney damage should not exceed 20 to 25 mcg/ml.
Concurrent and sequential use of other neurotoxic and/or nephrotoxic antibiotics, particularly neomycin, kanamycin, gentamicin, cephaloridine, paromomycin, viomycin, polymyxin B, colistin, vancomycin, tobramycin, and amikacin, should be avoided.
The neurotoxicity of streptomycin can result in respiratory paralysis from neuromuscular blockade, especially when the drug is given soon after the use of anesthesia or of muscle relaxants.
The administration of streptomycin in parenteral form should be reserved for situations in which adequate laboratory facilities are available and constant supervision of the patient is possible.

Description: Streptomycin is a water-soluble aminoglycoside derived from *Streptomyces griseus.* It is marketed as the sulfate salt of streptomycin.
Streptomycin in the dry form is relatively stable and may be stored at room temperature.

Continued on next page

*Identi-Code® symbol.

Lilly—Cont.

Sterile solutions of streptomycin should be used immediately. If necessary, they may be stored at room temperature for a period not to exceed 48 hours following reconstitution or may be refrigerated for a period not to exceed 14 days. The entire contents of the vial should be dissolved in 0.9% Sodium Chloride Injection or Sterile Water for Injection, and an appropriate aliquot of this solution should be used (*see* Table 1).
[See table below].
Streptomycin Sulfate Injection, USP, contains in each ml the equivalent of 0.5 gm streptomycin base, as streptomycin sulfate; sodium citrate, 1.5 percent; and monothioglycerol, 1 percent; with phenol, 0.25 percent, as a preservative. Sodium hydroxide and/or sulfuric acid may have been added during manufacture to adjust the *p*H.
Actions: Streptomycin sulfate is a bactericidal antibiotic in therapeutic dosage. Its mode of action is to interfere with normal protein synthesis and thereby produce "faulty proteins."
Following intramuscular injection of 1 gm of the drug, a peak serum level of 25 to 50 mcg/ml is reached within one hour; this diminishes slowly by about 50 percent after five to six hours. Appreciable concentrations are found in all organ tissues except the brain. Significant amounts have been found in pleural fluid and tuberculous cavities. Since streptomycin passes through the placenta, serum levels in the cord blood are similar to maternal levels. Small amounts are excreted in milk, saliva, and sweat.
Streptomycin is excreted rapidly in the urine by glomerular filtration. In patients with normal kidney function, between 29 and 89 percent of a single 0.6-gm dose is excreted within 24 hours. Any reduction of glomerular activity results in decreased excretion of the drug and concurrent rise in serum and tissue levels.
Susceptibility Testing—If the Bauer-Kirby method of disc susceptibility testing is used, a 10-mcg streptomycin disc should give a zone of more than 15 mm when tested against a streptomycin-sensitive bacterial strain.
Indications: 1. *Mycobacterium Tuberculosis*—Streptomycin may be indicated for all forms of this infection when the infecting organisms are susceptible. It should be used only in combination with other antituberculosis drugs.
2. *Nontuberculous Infections*—Streptomycin should be used only in those serious nontuberculous infections caused by organisms shown by in vitro susceptibility studies to be sensitive to it and when less potentially hazardous therapeutic agents are ineffective or contraindicated.

a. *Yersinia pestis* (plague)
b. *Francisella tularensis* (tularemia)
c. *Brucella*
d. Donovanosis (granuloma inguinale)
e. *Haemophilus ducreyi* (chancroid)
f. *H. influenzae* (in respiratory, endocardial, and meningeal infections—concomitantly with another antibacterial agent)
g. *Klebsiella pneumoniae* (in pneumonia—concomitantly with another antibacterial agent)
h. *Escherichia coli, Proteus, Enterobacter aerogenes, K. pneumoniae,* and *Streptococcus faecalis* in urinary tract infections
i. *Streptococcus* sp. (viridans group), *S. faecalis* (in endocardial infections—concomitantly with penicillin)
j. Gram-negative bacilli (in bacteremia—concomitantly with another antibacterial agent)

Contraindications: Streptomycin is contraindicated in those individuals who have shown previous toxic or hypersensitivity reactions to it.
Warnings: *Ototoxicity*—Streptomycin may frequently affect the vestibular branch of the auditory nerve and thus cause severe nausea, vomiting, and vertigo. The incidence of such side effects is directly proportional to the duration of therapy and amount of the drug administered. Advanced age and renal impairment predispose to ototoxicity. Symptoms subside and recovery is usually complete after discontinuance of the drug.
Loss of hearing has been reported following long-term therapy; however, ototoxic effect on the auditory branch of the eighth nerve is infrequent and usually is preceded by vestibular symptoms. Hearing loss, when extensive, is usually permanent.
Usage in Pregnancy—Since streptomycin readily crosses the placental barrier, cautious use of the drug is important to prevent ototoxicity in the fetus.
Precautions: Base-line and periodic caloric stimulation tests and audiometric tests are advisable for patients on extended streptomycin therapy. Tinnitus, roaring noises, or a sense of fullness in the ears indicates need for audiometric examination or termination of streptomycin therapy or both.
Care should be taken by individuals handling or preparing streptomycin for injection to avoid skin sensitivity reactions.
As is the case with other antibiotics, use of this drug may result in overgrowth of nonsusceptible organisms, including fungi. If superinfection occurs, appropriate therapy should be instituted.
Adverse Reactions: The following reactions are common: ototoxicity (nausea, vomiting, and vertigo), circumoral or peripheral paresthesias, rash, fever, urticaria, angioneurotic edema, and eosinophilia.
The following reactions are less frequent: deafness, exfoliative dermatitis, anaphylaxis, azotemia, leukopenia, thrombocytopenia, pancytopenia, hemolytic anemia, muscular weakness, amblyopia, myocarditis, and hepatic necrosis.
Administration and Dosage: Streptomycin is administered by the intramuscular route only.
1. *Tuberculosis*—All forms may be treated when the organisms are known or believed to be susceptible to the drug.
Combined therapy for adults includes 1 gm streptomycin and an appropriate dosage of one or more additional antitubercular drugs (usually isoniazid, ethambutol, or rifampin). Elderly patients should have a smaller daily dose of streptomycin in accordance with age, renal function, and eighth-nerve function. Ultimately, the streptomycin should be discontinued or reduced in dosage to 1 gm two or three times weekly. Therapy with streptomycin may be terminated when toxic symptoms have appeared, impending toxicity is feared, organisms have become resistant, or full therapeutic effect has been obtained. The total period of drug treatment of tuberculosis is a minimum of one year; however, as noted above, indications for terminating therapy with streptomycin may occur at any time.
2. *Tularemia*—1 to 2 gm daily in divided doses for seven to ten days until the patient is afebrile for five to seven days.
3. *Plague*—2 to 4 gm daily in divided doses until the patient is afebrile for at least three days.
4a. *Bacterial Endocarditis*—In endocarditis due to penicillin-sensitive alpha and nonhemolytic streptococci (sensitive to 0.1 mcg or less of penicillin per ml), streptomycin may be used for a two-week treatment concomitantly with penicillin. The streptomycin dosage is 1 gm b i d for one week and 0.5 gm b i d for the second week. If the patient is over 60 years of age, the dosage should be 0.5 gm b i d for the entire two-week period.
4b. *Enterococcal Endocarditis*—Streptomycin in doses of 1 gm b i d for two weeks and 0.5 gm b i d for four weeks is given in combination with penicillin. Ototoxicity may require termination of the streptomycin prior to completion of the six-week course of treatment.
5. *For Use Concomitantly with Other Agents to Which the Infecting Organism Is Also Sensitive*—Streptomycin in these conditions is considered a drug of secondary choice: gram-negative bacillary bacteremia, meningitis, and pneumonia; brucellosis; granuloma inguinale; chancroid; and urinary tract infection.
Adults:
a. For severe fulminating infections, 2 to 4 gm daily, administered intramuscularly in divided doses every six to 12 hours.
b. For less severe infections and highly susceptible organisms, 1 to 2 gm daily.
Children:
20 to 40 mg/kg of body weight daily (8 to 20 mg/lb) in divided doses every six to 12 hours. (Particular care should be taken to avoid excessive dosage in children.)

How Supplied: (℞) *Ampoules (Vials) Sterile Streptomycin Sulfate, USP,* rubber-stoppered (Dry Powder): *No. 431,* 1 gm (equivalent to base), 5-ml size, and *No. 692,* 5 gm (equivalent to base), 30-ml size, in singles (10 per carton).
(℞) *Ampoules (Vials) Streptomycin Sulfate Injection, USP,* rubber-stoppered: *No. 587,* 1 gm (equivalent to base) in 2 ml, in packages of 1 (10 per carton) and 100; *No. 588,* 0.5 gm (equivalent to base) per ml, 10 ml, in singles (10 per carton).
[101579]

TABLE 1. DILUTION TABLE

Diluent added to 1-gm vial	Concentration (approx.)	Diluent added to 5-gm vial	Concentration (approx.)
4.5 ml	200 mg per ml	17 ml	250 mg per ml
3.5 ml	250 mg per ml	6.5 ml	500 mg per ml

SURFACAINE® ℞
(cyclomethycaine sulfate)
Jelly, 0.75 Percent, NF

Description: Surfacaine® (Cyclomethycaine Sulfate, NF, Lilly) is a topical anesthetic. It is a substituted piperidino-alkyl benzoate and is not a derivative of *p*-aminobenzoic acid. Each gram of Jelly Surfacaine contains 7.5 mg (0.75 percent) cyclomethycaine sulfate, dried sodium phosphate, hydroxypropylmethylcellulose 1500, polysorbate 80, propylene glycol, thimerosal, and purified water.
Action: Surfacaine® (cyclomethycaine sulfate, Lilly) prevents the initiation and transmission of nerve impulses and thus effects local anesthetic action. Onset of anesthesia requires five to ten minutes. The vehicle provides lubrication for instrumentation.
Indications: For use as a topical anesthetic and lubricant on nontraumatized, accessible mucous membranes prior to clinical examination and instrumentation.
Contraindications: Jelly Surfacaine® (cyclomethycaine sulfate, Lilly) is contraindicated in persons with an idiosyncrasy or allergy to any of the ingredients. Do not use in the eyes.
Precautions: Avoid application to extensive skin areas. If prolonged or indefinite use of Surfacaine® (cyclomethycaine sulfate, Lilly) is undertaken, observe periodically to detect

possible development of allergic reaction. Increase in redness, itching, papules, or vesicles suggests possible allergy. Discontinue use if irritation or allergy develops.
Persons with a history of allergic asthma, rhinitis, or urticaria may have an increased risk of allergic reactions. One probable anaphylactoid reaction has occurred following the introduction of a cyclomethycaine sulfate suppository in a patient with a history of multiple allergies. No other case of systemic toxicity has been reported.
Urethral administration should be made only by the physician or persons under his direction. Extreme caution is imperative when any local anesthetic is injected into the traumatized urethra or under conditions in which trauma is likely to occur. Overdistention of the urethra by the jelly may produce trauma, with stinging and burning. These symptoms may recur following dissipation of the anesthetic effect if the injury to the mucosa is extensive.
Adverse Reactions: A transitory stinging and/or burning sensation is occasionally experienced before the onset of the anesthetic effect.
Contact dermatitis may occur in hypersensitive individuals. Unlike benzocaine and procaine, Surfacaine® (cyclomethycaine sulfate, Lilly) is not a *p*-aminobenzoic acid derivative, and allergic reactions are not common.
Administration and Dosage: To avoid contamination, employ only previously unused tubes.
Urethra—1. Sterilize tip of 3.5-gm tube with suitable antiseptic. See illustration in package literature.
2. Remove break-off tube.
For Surface Anesthesia of the Male Urethra—The outer orifice is washed and cleansed with a disinfectant. Before catheterization, instillation of small volumes (3.4 to 10 ml) of jelly is usually adequate.
If the 28-gm tube is to be used, the plastic urethral tip is sterilized for five minutes in boiling water, cooled, and attached to the tube. The tip may be gas sterilized or cold sterilized, if preferred. The jelly is instilled slowly into the urethra until the patient has a feeling of tension or until half the tube is emptied. A penile clamp is then applied for several minutes at the corona, and subsequently the remaining contents of the tube are instilled.
Prior to sounding or cystoscopy, a penile clamp should be applied for five to ten minutes to obtain adequate anesthesia. Thirty ml of the jelly are usually required to fill and dilate the male urethra.
For Surface Anesthesia of the Female Urethra—The outer orifice is washed and cleansed with a disinfectant. Three to 7 ml of the jelly are instilled slowly into the urethra. If desired, jelly may also be deposited on a cotton swab and introduced into the urethra.
If the 28-gm tube is to be used, the plastic urethral tip is sterilized for five minutes in boiling water, cooled, and attached to the tube. The tip may be gas sterilized or cold sterilized, if preferred.
In order to obtain adequate anesthesia, several minutes should be allowed before urologic procedures are performed.
Anus—Insert 10 ml into rectum five to ten minutes prior to anorectal, sigmoidoscopic, or prostatic examination. Apply a coating to gloved finger, anus, and instruments as needed for lubrication.
Vagina—Introduce 5 ml, using finger or vaginal applicator.
Nose and Throat—Apply to intubation apparatus, tracheal catheters, etc. Reflexes are reduced or abolished, and easier intubation may be achieved when the jelly is used in this manner. Jelly Surfacaine® (cyclomethycaine sulfate, Lilly) is not intended for use as the sole anesthetic agent prior to bronchoscopic examinations.
Maximum Dosage: No more than 30 ml should be given in any 12-hour period.
How Supplied: (℞) *Jelly No. 11, Surfacaine® (Cyclomethycaine Sulfate, NF), 0.75%,* in 3.5-gm (3.4-ml) tubes (packages of 25) and in 28-gm (26.9-ml) and 142-gm (136.5-ml) tubes. The 3.5-gm tubes have a special break-off urethral tip. The 28-gm package contains one nonsterile perforated urethral tip and one rectal pipe.

[081778]

TAPAZOLE® ℞
(methimazole)
Tablets, USP

Description: Tapazole (1-methyl-2-mercaptoimidazole) is a white crystalline substance that is freely soluble in water. It differs chemically from the drugs of the thiouracil series primarily in that it has a five instead of a six-membered ring.
Actions: Tapazole® (methimazole, Lilly) inhibits the synthesis of thyroid hormones and thus is effective in the treatment of hyperthyroidism. The drug does not inactivate existing thyroxine and triiodothyronine which is stored in colloid or is circulating in the blood, nor does it interfere with the effectiveness of thyroid hormones given by mouth or by injection.
Indications: Tapazole® (methimazole, Lilly) is indicated in the medical treatment of hyperthyroidism. Long-term therapy may lead to remission of the disease. Tapazole may also be used to ameliorate hyperthyroidism in preparation for subtotal thyroidectomy or radioactive iodine therapy.
Contraindication: Tapazole® (methimazole, Lilly) is contraindicated in the presence of hypersensitivity to the drug.
Warnings: *Pregnancy*—Tapazole® (methimazole, Lilly), used judiciously, is an effective drug in hyperthyroidism complicated by pregnancy. Because the drug readily crosses placental membranes and can induce goiter and even cretinism in the developing fetus, it is important that a sufficient, but not excessive, dose be given. In many pregnant women, the thyroid dysfunction diminishes as the pregnancy proceeds; consequently, a reduction of dosage may be possible. In some instances, Tapazole can be withdrawn two or three weeks before delivery.
The administration of thyroid along with Tapazole to the pregnant hyperthyroid woman is also recommended in order to prevent hypothyroidism in the mother and her fetus. Administration should continue throughout the pregnancy and after delivery. Postpartum patients receiving Tapazole should not nurse their babies.
Precautions: Patients who receive Tapazole® (methimazole, Lilly) should be under close surveillance and should be impressed with the necessity of reporting immediately any evidence of illness, particularly sore throat, skin eruptions, fever, headache, or general malaise. In such cases, white-blood-cell and differential counts should be made to determine whether agranulocytosis has developed. Particular care should be exercised with patients who are receiving additional drugs known to cause agranulocytosis.
Adverse Reactions: Adverse reactions probably occur in less than 3 percent of patients.
Minor adverse reactions include skin rash, urticaria, nausea, vomiting, epigastric distress, arthralgia, paresthesia, loss of taste, abnormal loss of hair, myalgia, headache, pruritus, drowsiness, neuritis, edema, vertigo, skin pigmentation, jaundice, sialadenopathy, and lymphadenopathy.
Major adverse reactions (much less common than the minor adverse reactions) include inhibition of myelopoiesis (agranulocytosis, granulopenia, and thrombocytopenia), drug fever, a lupuslike syndrome, hepatitis (jaundice may persist for several weeks after discontinuation of the drug), periarteritis, and hypoprothrombinemia.
It should be noted that about 10 percent of patients with untreated hyperthyroidism have leukopenia (white-blood-cell count of less than 4000 per cu mm), often with relative granulopenia.
Administration and Dosage: Tapazole® (methimazole, Lilly) is administered orally. It is usually given in three equal doses at approximately eight-hour intervals.
Adult—The initial daily dosage is 15 mg for mild hyperthyroidism, 30 to 40 mg for moderately severe hyperthyroidism, and 60 mg for severe hyperthyroidism, divided into three doses at eight-hour intervals. The maintenance dosage is 5 to 15 mg daily.
Pediatric—Initially, the daily dosage is 0.4 mg per kg of body weight divided into three doses and given at eight-hour intervals. The maintenance dosage is approximately one-half of the initial dose.
Overdosage: Agranulocytosis is the most serious effect. Rarely, exfoliative dermatitis, hepatitis, neuropathies, or C.N.S. stimulation or depression may occur.
Symptoms—Nausea, vomiting, epigastric distress, headache, fever, arthralgia, pruritus, edema, and pancytopenia. Prolonged therapy may result in hypothyroidism.
Treatment—For specific therapy, the drug should be discontinued in the presence of agranulocytosis, pancytopenia, hepatitis, fever, or exfoliative dermatitis.
For bone-marrow depression, use of an antibiotic, transfusions of fresh whole blood, and a corticosteroid should be considered. For hepatitis, rest and adequate diet and, in severe cases, corticosteroid therapy may be indicated. General management may consist in symptomatic and supportive therapy, including rest, analgesics, gastric lavage, intravenous fluids, and mild sedation.
How Supplied: (℞) *Tablets Tapazole® (Methimazole Tablets, USP)* (scored): *No. 1765, J94,** 5 mg, and *No. 1770, J95,** 10 mg, in bottles of 100 and 1000. [081678]

THERACEBRIN® ℞
(pan-vitamins)

Description: Each Pulvule® contains—
Thiamine (as the Mononitrate)
(Vitamin B_1) .... 15 mg
Riboflavin
(Vitamin B_2) .... 10 mg
Pyridoxine (as the Hydrochloride)
(Vitamin B_6) .... 2.5 mg
Pantothenic Acid (as *d*-Calcium Pantothenate) .... 20 mg
Niacinamide .... 150 mg
Vitamin B_{12} (Activity Equivalent) .... 10 mcg
Ascorbic Acid
(Vitamin C) .... 150 mg
dl-Alpha Tocopheryl Acetate
(Vitamin E) .... 18.5 IU (18.5 mg)
Vitamin A Synthetic .... 25,000 IU (7.5 mg)
Vitamin D Synthetic .... 1500 IU (37.5 mcg)
Indications: For the treatment of multiple vitamin deficiencies, especially in gastrointestinal surgery, severe burns, or infectious hepatitis.
Precautions: Rarely, vitamins A and D in large doses (respectively, 50,000 IU and 25,000 IU or more daily for several months or longer) cause toxicity.
Administration and Dosage: *Prophylaxis*—1 Pulvule daily. *Treatment*—1 Pulvule twice daily.
How Supplied: (℞) *Pulvules No. 200, Theracebrin® (pan-vitamins, Lilly), H72** (No. 0, Black Body, Black Cap), in bottles of 30 and 100.

[060776]

Continued on next page

*Identi-Code® symbol.

Lilly—Cont.

TOBRAMYCIN SULFATE, *see* Nebcin® (tobramycin sulfate, Lilly).

TRISOGEL® **OTC**
(magnesium trisilicate and aluminum hydroxide gel)

Description: A combination of rapid-acting aluminum hydroxide and long-acting magnesium trisilicate, available in Pulvules® or as a palatable, aromatized aqueous suspension.
Liquid Trisogel is an effective antacid with a creamy texture and fresh mint flavor; it is not gritty and leaves no chalky aftertaste. One teaspoonful contains 0.39 mEq of sodium.
Each 5 ml of the liquid contain—
Magnesium Trisilicate ....9 grs
Aluminum Hydroxide ....2.3 grs
(Equivalent to 3 grs Aluminum Hydroxide Gel, Desiccated)
Five ml neutralize at least 100 ml of 0.1 *N* hydrochloric acid.
Each Pulvule contains—
Magnesium Trisilicate ....4½ grs
Aluminum Hydroxide Gel,
Desiccated ....1½ grs
Indications: A nonsystemic antacid for acid indigestion, sour stomach, or heartburn.
Warning: This product should not be used by persons who have kidney disease. No more than 8 teaspoonfuls of the liquid should be taken in a 24-hour period, nor should the maximum dosage be used for more than two weeks except under the advice and supervision of a physician.
Drug Interaction Precaution: This product should not be used by individuals who are currently taking a prescription antibiotic drug containing any form of tetracycline.
Adverse Reactions: Trisogel may have a laxative effect or cause constipation.
Dosage: *Liquid*—Usual adult dose, 2 teaspoonfuls four times a day with water, or as directed by the physician.
Pulvules—4 four times a day with water.
Overdosage: In case of accidental overdose, professional assistance should be sought or a poison control center contacted immediately.
How Supplied: *Liquid No. 33, Trisogel® (magnesium trisilicate and aluminum hydroxide gel, Lilly),* in 12-fl-oz bottles. *Avoid freezing. Pulvules No. 290, Trisogel, F53** (No. 0, Pink), in bottles of 100. [060178]

TUBOCURARINE CHLORIDE ℞
Injection, USP
See also Metubine® Iodide (metocurine iodide, Lilly)

THIS DRUG SHOULD BE ADMINISTERED ONLY BY ADEQUATELY TRAINED INDIVIDUALS WHO ARE FAMILIAR WITH ITS ACTIONS, CHARACTERISTICS, AND HAZARDS.

Description: Tubocurarine Chloride Injection, USP, is a sterile isotonic solution for intravenous use. Each ml of the solution contains 3 mg (20 units) tubocurarine chloride, sodium bisulfite, 0.1 percent, and sodium chloride, 0.7 percent, with chlorobutanol (chloroform derivative), 0.5 percent, as a preservative. Sodium hydroxide and/or hydrochloric acid are sometimes added during manufacture to adjust the *p*H.
Actions: Tubocurarine chloride blocks nerve impulses to skeletal muscles at the myoneural junction. This is a nondepolarizing neuromuscular blockade. When it is administered intravenously (intramuscular injection is unpredictable), the onset of flaccid paralysis occurs within a few minutes.
Muscle paralysis may be expected for periods of 25 to 90 minutes. The use of repeated doses may be accompanied by a cumulative effect. Since tubocurarine chloride is excreted by the kidneys, severe renal disease or hypotension may result in a more prolonged action of this drug.
Concurrently administered general anesthetics, certain antibiotics, abnormal states (e.g., acidosis), electrolyte imbalance, and neuromuscular disease have been reported to cause a potentiation of this drug's activity.
Rapid intravenous injection may produce increased release of histamine with resultant decreased respiratory capacity due to bronchospasm and paralysis of the respiratory muscles. Hypotension may occur owing to ganglionic blockade, or it may be a complication of positive pressure respiration.
Tubocurarine chloride does not affect consciousness or cerebration, and it does not relieve pain. A patient in severe pain may not be able to communicate this to the anesthesiologist.
Indications: Tubocurarine chloride is indicated as an adjunct to anesthesia to induce skeletal-muscle relaxation. It may be employed to reduce the intensity of muscle contractions in pharmacologically or electrically induced convulsions. It may be used as a diagnostic agent for myasthenia gravis when the results of tests with neostigmine or edrophonium are inconclusive. It may also be employed to facilitate the management of patients undergoing mechanical ventilation.
Contraindications: Tubocurarine chloride is contraindicated in those persons who have shown an allergic reaction or hypersensitivity to the drug and in patients in whom histamine release is a definite hazard.
Warnings: TUBOCURARINE CHLORIDE IS A POTENT DRUG WHICH MAY CAUSE RESPIRATORY DEPRESSION. THEREFORE, IT SHOULD BE USED ONLY BY THOSE EXPERIENCED IN THE TECHNIQUE OF ARTIFICIAL RESPIRATION AND THE ADMINISTRATION OF OXYGEN UNDER POSITIVE PRESSURE. FACILITIES FOR THESE PROCEDURES SHOULD BE IMMEDIATELY AVAILABLE AT ALL TIMES.
Prolonged apnea with its attendant hazards due to hypoxia may result from overdosages of this preparation.
It should be employed with extreme caution in patients with known myasthenia gravis.
The administration of quinidine during postoperative recovery to patients who have received tubocurarine chloride may result in recurarization leading to respiratory paralysis.
Usage in Pregnancy—The safe use of tubocurarine chloride has not been established with respect to the possible adverse effects upon child development. Therefore, it should not be administered to women of childbearing potential and especially not during early pregnancy unless, in the judgment of the physician, the potential benefits outweigh the possible hazards.
Precautions: When sufficiently excessive dosage of curare has been administered, there is no antidote. It is again emphasized that dosage should be controlled so that emergency measures need not be instituted.
Tubocurarine chloride should be used with caution in patients with respiratory depression or with renal, hepatic, or pulmonary diseases. Hypotension can follow the administration of large doses.
Adverse Reactions: Adverse reactions consist primarily in extension of the drug's pharmacologic actions. Profound and prolonged muscle relaxation may occur, with consequent respiratory depression to the point of apnea. Hypersensitivity to the drug may exist in rare instances.
Idiosyncrasy, interference with physical signs of anesthesia, circulatory depression, ganglionic blockade, and release of histamine are complications that can result from the use of this medication.
Drug Interaction: The intensity of blockade and duration of action of tubocurarine chloride are increased in patients receiving patent inhalational anesthetics such as halothane, diethyl ether, methoxyflurane, and enflurane. No increased intensity of blockade or duration of action is noted from the use of thiobarbiturates, narcotic analgesics, nitrous oxide, or droperidol.
Prior administration of succinylcholine chloride, such as that used for endotracheal intubation, may enhance the relaxant effect of tubocurarine chloride. If succinylcholine chloride is used before tubocurarine, the administration of tubocurarine should be delayed until the succinylcholine shows signs of wearing off.
Administration and Dosage:
Conversion Table for Calculating Dosage
20 units are contained in each ml
1 mg equals 7 units
1 unit is contained in 0.05 ml of this solution
Tubocurarine chloride is administered intravenously as a sustained injection over a period of 1 to 1½ minutes. As a precaution, the initial dose should be reduced to 20 units below the calculated amount. The speed of injection of the drug influences the amount administered. Although rapid injection may be dangerous, curarization can be accomplished with a smaller dose than that mentioned above if this is given more rapidly.
Tubocurarine chloride should be administered only by or under the supervision of experienced clinicians. The dosage must be individualized in each case after evaluation of the patient and consideration of factors that might alter the action of the drug in a particular case. If inhalational anesthetics known to enhance the action of curariform drugs are being used, the initial dose should be reduced and the response noted as a guide to incremental doses. If enhanced sensitivity is suspected, fractional dosage is advised initially to avoid overdosage. The following doses are for average patients without altered sensitivity.
Surgery—In the patient of average weight, 40 to 60 units of Tubocurarine Chloride Injection are administered intravenously at the time the skin incision is made, and 20 to 30 units in three to five minutes if required for further relaxation. For long operations, supplemental doses of 20 units may be given as required. As a general rule, dosage may be calculated on the basis of ½ unit per pound of body weight.
Electroshock Therapy—Tubocurarine chloride is administered just before electroshock therapy in the treatment of mental diseases. It reduces the severity of the convulsions and is useful as a means of preventing fractures. The patient should be observed closely until consciousness is regained in case respiratory failure should develop. A dose of ½ unit per pound of body weight is given intravenously and slowly as a sustained 1 to 1 ½-minute injection. Rapid administration is dangerous. The initial dose is 20 units less than this.
Diagnosis of Myasthenia Gravis—Tubocurarine chloride has been useful as a diagnostic agent in patients suspected of having myasthenia gravis. When small doses are given, a profound exaggeration of this syndrome occurs. The dosage is 1/15 to 1/5 of the average adult electroshock-therapy dose administered intravenously.
Every effort should be made to control dosage to the end that emergencies do not arise. It is important that physicians familiarize themselves with the dangers involved in using the drug and that preparations be made in advance for treating the patient if unwarranted side effects occur (*see* Contraindications *and* Adverse Reactions).

Tubocurarine chloride is adjusted to a pH sufficiently low to assure full stability for indefinite periods without the need for refrigeration; therefore, because of the high pH of barbiturate solutions, a precipitate will form when tubocurarine chloride is combined with such agents as Brevital® Sodium (Methohexital Sodium for Injection, USP, Lilly) and Thiopental Sodium.

It is recommended that each component be given from a separate syringe to assure more uniform and predictable results with each of the drugs. A single needle and tube attached to a three-way stopcock apparatus can readily be adapted to this method if it is desirable to utilize as few of the patient's veins as possible.

Management of Adverse Reactions: If hypotension occurs, the etiology should be determined. When it is due to ganglionic blockade, hypotension may be treated with fluid and vasopressors which act at the adrenergic receptors as required. Apnea or prolonged curarization should be treated with controlled respiration. Edrophonium or neostigmine may antagonize the skeletal-muscle-relaxant action of tubocurarine chloride. Neostigmine injection should be accompanied or preceded by an injection of atropine sulfate or its equivalent. A nerve stimulator may be used to assess the nature and degree of the neuromuscular blockade. The optimum time to administer the antagonist is when the patient is being hyperventilated and the carbon-dioxide level of the blood is low. The effects of neostigmine given intravenously last from 30 to 90 minutes; the effects of edrophonium are usually dissipated within five minutes. The antagonists are merely adjuncts. Before they are used, the package inserts of these drugs should be consulted for prescribing information.

Pharmacology: Tubocurarine chloride blocks nervous impulses to skeletal muscles at the myoneural junction.

Renal excretion occurs fairly rapidly; therefore, the physiologic effect is of relatively short duration.

How Supplied: (℞) *Ampoules (Vials) No. 449, Tubocurarine Chloride Injection, USP,* 3 mg per ml (20 units per ml), 10 ml, rubber-stoppered, in singles (10 per carton).

[020679]

TUINAL® Ⓒ
(secobarbital sodium and amobarbital sodium)

Description: A combination of equal parts of Seconal® Sodium (secobarbital sodium, Lilly) and Amytal® Sodium (amobarbital sodium) Lilly) which results in a moderately long-acting, rapidly effective hypnotic.

Each Pulvule No. 302 contains 25 mg Seconal Sodium and 25 mg Amytal Sodium.

Each Pulvule No. 303 contains 50 mg Seconal Sodium and 50 mg Amytal Sodium.

Each Pulvule No. 304 contains 100 mg Seconal Sodium and 100 mg Amytal Sodium.

Indications: For use whenever prompt and moderately sustained hypnotic effect is required. Not suitable for continuous daytime sedation.

Contraindications: Tuinal is contraindicated in patients who are sensitive to the barbiturates and in those with a history of porphyria. Barbiturates should not be administered in the presence of uncontrolled pain, because excitement may be produced.

Warnings: May be habit-forming. Prolonged, uninterrupted use of barbiturates (particularly the short-acting drugs), even in therapeutic doses, may result in psychic and physical dependence.

The central-nervous-system depressant effect of secobarbital and amobarbital may be additive with that of other C.N.S. depressants, including alcohol.

Usage in Pregnancy—Safe use of Tuinal has not been established with respect to possible adverse effects on fetal development. Therefore, if this drug is to be given to pregnant women, particularly during early pregnancy, the potential benefits to the mother should be weighed against the possible risks to the fetus.

Usage in Ambulatory Patients—Tuinal may impair the mental and/or physical abilities required for the performance of potentially hazardous tasks, such as driving a car or operating machinery. The patient should be cautioned accordingly.

Precaution: Since the liver is the major site of degradation of sedative-hypnotics, caution should be observed when these drugs are given to patients with impaired liver function, and lower doses should be used initially.

Adverse Reactions: Idiosyncrasy, in the form of excitement, hangover, or pain, may appear. Hypersensitivity reactions occur in some patients, especially in those with asthma, urticaria, or angioneurotic edema.

Dosage: 50 to 200 mg at bedtime or one hour preoperatively.

Overdosage: C.N.S. depression. *Symptoms*—Respiratory depression, depression of superficial and deep reflexes, constriction of the pupils to a slight degree (though in severe poisoning they may dilate), decreased urine formation, lowered body temperature, and coma. *Treatment*—General management should consist in symptomatic and supportive therapy, including gastric lavage, administration of intravenous fluids, and maintenance of blood pressure, body temperature, and adequate respiratory exchange. Dialysis will increase the rate of removal of barbiturates from the body fluids.

How Supplied: (Ⓒ) *Pulvules® Tuinal® (secobarbital sodium and amobarbital sodium, Lilly): No. 302, F64,** 50 mg (No. 4, Blue Body, Orange Cap), in bottles of 100; *No. 303, F65,** 100 mg (No. 3, Blue Body, Orange Cap), in bottles of 100 and 1000, in 10 strips of 10 individually labeled blisters each containing 1 Pulvule (ID100), and in strip packages of individually sealed Pulvules (DS1000); *No. 304, F66,** 200 mg (No. 2, Blue Body, Orange Cap), in bottles of 100 and 1000 and in 10 strips of 10 individually labeled blisters each containing 1 Pulvule (ID100).

[062777]

[*Shown in Product Identification Section*]

TYLOSTERONE® ℞
(diethylstilbestrol and methyltestosterone) TABLETS

1. *PROLONGED USE OF ESTROGENS HAS BEEN REPORTED TO INCREASE THE RISK OF ENDOMETRIAL CARCINOMA*

Three independent case-control studies have reported an increased risk of endometrial cancer in postmenopausal women exposed to exogenous estrogens for prolonged periods. This risk was independent of other known risk factors for endometrial cancer. These studies are further supported by the finding that, since 1969, the incidence rate of endometrial cancer has increased sharply in eight different areas of the United States which have population-based cancer reporting systems.

The three case-control studies reported that the risk of endometrial cancer in estrogen users was about 4.5 to 13.9 times greater than in nonusers. The risk appears to depend on both the duration of treatment and the dose of estrogen. In view of these findings, the lowest dose that will control symptoms should be utilized when estrogens are used for the treatment of menopausal symptoms, and medication should be discontinued as soon as possible. When prolonged treatment is medically indicated, a reassessment should be made on at least a semiannual basis to determine the need for continued therapy. Although the evidence must be considered preliminary, one study suggests that cyclic administration of low doses of estrogen may carry less risk than does continuous administration; it therefore appears prudent to utilize such a regimen.

Close clinical surveillance of all women taking estrogens is important. In all cases of undiagnosed persistent or recurring abnormal vaginal bleeding, adequate diagnostic measures should be undertaken to rule out malignancy.

At present, there is no evidence that "natural" estrogens are more or less hazardous than "synthetic" estrogens at equivalent estrogenic doses.

2. *ESTROGENS SHOULD NOT BE USED DURING PREGNANCY*

The use of female sex hormones, both estrogens and progestogens, during early pregnancy may affect the offspring. It has been reported that females exposed *in utero* to diethylstilbestrol, a nonsteroidal estrogen, may have an increased risk of developing later in life a rare form of vaginal or cervical cancer. This risk has been estimated to be no greater than 4 per 1000 exposures. Furthermore, from 30 to 90 percent of such exposed women have been found to have vaginal adenosis and epithelial changes of the vagina and cervix. Although these changes are histologically benign, it is not known whether they are precursors of malignancy. Even though similar data are not available with the use of other estrogens, it cannot be presumed that they would not induce similar changes.

Several reports suggest that there is an association between intrauterine exposure to female sex hormones and congenital anomalies, including congenital heart defects and limb-reduction defects. One case-control study estimated a 4.7-fold increased risk of limb-reduction defects in infants exposed *in utero* to sex hormones (oral contraceptives, hormone withdrawal tests for pregnancy, or attempted treatment for threatened abortion). Some of these exposures were very short and involved only a few days of treatment. The data suggest that the risk of limb-reduction defects in exposed fetuses is somewhat less than 1 per 1000.

In the past, female sex hormones have been used during pregnancy in an attempt to treat threatened or habitual abortion; however, their efficacy was never conclusively proved or disproved.

If Tylosterone is administered during pregnancy or if the patient becomes pregnant while taking this drug, she should be apprised of the potential risks to the fetus and of the advisability of pregnancy continuation.

THIS DRUG PRODUCT SHOULD NOT BE USED AS A POSTCOITAL CONTRACEPTIVE

Description: Tablets Tylosterone contain 0.25 mg diethylstilbestrol and 5 mg methyltestosterone.

Diethylstilbestrol is a crystalline estrogenic substance capable of producing all the pharmacologic and therapeutic responses attributed to natural estrogens.

Methyltestosterone is a crystalline androgenic substance which, in adequate dosage, is capable of mediating the development of the male accessory organs, pubic hair and beard and

Continued on next page

*Identi-Code® symbol.

Lilly—Cont.

lowering of the voice, characteristic of puberty in men.

Indications: Tylosterone is indicated in the treatment of moderate to severe *vasomotor* symptoms associated with the menopause in those patients not improved by estrogen alone. (There is no evidence that estrogens are effective for nervous symptoms or depression which might occur during menopause, and they should not be used to treat these conditions.) TYLOSTERONE SHOULD NOT BE USED FOR ANY PURPOSE DURING PREGNANCY. ITS USE MAY CAUSE SEVERE HARM TO THE FETUS (*SEE* BOXED WARNING).

Contraindications: Estrogens should not be used in women (or men) with any of the following conditions:

1. Known or suspected cancer of the breast, except in appropriately selected patients being treated for metastatic disease
2. Known or suspected estrogen-dependent neoplasia
3. Known or suspected pregnancy (*see* boxed warning)
4. Undiagnosed abnormal genital bleeding
5. Active thrombophlebitis or thromboembolic disorders
6. A past history of thrombophlebitis, thrombosis, or thromboembolic disorders associated with previous use of estrogen (except when used in treatment of breast or prostatic malignancy)

Warnings: 1. *Induction of Malignant Neoplasms*—In certain animal species, long-term continuous administration of natural and synthetic estrogens increases the frequency of carcinomas of the breast, cervix, vagina, kidney, and liver. There are now reports that prolonged use of estrogens increases the risk of carcinoma of the endometrium in humans (*see* boxed warning).

At the present time, there is no satisfactory evidence that administration of estrogens to postmenopausal women increases the risk of cancer of the breast. This possibility, however, has been raised by a recent long-term follow-up of one physician's practice. Because of the animal data, there is a need for caution in prescribing estrogens for women with a family history of breast cancer or for women who have breast nodules, fibrocystic disease, or abnormal mammograms.

2. *Gallbladder Disease*—A recent study reported a two-to-threefold increase in the risk of gallbladder disease occurring in women receiving postmenopausal estrogen therapy, similar to the twofold increased risk previously noted in women using oral contraceptives. In the case of oral contraceptives, this increased risk appeared after two years of use.

3. *Effects Similar to Those Caused by Estrogen-Progestogen Oral Contraceptives*—There are several serious adverse effects associated with the use of oral contraceptives; however, most of these adverse effects have not as yet been documented as consequences of postmenopausal estrogen therapy. This may reflect the comparatively low doses of estrogen used in postmenopausal women. It would be expected that these adverse effects are more likely to occur following administration of the larger doses of estrogen used for treating prostatic or breast cancer. It has, in fact, been shown that there is an increased risk of thrombosis with the administration of estrogens for prostatic cancer in men and for postpartum breast engorgement in women.

a. *Thromboembolic Disease*—It is now well established that women taking oral contraceptives run an increased risk of various thromboembolic and thrombotic vascular diseases, such as thrombophlebitis, pulmonary embolism, stroke, and myocardial infarction. Cases of retinal thrombosis, mesenteric thrombosis, and optic neuritis have been reported in users of oral contraceptives. There is evidence that the risk of several of these adverse reactions is related to the dose of the drug. An increased risk of postsurgical thromboembolic complications has also been reported in users of oral contraceptives. If feasible, estrogen therapy should be discontinued at least four weeks before any surgery that may be associated with an increased risk of thromboembolism or may require periods of prolonged immobilization.

Although an increased rate of thromboembolic and thrombotic disease has not been noted in postmenopausal users of estrogen, this does not rule out the possibility that such an increase may be present or that it exists in subgroups of women who have underlying risk factors or who are receiving relatively large doses of estrogens. Therefore, estrogens should not be used in persons with active thrombophlebitis or thromboembolic disorders, nor should they be used (except in treatment of malignancy) in persons with a history of such disorders associated with estrogen therapy. Estrogens should be administered cautiously to patients with cerebral vascular or coronary artery disease and only when such therapy is clearly needed.

In a large prospective clinical trial in men, large doses of estrogen (5 mg of conjugated estrogens per day), comparable to those used to treat cancer of the prostate and breast, have been shown to increase the risk of nonfatal myocardial infarction, pulmonary embolism, and thrombophlebitis. When such large doses of estrogen are used, any of the thromboembolic and thrombotic adverse effects associated with the use of oral contraceptives should be considered a clear risk.

b. *Hepatic Adenoma*—Benign hepatic adenomas appear to be associated with the use of oral contraceptives. Although these adenomas are benign and rare, they may rupture and may cause death by intra-abdominal hemorrhage. Such lesions have not yet been reported in association with the administration of other estrogen or progestogen preparations, but they should be considered when abdominal pain and tenderness, abdominal mass, or hypovolemic shock occurs in persons receiving estrogen therapy. Hepatocellular carcinoma has also been reported in women taking estrogen-containing oral contraceptives. The relationship of this malignancy to such drugs is not known at present.

c. *Elevated Blood Pressure*—Increased blood pressure is not uncommon in women taking oral contraceptives. There is now one report that this may occur with use of estrogens in the menopause, and blood pressure should be monitored during estrogen therapy, especially if high doses are used.

d. *Glucose Tolerance*—A decrease in glucose tolerance has been observed in a significant percentage of patients on estrogen-containing oral contraceptives. For this reason, diabetic patients should be carefully observed while receiving estrogen.

4. *Hypercalcemia*—Administration of estrogens may lead to severe hypercalcemia in patients with breast cancer and bone metastases. If this occurs, the drug should be stopped and appropriate measures taken to reduce the serum calcium level.

Precautions: A. General Precautions

1. A complete medical and family history should be taken prior to initiation of any estrogen therapy. In the pretreatment and periodic physical examinations, special consideration should be given to blood pressure, breasts, abdomen, and pelvic organs, and a Papanicolaou smear should be performed. As a general rule, estrogen should not be prescribed for over a year without another physical examination.

2. Fluid retention—Because estrogens may cause some degree of fluid retention, conditions which might be influenced by this factor, such as epilepsy, migraine, and cardiac or renal dysfunction, require careful observation.

3. Certain patients may develop undesirable manifestations of excessive estrogenic stimulation, such as abnormal or excessive uterine bleeding, mastodynia, etc.

4. Oral contraceptives appear to be associated with an increased incidence of mental depression. Although it is not clear whether this is due to the estrogenic or progestogenic component of the contraceptive agent, patients with a history of depression should be carefully observed.

5. Preexisting uterine leiomyomata may increase in size with administration of estrogens.

6. The pathologist should be advised of estrogen therapy when relevant specimens are submitted.

7. Patients with a past history of jaundice during pregnancy run an increased risk of recurrence of jaundice while receiving estrogen-containing oral contraceptive therapy. If jaundice develops in any patient receiving estrogen, the medication should be discontinued while the cause is investigated.

8. Estrogens may be poorly metabolized in patients with impaired liver function, and they should therefore be administered with caution in such patients.

9. Because estrogens influence the metabolism of calcium and phosphorus, they should be used with caution in patients with metabolic bone diseases associated with hypercalcemia or in patients with renal insufficiency.

10. Because of the effects of estrogens on epiphyseal closure, they should be used judiciously in young patients in whom bone growth is not complete.

11. Certain endocrine and liver function tests may be affected by estrogen-containing oral contraceptives. The following similar changes may be expected with larger doses of estrogen:

a. Increased sulfobromophthalein retention.

b. Increased prothrombin and factors VII, VIII, IX, and X; decreased antithrombin 3; increased norepinephrine-induced platelet aggregability.

c. Increased thyroid binding globulin (TBG) leading to increased circulating total thyroid hormone, as measured by PBI, T^4 by column, or T^4 by radioimmunoassay. Free T^3 resin uptake is decreased, reflecting the elevated TBG; free T^4 concentration is unaltered.

d. Impaired glucose tolerance.

e. Decreased pregnanediol excretion.

f. Reduced response to metyrapone test.

g. Reduced serum folate concentration.

h. Increased serum triglyceride and phospholipid concentration.

B. Information for the Patient. See text of Patient Package Insert.

C. Pregnancy Category X—*See* Contraindications and boxed warning.

D. Nursing Mothers—As a general principle, any drug should be administered to nursing mothers only when clearly necessary, since many drugs are excreted in human milk.

Special caution is desirable in administering androgen to brunettes and to women who already have an unusually coarse growth of facial hair or other submasculine characteristics. When Tylosterone is administered in the dosage recommended for menopausal symptoms, such side effects of androgen are extremely unlikely. Should they occur, they can be expected to regress promptly if therapy is discontinued immediately.

Adverse Reactions: *Estrogen Related*—(*See* Warnings regarding induction of neoplasia, adverse effects on the fetus, increased incidence of gallbladder disease, and adverse effects similar to those of oral contraceptives, including thromboembolism.) The following additional adverse reactions have been reported with estrogenic therapy, including oral contraceptives:

1. *Genitourinary System*
   Breakthrough bleeding, spotting, change in menstrual flow
   Dysmenorrhea
   Premenstrual-like syndrome
   Amenorrhea during and after treatment
   Increase in size of uterine fibromyomata
   Vaginal candidiasis
   Change in cervical eversion and in degree of cervical secretion
   Cystitis-like syndrome
2. *Breasts*
   Tenderness, enlargement, secretion
3. *Gastrointestinal*
   Nausea, vomiting
   Abdominal cramps, bloating
   Cholestatic jaundice
4. *Skin*
   Chloasma or melasma which may persist when drug is discontinued
   Erythema multiforme
   Erythema nodosum
   Hemorrhagic eruption
   Loss of scalp hair
   Hirsutism
5. *Eyes*
   Steepening of corneal curvature
   Intolerance to contact lenses
6. *C.N.S.*
   Headache, migraine, dizziness
   Mental depression
   Chorea
7. *Miscellaneous*
   Increase or decrease in weight
   Reduced carbohydrate tolerance
   Aggravation of porphyria
   Edema
   Changes in libido

Androgen Related—The side effects of androgen are likewise dependent in large part on dosage. In women, excessive quantities tend to produce masculinizing effects (virilism), such as acne vulgaris, coarsening of body hair, growth of beard, baldness, hoarseness, deepening of the voice, and enlargement of the clitoris.

Androgens may produce symptoms resembling those of peptic ulcer.

BSP elevations, rises in transaminase levels, and cholestatic jaundice may be produced by steroid therapy. If tests show these abnormalities, it is recommended that they be repeated after the drug has been withdrawn for two months.

Significant alterations in libido have been reported.

Electrolyte and water retention may occur, with attendant possible complications such as edema, dyspnea, perspiring extremities, and confusion.

Acute Overdosage: Numerous reports indicate that serious ill effects do not occur when large doses of estrogen-containing oral contraceptives are ingested by young children. Overdosage of estrogen may cause nausea, and withdrawal bleeding may occur in females.

Administration and Dosage: For treatment of moderate to severe *vasomotor* symptoms associated with the menopause: The lowest dose that will control symptoms should be chosen, and medication should be discontinued as promptly as possible.

Administration should be cyclic (e.g., three weeks on and one week off).

Attempts to discontinue or taper medication should be made at three to six-month intervals. The usual initial dosage is 1 tablet daily. Two tablets daily may be given at first, but this dosage should not be continued longer than two weeks, nor should it be exceeded. As soon as possible, dosage or frequency of administration should be reduced. *Maintenance dosage is to be kept at all times at the minimum necessary for relief—½ tablet or less daily.*

Estrogen-withdrawal bleeding may occur about one week after discontinuance of the drug. Some clinicians may prefer to produce actual shedding of the endometrium, as in true menstruation, by giving 5 mg progesterone daily for five days just before the rest period. Any unscheduled bleeding should of course be investigated.

Patients with an intact uterus should be closely monitored for signs of endometrial cancer, and appropriate diagnostic measures should be taken to rule out malignancy in the event of persistent or recurring abnormal vaginal bleeding.

How Supplied: (℞) *Tablets No. 1779, Tylosterone® (diethylstilbestrol and methyltestosterone, Lilly), J96** (scored), in bottles of 100.

[112078]

ULTRALENTE® ILETIN® (extended insulin zinc suspension, Lilly), *see under* Iletin® (insulin, Lilly).

VANCOCIN® HCL ℞

(vancomycin hydrochloride)
Sterile, USP
IntraVenous

Description: Vancocin® HCl (vancomycin hydrochloride, Lilly), IntraVenous, is a glycopeptide antibiotic derived from *Streptomyces orientalis* which is bactericidal against many gram-positive bacteria. It should be administered intravenously, in dilute solution (*see* Administration and Dosage).

Actions: Vancocin® HCl (vancomycin hydrochloride, Lilly) is poorly absorbed by mouth, but an intravenous dose of 1 gm produces serum levels averaging 25 mcg/ml at two hours. Its half-life in the circulation is about six hours. Many strains of streptococci, staphylococci, and other gram-positive bacteria are susceptible in vitro to concentrations of 0.5 to 5 mcg/ml. Staphylococci are generally susceptible to less than 5 mcg of Vancocin HCl per ml, but a small proportion of *Staphylococcus aureus* strains require 10 or 20 mcg/ml for inhibition. If the Bauer-Kirby method of disc susceptibility testing is used, a 30-mcg disc of Vancocin HCl should produce a zone of more than 11 mm when tested against a vancomycin-susceptible bacterial strain.

Clinically effective concentrations of this antibiotic in the blood are usually achieved and maintained by its intravenous administration; moreover, inhibitory concentrations can be demonstrated in pleural, pericardial, ascitic, and synovial fluids and in urine. This antibiotic does not readily diffuse across normal meninges into the spinal fluid. However, when the meninges are inflamed as a result of infection, Vancocin HCl penetrates into the spinal fluid.

About 80 percent of injected Vancocin HCl is excreted by the kidneys. Concentrations are high in the urine. Impairment of renal function results in delayed excretion and in high blood levels associated with an increase in drug toxicity.

Indications: Vancocin® HCl (vancomycin hydrochloride, Lilly) is indicated in potentially life-threatening infections which cannot be treated with another effective, less toxic antimicrobial drug, including the penicillins and cephalosporins.

Vancocin HCl is useful in therapy of severe staphylococcal infections in patients who cannot receive or who have failed to respond to the penicillins and cephalosporins or who have infections with staphylococci that are resistant to other antibiotics.

Vancocin HCl has been used successfully alone in the treatment of staphylococcal endocarditis. Its effectiveness has been documented in other infections due to staphylococci, including osteomyelitis, pneumonia, septicemia, and soft-tissue infections. When staphylococcal infections are localized and purulent, antibiotics are used as adjuncts to appropriate surgical measures.

The parenteral form may be administered orally for treatment of staphylococcal enterocolitis. Parenteral antibiotic administration may be used concomitantly. Vancomycin is *not* effective by the oral route for other types of infection.

Contraindication: Vancocin® HCl (vancomycin hydrochloride, Lilly) is contraindicated in patients with known hypersensitivity to this antibiotic.

Warnings: Because of its ototoxicity and nephrotoxicity, Vancocin® HCl (vancomycin hydrochloride, Lilly) should be avoided in patients with renal insufficiency. The risk of toxicity is appreciably increased by high blood concentrations or prolonged therapy. If it is necessary to use Vancocin HCl in such patients, doses of less than 2 gm/day usually will provide satisfactory blood levels.

Vancocin HCl should also be avoided in patients with previous hearing loss. If it is used in such patients, the dose of Vancocin HCl should be regulated, if possible, by periodic determination of the drug level in the blood. Deafness may be preceded by tinnitus. The elderly are more susceptible to auditory damage. Experience with other antibiotics suggests that deafness may be progressive despite cessation of treatment.

Concurrent and sequential use of other neurotoxic and/or nephrotoxic antibiotics, particularly streptomycin, neomycin, kanamycin, gentamicin, cephaloridine, paromomycin, viomycin, polymyxin B, colistin, and tobramycin, should be avoided.

Precautions: Patients with borderline renal function and individuals over the age of 60 should be given serial tests of auditory function and of vancomycin blood levels. (Vancomycin serum levels may be determined by use of the modified Rammelkamp serial twofold-dilution technique with streptococcus C203 as the indicator organism.) All patients receiving the drug should have periodic hematologic studies, urinalyses, and liver and renal function tests.

Vancocin® HCl (vancomycin hydrochloride, Lilly) is very irritating to tissue and causes necrosis when injected intramuscularly; it must be administered intravenously. Pain and thrombophlebitis occur in many patients receiving Vancocin HCl and are occasionally severe. The frequency and severity of thrombophlebitis can be minimized if the drug is administered in a volume of at least 200 ml of glucose or saline solution and if the sites of injection are rotated.

Adverse Reactions: Nausea, chills, fever, urticaria, and macular rashes have been associated with the administration of Vancocin® HCl (vancomycin hydrochloride, Lilly). It may also produce eosinophilia and anaphylactoid reactions.

The use of Vancocin HCl may result in overgrowth of nonsusceptible organisms. If new infections due to bacteria or fungi appear during therapy with this product, appropriate measures should be taken.

Administration and Dosage: *Adults*—The usual intravenous dose is 500 mg (in 0.9% Sodium Chloride Injection or 5% glucose in Sterile Water for Injection) every six hours or 1 gm every 12 hours. The majority of patients with infections caused by organisms susceptible to the antibiotic show a therapeutic response by 48 to 72 hours. The total duration of therapy is determined by the type and severity of the infection and the clinical response of the patient.

Continued on next page

***Identi-Code® symbol.**

Lilly—Cont.

In staphylococcal endocarditis, therapy for three weeks or longer is recommended.

Children—The total daily dosage of Vancocin® HCl (vancomycin hydrochloride, Lilly), calculated on the basis of 20 mg per pound of body weight, can be divided and figured in with the child's 24-hour requirement of fluid.

PREPARATION OF SOLUTION:

At the time of use, add 10 ml of Sterile Water for Injection to the vial of dry, sterile Vancocin HCl powder.

FURTHER DILUTION IS REQUIRED. READ INSTRUCTIONS WHICH FOLLOW:

1. Intermittent Infusion (the preferred method of administration)
   The above solution (containing 500 mg Vancocin HCl) can be added to 100-200 ml of 0.9% Sodium Chloride Injection or 5% glucose in Sterile Water for Injection. This intravenous infusion may be given over a period of 20 to 30 minutes every six hours.
2. Continuous Infusion (should be used only when intermittent infusion is not feasible)
   Two to four vials of the above (1 to 2 gm) can be added to a sufficiently large volume of 0.9% Sodium Chloride Injection or 5% glucose in Sterile Water for Injection to permit the desired daily dose to be administered slowly by intravenous drip over a 24-hour period.

For Oral Administration—The contents of one vial (500 mg) may be diluted in one ounce of water and given to the patient to drink, or the diluted material may be administered via nasogastric tube. For convenience of oral administration, Vancocin HCl is also available in a screw-cap container (No. M-206).

Stability of Prepared Solution: After reconstitution, the solution may be stored in a refrigerator for 96 hours without significant loss of potency.

How Supplied: (℞) *Ampoules (Vials) No. 657, Vancocin® HCl (Sterile Vancomycin Hydrochloride, USP), IntraVenous,* equivalent to 500 mg vancomycin, 10-ml size, rubber-stoppered (Dry Powder), in singles (10 per carton).
[031778]

VANCOCIN® HCl ℞
(vancomycin hydrochloride)
For Oral Solution, NF

This preparation is for oral use only. If parenteral vancomycin therapy is desired, use Vancocin® HCl (Sterile Vancomycin Hydrochloride, USP), IntraVenous, and consult package insert accompanying that preparation.

Description: Vancocin® HCl (vancomycin hydrochloride, Lilly) is a glycopeptide antibiotic derived from *Streptomyces orientalis* which is bactericidal against many gram-positive bacteria.

Actions: Vancocin® HCl (vancomycin hydrochloride, Lilly) is poorly absorbed by mouth. Many strains of streptococci, staphylococci, and other gram-positive bacteria are susceptible in vitro to concentrations of 0.5 to 5 mcg/ml. Staphylococci are generally susceptible to less than 5 mcg of Vancocin HCl per ml, but a small proportion of *Staphylococcus aureus* strains require 10 or 20 mcg/ml for inhibition. If the Bauer-Kirby method of disc susceptibility testing is used, a 30-mcg disc of Vancocin HCl should produce a zone of more than 11 mm when tested against a vancomycin-susceptible bacterial strain.

Indication: Vancocin® HCl (vancomycin hydrochloride, Lilly) may be administered orally for treatment of staphylococcal enterocolitis. Parenteral antibiotic administration may be used concomitantly. Vancomycin is *not* effective by the oral route for other types of infection.

Contraindication: Vancocin® HCl (vancomycin hydrochloride, Lilly) is contraindicated in patients with known hypersensitivity to this antibiotic.

Warnings: Because of its ototoxicity and nephrotoxicity, Vancocin® HCl (vancomycin hydrochloride, Lilly) should be avoided in patients with renal insufficiency. During parenteral therapy, the risk of toxicity is appreciably increased by high blood concentrations or prolonged treatment. If it is necessary to use Vancocin HCl parenterally in such patients, doses of less than 2 gm/day usually will provide satisfactory blood levels.

Vancocin HCl should also be avoided in patients with previous hearing loss. If it is used in such patients, the dose of Vancocin HCl should be regulated, if possible, by periodic determination of the drug level in the blood. Deafness may be preceded by tinnitus. The elderly are more susceptible to auditory damage. Experience with other antibiotics suggests that deafness may be progressive despite cessation of treatment.

Concurrent and sequential use of other neurotoxic and/or nephrotoxic antibiotics, particularly streptomycin, neomycin, kanamycin, gentamicin, cephaloridine, paromomycin, viomycin, polymyxin B, colistin, and tobramycin, should be avoided.

Precautions: Patients with borderline renal function and individuals over the age of 60 should be given serial tests of auditory function and of vancomycin blood levels. (Vancomycin serum levels may be determined by use of the modified Rammelkamp serial twofold-dilution technique with streptococcus C203 as the indicator organism.) All patients receiving the drug should have periodic hematologic studies, urinalyses, and liver and renal function tests.

Adverse Reactions: Nausea, chills, fever, urticaria, and macular rashes have been associated with the administration of Vancocin HCl. It may also produce eosinophilia and anaphylactoid reactions.

The use of Vancocin® HCl (vancomycin hydrochloride, Lilly) may result in overgrowth of nonsusceptible organisms. If new infections due to bacteria or fungi appear during therapy with this product, appropriate measures should be taken.

Administration and Dosage: The contents of the container may be mixed with distilled or deionized water (115 ml) for oral administration. When mixed with 115 ml of water, each 6 ml provide approximately 500 mg of vancomycin. Mix thoroughly to dissolve. This mixture may be kept for one week in a refrigerator without significant loss of potency.

Adults—The usual dose is 500 mg every six hours or 1 gm every 12 hours.

Children—The total daily dose is 20 mg per pound of body weight in divided doses.

How Supplied: (℞) *Vancocin® HCl (Vancomycin Hydrochloride for Oral Solution, NF), M-206,* 10 gm (equivalent to vancomycin), in a screw-cap container. [010579]

VANCOMYCIN HYDROCHLORIDE, *see* Vancocin® HCl (vancomycin hydrochloride, Lilly).

V-CILLIN K® ℞
(penicillin V potassium)
USP

Description: V-Cillin K® (Penicillin V Potassium, USP, Lilly) is the potassium salt of V-Cillin® (Penicillin V, USP, Lilly). This chemically improved form combines acid stability with immediate solubility and rapid absorption.

Actions and Pharmacology: V-Cillin K® (penicillin V potassium, Lilly) is bactericidal against penicillin-sensitive microorganisms during the stage of active multiplication. It produces its effect by inhibiting biosynthesis of cell-wall mucopeptide. It is not active against the penicillinase-producing bacteria, which include many strains of staphylococci. The drug exerts high in vitro activity against staphylococci (except penicillinase-producing strains), streptococci (groups A, C, G, H, L, and M), and pneumococci. Other organisms sensitive in vitro to penicillin V are *Corynebacterium diphtheriae, Bacillus anthracis,* clostridia, *Actinomyces bovis, Streptobacillus moniliformis, Listeria monocytogenes, Leptospira,* and *Neisseria gonorrhoeae. Treponema pallidum* is extremely sensitive.

V-Cillin K has the distinct advantage over penicillin G in being resistant to inactivation by gastric acid. It may be given with meals; however, blood levels are slightly higher when the drug is given on an empty stomach. Average blood levels are two to five times higher than those following the same dose of oral penicillin G and also show much less individual variation.

Once absorbed, about 80 percent of V-Cillin K is bound to serum protein. Tissue levels are highest in the kidneys, and lesser amounts appear in the liver, skin, and intestines. Small concentrations are found in all other body tissues and the cerebrospinal fluid. The drug is excreted as rapidly as it is absorbed in individuals with normal kidney function; however, recovery of the drug from the urine indicates that only about 25 percent of the dose given is absorbed. In neonates, young infants, and individuals with impaired kidney function, excretion is considerably delayed.

Indications: V-Cillin K® (penicillin V potassium, Lilly) is indicated in the treatment of mild to moderately severe infections due to microorganisms whose sensitivity to penicillin G is within the range of serum levels common to this particular dosage form. Therapy should be guided by bacteriologic studies (including susceptibility tests) and by clinical response.

NOTE: Severe pneumonia, empyema, bacteremia, pericarditis, meningitis, and arthritis should not be treated with penicillin V during the acute stage.

Indicated surgical procedures should be performed.

The following infections will usually respond to adequate dosage of penicillin V:

Streptococcal Infections (without Bacteremia)—Mild to moderate infections of the upper respiratory tract, scarlet fever, and mild erysipelas.

NOTE: Streptococci in groups A, C, G, H, L, and M are very sensitive to penicillin. Other groups, including group D (enterococcus), are resistant.

Pneumococcal Infections—Mild to moderately severe infections of the respiratory tract.

Staphylococcal Infections Sensitive to Penicillin G—Mild infections of the skin and soft tissues.

NOTE: Reports indicate an increasing number of strains of staphylococci resistant to penicillin G, which emphasizes the need for culture and susceptibility studies in treating suspected staphylococcal infections.

Fusospirochetosis (Vincent's Gingivitis and Pharyngitis)—Mild to moderately severe infections of the oropharynx usually respond to therapy with oral penicillin.

NOTE: Necessary dental care should be accomplished in infections involving the gum tissue.

Medical Conditions in Which Oral Penicillin Therapy Is Indicated as Prophylaxis—To prevent recurrence following rheumatic fever and/or chorea. Prophylaxis with oral penicillin on a continuing basis has proved effective in preventing recurrence of these conditions.

To prevent bacterial endocarditis in patients with congenital and/or rheumatic heart lesions who are to undergo dental procedures or minor upper respiratory tract surgery or instrumentation. Prophylaxis should be instituted the day of the procedure and for two or more days afterward. Patients with a past history of rheumatic fever and receiving continuous prophylaxis may harbor increased numbers of penicillin-resistant organisms; use of another prophylactic anti-infective agent should be considered. If penicillin is to be used in these patients at surgery, the regular rheumatic fever program should be interrupted one week prior to the contemplated surgery. At the time of surgery, penicillin may be reinstituted as a prophylactic measure against the hazards of surgically induced bacteremia.

NOTE: Oral penicillin should not be used as adjunctive prophylaxis for genitourinary instrumentation or surgery, lower intestinal tract surgery, sigmoidoscopy, and childbirth.

Contraindication: A previous hypersensitivity reaction to any penicillin is a contraindication.

Warnings: Serious and occasionally fatal hypersensitivity (anaphylactoid) reactions have been reported in patients receiving penicillin therapy. Although anaphylaxis is more frequent following parenteral therapy, it has occurred in patients given oral penicillins. These reactions are more likely in individuals with a history of sensitivity to multiple allergens.

There have been well-documented reports of individuals with a history of penicillin hypersensitivity who have experienced severe reactions when treated with a cephalosporin. Before therapy with a penicillin, careful inquiry should be made concerning previous hypersensitivity reactions to penicillins, cephalosporins, and other allergens. If an allergic reaction occurs, the drug should be discontinued and the patient treated with the usual agents (e.g., epinephrine or other pressor amines, antihistamines, or corticosteroids).

Precautions: Penicillin should be used with caution in individuals with histories of significant allergies and/or asthma.

The oral route of administration should not be relied upon in patients with severe illness or with nausea, vomiting, gastric dilatation, cardiospasm, or intestinal hypermotility.

Occasional patients will not absorb therapeutic amounts of orally administered penicillin.

In streptococcal infections, therapy must be sufficient to eliminate the organism (a minimum of ten days); otherwise, the sequelae of streptococcal disease may occur. Cultures should be taken following completion of treatment to determine whether streptococci have been eradicated.

Prolonged use of antibiotics may promote the overgrowth of nonsusceptible organisms, including fungi. If superinfection occurs, appropriate measures should be taken.

Adverse Reactions: Although reactions have been reported much less frequently after oral than after parenteral penicillin therapy, it should be remembered that all degrees of hypersensitivity, including fatal anaphylaxis, have been observed with oral penicillin.

The most common reactions to oral penicillin are nausea, vomiting, epigastric distress, diarrhea, and black, hairy tongue. The hypersensitivity reactions noted are skin eruptions (ranging from maculopapular to exfoliative dermatitis); urticaria; reactions resembling serum sickness, including chills, fever, edema, arthralgia, and prostration; laryngeal edema; and anaphylaxis. Fever and eosinophilia may frequently be the only reactions observed. Hemolytic anemia, leukopenia, thrombocytopenia, neuropathy, and nephropathy are infrequent reactions and are usually associated with high doses of parenteral penicillin.

Administration and Dosage: The dosage of V-Cillin K® (penicillin V potassium, Lilly) should be determined according to the sensitivity of the causative microorganism and the severity of infection and should be adjusted to the clinical response of the patient.

The usual dosage recommendations for adults and children 12 years and over are as follows:

Streptococcal Infections—Mild to moderately severe infections of the upper respiratory tract, including scarlet fever and mild erysipelas: 200,000 to 500,000 units every six to eight hours for ten days.

Pneumococcal Infections—Mild to moderately severe infections of the respiratory tract, including otitis media: 400,000 to 500,000 units every six hours until the patient has been afebrile for at least two days.

Staphylococcal Infections—Mild infections of skin and soft tissue (culture and susceptibility tests should be performed): 400,000 to 500,000 units every six to eight hours.

Fusospirochetosis (Vincent's Infection) of the Oropharynx—Mild to moderately severe infections: 400,000 to 500,000 units every six to eight hours.

Prophylaxis in the Following Conditions—To prevent recurrence following rheumatic fever and/or chorea: 200,000 to 250,000 units twice daily on a continuing basis.

To prevent bacterial endocarditis in patients with rheumatic or congenital heart lesions who are to undergo dental or upper respiratory tract surgery or instrumentation: 500,000 units given the day of the procedure, 500,000 units of aqueous penicillin G intramuscularly one hour before the procedure, and 500,000 units every six hours for two days.

NOTE: Therapy for children under 12 years of age is calculated on the basis of body weight. For infants and small children, the suggested daily dose is 25,000 to 90,000 units (15 to 50 mg) per kg in three to six divided doses.

How Supplied: (℞) *For Oral Solution, V-Cillin K® (Penicillin V Potassium for Oral Solution, USP): M-126, W07,** 125 mg (200,000 units) (equivalent to penicillin V) per 5 ml of solution, in 40, 100, 150, and 200-ml-size packages and in unit-dose bottles of 100 (IDI00); *M-142, W16,** 250 mg (400,000 units) (equivalent to penicillin V) per 5 ml of solution, in 100, 150, and 200-ml-size packages and in unit-dose bottles of 100 (ID100).

Each package consists of a bottle containing penicillin V potassium equivalent to penicillin V in a dry, pleasantly flavored mixture, buffered with sodium citrate and citric acid.

After being mixed, the solution should be stored in a refrigerator. It may be kept for 14 days without significant loss of potency. *Shake well before using. Keep tightly closed.*

(℞) *Tablets V-Cillin K® (Penicillin V Potassium Tablets, USP),* Specially Coated: *No. 1830, C27,** 125 mg (200,000 units) (equivalent to penicillin V), in bottles of 50 and 100 and in 10 strips of 10 individually labeled blisters each containing 1 tablet (ID100); *No. 1831, C29,** 250 mg (400,000 units) (equivalent to penicillin V), and *No. 1832, C46,** 500 mg (800,000 units) (equivalent to penicillin V), in bottles of 24, 100, and 500 and in 10 strips of 10 individually labeled blisters each containing 1 tablet (ID100). [041879]

[*Shown in Product Identification Section*]

VELBAN® ℞

(vinblastine sulfate)
Sterile, USP

Description: Velban® (Vinblastine Sulfate, USP, Lilly) is the salt of an alkaloid extracted from *Vinca rosea* Linn., a common flowering herb known as the periwinkle (more properly known as *Catharanthus roseus* G. Don). Previously, the generic name was vincaleukoblastine, abbreviated VLB.

Chemical and physical evidence indicates that Velban has the empirical formula $C_{46}H_{58}O_9N_4 \cdot H_2SO_4$ and that it is a dimeric alkaloid containing both indole and dihydroindole moieties.

Vials of Velban contain 10 mg of vinblastine sulfate, in the form of a lyophilized plug, without excipients. When sodium chloride solution is added prior to injection, the pH of the resulting solution lies in the range of 3.5 to 5.

Actions: Velban® (vinblastine sulfate, Lilly) has been used for the palliative treatment of a variety of malignant neoplastic conditions. In susceptible clinical cases, Velban has produced temporary reduction in the size or temporary disappearance of some tumors. It has relieved pain and other symptoms and allowed some patients to regain appetite and weight.

Experimental data indicate that the action of Velban is different from that of other recognized antineoplastic agents. Tissue-culture studies suggest an interference with metabolic pathways of amino acids leading from glutamic acid to the citric acid cycle and to urea. In vivo experiments tend to confirm the in vitro results. A number of studies in vitro and in vivo have demonstrated that Velban produces a stathmokinetic effect and various atypical mitotic figures. The therapeutic responses, however, are not fully explained by the cytologic changes, since these changes are sometimes observed clinically and experimentally in the absence of any oncolytic effects.

Reversal of the antitumor effect of Velban by glutamic acid or tryptophan has been observed. In addition, glutamic acid and aspartic acid have protected mice from lethal doses of Velban. Aspartic acid was relatively ineffective in reversing the antitumor effect.

Other studies indicate that Velban has an effect on cell-energy production required for mitosis and interferes with nucleic acid synthesis.

Hematologic Effects—Clinically, leukopenia is an expected effect of Velban® (vinblastine sulfate, Lilly), and the level of the leukocyte count is an important guide to therapy with this drug. In general, the larger the dose employed, the more profound and longer lasting the leukopenia will be. The fact that the white-blood-cell count returns to normal levels after drug-induced leukopenia is an indication that the white-cell-producing mechanism is not permanently depressed. Usually, the white count has completely returned to normal after the virtual disappearance of white cells from the peripheral blood.

Following therapy with Velban, the nadir in white-blood-cell count may be expected to occur five to ten days after the last day of drug administration. Recovery of the white blood count is fairly rapid thereafter and is usually complete within another seven to 14 days. With the smaller doses employed for maintenance therapy, leukopenia may not be a problem.

Although the thrombocyte count ordinarily is not significantly lowered by therapy with Velban, patients whose bone marrow has been recently impaired by prior therapy with radiation or with other oncolytic drugs may show thrombocytopenia (less than 200,000 platelets per cu mm). When other chemotherapy or radiation has not been employed previously, thrombocyte reduction below the level of 200,000/cu mm is rarely encountered, even when Velban may be causing significant leukopenia. Rapid recovery from thrombocytopenia within a few days is the rule.

The effect of Velban upon the red-cell count and hemoglobin is usually insignificant when other therapy does not complicate the picture. It should be remembered, however, that patients with malignant disease may exhibit anemia even in the absence of any therapy.

Indications: Vinblastine sulfate is indicated in the palliative treatment of the following:

Continued on next page

*Identi-Code® symbol.

Lilly—Cont.

I. *Frequently Responsive Malignancies—*
Generalized Hodgkin's disease (Stages III and IV, Ann Arbor modification of Rye staging system)
Lymphocytic lymphoma (nodular and diffuse, poorly and well differentiated)
Histiocytic lymphoma
Mycosis fungoides (advanced stages)
Advanced carcinoma of the testis
Kaposi's sarcoma
Letterer-Siwe disease (histiocytosis X)

II. *Less Frequently Responsive Malignancies—*
Choriocarcinoma resistant to other chemotherapeutic agents
Carcinoma of the breast, unresponsive to appropriate endocrine surgery and hormonal therapy

Current principles of chemotherapy for many types of cancer include the concurrent administration of several antineoplastic agents. For enhanced therapeutic effect without additive toxicity, agents with different dose-limiting clinical toxicities and different mechanisms of action are generally selected. Therefore, although Velban® (vinblastine sulfate, Lilly) is effective as a single agent in the aforementioned indications, it is usually administered in combination with other antineoplastic drugs. Such combination therapy produces a greater percentage of response than does a single-agent regimen. These principles have been applied, for example, in the chemotherapy of Hodgkin's disease.

*Hodgkin's Disease—*Velban has been shown to be one of the most effective single agents for the treatment of Hodgkin's disease. Advanced Hodgkin's disease has also been successfully treated with several multiple-drug regimens that included Velban. Patients who had relapses after treatment with the MOPP program—mechlorethamine hydrochloride (nitrogen mustard), vincristine sulfate (Oncovin® [vincristine sulfate, Lilly]), prednisone, and procarbazine—have likewise responded to combination-drug therapy that included Velban. A protocol using cyclophosphamide in place of nitrogen mustard and Velban instead of Oncovin is an alternative therapy for previously untreated patients with advanced Hodgkin's disease.

Advanced testicular germinal-cell cancers (embryonal carcinoma, teratocarcinoma, and choriocarcinoma) are sensitive to Velban alone, but better clinical results are achieved when Velban is administered concomitantly with other antineoplastic agents. The effect of bleomycin is significantly enhanced if Velban is administered six to eight hours prior to the administration of bleomycin; this schedule permits more cells to be arrested during metaphase, the stage of the cell cycle in which bleomycin is active.

Contraindications: Velban® (vinblastine sulfate, Lilly) is contraindicated in patients who are leukopenic. It should not be used in the presence of bacterial infection. Such infections must be brought under control with antiseptics or antibiotics prior to the initiation of therapy with Velban.

Warnings: *Usage in Pregnancy—*Caution is necessary with the administration of all oncolytic drugs during pregnancy. Information on the use of Velban® (vinblastine sulfate, Lilly) during pregnancy is very limited. Although no abnormalities of the human fetus have been reported thus far, animal studies with Velban suggest that teratogenic effects may occur.

Aspermia has been reported in man. Animal studies show metaphase arrest and degenerative changes in germ cells.

Precautions: If leukopenia with less than 2000 white blood cells per cu mm occurs following a dose of Velban® (vinblastine sulfate, Lilly), the patient should be watched carefully for evidence of infection until the white-blood-cell count has returned to a safe level.

When cachexia or ulcerated areas of the skin surface are present, there may be a more profound leukopenic response to the drug; therefore, its use should be avoided in older persons suffering from either of these conditions.

In patients with malignant-cell infiltration of the bone marrow, the leukocyte and platelet counts have sometimes fallen precipitously after moderate doses of Velban. Further use of the drug in such patients is inadvisable.

The use of small amounts of Velban daily for long periods is not advised, even though the resulting total weekly dosage may be similar to that recommended. Little or no added therapeutic effect has been demonstrated when such regimens have been used. *Strict adherence to the recommended dosage schedule is very important.* When amounts equal to several times the recommended weekly dosage were given in seven daily installments for long periods, convulsions, severe and permanent central-nervous-system damage, and even death occurred.

Care must be taken to avoid contamination of the eye with concentrations of Velban used clinically. If accidental contamination occurs, severe irritation (or, if the drug was delivered under pressure, even corneal ulceration) may result. The eye should be washed with water immediately and thoroughly.

Adverse Reactions: *Prior to the use of the drug, patients should be advised of the possibility of untoward symptoms.*

In general, the incidence of adverse reactions attending the use of Velban® (vinblastine sulfate, Lilly) appears to be related to the size of the dose employed. With the exception of epilation, leukopenia, and neurologic side effects adverse reactions generally have not persisted for longer than 24 hours. Neurologic side effects are not common; but when they do occur, they often last for more than 24 hours. Leukopenia, the most common adverse reaction, is usually the dose-limiting factor.

The following are manifestations which have been reported as adverse reactions:

*Gastrointestinal—*Nausea, vomiting, constipation, vesiculation of the mouth, ileus, diarrhea, anorexia, abdominal pain, rectal bleeding, pharyngitis, hemorrhagic enterocolitis, bleeding from an old peptic ulcer

*Neurologic—*Numbness, paresthesias, peripheral neuritis, mental depression, loss of deep-tendon reflexes, headache, convulsions

*Miscellaneous—*Malaise, weakness, dizziness, pain in tumor site, vesiculation of the skin

Nausea and vomiting usually may be controlled with ease by antiemetic agents. When epilation develops, it frequently is not total; and, in some cases, hair regrows while maintenance therapy continues.

Extravasation during intravenous injection may lead to cellulitis and phlebitis. If the amount of extravasation is great, sloughing may occur.

Administration and Dosage: There are variations in the depth of the leukopenic response which follows therapy with Velban® (vinblastine sulfate, Lilly). For this reason, it is recommended that the drug be given no more frequently than *once every seven days.* It is wise to initiate therapy for adults by administering a single intravenous dose of 3.7 mg/m² of body surface area (bsa). Thereafter, white-blood-cell counts should be made to determine the patient's sensitivity to Velban.

A simplified and conservative incremental approach to dosage *at weekly intervals* may be outlined as follows:

	Adults	Children
First dose	3.7 mg/m² bsa	2.5 mg/m² bsa
Second dose	5.5 mg/m² bsa	3.75 mg/m² bsa
Third dose	7.4 mg/m² bsa	5.0 mg/m² bsa
Fourth dose	9.25 mg/m² bsa	6.25 mg/m² bsa
Fifth dose	11.1 mg/m² bsa	7.5 mg/m² bsa

The above-mentioned increases may be used until a maximum dose (not exceeding 18.5 mg/m² bsa for adults and 12.5 mg/m² bsa for children) is reached. The dose should not be increased after that dose which reduces the white-cell count to approximately 3000 cells/cu mm. In some adults, 3.7 mg/m² bsa may produce this leukopenia; other adults may require more than 11.1 mg/m² bsa; and, very rarely, as much as 18.5 mg/m² bsa may be necessary. For most adult patients, however, the weekly dosage will prove to be 5.5 to 7.4 mg/m² bsa.

When the dose of Velban which will produce the above degree of leukopenia has been established, a dose *one increment smaller* than this should be administered at weekly intervals for maintenance. Thus, the patient is receiving the maximum dose that does not cause leukopenia. *It should be emphasized that, even though seven days have elapsed, the next dose of Velban should not be given until the white-cell count has returned to at least 4000/cu mm.* In some cases, oncolytic activity may be encountered before leukopenic effect. When this occurs, there is no need to increase the size of subsequent doses.

The duration of maintenance therapy varies according to the disease being treated and the combination of antineoplastic agents being used. There are differences of opinion regarding the duration of maintenance therapy with the same protocol for a particular disease; for example, various durations have been used with the MOPP program in treating Hodgkin's disease. Prolonged chemotherapy for maintaining remissions involves several risks, among which are life-threatening infectious diseases, sterility, and possibly the appearance of other cancers through suppression of immune surveillance. In some disorders, survival following complete remission may not be as prolonged as that achieved with shorter periods of maintenance therapy. On the other hand, failure to provide maintenance therapy in some patients may lead to unnecessary relapse; complete remissions in patients with testicular cancer, unless maintained for at least two years, often result in early relapse.

To prepare a solution containing 1 mg of Velban per ml, add 10 ml of Sodium Chloride Injection (preserved with phenol or benzyl alcohol) to the 10 mg of Velban in the sterile vial. Other solutions are not recommended. The drug dissolves instantly to give a clear solution. After a solution has been made in this way and a portion of it has been removed from a vial, the remainder of the vial's contents may be stored in a refrigerator for future use for 30 days without significant loss of potency.

The dose of Velban (calculated to provide the desired amount) may be injected either into the tubing of a running intravenous infusion or directly into a vein. The latter procedure is readily adaptable to outpatient therapy. In either case, the injection may be completed in about one minute. If care is taken to insure that the needle is securely within the vein and that no solution containing Velban is spilled extravascularly, cellulitis and/or phlebitis will not occur. To minimize further the possibility of extravascular spillage, it is suggested that the syringe and needle be rinsed with venous blood before withdrawal of the needle. The dose should not be diluted in large volumes of diluent (i.e., 100 to 250 ml) or given intravenously for prolonged periods (ranging from 30 to 60 minutes or more), since this frequently results in irritation of the vein and increases the chance of extravasation.

Because of the enhanced possibility of thrombosis, it is considered inadvisable to inject a solution of Velban into an extremity in which the circulation is impaired or potentially impaired by such conditions as compressing or invading neoplasm, phlebitis, or varicosity.

Caution—If leakage into surrounding tissue should occur during intravenous administration of Velban® (vinblastine sulfate, Lilly), it may cause considerable irritation. The injection should be discontinued immediately, and any remaining portion of the dose should then be introduced into another vein. Local injection of hyaluronidase and the application of moderate heat to the area of leakage help disperse the drug and are thought to minimize discomfort and the possibility of cellulitis.

How Supplied: (℞) *Ampoules (Vials) No. 687, Velban® (Sterile Vinblastine Sulfate, USP),* 10 mg, 10-ml size, rubber-stoppered (Dry Powder), in singles (10 per carton). *The vials should be stored in a refrigerator (2° to 8° C, or 36° to 46° F) to insure extended stability.* [100278]

ZENTINIC® OTC
(multifactor hematinic with vitamins)

Description: Zentinic is a multifactor hematinic-vitamin formula.

Each Pulvule® contains—

Iron, Elemental (as Ferrous Fumarate)	100 mg
Folic Acid	0.05 mg
Thiamine Mononitrate (Vitamin B_1)	7.5 mg
Riboflavin (Vitamin B_2)	7.5 mg
Pyridoxine Hydrochloride (Vitamin B_6)	7.5 mg
Vitamin B_{12} (Activity Equivalent)	50 mcg
Pantothenic Acid (as Calcium Pantothenate)	15 mg
Niacinamide	30 mg
Ascorbic Acid (Vitamin C)	200 mg

Indications: For the prevention of iron-deficiency anemia and certain nutritional anemias and vitamin deficiencies of the B complex.

Contraindications: Hemochromatosis and hemosiderosis are contraindications to iron therapy.

Precautions: Anemia is a manifestation that requires appropriate investigation to determine its cause. The ingredients in Zentinic are not sufficient nor are they intended for the treatment of pernicious anemia. The use of folic acid without adequate vitamin B_{12} therapy in patients with pernicious anemia may result in hematologic remission but neurologic progression. Adequate doses of vitamin B_{12} usually prevent, halt, or improve the neurologic changes.

Adverse Reactions: Iron in therapeutic doses may occasionally cause gastrointestinal disturbances, such as nausea, vomiting, diarrhea, or constipation.

Dosage: 1 or 2 Pulvules a day, or as directed by the physician.

Overdosage: *Symptoms*—Those of iron intoxication, which may include pallor and cyanosis, vomiting, hematemesis, diarrhea, melena, shock, drowsiness, and coma. *Treatment*—For specific therapy, exchange transfusion and chelating agents. For general management, gastric and rectal lavage with sodium bicarbonate solution or milk, administration of intravenous fluids and electrolytes, and use of oxygen.

How Supplied: *Pulvules No. 4, Zentinic® (multifactor hematinic with vitamins, Lilly), G19**(No. 0, Dark-Red), in bottles of 60 and 500. [022379]

ZENTRON® OTC
and
ZENTRON® CHEWABLE
(iron, vitamin B complex, and vitamin C)

Description: Zentron is a liquid hematinic especially formulated for geriatric and pediatric patients. Zentron restores hemoglobin in patients with iron-deficiency anemia. It provides iron with B complex vitamins and vitamin C. A bright-yellow liquid with a wild-strawberry flavor, Zentron is readily accepted whether administered by spoon or mixed with formula, water, or fruit juice.

Each 5 ml (approximately one teaspoonful) of the liquid contain—

Iron, Elemental (as Ferrous Sulfate)	20 mg
Thiamine Hydrochloride (Vitamin B_1)	1 mg
Riboflavin (Vitamin B_2)	1 mg
Pyridoxine Hydrochloride (Vitamin B_6)	1 mg
Cyanocobalamin (Vitamin B_{12} Crystalline)	5 mcg
Pantothenic Acid (as *d*-Panthenol)	1 mg
Niacinamide	5 mg
Ascorbic Acid (Vitamin C)	100 mg

Alcohol, 2 percent.

Zentron Chewable is a hematinic in chewable tablet form, especially formulated for pediatric patients. Zentron Chewable restores hemoglobin in patients with iron-deficiency anemia. It provides iron with B complex vitamins and vitamin C. A strawberry-flavored tablet, Zentron Chewable may be chewed, dissolved in the mouth, taken with liquid, or swallowed alone.

Each tablet contains—

Iron, Elemental (as Ferrous Fumarate)	20 mg
Thiamine Mononitrate (Vitamin B_1)	1 mg
Riboflavin (Vitamin B_2)	1 mg
Pyridoxine Hydrochloride (Vitamin B_6)	1 mg
Cyanocobalamin (Vitamin B_{12} Crystalline)	5 mcg
Pantothenic Acid (as Panthenol)	1 mg
Niacinamide	5 mg
Ascorbic Acid (Vitamin C)	100 mg

Indications: For the prevention and treatment of iron-deficiency anemia and the prevention of vitamin B complex and vitamin C deficiencies. Liquid Zentron is equally useful for pediatric and geriatric patients who may prefer liquid medication.

Contraindications: Hemochromatosis and hemosiderosis are contraindications to iron therapy.

Precaution: Like all medications, Zentron and Zentron Chewable should be kept out of the reach of children.

Adverse Reactions: Iron in therapeutic doses may occasionally cause gastrointestinal disturbances, such as nausea, vomiting, diarrhea, or constipation.

Dosage: *Zentron*—Infants and children, ½ to 1 teaspoonful one to three times daily, or as directed by the physician. Adults, 1 or 2 teaspoonfuls three times daily, or as directed by the physician.

Zentron Chewable—Children two years and older, 1 tablet one to three times a day, or as directed by the physician. Adults, 1 or 2 tablets three times a day, or as directed by the physician.

Overdosage: *See under* Zentinic®.

How Supplied: *Liquid No. 34, Zentron® (iron, vitamin B complex, and vitamin C, Lilly),* in 8-fl-oz bottles.

*Tablets No. 14, Zentron Chewable, T01,** Pink, in bottles of 50. [060178]

[Shown in Product Identification Section]

ZINC-INSULIN CRYSTALS, *see under* Iletin® (insulin, Lilly).

Products are cross-indexed by generic and chemical names in the

YELLOW SECTION

Lincoln Laboratories, Inc.
HICKORY POINT ROAD
DECATUR, IL 62526

TUBERCULIN MONO-VACC® TEST ℞
(old tuberculin)
Multiple Puncture Device

For complete product information, consult Diagnostic Product Information Section.

Loma Linda Foods
RIVERSIDE, CALIFORNIA 92515

I-SOYALAC Ⓚ PAREVE
Concentrated Liquid and Ready-to-Serve

(See PDR For Nonprescription Drugs)

SOYALAC Liquid Concentrate, Ⓚ PAREVE
Ready-to-Serve and Powder

(See PDR For Nonprescription Drugs)

M² Ethicals, Inc.
P.O. BOX 174
WEST CHICAGO, IL 60185

DIZYME

Description: An effective digestive aid in capsule form containing: Glutamic Acid HCl 5 gr., Betaine HCl 3 gr., Pepsin 1 gr., and Pancreatin Enzyme Concentrate, enteric coated, 167 mg. in a base of comfrey leaf.

Indications: A formula designed to aid digestion and problems of nausea, burning or excessive flatulence which may be due to poor diet or imbalances in intestinal integrity.

Administration: For use as a digestive aid, adults, orally, one capsule with each meal or as otherwise directed by a physician.

Precaution: Keep out of reach of children.

How Supplied: Bottles of 100.

MAGACIN

Composition: Each capsule contains Vit. C 240 mg., Niacinamide 150 mg., Magnesium 80 mg., Niacin 10 mg., and 1-Glutamic Acid 50 mg.

Action and Uses: Designed to aid nervousness and tension resulting from nutritional deficient causes; stressful circumstances; emotional factors; hyperactivity; learning disabilities; or alcoholism.

Administration and Dosage: One to three capsules daily or as directed by a physician.

Adverse Reactions: No niacin flushing report to date, but higher dosage could cause a mild, transient flushing or warmth in sensitive individuals.

How Supplied: Bottles of 100.

Literature: Product information and dietary suggestions.

IDENTIFICATION PROBLEM?

Consult PDR's

Product Identification Section

where you'll find over 900

products pictured actual size

and in full color.

Macsil, Inc.
"A" STREET & LEHIGH AVE.
PHILADELPHIA, PA 19125

BALMEX® BABY POWDER

(See PDR For Nonprescription Drugs)

BALMEX® EMOLLIENT LOTION

(See PDR For Nonprescription Drugs)

BALMEX® OINTMENT

(See PDR For Nonprescription Drugs)

Mallard Incorporated
3021 WABASH AVE.
DETROIT, MI 48216

ALLERSONE OINTMENT ℞

Composition:
Representing:
Hydrocortisone 0.5%
Diperodon Hydrochloride 0.5%
Zinc Oxide 5.0%
Indications: Antiinflammatory, antipruritic and antiallergic, in the treatment of atopic dermatitis, dermatitis venenata or contact dermatitis, pruritus ani and vulvae, certain allergic skin diseases, eczemata, as infantile and chronic eczema of ear, neurodermatitides, intertrigo as chafing of opposing skin of thighs, axilla and below breasts. When used rectally, it helps to relieve discomfort due to uncomplicated hemmorrhoids as well as itching or pain associated with proctitis and pruritis ani.
Action: Hydrocortisone exhibits marked anti-inflammatory activity and is of benefit in pruritic, allergic and atopic dermatitis. Diperodon Hydrochloride is a local anesthetic with little or negligible incidence of sensitivity. Zinc Oxide is well known for its mild astringent and protective actions.
Dosage and Administration: Distribute a small amount by gentle application over the affected area two or three times a day; frequency of application to be reduced with improvement.
Contraindications: Do not apply in the presence of herpes simplex of the eye or skin tuberculosis; in case there is a coexisting bacterial infection an antibacterial should be used concurrently.
Precautions: In rare instances local sensitivity reactions might occur. The safety of the use of topical steroid preparations during pregnancy has not been fully established. Therefore, they should not be used extensively on pregnant patients, in large amounts or for prolonged periods of time.
Advantages: Contains a local anesthetic which quickly ameliorates pain—while hydrocortisone reduces inflammation.
Caution: Federal law prohibits dispensing without prescription.
How Supplied: 0-90 Allersone, ointment in 15 gm. tubes and in pound jars.
Literature Available: Yes.

Products are cross-indexed by
generic and chemical names
in the
YELLOW SECTION

Marion Laboratories, Inc.
Pharmaceutical Division
MARION INDUSTRIAL PARK
10236 BUNKER RIDGE ROAD
KANSAS CITY, MO 64137

AMBENYL® EXPECTORANT Ⓒ ℞

Each 5 ml contains:

Codeine sulfate (Warning —May be habit-forming)	10 mg
Bromodiphenhydramine hydrochloride	3.75 mg
Diphenhydramine hydrochloride	8.75 mg
Ammonium chloride	80 mg
Potassium guaiacolsulfonate	80 mg
Menthol	0.5 mg
Alcohol, 5%	

Action: Ambenyl is a combination of two antihistaminic agents, along with well-recognized agents exhibiting expectorant and antitussive properties.
Diphenhydramine hydrochloride, in addition to being a potent antihistaminic agent, also possesses an antitussive action.

Indications: Ambenyl is indicated as an antitussive and expectorant for control of cough due to colds or allergy.
Based on a review of this drug by the National Academy of Sciences—National Research Council and/or other information, FDA has classified this indication as follows: There is a lack of substantial evidence that this fixed combination drug has the effect purported.
Final classification of the less-than-effective indication requires further investigation.

Contraindications: This preparation should not be used in premature or newborn infants.
Do not use in patients with:
Hypersensitivity to any of the components;
Asthmatic attack;
Narrow-angle glaucoma;
Prostatic hypertrophy;
Stenosing peptic ulcer;
Pyloroduodenal obstruction;
Bladder-neck obstruction.
Preparations containing bromodiphenhydramine hydrochloride and diphenhydramine hydrochloride should not be given to patients receiving monomamine oxidase inhibitors.
Warnings: Overdosage or accidental ingestion of large quantities of antihistamines may produce convulsions or death, especially in infants and children.
As in the case of other preparations containing central nervous system depressant drugs, patients receiving Ambenyl should be cautioned about probable additive effects with alcohol and other central nervous system depressants (hypnotics, sedatives, and tranquilizers).
Serious toxicity, including central nervous system and respiratory depression, and rarely death have been reported in pediatric patients receiving overdosages of codeine, either alone or in combination with other CNS depressants.
Patients who become drowsy on antihistamine-containing preparations should be cautioned against engaging in activities requiring mental alertness, such as driving a car or operating heavy machinery or appliances when taking Ambenyl.
Pregnancy Warning: Although there is no evidence that the use of Ambenyl is detrimental to the mother or fetus, the use of any drug in pregnancy or lactation should be carefully assessed.
Because of the anticholinergic effect of diphenhydramine hydrochloride, an inhibitory effect on lactation may occur.
Precautions: Bromodiphenhydramine and diphenhydramine have an atropine-like action which should be considered when prescribing Ambenyl. Use with caution in patients with a history of asthma.
Adverse Reactions: The following side effects may occur in patients taking Ambenyl: drowsiness; confusion; nervousness; restlessness; nausea; vomiting; diarrhea; blurring of vision; diplopia; difficulty in urination; constipation; nasal stuffiness; vertigo; palpitation; headache; insomnia; urticaria; drug rash; tightness of the chest and wheezing; thickening of bronchial secretions; dryness of mouth, nose, and throat; tingling, heaviness, weakness of hands; photosensitivity; hemolytic anemia; hypotension; epigastric distress.
Dosage and Administration—Adults—One or two teaspoonfuls every four to six hours, not to exceed 12 teaspoonfuls in 24 hours. Children (total intake of codeine sulfate should not exceed 1 mg/kg/24 hours)—Six to under 12 years of age—one-half to one teaspoonful every six hours; Two to under 6 years of age—one-quarter to one-half teaspoonful every six hours. Not to be used in children under two years of age.
How Supplied: Ambenyl Expectorant is supplied in 4-fl.-oz., 1-pt., and 1-gal. bottles.
[*Shown in Product Identification Section*]

DEBROX® Drops OTC

Description: Carbamide peroxide 6.5% in specially prepared anhydrous glycerol.
Actions: DEBROX® penetrates, softens and facilitates removal of earwax, without causing the wax to swell.
Upon direct contact with earwax, carbamide peroxide releases oxygen to form a dense foam which helps to break up wax accumulations. These actions result in a chemomechanical cleansing, debriding effect. Any remaining wax may be removed by flushing with warm water, using a soft rubber bulb ear syringe. Avoid excessive pressure.
Indications: DEBROX provides a safe, nonirritating method of removing earwax. Aids in the prevention of ceruminosis. Used regularly, DEBROX Drops helps keep the ear canal free from blockage due to accumulated earwax.
Caution: Consult physician if redness, irritation, swelling or pain persists or increases.
Dosage and Administration: Use directly from bottle. Tilt head sideways and squeeze bottle gently so that 5-10 drops flow into ear. Tip of bottle should not enter ear canal. Keep drops in ear for several minutes while head remains tilted or by inserting cotton. Repeat twice daily for at least 3-4 days or as directed by physician. Any remaining wax may be removed by flushing with warm water, using a soft rubber bulb ear syringe.
Avoid contact with eyes. Keep out of reach of children. Protect from heat and direct sunlight.
How Supplied: DEBROX Drops in ½- or 1-fl.-oz. plastic squeeze bottles with applicator spouts.
[*Shown in Product Identification Section*]

DIA-QUEL™ Liquid Ⓒ OTC
antidiarrheal

Description: Each teaspoonful (5 ml) contains:

Tincture of opium	0.03 ml*
Homatropine methylbromide	0.15 mg
Pectin	24 mg
Alcohol 10% by volume	

*Equivalent to 0.75 ml of paregoric
Contains opium 18 mg (approx. ¼ grain) per fl. oz. (WARNING: May be habit-forming)
Indications: Multi-action, rapid control of common (non-specific) diarrhea; relief of associated cramping, colicky pain, and nausea. Dia-Quel soothes and protects the intestinal tract.

Caution: Children under 6 years of age or elderly persons should use only as directed by physician. Diarrhea may be serious. If symptoms are unusually severe or accompanied by high fever, or if they persist more than 2 days, see a physician. Do not exceed recommended dosage. Not for frequent or prolonged use. If excessive dryness of the mouth occurs, decrease dosage. Discontinue use if rapid pulse, dizziness, or blurring of vision occurs. Individuals with glaucoma or excessive pressure within the eye, and elderly persons (where undiagnosed glaucoma or excessive pressure within the eye may be present) should use only as directed by physician. Persons with undiagnosed glaucoma may experience eye pain; if this occurs, discontinue use and see physician immediately.
Usual Adult Dosage: 1 or 2 tablespoonfuls 3 or 4 times daily.
Usual Dosage for Children Six Years or Older: 1 or 2 teaspoonfuls 3 or 4 times daily. For children under six years of age, consult physician.
How Supplied: 4 fl. oz. bottle.

DITROPAN® Tablets ℞
(oxybutynin chloride) 5 mg

Description: Each biconvex, embossed blue DITROPAN® Tablet contains 5 mg of oxybutynin chloride. Chemically, oxybutynin chloride is the *dl*-(racemic) form of 4-diethylamino-2-butynyl-phenylcyclohexylglycolate hydrochloride. The empirical formula for oxybutynin chloride is $C_{22}H_{32}ClNO_3$.
Oxybutynin chloride is a white, crystalline solid with a molecular weight of 393.9. It is readily soluble in water and acids, but relatively insoluble in alkalis.
Action: DITROPAN® (oxybutynin chloride) exerts direct antispasmodic effect on smooth muscle and inhibits the muscarinic action of acetylcholine on smooth muscle. DITROPAN exhibits only one-fifth of the anticholinergic activity of atropine on the rabbit detrusor muscle, but four to ten times the antispasmodic activity. No blocking effects occur at skeletal neuromuscular junctions or autonomic ganglia (antinicotinic effects).
In patients with uninhibited neurogenic and reflex neurogenic bladder, cystometric studies have demonstrated that DITROPAN increases vesical capacity, diminishes the frequency of uninhibited contractions of the detrusor muscle and delays the initial desire to void. These effects are more consistently improved in patients with uninhibited neurogenic bladder.
DITROPAN was well tolerated in patients administered the drug in controlled studies of 30 days duration and in uncontrolled studies in which some of the patients received the drug for two years.
Indications: DITROPAN® (oxybutynin chloride) is indicated for the relief of symptoms associated with voiding in patients with uninhibited neurogenic and reflex neurogenic bladder.
Pre-treatment examination should include cystometry and other appropriate diagnostic procedures.
Cystometry should be repeated at appropriate intervals to evaluate response to therapy. The appropriate antimicrobial therapy should be instituted in the presence of infection.
Contraindications: DITROPAN® (oxybutynin chloride) is contraindicated in patients with glaucoma. It is also contraindicated in partial or complete obstruction of the gastrointestinal tract, paralytic ileus, intestinal atony of the elderly or debilitated patient, megacolon, toxic megacolon complicating ulcerative colitis, severe colitis and myasthenia gravis. It is contraindicated in patients with obstructive uropathy and in patients with unstable cardiovascular status in acute hemorrhage.
Warnings: DITROPAN® (oxybutynin chloride), when administered in the presence of high environmental temperature, can cause heat prostration (fever and heat stroke due to decreased sweating).
Diarrhea may be an early symptom of incomplete intestinal obstruction, especially in patients with ileostomy or colostomy. In this instance, treatment with DITROPAN would be inappropriate and possibly harmful.
DITROPAN may produce drowsiness or blurred vision. The patient should be cautioned regarding activities requiring mental alertness such as operating a motor vehicle or other machinery or performing hazardous work while taking this drug.
Pregnancy: Reproduction studies in the hamster, rabbit, rat and mouse have shown no definite evidence of impaired fertility or harm to the animal fetus. The safety of DITROPAN administered to women who are or who may become pregnant has not been established. Therefore, DITROPAN should not be given to pregnant women unless, in the judgement of the physician, the probable clinical benefits outweigh the possible hazards.
Usage in Children: The safety and efficacy of DITROPAN administration has been demonstrated for children five years of age and older (see "Dosage and Administration"). However, as there is insufficient clinical data for children under age five, DITROPAN is not recommended for this age group.
Precautions: DITROPAN® (oxybutynin chloride) should be used with caution in the elderly and in all patients with autonomic neuropathy, hepatic or renal disease. Administration of DITROPAN in large doses to patients with ulcerative colitis may suppress intestinal motility to the point of producing a paralytic ileus and precipitate or aggravate "toxic megacolon," a serious complication of the disease.
The symptoms of hyperthyroidism, coronary heart disease, congestive heart failure, cardiac arrhythmias, tachycardia, hypertension and prostatic hypertrophy may be aggravated following administration of DITROPAN. DITROPAN should be administered with caution to patients with hiatal hernia associated with reflux esophagitis, since anticholinergic drugs may aggravate this condition.
Adverse Reactions: Following administration of DITROPAN® (oxybutynin chloride), the symptoms that can be associated with the use of other anticholinergic drugs may occur: dry mouth, decreased sweating, urinary hesitance and retention, blurred vision, tachycardia, palpitations, dilatation of the pupil, cycloplegia, increased ocular tension, drowsiness, weakness, dizziness, insomnia, nausea, vomiting, constipation, bloated feeling, impotence, suppression of lactation, severe allergic reactions or drug idiosyncrasies including urticaria and other dermal manifestations.
Dosage and Administration:
Adults: The usual dose is one 5 mg tablet two to three times a day. The maximum recommended dose is one 5 mg tablet four times a day.
Children over 5 years of age: The usual dose is one 5 mg tablet two times a day.
The maximal recommended dose is one 5 mg tablet three times a day.
Overdosage: The symptoms of overdosage with DITROPAN® (oxybutynin chloride) progress from an intensification of the usual side effects of CNS disturbances (from restlessness and excitement to psychotic behavior), circulatory changes (flushing, fall in blood pressure, circulatory failure), respiratory failure, paralysis and coma.
Measures to be taken are (1) immediate lavage of the stomach and (2) injection of physostigmine 0.5 to 2 mg intravenously, and repeated as necessary up to a total of 5 mg. Fever may be treated symptomatically (alcohol sponging, ice packs). Excitement of a degree which demands attention may be managed with sodium thiopental 2% solution given slowly intravenously or chloral hydrate (100-200 ml of a 2% solution) by rectal infusion. In the event of progression of the curare-like effect to paralysis of the respiratory muscles, artificial respiration is required.
How Supplied: DITROPAN® (oxybutynin chloride) is supplied in bottles of 100 and 1000 tablets and in Unit Dose Identification Paks of 500 tablets. Blue tablets are embossed with Marion/1375.
[Shown in Product Identification Section]

DUOTRATE® and DUOTRATE® 45 ℞
Plateau CAPS®
(pentaerythritol tetranitrate)

Each sustained release capsule contains:
DUOTRATE® (pentaerythritol tetranitrate) ....30 mg.
White pellets in a black and clear capsule imprinted with MARION/1525.
DUOTRATE® 45 (pentaerythritol tetranitrate) ....45 mg.
White pellets in a black and light blue capsule imprinted with MARION/1530.
DUOTRATE® and DUOTRATE® 45 (pentaerythritol tetranitrate) are 2, 2-bishydroxymethyl-1, 3-propanediol tetranitrate.
Action: The mechanism of action in the relief of angina pectoris is unknown at this time, although the basic pharmacologic action is to relax smooth muscle. The effect of pentaerythritol tetranitrate is usually measured by its ability to reduce the frequency, duration and severity of anginal attacks and reduce the need for sublingual nitroglycerin.

> **Indications:**
> Based on a review of this drug by the National Academy of Sciences—National Research Council and/or other information, FDA has classified the indications as follows:
> Possibly effective:
> For the management, prophylaxis or treatment of anginal attacks.
> Final classification of the less-than-effective indications requires further investigation.

Contraindication: Idiosyncrasy to this drug.
Warnings: Data supporting the use of DUOTRATE® and DUOTRATE® 45 (pentaerythritol tetranitrate) during the early days of the acute phase of myocardial infarction (the period during which clinical and laboratory findings are unstable) are insufficient to establish safety.
Precautions: Intraocular pressure is increased; therefore, caution is required in administering to patients with glaucoma. Tolerance to this drug and cross-tolerance to other nitrites and nitrates may occur.
Adverse Reactions: Cutaneous vasodilation with flushing. Headache is common and may be severe and persistent. Transient episodes of dizziness and weakness, as well as other signs of cerebral ischemia associated with postural hypotension, may occasionally develop. This drug can act as a physiological antagonist to norepinephrine, acetylcholine, histamine, and many other agents. An occasional individual exhibits marked sensitivity to the hypotensive effects of nitrite and severe responses (nausea, vomiting, weakness, restlessness, pallor, perspiration and collapse) can occur, even with the usual therapeutic dose. Alcohol may enhance this effect. Drug rash and/or exfoliative dermatitis may occasionally occur.
Dosage and Administration: One capsule every 12 hours on an empty stomach. One capsule should be taken with an adequate amount of water before breakfast, and a second capsule approximately 12 hours later on an empty stomach. When medication is started, there is a delay from one to two hours before a signifi-

Continued on next page

Marion—Cont.

cant change in pain level occurs. The selection of DUOTRATE® should be based on the patient's need for approximately 30 mg of pentaerythritol tetranitrate during a twelve-hour period. The selection of DUOTRATE® 45 should be based on the patient's need for approximately 45 mg of pentaerythritol tetranitrate during a twelve-hour period. Use the smallest dose that proves effective.
How Supplied: Each of the products described is available in bottles of 100.
Caution: Federal law prohibits dispensing without a prescription.
[Shown in Product Identification Section]

GAVISCON® Antacid Tablets OTC

Composition: Each chewable tablet contains the following active ingredients:
Aluminum hydroxide dried gel ....80 mg
Magnesium trisilicate ....20 mg
and the following inactive ingredients: sucrose, alginic acid, sodium bicarbonate, starch, calcium stearate and flavoring.
Actions: Unique formulation produces soothing foam which floats on stomach contents. Foam containing antacid precedes stomach contents into the esophagus when reflux occurs to help protect the sensitive mucosa from further irritation. GAVISCON acts locally without neutralizing entire stomach contents to help maintain integrity of the digestive process. Endoscopic studies indicate that GAVISCON Antacid Tablets are equally as effective in the erect or supine patient.
Indications: For temporary relief of heartburn, sour stomach, and/or acid indigestion.
Directions: Chew two to four tablets four times a day or as directed by a physician. Tablets should be taken after meals and at bedtime or as needed. For best results follow by a half glass of water or other liquid. DO NOT SWALLOW WHOLE.
Warnings: Except under the advice and supervision of a physician: do not take more than 16 tablets in a 24-hour period or 16 tablets daily for more than 2 weeks; do not use this product if you are on a sodium restricted diet. Each GAVISCON Tablet contains approximately 0.8 mEq. sodium.
Drug Interaction Precautions: Do not take this product if you are presently taking a prescription antibiotic drug containing any form of tetracycline.
STORE AT A CONTROLLED ROOM TEMPERATURE IN A DRY PLACE.
KEEP THIS AND ALL DRUGS OUT OF THE REACH OF CHILDREN. In case of accidental overdose, seek professional assistance or contact a poison control center immediately.
How Supplied: Available in bottle of 100 tablets and in foil-wrapped 2's in box of 30 tablets.
[Shown in Product Identification Section]

GAVISCON® Liquid Antacid OTC

Each tablespoonful (15 ml) contains the following active ingredients:
Aluminum hydroxide dried gel ....160 mg
Magnesium trisilicate .... 40 mg
and the following inactive ingredients: water, sorbitol, glycerin, sodium alginate, sodium bicarbonate, flavoring, xanthan gum, disodium edetate, colors, and methylparaben and propylparaben as preservatives.
Indications: For temporary relief of heartburn, sour stomach, and/or acid indigestion.
Directions: Shake well before using. Take one to two tablespoonfuls four times a day or as directed by a physician. GAVISCON Liquid should be taken after meals and at bedtime, followed by a half glass of water.
Warnings: Except under the advice and supervision of a physician: do not take more than eight tablespoonfuls in a 24-hour period or eight tablespoonfuls daily for more than two weeks; do not use this product if you are on a sodium restricted diet. Each tablespoonful of GAVISCON Liquid contains approximately 3.5 mEq. sodium.
Drug Interaction Precautions: Do not take this product if you are presently taking a prescription antibiotic drug containing any form of tetracycline.
KEEP TIGHTLY CLOSED.
STORE AT A CONTROLLED ROOM TEMPERATURE.
AVOID FREEZING.
KEEP THIS AND ALL DRUGS OUT OF THE REACH OF CHILDREN. In case of accidental overdose, seek professional assistance or contact a poison control center immediately.
How Supplied: 12 fluid ounces (355 ml)
[Shown in Product Identification Section]

GAVISCON®-2 Antacid Tablets OTC

Each chewable tablet contains the following active ingredients:
Aluminum hydroxide dried gel ....160 mg
Magnesium trisilicate .... 40 mg
and the following inactive ingredients: sucrose, alginic acid, sodium bicarbonate, starch, calcium stearate and flavoring.
Indications: For temporary relief of heartburn, sour stomach, and/or acid indigestion.
Directions: Chew one to two tablets four times a day or as directed by a physician. Tablets should be taken after meals and at bedtime or as needed. For best results follow by a half glass of water or other liquid. DO NOT SWALLOW WHOLE.
Warnings: Except under the advice and supervision of a physician: do not take more than 8 tablets in a 24-hour period or 8 tablets daily for more than 2 weeks; do not use this product if you are on a sodium restricted diet. Each GAVISCON-2 Tablet contains approximately 1.6 mEq. sodium.
Drug Interaction Precautions: Do not take this product if you are presently taking a prescription antibiotic drug containing any form of tetracycline.
STORE AT A CONTROLLED ROOM TEMPERATURE IN A DRY PLACE.
KEEP THIS AND ALL DRUGS OUT OF THE REACH OF CHILDREN. In case of accidental overdose, seek professional assistance or contact a poison control center immediately.
How Supplied: Box of 48 foil-wrapped tablets.
[Shown in Product Identification Section]

GLY-OXIDE® Liquid OTC

Description: Carbamide peroxide 10% in specially prepared anhydrous glycerol. Artificial flavor added. Not NF—pH differs from NF specifications.
Actions: GLY-OXIDE® is a safe, stabilized oxygenating agent. Specifically formulated for topical oral administration, it provides unique chemomechanical cleansing and debriding action, which allows normal healing to occur.
Indications: Local treatment and hygienic prevention (as an aid to professional care) of minor oral inflammation such as canker sores, denture irritation and post-dental procedure irritation. GLY-OXIDE Liquid provides effective aid to oral hygiene when normal cleansing measures are inadequate or impossible (e.g., total-care geriatric patients). As an adjunct to oral hygiene (orthodontics, dental appliances) after regular brushing.
Precautions: Severe or persistent oral inflammation or denture irritation may be serious. If these or unexpected effects occur, consult physician or dentist promptly.
Dosage and Administration: DO NOT DILUTE—use directly from the bottle. Apply 4 times daily after meals and at bedtime, or as directed by a dentist or physician. Place several drops on affected area; expectorate after 2-3 minutes, or place 10 drops onto tongue, mix with saliva, swish for several minutes, expectorate. Do not rinse. Foams on contact with saliva.
Avoid contact with eyes. Protect from heat and direct sunlight. Keep out of reach of children.
How Supplied: GLY-OXIDE Liquid in ½-fl.-oz. and 2-fl.-oz. non-spill plastic squeeze bottles with applicator spouts.
[Shown in Product Identification Section]

METASEP® MEDICATED SHAMPOO CONCENTRATE OTC

Avoids drying hair. Will not discolor gray, blond or bleached hair.
Active Ingredient: Parachlorometaxylenol 2%.
Other Ingredients: Isopropyl alcohol NF 9%, sodium lauryl sulfate, water, lauramide DEA, laneth-10 acetate, citric acid USP, fragrance.
Indications: Use as an aid in relief of dandruff and associated conditions.
Directions: Wet hair thoroughly. Apply METASEP® Medicated Shampoo and massage to foamy lather. Allow lather to remain five minutes. Rinse hair thoroughly and repeat.
Caution: Avoid contact with eyes.
How Supplied: 4-fluid-ounce bottle.
Keep out of reach of children.

NAPRIL® Plateau CAPS® ℞

Composition: Each sustained release capsule contains:
Phenylpropanolamine HCl.....................25 mg.
Pyrilamine Maleate.................................25 mg.
Chlorpheniramine Maleate .... 4 mg.
Each in a special base to provide activity for 10 to 12 hours.
Phenylephrine HCl..................................15 mg.
Prepared for immediate release.
Actions and Uses: Napril provides the immediate release of the rapid acting sympathomimetic agent phenylephrine hydrochloride for rapid relief of nasal congestion, plus the sustained action of a second sympathomimetic agent phenylpropanolamine hydrochloride to continue the decongestant activity for 10 to 12 hours. Two antihistamines, pyrilamine maleate and chlorpheniramine maleate in sustained action form, reduce sneezing, rhinorrhea, and itching of the eyes.
Napril is recommended for prompt and prolonged relief of sinus and nasal congestion, associated with coryza, rhinorrhea, and allergic manifestations.
Precautions: The patient should be advised not to drive a car or operate dangerous machinery if he feels drowsy. Use only with caution in patients with hypertension, heart disease, diabetes, or thyrotoxicosis.
Adverse Reactions: In susceptible patients or in extreme overdose, drowsiness, nervousness, or rapid pulse may occur.
Administration and Dosage: For all patients 12 years and older, one capsule every morning and evening.
How Supplied: Napril Capsules are available in bottles of 50 capsules.
Caution: Federal law prohibits dispensing without prescription.

NICO-400® Plateau CAPS® ℞
(nicotinic acid) 400 mg

Description: Each capsule of timed-release pellets contains 400 mg of nicotinic acid.
Actions: The most prominent pharmacodynamic action of nicotinic acid is a direct effect on blood vessels. By relaxing the musculature of peripheral vessels, it produces vasodilatation. The effects of this drug are both prompt and prolonged. A portion of the pellets is released immediately and the initial effects are

observed within the hour. The remaining pellets release the nicotinic acid over time, providing a long-acting effect.
Indications: NICO-400® is recommended for all disease states in which nicotinic acid has been used. These include conditions associated with deficient circulation and for use in the correction of nicotinic acid deficiencies. Because NICO-400® releases slowly, it minimizes flushing, pruritus, gastrointestinal irritation, and permits adequate dosage with maximum patient cooperation.
Contraindications: Those individuals who have shown a hypersensitivity to nicotinic acid. Because of the vasodilatation produced by nicotinic acid, severe hypotension and hemorrhaging are obvious contraindications to nicotinic acid therapy.
Warnings: Use with caution in patients with a history of peptic ulcer, severe diabetes, and impaired gall bladder or liver functions.
Usage in Pregnancy: As with all therapeutic agents, use with caution in pregnant patients.
Precautions: Large oral doses of nicotinic acid may be accompanied by some impairment of hepatic function, including an abnormal glucose tolerance curve.
Adverse Reactions: Patients should be informed of the short-lived reactions experienced with nicotinic acid therapy: cutaneous flushing, a sensation of warmth, tingling and itching of the skin, increased gastrointestinal motility, and sebaceous gland activity. These reactions are coincidental to the vasodilatation produced by nicotinic acid. It is suggested that these reactions be regarded as desirable, being a physiological sign that the nicotinic acid is carrying out its intended function.
Dosage and Administration: One capsule every 12 hours or as directed by physician.
How Supplied: NICO-400® Plateau CAPS® are available in bottles of 100 capsules. Capsules are imprinted with Marion/1575.
Caution: Federal law prohibits dispensing without prescription.
[*Shown in Product Identification Section*]

NITRO-BID® Plateau CAPS® ℞
(nitroglycerin) 2.5 mg, 6.5 mg and 9 mg

Description: Each NITRO-BID® Controlled-Release Capsule contains:
2.5 mg nitroglycerin: Light purple and clear capsule with white beads; identification imprint MARION/1550.
6.5 mg nitroglycerin: Dark blue and yellow capsule with white beads; identification imprint MARION/1551.
9 mg nitroglycerin: Green and yellow capsule with white beads; identification imprint MARION/1553.
Action: The mechanism of action of nitroglycerin in the relief of angina pectoris is not as yet known. However, its main pharmacologic action is to relax smooth muscle, principally in the smaller blood vessels, thus dilating arterioles and capillaries, especially in the coronary circulation. In therapeutic doses, nitroglycerin is thought to increase the blood supply to the myocardium which may, in turn, relieve myocardial ischemia, the possible functional basis for the pain of angina pectoris. The sublingual administration of nitroglycerin is normally rapid and transient, but nitroglycerin in controlled-release NITRO-BID® 2.5, NITRO-BID® 6.5, and NITRO-BID® 9 produces a prolonged action.

Indications:
Based on a review of this drug and a related drug by the National Academy of Sciences—National Research Council and/or other information, FDA has classified the indications as follows:
"Possibly" effective:
For the management, prophylaxis or treatment of anginal attacks.
Final classification of the less-than-effective indications requires further investigation.

Contraindications: Acute or recent myocardial infarction, severe anemia, closed-angle glaucoma, postural hypotension, increased intracranial pressure, and idiosyncrasy to the drug.
Warnings: Capsules must be swallowed. FOR ORAL, NOT SUBLINGUAL, USE. NITRO-BID® 2.5, NITRO-BID® 6.5, and NITRO-BID® 9 Controlled-Release Capsules are not intended for immediate relief of anginal attacks.
Precautions: Intraocular pressure may be increased; therefore, caution is required in administering to patients with glaucoma. Tolerance to this drug and cross-tolerance to other organic nitrites and nitrates may occur. If blurring of vision, dryness of mouth, or lack of benefit occurs, the drug should be discontinued.
Adverse Reactions: Severe and persistent headaches, cutaneous flushing, dizziness and weakness. Occasionally, drug rash or exfoliative dermatitis and nausea and vomiting may occur; these responses may disappear with a decrease in dosage. Adverse effects are enhanced by ingestion of alcohol, which appears to increase absorption from the gastrointestinal tract.
Dosage and Administration: Administer the smallest effective dose two or three times daily at 8- to 12-hour intervals, unless clinical response suggests a different regimen. Patient should be titrated to anginal relief or hemodynamic response. Hemodynamic response can be measured by drop in systolic blood pressure. Discontinue if not effective.
How Supplied: NITRO-BID® 2.5 Controlled-Release Capsules and NITRO-BID® 6.5 Controlled-Release Capsules are each available in 60- and 100-count Uni-℞® Paks and in bottles of 60 and 100. NITRO-BID® 9 Controlled-Release Capsules are available in 60-count bottles.
[*Shown in Product Identification Section*]

NITRO-BID® Ointment ℞
(2% nitroglycerin)

Description: NITRO-BID® Ointment contains 2% nitroglycerin (glyceryl trinitrate) and lactose in a special lanolin petrolatum base. It is a prompt-acting vasodilator, which may be effective in the relief and prevention of anginal attacks.
Actions: When the ointment is spread on the skin, the active ingredient (nitroglycerin) is continuously absorbed through the skin into the circulation, thus exerting prolonged vasodilator effect. Nitroglycerin ointment is probably effective in the control of angina pectoris, regardless of the site of application.

Indications: "Possibly" Effective: Prevention and treatment of angina pectoris attacks, especially at night.

Contraindications: Nitroglycerin Ointment is contraindicated in patients with marked anemia, increased intraocular pressure, or increased intracranial pressure. Nitroglycerin Ointment should not be used in patients with known idiosyncrasies to nitrites.
Warnings: In terminating treatment of anginal patients, both the dosage and frequency of application must be gradually reduced over a period of 4 to 6 weeks to prevent sudden withdrawal reactions, which are characteristic of all vasodilators in the nitroglycerin class.
Precautions: A headache is a definite sign of overdosage and, therefore, dosage should be reduced. Occasionally elderly patients may have no untoward symptoms while recumbent but may develop postural hypotension with faintness upon suddenly arising.
Adverse Reactions: With use of nitrites, transient headache, postural hypotension, flushing, tachycardia and dizziness may occur.
Dosage and Administration: For angina pectoris the ointment may be applied every 3 to 4 hours as required. The usual dose is 1 to 2 inches, as squeezed from the tube, although some patients may require as much as 4 or 5 inches. The ointment should be spread in a thin uniform layer on the skin without massaging or rubbing it in. The optimum dosage is determined by starting with an application of ½ inch of ointment and increasing the dose in ½-inch increments each successive application until headache occurs, then decreasing to the largest dose which does not cause headache. The ointment can be applied to any convenient skin area, but psychologically, many patients prefer the chest. In applying the ointment, place the specially designed Dose Measuring Applicator supplied with the package printed side down, and squeeze the necessary amount of ointment from the tube onto the Dose Measuring Applicator. Then place the Dose Measuring Applicator, ointment side down, on the desired skin area, spreading it in a thin, uniform layer. The Dose Measuring Applicators serve the dual purpose of measuring the amount of ointment and preventing absorption of the ointment through the fingers while it is being applied. Keep the tube tightly closed and store in a cool place.
How Supplied: NITRO-BID® Ointment is available in 20-gram and 60-gram UNI-Rx® Paks (six tubes per pak) and in individual 20-gram and 60-gram tubes.
[*Shown in Product Identification Section*]

OS-CAL® Tablets OTC
calcium with vitamin D

Each tablet contains: 625 mg of calcium carbonate from oyster shell which provides:
Elemental calcium ....250 mg
Ergocalciferol (Vitamin D_2) .....125 USP Units
Indications: Os-Cal Tablets provide a source of calcium when it is desired to increase the dietary intake of this mineral. Os-Cal also contains Vitamin D_2 to aid in the absorption of calcium.
Directions: Take one tablet three times a day at mealtime. Three tablets daily provide:

	Quantity	%U.S.RDA* for Adults
Calcium	750 mg	75%
Vitamin D_2	375 units	94%

*Percent U.S. Recommended Daily Allowance
How Supplied: Bottles of 100, 240, 500, and 1000.
[*Shown in Product Identification Section*]

OS-CAL® 500 TABLETS OTC
calcium supplement

Each tablet contains:
1,250 mg of calcium carbonate from oyster shell which provides: Elemental calcium, 500 mg.
Indications: Os-Cal 500 Tablets provide a source of calcium where it is desired or recommended by a physician to increase the dietary intake of this mineral.
Directions: Take one tablet two or three times a day at mealtime or as directed. Two tablets daily provide:

	Quantity	%U.S.RDA†
Calcium	1,000 mg	100%*
		77%**

Three tablets daily provide:

	Quantity	%U.S.RDA†
Calcium	1,500 mg	150%*
		115%**

†Percent U.S. Recommended Daily Allowance.
*For adults and children 12 or more years of age.
**For pregnant and lactating women.
How Supplied: Bottles of 60.
[*Shown in Product Identification Section*]

Continued on next page

Marion—Cont.

OS-CAL FORTE® OTC
Multivitamin and Mineral Supplement

Each tablet contains:
Vitamin A (palmitate)............1668 USP Units
Ergocalciferol (Vitamin D_2).....125 USP Units
Thiamine mononitrate (Vitamin B_1).....1.7 mg
Riboflavin (Vitamin B_2)..........................1.7 mg
Pyridoxine hydrochloride
(Vitamin B_6).......2.0 mg
Cyanocobalamin (Vitamin B_{12}).............1.6 mcg
Ascorbic acid (Vitamin C)........................50 mg
dl-alpha-tocopherol acetate
(Vitamin E).....0.8 IU
Niacinamide...15 mg
Calcium (from oyster shell*)..................250 mg
Iron (as ferrous fumarate)..........................5 mg
Copper (as sulfate)..................................0.3 mg
Iodine (as potassium iodide)..................0.05 mg
Magnesium (as oxide)..............................1.6 mg
Manganese (as sulfate)............................0.3 mg
Zinc (as sulfate).......................................0.5 mg
*Trace minerals from oyster shell: copper, iron, magnesium, manganese, silica and zinc.
Indication: Multivitamin and mineral supplement.
Dosage: One tablet three times daily or as directed by physician.
How Supplied: Bottles of 100.
[*Shown in Product Identification Section*]

OS-CAL-GESIC® OTC
(antiarthritic)

Each tablet contains:
Salicylamide ....400 mg.
Calcium (from oyster shell)..................100 mg.
Ergocalciferol (Vitamin D_2)........50 USP Units
Indication: For temporary relief of symptoms associated with arthritis.
Dosage: Initially: 2 tablets hourly for 3 or 4 doses. Maintenance: 1 or 2 tablets 4 times daily.
How Supplied: OS-CAL-GESIC® is available in bottles of 100.
[*Shown in Product Identification Section*]

OS–CAL® Plus OTC
Multivitamin and Multimineral Supplement

Each tablet contains:
Calcium (from oyster shell*)..................250 mg
Ergocalciferol (Vitamin D_2).....125 USP Units
*Trace minerals from oyster shell: copper, iron, magnesium, manganese, silica and zinc.
Plus:
Vitamin A (palmitate)............1666 USP Units
Vitamin C (ascorbic acid)..........................33 mg
Vitamin B_2 (riboflavin)............................0.66 mg
Vitamin B_1 (thiamine mononitrate)......0.5 mg
Vitamin B_6 (pyridoxine HCl)....................0.5 mg
Vitamin B_{12} (cyanocobalamin)...........0.03 mcg
Niacinamide...3.33 mg
Iron (as ferrous fumarate)......................16.6 mg
Zinc (as the sulfate).................................0.75 mg
Manganese (as the sulfate)......................0.75 mg
Copper (as the sulfate)..........................0.036 mg
Iodine (as potassium iodide)..................0.036 mg
Indications: As a multivitamin and multimineral supplement.
Dosage: One (1) tablet three times a day before meals or as directed by a physician. For children under four years of age, consult a physician.
How supplied: Bottles of 100.
[*Shown in Product Identification Section*]

PAVABID® Plateau CAPS® ℞
(papaverine hydrochloride) 150 mg

Composition:
Each Pavabid capsule contains:
Papaverine hydrochloride.................. 150 mg.
In a specially prepared base to provide prolonged activity.
Actions and Uses: The main actions of papaverine are exerted on cardiac and smooth muscle. Like quinidine, papaverine acts directly on the heart muscle to depress conduction and prolong the refractory period. Papaverine relaxes various smooth muscles. This relaxation may be prominent if spasm exists. The muscle cell is not paralyzed by papaverine and still responds to drugs and other stimuli causing contraction. The antispasmodic effect is a direct one, and unrelated to muscle innervation. Papaverine is practically devoid of effects on the central nervous system.
Papaverine relaxes the smooth musculature of the larger blood vessels, especially coronary, systemic peripheral and pulmonary arteries. Perhaps by its direct vasodilating action on cerebral blood vessels papaverine increases cerebral blood flow and decreases cerebral vascular resistance in normal subjects; oxygen consumption is unaltered. These effects may explain the benefit reported from the drug in cerebral vascular encephalopathy.
The direct actions of papaverine on the heart to depress conduction and irritability and to prolong the refractory period of the myocardium provide the basis for its clinical trial in abrogating atrial and ventricular premature systoles and ominous ventricular arrhythmias. The coronary vasodilator action could be an additional factor of therapeutic value when such rhythms are secondary to insufficiency or occlusion of the coronary arteries.
In patients with acute coronary thrombosis, the occurrence of ventricular rhythms is serious and requires measures designed to decrease myocardial irritability. Papaverine may have advantages over quinidine, used for a similar purpose, in that it may be given in an emergency by the intravenous route, does not depress myocardial contraction or cause cinchonism, and produces coronary vasodilation.
Indications: For the relief of cerebral and peripheral ischemia associated with arterial spasm and myocardial ischemia complicated by arrhythmias.
Precaution: Use with caution in patients with glaucoma. Hepatic hypersensitivity has been reported with gastrointestinal symptoms, jaundice, eosinophilia and altered liver function tests. Discontinue medication if these occur.
Adverse Reactions: Although occurring rarely, the reported side effects of papaverine include nausea, abdominal distress, anorexia, constipation, malaise, drowsiness, vertigo, sweating, headache, diarrhea and skin rash.
Dosage and Administration: One capsule every 12 hours. In difficult cases administration may be increased to one capsule every 8 hours, or two capsules every 12 hours.
How Supplied: Pavabid® capsules are available in 60- and 100-count Uni-℞® Paks, in bottles of 100, 250, 1000 and 5000 and in Unit Dose Identification Paks of 500 capsules. Capsules are imprinted with Marion/1555.
Caution: Federal law prohibits dispensing without prescription.
[*Shown in Product Identification Section*]

PAVABID® HP Capsulets ℞
(papaverine hydrochloride) 300 mg

Composition: Each capsulet contains:
papaverine hydrochloride.....................300 mg.
Action and Uses: The main actions of papaverine are exerted on cardiac and smooth muscle. Like quinidine, papaverine acts directly on the heart muscle to depress conduction and prolong the refractory period. Papaverine relaxes various smooth muscles. This relaxation may be prominent if spasm exists. The muscle cell is not paralyzed by papaverine, and still responds to drugs and other stimuli causing contraction. The antispasmodic effect is a direct one, and unrelated to muscle innervation. Papaverine is practically devoid of effects on the central nervous system.
Papaverine relaxes the smooth musculature of the larger blood vessels, especially coronary, systemic peripheral, and pulmonary arteries. Perhaps by its direct vasodilating action on cerebral blood vessels, papaverine increases cerebral blood flow and decreases cerebral vascular resistance in normal subjects; oxygen consumption is unaltered. These effects may explain the benefit reported from the drug in cerebral vascular encephalopathy.
The direct actions of papaverine on the heart to depress conduction and irritability and to prolong the refractory period of the myocardium provide the basis for its clinical trial in abrogating atrial and ventricular premature systoles and ominous ventricular arrhythmias. The coronary vasodilator action could be an additional factor of therapeutic value when such rhythms are secondary to insufficiency or occlusion of the coronary arteries.
In patients with acute coronary thrombosis, the occurrence of ventricular rhythms is serious and requires measures designed to decrease myocardial irritability. Papaverine may have advantages over quinidine, used for a similar purpose, in that it may be given in an emergency by the intravenous route, does not depress myocardial contraction or cause cinchonism, and produces coronary vasodilation.
Indications: For the relief of cerebral and peripheral ischemia associated with arterial spasm and myocardial ischemia complicated by arrhythmias.
Precaution: Use with caution in patients with glaucoma. Hepatic hypersensitivity has been reported with gastrointestinal symptoms, jaundice, eosinophilia and altered liver function tests. Discontinue medication if these occur.
Adverse Reactions: Although occurring rarely, the reported side effects of papaverine include nausea, abdominal distress, anorexia, constipation, malaise, drowsiness, vertigo, sweating, headache, diarrhea and skin rash.
Dosage and Administration: In difficult cases, dosage is one capsulet every 8-12 hours.
How Supplied: PAVABID® HP Capsulets are available in 60-count bottles. Each light orange capsulet is imprinted with a raised M stamped MARION on one side and PAVABID-HP on the other side.
Caution: Federal law prohibits dispensing without prescription.
[*Shown in Product Identification Section*]

PRETTS® TABLETS OTC
Diet Control Adjunct

Each tablet contains:
Alginic acid...200 mg
Sodium carboxymethylcellulose...........100 mg
Sodium bicarbonate...................................70 mg
Contains FD&C Yellow No. 5 (tartrazine) as a color additive.
Indications: For use as an adjunct to diet control. PRETTS® Tablets provide bulk to help satisfy the feeling of hunger caused by emptiness, making it easier for you to adhere to your specific diet regimen.
Those on a sodium restricted diet should consult their physician.
Actions: PRETTS® Tablets, when chewed, introduce a bulky foam into the gastrointestinal tract to create a feeling of fullness and to help alleviate hunger pangs; this serves as an aid in helping the patient eat less.
Dosage and Administration: Take two to four tablets with a full glass of water three or four times a day, or as needed. Chew each tablet individually followed by small sips of water.

Do not swallow tablets whole!
How Supplied: Bottles of 60 tablets. Tablets are imprinted with MARION/1177.

SILVADENE® CREAM ℞
Brand of Silver Sulfadiazine (Micronized)

Description: SILVADENE Cream is a soft, white, water-miscible cream containing the antimicrobial agent, silver sulfadiazine in micronized form. Each gram of SILVADENE Cream contains 10 mg of micronized silver sulfadiazine. The cream vehicle consists of white petrolatum USP, stearyl alcohol USP, isopropyl myristate, sorbitan monooleate, polyoxyl 40 stearate USP, propylene glycol USP, and water, with methylparaben USP 0.3% as a preservative.
Actions: SILVADENE Cream (silver sulfadiazine) spreads easily and can be washed off readily with water.
Silver sulfadiazine, micronized, has broad antimicrobial activity. It is bactericidal for many Gram-negative and Gram-positive bacteria as well as being effective against yeast. Results from *in vitro* testing are listed below. Sufficient data have been obtained to demonstrate that silver sulfadiazine will inhibit bacteria that are resistant to other antimicrobial agents and that the compound is superior to sulfadiazine.

Number of Sensitive Strains/Total Strains Tested

Concentration of silver sulfadiazine

Genus & Species	50 μg/ml	100μg/ml
Pseudomonas aeruginosa	130/130	130/130
Pseudomonas maltophilia	7/7	7/7
Enterobacter species	48/50	50/50
Enterobacter cloacae	24/24	24/24
Klebsiella	53/54	54/54
Escherichia coli	63/63	63/63
Serratia	27/28	28/28
Proteus mirabilis	53/53	53/53
Proteus morganii	10/10	10/10
Proteus rettgeri	2/2	2/2
Proteus vulgaris	2/2	2/2
Providencia	1/1	1/1
Citrobacter	10/10	10/10
Herellea	8/9	9/9
Mima	2/2	2/2
Staphylococcus aureus	100/101	101/101
Staphylococcus epidermidis	51/51	51/51
β-hemolytic *Streptococcus*	4/4	4/4
Enterococcus (Group D *Streptococcus)*	52/53	53/53
Corynebacterium diphtheriae	2/2	2/2
Clostridium perfringens	0/2	2/2
Candida albicans	43/50	50/50

Studies utilizing radioactive micronized silver sulfadiazine, electron microscopy and elaborate biochemical techniques have revealed that the mechanism of action of silver sulfadiazine on bacteria differs from silver nitrate and sodium sulfadiazine. SILVADENE Cream (silver sulfadiazine) acts only on the cell membrane and cell wall to produce its bactericidal effect.
Silver sulfadiazine by its chemical nature is not a carbonic anhydrase inhibitor. **Acidosis in patients treated with SILVADENE Cream has not been reported.** Since it is not a carbonic anhydrase inhibitor, SILVADENE Cream may be particularly of value in treating pediatric burn patients.
Indications: SILVADENE Cream (silver sulfadiazine) is a topical antimicrobial drug indicated as an adjunct for the prevention and treatment of wound sepsis in patients with second and third degree burns.
Contraindications: Because sulfonamide therapy is known to increase the possibility of kernicterus, SILVADENE Cream should not be used at term pregnancy, on premature infants, or on newborn infants during the first month of life.
Warnings: SILVADENE Cream should be administered with great caution to patients with history of hypersensitivity to SILVADENE Cream. It is not known whether there is cross sensitivity to other sulfonamides. If allergic reactions attributable to treatment with SILVADENE Cream occur, discontinuation of SILVADENE Cream must be considered. The use of SILVADENE Cream in some cases of glucose-6-phosphate dehydrogenase deficient individuals may be hazardous, as hemolysis may occur.
Use in Pregnancy: Safe use of SILVADENE Cream during pregnancy has not been established. Therefore, the preparation is not recommended for the treatment of women of child-bearing potential, unless the burned area covers more than 20 percent of the total body surface area or the need for therapeutic benefit of SILVADENE Cream is, in the physician's judgment, greater than the possible risk to the fetus.
Fungal colonization in and below the eschar may occur concomitantly with reduction of bacterial growth in the burn wound. However, fungal dissemination is rare.
In the treatment of burn wounds involving extensive areas of the body, the serum sulfa concentration may approach adult therapeutic levels (8–12 mg%). Therefore, in these patients it would be advisable to monitor serum sulfa concentrations. Renal function should be carefully monitored and the urine should be checked for sulfa crystals.
Precautions: If hepatic and renal functions become impaired and elimination of drug decreases, accumulation may occur and discontinuation of SILVADENE Cream should be weighed against the therapeutic benefit being achieved.
In considering the use of topical proteolytic enzymes in conjunction with SILVADENE Cream, the possibility should be noted that silver may inactivate such enzymes.
Adverse Reactions: It is frequently difficult to distinguish between an adverse reaction due to SILVADENE Cream (silver sulfadiazine) and reactions that may occur due to the concomitant use of other therapeutic agents used in the treatment of a patient having a severe burn wound. In the aggregate of 2,297 patients treated with SILVADENE Cream, there were 59 drug related reactions (2.5%). Of these there were 51 cases of burning, 5 of rash, 2 of itching and 1 of interstitial nephritis. However, SILVADENE Cream therapy was discontinued in only 0.9% of the patient population.
Since significant quantities of silver sulfadiazine are absorbed, it is possible that any of the adverse reactions attributable to sulfonamides may occur.
Dosage and Administration: Prompt institution of appropriate regimens for care of the burned patient is of prime importance and includes the control of shock and pain. The burn wounds are then cleansed and debrided and SILVADENE Cream (silver sulfadiazine) is applied with sterile, gloved hand. The burn areas should be covered with SILVADENE Cream at all times. The cream should be applied once to twice daily to a thickness of approximately $^1/_{16}$ inch. Whenever necessary, the cream should be reapplied to any areas from which it has been removed by patient activity. Administration may be accomplished in minimal time because dressings are not required. However, if individual patient requirements make dressings necessary, they may be used.
When feasible, the patient should be bathed daily. This is an aid in debridement. A whirlpool bath is particularly helpful, but the patient may be bathed in bed or in a shower.
Reduction in bacterial growth after application of topical antibacterial agents has been reported to permit spontaneous healing of deep partial thickness burns by preventing conversion of the partial thickness to full thickness by sepsis. However, reduction in bacterial colonization has caused delayed separation, in some cases necessitating escharotomy in order to prevent contracture.
Treatment with SILVADENE Cream should be continued until satisfactory healing has occurred or until the burn site is ready for grafting. **The drug should not be withdrawn from the therapeutic regimen while there remains the possibility of infection except if a significant adverse reaction occurs.**
How Supplied: Jars containing 50 grams and 400 grams SILVADENE Cream (silver sulfadiazine).
Store at room temperature (59°F–86°F).
[*Shown in Product Identification Section*]

THROAT DISCS Throat Lozenges OTC

Description: Each lozenge contains Capsicum, Peppermint, Anise, Cubeb, Glycyrrhiza Extract (Licorice), and Linseed.
Indications: Effective for soothing, temporary relief of minor throat irritations from hoarseness and coughs due to colds.
Precautions: For severe or persistent cough or sore throat, or sore throat accompanied by high fever, headache, nausea, and vomiting, consult physician promptly. Not recommended for children under 3 years of age.
Dosage: Allow lozenge to dissolve slowly in mouth. One or two should give the desired relief. Do not use more than four lozenges per hour.
How Supplied: Box of 60.

THYROID STRONG TABLETS ℞
THYROID TABLETS, USP ℞

Description: Thyroid Tablets are prepared from defatted, desiccated thyroid glands of edible animals. Thyroid, USP is standardized to contain 0.2% iodine. Thyroid Strong is standardized to contain 0.3% iodine. The standard of 0.3% iodine was adopted before the USP Standard was established and is 50% stronger than the USP specification. Each grain of Thyroid Strong is equivalent to 1½ grains of Thyroid USP. Thyroid is assayed both chemically and biologically to assure uniform potency. In this preparation the active thyroid hormones, thyroxine and liothyronine, are available in their natural state.
Action: The activity of Thyroid is derived from its natural thyroid hormone content. Virtually every system of the body appears to be affected by the action of the thyroid hormones. The primary action of the thyroid hormones is the promotion of a generalized increase in the metabolic rate of the body tissues. The effect may be noted in increases in the following: oxygen consumption; respiratory rate; body temperature; cardiac output; heart rate; blood volume; rate of fat; protein and carbohydrate metabolism; enzyme system activity and growth and maturation. The basic mechanism of action is not yet understood.
Following the administration of thyroid hormones, rapid and almost complete absorption takes place, but their effects develop slowly with initial effects being observed in 24 hours

Continued on next page

Marion—Cont.

and full effect usually being achieved in 10 to 14 days.
The administration of small doses of thyroid to normal (euthyroid) individuals does not produce an increase in metabolic rate.
Indications: Thyroid is indicated for use in the treatment of thyroid deficiency states, especially cretinism and myxedema. In hypothyroidism, the administration of thyroid represents pure replacement therapy.
Thyroid is also indicated for administration as an adjunct to the use of thyroid-inhibiting agents when decreased release of thyrotrophic hormones is desired.
Contraindications: Thyroid preparations are contraindicated in the presence of uncorrected adrenal insufficiency and in acute myocardial infarction which is uncomplicated by hypothyroidism.
Warnings:

> Drugs with thyroid hormone activity, alone or together with other therapeutic agents, have been used for the treatment of obesity. In euthyroid patients, doses within the range of daily hormonal requirements are ineffective for weight reduction. Larger doses may produce serious or even life-threatening manifestations of toxicity, particularly when given in association with sympathomimetic amines such as those used for their anorectic effects.

The possibility of persons with coronary artery disease suffering an episode of coronary insufficiency following injections of epinephrine may be enhanced in persons on thyroid hormone.
Thyroid hormones may potentiate the effect of anticoagulant drugs and, consequently, special care is required in titrating the dosage for patients on such therapy.
Precautions: Patients with myxedema may be especially sensitive to the thyroid hormones. In such cases, treatment should be instituted with very small doses and the increments increasing dosage should be gradual.
Thyroid preparations should be administered with caution to persons with cardiovascular disease. If signs of aggravation of the cardiovascular disease develop, the dosage should be reduced.
The administration of thyroid preparations to persons with diabetes mellitus may affect insulin or hypoglycemic agent requirements and dosage of these agents should be adjusted as necessary.
Adverse Reactions: Excessive doses of thyroid produce signs and symptoms of thyrotoxicosis which include tachycardia, cardiac arrhythmias, palpitation, elevated pulse pressure, angina pectoris, tremors, nervousness, headache, insomnia, nausea, diarrhea, changes in appetite, excessive sweating, intolerance to heat and fever. Chronic overdosage causes emaciation.
Dosage and Administration: Each grain of Thyroid Strong is equivalent to 1½ grains of Thyroid USP. The following listing indicates the equivalent USP Thyroid potency that corresponds to each strength of Thyroid Strong.
½ gr Thyroid Strong is equivalent to ¾ gr Thyroid USP
1 gr Thyroid Strong is equivalent to 1½ gr Thyroid USP
2 gr Thyroid Strong is equivalent to 3 gr Thyroid USP
3 gr Thyroid Strong is equivalent to 4½ gr Thyroid USP
The dose of thyroid must be established on an individual basis for each patient beginning with a small dose and increasing gradually until the desired effect is obtained. In order to standardize the expression of thyroid dosage, the dosages indicated are given in terms of USP thyroid. Where Thyroid Strong is desired for convenience or more precise dosing, conversion to potencies of that product may be made in accordance with the preceding listing of equivalents.
The usual maintenance dose in thyroid-deficient patients is ½ to 2 grains daily. In some individuals, titrated dosage may be well in excess of the usual dose because of variations in individual response.
In cretinism it is desired to have early diagnosis and treatment, with prompt establishment of a maintenance dosage level. This may be achieved by administering ¼ grain daily, to be increased in ¼-grain increments every two weeks to a maximum level of 1 grain for each 6 months of age, not to exceed 4 grains per day.
In adult myxedema, replacement therapy is usually initiated at the rate of ½ grain per day and then increased at monthly intervals to 1 to 1½ grains daily, as the individual response dictates.
The effects of thyroid therapy are highly cumulative, and no advantage occurs from dividing the daily dose, nor administering at a particular time.
How Supplied:
Thyroid Tablets, USP are supplied as:
Compressed Tablets (plain)

NDC 0088-0775-58	15 mg	1000's
NDC 0088-0776-58	30 mg	1000's
NDC 0088-0777-47	60 mg	100's
NDC 0088-0777-58	60 mg	1000's
NDC 0088-0778-58	125 mg	1000's

Thyroid Strong Tablets are supplied as:
Compressed Tablets (plain)

NDC 0088-0686-47	½ gr (32.5 mg)	100's
NDC 0088-0686-58	½ gr (32.5 mg)	1000's
NDC 0088-0674-47	1 gr (65 mg)	100's
NDC 0088-0674-58	1 gr (65 mg)	1000's
NDC 0088-0675-47	2 gr (0.13 g)	100's
NDC 0088-0675-58	2 gr (0.13 g)	1000's

Compressed Tablets (sugar-coated)

NDC 0088-0626-47	½ gr (32.5 mg)	100's
NDC 0088-0626-58	½ gr (32.5 mg)	1000's
NDC 0088-0627-47	1 gr (65 mg)	100's
NDC 0088-0627-58	1 gr (65 mg)	1000's
NDC 0088-0628-47	2 gr (0.13 g)	100's
NDC 0088-0629-47	3 gr (0.2 g)	100's

References:

1. DiPalma, J.R.: "Drill's Pharmacology in Medicine," 3rd Edition, New York, McGraw-Hill, 1965.
2. "New Drugs," AMA Council on Drugs, 1966 Edition.
3. Goodman, L.S. & Gilman, A: "The Pharmacological Basis of Therapeutics," 3rd Edition, New York, MacMillan, 1965.
4. Sellman, T.H.: "A Manual of Pharmacology and Its Applications to Therapeutics and Toxicology," 8th Edition, Philadelphia, Saunders, 1957.
5. Beckman, H.: "Pharmacology: The Nature, Action and Use of Drugs," 2nd Edition, Philadelphia, W.B. Saunders Co, 1961.
6. Goth, A.: "Medical Pharmacology, Principles and Concepts" 3rd Edition, St. Louis, The C.V. Mosby Co., 1966.
7. Duncan, G.G.: "Diseases of Metabolism. Detailed Methods of Diagnosis and Treatment," 5th Edition, Philadelphia, W.B. Saunders Co., 1964.

Manufactured for
Pharmaceutical Division
Marion Laboratories Inc.
Kansas City, Missouri 64137
by
Parke, Davis & Co.
Detroit, MI 48232
[*Shown in Product Identification Section*]

TRITEN® Tablets ℞
(dimethindene maleate NF)
2.5 mg Tab-In™

Description: Triten is an antihistamine occurring as a white crystalline powder that is freely soluble in methanol, soluble in chloroform, and sparingly soluble in water. Chemically, it is 2-[1-[2-[2-(dimethylamino) ethyl] inden-3-yl]-ethyl] pyridine maleate.
Actions: Antihistamines are competitive antagonists of histamine, which also produce central nervous system effects (both stimulant and depressant) and peripheral anticholinergic, atropine-like effects (*eg*, drying).

> **Indications:**
> Based on a review of this drug by the National Academy of Sciences—National Research Council and/or other information, FDA has classified the indications as follows:
> "Probably" effective: Perennial and seasonal allergic rhinitis; vasomotor rhinitis; allergic conjunctivitis due to inhalant allergens and foods; mild, uncomplicated allergic skin manifestations of urticaria and angiodema; amelioration of allergic reactions to blood or plasma; dermographism; anaphylactic reactions as adjunctive therapy to epinephrine and other standard measures after the acute manifestations have been controlled.
> Final classification of the less-than-effective indications requires further investigation.

Contraindications: Triten should not be used in premature infants, neonates, or nursing mothers; patients receiving MAO inhibitors; patients with narrow angle glaucoma, stenosing peptic ulcer, symptomatic prostatic hypertrophy, bladder neck obstruction, pyloroduodenal obstruction, lower respiratory tract symptoms (including asthma), or hypersensitivity to dimethindene or related compounds.
Warnings: Antihistamines often produce drowsiness and may reduce mental alertness in children and adults. Patients should be warned about engaging in activities requiring mental alertness (*eg*, driving a car, operating machinery or hazardous appliances). In elderly patients, approximately 60 years or older, antihistamines are more likely to cause dizziness, sedation, and hypotension.
Patients should be warned that the central nervous system effects of Triten may be additive with those of alcohol and other CNS depressants (*eg*, hypnotics, sedatives, tranquilizers, antianxiety agents).
Antihistamines may produce excitation, particularly in children.
Usage in Pregnancy: Although no Triten-related teratogenic potential or other adverse effects on the fetus have been observed in limited animal reproduction studies, the safe use of this drug in pregnancy or during lactation has not been established. Therefore, the drug should not be used during pregnancy or lactation unless, in the judgment of the physician, the expected benefits outweigh the potential hazards.
Usage in Children: In infants and children particularly, antihistamines in overdosage may produce hallucinations, convulsions and/or death.
Precautions: Triten, like other antihistamines, has atropine-like, anticholinergic activity and should be used with caution in patients with increased intraocular pressure, hyperthyroidism, cardiovascular disease, hypertension, or history of bronchial asthma.
This product contains FD&C Yellow No. 5 (tartrazine) which may cause allergic-type reactions (including bronchial asthma) in certain susceptible individuals. Although the overall incidence of FD&C Yellow No. 5 (tartrazine) sensitivity in the general population is low, it is frequently seen in patients who also have aspirin hypersensitivity.
Adverse Reactions: The most frequent adverse reactions to antihistamines are sedation or drowsiness; sleepiness; dryness of the

mouth, nose, and throat; thickening of bronchial secretions; dizziness; disturbed coordination; epigastric distress.
Other adverse reactions which may occur are: fatigue; chills; confusion; restlessness; excitation; hysteria; nervousness; irritability; insomnia; euphoria; anorexia; nausea; vomiting; diarrhea; constipation; hypotension; tightness in the chest; wheezing; blurred vision; diplopia; vertigo; tinnitus; convulsions; headache; palpitations; tachycardia; extrasystoles; nasal stuffiness; urinary frequency; difficult urination; urinary retention; leukopenia; hemolytic anemia; thrombocytopenia; agranulocytosis; aplastic anemia; allergic or hypersensitivity reactions, including drug rash, urticaria, anaphylactic shock, and photosensitivity. Although the following may have been reported to occur in association with some antihistamines, they have not been known to result from the use of Triten: excessive perspiration, tremor, paresthesias, acute labyrinthitis, neuritis and early menses.

Dosage and Administration:
Dosage should be individualized.
Adults and Children Over 6 Years of Age: One 2.5-mg Tab-In™ once or twice daily.

Overdosage:
Signs and Symptoms
The greatest danger from acute overdosage with antihistamines is their central nervous system effects which produce depression and/or stimulation.
In children, stimulation predominates initially in a syndrome which may include excitement, hallucinations, ataxia, incoordination, athetosis, and convulsions followed by postictal depression. Dry mouth, fixed dilated pupils, flushing of the face, and fever are common and resemble the syndrome of atropine poisoning. In adults, CNS depression (*ie,* drowsiness, coma) is more common. CNS stimulation is rare; fever and flushing are uncommon.
In both children and adults, there can be a terminal deepening of coma and cardiovascular collapse; death can occur, especially in infants and children.

Treatment
There is no specific therapy for acute overdosage with antihistamines. General symptomatic and supportive measures should be instituted promptly and maintained for as long as necessary.
In the conscious patient, vomiting should be induced even though it may have occurred spontaneously. If vomiting cannot be induced, gastric lavage is indicated. Adequate precautions must be taken to protect against aspiration, especially in infants and children. Charcoal slurry or other suitable agent should be instilled into the stomach after vomiting or lavage. Saline cathartics or milk of magnesia may be of additional benefit.
In the unconscious patient, the airway should be secured with a cuffed endotracheal tube before attempting to evacuate the gastric contents. Intensive supportive and nursing care is indicated, as for any comatose patient.
If breathing is significantly impaired, maintenance of an adequate airway and mechanical support of respiration is the safest and most effective means of providing for adequate oxygenation of tissues to prevent hypoxia (especially brain hypoxia during convulsions).
Hypotension is an early sign of impending cardiovascular collapse and should be treated vigorously. Although general supportive measures are important, specific treatment with intravenous infusion of a vasopressor (*eg,* levarterenol bitartrate) titrated to maintain adequate blood pressure may be necessary.
Do *not* use CNS stimulants.
Convulsions should be controlled by careful titration of a short-acting barbiturate, repeated as necessary.
Ice packs and cooling sponge baths can aid in reducing the fever commonly seen in children.

How Supplied:
Tab-In™, 2.5 mg (yellow): bottles of 100.
Tab-In™ (Marion's brand of delayed release tablet)
Manufactured for
Pharmaceutical Division
Marion Laboratories, Inc.
Kansas City, Mo. 64137
by
Ciba-Geigy Corp.
Summit, N.J. 07901

Marlyn Pharmaceutical Co., Inc.
18261 ENTERPRISE LANE, BLDG. A
HUNTINGTON BEACH, CA 92648

HEP-FORTE® CAPSULES

Description: Hep Forte is a comprehensive formulation of nutritional factors which have proved to be important in maintenance and support of normal hepatic function and related estrogen/androgen imbalance.

Composition: Each HEP-FORTE capsule contains:

A fermentation extract equivalent in microbiological potency to Vitamin B-12	0.33 mcg.
Biotin	3.3 mcg.
Inositol	10.0 mg.
dl-Methionine	10.0 mg.
Choline Bitartrate	21.0 mg.
Yeast Dried, U S P	64.8 mg.
Mixed Tocopherols (Equivalent to 1.53 I.U. Vitamin E)	3.34 mg.

With excipients in an artificially colored gelatin capsule

Desiccated Liver, Undefatted, NF	198.4 mg.
Liver Concentrate, NF	64.8 mg.
Liver Fraction No. 2, NF	64.8 mg.
Vitamin A Palmitate	1667 USP Units
Thiamine Mononitrate	1 mg.
Riboflavin	1 mg.
Pyridoxine Hydrochloride	0.67 mg
Ascorbic Acid	6.67 mg.
Niacinamide	10 mg.
d-Panthenol	1.33 mg.

Indications: HEP-FORTE is indicated in the treatment of deficiencies caused by or associated with disordered hepatic function. It is particularly useful as supportive nutritional therapy in alcoholism and to improve fertility (male and female) due to estrogen/androgen imbalance.

Contraindications: There are no known contraindications to HEP-FORTE.

Dosage: Severe Cases: 6 to 10 capsules daily, in two or three divided doses.
Mild Cases or Borderline Deficiencies: 2 capsules, three times daily.

How Supplied: Bottles of 100 and 500 capsules.

MARLYN FORMULA 50

Composition: Each capsule contains:

Amino Acids	0.5 Gm*
Vitamin B6 (pyridoxine HCl)	1.0 mg.

*Approximate analysis of the amino acids: indispensable amino acids (lysine, tryptophan, phenylalanine, methionine, threonine, leucine, isoleucine, valine), 35.30%; semi-dispensable amino acids (arginine, histidine, tyrosine, cystine, glycine), 19.18%; dispensable amino acids (glutamic acid, alanine, aspartic acid, serine, proline), 45.56%.

Indications: For the treatment of brittle, splitting and peeling finger nails.

Dosage and Administration: The recommended daily dose is 6 capsules daily or as directed by the physician.

Supply: Bottles of 100, 250 and 1000 capsules.

Literature Available: File card (explanation of clinicals and illustration).

TEST-ESTRIN® ℞
Androgen-Estrogen Therapy Products

How Supplied:
Test-Estrin® Half Strength
Each buccal tablet contains:
Estradiol N.F., 0.25 mg., Testosterone (free) 1.25 mg.
Bottles of 100
NDC 10712-988-10
Test-Estrin® Full Strength
Each buccal tablet contains:
Estradiol N.F., 0.5 mg., Testosterone (free), 2.5 mg.
Bottles of 100.
NDC 10712-987-10
Test-Estrin® Capsules
Each capsule contains: Ethinyl Estradiol, 0.03 mg., Methyl Testosterone, 3.5 mg.
Bottles of 30, 100
NDC 10712-933-03; NDC 10712-933-10
Test-Estrin® Injectable (Aqueous Suspension)
Each cc. contains:
Estradiol, 1.0 mg., Testosterone (Crystalline) 10.0 mg.
Vials of 10 cc
NDC 10712-950-10

Mayrand, Inc.
P. O. BOX 20246
1026 E. LINDSAY STREET
GREENSBORO, NC 27420

ANAMINE T.D.* Caps ℞
ANAMINE Syrup
Sugar-Free/Alcohol-Free/Dye-Free

Composition:
ANAMINE T.D. Caps
Each Capsule Contains:

Chlorpheniramine Maleate	8 mg.
Pseudoephedrine Hydrochloride	120 mg.

ANAMINE Syrup
Each 5 ml (teaspoonful) contains:

Chlorpheniramine Maleate	2 mg.
Pseudoephedrine Hydrochloride	30 mg.

*Mayrand brand of timed disintegration capsules.

Indications: For symptomatic relief of upper respiratory congestion in seasonal and perennial allergic rhinitis, acute rhinitis, rhinosinusitis and eustachian tube congestion.

Chlorpheniramine Maleate in prolonged release form; based on a review of this drug by the National Academy of Sciences-National Research Council and/or other information, FDA has classified the indications as: "Probably Effective". Final classification of the less-than-effective indications requires further investigation.

Contraindications: Severe hypertension, coronary artery disease, pregnancy, nursing mothers, patients on MAO inhibitors, sensitivity to the ingredients.

Warnings: Alcohol and other CNS depressants, as hypnotics, sedatives and tranquilizers may cause additive effects. Driving, operation of machinery or hazardous occupations should be avoided since drowsiness may occur.

Precautions: Use with caution in hypertension, cardiovascular disease, glaucoma, prostatic hypertrophy, diabetes and hyperthyroidism.

Adverse Reactions: Side effects may include drowsiness, confusion, restlessness, nausea, vomiting, drug rash, vertigo, palpitation, anorexia, dizziness, dysuria, headache, insomnia, anxiety, tension, weakness, tachycardia,

Continued on next page

Mayrand—Cont.

angina, sweating, blood pressure elevation, mydriasis, GI distress or cramps, CNS stimulation or circulatory collapse.
Drug Interactions: MAO inhibitors and beta adrenergic blockers increase the effects of pseudoephedrine. The antihypertensive effects of methyldopa, mecamylamine, reserpine and veratrum may be reduced.
Dosage: ANAMINE T.D. Caps—Adults, one capsule every 8 to 12 hours. Not for use by children under 12 years of age. ANAMINE SYRUP—Adults, 2 teaspoonfuls every 4 to 6 hours. Children 6 to 12 years old, 1 teaspoonful every 4 to 6 hours. Children 1 to 6 years old, ½ to 1 teaspoonful every 6 hours. Children under 1 year, ¼ to ½ teaspoonful every 6 hours.
Supplied: ANAMINE T.D. Caps in bottles of 100. ANAMINE Syrup in bottles of 473 ml. (1 pint).
Literature and Samples: On request.

ANATUSS Tablets and Syrup ℞

Each green tablet contains: Acetaminophen 300 mg.; Guaifenesin 50 mg.; Dextromethorphan Hydrobromide 10 mg.; Phenylephrine Hydrochloride 5 mg.; Phenylpropanolamine Hydrochloride 25 mg.; Chlorpheniramine Maleate 2 mg.
Two teaspoonfuls of Anatuss Syrup are approximately equivalent to one Anatuss Tablet.
Supplied: Anatuss Tablets are available in bottles of 100 and 500 tablets. Anatuss Syrup is available in 4 fl. oz. (120 ml.) bottles.
Literature and Samples: On request.

BUFF-A COMP TABLETS ℞
Buffered Analgesic-Antitensive

Composition: Each tablet contains:

Aspirin (10 gr.)	648 mg.
Phenacetin	130 mg.
Caffeine	43.2 mg.
Butalbital	48.6 mg.

(Warning: May be habit forming.)
Buffered with calcium carbonate.
Action and Uses: BUFF-A COMP provides an effective buffered APC-antitensive combination with an exceptional ten grain dose of aspirin, along with the anxiety and tension reducing action of butalbital. BUFF-A COMP is useful in relieving pain, reducing fever and to allay tension and apprehension which accompany pain. It is buffered to minimize the occurrence of gastric distress. BUFF-A COMP is very effective in such conditions as simple headache, tension headache, neuralgic pains, rheumatic pains, dysmenorrhea, myalgia and arthralgia. It also renders the patient more comfortable in febrile states such as colds, grippe and influenza. EXEMPT from all DEA controls.
Average Dose: 1 tablet three or four times daily.
Caution: Phenacetin may cause renal damage in prolonged and excessive dosage.
Contraindications: Sensitivity to any of the components.
Supplied: Bottles of 100 tablets.
Also available as **BUFF-A COMP** Capsules and **BUFF-A COMP #3 Tablets** with Codeine 30 mg. (Warning: May be habit forming.)
Product identification: Imprinted "M/R".
Literature and Samples: On request.

ELDERCAPS ℞

Each capsule contains: Vitamin A 4,000 I.U.; Vitamin D_2 400 I.U.; Vitamin E 25 I.U.; Ascorbic Acid 200mg.; Thiamine Mononitrate 10mg.; Riboflavin 5mg.; Pyridoxine Hydrochloride 2mg.; Niacinamide 25mg.; d-Calcium Pantothenate 10mg.; Zinc Sulfate 110mg.; Magnesium Sulfate 70 mg.; Manganese Sulfate 5 mg.; Folic Acid 1 mg.
Indications: ELDERCAPS are indicated for the prophylaxis or treatment of vitamin and mineral deficiencies associated with restricted diets, improper food intake, and decreased absorption or utilization. ELDERCAPS are also indicated in patients with increased requirements for vitamins and minerals due to chronic disease, infection or the stress of surgery.
Warnings: Folic acid alone is improper therapy in the treatment of pernicious anemia and other megaloblastic anemias where vitamin B_{12} is deficient.
Precautions: Folic acid, especially in doses above 1 mg. daily, may obscure pernicious anemia, that is, hematological remission may occur while neurologic manifestations remain progressive.
Dosage: One capsule daily or as directed by the physician.
Supplied: Bottles of 100 capsules.
Literature and Samples: On request.

ELDERTONIC Elixir ℞

Each Fluid Ounce (30 ml.) contains: Thiamine Hydrochloride 2 mg.; Riboflavin 2 mg.; Pyridoxine Hydrochloride 0.5 mg.; Vitamin B-12 (as Cobalamin Conc.) 2 mcg.; Dexpanthenol 5 mg.; Niacinamide 10 mg.; Pentylenetetrazol 20 mg.; Alcohol 13.5%. In a Special Sherry Wine Base
Supplied: Pints and Gallons.
Literature and Samples: On request.

GLYTUSS Tablets
(Guaifenesin 200 mg.)

How Supplied: Bottles of 100 and 1,000.
Literature and Samples: On request.

HYDROTENSIN-25 Tablets ℞
HYDROTENSIN-50 Tablets ℞
(Hydrochlorothiazide 25 or 50 mg. and Reserpine 0.125 mg.)

How Supplied: Bottles of 100 and 1,000.
Literature and Samples: On request.

HYDRO-Z-25 Tablets ℞
HYDRO-Z-50 Tablets ℞
(Hydrochlorothiazide 25 or 50 mg.)

How Supplied: Bottles of 100 and 1,000.
Literature and Samples: On request.

NU-IRON 150 Caps
NU-IRON Elixir
(polysaccharide-iron complex)

Composition: NU-IRON is a highly water soluble complex of iron and a low molecular weight polysaccharide. Each NU-IRON 150 Capsule contains 150 mg. elemental iron. Each 5 ml. (teaspoonful) of NU-IRON Elixir contains 100 mg. elemental iron, alcohol 10% (Sugar free).
Action and Uses: NU-IRON is a non-ionic, easily assimilated, relatively non-toxic form of iron. Full therapeutic doses may be achieved with virtually no gastrointestinal side effects. There is no metallic aftertaste and no staining of teeth.
Indications: For treatment of uncomplicated iron deficiency anemia.
Contraindications: Hemochromatosis, hemosiderosis or a known hypersensitivity to any of the ingredients.
Dosage: ADULTS; One or two NU-IRON 150 Caps daily, or one or two teaspoonfuls NU-IRON Elixir daily. CHILDREN; 6 to 12 years old; one teaspoonful NU-IRON Elixir daily; 2 to 6 years old: ½ teaspoonful daily; under 2 years: ¼ teaspoonful daily.
Supplied: NU-IRON 150 Caps in bottles of 100. NU-IRON Elixir in 8 fl. oz. bottles.
Literature and Samples: On request.

NU-IRON-V Tablets ℞

Each maroon film-coated tablet contains: Iron (Elemental) 60 mg. (as POLYSACCHARIDE-IRON COMPLEX); Folic Acid 1 mg.; Ascorbic Acid 50 mg. (as sodium ascorbate); Cyanocobalamin (Vitamin B-12) 3 mcg.; Vitamin A 4000 I.U.; Vitamin D-2 400 I.U.; Thiamine Mononitrate 3 mg.; Riboflavin 3 mg.; Pyridoxine Hydrochloride 2 mg; Niacinamide 10 mg.; Calcium Carbonate 312 mg.
Indications: For the prevention and/or treatment of dietary vitamin and iron deficiencies.
Dosage: Prophylactic—one tablet daily. Therapeutic—two to four tablets daily.
Contraindications: Sensitivity to any of the ingredients.
Precautions: The use of folic acid in patients having or who may develop pernicious anemia involves the hazard of treating the anemia characteristic of the disease while permitting progressive development of combined system disease of the spinal cord.
Parenteral Vitamin B_{12} is the drug of choice in pernicious anemia and should be used in patients receiving folic acid unless pernicious anemia has been ruled out.
Supplied: Bottles of 100 tablets.
Literature and Samples: On request.

PAVATRAN TD* Capsules ℞
PAVATRAN-300 TD Capsules
(Papaverine Hydrochloride 150 mg. or 300 mg.)
***Mayrand brand of Timed Disintegration Capsules.**

How Supplied: Pavatran—Bottles of 100 and 500. Pavatran-300—Bottles of 100.
Literature and Samples: On request.

SEDAPAP-10 Tablets ℞

Composition: Each tablet contains acetaminophen 648 mg. (10 grains) and butabarbital 16 mg. (Warning: May be habit forming).
Action and Uses: An analgesic-antipyretic-antitensive to relieve pain as well as the anxiety that intensifies the perception of pain. EXEMPT from all DEA controls.
Indications: For symptomatic analgesic-antitensive-antipyretic relief in arthritic and rheumatic conditions involving musculoskeletal pain and in other conditions such as headache, tension headache, dysmenorrhea, myalgia, neuralgia and the common cold.
Dosage: Adults: One tablet 3 or 4 times daily. Children 6 to 12 years: one-half the adult dose.
Precautions: Observe the recommended dosage. Side effects may include nausea, dizziness or rash.
Contraindications: Hepatic disease or sensitivity to either component.
Supplied: Bottles of 100 tablets.
Also available as **SEDAPAP Elixir.** Each teaspoonful (5 ml.) contains: Acetaminophen 120 mg., Butabarbital 16 mg. and Alcohol 12%. Pints.
Literature and Samples: On request.

SORBIDE ℞
(Isosorbide Dinitrate)

Available as:
SORBIDE T.D. * Capsules 40 mg.
*MAYRAND brand of Timed Disintegration Capsules.
Supplied: Bottles of 100.
Literature and Samples: On request.

STERAPRED UNI-PAK ℞
(Prednisone 5 mg.)

Prednisone in convenient decremental dosage, for unit dispensing.
How Supplied: Box of 21 tablets.
Literature and Samples: On request.

TRIMTABS ℞
(Phendimetrazine Tartrate 35 mg.)

How Supplied: Bottles of 100 and 1000.
Literature and Samples: On request.

McNeil Consumer Products Company

McNEILAB, INC.
FORT WASHINGTON, PA 19034

COTYLENOL® Cold Formula Tablets OTC

Description: Each tablet contains acetaminophen 325 mg., chlorpheniramine maleate 2 mg., and pseudoephedrine hydrochloride 30 mg.

Actions and Indications: CoTylenol Cold Formula Tablets combine the non-salicylate analgesic-antipyretic acetaminophen with the decongestant pseudoephedrine hydrochloride and the antihistamine chlorpheniramine maleate to help relieve nasal congestion as well as the fever, aches, pains and general discomfort associated with colds and other upper respiratory infections.

While the acetaminophen component is equal to aspirin in analgesic and antipyretic effectiveness, it is unlikely to produce many of the side effects associated with aspirin and aspirin-containing products. Thus, CoTylenol Cold Formula Tablets are particularly well suited for relief of cold symptoms in patients who should avoid aspirin, such as those with ulcer, gastritis and hiatus hernia; those taking anticoagulants; and those allergic to aspirin.

Usual Dosage: Adults: Two tablets every four hours, not to exceed 12 tablets per day. Children (over 6): One tablet every four hours, not to exceed five tablets per day.

Note: Since CoTylenol Cold Formula Tablets are available without prescription, the following appears on the package label: "WARNING: Do not exceed the recommended dosage or administer to children under 6. Reduce dosage if nervousness, restlessness, or sleeplessness occurs. If you have asthma, glaucoma, high blood pressure, heart disease, diabetes, thyroid disease, enlargement of the prostate gland, or are presently taking a prescription drug for the treatment of high blood pressure or emotional disorders, do not take except under the advice and supervision of a physician. This preparation may cause drowsiness. Do not drive or operate machinery while taking this medication. If symptoms do not improve within seven days or are accompanied by high fever, consult a physician before continuing use. Keep this and all medication out of the reach of children. In case of accidental overdosage, contact a physician immediately."

Overdosage: IN ALL CASES OF SUSPECTED OVERDOSE, IMMEDIATELY CONTACT A POISON CONTROL CENTER OR McNEIL CONSUMER PRODUCTS COMPANY FOR ANTIDOTE INFORMATION. Acetaminophen in large overdosage may cause hepatic toxicity in some patients. Following the ingestion of a potentially toxic overdose of acetaminophen, early symptoms, if present, may include: nausea, vomiting, abdominal pain, diaphoresis, generalized weakness and lethargy.

The antidote, when required, should be administered as early as possible, preferably within 16 hours of the overdose ingestion. Whether antidote therapy is required depends upon acetaminophen plasma levels, since patients' estimates of the quantity of a drug ingested as an overdose are notoriously unreliable. When a patient's history suggests ingestion of an overdose of acetaminophen, blood should be drawn immediately for an acetaminophen plasma assay, without regard to the presence or absence of symptomatology. It is important to determine as accurately as possible the elapsed time from ingestion of an overdose to the time of the plasma acetaminophen assay, since plasma levels at specific time points following an overdose correlate with the probable occurrence of hepatic toxicity.

How Supplied: Tablets (colored yellow, imprinted "CoTylenol")—blister packs of 24's and 48's in bottles of 100.

Also Available: Children's CoTylenol Liquid Cold Formula; CoTylenol Liquid Cold Formula (with Cough Suppressant) for adults.

[Shown in Product Identification Section]

COTYLENOL® LIQUID COLD FORMULA (with Cough Suppressant) OTC

Description: Each 30 ml (1 fl. oz.) contains acetaminophen 650 mg, chlorpheniramine maleate 4 mg, pseudoephedrine hydrochloride 60 mg, and dextromethorphan hydrobromide 20 mg (alcohol 7.5%).

Actions and Indications: CoTylenol Liquid Cold Formula (with Cough Suppressant) combines the non-salicylate analgesic-antipyretic acetaminophen with the decongestant pseudoephedrine hydrochloride, the cough suppressant dextromethorphan hydrobromide and the antihistamine chlorpheniramine maleate to help relieve nasal congestion and coughing, as well as the fever, aches, pains and general discomfort associated with colds and other upper respiratory infections. While the acetaminophen component is equal to aspirin in analgesic and antipyretic effectiveness, it is unlikely to produce many of the side effects associated with aspirin and aspirin-containing products. Thus, CoTylenol Liquid Cold Formula (with Cough Suppressant) is particularly well suited for relief of cold symptoms in patients who should avoid aspirin, such as those with ulcer, gastritis and hiatus hernia; those taking anticoagulants and those allergic to aspirin.

Usual Dosage: Measuring cup is provided and marked for accurate dosing. Adults: 1 fluid ounce (2 tbsps.) every 4 hours as needed, not to exceed 6 doses in 24 hours. Children (6–12 yrs.): ½ fluid ounce (1 tbsp.) every 4 hours as needed, not to exceed 5 doses in 24 hours.

Note: Since CoTylenol Liquid Cold Formula (with Cough Suppressant) is available without a prescription, the following appears on the package label: "WARNING: Do not exceed the recommended dosage or administer to children under 6. Reduce dosage if nervousness, restlessness or sleeplessness occurs. Persistent cough may indicate a serious condition. Persons with a high fever, rash or persistent cough or headache or asthma, emphysema or with glaucoma, high blood pressure, heart disease, diabetes, thyroid disease, enlargement of the prostate gland, or who are presently taking a prescription drug for the treatment of high blood pressure or emotional disorders, do not take, except under the advice and supervision of a physician. This preparation may cause drowsiness. Do not drive or operate machinery while taking this medication. If symptoms do not improve within five days, consult a physician before continuing use. Keep this and all medication out of the reach of children. In case of accidental overdosage, contact a physician immediately."

Overdosage: IN ALL CASES OF SUSPECTED OVERDOSE, IMMEDIATELY CONTACT A POISON CONTROL CENTER OR McNEIL CONSUMER PRODUCTS COMPANY FOR ANTIDOTE INFORMATION. Acetaminophen in large overdosage may cause hepatic toxicity in some patients. Following the ingestion of a potentially toxic overdose of acetaminophen, early symptoms, if present, may include: nausea, vomiting, abdominal pain, diaphoresis, generalized weakness and lethargy.

The antidote, when required, should be administered as early as possible, preferably within 16 hours of the overdose ingestion. Whether antidote therapy is required depends upon acetaminophen plasma levels, since patients' estimates of the quantity of a drug ingested as an overdose are notoriously unreliable. When a patient's history suggests ingestion of an overdose of acetaminophen, blood should be drawn immediately for an acetaminophen plasma assay, without regard to the presence or absence of symptomatology. It is important to determine as accurately as possible the elapsed time from ingestion of an overdose to the time of the plasma acetaminophen assay, since plasma levels at specific time points following an overdose correlate with the probable occurrence of hepatic toxicity.

How Supplied: Cherry/mint flavored mentholated (colored amber) bottles of 5 and 10 oz. with child-resistant safety cap and special dosage cup graded in ounces and tablespoons.

SINE-AID® OTC
Sinus Headache Tablets

Description: Each SINE-AID Tablet contains acetaminophen 325 mg. and phenylpropanolamine hydrochloride 25 mg.

Actions: Acetaminophen is a clinically proven analgesic-antipyretic. Acetaminophen produces analgesia by elevation of the pain threshold and antipyresis through action on the hypothalamic heat regulating center. Phenylpropanolamine hydrochloride is a sympathomimetic amine and provides vasoconstriction to the nasopharyngeal mucosa. Although similar in action to ephedrine, phenylpropanolamine HCl is less likely to cause CNS stimulation.

Indications: SINE-AID provides effective symptomatic relief from sinus headache pain and pressure caused by sinusitis. Since it contains no antihistamine, SINE-AID will not produce the drowsiness that may interfere with work, driving an automobile or operating dangerous machinery. SINE-AID is particularly well suited in patients with aspirin allergy, hemostatic disturbances (including anticoagulant therapy), and bleeding diatheses (e.g. ulcer, gastritis, hiatus hernia).

Precautions and Adverse Reactions: Acetaminophen has rarely been found to produce any side effects. It is usually well tolerated by aspirin-sensitive patients. If a rare sensitivity occurs, the drug should be stopped. In patients with high blood pressure, diabetes, or thyroid disease, phenylpropanolamine hydrochloride should be used with caution and only as directed by a physician. Do not use in patients receiving MAO inhibitors.

Usual Dosage: Adult dosage: Two tablets every four hours, no more than 6 tablets in any 24-hour period.

Note: Since SINE-AID tablets are available without a prescription, the following appears on the package labels: "CAUTION: Individuals with high blood pressure, heart disease, diabetes, thyroid disease, and children under 12 should use only as directed by physician. Do not exceed recommended dosage unless directed by a physician. WARNING: If symptoms of sinusitis or colds persist after 3 days, consult a physician. Keep this and all medications out of the reach of children. In case of accidental overdose, contact a physician immediately."

Overdosage: IN ALL CASES OF SUSPECTED OVERDOSE, IMMEDIATELY CONTACT A POISON CONTROL CENTER OR McNEIL CONSUMER PRODUCTS COMPANY FOR ANTIDOTE INFORMATION. Acetaminophen in large overdosage may cause hepatic toxicity in some patients. Following the ingestion of a potentially toxic overdose of acetaminophen, early symptoms, if present, may include: nausea, vomiting, abdominal

Continued on next page

McNeil Consumer—Cont.

pain, diaphoresis, generalized weakness and lethargy.
The antidote, when required, should be administered as early as possible, preferably within 16 hours of the overdose ingestion. Whether antidote therapy is required depends upon acetaminophen plasma levels, since patients' estimates of the quantity of a drug ingested as an overdose are notoriously unreliable. When a patient's history suggests ingestion of an overdose of acetaminophen, blood should be drawn immediately for an acetaminophen plasma assay, without regard to the presence or absence of symptomatology. It is important to determine as accurately as possible the elapsed time from ingestion of an overdose to the time of the plasma acetaminophen assay, since plasma levels at specific time points following an overdose correlate with the probable occurrence of hepatic toxicity.
How Supplied: Tablets (colored white, imprinted "SINE-AID")—bottles of 24, 50 and 100.

TYLENOL® acetaminophen OTC
Chewable Tablets, Elixir, Drops

Description: Each TYLENOL Chewable Tablet contains 80 mg. acetaminophen in a fruit flavored tablet. TYLENOL acetaminophen Elixir and Drops are stable, cherry flavored, red in color and contain only 7% alcohol.
TYLENOL Elixir: Each 5 ml. contains 120 mg. acetaminophen.
TYLENOL Drops: Each 0.6 ml. (one calibrated dropperful) contains 60 mg. acetaminophen.
Actions: TYLENOL acetaminophen is an antipyretic and analgesic clinically proven in pediatric use. TYLENOL acetaminophen produces antipyresis through action on the hypothalamic heat regulating center and analgesia by elevation of the pain threshold.
Indications: TYLENOL Chewable Tablets, Elixir and Drops are designed for treatment of infants and children with conditions requiring reduction of fever or relief of pain—such as mild upper respiratory infections (tonsillitis, common cold, "grippe"), headache, myalgia, post-immunization reactions, post-tonsillectomy discomfort and gastroenteritis. In conjunction with antibiotics or sulfonamides, TYLENOL acetaminophen is useful as an analgesic and antipyretic in many bacterial or viral infections, such as bronchitis, pharyngitis, tracheobronchitis, sinusitis, pneumonia, otitis media, and cervical adenitis.
Precautions and Adverse Reactions: If a rare sensitivity reaction occurs, the drug should be stopped. TYLENOL acetaminophen has rarely been found to produce any side effects. It is usually well tolerated by aspirin-sensitive patients.
Usual Dosage: Doses may be repeated 3 or 4 times daily.
TYLENOL Chewable Tablets: 3 years: One and one-half tablets. 4–5 years: Two and one-half tablets. 6–8 years: Three tablets. 9–12 years: Four tablets.
TYLENOL Elixir: *Under 1 year:* One-half teaspoonful. *1 to 3 years:* One-half to one teaspoonful. 3 years: One teaspoonful. 4–5 years: One and one-half teaspoonfuls. 6–8 years: Two teaspoonfuls. 9–12 years: Three teaspoonfuls.
TYLENOL Drops: *Under 1 year:* 0.6 ml. *1 to 3 years:* 0.6 to 1.2 ml. 3 years: 1.2 ml. 4–5 years: 1.8 ml.
Note: Since TYLENOL acetaminophen Chewable Tablets, Elixir and Drops are available without prescription as an analgesic, the following appears on the package labels: "WARNING: Consult a physician for use by children under 3 or for use longer than 10 days. Keep this and all medication out of the reach of children. In cases of accidental overdosage, contact a physician immediately."
Overdosage: The occurrence of acetaminophen overdose toxicity is uncommon in the pediatric age group. Even with large overdoses, children appear to be less vulnerable than adults to developing hepatotoxicity. This may be due to age-related differences that have been demonstrated in the metabolism of acetaminophen. Despite these differences, the measures outlined below should be immediately initiated in any child reported to have ingested a large overdose of acetaminophen.
IN ALL CASES OF SUSPECTED OVERDOSE, IMMEDIATELY CONTACT A POISON CONTROL CENTER OR McNEIL CONSUMER PRODUCTS COMPANY FOR ANTIDOTE INFORMATION. Acetaminophen in large overdosage may cause hepatic toxicity in some patients. Following the ingestion of a potentially toxic overdose of acetaminophen, early symptoms, if present, may include: nausea, vomiting, abdominal pain, diaphoresis, generalized weakness and lethargy.
The antidote, when required, may be administered as early as possible, preferably within 16 hours of the overdose ingestion. Whether antidote therapy is required depends upon acetaminophen plasma levels, since patients' estimates of the quantity of a drug ingested as an overdose are notoriously unreliable. When a patient's history suggests ingestion of an overdose of acetaminophen, blood should be drawn immediately for an acetaminophen plasma assay, without regard to the presence or absence of symptomatology. It is important to determine as accurately as possible the elapsed time from ingestion of an overdose to the time of the plasma acetaminophen assay, since plasma levels at specific time points following an overdose correlate with the probable occurrence of hepatic toxicity.
How Supplied: Chewable Tablets (colored pink, scored, imprinted "TYLENOL")—Bottles of 30. Elixir (colored red)—bottles of 2 and 4 fl. oz. Drops (colored crimson)—bottles of ½ oz. (15 ml.) with calibrated plastic dropper.
All packages listed above have child-resistant safety caps.
[*Shown in Product Identification Section*]

TYLENOL® acetaminophen Tablets OTC

Description: Each TYLENOL Tablet contains acetaminophen 325 mg.
Actions: TYLENOL acetaminophen is a clinically proven analgesic and antipyretic. TYLENOL acetaminophen produces analgesia by elevation of the pain threshold and antipyresis through action on the hypothalamic heat-regulating center.
Indications: TYLENOL acetaminophen provides effective analgesia in a wide variety of arthritic and rheumatic conditions involving musculoskeletal pain, as well as in other painful disorders such as headache, dysmenorrhea, myalgias and neuralgias. In addition, TYLENOL is indicated as an analgesic and antipyretic in diseases accompanied by discomfort and fever, such as the common cold and other viral infections. TYLENOL is particularly well suited as an analgesic-antipyretic in the presence of aspirin allergy, hemostatic disturbances (including anticoagulant therapy), and bleeding diatheses (e.g., ulcer, gastritis, hiatus hernia).
Precautions and Adverse Reactions: If a rare sensitivity reaction occurs, the drug should be stopped. TYLENOL acetaminophen has rarely been found to produce any side effects. It is usually well tolerated by aspirin-sensitive patients.
Usual Dosage: *Adults:* One to two tablets every 4–6 hours. Not to exceed 12 tablets per day. *Children* (6 to 12): One-half to one tablet 3 or 4 times daily. (TYLENOL acetaminophen Chewable Tablets, Elixir and Drops are available for greater convenience in younger patients.)
Note: Since TYLENOL acetaminophen tablets are available without prescription as an analgesic, the following appears on the package labels: "Consult a physician for use by children under 6 or for use longer than 10 days. WARNING: Keep this and all medication out of the reach of children. In case of accidental overdosage, contact a physician immediately." In connection with its use for temporary relief of minor aches and pains of arthritis and rheumatism: "Caution: If pain persists for more than 10 days, or redness is present, or in arthritic or rheumatic conditions affecting children under 12 years, consult a physician immediately."
Overdosage: IN ALL CASES OF SUSPECTED OVERDOSE, IMMEDIATELY CONTACT A POISON CONTROL CENTER OR McNEIL CONSUMER PRODUCTS COMPANY FOR ANTIDOTE INFORMATION. Acetaminophen in large overdosage may cause hepatic toxicity in some patients. Following the ingestion of a potentially toxic overdose of acetaminophen, early symptoms, if present, may include: nausea, vomiting, abdominal pain, diaphoresis, generalized weakness and lethargy.
The antidote, when required, should be administered as early as possible, preferably within 16 hours of the overdose ingestion. Whether antidote therapy is required depends upon acetaminophen plasma levels, since patients' estimates of the quantity of a drug ingested as an overdose are notoriously unreliable. When a patient's history suggests ingestion of an overdose of acetaminophen, blood should be drawn immediately for an acetaminophen plasma assay, without regard to the presence or absence of symptomatology. It is important to determine as accurately as possible the elapsed time from ingestion of an overdose to the time of the plasma acetaminophen assay, since plasma levels at specific time points following an overdose correlate with the probable occurrence of hepatic toxicity.
How Supplied: Tablets (colored white, scored, imprinted "TYLENOL")—tins of 12; bottles of 24, 50, 100 and 200.
Also Available: For additional pain relief, Extra-Strength TYLENOL® Capsules and Tablets, 500 mg, and Extra-Strength TYLENOL® Adult Liquid Pain Reliever (1 fl. oz. = 1000 mg.)
[*Shown in Product Identification Section*]

Extra-Strength
TYLENOL® acetaminophen OTC
Capsules and Tablets

Description: Each capsule or tablet contains acetaminophen 500 mg.
Actions: TYLENOL acetaminophen is a clinically proven analgesic and antipyretic. Acetaminophen produces analgesia by elevation of the pain threshold and antipyresis through action on the hypothalamic heat-regulating center.
Indications: For relief of pain and fever. TYLENOL Extra-Strength Capsules and Tablets provide increased analgesic strength for minor conditions when the usual doses of mild analgesics are insufficient.
Precautions and Adverse Reactions: If a rare sensitivity reaction occurs, the drug should be stopped. TYLENOL acetaminophen has rarely been found to produce any side effects. It is usually well tolerated by aspirin-sensitive patients.
Usual Dosage: Adults: Two capsules or tablets 3 or 4 times daily. No more than a total of eight capsules or tablets in any 24-hour period.
Note: Since TYLENOL Extra-Strength Capsules and Tablets are available without a prescription, the following appears on the package labels: "Severe or recurrent pain or high or continued fever may be indicative of serious illness. Under these conditions, consult a physician. WARNING: Keep this and all medication out of the reach of children. In case of acciden-

tal overdosage, contact a physician immediately."

Overdosage: IN ALL CASES OF SUSPECTED OVERDOSE, IMMEDIATELY CONTACT A POISON CONTROL CENTER OR McNEIL CONSUMER PRODUCTS COMPANY FOR ANTIDOTE INFORMATION. Acetaminophen in large overdosage may cause hepatic toxicity in some patients. Following the ingestion of a potentially toxic overdose of acetaminophen, early symptoms, if present, may include: nausea, vomiting, abdominal pain, diaphoresis, generalized weakness and lethargy.

The antidote, when required, should be administered as early as possible, preferably within 16 hours of the overdose ingestion. Whether antidote therapy is required depends upon acetaminophen plasma levels, since patients' estimates of the quantity of a drug ingested as an overdose are notoriously unreliable. When a patient's history suggests ingestion of an overdose of acetaminophen, blood should be drawn immediately for an acetaminophen plasma assay, without regard to the presence or absence of symptomatology. It is important to determine as accurately as possible the elapsed time from ingestion of an overdose to the time of the plasma acetaminophen assay, since plasma levels at specific time points following an overdose correlate with the probable occurrence of hepatic toxicity.

How Supplied: Capsules (colored red and white, imprinted "TYLENOL 500 mg.")—bottles of 24, 50 and 100; Tablets (colored white, imprinted "TYLENOL" and "500")—bottles of 30, 60 and 100.

Also Available: For adults who prefer liquids or can't swallow solid medication, Extra-Strength TYLENOL® Adult Liquid Pain Reliever (1 fl. oz. = 1000 mg.).

[*Shown in Product Identification Section*]

Extra-Strength **OTC**
TYLENOL® acetaminophen
Adult Liquid Pain Reliever

Description: Each 15 ml. (½ fl. oz. or one tablespoonful) contains 500 mg. acetaminophen (alcohol 8 ½%).

Actions: TYLENOL acetaminophen is a clinically proven analgesic and antipyretic. Acetaminophen produces analgesia by elevation of the pain threshold and antipyresis through action on the hypothalamic heat-regulating center.

Indications: TYLENOL acetaminophen provides fast, effective relief of pain and/or fever for adults who prefer liquids or can't swallow solid medication, e.g., the aged, patients with easily triggered gag reflexes, extremely sore throats, or those on liquid diets.

Precautions and Adverse Reactions: If a rare sensitivity reaction occurs, the drug should be stopped. TYLENOL acetaminophen has rarely been found to produce any side effects. It is usually well tolerated by aspirin-sensitive patients.

Usual Dosage: Extra-Strength TYLENOL Adult Liquid is an adult preparation. Not for use in children under 12. Measuring cup is marked for accurate dosage.

Extra-Strength Dose—1 fl. oz. (1000 mg.), which is equivalent to two Extra-Strength TYLENOL tablets or capsules, every 4 to 6 hours, no more than 4 doses in any 24 hour period.

Note: Since TYLENOL Extra-Strength Adult Liquid Pain Reliever is available without a prescription, the following appears on the package labels: "Severe or recurrent pain or high or continued fever may be indicative of serious illness. Under these conditions, consult a physician. WARNING: Keep this and all medication out of the reach of children. In case of accidental overdosage, contact a physician immediately.

Overdosage: IN ALL CASES OF SUSPECTED OVERDOSE, IMMEDIATELY CONTACT A POISON CONTROL CENTER OR McNEIL CONSUMER PRODUCTS COMPANY FOR ANTIDOTE INFORMATION. Acetaminophen in large overdosage may cause hepatic toxicity in some patients. Following the ingestion of a potentially toxic overdose of acetaminophen, early symptoms, if present, may include: nausea, vomiting, abdominal pain, diaphoresis, generalized weakness and lethargy.

The antidote, when required, should be administered as early as possible, preferably within 16 hours of the overdose ingestion. Whether antidote therapy is required depends upon acetaminophen plasma levels, since patients' estimates of the quantity of a drug ingested as an overdose are notoriously unreliable. When a patient's history suggests ingestion of an overdose of acetaminophen, blood should be drawn immediately for an acetaminophen plasma assay, without regard to the presence or absence of symptomatology. It is important to determine as accurately as possible the elapsed time from ingestion of an overdose to the time of the plasma acetaminophen assay, since plasma levels at specific time points following an overdose correlate with the probable occurrence of hepatic toxicity.

How Supplied: Mint-flavored liquid (colored green), bottles of 8 and 16 fl. oz. with child resistent safety cap and special dosage cup.

McNeil Laboratories
McNEILAB, INC.
FORT WASHINGTON, PA 19034

BUTISOL SODIUM® ©
(sodium butabarbital) ℞
tablets, elixir
BUTICAPS® (sodium butabarbital) capsules
(Warning: May be habit forming.)

Description: Butabarbital is a barbituric acid derivative. The sodium salt occurs as a white, bitter powder which is freely soluble in water and alcohol but practically insoluble in benzene and ether.

Clinical Pharmacology: Following oral administration of BUTISOL SODIUM, peak plasma concentrations of butabarbital are reached on the average of 1.5 hours. Plasma elimination half-life following single oral dose has been estimated to be 100 hours. Less than 1% of the administered dose is excreted unmetabolized in the urine.

Actions: Butabarbital is a general depressant with the central nervous system being the most sensitive to this effect. In ordinary doses the drug acts as a sedative and hypnotic. The onset of action is approximately thirty minutes and the duration of action is from 5 to 6 hours. It is partially detoxified in the body and partly excreted unchanged in the urine.

Indications: For use as a sedative or hypnotic.

Hypnotic Use: The prolonged administration of BUTISOL SODIUM as a hypnotic is not recommended since it has not been shown to be effective for a period of more than 14 days. Should insomnia persist, drug-free intervals of one or more weeks should elapse before retreatment is considered. Attempts should be made to find alternative non-drug therapy in chronic insomnia.

Contraindications: This drug should not be given to patients with known sensitivity or idiosyncracy to barbiturates. It is contraindicated in patients with a history of manifest or latent porphyria or marked impairment of liver function, or with respiratory disease where dyspnea or obstruction is evident. It should not be administered to persons with known previous addiction to the sedative/hypnotic group, since ordinary doses may be ineffectual and may contribute to further addiction.

Warnings: BUTISOL SODIUM alone should not be administered in the presence of acute or chronic pain since paradoxical excitement may be induced or important symptoms might be masked.

This drug may impair the mental and/or physical abilities, required for the performance of potentially hazardous tasks such as driving a vehicle or operating machinery. The concomitant use of alcohol or other central nervous system depressants may have an additive effect. Patients should be warned accordingly.

Barbiturates induce liver microsomal enzyme activity. This accelerates the biotransformation of various drugs and is probably part of the mechanism of the tolerance which is seen with barbiturates. Butabarbital may decrease the potency of the coumarin anticoagulants so that patients receiving such concomitant therapy should have more frequent prothrombin determinations.

Usage in Pregnancy: The lack of adverse effects of this drug on fetal development has not been established. Therefore, its use in pregnancy is not recommended.

Drug Abuse and Dependence: Prolonged use of barbiturates, even in therapeutic dosages, may result in psychological dependence. These persons may increase dosage without consulting a physician and may subsequently develop a physical dependence on the drug. In such cases, abrupt discontinuance may precipitate typical withdrawal symptoms, including convulsions. Therefore, the drug should be withdrawn gradually from any patient known to be taking excessive dosages over long periods of time.

Precautions: As with other sedatives and hypnotics, elderly or debilitated patients may react to barbiturates with marked excitement or depression.

The systemic effects of exogenous hydrocortisone and endogenous hydrocortisone (cortisol) may be diminished by sodium butabarbital. Thus, BUTISOL SODIUM (sodium butabarbital) should be administered with caution to patients with borderline hypoadrenal function, whether of pituitary or primary adrenal origin.

Adverse Reactions: Adverse reactions reported include the following:

CNS depression: Residual sedation or "hangover," drowsiness, lethargy.

Respiratory/circulatory: Respiratory depression, apnea, circulatory collapse.

Allergic: Hypersensitivity reactions may occur, especially in those individuals with asthma, urticaria, angioneurotic edema, or similar conditions; skin eruptions.

Other: Nausea and vomiting, "headache."

Overdosage: This is manifested by coma, early hypothermia, later fever, sluggish or absent reflexes, respiratory depression, and gradual appearance of circulatory collapse and pulmonary edema. The treatment consists of:

a. Maintenance of an adequate airway, with assisted ventilation and oxygen administration as indicated.
b. Monitoring of vital signs and fluid balance.
c. Aspirate stomach contents, taking care to avoid pulmonary aspiration.
d. Fluid therapy and other standard treatment for shock, as required.
e. If renal function is normal, forced diuresis may aid in the elimination of the barbiturate.
f. Dialysis if indicated.
g. Antibiotics to control pulmonary complications when needed.

Dosage and Administration: For adults: as a daytime sedative, 15 mg. to 30 mg. 3 or 4 times daily; as a bedtime hypnotic or preoperative sedative, 50 mg. to 100 mg. For children: as a daytime sedative, dosage range is 7.5 mg. to 30 mg. depending on age, weight, and degree of

Continued on next page

McNeil Laboratories—Cont.

sedation desired; as a bedtime hypnotic or preoperative sedative the dose is to be determined by the physician according to age and weight.

How Supplied: BUTISOL SODIUM® (sodium butabarbital) 15 mg. Tablets, (colored lavender, imprinted "McNEIL" scored)—NDC 0045-0112, bottles of 100 and 1000. BUTISOL SODIUM® (sodium butabarbital) 30 mg. Tablets, (colored green, imprinted "McNEIL" scored)—NDC 0045-0113, bottles of 100 and 1000.

BUTISOL SODIUM® (sodium butabarbital) 50 mg. Tablets, (colored orange, imprinted "McNEIL" scored)—NDC 0045-0114, bottles of 100 and 1000.

BUTISOL SODIUM® (sodium butabarbital) 100 mg. Tablets, (colored pink, imprinted "McNEIL" scored)—NDC 0045-0115-60, bottles of 100.

BUTISOL SODIUM® (sodium butabarbital) elixir 30 mg./5 ml., alcohol 7% (colored green)—NDC 0045-0110, bottles of pints and gallons.

BUTICAPS® (sodium butabarbital) 15 mg. Capsules, (colored lavender and white, imprinted "McNEIL"). NDC 0045-0060-60 bottles of 100.

BUTICAPS® (sodium butabarbital) 30 mg. Capsules, (colored green and white, imprinted "McNEIL"). NDC 0045-0061-60 bottles of 100.

97412

COTYLENOL® Cold Formula Tablets OTC

(For Product Information, see McNeil Consumer Products Company)

COTYLENOL® Liquid Cold Formula (with Cough Suppressant) OTC

(For Product Information, see McNeil Consumer Products Company)

GRIFULVIN V® (griseofulvin microsize) tablets, suspension ℞

(For Product Information, see Ortho Pharmaceutical Corporation)

HALDOL® brand of haloperidol tablets, concentrate, injection ℞

1 mg (1000's):
Military NSN 6505-01-003-2415
VA NSN 6505-01-003-2415A
2 mg (1000's):
Military NSN 6505-00-876-7239
VA NSN 6505-00-876-7239A
5 mg (1000's):
Military NSN 6505-01-003-2416
VA NSN 6505-01-003-2416A
10 mg (1000's):
Military NSN 6505-01-003-2417
VA NSN 6505-01-003-2417A
Concentrate 120 ml:
VA NSN 6505-01-003-5341A
Injection 1 ml:
VA NSN 6505-00-268-8530A

Description: Haloperidol is the first of the butyrophenone series of major tranquilizers. The chemical designation for haloperidol is 4-[4-(p-chlorophenyl)-4-hydroxypiperidino]-4'-fluorobutyrophenone.

Actions: The precise mechanism of action has not been clearly established.

Indications: HALDOL haloperidol is indicated for use in the management of manifestations of psychotic disorders.

Haloperidol is indicated for the control of tics and vocal utterances of Gilles de la Tourette's Syndrome in children and adults.

Haloperidol is effective for the treatment of severe behavior problems in children of combative, explosive hyperexcitability (which cannot be accounted for by immediate provocation).

Haloperidol is effective in the short-term treatment of hyperactive children who show excessive motor activity with accompanying conduct disorders consisting of some or all of the following symptoms: impulsivity, difficulty sustaining attention, aggressivity, mood lability, and poor frustration tolerance.

Contraindications: HALDOL haloperidol is contraindicated in patients who are severely depressed, comatose, have CNS depression due to alcohol or other centrally-acting depressants or have Parkinson's disease.

HALDOL haloperidol is contraindicated in individuals who are hypersensitive to this drug.

Warnings: ***Usage in Pregnancy:*** Rodents given 2 to 20 times the usual maximum human dose of haloperidol by oral or parenteral routes showed an increased incidence of resorption, reduced fertility, delayed delivery and pup mortality. No teratogenic effect has been reported in rats, rabbits or dogs at dosages within this range, but cleft palate has been observed in mice given 15 times the usual maximum human dose. Cleft palate in mice appears to be a non-specific response to stress or nutritional imbalance as well as to a variety of drugs and there is no evidence to relate this phenomenon to predictable human risk for most of these agents.

There are no well controlled studies with haloperidol in pregnant women. There are reports, however, of two cases of limb malformations observed following maternal use of haloperidol along with other drugs which have suspected teratogenic potential during the first trimester of pregnancy. Causal relationships were not established in either case. Since such experience does not exclude the possibility of fetal damage due to haloperidol, this drug should be used during pregnancy or in women likely to become pregnant only if benefit clearly justifies a potential risk to the fetus. Infants should not be nursed during drug treatment.

Combined Use of HALDOL haloperidol and Lithium: An encephalopathic syndrome (characterized by weakness, lethargy, fever, tremulousness and confusion, extrapyramidal symptoms, leucocytosis, elevated serum enzymes, BUN and FBS) followed by irreversible brain damage has occurred in a few patients treated with lithium plus haloperidol. A causal relationship between these events and the concomitant administration of lithium and haloperidol has not been established; however, patients receiving such combined therapy should be monitored closely for early evidence of neurological toxicity and treatment discontinued promptly if such signs appear.

General: A number of cases of bronchopneumonia, some fatal, have followed the use of major tranquilizers, including haloperidol. It has been postulated that lethargy and decreased sensation of thirst due to central inhibition may lead to dehydration, hemoconcentration and reduced pulmonary ventilation. Therefore, if the above signs and symptoms appear, especially in the elderly, the physician should institute remedial therapy promptly.

Although not reported with HALDOL haloperidol, decreased serum cholesterol and/or cutaneous and ocular changes have been reported in patients receiving chemically-related drugs.

HALDOL haloperidol may impair the mental and/or physical abilities required for the performance of hazardous tasks such as operating machinery or driving a motor vehicle. The ambulatory patient should be warned accordingly.

The use of alcohol with this drug should be avoided due to possible additive effects and hypotension.

Precautions: HALDOL haloperidol should be administered cautiously to patients:

—with severe cardiovascular disorders, because of the possibility of transient hypotension and/or precipitation of anginal pain. Should hypotension occur and a vasopressor be required, epinephrine should not be used since HALDOL haloperidol may block its vasopressor activity and paradoxical further lowering of the blood pressure may occur.

—receiving anticonvulsant medication, because HALDOL haloperidol may lower the convulsive threshold. Adequate anticonvulsant therapy should be maintained concomitantly.

—with known allergies, or with a history of allergic reactions to drugs.

—receiving anticoagulants, since an isolated instance of interference occurred with the effects of one anticoagulant (phenindione).

If concomitant antiparkinson medication is required, it may have to be continued after HALDOL haloperidol is discontinued because of the difference in excretion rates. If both are discontinued simultaneously, extrapyramidal symptoms may occur. The physician should keep in mind the possible increase in intraocular pressure when anticholinergic drugs, including antiparkinson agents, are administered concomitantly with HALDOL haloperidol.

When HALDOL haloperidol is used to control mania in cyclic disorders, there may be a rapid mood swing to depression.

Severe neurotoxicity (rigidity, inability to walk or talk) may occur in patients with thyrotoxicosis who are also receiving antipsychotic medication, including HALDOL haloperidol.

Adverse Reactions: ***CNS Effects:*** *Extrapyramidal Reactions*—Neuromuscular (extrapyramidal) reactions during the administration of HALDOL haloperidol have been reported frequently, often during the first few days of treatment. In most patients, these reactions involved Parkinson-like symptoms which, when first observed, were usually mild to moderately severe and usually reversible. Other types of neuromuscular reactions (motor restlessness, dystonia, akathisia, hyperreflexia, opisthotonos, oculogyric crises) have been reported far less frequently, but were often more severe. Severe extrapyramidal reactions have been reported to occur at relatively low doses. Generally the occurrence and severity of most extrapyramidal symptoms are dose related since they occur at relatively high doses and have been shown to disappear or become less severe when the dose is reduced. Administration of antiparkinson drugs such as benztropine mesylate U.S.P. or trihexyphenidyl hydrochloride U.S.P. may be required for control of such reactions. It should be noted that persistent extrapyramidal reactions have been reported and that the drug may have to be discontinued in such cases.

Withdrawal Emergent Neurological Signs—Generally, patients receiving short term therapy experience no problems with abrupt discontinuation of antipsychotic drugs. However, some patients on maintenance treatment experience transient dyskinetic signs after abrupt withdrawal. In certain of these cases the dyskinetic movements are indistinguishable from the syndrome described below under "Persistent Tardive Dyskinesia" except for duration. It is not known whether gradual withdrawal of antipsychotic drugs will reduce the rate of occurrence of withdrawal emergent neurological signs but until further evidence becomes available, it seems reasonable to gradually withdraw use of haloperidol.

Persistent Tardive Dyskinesia—Although rarely reported with HALDOL halperidol, certain antipsychotic agents have been associated with persistent dyskinesias. Tardive dyskinesia may appear in some patients on long-term therapy or may occur after drug therapy has been discontinued. The risk appears to be greater in elderly patients on high-dose therapy, especially females. The symptoms are persistent and in some patients appear irreversible. The syndrome is characterized by rhythmical involuntary movements of tongue, face, mouth or jaw (e.g., protrusion of tongue, puffing of cheeks, puckering of mouth, chewing movements). Sometimes these may be accompanied by involuntary movements of extremities.

There is no known effective treatment for tardive dyskinesia; antiparkinson agents usually do not alleviate the symptoms of this syndrome. It is suggested that all antipsychotic agents be discontinued if these symptoms appear. Should it be necessary to reinstitute treatment, or increase the dosage of the agent, or switch to a different antipsychotic agent, this syndrome may be masked.

It has been reported that fine vermicular movement of the tongue may be an early sign of the syndrome and if the medication is stopped at that time the syndrome may not develop.

Other CNS Effects—Insomnia, restlessness, anxiety, euphoria, agitation, drowsiness, depression, lethargy, headache, confusion, vertigo, grand mal seizures, and exacerbation of psychotic symptoms including hallucinations.

Cardiovascular Effects: Tachycardia and hypotension.

Hematologic Effects: Reports have appeared citing the occurrence of mild and usually transient leukopenia and leukocytosis, minimal decreases in red blood cell counts, anemia, or a tendency toward lymphomonocytosis. Agranulocytosis has rarely been reported to have occurred with the use of haloperidol, and then only in association with other medication.

Liver Effects: Impaired liver function and/or jaundice have been reported.

Dermatologic Reactions: Maculopapular and acneiform skin reactions and isolated cases of photosensitivity and loss of hair.

Endocrine Disorders: Lactation, breast engorgement, mastalgia, menstrual irregularities, gynecomastia, impotence, increased libido, hyperglycemia and hypoglycemia.

Gastrointestinal Effects: Anorexia, constipation, diarrhea, hypersalivation, dyspepsia, nausea and vomiting.

Autonomic Reactions: Dry mouth, blurred vision, urinary retention and diaphoresis.

Respiratory Effects: Laryngospasm, bronchospasm and increased depth of respiration.

Dosage and Administration: There is considerable variation from patient to patient in the amount of medication required for therapy. As with all neuroleptic drugs, it is vitally important to titrate the dose of HALDOL haloperidol to the needs of each patient. Titration should be carried out as rapidly as practicable to achieve optimum therapeutic control.

To determine the initial dosage, consideration should be given to the patient's age, severity of illness, previous response to other neuroleptic drugs and any concomitant medication or disease state. Patients with previous adverse reactions to neuroleptic drugs and those who are elderly or debilitated may require less HALDOL haloperidol. The optimal response in such patients is usually obtained with more gradual titration and at lower dosage levels.

In severely disturbed nonpsychotic children or in hyperactive children with accompanying conduct disorders, it should be noted that since these behaviors may be short lived, short-term administration of HALDOL haloperidol may suffice. There is no evidence establishing a maximum effective dosage. There is little evidence that behavior improvement is further enhanced in dosages beyond 6 mg per day.

Clinical experience suggests the following recommendations:

Oral Administration

Initial Dosage Range

Moderate Symptomatology	0.5 mg. to 2.0 mg. b.i.d. or t.i.d.
Severe Symptomatology	3.0 mg. to 5.0 mg. b.i.d. or t.i.d.

To achieve prompt control, higher doses may be required in some cases.

Geriatric or Debilitated Patients	0.5 mg. to 2.0 mg. b.i.d. or t.i.d.
Chronic or Resistant Patients	3.0 mg. to 5.0 mg. b.i.d. or t.i.d.

Patients who remain severely disturbed or inadequately controlled may occasionally require further titration of dosage. Daily dosages up to 100 mg. may be necessary in some cases to achieve an optimal response. Infrequently HALDOL haloperidol has been used in doses above 100 mg. for severely resistant patients; however, the limited clinical usage has not demonstrated the safety of prolonged administration of such doses.

Maintenance Dosage

Upon achieving a satisfactory therapeutic response, dosage should then be gradually reduced to the lowest effective maintenance level.

Intramuscular Administration

Parenteral medication, administered intramuscularly in doses of 2 to 5 mg., is utilized for prompt control of the acutely agitated patient with moderately severe to very severe symptoms. Depending on the response of the patient, subsequent doses may be given, administered as often as every hour, although 4 to 8 hour intervals may be satisfactory. The oral form should supplant the injectable as soon as practicable.

Overdosage: ***Manifestations:*** In general, the symptoms of overdosage would be an exaggeration of known pharmacologic effects and adverse reactions, the most prominent of which would be: 1) severe extrapyramidal reactions, 2) hypotension, or 3) sedation. The patient would appear comatose with respiratory depression and hypotension which could be severe enough to produce a shock-like state. The extrapyramidal reaction would be manifest by muscular weakness or rigidity and a generalized or localized tremor as demonstrated by the akinetic or agitans types respectively. With accidental overdosage, hypertension rather than hypotension occurred in a two-year-old child.

Treatment: Gastric lavage or induction of emesis should be carried out immediately followed by administration of activated charcoal. Since there is no specific antidote, treatment is primarily supportive. A patent airway must be established by use of an oropharyngeal airway or endotracheal tube or, in prolonged cases of coma, by tracheostomy. Respiratory depression may be counteracted by artificial respiration and mechanical respirators. Hypotension and circulatory collapse may be counteracted by use of intravenous fluids, plasma, or concentrated albumin, and vasopressor agents such as norepinephrine. Epinephrine should not be used. In case of severe extrapyramidal reactions antiparkinson medication should be administered.

How Supplied: HALDOL® brand of haloperidol Tablets Scored, Imprinted "McNEIL"—½ mg (Colored White) **NDC** 0045-0240; 1 mg (Colored Yellow) **NDC** 0045-0241; 2 mg (Colored Pink) **NDC** 0045-0242—Bottles of 100 and 1000 and 1000 in Unit Dose; 5 mg (Colored Green) **NDC** 0045-0245 and 10 mg (Colored Aqua) **NDC** 0045-0246—Bottles of 50, 100 and 1000 and 1000 in Unit Dose.

HALDOL® brand of haloperidol Concentrate 2 mg per ml (as the lactate) Colorless, Odorless, and Tasteless Solution—**NDC** 0045-0250-15, bottles of 15 ml and **NDC** 0045-0250-04, bottles of 120 ml.

HALDOL® brand of haloperidol Injection 5 mg per ml (as the lactate)—**NDC** 0045-0255-01, units of 10 × 1 ml ampuls; **NDC** 0045-0255-49, 10 ml multiple-dose vial.

HALDOL tablets are manufactured by McNeil Laboratories Co., Dorado, Puerto Rico 00646.

[*Shown in Product Identification Section*]

INAPSINE® (droperidol) injection ℞

(For Product Information, see Janssen Pharmaceutica Inc.)

INNOVAR® injection Ⓒ ℞

(For Product Information, see Janssen Pharmaceutica Inc.)

PARAFLEX® (chlorzoxazone) tablets ℞

Description: Each tablet contains chlorzoxazone 250 mg.

Actions: Chlorzoxazone is a centrally-acting agent for painful musculoskeletal conditions. Data available from animal experiments as well as human study indicate that chlorzoxazone acts primarily at the level of the spinal cord and subcortical areas of the brain where it inhibits multisynaptic reflex arcs involved in producing and maintaining skeletal muscle spasm of varied etiology. The clinical result is a reduction of the skeletal muscle spasm with relief of pain and increased mobility of the involved muscles. Blood levels of chlorzoxazone can be detected in man during the first hour after administration and reach peak levels in the third and fourth hours. Chlorzoxazone is rapidly metabolized and excreted in the urine, primarily in a conjugated form as the glucuronide. Less than one percent of a dose of chlorzoxazone is excreted unchanged in the urine in 24 hours.

Indications: PARAFLEX chlorzoxazone is indicated as an adjunct to rest, physical therapy, and other measures for the relief of discomfort associated with acute, painful musculoskeletal conditions. The mode of action of this drug has not been clearly identified, but may be related to its sedative properties. Chlorzoxazone does not directly relax tense skeletal muscles in man.

Contraindications: PARAFLEX chlorzoxazone is contraindicated in patients with known intolerance to the drug.

Warnings: *Usage in Pregnancy:* The safe use of PARAFLEX chlorzoxazone has not been established with respect to the possible adverse effects upon fetal development. Therefore, it should be used in women of childbearing potential only when, in the judgment of the physician, the potential benefits outweigh the possible risks.

Precautions: PARAFLEX chlorzoxazone should be used with caution in patients with known allergies or with a history of allergic reactions to drugs. If a sensitivity reaction occurs such as urticaria, redness, or itching of the skin, the drug should be stopped.

If any signs or symptoms suggestive of liver dysfunction are observed, the drug should be discontinued.

Adverse Reactions: After more than twenty-one years of extensive clinical use of PARAFLEX chlorzoxazone and other chlorzoxazone-containing products in an estimated twenty-three million patients, it is apparent that the drug is well tolerated and seldom produces undesirable side effects. Occasional patients may develop gastrointestinal disturbances. It is possible in rare instances that PARAFLEX chlorzoxazone may have been associated with gastrointestinal bleeding. Drowsiness, dizziness, lightheadedness, malaise, or overstimulation may be noted by an occasional patient. Rarely, allergic-type skin rashes, petechiae, or ecchymoses may develop during treatment. Angioneurotic edema or anaphylactic reactions are extremely rare. There is no evi-

Continued on next page

McNeil Laboratories—Cont.

dence that the drug will cause renal damage. Rarely, a patient may note discoloration of the urine resulting from a phenolic metabolite of chlorzoxazone. This finding is of no known clinical significance.
Approximately twenty-seven patients have been reported in whom the administration of PARAFLEX chlorzoxazone or other chlorzoxazone-containing products was suspected as being the cause of liver damage. In one case, the jaundice was subsequently considered to be due to a carcinoma of the head of the pancreas rather than to the drug. In a second case, there was no jaundice but an elevated alkaline phosphatase and BSP retention. In this patient there was a malignancy with bony and liver metastases. The role of the drug was difficult to determine. A third and fourth case had cholelithiasis. Diagnosis in a fifth case was submassive hepatic necrosis possibly due to abusive use of the drug for approximately one year. The remaining cases had a clinical picture compatible with either a viral hepatitis or a drug-induced hepatitis. In all these latter cases the drug was stopped, and, with one exception, the patients recovered. It is not possible to state that the hepatitis in these patients was or was not drug-induced.
Dosage and Administration: ***Usual Adult Dosage:*** One tablet (250 mg.) three or four times daily. Initial dosage for painful musculoskeletal conditions should be two tablets (500 mg.) three or four times daily. If adequate response is not obtained with this dose, it may be increased to three tablets (750 mg.) three or four times daily. As improvement occurs dosage can usually be reduced.
Usual Child's Dosage: One-half to two tablets (125 mg. to 500 mg.) three or four times daily given according to age and weight. The tablets may be crushed and mixed with food or a suitable vehicle for administration to children.
How Supplied: Tablets (colored orange, scored, imprinted "McNEIL")—bottles of 100 **NDC** 0045-0317-60.

PARAFON FORTE® tablets ℞
500's:
Military NSN 6505-00-764-3313
VA NSN 6505-00-764-3313A

Description: Each tablet contains chlorzoxazone 250 mg. and acetaminophen 300 mg.
Actions: PARAFON FORTE tablets provide symptomatic relief of pain, stiffness, and limitation of motion associated with most musculoskeletal disorders through (a) relaxation of muscle spasm by chlorzoxazone, an effective and well-tolerated centrally-acting agent; and (b) analgesia by acetaminophen, a nonsalicylate analgesic useful in skeletal muscle pain.
Data available from animal experiments, as well as human study, indicate that chlorzoxazone acts primarily at the level of the spinal cord and subcortical areas of the brain where it inhibits multisynaptic reflex arcs involved in producing and maintaining skeletal muscle spasm of varied etiology. Blood levels of chlorzoxazone can be detected in man during the first hour after administration and reach peak levels by the third to fourth hour. Chlorzoxazone is rapidly metabolized and is excreted in the urine, primarily in a conjugated form as the glucuronide. Less than one percent of a dose of chlorzoxazone is excreted unchanged in the urine in 24 hours.
Acetaminophen provides analgesic action to supplement that which results secondarily from muscle relaxation. Acetaminophen is rapidly absorbed after oral administration, with peak plasma levels occurring in one to two hours. After eight hours, only negligible amounts remain in the blood. Only 4 percent is excreted unchanged; 85 percent of the ingested dose is recovered in the urine in conjugated form as the glucuronide.

> **Indications:** Based on a review of this drug by the National Academy of Sciences-National Research Council and/or other information, FDA has classified the indications as follows:
> "Probably" effective as an adjunct to rest and physical therapy for the relief of discomfort associated with acute, painful musculoskeletal conditions. The mode of action of this drug has not been clearly identified, but may be related to its sedative properties. Chlorzoxazone does not directly relax tense skeletal muscles in man.

Contraindications: PARAFON FORTE tablets are contraindicated in patients sensitive to either component.
Warnings: *Usage in Pregnancy:* The safe use of PARAFON FORTE tablets has not been established with respect to the possible adverse effects upon fetal development. Therefore, it should be used in women of childbearing potential only when, in the judgment of the physician, the potential benefits outweigh the possible risks.
Precautions: PARAFON FORTE tablets should be used with caution in patients with known allergies or with a history of allergic reactions to drugs. If a sensitivity reaction occurs such as urticaria, redness, or itching of the skin, the drug should be stopped.
If any signs or symptoms suggestive of liver dysfunction are observed, the drug should be discontinued.
Adverse Reactions: After more than twenty-one years of extensive clinical use of PARAFLEX® (chlorzoxazone) tablets and other chlorzoxazone-containing products in an estimated twenty-three million patients, it is apparent that the drug is well tolerated and seldom produces undesirable side effects. Occasional patients may develop gastrointestinal disturbances. It is possible in rare instances that chlorzoxazone may have been associated with gastrointestinal bleeding. Drowsiness, dizziness, lightheadedness, malaise, or overstimulation may be noted by an occasional patient. Rarely, allergic-type skin rashes, petechiae, or ecchymoses may develop during treatment. Angioneurotic edema or anaphylactic reactions are extremely rare. There is no evidence that the drug will cause renal damage. Rarely, a patient may note discoloration of the urine resulting from a phenolic metabolite of chlorzoxazone. This finding is of no known clinical significance.
Approximately twenty-seven patients have been reported in whom the administration of PARAFLEX chlorzoxazone or other chlorzoxazone-containing products was suspected as being the cause of liver damage. In one case, the jaundice was subsequently considered to be due to a carcinoma of the head of the pancreas rather than to the drug. In a second case, there was no jaundice but an elevated alkaline phosphatase and BSP retention. In this patient there was a malignancy with bony and liver metastases. The role of the drug was difficult to determine. A third and fourth case had cholelithiasis. Diagnosis in a fifth case was submassive hepatic necrosis possibly due to abusive use of the drug for approximately one year. The remaining cases had a clinical picture compatible with either a viral hepatitis or a drug-induced hepatitis. In all these latter cases the drug was stopped, and, with one exception, the patients recovered. It is not possible to state that the hepatitis in these patients was or was not drug induced.
Acetaminophen has rarely been found to produce any side effects.
Dosage and Administration *Usual Adult Dosage:* Two tablets 4 times daily.
Overdosage: Acetaminophen in massive overdosage may cause hepatotoxicity in some patients. Clinical and laboratory evidence of hepatotoxicity may be delayed for up to one week. Close clinical monitoring and serial hepatic enzyme determinations are therefore recommended.
How Supplied: Tablets (colored green, scored, imprinted "McNEIL")—bottles of 100 **NDC** 0045-0322-60 and 500 **NDC** 0045-0322-70; Unit dose of 200 **NDC** 0045-0322-58.
Manufactured by McNeil Laboratories Co., Dorado, Puerto Rico 00646
[*Shown in Product Identification Section*]

SUBLIMAZE® (fentanyl) injection Ⓒ ℞
(For Product Information, see Janssen Pharmaceutica Inc.)

TOLECTIN® DS (tolmetin sodium) capsules ℞
TOLECTIN® (tolmetin sodium) tablets for oral administration
200 mg. tablets—500's:
Military NSN 6505-01-030-3241
VA NSN 6505-01-030-3241A

Description: TOLECTIN DS (tolmetin sodium) capsules for oral administration contain tolmetin sodium as the dihydrate in an amount equivalent to 400 mg. of tolmetin. Each capsule contains 36 mg. (1.568 mEq.) of sodium.
TOLECTIN (tolmetin sodium) tablets for oral administration contain tolmetin sodium as the dihydrate in an amount equivalent to 200 mg. of tolmetin (scored for 100 mg.). Each tablet contains 18 mg. (0.784 mEq.) of sodium.
Tolmetin sodium is a non-steroidal anti-inflammatory agent.
Clinical Pharmacology: Studies in animals have shown TOLECTIN (tolmetin sodium) to possess anti-inflammatory, analgesic and antipyretic activity. In the rat, TOLECTIN prevents the development of experimentally induced polyarthritis and also decreases established inflammation.
The mode of action of TOLECTIN is not known. However, studies in laboratory animals and man have demonstrated that the anti-inflammatory action of TOLECTIN is *not* due to pituitary-adrenal stimulation. TOLECTIN inhibits prostaglandin synthetase *in vitro* and lowers the plasma level of prostaglandin E in man. This reduction in prostaglandin synthesis may be responsible for the anti-inflammatory action. TOLECTIN does not appear to alter the course of the underlying disease in man.
In patients with rheumatoid arthritis and in normal volunteers, TOLECTIN is rapidly and almost completely absorbed with peak plasma levels being reached within 30–60 minutes after an oral therapeutic dose. The drug is eliminated from the plasma with a mean half-life of one hour. Peak plasma levels of approximately 40 μg./ml. are obtained with a 400 mg. oral dose. Essentially, all of the administered dose is recovered in the urine in 24 hours either as an inactive oxidative metabolite or as conjugates of TOLECTIN.
In two fecal blood loss studies of 4 to 6 days duration involving 15 subjects each, TOLECTIN did not induce an increase in blood loss over that observed during a 4-day drug-free control period. In the same studies, aspirin produced a greater blood loss than occurred during the drug-free control period, and a greater blood loss than occurred during the TOLECTIN treatment period. In one of the two studies, indomethacin produced a greater fecal blood loss than occurred during the drug-free control period; in the second study, indomethacin did not induce a significant increase in blood loss.
TOLECTIN does not interfere with the clinical assessment of the tuberculin skin test or the immediate-type hypersensitivity skin test. It appears that the drug does not interfere with

the immune mechanism as measured by skin testing.

Indications and Usage: TOLECTIN (tolmetin sodium) is indicated for the relief of signs and symptoms of rheumatoid arthritis and osteoarthritis. TOLECTIN is indicated in the treatment of acute flares and the long-term management of the chronic disease. TOLECTIN is also indicated for treatment of juvenile rheumatoid arthritis.

The safety and effectiveness of TOLECTIN have not been established in those patients with rheumatoid arthritis who are designated by the American Rheumatism Association as Functional Class IV (incapacitated, largely or wholly bedridden or confined to a wheelchair; little or no self-care).

Improvement in patients treated with TOLECTIN for rheumatoid arthritis has been demonstrated by a reduction in joint swelling, a reduction in pain, a reduction in the number of inflamed joints, a reduction in the duration of morning stiffness, a decrease in disease activity as assessed by both the investigator and the patient, and improved functional capability as demonstrated by an increase in grip strength, a delay in the time to onset of fatigue and a decrease in the time to walk 50 feet.

Improvement in patients treated with TOLECTIN for osteoarthritis has been demonstrated by a reduction of pain at rest and pain on motion, a reduction of swelling, redness and tenderness, a reduction in the duration of morning stiffness and in the inflammation of Heberden's Nodes, a decrease in disease activity as assessed by both the investigator and patient, an increase in range of motion of affected joints, a decrease in the time to walk 50 feet and an improved functional capability as demonstrated by an increase in grip strength and performance of daily activities.

In clinical studies in patients with either rheumatoid arthritis or osteoarthritis, TOLECTIN has been shown to be comparable to aspirin and to indomethacin in controlling disease activity but the frequency of the milder gastrointestinal adverse effects and tinnitus was less than in aspirin-treated patients and the incidence of central nervous system adverse effects was less than in indomethacin-treated patients. It is not known whether TOLECTIN causes less peptic ulceration than aspirin or indomethacin.

Clinical studies have shown that, when added to a regimen of gold salts or corticosteroids, TOLECTIN has produced additional therapeutic benefit, although this effect was somewhat less when patients were receiving gold salts than when they were receiving corticosteroids. The use of TOLECTIN in conjunction with salicylates is not recommended since there does not appear to be any greater benefit from the combination over that achieved with aspirin alone and the potential for adverse reactions is increased.

In clinical studies in patients with juvenile rheumatoid arthritis, TOLECTIN has been shown to be comparable to aspirin in controlling disease activity, with a similar incidence of adverse reactions. In liver function tests, mean SGOT values, initially elevated in patients on previous aspirin therapy, remained elevated in the aspirin group and decreased in the TOLECTIN group. The safety and effectiveness of TOLECTIN have not been established in infants under two years of age.

Contraindications: TOLECTIN (tolmetin sodium) should not be used in patients who have previously exhibited intolerance to it. Because the potential exists for cross sensitivity to aspirin and other non-steroidal anti-inflammatory drugs, TOLECTIN should not be given to patients in whom aspirin and other non-steroidal anti-inflammatory drugs induce symptoms of asthma, rhinitis or urticaria.

Warnings: TOLECTIN (tolmetin sodium) should be given under close supervision to patients with a history of upper gastrointestinal tract disease and only after consulting the "Adverse Reactions" section. Peptic ulceration and gastrointestinal bleeding, sometimes severe, have been reported in patients receiving TOLECTIN.

In patients with active peptic ulcer, attempts should be made to treat the arthritis with nonulcerogenic drugs, such as gold. If TOLECTIN must be given, the patient should be under close supervision for signs of ulcer perforation or severe gastrointestinal bleeding.

Precautions: ***General:*** Clinical studies of up to two years duration have shown no changes in the eyes attributable to TOLECTIN (tolmetin sodium) administration; however, because of microscopic changes in the lens in rats receiving TOLECTIN at doses about twice the maximum recommended dose in man and because of ocular changes observed clinically with other non-steroidal anti-inflammatory drugs, it is recommended that ophthalmologic examinations be carried out within a reasonable time after starting chronic therapy and at periodic intervals thereafter.

In a chronic study in rats, lesions of the renal papillae were observed at doses of TOLECTIN approximately twice the maximum recommended human dose. In a chronic study in mice, chronic nephritis and glomerular sclerosis occurred in animals receiving doses of one and a half times the human dose. In a chronic study in monkeys, a single instance (one in eight) of renal papillary necrosis was observed at a dose more than three times the maximum recommended human dosage. There has been no evidence of renal toxicity to date in clinical studies; however, since TOLECTIN is eliminated primarily by the kidneys, patients with impaired renal function should be closely monitored and they may require lower doses.

TOLECTIN prolongs bleeding time. Patients who may be adversely affected by prolongation of bleeding time should be carefully observed when TOLECTIN is administered.

In patients receiving concomitant TOLECTIN-steroid therapy, any reduction in steroid dosage should be gradual to avoid the possible complications of sudden steroid withdrawal.

TOLECTIN has been shown to cause some retention of water and sodium, and mild peripheral edema has been reported in about 7% of patients receiving TOLECTIN. Therefore, TOLECTIN should be used with caution in patients with compromised cardiac function.

The metabolites of tolmetin in urine have been found to give positive tests for proteinuria using tests which rely on acid precipitation as their endpoint (e.g. sulfosalicylic acid). No interference is seen in the tests for proteinuria using dye-impregnated commercially available reagent strips (e.g. Albustix®, Uristix®, etc.).

Usage in Pregnancy: Since TOLECTIN has not been studied in pregnant women, the use of TOLECTIN during pregnancy is not recommended. Reproduction studies in rats and rabbits at doses up to 1.7 times the maximum clinical dose revealed no evidence of impaired fertility or teratogenesis due to TOLECTIN. However, as with other non-steroidal anti-inflammatory drugs known to inhibit prostaglandin synthesis, an increased incidence of dystocia and delayed parturition occurs in rats. These effects were absent when TOLECTIN was discontinued 24 hours prior to expected delivery.

Nursing Mothers: It is not known whether TOLECTIN is secreted in human milk; however, it is secreted in the milk of lactating rats. As a general rule nursing should not be undertaken while a patient is on TOLECTIN since it may be excreted in human milk.

Drug Interactions: Although TOLECTIN has been found *in vitro* to bind extensively to plasma protein, it does not alter the dosage of warfarin required to maintain a uniform prothrombin time.

In adult diabetic patients under treatment with either sulfonylureas or insulin there is no change in the clinical effects of either TOLECTIN or the hypoglycemic agents.

Adverse Reactions: ***Gastrointestinal System:*** The most frequent adverse reactions which occurred with TOLECTIN (tolmetin sodium) were gastrointestinal. The most frequent single adverse reaction was nausea, which occurred in approximately 1 in 9 patients. Other adverse reactions which occurred less frequently were dyspepsia (1 in 10 patients), abdominal pain (1 in 15 patients), gastrointestinal distress (1 in 15 patients), flatulence (1 in 25 patients), diarrhea (1 in 25 patients), constipation (1 in 40 patients), vomiting (1 in 30 patients) and gastritis (1 in 55 patients).

In clinical studies in about 3000 patients treated up to two years, the incidence of peptic ulcer was about 1 in 50 patients. Thirty-four percent of the ulcer patients had a prior history of peptic ulcer disease and/or were receiving concomitant anti-inflammatory drugs, including corticosteroids, known to produce peptic ulceration.

Significant gastrointestinal bleeding without evidence of peptic ulceration has been reported with an incidence of about 1 in 240 patients following administration of TOLECTIN.

In clinical trials with TOLECTIN (tolmetin sodium), about 10% of patients dropped out because of adverse reactions, mostly gastrointestinal in nature.

Body As A Whole: The most frequent adverse reaction in this body system was headache, occurring in approximately 1 in 10 patients. Other adverse reactions which occurred less frequently were asthenia, chest pain and, rarely, anaphylactoid reactions.

Cardiovascular: The most frequent adverse reaction in this body system was edema, occurring in approximately 1 in 15 patients. Hypertension occurred less frequently.

Central Nervous System/Psychiatric: The most frequent adverse reaction in these body systems was dizziness or lightheadedness, occurring in approximately 1 in 20 patients. Tension or nervousness occurred in 1 in 50 patients and drowsiness in 1 in 60 patients. Insomnia and depression occurred less frequently.

Dermatologic: The most frequent adverse reaction related to skin was rash, occurring in approximately 1 in 40 patients. Pruritus (1 in 60 patients) and skin irritation (1 in 55 patients) occurred less frequently.

Special Senses: The most frequent adverse reaction in this category was tinnitus, occurring in approximately 1 in 65 patients.

Hematologic: Small and transient decreases in hemoglobin and hematocrit not associated with gastrointestinal bleeding have occurred. This is similar to that reported with other non-steroidal anti-inflammatory drugs. A few cases of granulocytopenia have been observed.

Management of Overdosage: In the event of overdosage, the stomach should be emptied by inducing vomiting or by gastric lavage followed by the administration of activated charcoal. Studies in rats indicate that the urinary excretion of the drug is enhanced when the urine is made alkaline with sodium bicarbonate.

Dosage and Administration: The recommended starting dose for adults is 400 mg. three times daily (1200 mg. daily), preferably including a dose on arising and a dose at bedtime. To achieve optimal therapeutic effect the dose should be adjusted according to the patient's response. For rheumatoid arthritis control is usually achieved at doses of 600–1800 mg. daily in divided doses (t.i.d. or q.i.d.). For osteoarthritis control is usually achieved at doses of 600–1600 mg. daily in divided doses (t.i.d. or q.i.d.). Doses larger than 2000 mg./day for rheumatoid arthritis and 1600 mg./day for

Continued on next page

McNeil Laboratories—Cont.

osteoarthritis have not been studied and therefore are not recommended.
The recommended starting dose for children (two years and older) is 20 mg/kg/day in divided doses (t.i.d. or q.i.d.). When control has been achieved the usual dose ranges from 15 to 30 mg/kg/day. Doses higher than 30 mg/kg/day have not been studied and therefore are not recommended.
A therapeutic response to TOLECTIN (tolmetin sodium) can be expected in a few days to a week. Progressive improvement can be anticipated during succeeding weeks of therapy. If gastrointestinal symptoms occur, administer TOLECTIN with meals, milk or antacids, other than sodium bicarbonate.
How Supplied:
TOLECTIN® DS (tolmetin sodium) capsules 400 mg. (colored orange opaque, imprinted "McNEIL"), **NDC** 0045-0414-60, bottles of 100.
TOLECTIN® (tolmetin sodium) tablets 200 mg. (colored white, scored, imprinted "200" and "McNEIL"), bottles of 100 (**NDC** 0045-0412-60); bottles of 500 (**NDC** 0045-0412-70). 972201
[*Shown in Product Identification Section*]

TYLENOL® acetaminophen OTC
Chewable Tablets, Elixir, Drops

(For Product Information, see McNeil Consumer Products Company)

TYLENOL® acetaminophen Tablets OTC

(For Product Information, see McNeil Consumer Products Company)

Extra-Strength
TYLENOL® acetaminophen OTC
Capsules and Tablets

(For Product Information, see McNeil Consumer Products Company)

TYLENOL® with Codeine tablets© ℞
and elixir©
No. 3 (100's):
VA NSN 6505-00-400-2054
No. 3 (unit dose 20 × 25):
VA NSN 6505-00-406-2788
No. 3 (500's):
Military & VA
NSN 6505-00-147-8347

Description:
Tablets:

No. 1 Codeine Phosphate*	7.5 mg.	(1/8 gr.)
Acetaminophen	300 mg.	
No. 2 Codeine Phosphate*	15 mg.	(1/4 gr.)
Acetaminophen	300 mg.	
No. 3 Codeine Phosphate*	30 mg.	(1/2 gr.)
Acetaminophen	300 mg.	
No. 4 Codeine Phosphate*	60 mg.	(1 gr.)
Acetaminophen	300 mg.	

Elixir:
Each 5 ml. elixir contains:

Codeine Phosphate*	12 mg.
Acetaminophen	120 mg.
Alcohol 7%	

* *Warning*—May be habit forming.
Actions: Acetaminophen is a non-narcotic analgesic and antipyretic; codeine is a narcotic with analgesic and antitussive action. Codeine retains at least one-half of its analgesic activity when administered orally.
Indications: TYLENOL with Codeine No. 1, No. 2, and No. 3 are indicated for the relief of mild to moderate pain. TYLENOL with Codeine No. 4 is indicated for the relief of moderate to severe pain. TYLENOL with Codeine elixir is indicated for the relief of mild to moderate pain.
Contraindications: Hypersensitivity to acetaminophen or codeine.
Warnings:
Drug Dependence: Codeine can produce drug dependence of the morphine type, and therefore, has the potential for being abused. Psychic dependence, physical dependence and tolerance may develop upon repeated administration of this drug and it should be prescribed and administered with the same degree of caution appropriate to the use of other oral narcotic-containing medications. Like other narcotic-containing medications, the drug is subject to the Federal Controlled Substances Act.
Usage in Ambulatory Patients: Codeine may impair the mental and/or physical abilities required for the performance of potentially hazardous tasks such as driving a car or operating machinery. The patient using this drug should be cautioned accordingly.
Interaction with other central nervous system depressants: Patients receiving other narcotic analgesics, general anesthetics, phenothiazines, other tranquilizers, sedative-hypnotics or other CNS depressants (including alcohol) concomitantly with this drug may exhibit an additive CNS depression. When such combined therapy is contemplated, the dose of one or both agents should be reduced.
Usage in Pregnancy: Safe use in pregnancy has not been established relative to possible adverse effects on fetal development. Therefore this drug should not be used in pregnant women unless, in the judgment of the physician, the potential benefits outweigh the possible hazards.
Pediatric use: Safe dosage of this combination has not been established in children below the age of three.
Precautions:
Head injury and increased intracranial pressure: The respiratory depressant effects of narcotics and their capacity to elevate cerebrospinal fluid pressure may be markedly exaggerated in the presence of head injury, other intracranial lesions or a pre-existing increase in intracranial pressure. Furthermore, narcotics produce adverse reactions which may obscure the clinical course of patients with head injuries.
Acute abdominal conditions: The administration of this product or other narcotics may obscure the diagnosis or clinical course of patients with acute abdominal conditions.
Special risk patients: This drug should be given with caution to certain patients such as the elderly or debilitated, and those with severe impairment of hepatic or renal function, hypothyroidism, Addison's disease, and prostatic hypertrophy or urethral stricture.
Adverse Reactions: The most frequently observed adverse reactions include lightheadedness, dizziness, sedation, nausea and vomiting. These effects seem to be more prominent in ambulatory than in nonambulatory patients, and some of these adverse reactions may be alleviated if the patient lies down.
Other adverse reactions include euphoria, dysphoria, constipation, skin rash, and pruritus.
Dosage and Administration: Dosage should be adjusted according to the severity of the pain and the response of the patient. It may occasionally be necessary to exceed the usual dosage recommended below in cases of more severe pain or in those patients who have become tolerant to the analgesic effect of narcotics. TYLENOL with Codeine tablets are given orally. The usual adult dose is: Tablets No. 1, No. 2, and No. 3: One or two tablets every four hours as required. Tablets No. 4: One tablet every four hours as required.
TYLENOL with Codeine elixir is given orally. The usual doses are: *Children (3 to 6 years):* 1 teaspoonful (5 ml.) 3 or 4 times daily; *(7 to 12 years):* 2 teaspoonsful (10 ml.) 3 or 4 times daily; *(under 3 years):* safe dosage has not been established. *Adults:* 1 tablespoonful (15 ml.) every 4 hours as needed.
Drug Interactions: The CNS depressant effects of this drug may be additive with that of other CNS depressants. See WARNINGS.
Management of Overdosage: *Signs and Symptoms:* Serious overdose with this product is characterized by respiratory depression (a decrease in respiratory rate and/or tidal volume, Cheyne-Stokes respiration, cyanosis), extreme somnolence progressing to stupor or coma, skeletal muscle flaccidity, cold and clammy skin, and sometimes bradycardia and hypotension. In severe overdosage, apnea, circulatory collapse, cardiac arrest and death may occur. The ingestion of very large amounts of this drug may, in addition, result in acute hepatic toxicity.
Treatment: Primary attention should be given to the reestablishment of adequate respiratory exchange through provision of a patent airway and the institution of assisted or controlled ventilation. The narcotic antagonist naloxone is a specific antidote against respiratory depression which may result from overdosage or unusual sensitivity to narcotics, including codeine. Therefore, an appropriate dose of naloxone (see package insert) should be administered, perferably by the intravenous route, and simultaneously with efforts at respiratory resuscitation. Since the duration of action of codeine may exceed that of the antagonist, the patient should be kept under continued surveillance and repeated doses of the antagonist should be administered as needed to maintain adequate respiration.
An antagonist should not be administered in the absence of clinically significant respiratory or cardiovascular depression.
Oxygen, intravenous fluids, vasopressors and other supportive measures should be employed as indicated.
Gastric emptying may be useful in removing unabsorbed drug.
Acetaminophen in massive overdosage may cause hepatotoxicity in some patients. Clinical and laboratory evidence of hepatotoxicity may be delayed for up to one week. Close clinical monitoring and serial hepatic enzyme determinations are, therefore, recommended.
Treatment of acute acetaminophen overdosage is purely symptomatic.
How Supplied:
TYLENOL® with Codeine tablets (colored white, imprinted "McNEIL," "TYLENOL CODEINE," and either "1", "2", "3", "4"). No. 1 **NDC** 0045-0510—bottles of 100 and 500; No. 2 **NDC** 0045-0511, No. 3 **NDC** 0045-0513, and No. 4 **NDC** 0045-0515—bottles of 100, 500, and a Unit Dose Dispensit (20 × 25); No. 3 also available in bottles of 1000.
Manufactured by McNeil Laboratories Co., Dorado, P R 00646
TYLENOL® with Codeine elixir (colored amber, cherry flavored) bottles of 1 pint **NDC** 0045-0508-16.
[*Tablets shown in Product Identification Section*]

TYLOX® capsules © ℞
(oxycodone and acetaminophen)

Description: Each capsule contains:

Oxycodone Hydrochloride	4.5 mg.
Warning—May be habit forming.	
Oxycodone Terephthalate	0.38 mg.
Warning—May be habit forming.	
Acetaminophen	500 mg.

Actions: The principal analgesic ingredient, oxycodone, is a semisynthetic narcotic with multiple actions qualitatively similar to those of morphine; the most prominent of these involve the central nervous system and organs composed of smooth muscle. The principal actions of therapeutic value of the oxycodone in TYLOX capsules are analgesia and sedation.

Oxycodone is similar to codeine and methadone in that it retains at least one half of its analgesic activity when administered orally.

TYLOX capsules also contain the non-narcotic antipyretic-analgesic acetaminophen.

Indications: TYLOX capsules are indicated for the relief of moderate to moderately severe pain.

Contraindications: Hypersensitivity to oxycodone or acetaminophen.

Warnings:

Drug Dependence: Oxycodone can produce drug dependence of the morphine type and, therefore, has the potential for being abused. Psychic dependence, physical dependence, and tolerance may develop upon repeated administration of TYLOX capsules, and they should be prescribed and administered with the same degree of caution appropriate to the use of other oral narcotic-containing medications. Like other narcotic-containing medications, TYLOX capsules are subject to the Federal Controlled Substances Act.

Usage in Ambulatory Patients: Oxycodone may impair the mental and/or physical abilities required for the performance of potentially hazardous tasks such as driving a car or operating machinery. The patient using TYLOX capsules should be cautioned accordingly.

Interaction with Other Central Nervous System Depressants: Patients receiving other narcotic analgesics, general anesthetics, phenothiazines, other tranquilizers, sedative-hypnotics or other CNS depressants (including alcohol) concomitantly with TYLOX capsules may exhibit an additive CNS depression. When such combined therapy is contemplated, the dose of one or both agents should be reduced.

Usage in Pregnancy: Safe use in pregnancy has not been established relative to possible adverse effects on fetal development. Therefore, TYLOX capsules should not be used in pregnant women unless, in the judgment of the physician, the potential benefits outweigh the possible hazards.

Usage in Children: TYLOX capsules should not be administered to children.

Precautions:

Head Injury and Increased Intracranial Pressure: The respiratory depressant effects of narcotics and their capacity to elevate cerebrospinal fluid pressure may be markedly exaggerated in the presence of head injury, other intracranial lesions or a pre-existing increase in intracranial pressure. Furthermore, narcotics produce adverse reactions which may obscure the clinical course of patients with head injury.

Acute Abdominal Conditions: The administration of TYLOX capsules or other narcotics may obscure the diagnosis or clinical course in patients with acute abdominal conditions.

Special Risk Patients: TYLOX capsules should be given with caution to certain patients such as the elderly or debilitated, and those with severe impairment of hepatic or renal function, hypothyroidism, Addison's disease, and prostatic hypertrophy or urethral stricture.

Adverse Reactions: The most frequently observed adverse reactions include lightheadedness, dizziness, sedation, nausea and vomiting. These effects seem to be more prominent in ambulatory than in non-ambulatory patients, and some of these adverse reactions may be alleviated if the patient lies down.

Other adverse reactions include euphoria, dysphoria, constipation, skin rash and pruritis.

Dosage and Administration: Dosage should be adjusted according to the severity of the pain and the response of the patient. It may occasionally be necessary to exceed the usual dosage recommended below in cases of more severe pain or in those patients who have become tolerant to the analgesic effect of narcotics.

TYLOX capsules are given orally. The usual adult dose is 1 TYLOX capsule every 6 hours as needed for pain.

Drug Interactions: The CNS depressant effects of TYLOX capsules may be additive with that of other CNS depressants. See Warnings.

Management of Overdosage:

Signs and Symptoms: Serious overdosage with TYLOX capsules is characterized by respiratory depression (a decrease in respiratory rate and/or tidal volume, Cheyne-Stokes respiration, cyanosis), extreme somnolence progressing to stupor or coma, skeletal muscle flaccidity, cold and clammy skin, and sometimes bradycardia and hypotension. In severe overdosage, apnea, circulatory collapse, cardiac arrest and death may occur. The ingestion of very large amounts of TYLOX capsules may, in addition, result in acute hepatic toxicity.

Treatment: Primary attention should be given to the reestablishment of adequate respiratory exchange through provision of a patent airway and the institution of assisted or controlled ventilation. The narcotic antagonist naloxone is a specific antidote against respiratory depression which may result from overdosage or unusual sensitivity to narcotics, including oxycodone. Therefore, an appropriate dose of naloxone should be administered (usual adult dose: 0.4 mg), preferably by the intravenous route, simultaneously with efforts at respiratory resuscitation. Since the duration of action of oxycodone may exceed that of the antagonist, the patient should be kept under continued surveillance and repeated doses of the antagonist should be administered as needed to maintain adequate respiration.

An antagonist should not be administered in the absence of clinically significant respiratory or cardiovascular depression.

Oxygen, intravenous fluids, vasopressors and other supportive measures should be employed as indicated.

Gastric emptying may be useful in removing unabsorbed drug.

Acetaminophen in massive overdosage may cause hepatotoxicity in some patients. Clinical and laboratory evidence of hepatotoxicity may be delayed for up to one week. Close clinical monitoring and serial hepatic enzyme determinations are therefore recommended.

Treatment of acute acetaminophen overdosage is purely symptomatic.

How Supplied: TYLOX® capsules (colored red, imprinted "TYLOX McNEIL") **NDC** 0045-0525—bottles of 100 and unit dose 25's.

[Shown in Product Indentification Section]

Mead Johnson Nutritional Division

Mead Johnson & Company
2404 W. PENNSYLVANIA ST.
EVANSVILLE, INDIANA 47721

CASEC® powder
Calcium caseinate
Protein modifier

(See PDR For Nonprescription Drugs)

CE-VI-SOL®
Vitamin C supplement drops
For Infants

(See PDR For Nonprescription Drugs)

ENFAMIL® concentrated liquid • powder
Infant formula

(See PDR For Nonprescription Drugs)

ENFAMIL® with Iron
concentrated liquid • powder
Infant formula

(See PDR For Nonprescription Drugs)

ENFAMIL NURSETTE®
Infant formula

(See PDR For Nonprescription Drugs)

ENFAMIL® ready-to-use
Infant formula

(See PDR For Nonprescription Drugs)

ENFAMIL® with Iron ready-to-use
Infant formula

(See PDR For Nonprescription Drugs)

FEMININS® tablets
Multivitamin-mineral supplement for women taking oral contraceptives

(See PDR For Nonprescription Drugs)

FER-IN-SOL®
Iron supplement
- **drops**
- **syrup**
- **capsules**

Ferrous sulfate, Mead Johnson

(See PDR For Nonprescription Drugs)

FLEXICAL®
Nutritionally balanced elemental diet

(See PDR For Nonprescription Drugs)

ISOCAL®
Complete liquid diet

(See PDR For Nonprescription Drugs)

LOFENALAC® powder
Low phenylalanine food

(See PDR For Nonprescription Drugs)

LONALAC® powder
Low sodium, high protein beverage mix

(See PDR For Nonprescription Drugs)

LYTREN®
Oral electrolyte solution

(See PDR For Nonprescription Drugs)

MCT® Oil
Medium chain triglycerides oil

(See PDR For Nonprescription Drugs)

NUTRAMIGEN® powder
Protein hydrolysate formula

(See PDR For Nonprescription Drugs)

POLY-VI-FLOR® ℞
Multivitamin and fluoride supplement drops • chewable tablets

Composition: Usual daily doses supply:

	Drops 1.0 ml.	Chewable Tablets 1 tablet
Vitamin A, I.U.	1500	2500
Vitamin D, I.U.	400	400
Vitamin E, I.U.	5	15
Vitamin C, mg.	35	60
Folic acid, mg.	—	0.3
Thiamine, mg.	0.5	1.05
Riboflavin, mg.	0.6	1.2
Niacin, mg.	8	13.5
Vitamin B_6, mg.	0.4	1.05
Vitamin B_{12}, mcg.	2	4.5
Fluoride, mg.	0.5	1.0

Action and Uses: Supplementation of the diet with nine (drops) or ten (tablets) vitamins. Supplementation of the diet with the important mineral, fluoride, for caries prophylaxis

Continued on next page

Mead Johnson—Cont.

when fluoride of water supply does not exceed 0.7 p.p.m.
Administration and Dosage: For infants and children from birth to 3 years of age, 1.0 ml. of drops daily. From age 3, one chewable tablet daily. Continue administration throughout childhood.
Contraindications and Precautions: Should not be used when fluoride content of drinking water is 0.7 p.p.m. or more. Do not exceed recommended dose or give other fluoride-containing drugs concurrently—since prolonged excessive fluoride intake may cause dental fluorosis in children. Do not use in presence of frank dental fluorosis. Keep out of reach of children.
Side Effects: Allergic rash and other idiosyncrasies have rarely been reported.
How Supplied: Poly-Vi-Flor® drops: Plastic bottles with dropper marked to deliver 1.0 ml. (To be dispensed in original plastic bottles.)
NDC 0087-0472-01 Bottles of 1 fl. oz. (30 ml.)
NDC 0087-0472-02 Bottles of 1⅔ fl. oz. (50 ml.)
FSN 6505-080-0967 (50 ml.)
Poly-Vi-Flor® chewable tablets
NDC 0087-0474-02 Bottles of 100
NDC 0087-0474-03 Bottles of 1000
Literature Available: Yes.

POLY-VI-FLOR® 0.25 mg. ℞
Multivitamin and fluoride supplement drops

Composition: Each 1.0 ml. supplies:

		Percentage of U.S. Recommended Daily Allowance Infants
Vitamin A, I.U.	1500	100
Vitamin D, I.U.	400	100
Vitamin E, I.U.	5	100
Vitamin C (Ascorbic acid), mg.	35	100
Thiamine (Vitamin B_1), mg.	0.5	100
Riboflavin (Vitamin B_2), mg.	0.6	100
Niacin, mg.	8	100
Vitamin B_6, mg.	0.4	100
Vitamin B_{12}, mcg.	2	100
Fluoride, mg.	0.25	*

*U.S. Recommended Daily Allowance has not been established.
This product does not contain the essential vitamin folic acid.
Ingredients: Vitamin A palmitate, ergocalciferol, D-alpha-tocopheryl succinate, ascorbic acid, thiamine hydrochloride, riboflavin-5-phosphate sodium, niacinamide, pyridoxine, hydrochloride, cyanocobalamin, and sodium fluoride.
Made with natural sweeteners.
Indications:
Supplementation of the diet with nine essential vitamins.
Supplementation of the diet with the important mineral, fluoride, for caries prophylaxis.
Poly-Vi-Flor 0.25 mg. infants' drops supply significant amounts of vitamins A, D, E, C, thiamine, riboflavin, niacin, pyridoxine, and cyanocobalamin to supplement the diet, and to help assure that nutritional deficiencies of these vitamins will not develop. It is well established that fluoridation of the water supply (1 p.p.m. fluoride) during the period of tooth development leads to a significant decrease in the incidence of dental caries. Poly-Vi-Flor 0.25 mg. infants' drops were developed to provide fluoride in drop form for infants and young children from birth to 2 years of age in areas where the water fluoride level is less than 0.3 p.p.m. and for children ages 2–3 years in areas where the water fluoride level is 0.3 p.p.m. thru 0.7 p.p.m. Thus, in a single easy-to-use preparation, infants obtain nine essential vitamins and the important mineral, fluoride.
Action: Each 1.0 ml. supplies sodium fluoride (0.25 mg. fluoride) plus nine essential vitamins.
Hydroxyapatite is the principal crystal for all calcified tissue in the human body. The fluoride ion reacts with the *hydroxyapatite* in the tooth as it is formed to produce the more caries-resistant crystal, *fluorapatite*. The reaction may be expressed by the equation:[1]

$$Ca_{10}(PO_4)_6(OH)_2 + 2F^- \rightarrow Ca_{10}(PO_4)_6F_2 + 2OH^-$$

(Hydroxyapatite) (Fluorapatite)
Three stages of fluoride deposition in tooth enamel can be distinguished.[1]

1. Small amounts (reflecting the low levels of fluoride in tissue fluids) are incorporated into the enamel crystals while they are being formed.
2. After enamel has been laid down, fluoride deposition continues in the surface enamel. Diffusion of fluoride from the surface inward is apparently restricted.
3. After eruption, the surface enamel acquires fluoride from water, food, supplementary fluoride and smaller amounts from saliva.

Contraindications: Poly-Vi-Flor 0.25 mg. (multivitamin and fluoride supplement) drops should not be used by infants from birth to 2 years of age in areas where the drinking water contains 0.3 p.p.m. or more of fluoride; nor for children ages 2–3 years in areas where the drinking water contains more than 0.7 p.p.m. of fluoride. When prescribing Poly-Vi-Flor 0.25 mg. infants' drops, the physician should:
1. determine the fluoride content of the drinking water.
2. make sure the child is not receiving significant amounts of fluoride from other medications.
3. periodically check to make sure that the child does not develop significant dental fluorosis.

Warnings: Do not use Poly-Vi-Flor 0.25 mg. infants' drops for infants and young children from birth to 2 years of age in areas where the drinking water contains 0.3 p.p.m. or more of fluoride; nor for children ages 2–3 years in areas where the drinking water contains more than 0.7 p.p.m. fluoride. As in the case of all medications, keep out of the reach of children.
Precautions: Prolonged daily ingestion of excessive fluoride will result in varying degrees of dental fluorosis.
Poly-Vi-Flor 0.25 mg. infants' drops should be dispensed in the original plastic container, since contact with glass leads to instability and precipitation. (The amount of sodium fluoride in the 50-ml. size is well below the maximum to be dispensed at one time according to recommendations of the American Dental Association.)
Side Effects: Allergic rash and other idiosyncrasies have been rarely reported.
Dosage: 1.0 ml. daily or as prescribed by the physician. May be dropped directly into mouth with 'Safti-Dropper,' or mixed with cereal, fruit juice or other food.
How Supplied: Poly-Vi-Flor 0.25 mg. drops: Plastic bottles with dropper marked to deliver 1.0 ml.
NDC 0087-0451-41 Bottles of 50 ml.
References: 1. Brudevold, F., and McCann, H. G.: Fluoride and Caries Control—Mechanism of Action, in Nizel, A. E.: The Science of Nutrition and Its Application in Clinical Dentistry, Philadelphia, W. B. Saunders Company, 1966, pp. 331–347.

POLY-VI-FLOR® 0.5 mg. ℞
Multivitamin and fluoride supplement chewable tablets

Composition: Each tablet supplies:

		Percentage of U.S. Recommended Daily Allowances: Children Under 4 Years of Age	Adults and Children 4 or More Years of Age
Vitamin A, I.U.	2500	100	50
Vitamin D, I.U.	400	100	100
Vitamin E, I.U.	15	150	50
Vitamin C (Ascorbic acid), mg.	60	150	100
Folic acid (Folacin), mg.	0.3	150	75
Thiamine (Vitamin B_1), mg.	1.05	150	70
Riboflavin (Vitamin B_2), mg.	1.2	150	70
Niacin, mg.	13.5	150	68
Vitamin B_6, mg.	1.05	150	53
Vitamin B_{12}, mcg.	4.5	150	75
Fluoride, mg.	0.5	*	*

*U.S. Recommended Daily Allowance has not been established.
Ingredients: Vitamin A acetate, ergocalciferol, dl-alpha-tocopheryl acetate, ascorbic acid, sodium ascorbate, folic acid, thiamine mononitrate, riboflavin, niacinamide, pyridoxine hydrochloride, cyanocobalamin, and sodium fluoride. Made with natural sweeteners.
Indications: Supplementation of the diet with ten essential vitamins. Supplementation of the diet with the important mineral, fluoride, for caries prophylaxis.
Poly-Vi-Flor 0.5 mg. chewable tablets are indicated for children between the ages of 2–3 years where the water has a fluoride level of 0.3 p.p.m. or less and for children 3 years and above where the water has a fluoride level greater than 0.3 p.p.m. and not more than 0.7 p.p.m.
Contraindications: Poly-Vi-Flor 0.5 mg. (multivitamin and fluoride) supplement tablets should not be administered to infants and children under two.
Poly-Vi-Flor 0.5 mg. tablets are not to be used for children 2–3 years of age who regularly consume drinking water with a fluoride content greater than 0.3 p.p.m., or by children 3 years of age and above who consume drinking water containing more than 0.7 p.p.m. fluoride. Before prescribing Poly-Vi-Flor 0.5 mg. tablets, the physician should:
1. determine the fluoride content of the drinking water.
2. make sure that the child is not taking fluoride-containing drugs, and
3. the physician should also periodically check to make sure that the child does not develop significant dental fluorosis.

Warnings: As in the case of all medications, keep out of the reach of children.
Precautions: The suggested dose of Poly-Vi-Flor 0.5 mg. chewable tablets should not be exceeded, since dental fluorosis may result from continued ingestion of large amounts of fluoride.
Side Effects: Allergic rash and other idiosyncrasies have been rarely reported.
Dosage: One Poly-Vi-Flor 0.5 mg. (vitamins and fluoride) chewable tablet daily or as prescribed by the physician, for children two years of age or older. Because of the 0.5 mg. fluoride content of these tablets, they are not recommended for children under two years of age.

How Supplied: Poly-Vi-Flor® 0.5 mg. (vitamins and fluoride) chewable tablets are available on prescription only in 100 tablet bottles. NDC 0087-0468-41 Bottles of 100

POLY-VI-FLOR® with Iron ℞
Multivitamin, iron and fluoride supplement chewable tablets

Composition: Each tablet supplies same vitamins and fluoride as in Poly-Vi-Flor chewable tablets (see above) plus 12 mg. iron (from 40 mg. ferrous fumarate).
Action and Uses: Supplementation of the diet with iron and nine (drops) or ten (tablets) vitamins. Supplementation of the diet with the important mineral, fluoride, for caries prophylaxis.
Contraindications and Precautions: Same as Poly-Vi-Flor.
Administration and Dosage: 1 tablet daily.
How Supplied: Poly-Vi-Flor® with Iron chewable tablets
NDC 0087-0476-03 Bottles of 100
NDC 0087-0476-04 Bottles of 1000

POLY-VI-FLOR® with Iron ℞
Multivitamin, iron and fluoride supplement drops

Composition: Each 1.0 ml. dose supplies:

Vitamin A, I.U.	1500
Vitamin D, I.U.	400
Vitamin E, I.U.	5
Vitamin C, mg.	35
Thiamine, mg.	0.5
Riboflavin, mg.	0.6
Niacin, mg.	8
Vitamin B_6, mg.	0.4
Iron, mg.	10
Fluoride, mg.	0.5

Action and Uses: Supplementation of the diet with eight vitamins and iron. And, supplementation of the diet with the important mineral, fluoride, for caries prophylaxis.
Contraindications and Precautions: Same as Poly-Vi-Flor
Administration and Dosage: Drop into mouth with 'Safti-Dropper.'
Dose: 1.0 ml. daily, or as indicated.
How Supplied: Poly-Vi-Flor® with Iron drops: Plastic bottles with dropper marked to deliver 1.0 ml. (To be dispensed in original plastic bottle.)
NDC 0087-0469-41 Bottles of 1⅔ fl. oz. (50 ml.)

POLY-VI-SOL®
Multivitamin supplement drops • chewable tablets

(See PDR For Nonprescription Drugs)

POLY-VI-SOL® with Iron
Multivitamin and Iron supplement chewable tablets

(See PDR For Nonprescription Drugs)

POLY-VI-SOL® with Iron
Multivitamin and Iron supplement drops

(See PDR For Nonprescription Drugs)

PORTAGEN®
Nutritionally complete dietary with Medium Chain Triglycerides and "Lactose-Free" (Less than 0.15% w/w Lactose)
U.S. Patent No. 3,450,819

(See PDR For Nonprescription Drugs)

PREGESTIMIL®
Protein hydrolysate formula with medium chain triglycerides and added amino acids

(See PDR For Nonprescription Drugs)

PROBANA® powder
High protein formula with banana powder

(See PDR For Nonprescription Drugs)

PROSOBEE® concentrated liquid • ready-to-use
Milk-free formula with soy isolate

(See PDR For Nonprescription Drugs)

SUSTACAL®
• liquid (ready to use)
• powder (mix with milk)
• pudding (ready-to-eat)
Nutritionally complete food

(See PDR For Nonprescription Drugs)

SUSTAGEN® powder
Nutritional supplement

(See PDR For Nonprescription Drugs)

TEMPRA®
Acetaminophen

(See PDR For Nonprescription Drugs)

TRIND® syrup
expectorant • nasal decongestant • analgesic/antipyretic

(See PDR For Nonprescription Drugs)

TRIND-DM® syrup
decongestant • analgesic/antipyretic cough suppressant • expectorant

(See PDR For Nonprescription Drugs)

TRI-VI-FLOR® ℞
Vitamins A, D, C and Fluoride drops • chewable tablets

Composition: Usual daily doses supply:

	Drops 1.0 ml.	Chewable Tablet 1 tablet
Vitamin A, I.U.	1500	2500
Vitamin D, I.U.	400	400
Vitamin C., mg.	35	60
Fluoride, mg.	0.5	1.0

Action and Uses: Supplementation of the diet with vitamins A, D and C. Supplementation of the diet with the important mineral, fluoride, for caries prophylaxis when fluoride of water supply does not exceed 0.7 ppm.
Administration and Dosage: *Drops:* 1.0 ml. daily for infants and children from birth to 3 years of age. *Tablets:* From age 3, 1 chewable tablet daily. Administration should be continued throughout childhood.
Contraindications and Precautions: Should not be used when fluoride content of drinking water is 0.7 p.p.m. or greater. Do not exceed recommended dose or give other fluoride-containing drugs concurrently—since prolonged excessive fluoride intake may cause dental fluorosis in children. Do not use in presence of frank dental fluorosis. Keep out of reach of children.
Side Effects: Allergic rash and other idiosyncrasies have rarely been reported.
How Supplied: Tri-Vi-Flor® drops: (To be dispensed in original plastic bottles with dropper marked to deliver 1 ml.)
NDC 0087-0473-01 Bottles of 1 fl. oz. (30 ml.)
NDC 0087-0473-02 Bottles of 1⅔ fl. oz. (50 ml.)
Tri-Vi-Flor® tablets:
NDC 0087-0477-01 Bottles of 100
NDC 0087-0477-02 Bottles of 1000
Literature Available: Yes.

TRI-VI-FLOR® 0.25 mg. ℞
Vitamins A, D, C and Fluoride drops

Composition: Each 1.0 ml. supplies:

		Percentage of U.S. Recommended Daily Allowance Infants
Vitamin A, I.U.	1500	100
Vitamin D, I.U.	400	100
Vitamin C (Ascorbic acid), mg.	35	100
Fluoride, mg.	0.25	*

*U.S. Recommended Daily Allowance has not been established.
Ingredients: Vitamin A palmitate, ergocalciferol, ascorbic acid and sodium fluoride. Made with natural sweeteners.
Indications: Tri-Vi-Flor 0.25 mg. drops may be useful for infants whose diets are lacking in vitamins A, D and C.
Tri-Vi-Flor 0.25 mg. infants' drops also provide the important mineral fluoride for caries prophylaxis.
Action: It is well established that fluoridation of the water supply (1 p.p.m. fluoride) during the period of tooth development leads to a significant decrease in the incidence of dental caries. Tri-Vi-Flor 0.25 mg. (vitamins A, D, C and fluoride supplement) drops were developed to provide fluoride in drop form for infants and young children from birth to 2 years of age in areas where the drinking water contains less than 0.3 p.p.m. of fluoride; and for children ages 2–3 years in areas where the drinking water contains 0.3 thru 0.7 p.p.m. of fluoride. Each 1.0 ml. supplies sodium fluoride (0.25 mg. fluoride) plus three basic vitamins.
Hydroxyapatite is the principal crystal for all calcified tissue in the human body. The fluoride ion reacts with the *hydroxyapatite* in the tooth as it is formed to produce the more caries-resistant crystal, *fluorapatite.* The reaction may be expressed by the equation:[1]

$$Ca_{10}(PO_4)_6(OH)_2 + 2F^- \rightarrow Ca_{10}(PO_4)_6F_2 + 2OH^-$$
(Hydroxyapatite) (Fluorapatite)

Three stages of fluoride deposition in tooth enamel can be distinguished:[1]

1. Small amounts (reflecting the low levels of fluoride in tissue fluids) are incorporated into the enamel crystals while they are being formed.
2. After enamel has been laid down, fluoride deposition continues in the surface enamel. Diffusion of fluoride from the surface inward is apparently restricted.
3. After eruption, the surface enamel acquires fluoride from water, food, supplementary fluoride and smaller amounts from saliva.

Contraindications: Tri-Vi-Flor 0.25 mg. (vitamins A, D, C and fluoride) drops should not be used by infants from birth to 2 years of age in areas where the drinking water contains 0.3 p.p.m. or more of fluoride; nor for children ages 2–3 years in areas where the drinking water contains more than 0.7 p.p.m. of fluoride. When prescribing Tri-Vi-Flor 0.25 mg. infants' drops, the physician should:

1. determine the fluoride content of the drinking water.
2. make sure the child is not receiving significant amounts of fluoride from other medications.
3. periodically check to make sure that the child does not develop significant dental fluorosis.

Warnings: Do not use Tri-Vi-Flor 0.25 mg. infants' drops for infants and young children from birth to 2 years of age in areas where the drinking water contains 0.3 p.p.m. or more of fluoride; nor for children ages 2–3 years in areas where the drinking water contains more than 0.7 p.p.m. of fluoride. As in the case of all medications, keep out of the reach of children.

Continued on next page

Mead Johnson Pharm.—Cont.

Precautions: Prolonged daily ingestion of excessive fluoride may result in varying degrees of dental fluorosis.
Tri-Vi-Flor 0.25 mg. infants' drops should be dispensed in the original plastic container, since contact with glass leads to instability and precipitation. (The amount of sodium fluoride in the 50-ml. size is well below the maximum to be dispensed at one time according to recommendations of the American Dental Association.)
Side Effects: Allergic rash and other idiosyncrasies have been rarely reported.
Dosage: 1.0 ml. daily for infants and children under three years of age, or as prescribed by the physician. May be dropped directly into mouth with 'Safti-Dropper,' or mixed with cereal, fruit juice or other food.
How Supplied: Tri-Vi-Flor® 0.25 mg. drops: Plastic bottles with dropper marked to deliver 1.0 ml
NDC 0087-0452-41 Bottles of 50 ml.

References: 1. Brudevold, F., and McCann, H. G.: Fluoride and Caries Control—Mechanism of Action, in Nizel, A.E.: The Science of Nutrition and Its Application in Clinical Dentistry, Philadelphia, W. B. Saunders Company, 1966, pp. 331–347.

TRI-VI-FLOR® 0.25 mg. with Iron ℞
Vitamins A, D, C, Iron and Fluoride drops

Composition: Each 1.0 ml. dose supplies:

		Percentage of U.S. Recommended Daily Allowance Infants
Vitamin A, I. U.	1500	100
Vitamin D, I.U.	400	100
Vitamin C (Ascorbic acid), mg.	35	100
Iron, mg.	10	67
Fluoride, mg.	0.25	*

*U.S. Recommended Daily Allowance has not been established.
Ingredients: Vitamin A palmitate, ergocalciferol, ascorbic acid, ferrous sulfate and sodium fluoride. Made with natural sweeteners.
Indications: Tri-Vi-Flor 0.25 mg. with Iron drops may be useful for infants whose diets are lacking in vitamins A, D, C and iron.
Tri-Vi-Flor 0.25 mg. with Iron infants' drops also provide the important mineral fluoride for caries prophylaxis.
Contraindications: Tri-Vi-Flor 0.25 mg. with Iron (vitamins A, D, C, iron and fluoride) drops should not be used by infants from birth to 2 years of age in areas where the drinking water contains 0.3 p.p.m. or more of fluoride; nor for children ages 2–3 years in areas where the drinking water contains more than 0.7 p.p.m. of fluoride. When prescribing Tri-Vi-Flor 0.25 mg. with Iron infants' drops, the physician should:

1. Determine the fluoride content of the drinking water.
2. Make sure the child is not receving significant amounts of fluoride from other medications.
3. Periodically check to make sure that the child does not develop significant dental fluorosis.

Warnings: Do not use Tri-Vi-Flor 0.25 mg. with Iron infants' drops for infants and young children from birth to 2 years of age in areas where the drinking water contains 0.3 p.p.m. or more of fluoride; nor for children ages 2–3 years in areas where the drinking water contains more than 0.7 p.p.m. of fluoride. As in the case of all medications, keep out of the reach of children.
Precautions: Prolonged daily ingestion of excessive fluoride will result in varying degrees of dental fluorosis.
Tri-Vi-Flor 0.25 mg. with Iron infants' drops should be dispensed in the original plastic container, since contact with glass leads to instability and precipitation. (The amount of sodium fluoride in the 50-ml. size is well below the maximum to be dispensed at one time according to recommendations of the American Dental Association.)
Side Effects: Allergic rash and other idiosyncrasies have been rarely reported.
Dosage: 1.0 ml. daily for infants and children under three years of age, or as prescribed by the physician. May be dropped directly into mouth with 'Safti-Dropper' or mixed with cereal, fruit juice or other food.
How Supplied: Tri-Vi-Flor® 0.25 mg. with Iron drops: Plastic bottle with dropper marked to deliver 1.0 ml.
NDC 0087-0478-41 Bottles of 50 ml.

TRI-VI-SOL®
Vitamin A, D and C Supplement infants' drops • chewable tablets

(See PDR For Nonprescription Drugs)

TRI-VI-SOL® with Iron
Vitamins A, D, C and Iron Infants' Drops

(See PDR For Nonprescription Drugs)

Mead Johnson Pharmaceutical Division

Mead Johnson & Company
2404 W. PENNSYLVANIA ST.
EVANSVILLE, INDIANA 47721

COLACE®
Dioctyl sodium sulfosuccinate, Mead Johnson capsules • syrup • liquid (drops)

Description: Colace (dioctyl sodium sulfosuccinate) is a stool softener.
Actions and Uses: Colace, a surface-active agent, helps to keep stools soft for easy, natural passage. Not a laxative, thus not habit forming. Useful in constipation due to hard stools, in painful anorectal conditions, in cardiac and other conditions in which maximum ease of passage is desirable to avoid difficult or painful defecation, and when peristaltic stimulants are contraindicated. *Note:* When peristaltic stimulation is needed due to inadequate bowel motility, see Peri-Colace® (laxative and stool softener).
Contraindications: There are no known contraindications to Colace.
Side Effects: The incidence of side effects—none of a serious nature—is exceedingly small. Bitter taste, throat irritation, and nausea (primarily associated with the use of the syrup and liquid) are the main side effects reported. Rash has occurred.
Administration and Dosage: *Orally*—Suggested daily Dosage: *Adults and older children:* 50 to 200 mg. *Children 6 to 12:* 40 to 120 mg. *Children 3 to 6:* 20 to 60 mg. *Infants and children under 3:* 10 to 40 mg. The higher doses are recommended for initial therapy. Dosage should be adjusted to individual response. The effect on stools is usually apparent one to three days after the first dose. Give Colace liquid in half a glass of milk or fruit juice or in infant formula, to mask bitter taste. *In enemas*—Add 50 to 100 mg. Colace (5 to 10 ml. Colace liquid) to a retention or flushing enema.
How Supplied: Colace® capsules, 50 mg.
NDC 0087-0713-01 Bottles of 30
NDC 0087-0713-02 Bottles of 60
NDC 0087-0713-03 Bottles of 250
NDC 0087-0713-05 Bottles of 1000
NDC 0087-0713-07 Cartons of 100 single unit packs
Colace® capsules, 100 mg.
NDC 0087-0714-43 Cartons of 10 single unit packs
NDC 0087-0714-01 Bottles of 30
NDC 0087-0714-02 Bottles of 60
NDC 0087-0714-03 Bottles of 250
NDC 0087-0714-05 Bottles of 1000
NDC 0087-0714-07 Cartons of 100 single unit packs
VA 6505-00-582-5282A (Bottles of 250)
6505-00-809-0241 (Bottles of 1000) Defense
Note: Colace capsules should be stored at controlled room temperature (15°–30°C. or 59°–86°F.)
Colace® liquid, 1% solution; 10 mg./ml. (with calibrated dropper)
NDC 0087-0717-04 Bottles of 16 fl. oz.
NDC 0087-0717-02 Bottles of 30 ml.
6505-00-045-7786 (Bottle of 30 ml) Defense
Colace® syrup, 20 mg./5-ml. teaspoon; contains not more than 1% alcohol
NDC 0087-0720-01 Bottles of 8 fl. oz.
NDC 0087-0720-02 Bottles of 16 fl. oz.
[*Shown in Product Identification Section*]

CYTOXAN® Oral tablets • injections ℞
(Cyclophosphamide)

Description: Cytoxan is a synthetic antineoplastic drug chemically related to the nitrogen mustards. It is a white crystalline powder which is soluble in water, physiological saline, or alcohol. **Store Cytoxan products at a temperature between 2° and 32° C. (36° and 90° F.).**
Actions: Although it is classified generally as an alkylating agent, Cytoxan itself is not an alkylating agent or irritant. It interferes with the growth of susceptible neoplasms and, to some extent, certain normal tissues. Its mechanism of action is not known.
Cytoxan is absorbed from the gastrointestinal tract and parenteral sites. It is metabolized (the details of metabolism are not fully known) and the drug and its metabolites are distributed throughout the body, including the brain. Intravenously administered Cytoxan is reported to have a serum half-life of about four hours; however the drug and/or its metabolites may be detected in plasma up to seventy-two hours. Cytoxan and its metabolites are excreted by the kidneys, but the extent to which they are excreted by other routes is not known. Of three alkylating metabolites found in urine, only one (nor-nitrogen mustard) has been identified definitely.
Indications:
A. Frequently responsive myeloproliferative and lymphoproliferative disorders:
1. Malignant lymphomas (Stages III and IV, Peter's Staging System).
   a. Hodgkin's disease.
   b. Follicular lymphoma.
   c. Lymphocytic lymphosarcoma.
   d. Reticulum cell sarcoma.
   e. Lymphoblastic lymphosarcoma.
   f. Burkitt's lymphoma.
2. Multiple myeloma.
3. Leukemias:
   a. Chronic lymphocytic leukemia.
   b. Chronic granulocytic leukemia (it is ineffective in acute blastic crises).
   c. Acute myelogenous and monocytic leukemia.
   d. Acute lymphoblastic (stem-cell) leukemia in children (cyclophosphamide given during remission is effective in prolonging its duration).
4. Mycosis fungoides (advanced disease).

B. Frequently responsive solid malignancies:
1. Neuroblastoma (in patients with disseminated disease).
2. Adenocarcinoma of the ovary.
3. Retinoblastoma.

C. Infrequently responsive malignancies:
1. Carcinoma of the breast.
2. Malignant neoplasms of the lung.

Warnings: Since Cytoxan has been reported to be more toxic in adrenalectomized dogs, adjustment of the doses of both replacement steroids and Cytoxan may be necessary for the adrenalectomized patient.

The rate of metabolism and the leukopenic activity of Cytoxan reportedly are increased by chronic administration of high doses of phenobarbital. The physician should be alert for possible combined drug actions, desirable or undesirable, involving Cytoxan even though Cytoxan has been used successfully concurrently with other drugs, including other cytotoxic drugs.

Cytoxan may interfere with normal wound healing.

Usage in Pregnancy. Cytoxan can be teratogenic or cause fetal resorption in experimental animals. It should not be used in pregnancy, particularly in early pregnancy, unless in the judgment of the physician the potential benefits outweigh the possible risks. Cytoxan is excreted in breast milk and breast-feeding should be terminated prior to institution of Cytoxan therapy.

Patients, male or female, capable of conception ordinarily should be advised of the mutagenic potential of Cytoxan. Adequate methods of contraception appear desirable for such patients receiving Cytoxan.

Precautions: Cytoxan should be given cautiously to patients with any of the following conditions.

1. Leukopenia
2. Thrombocytopenia
3. Tumor cell infiltration of bone marrow
4. Previous X-ray therapy
5. Previous therapy with other cytotoxic agents
6. Impaired hepatic function
7. Impaired renal function

Because Cytoxan may exert a suppressive action on immune mechanisms, the interruption or modification of dosage should be considered for patients who develop bacterial, fungal or viral infections. This is especially true for patients receiving concomitant steroid therapy and perhaps those with a recent history of steroid therapy, since infections in some of these patients have been fatal. Varicella-zoster infections appear to be particularly dangerous under these circumstances.

Cytoxan 25 mg and 50 mg tablets contain FD&C Yellow No. 5 (tartrazine) which may cause allergic-type reactions (including bronchial asthma) in certain susceptible individuals. Although the overall incidence of FD&C Yellow No. 5 (tartrazine) sensitivity in the general population is low, it is frequently seen in patients who also have aspirin hypersensitivity.

Adverse Reactions:

Secondary Neoplasia. Secondary malignancies have developed in some patients treated with cyclophosphamide alone or in association with other antineoplastic drugs and/or modalities. These malignancies most frequently have been urinary bladder, myeloproliferative, and lymphoproliferative malignancies. Secondary malignancies most frequently have developed in the cyclophosphamide-treated patients with primary myeloproliferative and lymphoproliferative malignancies and primary nonmalignant diseases in which immune processes are believed to be involved pathologically. In some cases, the secondary malignancy was detected up to several years after cyclophosphamide treatment was discontinued. The secondary urinary bladder malignancies generally have occurred in patients who previously developed hemorrhagic cystitis (see Genitourinary under Adverse Reactions). Although no cause-effect relationship has been established between cyclophosphamide and the development of malignancy in humans, the possibility of secondary malignancy, based on available data, should be considered in any benefit-to-risk assessment for the use of the drug.

Hematopoietic. Leukopenia is an expected effect and ordinarily is used as a guide to therapy. Thrombocytopenia or anemia may occur in a few patients. These effects are almost always reversible when therapy is interrupted.

Gastrointestinal. Anorexia, nausea, or vomiting are common and related to dose as well as individual susceptibility. There are isolated reports of hemorrhagic colitis, oral mucosal ulceration and jaundice occurring during therapy.

Genitourinary. Sterile hemorrhagic cystitis can result from the administration of Cytoxan. **This can be severe, even fatal, and is probably due to metabolites in the urine.** Nonhemorrhagic cystitis and/or fibrosis of the bladder also have been reported to result from Cytoxan administration. Atypical epithelial cells may be found in the urinary sediment. **Ample fluid intake and frequent voiding help to prevent the development of cystitis,** but when it occurs it is ordinarily necessary to interrupt Cytoxan therapy. Hematuria usually resolves spontaneously within a few days after Cytoxan therapy is discontinued, but may persist for several months. In severe cases replacement of blood loss may be required. The application of electrocautery to telangiectatic areas of the bladder and diversion of urine flow have been successful methods used in treatment of protracted cases. Cryosurgery has also been used. (See also Secondary Neoplasia under Adverse Reactions.) Nephrotoxicity, including hemorrhage and clot formation in the renal pelvis, have been reported.

Gonadal suppression, resulting in amenorrhea or azoospermia, has been reported in a number of patients treated with cyclophosphamide and appears to be related to dosage and duration of therapy. This side effect, possibly irreversible, should be anticipated in patients treated with Cytoxan. It is not known to what extent Cytoxan may affect prepuberal gonads. Fibrosis of the ovary following Cytoxan therapy has been reported also.

Integument. It is ordinarily advisable to inform patients in advance of possible alopecia, a frequent complication of Cytoxan therapy. Regrowth of hair can be expected although occasionally the new hair may be of a different color or texture. The skin and fingernails may become darker during therapy. Non-specific dermatitis has been reported to occur with Cytoxan.

Pulmonary. Interstitial pulmonary fibrosis has been reported in patients receiving high doses of Cytoxan over a prolonged period.

Dosage and Administration: Chemotherapy with Cytoxan, as with other drugs used in cancer chemotherapy, is potentially hazardous and fatal complications can occur. It is recommended that it be administered only by physicians aware of the associated risks. Therapy may be aimed at either induction or maintenance of remission.

Induction Therapy. The usual initial intravenous loading dose for patients with no hematologic deficiency is 40–50 mg/kg. This total initial intravenous loading dose usually is given in divided doses over a period of two to five days.

Patients with any previous treatment that may have compromised the functional capacity of the bone marrow, such as X ray or cytotoxic drugs, and patients with tumor infiltration of the bone marrow may require reduction of the initial loading dose by ⅓ to ½.

A marked leukopenia is usually associated with the above doses, but recovery usually begins after 7–10 days. The white blood cell count should be monitored closely during induction therapy.

If initial therapy is given orally, a dose of 1–5 mg/kg/day can be administered depending on tolerance by the patient.

Maintenance Therapy. It is frequently necessary to maintain chemotherapy in order to suppress or retard neoplastic growth. A variety of schedules has been used:

(1) 1–5 mg/kg p.o. daily
(2) 10–15 mg/kg i.v. every 7–10 days
(3) 3–5 mg/kg i.v. twice weekly

Unless the disease is unusually sensitive to Cytoxan, it is advisable to give the largest maintenance dose that can be reasonably tolerated by the patient. The total leukocyte count is a good objective guide for regulating the maintenance dose. Ordinarily a leukopenia of 3000–4000 cells/cu. mm. can be maintained without undue risk of serious infection or other complications.

Preparation and Handling of Solutions. Cytoxan for Injection should be prepared for parenteral use by adding **Sterile Water for Injection, U.S.P.** or **Bacteriostatic Water for Injection, U.S.P. (paraben preserved only)** to the vial and shaking to dissolve. Use 5 ml. for the 100-mg. vial, 10 ml. for the 200-mg. vial, or 25 ml. for the 500-mg. vial. Solutions of Cytoxan for Injection may be injected intravenously, intramuscularly, intraperitoneally or intrapleurally or they may be infused intravenously in Dextrose Injection, U.S.P. (5% dextrose) or Dextrose and Sodium Chloride Injection, U.S.P. (5% dextrose and 0.9% sodium chloride). These solutions should be used within 24 hours if stored at room temperature or within 6 days if stored under refrigeration. Cytoxan for Injection does not contain an antimicrobial agent and **care must be taken to insure the sterility of prepared solutions.**

Extemporaneous liquid preparations of Cytoxan for oral administration may be prepared by dissolving Cytoxan for Injection in Aromatic Elixir, U.S.P. Such preparations should be stored under refrigeration and used within 14 days.

Overdosage: No specific antidote for Cytoxan is known. Management of overdosage would include general supportive measures to sustain the patient through any period of toxicity that might occur.

How Supplied: Cytoxan® (cyclophosphamide) for Injection. With sodium chloride.

NDC 0087-0500-01	100 mg vials, cartons of 12
NDC 0087-0501-01	200 mg vials, cartons of 12
NDC 0087-0502-01	500 mg vials, cartons of 12
6505-00-767-3578	(200 mg, 20 ml vial) Defense
6505-01-037-9356	(500 mg, 30 ml vial) Defense
VA6505-00-767-3572A	(200 mg, 20 ml vial)
VA6505-00-869-2980A	(500 mg, 30 ml vial)

Cytoxan® (cyclophosphamide) tablets.

NDC 0087-0503-01	50 mg, bottles of 100
NDC 0087-0503-02	50 mg, bottles of 1000
NDC 0087-0503-03	50 mg, Unit Dose cartons of 100
NDC 0087-0504-01	25 mg, bottles of 100
6505-00-733-5246	(50 mg, 100's) Defense
VA6505-00-733-5246A	(50 mg, 100's)

References: References on selected topics are available by writing to: Medical Affairs Department, Mead Johnson Pharmaceutical Division, Evansville, Indiana 47721.

July, 1979

[*Shown in Product Identification Section*]

DEAPRIL-ST®* ℞
***Sublingual tablets**

Description: Each 1.0 mg sublingual tablet contains dihydroergocornine 0.333 mg, dihydroergocristine 0.333 mg and dihydroergocryptine 0.333 mg (Dihydro-alpha-ergocryptine and Dihydro-beta-ergocryptine in the proportion of 2:1) as the methanesulfonates (mesylates), representing a total of 1.0 mg.

Actions: There is no specific evidence which clearly establishes the mechanism by which Deapril-ST produces its mental effects, nor is there conclusive evidence that it particularly

Continued on next page

Mead Johnson Pharm.—Cont.

affects cerebral arteriosclerosis or cerebrovascular insufficiency.

Indications: Deapril-ST is indicated for the treatment of selected symptoms in elderly patients. Short term clinical studies have demonstrated modest improvement in levels of performance of self-care and such symptoms as mood depression, confusion, unsociability and dizziness. These symptoms are of unknown etiology and are not specific to any age group or disease. However, to date, only short term studies conducted with elderly patients have been reported.

Contraindications: Deapril-ST is contraindicated in individuals who have previously shown hypersensitivity of the drug.

Precautions: *Practitioners are advised that because the target symptoms are of unknown etiology, careful diagnosis should be attempted before prescribing Deapril-ST.*

This product contains FD&C Yellow No. 5 (tartrazine) which may cause allergic-type reactions (including bronchial asthma) in certain susceptible individuals. Although the overall incidence of FD&C Yellow No. 5 (tartrazine) sensitivity in the general population is low, it is frequently seen in patients who also have aspirin hypersensitivity.

Adverse Reactions: Deapril-ST sublingual tablets have not been found to produce serious side effects. Some sublingual irritation, transient nausea, and gastric disturbances have been reported. Deapril-ST does not possess the vasoconstrictor properties of the natural ergot alkaloids.

Dosage and Administration: One 1 mg. sublingual tablet three times daily. Alleviation of symptoms is usually gradual and results may not be observed for 3–4 weeks.

How Supplied: Deapril-ST 1 mg, Sublingual Tablets.

NDC 0087-0555-41 Bottles of 100

[*Shown in Product Identification Section*]

DURICEF® ℞
(Cefadroxil Monohydrate)

Description: DURICEF® (cefadroxil monohydrate) is a semisynthetic cephalosporin antibiotic intended for oral administration. It is a white to yellowish-white crystalline powder. It is soluble in water and it is acid-stable. It is chemically designated as 7-[[D-2-amino-2-(4-hydroxyphenyl) acetyl]amino]-3-methyl-8-oxo-5-thia-1-azabicyclo[4.2.0]oct-2-ene-2-carboxylic acid monohydrate.

Clinical Pharmacology—DURICEF (Cefadroxil monohydrate) is rapidly absorbed after oral administration. Following single doses of 500 and 1000 mg., average peak serum concentrations were approximately 16 and 28 mcg./ml., respectively. Measurable levels were present 12 hours after administration. Over 90 percent of the drug is excreted unchanged in the urine within eight hours. Peak urine concentrations are approximately 1800 mcg./ml. during the period following a single 500 mg. oral dose. Increases in dosage generally produce a proportionate increase in DURICEF urinary concentration. The urine antibiotic concentration, following a 1 gm. dose, was maintained well above the MIC of susceptible urinary pathogens for 20 to 22 hours.

Microbiology: *In vitro* tests demonstrate that the cephalosporins are bactericidal because of their inhibition of cell-wall synthesis. DURICEF is active against the following organisms *in vitro:*

Beta-hemolytic streptococci
Staphylococci, including coagulase-positive, coagulase-negative, and penicillinase-producing strains
Streptococcus (Diplococcus) pneumoniae
Escherichia coli
Proteus mirabilis
Klebsiella species

Note—Most strains of *Enterococci (Streptococcus faecalis* and *S. faecium)* are resistant to DURICEF. It is not active against most strains of *enterobacter species, P. morganii* and *P. vulgaris.* It has no activity against Pseudomonas or *Herella species.*

Disc Susceptibility Tests—Quantitative methods that require measurement of zone diameters give the most precise estimates of antibiotic susceptibility. One recommended procedure (CFR Section 460.1) uses cephalosporin class disc for testing susceptibility; interpretations correlate zone diameters of this disc test with MIC values for DURICEF. With this procedure, a report from the laboratory of "resistant" indicates that the infecting organism is not likely to respond to therapy. A report of "intermediate susceptibility" suggests that the organism would be susceptible if the infection is confined to the urinary tract, as DURICEF produces high antibiotic levels in the urine.

Indications DURICEF (cefadroxil monohydrate) is indicated for the treatment of the following infections when caused by susceptible strains of the designated microorganisms:

Urinary tract infections caused by *E. coli, P. mirabilis,* and *Klebsiella* species

Skin and skin structure infections caused by staphylococci and/or streptococci

Note—Culture and susceptibility tests should be initiated prior to and during therapy. Renal function studies should be performed when indicated.

Contraindication: DURICEF (cefadroxil monohydrate) is contraindicated in patients with known allergy to the cephalosporin group of antibiotics.

WARNING: IN PENICILLIN-ALLERGIC PATIENTS, CEPHALOSPORIN ANTIBIOTICS SHOULD BE USED WITH GREAT CAUTION. THERE IS CLINICAL AND LABORATORY EVIDENCE OF PARTIAL CROSS-ALLERGENICITY OF THE PENICILLINS AND THE CEPHALOSPORINS, AND THERE ARE INSTANCES OF PATIENTS WHO HAVE HAD REACTIONS TO BOTH DRUGS (INCLUDING FATAL ANAPHALAXIS AFTER PARENTERAL USE).

Any patient who has demonstrated a history of some form of allergy, particularly to drugs, should receive antibiotics cautiously and then only when absolutely necessary. No exception should be made with regard to DURICEF (cefadroxil monohydrate).

Precautions: Patients should be followed carefully so that any side-effects or unusual manifestations of drug idiosyncrasy may be detected. If a hypersensitivity reaction occurs, the drug should be discontinued and the patient treated with the usual agents (e.g., epinephrine or other pressor amines, antihistamines, or corticosteroids.

DURICEF (cefadroxil monohydrate) should be used with caution in the presence of markedly impaired renal function (creatinine clearance rate of less than 50 ml/min/1.73 M^2). (See Dosage and Administration.) In patients with known or suspected renal impairment, careful clinical observation and appropriate laboratory studies should be made prior to and during therapy.

Prolonged use of DURICEF may result in the overgrowth of nonsusceptible organisms. Careful observation of the patient is essential. If superinfection occurs during therapy, appropriate measures should be taken.

Positive direct Coombs tests have been reported during treatment with the cephalosporin antibiotics. In hematologic studies or in transfusion cross-matching procedures when antiglobulin tests are performed on the minor side or in Coombs testing of newborns whose mothers have received cephalosporin antibiotics before parturition, it should be recognized that a positive Coombs test may be due to the drug.

Usage in Pregnancy: Although no teratogenic or anti-fertility effects were seen in reproductive studies in mice and rats receiving dosages greater than the normal human dose, the safety of this drug for use in human pregnancy has not been established. The benefits of the drug in pregnant women should be weighed against a possible risk to the fetus.

Adverse Reactions: Gastrointestinal—The most frequent side-effect has been nausea. It was infrequently severe enough to warrant cessation of therapy. Administration with food decreases nausea and does not decrease absorption. Diarrhea and dysuria have also occurred.

Hypersensitivity—Allergies (in the form of rash, urticaria, and angioedema) have been observed. These reactions usually subsided upon discontinuation of the drug.

Other reactions have included genital pruritus, genital moniliasis, vaginitis, and moderate transient neutropenia.

Dosage and Administration: DURICEF (cefadroxil monohydrate) is acid stable and may be administered orally without regard to meals. Administration with food may be helpful in diminishing potential gastrointestinal complaints occasionally associated with oral cephalosporin therapy.

Adults—For urinary tract infections the usual adult dosage is one gm (two 500 mg capsules) two times per day. For skin and skin structure infections the usual dose is 500 mg two times per day or 1 gm once a day.

In patients with renal impairment, the dosage of cefadroxil should be adjusted according to creatinine clearance rates to prevent drug accumulation. The following schedule is suggested. In adults, the initial dose is 1000 mg. of DURICEF (cefadroxil monohydrate) and the maintenance dose (based on the creatinine clearance rate [ml/min/1.73M^2]) is 500 mg. at the time intervals listed below.

Creatinine Clearances	Dosage Interval
0-10 ml/min	36 hours
10-25 ml/min	24 hours
25-50 ml/min	12 hours

Patients with creatinine clearance rates over 50 ml/min may be treated as if they were patients having normal renal function.

Children—Dosage and safety have not yet been established in children.

How Supplied: DURICEF® (cefadroxil monohydrate) capsules 500 mg. for oral administration in an opaque maroon cap and opaque white body No. 0 hard gelatin capsule. On each half capsule printed in black is "MJ" and "500." Available in bottles of 24 capsules (NDC 0087-0784-41) and 100 capsules (NDC 0087-0784-42).

U.S. Patent Re. 29,164
August, 1979

ESTRACE® ℞
(Estradiol)

WARNING

1. ESTROGENS HAVE BEEN REPORTED TO INCREASE THE RISK OF ENDOMETRIAL CARCINOMA.

Three independent case control studies have shown an increased risk of endometrial cancer in postmenopausal women exposed to exogenous estrogens for prolonged periods. This risk was independent of the other known risk factors for endometrial cancer. These studies are further supported by the finding that incidence rates of endometrial cancer have increased sharply since 1969 in eight different areas of the United States with population based cancer reporting systems, an increase which may be related to the rapidly expanding use of estrogens during the last decade.

The three case control studies reported that the risk of endometrial cancer in estrogen users was about 4.5 to 13.9 times greater than in nonusers. The risk appears to depend on both duration of treatment and on estrogen dose. In view of these findings, when estrogens are used for the treatment of menopausal symptoms, the lowest dose that will control symptoms should be utilized and medication should be discontinued as soon as possible. When prolonged treatment is medically indicated, the patient should be reassessed on at least a semiannual basis to determine the need for continued therapy. Although the evidence must be considered preliminary, one study suggests that cyclic administration of low doses of estrogen may carry less risk than continuous administration, it therefore appears prudent to utilize such a regimen.

Close clinical surveillance of all women taking estrogens is important. In all cases of undiagnosed persistent or recurring abnormal vaginal bleeding, adequate diagnostic measures should be undertaken to rule out malignancy.

There is no evidence at present that "natural" estrogens are more or less hazardous than "synthetic" estrogens at equiestrogenic doses.

2. ESTROGENS SHOULD NOT BE USED DURING PREGNANCY.

The use of female sex hormones, both estrogens and progestogens, during early pregnancy may seriously damage the offspring. It has been shown that females exposed *in utero* to diethylstilbestrol, a non-steroidal estrogen, have an increased risk of developing in later life a form of vaginal or cervical cancer that is ordinarily extremely rare. This risk has been estimated as not greater than 4 per 1000 exposures. Furthermore, a high percentage of such exposed women (from 30 to 90 percent) have been found to have vaginal adenosis, epithelial changes of the vagina and cervix. Although these changes are histologically benign, it is not known whether they are precursors of malignancy. Although similar data are not available with the use of other estrogens, it cannot be presumed they would not induce similar changes.

Several reports suggest an association between intrauterine exposure to female sex hormones and congenital anomalies, including congenital heart defects and limb reduction defects. One case control study estimated a 4.7-fold increased risk of limb reduction defects in infants exposed *in utero* to sex hormones (oral contraceptives, hormone withdrawal tests for pregnancy, or attempted treatment for threatened abortion). Some of these exposures were very short and involved only a few days of treatment. The data suggest that the risk of limb reduction defects in exposed fetuses is somewhat less than 1 per 1000.

In the past, female sex hormones have been used during pregnancy in an attempt to treat threatened or habitual abortion. There is considerable evidence that estrogens are ineffective for these indications, and there is no evidence from well controlled studies that progestogens are effective for these uses.

If Estrace® is used during pregnancy, or if the patient becomes pregnant while taking this drug, she should be apprised of the potential risks to the fetus and the advisability of pregnancy continuation.

Description: Estrace® oral tablets contain 1 or 2 mg. of micronized estradiol. Estradiol (17β-estradiol) is a white, crystalline solid, chemically described as estra-1,3,5(10)-triene-3,17β-diol. Estrace® oral tablets provide estrogen replacement therapy.

Clinical Pharmacology

17β-Estradiol is the most potent physiologic estrogen and, in fact, is the major estrogenic hormone secreted by the human. Estradiol in Estrace® has been micronized and demonstrated to be rapidly and effectively absorbed from the gastrointestinal tract.

Indications: Estrace® is indicated in the treatment of:

1. Moderate to severe *vasomotor* symptoms associated with the menopause. (There is no evidence that estrogens are effective for nervous symptoms or depression which might occur during menopause, and they should not be used to treat these conditions.)
2. Atrophic vaginitis.
3. Kraurosis vulvae.
4. Female hypogonadism.
5. Female castration.
6. Primary ovarian failure.

ESTRACE® HAS NOT BEEN SHOWN TO BE EFFECTIVE FOR ANY PURPOSE DURING PREGNANCY AND ITS USE MAY CAUSE SEVERE HARM TO THE FETUS (SEE BOXED WARNING).

Contraindications: Estrogens should not be used in women (or men) with any of the following conditions:

1. Known or suspected cancer of the breast except in appropriately selected patients being treated for metastatic disease.
2. Known or suspected estrogen-dependent neoplasia.
3. Known or suspected pregnancy (See Boxed Warning).
4. Undiagnosed abnormal genital bleeding.
5. Active thrombophlebitis or thromboembolic disorders.
6. A past history of thrombophlebitis, thrombosis or thromboembolic disorders associated with previous estrogen use (except when used in treatment of breast or prostatic malignancy).

Warnings:

1. **Induction of malignant neoplasms.** Long term continuous administration of natural and synthetic estrogens in certain animal species increases the frequency of carcinomas of the breast, cervix, vagina, and liver. There is now evidence that estrogens increase the risk of carcinoma of the endometrium in humans. (See Boxed Warning).

At the present time there is no satisfactory evidence that estrogens given to postmenopausal women increase the risk of cancer of the breast, although a recent long-term followup of a single physician's practice has raised this possibility. Because of the animal data there is a need for caution in prescribing estrogens for women with a strong family history of breast cancer or who have breast nodules, fibrocystic disease, or abnormal mammograms.

2. **Gall bladder disease.** A recent study has reported a 2 to 3-fold increase in the risk of surgically confirmed gall bladder disease in women receiving postmenopausal estrogens, similar to the 2-fold increase previously noted in users of oral contraceptives. In the case of oral contraceptives, the increased risk appeared after two years of use.

3. **Effects similar to those caused by estrogen-progestogen oral contraceptives.** There are several serious adverse effects of oral contraceptives, most of which have not, up to now, been documented as consequences of postmenopausal estrogen therapy. This may reflect the comparatively low doses of estrogen used in postmenopausal women. It would be expected that the larger doses of estrogen used to treat prostatic or breast cancer or postpartum breast engorgement are more likely to result in these adverse effects, and, in fact, it has been shown that there is an increased risk of thrombosis in men receiving estrogens for prostatic cancer and women for postpartum breast engorgement.

a. **Thromboembolic disease.** It is now well established that users of oral contraceptives have an increased risk of various thromboembolic and thrombotic vascular diseases, such as thrombophlebitis, pulmonary embolism, stroke, and myocardial infarction. Cases of retinal thrombosis, mesenteric thrombosis, and optic neuritis have been reported in oral contraceptive users. There is evidence that the risk of several of these adverse reactions is related to the dose of the drug. An increased risk of post-surgery thromboembolic complications has also been reported in users of oral contraceptives. If feasible, estrogen should be discontinued at least 4 weeks before surgery of the type associated with an increased risk of thromboembolism, or during periods of prolonged immobilization.

While an increased rate of thromboembolic and thrombotic disease in postmenopausal users of estrogens has not been found, this does not rule out the possibility that such an increase may be present or that subgroups of women who have underlying risk factors or who are receiving relatively large doses of estrogens may have increased risk. Therefore estrogens should not be used in persons with active thrombophlebitis or thromboembolic disorders, and they should not be used (except in treatment of malignancy) in persons with a history of such disorders in association with estrogen use. They should be used with caution in patients with cerebral vascular or coronary artery disease and only for those in whom estrogens are clearly needed.

Large doses of estrogen (5 mg conjugated estrogens per day), comparable to those used to treat cancer of the prostate and breast, have been shown in a large prospective clinical trial in men to increase the risk of nonfatal myocardial infarction, pulmonary embolism and thrombophlebitis. When estrogen doses of this size are used, any of the thromboembolic and thrombotic adverse effects associated with oral contraceptive use should be considered a clear risk.

b. **Hepatic adenoma.** Hepatic adenomas appear to be associated with the use of oral contraceptives. Although rare, these may rupture and may cause death through intraabdominal hemorrhage. Such lesions have not yet been reported in association with other estrogen or progestogen preparations but should be considered in estrogen users having abdominal pain and tenderness, abdominal mass, or hypovolemic shock. Hepatocellular carcinoma has also been reported in women taking estrogen-containing oral contraceptives. The relationship of this malignancy to these drugs is not known at this time.

c. **Elevated blood pressure.** Increased blood pressure is not uncommon in women using oral contraceptives. There is now a report that this may occur with use of estrogens in the menopause and blood pressure should be monitored with estrogen use, especially if high doses are used.

d. **Glucose tolerance.** A worsening of glucose tolerance has been observed in a significant percentage of patients on estrogen-containing oral contraceptives. For this reason, diabetic patients should be carefully observed while receiving estrogen.

4. **Hypercalcemia.** Administration of estrogens may lead to severe hypercalcemia in patients with breast cancer and bone metastases. If this occurs, the drug should be stopped and appropriate measures taken to reduce the serum calcium level.

Precautions:

A. General Precautions.

1. A complete medical and family history should be taken prior to the initiation of any estrogen therapy. The pretreatment and periodic physical examinations should include spe-

Continued on next page

Mead Johnson Pharm.—Cont.

cial reference to blood pressure, breasts, abdomen, and pelvic organs, and should include a Papanicolaou smear. As a general rule, estrogen should not be prescribed for longer than one year without another physical examination being performed.

2. Fluid retention—Because estrogens may cause some degree of fluid retention, conditions which might be influenced by this factor such as epilepsy, migraine, and cardiac or renal dysfunction, require careful observation.

3. Certain patients may develop undesirable manifestations of excessive estrogenic stimulation, such as abnormal or excessive uterine bleeding, mastodynia, etc.

4. Oral contraceptives appear to be associated with an increased incidence of mental depression. Although it is not clear whether this is due to the estrogenic or progestogenic component of the contraceptive, patients with a history of depression should be carefully observed.

5. Preexisting uterine leiomyomata may increase in size during estrogen use.

6. The pathologist should be advised of estrogen therapy when relevant specimens are submitted.

7. Patients with a past history of jaundice during pregnancy have an increased risk of recurrence of jaundice while receiving estrogen-containing oral contraceptive therapy. If jaundice develops in any patient receiving estrogen, the medication should be discontinued while the cause is investigated.

8. Estrogens may be poorly metabolized in patients with impaired liver function and they should be administered with caution in such patients.

9. Because estrogens influence the metabolism of calcium and phosphorus, they should be used with caution in patients with metabolic bone diseases that are associated with hypercalcemia or in patients with renal insufficiency.

10. Because of the effects of estrogens on epiphyseal closure, they should be used judiciously in young patients in whom bone growth is not complete.

11. Certain endocrine and liver function tests may be affected by estrogen-containing oral contraceptives. The following similar changes may be expected with larger doses of estrogen:

a. Increased sulfobromophthalein retention.

b. Increased prothrombin and factors VII and VIII, IX, and X; decreased antithrombin 3; increased norepinephrine-induced platelet aggregability.

c. Increased thyroid binding globulin (TBG) leading to increased circulating total thyroid hormone, as measured by PBI, T4 by column, or T4 by radioimmunoassay. Free T3 resin uptake is decreased, reflecting the elevated TBG; free T4 concentration is unaltered.

d. Impaired glucose tolerance.

e. Decreased pregnanediol excretion.

f. Reduced response to metyrapone test.

g. Reduced serum folate concentration.

h. Increased serum triglyceride and phospholipid concentration.

B. Information for the Patient. See text of Patient Package Insert.

C. Pregnancy Category X. See Contraindications and Boxed Warning.

D. Nursing Mothers. As a general principle, the administration of any drug to nursing mothers should be done only when clearly necessary since many drugs are excreted in human milk.

Estrace 2 mg tablets contain FD&C Yellow No. 5 (tartrazine) which may cause allergic-type reactions (including bronchial asthma) in certain susceptible individuals. Although the overall incidence of FD&C Yellow No. 5 (tartrazine) sensitivity in the general population is low, it is frequently seen in patients who also have aspirin hypersensitivity.

Adverse Reactions: (See Warnings regarding induction of neoplasia, adverse effects on the fetus, increased incidence of gall bladder disease, and adverse effects similar to those of oral contraceptives, including thromboembolism.) The following additional adverse reactions have been reported with estrogenic therapy, including oral contraceptives:

1. **Genitourinary system.**
   Breakthrough bleeding, spotting, change in menstrual flow.
   Dysmenorrhea.
   Premenstrual-like syndrome.
   Amenorrhea during and after treatment.
   Increase in size of uterine fibromyomata.
   Vaginal candidiasis.
   Change in cervical eversion and in degree of cervical secretion.
   Cystitis-like syndrome.
2. **Breast.**
   Tenderness, enlargement, secretion.
3. **Gastrointestinal.**
   Nausea, vomiting.
   Abdominal cramps, bloating.
   Cholestatic jaundice.
4. **Skin.**
   Chloasma or melasma which may persist when drug is discontinued.
   Erythema multiforme.
   Erythema nodosum.
   Hemorrhagic eruption.
   Loss of scalp hair.
   Hirsutism.
5. **Eyes.**
   Steepening of corneal curvature.
   Intolerance to contact lenses.
6. **CNS.**
   Headache, migraine, dizziness.
   Mental depression.
   Chorea.
7. **Miscellaneous.**
   Increase or decrease in weight.
   Reduced carbohydrate tolerance.
   Aggravation of porphyria.
   Edema.
   Changes in libido.

Acute Overdosage: Numerous reports of ingestion of large doses of estrogen-containing oral contraceptives by young children indicate that serious ill effects do not occur. Overdosage of estrogen may cause nausea, and withdrawal bleeding may occur in females.

Dosage and Administration:

1. **Given cyclically for short term use only:**
   For treatment of moderate to severe **vasomotor** symptoms, atrophic vaginitis, or kraurosis vulvae associated with the menopause.
   The lowest dose that will control symptoms should be chosen and medication should be discontinued as promptly as possible.
   Administration should be cyclic (e.g., 3 weeks on and 1 week off).
   Attempts to discontinue or taper medication should be made at 3 to 6 month intervals.
   The usual initial dosage range is 1 or 2 mg. daily of micronized estradiol adjusted as necessary to control presenting symptoms. The minimal effective dose for maintenance therapy should be determined by titration.
2. **Given cyclically:**
   Female hypogonadism.
   Female castration.
   Primary ovarian failure.
   Treatment is usually initiated with a dose of 1 or 2 mg. daily of micronized estradiol, adjusted as necessary to control presenting symptoms; the minimal effective dose for maintenance therapy should be determined by titration.

Treated patients with an intact uterus should be monitored closely for signs of endometrial cancer and appropriate diagnostic measures should be taken to rule out malignancy in the event of persistent or recurring abnormal vaginal bleeding.

How Supplied:
Estrace 1 mg; lavender scored tablets
NDC 0087-0755-01 Bottles of 100
Estrace 2 mg; turquoise scored tablets
NDC 0087-0756-01 Bottles of 100

PATIENT LABELING

What You Should Know About Estrogens: Estrogens are female hormones produced principally by the ovaries. The ovaries make several different kinds of estrogens. In addition, scientists have been able to make a variety of synthetic estrogens. As far as we know, all these estrogens have the same properties and therefore much the same usefulness, side effects, and risks. This leaflet is intended to help you understand what estrogens are used for, the risks involved in their use, and how to use them as safely as possible.

This leaflet includes important information about Estrace® (estradiol) and estrogens in general, but not all the information. If you want to know more you can ask your doctor or pharmacist to let you read the professional package insert.

Uses of Estrogen: Estrogens are prescribed by doctors for a number of purposes, including:

1. To provide estrogen during a period of adjustment when a woman's ovaries no longer produce it, in order to prevent certain uncomfortable symptoms of estrogen deficiency. (All women normally experience a decrease in the production of estrogens, generally between 45–55; this is called the menopause.)
2. To prevent symptoms of estrogen deficiency when a woman's ovaries have been removed surgically before the natural menopause.
3. To prevent pregnancy. (Some estrogens are given along with a progestogen, another female hormone; these combinations are called oral contraceptives or birth control pills. They will not be discussed in this leaflet.) However, Estrace is not intended for this use.
4. To treat certain cancers in women and men.
5. To prevent painful swelling of the breasts after pregnancy in women who choose not to nurse their babies.

THERE IS NO PROPER USE OF ESTROGENS IN A PREGNANT WOMAN.

Estrogens in The Menopause: In the natural course of their lives, all women eventually experience a decrease in estrogen production. This usually occurs between ages 45 and 55 but may occur earlier or later. Sometimes the ovaries may need to be removed before natural menopause by an operation, producing a "surgical menopause."

When the amount of estrogen in the blood begins to decrease, many women may develop typical symptoms: feelings of warmth in the face, neck, and chest or sudden intense episodes of heat and sweating throughout the body (called "hot flashes" or "hot flushes"). These symptoms are sometimes very uncomfortable. A few women eventually develop changes in the vagina (called "atrophic vaginitis") which cause discomfort, especially during and after intercourse.

Estrogens can be prescribed to treat these symptoms of the menopause. It is estimated that considerably more than half of all women undergoing the menopause have only mild symptoms or no symptoms at all and therefore do not need estrogens. Other women may need estrogens for a few months, while their bodies adjust to lower estrogen levels. Sometimes the need will be for periods longer than six months. In an attempt to avoid over-stimulation of the uterus (womb), estrogens are usually given cyclically during each month of use, that is three weeks of pills followed by one week without pills.

Sometimes women experience nervous symptoms or depression during menopause. There is no evidence that estrogens are effective for such symptoms and they should not be used to treat them, although other treatment may be needed.

You may have heard that taking estrogens for long periods (years) after the menopause will keep your skin soft and supple and keep you feeling young. There is no evidence that this is so, however, and such long-term treatment carries additional risks.

Estrogens To Prevent Swelling of The Breasts After Pregnancy: If you do not breast feed your baby after delivery, your breasts may fill up with milk and become painful and engorged. This usually begins about three to four days after delivery and may last for a few days to up to a week or more. Sometimes the discomfort is severe, but usually it is not and can be controlled by pain-relieving drugs such as aspirin and by binding the breasts up tightly. Estrogens can sometimes be used successfully to try to prevent the breasts from filling up. While this treatment is sometimes successful, in many cases the breasts fill up to some degree in spite of treatment. The dose of estrogens needed to prevent pain and swelling of the breasts is much larger than the dose needed to treat symptoms of the menopause and this may increase your chances of developing blood clots in the legs or lungs or other parts of the body (see below, 4. Abnormal Blood Clotting). Therefore, it is important that you discuss the benefits and the risks of estrogen use with your doctor, before using estrogen, if you have decided not to breast feed your baby.

The Dangers of Estrogens:

1. **Cancer of the uterus.** If estrogens are used in the postmenopausal period for more than a year, there is an increased risk of **cancer of the endometrium** (uterine lining). Women taking estrogens have roughly 5 to 15 times as great a chance of getting this cancer as women who take no estrogens. To put this another way, while a postmenopausal woman not taking estrogens has one chance in 1,000 each year of getting cancer of the uterus, a woman taking estrogens has 5 to 15 chances in 1,000 each year. For this reason **it is important to take estrogens only when you really need them.**
The risk of this cancer is greater the longer estrogens are used and also seems to be greater when larger doses are taken. For this reason **it is important to take the lowest dose of estrogen that will control symptoms and to take it only as long as it is needed.** If estrogens are needed for longer periods of time, your doctor will want to reevaluate your need for estrogens at least every six months.
Women using estrogens should report any irregular vaginal bleeding to their doctors; such bleeding may be of no importance, but it can be an early warning of cancer of the uterus. If you have undiagnosed vaginal bleeding, you should not use estrogens until a diagnosis is made and you are certain there is no cancer of the uterus. If you have had your uterus completely removed (total hysterectomy), there is no danger of developing cancer of the uterus.
2. **Other possible cancers.** Estrogens can cause development of other tumors in animals, such as tumors of the breast, cervix, vagina, or liver, when given for a long time. At present there is no satisfactory evidence that women using estrogens in the menopause have an increased risk of such tumors, but there is no way yet to be sure they do not; and one study raises the possibility that use of estrogens in the menopause may increase the risk of breast cancer many years later. This is a further reason to use estrogens only when clearly needed. While you are taking estrogens, it is important that you go to your doctor at least once a year for a physical examination. Also, if members of your family have had breast cancer or if you have breast nodules or abnormal mammograms (breast x-rays), your doctor may wish to carry out more frequent examinations.
3. **Gall bladder disease.** Women who use estrogens after menopause are two or three times more likely to develop gall bladder disease needing surgery than women who do not use estrogens. Birth control pills have a similar effect.
4. **Abnormal blood clotting.** Oral contraceptives increase the risk of blood clotting in various parts of the body. This can occur in different parts of the circulatory system causing thrombophlebitis (clot in the legs or pelvis), retinal thrombosis or optic neuritis (clots affecting vision, including blindness), mesenteric thrombosis (clots in the intestinal blood vessels), stroke (clot in the brain), heart attack (clot in a vessel of the heart) or a pulmonary embolism (clot which eventually lodges in the lungs). These can be fatal.
At this time use of estrogens in the menopause is not known to cause increased blood clotting, this has not been fully studied and there could still prove to be such a risk. It is recommended that if you have had clotting in the legs or lungs or a heart attack or stroke while you were using estrogens or birth control pills, you should not use estrogens (unless they are being used to treat cancer of the breast or prostate). If you have had a stroke or heart attack or if you have angina pectoris, estrogens should be used with great caution and only if clearly needed (for example, if you have severe symptoms of the menopause).
The larger doses of estrogen used to prevent swelling of the breasts after pregnancy have been reported to cause abnormal blood clotting **as indicated above.**

Special Warning About Pregnancy: You should not receive estrogen if you are pregnant.

If this should occur, there is a greater than usual chance that the developing child will be born with a birth defect, although the possibility remains fairly small. A female child may have an increased risk of developing cancer of the vagina or cervix later in life (in the teens or twenties). Every possible effort should be made to avoid exposure to estrogens during pregnancy. If exposure occurs, see your doctor.

Other Effects of Estrogens: In addition to the serious known risks of estrogens described above, estrogens have the following side effects and potential risks which, if occurring, should be discussed promptly with your doctor.

1. **Nausea and vomiting.** The most common side effect of estrogen therapy is nausea. Vomiting is less common.
2. **Effects on breasts.** Estrogens may cause breast tenderness or enlargement and may cause the breasts to secrete a liquid.
3. **Effects on the uterus.** Estrogens may cause benign fibroid tumors of the uterus to get larger. Some women will have menstrual bleeding when estrogens are stopped. But if the bleeding occurs on days you are still taking estrogens, you should report this to your doctor.
4. **Effects on liver.** Women taking oral contraceptives develop on rare occasions a tumor of the liver which can rupture, bleed into the abdomen, and cause death. So far, these tumors have not been reported in women using estrogens in the menopause, but you should report any swelling or unusual pain or tenderness in the abdomen to your doctor immediately.
Women with a past history of jaundice (yellowing of the skin and white parts of the eyes) may get jaundice again during estrogen use. If this occurs, stop taking estrogens and see your doctor.
5. **Other effects.** Estrogens may cause excess fluid to be retained in the body. This may make some conditions worse, such as epilepsy, migraine, heart disease, or kidney disease. Mental depression or high blood pressure may occur. A spotty darkening of the skin, particularly of the face, is possible and may persist.

Summary: Estrogens have important uses, and they may have serious risks as well. You must decide, with your doctor, whether the risks are acceptable to you in view of the benefits of treatment. Except where your doctor has prescribed estrogens for use in special cases of cancer of the breast or prostate, you should not use estrogens if you have cancer of the breast or uterus, are pregnant, have undiagnosed abnormal vaginal bleeding, clotting in the legs or lungs or have had a stroke, heart attack or angina, or clotting in the legs or lungs in the past while you were taking estrogens.

You can use estrogens as safely as possible by understanding that your doctor will require regular physical examinations while you are taking them and will try to discontinue the drug as soon as possible and use the smallest dose possible. Be alert for signs of trouble including:

1. Abnormal bleeding from the vagina.
2. Pains in the calves or chest or sudden shortness of breath, or coughing blood (indicating possible clots in the legs, heart, or lungs).
3. Severe headache, dizziness, faintness, or changes in vision (indicating possible developing clots in the brain or eye).
4. Breast lumps (you should ask your doctor how to examine your own breasts).
5. Jaundice (yellowing of the skin).
6. Mental depression.

Based on his or her assessment of your medical needs, your doctor has prescribed this drug for you. Do not give the drug to anyone else.

List of references available upon request.

[*Shown in Product Identification Section*]

K-LYTE® ℞

Effervescent Tablets
Each tablet in solution
supplies 25 mEq. potassium
as bicarbonate and citrate

K-LYTE® DS ℞

Effervescent Tablets
Each tablet in solution
supplies 50 mEq potassium
as bicarbonate and citrate

Indications: K-LYTE DS and K-LYTE are oral potassium supplements for therapy or prophylaxis of potassium deficiency. They are particularly useful when thiazide diuretics, corticosteroids, or severe vomiting and diarrhea cause excessive excretory potassium losses; and when dietary potassium is low. Carefully monitored, K-LYTE DS and K-LYTE may also be useful for potassium replacement where digitalis intoxication results in cardiac arrhythmias.

Contraindications: Impaired renal function with oliguria or azotemia; Addison's disease; hyperkalemia from any cause.

Warnings and Precautions: Since the amount of potassium deficiency may be difficult to determine accurately, supplements should be administered with caution, and dosages adjusted to the requirements of the individual patient. Potassium intoxication rarely occurs in patients with normal kidney function. Symptoms of potassium intoxication are variable. They include listlessness, mental confusion, and tingling of the extremities. Frequent checks of the clinical status of the patient, ECG, and serum potassium level are desirable. In established hypokalemia, attention should also be directed toward other potential electrolyte disturbances. Potassium supplements should be given cautiously to digitalized patients and such patients should be monitored by ECG for cardiac irregularities. To minimize the possibility of gastrointestinal

Continued on next page

Mead Johnson Pharm.—Cont.

irritation associated with the oral ingestion of concentrated potassium salt preparations, **patients should be carefully directed to dissolve each dose completely in the stated amount of water.**

Adverse Reactions: Nausea, vomiting, diarrhea, and abdominal discomfort may occur with the use of potassium salts.

Dosage and Administration: Adults—1 K-LYTE DS tablet completely dissolved 1 to 2 times daily depending upon the requirements of the patient. 1 K-LYTE tablet completely dissolved 2 to 4 times daily depending upon the requirements of the patient: 1 K-LYTE DS tablet (50 mEq potassium) dissolved in 6 to 8 ounces of cold or ice water; 1 K-LYTE tablet (25 mEq potassium) dissolved in 3 to 4 ounces of cold or ice water.

Note: It is suggested that K-LYTE DS and K-LYTE be taken with meals and sipped slowly over a 5 to 10 minute period.

How Supplied:

K-LYTE

NDC 0087-0760-01 Lime-flavored, Boxes of 30

NDC 0087-0760-02 Lime-flavored, Boxes of 250

NDC 0087-0761-01 Orange-flavored, Boxes of 30

NDC 0087-0761-02 Orange-flavored, Boxes of 250

6505-00-934-3477 (Box of 30) (Defense)

VA 6505-00-934-3477A (Box of 30) Lime

VA 6505-00-153-6904A (Box of 30) Orange

K-LYTE DS

NDC 0087-0772-41 Lime-flavored, Boxes of 30

NDC 0087-0771-41 Orange-flavored, Boxes of 30

NDC 0087-0771-42 Orange-flavored, Boxes of 100

NDC 0087-0772-42 Lime-Flavored, Boxes of 100

VA 6505-01-081-7650A (Box of 100) Lime

VA 6505-01-082-2931A (Box of 100) Orange

[Shown in Product Identification Section]

K-LYTE/CL® Effervescent Tablets and Powder ℞

Each dose in solution supplies 25 mEq. potassium chloride

Indications: K-Lyte/Cl is an oral potassium supplement for therapy or prophylaxis of potassium deficiency. It is particularly useful when thiazide diuretics, corticosteroids, or severe vomiting and diarrhea cause excessive excretory potassium losses; and when dietary potassium is low. Carefully monitored, K-Lyte/Cl may also be useful for potassium replacement where digitalis intoxication results in cardiac arrhythmias.

Contraindications: See K-LYTE® effervescent tablets.

Warnings and Precautions: See K-LYTE effervescent tablets. Also note: K-LYTE/CL powder contains approximately 20–25 kilocalories (as sucrose) per dose which should be considered for patients with restriction of caloric intake.

Adverse Reactions: See K-LYTE effervescent tablets.

Dosage and Administration: K-LYTE/CL Effervescent Tablets, Adults: 1 tablet **completely dissolved** 2 to 4 times daily, depending upon the requirements of the patient: 1 tablet (25 mEq. potassium chloride) in 3 to 4 ounces of cold or ice water. K-LYTE/CL Powder, Adults: 1 dose **completely dissolved** 2 to 4 times daily, depending upon the requirements of the patient; 1 dose (25 mEq. potassium chloride) in **6 ounces of cold or ice water.** The normal adult daily requirement is approximately 50 mEq. of elemental potassium.

NOTE: It is suggested that K-LYTE/CL be taken with meals and sipped slowly over a 5–10 minute period.

How Supplied: K-Lyte/CL Effervescent Tablets

NDC 0087-0766-41 Citrus-flavored, Boxes of 30

NDC 0087-0766-42 Citrus-flavored, Boxes of 250

NDC 0087-0767-41 Fruit Punch-flavored, Boxes of 30

NDC 0087-0767-42 Fruit Punch-flavored, Boxes of 250

K-Lyte/CL Powder

NDC 0087-0763-01 Fruit Punch-flavored, 225 g. can (30 measured doses with scoop)

[Shown in Product Identification Section]

MEGACE® tablets ℞

(megestrol acetate)

U.S. Patent No. 3,356,573

Description: Megestrol acetate is a white, crystalline solid chemically described as 17α-acetoxy-6-methylpregna-4, 6-diene-3, 20-dione. Its molecular weight is 384.5. The empirical formula is $C_{24}H_{32}O_4$.

Actions: While the precise mechanism by which Megace (megestrol acetate) produces its antineoplastic effects against endometrial carcinoma is unknown at the present time, an antiluteinizing effect mediated via the pituitary has been postulated. There is also evidence to suggest a local effect as a result of the marked changes brought about by the direct instillation of progestational agents into the endometrial cavity. Likewise, the antineoplastic action of Megace (megestrol acetate) on carcinoma of the breast is unclear.

Indications: Megace (megestrol acetate) is indicated for the palliative treatment of advanced carcinoma of the breast or endometrium (i.e., recurrent, inoperable, or metastatic disease). It should not be used in lieu of currently accepted procedures such as surgery, radiation, etc.

Contraindications: As a diagnostic test for pregnancy.

Warnings

THE USE OF PROGESTATIONAL AGENTS DURING THE FIRST FOUR MONTHS OF PREGNANCY IS NOT RECOMMENDED

Progestational agents have been used beginning with the first trimester of pregnancy in an attempt to prevent habitual abortion or treat threatened abortion. There is no adequate evidence that such use is effective and there is evidence of potential harm to the fetus when such drugs are given during the first four months of pregnancy.

Furthermore, in the vast majority of women, the cause of abortion is a defective ovum, which progestational agents could not be expected to influence. In addition, the use of progestational agents, with their uterine-relaxant properties, in patients with fertilized defective ova may cause a delay in spontaneous abortion. Therefore, the use of such drugs during the first four months of pregnancy is not recommended.

Several reports suggest an association between intrauterine exposure to female sex hormones and congenital anomalies, including congenital heart defects and limb reduction defects.[1–5] One study[4] estimated a 4.7-fold increased risk of limb reduction defects in infants exposed *in utero* to sex hormones (oral contraceptives, hormone withdrawal tests for pregnancy, or attempted treatment for threatened abortion).

Some of these exposures were very short and involved only a few days of treatment. The data suggest that the risk of limb reduction defects in exposed fetuses is somewhat less than 1 to 1,000.

If the patient is exposed to Megace during the first four months of pregnancy or if she becomes pregnant while taking this drug, she should be apprised of the potential risks to the fetus.

Administration for up to 7 years of megestrol acetate to female dogs is associated with an increased incidence of both benign and malignant tumors of the breast. Comparable studies in rats and ongoing studies in monkeys are not associated with an increased incidence of tumors. The relationship of the dog tumors to humans is unknown but should be considered in assessing the benefit-to-risk ratio when prescribing Megace and in surveillance of patients on therapy.

The use of Megace (megestrol acetate) in other types of neoplastic disease is not recommended.

Precautions: There are no specific precautions identified for the use of Megace (megestrol acetate) when used as recommended. Close, customary surveillance is indicated for any patient being treated for recurrent or metastatic cancer. Use with caution in patients with a history of thrombophlebitis.

This product contains FD&C Yellow No. 5 (tartrazine) which may cause allergic-type reactions (including bronchial asthma) in certain susceptible individuals. Although the overall incidence of FD&C Yellow No. 5 (tartrazine) sensitivity in the general population is low, it is frequently seen in patients who also have aspirin hypersensitivity.

Adverse Reactions: No untoward effects have been ascribed to Megace therapy. Reports have been received of patients developing carpal tunnel syndrome, deep vein thrombophlebitis and alopecia while taking megestrol acetate.

Overdosage: No serious side effects have resulted from studies involving Megace (megestrol acetate) administered in dosages as high as 800 mg/day.

Dosage and Administration:

Breast cancer: 160 mg/day (40 q.i.d.)

Endometrial carcinoma: 40—320 mg/day in divided doses.

At least two months of continuous treatment is considered an adequate period for determining the efficacy of Megace (megestrol acetate).

How Supplied: Megace® is available as light blue, scored tablets containing 20 mg or 40 mg megestrol acetate in bottles of 100 tablets each.

NDC 0087-0595-01, Bottles of 100 20 mg tablet

NDC 0087-0596-41, Bottles of 100 40 mg tablet

6505-01-070-1493 (Bottles of 100) (Defense)

References:

1. Gal I, Kirman B and Stern J: "Hormonal Pregnancy Tests and Congenital Malformation," Nature 216:83, 1967.
2. Levy EP, Cohen A and Fraser FC: "Hormone Treatment During Pregnancy and Congenital Heart Defects," Lancet 1:611, 1973.
3. Nora J and Nora A: "Birth Defects and Oral Contraceptives," Lancet 1:941, 1973.
4. Janerich DT, Piper JM and Glebatis DM: "Oral Contraceptives and Congenital Limb-Reduction Defects," N Eng J Med, 291:697, 1974.
5. Heinonen OP, Slone D, Monson RR, Hook EB and Shapiro S: "Cardiovascular Birth Defects and Antenatal Exposure to Female Sex Hormones," N Eng J Med, 296:67, 1977.

Patient labeling For Megace®

Warning For Women

There is an increased risk of birth defects in children whose mothers take this drug during the first four months of pregnancy.

MEGACE is similar to the progesterone hormones naturally produced by the body. Progesterone and progesterone-like drugs are used to treat menstrual disorders, to test if the body is

producing certain hormones, and to treat some forms of cancer in women.
They have been used as a test for pregnancy but such use is no longer considered safe because of possible damage to a developing baby. Also, more rapid methods for testing for pregnancy are now available.
These drugs have also been used to prevent miscarriage in the first few months of pregnancy. No adequate evidence is available to show that they are effective for this purpose and there is evidence of an increased risk of birth defects, such as heart or limb defects, if these drugs are taken during the first four months of pregnancy. Furthermore, most cases of early miscarriage are due to causes which could not be helped by these drugs.
The exact risk of taking this drug early in pregnancy and having a baby with a birth defect is not known. However, one study found that babies born to women who had taken sex hormones (such as progesterone-like drugs) during the first three months of pregnancy were 4 to 5 times more likely to have abnormalities of the arms or legs than if their mothers had not taken such drugs. Some of these women had taken these drugs for only a few days.
The chance that an infant whose mother had taken this drug will have this type of defect is about 1 in 1,000.
If you take MEGACE and later find you were pregnant when you took it, be sure to discuss this with your doctor as soon as possible.

[*Shown in Product Identification Section*]

MUCOMYST® ℞
(Acetylcysteine)
U.S. Patent No. 3,091,569

Description: Acetylcysteine is the nonproprietary name for the N-acetyl derivative of the naturally occurring amino acid, L-cysteine. Chemically, it is N-acetyl-L-cysteine. The compound is a white crystalline powder which melts at 104–110°C and has a very slight odor. It has a molecular weight of 163.2. The agent is supplied in vials containing a 10% or 20% solution of acetylcysteine as the sodium salt.
Actions: The viscosity of pulmonary mucous secretions depends on the concentrations of mucoprotein and to a lesser extent deoxyribonucleic acid (DNA). The latter increases with increasing purulence owing to cellular debris. The mucolytic action of acetylcysteine is related to the sulfhydryl group in the molecule. This group probably "opens" disulfide linkages in mucus thereby lowering the viscosity. The mucolytic activity of acetylcysteine is unaltered by the presence of DNA, and increases with increasing pH. Significant mucolysis occurs between pH 7 and 9.
Indications: Mucomyst (acetylcysteine) is indicated as adjuvant therapy for patients with abnormal, viscid, or inspissated mucous secretions in such conditions as:

- Chronic bronchopulmonary disease (chronic emphysema, emphysema with bronchitis, chronic asthmatic bronchitis, tuberculosis, bronchiectasis and primary amyloidosis of the lung)
- Acute bronchopulmonary disease (pneumonia, bronchitis, tracheobronchitis)
- Pulmonary complications of cystic fibrosis
- Tracheostomy care
- Pulmonary complications associated with surgery
- Use during anesthesia
- Post-traumatic chest conditions
- Atelectasis due to mucous obstruction
- Diagnostic bronchial studies (bronchograms, bronchospirometry, and bronchial wedge catheterization)

Contraindications: Mucomyst (acetylcysteine) is contraindicated in those patients who are sensitive to it.
Warnings: After proper administration of acetylcysteine, an increased volume of liquefied bronchial secretions may occur. When cough is inadequate, the open airway must be maintained by mechanical suction if necessary. When there is a large mechanical block due to foreign body or local accumulation, the airway should be cleared by endotracheal aspiration, with or without bronchoscopy.
Asthmatics under treatment with Mucomyst (acetylcysteine) should be watched carefully. If bronchospasm progresses, this medication should be immediately discontinued.
Precautions: With the administration of Mucomyst, the patient may observe initially a slight odor that is soon not noticeable. With a face mask there may be stickiness on the face after nebulization which is easily removed by washing with water. Under certain conditions, a light purple color may develop in the solution of acetylcysteine. This does not significantly affect safety or mucolytic effectiveness. To prevent the concentration of acetylcysteine in the solution remaining after prolonged nebulization, dilute with an equal volume of Sterile Water for Injection, U.S.P., when three-fourths of the initial volume has been nebulized.
Adverse Effects: Adverse effects have included stomatitis, nausea and rhinorrhea. Sensitivity and sensitization to Mucomyst have been reported very rarely. A few susceptible patients, particularly asthmatics (see Warnings), may experience varying degrees of bronchospasm associated with the administration of nebulized acetylcysteine. Most patients with bronchospasm are quickly relieved by the use of a bronchodilator given by nebulization.
Dosage and Administration: Mucomyst (acetylcysteine) is available in plastic stoppered glass vials containing 4, 10, or 30 ml. The 20% solution may be diluted to a lesser concentration with either sterile normal saline or Sterile Water for Injection, U.S.P. The 10% solution may be used undiluted.

Nebulization—face mask, mouth piece, tracheostomy
When nebulized into a face mask, mouth piece, or tracheostomy, 1–10 ml. of the 20% solution or 2–20 ml. of the 10% solution may be given every 2–6 hours; the recommended dose for most patients is 3–5 ml. of the 20% solution or 6–10 ml. of the 10% solution 3 to 4 times a day.

Nebulization—tent, Croupette
In special circumstances it may be necessary to nebulize into a tent or Croupette, and this method of use must be individualized to take into account the available equipment and the patient's particular needs. This form of administration requires very large volumes of the solution, occasionally as much as 300 ml. during a single treatment period. If a tent or Croupette must be used, the recommended dose is the volume of solution (using 10% or 20% acetylcysteine) that will maintain a very heavy mist in the tent or Croupette for the desired period. Administration for intermittent or continuous prolonged periods, including overnight, may be desirable.

Direct Instillation
When used by direct instillation, 1–2 ml. of a 10 to 20% solution may be given as often as every hour.
When used for the routine nursing care of patients with tracheostomy, 1 to 2 ml. of a 10 to 20% solution may be given every 1 to 4 hours by instillation into the tracheostomy.
Acetylcysteine may be introduced directly into a particular segment of the bronchopulmonary tree by inserting (under local anesthesia and direct vision) a small plastic catheter into the trachea. Two to 5 ml. of the 20% solution may then be instilled by means of a syringe connected to the catheter.
Acetylcysteine may also be given through a percutaneous intratracheal catheter. One to 2 ml. of the 20% or 2–4 ml. of the 10% solution every 1 to 4 hours may then be given by a syringe attached to the catheter.

Diagnostic Bronchograms
For diagnostic bronchial studies, 2 or 3 administrations of 1 to 2 ml. of the 20% solution or 2–4 ml. of the 10% solution should be given by nebulization or by instillation intratracheally, prior to the procedure.

Administration of Aerosol:

Materials
Mucomyst may be administered using conventional nebulizers made of plastic or glass. Certain materials used in nebulization equipment react with acetylcysteine. The most reactive of these are certain metals (notably iron and copper) and rubber. Where materials may come into contact with acetylcysteine solution, parts made of the following acceptable materials should be used: glass, plastic, aluminum, anodized aluminum, chromed metal, tantalum, sterling silver, or stainless steel. Silver may become tarnished after exposure, but this is not harmful to the drug action nor to the patient.

Nebulizing Gases
Compressed tank gas (air) or an air compressor should be used to provide pressure for nebulizing the solution. Oxygen may also be used but should be used with usual caution in patients with severe respiratory disease and CO_2 retention.
Apparatus: Mucomyst (acetylcysteine) is usually administered as fine nebulae for its local effect, and the nebulizer used should be capable of providing optimal quantities of a suitable range of particle sizes.
The selection of apparatus for nebulization depends upon the desired particle size and rate of administration. Commercially available nebulizers will produce nebulae of acetylcysteine satisfactory for retention in the respiratory tract. Most of the nebulizers tested will supply a high proportion of the drug solution as particles of less than 10 microns in diameter. Mitchell[a] has shown that a range of particle size up to 10 microns should be satisfactorily retained in the respiratory tract.
Hand bulbs may be used but are not recommended for routine use for nebulizing Mucomyst (acetylcysteine) because their output is generally too small. Some handoperated nebulizers deliver particles that are larger than optimum for inhalation therapy.

Heated (hot pot) Nebulizer
Mucomyst should not be placed directly into the chamber of a heated (hot pot) nebulizer. A heated nebulizer may be part of the nebulization assembly to provide a warm saturated atmosphere if the Mucomyst aerosol is introduced by means of a separate unheated nebulizer. Usual precautions for administration of warm saturated nebulae should be observed.
The nebulized solution may be breathed directly from the nebulizer. Nebulizers may also be attached to plastic face masks, plastic face tents, plastic mouth pieces, conventional plastic oxygen tents, or head tents. Suitable nebulizers may also be fitted for use with the various intermittent positive pressure breathing (IPPB) machines.
The nebulizing equipment should be cleaned immediately after use; the residues may occlude the fine orifices or corrode metal parts.

Storage of Opened Vials
If only a portion of the solution in the vial is used, to minimize contamination the remainder should be stored in a refrigerator and used within 96 hours.
How Supplied: Mucomyst® 20% acetylcysteine solution. Sterile.

NDC 0087-0570-03 Cartons of three 10 ml. vials, 1 plastic dropper
NDC 0087-0570-09 Cartons of three 30 ml. vials
NDC 0087-0570-07 Cartons of twelve 4 ml. vials

Continued on next page

Mead Johnson Pharm.—Cont.

6505-00-767-9111 (10 ml.) Defense
VA 6505-00-767-9111A (10 ml.)
6505-00-782-2688 (30 ml.) Defense
VA 6505-00-782-2688A (30 ml.)

Mucomyst®-10 10% acetylcysteine solution. Sterile.
NDC 0087-0572-01 Cartons of three 10 ml. vials, 1 plastic dropper
NDC 0087-0572-02 Cartons of three 30 ml. vials
NDC 0087-0572-03 Cartons of twelve 4 ml. vials

Literature Available: Yes.
July, 1979

a. Amer Rev Resp Dis 82:627-639, 1960

MUCOMYST® WITH ISOPROTERENOL ℞
(10% acetylcysteine—0.05% isoproterenol HCl solution)

Description: Mucomyst with Isoproterenol (10% acetylcysteine—0.05% isoproterenol HCl) is a ready-to-use sterile aqueous solution of a mucolytic agent and a bronchodilator available as a convenience to physicians who wish to prescribe these agents concomitantly for use by nebulization into a face mask or mouthpiece.

Acetylcysteine, N.F., is the N-acetyl derivative of the naturally occurring amino acid, L-cysteine. Chemically, it is N-acetyl-L-cysteine. Acetylcysteine is a white crystalline powder that melts at 104–110°C. It has a molecular weight of 163.2.

Isoproterenol Hydrochloride, U.S.P., is the nonproprietary name for the adrenergic bronchodilator 3,4-dihydroxy-a-[(isopropyl-amino)-methyl] benzyl alcohol hydrochloride. It is a nearly white, odorless, crystalline powder with a slightly bitter taste. It has a molecular weight of 247.72 and a melting range of 165—170°C. The amount of isoproterenol present in 5 ml. of this 10% acetylcysteine solution is equivalent to 0.5 ml. of a 1:200 solution of isoproterenol. The pH of the acetylcysteine-isoproterenol solution is 6.5.

Actions: The viscosity of pulmonary mucous secretions depends on the concentrations of mucoprotein and, to a lesser extent, deoxyribonucleic acid (DNA). The mechanism of the mucolytic action of acetylcysteine is related to its sulfhydryl (-SH) group which probably breaks disulfide (-S-S-) linkages in mucoprotein, thereby lowering the viscosity. Significant mucolysis occurs between pH 6 and 9. This mucolytic activity is unaltered by the presence of DNA. Thus acetylcysteine is effective against both purulent and nonpurulent sputum.

Occasionally, patients exposed to the inhalation of an acetylcysteine aerosol respond with the development of increased airways obstruction of varying and unpredictable severity. Those patients who are reactors cannot be identified *a priori* from a random patient population. Even when patients are known to have reacted previously to the inhalation of an acetylcysteine aerosol, they may not react during a subsequent treatment. The converse is also true; patients who have had inhalation treatments of acetylcysteine without incident may still react to a subsequent inhalation with increased airways obstruction. The presence of isoproterenol hydrochloride in the inhalation mixture generally reduces the severity of such reactions. However, it should be noted that (a) the isoproterenol in some patients may not reduce the acetylcysteine-induced airway obstruction and (b) in some patients the airway obstruction may return if the effect of the isoproterenol is dissipated prior to that of the acetylcysteine.

Indications and Usage: Mucomyst with Isoproterenol is indicated as adjuvant therapy for patients with viscid or inspissated mucous secretions who might react to an inhaled acetylcysteine aerosol with increased airways obstruction. Included among these patients are those with any of the following conditions who in the judgment of the physician may be placed at the risk of increased airways obstruction by inhalation therapy treatments using acetylcysteine:

Chronic bronchopulmonary disease (chronic emphysema, emphysema with bronchitis, chronic asthmatic bronchitis, tuberculosis, bronchiectasis and primary amyloidosis of the lung)
Acute bronchopulmonary disease (pneumonia, bronchitis, tracheobronchitis)
Pulmonary complications of cystic fibrosis
Pulmonary complications associated with surgery
Post-traumatic chest conditions
Atelectasis due to mucous obstruction

Mucomyst with Isoproterenol is not to be used as a routine bronchodilator since the isoproterenol component is only present to decrease possible increased airways obstruction caused by the acetylcysteine.

Contraindications: Mucomyst with Isoproterenol is contraindicated in those patients who are sensitive to it.

Use of isoproterenol in patients with a history of cardiac arrhythmias associated with tachycardia is generally contraindicated because the cardiac stimulant effect of the drug may aggravate such disorders.

Warnings:

After proper administration of Mucomyst with Isoproterenol an increased volume of liquefied bronchial secretions may occur. When cough is inadequate, an open airway must be maintained by mechanical suction, if necessary. When there is a large mechanical block due to a foreign body or local accumulation, the airway should be cleared by endotracheal aspiration, with or without bronchoscopy.

Asthmatics under treatment with Mucomyst with Isoproterenol should be observed carefully. If bronchospasm progresses, the medication should be discontinued immediately.

Excessive or repetitive use of an adrenergic aerosol such as the isoproterenol in Mucomyst with Isoproterenol should be discouraged because it may lose its effectiveness.

Occasional patients have been reported to develop severe, paradoxical airway resistance following repeated, excessive use of isoproterenol inhalation preparations. The cause of this refractory state is unknown. It is advisable that in such instances the use of this preparation be discontinued immediately and alternative therapy instituted, since in the reported cases the patients did not respond to other forms of therapy until the drug was withdrawn.

Deaths have been reported following excessive use of isoproterenol inhalation preparations and the exact cause is unknown. Cardiac arrest was noted in several instances.

Because insufficient experience exists with administration of Mucomyst with Isoproterenol by direct instillation or in tents or Croupettes, its use should be limited to nebulization and inhalation only using a face mask or mouthpiece delivery system.

Precautions: Continued nebulization of an acetylcysteine solution with a dry gas will result in an increased concentration of the drug in the nebulizer because of evaporation of the solvent. Extreme concentration may impede nebulization and efficient delivery of the drug. As concentration occurs, dilution of the nebulizing solution with Sterile Water for Injection, U.S.P., will obviate this problem.

With the administration of acetylcysteine, the patient may initially notice a slightly disagreeable sulfurous odor. With a face mask, any stickiness remaining on the face after nebulization may be removed easily by washing with water.

Epinephrine should not be administered with isoproterenol because both drugs are direct cardiac stimulants, and their combined effects may induce serious arrhythmia. However, if desired, they may be alternated, provided an interval of at least four hours has elapsed between agents.

Isoproterenol should be used with caution in patients with hypertension, cardiovascular disorders including coronary insufficiency, diabetes, or hyperthyroidism, and in persons sensitive to sympathomimetic amines.

Patients should be screened by exposure to an isoproterenol aerosol prior to the administration of Mucomyst with Isoproterenol to detect those patients whose bronchospasm may paradoxically worsen with isoproterenol.

It has not been determined whether the administration of isoproterenol prior to acetylcysteine inhalation might be more advantageous to a given patient than the concomitant administration of the two medications.

Usage in Pregnancy: Reproduction studies have been performed in rats and rabbits. In pregnant rabbits exposure to nebulized Mucomyst with Isoproterenol for 35 minutes daily resulted in a decreased number of live pups per litter. In rats exposed to nebulized Mucomyst with Isoproterenol for the same period of time there was no evidence of impaired fertility or harm to the fetus.

There are no well controlled studies in pregnant women but clinical experience does not include any positive evidence of adverse effects on the fetus. Although there is no clearly defined risk, such experience cannot exclude the possibility of infrequent or subtle damage to the fetus. Mucomyst with Isoproterenol should be used in pregnant women only when clearly needed.

Adverse Reactions: With acetylcysteine adverse effects have included stomatitis, nausea, vomiting, fever, rhinorrhea, drowsiness, clamminess, chest tightness, and bronchoconstriction. Clinically overt acetylcysteine induced bronchospasm occurs infrequently and unpredictably even in patients with asthmatic bronchitis or bronchitis complicating bronchial asthma. Acquired sensitization to acetylcysteine has been reported rarely. Reports of sensitization in patients have not been confirmed by patch testing. Sensitization has been confirmed in several inhalation therapists who reported a history of dermal eruptions after frequent and extended exposure to acetylcysteine. Reports of irritation to the tracheal and bronchial tracts have been received and although hemoptysis has occurred in patients receiving acetylcysteine such findings are not uncommon in patients with bronchopulmonary disease and a causal relationship has not been established.

As with other sympathomimetic drugs, isoproterenol may produce some undesirable side effects such as nervousness, dizziness, palpitation, nausea, vomiting, headache, tremor, flushing, weakness, tachycardia, sweating, precordial distress, or anginal-type pain.

With Mucomyst with Isoproterenol adverse effects have included drowsiness, jitteriness, lightheadedness, and increased airways obstruction.

Dosage and Administration: Mucomyst with Isoproterenol is available in plastic stoppered glass vials containing 4 ml. of solution. Should the solution require dilution, Sterile Water for Injection, U.S.P., may be used.

A critical determination in calculating the volume of Mucomyst with Isoproterenol to be given is the amount of isoproterenol contained in the volume of solution. The amount of isoproterenol present in 5 ml. of this 10% acetylcysteine solution is equivalent to 0.5 ml. of a 1:200 solution of isoproterenol.

Adult's Dosage: When nebulized into a face mask or mouthpiece, 3 to 5 ml. of the solution may be given every 3–6 hours up to 4 times daily. Recommended dose, 4 ml. qid.

CHILDREN'S DOSAGE—DUE TO THE ISOPROTERENOL COMPONENT, CAUTION SHOULD BE USED IN ADMINISTERING MUCOMYST WITH ISOPROTERENOL TO CHILDREN SIX YEARS AND YOUNGER.

While no formal studies have been undertaken to determine the optimal dosage in children of less than 15 years of age, retrospective studies have shown that combinations of acetylcysteine and isoproterenol are well tolerated by children. These studies and prior experience with the individual components of Mucomyst with Isoproterenol indicate the following dosages can serve as guides:

Children 2 to 6 years of age, 2 to 3 ml. bid.
Children 7 to 14 years of age, 2 to 3 ml. 2 or 3 times a day.

The duration of each treatment will vary with the type of nebulizing equipment and the capabilities and respiratory status of the patient but most often will be 15 to 30 minutes.

Because insufficient experience exists with administration of Mucomyst with Isoproterenol by direct instillation or in tents or Croupettes, it's use should be limited to nebulization and inhalation only using a face mask or mouthpiece.

For direct instillation or for use in tents or Croupettes, Mucomyst® or Mucomyst® -10 should be used.

Administration of Aerosol:

Materials

Mucomyst with Isoproterenol may be administered using conventional nebulizers made of plastic or glass. Certain materials used in nebulization equipment react with acetylcysteine. The most reactive of these are certain metals (notably iron and copper) and most rubbers. Where materials may come into contact with acetylcysteine solution, parts made of the following acceptable materials should be used: glass, plastic, aluminum, anodized aluminum, chromed metal, tantalum, sterling silver, or stainless steel. Silver may become tarnished after exposure, but this is not deleterious to the drug action or the patient.

Nebulizing Gases

Compressed tank gas (air) or an air compressor should be used to provide pressure for nebulizing the solution. Oxygen may also be used but should be used with usual caution in patients with severe respiratory disease and CO_2 retention.

Apparatus

Mucomyst with Isoproterenol is usually administered as a fine nebula and the nebulizer used should be capable of providing optimal quantities of a suitable range of particle sizes. Commercially available nebulizers will produce nebulae of Mucomyst with Isoproterenol satisfactory for retention in the respiratory tract. Most of the nebulizers tested will supply a high proportion of the drug solution as particles of less than 10 microns in diameter. Mitchell[a] has shown that a range of particle size up to 10 microns should be retained in the respiratory tract satisfactorily.

Units that nebulized in this solution with a satisfactory efficiency were the Maxi-Myst® Nebulizer (Mead Johnson Pharmaceutical Division, Evansville, Indiana), Hand-E-Vent intermittent positive pressure breathing device (Ohio Medical Products, 3030 Airco Drive, Madison, Wisconsin), and various other intermittent positive pressure breathing devices, No. 40 De Vilbiss (The De Vilbiss Co., Somerset, Pennsylvania), Bennett Twin-Jet Nebulizer (Puritan Bennett Corp. Oak at 13th St., Kansas City, Missouri).

The nebulized solution may be inhaled directly from the nebulizer. Nebulizers may also be attached to plastic face masks or plastic mouthpieces. Suitable nebulizers may also be fitted for use with the various intermittent positive pressure breathing (IPPB) machines. The nebulizing equipment should be cleaned immediately after use because the residues may clog the smaller orifices or corrode metal parts.

Hand bulbs are not recommended for routine use for nebulizing Mucomyst with Isoproterenol because their output is generally too small. Also, some hand-operated nebulizers deliver particles that are larger than optimum for inhalation therapy.

Heated (hot pot) Nebulizer

Mucomyst with Isoproterenol should not be placed directly into the chamber of a heated (hot pot) nebulizer.

A heated nebulizer may be part of the nebulization assembly to provide a warm saturated atmosphere if the aerosol is introduced by means of a separate unheated nebulizer. Usual precautions for administration of warm saturated nebulae should be observed.

Prolonged Nebulization

When three-fourths of the initial volume of Mucomyst with Isoproterenol solution have been nebulized, a quantity of Sterile Water for Injection USP (approximately equal to the volume of solution remaining) should be added to the nebulizer. This minimizes any concentration of the agent in the residual solvent remaining after prolonged nebulization.

Storage of Opened Vials

If only a portion of the solution in the vial is used, to minimize contamination the remainder should be capped and stored in a refrigerator and used within 96 hours.

Storage of Unopened Vials

Store unopened vials at room temperature (15° to 30°C, 59° to 86°F).

Avoid exposure to higher temperature.

Compatibility: The physical and chemical compatibility of Mucomyst with Isoproterenol with other drugs commonly administered by nebulization, direct instillation or topical application has not been studied as it has for Mucomyst® (acetylcysteine). Nevertheless, all of the known incompatibilities of Mucomyst apply. These are listed in the following table.

EXPECTED IN VITRO INCOMPATIBILITIES OF MUCOMYST WITH ISOPROTERENOL

Product and/or Agent(s)	Manufacturer (Trademark)
Amphotericin B	Squibb (Fungizone® (Intravenous)
Chlortetracycline HCl	Lederle (Aureomycin®)
Erythromycin lactobionate	(Abbott (Erythrocin®)
Oxytetracycline HCl	Pfizer (Terramycin®)
Sodium Ampicillin	Bristol (Polycillin-N®)
Tetracycline HCl	Lederle (Achromycin®)
Iodized Oil USP	Fougera (Lipiodol®)
Chymotrypsin	Armour
Trypsin	Armour
Hydrogen peroxide	

The rating incompatible is based on the formation of a precipitate, a change in color or clarity, immiscibility, or rapid loss of potency of acetylcysteine or the active ingredient of the product and/or agent in the admixture. These data are intended to serve only as a guide to predicting compounding problems.

How Supplied: Mucomyst with Isoproterenol: 10% acetylcysteine and 0.05% isoproterenol HCl solution. Sterile.

NDC 0087-0573-47 Carton of twelve 4 ml. vials

Also available:

Mucomyst® 20% acetylcysteine solution. Sterile.

NDC 0087-0570-04 Carton of twelve 4 ml. vials
NDC 0087-0570-03 Carton of three 10 ml. vials 1 plastic dropper
NDC 0087-0570-09 Carton of three 30 ml. vials

Mucomyst® -10 10% acetylcysteine solution. Sterile.

NDC 0087-0572-03 Carton of twelve 4 ml. vials
NDC 0087-0572-01 Carton of three 10 ml. vials 1 plastic dropper
NDC 0087-0572-02 Carton of three 30 ml. vials

Note to Pharmacist: Additional Warning To Patients

It is necessary for the protection of users that warning information to patients be included as part of the label and as part of any instructions to patients included in the package dispensed to the patient as follows:

Warning: Do not exceed the dose prescribed by your physician. If difficulty in breathing persists, contact your physician immediately.

References: A bibliography on Mucomyst with Isoproterenol is available on request.

Acetylcysteine: U.S. Patent No. 3,091,569

NATALINS® tablets

Multivitamin and multimineral supplement

Composition: Each Natalins tablet supplies:

		% U.S. RDA Pregnant or Lactating Women
Vitamins		
Vitamin A, I.U.	8,000	100
Vitamin D, I.U.	400	100
Vitamin E, I.U.	30	100
Vitamin C (Ascorbic acid), mg.	90	150
Folic acid (Folacin), mg.	0.8	100
Thiamine (Vitamin B_1), mg.	1.7	100
Riboflavin (Vitamin B_2), mg.	2.0	100
Niacin, mg.	20	100
Vitamin B_6, mg.	4.0	160
Vitamin B_{12}, mcg.	8	100
Minerals		
Calcium, mg.	200	15
Iodine, mcg.	150	100
Iron, mg.	45	250
Magnesium, mg.	100	22

Ingredients: Calcium carbonate, magnesium hydroxide, polyvinylpyrrolidone USP, gum arabic, ion exchange resin, methyl cellulose, magnesium stearate, artificial color, ethyl cellulose, silicon dioxide, glycerin, titanium dioxide, artificial flavor, vitamin A acetate, ergocalciferol, dl-alpha-tocopheryl acetate, sodium ascorbate, folic acid, thiamine mononitrate, riboflavin, niacinamide, pyridoxine hydrochloride, cyanocobalamin, calcium iodate and ferrous fumarate.

Action and Uses: Diet supplementation during pregnancy or lactation.

Administration and Dosage: One tablet a day or as indicated.

How Supplied:

Natalins® tablets
NDC 0087-0700-01 Bottles of 100
NDC 0087-0700-06 Bottles of 1000

[*Shown in Product Identification Section*]

NATALINS® RX ℞

Multivitamin and Multimineral Supplement Tablets with 1 mg. folic acid and 60 mg. Iron

Composition: Each Natalins Rx tablet supplies:

		% U.S. RDA Pregnant Or Lactating Women
Vitamins		
Vitamin A, I.U.	8,000	100
Vitamin D, I.U.	400	100

Continued on next page

Mead Johnson Pharm.—Cont.

Vitamin E, I.U.	30	100
Vitamin C (Ascorbic acid), mg.	90	150
Folic acid (Folacin), mg.	1.0	125
Thiamine (Vitamin B_1), mg.	2.55	150
Riboflavin (Vitamin B_2), mg.	3.0	150
Niacin, mg.	20	100
Vitamin B_6, mg.	10.0	400
Vitamin B_{12}, mcg.	8	100
Biotin, mg.	0.05	16
Pantothenic acid, mg.	15.0	150
Minerals		
Calcium, mg.	200	15
Iodine, mcg.	150	100
Iron, mg.	60	333
Magnesium, mg.	100	22
Copper, mg.	2.0	100
Zinc, mg.	15.0	100

Ingredients: Vitamin A acetate, ergocalciferol, dl-alpha-tocopheryl acetate, sodium ascorbate, folic acid, thiamine mononitrate, riboflavin, niacinamide, pyridoxine hydrochloride, cyanocobalamin, biotin, calcium pantothenate, calcium carbonate, calcium iodate, ferrous fumarate, magnesium hydroxide, cupric oxide and zinc oxide.

Indications for Use: Natalins Rx tablets help assure an adequate intake of the vitamins and minerals listed above.
The folic acid helps prevent the development of megaloblastic anemia during pregnancy.
Contraindications: Natalins Rx tablets should be used only by those people for whom supplemental vitamins and minerals are appropriate. Thus, Natalins Rx tablets should not be prescribed in
- patients with hemochromatosis
- patients with Wilson's disease

Warning: Keep Natalins Rx tablets out of the reach of children.
Caution: Pernicious anemia should be excluded before using this product. Folic acid may mask the symptoms of pernicious anemia by correcting the hematological picture while the neurological damage continues to progress. In patients with kidney stones, the calcium content of Natalins Rx tablets should be considered before prescribing.
Do not exceed the recommended dose of Natalins Rx tablets.
Adverse Reactions: No adverse reactions or undesirable side effects have been reported with the use of Natalins Rx tablets.
Daily Dose: One tablet, or as prescribed.
How Supplied:
Natalins® Rx Tablets: (Available on prescription.)
NDC 0087-0702-01 Bottles of 100
NDC 0087-0702-02 Bottles of 1000
[*Shown in Product Identification Section*]

OVCON®-50 ℞

21 tablets of norethindrone 1 mg and ethinyl estradiol 0.05 mg. Each green tablet in the 28 day regimen contains inert ingredients.

OVCON®-35 ℞

21 tablets of norethindrone 0.4 mg and ethinyl estradiol 0.035 mg. Each green tablet in the 28 day regimen contains inert ingredients.

Oral contraceptives

Description: 28-Day OVCON®-50 and OVCON®-35 tablets provide a continuous regimen for oral contraception derived from 21 tablets composed of norethindrone and ethinyl estradiol to be followed by 7 green tablets of inert ingredients.
21-Day OVCON®-50 and OVCON®-35 tablets provide a regimen for oral contraception derived from 21 tablets composed of norethindrone and ethinyl estradiol. The chemical name for norethindrone is 17-Hydroxy-19-nor-17α-pregn-4-en-20-yn-3-one and for ethinyl estradiol the chemical name is 19-Nor-17α-pregna-1,3,5 (10)-trien-20-yne-3, 17-diol.
Clinical Pharmacology: Combination oral contraceptives act primarily through the mechanism of gonadotropin suppression due to the estrogenic and progestational activity of the ingredients. Although the primary mechanism of action is inhibition of ovulation, alterations in the genital tract including changes in the cervical mucus (which increase the difficulty of sperm penetration) and the endometrium (which reduce the likelihood of implantation) may also contribute to contraceptive effectiveness.
Indications and Usage: OVCON is indicated for the prevention of pregnancy in women who elect to use oral contraceptives as a method of contraception.
Oral contraceptives are highly effective. The pregnancy rate in women using conventional combination oral contraceptives (containing 35 mcg or more of ethinyl estradiol or 50 mcg or more of mestranol) is generally reported as less than one pregnancy per 100 woman-years of use. Slightly higher rates (somewhat more than 1 pregnancy per 100 woman-years of use) are reported for some combination products containing 35 mcg or less of ethinyl estradiol, and rates on the order of 3 pregnancies per 100 woman-years are reported for the progestin-only oral contraceptives.
These rates are derived from separate studies conducted by different investigators in several population groups and cannot be compared precisely. Furthermore, pregnancy rates tend to be lower as clinical studies are continued, possibly due to selective retention in the longer studies of those patients who accept the treatment regimen and do not discontinue as a result of adverse reactions, pregnancy, or other reasons.
In clinical trials with OVCON-50, 1,252 patients completed 8,159 cycles and a total of 4 pregnancies were reported. This represents a pregnancy rate of 0.58 per 100 woman-years. In clinical trials with OVCON-35, 2493 patients completed 35,881 cycles and a total of 33 pregnancies were reported. This represents a pregnancy rate of 1.10 per 100 woman-years. The following table gives ranges of pregnancy rates reported in a standard textbook for other means of contraception. An individual patient may achieve higher or lower rates with any given method (except the IUD), depending upon the degree of adherence to the method.
Pregnancies per 100 Woman-Years: IUD, less than 1–6; Diaphragm with spermicidal product (creams or jellies), 2–20; Condom, 3–36; Aerosol foams, 2–29; Jellies and creams, 4–36; Rhythm (all types), less than 1–47: 1. Calendar method, 14–47; 2. Temperature method, 1–20; 3. Temperature method—intercourse only in post-ovulatory phase, less than 1–7; 4. Mucus method, 1–25; No contraception, 60–80.
Dose-Related Risk of Thromboembolism from Oral Contraceptives: Two studies have shown a positive association between the dose of estrogens in oral contraceptives and the risk of thromboembolism. For this reason, it is prudent and in keeping with good principles of therapeutics to minimize exposure to estrogen. The oral contraceptive product prescribed for any given patient should be that product which contains the least amount of estrogen that is compatible with an acceptable pregnancy rate and patient acceptance. It is recommended that new acceptors of oral contraceptives be started on preparations containing 50 mcg or less of estrogen.
Contraindications: Oral contraceptives should not be used in women with any of the following conditions:
1. Thrombophlebitis or thromboembolic disorders.
2. A past history of deep vein thrombophlebitis or thromboembolic disorders.
3. Cerebral vascular or coronary artery disease.
4. Known or suspected carcinoma of the breast.
5. Known or suspected estrogen dependent neoplasia.
6. Undiagnosed abnormal genital bleeding.
7. Known or suspected pregnancy (see warning No. 5).

Warnings:

Cigarette smoking increases the risk of serious cardiovascular side effects from oral contraceptive use. This risk increases with age and with heavy smoking (15 or more cigarettes per day) and is quite marked in women over 35 years of age. Women who use oral contraceptives should be strongly advised not to smoke.
The use of oral contraceptives is associated with increased risk of several serious conditions including thromboembolism, stroke, myocardial infarction, hepatic adenoma, gall bladder disease, hypertension. Practitioners prescribing oral contraceptives should be familiar with the following information relating to these risks.

1. *Thromboembolic Disorders and Other Vascular Problems* An increased risk of thromboembolic and thrombotic disease associated with the use of oral contraceptives is well established. Three principal studies in Great Britain and three in the United States have demonstrated an increased risk of fatal and nonfatal venous thromboembolism and stroke, both hemorrhagic and thrombotic. These studies estimate that users of oral contraceptives are 4 to 11 times more likely than nonusers to develop these diseases without evident cause (Table 2).
Cerebrovascular Disorders: In a collaborative American study of cerebrovascular disorders in women with and without predisposing causes, it was estimated that the risk of hemorrhagic stroke was 2.0 times greater in users than nonusers and the risk of thrombotic stroke was 4 to 9.5 times greater in users than in nonusers (Table 2).

TABLE 2
SUMMARY OF RELATIVE RISK OF THROMBOEMBOLIC DISORDERS AND OTHER VASCULAR PROBLEMS IN ORAL CONTRACEPTIVE USERS COMPARED TO NONUSERS

	Relative risk, times greater
Idiopathic thromboembolic disease	4–11
Post surgery thromboembolic complications	4–6
Thrombotic stroke	4–9.5
Hemorrhagic stroke	2
Myocardial infarction	2–12

Myocardial Infarction: An increased risk of myocardial infarction associated with the use of oral contraceptives has been reported confirming a previously suspected association. These studies, conducted in the United Kingdom, found, as expected, that the greater the number of underlying risk factors for coronary artery disease (cigarette smoking, hypertension, hypercholesterolemia, obesity, diabetes, history of preeclamptic toxemia) the higher the risk of developing myocardial infarction, regardless of whether the patient was an oral contraceptive user or not. Oral contraceptives, however, were found to be a clear additional risk factor.

In terms of relative risk, it has been estimated that oral contraceptive users who do not smoke (smoking is considered a major predisposing condition to myocardial infarction) are about twice as likely to have a fatal myocardial infarction as nonusers who do not smoke. Oral contraceptive users who are also smokers have about a 5-fold increased risk of fatal infarction compared to users who do not smoke, but about a 10- to 12-fold increased risk compared to nonusers who do not smoke. Furthermore, the amount of smoking is also an important factor. In determining the importance of these relative risks, however, the baseline rates for various age groups, as shown in Table 3, must be given serious consideration. The importance of other predisposing conditions mentioned above in determining relative and absolute risks has not as yet been quantified; it is quite likely that the same synergistic action exists, but perhaps to a lesser extent.

TABLE 3

ESTIMATED ANNUAL MORTALITY RATE PER 100,000 WOMEN FROM MYOCARDIAL INFARCTION BY USE OF ORAL CONTRACEPTIVES, SMOKING HABITS, AND AGE (IN YEARS)

	Myocardial infarction			
	Women aged 30–39		Women aged 40–44	
Smoking habits	Users	Non Users	Users	Non Users
All smokers	10.2	2.6	62.0	15.9
Heavy[1]	13.0	5.1	78.7	31.3
Light	4.7	.9	28.6	5.7
Nonsmokers	1.8	1.2	10.7	7.4
Smokers and nonsmokers	5.4	1.9	32.8	11.7

[1]Heavy smoker: 15 or more cigarettes per day. From Jain, A.K., Studies in Family Planning, 8:50, 1977.

Risk of Dose: In an analysis of data derived from several national adverse reaction reporting systems, British investigators concluded that the risk of thromboembolism including coronary thrombosis is directly related to the dose of estrogen used in oral contraceptives. Preparations containing 100 mcg or more of estrogen were associated with a higher risk of thromboembolism than those containing 50–80 mcg of estrogen. Their analysis did suggest, however, that the quantity of estrogen may not be the sole factor involved. This finding has been confirmed in the United States. Careful epidemiological studies to determine the degree of thromboembolic risk associated with progestogen-only oral contraceptives have not been performed. Cases of thromboembolic disease have been reported in women using these products, and they should not be presumed to be free of excess risk.

Estimate of Excess Mortality from Circulatory Diseases: A large prospective study carried out in the U.K. estimated the mortality rate per 100,000 women per year from diseases of the circulatory system for users and nonusers of oral contraceptives according to age, smoking habits, and duration of use. The overall excess death rate annually from circulatory diseases for oral contraceptive users was estimated to be 20 per 100,000 (ages 15–34—5/100,000; ages 35–44—33/100,000; ages 45–49—140/100,000), the risk being concentrated in older women, in those with a long duration of use, and in cigarette smokers. It was not possible, however, to examine the interrelationships of age, smoking and duration of use, nor to compare the effects of continuous versus intermittent use. Although the study showed a 10-fold increase in death due to circulatory diseases in users for 5 or more years, all of these deaths occurred in women 35 or older. Until larger numbers of women under 35 with continuous use for 5 or more years are available, it is not possible to assess the magnitude of the relative risk for this younger age group. The available data from a variety of sources have been analyzed to estimate the risk of death associated with various methods of contraception. The estimates of risk of death for each method include the combined risk of the contraceptive method (e.g., thromboembolic and thrombotic disease in the case of oral contraceptives) plus the risk attributable to pregnancy or abortion in the event of method failure. This latter risk varies with the effectiveness of the contraceptive method. The findings of this analysis are shown in Figure 1 below.

Figure 1. Estimated annual number of deaths associated with control of fertility and no control per 100,000 nonsterile women, by regimen of control and age of women.

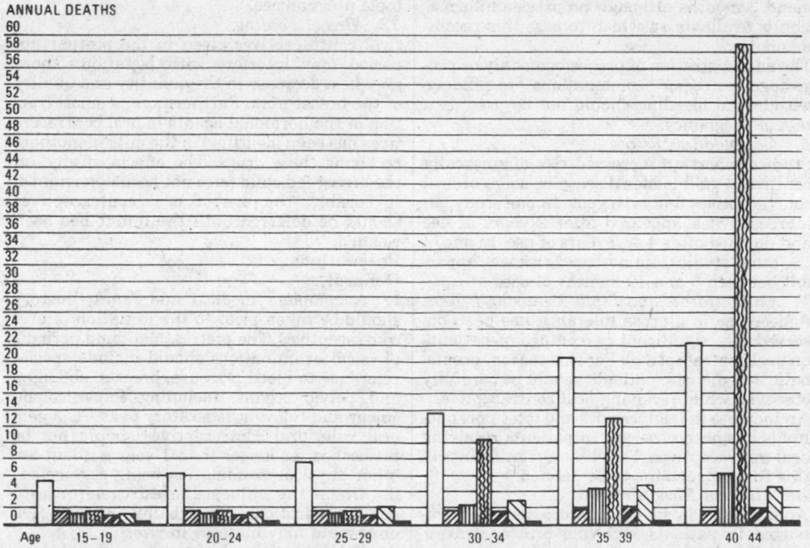

The study concluded that the mortality associated with all methods of birth control is low and below that associated with childbirth, with the exception of oral contraceptives in women over 40 who smoke. (The rates given for pill only/smokers for each age group are for smokers as a class. For "heavy" smokers [more than 15 cigarettes a day], the rates given would be about double; for "light" smokers [less than 15 cigarettes a day], about 50 percent.) The lowest mortality is associated with the condom or diaphragm backed up by early abortion.

The risk of thromboembolic and thrombotic disease associated with oral contraceptives increases with age after approximately age 30 and, for myocardial infarction, is further increased by hypertension, hypercholesterolemia, obesity, diabetes, or history of preeclamptic toxemia and especially by cigarette smoking.

Based on the data currently available, the following chart gives a gross estimate of the risk of death from circulatory disorders associated with the use of oral contraceptives:

SMOKING HABITS AND OTHER PREDISPOSING CONDITIONS—RISK ASSOCIATED WITH USE OF ORAL CONTRACEPTIVES

Age	Below 30	30–39	40+
Heavy smokers	C	B	A
Light smokers	D	C	B
Nonsmokers (no predisposing conditions) ..	D	C,D	C
Nonsmokers (other predisposing conditions) ..	C	C,B	B,A

A—Use associated with very high risk.
B—Use associated with high risk.
C—Use associated with moderate risk.
D—Use associated with low risk.

The physician and the patient should be alert to the earliest manifestations of thromboembolic and thrombotic disorders (e.g., thrombophlebitis, pulmonary embolism, cerebrovascular insufficiency, coronary occlusion, retinal thrombosis, and mesenteric thrombosis). Should any of these occur or be suspected, the drug should be discontinued immediately.

A four- to six-fold increased risk of post surgery thromboembolic complications has been reported in oral contraceptive users. If feasible, oral contraceptives should be discontinued at least 4 weeks before surgery of a type associated with an increased risk of thromboembolism or prolonged immobilization.

2. *Ocular Lesions.* There have been reports of neuro-ocular lesions such as optic neuritis or retinal thrombosis associated with the use of oral contraceptives. Discontinue oral contraceptive medication if there is unexplained, sudden or gradual, partial or complete loss of vision; onset of proptosis or diplopia; papilledema; or retinal vascular lesions and institute appropriate diagnostic and therapeutic measures.

3. *Carcinoma.* Long-term continuous administration of either natural or synthetic estrogen in certain animal species increases the frequency of carcinoma of the breast, cervix, vagina, and liver. Certain synthetic progestogens, none currently contained in oral contraceptives, have been noted to increase the incidence of mammary nodules, benign and malignant, in dogs.

In humans, three case control studies have reported an increased risk of endometrial carcinoma associated with the prolonged use of exogenous estrogen in post menopausal women. One publication reported on the first 21 cases submitted by physicians to a registry of cases of adenocarcinoma of the endome-

Continued on next page

Mead Johnson Pharm.—Cont.

trium in women under 40 on oral contraceptives. Of the cases found in women without predisposing risk factors for adenocarcinoma of the endometrium (e.g., irregular bleeding at the time oral contraceptives were first given, polycystic ovaries), nearly all occurred in women who had used a sequential oral contraceptive. These products are no longer marketed. No evidence has been reported suggesting an increased risk of endometrial cancer in users of conventional combination or progestogen-only oral contraceptives.

Several studies have found no increase in breast cancer in women taking oral contraceptives or estrogens. One study however, while also noting no overall increased risk of breast cancer in women treated with oral contraceptives, found an excess risk in the subgroups of oral contraceptive users with documented benign breast disease. A reduced occurrence of benign breast tumors in users of oral contraceptives has been well-documented.

In summary, there is at present no confirmed evidence from human studies of an increased risk of cancer associated with oral contraceptives. Close clinical surveillance of all women taking oral contraceptives is, nevertheless, essential. In all cases of undiagnosed persistent or recurrent abnormal vaginal bleeding, appropriate diagnostic measures should be taken to rule out malignancy. Women with a strong family history of breast cancer or who have breast nodules, fibrocystic disease or abnormal mammograms should be monitored with particular care if they elect to use oral contraceptives instead of other methods of contraception.

4. Hepatic Tumors. Benign hepatic adenomas have been found to be associated with the use of oral contraceptives. One study showed that oral contraceptive formulations with high hormonal potency were associated with a higher risk than lower potency formulations. Although benign, hepatic adenomas may rupture and may cause death through intra-abdominal hemorrhage. This has been reported in short-term as well as long-term users of oral contraceptives. Two studies relate risk with duration of use of the contraceptive, the risk being much greater after 4 or more years of oral contraceptive use. While hepatic adenoma is a rare lesion, it should be considered in women presenting abdominal pain and tenderness, abdominal mass or shock.

A few cases of hepatocellular carcinoma have been reported in women taking oral contraceptives. The relationship of these drugs to this type of malignancy is not known at this time.

5. Use in or Immediately Preceding Pregnancy, Birth Defects in Offspring, and Malignancy in Female Offspring.

The use of female sex hormones—both estrogenic and progestational agents—during early pregnancy may seriously damage the offspring. It has been shown that females exposed **in utero** to diethylstilbestrol, a nonsteroidal estrogen, have an increased risk of developing in later life a form of vaginal or cervical cancer that is ordinarily extremely rare. This risk has been estimated to be of the order of 1 in 1,000 exposures or less. Although there is no evidence at the present time that oral contraceptives further enhance the risk of developing this type of malignancy, such patients should be monitored with particular care if they elect to use oral contraceptives instead of other methods of contraception.

Furthermore, a high percentage of such exposed women (from 30 to 90%) have been found to have epithelial changes of the vagina and cervix. Although these changes are histologically benign, it is not known whether this condition is a precursor of vaginal malignancy. Male children so exposed may develop abnormalities of the urogenital tract. Although similar data are not available with the use of other estrogens, it cannot be presumed that they would not induce similar changes.

An increased risk of congenital anomalies, including heart defects and limb defects, has been reported with the use of sex hormones, including oral contraceptives, in pregnancy. One case control study has estimated a 4.7-fold increase in risk of limb-reduction defects in infants exposed **in utero** to sex hormones (oral contraceptives, hormonal withdrawal tests for pregnancy or attempted treatment for threatened abortion). Some of these exposures were very short and involved only a few days of treatment. The data suggest that the risk of limb-reduction defects in exposed fetuses is somewhat less than one in 1,000 live births.

In the past, female sex hormones have been used during pregnancy in an attempt to treat threatened or habitual abortion. There is considerable evidence that estrogens are ineffective for these indications, and there is no evidence from well controlled studies that progestogens are effective for these uses.

There is some evidence that triploidy and possibly other types of polyploidy are increased among abortuses from women who become pregnant soon after ceasing oral contraceptives. Embryos with these anomalies are virtually always aborted spontaneously. Whether there is an overall increase in spontaneous abortion of pregnancies conceived soon after stopping oral contraceptives is unknown.

It is recommended that for any patient who has missed two consecutive periods, pregnancy should be ruled out before continuing the contraceptive regimen. If the patient has not adhered to the prescribed schedule, the possibility of pregnancy should be considered at the time of the first missed period (or after 45 days from the last menstrual period if the progestogen-only oral contraceptives are used), and further use of oral contraceptives should be withheld until pregnancy has been ruled out. If pregnancy is confirmed, the patient should be apprised of the potential risks to the fetus and the advisability of continuation of the pregnancy should be discussed in the light of these risks.

It is also recommended that women who discontinue oral contraceptives with the intent of becoming pregnant use an alternate form of contraception for a period of time before attempting to conceive. Many clinicians recommend 3 months although no precise information is available on which to base this recommendation.

The administration of progestogen-only or progestogen-estrogen combinations to induce withdrawal bleeding should not be used as a test of pregnancy.

6. Gallbladder Disease.

Studies report an increased risk of surgically confirmed gallbladder disease in users of oral contraceptives and estrogens. In one study, an increased risk appeared after 2 years of use and doubled after 4 or 5 years of use. In one of the other studies, an increased risk was apparent between 6 and 12 months of use.

7. Carbohydrate and Lipid Metabolic Effects.

A decrease in glucose tolerance has been observed in a significant percentage of patients on oral contraceptives. For this reason, prediabetic and diabetic patients should be carefully observed while receiving oral contraceptives.

An increase in triglycerides and total phospholipids has been observed in patients receiving oral contraceptives. The clinical significance of this finding remains to be defined.

8. Elevated Blood Pressure.

An increase in blood pressure has been reported in patients receiving oral contraceptives. In some women, hypertension may occur within a few months of beginning oral contraceptive use. In the first year of use, the prevalence of women with hypertension is low in users and may be no higher than that of a comparable group of nonusers. The prevalence in users increases, however, with longer exposure, and in the fifth year of use is two and a half to three times the reported prevalence in the first year. Age is also strongly correlated with the development of hypertension in oral contraceptive users. Women who previously have had hypertension during pregnancy may be more likely to develop elevation of blood pressure when given oral contraceptives. Hypertension that develops as a result of taking oral contraceptives usually returns to normal after discontinuing the drug.

9. Headache.

The onset or exacerbation of migraine or development of headache of a new pattern which is recurrent, persistent, or severe, requires discontinuation of oral contraceptives and evaluation of the cause.

10. Bleeding Irregularities.

Breakthrough bleeding, spotting, and amenorrhea are frequent reasons for patients discontinuing oral contraceptives. In breakthrough bleeding, as in all cases of irregular bleeding from the vagina, nonfunctional causes should be borne in mind. In undiagnosed persistent or recurrent abnormal bleeding from the vagina, adequate diagnostic measures are indicated to rule out pregnancy or malignancy. If pathology has been excluded, time or a change to another formulation may solve the problem. Changing to an oral contraceptive with a higher estrogen content, while potentially useful in minimizing menstrual irregularity, should be done only if necessary since this may increase the risk of thromboembolic disease.

Women with a past history of oligomenorrhea or secondary amenorrhea or young women without regular cycles may have a tendency to remain anovulatory or to become amenorrheic after discontinuation of oral contraceptives. Women with these preexisting problems should be advised of this possibility and encouraged to use other contraceptive methods. Post-use anovulation, possibly prolonged, may also occur in women without previous irregularities.

11. Ectopic Pregnancy.

Ectopic as well as intrauterine pregnancy may occur in contraceptive failures. However, in progestogen-only oral contraceptive failures, the ratio of ectopic to intrauterine pregnancies is higher than in women who are not receiving oral contraceptives, since the drugs are more effective in preventing intrauterine than ectopic pregnancies.

12. Breast Feeding.

Oral contraceptives given in the postpartum period may interfere with lactation. There may be a decrease in the quantity and quality of the breast milk. Furthermore, a small fraction of the hormonal agents in oral contraceptives has been identified in the milk of mothers receiving these drugs. The effects, if any, on the breast-fed child have not been determined. If feasible, the use of oral contraceptives should be deferred until the infant has been weaned.

Precautions:

General

1. A complete medical and family history should be taken prior to the initiation of oral contraceptives. The pretreatment and periodic physical examinations should include special reference to blood pressure, breasts, abdomen and pelvic organs, including Papanicolaou smear and relevant laboratory tests. As a general rule, oral contraceptives should not be prescribed for longer than 1 year without another physical examination being performed.
2. Under the influence of estrogen-progestogen preparations, preexisting uterine leiomyomata may increase in size.
3. Patients with a history of psychic depression should be carefully observed and the drug discontinued if depression recurs to a serious degree. Patients becoming significantly depressed while taking oral contraceptives

should stop the medication and use an alternate method of contraception in an attempt to determine whether the symptom is drug related.

4. Oral contraceptives may cause some degree of fluid retention. They should be prescribed with caution, and only with careful monitoring, in patients with conditions which might be aggravated by fluid retention, such as convulsive disorders, migraine syndrome, asthma, or cardiac or renal insufficiency.

5. Patients with a past history of jaundice during pregnancy have an increased risk of recurrence of jaundice while receiving oral contraceptive therapy. If jaundice develops in any patient receiving such drugs, the medication should be discontinued.

6. Steroid hormones may be poorly metabolized in patients with impaired liver function and should be administered with caution in such patients.

7. Oral contraceptive users may have disturbances in normal tryptophan metabolism which may result from a relative pyridoxine deficiency. The clinical significance of this is yet to be determined.

8. Serum folate levels may be depressed by oral contraceptive therapy. Since the pregnant woman is predisposed to the development of folate deficiency and the incidence of folate deficiency increases with increasing gestation, it is possible that if a woman becomes pregnant shortly after stopping oral contraceptives, she may have a greater chance of developing folate deficiency, and complications attributed to this deficiency.

9. The pathologist should be advised of oral contraceptive therapy when relevant specimens are submitted.

10. Certain endocrine and liver function tests and blood components may be affected by estrogen-containing oral contraceptives:

a. Increased sulfobromophthalein-retention.

b. Increased prothrombin and factors VII, VIII, IX, and X; decreased antithrombin 3; increased norepinephrine-induced platelet aggregability.

c. Increased thyroid binding globulin (TBG) leading to increased circulating total thyroid hormone, as measured by protein-bound iodine (PBI), T4 by column, or T4 by radioimmunoassay. Free T3 resin uptake is decreased, reflecting the elevated TBG, free T4 concentration is unaltered.

d. Decreased pregnanediol excretion.

e. Reduced response to metyrapone test.

11. OVCON-50 (28 Day and 21 Day) and OVCON-35 (21 Day) contain FD&C Yellow No. 5 (tartrazine) which may cause allergic-type reactions (including bronchial asthma) in certain susceptible individuals. Although the overall incidence of FD&C Yellow No. 5 (tartrazine) sensitivity in the general population is low, it is frequently seen in patients who also have aspirin hypersensitivity.

Information for the Patient: See Patient Labeling Printed below

Drug Interactions: Reduced efficacy and increased incidence of breakthrough bleeding have been associated with concomitant use of rifampin. A similar association has been suggested with barbiturates, phenylbutazone, phenytoin sodium, and ampicillin.

Carcinogenesis: See Warning section for information on the carcinogenic potential of oral contraceptives.

Pregnancy: Pregnancy category X. See Contraindications and Warnings.

Nursing Mothers: See Warnings.

Adverse Reactions: An increased risk of the following serious adverse reactions has been associated with the use of oral contraceptives (see Warnings):

Thrombophlebitis.
Pulmonary embolism.
Coronary thrombosis.
Cerebral thrombosis.
Cerebral hemorrhage.
Hypertension.
Gallbladder disease.
Benign hepatomas.
Congenital anomalies.

There is evidence of an association between the following conditions and the use of oral contraceptives, although additional confirmatory studies are needed:

Mesenteric thrombosis.
Neuro-ocular lesions, e.g., retinal thrombosis and optic neuritis.

The following adverse reactions have been reported in patients receiving oral contraceptives and are believed to be drug related:

Nausea and/or vomiting, usually the most common adverse reactions, occur in approximately 10% or less of patients during the first cycle. Other reactions, as a general rule, are seen much less frequently or only occasionally.

Gastrointestinal symptoms (such as abdominal cramps and bloating).
Breakthrough bleeding.
Spotting.
Change in menstrual flow.
Dysmenorrhea.
Amenorrhea during and after treatment.
Temporary infertility after discontinuance of treatment.
Edema.
Chloasma or melasma which may persist.
Breast changes: tenderness, enlargement, and secretion.
Change in weight (increase or decrease).
Change in cervical erosion and cervical secretion.
Possible diminution in lactation when given immediately postpartum.
Cholestatic jaundice.
Migraine.
Increase in size of uterine leiomyomata.
Rash (allergic).
Mental depression.
Reduced tolerance to carbohydrates.
Vaginal candidiasis.
Change in corneal curvature (steepening).
Intolerance to contact lenses.

The following adverse reactions have been reported in users of oral contraceptives, and the association has been neither confirmed nor refuted:

Premenstrual-like syndrome.
Cataracts.
Changes in libido.
Chorea.
Changes in appetite.
Cystitis-like syndrome.
Headache.
Nervousness.
Dizziness.
Hirsutism.
Loss of scalp hair.
Erythema multiforme.
Erythema nodosum.
Hemorrhagic Eruption.
Vaginitis.
Porphyria.

Acute Overdose: Serious ill effects have not been reported following acute ingestion of large doses of oral contraceptives by young children. Overdosage may cause nausea, and withdrawal bleeding may occur in females.

Dosage and Administration: To achieve maximum contraceptive effectiveness, OVCON-50 or OVCON-35 must be taken exactly as directed and at intervals not exceeding 24 hours.

28-DAY REGIMEN

The patient takes one tablet daily from a convenient package as follows: (yellow or peach tablet containing active ingredients, green tablet containing inert ingredients)

For the first cycle of use only, the first yellow or peach tablet is taken on day 5 of the menstrual cycle, counting the first day of bleeding as day 1. One tablet is taken daily in the same sequence as in the package—first the yellow or peach, then the green tablets. After the last green tablet is taken, the first yellow or peach tablet from a new package is taken **the following day.** Withdrawal bleeding will usually begin while the patient is taking the green tablets and may continue during the first few tablets from the next package.

21-DAY REGIMEN

The patient takes one tablet daily from a convenient package as follows: (yellow or peach)

For the first cycle of use only, the first yellow or peach tablet is taken on day 5 of the menstrual cycle, counting the first day of bleeding as day 1. Continue taking one tablet daily from the 5th through the 25th day of the menstrual cycle. If the first tablet is taken later than the fifth day of the first menstrual cycle an additional form of contraception should be used for at least one week. Withdrawal bleeding will normally begin within 2–3 days after taking the last tablet. The first tablet of the next package should be taken seven days after the last tablet even if menstrual bleeding has not ceased. The dosage regimen then continues with one tablet daily for 21 days followed by 7 days of no medication, thus a cycle of three-weeks-on and one-week-off.

Patients should be cautioned to follow the dosage schedule strictly.

Evening administration is suggested. If the regimen is interrupted, an additional contraceptive method is recommended for the rest of the cycle. Should spotting or breakthrough bleeding occur, it is recommended that the patient continue medication. If bleeding is persistent or recurrent, the patient should consult her physician.

Use of oral contraceptives in the event of a missed menstrual period:

1. If the patient has not adhered to the prescribed dosage regimen, the possibility of pregnancy should be considered after the first missed period and oral contraceptives should be withheld until pregnancy has been ruled out.

2. If the patient has adhered to the prescribed regimen and misses two consecutive periods, pregnancy should be ruled out before continuing the contraceptive regimen.

How Supplied:

OVCON®-50 is available in 21 and 28 day regimens. Each package contains 21 yellow tablets of 1.0 mg. norethindrone and 0.05 mg. ethinyl estradiol. Each green tablet in the 28 day regimen contains inert ingredients.

NDC 0087-0584-40	Package of 21 tablets
NDC 0087-0584-42	Carton of 6 packages
NDC 0087-0579-40	Package of 28 tablets
NDC 0087-0579-41	Carton of 6 packages

OVCON®-35 is available in 21 and 28 day regimens. Each package contains 21 peach tablets of 0.4 mg. norethindrone and 0.035 mg. ethinyl estradiol. Each green tablet in the 28 day regimen contains inert ingredients.

NDC 0087-0583-40	Package of 21 tablets
NDC 0087-0583-42	Carton of 6 packages
6505-01-084-2667 (Pkg of 21) (Defense)	
NDC 0087-0578-40	Package of 28 tablets
NDC 0087-0578-41	Carton of 6 packages

The Patient Labeling for oral contraceptive drug products is set forth below:

BRIEF SUMMARY
PATIENT PACKAGE INSERT

Warning:

Cigarette smoking increases the risk of serious adverse effects on the heart and blood vessels from oral contraceptive use. This risk increases with age and with heavy smoking (15 or more cigarettes per day) and is quite marked in women over 35 years of age. Women who use oral contraceptives should not smoke.

Continued on next page

Mead Johnson Pharm.—Cont.

Oral contraceptives taken as directed are about 99% effective in preventing pregnancy. (The mini-pill, however, is somewhat less effective.) Forgetting to take your pills increases the chance of pregnancy.

Women who have or have had clotting disorders, cancer of the breast or sex organs, unexplained vaginal bleeding, a stroke, heart attack, angina pectoris, or who suspect they may be pregnant should not use oral contraceptives.

Most side effects of the pill are not serious. The most common side effects are nausea, vomiting, bleeding between menstrual periods, weight gain, and breast tenderness. However, proper use of oral contraceptives requires that they be taken under your doctor's continuous supervision, because they can be associated with serious side effects which may be fatal. Fortunately, these occur very infrequently. The serious side effects are:

1. Blood clots in the legs, lungs, brain, heart or other organs and hemorrhage into the brain due to bursting of a blood vessel.
2. Liver tumors, which may rupture and cause severe bleeding.
3. Birth defects if the pill is taken while you are pregnant.
4. High blood pressure.
5. Gallbladder disease.

The symptoms associated with these serious side effects are discussed in the detailed leaflet given you with your supply of pills. Notify your doctor if you notice any unusual physical disturbance while taking the pill.

The estrogen in oral contraceptives has been found to cause breast cancer and other cancers in certain animals. These findings suggest that oral contraceptives may also cause cancer in humans. However, studies to date in women taking currently marketed oral contraceptives have not confirmed that oral contraceptives cause cancer in humans.

The detailed leaflet describes more completely the benefits and risks of oral contraceptives. It also provides information on other forms of contraception. Read it carefully. If you have any questions, consult your doctor.

Caution: Oral contraceptives are of no value in the prevention or treatment of venereal disease.

Detailed Patient Labeling

What You Should Know About Oral Contraceptives: Oral contraceptives ("the pill") are the most effective way (except for sterilization) to prevent pregnancy. They are also convenient and, for most women, free of serious or unpleasant side effects. Oral contraceptives must always be taken under the continuous supervision of a physician.

It is important that any woman who considers using an oral contraceptive understand the risks involved. Although the oral contraceptives have important advantages over other methods of contraception, they have certain risks that no other method has. Only you can decide whether the advantages are worth these risks. This leaflet will tell you about the most important risks. It will explain how you can help your doctor prescribe the pill as safely as possible by telling him about yourself and being alert for the earliest signs of trouble. And it will tell you how to use the pill properly, so that it will be as effective as possible. There is more detailed information available in the leaflet prepared for doctors. Your pharmacist can show you a copy; you may need your doctor's help in understanding parts of it.

Who Should Not Use Oral Contraceptives:

A. If you have any of the following conditions you should not use the pill:

1. Clots in the legs or lungs.
2. Angina pectoris.
3. Known or suspected cancer of the breast or sex organs.
4. Unusual vaginal bleeding that has not yet been diagnosed.
5. Known or suspected pregnancy.

B. If you have had any of the following conditions you should not use the pill:

1. Heart attack or stroke.
2. Clots in the legs or lungs.

Warning:

> **C. Cigarette smoking increases the risk of serious adverse effects on the heart and blood vessels from oral contraceptive use. This risk increases with age and with heavy smoking (15 or more cigarettes per day) and is quite marked in women over 35 years of age. Women who use oral contraceptives should not smoke.**

D. If you have scanty or irregular periods or are a young woman without a regular cycle, you should use another method of contraception because, if you use the pill, you may have difficulty becoming pregnant or may fail to have menstrual periods after discontinuing the pill.

Deciding to Use Oral Contraceptives: If you do not have any of the conditions listed above and are thinking about using oral contraceptives, to help you decide, you need information about the advantages and risks of oral contraceptives and of other contraceptive methods as well. This leaflet describes the advantages and risks of oral contraceptives. Except for sterilization, the IUD and abortion, which have their own exclusive risks, the only serious risks of other methods of contraception are those due to pregnancy should the method fail. Your doctor can answer questions you may have with respect to other methods of contraception. He can also answer any questions you may have after reading this leaflet on oral contraceptives.

1. What Oral Contraceptives Are and How They Work. Oral Contraceptives are of two types. The most common, often simply called "the pill" is a combination of an estrogen and a progestogen, the two kinds of female hormones. The amount of estrogen and progestogen can vary, but the amount of estrogen is most important because both the effectiveness and some of the dangers of oral contraceptives are related to the amount of estrogen. This kind of oral contraceptive works principally by preventing release of an egg from the ovary. When the amount of estrogen is 50 micrograms or more of mestranol or 35 micrograms or more of ethinyl estradiol and the pill is taken as directed, oral contraceptives are more than 99% effective (i.e., there would be less than one pregnancy if 100 women used the pill for 1 year). Pills that contain 20 to 35 micrograms of estrogen vary slightly in effectiveness, ranging from 98% to more than 99% effective.

The second type of oral contraceptive, often called the "mini-pill", contains only a progestogen. It works in part by preventing release of an egg from the ovary but also by keeping sperm from reaching the egg and by making the uterus (womb) less receptive to any fertilized egg that reaches it. The mini-pill is less effective than the combination oral contraceptive, about 97% effective. In addition, the progestogen-only pill has a tendency to cause irregular bleeding which may be quite inconvenient, or cessation of bleeding entirely. The progestogen-only pill is used despite its lower effectiveness in the hope that it will prove not to have some of the serious side effects of the estrogen-containing pill (see below) but it is not yet certain that the mini-pill does in fact have fewer serious side effects. The discussion below, while based mainly on information about the combination pills, should be considered to apply as well to the mini-pill.

2. Other Nonsurgical Ways to Prevent Pregnancy. As this leaflet will explain, oral contraceptives have several serious risks. Other methods of contraception have lesser risks or none at all. They are also less effective than oral contraceptives, but, used properly, may be effective enough for many women. The following table gives reported pregnancy rates (the number of women out of 100 who would become pregnant in 1 year) for these methods:

Pregnancies per 100 Women per year:
Intrauterine device (IUD), less than 1–6;
Diaphragm with spermicidal products (creams or jellies), 2–20;
Condom (rubber), 3–36;
Aerosol foams, 2–29;
Jellies and creams, 4–36;
Periodic abstinence (rhythm) all types, less than 1–47:

1. Calendar method, 14–47;
2. Temperature method, 1–20;
3. Temperature method—intercourse only in post-ovulatory phase, less than 1–7;
4. Mucus method, 1–25;

No contraception, 60–80.

The figures (except for the IUD) vary widely because people differ in how well they use each method. Very faithful users of the various methods obtain very good results, except for users of the calendar method of periodic abstinence (rhythm). Except for the IUD, effective use of these methods requires somewhat more effort than simply taking a single pill every morning, but it is an effort that many couples undertake successfully. Your doctor can tell you a great deal more about these methods of contraception.

3. The Dangers of Oral Contraceptives.

a. Circulatory disorders (abnormal blood clotting and stroke due to hemorrhage). Blood clots (in various blood vessels of the body) are the most common of the serious side effects of oral contraceptives. A clot can result in a stroke (if the clot is in the brain), a heart attack (if the clot is in a blood vessel of the heart), or a pulmonary embolus (a clot which forms in the legs or pelvis, then breaks off and travels to the lungs). Any of these can be fatal. Clots also occur rarely in the blood vessels of the eye, resulting in blindness or impairment of vision in that eye. There is evidence that the risk of clotting increases with higher estrogen doses. It is therefore important to keep the dose of estrogen as low as possible, so long as the oral contraceptive used has an acceptable pregnancy rate and doesn't cause unacceptable changes in the menstrual pattern. Furthermore, cigarette smoking by oral contraceptive users increases the risk of serious adverse effects on the heart and blood vessels. This risk increases with age and with heavy smoking (15 or more cigarettes per day) and begins to become quite marked in women over 35 years of age. For this reason women who use oral contraceptives should not smoke.

The risk of abnormal clotting increases with age in both users and nonusers of oral contraceptives, but the increased risk from the contraceptive appears to be present at all ages. For oral contraceptive users in general, it has been estimated that in women between the ages of 15 and 34 the risk of death due to a circulatory disorder is about 1 in 12,000 per year, whereas for nonusers the rate is about 1 in 50,000 per year. In the age group 35 to 44, the risk is estimated to be about 1 in 2,500 per year for oral contraceptive users and about 1 in 10,000 per year for nonusers.

Even without the pill the risk of having a heart attack increases with age and is also increased by such heart attack risk factors as high blood pressure, high cholesterol, obesity, diabetes, and cigarette smoking. Without any risk factors present, the use of oral contraceptives alone may double the risk of heart attack. However, the combination of cigarette smoking, especially heavy smoking, and oral contraceptive use greatly increases the risk of heart attack. Oral contraceptive users who smoke are about 5 times more likely to have a heart attack than users who do not smoke and about

10 times more likely to have a heart attack than nonusers who do not smoke. It has been estimated that users between the ages of 30 and 39 who smoke have about a 1 in 10,000 chance each year of having a fatal heart attack compared to about a 1 in 50,000 chance in users who do not smoke, and about a 1 in 100,000 chance in nonusers who do not smoke. In the age group 40 to 44, the risk is about 1 in 1,700 per year for users who smoke compared to about 1 in 10,000 for users who do not smoke and to about 1 in 14,000 per year for nonusers who do not smoke. Heavy smoking (about 15 cigarettes or more a day) further increases the risk. If you do not smoke and have none of the other heart attack risk factors described above, you will have a smaller risk than listed. If you have several heart attack risk factors, the risk may be considerably greater than listed.

In addition to blood-clotting disorders, it has been estimated that women taking oral contraceptives are twice as likely as nonusers to have a stroke due to rupture of a blood vessel in the brain.

b. Formation of tumors. Studies have found that when certain animals are given the female sex hormone estrogen, which is an ingredient of oral contraceptives, continuously for long periods, cancers may develop in the breast, cervix, vagina, and liver.

These findings suggest that oral contraceptives may cause cancer in humans. However, studies to date in women taking currently marketed oral contraceptives have not confirmed that oral contraceptives cause cancer in humans. Several studies have found no increase in breast cancer in users, although one study suggested oral contraceptives might cause an increase in breast cancer in women who already have benign breast disease (e.g., cysts).

Women with a strong family history of breast cancer or who have breast nodules, fibrocystic disease, or abnormal mammograms or who were exposed to DES (diethylstilbestrol), an estrogen, during their mother's pregnancy must be followed very closely by their doctors if they choose to use oral contraceptives instead of another method of contraception. Many studies have shown that women taking oral contraceptives have less risk of getting benign breast disease than those who have not used oral contraceptives. Recently, strong evidence has emerged that estrogens (one component of oral contraceptives), when given for periods of more than one year to women after the menopause, increase the risk of cancer of the uterus (womb). There is also some evidence that a kind of oral contraceptive which is no longer marketed, the sequential oral contraceptive, may increase the risk of cancer of the uterus. There remains no evidence, however, that the oral contraceptives now available increase the risk of this cancer.

Oral contraceptives do cause, although rarely, a benign (non-malignant) tumor of the liver. These tumors do not spread, but they may rupture and cause internal bleeding, which may be fatal. A few cases of cancer of the liver have been reported in women using oral contraceptives, but it is not yet known whether the drug caused them.

c. Dangers to a developing child if oral contraceptives are used in or immediately preceding pregnancy. Oral contraceptives should not be taken by pregnant women because they may damage the developing child. An increased risk of birth defects, including heart defects and limb defects, has been associated with the use of sex hormones, including oral contraceptives, in pregnancy. In addition, the developing female child whose mother has received DES (diethylstilbestrol), an estrogen, during pregnancy has a risk of getting cancer of the vagina or cervix in her teens or young adulthood. This risk is estimated to be about 1 in 1,000 exposures or less. Abnormalities of the urinary and sex organs have been reported in male offspring so exposed. It is possible that other estrogens, such as the estrogens in oral contraceptives, could have the same effect in the child if the mother takes them during pregnancy.

If you stop taking oral contraceptives to become pregnant, your doctor may recommend that you use another method of contraception for a short while. The reason for this is that there is evidence from studies in women who have had "miscarriages" soon after stopping the pill, that the lost fetuses are more likely to be abnormal. Whether there is an overall increase in "miscarriage" in women who become pregnant soon after stopping the pill as compared with women who do not use the pill is not known, but it is possible that there may be. If, however, you do become pregnant soon after stopping oral contraceptives, and do not have a miscarriage, there is no evidence that the baby has an increased risk of being abnormal.

d. Gallbladder disease. Women who use oral contraceptives have a greater risk than nonusers of having gallbladder disease requiring surgery. The increased risk may first appear within 1 year of use and may double after 4 or 5 years of use.

e. Other side effects of oral contraceptives. Some women using oral contraceptives experience unpleasant side effects that are not dangerous and are not likely to damage their health. Some of these may be temporary. Your breasts may feel tender, nausea and vomiting may occur, you may gain or lose weight and your ankles may swell. A spotty darkening of the skin, particularly of the face, is possible and may persist. You may notice unexpected vaginal bleeding or changes in your menstrual period. Irregular bleeding is frequently seen when using the mini-pill or combination oral contraceptives containing less than 50 micrograms of estrogen.

More serious side effects include worsening of migraine, asthma, epilepsy, and kidney or heart disease because of a tendency for water to be retained in the body when oral contraceptives are used. Other side effects are growth of preexisting fibroid tumors of the uterus; mental depression; and liver problems with jaundice (yellowing of the skin). Your doctor may find that levels of sugar and fatty substances in your blood are elevated; the long-term effects of these changes are not known. Some women develop high blood pressure while taking oral contraceptives, which ordinarily returns to the original levels when the oral contraceptive is stopped.

Other reactions, although not proved to be caused by oral contraceptives, are occasionally reported. These include more frequent urination and some discomfort when urinating, nervousness, dizziness, some loss of scalp hair, an increase in body hair, an increase or decrease in sex drive, appetite changes, cataracts, and a need for a change in contact lens prescription or inability to use contact lenses.

After you stop using oral contraceptives there may be a delay before you are able to become pregnant or before you resume having menstrual periods. This is especially true of women who had irregular menstrual cycles prior to the use of oral contraceptives. As discussed previously, your doctor may recommend that you wait a short while after stopping the pill before you try to become pregnant. During this time, use another form of contraception. You should consult your physician before resuming use of oral contraceptives after childbirth, especially if you plan to nurse your baby. Drugs in oral contraceptives are known to appear in the milk, and the long-range effects on infants is not known at this time. Furthermore, oral contraceptives may cause a decrease in your milk supply as well as in the quality of the milk.

4. Comparison of the Risks of Oral Contraceptives and Other Contraceptive Methods. The many studies on the risks and effectiveness of oral contraceptives and other methods of contraception have been analyzed to estimate the risk of death associated with various methods of contraception. This risk has two parts: (a) the risk of the method itself (e.g., the risk that oral contraceptives will cause death due to abnormal clotting), and (b) the risk of death due to pregnancy or abortion in the event the method fails. The results of this analysis are shown in the bar graph below. The height of the bars is the number of deaths per 100,000 women each year. There are six sets of bars, each set referring to specific age groups of women. Within each set of bars there is a single bar for each of the different contraceptive methods. For oral contraceptives, there are two bars—one for smokers and the other for nonsmokers. The analysis is based on present knowledge and new information could, of course, alter it. The analysis shows that the risk of death from all methods of birth control is low and below that associated with child birth, except for oral contraceptives in women over 40 who smoke. It shows that the lowest risk of death is associated with the condom or diaphragm (traditional contraception) backed up by early abortion in case of failure of the condom or diaphragm to prevent pregnancy. Also, at any age the risk of death (due to unexpected pregnancy) from the use of traditional contraception, even without a backup of abortion, is generally the same as or less than that from use of oral contraceptives. (See Figure 1 next page)

How to Use Oral Contraceptives as Safely and Effectively as Possible, Once You Have Decided to Use Them:

1. What to Tell your Doctor.

You can make use of the pill as safe as possible by telling your doctor if you have any of the following:

a. Conditions that mean you should not use oral contraceptives:

Clots in the legs or lungs.

Clots in the legs or lungs in the past.

A stroke, heart attack, or angina pectoris.

Known or suspected cancer of the breast or sex organs.

Unusual vaginal bleeding that has not yet been diagnosed.

Known or suspected pregnancy.

b. Conditions that your doctor will want to watch closely or which might cause him to suggest another method of contraception:

A family history of breast cancer.

Breast nodules, fibrocystic disease of the breast, or an abnormal mammogram.

Diabetes.

High blood pressure.

High cholesterol.

Cigarette smoking.

Migraine headaches.

Heart or kidney disease.

Epilepsy.

Mental depression.

Fibroid tumors of the uterus.

Gallbladder disease.

c. Once you are using oral contraceptives, you should be alert for signs of a serious adverse effect and call your doctor if they occur:

Sharp pain in the chest, coughing blood, or sudden shortness of breath (indicating possible clots in the lungs).

Pain in the calf (possible clot in the leg).

Crushing chest pain or heaviness (indicating possible heart attack).

Sudden severe headache or vomiting, dizziness or fainting, disturbance of vision or speech or weakness or numbness in an arm or leg (indicating a possible stroke).

Sudden partial or complete loss of vision (indicating a possible clot in the eye).

Breast lumps (you should ask your doctor to show you how to examine your own breasts).

Severe pain in the abdomen (indicating a possible ruptured tumor of the liver).

Continued on next page

Mead Johnson Pharm.—Cont.

Severe depression.
Yellowing of the skin (jaundice).

2. How to Take the Pill So That It Is Most Effective.

Dosage and Administration: To achieve maximum contraceptive effectiveness, OVCON-50 or OVCON-35 must be taken exactly as directed and at intervals not exceeding 24 hours.

28-DAY REGIMEN

The patient takes one tablet daily from a convenient package as follows: (yellow or peach tablet containing active ingredients, green tablet containing inert ingredients)

For the first cycle of use only, the first yellow or peach tablet is taken on day 5 of the menstrual cycle, counting the first day of bleeding as day 1. One tablet is taken daily in the same sequence as in the package—first the yellow or peach, and then the green tablets. After the last green tablet is taken, the first yellow or peach tablet from a new package is taken **the following day.** Withdrawal bleeding will usually begin while the patient is taking the green tablets and may continue during the first few tablets from the next package.

21-DAY REGIMEN

The patient takes one tablet daily from a convenient package as follows: (yellow or peach)

For the first cycle of use only, the first yellow or peach tablet is taken on day 5 of the menstrual cycle, counting the first day of bleeding as day 1. Continue taking one tablet daily from the 5th through the 25th day of the menstrual cycle. If the first tablet is taken later than the fifth day of the first menstrual cycle an additional form of contraception should be used for at least one week. Withdrawal bleeding will normally begin within 2-3 days after taking the last tablet. The first tablet of the next package should be taken seven days after the last tablet even if menstrual bleeding has not ceased. The dosage regimen then continues with one tablet daily for 21 days followed by 7 days of no medication, thus a cycle of three-weeks-on and one-week-off.

Patients should be cautioned to follow the dosage schedule strictly.

Evening administration is suggested. If the regimen is interrupted, an additional contraceptive method is recommended for the rest of the cycle. Should spotting or breakthrough bleeding occur, it is recommended that the patient continue medication. If bleeding is persistent or recurrent, the patient should consult her physician.

Use of oral contraceptives in the event of a missed menstrual period:

1. If the patient has not adhered to the prescribed dosage regimen, the possibility of pregnancy should be considered after the first missed period and oral contraceptives should be withheld until pregnancy has been ruled out.
2. If the patient has adhered to the prescribed regimen and misses two consecutive periods, pregnancy should be ruled out before continuing the contraceptive regimen.

At times there may be no menstrual period after a cycle of pills. Therefore, if you miss one menstrual period but have taken the pills **exactly as you were supposed to,** continue as usual into the next cycle. If you have not taken the pills correctly and miss a menstrual period, you may be pregnant and should stop taking oral contraceptives until your doctor determines whether or not you are pregnant. Until you can get to your doctor, use another form of contraception. If two consecutive menstrual periods are missed, you should stop taking pills until it is determined whether you are pregnant. If you do become pregnant while using oral contraceptives, you should discuss the risks to the developing child with your doctor.

3. Periodic Examination.

Your doctor will take a complete medical and family history before prescribing oral contraceptives. At that time and about once a year thereafter, he will generally examine your blood pressure, breasts, abdomen, and pelvic organs (including a Papanicolaou smear, i.e., test for cancer).

Summary: Oral contraceptives are the most effective method, except sterilization, for preventing pregnancy. Other methods, when used conscientiously, are also very effective and have fewer risks. The serious risks of oral contraceptives are uncommon and the "pill" is a very convenient method of preventing pregnancy.

If you have certain conditions or have had these conditions in the past, you should not use oral contraceptives because the risk is too great. These conditions are listed in the leaflet. If you do not have these conditions, and decide to use the "pill," please read the leaflet carefully so that you can use the "pill" most safely and effectively.

Based on his or her assessment of your medical needs, your doctor has prescribed this drug for you. Do not give the drug to anyone else.

July, 1979

[*Shown in Product Identification Section*]

Figure 1. Estimated annual number of deaths associated with control of fertility and no control per 100,000 nonsterile women, by regimen of control and age of women.

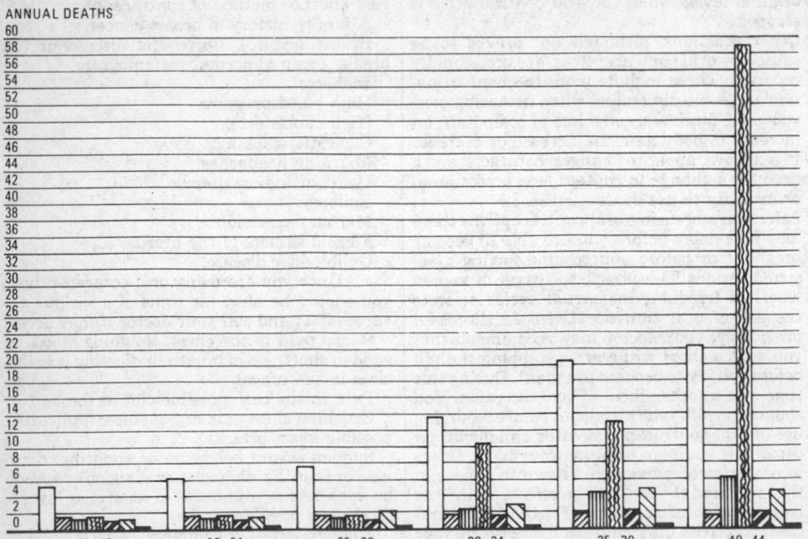

PERI-COLACE® capsules • syrup
Casanthranol and dioctyl sodium sulfosuccinate,

Description: Peri-Colace is a combination of the mild stimulant laxative Peristim (casanthranol, Mead Johnson) and the stool-softener Colace (dioctyl sodium sulfosuccinate, Mead Johnson). Each capsule contains 30 mg of Peristim and 100 mg of Colace; the syrup contains 30 mg of Peristim and 60 mg of Colace per 15-ml tablespoon (10 mg of Peristim and 20 mg of Colace per 5-ml teaspoon) and 10% alcohol.

Action and Uses: Peri-Colace provides gentle peristaltic stimulation and helps to keep stools soft for easier passage. Bowel movement is induced gently—usually overnight or in 8 to 12 hours. Nausea, griping, abnormally loose stools, and constipation rebound are minimized. Useful in management of chronic or temporary constipation.

Note: To prevent hard stools when laxative stimulation is not needed or undesirable, see Colace (stool softener).

Side Effects: The incidence of side effects—none of a serious nature—is exceedingly small. Nausea, abdominal cramping or discomfort, diarrhea, and rash are the main side effects reported.

Administration and Dosage: *Adults*—1 or 2 capsules, or 1 or 2 tablespoons syrup at bedtime, or as indicated. In severe cases, dosage may be increased to 2 capsules or 2 tablespoons twice daily, or 3 capsules at bedtime. *Children*—1 to 3 teaspoons of syrup at bedtime, or as indicated.

Warning: Do not use when abdominal pain, nausea, or vomiting are present. Frequent or prolonged use of this preparation may result in dependence on laxatives.

Overdosage: In addition to symptomatic treatment, gastric lavage, if timely, is recommended in cases of large overdosage.

How Supplied: Peri-Colace® Capsules

NDC 0087-0715-43 Cartons of 10 single unit packs
NDC 0087-0715-01 Bottles of 30
NDC 0087-0715-02 Bottles of 60
NDC 0087-0715-03 Bottles of 250
NDC 0087-0715-05 Bottles of 1000
NDC 0087-0715-07 Cartons of 100 single unit packs
VA 6505-00-880-4390A (1000's)

Note: Peri-Colace capsules should be stored at controlled room temperatures (15°-30° C or 59°-86° F).

Peri-Colace® Syrup

NDC 0087-0721-01 Bottles of 8 fl. oz.
NDC 0087-0721-02 Bottles of 16 fl. oz.

[*Shown in Product Identification Section*]

QUESTRAN® ℞
(Cholestyramine)
U.S. Patent No. 3,383,281

Description: The active ingredient in Questran Powder is cholestyramine, the chloride salt of a basic anion exchange resin. Cholestyramine is quite hydrophilic, but water insoluble. The cholestyramine in Questran is not absorbed from the digestive tract. Each 9 grams of Questran contain 4 grams of cholestyramine.

Clinical Pharmacology: Cholesterol is probably the sole precursor of bile acids. During normal digestion, bile acids are secreted into the intestines. A major portion of the bile acids is absorbed from the intestinal tract and returned to the liver via the enterohepatic circulation. Only very small amounts of bile acids are found in normal serum.

Cholestyramine resin adsorbs and combines with the bile acids in the intestine to form an insoluble complex which is excreted in the feces. This results in a partial removal of bile acids from the enterohepatic circulation by preventing their absorption.

The increased fecal loss of bile acids due to Questran administration leads to an increased oxidation of cholesterol to bile acids, a decrease in beta lipoprotein or low density lipoprotein plasma levels and a decrease in serum cholesterol levels. Although in man cholestyramine produces an increase in hepatic synthesis of cholesterol, plasma cholesterol levels fall.

In patients with partial biliary obstruction, the reduction of serum bile acid levels by cholestyramine resin reduces excess bile acids deposited in the dermal tissue with resultant decrease in pruritus.

Indications: Since no drug is innocuous, strict attention should be paid to the indications and contraindications, particularly when selecting drugs for chronic long term use.

1) Questran is indicated as adjunctive therapy to diet for the reduction of elevated serum cholesterol in patients with primary hypercholesterolemia (elevated low density lipoproteins). Questran may be useful to lower elevated cholesterol that occurs in patients with combined hypercholesterolemia and hypertriglyceridemia, but it is not indicated where hypertriglyceridemia is the abnormality of most concern.

It has not been established whether the drug-induced lowering of serum cholesterol or triglyceride levels has a beneficial effect, no effect, or a detrimental effect on the morbidity or mortality due to atherosclerosis including coronary heart disease. Current investigations now in progress may yield an answer to this question.

2) For the relief of pruritus associated with partial biliary obstruction. Cholestyramine has been shown to have a variable effect on serum cholesterol in these patients. Patients with primary biliary cirrhosis may exhibit an elevated cholesterol as part of their desease.

Contraindications: Questran is contraindicated in patients with complete biliary obstruction where bile is not secreted into the intestine and in those individuals who have shown hypersensitivity to any of its components.

Precautions

Before instituting therapy with Questran an attempt should be made to control serum cholesterol by appropriate dietary regimen, weight reduction, and the treatment of any underlying disorder which might be the cause of the hypercholesterolemia. Serum cholesterols should be determined frequently during the first few months of therapy and periodically thereafter. A favorable trend in cholesterol reduction should occur during the first month of Questran therapy. The therapy should be continued to sustain cholesterol reduction. Serum triglyceride levels should be measured periodically to detect whether significant changes have occurred.

Because cholestyramine binds bile acids, it may interfere with normal fat digestion and absorption and thus may prevent absorption of fat soluble vitamins such as A, D and K. When Questran is given for long periods of time, supplemental Vitamin A and D should be given daily in a water-miscible form (or administered parenterally). Chronic use of Questran may be associated with increased bleeding tendency due to hypoprothrombinemia associated with Vitamin K deficiency. This will usually respond promptly to parenteral Vitamin K_1 and recurrences can be prevented by oral administration of Vitamin K_1. Reduction of serum or red cell folate has been reported over long term administration of Questran. Supplementation with folic acid should be considered in these cases.

There is a possibility that prolonged use of Questran, since it is a chloride form of anion exchange resin, may produce hyperchloremic acidosis. This would especially be true in younger and smaller patients where the relative dosage may be higher.

Questran may produce or worsen pre-existing constipation. Dosage should be reduced or discontinued in such cases. Fecal impaction and aggravated hemorrhoids may occur. Every effort should be made to avert severe constipation and its inherent problems in those patients with clinically symptomatic coronary artery disease.

This product contains FD&C Yellow No. 5 (tartrazine) which may cause allergic-type reactions (including bronchial asthma) in certain susceptible individuals. Although the overall incidence of FD&C Yellow No. 5 (tartrazine) sensitivity in the general population is low, it is frequently seen in patients who also have aspirin hypersensitivity.

Drug Interactions

Questran may delay or reduce the absorption of concomitant oral medication such as phenylbutazone, warfarin, chlorothiazide (acidic), as well as tetracycline, phenobarbital, thyroid and thyroxine preparations, and digitalis. The discontinuance of the cholestyramine resin could pose a hazard to health if a potentially toxic drug such as digitalis has been titrated to a maintenance level while the patient was taking Questran.

SINCE QUESTRAN MAY BIND OTHER DRUGS GIVEN CONCURRENTLY, PATIENTS SHOULD TAKE OTHER DRUGS AT LEAST ONE HOUR BEFORE OR 4–6 HOURS AFTER QUESTRAN TO AVOID IMPEDING THEIR ABSORPTION OR AT AS GREAT AN INTERVAL AS POSSIBLE.

Adverse Reactions: The most common adverse reaction is constipation. Predisposing factors for most of these complaints when used as cholesterol lowering agent are high dose and increased age (more than 60 years old). Most instances of constipation are mild, transient, and controlled with conventional therapy. Some patients require a temporary decrease in dosage or discontinuation of therapy.

Less Frequent Adverse Reactions: Abdominal discomfort, flatulence, nausea, vomiting, diarrhea, heartburn, anorexia, indigestive feeling and steatorrhea, bleeding tendencies due to hypoprothrombinemia (Vitamin K deficiency) as well as Vitamin A (one case of night blindness reported) and D deficiencies, hyperchloremic acidosis in children, osteoporosis. Rash and irritation of the skin, tongue and perianal area. One ten month old baby with biliary atresia had an impaction presumed to be due to cholestyramine resin after three days administration of 9 grams daily. She developed acute intestinal sepsis and died.

Occasional calcified material has been observed in the biliary tree, including calcification of the gall bladder, in patients to whom cholestyramine resin has been given. However, this may be a manifestation of the liver disease and not drug related.

One patient experienced biliary colic on each of three occasions on which he took Questran. One patient diagnosed as acute abdominal symptom complex was found to have a "pasty mass" in the transverse colon on x-ray.

Other events (not necessarily drug-related) reported in patients taking Questran include: GI-rectal bleeding, black stools, hemorrhoidal bleeding, bleeding from known duodenal ulcer, dysphagia, hiccups, ulcer attack, sour taste, pancreatitis, rectal pain, diverticulitis.

Hematologic—Decreased prothrombin time, ecchymosis, anemia.

Hypersensitivity—Urticaria, asthma, wheezing, shortness of breath.

Musculoskeletal—Backache, muscle and joint pains, arthritis.

Neurologic—Headache, anxiety, vertigo, dizziness, fatigue, tinnitus, syncope, drowsiness, femoral nerve pain, paresthesia.

Eye—Uveitis.

Renal—Hematuria, dysuria, burnt odor to urine, diuresis.

Miscellaneous—Weight loss, weight gain, increased libido, swollen glands, edema, dental bleeding.

Overdosage: Overdosage of Questran (cholestyramine) has not been reported. Should overdosage occur, however, the chief potential harm would be obstruction of the gastrointestinal tract. The location of such potential obstruction, the degree of obstruction, and the presence or absence of normal gut motility would determine treatment.

Dosage and Administration: The recommended adult dose is one packet or one scoopful (containing 4 gm. of cholestyramine resin in 9 grams of Questran) three or four times daily. Dosage may be adjusted as required to meet the patient's needs.

Questran should not be taken in its dry form. Always mix Questran powder with water or other fluids before ingesting. See Preparation Instructions.

Use in children:

As experience in infants and children is limited, a practical dosage schedule has not been established.

The effects of long term drug administration, as well as its effect in maintaining lowered cholesterol levels in pediatric patients, are unknown.

Use in Pregnancy

The safe use of cholestyramine resin by pregnant or lactating women or women of childbearing age has not been established.

Preparation: Mix contents of one packet or one level scoopful of Questran with 2–6 fluid ounces of the preferred beverage (water, milk, fruit juice or other noncarbonated beverage). Questran may also be mixed with highly fluid soups or pulpy fruits with a high moisture content, such as applesauce or crushed pineapple.

How Supplied: Questran is available in cartons of fifty 9-gram packets and in cans containing 378 grams. Each 9 grams of Questran supplies 4 grams of cholestyramine.

NDC0087-0580-01 Cartons of 50 packets
NDC0087-0580-05 Cans, 378 gm
6505-00-105-0372 (Cartons of 50 packets)
Defense
VA6505-00-502-9602A (Cartons of 50 packets)

Bibliography available by writing to Director, Medical Services, Mead Johnson Pharmaceutical Division, Evansville, Indiana 47721.

QUIBRON® ℞
(Theophylline-Guaifenesin)

Description: Each Quibron® soft gelatin capsule or tablespoon (15 ml) of liquid contains 150 mg of theophylline (anhydrous) and 90 mg of guaifenesin, as an oral bronchodilator-expectorant.

Quibron Liquid contains no alcohol and is dye-free.

QUIBRON®-300 ℞
(Theophylline-Guaifenesin)

Description: Each Quibron®-300 soft gelatin capsule contains 300 mg of theophylline (anhydrous) and 180 mg of guaifenesin, as an oral bronchodilator-expectorant.

Theophylline, a xanthine compound, is a white, odorless crystalline powder, having a bitter taste.

Continued on next page

Mead Johnson Pharm.—Cont.

Guaifenesin, a guaiacol compound, is a white to slightly yellow crystalline powder with a bitter, aromatic taste.

Clinical Pharmacology:

Theophylline

Mode of Action

Theophylline acts as a bronchodilator by direct relaxation of bronchial smooth muscle. Theophylline is a competitive inhibitor of cyclic nucleotide phosphodiesterase resulting in increased intracellular levels of cAMP which mediates smooth muscle relaxation. Like some other xanthines, theophylline acts as a coronary vasodilator, cardiac stimulant, skeletal muscle stimulant, central nervous system stimulant and diuretic.

Pharmacokinetics

As theophylline is released from the formulation it is, under usual conditions, absorbed completely and fairly rapidly. Excretion, principally as inactive metabolites, is primarily via the kidney. The half-life of theophylline varies among individuals with a wide range having been documented. Theophylline half-life is shortened in cigarette smokers. Half-life is prolonged in alcoholism, reduced hepatic or renal function, congestive heart failure and patients receiving antibiotics such as troleandomycin, erythromycin and clindamycin. High fever for prolonged periods may decrease theophylline elimination. The theophylline half-life is generally shorter in children.

Therapeutic serum theophylline levels are usually 10–20 μg/ml.

Binding to plasma proteins is not extensive and theophylline is not preferentially taken up by any particular organ.

Apparently no development of tolerance occurs with chronic use of theophylline.

Clinical Pharmacology:

Guaifenesin

Mode of Action

Guaifenesin increases respiratory tract secretions, possibly by stimulating the Goblet cells.

Pharmacokinetics

Guaifenesin appears to be well absorbed, but its pharmacokinetics have not been well studied.

Indications and Usage: Quibron and Quibron-300 are indicated for the symptomatic treatment of bronchospasm associated with such conditions as bronchial asthma, chronic bronchitis and pulmonary emphysema.

Contraindications: Quibron products are contraindicated in individuals who have shown hypersensitivity to any of their components or xanthine derivatives.

Warnings: Excessive theophylline doses may be associated with toxicity; thus serum theophylline levels should be monitored to assure maximal benefit without excessive risk.

Serum levels of theophylline above the accepted therapeutic range (10–20 μg/ml) are associated with an increased incidence of toxicity. Such levels may be reached with customary doses in individuals who metabolize the drug slowly, especially patients (1) with lowered body plasma clearance (2) with liver dysfunction or chronic obstructive pulmonary disease (3) older than 55 years of age, particularly males.

Serious toxicity, such as seizure or ventricular arrhythmias, is not necessarily preceded by less serious side-effects such as nausea, irritability or restlessness.

Many patients who have higher (greater than 20 μg/ml) theophylline serum levels exhibit a tachycardia. Theophylline products may exacerbate pre-existing arrhythmias.

Precautions:

General: Theophylline

Use with caution in patients with severe cardiac disease, hypertension, acute myocardial injury, congestive heart failure, cor pulmonale, severe hypoxemia, hyperthyroidism, hepatic impairment, history of peptic ulcer, alcoholism and in the elderly. Concurrent administration with certain antibiotics (troleandomycin, erythromycin, clindamycin) may result in increased serum theophylline levels.

General: Guaifenesin

Plasma prothrombin and factor V may increase, but any resulting clinical effect is likely to be small.

Usage in Pregnancy

Teratogenic effects: Pregnancy Category C. Animal reproduction studies have not been conducted with Quibron products. It is also not known whether Quibron products can cause fetal harm when administered to a pregnant woman or can affect reproduction capacity. Quibron products should be given to a pregnant woman only if clearly indicated.

Nonteratogenic effects: It is not known whether use of this drug during labor or delivery has immediate or delayed adverse effects on the fetus, or whether it prolongs the duration of labor or increases the possibility of forceps delivery or other obstetrical intervention. It is not known whether this drug is excreted in human milk. Because many drugs are excreted in human milk, caution should be exercised when Quibron products are administered to a nursing woman.

Drug Interactions

Drug	Effect
Theophylline with furosemide	Increased diuresis
Theophylline with reserpine	Tachycardia
Theophylline with chlordiazepoxide	Fatty acid mobilization
Theophylline with troleandomycin, erythromycin, or clindamycin	Increased theophylline plasma levels

Drug/Laboratory Test Interactions

Theophylline may increase uric acid levels and urinary catecholamines. Metabolites of guaifenesin may contribute to increased urinary 5-hydroxyindoleacetic acid readings, when determined with nitrosonaphthol reagent.

Adverse Reactions: The frequency of adverse reactions is related to serum theophylline levels and is usually not a problem at levels below 20 μg/ml. The most consistent adverse reactions are usually due to overdosage and, while all have not been reported with Quibron or Quibron-300, the following reactions may be considered when theophylline is administered. Central nervous system: clonic and tonic generalized convulsions, muscle twitching, reflex hyperexcitability, headaches, insomnia, restlessness, and irritability. Cardiovascular: circulatory failure, ventricular arrhythmias, hypotension, extrasystoles, tachycardia, palpitation, and flushing. Gastrointestinal: hematemesis, vomiting, diarrhea, epigastric pain, and nausea. Renal: increased excretion of renal tubular cells and red blood cells, albuminuria, and diuresis. Respiratory: tachypnea. Others: hyperglycemia and inappropriate ADH syndrome.

Overdosage:

Symptoms

Nervousness, agitation, headache, insomnia, vomiting, tachycardia, extrasystoles, hyperreflexia, fasciculations and clonic and tonic convulsions. Children may be particularly prone to restlessness and hyperactivity that can proceed to convulsions.

Management

If potential oral overdose is established and seizure has *not* occurred.

1. Induce vomiting.
2. Administer a cathartic (this is particularly important if sustained release preparations have been taken).
3. Administer activated charcoal.
4. Monitor vital signs, maintain blood pressure and provide adequate hydration.

If patient is having seizure

1. Establish an airway.
2. Administer O_2.
3. Treat the seizure with intravenous diazepam 0.1 to 0.3 mg/kg up to 10 mg.
4. Monitor vital signs, maintain blood pressure and provide adequate hydration.

Post-Seizure Coma

1. Maintain airway and oxygenation.
2. If a result of oral medication, follow above recommendations to prevent absorption of drug, but intubation and lavage will have to be performed instead of inducing emesis and the cathartic and charcoal will need to be introduced via a large bore gastric lavage tube.
3. Continue to provide full supportive care and adequate hydration while waiting for drug to be metabolized. In general, the drug is metabolized rapidly enough so as to not warrant consideration of dialysis.

General

The oral LD_{50} of theophylline in mice is 350 mg/kg. The oral LD_{50} of guaifenesin in mice is 1725 mg/kg. In humans, adverse reactions often occur when serum theophylline levels exceed 20 μg/ml. Information on physiological variables which influence excretion of theophylline can be found under the heading "Clinical Pharmacology."

Dosage and Administration

General

Therapeutic serum levels associated with optimal likelihood for benefit and minimal risk of toxicity are considered to be between 10 μg/ml and 20 μg/ml. Levels above 20 μg/ml may produce toxic effects. There is great variation from patient to patient and dosage must be individualized because there is a relatively narrow range between therapeutic and toxic levels of theophylline. Monitoring of serum theophylline levels is highly recommended. Since theophylline does not distribute into fatty tissue, dosage should be calculated on the basis of ideal body weight.

Giving theophylline with food may prevent the rare case of stomach irritation and, although absorption may be slower, it is still complete.

Quibron

Treatment should be initiated at 150 mg theophylline every 6 hours for adults and 4 mg/kg every 6 hours for children. The usual recommended dosages are—Adults: 1–2 capsules or 1–2 tablespoons (15 ml) liquid every 6–8 hours. Children 9 to 12: 4–5 mg theophylline/kg body weight every 6–8 hours. Children under 9: 4–6 mg theophylline/kg body weight every 6–8 hours.

Approximate mg/kg dosage by TEASPOON (5 ml) of Quibron Liquid may be determined from the following table:

BODY WEIGHT		AVERAGE DOSAGE IN TEASPOONS (5 ml) TO PROVIDE THE FOLLOWING MG OF THEOPHYLLINE/ KG BODY WEIGHT/DOSE		
Lbs	Kgs	4 mg/kg	5 mg/kg	6 mg/kg
20	9	3/4	1	1
30	14	1	1 1/2	1 3/4
40	18	1 1/2	2	2 1/4
50	23	1 3/4	2 1/4	2 3/4
60	27	2	2 3/4	3 1/4
70	32	2 1/2	3	3 3/4
80	36	3	3 1/2	4 1/4
90	41	3 1/4	4	5
100	46	3 1/2	4 1/2	5 1/2

If the desired response is not achieved with the recommended initial dose, and there are no adverse reactions, the dose may be cautiously adjusted upward in increments of no more than 25 percent at 2–3 day intervals until the following MAXIMUM DOSE WITHOUT MEASUREMENT OF SERUM CONCENTRATION or a maximum of 900 mg in any 24 hour period (whichever is less) is attained:

MAXIMUM DAILY DOSE WITHOUT MEASUREMENT OF SERUM CONCENTRATION

	mg per kg Body Weight*
Children (under 9)	24
Children (9–12)	20
Adolescents (12–16)	18
Adults	13

*Use ideal body weight for obese patients

Do not attempt to maintain any dose that is not tolerated. If higher doses than those contained in the above MAXIMUM DOSE WITHOUT MEASUREMENT OF SERUM CONCENTRATION are necessary, it is recommended that serum theophylline levels be monitored. For therapeutic levels, draw blood sample just before next dose is due; for toxic levels, draw blood sample when last dose peaks (~2 hours after dosing). It is important that the patient has missed no doses during the previous 72 hours and that dosing intervals have been reasonably typical with no added doses during that period of time. DOSAGE ADJUSTMENT BASED ON SERUM THEOPHYLLINE MEASUREMENTS WHEN THESE INSTRUCTIONS HAVE *NOT* BEEN FOLLOWED, MAY RESULT IN RECOMMENDATIONS THAT PRESENT RISK OF TOXICITY TO THE PATIENT.

Quibron-300 Capsules

Quibron-300 is appropriate therapy when higher theophylline dosages are required. The usual recommended dosages for Quibron-300 are **Adults:** 1 capsule every 6–8 hours for patients whose dosage has been adjusted upward to achieve therapeutic serum levels.

How Supplied:

Quibron Capsules (yellow)

NDC 0087-0516-01	Bottles of 100
NDC 0087-0516-02	Bottles of 1000
NDC 0087-0516-03	Unit Dose 100's
VA6505-00-764-3367A	(Bottles of 100)
VA6505-00-764-3366A	(Bottles of 1000)
6505-00-764-3366	(Bottles of 1000) Defense

Quibron Liquid

NDC 0087-0510-03	Bottles of 1 pint
NDC 0087-0510-01	1 gallon

Quibron-300 Capsules (yellow and white)

NDC 0087-0515-41	Bottles of 100

July, 1979

Shown in Product Identification Section]

QUIBRON PLUS® ℞

Each capsule or tablespoon (15 ml) elixir contains theophylline (anhydrous) 150 mg., glyceryl guaiacolate (guaifenesin) 100 mg., ephedrine HCl 25 mg., and butabarbital 20 mg. (**Warning: May be habit-forming**) *Elixir:* alcohol 15%

Composition: Capsules are liquid-filled soft gelatin capsules. Elixir supplies the active ingredients in a flavored liquid.

Indications

Based on a review of a similar drug by the National Academy of Sciences—National Research Council and/or other information, FDA has classified the indications as follows:

"Possibly" effective: bronchial asthma; bronchitis, bronchiectasis, and emphysema in which bronchospasm is present or for the relief of brochospasm.

Final classification of the less-than-effective indications requires further investigation.

Dosage: *Adults:* 1–2 capsules or 1–2 tablespoons elixir 2–3 times daily.

Children 8 to 12: 1 capsule or 1 tablespoon elixir 2–3 times daily.

Children under 8: Up to ½ teaspoon elixir per 10 lb. body weight, 2–3 times daily. Dosage should be adjusted on an individual basis.

Contraindications: Contraindicated in patients who are sensitive to any ingredient of the formulation.

Warnings: Do not administer more frequently than every 6 hours or within 12 hours after rectal dose of any preparation containing theophylline or its derivatives such as aminophylline. Do not give other preparations containing xanthine derivatives concurrently. Be aware of the possible effects from concomitant doses of other sympathomimetic amines. Use in pregnancy only when clearly needed.

Precautions: Use cautiously in patients with cardiac disease, hypertension, hyperthyroidism, prostatic hypertrophy, hepatic disease, renal impairment, glaucoma, diabetes or peptic ulcer.

Adverse Reactions: While all have not been reported with Quibron Plus, the following reactions may be considered when theophylline and ephedrine are administered: gastric discomfort, nausea, vomiting, tremulousness, insomnia, convulsions, palpitation, tachycardia, flushing, extra systoles, arrhythmias, tachypnea, albuminuria, dehydration and precordial pain.

Overdosage: Treatment should include: drug discontinuance; appropriate supportive treatment for hypotension, seizure, arrhythmias or dehydration; airway and oxygenation maintenance.

How Supplied:

Quibron Plus® capsules

NDC 0087-0518-01 Bottles of 100

Quibron Plus® elixir

NDC 0087-0511-01 Bottles of 1 pint

July, 1979

[*Shown in Product Identification Section*]

VASODILAN® ℞

(Isoxsuprine HCl)
tablets • injection
U.S. Patent No. 3,056,836

Indications

Based on a review of this drug by the National Academy of Sciences—National Research Council and/or other information, the FDA has classified the indications as follows:

Possibly Effective:

1. For the relief of symptoms associated with cerebral vascular insufficiency.
2. In peripheral vascular disease of arteriosclerosis obliterans, thromboangiitis obliterans (Buerger's Disease) and Raynaud's disease.

Final classification of the less-than-effective indications requires further investigation.

Composition:

Vasodilan tablets, isoxsuprine HCl, 10 mg. and 20 mg.

Vasodilan injection, isoxsuprine HCl, 5 mg. per ml.

Dosage and Administration:

Oral: 10 to 20 mg. three or four times daily.

Intramuscular: 5 to 10 mg. (1 to 2 ml.) two or three times daily. Intramuscular administration may be used initially in severe or acute conditions.

Contraindications and Cautions: There are no known contraindications to oral use when administered in recommended doses. Should not be given immediately postpartum or in the presence of arterial bleeding.

Parenteral administration is not recommended in the presence of hypotension or tachycardia.

Intravenous administration should not be given because of increased likelihood of side effects.

Adverse Reactions: On rare occasions oral administration of the drug has been associated in time with the occurrences of hypotension, tachycardia, nausea, vomiting, dizziness, abdominal distress, and severe rash. If rash appears the drug should be discontinued.

Although available evidence suggests a temporal association of these reactions with isoxsuprine, a causal relationship can be neither confirmed nor refuted.

Administration of single dose of 10 mg intramuscularly may result in hypotension and tachycardia. These symptoms are more pronounced in higher doses. For these reasons single intramuscular doses exceeding 10 mg are not recommended. Repeated administration of 5 to 10 mg intramuscularly at suitable intervals may be employed.

How Supplied: Tablets, 10 mg.

NDC 0087-0543-01 Bottles of 100
NDC 0087-0543-02 Bottles of 1000
NDC 0087-0543-07 Bottles of 5000
NDC 0087-0543-05 Unit Dose
6505-00-890-1321 (1000's) Defense
VA 6505-00-890-1321A (1000's)

Tablets, 20 mg.

NDC 0087-0544-01 Bottles of 100
NDC 0087-0544-02 Bottles of 500
NDC 0087-0544-06 Bottles of 1000
NDC 0087-0544-47 Bottles of 5000
NDC 0087-0544-03 Unit Dose
VA 6505-00-173-5036A (500's)

Injection, 10 mg. per 2 ml. ampul

NDC 0087-0540-01 Boxes of six 2 ml. ampuls

July, 1979

[*Shown in Product Identification Section*]

Medical Products Panamericana, Inc.

P.O. BOX 771
CORAL GABLES, FLA. 33134

V G CAPSULES™ ℞

Composition: Each capsule contains: Vitamin C (Ascorbic Acid) 500 mg.; Vitamin B1 (Thiamine) 15 mg.; Vitamin B2 (Riboflavin) 15 mg.; Niacinamide 100 mg.; Vitamin B6 (Pyridoxine) 5 mg.; Vitamin B12 5 mcg.; Calcium Pantothenate 20 mg.; Folic Acid 0.5 mg.; Vitamin E (d-alpha tocopheryl acetate) 30 I.U.; 1-lysine Hydrochloride (need in human nutrition established, but no U.S. RDA established) 25 mg.; Manganese Sulfate 4 mg.; Magnesium Sulfate 35 mg. (equivalent to 25 mg. dried $MgSO_4$); Zinc Sulfate 80 mg. (equivalent to 25 mg. dried $ZnSO_4$).

Indications: Indicated in the treatment of patients with deficiencies of, or increased requirements for Vitamin C and/or B-Complex Vitamins including Folic Acid, Zinc, Magnesium and/or Manganese.

Suggested Dosage: One Capsule Daily or as directed by a physician.

Precautions: Folic Acid may obscure pernicious anemia; the peripheral blood picture may revert to normal while neurological manifestations remain progressive.

Caution: Federal Law prohibits dispensing without prescription.

Supplied: NDC 0576-0506-30 Bottle of 30 Capsules.

Over 7,000 products are

listed alphabetically

in the

PINK SECTION.

Medicone Company
**225 VARICK ST.
NEW YORK, NY 10014**

DERMA MEDICONE® Ointment

Composition: Each gram contains:

Benzocaine	20.0 mg.
Oxyquinoline sulfate	10.5 mg.
Menthol	4.8 mg.
Ichthammol	10.0 mg.
Zinc oxide	137.3 mg.
Petrolatum, Lanolin, perfume	q.s.

Action and Uses: For prompt, temporary relief of intolerable itching, burning and pain associated with minor skin irritations. A bland, non-toxic, well balanced formula in a non-drying base which will not disintegrate or liquefy at body temperature and is not washed away by urine, perspiration or exudate. Exerts a soothing, cooling influence on irritated skin surfaces by affording mild anesthesia to control the scratch reflex, promotes healing of the affected area and checks the spread of infection. Useful for symptomatic relief in a wide variety of pruritic skin irritations resulting from insect bites, prickly heat, eczema, chafed and raw skin surfaces, sunburn, fungus infections, plant poisoning, pruritus ani and pruritus vulvae—mouth sores, cracked lips, under dentures.
Administration and Dosage: Apply liberally directly to site of irritation and gently rub into affected area for better penetration and absorption. Cover area with gauze if necessary.
Precautions: Do not use in the eyes. If the condition for which this preparation is used persists, or if rash or irritation develops, discontinue use and consult physician.
How Supplied: 1 ounce tubes and one pound jars.

DERMA MEDICONE®-HC Ointment ℞

Composition: Each gram contains:

Hydrocortisone acetate	10.0 mg.
Benzocaine	19.8 mg.
Oxyquinoline sulfate	10.4 mg.
Ephedrine hydrochloride	1.1 mg.
Menthol	4.8 mg.
Ichthammol	9.9 mg.
Zinc oxide	135.8 mg.
Petrolatum, Lanolin, perfume	q.s.

Action and Uses: Offers the advantage of quick, lasting comfort during treatment of severely inflamed dermatoses by affording prompt temporary local anesthetic action, inhibiting pain, burning, itching and controlling the scratch reflex. The hydrocortisone acetate reduces inflammation and swelling, aiding the normal healing process. The non-drying base will not disintegrate or liquefy at body temperature and is not washed off by exudate, perspiration or urine. Effectively suppresses inflammation, pain, swelling, burning and itching in contact dermatitis, eczematoid dermatitis, atopic dermatitis, neurodermatitis, seborrheic dermatitis, allergic dermatitis, rhus dermatitis, pruritus ani and pruritus vulvae.
Administration and Dosage: Apply to affected area 2 to 4 times daily. When adequate improvement is noted, reduce frequency of application or continue maintenance control with regular Derma Medicone ointment.
Precautions: Observe the usual adrenocorticosteroid precautions. Exercise care if the patient is on other corticosteroid therapy or if infection is present or if rash or irritation develops. Do not use in the eyes.
Contraindications: Do not use in the presence of tuberculosis of the skin.
How Supplied: 7 gram and 20 gram tubes.

DioMEDICONE® Tablets

Composition: Each tablet contains:
50 mg. dioctyl sodium sulfosuccinate (a surface tension reducing wetting agent) and excipient q.s. to prevent hard stool formation.
Action and Uses: A gentle-acting, non-habit forming stool-softener for effective management of simple constipation due to hard, dry fecal matter. A medically accepted, clinically proven mode of treatment in preventing hard stool formation. Reduces surface tension of intestinal fluids, permitting better infiltration of waste matter, producing a soft pliable fecal mass, making evacuation easy and comfortable. Reduces straining. Does not irritate the intestinal tract or produce peristalsis. Useful in hemorrhoidal and anorectal conditions, during and after pregnancy and whenever smooth, easy bowel evacuation is essential such as in cardiac conditions and before and following surgery. May be safely used as directed, by anyone over 6 years of age.
Administration and Dosage: Children 6 to 12 years: 1 or 2 tablets (50 to 100 mg.) daily with water. Adults and older children: 1 to 4 tablets (50 to 200 mg.) daily with water. Initial dosages may be reduced as normal bowel function is restored. Note: The effect of DioMEDICONE in producing soft, pliable stools usually takes 2 to 3 days.
How Supplied: 50 mg. tablets in vials of 50 tablets.

MEDICONE® DRESSING Cream

Composition: Each gram contains:

Benzocaine	5.0 mg.
8-Hydroxyquinoline sulfate	0.5 mg.
Cod liver oil	125.0 mg.
Zinc oxide	125.0 mg.
Menthol	1.8 mg.
Petrolatum, Lanolin, talcum, paraffin & perfume	q.s.

Action and Uses: Meets the first requisite in the treatment of minor burns, wounds and other denuded skin lesions by exerting mild, cooling anesthetic action for the prompt temporary relief of pain, burning and itching. A stable, non-toxic anesthetic dressing which does not liquefy or wash off at body temperature, nor is it decomposed by exudate, urine or perspiration. Promotes granulation and aids epithelization of affected tissue. The anesthetic, antipruritic, antibacterial properties make Medicone Dressing ideal for the treatment of 1st and 2nd degree burns, minor wounds, abrasions, diaper rashes and a wide variety of pruritic skin irritations.
Administration and Dosage: The smooth, specially formulated consistency allows comfortable application directly to the painful, irritated affected area. It may be spread on gauze before application or covered with gauze as desired.
Precautions: Do not use in the eyes. If the condition for which this preparation is used persists or if a rash or irritation develops, discontinue use and consult physician.
How Supplied: Tubes of 1 ounce and 1 lb. jars.

MEDICONET®
(medicated rectal wipes)

Composition: Each cloth wipe medicated with Benzalkonium chloride, 0.02%; Ethoxylated lanolin, 0.5%; Methylparaben, 0.15%; Hamamelis water, 50%; Glycerin, 10%; Purified water, USP and Perfume, q.s.
Action and Uses: Soft disposable cloth wipes which fulfill the important requisite in treating anal discomfort by providing the facility for gently and thoroughly cleansing the affected area. For the temporary relief of intolerable pain, itching and burning in minor external hemorrhoidal, anal and outer vaginal discomfort. Lanolized, delicately scented, durable and delightfully soft. Antiseptic, antipruritic, astringent. Useful as a substitute for harsh, dry toilet tissue. May also be used as a compress in the pre- and post-operative management of anorectal discomfort. The hygienic Mediconet pad is generally useful in relieving pain, burning and itching in diaper rash, sunburn, heat rash, minor burns and insect bites.
How Supplied: Boxes of 20 individually packaged, pre-moistened cleansing cloths.

RECTAL MEDICONE® SUPPOSITORIES

Composition: Each suppository contains:

Benzocaine	2 gr.
Oxyquinoline sulfate	1/4 gr.
Zinc oxide	3 gr.
Menthol	1/7 gr.
Balsam Peru	1 gr.
Cocoa butter—vegetable & petroleum oil base, Certified color added	q.s.

Action and Uses: A soothing, non-toxic, comprehensive formula carefully designed to meet the therapeutic requirements in adequately treating simple hemorrhoids and minor anorectal disorders. Performs the primary function of promptly alleviating pain, burning and itching temporarily by exerting satisfactory local anesthesia. The muscle spasm, present in many cases of painful anal and rectal conditions, is controlled and together with the emollients provided, helps the patient to evacuate the bowel comfortably and normally. The active ingredients reduce congestion and afford antisepsis, accelerating the normal healing process. Used pre- and post-surgically in hemorrhoidectomy, in prenatal and postpartum care and whenever surgery is contraindicated for the comfort and well-being of the patient during treatment of an underlying cause.
Administration and Dosage: One suppository in the morning and one at night and after each stool, or as directed. Use of the suppositories should be continued for 10 to 15 days after cessation of discomfort to help protect against recurrence of symptoms. See Rectal Medicone Unguent for concurrent internal-external use.
Precautions: If a rash or irritation develops, or bleeding from the rectum occurs, discontinue use and consult physician.
How Supplied: Boxes of 12 and 24 individually foil-wrapped green suppositories.
[*Shown in Product Identification Section*]

RECTAL MEDICONE®-HC SUPPOSITORIES ℞

Composition: Each suppository contains:

Hydrocortisone acetate	10 mg.
Benzocaine	2 gr.
Oxyquinoline sulfate	1/4 gr.
Zinc oxide	3 gr.
Menthol	1/7 gr.
Balsam Peru	1 gr.
Cocoa butter—vegetable & petroleum oil base, Certified color added	q.s.

Action and Uses: The hydrocortisone acetate reduces and controls severe anorectal inflammation and swelling, effecting better management of the basic condition. Provides prompt, temporary relief from pain, burning and itching. Soothes, lubricates and protects; makes bowel evacuation more comfortable while accelerating the normal healing process. Useful as initial therapy in hemorrhoids, acute and chronic proctitis, post-operative edema, cryptitis, pruritus ani and inflamed post-operative scar tissue.
ANESTHETIC—ANTI-INFLAMMATORY
ANTIPRURITIC—ANTIBACTERIAL
Administration and Dosage: Start therapy with one Rectal Medicone-HC Suppository twice daily for a recommended period of three to six days. Continue maintenance control against recurring symptoms with regular Rectal Medicone Suppositories and/or Unguent as required.
Precautions: A thorough proctologic diagnosis should be made when use of hydrocortisone

is considered. Care should be exercised if the patient is on other corticosteroid therapy or if infection is present or if rash or irritation develops.
Contraindications: Do not use in the presence of tuberculosis of the rectum.
How Supplied: Boxes of 12 individually foil-wrapped pink suppositories.
[*Shown in Product Identification Section*]

RECTAL MEDICONE® UNGUENT

Composition: Each gram contains:

Benzocaine	20 mg.
Oxyquinoline sulfate	5 mg.
Menthol	4 mg.
Zinc oxide	100 mg.
Balsam Peru	12.5 mg.
Petrolatum	625 mg.
Lanolin	210 mg.

Certified color added
Action and Uses: A soothing, effective formulation which affords prompt, temporary relief of pain, burning and itching by exerting surface anesthetic action on the affected area in minor internal-external hemorrhoids and anorectal disorders. The active ingredients promote healing and protect against irritation, aiding inflamed tissue to retrogress to normal. The emollient petrolatum-lanolin base provides lubrication making bowel movements easier and more comfortable. Accelerates the normal healing process. Non-toxic. Rectal Medicone Unguent and Rectal Medicone Suppositories are excellent for concurrent management of internal-external irritations.
Administration and Dosage: For internal use—attach pliable applicator and lubricate tip with a small amount of Unguent to ease insertion. Apply liberally into affected area morning and night and after each stool or as directed. When used externally, cover area with gauze. When used with Rectal Medicone Suppositories, insert a small amount of Unguent into the rectum before inserting suppository.
Precautions: If a rash or irritation develops or rectal bleeding occurs, discontinue use and consult physician.
How Supplied: 1½ ounce tubes with pliable rectal applicator.

Medics Pharmaceutical Corporation
203 RIO CIRCLE
DECATUR, GEORGIA 30030

CERVEX™ Vaginal Cream ℞

Description: Sulfanilamide 15%, Aminacrine hydrochloride 0.2% and Allantoin 2.0%, in a dispersible base containing Triethanolamine, Propylene Glycol, Stearic Acid, Diglycol Stearate, Water.
How Supplied: 4 oz. tube and applicator NDC 0184-0046-40.

ESSENTIAL–8 CAPSULES OTC
Liquid Predigested Protein

How Supplied: Bottles of 120 NDC 0184-0040-70.

HEMOCYTE Injection ℞
Hematinic-Vitamin

Description: Each 2 ml. contains: Peptonized Iron 50 mg., Folic Acid 2 mg. (as Sodium Salt), Liver Injection (activity equivalent to 2 mcg. of cyanocobalamin), Cyanocobalamin 50 mcg., Benzyl Alcohol 1.5%, Phenol 0.5%.
How Supplied: 10 mg. multiple dose vial NDC 0184-0179-10.

HEMOCYTE Tablets OTC
(ferrous fumarate 324 mg.)

How Supplied:
Bottles of 100 NDC 0184-0307-60.
Bottles of 1000 NDC 0184-0307-80.

HEMOCYTE PLUS™ Tabules ℞
Iron-Vitamin-Mineral Complex

Description: Each tabule contains:

Ferrous Fumarate (anhydrous)	324 mg.
[Equivalent to about 106 mg. of Elemental Iron]	
Sodium Ascorbate (Vit. C)	200 mg.
Vit. B-1—Thiamine Mononitrate	10 mg.
Vit. B-2—Riboflavin	6 mg.
Vit. B-6—Pyridoxine HCl	5 mg.
Vit. B-12—Cyanocobalamin Concentrate	15mcg.
Folic Acid	1 mg.
Niacinamide	30 mg.
Calcium Pantothenate	10 mg.
Zinc Sulfate	80 mg.
Magnesium Sulfate	70 mg.
Manganese Sulfate	4 mg.
Copper Sulfate	2 mg.

How Supplied: Bottles of 100 NDC 0184-0308-60.

HEMOCYTE–F TABLETS ℞

Description: Each tablet contains:

Ferrous Fumarate	324 mg.
Folic Acid	1 mg.

How Supplied: Bottles of 100 NDC 0184-0306-60.

ISOVEX®–100 Capsules ℞
(ethaverine hydrochloride 100 mg.)

How Supplied:
Bottles of 100 NDC 0184-0203-60.
Bottles of 1000 NDC 0184-0203-80.

MEDIGESIC PLUS® Capsules ℞
Analgesic-Sedative

Description: Each capsule contains:

Butalbital*	50 mg
Warning: May be habit forming	
Acetaminophen	400 mg
Caffeine	30 mg

*Derivative of Barbituric Acid
How Supplied: Bottles of 100 NDC 0184-0211-60.

MEDIZINC Scored Tablets ℞
(zinc sulfate 220 mg.)

How Supplied: Bottles of 100 NDC 0184-0310-60.

NOREL PLUS Capsules ℞
Antihistamine-Analgesic-Decongestant

Description: Each capsule contains: Acetaminophen 325 mg., Phenyltoloxamine Dihydrogen Citrate 25 mg., Phenylpropanolamine HCl. 25 mg. and Chlorpheniramine Maleate 4 mg.
How Supplied: Bottles of 100 NDC 0184-0128-60.

NOREL PLUS Injection ℞
Antihistamine-Decongestant

Description: Each ml. contains: Atropine Sulfate 0.2 mg., Phenylpropanolamine HCl. 12.5 mg., Chlorpheniramine Maleate 5.0 mg., Benzyl Alcohol 2% as preservative in Water for Injection q.s.
How Supplied: 10 ml. multiple dose vial NDC 0184-0130-10.

W. F. Merchant Pharmaceutical Co., Inc.
P.O. BOX 6
MT. RAINIER, MD 20822

ADATUSS–D.C.™ ℞ Ⓒ
Expectorant cough syrup

Actions: Hydrocodone bitartrate is an effective semisynthetic narcotic antitussive. Guaifenesin (glyceryl guaiacolate) is an expectorant which enhances the output of lower respiratory tract fluid.
Indications: Indicated in non-productive cough spasm. It is useful in the symptomatic relief of the upper respiratory tract due to allergic conditions, the common cold, and acute bronchitis.
Contraindications: Hypersensitivity to any of the ingredients.
Precautions: Continuous dosage over an extended period is generally contraindicated since Hydrocone may cause addiction. Since drowsiness may occur, patients should be cautioned about driving or operating machinery.
Adverse Reactions: ADATUSS DC™ Expectorant is generally well tolerated. Occasional drowsiness, dizziness, gastrointestinal upset, nausea or constipation may occur.
Dosage and Administration: Adults and children over 90 lbs., one to two teaspoonful; children 50 to 90 lbs., ½ to one teaspoonful; children 25 to 50 lbs., ¼ to ½ teaspoonful. May be given three or four times a day as needed.
Supplied: As a black raspberry-flavored syrup containing sugar. Comes in pints NDC-12814-301-16 and in gallons NDC-12814-301-28.

CIRCUBID™ ℞
(ethaverine hydrochloride)
capsules*

Description: Each capsule contains Ethaverine HCl 150 mg.
Actions: Ethaverine HCl acts directly on the smooth muscle cells without involving the autonomic nervous system or its receptors.
Indications: In peripheral and cerebral vascular insufficiency associated with arterial spasm, in spastic conditions of the gastro-intestinal and genitourinary tracts.
Contraindications: Contraindicated in the presence of complete atrioventricular dissociation.
Precautions: It should be administered with caution in patients with glaucoma. It should not be used in pregnant women or in women of childbearing age unless directed by a physician.
Adverse Reactions: Even though the incidence of side effects as reported in literature is very low, it is possible for a patient to evidence nausea, anorexia, abdominal distress, dryness of the throat, hypotension, flushing, sweating, vertigo, respiratory depression, cardiac depression, cardiac arrhythmia and headache. If these side effects occur, reduce dosage or discontinue medication.
Dosage: The usual adult dose is 300 mg. daily, one capsule every 12 hours. In more difficult cases the dosage may be increased to 600 mg. daily as determined by the physician. It is most effective given early in the course of the vascular disorder. Because of the chronic nature of the disease long term therapy is required.
How Supplied: Bottles of 100 NDC-12814-101-01 and 1000 NDC-12814-101-10.
*Manufactured to provide a prolonged therapeutic effect.

Continued on next page

Merchant—Cont.

DECUBITEX™ ℞
ointment
Ingredients: Biebrich Scarlet Red, Sulfonated, Water Soluble 0.1% in an ointment base containing Peruvian Balsam, Zinc Oxide, Starch, Castor Oil, Petrolatum, Sodium Propionate, Methylparaben, Propylparaben, Propylene Glycol and Water.
Indications: As an aid in the management of decubitus ulcers.
Administration: Pour a small amount of 3% Hydrogen Peroxide or Sterile Normal Saline onto the affected area. Cleanse thoroughly and apply ointment. Cover with dry sterile gauze. Dressing should be changed twice daily.
Contraindications: Known hypersensitivity to any of the ingredients.
Adverse Reactions: Gastroenteritis and renal irritation have been reported following percutaneous absorption over a massive area.
Caution: Federal law prohibits dispensing without prescription.
How Supplied: Jars ½ oz. NDC-12814-501-04, 2 oz. NDC-12814-501-60, ½ oz. in 4 oz. pack of 8 × ½ oz. NDC-12814-501-14, 4 oz. BULK NDC-12814-501-12, ½ oz. in 16 oz. pack of 32 × ½ oz. NDC-12814-501-44, 16 oz. BULK NDC-12814-501-48.

HISTORAL™ ℞
Ingredients: Chlorpheniramine Maleate 12 mg., Pseudoephedrine HCl 60 mg., Methscopolamine Nitrate 2.5 mg.
Action: Antihistaminic-Decongestant; Chlorpheniramine Maleate is a potent antihistamine with an excellent therapeutic index and low incidence of side effects, particularly the sedation associated with many other antihistamines. Pseudoephedrine hydrochloride provides a rapid and sustained decongestant effect on swollen mucosa of the respiratory tract. It does this by vasoconstriction and opens obstructed airways through direct action on the smooth muscle of the bronchi. The vasoconstrictor action of pseudoephedrine is similar to that of ephedrine. In the usual oral dosage, it has minimal vasopressor effects. Methscopolamine Nitrate affords atropine-like action without the deep CNS stimulation associated with scopolamine (Goodman and Gilman: "Pharmacological Basic of Therapeutics") September, 1969.
Indication: For relief of upper respiratory and bronchial congestion associated with; the common cold, hay fever and allergies, sinusitis, influenza, and vasomotor and allergic rhinitis.
Contraindications: Sensitivity to antihistamines or sympathomimetic agents. It should not be used in patients with severe hypertension or coronary artery disease. Capsules should not be given to children under 12 years of age.
Warnings: Use with caution in patients suffering from hypertension, cardiac disease, or hyperthyroidism. Patients susceptible to the soporific effects of chlorpheniramine should be warned against driving or operating machinery should drowsiness occur.
Precautions: Use with caution in the presence of hypertension, coronary artery disease, narrow-angle glaucoma, prostatic hypertrophy, hyperthyroidism and diabetes. Patients should be cautioned about possible additive effects with alcohol and other central nervous system depressants (hypnotics, sedatives, tranquilizers), and should be cautioned against hazardous occupations requiring complete mental alertness such as operating machinery or driving a motor vehicle. If a sensitivity reaction or idiosyncrasy should occur, withdraw the drug.
Adverse Reactions: Most patients will have no side effects at the usual dosage. However, certain patients may exhibit mild stimulation or mild sedation. Although rare, hypersensitivity to either the antihistamine or decongestant may occur.
Dosage: Capsules—Adults and children over 12, one capsule every 12 hours. Liquid—Adults and children over 12, 1 or 2 teaspoonsful; children 6 to 12, 1 teaspoonful; children 3 to 6 years, ½ teaspoonful. May be repeated in 4 to 6 hours if required for relief.
How Supplied: Bottles of 100 NDC-12814-102-01 and 1000 NDC-12814-102-10. Liquid in 16 oz. NDC-12814-302-16 and gallon NDC-12814-302-28.

MAXIGESIC™ Capsules ℞ Ⓒ
Description: Each gray and white capsule contains; Codeine Phosphate 30 mg., Acetaminophen 325 mg., Promethazine HCl 6.25 mg.
Actions: Provide enhanced analgesia plus mild sedation. Codeine provides analgesic and antitussive actions. Acetaminophen is an effective analgesic and antipyretic. Promethazine has antiemetic and antihistaminic actions.
Indications: Provides enhanced analgesia for the relief from the discomfort of moderate acute pain such as may be associated with arthritis, bursitis, dysmenorrhea, myalgias, neuralgias, sinusitis, rheumatoid conditions, headache, tension headache, toothache and pain associated with dental procedures. It may also be useful in the temporary relief of symptoms of the common cold and fever.
Contraindications: Hypersensitivity to any of the ingredients.
Warnings: As with other codeine-containing preparations which may be habit forming, administration is not recommended over an extended period.
Precautions: May produce drowsiness or dizziness which may impair ability to drive or perform other tasks requiring alertness. Patients should be warned not to drive an automobile or operate machinery should they experience such reactions while taking this drug. In such cases, reduction in dosage or discontinuance of the drug should be considered. Avoid alcoholic beverages. As with all narcotic medications, care should be exercised in prescribing this product in view of the possibility of suppression of productive cough.
Adverse Reactions: As with other narcotic-containing products, drowsiness, constipation, miosis, nausea and vomiting may occur.
Dosage and Administration: Adults: 1 to 2 capsules every 4 hours as needed for pain. Children, 6 to 12 years of age: 1 capsule every 4 hours.
How Supplied: Bottles of 100 NDC-12814-202-01 and 1000 NDC-12814-202-10.

Merck Sharp & Dohme
DIVISION OF MERCK & CO., INC.
WEST POINT, PA 19486

Product Identification Codes

To provide quick and positive identification of Merck Sharp & Dohme products, we have imprinted a code number on tablet and capsule products. In order that you may identify a product by its code number, we have compiled below a numerical list of code numbers with their corresponding product names. We are also listing the code numbers by alphabetical listing of products as a cross reference.
The code number as it appears on tablets and capsules bears the letters MSD plus the numerical code. Decadron® (Dexamethasone, MSD) tablets 0.25 mg is identified MSD 20.

Numerical Listing

MSD Code No.	Product	Product No.
20	Decadron® (Dexamethasone, MSD) Tablets 0.25 mg.	7592
21	Cogentin® (Benztropine Mesylate, MSD) Tablets 0.5 mg.	3297
23	Elavil® (Amitriptyline HCl, MSD) Tablets 10 mg.	3287
25	Indocin® (Indomethacin, MSD) Capsules 25 mg.	3316
26	Vivactil® (Protriptyline HCl, MSD) Tablets 5 mg.	3313
41	Decadron® (Dexamethasone, MSD) Tablets 0.5 mg.	7598
42	HydroDIURIL® (Hydrochlorothiazide, MSD) Tablets 25 mg.	3263
43	Mephyton® (Phytonadione, MSD) Tablets 5 mg.	7776
45	Elavil® (Amitriptyline HCl, MSD) Tablets 25 mg.	3288
47	Vivactil® (Protriptyline HCl, MSD) Tablets 10 mg.	3314
49	Daranide® (Dichlorphenamide, MSD) Tablets	3256
50	Indocin® (Indomethacin, MSD) Capsules 50 mg.	3317
52	Inversine® (Mecamylamine HCl, MSD) Tablets 2.5 mg.	3219
53	Hydropres®-25 Tablets	3265
60	Cogentin® (Benztropine Mesylate, MSD) Tablets 2 mg.	3172
62	Periactin® (Cyproheptadine HCl, MSD) Tablets 4 mg.	3276
63	Decadron® (Dexamethasone, MSD) Tablets 0.75 mg.	7601
65	Edecrin® (Ethacrynic Acid, MSD) Tablets 25 mg.	3321
90	Edecrin® (Ethacrynic Acid, MSD) Tablets 50 mg.	3322
95	Decadron® (Dexamethasone, MSD) Tablets 1.5 mg.	7638
97	Decadron® (Dexamethasone, MSD) Tablets 4 mg.	7645
102	Elavil® (Amitriptyline HCl, MSD) Tablets 50 mg.	3320
105	HydroDIURIL® (Hydrochlorothiazide, MSD) Tablets 50 mg.	3264
120	Inversine® (Mecamylamine HCl, MSD) Tablets 10 mg.	3220
126	Cortone® (Cortisone Acetate, MSD) Tablets 5 mg.	7067
127	Hydropres®-50 Tablets	3266
135	Aldomet® (Methyldopa, MSD) Tablets 125 mg.	3341
214	Diuril® (Chlorothiazide, MSD) Tablets 250 mg.	3244
219	Cortone® (Cortisone Acetate, MSD) Tablets 25 mg.	7063
230	Diupres®-250 Tablets	3261
401	Aldomet® (Methyldopa, MSD) Tablets 250 mg.	3290
403	Urecholine® (Bethanechol Chloride, MSD) Tablets 5 mg.	7785
405	Diupres®-500 Tablets	3262
410	HydroDIURIL® (Hydrochlorothiazide, MSD) Tablets 100 mg.	3340
412	Urecholine® (Bethanechol Chloride, MSD) Tablets 10 mg.	7787
423	Aldoril®-15 Tablets	3294
430	Elavil® (Amitriptyline HCl, MSD) Tablets 75 mg.	3348
432	Diuril® (Chlorothiazide, MSD) Tablets 500 mg.	3245
435	Elavil® (Amitriptyline HCl, MSD) Tablets 100 mg.	3349
456	Aldoril®-25 Tablets	3295
457	Urecholine® (Bethanechol Chloride, MSD) Tablets 25 mg.	7788
501	Benemid® (Probenecid, MSD) Tablets 0.5 g.	3337
512	Sulfathalidine® (Phthalylsulfathiazole, MSD) Tablets 0.5 g.	2295
516	Aldomet® (Methyldopa, MSD) Tablets 500 mg.	3292
517	Triavil® 4-50 Tablets	3364
602	Cuprimine® (Penicillamine, MSD) Capsules 250 mg.	3299
605	Propadrine® (Phenylpropanolamine HCl, MSD) Capsules 25 mg.	2197
612	Aldoclor®-150 Tablets	3318

613	Propadrine® (Phenylpropanolamine HCl, MSD) Capsules 50 mg.	2198
614	ColBENEMID® Tablets	3283
619	Hydrocortone® (Hydrocortisone, MSD) Tablets 10 mg.	7604
625	Hydrocortone® (Hydrocortisone, MSD) Tablets 20 mg.	7602
634	Aldoclor®-250 Tablets	3319
635	Cogentin® (Benztropine Mesylate, MSD) Tablets 1 mg.	3334
647	Sinemet®-10/100 Tablets	3346
654	Sinemet®-25/250 Tablets	3347
672	Cuprimine® (Penicillamine, MSD) Capsules 125 mg	3350
673	Elavil® (Amitriptyline HCl, MSD) Tablets 150 mg.	3351
694	Aldoril® D30 Tablets	3362
907	Mintezol (Thiabendazole, MSD) Chewable Tablets 500 mg.	3332
914	Triavil® 2-10 Tablets	3328
921	Triavil® 2-25 Tablets	3311
931	Flexeril® (Cyclobenzaprine HCl, MSD) Tablets 10 mg.	3358
934	Triavil® 4-10 Tablets	3310
935	Aldoril® D50 Tablets	3363
941	Clinoril® (Sulindac, MSD) Tablets 150 mg.	3360
942	Clinoril® (Sulindac, MSD) Tablets 200 mg.	3353
946	Triavil® 4-25 Tablets	3312

Alphabetical Listing

MSD Code No.	Product	Product No.
612	Aldoclor®-150 Tablets	3318
634	Aldoclor®-250 Tablets	3319
135	Aldomet® (Methyldopa, MSD) Tablets 125 mg.	3341
401	Aldomet® (Methyldopa, MSD) Tablets 250 mg.	3290
516	Aldomet® (Methyldopa, MSD) Tablets 500 mg.	3292
423	Aldoril®-15 Tablets	3294
456	Aldoril®-25 Tablets	3295
694	Aldoril® D30 Tablets	3362
935	Aldoril® D50 Tablets	3363
501	Benemid® (Probenecid, MSD) Tablets 0.5 g.	3337
941	Clinoril® (Sulindac, MSD) Tablets 150 mg.	3360
942	Clinoril® (Sulindac, MSD) Tablets 200 mg.	3353
21	Cogentin® (Benztropine Mesylate, MSD) Tablets 0.5 mg.	3297
635	Cogentin® (Benztropine Mesylate, MSD) Tablets 1 mg.	3334
60	Cogentin® (Benztropine Mesylate, MSD) Tablets 2 mg.	3172
614	ColBENEMID® Tablets	3283
126	Cortone® (Cortisone Acetate, MSD) Tablets 5 mg.	7067
219	Cortone® (Cortisone Acetate, MSD) Tablets 25 mg.	7063
672	Cuprimine® (Penicillamine, MSD) Capsules 125 mg	3350
602	Cuprimine® (Penicillamine, MSD) Capsules 250 mg.	3299
49	Daranide® (Dichlorphenamide, MSD) Tablets	3256
20	Decadron® (Dexamethasone, MSD) Tablets 0.25 mg.	7592
41	Decadron® (Dexamethasone, MSD) Tablets 0.5 mg.	7598
63	Decadron® (Dexamethasone, MSD) Tablets 0.75 mg.	7601
95	Decadron® (Dexamethasone, MSD) Tablets 1.5 mg.	7638
97	Decadron® (Dexamethasone, MSD) Tablets 4 mg.	7645
230	Diupres®-250 Tablets	3261
405	Diupres®-500 Tablets	3262
214	Diuril® (Chlorothiazide, MSD) Tablets 250 mg.	3244
432	Diuril® (Chlorothiazide, MSD) Tablets 500 mg.	3245
65	Edecrin® (Ethacrynic Acid, MSD) Tablets 25 mg.	3321
90	Edecrin® (Ethacrynic Acid, MSD) Tablets 50 mg.	3322
23	Elavil® (Amitriptyline HCl, MSD) Tablets 10 mg.	3287
45	Elavil® (Amitriptyline HCl, MSD) Tablets 25 mg.	3288
102	Elavil® (Amitriptyline HCl, MSD) Tablets 50 mg.	3320
430	Elavil® (Amitriptyline HCl, MSD) Tablets 75 mg.	3348
435	Elavil® (Amitriptyline HCl, MSD) Tablets 100 mg.	3349
673	Elavil® (Amitriptyline HCl, MSD) Tablets 150 mg	3351
931	Flexeril® (Cyclobenzaprine HCl, MSD) Tablets 10 mg.	3358
619	Hydrocortone® (Hydrocortisone, MSD) Tablets 10 mg.	7604
625	Hydrocortone® (Hydrocortisone, MSD) Tablets 20 mg.	7602
42	HydroDIURIL® (Hydrochlorothiazide, MSD) Tablets 25 mg.	3263
105	HydroDIURIL® (Hydrochlorothiazide, MSD) Tablets 50 mg.	3264
410	HydroDIURIL® (Hydrochlorothiazide, MSD) Tablets 100 mg.	3340
53	Hydropres®-25 Tablets	3265
127	Hydropres®-50 Tablets	3266
25	Indocin® (Indomethacin, MSD) Capsules 25 mg.	3316
50	Indocin® (Indomethacin, MSD) Capsules 50 mg.	3317
52	Inversine® (Mecamylamine HCl, MSD) Tablets 2.5 mg.	3219
120	Inversine® (Mecamylamine HCl, MSD) Tablets 10 mg.	3220
43	Mephyton® (Phytonadione, MSD) Tablets 5 mg.	7776
907	Mintezol (Thiabendazole, MSD) Chewable Tablets 500 mg.	3332
62	Periactin® (Cyproheptadine HCl, MSD) Tablets 4 mg.	3276
605	Propadrine® (Phenylpropanolamine HCl, MSD) Capsules 25 mg.	2197
613	Propadrine® (Phenylpropanolamine HCl, MSD) Capsules 50 mg.	2198
647	Sinemet®-10/100 Tablets	3346
654	Sinemet®-25/250 Tablets	3347
512	Sulfathalidine® (Phthalylsulfathiazole, MSD) Tablets 0.5 g.	2295
914	Triavil® 2-10 Tablets	3328
921	Triavil® 2-25 Tablets	3311
934	Triavil® 4-10 Tablets	3310
946	Triavil® 4-25 Tablets	3312
517	Triavil® 4-50 Tablets	3364
403	Urecholine® (Bethanechol Chloride, MSD) Tablets 5 mg.	7785
412	Urecholine® (Bethanechol Chloride, MSD) Tablets 10 mg.	7787
457	Urecholine® (Bethanechol Chloride, MSD) Tablets 25 mg.	7788
26	Vivactil® (Protriptyline HCl, MSD) Tablets 5 mg.	3313
47	Vivactil® (Protriptyline HCl, MSD) Tablets 10 mg.	3314

ALDOCLOR® Tablets ℞
Antihypertensive

WARNING

This fixed combination drug is not indicated for initial therapy of hypertension. Hypertension requires therapy titrated to the individual patient. If the fixed combination represents the dosage so determined, its use may be more convenient in patient management. The treatment of hypertension is not static, but must be reevaluated as conditions in each patient warrant.

Description

ALDOCLOR® is a combination of methyldopa and chlorothiazide. The chemical name for methyldopa is levo-3-(3,4-dihydroxyphenyl)-2-methylalanine. Chlorothiazide is 6-chloro-*2H*-1, 2, 4-benzothiadiazine-7-sulfonamide 1, 1-dioxide.

Actions

ALDOMET® (Methyldopa, MSD)
Methyldopa, a unique antihypertensive, is an aromatic-amino-acid decarboxylase inhibitor in animals and in man. Although the mechanism of action has yet to be conclusively demonstrated, the antihypertensive effect of methyldopa probably is due to its metabolism to alpha-methylnorepinephrine, which then lowers arterial pressure by stimulation of central inhibitory alpha-adrenergic receptors, false neurotransmission, and/or reduction of plasma renin activity. Methyldopa has been shown to cause a net reduction in the tissue concentration of serotonin, dopamine, norepinephrine, and epinephrine.
Only methyldopa, the *L*-isomer of alpha-methyldopa, has the ability to inhibit dopa decarboxylase and to deplete animal tissues of norepinephrine. In man, the antihypertensive activity appears to be due solely to the *L*-isomer. About twice the dose of the racemate (*DL*-alpha-methyldopa) is required for equal antihypertensive effect.
Methyldopa has no direct effect on cardiac function and usually does not reduce glomerular filtration rate, renal blood flow, or filtration fraction. Cardiac output usually is maintained without cardiac acceleration. In some patients the heart rate is slowed.
Normal or elevated plasma renin activity may decrease in the course of methyldopa therapy.
Methyldopa reduces both supine and standing blood pressure. It usually produces highly effective lowering of the supine pressure with infrequent symptomatic postural hypotension. Exercise hypotension and diurnal blood pressure variations rarely occur.
DIURIL® (Chlorothiazide, MSD)
Chlorothiazide is a diuretic and antihypertensive. It affects the renal tubular mechanism of electrolyte reabsorption. At maximal therapeutic dosage all thiazides are approximately equal in their diuretic efficacy.
Chlorothiazide increases excretion of sodium and chloride in approximately equivalent amounts. Natriuresis may be accompanied by some loss of potassium and bicarbonate.
The mechanism of the antihypertensive effect of thiazides is unknown. Chlorothiazide does not affect normal blood pressure.
Chlorothiazide is eliminated rapidly by the kidney.
ALDOCLOR
The concomitant use of methyldopa and chlorothiazide, as provided in ALDOCLOR, frequently produces a more pronounced antihypertensive response than when either compound is the sole therapeutic agent. Particularly in those cases of hypertensive vascular disease where sodium and water retention is a problem, the coadministration of these two drugs in the form of ALDOCLOR will help control the fluid imbalance.
In severe essential hypertension and in malignant hypertension, ALDOCLOR may achieve

Continued on next page

Information on the Merck Sharp & Dohme products listed on these pages is the full prescribing information from package circulars in use October 31, 1979.

Merck Sharp & Dohme—Cont.

effective lowering of blood pressure with fewer side effects than occur with other compounds used for this purpose.
ALDOCLOR reduces both supine and standing blood pressure; more effective lowering of the supine pressure with less frequent symptomatic postural hypotension can be obtained with ALDOCLOR than with most other antihypertensive agents. In patients treated with ALDOCLOR, exercise hypotension and diurnal blood pressure variations rarely occur.

Indication

Hypertension (see box warning).

Contraindications

Active hepatic disease, such as acute hepatitis and active cirrhosis.
If previous methyldopa therapy has been associated with liver disorders (see WARNINGS).
Anuria.
Hypersensitivity to methyldopa, or to chlorothiazide or other sulfonamide-derived drugs.

Warnings

Methyldopa
It is important to recognize that a positive Coombs test, hemolytic anemia, and liver disorders may occur with methyldopa therapy. The rare occurrences of hemolytic anemia or liver disorders could lead to potentially fatal complications unless properly recognized and managed. Read this section carefully to understand these reactions.
With prolonged methyldopa therapy, 10 to 20 percent of patients develop a positive direct Coombs test which usually occurs between 6 and 12 months of methyldopa therapy. Lowest incidence is at daily dosage of 1 g or less. This on rare occasions may be associated with hemolytic anemia, which could lead to potentially fatal complications. One cannot predict which patients with a positive direct Coombs test may develop hemolytic anemia.
Prior existence or development of a positive direct Coombs test is not in itself a contraindication to use of methyldopa. If a positive Coombs test develops during methyldopa therapy, the physician should determine whether hemolytic anemia exists and whether the positive Coombs test may be a problem. For example, in addition to a positive direct Coombs test there is less often a positive indirect Coombs test which may interfere with cross matching of blood.
At the start of methyldopa therapy, it is desirable to do a blood count (hematocrit, hemoglobin, or red cell count) for a baseline or to establish whether there is anemia. Periodic blood counts should be done during therapy to detect hemolytic anemia. It may be useful to do a direct Coombs test before therapy and at 6 and 12 months after the start of therapy.
If Coombs-positive hemolytic anemia occurs, the cause may be methyldopa and the drug should be discontinued. Usually the anemia remits promptly. If not, corticosteroids may be given and other causes of anemia should be considered. If the hemolytic anemia is related to methyldopa, the drug should not be reinstituted.
When methyldopa causes Coombs positivity alone or with hemolytic anemia, the red cell is usually coated with gamma globulin of the IgG (gamma G) class only. The positive Coombs test may not revert to normal until weeks to months after methyldopa is stopped.
Should the need for transfusion arise in a patient receiving methyldopa, both a direct and an indirect Coombs test should be performed on his blood. In the absence of hemolytic anemia, usually only the direct Coombs test will be positive. A positive direct Coombs test alone will not interfere with typing or cross matching. If the indirect Coombs test is also positive, problems may arise in the major cross match and the assistance of a hematologist or transfusion expert will be needed.
Occasionally, fever has occurred within the first three weeks of methyldopa therapy, associated in some cases with eosinophilia or abnormalities in one or more liver function tests, such as serum alkaline phosphatase, serum transaminases (SGOT, SGPT), bilirubin, cephalin cholesterol flocculation, prothrombin time, and bromsulphalein retention. Jaundice, with or without fever, may occur with onset usually within the first two to three months of therapy. In some patients the findings are consistent with those of cholestasis.
Rarely fatal hepatic necrosis has been reported after use of methyldopa. These hepatic changes may represent hypersensitivity reactions. Periodic determination of hepatic function should be done particularly during the first 6 to 12 weeks of therapy or whenever an unexplained fever occurs. If fever, abnormalities in liver function tests, or jaundice appear, stop therapy with methyldopa. If caused by methyldopa, the temperature and abnormalities in liver function characteristically have reverted to normal when the drug was discontinued. Methyldopa should not be reinstituted in such patients.
Rarely, a reversible reduction of the white blood cell count with a primary effect on the granulocytes has been seen. The granulocyte count returned promptly to normal on discontinuance of the drug. Rare cases of granulocytopenia have been reported. In each instance, upon stopping the drug, the white cell count returned to normal. Reversible thrombocytopenia has occurred rarely.
When methyldopa is used with other antihypertensive drugs, potentiation of antihypertensive effect may occur. Patients should be followed carefully to detect side reactions or unusual manifestations of drug idiosyncrasy.
Chlorothiazide
Use with caution in severe renal disease. In patients with renal disease, thiazides may precipitate azotemia. Cumulative effects of the drug may develop in patients with impaired renal function.
Thiazides should be used with caution in patients with impaired hepatic function or progressive liver disease, since minor alterations of fluid and electrolyte balance may precipitate hepatic coma.
Thiazides may add to or potentiate the action of other antihypertensive drugs.
Sensitivity reactions may occur in patients with or without a history of allergy or bronchial asthma.
The possibility of exacerbation or activation of systemic lupus erythematosus has been reported.
Lithium generally should not be given with diuretics because they reduce its renal clearance and add a high risk of lithium toxicity. Read circulars for lithium preparations before use of such concomitant therapy.

Pregnancy and Nursing

Use of any drug in women who are or may become pregnant requires that anticipated benefits be weighed against possible risks.
Methyldopa crosses the placental barrier and appears in cord blood. No unusual adverse reactions have been reported in association with the use of methyldopa during pregnancy. Though no obvious teratogenic effects have been reported, the possibility of fetal injury cannot be excluded.
Thiazides also cross the placental barrier and appear in cord blood. Hazards include fetal or neonatal jaundice, thrombocytopenia, and possibly other adverse reactions which have occurred in the adult.
Methyldopa and thiazides appear in breast milk. Patients taking ALDOCLOR should not nurse.

Precautions

Methyldopa
Methyldopa should be used with caution in patients with a history of previous liver disease or dysfunction (see WARNINGS).
Methyldopa may interfere with measurement of: urinary uric acid by the phosphotungstate method, serum creatinine by the alkaline picrate method, and SGOT by colorimetric methods. Interference with spectrophotometric methods for SGOT analysis has not been reported.
Since methyldopa causes fluorescence in urine samples at the same wave lengths as catecholamines, falsely high levels of urinary catecholamines may be reported. This will interfere with the diagnosis of pheochromocytoma. It is important to recognize this phenomenon before a patient with a possible pheochromocytoma is subjected to surgery. Methyldopa does not interfere with measurement of VMA (vanillylmandelic acid), a test for pheochromocytoma, by those methods which convert VMA to vanillin. Methyldopa is not recommended for the treatment of patients with pheochromocytoma. Rarely, when urine is exposed to air after voiding, it may darken because of breakdown of methyldopa or its metabolites.
Rarely, involuntary choreoathetotic movements have been observed during therapy with methyldopa in patients with severe bilateral cerebrovascular disease. Should these movements occur, stop therapy.
Patients may require reduced doses of anesthetics when on methyldopa. If hypotension does occur during anesthesia, it usually can be controlled by vasopressors. The adrenergic receptors remain sensitive during treatment with methyldopa.
Hypertension has recurred occasionally after dialysis in patients given methyldopa because the drug is removed by this procedure.
Chlorothiazide
Periodic determination of serum electrolytes to detect possible electrolyte imbalance should be performed at appropriate intervals.
All patients receiving diuretic therapy should be observed for evidence of fluid or electrolyte imbalance: namely, hyponatremia, hypochloremic alkalosis, and hypokalemia. Serum and urine electrolyte determinations are particularly important when the patient is vomiting excessively or receiving parenteral fluids. Warning signs or symptoms of fluid and electrolyte imbalance include dryness of mouth, thirst, weakness, lethargy, drowsiness, restlessness, muscle pains or cramps, muscular fatigue, hypotension, oliguria, tachycardia, and gastrointestinal disturbances such as nausea and vomiting.
Hypokalemia may develop, especially with brisk diuresis, when severe cirrhosis is present, during concomitant use of corticosteroids or ACTH, or after prolonged therapy.
Interference with adequate oral electrolyte intake will also contribute to hypokalemia. Hypokalemia can sensitize or exaggerate the response of the heart to the toxic effects of digitalis (e.g., increased ventricular irritability). Hypokalemia may be avoided or treated by use of potassium supplements such as foods with a high potassium content.
Although any chloride deficit is generally mild and usually does not require specific treatment except under extraordinary circumstances (as in liver disease or renal disease), chloride replacement may be required in the treatment of metabolic alkalosis.
Dilutional hyponatremia may occur in edematous patients in hot weather; appropriate therapy is water restriction, rather than administration of salt, except in rare instances when the hyponatremia is life threatening. In actual

salt depletion, appropriate replacement is the therapy of choice.
Hyperuricemia may occur or acute gout may be precipitated in certain patients receiving thiazide therapy.
Insulin requirements in diabetic patients may be increased, decreased, or unchanged. Diabetes mellitus which has been latent may become manifest during thiazide administration.
Thiazide drugs may increase the responsiveness to tubocurarine.
The antihypertensive effects of the drug may be enhanced in the postsympathectomy patient. Thiazides may decrease arterial responsiveness to norepinephrine. This diminution is not sufficient to preclude effectiveness of the pressor agent for therapeutic use.
If progressive renal impairment becomes evident, consider withholding or discontinuing diuretic therapy.
Thiazides may decrease serum PBI levels without signs of thyroid disturbance.
Calcium excretion is decreased by thiazides. Pathological changes in the parathyroid glands with hypercalcemia and hypophosphatemia have been observed in a few patients on prolonged thiazide therapy. The common complications of hyperparathyroidism such as renal lithiasis, bone resorption, and peptic ulceration have not been seen. Thiazides should be discontinued before carrying out tests for parathyroid function.

Adverse Reactions

Methyldopa
Sedation, usually transient, may occur during the initial period of therapy or whenever the dose is increased. Headache, asthenia, or weakness may be noted as early and transient symptoms. However, significant adverse effects due to methyldopa have been infrequent and this agent usually is well tolerated.
Central nervous system: Sedation, headache, asthenia or weakness, dizziness, lightheadedness, symptoms of cerebrovascular insufficiency, paresthesias, parkinsonism, Bell's palsy, decreased mental acuity, involuntary choreoathetotic movements. Psychic disturbances including nightmares and reversible mild psychoses or depression.
Cardiovascular: Bradycardia, aggravation of angina pectoris. Orthostatic hypotension (decrease daily dosage). Edema (and weight gain) usually relieved by use of a diuretic. (Discontinue methyldopa if edema progresses or signs of heart failure appear.)
Gastrointestinal: Nausea, vomiting, distention, constipation, flatus, diarrhea, mild dryness of mouth, sore or "black" tongue, pancreatitis, sialadenitis.
Hepatic: Abnormal liver function tests, jaundice, liver disorders.
Hematologic: Positive Coombs test, hemolytic anemia. Leukopenia, granulocytopenia, thrombocytopenia. Positive tests for antinuclear antibody, LE cells, and rheumatoid factor.
Allergic: Drug-related fever, lupus-like syndrome, myocarditis.
Other: Nasal stuffiness, rise in BUN, breast enlargement, gynecomastia, lactation, impotence, decreased libido, dermatologic reactions including eczema and lichenoid eruptions, mild arthralgia, myalgia.
Chlorothiazide
Gastrointestinal system: Anorexia, gastric irritation, nausea, vomiting, cramping, diarrhea, constipation, jaundice (intrahepatic cholestatic jaundice), pancreatitis, sialadenitis.
Central nervous system: Dizziness, vertigo, paresthesias, headache, xanthopsia.
Hematologic: Leukopenia, agranulocytosis, thrombocytopenia, aplastic anemia, hemolytic anemia.
Cardiovascular: Orthostatic hypotension (may be aggravated by alcohol, barbiturates, or narcotics).
Hypersensitivity: Purpura, photosensitivity, rash, urticaria, necrotizing angiitis (vasculitis) (cutaneous vasculitis), fever, respiratory distress including pneumonitis, anaphylactic reactions.
Other: Hyperglycemia, glycosuria, hyperuricemia, muscle spasm, weakness, restlessness, transient blurred vision.
Whenever adverse reactions are moderate or severe, thiazide dosage should be reduced or therapy withdrawn.

Dosage and Administration

Dosage: As determined by individual titration (see box warning).
The usual starting dosage is 1 tablet of ALDOCLOR-150 or 1 tablet of ALDOCLOR-250 two or three times a day in the first 48 hours. The daily dosage then may be increased or decreased, preferably at intervals of not less than two days, until an adequate response is achieved. To minimize the sedation associated with methyldopa, start dosage increases in the evening. By adjustment of dosage, morning hypotension may be prevented without sacrificing control of afternoon blood pressure.
When ALDOCLOR is given to patients on other antihypertensives, the dose of these agents may need to be adjusted to effect a smooth transition. When ALDOCLOR is given with antihypertensives other than thiazides, the initial dosage of methyldopa should be limited to 500 mg daily in divided doses.
Although occasional patients have responded to higher doses, the maximum recommended daily dosage is 3.0 g of methyldopa and 1.0 to 2.0 g of chlorothiazide. Once an effective dosage range is attained, a smooth blood pressure response occurs in most patients in 12 to 24 hours. If ALDOCLOR alone does not adequately control blood pressure, additional methyldopa may be given separately to obtain the maximum blood pressure response.
Since both components of ALDOCLOR have a relatively short duration of action, withdrawal is followed by return of hypertension usually within 48 hours. This is not complicated by an overshoot of blood pressure.
Occasionally tolerance may occur, usually between the second and third month of therapy. Increasing the dosage of either methyldopa or chlorothiazide separately or together frequently will restore effective control of blood pressure.
Methyldopa is largely excreted by the kidney and patients with impaired renal function may respond to smaller doses of ALDOCLOR. Syncope in older patients may be related to an increased sensitivity and advanced arteriosclerotic vascular disease. This may be avoided by lower doses.

How Supplied

No. 3318—Tablets ALDOCLOR-150 are beige, oval, film coated tablets coded MSD 612. Each tablet contains 250 mg of methyldopa and 150 mg of chlorothiazide. They are supplied as follows:
NDC 0006-0612-68 bottles of 100.
[*Shown in Product Identification Section*]
No. 3319—Tablets ALDOCLOR-250 are green, oval, film coated tablets coded MSD 634. Each tablet contains 250 mg of methyldopa and 250 mg of chlorothiazide. They are supplied as follows:
NDC 0006-0634-68 bottles of 100.
[*Shown in Product Identification Section*]
A.H.F.S. 24:08
DC 6078617 Issued June 1979

ALDOMET® Tablets (methyldopa, MSD), U.S.P. ℞

Description

Methyldopa is the L-isomer of alpha-methyldopa. Its chemical name is levo-3-(3,4-dihydroxyphenyl)-2-methylalanine.

Actions

ALDOMET (Methyldopa, MSD), a unique antihypertensive, is an aromatic-amino-acid decarboxylase inhibitor in animals and in man. Although the mechanism of action has yet to be conclusively demonstrated, the antihypertensive effect of methyldopa probably is due to its metabolism to alpha-methylnorepinephrine, which then lowers arterial pressure by stimulation of central inhibitory alpha-adrenergic receptors, false neurotransmission, and/or reduction of plasma renin activity. Methyldopa has been shown to cause a net reduction in the tissue concentration of serotonin, dopamine, norepinephrine, and epinephrine.
Only methyldopa, the L-isomer of alpha-methyldopa, has the ability to inhibit dopa decarboxylase and to deplete animal tissues of norepinephrine. In man the antihypertensive activity appears to be due solely to the L-isomer. About twice the dose of the racemate (DL-alpha-methyldopa) is required for equal antihypertensive effect.
Methyldopa has no direct effect on cardiac function and usually does not reduce glomerular filtration rate, renal blood flow, or filtration fraction. Cardiac output usually is maintained without cardiac acceleration. In some patients the heart rate is slowed.
Normal or elevated plasma renin activity may decrease in the course of methyldopa therapy. ALDOMET reduces both supine and standing blood pressure. Methyldopa usually produces highly effective lowering of the supine pressure with infrequent symptomatic postural hypotension. Exercise hypotension and diurnal blood pressure variations rarely occur.

Indication

Hypertension.

Contraindications

Active hepatic disease, such as acute hepatitis and active cirrhosis.
If previous methyldopa therapy has been associated with liver disorders (see WARNINGS).
Hypersensitivity.

Warnings

It is important to recognize that a positive Coombs test, hemolytic anemia, and liver disorders may occur with methyldopa therapy. The rare occurrences of hemolytic anemia or liver disorders could lead to potentially fatal complications unless properly recognized and managed. Read this section carefully to understand these reactions.
With prolonged methyldopa therapy, 10 to 20 percent of patients develop a positive direct Coombs test which usually occurs between 6 and 12 months of methyldopa therapy. Lowest incidence is at daily dosage of 1 g or less. This on rare occasions may be associated with hemolytic anemia, which could lead to potentially fatal complications. One cannot predict which patients with a positive direct Coombs test may develop hemolytic anemia.
Prior existence or development of a positive direct Coombs test is not in itself a contraindication to use of methyldopa. If a positive Coombs test develops during methyldopa therapy, the physician should determine whether hemolytic anemia exists and whether the posi-

Continued on next page

Information on the Merck Sharp & Dohme products listed on these pages is the full prescribing information from package circulars in use October 31, 1979.

Merck Sharp & Dohme—Cont.

tive Coombs test may be a problem. For example, in addition to a positive direct Coombs test there is less often a positive indirect Coombs test which may interfere with cross matching of blood.
At the start of methyldopa therapy, it is desirable to do a blood count (hematocrit, hemoglobin, or red cell count) for a baseline or to establish whether there is anemia. Periodic blood counts should be done during therapy to detect hemolytic anemia. It may be useful to do a direct Coombs test before therapy and at 6 and 12 months after the start of therapy.
If Coombs-positive hemolytic anemia occurs, the cause may be methyldopa and the drug should be discontinued. Usually the anemia remits promptly. If not, corticosteroids may be given and other causes of anemia should be considered. If the hemolytic anemia is related to methyldopa, the drug should not be reinstituted.
When methyldopa causes Coombs positivity alone or with hemolytic anemia, the red cell is usually coated with gamma globulin of the IgG (gamma G) class only. The positive Coombs test may not revert to normal until weeks to months after methyldopa is stopped.
Should the need for transfusion arise in a patient receiving methyldopa, both a direct and an indirect Coombs test should be performed on his blood. In the absence of hemolytic anemia, usually only the direct Coombs test will be positive. A positive direct Coombs test alone will not interfere with typing or cross matching. If the indirect Coombs test is also positive, problems may arise in the major cross match and the assistance of a hematologist or transfusion expert will be needed.
Occasionally, fever has occurred within the first 3 weeks of methyldopa therapy, associated in some cases with eosinophilia or abnormalities in one or more liver function tests, such as serum alkaline phosphatase, serum transaminases (SGOT, SGPT), bilirubin, cephalin cholesterol flocculation, prothrombin time, and bromsulphalein retention. Jaundice, with or without fever, may occur with onset usually within the first 2 to 3 months of therapy. In some patients the findings are consistent with those of cholestasis.
Rarely fatal hepatic necrosis has been reported after use of methyldopa. These hepatic changes may represent hypersensitivity reactions. Periodic determinations of hepatic function should be done particularly during the first 6 to 12 weeks of therapy or whenever an unexplained fever occurs. If fever, abnormalities in liver function tests, or jaundice appear, stop therapy with methyldopa. If caused by methyldopa, the temperature and abnormalities in liver function characteristically have reverted to normal when the drug was discontinued. Methyldopa should not be reinstituted in such patients.
Rarely, a reversible reduction of the white blood cell count with a primary effect on the granulocytes has been seen. The granulocyte count returned promptly to normal on discontinuance of the drug. Rare cases of granulocytopenia have been reported. In each instance, upon stopping the drug, the white cell count returned to normal. Reversible thrombocytopenia has occurred rarely.
When methyldopa is used with other antihypertensive drugs, potentiation of antihypertensive effect may occur. Patients should be followed carefully to detect side reactions or unusual manifestations of drug idiosyncrasy.

Pregnancy and Nursing
Use of any drug in women who are or may become pregnant or intend to nurse requires that anticipated benefits be weighed against possible risks.
Methyldopa crosses the placental barrier, appears in cord blood, and appears in breast milk. No unusual adverse reactions have been reported in association with the use of methyldopa during pregnancy. Though no obvious teratogenic effects have been reported, the possibility of fetal injury cannot be excluded. Also, the possibility of injury to a nursing infant cannot be excluded.

Precautions

Methyldopa should be used with caution in patients with a history of previous liver disease or dysfunction (see WARNINGS).
Methyldopa may interfere with measurement of: urinary uric acid by the phosphotungstate method, serum creatinine by the alkaline picrate method, and SGOT by colorimetric methods. Interference with spectrophotometric methods for SGOT analysis has not been reported.
Since methyldopa causes fluorescence in urine samples at the same wave lengths as catecholamines, falsely high levels of urinary catecholamines may be reported. This will interfere with the diagnosis of pheochromocytoma. It is important to recognize this phenomenon before a patient with a possible pheochromocytoma is subjected to surgery. Methyldopa does not interfere with measurement of VMA (vanillylmandelic acid), a test for pheochromocytoma, by those methods which convert VMA to vanillin. Methyldopa is not recommended for the treatment of patients with pheochromocytoma. Rarely, when urine is exposed to air after voiding, it may darken because of breakdown of methyldopa or its metabolites.
Rarely involuntary choreoathetotic movements have been observed during therapy with methyldopa in patients with severe bilateral cerebrovascular disease. Should these movements occur, stop therapy.
Patients may require reduced doses of anesthetics when on methyldopa. If hypotension does occur during anesthesia, it usually can be controlled by vasopressors. The adrenergic receptors remain sensitive during treatment with methyldopa.
Hypertension has recurred occasionally after dialysis in patients given methyldopa because the drug is removed by this procedure.

Adverse Reactions

Sedation, usually transient, may occur during the initial period of therapy or whenever the dose is increased. Headache, asthenia, or weakness may be noted as early and transient symptoms. However, significant adverse effects due to ALDOMET have been infrequent and this agent usually is well tolerated.
Central nervous system: Sedation, headache, asthenia or weakness, dizziness, light-headedness, symptoms of cerebrovascular insufficiency, paresthesias, parkinsonism, Bell's palsy, decreased mental acuity, involuntary choreoathetotic movements. Psychic disturbances including nightmares and reversible mild psychoses or depression.
Cardiovascular: Bradycardia, aggravation of angina pectoris. Orthostatic hypotension (decrease daily dosage). Edema (and weight gain) usually relieved by use of a diuretic. (Discontinue methyldopa if edema progresses or signs of heart failure appear).
Gastrointestinal: Nausea, vomiting, distention, constipation, flatus, diarrhea, mild dryness of mouth, sore or "black" tongue, pancreatitis, sialadenitis.
Hepatic: Abnormal liver function tests, jaundice, liver disorders.
Hematologic: Positive Coombs test, hemolytic anemia. Leukopenia, granulocytopenia, thrombocytopenia. Positive tests for antinuclear antibody, LE cells, and rheumatoid factor.
Allergic: Drug-related fever, lupus-like syndrome, myocarditis.
Other: Nasal stuffiness, rise in BUN, breast enlargement, gynecomastia, lactation, impotence, decreased libido, dermatologic reactions including eczema and lichenoid eruptions, mild arthralgia, myalgia.

Dosage and Administration

ADULTS

Initiation of Therapy
The usual starting dosage of ALDOMET is 250 mg two or three times a day in the first 48 hours. The daily dosage then may be increased or decreased, preferably at intervals of not less than two days, until an adequate response is achieved. To minimize the sedation, start dosage increases in the evening. By adjustment of dosage, morning hypotension may be prevented without sacrificing control of afternoon blood pressure.
When methyldopa is given to patients on other antihypertensives, the dose of these agents may need to be adjusted to effect a smooth transition. When ALDOMET is given with antihypertensives other than thiazides, the initial dosage of ALDOMET should be limited to 500 mg daily in divided doses; when ALDOMET is added to a thiazide, the dosage of thiazide need not be changed.

Maintenance Therapy
The usual daily dosage of ALDOMET is 500 mg to 2.0 g in two to four doses. Although occasional patients have responded to higher doses, the maximum recommended daily dosage is 3.0 g. Once an effective dosage range is attained, a smooth blood pressure response occurs in most patients in 12 to 24 hours. Since methyldopa has a relatively short duration of action, withdrawal is followed by return of hypertension usually within 48 hours. This is not complicated by an overshoot of blood pressure.
Occasionally tolerance may occur, usually between the second and third month of therapy. Adding a diuretic or increasing the dosage of methyldopa frequently will restore effective control of blood pressure. A thiazide may be added at any time during methyldopa therapy and is recommended if therapy has not been started with a thiazide or if effective control of blood pressure cannot be maintained on 2.0 g of methyldopa daily.
Methyldopa is largely excreted by the kidney and patients with impaired renal function may respond to smaller doses. Syncope in older patients may be related to an increased sensitivity and advanced arteriosclerotic vascular disease. This may be avoided by lower doses.

CHILDREN

Initial dosage is based on 10 mg/kg of body weight daily in two to four doses. The daily dosage then is increased or decreased until an adequate response is achieved. The maximum dosage is 65 mg/kg or 3.0 g daily, whichever is less.

How Supplied

No. 3341—Tablets ALDOMET, 125 mg, are yellow, film coated, round tablets, coded MSD 135. They are supplied as follows:
NDC 0006-0135-68 bottles of 100
[*Shown in Product Identification Section*]
No. 3290—Tablets ALDOMET, 250 mg, are yellow, film coated, round tablets, coded MSD 401. They are supplied as follows:
NDC 0006-0401-68 bottles of 100
(6505-00-890-1856, 250 mg 100's)
NDC 0006-0401-28 single unit packages of 100
(6505-00-149-0090, 250 mg individually sealed 100's)
NDC 0006-0401-82 bottles of 1000
(6505-00-931-6646, 250 mg 1000's)
[*Shown in Product Identification Section*]
No. 3292—Tablets ALDOMET, 500 mg, are yellow, film coated, round tablets, coded MSD 516. They are supplied as follows:

NDC 0006-0516-68 bottles of 100
NDC 0006-0516-28 single unit packages of 100
NDC 0006-0516-74 bottles of 500.
[*Shown in Product Identification Section*]
A.H.F.S. 24:08
DC 6649709 Issued June 1977

ALDOMET® Ester HCl Injection ℞
(methyldopate hydrochloride, MSD), U.S.P.

Description

Injection ALDOMET ester hydrochloride (Methyldopate Hydrochloride, MSD) is an antihypertensive agent for intravenous use, each 5 ml of which contains:

Methyldopate hydrochloride	250.0 mg
Citric acid anhydrous	25.0 mg
Sodium bisulfite	16.0 mg
Disodium edetate	2.5 mg
Monothioglycerol	10.0 mg
Sodium hydroxide to adjust pH	
Water for Injection, q.s. to	5.0 ml

Methylparaben 0.15% and propylparaben 0.02% added as preservatives.
Methyldopate hydrochloride [levo-3-(3,4-dihydroxyphenyl)-2-methylalanine, ethyl ester hydrochloride] is the ethyl ester of methyldopa, supplied as the hydrochloride salt. Methyldopate hydrochloride is more soluble and stable in solution than methyldopa and is the preferred form for intravenous use.

Actions

ALDOMET (Methyldopa, MSD), a unique antihypertensive, is an aromatic-amino-acid decarboxylase inhibitor in animals and in man. Although the mechanism of action has yet to be conclusively demonstrated, the antihypertensive effect of methyldopa probably is due to its metabolism to alpha-methylnorepinephrine, which then lowers arterial pressure by stimulation of central inhibitory alpha-adrenergic receptors, false neurotransmission, and/or reduction of plasma renin activity. Methyldopa has been shown to cause a net reduction in the tissue concentration of serotonin, dopamine, norepinephrine, and epinephrine.
Only methyldopa, the L-isomer of alphamethyldopa, has the ability to inhibit dopa decarboxylase and to deplete animal tissues of norepinephrine. In man the antihypertensive activity appears to be due solely to the L-isomer. About twice the dose of the racemate (DL-alpha-methyldopa) is required for equal antihypertensive effect.
Methyldopa has no direct effect on cardiac function and usually does not reduce glomerular filtration rate, renal blood flow, or filtration fraction. Cardiac output usually is maintained without cardiac acceleration. In some patients the heart rate is slowed.
Normal or elevated plasma renin activity may decrease in the course of methyldopa therapy.
Methyldopa reduces both supine and standing blood pressure. It usually produces highly effective lowering of the supine pressure with infrequent symptomatic postural hypotension. Exercise hypotension and diurnal blood pressure variations rarely occur.
Methyldopate hydrochloride is the ethyl ester of methyldopa hydrochloride and possesses the same pharmacologic attributes.

Indication

Hypertension, when parenteral medication is indicated.
The treatment of hypertensive crises may be initiated with injection ALDOMET ester hydrochloride.

Contraindications

Active hepatic disease, such as acute hepatitis and active cirrhosis.
If previous methyldopa therapy has been associated with liver disorders (see WARNINGS).
Hypersensitivity to any component of this product.

Warnings

It is important to recognize that a positive Coombs test, hemolytic anemia, and liver disorders may occur with methyldopa therapy. The rare occurrences of hemolytic anemia or liver disorders could lead to potentially fatal complications unless properly recognized and managed. Read this section carefully to understand these reactions.
With prolonged methyldopa therapy, 10 to 20 percent of patients develop a positive direct Coombs test which usually occurs between 6 and 12 months of methyldopa therapy. Lowest incidence is at daily dosage of 1 g or less. This on rare occasions may be associated with hemolytic anemia, which could lead to potentially fatal complications. One cannot predict which patients with a positive direct Coombs test may develop hemolytic anemia.
Prior existence or development of a positive direct Coombs test is not in itself a contraindication to use of methyldopa. If a positive Coombs test develops during methyldopa therapy, the physician should determine whether hemolytic anemia exists and whether the positive Coombs test may be a problem. For example, in addition to a positive direct Coombs test there is less often a positive indirect Coombs test which may interfere with cross matching of blood.
At the start of methyldopa therapy, it is desirable to do a blood count (hematocrit, hemoglobin, or red cell count) for a baseline or to establish whether there is anemia. Periodic blood counts should be done during therapy to detect hemolytic anemia. It may be useful to do a direct Coombs test before therapy and at 6 and 12 months after the start of therapy.
If Coombs-positive hemolytic anemia occurs, the cause may be methyldopa and the drug should be discontinued. Usually the anemia remits promptly. If not, corticosteroids may be given and other causes of anemia should be considered. If the hemolytic anemia is related to methyldopa, the drug should not be reinstituted.
When methyldopa causes Coombs positivity alone or with hemolytic anemia, the red cell is usually coated with gamma globulin of the lgG (gamma G) class only. The positive Coombs test may not revert to normal until weeks to months after methyldopa is stopped.
Should the need for transfusion arise in a patient receiving methyldopa, both a direct and an indirect Coombs test should be performed on his blood. In the absence of hemolytic anemia, usually only the direct Coombs test will be positive. A positive direct Coombs test alone will not interfere with typing or cross matching. If the indirect Coombs test is also positive, problems may arise in the major cross match and the assistance of a hematologist or transfusion expert will be needed.
Occasionally, fever has occurred within the first three weeks of methyldopa therapy, associated in some cases with eosinophilia or abnormalities in one or more liver function tests, such as serum alkaline phosphatase, serum transaminases (SGOT, SGPT), bilirubin, cephalin cholesterol flocculation, prothrombin time, and bromsulphalein retention. Jaundice, with or without fever, may occur with onset usually within the first two to three months of therapy. In some patients the findings are consistent with those of cholestasis.
Rarely fatal hepatic necrosis has been reported after use of methyldopa. These hepatic changes may represent hypersensitivity reactions. Periodic determination of hepatic function should be done particularly during the first 6 to 12 weeks of therapy or whenever an unexplained fever occurs. If fever, abnormalities in liver function tests, or jaundice appear, stop therapy with methyldopa. If caused by methyldopa, the temperature and abnormalities in liver function characteristically have reverted to normal when the drug was discontinued. Methyldopa should not be reinstituted in such patients.
Rarely, a reversible reduction of the white blood cell count with a primary effect on the granulocytes has been seen. The granulocyte count returned promptly to normal on discontinuance of the drug. Rare cases of granulocytopenia have been reported. In each instance, upon stopping the drug, the white cell count returned to normal. Reversible thrombocytopenia has occurred rarely.
When methyldopa is used with other antihypertensive drugs, potentiation of antihypertensive effect may occur. Patients should be followed carefully to detect side reactions or unusual manifestations of drug idiosyncrasy.
Pregnancy and Nursing
Use of any drug in women who are or may become pregnant or intend to nurse requires that anticipated benefits be weighed against possible risks.
Methyldopa crosses the placental barrier, appears in cord blood, and appears in breast milk. No unusual adverse reactions have been reported in association with the use of methyldopa during pregnancy. Though no obvious teratogenic effects have been reported, the possibility of fetal injury cannot be excluded. Also, the possibility of injury to a nursing infant cannot be excluded.

Precautions

Methyldopa should be used with caution in patients with a history of previous liver disease or dysfunction (see WARNINGS).
Methyldopa may interfere with measurement of: urinary uric acid by the phosphotungstate method, serum creatinine by the alkaline picrate method, and SGOT by colorimetric methods. Interference with spectrophotometric methods for SGOT analysis has not been reported.
A paradoxical pressor response has been reported with intravenous administration of ALDOMET ester hydrochloride.
Since methyldopa causes fluorescence in urine samples at the same wave lengths as catecholamines, falsely high levels of urinary catecholamines may be reported. This will interfere with the diagnosis of pheochromocytoma. It is important to recognize this phenomenon before a patient with a possible pheochromocytoma is subjected to surgery. Methyldopa does not interfere with measurement of VMA (vanillylmandelic acid), a test for pheochromocytoma, by those methods which convert VMA to vanillin. Methyldopa is not recommended for the treatment of patients with pheochromocytoma. Rarely, when urine is exposed to air after voiding, it may darken because of breakdown of methyldopa or its metabolites.
Rarely involuntary choreoathetotic movements have been observed during therapy with methyldopa in patients with severe bilateral cerebrovascular disease. Should these movements occur, stop therapy.
Patients may require reduced doses of anesthetics when on methyldopa. If hypotension does occur during anesthesia, it usually can be controlled by vasopressors. The adrenergic receptors remain sensitive during treatment with methyldopa.

Continued on next page

Information on the Merck Sharp & Dohme products listed on these pages is the full prescribing information from package circulars in use October 31, 1979.

Merck Sharp & Dohme—Cont.

Hypertension has recurred occasionally after dialysis in patients given methyldopa because the drug is removed by this procedure.

Adverse Reactions

Sedation, usually transient, may occur during the initial period of therapy or whenever the dose is increased. Headache, asthenia, or weakness may be noted as early and transient symptoms. However, significant adverse effects due to methyldopa have been infrequent and this agent usually is well tolerated.
Central nervous system: Sedation, headache, asthenia or weakness, dizziness, lightheadedness, symptoms of cerebrovascular insufficiency, paresthesias, parkinsonism, Bell's palsy, decreased mental acuity, involuntary choreoathetotic movements. Psychic disturbances including nightmares and reversible mild psychoses or depression.
Cardiovascular: Bradycardia, aggravation of angina pectoris. Paradoxical pressor response with intravenous use. Orthostatic hypotension (decrease daily dosage). Edema (and weight gain) usually relieved by use of a diuretic. (Discontinue methyldopa if edema progresses or signs of heart failure appear.)
Gastrointestinal: Nausea, vomiting, distention, constipation, flatus, diarrhea, mild dryness of mouth, sore or "black" tongue, pancreatitis, sialadenitis.
Hepatic: Abnormal liver function tests, jaundice, liver disorders.
Hematologic: Positive Coombs test, hemolytic anemia. Leukopenia, granulocytopenia, thrombocytopenia. Positive tests for antinuclear antibody, LE cells, and rheumatoid factor.
Allergic: Drug-related fever, lupus-like syndrome, myocarditis.
Other: Nasal stuffiness, rise in BUN, breast enlargement, gynecomastia, lactation, impotence, decreased libido, dermatologic reactions including eczema and lichenoid eruptions, mild arthralgia, myalgia.

Dosage and Administration

Injection ALDOMET ester hydrochloride, when given intravenously in effective doses, causes a decline in blood pressure that may begin in four to six hours and last 10 to 16 hours after injection.
Add the desired dose of injection ALDOMET ester hydrochloride to 100 ml of 5 percent Dextrose Injection U.S.P. (sterile solution containing 5 percent dextrose in water). Give this intravenous infusion slowly over a period of 30 to 60 minutes.

ADULTS

The usual adult dosage intravenously is 250 to 500 mg at six hour intervals as required. The maximum recommended intravenous dose is 1.0 g every six hours.
When control has been obtained, oral therapy with tablets ALDOMET (Methyldopa, MSD) may be substituted for intravenous therapy, starting with the same dosage schedule used for the parenteral route. The effectiveness and anticipated responses are described in the circular for tablets ALDOMET (Methyldopa, MSD).
Since methyldopa has a relatively short duration of action, withdrawal is followed by return of hypertension usually within 48 hours. This is not complicated by an overshoot of blood pressure.
Occasionally tolerance may occur, usually between the second and third month of therapy. Adding a diuretic or increasing the dosage of methyldopa frequently will restore effective control of blood pressure. A thiazide may be added at any time during methyldopa therapy and is recommended if therapy has not been started with a thiazide or if effective control of blood pressure cannot be maintained on 2.0 g of methyldopa daily.
Methyldopa is largely excreted by the kidney and patients with impaired renal function may respond to smaller doses. Syncope in older patients may be related to an increased sensitivity and advanced arteriosclerotic vascular disease. This may be avoided by lower doses.

CHILDREN

The recommended dosage is 20 to 40 mg/kg of body weight in divided doses every six hours. The maximum dosage is 65 mg/kg or 3.0 g daily, whichever is less. When the blood pressure is under control, continue with oral therapy using tablets ALDOMET (Methyldopa, MSD) in the same dosage as for the parenteral route.

How Supplied

No. 3293—Injection ALDOMET ester hydrochloride, 250 mg per 5 ml, is a clear, colorless solution and is supplied as follows:
NDC 0006-3293-05 in 5 ml vials.
A.H.F.S. 24:08
DC 6112020 Issued December 1977

ALDORIL® Tablets ℞
Antihypertensive

WARNING

This fixed combination drug is not indicated for initial therapy of hypertension. Hypertension requires therapy titrated to the individual patient. If the fixed combination represents the dosage so determined, its use may be more convenient in patient management. The treatment of hypertension is not static, but must be reevaluated as conditions in each patient warrant.

Description

ALDORIL® is a combination of methyldopa and hydrochlorothiazide. The chemical name for methyldopa is levo - 3 - (3,4-dihydroxyphenyl)-2-methylalanine. Hydrochlorothiazide is 6-chloro-3, 4-dihydro-*2H*-1, 2, 4-benzothiadiazine-7-sulfonamide 1,1-dioxide.

Actions

ALDOMET® (Methyldopa, MSD)
Methyldopa, a unique antihypertensive, is an aromatic-amino-acid decarboxylase inhibitor in animals and in man. Although the mechanism of action has yet to be conclusively demonstrated, the antihypertensive effect of methyldopa probably is due to its metabolism to alpha-methylnorepinephrine, which then lowers arterial pressure by stimulation of central inhibitory alpha-adrenergic receptors, false neurotransmission, and/or reduction of plasma renin activity. Methyldopa has been shown to cause a net reduction in the tissue concentration of serotonin, dopamine, norepinephrine, and epinephrine.
Only methyldopa, the *L*-isomer of alpha-methyldopa, has the ability to inhibit dopa decarboxylase and to deplete animal tissues of norepinephrine. In man, the antihypertensive activity appears to be due solely to the *L*-isomer. About twice the dose of the racemate (*DL*-alpha-methyldopa) is required for equal antihypertensive effect.
Methyldopa has no direct effect on cardiac function and usually does not reduce glomerular filtration rate, renal blood flow, or filtration fraction. Cardiac output usually is maintained without cardiac acceleration. In some patients the heart rate is slowed.
Normal or elevated plasma renin activity may decrease in the course of methyldopa therapy.
Methyldopa reduces both supine and standing blood pressure. It usually produces highly effective lowering of the supine pressure with infrequent symptomatic postural hypotension. Exercise hypotension and diurnal blood pressure variations rarely occur.
HydroDIURIL®
(Hydrochlorothiazide, MSD)
Hydrochlorothiazide is a diuretic and antihypertensive. It affects the renal tubular mechanism of electrolyte reabsorption. At maximal therapeutic dosage all thiazides are approximately equal in their diuretic efficacy.
Hydrochlorothiazide increases excretion of sodium and chloride in approximately equivalent amounts. Natriuresis may be accompanied by some loss of potassium and bicarbonate.
The mechanism of the antihypertensive effect of thiazides is unknown. Hydrochlorothiazide does not affect normal blood pressure.
Hydrochlorothiazide is eliminated rapidly by the kidney.
ALDORIL
The concomitant use of methyldopa and hydrochlorothiazide, as provided in ALDORIL, frequently produces a more pronounced antihypertensive response than when either compound is the sole therapeutic agent. Particularly in those cases of hypertensive vascular disease where sodium and water retention is a problem, the coadministration of these two drugs in the form of ALDORIL will help control the fluid imbalance.
In severe essential hypertension and in malignant hypertension ALDORIL may achieve effective lowering of blood pressure with fewer side effects than occur with other compounds used for this purpose.
ALDORIL reduces both supine and standing blood pressure; more effective lowering of the supine pressure with less frequent symptomatic postural hypotension can be obtained with ALDORIL than with most other antihypertensive agents. In patients treated with ALDORIL, exercise hypotension and diurnal blood pressure variations rarely occur.

Indication

Hypertension (see box warning).

Contraindications

Active hepatic disease, such as acute hepatitis and active cirrhosis.
If previous methyldopa therapy has been associated with liver disorders (see WARNINGS).
Anuria.
Hypersensitivity to methyldopa, or to hydrochlorothiazide or other sulfonamide-derived drugs.

Warnings

Methyldopa
It is important to recognize that a positive Coombs test, hemolytic anemia, and liver disorders may occur with methyldopa therapy. The rare occurrences of hemolytic anemia or liver disorders could lead to potentially fatal complications unless properly recognized and managed. Read this section carefully to understand these reactions.
With prolonged methyldopa therapy, 10 to 20 percent of patients develop a positive direct Coombs test which usually occurs between 6 and 12 months of methyldopa therapy. Lowest incidence is at daily dosage of 1 g or less. This on rare occasions may be associated with hemolytic anemia, which could lead to potentially fatal complications. One cannot predict which patients with a positive direct Coombs test may develop hemolytic anemia.
Prior existence or development of a positive direct Coombs test is not in itself a contraindication to use of methyldopa. If a positive Coombs test develops during methyldopa ther-

apy, the physician should determine whether hemolytic anemia exists and whether the positive Coombs test may be a problem. For example, in addition to a positive direct Coombs test there is less often a positive indirect Coombs test which may interfere with cross matching of blood.

At the start of methyldopa therapy, it is desirable to do a blood count (hematocrit, hemoglobin, or red cell count) for a baseline or to establish whether there is anemia. Periodic blood counts should be done during therapy to detect hemolytic anemia. It may be useful to do a direct Coombs test before therapy and at 6 and 12 months after the start of therapy.

If Coombs-positive hemolytic anemia occurs, the cause may be methyldopa and the drug should be discontinued. Usually the anemia remits promptly. If not, corticosteroids may be given and other causes of anemia should be considered. If the hemolytic anemia is related to methyldopa, the drug should not be reinstituted.

When methyldopa causes Coombs positivity alone or with hemolytic anemia, the red cell is usually coated with gamma globulin of the IgG (gamma G) class only. The positive Coombs test may not revert to normal until weeks to months after methyldopa is stopped.

Should the need for transfusion arise in a patient receiving methyldopa, both a direct and an indirect Coombs test should be performed on his blood. In the absence of hemolytic anemia, usually only the direct Coombs test will be positive. A positive direct Coombs test alone will not interfere with typing or cross matching. If the indirect Coombs test is also positive, problems may arise in the major cross match and the assistance of a hematologist or transfusion expert will be needed.

Occasionally, fever has occurred within the first three weeks of methyldopa therapy, associated in some cases with eosinophilia or abnormalities in one or more liver function tests, such as serum alkaline phosphatase, serum transaminases (SGOT, SGPT), bilirubin, cephalin cholesterol flocculation, prothrombin time, and bromsulphalein retention. Jaundice, with or without fever, may occur with onset usually within the first two to three months of therapy. In some patients the findings are consistent with those of cholestasis.

Rarely fatal hepatic necrosis has been reported after use of methyldopa. These hepatic changes may represent hypersensitivity reactions. Periodic determination of hepatic function should be done particularly during the first 6 to 12 weeks of therapy or whenever an unexplained fever occurs. If fever, abnormalities in liver function tests, or jaundice appear, stop therapy with methyldopa. If caused by methyldopa, the temperature and abnormalities in liver function characteristically have reverted to normal when the drug was discontinued. Methyldopa should not be reinstituted in such patients.

Rarely, a reversible reduction of the white blood cell count with a primary effect on the granulocytes has been seen. The granulocyte count returned promptly to normal on discontinuance of the drug. Rare cases of granulocytopenia have been reported. In each instance, upon stopping the drug, the white cell count returned to normal. Reversible thrombocytopenia has occurred rarely.

When methyldopa is used with other antihypertensive drugs, potentiation of antihypertensive effect may occur. Patients should be followed carefully to detect side reactions or unusual manifestations of drug idiosyncrasy.

Hydrochlorothiazide

Use with caution in severe renal disease. In patients with renal disease, thiazides may precipitate azotemia. Cumulative effects of the drug may develop in patients with impaired renal function.

Thiazides should be used with caution in patients with impaired hepatic function or progressive liver disease, since minor alterations of fluid and electrolyte balance may precipitate hepatic coma.

Thiazides may add to or potentiate the action of other antihypertensive drugs.

Sensitivity reactions may occur in patients with or without a history of allergy or bronchial asthma.

The possibility of exacerbation or activation of systemic lupus erythematosus has been reported.

Lithium generally should not be given with diuretics because they reduce its renal clearance and add a high risk of lithium toxicity. Read circulars for lithium preparations before use of such concomitant therapy.

Pregnancy and Nursing

Use of any drug in women who are or may become pregnant requires that anticipated benefits be weighed against possible risks.

Methyldopa crosses the placental barrier and appears in cord blood. No unusual adverse reactions have been reported in association with the use of methyldopa during pregnancy. Though no obvious teratogenic effects have been reported, the possibility of fetal injury cannot be excluded.

Thiazides also cross the placental barrier and appear in cord blood. Hazards include fetal or neonatal jaundice, thrombocytopenia, and possibly other adverse reactions which have occurred in the adult.

Methyldopa and thiazides appear in breast milk. Patients taking ALDORIL should not nurse.

Precautions

Methyldopa

Methyldopa should be used with caution in patients with a history of previous liver disease or dysfunction (see WARNINGS).

Methyldopa may interfere with measurement of: urinary uric acid by the phosphotungstate method, serum creatinine by the alkaline picrate method, and SGOT by colorimetric methods. Interference with spectrophotometric methods for SGOT analysis has not been reported.

Since methyldopa causes fluorescence in urine samples at the same wave lengths as catecholamines, falsely high levels of urinary catecholamines may be reported. This will interfere with the diagnosis of pheochromocytoma. It is important to recognize this phenomenon before a patient with a possible pheochromocytoma is subjected to surgery. Methyldopa does not interfere with measurement of VMA (vanillylmandelic acid), a test for pheochromocytoma, by those methods which convert VMA to vanillin. Methyldopa is not recommended for the treatment of patients with pheochromocytoma. Rarely, when urine is exposed to air after voiding, it may darken because of breakdown of methyldopa or its metabolites.

Rarely, involuntary choreoathetotic movements have been observed during therapy with methyldopa in patients with severe bilateral cerebrovascular disease. Should these movements occur, stop therapy.

Patients may require reduced doses of anesthetics when on methyldopa. If hypotension does occur during anesthesia, it usually can be controlled by vasopressors. The adrenergic receptors remain sensitive during treatment with methyldopa.

Hypertension has recurred occasionally after dialysis in patients given methyldopa because the drug is removed by this procedure.

Hydrochlorothiazide

Periodic determination of serum electrolytes to detect possible electrolyte imbalance should be performed at appropriate intervals.

All patients receiving diuretic therapy should be observed for evidence of fluid or electrolyte imbalance: namely, hyponatremia, hypochloremic alkalosis, and hypokalemia. Serum and urine electrolyte determinations are particularly important when the patient is vomiting excessively or receiving parenteral fluids. Warning signs or symptoms of fluid and electrolyte imbalance include dryness of mouth, thirst, weakness, lethargy, drowsiness, restlessness, muscle pains or cramps, muscular fatigue, hypotension, oliguria, tachycardia, and gastrointestinal disturbances such as nausea and vomiting.

Hypokalemia may develop, especially with brisk diuresis, when severe cirrhosis is present, during concomitant use of corticosteroids or ACTH, or after prolonged therapy.

Interference with adequate oral electrolyte intake will also contribute to hypokalemia. Hypokalemia can sensitize or exaggerate the response of the heart to the toxic effects of digitalis (e.g., increased ventricular irritability). Hypokalemia may be avoided or treated by use of potassium supplements such as foods with a high potassium content.

Although any chloride deficit is generally mild and usually does not require specific treatment except under extraordinary circumstances (as in liver disease or renal disease), chloride replacement may be required in the treatment of metabolic alkalosis.

Dilutional hyponatremia may occur in edematous patients in hot weather; appropriate therapy is water restriction, rather than administration of salt, except in rare instances when the hyponatremia is life threatening. In actual salt depletion, appropriate replacement is the therapy of choice.

Hyperuricemia may occur or acute gout may be precipitated in certain patients receiving thiazide therapy.

Insulin requirements in diabetic patients may be increased, decreased, or unchanged. Diabetes mellitus which has been latent may become manifest during thiazide administration.

Thiazide drugs may increase the responsiveness to tubocurarine.

The antihypertensive effects of the drug may be enhanced in the postsympathectomy patient. Thiazides may decrease arterial responsiveness to norepinephrine. This diminution is not sufficient to preclude effectiveness of the pressor agent for therapeutic use.

If progressive renal impairment becomes evident, consider withholding or discontinuing diuretic therapy.

Thiazides may decrease serum PBI levels without signs of thyroid disturbance.

Calcium excretion is decreased by thiazides. Pathological changes in the parathyroid glands with hypercalcemia and hypophosphatemia have been observed in a few patients on prolonged thiazide therapy. The common complications of hyperparathyroidism such as renal lithiasis, bone resorption, and peptic ulceration have not been seen. Thiazides should be discontinued before carrying out tests for parathyroid function.

Adverse Reactions

Methyldopa

Sedation, usually transient, may occur during the initial period of therapy or whenever the dose is increased. Headache, asthenia, or weakness may be noted as early and transient symptoms. However, significant adverse effects due to methyldopa have been infrequent and this agent usually is well tolerated.

Central nervous system: Sedation, headache, asthenia or weakness, dizziness, lightheaded-

Continued on next page

Information on the Merck Sharp & Dohme products listed on these pages is the full prescribing information from package circulars in use October 31, 1979.

Merck Sharp & Dohme—Cont.

ness, symptoms of cerebrovascular insufficiency, paresthesias, parkinsonism, Bell's palsy, decreased mental acuity, involuntary choreoathetotic movements. Psychic disturbances including nightmares and reversible mild psychoses or depression.
Cardiovascular: Bradycardia, aggravation of angina pectoris. Orthostatic hypotension (decrease daily dosage). Edema (and weight gain) usually relieved by use of a diuretic. (Discontinue methyldopa if edema progresses or signs of heart failure appear.)
Gastrointestinal: Nausea, vomiting, distention, constipation, flatus, diarrhea, mild dryness of mouth, sore or "black" tongue, pancreatitis, sialadenitis.
Hepatic: Abnormal liver function tests, jaundice, liver disorders.
Hematologic: Positive Coombs test, hemolytic anemia. Leukopenia, granulocytopenia, thrombocytopenia. Positive tests for antinuclear antibody, LE cells, and rheumatoid factor.
Allergic: Drug-related fever, lupus-like syndrome, myocarditis.
Other: Nasal stuffiness, rise in BUN, breast enlargement, gynecomastia, lactation, impotence, decreased libido, dermatologic reactions including eczema and lichenoid eruptions, mild arthralgia, myalgia.
Hydrochlorothiazide
Gastrointestinal system: Anorexia, gastric irritation, nausea, vomiting, cramping, diarrhea, constipation, jaundice (intrahepatic cholestatic jaundice), pancreatitis, sialadenitis.
Central nervous system: Dizziness, vertigo, paresthesias, headache, xanthopsia.
Hematologic: Leukopenia, agranulocytosis, thrombocytopenia, aplastic anemia, hemolytic anemia.
Cardiovascular: Orthostatic hypotension (may be aggravated by alcohol, barbiturates, or narcotics).
Hypersensitivity: Purpura, photosensitivity, rash, urticaria, necrotizing angiitis (vasculitis) (cutaneous vasculitis), fever, respiratory distress including pneumonitis, anaphylactic reactions.
Other: Hyperglycemia, glycosuria, hyperuricemia, muscle spasm, weakness, restlessness, transient blurred vision.
Whenever adverse reactions are moderate or severe, thiazide dosage should be reduced or therapy withdrawn.

Dosage and Administration

Dosage: As determined by individual titration (see box warning).
The usual dosage is 1 tablet of ALDORIL-15, ALDORIL-25, ALDORIL D30, or ALDORIL D50 two or three times a day in the first 48 hours. The daily dosage then may be increased or decreased, preferably at intervals of not less than two days, until an adequate response is achieved. To minimize the sedation associated with methyldopa, start dosage increases in the evening. By adjustment of dosage, morning hypotension may be prevented without sacrificing control of afternoon blood pressure.
When ALDORIL is given to patients on other antihypertensives, the dose of these agents may need to be adjusted to effect a smooth transition. When ALDORIL is given with antihypertensives other than thiazides, the initial dosage of methyldopa should be limited to 500 mg daily in divided doses.
Although occasional patients have responded to higher doses, the maximum recommended daily dosage is 3.0 g of methyldopa and 100 to 200 mg of hydrochlorothiazide. Once an effective dosage range is attained, a smooth blood pressure response occurs in most patients in 12 to 24 hours. If ALDORIL alone does not adequately control blood pressure, additional methyldopa may be given separately to obtain the maximum blood pressure response.
Since both components of ALDORIL have a relatively short duration of action, withdrawal is followed by return of hypertension usually within 48 hours. This is not complicated by an overshoot of blood pressure.
Occasionally tolerance may occur, usually between the second and third month of therapy. Increasing the dosage of either methyldopa or hydrochlorothiazide separately or together frequently will restore effective control of blood pressure.
Methyldopa is largely excreted by the kidney and patients with impaired renal function may respond to smaller doses of ALDORIL. Syncope in older patients may be related to an increased sensitivity and advanced arteriosclerotic vascular disease. This may be avoided by lower doses.

How Supplied

No. 3294—Tablets ALDORIL-15 are salmon, round, film coated tablets, coded MSD 423. Each tablet contains 250 mg of methyldopa and 15 mg of hydrochlorothiazide. They are supplied as follows:
NDC 0006-0423-68 bottles of 100
NDC 0006-0423-82 bottles of 1000
[*Shown in Product Identification Section*]
No. 3295—Tablets ALDORIL-25 are white, round, film coated tablets, coded MSD 456. Each tablet contains 250 mg of methyldopa and 25 mg of hydrochlorothiazide. They are supplied as follows:
NDC 0006-0456-68 bottles of 100
NDC 0006-0456-82 bottles of 1000.
[*Shown in Product Identification Section*]
No. 3362—Tablets ALDORIL D30 are salmon, oval, film coated tablets, coded MSD 694. Each tablet contains 500 mg of methyldopa and 30 mg of hydrochlorothiazide. They are supplied as follows:
NDC 0006-0694-68 bottles of 100.
NDC 0006-0694-28 single unit package of 100.
[*Shown in Product Identification Section*]
No. 3363—Tablets ALDORIL D50 are white, oval, film coated tablets, coded MSD 935. Each tablet contains 500 mg of methyldopa and 50 mg of hydrochlorothiazide. They are supplied as follows:
NDC 0006-0935-68 bottles of 100.
NDC 0006-0935-28 single unit package of 100.
[*Shown in Product Identification Section*]
A.H.F.S. 24:08
DC 6086026 Issued June 1979

ANTIVENIN ℞
(latrodectus mactans), MSD
Black Widow Spider Antivenin
Equine Origin

Indications

Antivenin (Latrodectus mactans), MSD is used to treat patients with symptoms due to bites by the black widow spider (Latrodectus mactans). Early use of the Antivenin is emphasized for prompt relief.
Local muscular cramps begin from 15 minutes to several hours after the bite which usually produces a sharp pain similar to that caused by puncture with a needle. The exact sequence of symptoms depends somewhat on the location of the bite. The venom acts on the myoneural junctions or on the nerve endings, causing an ascending motor paralysis or destruction of the peripheral nerve endings. The groups of muscles most frequently affected at first are those of the thigh, shoulder, and back. After a varying length of time, the pain becomes more severe, spreading to the abdomen, and weakness and tremor usually develop. The abdominal muscles assume a boardlike rigidity, but tenderness is slight. Respiration is thoracic. The patient is restless and anxious. Feeble pulse, cold, clammy skin, labored breathing and speech, light stupor, and delirium may occur. Convulsions also may occur, particularly in small children. The temperature may be normal or slightly elevated. Urinary retention, shock, cyanosis, nausea and vomiting, insomnia, and cold sweats also have been reported. The syndrome following the bite of the black widow spider may be confused easily with any medical or surgical condition with acute abdominal symptoms.
The symptoms of black widow spider bite increase in severity for several hours, perhaps a day, and then very slowly become less severe, gradually passing off in the course of two or three days except in fatal cases. Residual symptoms such as general weakness, tingling, nervousness, and transient muscle spasm may persist for weeks or months after recovery from the acute stage.
If possible, the patient should be hospitalized. Other additional measures giving greatest relief are prolonged warm baths and intravenous injection of 10 ml of 10 percent solution of calcium gluconate repeated as necessary to control muscle pain. Morphine also may be required to control pain. Barbiturates may be used for extreme restlessness. However, as the venom is a neurotoxin, it can cause respiratory paralysis. This must be borne in mind when considering use of morphine or a barbiturate. Adrenocorticosteroids have been used with varying degrees of success. Supportive therapy is indicated by the condition of the patient. Local treatment of the site of the bite is of no value. Nothing is gained by applying a tourniquet or by attempting to remove venom from the site of the bite by incision and suction.
In otherwise healthy individuals between the ages of 16 and 60, the use of Antivenin may be deferred and treatment with muscle relaxants may be considered.

Precautions

Prior to treatment with any product prepared from horse serum, a careful review of the patient's history should be taken emphasizing prior exposure to horse serum or any allergies. Serious sickness and even death could result from the use of horse serum in a sensitive patient. A skin or conjunctival test should be performed prior to administration of Antivenin.
Skin test: Inject into (not under) the skin not more than 0.02 ml of the test material (1:10 dilution of normal horse serum in physiologic saline). Evaluate result in 10 minutes. A positive reaction is an urticarial wheal surrounded by a zone of erythema. A control test using Sodium Chloride Injection facilitates interpretation of the results.
Conjunctival test: For adults instill into the conjunctival sac one drop of a 1:10 dilution of horse serum and for children one drop of 1:100 dilution. Itching of the eye and reddening of the conjunctiva indicate a positive reaction, usually within 10 minutes.
Patients should be observed for serum sickness for an average of 8 to 12 days following administration of Antivenin.
Desensitization should be attempted only when the administration of Antivenin is considered necessary to save life. Epinephrine must be available in case of untoward reaction.
Desensitization: If the history is positive or the results of the sensitivity tests are mildly or questionably positive, Antivenin should be administered as follows to reduce the risk of an immediate severe allergic reaction:
1. In separate sterile vials or syringes prepare 1:10 or 1:100 dilutions of Antivenin in Sodium Chloride for Injection.
2. Allow at least 15 but preferably 30 minutes between injections and only proceed with the next dose if no reactions occurred following the previous dose.
3. Using a tuberculin syringe, inject subcutaneously 0.1, 0.2 and 0.5 ml of the 1:100

dilution at 15 or 30 minute intervals; repeat with the 1:10 dilution, and finally the undiluted Antivenin.

4. If there is a reaction after any of the injections, place a tourniquet proximal to the sites of injection and administer epinephrine, 1:1000 (0.3 to 1.0 ml subcutaneously, 0.05 to 0.1 ml intravenously), proximal to the tourniquet or into another extremity. Wait at least 30 minutes before giving another injection of Antivenin, the amount of which should be the same as the last one not evoking a reaction.
5. If no reaction has occurred after 0.5 ml of undiluted Antivenin has been given, it is probably safe to continue the dose at 15 minute intervals until the entire dose has been injected.

Method of Preparation

Antivenin (Latrodectus mactans), MSD is prepared from the blood serum of horses immunized against the venom of the black widow spider.
Each vial contains not less than 6000 Antivenin units. One unit of Antivenin will neutralize one average mouse lethal dose of black widow spider venom when the Antivenin and the venom are injected simultaneously in mice under suitable conditions.
Using a sterile syringe, remove from the accompanying vial 2.5 ml of Sterile Water for Injection and inject into the vial of Antivenin. With the needle still in the rubber stopper, shake the vial to dissolve the contents completely.

Dosage and Administration

The dose for adults and children is the entire contents of a restored vial (2.5 ml) of Antivenin. It may be given intramuscularly, preferably in the region of the anterolateral thigh so that a tourniquet may be applied in the event of a systemic reaction. Symptoms usually subside in 1 to 3 hours. Although one dose of Antivenin usually is adequate, a second dose may be necessary in some cases.
Antivenin also may be given intravenously in 10 to 50 ml of saline solution over a 15 minute period. It is the preferred route in severe cases, or when the patient is under 12, or in shock. One restored vial usually is enough.

How Supplied

No. 4084—Antivenin (latrodectus mactans), MSD equine origin is supplied in a vial containing not less than 6000 Antivenin units. Thimerosal (mercury derivative) 1:10,000 is added as preservative, **NDC** 0006-4084-00. A 2.5 ml vial of Sterile Water for Injection is included. Also supplied is a 1 ml vial of normal horse serum (1:10 dilution) for sensitivity testing. Thimerosal (mercury derivative) 1:10,000 is added as preservative.

A.H.F.S. 80:04
DC 6145210 Issued April 1975

AQUAMEPHYTON® Injection ℞
(phytonadione, MSD), U.S.P.
Aqueous Colloidal Solution of Vitamin K_1

WARNING—INTRAVENOUS USE

Severe reactions, including fatalities, have occurred during and immediately after INTRAVENOUS injection of AquaMEPHYTON® (Phytonadione, MSD), even when precautions have been taken to dilute the AquaMEPHYTON and to avoid rapid infusion. Typically these severe reactions have resembled hypersensitivity or anaphylaxis, including shock and cardiac and/or respiratory arrest. Some patients have exhibited these severe reactions on receiving AquaMEPHYTON for the first time. Therefore the INTRAVENOUS route should be restricted to those situations where other routes are not feasible and the serious risk involved is considered justified.

Description

AquaMEPHYTON injection is a yellow, sterile, aqueous colloidal solution of vitamin K_1, available for injection by the intravenous, intramuscular, and subcutaneous routes. Each milliliter contains:

Phytonadione	2 mg or 10 mg
Inactive ingredients:	
Polyoxyethylated fatty acid derivative	70 mg
Dextrose	37.5 mg
Water for Injection, q.s.	1 ml
Added as preservative:	
Benzyl alcohol	0.9%

Actions

AquaMEPHYTON aqueous colloidal solution of vitamin K_1 for parenteral injection, possesses the same type and degree of activity as does naturally-occurring vitamin K, which is necessary for the production via the liver of active prothrombin (factor II), proconvertin (factor VII), plasma thromboplastin component (factor IX), and Stuart factor (factor X). The prothrombin test is sensitive to the levels of three of these four factors—II, VII, and X. The mechanism by which vitamin K promotes formation of these clotting factors in the liver is not known.
The action of the aqueous colloidal solution, when administered intravenously, is generally detectable within an hour or two and hemorrhage is usually controlled within 3 to 6 hours. A normal prothrombin level may often be obtained in 12 to 14 hours.
In the prophylaxis and treatment of hemorrhagic disease of the newborn, phytonadione has demonstrated a greater margin of safety than that of the water-soluble vitamin K analogues.

Indications

AquaMEPHYTON is indicated in the following coagulation disorders which are due to faulty formation of factors II, VII, IX and X when caused by vitamin K deficiency or interference with vitamin K activity.
AquaMEPHYTON injection is indicated in:
- anticoagulant-induced prothrombin deficiency;
- prophylaxis and therapy of hemorrhagic disease of the newborn;
- hypoprothrombinemia due to antibacterial therapy;
- hypoprothrombinemia secondary to factors limiting absorption or synthesis of vitamin K, e.g., obstructive jaundice, biliary fistula, sprue, ulcerative colitis, celiac disease, intestinal resection, cystic fibrosis of the pancreas, and regional enteritis;
- other drug-induced hypoprothrombinemia where it is definitely shown that the result is due to interference with vitamin K metabolism, e.g., salicylates.

Contraindication

Hypersensitivity to any component of this medication.

Warnings

An immediate coagulant effect should not be expected after administration of phytonadione. It takes a minimum of 1 to 2 hours for measurable improvement in the prothrombin time. Whole blood or component therapy may also be necessary if bleeding is severe.
Phytonadione will not counteract the anticoagulant action of heparin.
When vitamin K_1 is used to correct excessive anticoagulant-induced hypoprothrombinemia, anticoagulant therapy still being indicated, the patient is again faced with the clotting hazards existing prior to starting the anticoagulant therapy. Phytonadione is not a clotting agent, but overzealous therapy with vitamin K_1 may restore conditions which originally permitted thromboembolic phenomena. Dosage should be kept as low as possible, and prothrombin time should be checked regularly as clinical conditions indicate.
Repeated large doses of vitamin K are not warranted in liver disease if the response to initial use of the vitamin is unsatisfactory. Failure to respond to vitamin K may indicate that the condition being treated is inherently unresponsive to vitamin K.
Reproduction studies have not been performed in animals. There is no adequate information of whether this drug may affect fertility in human males or females or have a teratogenic potential or other adverse effect on the fetus.

Precautions

Protect from light at all times.
Temporary resistance to prothrombin-depressing anticoagulants may result, especially when larger doses of phytonadione are used. If relatively large doses have been employed, it may be necessary when reinstituting anticoagulant therapy to use somewhat larger doses of the prothrombin-depressing anticoagulant, or to use one which acts on a different principle, such as heparin sodium.

Adverse Reactions

Deaths have occurred after intravenous administration. (See Box Warning at beginning of circular).
Transient "flushing sensations" and "peculiar" sensations of taste have been observed, as well as rare instances of dizziness, rapid and weak pulse, profuse sweating, brief hypotension, dyspnea, and cyanosis.
Pain, swelling, and tenderness at the injection site may occur. The possibility of allergic sensitivity, including an anaphylactoid reaction, should be kept in mind.
Rarely, after repeated injections, reactions resembling erythema perstans have been reported.
Hyperbilirubinemia has been observed in the newborn following administration of phytonadione. This has occurred rarely and primarily with doses above those recommended.

Dosage and Administration

Whenever possible, AquaMEPHYTON should be given by the subcutaneous or intramuscular route. When intravenous administration is considered unavoidable, the drug should be injected very slowly, not exceeding 1 mg per minute.
The human minimum daily requirements for vitamin K have not been established officially but they have been estimated to be 1 to 5 mcg/kg of body weight for infants and 0.03 mcg/kg for adults. Usually, the dietary abundance of vitamin K will satisfy these requirements, except during the first five to eight days of the neonatal period.

Anticoagulant-Induced Prothrombin Deficiency
To correct excessively prolonged prothrombin time caused by oral anticoagulant thera-

Continued on next page

Information on the Merck Sharp & Dohme products listed on these pages is the full prescribing information from package circulars in use October 31, 1979.

Merck Sharp & Dohme—Cont.

py—2.5 to 10 mg or up to 25 mg initially is recommended. In rare instances 50 mg may be required. Frequency and amount of subsequent doses should be determined by prothrombin time response or clinical condition. If in 6 to 8 hours after parenteral administration the prothrombin time has not been shortened satisfactorily, the dose should be repeated.
In the event of shock or excessive blood loss, the use of whole blood or component therapy is indicated.
Smaller doses are recommended for patients being treated with the shorter-acting anticoagulants, and for those in need of continued anticoagulant therapy. The smallest effective dose should be sought to obviate the possibility of temporary refractoriness to further anticoagulant therapy, and to avoid lowering the prothrombin time too far below that indicating an effective level of anticoagulant activity.
Larger doses are recommended for patients on the longer-acting anticoagulants, for those with severe bleeding, and for those not needing further anticoagulant therapy. Although more than 25 mg may be necessary and a dose may need to be repeated, these courses of action are indicated *only rarely.*
Prophylaxis and Treatment of Hemorrhagic Disease of the Newborn
Prophylaxis
The Committee on Nutrition of the American Academy of Pediatrics recommends that vitamin K_1 be given to the newborn. A single intramuscular dose of AquaMEPHYTON 0.5 to 1.0 mg is recommended. Although less desirable, AquaMEPHYTON 1 to 5 mg may be given to the mother 12 to 24 hours before delivery.
Treatment
AquaMEPHYTON 1.0 mg should be given either subcutaneously or intramuscularly. Higher doses mg be necessary if the mother has been receiving oral anticoagulants.
Empiric administration of vitamin K_1 should not replace proper laboratory evaluation of the coagulation mechanism. A prompt response (shortening of the prothrombin time in 2 to 4 hours) following administration of vitamin K_1 is usually diagnostic of hemorrhagic disease of the newborn, and failure to respond indicates another diagnosis or coagulation disorder.
Whole blood or component therapy may be indicated if bleeding is excessive. This therapy, however, does not correct the underlying disorder and AquaMEPHYTON should be given concurrently.
Hypoprothrombinemia Due to Other Causes
A dosage of 2.5 to 25 mg or more (rarely up to 50 mg) is recommended, the amount and route of administration depending upon the severity of the condition and response obtained.
If possible, discontinuation or reduction of the dosage of drugs interfering with coagulation mechanisms (such as salicylates, antibiotics) is suggested as an alternative to administering concurrent AquaMEPHYTON. The severity of the coagulation disorder should determine whether the immediate administration of AquaMEPHYTON is required in addition to discontinuation or reduction of interfering drugs.

Directions for Dilution

AquaMEPHYTON may be diluted with 0.9% Sodium Chloride Injection, 5% Dextrose Injection, or 5% Dextrose and Sodium Chloride Injection. *Other diluents should not be used.* When dilutions are indicated, administration should be started immediately after mixture with the diluent, and unused portions of the dilution should be discarded, as well as unused contents of the ampul.

How Supplied

Injection AquaMEPHYTON is a yellow, sterile, aqueous colloidal solution and is supplied in the following concentrations:
No. 7780—10 mg of vitamin K_1 per ml
NDC 0006-7780-64 boxes of 6–1 ml ampuls (6505-00-854-2499 10 mg 1.0 ml 6's)
NDC 0006-7780-66 boxes of 25–1 ml ampuls.
No. 7782—10 mg of vitamin K_1 per ml
NDC 0006-7782-30 in 2.5 ml multiple dose vials
NDC 0006-7782-03 in 5 ml multiple dose vials.
No. 7784—1 mg of vitamin K_1 per 0.5 ml
NDC 0006-7784-33 boxes of 25–0.5 ml ampuls (6505-00-180-6372 1 mg 0.5 ml 25's).

A.H.F.S. 88:24
DC 6136712 Issued October 1975

ARAMINE® Injection ℞
(metaraminol bitartrate, MSD), U.S.P.

Description

Injection ARAMINE (Metaraminol Bitartrate, MSD) is a sterile solution, each ml of which contains:

Metaraminol bitartrate equivalent to metaraminol	10.0 mg
Inactive ingredients:	
Sodium chloride	4.4 mg
Water for Injection q.s. ad	1.0 ml

Methylparaben 0.15%, propylparaben 0.02%, and sodium bisulfite 0.2% added as preservatives.
Metaraminol bitartrate is the generic name for levo-1-(m-hydroxyphenyl)-2-amino-1-propanol hydrogen D-tartrate. Metaraminol bitartrate is a white, crystalline powder, freely soluble in water, slightly soluble in alcohol, and practically insoluble in chloroform and in ether.

Actions

ARAMINE is a potent sympathomimetic amine that increases both systolic and diastolic blood pressure.
The pressor effect of ARAMINE begins in 1 to 2 minutes after intravenous infusion, in about 10 minutes after intramuscular injection, and in 5 to 20 minutes after subcutaneous injection. The effect lasts from about 20 minutes to one hour. ARAMINE has a positive inotropic effect on the heart and a peripheral vasoconstrictor action.
Renal, coronary, and cerebral blood flow are a function of perfusion pressure and regional resistance. In most instances of cardiogenic shock, the beneficial effect of sympathomimetic amines is attributable to their positive inotropic effect. In patients with insufficient or failing vasoconstriction, there is additional advantage to the peripheral action of ARAMINE, but in most patients with shock, vasoconstriction is adequate and any further increase is unnecessary. Therefore, blood flow to vital organs may decrease with ARAMINE if regional resistance increases excessively.
The pressor effect of ARAMINE is decreased but not reversed by alpha-adrenergic blocking agents. Primary or secondary fall in blood pressure and tachyphylactic response to repeated use are uncommon.

INDICATIONS

Based on a review of this drug by the National Academy of Sciences-National Research Council and/or other information, FDA has classified the indications as follows:
Effective: ARAMINE is indicated for prevention and treatment of the acute hypotensive state occurring with spinal anesthesia. Adjunctive treatment of hypotension due to hemorrhage; reactions to medications; surgical complications; and shock associated with brain damage due to trauma or tumor.
"Probably" effective: It may also be useful as an adjunct in the treatment of hypotension due to cardiogenic shock or septicemia.
Final classification of the less-than-effective indications requires further investigation.

Contraindications

Use of ARAMINE with cyclopropane or halothane anesthesia should be avoided, unless clinical circumstances demand such use.
Hypersensitivity to any component of this product.

Precautions

Caution should be used to avoid excessive blood pressure response. Rapidly induced hypertensive responses have been reported to cause acute pulmonary edema, arrhythmias, and cardiac arrest. ARAMINE should be used with caution in digitalized patients, since the combination of digitalis and sympathomimetic amines is capable of causing ectopic arrhythmic activity.
Patients with cirrhosis should be treated with caution, with adequate restoration of electrolytes if diuresis ensues. Fatal ventricular arrhythmia has been reported in one patient with Laennec's cirrhosis while receiving metaraminol bitartrate. In several instances, ventricular extrasystoles that appeared during infusion of this vasopressor subsided promptly when the rate of infusion was reduced.
With the prolonged action of ARAMINE, a cumulative effect is possible, and with an excessive vasopressor response there may be a prolonged elevation of blood pressure even with discontinuation of therapy. Monoamine oxidase inhibitors have been reported to potentiate the action of sympathomimetic amines.
When vasopressor amines are used for long periods, the resulting vasoconstriction may prevent adequate expansion of circulating volume and may cause perpetuation of the shock state. There is evidence that plasma volume may be reduced in all types of shock, and that the measurement of central venous pressure is useful in assessing the adequacy of the circulating blood volume. Therefore, blood or plasma volume expanders should be employed when the principal reason for hypotension or shock is decreased circulating volume.
Because of its vasoconstrictor effect ARAMINE should be given with caution in heart or thyroid disease, hypertension, or diabetes. Sympathomimetic amines may provoke a relapse in patients with a history of malaria.

Adverse Reactions

Sympathomimetic amines, including ARAMINE, may cause sinus or ventricular tachycardia, or other arrhythmias, especially in patients with myocardial infarction. See also PRECAUTIONS.
Also, in patients with a history of malaria, these compounds may provoke a relapse.
Abscess formation, tissue necrosis, or sloughing rarely may follow the use of ARAMINE. In choosing the site of injection, it is important to avoid those areas recognized as *not* suitable for use of any pressor agent and to discontinue the infusion immediately if infiltration or thrombosis occurs. Although the physician may be forced by the urgent nature of the patient's condition to choose injection sites that are not recognized as suitable, he should, when possible, use the preferred areas of injection. The larger veins of the antecubital fossa or the thigh are preferred to veins in the dorsum of the hand or ankle veins, particularly in patients with peripheral vascular disease, diabetes mellitus, Buerger's disease, or conditions with coexistent hypercoagulability.

Dosage and Administration

ARAMINE may be given intramuscularly, subcutaneously, or intravenously, the route depending on the nature and severity of the indication.
Allow at least 10 minutes to elapse before increasing the dose because the maximum effect is not immediately apparent. When the vasopressor is discontinued, observe the patient carefully as the effect of the drug tapers off, so that therapy can be reinitiated promptly if the blood pressure falls too rapidly. The response to vasopressors may be poor in patients with coexistent shock and acidosis. Established methods of shock management, such as blood or fluid replacement when indicated, and other measures directed to the specific cause of the shock state also should be used.
Intramuscular or Subcutaneous Injection (for prevention of hypotension—see INDICATIONS):
The recommended dose is 2 to 10 mg (0.2 to 1 ml). As with other agents given subcutaneously, only the preferred sites of injection, as set forth in standard texts, should be used.
Intravenous Infusion (for adjunctive treatment of hypotension—see INDICATIONS):
The recommended dose is 15 to 100 mg (1.5 to 10 ml) in 500 ml of Sodium Chloride Injection or 5% Dextrose Injection, adjusting the rate of infusion to maintain the blood pressure at the desired level. Higher concentrations of ARAMINE, 150 to 500 mg per 500 ml of infusion fluid, have been used.
If the patient needs more saline or dextrose solution at a rate of flow that would provide an excessive dose of the vasopressor, the recommended volume of infusion fluid (500 ml) should be increased accordingly. ARAMINE may also be added to *less* than 500 ml of infusion fluid if a smaller volume is desired.
Compatibility Information
In addition to Sodium Chloride Injection* and Dextrose Injection 5%*, the following infusion solutions were found physically and chemically compatible with injection ARAMINE when 5 ml of injection ARAMINE, 10 mg/ml (metaraminol equivalent), was added to 500 ml of infusion solution: Ringer's Injection*, Lactated Ringer's Injection*, Dextran 6% in Saline†, Normosol®-R pH 7.4†, and Normosol®-M in D5-W†.
When injection ARAMINE is mixed with an infusion solution, sterile precautions should be observed. Since infusion solutions generally do not contain preservatives, mixtures should be used within 24 hours.
Direct Intravenous Injection: In severe shock, where time is of great importance, this agent should be given by direct intravenous injection. The suggested dose is 0.5 to 5 mg (0.05 to 0.5 ml), followed by an infusion of 15 to 100 mg (1.5 to 10 ml) in 500 ml of infusion fluid as described previously.
If necessary, vials may be sterilized by autoclaving or by immersion in a sterilizing solution.

How Supplied

No. 3222X—Injection ARAMINE 1%, containing metaraminol bitartrate equivalent to 10 mg of metaraminol per ml, is a clear, colorless solution and is supplied as follows:
NDC 0006-3222-10 in 10 ml vials (6505-00-753-9601 10 ml vial)
NDC 0006-3222-17 in 12 × 1 ml vials.
A.H.F.S. 12:12
DC 6019019 Issued December 1977

*U.S.P.
†Product of Abbott Laboratories

ATTENUVAX® ℞
(measles virus vaccine, live, attenuated, MSD), U.S.P.
(More Attenuated Enders' Line)
Prepared in Cell Cultures of Chick Embryo

Description

ATTENUVAX (Measles Virus Vaccine, Live, Attenuated, MSD) is a live virus vaccine for immunization against measles (rubeola).
ATTENUVAX is a lyophilized preparation of a more attenuated line of measles virus derived from Enders' attenuated Edmonston strain. The further modification of the virus in ATTENUVAX was achieved in the Merck Institute for Therapeutic Research by multiple passage of Edmonston virus in cell cultures of chick embryo at low temperature.
When reconstituted as directed, the dose for injection contains not less than the equivalent of 1,000 $TCID_{50}$ (tissue culture infectious doses) of measles virus vaccine expressed in terms of the assigned titer of the FDA Reference Measles Virus. Each dose also contains approximately 25 mcg of neomycin.

Actions

ATTENUVAX produces a modified measles infection in susceptible persons. Fever and rash may appear. Extensive clinical trials have demonstrated that ATTENUVAX is highly immunogenic and generally well tolerated. A single injection of the vaccine has been shown to induce measles hemagglutination-inhibiting (HI) antibodies in 97 percent or more of susceptible persons. Vaccine-induced antibody levels have been shown to persist for at least eight years without substantial decline. If the present pattern continues, it will provide a basis for the expectation that immunity following the vaccine will be permanent. However, continued surveillance will be required to demonstrate this point.

Indications

ATTENUVAX is recommended for active immunization of children 15 months of age or older against measles (rubeola). A booster is not needed. Infants who are less than 15 months of age may fail to respond to the vaccine due to presence in the circulation of residual measles antibody of maternal origin; the younger the infant, the lower the likelihood of seroconversion. In geographically isolated or other relatively inaccessible populations for whom immunization programs are logistically difficult, and in population groups in which natural measles infection may occur in a significant proportion of infants before 15 months of age, it may be desirable to give the vaccine to infants at an earlier age. The advantage of early protection must be weighed against the chance for failure of response; infants vaccinated under these conditions should be revaccinated after reaching 15 months of age.
Recent serologic evidence shows that when M-M-R® (Measles, Mumps and Rubella Virus Vaccine, Live, MSD) is given simultaneously with trivalent oral poliovirus vaccine, antibody responses can be expected to be comparable to those which follow administration of the vaccines at different times. From this it follows that when ATTENUVAX is given simultaneously with either monovalent or trivalent oral poliovirus vaccine, MERUVAX® (Rubella Virus Vaccine, Live, MSD), and/or MUMPSVAX® (Mumps Virus Vaccine, Live, MSD), antibody responses can be expected to be comparable to those which follow administration of the vaccines at different times.
Children for whom ATTENUVAX is strongly recommended include those living in schools, orphanages, and similar institutions. It is also recommended for children with inactive tuberculosis or active tuberculosis under treatment, as well as for those with chronic diseases such as cystic fibrosis, heart disease, asthma, and other chronic pulmonary diseases, to minimize the risk of serious complications of natural measles.
ATTENUVAX given immediately after exposure to natural measles may provide some protection. If, however, the vaccine is given a few days before exposure, substantial protection may be provided.
Ordinarily, adults need not be immunized, since most are immune to measles. However, vaccination may be advisable for high school and college persons in epidemic situations and for adults in isolated communities where measles is not endemic.
Revaccination: Children vaccinated before 12 months of age—particularly if vaccine was administered with immune serum globulin or measles immune globulin, a standardized globulin preparation—should be revaccinated with live measles vaccine at about 15 months of age for optimal protection.
Based on available evidence, there is no reason to routinely revaccinate children originally vaccinated when 12 months of age or older. The decision to revaccinate should be based on evaluation of each individual case.
Despite the risk of local reaction (see Adverse Reactions), children who have previously been given inactivated vaccine alone or followed by live vaccine within 3 months should be revaccinated with live vaccine to avoid the severe atypical form of natural measles that may occur.

Contraindications

ATTENUVAX is contraindicated in the following conditions:
- Hypersensitivity to neomycin (each dose of reconstituted vaccine contains approximately 25 mcg of neomycin).
- Any febrile respiratory illness, or other active febrile infection.
- Active untreated tuberculosis.
- Patients receiving therapy with ACTH, corticosteroids, irradiation, alkylating agents or antimetabolites.
  This contraindication does not apply to patients who are receiving corticosteroids as replacement therapy, e.g., for Addison's disease.
- Individuals with blood dyscrasias, leukemia, lymphomas of any type, or other malignant neoplasms affecting the bone marrow or lymphatic systems.
- Primary immuno-deficiency states, including cellular immune deficiencies, hypogammaglobulinemic and dysgammaglobulinemic states.

Hypersensitivity to Eggs, Chicken, or Chicken Feathers

This vaccine is essentially devoid of potentially allergenic substances derived from host tissues (chick embryo).* However, since this vaccine is propagated in cell cultures of chick embryo, in considering its use in patients hypersensitive to eggs, chicken, or chicken feathers, the attending physician must weigh the benefits of immunization against the potential risks of hypersensitivity reactions.

Pregnancy

The effects of ATTENUVAX on fetal development are unknown at this time. Therefore, live attenuated measles virus vaccine should not be given to persons known to be pregnant; fur-

Continued on next page

Information on the Merck Sharp & Dohme products listed on these pages is the full prescribing information from package circulars in use October 31, 1979.

Merck Sharp & Dohme—Cont.

thermore, pregnancy should be avoided for three months following vaccination.
Reports have indicated that contracting of natural measles during pregnancy enhances fetal risk. Increased rates of spontaneous abortion, stillbirth, congenital defects and prematurity have been observed subsequent to natural measles during pregnancy. There are no adequate studies of the attenuated (vaccine) strain of measles virus in pregnancy. However, it would be prudent to assume that the vaccine strain of virus is also capable of inducing adverse fetal effects for up to three months following vaccination.
Vaccine administration to post-pubertal females entails a potential for inadvertent immunization during pregnancy. Theoretical risks involved should be weighed against the risks that measles poses to the unimmunized adolescent or adult. Advisory committees reviewing this matter have recommended vaccination of post-pubertal females who are presumed to be susceptible to measles and not known to be pregnant. If a measles exposure occurs during pregnancy, one should consider the possibility of providing temporary passive immunity through the administration of immune serum globulin (human).

Precautions

For subcutaneous administration; *do not give intravenously.*
Epinephrine should be available for immediate use should an anaphylactoid reaction occur.
ATTENUVAX may be given simultaneously with monovalent or trivalent poliovirus vaccine, live, oral, with MERUVAX (Rubella Virus Vaccine, Live, MSD) and/or MUMPSVAX (Mumps Virus Vaccine, Live, MSD). It should not be given less than one month before or after immunization with other live virus vaccines.
Due caution should be employed in administration of measles vaccine to children with a history of febrile convulsions, or cerebral injury, or of any other condition in which stress due to fever should be avoided. The physician should be alert to the temperature elevation which may occur following vaccination.
The occurrence of thrombocytopenia and purpura associated with live virus measles vaccines has been extremely rare.
Vaccination should be deferred for at least 3 months following blood or plasma transfusions, or administration of more than 0.02 ml of human immune serum globulin per pound of body weight.
It has been reported that attenuated measles virus vaccine, live, may result in a temporary depression of tuberculin skin sensitivity. Therefore, if a tuberculin test is to be done, it should be administered either before or simultaneously with ATTENUVAX.
Children under treatment for tuberculosis have not experienced exacerbation of the disease when immunized with live measles virus vaccine; no studies have been reported to date of the effect of measles virus vaccines on untreated tuberculous children.

Adverse Reactions

Occasional
Moderate fever (101–102.9°F) may occur during the month after vaccination. Generally, fever, rash, or both appear between the 5th and the 12th days. Rash, when it occurs, is usually minimal without generalized distribution.
Less Common
High fever (over 103°F).
Rare
Reactions at injection site.
Children developing fever may, on rare occasions, exhibit febrile convulsions.
Experience from more than 80 million doses of all live measles vaccines given in the U.S. through 1975 indicates that significant central nervous system reactions such as encephalitis and encephalopathy, occurring within 30 days after vaccination, have been temporally associated with measles vaccine approximately once for every million doses. In no case has it been shown that reactions were actually caused by vaccine. The Center for Disease Control has pointed out that "a certain number of cases of encephalitis may be expected to occur in a large childhood population in a defined period of time even when no vaccines are administered." However, the data suggest the possibility that some of these cases may have been caused by measles vaccines. The risk of such serious neurological disorders following live measles virus vaccine administration remains far less than that for encephalitis and encephalopathy with natural measles (one per thousand reported cases).
There have been reports of subacute sclerosing panencephalitis (SSPE) in children who did not have a history of natural measles but did receive measles vaccine. Some of these cases may have resulted from unrecognized measles in the first year of life or possibly from the measles vaccination. Based on estimated nationwide measles vaccine distribution, the association of SSPE cases to measles vaccination is about one case per million vaccine doses distributed. This is far less than the association with natural measles, 5–10 cases of SSPE per million cases of measles. The results of a retrospective case-controlled study conducted by the Center for Disease Control suggest that the overall effect of measles vaccine has been to protect against SSPE by preventing measles with its inherent higher risk of SSPE.
Local reactions characterized by marked swelling, redness and vesiculation at the injection site of attenuated live virus measles vaccines have occurred in children who have previously received killed measles vaccine.

Dosage and Administration

After suitable cleansing of the immunization site, inject the total volume of reconstituted vaccine subcutaneously, preferably into the outer aspect of the upper arm. Do not inject intravenously.
The dosage of vaccine is the same for all patients. Inject the entire contents of the syringe (about 0.5 ml).
CAUTION: A new unused sterile disposable syringe with a 25 gauge ⅝″ needle should be used for each injection of the vaccine because certain preservatives, antiseptics, and detergents will inactivate the live measles virus vaccine.

Shipment, Storage and Reconstitution

During shipment, to insure that there is no loss of potency, the vaccine must be maintained at a temperature of 10°C (50°F) or less.
Prior to reconstitution, store the vaccine in a refrigerator at 2–8° C (35.6–46.4° F). *Protect from light.*
The reconstituted vaccine should be protected from light, since such exposure may inactivate the virus.
To reconstitute, inject all the diluent in the syringe into the vial of lyophilized vaccine. Agitate to insure thorough mixing. Draw the entire volume of reconstituted vaccine into the syringe. Each dose of ATTENUVAX contains not less than 1,000 $TCID_{50}$ (tissue culture infectious doses) of measles virus vaccine expressed in terms of the assigned titer of the FDA Reference Measles Virus.
Use only the diluent supplied and reconstitute ATTENUVAX just before using. Protect the vaccine from light at all times. If not used immediately, return the reconstituted vaccine to a dark place at 2–8° C (35.6–46.4° F). Discard if not used within eight hours.
Color: The color of the vaccine when reconstituted is yellow. It is acceptable for use only if clear.

How Supplied

No. 4588X—ATTENUVAX is supplied as a single-dose vial of lyophilized vaccine, **NDC** 0006-4588-00, and a diluent-containing disposable syringe with affixed 25 gauge, ⅝″ needle.
No. 4589X/4590—ATTENUVAX is supplied as follows: (1) a box of 10 single-dose vials of lyophilized vaccine, **NDC** 0006-4589-00; and (2) a box of 10 diluent-containing disposable syringes with affixed 25 gauge, ⅝″ needles. To conserve refrigerator space, the syringes may be stored separately at room temperature.
(6505-01-038-0794 Ten Pack)

*Morbidity and Mortality Weekly Report *25* (44): 350, Nov. 12, 1976.
A.H.F.S. 80:12
DC 7075500 Issued October 1978

BENEMID® Tablets (probenecid, MSD), U.S.P. ℞

Description

Probenecid is the generic name for 4-[(dipropylamino)sulfonyl] benzoic acid (molecular weight 285.36).
Probenecid is a white or nearly white, fine, crystalline powder. Probenecid is soluble in dilute alkali, in alcohol, in chloroform, and in acetone; it is practically insoluble in water and in dilute acids.

Actions

BENEMID (Probenecid, MSD) is a uricosuric and renal tubular blocking agent. It inhibits the tubular reabsorption of urate, thus increasing the urinary excretion of uric acid and decreasing serum urate levels. Effective uricosuria reduces the miscible urate pool, retards urate deposition, and promotes resorption of urate deposits.
BENEMID inhibits the tubular secretion of penicillin and usually increases penicillin plasma levels by any route the antibiotic is given. A 2-fold to 4-fold elevation has been demonstrated for various penicillins.
BENEMID also has been reported to inhibit the renal transport of many other compounds including aminohippuric acid (PAH), aminosalicylic acid (PAS), indomethacin, sodium iodomethamate and related iodinated organic acids, 17-ketosteroids, pantothenic acid, phenolsulfonphthalein (PSP), sulfonamides, and sulfonylureas. See also DRUG INTERACTIONS.
BENEMID decreases both hepatic and renal excretion of sulfobromophthalein (BSP). The tubular reabsorption of phosphorus is inhibited in hypoparathyroid but not in euparathyroid individuals.
BENEMID does not influence plasma concentrations of salicylates, nor the excretion of streptomycin, chloramphenicol, chlortetracycline, oxytetracycline, or neomycin.

Indications

For treatment of the hyperuricemia associated with gout and gouty arthritis.
As an adjuvant to therapy with penicillin or with ampicillin, methicillin, oxacillin, cloxacillin, or nafcillin, for elevation and prolongation of plasma levels by whatever route the antibiotic is given.

Contraindications

Hypersensitivity to this product.
Children under 2 years of age.
Not recommended in persons with known blood dyscrasias or uric acid kidney stones.
Therapy with BENEMID should not be started until an acute gouty attack has subsided.

Warnings

Exacerbation of gout following therapy with BENEMID may occur; in such cases colchicine or other appropriate therapy is advisable.
BENEMID increases plasma concentrations of methotrexate in both animals and humans. In animal studies, increased methotrexate toxicity has been reported. If BENEMID is given with methotrexate, the dosage of methotrexate should be reduced and serum levels may need to be monitored.
In patients on BENEMID the use of salicylates in either small or large doses is contraindicated because it antagonizes the uricosuric action of BENEMID. The biphasic action of salicylates in the renal tubules accounts for the so-called "paradoxical effect" of uricosuric agents. In patients on BENEMID who require a mild analgesic agent the use of acetaminophen rather than small doses of salicylates would be preferred.
The appearance of hypersensitivity reactions requires cessation of therapy with BENEMID.
Use in Pregnancy: BENEMID crosses the placental barrier and appears in cord blood. The use of any drug in women of childbearing potential requires that the anticipated benefit be weighed against possible hazards.

Precautions

Hematuria, renal colic, costovertebral pain, and formation of uric acid stones associated with the use of BENEMID in gouty patients may be prevented by alkalization of the urine and a liberal fluid intake (*see* DOSAGE AND ADMINISTRATION). In these cases when alkali is administered, the acid-base balance of the patient should be watched.
Use with caution in patients with a history of peptic ulcer.
BENEMID has been used in patients with some renal impairment but dosage requirements may be increased. BENEMID may not be effective in chronic renal insufficiency particularly when the glomerular filtration rate is 30 ml/minute or less. Because of its mechanism of action, BENEMID is not recommended in conjunction with a penicillin in the presence of *known* renal impairment.
A reducing substance may appear in the urine of patients receiving BENEMID. This disappears with discontinuance of therapy. Suspected glycosuria should be confirmed by using a test specific for glucose.

Adverse Reactions

Headache, gastrointestinal symptoms (e.g., anorexia, nausea, vomiting), urinary frequency, hypersensitivity reactions (including anaphylaxis, dermatitis, pruritus, and fever), sore gums, flushing, dizziness, and anemia have occurred.
In gouty patients exacerbation of gout, and uric acid stones with or without hematuria, renal colic, or costovertebral pain, have been observed. Nephrotic syndrome, hepatic necrosis, and aplastic anemia occur rarely. Hemolytic anemia which in some instances could be related to genetic deficiency of glucose-6-phosphate dehydrogenase in red blood cells has been reported.

Drug Interactions

The use of salicylates antagonizes the uricosuric action of BENEMID (*see* WARNINGS). The uricosuric action of BENEMID is also antagonized by pyrazinamide.
BENEMID produces an insignificant increase in free sulfonamide plasma concentrations but a significant increase in total sulfonamide plasma levels. Since BENEMID decreases the renal excretion of conjugated sulfonamides, plasma concentrations of the latter should be determined from time to time when a sulfonamide and BENEMID are coadministered for prolonged periods. BENEMID may prolong or enhance the action of oral sulfonylureas and thereby increase the risk of hypoglycemia.
When BENEMID is given to patients receiving indomethacin, the plasma levels of indomethacin are likely to be increased. Therefore, a lower dosage of indomethacin may be required to produce a therapeutic effect, and increases in the dosage of indomethacin should be made cautiously and in small increments. BENEMID may increase plasma levels of rifampin. The clinical significance of this is not known.
In animals and in humans, BENEMID has been reported to increase plasma concentrations of methotrexate (*see* WARNINGS).
Falsely high readings for theophylline have been reported in an *in vitro* study, using the Schack and Waxler technic, when therapeutic concentrations of theophylline and BENEMID® were added to human plasma.

Dosage and Administration

Gout
Therapy with BENEMID should not be *started* until an acute gouty attack has subsided. However, if an acute attack is precipitated *during* therapy, BENEMID may be continued without changing the dosage, and full therapeutic dosage of colchicine or other appropriate therapy should be given to control the acute attack.
The recommended adult dosage is 0.25 g (½ tablet of BENEMID) twice a day for one week, followed by 0.5 g (1 tablet) twice a day thereafter.
Some degree of renal impairment may be present in patients with gout. A daily dosage of 1 g may be adequate. However, if necessary, the daily dosage may be increased by 0.5 g increments every 4 weeks within tolerance (and usually not above 2 g per day) if symptoms of gouty arthritis are not controlled or the 24 hour uric acid excretion is not above 700 mg.
As noted, BENEMID may not be effective in chronic renal insufficiency particularly when the glomerular filtration rate is 30 ml/minute or less.
Gastric intolerance may be indicative of overdosage, and may be corrected by decreasing the dosage.
As uric acid tends to crystallize out of an acid urine, a liberal fluid intake is recommended, as well as sufficient sodium bicarbonate (3 to 7.5 g daily) or potassium citrate (7.5 g daily) to maintain an alkaline urine (*see* PRECAUTIONS).
Alkalization of the urine is recommended until the serum urate level returns to normal limits and tophaceous deposits disappear, i.e., during the period when urinary excretion of uric acid is at a high level. Thereafter, alkalization of the urine and the usual restriction of purine-producing foods may be somewhat relaxed.
BENEMID should be continued at the dosage that will maintain normal serum urate levels. When acute attacks have been absent for 6 months or more and serum urate levels remain within normal limits, the daily dosage may be decreased by 0.5 g every 6 months. The maintenance dosage should not be reduced to the point where serum urate levels tend to rise.
BENEMID *and Penicillin Therapy (General)*
Adults:
The recommended dosage is 2 g (4 tablets of BENEMID) daily in divided doses. This dosage should be reduced in older patients in whom renal impairment may be present.
Children 2-14 years of age:
Initial dose: 25 mg/kg body weight (*or* 0.7 g/square meter body surface).
Maintenance dose: 40 mg/kg body weight (*or* 1.2 g/square meter body surface) per day, divided into 4 doses.
For children weighing more than 50 kg (110 lb) the adult dosage is recommended.
BENEMID is contraindicated in children under 2 years of age.
The PSP excretion test may be used to determine the effectiveness of BENEMID in retarding penicillin excretion and maintaining therapeutic levels. The renal clearance of PSP is reduced to about one-fifth the normal rate when dosage of BENEMID is adequate.
Penicillin Therapy (Gonorrhea)
[See table above].
[See table on next page].

How Supplied

No. 3337—Tablets BENEMID, 0.5 g, are yellow, capsule shaped, scored, film coated tablets, coded MSD 501. They are supplied as follows:
NDC 0006-0501-68 bottles of 100
(6505-00-104-9735 100's)
NDC 0006-0501-28 single unit packages of 100.
NDC 0006-0501-82 bottles of 1000.
(6505-00-181-8387 1000's)
[*Shown in Product Identification Section*]
A.H.F.S. 40:40
DC 6103915 Issued September 1978

BIAVAX®II ℞
(rubella and mumps virus vaccine, live, MSD), U.S.P.

Description

BIAVAX II (Rubella and Mumps Virus Vaccine, Live, MSD) is a live virus vaccine for immunization against rubella (German measles) and mumps.
BIAVAX II is a lyophilized preparation of MERUVAX®II (Rubella Virus Vaccine, Live, MSD), the Wistar RA 27/3 strain of live attenuated rubella virus grown in human diploid cell (WI-38) culture; and MUMPSVAX® (Mumps Virus Vaccine, Live, MSD), the Jeryl Lynn (B level) mumps strain grown in cell cultures of chick embryo. The two viruses are mixed before being lyophilized. The product contains no preservative.
When reconstituted as directed, the dose for injection is 0.5 ml and contains not less than 1,000 $TCID_{50}$ (tissue culture infectious doses) of Rubella Virus Vaccine, Live, and 5,000 $TCID_{50}$ of Mumps Virus Vaccine, Live, expressed in terms of the assigned titer of the FDA Reference Rubella and Mumps Viruses. Each dose contains approximately 25 mcg of neomycin.

Actions

Clinical studies of 73 double seronegative children 12 months to 2 years of age demonstrated that BIAVAX II is highly immunogenic and generally well tolerated. In these studies, a single injection of the vaccine induced rubella hemagglutination inhibition (HI) antibodies in 100 percent, and mumps neutralizing antibodies in 97 percent of the susceptible children. The RA 27/3 rubella strain in BIAVAX II elicits higher immediate post-vaccination HI, complement-fixing and neutralizing antibody levels than other strains of rubella vaccine and has been shown to induce a broader profile of circulating antibodies including anti-theta and anti-iota precipitating antibodies. The RA 27/3 rubella strain simulates natural infection more closely than other rubella vaccine

Continued on next page

Information on the Merck Sharp & Dohme products listed on these pages is the full prescribing information from package circulars in use October 31, 1979.

Merck Sharp & Dohme—Cont.

viruses. The broader profile of antibodies produced by RA 27/3 strain rubella virus vaccine appears to correlate with greater resistance to subclinical reinfection with the wild virus.
Data relating to persistence of vaccine-induced antibodies are not available for BIAVAX II at this time; however, it is expected that the antibodies against rubella and mumps will be just as durable following administration of BIAVAX II as after the single vaccines given separately. Antibody levels after immunization with RA 27/3 strain rubella virus vaccine have persisted for at least six years without substantial decline, and for ten years after MUMPSVAX (Mumps Virus Vaccine, Live, MSD).

Indications

BIAVAX II is indicated for simultaneous immunization against rubella and mumps in children from 15 months of age to puberty. It may be given as early as 12 months, if that offers greater convenience in scheduling.
The vaccine is not recommended for infants less than 12 months of age because they may retain maternal rubella and mumps neutralizing antibodies which may interfere with the immune response.
Revaccination: Based on available evidence, there is no reason to routinely revaccinate children originally vaccinated when 12 months of age or older; however, children vaccinated when younger than 12 months of age should be revaccinated. The decision to revaccinate should be based on evaluation of each individual case.

Contraindications

Do not give BIAVAX II to pregnant females; the possible effects of the vaccine on fetal development are unknown at this time. When vaccination of post-pubertal females is undertaken, pregnancy must be avoided for three months following vaccination.
Previously unimmunized children of susceptible pregnant women should receive live attenuated rubella vaccine, because an immunized child will be less likely to acquire natural rubella and introduce the virus into the household.
Hypersensitivity to neomycin (each dose of reconstituted vaccine contains approximately 25 mcg of neomycin).
Any febrile respiratory illness or other active febrile infection.
Patients receiving therapy with ACTH, corticosteroids, irradiation, alkylating agents or antimetabolites. This contraindication does not apply to patients who are receiving corticosteroids as replacement therapy, e.g., for Addison's disease.
Individuals with blood dyscrasias, leukemia, lymphomas of any type, or other malignant neoplasms affecting the bone marrow or lymphatic systems.
Primary immuno-deficiency states, including cellular immune deficiencies, hypogammaglobulinemic and dysgammaglobulinemic states.

Hypersensitivity to Eggs, Chicken, or Chicken Feathers

This vaccine is essentially devoid of potentially allergenic substances derived from host tissues

BENEMID® (Probenecid, MSD) Penicillin Therapy (Gonorrhea)*

	Recommended Regimens**	Remarks
Uncomplicated gonoococcal infection in men and women (urethral, cervical, rectal)	4.8 million units of aqueous procaine penicillin G† I.M., in at least 2 doses injected at different sites at one visit + 1 g of BENEMID (Probenecid, MSD) orally just before injections *or* 3.5 g of ampicillin† orally + 1 g of BENEMID orally given simultaneously.	Follow-up: Obtain urethral and other appropriate cultures from men, and cervical, anal, and other appropriate cultures from women, 7 to 14 days after completion of treatment. Treatment of sexual partners: Persons with known recent exposure to gonorrhea should receive same treatment as those known to have gonorrhea. Examination and treatment of male sex partners of persons with gonorrhea are essential because of high prevalence of nonsymptomatic urethral gonococcal infection in such men.
Pharyngeal gonococcal infection in men and women	4.8 million units of aqueous procaine penicillin G† I.M., in at least 2 doses injected at different sites at one visit + 1 g of BENEMID orally just before injections	Pharyngeal gonococcal infections may be more difficult to treat than anogenital gonorrhea. Posttreatment cultures are essential.
Uncomplicated gonorrhea in pregnant patients	4.8 million units of aqueous procaine penicillin G† I.M., in at least 2 doses injected at different sites at one visit *or* 3.5 g of ampicillin† orally + 1 g of BENEMID orally given simultaneously	
Acute gonococcal salpingitis	*Outpatients:* Aqueous procaine penicillin G† or ampicillin† with BENEMID as for gonorrhea in pregnancy, followed by 500 mg of ampicillin 4 times a day for 10 days *Hospitalized patients:* See details in CDC recommendations	Follow-up of patients with acute salpingitis is essential. All patients should receive repeat pelvic examinations and cultures for *Neisseria gonorrhoeae* after treatment. Examination and appropriate treatment of male sex partners are essential because of high prevalence of nonsymptomatic urethral gonorrhea in such men.
Disseminated gonococcal infection (arthritis-dermatitis syndrome)	10 million units of aqueous crystalline penicillin G† I.V. a day for 3 days or till significant clinical improvement occurs. May be followed with 500 mg of ampicillin† 4 times a day orally to complete 7 days of treatment *or* 3.5 g of ampicillin† orally with 1 g of BENEMID, followed by 500 mg of ampicillin† 4 times a day for at least 7 days	
Gonococcal infection in children	For postpubertal children and/or those weighing over 45 kg (100 lb) use the dosage regimens given above for adults Uncomplicated vulvovaginitis and urethritis: aqueous procaine penicillin G† 75,000—100,000 units/kg I.M., with BENEMID 23 mg/kg orally	See CDC recommendations for detailed information about prevention and treatment of neonatal gonococcal infection and gonococcal ophthalmia.

Note: Before treating gonococcal infections in patients with suspected primary or secondary syphilis, perform proper diagnostic procedures including darkfield examinations. If concomitant syphilis is suspected, perform monthly serological tests for at least 4 months.
* Recommended by Venereal Disease Control Advisory Committee, Center for Disease Control, U.S. Department of Health, Education, and Welfare, Public Health Service (Morbidity and Mortality Weekly Report, Vol. *23:* 341, 342, 347, 348, Oct. 11, 1974).
** See CDC recommendations for definition of regimens of choice, alternative regimens, treatment of hypersensitive patients, and other aspects of therapy.
† See package circulars of manufacturers for detailed information about contraindications, warnings, precautions, and adverse reactions.

(chick embryos).* However, since the mumps component is propagated in cell cultures of chick embryo, in considering vaccine use in patients hypersensitive to chicken or chicken eggs or feathers, the attending physician must weigh the benefits of immunization against the potential risks of hypersensitivity reactions.

Precautions

Administer BIAVAX II subcutaneously; *do not give intravenously.*

Epinephrine should be available for immediate use in case an anaphylactoid reaction occurs.

BIAVAX II should not be given less than one month before or after immunization with other *live* virus vaccines, with the exception of ATTENUVAX® (Measles Virus Vaccine, Live, Attenuated, MSD). There are no data available concerning simultaneous use of BIAVAX II with monovalent or trivalent poliovirus vaccine, live, oral.

Vaccination should be deferred for at least 3 months following blood or plasma transfusions, or administration of more than 0.02 ml of human immune serum globulin per pound of body weight.

Excretion of small amounts of the live attenuated rubella virus from the nose and throat has occurred in the majority of susceptible individuals 7–28 days after vaccination. There is no confirmed evidence to indicate that such virus is transmitted to susceptible persons who are in contact with the vaccinated individuals. Consequently, transmission, while accepted as a theoretical possibility, is not regarded as a significant risk.**

There are no reports of transmission of live attenuated mumps virus from vaccinees to susceptible contacts.

It has been reported that live attenuated rubella and mumps virus vaccines given individually may result in a temporary depression of tuberculin skin sensitivity. Therefore, if a tuberculin test is to be done, it should be administered either before or simultaneously with BIAVAX II.

As for any vaccine, vaccination with BIAVAX II may not result in seroconversion in 100% of susceptible subjects given the vaccine.

Adverse Reactions

The adverse clinical reactions associated with the use of BIAVAX II are those expected to follow administration of the monovalent vaccines given separately. These may include malaise, sore throat, headache, fever, and rash; mild local reactions such as erythema, induration, tenderness and regional lymphadenopathy; parotitis; orchitis; thrombocytopenia and purpura; allergic reactions such as urticaria; and arthritis, arthralgia and polyneuritis.

Moderate fever [101–102.9°F (38.3–39.4°C)] occurs occasionally, and high fever [above 103°F (39.4°C)] occurs less commonly. On rare occasions, children developing fever may exhibit febrile convulsions. Rash occurs infrequently and is usually minimal without generalized distribution.

Clinical experience with live attenuated rubella and mumps virus vaccines given individually indicates that encephalitis and other nervous system reactions have occurred very rarely. These might occur also with BIAVAX II.

Transient arthritis, arthralgia and polyneuritis are features of natural rubella and vary in frequency and severity with age and sex, being greatest in adult females and least in prepubertal children. This type of involvement has also been reported following administration of MERUVAX II (Rubella Virus Vaccine, Live, MSD). In children, joint reactions are rare and of brief duration if they do occur. In women, incidence rates for arthritis and arthralgia are generally higher than those seen in children (children: 0–3%; women: 12–20%), and the reactions tend to be more marked and of longer duration. Rarely, symptoms may persist for a matter of months. In adolescent girls, the reactions appear to be intermediate in incidence between those seen in children and in adult women. Even in older women (35–45 years), these reactions are generally well tolerated and rarely interfere with normal activities.

Dosage and Administration

After suitably cleansing the immunization site, inject the total volume of reconstituted vaccine subcutaneously, preferably into the outer aspect of the upper arm. Do not inject BIAVAX II intravenously.

Shipment, Storage, and Reconstitution

During shipment, to insure that there is no loss of potency, the vaccine must be maintained at a temperature of 10°C (50°F) or less.

Before reconstitution, store BIAVAX II at 2–8°C (35.6–46.4°F). *Protect from light.*

To reconstitute, use only the diluent supplied, since it is free of preservatives or other antiviral substances which might inactivate the vaccine. Inject all the diluent in the syringe into the vial of lyophilized vaccine, and agitate to mix thoroughly. Withdraw the entire contents into the syringe and inject the total volume of restored vaccine subcutaneously.

It is important to use a separate sterile syringe and needle for each individual patient to prevent transmission of hepatitis B and other infectious agents from one person to another.

The color of the vaccine when reconstituted is yellow.

It is recommended that the vaccine be used as soon as possible after reconstitution. Protect the vaccine from light at all times. Store reconstituted vaccine in a dark place at 2–8°C (35.6–46.4°F) and discard if not used within eight hours.

How Supplied

No. 4668—BIAVAX II is supplied as a single-dose vial of lyophilized vaccine with a disposable syringe containing diluent, and fitted with a 25 gauge, ⅝" needle, **NDC** 0006-4668-00.

No. 4669/4590—BIAVAX II is supplied as follows: (1) a box of ten single-dose vials of lyophilized vaccine, **NDC** 0006-4669-00; and (2) a box of ten diluent-containing disposable syringes with affixed 25 gauge, ⅝" needles. To conserve refrigerator space, the syringes may be stored separately at room temperature.

* Morbidity and Mortality Weekly Report *25*(44): 350, Nov. 12, 1976.

** Recommendation of the Public Health Service Advisory Committee on Immunization Practices, Morbidity and Mortality Weekly Report, *26*(47): 385, 386, 391, Nov. 25, 1977.

A.H.F.S. 80:12

DC 7032301 Issued October 1978

CLINORIL® Tablets ℞
(sulindac, MSD)

Description

Sulindac is a nonsteroidal, anti-inflammatory indene derivative designated chemically as (Z)-5-fluoro-2-methyl-1- [[*p*-(methylsulfinyl) phenyl]methylene]- 1*H*- indene-3-acetic acid. It is not a salicylate, pyrazolone or propionic acid derivative. Its empirical formula is $C_{20}H_{17}FO_3S$, with a molecular weight of 356.42. Sulindac, a yellow crystalline compound, is a weak organic acid practically insoluble in water below pH 4.5, but soluble as the sodium salt or in buffers of pH 6 or higher.

Following absorption, sulindac undergoes two major biotransformations—reversible reduction to the sulfide metabolite, and irreversible oxidation to the sulfone metabolite. Available evidence indicates that the biological activity resides with the sulfide metabolite.

Clinical Pharmacology

CLINORIL (Sulindac, MSD) is a nonsteroidal anti-inflammatory drug, also possessing analgesic and antipyretic activities. Its mode of action, like that of other nonsteroidal, anti-inflammatory agents, is not known; however, its therapeutic action is not due to pituitary-adrenal stimulation. Inhibition of prostaglandin synthesis by the sulfide metabolite may be involved in the anti-inflammatory action of CLINORIL.

Sulindac is approximately 90% absorbed in man after oral administration. The peak plasma concentrations of the biologically active sulfide metabolite are achieved in about two hours when sulindac is administered in the fasting state, and in about three to four hours when sulindac is administered with food. The mean half-life of sulindac is 7.8 hours while the mean half-life of the sulfide metabolite is 16.4 hours. Sustained plasma levels of the sulfide metabolite are consistent with a prolonged anti-inflammatory action which is the rationale for a twice per day dosage schedule.

Sulindac and its two metabolites undergo extensive enterohepatic circulation in animals. Similar enterohepatic circulation together with the reversible metabolism are probably major contributors to sustained plasma levels of the active drug in man.

The primary route of excretion in man is via the urine as both sulindac and its sulfone metabolite (free as well as glucuronides). Approximately 50% of the administered dose is excreted in the urine, with the sulfone metabolite accounting for the major portion. Less than 1% of the administered dose of sulindac appears in the urine as the sulfide metabolite. Approximately 25% is found in the feces, primarily as the sulfone and sulfide metabolites.

The bioavailability of sulindac, as assessed by urinary excretion, was not changed by concomitant administration of an antacid containing magnesium and aluminum hydroxides (MAALOX®).

In healthy men, the average fecal blood loss, measured over a two-week period during administration of 400 mg per day of CLINORIL, was similar to that for placebo, and was statistically significantly less than that resulting from 4800 mg per day of aspirin.

In controlled clinical studies CLINORIL was evaluated in the following five conditions:

1. *Osteoarthritis*

In patients with osteoarthritis of the hip and knee, the anti-inflammatory and analgesic activity of CLINORIL was demonstrated by clinical measurements that included: assessments by both patient and investigator of overall response; decrease in disease activity as assessed by both patient and investigator; improvement in ARA Functional Class; relief of night pain; improvement in overall evaluation of pain, including pain on weight bearing and pain on active and passive motion; improvement in joint mobility, range of motion, and functional activities; decreased swelling and tenderness; and decreased duration of stiffness following prolonged inactivity.

In clinical studies in which dosages were adjusted according to patient needs, CLINORIL 200 to 400 mg daily was shown to be comparable in effectiveness to aspirin 2400 to 4800 mg daily. CLINORIL was generally well tolerated, and patients on it had a lower overall incidence of total adverse effects, of milder gastrointesti-

Continued on next page

Information on the Merck Sharp & Dohme products listed on these pages is the full prescribing information from package circulars in use October 31, 1979.

Merck Sharp & Dohme—Cont.

nal reactions, and of tinnitus than did patients on aspirin. (See ADVERSE REACTIONS.)

2. *Rheumatoid Arthritis*

In patients with rheumatoid arthritis, the anti-inflammatory and analgesic activity of CLINORIL was demonstrated by clinical measurements that included: assessments by both patient and investigator of overall response; decrease in disease activity as assessed by both patient and investigator; reduction in overall joint pain; reduction in duration and severity of morning stiffness; reduction in day and night pain; decrease in time required to walk 50 feet; decrease in general pain as measured on a visual analog scale; improvement in the Ritchie articular index; decrease in proximal interphalangeal joint size; improvement in ARA Functional Class; increase in grip strength; reduction in painful joint count and score; reduction in swollen joint count and score; and increased flexion and extension of the wrist.

In clinical studies in which dosages were adjusted according to patient needs, CLINORIL 300 to 400 mg daily was shown to be comparable in effectiveness to aspirin 3600 to 4800 mg daily. CLINORIL was generally well tolerated, and patients on it had a lower overall incidence of total adverse effects, of milder gastrointestinal reactions, and of tinnitus than did patients on aspirin. (See ADVERSE REACTIONS.)

In patients with rheumatoid arthritis, CLINORIL may be used in combination with gold salts at usual dosage levels. In clinical studies, CLINORIL added to the regimen of gold salts usually resulted in additional symptomatic relief but did not alter the course of the underlying disease.

3. *Ankylosing spondylitis*

In patients with ankylosing spondylitis, the anti-inflammatory and analgesic activity of CLINORIL was demonstrated by clinical measurements that included: assessments by both patient and investigator of overall response; decrease in disease activity as assessed by both patient and investigator; improvement in ARA Functional Class; improvement in patient and investigator evaluation of spinal pain, tenderness and/or spasm; reduction in the duration of morning stiffness; increase in the time to onset of fatigue; relief of night pain; increase in chest expansion; and increase in spinal mobility evaluated by fingers-to-floor distance, occiput to wall distance, the Schober Test, and the Wright Modification of the Schober Test. In a clinical study in which dosages were adjusted according to patient need, CLINORIL 200 to 400 mg daily was as effective as indomethacin 75 to 150 mg daily. In a second study, CLINORIL 300 to 400 mg daily was comparable in effectiveness to phenylbutazone 400 to 600 mg daily. CLINORIL was better tolerated than phenylbutazone. (See ADVERSE REACTIONS.)

4. *Acute painful shoulder (Acute subacromial bursitis/supraspinatus tendinitis)*

In patients with acute painful shoulder (acute subacromial bursitis/supraspinatus tendinitis), the anti-inflammatory and analgesic activity of CLINORIL was demonstrated by clinical measurements that included: assessments by both patient and investigator of overall response; relief of night pain, spontaneous pain, and pain on active motion; decrease in local tenderness; and improvement in range of motion measured by abduction, and internal and external rotation. In clinical studies in acute painful shoulder, CLINORIL 300 to 400 mg daily and oxyphenbutazone 400 to 600 mg daily were shown to be equally effective and well tolerated.

5. *Acute gouty arthritis*

In patients with acute gouty arthritis, the anti-inflammatory and analgesic activity of CLINORIL was demonstrated by clinical measurements that included: assessments by both the patient and investigator of overall response; relief of weight-bearing pain; relief of pain at rest and on active and passive motion; decrease in tenderness; reduction in warmth and swelling; increase in range of motion; and improvement in ability to function. In clinical studies, CLINORIL at 400 mg daily and phenylbutazone at 600 mg daily were show to be equally effective. In these short-term studies in which reduction of dosage was permitted according to response, both drugs were equally well tolerated.

Indications and Usage

CLINORIL is indicated for acute or long-term use in the relief of signs and symptoms of the following:

1. Osteoarthritis
2. Rheumatoid arthritis*
3. Ankylosing spondylitis
4. Acute painful shoulder (Acute subacromial bursitis/supraspinatus tendinitis)
5. Acute gouty arthritis

Contraindications

CLINORIL should not be used in:

Patients who are hypersensitive to this product.

Patients in whom acute asthmatic attacks, urticaria, or rhinitis are precipitated by aspirin or other nonsteroidal anti-inflammatory agents.

Warnings

Peptic ulceration and gastrointestinal bleeding have been reported in patients receiving CLINORIL. In patients with active gastrointestinal bleeding or an active peptic ulcer, an appropriate ulcer regimen should be instituted, and the physician must weigh the benefits of therapy with CLINORIL against possible hazards, and carefully monitor the patient's progress. When CLINORIL is given to patients with a history of upper gastrointestinal tract disease, it should be given under close supervision and only after consulting the ADVERSE REACTIONS section.

Precautions

General

Although CLINORIL has less effect on platelet function and bleeding time than aspirin, it is an inhibitor of platelet function; therefore, patients who may be adversely affected should be carefully observed when CLINORIL is administered.

Abnormalities in liver function tests, particularly elevated alkaline phosphatase, may occur. These are usually transient. If an abnormal liver function test occurs, it should be monitored until it returns to normal. If a significant abnormality persists, CLINORIL should be discontinued.

Because of reports of adverse eye findings with nonsteroidal anti-inflammatory agents, it is recommended that patients who develop eye complaints during treatment with CLINORIL have ophthalmologic studies.

Since CLINORIL is eliminated primarily by the kidneys, patients with significantly impaired renal function should be closely monitored and a reduction of daily dosage may be anticipated to avoid excessive drug accumulation.

*The safety and effectiveness of CLINORIL have not been established in rheumatoid arthritis patients who are designated in the American Rheumatism Association classification as Functional Class IV (incapacitated, largely or wholly bedridden, or confined to wheelchair; little or no self-care).

In chronic studies in mice, rats and monkeys at high dosages, there were occasional occurrences of mild renal toxicity as evidenced by papillary edema or mild interstitial nephritis in some animals. Papillary necrosis occurred infrequently in mice and rats. However, there has been no evidence to date of renal toxicity in clinical studies.

Peripheral edema has been observed in some patients taking CLINORIL. Therefore, as with other non-steroidal anti-inflammatory drugs, CLINORIL should be used with caution in patients with compromised cardiac function, hypertension, or other conditions predisposing to fluid retention.

CLINORIL may allow a reduction in dosage or the elimination of chronic corticosteroid therapy in some patients with rheumatoid arthritis. However, it is generally necessary to reduce corticosteroids gradually over several months in order to avoid an exacerbation of disease or signs and symptoms of adrenal insufficiency. Abrupt withdrawal of chronic corticosteroid treatment is generally not recommended even when patients have had a serious complication of chronic corticosteroid therapy.

Use in Pregnancy

CLINORIL is not recommended for use in pregnant women, since safety for use has not been established. In reproduction studies in the rat, a decrease in average fetal weight and an increase in numbers of dead pups were observed on the first day of the postpartum period at dosage levels of 20 and 40 mg/kg/day (2½ and 5 times the usual maximum daily dose in humans), although there was no adverse effect on the survival and growth during the remainder of the postpartum period. CLINORIL prolongs the duration of gestation in rats, as do other compounds of this class which also may cause dystocia and delayed parturition in pregnant animals. Visceral and skeletal malformations observed in low incidence among rabbits in some teratology studies did not occur at the same dosage levels in repeat studies, nor at a higher dosage level in the same species.

Nursing Mothers

Nursing should not be undertaken while a patient is on CLINORIL. It is not known whether sulindac is secreted in human milk; however, it is secreted in the milk of lactating rats.

Use in Children

Pediatric indications and dosage have not been established, but studies in juvenile rheumatoid arthritis are in progress.

Drug Interactions

Although sulindac and its sulfide metabolite are highly bound to protein, studies have shown no clinically significant interaction with oral anticoagulants or oral hypoglycemic agents. However, until wider clinical experience is obtained, CLINORIL should be used with caution in patients receiving such agents.

The concomitant administration of aspirin with sulindac significantly depressed the plasma levels of the active sulfide metabolite. Clinical studies to demonstrate whether or not there is any beneficial effect or harmful interaction with the use of CLINORIL in conjunction with aspirin have not been completed. Therefore, the combination cannot be recommended.

Probenecid given concomitantly with sulindac had only a slight effect on plasma sulfide levels, while plasma levels of sulindac and sulfone were increased. Sulindac was shown to produce a modest reduction in the uricosuric action of probenecid, which probably is not significant under most circumstances.

Neither propoxyphene hydrochloride nor acetaminophen had any effect on the plasma levels of sulindac or its sulfide metabolite.

Adverse Reactions

The adverse reactions which have been observed in clinical trials encompass observations in 1,865 patients, including 232 observed for at least 48 weeks.

Incidence Greater Than 1%

Gastrointestinal

The most frequent types of adverse reactions occurring with CLINORIL are gastrointestinal; these include gastrointestinal pain (10%), dyspepsia*, nausea* with or without vomiting, diarrhea*, constipation*, flatulence, anorexia and gastrointestinal cramps.

Dermatologic

Rash*, pruritus.

Central Nervous System

Dizziness*, headache*, nervousness.

Special Senses

Tinnitus.

Miscellaneous

Edema.

Incidence Less Than 1 in 100

The following adverse reactions, occurring less frequently than one in 100, were reported in clinical trials or have been reported since the drug was marketed. The probability exists of a causal relationship between CLINORIL and these adverse reactions.

Gastrointestinal

Gastritis or gastroenteritis. Peptic ulcer was reported in seven patients (1 in 250). Gastrointestinal bleeding was reported in three patients (1 in 600).

Liver function abnormalities associated with jaundice have been reported rarely.

Dermatologic

Stomatitis, sore or dry mucous membranes.

Nervous System

Vertigo.

Miscellaneous

Hypersensitivity, including fever, which may be accompanied by chills, skin rash, leukopenia or eosinophilia.

Causal Relationship Unknown

Other reactions have been reported but occurred under circumstances where a causal relationship could not be established. However, in these rarely reported events, that possibility cannot be excluded. Therefore, these observations are listed to serve as alerting information to physicians.

Dermatologic

Toxic epidermal necrolysis.

Cardiovascular

Hypertension.

Nervous System

Paresthesias, neuritis.

Special Senses

Transient visual disturbances, decreased hearing.

Respiratory

Epistaxis.

Psychiatric

Depression.

Management of Overdosage

In the event of overdosage, the stomach should be emptied by inducing vomiting or by gastric lavage, and the patient carefully observed and given symptomatic and supportive treatment.

Dosage and Administration

CLINORIL should be administered orally twice a day with food. In clinical studies to date, the usual maximum dosage was 400 mg per day. Although a few patients have received higher dosages, until further clinical experience is obtained, dosages above 400 mg per day are not recommended.

In osteoarthritis, rheumatoid arthritis, and ankylosing spondylitis, the recommended starting dosage is 150 mg twice a day. The dosage may be lowered or raised depending on the response.

In acute painful shoulder (acute subacromial bursitis/supraspinatus tendinitis) and acute gouty arthritis, the recommended dosage is 200 mg twice a day. After a satisfactory response has been achieved, the dosage may be reduced according to the response. In acute painful shoulder, therapy for 7–14 days is usually adequate. In acute gouty arthritis, therapy for 7 days is usually adequate.

How Supplied

CLINORIL is available for oral administration as 150 mg yellow tablets, and as 200 mg scored yellow tablets.

No. 3360—Tablets CLINORIL 150 mg are yellow, hexagon-shaped, compressed tablets, coded MSD 941. They are supplied as follows:
NDC 0006-0941-68 in bottles of 100.

No. 3353—Tablets CLINORIL 200 mg are yellow, hexagon-shaped, scored, compressed tablets, coded MSD 942. They are supplied as follows:
NDC 0006-0942-68 in bottles of 100.

[*Shown in Product Identification Section*]

A.H.F.S. 28:08

DC 7020001 Issued March 1979

*Incidence between 3% and 9%. Those reactions occurring in 1 to 3% of patients are not marked with an asterisk.

COGENTIN® Tablets ℞
(benztropine mesylate, MSD), U.S.P.
COGENTIN® Injection ℞
(benztropine mesylate, MSD), U.S.P.

Description

Benztropine mesylate is a synthetic compound resulting from the combination of the active portions of atropine and diphenhydramine.

It is a crystalline white powder, very soluble in water.

If its formula is compared with that of atropine, and that of diphenhydramine, it can be seen that benztropine contains the tropine portion of the atropine molecule and the benzohydryl portion of diphenhydramine.

COGENTIN (Benztropine Mesylate, MSD) is supplied as tablets in three strengths (0.5 mg, 1 mg, and 2 mg per tablet), and as an injection for intravenous and intramuscular use.

Each milliliter of the injection contains:

Benztropine mesylate	1.0 mg
Sodium chloride	9.0 mg
Water for injection q.s.	1.0 ml

Actions

COGENTIN possesses both anticholinergic and antihistaminic effects, although only the former have been established as therapeutically significant in the management of parkinsonism.

In the isolated guinea pig ileum, the anticholinergic activity of this drug is about equal to that of atropine; however, when administered orally to unanesthetized cats, it is only about half as active as atropine.

In laboratory animals, its antihistaminic activity and duration of action approach those of pyrilamine maleate.

Indications

For use as an adjunct in the therapy of all forms of parkinsonism.

Useful also in the control of extrapyramidal disorders (except tardive dyskinesia—see PRECAUTIONS) due to neuroleptic drugs (e.g., phenothiazines).

Contraindications

Hypersensitivity to COGENTIN tablets or to any component of COGENTIN injection.

Because of its atropine-like side effects, this drug is contraindicated in children under three years of age, and should be used with caution in older children.

Warnings

Safe use in pregnancy has not been established.

COGENTIN may impair mental and/or physical abilities required for performance of hazardous tasks, such as operating machinery or driving a motor vehicle.

When COGENTIN is given concomitantly with phenothiazines or other drugs with anticholinergic activity, patients should be advised to report gastrointestinal complaints promptly. Paralytic ileus, sometimes fatal, has occurred in patients taking anticholinergic-type antiparkinsonism drugs, including COGENTIN, in combination with phenothiazines and/or tricyclic antidepressants.

Since COGENTIN contains structural features of atropine, it may produce anhidrosis. For this reason, it should be administered with caution during hot weather, especially when given concomitantly with other atropine-like drugs to the chronically ill, the alcoholic, those who have central nervous system disease, and those who do manual labor in a hot environment. Anhidrosis may occur more readily when some disturbance of sweating already exists. If there is evidence of anhidrosis, the possibility of hyperthermia should be considered. Dosage should be decreased at the discretion of the physician so that the ability to maintain body heat equilibrium by perspiration is not impaired. Severe anhidrosis and fatal hyperthermia have occurred.

Precautions

Since COGENTIN has cumulative action, continued supervision is advisable. Patients with a tendency to tachycardia and patients with prostatic hypertrophy should be observed closely during treatment.

Dysuria may occur, but rarely becomes a problem.

In large doses, the drug may cause complaints of weakness and inability to move particular muscle groups. For example, if the neck has been rigid and suddenly relaxes, it may feel weak, causing some concern. In this event, dosage adjustment is required.

Mental confusion and excitement may occur with large doses, or in susceptible patients. Visual hallucinations have been reported occasionally. Furthermore, in the treatment of extrapyramidal disorders due to neuroleptic drugs (e.g., phenothiazines), in patients with mental disorders, occasionally there may be intensification of mental symptoms. In such cases, at times, increased doses of antiparkinsonian drugs can precipitate a toxic psychosis. These patients should be kept under careful observation, especially at the beginning of treatment or if dosage is increased.

Tardive dyskinesia may appear in some patients on long-term therapy with phenothiazines and related agents, or may occur after therapy with these drugs has been discontinued. Antiparkinsonism agents do not alleviate the symptoms of tardive dyskinesia, and in some instances may aggravate them. COGENTIN is not recommended for use in patients with tardive dyskinesia.

The physician should be aware of the possible occurrence of glaucoma. Although the drug does not appear to have any adverse effect on

Continued on next page

Information on the Merck Sharp & Dohme products listed on these pages is the full prescribing information from package circulars in use October 31, 1979.

Merck Sharp & Dohme—Cont.

simple glaucoma, it probably should not be used in angle-closure glaucoma.

Adverse Reactions

Adverse reactions may be anticholinergic or antihistaminic in nature.
Dry mouth, blurred vision, nausea, and nervousness may develop. Adjustment of dosage or time of administration sometimes helps to control these reactions. If dry mouth is so severe that there is difficulty in swallowing or speaking, or loss of appetite and weight, reduce dosage, or discontinue the drug temporarily.
Vomiting occurs infrequently. Nausea unaccompanied by vomiting usually can be disregarded. Slight reduction in dosage may control the nausea and still give sufficient relief of symptoms. Vomiting may be controlled by temporary discontinuation, followed by resumption at a lower dosage.
Other adverse reactions include constipation, numbness of the fingers, listlessness and depression.
Occasionally, an allergic reaction, e.g., skin rash, develops. Sometimes this can be controlled by reducing dosage, but occasionally medication has to be discontinued.

Dosage and Administration

COGENTIN tablets should be used when patients are able to take oral medication.
The injection is especially useful for psychotic patients with acute dystonic reactions or other reactions that make oral medication difficult or impossible. It is recommended also when a more rapid response is desired than can be obtained with the tablets.
Since there is no significant difference in onset of effect after intravenous or intramuscular injection, usually there is no need to use the intravenous route. The drug is quickly effective after either route, with improvement sometimes noticeable a few minutes after injection. In emergency situations, when the condition of the patient is alarming, 1 to 2 ml of the injection normally will provide quick relief. If the parkinsonian effect begins to return, the dose can be repeated.
Because of cumulative action, therapy should be initiated with a low dose which is increased gradually at five or six-day intervals to the smallest amount necessary for optimal relief. Increases should be made in increments of 0.5 mg, to a maximum of 6 mg, or until optimal results are obtained without excessive adverse reactions.
Postencephalitic and Idiopathic Parkinsonism—
The usual daily dose is 1 to 2 mg, with a range of 0.5 to 6 mg orally or parenterally.
As with any agent used in parkinsonism, dosage must be individualized according to age and weight, and the type of parkinsonism being treated. Generally, older patients and thin patients cannot tolerate large doses. Most patients with postencephalitic parkinsonism need fairly large doses and tolerate them well. Patients with a poor mental outlook are usually poor candidates for therapy.
In idiopathic parkinsonism, therapy may be initiated with a single daily dose of 0.5 to 1 mg at bedtime. In some patients, this will be adequate; in others 4 to 6 mg a day may be required.
In postencephalitic parkinsonism, therapy may be initiated in most patients with 2 mg a day in one or more doses. In highly sensitive patients, therapy may be initiated with 0.5 mg at bedtime, and increased as necessary.
Some patients experience greatest relief by taking the entire dose at bedtime; others react more favorably to divided doses, two to four times a day. Frequently, one dose a day is sufficient, and divided doses may be unnecessary or undesirable.
The long duration of action of this drug makes it particularly suitable for bedtime medication when its effects may last throughout the night, enabling patients to turn in bed during the night more easily, and to rise in the morning.
When COGENTIN is started, do not terminate therapy with other antiparkinsonian agents abruptly. If the other agents are to be reduced or discontinued, it must be done gradually.
Many patients obtain greatest relief with combination therapy.
COGENTIN may be used concomitantly with SINEMET® (a combination of carbidopa and levodopa), or with levodopa, in which case periodic dosage adjustment may be required in order to maintain optimum response.
Drug-Induced Extrapyramidal Disorders—In treating extrapyramidal disorders due to neuroleptic drugs (e.g., phenothiazines), the recommended dosage is 1 to 4 mg once or twice a day orally or parenterally. Dosage must be individualized according to the need of the patient. Some patients require more than recommended; others do not need as much.
In acute dystonic reactions, 1 to 2 ml of the injection usually relieves the condition quickly. After that, the tablets, 1 to 2 mg twice a day, usually prevent recurrence.
When extrapyramidal disorders develop soon after initiation of treatment with neuroleptic drugs (e.g., phenothiazines), they are likely to be transient. One to 2 mg of COGENTIN tablets two or three times a day usually provides relief within one or two days. After one or two weeks, the drug should be withdrawn to determine the continued need for it. If such disorders recur, COGENTIN can be reinstituted.
Certain drug-induced extrapyramidal disorders that develop slowly may not respond to COGENTIN.

Overdosage

Manifestations—May be any of those seen in atropine poisoning or antihistamine overdosage: CNS depression, preceded or followed by stimulation; confusion; nervousness; listlessness; intensification of mental symptoms or toxic psychosis in patients with mental illness being treated with neuroleptic drugs (e.g., phenothiazines); hallucinations (especially visual); dizziness; muscle weakness; ataxia; dry mouth; mydriasis; blurred vision; palpitations; nausea; vomiting; dysuria; numbness of fingers; dysphagia; allergic reactions, e.g., skin rash; headache; hot, dry, flushed skin; delirium; coma; shock; convulsions; respiratory arrest; anhidrosis; hyperthermia; glaucoma; constipation.
Treatment—Physostigmine salicylate, 1 to 2 mg, sc or iv, reportedly will reverse symptoms of anticholinergic intoxication (Duvoisin, R.C.; Katz, R.: J. Amer. Med. Ass. *206*:1963-1965, Nov. 25, 1968). A second injection may be given after 2 hours if required. Otherwise treatment is symptomatic and supportive. Induce emesis or perform gastric lavage (contraindicated in precomatose, convulsive, or psychotic states). Maintain respiration. A short-acting barbiturate may be used for CNS excitement, but with caution to avoid subsequent depression; supportive care for depression (avoid convulsant stimulants such as picrotoxin, pentylenetetrazol, or bemegride); artificial respiration for severe respiratory depression; a local miotic for mydriasis and cycloplegia; ice bags or other cold applications and alcohol sponges for hyperpyrexia, a vasopressor and fluids for circulatory collapse. Darken room for photophobia.

How Supplied

No. 3297—Tablets COGENTIN, 0.5 mg, are white, round, scored, compressed tablets, coded MSD 21. They are supplied as follows:
NDC 0006-0021-68 in bottles of 100.
[*Shown in Product Identification Section*]
No. 3334—Tablets COGENTIN, 1 mg, are white, oval shaped, scored, compressed tablets, coded MSD 635. They are supplied as follows:
NDC 0006-0635-68 in bottles of 100.
NDC 0006-0635-28 single unit packages of 100.
[*Shown in Product Identification Section*]
No. 3172—Tablets COGENTIN, 2 mg, are white, round, scored, compressed tablets, coded MSD 60. They are supplied as follows:
NDC 0006-0060-68 in bottles of 100.
(6505-00-680-1907 2 mg 100's)
NDC 0006-0060-28 single unit packages of 100.
NDC 0006-0060-82 in bottles of 1000.
[*Shown in Product Identification Section*]
No. 3275—Injection COGENTIN, 1 mg per ml, is a clear, colorless solution and is supplied as follows:
NDC 0006-3275-16 in boxes of 6×2 ml ampuls.
A.H.F.S. 12:08
DC 6460713 Issued September 1978

ColBENEMID® Tablets ℞
Uricosuric

Description

ColBENEMID® contains BENEMID® (Probenecid, MSD) and colchicine.
Probenecid is the generic name for 4-[(dipropylamino) sulfonyl] benzoic acid (molecular weight 285.36).
Probenecid is a white or nearly white, fine, crystalline powder. It is soluble in dilute alkali, in alcohol, in chloroform, and in acetone; it is practically insoluble in water and in dilute acids.
Colchicine is an alkaloid obtained from various species of Colchicum. The chemical name for colchicine is (*S*)-*N*-(5,6,7,9-tetrahydro-1,2,3,10-tetramethoxy-9-oxobenzo [*a*] heptalen-7-yl) acetamide (molecular weight 399.43). Colchicine consists of pale yellow scales or powder; it darkens on exposure to light. Colchicine is soluble in water, freely soluble in alcohol and in chloroform, and slightly soluble in ether.

Actions

Probenecid is a uricosuric and renal tubular blocking agent. It inhibits the tubular reabsorption of urate, thus increasing the urinary excretion of uric acid and decreasing serum urate levels. Effective uricosuria reduces the miscible urate pool, retards urate deposition, and promotes resorption of urate deposits.
Probenecid inhibits the tubular secretion of penicillin and usually increases penicillin plasma levels by any route the antibiotic is given. A 2-fold to 4-fold elevation has been demonstrated for various penicillins.
Probenecid also has been reported to inhibit the renal transport of many other compounds including aminohippuric acid (PAH), aminosalicylic acid (PAS), indomethacin, sodium iodomethamate and related iodinated organic acids, 17-ketosteroids, pantothenic acid, phenolsulfonphthalein (PSP), sulfonamides, and sulfonylureas. See also DRUG INTERACTIONS.
Probenecid decreases both hepatic and renal excretion of sulfobromophthalein (BSP). The tubular reabsorption of phosphorus is inhibited in hypoparathyroid but not in euparathyroid individuals.
Probenecid does not influence plasma concentrations of salicylates, nor the excretion of streptomycin, chloramphenicol, chlortetracycline, oxytetracycline, or neomycin.
The mode of action of colchicine in gout is unknown. It is not an analgesic, though it relieves pain in acute attacks of gout. It is not a uricosuric agent and will not prevent progression of gout to chronic gouty arthritis. It does have a prophylactic, suppressive effect that helps to reduce the incidence of acute attacks and to

relieve the residual pain and mild discomfort that patients with gout occasionally feel.
In man and certain other animals, colchicine can produce a temporary leukopenia that is followed by leukocytosis.
Colchicine has other pharmacologic actions in animals: It alters neuromuscular function, intensifies gastrointestinal activity by neurogenic stimulation, increases sensitivity to central depressants, heightens response to sympathomimetic compounds, depresses the respiratory center, constricts blood vessels, causes hypertension by central vasomotor stimulation, and lowers body temperature.

Indications

For the treatment of chronic gouty arthritis when complicated by frequent, recurrent acute attacks of gout.

Contraindications

Hypersensitivity to this product or to probenecid or colchicine.
Children under 2 years of age.
Not recommended in persons with known blood dyscrasias or uric acid kidney stones.
Therapy with ColBENEMID should not be started until an acute gouty attack has subsided.
Pregnancy: Probenecid crosses the placental barrier and appears in cord blood. Colchicine can arrest cell division in animals and plants. In certain species of animal under certain conditions, colchicine has produced teratogenic effects. The possibility of such effects in humans also has been reported. Because of the colchicine component, ColBENEMID is contraindicated in pregnant patients. The use of any drug in women of childbearing potential requires that the anticipated benefit be weighed against possible hazards.

Warnings

Exacerbation of gout following therapy with ColBENEMID may occur; in such cases additional colchicine or other appropriate therapy is advisable.
Probenecid increases plasma concentrations of methotrexate in both animals and humans. In animal studies, increased methotrexate toxicity has been reported. If ColBENEMID is given with methotrexate, the dosage of methotrexate should be reduced and serum levels may need to be monitored.
In patients on ColBENEMID the use of salicylates in either small or large doses is contraindicated because it antagonizes the uricosuric action of probenecid. The biphasic action of salicylates in the renal tubules accounts for the so-called "paradoxical effect" of uricosuric agents. In patients on ColBENEMID who require a mild analgesic agent the use of acetaminophen rather than small doses of salicylates would be preferred.
The appearance of hypersensitivity reactions requires cessation of therapy with ColBENEMID.
Colchicine has been reported to adversely affect spermatogenesis in animals. Reversible azoospermia has been reported in one patient.

Precautions

Hematuria, renal colic, costovertebral pain, and formation of uric acid stones associated with the use of ColBENEMID in gouty patients may be prevented by alkalization of the urine and a liberal fluid intake (*see* DOSAGE AND ADMINISTRATION). In these cases when alkali is administered, the acid-base balance of the patient should be watched.
Use with caution in patients with a history of peptic ulcer.
ColBENEMID has been used in patients with some renal impairment but dosage requirements may be increased. ColBENEMID may not be effective in chronic renal insufficiency particularly when the glomerular filtration rate is 30 ml/minute or less.
A reducing substance may appear in the urine of patients receiving probenecid. This disappears with discontinuance of therapy. Suspected glycosuria should be confirmed by using a test specific for glucose.

Adverse Reactions

Headache, gastrointestinal symptoms (e.g., anorexia, nausea, vomiting), urinary frequency, hypersensitivity reactions (including anaphylaxis, dermatitis, pruritus, and fever), sore gums, flushing, dizziness, and anemia have occurred following the use of probenecid. In gouty patients exacerbation of gout, and uric acid stones with or without hematuria, renal colic, or costovertebral pain, have been observed. Nephrotic syndrome, hepatic necrosis, and aplastic anemia occur rarely. Hemolytic anemia which in some instances could be related to genetic deficiency of glucose-6-phosphate dehydrogenase in red blood cells has been reported.
Side effects due to colchicine appear to be a function of dosage. The most prominent symptoms are referable to the gastrointestinal tract (e.g., nausea, vomiting, abdominal pain, diarrhea) and may be particularly troublesome in the presence of peptic ulcer or spastic colon. At toxic doses colchicine may cause severe diarrhea, generalized vascular damage, and renal damage with hematuria and oliguria. Muscular weakness, which disappears with discontinuance of therapy, urticaria, dermatitis, and purpura have also been reported. Hypersensitivity to colchicine is a very rare occurrence, but should be borne in mind. The appearance of any of the aforementioned symptoms may require reduction of dosage or discontinuance of the drug.
When given for prolonged periods, colchicine may cause agranulocytosis, aplastic anemia, and peripheral neuritis. Loss of hair attributable to colchicine therapy has been reported. The possibility of increased colchicine toxicity in the presence of hepatic dysfunction should be considered.

Drug Interactions

The use of salicylates antagonizes the uricosuric action of probenecid (*see* WARNINGS).
Probenecid produces an insignificant increase in free sulfonamide plasma concentrations but a significant increase in total sulfonamide plasma levels. Since probenecid decreases the renal excretion of conjugated sulfonamides, plasma concentrations of the latter should be determined from time to time when a sulfonamide and ColBENEMID are coadministered for prolonged periods. Probenecid may prolong or enhance the action of oral sulfonylureas and thereby increase the risk of hypoglycemia.
When probenecid is given to patients receiving indomethacin, the plasma levels of indomethacin are likely to be increased. Therefore, a lower dosage of indomethacin may be required to produce a therapeutic effect, and increases in the dosage of indomethacin should be made cautiously and in small increments. Probenecid may increase plasma levels of rifampin. The clinical significance of this is not known.
In animals and in humans, probenecid has been reported to increase plasma concentrations of methotrexate (see WARNINGS).
Falsely high readings for theophylline have been reported in an *in vitro* study, using the Schack and Waxler technic, when therapeutic concentrations of theophylline and probenecid were added to human plasma.

Dosage and Administration

Therapy with ColBENEMID should not be *started* until an acute gouty attack has subsided. However, if an acute attack is precipitated *during* therapy, ColBENEMID may be continued without changing the dosage, and additional colchicine or other appropriate therapy should be given to control the acute attack.
The recommended adult dosage is 1 tablet of ColBENEMID daily for one week, followed by 1 tablet twice a day thereafter.
Some degree of renal impairment may be present in patients with gout. A daily dosage of 2 tablets may be adequate. However, if necessary, the daily dosage may be increased by 1 tablet every four weeks within tolerance (and usually not above 4 tablets per day) if symptoms of gouty arthritis are not controlled or the 24 hour uric acid excretion is not above 700 mg.
As noted, probenecid may not be effective in chronic renal insufficiency particularly when the glomerular filtration rate is 30 ml/minute or less.
Gastric intolerance may be indicative of overdosage, and may be corrected by decreasing the dosage.
As uric acid tends to crystallize out of an acid urine, a liberal fluid intake is recommended, as well as sufficient sodium bicarbonate (3 to 7.5 g daily) or potassium citrate (7.5 g daily) to maintain an alkaline urine (*see* PRECAUTIONS).
Alkalization of the urine is recommended until the serum urate level returns to normal limits and tophaceous deposits disappear, i.e., during the period when urinary excretion of uric acid is at a high level. Thereafter, alkalization of the urine and the usual restriction of purine-producing foods may be somewhat relaxed.
ColBENEMID (or probenecid) should be continued at the dosage that will maintain normal serum urate levels. When acute attacks have been absent for six months or more and serum urate levels remain within normal limits, the daily dosage of ColBENEMID may be decreased by 1 tablet every six months. The maintenance dosage should not be reduced to the point where serum urate levels tend to rise.

How Supplied

No. 3283—Tablets ColBENEMID are white to off-white, capsule-shaped, scored tablets, coded MSD 614. Each tablet contains 0.5 g of probenecid and 0.5 mg of colchicine. They are supplied as follows:
NDC 0006-0614-68 bottles of 100.
[*Shown in Product Identification Section*]
A.H.F.S. 40:40
DC 6213019 Issued September 1978

COSMEGEN® Injection ℞
(dactinomycin, MSD), U.S.P.

WARNING

Dactinomycin is extremely corrosive to soft tissue. If extravasation occurs during intravenous use, severe damage to soft tissues will occur. In at least one instance, this has led to contracture of the arms.

DOSAGE

The dosage of COSMEGEN (Dactinomycin, MSD) is calculated in micrograms (mcg). The usual adult dosage is 500 micrograms (0.5 mg) daily intravenously for a maximum of five days. The dosage for adults or children should not exceed 15 mcg/kg or 400–600 mcg/square meter of body surface daily intravenously for five days. Calculation of the dosage for obese or

Continued on next page

Information on the Merck Sharp & Dohme products listed on these pages is the full prescribing information from package circulars in use October 31, 1979.

Merck Sharp & Dohme—Cont.

edematous patients should be on the basis of surface area in an effort to relate dosage to lean body mass.

Description

Dactinomycin is one of the actinomycins, a group of antibiotics produced by various species of *Streptomyces.* Dactinomycin is the principal component of the mixture of actinomycins produced by *Streptomyces parvullus.* Unlike other species of *Streptomyces,* this organism yields an essentially pure substance that contains only traces of similar compounds differing in the amino acid content of the peptide side chains.

Actions

Generally, the actinomycins exert an inhibitory effect on gram-positive and gram-negative bacteria and on some fungi. However, the toxic properties of the actinomycins (including dactinomycin) in relation to antibacterial activity are such as to preclude their use as antibiotics in the treatment of infectious diseases.
Because the actinomycins are cytotoxic, they have an antineoplastic effect which has been demonstrated in experimental animals with various types of tumor implant. This cytotoxic action is the basis for their use in the palliative treatment of certain types of cancer.
Dactinomycin is minimally metabolized. Its plasma clearance half-life is 36 hours. It tends to concentrate in nucleated cells and does not cross the blood brain barrier.

Indications

Wilms's Tumor
The neoplasm responding most frequently to COSMEGEN is Wilms's tumor. With low doses of both dactinomycin and radiotherapy, temporary objective improvement may be as good as and may last longer than with higher doses of each given alone. In the National Wilms's Tumor study, combination therapy with dactinomycin and vincristine together with surgery and radiotherapy, was shown to have significantly improved the prognosis of patients in groups II and III. Dactinomycin and vincristine were given for a total of seven cycles, so that maintenance therapy continued for approximately 15 months.
Postoperative radiotherapy in group I patients and optimal combination chemotherapy for those in group IV are unsettled issues. About 70 percent of lung metastases have disappeared with an appropriate combination of radiation, dactinomycin and vincristine.
Rhabdomyosarcoma
Temporary regression of the tumor and beneficial subjective results have occurred with dactinomycin in rhabdomyosarcoma which, like most soft tissue sarcomas, is comparatively radio-resistant.
Several groups have reported successful use of cyclophosphamide, vincristine, dactinomycin and doxorubicin hydrochloride in various combinations. Effective combinations have included vincristine and dactinomycin; vincristine, dactinomycin and cyclophosphamide (VAC therapy) and all four drugs in sequence. At present, the most effective treatment for children with inoperable or metastatic rhabdomyosarcoma has been VAC chemotherapy. Two thirds of these children were doing well without evidence of disease at a median time of three years after diagnosis.
Carcinoma of Testis and Uterus
The sequential use of dactinomycin and methotrexate, along with meticulous monitoring of human chorionic gonadotropin levels until normal, has resulted in survival in the majority of women with metastatic choriocarcinoma. Sequential therapy is used if there is:

1. Stability in gonadotropin titers following two successive courses of an agent.
2. Rising gonadotropin titers during treatment.
3. Severe toxicity preventing adequate therapy.

In patients with nonmetastatic choriocarcinoma, dactinomycin or methotrexate or both, have been used successfully, with or without surgery.
Dactinomycin has been beneficial as a single agent in the treatment of metastatic nonseminomatour testicular carcinoma when used in cycles of 500 mcg/day for five consecutive days, every 6–8 weeks for periods of four months or longer.
Other Neoplasms
Dactinomycin has been given intravenously or by regional perfusion, either alone or with other antineoplastic compounds or x-ray therapy, in the palliative treatment of Ewing's sarcoma and sarcoma botryoides. For nonmetastatic Ewing's sarcoma, promising results were obtained when dactinomycin (45 mcg/m^2) and cyclophosphamide (1200 mg/m^2) were given sequentially and with radiotherapy, over an 18 month period. Those with metastatic disease remain the subject of continued investigation with a more aggressive chemotherapeutic regimen employed initially.
Temporary objective improvement and relief of pain and discomfort have followed the use of dactinomycin usually in conjunction with radiotherapy for sarcoma botryoides. This palliative effect ranges from transitory inhibition of tumor growth to a considerable but temporary regression in tumor size.
COSMEGEN (Dactinomycin, MSD) and Radiation Therapy
Much evidence suggests that dactinomycin potentiates the effects of x-ray therapy. The converse also appears likely; i.e., dactinomycin may be more effective when radiation therapy also is given.
With combined dactinomycin-radiation therapy, the normal skin, as well as the buccal and pharyngeal mucosa, show early erythema. A smaller than usual x-ray dose when given with dactinomycin causes erythema and vesiculation, which progress more rapidly through the stages of tanning and desquamation. Healing may occur in four to six weeks rather than two to three months. Erythema from previous x-ray therapy may be reactivated by dactinomycin alone, even when irradiation occurred many months earlier, and especially when the interval between the two forms of therapy is brief. This potentiation of radiation effect represents a special problem when the irradiation treatment area includes the mucous membrane. When irradiation is directed toward the nasopharynx, the combination may produce severe oropharyngeal mucositis. *Severe reactions may ensue if high doses of both dactinomycin and radiation therapy are used or if the patient is particularly sensitive to such combined therapy.*
Because of this potentiating effect, dactinomycin may be tried in radio-sensitive tumors not responding to doses of x-ray therapy that can be tolerated. Objective improvement in tumor size and activity may be observed when lower, better tolerated doses of both types of therapy are employed.
COSMEGEN (Dactinomycin, MSD) and Perfusion Technic
Dactinomycin alone or with other antineoplastic agents has also been given by the isolation-perfusion technic, either as palliative treatment or as an adjunct to resection of a tumor. Some tumors considered resistant to chemotherapy and radiation therapy may respond when the drug is given by the perfusion technic. Neoplasms in which dactinomycin has been tried by this technic include various types of sarcoma, carcinoma, and adenocarcinoma. In some instances tumors regressed, pain was relieved for variable periods, and surgery made possible. On other occasions, however, the outcome has been less favorable. Nevertheless, in selected cases, the drug by perfusion may provide more effective palliation than when given systemically.
Dactinomycin by the isolation-perfusion technic offers certain advantages, provided leakage of the drug through the general circulation into other areas of the body is minimal. By this technic the drug is in continuous contact with the tumor for the duration of treatment. The dose may be increased well over that used by the systemic route, usually without adding to the danger of toxic effects. If the agent is confined to an isolated part, it should not interfere with the patient's defense mechanism. Systemic absorption of toxic products from neoplastic tissue can be minimized by removing the perfusate when the procedure is finished.

Contraindications

If dactinomycin is given at or about the time of infection with chicken pox, a severe generalized disease, which may result in death, may occur.

Warning

COSMEGEN should be administered only under the supervision of a physician who is experienced in the use of cancer chemotherapeutic agents.

Precautions

As with all antineoplastic agents, dactinomycin is a toxic drug and very careful and frequent observation of the patient for adverse reactions is necessary. These reactions may involve any tissue of the body. The possibility of an anaphylactoid reaction should be borne in mind.
The greater frequency of toxic effects of dactinomycin peculiar to infants suggest that this drug should be given to infants only over the age of 6 to 12 months.
A variety of abnormalities of renal, hepatic, and bone marrow function have been reported in patients with neoplastic disease and receiving dactinomycin. It is advisable to make frequent checks of renal, hepatic, and bone marrow function.
Increased incidence of gastrointestinal toxicity and marrow suppression has been reported when dactinomycin was given with x-ray therapy.
Particular caution is necessary when administering dactinomycin in the first two months after irradiation for the treatment of right-sided Wilms's tumor, since hepatomegaly and elevated SGOT levels have been noted.
Nausea and vomiting due to dactinomycin make it necessary to give this drug intermittently. It is extremely important to observe the patient daily for toxic side effects when multiple chemotherapy is employed, since a full course of therapy occasionally is not tolerated. If stomatitis, diarrhea, or severe hemopoietic depression appear during therapy, these drugs should be discontinued until the patient has recovered.
Use in pregnancy: When administration of this drug during pregnancy is considered necessary, the danger for the fetus should be taken into consideration. The need for this precaution is based on published data showing teratogenic effects of dactinomycin in animals.
Nursing Mothers
Although breast milk studies have not been performed in animals or humans, breast feeding should be stopped before beginning treatment with COSMEGEN.

Adverse Reactions

Toxic effects (excepting nausea and vomiting) usually do not become apparent until two to four days after a course of therapy is stopped, and may not be maximal before one to two weeks have elapsed. Deaths have been reported. However, adverse reactions are usually reversible on discontinuance of therapy. They include the following:
Miscellaneous (malaise, fatigue, lethargy, fever, myalgia, proctitis, hypocalcemia).
Oral (cheilitis, dysphagia, esophagitis, ulcerative stomatitis, pharyngitis).
Gastrointestinal (anorexia, nausea, vomiting, abdominal pain, diarrhea, gastrointestinal ulceration). Nausea and vomiting, which occur early during the first few hours after administration, may be alleviated by giving antiemetics.
Hematologic (anemia, even to the point of aplastic anemia, agranulocytosis, leukopenia, thrombopenia, pancytopenia, reticulopenia). Platelet and white cell counts should be done *daily* to detect severe hemopoietic depression. If either count markedly decreases, the drug should be withheld to allow marrow recovery. This often takes up to three weeks.
Dermatologic (alopecia, skin eruptions, acne, flare-up of erythema or increased pigmentation of previously irradiated skin).
Soft tissues. Dactinomycin is extremely corrosive. If extravasation occurs during intravenous use, severe damage to soft tissues will occur. In at least one instance, this has led to contracture of the arms.

Dosage and Administration

Toxic reactions due to dactinomycin are frequent and may be severe (see ADVERSE REACTIONS), thus limiting in many instances the amount that may be given. However, the severity of toxicity varies markedly and is only partly dependent on the dose employed. The drug must be given in short courses.
Intravenous Use
The dosage of dactinomycin varies depending on the tolerance of the patient, the size and location of the neoplasm, and the use of other forms of therapy. It may be necessary to decrease the usual dosages suggested below when other chemotherapy or x-ray therapy is used concomitantly or has been used previously.
The dosage for adults or children should not exceed 15 mcg/kg or 400–600 mcg/square meter of body surface daily intravenously for five days. Calculation of the dosage for obese or edematous patients should be on the basis of surface area in an effort to relate dosage to lean body mass.
Adults: The usual adult dosage is 500 mcg (0.5 mg) daily intravenously for a maximum of five days.
Children: In children 15 mcg (0.015 mg) per kilogram of body weight is given intravenously daily for five days. An alternative schedule is a total dosage of 2500 mcg (2.5 mg) per square meter of body surface given intravenously over a one week period.
In both adults and children, a second course may be given after at least three weeks have elapsed, provided all signs of toxicity have disappeared.
Reconstitute COSMEGEN by adding 1.1 ml of **Sterile Water for Injection (without preservative)** using aseptic precautions. The resulting solution of dactinomycin will contain approximately 500 mcg or 0.5 mg per ml.
Once reconstituted, the solution of dactinomycin can be added to infusion solutions of Dextrose Injection 5 percent or Sodium Chloride Injection either directly or to the tubing of a running intravenous infusion.
Although reconstituted COSMEGEN is chemically stable, the product does not contain a preservative and accidental microbial contamination might result. Any unused portion should be discarded. Use of water containing preservatives (benzyl alcohol or parabens) to reconstitute COSMEGEN for injection, results in the formation of a precipitate.
Partial removal of dactinomycin from intravenous solutions by cellulose ester membrane filters used in some intravenous in-line filters has been reported.
Since dactinomycin is extremely corrosive to soft tissue, precautions for materials of this nature should be observed.
If the drug is given directly into the vein without the use of an infusion, the "two-needle technic" should be used. Reconstitute and withdraw the calculated dose from the vial with one sterile needle. Use another sterile needle for direct injection into the vein.
Discard any unused portion of the dactinomycin solution.
Isolation-Perfusion Technic
The dosage schedules and the technic itself vary from one investigator to another; the published literature, therefore, should be consulted for details. In general, the following doses are suggested:
50 mcg (0.05 mg) per kilogram of body weight for lower extremity or pelvis.
35 mcg (0.035 mg) per kilogram of body weight for upper extremity.
It may be advisable to use lower doses in obese patients, or when previous chemotherapy or radiation therapy has been employed.
Complications of the perfusion technic are related mainly to the amount of drug that escapes into the systemic circulation and may consist of hemopoietic depression, absorption of toxic products from massive destruction of neoplastic tissue, increased susceptibility to infection, impaired wound healing, and superficial ulceration of the gastric mucosa. Other side effects may include edema of the extremity involved, damage to soft tissues of the perfused area, and (potentially) venous thrombosis.

How Supplied

No. 3298—Injection COSMEGEN is a lyophilized powder and is supplied as follows: **NDC** 0006-3298-22 in vials containing 0.5 mg (500 micrograms) of dactinomycin with 20.0 mg of mannitol. In the dry form the compound is an amorphous yellow powder. The solution is clear and gold-colored.

A.H.F.S. 10:00
DC 6059218 Issued June 1979

CUPRIMINE® Capsules (penicillamine, MSD), U.S.P. ℞

Physicians planning to use penicillamine should thoroughly familiarize themselves with its toxicity, special dosage considerations, and therapeutic benefits. Penicillamine should never be used casually. Each patient should remain constantly under the close supervision of the physician. Patients should be warned to report promptly any symptoms suggesting toxicity.

Description

Penicillamine is the D-isomer of 3-mercaptovaline. It is a white or practically white, crystalline powder, freely soluble in water, slightly soluble in alcohol, and insoluble in ether, acetone, benzene, and carbon tetrachloride. Although its configuration is D, it is levorotatory as usually measured:

$$[\alpha]^{25^\circ}_{D} = -63^\circ \pm 5^\circ \ (C = 1, 1\,N\,\text{NaOH}).$$

The empirical formula is $C_5H_{11}NO_2S$, giving it a molecular weight of 149.21.
It reacts readily with formaldehyde or acetone to form a thiazolidine-carboxylic acid.

Clinical Pharmacology

Penicillamine is a chelating agent recommended for the removal of excess copper in patients with Wilson's disease. From *in vitro* studies which indicate that one atom of copper combines with two molecules of penicillamine, it would appear that one gram of penicillamine should be followed by the excretion of about 200 milligrams of copper; however, the actual amount excreted is about one percent of this.
Penicillamine also reduces excess cystine excretion in cystinuria. This is done, at least in part, by disulfide interchange between penicillamine and cystine, resulting in formation of penicillamine-cysteine disulfide, a substance that is much more soluble than cystine and is excreted readily.
Penicillamine interferes with the formation of cross-links between tropocollagen molecules and cleaves them when newly formed.
The mechanism of action of penicillamine in rheumatoid arthritis is unknown although it appears to suppress disease activity. Unlike cytotoxic immunosuppressants, penicillamine markedly lowers IgM rheumatoid factor but produces no significant depression in absolute levels of serum immunoglobulins. Also unlike cytotoxic immunosuppressants which act on both, penicillamine *in vitro* depresses T-cell activity but not B-cell activity.
In vitro, penicillamine dissociates macroglobulins (rheumatoid factor) although the relationship of the activity to its effect in rheumatoid arthritis is not known.
In rheumatoid arthritis, the onset of therapeutic response to CUPRIMINE (Penicillamine, MSD) may not be seen for two or three months. In those patients who respond, however, the first evidence of suppression of symptoms such as pain, tenderness, and swelling is generally apparent within three months. The optimum duration of therapy has not been determined. If remissions occur, they may last from months to years, but usually require continued treatment (see DOSAGE AND ADMINISTRATION).
In patients with rheumatoid arthritis, it is important that CUPRIMINE be given on an empty stomach, at least one hour before meals and at least one hour apart from any other drug, food, or milk. This permits maximum absorption and reduces the likelihood of inactivation by metal binding.
Methodology for determining the bioavailability of penicillamine is not available; however, penicillamine is known to be a very soluble substance.

Indications

CUPRIMINE is indicated in the treatment of Wilson's disease, cystinuria, and in patients with severe, active rheumatoid arthritis who have failed to respond to an adequate trial of conventional therapy. Available evidence suggests that CUPRIMINE is not of value in ankylosing spondylitis.
Wilson's Disease—Wilson's disease (hepatolenticular degeneration) results from the interaction of an inherited defect and an abnormality in copper metabolism. The metabolic defect, which is the consequence of the autosomal inheritance of one abnormal gene from each parent, manifests itself in a greater positive copper balance than normal. As a result, copper is deposited in several organs and appears even-

Continued on next page

Information on the Merck Sharp & Dohme products listed on these pages is the full prescribing information from package circulars in use October 31, 1979.

tually to produce pathologic effects most prominently seen in the brain, where degeneration is widespread; in the liver, where fatty infiltration, inflammation, and hepatocellular damage progress to postnecrotic cirrhosis; in the kidney, where tubular and glomerular dysfunction results; and in the eye, where characteristic corneal copper deposits are known as Kayser-Fleischer rings.
Two types of patients require treatment for Wison's disease: (1) the symptomatic, and (2) the asymptomatic in whom it can be assumed the disease will develop in the future if the patient is not treated.
Diagnosis, suspected on the basis of family or individual history, physical examination, or a low serum concentration of ceruloplasmin*, is confirmed by the demonstration of Kayser-Fleischer rings or, particularly in the asymptomatic patient, by the quantitative demonstration in a liver biopsy specimen of a concentration of copper in excess of 250 mcg/g dry weight.

Treatment has two objectives:
(1) to minimize dietary intake and absorption of copper.
(2) to promote excretion of copper deposited in tissues.
The first objective is attained by a daily diet that contains no more than one or two milligrams of copper. Such a diet should exclude, most importantly, chocolate, nuts, shellfish, mushrooms, liver, molasses, broccoli, and cereals enriched with copper, and be composed to as great an extent as possible of foods with a low copper content. Distilled or demineralized water should be used if the patient's drinking water contains more than 0.1 mg of copper per liter.
For the second objective, a copper chelating agent is used. Penicillamine is the only one of these agents that is orally effective.
In symptomatic patients this treatment usually produces marked neurologic improvement, fading of Kayser-Fleischer rings, and gradual amelioration of hepatic dysfunction and psychic disturbances.
Clinical experience to date suggests that life is prolonged with the above regimen.
Noticeable improvement may not occur for one to three months. Occasionally, neurologic symptoms become worse during initiation of therapy with CUPRIMINE. Despite this, the drug should not be discontinued permanently, although temporary interruption may result in clinical improvement of the neurological symptoms but it carries an increased risk of developing a sensitivity reaction upon resumption of therapy (see WARNINGS).
Treatment of asymptomatic patients has been carried out for over ten years. Symptoms and signs of the disease appear to be prevented indefinitely if daily treatment with CUPRIMINE can be continued.
Cystinuria—Cystinuria is characterized by excessive urinary excretion of the dibasic amino acids, arginine, lysine, ornithine, and cystine, and the mixed disulfide of cysteine and homocysteine. The metabolic defect that leads to cystinuria is inherited as an autosomal, recessive trait. Metabolism of the affected amino acids is influenced by at least two abnormal factors: (1) defective gastrointestinal absorption and (2) renal tubular dysfunction.

*For quantitative test for serum ceruloplasmin see: Morell, A.G.; Windsor, J.; Sternlieb, I.; Scheinberg, I.H.: Measurement of the concentration of ceruloplasmin in serum by determination of its oxidase activity, in "Laboratory Diagnosis of Liver Disease", F.W. Sunderman; F.W. Sunderman, Jr. (eds.), St. Louis, Warren H. Green, Inc., 1968, pp. 193-195.

Arginine, lysine, ornithine, and cysteine are soluble substances, readily excreted. There is no apparent pathology connected with their excretion in excessive quantities.
Cystine, however, is so slightly soluble at the usual range of urinary pH that it is not excreted readily, and so crystallizes and forms stones in the urinary tract. Stone formation is the only known pathology in cystinuria.
Normal daily output of cystine is 40 to 80 mg. In cystinuria, output is greatly increased and may exceed 1 g/day. At 500 to 600 mg/day, stone formation is almost certain. When it is more than 300 mg/day, treatment is indicated.
Conventional treatment is directed at keeping urinary cystine diluted enough to prevent stone formation, keeping the urine alkaline enough to dissolve as much cystine as possible, and minimizing cystine production by a diet low in methionine (the major dietary precursor of cystine). Patients must drink enough fluid to keep urine specific gravity below 1.010, take enough alkali to keep urinary pH at 7.5 to 8, and maintain a diet low in methionine. This diet is not recommended in growing children and probably is contraindicated in pregnancy because of its low protein content (see PRECAUTIONS).
When these measures are inadequate to control recurrent stone formation, CUPRIMINE may be used as additional therapy. When patients refuse to adhere to conventional treatment, CUPRIMINE may be a useful substitute. It is capable of keeping cystine excretion to near normal values, thereby hindering stone formation and the serious consequences of pyelonephritis and impaired renal function that develop in some patients.
Bartter and colleagues depict the process by which penicillamine interacts with cystine to form penicillamine-cysteine mixed disulfide as:

$$\text{CSSC} + \text{PS}' \rightleftharpoons \text{CS}' + \text{CSSP}$$
$$\text{PSSP} + \text{CS}' \rightleftharpoons \text{PS}' + \text{CSSP}$$
$$\text{CSSC} + \text{PSSP} \rightleftharpoons 2\text{CSSP}$$

CSSC = cystine
CS′ = deprotonated cysteine
PSSP = penicillamine
PS′ = deprotonated penicillamine sulfhydryl
CSSP = penicillamine-cysteine mixed disulfide

In this process, it is assumed that the deprotonated form of penicillamine, PS′, is the active factor in bringing about the disulfide interchange.
Rheumatoid Arthritis—Because CUPRIMINE can cause severe adverse reactions, its use in rheumatoid arthritis should be restricted to patients who have severe, active disease and who have failed to respond to an adequate trial of conventional therapy. Even then, benefit-to-risk ratio should be carefully considered. Other measures, such as rest, physiotherapy, salicylates, and corticosteroids should be used, when indicated, in conjunction with CUPRIMINE (see PRECAUTIONS).

Contraindications

Penicillamine should not be administered to patients with rheumatoid arthritis who are pregnant (see PRECAUTIONS).
Patients with a history of penicillamine-related aplastic anemia or agranulocytosis should not be restarted on penicillamine (see WARNINGS and ADVERSE REACTIONS).
Because of its potential for causing renal damage, penicillamine should not be administered to rheumatoid arthritis patients with a history or other evidence of renal insufficiency.

Warnings

The use of penicillamine has been associated with fatalities due to certain diseases such as aplastic anemia, agranulocytosis, thrombocytopenia, Goodpasture's syndrome, and myasthenic syndrome.
Because of the potential for serious hematological and renal adverse reactions, routine urinalysis, white and differential blood cell count, hemoglobin determination, and direct platelet count must be done every two weeks for the first six months of penicillamine therapy and monthly thereafter. Patients should be instructed to report promptly the development of signs and symptoms of granulocytopenia and/or thrombocytopenia such as fever, sore throat, chills, bruising or bleeding. The above laboratory studies should then be promptly repeated.
Leukopenia and thrombocytopenia have been reported to occur in up to five percent of patients during penicillamine therapy. Leukopenia is of the granulocytic series and may or may not be associated with an increase in eosinophils. A confirmed reduction in WBC below 3500 mandates discontinuance of penicillamine therapy. Thrombocytopenia may be on an idiosyncratic basis, with decreased or absent megakaryocytes in the marrow, when it is part of an aplastic anemia. In other cases the thrombocytopenia is presumably on an immune basis since the number of megakaryocytes in the marrow has been reported to be normal or sometimes increased. The development of a platelet count below 100,000, even in the absence of clinical bleeding, requires at least temporary cessation of penicillamine therapy. A progressive fall in either platelet count or WBC in three successive determinations, even though values are still within the normal range, likewise requires at least temporary cessation.
Proteinuria and/or hematuria may develop during therapy and may be warning signs of membranous glomerulopathy which can progress to a nephrotic syndrome. Close observation of these patients is essential. In some patients the proteinuria disappears with continued therapy; in others, penicillamine must be discontinued. When a patient develops proteinuria or hematuria the physician must ascertain whether it is a sign of drug-induced glomerulopathy or is unrelated to penicillamine.
Rheumatoid arthritis patients who develop moderate degrees of proteinuria may be continued cautiously on penicillamine therapy, provided that quantitative 24-hour urinary protein determinations are obtained at intervals of one to two weeks. Penicillamine dosage should not be increased under these circumstances. Proteinuria which exceeds 1 g/24 hours, or proteinuria which is progressively increasing, requires either discontinuance of the drug or a reduction in the dosage. In some patients, proteinuria has been reported to clear following reduction in dosage.
In rheumatoid arthritis patients, penicillamine should be discontinued if unexplained gross hematuria or persistent microscopic hematuria develops.
In patients with Wilson's disease or cystinuria the risks of continued penicillamine therapy in patients manifesting potentially serious urinary abnormalities must be weighed against the expected therapeutic benefits.
When penicillaminne is used in cystinuria, an annual x-ray for renal stones is advised. Cystine stones form rapidly, sometimes in six months.
Up to one year or more may be required for any urinary abnormalities to disappear after penicillamine has been discontinued.
Because of rare reports of intrahepatic cholestasis and toxic hepatitis, liver function tests are recommended every six months during the first year and a half of therapy.
Goodpasture's syndrome has occurred rarely. The development of abnormal urinary findings associated with hemoptysis and pulmonary infiltrates on x-ray requires immediate cessation of penicillamine.
A myasthenic syndrome has been reported. In the majority of cases, symptoms of myasthenia

have receded after withdrawal of penicillamine.

Pemphigoid-type reactions characterized by bullous lesions clinically indistinguishable from pemphigus have occurred and have required discontinuation of penicillamine and treatment with corticosteroids.

Once instituted for Wilson's disease or cystinuria, treatment with penicillamine should, as a rule, be continued on a daily basis. Interruptions for even a few days have been followed by sensitivity reactions after reinstitution of therapy.

Precautions

Some patients may experience drug fever, a marked febrile response to penicillamine, usually in the second to third week following initiation of therapy. Drug fever may sometimes be accompanied by a macular cutaneous eruption.

In the case of drug fever in patients with Wilson's disease or cystinuria, because no alternative treatment is available, penicillamine should be temporarily discontinued until the reaction subsides. Then penicillamine should be reinstituted with a small dose that is gradually increased until the desired dosage is attained. Systemic steroid therapy may be necessary, and is usually helpful, in such patients in whom toxic reactions develop a second or third time.

In the case of drug fever in rheumatoid arthritis patients, because other treatments are available, penicillamine should be discontinued and another therapeutic alternative tried since experience indicates that the febrile reaction will recur in a very high percetage of patients upon readministration of penicillamine.

The skin and mucous membranes should be observed for allergic reactions. Early and late rashes have occurred. Early rash occurs during the first few months of treatment and is more common. It is usually a generalized pruritic, erythematous, maculopapular or morbilliform rash and resembles the allergic rash seen with other drugs. Early rash usually disappears within days after stopping penicillamine and seldom recurs when the drug is restarted at a lower dosage. Pruritus and early rash may often be controlled by the concomitant administration of antihistamines. Less commonly, a late rash may be seen, usually after six months or more of treatment, and requires discontinuation of penicillamine. It is usually on the trunk, is accompanied by intense pruritus, and is usually unresponsive to topical corticosteroid therapy. Late rash may take weeks to disappear after penicillamine is stopped and usually recurs if the drug is restarted.

The appearance of a drug eruption accompanied by fever, arthralgia, lymphadenopathy or other allergic manifestations usually requires discontinuation of penicillamine.

Certain patients will develop a positive antinuclear antibody (ANA) test and some of these may show a lupus erythematosus-like syndrome similar to drug-induced lupus associated with other drugs. The lupus erythematosus-like syndrome is not associated with hypocomplementemia and may be present without nephropathy. The development of a positive ANA test does not mandate discontinuance of the drug; however, the physician should be alerted to the possibility that a lupus erythematosus-like syndrome may develop in the future.

Some patients may develop oral ulcerations which in some cases have the appearance of aphthous stomatitis. The stomatitis usually recurs on rechallenge but often clears on a lower dosage. Although rare, cheilosis, glossitis and gingivostomatitis have also been reported. These oral lesions are frequently dose-related and may preclude further increase in penicillamine dosage or require discontinuation of the drug.

Hypogeusia (a blunting or diminution in taste perception) has occurred in some patients. This may last two to three months or more and may develop into a total loss of taste; however, it is usually self-limited despite continued penicillamine treatment. Such taste impairment is rare in patients with Wilson's disease.

Penicillamine should not be used in patients who are receiving concurrently gold therapy, antimalarial or cytotoxic drugs, oxyphenbutazone or phenylbutazone because these drugs are also associated with similar serious hematologic and renal adverse reactions.

Patients who are allergic to penicillin may theoretically have cross-sensitivity to penicillamine. The possibility of reactions from contamination of penicillamine by trace amounts of penicillin has been eliminated now that penicillamine is being produced synthetically rather than as a degradation product of penicillin.

Because of their dietary restrictions, patients with Wilson's disease and cystinuria should be given 25 mg/day of pyridoxine during therapy, since penicillamine increases the requirement for this vitamin. Patients also may receive benefit from a multivitamin preparation, although there is no evidence that deficiency of any vitamin other than pyridoxine is associated with penicillamine. In Wilson's disease, multivitamin preparations must be copper-free.

Rheumatoid arthritis patients whose nutrition is impaired should also be given a daily supplement of pyridoxine. Mineral supplements should not be given, since they may block the response to penicillamine.

Iron deficiency may develop, especially in children and in menstruating women. In Wilson's disease, this may be a result of adding the effects of the low copper diet, which is probably also low in iron, and the penicillamine to the effects of blood loss or growth. In cystinuria, a low methionine diet may contribute to iron deficiency, since it is necessarily low in protein. If necessary, iron may be given in short courses, but a period of two hours should elapse between administration of penicillamine and iron, since orally administered iron has been shown to reduce the effects of penicillamine.

Penicillamine causes an increase in the amount of soluble collagen. In the rat this results in inhibition of normal healing and also a decrease in tensile strength of intact skin. In man this may be the cause of increased skin friability at sites especially subject to pressure or trauma, such as shoulders, elbows, knees, toes, and buttocks. Extravasations of blood may occur and may appear as purpuric areas, with external bleeding if the skin is broken, or as vesicles containing dark blood. Neither type is progressive. There is no apparent association with bleeding elsewhere in the body and no associated coagulation defect has been found. Therapy with penicillamine may be continued in the presence of these lesions. They may not recur if dosage is reduced. Other reported effects probably due to the action of penicillamine on collagen are excessive wrinkling of the skin and development of small, white papules at venipuncture and surgical sites.

The effects of penicillamine on collagen and elastin make it advisable to consider a reduction in dosage to 250 mg/day, when surgery is contemplated. Reinstitution of full therapy should be delayed until wound healing is complete.

Carcinogenesis—Long-term animal carcinogenicity studies have not been done with penicillamine. There is a report that five of ten autoimmune disease-prone NZB hybrid mice developed lymphocytic leukemia after 6 months' intraperitoneal treatment with a dose of 400 mg/kg penicillamine 5 days per week.

Use in Pregnancy—Penicillamine has been shown to be teratogenic in rats when given in doses several times higher than the highest dose recommended for human use. Skeletal defects, cleft palates and fetal toxicity (resorptions) have been reported.

Wilson's Disease—There are no controlled studies in pregnant women with Wilson's disease, but experience does not include any positive evidence of adverse effects on the fetus. Reported experience* shows that continued treatment with penicillamine throughout pregnancy protects the mother against relapse of the Wilson's disease, and that discontinuation of penicillamine has deleterious effects on the mother. It indicates that the drug does not increase the risks of fetal abnormalities, but it does not exclude the possibility of infrequent or subtle damage to the fetus.

*Scheinberg, I.H., Sternlieb, I.: N Engl J Med *293*: 1300-1302, Dec. 18, 1975.

If penicillamine is administered during pregnancy to patients with Wilson's disease, it is recommended that the daily dosage be limited to 1 g. If cesarean section is planned, the daily dosage should be limited to 250 mg during the last six weeks of pregnancy and postoperatively until wound healing is complete.

Cystinuria—If possible, penicillamine should not be give during pregnancy to women with cystinuria. There is a report of a woman with cystinuria treated with 2 g/day of penicillamine during pregnancy who gave birth to a child with a generalized connective tissue defect that may have been caused by penicillamine. If stones continue to form in these patients, the benefits of therapy to the mother must be evaluated against the risk to the fetus.

Rheumatoid Arthritis—Penicillamine should not be administered to rheumatoid arthritis patients who are pregnant (see CONTRAINDICATIONS) and should be discontinued promptly in patients in whom pregnancy is suspected or diagnosed. Penicillamine should be used in women of childbearing potential only when the expected benefits outweigh possible hazards. Women of childbearing potential should be informed of the possible hazards of penicillamine to the developing fetus and should be advised to report promptly any missed menstrual periods or other indications of possible pregnancy.

There is a report that a woman with rheumatoid arthritis treated with less than one gram a day of penicillamine during pregnancy gave birth (cesarean delivery) to an infant with growth retardation, flattened face with broad nasal bridge, low set ears, short neck with loose skin folds, and unusually lax body skin.

Usage in Children—The efficacy of CUPRIMINE in juvenile rheumatoid arthritis has not been established.

Adverse Reactions

Penicillamine is a drug with a high incidence of untoward reactions, some of which are potentially fatal. Therefore, it is mandatory that patients receiving penicillamine therapy remain under close medical supervision throughout the period of drug administration (see WARNINGS and PRECAUTIONS).

Reported incidences (%) for the most commonly occurring adverse reactions in rheumatoid arthritis patients are noted, based on 17 representative clinical trials reported in the literature (1270 patients).

Allergic—Generalized pruritus, early and late rashes (5%), pemphigoid-type reactions, and drug eruptions which may be accompanied by fever, arthralgia, or lymphadenopathy have occurred (see WARNINGS and PRECAU-

Continued on next page

Information on the Merck Sharp & Dohme products listed on these pages is the full prescribing information from package circulars in use October 31, 1979.

Merck Sharp & Dohme—Cont.

TIONS). Some patients may show a lupus erythematosus-like syndrome similar to drug-induced lupus produced by other pharmacological agents (see PRECAUTIONS).

Urticaria and exfoliative dermatitis have occurred.

Thyroiditis has been reported but is extremely rare.

Some patients may develop a migratory polyarthralgia, often with objective synovitis (see DOSAGE AND ADMINISTRATION).

Gastrointestinal—Anorexia, epigastric pain, nausea, vomiting, or occasional diarrhea may occur (17%).

Isolated cases of reactivated peptic ulcer have occurred, as have hepatic dysfunction, cholestatic jaundice, and pancreatitis. There have been a few reports of increased serum alkaline phosphatase, lactic dehydrogenase, and positive cephalin flocculation and thymol turbidity tests.

Some patients may report a blunting, diminution, or total loss of taste perception (12%), or may develop oral ulcerations. Although rare, cheilosis, glossitis, and gingivostomatitis have been reported (see PRECAUTIONS).

Gastrointestinal side effects are usually reversible following cessation of therapy.

Hematological—Penicillamine can cause bone marrow depression (see WARNINGS). Leukopenia (2%) and thrombocytopenia (4%) have occurred. Fatalities have been reported as a result of thrombocytopenia, agranulocytosis, and aplastic anemia.

Thrombotic thrombocytopenic purpura, hemolytic anemia, red cell aplasia, monocytosis, leukocytosis, eosinophilia, and thrombocytosis have also been reported.

Renal—Patients on penicillamine therapy may develop proteinuria (6%) and/or hematuria which, in some, may progress to the development of the nephrotic syndrome as a result of an immune complex membranous glomerulopathy (see WARNINGS).

Central Nervous System—Tinnitus has been reported. Reversible optic neuritis has been reported with the administration of the racemic penicillamine (dl-form) and may be related to pyridoxine deficiency.

Other—Adverse reactions that have been reported rarely include thrombophelebitis; hyperpyrexia (see PRECAUTIONS); falling hair or alopecia; myasthenic syndrome (see WARNINGS); polymyositis; mammary hyperplasia; elastosis perforans serpiginosa; toxic epidermal necrolysis; anetoderma (cutaneous macular atrophy); and Goodpasture's syndrome, a severe and ultimately fatal glomerulonephritis associated with intra-alveolar hemorrhage (see WARNINGS). Allergic alveolitis and obliterative bronchiolitis have been reported in patients with severe rheumatoid arthritis, some of whom were receiving penicillamine.

Increased skin friability, excessive wrinkling of skin, and development of small white papules at venipuncture and surgical sites have been reported (see PRECAUTIONS).

The chelating action of the drug may cause increased excretion of other heavy metals such as zinc, mercury and lead.

Dosage and Administration

Wilson's Disease—CUPRIMINE capsules should be given on an empty stomach, four times a day; one-half to one hour before meals and at bedtime–at least two hours after the evening meal.

Optimal dosage can be determined only by measurement of urinary copper excretion. The urine must be collected in copper-free glassware, and should be quantitatively analyzed for copper before and soon after initiation of therapy with CUPRIMINE. Continued therapy should be monitored by doing a 24-hour urinary copper analysis every three months or so for the duration of therapy. Since a low copper diet should keep copper absorption down to less than one milligram a day, the patient probably will be in negative copper balance if 0.5 to one milligram of copper is present in a 24-hour collection of urine.

To achieve this, the suggested initial dosage of CUPRIMINE in the treatment of Wilson's disease is 1 g/day for children or adults. This may be increased, as indicated by the urinary copper analyses, but it is seldom necessary to exceed a dosage of 2 g/day.

In patients who cannot tolerate as much as 1 g/day initially, initiating dosage with 250 mg/day, and increasing gradually to the requisite amount, gives closer control of the effects of the drug and may help to reduce the incidence of adverse reactions.

Cystinuria—It is recommended that CUPRIMINE be used along with conventional therapy. By reducing urinary cystine, it decreases crystalluria and stone formation. In some instances, it has been reported to decrease the size of, and even to dissolve, stones already formed.

The usual dosage of CUPRIMINE in the treatment of cystinuria is 2 g/day for adults, with a range of 1 to 4 g/day. For children, dosage can be based on 30 mg/kg/day. The total daily amount should be divided into four doses. If four equal doses are not feasible, give the larger portion at bedtime. If adverse reactions necessitate a reduction in dosage, it is important to retain the bedtime dose.

Initiating dosage with 250 mg/day, and increasing gradually to the requisite amount, gives closer control of the effects of the drug and may help to reduce the incidence of adverse reactions.

In addition to taking CUPRIMINE, patients should drink copiously. It is especially important to drink about a pint of fluid at bedtime and another pint once during the night when urine is more concentrated and more acid than during the day. The greater the fluid intake, the lower the required dosage of CUPRIMINE.

Dosage must be individualized to an amount that limits cystine excretion to 100–200 mg/day in those with no history of stones, and below 100 mg/day in those who have had stone formation and/or pain. Thus, in determining dosage, the inherent tubular defect, the patient's size, age, and rate of growth, and his diet and water intake all must be taken into consideration.

The standard nitroprusside cyanide test has been reported useful as a qualitative measure of the effective dose *: Add 2 ml of freshly prepared 5 percent sodium cyanide to 5 ml of a 24-hour aliquot of protein-free urine and let stand ten minutes. Add 5 drops of freshly prepared 5 percent sodium nitroprusside and mix. Cystine will turn the mixture magenta. If the result is negative, it can be assumed that cystine excretion is less than 100 mg/g creatinine.

*Lotz, M., Potts, J.T. and Bartter, F.C.: Brit Med J *2*:521, Aug. 28, 1965 (in Medical Memoranda).

Although penicillamine is rarely excreted unchanged, it also will turn the mixture magenta. If there is any question as to which substance is causing the reaction, a ferric chloride test can be done to eliminate doubt: Add 3 percent ferric chloride dropwise to the urine. Penicillamine will turn the urine an immediate and quickly fading blue. Cystine will not produce any change in appearance.

Rheumatoid Arthritis—The principal rule of treatment with CUPRIMINE in rheumatoid arthritis is patience. The onset of therapeutic response is typically delayed. Two or three months may be required before the first evidence of a clinical response is noted (see CLINICAL PHARMACOLOGY).

When treatment with CUPRIMINE has been interrupted because of adverse reactions or other reasons, the drug should be reintroduced cautiously by starting with a lower dosage and increasing slowly.

Initial Therapy—The currently recommended dosage regimen in rheumatoid arthritis begins with a single daily dose of 125 mg or 250 mg which is thereafter increased at one to three month intervals, by 125 mg or 250 mg/day, as patient reponse and tolerance indicate. If a satisfactory remission of symptoms is achieved, the dose associated with the remission should be continued (see *Maintenance Therapy*). If there is no improvement and there are no signs of potentially serious toxicity after two to three months of treatment with doses of 500–750 mg/day, increases of 250 mg/day at two to three month intervals may be continued until a satisfactory remission occurs (see *Maintenance Therapy*) or signs of toxicity develop (see WARNINGS and PRECAUTIONS). If there is no discernible improvement after three to four months of treatment with 1000 to 1500 mg of penicillamine/day, it may be assumed the patient will not respond and CUPRIMINE should be discontinued.

It is important that CUPRIMINE be given on an empty stomach at least one hour before meals and at least one hour apart from any other drug, food or milk (see CLINICAL PHARMACOLOGY).

Maintenance Therapy—The maintenance dosage of CUPRIMINE must be individualized, and may require adjustment during the course of treatment. Many patients respond satisfactorily to a dosage within the 500–750 mg/day range. Some need less.

Changes in maintenance dosage levels may not be reflected clinically or in the erythrocyte sedimentation rate for two to three months after each dosage adjustment.

Some patients will subsequently require an increase in the maintenance dosage to achieve maximal disease suppression. In those patients who do respond, but who evidence incomplete suppression of their disease after the first six to nine months of treatment, the daily dosage of CUPRIMINE may be increased by 125 mg or 250 mg/day at three-month intervals. It is unusual in current practice to employ a dosage in excess of 1 g/day, but up to 1.5 g/day has sometimes been required.

Management of Exacerbations—During the course of treatment some patients may experience an exacerbation of disease activity following an initial good response. These may be self-limited and can subside within twelve weeks. They are usually controlled by the addition of nonsteroidal anti-inflammatory drugs, and only if the patient has demonstrated a true "escape" phenomenon (as evidenced by failure of the flare to subside within this time period) should an increase in the maintenance dose ordinarily be considered.

In the rheumatoid patient, migratory polyarthralgia due to penicillamine is extremely difficult to differentiate from an exacerbation of the rheumatoid arthritis. Discontinuance or a substantial reduction in dosage of CUPRIMINE therapy for up to several weeks will usually determine which of these processes is responsible for the arthralgia.

Duration of Therapy—The optimum duration of CUPRIMINE therapy in rheumatoid arthritis has not been determined. If the patient has been in remission for six months or more, a gradual, stepwise dosage reduction in decrements of 125 mg or 250 mg/day at approximately three month intervals may be attempted.

Concomitant Drug Therapy—CUPRIMINE should not be used in patients who are receiving gold therapy, antimalarial or cytotoxic drugs, oxyphenbutazone, or phenylbutazone (see PRECAUTIONS). Other measures, such as salicylates, other nonsteroidal anti-inflammatory drugs, or systemic corticosteroids, may be continued when penicillamine is initiated. After improvement commences, analgesic and anti-inflammatory drugs may be slowly discontinued as symptoms permit. Steroid withdrawal must be done gradually, and many months of CUPRIMINE treatment may be required before steroids can be completely eliminated.

Dosage Frequency—Based on clinical experience dosages up to 500 mg/day can be given as a single daily dose. Dosages in excess of 500 mg/day should be administered in divided doses.

How Supplied

No. 3299—Capsules CUPRIMINE, 250 mg, are ivory-colored capsules containing a white or nearly white powder, and are coded MSD 602. They are supplied as follows:
NDC 0006-0602-68 in bottles of 100.
[*Shown in Product Identification Section*]
No. 3350—Capsules CUPRIMINE, 125 mg, are opaque yellow and gray capsules containing a white or nearly white powder, and are coded MSD 672. They are supplied as follows:
NDC 0006-0672-68 in bottles of 100.
[*Shown in Product Identification Section*]
A.H.F.S. 64:00
DC 6177824 Issued May 1978

DECADRON® Elixir (dexamethasone, MSD), U.S.P. ℞

Description

Glucocorticoids are adrenocortical steroids, both naturally occurring and synthetic, which are readily absorbed from the gastrointestinal tract.
Dexamethasone, a synthetic adrenocortical steroid, is a white to practically white, odorless, crystalline powder. It is stable in air. It is practically insoluble in water. The molecular weight is 392.47. It is designated chemically as 9-fluoro-11β, 17, 21-trihydroxy-16α-methylpregna-1,4-diene-3,20-dione. The empirical formula is $C_{22}H_{29}FO_5$.
DECADRON (Dexamethasone, MSD) elixir contains 0.5 mg of dexamethasone in each 5 ml. Benzoic acid, 0.1%, is added as a preservative. It also contains alcohol 5%.

Actions

Naturally occurring glucocorticoids (hydrocortisone and cortisone), which also have salt-retaining properties, are used as replacement therapy in adrenocortical deficiency states. Their synthetic analogs, including dexamethasone, are primarily used for their potent anti-inflammatory effects in disorders of many organ systems.
Glucocorticoids cause profound and varied metabolic effects. In addition, they modify the body's immune responses to diverse stimuli.
At equipotent anti-inflammatory doses, dexamethasone almost completely lacks the sodium retaining property of hydrocortisone and closely related derivatives of hydrocortisone.

Indications

1. *Endocrine Disorders*
Primary or secondary adrenocortical insufficiency (hydrocortisone or cortisone is the first choice; synthetic analogs may be used in conjunction with mineralocorticoids where applicable; in infancy mineralocorticoid supplementation is of particular importance)
Congenital adrenal hyperplasia
Nonsuppurative thyroiditis
Hypercalcemia associated with cancer
2. *Rheumatic Disorders*
As adjunctive therapy for short-term administration (to tide the patient over an acute episode or exacerbation) in:
Psoriatic arthritis
Rheumatoid arthritis, including juvenile rheumatoid arthritis (selected cases may require low-dose maintenance therapy)
Ankylosing spondylitis
Acute and subacute bursitis
Acute nonspecific tenosynovitis
Acute gouty arthritis
Post-traumatic osteoarthritis
Synovitis of osteoarthritis
Epicondylitis
3. *Collagen Diseases*
During an exacerbation or as maintenance therapy in selected cases of—
Systemic lupus erythematosus
Acute rheumatic carditis
4. *Dermatologic Diseases*
Pemphigus
Bullous dermatitis herpetiformis
Severe erythema multiforme (Stevens-Johnson syndrome)
Exfoliative dermatitis
Mycosis fungoides
Severe psoriasis
Severe seborrheic dermatitis
5. *Allergic States*
Control of severe or incapacitating allergic conditions intractable to adequate trials of conventional treatment:
Seasonal or perennial allergic rhinitis
Bronchial asthma
Contact dermatitis
Atopic dermatitis
Serum sickness
Drug hypersensitivity reactions
6. *Ophthalmic Diseases*
Severe acute and chronic allergic and inflammatory processes involving the eye and its adnexa, such as—
Allergic conjunctivitis
Keratitis
Allergic corneal marginal ulcers
Herpes zoster ophthalmicus
Iritis and iridocyclitis
Chorioretinitis
Anterior segment inflammation
Diffuse posterior uveitis and choroiditis
Optic neuritis
Sympathetic ophthalmia
7. *Respiratory Diseases*
Symptomatic sarcoidosis
Loeffler's syndrome not manageable by other means
Berylliosis
Fulminating or disseminated pulmonary tuberculosis when used concurrently with appropriate antituberculous chemotherapy
Aspiration pneumonitis
8. *Hematologic Disorders*
Idiopathic thrombocytopenic purpura in adults
Secondary thrombocytopenia in adults
Acquired (autoimmune) hemolytic anemia
Erythroblastopenia (RBC anemia)
Congenital (erythroid) hypoplastic anemia
9. *Neoplastic Diseases*
For palliative management of:
Leukemias and lymphomas in adults
Acute leukemia of childhood
10. *Edematous States*
To induce a diuresis or remission of proteinuria in the nephrotic syndrome, without uremia, of the idiopathic type or that due to lupus erythematosus
11. *Gastrointestinal Diseases*
To tide the patient over a critical period of the disease in:
Ulcerative colitis
Regional enteritis
12. *Miscellaneous*
Tuberculous meningitis with subarachnoid block or impending block when used concurrently with appropriate antituberculous chemotherapy
Trichinosis with neurologic or myocardial involvement
13. *Diagnostic testing of adrenocortical hyperfunction.*

Contraindications

Systemic fungal infections
Hypersensitivity to this product

Warnings

In patients on corticosteroid therapy subjected to unusual stress, increased dosage of rapidly acting corticosteroids before, during, and after the stressful situation is indicated.
Drug-induced secondary adrenocortical insufficiency may result from too rapid withdrawal of corticosteroids and may be minimized by gradual reduction of dosage. This type of relative insufficiency may persist for months after discontinuation of therapy; therefore, in any situation of stress occurring during that period, hormone therapy should be reinstituted. If the patient is receiving steroids already, dosage may have to be increased. Since mineralocorticoid secretion may be impaired, salt and/or a mineralocorticoid should be administered concurrently.
Corticosteroids may mask some signs of infection, and new infections may appear during their use. There may be decreased resistance and inability to localize infection when corticosteroids are used. Moreover, corticosteroids may affect the nitroblue-tetrazolium test for bacterial infection and produce false negative results.
Corticosteroids may activate latent amebiasis. Therefore, it is recommended that latent or active amebiasis be ruled out before initiating corticosteroid therapy in any patient who has spent time in the tropics or any patient with unexplained diarrhea.
Prolonged use of corticosteroids may produce posterior subcapsular cataracts, glaucoma with possible damage to the optic nerves, and may enhance the establishment of secondary ocular infections due to fungi or viruses.
Usage in pregnancy: Since adequate human reproduction studies have not been done with corticosteroids, use of these drugs in pregnancy or in women of childbearing potential requires that the anticipated benefits be weighed against the possible hazards to the mother and embryo or fetus. Infants born of mothers who have received substantial doses of corticosteroids during pregnancy, should be carefully observed for signs of hypoadrenalism.
Corticosteroids appear in breast milk and could suppress growth, interfere with endogenous corticosteroid production, or cause other unwanted effects. Mothers taking pharmacologic doses of corticosteroids should be advised not to nurse.
Average and large doses of hydrocortisone or cortisone can cause elevation of blood pressure, salt and water retention, and increased excretion of potassium. These effects are less likely to occur with the synthetic derivatives except when used in large doses. Dietary salt restriction and potassium supplementation may be necessary. All corticosteroids increase calcium excretion.
While on corticosteroid therapy patients should not be vaccinated against smallpox. Other immunization procedures should not be undertaken in patients who are on corticosteroids, especially on high doses, because of possible hazards of neurologic complications and a lack of antibody response. However, immunization procedures may be undertaken in pa-

Continued on next page

Information on the Merck Sharp & Dohme products listed on these pages is the full prescribing information from package circulars in use October 31, 1979.

Merck Sharp & Dohme—Cont.

tients who are receiving corticosteroids as replacement therapy, e.g., for Addison's disease.
The use of DECADRON elixir in active tuberculosis should be restricted to those cases of fulminating or disseminated tuberculosis in which the corticosteroid is used for the management of the disease in conjunction with an appropriate antituberculous regimen.
If corticosteroids are indicated in patients with latent tuberculosis or tuberculin reactivity, close observation is necessary as reactivation of the disease may occur. During prolonged corticosteroid therapy, these patients should receive chemoprophylaxis.

Precautions

Following prolonged therapy, withdrawal of corticosteroids may result in symptoms of the corticosteroid withdrawal syndrome including fever, myalgia, arthralgia, and malaise. This may occur in patients even without evidence of adrenal insufficiency.
There is an enhanced effect of corticosteroids in patients with hypothyroidism and in those with cirrhosis.
Corticosteroids should be used cautiously in patients with ocular herpes simplex because of possible corneal perforation.
The lowest possible dose of corticosteroid should be used to control the condition under treatment, and when reduction in dosage is possible, the reduction should be gradual.
Psychic derangements may appear when corticosteroids are used, ranging from euphoria, insomnia, mood swings, personality changes, and severe depression, to frank psychotic manifestations. Also, existing emotional instability or psychotic tendencies may be aggravated by corticosteroids.
Aspirin should be used cautiously in conjunction with corticosteroids in hypoprothrombinemia.
Steroids should be used with caution in nonspecific ulcerative colitis, if there is a probability of impending perforation, abscess, or other pyogenic infection; diverticulitis; fresh intestinal anastomoses; active or latent peptic ulcer; renal insufficiency; hypertension; osteoporosis; and myasthenia gravis. Fat embolism has been reported as a possible complication of hypercortisonism.
When large doses are given, some authorities advise that corticosteroids be taken with meals and antacids taken between meals to help to prevent peptic ulcer.
Growth and development of infants and children on prolonged corticosteroid therapy should be carefully observed.
Steroids may increase or decrease motility and number of spermatozoa in some patients.
Phenytoin, phenobarbital, ephedrine, and rifampin may enhance the metabolic clearance of corticosteroids, resulting in decreased blood levels and lessened physiologic activity, thus requiring adjustment in corticosteroid dosage. These interactions may interfere with dexamethasone suppression tests which should be interpreted with caution during administration of these drugs.
The prothrombin time should be checked frequently in patients who are receiving corticosteroids and coumarin anticoagulants at the same time because of reports that corticosteroids have altered the response to these anticoagulants. Studies have shown that the usual effect produced by adding corticosteroids is inhibition of response to coumarins, although there have been some conflicting reports of potentiation not substantiated by studies.
When corticosteroids are administered concomitantly with potassium-depleting diuretics, patients should be observed closely for development of hypokalemia.

Adverse Reactions

Fluid and Electrolyte Disturbances
- Sodium retention
- Fluid retention
- Congestive heart failure in susceptible patients
- Potassium loss
- Hypokalemic alkalosis
- Hypertension

Musculoskeletal
- Muscle weakness
- Steroid myopathy
- Loss of muscle mass
- Osteoporosis
- Vertebral compression fractures
- Aseptic necrosis of femoral and humeral heads
- Pathologic fracture of long bones
- Tendon rupture

Gastrointestinal
- Peptic ulcer with possible perforation and hemorrhage
- Pancreatitis
- Abdominal distention
- Ulcerative esophagitis

Dermatologic
- Impaired wound healing
- Thin fragile skin
- Petechiae and ecchymoses
- Erythema
- Increased sweating
- May suppress reactions to skin tests
- Other cutaneous reactions, such as allergic dermatitis, urticaria, angioneurotic edema

Neurologic
- Convulsions
- Increased intracranial pressure with papilledema (pseudotumor cerebri) usually after treatment
- Vertigo
- Headache

Endocrine
- Menstrual irregularities
- Development of cushingoid state
- Suppression of growth in children
- Secondary adrenocortical and pituitary unresponsiveness, particularly in times of stress, as in trauma, surgery, or illness
- Decreased carbohydrate tolerance
- Manifestations of latent diabetes mellitus
- Increased requirements for insulin or oral hypoglycemic agents in diabetics

Ophthalmic
- Posterior subcapsular cataracts
- Increased intraocular pressure
- Glaucoma
- Exophthalmos

Metabolic
- Negative nitrogen balance due to protein catabolism

Other
- Hypersensitivity
- Thromboembolism
- Weight gain
- Increased appetite
- Nausea
- Malaise

Dosage and Administration

For oral administration
DOSAGE REQUIREMENTS ARE VARIABLE AND MUST BE INDIVIDUALIZED ON THE BASIS OF THE DISEASE AND THE RESPONSE OF THE PATIENT.
The initial dosage varies from 0.75 to 9 mg a day depending on the disease being treated. In less severe diseases doses lower than 0.75 mg may suffice, while in severe diseases doses higher than 9 mg may be required. The initial dosage should be maintained or adjusted until the patient's response is satisfactory. If satisfactory clinical response does not occur after a reasonable period of time, discontinue DECADRON elixir and transfer the patient to other therapy.
After a favorable initial response, the proper maintenance dosage should be determined by decreasing the initial dosage in small amounts to the lowest dosage that maintains an adequate clinical response.
Patients should be observed closely for signs that might require dosage adjustment, including changes in clinical status resulting from remissions or exacerbations of the disease, individual drug responsiveness, and the effect of stress (e.g., surgery, infection, trauma). During stress it may be necessary to increase dosage temporarily.
If the drug is to be stopped after more than a few days of treatment, it usually should be withdrawn gradually.
The following milligram equivalents facilitate changing to DECADRON from other glucocorticoids:

DECADRON	Methylprednisolone and Triamcinolone	Prednisolone and Prednisone	Hydrocortisone	Cortisone
0.75 mg =	4 mg =	5 mg =	20 mg =	25 mg

Dexamethasone suppression tests
1. Tests for Cushing's syndrome
   Give 1.0 mg of DECADRON orally at 11:00 p.m. Blood is drawn for plasma cortisol determination at 8:00 a.m. the following morning.
   For greater accuracy, give 0.5 mg of DECADRON orally every 6 hours for 48 hours. Twenty-four hour urine collections are made for determination of 17-hydroxycorticosteroid excretion.
2. Test to distinguish Cushing's syndrome due to pituitary ACTH excess from Cushing's syndrome due to other causes
   Give 2.0 mg of DECADRON orally every 6 hours for 48 hours. Twenty-four hour urine collections are made for determination of 17-hydroxycorticosteroid excretion.

How Supplied

No. 7622—Elixir DECADRON, 0.5 mg dexamethasone per 5 ml, is a clear, red liquid and is supplied as follows:
NDC 0006-7622-55 bottles of 100 ml with calibrated dropper assembly.
NDC 0006-7622-66 bottles of 237 ml without dropper assembly.
A.H.F.S. 68:04
DC 6030722 Issued May 1979

DECADRON® Tablets ℞
(dexamethasone, MSD), U.S.P.

Description

Glucocorticoids are adrenocortical steroids, both naturally occurring and synthetic, which are readily absorbed from the gastrointestinal tract.
Dexamethasone, a synthetic adrenocortical steroid, is a practically white, odorless, crystalline powder. It is stable in air. It is practically insoluble in water. The molecular weight is 392.47. It is designated chemically as 9-fluoro-11β,17,21-trihydroxy-16α-methylpregna-1, 4-diene-3,20-dione. The empirical formula is $C_{22}H_{29}FO_5$.
DECADRON (Dexamethasone, MSD) tablets are supplied in five potencies, 0.25 mg, 0.5 mg, 0.75 mg, 1.5 mg, and 4 mg.

Actions

Naturally occurring glucocorticoids (hydrocortisone and cortisone), which also have salt-retaining properties, are used as replacement therapy in adrenocortical deficiency states. Their synthetic analogs including dexamethasone are primarily used for their potent anti-inflammatory effects in disorders of many organ systems.
Glucocorticoids cause profound and varied metabolic effects. In addition, they modify the body's immune responses to diverse stimuli.
At equipotent anti-inflammatory doses, dexamethasone almost completely lacks the sodium retaining property of hydrocortisone and closely related derivatives of hydrocortisone.

Indications

1. *Endocrine Disorders*
Primary or secondary adrenocortical insufficiency (hydrocortisone or cortisone is the first choice; synthetic analogs may be used in conjunction with mineralocorticoids where applicable; in infancy mineralocorticoid supplementation is of particular importance).
Congenital adrenal hyperplasia
Nonsuppurative thyroiditis
Hypercalcemia associated with cancer
2. *Rheumatic Disorders*
As adjunctive therapy for short-term administration (to tide the patient over an acute episode or exacerbation) in:
Psoriatic arthritis
Rheumatoid arthritis, including juvenile rheumatoid arthritis (selected cases may require low-dose maintenance therapy)
Ankylosing spondylitis
Acute and subacute bursitis
Acute nonspecific tenosynovitis
Acute gouty arthritis
Post-traumatic osteoarthritis
Synovitis of osteoarthritis
Epicondylitis
3. *Collagen Diseases*
During an exacerbation or as maintenance therapy in selected cases of—
Systemic lupus erythematosus
Acute rheumatic carditis
4. *Dermatologic Diseases*
Pemphigus
Bullous dermatitis herpetiformis
Severe erythema multiforme (Stevens-Johnson syndrome)
Exfoliative dermatitis
Mycosis fungoides
Severe psoriasis
Severe seborrheic dermatitis
5. *Allergic States*
Control of severe or incapacitating allergic conditions intractable to adequate trials of conventional treatment:
Seasonal or perennial allergic rhinitis
Bronchial asthma
Contact dermatitis
Atopic dermatitis
Serum sickness
Drug hypersensitivity reactions
6. *Ophthalmic Diseases*
Severe acute and chronic allergic and inflammatory processes involving the eye and its adnexa, such as—
Allergic conjunctivitis
Keratitis
Allergic corneal marginal ulcers
Herpes zoster ophthalmicus
Iritis and iridocyclitis
Chorioretinitis
Anterior segment inflammation
Diffuse posterior uveitis and choroiditis
Optic neuritis
Sympathetic ophthalmia
7. *Respiratory Diseases*
Symptomatic sarcoidosis
Loeffler's syndrome not manageable by other means
Berylliosis
Fulminating or disseminated pulmonary tuberculosis when used concurrently with appropriate antituberculous chemotherapy
Aspiration pneumonitis
8. *Hematologic Disorders*
Idiopathic thrombocytopenic purpura in adults
Secondary thrombocytopenia in adults
Acquired (autoimmune) hemolytic anemia
Erythroblastopenia (RBC anemia)
Congenital (erythroid) hypoplastic anemia
9. *Neoplastic Diseases*
For palliative management of:
Leukemias and lymphomas in adults
Acute leukemia of childhood
10. *Edematous States*
To induce a diuresis or remission of proteinuria in the nephrotic syndrome, without uremia, of the idiopathic type or that due to lupus erythematosus
11. *Gastrointestinal Diseases*
To tide the patient over a critical period of the disease in:
Ulcerative colitis
Regional enteritis
12. *Cerebral Edema* associated with primary or metastatic brain tumor, craniotomy, or head injury. Use in cerebral edema is not a substitute for careful neurosurgical evaluation and definitive management such as neurosurgery or other specific therapy.
13. *Miscellaneous*
Tuberculous meningitis with subarachnoid block or impending block when used concurrently with appropriate antituberculous chemotherapy
Trichinosis with neurologic or myocardial involvement
14. *Diagnostic testing of adrenocortical hyperfunction.*

Contraindications

Systemic fungal infections
Hypersensitivity to this drug

Warnings

In patients on corticosteroid therapy subjected to unusual stress, increased dosage of rapidly acting corticosteroids before, during, and after the stressful situation is indicated.
Drug-induced secondary adrenocortical insufficiency may result from too rapid withdrawal of corticosteroids and may be minimized by gradual reduction of dosage. This type of relative insufficiency may persist for months after discontinuation of therapy; therefore, in any situation of stress occurring during that period, hormone therapy should be reinstituted. If the patient is receiving steroids already, dosage may have to be increased. Since mineralocorticoid secretion may be impaired, salt and/or a mineralocorticoid should be administered concurrently.
Corticosteroids may mask some signs of infection, and new infections may appear during their use. There may be decreased resistance and inability to localize infection when corticosteroids are used. Moreover, corticosteroids may affect the nitroblue-tetrazolium test for bacterial infection and produce false negative results.
Corticosteroids may activate latent amebiasis. Therefore, it is recommended that latent or active amebiasis be ruled out before initiating corticosteroid therapy in any patient who has spent time in the tropics or any patient with unexplained diarrhea.
Prolonged use of corticosteroids may produce posterior subcapsular cataracts and glaucoma with possible damage to the optic nerves, and may enhance the establishment of secondary ocular infections due to fungi or viruses.
Usage in pregnancy: Since adequate human reproduction studies have not been done with corticosteroids, use of these drugs in pregnancy or in women of childbearing potential requires that the anticipated benefits be weighed against the possible hazards to the mother and embryo or fetus. Infants born of mothers who have received substantial doses of corticosteroids during pregnancy should be carefully observed for signs of hypoadrenalism.
Corticosteroids appear in breast milk and could suppress growth, interfere with endogenous corticosteroid production, or cause other unwanted effects. Mothers taking pharmacologic doses of corticosteroids should be advised not to nurse.
Average and large doses of hydrocortisone or cortisone can cause elevation of blood pressure, salt and water retention, and increased excretion of potassium. These effects are less likely to occur with the synthetic derivatives except when used in large doses. Dietary salt restriction and potassium supplementation may be necessary. All corticosteroids increase calcium excretion.
While on corticosteroid therapy patients should not be vaccinated against smallpox. Other immunization procedures should not be undertaken in patients who are on corticosteroids, especially on high doses, because of possible hazards of neurologic complications and a lack of antibody response. However, immunization procedures may be undertaken in patients who are receiving corticosteroids as replacement therapy, e.g., for Addison's disease.
The use of DECADRON tablets in active tuberculosis should be restricted to those cases of fulminating or disseminated tuberculosis in which the corticosteroid is used for the management of the disease in conjunction with an appropriate antituberculous regimen.
If corticosteroids are indicated in patients with latent tuberculosis or tuberculin reactivity, close observation is necessary as reactivation of the disease may occur. During prolonged corticosteroid therapy, these patients should receive chemoprophylaxis.

Precautions

Following prolonged therapy, withdrawal of corticosteroids may result in symptoms of the corticosteroid withdrawal syndrome including fever, myalgia, arthralgia, and malaise. This may occur in patients even without evidence of adrenal insufficiency.
There is an enhanced effect of corticosteroids in patients with hypothyroidism and in those with cirrhosis.
Corticosteroids should be used cautiously in patients with ocular herpes simplex because of possible corneal perforation.
The lowest possible dose of corticosteroid should be used to control the condition under treatment, and when reduction in dosage is possible, the reduction should be gradual.
Psychic derangements may appear when corticosteroids are used, ranging from euphoria, insomnia, mood swings, personality changes, and severe depression, to frank psychotic manifestations. Also, existing emotional instability or psychotic tendencies may be aggravated by corticosteroids.
Aspirin should be used cautiously in conjunction with corticosteroids in hypoprothrombinemia.
Steroids should be used with caution in nonspecific ulcerative colitis, if there is a probability of impending perforation, abscess, or other pyogenic infection, diverticulitis, fresh intestinal anastomoses, active or latent peptic ulcer, renal insufficiency, hypertension, osteoporosis,

Continued on next page

Information on the Merck Sharp & Dohme products listed on these pages is the full prescribing information from package circulars in use October 31, 1979.

Merck Sharp & Dohme—Cont.

and myasthenia gravis. Fat embolism has been reported as a possible complication of hypercortisonism.

When large doses are given, some authorities advise that corticosteroids be taken with meals and antacids taken between meals to help to prevent peptic ulcer.

Growth and development of infants and children on prolonged corticosteroid therapy should be carefully observed.

Steroids may increase or decrease motility and number of spermatozoa in some patients.

Phenytoin, phenobarbital, ephedrine, and rifampin may enhance the metabolic clearance of corticosteroids, resulting in decreased blood levels and lessened physiologic activity, thus requiring adjustment in corticosteroid dosage. These interactions may interfere with dexamethasone suppression tests which should be interpreted with caution during administration of these drugs.

The prothrombin time should be checked frequently in patients who are receiving corticosteroids and coumarin anticoagulants at the same time because of reports that corticosteroids have altered the response to these anticoagulants. Studies have shown that the usual effect produced by adding corticosteroids is inhibition of response to coumarins, although there have been some conflicting reports of potentiation not substantiated by studies.

When corticosteroids are administered concomitantly with potassium-depleting diuretics, patients should be observed closely for development of hypokalemia.

Adverse Reactions

Fluid and Electrolyte Disturbances

Sodium retention
Fluid retention
Congestive heart failure in susceptible patients
Potassium loss
Hypokalemic alkalosis
Hypertension

Musculoskeletal

Muscle weakness
Steroid myopathy
Loss of muscle mass
Osteoporosis
Vertebral compression fractures
Aseptic necrosis of femoral and humeral heads
Pathologic fracture of long bones
Tendon rupture

Gastrointestinal

Peptic ulcer with possible perforation and hemorrhage
Pancreatitis
Abdominal distention
Ulcerative esophagitis

Dermatologic

Impaired wound healing
Thin fragile skin
Petechiae and ecchymoses
Erythema
Increased sweating
May suppress reactions to skin tests
Other cutaneous reactions, such as allergic dermatitis, urticaria, angioneurotic edema

Neurologic

Convulsions
Increased intracranial pressure with papilledema (pseudotumor cerebri) usually after treatment
Vertigo
Headache

Endocrine

Menstrual irregularities
Development of cushingoid state
Suppression of growth in children
Secondary adrenocortical and pituitary unresponsiveness, particularly in times of stress, as in trauma, surgery, or illness
Decreased carbohydrate tolerance
Manifestations of latent diabetes mellitus
Increased requirements for insulin or oral hypoglycemic agents in diabetics

Ophthalmic

Posterior subcapsular cataracts
Increased intraocular pressure
Glaucoma
Exophthalmos

Metabolic

Negative nitrogen balance due to protein catabolism

Other

Hypersensitivity
Thromboembolism
Weight gain
Increased appetite
Nausea
Malaise

Dosage and Administration

For oral administration

DOSAGE REQUIREMENTS ARE VARIABLE AND MUST BE INDIVIDUALIZED ON THE BASIS OF THE DISEASE AND THE RESPONSE OF THE PATIENT.

The initial dosage varies from 0.75 to 9 mg a day depending on the disease being treated. In less severe diseases doses lower than 0.75 mg may suffice, while in severe diseases doses higher than 9 mg may be required. The initial dosage should be maintained or adjusted until the patient's response is satisfactory. If satisfactory clinical response does not occur after a reasonable period of time, discontinue DECADRON tablets and transfer the patient to other therapy.

After a favorable initial response, the proper maintenance dosage should be determined by decreasing the initial dosage in small amounts to the lowest dosage that maintains an adequate clinical response.

Patients should be observed closely for signs that might require dosage adjustment, including changes in clinical status resulting from remissions or exacerbations of the disease, individual drug responsiveness, and the effect of stress (e.g., surgery, infection, trauma). During stress it may be necessary to increase dosage temporarily.

If the drug is to be stopped after more than a few days of treatment, it usually should be withdrawn gradually.

The following milligram equivalents facilitate changing to DECADRON from other glucocorticoids:

DECADRON	Methylprednisolone and Triamcinolone	Prednisolone and Prednisone	Hydrocortisone	Cortisone
0.75 mg =	4 mg =	5 mg =	20 mg =	25 mg

In *acute, self-limited allergic disorders or acute exacerbations of chronic allergic disorders,* the following dosage schedule combining parenteral and oral therapy is suggested:

DECADRON phosphate (Dexamethasone Sodium Phosphate, MSD) injection, 4 mg per ml:

First Day
1 or 2 ml, intramuscularly

DECADRON tablets, 0.75 mg:

Second Day
4 tablets in two divided doses
Third Day
4 tablets in two divided doses
Fourth Day
2 tablets in two divided doses
Fifth Day
1 tablet
Sixth Day
1 tablet
Seventh Day
No treatment
Eighth Day
Follow-up visit

This schedule is designed to ensure adequate therapy during acute episodes, while minimizing the risk of overdosage in chronic cases.

In *cerebral edema,* DECADRON phosphate (Dexamethasone Sodium Phosphate, MSD) injection is generally administered initially in a dosage of 10 mg intravenously followed by 4 mg every six hours intramuscularly until the symptoms of cerebral edema subside. Response is usually noted within 12 to 24 hours and dosage may be reduced after two to four days and gradually discontinued over a period of five to seven days. For palliative management of patients with recurrent or inoperable brain tumors, maintenance therapy with either DECADRON phosphate (Dexamethasone Sodium Phosphate, MSD) injection or DECADRON tablets in a dosage of two mg two or three times daily may be effective.

Dexamethasone suppression tests

1. Tests for Cushing's syndrome
   Give 1.0 mg of DECADRON orally at 11:00 p.m. Blood is drawn for plasma cortisol determination at 8:00 a.m. the following morning.
   For greater accuracy, give 0.5 mg of DECADRON orally every 6 hours for 48 hours. Twenty-four hour urine collections are made for determination of 17-hydroxycorticosteroid excretion.
2. Test to distinguish Cushing's syndrome due to pituitary ACTH excess from Cushing's syndrome due to other causes
   Give 2.0 mg of DECADRON orally every 6 hours for 48 hours. Twenty-four hour urine collections are made for determination of 17-hydroxycorticosteroid excretion.

How Supplied

Tablets DECADRON are compressed, pentagonal-shaped tablets, colored to distinguish potency. They are scored on one side and are available as follows:

No. 7645—4 mg, white in color and coded MSD 97.
NDC 0006-0097-50 bottles of 50.
NDC 0006-0097-28 single unit packages of 100.
[*Shown in Product Identification Section*]

No. 7638—1.5 mg, pink in color and coded MSD 95.
NDC 0006-0095-50 bottles of 50.
NDC 0006-0095-28 single unit packages of 100.
[*Shown in Product Identification Section*]

No. 7601—0.75 mg, bluish-green in color and coded MSD 63.
NDC 0006-0063-12 5-12 PAK (package of 12).
NDC 0006-0063-68 bottles of 100.
NDC 0006-0063-28 single unit packages of 100.
NDC 0006-0063-82 bottles of 1000.
[*Shown in Product Identification Section*]

No. 7598—0.5 mg, yellow in color and coded MSD 41.
NDC 0006-0041-68 bottles of 100.
(6505-00-687-8482 0.5 mg 100's).
NDC 0006-0041-28 single unit packages of 100.
NDC 0006-0041-82 bottles of 1000.
[*Shown in Product Identification Section*]

No. 7592—0.25 mg, orange in color and coded MSD 20.
NDC 0006-0020-68 bottles of 100.
[*Shown in Product Identification Section*]

A.H.F.S. 68:04
DC 6025237 Issued May 1979

DECADRON® Phosphate Injection ℞
(dexamethasone sodium phosphate, MSD), U.S.P.

Description

Dexamethasone sodium phosphate, a synthetic adrenocortical steroid, is a white or slightly yellow, crystalline powder. It is freely soluble in water and is exceedingly hygroscopic. The molecular weight is 516.14. It is designated chemically as 9-fluoro-11β, 17-dihydroxy-16α-methyl-21-(phosphonooxy)pregna-1, 4-diene-3, 20-dione disodium salt. The empirical formula is $C_{22}H_{28}FNa_2O_8P$.

DECADRON phosphate (Dexamethasone Sodium Phosphate, MSD) injection is a sterile solution (pH 7.0 to 8.5) of dexamethasone sodium phosphate, and is supplied in two concentrations: 4 mg/ml and 24 mg/ml. The 24 mg/ml concentration offers the advantage of less volume in indications where high doses of corticosteroids by the intravenous route are needed.

Each milliliter of DECADRON phosphate injection, 4 mg/ml, contains dexamethasone sodium phosphate equivalent to 4 mg dexamethasone phosphate or 3.33 mg dexamethasone. Inactive ingredients per ml: 8 mg creatinine, 10 mg sodium citrate, sodium hydroxide to ajust pH, and Water for Injection q.s., with 1 mg sodium bisulfite, 1.5 mg methylparaben, and 0.2 mg propylparaben added as preservatives.

Each milliliter of DECADRON phosphate injection, 24 mg/ml, contains dexamethasone sodium phosphate equivalent to 24 mg dexamethasone phosphate or 20 mg dexamethasone. Inactive ingredients per ml: 8 mg creatinine, 10 mg sodium citrate, 0.5 mg disodium edetate, sodium hydroxide to adjust pH, and Water for Injection q.s., with 1 mg sodium bisulfite, 1.5 mg methylparaben, and 0.2 mg propylparaben added as preservatives.

Actions

DECADRON phosphate injection has a rapid onset but short duration of action when compared with less soluble preparations. Because of this, it is suitable for the treatment of acute disorders responsive to adrenocortical steroid therapy.

Naturally occurring glucocorticoids (hydrocortisone and cortisone), which also have salt-retaining properties, are used as replacement therapy in adrenocortical deficiency states. Their synthetic analogs, including dexamethasone, are primarily used for their potent anti-inflammatory effects in disorders of many organ systems.

Glucocorticoids cause profound and varied metabolic effects. In addition, they modify the body's immune responses to diverse stimuli.

At equipotent anti-inflammatory doses, dexamethasone almost completely lacks the sodium-retaining property of hydrocortisone and closely related derivatives of hydrocortisone.

Indications

A. By intravenous or intramuscular injection when oral therapy is not feasible:

1. *Endocrine disorders*

Primary or secondary adrenocortical insufficiency (hydrocortisone or cortisone is the drug of choice; synthetic analogs may be used in conjunction with mineralocorticoids where applicable; in infancy, mineralocorticoid supplementation is of particular importance)

Acute adrenocortical insufficiency (hydrocortisone or cortisone is the drug of choice; mineralocorticoid supplementation may be necessary, particularly when synthetic analogs are used)

Preoperatively, and in the event of serious trauma or illness, in patients with known adrenal insufficiency or when adrenocortical reserve is doubtful

Shock unresponsive to conventional therapy if adrenocortical insufficiency exists or is suspected

Congenital adrenal hyperplasia

Nonsuppurative thyroiditis

Hypercalcemia associated with cancer

2. *Rheumatic disorders*

As adjunctive therapy for short-term administration (to tide the patient over an acute episode or exacerbation) in:

Post-traumatic osteoarthritis

Synovitis of osteoarthritis

Rheumatoid arthritis, including juvenile rheumatoid arthritis (selected cases may require low-dose maintenance therapy)

Acute and subacute bursitis

Epicondylitis

Acute nonspecific tenosynovitis

Acute gouty arthritis

Psoriatic arthritis

Ankylosing spondylitis

3. *Collagen diseases*

During an exacerbation or as maintenance therapy in selected cases of:

Systemic lupus erythematosus

Acute rheumatic carditis

4. *Dermatologic diseases*

Pemphigus

Severe erythema multiforme (Stevens-Johnson syndrome)

Exfoliative dermatitis

Bullous dermatitis herpetiformis

Severe seborrheic dermatitis

Severe psoriasis

Mycosis fungoides

5. *Allergic states*

Control of severe or incapacitating allergic conditions intractable to adequate trials of conventional treatment in:

Bronchial asthma

Contact dermatitis

Atopic dermatitis

Serum sickness

Seasonal or perennial allergic rhinitis

Drug hypersensitivity reactions

Urticarial transfusion reactions

Acute noninfectious laryngeal edema (epinephrine is the drug of first choice)

6. *Ophthalmic diseases*

Severe acute and chronic allergic and inflammatory processes involving the eye, such as:

Herpes zoster ophthalmicus

Iritis, iridocyclitis

Chorioretinitis

Diffuse posterior uveitis and choroiditis

Optic neuritis

Sympathetic ophthalmia

Anterior segment inflammation

Allergic conjunctivitis

Keratitis

Allergic corneal marginal ulcers

7. *Gastrointestinal diseases*

To tide the patient over a critical period of the disease in:

Ulcerative colitis (Systemic therapy)

Regional enteritis (Systemic therapy)

8. *Respiratory diseases*

Symptomatic sarcoidosis

Berylliosis

Fulminating or disseminated pulmonary tuberculosis when used concurrently with appropriate antituberculous chemotherapy

Loeffler's syndrome not manageable by other means

Aspiration pneumonitis

9. *Hematologic disorders*

Acquired (autoimmune) hemolytic anemia

Idiopathic thrombocytopenic purpura in adults (I.V. only; I.M. administration is contraindicated)

Secondary thrombocytopenia in adults

Erythroblastopenia (RBC anemia)

Congenital (erythroid) hypoplastic anemia

10. *Neoplastic diseases*

For palliative management of:

Leukemias and lymphomas in adults

Acute leukemia of childhood

11. *Edematous states*

To induce diuresis or remission of proteinuria in the nephrotic syndrome, without uremia, of the idiopathic type, or that due to lupus erythematosus

12. *Miscellaneous*

Tuberculous meningitis with subarachnoid block or impending block when used concurrently with appropriate antituberculous chemotherapy

Trichinosis with neurologic or myocardial involvement

13. *Diagnostic testing of adrenocortical hyperfunction*

14. *Cerebral Edema* associated with primary or metastatic brain tumor, craniotomy, or head injury. Use in cerebral edema is not a substitute for careful neurosurgical evaluation and definitive management such as neurosurgery or other specific therapy.

B. By intra-articular or soft tissue injection:

As adjunctive therapy for short-term administration (to tide the patient over an acute episode or exacerbation) in:

Synovitis of osteoarthritis

Rheumatoid arthritis

Acute and subacute bursitis

Acute gouty arthritis

Epicondylitis

Acute nonspecific tenosynovitis

Post-traumatic osteoarthritis

C. By intralesional injection:

Keloids

Localized hypertrophic, infiltrated, inflammatory lesions of: lichen planus, psoriatic plaques, granuloma annulare, and lichen simplex chronicus (neurodermatitis)

Discoid lupus erythematosus

Necrobiosis lipoidica diabeticorum

Alopecia areata

May also be useful in cystic tumors of an aponeurosis or tendon (ganglia)

Contraindications

Systemic fungal infections (See WARNINGS re amphotericin B)

Hypersensitivity to any component of this product

Warnings

Corticosteroids may exacerbate systemic fungal infections and therefore should not be used in the presence of such infections unless they are needed to control drug reactions due to amphotericin B. Moreover, there have been cases reported in which concomitant use of amphotericin B and hydrocortisone was followed by cardiac enlargement and congestive failure.

In patients on corticosteroid therapy subjected to any unusual stress, increased dosage of rapidly acting corticosteroids before, during, and after the stressful situation is indicated.

Drug-induced secondary adrenocortical insufficiency may result from too rapid withdrawal of corticosteroids and may be minimized by gradual reduction of dosage. This type of relative insufficiency may persist for months after discontinuation of therapy; therefore, in any situation of stress occurring during that period, hormone therapy should be reinstituted. If the patient is receiving steroids already, dosage may have to be increased. Since mineralocorticoid secretion may be impaired, salt and/or a mineralocorticoid should be administered concurrently.

Continued on next page

Information on the Merck Sharp & Dohme products listed on these pages is the full prescribing information from package circulars in use October 31, 1979.

Merck Sharp & Dohme—Cont.

Corticosteroids may mask some signs of infection, and new infections may appear during their use. There may be decreased resistance and inability to localize infection when corticosteroids are used. Moreover, corticosteroids may affect the nitroblue-tetrazolium test for bacterial infection and produce false negative results.
Corticosteroids may activate latent amebiasis. Therefore, it is recommended that latent or active amebiasis be ruled out before initiating corticosteroid therapy in any patient who has spent time in the tropics or any patient with unexplained diarrhea.
Prolonged use of corticosteroids may produce posterior subcapsular cataracts, glaucoma with possible damage to the optic nerves, and may enhance the establishment of secondary ocular infections due to fungi or viruses.
Usage in pregnancy. Since adequate human reproduction studies have not been done with corticosteroids, use of these drugs in pregnancy or in women of childbearing potential requires that the anticipated benefits be weighed against the possible hazards to the mother and embryo or fetus. Infants born of mothers who have received substantial doses of corticosteroids during pregnancy should be carefully observed for signs of hypoadrenalism.
Corticosteroids appear in breast milk and could suppress growth, interfere with endogenous corticosteroid production, or cause other unwanted effects. Mothers taking pharmacologic doses of corticosteroids should be advised not to nurse.
Average and large doses of cortisone or hydrocortisone can cause elevation of blood pressure, salt and water retention, and increased excretion of potassium. These effects are less likely to occur with the synthetic derivatives except when used in large doses. Dietary salt restriction and potassium supplementation may be necessary. All corticosteroids increase calcium excretion.
While on corticosteroid therapy patients should not be vaccinated against smallpox. Other immunization procedures should not be undertaken in patients who are on corticosteroids, especially on high doses, because of possible hazards of neurologic complications and lack of antibody response. However, immunization procedures may be undertaken in patients who are receiving corticosteroids as replacement therapy, e.g., for Addison's disease.
The use of DECADRON phosphate injection in active tuberculosis should be restricted to those cases of fulminating or disseminated tuberculosis in which the corticosteroid is used for the management of the disease in conjunction with an appropriate antituberculous regimen.
If corticosteroids are indicated in patients with latent tuberculosis or tuberculin reactivity, close observation is necessary as reactivation of the disease may occur. During prolonged corticosteroid therapy, these patients should receive chemoprophylaxis.
Because rare instances of anaphylactoid reactions have occurred in patients receiving parenteral corticosteroid therapy, appropriate precautionary measures should be taken prior to administration, especially when the patient has a history of allergy to any drug.

Precautions

This product, like many other steroid formulations, is sensitive to heat. Therefore, it should not be autoclaved when it is desirable to sterilize the exterior of the vial.
Following prolonged therapy, withdrawal of corticosteroids may result in symptoms of the corticosteroid withdrawal syndrome including fever, myalgia, arthralgia, and malaise. This may occur in patients even without evidence of adrenal insufficiency.
There is an enhanced effect of corticosteroids in patients with hypothyroidism and in those with cirrhosis.
Corticosteroids should be used cautiously in patients with ocular herpes simplex for fear of corneal perforation.
The lowest possible dose of corticosteroid should be used to control the condition under treatment, and when reduction in dosage is possible, the reduction must be gradual.
Psychic derangements may appear when corticosteroids are used, ranging from euphoria, insomnia, mood swings, personality changes, and severe depression to frank psychotic manifestations. Also, existing emotional instability or psychotic tendencies may be aggravated by corticosteroids.
Aspirin should be used cautiously in conjunction with corticosteroids in hypoprothrombinemia.
Steroids should be used with caution in nonspecific ulcerative colitis, if there is a probability of impending perforation, abscess, or other pyogenic infection, also in diverticulitis, fresh intestinal anastomoses, active or latent peptic ulcer, renal insufficiency, hypertension, osteoporosis, and myasthenia gravis. Fat embolism has been reported as a possible complication of hypercortisonism.
When large doses are given, some authorities advise that antacids be administered between meals to help to prevent peptic ulcer.
Growth and development of infants and children on prolonged corticosteroid therapy should be carefully followed.
Steroids may increase or decrease motility and number of spermatozoa in some patients.
Phenytoin, phenobarbital, ephedrine, and rifampin may enhance the metabolic clearance of corticosteroids, resulting in decreased blood levels and lessened physiologic activity, thus requiring adjustment in corticosteroid dosage. These interactions may interfere with dexamethasone suppression tests which should be interpreted with caution during administration of these drugs.
The prothrombin time should be checked frequently in patients who are receiving corticosteroids and coumarin anticoagulants at the same time because of reports that corticosteroids have altered the response to these anticoagulants. Studies have shown that the usual effect produced by adding corticosteroids is inhibition of response to coumarins, although there have been some conflicting reports of potentiation not substantiated by studies.
When corticosteroids are administered concomitantly with potassium-depleting diuretics, patients should be observed closely for development of hypokalemia.
Intra-articular injection of a corticosteroid may produce systemic as well as local effects.
Appropriate examination of any joint fluid present is necessary to exclude a septic process.
A marked increase in pain accompanied by local swelling, further restriction of joint motion, fever, and malaise is suggestive of septic arthritis. If this complication occurs and the diagnosis of sepsis is confirmed, appropriate antimicrobial therapy should be instituted.
Injection of a steroid into an infected site is to be avoided.
Corticosteroids should not be injected into unstable joints.
Patients should be impressed strongly with the importance of not overusing joints in which symptomatic benefit has been obtained as long as the inflammatory process remains active.
Frequent intra-articular injection may result in damage to joint tissues.
The slower rate of absorption by intramuscular administration should be recognized.

Adverse Reactions

Fluid and electrolyte disturbances
Sodium retention
Fluid retention
Congestive heart failure in susceptible patients
Potassium loss
Hypokalemic alkalosis
Hypertension

Musculoskeletal
Muscle weakness
Steroid myopathy
Loss of muscle mass
Osteoporosis
Vertebral compression fractures
Aseptic necrosis of femoral and humeral heads
Pathologic fracture of long bones
Tendon rupture

Gastrointestinal
Peptic ulcer with possible subsequent perforation and hemorrhage
Pancreatitis
Abdominal distention
Ulcerative esophagitis

Dermatologic
Impaired wound healing
Thin fragile skin
Petechiae and ecchymoses
Erythema
Increased sweating
May suppress reactions to skin tests
Burning or tingling, especially in the perineal area (after I.V. injection)
Other cutaneous reactions, such as allergic dermatitis, urticaria, angioneurotic edema

Neurologic
Convulsions
Increased intracranial pressure with papilledema (pseudotumor cerebri) usually after treatment
Vertigo
Headache

Endocrine
Menstrual irregularities
Development of cushingoid state
Suppression of growth in children
Secondary adrenocortical and pituitary unresponsiveness, particularly in times of stress, as in trauma, surgery, or illness
Decreased carbohydrate tolerance
Manifestations of latent diabetes mellitus
Increased requirements for insulin or oral hypoglycemic agents in diabetics

Ophthalmic
Posterior subcapsular cataracts
Increased intraocular pressure
Glaucoma
Exophthalmos

Metabolic
Negative nitrogen balance due to protein catabolism

Other
Anaphylactoid or hypersensitivity reactions
Thromboembolism
Weight gain
Increased appetite
Nausea
Malaise

The following *additional* adverse reactions are related to parenteral corticosteroid therapy:
Rare instances of blindness associated with intralesional therapy around the face and head
Hyperpigmentation or hypopigmentation
Subcutaneous and cutaneous atrophy
Sterile abscess
Postinjection flare (following intra-articular use)
Charcot-like arthropathy

Dosage and Administration

DECADRON phosphate injection, 4 mg/ml—*For intravenous, intramuscular, intra-articular, intralesional, and soft tissue injection.*
DECADRON phosphate injection, 24 mg/ml—*For intravenous injection only.*

DOSAGE REQUIREMENTS ARE VARIABLE AND MUST BE INDIVIDUALIZED ON THE BASIS OF THE DISEASE AND THE RESPONSE OF THE PATIENT.

Intravenous and Intramuscular Injection

The initial dosage of DECADRON phosphate injection varies from 0.5 to 9 mg a day depending on the disease being treated. In less severe diseases doses lower than 0.5 mg may suffice, while in severe diseases doses higher than 9 mg may be required.

The initial dosage should be maintained or adjusted until the patient's response is satisfactory. If a satisfactory clinical response does not occur after a reasonable period of time, discontinue DECADRON phosphate injection and transfer the patient to other therapy.

After a favorable initial response, the proper maintenance dosage should be determined by decreasing the initial dosage in small amounts to the lowest dosage that maintains an adequate clinical response.

Patients should be observed closely for signs that might require dosage adjustment, including changes in clinical status resulting from remissions or exacerbations of the disease, individual drug responsiveness, and the effect of stress (e.g., surgery, infection, trauma). During stress it may be necessary to increase dosage temporarily.

If the drug is to be stopped after more than a few days of treatment, it usually should be withdrawn gradually.

When the intravenous route of administration is used, dosage usually should be the same as the oral dosage. In certain overwhelming, acute, life-threatening situations, however, administration in dosages exceeding the usual dosages may be justified and may be in multiples of the oral dosages. The slower rate of absorption by intramuscular administration should be recognized.

Shock

There is a tendency in current medical practice to use high (pharmacologic) doses of corticosteroids for the treatment of unresponsive shock. The following dosages of DECADRON phosphate injection have been suggested by various authors:

*Author**	*Dosage*
Cavanagh[1]	3 mg/kg of body weight per 24 hours by constant intravenous infusion after an initial intravenous injection of 20 mg
Dietzman[2]	2 to 6 mg/kg of body weight as a single intravenous injection
Frank[3]	40 mg initially followed by repeat intravenous injection every 4 to 6 hours while shock persists
Oaks[4]	40 mg initially followed by repeat intravenous injection every 2 to 6 hours while shock persists
Schumer[5]	1 mg/kg of body weight as a single intravenous injection

Administration of high dose corticosteroid therapy should be continued only until the patient's condition has stabilized and usually not longer than 48 to 72 hours.

Although adverse reactions associated with high dose, short term corticosteroid therapy are uncommon, peptic ulceration may occur.

*1. Cavanagh, D.; Singh, K. B.: Endotoxin shock in pregnancy and abortion, in "Corticosteroids in the Treatment of Shock", Schumer, W.; Nyhus, L. M., Editors, Urbana, University of Illinois Press, 1970, pp. 86-96.

2. Dietzman, R. H.; Ersek, R. A.; Bloch, J. M.; Lillehei, R. C.: High-output, low-resistance gram-negative septic shock in man, Angiology *20:*691-700, Dec. 1969.

3. Frank, E.: Clinical observations in shock and management (In: Shields, T. F., ed.: Symposium on current concepts and management of shock), J. Maine Med. Ass. *59:*195-200, Oct. 1968.

4. Oaks, W. W.; Cohen, H. E.: Endotoxin shock in the geriatric patient, Geriat. *22:*120-130, Mar. 1967.

5. Schumer, W.; Nyhus, L. M.: Corticosteroid effect on biochemical parameters of human oligemic shock, Arch. Surg. *100:*405-408, Apr. 1970.

Cerebral Edema

DECADRON phosphate injection is generally administered initially in a dosage of 10 mg intravenously followed by 4 mg every six hours intramuscularly until the symptoms of cerebral edema subside. Response is usually noted within 12 to 24 hours and dosage may be reduced after two to four days and gradually discontinued over a period of five to seven days. For palliative management of patients with recurrent or inoperable brain tumors, maintenance therapy with two mg two or three times a day may be effective.

Acute Allergic Disorders

In acute, self-limited allergic disorders or acute exacerbations of chronic allergic disorders, the following dosage schedule combining parenteral and oral therapy is suggested:

DECADRON phosphate injection, 4 mg/ml,: *first day,* 1 or 2 ml (4 or 8 mg), intramuscularly.

DECADRON (Dexamethasone, MSD) tablets, 0.75 mg: *second and third days,* 4 tablets in two divided doses each day; *fourth day,* 2 tablets in two divided doses; *fifth and sixth days,* 1 tablet each day; *seventh day,* no treatment; *eighth day,* follow-up visit.

This schedule is designed to ensure adequate therapy during acute episodes, while minimizing the risk of overdosage in chronic cases.

Intra-articular, Intralesional, and Soft Tissue Injection

Intra-articular, intralesional, and soft tissue injections are generally employed when the affected joints or areas are limited to one or two sites. Dosage and frequency of injection varies depending on the condition and the site of injection. The usual dose is from 0.2 to 6 mg. The frequency usually ranges from once every three to five days to once every two to three weeks. Frequent intra-articular injection may result in damage to joint tissues.

Some of the usual single doses are:

Site of Injection	Amount of Dexamethasone Phosphate (mg)
Large Joints (e.g., Knee)	2 to 4
Small Joints (e.g., Interphalangeal, Temporomandibular)	0.8 to 1
Bursae	2 to 3
Tendon Sheaths	0.4 to 1
Soft Tissue Infiltration	2 to 6
Ganglia	1 to 2

DECADRON phosphate injection is particularly recommended for use in conjunction with one of the less soluble, longer-acting steroids for intra-articular and soft tissue injection.

How Supplied

No. 7628X—Injection DECADRON phosphate, 4 mg per ml, is a clear, colorless solution, and is available in 1 ml disposable syringes and in 1 ml, 5 ml, and 25 ml vials as follows:

NDC 0006-7628-01, 1 ml disposable syringe (6505-00-935-4117, 1 ml syringe)

NDC 0006-7628-66, boxes of 25 × 1 ml vials

NDC 0006-7628-03, 5 ml vial (6505-00-963-5355, 5 ml vial)

NDC 0006-7628-25, 25 ml vial

FOR INTRAVENOUS USE ONLY:

No. 7646—Injection DECADRON phosphate, 24 mg per ml, is a clear, colorless to light yellow solution and is available in 5 ml and 10 ml vials as follows:

NDC 0006-7646-03, 5 ml vial

NDC 0006-7646-10, 10 ml vial.

A.H.F.S. 68:04

DC 6597116 Issued May 1979

DECADRON® Phosphate ℞
(dexamethasone sodium phosphate, MSD), U.S.P.
0.05% Dexamethasone Phosphate Equivalent
Sterile Ophthalmic Ointment

Description

Sterile Ophthalmic Ointment DECADRON Phosphate (Dexamethasone Sodium Phosphate, MSD) is a topical steroid ointment containing dexamethasone sodium phosphate equivalent to 0.5 mg (0.05%) dexamethasone phosphate in each gram. Inactive ingredients: white petrolatum and mineral oil.

Dexamethasone sodium phosphate is an inorganic ester of dexamethasone.

Action

Inhibition of inflammatory response to inciting agents of mechanical, chemical or immunological nature. No generally accepted explanation of this steroid property has been advanced.

Indications

For the treatment of the following conditions: Steroid responsive inflammatory conditions of the palpebral and bulbar conjunctiva, cornea, and anterior segment of the globe, such as allergic conjunctivitis, acne rosacea, superficial punctate keratitis, herpes zoster keratitis, iritis, cyclitis, selected infective conjunctivitis when the inherent hazard of steroid use is accepted to obtain an advisable diminution in edema and inflammation; corneal injury from chemical or thermal burns, or penetration of foreign bodies.

Contraindications

Acute superficial herpes simplex keratitis.
Fungal diseases of ocular structures.
Vaccinia, varicella and most other viral diseases of the cornea and conjunctiva.
Tuberculosis of the eye.
Hypersensitivity to a component of this medication.

Warning

Employment of steroid medication in the treatment of stromal herpes simplex requires great caution; frequent slit-lamp microscopy is mandatory.

Prolonged use may result in glaucoma, damage to the optic nerve, defects in visual acuity and fields of vision, posterior subcapsular cataract formation, or may aid in the establishment of secondary ocular infections from pathogens liberated from ocular tissues.

In those diseases causing thinning of the cornea or sclera, perforation has been known to occur with the use of topical steroids.

Continued on next page

Information on the Merck Sharp & Dohme products listed on these pages is the full prescribing information from package circulars in use October 31, 1979.

Merck Sharp & Dohme—Cont.

Acute purulent untreated infection of the eye may be masked or activity enhanced by the presence of steroid medication.
Usage in Pregnancy
Safety of intensive or protracted use of topical steroids during pregnancy has not been substantiated.

Precautions

As fungal infections of the cornea are particularly prone to develop coincidentally with long-term local steroid applications, fungus invasion must be considered in any persistent corneal ulceration where a steroid has been used or is in use.
Intraocular pressure should be checked frequently.

Adverse Reactions

Glaucoma with optic nerve damage, visual acuity and field defects, posterior subcapsular cataract formation, secondary ocular infection from pathogens including herpes simplex liberated from ocular tissues, perforation of the globe.
Rarely, filtering blebs have been reported when topical steroids have been used following cataract surgery.
Viral and fungal infections of the cornea may be exacerbated by the application of steroids.
Rarely, stinging or burning may occur.

Dosage and Administration

The duration of treatment will vary with the type of lesion and may extend from a few days to several weeks, according to therapeutic response. Relapses, more common in chronic active lesions than in self-limited conditions, usually respond to retreatment.
Apply a thin coating of ointment three or four times a day. When a favorable response is observed, reduce the number of daily applications to two, and later to one a day as a maintenance dose if this is sufficient to control symptoms.
Ophthalmic ointment DECADRON phosphate is particularly convenient when an eye pad is used. It may also be the preparation of choice for patients in whom therapeutic benefit depends on prolonged contact of the active ingredients with ocular tissues.

How Supplied

No. 7615—0.05% Sterile Ophthalmic Ointment DECADRON phosphate is a clear unctuous ointment and is supplied as follows:
NDC 0006-7615-04 in 3.5 g tubes.
A.H.F.S. 52:08
DC 6033123 Issued November 1975

DECADRON® Phosphate ℞
(dexamethasone sodium phosphate, MSD), U.S.P.
0.1% Dexamethasone Phosphate Equivalent
Sterile Ophthalmic Solution

Description

Ophthalmic Solution DECADRON Phosphate (Dexamethasone Sodium Phosphate, MSD) in the 2.5 ml and 5 ml glass bottles with dropper assembly is a topical steroid solution containing dexamethasone sodium phosphate equivalent to 1 mg (0.1%) dexamethasone phosphate in each milliliter of buffered solution. Inactive ingredients: creatinine, sodium citrate, sodium borate, polysorbate 80, sodium hydroxide to adjust pH, and water for injection. Sodium bisulfite 0.32%, phenylethanol 0.25%, and benzalkonium chloride 0.02% added as preservatives.
Each milliliter of buffered ophthalmic solution DECADRON phosphate in the OCUMETER® ophthalmic dispenser contains: dexamethasone sodium phosphate equivalent to 1 mg (0.1%) dexamethasone phosphate. Inactive ingredients: creatinine, sodium citrate, sodium borate, polysorbate 80, disodium edetate, hydrochloric acid to adjust pH, and water for injection. Sodium bisulfite 0.1%, phenylethanol 0.25% and benzalkonium chloride 0.02% added as preservatives.
Dexamethasone sodium phosphate is a water soluble, inorganic ester of dexamethasone. It is approximately three thousand times more soluble in water at 25°C than hydrocortisone.

Action

Inhibition of inflammatory response to inciting agents of mechanical, chemical or immunological nature. No generally accepted explanation of this steroid property has been advanced.

Indications

For the treatment of the following conditions:
Ophthalmic:
Steroid responsive inflammatory conditions of the palpebral and bulbar conjunctiva, cornea, and anterior segment of the globe, such as allergic conjunctivitis, acne rosacea, superficial punctate keratitis, herpes zoster keratitis, iritis, cyclitis, selected infective conjunctivitis when the inherent hazard of steroid use is accepted to obtain an advisable diminution in edema and inflammation; corneal injury from chemical or thermal burns, or penetration of foreign bodies.
Otic:
Steroid responsive inflammatory conditions of the external auditory meatus, such as allergic otitis externa, selected purulent and nonpurulent infective otitis externa when the hazard of steroid use is accepted to obtain an advisable diminution in edema and inflammation.

Contraindications

Acute superficial herpes simplex keratitis.
Fungal diseases of ocular or auricular structures.
Vaccinia, varicella and most other viral diseases of the cornea and conjunctiva.
Tuberculosis of the eye.
Hypersensitivity to a component of this medication.
Perforation of a drum membrane.

Warnings

Employment of steroid medication in the treatment of stromal herpes simplex requires great caution; frequent slit-lamp microscopy is mandatory.
Prolonged use may result in glaucoma, damage to the optic nerve, defects in visual acuity and fields of vision, posterior subcapsular cataract formation, or may aid in the establishment of secondary ocular infections from pathogens liberated from ocular tissues.
In those diseases causing thinning of the cornea or sclera, perforation has been known to occur with the use of topical steroids.
Acute purulent untreated infection of the eye or ear may be masked or activity enhanced by the presence of steroid medication.
Usage in Pregnancy
Safety of intensive or protracted use of topical steroids during pregnancy has not been substantiated.

Precautions

As fungal infections of the cornea are particularly prone to develop coincidentally with long-term local steroid applications, fungus invasion must be considered in any persistent corneal ulceration where a steroid has been used or is in use.
Intraocular pressure should be checked frequently.

Adverse Reactions

Glaucoma with optic nerve damage, visual acuity and field defects, posterior subcapsular cataract formation, secondary ocular infection from pathogens including herpes simplex liberated from ocular tissues, perforation of the globe.
Rarely, filtering blebs have been reported when topical steroids have been used following cataract surgery.
Viral and fungal infections of the cornea may be exacerbated by the application of steroids.
Rarely, stinging or burning may occur.

Dosage and Administration

The duration of treatment will vary with the type of lesion and may extend from a few days to several weeks, according to therapeutic response. Relapses, more common in chronic active lesions than in self-limited conditions, usually respond to retreatment.
Eye—Instill one or two drops of solution into the conjunctival sac every hour during the day and every two hours during the night as initial therapy. When a favorable response is observed, reduce dosage to one drop every four hours. Later, further reduction in dosage to one drop three or four times daily may suffice to control symptoms.
Ear—Clean the aural canal thoroughly and sponge dry. Instill the solution directly into the aural canal. A suggested initial dosage is three or four drops two or three times a day. When a favorable response is obtained, reduce dosage gradually and eventually discontinue.
If preferred, the aural canal may be packed with a gauze wick saturated with solution. Keep the wick moist with the preparation and remove from the ear after 12 to 24 hours. Treatment may be repeated as often as necessary at the discretion of the physician.

How Supplied

Sterile ophthalmic solution DECADRON phosphate is a clear, colorless to pale yellow solution.
No. 7610—Ophthalmic solution DECADRON phosphate is supplied as follows:
NDC 0006-7610-30 in 2.5 ml glass bottles with dropper assembly.
NDC 0006-7610-03 in 5 ml glass bottles with dropper assembly.
No. 7643—Ophthalmic solution DECADRON phosphate is supplied as follows:
NDC 0006-7643-03 in 5 ml white, opaque, plastic OCUMETER ophthalmic dispenser with a controlled drop tip.
A.H.F.S. 52:08
DC 6460009 Issued November 1975

DECADRON® Phosphate TURBINAIRE® ℞
(dexamethasone sodium phosphate, MSD)

Description

TURBINAIRE DECADRON Phosphate (Dexamethasone Sodium Phosphate, MSD) is an aerosol for intranasal application. The inactive ingredients are fluorochlorohydrocarbons as propellants and alcohol 2%. One cartridge delivers an amount sufficient to ensure delivery of 170 metered sprays, each containing dexamethasone sodium phosphate equivalent to approximately 0.1 mg dexamethasone phosphate or to approximately 0.084 mg dexamethasone. Twelve sprays deliver a theoretical maximum of 1.0 mg dexamethasone.
Dexamethasone sodium phosphate, a synthetic adrenocortical steroid, is a white or slightly yellow, crystalline powder. It is freely soluble in water and is exceedingly hygroscopic. The molecular weight is 516.41. It is designated

chemically as 9-fluoro-11β, 17-dihydroxy-16α-methyl-21-(phosphonooxy) pregna-1, 4-diene-3, 20-dione disodium salt. The empirical formula is $C_{22}H_{28}FNa_2O_8P$.

Action

Inhibition of inflammatory response to inciting agents of mechanical, chemical or immunological nature.

Indications

Allergic or inflammatory nasal conditions, and nasal polyps (excluding polyps originating within the sinuses).

Contraindications

Systemic fungal infections.
Hypersensitivity to components.
Tuberculous, viral and fungal nasal conditions, ocular herpes simplex.

Warnings

In patients on therapy with TURBINAIRE DECADRON Phosphate subjected to unusual stress, increased dosage of rapidly acting corticosteroids before, during, and after the stressful situation is indicated.
Drug-induced secondary adrenocortical insufficiency may result from too rapid withdrawal of corticosteroids and may be minimized by gradual reduction of dosage. This type of relative insufficiency may persist for months after discontinuation of therapy; therefore, in any situation of stress occurring during that period, hormone therapy should be reinstituted. If the patient is receiving steroids already, dosage may have to be increased. Since mineralocorticoid secretion may be impaired, salt and/or a mineralocorticoid should be administered concurrently.
Dexamethasone may mask some signs of infection, and new infections may appear during its use. There may be decreased resistance and inability to localize infection when corticosteroids are used. Moreover, dexamethasone may affect the nitroblue-tetrazolium test for bacterial infection and produce false negative results.
Corticosteroids may activate latent amebiasis. Therefore, it is recommended that latent or active amebiasis be ruled out before initiating corticosteroid therapy in any patient who has spent time in the tropics or any patient with unexplained diarrhea.
Prolonged use of TURBINAIRE DECADRON Phosphate may produce posterior subcapsular cataracts, glaucoma with possible damage to the optic nerves, and may enhance the establishment of secondary ocular infections due to fungi or viruses.
Usage in pregnancy: Since adequate human reproduction studies have not been done with TURBINAIRE DECADRON Phosphate, use of this drug in pregnancy or in women of childbearing potential requires that the anticipated benefits be weighed against the possible hazards to the mother and embryo or fetus. Infants born of mothers who have received substantial doses of dexamethasone during pregnancy, should be carefully observed for signs of hypoadrenalism.
Dexamethasone appears in breast milk and could suppress growth, interfere with endogenous corticosteroid production, or cause other unwanted effects. Mothers taking pharmacologic doses of dexamethasone should be advised not to nurse.
Average and large doses of hydrocortisone or cortisone can cause elevation of blood pressure, salt and water retention, and increased excretion of potassium. These effects are less likely to occur with the synthetic derivatives and with TURBINAIRE DECADRON Phosphate, except when used in large doses. Dietary salt restriction and potassium supplementation may be necessary. All corticosteroids increase calcium excretion.
While on therapy with TURBINAIRE DECADRON Phosphate, patients should not be vaccinated against smallpox. Other immunization procedures should not be undertaken in patients who are on TURBINAIRE DECADRON Phosphate, especially on high doses, because of possible hazards of neurological complications and a lack of antibody response.
If TURBINAIRE DECADRON Phosphate is indicated in patients with latent tuberculosis or tuberculin reactivity, close observation is necessary as reactivation of the disease may occur. During prolonged therapy with TURBINAIRE DECADRON Phosphate, these patients should receive chemoprophylaxis.

Precautions

Although systemic absorption is low when TURBINAIRE DECADRON Phosphate is used in the recommended dosage, adrenal suppression may occur. In addition, other systemic effects of steroid administration must be considered as a possibility.
Following prolonged therapy, withdrawal of corticosteroids may result in symptoms of the corticosteroid withdrawal syndrome including fever, myalgia, arthralgia, and malaise. This may occur in patients even without evidence of adrenal insufficiency.
There is an enhanced effect of dexamethasone in patients with hypothyroidism and in those with cirrhosis.
TURBINAIRE DECADRON Phosphate should be used cautiously in patients with ocular herpes simplex for fear of corneal perforation.
The lowest possible dose of TURBINAIRE DECADRON Phosphate should be used to control the condition under treatment, and when reduction in dosage is possible, the reduction must be gradual.
Psychic derangements may appear when dexamethasone is used, ranging from euphoria, insomnia, mood swings, personality changes, and severe depression, to frank psychotic manifestations. Also, existing emotional instability or psychotic tendencies may be aggravated.
Aspirin should be used cautiously in conjunction with TURBINAIRE DECADRON Phosphate in hypoprothrombinemia.
TURBINAIRE DECADRON Phosphate should be used with caution in nonspecific ulcerative colitis, if there is a probability of impending perforation, abscess or other pyogenic infection; also in diverticulitis; fresh intestinal anastomoses; active or latent peptic ulcer; renal insufficiency; hypertension; osteoporosis; and myasthenia gravis. Fat embolism has been reported as a possible complication of hypercortisonism.
Growth and development of infants and children on prolonged therapy with TURBINAIRE DECADRON Phosphate should be carefully followed.
Dexamethasone may increase or decrease motility and number of spermatozoa in some patients.
Phenytoin, phenobarbital, ephedrine and rifampin may enhance the metabolic clearance of dexamethasone, resulting in decreased blood levels and lessened physiologic activity, thus requiring adjustment in dexamethasone dosage.
The prothrombin time should be checked frequently in patients who are receiving TURBINAIRE DECADRON Phosphate and coumarin anticoagulants at the same time because of reports that corticosteroids have altered the response to these anticoagulants. Studies have shown that the usual effect produced by adding corticosteroids is inhibition of response to coumarins, although there have been some conflicting reports of potentiation, not substantiated by studies.
When TURBINAIRE DECADRON Phosphate is used concomitantly with potassium-depleting diuretics, patients should be observed closely for development of hypokalemia.
Since the contents of TURBINAIRE DECADRON Phosphate are under pressure, the container should not be broken, stored in extreme heat, or incinerated. It should be stored at a temperature below 120°F.

Adverse Reactions

Nasal irritation and dryness are the most common adverse reactions. The following have been reported: headache, lightheadedness, urticaria, nausea, epistaxis, rebound congestion, bronchial asthma, perforation of the nasal septum, and anosmia. Signs of adrenal hypercorticism may occur in some patients, especially with overdosage.
Systemic effects from therapy with TURBINAIRE DECADRON Phosphate are less likely to occur than with oral or parenteral corticosteroid therapy because of a lower total dose administered. Nevertheless, patients should be observed for the hormonal effects described below because of absorption of dexamethasone from the nasal mucosa.

Fluid and Electrolyte Disturbances
- Sodium retention
- Fluid retention
- Congestive heart failure in susceptible patients
- Potassium loss
- Hypokalemic alkalosis
- Hypertension

Musculoskeletal
- Muscle weakness
- Steroid myopathy
- Loss of muscle mass
- Osteoporosis
- Vertebral compression fractures
- Aseptic necrosis of femoral and humeral heads
- Pathologic fracture of long bones
- Tendon rupture

Gastrointestinal
- Peptic ulcer with possible subsequent perforation and hemorrhage
- Pancreatitis
- Abdominal distention
- Ulcerative esophagitis

Dematologic
- Impaired wound healing
- Thin fragile skin
- Petechiae and ecchymoses
- Erythema
- Increased sweating
- May suppress reactions to skin tests
- Other cutaneous reactions, such as allergic dermatitis, urticaria, angioneurotic edema.

Neurologic
- Convulsions
- Increased intracranial pressure with papilledema (pseudotumor cerebri) usually after treatment
- Vertigo
- Headache

Endocrine
- Menstrual irregularities
- Development of cushingoid state
- Suppression of growth in children
- Secondary adrenocortical and pituitary unresponsiveness, particularly in times of stress, as in trauma, surgery, or illness
- Decreased carbohydrate tolerance
- Manifestations of latent diabetes mellitus
- Increased requirements for insulin or oral hypoglycemic agents in diabetics

Continued on next page

Information on the Merck Sharp & Dohme products listed on these pages is the full prescribing information from package circulars in use October 31, 1979.

Merck Sharp & Dohme—Cont.

Ophthalmic
Posterior subcapsular cataracts
Increased intraocular pressure
Glaucoma
Exophthalmos
Metabolic
Negative nitrogen balance due to protein catabolism
Other
Hypersensitivity
Thromboembolism
Weight gain
Increased appetite
Nausea
Malaise

Dosage and Administration

DO NOT EXCEED THE RECOMMENDED DOSAGE.
The usual initial dosage of TURBINAIRE DECADRON Phosphate is:
Adults—2 sprays in each nostril 2 or 3 times a day.
Children (6 to 12 years of age)—1 or 2 sprays in each nostril 2 times a day depending on age.
See accompanying instructions on the proper use of TURBINAIRE.
When improvement occurs the dosage should be gradually reduced. Some patients will be symptom-free on one spray in each nostril 2 times a day. The maximum daily dosage for adults is 12 sprays, and for children, 8 sprays. Therapy should be discontinued as soon as feasible. It may be reinstituted if recurrence of symptoms occurs.

How Supplied

No. 7634—TURBINAIRE DECADRON Phosphate, aerosol for intranasal application, is supplied as follows: **NDC** 0006-7634-13 in a pressurized container and includes a plastic adapter.
(6505-00-885-6302, 12.6 Grams, 170 Metered Doses)
No. 7642—Refill unit for TURBINAIRE DECADRON Phosphate aerosol for intranasal application is supplied as follows: **NDC** 0006-7642-13 in a pressurized container.
A.H.F.S. 52:08
DC 6006415 Issued May 1979

DECADRON-LA® Suspension ℞
(dexamethasone acetate, MSD)

NOT FOR INTRAVENOUS USE

Description

Dexamethasone acetate, a synthetic adrenocortical steroid, is a white to practically white, odorless powder. It is a practically insoluble ester of dexamethasone.
Dexamethasone acetate is present in DECADRON-LA (Dexamethasone Acetate, MSD) suspension as the monohydrate, with the empirical formula, $C_{24}H_{31}FO_6 \cdot H_2O$, and molecular weight, 452.52. Dexamethasone acetate is designated chemically as 21-(acetyloxy)-9-fluoro-11β, 17-dihydroxy-16α-methylpregna-1,4-diene-3,20-dione.
DECADRON-LA suspension is a sterile white suspension (pH 5.0 to 7.5) that settles on standing, but is easily resuspended by mild shaking. Each milliliter contains dexamethasone acetate equivalent to 8 mg dexamethasone. Inactive ingredients per ml: 6.67 mg sodium chloride; 5 mg creatinine; 0.5 mg disodium edetate; 5 mg sodium carboxymethylcellulose; 0.75 mg polysorbate 80; sodium hydroxide to adjust pH; and Water for Injection, q.s. 1 ml with 9 mg benzyl alcohol, and 1 mg sodium bisulfite added as preservatives.

Actions

DECADRON-LA suspension is a long-acting, repository adrenocorticosteroid preparation with a prompt onset of action. It is suitable for intramuscular or local injection, but not when an immediate effect of short duration is desired.
Naturally occurring glucocorticoids (hydrocortisone and cortisone), which also have salt-retaining properties, are used as replacement therapy in adrenocortical deficiency states. Their synthetic analogs, including dexamethasone, are primarily used for their potent anti-inflammatory effects in disorders of many organ systems.
Glucocorticoids cause profound and varied metabolic effects. In addition, they modify the body's immune responses to diverse stimuli.
At equipotent anti-inflammatory doses, dexamethasone almost completely lacks the sodium-retaining property of hydrocortisone.

Indications

A. By intramuscular injection when oral therapy is not feasible:
1. *Endocrine disorders*
Congenital adrenal hyperplasia
Nonsuppurative thyroiditis
Hypercalcemia associated with cancer
2. *Rheumatic disorders*
As adjunctive therapy for short-term administration (to tide the patient over an acute episode or exacerbation) in:
Post-traumatic osteoarthritis
Synovitis of osteoarthritis
Rheumatoid arthritis, including juvenile rheumatoid arthritis (selected cases may require low-dose maintenance therapy)
Acute and subacute bursitis
Epicondylitis
Acute nonspecific tenosynovitis
Acute gouty arthritis
Psoriatic arthritis
Ankylosing spondylitis
3. *Collagen diseases*
During an exacerbation or as maintenance therapy in selected cases of:
Systemic lupus erythematosus
Acute rheumatic carditis
4. *Dermatologic diseases*
Pemphigus
Severe erythema multiforme (Stevens-Johnson syndrome)
Exfoliative dermatitis
Bullous dermatitis herpetiformis
Severe seborrheic dermatitis
Severe psoriasis
Mycosis fungoides
5. *Allergic states*
Control of severe or incapacitating allergic conditions intractable to adequate trials of conventional treatment in:
Bronchial asthma
Contact dermatitis
Atopic dermatitis
Serum sickness
Seasonal or perennial allergic rhinitis
Drug hypersensitivity reactions
Urticarial transfusion reactions
6. *Ophthalmic diseases*
Severe acute and chronic allergic and inflammatory processes involving the eye, such as:
Herpes zoster ophthalmicus
Iritis, Iridocyclitis
Chorioretinitis
Diffuse posterior uveitis and choroiditis
Optic neuritis
Sympathetic ophthalmia
Anterior segment inflammation
Allergic conjunctivitis
Keratitis
Allergic corneal marginal ulcers
7. *Gastrointestinal diseases*
To tide the patient over a critical period of the disease in:
Ulcerative colitis (Systemic therapy)
Regional enteritis (Systemic therapy)
8. *Respiratory diseases*
Symptomatic sarcoidosis
Berylliosis
Loeffler's syndrome not manageable by other means
Aspiration pneumonitis
9. *Hematologic disorders*
Acquired (autoimmune) hemolytic anemia
Secondary thrombocytopenia in adults
Erythroblastopenia (RBC anemia)
Congenital (erythroid) hypoplastic anemia
10. *Neoplastic diseases*
For palliative management of:
Leukemias and lymphomas in adults
Acute leukemia of childhood
11. *Edematous states*
To induce diuresis or remission of proteinuria in the nephrotic syndrome, without uremia, of the idiopathic type, or that due to lupus erythematosus
12. *Miscellaneous*
Trichinosis with neurologic or myocardial involvement

B. By intra-articular or soft tissue injection as adjunctive therapy for short-term administration (to tide the patient over an acute episode or exacerbation) in:
Synovitis of osteoarthritis
Rheumatoid arthritis
Acute and subacute bursitis
Acute gouty arthritis
Epicondylitis
Acute nonspecific tenosynovitis
Post-traumatic osteoarthritis

C. By intralesional injection in:
Keloids
Localized hypertrophic, infiltrated, inflammatory lesions of: lichen planus, psoriatic plaques, granuloma annulare, and lichen simplex chronicus (neurodermatitis)
Discoid lupus erythematosus
Necrobiosis lipoidica diabeticorum
Alopecia areata
May also be useful in cystic tumors of an aponeurosis or tendon (ganglia)

Contraindications

Systemic fungal infections
Hypersensitivity to any component of this product

Warnings

DO NOT INJECT INTRAVENOUSLY.
In patients on corticosteroid therapy subjected to any unusual stress, increased dosage of rapidly acting corticosteroids before, during, and after the stressful situation is indicated.
Drug-induced secondary adrenocortical insufficiency may result from too rapid withdrawal of corticosteroids and may be minimized by gradual reduction of dosage. This type of relative insufficiency may persist for months after discontinuation of therapy; therefore, in any situation of stress occurring during that period, hormone therapy should be reinstituted. If the patient is receiving steroids already, dosage may have to be increased. Since mineralocorticoid secretion may be impaired, salt and/or a mineralocorticoid should be administered concurrently.
Corticosteroids may mask some signs of infection, and new infections may appear during their use. There may be decreased resistance and inability to localize infection when corticosteroids are used. Moreover, corticosteroids may affect the nitroblue-tetrazolium test for bacterial infection and produce false negative results.
Corticosteroids may activate latent amebiasis. Therefore, it is recommended that latent or active amebiasis be ruled out before initiating corticosteroid therapy in any patient who has spent time in the tropics or any patient with unexplained diarrhea.

Prolonged use of corticosteroids may produce posterior subcapsular cataracts, glaucoma with possible damage to the optic nerves, and may enhance the establishment of secondary ocular infections due to fungi or viruses.

Usage in pregnancy. Since adequate human reproduction studies have not been done with corticosteroids, use of these drugs in pregnancy or in women of childbearing potential requires that the anticipated benefits be weighed against the possible hazards to the mother and embryo or fetus. Infants born of mothers who have received substantial doses of corticosteroids during pregnancy should be carefully observed for signs of hypoadrenalism.

Corticosteroids appear in breast milk and could suppress growth, interfere with endogenous corticosteroid production, or cause other unwanted effects. Mothers taking pharmacologic doses of corticosteroids should be advised not to nurse.

Average and large doses of cortisone or hydrocortisone can cause elevation of blood pressure, salt and water retention, and increased excretion of potassium. These effects are less likely to occur with the synthetic derivatives except when used in large doses. Dietary salt restriction and potassium supplementation may be necessary. All corticosteroids increase calcium excretion.

While on corticosteroid therapy patients should not be vaccinated against smallpox. Other immunization procedures should not be undertaken in patients who are on corticosteroids, especially on high doses, because of possible hazards of neurologic complications and lack of antibody response.

If corticosteroids are indicated in patients with latent tuberculosis or tuberculin reactivity, close observation is necessary as reactivation of the disease may occur. During prolonged corticosteroid therapy, these patients should receive chemoprophylaxis.

Because rare instances of anaphylactoid reactions have occurred in patients receiving parenteral corticosteroid therapy, appropriate precautionary measures should be taken prior to administration, especially when the patient has a history of allergy to any drug.

Repository adrenocorticosteroid preparations may cause atrophy at the site of injection. To minimize the likelihood and/or severity of atrophy, do not inject subcutaneously, avoid injection into the deltoid muscle, and avoid repeated intramuscular injections into the same site if possible.

Dosage in children under 12 has not been established.

Precautions

DECADRON-LA suspension is not recommended as initial therapy in acute, life-threatening situations.

This product, like many other steroid formulations, is sensitive to heat. Therefore, it should not be autoclaved when it is desirable to sterilize the exterior of the vial.

Following prolonged therapy, withdrawal of corticosteroids may result in symptoms of the corticosteroid withdrawal syndrome including fever, myalgia, arthralgia, and malaise. This may occur in patients even without evidence of adrenal insufficiency.

There is an enhanced effect of corticosteroids in patients with hypothyroidism and in those with cirrhosis.

Corticosteroids should be used cautiously in patients with ocular herpes simplex for fear of corneal perforation.

Psychic derangements may appear when corticosteroids are used, ranging from euphoria, insomnia, mood swings, personality changes, and severe depression to frank psychotic manifestations. Also, existing emotional instability or psychotic tendencies may be aggravated by corticosteroids.

Aspirin should be used cautiously in conjunction with corticosteroids in hypoprothrombinemia.

Steroids should be used with caution in nonspecific ulcerative colitis, if there is a probability of impending perforation, abscess, or other pyogenic infection, also in diverticulitis, fresh intestinal anastomoses, active or latent peptic ulcer, renal insufficiency, hypertension, osteoporosis, and myasthenia gravis. Fat embolism has been reported as a possible complication of hypercortisonism.

When large doses are given, some authorities advise that antacids be administered between meals to help to prevent peptic ulcer.

Growth and development of infants and children on prolonged corticosteroid therapy should be carefully followed.

Steroids may increase or decrease motility and number of spermatozoa in some patients.

Phenytoin, phenobarbital, ephedrine, and rifampin may enhance the metabolic clearance of corticosteroids, resulting in decreased blood levels and lessened physiologic activity, thus requiring adjustment in corticosteroid dosage.

The prothrombin time should be checked frequently in patients who are receiving corticosteroids and coumarin anticoagulants at the same time because of reports that corticosteroids have altered the response to these anticoagulants. Studies have shown that the usual effect produced by adding corticosteroids is inhibition of response to coumarins, although there have been some conflicting reports of potentiation not substantiated by studies.

When corticosteroids are administered concomitantly with potassium-depleting diuretics, patients should be observed closely for development of hypokalemia.

Intra-articular injection of a corticosteroid may produce systemic as well as local effects.

Appropriate examination of any joint fluid present is necessary to exclude a septic process.

A marked increase in pain accompanied by local swelling, further restriction of joint motion, fever, and malaise is suggestive of septic arthritis. If this complication occurs and the diagnosis of sepsis is confirmed, appropriate antimicrobial therapy should be instituted.

Injection of a steroid into an infected site is to be avoided.

Corticosteroids should not be injected into unstable joints.

Patients should be impressed strongly with the importance of not overusing joints in which symptomatic benefit has been obtained as long as the inflammatory process remains active.

Frequent intra-articular injection may result in damage to joint tissues.

Adverse Reactions

Fluid and electrolyte disturbances
Sodium retention
Fluid retention
Congestive heart failure in susceptible patients
Potassium loss
Hypokalemic alkalosis
Hypertension

Musculoskeletal
Muscle weakness
Steroid myopathy
Loss of muscle mass
Osteoporosis
Vertebral compression fractures
Aseptic necrosis of femoral and humeral heads
Pathologic fracture of long bones
Tendon rupture

Gastrointestinal
Peptic ulcer with possible subsequent perforation and hemorrhage
Pancreatitis
Abdominal distention
Ulcerative esophagitis

Dermatologic
Impaired wound healing
Thin fragile skin
Petechiae and ecchymoses
Erythema
Increased sweating
May suppress reactions to skin tests
Other cutaneous reactions, such as allergic dermatitis, urticaria, angioneurotic edema

Neurologic
Convulsions
Increased intracranial pressure with papilledema (pseudotumor cerebri) usually after treatment
Vertigo
Headache

Endocrine
Menstrual irregularities
Development of cushingoid state
Suppression of growth in children
Secondary adrenocortical and pituitary unresponsiveness, particularly in times of stress, as in trauma, surgery, or illness
Decreased carbohydrate tolerance
Manifestations of latent diabetes mellitus
Increased requirements for insulin or oral hypoglycemic agents in diabetics

Ophthalmic
Posterior subcapsular cataracts
Increased intraocular pressure
Glaucoma
Exophthalmos

Metabolic
Negative nitrogen balance due to protein catabolism

Other
Anaphylactoid or hypersensitivity reactions
Thromboembolism
Weight gain
Increased appetite
Nausea
Malaise

The following *additional* adverse reactions are related to parenteral corticosteroid therapy:
Rare instances of blindness associated with intralesional therapy around the face and head
Hyperpigmentation or hypopigmentation
Subcutaneous and cutaneous atrophy
Sterile abscess
Postinjection flare (following intra-articular use)
Charcot-like arthropathy
Scarring
Induration
Inflammation
Paresthesia
Delayed pain or soreness
Muscle twitching, ataxia, hiccups, and nystagmus have been reported in low incidence after injection of DECADRON-LA suspension.

Dosage and Administration

For intramuscular, intralesional, intra-articular, and soft tissue injection.

Dosage Requirements Are Variable and Must Be Individualized on the Basis of the Disease and the Response of the Patient.

Dosage in children under 12 has not been established.

Intramuscular Injection
Dosage ranges from 1 to 2 ml, equivalent to 8 to 16 mg of dexamethasone. If further treatment is needed, dosage may be repeated at intervals of 1 to 3 weeks.

Intralesional Injection
The usual dose is 0.1 to 0.2 ml, equivalent to 0.8 to 1.6 mg of dexamethasone, per injection site.

Intra-articular and Soft Tissue Injection
The dose varies, depending on the location and the severity of inflammation. The usual dose is 0.5 to 2 ml, equivalent to 4 to 16 mg of dexamethasone. If further treatment is needed,

Continued on next page

Information on the Merck Sharp & Dohme products listed on these pages is the full prescribing information from package circulars in use October 31, 1979.

Merck Sharp & Dohme—Cont.

dosage may be repeated at intervals of 1 to 3 weeks. Frequent intra-articular injection may result in damage to joint tissues.

How Supplied

No. 7644—Suspension DECADRON-LA, 8 mg dexamethasone equivalent per ml, is a sterile white suspension, and is supplied as follows:
NDC 0006-7644-01 in 1 ml vials
NDC 0006-7644-03 in 5 ml vials.

A.H.F.S. 68:04
DC 6626710 Issued May 1979

DECASPRAY® Topical Aerosol ℞
(dexamethasone, MSD), N.F.

Description

Topical Aerosol DECASPRAY (Dexamethasone, MSD) is a topical steroid preparation that is virtually odorless, colorless, stainless, and invisible. The spray has a cooling effect.
Each 25 g of DECASPRAY contains 10 mg of dexamethasone. The inactive ingredients are isopropyl myristate, and isobutane. Each second of spray dispenses approximately 0.075 mg of dexamethasone.

Actions

Topical steroids are primarily effective because of their anti-inflammatory, antipruritic and vasoconstrictive actions.

Indications

DECASPRAY Topical Aerosol is indicated for relief of the inflammatory manifestations of corticosteroid-responsive dermatoses.

Contraindications

Topical steroids are contraindicated in those patients with a history of hypersensitivity to any of the components of the preparation.
Topical steroids are contraindicated in vaccinia and varicella; herpes simplex; in fungal infections; when tuberculosis of the skin is present; and in the ear if the drum is perforated.

Warnings

Avoid spraying in eyes or nose. Contents under pressure. Do not puncture or burn. Keep out of reach of children. Use only as directed. Intentional misuse by deliberately concentrating and inhaling the contents can be harmful or fatal.

Precautions

If irritation develops, the product should be discontinued and appropriate therapy instituted.
In the presence of an infection, the use of an appropriate antifungal or antibacterial agent should be instituted. If a favorable response does not occur promptly, the corticosteroid should be discontinued until the infection has been adequately controlled.
If extensive areas are treated or if the occlusive technique is used, there will be increased systemic absorption of the corticosteroid and suitable precautions should be taken, particularly in children and infants.
Although topical steroids have not been reported to have an adverse effect on human pregnancy, the safety of their uses in pregnant women has not absolutely been established. In laboratory animals, increases in incidence of fetal abnormalities have been associated with exposure of gestating females to topical corticosteroids, in some cases at rather low dosage levels. Therefore, drugs of this class should not be used extensively on pregnant patients, in large amounts, or for prolonged periods of time.
The product is not for ophthalmic use.
A few individuals may be sensitive to one or more of the components of this product. If any reaction indicating sensitivity is observed, discontinue use.
Generally, occlusive dressings should not be used on weeping or exudative lesions.
If the occlusive dressing technique is employed, caution should be exercised with regard to the use of plastic films which are often flammable and may pose a suffocation hazard for children.
If occlusive dressing therapy is used, inspect lesions between dressings for development of infection. If infection develops, the technique should be discontinued and appropriate antimicrobial therapy instituted.
When large areas of the body are covered with an occlusive dressing, thermal homeostasis may be impaired. If elevation of body temperature occurs, use of the occlusive dressing should be discontinued.
CAUTION: Flammable. Do not use around open flame or while smoking.

Adverse Reactions

The following local adverse reactions have been reported with topical corticosteroids: burning, itching, irritation, dryness, folliculitis, hypertrichosis, acneiform eruptions, hypopigmentation, perioral dermatitis, allergic contact dermatitis, maceration of the skin, secondary infection, skin atrophy, striae, and miliaria.
Contact sensitivity to a particular dressing or adhesive may occur occasionally.

Dosage and Administration

Patients should be instructed in the correct way to use DECASPRAY. The preparation is readily applied, even on hairy areas. It does not have to be rubbed into the skin.
Optimal effects will be obtained with DECASPRAY when these directions are followed:

1. Keep the affected area clean to reduce the possibility of infection.
2. Shake the container *gently* once or twice each time before using. Hold it about six inches from the area to be treated. Effective medication may be obtained with the container held either upright or inverted, since it is fitted with a special valve that dispenses approximately the same dosage in either position.
3. Spray each four inch square of affected area for one or two seconds three or four times a day, depending on the nature of the condition and the response to therapy.
4. When a favorable response is obtained, reduce dosage gradually and eventually discontinue.

How Supplied

No. 7623X—DECASPRAY is supplied as follows:
NDC 0006-7623-25 in a 25 g pressurized container.

A.H.F.S. 84:06
DC 6005316 Issued December 1978

DIUPRES® Tablets ℞
Antihypertensive

WARNING

This fixed combination drug is not indicated for initial therapy of hypertension. Hypertension requires therapy titrated to the individual patient. If the fixed combination represents the dosage so determined, its use may be more convenient in patient management. The treatment of hypertension is not static, but must be reevaluated as conditions in each patient warrant.

Description

DIUPRES combines two antihypertensive agents: DIURIL (Chlorothiazide, MSD) and reserpine. The chemical name for chlorothiazide is 6-chloro-2H-1,2,4-benzothiadiazine-7-sulfonamide 1,1-dioxide. Reserpine (11,17α-dimethoxy-18β-[(3,4,5-trimethoxybenzoyl)oxy]-3β,20α-yohimban-16β-carboxylic acid methyl ester) is a crystalline alkaloid derived from Rauwolfia serpentina.

Actions

Chlorothiazide
Chlorothiazide is a diuretic and antihypertensive. It affects the renal tubular mechanism of electrolyte reabsorption. At maximal therapeutic dosage all thiazides are approximately equal in their diuretic efficacy.
Chlorothiazide increases excretion of sodium and chloride in approximately equivalent amounts. Natriuresis may be accompanied by some loss of potassium and bicarbonate.
The mechanism of the antihypertensive effect of thiazides is unknown. Chlorothiazide does not affect normal blood pressure.
Chlorothiazide is eliminated rapidly by the kidney.
Reserpine
Reserpine has antihypertensive, bradycardic, and tranquilizing properties. It lowers arterial blood pressure by depletion of catecholamines. Reserpine is beneficial in relieving anxiety, tension, and headache in the hypertensive patient. It acts at the hypothalamic level of the central nervous system to promote relaxation without hypnosis or analgesia. The sleep pattern shown by the electroencephalogram following barbiturates does not occur with this drug. In laboratory animals spontaneous activity and response to external stimuli are decreased, but confusion or difficulty of movement is not evident.
The bradycardic action of reserpine promotes relaxation and may eliminate sinus tachycardia. It is most pronounced in subjects with sinus tachycardia and usually is not prominent in persons with a normal pulse rate.
Miosis, relaxation of the nictitating membrane, ptosis, hypothermia, and increased gastrointestinal activity are noted in animals given reserpine, sometimes in subclinical doses. None of these effects, except increased gastrointestinal activity, has been found to be clinically significant in man with therapeutic doses.

Indication

Hypertension (see box warning)

Contraindications

Chlorothiazide is contraindicated in anuria.
DIUPRES is contraindicated in hypersensitivity to chlorothiazide or other sulfonamide-derived drugs or to reserpine.
Electroshock therapy should not be given to patients while on reserpine, as severe and even fatal reactions have been reported with minimal convulsive electroshock dosage. After discontinuing reserpine, allow at least seven days before starting electroshock therapy.
Active peptic ulcer, ulcerative colitis, and active mental depression, especially suicidal tendencies, are contraindications to reserpine therapy.

Warnings

Chlorothiazide

Use with caution in severe renal disease. In patients with renal disease, thiazides may precipitate azotemia. Cumulative effects of the drug may develop in patients with impaired renal function.

Thiazides should be used with caution in patients with impaired hepatic function or progressive liver disease, since minor alterations of fluid and electrolyte balance may precipitate hepatic coma.

Thiazides may add to or potentiate the action of other antihypertensive drugs.

Sensitivity reactions may occur in patients with or without a history of allergy or bronchial asthma.

The possibility of exacerbation or activation of systemic lupus erythematosus has been reported.

Lithium generally should not be given with diuretics because they reduce its renal clearance and add a high risk of lithium toxicity. Read circulars for lithium preparations before use of such concomitant therapy.

Reserpine

The occurrence of mental depression due to reserpine in doses of 0.25 mg daily or less is unusual. In any event, DIUPRES should be discontinued at the first sign of depression.

Use in Pregnancy

Reserpine has been demonstrated to cross the placental barrier in guinea pigs with depression of adrenal catecholamine stores in the newborn. There is some evidence that side effects such as nasal congestion, lethargy, depressed Moro reflex, and bradycardia may appear in infants born of reserpine-treated mothers.

Thiazides cross the placental barrier and appear in cord blood. The use of thiazides in pregnancy requires that the anticipated benefit be weighed against possible hazards to the fetus. These hazards include fetal or neonatal jaundice, thrombocytopenia, and possibly other adverse reactions which have occurred in the adult.

Nursing Mothers

Thiazides and reserpine appear in breast milk. If use of the drug is deemed essential, the patient should stop nursing.

Precautions

Chlorothiazide

Periodic determination of serum electrolytes to detect possible electrolyte imbalance should be performed at appropriate intervals.

All patients receiving diuretic therapy should be observed for evidence of fluid or electrolyte imbalance: namely, hyponatremia, hypochloremic alkalosis, and hypokalemia. Serum and urine electrolyte determinations are particularly important when the patient is vomiting excessively or receiving parenteral fluids. Warning signs or symptoms of fluid and electrolyte imbalance include dryness of mouth, thirst, weakness, lethargy, drowsiness, restlessness, muscle pains or cramps, muscular fatigue, hypotension, oliguria, tachycardia, and gastrointestinal disturbances such as nausea and vomiting.

Hypokalemia may develop, especially with brisk diuresis, when severe cirrhosis is present, during concomitant use of corticosteroids or ACTH, or after prolonged therapy.

Interference with adequate oral electrolyte intake will contribute to hypokalemia. Hypokalemia can sensitize or exaggerate the response of the heart to the toxic effects of digitalis (e.g., increased ventricular irritability). Hypokalemia may be avoided or treated by use of potassium supplements such as foods with a high potassium content.

Although any chloride deficit is generally mild and usually does not require specific treatment except under extraordinary circumstances (as in liver disease or renal disease), chloride replacement may be required in the treatment of metabolic alkalosis.

Dilutional hyponatremia may occur in edematous patients in hot weather. Appropriate therapy is water restriction, rather than administration of salt, except in rare instances when the hyponatremia is life threatening. In actual salt depletion, appropriate replacement is the therapy of choice.

Hyperuricemia may occur or acute gout may be precipitated in certain patients receiving thiazide therapy.

Insulin requirements in diabetic patients may be increased, decreased, or unchanged. Diabetes mellitus which has been latent may become manifest during thiazide administration.

Thiazide drugs may increase the responsiveness to tubocurarine.

The antihypertensive effect of the drug may be enhanced in the postsympathectomy patient.

Thiazides may decrease arterial responsiveness to norepinephrine. This diminution is not sufficient to preclude effectiveness of the pressor agent for therapeutic use.

If progressive renal impairment becomes evident, consider withholding or discontinuing diuretic therapy.

Thiazides may decrease serum PBI levels without signs of thyroid disturbance.

Calcium excretion is decreased by thiazides. Pathological changes in the parathyroid glands with hypercalcemia and hypophosphatemia have been observed in a few patients on prolonged thiazide therapy. The common complications of hyperparathyroidism such as renal lithiasis, bone resorption, and peptic ulceration have not been seen. Thiazides should be discontinued before carrying out tests for parathyroid function.

Reserpine

Since reserpine may increase gastric secretion and motility, it should be used cautiously in patients with a history of peptic ulcer, ulcerative colitis, or other gastrointestinal disorder. This compound may precipitate biliary colic in patients with gallstones, or bronchial asthma in susceptible persons.

Reserpine may case hypotension including orthostatic hypotension.

In hypertensive patients on reserpine therapy significant hypotension and bradycardia may develop during surgical anesthesia. The anesthesiologist should be aware that reserpine has been taken, since it may be necessary to give vagal blocking agents parenterally to prevent or reverse hypotension and/or bradycardia.

Anxiety or depression, as well as psychosis, may develop during reserpine therapy. If depression is present when therapy is begun, it may be aggravated. Mental depression is unusual with reserpine doses of 0.25 mg daily or less. In any case, DIUPRES should be discontinued at the first sign of depression. Extreme caution should be used in treating patients with a history of mental depression, and the possibility of suicide should be kept in mind.

As with most antihypertensive therapy, caution should be exercised when treating hypertensive patients with renal insufficiency, since they adjust poorly to lowered blood pressure levels. Use reserpine cautiously with digitalis and quinidine; cardiac arrhythmias have occurred with reserpine preparations.

When two or more antihypertensives are given, the individual dosages may have to be reduced to prevent excessive drop in blood pressure. In hypertensive patients with coronary artery disease, it is important to avoid a precipitous drop in blood pressure.

Adverse Reactions

Chlorothiazide

Gastrointestinal: Anorexia, gastric irritation, nausea, vomiting, cramping, diarrhea, constipation, jaundice (intrahepatic cholestatic jaundice), pancreatitis, sialadenitis.

Central nervous system: Dizziness, vertigo, paresthesias, headache, xanthopsia.

Hematologic: Leukopenia, agranulocytosis, thrombocytopenia, aplastic anemia, hemolytic anemia.

Cardiovascular: Orthostatic hypotension (may be aggravated by alcohol, barbiturates, or narcotics).

Allergic: Purpura, photosensitivity, rash, urticaria, necrotizng angiitis (vasculitis) (cutaneous vasculitis), fever, respiratory distress including pneumonitis, anaphylactic reactions.

Other: Hyperglycemia, glycosuria, hyperuricemia, muscle spasm, weakness, restlessness, transient blurred vision.

Whenever adverse reactions are moderate or severe, thiazide dosage should be reduced or therapy withdrawn.

Reserpine

Central nervous system: Excessive sedation, mental depression, nightmares, headache, dizziness, syncope, nervousness, paradoxical anxiety, central nervous system sensitization (dull sensorium, deafness, glaucoma, uveitis, optic atrophy), parkinsonism (usually reversible with decreased dosage or discontinuance of therapy).

Respiratory: Nasal congestion, dyspnea, epistaxis.

Cardiovascular: Bradycardia, angina pectoris, arrhythmia, premature ventricular contractions, and other direct cardiac effects (e.g., fluid retention, congestive failure).

Gastrointestinal: Hypersecretion and increased motility, nausea, vomiting, anorexia, diarrhea, dryness of mouth, increased salivation.

Hematologic: Excessive bleeding following prostatic surgery, thrombocytopenic purpura.

Allergic: Flushing of skin, pruritus, rash.

Other: Conjunctival injection, enhanced susceptibility to colds, muscular aches, weight gain, blurred vision, dysuria, nonpuerperal lactation, impotence, decreased libido.

Dosage and Administration

The initial dosage of DIUPRES should conform to the dosages of the individual components established during titration (see box warning). The usual adult dosage of DIUPRES-250 is 1 or 2 tablets once or twice a day; that of DIUPRES-500 is 1 tablet once or twice a day. Dosage may require adjustment according to the blood pressure response of the patient.

Careful observations for changes in blood pressure must be made when DIUPRES is used with other antihypertensive drugs.

How Supplied

No. 3261—Tablets DIUPRES-250 are pink, round, scored, compressed tablets, coded MSD 230. Each tablet contains 250 mg of chlorothiazide and 0.125 mg of reserpine. They are supplied as follows:

NDC 0006-0230-68 in bottles of 100
NDC 0006-0230-82 in bottles of 1000.

[*Shown in Product Identification Section*]

No. 3262—Tablets DIUPRES-500 are pink, round, scored, compressed tablets, coded MSD 405. Each tablet contains 500 mg of chlorothiazide and 0.125 mg of reserpine. They are supplied as follows:

NDC 0006-0405-68 in bottles of 100
NDC 0006-0405-82 in bottles of 1000.

[*Shown in Product Identification Section*]

A.H.F.S. 24:08
DC 6053127 Issued June 1979

Continued on next page

Information on the Merck Sharp & Dohme products listed on these pages is the full prescribing information from package circulars in use October 31, 1979.

Merck Sharp & Dohme—Cont.

DIURIL® Intravenous Sodium (chlorothiazide sodium, MSD), N.F. ℞

Description

DIURIL (Chlorothiazide, MSD) is 6-chloro-2H-1,2,4-benzothiadiazine-7-sulfonamide 1,1-dioxide. It is a white, or practically white, crystalline compound very slightly soluble in water, but readily soluble in dilute aqueous sodium hydroxide. It is soluble in urine to the extent of about 150 mg per 100 ml at pH 7.

Intravenous Sodium DIURIL (Chlorothiazide Sodium, MSD) is supplied in a vial containing:

Chlorothiazide sodium equivalent to chlorothiazide................................0.5 g

Inactive ingredients:

Mannitol ....0.25 g

Sodium hydroxide to adjust pH, with 0.4 mg thimerosal added as preservative.

Actions

DIURIL is a diuretic and antihypertensive.

DIURIL affects the renal tubular mechanism of electrolyte reabsorption. At maximal therapeutic dosage all thiazides are approximately equal in their diuretic efficacy.

DIURIL increases excretion of sodium and chloride in approximately equivalent amounts. Natriuresis may be accompanied by some loss of potassium and bicarbonate.

Onset of the diuretic action of DIURIL after oral use occurs in 2 hours and the peak action in about 4 hours. Diuretic activity lasts about 6 to 12 hours. Following intravenous use of Sodium DIURIL, onset of the diuretic action occurs in 15 minutes and the maximal action in 30 minutes. DIURIL is eliminated rapidly by the kidney.

The mechanism of the antihypertensive effect of thiazides is unknown. DIURIL does not affect normal blood pressure.

Indications

Intravenous Sodium DIURIL is indicated as adjunctive therapy in edema associated with congestive heart failure, hepatic cirrhosis, and corticosteroid and estrogen therapy.

Intravenous Sodium DIURIL has also been found useful in edema due to various forms of renal dysfunction such as nephrotic syndrome, acute glomerulonephritis, and chronic renal failure.

Use in Pregnancy. Routine use of diuretics during normal pregnancy is inappropriate and exposes mother and fetus to unnecessary hazard. Diuretics do not prevent development of toxemia of pregnancy and there is no satisfactory evidence that they are useful in the treatment of toxemia.

Edema during pregnancy may arise from pathologic causes or from the physiologic and mechanical consequences of pregnancy. Thiazides are indicated in pregnancy when edema is due to pathologic causes, just as they are in the absence of pregnancy (however, see WARNINGS, below). Dependent edema in pregnancy, resulting from restriction of venous return by the gravid uterus, is properly treated through elevation of the lower extremities and use of support stockings. Use of diuretics to lower intravascular volume in this instance is inappropriate. During normal pregnancy there is hypervolemia which is not harmful to the fetus or the mother in the absence of cardiovascular disease. However, it may be associated with edema, rarely generalized edema. If such edema causes discomfort, increased recumbency will often provide relief. Rarely this edema may cause extreme discomfort which is not relieved by rest. In these instances, a short course of diuretic therapy may provide relief and be appropriate.

Contraindications

Anuria.

Hypersensitivity to any component of this product or to other sulfonamide-derived drugs.

Warnings

Intravenous use in infants and children has been limited and is not generally recommended.

Use with caution in severe renal disease. In patients with renal disease, thiazides may precipitate azotemia. Cumulative effects of the drug may develop in patients with impaired renal function.

Thiazides should be used with caution in patients with impaired hepatic function or progressive liver disease, since minor alterations of fluid and electrolyte balance may precipitate hepatic coma.

Thiazides may add to or potentiate the action of other antihypertensive drugs.

Sensitivity reactions may occur in patients with or without a history of allergy or bronchial asthma.

The possibility of exacerbation or activation of systemic lupus erythematosus has been reported.

Lithium generally should not be given with diuretics because they reduce its renal clearance and add a high risk of lithium toxicity. Read circulars for lithium preparations before use of such concomitant therapy.

Use in Pregnancy. Thiazides cross the placental barrier and appear in cord blood. The use of thiazides in pregnancy requires that the anticipated benefit be weighed against possible hazards to the fetus. These hazards include fetal or neonatal jaundice, thrombocytopenia, and possibly other adverse reactions which have occurred in the adult.

Nursing Mothers. Thiazides appear in breast milk. If use of the drug is deemed essential, the patient should stop nursing.

Precautions

Periodic determination of serum electrolytes to detect possible electrolyte imbalance should be performed at appropriate intervals.

All patients receiving diuretic therapy should be observed for evidence of fluid or electrolyte imbalance: namely, hyponatremia, hypochloremic alkalosis, and hypokalemia. Serum and urine electrolyte determinations are particularly important when the patient is vomiting excessively or receiving parenteral fluids. Warning signs or symptoms of fluid and electrolyte imbalance include dryness of mouth, thirst, weakness, lethargy, drowsiness, restlessness, muscle pains or cramps, muscular fatigue, hypotension, oliguria, tachycardia, and gastrointestinal disturbances such as nausea and vomiting.

Hypokalemia may develop especially with brisk diuresis, when severe cirrhosis is present, during concomitant use of corticosteroids or ACTH, or after prolonged therapy.

Interference with adequate oral electrolyte intake will also contribute to hypokalemia. Hypokalemia can sensitize or exaggerate the response of the heart to the toxic effects of digitalis (e.g., increased ventricular irritability). Hypokalemia may be avoided or treated by use of potassium supplements such as foods with a high potassium content.

Although any chloride deficit is generally mild and usually does not require specific treatment except under extraordinary circumstances (as in liver disease or renal disease), chloride replacement may be required in the treatment of metabolic alkalosis.

Dilutional hyponatremia may occur in edematous patients in hot weather; appropriate therapy is water restriction, rather than administration of salt, except in rare instances when the hyponatremia is life threatening. In actual salt depletion, appropriate replacement is the therapy of choice.

Hyperuricemia may occur or acute gout may be precipitated in certain patients receiving thiazide therapy.

Insulin requirements in diabetic patients may be increased, decreased, or unchanged. Diabetes mellitus which has been latent may become manifest during thiazide administration.

Thiazide drugs may increase the responsiveness to tubocurarine.

The antihypertensive effects of the drug may be enhanced in the postsympathectomy patient. Thiazides may decrease arterial responsiveness to norepinephrine. This diminution is not sufficient to preclude effectiveness of the pressor agent for therapeutic use.

If progressive renal impairment becomes evident, consider withholding or discontinuing diuretic therapy.

Thiazides may decrease serum PBI levels without signs of thyroid disturbance.

Calcium excretion is decreased by thiazides. Pathologic changes in the parathyroid glands with hypercalcemia and hypophosphatemia have been observed in a few patients on prolonged thiazide therapy. The common complications of hyperparathyroidism such as renal lithiasis, bone resorption, and peptic ulceration have not been seen. Thiazides should be discontinued before carrying out tests for parathyroid function.

Adverse Reactions

A. *Gastrointestinal System*
1. anorexia
2. gastric irritation
3. nausea
4. vomiting
5. cramping
6. diarrhea
7. constipation
8. jaundice (intrahepatic cholestatic jaundice)
9. pancreatitis
10. sialadenitis

B. *Central Nervous System*
1. dizziness
2. vertigo
3. paresthesias
4. headache
5. xanthopsia

C. *Hematologic*
1. leukopenia
2. agranulocytosis
3. thrombocytopenia
4. aplastic anemia
5. hemolytic anemia

D. *Cardiovascular*
Orthostatic hypotension (may be aggravated by alcohol, barbiturates, or narcotics)

E. *Hypersensitivity*
1. purpura
2. photosensitivity
3. rash
4. urticaria
5. necrotizing angiitis (vasculitis) (cutaneous vasculitis)
6. fever
7. respiratory distress including pneumonitis
8. anaphylactic reactions

F. *Other*
1. hyperglycemia
2. glycosuria
3. hyperuricemia
4. muscle spasm
5. weakness
6. restlessness
7. transient blurred vision
8. hematuria (one case following intravenous use)

Whenever adverse reactions are moderate or severe, thiazide dosage should be reduced or therapy withdrawn.

Dosage and Administration

Intravenous Sodium DIURIL should be reserved for patients unable to take oral medication or for emergency situations.
Therapy should be individualized according to patient response. Use the smallest dosage necessary to achieve the required response.
Intravenous use in infants and children has been limited and is not generally recommended.
When medication can be taken orally, therapy with DIURIL tablets or oral suspension may be substituted for intravenous therapy, using the same dosage schedule as for the parenteral route.
Add 18 ml of Sterile Water for Injection to the vial to form an isotonic solution for intravenous injection. Never add less than 18 ml. Unused solution may be stored at room temperature for 24 hours, after which it must be discarded. The solution is compatible with dextrose or sodium chloride solutions for intravenous infusion. Avoid simultaneous administration of solutions of chlorothiazide with whole blood or its derivatives.
Extravasation must be rigidly avoided. Do not give subcutaneously or intramuscularly.
The usual adult dosage is 0.5 to 1.0 g once or twice a day. Many patients with edema respond to intermittent therapy, i.e., administration on alternate days or on three to five days each week. With an intermittent schedule, excessive response and the resulting undesirable electrolyte imbalance are less likely to occur.

How Supplied

No. 3250—Intravenous Sodium DIURIL is a dry, white powder usually in plug form, supplied in vials containing chlorothiazide sodium equivalent to 0.5 g of chlorothiazide. **NDC** 0006-3250-32.

A.H.F.S. 40:28
DC 6435017 Issued June 1979

DIURIL® Tablets ℞
(chlorothiazide, MSD), U.S.P.
DIURIL® Oral Suspension ℞
(chlorothiazide, MSD), U.S.P.

Description

DIURIL (Chlorothiazide, MSD) is 6-chloro-2H-1,2,4-benzothiadiazine-7-sulfonamide 1,1-dioxide. It is a white, or practically white, crystalline compound very slightly soluble in water, but readily soluble in dilute aqueous sodium hydroxide. It is soluble in urine to the extent of about 150 mg per 100 ml at pH 7.
DIURIL is supplied as 250 mg and 500 mg tablets, and as an oral suspension containing 250 mg per 5 ml, alcohol 0.5 percent, with methylparaben 0.12 percent, propylparaben 0.02 percent, and benzoic acid 0.1 percent added as preservatives.

Actions

DIURIL is a diuretic and antihypertensive.
DIURIL affects the renal tubular mechanism of electrolyte reabsorption. At maximal therapeutic dosage all thiazides are approximately equal in their diuretic efficacy.
DIURIL increases excretion of sodium and chloride in approximately equivalent amounts. Natriuresis may be accompanied by some loss of potassium and bicarbonate.
Onset of the diuretic action of DIURIL after oral use occurs in 2 hours and the peak action in about 4 hours. Diuretic activity lasts about 6 to 12 hours. DIURIL is eliminated rapidly by the kidney.
The mechanism of the antihypertensive effect of thiazides is unknown. DIURIL does not affect normal blood pressure.

Indications

DIURIL is indicated as adjunctive therapy in edema associated with congestive heart failure, hepatic cirrhosis, and corticosteroid and estrogen therapy.
DIURIL has also been found useful in edema due to various forms of renal dysfunction such as nephrotic syndrome, acute glomerulonephritis, and chronic renal failure.
DIURIL is indicated in the management of hypertension either as the sole therapeutic agent or to enhance the effectiveness of other antihypertensive drugs in the more severe forms of hypertension.
Use in Pregnancy. Routine use of diuretics during normal pregnancy is inappropriate and exposes mother and fetus to unnecessary hazard. Diuretics do not prevent development of toxemia of pregnancy and there is no satisfactory evidence that they are useful in the treatment of toxemia.
Edema during pregnancy may arise from pathologic causes or from the physiologic and mechanical consequences of pregnancy. Thiazides are indicated in pregnancy when edema is due to pathologic causes, just as they are in the absence of pregnancy (however, see WARNINGS, below). Dependent edema in pregnancy, resulting from restriction of venous return by the gravid uterus, is properly treated through elevation of the lower extremities and use of support stockings. Use of diuretics to lower intravascular volume in this instance is illogical and unnecessary. During normal pregnancy there is hypervolemia which is not harmful to the fetus or the mother in the absence of cardiovascular disease. However, it may be associated with edema, rarely generalized edema. If such edema causes discomfort, increased recumbency will often provide relief. Rarely this edema may cause extreme discomfort which is not relieved by rest. In these instances, a short course of diuretic therapy may provide relief and be appropriate.

Contraindications

Anuria.
Hypersensitivity to this product or to other sulfonamide-derived drugs.

Warnings

Use with caution in severe renal disease. In patients with renal disease, thiazides may precipitate azotemia. Cumulative effects of the drug may develop in patients with impaired renal function.
Thiazides should be used with caution in patients with impaired hepatic function or progressive liver disease, since minor alterations of fluid and electrolyte balance may precipitate hepatic coma.
Thiazides may add to or potentiate the action of other antihypertensive drugs.
Sensitivity reactions may occur in patients with or without a history of allergy or bronchial asthma.
The possibility of exacerbation or activation of systemic lupus erythematosus has been reported.
Lithium generally should not be given with diuretics because they reduce its renal clearance and add a high risk of lithium toxicity. Read circulars for lithium preparations before use of such concomitant therapy.
Use in Pregnancy. Thiazides cross the placental barrier and appear in cord blood. The use of thiazides in pregnancy requires that the anticipated benefit be weighed against possible hazards to the fetus. These hazards include fetal or neonatal jaundice, thrombocytopenia, and possibly other adverse reactions which have occurred in the adult.
Nursing Mothers. Thiazides appear in breast milk. If use of the drug is deemed essential, the patient should stop nursing.

Precautions

Periodic determination of serum electrolytes to detect possible electrolyte imbalance should be performed at appropriate intervals.
All patients receiving diuretic therapy should be observed for evidence of fluid or electrolyte imbalance: namely, hyponatremia, hypochloremic alkalosis, and hypokalemia. Serum and urine electrolyte determinations are particularly important when the patient is vomiting excessively or receiving parenteral fluids. Warning signs or symptoms of fluid and electrolyte imbalance include dryness of mouth, thirst, weakness, lethargy, drowsiness, restlessness, muscle pains or cramps, muscular fatigue, hypotension, oliguria, tachycardia, and gastrointestinal disturbances such as nausea and vomiting.
Hypokalemia may develop, especially with brisk diuresis, when severe cirrhosis is present, during concomitant use of corticosteroids or ACTH, or after prolonged therapy.
Interference with adequate oral electrolyte intake will also contribute to hypokalemia. Hypokalemia can sensitize or exaggerate the response of the heart to the toxic effects of digitalis (e.g., increased ventricular irritability). Hypokalemia may be avoided or treated by use of potassium supplements such as foods with a high potassium content.
Although any chloride deficit is generally mild and usually does not require specific treatment except under extraordinary circumstances (as in liver disease or renal disease), chloride replacement may be required in the treatment of metabolic alkalosis.
Dilutional hyponatremia may occur in edematous patients in hot weather; appropriate therapy is water restriction, rather than administration of salt, except in rare instances when the hyponatremia is life threatening. In actual salt depletion, appropriate replacement is the therapy of choice.
Hyperuricemia may occur or acute gout may be precipitated in certain patients receiving thiazide therapy.
Insulin requirements in diabetic patients may be increased, decreased, or unchanged. Diabetes mellitus which has been latent may become manifest during thiazide administration.
Thiazide drugs may increase the responsiveness to tubocurarine.
The antihypertensive effects of the drug may be enhanced in the postsympathectomy patient. Thiazides may decrease arterial responsiveness to norepinephrine. This diminution is not sufficient to preclude effectiveness of the pressor agent for therapeutic use.
If progressive renal impairment becomes evident, consider withholding or discontinuing diuretic therapy.
Thiazides may decrease serum PBI levels without signs of thyroid disturbance.
Calcium excretion is decreased by thiazides. Pathologic changes in the parathyroid glands with hypercalcemia and hypophosphatemia have been observed in a few patients on prolonged thiazide therapy. The common complications of hyperparathyroidism such as renal lithiasis, bone resorption, and peptic ulceration have not been seen. Thiazides should be discontinued before carrying out tests for parathyroid function.

Adverse Reactions

A. *Gastrointestinal System*
 1. anorexia
 2. gastric irritation

Continued on next page

Information on the Merck Sharp & Dohme products listed on these pages is the full prescribing information from package circulars in use October 31, 1979.

Merck Sharp & Dohme—Cont.

3. nausea
4. vomiting
5. cramping
6. diarrhea
7. constipation
8. jaundice (intrahepatic cholestatic jaundice)
9. pancreatitis
10. sialadenitis

B. *Central Nervous System*
1. dizziness
2. vertigo
3. paresthesias
4. headache
5. xanthopsia

C. *Hematologic*
1. leukopenia
2. agranulocytosis
3. thrombocytopenia
4. aplastic anemia
5. hemolytic anemia

D. *Cardiovascular*
Orthostatic hypotension (may be aggravated by alcohol, barbiturates, or narcotics)

E. *Hypersensitivity*
1. purpura
2. photosensitivity
3. rash
4. urticaria
5. necrotizing angiitis (vasculitis) (cutaneous vasculitis)
6. fever
7. respiratory distress including pneumonitis
8. anaphylactic reactions

F. *Other*
1. hyperglycemia
2. glycosuria
3. hyperuricemia
4. muscle spasm
5. weakness
6. restlessness
7. transient blurred vision

Whenever adverse reactions are moderate or severe, thiazide dosage should be reduced or therapy withdrawn.

Dosage and Administration

Therapy should be individualized according to patient response. Use the smallest dosage necessary to achieve the required response.

Adults

For Diuresis

The usual adult dosage is 0.5 to 1.0 g once or twice a day. Many patients with edema respond to intermittent therapy, i.e., administration on alternate days or on three to five days each week. With an intermittent schedule, excessive response and the resulting undesirable electrolyte imbalance are less likely to occur.

For Control of Hypertension

The usual adult starting dosage is 0.5 or 1.0 g a day as a single or divided dose. Dosage is increased or decreased according to blood pressure response. Rarely some patients may require up to 2.0 g a day in divided doses.

When thiazides are used with other antihypertensives, the dose of the latter may need to be reduced to prevent excessive decrease in blood pressure.

Infants and Children

The usual oral pediatric dosage is based on 10 mg of DIURIL per pound of body weight per day in two doses. Infants under 6 months of age may require up to 15 mg per pound per day in two doses.

On this basis, infants up to 2 years of age may be given 125 to 375 mg daily in two doses (2.5 to 7.5 ml, or ½ to 1½ teaspoonfuls of the oral suspension daily). Children from 2 to 12 years of age may be given 375 mg to 1.0 g daily in two doses (7.5 to 20 ml, or 1½ to 4 teaspoonfuls of oral suspension daily). Dosage in both age groups should be based on body weight.

How Supplied

No. 3244—Tablets DIURIL, 250 mg, are white, round, scored, compressed tablets, coded MSD 214. They are supplied as follows:

NDC 0006-0214-68 bottles of 100
NDC 0006-0214-28 single unit packages of 100
NDC 0006-0214-82 bottles of 1000

[*Shown in Product Identification Section*]

No. 3245—Tablets DIURIL, 500 mg, are white, round, scored, compressed tablets, coded MSD 432. They are supplied as follows:

NDC 0006-0432-68 bottles of 100
NDC 0006-0432-28 single unit packages of 100
NDC 0006-0432-82 bottles of 1000
NDC 0006-0432-86 bottles of 5000

[*Shown in Product Identification Section*]

No. 3239—Oral Suspension DIURIL, 250 mg per 5 ml, is a yellow, creamy suspension, and is supplied as follows:

NDC 0006-3239-66 bottles of 237 ml.

A.H.F.S. 40:28

DC 6020740 Issued June 1979

EDECRIN® Tablets ℞
(ethacrynic acid, MSD), U.S.P.

Intravenous

SODIUM EDECRIN® ℞
(ethacrynate sodium, MSD), U.S.P.

Warning

EDECRIN (Ethacrynic Acid, MSD) is a potent diuretic which, if given in excessive amounts, may lead to profound diuresis with water and electrolyte depletion. Therefore, careful medical supervision is required, and dose and dose schedule must be adjusted to the individual patient's needs (see Dosage and Administration).

Description

Ethacrynic acid is an unsaturated ketone derivative of an aryloxyacetic acid. Its chemical name is [2,3-dichloro-4-(2-methylenebutyryl) phenoxy]acetic acid. It is a white, or practically white, crystalline powder, only very slightly soluble in water, but is soluble in most organic solvents such as alcohols, chloroform, and benzene. The sodium salt of ethacrynic acid is soluble in water at 25°C to the extent of about 7 percent. Solutions of the sodium salt are relatively stable at about pH 7 at room temperature for short periods, but as the pH or temperature increases the solutions are less stable.

Actions

EDECRIN acts on the ascending limb of the loop of Henle and on the proximal and distal tubules. Urinary output is usually dose dependent and related to the magnitude of fluid accumulation. Water and electrolyte excretion may be increased several times over that observed with thiazide diuretics, since EDECRIN inhibits reabsorption of a much greater proportion of filtered sodium than most other diuretic agents. Therefore, EDECRIN is effective in many patients who have significant degrees of renal insufficiency. EDECRIN has little or no effect on glomerular filtration or on renal blood flow, except following pronounced reductions in plasma volume when associated with rapid diuresis.

The electrolyte excretion pattern of ethacrynic acid varies from that of the thiazides and mercurial diuretics. Initial sodium and chloride excretion is usually substantial and chloride loss exceeds that of sodium. With prolonged administration, chloride excretion declines, and potassium and hydrogen ion excretion may increase. EDECRIN is effective whether or not there is clinical acidosis or alkalosis.

Although EDECRIN, in carefully controlled studies in animals and experimental subjects, produces a more favorable sodium/potassium excretion ratio than the thiazides, in patients with increased diuresis excessive amounts of potassium may be excreted.

Onset of action is rapid, usually within 30 minutes after an oral dose of EDECRIN or within 5 minutes after an intravenous injection of SODIUM EDECRIN (Ethacrynate Sodium, MSD). Duration of action following oral administration is 6 to 8 hours, with peak activity occurring in about 2 hours.

The sulfhydryl binding propensity of ethacrynic acid differs somewhat from that of the organomercurials; its mode of action is not by carbonic anhydrase inhibition.

Indications

EDECRIN is especially useful in patients who require an agent with greater diuretic potential than those commonly employed.

1. Treatment of the edema associated with congestive heart failure, cirrhosis of the liver, and renal disease, including the nephrotic syndrome.
2. Short term management of ascites due to malignancy, idiopathic edema, and lymphedema.
3. Short term management of hospitalized pediatric patients with congenital heart disease or the nephrotic syndrome. Information in infants is insufficient to recommend therapy with EDECRIN.
4. Intravenous administration of SODIUM EDECRIN is indicated when a rapid onset of diuresis is desired, e.g., in acute pulmonary edema, or when gastrointestinal absorption is impaired or oral medication is not practicable.

Contraindications

All diuretics, including ethacrynic acid, are contraindicated in anuria. If increasing electrolyte imbalance, azotemia, and/or oliguria occur during treatment of severe, progressive renal disease, the diuretic should be discontinued.

In a few patients this diuretic has produced severe, watery diarrhea. If this occurs, it should be discontinued and not readministered.

Until further experience in infants is accumulated, therapy with oral and parenteral EDECRIN is contraindicated.

See also *Use in Pregnancy* under ADDITIONAL WARNINGS.

Hypersensitivity to any component of this product.

Additional Warnings

Frequent serum electrolyte, CO_2 and BUN determinations should be performed early in therapy and periodically thereafter during active diuresis. Any electrolyte abnormalities should be corrected or the drug temporarily withdrawn.

Initiation of diuretic therapy with EDECRIN in the cirrhotic patient with ascites is best carried out in the hospital. When maintenance therapy has been established, the individual can be satisfactorily followed as an outpatient.

EDECRIN should be given with caution to patients with advanced cirrhosis of the liver, particularly those with a history of previous episodes of electrolyte imbalance or hepatic encephalopathy. Like other diuretics it may precipitate hepatic coma and death.

Too vigorous a diuresis, as evidenced by rapid and excessive weight loss, may induce an acute hypotensive episode. In elderly cardiac patients, rapid contraction of plasma volume and the resultant hemoconcentration should be avoided to prevent the development of thromboembolic episodes, such as cerebral vascular thromboses and pulmonary emboli which may be fatal. Excessive loss of potassium in patients receiving digitalis glycosides may precipitate digitalis toxicity. Care should also be exercised in patients receiving potassium-depleting steroids.

The effects of EDECRIN on electrolytes are related to its renal pharmacologic activity and are dose dependent. The possibility of profound electrolyte and water loss may be avoided by weighing the patient throughout the treatment period, by careful adjustment of dosage, by initiating treatment with small doses, and by using the drug on an intermittent schedule when possible. When excessive diuresis occurs, the drug should be withdrawn until homeostasis is restored. When excessive electrolyte loss occurs, the dosage should be reduced or the drug temporarily withdrawn.

A number of possibly drug-related deaths have occurred in critically ill patients refractory to other diuretics. These generally have fallen into two categories: (1) patients with severe myocardial disease who have been receiving digitalis and presumably developed acute hypokalemia with fatal arrhythmia; (2) patient with severely decompensated hepatic cirrhosis with ascites, with or without accompanying encephalopathy, who were in electrolyte imbalance and died because of intensification of the electrolyte defect.

Lithium generally should not be given with diuretics because they reduce its renal clearance and add a high risk of lithium toxicity. Read circulars for lithium preparations before use of such concomitant therapy.

Nonspecific small bowel lesions consisting of stenosis with or without ulceration may occur in association with administration of enteric coated potassium tablets alone or in conjunction with diuretic therapy. Surgery was frequently required and deaths have occurred. Therefore, enteric coated potassium tablets should not be used when supplementary potassium administration is needed.

Use in Pregnancy

EDECRIN is not recommended for use in pregnant patients. Use of the drug in women of the childbearing age requires that its potential benefits be weighed against the possible hazards to the fetus. The safety and efficacy of the drug in toxemia of pregnancy have not been established. EDECRIN is contraindicated in nursing mothers. If use of the drug is deemed essential, the patient should stop nursing.

Precautions

Weakness, muscle cramps, paresthesias, thirst, anorexia, and signs of hyponatremia, hypokalemia, and/or hypochloremic alkalosis may occur following vigorous or excessive diuresis and these may be accentuated by rigid salt restriction. Rarely tetany has been reported following vigorous diuresis. *During therapy with ethacrynic acid, liberalization of salt intake and supplementary potassium chloride are often necessary.*

When a metabolic alkalosis may be anticipated, e.g., in cirrhosis with ascites, the use of potassium chloride with or without an aldosterone antagonist before and continuously during therapy with EDECRIN may mitigate or prevent the hypokalemia.

The safety and efficacy of ethacrynic acid in hypertension have not been established. However, the dosage of coadministered antihypertensive agents may require adjustment.

Orthostatic hypotension may occur in patients receiving other antihypertensive agents when given ethacrynic acid.

EDECRIN has little or no effect on glomerular filtration or on renal blood flow, except following pronounced reductions in plasma volume when associated with rapid diuresis. A transient increase in serum urea nitrogen may occur. Usually, this is readily reversible when the drug is discontinued.

As with other diuretics used in the treatment of renal edema, hypoproteinemia may reduce responsiveness to ethacrynic acid and the use of salt-poor albumin should be considered.

Vertigo, deafness, and tinnitus with a sense of fullness in the ears have occurred, most frequently in patients with severe impairment of renal function. These symptoms have been associated most often with intravenous administration and with doses in excess of those recommended. The deafness has usually been reversible and of short duration (one to 24 hours). However, in some critically ill patients the hearing loss has been permanent. A number of these patients were also receiving drugs known to be ototoxic.

A number of drugs, including ethacrynic acid, have been shown to displace warfarin from plasma protein; a reduction in the usual anticoagulant dosage may be required in patients receiving both drugs.

Adverse Reactions

Gastrointestinal

Anorexia, malaise, abdominal discomfort or pain, dysphagia, nausea, vomiting, and diarrhea have occurred. These are more frequent with large doses or after one to three months of continuous therapy. A few patients have had sudden onset of watery, profuse diarrhea. Discontinue EDECRIN if diarrhea is severe and do not readminister it. Gastrointestinal bleeding has occurred in some patients.

Rarely, acute pancreatitis has been reported in patients receiving diuretics, including EDECRIN.

Renal

Reversible hyperuricemia and acute gout have been reported. Acute symptomatic hypoglycemia with convulsions occurred in two uremic patients who received doses above those recommended.

Carbohydrate Metabolism

Hyperglycemia has been reported in a few patients, most of whom had decompensated cirrhosis. However, patients who developed hyperglycemia on thiazide therapy have not done so when given EDECRIN.

Hemopoietic System

Agranulocytosis or severe neutropenia has been reported in a few critically ill patients also receiving agents known to produce this effect. Thrombocytopenia has been reported rarely. Rare instances of Henoch-Schönlein purpura have been reported in patients with rheumatic heart disease receiving many drugs, including EDECRIN.

Hepatic

Rarely, jaundice and abnormal liver function tests have been reported in seriously ill patients on multiple drug therapy that included EDECRIN.

Miscellaneous

Vertigo, deafness, and tinnitus, with a sense of fullness in the ears, have occurred (see PRECAUTIONS). Infrequently, skin rash, headache, fever, chills, hematuria, blurred vision, fatigue, apprehension, and confusion have occurred.

SODIUM EDECRIN occasionally has caused local irritation and pain after intravenous use.

Dosage and Administration

Dosage must be regulated carefully to prevent a more rapid or substantial loss of fluid or electrolyte than is indicated or necessary. The magnitude of diuresis and natriuresis is largely dependent on the degree of fluid accumulation present in the patient. Similarly, the extent of potassium excretion is determined in large measure by the presence and magnitude of aldosteronism.

Oral Use

EDECRIN is available for oral use as 25 mg and 50 mg tablets.

Dosage: To Initiate Diuresis

The smallest dose required to produce gradual weight loss (about 1 to 2 pounds per day) is recommended. Onset of diuresis usually occurs at 50 to 100 mg for adults. After diuresis has been achieved, the minimally effective dose (usually from 50 to 200 mg daily) may be given on a continuous or intermittent dosage schedule. Dosage adjustments are usually in 25 to 50 mg increments to avoid derangement of water and electrolyte excretion.

The patient should be weighed under standard conditions before and during the institution of diuretic therapy with this compound. Small alterations in dose should effectively prevent a massive diuretic response. The following schedule may be helpful in determining the smallest effective dose.

Day 1— 50 mg (single dose) after a meal
Day 2— 50 mg twice daily after meals, if necessary
Day 3— 100 mg in the morning and 50 to 100 mg following the afternoon or evening meal, depending upon response to the morning dose

A few patients may require initial and maintenance doses as high as 200 mg twice daily. These higher doses, which should be achieved gradually, are most often required in patients with severe, refractory edema.

In children, the initial dose should be 25 mg. Careful stepwise increments in dosage of 25 mg should be made to achieve effective maintenance. A dosage for *infants* has not been established.

Maintenance Therapy

It is usually possible to reduce the dosage and frequency of administration once dry weight has been achieved.

EDECRIN (Ethacrynic Acid, MSD) may be given intermittently after an effective diuresis is obtained with the regimen outlined above. Dosage may be on an alternate daily schedule or more prolonged periods of diuretic therapy may be interspersed with rest periods. Such an intermittent dosage schedule allows time for correction of any electrolyte imbalance and may provide a more efficient diuretic response.

The chloruretic effect of this agent may give rise to retention of bicarbonate and a metabolic alkalosis. This may be corrected by giving chloride (ammonium chloride or arginine chloride). Ammonium chloride should not be given to cirrhotic patients.

EDECRIN has additive effects when used with other diuretics. For example, a patient who is on maintenance dosage of an oral diuretic may require additional intermittent diuretic therapy, such as an organomercurial, for the maintenance of basal weight. The intermittent use of EDECRIN orally may eliminate the need for injections of organomercurials. Small doses of EDECRIN may be added to existing diuretic regimens to maintain basal weight. This drug may potentiate the action of carbonic anhydrase inhibitors, with augmentation of natriuresis and kaliuresis. Therefore, when adding EDECRIN the initial dose and changes of dose should be in 25 mg increments, to avoid electrolyte depletion. Rarely, patients who failed to respond to ethacrynic acid have responded to older established agents.

While many patients do not require supplemental potassium, the use of potassium chloride or aldosterone antagonists, or both, during treatment with EDECRIN is advisable, especially in cirrhotic or nephrotic patients and in patients receiving digitalis.

Continued on next page

Information on the Merck Sharp & Dohme products listed on these pages is the full prescribing information from package circulars in use October 31, 1979.

Merck Sharp & Dohme—Cont.

Salt liberalization usually prevents the development of hyponatremia and hypochloremia. During treatment with EDECRIN, salt may be liberalized to a greater extent than with other diuretics. Cirrhotic patients, however, usually require at least moderate salt restriction concomitant with diuretic therapy.

Intravenous Use

INTRAVENOUS SODIUM EDECRIN is for intravenous use when oral intake is impractical or in urgent conditions, such as acute pulmonary edema.

Each vial contains:

Ethacrynate sodium equivalent to ethacrynate acid .... 50 mg

Inactive ingredients:

Mannitol ....62.5 mg

with 0.1 mg thimerosal added as preservative

The usual intravenous dose for the average sized adult is 50 mg, or 0.5 to 1.0 mg per kg. of body weight. Usually only one dose has been necessary; occasionally a second dose at a new injection site, to avoid possible thrombophlebitis, may be required. A single intravenous dose not exceeding 100 mg has been used in critical situations. Insufficient pediatric experience precludes recommendation for this age group.

To reconstitute the dry material, add 50 ml of 5 percent Dextrose Injection, or Sodium Chloride Injection to the vial. Occasionally, some 5 percent Dextrose Injection solutions may have a low pH (below 5). The resulting solution with such a diluent may be hazy or opalescent. Intravenous use of such a solution is not recommended.

The solution may be given slowly through the tubing of a running infusion or by direct intravenous injection over a period of several minutes. Do not mix this solution with whole blood or its derivatives. Discard unused reconstituted solution after 24 hours.

SODIUM EDECRIN should not be given subcutaneously or intramuscularly because of local pain and irritation.

How Supplied

No. 3321—Tablets EDECRIN, 25 mg are white, capsule shaped, scored tablets, coded MSD 65. They are supplied as follows:

NDC 0006-0065-68 in bottles of 100

[*Shown in Product Identification Section*]

No. 3322—Tablets EDECRIN, 50 mg are green, capsule shaped, scored tablets, coded MSD 90. They are supplied as follows:

NDC 0006-0090-68 in bottles of 100

(6505-00-834-0473 50 mg 100's)

[*Shown in Product Identification Section*]

No. 3330—INTRAVENOUS SODIUM EDECRIN is a dry white material either in a plug form or as a powder. It is supplied in vials containing ethacrynate sodium equivalent to 50 mg of ethacrynic acid, **NDC** 0006-3330-50.

(6505-00-875-7941 50 mg 50 ml vial)

A.H.F.S. 40:28

DC 6073017 Issued January 1978

ELAVIL® Tablets ℞
(amitriptyline HCl, MSD), U.S.P.
ELAVIL® Injection ℞
(amitriptyline HCl, MSD), U.S.P.

Description

Amitriptyline HCl, a dibenzocycloheptadiene derivative, is a white or practically white, crystalline compound that is freely soluble in water.

It is designated chemically as 10,11-dihydro-*N,N*-dimethyl-5*H*-dibenzo [*a,d*] cycloheptene-$^{\Delta 5\gamma}$-propylamine hydrochloride. The molecular weight is 313.87. The empirical formula is $C_{20}H_{23}N \cdot HCl$.

ELAVIL (Amitriptyline HCl, MSD) is supplied as 10 mg, 25 mg, 50 mg, 75 mg, 100 mg, and 150 mg tablets and as a sterile solution for intramuscular use. Each milliliter of the sterile solution contains:

Amitriptyline hydrochloride.........................10 mg
Dextrose..44 mg
Water for Injection, q.s. ....1 ml
Added as preservatives:
Methylparaben ....1.5 mg
Propylparaben ....0.2 mg

Actions

ELAVIL is an antidepressant with an anxiety-reducing, sedative component to its action. Its mechanism of action in man is not known. It is not a monoamine oxidase inhibitor and it does not act primarily by stimulation of the central nervous system.

Amitriptyline inhibits the membrane pump mechanism responsible for reuptake of norepinephrine into adrenergic neurons. Pharmacologically this action may potentiate or prolong sympathetic activity, since reuptake of norepinephrine is important physiologically in terminating its transmitting actions. This interference with reuptake of norepinephrine is believed by some to underlie the antidepressant activity of amitriptyline.

Indications

For the relief of symptoms of depression. Endogenous depression is more likely to be alleviated than are other depressive states.

Depression accompanied by anxiety.

Contraindications

ELAVIL is contraindicated in patients who have shown prior hypersensitivity to it.

It should not be given concomitantly with monoamine oxidase inhibitors. Hyperpyretic crises, severe convulsions, and deaths have occurred in patients receiving tricyclic antidepressant and monoamine oxidase inhibiting drugs simultaneously. When it is desired to replace a monoamine oxidase inhibitor with ELAVIL, a minimum of 14 days should be allowed to elapse after the former is discontinued. ELAVIL should then be initiated cautiously with gradual increase in dosage until optimum response is achieved.

This drug is not recommended for use during the acute recovery phase following myocardial infarction.

Warnings

ELAVIL may block the antihypertensive action of guanethidine or similarly acting compounds.

It should be used with caution in patients with a history of seizures and, because of its atropine-like action, in patients with a history of urinary retention, angle-closure glaucoma or increased intraocular pressure. In patients with angle-closure glaucoma, even average doses may precipitate an attack.

Patients with cardiovascular disorders should be watched closely. Tricyclic antidepressant drugs, including ELAVIL, particularly when given in high doses, have been reported to produce arrhythmias, sinus tachycardia, and prolongation of the conduction time. Myocardial infarction and stroke have been reported with drugs of this class.

Close supervision is required when ELAVIL is given to hyperthyroid patients or those receiving thyroid medication.

This drug may impair mental and/or physical abilities required for performance of hazardous tasks, such as operating machinery or driving a motor vehicle.

In patients who may use alcohol excessively, it should be borne in mind that the potentiation may increase the danger inherent in any suicide attempt or overdosage.

Usage in Pregnancy—Safe use of ELAVIL during pregnancy and lactation has not been established; therefore, in administering the drug to pregnant patients, nursing mothers, or women who may become pregnant, the possible benefits must be weighed against the possible hazards to mother and child.

Animal reproduction studies have been inconclusive and clinical experience has been limited.

Usage in Children—In view of the lack of experience with the use of this drug in children, it is not recommended at the present time for patients under 12 years of age.

Precautions

Schizophrenic patients may develop increased symptoms of psychosis; patients with paranoid symptomatology may have an exaggeration of such symptoms; manic depressive patients may experience a shift to the manic phase.

In these circumstances the dose of amitriptyline may be reduced or a major tranquilizer such as perphenazine may be administered concurrently.

When ELAVIL is given with anticholinergic agents or sympathomimetic drugs, including epinephrine combined with local anesthetics, close supervision and careful adjustment of dosages are required.

Paralytic ileus may occur in patients taking tricyclic antidepressants in combination with anticholinergic-type drugs.

Caution is advised if patients receive large doses of ethchlorvynol concurrently. Transient delirium has been reported in patients who were treated with one g of ethchlorvynol and 75-150 mg of ELAVIL.

ELAVIL may enhance the response to alcohol and the effects of barbiturates and other CNS depressants.

The possibility of suicide in depressed patients remains until significant remission occurs. Potentially suicidal patients should not have access to large quantities of this drug. Prescriptions should be written for the smallest amount feasible.

Concurrent administration of ELAVIL and electroshock therapy may increase the hazards associated with such therapy. Such treatment should be limited to patients for whom it is essential.

When possible, the drug should be discontinued several days before elective surgery.

Both elevation and lowering of blood sugar levels have been reported.

ELAVIL should be used with caution in patients with impaired liver function.

Adverse Reactions

Note: Included in the listing which follows are a few adverse reactions which have not been reported with this specific drug. However, pharmacological similarities among the tricyclic antidepressant drugs require that each of the reactions be considered when amitriptyline is administered.

Cardiovascular: Hypotension, hypertension, tachycardia, palpitation, myocardial infarction, arrhythmias, heart block, stroke.

CNS and Neuromuscular: Confusional states; disturbed concentration; disorientation; delusions; hallucinations; excitement; anxiety; restlessness; insomnia; nightmares; numbness, tingling, and paresthesias of the extremities; peripheral neuropathy; incoordination; ataxia; tremors; seizures; alteration in EEG patterns; extrapyramidal symptoms; tinnitus; syndrome of inappropriate ADH (antidiuretic hormone) secretion.

Anticholinergic: Dry mouth, blurred vision, disturbance of accommodation, increased intraocular pressure, constipation, paralytic ileus, urinary retention, dilatation of urinary tract.

Allergic: Skin rash, urticaria, photosensitization, edema of face and tongue.

Hematologic: Bone marrow depression including agranulocytosis, leukopenia, eosinophilia, purpura, thrombocytopenia.
Gastrointestinal: Nausea, epigastric distress, vomiting, anorexia, stomatitis, peculiar taste, diarrhea, parotid swelling, black tongue. Rarely hepatitis (including altered liver function and jaundice).
Endocrine: Testicular swelling and gynecomastia in the male, breast enlargement and galactorrhea in the female, increased or decreased libido, elevation and lowering of blood sugar levels.
Other: Dizziness, weakness, fatigue, headache, weight gain or loss, increased perspiration, urinary frequency, mydriasis, drowsiness, alopecia.
Withdrawal Symptoms: Abrupt cessation of treatment after prolonged administration may produce nausea, headache, and malaise. These are not indicative of addiction.

Dosage and Administration

Oral Dosage
Dosage should be initiated at a low level and increased gradually, noting carefully the clinical response and any evidence of intolerance.
Initial Dosage for Adults—For outpatients 75 mg of amitriptyline HCl a day in divided doses usually is satisfactory. If necessary, this may be increased to a total of 150 mg per day. Increases are made preferably in the late afternoon and/or bedtime doses. A sedative effect may be apparent before the antidepressant effect is noted, but an adequate therapeutic effect may take as long as 30 days to develop. An alternate method of initiating therapy in outpatients is to begin with 50 to 100 mg amitriptyline HCl at bedtime. This may be increased by 25 or 50 mg as necessary in the bedtime dose to a total of 150 mg per day.
Hospitalized patients may require 100 mg a day initially. This can be increased gradually to 200 mg a day if necessary. A small number of hospitalized patients may need as much as 300 mg a day.
Adolescent and Elderly Patients—In general, lower dosages are recommended for these patients. Ten mg 3 times a day with 20 mg at bedtime may be satisfactory in adolescent and elderly patients who do not tolerate higher dosages.
Maintenance—The usual maintenance dosage of amitriptyline HCl is 50 to 100 mg per day. In some patients 40 mg per day is sufficient. For maintenance therapy the total daily dosage may be given in a single dose preferably at bedtime. When satisfactory improvement has been reached, dosage should be reduced to the lowest amount that will maintain relief of symptoms. It is appropriate to continue maintenance therapy 3 months or longer to lessen the possibility of relapse.
Intramuscular Dosage
Initially, 20 to 30 mg (2 to 3 ml) four times a day.
When ELAVIL injection is administered intramuscularly, the effects may appear more rapidly than with oral administration.
When ELAVIL injection is used for initial therapy in patients unable or unwilling to take ELAVIL tablets, the tablets should replace the injection as soon as possible.
Usage in Children
In view of the lack of experience with the use of this drug in children, it is not recommended at the present time for patients under 12 years of age.

Overdosage

Manifestations—High doses may cause temporary confusion, disturbed concentration, or transient visual hallucinations. Overdosage may cause drowsiness; hypothermia; tachycardia and other arrhythmic abnormalities, such as bundle branch block; ECG evidence of impaired conduction; congestive heart failure; dilated pupils; convulsions; severe hypotension; stupor; and coma. Other symptoms may be agitation, hyperactive reflexes, muscle rigidity, vomiting, hyperpyrexia, or any of those listed under ADVERSE REACTIONS.
All patients suspected of having taken an overdosage should be admitted to a hospital as soon as possible. *Treatment* is symptomatic and supportive. Empty the stomach as quickly as possible by emesis followed by gastric lavage upon arrival at the hospital. Following gastric lavage, activated charcoal may be administered. Twenty to 30 g of activated charcoal may be given every four to six hours during the first 24 to 48 hours after ingestion. An ECG should be taken and close monitoring of cardiac function instituted if there is any sign of abnormality. Maintain an open airway and adequate fluid intake; regulate body temperature.
The intravenous administration of 1–3 mg of physostigmine salicylate is reported to reverse the symptoms of tricyclic antidepressant poisoning. Because physostigmine is rapidly metabolized, the dosage of physostigmine should be repeated as required particularly if life threatening signs such as arrhythmias, convulsions, and deep coma recur or persist after the initial dosage of physostigmine.
Standard measures should be used to manage circulatory shock and metabolic acidosis. Cardiac arrhythmias may be treated with neostigmine, pyridostigmine, or propranolol. Should cardiac failure occur, the use of digitalis should be considered. Close monitoring of cardiac function for not less than five days is advisable.
Anticonvulsants may be given to control convulsions. Amitriptyline increases the CNS depressant action but not the anticonvulsant action of barbiturates; therefore, an inhalation anesthetic, diazepam, or paraldehyde is recommended for control of convulsions.
Dialysis is of no value because of low plasma concentrations of the drug.
Since overdosage is often deliberate, patients may attempt suicide by other means during the recovery phase.
Deaths by deliberate or accidental overdosage have occurred with this class of drugs.

How Supplied

No. 3287—Tablets ELAVIL, 10 mg, are blue, round, film coated tablets, coded MSD 23. They are supplied as follows:
NDC 0006-0023-68 bottles of 100
(6505-00-079-7453, 10 mg 100's)
NDC 0006-0023-28 single unit packages of 100
NDC 0006-0023-82 bottles of 1000
NDC 0006-0023-86 bottles of 5000.
[*Shown in Product Identification Section*]
No. 3288—Tablets ELAVIL, 25 mg, are yellow, round, film coated tablets, coded MSD 45. They are supplied as follows:
NDC 0006-0045-68 bottles of 100
(6505-00-082-2659, 25 mg 100's)
NDC 0006-0045-28 single unit packages of 100
(6505-00-118-2509, 25 mg individually sealed 100's)
NDC 0006-0045-82 bottles of 1000
(6505-00-724-6358, 25 mg 1000's)
NDC 0006-0045-86 bottles of 5000.
[*Shown in Product Identification Section*]
No. 3320—Tablets ELAVIL, 50 mg, are beige, round, film coated tablets, coded MSD 102. They are supplied as follows:
NDC 0006-0102-68 bottles of 100
NDC 0006-0102-28 single unit packages of 100
NDC 0006-0102-82 bottles of 1000.
[*Shown in Product Identification Section*]
No. 3348—Tablets ELAVIL, 75 mg, are orange, round, film coated tablets, coded MSD 430. They are supplied as follows:
NDC 0006-0430-68 bottles of 100
NDC 0006-0430-28 single unit packages of 100.
[*Shown in Product Identification Section*]
No. 3349—Tablets ELAVIL, 100 mg, are mauve, round, film coated tablets, coded MSD 435. They are supplied as follows:
NDC 0006-0435-68 bottles of 100
NDC 0006-0435-28 single unit packages of 100.
[*Shown in Product Identification Section*]
No. 3351—Tablets ELAVIL, 150 mg, are blue, capsule shaped, film coated tablets, coded MSD 673. They are supplied as follows:
NDC 0006-0673-30 bottles of 30
NDC 0006-0673-68 bottles of 100
NDC 0006-0673-28 single unit packages of 100.
[*Shown in Product Identification Section*]
No. 3286—Injection ELAVIL, 10 mg/ml, is a clear, colorless solution, and is supplied as follows:
NDC 0006-3286-10 in 10 ml vials.
A.H.F.S. 28:16:04
DC 6613116 Issued December 1976

ELSPAR® ℞
(asparaginase, MSD)

Warning

IT IS RECOMMENDED THAT ASPARAGINASE BE ADMINISTERED TO PATIENTS ONLY IN A HOSPITAL SETTING UNDER THE SUPERVISION OF A PHYSICIAN WHO IS QUALIFIED BY TRAINING AND EXPERIENCE TO ADMINISTER CANCER CHEMOTHERAPEUTIC AGENTS, BECAUSE OF THE POSSIBILITY OF SEVERE REACTIONS, INCLUDING ANAPHYLAXIS AND SUDDEN DEATH. THE PHYSICIAN MUST BE PREPARED TO TREAT ANAPHYLAXIS AT EACH ADMINISTRATION OF THE DRUG.
IN THE TREATMENT OF EACH PATIENT THE PHYSICIAN MUST WEIGH CAREFULLY THE POSSIBILITY OF ACHIEVING THERAPEUTIC BENEFIT VERSUS THE RISK OF TOXICITY. THE FOLLOWING DATA SHOULD BE THOROUGHLY REVIEWED BEFORE ADMINISTERING THE COMPOUND.

Description

ELSPAR (Asparaginase, MSD) contains the enzyme L-asparagine amidohydrolase, type EC-2, derived from *Escherichia coli.* Its activity is expressed in terms of International Units (I.U.) according to the recommendation of the International Union of Biochemistry. The specific activity of ELSPAR is at least 225 I.U. per milligram of protein and each vial contains 10,000 I.U. of asparaginase and 80 mg of mannitol, an inactive ingredient, as a sterile, lyophilized plug or powder.

Actions

In a significant number of patients with acute leukemia, particularly lymphocytic, the malignant cells are dependent on an exogenous source of asparagine for survival. Normal cells, however, are able to synthesize asparagine and thus are affected less by the rapid depletion produced by treatment with the enzyme asparaginase. This is a unique approach to therapy based on a metabolic defect in asparagine synthesis of some malignant cells. ELSPAR, derived from *Escherichia coli,* is effective in inducing remissions in some patients with acute lymphocytic leukemia.

Continued on next page

Information on the Merck Sharp & Dohme products listed on these pages is the full prescribing information from package circulars in use October 31, 1979.

Merck Sharp & Dohme—Cont.

Asparagine Dependence Test
An asparagine dependence test has been utilized during the investigational studies. In this test leukemic cells obtained from some marrow cultures could be shown to require asparagine *in vitro*, suggesting sensitivity to asparaginase therapy in *vivo*. However, present data indicate that the correlation between asparagine dependence in such tests and the final response to therapy is sufficiently poor that the test is not recommended as a basis for selection of patients for treatment.

Indications

ELSPAR is indicated in the therapy of patients with acute lymphocytic leukemia. This agent is useful primarily in combination with other chemotherapeutic agents in the induction of remissions of the disease in children. ELSPAR should not be used as the sole induction agent unless combination therapy is deemed inappropriate. ELSPAR is not recommended for maintenance therapy.

Contraindications

ELSPAR is contraindicated in patients with pancreatitis or a history of pancreatitis. Acute hemorrhagic pancreatitis, in some instances fatal, has been reported following asparaginase administration. Asparaginase is also contraindicated in patients who have had previous anaphylactic reactions to it.

Warnings

Allergic reactions to asparaginase are frequent and may occur during the primary course of therapy. They are not completely predictable on the basis of the intradermal skin test. Anaphylaxis and death have occurred even in a hospital setting with experienced observers.
Once a patient has received ELSPAR as part of a treatment regimen, retreatment with this agent at a later time is associated with increased risk of hypersensitivity reactions. In patients found by skin testing to be hypersensitive to asparaginase, and in any patient who has received a previous course of therapy with asparaginase, therapy with this agent should be instituted or reinstituted only after successful desensitization, and then only if in the judgement of the physician the possible benefit is greater than the increased risk. Desensitization itself may be hazardous. (See DOSAGE AND ADMINISTRATION, *Intradermal Skin Test.*)
In view of the unpredictability of the adverse reactions to asparaginase, it is recommended that this product be used in a hospital setting.
Asparaginase has an adverse effect on liver function in the majority of patients. Therapy with asparaginase may increase pre-existing liver impairment caused by prior therapy or the underlying disease. Because of this there is a possibility that asparaginase may increase the toxicity of other medications.
The administration of ELSPAR *intravenously concurrently with* or *immediately before* a course of vincristine and prednisone may be associated with increased toxicity.

Precautions

The fall in circulating lymphoblasts often is quite marked; normal or below normal leukocyte counts are noted frequently within the first several days after initiating therapy. This may be accompanied by a marked rise in serum uric acid. The possible development of uric acid nephropathy should be borne in mind. Appropriate preventive measures should be taken, e.g., allopurinol, increased fluid intake, alkalization of urine. As a guide to the effects of therapy, the patient's peripheral blood count and bone marrow should be monitored frequently.
Frequent serum amylase determinations should be obtained to detect early evidence of pancreatitis. If pancreatitis occurs, therapy should be stopped and not reinstituted.
Blood sugar should be monitored during therapy with ELSPAR because hyperglycemia may occur.
Since teratogenic effects have occurred in animals, ELSPAR must be considered potentially teratogenic in humans.
Asparaginase has been reported to have immunosuppressive activity in animal experiments. Accordingly, the possibility that use of the drug in man may predispose to infection should be considered.
Asparaginase toxicity is reported to be greater in adults than in children.
Animal Toxicology
The acute intravenous LD_{50} of ELSPAR for mice was about 500,000 I.U./kg and for rabbits about 22,000 I.U./kg. A one-month intravenous toxicity study of ELSPAR in dogs at doses of 250, 1000, and 2000 I.U./kg/day revealed reduced serum total protein and albumin with loss of body weight at the highest dose level and anorexia, emesis, and diarrhea at all dosage levels. A similar study in monkeys at doses of 100, 300, and 1000 I.U./kg/day also revealed reduction of serum total protein and albumin and body weight loss at all dosage levels. Bromsulfalein retention and fatty changes in the liver were noted in monkeys that were given 300 and 1000 I.U./kg/day. The rabbit was unusually sensitive to ELSPAR since a single intravenous dose of 1000 I.U./kg caused hypocalcemia associated with necrosis of the parathyroid cells, convulsions, and death in about one third of the animals. Some rabbits that died showed small thymic and lymph node hemorrhages and necrosis of the germinal centers in the lymph nodes and spleen. The intravenous administration of calcium gluconate alleviated or prevented the adverse effects.
Changes in the pancreatic islets (not pancreatitis) ranging from edema to necrosis were observed in the rabbits in the acute intravenous toxicity studies (doses of 12,500 to 50,000 I.U./kg) but not in rabbits that received 1000 I.U./kg. The anatomical changes and the hypocalcemia found in the rabbits were not observed in the subacute intravenous studies in the dogs and monkeys.
Tissue culture and animal studies indicate that ELSPAR can diminish or abolish the effect of methotrexate on malignant cells. This effect on methotrexate activity persists as long as plasma asparagine levels are suppressed. These results would seem to dictate against the clinical use of methotrexate with ELSPAR, or during the period following ELSPAR therapy when plasma asparagine levels are below normal.

Adverse Reactions

Allergic reactions, including skin rashes, urticaria, arthralgia, respiratory distress, and acute anaphylaxis have been reported. (See WARNINGS.) Acute reactions have occurred in the absence of a positive skin test and during continued maintenance of therapeutic serum levels of ELSPAR.
Fatal hyperthermia has been reported.
Pancreatitis, sometimes fulminant, has occurred during or following therapy with ELSPAR.
Hyperglycemia with glucosuria and polyuria has been reported in low incidence. Serum and urine acetone usually have been absent or negligible in these patients; this syndrome thus resembles hyperosmolar, nonketotic, hyperglycemia induced by a variety of other agents. This complication usually responds to discontinuance of ELSPAR, judicious use of intravenous fluid, and insulin, but may be fatal on occasion.
In addition to hypofibrinogenemia, depression of various other clotting factors has been reported. Most marked has been a decrease in plasma levels of factors V and VIII with a variable decrease in factors VII and IX. A decrease in circulating platelets has occurred in low incidence which, together with the increased levels of fibrin degradation products in the serum, may indicate development of a consumption coagulopathy. Bleeding has been a problem in only a minority of patients with demonstrable coagulopathy. However, fatal bleeding associated with low fibrinogen levels has been reported. Increased fibrinolytic activity, apparently compensatory in nature, also has occurred.
Some patients have shown central nervous system effects consisting of depression, somnolence, fatigue, coma, confusion, agitation, and hallucinations varying from mild to severe. Rarely, a Parkinson-like syndrome has occurred, with tremor and a progressive increase in muscular tone. These side effects usually have reversed spontaneously after treatment was stopped. Therapy with ELSPAR is associated with an increase in blood ammonia during the conversion of asparagine to asparatic acid by the enzyme. No clear correlation exists between the degree of elevation of blood ammonia levels and the appearance of CNS changes.
Chills, fever, nausea, vomiting, anorexia, abdominal cramps, weight loss, headache, and irritability may occur and usually are mild.
Azotemia, usually pre-renal, occurs frequently. Acute renal shut down and fatal renal insufficiency have been reported during treatment. Proteinuria has occurred infrequently.
A variety of liver function abnormalities have been reported, including elevations of SGOT, SGPT, alkaline phosphatase, bilirubin (direct and indirect), and depression of serum albumin, cholesterol (total and esters), and plasma fibrinogen. Increases and decreases of total lipids have occurred. Marked hypoalbuminemia associated with peripheral edema has been reported. However, these abnormalities usually are reversible on discontinuance of therapy and some reversal may occur during the course of therapy. Fatty changes in the liver have been documented by biopsy. Malabsorption syndrome has been reported.
Rarely, transient bone marrow depression has been observed, as evidenced by a delay in return of hemoglobin or hematocrit levels to normal in patients undergoing hematologic remission of leukemia. Marked leukopenia has been reported.

Dosage and Administration

As a component of selected multiple agent induction regimens, ELSPAR may be administered by either the intravenous or the intramuscular route. When administered intravenously this enzyme should be given over a period of not less than thirty minutes through the side arm of an already running infusion of Sodium Chloride Injection or Dextrose Injection 5% (D_5W). ELSPAR has little tendency to cause phlebitis when given intravenously. Anaphylactic reactions require the immediate use of epinephrine, oxygen, and intravenous steroids.
When administering ELSPAR intramuscularly, the volume at a single injection site should be limited to 2 ml. If a volume greater than 2 ml is to be administered two injection sites should be used.
Unfavorable interactions of ELSPAR with some antitumor agents have been demonstrated. It is recommended therefore, that ELSPAR be used in combination regimens only by physicians familiar with the benefits and risks of a given regimen. During the period of its inhibition of protein synthesis and cell replication ELSPAR may interfere with the action of drugs such as methotrexate which require cell replication for their lethal effect. ELSPAR

may interfere with the enzymatic detoxification of other drugs, particularly in the liver.

Recommended Induction Regimens:

When using chemotherapeutic agents in combination for the induction of remissions in patients with acute lymphocytic leukemia, regimens are sought which provide maximum chance of success while avoiding excessive cumulative toxicity or negative drug interactions.

One of the following combination regimens incorporating ELSPAR is recommended for acute lymphocytic leukemia in children:

In the regimens below, Day 1 is considered to be the first day of therapy.

Regimen I

Prednisone 40 mg/square meter of body surface area per day orally in three divided doses for 15 days, followed by tapering of the dosage as follows:

20 mg/square meter for 2 days, 10 mg/square meter for 2 days, 5 mg/square meter for 2 days, 2.5 mg/square meter for 2 days and then discontinue.

Vincristine sulfate 2 mg/square meter of body surface area intravenously once weekly on Days 1, 8, and 15 of the treatment period. The maximum single dose should not exceed 2.0 mg.

Asparaginase 1,000 I.U./kg/day intravenously for ten successive days beginning on Day 22 of the treatment period.

Regimen II

Prednisone 40 mg/square meter of body surface area per day orally in three divided doses for 28 days (the total daily dose should be to the nearest 2.5 mg), following which the dosage of prednisone should be discontinued gradually over a 14 day period.

Vincristine sulfate 1.5 mg/square meter of body surface area intravenously weekly for four doses, on Days 1, 8, 15, and 22 of the treatment period. The maximum single dose should not exceed 2.0 mg.

Asparaginase 6,000 I.U./square meter of body surface area intramuscularly on Days 4, 7, 10, 13, 16, 19, 22, 25, and 28 of the treatment period. When a remission is obtained with either of the above regimens, appropriate maintenance therapy must be instituted. ELSPAR should not be used as part of a maintenance regimen. The above regimens do not preclude a need for special therapy directed toward the prevention of central nervous system leukemia.

It should be noted that ELSPAR has been used in combination regimens other than those recommended above. It is important to keep in mind that ELSPAR administered intravenously concurrently with or immediately before a course of vincristine and prednisone may be associated with increased toxicity. Physicians using a given regimen should be thoroughly familiar with its benefits and risks. Clinical data are insufficient for a recommendation concerning the use of combination regimens in adults. Asparaginase toxicity is reported to be greater in adults than in children. Use of ELSPAR as the sole induction agent should be undertaken only in an unusual situation when a combined regimen is inappropriate because of toxicity or other specific patient-related factors, or in cases refractory to other therapy. When ELSPAR is to be used as the sole induction agent for children or adults the recommended dosage regimen is 200 I.U./kg/day intravenously for 28 days. When complete remissions were obtained with this regimen, they were of short duration, 1 to 3 months. ELSPAR has been used as the sole induction agent in other regimens. Physicians using a given regimen should be thoroughly familiar with its benefits and risks.

Patients undergoing induction therapy must be carefully monitored and the therapeutic regimen adjusted according to response and toxicity. Such adjustments should always involve decreasing dosages of one or more agents or discontinuation depending on the degree of toxicity. Patients who have received a course of ELSPAR, if retreated, have an increased risk of hypersensitivity reactions. Therefore, retreatment should be undertaken only when the benefit of such therapy is weighed against the increased risk.

Intradermal Skin Test:

Because of the occurrence of allergic reactions, an intradermal skin test should be performed prior to the initial administration of ELSPAR and when ELSPAR is given after an interval of a week or more has elapsed between doses. The skin test solution may be prepared as follows: Reconstitute the contents of a 10,000 I.U. vial with 5.0 ml of diluent. From this solution (2,000 I.U./ml) withdraw 0.1 ml and inject it into another vial containing 9.9 ml of diluent, yielding a skin test solution of approximately 20.0 I.U./ml. Use 0.1 ml of this solution (about 2.0 I.U.) for the intradermal skin test. The skin test site should be observed for at least one hour for the appearance of a wheal or erythema either of which indicates a positive reaction. An allergic reaction even to the skin test dose in certain sensitized individuals may rarely occur. A negative skin test reaction does not preclude the possibility of the development of an allergic reaction.

Desensitization:

Desensitization should be performed before administering the first dose of ELSPAR on initiation of therapy in positive reactors, and on retreatment of any patient in whom such therapy is deemed necessary after carefully weighing the increased risk of hypersensitivity reactions. Rapid desensitization of the patient may be attempted with progressively increasing amounts of intravenously administered ELSPAR provided adequate precautions are taken to treat an acute allergic reaction should it occur. One reported schedule begins with a total of 1 I.U. given intravenously and doubles the dose every 10 minutes, provided no reaction has occurred, until the accumulated total amount given equals the planned doses for that day.

For convenience the following table is included to calculate the number of doses necessary to reach the patient's total dose for that day:

Injection Number	ELSPAR Dose in I.U.	Accumulated Total Dose
1	1	1
2	2	3
3	4	7
4	8	15
5	16	31
6	32	63
7	64	127
8	128	255
9	256	511
10	512	1023
11	1024	2047
12	2048	4095
13	4096	8191
14	8192	16383
15	16384	32767
16	32768	65535
17	65536	131071
18	131072	262143

For example: A patient weighing 20 kg who is to receive 200 I.U./kg (total dose 4000 I.U.) would receive injections 1 through 12 during desensitization.

Directions for Reconstitution

For Intravenous Use

Reconstitute with Sterile Water for Injection or with Sodium Chloride Injection. The resultant solution should be clear. If not, discard. The volume recommended for reconstitution is 5 ml for the 10,000 unit vials. Ordinary shaking during reconstitution does not inactivate the enzyme. As long as this solution remains clear, it may be used for direct intravenous administration within an eight hour period following restoration. For administration by infusion, solutions should be diluted with the isotonic solutions, Sodium Chloride Injection or Dextrose Injection 5%. These solutions also should be infused within eight hours and only if clear.

For Intramuscular Use

When ELSPAR is administered intramuscularly according to the schedule cited in the induction regimen, reconstitution is carried out by adding 2 ml Sodium Chloride Injection to the 10,000 unit vial. The resulting solution should be used within eight hours and only if clear.

Storage

Store below 8°C (46°F). ELSPAR does not contain a preservative. Unused, reconstituted solution should be stored at 2 to 8°C (36 to 46°F) and discarded after eight hours, or sooner if it becomes cloudy.

How Supplied

No. 4612 — ELSPAR is a white lyophilized plug or powder supplied as follows:

NDC 0006-4612-00 in a sterile 10 ml vial containing 10,000 I.U. of asparaginase and 80 mg mannitol, an inactive ingredient.

Clinical Pharmacology

Plasma asparaginase levels are dose dependent and show a cumulative effect on repeated administration. The plasma half-life varies from 8 to 30 hours. The half-life is not influenced by dosage, either single or repetitive, and cannot be correlated with age, sex, surface area, renal or hepatic function, diagnosis or extent of disease. Some movement out of the intravascular compartment is indicated by a distribution volume greater than the calculated plasma volume and a polyphasic plasma disappearance curve after discontinuing therapy. It has been detected in thoracic and cervical lymph. Cerebrospinal fluid levels usually are less than 1% of concurrent plasma levels. Trace amounts appear in the urine.

A.H.F.S. 44:00

DC 6680202 Issued November 1977

FLEXERIL® Tablets ℞
(cyclobenzaprine HCl, MSD)

Description

Cyclobenzaprine hydrochloride is a white, crystalline tricyclic amine salt with the empirical formula $C_{20}H_{21}N \cdot HCl$ and a molecular weight of 311.9. It is freely soluble in water and alcohol, sparingly soluble in isopropanol, and insoluble in hydrocarbon solvents. If aqueous solutions are made alkaline, the free base separates. Cyclobenzaprine HCl is designated chemically as 3-(5*H*-dibenzo[*a*, *d*]cyclohepten-

Continued on next page

Information on the Merck Sharp & Dohme products listed on these pages is the full prescribing information from package circulars in use October 31, 1979.

Merck Sharp & Dohme—Cont.

5-ylidene)-*N*, *N*-dimethyl-1-propanamine hydrochloride.
FLEXERIL® (Cyclobenzaprine HCl, MSD) is supplied as 10 mg tablets.

Clinical Pharmacology

Cyclobenzaprine HCl relieves skeletal muscle spasm of local origin without interfering with muscle function. It is ineffective in muscle spasm due to central nervous system disease.
Cyclobenzaprine reduced or abolished skeletal muscle hyperactivity in several animal models. Animal studies indicate that cyclobenzaprine does not act at the neuromuscular junction or directly on skeletal muscle. Such studies show that cyclobenzaprine acts primarily within the central nervous system at brain stem as opposed to spinal cord levels, although its action on the latter may contribute to its overall skeletal muscle relaxant activity. Evidence suggests that the net effect of cyclobenzaprine is a reduction of tonic somatic motor activity, influencing both gamma (γ) and alpha (α) motor systems.
Pharmacological studies in animals showed a similarity between the effects of cyclobenzaprine and the structurally related tricyclic antidepressants, including reserpine antagonism, norepinephrine potentiation, potent peripheral and central anticholinergic effects, and sedation. Cyclobenzaprine caused slight to moderate increase in heart rate in animals.
Controlled clinical studies show that FLEXERIL significantly improves the signs and symptoms of skeletal muscle spasm as compared with placebo. The clinical responses include improvement in muscle spasm as determined by palpation, reduction in local pain and tenderness, increased range of motion, and less restriction in activities of daily living. When daily observations were made, clinical improvement was observed as early as the first day of therapy.
Eight double-blind controlled clinical studies were performed in 642 patients comparing FLEXERIL, diazepam*, and placebo. Muscle spasm, local pain and tenderness, limitation of motion, and restriction in activities of daily living were evaluated. In three of these studies there was a significantly greater improvement with FLEXERIL than with diazepam, while in the other studies the improvement following both treatments was comparable.
Although the frequency and severity of adverse reactions observed in patients treated with FLEXERIL were comparable to those observed in patients treated with diazepam, dry mouth was observed more frequently in patients treated with FLEXERIL and dizziness more frequently in those treated with diazepam. The incidence of drowsiness, the most frequent adverse reaction, was similar with both drugs.
Analysis of the data from controlled studies shows that FLEXERIL produces clinical improvement whether or not sedation occurs.
Cyclobenzaprine is well absorbed after oral administration, but there is a large intersubject variation in plasma levels. Cyclobenzaprine is eliminated quite slowly with a half-life as long as one to three days. It is highly bound to plasma proteins, is extensively metabolized primarily to glucuronide-like conjugates, and is excreted primarily via the kidneys.
In one study, no effect on the plasma levels or bioavailability of FLEXERIL was noted with acute administration of aspirin. However, adequate studies have not been done to determine whether there is a drug interaction between FLEXERIL and concomitantly administered analgesics, including chronic administration of aspirin. No studies have been performed to indicate whether FLEXERIL enhances the clinical effect of aspirin or other analgesics, or whether analgesics enhance the clinical effect of FLEXERIL in acute musculoskeletal conditions.

Indications

FLEXERIL is indicated as an adjunct to rest and physical therapy for relief of muscle spasm associated with acute, painful musculoskeletal conditions.
Improvement is manifested by relief of muscle spasm and its associated signs and symptoms, namely, pain, tenderness, limitation of motion, and restriction in activities of daily living.
FLEXERIL (Cyclobenzaprine HCl, MSD) should be used only for short periods (up to two or three weeks) because adequate evidence of effectiveness for more prolonged use is not available and because muscle spasm associated with acute, painful musculoskeletal conditions is generally of short duration and specific therapy for longer periods is seldom warranted.
FLEXERIL has not been found effective in the treatment of spasticity associated with cerebral or spinal cord disease, or in children with cerebral palsy.

Contraindications

Hypersensitivity to the drug.
Concomitant use of monoamine oxidase inhibitors or within 14 days after their discontinuation.
Acute recovery phase of myocardial infarction, and patients with arrhythmias, heart block or conduction disturbances, or congestive heart failure.
Hyperthyroidism.

Warnings

Use of FLEXERIL (Cyclobenzaprine HCl, MSD) for periods longer than two or three weeks is not recommended (see INDICATIONS).
FLEXERIL is closely related to the tricyclic antidepressants, e.g., amitriptyline and imipramine. In short term studies for indications other than muscle spasm associated with acute musculoskeletal conditions, and usually at doses somewhat greater than those recommended for skeletal muscle spasm, some of the more serious central nervous system reactions noted with the tricyclic antidepressants have occurred (see WARNINGS, below, and ADVERSE REACTIONS).
FLEXERIL may interact with monoamine oxidase (MAO) inhibitors. Hyperpyretic crisis, severe convulsions, and deaths have occurred in patients receiving tricyclic antidepressants and MAO inhibitor drugs.
Tricyclic antidepressants have been reported to produce arrhythmias, sinus tachycardia, prolongation of the conduction time leading to myocardial infarction and stroke.
FLEXERIL may enhance the effects of alcohol, barbiturates, and other CNS depressants.

Precautions

FLEXERIL may impair mental and/or physical abilities required for performance of hazardous tasks, such as operating machinery or driving a motor vehicle.
Because of its atropine-like action, FLEXERIL should be used with caution in patients with a history of urinary retention, angle-closure glaucoma, increased intraocular pressure, and in patients taking anticholinergic medication.
Tricyclic antidepressants may block the antihypertensive action of guanethidine and similarly acting compounds.
In rats treated with FLEXERIL for up to 67 weeks at doses of 5 to 50 mg/kg, pale, sometimes enlarged, livers were noted and there was a dose-related hepatocyte vacuolation with lipidosis. In the higher dose groups this microscopic change was seen after 26 weeks and even earlier in rats which died prior to 26 weeks; at lower doses, the change was not seen until after 26 weeks. In clinical trials with FLEXERIL, most of which were short-term, no liver function abnormalities were noted.
Use in Pregnancy: In female rats reproduction studies were conducted with oral doses of 5 to 20 mg/kg/day. Pups of rats given 20 mg/kg/day weighed less than corresponding controls up to 21 days postpartum. Oral doses of up to 20 mg/kg/day given to pregnant mice and rabbits produced no evidence of external, visceral, or skeletal abnormalities in the offspring.
The safe use of FLEXERIL in pregnant women has not been established. Therefore, the anticipated benefits must be weighed against possible hazards to mother and child.
Use in Nursing Mothers: Because it is likely that FLEXERIL is excreted in milk, it should not be given to nursing mothers.
Use in Children: Safety and effectiveness of FLEXERIL in children below the age of 15 have not been established.

Adverse Reactions

The following adverse reactions have been reported with FLEXERIL:
Most frequent: Drowsiness (40%), dry mouth (28%), dizziness (11%).
Less frequent: Increased heart rate (and several cases of tachycardia), weakness, fatigue, dyspepsia, nausea, paresthesia, unpleasant taste, blurred vision, and insomnia.
Rare: Sweating, myalgia, dyspnea, abdominal pain, constipation, coated tongue, tremors, dysarthria, euphoria, nervousness, disorientation, confusion, headache, urinary retention, decreased bladder tonus; ataxia; depressed mood; hallucinations; and allergic reactions including skin rash, urticaria, and edema of the face and tongue.
Pharmacologic similarities among the tricyclic drugs require that each of the following reactions be considered when FLEXERIL is administered:
Cardiovascular: Hypotension, hypertension, palpitation, myocardial infarction, arrhythmias, heart block, stroke.
CNS and Neuromuscular: Disturbed concentration, delusions, excitement, anxiety, restlessness, nightmares, peripheral neuropathy, incoordination, seizures, alteration in EEG patterns, extrapyramidal symptoms, tinnitus, syndrome of inappropriate ADH (antidiuretic hormone) secretion.
Anticholinergic: Disturbance of accommodation, paralytic ileus, dilatation of urinary tract.
Allergic: Photosensitization.
Hematologic: Bone marrow depression including agranulocytosis, leukopenia, eosinophilia, purpura, thrombocytopenia.
Gastrointestinal: Vomiting, anorexia, stomatitis, diarrhea, parotid swelling, black tongue. Rarely hepatitis (including altered liver function and jaundice).
Endocrine: Testicular swelling and gynecomastia in the male, breast enlargement and galactorrhea in the female, increased or decreased libido, elevation and lowering of blood sugar levels.
Other: Weight gain or loss, urinary frequency, mydriasis, jaundice, alopecia.
Withdrawal Symptoms: Abrupt cessation of treatment after prolonged administration may produce nausea, headache, and malaise. These are not indicative of addiction.

Overdosage

Manifestations: High doses may cause temporary confusion, disturbed concentration, transient visual hallucinations, agitation, hyperactive reflexes, muscle rigidity, vomiting, or hyperpyrexia, in addition to anything listed under ADVERSE REACTIONS. Based on the known pharmacologic actions of the drug, overdosage may cause drowsiness, hypothermia, tachycardia and other cardiac rhythm abnormalities such as bundle branch block, ECG evidence of impaired conduction, and congestive heart failure. Other manifestations may be dilated pupils, convulsions, severe hypotension, stupor, and coma.

Treatment: Treatment is symptomatic and supportive. Empty the stomach as quickly as possible by emesis, followed by gastric lavage. After gastric lavage, activated charcoal may be administered. Twenty to 30 g of activated charcoal may be given every four to six hours during the first 24 to 48 hours after ingestion. An ECG should be taken and close monitoring of cardiac function must be instituted if there is any evidence of dysrhythmia. Maintenance of an open airway, adequate fluid intake, and regulation of body temperature are necessary. The intravenous administration of 1-3 mg of physostigmine salicylate is reported to reverse symptoms of poisoning by atropine and other drugs with anticholinergic activity. Physostigmine may be helpful in the treatment of cyclobenzaprine overdose. Because physostigmine is rapidly metabolized, its dosage should be repeated as often as required when life-threatening signs such as arrhythmias, convulsions, and deep coma recur or persist.

Standard medical measures should be used to manage circulatory shock and metabolic acidosis. Cardiac arrhythmias may be treated with neostigmine, pyridostigmine, or propranolol. When signs of cardiac failure occur, the use of a short-acting digitalis preparation should be considered. Close monitoring of cardiac function for not less than five days is advisable.

Anticonvulsants may be given to control seizures.

Dialysis is probably of no value because of low plasma concentrations of the drug.

Since overdosage is often deliberate, patients may attempt suicide by other means during the recovery phase. Deaths by deliberate or accidental overdosage have occurred with this class of drugs.

Dosage and Administration

The usual dosage of FLEXERIL is 10 mg three times a day, with a range of 20 to 40 mg a day in divided doses. Dosage should not exceed 60 mg a day. Use of FLEXERIL for periods longer than two or three weeks is not recommended.

How Supplied

No. 3358—Tablets FLEXERIL, 10 mg, are butterscotch yellow, D-shaped, film coated tablets, coded MSD 931. They are supplied as follows:
NDC 0006-0931-68 in bottles of 100.
NDC 0006-0931-28 single unit packages of 100.

[*Shown in Product Identification Section*]

A.H.F.S. 12:20

DC 6919204 Issued May 1978

*VALIUM® (diazepam, Roche)

HEP-B-GAMMAGEE® ℞

(hepatitis B immune globulin [human], MSD)

Description

HEP-B-GAMMAGEE [Hepatitis B Immune Globulin (Human), MSD] is a sterile solution of human immunoglobulin (10–18% protein) prepared by Cohn cold ethanol fractionation of pooled plasma drawn from individuals with high titers of antibody to the hepatitis B surface antigen (anti-HBs). HEP-B-GAMMAGEE is prepared from human plasma that was nonreactive when tested for hepatitis B surface antigen (HBsAg). The product is dissolved in 0.3 molar glycine and contains thimerosal (mercury derivative) 1:10,000 added as a preservative. The solution has a pH of 6.8 ± 0.4 adjusted with hydrochloric acid or sodium hydroxide. Each vial of HEP-B-GAMMAGEE contains anti-HBs equivalent to or exceeding the potency of anti-HBs in a U.S. reference Hepatitis B Immune Globulin (Bureau of Biologics, FDA).

Actions

Hepatitis B Immune Globulin (Human) provides passive immunization for individuals exposed to the hepatitis B virus (HBV) as evidenced by a reduction in the attack rate of hepatitis B following its use. The administration of the usual recommended dose of HEP-B-GAMAGEE generally results in a detectable level of circulating antibody to hepatitis B surface antigen (anti-HBs) which persists for approximately 2 months or longer. The possibility of hepatitis B transmission is remote, as it is with other immune globulins prepared by the cold ethanol process.

Indications

HEP-B-GAMMAGEE is indicated for post-exposure prophylaxis following either parenteral exposure, direct mucous membrane contact, or oral ingestion involving HBsAg positive materials such as blood, plasma or serum. Such exposures might occur by accidental "needlestick", accidental splash, or a pipetting accident.

Use of Hepatitis B Immune Globulin (Human) has been and continues to be evaluated in other situations which include nonparenteral exposure to hepatitis B, in dialysis patients and among hospital staffs, and in infants born to hepatitis B-positive mothers. In addition, it has been tested as a prophylactic measure for susceptible individuals in close association with HBsAg-positive persons. These studies are still in progress and there are insufficient data at present on effectiveness, dosage and schedule for any of these uses to be included as definite indications.

Warnings

Persons with isolated immunoglobulin A deficiency have the potential for developing antibodies to immunoglobulin A and could have anaphylactic reactions to subsequent administration of blood products that contain immunoglobulin A. Therefore, Hepatitis B Immune Globulin (Human) should be given to such persons only if the expected benefits outweigh the potential risks.

In patients who have severe thrombocytopenia or any coagulation disorder that would contraindicate intramuscular injections, Hepatitis B Immune Globulin (Human) should be given only if the expected benefits outweigh the potential risks.

Precautions

HEP-B-GAMMAGEE should be given with caution to patients with a history of prior systemic allergic reactions following the administration of human immune globulin preparations. Hypersensitivity reactions to injections of immune serum globulin occur rarely. The incidence of these reactions may be increased in patients receiving large intramuscular doses or in patients receiving repeated injections of immune serum globulin.

HEP-B-GAMMAGEE *must not be administered intravenously* because of the potential for serious reactions. Injections should be made intramuscularly. Care should be taken to draw back on the plunger of the syringe before injection in order to be certain that the needle is not in a blood vessel.

Epinephrine should be available for treatment of acute allergic symptoms.

Clinically Significant Product Interactions

Antibodies present in immune globulin preparations may interfere with the immune response to live virus vaccines such as measles, mumps, and rubella. Therefore, vaccination with live virus vaccines should be deferred until approximately three months after administration of Hepatitis B Immune Globulin. It may be necessary to revaccinate persons who received Hepatitis B Immune Globulin shortly after live virus vaccination.

Pregnancy

Pregnancy is not a contraindication to the administration of Hepatitis B Immune Globulin (Human). No studies have been conducted in pregnant patients. Clinical experience with other immunoglobulin preparations administered during pregnancy suggests that there are no known adverse effects on the fetus from immune globulins per se. However, there are no reported studies indicating whether or not such adverse effects occur.

Adverse Reactions

Local pain and tenderness at the injection site, urticaria and angioedema may occur. Anaphylactic reactions, although rare, have been reported following the injection of human immune globulin preparations. Anaphylaxis is more likely to occur if Hepatitis B Immune Globulin (Human) is given intravenously; therefore, Hepatitis B Immune Globulin (Human) must be administered *only* intramuscularly. In highly allergic individuals, repeated injections may lead to anaphylactic shock.

Dosage and Administration

HEP-B-GAMMAGEE is administered *intramuscularly,* preferably in the gluteal or deltoid region. *It must not be injected intravenously.* The recommended dose is 0.06 ml per kilogram of body weight; the usual adult dose is 3 to 5 ml. The appropriate dose should be administered as soon after exposure as possible (preferably within 7 days) and repeated 28–30 days after exposure.

It is important to use a separate sterile syringe and needle for each individual patient to prevent transmission of hepatitis B and other infectious agents from one person to another.

Overdosage

Although no data are available, clinical experience with other immunoglobulin preparations suggests that the only manifestations would be pain and tenderness at the injection site.

Storage

Store at 2–8°C (35.6–46.4°F). Do not freeze.

How Supplied

HEP-B-GAMMAGEE is supplied as follows:
No. 4692–one 5 ml vial.
NDC 0006-4692-00

A.H.F.S. 80:04

DC 7062001 Issued October 1978

Continued on next page

Information on the Merck Sharp & Dohme products listed on these pages is the full prescribing information from package circulars in use October 31, 1979.

Merck Sharp & Dohme—Cont.

HydroDIURIL® Tablets ℞
(hydrochlorothiazide, MSD), U.S.P.

Description

HydroDIURIL (Hydrochlorothiazide, MSD) is the 3,4-dihydro derivative of chlorothiazide. Its chemical name is 6-chloro-3,4-dihydro- 2H-1,2,4-benzothiadiazine-7-sulfonamide 1,1- dioxide. It is a white, or practically white, crystalline compound slightly soluble in water, but freely soluble in sodium hydroxide solution.

Actions

HydroDIURIL is a diuretic and antihypertensive.
HydroDIURIL affects the renal tubular mechanism of electrolyte reabsorption. At maximal therapeutic dosage all thiazides are approximately equal in their diuretic efficacy.
HydroDIURIL increases excretion of sodium and chloride in approximately equivalent amounts. Natriuresis may be accompanied by some loss of potassium and bicarbonate.
Onset of the diuretic action of HydroDIURIL after oral use occurs in 2 hours and the peak action in about 4 hours. Diuretic activity lasts about 6 to 12 hours. HydroDIURIL is eliminated rapidly by the kidney.
The mechanism of the antihypertensive effect of thiazides is unknown. HydroDIURIL does not affect normal blood pressure.

Indications

HydroDIURIL is indicated as adjunctive therapy in edema associated with congestive heart failure, hepatic cirrhosis, and corticosteroid and estrogen therapy.
HydroDIURIL has also been found useful in edema due to various forms of renal dysfunction such as nephrotic syndrome, acute glomerulonephritis, and chronic renal failure.
HydroDIURIL is indicated in the management of hypertension either as the sole therapeutic agent or to enhance the effectiveness of other antihypertensive drugs in the more severe forms of hypertension.
Use in Pregnancy. Routine use of diuretics during normal pregnancy is inappropriate and exposes mother and fetus to unnecessary hazard. Diuretics do not prevent development of toxemia of pregnancy and there is no satisfactory evidence that they are useful in the treatment of toxemia.
Edema during pregnancy may arise from pathologic causes or from the physiologic and mechanical consequences of pregnancy. Thiazides are indicated in pregnancy when edema is due to pathologic causes, just as they are in the absence of pregnancy (however, see WARNINGS, below). Dependent edema in pregnancy, resulting from restriction of venous return by the gravid uterus, is properly treated through elevation of the lower extremities and use of support stockings. Use of diuretics to lower intravascular volume in this instance is illogical and unnecessary. During normal pregnancy there is hypervolemia which is not harmful to the fetus or the mother in the absence of cardiovascular disease. However, it may be associated with edema, rarely generalized edema. If such edema causes discomfort, increased recumbency will often provide relief. Rarely this edema may cause extreme discomfort which is not relieved by rest. In these instances, a short course of diuretic therapy may provide relief and be appropriate.

Contraindications

Anuria.
Hypersensitivity to this product or to other sulfonamide-derived drugs.

Warnings

Use with caution in severe renal disease. In patients with renal disease, thiazides may precipitate azotemia. Cumulative effects of the drug may develop in patients with impaired renal function.
Thiazides should be used with caution in patients with impaired hepatic function or progressive liver disease, since minor alterations of fluid and electrolyte balance may precipitate hepatic coma.
Thiazides may add to or potentiate the action of other antihypertensive drugs.
Sensitivity reactions may occur in patients with or without a history of allergy or bronchial asthma.
The possibility of exacerbation or activation of systemic lupus erythematosus has been reported.
Lithium generally should not be given with diuretics because they reduce its renal clearance and add a high risk of lithium toxicity. Read circulars for lithium preparations before use of such concomitant therapy.
Use in Pregnancy. Thiazides cross the placental barrier and appear in cord blood. The use of thiazides in pregnancy requires that the anticipated benefit be weighed against possible hazards to the fetus. These hazards include fetal or neonatal jaundice, thrombocytopenia, and possibly other adverse reactions which have occurred in the adult.
Nursing Mothers. Thiazides appear in breast milk. If use of the drug is deemed essential, the patient should stop nursing.

Precautions

Periodic determination of serum electrolytes to detect possible electrolyte imbalance should be performed at appropriate intervals.
All patients receiving diuretic therapy should be observed for evidence of fluid or electrolyte imbalance: namely, hyponatremia, hypochloremic alkalosis, and hypokalemia. Serum and urine electrolyte determinations are particularly important when the patient is vomiting excessively or receiving parenteral fluids. Warning signs or symptoms of fluid and electrolyte imbalance include dryness of mouth, thirst, weakness, lethargy, drowsiness, restlessness, muscle pains or cramps, muscular fatigue, hypotension, oliguria, tachycardia, and gastrointestinal disturbances such as nausea and vomiting.
Hypokalemia may develop, especially with brisk diuresis, when severe cirrhosis is present, during concomitant use of corticosteroids or ACTH, or after prolonged therapy.
Interference with adequate oral electrolyte intake will also contribute to hypokalemia. Hypokalemia can sensitize or exaggerate the response of the heart to the toxic effects of digitalis (e.g., increased ventricular irritability). Hypokalemia may be avoided or treated by use of potassium supplements such as foods with a high potassium content.
Although any chloride deficit is generally mild and usually does not require specific treatment except under extraordinary circumstances (as in liver disease or renal disease), chloride replacement may be required in the treatment of metabolic alkalosis.
Dilutional hyponatremia may occur in edematous patients in hot weather; appropriate therapy is water restriction, rather than administration of salt, except in rare instances when the hyponatremia is life threatening. In actual salt depletion, appropriate replacement is the therapy of choice.
Hyperuricemia may occur or acute gout may be precipitated in certain patients receiving thiazide therapy.
Insulin requirements in diabetic patients may be increased, decreased, or unchanged. Diabetes mellitus which has been latent may become manifest during thiazide administration.
Thiazide drugs may increase the responsiveness to tubocurarine.
The antihypertensive effects of the drug may be enhanced in the postsympathectomy patient. Thiazides may decrease arterial responsiveness to norepinephrine. This diminution is not sufficient to preclude effectiveness of the pressor agent for therapeutic use.
If progressive renal impairment becomes evident, consider withholding or discontinuing diuretic therapy.
Thiazides may decrease serum PBI levels without signs of thyroid disturbance.
Calcium excretion is decreased by thiazides. Pathologic changes in the parathyroid glands with hypercalcemia and hypophosphatemia have been observed in a few patients on prolonged thiazide therapy. The common complications of hyperparathyroidism such as renal lithiasis, bone resorption, and peptic ulceration have not been seen. Thiazides should be discontinued before carrying out tests for parathyroid function.

Adverse Reactions

A. *Gastrointestinal System*
1. anorexia
2. gastric irritation
3. nausea
4. vomiting
5. cramping
6. diarrhea
7. constipation
8. jaundice (intrahepatic cholestatic jaundice)
9. pancreatitis
10. sialadenitis

B. *Central Nervous System*
1. dizziness
2. vertigo
3. paresthesias
4. headache
5. xanthopsia

C. *Hematologic*
1. leukopenia
2. agranulocytosis
3. thrombocytopenia
4. aplastic anemia
5. hemolytic anemia

D. *Cardiovascular*
Orthostatic hypotension (may be aggravated by alcohol, barbiturates, or narcotics)

E. *Hypersensitivity*
1. purpura
2. photosensitivity
3. rash
4. urticaria
5. necrotizing angiitis (vasculitis) (cutaneous vasculitis)
6. fever
7. respiratory distress including pneumonitis
8. anaphylactic reactions

F. *Other*
1. hyperglycemia
2. glycosuria
3. hyperuricemia
4. muscle spasm
5. weakness
6. restlessness
7. transient blurred vision

Whenever adverse reactions are moderate or severe, thiazide dosage should be reduced or therapy withdrawn.

Dosage and Administration

Therapy should be individualized according to patient response. Use the smallest dosage necessary to achieve the required response.

Adults
For Diuresis
The usual adult dosage is 50 to 100 mg once or twice a day. Many patients with edema respond to intermittent therapy, i.e., administration on alternate days or on three to five days

each week. With an intermittent schedule, excessive response and the resulting undesirable electrolyte imbalance are less likely to occur.

For Control of Hypertension

The usual adult starting dosage is 50 or 100 mg a day as a single or divided dose. Dosage is increased or decreased according to blood pressure response. Rarely some patients may require up to 200 mg a day in divided doses. When thiazides are used with other antihypertensives, the dose of the latter may need to be reduced to prevent excessive decrease in blood pressure.

Infants and Children

The usual pediatric dosage is based on 1.0 mg of HydroDIURIL per pound of body weight per day in two doses. Infants under 6 months of age may require up to 1.5 mg per pound per day in two doses.

On this basis, infants up to 2 years of age may be given 12.5 to 37.5 mg daily in two doses. Children from 2 to 12 years of age may be given 37.5 to 100 mg daily in two doses. Dosage in both age groups should be based on body weight.

How Supplied

No. 3263—Tablets HydroDIURIL, 25 mg, are peach-colored, round, scored, compressed tablets, coded MSD 42. They are supplied as follows:

NDC 0006-0042-68 bottles of 100
NDC 0006-0042-28 single unit packages of 100
NDC 0006-0042-82 bottles of 1000

[*Shown in Product Identification Section*]

No. 3264—Tablets HydroDIURIL, 50 mg, are peach-colored, round, scored, compressed tablets, coded MSD 105. They are supplied as follows:

NDC 0006-0105-68 bottles of 100
NDC 0006-0105-28 single unit packages of 100
NDC 0006-0105-82 bottles of 1000
NDC 0006-0105-86 bottles of 5000

[*Shown in Product Identification Section*]

No. 3340—Tablets HydroDIURIL, 100 mg, are peach-colored, round, scored, compressed tablets, coded MSD 410. They are supplied as follows:

NDC 0006-0410-68 bottles of 100.

[*Shown in Product Identification Section*]

A.H.F.S. 40:28

DC 6028531 Issued June 1979

HYDROPRES® Tablets ℞
Antihypertensive

WARNING

This fixed combination drug is not indicated for initial therapy of hypertension. Hypertension requires therapy titrated to the individual patient. If the fixed combination represents the dosage so determined, its use may be more convenient in patient management. The treatment of hypertension is not static, but must be reevaluated as conditions in each patient warrant.

Description

HYDROPRES combines two antihypertensive agents: HydroDIURIL (Hydrochlorothiazide, MSD) and reserpine. The chemical name for hydrochlorothiazide is 6-chloro-3, 4-dihydro-2*H*-1, 2, 4 - benzothiadiazine - 7 - sulfonamide 1,1-dioxide. Reserpine (11,17α-dimethoxy-18β-[(3,4,5-trimethoxybenzoyl) oxy]-3β,20α-yohimban-16β-carboxylic acid methyl ester) is a crystalline alkaloid derived from Rauwolfia serpentina.

Actions

Hydrochlorothiazide

Hydrochlorothiazide is a diuretic and antihypertensive. It affects the renal tubular mechanism of electrolyte reabsorption. At maximal therapeutic dosage all thiazides are approximately equal in their diuretic efficacy. Hydrochlorothiazide increases excretion of sodium and chloride in approximately equivalent amounts. Natriuresis may be accompanied by some loss of potassium and bicarbonate.

The mechanism of the antihypertensive effect of thiazides is unknown. Hydrochlorothiazide does not affect normal blood pressure.

Hydrochlorothiazide is eliminated rapidly by the kidney.

Reserpine

Reserpine has antihypertensive, bradycardic, and tranquilizing properties. It lowers arterial blood pressure by depletion of catecholamines. Reserpine is beneficial in relieving anxiety, tension, and headache in the hypertensive patient. It acts at the hypothalamic level of the central nervous system to promote relaxation without hypnosis or analgesia. The sleep pattern shown by the electroencephalogram following barbiturates does not occur with this drug. In laboratory animals spontaneous activity and response to external stimuli are decreased, but confusion or difficulty of movement is not evident.

The bradycardic action of reserpine promotes relaxation and may eliminate sinus tachycardia. It is most pronounced in subjects with sinus tachycardia and usually is not prominent in persons with a normal pulse rate.

Miosis, relaxation of the nictitating membrane, ptosis, hypothermia, and increased gastrointestinal activity are noted in animals given reserpine, sometimes in subclinical doses. None of these effects, except increased gastrointestinal activity, has been found to be clinically significant in man with therapeutic doses.

Indication

Hypertension (see box warning).

Contraindications

Hydrochlorothiazide is contraindicated in anuria.

HYDROPRES is contraindicated in hypersensitivity to hydrochlorothiazide or other sulfonamide-derived drugs or to reserpine.

Electroshock therapy should not be given to patients while on reserpine, as severe and even fatal reactions have been reported with minimal convulsive electroshock dosage. After discontinuing reserpine, allow at least seven days before starting electroshock therapy.

Active peptic ulcer, ulcerative colitis, and active mental depression, especially suicidal tendencies, are contraindications to reserpine therapy.

Warnings

Hydrochlorothiazide

Use with caution in severe renal disease. In patients with renal disease, thiazides may precipitate azotemia. Cumulative effects of the drug may develop in patients with impaired renal function.

Thiazides should be used with caution in patients with impaired hepatic function or progressive liver disease, since minor alterations of fluid and electrolyte balance may precipitate hepatic coma.

Thiazides may add to or potentiate the action of other antihypertensive drugs.

Sensitivity reactions may occur in patients with or without a history of allergy or bronchial asthma.

The possibility of exacerbation or activation of systemic lupus erythematosus has been reported.

Lithium generally should not be given with diuretics because they reduce its renal clearance and add a high risk of lithium toxicity. Read circulars for lithium preparations before use of such concomitant therapy.

Reserpine

The occurrence of mental depression due to reserpine in doses of 0.25 mg daily or less is unusual. In any event, HYDROPRES should be discontinued at the first sign of depression.

Use in Pregnancy

Reserpine has been demonstrated to cross the placental barrier in guinea pigs with depression of adrenal catecholamine stores in the newborn. There is some evidence that side effects such as nasal congestion, lethargy, depressed Moro reflex, and bradycardia may appear in infants born of reserpine-treated mothers.

Thiazides cross the placental barrier and appear in cord blood. The use of thiazides in pregnancy requires that the anticipated benefit be weighed against possible hazards to the fetus. These hazards include fetal or neonatal jaundice, thrombocytopenia, and possibly other adverse reactions which have occurred in the adult.

Nursing Mothers

Thiazides and reserpine appear in breast milk. If use of the drug is deemed essential, the patient should stop nursing.

Precautions

Hydrochlorothiazide

Periodic determination of serum electrolytes to detect possible electrolyte imbalance should be performed at appropriate intervals.

All patients receiving diuretic therapy should be observed for evidence of fluid or electrolyte imbalance: namely, hyponatremia, hypochloremic alkalosis, and hypokalemia. Serum and urine electrolyte determinations are particularly important when the patient is vomiting excessively or receiving parenteral fluids. Warning signs or symptoms of fluid and electrolyte imbalance include dryness of mouth, thirst, weakness, lethargy, drowsiness, restlessness, muscle pains or cramps, muscular fatigue, hypotension, oliguria, tachycardia, and gastrointestinal disturbances such as nausea and vomiting.

Hypokalemia may develop, especially with brisk diuresis, when severe cirrhosis is present, during concomitant use of corticosteroids or ACTH, or after prolonged therapy.

Interference with adequate oral electrolyte intake will contribute to hypokalemia. Hypokalemia can sensitize or exaggerate the response of the heart to the toxic effects of digitalis (e.g., increased ventricular irritability). Hypokalemia may be avoided or treated by use of potassium supplements such as foods with a high potassium content.

Although any chloride deficit is generally mild and usually does not require specific treatment except under extraordinary circumstances (as in liver disease or renal disease), chloride replacement may be required in the treatment of metabolic alkalosis.

Dilutional hyponatremia may occur in edematous patients in hot weather. Appropriate therapy is water restriction, rather than administration of salt, except in rare instances when the hyponatremia is life threatening. In actual salt depletion, appropriate replacement is the therapy of choice.

Continued on next page

Information on the Merck Sharp & Dohme products listed on these pages is the full prescribing information from package circulars in use October 31, 1979.

Merck Sharp & Dohme—Cont.

Hyperuricemia may occur or acute gout may be precipitated in certain patients receiving thiazide therapy.
Insulin requirements in diabetic patients may be increased, decreased, or unchanged. Diabetes mellitus which has been latent may become manifest during thiazide administration.
Thiazide drugs may increase the responsiveness to tubocurarine.
The antihypertensive effect of the drug may be enhanced in the postsympathectomy patient.
Thiazides may decrease arterial responsiveness to norepinephrine. This diminution is not sufficient to preclude effectiveness of the pressor agent for therapeutic use.
If progressive renal impairment becomes evident, consider withholding or discontinuing diuretic therapy.
Thiazides may decrease serum PBI levels without signs of thyroid disturbance.
Calcium excretion is decreased by thiazides. Pathological changes in the parathyroid glands with hypercalcemia and hypophosphatemia have been observed in a few patients on prolonged thiazide therapy. The common complications of hyperparathyroidism such as renal lithiasis, bone resorption, and peptic ulceration have not been seen. Thiazides should be discontinued before carrying out tests for parathyroid function.
Reserpine
Since reserpine may increase gastric secretion and motility, it should be used cautiously in patients with a history of peptic ulcer, ulcerative colitis, or other gastrointestinal disorder. This compound may precipitate biliary colic in patients with gallstones, or bronchial asthma in susceptible persons.
Reserpine may cause hypotension including orthostatic hypotension.
In hypertensive patients on reserpine therapy significant hypotension and bradycardia may develop during surgical anesthesia. The anesthesiologist should be aware that reserpine has been taken, since it may be necessary to give vagal blocking agents parenterally to prevent or reverse hypotension and/or bradycardia.
Anxiety or depression, as well as psychosis, may develop during reserpine therapy. If depression is present when therapy is begun, it may be aggravated. Mental depression is unusual with reserpine doses of 0.25 mg daily or less. In any case, HYDROPRES should be discontinued at the first sign of depression. Extreme caution should be used in treating patients with a history of mental depression, and the possibility of suicide should be kept in mind.
As with most antihypertensive therapy, caution should be exercised when treating hypertensive patients with renal insufficiency, since they adjust poorly to lowered blood pressure levels. Use reserpine cautiously with digitalis and quinidine; cardiac arrhythmias have occurred with reserpine preparations.
When two or more antihypertensives are given, the individual dosages may have to be reduced to prevent excessive drop in blood pressure. In hypertensive patients with coronary artery disease, it is important to avoid a precipitous drop in blood pressure.

Adverse Reactions

Hydrochlorothiazide
Gastrointestinal: Anorexia, gastric irritation, nausea, vomiting, cramping, diarrhea, constipation, jaundice (intrahepatic cholestatic jaundice), pancreatitis, sialadenitis.
Central nervous system: Dizziness, vertigo, paresthesias, headache, xanthopsia.
Hematologic: Leukopenia, agranulocytosis, thrombocytopenia, aplastic anemia, hemolytic anemia.
Cardiovascular: Orthostatic hypotension (may be aggravated by alcohol, barbiturates, or narcotics).
Allergic: Purpura, photosensitivity, rash, urticaria, necrotizing angiitis (vasculitis) (cutaneous vasculitis), fever, respiratory distress including pneumonitis, anaphylactic reactions.
Other: Hyperglycemia, glycosuria, hyperuricemia, muscle spasm, weakness, restlessness, transient blurred vision.
Whenever adverse reactions are moderate or severe, the thiazide dosage should be reduced or therapy withdrawn.
Reserpine
Central nervous system: Excessive sedation, mental depression, nightmares, headache, dizziness, syncope, nervousness, paradoxical anxiety, central nervous system sensitization (dull sensorium, deafness, glaucoma, uveitis, optic atrophy), parkinsonism (usually reversible with decreased dosage or discontinuance of therapy).
Respiratory: Nasal congestion, dyspnea, epistaxis.
Cardiovascular: Bradycardia, angina pectoris, arrhythmia, premature ventricular contractions, and other direct cardiac effects (e.g., fluid retention, congestive failure).
Gastrointestinal: Hypersecretion and increased motility, nausea, vomiting, anorexia, diarrhea, dryness of mouth, increased salivation.
Hematologic: Excessive bleeding following prostatic surgery, thrombocytopenic purpura.
Allergic: Flushing of skin, pruritus, rash.
Other: Conjunctival injection, enhanced susceptibility to colds, muscular aches, weight gain, blurred vision, dysuria, nonpuerperal lactation, impotence, decreased libido.

Dosage and Administration

The initial dosage of HYDROPRES should conform to the dosages of the individual components established during titration (see box warning).
The usual adult dosage of HYDROPRES-25 is 1 or 2 tablets once or twice a day; that of HYDROPRES-50 is 1 tablet once or twice a day. Dosage may require adjustment according to the blood pressure response of the patient.
Careful observations for changes in blood pressure must be made when HYDROPRES is used with other antihypertensive drugs.

How Supplied

No. 3265—Tablets HYDROPRES-25 are green, round, scored, compressed tablets, coded MSD 53. Each tablet contains 25 mg of hydrochlorothiazide and 0.125 mg of reserpine. They are supplied as follows:
NDC 0006-0053-68 in bottles of 100.
NDC 0006-0053-82 in bottles of 1000.
[*Shown in Product Identification Section*]
No. 3266—Tablets HYDROPRES-50 are green, round, scored, compressed tablets, coded MSD 127. Each tablet contains 50 mg of hydrochlorothiazide and 0.125 mg of reserpine. They are supplied as follows:
NDC 0006-0127-68 in bottles of 100.
NDC 0006-0127-82 in bottles of 1000.
[*Shown in Product Identification Section*]
A.H.F.S. 24:08
DC 6053226 Issued June 1979

INDOCIN® Capsules ℞
(indomethacin, MSD), N.F.

Description

INDOCIN (Indomethacin, MSD) cannot be considered a simple analgesic and should not be used in conditions other than those recommended under INDICATIONS.
Capsules INDOCIN for oral administration are provided in two dosage strengths which contain either 25 mg or 50 mg of indomethacin. Indomethacin is a non-steroidal anti-inflammatory indole derivative designated chemically as 1-(p-chlorobenzoyl)-5-methoxy-2-methylindole-3-acetic acid.

Clinical Pharmacology

INDOCIN is a non-steroidal drug with anti-inflammatory, antipyretic and analgesic properties. Its mode of action, like that of other anti-inflammatory drugs, is not known. However, its therapeutic action is not due to pituitary-adrenal stimulation.
INDOCIN is a potent inhibitor of prostaglandin synthesis *in vitro*. Concentrations are reached during therapy which have been demonstrated to have an effect *in vivo* as well. Inhibition of prostaglandin synthesis may be involved in the anti-flammatory action of INDOCIN.
INDOCIN has been shown to be an effective anti-inflammatory agent, appropriate for long-term use in rheumatoid arthritis, ankylosing spondylitis, and osteoarthritis.
INDOCIN affords relief of symptoms; it does not alter the progressive course of the underlying disease.
INDOCIN suppresses inflammation in rheumatoid arthritis as demonstrated by relief of pain, and reduction of fever, swelling and tenderness. Improvement in patients treated with INDOCIN for rheumatoid arthritis has been demonstrated by a reduction in joint swelling, average number of joints involved, and morning stiffness; by increased mobility as demonstrated by a decrease in walking time; and by improved functional capability as demonstrated by an increase in grip strength.
INDOCIN has been found effective in relieving the pain, reducing the fever, swelling, redness, and tenderness of acute gouty arthritis.
Indomethacin is readily absorbed, attaining peak plasma concentrations of about 1 and 2 mcg/ml following single oral doses of 25 and 50 mg, respectively. Orally administered indomethacin is virtually 100% bioavailable. Indomethacin is eliminated via renal excretion, metabolism, and biliary excretion. Indomethacin undergoes appreciable enterohepatic circulation. The mean half-life of indomethacin is estimated to be about 4.5 hours. With a typical therapeutic regimen of 25 or 50 mg t.i.d., the steady-state plasma concentrations of indomethacin are an average 1.4 times those following the first dose.
Indomethacin exists in the plasma as the parent drug and its desmethyl, desbenzoyl, and desmethyl-desbenzoyl metabolites, all in the unconjugated form. About 60 percent of an oral dosage is recovered in urine as drug and metabolites (26 percent as indomethacin and its glucuronide), and 33 percent is recovered in feces (1.5 percent as indomethacin).
About 90% of indomethacin is bound to protein in plasma over the expected range of therapeutic plasma concentrations.

Indications

Because of its potential to cause adverse reactions, particularly at high dose levels, the use of INDOCIN in rheumatoid arthritis and osteoarthritis in adults should be carefully considered for active disease unresponsive to adequate trial with salicylates and other measures of established value, such as appropriate rest.
In accord with this important concept INDOCIN has been found effective in active stages of the following:
1. Moderate to severe rheumatoid arthritis including acute flares of chronic disease.
2. Moderate to severe ankylosing spondylitis.
3. Moderate to severe osteoarthritis of large joints (hips, knees and shoulders).
4. Acute gouty arthritis.

INDOCIN may enable the reduction of steroid dosage in patients receiving steroids for the more severe forms of rheumatoid arthritis. In such instances the steroid dosage should be reduced slowly and the patients followed very closely for any possible adverse effects.

The use of INDOCIN in conjunction with aspirin or other salicylates is not recommended. Controlled clinical studies have shown that the combined use of INDOCIN and aspirin does not produce any greater therapeutic effect than the use of INDOCIN alone. Furthermore, in one of these clinical studies, the incidence of gastrointestinal side effects was significantly increased with combined therapy. (See DRUG INTERACTIONS)

Contraindications

INDOCIN is contraindicated in patients who are allergic to INDOCIN or who have nasal polyps associated with angioedema or a bronchospastic reaction to aspirin or other non-steroidal anti-inflammatory drugs.

Warnings

General:

Because of the variability of the potential of INDOCIN to cause adverse reactions in the individual patient, the following are strongly recommended:

1. The lowest possible effective dose for the individual patient should be prescribed. Increased dosage tends to increase adverse effects, particularly in doses over 150–200 mg/day, without corresponding increase in clinical benefits.
2. Careful instructions to, and observations of, the individual patient are essential to the prevention of serious adverse reactions. As advancing years appear to increase the possibility of adverse reactions, INDOCIN should be used with greater care in the aged.
3. Safe conditions for use in children have not been established; therefore, INDOCIN should not be prescribed for children 14 years of age and under except under circumstances where lack of efficacy or toxicity associated with other drugs warrants the risk. Such patients should be monitored closely.

Gastrointestinal Effects:

Single or multiple ulcerations, including perforation and hemorrhage of the esophagus, stomach, duodenum or small intestine, have been reported to occur with INDOCIN. Fatalities have been reported in some instances. Rarely, intestinal ulceration has been associated with stenosis and obstruction.

Gastrointestinal bleeding without obvious ulcer formation and perforation of pre-existing sigmoid lesions (diverticulum, carcinoma, etc.) have occurred. Increased abdominal pain in ulcerative colitis patients or the development of ulcerative colitis and regional ileitis have been reported to occur rarely.

Because of the occurrence, and at times severity, of gastrointestinal reactions to INDOCIN, the prescribing physician must be continuously alert for any sign or symptom signaling a possible gastrointestinal reaction. The risks of continuing therapy with INDOCIN in the face of such symptoms must be weighed against the possible benefits to the individual patient.

INDOCIN should not be given to patients with active gastrointestinal lesions or with a history of recurrent gastrointestinal lesions except under circumstances which warrant the very high risk and where patients can be monitored very closely.

The gastrointestinal effects may be reduced by giving the drug immediately after meals, with food, or with antacids.

Ocular Effects:

Corneal deposits and retinal disturbances, including those of the macula, have been observed in some patients who had received prolonged therapy with INDOCIN. The prescribing physician should be alert to the possible association between the changes noted and INDOCIN. It is advisable to discontinue therapy if such changes are observed. Blurred vision may be a significant symptom and warrants a thorough ophthalmological examination. Since these changes may be asymptomatic, ophthalmologic examination at periodic intervals is desirable in patients where therapy is prolonged.

Central Nervous System Effects:

INDOCIN may aggravate psychiatric disturbances, epilepsy, and parkinsonism, and should be used with considerable caution in patients with these conditions. If severe CNS adverse reactions develop, INDOCIN should be discontinued.

INDOCIN may cause drowsiness; therefore, patients should be cautioned about engaging in activities requiring mental alertness and motor coordination, such as driving a car. INDOCIN may also cause headache. Headache which persists despite dosage reduction requires cessation of therapy with INDOCIN.

Use in Pregnancy

The safe use of INDOCIN in pregnant women has not been etablished. Administration of INDOCIN is not recommended during pregnancy.

Teratogenic studies were conducted in mice and rats at dosages of 0.5, 1.0, 2.0 and 4.0 mg/kg/day. The 4.0 mg/kg/day dosage was toxic in both species as evidenced by gastrointestinal ulceration and decreased average maternal weight gain. However, no increase in visceral or skeletal malformations was noted in any treatment group as compared with control groups. Decreased average fetal weights were noted in the offspring of mice receiving 4.0 mg/kg/day. In this dosage group, an increase in skeletal variations resulting from retarded ossification was considered secondary to the decreased average fetal weights.

Indomethacin has been found to delay parturition in rats. This effect has been described with other non-steroidal anti-inflammatory agents which inhibit prostaglandin synthesis.

In rats, 4.0 mg/kg/day given during the last three days of gestation caused some maternal and fetal deaths. An increased incidence of neuronal necrosis in the diencephalon in the live-born fetuses was observed. At 2.0 mg/kg/day, no increase in neuronal necrosis was observed as compared to the control groups.

Use in Nursing Mothers

INDOCIN is excreted in the milk of lactating mothers. INDOCIN is not recommended for use in nursing mothers.

Precautions

INDOCIN may mask the usual signs and symptoms of infection. Therefore, the physician must be continually on the alert for this and should use the drug with extra care in the presence of existing controlled infection.

INDOCIN, like other non-steroidal anti-inflammatory agents, can inhibit platelet aggregation. This effect is of shorter duration than that seen with aspirin and usually disappears within 24 hours after discontinuation of INDOCIN. INDOCIN has been shown to prolong bleeding time (but within the normal range) in normal subjects. Because this effect may be exaggerated in patients with underlying hemostatic defects, INDOCIN should be used with caution in persons with coagulation defects.

Drug Interactions

In a study in normal volunteers, it was found that chronic concurrent administration of 3.6 gm of aspirin per day decreases indomethacin blood levels approximately 20%.

Clinical studies have shown that INDOCIN does not influence the hypoprothrombinemia produced by anticoagulants. However, when any additional drug, including INDOCIN, is added to the treatment of patients on anticoagulant therapy, the patients should be observed for alterations of the prothrombin time.

When INDOCIN is given to patients receiving probenecid, the plasma levels of indomethacin are likely to be increased. Therefore, a lower total daily dosage of INDOCIN may produce a satisfactory therapeutic effect. When increases in the dose of INDOCIN are made, they should be made carefully and in small increments.

Clinical studies have shown that the administraton of INDOCIN can reduce the natriuretic and anti-hypertensive effect of furosemide in some patients. This response has been attributed to inhibition of prostaglandin synthesis by INDOCIN. Therefore, when INDOCIN is added to the treatment of a patient receiving furosemide, or furosemide is added to the treatment of a patient receiving INDOCIN, the patient should be observed closely to determine if the desired effect of furosemide is obtained.

INDOCIN blocks the furosemide-induced increase in plasma renin activity. This fact should be kept in mind when evaluating plasma renin activity in hypertensive patients.

Adverse Reactions

The adverse reactions listed in the following table have been arranged into two groups: (1) incidence greater than 1%; and (2) incidence less than 1%. The incidence for group (1) was obtained from 33 double-blind controlled clinical trials reported in the literature (1,092 patients). The incidence for group (2) was based on reports in clinical trials, in the literature, and on voluntary reports since marketing. The probability of a causal relationship exists between INDOCIN and these adverse reactions, some of which have been reported only rarely. [See table on next page].

Causal relationship unknown: Other reactions have been reported but occurred under circumstances where a causal relationship could not be established. However, in these rarely reported events, the possibility cannot be excluded. Therefore, these observations are being listed to serve as alerting information to physicians:

Hematologic: Although there have been several reports of leukemia, the supporting information is weak.

Genitourinary Reactions: Urinary frequency.

Miscellaneous: Breast changes including enlargement and tenderness.

Dosage and Administration

Adverse reactions appear to correlate with the size of the dose of INDOCIN in most patients but not all. Therefore, every effort should be made to determine the smallest effective dosage for the individual patient.

Always give the drug with food, immediately after meals, or with antacids to reduce gastric irritation.

INDOCIN should not ordinarily be prescribed for children 14 years of age and under because safe conditions for use have not been established. (See Warnings.)

Dosage Recommendations for Active Stages of the Following:

1. Moderate to severe rheumatoid arthritis including acute flares of chronic disease; moderate to severe ankylosing spondylitis, and moderate to severe osteoarthritis of large joints (hips, knees and shoulders).

   Suggested Dosage:

   25 mg b.i.d. or t.i.d. If this is well tolerated, increase the daily dosage by 25 or by 50 mg, if required by continuing symptoms, at weekly intervals until a satisfactory response is obtained or until a total daily dose of 150–200 mg is reached. DOSES ABOVE THIS AMOUNT GENERALLY DO NOT INCREASE THE EFFECTIVENESS OF THE DRUG.

In patients who have persistent night pain and/or morning stiffness, the giving of a large portion, up to a maximum of 100 mg, of the

Continued on next page

Information on the Merck Sharp & Dohme products listed on these pages is the full prescribing information from package circulars in use October 31, 1979.

Merck Sharp & Dohme—Cont.

total daily dose at bedtime may be helpful in affording relief. The total daily dose should not exceed 200 mg. In acute flares of chronic rheumatoid arthritis, it may be necessary to increase the dosage by 25 mg or, if required, by 50 mg daily. If minor adverse effects develop as the dosage is increased, reduce the dosage rapidly to a tolerated dose and OBSERVE THE PATIENT CLOSELY.

If severe adverse reactions occur, STOP THE DRUG. After the acute phase of the disease is under control, an attempt to reduce the daily dose should be made repeatedly until the patient is receiving the smallest effective dose or the drug is discontinued.

Careful instruction to, and observations of, the individual patient are essential to the prevention of serious, irreversible, including fatal, adverse reactions.

As advancing years appear to increase the possiblity of adverse reactions, INDOCIN should be used with greater care in the aged.

2. Acute gouty arthritis.

Suggested Dosage:

50 mg t.i.d. until pain is tolerable. The dose should then be rapidly reduced to complete cessation of the drug. Definite relief of pain has been reported within 2 to 4 hours. Tenderness and heat usually subside in 24 to 36 hours, and swelling gradually disappears in 3 to 5 days.

How Supplied

No. 3316—Capsules INDOCIN, 25 mg are opaque blue and white capsules, coded MSD 25. They are supplied as follows:

NDC 0006-0025-68 bottles of 100 (6505-00-926-2154, 25 mg 100's)

NDC 0006-0025-28 single unit packages of 100 (6505-00-118-2776, 25 mg individually sealed 100's)

NDC 0006-0025-82 bottles of 1000 (6505-00-931-0680, 25 mg 1000's)

[*Shown in Product Identification Section*]

No. 3317—Capsules INDOCIN, 50 mg are opaque blue and white capsules, coded MSD 50. They are supplied as follows:

NDC 0006-0050-68 bottles of 100

NDC 0006-0050-28 single unit packages of 100.

[*Shown in Product Identification Section*]

A.H.F.S. 28:08

DC 6473215 Issued February 1978

M-M-R®$_{II}$ ℞

(measles, mumps and rubella virus vaccine, live, MSD), U.S.P.

Description

M-M-R$_{II}$ (Measles, Mumps and Rubella Virus Vaccine, Live, MSD) is a live virus vaccine for immunization against measles (rubeola), mumps and rubella (German measles).

M-M-R$_{II}$ is a lyophilized preparation of (1) ATTENUVAX® (Measles Virus Vaccine, Live, Attenuated, MSD), a more attenuated line of measles virus, derived from Enders' attenuated Edmonston strain and grown in cell cultures of chick embryo; (2) MUMPSVAX® (Mumps Virus Vaccine, Live, MSD), the Jeryl Lynn (B level) mumps strain grown in cell cultures of chick embryo; and (3) MERUVAX®$_{II}$ (Rubella Virus Vaccine, Live, MSD), the Wistar RA 27/3 strain of live attenuated rubella virus grown in human diploid cell (WI-38) culture. The three viruses are mixed before being lyophilized. The product contains no preservative.

When reconstituted as directed, the dose for injection is 0.5 ml and contains not less than 1,000 $TCID_{50}$ (tissue culture infectious doses) of Measles Virus Vaccine, Live, Attenuated; 5,000 $TCID_{50}$ of Mumps Virus Vaccine, Live; and 1,000 $TCID_{50}$ of Rubella Virus Vaccine, Live, expressed in terms of the assigned titer of the FDA Reference Measles, Mumps and Rubella Viruses. Each dose contains approximately 25 mcg of neomycin.

Actions

Clinical studies of 279 triple seronegative children, 11 months to 7 years of age, demonstrated that M-M-R$_{II}$ is highly immunogenic and generally well tolerated. In these studies, a single injection of the vaccine induced measles

Incidence greater than 1%	Incidence less than 1%	
GASTROINTESTINAL		
nausea* with or without vomiting dyspepsia* (including indigestion, heartburn and epigastric pain) diarrhea abdominal distress or pain constipation	anorexia bloating (includes distention) flatulence peptic ulcer gastro-enteritis rectal bleeding proctitis perforation and hemorrhage of the esophagus, stomach, duodenum or small intestines intestinal ulceration associated with stenosis and obstruction	gastrointestinal bleeding without obvious ulcer formation and perforation of pre-existing sigmoid lesions (diverticulum, carcinoma, etc.) development of ulcerative colitis and regional ileitis ulcerative stomatitis toxichepatitis and jaundice (some fatal cases have been reported)
CENTRAL NERVOUS SYSTEM		
headache** dizziness* vertigo somnolence depression and fatigue (including malaise and listlessness)	anxiety (includes nervousness) muscle weakness involuntary muscle movements insomnia muzziness psychic disturbances including psychotic episodes mental confusion drowsiness	light-headedness syncope paresthesia aggravation of epilepsy and parkinsonism depersonalization coma peripheral neuropathy convulsions
SPECIAL SENSES		
tinnitus	ocular-corneal deposits and retinal disturbances, including those of the macula, have been reported in some patients on prolonged therapy with INDOCIN	blurred vision hearing disturbances, deafness
CARDIOVASCULAR		
none	hypertension tachycardia chest pain	arrhythmia, palpitations BUN elevation
METABOLIC		
none	edema weight gain flushing or sweating	hyperglycemia glycosuria
INTEGUMENTARY		
none	pruritus rash, urticaria petechiae or ecchymosis	exfoliative dermatitis erythema nodosum loss of hair
HEMATOLOGIC		
none	leukopenia bone marrow depression anemia secondary to obvious or occult gastrointestinal bleeding	aplastic anemia hemolytic anemia agranulocytosis thrombocytopenic purpura
HYPERSENSITIVITY		
none	acute respiratory distress rapid fall in blood pressure resembling a shock-like state angioedema	dyspnea asthma purpura angiitis
GENITOURINARY		
none	hematuria vaginal bleeding	
MISCELLANEOUS		
none	epistaxis	

* Reactions occurring in 3% to 9% of patients treated with INDOCIN. (Those reactions occurring in less than 3% of the patients are unmarked.)

** Reactions occurring in over 10% of patients treated with INDOCIN.

hemagglutination-inhibition (HI) antibodies in 95 percent, mumps neutralizing antibodies in 96 percent, and rubella HI antibodies in 99 percent of susceptible persons.
The RA 27/3 rubella strain in M-M-R_{II} elicits higher immediate postvaccination HI, complement-fixing and neutralizing antibody levels than other strains of rubella vaccine and has been shown to induce a broader profile of circulating antibodies including anti-theta and anti-iota precipitating antibodies. The RA 27/3 rubella strain simulates natural infection more closely than other rubella vaccine viruses. The broader profile of antibodies produced by RA 27/3 strain rubella virus vaccine appears to correlate with greater resistance to subclinical reinfection with the wild virus.
Data relating to persistence of vaccine-induced antibodies are not available for M-M-R_{II} at this time; however, it is expected that the antibodies against measles, mumps and rubella will be just as durable following administration of M-M-R_{II} as after the single vaccines given separately. Antibody levels after immunization with ATTENUVAX (Measles Virus Vaccine, Live, Attenuated, MSD) have persisted for at least eight years without substantial decline; for ten years after MUMPSVAX (Mumps Virus Vaccine, Live, MSD); and for at least six years after administration of RA 27/3 strain rubella virus vaccine.

Indications

M-M-R_{II} is indicated for simultaneous immunization against measles, mumps, and rubella in children from 15 months of age to puberty.
Infants who are less than 15 months of age may fail to respond to one or all three components of the vaccine due to presence in the circulation of residual measles and/or mumps and/or rubella antibody of maternal origin; the younger the infant, the lower the likelihood of seroconversion. In geographically isolated or other relatively inaccessible populations for whom immunization programs are logistically difficult, and in population groups in which natural measles infection may occur in a significant proportion of infants before 15 months of age, it may be desirable to give the vaccine to infants at an earlier age. The advantage of early protection must be weighed against the chance for failure of response; infants vaccinated under these conditions should be revaccinated after reaching 15 months of age.
Revaccination: Based on available evidence, there is no reason to routinely revaccinate children originally vaccinated when 12 months of age or older; however, children vaccinated when younger than 12 months of age should be revaccinated. The decision to revaccinate should be based on evaluation of each individual case.

Contraindications

Do not give M-M-R_{II} to pregnant females; the possible effects of the vaccine on fetal development are unknown at this time. When vaccination of post-pubertal females is undertaken, pregnancy must be avoided for three months following vaccination.
Previously unimmunized children of susceptible pregnant women should receive live attenuated rubella vaccine, because an immunized child will be less likely to acquire natural rubella and introduce the virus into the household.
Hypersensitivity to neomycin (each dose of reconstituted vaccine contains approximately 25 mcg of neomycin).
Any febrile respiratory illness or other active febrile infection.
Active untreated tuberculosis.
Patients receiving therapy with ACTH, corticosteroids, irradiation, alkylating agents or antimetabolites. This contraindication does not apply to patients who are receiving corticosteroids as replacement therapy, e.g., for Addison's disease.
Individuals with blood dyscrasias, leukemia, lymphomas of any type, or other malignant neoplasms affecting the bone marrow or lymphatic systems.
Primary immuno-deficiency states, including cellular immune deficiencies, hypogammaglobulinemic and dysgammaglobulinemic states.

Hypersensitivity to Eggs, Chicken, or Chicken Feathers

This vaccine is essentially devoid of potentially allergenic substances derived from host tissues (chick embryos).* However, since the measles and mumps components are propagated in cell cultures of chick embryo, in considering vaccine use in patients hypersensitive to chicken or chicken eggs or feathers, the attending physician must weigh the benefits of immunization against the potential risks of hypersensitivity reactions.

Precautions

Administer M-M-R_{II} subcutaneously; *do not give intravenously.*
Epinephrine should be available for immediate use in case an anaphylactoid reaction occurs.
M-M-R_{II} should not be given less than one month before or after immunization with other *live* virus vaccines. There are no data available concerning simultaneous use of M-M-R_{II} with monovalent or trivalent poliovirus vaccine, live, oral.
Due caution should be employed in administration of M-M-R_{II} to children with a history of febrile convulsions, cerebral injury or any other condition in which stress due to fever should be avoided. The physician should be alert to the temperature elevation which may occur 5 to 12 days following vaccination.
Vaccination should be deferred for at least 3 months following blood or plasma transfusions, or administration of more than 0.02 ml of human immune serum globulin per pound of body weight.
Excretion of small amounts of the live attenuated rubella virus from the nose or throat has occurred in the majority of susceptible individuals 7–28 days after vaccination. There is no confirmed evidence to indicate that such virus is transmitted to susceptible persons who are in contact with the vaccinated individuals. Consequently, transmission, while accepted as a theoretical possibility, is not regarded as a significant risk.**
There are no reports of transmission of live attenuated measles or mumps viruses from vaccinees to susceptible contacts.
It has been reported that live attenuated measles, mumps and rubella virus vaccines given individually may result in a temporary depression of tuberculin skin sensitivity. Therefore, if a tuberculin test is to be done, it should be administered either before or simultaneously with M-M-R_{II}.
As for any vaccine, vaccination with M-M-R_{II} may not result in seroconversion in 100% of susceptible subjects given the vaccine.

Adverse Reactions

The adverse clinical reactions associated with the use of M-M-R_{II} are those expected to follow administration of the monovalent vaccines given separately. These may include malaise, sore throat, headache, fever, and rash; mild local reactions such as erythema, induration, tenderness and regional lymphadenopathy; parotitis; orchitis; thrombocytopenia and purpura; allergic reactions such as urticaria; and arthritis, arthralgia and polyneuritis.
Moderate fever [101–102.9°F (38.3–39.4°C)] occurs occasionally, and high fever [above 103°F (39.4°C)] occurs less commonly. On rare occasions, children developing fever may exhibit febrile convulsions. Rash occurs infrequently and is usually minimal without generalized distribution.
Clinical experience with live attenuated measles, mumps and rubella virus vaccines given individually indicates that encephalitis and other nervous system reactions have occurred very rarely. These might occur also with M-M-R_{II}.
Experience from more than 80 million doses of all live measles vaccines given in the U.S. through 1975 indicates that significant central nervous system reactions such as encephalitis and encephalopathy, occurring within 30 days after vaccination, have been temporally associated with measles vaccine approximately once for every million doses. In no case has it been shown that reactions were actually caused by vaccine. The Center for Disease Control has pointed out that "a certain number of cases of encephalitis may be expected to occur in a large childhood population in a defined period of time even when no vaccines are administered". However, the data suggest the possibility that some of these cases may have been caused by measles vaccines. The risk of such serious neurological disorders following live measles virus vaccine administration remains far less than that for encephalitis and encephalopathy with natural measles (one per thousand reported cases).
There have been reports of subacute sclerosing panencephalitis (SSPE) in children who did not have a history of natural measles but did receive measles vaccine. Some of these cases may have resulted from unrecognized measles in the first year of life or possibly from the measles vaccination. Based on estimated nationwide measles vaccine distribution, the association of SSPE cases to measles vaccination is about one case per million vaccine doses distributed. This is far less than the association with natural measles, 5–10 cases of SSPE per million cases of measles. The results of a retrospective case-controlled study conducted by the Center for Disease Control suggest that the overall effect of measles vaccine has been to protect against SSPE by preventing measles with its inherent higher risk of SSPE.
Local reactions characterized by marked swelling, redness and vesiculation at the injection site of attenuated live measles virus vaccines have occurred in children who received killed measles vaccine previously. M-M-R_{II} was not given under this condition in clinical trials.
Transient arthritis, arthralgia and polyneuritis are features of natural rubella and vary in frequency and severity with age and sex, being greatest in adult females and least in prepubertal children. This type of involvement has also been reported following administration of MERUVAX$_{II}$ (Rubella Virus Vaccine, Live, MSD). In children, joint reactions are rare and of brief duration if they do occur. In women, incidence rates for arthritis and arthralgia are generally higher than those seen in children (children: 0–3%; women: 12–20%), and the reactions tend to be more marked and of longer duration. Rarely, symptoms may persist for a matter of months. In adolescent girls, the reactions appear to be intermediate in incidence between those seen in children and in adult women. Even in older women (35–45 years), these reactions are generally well tolerated and rarely interfere with normal activities.

Continued on next page

Information on the Merck Sharp & Dohme products listed on these pages is the full prescribing information from package circulars in use October 31, 1979.

Merck Sharp & Dohme—Cont.

Dosage and Administration

After suitably cleansing the immunization site, inject the total volume of reconstituted vaccine subcutaneously, preferably into the outer aspect of the upper arm. Do not inject M-M-R_{II} intravenously.

Shipment, Storage, and Reconstitution

During shipment, to insure that there is no loss of potency, the vaccine must be maintained at a temperature of 10°C (50°F) or less.
Before reconstitution, store M-M-R_{II} at 2–8°C (35.6–46.4°F). *Protect from light.*
To reconstitute, use only the diluent supplied, since it is free of preservatives or other antiviral substances which might inactivate the vaccine. Inject all the diluent in the syringe into the vial of lyophilized vaccine, and agitate to mix thoroughly. Withdraw the entire contents into the syringe and inject the total volume of restored vaccine subcutaneously.
It is important to use a separate sterile syringe and needle for each individual patient to prevent transmission of hepatitis B and other infectious agents from one person to another.
The color of the vaccine when reconstituted is yellow.
It is recommended that the vaccine be used as soon as possible after reconstitution. Protect vaccine from light at all times. Store reconstituted vaccine in a dark place at 2–8°C (35.6–46.4°F) and discard if not used within 8 hours.

How Supplied

No. 4680—M-M-R_{II} is supplied as a single-dose vial of lyophilized vaccine with a disposable syringe containing diluent, and fitted with a 25 gauge, 5/8" needle, **NDC** 0006-4680-00.
No. 4681/4590—M-M-R_{II} is supplied as follows: (1) a box of ten single-dose vials of lyophilized vaccine, **NDC** 0006-4681-00; and (2) a box of ten diluent-containing disposable syringes with affixed 25 gauge, 5/8" needles. To conserve refrigerator space, the syringes may be stored separately at room temperature.

* Morbidity and Mortality Weekly Report *25*(44): 350, Nov. 12, 1976.
** Recommendation of the Public Health Service Advisory Committee on Immunization Practices, Morbidity and Mortality Weekly Report, *26*(47): 385, 386, 391, Nov. 25, 1977.

A.H.F.S. 80:12
DC 7034400 Issued October 1978

M-R-VAX®$_{II}$ ℞
(measles and rubella virus vaccine, live, MSD), U.S.P.

Description

M-R-VAX$_{II}$ (Measles and Rubella Virus Vaccine, Live, MSD) is a live virus vaccine for immunization against measles (rubeola) and rubella (German measles).
M-R-VAX$_{II}$ is a lyophilized preparation of (1) ATTENUVAX® (Measles Virus Vaccine, Live, Attenuated, MSD), a more attenuated line of measles virus, derived from Enders' attenuated Edmonston strain and grown in cell cultures of chick embryo; and (2) MERUVAX®$_{II}$ (Rubella Virus Vaccine, Live, MSD), the Wistar RA 27/3 strain of live attenuated rubella virus grown in human diploid cell (WI-38) culture. The two viruses are mixed before being lyophilized. The product contains no preservative.
When reconstituted as directed, the dose for injection is 0.5 ml and contains not less than 1,000 $TCID_{50}$ (tissue culture infectious doses) of Measles Virus Vaccine, Live, Attenuated; and 1,000 $TCID_{50}$ of Rubella Virus Vaccine, Live, expressed in terms of the assigned titer of the FDA Reference Measles and Rubella Viruses. Each dose contains approximately 25 mcg of neomycin.

Actions

Clinical studies of 237 double seronegative children, 10 months to 10 years of age, demonstrated that M-R-VAX$_{II}$ is highly immunogenic and generally well tolerated. In these studies, a single injection of the vaccine induced measles hemagglutination-inhibition (HI) antibodies in 95 percent and rubella HI antibodies in 99 percent of susceptible persons.
The RA 27/3 rubella strain in M-R-VAX$_{II}$ elicits higher immediate post-vaccination HI, complement-fixing and neutralizing antibody levels than other strains of rubella vaccine and has been shown to induce a broader profile of circulating antibodies including anti-theta and anti-iota precipitating antibodies. The RA 27/3 rubella strain simulates natural infection more closely than other rubella vaccine viruses. The broader profile of antibodies produced by RA 27/3 strain rubella virus vaccine appears to correlate with greater resistance to subclinical reinfection with the wild virus.
Data relating to persistence of vaccine-induced antibodies are not available for M-R-VAX$_{II}$ at this time; however, it is expected that the antibodies against measles and rubella will be just as durable following administration of M-R-VAX$_{II}$ as after the single vaccines given separately. Antibody levels after immunization with ATTENUVAX (Measles Virus Vaccine, Live, Attenuated, MSD) have persisted for at least eight years without substantial decline; and for at least six years after administration of RA 27/3 strain rubella virus vaccine.

Indications

M-R-VAX$_{II}$ is indicated for simultaneous immunization against measles and rubella in children from 15 months of age to puberty.
Infants who are less than 15 months of age may fail to respond to one or both components of the vaccine due to presence in the circulation of residual measles and/or rubella antibody of maternal origin; the younger the infant, the lower the likelihood of seroconversion. In geographically isolated or other relatively inaccessible populations for whom immunization programs are logistically difficult, and in population groups in which natural measles infection may occur in a significant proportion of infants before 15 months of age, it may be desirable to give the vaccine to infants at an earlier age. The advantage of early protection must be weighed against the chance for failure of response; infants vaccinated under these conditions should be revaccinated after reaching 15 months of age.
Revaccination: Based on available evidence, there is no reason to routinely revaccinate children originally vaccinated when 12 months of age or older; however, children vaccinated when younger than 12 months of age should be revaccinated. The decision to revaccinate should be based on evaluation of each individual case.

Contraindications

Do not give M-R-VAX$_{II}$ to pregnant females; the possible effects of the vaccine on fetal development are unknown at this time. When vaccination of post-pubertal females is undertaken, pregnancy must be avoided for three months following vaccination.
Previously unimmunized children of susceptible pregnant women should receive live attenuated rubella vaccine, because an immunized child will be less likely to acquire natural rubella and introduce the virus into the household.
Hypersensitivity to neomycin (each dose of reconstituted vaccine contains approximately 25 mcg of neomycin).
Any febrile respiratory illness or other active febrile infection.
Active untreated tuberculosis.
Patients receiving therapy with ACTH, corticosteroids, irradiation, alkylating agents or antimetabolites. This contraindication does not apply to patients who are receiving corticosteroids as replacement therapy, e.g., for Addison's disease.
Individuals with blood dyscrasias, leukemia, lymphomas of any type, or other malignant neoplasms affecting the bone marrow or lymphatic systems.
Primary immuno-deficiency states, including cellular immune deficiencies, hypogammaglobulinemic and dysgammaglobulinemic states.

Hypersensitivity to Eggs, Chicken, or Chicken Feathers

This vaccine is essentially devoid of potentially allergenic substances derived from host tissues (chick embryos).* However, since the measles component is propagated in cell cultures of chick embryo, in considering vaccine use in patients hypersensitive to chicken or chicken eggs or feathers, the attending physician must weigh the benefits of immunization against the potential risks of hypersensitivity reactions.

Precautions

Administer M-R-VAX$_{II}$ subcutaneously; *do not give intravenously.*
Epinephrine should be available for immediate use in case an anaphylactoid reaction occurs.
M-R-VAX$_{II}$ should not be given less than one month before or after immunization with other *live* virus vaccines, with the exception of MUMPSVAX® (Mumps Virus Vaccine, Live, MSD) which may be given simultaneously.
There are no data available concerning simultaneous use of M-R-VAX$_{II}$ with monovalent or trivalent poliovirus vaccine, live, oral.
Due caution should be employed in administration of M-R-VAX$_{II}$ to children with a history of febrile convulsions, cerebral injury or any other condition in which stress due to fever should be avoided. The physician should be alert to the temperature elevation which may occur 5 to 12 days following vaccination.
Vaccination should be deferred for at least 3 months following blood or plasma transfusions, or administration of more than 0.02 ml of human immune serum globulin per pound of body weight.
Excretion of small amounts of the live attenuated rubella virus from the nose or throat has occurred in the majority of susceptible individuals 7–28 days after vaccination. There is no confirmed evidence to indicate that such virus is transmitted to susceptible persons who are in contact with the vaccinated individuals. Consequently, transmisson, while accepted as a theoretical possibility, is not regarded as a significant risk.**
There are no reports of transmission of live attenuated measles virus from vaccinees to susceptible contacts.
It has been reported that live attenuated measles and rubella virus vaccines given individually may result in a temporary depression of tuberculin skin sensitivity. Therefore, if a tuberculin test is to be done, it should be administered either before or simultaneously with M-R-VAX$_{II}$.
As for any vaccine, vaccination with M-R-VAX$_{II}$ may not result in seroconversion in 100% of susceptible subjects given the vaccine.

Adverse Reactions

The adverse clinical reactions associated with the use of M-R-VAX$_{II}$ are those expected to follow administration of the monovalent vaccines given separately. These may include malaise, sore throat, headache, fever and rash; mild local reactions such as erythema, induration, tenderness and regional lymphadenopathy; thrombocytopenia and purpura; allergic reactions such as urticaria; and arthritis, arthralgia and polyneuritis.
Moderate fever (101–102.9°F) occurs occasionally, and high fever (above 103°F) occurs less commonly. On rare occasions, children developing fever may exhibit febrile convulsions. Rash occurs infrequently and is usually minimal without generalized distribution.
Clinical experience with live attenuated measles and rubella virus vaccines given individually indicates that encephalitis and other nervous system reactions have occurred very rarely. These might occur also with M-R-VAX$_{II}$.
Experience from more than 80 million doses of all live measles vaccines given in the U.S. through 1975 indicates that significant central nervous system reactions such as encephalitis and encephalopathy, occurring within 30 days after vaccination, have been temporally associated with measles vaccine approximately once for every million doses. In no case has it been shown that reactions were actually caused by vaccine. The Center for Disease Control has pointed out that "a certain number of cases of encephalitis may be expected to occur in a large childhood population in a defined period of time even when no vaccines are administered". However, the data suggest the possibility that some of these cases may have been caused by measles vaccines. The risk of such serious neurological disorders following live measles virus vaccine administration remains far less than that for encephalitis and encephalopathy with natural measles (one per thousand reported cases).
There have been reports of subacute sclerosing panencephalitis (SSPE) in children who did not have a history of natural measles but did receive measles vaccine. Some of these cases may have resulted from unrecognized measles in the first year of life or possibly from the measles vaccination. Based on estimated nationwide measles vaccine distribution, the association of SSPE cases to measles vaccination is about one case per million vaccine doses distributed. This is far less than the association with natural measles, 5–10 cases of SSPE per million cases of measles. The results of a retrospective case-controlled study conducted by the Center for Disease Control suggest that the overall effect of measles vaccine has been to protect against SSPE by preventing measles with its inherent higher risk of SSPE.
Local reactions characterized by marked swelling, redness and vesiculation at the injection site of attenuated live measles virus vaccines have occurred in children who received killed measles vaccine previously. M-R-VAX$_{II}$ was not given under this condition in clinical trials.
Transient arthritis, arthralgia and polyneuritis are features of natural rubella and vary in frequency and severity with age and sex, being greatest in adult females and least in prepubertal children. This type of involvement has also been reported following administration of MERUVAX$_{II}$ (Rubella Virus Vaccine, Live, MSD). In children, joint reactions are rare and of brief duration if they do occur. In women, incidence rates for arthritis and arthralgia are generally higher than those seen in children (children: 0–3%; women: 12–20%), and the reactions tend to be more marked and of longer duration. Rarely, symptoms may persist for a matter of months. In adolescent girls, the reactions appear to be intermediate in incidence between those seen in children and in adult women. Even in older women (35–45 years), these reactions are generally well tolerated and rarely interfere with normal activities.

Dosage and Administration

After suitably cleansing the immunization site, inject the total volume of reconstituted vaccine subcutaneously, preferably into the outer aspect of the upper arm. Do not inject M-R-VAX$_{II}$ intravenously.

Shipment, Storage, and Reconstitution

During shipment, to insure that there is no loss of potency, the vaccine must be maintained at a temperature of 10°C (50°F) or less.
Before reconstitution, store M-R-VAX$_{II}$ at 2–8°C (35.6–46.4°F). *Protect from light.*
To reconstitute, use only the diluent supplied, since it is free of preservatives or other antiviral substances which might inactivate the vaccine. Inject all the diluent in the syringe into the vial of lyophilized vaccine, and agitate to mix thoroughly. Withdraw the entire contents into the syringe and inject the total volume of restored vaccine subcutaneously.
It is important to use a separate sterile syringe and needle for each individual patient to prevent transmission of hepatitis B and other infectious agents from one person to another.
The usual color of the vaccine when reconstituted is yellow.
It is recommended that the vaccine be used as soon as possible after reconstitution. Protect vaccine from light at all times. Store reconstituted vaccine in a dark place at 2–8°C (35.6–46.4°F) and discard if not used within 8 hours.

How Supplied

No. 4676—M-R-VAX$_{II}$ is supplied as a single-dose vial of lyophilized vaccine with a disposable syringe containing diluent, and fitted with a 25 gauge, 5/8" needle, **NDC** 0006-4676-00.
No. 4677/4590—M-R-VAX$_{II}$ is supplied as follows: (1) a box of ten single-dose vials of lyophilized vaccine, **NDC** 0006-4677-00; and (2) a box of ten diluent-containing disposable syringes with affixed 25 gauge, 5/8" needles. To conserve refrigerator space, the syringes may be stored separately at room temperature.

---

* Morbidity and Mortality Weekly Report *25*(44): 350, Nov. 12, 1976.
** Recommendation of the Public Health Service Advisory Committee on Immunization Practices, Morbidity and Mortality Weekly Report, *26*(47): 385, 386, 391, Nov. 25, 1977.

A.H.F.S. 80:12
DC 7032900 Issued October 1978

MEFOXIN® ℞
(cefoxitin sodium, MSD)

Description

MEFOXIN (Sterile Cefoxitin Sodium, MSD) is a semi-synthetic, broad-spectrum cepha antibiotic for parenteral administration. It is derived from cephamycin C, which is produced by *Streptomyces lactamdurans.* It is the sodium salt of 3-(hydroxymethyl)-7α-methoxy-8-oxo-7-[2- (2-thienyl) acetamido]-5-thia-1-azabicyclo [4.2.0] oct-2-ene-2-carboxylate carbamate (ester). MEFOXIN contains approximately 53.8 mg (2.3 milliequivalents) of sodium per gram of cefoxitin activity. Solutions of MEFOXIN range from clear to light amber in color. The pH of freshly constituted solutions usually ranges from 4.2 to 7.0.

Actions

Clinical Pharmacology
After intramuscular administration of a 1 gram dose of MEFOXIN to normal volunteers, the mean peak serum concentration was 24 mcg/ml. The peak occurred at 20 to 30 minutes. Following an intravenous dose of 1 gram, serum concentrations were 110 mcg/ml at 5 minutes, declining to less than 1 mcg/ml at 4 hours. The half-life after an intravenous dose is 41 to 59 minutes; after intramuscular administration, the half-life is 64.8 minutes. Approximately 85 percent of cefoxitin is excreted unchanged by the kidneys over a 6-hour period, resulting in high urinary concentrations. Following an intramuscular dose of 1 gram, urinary concentrations greater than 3000 mcg/ml were observed. Probenecid slows tubular excretion and produces higher serum levels and increases the duration of measurable serum concentrations.

Cefoxitin passes into pleural and joint fluids and is detectable in antibacterial concentrations in bile.

Clinical experience has demonstrated that MEFOXIN can be administered to patients who are also receiving carbenicillin, kanamycin, gentamicin, tobramycin, or amikacin (see PRECAUTIONS and ADMINISTRATION).

Microbiology
The bactericidal action of cefoxitin results from inhibition of cell wall synthesis. Cefoxitin has *in vitro* activity against a wide range of gram-positive and gram-negative organisms. The methoxy group in the 7α position provides MEFOXIN with a high degree of stability in the presence of beta-lactamases, both penicillinases and cephalosporinases, of gram-negative bacteria. Cefoxitin is usually active against the following organisms *in vitro* and in clinical infections:

Gram-positive
- *Staphylococcus aureus,* including penicillinase and non-penicillinase producing strains.
- *Staphylococcus epidermidis*
- Beta-hemolytic and other streptococci (most strains of enterococci, e.g., *Streptococcus faecalis,* are resistant)
- *Streptococcus pneumoniae* (formerly *Diplococcus pneumoniae)*

Gram-negative
- *Escherichia coli*
- *Klebsiella* species (including *K. pneumoniae)*
- *Hemophilus influenzae*
- *Neisseria gonorrhoeae*
- *Proteus mirabilis*
- *Proteus rettgeri*
- *Proteus morganii*
- *Proteus vulgaris*
- *Providencia* species

Anaerobic organisms
- *Peptococcus* species
- *Peptostreptococcus* species
- *Clostridium* species
- *Bacteroides* species, including the *B. fragilis* group (includes *B. fragilis, B. distasonis, B. ovatus, B. thetaiotaomicron, B. vulgatus)*

MEFOXIN is inactive *in vitro* against most strains of *Pseudomonas aeruginosa* and enterococci and many strains of *Enterobacter cloacae.* Methicillin-resistant staphylococci are almost uniformly resistant to MEFOXIN.

Susceptibility Tests
For fast-growing aerobic organisms, quantitative methods that require measurements of zone diameters give the most precise estimates of antibiotic susceptibility. One such proce-

Continued on next page

Information on the Merck Sharp & Dohme products listed on these pages is the full prescribing information from package circulars in use October 31, 1979.

Merck Sharp & Dohme—Cont.

dure* has been recommended for use with discs to test susceptibility to cefoxitin. Interpretation involves correlation of the diameters obtained in the disc test with minimal inhibitory concentration (MIC) values for cefoxitin.
Reports from the laboratory giving results of the standardized single disc susceptibility test* using a 30 mcg cefoxitin disc should be interpreted according to the following criteria:
Organisms producing zones of 18 mm or greater are considered susceptible, indicating that the tested organism is likely to respond to therapy.
Organisms of intermediate susceptibility produce zones of 15 to 17 mm, indicating that the tested organism would be susceptible if high dosage is used or if the infection is confined to tissues and fluids (e.g., urine) in which high antibiotic levels are attained.
Resistant organisms produce zones of 14 mm or less, indicating that other therapy should be selected.
The cefoxitin disc should be used for testing cefoxitin susceptibility.
Cefoxitin has been shown by *in vitro* tests to have activity against certain strains of *Enterobacteriaceae* found resistant when tested with the cephalosporin class disc. For this reason, the cefoxitin disc should not be used for testing susceptibility to cephalosporins, and cephalosporin discs should not be used for testing susceptibility to cefoxitin.
Dilution methods, preferably the agar plate dilution procedure, are most accurate for susceptibility testing of obligate anaerobes.

A bacterial isolate may be considered susceptible if the MIC value for cefoxitin† is not more than 16 mcg/ml. Organisms are considered resistant if the MIC is greater than 32 mcg/ml.

Indications

MEFOXIN is indicated for the treatment of serious infections caused by susceptible strains of the designated microorganisms in the diseases listed below.
(1) Lower respiratory tract infections, including pneumonia and lung abscess, caused by *Streptococcus pneumoniae* (formerly *Diplococcus pneumoniae),* other streptococci (excluding enterococci, e.g., *Streptococcus faecalis), Staphylococcus aureus* (penicillinase and non-penicillinase producing), *Escherichia coli, Klebsiella* species, *Hemophilus influenzae,* and *Bacteroides* species.
(2) Genitourinary infections. Urinary tract infections caused by *Escherichia coli, Klebsiella* species, *Proteus mirabilis,* indole-positive Proteus (i.e., *Proteus morganii, rettgeri,* and *vulgaris*), and *Providencia* species. Uncomplicated gonorrhea due to *Neisseria gonorrhoeae.*
(3) Intra-abdominal infections, including peritonitis and intra-abdominal abscess, caused by *Escherichia coli, Klebsiella* species, *Bacteroides* species including the *Bacteroides fragilis* group**, and *Clostridium* species.
(4) Gynecological infections, including endometritis, pelvic cellulitis, and pelvic inflammatory disease caused by *Escherichia coli, Neisseria gonorrhoeae, Bacteroides* species including the *Bacteroides fragilis* group**, *Clostridium* species, *Peptococcus* species, *Peptostreptococcus* species, and Group B streptococci.
(5) Septicemia caused by *Streptococcus pneumoniae* (formerly *Diplococcus pneumoniae), Staphylococcus aureus* (penicillinase and non-penicillinase producing), *Escherichia coli, Klebsiella* species, and *Bacteroides* species including the *Bacteroides fragilis* group.**
(6) Bone and joint infections caused by *Staphylococcus aureus* (penicillinase and non-penicillinase producing).
(7) Skin and skin structure infections caused by *Staphylococcus aureus* (penicillinase and non-penicillinase producing), *Staphylococcus epidermidis,* streptococci (excluding enterococci, e.g., *Streptococcus faecalis), Escherichia coli, Proteus mirabilis, Klebsiella* species, *Bacteroides* species including the *Bacteroides fragilis* group**, *Clostridium* species, *Peptococcus* species, and *Peptostreptococcus* species.
Appropriate culture and susceptibility studies should be performed to determine the susceptibility of the causative organisms to MEFOXIN. Therapy may be started while awaiting the results of these studies.
In randomized comparative studies, MEFOXIN and cephalothin were comparably safe and effective in the management of infections caused by gram-positive cocci and gram-negative rods susceptible to the cephalosporins. MEFOXIN has a high degree of stability in the presence of bacterial beta-lactamases, both penicillinases and cephalosporinases.
Many infections caused by aerobic and anaerobic gram-negative bacteria resistant to some cephalosporins respond to MEFOXIN. Similarly, many infections caused by aerobic and anaerobic bacteria resistant to some penicillin antibiotics (ampicillin, carbenicillin, penicillin G) respond to treatment with MEFOXIN. Many infections caused by mixtures of susceptible aerobic and anaerobic bacteria respond to treatment with MEFOXIN.

Contraindications

MEFOXIN is contraindicated in patients who have shown hypersensitivity to cefoxitin and the cephalosporin group of antibiotics.

Warnings

BEFORE THERAPY WITH MEFOXIN IS INSTITUTED, CAREFUL INQUIRY SHOULD BE MADE TO DETERMINE WHETHER THE PATIENT HAS HAD PREVIOUS HYPERSENSITIVITY REACTIONS TO CEFOXITIN, CEPHALOSPORINS, PENICILLINS, OR OTHER DRUGS. THIS PRODUCT SHOULD BE GIVEN WITH CAUTION TO PENICILLIN-SENSITIVE PATIENTS. ANTIBIOTICS SHOULD BE ADMINISTERED WITH CAUTION TO ANY PATIENT WHO HAS DEMONSTRATED SOME FORM OF ALLERGY, PARTICULARLY TO DRUGS. IF AN ALLERGIC REACTION TO MEFOXIN OCCURS, DISCONTINUE THE DRUG. SERIOUS HYPERSENSITIVITY REACTIONS MAY REQUIRE EPINEPHRINE AND OTHER EMERGENCY MEASURES.

Precautions

The total daily dose should be reduced when MEFOXIN is administered to patients with transient or persistent reduction of urinary output due to renal insufficiency (see DOSAGE), because high and prolonged serum antibiotic concentrations can occur in such individuals from usual doses.
As with other antibiotics, prolonged use of MEFOXIN may result in overgrowth of nonsusceptible organisms. Repeated evaluation of the patient's condition is essential. If superinfection occurs during therapy, appropriate measures should be taken.
Increased nephrotoxicity has been reported following concomitant administration of cephalosporins and aminoglycoside antibiotics.
Interference with Laboratory Tests
As with cephalothin, high concentrations of cefoxitin (> 100 micrograms/ml) may interfere with measurement of serum and urine creatinine levels by the Jaffé reaction, and produce false increases of modest degree in the levels of creatinine reported. Serum samples from patients treated with cefoxitin should not be analyzed for creatinine if withdrawn within 2 hours of drug administration.
A false-positive reaction for glucose in the urine may occur. This has been observed with CLINITEST* reagent tablets.
Pregnancy
Reproduction and teratologic studies have been performed in mice and rats and have revealed no evidence of impaired fertility or harm to the fetus due to MEFOXIN. There are no well controlled studies with MEFOXIN in pregnant women. Use of the drug in women of childbearing potential requires that the anticipated benefit be weighed against the possible risks.
Nursing Mothers
MEFOXIN is excreted in human milk in low concentrations.
Infants and Children
Safety and efficacy in infants and children have not yet been established.

Adverse Reactions

MEFOXIN is generally well tolerated. The most common adverse reactions have been local reactions following intravenous or intramuscular injection. Other adverse reactions have been encountered infrequently.
Local Reactions
Thrombophlebitis has occurred with intravenous administration. Pain, induration, and tenderness after intramuscular injections have been reported.
Allergic Reactions
Rash, pruritus, eosinophilia, fever, and other allergic reactions have been noted.
Gastrointestinal
Nausea, vomiting, and diarrhea have been reported rarely.
Blood
Transient leukopenia, neutropenia, and hemolytic anemia have been reported. A positive direct Coombs test may develop in some individuals, especially those with azotemia.
Liver Function
Transient elevations in SGOT, SGPT, serum LDH, and serum alkaline phosphatase have been reported.
Renal Function
Elevations in serum creatinine and/or blood urea nitrogen levels have been observed. The role of MEFOXIN in changes in renal function tests is difficult to assess, since factors predisposing to prerenal azotemia or to impaired renal function usually have been present.

Dosage

The usual adult dosage range is 1 gram to 2 grams every six to eight hours. Dosage and route of administration should be determined by susceptibility of the causative organisms, severity of infection, and the condition of the patient (see Table 1 for dosage guidelines).
[See table on next page].
MEFOXIN may be used in patients with reduced renal function with the following dosage adjustments:
In adults with renal insufficiency, an initial loading dose of 1 gram to 2 grams may be given.

*Bauer, A. W.; Kirby, W. M. M.; Sherris, J. C.; Turck, M.: Antibiotic susceptibility testing by a standardized single disk method, Amer. J. Clin. Path. *45*: 493–496, Apr. 1966. Standardized disc susceptibility test, Federal Register *37*: 20527–20529, 1972. National Committee for Clinical Laboratory Standards: Approved Standard: ASM-2, Performance Standards for Antimicrobial Disc Susceptibility Tests, July 1975.

†Determined by the ICS agar dilution method (Ericsson and Sherris, Acta Path. Microbiol. Scand. (B) Suppl. No. 217, 1971) or any other method that has been shown to give equivalent results.

** *B. fragilis, B. distasonis, B. ovatus, B. thetaiotaomicron, B. vulgatus.*

*Registered trademark of Ames Company, Division of Miles Laboratories, Inc.

After a loading dose, the recommendations for *maintenance dosage* (Table 2) may be used as a guide.
(See table top right)

When only the serum creatinine level is available, the following formula (based on sex, weight, and age of the patient) may be used to convert this value into creatinine clearance. The serum creatinine should represent a steady state of renal function.

$$\text{Males: } \frac{\text{Weight (kg)} \times (140 - \text{age})}{72 \times \text{serum creatinine (mg/100 ml)}}$$

Females: 0.85 × above value

In patients undergoing hemodialysis, the loading dose of 1 to 2 grams should be given after each hemodialysis, and the maintenance dose should be given as indicated in Table 2.
Antibiotic therapy for group A beta-hemolytic streptococcal infections should be maintained for at least 10 days to guard against the risk of rheumatic fever or glomerulonephritis. In staphylococcal and other infections involving a collection of pus, surgical drainage should be carried out where indicated.
The recommended dosage of MEFOXIN **for uncomplicated gonorrhea** is 2 grams intramuscularly, with 1 gram of BENEMID® (Probenecid, MSD) given by mouth at the same time or up to ½ hour before MEFOXIN.

Preparation of Solution

Table 3 is provided for convenience in constituting MEFOXIN for both intravenous and intramuscular administration.
[See table on next page].
For intravenous use, 1 gram should be constituted with at least 10 ml of Sterile Water for Injection, and 2 grams, with 10 or 20 ml. One or 2 grams of MEFOXIN may be constituted with 50 or 100 ml of 0.9 percent Sodium Chloride Injection, 5 percent or 10 percent Dextrose Injection, or any of the solutions listed under the *Intravenous* portion of the COMPATIBILITY AND STABILITY section.
For intramuscular use, each gram of MEFOXIN may be constituted with 2 ml of Sterile Water for Injection *or*
For intramuscular use ONLY: each gram of MEFOXIN may be constituted with 2 ml of 0.5 percent lidocaine hydrochloride solution* (without epinephrine) to minimize the discomfort of intramuscular injection.

Administration

MEFOXIN may be administered intravenously or intramuscularly after constitution.
Intravenous Administration
The intravenous route is preferable for patients with bacteremia, bacterial septicemia, or other severe or life-threatening infections, or for patients who may be poor risks because of lowered resistance resulting from such debilitating conditions as malnutrition, trauma, surgery, diabetes, heart failure, or malignancy, particularly if shock is present or impending.
For intermittent intravenous administration, a solution containing 1 gram or 2 grams in 10 ml of Sterile Water for Injection can be injected over a period of three to five minutes. Using an infusion system, it may also be given over a longer period of time through the tubing system by which the patient may be receiving other intravenous solutions. However, during infusion of the solution containing MEFOXIN, it is advisable to temporarily discontinue administration of any other solutions at the same site.
For the administration of higher doses by continuous intravenous infusion, a solution of MEFOXIN may be added to an intravenous bottle containing 5 percent Dextrose Injection, 0.9 percent Sodium Chloride Injection, 5 percent Dextrose and 0.9 percent Sodium Chloride Injection, or 5 percent Dextrose Injection with 0.02 percent sodium bicarbonate solution. BUTTERFLY** or scalp vein-type needles are preferred for this type of infusion.
Solutions of MEFOXIN, like those of most beta-lactam antibiotics, should not be added to aminoglycoside solutions (e.g., gentamicin sulfate, tobramycin sulfate, amikacin sulfate) because of potential interaction. However, MEFOXIN and aminoglycosides may be administered separately to the same patient.
Intramuscular Administration
As with all intramuscular preparations, MEFOXIN should be injected well within the body of a relatively large muscle such as the upper outer quadrant of the buttock (i.e., gluteus maximus); aspiration is necessary to avoid inadvertent injection into a blood vessel.

Compatibility and Stability

Intravenous
MEFOXIN, as constituted to 1 gram/10 ml with Sterile Water for Injection, Bacteriostatic Water for Injection, 0.9 percent Sodium Chloride Injection, or 5 percent Dextrose Injection, maintains satisfactory potency for 24 hours at room temperature, for one week under refrigeration (below 5°C), and for at least 26 weeks in the frozen state.
These primary solutions may be further diluted in 50 to 1000 ml of the following solutions and maintain potency for 24 hours at room temperature and at least 48 hours under refrigeration:
Sterile Water for Injection
0.9 percent Sodium Chloride Injection
5 percent or 10 percent Dextrose Injection
5 percent Dextrose and 0.9 percent Sodium Chloride Injection
5 percent Dextrose Injection with 0.02 percent sodium bicarbonate solution
5 percent Dextrose Injection with 0.2 percent or 0.45 percent saline solution
Ringer's Injection
Lactated Ringer's Injection
5 percent dextrose in Lactated Ringer's Injection
5 percent or 10 percent invert sugar in water
10 percent invert sugar in saline solution
5 percent Sodium Bicarbonate Injection
M/6 sodium lactate solution
AMINOSOL** 5 percent Solution
NORMOSOL-M in D5-W**
IONOSOL B w/Dextrose 5 percent**
POLYONIC M 56 in 5 percent Dextrose*
Limited studies with solutions of MEFOXIN in 0.9 percent Sodium Chloride Injection, Lactated Ringer's Injection, and 5 percent Dextrose Injection in VIAFLEX† intravenous bags show stability for 24 hours at room temperature and 48 hours under refrigeration. Also, solutions of MEFOXIN in 0.9 percent Sodium Chloride Injection show similar stability in plastic tubing, drip chambers, and volume control devices of common intravenous infusion sets.
After constitution with Sterile Water for Injection and subsequent storage in disposable plastic syringes, MEFOXIN is stable for 24 hours at room temperature and 48 hours under refrigeration.
After the periods mentioned above, any unused solutions or frozen material should be discarded. Do not refreeze.
Intramuscular
MEFOXIN, as constituted with Sterile Water for Injection, Bacteriostatic Water for Injection, or 0.5 percent or 1 percent lidocaine hydrochloride solution (without epinephrine), maintains satisfactory potency for 24 hours at room temperature, for one week under refrigeration (below 5°C), and for at least 26 weeks in the frozen state.
After the periods mentioned above, any unused solutions or frozen material should be discarded. Do not refreeze.
Note: MEFOXIN in the dry state should be stored below 30°C. Avoid exposure to temperatures above 50°C. The dry material as well as solutions tend to darken, depending on storage

Table 1—Guidelines for Dosage of MEFOXIN

Type of Infection	Daily Dosage	Frequency and Route
Uncomplicated forms* of infections such as pneumonia, urinary tract infection, cutaneous infection	3–4 grams	1 gram every 6–8 hours IV or IM
Moderately severe or severe infections	6–8 grams	1 gram every 4 hours *or* 2 grams every 6–8 hours IV
Infections commonly needing antibiotics in higher dosage (e.g., gas gangrene)	12 grams	2 grams every 4 hours *or* 3 grams every 6 hours IV

*Including patients in whom bacteremia is absent or unlikely

Table 2—Maintenance Dosage of MEFOXIN in Adults with Reduced Renal Function

Renal Function	Creatinine Clearance (ml/min)	Dose (grams)	Frequency
Mild impairment	50–30	1–2	every 8–12 hours
Moderate impairment	29–10	1–2	every 12–24 hours
Severe impairment	9–5	0.5–1	every 12–24 hours
Essentially no function	<5	0.5–1	every 24–48 hours

*See package circular of manufacturer for detailed information concerning contraindications, warnings, precautions, and adverse reactions.

**Registered trademark of Abbott Laboratories.

**Registered trademark of Abbott Laboratories
* Registered trademark of Cutter Laboratories, Inc.
† Registered trademark of Travenol Laboratories, Inc.

Continued on next page

Information on the Merck Sharp & Dohme products listed on these pages is the full prescribing information from package circulars in use October 31, 1979.

Merck Sharp & Dohme—Cont.

conditions; product potency, however, is not adversely affected.

How Supplied

Sterile MEFOXIN is a dry white to off-white powder supplied in vials and infusion bottles containing cefoxitin sodium as follows:

1 gram cefoxitin equivalent
NDC 0006-3356-02 in vials
NDC 0006-3368-02 in infusion bottles
2 gram cefoxitin equivalent
NDC 0006-3357-03 in vials
NDC 0006-3369-03 in infusion bottles

A.H.F.S. 8:12.28

DC 7057106 Issued May 1979

Table 3—Preparation of Solution

Strength	Amount of Diluent to be Added (ml)*	Approximate Withdrawable Volume (ml)	Approximate Average Concentration (mg/ml)
1 gram Vial	2 (intramuscular)	2.5	400
1 gram Vial	10 (IV)	10.5	95
2 gram Vial	10 or 20 (IV)	11.1 or 21.0	180 or 95
1 gram Infusion Bottle	50 to 100 (IV)	50 to 100	20 to 10
2 gram Infusion Bottle	50 to 100 (IV)	50 to 100	40 to 20

*Shake to dissolve and let stand until clear.

MERUVAX® II ℞

(rubella virus vaccine, live, MSD), U.S.P.
(Wistar RA 27/3 Strain
Prepared in WI-38 Human Diploid Cells)

Description

MERUVAX II (Rubella Virus Vaccine, Live, MSD) is a live virus vaccine for immunization against rubella (German measles).
MERUVAX II is a lyophilized preparation of the Wistar Institute RA 27/3 strain of live attenuated rubella virus. The virus was adapted to and propagated in human diploid cell (WI-38) culture.
When reconstituted as directed, the dose for injection is 0.5 ml and contains not less than the equivalent of 1,000 $TCID_{50}$ (tissue culture infective doses) of rubella virus vaccine expressed in terms of the assigned titer of the FDA Reference Rubella Virus. Each dose also contains approximately 25 mcg of neomycin.

Actions

Extensive clinical trials of rubella virus vaccines, prepared using RA 27/3 strain rubella virus, have been carried out in more than 28,000 human subjects (approximately 11,000 with MERUVAX II) in the U.S.A. and more than 20 additional countries. Following subcutaneous inoculation, the vaccines have been shown to induce rubella hemagglutination-inhibiting (HI) antibodies in over 97% of susceptible subjects. The RA 27/3 rubella strain elicits higher immediate post-vaccination HI, complement-fixing and neutralizing antibody levels than other strains of rubella vaccine and has been shown to induce a broader profile of circulating antibodies including anti-theta and anti-iota precipitating antibodies. The RA 27/3 rubella strain simulates natural infection more closely than other rubella vaccine viruses. The broader profile of antibodies produced by RA 27/3 strain rubella virus vaccine appears to correlate with greater resistance to subclinical reinfection with the wild virus.
Vaccine induced antibody levels have been shown to persist for at least six years without substantial decline. If the present pattern continues, it will provide a basis for the expectation that immunity following the vaccine will be permanent. However, continued surveillance will be required to demonstrate this point.

Indications†

1. *Children Between 15 Months of Age and Puberty*
MERUVAX II is indicated for immunization against rubella in boys and girls from 15 months of age to puberty. It may be given as early as 12 months, if that offers greater convenience in scheduling. No booster is needed. It is not recommended for infants less than 12 months of age because persons of that age may retain maternal rubella neutralizing antibodies that may interfere with the immune response. Children in kindergarten and the first grades of elementary school deserve priority for vaccination because often they are epidemiologically the major source of virus dissemination in the community. A history of rubella illness is usually not reliable enough to exclude children from immunization.
2. *Adolescent and Adult Males*
Vaccination of adolescent or adult males may be a useful procedure in preventing or controlling outbreaks of rubella in circumscribed population groups.
3. *Non-Pregnant Adolescent and Adult Females*
Pregnant females *must not* be given live attenuated rubella virus vaccine.
Since it is not known to what extent infection of the fetus with attenuated virus might take place following vaccination, or whether damage to the fetus could result, *routine immunization* of postpubertal females of unknown rubella immune status should not be undertaken because of the danger of inadvertently administering vaccine before pregnancy becomes evident.
Postpubertal females should be considered for vaccination individually. Vaccine should only be given if subjects are shown to be rubella-susceptible by serologic testing (see below), if they are not pregnant at the time of vaccination, and if they agree that they will not become pregnant within three months following vaccination.
This cautious approach to the vaccination of postpubertal females is indicated because of the potential risk from vaccination during pregnancy, and because congenital abnormalities occur in up to 7% of *all* live births. Their chance appearance after vaccination could lead to serious misinterpretation.
It has been found convenient, in many instances, to vaccinate rubella-susceptible women in the immediate post-partum period.
If vaccination of a postpubertal female is contemplated, the following is recommended:

a. She should be tested for susceptibility to rubella by the HI (Hemagglutination Inhibition) test.
b. If immune, as evidenced by a specific rubella antibody titer of 1:8 or greater, vaccination is unnecessary.
c. If susceptible, she may be vaccinated only if she agrees not to become pregnant for the next three months. (This precaution also applies to women in the immediate post-partum period.)
d. She should be informed of the frequent occurrence of self-limited arthralgia and possible arthritis beginning 2 to 4 weeks after vaccination.

As with any vaccine, inoculation of susceptibles does not result in seroconversion in 100 percent of the vaccinees.
Revaccination
Based on available evidence, there is no reason to revaccinate children who were vaccinated originally when 12 months of age or older; however, children vaccinated when younger than 12 months of age should be revaccinated.

Contraindications

Do not give MERUVAX II to pregnant females; the possible effects of the vaccine on fetal development are unknown at this time. When vaccination of post-pubertal females is undertaken, pregnancy must be avoided for three months following vaccination.
Previously unimmunized children of susceptible pregnant women should receive live attenuated rubella vaccine, because an immunized child will be less likely to acquire natural rubella and introduce the virus into the household.
Hypersensitivity to neomycin (each dose of reconstituted vaccine contains approximately 25 mcg of neomycin).
Any febrile respiratory illness, or other active febrile infection.
Patients receiving therapy with ACTH, corticosteroids, irradiation, alkylating agents or antimetabolites. This contraindication does not apply to patients who are receiving corticosteroids as replacement therapy, e.g., for Addison's disease.
Individuals with blood dyscrasias, leukemia, lymphomas of any type, or other malignant neoplasms affecting the bone marrow or lymphatic systems.
Primary immuno-deficiency states, including cellular immune deficiencies, hypogammaglobulinemic and dysgammaglobulinemic states.

Precautions

The vaccine is to be given subcutaneously; *do not give intravenously.*
Epinephrine should be available for immediate use should an anaphylactoid reaction occur.
MERUVAX II should not be given less than one month before or after immunization with other *live* virus vaccines, with the exception of ATTENUVAX® (Measles Virus Vaccine, Live, Attenuated, MSD), and/or MUMPSVAX® (Mumps Virus Vaccine, Live, MSD), which may be administered simultaneously.
Excretion of small amounts of the live attenuated rubella virus from the nose or throat has occurred in the majority of susceptible individuals 7–28 days after vaccination. There is no confirmed evidence to indicate that such virus is transmitted to susceptible persons who are in contact with the vaccinated individuals. Consequently, transmission, while accepted as a theoretical possibility, is not regarded as a significant risk.*
There is no evidence that live rubella virus vaccine given after exposure to natural rubella virus will prevent illness. There is, however, no contraindication to vaccinating children already exposed to natural rubella.
Vaccination should be deferred for at least three months following blood or plasma transfusions, or administration of more than 0.02 ml of human immune serum globulin per pound of body weight. However, susceptible post-partum patients who received blood products may receive MERUVAX II prior to discharge provided that a repeat HI titer is drawn 6–8 weeks after vaccination to insure seroconversion. Similarly, although studies with other live

rubella virus vaccines suggest that MERUVAX II may be given in the immediate postpartum period to those non-immune women who have received anti-Rho (D) globulin (human) without interfering with vaccine effectiveness, a follow-up post-vaccination HI titer should also be determined.
It has been reported that attenuated rubella virus vaccine, live, may result in a temporary depression of tuberculin skin sensitivity. Therefore, if a tuberculin test is to be done, it should be administered either before or simultaneously with MERUVAX II.
As for any vaccine, vaccination with MERUVAX II may not result in seroconversion in 100% of susceptible subjects given the vaccine.

Adverse Reactions

Adverse reactions are uncommon, but symptoms of the same kind as those seen following natural rubella may occur after vaccination. These include regional lymphadenopathy, urticaria, rash, malaise, sore throat, fever, headache, polyneuritis, and occasionally temporary arthralgia that is infrequently associated with signs of inflammation. Local pain, induration, and erythema may occur at the site of injection.
Moderate fever (101–102.9°F) occurs occasionally, and high fever (103°F) occurs less commonly.
Reactions are usually mild and transient.
In children, joint reactions are rare and of brief duration if they do occur. In women, incidence rates for arthritis and arthralgia are generally higher than those seen in children (children: 0–3%; women: 12–20%) and the reactions tend to be more marked and of longer duration. Rarely, symptoms may persist for a matter of months. In adolescent girls, the reactions appear to be intermediate in incidence between those seen in children and in adult women. Even in older women (35–45 years), these reactions are generally well tolerated and rarely interfere with normal activities.
Clinical experience with live virus rubella vaccines thus far indicates that encephalitis and other nervous system reactions have occurred very rarely in subjects who were given the vaccines, but a cause and effect relationship has not been established.
In view of the decreases in platelet counts that have been reported, thrombocytopenic purpura is a theoretical hazard.

Dosage and Administration

Inject the total volume of reconstituted vaccine subcutaneously, preferably into the outer aspect of the upper arm, after suitable cleansing of the immunization site. MERUVAX II should not be injected intravenously, or administered intranasally.

Shipment, Storage and Reconstitution

To insure that there is no loss of potency during shipment, the vaccine must be maintained at a temperature of 10°C (50°F) or less.
Before reconstitution, store MERUVAX II at 2–8°C (35.6–46.4°F). *Protect from light.*
To reconstitute, inject all of the diluent in the syringe into the vial of lyophilized vaccine, and agitate to ensure thorough mixing. Withdraw the entire contents into the syringe and inject the total volume of restored vaccine subcutaneously.
It is important to use a separate sterile syringe and needle for each individual patient to prevent transmission of hepatitis B and other infectious agents from one person to another.
Each dose of reconstituted vaccine contains not less than 1000 $TCID_{50}$ (tissue culture infectious doses) of rubella virus vaccine expressed in terms of the assigned titer of the FDA Reference Rubella Virus.
The color of the vaccine when reconstituted is yellow.
Use only the diluent supplied to reconstitute the vaccine. It is recommended that the vaccine be used as soon as possible after reconstitution. Protect vaccine from light, at all times. Store reconstituted vaccine in a dark place at 2–8°C (35.6–46.4°F) and discard if not used within 8 hours.

How Supplied

No. 4672 MERUVAX II is supplied as a single-dose vial of lyophilized vaccine, **NDC** 0006-4672-00, with a disposable syringe containing diluent and fitted with a 25 gauge, 5/8″ needle.
No. 4673/4590 MERUVAX II is supplied as follows: (1) a box of 10 single-dose vials of lyophilized vaccine, **NDC** 0006-4673-00, and (2) a box of 10 diluent-containing disposable syringes with affixed 25 gauge, 5/8″ needles. To conserve refrigerator space, the syringes may be stored separately at room temperature.

†Based in part on the recommendation for rubella vaccine use of the Public Health Service Advisory Committee on Immunization Practices, Morbidity and Mortality Weekly Report *26*(47): 385, 386, 391, Nov. 25, 1977.
*Recommendation of the Public Health Service Advisory Committee on immunization Practices, Morbidity and Mortality Weekly Report, *26*(47): 385, 386, 391, Nov. 25, 1977.

A.H.F.S. 80:12
DC 7030802 Issued October 1978

MUMPSVAX® ℞
(mumps virus vaccine, live, MSD), U.S.P.
Jeryl Lynn Strain

Usually, mumps is a mild disease. However, it may occasionally be severe and produce serious complications. For example, meningoencephalitis has been estimated to occur in about 10 percent of patients, and unilateral orchitis in about 20 to 30 percent of postpubertal males. Post-infectious encephalitis, oophoritis, pancreatitis, muscular weakness, myelitis, myocarditis, facial neuritis, arthritis, hepatitis, and deafness may also occur. The relationship of endocardial fibroelastosis in infants, and mumps in the mother during pregnancy, has not been conclusively established.
Studies in susceptible children and adults have assessed the safety and efficacy of MUMPSVAX (Mumps Virus Vaccine, Live, MSD). A single dose induced an effective antibody response in approximately 97 percent of susceptible children and approximately 93 percent of susceptible adults. There were few reports of soreness at the site of injection during clinical studies. There was no significant difference in the incidence of fever in clinical trials when children vaccinated with mumps vaccine were compared with unvaccinated subjects studied concurrently. In studies which included more than 200 susceptible male adults inoculated with mumps vaccine, no significant clinical side effects were reported. (See ADVERSE REACTIONS.)
No reports have been received of transmission of mumps from vaccinees to susceptible contacts.
Adequate antibody levels, with continuing protection of vaccinated children exposed to mumps, have persisted for ten years without substantial decline. The pattern of antibody closely resembles that observed for natural mumps although the antibody level is significantly lower than that following the natural infection. If this pattern continues it will provide a basis for expectation that immunity following the vaccine will be permanent. However, continued surveillance will be required to demonstrate this point.

Preparation

This vaccine is prepared from the Jeryl Lynn (B level) strain, named after the patient from whom the virus was initially recovered.
MUMPSVAX is grown in cell cultures of chick embryos, free of Avian leukosis, according to the general procedures used to prepare Enders' measles virus vaccine, live, attenuated. The vaccine is tested for safety and efficacy.

Indications

MUMPSVAX induces protective antibodies in essentially all non-immune recipients, provides protection against natural mumps in most cases, and has not been shown to cause significant systemic or local reactions. Evidence indicates that the mumps virus infection initiated by the vaccine is not contagious.
The vaccine is indicated for immunization against mumps in children 15 months of age or older, and adults. It may be given as early as 12 months, if that offers greater convenience in scheduling. However, it is not recommended for infants less than 12 months of age because they may retain maternal mumps neutralizing antibodies which may interfere with the immune response.
Recent serologic evidence shows that when M-M-R® (Measles, Mumps and Rubella Virus Vaccine, Live, MSD) is given simultaneously with trivalent oral poliovirus vaccine, antibody responses can be expected to be comparable to those which follow administration of the vaccines at different times. From this it follows that when MUMPSVAX is given simultaneously with either monovalent or trivalent oral poliovirus vaccine, antibody responses can be expected to be comparable to those which follow administration of the vaccines at different times.
Evidence indicates that the vaccine will not offer protection when given after exposure to natural mumps. It has been reported that immune serum globulin (human) in a dosage of .01 to .02 ml/lb did not prevent the antibody response to the live vaccine when the two were administered simultaneously in opposite arms. However, protection afforded with this regimen has not been established.
Revaccination: Based on available evidence, there is no reason to routinely revaccinate children originally vaccinated when 12 months of age or older.

Contraindications

Hypersensitivity to neomycin (each dose of reconstituted vaccine contains approximately 25 micrograms of neomycin).
Individuals with blood dyscrasias, leukemia, lymphomas of any type, or other malignant neoplasms affecting the bone marrow or lymphatic systems.
Patients receiving therapy with ACTH, corticosteroids, irradiation, alkylating agents or antimetabolites.
This contraindication does not apply to patients who are receiving corticosteroids as replacement therapy, e.g., for Addison's disease.
Primary immuno-deficiency states, including cellular immune deficiencies, hypogammaglobulinemic and dysgammaglobulinemic states.
Any active infection is reason for delaying mumps vaccination.

Hypersensitivity to Eggs, Chicken, or Chicken Feathers

Continued on next page

Information on the Merck Sharp & Dohme products listed on these pages is the full prescribing information from package circulars in use October 31, 1979.

Merck Sharp & Dohme—Cont.

This vaccine is essentially devoid of potentially allergenic substances derived from host tissues (chick embryo)*. However, since this vaccine is propagated in cell cultures of chick embryo, in considering its use in patients hypersensitive to eggs, chicken, or chicken feathers, the attending physician must weigh the benefits of immunization against the potential risks of hypersensitivity reactions.

Pregnancy

Do not give MUMPSVAX to pregnant females; the possible effects of the vaccine on fetal development are unknown at this time. When vaccination of post-pubertal females is undertaken, pregnancy at the time of vaccination must be ruled out and in addition, the possibility of pregnancy occurring in the three months following vaccination must be eliminated by medically acceptable methods.

Precautions

For subcutaneous use; *do not give intravenously.*
MUMPSVAX should not be given less than one month before or after immunization with other live virus vaccines, with the exception of ATTENUVAX® (Measles Virus Vaccine, Live, Attenuated, MSD), MERUVAX® (Rubella Virus Vaccine, Live, MSD), and/or monovalent or trivalent poliovirus vaccine, live, oral, which may be administered simultaneously.
Vaccination should be deferred for at least 3 months following blood or plasma transfusions, or administration of more than 0.02 ml of human immune serum globulin per pound of body weight.
It has been reported that mumps virus vaccine, live, may result in a temporary depression of tuberculin skin sensitivity. Therefore, if a tuberculin test is to be done, it should be administered either before or simultaneously with MUMPSVAX.
Epinephrine should be available for immediate use if needed.

Adverse Reactions

Mild fever occurs occasionally. Fever above 103°F is uncommon.
Parotitis has been reported to occur in very low incidence, and orchitis rarely, in persons who were vaccinated. In most instances investigated, prior exposure to natural mumps was established. In other instances, whether or not this was due to vaccine or to prior natural mumps exposure or to other causes has not been established.
Reports of purpura and allergic reactions such as urticaria have been extremely rare.
Very rarely encephalitis and other nervous system reactions have occurred in vaccinees. A cause-effect relationship has not been established.

Shipment, Storage, and Reconstitution

During shipment, to insure that there is no loss of potency, the vaccine must be maintained at a temperature of 10°C (50°F) or less.
Prior to reconstitution, store the vaccine in a refrigerator at 2–8°C (35.6–46.4°F). *Protect from light.*
To reconstitute the vaccine, inject all the diluent in the syringe into the vial of lyophilized vaccine, and agitate to ensure thorough mixing. Draw back entire contents into the syringe and inject total volume of restored vaccine subcutaneously. Each dose of reconstituted vaccine contains not less than 5,000 $TCID_{50}$ (tissue culture infectious doses) of mumps virus vaccine expressed in terms of the assigned titer of the FDA Reference Mumps Virus.
Use only the diluent supplied and reconstitute the vaccine just before using. It is recommended that the vaccine be used as soon as possible after reconstitution. Protect the vaccine from light at all times. Store the reconstituted vaccine in a dark place at 2–8°C (35.6–46.4°F) and discard if not used within 8 hours.
Color: The color of the vaccine when reconstituted is yellow.

Dosage and Administration

After suitably cleansing the immunization site, inject total volume of reconstituted vaccine subcutaneously, preferably into the outer aspect of the upper arm. Do not inject intravenously.
The dosage of vaccine is the same for all patients.

How Supplied

No. 4582X—MUMPSVAX—a single-dose vial of lyophilized vaccine packed with a disposable syringe containing diluent, **NDC** 0006-4582-00. (6505-00-142-9203 Single dose).
No. 4584X/4590—MUMPSVAX—a box of 10 single dose vials of lyophilized vaccine, **NDC** 0006-4584-00; and a box of 10 diluent-containing disposable syringes with affixed 25 gauge, ⅝" needles supplied in an accompanying separate package. To conserve refrigerator space, the syringes may be stored at room temperature.

*Morbidity and Mortality Weekly Report *25*(44): 350, Nov. 12, 1976.

A.H.F.S. 80:12
DC 7075400 Issued October 1978

MUSTARGEN®, Trituration of (mechlorethamine HCl for injection, MSD), U.S.P. ℞

Description

MUSTARGEN (Mechlorethamine HCl, MSD) a nitrogen mustard also known as HN2 hydrochloride, is a nitrogen analog of sulfur mustard. It is a white, crystalline, hygroscopic powder that is very soluble in water and also soluble in alcohol.
MUSTARGEN is designated chemically as 2-chloro- *N*-(2-chloroethyl)- *N*-methylethanamine hydrochloride. The molecular weight is 192.52 and the melting point is 109–110°C. The empirical formula is $C_5H_{11}Cl_2N{\bullet}HCl$, and the structural formula is: $CH_3N(CH_2CH_2Cl)_2{\bullet}HCl$.
Trituration of MUSTARGEN is a white crystalline powder. Each vial of MUSTARGEN contains 10 mg of mechlorethamine hydrochloride triturated with sodium chloride.

Actions

Mechlorethamine, a biologic alkylating agent, has a cytotoxic action which inhibits rapidly proliferating cells.

Indications

Before using MUSTARGEN *see Contraindications, Warnings, Precautions, Adverse Reactions, and Dosage and Administration.*
MUSTARGEN, administered intravenously, is indicated for the palliative treatment of Hodgkin's disease (Stages III and IV), lymphosarcoma, chronic myelocytic or chronic lymphocytic leukemia, polycythemia vera, mycosis fungoides, and bronchogenic carcinoma.
MUSTARGEN, administered intrapleurally, intraperitoneally, or intrapericardially, is indicated for the palliative treatment of metastatic carcinoma resulting in effusion.

Contraindications

Because of the toxicity of MUSTARGEN, and the unpleasant side effects following its use, the potential risk and discomfort from the use of this drug in patients with inoperable neoplasms or in the terminal stage of the disease must be balanced against the limited gain obtainable. These gains will vary with the nature and the status of the disease under treatment.
The routine use of MUSTARGEN in all cases of widely disseminated neoplasms is to be discouraged.
The use of MUSTARGEN in patients with leukopenia, thrombocytopenia, and anemia, due to invasion of the bone marrow by tumor carries a greater risk. In such patients a good response to treatment with disappearance of the tumor from the bone marrow may be associated with improvement of bone marrow function. However, in the absence of a good response or in patients who have been previously treated with chemotherapeutic agents, hematopoiesis may be further compromised, and leukopenia, thrombocytopenia and anemia may become more severe and lead to the demise of the patient.
Tumors of bone and nervous tissue have responded poorly to therapy. Its use is contraindicated in the presence of known infectious diseases. Results are unpredictable in disseminated and malignant tumors of different types.

WARNINGS

Extravasation of the drug into subcutaneous tissues results in a painful inflammation. The area usually becomes indurated and sloughing may occur. If leakage of drug is obvious, prompt infiltration of the area with sterile isotonic sodium thiosulfate (⅙ molar) and application of an ice compress for 6 to 12 hours may minimize the local reaction. For a ⅙ molar solution of sodium thiosulfate, use 4.14 g of sodium thiosulfate per 100 ml of Sterile Water for Injection or 2.64 g of anhydrous sodium thiosulfate per 100 ml, or dilute 4 ml of Sodium Thiosulfate Injection U.S.P. (10%) with 6 ml of Sterile Water for Injection U.S.P.

Before using MUSTARGEN, *an accurate histologic diagnosis of the disease, a knowledge of its natural course, and an adequate clinical history are important. The hematologic status of the patient must first be determined. It is essential to understand the hazards and therapeutic effects to be expected. Careful clinical judgment must be exercised in selecting patients. If the indication for its use is not clear, the drug should not be used.*
As nitrogen mustard therapy may contribute to extensive and rapid development of amyloidosis, it should be used only if foci of acute and chronic suppurative inflammation are absent.
Usage in Pregnancy
There is evidence that the nitrogen mustards have induced fetal abnormalities particularly when used early in pregnancy. The possible benefits of administration of MUSTARGEN in women of childbearing potential must be weighed against the considered risks; patients should be apprised of the risks involved. In pregnant patients requiring treatment for a life-threatening progressive tumor, use of MUSTARGEN should be avoided at least until the third trimester.

Precautions

This drug is highly toxic and both powder and solution must be handled and administered with care. Since MUSTARGEN is a powerful vesicant, it is intended primarily for intravenous use, and in most instances is given by this route. Inhalation of dust or vapors and contact with skin or mucous membranes, especially that of the eyes, must be avoided. Should accidental eye contact occur, copious irrigation with normal saline or a balanced salt ophthalmic irrigating solution should be instituted immediately, followed by prompt ophthalmologic consultation. Should accidental skin contact occur, the affected part must be irrigated immediately with copious amounts of water, for at least 15 minutes, followed by 2 percent sodium thiosulfate solution. (See also box warning.)

Do not use if the solution is discolored or if droplets of water are visible within the vial. Prepare fresh solution for injection and dispose of the unused portion after neutralization. (See DOSAGE AND ADMINISTRATION.)

Precautions must be observed with the use of MUSTARGEN and x-ray therapy or other chemotherapy in alternating courses. Hematopoietic function is characteristically depressed by either form of therapy, and neither MUSTARGEN following x-ray therapy nor x-ray therapy subsequent to the drug should be given until bone marrow function has recovered. In particular, irradiation of such areas as sternum, ribs, and vertebrae shortly after a course of nitrogen mustard may lead to hematologic complications.

Therapy with alkylating agents such as MUSTARGEN may be associated with an increased incidence of a second malignant tumor, especially when such therapy is combined with other antineoplastic agents or radiation therapy.

Hyperuricemia may develop during therapy with MUSTARGEN. The problem of urate precipitation should be anticipated, particularly in the treatment of the lymphomas, and adequate methods for control of hyperuricemia should be instituted and careful attention directed toward adequate fluid intake before treatment.

Since drug toxicity, especially sensitivity to bone marrow failure, seems to be more common in chronic lymphatic leukemia than in other conditions, the drug should be given in this condition with great caution, if at all.

Adverse Reactions

Clinical use of MUSTARGEN *usually is accompanied by toxic manifestations.*

Local Toxicity

Thrombosis and thrombophlebitis may result from direct contact of the drug with the intima of the injected vein. Avoid high concentration and prolonged contact with the drug, especially in cases of elevated pressure in the antebrachial vein (e.g., in mediastinal tumor compression from severe vena cava syndrome).

Systemic Toxicity

Nausea, vomiting and depression of formed elements in the circulating blood are dose-limiting side effects and usually occur with the use of full doses of MUSTARGEN. Jaundice, alopecia, vertigo, tinnitus and diminished hearing may occur infrequently. Rarely, hemolytic anemia associated with such diseases as the lymphomas and chronic lymphocytic leukemia may be precipitated by treatment with alkylating agents including MUSTARGEN. Also, various chromosomal abnormalities have been reported in association with nitrogen mustard therapy.

MUSTARGEN is given preferably at night in case sedation for side effects is required. Nausea and vomiting usually occur 1 to 3 hours after use of the drug. Emesis may disappear in the first 8 hours, but nausea may persist for 24 hours. Nausea and vomiting may be so severe as to precipitate vascular accidents in patients with a hemorrhagic tendency. Premedication with antiemetics, in addition to sedatives, may help control severe nausea and vomiting. Anorexia, weakness and diarrhea may also occur.

The usual course of MUSTARGEN (total dose of 0.4 mg/kg either given as a single intravenous dose or divided into two or four daily doses of 0.2 or 0.1 mg/kg respectively) generally produces a lymphocytopenia within 24 hours after the first injection; significant granulocytopenia occurs within 6 to 8 days and lasts for 10 days to 3 weeks. Agranulocytosis appears to be relatively infrequent and recovery from leukopenia in most cases is complete within two weeks of the maximum reduction. Thrombocytopenia is variable but the time course of the appearance and recovery from reduced platelet counts generally parallels the sequence of granulocyte levels. In some cases severe thrombocytopenia may lead to bleeding from the gums and gastrointestinal tract, petechiae, and small subcutaneous hemorrhages; these symptoms appear to be transient and in most cases disappear with return to a normal platelet count. However, a severe and even uncontrollable depression of the hematopoietic system occasionally may follow the usual dose of MUSTARGEN, particularly in patients with widespread disease and debility and in patients previously treated with other antineoplastic agents or x-ray. Persistent pancytopenia has been reported. In rare instances, hemorrhagic complications may be due to hyperheparinemia. Erythrocyte and hemoglobin levels may decline during the first 2 weeks after therapy but rarely significantly. Depression of the hematopoietic system may be found up to 50 days or more after starting therapy.

MUSTARGEN has been reported to have immunosuppressive activity. Therefore, it should be borne in mind that use of the drug may predispose the patient to bacterial, viral or fungal infection. This is more likely to occur when concomitant steroid therapy is employed.

Occasionally, a maculopapular skin eruption occurs, but this may be idiosyncratic and does not necessarily recur with subsequent courses of the drug. In one patient erythema multiforme has been observed. Herpes zoster, a common complicating infection in patients with lymphomas, may first appear after therapy is instituted and on occasion may be precipitated by treatment. Further treatment should be discontinued during the acute phase of this illness to avoid progression to generalized herpes zoster.

Since the gonads are susceptible to MUSTARGEN, treatment may be followed by delayed catamenia, oligomenorrhea, or temporary or permanent amenorrhea. Impaired spermatogenesis, azoospermia, and total germinal aplasia have been reported in male patients treated with alkylating agents, especially in combination with other drugs. In some instances spermatogenesis may return in patients in remission, but this may occur only several years after intensive chemotherapy has been discontinued. Patients should be warned of the potential risk to their reproductive capacity.

With total doses exceeding 0.4 mg/kg of body weight for a single course, severe leukopenia, anemia, thrombocytopenia and a hemorrhagic diathesis with subsequent delayed bleeding may develop. Death may follow. The only treatment in instances of excessive dosage appears to be repeated blood product transfusions, antibiotic treatment of complicating infections and general supportive measures. *Extreme caution must be used in exceeding the average recommended dose.*

Dosage and Administration

Intravenous Administration

The dosage of MUSTARGEN varies with the clinical situation, the therapeutic response and the magnitude of hematologic depression. A total dose of 0.4 mg/kg of body weight for each course usually is given either as a single dose or in divided doses of 0.1 to 0.2 mg/kg per day. Dosage should be based on ideal dry body weight. The presence of edema or ascites must be considered so that dosage will be based on actual weight unaugmented by these conditions.

Within a few minutes after intravenous injection, MUSTARGEN undergoes chemical transformation, combines with reactive compounds, and is no longer present in its active form in the blood stream. Subsequent courses should not be given until the patient has recovered hematologically from the previous course; this is best determined by repeated studies of the peripheral blood elements awaiting their return to normal levels. It is often possible to give repeated courses of MUSTARGEN as early as three weeks after treatment.

The margin of safety in therapy with MUSTARGEN *is narrow and considerable care must be exercised in the matter of dosage.* Repeated examinations of blood are *mandatory* as a guide to subsequent therapy.

Preparation of Solution and Intravenous Administration

Each vial of MUSTARGEN contains 10 mg of mechlorethamine hydrochloride triturated with sodium chloride q.s. 100 mg. In neutral or alkaline aqueous solution it undergoes rapid chemical transformation and is highly unstable. Although solutions prepared according to instructions are acidic and do not decompose as rapidly, they should be prepared immediately before each injection since they will decompose on standing.

Using a sterile 10 ml syringe, inject 10 ml of Sterile Water for Injection or 10 ml Sodium Chloride Injection into a vial of MUSTARGEN. With the needle still in the rubber stopper, shake the vial several times to dissolve the drug completely. The resultant solution contains 1 mg of mechlorethamine hydrochloride per ml.

Withdraw into the syringe the calculated volume of solution required for a single injection. *Dispose of any remaining solution after neutralization* (see below). Although the drug may be injected directly into any suitable vein, it is injected preferably into the rubber or plastic tubing of a flowing intravenous infusion set. This reduces the possibility of severe local reactions due to extravasation or high concentration of the drug. Injecting the drug into the tubing rather than adding it to the entire volume of the infusion fluid minimizes a chemical reaction between the drug and the solution. The rate of injection apparently is not critical provided it is completed within a few minutes.

Intracavitary Administration

Nitrogen mustard has been used by intracavitary administration with varying success in certain malignant conditions for the control of pleural, peritoneal, and pericardial effusions caused by malignant cells.

The technic and the dose used by any of these routes varies. Therefore, if MUSTARGEN is given by the intracavitary route, the published articles concerning such use should be consulted. *Because of the inherent risks involved, the physician should be experienced in the appropriate injection technics, and be thoroughly aware of the indications, dosages, hazards, and precautions as set forth in the published literature. When using* MUSTARGEN *by the intracavitary route, the general precautions concerning this agent should be borne in mind.*

As a general guide, reference is made especially to the technics of Weisberger et al. Intracavitary use is indicated in the presence of pleural, peritoneal, or pericardial effusion due to metastatic tumors. Local therapy with nitrogen mustard is used only when malignant cells

Continued on next page

Information on the Merck Sharp & Dohme products listed on these pages is the full prescribing information from package circulars in use October 31, 1979.

are demonstrated in the effusion. Intracavitary injection is not recommended when the accumulated fluid is chylous in nature, since results are likely to be poor.
Paracentesis is first performed with most of the fluid being removed from the pleural or peritoneal cavity. The intracavitary use of MUSTARGEN may exert at least some of its effect through production of a chemical poudrage. Therefore, the removal of excess fluid allows the drug to more easily contact the peritoneal and pleural linings. For intrapleural or intrapericardial injection nitrogen mustard is introduced directly through the thoracentesis needle. For intraperitoneal injection it is given through a rubber catheter inserted into the trocar used for paracentesis or through a No. 18 gauge needle inserted at another site. This drug should be injected slowly, with frequent aspiration to ensure that a free flow of fluid is present. If fluid cannot be aspirated, pain and necrosis due to injection of solution outside the cavity may occur. Free flow of fluid also is necessary to prevent injection into a loculated pocket and to ensure adequate dissemination of nitrogen mustard.
The usual dose of nitrogen mustard for intracavitary injection is 0.4 mg/kg of body weight, though 0.2 mg/kg (or 10 to 20 mg) has been used by the intrapericardial route. The solution is prepared, as previously described for intravenous injection, by adding 10 ml of Sterile Water for Injection or 10 ml of Sodium Chloride Injection to the vial containing 10 mg of mechlorethamine hydrochloride. (Amounts of diluent of 50 to 100 ml of normal saline have also been used.) The position of the patient should be changed every 5 to 10 minutes for an hour after injection to obtain more uniform distribution of the drug throughout the serous cavity. The remaining fluid may be removed from the pleural or peritoneal cavity by paracentesis 24 to 36 hours later. The patient should be followed carefully by clinical and x-ray examination to detect reaccumulation of fluid.
Pain occurs rarely with intrapleural use; it is common with intraperitoneal injection and is often associated with nausea, vomiting, and diarrhea of 2 to 3 days duration. Transient cardiac irregularities may occur with intrapericardial injection. Death, possibly accelerated by nitrogen mustard, has been reported following the use of this agent by the intracavitary route. Although absorption of MUSTARGEN when given by the intracavitary route is probably not complete because of its rapid deactivation by body fluids, the systemic effect is unpredictable. The acute side effects such as nausea and vomiting are usually mild. Bone marrow depression is generally milder than when the drug is given intravenously. Care should be taken to avoid use by the intracavitary route when other agents which may suppress bone marrow function are being used systemically.
Neutralization of Equipment and Unused Solution
To clean rubber gloves, tubing, glassware, etc., after giving MUSTARGEN, soak them in an aqueous solution containing equal volumes of sodium thiosulfate (5%) and sodium bicarbonate (5%) for 45 minutes. Excess reagents and reaction products are washed away easily with water. Any unused injection solution should be neutralized by mixing with an equal volume of sodium thiosulfate/sodium bicarbonate solution. Allow the mixture to stand for 45 minutes. Vials that have contained MUSTARGEN should be treated in the same way with thiosulfate/bicarbonate solution before disposal.

How Supplied

No. 7753—Trituration of MUSTARGEN is a white crystalline powder, each vial containing 10 mg mechlorethamine hydrochloride with sodium chloride q.s. 100 mg, and is supplied as follows:
NDC 0006-7753-31 in treatment sets of 4 vials.
A.H.F.S. 10:00
DC 6382422 Issued November 1977

MYOCHRYSINE® Injection ℞
(gold sodium thiomalate, MSD), U.S.P.

Description

MYOCHRYSINE (Gold Sodium Thiomalate, MSD) is a sterile aqueous solution of gold sodium thiomalate, prepared for intramuscular injection. It contains 0.5 percent benzyl alcohol as a preservative.
Gold sodium thiomalate is [mercaptobutanedioato(1-)] gold, disodium salt, monohydrate.
The molecular weight is 408.1. The gold content of gold sodium thiomalate is approximately 50 percent. It is a white to yellowish white powder, very soluble in water. The pH of a 1 in 10 solution is about 6.

Actions

The mode of action of gold sodium thiomalate is unknown. The predominant action appears to be a suppressive effect on the synovitis of active rheumatoid disease.

Indications

MYOCHRYSINE is indicated in the treatment of selected cases of active rheumatoid arthritis—both adult and juvenile type. The greatest benefit occurs in the early active stage. In late stages of the illness when cartilage and bone damage have occurred, gold can only check the progression of rheumatoid arthritis and prevent further structural damage to joints. It cannot repair damage caused by previously active disease.
MYOCHRYSINE should be used only as *one part* of a complete program of therapy; alone it is not a complete treatment.

Contraindications

Severe toxicity resulting from previous exposure to gold or other heavy metals.
Severe debilitation.
Systemic lupus erythematosus.
Sjögren's syndrome in rheumatoid arthritis.
Usage in Pregnancy
MYOCHRYSINE has been shown to be teratogenic in rats and rabbits. Therefore, MYOCHRYSINE should be used in patients who are pregnant or in women of childbearing potential only when the expected benefits outweigh the possible hazards.

Warnings

Physicians planning to use MYOCHRYSINE *should thoroughly familiarize themselves with its toxicity and its benefits. The possibility of toxic reactions should always be explained to the patient before starting therapy. Patients should be warned to promptly report any symptoms suggesting toxicity. Before each injection of* MYOCHRYSINE, *the physician should see the patient to determine the presence or absence of adverse reactions.*
Before treatment is started, the patient's hemoglobin, erythrocyte, white blood cell, differential and platelet counts should be determined, and urinalysis should be done to serve as basic reference. Urine should be analyzed for protein and sediment changes prior to each injection. Complete blood counts including platelet estimation should be made before every second injection throughout treatment. Purpura or ecchymoses at any time always require a platelet count.
Rapid reduction of hemoglobin, leukopenia below 4000 WBC/cu ml, eosinophilia above 5 percent, platelet decrease below 100,000/cu ml, albuminuria, hematuria, pruritus, skin eruption or stomatitis are to be considered danger signals of possible gold toxicity. No additional injections of MYOCHRYSINE should be given unless further studies show these abnormalities to be caused by conditions other than gold toxicity.
Diabetes mellitus or congestive heart failure should be under control before gold therapy is instituted.
Extreme caution is indicated in the use of MYOCHRYSINE in patients with the following:
1. a history of blood dyscrasias such as granulocytopenia or anemia caused by drug sensitivity,
2. allergy or hypersensitivity to medications,
3. skin rash,
4. previous kidney or liver disease,
5. marked hypertension,
6. compromised cerebral or cardiovascular circulation.

Renal adenomas have been reported in long-term toxicity studies of rats receiving MYOCHRYSINE at high dose levels (2 mg/kg weekly for 45 weeks, followed by 6 mg/kg daily for 47 weeks). These adenomas are histologically similar to those produced in rats by chronic administration of experimental gold compounds and other heavy metals, such as lead. No reports have been received of renal adenomas in man in association with the use of MYOCHRYSINE.

Adverse Reactions

A variety of adverse reactions may develop during the initial phase (weekly injections) of therapy or during maintenance treatment. Adverse reactions are observed most frequently when the cumulative dose of MYOCHRYSINE administered is between 400 and 800 mg. Very uncommonly, complications occur days to months after cessation of treatment.
Cutaneous reactions: Dermatitis is the most common reaction. *Any eruption, especially if pruritic, that develops during treatment with* MYOCHRYSINE *should be considered a reaction to gold until proven otherwise.* Pruritus often exists before dermatitis becomes apparent, and therefore should be considered a warning signal of impending cutaneous reaction. The most serious form of cutaneous reaction is generalized exfoliative dermatitis which may lead to alopecia and shedding of nails. Gold dermatitis may be aggravated by exposure to sunlight or an actinic rash may develop.
Mucous membrane reactions: Stomatitis is the second most common adverse reaction. Shallow ulcers on the buccal membranes, on the borders of the tongue, and on the palate or in the pharynx may occur as the only adverse reaction, or along with dermatitis. Sometimes diffuse glossitis or gingivitis develops. A metallic taste may precede these oral mucous membrane reactions and should be considered a warning signal.
Conjunctivitis is a rare reaction.
Renal reactions: Gold may be toxic to the kidney and produce a nephrotic syndrome or glomerulitis with hematuria. These renal reactions are usually relatively mild and subside completely if recognized early and treatment is discontinued. They may become severe and chronic if treatment is continued after onset of the reaction. Therefore, it is important to perform a *urinalysis before every injection,* and to discontinue treatment promptly if proteinuria or hematuria develops.
Hematologic reactions: Blood dyscrasia due to gold toxicity is rare, but because of the potential serious consequences it must be constantly

watched for and recognized early by frequent blood examinations done throughout treatment. Granulocytopenia; thrombocytopenia, with or without purpura; hypoplastic and aplastic anemia have all been reported. These hematologic disorders may occur separately or in combinations.

Nitritoid and allergic reactions: Reactions of the "nitritoid type" which may resemble anaphylactoid effects have been reported. Flushing, fainting, dizziness and sweating are most frequently reported. Other symptoms that may occur include: nausea, vomiting, malaise and weakness.

More severe, but less common effects include: anaphylactic shock, syncope, bradycardia, thickening of the tongue, difficulty in swallowing and breathing, and angioneurotic edema. These effects may occur almost immediately after injection or as late as 10 minutes following injection. They may occur at any time during the course of therapy and if observed, discontinue treatment with MYOCHRYSINE.

Miscellaneous reactions: Gastrointestinal reactions have been reported, including nausea, vomiting, anorexia, abdominal cramps, diarrhea, and ulcerative enterocolitis. Some of these reactions can be severe or even fatal.

There have been rare reports of reactions involving the eye such as iritis, corneal ulcers, and gold deposits in ocular tissues.

Hepatitis with jaundice, peripheral neuritis, gold bronchitis, pulmonary injury manifested by interstitial pneumonitis and fibrosis, partial or complete hair loss and fever have also been reported.

Sometimes arthralgia occurs for a day or two after an injection of MYOCHRYSINE; this reaction usually subsides after the first few injections.

Management of Adverse Reactions

Treatment with MYOCHRYSINE should be discontinued immediately when toxic reactions occur. Minor complications such as localized dermatitis, mild stomatitis, or slight proteinuria generally require no other therapy and resolve spontaneously with suspension of MYOCHRYSINE. Moderately severe skin and mucous membrane reactions often benefit from topical corticosteroids, oral antihistaminics, and soothing or anesthetic lotions.

If stomatitis or dermatitis becomes severe or more generalized, systemic corticosteroids (generally, 10 to 40 mg prednisone daily in divided doses) may provide symptomatic relief.

For serious renal, hematologic, pulmonary, and enterocolitic complications, high doses of systemic corticosteroids (40 to 100 mg prednisone daily in divided doses) are recommended. The optimum duration of corticosteroid treatment varies with the response of the individual patient. Therapy may be required for many months when adverse effects are unusually severe or progressive.

In patients whose complications do not improve with high-dose corticosteroid treatment, or who develop significant steroid-related adverse reactions, a chelating agent may be given to enhance gold excretion. Dimercaprol (BAL) has been used successfully, but patients must be monitored carefully as numerous untoward reactions may attend its use. Corticosteroids and a chelating agent may be used concomitantly.

MYOCHRYSINE *should not be reinstituted after severe or idiosyncratic reactions.*

MYOCHRYSINE may be readministered following resolution of mild reactions, using a reduced dosage schedule. If an initial test dose of 5 mg MYOCHRYSINE is well-tolerated, progressively larger doses (5 to 10 mg increments) may be given at weekly to monthly intervals until a dose of 25 to 50 mg is reached.

Dosage and Administration

MYOCHRYSINE should be administered only by intramuscular injection, preferably intragluteally. It should be given with the patient lying down. He should remain recumbent for approximately 10 minutes after the injection. Therapeutic effects from MYOCHRYSINE occur slowly. Early improvement, often limited to a reduction in morning stiffness, may begin after six to eight weeks of treatment, but beneficial effects may not be observed until after months of therapy.

Do not use if material has darkened. Color should not exceed pale yellow.

For the adult of average size the following dosage schedule is suggested:

Weekly Injections

1st injection	10 mg
2nd injection	25 mg

3rd and subsequent injections, 25 to 50 mg until there is toxicity or major clinical improvement, or, in the absence of either of these, the cumulative dose of MYOCHRYSINE reaches one gram.

MYOCHRYSINE is continued until the cumulative dose reaches one gram unless toxicity or major clinical improvement occurs. If significant clinical improvement occurs before a cumulative dose of one gram has been administered, the dose may be decreased or the interval between injections increased as with maintenance therapy. Maintenance doses of 25 to 50 mg every other week for two to 20 weeks are recommended. If the clinical course remains stable, injections of 25 to 50 mg may be given every third and subsequently every fourth week indefinitely. Some patients may require maintenance treatment at intervals of one to three weeks. Should the arthritis exacerbate during maintenance therapy, weekly injections may be resumed temporarily until disease activity is suppressed.

Should a patient fail to improve during initial therapy (cumulative dose of one gram), several options are available:

1— the patient may be considered to be unresponsive and MYOCHRYSINE is discontinued
2— the same dose (25 to 50 mg) of MYOCHRYSINE may be continued for approximately ten additional weeks
3— the dose of MYOCHRYSINE may be increased by increments of 10 mg every one to four weeks, not to exceed 100 mg in a single injection.

If significant clinical improvement occurs using option 2 or 3, the maintenance schedule described above should be initiated. If there is no significant improvement or if toxicity occurs, therapy with MYOCHRYSINE should be stopped. The higher the individual dose of MYOCHRYSINE, the greater the risk of gold toxicity. Selection of one of these options for chrysotherapy should be based upon a number of factors, including the physician's experience with gold salt therapy, the course of the patient's condition, the choice of alternative treatments, and the availability of the patient for the close supervision required.

Juvenile Rheumatoid Arthritis

The pediatric dose of MYOCHRYSINE is proportional to the adult dose on a weight basis. After the initial test dose of 10 mg, the recommended dose for children is one mg per kilogram body weight, not to exceed 50 mg for a single injection. Otherwise, the guidelines given above for administration to adults also apply to children.

How Supplied

Injection MYOCHRYSINE, a clear light yellow to yellow solution, is supplied as follows:

No. 7763—10 mg of gold sodium thiomalate per ml as
NDC 0006-7763-64 in boxes of 6 × 1 ml ampuls.

No. 7764—25 mg of gold sodium thiomalate per ml as
NDC 0006-7764-64 in boxes of 6 × 1 ml ampuls.

No. 7762—50 mg of gold sodium thiomalate per ml as
NDC 0006-7762-64 in boxes of 6 × 1 ml ampuls
NDC 0006-7762-10 in 10 ml vials.

No. 7761—100 mg of gold sodium thiomalate per ml as
NDC 0006-7761-64 in boxes of 6 × 1 ml ampuls.

A.H.F.S. 60:00
DC 6015518 Issued March 1979

PERIACTIN® Tablets ℞
(cyproheptadine HCl, MSD), N.F.
PERIACTIN® Syrup ℞
(cyproheptadine HCl, MSD), N.F.

Description

Cyproheptadine hydrochloride is a white to slightly yellowish, crystalline solid. It is the sesquihydrate of 4-(5*H*-dibenzo[*a,d*]cyclohepten-5-ylidene)-1-methylpiperidine hydrochloride. The empirical formula of the anhydrous salt is $C_{21}H_{21}N \cdot HCl$.

Actions

PERIACTIN (Cyproheptadine HCl, MSD) is a serotonin and histamine antagonist with anticholinergic and sedative effects.

Antiserotonin and antihistamine drugs appear to compete with serotonin and histamine, respectively, for receptor sites.

Indications

Perennial and seasonal allergic rhinitis
Vasomotor rhinitis
Allergic conjunctivitis due to inhalant allergens and foods
Mild, uncomplicated allergic skin manifestations of urticaria and angioedema
Amelioration of allergic reactions to blood or plasma
Cold urticaria
Dermatographism
As therapy for anaphylactic reactions *adjunctive* to epinephrine and other standard measures after the acute manifestations have been controlled

Contraindications

Newborn or Premature Infants
This drug should *not* be used in newborn or premature infants.

Nursing Mothers
Because of the higher risk of antihistamines for infants generally and for newborns and prematures in particular, antihistamine therapy is contraindicated in nursing mothers.

Lower Respiratory Disease
Antihistamines should not be used to treat lower respiratory tract symptoms including asthma.

Other Conditions
Hypersensitivity to cyproheptadine and other drugs of similar chemical structure:
Monoamine oxidase inhibitor therapy (see DRUG INTERACTIONS)
Angle-closure glaucoma
Stenosing peptic ulcer
Symptomatic prostatic hypertrophy
Bladder neck obstruction

Continued on next page

Information on the Merck Sharp & Dohme products listed on these pages is the full prescribing information from package circulars in use October 31, 1979.

Merck Sharp & Dohme—Cont.

Pyloroduodenal obstruction
Elderly, debilitated patients

Warnings

Children
Overdosage of antihistamines, particularly in infants and children, may produce hallucinations, central nervous system depression, convulsions, and death.
Antihistamines may diminish mental alertness; conversely, particularly, in the young child, they may occasionally produce excitation.
Pregnancy
The use of any drug in pregnancy or in women of childbearing potential requires that the anticipated benefit be weighed against possible hazards to the embryo or fetus.
CNS Depressants
Antihistamines may have additive effects with alcohol and other CNS depressants, e.g., hypnotics, sedatives, tranquilizers, antianxiety agents.
Activities Requiring Mental Alertness
Patients should be warned about engaging in activities requiring mental alertness and motor coordination, such as driving a car or operating machinery.
Antihistamines are more likely to cause dizziness, sedation, and hypotension in elderly patients.

Precautions

Cyproheptadine has an atropine-like action and, therefore, should be used with caution in patients with:
History of bronchial asthma
Increased intraocular pressure
Hyperthyroidism
Cardiovascular disease
Hypertension

Drug Interactions

MAO Inhibitors prolong and intensify the anticholinergic effects of antihistamines.

Adverse Reactions

The most frequent adverse reactions to antihistamines are:
Sedation and sleepiness (often transient); dryness of mouth, nose, and throat; thickening of bronchial secretions, dizziness, epigastric distress, disturbed coordination.
Other adverse reactions which may occur with antihistamines:
Fatigue, confusion, restlessness, excitation, nervousness, tremor, irritability, paresthesias, acute labyrinthitis, hysteria, neuritis, convulsions, excessive perspiration, chills, hallucinations, insomnia, euphoria, anorexia, nausea, vomiting, diarrhea, constipation, faintness, hypotension, extrasystoles, tightness of chest and wheezing, urticaria, allergic manifestations of rash and edema, anaphylactic shock, blurred vision, diplopia, vertigo, tinnitus, headache, palpitation, tachycardia, nasal stuffiness, urinary frequency, difficult urination, urinary retention, early menses, photosensitivity, hemolytic anemia, leukopenia, agranulocytosis, thrombocytopenia.

Management of Overdosage

Antihistamine overdosage reactions may vary from central nervous system depression to stimulation especially in children. Also, atropine-like signs and symptoms (dry mouth; fixed, dilated pupils; flushing, etc.) as well as gastrointestinal symptoms may occur.
If vomiting has not occurred spontaneously the patient should be induced to vomit. This is best done by having him drink a glass of water after which he should be made to gag. Precautions against aspiration must be taken especially in infants and children.
If patient is unable to vomit, gastric lavage is indicated. Isotonic or ½ isotonic saline is the lavage of choice.
Saline cathartics, as milk of magnesia, by osmosis draw water into the bowel and, therefore, are valuable for their action in rapid dilution of bowel content.
Stimulants should *not* be used.
Vasopressors may be used to treat hypotension.

Dosage and Administration

DOSAGE SHOULD BE INDIVIDUALIZED ACCORDING TO THE NEEDS AND THE RESPONSE OF THE PATIENT.
Each PERIACTIN tablet contains 4 mg of cyproheptadine hydrochloride. Each 5 ml of PERIACTIN syrup contains 2 mg of cyproheptadine hydrochloride.
Although intended primarily for administration to children, the syrup is also useful for administration to adults who cannot swallow tablets.
Children
The total daily dosage for children may be calculated on the basis of body weight or body area using approximately 0.25 mg/kg/day (0.11 mg/lb/day) or 8 mg per square meter of body surface (8 mg/M^2). In small children for whom the calculation of dosage based upon body size is most important, it may be necessary to use PERIACTIN syrup to permit accurate dosage.
Age 2 to 6 years
The usual dose is 2 mg (½ tablet or 1 teaspoon) two or three times a day, adjusted as necessary to the size and response of the patient. The dose is not to exceed 12 mg a day.
Age 7 to 14 years
The usual dose is 4 mg (1 tablet or 2 teaspoons) two or three times a day, adjusted as necessary to the size and response of the patient. The dose is not to exceed 16 mg a day.
Adults
The total daily dose for adults should not exceed 0.5 mg/kg/day (0.23 mg/lb/day).
The therapeutic range is 4 to 20 mg a day, with the majority of patients requiring 12 to 16 mg a day. An occasional patient may require as much as 32 mg a day for adequate relief. It is suggested that dosage be initiated with 4 mg (1 tablet or 2 teaspoons) three times a day and adjusted according to the size and response of the patient.

How Supplied

No. 3276—Tablets PERIACTIN, containing 4 mg of cyproheptadine hydrochloride each, are white, round, scored compressed tablets, coded MSD 62. They are supplied as follows:
NDC 0006-0062-68 bottles of 100.
(6505-00-890-1884 4 mg 100's)
[*Shown in Product Identification Section*]
No. 3289X—Syrup PERIACTIN, 2 mg per 5 ml is a clear, yellow, syrupy liquid. Contains alcohol 5%, with sorbic acid 0.1% added as preservative and is supplied as follows:
NDC 0006-3289-74 bottles of 473 ml.
A.H.F.S. 4:00
DC 6589611 Issued August 1978

PNEUMOVAX® ℞
(pneumococcal vaccine, polyvalent, MSD)

Description

PNEUMOVAX (Pneumococcal Vaccine, Polyvalent, MSD), is derived from the capsules of cultured pneumococci. This vaccine is indicated for immunization against infections caused by pneumococci. The vaccine affords protection against the 14 most prevalent or invasive capsular types accounting for at least 80% of pneumococcal disease isolates as determined by on-going surveillance. Protective capsular type-specific antibody levels develop by the third week following vaccination.
PNEUMOVAX consists of polysaccharides isolated from the capsules of bacteria of the individual types and is manufactured according to methods developed by the MERCK SHARP & DOHME Research Laboratories. The vaccine is formulated so that each 0.5 ml dose contains 50 μg of each polysaccharide type dissolved in isotonic saline solution containing phenol 0.25% added as preservative.

14 Pneumococcal Capsular Types Included in PNEUMOVAX

Nomenclature	Pneumococcal Types						
U.S.	1	2	3	4	6	8	9
	12	14	19	23	25	51	56
Danish	1	2	3	4	6A	8	9N
	12F	14	19F	23F	25	7F	18C

Actions

Pneumococcal infection is a leading cause of death throughout the world and a major cause of pneumonia, meningitis, and otitis media. The exact incidence of pneumococcal infection is not known. On the basis of the limited epidemiological data obtained from studies in municipal hospitals where the incidence might be higher than that found in the average population, it is estimated that there are annually 200,000 to 1,000,000 cases of pneumococcal pneumonia in the United States, and between 13,200 and 66,000 deaths resulting therefrom. Thus, the attack rate for pneumococcal pneumonia is estimated to be between 1 and 5 cases per 1,000 persons per year, and death is estimated to occur in about 1 of 15 cases. Based on these same data, about 25% of all persons with pneumococcal pneumonia develop bacteremia. Death occurs in about 28% of these bacteremic patients more than 50 years of age.
In the United States, pneumococcal meningitis occurs principally in young children, with annual rates of about 3 to 11 per 100,000 children less than 5 years old. Within the first two years of life, about 15 to 20% of all children develop otitis media caused by pneumococci, and 50% of all children develop such illness within the first 10 years of life (see under INDICATIONS).
Invasive pneumococcal disease causes high morbidity and mortality in spite of effective antimicrobial control by antibiotics. These effects of pneumococcal disease appear due to irreversible physiologic damage caused by the bacteria during the first 5 days following onset of illness, and irrespective of antimicrobial therapy. Older persons, individuals with chronic debilitating diseases, and persons with absent or impaired splenic function, including those with homozygous sickle cell anemia and sickle thalassemia, are especially susceptible to severe pneumococcal disease.
Presently, there are 83 known pneumococcal capsular types. However, the preponderance of pneumococcal disease is caused by only some capsular types. For example, a 10-year (1952–1962) surveillance at a New York medical center showed that 56% of all deaths due to pneumococcal pneumonia were caused by 6 capsular types and that approximately 78% of all pneumococcal pneumonias were caused by 12 capsular types. Such unequal distribution of pneumococcal capsular types causing disease has been shown throughout the world. It is on the basis of this information that the pneumococcal vaccine is composed of 14 capsular types.
It has been established that the purified pneumococcal capsular polysaccharides induce antibody production and that such antibody is effective in preventing pneumococcal disease.
PNEUMOVAX consists of 14 different capsular polysaccharides which represent at least 80% of pneumococcal disease isolates in the U.S.A. and Europe. Studies in humans have demonstrated the immunogenicity (antibody-

stimulating capability) of each of the 14 capsular types when tested in polyvalent vaccines. Adults of all ages and children of 2 years of age or older responded immunologically to the vaccines. In a recent study of PNEUMOVAX, at least 90% of all adults showed a fourfold or greater increase in type-specific antibody for each vaccine capsular type.

The protective efficacy of pneumococcal vaccines containing 6 and 12 capsular polysaccharides was investigated in controlled studies of gold miners in South Africa, in whom there is a high attack rate for pneumococcal pneumonia. Capsular type-specific attack rates for pneumococcal pneumonia were observed for the period from 2 weeks through about 1 year after vaccination. The rates for pneumonia caused by the same capsular types represented in the vaccines are given in the table. Protective efficacy was 76% and 92%, respectively, in the two studies for the capsular types represented. [See table above].

Number of Capsular Types in Pneumococcal Vaccine	Rate/1000 for Pneumonia Caused by Homologous Capsular Types: Vaccinated Group	Control Group	Protective Efficacy
6	9.2	38.3	76%
12	1.4	16.7	92%

In similar studies carried out by Dr. R. Austrian and associates using similar pneumococcal vaccines, prepared for the National Institute of Allergy and Infectious Diseases by a different source, the reduction in pneumonias caused by the vaccine capsular types was 79%. Type-specific reduction in pneumococcal bacteremia was 82%. A preliminary report suggests efficacy of the vaccine in persons over two years of age in preventing severe pneumococcal disease and bacteremia in patients with sickle cell anemia and in individuals without spleens or those who have impaired splenic function.

The duration of protective effect of PNEUMOVAX is presently unknown, but it has been shown in previous studies with other pneumococcal vaccines that antibody induced by the vaccine may persist for as long as 5 years. Type-specific antibody levels induced by PNEUMOVAX have been observed to decline over a 20-month period of observation, but remain significantly above prevaccination levels in almost all recipients who manifest an initial response.

Because of the decline in antibody levels, revaccination may be considered. Available data suggest that revaccination should not be carried out at less than 3-year intervals so as to minimize the frequency and severity of local reactions, especially in persons who have retained high antibody levels. Long-term surveillance of antibody levels in immunized individuals is continuing.

Indications

PNEUMOVAX is indicated for immunization against lobar pneumonia and bacteremia, caused by those types of pneumococci included in the vaccine, in all persons two years of age or older in whom there is an increased risk of morbidity and mortality from pneumococcal pneumonia. These include: (1) persons having chronic physical conditions such as chronic heart disease of any etiology, chronic bronchopulmonary diseases, chronic renal failure, and diabetes mellitus or other chronic metabolic disorders; (2) persons in chronic care facilities; (3) persons convalescing from severe disease; (4) persons 50 years of age or older.

Preliminary data suggest the vaccine is efficacious for preventing severe pneumonic disease and bacteremia in persons over two years of age with sickle cell anemia and in individuals who have had a splenectomy or who have impaired splenic function, and in pediatric patients over two years of age with nephrotic syndrome. It is expected also that the vaccine will be found effective in preventing pneumococcal meningitis of bacteremic origin. However, PNEUMOVAX may not be effective in preventing infection resulting from basilar skull fracture or from external communication with cerebrospinal fluid. Studies are under way to determine the effectiveness of the vaccine for preventing pneumococcal otitis media in infants.

Contraindications

Hypersensitivity to any component of the vaccine. Epinephrine injection (1:1000) must be immediately available should an acute anaphylactoid reaction occur due to any component of the vaccine.

Do not give PNEUMOVAX to pregnant females; the possible effects of the vaccine on fetal development are unknown.

Children less than 2 years of age do not respond satisfactorily to the capsular types of PNEUMOVAX that are most often the cause of pneumococcal disease in this age group. Accordingly, PNEUMOVAX is not recommended in this age group.

Patients with Hodgkin's disease who have received extensive chemotherapy and/or nodal irradiation have been shown to have an impaired antibody response to a 12-valent pneumococcal vaccine. Because, in some intensively treated patients, administration of that vaccine depressed pre-existing levels of antibody to some pneumococcal types, PNEUMOVAX is not recommended at this time for patients who have received these forms of therapy for Hodgkin's disease.

Warnings

PNEUMOVAX *will not immunize against capsular types of pneumococcus other than those contained in the vaccine* (see above).

If the vaccine is used in persons receiving immunosuppressive therapy, the expected serum antibody response may not be obtained.

Intradermal administration may cause severe local reactions.

Precautions

Any febrile respiratory illness or other active infection is reason for delaying use of PNEUMOVAX, except when, in the opinion of the physician, withholding the agent entails even greater risk.

Caution and appropriate care should be exercised in administering PNEUMOVAX to individuals with severely compromised cardiac and/or pulmonary function in whom a systemic reaction would pose a significant risk.

Patients who have had episodes of pneumococcal pneumonia or other pneumococcal infection in the preceding three years may have high levels of pre-existing pneumococcal antibodies which may result in increased reactions to PNEUMOVAX, mostly local but occasionally systemic. Caution should be exercised if such patients are considered for vaccination with PNEUMOVAX.

Available data suggest that revaccination before 3 years may result in more frequent and severe local reactions at the site of injection, especially in persons who have retained high antibody levels (see DOSAGE AND ADMINISTRATION).

Children under 2 years of age may not obtain a satisfactory antibody response to some pneumococcal capsular types. Therefore, the vaccine should not be used in this age group.

Adverse Reactions

Local erythema and soreness at the injection site, usually of less than 48 hours duration, occurs commonly; local induration occurs less commonly. In a study of PNEUMOVAX (containing 14 capsular types) in 26 adults, 24 (92%) showed local reaction characterized principally by local soreness and/or induration at the injection site within 2 days after vaccination.

Low grade fever (less than 100.9°F) occurs occasionally and is usually confined to the 24-hour period following vaccination.

Although rare, fever over 102°F has been reported.

Reactions of greater severity, duration, or extent are unusual. Rarely, anaphylactoid reactions have been reported.

Dosage and Administration

Do not inject intravenously.

Administer a single 0.5 ml dose of PNEUMOVAX subcutaneously or intramuscularly (preferably in the deltoid muscle or lateral midthigh), with appropriate precautions to avoid intravascular administration. (See INDICATIONS.) *Intradermal* administration should be avoided.

Until further information on duration of immunity becomes available, revaccination should not be considered at less than 3 year intervals, since protective antibody levels are believed to persist for substantial periods in most vaccinated persons. Available data suggest that revaccination before 3 years may result in more frequent and severe local reactions at the site of injection, especially in persons who have retained high antibody levels (see ACTIONS).

Storage and Use

Store single-dose prefilled syringes and unopened and opened vials at 2–8°C (35.6–46.4°F). The vaccine is used directly as supplied. No dilution or reconstitution is necessary. Phenol 0.25% added as preservative.

It is important to use a separate sterile syringe and needle for each individual patient to prevent transmission of hepatitis B and other infectious agents from one person to another. All vaccine must be discarded after the expiration date.

Single-Dose Prefilled Syringe

Inject contents of syringe to effect a single dose.

Single-Dose and 5-Dose Vials

For Syringe Use Only: Withdraw 0.5 ml from the vial using a sterile needle and syringe free of preservatives, antiseptics and detergents.

How Supplied

No. 4666—PNEUMOVAX contains one 5-dose vial of liquid vaccine, **NDC** 0006-4666-00. For use with syringe only.

No. 4689—PNEUMOVAX is supplied as follows: **NDC** 0006-4689-00. A box of 5 individual cartons, each containing a single dose vial of vaccine.

No. 4670—PNEUMOVAX contains five single-dose 0.5 ml prefilled syringes, **NDC** 0006-4670-38.

A.H.F.S. 80:12

DC7014803 Issued November 1978

Continued on next page

Information on the Merck Sharp & Dohme products listed on these pages is the full prescribing information from package circulars in use October 31, 1979.

Merck Sharp & Dohme—Cont.

SINEMET® Tablets ℞

Description

SINEMET is a combination of carbidopa and levodopa. Before instituting therapy with SINEMET, physicians should be familiar with directions for its use.

When SINEMET is to be given to patients who are being treated with levodopa, levodopa must be discontinued at least eight hours before therapy with SINEMET is started. In order to reduce adverse reactions, it is necessary to individualize therapy. See the WARNINGS and DOSAGE AND ADMINISTRATION sections before initiating therapy.

Carbidopa, an inhibitor of aromatic amino acid decarboxylation, is a white, crystalline compound, slightly soluble in water, with a molecular weight of 244.3. It is designated chemically as (—)-L-α-hydrazino-α-methyl-β-(3,4-dihydroxybenzene) propanoic acid monohydrate. Tablet content is expressed in terms of anhydrous carbidopa which has a molecular weight of 226.3.

Levodopa, an aromatic amino acid, is a white, crystalline compound, slightly soluble in water, with a molecular weight of 197.2. It is designated chemically as (—)-L-α-amino-β-(3,4-dihydroxybenzene) propanoic acid.

SINEMET, a combination of carbidopa and levodopa, is supplied as tablets in three strengths:

SINEMET-10/100, containing 10 mg of carbidopa and 100 mg of levodopa

SINEMET-25/100, containing 25 mg of carbidopa and 100 mg of levodopa

SINEMET-25/250, containing 25 mg of carbidopa and 250 mg of levodopa

Actions

Current evidence indicates that symptoms of Parkinson's disease are related to depletion of dopamine in the corpus striatum. Administration of dopamine is ineffective in the treatment of Parkinson's disease apparently because it does not cross the blood-brain barrier. However, levodopa, the metabolic precursor of dopamine, does cross the blood-brain barrier, and presumably is converted to dopamine in the basal ganglia. This is thought to be the mechanism whereby levodopa relieves symptoms of Parkinson's disease.

When levodopa is administered orally it is rapidly converted to dopamine in extracerebral tissues so that only a small portion of a given dose is transported unchanged to the central nervous system. For this reason, large doses of levodopa are required for adequate therapeutic effect and these may often be attended by nausea and other adverse reactions, some of which are attributable to dopamine formed in extracerebral tissues.

Carbidopa inhibits decarboxylation of peripheral levodopa. It does not cross the blood-brain barrier and does not affect the metabolism of levodopa within the central nervous system.

Since its decarboxylase inhibiting activity is limited to extracerebral tissues, administration of carbidopa with levodopa makes more levodopa available for transport to the brain.

In dogs, reduced formation of dopamine in extracerebral tissues, such as the heart, provides protection against the development of dopamine-induced cardiac arrhythmias. Clinical studies tend to support the hypothesis of a similar protective effect in humans although controlled data are too limited at the present time to draw firm conclusions.

Carbidopa reduces the amount of levodopa required by about 75 percent and, when administered with levodopa, increases both plasma levels and the plasma half-life of levodopa, and decreases plasma and urinary dopamine and homovanillic acid.

In clinical pharmacologic studies, simultaneous administration of carbidopa and levodopa produced greater urinary excretion of levodopa in proportion to the excretion of dopamine than administration of the two drugs at separate times.

Pyridoxine hydrochloride (vitamin B_6), in oral doses of 10 mg to 25 mg, may reverse the effects of levodopa by increasing the rate of aromatic amino acid decarboxylation. Carbidopa inhibits this action of pyridoxine.

Indications

SINEMET, a combination of carbidopa and levodopa, is indicated in the treatment of the symptoms of idiopathic Parkinson's disease (paralysis agitans), postencephalitic parkinsonism, and symptomatic parkinsonism which may follow injury to the nervous system by carbon monoxide intoxication and manganese intoxication. SINEMET is indicated in these conditions to permit the administration of lower doses of levodopa with reduced nausea and vomiting, with more rapid dosage titration, with a somewhat smoother response, and with supplemental pyridoxine (vitamin B_6).

The incidence of levodopa-induced nausea and vomiting is less with SINEMET than with levodopa. In many patients this reduction in nausea and vomiting will permit more rapid dosage titration.

In some patients a somewhat smoother antiparkinsonian effect results from therapy with SINEMET than with levodopa. However, patients with markedly irregular ("on-off") responses to levodopa have not been shown to benefit from SINEMET.

Since carbidopa prevents the reversal of levodopa effects caused by pyridoxine, SINEMET can be given to patients receiving supplemental pyridoxine (vitamin B_6).

Although the administration of carbidopa permits control of parkinsonism and Parkinson's disease with much lower doses of levodopa, there is no conclusive evidence at present that this is beneficial other than in reducing nausea and vomiting, permitting more rapid titration, and providing a somewhat smoother response to levodopa. *Carbidopa does not decrease adverse reactions due to central effects of levodopa. By permitting more levodopa to reach the brain, particularly when nausea and vomiting is not a dose-limiting factor, certain adverse CNS effects, e.g., dyskinesias, may occur at lower dosages and sooner during therapy with* SINEMET *than with levodopa.*

Certain patients who responded poorly to levodopa have improved when SINEMET was substituted. This is most likely due to decreased peripheral decarboxylation of levodopa which results from administration of carbidopa rather than to a primary effect of carbidopa on the nervous system. Carbidopa has not been shown to enhance the intrinsic efficacy of levodopa in parkinsonian syndromes.

In considering whether to give SINEMET to patients already on levodopa who have nausea and/or vomiting, the practitioner should be aware that, while many patients may be expected to improve, some do not. Since one cannot predict which patients are likely to improve, this can only be determined by a trial of therapy. It should be further noted that in controlled trials comparing SINEMET with levodopa, about half of the patients with nausea and/or vomiting on levodopa improved spontaneously despite being retained on the same dose of levodopa during the controlled portion of the trial.

Contraindications

Monoamine oxidase inhibitors and SINEMET should not be given concomitantly. These inhibitors must be discontinued at least two weeks prior to initiating therapy with SINEMET.

SINEMET is contraindicated in patients with known hypersensitivity to this drug, and in narrow angle glaucoma.

Because levodopa may activate a malignant melanoma, it should not be used in patients with suspicious, undiagnosed skin lesions or a history of melanoma.

Warnings

When patients are receiving levodopa, it must be discontinued at least eight hours before SINEMET is started. SINEMET should be substituted at a dosage that will provide approximately 25 percent of the previous levodopa dosage (see DOSAGE AND ADMINISTRATION). Patients who are taking SINEMET should be instructed not to take additional levodopa unless it is prescribed by the physician.

As with levodopa, SINEMET may cause involuntary movements and mental disturbances. These reactions are thought to be due to increased brain dopamine following administration of levodopa. All patients should be observed carefully for the development of depression with concomitant suicidal tendencies. Patients with past or current psychoses should be treated with caution. *Because carbidopa permits more levodopa to reach the brain and, thus, more dopamine to be formed, dyskinesias may occur at lower dosages and sooner with* SINEMET *than with levodopa.* The occurrence of dyskinesias may require dosage reduction.

SINEMET should be administered cautiously to patients with severe cardiovascular or pulmonary disease, bronchial asthma, renal, hepatic or endocrine disease.

Care should be exercised in administering SINEMET, as with levodopa, to patients with a history of myocardial infarction who have residual atrial, nodal, or ventricular arrhythmias. In such patients, cardiac function should be monitored with particular care during the period of initial dosage adjustment, in a facility with provisions for intensive cardiac care.

As with levodopa there is a possibility of upper gastrointestinal hemorrhage in patients with a history of peptic ulcer.

Usage in Pregnancy and Lactation: Although the effects of SINEMET on human pregnancy and lactation are unknown, both levodopa and combinations of carbidopa and levodopa have caused visceral and skeletal malformations in rabbits. Use of SINEMET in women of childbearing potential requires that the anticipated benefits of the drug be weighed against possible hazards to mother and child. SINEMET should not be given to nursing mothers.

Usage in Children: The safety of SINEMET in patients under 18 years of age has not been established.

Precautions

As with levodopa, periodic evaluations of hepatic, hematopoietic, cardiovascular, and renal function are recommended during extended therapy.

Patients with chronic wide angle glaucoma may be treated cautiously with SINEMET provided the intraocular pressure is well controlled and the patient is monitored carefully for changes in intraocular pressure during therapy.

Symptomatic postural hypotension can occur. For this reason, SINEMET should be given cautiously to patients on antihypertensive drugs. When SINEMET is started, dosage adjustment of the antihypertensive drug may be required. (For patients receiving pargyline, see the contraindication on monoamine oxidase inhibitors.)

Since phenothiazines and butyrophenones may reduce the therapeutic effects of levodopa, they should be administered with caution if concomitant administration with SINEMET is necessary. Also, the beneficial effects of levodopa in Parkinson's disease have been reported to be reversed by phenytoin and papaverine. Patients taking these drugs with SINEMET should be carefully observed for loss of antiparkinsonian effect.

Adverse Reactions

The most common serious adverse reactions occurring with SINEMET are choreiform, dystonic, and other involuntary movements. Other serious adverse reactions are mental changes including paranoid ideation and psychotic episodes, depression with or without development of suicidal tendencies, and dementia. Convulsions also have occurred; however, a causal relationship with SINEMET has not been established.

A common but less serious effect is nausea.

Less frequent adverse reactions are cardiac irregularities and/or palpitations, orthostatic hypotensive episodes, bradykinetic episodes (the "on-off" phenomenon), anorexia, vomiting, and dizziness.

Rarely, gastrointestinal bleeding, development of duodenal ulcer, hypertension, phlebitis, hemolytic anemia, leukopenia, and agranulocytosis have occurred.

Other adverse reactions that have been reported with levodopa include dry mouth, dysphagia, sialorrhea, abdominal pain and distress, ataxia, increased hand tremor, headache, numbness, weakness and faintness, bruxism, confusion, insomnia and nightmares, hallucinations and delusions, agitation and anxiety, malaise, fatigue, euphoria, muscle twitching, and blepharospasm (which may be taken as an early sign of excess dosage; consideration of dosage reduction may be made at this time), trismus, burning sensation of tongue, bitter taste, diarrhea, constipation, flatulence, flushing, skin rash, increased sweating, bizarre breathing patterns, urinary retention, urinary incontinence, diplopia, blurred vision, dilated pupils, hot flashes, weight gain or loss, dark sweat and/or urine, oculogyric crises, sense of stimulation, hiccups, edema, loss of hair, hoarseness, priapism, and activation of latent Horner's syndrome.

Abnormalities in laboratory tests may include elevations of blood urea nitrogen, SGOT, SGPT, lactic dehydrogenase, bilirubin, alkaline phosphatase, protein-bound iodine and positive Coombs test. More commonly, levels of blood urea nitrogen, creatinine, and uric acid are lower during administration of SINEMET than with levodopa.

Dosage and Administration

The optimum daily dosage of SINEMET must be determined by careful titration for each patient. SINEMET tablets are available in a 1:10 ratio of carbidopa to levodopa (SINEMET-10/100 and SINEMET-25/250) and a 1:4 ratio (SINEMET-25/100). Tablets of the two ratios may be given separately or combined as needed to provide the optimum dosage. Certain patients receiving low doses of SINEMET may require a relatively higher proportion of carbidopa. In such patients SINEMET-25/100 may be given with or without SINEMET-10/100 or SINEMET-25/250 to attain the proportion that provides the greatest clinical benefit.

Studies show that peripheral dopa decarboxylase is saturated by carbidopa at approximately 70 to 100 mg per diem. Patients who require only low doses of levodopa, e.g., less than 700 mg when given as SINEMET-10/100, will receive doses of carbidopa which theoretically do not saturate peripheral dopa decarboxylase. SINEMET-25/100 may be helpful in these patients especially if they have nausea and vomiting. Most patients can be maintained on three to six tablets of SINEMET-25/250 a day given in divided doses.

The maximum dosage should not exceed eight tablets of SINEMET-25/250 or SINEMET-25/100 a day, since experience with total daily dosages of carbidopa greater than 200 mg is limited. If patients show need for higher doses, levodopa should be added to the treatment regimen.

Patients Not Presently Receiving Levodopa:

Dosage may be initiated with one tablet of SINEMET-10/100 or SINEMET-25/100 three times a day, and increased by one tablet every day or every other day until a dosage of six tablets a day is reached. When patients have nausea and vomiting on low daily dosages of SINEMET-10/100, one tablet of SINEMET-25/100 may be substituted for one tablet of SINEMET-10/100. When it is evident that patients need more levodopa, SINEMET-25/250, at a dosage of one tablet three or four times a day, should be substituted.

If still further titration is necessary, dosage with SINEMET-25/250 may be increased by one-half or one tablet every day or every other day to a maximum of eight tablets a day. Alternatively, dosage may be titrated to six tablets of SINEMET-25/250 a day, and further adjusted with increments of levodopa.

Because both therapeutic and adverse responses occur more rapidly with SINEMET than when levodopa is given, patients should be monitored closely during the dose adjustment period. Specifically, involuntary movements will occur more rapidly with SINEMET than with levodopa. The occurrence of involuntary movements may require dosage reduction. Blepharospasm may be a useful early sign of excess dosage in some patients.

Patients Receiving Levodopa:

Levodopa must be discontinued before SINEMET is started. The easiest way to change patients from therapy with levodopa to SINEMET is to start SINEMET with the morning dose after a night (at least eight hours) when the patient has not received any levodopa. A daily dosage of SINEMET should be chosen that will provide approximately 25 percent of the previous levodopa daily dosage. The suggested starting dosage for most patients is one tablet of SINEMET-25/250 three or four times a day. Patients who required less than 1500 mg of levodopa a day should be started on one tablet of SINEMET-10/100 or SINEMET-25/100 three or four times a day.

Adjustment in dosage may be made as necessary by adding or omitting one-half or one tablet a day.

Current evidence indicates that other standard antiparkinsonian drugs may be continued while SINEMET is being administered although their dosage may have to be adjusted.

If general anesthesia is required, therapy with SINEMET may be continued as long as the patient is permitted to take fluids and medication by mouth. If therapy is interrupted temporarily, the usual daily dosage may be administered as soon as the patient is able to take oral medication.

Overdosage

Management of acute overdosage with SINEMET is basically the same as management of acute overdosage with levodopa; however, pyridoxine is not effective in reversing the actions of SINEMET.

General supportive measures should be employed, along with immediate gastric lavage. Intravenous fluids should be administered judiciously and an adequate airway maintained. Electrocardiographic monitoring should be instituted and the patient carefully observed for the development of arrhythmias; if required, appropriate antiarrhythmic therapy should be given. The possibility that the patient may have taken other drugs as well as SINEMET should be taken into consideration. To date, no experience has been reported with dialysis; hence, its value in overdosage is not known.

How Supplied

No. 3346—Tablets SINEMET-10/100 are dark dapple-blue, oval, scored, uncoated tablets, coded MSD 647. They are supplied as follows:

NDC 0006-0647-68 bottles of 100 (6505-01-020-8280 100's)

NDC 0006-0647-28 single unit packages of 100.

[*Shown in Product Identification Section*]

No. 3365—Tablets SINEMET-25/100 are yellow, oval, scored tablets, coded MSD 650. They are supplied as follows:

NDC 0006-0650-68 bottles of 100.

[*Shown in Product Identification Section*]

No. 3347—Tablets SINEMET-25/250 are light dapple-blue, oval, scored, uncoated tablets, coded MSD 654. They are supplied as follows:

NDC 0006-0654-68 bottles of 100 (6505-01-020-8279 100's)

NDC 0006-0654-28 single unit packages of 100.

[*Shown in Product Identification Section*]

A.H.F.S. 92:00

DC6834805 Issued July 1977

TIMOPTIC® Sterile Ophthalmic Solution (timolol maleate, MSD) ℞

Description

TIMOPTIC (Timolol Maleate, MSD) Ophthalmic Solution is supplied as a sterile, isotonic, buffered, aqueous solution of timolol maleate in two dosage strengths: Each ml of TIMOPTIC 0.25% contains 2.5 mg of timolol (3.4 mg of timolol maleate). Each ml of TIMOPTIC 0.5% contains 5.0 mg of timolol (6.8 mg of timolol maleate). Inactive ingredients: monobasic and dibasic sodium phosphate, sodium hydroxide to adjust pH, and water for injection. Benzalkonium chloride 0.01% is added as preservative. TIMOPTIC is stable at room temperature.

Timolol maleate is a beta-adrenergic receptor blocking agent. Its chemical name is (S)-1-[(1,1-dimethyl-ethyl) amino]-3-[[4- (4-morpholinyl)-1, 2, 5-thiadiazol-3 -yl] oxy] - 2 - propanol, (Z)-butenedioate (1:1) salt. Timolol maleate possesses an asymmetric carbon atom in its structure and is provided as the levo isomer. The nominal optical rotation of timolol maleate is $[\alpha]^{25^\circ}_{405nm}$ in 0.1N HCl (C = 5%) = −12.2°.

Actions

Timolol maleate is a general beta-adrenergic receptor blocking agent that does not have significant intrinsic sympathomimetic, direct myocardial depressant, or local anesthetic (membrane-stabilizing) activity.

TIMOPTIC Ophthalmic Solution, when applied topically in the eye, has the action of reducing elevated as well as normal intraocular pressure, whether or not accompanied by glaucoma. Elevated intraocular pressure is a major risk factor in the pathogenesis of glaucomatous visual field loss. The higher the level of intraocular pressure, the greater the likelihood of glaucomatous visual field loss and optic nerve damage.

The onset of reduction in intraocular pressure following administration of TIMOPTIC can usually be detected within one-half hour after a single dose. The maximum effect usually occurs in one to two hours and significant lowering of intraocular pressure can be maintained for periods as long as 24 hours with a single dose. Repeated observations over a period of one year indicate that the intraocular pressure-lowering effect of TIMOPTIC is well maintained.

Continued on next page

Information on the Merck Sharp & Dohme products listed on these pages is the full prescribing information from package circulars in use October 31, 1979.

Merck Sharp & Dohme—Cont.

The precise mechanism of the ocular hypotensive action of TIMOPTIC is not clearly established at this time. Tonography and fluorophotometry studies in man suggest that its predominant action may be related to reduced aqueous formation. However, in some studies a slight increase in outflow facility was also observed. Unlike miotics, TIMOPTIC reduces intraocular pressure with little or no effect on pupil size or visual acuity due to increased accommodation. Thus, dim or blurred vision and night blindness produced by miotics are not evident. In addition, in patients with cataracts the inability to see around lenticular opacities when the pupil is constricted is avoided.
In controlled multiclinic studies in patients with untreated intraocular pressures of 22 mmHg or greater, TIMOPTIC 0.25 percent or 0.5 percent administered twice a day produced a greater reduction in intraocular pressure than 1, 2, 3, or 4 percent pilocarpine solution administered four times a day or 0.5, 1, or 2 percent epinephrine hydrochloride solution administered twice a day.
In the multiclinic studies comparing TIMOPTIC with pilocarpine, 61 percent of patients treated with TIMOPTIC had intraocular pressure reduced to less than 22 mmHg compared to 32 percent of patients treated with pilocarpine. For patients completing these studies, the mean reduction in pressure at the end of the study from pretreatment was 30.7 percent for patients treated with TIMOPTIC and 21.7 percent for patients treated with pilocarpine.
In the multiclinic studies comparing TIMOPTIC with epinephrine, 69 percent of patients treated with TIMOPTIC had intraocular pressure reduced to less than 22 mmHg compared to 42 percent of patients treated with epinephrine. For patients completing these studies, the mean reduction in pressure at the end of the study from pretreatment was 33.2 percent for patients treated with TIMOPTIC and 28.1 percent for patients treated with epinephrine.
TIMOPTIC was generally well tolerated and produced fewer and less severe side effects than either pilocarpine or epinephrine.
TIMOPTIC has also been used in patients with glaucoma wearing conventional (PMMA) hard contact lenses, and has generally been well tolerated. TIMOPTIC has not been studied in patients wearing lenses made with materials other than PMMA.

Indications and Usage

TIMOPTIC Ophthalmic Solution has been shown to be effective for the reduction of elevated intraocular pressure. In clinical trials it has been shown to reduce intraocular pressure in:
Patients with chronic open-angle glaucoma
Patients with aphakic glaucoma
Some patients with secondary glaucoma
Patients with ocular hypertension
Clinical trials have also shown that in patients who respond inadequately to multiple antiglaucoma drug therapy the addition of TIMOPTIC may produce a further reduction of intraocular pressure.

Contraindications

TIMOPTIC Ophthalmic Solution is contraindicated in patients who are hypersensitive to any component of this product.

Precautions

TIMOPTIC Ophthalmic Solution should be used with caution in patients with known contraindications to systemic use of beta-adrenergic receptor blocking agents. These include bronchial asthma; sinus bradycardia and greater than first degree block; cardiogenic shock; right ventricular failure secondary to pulmonary hypertension; congestive heart failure; concomitant use with adrenergic-augmenting psychotropic drugs. In patients with a history of severe cardiac disease, pulse rates should be checked.
Patients who are already receiving a beta-adrenergic blocking agent orally and who are given TIMOPTIC should be observed for a potential additive effect either on the intraocular pressure or on the known systemic effects of beta blockade.
Sufficient clinical data have not been obtained to show safety or efficacy in narrow-angle or angle-closure glaucoma.
With the use of other antiglaucoma drugs, tolerance to drug therapy may occur. No evidence of diminished responsiveness to TIMOPTIC has been reported in 102 patients treated for at least two years.
Pregnancy
TIMOPTIC has not been studied in human pregnancy. The use of TIMOPTIC in pregnant women requires that the anticipated benefit be weighed against possible hazards.
Use in Children
Since clinical studies in children have not been done, TIMOPTIC is not recommended for use in children at this time.
Animal Studies
No adverse ocular effects were observed in rabbits and dogs administered TIMOPTIC topically in studies lasting one and two years respectively. In long-term safety assessment studies of oral timolol in rats and mice at dosage levels of 5, 10, and 25 mg/kg per day, and 5, 15, and 45 mg/kg per day respectively, mammary fibroadenomas in rats and hepatomas in mice were observed significantly more frequently in the animals given timolol than in the control animals. However, the incidence of these neoplasms was within the range observed in control animals in concurrent studies of other compounds. The oral rodent studies with timolol are being repeated at higher dosage levels (25, 100, and 300 mg/kg per day in rats and 5, 50, and 500 mg/kg per day in mice).

Adverse Reactions

TIMOPTIC Ophthalmic Solution is usually well tolerated. Occasionally, signs and symptoms of mild ocular irritation have been reported. Local hypersensitivity reactions, including localized and generalized rash, have occurred rarely.
Slight reduction of the resting heart rate (mean reduction 2.9 beats/minute, standard deviation 10.2) has been observed in some patients. Rarely, episodes of acute bronchospasm have been reported in patients with bronchospastic disease (see PRECAUTIONS).

Dosage and Administration

TIMOPTIC Ophthalmic Solution is available in concentrations of 0.25 and 0.5 percent. The usual starting dose is one drop of 0.25 percent TIMOPTIC in each eye twice a day. If the clinical response is not adequate, the dosage may be changed to one drop of 0.5 percent solution in each eye twice a day. If the intraocular pressure is maintained at satisfactory levels, the dosage schedule may be changed to one drop once a day in each eye. Because of diurnal variations in intraocular pressure, satisfactory response to the once-a-day dose is best determined by measuring the intraocular pressure at different times during the day.
Dosages above one drop of 0.5 percent TIMOPTIC twice a day generally have not been shown to produce further reduction in intraocular pressure. If the patient's intraocular pressure is still not at a satisfactory level on this regimen, concomitant therapy with pilocarpine and other miotics, and/or epinephrine, and/or systemically administered carbonic anhydrase inhibitors, such as acetazolamide, can be instituted.
When a patient is transferred from a single antiglaucoma agent, continue the agent already being used and add one drop of 0.25 percent TIMOPTIC in each eye twice a day. On the following day, discontinue the previously used antiglaucoma agent completely and continue with TIMOPTIC. If a higher dosage of TIMOPTIC is required, substitute one drop of 0.5 percent solution in each eye twice a day.
When a patient is transferred from several concomitantly administered antiglaucoma agents, individualization is required. Adjustments should involve one agent at a time and usually should be made at intervals of not less than one week. A recommended approach is to continue the agents being used and to add 0.25 percent TIMOPTIC in each eye twice a day. On the following day, discontinue one of the other antiglaucoma agents. The remaining antiglaucoma agents may be decreased or discontinued according to the patient's response to treatment. If a higher dosage of TIMOPTIC is required, substitute one drop of 0.5 percent solution in each eye twice a day. The physician may be able to discontinue some or all of the other antiglaucoma agents.

How Supplied

Sterile Ophthalmic Solution TIMOPTIC is a clear, colorless to light yellow solution.
No. 3366—TIMOPTIC Ophthalmic Solution, 0.25% timolol is supplied as follows:
NDC 0006-3366-03 in 5 ml white, opaque, plastic OCUMETER® ophthalmic dispenser with a controlled drop tip.
NDC 0006-3366-10 in 10 ml white, opaque, plastic OCUMETER ophthalmic dispenser with a controlled drop tip.
No. 3367—TIMOPTIC Ophthalmic Solution, 0.5% timolol, is supplied as follows:
NDC 0006-3367-03 in 5 ml white, opaque, plastic OCUMETER ophthalmic dispenser with a controlled drop tip.
NDC 0006-3367-10 in 10 ml white, opaque, plastic OCUMETER ophthalmic dispenser with a controlled drop tip.
A.H.F.S. 52:36
DC7046008 Issued July 1979

TRIAVIL® Tablets ℞
Tranquilizer-antidepressant

Description

TRIAVIL, a broad-spectrum psychotherapeutic agent for the management of outpatients and hospitalized patients with psychoses or neuroses characterized by mixtures of anxiety or agitation with symptoms of depression, is a combination of perphenazine and ELAVIL® (Amitriptyline HCl, MSD). Since such mixed syndromes can occur in patients with various degrees of intensity of mental illness, TRIAVIL tablets are provided in multiple combinations to afford dosage flexibility for optimum management.

Actions

Perphenazine—In common with all members of the piperazine group of phenothiazine derivatives, perphenazine has greater behavioral potency than phenothiazine derivatives of other groups without a corresponding increase in autonomic, hematologic, or hepatic side effects.
Extrapyramidal effects, however, may occur more frequently. These effects are interpreted as neuropharmacologic. They usually regress after discontinuation of the drug.
Perphenazine is a potent tranquilizer and also a potent antiemetic. Orally, its milligram potency is about five or six times that of chlorpro-

mazine with respect to behavorial effects. It is capable of alleviating symptoms of anxiety, tension, psychomotor excitement, and other manifestations of emotional stress without apparent dulling of mental acuity.
ELAVIL (Amitriptyline HCl, MSD) is an antidepressant with an anxiety-reducing, sedative component to its action. Its mechanism of action in man is not known. It is not a monoamine oxidase inhibitor and it does not act primarily by stimulation of the central nervous system.

Indications

TRIAVIL is recommended for treatment of (1) patients with *moderate to severe anxiety and/or agitation and depressed mood,* (2) patients with *depression in whom anxiety and/or agitation are severe,* and (3) patients with *depression and anxiety in association with chronic physical disease.* In many of these patients, anxiety masks the depressive state so that, although therapy with a tranquilizer appears to be indicated, the administration of a tranquilizer alone will not be adequate.
Schizophrenic patients who have associated depressive symptoms should be considered for therapy with TRIAVIL.
Many patients presenting symptoms such as agitation, anxiety, insomnia, psychomotor retardation, functional somatic complaints, a feeling of tiredness, loss of interest, and anorexia have responded well to therapy with TRIAVIL.

Contraindications

TRIAVIL is contraindicated in depression of the central nervous system from drugs (barbiturates, alcohol, narcotics, analgesics, antihistamines); in the presence of evidence of bone marrow depression; and in patients known to be hypersensitive to phenothiazines or amitriptyline.
It should not be given concomitantly with monoamine oxidase inhibitors. Hyperpyretic crises, severe convulsions, and deaths have occurred in patients receiving tricyclic antidepressants and monoamine oxidase inhibitors simultaneously. When it is desired to replace a monoamine oxidase inhibitor with TRIAVIL, a minimum of 14 days should be allowed to elapse after the former is discontinued. TRIAVIL should then be initiated cautiously with gradual increase in dosage until optimum response is achieved.
Amitriptyline HCl is not recommended for use during the acute recovery phase following myocardial infarction.

Warnings

TRIAVIL should not be given concomitantly with guanethidine or similarly acting compounds, since amitriptyline, like other tricyclic antidepressants, may block the antihypertensive effect of these compounds.
Because of the atropine-like activity of amitriptyline, TRIAVIL should be used with caution in patients with a history of urinary retention, or with angle-closure glaucoma or increased intraocular pressure. In patients with angle-closure glaucoma, even average doses may precipitate an attack.
It should be used with caution also in patients with convulsive disorders. Dosage of anticonvulsive agents may have to be increased.
Patients with cardiovascular disorders should be watched closely. Tricyclic antidepressants, including amitriptyline HCl, particularly when given in high doses, have been reported to produce arrhythmias, sinus tachycardia, and prolongation of the conduction time. Myocardial infarction and stroke have been reported with drugs of this class.
Close supervision is required when amitriptyline HCl is given to hyperthyroid patients or those receiving thyroid medication.
This drug may impair mental and/or physical abilities required for performance of hazardous tasks, such as operating machinery or driving a motor vehicle.
In patients who may use alcohol excessively, it should be borne in mind that the potentiation may increase the danger inherent in any suicide attempt or overdosage.
Usage in Pregnancy—TRIAVIL is not recommended for use in pregnant patients at this time. Reproduction studies in rats have shown no fetal abnormalities; however, clinical experience and follow-up in pregnancy have been limited, and the possibility of adverse effects on fetal development must be considered.
Usage in Children—Since dosage for children has not been established, TRIAVIL is not recommended for use in children.

Precautions

The possibility of suicide in depressed patients remains during treatment and until significant remission occurs. Such patients should not have access to large quantities of this drug.

Perphenazine
As with all phenothiazine compounds, perphenazine should not be used indiscriminately. Caution should be observed in giving it to patients who have previously exhibited severe adverse reactions to other phenothiazines.
Some of the untoward actions of perphenazine tend to appear more frequently when high doses are used. However, as with other phenothiazine compounds, patients receiving perphenazine in any dosage should be kept under close supervision.
The antiemetic effect of perphenazine may obscure signs of toxicity due to overdosage of other drugs, or render more difficult the diagnosis of disorders such as brain tumors or intestinal obstruction.
A significant, not otherwise explained, rise in body temperature may suggest individual intolerance to perphenazine, in which case TRIAVIL should be discontinued.
If hypotension develops, epinephrine should not be employed, as its action is blocked and partially reversed by perphenazine.
Phenothiazines may potentiate the action of central nervous system depressants (opiates, analgesics, antihistamines, barbiturates, alcohol) and atropine. In concurrent therapy with any of these, TRIAVIL should be given in reduced dosage. Phenothiazines also may potentiate the action of heat and phosphorous insecticides.
There is sufficient experimental evidence to conclude that chronic administration of antipsychotic drugs which increase prolactin secretion has the potential to induce mammary neoplasms in rodents under the appropriate conditions. There are recognized differences in the physiological role of prolactin between rodents and humans. Since there are, at present, no adequate epidemiological studies, the relevance to human mammary cancer risk from prolonged exposure to perphenazine and other antipsychotic drugs is not known.

ELAVIL (Amitriptyline HCl, MSD)
In manic-depressive psychosis, depressed patients may experience a shift toward the manic phase if they are treated with an antidepressant. Patients with paranoid symptomatology may have an exaggeration of such symptoms. The tranquilizing effect of TRIAVIL seems to reduce the likelihood of this effect.
When ELAVIL (Amitriptyline HCl, MSD) is given with anticholinergic agents or sympathomimetic drugs, including epinephrine combined with local anesthetics, close supervision and careful adjustment of dosages are required.
Paralytic ileus may occur in patients taking tricyclic antidepressants in combination with anticholinergic-type drugs.
Caution is advised if patients receive large doses of ethchlorvynol concurrently. Transient delirium has been reported in patients who were treated with 1 g of ethchlorvynol and 75-150 mg of ELAVIL (Amitriptyline HCl, MSD).
ELAVIL (Amitriptyline HCl, MSD) may enhance the response to alcohol and the effects of barbiturates and other CNS depressants.
Concurrent administration of amitriptyline HCl and electroshock therapy may increase the hazards associated with such therapy. Such treatment should be limited to patients for whom it is essential.
Discontinue the drug several days before elective surgery if possible.
Both elevation and lowering of blood sugar levels have been reported.
ELAVIL (Amitriptyline HCl, MSD) should be used with caution in patients with impaired liver function.

Adverse Reactions

To date, clinical evaluation of TRIAVIL has not revealed any adverse reactions peculiar to the combination. The adverse reactions that occurred were limited to those that have been reported previously for perphenazine and amitriptyline.

Perphenazine
Extrapyramidal symptoms (opisthotonus, oculogyric crisis, hyper-reflexia, dystonia, akathisia, acute dyskinesia, ataxis, parkinsonism) have been reported. Their incidence and severity usually increase with an increase in dosage, but there is considerable individual variation in the tendency to develop such symptoms. Extrapyramidal symptoms can usually be controlled by the concomitant use of effective antiparkinsonian drugs, such as benztropine mesylate, and/or by reduction in dosage. In some instances, they may persist after discontinuation of the drug.
Tardive dyskinesia may appear in some patients on long-term therapy or may occur after drug therapy with phenothiazines and related agents has been discontinued. The risk appears to be greater in elderly patients on high-dose therapy, especially females. The symptoms are persistent and in some patients appear to be irreversible. The syndrome is characterized by rhythmical involuntary movements of the tongue, face, mouth or jaw (e.g., protrusion of tongue, puffing of cheeks, puckering of mouth, chewing movements). Involuntary movements of the extremities sometimes occur. There is no known treatment for tardive dyskinesia; antiparkinsonism agents usually do not alleviate the symptoms. It is advised that all antipsychotic agents be discontinued if the above symptoms appear. If treatment is reinstituted, or dosage of the particular drug increased, or another drug substituted, the syndrome may be masked. It has been suggested that fine vermicular movements of the tongue may be an early sign of the syndrome, and that the full-blown syndrome may not develop if medication is stopped when lingual vermiculation appears.
Skin disorders have occurred with phenothiazine compounds (photosensitivity, itching, erythema, urticaria, eczema, up to exfoliative dermatitis); as well as other allergic reactions (asthma, laryngeal edema, angioneurotic edema, anaphylactoid reactions); peripheral edema; reversed epinephrine effect; hyperglycemia; endocrine disturbances (lactation, galactorrhea, gynecomastia, disturbances in the menstrual cycle); altered cerebrospinal fluid

Continued on next page

Information on the Merck Sharp & Dohme products listed on these pages is the full prescribing information from package circulars in use October 31, 1979.

Merck Sharp & Dohme—Cont.

proteins; paradoxical excitement; hypertension, hypotension, tachycardia, and EKG abnormalities (quinidine-like effect). Reactivation of psychotic processes and the production of catatonic-like states have been described.
Autonomic reactions, such as dry mouth or salivation, headache, anorexia, nausea, vomiting, constipation, obstipation, urinary frequency or incontinence, blurred vision, nasal congestion, and a change in the pulse rate occasionally may occur.
Other adverse reactions reported with various phenothiazine compounds, but not with perphenazine, include grand mal convulsions, cerebral edema, polyphagia, photophobia, skin pigmentation, and failure of ejaculation.
The phenothiazine compounds have produced blood dyscrasias (pancytopenia, thrombocytopenic purpura, leukopenia, agranulocytosis, eosinophilia); and liver damage (jaundice, biliary stasis).
Pigmentary retinopathy has been reported to occur after administration of some phenothiazines with a piperidylethyl side chain, but not with perphenazine which has a piperazine side chain.
Pigmentation of the cornea and lens has been reported to occur after long-term administration of some phenothiazines. Although it has not been reported in patients receiving TRIAVIL, the possibility that it might occur should be considered.
Hypnotic effects appear to be minimal, particularly in patients who are permitted to remain active.
A few patients have reported lassitude, muscle weakness, and mild insomnia.

ELAVIL (Amitriptyline HCl, MSD)
Note: Included in the listing which follows are a few adverse reactions which have not been reported with this specific drug. However, pharmacological similarities among the tricyclic antidepressant drugs require that each of the reactions be considered when amitriptyline is administered.
Cardiovascular: Hypotension, hypertension, tachycardia, palpitation, myocardial infarction, arrhythmias, heart block, stroke.
CNS and Neuromuscular: Confusional states; disturbed concentration; disorientation; delusions; hallucinations; excitement; anxiety; restlessness; insomnia; nightmares; numbness, tingling, and paresthesias of the extremities; peripheral neuropathy; incoordination; ataxia; tremors; seizures; alteration in EEG patterns; extrapyramidal symptoms; tinnitus; syndrome of inappropriate ADH (antidiuretic hormone) secretion.
Anticholinergic: Dry mouth, blurred vision, disturbance of accommodation, constipation, paralytic ileus, urinary retention, dilatation of urinary tract.
Allergic: Skin rash, urticaria, photosensitization, edema of face and tongue.
Hematologic: Bone marrow depression including agranulocytosis, leukopenia, eosinophilia, purpura, thrombocytopenia.
Gastrointestinal: Nausea, epigastric distress, vomiting, anorexia, stomatitis, peculiar taste, diarrhea, parotid swelling, black tongue. Rarely hepatitis (including altered liver function and jaundice).
Endocrine: Testicular swelling and gynecomastia in the male, breast enlargement and galactorrhea in the female, increased or decreased libido, elevation and lowering of blood sugar levels.
Other: Dizziness, weakness, fatigue, headache, weight gain or loss, increased perspiration, urinary frequency, mydriasis, drowsiness, alopecia.
Withdrawal Symptoms: Abrupt cessation of treatment after prolonged administration may produce nausea, headache, and malaise. These are not indicative of addiction.

Dosage and Administration

TRIAVIL tablets are provided as:
TRIAVIL 2-25, containing 2 mg of perphenazine and 25 mg of amitriptyline HCl.
TRIAVIL 4-25, containing 4 mg of perphenazine and 25 mg of amitriptyline HCl.
TRIAVIL 4-50, containing 4 mg of perphenazine and 50 mg of amitriptyline HCl.
TRIAVIL 2-10, containing 2 mg of perphenazine and 10 mg of amitriptyline HCl.
TRIAVIL 4-10, containing 4 mg of perphenazine and 10 mg of amitriptyline HCl.
Since dosage for children has not been established, TRIAVIL is not recommended for use in children.
The total daily dose of TRIAVIL should not exceed four tablets of the 4-50 or eight tablets of any other dosage strength.

Initial Dosage
In psychoneurotic patients when anxiety and depression are of such a degree as to warrant combined therapy, one tablet of TRIAVIL 2-25 or TRIAVIL 4-25 three or four times a day or one tablet of TRIAVIL 4-50 twice a day is recommended.

In more severely ill patients with schizophrenia, TRIAVIL 4-25 is recommended in an initial dose of two tablets three times a day. If necessary, a fourth dose may be given at bedtime.
In elderly patients and adolescents, and some other patients in whom anxiety tends to predominate, TRIAVIL 4-10 may be administered three or four times a day initially, then adjusted as required for subsequent adequate therapy.

Maintenance Dosage
Depending on the condition being treated, therapeutic response may take from a few days to a few weeks or even longer. After a satisfactory response is noted, dosage should be reduced to the smallest amount necessary to obtain relief from the symptoms for which TRIAVIL is being administered. A useful maintenance dosage is one tablet of TRIAVIL 2-25 or 4-25 two to four times a day or one tablet of TRIAVIL 4-50 twice a day. TRIAVIL 2-10 and 4-10 can be used to increase flexibility in adjusting maintenance dosage to the lowest amount consistent with relief of symptoms. In some patients, maintenance dosage is required for many months.

Overdosage

Manifestations—High doses may cause temporary confusion, disturbed concentration, or transient visual hallucinations. Overdosage may cause drowsiness; hypothermia; tachycardia and other arrhythmic abnormalities, such as bundle branch block; ECG evidence of impaired conduction; congestive heart failure; dilated pupils; convulsions; severe hypotension; stupor; and coma. Other symptoms may be agitation, hyperactive reflexes, muscle rigidity, vomiting, hyperpyrexia, or any of the adverse reactions listed for perphenazine or amitriptyline.
Levarterenol (norepinephrine) may be used to treat hypotension, but not epinephrine.
All patients suspected of having taken an overdosage should be admitted to a hospital as soon as possible. *Treatment* is symptomatic and supportive. Empty the stomach as quickly as possible by emesis followed by gastric lavage upon arrival at the hospital. Saline emetics should not be used as the antiemetic effect of perphenazine may cause retention of the saline load and subsequent hypernatremia. Following gastric lavage, activated charcoal may be administered. Twenty to 30 g of activated charcoal may be given every four to six hours during the first 24 to 48 hours after ingestion. An ECG should be taken and close monitoring of cardiac function instituted if there is any sign of abnormality. Maintain an open airway and adequate fluid intake; regulate body temperature.
The intravenous administration of 1–3 mg of physostigmine salicylate is reported to reverse the symptoms of tricyclic antidepressant poisoning. Because physostigmine is rapidly metabolized, the dosage of physostigmine should be repeated as required particularly if life threatening signs such as arrhythmias, convulsions, and deep coma recur or persist after the initial dosage of physostigmine. On this basis, in severe overdosage with perphenazine-amitriptyline combinations, symptomatic treatment of central anticholinergic effects with physostigmine salicylate should be considered.
Standard measures should be used to manage circulatory shock and metabolic acidosis. Cardiac arrhythmias may be treated with neostigmine, pyridostigmine, or propranolol. Should cardiac failure occur, the use of digitalis should be considered. Close monitoring of cardiac function for not less than five days is advisable.
Anticonvulsants may be given to control convulsions. Amitriptyline and perphenazine increase the CNS depressant action but not the anticonvulsant action of barbiturates; therefore, an inhalation anesthetic, diazepam, or paraldehyde is recommended for control of convulsions. The management of acute symptoms of parkinsonism resulting from perphenazine intoxication may be treated with appropriate doses of COGENTIN® (Benztropine Mesylate, MSD) or diphenhydramine hydrochloride.*
Dialysis is of no value because of low plasma concentrations of the drug.
Since overdosage is often deliberate, patients may attempt suicide by other means during the recovery phase.
Deaths by deliberate or accidental overdosage have occurred with this class of drugs.

How Supplied

No. 3328—Tablets TRIAVIL 2–10 are blue, triangular, film coated tablets, coded MSD 914.
They are supplied as follows:
NDC 0006-0914-68 bottles of 100
NDC 0006-0914-28 single unit package of 100
NDC 0006-0914-74 bottles of 500.
[*Shown in Product Identification Section*]
No. 3311—Tablets TRIAVIL 2–25 are orange, triangular, film coated tablets, coded MSD 921.
They are supplied as follows:
NDC 0006-0921-68 bottles of 100
NDC 0006-0921-28 single unit package of 100
NDC 0006-0921-74 bottles of 500
(6505-00-931-4303 500's)
[*Shown in Product Identification Section*]
No. 3310—Tablets TRIAVIL 4–10 are salmon, triangular, film coated tablets, coded MSD 934.
They are supplied as follows:
NDC 0006-0934-68 bottles of 100
NDC 0006-0934-28 single unit package of 100
NDC 0006-0934-74 bottles of 500.
[*Shown in Product Identification Section*]
No. 3312—Tablets TRIAVIL 4–25 are yellow, triangular, film coated tablets, coded MSD 946.
They are supplied as follows:
NDC 0006-0946-68 bottles of 100
NDC 0006-0946-28 single unit package of 100
NDC 0006-0946-74 bottles of 500.
[*Shown in Product Identification Section*]
No. 3364—Tablets TRIAVIL 4-50 are orange, diamond shaped, film coated tablets, coded MSD 517.
They are supplied as follows:
NDC 0006-0517-60 bottles of 60
NDC 0006-0517-68 bottles of 100
NDC 0006-0517-28 single unit package of 100
[*Shown in Product Identification Section*]
A.H.F.S. 28:16:04, 28:16:08
DC 6613215 Issued June 1978

*BENADRYL® (Diphenhydramine Hydrochloride), Parke, Davis & Co.

TURBINAIRE®—see under DECADRON® Phosphate, TURBINAIRE® (dexamethasone sodium phosphate, MSD)

URECHOLINE® Tablets ℞
(bethanechol chloride, MSD), N.F.
URECHOLINE® Injection ℞
(bethanechol chloride, MSD), N.F.

Description

Bethanechol chloride is an ester of a choline-like compound.
It is designated chemically as 2-[(aminocarbonyl) oxy] -*N, N, N*-trimethyl-1-propanaminium chloride.
It is a white, hygroscopic crystalline compound having a slight amine-like odor and is freely soluble in water.
URECHOLINE (Bethanechol Chloride, MSD) is available as 5 mg, 10 mg, and 25 mg tablets for oral use, and as a sterile solution for subcutaneous use only.
The sterile solution is essentially neutral. Each milliliter contains bethanechol chloride, 5 mg, and Water for Injection, q.s., 1 ml. It may be autoclaved at 120° C for 20 minutes without discoloration or loss of potency.

Actions

Bethanechol chloride acts principally by producing the effects of stimulation of the parasympathetic nervous system. It increases the tone of the detrusor urinae muscle, usually producing a contraction sufficiently strong to initiate micturition and empty the bladder. It stimulates gastric motility, increases gastric tone, and often restores impaired rhythmic peristalsis.
Stimulation of the parasympathetic nervous system releases acetylcholine at the nerve endings. When spontaneous stimulation is reduced and therapeutic intervention is required, acetylcholine can be given, but it is rapidly hydrolyzed by cholinesterase, and its effects are transient. Bethanechol chloride is not destroyed by cholinesterase and its effects are more prolonged than those of acetylcholine.
It has predominant muscarinic action and only feeble nicotinic action. Doses that stimulate micturition and defecation and increase peristalsis do not ordinarily stimulate ganglia or voluntary muscles. Therapeutic test doses in normal human subjects have little effect on heart rate, blood pressure, or peripheral circulation.

Indications

For the treatment of acute postoperative and postpartum nonobstructive (functional) urinary retention and for neurogenic atony of the urinary bladder with retention.

Contraindications

Hypersensitivity to URECHOLINE tablets or to any component of URECHOLINE injection, hyperthyroidism, pregnancy, peptic ulcer, latent or active bronchial asthma, pronounced bradycardia or hypotension, vasomotor instability, coronary artery disease, epilepsy, and parkinsonism.
URECHOLINE should not be employed when the strength or integrity of the gastrointestinal or bladder wall is in question, or in the presence of mechanical obstruction; when increased muscular activity of the gastrointestinal tract or urinary bladder might prove harmful, as following recent urinary bladder surgery, gastrointestinal resection and anastomosis, or when there is possible gastrointestinal obstruction; in bladder neck obstruction, spastic gastrointestinal disturbances, acute inflammatory lesions of the gastrointestinal tract, or peritonitis; or in marked vagotonia.

Warning

The sterile solution is for subcutaneous use only. It should never be given intramuscularly or intravenously. Violent symptoms of cholinergic over-stimulation, such as circulatory collapse, fall in blood pressure, abdominal cramps, bloody diarrhea, shock, or sudden cardiac arrest are likely to occur if the drug is given by either of these routes. Although rare, these same symptoms have occurred after subcutaneous injection, and may occur in cases of hypersensitivity or overdosage.

Precautions

Special care is required if this drug is given to patients receiving ganglion blocking compounds because a critical fall in blood pressure may occur. Usually, severe abdominal symptoms appear before there is such a fall in the blood pressure.
In urinary retention, if the sphincter fails to relax as URECHOLINE contracts the bladder, urine may be forced up the ureter into the kidney pelvis. If there is bacteriuria, this may cause reflux infection.

Adverse Reactions

Abdominal discomfort, salivation, flushing of the skin ("hot feeling"), sweating.
Large doses more commonly result in effects of parasympathetic stimulation, such as malaise, headache, sensation of heat about the face, flushing, colicky pain, diarrhea, nausea and belching, abdominal cramps, borborygmi, asthmatic attacks, and fall in blood pressure.
Atropine is a specific antidote. The recommended dose for adults is 0.6 mg (1/100 grain). Use proportionately smaller amounts for children. Subcutaneous injection of atropine is preferred except in emergencies when the intravenous route may be employed.
When URECHOLINE is administered subcutaneously, a syringe containing a dose of atropine sulfate should always be available to treat symptoms of toxicity.

Dosage and Administration

Dosage and route of administration must be individualized, depending on the type and severity of the condition to be treated.
Preferably give the drug when the stomach is empty. If taken soon after eating, nausea and vomiting may occur.
Oral—The usual adult dosage is 10 to 50 mg three or four times a day. The minimum effective dose is determined by giving 5 or 10 mg initially and repeating the same amount at hourly intervals until satisfactory response occurs or until a maximum of 50 mg has been given. The effects of the drug sometimes appear within 30 minutes and usually within 60 to 90 minutes. They persist for about an hour.
Subcutaneous—The usual dose is 1 ml (5 mg), although some patients respond satisfactorily to as little as 0.5 ml (2.5 mg). The minimum effective dose is determined by injecting 0.5 ml (2.5 mg) initially and repeating the same amount at 15 to 30 minute intervals to a maximum of four doses until satisfactory response is obtained, unless disturbing reactions appear. The minimum effective dose may be repeated thereafter three or four times a day as required.
Rarely, single doses up to 2 ml (10 mg) may be required. Such large doses may cause severe reactions and should be used only after adequate trial of single doses of 0.5 to 1 ml (2.5 to 5 mg) has established that smaller doses are not sufficient.
URECHOLINE is usually effective in 5 to 15 minutes after subcutaneous injection.
If necessary, the effects of the drug can be abolished promptly by atropine (see ADVERSE REACTIONS).

How Supplied

Tablets URECHOLINE are round, compressed tablets, scored on one side. They are supplied as follows:
No. 7785—5 mg, white in color, coded MSD 403.
NDC 0006-0403-68 in bottles of 100.
NDC 0006-0403-28 single unit packages of 100.
[*Shown in Product Identification Section*]
No. 7787—10 mg, pink in color, coded MSD 412.
NDC 0006-0412-68 in bottles of 100.
(6505-00-616-7856 10 mg 100's)
NDC 0006-0412-28 single unit packages of 100.
[*Shown in Product Identification Section*]
No. 7788—25 mg, yellow in color, coded MSD 457.
NDC 0006-0457-68 in bottles of 100.
NDC 0006-0457-28 single unit packages of 100.
[*Shown in Product Identification Section*]
No. 7786—Injection URECHOLINE, 5 mg per ml, is a clear, colorless solution, and is supplied as follows:
NDC 0006-7786-29 in box of 6 × 1 ml vials.
A.H.F.S. 12:04
DC 6208424 Issued July 1979

VIVACTIL® Tablets ℞
(protriptyline HCl, MSD), N.F.

Description

Protriptyline HCl, a dibenzocycloheptene derivative, is a white to yellowish powder freely soluble in water.
It is designated chemically as N-methyl-5H-dibenzo[a,d]cycloheptene-5-propylamine hydrochloride.
The molecular weight is 299.8. The empirical formula is $C_{19}H_{21}N \bullet HCl$.
VIVACTIL (Protriptyline HCl, MSD) is supplied as 5 mg. and 10 mg. film coated tablets.

Actions

VIVACTIL is an antidepressant agent. The mechanism of its antidepressant action in man is not known. It is not a monoamine oxidase inhibitor, and it does not act primarily by stimulation of the central nervous system.
VIVACTIL has been found in some studies to have a more rapid onset of action than imipramine or amitriptyline. The initial clinical effect may occur within one week. Sedative and tranquilizing properties are lacking. The rate of excretion is slow.

Indications

VIVACTIL is indicated for the treatment of symptoms of mental depression in patients who are under close medical supervision. Its activating properties make it particularly suitable for withdrawn and anergic patients.

Contraindications

VIVACTIL is contraindicated in patients who have shown prior hypersensitivity to it.
It should not be given concomitantly with a monoamine oxidase inhibiting compound. Hyperpyretic crises, severe convulsions, and deaths have occurred in patients receiving tricyclic antidepressant and monoamine oxidase inhibiting drugs simultaneously. When it is desired to substitute VIVACTIL for a mono-

Continued on next page

Information on the Merck Sharp & Dohme products listed on these pages is the full prescribing information from package circulars in use October 31, 1979.

Merck Sharp & Dohme—Cont.

amine oxidase inhibitor, a minimum of 14 days should be allowed to elapse after the latter is discontinued. VIVACTIL should then be initiated cautiously with gradual increase in dosage until optimum response is achieved.
This drug should not be used during the acute recovery phase following myocardial infarction.

Warnings

VIVACTIL may block the antihypertensive effect of guanethidine or similarly acting compounds.
It may impair mental and/or physical abilities required for the performance of hazardous tasks, such as operating machinery or driving a motor vehicle.
VIVACTIL should be used with caution in patients with a history of seizures, and, because of its autonomic activity, in patients with a tendency to urinary retention, or increased intraocular tension.
Tachycardia and postural hypotension may occur more frequently with VIVACTIL than with other antidepressant drugs. VIVACTIL should be used with caution in elderly patients and patients with cardiovascular disorders; such patients should be observed closely because of the tendency of the drug to produce tachycardia, hypotension, arrhythmias, and prolongation of the conduction time. Myocardial infarction and stroke have occurred with drugs of this class.
On rare occasions, hyperthyroid patients or those receiving thyroid medication may develop arrhythmias when this drug is given.
In patients who may use alcohol excessively, it should be borne in mind that the potentiation may increase the danger inherent in any suicide attempt or overdosage.

Usage in Children
This drug is not recommended for use in children because safety and effectiveness in the pediatric age group have not been established.

Usage in Pregnancy
Safe use in pregnancy and lactation has not been established; therefore, use in pregnant women, nursing mothers or women who may become pregnant requires that possible benefits be weighed against possible hazards to mother and child.
In mice, rats, and rabbits, doses about ten times greater than the recommended human doses had no apparent adverse effects on reproduction.

Precautions

When protriptyline HCl is used to treat the depressive component of schizophrenia, psychotic symptoms may be aggravated. Likewise, in manic-depressive psychosis, depressed patients may experience a shift toward the manic phase if they are treated with an antidepressant drug. Paranoid delusions, with or without associated hostility, may be exaggerated. In any of these circumstances, it may be advisable to reduce the dose of VIVACTIL or to use a major tranquilizing drug concurrently.
Symptoms, such as anxiety or agitation, may be aggravated in overactive or agitated patients.
When VIVACTIL is given with anticholinergic agents or sympathomimetic drugs, including epinephrine combined with local anesthetics, close supervision and careful adjustment of dosages are required.
It may enhance the response to alcohol and the effects of barbiturates and other CNS depressants.
The possibility of suicide in depressed patients remains during treatment and until significant remission occurs. This type of patient should not have access to large quantities of the drug.
Concurrent administration of VIVACTIL and electroshock therapy may increase the hazards of therapy. Such treatment should be limited to patients for whom it is essential.
Discontinue the drug several days before elective surgery, if possible.
Both elevation and lowering of blood sugar levels have been reported.

Adverse Reactions

Note: Included in the listing which follows are a few adverse reactions which have not been reported with this specific drug. However, the pharmacological similarities among the tricyclic antidepressant drugs require that each of the reactions be considered when protriptyline is administered. VIVACTIL is more likely to aggravate agitation and anxiety and produce cardiovascular reactions such as tachycardia and hypotension.
Cardiovascular: hypotension, hypertension, tachycardia, palpitation, myocardial infarction, arrhythmias, heart block, stroke.
Psychiatric: confusional states (especially in the elderly) with hallucinations, disorientation, delusions, anxiety, restlessness, agitation; insomnia, panic, and nightmares; hypomania; exacerbation of psychosis.
Neurological: numbness, tingling, and paresthesias of extremities; incoordination, ataxia, tremors, peripheral neuropathy; extrapyramidal symptoms; seizures; alteration in EEG patterns, tinnitus.
Anticholinergic: dry mouth and rarely associated sublingual adenitis; blurred vision, disturbance of accommodation, mydriasis; constipation, paralytic ileus; urinary retention, delayed micturition, dilatation of the urinary tract.
Allergic: skin rash, petechiae, urticaria, itching, photosensitization (avoid excessive exposure to sunlight), edema (general, or of face and tongue), drug fever.
Hematologic: bone marrow depression; agranulocytosis; leukopenia; eosinophilia; purpura; thrombocytopenia.
Gastrointestinal: nausea and vomiting, anorexia, epigastric distress, diarrhea, peculiar taste, stomatitis, abdominal cramps, black tongue.
Endocrine: gynecomastia in the male; breast enlargement and galactorrhea in the female; increased or decreased libido, impotence; testicular swelling; elevation or depression of blood sugar levels.
Other: jaundice (simulating obstructive); altered liver function; weight gain or loss; perspiration; flushing; urinary frequency, nocturia; drowsiness, dizziness, weakness and fatigue; headache; parotid swelling; alopecia.
Withdrawal Symptoms: Though not indicative of addiction, abrupt cessation of treatment after prolonged therapy may produce nausea, headache, and malaise.

Dosage and Administration

Dosage should be initiated at a low level and increased gradually, noting carefully the clinical response and any evidence of intolerance.
Usual Adult Dosage—Fifteen to 40 mg. a day divided into 3 or 4 doses. If necessary, dosage may be increased to 60 mg. a day. Dosages above this amount are not recommended. Increases should be made in the morning dose.
Adolescent and Elderly Patients—In general, lower dosages are recommended for these patients. Five mg. 3 times a day may be given initially, and increased gradually if necessary. In elderly patients, the cardiovascular system must be monitored closely if the daily dose exceeds 20 mg.
When satisfactory improvement has been reached, dosage should be reduced to the smallest amount that will maintain relief of symptoms.
Minor adverse reactions require reduction in dosage. Major adverse reactions or evidence of hypersensitivity require prompt discontinuation of the drug.
Usage in Children—This drug is not recommended for use in children because safety and effectiveness in the pediatric age group have not been established.

Overdosage

Manifestations—High doses may cause temporary confusion, disturbed concentration, or transient visual hallucinations. Overdosage may cause drowsiness; hypothermia; tachycardia and other arrhythmic abnormalities, for example, bundle branch block; ECG evidence of impaired conduction; congestive heart failure; dilated pupils; convulsions; severe hypotension; stupor; and coma. Other symptoms may be agitation, hyperactive reflexes, muscle rigidity, vomiting, hyperpyrexia, or any of those listed under ADVERSE REACTIONS.
Experience in the management of overdosage with protriptyline is limited. The following recommendations are based on the management of overdosage with other tricyclic antidepressants.
All patients suspected of having taken an overdosage should be admitted to a hospital as soon as possible. *Treatment* is symptomatic and supportive. Empty the stomach as quickly as possible by emesis followed by gastric lavage upon arrival at the hospital. Following gastric lavage, activated charcoal may be administered. Twenty to 30 g of activated charcoal may be given every four to six hours during the first 24 to 48 hours after ingestion. An ECG should be taken and close monitoring of cardiac function instituted if there is any sign of abnormality. Maintain an open airway and adequate fluid intake; regulate body temperature.
The intravenous administration of 1-3 mg. of physostigmine salicylate is reported to reverse the symptoms of other tricyclic antidepressant poisoning in humans. Because physostigmine is rapidly metabolized, the dosage of physostigmine should be repeated as required particularly if life threatening signs such as arrhythmias, convulsions, and deep coma recur or persist after the initial dosage of physostigmine.
Standard measures should be used to manage circulatory shock and metabolic acidosis. Cardiac arrhythmias may be treated with neostigmine, pyridostigmine, or propranolol. Should cardiac failure occur, the use of digitalis should be considered. Close monitoring of cardiac function for not less than five days is advisable. Anticonvulsants may be given to control convulsions.
Dialysis is of no value because of low plasma concentrations of the drug.
Since overdosage is often deliberate, patients may attempt suicide by other means during the recovery phase.
Deaths by deliberate or accidental overdosage have occurred with this class of drugs.

How Supplied

No. 3313—Tablets VIVACTIL, 5 mg., are orange, oval, film coated tablets, coded MSD 26. They are supplied as follows:
NDC 0006-0026-68 bottles of 100
NDC 0006-0026-28 single unit packages of 100
NDC 0006-0026-82 bottles of 1000.
[*Shown in Product Identification Section*]
No. 3314—Tablets VIVACTIL, 10 mg., are yellow, oval, film coated tablets, coded MSD 47. They are supplied as follows:
NDC 0006-0047-68 bottles of 100
NDC 0006-0047-28 single unit packages of 100
NDC 0006-0047-82 bottles of 1000.
[*Shown in Product Identification Section*]

Metabolism

Metabolic studies indicate that protriptyline is well absorbed from the gastrointestinal tract and is rapidly sequestered in tissues. Relatively low plasma levels are found after administration, and only a small amount of unchanged drug is excreted in the urine of dogs and rabbits. Preliminary studies indicate that demethylation of the secondary amine moiety occurs to a significant extent, and that metabolic transformation probably takes place in the liver. It penetrates the brain rapidly in mice and rats, and moreover that which is present in the brain is almost all unchanged drug. Studies on the disposition of radioactive protriptyline in human test subjects showed significant plasma levels within 2 hours, peaking at 8 to 12 hours, then declining gradually. Urinary excretion studies in the same subjects showed significant amounts of radioactivity in 2 hours. The rate of excretion was slow. Cumulative urinary excretion during 16 days accounted for approximately 50% of the drug. The fecal route of excretion did not seem to be important.

A.H.F.S. 28:16:04
DC 6380612 Issued October 1977

Information on the Merck Sharp & Dohme products listed on these pages is the full prescribing information from package circulars in use October 31, 1979.

Mericon Industries, Inc.
420 SOUTH WEST WASHINGTON STREET
PEORIA, ILLINOIS 61602

ORAZINC CAPSULES **OTC**
(zinc sulfate USP)

(See PDR For Nonprescription Drugs)

ZINC TABLETS **OTC**
(zinc sulfate USP)

(See PDR For Nonprescription Drugs)

Merrell-National Laboratories
Division of Richardson-Merrell Inc.
CINCINNATI, OHIO 45215

Merrell-National Laboratories Inc.
CAYEY, PUERTO RICO 00633

AVC™ Cream/Suppositories ℞

AVAILABLE ONLY ON PRESCRIPTION

Description:
AVC Cream
Each tube contains:
Sulfanilamide 15.0%
Aminacrine hydrochloride 0.2%
Allantoin 2.0%
with lactose, in a water-miscible base made from propylene glycol, stearic acid, diglycol stearate, and triethanolamine; buffered with lactic acid to an acid pH.
AVC Suppositories
Each suppository contains:
Sulfanilamide ....1.05 g.
Aminacrine hydrochloride ....0.014 g.
Allantoin ....0.14 g.
with lactose, in a base made from polyethylene glycol 400, polysorbate 80, polyethylene glycol 4000, and glycerin; buffered with lactic acid to an acid pH. AVC Suppositories have an inert covering, which dissolves promptly in the vagina. The covering is composed of gelatin, glycerin, water, methylparaben, propylparaben, and coloring.
Actions: AVC is a vaginal preparation combining aminacrine hydrochloride and sulfanilamide. Sulfanilamide is believed to block certain metabolic processes essential for the growth of susceptible bacteria.
Aminacrine hydrochloride, a highly ionized acridine derivative, is thought to act by interfering or competing with certain hydrogen ions in microbial enzyme systems.
These ingredients are combined in a specially compounded base buffered to the pH of the normal vagina to encourage the presence of the normally occurring Döderlein's bacilli of the vagina.

Indications
Based on a review of AVC by the National Academy of Sciences—National Research Council and/or other information, FDA has classified the indications as follows:
"Probably" effective: For the relief of symptoms of vulvovaginitis where isolation of the specific organism responsible (usually *Trichomonas vaginalis, Candida albicans,* or *Hemophilus vaginalis*) is not possible.
NOTE: When the offending organism is known, treatment with a specific agent known to be active against that microorganism is preferred.
"Possibly" effective: For the treatment of trichomoniasis, vulvovaginal candidiasis, and vaginitis due to *Hemophilus vaginalis* or other susceptible bacteria.
Final classification of the less-than-effective indications requires further investigation.

Contraindications: AVC should not be used in patients known to be sensitive to the sulfonamides.
Precautions: As with all sulfonamides, the usual precautions apply. Patients should be observed for manifestations such as skin rash or other evidence of systemic toxicity, and if these develop, the medication should be discontinued.
Adverse Reactions: Although some absorption of sulfanilamide may occur through the vaginal mucosa, systemic manifestations attributable to this drug are infrequent. Local sensitivity reactions such as increased discomfort or a burning sensation have occasionally been reported following the use of topical sulfonamides. Treatment should be discontinued if either local or systemic manifestations of sulfonamide toxicity or sensitivity occur.
Dosage and Administration: 1 applicatorful (about 6 g.) or 1 suppository intravaginally once or twice daily. Improvements in symptoms should occur within a few days, but treatment should be continued through one complete menstrual cycle unless a definite diagnosis is made and specific therapy initiated.
If there is no response within a few days or if symptoms recur, AVC should be discontinued and another attempt made by appropriate laboratory methods to isolate the organism responsible (*Trichomonas vaginalis, Candida albicans, Hemophilus vaginalis*) and institute specific therapy.
Douching with a suitable solution before insertion may be recommended for hygienic purposes. A pad may be used to prevent staining of clothing.
How Supplied:
AVC Cream
0068-0110-13: 4 oz. tube with applicator
0068-0110-15: 24 unit dose package containing ¼ oz. tube with applicator
AVC Suppositories
0068-0111-16: Box of 16 suppositories with inserter

Product Information as of November, 1974
(Package Information amended as of February, 1977)

Suppositories are
Manufactured by
R. P. Scherer Corporation
Detroit, Michigan 48213
Distributed by
MERRELL-NATIONAL LABORATORIES
Division of Richardson-Merrell Inc.
Cincinnati, Ohio 45215, U.S.A.

BENDECTIN® ℞

Description:
Each specially coated tablet contains:
Decapryn® (doxylamine succinate)
—antihistamine ....10 mg.
Pyridoxine hydrochloride ....10 mg.
Actions: Bendectin provides the action of 2 unrelated compounds. Doxylamine succinate, an antihistamine, provides anti-nauseant and anti-emetic activity; the pyridoxine hydrochloride provides vitamin B_6 supplementation to help avoid pyridoxine deficiency that may occur during pregnancy. Also, studies indicate B_6 has an anti-nauseant activity. The anti-emetic action of Bendectin is delayed by a special coating that permits the nighttime dose to be effective in the morning hours—when the patient needs it most.
Indication: Nausea and vomiting of pregnancy
Precautions: Because of potential drowsiness, Bendectin should be prescribed with caution for patients who must drive automobiles or operate machinery.
Studies in rats and rabbits have revealed no suggestion of drug-induced fetal abnormalities at doses of Bendectin up to 90 times the maximum human dose. In addition, several epidemiologic studies in women who received Bendectin during pregnancy have shown that the incidence of birth defects in their offspring is no higher than in women not taking the drug during pregnancy. Nevertheless, like all drugs considered for use during pregnancy, particularly during the first trimester, Bendectin should be used only when clearly needed.
Adverse Reactions: The adverse reactions that may occur are those of the individual ingredients. Doxylamine succinate may cause drowsiness, vertigo, nervousness, epigastric pain, headache, palpitation, diarrhea, disorientation, or irritability.
Pyridoxine hydrochloride is a vitamin that is generally recognized as having no adverse effects.
Dosage and Administration: 2 Bendectin tablets at bedtime. In severe cases or when nausea occurs during the day: 1 additional Bendectin tablet in the morning and another in midafternoon.
How Supplied: Bottles of 100

Product Information as of January, 1978
[*Shown in Product Identification Section*]

BENTYL® ℞
(dicyclomine hydrochloride USP)
Capsules, Tablets, Syrup, Injection

Description:
1. Bentyl 10 mg. capsules
   10 mg. dicyclomine hydrochloride USP in each blue capsule.
2. Bentyl 20 mg. tablets
   20 mg. dicyclomine hydrochloride USP in each blue tablet.
3. Bentyl syrup
   10 mg. dicyclomine hydrochloride USP in each 5 ml. (1 teaspoonful) pink syrup.

Continued on next page

Merrell-National—Cont.

4. Bentyl Injection
   Ampul—2 ml.—Each ml. contains 10 mg. dicyclomine hydrochloride USP, in water for injection, made isotonic with sodium chloride.
   Vial—10 ml.—Each ml. contains 10 mg. dicyclomine hydrochloride USP, in water for injection, made isotonic with sodium chloride. 0.5% chlorobutanol hydrous (chloral derivative) added as a preservative.
   Prefilled Syringe—2 ml.—Each ml. contains 10 mg. dicyclomine hydrochloride USP, in water for injection, made isotonic with sodium chloride.

Actions: Bentyl relieves smooth muscle spasm of the gastrointestinal tract.

Indications
Based on a review of this drug by the National Academy of Sciences—National Research Council and/or other information, FDA has classified the following indications as "probably" effective:
For the treatment of functional bowel/irritable bowel syndrome (irritable colon, spastic colon, mucous colitis) and acute enterocolitis.
THESE FUNCTIONAL DISORDERS ARE OFTEN RELIEVED BY VARYING COMBINATIONS OF SEDATIVE, REASSURANCE, PHYSICIAN INTEREST, AMELIORATION OF ENVIRONMENTAL FACTORS.
For use in the treatment of infant colic (syrup).
Final classification of the less-than-effective indications requires further investigation.

Contraindications: Obstructive uropathy (for example, bladder neck obstruction due to prostatic hypertrophy); obstructive disease of the gastrointestinal tract (as in achalasia, pyloroduodenal stenosis); paralytic ileus, intestinal atony of the elderly or debilitated patient; unstable cardiovascular status in acute hemorrhage; severe ulcerative colitis; toxic megacolon complicating ulcerative colitis; myasthenia gravis.

Warnings: In the presence of a high environmental temperature, heat prostration can occur with drug use (fever and heat stroke due to decreased sweating).
Diarrhea may be an early symptom of incomplete intestinal obstruction, especially in patients with ileostomy or colostomy. In this instance treatment with this drug would be inappropriate and possibly harmful.
Bentyl may produce drowsiness or blurred vision. In this event, the patient should be warned not to engage in activities requiring mental altertness such as operating a motor vehicle or other machinery or perform hazardous work while taking this drug.

Precautions: Although studies have failed to demonstrate adverse effects of dicyclomine hydrochloride in glaucoma or in patients with prostatic hypertrophy, it should be prescribed with caution in patients known to have or suspected of having glaucoma or prostatic hypertrophy.
Use with caution in patients with:
- Autonomic neuropathy.
- Hepatic or renal disease.
- Ulcerative colitis. Large doses may suppress intestinal motility to the point of producing a paralytic ileus and the use of this drug may precipitate or aggravate the serious complication of toxic megacolon.
- Hyperthyroidism, coronary heart disease, congestive heart failure, cardiac arrhythmias, and hypertension.
- Hiatal hernia associated with reflux esophagitis since anticholinergic drugs may aggravate this condition.

Do not rely on the use of the drug in the presence of complication of biliary tract disease.
Investigate any tachycardia before giving anticholinergic (atropine-like) drugs since they may increase the heart rate.
With overdosage, a curare-like action may occur.

Adverse Reactions: Anticholinergics/antispasmodics produce certain effects which may be physiologic or toxic depending upon the individual patient's response. The physician must delineate these.
Adverse reactions may include xerostomia; urinary hesitancy and retention; blurred vision and tachycardia; palpitations; mydriasis; cycloplegia; increased ocular tension; loss of taste; headache; nervousness; drowsiness; weakness; dizziness; insomnia; nausea; vomiting; impotence; suppression of lactation; constipation; bloated feeling; severe allergic reaction or drug idiosyncrasies including anaphylaxis; urticaria and other dermal manifestations; some degree of mental confusion and/or excitement, especially in elderly persons; and decreased sweating.
With the injectable form there may be a temporary sensation of lightheadedness and occasionally local irritation.

Dosage and Administration: Dosage must be adjusted to individual patient's needs.
Usual Dosage
Bentyl 10 mg. capsule and syrup:
- Adults: 1 or 2 capsules or teaspoonfuls syrup three or four times daily.
- Children: 1 capsule or teaspoonful syrup three or four times daily.
- Infants: ½ teaspoonful syrup three or four times daily. (May be diluted with equal volume of water.)

Bentyl 20 mg.:
- Adults: 1 tablet three or four times daily.

Bentyl Injection:
- Adults: 2 ml. (20 mg.) every four to six hours intramuscularly only.
  NOT FOR INTRAVENOUS USE.

Management of Overdose: The signs and symptoms of overdose are headache, nausea, vomiting, blurred vision, dilated pupils, hot, dry skin, dizziness, dryness of the mouth, difficulty in swallowing, CNS stimulation. Treatment should consist of gastric lavage, emetics, and activated charcoal. Barbiturates may be used either orally or intramuscularly for sedation but they should not be used if Bentyl with Phenobarbital has been ingested. If indicated, parenteral cholinergic agents such as Urecholine® (bethanecol chloride USP) should be used.

How Supplied:
10 mg. Capsules
  Bottles of 100, 500, and 1000 and unit dose dispenser of 100
Syrup
  16-ounce bottles
20 mg. Tablets
  Bottles of 100, 500, and 1000 and unit dose dispenser of 100
Injection
  10 ml. multiple dose vials
  Boxes of five 2 ml. ampuls
  Cartons of five 2 ml. prefilled syringes

Product Information as of October, 1978
(Shown in Product Identification Section)

Injectable dosage forms manufactured by
CONNAUGHT LABORATORIES, INC.
Swiftwater, Pennsylvania 18370 or
TAYLOR PHARMACAL COMPANY
Decatur, Illinois 62525 for
MERRELL-NATIONAL LABORATORIES
Division of Richardson-Merrell Inc.
Cincinnati, Ohio 45215, U.S.A.

CANTIL® ℞
(mepenzolate bromide NF)
Tablets

Caution: Federal law prohibits dispensing without prescription.

Description: Cantil (mepenzolate bromide NF) chemically is 3-[(hydroxydiphenylacetyl) oxy]-1,1-dimethylpiperidinium bromide.
Mepenzolate bromide occurs as a white or light cream-colored powder, which is freely soluble in methanol, slightly soluble in water and chloroform, and practically insoluble in ether.
Each yellow tablet contains 25 mg. mepenzolate bromide NF.

Clinical Pharmacology: Cantil diminishes gastric acid and pepsin secretion. Cantil also suppresses spontaneous contractions of the colon. Pharmacologically, it is a post-ganglionic parasympathetic inhibitor.
Radiotracer studies in which Cantil-^{14}C was used in animals and humans indicate that absorption following oral administration, as with other quaternary ammonium compounds, is low. Between 3 and 22% of an orally administered dose is excreted in the urine over a 5-day period, with the majority of the radioactivity appearing on Day 1. The remainder appears in the next 5 days in the feces and presumably has not been absorbed.

Indication: Cantil is indicated for use as adjunctive therapy in the treatment of peptic ulcer. Cantil has not been shown to be effective in contributing to the healing of peptic ulcer, decreasing the rate of recurrence or preventing complications.

Contraindications: Glaucoma, obstructive uropathy (for example, bladder neck obstruction due to prostatic hypertrophy), obstructive disease of the gastrointestinal tract (for example, pyloroduodenal stenosis, achalasia), paralytic ileus, intestinal atony of the elderly or debilitated patient, unstable cardiovascular status in acute hemorrhage, severe ulcerative colitis, toxic megacolon complicating ulcerative colitis, myasthenia gravis, allergic or idiosyncratic reactions to Cantil or related compounds.

Warnings: In the presence of high environmental temperature, heat prostration (fever and heat stroke due to decreased sweating) can occur with use of Cantil.
Cantil may produce drowsiness or blurred vision. The patient should be cautioned regarding activities requiring mental alertness such as operating a motor vehicle or other machinery or performing hazardous work while taking this drug.
With overdosage, a curare-like action may occur, i.e., neuromuscular blockade leading to muscular weakness and possible paralysis.
It should be noted that the use of anticholinergic drugs in the treatment of gastric ulcer may produce a delay in gastric emptying time and may complicate such therapy (antral stasis).

Pregnancy
Reproduction studies in rats and rabbits have shown no evidence of impaired fertility or harm to the animal fetus. Information on possible adverse effects in the pregnant female is limited to uncontrolled data derived from marketing experience. Such experience has revealed no reports of the effect of Cantil on human pregnancies. No controlled studies to establish the safety of the drug in pregnancy have been performed.

Pediatric Use
Since there is no adequate experience in children who have received this drug, safety and efficacy in children have not been established. Newborn animal studies have been undertaken that show that younger animals are more sensitive to the toxic effects of mepenzolate bromide than are older animals.

Precautions: Use Cantil with caution in the elderly and in all patients with:

Autonomic neuropathy
Hepatic or renal disease
Ulcerative colitis. Large doses may suppress intestinal motility to the point of producing a paralytic ileus and for this reason precipitate or aggravate "toxic megacolon," a serious complication of the disease.

Hyperthyroidism, coronary heart disease, congestive heart failure, "cardiac tachyarrhythmias," tachycardia, hypertension, and prostatic hypertrophy.

Hiatal hernia associated with reflux esophagitis, since anticholinergic drugs may aggravate this condition.

This product contains FD&C Yellow No. 5 (tartrazine), which may cause allergic-type reactions (including bronchial asthma) in certain susceptible individuals. Although the overall incidence of FD&C Yellow No. 5 (tartrazine) sensitivity in the general population is low, it is frequently seen in patients who also have aspirin hypersensitivity.

Nursing Mothers

It is not known whether this drug is secreted in human milk. As a general rule, nursing sould not be undertaken while a patient is on a drug since many drugs are excreted in human milk.

Adverse Reactions: Xerostomia, decreased sweating, urinary hesitancy and retention, blurred vision, tachycardia, palpitations, dilatation of the pupil, cycloplegia, increased ocular tension, loss of taste, headaches, nervousness, mental confusion, drowsiness, weakness, dizziness, insomnia, nausea, vomiting, constipation, bloated feeling, impotence, suppression of lactation, severe allergic reaction or drug idiosyncrasies including anaphylaxis, urticaria and other dermal manifestations.

Overdosage: The symptoms of overdosage with Cantil progress from an intensification of the usual adverse effects to CNS disturbances (from restlessness and excitement to psychotic behavior), circulatory changes (flushing, fall in blood pressure, circulatory failure), respiratory failure, paralysis, and coma.

Measures to be taken are (1) immediate lavage of the stomach and (2) injection of physostigmine 0.5 to 2 mg. intravenously, repeated as necessary up to a total of 5 mg. Fever may be treated symptomatically (alcohol sponging, ice packs). Excitement of a degree that demands attention may be managed with sodium thiopental 2% solution given slowly intravenously or chloral hydrate (100–200 ml. of a 2% solution) by rectal infusion. In the event of progression of the curare-like effect to paralysis of the respiratory muscles, artificial respiration should be instituted and maintained until effective respiratory action returns.

Dosage and Administration: Usual Adult Dose: 1 or 2 tablets three times a day preferably with meals and 1 or 2 tablets at bedtime. Begin with the lower dosage when possible and adjust subsequently according to the patient's response.

Since there is no adequate experience in children who have received this drug, safety and efficacy in children have not been established.

Drug Interactions: Concomitant administration of anticholinergic drugs and any other drugs which would increase the anticholinergic effects of Cantil is to be avoided.

How Supplied: Tablets (25 mg.): bottles of 100, 250, and 1000

Product Information as of July, 1979

[*Shown in Product Identification Section*]

CĒPACOL® Mouthwash/Gargle

Description:

Ceepryn® (cetylpyridinium chloride) 1:2000
Alcohol 14%
Phosphate buffers and aromatics

Cēpacol is a soothing, pleasant tasting mouthwash/gargle. It has a low surface tension, approximately ½ that of water. This property is the basis of the spreading action in the oral cavity as well as its foaming action. Cēpacol leaves the mouth feeling fresh and clean and helps provide soothing, temporary relief of dryness and minor irritations.

Uses: Recommended as a mouthwash and gargle for daily oral care; as an aromatic mouth freshener to provide a clean feeling in the mouth; as a soothing, foaming rinse to freshen the mouth.

Used routinely before dental procedures, helps give patient confidence of not offending with mouth odor. Often employed as a foaming and refreshing rinse before, during, and after instrumentation and dental prophylaxis. Convenient as a mouth-freshening agent after taking dental impressions. Helpful in reducing the unpleasant taste and odor in the mouth following gingivectomy.

Used in hospitals as a mouthwash and gargle for daily oral care. Also used to refresh and soothe the mouth following emesis; inhalation therapy, and intubations, and for swabbing the mouths of patients incapable of personal care.

Warning: Keep out of reach of children.

Instructions For Use: Rinse vigorously after brushing or any time to freshen the mouth. Particularly useful after meals or before social engagements. Aromatic Cēpacol leaves the mouth feeling refreshingly clean.

Use full strength every two or three hours as a soothing, foaming gargle, or as directed by a physician or dentist. May also be mixed with warm water.

How Supplied:

6 oz., 12 oz., 18 oz., 24 oz., and a unit package of 4/2-quart bottles
3 oz. Hospital Bedside Bottles (not for retail sale)
3 oz. Dental Chairside Bottles (not for retail sale)
5 oz. Hospital Bedside Bottle (not for retail sale)
14 oz. Direct Stream Dispenser (not for retail sale)
Professional Unit of 4/2-quart bottles with dispensing pump (not for retail sale)

Product Information as of October, 1971
(Package Information amended April, 1977)

CĒPACOL® Throat Lozenges

Description:

Ceepryn® (cetylpyridinium chloride) 1:1500
Benzyl alcohol 0.3%
Aromatics
Yellow mint-flavored hard candy base

Cetylpyridinium chloride (Ceepryn) is a cationic quaternary ammonium compound. This is a surface-active agent, which in aqueous solution, has a surface tension lower than that of water.

Cetylpyridinium chloride in the concentration used in Cēpacol is non-irritating to tissues.

Indications: Cēpacol Lozenges stimulate salivation to help provide soothing temporary relief of dryness and minor irritation of mouth and throat and resulting cough.

Warning: Severe sore throat or sore throat accompanied by high fever or headache or nausea and vomiting, or any sore throat persisting more than two days may be serious. Consult a physician promptly. Persons with a high fever or persistent cough should not use this preparation unless directed by physician. Do not administer to children under 3 years of age unless directed by physician. Keep this and all medication out of children's reach.

Instructions For Use: May be used as needed. Allow to dissolve slowly in the mouth.

How Supplied:

Boxes of 24 Lozenges, 6 Foil Strips of 4 Lozenges Each
Boxes of 400 Lozenges, 100 Foil Strips of 4 Lozenges Each

Product Information as of October, 1971

CĒPACOL® Anesthetic Troches

Description:

Ceepryn® (cetylpyridinium chloride) 1:1500
Benzocaine
Aromatics
Green citrus-flavored hard candy base

Cetylpyridinium chloride (Ceepryn) is a cationic quaternary ammonium compound, which is a surface-active agent. Aqueous solutions of cetylpyridinium chloride have a surface tension lower than that of water.

Cetylpyridinium chloride in the concentration used in Cēpacol is non-irritating to tissues.

Actions:

Anesthetic effect for pain relief
Stimulates salivation—Relieves dryness

Indications: *Sore Throat:* For fast, temporary relief of pain and discomfort due to minor sore throat. For temporary relief of pain and discomfort associated with tonsillitis and pharyngitis. *Mouth Irritations:* For fast, temporary relief of pain and discomfort due to minor mouth irritations. For temporary relief of discomfort associated with stomatitis. For adjunctive, temporary relief of pain and discomfort following periodontal procedures and minor surgery of the mouth.

Warning: Severe sore throat or sore throat accompanied by high fever or headache or nausea and vomiting, or any sore throat persisting more than two days may be serious. Consult a physician promptly. Do not administer to children under 3 years of age unless directed by physician. Keep this and all medication out of children's reach.

Instructions For Use: May be used as needed. Allow to dissolve slowly in the mouth.

How Supplied:

Boxes of 16 Troches, 4 foil strips of 4 Troches each
Boxes of 200 Troches, 50 foil strips of 4 Troches each

Product Information as of July, 1972

CĒPASTAT®
mouthwash/gargle and lozenges

Description:

Mouthwash/Gargle

A soothing mouthwash/gargle containing phenol (1.4%) and glycerin in a slightly alkaline aqueous solution, pleasantly flavored with eugenol and menthol.

Lozenges

Cooling sugar-free lozenges containing phenol (1.45%) and menthol (0.12%) in a sorbitol base flavored with eucalyptus oil.

Indications:

Mouthwash/Gargle and Lozenges

1. Sore throat:
   For prompt temporary relief of local pain or discomfort associated with pharyngitis or tonsillitis or following tonsillectomy.
2. Sore mouth or gums:
   For prompt temporary relief of local pain or discomfort associated with pericoronitis or periodontitis or with dental procedures such as extractions, gingivectomies, and other minor oral surgery.
3. Breath-freshening:
   For prompt temporary breath-freshening.

Action:

Mouthwash/Gargle

Phenol is a recognized topical anesthetic. Glycerine provides a soothing effect.

Lozenge

Phenol is a recognized topical anesthetic. Menthol provides a cooling sensation to aid in symptomatic relief and adds to the lozenge effect in stimulating salivary flow.

Caution*:

Mouthwash/Gargle

Not for use for children under 6 years of age unless directed by physician or dentist. Do not

Continued on next page

Merrell-National—Cont.

swallow or exceed recommended dose. If soreness or discomfort is severe or persists for more than 2 days or is accompanied by high fever, headache, nausea, or vomiting, it may be serious. Consult your physician or dentist promptly. CEPASTAT mouthwash/gargle should not be used for more than 10 days at a time.

Warning*:

Mouthwash/Gargle and Lozenges

KEEP OUT OF REACH OF CHILDREN.

Lozenges

Do not exceed recommended dosage. Consult physician or dentist promptly if throat soreness or discomfort is severe or persists for more than 2 days or is accompanied by high fever, headache, nausea, or vomiting. Do not give to children under 6 years of age unless directed by physician or dentist. Not to be used for more than 10 days at a time. Not a diabetic product.

Instructions For Use:

Mouthwash/Gargle

For minor sore throat:

As gargle, use full strength. Limit gargling to 15 seconds and expel.

As spray, spray 5 times (children 6 to 12 years, spray 3 times) and expel.

Repeat either gargle or spray every 2 hours, if necessary.

For discomforts of mouth or gums:

Use full strength. Swish around sore or painful areas for 15 seconds and expel. DO NOT SWALLOW. Repeat every 2 hours, if necessary.

For temporary breath-freshening effect:

Use as full strength or dilute to half strength with water. Swish and gargle, as needed. Expel. DO NOT SWALLOW. Not intended for routine daily hygiene.

Lozenges

Adults

Dissolve 1 lozenge in mouth every 2 hours. Do not exceed 9 lozenges per day.

Children (6 to 12 years of age)

Dissolve 1 lozenge in mouth every 3 hours. Do not exceed 4 lozenges per day.

How Supplied:

Mouthwash/Gargle

3-ounce bottles with sprayer

7-ounce bottles with and without sprayer

14-ounce bottles without sprayer

All bottles are shatterproof plastic.

Lozenges

300 lozenges in 100 strips of 3 each

Boxes of 18 lozenges as 2 pocket packs of 9 lozenges each

Product Information as of May, 1977

*This section appears on the label for the consumer.

CEPHULAC® ℞
(lactulose)
Syrup

For Oral Administration

Description: Lactulose is 4-O-β-D-galactopyranosyl-D-fructofuranose.

The molecular formula is $C_{12}H_{22}O_{11}$ and the molecular weight is 342.30. Each 15 ml. of Cephulac contains: 10 g. lactulose (and less than 2.2 g. galactose, less than 1.2 g. lactose, and 1.2 g. or less of other sugars), water, flavoring, and coloring. Sodium hydroxide used to adjust pH.

Clinical Pharmacology: Lactulose causes a decrease in blood ammonia concentration and reduces the degree of portal-systemic encephalopathy. These actions are considered to be results of the following:

Bacterial degradation of lactulose in the colon acidifies the colonic contents.

This acidification of colonic contents results in the retention of ammonia in the colon as the ammonium ion. Since the colonic contents are then more acid than the blood, ammonia can be expected to migrate from the blood into the colon to form the ammonium ion.

The acid colonic contents convert NH_3 to the ammonium ion $[NH_4]^+$, trapping it and preventing its absorption.

The laxative action of the metabolites of lactulose then expels the trapped ammonium ion from the colon.

Experimental data indicate that lactulose is poorly absorbed. Lactulose given orally to man and experimental animals resulted in only small amounts reaching the blood. Urinary excretion has been determined to be 3% or less and is essentially complete within 24 hours.

When incubated with extracts of human small intestinal mucosa, lactulose was not hydrolyzed during a 24-hour period and did not inhibit the activity of these extracts on lactose. Lactulose reaches the colon essentially unchanged. There it is metabolized by bacteria with the formation of low molecular weight acids that acidify the colonic contents.

Indications: For the prevention and treatment of portal-systemic encephalopathy, including the stages of hepatic pre-coma and coma.

Controlled studies have shown that lactulose syrup therapy reduces the blood ammonia levels by 25–50%; this is generally paralleled by an improvement in the patients' mental state and by an improvement in EEG patterns. The clinical response has been observed in about 75% of patients, which is at least as satisfactory as that resulting from neomycin therapy. An increase in patients' protein tolerance is also frequently observed with lactulose therapy. In the treatment of chronic portal-systemic encephalopathy, Cephulac has been given for over 2 years in controlled studies.

Contraindications: Since Cephulac contains galactose (less than 2.2 g./15 ml.), it is contraindicated in patients who require a low galactose diet.

Warnings:

Use in Pregnancy

Studies in laboratory animals have not revealed a teratogenic potential of lactulose. The safety of lactulose syrup during pregnancy and its effect on the mother or the fetus have not been evaluated in humans. The physician and patient should understand that the possibility that lactulose syrup might cause damage to the human fetus cannot be excluded. Lactulose syrup should not be given during pregnancy unless, in the opinion of the physician, the possible benefits outweigh the possible risks.

Precautions: Lactulose syrup contains galactose (less than 2.2 g./15 ml.) and lactose (less than 1.2 g./15 ml.) and it should be used with caution in diabetics.

There have been conflicting reports about the concomitant use of neomycin and lactulose syrup. Theoretically, the elimination of certain colonic bacteria by neomycin and possibly other anti-infective agents may interfere with the desired degradation of lactulose and thus prevent the acidification of colonic contents. Thus the status of the lactulose-treated patient should be closely monitored in the event of concomitant oral anti-infective therapy.

Other laxatives should not be used especially during the initial phase of therapy for portal-systemic encephalopathy because the loose stools resulting from their use may falsely suggest that adequate Cephulac dosage has been achieved.

In the overall management of portal-systemic encephalopathy it should be recognized that there is serious underlying liver disease with complications such as electrolyte disturbance (e.g., hypokalemia) for which other specific therapy may be required.

Adverse Reactions: Cephulac may produce gaseous distention with flatulence or belching and abdominal discomfort such as cramping in about 20% of patients. Excessive dosage can lead to diarrhea. Nausea and vomiting have been reported infrequently.

Overdosage: There have been no reports of accidental overdosage. In the event of overdosage it is expected that diarrhea and abdominal cramps would be the major symptoms.

Dosage and Administration:

Adult: The usual adult, oral dosage is 2 to 3 tablespoonfuls (30 to 45 ml., containing 20 g. to 30 g. of lactulose) three or four times daily. The dosage may be adjusted every day or two to produce 2 or 3 soft stools daily.

Hourly doses of 30 to 45 ml. of Cephulac may be used to induce the rapid laxation indicated in the initial phase of the therapy of portal-systemic encephalopathy. When the laxative effect has been achieved, the dose of Cephulac may then be reduced to the recommended daily dose. Improvement in the patient's condition may occur within 24 hours but may not begin before 48 hours or even later.

Continuous long-term therapy is indicated to lessen the severity and prevent the recurrence of portal-systemic encephalopathy. The dose of Cephulac for this purpose is the same as the recommended daily dose.

Pediatric: Very little information on the use of lactulose in young children and adolescents has been recorded. As with adults, the subjective goal in proper treatment is to produce 2 or 3 soft stools daily. On the basis of information available, the recommended initial daily oral dose in infants is 2.5 to 10 ml. in divided doses. For older children and adolescents the total daily dose is 40 to 90 ml. If the initial dose causes diarrhea, the dose should be reduced immediately. If diarrhea persists, lactulose should be discontinued.

How Supplied:

1 pint (473 ml. containing 315 g. of lactulose)

2 quarts (1.89 liters containing 1260 g. or 1.26 kg. of lactulose)

15 ml. (containing 10 g. of lactulose) unit dose containers

30 ml. (containing 20 g. of lactulose) unit dose containers

45 ml. (containing 30 g. of lactulose) unit dose containers

Product Information as of March, 1978

Store at room temperature, perferably below 86°. Do not freeze.

Unit dose cup containers are packaged by Ivers-Lee

West Caldwell, New Jersey 07006 for

MERRELL-NATIONAL LABORATORIES

Division of Richardson-Merrell Inc.

Cincinnati, Ohio 45215, U.S.A.

[*Shown in Product Identification Section*]

CHRONULAC® ℞
(lactulose)
Syrup

Caution: Federal law prohibits dispensing without a prescription.

Description: Chronulac is 4-O-β-D-galactopyranosyl-D-fructofuranose.

The molecular formula is $C_{12}H_{22}O_{11}$ and the molecular weight is 342.30. Each 15 ml. of Chronulac contains: 10 g. lactulose (and less than 2.2 g. galactose, less than 1.2 g. lactose, and 1.2 g. or less of other sugars).

Clinical Pharmacology: Chronulac is poorly absorbed from the gastrointestinal tract and no enzyme capable of hydrolysis of this disaccharide is present in human gastrointestinal tissue. As a result, oral doses of Chronulac reach the colon virtually unchanged. In the colon, Chronulac is broken down primarily to lactic acid, and also to small amounts of formic and acetic acids, by the action of colonic bacteria, which results in an increase in osmotic pressure and slight acidification of the colonic contents. This in turn causes an increase in stool water content and softens the stool.

Since Chronulac does not exert its effect until it reaches the colon, and since transit time through the colon may be slow, 24 to 48 hours may be required to produce a normal bowel movement.

Chronulac given orally to man and experimental animals resulted in only small amounts reaching the blood. Urinary excretion has been determined to be 3% or less and is essentially complete within 24 hours.

Indication: For the treatment of constipation. In patients with a history of chronic constipation, lactulose syrup (Chronulac) therapy increases the number of bowel movements per day and the number of days on which bowel movements occur.

Contraindications: Since Chronulac contains galactose (less than 2.2 g./15 ml.), it is contraindicated in patients who require a low galactose diet.

Warnings:

Use in Pregnancy

Studies in laboratory animals (mice, rats, rabbits) have not revealed a teratogenic potential of Chronulac. The safety of Chronulac Syrup during pregnancy and its effect on the mother or the fetus have not been evaluated in humans.

The physician and patient should understand that the possibility that Chronulac might cause damage to the human fetus cannot be excluded. Chronulac should not be given during pregnancy unless, in the opinion of the physician, the possible benefits outweigh the possible risks.

Use in Nursing Mothers

There are no data on secretion of Chronulac in human milk or effect on the nursing infant.

Use in Children

There is insufficient experience to recommend a dose of Chronulac that is safe and effective for treatment of constipation in children.

Precautions: Elderly, debilitated patients who receive Chronulac for more than six months should have serum electrolytes (potassium, chloride, carbon dioxide) measured periodically. Also, since Chronulac contains galactose (less than 2.2 g./15 ml.) and lactose (less than 1.2 g./15 ml.), it should be used with caution in diabetics.

Adverse Reactions: Initial dosing may produce flatulence and intestinal cramps, which are usually transient. Excessive dosage can lead to diarrhea. Nausea has been reported.

Overdosage: There have been no reports of accidental overdosage. In the event of overdosage it is expected that diarrhea and abdominal cramps would be the major symptoms. Medication should be terminated.

Dosage and Administration: The usual dose is 1 to 2 tablespoonfuls (15 to 30 ml., containing 10 g. to 20 g. of lactulose) daily. The dose may be increased to 60 ml. daily if necessary. Twenty-four to 48 hours may be required to produce a normal bowel movement.

Note: Some patients have found that Chronulac may be more acceptable when mixed with fruit juice, water, or milk.

How Supplied: Bottles containing 8 fl. oz. (237 ml. containing 158 g. of lactulose)

Product Information as of April, 1979

Store at room temperature, preferably below 86°F. Do not freeze.

Prolonged high-temperature storage may cause darkening and loss of clarity, but therapeutic action is not affected. Freezing may cause change to a semisolid, too viscous to pour. (Viscosity will return to normal upon warming to room temperature.)

[*Shown in Product Identification Section*]

CLOMID® ℞
(clomiphene citrate)

For prescribing information, write to:
Manager, Professional Services
MERRELL-NATIONAL LABORATORIES
Division of Richardson-Merrell Inc.
110 E. Amity Road
Cincinnati, Ohio 45215

DV® (dienestrol NF) ℞
Cream/Suppositories

AVAILABLE ONLY ON PRESCRIPTION

Warnings:

1. ESTROGENS HAVE BEEN REPORTED TO INCREASE THE RISK RATIO FOR ENDOMETRIAL CARCINOMA.
Three independent case control studies have reported an increased risk ratio of endometrial cancer in postmenopausal women exposed to exogenous estrogens for prolonged periods.[1–3] This reported risk was independent of the other risk factors studied. Additionally, the incidence rates of endometrial cancer have increased since 1969 in 8 different areas of the United States with population-based cancer reporting systems, an increase that may [or may not] be related to the expanded use of estrogens during the last decade.[4]

The 3 case control studies reported that the estimated risk ratio for endometrial cancer in estrogen users was about 4.5 to 13.9 times greater than in nonusers. The risk appeared to depend on both duration of treatment[1] and on estrogen dose.[3] In view of these reports, when estrogens are used for the treatment of menopausal symptoms, the lowest dose that will control symptoms should be utilized and medication should be discontinued as soon as possible. When prolonged treatment is medically indicated, the patient should be reassessed on at least a semiannual basis to determine the need for continued therapy. Although the evidence must be considered preliminary, one study suggests that cyclic administration of low doses of estrogen may carry less risk than continuous administration;[3] it therefore appears prudent to utilize such a regimen.

Close clinical surveillance of all women taking estrogens is important. In all cases of undiagnosed persistent or recurring abnormal vaginal bleeding, adequate diagnostic measures should be undertaken to rule out malignancy.

There is no evidence at present that "natural" estrogens are more or less hazardous than "synthetic" estrogens at equiestrogenic doses.

2. ESTROGENS SHOULD NOT BE USED DURING PREGNANCY.
The use of exogenous estrogens and progestagens during early pregnancy has been reported to damage the offspring. An association has been reported between *in utero* exposure of the female fetus to diethylstilbestrol, a non-steroidal estrogen, and an increased risk of the post-pubertal development of an ordinarily rare form of vaginal or cervical cancer.[5,6] This risk for diethylstilbestrol was recently estimated to be in the range of 0.14 to 1.4 per 1000 exposures,[7] consistent with a previous risk estimate of not greater than 4 per 1000 exposures.[8] Furthermore, a high percentage of such females exposed *in utero* (30 to over 90%) has been reported to have vaginal adenosis, epithelial changes of the vagina and cervix.[9–12] Although these changes are histologically benign, it is not known whether they are precursors of adenocarcinoma. Although similar data are not available with the use of other estrogens, it cannot be presumed they would not induce similar changes.

Several reports suggest a possible association between fetal exposure to exogenous estrogens and progestagens and congenital anomalies, including congenital heart defects and limb reduction defects.[13–16] One case control study[16] estimated a 4.7 fold increased risk of limb reduction defects in infants exposed *in utero* to exogenous steroids (oral contraceptives, hormone withdrawal tests for pregnancy, or attempted treatment for threatened abortion). Some of these exposures were very short and involved only a few days of treatment. The data suggest that the risk of limb reduction defects in exposed fetuses is somewhat less than 1 per 1000.

This product is not for use in therapy of threatened or habitual abortion.

If DV (dienestrol NF) Cream or Suppositories are used during pregnancy, or if the patient becomes pregnant while using this drug, she should be apprised of the potential risks to the fetus, and the advisability of pregnancy continuation.

Description: DV (dienestrol NF) is a synthetic estrogen in cream and suppository form suitable for vaginal administration.

DV Cream (dienestrol cream NF)—Each tube contains:

Dienestrol NF 0.01%

with lactose, in a water-miscible base made from propylene glycol, stearic acid, diglycol stearate, triethanolamine, benzoic acid, butylated hydroxytoluene and disodium edetate; buffered with lactic acid to an acid pH.

DV Suppositories—Each suppository contains:

Dienestrol NF ....0.70 mg.

with lactose, in a base made from polyethylene glycol 400, polysorbate 80, polyethylene glycol 4000, glycerin, and butylated hydroxytoluene; buffered with lactic acid to an acid pH. DV Suppositories have an inert covering, which dissolves promptly in the vagina. The covering is composed of gelatin, glycerin, water, methylparaben, and propylparaben. Contains color additives including FD&C Yellow No. 5 (tartrazine).

Chemistry

Generic name: Dienestrol NF

Chemical name: Phenol, 4, 4-(1,2-diethylidene-1,2-ethanediyl)bis-4,4'-(Diethylideneethylene) diphenol

Dienestrol occurs as colorless, white, or practically white needlelike crystals or as a white or practically white crystalline powder. It is odorless. It is practically insoluble in water, is slightly soluble in chloroform and fatty oils, and is soluble in alcohol, acetone, ether, and propylene glycol.

Indications: For the treatment of atrophic vaginitis and kraurosis vulvae.

DV (dienestrol NF) CREAM AND SUPPOSITORIES HAVE NOT BEEN SHOWN TO BE EFFECTIVE FOR ANY PURPOSE DURING PREGNANCY AND THE USE MAY HAVE POTENTIAL RISKS TO THE FETUS. (SEE BOXED WARNING.)

Contraindications: DV (dienestrol NF) should not be used in patients with any of the following conditions:

1. Known or suspected cancer of the breast except in appropriately selected patients being treated for metastatic disease.
2. Known or suspected estrogen-dependent neoplasia.
3. Known or suspected pregnancy. (See Boxed Warning.)
4. Undiagnosed abnormal genital bleeding.
5. Active thrombophlebitis or thromboembolic disorders.
6. A past history of thrombophlebitis, thrombosis, or thromboembolic disorders.
7. Hypersensitivity to the ingredients of the cream or suppositories.

Warnings:

1. *Induction of malignant neoplasms.* Long-term continuous administration of natural and synthetic estrogens in certain animal species increases the frequency of carcinomas of the breast, cervix, vagina, and liver. There are now reports that estrogens increase the risk of car-

Continued on next page

Merrell-National—Cont.

cinoma of the endometrium in humans. (See Boxed Warning.)

At the present time there is no satisfactory evidence that estrogens given to postmenopausal women increase the risk of cancer of the breast,[17] although a recent long-term followup of a single physician's practice has raised this possibility.[18] Because of the animal data, there is a need for caution in prescribing estrogens for women with a strong family history of breast cancer or who have breast nodules, fibrocystic disease, or abnormal mammograms.

2. *Gallbladder disease.* A recent study has reported a two to threefold increase in the risk of surgically confirmed gallbladder disease in women receiving postmenopausal estrogens,[17] similar to the twofold increase previously noted in users of oral contraceptives.[19] In the case of oral contraceptives the increased risk appeared after a period of use.[19]

3. *Effects similar to those caused by estrogen-progestagen oral contraceptives.* There are several adverse effects reported in association with oral contraceptives, most of which have not been documented as consequences of postmenopausal estrogen therapy, although it has been reported that there is an increased risk of thrombosis in men receiving high doses of estrogens for prostatic cancer and in women receiving estrogens for postpartum breast engorgement.[20–23] The possibility that the adverse effects reported in association with oral contraceptives may be associated with larger doses of estrogen cannot be excluded.

a. *Thromboembolic disease.* Studies have now shown that users of oral contraceptives have an increased risk of various thromboembolic, thrombotic, and vascular diseases, such as thrombophlebitis, pulmonary embolism, stroke, and myocardial infarction.[24–31] Cases of retinal thrombosis, mesenteric thrombosis, and optic neuritis have been reported in oral contraceptive users. There is evidence that the risk of several of these adverse reactions is related to the dose of the drug.[32,33] An increased risk of post-surgery thromboembolic complications has also been reported in users of oral contraceptives.[34,35] If feasible, estrogen should be discontinued at least 4 weeks before surgery of the type associated with an increased risk of thromboembolism, or during periods of prolonged immobilization.

While an increased rate of thromboembolic and thrombotic disease in postmenopausal users of estrogens has not been found,[17,36] this does not rule out the possibility that such an increase may be present, or that subgroups of women who have underlying risk factors, or who are receiving relatively large doses of estrogens may have an increased risk. Therefore, estrogens should not be used in persons with active thrombophlebitis or thromboembolic disorders, and they should not be used (except in treatment of malignancy) in persons with a history of such disorders. They should be used with caution in patients with cerebral vascular or coronary artery disease and only for those in whom estrogens are needed.

Doses of estrogen (5 mg. conjugated estrogens per day), comparable to those used to treat cancer of the prostate and breast, have been reported in a large prospective clinical trial in men[37] to increase the risk of nonfatal myocardial infarction, pulmonary embolism, and thrombophlebitis. When estrogen doses of this size are used, any of the thromboembolic and thrombotic adverse effects associated with oral contraceptive use should be considered as a risk.

b. *Hepatic adenoma.* Benign hepatic adenomas have been reported to be associated with the use of oral contraceptives.[38–40] Although benign and rare, these may rupture and may cause death through intra-abdominal hemorrhage. Such lesions have not yet been reported in association with other estrogen or progestagen preparations but should be considered in estrogen users having abdominal pain and tenderness, abdominal mass, or hypovolemic shock. Hepatocellular carcinoma has also been reported in women taking estrogen-containing oral contraceptives.[39] The relationship of this malignancy to these drugs is not known at this time.

c. *Elevated blood pressure.* Increased blood pressure is not uncommon in women using oral contraceptives and there is now a report that this may occur with use of estrogens in the menopause[41] and blood pressure should be monitored with estrogen use, especially if high doses are used.

d. *Glucose tolerance.* A worsening of glucose tolerance has been observed in a significant percentage of patients on estrogen-containing oral contraceptives. For this reason diabetic patients should be carefully observed while receiving estrogen.

4. *Hypercalcemia.* Administration of estrogens may lead to hypercalcemia in patients with breast cancer and bone metastases. If this occurs, the drug should be stopped and appropriate measures taken to reduce the serum calcium level.

Precautions:

A. General Precautions

1. A complete medical and family history should be taken prior to the initiation of any estrogen therapy. The pretreatment and periodic physical examinations should include special reference to blood pressure, breasts, abdomen, and pelvic organs, and should include a Papanicolaou smear. As a general rule, estrogen should not be prescribed for longer than 1 year without another physical examination being performed.

2. For conditions due to infection with known organisms, specific treatment should be given for the organism responsible.

3. Fluid retention—Because estrogens may cause some degree of fluid retention, conditions that might be influenced by this factor such as epilepsy, migraine, and cardiac or renal dysfunction require careful observation.

4. Certain patients may develop undesirable manifestations of excessive estrogenic stimulation, such as abnormal or excessive uterine bleeding, mastodynia, etc. In order to avoid this, the dosage should be reduced or the estrogens should be administered intermittently in the menopausal or hypogonadal patient.

5. The age of the patient constitutes no absolute limiting factor, although treatment with estrogens may mask the onset of the climacteric.

6. Oral contraceptives have been reported to be associated with an increased incidence of mental depression. Although it is not clear whether this is possibly due to the estrogenic or progestagenic component of the contraceptive, patients with a history of depression should be carefully observed.

7. Patients having pre-existing uterine leiomyomata should be observed for increased growth of myomata during estrogen therapy.

8. The pathologist should be advised of estrogen therapy when relevant specimens are submitted.

9. Patients with a past history of jaundice during pregnancy have an increased risk of recurrence of jaundice while receiving estrogen-containing oral contraceptive therapy. If jaundice develops in any patient receiving estrogen, the medication should be discontinued while the cause is investigated.

10. Estrogens may be poorly metabolized in patients with impaired liver function and they should be administered with caution in such patients.

11. Because estrogens influence the metabolism of calcium and phosphorus, they should be used with caution in patients with metabolic bone diseases that are associated with hypercalcemia or in patients with renal insufficiency.

12. Because of the effects of estrogens on epiphyseal closure, they should be used judiciously in young patients in whom bone growth is not complete.

13. Judicious assessment of the following changes in certain endocrine and liver function tests is necessary for patients receiving large doses of estrogen:

a. Increased sulfobromophthalein retention.
b. Increased prothrombin and factors VII, VIII, IX, and X; decreased antithrombin 3; increased norepinephrine-induced platelet aggregability.
c. Increased thyroid binding globulin (TBG) leading to increased circulating total thyroid hormone, as measured by PBI, T4 by column, or T4 by radioimmunoassay. Free T3 resin uptake is decreased, reflecting the elevated TBG; free T4 concentration is unaltered.
d. Impaired glucose tolerance.
e. Decreased pregnanediol excretion.
f. Reduced response to metyrapone test.
g. Reduced serum folate concentration.
h. Increased serum triglyceride, phospholipid, or cholesterol.

14. DV Suppositories contain FD&C Yellow No. 5 (tartrazine), which may cause allergic-type reactions (including bronchial asthma) in certain susceptible individuals. Although the overall incidence of FD&C Yellow No. 5 (tartrazine) sensitivity in the general population is low, it is frequently seen in patients who also have aspirin hypersensitivity.

B. Information For The Patient

A patient package insert accompanies this drug product. This insert is available from pharmacists who carry this product and from the company upon request.

C. Pregnancy Category X

See Contraindications and Boxed Warning.

D. Nursing Mothers

As a general principle, the administration of any drug to nursing mothers should be done only when clearly necessary since many drugs are excreted in human milk.

Adverse Reactions: (See Warnings regarding reports of induction of neoplasia, adverse effects on the fetus, increased incidence of gallbladder disease, and adverse effects similar to those of oral contraceptives, including thromboembolism.)

Since there is a possibility of dienestrol absorption through the vaginal mucosa, uterine bleeding might be provoked by excessive administration of dienestrol in menopausal women. Cytologic study or D & C may be required to differentiate this uterine bleeding from carcinoma. Tenderness of the breasts and vaginal discharge due to mucus hypersecretion may result from excessive estrogenic stimulation; endometrial withdrawal bleeding may occur if use of dienestrol is suddenly discontinued. Such reactions indicate overdosage.

Menstrual irregularity may be made worse by dienestrol if a sufficient amount is absorbed. Dienestrol may cause serious bleeding in a woman sterilized because of endometriosis and in whom remaining foci of endometrium could be activated.

The following additional adverse reactions have been reported with estrogenic therapy including oral contraceptives:

1. *Genitourinary system*

Breakthrough bleeding, spotting, change in menstrual flow and cycle.
Dysmenorrhea.
Premenstrual-like syndrome.
Amenorrhea during and after treatment.
Increase in size of uterine fibromyomata.
Vaginal candidiasis.
Change in cervical eversion and in degree of cervical secretion.
Cystitis-like syndrome.

2. *Breasts*

Tenderness, enlargement, secretion.

3. *Gastrointestinal*
Nausea, vomiting.
Abdominal cramps, bloating.
Cholestatic jaundice.
4. *Skin*
Chloasma or melasma which may persist when drug is discontinued.
Erythema multiforme.
Erythema nodosum.
Hemorrhagic eruption.
Loss of scalp hair.
Hirsutism.
Urticaria.
5. *Eyes*
Steepening of corneal curvature.
Intolerance to contact lenses.
6. *CNS*
Headache, migraine, dizziness.
Mental depression.
Chorea.
7. *Miscellaneous*
Increase or decrease in weight.
Reduced carbohydrate tolerance.
Aggravation of porphyria.
Edema.
Changes in libido and/or potency.

Acute Overdosage: Numerous reports of ingestion of large doses of estrogen-containing oral contraceptives by young children indicate that serious ill effects usually do not occur. Overdosage of estrogen may cause nausea, and withdrawal bleeding may occur in females.

Dosage and Administration: 1 or 2 applicatorfuls of cream or 1 or 2 suppositories intravaginally per day for 1 or 2 weeks, then reduced to either one-half initial dosage or 1 applicatorful (about 6 g.) or 1 suppository every other day for a similar period.

Maintenance Dose
1 applicatorful of cream or 1 suppository one to three times a week may be used after restoration of the vaginal mucosa has been effected.

How Supplied:
DV Cream
NDC 0068-0293-13: 3 oz. tube with applicator
DV Suppositories
NDC 0068-0294-16: box of 16 with inserter

References:

1. Ziel, H.K. and Finkel, W.D.: Increased risk of endometrial carcinoma among users of conjugated estrogens. New Eng. J. Med. 293:1167-1170, 1975.
2. Smith, D.C., Prentice, R., Thompson, D.J., and Hermann, W.L.: Association of exogenous estrogen and endometrial carcinoma. New Eng. J. Med. 293:1164-1167, 1975.
3. Mack, T.M., Pike, M.C., Henderson, B.E., Pfeffer, R.I., Gerkins, V.R., Arthur, M., and Brown, S.E.: Estrogens and endometrial cancer in a retirement community. New Eng. J. Med. 294:1262-1267, 1976.
4. Weiss, N.S., Szekely, D.R., and Austin, D.F.: Increasing incidence of endometrial cancer in the United States. New Eng. J. Med. 294:1259-1262, 1976.
5. Herbst, A.L., Ulfelder, H., and Poskanzer, D.C.: Adenocarcinoma of the vagina. New Eng. J. Med. 284:878-881, 1971.
6. Greenwald, P., Barlow, J.J., Nasca, P.C., and Burnett, W.S.: Vaginal cancer after maternal treatment with synthetic estrogens. New Eng. J. Med. 285:390-392, 1971.
7. Herbst, A.L., Cole, P., Colton, T., Robboy, S.J., and Scully, R.E.: Latency period and incidence aspects of DES-related clear cell adenocarcinoma of the vagina and cervix. In press. Amer. J. Obstet. Gynec.
8. Lanier, A.P., Noller, K.L., Decker, D.G., Elveback, L.R., and Kurland, L.T.: Cancer and stilbestrol. A follow-up of 1719 persons exposed to estrogens in utero and born 1943-1959. Mayo Clin. Proc. 48:793-799, 1973.
9. Herbst, A.L., Kurman, R.J., and Scully, R.E.: Vaginal and cervical abnormalities after exposure to stilbestrol in utero. Obstet. Gynec. 40:287-298, 1972.
10. Herbst, A.L., Poskanzer, D.C., Robboy, S.J., Friedlander, L., and Scully, R.E.: Prenatal exposure to stilbestrol. A prospective comparison of exposed female offspring with unexposed controls. New Eng. J. Med. 292:334-339, 1975.
11. Stafl, A., Mattingly, R.F., Foley, D.V., and Fetherston, W.C.: Clinical diagnosis of vaginal adenosis. Obstet. Gynec. 43:118-128, 1974.
12. Sherman, A.I., Goldrath, M., Berlin, A., Vakhariya, V., Banooni, F., Michaels, W., Goodman, P., and Brown, S.: Cervical-vaginal adenosis after *in utero* exposure to synthetic estrogens. Obstet. Gynec. 44:531-545, 1974.
13. Gal, I., Kirman, B., and Stern, J.: Hormone pregnancy tests and congenital malformation. Nature 216:83, 1967.
14. Levy, E.P., Cohen, A., and Fraser, F.C.: Hormone treatment during pregnancy and congenital heart defects. Lancet 1:611, 1973.
15. Nora, J.J. and Nora, A.H.: Birth defects and oral contraceptives. Lancet 1:941-942, 1973.
16. Janerich, D.T., Piper, J.M., and Glebatis, D.M.: Oral contraceptives and congenital limb-reduction defects. New Eng. J. Med. 291:697-700, 1974.
17. Boston Collaborative Drug Surveillance Program: Surgically confirmed gall bladder disease, venous thromboembolism, and breast tumors in relation to post menopausal estrogen therapy. New Eng. J. Med. 290:15-19, 1974.
18. Hoover, R., Gray, L.A., Sr., Cole, P., and MacMahon, B.: Menopausal estrogens and breast cancer. New Eng. J. Med. 295:401-405, 1976.
19. Boston Collaborative Drug Surveillance Program: Oral contraceptives and venous thromboembolic disease, surgically confirmed gall-bladder disease, and breast tumors. Lancet 1:1399-1404, 1973.
20. Daniel, D.G., Campbell, H., and Turnbull, A.C.: Puerperal thromboembolism and suppression of lactation. Lancet 2:287-289, 1967.
21. Bailar, J.C., III: Thromboembolism and oestrogen therapy. Lancet 2:560, 1967.
22. The Veterans Administration Cooperative Urological Research Group: Carcinoma of the prostate: Treatment comparisons. J. Urol. 98:516-522, 1967.
23. Blackard, C.E., Doe, R.P., Mellinger, G.T., and Byar, D.P.: Incidence of cardiovascular disease and death in patients receiving diethylstilbestrol for carcinoma of the prostate. Cancer 26:249-256, 1970.
24. Royal College of General Practitioners: Oral contraception and thromboembolic disease. J. Roy. Coll. Gen. Pract. 13:267-269, 1967.
25. Inman, W.H.W. and Vessey, M.P.: Investigation of deaths from pulmonary, coronary, and cerebral thrombosis and embolism in women of child-bearing age. Brit. Med. J. 2:193-199, 1968.
26. Vessey, M.P. and Doll, R.: Investigation of relation between use of oral contraceptives and thromboembolic disease. A further report. Brit. Med. J. 2:651-657, 1969.
27. Sartwell, P.E., Masi, A.T., Arthes, F.G., Greene, G.R., and Smith, H.E.: Thromboembolism and oral contraceptives: An epidemiological case-control study. Amer. J. Epidem. 90:365-380, 1969.
28. Collaborative Group for the Study of Stroke in Young Women: Oral contraception and increased risk of cerebral ischemia or thrombosis. New Eng. J. Med. 288:871-878, 1973.
29. Collaborative Group for the Study of Stroke in Young Women: Oral contraceptives and stroke in young women: Associated risk factors. J.A.M.A. 231:718-722, 1975.
30. Mann, J.I. and Inman, W.H.W.: Oral contraceptives and death from myocardial infarction. Brit. Med. J. 2:245-248, 1975.
31. Mann, J.I., Vessey, M.P., Thorogood, M., and Doll, R.: Myocardial infarction in young women with special reference in oral contraceptive practice. Brit. Med. J. 2:241-245, 1975.
32. Inman, W.H.W., Vessey, M.P., Westerholm, B., and Engelund, A.: Thromboembolic disease and the steroidal content of oral contraceptives. A report to the Committee on Safety of Drugs. Brit. Med. J. 2:203-209, 1970.
33. Stolley, P.D., Tonascia, J.A., Tockman, M.S., Sartwell, P.E., Rutledge, A.H., and Jacobs, M.P.: Thrombosis with low-estrogen oral contraceptives. Amer. J. Epidem. 102:197-208, 1975.
34. Vessey, M.P., Doll, R., Fairbairn, A.S., and Glober, G.: Post-operative thromboembolism and the use of the oral contraceptives. Brit. Med. J. 3:123-126, 1970.
35. Greene, G.R. and Sartwell, P.E.: Oral contraceptive use in patients with thromboembolism following surgery, trauma, or infection. Amer. J. Public Health 62:680-685, 1972.
36. Rosenberg, L., Armstrong, B., Phil, D., and Jick, H.: Myocardial infarction and estrogen therapy in post-menopausal women. New Eng. J. Med. 294:1256-1259, 1976.
37. Coronary Drug Project Research Group: The coronary drug project: Initial findings leading to modifications of its research protocol. J.A.M.A. 214:1303-1313, 1970.
38. Baum, J., Holtz, F., Bookstein, J.J., and Klein, E.W.: Possible association between benign hepatomas and oral contraceptives. Lancet 2:926-928, 1973.
39. Mays, E.T., Christopherson, W.M., Mahr, M.M., and Williams, H.C.: Hepatic changes in young women ingesting contraceptive steroids. Hepatic hemorrhage and primary hepatic tumors. J.A.M.A. 235:730-732, 1976.
40. Edmondson, H., Henderson, A.B., and Benton, B.: Liver-cell adenomas associated with the use of oral contraceptives. New Eng. J. Med. 294:470-472, 1976.
41. Pfeffer, R.I. and Van Den Noort, S.: Estrogen use and stroke risk in postmenopausal women. Amer. J. Epidem. 103:445-456, 1976.

Product Information as of August, 1979

DV Suppositories are manufactured by
R. P. Scherer Corporation
Detroit, Michigan 48213
Distributed by
MERRELL-NATIONAL LABORATORIES
Division of Richardson-Merrell Inc.
Cincinnati, Ohio 45215, U.S.A.

DELCID®

Description: Each teaspoonful (5 ml.) contains a balanced combination of 600 mg. aluminum hydroxide [Al $(OH)_3$] and 665 mg. magnesium hydroxide [Mg $(OH)_2$]. The sodium content is not more than 15 mg. per teaspoonful.

Actions: The balanced ratio of antacids provides reduction of gastric acidity and gives symptomatic comfort to the patient. The acid neutralizing capacity is 42 mEq. for each 5 ml.

Indications: Delcid is used to relieve the symptoms of hyperacidity associated with peptic ulcer, gastritis, peptic esophagitis, gastric hyperacidity, and hiatal hernia, and to relieve the following symptoms: heartburn, sour stomach, or acid indigestion.

Warnings*: Do not take more than 6 teaspoonfuls in a 24-hour period or use the maximum dosage of this product for more than 2 weeks, except under the advice and supervision of a physician. May have laxative effect. Do not use this product except under the advice and supervision of a physician if you have kidney disease. Keep this and all drugs out of the reach of children. In case of accidental overdose, seek professional assistance or contact a poison control center immediately.

Drug Interaction Precautions*: Do not take this product if you are presently taking a prescription antibiotic drug containing any form of tetracycline.

Adverse Reactions: Miscellaneous reports include diarrhea, nausea, and vomiting.

Dosage and Administration: 1 teaspoonful, ½ to 1 hour after meals and at bedtime or as directed.

Continued on next page

Merrell-National—Cont.

Directions : Take as needed to alleviate symptoms: 1 teaspoonful every 4 hours, or as directed by a physician.
How Supplied: 8 fl. oz. plastic bottles

*This section appears on the label for the consumer.

Product Information as of April, 1977

HIPREX® ℞
(methenamine hippurate)

Description: Hiprex (methenamine hippurate) is the hippuric acid salt of methenamine (hexamethylenetetramine).
Actions: Microbiology: Hiprex (methenamine hippurate) has antibacterial activity because the methenamine component is hydrolyzed to formaldehyde in acid urine. Hippuric acid, the other component, has some antibacterial activity and also acts to keep the urine acid. The drug is generally active against *E. coli,* enterococci and staphylococci. *Enterobacter aerogenes* is generally resistant. The urine must be kept sufficiently acid for urea-splitting organisms such as *Proteus* and *Pseudomonas* to be inhibited.
Human Pharmacology: Within ½ hour after ingestion of a single 1-gram dose of Hiprex, antibacterial activity is demonstrable in the urine. Urine has continuous antibacterial activity when Hiprex is administered at the recommended dosage schedule of 1 gram twice daily. Over 90% of methenamine moiety is excreted in the urine within 24 hours after administration of a single 1-gram dose. Similarly, the hippurate moiety is rapidly absorbed and excreted, and it reaches the urine by both tubular secretion and glomerular filtration. This action may be important in older patients or in those with some degree of renal impairment.
Indications: Hiprex is indicated for prophylactic or suppressive treatment of frequently recurring urinary tract infections when long-term therapy is considered necessary. This drug should only be used after eradication of the infection by other appropriate antimicrobial agents.
Contraindications: Hiprex (methenamine hippurate) is contraindicated in patients with renal insufficiency, severe hepatic insufficiency, or severe dehydration. Methenamine preparations should not be given to patients taking sulfonamides because some sulfonamides may form an insoluble precipitate with formaldehyde in the urine.
Warning: Large doses of methenamine (8 grams daily for 3 to 4 weeks) have caused bladder irritation, painful and frequent micturition, albuminuria, and gross hematuria.
Precautions:
1. Care should be taken to maintain an acid pH of the urine, especially when treating infections due to urea-splitting organisms such as *Proteus* and strains of *Pseudomonas.*
2. In a few instances in one study, the serum transaminase levels were slightly elevated during treatment but returned to normal while the patients were still taking Hiprex. Because of this report, it is recommended that liver function studies be performed periodically on patients taking the drug, especially those with liver dysfunction.
3. Use in pregnancy: In early pregnancy the safe use of Hiprex is not established. In the last trimester, safety is suggested, but not definitely proved. No adverse effects on the fetus were seen in studies in pregnant rats and rabbits.

Adverse Reactions: Minor adverse reactions have been reported in less than 3.5% of patients treated. These reactions have included nausea, upset stomach, dysuria, and rash.
Dosage and Administration: 1 tablet (1.0 g.) twice daily (morning and night) for adults and children over 12 years of age.
½ to 1 tablet (0.5 to 1.0 g.) twice daily (morning and night) for children 6 to 12 years of age.
Since the antibacterial activity of Hiprex is greater in acid urine, restriction of alkalinizing foods and medications is desirable. If necessary, as indicated by urinary pH and clinical response, supplemental acidification of the urine should be instituted. The efficacy of therapy should be monitored by repeated urine cultures.
How Supplied: 1-gram scored, yellow tablets in bottles of 100 and 500

Product Information as of April, 1976

[*Shown in Product Identification Section*]

IMFERON® ℞
(iron dextran injection USP)

Warning:

THE PARENTERAL USE OF COMPLEXES OF IRON AND CARBOHYDRATES HAS RESULTED IN FATAL ANAPHYLACTIC-TYPE REACTIONS. DEATHS ASSOCIATED WITH SUCH ADMINISTRATION HAVE BEEN REPORTED. THEREFORE, IMFERON SHOULD BE USED ONLY IN THOSE PATIENTS WHERE CLEARLY ESTABLISHED INDICATIONS EXIST, CONFIRMED BY APPROPRIATE LABORATORY INVESTIGATIONS CORROBORATING IRON DEFICIENCY ANEMIA NOT AMENABLE TO ORAL IRON THERAPY.

Description: Imferon® (iron dextran injection USP)—a dark brown, slightly viscous liquid complex of ferric hydroxide and dextran in a 0.9% sodium chloride solution for injection. It contains 50 mg. of elemental iron per ml. Multiple dose vial also contains 0.5% phenol.
Action: The iron dextran complex is dissociated by the reticuloendothelial system, and the ferric iron is transported by transferrin and incorporated into hemoglobin.
Indications: For the treatment of iron deficiency anemia: intramuscular or intravenous injections of iron are advisable solely for use in those patients in whom iron deficiency anemia is present, its cause has been determined and, if possible, corrected, and in whom oral administration of iron is unsatisfactory or impossible; for example: intolerance to oral preparation; resistance to oral iron therapy; rapid replenishment of iron stores in selected patients in whom oral therapy is ineffective, such as hypochromic anemia of infancy and hypochromic anemia of the last trimester of pregnancy; selected hemorrhagic cases (appropriate steps should be taken to correct and prevent any excessive blood loss that may have been revealed as an etiologic factor); to replace postoperative transfusion to some degree; in those patients who cannot be relied upon to take oral medication.
Imferon (iron dextran injection) injected intramuscularly is the preferred and recommended route of administration. Intravenous use of Imferon should be limited to the following circumstances:

a. insufficient muscle mass for deep intramuscular injection
b. impaired absorption from the muscle due to stasis or edema
c. the possibility of uncontrolled intramuscular bleeding due to trauma as may occur in hemophilia
d. where massive and prolonged parenteral therapy is indicated as may be necessary in instances of chronic substantial blood loss, such as familial telangiectasia
e. in those circumstances where, in the opinion of the physician, the benefit of intravenous administration substantially outweighs the risk.

Contraindications: Hypersensitivity to the product. All anemias other than iron deficiency anemia.
Warnings: This preparation should be used with extreme care in the presence of serious impairment of liver function.
A risk of carcinogenesis may attend the intramuscular injection of iron-carbohydrate complexes. Such complexes have been found under experimental conditions to produce sarcomas when injected in rats, mice and rabbits, and possibly in hamsters, in very large doses. The number of tumors produced was relatively small, and such tumors have not been produced in guinea pigs. The long latent period between the injection of a potential carcinogen and the appearance of a tumor makes it impossible as yet to measure the risk in man. However, the risk of carcinogenesis in man, following recommended therapy, appears to be extremely small.
Usage in Pregnancy: in animals, fetal abnormalities have been demonstrated when Imferon (iron dextran injection) was given early in pregnancy. Safe use of Imferon (iron dextran injection) has not been established with respect to adverse effects on human fetal development. Imferon should not be used in early pregnancy and should be used in women of child-bearing potential only when, in the judgment of the physician, the potential benefits outweigh the possible hazards.
Precautions: Unwarranted therapy with parenteral iron will cause excess storage of iron with the consequent possibility of exogenous hemosiderosis. Such iron overload is particularly apt to occur in patients with hemoglobinopathies and other refractory anemias which might be erroneously diagnosed as iron deficiency anemias.
Patients with iron deficiency anemia and rheumatoid arthritis may have an acute exacerbation of joint pain and swelling following the intravenous administration of Imferon (iron dextran injection).
Adverse Reactions: Anaphylactic reactions including fatal anaphylaxis; severe febrile reactions; arthralgia and myalgia; variable degree of soreness and inflammation at injection site (IM injection); brown skin discoloration at injection site (IM injection); local phlebitis at injection site (IV injection); peripheral vascular "flushing" with overly rapid IV administration; hypotensive reaction; possible arthritic reactivation in patients with quiescent rheumatoid arthritis; minor reactions may include headache, transitory paresthesias, nausea, shivering, itching, and rash.
Dosage and Administration: Periodic hematologic determinations are to be used as a guide in therapy, bearing in mind that iron storage may lag behind the appearance of normal blood morphology.
The following table provides a convenient method of determining the approximate quantity (in ml.) of Imferon (iron dextran injection) needed for restoration of the hemoglobin and body stores of iron.
The requirements for individuals weighing 30 pounds or less have been reduced to 80% of the formula cited; such patients may be considered to be infants whose "normal hemoglobin" between 6 months and 30 months of age is roughly 12 Gm., rather than the 14.8 Gm. on which the rest of the table is based.
[See table on next page].
Dosage For Intramuscular Use: The total amount of Imferon (iron dextran injection) required is calculated from the formula or table. Inject a test dose of 0.5 ml. the first day. If no indications of adverse reactions are apparent, proceed to administer Imferon according to the following schedule until the calculated total amount required has been reached. Each day's dose should ordinarily not exceed 0.5 ml. (25 mg. of iron) for infants under 10 lbs., 1.0 ml.

(50 mg. of iron) for children under 20 lbs., 2.0 ml. (100 mg. of iron) for patients under 110 lbs., and 5 ml. (250 mg. of iron) for others.

Inject only into the upper outer quadrant of the buttock—never into the arm or other exposed area. Inject deeply, with a two- or three-inch 19 or 20 gauge needle. If the patient is standing, he should be bearing his weight on the leg opposite the injection site, or if in bed, he should be in the lateral position with injection site uppermost. To avoid injection or leakage into the subcutaneous tissue, a Z-track technique (displacement of the skin laterally prior to injection) is recommended.

Dosage For Intravenous Use: The total amount of Imferon (iron dextran injection) required is calculated from the formula or table (see above). This is given in a dose of 0.5 ml. the first day to test for and minimize the chance of toxic reactions. Within two or three days the dosage may be raised to 2 ml. per day, and given thus until the calculated total amount required has been reached. The Imferon is given undiluted, and slowly (one minute per ml. or fraction thereof).

Supplied: For intravenous or intramuscular use:
NDC 0068-0050-09 2 ml. ampuls, boxes of 10
NDC 0068-0050-55 5 ml. ampuls, boxes of 5
For intramuscular use ONLY:
NDC 0068-0052-22 10 ml. multiple dose vial containing phenol 0.5% as preservative, boxes of 2

Imferon® (iron dextran injection USP) is distributed under license from Fisons Limited—Pharmaceutical Division, England.

Revised February, 1975

Manufactured by
Fisons Limited
Pharmaceutical Division, England for
MERRELL-NATIONAL LABORATORIES
Division of Richardson-Merrell Inc.
Cincinnati, Ohio 45215, U.S.A.

TABLE: TOTAL NUMBER OF ml. OF IMFERON (iron dextran injection) REQUIRED IN A COURSE OF TREATMENT

Patient's Weight in Pounds	OBSERVED HEMOGLOBIN 30% (4.4 Gm. 100 ml.)	40% (5.9 Gm. 100 ml.)	50% (7.4 Gm. 100 ml.)	60% (8.9 Gm. 100 ml.)	70% (10.4 Gm. 100 ml.)
10	4 ml.	3 ml.	2 ml.	2 ml.	2 ml.
20	7	6	5	4	3
30	10	9	7	6	5
40	17	15	12	10	7
50	21	18	15	12	9
60	25	22	18	15	11
70	30	25	21	17	13
80	34	29	24	19	15
90	38	32	27	22	16
100	42	36	30	24	18
110	46	39	33	26	20
120	51	43	36	29	22
130	55	47	39	31	23
140	59	50	42	34	25
150	63	54	45	36	27
160	68	57	48	38	29
170	72	61	51	41	31
180	76 ml.	64 ml.	54 ml.	43 ml.	32 ml.

The total cumulative amount required to restore hemoglobin and replenish iron stores may be approximated from the formula:

$$0.3 \times \text{Body weight in pounds} \times \left(100 - \frac{\text{Patient's hemoglobin in gram percent} \times 100}{14.8}\right) = \text{Milligrams}$$

total iron to be injected (To calculate dose in ml. of Imferon, divide this result by 50)

KOLANTYL®

Description: Each teaspoonful (5 ml.) of Kolantyl Gel contains:
Aluminum hydroxide [Al $(OH)_3$] ......150 mg.
Magnesium hydroxide [Mg $(OH)_2$] ....150 mg.
Each Kolantyl Wafer contains:
Aluminum hydroxide ....180 mg.
(supplied as dried aluminum hydroxide gel)
Magnesium hydroxide ....170 mg.

Actions: The balanced ratio of antacids provides reduction of gastric acidity and gives symptomatic comfort to the patient. The acid neutralizing capacity is 10.5 mEq. for each 5 ml. of gel and 10.8 mEq. for each wafer.

Indications: Kolantyl is used to relieve the symptoms of hyperacidity associated with peptic ulcer, gastritis, peptic esophagitis, gastric hyperacidity, and hiatal hernia, and to relieve the following symptons: heartburn, sour stomach, or acid indigestion.

Warnings*: Do not take more than 12 teaspoonfuls of gel or 12 wafers in a 24-hour period or use the maximum dosage of this product for more than 2 weeks, except under the advice and supervision of a physician. May have laxative effect. Do not use this product except under the advice and supervision of a physician if you have kidney disease. Keep this and all drugs out of the reach of children. In case of accidental overdose, seek professional assistance or contact a poison control center immediately.

Drug Interaction Precautions*: Do not take this product if you are presently taking a prescription antibiotic drug containing any form of tetracycline.

Adverse Reactions: Miscellaneous reports include nausea and vomiting, abdominal discomfort, stomatitis, rash, dizziness, and diarrhea.

Dosage and Administration:
Kolantyl Gel: 1 to 4 teaspoonfuls ½ to 1 hour after meals and at bedtime or as directed. May be taken undiluted or mixed with milk or water, particularly if the patient is on a regular milk regimen.
Kolantyl Wafers: 1 to 4 wafers ½ to 1 hour after meals and at bedtime or as directed. Wafers may be chewed or allowed to dissolve in the mouth.

Directions*:
Kolantyl Gel—Take as needed to alleviate symptoms: 1 to 4 teaspoonfuls every 4 hours, or as directed by a physician.
Kolantyl Wafers—Take as needed to alleviate symptoms: 1 to 4 wafers every 4 hours, or as directed by a physician. Wafers may be chewed or allowed to dissolve in the mouth.

How Supplied:
Kolantyl Gel: 6 oz. and 12 oz. bottles
Kolantyl Wafers: boxes of 32 wafers, boxes of 96 wafers, and boxes of 400 wafers in sealed strips of 4 wafers each

*This section appears on the label for the consumer.

Product Information as of November, 1976

METAHYDRIN® ℞
(trichlormethiazide NF)

AVAILABLE ONLY ON PRESCRIPTION

Description: Metahydrin is an oral diuretic and antihypertensive of the thiazide class. Differing from other thiazides by the inclusion of a dichloromethyl radical at the 3 position on the benzothiadiazine structure.

Action: The mechanism of action results in an interference with the renal tubular mechanism of electrolyte reabsorption. At maximal therapeutic dosage all thiazides are approximately equal in their diuretic potency. The mechanism whereby thiazides function in the control of hypertension is unknown.

Indications: Metahydrin is indicated as adjunctive therapy in edema associated with congestive heart failure, hepatic cirrhosis, and corticosteroid and estrogen therapy.

Metahydrin has also been found useful in edema due to various forms of renal dysfunction as:
Nephrotic syndrome;
Acute glomerulonephritis; and
Chronic renal failure.

Metahydrin is indicated in the management of hypertension either as the sole therapeutic agent or to enhance the effectiveness of other antihypertensive drugs in the more severe forms of hypertension.

Usage in Pregnancy. The routine use of diuretics in an otherwise healthy woman is inappropriate and exposes mother and fetus to unnecessary hazard. Diuretics do not prevent development of toxemia of pregnancy, and there is no satisfactory evidence that they are useful in the treatment of developed toxemia. Edema during pregnancy may arise from pathologic causes or from the physiologic and mechanical consequences of pregnancy. Thiazides are indicated in pregnancy when edema is due to pathologic causes, just as they are in the absence of pregnancy. (However, see Warnings, below.) Dependent edema in pregnancy, resulting from restriction of venous return by the expanded uterus, is properly treated through elevation of the lower extremities and use of support hose; use of diuretics to lower intravascular volume in this case is illogical and unnecessary. There is hypervolemia during normal pregnancy, which is harmful to neither the fetus nor the mother (in the absence of cardiovascular disease), but which is associated with edema, including generalized edema, in the majority of pregnant women. If this edema produces discomfort, increased recumbency will often provide relief. In rare instances, this edema may cause extreme discomfort which is not relieved by rest. In these cases, a short course of diuretics may provide relief and may be appropriate.

Contraindications:
Anuria.
Hypersensitivity to this or other sulfonamide-derived drugs.

Warnings: Thiazides should be used with caution in severe renal disease. In patients with renal disease, thiazides may precipitate azotemia. Cumulative effects of the drug may develop in patients with impaired renal function.

Thiazides should be used with caution in patients with impaired hepatic function or progressive liver disease, since minor alterations

Continued on next page

Merrell-National—Cont.

of fluid and electrolyte balance may precipitate hepatic coma.
Thiazides may add to or potentiate the action of other antihypertensive drugs. Potentiation occurs with ganglionic or peripheral adrenergic blocking drugs.
Sensitivity reactions may occur in patients with a history of allergy or bronchial asthma. The possibility of exacerbation or activation of systemic lupus erythematosus has been reported.
Usage in Pregnancy. Thiazides cross the placental barrier and appear in cord blood. The use of thiazides in pregnant women requires that the anticipated benefit be weighed against possible hazards to the fetus. These hazards include fetal or neonatal jaundice, thrombocytopenia, and possibly other adverse reactions which have occurred in the adult.
Nursing Mothers. Thiazides appear in the breast milk. If use of the drug is deemed essential, the patient should stop nursing.
Precautions: Periodic determination of serum electrolytes to detect possible electrolyte imbalance should be performed at appropriate intervals.
All patients receiving thiazide therapy should be observed for clinical signs of fluid or electrolyte imbalance; namely, hyponatremia, hypochloremic alkalosis, and hypokalemia. Serum and urine electrolyte determinations are particularly important when the patient is vomiting excessively or receiving parenteral fluids. Medication such as digitalis may also influence serum electrolytes. Warning signs, irrespective of cause, are: dryness of mouth, thirst, weakness, lethargy, drowsiness, restlessness, muscle pains or cramps, muscular fatigue, hypotension, oliguria, tachycardia, and gastrointestinal disturbances such as nausea and vomiting.
Hypokalemia may develop with thiazides as with any other potent diuretic, especially with brisk diuresis, when severe cirrhosis is present, or during concomitant use of corticosteroids or ACTH.
Interference with adequate oral electrolyte intake will also contribute to hypokalemia. Digitalis therapy may exaggerate metabolic effects of hypokalemia especially with reference to myocardial activity.
Any chloride deficit is generally mild and usually does not require specific treatment except under extraordinary circumstances (as in liver disease or renal disease). Dilutional hyponatremia may occur in edematous patients in hot weather; appropriate therapy is water restriction, rather than administration of salt except in rare instances when the hyponatremia is life threatening. In actual salt depletion, appropriate replacement is the therapy of choice.
Hyperuricemia may occur or frank gout may be precipitated in certain patients receiving thiazide therapy.
Insulin requirements in diabetic patients may be increased, decreased, or unchanged. Latent diabetes mellitus may become manifest during thiazide administration.
Thiazide drugs may increase the responsiveness to tubocurarine.
The antihypertensive effects of the drug may be enhanced in the postsympathectomy patient.
Thiazides may decrease arterial responsiveness to norepinephrine. This diminution is not sufficient to preclude effectiveness of the pressor agent for therapeutic use.
If progressive renal impairment becomes evident, as indicated by a rising nonprotein nitrogen or blood urea nitrogen, a careful reappraisal of therapy is necessary with consideration given to withholding or discontinuing diuretic therapy.
Thiazides may decrease serum PBI levels without signs of thyroid disturbance.
This product contains FD&C Yellow No. 5 (tartrazine), which may cause allergic-type reactions (including bronchial asthma) in certain susceptible individuals. Although the overall incidence of FD&C Yellow No. 5 (tartrazine) sensitivity in the general population is low, it is frequently seen in patients who also have aspirin hypersensitivity.
Adverse Reactions:
1. Gastrointestinal System Reactions: anorexia, gastric irritation, nausea, diarrhea, constipation, jaundice (intrahepatic cholestatic jaundice), vomiting, cramping, pancreatitis.
2. Central Nervous System Reactions: dizziness, vertigo, parasthesias, headache, xanthopsia.
3. Hematologic Reactions: leukopenia, agranulocytosis, thrombocytopenia, aplastic anemia.
4. Dermatologic-Hypersensitivity Reactions: purpura, photosensitivity, rash, urticaria, necrotizing angiitis (vasculitis) (cutaneous vasculitis).
5. Cardiovascular Reaction: orthostatic hypotension may occur and may be aggravated by alcohol, barbiturates, or narcotics.
6. Other: hyperglycemia, glycosuria, hyperuricemia, muscle spasm, weakness, restlessness.
Whenever adverse reactions are moderate or severe, Metahydrin dosage should be reduced or therapy withdrawn.
Dosage and Administration: Therapy should be individualized according to patient response. This therapy should be titrated to gain maximal therapeutic response as well as the minimal dose possible to maintain that therapeutic response.
The usual daily doses of Metahydrin for antihypertensive and diuretic effect are as follows:
The usual dose is one 2 mg. or 4 mg. tablet once daily.
In initiating therapy, these doses may be given twice daily.
How Supplied: 2 mg. pink tablets: bottles of 100 and 1000
4 mg. aqua blue tablets: bottles of 100 and 1000
Product Information as of August, 1979
[*Shown in Product Identification Section*]

METATENSIN® ℞
(trichlormethiazide NF and reserpine)

Warning
This fixed combination drug is not indicated for initial therapy of hypertension. Hypertension requires therapy titrated to the individual patient. If the fixed combination represents the dosage so determined, its use may be more convenient in patient management. The treatment of hypertension is not static, but must be reevaluated as conditions in each patient warrant.

Description: Each tablet contains Metahydrin® (trichlormethiazide NF) 2 mg. or 4 mg. and reserpine 0.1 mg.
Metahydrin (trichlormethiazide NF) is an orally effective diuretic and antihypertensive of the thiazide class. Differing from other thiazides by the inclusion of a dichloromethyl radical at the 3 position on the benzothiadiazine structure.
Reserpine is a pure crystalline alkaloid derived from the root of Rauwolfia serpentina.
Action:
Trichlormethiazide
The mechanism of action results in an interference with the renal tubular mechanism of electrolyte reabsorption. At maximal therapeutic dosage all thiazides are approximately equal in their diuretic potency. The mechanism whereby thiazides function in the control of hypertension is unknown.
Reserpine
Reserpine probably produces its antihypertensive effects through depletion of tissue stores of epinephrine and norepinephrine from peripheral sites. By contrast, its sedative and tranquilizing properties are thought to be related to depletion of 5-hydroxytryptamine from the brain.
Reserpine is characterized by slow onset of action and sustained effect. Both its cardiovascular and central nervous system effects may persist following withdrawal of the drug.
Indications: Hypertension (See box Warning.)
Usage in Pregnancy. The routine use of diuretics in an otherwise healthy woman is inappropriate and exposes mother and fetus to unnecessary hazard. Diuretics do not prevent development of toxemia of pregnancy, and there is no satisfactory evidence that they are useful in the treatment of developed toxemia.

Edema during pregnancy may arise from pathologic causes or from the physiologic and mechanical consequences of pregnancy. Thiazides are indicated in pregnancy when edema is due to pathologic causes, just as they are in the absence of pregnancy. (However, see Warnings, below.) Dependent edema in pregnancy, resulting from restriction of venous return by the expanded uterus, is properly treated through elevation of the lower extremities and use of support hose; use of diuretics to lower intravascular volume in this case is illogical and unnecessary. There is hypervolemia during normal pregnancy, which is harmful to neither the fetus nor the mother (in the absence of cardiovascular disease), but which is associated with edema, including generalized edema, in the majority of pregnant women. If this edema produces discomfort, increased recumbency will often provide relief. In rare instances, this edema may cause extreme discomfort which is not relieved by rest. In these cases, a short course of diuretics may provide relief and may be appropriate.
Contraindications:
Trichlormethiazide
Trichlormethiazide is contraindicated in patients with anuria and in patients known to be hypersensitive to this or other sulfonamide derived drugs.
Reserpine
Hypersensitivity, mental depression especially with suicidal tendencies, active peptic ulcer and ulcerative colitis.
Warnings:
Trichlormethiazide
Use with caution in severe renal disease. In patients with renal disease, thiazides may precipitate azotemia. Cumulative effects of the drug may develop in patients with impaired renal function.
Thiazides should be used with caution in patients with impaired hepatic function or progressive liver disease, since minor alterations of fluid and electrolyte balance may precipitate hepatic coma.
Thiazides may add to or potentiate the action of other antihypertensive drugs. Potentiation occurs with ganglionic or peripheral adrenergic blocking drug.
Sensitivity reactions may occur in patients with a history of allergy or bronchial asthma. Exacerbation or activation of systemic lupus erythematosis has been reported.
Reserpine
As suicide is always a possible result of mental depression, discontinue treatment if mood depression develops.
Reserpine may induce peptic ulceration; discontinue use if peptic ulcer develops.
Electroshock therapy should not be given to patients taking reserpine, since severe and even fatal reactions have been reported. The drug should be discontinued for two weeks before giving electroshock therapy.

Usage in Pregnancy. Thiazides and reserpine cross the placental barrier and appear in cord blood. The use of thiazides in pregnant women requires that the anticipated benefit be weighed against possible hazards to the fetus. These hazards include fetal or neonatal jaundice, thrombocytopenia, and possibly other adverse reactions which have occurred in the adult.
Increased respiratory secretions, nasal congestion, cyanosis, and anorexia may occur in infants born to reserpine-treated mothers.
Nursing Mothers. Thiazides and reserpine appear in breast milk. If use of Metatensin is deemed essential, the patient should stop nursing.

Precautions:
Trichlormethiazide
Periodic determinations of serum electrolytes to detect possible electrolyte imbalance should be performed at appropriate intervals.
All patients receiving thiazide therapy should be observed for clinical signs of fluid or electrolyte imbalance; namely, hyponatremia, hypochloremic alkalosis, and hypokalemia. Serum and urine electrolyte determinations are particularly important when the patient is vomiting excessively or receiving parenteral fluids. Medication such as digitalis may also influence serum electrolytes. Warning signs, irrespective of cause, are: dryness of mouth, thirst, weakness, lethargy, drowsiness, restlessness, muscle pains or cramps, muscular fatigue, hypotension, oliguria, tachycardia, and gastrointestinal disturbances such as nausea and vomiting.
Hypokalemia may develop with thiazides as with any other potent diuretic, especially with brisk diuresis, when severe cirrhosis is present, or during concomitant use of corticosteroids or ACTH.
Interference with adequate oral electrolyte intake will also contribute to hypokalemia. Digitalis therapy may exaggerate metabolic effects of hypokalemia especially with reference to myocardial activity.
Any chloride deficit is generally mild and usually does not require specific treatment except under extraordinary circumstances (as in liver disease or renal disease). Dilutional hyponatremia may occur in edematous patients in hot weather; appropriate therapy is water restriction, rather than administration of salt except in rare instances when the hyponatremia is life threatening. In actual salt depletion, appropriate replacement is the therapy of choice.
Hyperuricemia may occur or frank gout may be precipitated in certain patients receiving thiazide therapy.
Insulin requirements in diabetic patients may be increased, decreased, or unchanged. Latent diabetes mellitus may become manifest during thiazide administration.
Thiazide drugs may increase the responsiveness to tubocurarine.
The antihypertensive effects of the drug may be enhanced in the postsympathectomy patient.
Thiazides may decrease arterial responsiveness to norepinephrine. This diminution is not sufficient to preclude effectiveness of the pressor agent for therapeutic use.
If progressive renal impairment becomes evident, as indicated by a rising nonprotein nitrogen or blood urea nitrogen, a careful reappraisal of therapy is necessary with consideration given to withholding or discontinuing diuretic therapy.
Thiazides may decrease serum PBI levels without signs of thyroid disturbance.

Reserpine
Caution should be used in treating hypertensive patients with renal insufficiency.
Cardiac arrhythmias have occurred in patients receiving digitalis and quinidine with reserpine.
Reserpine potentiates many anesthetic agents; hypotension and bradycardia have been noted during anesthesia. In addition, a relative sensitivity to norepinephrine or other pressor agents may exist due to the previous action of reserpine thus usual amounts of the pressor agent may be excessive.
Use with caution in patients with a previous history of depression, peptic ulcer or other gastrointestinal disorders and in hypertensive patients with functionally severe coronary artery disease.

Adverse Reactions:
Trichlormethiazide
1. Gastrointestinal System Reactions: anorexia, gastric irritation, nausea, diarrhea, constipation, jaundice (intrahepatic cholestatic jaundice), vomiting, cramping, pancreatitis.
2. Central Nervous System Reactions: dizziness, vertigo, paresthesias, headache, xanthopsia.
3. Hematologic Reactions: leukopenia, agranulocytosis, thrombocytopenia, aplastic anemia.
4. Dermatologic-Hypersensitivity Reactions: purpura, photosensitivity, rash, urticaria, necrotizing angiitis (vasculitis) (cutaneous vasculitis).
5. Cardiovascular Reaction: orthostatic hypotension may occur and may be aggravated by alcohol, barbiturates, or narcotics.
6. Other: hyperglycemia, glycosuria, hyperuricemia, muscle spasm, weakness, restlessness.

Reserpine
Gastric hypersecretion; vomiting; nervousness; paradoxical anxiety, CNS sensitization manifested by deafness, glaucoma, uveitis, and optic atrophy; purpura; nasal stuffiness; loose stools; reversible parkinsonism; muscular fatigue and weakness; and nightmares. Mental depression particularly when doses of reserpine of over 1.0 mg daily are used has been reported. Other side effects of reserpine reported include anorexia, nausea, dizziness, headaches, impotence, flushing of the skin, dryness of the mouth, biliary colic, blurring of vision, muscular aches and pruritus. Hypotension, including the orthostatic variety, may occur in some patients. Angina pectoris, arrhythmias and congestive heart failure have also been reported but are uncommon. After the onset of therapy with reserpine, a turbulent phase of short duration may occur. Very rare additional adverse effects that have been observed in association with reserpine therapy include epistaxis, skin eruptions and edema due to sodium retention. Bradycardia may occur as an exaggerated response related to the pharmacodynamic effect of reserpine.

Dosage: As determined by individual titration (see box warning).
In the stabilized hypertensive patient, administration may be continued on a once-daily basis administered in the morning. The maximum single effective dose of Metatensin is 8 mg (in some patients 4 mg). Doses in excess of 8 mg normally will not produce any increase in sodium and water excretion and in refractory patients may increase excretion of potassium.

How Supplied:
Metatensin 2 mg.
Bottles of 100 and 1000 yellow tablets
Metatensin 4 mg.
Bottles of 100 and 1000 lavender tablets

Product Information as of September, 1977
[Shown in Product Identification Section]

NORPRAMIN® ℞
(desipramine hydrochloride tablets NF)

AVAILABLE ONLY ON PRESCRIPTION

Description: Norpramin (desipramine hydrochloride NF) is an antidepressant drug of the tricyclic type.

Clinical Pharmacology:
Mechanism of Action
Available evidence suggests that many depressions have a biochemical basis in the form of a relative deficiency of neurotransmitters such as norepinephrine and serotonin. Norepinephrine deficiency may be associated with relatively low urinary 3-methoxy-4-hydroxyphenyl glycol (MHPG) levels, while serotonin deficiencies may be associated with low spinal fluid levels of 5-hydroxyindolacetic acid.
While the precise mechanism of action of the tricyclic antidepressants is unknown, a leading theory suggests that they restore normal levels of neurotransmitters by blocking the re-uptake of these substances from the synapse in the central nervous system. Evidence indicates that the secondary amine tricyclic antidepressants, including Norpramin, may have greater activity in blocking the re-uptake of norepinephrine. Tertiary amine tricyclic antidepressants, such as amitriptyline, may have greater effect on serotonin re-uptake.
Norpramin (desipramine hydrochloride) is not a monoamine oxidase (MAO) inhibitor and does not act primarily as a central nervous system stimulant. It has been found in some studies to have a more rapid onset of action than imipramine. Earliest therapeutic effects may occasionally be seen in 2 to 5 days, but full treatment benefit usually requires 2 to 3 weeks to obtain.

Metabolism
Tricyclic antidepressants, such as desipramine hydrochloride, are rapidly absorbed from the gastrointestinal tract. Tricyclic antidepressants or their metabolites are to some extent excreted through the gastric mucosa and reabsorbed from the gastrointestinal tract. Desipramine is metabolized in the liver and approximately 70% is excreted in the urine.
The rate of metabolism of tricyclic antidepressants varies widely from individual to individual, chiefly on a genetically determined basis. Up to a thirty-sixfold difference in plasma level may be noted among individuals taking the same oral dose of desipramine. In general, the elderly metabolize tricyclic antidepressants more slowly than do younger adults.
Certain drugs, particularly the psychostimulants and the phenothiazines, increase plasma levels of concomitantly administered tricyclic antidepressants through competition for the same metabolic enzyme systems. Other substances, particularly barbiturates and alcohol, induce liver enzyme activity and thereby reduce tricyclic antidepressant plasma levels. Similar effects have been reported with tobacco smoke.
The usual therapeutic plasma level for most tricyclic antidepressants has been reported to be in the range of 50 to 250 nanograms per milliliter.

Indications: Norpramin (desipramine hydrochloride) is indicated for relief of symptoms in various depressive syndromes, especially endogenous depression.

Contraindications: Desipramine hydrochloride should not be given in conjunction with, or within 2 weeks of, treatment with an MAO inhibitor drug; hyperpyretic crises, severe convulsions, and death have occurred in patients taking MAO inhibitors and tricyclic antidepressants. When Norpramin (desipramine hydrochloride) is substituted for an MAO inhibitor, at least 2 weeks should elapse between treatments. Norpramin should then be started cautiously and should be increased gradually.
The drug is contraindicated in the acute recovery period following myocardial infarction. It should not be used in those who have shown prior hypersensitivity to the drug. Cross sensitivity between this and other dibenzazepines is a possibility.

Warnings:
1. Extreme caution should be used when this drug is given in the following situations:
   a. In patients with cardiovascular disease, because of the possibility of conduction de-

Continued on next page

Merrell-National—Cont.

fects, arrhythmias, tachycardias, strokes, and acute myocardial infarction.
b. In patients with a history of urinary retention or glaucoma, because of the anticholinergic properties of the drug.
c. In patients with thyroid disease or those taking thyroid medication, because of the possibility of cardiovascular toxicity, including arrhythmias.
d. In patients with a history of seizure disorder, because this drug has been shown to lower the seizure threshold.
2. This drug is capable of blocking the antihypertensive effect of guanethidine and similarly acting compounds.
3. USE IN PREGNANCY
Safe use of desipramine hydrochloride during pregnancy and lactation has not been established; therefore, if it is to be given to pregnant patients, nursing mothers, or women of childbearing potential, the possible benefits must be weighed against the possible hazards to mother and child. Animal reproductive studies have been inconclusive.
4. USE IN CHILDREN
Norpramin (desipramine hydrochloride) is not recommended for use in children since safety and effectiveness in the pediatric age group have not been established.
5. The patient should be cautioned that this drug may impair the mental and/or physical abilities required for the performance of potentially hazardous tasks such as driving a car or operating machinery.
6. In patients who may use alcohol excessively, it should be borne in mind that the potentiation may increase the danger inherent in any suicide attempt or overdosage.

Precautions:
1. It is important that this drug be dispensed in the least possible quantities to depressed outpatients, since suicide has been accomplished with this class of drug. Ordinary prudence requires that children not have access to this drug or to potent drugs of any kind; if possible this drug should be dispensed in containers with child-resistant safety closures. Storage of this drug in the home must be supervised responsibly.
2. If serious adverse effects occur, dosage should be reduced or treatment should be altered.
3. Norpramin (desipramine hydrochloride) therapy in patients with manic-depressive illness may induce a hypomanic state after the depressive phase terminates.
4. The drug may cause exacerbation of psychosis in schizophrenic patients.
5. Close supervision and careful adjustment of dosage are required when this drug is given concomitantly with anticholinergic or sympathomimetic drugs.
6. Patients should be warned that while taking this drug their response to alcoholic beverages may be exaggerated.
7. Clinical experience in the concurrent administration of ECT and antidepressant drugs is limited. Thus, if such treatment is essential, the possibility of increased risk relative to benefits should be considered.
8. The sedative effects of Norpramin and benzodiazepines (*e.g.,* chlordiazepoxide or diazepam) are additive. Both the sedative and anticholinergic effects of the major tranquilizers are additive to those of Norpramin.
9. This drug should be discontinued as soon as possible prior to elective surgery because of the possible cardiovascular effects. Hypertensive episodes have been observed during surgery in patients taking desipramine hydrochloride.
10. Both elevation and lowering of blood sugar levels have been reported.
11. Leukocyte and differential counts should be performed in any patient who develops fever and sore throat during therapy; the drug should be discontinued if there is evidence of pathologic neutrophil depression.
12. Norpramin 25, 50, 75, and 100 mg. tablets contain FD&C Yellow No. 5 (tartrazine), which may cause allergic-type reactions (including bronchial asthma) in certain susceptible individuals. Although the overall incidence of FD&C Yellow No. 5 (tartrazine) sensitivity in the general population is low, it is frequently seen in patients who also have aspirin hypersensitivity.

Adverse Reactions:
Note: Included in the following listing are a few adverse reactions that have not been reported with this specific drug. However, the pharmacologic similarities among the tricyclic antidepressant drugs require that each of the reactions be considered when Norpramin (desipramine hydrochloride) is given.
Cardiovascular: hypotension, hypertension, tachycardia, palpitation, arrhythmias, heart block, myocardial infarction, stroke.
Psychiatric: confusional states (especially in the elderly) with hallucinations, disorientation, delusions; anxiety, restlessness, agitation; insomnia and nightmares; hypomania; exacerbation of psychosis.
Neurologic: numbness, tingling, paresthesias of extremities; incoordination, ataxia, tremors; peripheral neuropathy; extrapyramidal symptoms; seizures; alteration in EEG patterns; tinnitus.
Anticholinergic: dry mouth, and rarely associated sublingual adenitis; blurred vision, disturbance of accommodation, mydriasis, increased intraocular pressure; constipation, paralytic ileus; urinary retention, delayed micturition, dilatation of urinary tract.
Allergic: skin rash, petechiae, urticaria, itching, photosensitization (avoid excessive exposure to sunlight), edema (of face and tongue or general), drug fever, cross sensitivity with other tricyclic drugs.
Hematologic: bone marrow depressions including agranulocytosis, eosinophilia, purpura, thrombocytopenia.
Gastrointestinal: anorexia, nausea and vomiting, epigastric distress, peculiar taste, abdominal cramps, diarrhea, stomatitis, black tongue.
Endocrine: gynecomastia in the male, breast enlargement and galactorrhea in the female; increased or decreased libido, impotence, testicular swelling; elevation or depression of blood sugar levels.
Other: jaundice (simulating obstructive), altered liver function; weight gain or loss; perspiration, flushing; urinary frequency, nocturia; parotid swelling; drowsiness, dizziness, weakness and fatigue, headache; alopecia.
Withdrawal Symptoms: Though not indicative of addiction, abrupt cessation of treatment after prolonged therapy may produce nausea, headache, and malaise.

Dosage and Administration: Not recommended for use in children.
Lower dosages are recommended for elderly patients and adolescents. Lower dosages are also recommended for outpatients compared to hospitalized patients, who are closely supervised. Dosage should be initiated at a low level and increased according to clinical response and any evidence of intolerance. Following remission, maintenance medication may be required for a period of time and should be at the lowest dose that will maintain remission.
Usual Adult Dose:
The usual adult dose is 100 to 200 mg. per day. In more severely ill patients, dosage may be further increased gradually to 300 mg./day if necessary. Dosages above 300 mg./day are not recommended.
Dosage should be initiated at a lower level and increased according to tolerance and clinical response.
Treatment of patients requiring as much as 300 mg. should generally be initiated in hospitals, where regular visits by the physician, skilled nursing care, and frequent electrocardiograms (ECG's) are available.
The best available evidence of impending toxicity from very high doses of Norpramin is prolongation of the QRS or QT intervals on the ECG. Prolongation of the PR interval is also significant, but less closely correlated with plasma levels. Clinical symptoms of intolerance, especially drowsiness, dizziness, and postural hypotension, should also alert the physician to the need for reduction in dosage. Plasma desipramine measurement would constitute the optimal guide to dosage monitoring.
Initial therapy may be administered in divided doses or a single daily dose.
Maintenance therapy may be given on a once-daily schedule for patient convenience and compliance.
Adolescent and Geriatric Dose:
The usual adolescent and geriatric dose is 25 to 100 mg. daily.
Dosage should be initiated at a lower level and increased according to tolerance and clinical response to a usual maximum of 100 mg. daily. In more severely ill patients, dosage may be further increased to 150 mg./day. Doses above 150 mg./day are not recommended in these age groups.
Initial therapy may be administered in divided doses or a single daily dose.
Maintenance therapy may be given on a once-daily schedule for patient convenience and compliance.

Overdosage: There is no specific antidote for desipramine, nor are there specific phenomena of diagnostic value characterizing poisoning by the drug.
Within an hour of ingestion the patient may become agitated or stuporous and then comatose. Hypotension, shock, and renal shutdown may ensue. Grand mal seizures, both early and late after ingestion, have been reported. Hyperactive reflexes, hyperpyrexia, muscle rigidity, vomiting, and ECG evidence of impaired conduction may occur. Serious disturbances of cardiac rate, rhythm, and output can occur.
The precepts of early evacuation of the ingested material and subsequent support of respiration (airway and movement), circulation, and renal output apply.
The principles of management of coma and shock by means of the mechanical respirator, cardiac pacemaker, monitoring of central venous pressure, and regulation of fluid and acid-base balance are well known in most medical centers and are not further discussed here.
Because CNS involvement, respiratory depression, and cardiac arrhythmia can occur suddenly, hospitalization and close observation are generally advisable, even when the amount ingested is thought to be small or the initial degree of intoxication appears slight or moderate. Most patients with ECG abnormalities should have continuous cardiac monitoring for at least 72 hours and be closely observed until well after cardiac status has returned to normal; relapses may occur after apparent recovery.
The slow intravenous administration of physostigmine salicylate has been reported to reverse most of the anticholinergic cardiovascular and CNS effects of overdose with tricyclic antidepressants. In adults, 1 to 3 mg. has been reported to be effective. In children, the dose should be started with 0.5 mg. and repeated at 5-minute intervals to determine the minimum effective dose; no more than 2 mg. should be given. Because of the short duration of action of physostigmine, the effective dose should be repeated at 30-minute to 60-minute intervals, as necessary. Rapid injection should be avoided to reduce the possibility of physostigmine-induced convulsions.
Other possible therapeutic considerations include:

(a) Dialysis: Desipramine is found in low concentration in the serum, even after a massive oral dose. *In vitro* experiments in which blood bank blood was used indicate that it is very poorly dialyzed. Because of indications that the drug is secreted in gastric juice, constant gastric lavage has been suggested.
(b) Pharmacologic treatment of shock: Since desipramine potentiates the action of such vasopressor agents as levarterenol and metaraminol, they should be used only with caution.
(c) Pharmacologic control of seizures: Intravenous barbiturates are the treatment of choice for the control of grand mal seizures. One may, alternately, consider the parenteral use of diphenylhydantoin, which has less central depressant effect but also has an effect on heart rhythm that has not yet been fully defined.
(d) Pharmacologic control of cardiac function: Severe disturbances of cardiac rate, rhythm, and output are probably the initiating events in shock. Intravascular volume must be maintained by i.v. fluids. Digitalization should be carried out early in view of the fact that a positive inotropic effect can be achieved without increase in cardiac work. Many of the cardiodynamic effects of digitalis are the exact opposite of those of massive doses of desipramine (animal studies).

How Supplied:
25 mg. yellow coated tablets
Bottles of 100, 500, and 1000 and unit dose dispenser of 100
50 mg. green coated tablets
Bottles of 100, 500, and 1000 and unit dose dispenser of 100
75 mg. orange coated tablets
Bottles of 50 and 1000 and unit dose dispenser of 100
100 mg. peach coated tablets
Bottles of 50 and 1000 and unit dose dispenser of 100
150 mg. white coated tablets
Bottles of 50 and 1000 and unit dose dispenser of 100
U.S. Patent Numbers 3,454,554
3,454,698
Product Information as of July, 1979
[*Shown in Product Identification Section*]

ORENZYME® ℞
(Oral enteric coated enzyme tablet)
ORENZYME® BITABS™
(Double strength oral enteric coated enzyme tablet)

AVAILABLE ONLY ON PRESCRIPTION

Description:
Orenzyme
Each red, enteric coated tablet of Orenzyme contains:
trypsin ....50,000 NF Units
chymotrypsin ....4,000 USP Units
equivalent in tryptic activity to 20 mg. of NF trypsin.
Orenzyme Bitabs
Each yellow, enteric coated tablet of Orenzyme Bitabs contains:
trypsin ....100,000 NF Units
chymotrypsin ....8,000 USP Units
equivalent in tryptic activity to 40 mg. of NF trypsin.
The tablets have a special enteric coating designed to permit intact passage through the stomach, followed by disintegration in the intestinal tract.
Action: The mode of action of Orenzyme has not been established.

Indications:
Based on a review of this drug by the National Academy of Sciences—National Research Council and/or other information, FDA has classified the indications as follows:
"Possibly" effective: Relief of symptomatology related to episiotomy.
Lack of substantial evidence of effectiveness: Adjunctive therapy for the resolution of inflammation and edema resulting from serious accidental trauma or surgical trauma.
Final classification of the less-than-effective indications requires further investigation.

Contraindications: Orenzyme should not be given to patients with a known sensitivity to trypsin or chymotrypsin.
Precautions: Orenzyme should be used with caution in patients with abnormality of the blood clotting mechanism such as hemophilia or with severe hepatic or renal disease. Safe use in pregnancy has not been established.
This product contains FD&C Yellow No. 5 (tartrazine), which may cause allergic-type reactions (including bronchial asthma) in certain susceptible individuals. Although the overall incidence of FD&C Yellow No. 5 (tartrazine) sensitivity in the general population is low, it is frequently seen in patients who also have aspirin hypersensitivity.
Adverse Reactions: Adverse reactions with Orenzyme have been reported infrequently. Reports include allergic manifestations (rash, urticaria, itching), gastrointestinal upset, and increased speed of dissolution of animal-origin surgical sutures. There have been isolated reports of anaphylactic shock, albuminuria, and hematuria. Increased tendency to bleed has also been reported, but in controlled studies it has been seen with equal incidence in placebo-treated groups. (See Precautions.)
It is recommended that if side effects occur, medication be discontinued.
Dosage and Administration:
Orenzyme: 1 or 2 tablets q.i.d.
Orenzyme Bitabs: 1 tablet q.i.d.
How Supplied:
Orenzyme
NDC 0068-0441-13: bottles of 48
NDC 0068-0441-16: bottles of 500
Orenzyme Bitabs
NDC 0068-0442-15: bottles of 100
Product Information as of August, 1979

QUINAMM™ ℞

Description:
Each white, beveled, compressed tablet contains:
Quinine sulfate.......................................260 mg.
Aminophylline ....195 mg.
Actions: Quinine acts on skeletal muscle by two mechanisms; it increases the refractory period by direct action on the muscle fiber, and it also decreases the excitability of the motor end-plate by a curariform action. The mechanism of action of aminophylline is not fully established; it may be due to increase in blood flow, a depolarization of the muscle membrane, or an increase in metabolic rate of muscle.
Indications: For the prevention and treatment of nocturnal recumbency leg muscle cramps, including those associated with arthritis, diabetes, varicose veins, thrombophlebitis, arteriosclerosis, and static foot deformities.
Contraindications: Because of the quinine content, Quinamm is contraindicated in women of childbearing potential, in pregnancy, in patients with known quinine sensitivity, and in patients with glucose-6-phosphate dehydrogenase deficiency. Hemolysis (with the potential for hemolytic anemia) has been associated with a G-6-PD deficiency in patients taking quinine.
Precautions: Thrombocytopenic purpura may follow the administration of quinine in highly sensitive patients. Recovery will follow withdrawal of the medication.
Cinchona alkaloids, including quinine, have the potential to depress the hepatic enzyme system that synthesizes the vitamin K-dependent factors. The resulting hypoprothrombinemic effect may enhance the action of warfarin and other oral anticoagulants.
Adverse Reactions: Aminophylline may produce intestinal cramps in some instances, and quinine may produce symptoms of cinchonism, such as tinnitus, dizziness, and gastrointestinal disturbance. If ringing in the ears, deafness, skin rash, or visual disturbances occur, the drug should be discontinued.
Dosage and Administration: 1 tablet upon retiring. When necessary, 1 additional tablet may be taken following the evening meal.
How Supplied: Bottles of 100 and 500 tablets
U.S. Patent 2,985,558
Product Information as of September, 1977
MERRELL-NATIONAL LABORATORIES Inc.
Cayey, Puerto Rico 00633

Direct Medical Inquiries to:
MERRELL-NATIONAL LABORATORIES
Division of Richardson-Merrell Inc.
Cincinnati, Ohio 45215

Licensor of Merrell®
[*Shown in Product Identification Section*]

SIMRON™

Description:
Each maroon, soft-gelatin Simron capsule contains:
Elemental iron...10 mg.
(supplied as ferrous gluconate)
Sagacen™ (polysorbate 20)...............400 mg.
Actions: Ferrous gluconate provides a source of elemental iron that will prevent and correct iron deficiency and iron-deficiency anemia. Sagacen (polysorbate 20) is polyoxyethylene 20 sorbitan monolaurate. It is an amber-colored liquid intended to enhance iron absorption and, as a surfactant, aids in the prevention of constipation.
Indications: For the prevention and treatment of iron deficiency and iron-deficiency anemia.
Simron is unusually well tolerated in patients who cannot tolerate other oral iron preparations and in patients with gastrointestinal disease, including peptic ulcer and ulcerative colitis.
Simron is indicated in the treatment of iron-deficiency anemia of patients with a potential for upper gastrointestinal bleeding because it rarely produces black stools, which could mask evidence of bleeding. Simron is indicated in the treatment of iron-deficiency anemia of patients with ulcerative colitis because only small amounts of unabsorbed irritant iron salts are present in the stool. Simron is indicated in the prevention and treatment of iron deficiency and iron-deficiency anemia of pregnancy.
Contraindications: Simron is contraindicated in the treatment of patients with disease associated with increased iron storage (hemochromatosis).
Warnings: Simron should be stored out of the reach of children because of the possibility of iron intoxication from accidental overdosage. Individuals with normal iron balance should not chronically take iron.
Precautions: When anemia is diagnosed, the type of anemia should be established. When iron-deficiency anemia is diagnosed, the cause of the iron deficiency should be established.
Ferrous iron compounds taken by mouth can impair the absorption of tetracycline and tetracycline derivatives. Antacids given concomi-

Continued on next page

Merrell-National—Cont.

tantly with iron compounds will decrease the absorption of iron.

Adverse Reactions: The incidence of adverse gastrointestinal reactions is reduced with Simron. Gastric irritation, nausea, constipation, and diarrhea are rarely observed.

Dosage and Administration: For the prevention and treatment of iron deficiency and iron-deficiency anemia the recommended dose is 1 Simron capsule three times a day *between meals.* This supplies 30 mg. elemental iron. It should be noted that in patients with continued blood loss it may be necessary to exceed the recommended dose of Simron to obtain optimum therapeutic effect.

Overdosage: As little as 1 gram of elemental iron ingested orally may be toxic. Onset of symptoms usually occurs approximately 30 minutes after ingestion. Initially, gastrointestinal symptoms predominate (vomiting, diarrhea, melena). Shock, dyspnea, lethargy, and coma may follow. Metabolic acidosis may then occur.

Standard measures used to treat acute iron intoxication may include the following: 1) induced vomiting, 2) gastric lavage with 1% sodium bicarbonate, 3) general supportive measures for the treatment of shock and acidosis. Deferoxamine mesylate (Desferal®) should be given intramuscularly for patients not in shock, and intravenously for patients in shock. The manufacturer's recommendations should be consulted for details of administration. Some authors recommend 8000 mg. deferoxamine in 50 ml. of water via nasogastric tube.

How Supplied: Bottles of 100 soft-gelatin capsules

Product Information as of November, 1974

SIMRON PLUS®

Description: Each maroon, soft-gelatin capsule contains:

Elemental iron	10 mg.
(supplied as ferrous gluconate)	
Sacagen™ (polysorbate 20)	400 mg.
Ascorbic acid	50 mg.
(supplied as sodium ascorbate)	
Pyridoxine hydrochloride	1.0 mg.
Folic acid	0.1 mg.
Vitamin B_{12}	3.33 mcg.
(supplied as cyanocobalamin)	

TACE® ℞
(CHLOROTRIANISENE NF)
12 mg. and 25 mg. Capsules

AVAILABLE ONLY ON PRESCRIPTION

Warnings:

1. ESTROGENS HAVE BEEN REPORTED TO INCREASE THE RISK RATIO FOR ENDOMETRIAL CARCINOMA.

Three independent case control studies have reported an increased risk ratio of endometrial cancer in postmenopausal women exposed to exogenous estrogens for prolonged periods.[1–3] This reported risk was independent of the other risk factors studied. Additionally, the incidence rates of endometrial cancer have increased since 1969 in 8 different areas of the United States with population-based cancer reporting systems, an increase that may [or may not] be related to the expanded use of estrogens during the last decade.[4]

The 3 case control studies reported that the estimated risk ratio for endometrial cancer in estrogen users was about 4.5 to 13.9 times greater than in nonusers. The risk appeared to depend on both duration of treatment[1] and on estrogen dose.[3] In view of these reports, when estrogens are used for the treatment of menopausal symptoms, the lowest dose that will control symptoms should be utilized and medication should be discontinued as soon as possible. When prolonged treatment is medically indicated, the patient should be reassessed on at least a semiannual basis to determine the need for continued therapy. Although the evidence must be considered preliminary, one study suggests that cyclic administration of low doses of estrogen may carry less risk than continuous administration;[3] it therefore appears prudent to utilize such a regimen.

Close clinical surveillance of all women taking estrogens is important. In all cases of undiagnosed persistent or recurring abnormal vaginal bleeding, adequate diagnostic measures should be undertaken to rule out malignancy.

There is no evidence at present that "natural" estrogens are more or less hazardous than "synthetic" estrogens at equiestrogenic doses.

2. ESTROGENS SHOULD NOT BE USED DURING PREGNANCY.

The use of exogenous estrogens and progestagens during early pregnancy has been reported to damage the offspring. An association has been reported between *in utero* exposure of the female fetus to diethylstilbestrol, a non-steroidal estrogen, and an increased risk of the post-pubertal development of an ordinarily rare form of vaginal or cervical cancer.[5,6] This risk for diethylstilbestrol was recently estimated to be in the range of 0.14 to 1.4 per 1000 exposures,[7] consistent with a previous risk estimate of not greater than 4 per 1000 exposures.[8] Furthermore, a high percentage of such females exposed *in utero* (30 to over 90%) has been reported to have vaginal adenosis, epithelial changes of the vagina and cervix.[9–12] Although these changes are histologically benign, it is not known whether they are precursors of adenocarcinoma. Although similar data are not available with the use of other estrogens, it cannot be presumed they would not induce similar changes.

Several reports suggest a possible association between fetal exposure to exogenous estrogens and progestagens and congenital anomalies, including congenital heart defects and limb reduction defects.[13–16] One case control study[16] estimated a 4.7 fold increased risk of limb reduction defects in infants exposed *in utero* to exogenous steroids (oral contraceptives, hormone withdrawal tests for pregnancy, or attempted treatment for threatened abortion). Some of these exposures were very short and involved only a few days of treatment. The data suggest that the risk of limb reduction defects in exposed fetuses is somewhat less than 1 per 1000.

This product is not for use in therapy of threatened or habitual abortion.

If TACE (CHLOROTRIANISENE NF) is used during pregnancy, or if the patient becomes pregnant while taking this drug, she should be apprised of the potential risks to the fetus, and the advisability of pregnancy continuation.

Description: TACE (CHLOROTRIANISENE NF) is a long-acting, synthetic estrogen in capsule form suitable for oral administration.

Each green, soft gelatin capsule contains 12 mg. of chlorotrianisene in corn oil. Each two-tone green, hard gelatin capsule contains 25 mg. of chlorotrianisene in tristearin.

Chemistry

Generic name: Chlorotrianisene NF

Chemical name: Benzene, 1,1′,1″-(1-chloro-1-ethenyl-2-ylidene)tris[4-methoxy-Chlorotris(*p*-methoxyphenyl)ethylene

Chlorotrianisene occurs as small, white crystals or as a crystalline powder. It is odorless. It is slightly soluble in alcohol and very slightly soluble in water.

Indications:

1. Postpartum breast engorgement—Although estrogens have been widely used for the prevention of postpartum breast engorgement, controlled studies have demonstrated that the incidence of significant painful engorgement in patients not receiving such hormonal therapy is low and usually responsive to appropriate analgesic or other supportive therapy. Consequently, the benefit to be derived from estrogen therapy for this indication must be carefully weighed against the potential risk of puerperal thromboembolism associated with the use of estrogens.[17]
2. Prostatic carcinoma—palliative therapy of advanced disease.
3. Moderate to severe *vasomotor* symptoms associated with the menopause. (There is no well-documented evidence that estrogens are effective for nervous symptoms or depression which might occur during menopause and they should not be used to treat these conditions.)
4. Atrophic vaginitis.
5. Kraurosis vulvae.
6. Female hypogonadism.

TACE (CHLOROTRIANISENE NF) HAS NOT BEEN SHOWN TO BE EFFECTIVE FOR ANY PURPOSE DURING PREGNANCY, AND ITS USE MAY HAVE POTENTIAL RISKS TO THE FETUS. (SEE BOXED WARNING.)

Contraindications: TACE (CHLOROTRIANISENE NF) should not be used in women or men with any of the following conditions:

1. Known or suspected cancer of the breast except in appropriately selected patients being treated for metastatic disease.
2. Known or suspected estrogen-dependent neoplasia.
3. Known or suspected pregnancy. (See Boxed Warning.)
4. Undiagnosed abnormal genital bleeding.
5. Active thrombophlebitis or thromboembolic disorders.
6. A past history of thrombophlebitis, thrombosis, or thromboembolic disorders (except when used in treatment of prostatic malignancy).

Warnings:

1. *Induction of malignant neoplasms.* Long-term continuous administration of natural and synthetic estrogens in certain animal species increases the frequency of carcinomas of the breast, cervix, vagina, and liver. There are now reports that estrogens increase the risk of carcinoma of the endometrium in humans. (See Boxed Warning.)
   At the present time there is no satisfactory evidence that estrogens given to postmenopausal women increase the risk of cancer of the breast,[18] although a recent long-term followup of a single physician's practice has raised this possibility.[19] Because of the animal data, there is a need for caution in prescribing estrogens for women with a strong family history of breast cancer or who have breast nodules, fibrocystic disease, or abnormal mammograms.
2. *Gallbladder disease.* A recent study has reported a two to threefold increase in the risk of surgically confirmed gallbladder disease in women receiving postmenopausal estrogens,[18] similar to the twofold increase previously noted in users of oral contraceptives.[20] In the case of oral contraceptives the increased risk appeared after a period of use.[20]
3. *Effects similar to those caused by estrogen-progestagen oral contraceptives.* There are several adverse effects reported in associa-

tion with oral contraceptives, most of which have not been documented as consequences of postmenopausal estrogen therapy, although it has been reported that there is an increased risk of thrombosis in men receiving high doses of estrogens for prostatic cancer and in women receiving estrogens for postpartum breast engorgement.[17,21–23] The possibility that the adverse effects reported in association with oral contraceptives may be associated with larger doses of estrogen cannot be excluded.

a. *Thromboembolic disease.* Studies have now shown that users of oral contraceptives have an increased risk of various thromboembolic, thrombotic, and vascular diseases, such as thrombophlebitis, pulmonary embolism, stroke, and myocardial infarction.[24–31] Cases of retinal thrombosis, mesenteric thrombosis, and optic neuritis have been reported in oral contraceptive users. There is evidence that the risk of several of these adverse reactions is related to the dose of the drug.[32,33] An increased risk of post-surgery thromboembolic complications has also been reported in users of oral contraceptives.[34,35] If feasible, estrogen should be discontinued at least 4 weeks before surgery of the type associated with an increased risk of thromboembolism, or during periods of prolonged immobilization.

While an increased rate of thromboembolic and thrombotic disease in postmenopausal users of estrogens has not been found,[18,36] this does not rule out the possibility that such an increase may be present, or that subgroups of women who have underlying risk factors, or who are receiving relatively large doses of estrogens may have an increased risk. Therefore, estrogens should not be used in persons with active thrombophlebitis or thromboembolic disorders, and they should not be used (except in treatment of malignancy) in persons with a history of such disorders. They should be used with caution in patients with cerebral vascular or coronary artery disease and only for those in whom estrogens are needed.

Doses of estrogen (5 mg. conjugated estrogens per day), comparable to those used to treat cancer of the prostate and breast, have been reported in a large prospective clinical trial in men[37] to increase the risk of nonfatal myocardial infarction, pulmonary embolism, and thrombophlebitis. When estrogen doses of this size are used, any of the thromboembolic and thrombotic adverse effects associated with oral contraceptive use should be considered as a risk.

b. *Hepatic adenoma.* Benign hepatic adenomas have been reported to be associated with the use of oral contraceptives.[38–40] Although benign and rare, these may rupture and may cause death through intra-abdominal hemorrhage. Such lesions have not yet been reported in association with other estrogen or progestagen preparations but should be considered in estrogen users having abdominal pain and tenderness, abdominal mass, or hypovolemic shock. Hepatocellular carcinoma has also been reported in women taking estrogen-containing oral contraceptives.[39] The relationship of this malignancy to these drugs is not known at this time.

c. *Elevated blood pressure.* Increased blood pressure is not uncommon in women using oral contraceptives and there is now a report that this may occur with use of estrogens in the menopause[41] and blood pressure should be monitored with estrogen use, especially if high doses are used.

d. *Glucose tolerance.* A worsening of glucose tolerance has been observed in a significant percentage of patients on estrogen-containing oral contraceptives. For this reason diabetic patients should be carefully observed while receiving estrogen.

4. *Hypercalcemia.* Administration of estrogens may lead to hypercalcemia in patients with breast cancer and bone metastases. If this occurs, the drug should be stopped and appropriate measures taken to reduce the serum calcium level.

Precautions:

A. General Precautions

1. A complete medical and family history should be taken prior to the initiation of any estrogen therapy. The pretreatment and periodic physical examinations should include special reference to blood pressure, breasts, abdomen, and pelvic organs, and should include a Papanicolaou smear. As a general rule, estrogen should not be prescribed for longer than 1 year without another physical examination being performed.
2. Fluid retention—Because estrogens may cause some degree of fluid retention, conditions that might be influenced by this factor such as epilepsy, migraine, and cardiac or renal dysfunction require careful observation.
3. Certain patients may develop undesirable manifestations of excessive estrogenic stimulation, such as abnormal or excessive uterine bleeding, mastodynia, etc.
4. Oral contraceptives have been reported to be associated with an increased incidence of mental depression. Although it is not clear whether this is possibly due to the estrogenic or progestagenic component of the contraceptive, patients with a history of depression should be carefully observed.
5. Patients having pre-existing uterine leiomyomata should be observed for increased growth of myomata during estrogen therapy.
6. The pathologist should be advised of estrogen therapy when relevant specimens are submitted.
7. Patients with a past history of jaundice during pregnancy have an increased risk of recurrence of jaundice while receiving estrogen-containing oral contraceptive therapy. If jaundice develops in any patient receiving estrogen, the medication should be discontinued while the cause is investigated.
8. Estrogens may be poorly metabolized in patients with impaired liver function and they should be administered with caution in such patients.
9. Because estrogens influence the metabolism of calcium and phosphorus, they should be used with caution in patients with metabolic bone diseases that are associated with hypercalcemia or in patients with renal insufficiency.
10. Because of the effects of estrogens on epiphyseal closure, they should be used judiciously in young patients in whom bone growth is not complete.
11. Judicious assessment of the following changes in certain endocrine and liver function tests is necessary for patients receiving large doses of estrogen:
    a. Increased sulfobromophthalein retention.
    b. Increased prothrombin and factors VII, VIII, IX, and X; decreased antithrombin 3; increased norepinephrine-induced platelet aggregability.
    c. Increased thyroid binding globulin (TBG) leading to increased circulating total thyroid hormone, as measured by PBI, T4 by column, or T4 by radioimmunoassay. Free T3 resin uptake is decreased, reflecting the elevated TBG; free T4 concentration is unaltered.
    d. Impaired glucose tolerance.
    e. Decreased pregnanediol excretion.
    f. Reduced response to metyrapone test.
    g. Reduced serum folate concentration.
    h. Increased serum triglyceride, phospholipid, or cholesterol.
12. This product contains FD&C Yellow No. 5 (tartrazine), which may cause allergic-type reactions (including bronchial asthma) in certain susceptible individuals. Although the overall incidence of FD&C Yellow No. 5 (tartrazine) sensitivity in the general population is low, it is frequently seen in patients who also have aspirin hypersensitivity.

B. Information For The Patient
A patient package insert accompanies this drug product. This insert is available from pharmacists who carry this product and from the company upon request.

C. Pregnancy Category X
See Contraindications and Boxed Warning.

D. Nursing Mothers
As a general principle, the administration of any drug to nursing mothers should be done only when clearly necessary since many drugs are excreted in human milk.

Adverse Reactions: (See Warnings regarding reports of induction of neoplasia, adverse effects on the fetus, increased incidence of gallbladder disease, and adverse effects similar to those of oral contraceptives, including thromboembolism.) The following additional adverse reactions have been reported with estrogenic therapy including oral contraceptives:

1. *Genitourinary system*
   Breakthrough bleeding, spotting, change in menstrual flow and cycle.
   Dysmenorrhea.
   Premenstrual-like syndrome.
   Amenorrhea during and after treatment.
   Increase in size of uterine fibromyomata.
   Vaginal candidiasis.
   Change in cervical eversion and in degree of cervical secretion.
   Cystitis-like syndrome.
2. *Breasts*
   Tenderness, enlargement, secretion.
3. *Gastrointestinal*
   Nausea, vomiting.
   Abdominal cramps, bloating.
   Cholestatic jaundice.
4. *Skin*
   Chloasma or melasma, which may persist when drug is discontinued.
   Erythema multiforme.
   Erythema nodosum.
   Hemorrhagic eruption.
   Loss of scalp hair.
   Hirsutism.
   Urticaria.
5. *Eyes*
   Steepening of corneal curvature.
   Intolerance to contact lenses.
6. *CNS*
   Headache, migraine, dizziness.
   Mental depression.
   Chorea.
7. *Miscellaneous*
   Increase or decrease in weight.
   Reduced carbohydrate tolerance.
   Aggravation of porphyria.
   Edema.
   Changes in libido and/or potency.

Acute Overdosage: Numerous reports of ingestion of large doses of estrogen-containing oral contraceptives by young children indicate that serious ill effects usually do not occur. Overdosage of estrogen may cause nausea, and withdrawal bleeding may occur in females.

Continued on next page

Merrell-National—Cont.

Dosage and Administration:

Given for a few days

Prevention of postpartum breast engorgement.

The usual dosage is one 12 mg. capsule four times daily for 7 days, or two 25 mg. capsules every six hours for 6 doses. For immediate postpartum use, the first dose should be given within 8 hours after delivery.

Given chronically

Inoperable progressing prostatic cancer.

The usual dosage is 12 to 25 mg. daily (one or two 12 mg. capsules or one 25 mg. capsule).

Given cyclically for short-term use only

For treatment of moderate to severe *vasomotor* symptoms, atrophic vaginitis, or kraurosis vulvae associated with the menopause.

The lowest dose that will control symptoms should be chosen and medication should be discontinued as promptly as possible.

Administration should be cyclic (*e.g.,* 3 weeks on and 1 week off).

Attempts to discontinue or taper medication should be made at 3-month to 6-month intervals.

The usual dosage range for vasomotor symptoms associated with the menopause is 12 to 25 mg. daily (one or two 12 mg. capsules or one 25 mg. capsule) for 30 days; one or more courses may be prescribed.

The usual dosage range for atrophic vaginitis or kraurosis vulvae is 12 to 25 mg. daily (one or two 12 mg. capsules or one 25 mg. capsule) for 30 to 60 days.

Given cyclically

For female hypogonadism.

The usual dosage is 12 to 25 mg. daily (one or two 12 mg. capsules or one 25 mg. capsule) for 21 days. This course may, if desired, be followed immediately by the intramuscular injection of 100 mg. of progesterone; alternatively, an oral progestogen such as medroxyprogesterone may be given during the last 5 days of TACE (CHLOROTRIANISENE NF) therapy. The next course may begin on the 5th day of the induced uterine bleeding.

Treated patients with an intact uterus should be monitored closely for signs of endometrial cancer, and appropriate diagnostic measures should be taken to rule out malignancy in the event of persistent or recurrent abnormal vaginal bleeding.

How Supplied:

TACE 12 mg. (CHLOROTRIANISENE CAPSULES NF)

NDC 0068-0690-28:	bottles of 28
NDC 0068-0690-61:	bottles of 100
NDC 0068-0690-65:	bottles of 500

TACE 25 mg. (CHLOROTRIANISENE CAPSULES NF)

NDC 0068-0691-60:	bottles of 60

References

1. Ziel, H.K. and Finkel, W.D.: Increased risk of endometrial carcinoma among users of conjugated estrogens. New Eng. J. Med. 293:1167–1170, 1975.
2. Smith, D.C., Prentice, R., Thompson, D.J., and Hermann, W.L.: Association of exogenous estrogen and endometrial carcinoma. New Eng. J. Med. 293:1164–1167, 1975.
3. Mack, T.M., Pike, M.C., Henderson, B.E., Pfeffer, R.I., Gerkins, V.R., Arthur, M., and Brown, S.E.: Estrogens and endometrial cancer in a retirement community. New Eng. J. Med. 294:1262–1267, 1976.
4. Weiss, N.S., Szekely, D.R., and Austin, D.F.: Increasing incidence of endometrial cancer in the United States. New Eng. J. Med. 294:1259–1262, 1976.
5. Herbst, A.L., Ulfelder, H., and Poskanzer, D.C.: Adenocarcinoma of the vagina. New Eng. J. Med. 284:878–881, 1971.
6. Greenwald, P., Barlow, J.J., Nasca, P.C., and Burnett, W.S.: Vaginal cancer after maternal treatment with synthetic estrogens. New Eng. J. Med. 285:390–392, 1971.
7. Herbst, A.L., Cole, P., Colton, T., Robboy, S.J., and Scully, R.E.: Latency period and incidence aspects of DES-related clear cell adenocarcinoma of the vagina and cervix. Amer. J. Obstet. Gynec. In press.
8. Lanier, A.P., Noller, K.L., Decker, D.G., Elveback, L.R., and Kurland, L.T.: Cancer and stilbestrol. A follow-up of 1719 persons exposed to estrogens in utero and born 1943–1959. Mayo Clin. Proc. 48:793–799, 1973.
9. Herbst, A.L., Kurman, R.J., and Scully, R.E.: Vaginal and cervical abnormalities after exposure to stilbestrol in utero. Obstet. Gynec. 40:287–298, 1972.
10. Herbst, A.L., Poskanzer, D.C., Robboy, S.J., Friedlander, L., and Scully, R.E.: Prenatal exposure to stilbestrol. A prospective comparison of exposed female offspring with unexposed controls. New Eng. J. Med. 292:334–339, 1975.
11. Stafl, A., Mattingly, R.F., Foley, D.V., and Fetherston, W.C.: Clinical diagnosis of vaginal adenosis. Obstet. Gynec. 43:118–128, 1974.
12. Sherman, A.I., Goldrath, M., Berlin, A., Vakhariya, V., Banooni, F., Michaels, W., Goodman, P., and Brown, S.: Cervical-vaginal adenosis after *in utero* exposure to synthetic estrogens. Obstet. Gynec. 44:531–545, 1974.
13. Gal, I., Kirman, B., Stern, J.: Hormone pregnancy tests and congenital malformation. Nature 216:83, 1967.
14. Levy, E.P., Cohen, A., and Fraser, F.C.: Hormone treatment during pregnancy and congenital heart defects. Lancet 1:611, 1973.
15. Nora, J.J. and Nora, A.H.: Birth defects and oral contraceptives. Lancet 1:941–942, 1973.
16. Janerich, D.T., Piper, J.M., and Glebatis, D.M.: Oral contraceptives and congenital limb-reduction defects. New Eng. J. Med. 291:697–700, 1974.
17. Daniel, D.G., Campbell, H., and Turnbull, A.C.: Puerperal thromboembolism and suppression of lactation. Lancet 2:287–289, 1967.
18. Boston Collaborative Drug Surveillance Program: Surgically confirmed gall bladder disease, venous thromboembolism, and breast tumors in relation to post menopausal estrogen therapy. New Eng. J. Med. 290:15–19, 1974.
19. Hoover, R., Gray, L.A., Sr., Cole, P., and MacMahon, B.: Menopausal estrogens and breast cancer. New Eng. J. Med. 295:401–405, 1976.
20. Boston Collaborative Drug Surveillance Program: Oral contraceptives and venous thromboembolic disease, surgically confirmed gall-bladder disease, and breast tumors. Lancet 1:1399–1404, 1973.
21. Bailar, J.C., III: Thromboembolism and oestrogen therapy. Lancet 2:560, 1967.
22. The Veterans Administration Cooperative Urological Research Group: Carcinoma of the prostate: Treatment comparisons. J. Urol. 98:516–522, 1967.
23. Blackard, C.E., Doe, R.P., Mellinger, G.T., and Byar, D.P.: Incidence of cardiovascular disease and death in patients receiving diethylstilbestrol for carcinoma of the prostate. Cancer 26:249–256, 1970.
24. Royal College of General Practitioners: Oral contraception and thromboembolic disease. J. Roy. Coll. Gen. Pract. 13:267–269, 1967.
25. Inman, W.H.W. and Vessey, M.P.: Investigation of deaths from pulmonary, coronary, and cerebral thrombosis and embolism in women of child-bearing age. Brit. Med. J. 2:193–199, 1968.
26. Vessey, M.P. and Doll, R.: Investigation of relation between use of oral contraceptives and thromboembolic disease. A further report. Brit. Med. J. 2:651–657, 1969.
27. Sartwell, P.E., Masi, A.T., Arthes, F.G., Greene, G.R., and Smith, H.E.: Thromboembolism and oral contraceptives: An epidemiological case-control study. Amer. J. Epidem. 90:365–380, 1969.
28. Collaborative Group for the Study of Stroke in Young Women: Oral contraception and increased risk of cerebral ischemia or thrombosis. New Eng. J. Med. 288:871–878, 1973.
29. Collaborative Group for the Study of Stroke in Young Women: Oral contraceptives and stroke in young women: Associated risk factors. J.A.M.A. 231:718–722, 1975.
30. Mann, J.I. and Inman, W.H.W.: Oral contraceptives and death from myocardial infarction. Brit. Med. J. 2:245–248, 1975.
31. Mann, J.I., Vessey, M.P., Thorogood, M., and Doll, R.: Myocardial infarction in young women with special reference in oral contraceptive practice. Brit. Med. J. 2:241–245, 1975.
32. Inman, W.H.W., Vessey, M.P., Westerholm, B., and Engelund, A.: Thromboembolic disease and the steroidal content of oral contraceptives. A report to the Committee on Safety of Drugs. Brit. Med. J. 2:203–209, 1970.
33. Stolley, P.D., Tonascia, J.A., Tockman, M.S., Sartwell, P.E., Rutledge, A.H., and Jacobs, M.P.: Thrombosis with low-estrogen oral contraceptives. Amer. J. Epidem. 102:197–208, 1975.
34. Vessey, M.P., Doll, R., Fairbairn, A.S., and Glober, G.: Post-operative thromboembolism and the use of the oral contraceptives. Brit. Med. J. 3:123–126, 1970.
35. Greene, G.R. and Sartwell, P.E.: Oral contraceptive use in patients with thromboembolism following surgery, trauma, or infection. Amer. J. Public Health 62:680–685, 1972.
36. Rosenberg, L., Armstrong, B., Phil, D., and Jick, H.: Myocardial infarction and estrogen therapy in post-menopausal women. New Eng. J. Med. 294:1256–1259, 1976.
37. Coronary Drug Project Research Group: The coronary drug project: Initial findings leading to modifications of its research protocol. J.A.M.A. 214:1303–1313, 1970.
38. Baum, J., Holtz, F., Bookstein, J.J., and Klein, E.W.: Possible association between benign hepatomas and oral contraceptives. Lancet 2:926–928, 1973.
39. Mays, E.T., Christopherson, W.M., Mahr, M.M., and Williams, H.C.: Hepatic changes in young women ingesting contraceptive steroids. Hepatic hemorrhage and primary hepatic tumors. J.A.M.A. 235:730–732, 1976.
40. Edmondson, H., Henderson, A.B., and Benton, B.: Liver-cell adenomas associated with the use of oral contraceptives. New Eng. J. Med. 294:470–472, 1976.
41. Pfeffer, R.I. and Van Den Noort, S.: Estrogen use and stroke risk in postmenopausal women. Amer. J. Epidem. 103:445–456, 1976.

Product Information as of August, 1979

TACE 12 mg. Capsules are jointly manufactured by
R. P. Scherer Corporation
Detroit, Michigan 48213 and
MERRELL-NATIONAL LABORATORIES
Division of Richardson-Merrell Inc.
Cincinnati, Ohio 45215, U.S.A.

[*Shown in Product Identification Section*]

TACE® ℞
(CHLOROTRIANISENE NF)
72 mg. Capsules

Description: TACE (CHLOROTRIANISENE NF) is a long-acting, synthetic estrogen in capsule form suitable for oral administration.

Each two-tone green and yellow soft gelatin capsule contains 72 mg. of TACE (CHLOROTRIANISENE) in Dispex®, an emulsifiable vehicle containing corn oil, sorbitan trioleate, polysorbate 80, and benzyl benzoate.

Chemistry

Generic name: Chlorotrianisene NF

Chemical name: Benzene, 1,1′,1″-(1-chloro-1-ethenyl-2-ylidene)tris[4- methoxy- Chlorotris-(*p*-methoxyphenyl)ethylene

Chlorotrianisene occurs as small, white crystals or as a crystalline powder. It is odorless. It is slightly soluble in alcohol and very slightly soluble in water.

Indications: Postpartum breast engorgement—Although estrogens have been widely used for the prevention of postpartum breast engorgement, controlled studies have demonstrated that the incidence of significant painful engorgement in patients not receiving such hormonal therapy is low and usually responsive to appropriate analgesic or other supportive therapy. Consequently, the benefit to be derived from estrogen therapy for this indication must be carefully weighed against the potential risk of puerperal thromboembolism associated with the use of estrogens.[17]

TACE (CHLOROTRIANISENE NF) HAS NOT BEEN SHOWN TO BE EFFECTIVE FOR ANY PURPOSE DURING PREGNANCY, AND ITS USE MAY HAVE POTENTIAL RISKS TO THE FETUS. (SEE BOXED WARNING.)

Dosage and Administration:

Given for a few days

Prevention of postpartum breast engorgement. The usual dosage is 1 TACE 72 mg. capsule twice daily for 2 days. The first dose should be given as soon as possible after delivery but within 8 hours.

How Supplied:

TACE 72 mg. (CHLOROTRIANISENE CAPSULES NF)

NDC 0068-0692-48: packages of 48 capsules in foil strips in dispensing units of 4 capsules.

For additional prescribing information, please see listing for TACE 12 & 25 mg.

[*Shown in Product Identification Section*]

TENUATE® Ⓒ ℞
(diethylpropion hydrochloride NF)
TENUATE DOSPAN®
(diethylpropion hydrochloride NF)
controlled-release tablets

Description: Diethylpropion hydrochloride, a sympathomimetic agent, is 1-phenyl-2-diethylamino-1-propanone hydrochloride.

In Tenuate Dospan tablets, diethylpropion hydrochloride is dispersed in a hydrophilic matrix. On exposure to water the diethylpropion hydrochloride is released at a relatively uniform rate as a result of slow hydration of the matrix. The result is controlled release of the anorexic agent.

Actions: Tenuate is a sympathomimetic amine with some pharmacologic activity similar to that of the prototype drugs of this class used in obesity, the amphetamines. Actions include some central nervous system stimulation and elevation of blood pressure. Tolerance has been demonstrated with all drugs of this class in which these phenomena have been looked for.

Drugs of this class used in obesity are commonly known as "anorectics" or "anorexigenics." It has not been established, however, that the action of such drugs in treating obesity is primarily one of appetite suppression. Other central nervous system actions, or metabolic effects may be involved, for example.

Adult obese subjects instructed in dietary management and treated with "anorectic" drugs lose more weight on the average than those treated with placebo and diet, as determined in relatively short-term clinical trials.

The magnitude of increased weight loss of drug-treated patients over placebo-treated patients is some fraction of a pound a week. However, some patients lose more weight than this and some lose less. The rate of weight loss is greatest in the first weeks of therapy for both drug and placebo subjects and tends to decrease in succeeding weeks. The possible origins of the increased weight loss due to the various drug effects are not established. The amount of weight loss associated with the use of an "anorectic" drug varies from trial to trial, and the increased weight loss appears to be related in part to variables other than the drug prescribed, such as the physician-investigator, the population treated, and the diet prescribed. Studies do not permit conclusions as to the relative importance of the drug and non-drug factors on weight loss.

The natural history of obesity is measured in years, whereas most studies cited are restricted to a few weeks duration; thus, the total impact of drug-induced weight loss over that of diet alone must be considered clinically limited.

The controlled-release characteristics of Tenuate Dospan have been demonstrated by studies in humans in which plasma levels of diethylpropion-related material were measured by phosphorescence analysis. Plasma levels obtained with the 75 mg. Dospan formulation administered once daily indicated a more gradual release than the standard formulation. The formulation has not been shown superior in effectiveness to the same dosage of the standard, noncontrolled-release formulation.

Indication: Tenuate and Tenuate Dospan are indicated in the management of exogenous obesity as a short-term adjunct (a few weeks) in a regimen of weight reduction based on caloric restriction. The limited usefulness of agents of this class (see ACTIONS) should be measured against possible risk factors inherent in their use such as those described below.

Contraindications: Advanced arteriosclerosis, hyperthyroidism, known hypersensitivity, or idiosyncrasy to the sympathomimetic amines, glaucoma.

Agitated states.

Patients with a history of drug abuse.

During or within 14 days following the administration of monoamine oxidase inhibitors, (hypertensive crises may result).

Warnings: If tolerance develops, the recommended dose should not be exceeded in an attempt to increase the effect; rather, the drug should be discontinued. Tenuate may impair the ability of the patient to engage in potentially hazardous activities such as operating machinery or driving a motor vehicle; the patient should therefore be cautioned accordingly.

Drug Dependence

Tenuate has some chemical and pharmacologic similarities to the amphetamines and other related stimulant drugs that have been extensively abused. There have been reports of subjects becoming psychologically dependent on diethylpropion. The possibility of abuse should be kept in mind when evaluating the desirability of including a drug as part of a weight reduction program. Abuse of amphetamines and related drugs may be associated with varying degrees of psychologic dependence and social dysfunction which, in the case of certain drugs, may be severe. There are reports of patients who have increased the dosage to many times that recommended. Abrupt cessation following prolonged high dosage administration results in extreme fatigue and mental depression; changes are also noted on the sleep EEG. Manifestations of chronic intoxication with anorectic drugs include severe dermatoses, marked insomnia, irritability, hyperactivity, and personality changes. The most severe manifestation of chronic intoxications is psychosis, often clinically indistinguishable from schizophrenia.

Use in Pregnancy

Although rat and human reproductive studies have not indicated adverse effects, the use of Tenuate by women who are pregnant or may become pregnant requires that the potential benefits be weighed against the potential risks.

Use in Children

Tenuate is not recommended for use in children under 12 years of age.

Precautions: Caution is to be exercised in prescribing Tenuate for patients with hypertension or with symptomatic cardiovascular disease, including arrhythmias. Tenuate should not be administered to patients with severe hypertension.

Insulin requirements in diabetes mellitus may be altered in association with the use of Tenuate and the concomitant dietary regimen.

Tenuate may decrease the hypotensive effect of guanethidine.

The least amount feasible should be prescribed or dispensed at one time in order to minimize the possibility of overdosage.

Reports suggest that Tenuate may increase convulsions in some epileptics. Therefore, epileptics receiving Tenuate should be carefully monitored. Titration of dose or discontinuance of Tenuate may be necessary.

Adverse Reactions: *Cardiovascular:* Palpitation, tachycardia, elevation of blood pressure, precordial pain, arrhythmia. One published report described T-wave changes in the ECG of a healthy young male after ingestion of diethylpropion hydrochloride.

Central Nervous System: Overstimulation, nervousness, restlessness, dizziness, jitteriness, insomnia, anxiety, euphoria, depression, dysphoria, tremor, dyskinesia, mydriasis, drowsiness, malaise, headache; rarely psychotic episodes at recommended doses. In a few epileptics an increase in convulsive episodes has been reported.

Gastrointestinal: Dryness of the mouth, unpleasant taste, nausea, vomiting, abdominal discomfort, diarrhea, constipation, other gastrointestinal disturbances.

Allergic: Urticaria, rash, ecchymosis, erythema.

Endocrine: Impotence, changes in libido, gynecomastia, menstrual upset.

Hematopoietic System: Bone marrow depression, agranulocytosis, leukopenia.

Miscellaneous: A variety of miscellaneous adverse reactions has been reported by physicians. These include complaints such as dyspnea, hair loss, muscle pain, dysuria, increased sweating, and polyuria.

Dosage and Administration:

Tenuate (diethylpropion hydrochloride):

One 25 mg. tablet three times daily, one hour before meals, and in midevening if desired to overcome night hunger.

Tenuate Dospan (diethylpropion hydrochloride) controlled-release:

One 75 mg. tablet daily, swallowed whole, in midmorning.

Tenuate is not recommended for use in children under 12 years of age.

Overdosage: Manifestations of acute overdosage include restlessness, tremor, hyperreflexia, rapid respiration, confusion, assaultiveness, hallucinations, panic states.

Fatigue and depression usually follow the central stimulation.

Cardiovascular effects include arrhythimas, hypertension or hypotension and circulatory collapse. Gastrointestinal symptoms include

Continued on next page

Merrell-National—Cont.

nausea, vomiting, diarrhea, and abdominal cramps. Overdose of pharmacologically similar compounds has resulted in fatal poisoning, usually terminating in convulsions and coma. Management of acute Tenuate intoxication is largely symptomatic and includes lavage and sedation with a barbiturate. Experience with hemodialysis or peritoneal dialysis is inadequate to permit recommendation in this regard. Intravenous phentolamine (Regitine®) has been suggested on pharmacologic grounds for possible acute, severe hypertension, if this complicates Tenuate overdosage.

How Supplied: Light blue 25 mg. Tenuate tablets: bottles of 100 and 1000

White capsule-shaped 75 mg. Tenuate Dospan tablets: bottles of 100 and 250

Product Information as of April, 1976

MERRELL-NATIONAL LABORATORIES Inc.
Cayey, Puerto Rico 00633
Direct Medical Inquiries to:
MERRELL-NATIONAL LABORATORIES
Division of Richardson-Merrell Inc.
Cincinnati, Ohio 45215
Licensor of Merrell®

[*Shown in Product Indentification Section*]

TRICLOS® ℞
(triclofos sodium)

Description: Triclos is a phosphate ester of trichlorethanol with hypnotic properties. Triclofos sodium is the sodium salt of trichlorethyl phosphate.

Actions: Triclos is rapidly dephosphorylated, principally in the gut, yielding high blood levels of trichlorethanol which is the same pharmacologically active metabolite obtained from chloral hydrate by enzymatic reduction. Triclos produces a peak serum level of trichlorethanol in about one hour and has a half-life of approximately eleven hours.

Triclos has minimal effects on the various stages of normal sleep, including REM sleep. The exact clinical significance of changes in REM sleep have not been established.

In animal studies Triclos increased the content of slow wave, high voltage spontaneous corticol EEG activity concomitant with behavioral sleep. The arousal threshold on electrical stimulation of the midbrain reticular formation was increased. Whether the latter effect is responsible for the hypnotic action of Triclos is not known.

Indications: Triclos is a hypnotic agent useful in the treatment of insomnia characterized by difficulty in falling asleep, frequent nocturnal awakenings and/or early morning awakening. Triclos has not been shown effective for more than 14 days except in persons over age 65 where it was effective for up to 42 days in one inpatient study.

Also, Triclos can be used as a pre-medication for obtaining sleep records in electroencephalography.

Contraindications: Triclos is contraindicated in patients with marked renal or hepatic impairment and in patients known to be sensitive or allergic to chloral hydrate or triclofos sodium.

Triclos is also contraindicated in women at labor and in the neonate because trichloroacetic acid, the principal metabolite in man of Triclos, frees bilirubin from albumin. Thus, by displacing protein-bound bilirubin, kernicterus could occur in the neonate.

Warnings:

Drug Dependency: Triclos may be habit forming. The relationship of Triclos to chloral hydrate suggests that the addiction liability would be similar. Therefore, caution should be exercised in administering Triclos to patients known to be addiction prone and repeated prescriptions are only advisable under careful medical supervision.

Drug Interactions: Response to concomitantly administered oral anticoagulants may be modified by Triclos in some patients; the anticoagulant effect may be either increased or decreased. Therefore, careful monitoring of prothrombin time with adjustment of anticoagulant dosage is advised throughout Triclos administration and following withdrawal of this drug.

Usage in Pregnancy: Triclos has been administered to three species of animals at various stages of pregnancy at levels as high as 700 mg/kg/day. No dose related effects were observed in these reproductive studies. The relevance to the human is not known. Since there is no experience in pregnant women who have received the drug, safety in pregnancy has not been established.

Nursing Mothers: There are no data on secretion of the drug in human milk or effect on the nursing infant.

Usage in Children: Except for single dose administration of Triclos Liquid for sleep induction in electroencephalography, the drug is not currently recommended for use in persons under 12 years of age.

Precautions: Triclos, like chloral hydrate, may increase the CNS depressant effects of other drugs such as alcohol, barbiturates, and tranquilizers. Therefore, patients taking Triclos should be cautioned accordingly.

Since Triclos may reduce alertness, it should be used cautiously in patients operating vehicles or machinery.

Triclos should be used with caution in patients with cardiac arrhythmias and with severe cardiac disease.

Most insomnias will be of brief duration and therefore long term chronic administration of Triclos is neither advised nor recommended. In cases where prolonged therapy with Triclos is necessary for treatment of insomnia, it is recommended that periodic blood counts be done. Studies of the efficacy of Triclos for periods exceeding six weeks have not been carried out.

Adverse Reactions: The following undesirable reactions have been reported in patients taking Triclos: headache, hangover, drowsiness, gastrointestinal upset, "gas," flatulence, nausea and vomiting, staggering gait, ataxia, "bad taste," ketonuria, relative eosinophilia, urticaria, light-headedness, vertigo, nightmares, malaise, and reduction in total white blood cell count. Excitement and delirium, since they have been observed with chloral hydrate, are possible.

Dosage and Administration: The usual hypnotic dosage of Triclos is 1500 mg. (two 750 mg. tablets or 15 ml. of liquid) taken 15 to 30 minutes before bedtime.

The usual dose for sleep induction in electroencephalography in children under 12 years of age is 0.1 ml. of Triclos Liquid per pound of body weight.

Overdosage: Accidental overdosage should be treated with gastric lavage or induce vomiting to empty the stomach. Supportive measures may be used.

How Supplied: TRICLOS (triclofos sodium), 750 mg. film coated tablets, orange, capsule shaped.

NDC 0068-0085-01: bottles of 100 tablets.
NDC 0068-0085-05: bottles of 500 tablets.
TRICLOS (triclofos sodium) Liquid, 1.5 g./15 ml. (100 mg./ml.).
NDC 0068-0086-08: bottles containing 8 fl. oz.

Revised July, 1978

(*Shown in Product Identification Section*)

VANOBID® ℞
(candicidin NF)
Vaginal Ointment/Tablets

Description: Vanobid Vaginal Ointment and Vanobid Vaginal Tablets contain candicidin, a conjugated heptaene antibiotic complex, produced by a soil actinomycete similar to *Streptomyces griseus*. Vanobid Vaginal Ointment is a dispersion of candicidin in U.S.P. petrolatum. It contains 0.6 mg. candicidin activity per 1 gram of ointment. Each Vanobid Vaginal Tablet contains 3 mg. candicidin activity dispersed in starch, lactose, and magnesium stearate.

Action: Vanobid Vaginal Ointment and Vanobid Vaginal Tablets have anti-*Candida* activity.

Indications: For the treatment of vaginitis due to *Candida albicans* and other *Candida* species. Vanobid Vaginal Tablets are particularly suited for gravid patients.

Contraindications: Contraindicated for patients known to be sensitive to any of the components of Vanobid Vaginal Ointment and Vanobid Vaginal Tablets. During pregnancy, the use of an applicator may be contraindicated. The tablet inserter should be used only on advice of physician. Manual tablet insertion may be preferred.

Precautions: During treatment it is recommended that the patient refrain from sexual intercourse or the husband wear a condom to avoid re-infection.

A contraceptive diaphragm may deteriorate during prolonged contact with petrolatum-based products. The patient using a diaphragm should be advised to substitute another form of contraception during treatment with Vanobid Vaginal Ointment.

Adverse Reactions: Clinical reports of sensitization or temporary irritation with candicidin ointment or tablets have been extremely rare.

Dosage and Administration: 1 vaginal applicatorful of Vanobid Vaginal Ointment or 1 Vanobid Vaginal Tablet inserted high in the vagina twice daily, in the morning and at bedtime, for 14 days. Treatment may be repeated if symptoms persist or reappear.

How Supplied: A 14-day course of therapy of Vanobid Vaginal Ointment is supplied in a package containing two 75-gram tubes, two vaginal applicators, and patient instructions.

A 14-day course of therapy of Vanobid Tablets is supplied in packages of 28 individually foil-wrapped tablets with vaginal inserter and patient instructions.

A pad may be used to protect clothing.

Store under refrigeration to ensure full potency.

Product Information as of November, 1974

[*Shown in Product Identification Section*]

Metabolic Products Corporation
37 HURLEY STREET
CAMBRIDGE, MA 02141

PROSTALL®

Composition: Each capsule contains 6 gr. of a combination of glutamic acid, alanine and aminoacetic acid (glycine).

Action and Uses: Symptomatic relief of benign prostatic hypertrophy (urgency, frequency, nocturia, dribbling and delayed urination).

Contraindications and Side Effects: No known side effects.

Administration and Dosage: 2 capsules t.i.d. after meals for 3 weeks, thereafter 1 capsule t.i.d. after meals for not less than 2 months.

How Supplied: In bottles of 100 and 250 capsules.

TE TREE® OINTMENT

Composition: Australian oil of melaleuca alternifolia in a special ointment base.

Action and Uses: Promotes the healing of minor abrasions, cuts, scrapes and burns.

Gives relief of chapped skin, chapped lips, and non-poisonous insect bites. Promotes the healing of poison ivy, oak and sumac. Do not apply to these open lesions.
Administration: Apply ointment without excessive rubbing and leave on for at least 4 hours. Bandage only if needed.
How Supplied: In 1 oz. tubes

Metro Med, Inc.
5400 HUDSON BEND ROAD
AUSTIN, TEXAS 78734

DIGESTAMIC

Description: Each tablet contains: Pancrelipase N.F., 162mg. representing 3888 N.F. Units of lipase activity, 16,200 N.F. Units of amylase activity, 16,200 N.F. Units of protease activity.

Papain	97.2mg.
Atropine Sulfate	0.024mg.
Hyoscine Hydrobromide	0.014mg.
Hyoscyamine Sulfate	0.122mg.

(Total Belladonna alkaloidal salts, 0.16mg.)
Precautions: Use with caution in patients known to be sensitive to pork or enzymes. Discontinue use in patients with symptoms of sensitivity. High dosages may cause nausea or diarrhea in certain patients.
Warning: Not to be used by persons having glaucoma or excessive pressure within the eye, by elderly persons (where undiagnosed glaucoma or excessive pressure within the eye occurs most frequently), or by children under 12 years of age, unless directed by a physician. Discontinue use if blurring of vision, rapid pulse, or dizziness occurs. Do not exceed recommended dosage. If eye pain occurs, discontinue use and see your physician immediately as this may indicate undiagnosed glaucoma.
Directions For Use: As digestive aid; adults; 2 to 4 tablets with meals and 1 tablet with any food eaten between meals or as directed by a physician.
How Supplied: Bottles of 50 and 500 Tablets.
KEEP THIS AND ALL DRUGS OUT OF THE REACH OF CHILDREN. IN CASE OF ACCIDENTAL OVERDOSE, SEEK PROFESSIONAL ASSISTANCE OR CONTACT A POISON CONTROL CENTER IMMEDIATELY.

SPAN–FF OTC

Description: Each capsule contains: FERROUS FUMARATE 5 gr. 325 mg—106 mg Elemental Iron.
Each capsule provides for the following Minimum Daily Requirement of Iron.
Adults and Children over 6 years 1060%, Children under six years 1443%.
Indications: For use in the treatment of simple (iron deficiency) anemia.
Warning: Keep this and all medications out of the reach of children.
Dosage: Adults—One capsule in the morning and one capsule in the evening.
Children—The contents of one capsule daily in any vehicle or food
How Supplied: Bottles of 60 (NDC 0454-3002-06) and 500 (NDC 0454-3002-50) capsules.

Products are cross-indexed

by product classifications

in the

BLUE SECTION

Meyer Laboratories, Inc.
1900 WEST COMMERCIAL BLVD.
FT. LAUDERDALE, FLA. 33309

(See product listings under Glaxo Inc.)

Miles Laboratories, Inc.
P. O. BOX 340
ELKHART, INDIANA 46515

ALKA-SELTZER® Effervescent Pain Reliever & Antacid
(See PDR for Nonprescription Drugs)

ALKA-SELTZER® Effervescent Antacid
(See PDR For Nonprescription Drugs)

ALKA-2® Chewable Antacid Tablets
(See PDR For Nonprescription Drugs)

ALKA-SELTZER PLUS® Cold Medicine
(See PDR For Nonprescription Drugs)

FLINTSTONES® PLUS IRON MULTIVITAMIN SUPPLEMENT
(Multivitamin Supplement with Iron)

FLINTSTONES® MULTIVITAMIN SUPPLEMENT
(Multivitamin Supplement)

CHOCKS® BUGS BUNNY® MULTIVITAMIN SUPPLEMENT
(Multivitamin Supplement)

CHOCKS® BUGS BUNNY® PLUS IRON MULTIVITAMIN SUPPLEMENT
(Multivitamin Supplement with Iron)

CHOCKS® PLUS IRON MULTIVITAMIN SUPPLEMENT
(Multivitamin Supplement with Iron)

CHOCKS® MULTIVITAMIN SUPPLEMENT
(Multivitamin Supplement)

(See PDR For Nonprescription Drugs)

ONE-A-DAY® BRAND VITAMINS PLUS MINERALS
(Multivitamin/Multimineral Supplement)

ONE-A-DAY® BRAND VITAMINS PLUS IRON
(Multivitamin Supplement with Iron)

ONE-A-DAY® BRAND VITAMINS
(Multivitamin Supplement)

(See PDR For Nonprescription Drugs)

Important Notice

Before prescribing or administering

any product described in

PHYSICIANS' DESK REFERENCE

always consult the PDR Supplement for

possible new or revised information.

Milex Products, Inc.
5915 NORTHWEST HIGHWAY
CHICAGO, ILLINOIS 60631

AMINO-CERV™ ℞
pH 5.5 Cervical Creme

Active Ingredients: Urea 8.34%, Sodium Propionate 0.50%, Methionine 0.83%, Cystine 0.35%, Inositol 0.83%, Benzalkonium Chloride 0.000004%. Buffered to pH of 5.5 in a water-miscible creme base.
Description: An AMINO-ACID and UREA creme specifically formulated for cervical treatment: Cervicitis (mild), postpartum cervicitis, postpartum cervical tears, post cauterization, post cryosurgery and post conization.
Advantages: METHIONINE and CYSTINE are amino-acids necessary for wound healing and forming of epithelial tissue. INOSITOL acts as an essential growth factor and promotes epithelialization.
UREA aids in debridement, dissolves the coagulum and promotes epithelialization. Its solvent action on fibroblasts prevents the formation of excessive tissue—thus preventing stenosis when used as directed.
BENZALKONIUM CHLORIDE serves to lower surface tension and thus aids in spreading the medication. Along with SODIUM PROPIONATE it also exerts a bacteriostatic effect.
AMINO-CERV is geared to the higher pH of the healthy cervix in contrast with pH 4 vaginal preparations. With its pH factor of 5.5 Amino-Cerv promotes faster healing of the cervix, yet will not adversely affect a healthy vagina.
Directions: When immediate postpartum bleeding has subsided (usually from 24 to 48 hours after delivery), one Milex-Jector full of AMINO-CERV creme should be applied nightly for four weeks. In mild CERVICITIS (not requiring cautery or cryosurgery) one applicatorful of AMINO-CERV should be injected in the vagina nightly upon retiring for 2 weeks.
A small amount of AMINO-CERV should be applied immediately after HOT CAUTERIZATION, HOT CONIZATION and CRYOSURGERY. One applicatorful should be injected nightly upon retiring for 2 to 4 weeks (the duration of treatment depends on extent of cauterization or hot conization or cryosurgery). During the weekly office visit for (2 to 4 visits) the physician should again apply a small amount of AMINO-CERV with a probe or applicator. The canal is to be completely probed on the last visit.
After COLD CONING, one applicatorful should be injected upon retiring about 24 hours after surgery and nightly thereafter for four weeks. During the four weekly office visits following cold coning, a small amount of AMINO-CERV should be applied with a probe or applicator into the canal by the physician. The canal is to be completely probed on the last visit.
Reasons For Variation of Directions:
(1) After hot conization, cauterization and cryosurgery immediate use of AMINO-CERV is indicated to aid in dissolving dead or burned tissue.
(2) After cold coning, there is no dead tissue to slough off. Therefore, a wait of 24 hours or longer is desirable for normal healing to take place and for some fibroblasts to be laid down before applying the AMINO-CERV (which has a solvent action on both the fibroblasts and the absorbable sutures). When NONABSORBABLE sutures are used, AMINO-CERV can be used immediately.
Contraindications: Deleterious side effects have not been a problem at the doses recommended. The usual precautions against allergic reactions should be observed.

Continued on next page

Milex—Cont.

Storage: Store at room temperature.
Packaging: 2¾ oz. tube with Milex-Jector (2 weeks supply, 14 applications).
Available only on hospital direct orders: 5½ oz. tube with MILEX-JECTOR (4 weeks supply, 28 applications).

PRO-CEPTION

Description: PRO-CEPTION is a precoital douche to help promote conception. It provides in a convenient form supplementary nutrient immediately available to the sperm for metabolism and movement. Also effective for removal of a thick tenacious mucous plug of the cervix.
Directions: The screw cap is used as a measuring device and filled level with the powder which is then dissolved in eight ounces of lukewarm water. The woman is told to douche while in a recombent position and to retain the solution (10 to 15 minutes). Following coitus the patient should remain recumbent for two hours or more. May be used as a companion with Milex Oligospermia Cups. Frequently used in connection with PRO-CEPTION Basal Thermometers.
Contraindications: None.
Packaging: Available in 12 douche container.

Miller Pharmacal

Div. of Medical Modalities Associates, Inc.
An AKORN Company
1425 MELODY DRIVE
METAIRIE, LA 70002

A/G-PRO

Composition: Each 6 tablets contain: Protein Hydrolysate (45% Amino Acids) 50 gr.; L-Lysine Monohydrochloride 300 mg.; dl-Methionine 75 mg.; Iron* 10 mg.; Copper* 1 mg.; Iodine* .015 mg.; Manganese* 2 mg.; Potassium 20 mg.; Zinc* 2 mg.; Magnesium* 30 mg. Zinc, copper, iron, manganese and magnesium complexed from sulfate.
*These minerals are present as a complex with a portion of the amino acids. Approximate amino acid content: 6 tablets will supply the following amounts of essential and non-essential amino acids: Aspartic Acid 179 mg.; Serine 115 mg.; Glycine 107 mg.; Alanine 68 mg.; Arginine 74 mg.; Histidine 45 mg.; Lysine 425 mg.; Tyrosine 74 mg.; Tryptophan 27 mg.; Phenylalanine 103 mg.; Cystine 16 mg.; Methionine 110 mg.; Threonine 84 mg.; Leucine 136 mg.; Isoleucine 101 mg.; Valine 117 mg.; Glutamic Acid 226 mg.
Action and Uses: An adjunct in the treatment of tissue repair in pre- and post-operative build-up, post pathologic therapy and in tissue detoxification.
Administration and Dosage: The usual dose, as a dietary supplement of amino acids and minerals for adults and children, is 2 tablets 3 times daily before meals, or as otherwise directed by a physician.
Side Effects: None reported.
Precautions: None.
How Supplied: In bottles of 180 tablets.
Literature Available: File card.

Ca-PLUS

Composition: Each tablet contains: Calcium (as contained in a calcium-protein complex made with specially isolated soy protein and Torula Yeast) 280 mg.
Action and Uses: For better absorption. Wherever Calcium deficiency is indicated.
Administration and Dosage: As a dietary supplement, 1 tablet 4 times daily, or as otherwise directed by a physician. The suggested dose of 4 tablets supplies 150% of the Minimum Adult Daily requirement of Calcium.
Precaution: When diet contains excessive oxalic acid. Avoid use when Calcium blood levels are excessively high or where conditions favor kidney stones.
How Supplied: In bottles of 100 tablets.
Literature Available: File cards.

CARDENZ®

Composition: Each tablet contains: Magnesium Ascorbic Acid Complex, Magnesium Oxide, Magnesium p-Aminobenzoate, Vitamin E Succinate, Inositol, Magnesium Gluconate, Potassium Gluconate, Vitamin A Palmitate, Irradiated Ergosterol, Pyridoxine HCl, Cyanocobalamin, Niacinamide, Potassium Iodide, supplying the following nutrients: Vitamin A 2000 IU; Vitamin D 100 Units; Vitamin E 5 IU; Vitamin B_6 1.5 mg.; Vitamin B_{12} 1 mcg.; Niacinamide 20 mg.; Vitamin C 25 mg.; Inositol 30 mg.; p-Aminobenzoic Acid 9 mg.; Magnesium 23 mg.; Potassium 8 mg.; Iodine .05 mg.
Administration and Dosage: One or two tablets three times daily with meals, or as directed by a physician.
How Supplied: Tablets of 100 per bottle.
Literature Available: File cards and dietary suggestions.

CHENATAL ℞

Composition: Each 2 tablets contains: Magnesium (as Magnesium Gluconate, Magnesium-Ascorbic Acid Complex and Magnesium p-Aminobenzoate) 27 mg.; Vitamin C (as Magnesium-Ascorbic Acid Complex) 100 mg.; Calcium (as Dicalcium Phosphate) 580 mg.; Phosphorus (as Dicalcium Phosphate) 450 mg.; L-Lysine 25 mg.; D, L-Methionine 30 mg.; Vitamin A 5000 Units; Vitamin D 400 Units; Vitamin E 10 mg.; Vitamin B_1 3 mg.; Vitamin B_2 3 mg.; Vitamin B_6 5 mg.; Vitamin B_{12} 9 mcg.; Niacinamide 30 mg.; Pantothenic Acid (as Cal. Pantothenate) 5 mg.; Iron (as Ferrous Gluconate) 20 mg.; Copper (as Copper Gluconate) 1 mg.; Manganese (as Manganese Gluconate) 2 mg.; Potassium (as Potassium Gluconate) 10 mg.; Zinc (as Zinc Gluconate) 2 mg.; Iodine (as Potassium Iodide) 0.1 mg.; Folic Acid 1.0 or 1 mg.
Action and Uses: High calcium multivitamin mineral prenatal combination.
Administration and Dosage: As a dietary adjunct in nutritional stress associated with pregnancy and lactation, 2 to 3 tablets daily, taken before meals, or as directed by physician.
How Supplied: Bottles of 100 tablets.
Literature Available: File cards and dietary suggestions.

DEQUAsine OTC

Composition: Each tablet contains: magnesium 40 mg; copper 1 mg; iodine (potassium iodide) .015 mg; iron 5 mg; manganese 2 mg; zinc 2 mg; 1-lysine (monohydrochloride) 20 mg; vitamin C 200 mg; dl-Methionine 50 mg; 1-Cysteine 100 mg. In a base of specially prepared yeast culture and amino acids.
Action and Uses: Adults, orally as a dietary supplement.
Administration and Dosage: 1 tablet daily or as prescribed by a physician.
Side Effects: None.
Precautions: None.
Contraindications: No reported contraindications to this date.
Antidote: None.
How Supplied: Bottles of 100.
Literature Available: File cards and dietary suggestions.

DǒFUS

Composition: Each capsule contains a minimum of 100,000,000 viable organisms acidophilus when packaged.
Action and Uses: As a corrective for constipation and diarrhea, and restorative for normal intestinal flora.
Administration and Dosage: One tablet daily with water before meals or as directed by a physician.
Side Effects: None.
Precautions: None.
How Supplied: Packed in bottles of 100.
Literature Available: File card.

Fe-PLUS

Composition: Each tablet contains: Iron (as an iron-protein complex made with specially isolated soy protein) 50 mg.
Action and Uses: Iron protein complex hematinic indicated for simple iron deficiency anemia. Easy to take—preferably with meals.
Administration and Dosage: Oral. One tablet three times daily, or as directed by physician. Swallow with water.
Precaution: Physician should check hemoglobin level monthly.
How Supplied: In bottles of 100 tablets.
Literature Available: File cards.

HYALEX®

Composition: Each tablet contains magnesium salicylate 4 gr.; magnesium p-aminobenzoate 2½ gr.; vitamin A palmitate 1500 i.u.; vitamin D (irradiated ergosterol) 100 i.u.; vitamin E (D,L-alpha tocopherol acetate 3 i.u.); vitamin B_{12} N.F. 2 mcg.; vitamin C (as magnesium ascorbic acid complex) 30 mg.; calcium pantothenate 5 mg.; zinc (as gluconate) 0.7 mg.; magnesium oxide 5.0 mg.
Action and Uses: HYALEX for temporary relief of minor aches and pains associated with arthritis, neuritis, bursitis, rheumatism, and for nutritional support of affected structures.
Administration and Dosage: For adults and children over 12 yrs.: One or two tablets with each meal, or as directed by a physician.
Precautions: If pain persists for more than 10 days or redness is present, or conditions affecting children under 12 years of age, consult a physician immediately. Keep out of reach of children.
How Supplied: Tablets, bottles of 100.
Literature Available: File cards and dietary suggestions.

LYSMINS™ OTC

Composition: Each tablet contains: L-Lysine 20.0 mg.; D, L-Methionine 150.0 mg.; copper 1.0 mg.; iodine 0.015 mg.; manganese 2.0 mg.; iron 10.0 mg.; potassium 20.0 mg.; zinc 2.0 mg.; magnesium 20.0 mg. Iron, manganese, magnesium, copper and zinc complexed from sulfate.
Other factors natural to Yeast Extract (biotin, folinic acid, etc.) L-Lysine and D, L-Methionine in admixture and fortification of a concentrated source of minerals, plus micronutrients in chemical combination with amino acids and polypeptides of a special yeast extract.
Action and Uses: Adults, orally as a dietary supplement. Used with HYALEX for nutritional supplementation in osteoporosis.
Administration and Dosage: 1 to 3 tablets a day or as prescribed by a physician.
Side Effects: None.
Precautions: None.
Contraindications: No reported contraindications to this date.
Antidote: None.
How Supplied: Bottles of 100.
Literature Available: File cards and dietary suggestions.

Mg-PLUS

EACH TABLET CONTAINS:
Magnesium (as a Magnesium-Protein complex made with specially isolated Soy Protein and Torula Yeast)..133 mg.
Action and Uses: A convenient source of Magnesium for patients deficient in this essential element.
Administration and Dosage: As a dietary supplement—One tablet—1 to 3 times daily—or as prescribed by a physician.
Side Effects: None Reported.
Precautions: Excessive dosage might cause laxation.
How Supplied: Bottles of 100's.
Literature Available: File cards.

NIARB-SUPER

Composition: Each tablet contains: Vitamin C (as Ascorbate Complexes) 300 mg.; Niacinamide (as Niacinamide Ascorbate Complexes) 200 mg.; Magnesium (as Magnesium Ascorbate) 50 mg.
Action and Uses: As a dietary supplement designed to prevent deficiencies of niacinamide, ascorbic acid, and magnesium.
Administration and Dosage: 1 tablet before each meal or as directed by a physician.
Side Effects: Temporary, mild flushing.
Precautions: None, if taken as directed.
How Supplied: Packed in bottles of 100.
Literature Available: File Card.

NUCLOMIN

Composition: Each two tablets contain: amino acid complexed trace minerals with multi-vitamins: vitamin A 5000 units; vitamin D 400 units; vitamin E 25 units; vitamin B-1,2.25 mg.; vitamin B-2,2.25 mg.; vitamin B-6,, 3 mg.; niacinamide 25.0 mg.; pantothenic acid (as calcium pantothenate) 15.0 mg.; vitamin C 50.0 mg.; vitamin B-12, 6 mcg.; other factors natural to yeast extract (biotin, folinic acid, etc.). Minerals: copper 1.0 mg.; iodine 0.075 mg.; manganese 3.0 mg.; iron 10.0 mg.; zinc 7.5 mg.; magnesium 100.0 mg. Iron, manganese, magnesium, copper and zinc complexed from sulfate.
Action and Uses: Amino acid complexed minerals with multi-vitamins and calcium succinate all-in-one tablet as a dietary supplement.
Administration and Dosage: 1 or 2 tablets daily or as prescribed by a physician.
How Supplied: Bottles of 100.
Literature Available: File card and dietary suggestions.

RAGUS

Composition: Each 3 tablets contain: Magnesium (as Magnesium Gluconate, Magnesium-Ascorbic Acid Complex and Magnesium p-Aminobenzoate) 27 mg.; Vitamin C (as Magnesium-Ascorbic Acid Complex) 100 mg.; Calcium (as Dicalcium Phosphate) 580 mg.; Phosphorus (as Dicalcium Phosphate) 450 mg.; L-Lysine 25 mg.; D, L-Methionine 50 mg.; Vitamin A 5000 Units; Vitamin D 400 Units; Vitamin E 10 mg.; Vitamin B_1 20 mg.; Vitamin B_2 3 mg.; Vitamin B_6 5 mg.; Vitamin B_{12} 9 mcg.; Niacinamide 80 mg.; Pantothenic Acid (as Cal. Pantothenate) 5 mg.; Iron (as Ferrous Gluconate) 20 mg.; Copper (as Copper Gluconate) 1 mg.; Manganese (as Manganese Gluconate) 2 mg.; Potassium (as Potassium Gluconate) 10 mg.; Zinc (as Zinc Gluconate) 2 mg.; Iodine (as Potassium Iodide) 0.1 mg.
Action and Uses: A concentrated source of vitamins, minerals and other nutritional factors for use as a dietary supplement.
Administration and Dosage: *Adults*—as a dietary adjunct 3 or 4 tablets daily before meals, or as directed by a physician.
How Supplied: Bottles of 100.
Literature Available: File card and dietary suggestions.

SCLEREX®

Composition: Each 3 tablets contain: inositol 2 gm.; glutamic acid magnesium complex, 19 mg.; magnesium gluconate 7.5 mg.; vitamin C (as magnesium ascorbic acid complex) 100 mg.; calcium succinate 25 mg.; vitamin A 2500 units; vitamin D 200 units; vitamin E 6 I.U.; vitamin B_1 5 mg.; vitamin B_2 2 mg.; vitamin B_6 4 mg.; vitamin B_{12} 3 mcg.; niacin 5 mg.; niacinamide 30 mg.; calcium pantothenate 7.5 mg.; iron (as gluconate)10 mg.; copper (as gluconate) 1 mg.; manganese (as gluconate) 1 mg.; zinc (as gluconate) 3 mg.; iodine (as potassium iodide) 0.10 mg.
Action and Uses: A concentrated source of vitamins, minerals and other nutritional factors for use as a dietary supplement.
For Alcoholism (SCLEREX, LYSMINS, ULCIMINS, MG-PLUS combination) information available.
Administration and Dosage: *Adults*—orally two to three tablets at mealtime, or as prescribed by a physician.
How Supplied: Bottles of 100 tablets.
Literature Available: File cards and dietary suggestions.

Zn-PLUS

Each Tablet Contains:
Zinc (as contained in a Zinc-protein complex made with specially isolated soy protein and Torula yeast)..15 mg.
Action and Uses: A convenient source of Zinc for patients deficient in this essential element.
Administration and Dosage: As a dietary supplement, 1 tablet 3 times daily, or as otherwise directed by a physician.
Side Effects: None Reported.
How Supplied: Bottles of 100's.
Literature Available: File Cards.

Mission Pharmacal Company
1325 E. DURANGO ST.
SAN ANTONIO, TEXAS 78210

CALCET®
Calcium Supplement
NDC-0178-0251-01

Composition: Each tablet contains:

	% US RDA*	
Calcium Lactate		240 mg.
Calcium Gluconate		240 mg.
Calcium Carbonate		240 mg.
(Calcium	15	152.8 mg.)
Vitamin D2	25	100. Units

* Percent of U.S. Recommended Daily Allowance for adults and children 4 or more years of age.
Indications: CALCET® tablets are indicated as a daily supplement to provide a dietary source of calcium. CALCET® tablets are of particular value in people who have milk allergies, in people who have low calcium leg cramps or calcium deficiencies due to low dietary calcium.
Dosage: TWO CALCET® TABLETS AT BEDTIME as a general or prenatal supplement. In calcium deficiency states or in nocturnal leg cramping, dosage should be increased to TWO CALCET® TABLETS AT BEDTIME plus one tablet mid-morning and one tablet mid-afternoon.
How Supplied: CALCET® tablets are supplied as yellow, oval shaped, coated tablets in bottles of 100 tablets.
Literature Available: Yes.

DILAX®-250
Dioctyl Sodium Sulfosuccinate 250 mg.
NDC 0178-0242-01

Indications: DILAX® is a stool softener which works by softening and homogenizing bowel contents. DILAX® is safe because it has no systemic drug action and is not habit forming. DILAX® does not cause irritation of the bowel and is recommended by physicians for the prevention of constipation in heart conditions, anorectal conditions, in obstetrical patients and following surgical procedures. DILAX® is also helpful in ulcerative colitis, diverticulitis and in bedridden or hospitalized patients who must avoid constipation. DILAX® provides formation of soft easily evacuated stools without discomfort, oily leakage or interference with vitamin absorption.
Contraindications: DILAX® does not cause known side effects and overdosage does not cause toxic effect.
Dosage and Administration: Take one DILAX®-250 capsule at bedtime with a full glass of water. Dosage may be adjusted upward if necessary to achieve the desired result. In some individuals several days dosage may be necessary to provide proper softening actions.

EQUILET®
Antacid Compound
NDC-0178-0010-01

Composition: Each tablet contains:
Calcium Carbonate................................500 mg.
Action and Uses: High capacity gastric antacid.
Administration and Dosage: One or two EQUILET® tablets as needed preferably between meals and at bedtime. EQUILET® tablets may be chewed or swallowed with water with equal effect according to the convenience or desire of the individual. Do not take more than 16 tablets in a 24-hour period except as may be directed by your physician.
How Supplied: EQUILET® is supplied as light yellow scored tablets in packages of 50 and 100 film stripped tablets.
Literature Available: Yes.

FERRALET®
Ferrous Gluconate
NDC-0178-0082-01

Composition: Each tablet contains:

		% US RDA*
Ferrous Gluconate	320 mg	
(Iron	37.0 mg.)	206.0

*Percent of U.S. recommended daily allowance for adults and children 4 or more years of age.
Description: The FERRALET® tablet contains only one active ingredient, iron, as ferrous gluconate. FERRALET® is particularly well tolerated in most patients because ferrous gluconate is non-astringent, non-irritating, and will not precipitate protein from aqueous media. FERRALET® provides a more efficient source of ferrous ion because of the low ionization constant of ferrous gluconate, coupled with high solubility and stability over the entire pH range of the gastrointestinal tract. FERRALET® provides utilizable iron throughout the entire length of the intestinal absorption bed. With FERRALET®, heavy iron loading is not necessary due to the superior efficiency of the iron component. The result of moderate ferrous ion dosage is usually improved patient acceptance and excellent dosage continuity. FERRALET® is manufactured in a unique, easy to swallow shape, to further enhance patient acceptance of the product. FERRALET® has a tailored disintegration rate to minimize gastric intoleration with a rapid dissolution rate to assure rapid availability for absorption.
Indications: Anemias amenable to iron therapy.

Continued on next page

Mission—Cont.

Dosage: One to three tablets a day depending upon the severity of the anemia and the particular toleration of the patient.
How Supplied: FERRALET® is packaged in bottles of 100 tablets.
Literature Available: Yes.

FOSFREE®
Calcium—Vitamins—Iron
NDC-0178-0031-01

Composition: Each tablet contains:

	One Tablet	% US RDA
Calcium Lactate	250.0 mg.	
Calcium Gluconate	250.0 mg.	
Calcium Carbonate	300.0 mg.	
(Calcium	175.7 mg.)	17
Ferrous Gluconate	125.0 mg.	
(Iron	14.5 mg.)	80
Vitamin D_2	150.0 USP U.	optional
Vitamin A Acetate	1500.0 USP U.	30
Ascorbic Acid (C)	50.0 mg.	83
Pyridoxine HCl (B_6)	3.0 mg.	150
Thiamine Mononitrate (B_1)	5.0 mg.	333
Riboflavin (B_2)	2.0 mg.	117
Niacinamide (B_3)	10.0 mg.	50
d-Calcium Pantothenate (B_5)	1.0 mg.	10
Vitamin B_{12} (Crystalline on resin)	2.0 mcg.	33

Action and Uses: FOSFREE® tablets are primarily indicated as a prenatal, postpartum or geriatric supplement particularly when soluble calcium salt supplementation is desired. FOSFREE® is a specific for hypocalcemic tetany (nocturnal leg cramping).
Administration and Dosage: One or two FOSFREE® tablets at bedtime as a general or prenatal supplement. In calcium deficiency states or in nocturnal leg cramping, dosage should be increased to two FOSFREE® tablets at bedtime plus one tablet mid-morning and one tablet mid-afternoon.
How Supplied: FOSFREE® is supplied as yellow capsule shaped coated tablets in bottles of 100 tablets.
Literature Available: Yes.

IROMIN-G®
Hematinic Supplement
NDC-0178-0081-01

Composition: Each tablet contains:

	% US RDA	
Ferrous Gluconate		333.3 mg.
(Iron	214	38.6 mg.)
Ascorbic Acid (C)	166	100.0 mg.
Thiamine Mononitrate (B_1)	333	5.0 mg.
Pyridoxine HCl (B_6)	150	3.0 mg.
Riboflavin (B_2)	117	2.0 mg.
Niacinamide	50	10.0 mg.
d-Calcium Pantothenate	10	1.0 mg.
Vitamin B_{12} (Crystalline on resin)	33	2.0 mcg.
Vitamin A Acetate	80	4000.0 USP U.
Vitamin D_2	Optional	400.0 USP U.
Calcium Carbonate		70.0 mg.
Calcium Gluconate		100.0 mg.
Calcium Lactate		100.0 mg.
(Calcium	5	50.0 mg.)

Action and Uses: Secondary anemias, and as a supplement for the prenatal, teenage and geriatric diet.
Administration and Dosage: One to three tablets daily after meals or as directed by a physician.
Side Effects: IROMIN-G® is virtually free of side effects when given in the recommended dosage. The rare constipation, diarrhea, or gastric upset can usually be controlled by dosage adjustment.
How Supplied: IROMIN-G® is supplied as red football shaped coated tablets in bottles of 100 tablets.
Literature Available: Yes.

MISSION PRENATAL SERIES

MISSION PRENATAL®
Vitamins—Iron—Calcium—.4 mg. Folic Acid
NDC 0178-132-01

MISSION PRENATAL® F.A.
Vitamins—Iron—Calcium—.8 mg. Folic Acid and Zinc
NDC 0178-0153-01

MISSION PRENATAL® H.P. ℞
Vitamins—Iron—Calcium—1.0 mg. Folic Acid
NDC 0178-0161-01

Composition: Each tablet contains:

	%U.S.R.D.A.	
Ferrous Gluconate		333.3 mg.
(Iron	214	38.6 mg.)
Ascorbic Acid (C)	167	100.0 mg.
Thiamine Mononitrate (B_1)	270	5.0 mg.
*† Pyridoxine HCl (B_6)	99	3.0 mg.
Riboflavin (B_2)	100	2.0 mg.
Niacinamide	50	10.0 mg.
d-Calcium Pantothenate	9	1.0 mg.
Vitamin B_{12} (Crystalline on Resin)	25	2.0 mcg.
*† Folic Acid	50	0.4 mg.
Vitamin A Acetate	50	4000.0 USPU
Vitamin D_2	100	400.0 USPU
Calcium Carbonate		70.0 mg.
Calcium Gluconate		100.0 mg.
Calcium Lactate		100.0 mg.
(Calcium	4	50.0 mg.)
Zinc (as Zinc Sulfate)		15.0 mg.

*Pyridoxine HCL—Mission® Prenatal F.A. =10mg., 329%U.S.R.D.A.
*Folic Acid—Mission® Prenatal F.A. =.8mg., 100%U.S.R.D.A.
†Pyridoxine HCL—Mission®Prenatal H.P. =25 mg., 1250%U.S.R.D.A.
†Folic Acid—Mission® Prenatal H.P. =1.0 mg., 125%U.S.R.D.A.
Zinc—only in Mission® Prenatal F.A.
Indications: ALL MISSION® PRENATALS are prenatal and postpartum supplements.
Dosage: Take one tablet at bedtime or as directed by your physician. Keep this and all medications out of the reach of children.
Caution: MISSION® PRENATAL H.P. prohibits dispensing without a prescription.
Precaution: Folic acid may obscure pernicious anemia in that the peripheral blood picture may revert to normal while the neurological changes remain progressive.
How Supplied: MISSION® PRENATAL is supplied as pink, football-shaped, sugar-coated tablets in bottles of 100.
MISSION® PRENATAL F.A. is supplied as blue, football-shaped, sugar coated tablets in bottles of 100.
MISSION® PRENATAL H.P. is supplied as green, football-shaped, sugar-coated tablets in bottles of 100.

PRULET®
White Phenolphthalein tablets N.F.
NDC 0178-0090-01

Composition: Each tablet contains:
White phenolphthalein N.F. .... 60 mg.
Action and Uses: PRULET® is a mild and gentle, effective laxative for patients with atonic or hypotonic bowel syndrome.
PRULET® is a chewable tablet in lemon—lime flavor.
Administration and Dosage: Take one to three tablets administered at bedtime; then adjust to need.
Contraindications: Not to be taken in the presence of nausea, vomiting, abdominal pains, or other symptoms of appendicitis.
Precautions: Phenolphthalein is known to produce skin eruptions in sensitized individuals. If a skin rash or eruption appears, do not take this or any other preparation containing phenolphthalein. PRULET® may cause pink to red urine coloration in patients with an alkaline urine.
How Supplied: PRULET® is supplied in green scored tablets in film strip packages of 12 and 50 tablets.
Literature Available: Yes.

PRULET® LIQUITAB®
White phenolphthalein tablets N.F.
NDC 0178-0120-50

Composition: Each tablet contains:
White phenolphtalein N.F. .... 30 mg.
Action and Uses: The PRULET® LIQUITAB® is a delicious fruit flavored, chewable laxative for adults and children (see PRULET®).
Administration and Dosage: Children: Chew or allow to dissolve in mouth 1 to 2 tablets at bedtime. Adults: Chew or allow to dissolve in mouth 1 to 3 tablets at bedtime. Adjust dosage to optimum level on following evening.
Contraindications: (See PRULET®)
Precautions: (See PRULET®)
How Supplied: PRULET® LIQUITABS® are supplied in film strip packages of 50 tablets.
Literature Available: Yes.

SUPAC®
Analgesic Compound
NDC-0178-0100-01

Composition: Each tablet contains:

Acetaminophen	160 mg.
Aspirin	230 mg.
Caffeine	33 mg.
Calcium Gluconate	60 mg.

Action and Uses: For temporary relief of pain accompanying simple head colds, temporary relief of pain accompanying menstruation, sinus and tension headache, minor traumatic pain, tooth extractions, arthritic and rheumatic pain syndromes.
Administration and Dosage: Adults—One or two tablets. This dose may be repeated in 4 hours. Do not exceed 4 tablets at a single dose or 16 tablets in a 24 hour period. Children—6 to 12 years of age, ½ of the maximum adult dose or dosage; 3 to 6 years of age, ⅓ of the maximum adult dose or dosage.
Precautions: If pain persists for more than 10 days, or redness is present, or in conditions affecting children under 12 years of age, physicians should be alert to other possible complications.
How Supplied: SUPAC® is supplied as white scored tablets in film strips of 24's and 100's and in bottles of 1000 tablets.
Literature Available: Yes.

THERABID®

Therapeutic Multivitamin

NDC 0178-0171-01

Composition: Each Tablet Contains:

		% US RDA
Ascorbic Acid (Vitamin C)	500 mg.	833
Thiamine Mononitrate (Vitamin B_1)	15 mg.	1000
Riboflavin (Vitamin B_2)	10 mg.	588
Niacinamide (Vitamin B_3)	100 mg.	500
Calcium Pantothenate (Vitamin B_5)	20 mg.	200
Pyridoxine Hydrochloride (Vitamin B_6)	10 mg.	500
Vitamin B_{12}	5 mcg.	83
Vitamin A Acetate	5,000 U.	100
Vitamin D_2	200 U.	optional
Vitamin E (as a-tocopheryl acetate)	30 IU	100

Action and Uses: THERABID® is a therapeutic multivitamin preparation.

Administration and Dosage: One to two tablets per day or at the discretion of the physician.

Precautions: Do not exceed a dosage of four tablets per day.

How Supplied: THERABID® is supplied as green capsule shaped sugar coated tablets in bottles of 100 tablets.

Literature Available: Yes.

Muro Pharmacal Laboratories, Inc.

Muro-Derm
890 EAST STREET
TEWKSBURY, MA 01876

DERMODEX™ 5 ℞
DERMODEX™ 10
(Benzoyl Peroxide)

Composition: Dermodex 5 contains 5% benzoyl peroxide, 20% alcohol, polyoxyethylene lauryl ether, colloidal magnesium aluminum silicate, hydroxypropylmethylcellulose, citric acid, and purified water.
Dermodex 10 contains 10% benzoyl peroxide, 20% alcohol, polyoxyethylene lauryl ether, colloidal magnesium aluminum silicate, hydroxypropylmethylcellulose, citric acid, and purified water.
Caution: Federal Law prohibits dispensing without a prescription.
Action and Uses: The topical use of Dermodex 5 and Dermodex 10 provides therapeutic control of acne through drying and desquamative action, as well as providing antiseptic activity.
Indications: Use as an aid in the treatment of acne.
Dosage and Administration: Apply 1 or more times daily to affected areas. Washing the face with soap and water prior to application greatly enhances the efficacy of the medication.
Contraindications: Patients with a known sensitivity to Benzoyl Peroxide should not employ these medications.
Precautions: For topical use only. Do not permit products to come in contact with the eyes or mucosal membranes. Keep this and all drugs out of reach of children. Very fair individuals should always be started on a single application at bedtime, allowing the medication to remain on the skin overnight. Dermodex may bleach hair and colored fabrics. Store below 80°F.
How Supplied: Dermodex 5 and Dermodex 10 are supplied in 2.0 ounce plastic tubes.

Dermodex 5	NDC 0451-1350-05
Dermodex 10	NDC 0451-1360-05

TEEN™ 5 LOTION OTC
TEEN™ 10 LOTION
TEEN™ 5 WASH
(Benzoyl Peroxide)

Contents: Benzoyl Peroxide 5% or 10% in a washable, grease-free, vanishing lotion base.
Indications: Antibacterial, antiseptic acne lotion medication for use as an aid in the treatment of the blemishes and pimples associated with acne. May also be used to dry up oily skin.
Directions: Shake well before use. Wash affected areas with a mild soap before using. Using the fingertips, apply one to three times a day or as directed by physician.
Caution: EXTERNAL USE ONLY. Avoid contact with eyes, lips, mouth and sensitive areas of the neck. Colored clothing or hair may become bleached. Keep tightly closed and avoid excessive heat. Keep out of the reach of children. KEEP FROM HEAT.
How Supplied: Teen 5 and Teen 10 Lotion in one ounce plastic bottles. Also, Teen 5 Wash in 6 fl. ounce plastic bottle.

Teen 5 Lotion	NDC 0451-1450-05
Teen 10 Lotion	NDC 0451-1460-05
Teen 5 Wash	NDC 0451-1600-03

MEMORANDUM

Nature's Bounty, Inc.

105 ORVILLE DRIVE
BOHEMIA, NY 11716

ACEROLA "C" 100 mg.
Tablets, Bottles of 100, 500

ACIDOPHILUS
Capsules, Bottles of 100

ALFALFA 500 mg.
Tablets, Bottles of 500 & 1000

B–1 (THIAMINE HCl) 100 mg.
B–1 (THIAMINE HCl) 250 mg.
B–1 (THIAMINE HCl) 500 mg.
Tablets, Bottles of 100, 500

B–2 (RIBOFLAVIN) 100 mg.
Tablets, Bottles of 100

B–6 (PYRIDOXINE HCl) 100 mg.
B–6 (PYRIDOXINE HCl) 500 mg.
Tablets, Bottles of 100, 250, 500

B–12 (COBALAMIN CONCENTRATE) 100 mcg.
Tablets, Bottles of 100, 250

B–12 (COBALAMIN CONCENTRATE) 250 mcg.
Tablets, Bottles of 100, 250, 500

B–12 (COBALAMIN CONCENTRATE) 500 mcg.
Tablets, Bottles of 100, 250

B–12 (COBALAMIN CONCENTRATE) 1000 mcg.
Tablets, Bottles of 100, 250

B–50®
Tablets, Bottles of 100, 250, 500

B–100®
Tablets, Bottles of 50, 100, 250

B-100® TIME RELEASE
Tablets, Bottles of 50, 100, 250

B–125®
Tablets, Bottles of 50, 100, 250

B & C LIQUID
Liquid, 4 oz. Bottles

B-COMPLEX & B-12
Tablets, Bottles of 90

B-COMPLEX & C
Time Release Capsules, Bottles of 100, 500

BEE POLLEN 500 mg.
Tablets, Bottles of 100, 250

BIOTIN .3 mg.
Tablets, Bottles of 100, 500

BONE MEAL WITH VITAMIN D
Tablets, Bottles of 100, 250, 500, 1000

BREWER'S YEAST 7½ gr.
Tablets, Bottles of 250, 500, 1000

BREWER'S YEAST
Powder, 16 oz. cans

CALCIUM ASCORBATE 500 mg.
Tablets, Bottles of 100, 250, 500

CALCIUM LACTATE (10 gr.)
Tablets, Bottles of 100, 250, 500, 1000

CALCIUM PANGAMATE (50 mg.)
Tablets, 100, 250, 500

CHILDREN'S CHEWABLES
Tablets, Bottles of 100, 250, 500

CHOLINE (650 mg.)
Tablets, Bottles of 100, 500

COD LIVER OIL
Capsules, Bottles of 100, 250

COPPER (3 mg.)
Tablets, Bottles of 100

C–1000 mg.
Tablets, Bottles of 100, 250, 500

C-TIME 1500 mg. TIME RELEASE
Tablets, Bottles of 30, 100, 250

C–LIQUID (300 mg.)
Liquid, 4 oz. Bottles

DOLOMITE
Tablets, Bottles of 100, 250, 500, 1000

VITAMIN E (D–ALPHA TOCOPHERYL)
Capsules 100 I.U. Bottles of 100, 250
200 I.U. Bottles of 100, 250, 500, 1000
400 I.U. Bottles of 100, 250, 500, 1000
600 I.U. Bottles of 50, 100, 250
1000 I.U. Bottles of 50, 100, 250

VITAMIN E–OIL
24,000 I.U.
Bottles of 2 oz.

FRUCTOSE
Tablets, Bottles of 100

GARLIC OIL CAPSULES (15 gr.)
GARLIC OIL CAPSULES (77 gr.)
Bottles of 100, 500

GARLIC & PARSLEY
Capsules, Bottles of 100, 250, 500

GINSENG, MANCHURIAN 250 mg.
Capsules, Bottles of 50, 100, 250, 500

GLUTAMIC ACID 500 mg.
Tablets, Bottles of 100, 500

GOTU KOLA (250 mg.)
Tablets, Bottles of 100, 500

INOSITOL (650 mg.)
Tablets, Bottles of 100, 500

KELP (6.5 gr.)
Tablets, Bottles of 500, 1000

LECITHIN (19 gr.) 1200 mg.
Capsules, Bottles of 100, 250

LECITHIN GRANULES
Bottles of 14 oz.

L-GLUTAMINE 500 mg.
Tablets, Bottles of 50, 100, 250

L-LYSINE 500 mg.
Tablets, Bottles of 100, 500

MAGNESIUM (30 mg.)
Tablets, Bottles of 100

MANGANESE (50 mg.)
Tablets, Bottles of 100

MEGA V & M®
Tablets, Bottles of 30, 60, 100, 250

MULTI–MINERAL
Tablets, Bottles of 100, 250

NIACIN (50 mg., 100 mg. & 250 mg.)
Tablets, Bottles of 100, 500

NIACINAMIDE (500 mg.)
Tablets, Bottles of 100, 250

OYSTER CALCIUM
Tablets, Bottles of 100, 500

PABA (PARA–AMINO BENZOIC ACID) (100 mg. & 500 mg.)
Tablets, 100, 250, 500, 1000

PANTOTHENIC ACID (100 mg. & 200 mg.)
Tablets, Bottles of 100, 250

POTASSIUM (83.5 mg.)
Tablets, Bottles of 100, 250

PROTEIN CAPSULES (500 mg.)
Bottles of 100, 500

PROTEIN LIQUID
Bottles of 16 ozs., 32 ozs.

PROTEIN POWDER
16 oz. cans

PROTEIN TABLETS (250 mg.)
Bottles of 100, 250, 500

RNA 100 mg. (NUCLEIC ACID)
Tablets, Bottles of 100, 250

RUTIN (50 mg.)
Tablets, Bottles of 250, 500

SAFFLOWER OIL (750 mg.)
Capsules, Bottles of 100, 250

SELENIUM (50 mcg.)
Tablets, Bottles of 100, 250

TRYPTOPHANE (200 mg.)
TRYPTOPHANE (667 mg.)
Tablets, Bottles of 30, 100

ULTRA "A" (25,000 USP UNITS)
Capsules & Tablets, Bottles of 250, 500

ULTRA "A & D"
(25,000 USP UNITS VITAMIN A)
(1,000 USP UNITS VITAMIN D)
Tablets, Bottles of 100, 500, 1000

ULTRA "D" (1000 USP UNITS)
Tablets, Bottles of 100, 500, 1000

VITAMIN A & D
(10,000 USP UNITS VITAMIN A)
(400 USP UNITS VITAMIN D)
Bottles of 100, 250, 500, 1000

WHEAT BRAN (500 mg.)
Tablets, Bottles of 250, 500

WHEAT GERM OIL
Capsules, 6 minim, 14 minim, 20 minim, Bottles of 100, 250

ZACNE®
Tablets, Bottles of 100, 250

ZINC (10 mg., 25 mg., 50 mg., 100 mg.)
Tablets, Bottles of 100, 250, 500, 1000

Neutrogena Corporation

5755 W. 96TH STREET
P.O. BOX 45036
LOS ANGELES, CA 90045

NEUTROGENA® Acne-Drying Gel

Composition: A clear gel base containing witch hazel, isopropyl alcohol, propylene glycol, carbomer 940, triethanolamine, EDTA, methylparaben, propylparaben, benzophenone-2, FD&C Yellow #5, FD&C Red #40, FD&C Blue #1. Contains 46% isopropyl alcohol, 7.5% alcohol (derived from witch hazel).
Actions and Uses: For use as a drying adjunct to acne treatment for the acne patient with sensitive skin. Helps degrease and reduce oily secretions on the skin, combining antisepsis and astringency. Neutrogena Acne-Drying Gel contains no perfume, is non-medicated and has a fresh, natural witch hazel scent. Can be applied under makeup.
Caution: Avoid contact with eyes and mouth. Should irritation occur, discontinue use.
Administration and Dosage: First wash with Neutrogena Acne-Cleansing Soap then apply Neutrogena Acne-Drying Gel. For mild to moderate drying affect, use once or twice a

day; for more intensive drying, use three times a day; or use as physician directs.
How Supplied: 3/4 oz. plastic tube.

NEUTROGENA®
Norwegian Formula Hand Cream

Composition: Neutrogena® Hand Cream is a highly concentrated, heavy duty protective cream containing water, glycerin, cetearyl alcohol, sodium cetearyl sulfate, fragrance (deleted for unscented formula), stearic acid, methylparaben, propylparaben, sodium sulfate, and dilauryl thiodipropionate.
Action and Uses: For use in dermatoses caused by over-exposure to water and weather and for extremely dry, chapped hands and skin. Effective as an industrial, non-silicone barrier cream to protect hands and skin from detergents and chemicals. Useful in the treatment of hand eczemas, as an adjunct to topical steroids.
Administration and Dosage: Highly concentrated, use sparingly. Apply in small quantity and rub in gently or as physician directs.
How Supplied: 2 oz. plastic tube. Scented or Unscented.

NEUTROGENA® Rainbath® Shower Gel

Composition: Rainbath is a gentle, soapless cleanser containing water, sodium laureth sulfate, oleyl betaine, lauramide DEA, polysorbate 20, fragrance (deleted from unscented formula), propylene glycol, methylparaben, propylparaben and sodium chloride.
Action and Uses: A lipid-free foaming gel cleanser for use in bath or shower. Indicated as a cleansing adjunct in atopic dermatitis and other conditions where soap is contraindicated. Produces a rich lather and cleanses with uncommon mildness. Satisfies patients that they are getting the cleansing quality of soap without soap, leaving skin smooth to touch.
Caution: Avoid contact with eyes.
Administration and Dosage: For shower, apply directly to wet skin and lather. Rinse and pat dry. May be used for foaming bath; pour one tablespoon into running water. Or use as physician directs.
How Supplied: 4 oz. plastic tube, 8 oz. and 32 oz. shatterproof plastic bottle in Scented formula. 8 oz. shatterproof plastic bottle in Unscented formula.

NEUTROGENA® Sesame Seed Body Oil

Composition: A light, non-greasy, easily applied oil with excellent patient acceptance. Contains isopropyl myristate, sesame oil, PEG-40 sorbitan peroleate and fragrance (deleted for unscented formula).
Action and Uses: Effective as an adjunct in the management and maintenance therapy of xerotic dermatosis, pruritus, geriatric skin problems, and lichenification of the skin due to inflammation from chronic scratching or irritation. Neutrogena Body Oil helps skin retain its normal lipid/aqueous balance by retarding evaporation of moisture. Acts as an effective, easy-to-use adjunct in the nursing care of bedridden and/or elderly patients. Neutrogena Body Oil may be applied directly to wet skin and rinsing is not necessary.
Administration and Dosage: Apply directly to the skin immediately after bath, shower or sponge-bath, while the skin is still damp. Rub in gently. For use in the bath, pour two or three capfuls in the tub as it fills. Neutrogena Body Oil is easily dispersible in water. Will not leave the tub oily and slippery.
How Supplied: 8 oz. and 32 oz. shatterproof plastic bottle in Scented formula. 8 oz. shatterproof plastic bottle in Unscented formula.

NEUTROGENA® Soap for Normal-to-Dry Skin

Composition: A mild, transparent, ethanolamine base soap containing no free alkali. Contains triethanolamine, stearic acid, tallow, glycerin, water, coconut oil, castor oil, sodium hydroxide, oleic acid, laneth-10-acetate, nonoxynol-14 and PEG-4 octoate, cocamide DEA, fragrance (deleted for unscented formula), BHT, and O-tolyl biguanide.
Action and Uses: Neutrogena Dry-Skin Soap is specifically formulated to aid dry skin problems. Formulation is based on the original Neutrogena Soap formula with two added superfatting agents, nonoxynol-14 and PEG-4 octoate, plus laneth-10-acetate, and fatty acid esters to help retain mositure.
Administration and Dosage: Use daily in place of other soaps or as physician directs.
How Supplied: 3.5 and 5.5 oz. bars in Scented formula; 3.5 oz. bars in Unscented formula.

NEUTROGENA® Soap for Normal-to-Oily Skin

Composition: A mild, transparent, ethanolamine base soap with no free alkali. Contains triethanolamine, stearic acid, tallow, water, glycerin, coconut oil, caster oil, sodium hydroxide, oleic acid, cocamide DEA and fragrance (deleted for unscented formula).
Action and Uses: Neutrogena Soap is formulated to gently cleanse sensitive skin. It is well tolerated in the cleansing care of post-dermatosis cutaneous irritation and inflammation, especially when washing with soap is contraindicated. Neutrogena Soap contains no free alkali and affects the pH of the skin no more than rinsing with plain water. It is extremely water soluble, resulting in reduced possibility of irritation due to soap residue on the skin. The heavy molecular structure of Neutrogena Soap minimizes epidermal penetration and therefore skin irritation.
Administration and Dosage: Use daily or as physician directs.
How Supplied: 3.5 and 5.5 oz. Bars. Scented or Unscented.

NEUTROGENA® Soap for Skin with Acne

Composition: A mild, transparent, ethanolamine base soap containing no free alkali. Contains triethanolamine, stearic acid, tallow, water, glycerin, coconut oil, castor oil, TEA lauryl sulfate, sodium hydroxide, oleic acid, acetylated lanolin alcohol, cocamide DEA, alcohol, and fragrance.
Actions and Uses: For use as a cleansing and drying adjunct to acne treatment. Neutrogena Soap for Skin with Acne is based on the original Neutrogena Soap formulation with the addition of a lipid solvent, acetylated lanolin alcohol, and a surfactant, TEA lauryl sulfate. Aids in the cleansing and degreasing of the skin, and helps remove fatty or oily secretions. Extremely water soluble and biodegradable, Neutrogena Soap for Skin with Acne is also non-medicated and will not interfere with other acne treatment, systemic or topical.
Administration and Dosage: For a mild drying affect, use once a day; for moderate drying, use twice a day; for more intensive drying, use three times a day; or use as physician directs.
How Supplied: 3.5 oz. Bar.

NEUTROGENA® Vehicle/N®

Composition: Neutrogena® Vehicle/N® with Appliderm™ Filter/Applicator Unit is a topical vehicle system for extemporaneous compounding. Neutrogena® Vehicle/N® contains ethyl alcohol 47.5%, purified water, laureth-4, isopropyl alcohol 4%, and propylene glycol, a formulation which solubilizes selected dermatologic drugs and provides mild astringent and drying actions.
Action and Uses: Neutrogena® Vehicle/N® provides topical compounding convenience, economy and cosmetic elegance in an easy-to-use delivery system that greatly enhances patient acceptance.
The following drugs have been found to be compatible with and soluble in Neutrogena® Vehicle/N® in concentrations normally used in dermatology: hydroquinone (with 100 mg ascorbic acid to stabilize), menthol, camphor, hydrocortisone alcohol (up to 1.5%), clindamycin HCl, lincomycin, LCD, triamcinolone acetonide and erythromycin. (Note that hydrocortisone acetate is insoluble in Vehicle/N®). The antibiotics commonly prescribed for topical use have been shown to be stable in Vehicle/N® for a minimum of two months without refrigeration.
Dosage and Administration: As physician directs. The Appliderm™ Filter/Applicator Unit removes any insoluble excipients from the compounded preparation and provides a convenient spill-proof container and topical application device which assures even, efficient coverage. The solution is applied directly to the skin by tilting the bottle and rubbing the Appliderm™ Applicator over the affected area.
Note: Laboratory and clinical evaluations necessary to determine the safety and efficacy of the preparations resulting from the addition of the drugs described to Neutrogena® Vehicle/N® have not been conducted. Neutrogena Corporation makes no claims regarding the safety or efficacy of extemporaneously prepared products utilizing Vehicle/N®.
Precautions: Do not use near fire or flame due to alcohol content. Neutrogena® Vehicle/N® contains substantial alcohol and is not suitable for use in acute dermatoses. Stinging may be noted if used on irritated or abraded skin. Avoid contact with eyes or eyelids. If the product accidentally comes in contact with eyes, rinse thoroughly with water, and consult physician. For external use only. Keep out of the reach of children.
Availability: 50 ml in plastic bottle with Appliderm™ Applicator.
NDC # 10812-9100-1
Patent Pending

Norcliff Thayer Inc.
ONE SCARSDALE ROAD
TUCKAHOE, NEW YORK 10707

A-200 Pyrinate® Liquid, Gel

(See PDR For Nonprescription Drugs)

CO-SALT®
Salt Substitute

(See PDR For Nonprescription Drugs)

DICARBOSIL® Antacid Tablets

(See PDR For Nonprescription Drugs)

LIQUIPRIN®
(acetaminophen)

(See PDR For Nonprescription Drugs)

Continued on next page

Norcliff Thayer—Cont.

OXY-5® LOTION
OXY-10™ LOTION
Benzoyl Peroxide Lotion 5% and 10%

(See PDR For Nonprescription Drugs)

Norgine Laboratories, Inc.

420 LEXINGTON AVENUE
NEW YORK, NY 10017

ENZYPAN® Tablets

Composition: Each tablet contains pancreatin sufficient to digest in 2 hours time: 19 g. of protein, 43 g. of starch and 10 g. of fat; in addition it provides Ox Bile (des.), 0.056 g. and peptic potency equivalent to Pepsin 1-3,000, 9 mg.
Action and Uses: Releases the principal digestive enzymes consecutively from two specially constructed tablet sections. Valuable in digestive enzyme deficiencies leading to fat, protein or starch intolerance and such enzyme-deficiency-linked symptoms as fermentative or putrefactive dyspepsia, postprandial distress, epigastric fullness, flatulence, regurgitation.
Administration and Dosage: *Adults*—2 to 3 tablets during or after each meal. To be taken whole, with water.
How Supplied: Containers of 120, 500.

HEPP-IRON DROPS

Composition: Each ml. contains vitamin B_{12} (Cyanocobalamin) 25 mcg., iron ammonium citrate (equiv. to 20 mg. of iron) 120 mg., thiamine hydrochloride 10 mg., pyridoxine hydrochloride 2 mg., biotin 2.5 mcg.
Action and Uses: Hematinic; for iron-deficiency anemias.
Administration and Dosage: *Infants up to 1 year*—1-5 drops (0.06-0.3 ml.) daily. *Children and adults*—10 drops (0.6 ml.) daily. Directly on tongue, or diluted in fluid.
How Supplied: 30 ml. bottles; dropper calibrated to 0.3 and 0.6 ml. doses.

MOVICOL® Granules

Composition: Gum Karaya and cortex rhamni frangulae in a pleasantly sweetened mixture.
Action and Uses: Treatment of constipation with natural mucilage (for bulk formation) and small amounts of well-aged frangula (for initial peristalsis). Especially in cardiovascular, hernial, rectal cases; diverticulosis; invalid, surgical, convalescent cases; geriatric patients; dieters; patients with sedentary habits. In bulk-producing capacity, 1 teaspoonful of Movicol equals 2 lbs. of consumed vegetables.
Administration and Dosage: *Adults*—1 or 2 heaped teaspoonfuls once or twice daily after the main meals, or on retiring. Dry granules are placed on the tongue in small amounts and, without chewing or crushing, swallowed with plenty of water. As bowel tone and rhythm are gradually restored, dosage may be reduced and ultimately discontinued.
Warning: Not to be used if abdominal pain, nausea or vomiting are present. Frequent or prolonged use may result in dependence on laxatives.
Contraindications: Intestinal obstruction, fecal impaction.
How Supplied: 250 Gram container.

MURIPSIN® Tablets

Composition: Each tablet contains: glutamic acid hydrochloride 500 mg.; pepsin 35 mg.; in a special base.*
Action and Uses: Gastric hydrochloric acid therapy in a solid tablet. Muripsin avoids corrosive unpleasantness and uncontrolled acid release; formulated with glutamic acid hydrochloride, it not only substitutes hydrochloric acid but also stimulates secretagogue action. Each tablet provides the equivalent of 15 minims of dilute hydrochloric acid. Useful in hydrochloric acid deficiencies, primary or secondary.
Administration and Dosage: For adults one to two tablets with each meal to be swallowed whole with water.
Contraindications: Hyperacidity or if peptic ulcers are present.
How Supplied: Containers of 100 and 500.
*U.S. Patent 2,958,627

North American Pharmacal, Inc.

6851 CHASE ROAD
DEARBORN, MICH. 48126

BAUMODYNE GEL AND OINTMENT

Composition: Ointment—Methyl Salicylate, Oil of Eucalyptus and Menthol in a greaseless base.
Gel—Methyl Salicylate, Oil of Eucalyptus and Menthol in Isopropyl Alcohol Gel. Preservatives are Methylparaben and Butylparaben.
Actions and Uses: Baumodyne, which comes in either a greaseless ointment/balm or a gel/liniment form, helps reduce soreness and tightness in muscles and tendons. Its absorptive qualities produce a soothing heat, penetrating the ache or pain and inducing a beneficial hyperemia. Baumodyne's analgesic action helps relieve arthritic and rheumatic conditions, bursitis and arthralgia. It stimulates the circulation and helps to relieve minor aches and pains due to exertion and fatigue, e.g. sprains, sore feet.
Administration: Apply freely as needed, rubbing and massaging in well. Bandaging or wrapping is not recommended.
Caution: For topical use only. Discontinue use if excessive irritation of the skin develops.
Precaution: Avoid getting into the eyes or on mucous membranes. In case of accidental ingestion, seek professional assistance or contact a poison control center immediately. Do not use on sunburned membranes. Keep out reach of children.
How Supplied: Ointment, 2 oz. and 1 lb. jars. Gel, 4 oz., 8 oz., pint and ½ gal. plastic bottles.

Norwich Products Division

See NORWICH-EATON PHARMACEUTICALS
Consumer Products Group

Norwich-Eaton Pharmaceuticals

Professional Products Group
(formerly Eaton Laboratories)
Consumer Products Group
(formerly Norwich Products)
Division of Morton-Norwich Products, Inc.
NORWICH, NY 13815

Literature on Norwich-Eaton products sent to physicians on request.

Norwich-Eaton Product Identification

The word EATON is imprinted or embossed on each solid-dosage unit, as well as a code number, which corresponds to the last three digits of the middle portion of the National Drug Code Numbers, as follows:

NDC 0149-0705-12 (51)
Alphaderm® Cream (hydrocortisone)
NDC 0149-0792-48 (61, 82, 11)
Menthol Chloraseptic® Mouthwash & Gargle
NDC 0149-0791-48 (61, 11)
Cherry Chloraseptic Mouthwash & Gargle
NDC 0149-0793-45
Menthol Chloraseptic Spray
NDC 0149-0797-45
Cherry Chloraseptic Spray
NDC 0149-0794-18 (45, 70)
Menthol Chloraseptic Lozenges
NDC 0149-0798-18 (45, 50)
Cherry Chloraseptic Lozenges
NDC 0149-0790-01
Children's Chloraseptic Lozenges
NDC 0149-0799-01
Chloraseptic DM Cough Control Lozenges
NDC 0149-0795-24 (25)
Chloraseptic Gel
NDC 0149-0030-05 (66)
Dantrium® Capsules 25 mg (dantrolene sodium)
NDC 0149-0031-05
Dantrium Capsules 50 mg
NDC 0149-0033-05
Dantrium Capsules 100 mg
NDC 0149-0030-77
Dantrium Unit Dose 25 mg
NDC 0149-0030-77
Dantrium Unit Dose 100 mg
NDC 0149-0734-01
Dantrium® Intravenous (dantrolene sodium)
NDC 0149-0013-05
Dopar® Capsules 100 mg(levodopa)
NDC 0149-0014-05
Dopar Capsules 250 mg
NDC 0149-0015-05 (77)
Dopar Capsules 500 mg
NDC 0149-0045-05
Duvoid® Tablets 10 mg (bethanechol chloride)
NDC 0149-0046-05
Duvoid Tablets 25 mg
NDC 0149-0047-05
Duvoid Tablets 50 mg
NDC 0149-0045-77
Duvoid Unit Dose 10 mg
NDC 0149-0046-77
Duvoid Unit Dose 25 mg
NDC 0149-0047-77
Duvoid Unit Dose 50 mg
NDC 0390-0021-12
Encare®
NDC 0149-0704-12 (11, 51, 61, 90)
Furacin® Soluble Dressing (nitrofurazone)
NDC 0149-0723-11
Furacin Soluble Powder
NDC 0149-0777-12 (15, 61)
Furacin Topical Cream
NDC 0149-0735-15 (61)
Furadantin® Oral Suspension (nitrofurantoin)
NDC 0149-0036-01 (05)
Furadantin Tablets 50 mg
NDC 0149-0037-05 (07)
Furadantin Tablets 100 mg
NDC 0149-0036-06
Furadantin Unit Dose 50 mg
NDC 0149-0037-07
Furadantin Unit Dose 100 mg
NDC 0149-0784-15
Ivadantin® (nitrofurantoin sodium)
NDC 0149-0007-05
Macrodantin® Capsules 25 mg (nitrofurantoin macrocrystals)
NDC 0149-0008-01 (05, 10)
Macrodantin Capsules 50 mg
NDC 0149-0009-01 (05, 10)
Macrodantin Capsules 100 mg
NDC 0149-0008-77
Macrodantin Unit Dose 50 mg

NDC 0149-0009-05
Macrodantin Unit Dose 100 mg
NDC 0149-0052-01
Vivonex® Chemically Defined Elemental Standard Diet/Soluble Powder (Unflavored)
NDC 0149-0050-10
Vivonex Delivery System
NDC 0149-0051-01
Vivonex HN Chemically Defined Elemental High Nitrogen Diet/Soluble Powder (Unflavored)
NDC 0149-0058-02
Orange-Pineapple
NDC 0149-0054-02
Vanilla
NDC 0149-0057-02
Lemon-Lime
NDC 0149-0056-02
Strawberry

ALPHADERM® ℞
(1% hydrocortisone)
CREAM

Description: Contains hydrocortisone 1% in a powder-in-cream base incorporating a hypermolar solution of urea 10% (carbamide), purified water, sorbitol, polyoxyethylene fatty glyceride, starch, white petrolatum, triglycerides of saturated fatty acids, isopropyl myristate, and sorbitan monolaurate. The near neutral pH of the formulation is made possible by the stabilized delivery system in which urea is absorbed by a polysaccharide powder matrix. Alphaderm (1% hydrocortisone) Cream is hypoallergenic and contains no parabens or lanolin.
Action: Topical steroids are primarily effective because of their anti-inflammatory, antipruritic and vasoconstrictive actions.
Indications: For relief of the inflammatory manifestations of corticosteroid-responsive dermatoses.
Contraindications: Topical steroids are contraindicated in those patients with a history of hypersensitivity to any of the components of the preparation.
Precautions: If irritation develops, the product should be discontinued and appropriate therapy instituted.
In the presence of an infection, the use of an appropriate antifungal or antibacterial agent should be instituted. If a favorable response does not occur promptly, the corticosteroid should be discontinued until the infection has been adequately controlled.
If extensive areas are treated or if the occlusive technique is used, there will be increased systemic absorption of the corticosteroid and suitable precautions should be taken, particularly in children and infants.
Although topical steroids have not been reported to have an adverse effect on human pregnancy, the safety of their use in pregnant women has not absolutely been established. In laboratory animals, increases in incidence of fetal abnormalities have been associated with exposure of gestating females to topical corticosteroids, in some cases at rather low dosage levels. Therefore, drugs of this class should not be used extensively on pregnant patients, in large amounts, or for prolonged periods of time.
The product is not for ophthalmic use.
Adverse Reactions: The following local adverse reactions have been reported with topical corticosteroids, especially under occlusive dressings:
1. burning; 2. itching; 3. irritation; 4. dryness; 5. folliculitis; 6. hypertrichosis; 7. acneiform eruptions; 8. hypopigmentation; 9. perioral dermatitis; 10. allergic contact dermatitis; 11. maceration of the skin; 12. secondary infection; 13. skin atrophy; 14. striae; 15. miliaria.
Dosage and Administration: Apply a small quantity of Alphaderm (1% hydrocortisone) Cream to affected areas twice daily.
How Supplied: Alphaderm (1% hydrocortisone) Cream is available in
NDC 0149-0705-12 tubes of 30 grams
NDC 0149-0705-51 tubes of 100 grams

MENTHOL CHLORASEPTIC®
MOUTHWASH AND GARGLE
CHERRY CHLORASEPTIC®
MOUTHWASH AND GARGLE
MENTHOL CHLORASEPTIC®
SPRAY
CHERRY CHLORASEPTIC®
SPRAY
(oral anesthetic, antiseptic)

Description: An alkaline solution containing phenol and sodium phenolate (total phenol 1.4%). In addition, Menthol Chloraseptic and Cherry Chloraseptic 1.5-oz Spray contain compressed nitrogen as a propellant.
Indications: Pleasant-tasting Chloraseptic is an antiseptic, anesthetic, deodorizing mouthwash and gargle. It is an alkaline solution designed specifically to maintain oral hygiene and to relieve local soreness and irritation without "caines." Chloraseptic may be used as a topical anesthetic while antibacterials are used systemically in the treatment of infection. Chloraseptic acts promptly, often providing effective surface anesthesia in minutes. It is a valuable adjunct for temporary relief of pain and discomfort and will reduce oral bacterial flora temporarily to improve oral hygiene.
Chloraseptic is indicated for prompt temporary relief of discomfort due to the following conditions: *Medical*—oropharyngitis and throat infections; acute tonsillitis; posttonsillectomy soreness; peritonsillar abscess; oropharyngeal manifestations of postnasal drip; throat and mouth dryness (smoker's cough); and before intubation (anti-gag) and after (for soreness); *Dental*—after oral surgery or extractions; aphthous ulcers and infectious stomatitis; Vincent's infection; gingivitis; preinjection topical anesthesia; insertion of immediate denture; pericoronitis; and x-rays and impressions (anti-gag).
Administration and Dosage: Chloraseptic Mouthwash and Gargle—*Irritated throat:* Advise patient to spray 5 times (children 6-12 years of age, 3 times) and swallow. May be used as a gargle. Repeat every 2 hours if necessary. *After oral surgery:* Advise patient to allow full-strength solution to run over affected areas for 15 seconds without swishing, then expel remainder. Repeat every 2 hours if necessary. Not for children under 6 years of age unless directed by a physician or dentist. *Adjunctive gingival therapy:* Rinse vigorously with full-strength solution for 15 seconds, working between teeth, then expel remainder. Repeat every 2 hours if necessary. *Daily deodorizing mouthwash and gargle:* Dilute with equal parts of water and rinse thoroughly, or spray full strength, then expel remainder.
Chloraseptic Spray: *Irritated throat:* Advise patient to spray throat about 2 seconds (children 6 to 12 years about 1 second) and swallow. Repeat every 2 hours if necessary. *After oral surgery:* Advise patient to spray affected area for 1 to 2 seconds, allow solution to remain for 15 seconds without swishing, then expel remainder. Repeat every 2 hours if necessary. *Adjunctive gingival therapy:* Spray affected area for about 2 seconds, swish for 15 seconds working between teeth, then expel remainder. Repeat every 2 hours if necessary. *Daily deodorizing spray:* Spray, rinse thoroughly, and expel remainder. Not for children under 6 years of age unless directed by a physician or dentist.
Packaging: Menthol Chloraseptic—85-ml bottle with sprayer, 6-oz bottle with sprayer, 8- and 12-oz bottles without sprayer, and 1.5-oz spray can. Cherry Chloraseptic—85-ml bottle with sprayer, 6-oz bottle with sprayer, 12-oz bottle without sprayer, and 1.5-oz spray can. No prescription necessary.

MENTHOL CHLORASEPTIC®
LOZENGES
CHERRY CHLORASEPTIC® LOZENGES

Description: Each Chloraseptic Lozenge contains phenol, sodium phenolate (total phenol 32.5 mg).
Action and Uses: Chloraseptic Lozenges provide prompt temporary relief of discomfort due to mouth and gum irritations and of minor sore throat due to colds. They are anesthetic and antiseptic—and also may be used as a topical adjunct to systemic antibacterial therapy for severe cases. For prompt temporary relief of pain and discomfort associated with the following conditions: *Medical*—oropharyngitis and throat infections; acute tonsillitis; posttonsillectomy soreness; peritonsillar abscess; oropharyngeal manifestations of postnasal drip; and throat and mouth dryness (smoker's cough); *Dental*—after oral surgery; aphthous ulcers and infectious stomatitis; Vincent's infection; gingivitis; and pericoronitis.
Administration and Dosage: Adults: Dissolve 1 lozenge in the mouth every 2 hours; do not exceed 8 lozenges per day. Children 6-12 years: Dissolve 1 lozenge in the mouth every 3 hours; do not exceed 4 lozenges per day. Not for children under 6 unless directed by a physician or dentist.
Packaging: Menthol and Cherry Chloraseptic Lozenges—packages of 18, 45, and 50 lozenges.
No prescription necessary.

CHILDREN'S CHLORASEPTIC®
LOZENGES

Description: Each 5 mg. Children's Chloraseptic Lozenge contains benzocaine as anesthetic in a grape flavored base of sugar and corn syrup solids.
Action and Use: Children's Chloraseptic Lozenges provide prompt, temporary relief of minor sore throat pain which may accompany conditions such as tonsillitis, pharyngitis and in post tonsillectomy soreness, and discomfort of minor mouth and gum irritations.
Administration & Dosage: Allow one lozenge to dissolve slowly in the mouth. Repeat hourly if needed. Do not take more than 12 lozenges per day. Not for children under 3 unless directed by a physician.
Packaging: Carton of 18 lozenges.

CHLORASEPTIC® DM COUGH
CONTROL LOZENGES

Description: Each CHLORASEPTIC DM Cough Control Lozenge contains phenol and sodium phenolate (total phenol 32.5 mg), and a 10-mg therapeutic dose of dextromethorphan hydrobromide.
Action and Uses: CHLORASEPTIC DM Cough Control Lozenges provide fast relief of minor sore throat pain and control coughs due to colds. Each lozenge contains two active ingredients. One is the same agent contained in CHLORASEPTIC, a widely used medication for relief of minor sore throat pain. This ingredient acts as a local anesthetic stopping sore throat pain by temporarily blocking the nerve impulse transmission to the ninth cranial nerve. The second agent, dextromethorphan hydrobromide, a nonnarcotic antitussive, acts by selective suppression of the central cough mechanism. Dual-active CHLORASEPTIC DM Cough Control Lozenges provide temporary symptomatic relief of coughs and minor sore throat pain.
Administration and Dosage: Adults: Dissolve one lozenge slowly in mouth every two hours; do not exceed eight lozenges per day. Children 6 to 12 years: Dissolve one lozenge slowly in mouth every four hours; do not exceed four lozenges per day. Do not administer

Continued on next page

Norwich-Eaton—Cont.

to children under 6 years of age unless directed by a physician.
Caution: Persistent cough may indicate the presence of a serious condition. Persons with a high fever or persistent cough should not use this preparation unless directed by physician. Consult physician promptly if sore throat is severe or lasts more than two days, or if accompanied by high fever, headache, nausea or vomiting.
Warning: Do not take this product for persistent cough such as occurs with smoking, asthma, emphysema, or where cough is accompanied by excessive secretions except with the advice and supervision of a physician.
Packaging: Pocket-size box of 10 lozenges.

CHLORASEPTIC® GEL

Description: Chloraseptic Gel contains phenol, sodium phenolate (total phenol 1.4%) in a special adherent base.
Indications: For prompt, temporary relief of discomfort from minor mouth and gum irritations.
Warnings: If irritation or pain persists, discontinue use and consult physician or dentist. Do not administer to children under 6 years of age unless directed by a physician.
Administration: Apply directly to the affected area. Repeat as necessary.
How Supplied: Chloraseptic Gel is available in ¼-oz tubes.

DANTRIUM® Capsules ℞
(dantrolene sodium)

> DANTRIUM (dantrolene sodium) has a potential for hepatotoxicity, and should not be used in conditions other than those recommended. Symptomatic hepatitis (fatal and non-fatal) has been reported at various dose levels of the drug. The incidence reported in patients taking up to 400 mg/day is much lower than in those taking doses of 800 mg or more per day. Even sporadic short courses of these higher dose levels within a treatment regimen markedly increased the risk of serious hepatic injury. Liver dysfunction, as evidenced by blood chemical abnormalities alone (liver enzyme elevations), have been observed in patients exposed to Dantrium for varying periods of time. Overt hepatitis has occurred at varying intervals after initiation of therapy, but has been most frequently observed between the third and twelfth months of therapy. The risk of hepatic injury appears to be greater in females, in patients over 35 years of age, and in patients taking other medication(s) in addition to Dantrium (dantrolene sodium). Dantrium should be used only in conjunction with appropriate monitoring of hepatic function including frequent determination of SGOT or SGPT. If no observable benefit is derived from the administration of Dantrium after a total of 45 days, therapy should be discontinued.
> The lowest possible effective dose for the individual patient should be prescribed.

Description: Dantrium is dantrolene sodium, chemically 1-{[5-(p-nitrophenyl)furfurylidene]amino}hydantion sodium hydrate. It is an orange powder, slightly soluble in water, but due to its slightly acidic nature the solubility increases somewhat in alkaline solution. The anhydrous salt has a molecular weight of 336. The hydrated salt contains approximately 15% water (3½ moles) and has a molecular weight of 399.
Dantrium (dantrolene sodium) is supplied in capsules of 25-mg, 50-mg and 100-mg.
Actions: In isolated nerve-muscle preparation, Dantrium (dantrolene sodium) has been shown to produce relaxation by affecting the contractile response of the skeletal muscle at a site beyond the myoneural junction, directly on the muscle itself. In skeletal muscle, Dantrium (dantrolene sodium) dissociates the excitation-contraction coupling, probably by interfering with the release of Ca^{++} from the sarcoplasmic reticulum. This effect appears to be more pronounced in fast muscle fibers as compared to slow ones, but generally affects both. A central nervous system effect occurs, with drowsiness, dizziness and generalized weakness occasionally present. Although Dantrium (dantrolene sodium) does not appear to directly affect the CNS, the extent of its indirect effect is unknown. The absorption of Dantrium (dantrolene sodium) after oral administration in humans is incomplete and slow but consistent, and dose-related blood levels are obtained. The duration and intensity of skeletal muscle relaxation is related to the dosage and blood levels. The mean biologic half-life of Dantrium (dantrolene sodium) in adults is 8.7 hours after a 100-mg dose. Specific metabolic pathways in the degradation and elimination of Dantrium (dantrolene sodium) in human subjects have been established. Metabolic patterns are similar in adults and children. In addition to the parent compound, dantrolene, which is found in measurable amounts in blood and urine, the major metabolites noted in body fluids are the 5-hydroxy analog and the acetamido analog. Since Dantrium (dantrolene sodium) is probably metabolized by hepatic microsomal enzymes, enhancement of its metabolism by other drugs is possible. However, neither phenobarbital nor diazepam appears to affect Dantrium (dantrolene sodium) metabolism.
Indications: Dantrium (dantrolene sodium) is indicated in controlling the manifestations of clinical spasticity resulting from upper motor neuron disorders (e.g. spinal cord injury, stroke, cerebral palsy, or multiple sclerosis). It is of particular benefit to the patient whose functional rehabilitation has been retarded by the sequelae of spasticity. Such patients must have presumably reversible spasticity where relief of spasticity will aid in restoring residual function. Dantrium (dantrolene sodium) is not indicated in the treatment of skeletal muscle spasm resulting from rheumatic disorders.
If improvement occurs, it will ordinarily occur within the dosage titration (see dosage and administration), and will be manifested by a decrease in the severity of spasticity and the ability to resume a daily function not quite attainable without Dantrium (dantrolene sodium).
Occasionally, subtle but meaningful improvement in spasticity may occur with Dantrium (dantrolene sodium) therapy. In such instances information regarding improvement should be solicited from the patient and those who are in constant daily contact and attendance with him. Brief withdrawal of Dantrium (Dantrolene sodium) for a period of 2 to 4 days will frequently demonstrate exacerbation of the manifestations of spasticity and may serve to confirm a clinical impression.
A decision to continue the administration of Dantrium (dantrolene sodium) on a long-term basis is justified if introduction of the drug into the patient's regimen:

produces a significant reduction in painful and/or disabling spasticity such as clonus, or permits a significant reduction in the intensity and/or degree of nursing care required, or
rids the patient of any annoying manifestation of spasticity considered important by the patient himself.

Contraindications: Active hepatic disease, such as hepatitis and cirrhosis, is a contraindication for use of Dantrium (dantrolene sodium). Dantrium (dantrolene sodium) is contraindicated where spasticity is utilized to sustain upright posture and balance in locomotion or whenever spasticity is utilized to obtain or maintain increased function.
Warnings: It is important to recognize that fatal and non-fatal liver disorders of an idiosyncratic or hypersensitivity type may occur with Dantrium (dantrolene sodium) therapy.
At the start of Dantrium (dantrolene sodium) therapy, it is desirable to do liver function studies (SGOT, SGPT, alkaline phosphatase, total bilirubin) for a baseline or to establish whether there is pre-existing liver disease. If baseline liver abnormalities exist and are confirmed, there is a clear possibility that the potential for Dantrium (dantrolene sodium) hepatotoxicity could be enhanced, although such a possibility has not yet been established.
Liver function studies (e.g. SGOT or SGPT) should be performed at appropriate intervals during Dantrium (dantrolene sodium) therapy. If such studies reveal abnormal values, therapy should generally be discontinued. Only where benefits of the drug have been of major importance to the patient, should reinitiation or continuation of therapy be considered. Some patients have revealed a return to normal laboratory values in the face of continued therapy while others have not.
If symptoms compatible with hepatitis, accompanied by abnormalities in liver function tests or jaundice appear, Dantrium (dantrolene sodium) should be discontinued. If caused by Dantrium (dantrolene sodium) and detected early, the abnormalities in liver function characteristically have reverted to normal when the drug was discontinued.
Dantrium (dantrolene sodium) therapy has been reinstituted in a few patients who have developed clinical and/or laboratory evidence of hepatocellular injury. If such reinstitution of therapy is done, it should be attempted only in patients who clearly need Dantrium (dantrolene sodium) and only after previous symptoms and laboratory abnormalities have cleared. The patient should be hospitalized and the drug should be restarted in very small and gradually increasing doses. Laboratory monitoring should be frequent and the drug should be withdrawn immediately if there is any indication of recurrent liver involvement. Some patients have reacted with unmistakable signs of liver abnormality upon administration of a challenge dose, while others have not.
Dantrium (dantrolene sodium) should be used with particular caution in females and in patients over 35 years of age in view of apparent greater likelihood of drug-induced, potentially fatal, hepatocellular disease in these groups.
Long-term safety of Dantrium (dantrolene sodium) in humans has not been established. Chronic studies in rats, dogs and monkeys at dosages greater than 30 mg/kg/day showed growth or weight depression and signs of hepatopathy and possible occlusion nephropathy, all of which were reversible upon cessation of treatment. Sprague-Dawley female rats fed dantrolene sodium for 18 months at dosage levels of 15, 30 and 60 mg/kg/day showed an increased incidence of benign and malignant mammary tumors compared with concurrent controls and, at the highest dosage, an increase in the incidence of hepatic lymphangiomas and hepatic angiosarcomas. These effects were not seen in 2½ year studies in Sprague-Dawley or Fischer 344 rats or in 2 year studies in mice of the HaM/ICR strain. Carcinogenicity in humans cannot be fully excluded, so that this possible risk of chronic administration must be weighed against the benefits of the drug (i.e., after a brief trial) for the individual patient.
Usage in Pregnancy: The safety of Dantrium (dantrolene sodium) for use in women who are or who may become pregnant has not been established. Dantrium (dantrolene sodium) should not be used in nursing mothers.

Usage in Children: The long-term safety of Dantrium (dantrolene sodium) in children under the age of 5 years has not been established. Because of the possibility that adverse effects of the drug could become apparent only after many years, a benefit-risk consideration of the long-term use of Dantrium (dantrolene sodium) is particularly important in pediatric patients.

Drug Interactions: While a definite drug interaction with estrogen therapy has not yet been established, caution should be observed if the two drugs are to be given concomitantly. Hepatotoxicity has occurred more often in women over 35 years of age receiving concomitant estrogen therapy.

Precautions: Dantrium (dantrolene sodium) should be used with caution in patients with impaired pulmonary function, particularly those with obstructive pulmonary disease, and in patients with severely impaired cardiac function due to myocardial disease. It should be used with caution in patients with a history of previous liver disease or dysfunction (See Warnings).

Patients should be cautioned against driving a motor vehicle or participating in hazardous occupations while taking Dantrium (dantrolene sodium) Caution should be exercised in the concomitant administration of tranquilizing agents.

Dantrium (dantrolene sodium) might possibly evoke a photosensitivity reaction; patients should be cautioned about exposure to sunlight while taking it.

Adverse Reactions: The most frequently occurring side effects of Dantrium have been drowsiness, dizziness, weakness, general malaise, fatigue, and diarrhea. These are generally transient, occuring early in treatment, and can often be obviated by beginning with a low dose and increasing dosage gradually until an optimal regimen is established. Diarrhea may be severe and may necessitate temporary withdrawal of Dantrium therapy. If diarrhea recurs upon readministration of Dantrium, therapy should probably be withdrawn permanently.

Other less frequent side effects, listed according to system, are:

Gastrointestinal: Constipation, G.I. bleeding, anorexia, swallowing difficulty, gastric irritation, abdominal cramps
Hepatobiliary: Hepatitis (See Warnings)
Neurologic: Speech disturbance, seizure, headache, light-headedness, visual disturbance, diplopia, alteration of taste, insomnia
Cardiovascular: Tachycardia, erratic blood pressure, phlebitis
Psychiatric: Mental depression, mental confusion, increased nervousness
Urogenital: Increased urinary frequency, crystalluria, hematuria, difficult erection, urinary incontinence and/or nocturia, difficult urination and/or urinary retention
Integumentary: Abnormal hair growth, acne-like rash, pruritus, urticaria, eczematoid eruption, sweating
Musculoskeletal: Myalgia, backache
Respiratory: Feeling of suffocation
Special Senses: Excessive tearing
Hypersensitivity: Pleural effusion with pericarditis
Other: Chills and fever

Dosage and Administration: Prior to the administration of Dantrium (dantrolene sodium), consideration should be given to the potential response to treatment. A decrease in spasticity sufficient to allow a daily function not otherwise attainable should be the therapeutic goal of treatment with Dantrium (dantrolene sodium). Refer to Indications section for description of response to be anticipated.

It is important to establish a therapeutic goal (regain and maintain a specific function such as therapeutic exercise program, utilization of braces, transfer maneuvers, etc.) before beginning Dantrium (dantrolene sodium) therapy. Dosage should be increased until the maximum performance compatible with the dysfunction due to underlying disease is achieved. No further increase in dosage is then indicated.

Usual Dosage: It is important that the dosage be titrated and individualized for maximum effect. The lowest dose compatible with optimal response is recommended.

In view of the potential for liver damage in long-term Dantrium (dantrolene sodium) use, therapy should be stopped if benefits are not evident within 45 days.

Adults: Begin therapy with 25 mg once daily; increase to 25 mg two, three, or four times daily and then by increments of 25 mg up to as high as 100 mg two, three, or four times daily if necessary. As most patients will respond to a dose of 400 mg/day or less, rarely should doses higher than 400 mg/day be used. (See Box Warning.)

Each dosage level should be maintained for four to seven days to determine the patient's response. The dose should not be increased beyond, and may even have to be reduced to, the amount at which the patient received maximal benefit without adverse effects.

Children: A similar approach should be utilized, starting with 0.5 mg/kg of body weight twice daily; this is increased to 0.5 mg/kg three or four times daily and then by increments of 0.5 mg/kg up to as high as 3.0 mg/kg two, three, or four times daily, if necessary. Doses higher than 100 mg four times daily should not be used in children.

Overdosage: For acute overdosage general supportive measures should be employed along with immediate gastric lavage.

Intravenous fluids should be administered in fairly large quantities to avert the possibility of crystalluria. An adequate airway should be maintained and artificial resuscitation equipment should be at hand. Electrocardiographic monitoring should be instituted, and the patient carefully observed. To date, no experience has been reported with dialysis; its value in Dantrium overdosage is not known.

How Supplied: Dantrium (dantrolene sodium) is available in:

25 mg: opaque, orange and light brown capsules coded "Eaton 030" in black
NDC 0149-0030-05 bottles of 100
NDC 0149-0030-66 bottles of 500
NDC 0149-0030-05 hospital unit-dose strips in boxes of 100
50 mg: opaque, orange and dark brown capsules coded "Eaton 031" in white
NDC 0149-0031-05 bottles of 100
100 mg: opaque, orange and light brown capsules coded "Eaton 033" in white
NDC 0149-0033-05 bottles of 100
NDC 0149-0033-77 hospital unit-dose strips in boxes of 100

Address medical inquiries to:
Norwich-Eaton Pharmaceuticals
Medical Department
Norwich, NY 13815

DANTRIUM® ℞
(dantrolene sodium)
INTRAVENOUS

Description: Dantrium Intravenous is a sterile lyophilized formulation of dantrolene sodium, and in this form provides a preparation for intravenous use. Each 70 ml vial contains 20 mg dantrolene sodium, 3,000 mg mannitol, and sufficient sodium hydroxide to yield a pH of approximately 9.5 when reconstituted with 60 ml sterile water. Dantrolene sodium is classified as a direct-acting skeletal muscle relaxant. Chemically, the drug is hydrated 1-[[[5-(4-nitrophenyl)-2-furanyl] methylene] amino]-2,4-imidazolidinedione sodium salt. The hydrated salt contains approximately 15% water (3½ moles) and has a molecular weight of 399. The anhydrous salt (dantrolene) has a molecular weight of 336.

Actions: Dantrolene sodium is a muscle relaxant acting specifically on skeletal muscle. It does not affect neuromuscular transmission nor does it have measurable effects on the electrically excitable surface membrane. Studies have shown that in the presence of dantrolene sodium, the responses of the muscle to caffeine are decreased or delayed.

In isolated muscle preparations, dantrolene sodium uncouples the excitation and contraction of skeletal muscle, probably by interfering with the release of calcium from the sarcoplasmic reticulum.

In the anesthetic-induced malignant hyperthermia syndrome, evidence points to an intrinsic abnormality of muscle tissue. In affected humans and swine, it has been postulated that "triggering agents" induce a sudden rise in myoplasmic calcium either by preventing the sarcoplasmic reticulum from accumulating calcium adequatelty, or by accelerating its release. This rise in myoplasmic calcium activates acute catabolic processes common to the malignant hyperthermia crisis.

Dantrolene sodium may prevent the increase in myoplasmic calcium and the acute catabolism within the muscle cell by interfering with the release of calcium from the sarcoplasmic reticulum to the myoplasm. Thus, the physiologic, metabolic, and biochemical changes associated with the crisis may be reversed or attenuated.

Specific metabolic pathways in the degradation and elimination of dantrolene sodium in humans have been established. Dantrolene is found in measurable amounts in blood and urine. In addition, its major metabolites in body fluids are the 5-hydroxy analog and the acetamido analog. Another metabolite with an unknown structure appears related to acetylamino-dantrolene. Dantrolene sodium may also undergo hydrolysis and subsequent oxidation forming nitrophenylfuroic acid.

Since dantrolene sodium is metabolized by the liver, enhancement of its metabolism by other drugs is possible. However, neither phenobarbital nor diazepam appears to affect dantrolene sodium metabolism.

The mean biologic half-life of dantrolene sodium after intravenous administration is about 5 hours. Based on assays of whole blood and plasma, slightly greater amounts of dantrolene are associated with red blood cells than with the plasma fraction of blood. Significant amounts of dantrolene are bound to plasma proteins, mostly albumin, and this binding is readily reversible. Binding to plasma protein is not significantly altered by diazepam, diphenylhydantoin, or phenylbutazone. Binding to plasma proteins is reduced by warfarin and clofibrate and increased by tolbutamide.

In animals, dantrolene sodium given intravenously has no appreciable effect on the cardiovascular system or on respiratory function. A transient inconsistent effect on smooth muscles has been observed at high doses.

Because of the low drug concentration requiring the administration of large volumes of fluid, acute toxicity of a dantrolene sodium intravenous formulation could not be assessed. In 14-day (subacute) studies, the intravenous formulation of dantrolene sodium was relatively non-toxic to rats at doses of 10 mg/kg/day and 20 mg/kg/day. While 10 mg/kg/day in dogs for 14 days evoked little toxicity, 20 mg/kg/day for 14 days caused hepatic changes of questionable biologic significance.

Indications: Dantrium Intravenous is indicated, along with appropriate supportive measures, for the management of the fulminant hypermetabolism of skeletal muscle characteristic of malignant hyperthermia crisis. It should be administered by intravenous injection as soon as the malignant hyperthermia

Continued on next page

Norwich-Eaton—Cont.

reaction is recognized (i.e. tachycardia, tachypnea, central venous desaturation, hypercarbia, metabolic acidosis, skeletal muscle rigidity, increased utilization of anesthesia circuit carbon dioxide absorber, cyanosis and mottling of the skin, and, in many cases, fever).

Contraindications: None.

Warnings: *The use of Dantrium Intravenous in the management of malignant hyperthermia crisis is not a substitute for previously known supportive measures. These measures must be individualized, but it will usually be necessary to discontinue the suspect triggering agents, attend to increased oxygen requirements, manage the metabolic acidosis, institute cooling when necessary, attend to urinary output monitor for electrolyte imbalance.*

Precautions:

a) Because of the high pH of the intravenous formulation of Dantrium, care must be taken to prevent extravasation of the intravenous solution into the surrounding tissues.

b) Pregnancy: The safety of Dantrium Intravenous in women who are or who may become pregnant has not been established; it should be given only when the potential benefits have been weighed against the possible risk to mother and child.

Adverse Reactions: The serious reactions reported with chronic oral Dantrium use have been hepatitis, seizures, and pleural effusion with pericarditis. Hypersensitivity with attendant skin reactions has been infrequently noted. None of the reactions reported in patients taking oral Dantrium have been reported in patients treated with short-term Dantrium Intravenous therapy for malignant hyperthermia.

Dosage and Administration: As soon as the malignant hyperthermia reactions is recognized, all anesthetic agents should be discontinued. An initial Dantrium Intravenous dose of 1 mg/kg should be given rapidly. If the physiologic and metabolic abnormalities persist or reappear, this dose may be repeated up to a cumulative dose of 10 mg/kg. Based on clinical experience to date, reversal of the manifestations of malignant hyperthermia may be achieved with an average cumulative dose of 2.5 mg/kg of Dantrium Intravenous. It may be necessary to administer oral Dantrium in doses of 1 to 2 mg/kg q.i.d. for a one to three day period to prevent recurrence of the manifestations of malignant hyperthermia.

Children's Dose: Experience to date indicates that the dose for children is the same as for adults, with an initial Dantrium Intravenous dose of 1 mg/kg given rapidly.

Preparation: Each vial of Dantrium Intravenous should be reconstituted by adding 60 ml of sterile water for injection U.S.P. (without a bacteriostatic agent), and the vial shaken until the solution is clear. The contents of the vial must be *protected from direct light* and *used within 6 hours* after reconstitution. Protect the reconstituted solutions from temperatures above 86°F (30°C) and below 59°F (15°C).

How Supplied: Dantrium Intravenous (NDC 0149-0734-01) is available in vials containing a sterile lyophilized mixture of 20 mg dantrolene sodium, 3,000 mg mannitol, and sufficient sodium hydroxide to yield a pH of approximately 9.5 when reconstituted with 60 ml sterile water.

Address medical inquiries to Norwich-Eaton Pharmaceuticals, Medical Department, Norwich, NY 13815.

Manufactured by:
Eaton Laboratories, Inc.
Manati, Puerto Rico 00701
Distributed by:
Norwich-Eaton Pharmaceuticals
Divison of Morton-Norwich Products, Inc.
Norwich, New York 13815

DUVOID® ℞
(bethanechol chloride-oral)

Description: Bethanechol chloride is an ester of a choline-like compound.

Actions: Bethanechol chloride acts principally by producing the effects of stimulation of the parasympathetic nervous system. It increases the tone of the detrusor urinae muscle, usually producing a contraction sufficiently strong to initiate micturition and empty the bladder. It stimulates gastric motility, increases gastric tone, and often restores impaired rhythmic peristalsis.

Stimulation of the parasympathetic nervous system releases acetylcholine at the nerve endings. When spontaneous stimulation is reduced and therapeutic intervention is required, acetylcholine can be given, but it is rapidly hydrolyzed by cholinesterase, and its effects are transient. Bethanechol chloride is not destroyed by cholinesterase and its effects are more prolonged than those of acetylcholine.

It has predominant muscarinic action and only feeble nicotinic action. Doses that stimulate micturition and defecation and increase peristalsis do not ordinarily stimulate ganglia or voluntary muscles. Therapeutic test doses in normal human subjects have little effect on heart rate, blood pressure, or peripheral circulation.

Indications: Acute postoperative and postpartum nonobstructive (functional) urinary retention, and neurogenic atony of the urinary bladder with retention.

Contraindications: Bethanechol chloride is contraindicated in the presence of mechanical obstruction of the gastrointestinal or urinary tracts, or in conditions where the integrity of the gastrointestinal or bladder wall is questionable. Also, it is contraindicated in spastic gastrointestinal disturbances, peptic ulcer, acute inflammatory conditions of the gastrointestinal tract, or peritonitis, or in marked vagotonia.

Other major contraindications to the use of bethanechol chloride are latent or active asthma, pregnancy, hyperthyroidism, and coronary occlusion. Additional contraindications are bradycardia, atrioventricular conduction defects, vasomotor instability, hypotension, hypertension, coronary artery disease, epilepsy, and parkinsonism.

Precautions: Special care and consideration are required when bethanechol chloride is administered to patients concomitantly being treated with other drugs with which pharmacologic interactions may occur. Examples of drugs with potentials for such interactions are: quinidine and procainamide, which may antagonize cholinergic effects; cholinergic drugs, particularly cholinesterase inhibitors, where additive effects may occur. When administered to patients receiving ganglionic blocking compounds a critical fall in blood pressure may occur which usually is preceded by severe abdominal symptoms.

In urinary retention, if the sphincter fails to relax as Duvoid (bethanechol chloride) contracts the bladder, urine may be forced up the ureter into the kidney pelvis. If there is bacteriuria, this may cause a reflux infection.

Adverse Reactions: Untoward effects are usually due to overdosage but occur infrequently with the oral administration of bethanechol chloride. Abdominal discomfort, salivation, flushing of the skin ("hot feeling"), sweating, nausea and vomiting are early signs of overdosage. Asthmatic attacks, especially in asthmatic individuals, may be precipitated. Substernal pressure or pain may occur, however, it is uncertain whether this is due to bronchoconstriction, or spasm of the esophagus. Myocardial hypoxia must be considered if a marked fall in blood pressure occurs. Transient syncope with cardiac arrest, transient complete heart block, dyspnea, and orthostatic hypotension may be associated with large doses. Patients with hypertension may react to the drug with a precipitous fall in blood pressure. Short periods of atrial fibrillation have been observed in hyperthyroid individuals following the administration of cholinergic drugs. Also, involuntary defecation and urinary urgency may occur after large doses.

Atropine sulfate is a specific antidote. A dose of 0.6 mg–1.2 mg (1/100 grain–1/50 grain), for intramuscular or intravenous administration should be readily available to counteract severe toxic cardiovascular or bronchoconstrictor responses to bethanechol chloride.

Dosage and Administration: Dosage must be individualized, depending on type of severity of the conditions to be treated.

The usual adult oral dose is administered with 10-mg, 25-mg and 50-mg tablets 2, 3, or 4 times daily to a maximum dosage of 120 mg. The minimum effective dose is determined by giving 10 mg initially, and repeating with 25 mg, and then 50 mg at six hour intervals, until the desired response is obtained. The drug's effects appear within 60 to 90 minutes and persist for up to six hours. Individual doses should, therefore, be spaced at least six hours apart.

How Supplied: Duvoid (bethanechol chloride) is available in:

10-mg pale orange tablets coded "Eaton 045"
NDC 0149-0045-05 Unit-of-Use bottles of 100
NDC 0149-0045-77 hospital unit-dose strips in box of 100
25-mg white tablets coded "Eaton 046"
NDC 0149-0046-05 Unit-of-Use bottles of 100
NDC 0149-0046-77 hospital unit-dose strips in box of 100
50-mg tan tablets coded "Eaton 047"
NDC 0149-0047-05 Unit-of-Use bottles of 100
NDC 0149-0047-77 hospital unit-dose strips in box of 100

Clinical Studies: Bethanechol chloride has been extensively used in the therapy of nonobstructive urinary retention. Although the dose of bethanechol chloride varies from individual to individual and depends upon the condition under therapy, oral doses of 10 mg to 30 mg given three or four times daily are often suggested.[1]

However, it has been reported that these doses are often inadequate in the treatment of nonobstructive urinary retention[2] and that the commonly used oral doses of 5 mg or 10 mg "achieves a purely placebo effect."[3] Even in those individuals considered to have detrusor super-sensitivity to bethanechol chloride an initial dose of 25 mg is suggested.[4] More recently it has been suggested that single oral doses of at least 50 mg, with total daily doses of 200 mg to 450 mg, may be necessary to meaningfully reduce residual urine volumes.[4-8]

The effects of oral and subcutaneous bethanechol chloride upon detrusor function have previously been evaluated by cystometry.[8,9] In general, the onset of subcutaneous dosage activity is more rapid and of shorter duration than oral medication.[8,9] In the comparison of oral and subcutaneous bethanechol chloride in patients with decompensated bladders, 5-mg subcutaneous drug produced maximum mean changes in cystometric pressure greater than did a single oral dose of 200 mg.[9]

Recently, the activity of 50-mg oral doses of Duvoid, Eaton brand of bethanechol chloride, was compared to that produced by 2 mg subcutaneous bethanechol chloride.[10] Both Duvoid (bethanechol chloride) and subcutaneous bethanechol chloride were associated with decreased bladder capacities and increased intravesical pressure. In addition, the 50-mg Duvoid (bethanechol chloride) dose appeared to cause little unwanted cholinergic activity in these individuals.

References (Clinical Studies):

1. Physicians' Desk Reference, ed. 31, Oradell, N.J.: Medical Economics Company, 1977; p 846-847, 1105.
2. Lapides J, Hodgson NB, Boyd RE, Shook EL, Lichtwardt JR. Further Observations

on Pharmacologic Reactions of the Bladder. J Urol 79:707, 1958.
3. Kendall AR, Karafin L. Understanding and Rehabilitating the Atonic Neurogenic Bladder. Geriatrics 28:110, 1973.
4. Diokno AC, Koppenhoefer R. Bethanechol Chloride in Neurogenic Bladder Dysfunction. Urology 8:455, 1976.
5. Lapides J. Neurogenic Bladder: Principles of Treatment. Urol Clin North Am 1:81, 1974.
6 Smith DR. The Neurogenic Bladder. In General Urology, ed 9, Los Altos, Cal.: Lange Medical Publications, 1976; p 315.
7. Bors E, Comarr AE. Disturbances of Micturition. In Neurological Urology: Baltimore, University Park Press, 1971; p 215.
8. Lapides J, Friend CR, Ajemian EP, Sonda LP. Comparison of Action of Oral and Parenteral Bethanechol Chloride upon the Urinary Bladder. Invest Urol 1:94, 1963.
9. Diokno AC, Lapides J. Action of Oral and Parenteral Bethanechol on Decompensated Bladder. Urology 10:23, 1977.
10. Data on file, Medical Department, Norwich-Eaton Pharmaceuticals.

ENCARE®

Description: ENCARE is a small, ovoid vaginal contraceptive insert containing the potent spermicide nonoxynol 9.

Actions: ENCARE is a highly reliable contraceptive. In the vagina, ENCARE gently effervesces to disperse a spermicidal foam within. As the product effervesces there may be some sensation of warmth; however, this should not be a cause for concern. Each ENCARE insert contains a premeasured dose of the most widely used spermicide, nonoxynol 9, which kills sperm on contact.

Because ENCARE contains no hormones, it is free of the serious side effects associated with oral contraceptives. The product can be used by most women during all their fertile years.

Dosage and Administration: The smooth white ENCARE is inserted with the index finger into the vagina. The best protection will occur when the ENCARE insert is placed deep in the vagina close to the cervix. After insertion, it is necessary to wait ten minutes to assure proper dispersion, which is necessary for contraceptive protection. ENCARE provides protection for up to one hour for one act of intercourse. To provide the same reliable protection, a new ENCARE must be inserted each time intercourse is repeated. The patient should wait for at least six hours after intercourse before douching, if a douch is desired.

Precautions: WHEN PREGNANCY IS CONTRAINDICATED, THE CONTRACEPTIVE PROGRAM SHOULD BE PRESCRIBED BY A PHYSICIAN.

IF ALLERGIC REACTIONS TO CREAM, FOAM, TABLET, OR SUPPOSITORY TYPE CONTRACEPTIVES HAVE BEEN EXPERIENCED, A PHYSICIAN SHOULD BE CONSULTED BEFORE USE.

BURNING AND/OR IRRITATION OF THE VAGINA OR PENIS HAVE BEEN REPORTED IN A LIMITED NUMBER OF USERS; IF THIS OCCURS, DISCONTINUE USE.

DO NOT TAKE BY MOUTH.

ENCARE AFFORDS A HIGH DEGREE OF CONTRACEPTIVE PROTECTION WHEN PROPERLY USED; HOWEVER, NO CONTRACEPTIVE PROVIDES AN ABSOLUTE GUARANTEE AGAINST BECOMING PREGNANT.

ENCARE should be stored at a temperature below 86° F (30° C). Should the product inadvertently be exposed to higher temperatures, hold under cold water for two minutes before removing protective wrap.

How Supplied: Boxes of 12 inserts.

Eaton-Merz Laboratories, Inc.
Distributed by Eaton-Merz Laboratories, Inc.
Manufactured by Norwich-Eaton Pharmaceuticals
Division of Morton-Norwich Products, Inc.
Norwich, NY 13815

FURACIN® PREPARATIONS ℞
(nitrofurazone)

Description: Chemically, Furacin is nitrofurazone, 5-nitro-2-furaldehyde semicarbazone. **Furacin** is available in the following formulations: **Furacin** (nitrofurazone) **Soluble Dressing:** Contains 0.2% Furacin (nitrofurazone) in Solubase® (a water-soluble base of polyethylene glycols 4000, 1000, and 300).

Furacin (nitrofurazone) **Soluble Powder:** Contains 0.2% Furacin (nitrofurazone) in a water-soluble powder of polyethylene glycol 6000.

Furacin (nitrofurazone) **Topical Cream:** Contains 0.2% Furacin (nitrofurazone) in a water-miscible base consisting of glycerin, cetyl alcohol, mineral oil, an ethoxylated fatty alcohol, methylparaben, propylparaben, and water.

The discoloration of these preparations by light does not indicate loss of efficacy.

Actions: Nitrofurazone is a synthetic nitrofuran with a broad antibacterial spectrum. It is bactericidal against most bacteria commonly causing surface infections, including many that have become antibiotic resistant.

It acts by inhibiting enzymes necessary for carbohydrate metabolism in bacteria. This action occurs in both the aerobic and anaerobic cycles of carbohydrate metabolism, explaining its bactericidal effect in aerobic, anaerobic, and facultative bacteria. Topically it is without appreciable toxicity to human cells.

Indications: Nitrofurazone is a topical antibacterial agent indicated for adjunctive therapy of patients with second- and third-degree burns when bacterial resistance to other agents is a real or potential problem.

It is also indicated in skin grafting where bacterial contamination may cause graft rejection and/or donor site infection particularly in hospitals with historical resistant-bacteria epidemics.

There is no known evidence of effectiveness of this product in the treatment of minor burns or surface bacterial infections involving wounds, cutaneous ulcers or the various pyodermas.

Contraindications: Known prior sensitization is a contraindication to the use of nitrofurazone.

Warnings: Nitrofurazone has been shown to produce mammary tumors when fed at high doses to female Sprague-Dawley rats. The relevance of this to topical use in humans is unknown.

Usage in Pregnancy: Safe use of nitrofurazone during pregnancy has not been established. Therefore, the drug is not recommended for the treatment of women of childbearing potential, unless the need for the therapeutic benefit of nitrofurazone is, in the attending physician's judgment, greater than the possible risk.

Precautions: Use of topical antimicrobials occasionally allows overgrowth of nonsusceptible organisms including fungi. If this occurs or if irritation, sensitization or superinfection develop, treatment with nitrofurazone should be discontinued and appropriate therapy instituted.

Adverse Reactions: Nitrofurazone has not been significantly toxic in man by topical application. In quantitative studies published in the period 1945-70, 206 instances of clinical skin reaction were reported out of 18,249 patients treated with nitrofurazone topical formulations, an overall incidence of 1.1 percent. The treatment of nitrofurazone sensitization is not distinctive; general measures commonly used for a variety of sensitization reactions are adequate, except for the rare instance of severe contact dermatitis in which steroid administration may be indicated.

Dosage and Administration:

Furacin Soluble Dressing: BURNS. Apply directly to the lesion as with a spatula, or first place on gauze. Impregnated gauze may be used. Reapply once daily or once weekly, depending on the preferred dressing technique. SKIN GRAFTS. The dressing is used both to prepare burns and other lesions for grafting, and postoperatively as a prophylactic measure. By rapid eradication of the infection, it can produce clean, firm granulation tissue. Because it is water-soluble and has negligible tissue toxicity, it does not interfere with successful takes. Flushing the gauze with sterile saline facilitates removal.

Furacin Soluble Powder: Apply to the lesion directly from the shaker top vial or by means of a non-metallic powder insufflator such as De Vilbiss 119 or 288. To open vial, tear off aluminum top and lift off plastic cap.

Furacin Topical Cream: Apply directly to the lesion, or first place on gauze. Reapply once daily or every few days, depending on the usual dressing technique.

How Supplied:

Furacin soluble Dressing is available in:
NDC 0149-0704-12 tubes of 28 grams
NDC 0149-0704-11 tubes of 56 grams
NDC 0149-0704-51 tubes of 135 grams
NDC 0149-0704-61 jars of 454 grams
NDC 0149-0704-90 jars of 5 lb.

Furacin Soluble Powder is available in:
NDC 0149-0723-11 Shaker top vials of 14 grams

Furacin Topical Cream is available in:
NDC 0149-0777-15 tubes of 14 grams
NDC 0149-0777-12 tubes of 28 grams
NDC 0149-0777-61 jars of 368 grams

Animal Toxicology: The oral administration of nitrofurazone for 7 days to rats at extremely high dosage levels of 250 mg/kg/day produced severe hepatorenal lesions whereas only renal changes were seen when the dosage level was reduced to 60 mg/kg/day for 60 days.

Dosage levels of 60 and 30 mg/kg/day shortened the time of appearance of the typical mammary gland tumor associated with older female rats. These tumors exhibited the same histological characteristics seen in the spontaneously occurring tumors and were seen only in the female animals. No mammary tumors were seen in rats treated with nitrofurazone orally for 1 year at levels of approximately 11 mg/kg/day. Spermatogenic arrest was noted in the male rats at dosage levels of 30 mg/kg/day and above.

Dogs treated orally with nitrofurazone for 400 days at levels of 11 mg/kg/day showed no toxic effects related to drug treatment. The single intravenous administration in dogs of 20, 35, or 75 mg/kg nitrofurazone produced clinical signs of lacrimation, salivation, emesis, diarrhea, excitation, weakness, ataxia and weight loss, whereas 100 mg/kg produced convulsions and death.

There was no evidence of toxicosis in rhesus monkeys treated with doses of nitrofurazone as high as 58 mg/kg/day for 10 weeks and 23 mg/kg/day for 63 weeks.

Finally, when 30 mg/kg of nitrofurazone was administered to pregnant rabbits once daily on days 7 through 15 of pregnancy there was a slight increase in the frequency of stillbirths, but no teratogenetic effects were seen.

Preparation of Impregnated Gauze: Sterile gauze strips are placed in a tray and covered with Furacin Soluble Dressing. Repeat the procedure, adding several layers of gauze for each layer of Soluble Dressing. Sprinkling a little sterile water on each layer of dressing will minimize any color change from autoclaving. Cover the tray very loosely and autoclave at 121° C for 30 minutes at 15 to 20 pounds pressure.

Continued on next page

Norwich-Eaton—Cont.

To impregnate bandage rolls, place some Soluble Dressing in the bottom of a glass jar. Stand rolls on end. Place more Dressing on top. Cover top of jar with aluminum foil. Autoclave at 121° C for 45 minutes at 15 to 20 pounds of pressure.
Autoclaving more than once is not recommended.
For bacterial sensitivity tests: Furacin (nitrofurazone) Sensi-Discs are available from BBL, Division of BioQuest.

FURADANTIN® ORAL SUSPENSION ℞
(nitrofurantoin)
FURADANTIN® TABLETS
(nitrofurantoin)

Description: Furadantin is 1-[(5-nitrofurfurylidene) amino]hydantoin, a synthetic antimicrobial agent. It is supplied as round, yellow, bisected tablets containing 50 mg or 100 mg of nitrofurantoin, and as Furadantin Oral Suspension, containing 25 mg Furadantin (nitrofurantoin) per 5-ml teaspoonful, suspended in a palatable banana-raspberry-mint flavored gel for administration to infants and young children. The suspension is readily miscible with water, milk, fruit juices, or infants' formulas.
Actions, Indications, Contraindications, Warnings, Usage in Pregnancy, Precautions, Adverse Reactions and **Administration:** Same as for Macrodantin® (nitrofurantoin macrocrystals) Capsules.
Dosage: *Adults:* 50 to 100 mg 4 times a day. *Children:* Should be calculated on the basis of 5 to 7 mg/kg of body weight per 24 hr, to be given in divided doses 4 times a day (contraindicated under 1 month).

AVERAGE DOSE FOR CHILDREN

Body Weight lb	Body Weight kg	No. Teaspoonfuls 4 times a day
15-26	7-11	½ (2.5 ml)
27-46	12-21	1 (5 ml)
47-68	22-30	1½ (7.5 ml)
69-91	31-41	2 (10 ml)

How Supplied: Furadantin (nitrofurantoin) is available in:
50-mg scored, yellow tablets coded "Eaton 036"
NDC-0149-0036-05 bottle of 100
NDC-0149-0036-66 bottle of 500
NDC-0149-0036-06 hospital unit-dose strips in box of 100
100-mg scored, yellow tablets coded "Eaton 037"
NDC-0149-0037-05 bottle of 100
NDC-0149-0037-66 bottle of 500
NDC-0149-0037-07 hospital unit-dose strips in box of 100
Furadantin (nitrofurantoin) Oral Suspension is available in:
NDC 0149-0735-15 amber bottle of 60 ml
NDC 0149-0735-61 amber bottle of 470 ml
Avoid exposure to strong light which may darken the drug. It is stable in storage. It should be dispensed in amber bottles.
Military FNS#:
Furadantin Oral Suspension, 470 ml, 6506-082-2658
Laboratory sensitivity testing and nitrofurantoin assay: see Macrodantin® (nitrofurantoin macrocrystals) Capsules.
Eaton Laboratories Inc.
a subsidiary of Morton-Norwich Products, Inc.
Manati, Puerto Rico 00701
Address medical inquiries to:
Norwich-Eaton Pharmaceuticals
Medical Department
Norwich, NY 13815

IVADANTIN® ℞
(nitrofurantoin sodium)
STERILE—For Intravenous Use

Description: Ivadantin is a synthetic antibacterial agent for intravenous use. Each vial contains sufficient sterile powder to permit withdrawal, when reconstituted, of 180 mg (one adult dose) of nitrofurantoin.
Actions: Clinical Pharmacology: Following intravenous administration of Ivadantin, nitrofurantoin is readily excreted in the urine. Under these conditions, about 45% of the drug dose is excreted unchanged in the urine. It is highly soluble in urine, to which it may impart a brown color. Usually, the blood drug levels present are low, and nitrofurantoin has a half-life of about 0.3 hours in whole blood.
Microbiology: Nitrofurantoin is an antibacterial agent for specific urinary tract infections. It is bacteriostatic in low concentrations (10 mcg/ml to 5 mcg/ml) and *in vitro* is considered to be bactericidal in higher concentrations. Its presumed mode of action is based upon its interference with several bacterial enzyme systems. Bacteria develop only a limited resistance to furan derivatives clinically.
Ivadantin is usually active against the following organisms *in vitro: Escherichia coli*, enterococci (e.g. *Streptococcus fecalis*), *Staphylococcus aureus.*
Note: Some strains of *Enterobacter* species and *Klebsiella* species are resistant to Ivadantin. It is not active against most strains of *Proteus* species, and *Serratia* species. It has no activity against *Pseudomonas* species.
Susceptibility Tests—Quantitative methods that require measurement of zone diameters give the most precise estimates of antimicrobial susceptibility. One recommended procedure, (NCCLS, ASM-2)*, uses a disc containing 300 micrograms for testing susceptibility; interpretations correlate zone diameters of this disc test with MIC values for nitrofurantoin.
Reports from the laboratory should be interpreted according to the following criteria:
Susceptible organisms produce zones of 17 mm or greater, indicating that the tested organism is likely to respond to therapy.
Organisms of intermediate susceptibility produce zones of 15 to 16 mm, indicating that the tested organism would be susceptible if high dosage is used.
Resistant organisms produce zones of 14 mm or less, indicating that other therapy should be selected.
A bacterial isolate may be considered susceptible if the MIC value for nitrofurantoin is not more than 25 micrograms per ml. Organisms are considered resistant if the MIC is not less than 100 micrograms per ml.
Indications: Ivadantin should be used only in patients with clinically significant urinary tract infections when oral nitrofurantoin or nitrofurantoin macrocrystal therapy cannot be given.
Ivadantin is indicated for the treatment of urinary tract infections when due to susceptible strains of *E. coli*, enterococci, *S. aureus* (it is not indicated for the treatment of associated renal cortical or perinephric abscesses), and certain susceptible strains of *Klebsiella* species, *Enterobacter* species, and *Proteus* species.
Note: Specimens for culture and susceptibility testing should be obtained prior to and during drug administration.
Contraindications: Anuria, oliguria, or significant impairment of renal function (creatinine clearance under 40 ml per minute) are contraindications to therapy with this drug. Treatment of this type of patient carries an increased risk of toxicity because of impaired excretion of the drug. For the same reason, this drug is much less effective under these circumstances.
The drug is contraindicated in pregnant patients at term as well as in infants under one month of age because of the possibility of hemolytic anemia due to immature enzyme systems (glutathione instability).
The drug is also contraindicated in those patients with known hypersensitivity to Ivadantin, Macrodantin® (nitrofurantoin macrocrystals), Furadantin® (nitrofurantoin), and other nitrofurantoin preparations.
Warnings: Acute, subacute and chronic pulmonary reactions have been observed in patients treated with nitrofurantoin products. If these reactions occur, the drug should be withdrawn and appropriate measures should be taken.
An insidious onset of pulmonary reactions (diffuse interstitial pneumonitis or pulmonary fibrosis, or both) in patients on long-term therapy warrants close monitoring of these patients.
There have been isolated reports giving pulmonary reactions as a contributing cause of death. (See Hypersensitivity reactions).
Cases of hemolytic anemia of the primaquine sensitivity type have been induced by nitrofurantoin. The hemolysis appears to be linked to a glucose-6-phosphate dehydrogenase deficiency in the red blood cells of the affected patients. This deficiency is found in 10 percent of Negroes and a small percentage of ethnic groups of Mediterranean and Near-Eastern origin. Any sign of hemolysis is an indication to discontinue the drug. Hemolysis ceases when the drug is withdrawn.
Pseudomonas is the organism most commonly implicated in superinfections in patients treated with nitrofurantoin.
Precautions: Peripheral neuropathy may occur with nitrofurantoin therapy; this may become severe or irreversible. Fatalities have been reported. Predisposing conditions such as renal impairment (creatinine clearance under 40 ml per minute), anemia, diabetes, electrolyte imbalance, vitamin B deficiency, and debilitating disease may enhance such occurrence.
Usage in Pregnancy: The safety of nitrofurantoin during pregnancy and lactation has not been established. Use of the drug in women of childbearing potential requires that the anticipated benefit be weighed against the possible risks.
Usage in Children: Safety has not been established in children under 12 years.
Adverse Reactions: Gastrointestinal reactions: Anorexia, nausea, and emesis are the most frequent reactions and these are related to the drip speed; abdominal pain and diarrhea occur less frequently. Hepatitis occurs rarely.
Hypersensitivity Reactions: Pulmonary sensitivity reactions may occur which can be acute, subacute, or chronic.
Acute reactions are commonly manifested by fever, chills, cough, chest pain, dyspnea, pulmonary infiltration with consolidation or pleural effusion on x-ray, and eosinophilia. The acute reactions usually occur within the first week of treatment and are reversible with cessation of therapy. Resolution may be dramatic.
In subacute reactions, fever and eosinophilia are observed less often. Recovery is somewhat slower, perhaps as long as several months. If the symptoms are not recognized as being drug related and nitrofurantoin is not withdrawn, symptoms may become more severe.
Chronic pulmonary reactions are more likely to occur in patients who have been on continuous nitrofurantoin therapy for six months or longer. The insidious onset of malaise, dyspnea on exertion, cough, and altered pulmonary function are common manifestations. Roentgenographic and histologic findings of diffuse interstitial pneumonitis or fibrosis, or both, are also common manifestations. Fever is rarely prominent.
The severity of these chronic pulmonary reactions and the degree of their resolution appear to be related to the duration of therapy after the first clinical signs appear. Pulmonary function may be permanently impaired even after

cessation of nitrofurantoin therapy. This risk is greater when pulmonary reactions are not recognized early.

Dermatologic reactions: Maculopapular, erythematous, or eczematous eruption, pruritus, urticaria, and angioedema.

Other sensitivity reactions: Anaphylaxis, asthmatic attack in patients with history of asthma, cholestatic jaundice, drug fever, and arthralgia.

Hematologic reactions: Hemolytic anemia, granulocytopenia, leukopenia, eosinophilla, and megaloblastic anemia. Return of the blood picture to normal has followed cessation of therapy.

Neurological reactions: Peripheral neuropathy, headache, dizziness, nystagmus, and drowsiness.

Miscellaneous reactions: Transient alopecia. As with other antimicrobial agents, superinfections by resistant organisms may occur. With nitrofurantoin, however, these are limited to the genitourinary tract because suppression of normal bacterial flora elsewhere in the body does not occur.

Dosage and Administration: Dosage: Patients weighing over 120 pounds: 180 mg of nitrofurantoin twice daily.

Patients weighing less than 120 pounds: 3 mg per pound of body weight per day in two equal doses.

Intravenous Administration: Dissolve just prior to use as follows: Add 20 ml of 5% dextrose injection, USP, or sterile water for injection, USP, to the vial of dry, sterile Ivadantin. To prepare the final solution, each ml of the initial dilution should be added to a minimum of 25 ml of parenteral fluid, e.g. 20 ml = 180 mg in at least 500 ml. (Do not use solutions containing methyl- and propyl-parabens, phenol or cresol as preservatives, since these compounds cause the Ivadantin to be precipitated out of solution.) Shake well to insure complete solution.

This final solution is to be given by intravenous drip at the rate of 50–60 drops (2–3 ml) per minute. The final solution should be used within 24 hours. It should be protected from ultraviolet light and excessive heat. Mixing other antibacterials in the same solution with nitrofurantoin sodium is not recommended. A list of known physical compatabilities will be supplied on request.

Therapy with peroral Macrodantin (nitrofurantoin macrocrystals) should replace the intravenous form when possible. The drug should be continued for at least one week and for at least three days after sterility of the urine is obtained. Continued infection indicates the need for reevaluation.

How Supplied: Sterile 20 ml vials containing one adult dose of sterile Ivadantin equivalent to 180 mg of nitrofurantoin.

Note: Mix just prior to use. Do not use intravenously without further dilution.

Furadantin (nitrofurantoin)/Macrodantin (nitrofurantoin macrocrystals) 300 mcg Sensi-Discs for the laboratory determination of bacterial sensitivity are available from BBL, Division of BioQuest. For information on simple Furadantin (nitrofurantoin) assays in blood, serum, and urine, write or call the Medical Department.

Literature sent to physicians on request.

Manufactured for
Norwich-Eaton Pharmaceuticals
Division of Morton-Norwich Products, Inc.
Norwich, New York 13815
by **Boehringer-Mannheim**
68 Mannheim 31
Germany

* National Committee for Clinical Laboratory Standards. Approved Standard: ASM-2, Performance Standards for Antimicrobial Disc Susceptibility Tests, July, 1975.

MACRODANTIN® ℞
(nitrofurantoin macrocrystals)
CAPSULES

Description: Macrodantin is a synthetic chemical of controlled crystal size. It is a stable, yellow crystalline compound. It is supplied in capsules containing 25 mg, 50 mg, and 100 mg.

Actions: Clinical Pharmacology: Macrodantin is a larger crystal form of Furadantin (nitrofurantoin). The absorption of macrodantin is slower and its excretion somewhat less when compared to Furadantin. During therapeutic drug dosage, only low blood drug concentrations are usually present. A number of patients who cannot tolerate Furadantin (nitrofurantoin) Tablets are able to take Macrodantin Capsules without nausea. It is highly soluble in urine, to which it may impart a brown color. Following a therapeutic dose regimen (100 mg qid for 7 days) average urinary drug recoveries (0–24 hours) on day 1 and 7 were 37.9% and 35.0%, respectively, for Macrodantin.

Microbiology: Macrodantin is an antibacterial agent for specific urinary tract infections. It is bacteriostatic in low concentrations (10 mcg/ml to 5 mcg/ml) and *in vitro* is considered to be bactericidal in higher concentrations. Its presumed mode of action is based upon its inheritance with several bacterial enzyme systems. Bacteria develop only a limited resistance to furan derivatives clinically.

Macrodantin is usually active against the following organisms *in vitro: Escherichia coli,* enterococci (e.g., *Streptococcus fecalis*) *Staphylococcus aureus.*

Note: Some strains of *Enterobacter* species and *Klebsiella* species are resistant to Macrodantin. It is not active against most strains of *Proteus* species, and *Serratia* species. It has no activity against *Pseudomonas* species.

Susceptibility Tests—Quantitative methods that require measurement of zone diameters give the most precise estimates of antimicrobial susceptibility. One recommended procedure, (NCCLS, ASM-2)*, uses a disc containing 300 micrograms for testing susceptibility, interpretations correlate zone diameters of this disc test with MIC values for nitrofurantoin. Reports from the laboratory should be interpreted according to the following criteria.

Susceptible organisms produce zones of 17 mm or greater, indicating that the tested organism is likely to respond to therapy.

Organisms of intermediate susceptibility produce zones of 15 to 16 mm, indicating that the tested organism would be susceptible if high dosage is used.

Resistant organisms produce zones of 14 mm or less, indicating that other therapy should be selected.

A bacterial isolate may be considered susceptible if the MIC value for nitrofurantoin is not more than 25 micrograms per ml. Organisms are considered resistant if the MIC is not less than 100 micrograms per ml.

Indications: Macrodantin is indicated for the treatment of uninary tract infections when due to susceptible strains of *E. coli,* enteroccoci, *S. aureus* (it is not indicated for the treatment of associated renal cortical or perinephric abscesses), and certain susceptible strains of *Klebsiella* species, *Enterobacter* species, and *Proteus* species.

Note: Specimens for culture and susceptibility testing should be obtained prior to and during drug administration.

Contraindications: Anuria, oliguria, or significant impairment of renal function (creatinine clearance under 40 ml per minute) are contraindications to therapy with this drug. Treatment of this type of patient carries an increased risk of toxicity because of impaired excretion of the drug. For the same reason, this drug is much less effective under these circumstances.

The drug is contraindicated in pregnant patients at term as well as in infants under one month of age because of the possibility of hemolytic anemia due to immature enzyme systems (glutathione instability).

The drug is also contraindicated in those patients with known hypersensitivity to Macrodantin, Furadantin® (nitrofurantoin), and other nitrofurantoin preparations.

Warnings: Acute, subacute and chronic pulmonary reactions have been observed in patients treated with nitrofurantoin products. If these reactions occur, the drug should be withdrawn and appropriate measures should be taken.

An insidious onset of pulmonary reactions (diffuse interstitial pneumonitis or pulmonary fibrosis, or both) in patients on long-term therapy warrants close monitoring of these patients.

There have been isolated reports giving pulmonary reactions as a contributing cause of death. (See Hypersensitivity reactions.)

Cases of hemolytic anemia of the primaquine sensitivity type have been induced by Macrodantin. The hemolysis appears to be linked to a glucose-6-phosphate dehydrogenase deficiency in the red blood cells of the affected patients. This deficiency is found in 10 percent of Negroes and a small percentage of ethnic groups of Mediterranean and near-Eastern origin. Any sign of hemolysis is an indication to discontinue the drug. Hemolysis ceases when the drug is withdrawn.

Pseudomonas is the organism most commonly implicated in superinfections in patients treated with Macrodantin.

Precautions: Peripheral neuropathy may occur with Macrodantin therapy; this may become severe or irreversible. Fatalities have been reported. Predisposing conditions such as renal impairment (creatinine clearance under 40 ml per minute) anemia, diabetes, electrolyte imbalance, vitamin B deficiency, and debilitating disease may enhance such occurrence.

Usage in Pregnancy: The safety of Macrodantin during pregnancy and lactation has not been established. Use of this drug in women of childbearing potential requires that the anticipated benefit be weighed against the possible risks.

Adverse Reactions: Gastrointestinal reactions: Anorexia, nausea and emesis are the most frequent reactions; abdominal pain and diarrhea occur less frequently. These dose-related toxicity reactions can be minimized by reduction of dosage, especially in the female patient. Hepatitis occurs rarely.

Hypersensitivity reactions: Pumonary sensitivity reactions may occur, which can be acute, subacute, or chronic.

Acute reactions are commonly manifested by fever, chills, cough, chest pain, dyspnea, pulmonary infiltration with consolidation or pleural effusion on x-ray, and eosinophilia. The acute reactions usually occur within the first week of treatment and are reversible with cessation of therapy. Resolution may be dramatic. In subacute reactions, fever and eosinophilia are observed less often. Recovery is somewhat slower, perhaps as long as several months. If the symptoms are not recognized as being drug related and nitrofurantoin is not withdrawn, symptoms may become more severe.

Chronic pulmonary reactions are more likely to occur in patients who have been on continuous nitrofurantoin therapy for six months or longer. The insidious onset of malaise, dyspnea on exertion, cough, and altered pulmonary function are common manifestations. Roentgenographic and histologic findings of diffuse interstitial pneumonitis or fibrosis, or both, are also common manifestations. Fever is rarely prominent.

Continued on next page

Norwich-Eaton—Cont.

The severity of these chronic pulmonary reactions and the degree of their resolution appear to be related to the duration of therapy after the first clinical signs appear. Pulmonary function may be permanently impaired even after cessation of nitrofurantoin therapy. This risk is greater when pulmonary reactions are not recognized early.

Dermatologic reactions: Maculopapular, erythematous, or eczematous eruption, pruritus, urticaria, and angioedema.

Other sensitivity reactions: Anaphylaxis, asthmatic attack in patients with history of asthma, cholestatic jaundice, drug fever, and arthralgia.

Hematologic reactions: Hemolytic anemia, granulocytopenia, leukopenia, eosinophilia, and megaloblastic anemia. Return of the blood picture to normal has followed cessation of therapy.

Neurological reactions: Peripheral neuropathy, headache, dizziness, nystagmus, and drowsiness.

Miscellaneous reactions: Transient alopecia. As with other antimicrobial agents, superinfections by resistant organisms may occur. With Macrodantin, however, these are limited to the genitourinary tract because suppression of normal bacterial flora elsewhere in the body does not occur.

Dosage and Administration:

Dosage—Adults: 50–100 mg four times a day. **Children:** Should be calculated on the basis of 5–7 mg/kg of body weight per 24 hours to be given in divided doses four times a day (contraindicated under one month).

Administration: Macrodantin may be given with food or milk to further minimize gastric upset.

Therapy should be continued for at least one week and for at least 3 days after sterility of the urine is obtained. Continued infection indicates the need for reevaluation.

If the drug is to be used for long-term suppressive therapy, a reduction of dosage should be considered.

How Supplied: Macrodantin is available in:

100-mg; opaque, yellow capsules coded "Eaton 009"

NDC 0149-0009-01 bottle of 30
NDC 0149-0009-05 bottle of 100
NDC 0149-0009-66 bottle of 500
NDC 0149-0009-67 bottle of 1000
NDC 0149-0009-77 hospital unit-dose strips in box of 100

50-mg: opaque, yellow and white capsules coded "Eaton 008"

NDC 0149-0008-01 bottle of 30
NDC 0149-0008-05 bottle of 100
NDC 0149-0008-66 bottle of 500
NDC 0149-0008-67 bottle of 1000
NDC 0149-0008-77 hospital unit-dose strips in box of 100

25-mg: opaque, white capsules coded "Eaton 007"

NDC 1049-0007-05 bottle of 100

Furadantin (nitrofurantoin)/Macrodantin Sensi-Discs for the laboratory determination of bacterial sensitivity are available from BBL, Division of BioQuest. For information on simple nitrofurantoin assays in blood, serum, and urine, write or call the Medical Department.

Literature sent to physicians on request.

Address medical inquiries to Norwich-Eaton Pharmaceuticals, Medical Department, Norwich, NY 13815.

Manufactured by
Eaton Laboratories Inc.
Manati, Puerto Rico 00701
Distributed by
Norwich-Eaton Pharmaceuticals
Division of Morton-Norwich Products, Inc.
Norwich, New York 13815

* National Committee for Clinical Laboratory Standards. Approved Standard: ASM-2, Performance Standards for Antimicrobial Disc Susceptibility Tests, July, 1975.

VIVONEX® STANDARD DIET
Elemental Standard Diet/Soluble Powder
VIVONEX® HN
Elemental High Nitrogen Diet/Soluble Powder

What an elemental diet is: Elemental, chemically defined or molecular diets differ from conventional foods in that they are formulated from known chemical nutrients, such as purified amino acids, simple carbohydrates, vitamins, mineral salts and essential fat. They contain no protein hydrolysates, peptides or undefined peptone fractions which have been reported to cause a variety of undesirable effects. They contain no bulk and therefore produce a minimum of residue.

Clinical importance of the elemental diet:

Elemental diets are used—
- when there is a need for defined and balanced nutrition
- as an ultra low-residue food source
- when digestion is difficult and absorption questionable.

VIVONEX®
Elemental Standard Diet/Soluble Powder

Description: Vivonex is a unique, nutritionally complete enteral diet utilizing free crystalline L-amino acids as a nitrogen (protein) source. Vivonex is packaged as an unflavored powder. When mixed with water it may be tube fed, or when appropriately flavored, consumed as an oral beverage. Vivonex is formulated to contain minimum fat and has low viscosity. Vivonex is an ideal routine feeding for tube administration because the low fat content promotes fast stomach emptying and reduces the possibility of regurgitation/aspiration. Low viscosity permits feeding via small tubes to minimize patient discomfort.

Vivonex requires virtually no digestion and as little as 100 cm of functional intestine for absorption. Because it is almost totally absorbed it yields negligible residue. Accordingly, Vivonex feeding may be employed in the dietary management of diseases/impairments of the gastrointestinal tract.

Vivonex is also useful to fortify clear liquid regimens, increasing patient calorie and nitrogen intake, while supporting the diet objective of negligible residue.

Nutritional Information: Contents of one packet (diluted with water to total volume of 300 ml) supply 300 kcal and the following:

Available nitrogen in the form of pure amino acids ....0.98 gram (1.22%)
Fat as highly purified safflower oil (containing 80% linoleic acid)..........0.435 gram (0.54%)
Carbohydrate (glucose oligosaccharides ....69.0 grams (86.3%)

Caloric Contribution:
Amino Acids.......................................8.2%
Fat.......................................1.3%
Carbohydrates.......................................90.5%

Six packets in normal dilution supply 1800 kcal, 5.88 grams of available nitrogen (equivalent to approximately 37 g protein), 2.61 grams fat, 414 grams carbohydrates, and the following vitamins, minerals and amino acids (Table I at left):

ESSENTIAL AMINO ACIDS	% Total Amino Acids
L-Isoleucine	4.55
L-Leucine	7.20
L-Lysine	5.41
L-Methionine	4.66
L-Phenylalanine	5.18
L-Threonine	4.55
L-Tryptophan	1.41
L-Valine	5.02
Total essential amino acids	37.98

NONESSENTIAL AMINO ACIDS	
L-Alanine	4.85
L-Arginine	8.87
L-Aspartic Acid	10.35
L-Glutamine	17.07
Glycine	7.91
L-Histidine	2.21
L-Proline	6.48

Table I
QUANTITY AND PERCENTAGE OF ADULT US RECOMMENDED DAILY ALLOWANCES (US RDA)

	Units/Packet	Units/Liter	% US RDA in 6 packets
VITAMINS			
Vitamin A, IU	833.3	2777.8	100%
Vitamin D, IU	66.7	222.0	100%
Vitamin E, IU	5.0	16.7	100%
Vitamin C, mg	10.0	33.3	100%
Folic Acid, mg	0.067	0.2	100%
Thiamine, mg	0.25	0.83	100%
Riboflavin, mg	0.28	0.94	100%
Niacin, mg	3.3	11.1	100%
Vitamin B_6, mg	0.33	1.1	100%
Vitamin B_{12}, mcg	1.0	3.3	100%
Biotin, mg	0.05	0.17	100%
Pantothenic Acid, mg	1.67	5.6	100%
Vitamin K, mcg	11.17	37.2	*
Choline, mg	12.28	40.94	*
MINERALS			
Calcium, gm	0.17	0.56	100%
Phosphorus, gm	0.17	0.56	100%
Iodine, mcg	25.0	83.3	100%
Iron, mg	3.0	10.0	100%
Magnesium, mg	66.7	222.0	100%
Copper, mg	0.33	1.1	100%
Zinc, mg	2.5	8.3	100%

* No US RDA established.

L-Serine	3.34
L-Tyrosine	0.94
Total nonessential amino acids	62.02

Table II
Electrolytes in Vivonex
(in normal dilution—80 grams in 300 ml)

	mEq/ liter	mg/80 gram packet	mg/ liter
CATIONS			
Sodium	37.4	258.0	859.1
Potassium	29.9	351.5	1170.5
Calcium	27.7	166.7	555.1
Magnesium	18.3	66.67	222.0
Manganese	0.0567	0.468	1.6
Iron	0.358	3.0	10.0
Copper	0.035	0.333	1.1
Zinc	0.255	2.5	8.3
ANIONS			
Chloride	51.85	551.6	1836.8
Phosphate	54.0	166.6*	554.8*
Acetate	0.296	5.25	17.5
Iodide	0.00066	0.025	0.083

*Calculated as P

Mixing Instructions: For a normal dilution, put 8½ oz (255 ml) of water into a blender, then add an 80-gram packet of Vivonex Standard Diet. Blend at medium speed until in solution. To mix in a container (a pint or larger container is preferred), add one packet of Vivonex Standard Diet, and 2 oz (60 ml) of water. Shake or stir for approximately 30 seconds until lumps break up. Add the remaining water and shake or stir another 30 seconds until solution is achieved.

Flavoring: Vivonex Standard Diet is unflavored. When consumed as a beverage it should be flavored by the addition of one Vivonex Flavor Packet per 80 g of diet before blending. Flavor packets are available in orange, strawberry, grape, and vanilla. Fruit and vanilla flavors are best when served cold or over ice. The osmolality contribution of flavor packets is approximately 60 mOsm/kg; the nutrition contribution is negligible. For complete information refer to labeling for Vivonex Flavor Packets.

Vivonex may also be flavored by mixing with various agents such as natural or artificially sweetened carbonated beverages, fruit or vegetable flavored liquids, fruit flavor concentrates, flavoring extracts, and instant drink mixes. Consideration should be given to the resulting changes in calories, minerals, vitamins and osmolality, and to those beverages which may be contraindicated. Water used in mixing the diet should be reduced by the amount contributed by flavoring agents.

Feeding Instructions: Vivonex Standard Diet should be provided in quantities sufficient to meet nutritional needs of the patient. Volume, concentration and rate of administration should be adjusted according to patient tolerance. The diet can be consumed as a beverage or fed via nasogastric or gastrointestinal tube.

Tube Administration: This can be accomplished through a small 16 gauge catheter or a #5 French feeding tube placed nasogastrically or into a gastrostomy or jejunostomy. It is suggested that the diet be given at room temperature by constant gravity drip using the Vivonex Delivery System (List #71281) or by means of an infusion pump.

Initiate feeding with a dilute solution at a slow rate. Increase the rate and/or concentration gradually until maximum tolerated rate and full strength dilution is attained. Table III is a suggested feeding schedule to reach full strength in 2 days:

Table III

Day	No. of Packets	Dilute to Volume	Approximate Feeding Rate
1st 12 hours	3	1800 ml	75 ml/hr
2nd 12 hours	4	1800 ml	75 ml/hr
3rd 12 hours	5	1800 ml	75 ml/hr
4th 12 hours	6	1800 ml	75 ml/hr

Oral Feeding: Sip each serving slowly. Initiate feeding with dilute solution and gradually increase volume and concentration to maximum tolerated. Table IV is a suggested feeding schedule to reach full strength in 3 days:

Table IV

Day	No. of Packets	Dilute to Volume	No. of Servings/Day
1	3–4	1800 ml	7–10
2	4–5	1800 ml	6–8
3	5–6	1800 ml	6–8

Pediatric Feedings: Volume, concentration and feeding rate must be adjusted to the fluid, electrolyte and nutritional requirements of the pediatric patient. Infant feeding should be initiated with a concentration of 8% weight/volume and gradually increased, not to exceed 16%. Infants over 10 months of age may tolerate higher concentrations up to 25% weight/volume when fully adapted over a 5 to 7 day period. The initial feeding should not exceed 50 ml/kg of body weight per 24 hours using the 8% solution.

Osmolality: Full strength Vivonex Standard is hypertonic and has an osmolality of 550 mOsm/kg. Gastrointestinal distress, nausea, vomiting, gastric dumping and diarrhea, when encountered in sensitive patients, can be avoided by careful adjustments of feeding rate and dilution of the diet. If diarrhea is encountered, revert one step to a more dilute solution. Nausea, if encountered, is usually due to feeding speed. Stop feeding for one hour, then resume feeding at a slower rate. Table V shows the osmolality of Vivonex Standard Diet at various concentrations:

Table V

No. of Packets	Dilute to Volume	Osmolality
3	1800 ml	265 mOsm/kg
5	1800 ml	450 mOsm/kg
6	1800 ml	550 mOsm/kg

Storage: Store Vivonex Soluble powder at 68°F or less. In solution Vivonex is a perishable liquid food. A full day's supply may be prepared at one time and stored in the refrigerator for up to 24 hours. The diet may be stored in the Vivonex Delivery System in the refrigerator. For complete information, refer to labeling for the Vivonex Delivery System. Shake the liquid briefly before serving. Once removed from the refrigerator, the diet should be administered within 8 hours.

How Supplied: Six sealed packets per carton, each packet containing 80 grams (2.82 ounces) of water-soluble powder, yielding 300 kcal.

Precautions: For use only under medical supervision. Do not administer parenterally. Diabetics receiving this diet should be closely monitored. The electrolyte content of the diet is based on requirements of normal adults and should be monitored for patients with electrolyte imbalance. Use during pregnancy or lactation may require supplemental vitamins and minerals. Use for children may require adjusting the daily consumption to meet the Recommended Daily Allowance for the age group involved. Clinical data support nutritional adequacy of exclusive use for up to 12 months.

Please contact your local Norwich-Eaton representative for further information if you have any questions regarding preparation or feeding, or write Norwich-Eaton Pharmaceuticals, Medical Department, Norwich, NY 13815.

VIVONEX® Delivery System

Description: A complete, single component delivery system that allows continuous gravity-flow administration of Vivonex Diets. The single disposable component holds up to 1 liter of Vivonex Diet in its flexible 1000 ml-pouch. The sturdy pouch access can be opened and closed without weakening, permitting volume or concentration changes. The unique drip meter allows simple flow-rate monitoring and regulation (microdrops/minute equate to ml/hr for desired flow rate), facilitating continuous (24-hour) administration of Vivonex HN or Standard Elemental Diet. A red warning tag on the connecting tubing, in addition to the overall design, clearly differentiates this from comparable I.V. equipment.

Dosage and Administration: A full day's supply of Vivonex High Nitrogen or Standard Diet may be prepared at one time, divided into four pouches, and refrigerated for up to 24 hours. To fill pouches, grasp aperture ring of filling orifice and pull "back" of pouch away from orifice to create a larger opening. Then, fill with Vivonex Diet to desired level and seal securely. Close screw clamp fully and shake pouch well. For storage, the tubing may be wound around the filled pouch, with the distal end inserted into the hanger hole. Once removed from refrigerator, contents should be administered within 8 hours.

For continuous administration, divide total volume (ml) in each pouch by 8 and maintain flow rate to that number of drops per minute. Sixty drops is approximately equal to 1 ml; therefore, 60 drops per minute is equal to a flow rate of 60 ml per hour.

The filled pouch should be hung with the fluid level approximately 30 inches above patient. To expel air from the connecting tube, remove the protective cap from the male Luer at the distal end of the tubing and open the screw clamp. Then reclose the screw clamp. The male Luer should be inserted into the patient's indwelling enteral catheter (feeding tube). Release the screw clamp and adjust to the desired flow rate. Allow the flow rate of Vivonex Diet to stabilize for a few minutes. Thereafter, monitor occasionally, readjusting flow rate as needed with screw clamp.

THE VIVONEX DELIVERY SYSTEM SHOULD BE DISCARDED WHEN EMPTY; DO NOT REFILL.

Warning: Administration of high-nutrient solutions in plastic containers will result in a significant loss of fat-soluble vitamins - supplementation should be considered. (Reported losses ranged from 40% to 60%.)

How Supplied: Each individual Vivonex Delivery System is packaged in a polyethylene bag with instructions enclosed. There are 10 systems per carton and 12 cartons per case (120 systems per case).

VIVONEX® HN

Elemental High Nitrogen Diet/Soluble Powder

Description: Vivonex HN is a unique, nutritionally complete *high nitrogen* enteral diet utilizing free crystalline L-amino acids as a nitrogen (protein) source. The nitrogen-to-calorie ratio is 1 gram nitrogen to 150 kcal, an optimum ratio to spare the nitrogen for anabolic purposes. Vivonex HN is packaged as an unflavored powder. When mixed with water it may be tube fed, or when appropriately flavored, consumed as an oral beverage. Vivonex HN is formulated to contain minimum fat and has low viscosity.

Vivonex HN is an ideal feeding for tube administration because the low fat content promotes fast stomach emptying and reduces the possibility of regurgitation/aspiration. Low viscosity permits feeding via small tubes to minimize patient discomfort.

Continued on next page

Norwich-Eaton—Cont.

Vivonex HN requires virtually no digestion and as little as 100 cm of functional intestine for absorption. Because it is almost totally absorbed it yields negligible residue. Accordingly, Vivonex HN feeding may be employed in the dietary management of diseases/impairments of the gastrointestinal tract and as an enteral alternative to parenteral nutrition when the patient has at least minimal gastrointestinal function.

Vivonex HN is also useful to fortify clear liquid regimens, increasing patient calorie and nitrogen intake, while supporting the diet objective of negligible residue.

Nutritional Information: Contents of one packet (diluted with water to total volume of 300 ml) supply 300 kcal and the following:

Available nitrogen in the form of pure amino acids..........2.0 grams (2.5%)

Fat as highly purified safflower oil (containing 80% linoleic acid)..........0.261 gram (0.33%)

Carbohydrate as glucose oligosaccharides ....63.3 grams (79.1%)

Caloric Contribution:

Amino Acids..........17.7%

Fat..........0.78%

Carbohydrates..........81.5%

Ten packets of Vivonex HN supply 20.0 grams of available nitrogen (equivalent to approximately 130 g of protein), 2.61 grams fat, 633 grams carbohydrates, and the following vitamins, minerals and amino acids (Table I): [See table below].

ESSENTIAL AMINO ACIDS	% Total Amino Acids
L-Isoleucine	4.15
L-Leucine	6.57
L-Lysine	4.94
L-Methionine	4.58
L-Phenylalanine	7.10
L-Threonine	4.16
L-Tryptophan	1.28
L-Valine	4.58
Total essential amino acids	37.36
NONESSENTIAL AMINO ACIDS	
L-Alanine	5.18
L-Arginine	4.07
L-Aspartic Acid	11.06
L-Glutamine	18.22
Glycine	9.84
L-Histidine	2.36
L-Proline	6.92
L-Serine	4.15
L-Tyrosine	0.84
Total nonessential amino acids	62.64

Table II

Electrolytes in Vivonex HN:

	mEq/ liter	mg/80 gram packet	mg/ liter
CATIONS			
Sodium	33.5	231.3	770.2
Potassium	17.9	210.5	700.0
Calcium	16.6	100.0	333.0
Magnesium	10.97	40.0	133.2
Manganese	0.0341	0.281	0.94
Iron	0.2148	1.8	6.0
Copper	0.02098	0.2	0.67
Zinc	0.0153	1.5	5.0
ANIONS			
Chloride	52.4	557.3	1855.8
Phosphate	31.6	100.0*	333.0*
Acetate	0.178	3.15	10.5
Iodide	0.00039	0.015	0.05

*Calculated as P

Mixing Instructions: For a normal dilution, put 8½ oz (255 ml) of water into a blender, then add an 80-gram packet of Vivonex HN Diet. Blend at medium speed until in solution. To mix in a container (a pint or larger is preferred), add one packet of Vivonex HN Diet, and 2 oz (60 ml) of water. Shake or stir for approximately 30 seconds until lumps break up. Add the remaining water and shake or stir another 30 seconds until solution is achieved.

Flavoring: Vivonex HN Diet is unflavored. When consumed as a beverage it should be flavored by the addition of one Vivonex Flavor Packet per 80 g of diet before blending. Flavor packets are available in orange, strawberry, grape, and vanilla. Fruit and vanilla flavors are best when served cold or over ice. The osmolality contribution of flavor packets is approximately 60 mOsm/kg; the nutritional contribution is negligible. For complete information refer to labeling of Vivonex Flavor Packets.

Vivonex HN Diet may also be flavored by mixing with various agents such as natural or artificially sweetened carbonated beverages, fruit or vegetable flavored liquids, fruit flavor concentrates, flavoring extracts, and instant drink mixes. Consideration should be given to the resulting changes in calories, minerals, vitamins and osmolality, and to those beverages which may be contraindicated. Water used in mixing the diet should also be reduced by the amount contributed by the flavoring agent.

Feeding Instructions: Vivonex HN Diet should be provided in quantities sufficient to meet the nutritional needs of the patient. Volume, concentration and rate of administration should be adjusted according to patient tolerance. The diet can be consumed as a beverage or fed via nasogastric or gastrointestinal tube.

Tube Administration: This can be accomplished through a small 16 gauge catheter or a #5 French feeding tube placed nasogastrically or into a gastrostomy or jejunostomy. It is suggested that the diet be given at room temperature by constant gravity drip using the Vivonex Delivery System (List #71281), or by means of an infusion pump.

Initiate feeding with a dilute solution at a slow rate. Increase the rate and/or concentration gradually until maximum tolerated rate and full strength dilution is attained. Table III is a suggested feeding schedule to reach full strength in 3 to 4 days.

Table III

Day	No. of Packets	Dilute to Volume	Feeding Rate
1	2–3	1200ml	50 ml/hr
2	4–5	1800 ml	75 ml/hr
3	6–8	2400 ml	100 ml/hr
4	8–10	3000 ml	125 ml/hr

Oral Feeding: Sip each serving slowly. Initiate feeding with dilute solution and gradually increase volume and concentration to maximum tolerated. Table IV is a suggested feeding schedule to reach full strength in 3 to 4 days:

Table IV

Day	No. of Packets	Dilute to Volume	No of Servings day
1	2–3	1200 ml	4–6
2	4–5	1800 ml	6–8
3	6–8	2400 ml	8–10
4	8–10	3000 ml	8–10

Pediatric Feeding: Volume, concentration and feeding rate must be adjusted to the fluid, electrolyte and nutritional requirements of the pediatric patient. Infant feeding should be initiated with a concentration of 8% weight/volume and gradually increased, not to exceed 16%. Infants over 10 months of age may tolerate higher concentrations up to 25% weight/volume when fully adapted over a 5 to 7 day period. The initial feeding should not exceed 50 ml/kg of body weight per 24 hours using the 8% solution.

Osmolality: Full strength Vivonex HN is hypertonic and has an osmolality of 810 mOsm/kg. Gastrointestinal distress, nausea, vomiting, gastric dumping and diarrhea when encountered in sensitive patients can be avoided by careful adjustment of feeding rate and dilution of the diet. If diarrhea is encountered, revert one step to a more dilute solution. Nausea, if encountered, is usually due to feeding speed. Stop feeding for one hour, then resume feeding at a slower rate. Table V shows the osmolality of Vivonex HN Diet at various concentrations.

Table I

QUANTITY AND PERCENTAGE OF ADULT US RECOMMENDED DAILY ALLOWANCES (US RDA)

	Units/Packet	Units/Liter	% of US RDA in 10 packets
VITAMINS			
Vitamin A, IU	500.0	1667.0	100%
Vitamin D, IU	40.0	133.0	100%
Vitamin E, IU	3.0	10.0	100%
Vitamin C, mg	6.0	20.0	100%
Folic Acid, mg	0.04	0.13	100%
Thiamine, mg	0.15	0.5	100%
Riboflavin, mg	0.17	0.57	100%
Niacin, mg	2.0	6.7	100%
Vitamin B_6, mg	0.2	0.67	100%
Vitamin B_{12}, mcg	0.6	2.0	100%
Biotin, mg	0.03	0.1	100%
Pantothenic Acid, mg	1.0	3.3	100%
Vitamin K, mcg	6.7	22.3	*
Choline, mg	7.37	24.6	*

*No US RDA established.

MINERALS	Units/Packet	Units/Liter	% of US RDA in 10 packets
Calcium, gm	0.1	0.33	100%
Phosphorus, gm	0.1	0.33	100%
Iodine, mcg	15.0	50.0	100%
Iron, mg	1.8	6.0	100%
Magnesium, mg	40.0	133.0	100%
Copper, mg	0.2	0.67	100%
Zinc, mg	1.5	5.0	100%

Table V

No. of Packets	Dilute to Volume	Approximate Osmolality
3	1800 ml	370 mOsm/kg
4	2400 ml	370 mOsm/kg
6	2400 ml	510 mOsm/kg
10	3000 ml	810 mOsm/kg

Storage: Store Vivonex HN soluble powder at 68°F or less. In solution Vivonex HN is a perishable liquid food. A full day's supply may be prepared at one time and stored in the refrigerator for up to 24 hours. The diet may be stored in the Vivonex Delivery System in the refrigerator. For complete information, refer to the labeling for the Vivonex Delivery System. Shake the liquid briefly before serving. Once removed from the refrigerator, the diet should be administered within 8 hours.

How Supplied: Ten sealed packets per carton, each packet containing 80 grams (2.82 ounces) of water-soluble powder, yielding 300 kcal.

Precautions: For use only under medical supervision. Do not administer parenterally. Diabetics receiving this diet should be closely monitored. The electrolyte content of the diet is based on requirements of normal adults and should be monitored for patients with electrolyte imbalance. Use during pregnancy or lactation may require supplemental vitamins and minerals. Use for children may require adjusting the daily consumption to meet the Recommended Daily Allowance for the age group involved. Clinical data support nutritional adequacy of exclusive use for up to 4 months.

Please contact your local, Norwich-Eaton representative for further information if you have any questions regarding preparation or feeding, or write Norwich-Eaton Pharmaceuticals, Medical Department, Norwich, NY 13815.

VIVONEX® FLAVOR PACKETS

Mixing Instructions: Put 8-½ ounces of water into a blender; then add the contents of a flavor packet and an 80-gram packet of Vivonex Standard (unflavored) or Vivonex-HN High Nitrogen (unflavored). Blend at medium speed until in solution. Serve ice cold.

Storage: Store Vivonex Flavor Packets away from excessive heat. In normal dilution, Vivonex Elemental Diets are perishable liquid foods and refrigeration is necessary. No more than the amount for a single day should be prepared at a time.

Flavors: Additives for Vivonex Standard (unflavored) and Vivonex High Nitrogen (unflavored) are available in the following four flavors.

Lemon-Lime Flavor
Contributes:
- Calories 8
- Protein .... 0 gram
- Carbohydrate .... 0.77 gram
- Fat .... 0 gram
- Saccharin .... 20 milligrams

Ingredients: Citric acid, dextrose, artificial flavor, saccharin and silicon dioxide.

Osmolality: Standard diet with flavor added —approximately 595 mOsm/kg; High Nitrogen diet with flavor added—approximately 855 mOsm/kg.

Orange-Pineapple Flavor
Contributes:
- Calories 8
- Protein .... 0 gram
- Carbohydrate .... 0.93 gram
- Fat .... 0 gram
- Saccharin .... 20 milligrams

Ingredients: Citric acid, dextrose, artificial flavor, saccharin, ethyl maltol, artificial color, silicon dioxide.

Osmolality: Standard diet with flavor added—approximately 595 mOsm/kg; High Nitrogen diet with flavor added—approximately 855 mOsm/kg.

Strawberry Flavor
Contributes:
- Calories 8
- Protein .... 0 gram
- Carbohydrate .... 1.71 gram
- Fat .... 0 gram
- Saccharin .... 20 milligrams

Ingredients: Dextrose, artificial flavor, citric acid, saccharin, silicon dioxide, artificial color.

Osmolality: Standard diet with flavor added —approximately 595 mOsm/kg; High Nitrogen diet with flavor added—approximately 855 mOsm/kg.

Vanilla Flavor
Contributes:
- Calories 7
- Protein .... 0 gram
- Carbohydrate .... 1.7 grams
- Fat .... 0 gram
- Saccharin .... 20 milligrams

Ingredients: Anhydrous dextrose, artificial flavor, saccharin and silicon dioxide.

Osmolality: Standard diet with flavor added—610 mOsm/kg; High Nitrogen diet with flavor added—850 mOsm/kg.

Nutrition Control Products

Division of Pharmex Inc.
2113 LINCOLN STREET
P.O. BOX 151
HOLLYWOOD, FLORIDA 33022

BETACREST Improved
Super Potency B Complex Formula with Liver, Iron & Vitamin C

(See PDR For Nonprescription Drugs)

BIO–CREST Double Strength Bioflavonoid Complex with Rutin and Vitamin C.

(See PDR For Nonprescription Drugs)

CHELATED MINERALS

(See PDR For Nonprescription Drugs)

LETHOPHEROL® Improved Vitamin E

(See PDR For Nonprescription Drugs)

LEVOID® (L-Thyroxine Sod.) T-4 ℞

Composition: Each cc. injection contains L-thyroxine Sod. 100 mcg.; Sod. Formaldehyde Sulfoxylate 0.1%, Phenol 0.5%, Sod. Hydroxide/Glycine buffer in Water for Injection.

Action and Uses: Whenever thyroid is indicated: Myxedema, simple (non-toxic) goiter, hypothyroidism.

Administration and Dosage: Depending on age, the severity of the condition and the response of the patient, initial dosage is usually 100 mcg. L-thyroxine Sod. 100 mcg. L-Thyroxine Sod. is metabolically equivalent to 1 gr. thyroid extract.

Precautions: Side effects include tachycardia, nervousness and sweating which disappear on reduction of dosage.

Contraindications: Thyrotoxicosis, heart disease and hypertension.

How Supplied: 10 cc. vials, 100 mcg. per cc. for I.M. or I.V. use.

NUTRICOL B-Complex in Safflower oil base

(See PDR For Nonprescription Drugs)

VITACREST® Therapeutic Vitamin Formula with Ferrous Iron and Phosphorus-free Calcium in a Natural Base

(See PDR For Nonprescription Drugs)

ZINC SULFATE

(See PDR For Nonprescription Drugs)

OLC Laboratories, Inc.

99 N.W. MIAMI GRADENS DR.
MIAMI, FLORIDA 33169

TRYPTACIN
(brand of L.Tryptophan)

Description: TRYPTACIN — Chemically, L.Tryptophan, aminoindole-3-propionic acid is white to slightly yellowish white crystals or crystaline powder; taste slightly bitter. When dried, contains not less than 98.5% and not more than 100.5% of L.Tryptophan ($C11_{H12}N202$).

Action and Uses: For oral amino acid therapy. Claimed in latest research to be used as an antidepressant and to induce sleep.

Administration and Dosage: AS A DIETARY SUPPLEMENT; 125 mg—4 times a day, 250 mg—3 to 4 times a day, 500 mg—2 to 4 tablets after evening meal.

How Supplied:

Tablets:	125 mg	(NDC 48558-002)
	250 mg	(NDC 48558-004)
	500 mg	(NDC 48558-001)

Literature Available: Yes.

References:

American Journal Psych. *127*:7—January, 1971
Archives of Gen. Psych. Vol. 31—Sept., 1974
Diseases of the Nervous System, January, 1974
American Journal Psych. *134*:4, April, 1977
New England Journal of Med. Jan. 13, 1977

Obetrol Pharmaceuticals

(Division of Rexar Pharmacal Corp.)
396 ROCKAWAY AVE.
VALLEY STREAM, NY 11581

OBETROL™
OBETROL TABLETS ©

AMPHETAMINES HAVE A HIGH POTENTIAL FOR ABUSE. THEY SHOULD THUS BE TRIED ONLY IN WEIGHT REDUCTION PROGRAMS FOR PATIENTS IN WHOM ALTERNATIVE THERAPY HAS BEEN INEFFECTIVE. ADMINISTRATION OF AMPHETAMINES FOR PROLONGED PERIODS OF TIME IN OBESITY MAY LEAD TO DRUG DEPENDENCE AND MUST BE AVOIDED. PARTICULAR ATTENTION SHOULD BE PAID TO THE POSSIBILITY OF SUBJECTS OBTAINING AMPHETAMINES FOR NON-THERAPEUTIC USE OR DISTRIBUTION TO OTHERS, AND THE DRUGS SHOULD BE PRESCRIBED OR DISPENSED SPARINGLY.

Description: A single entity amphetamine product combining the neutral sulfate salts of dextroamphetamine and amphetamine, with the dextro isomer of amphetamine saccharate and d, l amphetamine aspartate.

Actions: Amphetamines are sympathomimetic amines with CNS stimulant activity. Peripheral actions include elevation of systolic and diastolic blood pressures and weak bronchodilator and respiratory stimulant action. Drugs of this class used in obesity are commonly known as "anorectics" or "anorexigenics". It has not been established, however, that the action of such drugs in treating obesity is primarily one of appetite suppression. Other central nervous system actions, or metabolic effects, may be involved, for example.

Continued on next page

Obetrol—Cont.

Adult obese subjects instructed in dietary management and treated with "anorectic" drugs, lose more weight on the average than those treated with placebo and diet, as determined in relatively short-term clinical trials.
The magnitude of increased weight loss of drug-treated patients over placebo-treated patients is only a fraction of a pound a week. The rate of weight loss is greatest in the first weeks of therapy for both drug and placebo subjects and tends to decrease in succeeding weeks. The origins of the increased weight loss due to the various possible drug effects are not established. The amount of weight loss associated with the use of an "anorectic" drug varies from trial to trial, and the increased weight loss appears to be related in part to variables other than the drug prescribed, such as the physician-investigator, the population treated, and the diet prescribed. Studies do not permit conclusions as to the relative importance of the drug and non-drug factors on weight loss.
The natural history of obesity is measured in years, whereas the studies cited are restricted to a few weeks duration; thus, the total impact of drug-induced weight loss over that of diet alone must be considered clinically limited.
There is neither specific evidence which clearly establishes the mechanism whereby Amphetamine products its mental and behavioral effects in children, nor conclusive evidence regarding how these effects relate to the condition of the central nervous system.
Indications: Amphetamine is indicated as an integral part of a total treatment program which typically includes other remedial measures (psychological, educational, social) for a stabilizing effect in children with a behavioral syndrome characterized by the following group of developmentally inappropriate symptoms: moderate to severe distractibility, short attention span, hyperactivity, emotional lability, and impulsivity. The diagnosis of this syndrome should not be made with finality when these symptoms are only of comparatively recent origin. Nonlocalizing (soft) neurological signs, learning disability and abnormal EEG may or may not be present, and a diagnosis of central nervous system dysfunction may or may not be warranted.
Exogenous Obesity as a short-term (a few weeks) adjunct in a regimen of weight reduction based on caloric restriction, for patients refractory to alternative therapy, e.g., repeated diets, group programs, and other drugs. The limited usefulness of amphetamines (see ACTIONS) should be weighed against possible risks inherent in use of the drug, such as those described below.
Narcolepsy
Contraindications: Advanced arteriosclerosis, symptomatic cardiovascular disease, moderate to severe hypertension, hyperthyroidism, known hypersensitivity or idiosyncrasy to the sympathomimetic amines, glaucoma.
Agitated states.
Patients with a history of drug abuse.
During or within 14 days following administration of monoamine oxidase inhibitors (hypertensive crises may result).
Warnings: When tolerance to the "anorectic" effect develops, the recommended dose should not be exceeded in an attempt to increase the effect; rather, the drug should be discontinued. Amphetamines may impair the ability of the patient to engage in potentially hazardous activities such as operating machinery or driving a motor vehicle; the patient should therefore be cautioned accordingly.
Clinical experience suggest that in psychotic children, administration of Amphetamine may exacerbate symptoms of behavior disturbance and thought disorder.
Data are inadequate to determine whether chronic administration of Amphetamine may be associated with growth inhibition; therefore, growth should be monitored during treatment.
Drug Dependence: Amphetamines have been extensively abused. Tolerance, extreme psychological dependence, and severe social disability have occurred. There are reports of patients who have increased the dosage to many times that recommended. Abrupt cessation following prolonged high dosage administration results in extreme fatigue and mental depression; changes are also noted on the sleep EEG. Manifestations of chronic intoxication with amphetamines include severe dermatoses, marked insomnia, irritability, hyperactivity, and personality changes. The most severe manifestation of chronic intoxication is psychosis, often clinically indistinguishable from schizophrenia.
Usage in Pregnancy: Safe use in pregnancy has not been established. Reproduction studies in mammals at high multiples of the human dose have suggested both an embryotoxic and a teratogenic potential. Use of amphetamines by women who are or who may become pregnant, and especially those in the first trimester of pregnancy, requires that the potential benefit be weighed against the possible hazard to mother and infant.
Usage in Children: Amphetamines are not recommended for use as anorectic agents in children under 12 years of age.
Precautions: Drug treatment is not indicated in all cases of this behavioral syndrome and should be considered only in light of the complete history and evaluation of the child. The decision to prescribe Amphetamine should depend on the physician's assessment of the chronicity and severity of the child's symptoms and their appropriateness for his/her age. Prescription should not depend solely on the presence of one or more of the behavioral characteristics.
When these symptoms are associated with acute stress reactions, treatment with Amphetamine is usually not indicated.
Long term effects of Amphetamine in children have not been well-established.
Caution is to be exercised in prescribing amphetamines for patients with even mild hypertension.
Insulin requirements in diabetes mellitus may be altered in association with the use of amphetamines and the concomitant dietary regimen.
Amphetamines may decrease the hypotensive effect of guanethidine.
The least amount feasible should be prescribed or dispensed at one time in order to minimize the possibility of overdosage.
Adverse Reactions:
Cardiovascular: Palpitation, tachycardia, elevation of blood pressure.
Central nervous system: Overstimulation, restlessness, dizziness, insomnia, euphoria, dysphoria, tremor, headache; rarely, psychotic episodes at recommended doses.
Gastrointestinal: Dryness of the mouth, unpleasant taste, diarrhea, constipation, other gastrointestinal disturbances. Anorexia and weight loss may occur as undesirable effects when amphetamines are used for other than the anorectic effect.
Allergic: Urticaria.
Endocrine: Impotence, changes in libido.
Dosage and Administration: Regardless of indication, amphetamines should be administered at the lowest effective dosage and dosage should be individually adjusted. Late evening medication should be avoided because of the resulting insomnia.

1. Narcolepsy: Usual dose 5 to 60 milligrams per day in divided doses.
2. Hyperkinesis:
   a. Not recommended for children under 3 years of age.
   b. Children from 3 to 5 years of age: 2.5 milligrams daily, raised in increments of 2.5 milligrams at weekly intervals until optimal response is obtained.
   c. Children 6 years of age and older: 5 milligrams once or twice daily, increased in increments of 5 milligrams at weekly intervals. Only in rare cases will it be necessary to exceed a total of 40 milligrams per day.
   Where possible, drug administration should be interrupted occasionally to determine if there is a recurrence of behavioral symptoms sufficient to require continued therapy.
3. Obesity: Usual adult dose 5 to 30 milligrams per day in divided doses.

Overdosage: Manifestations of acute overdosage with amphetamines include restlessness, tremor, hyperreflexia, rapid respiration, confusion, assaultiveness, hallucinations, panic states.
Fatigue and depression usually follow the central stimulation.
Cardiovascular effects include arrhythmias, hypertension or hypotension and circulatory collapse. Gastrointestinal symptoms include nausea, vomiting, diarrhea, and abdominal cramps. Fatal poisoning usually terminates in convulsions and coma.
Management of acute amphetamine intoxication is largely symptomatic and includes lavage and sedation with a barbiturate. Experience with hemodialysis or peritoneal dialysis is inadequate to permit recommendation in this regard. Acidification of the urine increases amphetamine excretion. Intravenous phentolamine (Regitine) has been suggested for possible acute, severe hypertension, if this complicates amphetamine overdosage.
Caution: FEDERAL LAW PROHIBITS DISPENSING WITHOUT PRESCRIPTION.
How Supplied:
OBETROL TABLETS

Each tablet contains:	10 mg.	20 mg.
Dextroamphetamine Saccharate	2.5 mg.	5 mg.
Amphetamine Aspartate	2.5 mg.	5 mg.
Dextroamphetamine Sulfate	2.5 mg.	5 mg.
Amphetamine Sulfate	2.5 mg.	5 mg.

Available in bottles of 100's, 500's and 1000's.
LC-NDC-0477 November 1978
[*Shown in Product Identification Section*]

O'Neal, Jones & Feldman Pharmaceuticals
2510 METRO BLVD.
MARYLAND HEIGHTS MO 63043

ANTILIRIUM AMPULES ℞
(physostigmine salicylate)

Each ml. contains:
Physostigmine Salicylate .... 1 mg.
Description: ANTILIRIUM (physostigmine salicylate) is OJF's brand of physostigmine salicylate.
Action: ANTILIRIUM (physostigmine salicylate) is a salicylic acid derivative of an alkaloid extracted from seeds of Physostigma Venenosum (calabar bean). The action of the parasympathetic nerves is intermediated by the formation of acetylcholine at the peripheral end of these nerves. The action of acetylcholine is normally very fleeting because of its hydrolysis by a specific enzyme. Physostigmine inhibits the destructive action of cholinesterase and thereby prolongs and exaggerates the effect of the acetylcholine. The changes in body function which are produced by the injection of physostigmine are, therefore, very similar to those which would occur from simultaneous stimulation of the parasympathetic nerves and include contraction of the pupil, increased tonus of the intestinal musculature, constriction

of the bronchi and stimulation of secretion of the salivary and sweat glands.
Indications: To reverse the toxic effects upon the central nervous system caused by drugs in clinical or toxic dosages capable of producing anticholinergic poisoning. Central toxic effects include:
Hallucinations
Delirium
Disorientation
Anxiety
Hyperactivity
Severe anticholinergic poisoning may produce:
Coma
Medullary Paralysis
Death
Contraindications: Physostigmine salicylate injections should not be used in the presence of asthma, gangrene, diabetes, cardiovascular disease, mechanical obstruction of the intestines or urogenital tract or any vagotonic state, and in patients receiving choline esters or depolarizing neuromuscular blocking agents (decamethonium, succinylcholine).
Warning: If excessive symptoms of salivation, emesis, urination and defecation occur, the use of ANTILIRIUM should be terminated. If excessive sweating or nausea occur, the dosage should be reduced.
Intravenous administration should be at a slow, controlled rate, no more than 1 mg. per minute (see dosage). Rapid administration can cause bradycardia, hypersalivation leading to respiratory difficulties and possibly convulsions.
An overdosage of ANTILIRIUM can cause a cholinergic crisis.
Precautions: Because of the possibility of hypersensitivity in an occasional patient, atropine sulfate injection should always be at hand since it is an antagonist and antidote for physostigmine.
Administration and Dosage: The usual adult dose of ANTILIRIUM is 0.5 to 2.0 mg. intramuscularly or intravenously. Intravenous administration should be at a slow, controlled rate of no more than 1 mg. per minute. It may be necessary to repeat dosages of 1 mg. to 4 mg. at intervals as life threatening signs such as arrhythmias, convulsions and deep coma recur. Physostigmine salicylate is rapidly metabolized in the body.
IN ALL CASES OF POISONING, THE USUAL SUPPORTIVE MEASURES SHOULD BE UNDERTAKEN.
How Supplied: 2 ml. ampules, packed 12 ampules per box.

BANALG® LINIMENT — OTC

Composition: Menthol, Camphor, Methyl Salicylate, and Eucalyptus Oil in a nongreasy base.
Action and Uses: For minor muscular aches and pains, athletic soreness, and temporary relief of minor pains of arthritis and rheumatism. Mild, effective, nongreasy, pleasant to use, quick action; no bandage needed.
Administration: Apply with gentle massage several times daily, or as needed.
Caution: If pain persists for more than 10 days, or redness is present, or in conditions affecting children under 12 years of age, consult a physician immediately. Do not apply covering or heat.
Warning: Keep out of the reach of children to avoid accidental poisoning.
Precautions: Avoid getting into eyes or on mucous membranes. Discontinue use if excessive irritation of the skin develops.

BANCAP CAPSULES — ℞
BANCAP c̄ CODEINE CAPSULES ©

BANCAP CAPSULES
Each capsule contains:
Salicylamide .... 200 mg.
Acetaminophen .... 300 mg.

BANCAP c̄ CODEINE CAPSULES
Each capsule contains:
Salicylamide .... 200 mg.
Acetaminophen .... 300 mg.
Codeine phosphate .... (½ gr.) 32 mg.
(Warning: May be habit forming)
Indications: BANCAP Capsules provide effective analgesia in a wide variety of conditions including headache, dysmenorrhea, myalgia, neuralgia and neuritis, toothache, pain following dental procedures, bursitis, arthritis and rheumatism as well as other conditions involving musculoskeletal pain. BANCAP Capsules are also indicated as an analgesic and antipyretic in diseases accompanied by minor pain and fever, such as the common cold, "flu", and other viral infections. BANCAP Capsules are especially useful in patients who must avoid the gastric irritation of aspirin while being treated for peptic ulcers, acute and chronic gastritis and those on steroid therapy. In conditions where pain is more severe, BANCAP c̄ CODEINE Capsules are indicated for a greater degree of analgesia. BANCAP c̄ CODEINE Capsules are also indicated as an analgesic-antipyretic-antitussive in the acute cold, cough, and other acute respiratory diseases.
Contraindications: BANCAP c̄ CODEINE Capsules are contraindicated in those patients sensitive to codeine.
Precautions: BANCAP Capsules have rarely been asssociated with the production of any side effects such as gastric discomfort. If a rare sensitivity reaction should occur, such as urticaria, dizziness, redness or itching, the drug should be discontinued.
Due to the codeine component of BANCAP c̄ CODEINE Capsules possible nausea, vomiting or constipation may occur. Dosage in excess of two BANCAP c̄ CODEINE Capsules may cause excitability.
Dosage: Adults and children over 12 years, one or two BANCAP capsules every 4 hours as needed. One or two BANCAP c̄ CODEINE Capsules every 4 hours as required.

CETANE TIMED CAPSULES® — OTC
(Ascorbic Acid U.S.P. 500 mg. – Timed Disintegrating)

Directions: One capsule daily as a dietary supplement.
How Supplied:
Bottles of 100 NDC 0456-0710-01
Bottles of 1000 NDC 0456-0710-00

CETANE INJECTION — ℞
(Vitamin C)
Ascorbic Acid and Sodium Ascorbate with and without preservative

How Supplied:
30 ml. vial 500 mg/ml.
Ascorbic Acid without preservative
50 ml. vial 250 mg/ml.
Sodium Ascorbate without preservative
30 ml. vial 250 mg/ml.
Sodium Ascorbate with preservative
30 ml. vial 250 mg/ml.
Sodium Ascorbate without preservative

DURADYNE DHC TABLET — © ℞

Each green, scored tablet contains:
Hydrocodone Bitartrate .... 5 mg.
(Warning: May be habit forming)
Aspirin .... 230 mg.
Acetaminophen .... 150 mg.
Caffeine .... 30 mg.
Action: Hydrocodone the principal ingredient of Duradyne DHC, has similar narcotic analgesic action to codeine, except it is more potent, and combines with the non-narcotic analgesic—antipyretic actions of aspirin and acetaminophen.
Indications: For continual relief of pain from moderate to severe, caused by headache and muscloskeletal problems.
Contraindications: Do not use in patients sensitive to any ingredient.
Warning: Drug Dependence: Hydrocodone like narcotics such as morphine, can be habit forming and can cause drug dependence if administered repeatedly. The same caution should be exercised as with other oral narcotic preparations.
Ambulatory Patients: Patient should be advised that mental and physical abilities required for driving a car or operating machinery may be impaired.
Pregnancy: Safe usage during pregnancy has not been established by formal clinical procedures.
Central Nervous System: Additive CNS depression may occur if used concurrently with other narcotic analgesics, tranquilizers, sedatives, or other CNS depressants. Any combined therapy should be carefully scrutinized by the physician.
Precautions: Care should be exercised that the depressant effects of narcotics do not interfere with the clinical care of patients with head injuries, or that the narcotic effects do not hide the diagnosis of severe abdominal conditions.
Adverse Reactions: Reactions that may occur include drowsiness, nausea, miosis, and vomiting, and constipation.
Dosage and Administration: Severity of pain and patient response should be taken into consideration, if it is necessary to exceed the recommended dosage, also the patient tolerance to oral narcotics.
For Adults: One or two tablets every four to six hours.
DEA Classification: Duradyne DHC is classified as a Schedule III Controlled Drug. Available on oral prescription, and may be refilled up to five times in six months, unless restricted by state law.

E-FEROL CAPSULES — OTC
(Vitamin E)
d-Alpha Tocopherol Acetate (Natural) and also d-Alpha Tocopherol Succinate (Natural)

How Supplied:

Acetate Capsules (SG)	Succinate Capsules (HS)
100 Int. Units	100 Int. Units
Bottles of 100's	
200 Int. Units	200 Int. Units
400 Int. Units	400 Int. Units
Bottles of 100's - 500's	

Ointment: 1 ½ oz. tubes, 2 oz. jars
Injectable: 200 mg./ml., 10 ml. vial

FEOSTAT Tablets — OTC
FEOSTAT Suspension
FEOSTAT Drops
(Ferrous Fumarate)

FEOSTAT Tablets
Each chocolate-flavored chewable tablet contains:
Ferrous fumarate .... 100 mg.
(Elemental iron .... 33 mg.)

FEOSTAT Suspension
Each 5 cc. (teaspoonful) contains:
Ferrous fumarate .... 100 mg.
(Elemental iron .... 33 mg.)

FEOSTAT Drops
Each 12 drops (0.6 cc.) contains:
Ferrous fumarate .... 45 mg.
(Elemental iron .... 15 mg.)

Actions and Uses: FEOSTAT products are convenient and pleasant tasting dosage forms of iron for the oral treatment of iron deficiency anemia in adults, children and infants.

Continued on next page

O'Neal, Jones & Feldman—Cont.

Administration and Dosage:
FEOSTAT Tablets
Adults: One tablet, one to four times daily.
Children 5 to 12 years: One tablet, one to three times daily.
FEOSTAT Suspension
Adults: 1 teaspoonful, one to four times daily.
Children 1 to 5 years: ½ teaspoonful, one to four times daily.
FEOSTAT Drops
Children under 1 year and infants: One to four drops, one to four times daily.
FEOSTAT products rarely produce side effects; however, diarrhea, constipation, stained teeth and gastric discomfort occasionally appear.
Warning: Discontinue if any symptoms of intolerance occur. Iron-containing products occasionally cause constipation or diarrhea. Oral iron products interfere with absorption of oral tetracycline antibiotics; these products should not be taken within two hours of each other.

IODO-NIACIN® TABLETS ℞

Each controlled action tablet contains:

Potassium Iodide	135 mg.
Niacinamide Hydroiodide	25 mg.

Indications: To facilitate cough and bronchial drainage in chronic bronchitis, bronchiectasis and asthma. For the prophylaxis of goiter and in the management of certain phases of hyperthyroidism.
Contraindications: Hypersensitivity or idiosyncrasy to iodides and in hyperkalemic states.
Precautions: Iodides should be administered with caution during pregnancy since iodides have been associated with abnormal thyroid function and/or goiter in the newborn. Iodides should be given with utmost caution, if at all, in the presence of tuberculosis.
Side Effects: Serious adverse side effects from the use of IODO-NIACIN are uncommon. Symptoms of iodism such as metallic taste, fever, skin rash, mucous membrane ulceration, salivary gland swelling, and gastric distress have occurred occasionally. These generally subside promptly when the drug is discontinued. Pulmonary tuberculosis is considered a contraindication to the use of iodides by some authorities, and the drug should be used with caution in such cases. Rare cases of goiter with hypothyroidism have been reported in adults who had taken iodides over a prolonged period of time, and in newborn infants whose mothers had taken iodides for prolonged periods. The signs and symptoms regressed spontaneously after iodides were discontinued. The causal relationship and exact mechanism of action of iodides in this phenomenon are unknown. Appropriate precautions should be followed in pregnancy and in individuals receiving IODO-NIACIN for prolonged periods.
Dosage: The average oral dose for adults is two tablets three times daily after meals taken with a glass of water. For children over eight years, one tablet after meals with water. The dosage should be individualized according to the needs of the patient on long-term therapy.
[*Shown in Product Identification Section*]

PEDAMETH® CAPSULE ℞
PEDAMETH® LIQUID ℞
(methionine)

Composition:
CAPSULES—200 mg. methionine.
LIQUID—75 mg. methionine per 5 cc. (teaspoon) in a fruit flavored base.
Indications:
CAPSULES—Control of urine odor, dermatitis and ulcerations caused by ammoniacal urine in the incontinent adult patient.
LIQUID—Diaper rash caused by ammoniacal urine.
Contraindication: Do not administer to patients with history of liver disease as large doses of methionine may exaggerate the toxemia of the disease.
Precautions: It has been pointed out by Goldstein and in animal studies that excessive dosage of methionine, added alone to the diet over extended periods, may result in a weight gain below normal when protein intake is insufficient. Thus, it is essential that adequate protein intake be maintained during therapy and that recommended dosage not be exceeded. Methionine should not be administered on an empty stomach.
Dosage and Administration:
Capsules—Adults: one capsule three or four times a day after meals.
Liquid—Infants: 2 months to 6 months—one teaspoon (5 cc.) three times per day for 3-5 days. May be added to formula, milk or juice; 6 months to 14 months—one teaspoon (5 cc.) four times per day for 3-5 days. In severe cases it may be necessary to double the dosage the first two days of treatment.
[*Shown in Product Identification Section*]

VERAZINC CAPSULES OTC
(Zinc Sulfate 220 mg.)

Composition: Each Pink and Blue capsule contains 220 mg. of Zinc sulfate (50 mg. elemental Zinc).
Actions and Uses: Nutritional Supplement.
Administration and Dosage: Adult dose (12 years and older)-one capsule daily with meal.
Precautions: As with all Zinc Sulfate, it is possible for nausea or vomiting to occur; discontinue use of capsule.
How Supplied:
Bottles of 100
Bottles of 1000

Organon Pharmaceuticals
A Division of Organon Inc
375 MT. PLEASANT AVE.
WEST ORANGE, NJ 07052

COTAZYM® ℞
(Pancrelipase, NF)

Description: Cotazym (Pancrelipase, NF) is a concentrate of pancreatic enzymes of porcine origin with standardized lipase activity. Each capsule (regular or cherry flavored) and each ¼ (.43g) teaspoon of Cotazym Powder contains:
Lipase-
8,000 NF Units
Protease-
30,000 NF Units
Amylase-
30,000 NF Units
plus other enzymes from whole hog pancreas with calcium carbonate, precipitated, USP, 25 mg. In addition to steapsin (lipase) sufficient to digest 17 Gm dietary fat, Cotazym (Pancrelipase, NF) provides protease, sufficient to digest 34 Gm dietary protein; and amylase, sufficient to digest 40 Gm dietary starch.
Each regular packet contains:
Lipase-
16,000 NF Units
Protease-
60,000 NF Units
Amylase-
60,000 NF Units
plus other enzymes from whole hog pancreas with calcium carbonate, precipitated, USP 50 mg.
Each cherry flavored packet contains:
Lipase-
40,000 NF Units
Protease-
150,000 NF Units
Amylase-
150,000 NF Units
plus other enzymes from whole hog pancreas with calcium carbonate, precipitated, USP 50 mg.
Indications: It is indicated in conditions where pancreatic enzymes are absent from or present in insufficient amount in the intestine (pancreatectomy, chronic pancreatitis with insufficiency), cystic fibrosis, steatorrhea, and in conditions in which fat digestion is inadequate due to deficiency of pancreatic enzymes.
Dosage: 1 to 3 capsules, ¼ to ¾ (.43g to 1.29g) teaspoons or 1 or 2 packets just prior to each meal or snack or as directed by physician. It should be used with caution in patients known to be sensitive to pork.
Precautions: A proper balance between fat, protein and starch intake must be maintained to avoid temporary indigestion. A careful ratio of Cotazym (Pancrelipase, NF) dosage to food intake is desirable. Use with caution in patients sensitive to pork protein.
How Supplied: Capsules (regular) bottles of 100 and 500. NDC # 0052-0381-91, NDC # 0052-0381-95
Capsules (cherry flavored) bottles of 100. NDC # 0052-0386-91
Powder bottles of 4 oz (113.5g) and 8 oz. (227g). NDC # 0052-0380-04, NDC # 0052-0380-08
Packets (regular) boxes of 250. NDC # 0052-0382-95
Packets (cherry flavored) boxes of 100. NDC # 0052-0387-92
[*Shown in Product Identification Section*]

DECA-DURABOLIN® ℞
(nandrolone decanoate injection N.F.)

Description: Deca-Durabolin is nandrolone decanoate, a long-acting anabolic agent, dissolved in sesame oil for intramuscular injection. Chemically it is 19 nor-Δ^4-androstene-17 beta-ol-3-one-decanoate.
Action: Anabolic steroids are synthetic derivatives of testosterone. The action of Deca-Durabolin (nandrolone decanoate injection N.F.) is primarily anabolic (protein sparing). It promotes body tissue-building processes and reverses catabolic or tissue depleting processes. Nitrogen balance is improved with anabolic agents but only when there is sufficient intake of calories and protein. Whether this positive nitrogen balance is of primary benefit in the utilization of protein building dietary substances has not been established.
Certain clinical effects and adverse reactions demonstrate the androgenic properties of this class of drugs. The deletion of the CH3 group from the C-19-position has resulted in reduction of its androgenic properties and retention and enhancement of its anabolic, tissue-building properties. Thus it is possible to employ doses that provide significant anabolic effects without undesired androgenic effects. Complete dissociation of anabolic and androgenic effects has not been achieved. The actions of anabolic steroids are therefore similar to those of male sex hormones with the possibility of causing serious disturbances of growth and sexual development if given to young children. Anabolic steroids suppress the gonadotropic functions of the pituitary and may exert a direct effect upon the testis.

Indications:
Based on a review of this drug by the National Academy of Sciences, National Research Council and/or other information, FDA has classified the indication(s) as follows:
Probably Effective: As adjunctive therapy in senile and post-menopausal osteoporosis. Anabolic steroids are without value as primary therapy but may be of value as adjunctive therapy. Equal or greater con-

sideration should be given to diet, calcium balance, physiotherapy and good general health-promoting measures. In pituitary dwarfism anabolic agents may be used with care until growth hormone is more available.
Possibly Effective: In the treatment of those conditions in which a potent tissue-building or protein-sparing action is desired (eg. pre and post surgical care, burns), in the control of metastatic breast cancer and as adjuvant therapy of certain types of refractory anemia.
Final classification of the less than effective indications require further investigation.

Contraindications:
1. Male patients with carcinoma of the prostate or breast.
2. Carcinoma of the breast in some females.
3. Pregnancy, because of masculinization of the fetus.
4. Nephrosis or the nephrotic phase of nephritis.

Warning: Anabolic steroids do not enhance athletic ability.

Precautions:
1. Hypercalcemia may develop both spontaneously and as a result of hormonal therapy in women with disseminated breast carcinoma. If it develops while on this agent, the drug should be stopped.
2. Caution is required in administering these agents to patients with cardiac, renal or hepatic disease. Edema may occur occasionally. Concomitant administration with adrenal steroids or ACTH may add to the edema.
3. If amenorrhea or menstrual irregularities develop the drug should be discontinued until the etiology is determined.
4. Anabolic steroids may increase sensitivity to oral anticoagulants. Dosage of the anticoagulant may have to be decreased in order to maintain the prothrombin time at the desired therapeutic level.
5. Anabolic steroids have been shown to alter glucose tolerance tests. Diabetics should be followed carefully and the insulin or oral hypoglycemic dosage adjusted accordingly.
6. Anabolic steroids should be used with caution in patients with benign prostatic hypertrophy.
7. Serum cholesterol may increase during therapy. Therefore, caution is required in administering these agents to patients with a history of myocardial infarction or coronary artery disease. Serial determinations of serum cholesterol should be made and therapy adjusted accordingly.

Adverse Reactions:
1. In Males
   a. Prepubertal
      1) Phallic enlargement
      2) Increased frequency of erections
   b. Post-pubertal
      1) Inhibition of testicular function and oligospermia
      2) Gynecomastia
2. In Females
   a. Hirsutism, male pattern baldness, deepening of the voice and clitoral enlargement. These changes are usually irreversible even after prompt discontinuance of therapy and are not prevented by concomitant use of estrogens.
   b. Menstrual irregularities
   c. Masculinization of the fetus.
3. In Both Sexes
   a. Nausea
   b. Increased or decreased libido
   c. Acne (especially in females and prepubertal males)
   d. Inhibition of gonadotropin secretion.
   e. Bleeding in patients on concomitant anticoagulant therapy.
   f. Premature closure of epiphysis in children.
4. Alterations in these clinical laboratory tests:
   a. The metyrapone test.
   b. Glucose tolerance test.
   c. The thyroid function tests: a decrease in the PBI, in thyroxine-binding capacity and radioactive iodine uptake.
   d. The electrolytes: retention of sodium, chlorides, water, potassium, phosphates and calcium.
   e. Liver function tests:
      1) Increased serum cholesterol.
      2) Suppression of clotting factors II, V, VII, AND X.
5. There have been rare reports of hepatocellular neoplasms and peliosis hepatis in association with long-term androgenic-anabolic steroid therapy.

Dosage and Administration: Deca-Durabolin (nandrolone decanoate injection N.F.) is intended for deep intramuscular injection into the gluteal muscle preferably. For general anabolic effects in adults, the average dosage recommended is 50 to 100 mg. every 3 to 4 weeks. For children from two to thirteen years of age, the average dose is 25 to 50 mg. every three to four weeks.
Higher doses may be required for the treatment of severe disease states such as metastatic breast cancer, refractory anemias, etc. The recommended dose is 100 to 200 mg. weekly based on therapeutic response, and consideration of the benefit-to-risk ratio.
Duration of therapy will depend on the response of the condition and the appearance of adverse reactions. If possible, therapy should be intermittent.
Deca-Durabolin should be regarded as adjunctive therapy and adequate quantities of nutrients should be consumed in order to obtain maximal therapeutic effects. When it is used in the treatment of refractory anemias, for example, adequate iron intake is required for a maximal response.

Supplied: Deca-Durabolin (in sterile sesame oil solution for intramuscular injection) is available in a potency of 50 mg./ml. with 10% benzyl alcohol (preservative):
1 ml. ampuls, box of 4. NDC 0052-0696-14
2 ml. multiple dose vial. NDC 0052-0696-02
1 ml. prefilled Rediject® syringe. NDC 0052-0696-71
Also available in a potency of 100 mg./ml. with 10% benzyl alcohol (preservative):
2 ml. multiple dose vial. NDC 0052-0697-02
1 ml. prefilled Rediject® syringe. NDC 0052-0697-71
2 ml. prefilled Rediject® syringe. NDC 0052-0697-72

DURABOLIN® ℞
(nandrolone phenpropionate injection, N.F.)

Description: Durabolin is nandrolone phenpropionate injection N.F. Chemically it is 19 nor-Δ^4- androstene- 17β-ol-3-one-β-phenylpropionate.

Actions: Anabolic steroids are synthetic derivatives of testosterone. The action of Durabolin (nandrolone phenpropionate) is primarily anabolic (protein-sparing). It promotes body tissue-building processes and reverses catabolic or tissue depleting processes. Nitrogen balance is improved with anabolic agents but only when there is sufficient intake of calories and protein. Whether this positive nitrogen balance is of primary benefit in the utilization of protein building dietary substances has not been established.
Certain clinical effects and adverse reactions demonstrate the androgenic properties of this class of drugs. The deletion of the CH3 group from the C-19-position has resulted in reduction of its androgenic properties and retention and enhancement of its anabolic, tissue-building properties. Thus it is possible to employ doses that provide significant anabolic effects without undesired androgenic effects. Complete dissociation of anabolic and androgenic effects has not been achieved. The actions of anabolic steroids are therefore similar to those of male sex hormones with the possibility of causing serious disturbances of growth and sexual development if given to young children. Anabolic steroids suppress the gonadotropic functions of the pituitary and may exert a direct effect upon the testis.

Indications:
Based on a review of this drug by the National Academy of Sciences, National Research Council and/or other information, FDA has classified the indications as follows:
Effective: Control of metastatic breast cancer.
Probably Effective: As adjunctive therapy in senile and postmenopausal osteoporosis. Anabolic steroids are without value as primary therapy but may be of value as adjunctive therapy. Equal or greater consideration should be given to diet, calcium balance, physiotherapy and good health promoting measures. In pituitary dwarfism anabolic agents may be used with care until growth hormone is more available.
Possibly Effective: For conditions in which a potent tissue building or protein sparing action is desired (eg., pre and post surgical care, burns), uremia and as adjuvant therapy of certain types of refractory anemia.
Final classification of the less than effective indications requires further investigation.

Contraindications:
1. Male patients with carcinoma of the prostate or breast.
2. Carcinoma of the breast in some females.
3. Pregnancy, because of masculinization of the fetus.
4. Nephrosis or the nephrotic phase of nephritis.

Warning: Anabolic steroids do not enhance athletic ability.

Precautions:
1. Hypercalcemia may develop both spontaneously and as a result of hormonal therapy in women with disseminated breast carcinoma. If it develops while on this agent, the drug should be stopped.
2. Caution is required in administering these agents to patients with cardiac, renal or hepatic disease. Edema may occur occasionally. Concomitant administration with adrenal steroids or ACTH may add to the edema.
3. If amenorrhea or menstrual irregularities develop the drug should be discontinued until the etiology is determined.
4. Anabolic steroids may increase sensitivity to oral anticoagulants. Dosage of the anticoagulant may have to be decreased in order to maintain the prothrombin time at the desired therapeutic level.
5. Anabolic steroids have been shown to alter glucose tolerance tests. Diabetics should be followed carefully and the insulin or oral hypoglycemic dosage adjusted accordingly.
6. Anabolic steroids should be used with caution in patients with benign prostatic hypertrophy.
7. Serum cholesterol may increase during therapy. Therefore, caution is required in administering these agents to patients with a history of myocardial infarction or coronary artery disease. Serial determi-

Continued on next page

Organon—Cont.

nations of serum cholesterol should be made and therapy adjusted accordingly.

Adverse Reactions:

1. In Males
   a. Prepubertal.
      1) Phallic enlargement
      2) Increased frequency of erections
   b. Post-pubertal.
      1) Inhibition of testicular function and oligospermia
      2) Gynecomastia
2. In Females
   a. Hirsutism, male pattern baldness, deepening of the voice and clitoral enlargement. These changes are usually irreversible even after prompt discontinuance of therapy and are not prevented by concomitant use of estrogens.
   b. Menstrual irregularities.
   c. Masculinization of the fetus.
3. In Both Sexes
   a. Nausea.
   b. Increased or decreased libido.
   c. Acne (especially in females and prepubertal males).
   d. Inhibition of gonadotropin secretion.
   e. Bleeding in patients on concomitant anticoagulant therapy.
   f. Premature closure of epiphysis in children.
4. Alterations in these clinical laboratory tests:
   a. The metyrapone test.
   b. Glucose tolerance test.
   c. The thyroid function tests: a decrease in the PBI, in thyroxine-binding capacity and radioactive iodine uptake.
   d. The electrolytes: retention of sodium, chlorides, water, potassium, phosphates and calcium.
   e. Liver function tests:
      1) Increased serum cholesterol.
      2) Suppression of clotting factors II, V, VII, AND X.
5. There have been rare reports of hepatocellular neoplasms and peliosis hepatis in association with long-term androgenic-anabolic steroid therapy.

Dosage and Administration: Durabolin (nandrolone phenpropionate injection, N.F.) is intended for deep intramuscular injection into the gluteal muscle preferably. For general anabolic effects in adults the recommended dose is 25 to 50 mg. weekly. For children from two to thirteen years of age the recommended dose is 12.5 to 25 mg. every two to four weeks.

Higher doses may be required for the treatment of severe disease states such as metastatic breast cancer, refractory anemias, etc. The recommended dose is 50 to 100 mg. weekly based on therapeutic response and consideration of the benefit-to-risk ratio. Duration of therapy will depend on the response of the condition and the appearance of adverse reactions. If possible, therapy should be intermittent.

Durabolin should be regarded as adjunctive therapy and adequate quantities of nutrients should be consumed in order to obtain maximal therapeutic effects. When it is used in the treatment of refractory anemias, for example, adequate iron intake is required for a maximal response.

Supplied: Durabolin (in sterile sesame oil solution for intramuscular injection) is available in a strength of 25 mg. per ml. in 5 ml. vials NDC 0052-0691-05 and 1 ml. ampuls NDC 0052-0691-13, with 5% benzyl alcohol and as Durabolin-50 containing 50 mg. per ml. in 2 ml. vials with 10% benzyl alcohol, NDC 0052-0695-02

HEXADROL® ℞
(dexamethasone U.S.P.)

Description: Hexadrol (dexamethasone U.S.P.) is an analogue of prednisolone. Its spectrum of anti-inflammatory activity is similar to other corticosteroids but it is clinically effective in much lower doses. Unlike earlier corticosteroids it has the added advantage of lacking significant mineralocorticoid activity so that salt and water retention are rarely observed. Dexamethasone, $C_{22}H_{29}FO_5$, has a molecular weight of 392.47, its chemical name is Pregna-1, 4-diene-3, 20-dione, 9 fluoro-11, 17, 21-trihydroxy-16-methyl-(11 β, 16 α). It is white to practically white crystalline powder which is practically insoluble in water and melts at about 250°C (with decomposition).

Actions: Naturally occurring glucocorticoids (hydrocortisone and cortisone), which also have salt-retaining properties, are used as replacement therapy in adrenocortical deficiency states. Their synthetic analogs are primarily used for their potent anti-inflammatory effects in disorders of many organ systems.

Glucocorticoids cause profound and varied metabolic effects. In addition, they modify the body's immune responses to diverse stimuli.

Indications:

1. Endocrine Disorders:
   Primary or secondary adrenocortical insufficiency (hydrocortisone or cortisone is the first choice; synthetic analogs may be used in conjunction with mineralocorticoids where applicable; in infancy mineralocorticoid supplementation is of particular importance).
   Congenital adrenal hyperplasia.
   Nonsuppurative thyroiditis.
   Hypercalcemia associated with cancer.
2. Rheumatic Disorders:
   As adjunctive therapy for short-term administration (to tide the patient over an acute episode or exacerbation) in:
   Psoriatic Arthritis.
   Rheumatoid arthritis (selected cases may require low-dose maintenance therapy).
   Ankylosing spondylitis.
   Acute and subacute bursitis.
   Acute nonspecific tenosynovitis.
   Acute gouty arthritis.
   Post-traumatic osteoarthritis.
   Synovitis of osteoarthritis.
   Epicondylitis.
3. Collagen Diseases:
   During an exacerbation or as maintenance therapy in selected cases of:
   Systemic lupus erythematosus.
   Acute rheumatic carditis.
4. Dermatologic Diseases:
   Pemphigus.
   Bullous dermatitis herpetiformis.
   Severe erythema multiforme (Stevens-Johnson syndrome).
   Exfoliative dermatitis.
   Mycosis fungoides.
   Severe psoriasis.
   Severe seborrheic dermatitis.
5. Allergic States:
   Control of severe or incapacitating allergic conditions intractable to adequate trials of conventional treatment:
   Seasonal or perennial allergic rhinitis.
   Serum sickness.
   Bronchial asthma.
   Contact dermatitis.
   Atopic dermatitis.
   Drug hypersensitivity reactions.
6. Ophthalmic Diseases:
   Severe, acute and chronic allergic and inflammatory processes involving the eye and its adnexa such as:
   Allergic conjunctivitis.
   Keratitis.
   Allergic corneal marginal ulcers.
   Herpes zoster ophthalmicus.
   Iritis and iridocyclitis.
   Chorioretinitis.
   Anterior segment inflammation.
   Diffuse posterior uveitis and choroiditis.
   Optic neuritis.
   Sympathetic ophthalmia.
7. Respiratory Diseases:
   Symptomatic sarcoidosis.
   Loeffler's syndrome not manageable by other means.
   Berylliosis.
   Fulminating or disseminated pulmonary tuberculosis when concurrently accompanied by appropriate antituberculous chemotherapy.
   Aspiration pneumonitis.
8. Hematologic Disorders:
   Idiopathic thrombocytopenic purpura in adults.
   Secondary thrombocytopenia in adults.
   Acquired (autoimmune) hemolytic anemia.
   Erythroblastopenia (RBC anemia).
   Congenital (erythroid) hypoplastic anemia.
9. Neoplastic Diseases:
   For palliative management of:
   Leukemias and lymphomas in adults.
   Acute leukemia of childhood.
10. Edematous States:
    To induce a diuresis or remission of proteinuria in the nephrotic syndrome, without uremia, of the idiopathic type or that due to lupus erythematosus.
11. Gastrointestinal diseases:
    To tide the patient over a critical period of the disease in:
    Ulcerative colitis.
    Regional enteritis.
12. Nervous System:
    Acute exacerbations of multiple sclerosis.
13. Miscellaneous:
    Tuberculous meningitis with subarachnoid block or impending block when concurrently accompanied by appropriate antituberculous chemotherapy.
    Trichinosis with neurologic or myocardial involvement.
    Diagnostic testing of adrenocortical hyperfunction.

Contraindications: Systemic fungal infections.

Warnings: In patients on corticosteroid therapy subjected to unusual stress, increased dosage of rapidly acting corticosteroids before, during, and after the stressful situation is indicated.

Corticosteroids may mask some signs of infection, and new infections may appear during their use. There may be decreased resistance and inability to localize infection when corticosteroids are used.

Prolonged use of corticosteroids may produce posterior subcapsular cataracts, glaucoma with possible damage to the optic nerves, and may enhance the establishment of secondary ocular infections due to fungi or viruses.

Usage in pregnancy: Since adequate human reproduction studies have not been done with corticosteroids, the use of these drugs in pregnancy, nursing mothers or women of childbearing potential requires that the possible benefits of the drug be weighed against the potential hazards to the mother and embryo or fetus. Infants born of mothers who have received substantial doses of corticosteroids during pregnancy, should be carefully observed for signs of hypoadrenalism. Average and large doses of hydrocortisone or cortisone can cause elevation of blood pressure, salt and water retention, and increased excretion of potassium. These effects are less likely to occur with the synthetic derivatives except when used in large doses. Dietary salt restriction and potassium supplementation may be necessary. All corticosteroids increase calcium excretion.

While on Corticosteroid Therapy Patients Should Not Be Vaccinated Against Smallpox. Other Immunization Procedures Should Not Be Undertaken in Patients Who are on Corticosteroids, Especially on High Dose, Because of Possible Hazards of Neurological Complications and a Lack of Antibody Response.

The use of Hexadrol in active tuberculosis should be restricted to those cases of fulminating or disseminated tuberculosis in which the corticosteroid is used for the management of the disease in conjunction with an appropriate antituberculous regimen.

If corticosteroids are indicated in patients with latent tuberculosis or tuberculin reactivity, close observation is necessary as reactivation of the disease may occur. During prolonged corticosteroid therapy, these patients should receive chemoprophylaxis.

Precautions: Drug-induced secondary adrenocortical insufficiency may be minimized by gradual reduction of dosage. This type of relative insufficiency may persist for months after discontinuation of therapy; therefore, in any situation of stress occurring during that period, hormone therapy should be reinstituted. Since mineralocorticoid secretion may be impaired, salt and/or a mineralocorticoid should be administered concurrently.

There is an enhanced effect of corticosteroids on patients with hypothyroidism and in those with cirrhosis.

Corticosteroids should be used cautiously in patients with ocular herpes simplex because of possible corneal perforation.

The lowest possible dose of corticosteroid should be used to control the condition under treatment, and when reduction in dosage is possible, the reduction should be gradual.

Psychic derangements may appear when corticosteroids are used, ranging from euphoria, insomnia, mood swings, personality changes, and severe depression, to frank psychotic manifestations. Also, existing emotional instability or psychotic tendencies may be aggravated by corticosteroids.

Aspirin should be used cautiously in conjunction with corticosteroids in hypoprothrombinemia.

Steroids should be used with caution in nonspecific ulcerative colitis, if there is a probability of impending perforation, abscess or other pyogenic infection; diverticulitis; fresh intestinal anastomoses; active or latent peptic ulcer; renal insufficiency; hypertension; osteoporosis; and myasthenia gravis.

Growth and development of infants and children on prolonged corticosteroid therapy should be carefully observed.

Although controlled clinical trials have shown corticosteroids to be effective in speeding the resolution of acute exacerbations of multiple sclerosis they do not show that they affect the ultimate outcome or natural history of the disease. The studies do show that relatively high doses of corticosteroids are necessary to demonstrate a significant effect. (See Dosage and Administration Section).

Since complications of treatment with glucocorticoid are dependent on the size of the dose and the duration of treatment a risk/benefit decision must be made in each individual case as to dose and duration of treatment and as to whether daily or intermittent therapy should be used.

Adverse Reactions:

Fluid and Electrolyte Disturbances.
- Sodium retention.
- Fluid retention.
- Congestive heart failure in susceptible patients.
- Potassium loss.
- Hypokalemic alkalosis.
- Hypertension.

Musculoskeletal.
- Muscle weakness.
- Steroid myopathy.
- Loss of muscle mass.
- Osteoporosis.
- Vertebral compression fractures.
- Aseptic necrosis of femoral and humeral heads.
- Pathologic fracture of long bones.

Gastrointestinal.
- Peptic ulcer with possible perforation and hemorrhage.
- Pancreatitis.
- Abdominal distention.
- Ulcerative esophagitis.

Dermatologic.
- Impaired wound healing.
- Thin fragile skin.
- Petechiae and ecchymoses.
- Facial erythema.
- Increased sweating.
- May suppress reactions to skin tests.

Neurological.
- Convulsions.
- Increased intracranial pressure with papilledema (pseudo-tumor cerebri) usually after treatment.
- Vertigo.
- Headache.

Endocrine.
- Menstrual irregularities.
- Development of Cushingoid state.
- Suppression of growth in children.
- Secondary adrenocortical and pituitary unresponsiveness, particularly in times of stress, as in trauma, surgery or illness.
- Decreased carbohydrate tolerance.
- Manifestations of latent diabetes mellitus.
- Increased requirements for insulin or oral hypoglycemic agents in diabetics.
- Posterior subcapsular cataracts.
- Increased intraocular pressure.
- Glaucoma.
- Exophthalmos.

Metabolic.
- Negative nitrogen balance due to protein catabolism.

Dosage and Administration: The initial dosage of Hexadrol (dexamethasone) may vary from 0.75 mg. to 9.0 mg. per day depending on the specific disease entity being treated. In situations of less severity lower doses will generally suffice while in selected patients higher initial doses may be required. The initial dosage should be maintained or adjusted until a satisfactory response is noted. If after a reasonable period of time there is a lack of satisfactory clinical response, Hexadrol (dexamethasone) should be discontinued and the patient transferred to other appropriate therapy. *IT SHOULD BE EMPHASIZED THAT DOSAGE REQUIREMENTS ARE VARIABLE AND MUST BE INDIVIDUALIZED ON THE BASIS OF THE DISEASE UNDER TREATMENT AND THE RESPONSE OF THE PATIENT.*

After a favorable response is noted, the proper maintenance dosage should be determined by decreasing the initial drug dosage in small decrements at appropriate time intervals until the lowest dosage which will maintain an adequate clinical response is reached. It should be kept in mind that constant monitoring is needed in regard to drug dosage. Included in the situations which may make dosage adjustments necessary are changes in clinical status secondary to remissions or exacerbations in the disease process, the patient's individual drug responsiveness, and the effect of patient exposure to stressful situations not directly related to the disease entity under treatment; in this latter situation it may be necessary to increase the dosage of Hexadrol (dexamethasone) for a period of time consistent with the patient's condition. If after long-term therapy the drug is to be stopped, it is recommended that it be withdrawn gradually rather than abruptly.

In treatment of acute exacerbations of multiple sclerosis daily doses of 200 mg of prednisolone for a week followed by 80 mg every other day or 4–8 mg dexamethasone every other day for 1 month have been shown to be effective.

Patients currently being treated with other corticosteroids may be transferred conveniently to this agent using the following dosage equivalents:

0.75 mg. dexamethasone equivalent to	25 mg. cortisone
	20 mg. hydrocortisone
	5 mg. prednisone or prednisolone
	4 mg. methylprednisolone
	4 mg. triamcinolone

How Supplied: Hexadrol (dexamethasone tablets, USP):

0.50 mg tablets (yellow, scored), bottles of 100 and 500; unit dose package of 100. NDC # 0052-0792-91, NDC # 0052-0792-95, NDC # 0052-0792-90.

0.75 mg tablets (white, scored), bottles of 100 and 500; unit dosage package of 100. NDC # 0052-0791-91, NDC # 0052-0791-95, NDC # 0052-0791-90.

1.5 mg tablets (peach, scored), bottles of 100; unit dose package of 100. NDC # 0052-0790-91, NDC # 0052-0790-90.

4.0 mg tablets (light green, scored), bottles of 100; unit dose package of 100. NDC # 0052-0798-91, NDC # 0052-0798-90.

Therapeutic Pack—package of six 1.5 mg and eight 0.75 mg tablets provides a one-week supply. NDC # 0052-0795-14.

[*Shown in Product Identification Section*]

HEXADROL® PHOSPHATE INJECTION ℞

(dexamethasone sodium phosphate U.S.P.)

Description: Hexadrol Phosphate Injection (dexamethasone sodium phosphate, U.S.P.) is a water-soluble inorganic ester of dexamethasone which produces a rapid response even when injected intramuscularly. Dexamethasone Sodium Phosphate, $C_{22}H_{28}FNa_2O_8P$, has a molecular weight of 516.41 and chemically is: Pregn-4-ene-3, 20-dione, 9-fluoro-11, 17-dihydroxy-16-methyl-21-(phosphonooxy)-, disodium salt, (11β, 16α)-. It occurs as a white to creamy white powder, is exceedingly hygroscopic, is soluble in water and its solutions have a pH between 7.5 and 10.5.

It is available in two potencies, 4mg/ml and 10mg/ml, in aqueous solution with 1% benzyl alcohol as preservative.

Actions: Naturally occurring glucocorticoids (hydrocortisone), which also have salt-retaining properties, are used as replacement therapy in adrenocortical deficiency states. Their synthetic analogs are primarily used for their potent anti-inflammatory effects in disorders of many organ systems.

Glucocorticoids cause profound and varied metabolic effects. In addition, they modify the body's immune responses to diverse stimuli.

Indications:

A. ***Intravenous or intramuscular administration.*** When oral therapy is not feasible and the strength, dosage form, and route of administration of the drug reasonably lend the preparation to the treatment of the condition, those products labeled for intravenous or intramuscular use are indicated as follows:

1. ***Endocrine disorders***

   Primary or secondary adrenocortical insufficiency (hydrocortisone or cortisone is the drug of choice; synthetic analogs may be used in conjunction with mineralocorticoids where applicable; in infancy, mineralocorticoid supplementation is of particular importance).

   Acute adrenocortical insufficiency (hydrocortisone or cortisone is the drug of choice; mineralocorticoid supplementation may be necessary, particularly when synthetic analogs are used).

   Preoperatively and in the event of serious trauma or illness, in patients with known adrenal insufficiency or when adrenocortical reserve is doubtful.

   Shock unresponsive to conventional therapy if adrenocortical insufficiency exists or is suspected.

Continued on next page

Organon—Cont.

Congenital adrenal hyperplasia.
Nonsuppurative thyroiditis.
Hypercalcemia associated with cancer.

2. ***Rheumatic disorders.*** As adjunctive therapy for short-term administration (to tide the patient over an acute episode or exacerbation) in:
Post-traumatic osteoarthritis.
Synovitis of osteoarthritis.
Rheumatoid arthritis, including juvenile rheumatoid arthritis (selected cases may require low-dose maintenance therapy).
Acute and subacute bursitis.
Epicondylitis.
Acute nonspecific tenosynovitis.
Acute gouty arthritis.
Psoriatic arthritis.
Ankylosing spondylitis.
3. ***Collagen diseases.*** During an exacerbation or as maintenance therapy in selected cases of:
Systemic lupus erythematosus.
Acute rheumatic carditis.
4. ***Dermatologic diseases:***
Pemphigus.
Severe erythema multiforme (Stevens-Johnson syndrome).
Exfoliative dermatitis.
Bullous dermatitis herpetiformis.
Severe seborrheic dermatitis.
Severe psoriasis.
Mycosis fungoides.
5. ***Allergic states.*** Control of severe or incapacitating allergic conditions intractable to adequate trials of conventional treatment in:
Bronchial asthma.
Contact dermatitis.
Atopic dermatitis.
Serum sickness.
Seasonal or perennial allergic rhinitis.
Drug hypersensitivity reactions.
Urticarial transfusion reactions.
Acute noninfectious laryngeal edema (epinephrine is the drug of first choice).
6. ***Ophthalmic diseases.*** Severe acute and chronic allergic and inflammatory processes involving the eye, such as:
Herpes zoster ophthalmicus.
Iritis, iridocyclitis.
Chorioretinitis.
Diffuse posterior uveitis and choroiditis.
Optic neuritis.
Sympathetic ophthalmia.
Anterior segment inflammation.
Allergic conjunctivitis.
Allergic corneal marginal ulcers.
Keratitis.
7. ***Gastrointestinal diseases.*** To tide the patient over a critical period of disease in:
Ulcerative colitis (systemic therapy).
Regional enteritis (systemic therapy).
8. ***Respiratory diseases:***
Symptomatic sarcoidosis.
Berylliosis.
Fulminating or disseminated pulmonary tuberculosis when used concurrently with appropriate antituberculous chemotherapy.
Loeffler's syndrome not manageable by other means.
Aspiration pneumonitis.
9. ***Hematologic disorders:***
Acquired (autoimmune) hemolytic anemia.
Idiopathic thrombocytopenic purpura in adults (I.V. only; I.M. administration is contraindicated).
Secondary thrombocytopenia in adults.
Erythroblastopenia (RBC anemia).
Congenital (erythroid) hypoplastic anemia.
10. ***Neoplastic diseases.*** For palliative management of:
Leukemias and lymphomas in adults.
Acute leukemia of childhood.
11. ***Edematous state.*** To induce diuresis or remission of proteinuria in the nephrotic syndrome, without uremia, of the idiopathic type or that due to lupus erythematosus.
12. ***Nervous System.***
Acute exacerbations of multiple sclerosis.
13. ***Miscellaneous:***
Tuberculous meningitis with subarachnoid block or impending block when used concurrently with appropriate antituberculous chemotherapy.
Trichinosis with neurologic or myocardial involvement.
Diagnostic testing of adrenocortical hyperfunction.
Cerebral edema of diverse etiologies in conjunction with adequate neurological evaluation and management.

B. ***Intra-articular or soft tissue administration.*** When the strength and dosage form of the drug lend the preparation to the treatment of the condition, those products labeled for intraarticular or soft tissue administration are indicated as adjunctive therapy for short-term administration (to tide the patient over an acute episode or exacerbation) in:
Synovitis of osteoarthritis.
Rheumatoid arthritis.
Acute and subacute bursitis.
Acute gouty arthritis.
Epicondylitis.
Acute nonspecific tenosynovitis.
Post-traumatic osteoarthritis.

C. ***Intralesional administration.*** When the strength and dosage form of the drug lend the preparation to the treatment of the condition, those products labeled for intralesional administration are indicated for:
Keloids.
Localized hypertrophic, infiltrated, inflammatory lesions of: lichen planus, psoriatic plaques, granuloma annulare, and lichen simplex chronicus (neurodermatitis).
Discoid lupus erythematosus.
Necrobiosis lipodica diabeticorum.
Alopecia areata.
They also may be useful in cystic tumors of an aponeurosis or tendon (ganglia).

Contraindications: Systemic fungal infections.

Warnings: In patients on corticosteroid therapy subject to any unusual stress, increased dosage of rapidly acting corticosteroids before, during and after the stressful situation is indicated. Corticosteroids may mask some signs of infection, and new infections may appear during their use. There may be decreased resistance and inability to localize infection when corticosteroids are used.

Prolonged use of corticosteroids may produce posterior subcapsular cataracts, glaucoma with possible damage to the optic nerves, and may enhance the establishment of secondary ocular infections due to fungi or viruses.

Usage in Pregnancy. Since adequate human reproduction studies have not been done with corticosteroids, the use of these drugs in pregnancy, nursing mothers or women of childbearing potential requires that the possible benefits of the drug be weighed against the potential hazards to the mother and embryo or fetus. Infants born of mothers who have received substantial doses of corticosteroids during pregnancy should be carefully observed for signs of hypoadrenalism.

Average and large doses of cortisone or hydrocortisone can cause elevation of blood pressure, salt and water retention, and increased excretion of potassium. These effects are less likely to occur with the synthetic derivatives except when used in large doses. Patients with a stressed myocardium should be observed carefully and the drug administered slowly since premature ventricular contractions may occur with rapid administration. Dietary salt restriction and potassium supplementation may be necessary. All corticosteroids increase calcium excretion.

While on Corticosteroid Therapy Patients Should Not Be Vaccinated Against Smallpox. Other Immunization Procedures Should Not Be Undertaken in Patients Who Are on Corticosteroids, Especially in High Doses, Because of Possible Hazards of Neurological Complications and Lack of Antibody Response.

The use of Hexadrol Phosphate Injection in active tuberculosis should be restricted to those cases of fulminating or disseminated tuberculosis in which the corticosteroid is used for the management of the disease in conjunction with appropriate anti-tuberculous regimen.

If corticosteroids are indicated in patients with latent tuberculosis or tuberculin reactivity, close observation is necessary as reactivation of the disease may occur. During prolonged corticosteroid therapy, these patients should receive chemoprophylaxis.

Because rare instances of anaphylactoid reactions have occurred in patients receiving parenteral corticosteroid therapy, appropriate precautionary measures should be taken prior to administration, especially when the patient has a history of allergy to any drug.

Precautions: Drug-induced secondary adrenocortical insufficiency may be minimized by gradual reduction of dosage. This type of relative insufficiency may persist for months after discontinuation of therapy; therefore, in any situation of stress occurring during that period, hormone therapy should be reinstituted. Since mineralocorticoid secretion may be impaired, salt and/or a mineralocorticoid should be administered concurrently.

There is an enhanced effect of corticosteroids in patients with hypothyroidism and in those with cirrhosis.

Corticosteroids should be used cautiously in patients with ocular herpes simplex for fear of corneal perforation.

The lowest possible dose of corticosteroid should be used to control the condition under treatment, and when reduction in dosage is possible, the reduction must be gradual.

Psychic derangements may appear when corticosteroids are used ranging from euphoria, insomnia, mood swings, personality changes, and severe depression to frank psychotic manifestations. Also, existing emotional instability or psychotic tendencies may be aggravated by corticosteroids.

Aspirin should be used cautiously in conjunction with corticosteroids in hypoprothrombinemia.

Steroids should be used with caution in nonspecific ulcerative colitis, if there is a probability of impending perforation, abscess or other pyogenic infection, also in diverticulitis, fresh intestinal anastomoses, active or latent peptic ulcer, renal insufficiency, hypertension, osteoporosis, and myasthenia gravis.

Growth and development of infants and children on prolonged corticosteroid therapy should be carefully followed.

Intra-articular injection of a corticosteroid may produce systemic as well as local effects. Appropriate examination of any joint fluid present is necessary to exclude a septic process. A marked increase in pain accompanied by local swelling, further restriction of joint motion, fever, and malaise are suggestive of septic arthritis. If this complication occurs and the diagnosis of sepsis is confirmed, appropriate antimicrobial therapy should be instituted.

Local injection of a steroid into a previously infected joint is to be avoided. Corticosteroids should not be injected into unstable joints.

Although controlled clinical trials have shown corticosteroids to be effective in speeding the resolution of acute exacerbations of multiple sclerosis they do not show that they affect the

ultimate outcome or natural history of the disease. The studies do show that relatively high doses of corticosteroids are necessary to demonstrate a significant effect. (See Dosage and Administration Section).
Since complications of treatment with glucorcorticoid are dependent on the size of the dose and the duration of treatment a risk/benefit decision must be made in each individual case as to dose and duration of treatment and as to whether daily or intermittent therapy should be used.

Adverse Reactions:

Fluid and electrolyte disturbances:
- Sodium retention
- Fluid retention
- Congestive heart failure in susceptible patients
- Potassium loss
- Hypokalemic alkalosis
- Hypertension

Musculoskeletal:
- Muscle weakness
- Steroid myopathy
- Loss of muscle mass
- Osteoporosis
- Vertebral compression fractures
- Aseptic necrosis of femoral and humeral heads
- Pathologic fracture of long bones

Gastrointestinal:
- Peptic ulcer with possible subsequent perforation and hemorrhage
- Pancreatitis
- Abdominal distention
- Ulcerative esophagitis

Dermatologic:
- Impaired wound healing
- Thin fragile skin
- Petechiae and ecchymoses
- Facial erythema
- Increased sweating
- May suppress reactions to skin tests

Neurological:
- Convulsions
- Increased intracranial pressure with papilledema (pseudotumor cerebri) usually after treatment
- Vertigo
- Headache

Endocrine:
- Menstrual irregularities
- Development of Cushingoid state
- Suppression of growth in children
- Secondary adrenocortical and pituitary unresponsiveness, particularly in times of stress, as in trauma, surgery, or illness
- Decreased carbohydrate tolerance
- Manifestations of latent diabetes mellitus
- Increased requirements for insulin or oral hypoglycemic agents in diabetics

Ophthalmic:
- Posterior subcapsular cataracts
- Increased intraocular pressure
- Glaucoma
- Exophthalmos

Metabolic:
- Negative nitrogen balance due to protein catabolism

Miscellaneous:
- Hyperpigmentation or hypopigmentation
- Subcutaneous and cutaneous atrophy
- Sterile abscess
- Postinjection flare, following intra-articular use
- Charcot-like arthropathy
- Itching, burning, tingling in the ano-genital region.

Dosage and Administration:

A. ***Intravenous or intramuscular administration.*** The initial dosage of Hexadrol Phosphate Injection may vary from 0.50 mg/day to 9.0 mg/day depending on the specific disease entity being treated. In situations of less severity, lower doses will generally suffice while in selected patients higher initial doses may be required. Usually the parenteral dosage ranges are one-third to one-half the oral dose given every 12 hours. However, in certain overwhelming, acute, life-threateing situations, administration in dosages exceeding the usual dosages may be justified and may be in multiples of the oral dosages.
For the treatment of unresponsive shock high pharmacologic doses of this product are currently recommended. Reported regimens range from 1 to 6 mg/kg of body weight as a single intravenous injection to 40 mg initially followed by repeat intravenous injection every 2 to 6 hours while shock persists.

For the treatment of cerebral edema in adults in initial intravenous dose of 10 mg. is recommended followed by 4 mg. intramuscularly every six hours until maximum response has been noted. This regimen may be continued for several days postoperatively in patients requiring brain surgery. Oral dexamethasone, 1 to 3 mg t.i.d., should be given as soon as possible and dosage tapered off over a period of five to seven days. Nonoperative cases may require continuous therapy to remain free of symptoms of increased intracranial pressure. The smallest effective dose should be used in children, preferably orally. This may approximate 0.2 mg/kg/24 hours in divided doses.

In treatment of acute exacerbations of multiple sclerosis daily doses of 200 mg of prednisolone for a week followed by 80 mg every other day or 4-8 mg dexamethasone every other day for 1 month have been shown to be effective.
The initial dosage should be maintained or adjusted until a satisfactory response is noted. If after a reasonable period of time there is a lack of satisfactory clinical response, Hexadrol Phosphate Injection should be discontinued and the patient transferred to other appropriate therapy. It Should Be Emphasized That Dosage Requirements Are Variable and Must Be Individualized on the Basis of the Disease Under Treatment and the Response of the Patient.

After a favorable response is noted, the proper maintenance dosage should be determined by decreasing the initial drug dosage in small decrements at appropriate time intervals until the lowest dosage which will maintain an adequate clinical response is reached. It should be kept in mind that constant monitoring is needed in regard to drug dosage. Included in the situations which may make dosage adjustments necessary are changes in clinical status secondary to remissions or exacerbations in the disease process, the patient's individual drug responsiveness and the effect of patient exposure to stressful situations not directly related to the disease entity under treatment; in this latter situation it may be necessary to increase the dosage of Hexadrol Phosphate Injection for a period of time consistent with the patient's condition. If after long-term therapy the drug is to be stopped, it is recommended that it be withdrawn gradually rather than abruptly.

B. ***Intra-articular, Soft Tissue and Intralesional Administration.*** The dose for intrasynovial administration is usually 2 to 4 mg. for large joints and 0.8 to 1 mg. for small joints. For soft tissue and bursal injections a dose of 2 to 4 mg. is recommended. Ganglia require a dose of 1 to 2 mg. A dose of 0.4 to 1 mg. is used for injection into tendon sheaths. Injection into intervertebral joints should not be attempted at any time and hip joint injection cannot be recommended as an office procedure. Intrasynovial and soft tissue injections should be employed only when affected areas are limited to 1 or 2 sites. It should be remembered that corticoids provide palliation only and that other conventional or curative methods of therapy should be employed when indicated.
Frequency of injection usually ranges from once every 3 to 5 days to once every 2 to 3 weeks. Frequent intra-articular injection may cause damage to joint tissue.

How Supplied—5-ml (4mg/ml) multiple dose vial NDC 0052-0796-05
1-ml (4mg/ml) vial, box of 25 NDC 0052-0796-25
10-ml (10mg/ml) vial, (for intravenous use or intramuscular use only) NDC 0052-0797-10.
1-ml (4mg/ml) Prefilled Disposable Syringe NDC 0052-0796-26

PAVULON® ℞
(pancuronium bromide)

THIS DRUG SHOULD ONLY BE ADMINISTERED BY ADEQUATELY TRAINED INDIVIDUALS FAMILIAR WITH ITS ACTIONS, CHARACTERISTICS, AND HAZARDS.

Description: Pavulon (pancuronium bromide) is the aminosteroid 2 beta, 16 beta-dipiperidine-5 alpha-androstane-3 alpha, 17-beta-diol diacetate dimethobromide.
Actions: Pavulon is a non-depolarizing neuromuscular blocking agent possessing all of the characteristic pharmacological actions of this class of drugs (curariform) on the myoneural junction.
Pavulon is approximately 5 times as potent as d-tubocurarine chloride.
The onset and duration of action of Pavulon is dose dependent. With the administration of 0.04 mg. per kg. the onset of action, as measured by a peripheral nerve stimulator, is usually within 45 seconds, and its peak effect is usually within 4½ minutes; recovery to 90% of control twitch height usually takes place in less than one hour. Larger doses, more suitable for endotracheal intubation, such as 0.08 mg. per kg. of Pavulon have an onset of action of about 30 seconds, and a peak effect within 3 minutes. Supplemental incremental doses of Pavulon, following the initial dose, slightly increase the magnitude of blockade, and significantly increase the duration of the blockade.
Pavulon has little effect upon the circulatory system. The most frequently reported observation is a slight rise in pulse rate.
Human histamine assays, and clinical observations, as well as in *vivo* guinea pig testing, and in *vitro* mast cell testing, indicate that histamine release rarely, if ever, occurs.
Pavulon (pancuronium bromide) is antagonized by acetylcholine, anticholinesterases, and potassium ion. Its action is increased by inhalational anesthetics such as halothane, diethyl ether, enflurane and methoxyflurane, as well as quinine, magnesium salts, hypokalemia, some carcinomas, and certain antibiotics such as neomycin, streptomycin, kanamycin, gentamicin and bacitracin. The action of Pavulon may be altered by dehydration, electrolyte imbalance, acid-base imbalance, renal disease, and concomitant administration of other neuromuscular agents.
Pavulon has no known effect on consciousness, the pain threshold, or cerebration.
Indications: Pavulon is indicated as an adjunct to anesthesia to induce skeletal muscle relaxation. It may also be employed to facilitate the management of patients undergoing mechanical ventilation.
Contraindications: Pavulon is contraindicated in patients known to be hypersensitive to the drug or to the bromide ion.
Warnings: PAVULON SHOULD BE ADMINISTERED IN CAREFULLY ADJUSTED DOSAGE BY OR UNDER THE SUPERVISION OF EXPERIENCED CLINICIANS, WHO ARE FAMILIAR WITH ITS ACTIONS AND THE POSSIBLE COMPLICATIONS THAT MIGHT OCCUR FOLLOWING ITS USE. THE DRUG SHOULD NOT BE ADMINISTERED UNLESS FACILITIES FOR INTU-

Continued on next page

Organon—Cont.

BATION, ARTIFICIAL RESPIRATION, OXYGEN THERAPY, AND REVERSAL AGENTS ARE IMMEDIATELY AVAILABLE. THE CLINICIAN MUST BE PREPARED TO ASSIST OR CONTROL RESPIRATION.
In patients who are known to have myasthenia gravis small doses of Pavulon may have profound effects. A peripheral nerve stimulator is especially valuable in assessing the effects of Pavulon in such patients.
Usage in Pregnancy: The safe use of pancuronium bromide has not been established with respect to the possible adverse effects upon fetal development. Therefore, it should not be used in women of childbearing potential and particularly during early pregnancy unless in the judgment of the physician the potential benefits outweigh the unknown hazards.
Pavulon may be used in operative obstetrics (Cesarean section), but reversal of pancuronium may be unsatisfactory in patients receiving magnesium sulfate for toxemia of pregnancy, because magnesium salts enhance neuromuscular blockade. Dosage should usually be reduced, as indicated, in such cases.
Precautions: Although Pavulon has been used successfully in many patients with preexisting pulmonary, hepatic, or renal disease, caution should be exercised in these situations. This is particularly true of renal disease since a major portion of administered Pavulon is excreted unchanged in the urine.
Adverse Reactions: Neuromuscular: the most frequently noted adverse reactions consist primarily of an extension of the drug's pharmacological actions beyond the time period needed for surgery and anesthesia. This may vary from skeletal muscle weakness to profound and prolonged skeletal muscle relaxation resulting in respiratory insufficiency or apnea. Inadequate reversal of the neuromuscular blockade by anticholinesterase agents has also been observed with Pavulon (pancuronium bromide) as with all curariform drugs. These adverse reactions are managed by manual or mechanical ventilation until recovery is judged adequate.
Cardiovascular: A slight increase in pulse rate is frequently noted.
Gastrointestinal: Salivation is sometimes noted during very light anesthesia, especially if no anticholinergic premedication is used.
Skin: An occasional transient rash is noted accompanying the use of Pavulon.
Respiratory: One case of wheezing, responding to deepening of the inhalational anesthetic, has been reported.
Drug Interaction: The intensity of blockade and duration of action of Pavulon is increased in patients receiving potent volatile inhalational anesthetics such as halothane, diethyl ether, enflurane and methoxyflurane. No increase in intensity of blockade or duration of action of Pavulon is noted from the use of thiobarbiturates, narcotic analgesics, nitrous oxide, or droperidol.
Prior administration of succinylcholine, such as that used for endotracheal intubation, enhances the relaxant effect of Pavulon and the duration of action. If succinylcholine is used before Pavulon, the administration of Pavulon should be delayed until the succinylcholine shows signs of wearing off.
Dosage and Administration: Pavulon should be administered only by or under the supervision of experienced clincians. DOSAGE MUST BE INDIVIDUALIZED IN EACH CASE. The dosage information which follows has been derived from dose-response studies based on body weight and is intended to serve as a guide only. Since potent inhalational agents or prior administration of succinylcholine enhance the intensity of blockade and duration of Pavulon (see DRUG INTERACTION), these factors should be taken into consideration in selection of initial and incremental dosage.
In adults the initial intravenous dosage range is 0.04 to 0.1 mg. per kg. Later incremental doses starting at 0.01 mg. per kg. may be used. These increments slightly increase the magnitude of the blockade, and significantly increase the duration of blockade, because a significant number of myoneural junctions are still blocked when there is clinical need for more drug.
If Pavulon is used to provide skeletal muscle relaxation for endotracheal intubation, doses of 0.06 to 0.1 mg. per kg. are recommended. Conditions satisfactory for intubation are usually present within 2 to 3 minutes. The ability of the anesthetist to intubate with Pavulon (pancuronium bromide) improves with experience.
Dosage in Children: Dose response studies in children indicate that, with the exception of neonates, dosage requirements are the same as for adults. Neonates are especially sensitive to non-depolarizing neuromuscular blocking agents, such as Pavulon, (pancuronium bromide) during the first month of life. It is recommended that a test dose of 0.02 mg. per kg. be given first in this group to measure responsiveness.
Cesarean Section: The dosage to provide relaxation for intubation and operation is the same as for general surgical procedures. The dosage to provide relaxation, following usage of succinylcholine for intubation (see DRUG INTERACTION), is the same as for general surgical procedures.
Management of Prolonged Neuromuscular Blockade: Residual neuromuscular blockade beyond the time period needed for surgery and anesthesia may occur with Pavulon as with other neuromuscular blockers. This may be manifested by skeletal muscle weakness, decreased respiratory reserve, low tidal volume or apnea. A peripheral nerve stimulator may be used to assess the degree of residual neuromuscular blockade. Under such circumstances the primary treatment is manual or mechanical ventilation and maintenance of a patent airway until complete recovery of normal respiration is assured. Regonol (pridostigmine bromide) or neostigmine, in conjunction with atropine, will usually antagonize the skeletal muscle relaxant action of Pavulon. These should be accompanied by or preceded by injection of atropine sulfate to minimize the incidence of cholinergic side effects, notably excessive secretions and bradycardia. Satisfactory reversal can be judged by adequacy of skeletal muscle tone, and by adequacy of respiration. A peripheral nerve stimulator may also be used to monitor restoration of twitch height. Failure of prompt reversal (within 30 minutes) may occur in the presence of extreme debilitation, carcinomatosis, and with concomitant use of certain broad spectrum antibiotics, or anesthetic agents and adjuncts which enhance neuromuscular blockade or cause respiratory depression of their own. Under such circumstances the management is the same as that of prolonged neuromuscular blockade; ventilation must be supported by artificial means until the patient has resumed control of his respiration. Prior to the use of reversal agents, reference to the specific package insert of the reversal agents should be made.
How Supplied:
2 ml. ampuls—2 mg./ml.—boxes of 25 NDC 0052-0444-26
5 ml. ampuls—2 mg./ml.—boxes of 25 NDC 0052-0444-25
10 ml. vials—1 mg./ml.—boxes of 25 NDC 0052-0443-25

REGONOL® ℞
(pyridostigmine bromide injection)

Description: Regonol (pyridostigmine bromide injection) is an active cholinesterase inhibitor. Chemically, pyridostigmine bromide is 3-hydroxy-1-methylpyridinium bromide dimethylcarbamate.
Each ml. contains 5 mg. pyridostigmine bromide compounded with 0.2% parabens (methyl and propyl) as preservatives, 0.02% sodium citrate and pH adjusted to approximately 5.0 with citric acid and sodium hydroxide.
Actions: Pyridostigmine bromide facilitates the transmission of impulses across the myoneural junction by inhibiting the destruction of acetylcholine by cholinesterase. Pyridostigmine is an analog of neostigmine but differs from it clinically by having fewer side effects. Currently available data indicate that pyridostigmine may have a significantly lower degree and incidence of bradycardia, salivation and gastroinestinal stimulation. Animal studies using the injectable form of pyridostigmine and human studies using the oral preparation have indicated that pyridostigmine has a longer duration of action than does neostigmine measured under similar circumstances.
Indications: Pyridostigmine bromide is useful as a reversal agent or antagonist to nondepolarizing muscle relaxants.
Contraindications: Known hypersensitivity to anticholinesterase agents; intestinal and urinary obstructions of mechanical type.
Warnings: Pyridostigmine bromide should be used with particular caution in patients with bronchial asthma or cardiac dysrhythmias. Transient bradycardia may occur and be relieved by atropine sulfate. Atropine should also be used with caution in patients with cardiac dysrhythmias. When large doses of pyridostigmine bromide are administered, as during reversal of muscle relaxants, prior or simultaneous injection of atropine sulfate is advisable. Because of the possibility of hypersensitivity in an occasional patient, atropine and antishock medication should always be readily available.
When used as an antagonist to nondepolarizing muscle relaxants, adequate recovery of voluntary respiration and neuromuscular transmission must be obtained prior to discontinuation of respiratory assistance and there should be continuous patient observation. Satisfactory recovery may be defined by a combination of clinical judgement, respiratory measurements and observation of the effects of peripheral nerve stimulation. If there is any doubt concerning the adequacy of recovery from the effects of the nondepolarizing muscle relaxant, artificial ventilation should be continued until all doubt has been removed.
Usage in Pregnancy—The safety of pyridostigmine bromide during pregnancy or lactation in humans has not been established. Therefore, its use in women who are pregnant requires weighing the drug's potential benefits against its possible hazards to mother and child.
Adverse Reactions: The side effects of pyridostigmine bromide are most commonly related to overdosage and generally are of two varieties, muscarinic and nicotinic. Among those in the former group are nausea, vomiting, diarrhea, abdominal cramps, increased peristalsis, increased salivation, increased bronchial secretions, miosis and diaphoresis. Nicotine side effects are comprised chiefly of muscle cramps, fasciculation and weakness, Muscarinic side effects can usually be counteracted by atropine. As with any compound containing the bromide radical, a skin rash may be seen in an occasional patient. Such reactions usually subside promptly upon discontinuance of the medication. Thrombophlebitis has been reported subsequent to intravenous administration.
Dosage and Administration: When pyridostigmine bromide is given intravenously to

reverse the action of muscle relaxant drugs, it is recommended that atropine sulfate (0.6 to 1.2 mg.) also be given intravenously immediately prior to its administration. Side effects, notably excessive secretions and bradycardia are thereby minimized. Usually 10 or 20 mg. of pyridostigmine bromide will be sufficient for antagonism of the effects of the nondepolarizing muscle relaxants. Although full recovery may occur within 15 minutes in most patients, others may require a half hour or more. Satisfactory reversal can be evident by adequate voluntary respiration, respiratory measurements and use of a peripheral nerve stimulator device. It is recommended that the patient be well ventilated and a patent airway maintained until complete recovery of normal respiration is assured. Once satisfactory reversal has been attained, recurarization has not been reported.

Failure of pyridostigmine bromide to provide prompt (within 30 minutes) reversal may occur, e.g. in the presence of extreme debilitation, carcinomatosis, or with concomitant use of certain broad spectrum antibiotics or anesthetic agents, notably ether. Under these circumstances ventilation must be supported by artificial means until the patient has resumed control of his respiration.

How Supplied: Regonol is available in: 2 ml. ampuls—5 mg./ml. boxes of 10—NDC 0052-0460-10

WIGRAINE® ℞

Description: Each Wigraine tablet and Wigraine rectal suppository contains:

Ergotamine tartrate	1 mg
Caffeine	100 mg
Belladonna Alkaloids (levorotatory)*	0.1 mg
Phenacetin	130 mg

Wigraine combines four ingredients specifically indicated for treatment of: severe throbbing head pain, nausea and vomiting and residual muscle pain of vascular headaches. The ergotamine and caffeine through their constricting action on dilated cerebral arteries relieve the throbbing head pain of vascular headaches. Belladonna alkaloids exert an inhibitory effect on the tone and peristaltic waves of the stomach and intestine, thus alleviating the nausea and vomiting. Phenacetin relieves residual skeletal muscle pain frequently accompanying a typical migraine attack.

Wigraine tablets are uncoated and prepared so they disintegrate rapidly to facilitate quick absorption. This is also true for the suppositories since rapid onset of effect is important for the satisfactory treatment of acute attacks of vascular headaches.

Indications: Wigraine is indicated for the treatment of acute attacks of vascular headaches such as migraine, frontal headache, migraine variants, histamine cephalalgia, occipital and throbbing type of headache.

Dosage: One or two Wigraine tablets or suppositories should be taken immediately upon the appearance of symptoms of headache, followed by one or two tablets or suppositories every 15 minutes until the pain subsides. No more than 6 Wigraine tablets or suppositories should be taken for one attack. If a patient requires more than one tablet or suppository to abort an attack, the initial dosage for the next attack of equal severity should be increased to obtain immediate relief. When possible, the patient should rest in a dark room for one hour after taking Wigraine tablets or suppositories to secure maximum effect. No more than 12 Wigraine tablets or suppositories should be administered during any seven day period.

Precaution: Wigraine tablets and suppositories are intended for the treatment of acute attacks and have no prophylactic value. Wigraine should not be used in the presence of peripheral vascular disease, coronary disease, angina pectoris, hypertension, renal or hepatic disease, pregnancy or septic states or incipient glaucoma.

It has been estimated ill effects follow ergotamine administration in only 0.01 per cent of the cases in which the alkaloid is used. Ergotamine is capable of producing all the symptoms of ergotism. When ergotamine is prescribed in the correct dosage (see dosage section) in the absence of contraindications it is a safe and useful drug. No serious complications have been reported when using the suggested dosage for the treatment of vascular headache.

How Supplied: Wigraine tablets are individually foil stripped and packaged in boxes of 20, NDC 0052-0541-20 and 100, NDC 0052-0541-91 Wigraine suppositories are individually foil wrapped and packaged in boxes of 12, NDC 0052-0546-12.

---

*Representing 87.5% hyoscyamine and 12.5% atropine as sulfates.

[*Shown in Product Identification Section*]

Ortho Diagnostics Inc.
ROUTE 202
RARITAN, NEW JERSEY 08869

MICRhoGAM™ ℞
Rh_o (D) Immune Globulin (Human)
For Intramuscular Use Only

Description: MICRhoGAM Rh_o (D) Immune Globulin (Human), Micro-Dose, is a sterile, concentrated solution of specific immunoglobulin (IgG) containing anti-Rh_o (D). This product is prepared from fractionated human plasma (cold alcohol method) and may include immunoglobulin, which does not contain anti-Rh_o (D), derived from an intermediate plasma fraction prepared by other Bureau of Biologics licensed manufacturers. All plasma used in the manufacture of this product was tested for hepatitis B surface antigen and found to be nonreactive.

Active Ingredient
Anti-Rh_o (D) in 15% ± 1.5% serum globulin

Inactive Ingredients
15 mg/ml glycine (approximately)
2.9 mg/ml sodium chloride (approximately)
Preservative 0.01% thimerosal (mercury derivative)

Action: MICRhoGAM is used to prevent the formation of anti-Rh_o (D) in Rh_o (D) negative and D^u negative women who are exposed to the Rh_o (D) antigen at the time of abortion or miscarriage (up to 12 weeks gestation). The probable mechanism of action is the binding of passive antibody to antigen in the circulation, thereby preventing the stimulation of antigen sensitive cells and subsequent production of anti-Rh_o (D).

Indication: MICRhoGAM is indicated for the prevention of maternal Rh immunization following abortion or miscarriage up to 12 weeks gestation. The material should be administered to the Rh_o (D) negative, D^u negative woman as soon as possible after the spontaneous passage or surgical removal of the products of conception.

Clinical trials indicated that MICRhoGAM was effective when administered following abortions and in these trials the product was routinely injected within three (3) hours. However, if MICRhoGAM is not given within this time period, consideration should still be given to the administration of the product, since it was shown to be effective in a male volunteer study when given as long as 72 hours after the infusion of Rh_o (D) positive red cells.

FOR ABORTIONS OR MISCARRIAGES OCCURRING AFTER 12 WEEKS GESTATION, A STANDARD DOSE OF RhoGAM™ Rh_o (D) Immune Globulin (Human) IS INDICATED.

MICRhoGAM prophylaxis should be considered for every woman undergoing abortion or miscarriage up to 12 weeks gestation unless:

It has been proven that she is Rh_o (D) positive or D^u positive. [See direction circular such as that accompanying ORTHO™ Blood Grouping Serum Anti-D (Anti-Rh_o) for Slide and Modified Tube Tests.]

It has been proven that she is immunized to the Rh_o (D) antigen as demonstrated by the presence of anti-Rh_o (D) in her serum. This testing may be performed in the laboratory using products such as SELECTOGEN™ and IDENTIGEN™ Reagent Red Blood Cells.

Or, it has been proven by Rh typing that the father and/or fetus is Rh negative.

Dosage: One vial of MICRhoGAM will suppress the immunogenic challenge of 2.5 ml of Rh_o (D) positive or D^u positive packed red blood cells (not whole blood), or the equivalent (5.0 ml) of whole blood in males. This dose will provide protection against maternal Rh isoimmunization for women undergoing abortion or miscarriage up to 12 weeks gestation.

Injection Control: After qualifying testing is performed, complete the injection control form included with the package of MICRhoGAM.

1. Separate the three-part form, remove the first copy and place it securely with the product.
2. The second copy should be retained in the laboratory for record.
3. Fold and place the card copy with the vial of MICRhoGAM, the direction circular and patient identification card.
4. Send the vial of MICRhoGAM, the direction circular and patient identification card to the patient's room for injection.
5. The empty vial of MICRhoGAM should be returned to the hospital or clinic laboratory with the card copy attached. The time of injection should be noted.

Injection Procedure

1. Verify the lot number of MICRhoGAM on the injection control form with the lot number printed on the vial of MICRhoGAM to be injected.
2. Establish complete patient identification.
3. Using a 1 ml capacity syringe and employing sterile technique, withdraw the entire contents of one vial of MICRhoGAM into the syringe.
4. Intramuscularly inject the entire contents of the vial into the post-abortion or post-miscarriage woman.
5. After injection, return the empty MICRhoGAM vial with its attached control form to the laboratory.

A patient identification card is included in the package for the physician's convenience and may be completed at his discretion.

INTRAMUSCULARLY INJECT THE ENTIRE CONTENTS OF ONE VIAL. DO NOT INJECT INTRAVENOUSLY.

Precautions: Reactions of Rh negative individuals given Rh_o (D) Immune Globulin (Human) are infrequent, of a mild nature and are mostly confined to the area of injection. A slight elevation of temperature has been noted in a small number of women who have received this material. Systemic reactions are rare and sensitization due to repeated injections of immune globulins is unusual. Immune Serum Globulin (Human) has not been reported to transmit hepatitis.

Packaging: MICRhoGAM is supplied in a package containing:

- one single-dose vial of MICRhoGAM
- direction circular
- patient injection control form
- patient identification card

MICRhoGAM is also supplied in a package containing:

Continued on next page

Ortho Diagnostics—Cont.

- 50 single-dose vials of MICRhoGAM
- direction circular
- 50 patient injection control forms
- 50 patient identification cards

Storage: Store at 2° to 8°C. DO NOT FREEZE.

RhoGAM™ ℞

Rh_0 (D) Immune Globulin (Human)
For Intramuscular Use Only

Description: RhoGAM Rh_0 (D) Immune Globulin (Human) is a sterile concentrated solution of specific immunoglobulin (IgG) containing anti-Rh_0(D). This product is prepared from fractionated human plasma (cold alcohol method) and may include immunoglobulin, which does not contain anti-Rh_0 (D), derived from an intermediate plasma fraction prepared by other Bureau of Biologics licensed manufacturers. All plasma used in the manufacture of this product was tested for hepatitis B surface antigen and found to be nonreactive.

Active Ingredient
Anti-Rh_0 (D) in 15% $\pm$ 1.5% serum globulin

Inactive Ingredients
15 mg/ml glycine—approximately
2.9 mg/ml sodium chloride—approximately
Preservative 0.01% Thimerosal (mercury derivative)

Action: RhoGAM is used to prevent the formation of active antibodies in the Rh_0 (D) negative, D^u negative individual who has received Rh positive blood as a result of delivering an Rh_0 (D) positive or D^u positive infant, or as a result of a transfusion accident. With an injection of passive Rh_0 (D) antibody (RhoGAM), to the postpartum mother or to the recipient of a transfusion accident, the person's antibody response to the foreign Rh_0 (D) positive cells is suppressed.
Active Rh_0 (D) antibody produced by the mother is the cause of Rh Hemolytic Disease of the Newborn in subsequent pregnancies. When the formation of active Rh_0 (D) antibody is prevented, Rh Hemolytic Disease of the Newborn has not been observed in the subsequent pregnancy. Clinical studies to date indicate that RhoGAM effectively prevents Rh_0 (D) Hemolytic Disease of the Newborn.

Indications

Full Term Delivery
RhoGAM has been shown to be effective in preventing the postpartum formation of antibodies to the Rh_0 (D) factor in the Rh_0 (D) negative, D^u negative woman. The material should be administered to the Rh_0 (D) negative, D^u negative postpartum mother within 72 hours of the birth of an Rh_0 (D) positive or D^u positive baby. (See note regarding miscarriage.) The postpartum mother should meet the following criteria in order to be considered a candidate for RhoGAM:

1. The mother must be Rh_0 (D) negative and D^u negative. [See direction circular such as accompanying ORTHO™ Blood Grouping Serum Anti-D (Anti-Rh_0) for Slide and Modified Tube Tests.]
2. The mother must not already be immunized to the Rh_0 (D) factor as determined by using Reagent Red Blood Cells which are designed for the detection and identification of atypical antibodies. These tests may be performed in the laboratory using products such as SELECTOGEN™ and IDENTIGEN™ Reagent Red Blood Cells.
3. Her baby must be Rh_0 (D) positive or D^u positive.
4. Her baby should have a negative direct Coombs test. (See direction circular such as accompanying ORTHO Anti-Human Serum.) Positive direct Coombs tests may be caused by antibodies other than Rh_0 (D); these are not significant as regards RhoGAM prophylaxis but should be investigated. A positive direct Coombs test due to anti-Rh_0 (D) should be considered significant and RhoGAM should not be administered.

Since ABO incompatibility between the Rh_0 (D) negative mother and her Rh_0 (D) positive fetus offers only incomplete protection against Rh isoimmunization, the use of immune prophylaxis in these cases is also advisable.

Miscarriages
It has been suggested that a miscarriage, abortion or ectopic pregnancy can serve as a primary immunizing stimulus by virtue of the entry of a small amount of Rh_0 (D) positive fetal cells into the Rh_0 (D) negative mother's bloodstream. Therefore, if an Rh_0 (D) negative mother has a miscarriage, abortion or ectopic pregnancy, she should be considered as a candidate for protective treatment with RhoGAM. The administration procedure should be followed as described. Since the fetus' blood type may not be known, one should assume that it was Rh_0 (D) positive [except when the father is known to be Rh_0 (D) negative and D^u negative] and extend RhoGAM to the mother within 72 hours after the spontaneous passage or surgical removal of the products of conception.

Transfusion Accidents
Rh positive blood transfused into an Rh_0 (D) negative, D^u negative individual (transfusion accident) can cause Rh immunization in the recipient. To prevent this, RhoGAM Rh_0 (D) Immune Globulin (Human) should be administered to the recipient of the blood in accordance with administration procedure described.

Pre-Administration—Laboratory Directions: In addition to the vial(s) of RhoGAM, each package contains a serum vial containing a 1:1000 dilution of the same lot number of RhoGAM. This crossmatch solution is provided so that the laboratory may perform a minor crossmatch to ensure that the individual is Rh_0 (D) negative and D^u negative. Incompatibility between the individual's red cells and the 1:1000 dilution of RhoGAM is not in itself a contraindication to RhoGAM prophylaxis but should serve to alert the technologist to the possibility that the person may be Rh_0 (D) positive or D^u positive.
In the case of incompatibility, repeat Rh typing of the person is advisable. If the individual can be shown to be Rh_0 (D) negative and D^u negative, RhoGAM can be administered safely.
When the crossmatch procedure is employed, it should be performed by an acceptable minor crossmatch procedure using:

- 1 drop of the patient's freshly drawn red cells—5% suspension in normal saline
- 2 drops of the 1:1000 dilution of RhoGAM.

A positive reaction in the minor crossmatch or in repeat Rh typing may be due to the following reasons:

1. The individual is D^u positive and therefore is not a candidate for RhoGAM prophylaxis.
2. There is an admixture of maternal Rh_0 (D) negative and Rh_0 (D) positive fetal erythrocytes due to a large transplacental hemorrhage. This type of agglutination appears as a mixed field (Ashby) agglutination which can be readily distinguished from a weakly positive D^u test when viewed under magnification. In the latter case, the woman should be considered a candidate for RhoGAM prophylaxis provided it can be established that the woman is Rh_0 (D) negative.
3. There is an admixture of recipient Rh_0 (D) negative and donor Rh_0 (D) positive red blood cells in the case of a transfusion accident. The recipient should be considered a candidate for RhoGAM prophylaxis provided it can be established that the recipient is Rh_0 (D) negative.

After the minor crossmatch is performed, complete the injection data form included with the package(s) of RhoGAM.

1. Separate the three-part form, remove the first copy and place it securely with the product.
2. The second copy should be retained in the laboratory for record.
3. Fold and place the card copy with the vial(s) of RhoGAM, the direction circular and patient identification card.
4. Send the vial(s) of RhoGAM, the direction circular and patient identification card to the patient's room for injection.
5. The empty vial(s) of RhoGAM should be returned to the hospital laboratory with the card copy attached. The time(s) of injection should be noted.

Dosage: One vial of RhoGAM will completely suppress immunity to 15 ml of Rh positive red blood cells (packed cells, not whole blood).
In deciding the dose of RhoGAM which is to be administered to an individual, the volume of Rh positive blood which entered that person's bloodstream is to be determined.

1. In the usual full term delivery, a single dose (one vial) of RhoGAM will be adequate to suppress immunity to the Rh_0 (D) antigen.
2. However, in the case of a large feto-maternal hemorrhage, the clinician must establish the magnitude of the bleed by an approved laboratory technique, e.g., acid elution test of Kleihauer-Betke.† In order to convert the volume of feto-maternal hemorrhage to packed red blood cells, multiply by 0.50 (approximate hematocrit). The volume of packed red blood cells is divided by 15 ml to provide the number of vials of RhoGAM to be administered.
3. In the case of a transfusion accident, the volume of Rh positive whole blood administered is multiplied by the hematocrit value of the donor unit. This value equals the volume of packed red blood cells transfused. The volume of packed red blood cells is divided by 15 ml to provide the number of vials of RhoGAM to be administered.

NOTE: If the dose calculation results in a fraction, administer the next whole number of vials of RhoGAM.

---

†The Kleihauer-Betke acid elution technique may be used to quantitate the magnitude of feto-maternal hemorrhage.

Reagents
Ethanol (80%)
Citric Phosphate Buffer (0.07M Citric Acid Monohydrate; 0.06M Na_2HPO_4,pH 3.5)
Hematoxylin (6.4 mg hematoxylin/ml)
Erythrosin (1.0 mg erythrosin/ml)

Smear
On an alcohol-cleaned glass slide, prepare a thin smear of capillary, citrate, or heparinized whole blood. Air dry the smear at room temperature for 30 to 60 minutes.

Fixation
Fix the smear in ethanol (80%) for 5 minutes. Gently rinse the smear in distilled water. Allow the smear to air dry at room temperature.

Elution
Place the smear in a Coplin jar containing citric phosphate buffer at 37° C for 5 minutes.
NOTE: In order to produce uniform laking of the adult hemoglobin, remove the smear from the Coplin jar after 2 minutes incubation and immediately replace it in the Coplin jar for the remainder of the incubation period.
Gently rinse the smear in distilled water.

Stain
Place 1.0 ml of filtered hematoxylin on the smear for 5 minutes. Gently rinse the smear under running tap water.
Place 1.0 ml of erythrosin on the smear for 5 minutes. Gently rinse the smear under running tap water.

Examination and Interpretation
Scan the smear for 5 minutes under low power (10X) magnification. Count the number of

eluted adult "ghost" cells and the number of stained fetal cells. When the ratio of fetal cells to maternal cells has been determined, and the total maternal blood volume has been estimated, the volume of feto-maternal hemorrhage can be calculated according to the following formula:

$$\frac{\text{number of fetal cells}}{\text{number of maternal cells}} = \frac{\text{X (volume of feto-maternal hemorrhage)}}{\text{total maternal blood volume}}$$

[See table above].

References: Kleihauer E, Braun H and Betke K: Demonstration of fetal hemoglobin in the erythrocytes of a blood smear. Klin Wschr 35:637, 1957.
Kleihauer E, Betke K: Practical use of the demonstration of cells containing hemoglobin F in blood smears. Der Internist 1:292, 1960.
Finn R. et al: Transplacental Hemorrhage. Transfusion 3:114, 1963.

Injection Procedure

Single Vial Dose

1. Verify the lot number of RhoGAM on the crossmatch form with the lot number printed on the vial of RhoGAM to be injected.
2. Establish complete patient identification.
3. Using a 2 ml capacity syringe and employing sterile technique, withdraw completely the contents of the vial of RhoGAM into the syringe.
4. INJECT THE ENTIRE CONTENTS OF ONE VIAL INTO THE INDIVIDUAL INTRAMUSCULARLY. DO NOT INJECT INTRAVENOUSLY. DO NOT INJECT INFANT.
5. After injection, return the empty RhoGAM vial with its attached identification form to the laboratory.

A patient identification card is included in the package for the physician's convenience and may be completed at his discretion.

Multiple Vial Dose

1. Ascertain that the patient is Rh_0 (D) and D^u negative (a minor crossmatch after a transfusion accident would probably be incompatible due to the large number of Rh positive cells in the circulation).
2. Establish complete patient identification.
3. Calculate the number of vials of RhoGAM which are to be administered. (See dosage section.)
4. Employing sterile technique, withdraw the entire contents of all vials of RhoGAM to be administered at one time, and inject them intramuscularly into the patient. For convenience and patient comfort, the total volume of RhoGAM to be given can be injected in divided doses at different sites at one time, or at 12-hour intervals, as long as the last dose is given within 72 hours of the transfusion accident or feto-maternal hemorrhage.

Cautions: Reactions of Rh_0 (D) negative individuals given Rh_0 (D) Immune Globulin (Human) are infrequent, of a mild nature and mostly confined to the area of injection. An occasional patient may react more strongly, both locally and generally. A slight elevation of temperature has been noted in a small number of postpartum women.

Approximately five out of 22 subjects, receiving the multi-dose regimen following mismatched transfusions, noted fever, myalgia and lethargy 24-36 hours after injection of several vials of RhoGAM. Bilirubin levels of 0.4-6.8 mg % were observed in some of the treated subjects. One subject had splenomegaly.

In either regimen, systemic reactions are rare and sensitization due to repeated injections of immune globulins is unusual. Immune Serum Globulin (Human) has not been reported to transmit hepatitis.

RhoGAM IS TO BE GIVEN TO THE RECIPIENT IN A TRANSFUSION ACCIDENT OR THE POSTPARTUM MOTHER OR POST-MISCARRIAGE WOMAN, ONLY. IT MUST NOT BE GIVEN TO THE INFANT.

Contraindications: Rh_0 (D) Immune Globulin (Human) should *not* be administered to:

1. An Rh_0 (D) positive or D^u positive individual.
2. An Rh_0(D) negative patient who has inadvertently received an Rh_0 (D) positive blood transfusion within three months of delivery.
3. A patient previously immunized to the Rh_0 (D) blood factor.

Packaging: RhoGAM is supplied in a package containing:

- one single-dose vial of RhoGAM
- one droppered vial of a 1:1000 dilution of RhoGAM for crossmatch
- direction circular
- patient crossmatch form
- patient identification card

RhoGAM is also supplied in a package containing:

- 25 single-dose vials of RhoGAM
- one droppered vial of a 1:1000 dilution of RhoGAM sufficient for 25 crossmatches
- direction circular
- 25 patient crossmatch forms
- 25 patient identification cards

Storage: Store at 2°-8° C. DO NOT FREEZE.
Licensed under U.S.P.H.S. Act 351 with a one year dating.
Manufactured using U.S. Patent 3,449,314.

Literature Available: Medical and Lay information available on request.

Ortho Pharmaceutical Corporation
RARITAN, NJ 08869

ACI-JEL® Therapeutic Vaginal Jelly ℞

Composition: A bland, nonirritant, water-dispersible, buffered acid jelly, containing acetic acid 0.92%, oxyquinoline sulfate 0.025%, ricinoleic acid 0.7%, boric acid 3% and glycerin 5%, compounded with tragacanth, acacia, propylparaben, potassium hydroxide, stannous chloride, egg albumen, potassium bitartrate, perfume and water.

Indications: In any case where the restoration and maintenance of vaginal acidity is desirable.

Contraindications: None known.

Dosage: In the average case, one applicatorful intravaginally in the morning and upon retiring.

The frequency of application and duration of treatment depend upon the type of case and degree of progress.

Packaging: 85 g tubes with the ORTHO® Measured-Dose Applicator.

CONCEPTROL® Birth Control Cream

(See PDR For Nonprescription Drugs)

DELFEN® Contraceptive Foam

(See PDR For Nonprescription Drugs)

DIENESTROL Cream ℞

(See ORTHO® Dienestrol Cream)

IMODIUM® Ⓒ
(loperamide HCl)
Capsules

Description: IMODIUM (loperamide hydrochloride), 4- (*p*-chlorophenyl) -4-hydroxy-N, N-dimethyl-α, α-diphenyl-1-piperidinebutyramide monohydrochloride, is a synthetic antidiarrheal for oral use. IMODIUM is available in 2 mg capsules.

Important Information: IMODIUM Capsules are classified as a Schedule V controlled substance by federal law (*see* Overdosage Section).

KEEP THIS AND ALL MEDICATIONS OUT OF THE REACH OF CHILDREN.

Clinical Pharmacology: *In vitro* and animal studies show that IMODIUM acts by slowing intestinal motility. It inhibits peristaltic activity by a direct effect on the circular and longitudinal muscles of the intestinal wall.

In man, IMODIUM prolongs the transit time of the intestinal contents. It reduces the daily fecal volume, increases the viscosity and bulk density, and diminishes the loss of fluid and electrolytes. Tolerance to the antidiarrheal effect has not been observed. Studies in morphine-dependent monkeys demonstrated that loperamide hydrochloride at doses above those recommended for humans prevented signs of morphine withdrawal. However, in humans, the naloxone challenge pupil test, which when positive indicates opiate-like effects, performed after a single high dose, or after more than two years of therapeutic use of IMODIUM was negative.

Clinical studies have indicated that the apparent elimination half-life of loperamide in man is 10.8 hours with a range of 9.1 - 14.4 hours. Unchanged drug remains below 2 nanograms per ml after the intake of a 2 mg capsule of IMODIUM. Plasma levels are highest approximately five hours after the administration of the capsule dosage form. Of the total excreted in urine and feces, most of the administered drug was excreted in feces.

In those patients in whom biochemical and hematological parameters were monitored during clinical trials, no trends toward abnormality during IMODIUM therapy were noted. Similarly, urinalyses, EKG and clinical ophthalmological examinations did not show trends toward abnormality. There was no evidence in clinical trials of drug interaction with concurrent medications.

Indications: IMODIUM is indicated for the control and symptomatic relief of acute nonspecific diarrhea and of chronic diarrhea associated with inflammatory bowel disease. IMODIUM is also indicated for reducing the volume of discharge from ileostomies.

Contraindications: IMODIUM is contraindicated in patients with known hypersensitivity to the drug and in those in whom constipation must be avoided.

Warnings: Antiperistaltic agents should not be used in acute diarrhea associated with organisms that penetrate the intestinal mucosa, e.g., toxigenic E. coli, salmonella, shigella, and in pseudomembranous colitis associated with broad-spectrum antibiotics.

Fluid and electrolyte depletion may occur in patients who have diarrhea. The use of IMODIUM does not preclude the administration of appropriate fluid and electrolyte therapy. In some patients with acute ulcerative colitis, agents which inhibit intestinal motility or delay intestinal transit time have been reported to induce toxic megacolon. IMODIUM therapy should be discontinued promptly if abdominal distention occurs or if other untoward symptoms develop in patients with acute ulcerative colitis.

Precautions: In acute diarrhea, if clinical improvement is not observed in 48 hours, the administration of IMODIUM should be discontinued.

Abuse and Dependence: Physical dependence to IMODIUM in humans has not been observed. However, studies in monkeys demonstrated that loperamide hydrochloride at high doses produced symptoms of physical dependence of the morphine type.

Continued on next page

Ortho Pharm.—Cont.

Carcinogenesis: In an 18 month rat study with doses up to 133 times the maximum human dose (on a mg/kg basis) there was no evidence of carcinogenesis.
Pregnancy: Safe use of IMODIUM during pregnancy has not been established. Reproduction studies performed in rats and rabbits with dosage levels up to 30 times the human therapeutic dose did not demonstrate evidence of impaired fertility or harm to the offspring due to IMODIUM. Higher doses impaired maternal and neonate survival, but no dose level up to 30 times the human dose demonstrated teratogenicity. Such experience cannot exclude the possibility of damage to the fetus. IMODIUM should be used in pregnant women only when clearly needed.
Nursing Mothers: It is not known whether IMODIUM is excreted in human milk. As a general rule, nursing should not be undertaken while a patient is on a drug since many drugs are excreted in human milk.
Pediatric Use: Safety and effectiveness in children have not been established. Therefore, use of IMODIUM is not recommended in the pediatric age group (under the age of 12). In case of accidental ingestion of IMODIUM by children, *see* Overdosage Section for suggested treatment.
Adverse Reactions: The adverse effects reported during clinical investigations of IMODIUM are difficult to distinguish from symptoms associated with the diarrheal syndrome. Adverse experiences recorded during clinical studies with IMODIUM were generally of a minor and self-limiting nature. They were more commonly observed during the treatment of chronic diarrhea.
The following patient complaints have been reported:

Abdominal pain, distention or discomfort
Constipation
Drowsiness or dizziness
Dry mouth
Nausea and vomiting
Tiredness

Hypersensitivity Reactions (including skin rash), however, have been reported with IMODIUM use.
Overdosage: Animal pharmacological and toxicological data indicate that overdosage in man may result in constipation, CNS depression, and gastrointestinal irritation. In clinical trials an adult who took three 20 mg doses within a 24-hour period was nauseated after the second dose and vomited after the third dose. If vomiting has occurred spontaneously, a slurry of 100 gms of activated charcoal should be administered orally as soon as fluids can be retained.
If vomiting has not occurred, gastric lavage should be performed followed by administration of 100 gms of the activated charcoal slurry through the gastric tube. In the event of overdosage, patients should be monitored for signs of CNS depression for at least 24 hours. If CNS depression is observed, naloxone may be administered. If responsive to naloxone, vital signs must be monitored carefully for recurrence of symptoms of drug overdose for at least 24 hours after the last dose of naloxone.
In view of the prolonged action of loperamide and the short duration (one to three hours) of naloxone, the patient must be monitored closely and treated repeatedly with naloxone as indicated. Based on the fact that relatively little drug is excreted in urine, forced diuresis is not expected to be effective for IMODIUM overdosage.
Dosage and Administration:
Acute diarrhea
The recommended initial dose of IMODIUM is two capsules (4 mg) followed by one capsule (2 mg) after each unformed stool. Daily dosage should not exceed eight capsules (16 mg). Clinical improvement is usually observed within 48 hours.
Chronic diarrhea
The recommended initial dosage of IMODIUM is two capsules (4 mg) followed by one capsule (2 mg) after each unformed stool until diarrhea is controlled, after which the dosage of IMODIUM should be reduced to meet individual requirements. When the optimal daily dosage has thus been established, this amount should then be administered as a single dose or in divided doses.
The average daily maintenance dosage in clinical trials was two to four capsules (4–8 mg). A dosage of eight capsules (16 mg) was rarely exceeded. If clinical improvement is not observed after treatment with eight capsules (16 mg) of IMODIUM per day for at least 10 days, symptoms are unlikely to be controlled by further administration. IMODIUM administration may be continued if diarrhea cannot be adequately controlled with diet or specific treatment.
How Supplied: IMODIUM is available as 2 mg capsules of loperamide hydrochloride. The capsules have a light green body and a dark green cap, with "ORTHO 1000" imprinted on each segment. IMODIUM capsules are supplied in bottles of 100 and 500.
IMODIUM (loperamide hydrochloride) is an original product of Janssen Pharmaceutica, Belgium and co-developed by Ortho Pharmaceutical Corporation.
[*Shown in Product Identification Section*]

LIPPES LOOP® ℞
Intrauterine Device

Description: The LIPPES LOOP is made of polyethylene in the shape of a double S. Four different sizes are manufactured to allow for the variability in the size of the uterus. (See below.) A fine, double thread or "tail" made of polyethylene suture (monofilament) is attached to the lower end to facilitate removal. In addition, palpation of the tail through the cervix by the patient, or visualization by the physician, can assist in determining whether or not an undetected expulsion has occurred. A LIPPES LOOP comes prepackaged and sterilized with an introducer, together with an insertion tube in a polyethylene pouch. The insertion tube is equipped with a flange to aid in gauging the depth to which the insertion tube should be inserted through the cervical canal and into the uterine cavity. The four available sizes are as follows:

Loop A—22.5 mm. Blue thread. For nulliparous females.
Loop B—27.5 mm. WITH REDUCED RADII. Black thread. Suggested for women who have had premature pregnancy losses and multiparous females whose uteri sound out less than 3 cm.
Loop C—30 mm. WITH REDUCED RADII. Yellow thread. Suggested for use when Loop D is removed for bleeding or pain. The physician is advised to wait two to four weeks between removing a loop for bleeding and reinserting a second loop.
Loop D—30 mm. White thread. Suggested for use in women with one or more children.

Mode of Action or Principles of IUD Design: The exact mechanism of action of the LIPPES LOOP is not known. However, it is believed to interfere in some manner with nidation in the endometrium, probably through foreign body reaction in the uterus.
Indications and Usage: LIPPES LOOP is indicated for contraception.
Contraindications: IUD's should not be inserted when the following conditions exist:

1. Pregnancy or suspicion of pregnancy.
2. Abnormalities of the uterus resulting in distortion of the uterine cavity.
3. Pelvic inflammatory disease or a history of repeated pelvic inflammatory disease.
4. Postpartum endometritis or infected abortion in the past three months.
5. Known or suspected uterine or cervical malignancy including unresolved, abnormal "Pap" smear.
6. Genital bleeding of unknown etiology.
7. Cervicitis until infection is controlled.

Warnings:
1. Pregnancy. a. Long-term effects. Long-term effects on the offspring when pregnancy occurs with LIPPES LOOP in place are unknown.
b. Septic abortion. Reports have indicated an increased incidence of septic abortion associated in some instances with septicemia, septic shock, and death in patients becoming pregnant with an IUD in place. Most of these reports have been associated with the mid-trimester of pregnancy. In some cases, the initial symptoms have been insidious and not easily recognized. If pregnancy should occur with an IUD in place, the IUD should be removed if the string is visible or, if removal proves to be or would be difficult, termination of the pregnancy should be considered and offered the patient as an option, bearing in mind that the risks associated with an elective abortion increases with gestational age.
c. Continuation of pregnancy. If the patient chooses to continue the pregnancy, she must be warned of the increased risk of spontaneous abortion and of the increased risk of sepsis, including death, if the pregnancy continues with the IUD in place. The patient must be closely observed and she must be advised to report all abnormal symptoms, such as flu-like syndrome, fever, abdominal cramping and pain, bleeding, or vaginal discharge, immediately because generalized symptoms of septicemia may be insidious.
2. Ectopic pregnancy. a. A pregnancy that occurs with an IUD in place is more likely to be ectopic than a pregnancy occuring without an IUD in place. Accordingly, patients who become pregnant while using the IUD should be carefully evaluated for the possibility of an ectopic pregnancy.
b. Special attention should be directed to patients with delayed menses, slight metrorrhagia and/or unilateral pelvic pain, and to those patients who wish to terminate a pregnancy because of IUD failure, to determine whether ectopic pregnancy has occurred.
3. Pelvic Infection. An increased risk of pelvic infection has been reported with the IUD in place. This, at times, results in the development of bilateral or unilateral tubo-ovarian abscesses or general peritonitis which may lead to hospitalization or surgery and infertility if untreated. Appropriate aerobic and anaerobic bacteriological studies should be done and antibiotic therapy initiated. The IUD should be removed and the continuing treatment reassessed based upon the results of culture and sensitivity tests.
4. Embedment. Partial penetration or lodging of the IUD in the endometrium can result in difficult removals.
5. Perforation. Partial or total perforation of the uterine wall or cervix may occur with the use of IUDs. The possibility of perforation must be kept in mind during insertion and at the time of any subsequent examination. If perforation occurs, the IUD should be removed. Adhesions, foreign body reactions, and intestinal obstruction may result if an IUD is left in the peritoneal cavity. There are a few reports that there has been migration after insertion apparently in the absence of perforation at insertion. In any event, it is possible for the IUD to perforate outside the uterus.
Precautions:
1. Patient counseling. Prior to insertion, the physician, nurse, or other trained health professional must provide the patient with the

Patient Brochure. The patient should be given the opportunity to read the brochure and discuss fully any questions she may have concerning the IUD as well as other methods of contraception.

2. Patient evaluation and clinical considerations. **a.** A complete medical history should be obtained to determine conditions that might influence the selection of an IUD. Physical examination should include a pelvic examination, "Pap" smear, gonorrhea culture and, if indicated, appropriate tests for other forms of venereal disease.

b. The uterus should be carefully sounded prior to insertion to determine the degree of patency of the endocervical canal and the internal os, and the direction and depth of the uterine cavity. In occasional cases, severe cervical stenosis may be encountered. Do not use excessive force to overcome this resistance.

c. The uterus should sound to a depth of 6 to 8 centimeters (cm). Insertion of an IUD into a uterine cavity measuring less than 6.5 cm by sounding may increase the incidence of expulsion, bleeding, pain and perforation.

d. The possibility of insertion in the presence of an existing undetermined pregnancy is reduced if insertion is performed during or shortly following a menstrual period. The IUD should not be inserted postpartum or postabortion until involution of the uterus is completed. The incidence of perforation and expulsion is greater if involution is not completed.

e. IUD's should be used with caution in those patients who have anemia or a history of menorrhagia or hypermenorrhea. Patients experiencing menorrhagia and/or metrorrhagia following IUD insertion may be at risk for the development of hypochromic microcytic anemia. Also, IUD's should be used with caution in patients receiving anticoagulants or having a coagulopathy.

f. Syncope, bradycardia, or other neurovascular episodes may occur during insertion or removal of IUD's, especially in patients with a previous disposition to these conditions.

g. Patients with valvular or congential heart disease are more prone to develop subacute bacterial endocarditis than patients who do not have valvular or congenital heart disease. Use of an IUD in these patients may represent a potential source of septic emboli.

h. Use of an IUD in those patients with cervicitis should be postponed until treatment has cured the infection (see CONTRAINDICATIONS Section).

i. Since an IUD may be expelled or displaced, patients should be reexamined and evaluated shortly after the first postinsertion menses, but definitely within three months after insertion. Thereafter, annual examination with appropriate medical and laboratory examination should be carried out.

j. The patient should be told that some bleeding and cramps may occur during the first few weeks after insertion, but if these symptoms continue or are severe, she should report them to her physician. The patient should be instructed on how to check to make certain that the thread still protrudes from the cervix, and she should be cautioned that there is no contraceptive protection if the IUD is expelled. She should be instructed to check the tail as often as possible, but at least after each menstrual period. The patient should be cautioned not to pull on the thread and displace the IUD. If partial expulsion occurs, removal is indicated and a new IUD may be inserted.

k. The use of medical diathermy (shortwave and microwave) in patients with metal-containing IUD's may cause heat injury to the surrounding tissue. Therefore, medical diathermy to the abdominal and sacral areas should not be used.

[LIPPES LOOP contains no metals. This section does not apply to LIPPES LOOP].

TABLE I

LIPPES LOOP Size	Number Woman/Months	Woman/Months of Use 1st Year After Insertion	Woman/Months of Use 2nd year After Insertion
A	13,453	8,751	4,702
B	12,463	9,660	2,803
C	50,775	31,032	19,743
D	121,566	72,046	49,520

Adverse Reactions: These adverse reactions are not listed in any order of frequency or severity.

Reported adverse reactions include: endometritis, spontaneous abortion, septic abortion, septicemia, perforation of the uterus and cervix, embedment, migration resulting in partial or complete perforation, fragmentation of the IUD, pelvic infection (pelvic inflammatory disease), vaginitis, leukorrhea, cervical erosion, pregnancy, ectopic pregnancy, difficult removal, complete or partial expulsion of the IUD, intermenstrual spotting, prolongation of menstrual flow, anemia, pain and cramping, dysmenorrhea, backaches, dyspareunia, neurovascular episodes, including bradycardia and syncope secondary to insertion. Perforation into the abdomen has been followed by abdominal adhesions, intestinal penetration, intestinal obstruction, and cystic masses in the pelvis.

Directions For Use:

Preinsertion

1. It is imperative that sterile technique be maintained throughout the insertion procedure.

2. Perform a thorough pelvic examination to determine freedom from overt disease and to determine position and shape of the uterus. RULE OUT PREGNANCY AND OTHER CONTRAINDICATIONS.

3. With a speculum in place, gently insert a sterile sound to determine the depth and direction of the uterine canal. Be sure to determine the position of the uterus before insertion.

Occasionally a tenaculum is required if the uterine canal needs to be straightened. If a stenotic cervix must be dilated, use a sterile Hank's dilator rather than a Hegar's; dilation to a Hank's 16 to 18 should be sufficient.

Insertion

Caution: It is generally felt that perforations are caused at the time of insertion, although the perforation may not be detected until some time later. The position of the uterus should be determined during the preinsertion examination. Great care must be exercised during the preinsertion sounding and subsequent insertion. No attempt should be made to force the insertion. There are a few reports, however, that there has been migration after insertion apparently in the absence of perforation at insertion. In any event, it is possible for the IUD to perforate outside the uterus.

1. How to prepare the LIPPES LOOP Intrauterine Double-S inserter.

Using sterile gloves, hold tube in one hand and with the other draw LOOP into inserter by pulling the push rod. Continue to pull the push rod until all but the bulbous tip of the LOOP is entirely within the inserter. At this point, insure that both the flat surface of the bulbous tip and the inserter flange are in a horizontal plane.

Do this not more than one minute before insertion.

2. How to insert LIPPES LOOP Intrauterine Double-S.

Insert the loaded inserter gently through the endocervical canal, with the flange in a horizontal plane. DO NOT FORCE THE INSERTION. If resistance is encountered, do not proceed; perforation of the uterus may occur. If the flange makes contact with the cervix WITHOUT the inserter touching the fundal wall, withdraw 1/4 inch before pressing the push rod to release the device in utero. Should the inserter touch the fundal wall BEFORE the flange makes contact, withdraw 1/2 inch prior to pressing the push rod to release the device in utero. With the inserter now in place, proceed, and WITHOUT UNDUE PRESSURE, Push the rod slowly as far as it will go. LIPPES LOOP Intrauterine Double-S should now be in place. Withdraw the inserter tube and push rod from the cervical os until the tail is visible. Cut the tail leaving it as long as possible.

Time of Insertion

LIPPES LOOP Intrauterine Double-S should be inserted perferably the last one or two days of a normal menstrual period or the two days following the last day.

The expulsion and perforation rate may be increased when insertions are made before normal uterine involution occurs (usually four to six weeks postpartum or postabortion).

To Remove

To remove LIPPES LOOP Intrauterine Double-S, pull gently on the exposed tail. On those rare occasions that the tail is not available, the device should be carefully removed.

Clinical Studies: Different event rates have been recorded with the use of different IUD's. Inasmuch as these rates are usually derived from separate studies conducted by different investigators in several population groups, they cannot be compared with precision. Furthermore, event rates tend to be lower as clinical experience is expanded, possibly due to retention in the cinical study of those patients who accept the treatment regimen and do not discontinue due to adverse reactions or pregnancy. In clinical trials conducted by The Population Council with the LIPPES LOOP, use effectiveness was determined as follows for women, as tabulated by the life table method. (Rates are expressed as events per 100 women through 12 and 24 months of use.) This experience is based on 198,257 woman/months of use, including 121,489 woman/months of use in first year after insertion, and 76,768 woman/months of use in second year after insertion. LIPPES LOOP Intrauterine Double-S devices are manufactured in four different sizes, and the figures given above represent the totals for the four sizes. The following table presents these figures individually for each size LOOP:

[See Table I above].

Tables II–V below give the pregnancy expulsion, medical removal and continuation rates for each individual size LOOP.

TABLE II
LOOP A
(Annual Rates Per 100 Users)

	12 Months	24 Months (cumulative)
Pregnancy	5.3	9.7
Expulsion	23.9	27.7
Medical Removal	12.2	20.0
Continuation Rate	75.2	63.6

TABLE III
LOOP B
(Annual Rates Per 100 Users)

	12 Months	24 Months (cumulative)
Pregnancy	3.4	6.3
Expulsion	18.9	24.9
Medical Removal	15.1	23.8
Continuation Rate	74.6	59.2

Continued on next page

Ortho Pharm.—Cont.

TABLE IV
LOOP C
(Annual Rates Per 100 Users)

	12 Months	24 Months (cumulative)
Pregnancy	3.0	4.8
Expulsion	19.1	24.6
Medical Removal	14.3	22.1
Continuation Rate	76.5	62.8

TABLE V
LOOP D
(Annual Rates Per 100 Users)

	12 Months	24 Months (cumulative)
Pregnancy	2.7	4.2
Expulsion	12.7	16.0
Medical Removal	15.2	23.3
Continuation Rate	77.4	65.6

MONISTAT® 7 Vaginal Cream ℞
(miconazole nitrate 2%)

Description: MONISTAT 7 Vaginal Cream (miconazole nitrate 2%) is a water-miscible, white cream containing as the active ingredient, 2% miconazole nitrate, 1-[2,4-dichloro-β-(2,4-dichlorobenzyloxy) phenethyl] imidazole nitrate.
Actions: MONISTAT 7 Vaginal Cream exhibits fungicidal activity *in vitro* against species of the genus *Candida*. The pharmacologic mode of action is unknown.
Indications: MONISTAT 7 Vaginal Cream is indicated for the local treatment of vulvovaginal candidiasis (moniliasis). As MONISTAT 7 Vaginal Cream is effective only for candidal vulvovaginitis, the diagnosis should be confirmed by KOH smears and/or cultures. Other pathogens commonly associated with vulvovaginitis (Trichomonas and *Haemophilus vaginalis*) should be ruled out by appropriate laboratory methods.
MONISTAT 7 is effective in both pregnant and non-pregnant women, as well as in women taking oral contraceptives. (See PRECAUTIONS.)
Contraindications: Patients known to be hypersensitive to this drug.
Precautions:
General: Discontinue drug if sensitization or irritation is reported during use. Laboratory Tests: If there is a lack of response to MONISTAT 7, appropriate microbiological studies should be repeated to confirm the diagnosis and rule out other pathogens.
Pregnancy: Since MONISTAT is absorbed in small amounts from the human vagina, it should be used in the first trimester of pregnancy only when the physician considers it essential to the welfare of the patient.
Clinical studies, during which MONISTAT was used for 14 days, included 209 pregnant patients. Follow-up reports now available in 117 of these patients reveal no adverse effects or complications attributable to MONISTAT therapy in infants born to these women.
Adverse Reactions: During clinical studies with MONISTAT for a 14-day regimen, 39 of the 528 patients (7.4%) treated with MONISTAT reported complaints during therapy that were possibly drug-related. Most complaints were reported during the first week of therapy. Vulvovaginal burning, itching or irritation occurred in 6.6%, while other complaints such as vaginal burning, pelvic cramps, hives, skin rash and headache occurred rarely (each less than 0.2% patient incidence). The therapy-related dropout rate was 0.9%.
Clinical: Statistical analysis of randomized clinical trials, conducted to determine the shortest effective course of therapy with MONISTAT, demonstrates that a regimen of seven or more days has a cure rate equivalent to the 14-day regimen.
The graphic representation of this conclusion plots days of therapy versus cure rates. The solid line represents the mean therapeutic cure rate and the shaded area represents the 95% confidence interval.

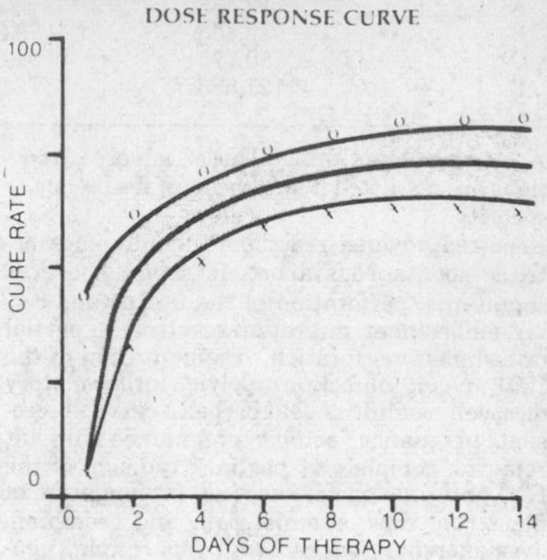

Dosage and Administration: One applicatorful is administered intravaginally once daily at bedtime for seven days. Course of therapy may be repeated after other pathogens have been ruled out by appropriate smears and cultures.
Supplied: MONISTAT 7 Vaginal Cream is available in 1.66 oz. (47 g) tubes with ORTHO® Measured-Dose Applicator.
MONISTAT Cream (miconazole nitrate 2%) is a development of Ortho Pharmaceutical Corporation and Janssen Pharmaceutica, Belgium.

NICKERSON'S® Medium

Diagnostic Aid: Members of the genus *Candida* will grow very dark brown to black colonies on this selective medium. Other yeasts and fungi may grow but will appear much lighter in color and so are easily differentiated from the genus *Candida*. This medium will not support bacterial growth. After inoculation, positive *Candida* cultures exhibit very dark brown to black colonies within two days' incubation at room temperature (growth appears more rapidly at 28° to 37°C.).
How Supplied: NICKERSON'S Medium 12's. Contains twelve vials NICKERSON'S Medium.

ORTHO-CREME® Contraceptive Cream

(See PDR For Nonprescription Drugs)

ORTHO® Diaphragm Kit—ALL-FLEX® ℞

Action and Uses: The ALL-FLEX Diaphragm is a molded, buff-colored, latex vaginal diaphragm containing a distortion-free, dual spring-within-a-spring which provides unique arcing action no matter where compressed. Ideal not only where ordinary diaphragms are indicated but also in patients with mild cystocele, rectocele or retroversion.
How Supplied: Available individually with tube of ORTHO-GYNOL Contraceptive Jelly. Each diaphragm is contained in an attractive plastic compact. Sizes 55, 60, 65, 70, 75, 80, 85, 90, 95 mm.

ORTHO® Diaphragm Kit—Coil Spring ℞

Action and Uses: The ORTHO Diaphragm (coil spring) is a molded latex vaginal diaphragm. The rim encases a tension-adjusted cadmium-plated coil spring. The diaphragm is used in conjunction with ORTHO-GYNOL Contraceptive Jelly or ORTHO-CREME Contraceptive Cream in conception control.
How Supplied: Available individually with tube of ORTHO-GYNOL Contraceptive Jelly. Each diaphragm is contained in an attractive plastic compact. Sizes 50, 55, 60, 65, 70, 75, 80, 85, 90, 95, 100, 105 mm.

ORTHO® Diaphragm Kit—Flat Spring ℞

Action and Uses: The ORTHO-WHITE® Diaphragm is a molded pure white latex vaginal diaphragm containing a flat watch-type spring which allows compressibility in one plane only, thus facilitating insertion.
How Supplied: Available individually with tube of ORTHO-GYNOL Contraceptive Jelly. Each diaphragm is contained in an attractive plastic compact. Sizes 55, 60, 65, 70, 75, 80, 85, 90, 95 mm.

ORTHO® Dienestrol Cream ℞

1. ESTROGENS HAVE BEEN REPORTED TO INCREASE THE RISK OF ENDOMETRIAL CARCINOMA.
Three independent case control studies have shown an increased risk of endometrial cancer in postmenopausal women exposed to exogenous estrogens for prolonged periods.[1–3] This risk was independent of the other known risk factors for endometrial cancer. These studies are further supported by the finding that incidence rates of endometrial cancer have increased sharply since 1969 in eight different areas of the United States with population-based cancer reporting systems, an increase which may be related to the rapidly expanding use of estrogens during the last decade.[4]
The three case control studies reported that the risk of endometrial cancer in estrogen users was about 4.5 to 13.9 times greater than in nonusers. The risk appears to depend on both duration of treatment[1] and on estrogen dose.[3] In view of these findings, when estrogens are used for the treatment of menopausal symptoms, the lowest dose that will control symptoms should be utilized and medication should be discontinued as soon as possible. When prolonged treatment is medically indicated, the patient should be reassessed on at least a semiannual basis to determine the need for continued therapy. Although the evidence must be considered preliminary, one study suggests that cyclic administration of low doses of estrogen may carry less risk than continuous administration;[3] it therefore appears prudent to utilize such a regimen.
Close clinical surveillance of all women taking estrogens is important. In all cases of undiagnosed persistent or recurring abnormal vaginal bleeding, adequate diagnostic measures should be undertaken to rule out malignancy.
There is no evidence at present that "natural" estrogens are more or less hazardous than "synthetic" estrogens at equiestrogenic doses.
2. ESTROGENS SHOULD NOT BE USED DURING PREGNANCY
The use of female sex hormones, both estrogens and progestogens, during early pregnancy may seriously damage the offspring. It has been shown that females exposed *in utero* to diethylstilbestrol, a non-steroidal estrogen, have an increased risk of developing in later life a form of vaginal or cervical cancer that ordinarily is extremely rare.[5,6] This risk has been estimated as not greater than 4 per 1000 exposures.[7] Furthermore, a high percentage of such exposed women (from 30 to 90 percent) have been found to have vaginal adenosis,[8,13] epithelial changes of the vagina and cervix. Although these changes are histologically benign, it is not known whether they are precursors of malig-

nancy. Although similar data are not available with the use of other estrogens, it cannot be presumed they would not induce similar changes.

Several reports suggest an association between intrauterine exposure to female sex hormones and congenital anomalies, including congenital heart defects and limb reduction defects.[13–16] One case control study[16] estimated a 4.7 fold increased risk of limb reduction defects in infants exposed in utero to sex hormones (oral contraceptives, hormone withdrawal tests for pregnancy, or attempted treatment for threatened abortion). Some of these exposures were very short and involved only a few days of treatment. The data suggest that the risk of limb reduction defects in exposed fetuses is somewhat less than 1 per 1000.

In the past, female sex hormones have been used during pregnancy in an attempt to treat threatened or habitual abortion. There is considerable evidence that estrogens are ineffective for these indications, and there is no evidence from well controlled studies that progestogens are effective for these uses.

If ORTHO Dienestrol Cream is used during pregnancy, or if the patient becomes pregnant while using this drug, she should be apprised of the potential risks to the fetus, and the advisability of pregnancy continuation.

Description:
ORTHO Dienestrol Cream
Cream for intravaginal use only
Active ingredient: Dienestrol 0.01%.
Compounded with: Glyceryl monostearate, peanut oil, glycerin, benzoic acid, glutamic acid and water.

Clinical Pharmacology: Systemic absorption and mode of action are undetermined.

Indications: Dienestrol Cream is indicated in the treatment of atrophic vaginitis and kraurosis vulvae.

ORTHO DIENESTROL CREAM HAS NOT BEEN SHOWN TO BE EFFECTIVE FOR ANY PURPOSE DURING PREGNANCY AND ITS USE MAY CAUSE SEVERE HARM TO THE FETUS (*SEE* BOXED WARNING).

Contraindications: Estrogens should not be used in women with any of the following conditions:
1. Known or suspected cancer of the breast.
2. Known or suspected estrogen-dependent neoplasia.
3. Known or suspected pregnancy (*See* Boxed Warning).
4. Undiagnosed abnormal genital bleeding.
5. Active thrombophlebitis or thromboembolic disorders.
6. A past history of thrombophlebitis, thrombosis, or thromboembolic disorders associated with previous estrogen use.

Warnings:
1. *Induction of malignant neoplasms.* Long-term continuous administration of natural and synthetic estrogens in certain animal species increases the frequency of carcinomas of the breast, cervix, vagina, and liver. There is now evidence that estrogens increase the risk of carcinoma of the endometrium in humans. (*See* Boxed Warning.)

At the present time there is no satisfactory evidence that estrogens given to postmenopausal women increase the risk of cancer of the breast,[18] although a recent long-term followup of a single physician's practice has raised this possibility.[18a] Because of the animal data, there is a need for caution in prescribing estrogens for women with a strong family history of breast cancer or who have breast nodules, fibrocystic disease, or abnormal mammograms.

2. *Gall bladder disease.* A recent study has reported a 2 to 3-fold increase in the risk of surgically confirmed gall bladder disease in women receiving postmenopausal estrogens,[18] similar to the 2-fold increase previously noted in users of oral contraceptives.[19–24] In the case of oral contraceptives the increased risk appeared after two years of use.[24]

3. *Effects similar to those caused by estrogen-progestogen oral contraceptives.* There are several serious adverse effects of oral contraceptives, most of which have not, up to now, been documented as consequences of postmenopausal estrogen therapy. This may reflect the comparatively low doses of estrogen used in postmenopausal women. It would be expected that the larger doses of estrogen used to treat prostatic or breast cancer or postpartum breast engorgement are more likely to result in these adverse effects, and, in fact, it has been shown that there is an increased risk of thrombosis in men receiving estrogens for prostatic cancer and women for postpartum breast engorgement.[20–23]

a. *Thromboembolic disease.* It is now well established that users of oral contraceptives have an increased risk of various thromboembolic and thrombotic vascular diseases, such as thrombophlebitis, pulmonary embolism, stroke, and myocardial infarction.[24–31] Cases of retinal thrombosis, mesenteric thrombosis, and optic neuritis have been reported in oral contraceptive users. There is evidence that the risk of several of these adverse reactions is related to the dose of the drug.[32,33] An increased risk of postsurgery thromboembolic complications has also been reported in users of oral contraceptives.[34,35] If feasible, estrogen should be discontinued at least 4 weeks before surgery of the type associated with an increased risk of thromboembolism, or during periods of prolonged immobilization.

While an increased risk of thromboembolic and thrombotic disease in postmenopausal users of estrogens has not been found,[18–36] this does not rule out the possibility that such an increase may be present or that subgroups of women who have underlying risk factors or who are receiving relatively large doses of estrogens may have increased risk. Therefore estrogens should not be used in persons with active thrombophlebitis or thromboembolic disorders, and they should not be used (except in treatment of malignancy) in persons with a history of such disorders in association with estrogen use. They should be used with caution in patients with cerebral vascular or coronary artery disease and only for those in whom estrogens are clearly needed.

Large doses of estrogen (5 mg conjugated estrogens per day), comparable to those used to treat cancer of the prostate and breast, have been shown in a large prospective clinical trial in men to increase the risk of nonfatal myocardial infarction, pulmonary embolism and thrombophlebitis. When estrogen doses of this size are used, any of the thromboembolic and thrombotic adverse effects associated with oral contraceptive use should be considered a clear risk.

b. *Hepatic adenoma.* Benign hepatic adenomas appear to be associated with the use of oral contraceptives.[38–40] Although benign, and rare, these may rupture and may cause death through intra-abdominal hemorrhage. Such lesions have not yet been reported in association with other estrogen or progestogen preparations but should be considered in estrogen users having abdominal pain and tenderness, abdominal mass, or hypovolemic shock. Hepatocellular carcinoma has also been reported in women taking estrogen-containing oral contraceptives.[39] The relationship of this malignancy to these drugs is not known at this time.

c. *Elevated blood pressure.* Increased blood pressure is not uncommon in women using oral contraceptives. There is now a report that this may occur with use of estrogens in the menopause[41] and blood pressure should be monitored with estrogen use, especially if high doses are used.

d. *Glucose tolerance.* A worsening of glucose tolerance has been observed in a significant percentage of patients on estrogen-containing oral contraceptives. For this reason, diabetic patients should be carefully observed while receiving estrogen.

4. *Hypercalcemia.* Administration of estrogens may lead to severe hypercalcemia in patients with breast cancer and bone metastases. If this occurs, the drug should be stopped and appropriate measures taken to reduce the serum calcium level.

Precautions:
A. General Precautions.
1. A complete medical and family history should be taken prior to the initiation of any estrogen therapy. The pretreatment and periodic physical examinations should include special reference to blood pressure, breasts, abdomen, and pelvic organs, and should include a Papanicolaou smear. As a general rule, estrogen should not be prescribed for longer than one year without another physical examination being performed.
2. Fluid retention—Because estrogens may cause some degree of fluid retention, conditions which might be influenced by this factor such as epilepsy, migraine, and cardiac or renal dysfunction, require careful observation.
3. Certain patients may develop undesirable manifestations of excessive estrogenic stimulation, such as abnormal or excessive uterine bleeding, mastodynia, etc.
4. Oral contraceptives appear to be associated with an increased incidence of mental depression.[24] Although it is not clear whether this is due to the estrogenic or progestogenic component of the contraceptive, patients with a history of depression should be carefully observed.
5. Preexisting uterine leiomyomata may increase in size during estrogen use.
6. The pathologist should be advised of estrogen therapy when relevant specimens are submitted.
7. Patients with a past history of jaundice during pregnancy have an increased risk of recurrence of jaundice while receiving estrogen-containing oral contraceptive therapy. If jaundice develops in any patient receiving estrogen, the medication should be discontinued while the cause is investigated.
8. Estrogens may be poorly metabolized in patients with impaired liver function and they should be administered with caution in such patients.
9. Because estrogens influence the metabolism of calcium and phosphorus, they should be used with caution in patients with metabolic bone diseases that are associated with hypercalcemia or in patients with renal insufficiency.
10. Because of the effects of estrogens on epiphyseal closure, they should be used judiciously in young patients in whom bone growth is not complete.
11. Certain endocrine and liver function tests may be affected by estrogen-containing oral contraceptives. The following similar changes may be expected with larger doses of estrogen:
a. Increased sulfobromophthalein retention.
b. Increased prothrombin and factors VII, VIII, IX, and X; decreased antithrombin 3; increased norepinephrine-induced platelet aggregability.
c. Increased thyroid binding globulin (TBG) leading to increased circulating total thyroid hormone, as measured by PBI, T4 by column, or T4 by radioimmunoassay. Free T3 resin uptake is decreased, reflecting the elevated TBG; free T4 concentration is unaltered.

Continued on next page

Ortho Pharm.—Cont.

d. Impaired glucose tolerance.
e. Decreased pregnanediol excretion.
f. Reduced response to metyrapone test.
g. Reduced serum folate concentration.
h. Increased serum triglyceride and phospholipid concentration.

B. Information for the Patient. See text of Patient Package Information which is reproduced below.

C. Pregnancy Category X
See Contraindications and Boxed Warning.

D. Nursing Mothers. As a general principle, the administration of any drug to nursing mothers should be done only when clearly necessary since many drugs are excreted in human milk.

Adverse Reactions: (*See* Warnings regarding induction of neoplasia, adverse effects on the fetus, increased incidence of gall bladder disease, and adverse effects similar to those of oral contraceptives, including thromboembolism.) The following additional adverse reactions have been reported with estrogenic therapy, including oral contraceptives:

1. *Genitourinary system.*
Breakthrough bleeding, spotting, change in menstrual flow.
Dysmenorrhea.
Premenstrual-like syndrome.
Amenorrhea during and after treatment.
Increase in size of uterine fibromyomata.
Vaginal candidiasis.
Change in cervical eversion and in degree of cervical secretion.
Cystitis-like syndrome.

2. *Breasts.*
Tenderness, enlargement, secretion.

3. *Gastrointestinal.*
Nausea, vomiting.
Abdominal cramps, bloating.
Cholestatic jaundice.

4. *Skin.*
Chloasma or melasma which may persist when drug is discontinued.
Erythema multiforme.
Erythema nodosum.
Hemorrhagic eruption.
Loss of scalp hair.
Hirsutism.

5. *Eyes.*
Steepening of corneal curvature.
Intolerance to contact lenses.

6. *CNS.*
Headache, migraine, dizziness.
Mental depression.
Chorea.

7. *Miscellaneous.*
Increase or decrease in weight.
Reduced carbohydrate tolerance.
Aggravation of porphyria.
Edema.
Changes in libido.

Acute Overdosage: Numerous reports of ingestion of large doses of estrogen-containing oral contraceptives by young children indicate that serious ill effects do not occur. Overdosage of estrogen may cause nausea, and withdrawal bleeding may occur in females.

Dosage and Administration: *Given cyclically for short term use only:*
For treatment of atrophic vaginitis, or kraurosis vulvae associated with the menopause.
The lowest dose that will control symptoms should be chosen and medication should be discontinued as promptly as possible.
Attempts to discontinue or taper medication should be made at 3 to 6 month intervals.
The usual dosage range is one or two applicatorsful per day for one or two weeks, then gradually reduced to one half initial dosage for a similar period. A maintenance dosage of one applicatorful, one to three times a week, may be used after restoration of the vaginal mucosa has been achieved.
Treated patients with an intact uterus should be monitored closely for signs of endometrial cancer and appropriate diagnostic measures should be taken to rule out malignancy in the event of persistent or recurring abnormal vaginal bleeding.

Supplied: Available in 2.75 oz. (78g) tubes with or without ORTHO® Measured-Dose Applicator.

Physician References:

1. Ziel, H.K. and W.D. Finkle, "Increased Risk of Endometrial Carcinoma Among Users of Conjugated Estrogens," *New England Journal of Medicine,* 293:1167–1170, 1975.
2. Smith, D.C., R. Prentic, D.J. Thompson, and W.L. Hermann, "Association of Exogenous Estrogen and Endometrial Carcinoma," *New England Journal of Medicine,* 293:1164–1167, 1975.
3. Mack, T.M., M.C. Pike, B.E. Henderson, R.I. Pfeffer, V.R. Gerkins, M. Arthur, and S.E. Brown, "Estrogens and Endometrial Cancer in a Retirement Community," *New England Journal of Medicine,* 294:1267–1287, 1976.
4. Weiss, N.S., D.R. Szekely and D.F. Austin, "Increasing Incidence of Endometrial Cancer in the United States," *New England Journal of Medicine,* 294:1259–1262, 1976.
5. Herbst, A.L., H. Ulfelder and D.C. Poskanzer, "Adenocarcinoma of Vagina," *New England Journal of Medicine,* 284:878–881, 1971.
6. Greenwald, P., J. Barlow, P. Nasca, and W. Burnett, "Vaginal Cancer after Maternal Treatment with Synthetic Estrogens," *New England Journal of Medicine,* 285:390–392, 1971.
7. Lanier, A., K. Noller, D. Decker, L. Elveback, and L. Kurland, "Cancer and Stilbestrol. A Follow-up of 1719 Persons Exposed to Estrogens in Utero and Born 1943–1959," *Mayo Clinic Proceedings,* 48:793–799, 1973.
8. Herbst, A., R. Kurman, and R. Scully, "Vaginal and Cervical Abnormalities After Exposure to Stilbestrol In Utero," *Obstetrics and Gynecology,* 40:287–298, 1972.
9. Herbst, A., S. Robboy, G. Macdonald, and R. Scully, "The Effects of Local Progesterone on Stilbestrol-Associated Vaginal Adenosis," *American Journal of Obstetrics and Gynecology* 118:607–615, 1974.
10. Herbst, A., D. Poskanzer, S. Robboy, L. Friedlander, and R. Scully, "Prenatal Exposure to Stilbestrol, A Prospective Comparison of Exposed Female Offspring with Unexposed Controls," *New England Journal of Medicine,* 292:334–339, 1975.
11. Staffi, A., R. Mattingly, D. Foley, and W. Fetherston, "Clinical Diagnosis of Vaginal Adenosis," *Obstetrics and Gynecology,* 43:118–128, 1974.
12. Sherman, A.I., M. Goldrath, A. Berlin, V. Vakhariya, F. Banooni, W. Michaels, P. Goodman, S. Brown, "Cervical-Vaginal Adenosis After *In Utero* Exposure to Synthetic Estrogens," *Obstetrics and Gynecology,* 44:531–545, 1974.
13. Gal, I., B. Kirman, and J. Stern, "Hormone Pregnancy Tests and Congenital Malformation," *Nature,* 216:83, 1967.
14. Levy, E.P., A. Cohen, and F.C. Fraser, "Hormone Treatment During Pregnancy and Congenital Heart Defects," *Lancet,* 1:611, 1973.
15. Nora, J. and A. Nora, "Birth Defects and Oral Contraceptives," *Lancet,* 1:941–942, 1973.
16. Janerich, D.T., J.M. Piper, and D.M. Glebatis, "Oral Contraceptives and Congenital Limb-Reduction Defects," *New England Journal of Medicine,* 291:697–700, 1974.
17. "Estrogens for Oral or Parenteral Use," *Federal Register,* 40:8212, 1975.
18. Boston Collaborative Drug Surveillance Program, "Surgically Confirmed Gall Bladder Disease, Venous Thromboembolism and Breast Tumors in Relation to Post-Menopausal Estrogen Therapy," *New England Journal of Medicine,* 290:15–19, 1974.
18a. Hoover, R., L.A. Gray, Sr., P. Cole, and B. MacMahon, "Menopausal Estrogens and Breast Cancer," *New England Journal of Medicine,* 295:401–405, 1976.
19. Boston Collaborative Drug Surveillance Program, "Oral Contraceptives and Venous Thromboembolic Disease, Surgically Confirmed Gall Bladder Disease, and Breast Tumors," *Lancet* 1:1399–1404, 1973.
20. Daniel, D.G., H. Campbell, and A.C. Turnbull, "Puerperal Thromboembolism and Suppression of Lactation," *Lancet,* 2:287–289, 1967.
21. The Veterans Administration Cooperative Urological Research Group, "Carcinoma of the Prostate: Treatment Comparisons," *Journal of Urology,* 98:516–522, 1967.
22. Bailer, J.C., "Thromboembolism and Oestrogen Therapy," *Lancet,* 2:560, 1967.
23. Blackard, C., R. Doe, G. Mellinger, and D. Byar, "Incidence of Cardiovascular Disease and Death In Patients Receiving Diethylstilbestrol for Carcinoma of the Prostate," *Cancer,* 26:249–256, 1970.
24. Royal College of General Practitioners, "Oral Contraception and Thromboembolic Disease," *Journal of the Royal College of General Practitioners,* 13:267–279, 1967.
25. Inman, W.H.W. and M.P. Vessey, "Investigation of Deaths from Pulmonary, Coronary, and Cerebral Thrombosis and Embolism in Women of Child-Bearing Age," *British Medical Journal,* 2:193–199, 1968.
26. Vessey, M.P. and R. Doll, "Investigation of Relation Between Use of Oral Contraceptives and Thromboembolic Disease, A Further Report," *British Medical Journal,* 2:651–657, 1969.
27. Sartwell, P.E., A.T. Masi, F.G. Arthes, G.R. Greene, and H.E. Smith, "Thromboembolism and Oral Contraceptives: An Epidemiological Case Control Study," *American Journal of Epidemiology,* 90:365–380, 1969.
28. Collaborative Group for the Study of Stroke In Young Women, "Oral Contraception and Increased Risk of Cerebral Ischemia or Thrombosis," *New England Journal of Medicine,* 288:871–878, 1973.
29. Collaborative Group for the Study of Stroke in Young Women, "Oral Contraceptives and Stroke in Young Women: Associated Risk Factors," *Journal of the American Medical Association,* 231:718–722, 1975.
30. Mann, J.I. and W.H.W. Inman, "Oral Contraceptives and Death from Myocardial Infarction," *British Medical Journal,* 2:245–248, 1975.
31. Mann, J.I., M.P. Vessey, M. Thorogood, and R. Doll., "Myocardial Infarction in Young Women with Special Reference to Oral Contraceptive Practice," *British Medical Journal,* 2:241–245, 1975.
32. Inman, W.H.W., V.P. Vessey, B. Westerholm, and A. Engelund, "Thromboembolic Disease and the Steroidal Content of Oral Contraceptives," *British Medical Journal,* 2:203–209, 1970.
33. Stolley, P.D., J.A. Tonascia, M.S. Tockman, P.E. Sartwell, A.H. Rutledge, and M.P. Jacobs, "Thrombosis with Low-Estrogen Oral Contraceptives," *American Journal of Epidemiology,* 102:197–208, 1975.
34. Vessey, M.P., R. Doll, A.S. Fairbairn, and G. Glober, "Post-Operative Thromboembolism and the Use of the Oral Contraceptives," *British Medical Journal,* 3:123–126, 1970.
35. Greene, G.R. and P.E. Sartwell, "Oral Contraceptive Use in Patients with Thromboembolism Following Surgery, Trauma or Infection," *American Journal of Public Health,* 62:680–685, 1972.
36. Rosenberg, L., M.B. Armstrong and H. Jick, "Myocardial Infarction and Estrogen Therapy is Postmenopausal Women," *New England Journal of Medicine,* 294:1256–1259, 1976.
37. Coronary Drug Project Research Group, "The Coronary Drug Project: Initial Findings

Leading to Modifications of Its Research Protocol, *Journal of the American Medical Association*, 214:1303–1313, 1970.
38. Baum, J., F. Holtz, J.J. Bookstein, and E.W. Klein, "Possible Association between Benign Hepatomas and Oral Contraceptives," *Lancet*, 2:926–928, 1973.
39. Mays, E.T., W.M. Christopherson, M.M. Mahr, and H.C. Williams, "Hepatic Changes in Young Women Ingesting Contraceptive Steroids, Hepatic Hemorrhage and Primary Hepatic Tumors." *Journal of the American Medical Association*, 235:730–782, 1976.
40. Edmondson, H.A., B. Henderson, and B. Benton, "Liver Cell Adenomas Associated with the Use of Oral Contraceptives," *New England Journal of Medicine*, 294:470–472, 1976.
41. Pfeffer, R.I. and S. Van Den Noore, "Estrogen Use and Stroke Risk in Postmenopausal Women," *American Journal of Epidemiology*, 103:445–456, 1976.

PATIENT INFORMATION ABOUT ESTROGENS

Estrogens are female hormones produced by the ovaries. The ovaries make several different kinds of estrogens. In addition, scientists have been able to make a variety of synthetic estrogens. As far as we know, all these synthetic estrogens have similar properties and therefore much the same usefulness, side effects, and risks. This leaflet is intended to help you understand what estrogens are used for, some of the risks involved in their use, and to help minimize these risks.

This leaflet includes important information about estrogens, but not all the information. If you want to know more, you can ask your doctor or pharmacist to let you read the package insert prepared for the doctor.

Uses of Estrogen: THERE IS NO PROPER USE OF ESTROGENS IN A PREGNANT WOMAN

Estrogens are prescribed by doctors for a number of purposes, including:

1. To provide estrogen during a period of adjustment when a woman's ovaries no longer produce it, in order to prevent certain uncomfortable symptoms of estrogen deficiency. (All women normally decrease the production of estrogens, generally between the ages of 45 and 55; this is called the menopause.)
2. To prevent symptoms of estrogen deficiency when a woman's ovaries have been removed surgically before the natural menopause.
3. To prevent pregnancy. (Estrogens are given along with a progestogen, another female hormone; these combinations are called oral contraceptives or birth control pills. Patient labeling is available to women taking oral contraceptives and they will not be discussed in this leaflet.)
4. To treat certain cancers in women and men.
5. To prevent painful swelling of the breasts after pregnancy in women who choose not to nurse their babies.

Estrogens in the Menopause: In the natural course of their lives, all women eventually experience a decrease in estrogen production. This usually occurs between ages 45 and 55 but may occur earlier or later. Sometimes the ovaries may need to be removed by an operation before natural menopause, producing a "surgical menopause."

When the amount of estrogen in the blood begins to decrease, many women may develop typical symptoms: Feelings of warmth in the face, neck, and chest or sudden intense episodes of heat and sweating throughout the body (called "hot flashes" or "hot flushes"). These symptoms are sometimes very uncomfortable. A few women eventually develop changes in the vagina (called "atrophic vaginitis") which cause discomfort, especially during and after intercourse.

Estrogens can be prescribed to treat these symptoms of the menopause. It is estimated that considerably more than half of all women undergoing the menopause have only mild symptoms or no symptoms at all and therefore do not need estrogens. Other women may need estrogens for a few months, while their bodies adjust to lower estrogen levels. Sometimes the need will be for periods longer than six months. In an attempt to avoid over-stimulation of the uterus (womb), estrogens are usually given cyclically during each month of use, that is three weeks of pills followed by one week without pills.

Sometimes women experience nervous symptoms or depression during menopause. There is no evidence that estrogens are effective for such symptoms and they should not be used to treat them, although other treatment may be needed.

You may have heard that taking estrogens for long periods (years) after the menopause will keep your skin soft and supple and keep you feeling young. There is no evidence that this is so, however, and such long-term treatment carries important risks.

Estrogens to Prevent Swelling of the Breasts After Pregnancy: If you do not breast-feed your baby after delivery, your breasts may fill up with milk and become painful and engorged. This usually begins about three to four days after delivery and may last for a few days to up to a week or more. Sometimes the discomfort is severe, but usually it is not and can be controlled by pain-relieving drugs such as aspirin and by binding the breasts up tightly. Estrogens can be used to try to prevent the breasts from filling up. While this treatment is sometimes successful, in many cases the breasts fill up to some degree in spite of treatment. The dose of estrogens needed to prevent pain and swelling of the breasts is much larger than the dose needed to treat symptoms of the menopause and this may increase your chances of developing blood clots in the legs or lungs (see below). Therefore, it is important that you discuss the benefits and the risks of estrogen use with your doctor if you have decided not to breast-feed your baby.

Some of the Dangers of Estrogen:

1. *Cancer of the uterus.* If estrogens are used in the postmenopausal period for more than a year, there is an increased risk of *endometrial cancer* (cancer of the uterus). Women taking estrogens have roughly five to ten times as great a chance of getting this cancer as women who take no estrogens. To put this another way, while a postmenopausal woman not taking estrogens has one chance in 1,000 each year of getting cancer of the uterus, a woman taking estrogens has five to ten chances in 1,000 each year. For this reason *it is important to take estrogens only when you really need them.*

The risk of this cancer is greater the longer estrogens are used and also seems to be greater when larger doses are taken. For this reason *it is important to take the lowest dose of estrogen that will control symptoms and to take it only as long as it is needed.* If estrogens are needed for longer periods of time, your doctor will want to reevaluate your need for estrogens at least every six months.

Women using estrogens should report any irregular vaginal bleeding to their doctors; such bleeding may be of no importance, but it can be an early warning of cancer of the uterus. If you have undiagnosed vaginal bleeding, you should not use estrogens until a diagnosis is made and you are certain there is no cancer of the uterus. If you have had your uterus completely removed (total hysterectomy), there is no danger of developing cancer of the uterus.

2. *Other possible cancers.* Estrogens can cause development of other tumors in animals, such as tumors of the breast, cervix, vagina, or liver, when given for a long time. At present there is no good evidence that women using estrogen in the menopause have an increased risk of such tumors, but there is no way yet to be sure they do not; and one study raises the possibility that use of estrogens in the menopause may increase the risk of breast cancer many years later. This is a further reason to use estrogens only when clearly needed. While you are taking estrogens, it is important that you go to your doctor at least once a year for a physical examination. Also, if members of your family have had breast cancer or if you have breast nodules or abnormal mammograms (breast x-rays), your doctor may wish to carry out more frequent examinations of your breasts.
3. *Gall bladder disease.* Women who use estrogens after menopause are more likely to develop gall bladder disease needing surgery than women who do not use estrogens. Birth control pills have a similar effect.
4. *Abnormal blood clotting.* Oral contraceptives, some of which contain estrogens, increase the risk of blood clotting in various parts of the body. This can result in a stroke (if the clot is in the brain), a heart attack (clot in a blood vessel of the heart), or a pulmonary embolus (a clot which forms in the legs or pelvis, then breaks off and travels to the lungs). Any of these can be fatal. Blood clots may result in the loss of a limb, paralysis or loss of sight, depending on where the blood clot is formed or lodges if it breaks loose.

The larger doses of estrogen used to prevent swelling of the breasts after pregnancy have been reported to cause clotting in the legs and lungs.

It is recommended that if you have had any blood clotting disorders including clotting in the legs or lungs, or a heart attack or stroke, you should not use estrogens.

Special Warning About Pregnancy: You should not receive estrogen if you are pregnant, If this should occur, there is a greater than usual chance that the developing child will be born with a birth defect, although the possibility remains fairly small. A female child may have an increased risk of developing cancer of the vagina or cervix later in life (in the teens or twenties). Every possible effort should be made to avoid exposure to estrogens during pregnancy. If exposure occurs, see your doctor.

Some Other Effects of Estrogens: In addition to the serious known risks of estrogens described above, estrogens have the following side effects and potential risks:

1. *Nausea and vomiting.* The most common side effect of estrogen therapy is nausea. Vomiting is less common.
2. *Effects on breasts.* Estrogens may cause breast tenderness or enlargement and may cause the breasts to secrete a liquid.
3. *Effects on the uterus.* Estrogens may cause benign fibroid tumors of the uterus to get larger.

Some women will have menstrual bleeding when estrogens are stopped. But if the bleeding occurs on days you are still taking estrogens you should report this to your doctor.

4. *Effects on liver.* Women taking estrogens develop on rare occasions a tumor of the liver which can rupture and bleed into the abdomen. You should report any swelling or unusual pain or tenderness in the abdomen to your doctor immediately.

Women with a past history of jaundice (yellowing of the skin and white parts of the eyes) may get jaundice again during estrogen use.

5. *Other effects.* Estrogens may cause excess fluid to be retained in the body. This may make some conditions worse, such as epilepsy, migraine, heart disease, or kidney disease.

If any of the above occur, stop taking estrogens and call your doctor.

Summary: Estrogens have important uses, but they have serious risks as well. You must decide, with your doctor, whether the risks are acceptable to you in view of the benefits of

Continued on next page

Ortho Pharm.—Cont.

treatment. Except where your doctor has prescribed estrogens for use in special cases of cancer of the breast or prostate, you should not use estrogens if you have cancer of the breast or uterus, are pregnant, have undiagnosed abnormal vaginal bleeding, blood clotting disorders including clotting in the legs or lungs, or have had a stroke, heart attack or angina.
You must understand that your doctor will require regular physical examinations while you are taking them and will try to discontinue the drug as soon as possible and use the smallest dose possible. You can help minimize the risk by being alert for signs of trouble including:
1. Abnormal bleeding from the vagina.
2. Pains in the calves or chest or sudden shortness of breath, or coughing blood (indicating possible clots in the legs, heart or lungs).
3. Severe headache, dizziness, faintness,, or changes in vision (indicating possible developing clots in the brain or eye).
4. Breast lumps (you should ask your doctor how to examine your own breasts).
5. Jaundice (yellowing of the skin).
6. Mental depression.
7. _Any_ other unusual condition or problem.

Based on his or her assessment of your medical needs, your doctor has prescribed this drug for you. Do not give the drug to anyone else.
How Supplied: Available in 2.75 oz. (78g) tubes with or without ORTHO® Measured-Dose Applicator.

ORTHO® Disposable Applicator

(See PDR For Nonprescription Drugs)

ORTHO-GYNOL® Contraceptive Jelly

(See PDR For Nonprescription Drugs)

ORTHO–NOVUM® Tablets ℞
and
MODICON® Tablets
MICRONOR® ℞

Description:
ORTHO-NOVUM 1/50□21 Tablets are a combination oral contraceptive. Each ORTHO-NOVUM 1/50□21 Tablet† contains 1 mg of the progestational compound, norethindrone (17-hydroxy-19-nor-17α-pregn-4-en-20-yn-3-one), together with 0.05 mg of the estrogenic compound, mestranol (3-methoxy-19-nor-17α-pregna-1,3,5 (10)-trien-20-yn-17-ol).
ORTHO-NOVUM 1/50□28 Tablets are a combination oral contraceptive. Each yellow ORTHO-NOVUM 1/50□28 Tablet† contains 1 mg of the progestational compound, norethindrone (17-hydroxy-19-nor-17α-pregn-4-en-20-yn-3-one), together with 0.05 mg of the estrogenic compound, mestranol (3-methoxy-19-nor-17α-pregna-1,3,5 (10)-trien-20-yn-17-ol). Each green tablet contains inert ingredients.
†Contains FD&C Yellow No. 5 (tartrazine) as a color additive.
ORTHO-NOVUM 1/80□21 Tablets are a combination oral contraceptive. Each ORTHO-NOVUM 1/80□21 Tablet contains 1 mg of the progestational compound, norethindrone (17-hydroxy-19-nor-17α-pregn-4-en-20-yn-3-one), together with 0.08 mg of the estrogenic compound, mestranol (3-methoxy-19-nor-17α-pregna-1,3,5 (10)-trien-20-yn-17-ol).
ORTHO-NOVUM 1/80□28 Tablets are a combination oral contraceptive. Each white ORTHO-NOVUM 1/80□28 Tablet contains 1 mg of the progestational compound, norethindrone (17-hydroxy-19-nor-17α-pregn-4-en-20-yn-3-one), together with 0.08 mg of the estrogenic compound, mestranol (3-methoxy-19-nor-17α-pregna-1,3,5 (10)-trien-20-yn-17-ol). Each green tablet contains inert ingredients.
ORTHO-NOVUM 2 mg□21 Tablets are a combination oral contraceptive. Each ORTHO-NOVUM 2 mg□21 Tablet contains 2 mg of the progestational compound, norethindrone (17-hydroxy-19-nor-17α-pregn-4-en-20-yn-3-one), together with 0.10 mg of the estrogenic compound, mestranol (3-methoxy-19-nor-17α-pregna-1,3,5 (10)-trien-20-yn-17-ol).
ORTHO-NOVUM 10 mg□21 Tablets are a combination oral contraceptive. Each ORTHO-NOVUM 10 mg□21 Tablet contains 10 mg of the progestational compound, norethindrone (17-hydroxy-19-nor-17α-pregn-4-en-20-yn-3-one), together with 0.06 mg of the estrogenic compound, mestranol (3-methoxy-19-nor-17α-pregna-1,3,5 (10)-trien-20-yn-17-ol).
MODICON Tablets are a combination oral contraceptive. Each MODICON Tablet contains 0.5 mg of the progestational compound, norethindrone (17-hydroxy-19-nor-17α-pregn-4-en-20-yn-3-one), together with 0.035 mg of the estrogenic compound, ethinyl estradiol (19-nor-17α-pregna-1,3,5 (10)-trien-20-yne-3,17-diol).
MODICON 28 Tablets are a combination oral contraceptive. Each white MODICON 28 Tablet contains 0.5 mg of the progestational compound, norethindrone (17-hydroxy-19-nor-17α-pregn-4-en-20-yn-3-one), together with 0.035 mg of the estrogenic compound, ethinyl estradiol (19-nor-17α-pregna-1,3,5 (10)-trien-20-yne-3,17-diol). Each green tablet contains inert ingredients.
MICRONOR Tablets are a progestogen-only oral contraceptive. Each MICRONOR tablet contains 0.35 mg of the purified crystalline compound, norethindrone (17-hydroxy-19-nor-17α-pregn-4-en-20-yn-3-one), a synthetic progestogen.
Clinical Pharmacology for Combination Oral Contraceptives Only: Combination oral contraceptives act primarily through the mechanism of gonadotropin suppression due to the estrogenic and progestational activity of the ingredients. Although the primary mechanism of action is inhibition of ovulation, alterations in the genital tract including changes in the cervical mucus (which increase the difficulty of sperm penetration) and the endometrium (which reduce the likelihood of implantation) may also contribute to contraceptive effectiveness.
Clinical Pharmacology Progestogen Oral Contraceptives: The primary mechanism through which MICRONOR prevents conception is not known, but progestogen-only contraceptives are known to alter the cervical mucus, exert a progestational effect on the endometrium, interfering with implantation, and, in some patients, suppress ovulation.
Indications and Usage: ORTHO-NOVUM 1/50 □ 21, ORTHO-NOVUM 1/50 □ 28, ORTHO-NOVUM 1/80□21, ORTHO-NOVUM 1/80□28, MODICON, MODICON 28 and MICRONOR are indicated for the prevention of pregnancy in women who elect to use oral contraceptives as a method of contraception.
ORTHO-NOVUM 2 mg □ 21 is indicated for the treatment of hypermenorrhea. ORTHO-NOVUM 2 mg□21 is indicated for the prevention of pregnancy in women who elect to use oral contraceptives as a method of contraception. (See first paragraph immediately following the opening WARNINGS statement.)
ORTHO-NOVUM 10 mg□21 is indicated for the treatment of endometriosis and hypermenorrhea. ORTHO-NOVUM 10 mg□21 is indicated for the prevention of pregnancy in women who elect to use oral contraceptives as a method of contraception. (See second paragraph immediately following the opening WARNINGS statement.)
Oral contraceptives are highly effective. The pregnancy rate in women using conventional combination oral contraceptives (containing 35 mcg or more of ethinyl estradiol or 50 mcg or more of mestranol) is generally reported as less than one pregnancy per 100 woman-years of use. Slightly higher rates (somewhat more than one pregnancy per 100 woman-years of use) are reported for some combination products containing 35 mcg or less of ethinyl estradiol, and rates on the order of three pregnancies per 100 woman-years are reported for the progestogen-only oral contraceptives.
These rates are derived from separate studies conducted by different investigators in several population groups and cannot be compared precisely. Furthermore, pregnancy rates tend to be lower as clinical studies are continued, possibly due to selective retention in the longer studies of those patients who accept the treatment regimen and do not discontinue as a result of adverse reactions, pregnancy or other reasons.
In clinical trials with ORTHO-NOVUM 1/50□21, 3,852 patients completed 45,937 cycles, and a total of 10 pregnancies was reported. This represents a pregnancy rate of 0.26 per 100 woman-years.
In clinical trials with ORTHO-NOVUM 1/50□28, 1,590 patients completed 7,330 cycles, and a total of three pregnancies was reported. This represents a pregnancy rate of 0.5 per 100 woman-years.
In clinical trials with ORTHO-NOVUM 1/80□21, and ORTHO-NOVUM 1/80□28, 3,464 patients completed 34,068 cycles, and a total of five pregnancies was reported. This represents a pregnancy rate of 0.18 per 100 woman-years.
In clinical trials with ORTHO-NOVUM 2 mg□20, 6,097 patients completed 121,233 cycles, and a total of 13 pregnancies was reported. This represents a pregnancy rate of 0.13 per 100 woman-years. In clinical trials with ORTHO-NOVUM 2 mg□21, 965 patients completed 3,743 cycles, and no pregnancies were reported. This represents a pregnancy rate of 0.0 per 100 woman-years.
In clinical trials with ORTHO-NOVUM 10 mg, 1,185 patients completed 32,906 cycles, and a total of one pregnancy was reported. This represents a pregnancy rate of 0.03 per 100 woman-years.
The dropout rate for medical reasons, as observed in the clinical trials conducted with MODICON, appears to be somewhat higher than observed with higher dose combination products. The dropout rate due to menstrual disorders and irregularities was also somewhat higher, dropouts being equally split between menstrual disorders and irregularities and other medical reasons attributable to the drug. In clinical trials with MODICON and MODICON 28, 1,168 patients completed 16,345 cycles of use, and a total of three pregnancies was reported. This represents a pregnancy rate of 0.22 per 100 woman-years.
In clinical trials with MICRONOR, 2,963 patients completed 25,901 cycles of therapy, and a total of 55 pregnancies was reported. This represents an average pregnancy rate of 2.54 per 100 woman-years.
A higher pregnancy rate of 3.72 was recorded in "fresh" patients (those who had never taken oral contraceptives prior to starting MICRONOR therapy) to a large extent because of incorrect tablet intake. This compares to the lower pregnancy rate of 1.95 recorded in "changeover" patients (those switched from other oral contraceptives).
This difference was found to be statistically significant. Furthermore, an even greater statistically significant difference in pregnancy rates between these two groups was found during the first six months of MICRONOR therapy. Therefore, it is especially important for "fresh" patients to strictly adhere to the regimen.
Table 1 gives ranges of pregnancy rates reported in the literature[1] for other means of contraception. The efficacy of these means of contraception (except the IUD) depends upon the degree of adherence to the method.

Table 1
Pregnancies Per 100 Women-Years

IUD, less than 1–6;
Diaphragm with spermicidal product (creams or jellies), 2–20;
Condom, 3–36; Aerosol foams, 2–29; Jellies and creams, 4–36;
Periodic abstinence (rhythm) all types, less than 1–47;
1. Calendar method, 14–47;
2. Temperature method, 1–20;
3. Temperature method—intercourse only in postovulatory phase, less than 1–7;
4. Mucus method, 1–25;
No contraception, 60–80.

Dose-Related Risk of Thromboembolism From Oral Contraceptives: Two studies have shown a positive association between the dose of estrogens in oral contraceptives and the risk of thromboembolism.[2,3] For this reason, it is prudent and in keeping with good principles of therapeutics to minimize exposure to estrogen. The oral contraceptive product prescribed for any given patient should be that product which contains the least amount of estrogen that is compatible with an acceptable pregnancy rate and patient acceptance. It is recommended that new acceptors of oral contraceptives be started on preparations containing .05 mg or less of estrogen.

Contraindications: Oral contraceptives should not be used in women with any of the following conditions:
1. Thrombophlebitis or thromboembolic disorders.
2. A past history of deep vein thrombophlebitis or thromboembolic disorders.
3. Cerebral vascular or coronary artery disease.
4. Known or suspected carcinoma of the breast.
5. Known or suspected estrogen-dependent neoplasia.
6. Undiagnosed, abnormal genital bleeding.
7. Known or suspected pregnancy (see WARNINGS, No. 5).

WARNINGS

Cigarette smoking increases the risk of serious cardiovascular side effects from oral contraceptive use. This risk increases with age and with heavy smoking (15 or more cigarettes per day) and is quite marked in women over 35 years of age. Women who use oral contraceptives should be strongly advised not to smoke. The use of oral contraceptives is associated with increased risk of several serious conditions including thromboembolism, stroke, myocardial infarction, hepatic adenoma, gallbladder disease, hypertension. Practitioners prescribing oral contraceptives should be familiar with the following information relating to these risks.

ORTHO-NOVUM 2 mg☐21 should only be used for contraception when lower dose formulations prove unacceptable.

ORTHO-NOVUM 10 mg☐21 should be used for contraception only when formulations with lower progestogen doses prove unacceptable.

1. THROMBOEMBOLIC DISORDERS AND OTHER VASCULAR PROBLEMS. An increased risk of thromboembolic and thrombotic disease associated with the use of oral contraceptives is well established. Four principal studies in Great Britain[4,5,6,26] and three in the United States[7–10] have demonstrated an increased risk of fatal and nonfatal venous thromboembolism and stroke, both hemorrhagic and thrombotic. These studies estimate that users of oral contraceptives are 4 to 11 times more likely than nonusers to develop these diseases without evident cause (Tables 2, 4) Overall excess mortality due to pulmonary embolism or stroke is on the order of 1.0 to 3.5 deaths annually per 100,000 users and increases with age (Table 3).

Table 2
Hospitalization Rates Due to Venous Thromboembolic Disease[6]

Admissions annually per 100,000 women, age 20–44

Users of oral contraceptives	45
Nonusers	5

Table 3
Death Rates Due To Pulmonary Embolism or Cerebral Thrombosis[5] —Deaths Annually Per 100,000 Nonpregnant Women

	Age 20 to 34	Age 35 to 44
Users of oral contraceptives	1.5	3.9
Nonusers	.2	.5

Cerebrovascular Disorders: In a collaborative American study[9,10] of cerebrovascular disorders in women with and without predisposing causes, it was estimated that the risk of hemorrhagic stroke was 2.0 times greater in users than in nonusers and the risk of thrombotic stroke was 4.0 to 9.5 times greater in users than in nonusers (Table 4).

Table 4
Summary of Relative Risk of Thromboembolic Disorders and Other Vascular Problems in Oral Contraceptive Users Compared to Nonusers

	Relative risk, times greater
Idiopathic thromboembolic disease	4–11
Post surgery thromboembolic complications	4–6
Thrombotic stroke	4–9.5
Hemorrhagic stroke	2
Myocardial infarction	2–12

Myocardial Infarction: An increased risk of myocardial infarction associated with the use of oral contraceptives has been reported[11,12,13] confirming a previously suspected association (Tables 5 & 6). These studies, conducted in the United Kingdom, found, as expected, that the greater the number of underlying risk factors for coronary artery disease (cigarette smoking, hypertension, hypercholesterolemia, obesity, diabetes, history of preeclamptic toxemia), the higher the risk of developing myocardial infarction, regardless of whether the patient was an oral contraceptive user or not. Oral contraceptives, however, were found to be a clear additional risk factor. The annual excess case rate (increased risk) of myocardial infarction (fatal and nonfatal) in oral contraceptive users was estimated to be approximately 7 cases per 100,000 women users in the 30–39 age group and 67 cases per 100,000 women users in the 40–44 age group. In terms of relative risk, it has been estimated[52] that oral contraceptive users who do not smoke (smoking is considered a major predisposing condition to myocardial infarction) are about twice as likely to have a fatal myocardial infarction as nonusers who do not smoke. Oral contraceptive users who are also smokers have about a 5-fold increased risk of fatal infarction compared to users who do not smoke, but about a 10-to 12-fold increased risk compared to nonusers who do not smoke. Furthermore, the amount of smoking is also an important factor. In determining the importance of these relative risks, however, the baseline rates for various age groups, as shown in Table 5, must be given serious consideration. The importance of other predisposing conditions mentioned above in determining relative and absolute risks has not as yet been quantified; it is quite likely that the same synergistic action exists, but perhaps to a lesser extent.

Table 5
Estimated Annual Mortality Rate Per 100,000 Women From Myocardial Infarction By Use Of Oral Contraceptives, Smoking Habits, And Age (in years)

	Myocardial Infarction			
	Women aged 30–39		Women aged 40–44	
Smoking habits	Users	Non-users	Users	Non-users
All smokers	10.2	2.6	62.0	15.9
Heavy[1]	13.0	5.1	78.7	31.3
Light	4.7	.9	28.6	5.7
Nonsmokers	1.8	1.2	10.7	7.4
Smokers and nonsmokers	5.4	1.9	32.8	11.7

[1]Heavy smoker: 15 or more cigarettes per day. From Jain, A.K., Studies in Family Planning, 8:50, 1977.

Table 6
Myocardial Infarction Rates In Users And Nonusers Of Oral Contraceptives In Britain[11,12,13]—Cases Annually Per 100,000 Women

	Nonfatal		Fatal	
	Age 30 to 39	Age 40 to 44	Age 30 to 39	Age 40 to 44
Users of oral contraceptives	5.6	56.9	5.4	32.0
Nonusers of oral contraceptives	2.1	9.9	1.9	12.0
Relative risk	2.7	5.7	2.8	2.8

Risk of Dose: In an analysis of data derived from several national adverse reaction reporting systems[2], British investigators concluded that the risk of thromboembolism including coronary thrombosis is directly related to the dose of estrogen used in oral contraceptives. Preparations containing 100 mcg or more of estrogen were associated with a higher risk of thromboembolism than those containing 50–80 mcg of estrogen. Their analysis did suggest, however, that the quantity of estrogen may not be the sole factor involved. This finding has been confirmed in the United States.[3] Careful epidemiological studies to determine the degree of thromboembolic risk associated with progestogen-only oral contraceptives have not been performed. Cases of thromboembolic disease have been reported in women using these products, and they should not be presumed to be free of excess risk.

The risk of thromboembolic and thrombotic disorders, in both users and nonusers of oral contraceptives, increases with age. Oral contraceptives are, however, an independent risk factor for these events.

Estimate of Excess Mortality From Circulatory Diseases: A large prospective study[53] carried out in the United Kingdom estimated the mortality rate per 100,000 women per year from diseases of the circulatory system for users and nonusers of oral contraceptives according to age, smoking habits, and duration of use. The overall excess death rate annually from circulatory diseases for oral contraceptive users was estimated to be 20 per 100,000 (ages 15–34—5/100,000; ages 35–44—33/100,000; ages 45–49—140/100,000), the risk being concentrated in older women, in those with a long duration of use, and in cigarette smokers. It was not possible, however, to examine the interrelationships of age, smoking, and duration

Continued on next page

Ortho Pharm.—Cont.

of use, nor to compare the effects of continuous versus intermittent use. Although the study showed a 10-fold increase in death due to circulatory diseases in users for five or more years, all of these deaths occurred in women 35 or older. Until larger numbers of women under 35 with continuous use for five or more years are available, it is not possible to assess the magnitude of the relative risk for this younger age group.

This study reports that the increased risk of circulatory diseases may persist after the pill is discontinued.

Another study published at the same time confirms a previously reported increase of mortality in pill users from cardiovascular diseases.[54]

The available data from a variety of sources have been analyzed[14] to estimate the risk of death associated with various methods of contraception. The estimates of risk of death for each method include the combined risk of the contraceptive method (e.g., thromboembolic and thrombotic disease in the case of oral contraceptives) plus the risk attributable to pregnancy or abortion in the event of method failure. This latter risk varies with the effectiveness of the contraceptive method. The findings of this analysis are shown in Figure 1 below.[14] The study concluded that the mortality associated with all methods of birth control is low and below that associated with childbirth, with the exception of oral contraceptives in women over 40 who smoke. (The rates given for pill only/smokers for each age group are for smokers as a class. For "heavy" smokers [more than 15 cigarettes a day], the rates given would be about double; for "light" smokers [less than 15 cigarettes a day], about 50 percent.)

The mortality associated with oral contraceptive use in nonsmokers over 40 is higher than with any other method of contraception in that age group.

The lowest mortality is associated with the condom or diaphragm backed up by early abortion.

The risk of thromboembolic and thrombotic disease associated with oral contraceptives increases with age after approximately age 30 and, for myocardial infarction, is further increased by hypertension, hypercholesterolemia, obesity, diabetes, or history of preeclamptic toxemia and especially by cigarette smoking. The risk of myocardial infarction in oral contraceptive users is substantially increased in women age 40 and over, especially those with other risk factors.

Based on the data currently available, the following chart gives a gross estimate of the risk of death from circulatory disorders associated with the use of oral contraceptives:

Smoking Habits And Other Predisposing Conditions—Risk Associated With Use Of Oral Contraceptives

Age	Below 30	30–39	40+
Heavy smokers	C	B	A
Light smokers	D	C	B
Nonsmokers (no predisposing conditions)	D	C,D	C
Nonsmokers (other predisposing conditions)	C	C,B	B,A

A—Use associated with very high risk.
B—Use associated with high risk.
C—Use associated with moderate risk.
D—Use associated with low risk.

The physician and the patient should be alert to the earliest manifestations of thromboembolic and thrombotic disorders (e.g., thrombophlebitis, pulmonary embolism, cerebrovascular insufficiency, coronary occlusion, retinal thrombosis, and mesenteric thrombosis). Should any of these occur or be suspected, the drug should be discontinued immediately.

A four- to six-fold increased risk of post surgery thromboembolic complications has been reported in oral contraceptive users.[15,16] If feasible, oral contraceptives should be discontinued at least four weeks before surgery of a type associated with an increased risk of thromboembolism or prolonged immobilization.

2. OCULAR LESIONS. There have been reports of neuro-ocular lesions such as optic neuritis or retinal thrombosis associated with the use of oral contraceptives. Discontinue oral contraceptive medication if there is unexplained, sudden or gradual, partial or complete loss of vision; onset of proptosis or diplopia; papilledema; or retinal vascular lesions and institute appropriate diagnostic and therapeutic measures.

3. CARCINOMA. Long-term continuous administration of either natural or synthetic estrogen in certain animal species increases the frequency of carcinoma of the breast, cervix, vagina, and liver. Certain synthetic progestogens, none currently contained in oral contraceptives, have been noted to increase the incidence of mammary nodules, benign and malignant, in dogs.

In humans, three case control studies have reported an increased risk of endometrial carcinoma associated with the prolonged use of exogenous estrogen in postmenopausal women.[17,18,19] One publication[20] reported on the first 21 cases submitted by physicians to a registry of cases of adenocarcinoma of the endometrium in women under 40 on oral contraceptives. Of the cases found in women without predisposing risk factors for adenocarcinoma of the endometrium (e.g., irregular bleeding at the time oral contraceptives were first given, polycystic ovaries), nearly all occurred in women who had used a sequential oral contraceptive. These products are no longer marketed. No evidence has been reported suggesting an increased risk of endometrial cancer in users of conventional combination or progestogen-only oral contraceptives.

Several studies[8,21,24] have found no increases in breast cancer in women taking oral contraceptives or estrogens. One study[25], however, while also noting no overall increased risk of breast cancer in women treated with oral contraceptives, found an excess risk in the subgroups of oral contraceptive users with documented benign breast disease. A reduced occurrence of benign breast tumors in users of oral contraceptives has been well-documented.[8,21,25,26,27]

In summary, there is at present no confirmed evidence from human studies of an increased risk of cancer associated with oral contraceptives. Close clinical surveillance of all women taking oral contraceptives is, nevertheless, essential. In all cases of undiagnosed persistent or recurrent abnormal vaginal bleeding, appropriate diagnostic measures should be taken to rule out malignancy. Women with a strong family history of breast cancer or who have breast nodules, fibrocystic disease or abnormal mammograms should be monitored with particular care if they elect to use oral contraceptives instead of other methods of contraception.

Figure 1. Estimated annual number of deaths associated with control of fertility and no control per 100,000 nonsterile women, by regimen of control and age of woman.

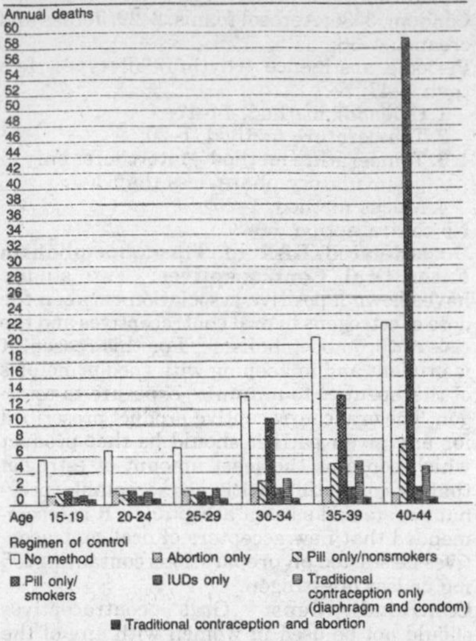

4. HEPATIC TUMORS. Benign hepatic adenomas have been found to be associated with the use of oral contraceptives.[28,29,30,46] One study[46] showed that oral contraceptive formulations with high hormonal potency were associated with a higher risk than lower potency formulations. Although benign, hepatic adenomas may rupture and may cause death through intra-abdominal hemorrhage. This has been reported in short-term as well as long-term users of oral contraceptives. Two studies relate risk with duration of use of the contraceptive, the risk being much greater after four or more years of oral contraceptive use.[30,46] While hepatic adenoma is a rare lesion, it should be considered in women presenting abdominal pain and tenderness, abdominal mass or shock.

A few cases of hepatocellular carcinoma have been reported in women taking oral contraceptives. The relationship of these drugs to this type of malignancy is not known at this time.

5. USE IN OR IMMEDIATELY PRECEDING PREGNANCY, BIRTH DEFECTS IN OFFSPRING, AND MALIGNANCY IN FEMALE OFFSPRING. The use of female sex hormones—both estrogenic and progestational agents—during early pregnancy may seriously damage the offspring. It has been shown that females exposed in utero to diethylstilbestrol, a nonsteroidal estrogen, have an increased risk of developing in later life a form of vaginal or cervical cancer that is ordinarily extremely rare.[31,32] This risk has been estimated to be of the order of 1 to 4 in 1000 exposures.[33,47] Although there is no evidence at the present time that oral contraceptives further enhance the risk of developing this type of malignancy, such patients should be monitored with particular care if they elect to use oral contraceptives instead of other methods of contraception. Furthermore, a high percentage of such exposed women (from 30 to 90%) have been found to have epithelial changes of the vagina and cervix.[34–38] Although these changes are histologically benign, it is not known whether this condition is a precursor of vaginal malignancy. Male children so exposed may develop abnormalities of the urogenital tract.[48,49,50] Although similar data are not available with the use of other estrogens, it cannot be presumed that they would not induce similar changes.

An increased risk of congenital anomalies, including heart defects and limb defects, has been reported with the use of sex hormones, including oral contraceptives, in pregnancy.[39–42,51] One case control study[42] has estimated a 4.7-fold increase in risk of limb-reduction defects in infants exposed in utero to sex hormones (oral contraceptives, hormonal withdrawal tests for pregnancy or attempted treatment for threatened abortion). Some of these exposures were very short and involved only a few days of treatment. The data suggest that the risk of limb-reduction defects in exposed fetuses is somewhat less than one in 1,000 live births.

In the past, female sex hormones have been used during pregnancy in an attempt to treat threatened or habitual abortion. There is considerable evidence that estrogens are ineffective for these indications, and there is no evidence from well-controlled studies that progestogens are effective for these uses.

There is some evidence that triploidy and possibly other types of polyploidy are increased among abortuses from women who become pregnant soon after ceasing oral contraceptives.[43] Embryos with these anomalies are virtually always aborted spontaneously. Whether there is an overall increase in spontaneous abortion of pregnancies conceived soon after stopping oral contraceptives is unknown. It is recommended that for any patient who has missed two consecutive periods, pregnancy should be ruled out before continuing the contraceptive regimen. If the patient has not adhered to the prescribed schedule, the possibility of pregnancy should be considered at the time of the first missed period (or after 45 days from the last menstrual period if the progestogen-only oral contraceptives are used), and further use of oral contraceptives should be withheld until pregnancy has been ruled out. If pregnancy is confirmed, the patient should be apprised of the potential risks to the fetus and the advisability of continuation of the pregnancy should be discussed in the light of these risks.

(See indications for use of ORTHO-NOVUM 10 mg☐21 in the treatment of endometriosis.)

It is also recommended that women who discontinue oral contraceptives with the intent of becoming pregnant use an alternate form of contraception for a period of time before attempting to conceive. Many clinicians recommend three months although no precise information is available on which to base this recommendation.

The administration of progestogen-only or progestogen-estrogen combinations to induce withdrawal bleeding should not be used as a test of pregnancy.

6. GALLBLADDER DISEASE. Studies[8,23,26] report an increased risk of surgically confirmed gallbladder disease in users of oral contraceptives and estrogens. In one study, an increased risk appeared after two years of use and doubled after four or five years of use. In one of the other studies, an increased risk was apparent between six and twelve months of use.

7. CARBOHYDRATE AND LIPID METABOLIC EFFECTS. A decrease in glucose tolerance has been observed in a significant percentage of patients on oral contraceptives. For this reason, prediabetic and diabetic patients should be carefully observed while receiving oral contraceptives.

An increase in triglycerides and total phospholipids has been observed in patients receiving oral contraceptives.[44] The clinical significance of this finding remains to be defined.

8. ELEVATED BLOOD PRESSURE. An increase in blood pressure has been reported in patients receiving oral contraceptives.[26] In some women hypertension may occur within a few months of beginning oral contraceptive use. In the first year of use, the prevalence of women with hypertension is low in users and may be no higher than that of a comparable group of nonusers. The prevalence in users increases, however, with longer exposure, and in the fifth year of use is two and a half to three times the reported prevalence in the first year. Age is also strongly correlated with the development of hypertension in oral contraceptive users. Women who previously have had hypertension during pregnancy may be more likely to develop elevation of blood pressure when given oral contraceptives. Hypertension that develops as a result of taking oral contraceptives usually returns to normal after discontinuing the drug.

9. HEADACHE. The onset or exacerbation of migraine or development of headache of a new pattern which is recurrent, persistent, or severe, requires discontinuation of oral contraceptives and evaluation of the cause.

10. BLEEDING IRREGULARITIES. Breakthrough bleeding, spotting, and amenorrhea are frequent reasons for patients discontinuing oral contraceptives. In breakthrough bleeding, as in all cases of irregular bleeding from the vagina, nonfunctional causes should be borne in mind. In undiagnosed persistent or recurrent abnormal bleeding from the vagina, adequate diagnostic measures are indicated to rule out pregnancy or malignancy. If pathology has been excluded, time or a change to another formulation may solve the problem. Changing to an oral contraceptive with a higher estrogen content, while potentially useful in minimizing menstrual irregularity, should be done only if necessary since this may increase the risk of thromboembolic disease.

An alteration in menstrual patterns is likely to occur in women using progestogen-only oral contraceptives. The amount and duration of flow, cycle length, breakthrough bleeding, spotting and amenorrhea will probably be quite variable. Bleeding irregularities occur more frequently with the use of progestogen-only oral contraceptives than with the combinations and the dropout rate due to such conditions is higher.

Women with a past history of oligomenorrhea or secondary amenorrhea or young women without regular cycles may have a tendency to remain anovulatory or to become amenorrheic after discontinuation of oral contraceptives. Women with these preexisting problems should be advised of this possibility and encouraged to use other contraceptive methods. Postuse anovulation, possibly prolonged, may also occur in women without previous irregularities.

11. ECTOPIC PREGNANCY. Ectopic as well as intrauterine pregnancy may occur in contraceptive failures. However, in progestogen-only oral contraceptive failures, the ratio of ectopic to intrauterine pregnancies is higher than in women who are not receiving oral contraceptives, since the drugs are more effective in preventing intrauterine than ectopic pregnancies.

12. BREAST FEEDING. Oral contraceptives given in the postpartum period may interfere with lactation. There may be a decrease in the quantity and quality of the breast milk. Furthermore, a small fraction of the hormonal agents in oral contraceptives has been identified in the milk of mothers receivng these drugs[45] The effects, if any, on the breast-fed child have not been determined. If feasible, the use of oral contraceptives should be deferred until the infant has been weaned.

Precautions:

General

1. A complete medical and family history should be taken prior to the initiation of oral contraceptives. The pretreatment and periodic physical examinations should include special reference to blood pressure, breasts, abdomen and pelvic organs, including Papanicolaou smear and relevant laboratory tests. As a general rule, oral contraceptives should not be prescribed for longer than one year without another physical examination being performed.

2. Under the influence of estrogen-progestogen preparations, preexisting uterine leiomyomata may increase in size.

3. Patients with a history of psychic depression should be carefully observed and the drug discontinued if depression recurs to a serious degree. Patients becoming significantly depressed while taking oral contraceptives should stop the medication and use an alternate method of contraception in an attempt to determine whether the symptom is drug-related.

4. Oral contraceptives may cause some degree of fluid retention. They should be prescribed with caution, and only with careful monitoring, in patients with conditions which might be aggravated by fluid retention, such as convulsive disorders, migraine syndrome, asthma, or cardiac or renal insufficiency.

5. Patients with a past history of jaundice during pregnancy have an increased risk of recurrence of jaundice while receiving oral contraceptive therapy. If jaundice develops in any patient receiving such drugs, the medication should be discontinued.

6. Steroid hormones may be poorly metabolized in patients with impaired liver function and should be administered with caution in such patients.

7. Oral contraceptive users may have disturbances in normal tryptophan metabolism which may result in a relative pyridoxine deficiency. The clinical significance of this is yet to be determined.

8. Serum folate levels may be depressed by oral contraceptive therapy. Since the pregnant woman is predisposed to the development of folate deficiency and the incidence of folate deficiency increases with increasing gestation, it is possible that if a woman becomes pregnant shortly after stopping oral contraceptives, she may have a greater chance of developing folate deficiency and complications attributed to this deficiency.

9. The pathologist should be advised of oral contraceptive therapy when relevant specimens are submitted.

10. Certain endocrine and liver function tests and blood components may be affected by estrogen-containing oral contraceptives.

a. Increased sulfobromophthalein retention.

b. Increased prothrombin and factors VII, VIII, IX, and X; decreased antithrombin 3; increased norepinephrine-induced platelet aggregability.

c. Increased thyroid-binding globulin (TBG) leading to increased circulating total thyroid hormone, as measured by protein-bound iodine (PBI), T4 by column, or T4 by radioimmunoassay. Free T3 resin uptake is decreased, reflecting the elevated TBG, free T4 concentration is unaltered.

d. Decreased pregnanediol excretion.

e. Reduced response to metyrapone test.

11. ORTHO-NOVUM 1/50 ☐21 and ORTHO-NOVUM 1/50☐28 contain FD&C Yellow No. 5 (tartrazine) which may cause allergic type reactions (including bronchial asthma) in certain susceptible individuals. Although the overall incidence of FD&C Yellow No. 5 (tartrazine) sensitivity in the general population is low, it is frequently seen in patients who also have aspirin hypersensitivity.

Information for the Patient

(See Patient Labeling printed below.)

Drug Interactions: Reduced efficacy and increased incidence of breakthrough bleeding have been associated with concomitant use of rifampin. A similar association has been suggested with barbiturates, phenylbutazone, phenytoin sodium, and ampicillin.

Carcinogenesis: See WARNINGS section for information on the carcinogenic potential of oral contraceptives.

Continued on next page

Ortho Pharm.—Cont.

Pregnancy: Pregnancy category X. See CONTRAINDICATIONS and WARNINGS.
Nursing Mothers: See WARNINGS.
Adverse Reactions: An increased risk of the following serious adverse reactions has been associated with the use of oral contraceptives (see WARNINGS):

- Thrombophlebitis.
- Pulmonary embolism.
- Coronary thrombosis.
- Cerebral thrombosis.
- Cerebral hemorrhage.
- Hypertension.
- Gallbladder disease.
- Liver tumors.
- Congenital anomalies.

There is evidence of an association between the following conditions and the use of oral contraceptives, although additional confirmatory studies are needed:

- Mesenteric thrombosis.
- Neuro-ocular lesions, e.g., retinal thrombosis and optic neuritis.

The following adverse reactions have been reported in patients receiving oral contraceptives and are believed to be drug-related:

- Nausea and/or vomiting, usually the most common adverse reactions occur in approximately 10% or less of patients during the first cycle. Other reactions, as a general rule, are seen much less frequently or only occasionally.
- Gastrointestinal symptoms (such as abdominal cramps and bloating).
- Breakthrough bleeding.
- Spotting.
- Change in menstrual flow.
- Dysmenorrhea.
- Amenorrhea during and after treatment.
- Temporary infertility after discontinuance of treatment.
- Edema.
- Chloasma or melasma which may persist.
- Breast changes: tenderness, enlargement, and secretion.
- Change in weight (increase or decrease).
- Change in cervical erosion and cervical secretion.
- Possible diminution in lactation when given immediately postpartum.
- Cholestatic jaundice.
- Migraine.
- Increase in size of uterine leiomyomata.
- Rash (allergic).
- Mental depression.
- Reduced tolerance to carbohydrates.
- Vaginal candidiasis.
- Change in corneal curvature (steepening).
- Intolerance to contact lenses.

The following adverse reactions have been reported in users of oral contraceptives, and the association has been neither confirmed nor refuted:

- Premenstrual-like syndrome.
- Cataracts.
- Changes in libido.
- Chorea.
- Changes in appetite.
- Cystitis-like syndrome.
- Headache.
- Nervousness.
- Dizziness.
- Hirsutism.
- Loss of scalp hair.
- Erythema multiforme.
- Erythema nodosum.
- Hemorrhagic eruption.
- Vaginitis.
- Porphyria.
- Impaired renal function.

Acute Overdose: Serious ill effects have not been reported following acute ingestion of large doses of oral contraceptives by young children. Overdosage may cause nausea, and withdrawal bleeding may occur in females.

Dosage and Administration: To achieve maximum contraceptive effectiveness, ORTHO-NOVUM Tablets, MODICON Tablets, and MICRONOR must be taken exactly as directed and at intervals not exceeding 24 hours.

21-DAY REGIMEN (21 days on, 7 days off)

The dosage of ORTHO-NOVUM 1/50□21, ORTHO-NOVUM 1/80□21, ORTHO-NOVUM 2 mg□21 and MODICON for the initial cycle of therapy is one tablet administered daily from the 5th day through the 25th day of the menstrual cycle, counting the first day of menstrual flow as "Day 1." The use of these products for contraception may be initiated postpartum. When the tablets are administered during the postpartum period, the increased risk of thromboembolic disease associated with the postpartum period must be considered. (See CONTRAINDICATIONS, WARNINGS, and PRECAUTIONS concerning thromboembolic disease.) If ORTHO-NOVUM 1/50□21, ORTHO-NOVUM 1/80□21, ORTHO-NOVUM 2 mg□21 and MODICON Tablets are first taken later than the fifth day of the first menstrual cycle of medication or postpartum, contraceptive reliance should not be placed on these products until after the first seven consecutive days of administration. For subsequent cycles, no tablets are taken for 7 days, then a new course is started of one tablet a day for 21 days. The dosage regimen then continues with 7 days of no medication, followed by 21 days of medication, instituting a three-weeks-on, one-week-off dosage regimen. The possibility of ovulation and conception prior to initiation of medication should be considered. If the patient misses more than one tablet, the patient should begin taking tablets again as soon as remembered and another method of contraception used for the balance of that tablet cycle.

ORTHO-NOVUM 2 mg□21: Following three months of treatment of hypermenorrhea, medication may be discontinued to determine the need for further therapy.

ORTHO-NOVUM 10 mg□21: In the initial cycle, the dosage of ORTHO-NOVUM 10 mg□21 for contraception and hypermenorrhea is one tablet administered daily from the 5th through the 25th day of the menstrual cycle, counting the first day of menstrual flow as "Day 1." The use of ORTHO-NOVUM 10 mg□21 for contraception may be initiated postpartum. When ORTHO-NOVUM 10 mg□21 is administered during the postpartum period, the increased risk of thromboembolic disease associated with the postpartum period must be considered. (See CONTRAINDICATIONS, WARNINGS, and PRECAUTIONS concerning thromboembolic disease.) If ORTHO-NOVUM 10 mg□21 is first taken later than the fifth day of the first menstrual cycle of medication or postpartum, contraceptive reliance should not be placed on ORTHO-NOVUM 10 mg□21 until after the first seven consecutive days of administration. The possibility of ovulation and conception prior to initiation of medication should be considered. If the patient misses more than one tablet, the patient should begin taking tablets again as soon as remembered and another method of contraception used for the balance of that tablet cycle. In all subsequent cycles the first tablet is taken on the 7th day following completion of the previous 21-day course, i.e., 7 days without medication. Following three months of treatment of hypermenorrhea, medication may be discontinued to determine the need for further therapy.

Clinical experience indicates that the use of ORTHO-NOVUM 10 mg indefinitely postpones menses and controls ovulation, resulting in symptomatic and clinical improvement in cases of endometriosis. (a) Suppressive therapy—ORTHO-NOVUM 10 mg□21 daily for 3 to 9 months is suggested with an increase in dose to 20 or 30 mg daily when indicated by the occurrence of breakthrough bleeding. Duration of treatment is determined on the basis of clinical findings. (b) Cyclic therapy—some cases of endometriosis apparently respond to cyclic therapy with ORTHO-NOVUM 10 mg□21, which suppresses ovulation. Administer one tablet daily for 21 days, (as described above for contraception).

(See discussion of Dose-Related Risk of Thromboembolism for Oral Contraceptives.)

28-DAY REGIMEN (Sunday Start)

When taking ORTHO-NOVUM 1/50□28, the first yellow tablet should be taken on the first Sunday after menstruation begins. When taking ORTHO-NOVUM 1/80□28 or MODICON 28, the first white tablet should be taken on the first Sunday after menstruation begins. If period begins on Sunday, the first yellow tablet or white tablet is taken on that day. Tablets are taken without interruption as follows: One yellow or white tablet daily for 21 days, then one green tablet daily for 7 days. After 28 tablets have been taken, a yellow or white tablet is then taken the next day (Sunday) etc. Contraceptive reliance should not be placed on these products until after the first 7 consecutive days of administration. The use of ORTHO-NOVUM 1/50□28, ORTHO-NOVUM 1/80□28, and MODICON 28 for contraception may be initiated portpartum. When the tablets are administered during the postpartum period, the increased risk of thromboembolic disease associated with the postpartum period must be considered. (See CONTRAINDICATIONS, WARNINGS, and PRECAUTIONS concerning thromboembolic disease.) The possibility of ovulation and conception prior to initiation of medication should be considered. If the patient misses more than one tablet, the patient should begin taking tablets against as soon as remembered and another method of contraception used for the balance of that tablet cycle.

MICRONOR (Continuous Regimen)

MICRONOR (norethindrone) is administered on a continuous daily dosage regimen starting on the first day of menstruation, i.e., one tablet each day, every day of the year. Tablets should be taken at the same time each day and continued daily. The patient should be advised that if prolonged bleeding occurs, she should consult her physician.

The use of MICRONOR for contraception may be initiated postpartum (see WARNINGS section). When MICRONOR is administered during the postpartum period, the increased risk of thromboembolic disease associated with the postpartum period must be considered. (See CONTRAINDICATIONS, WARNINGS, and PRECAUTIONS concerning thromboembolic disease.)

If the patient misses one tablet, MICRONOR should be discontinued immediately and a method of nonhormonal contraception should be used until mensis has appeared or pregnancy has been excluded.

Alternatively, if the patient has taken the tablets correctly, and if mensis does not appear when expected, a nonhormonal method of contraception should be substituted until an appropriate diagnostic procedure is performed to rule out pregnancy.

All Oral Contraceptives

Breakthrough bleeding, spotting, and amenorrhea are frequent reasons for patients discontinuing oral contraceptives. In breakthrough bleeding, as in all cases of irregular bleeding from the vagina, nonfunctional causes should be borne in mind. In undiagnosed persistent or recurrent abnormal bleeding from the vagina, adequate diagnostic measures are indicated to rule out pregnancy or malignancy. If pathology has been excluded, time or a change to another formulation may solve the problem. Changing to an oral contraceptive with a higher estrogen content, while potentially useful in minimizing menstrual irregularity,

should be done only if necessary since this may increase the risk of thromboembolic disease.
Use of oral contraceptives in the event of a missed menstrual period:
1. If the patient has not adhered to the prescribed dosage regimen, the possibility of pregnancy should be considered after the first missed period (or after 45 days from the last menstrual period if the progestogen-only oral contraceptives are used) and oral contraceptives should be withheld until pregnancy has been ruled out.
2. If the patient has adhered to the prescribed regimen and misses two consecutive periods, pregnancy should be ruled out before continuing the contraceptive regimen.

How Supplied: ORTHO-NOVUM 1/50□21 Tablets (as yellow unscored tablets with "Ortho" and "1" debossed on each side) are available in a DIALPAK* Tablet Dispenser containing 21 tablets and a dispensing unit which contains one DIALPAK and two refills of 21 tablets each. Each yellow ORTHO-NOVUM 1/50□21 Tablet† contains 1 mg of the progestational compound, norethindrone, together with 0.05 mg of the estrogenic compound, mestranol.
ORTHO-NOVUM 1/50□21 is available for clinic usage in a VERIDATE* Tablet Dispenser (unfilled) and VERIDATE Refills.
ORTHO-NOVUM 1/50□28 Tablets (as yellow unscored tablets with "Ortho" and "1" debossed on each side) are available in a DIALPAK Tablet Dispenser containing 28 tablets, 21 yellow norethindrone with mestranol tablets and 7 green tablets containing inert ingredients. Each yellow ORTHO-NOVUM 1/50□28 Tablet† contains 1 mg of the progestational compound, norethindrone, together with 0.05 mg of the estrogenic compound, mestranol.
ORTHO-NOVUM 1/50□28 is available for clinic usage in a VERIDATE Tablet Dispenser (unfilled) and VERIDATE Refills.
†Contains FD&C Yellow No. 5 (tartrazine) as a color additive.
ORTHO-NOVUM 1/80□21 Tablets (as white unscored tablets with "Ortho" and "1" debossed on each side) are available in a DIALPAK Tablet Dispenser containing 21 tablets and a dispensing unit which contains one DIALPAK and two refills of 21 tablets each. Each white ORTHO-NOVUM 1/80□21 Tablet contains 1 mg of the progestational compound, norethindrone, together with 0.08 mg of the estrogenic compound, mestranol.
ORTHO-NOVUM 1/80□21 is available for clinic usage in a VERIDATE Tablet Dispenser (unfilled) and VERIDATE Refills.
ORTHO-NOVUM 1/80□28 Tablets (as white unscored tablets with "Ortho" and "1" debossed on each side) are available in a DIALPAK Tablet Dispenser containing 28 tablets, 21 white norethindrone with mestranol tablets and 7 green tablets containing inert ingredients. Each white ORTHO-NOVUM 1/80□28 Tablet contains 1 mg of the progestational compound, norethindrone, together with 0.08 mg of the estrogenic compound, mestranol.
ORTHO-NOVUM 1/80□28 is available for clinic usage in a VERIDATE Tablet Dispenser (unfilled) and VERIDATE Refills.
ORTHO-NOVUM 2 mg□21 Tablets (as white unscored tablets with "Ortho" and "2" debossed on each side) are available in a DIALPAK Tablet Dispenser containing 21 tablets. Each white ORTHO-NOVUM 2 mg□21 Tablet contains 2 mg of the progestational compound, norethindrone, together with 0.10 mg of the estrogenic compound, mestranol.
ORTHO-NOVUM 2 mg□21 is available for clinic usage in a VERIDATE Tablet Dispenser (unfilled) and VERIDATE Refills.
ORTHO-NOVUM 10 mg□21 Tablets (as white unscored tablets with "Ortho" and "10" debossed on each side) are available in a DIALPAK Tablet Dispenser containing 21 tablets. Each white ORTHO-NOVUM 10 mg□21 Tablet contains 10 mg of the progestational compound, norethindrone, together with 0.06 mg of the estrogenic compound, mestranol.
MODICON Tablets (as white unscored tablets with "Ortho" appearing on each side) are available in a DIALPAK Tablet Dispenser containing 21 tablets. Each white tablet contains 0.5 mg of the progestational compound, norethindrone, together with 0.035 mg of the estrogenic compound, ethinyl estradiol.
MODICON is available for clinic usage in a VERIDATE Tablet Dispenser (unfilled) and VERIDATE Refills.
MODICON 28 Tablets (as white unscored tablets with "Ortho" appearing on each side) are available in a DIALPAK Tablet Dispenser containing 28 tablets, 21 white norethindrone with ethinyl estradiol tablets and 7 green tablets containing inert ingredients. Each white MODICON 28 Tablet contains 0.5 mg of the progestational compound, norethindrone, together with 0.035 mg of the estrogenic compound, ethinyl estradiol.
MODICON 28 is available for clinic usage in a VERIDATE Tablet Dispenser (unfilled) and VERIDATE Refills.
MICRONOR Tablets (as lime unscored tablets with "Ortho" and "0.35" debossed on each side) are available in a DIALPAK Tablet Dispenser containing 28 tablets. Each lime MICRONOR Tablet contains 0.35 mg of the progestational substance norethindrone.
MICRONOR is available for clinic usage in a VERIDATE Tablet Dispenser (unfilled) and VERIDATE Refills.

References:

1. "Population Reports," Series H, Number 2, May 1974; Series I, Number 1, June 1974; Series B, Number 2, January 1975; Series H, Number 3, 1975; Series H, Number 4, January 1976 (published by the Population Information Program, The George Washington University Medical Center, 2001 S St. NW, Washington, D.C.) **2.** Inman, W.H.W., M.P. Vessey, B. Westerholm, and A. Engelund, "Thromboembolic disease and the steroidal content of oral contraceptives. A report to the Committee on Safety of Drugs," Brit Med J *2*:203–209, 1970. **3.** Stolley, P.D., J.A. Tonascia, M.S. Tockman, P.E. Sartwell, A.H. Rutledge, and M.P. Jacobs, "Thrombosis with low-estrogen oral contraceptives," Am J Epidemiol *102*:197–208, 1975. **4.** Royal College of General Practitioners, "Oral contraception and thromboembolic disease," J Coll Gen Pract *13*:267–279, 1967. **5.** Inman, W.H.W. and M.P. Vessey, "Investigation of deaths from pulmonary, coronary, and cerebral thrombosis and embolism in women of childbearing age," Brit Med J *2*:193–199, 1968. **6.** Vessey, M.P. and R. Doll, "Investigation of relation between use of oral contraceptives and thromboembolic disease. A further report," Brit Med J *2*:651–657, 1969. **7.** Sartwell, P.E., A.T. Masi, F.G. Arthes, G.R. Greene, and H.E. Smith, "Thromboembolism and oral contraceptives: an epidemiological case control study." Am J Epidemiol *90*:365–380, 1969. **8.** Boston Collaborative Drug Surveillance Program, "Oral contraceptives and venous thromboembolic disease, surgically confirmed gall bladder disease and breast tumors," Lancet *1*:1399–1404, 1973. **9.** Collaborative Group for the Study of Stroke in Young Women, "Oral contraception and increased risk of cerebral ischemia or thrombosis," N Engl J Med *288*:871–878, 1973. **10.** Collaborative Group for the Study of Stroke in Young Women, "Oral contraceptives and strokes in young women: associated risk factors," JAMA *231*:718–722, 1975. **11.** Mann, J.I. and W.H.W. Inman, "Oral contraceptives and death from myocardial infarction," Brit Med J *2*:245–248, 1975. **12.** Mann, J.I., W.H.W. Inman, and M. Thorogood, "Oral contraceptive use in older women and fatal myocardial infarction," Brit Med J *2*:445–447, 1976. **13.** Mann, J.I., M.P. Vessey, M. Thorogood, and R. Doll, "Myocardial infarction in young women with special reference to oral contraceptive practice," Brit Med J *2*:241–245, 1975. **14.** Tietze, C., "New Estimate of Mortality Associated with Fertility Control," Family Planning Perspectives Vol. 9, No. 2, 74–76, 1977. **15.** Vessey, M.P., R. Doll, A.S. Fairbairn, and G. Glober, "Post-operative thromboembolism and the use of oral contraceptives," Brit Med J *3*:123–126, 1970. **16.** Greene, G.R., and P.E. Sartwell, "Oral contraceptive use in patients with thromboembolism following surgery, trauma, or infection," Am J Pub Health *62*:680–685, 1972. **17.** Smith, D.C., R. Prentice, D.J. Thompson, and W.L. Herrmann, "Association of exogenous estrogen and endometrial carcinoma," N Engl J Med *293*:1164–1167, 1975. **18.** Ziel, H.K. and W.D. Finkle, "Increased risk of endometrial carcinoma among users of conjugated estrogens," N Engl J Med *293*:1167–1170, 1975. **19.** Mack, T.N., M.C. Pike, B.E. Henderson, R.I. Pfeffer, V.R. Gerkins, M. Arthur, and S.E. Brown, "Estrogens and endometrial cancer in a retirement community," N Engl J Med *294*: 1262–1267, 1976.
20. Silverberg, S.G., and E.L. Makowski, "Endometrial carcinoma in young women taking oral contraceptive agents," Obstet Gynecol *46*:503–506, 1975. **21.** Vessey, M.P., R. Doll, and P.M. Sutton, "Oral contraceptives and breast neoplasia: a retrospective study," Brit Med J *3*:719–724, 1972. **22.** Vessey, M.P., R. Doll, and K. Jones, "Oral contraceptives and breast cancer. Progress report of an epidemiological study," Lancet *1*:941–943, 1975. **23.** Boston Collaborative Drug Surveillance Program, "Surgically confirmed gall bladder disease, venous thromboembolism and breast tumors in relation to postmenopausal estrogen therapy," N Engl J Med *290*:15–19, 1974. **24.** Arthes, F.G., P.E. Sartwell, and E.F. Lewison, "The pill, estrogens, and the breast. Epidemiological aspects," Cancer *28*:1391–1394, 1971. **25.** Fasal, E., and R.S. Paffenbarger, "Oral contraceptives as related to cancer and benign lesions of the breast," J Natl Cancer Inst *55*:767–773, 1975. **26.** Royal College of General Practitioners, "Oral Contraceptives and Health," London, Pitman, 1974. **27.** Ory, H., P. Cole, B. MacMahon and R. Hoover, "Oral contraceptives and reduced risk of benign breast diseases," N Engl J Med *294*:419–422, 1976. **28.** Baum, J., F. Holts, J.J. Bookstein and E.W. Klein, "Possible association between benign hepatomas and oral contraceptives," Lancet *2*:926–928, 1973. **29.** Mays, E.T., W.M. Christopherson, M.M. Mahr, and H.C. Williams, "Hepatic changes in young women ingesting contraceptive steroids. Hepatic hemorrhage and primary hepatic tumors," JAMA *235*:730–732, 1976.
30. Edmonsen, H.A., B. Henderson, and B. Benton, "Liver-cell adenomas associated with the use of oral contraceptives," N Engl J Med *294*:470–472, 1976. **31.** Herbst, A.L., H. Ulfelder, and D.C. Poskanzer, "Adenocarcinoma of the vagina," N Engl J Med *284*:878–881, 1971. **32.** Greenwald, P., J.J. Barlow, P.C. Nasca, and W. Burnett, "Vaginal cancer after maternal treatment with synthetic estrogens," N Engl J Med *285*:390–392, 1971. **33.** Lanier, A.P., K.L. Noller, D.G. Decker, L. Elveback, and L.T. Kurland, "Cancer and stilbestrol. A follow-up of 1719 persons exposed to estrogen in utero and born 1943–1959," Mayo Clinic Pro *48*:793–799, 1973. **34.** Herbst, A.L., R.J. Kurman, and R.E. Scully, "Vaginal and cervical abnormalities after exposure to stilbestrol in utero," Obstet Gynecol *40*:287–298, 1972. **35.** Herbst, A.L., S.J. Robboy, G.J. Macdonald, and R.E. Scully, "The effects of local progesterone on stilbestrol-associated vaginal adenosis," Am J Obstet Gynecol *118*:607–615, 1974. **36.** Herbst, A.L., D.C. Poskanzer, S.J.

Continued on next page

Ortho Pharm.—Cont.

Robboy, L. Friedlander, and R.E. Scully, "Prenatal exposure to stilbestrol: a prospective comparison of exposed female offspring with unexposed controls," N Engl J Med *292*:334–339, 1975. **37.** Stafi, A., R.F. Mattingly, D.V. Foley, W. Fetherston, "Clinical diagnosis of vaginal adenosis," Obstet Gynecol *43*:118–128, 1974. **38.** Sherman, A.I., M. Goldrath, A. Berlin, V. Vakhariya, F. Banooni, W. Michaels, P. Goodman, and S. Brown, "Cervical-vaginal adenosis after in utero exposure to synthetic estrogens," Obstet Gynecol *44*:531–545, 1974. **39.** Gal, I., B. Kirman, and J. Stern, "Hormone pregnancy tests and congenital malformation," Nature *216*:83, 1967. **40.** Levy, E.P., A. Cohen, and F.C. Fraser, "Hormone treatment during pregnancy and congenital heart defects," Lancet *1*:611, 1973. **41.** Nora, J.J. and A.H. Nora, "Birth defects and oral contraceptives," Lancet *1*:941–942, 1973. **42.** Janerich, D.T., J.M. Piper, and D.M. Glebatis, "Oral contraceptives and congenital limb-reduction defects," N Engl J Med *291*:697–700, 1974. **43.** Carr, D.H., "Chromosome studies in selected spontaneous abortions: I. Conception after oral contraceptives," Canad Med Assoc J *103*:343–348, 1970. **44.** Wynn, V., J.W.H. Doar, and G.L. Mills, "Some effects of oral contraceptives on serum-lipid and lipoprotein levels," Lancet *2*:720–723, 1966. **45.** Laumas, K.R., P.K. Malkani, S. Bhatnagar, and V. Laumas, "Radioactivity in the breast milk of lactating women after oral administration of 3 H-norethynodrel," Amer J Obstet Gynecol *98*:411–413, 1967. **46.** Center for Disease Control, "Increased Risk of Hepatocellular Adenoma in Women with Long-term use of Oral Contraceptives," Morbidity and Mortality Weekly Report, *26*:293–294, 1977. **47.** Herbst, A.L., P. Cole, T. Colton, S.J. Robboy, R.E. Scully, "Age-incidence and Risk of Diethylstilbestrol-related Clear Cell Adenocarcinoma of the Vagina and Cervix," Am J Obstet Gynecol, *128*:43–50, 1977. **48.** Bibbo, M., M. Al-Neqeeb, I. Baccarini, W. Gill, M. Newton, K.M. Sleeper, M. Sonek, G.L. Wied, "Follow-up Study of Male and Female Offspring of DES-treated Mothers. A Preliminary Report," Jour of Repro Med., *15*:29–32, 1975. **49.** Gill, W.B., G.F.B. Schumacher, M. Bibbo, "Structural and Functional Abnormalities in the Sex Organs of Male Offspring of Mothers Treated with Diethylstilbestrol (DES)," Jour of Repro Med., *16*:147–153, 1976. **50.** Henderson, B.E., B. Senton, M. Cosgrove, J. Baptista, J. Aldrich, D. Townsend, W. Hart, T. Mack, "Urogenital Tract Abnormalities in Sons of Women Treated with Diethylstilbestrol," Pediatrics, *58*:505–507, 1976. **51.** Heinonen, O.P., D. Slone, R.R. Nonson, E.B. Hook, S. Shapiro, "Cardiovascular Birth Defects and Antenatal Exposure to Female Sex Hormones," N Engl J Med, *296*:67–70, 1977. **52.** Jain, A.K., "Mortality Risk Associated with the Use of Oral Contraceptives," Studies in Family Planning, *8*:50–54, 1977. **53.** Berat, V., "Mortality Among Oral Contraceptive Users," Lancet *2*:727–731, 1977. **54.** Vessey, M.P., McPherson, K., and Johnson, B., "Mortality Among Women Participating in the Oxford/Family Planning Association Contraceptive Study," Lancet *2*:731–733, 1977.

The patient labeling for oral contraceptive drug products is set forth below:

Brief Summary Patient Package Insert:

Cigarette smoking increases the risk of serious adverse effects on the heart and blood vessels from oral contraceptive use. This risk increases with age and with heavy smoking (15 or more cigarettes per day) and is quite marked in women over 35 years of age. Women who use oral contraceptives should not smoke.

Oral contraceptives taken as directed are about 99% effective in preventing pregnancy. (The mini-pill, however, is somewhat less effective.) Forgetting to take your pills increases the chance of pregnancy.

Women who have or have had clotting disorders, cancer of the breast or sex organs, unexplained vaginal bleeding, a stroke, heart attack, angina pectoris, or who suspect they may be pregnant should not use oral contraceptives.

Most side effects of the pill are not serious. The most common side effects are nausea, vomiting, bleeding between menstrual periods, weight gain, and breast tenderness. However, proper use of oral contraceptives requires that they be taken under your doctor's continuous supervision, because they can be associated with serious side effects which may be fatal. Fortunately, these occur very infrequently. The serious side effects are:

1. Blood clots in the legs, lungs, brain, heart or other organs and hemorrhage into the brain due to bursting of a blood vessel.
2. Liver tumors, which may rupture and cause severe bleeding.
3. Birth defects if the pill is taken while you are pregnant.
4. High blood pressure.
5. Gallbladder disease.

Some of the symptoms associated with these serious side effects are discussed in the detailed leaflet given you with your supply of pills. Notify your doctor if you notice any unusual physical disturbance while taking the pill.

The estrogen in oral contraceptives has been found to cause breast cancer and other cancers in certain animals. These findings suggest that oral contraceptives may also cause cancer in humans. However, studies to date in women taking currently marketed oral contraceptives have not confirmed that oral contraceptives cause cancer in humans.

The detailed leaflet describes more completely the benefits and risks of oral contraceptives. It also provides information on other forms of contraception. Read it carefully. If you have any questions, consult your doctor.

Caution. Oral contraceptives are of no value in the prevention or treatment of venereal disease.

Detailed Patient Labeling

What You Should Know About Oral Contraceptives: Oral contraceptives ("the pill") are the most effective way (except for sterilization) to prevent pregnancy. They are also convenient and, for most women, free of serious or unpleasant side effects. Oral contraceptives must always be taken under the continuous supervision of a physician.

The information in this leaflet under the headings "Who Should Not Use Oral Contraceptives," "The Dangers of Oral Contraceptives," and "How to Use Oral Contraceptives As Effectively As Possible, Once You Have Decided to Use Them" is also applicable when these drugs are used for other indications.

ORTHO-NOVUM 2 mg☐21 may be prescribed for you for the treatment of hypermenorrhea. ORTHO-NOVUM 10 mg☐21 may be prescribed for you for the treatment of hypermenorrhea or endometriosis.

It is important that any woman who considers using an oral contraceptive understand the risks involved. Although the oral contraceptives have important advantages over other methods of contraception, they have certain risks that no other method has. Only you can decide whether the advantages are worth these risks. This leaflet will tell you about the most important risks. It will explain how you can help your doctor prescribe the pill as safely as possible by telling him about yourself and being alert for the earliest signs of trouble. And it will tell you how to use the pill properly, so that it will be as effective as possible. There is more detailed information available in the leaflet prepared for doctors. Your pharmacist can show you a copy; you may need your doctor's help in understanding parts of it.

Who Should Not Use Oral Contraceptives:

A. If you have now, or have had in the past, any of the following conditions you should not use the pill:
1. Heart attack or stroke
2. Clots in the legs or lungs
3. Angina pectoris
4. Known or suspected cancer of the breast or sex organs
5. Unusual vaginal bleeding that has not yet been diagnosed.

B. If you are pregnant or suspect that you are pregnant, do not use the pill.

C. Cigarette smoking increases the risk of serious adverse effects on the heart and blood vessels from oral contraceptive use. This risk increases with age and with heavy smoking (15 or more cigarettes per day) and is quite marked in women over 35 years of age. Women who use oral contraceptives should not smoke.

D. If you have scanty or irregular periods or are a young woman without a regular cycle, you should use another method of contraception because, if you use the pill, you may have difficulty becoming pregnant or may fail to have menstrual periods after discontinuing the pill.

Deciding To Use Oral Contraceptives: If you do not have any of the conditions listed above and are thinking about using oral contraceptives, to help you decide, you need information about the advantages and risks of oral contraceptives and of other contraceptive methods as well. This leaflet describes the advantages and risks of oral contraceptives. Except for sterilization, the IUD and abortion, which have their own exclusive risks, the only risks of other methods of contraception are those due to pregnancy should the method fail. Your doctor can answer questions you may have with respect to other methods of contraception. He can also answer any questions you may have after reading this leaflet on oral contraceptives.

1. What Oral Contraceptives Are and How They Work. Oral Contraceptives are of two types. The most common, often simply called "the pill", is a combination of an estrogen and a progestogen, the two kinds of female hormones. The amount of estrogen and progestogen can vary, but the amount of estrogen is most important because both the effectiveness and some of the dangers of oral contraceptives are related to the amount of estrogen. This kind of oral contraceptive works principally by preventing release of an egg from the ovary. When the amount of estrogen is 50 micrograms or more, and the pill is taken as directed, oral contraceptives are more than 99% effective (i.e., there would be less than one pregnancy if 100 women used the pill for one year.) Pills that contain 20 to 35 micrograms of estrogen vary slightly in effectiveness, ranging from 98% to more than 99% effective.

The second type of oral contraceptive, often caled the "mini-pill," contains only a progestogen. It works in part by preventing release of an egg from the ovary but also by keeping sperm from reaching the egg and by making the uterus (womb) less receptive to any fertilized egg that reaches it. The mini-pill is less effective than the combination oral contraceptive, about 97% effective. In addition, the progestogen-only pill has a tendency to cause irregular bleeding which may be quite inconvenient, or cessation of bleeding entirely. The progestogen-only pill is used despite its lower effectiveness in the hope that it will prove not to have some of the serious side effects of the estrogen-containing pill (see below) but it is not yet certain that the mini-pill does in fact have fewer serious side effects. The discussion below, while based mainly on information about the combination pills, should be considered to apply as well to the mini-pill.

2. Other Nonsurgical Ways to Prevent Pregnancy. As this leaflet will explain, oral contraceptives have several serious risks. Other methods of contraception have lesser risks or none at all. They are also less effective than oral contraceptives, but, used properly, may be effective enough for many women. The following table gives reported pregnancy rates (the number of women out of 100 who would become pregnant in one year) for these methods:

Pregnancies Per 100 Women Per Year

Intrauterine device (IUD), less than 1–6;
Diaphragm with spermicidal products (creams or jellies), 2–20;
Condom (rubber) 3–36; Aerosol foams, 2–29;
Jellies and creams, 4–36;
Periodic abstinence (rhythm) all types, less than 1–47;

1. Calendar method, 14–47;
2. Temperature method, 1–20;
3. Temperature method–intercourse only in postovulatory phase, less than 1–7;
4. Mucus method, 1–25;

No contraception, 60–80.

The figures (except for the IUD) vary widely because people differ in how well they use each method. Very faithful users of the various methods obtain very good results, except for users of the calendar method of perodic abstinence (rhythm). Except for the IUD, effective use of these methods requires somewhat more effort than simply taking a single pill every morning, but it is an effort that many couples undertake successfully. Your doctor can tell you a great deal more about these methods of contraception.

3. The Dangers of Oral Contraceptives.

a. *Circulatory disorders (abnormal blood clotting, heart attack, and stroke due to hemorrhage).* Blood clots (in various blood vessels of the body) are the most common of the serious side effects of oral contraceptives. A clot can result in a stroke (if the clot is in the brain), a heart attack (if the clot is in a blood vessel of the heart), or a pulmonary embolus (a clot which forms in the legs or pelvis, then breaks off and travels to the lungs). Any of these can be fatal. Clots also occur rarely in the blood vessels of the eye, resulting in blindness or impairment of vision in that eye. There is evidence that the risk of clotting increases with higher estrogen doses. It is therefore important to keep the dose of estrogen as low as possible, so long as the oral contraceptive used has an acceptable pregnancy rate and doesn't cause unacceptable changes in the menstrual pattern. Furthermore, cigarette smoking by oral contraceptive users increases the risk of serious adverse effects on the heart and blood vessels. This risk increases with age and with heavy smoking (15 or more cigarettes per day) and begins to become quite marked in women over 35 years of age. For this reason, women who use oral contraceptives should not smoke.
The risk of abnormal blood clotting increases with age in both users and nonusers of oral contraceptives, but the increased risk from the oral contraceptive appears to be present at all ages. For women aged 20 to 44 it is estimated that about 1 in 2,000 using oral contraceptives will be hospitalized each year because of abnormal clotting. Among nonusers in the same age group, about 1 in 20,000 would be hospitalized each year. For oral contraceptive users in general, it has been estimated that in women between the ages of 15 and 34 the risk of death due to circulatory disorder is about 1 in 12,000 per year, whereas for nonusers the rate is about 1 in 50,000 per year. In the age group 35 to 44, the risk is estimated to be about 1 in 2,500 per year for oral contraceptive users and about 1 in 10,000 per year for nonusers.
Even without the pill the risk of having a heart attack increases with age and is also increased by such heart attack risk factors as high blood pressure, high cholesterol, obesity, diabetes, and cigarette smoking. Without any risk factors present, the use of oral contraceptives alone may double the risk of heart attack. However, the combination of cigarette smoking, especially heavy smoking, and oral contraceptive use greatly increases the risk of heart attack. Oral contraceptive users who smoke are about five times more likely to have a heart attack than users who do not smoke and about ten times more likely to have a heart attack than nonusers who do not smoke. It has been estimated that users between the ages of 30 and 39 who smoke have about a 1-in-10,000 chance each year of having a fatal heart attack compared to about a 1-in-50,000 chance in users who do not smoke, and about a 1-in-100,000 chance in nonusers who do not smoke. In the age group 40 to 44, the risk is about 1 in 1,700 per year for users who smoke compared to about 1 in 10,000 for users who do not smoke and to about one in 14,000 per year for nonusers who do not smoke. Heavy smoking (about 15 cigarettes or more a day) further increases the risk. If you do not smoke and have none of the other heart attack risk factors described above, you will have a smaller risk than listed. If you have several heart attack risk factors, the risk may be considerably greater than listed.
In addition to blood-clotting disorders, it has been estimated that women taking oral contraceptives are twice as likely as nonusers to have a stroke due to rupture of blood vessel in the brain.
One report suggests that the risk of circulatory diseases appears to increase the longer you are on the pill and may continue after you stop.

b. *Formation of tumors.* Studies have found that when certain animals are given the female sex hormone estrogen, which is an ingredient of oral contraceptives, continuously for long periods, cancers may develop in the breast, cervix, vagina, and liver.
These findings suggest that oral contraceptives may cause cancer in humans. However, studies to date in women taking currently marketed oral contraceptives have not confirmed that oral contraceptives cause cancer in humans. Several studies have found no increase in breast cancer in users, although one study suggested oral contraceptives might cause an increase in breast cancer in women who already have benign breast disease (e.g., cysts).
Women with a strong family history of breast cancer or who have breast nodules, fibrocystic disease, or abnormal mammograms or who were exposed to DES (diethylstilbestrol), an estrogen, during their mother's pregnancy must be followed very closely by their doctors if they choose to use oral contraceptives instead of another method of contraception. Many studies have shown that women taking oral contraceptives have less risk of getting benign breast disease than those who have not used oral contraceptives. Recently, strong evidence has emerged that estrogens (one component of oral contraceptives), when given for periods of more than one year to women after the menopause, increase the risk of cancer of the uterus (womb). There is also some evidence that a kind of oral contraceptive which is no longer marketed, the sequential oral contraceptive, may increase the risk of cancer of the uterus. There remains no evidence, however, that the oral contraceptives now available increase the risk of this cancer.
Oral contraceptives do cause, although rarely, a benign (non-malignant) tumor of the liver. These tumors do not spread, but they may rupture and cause internal bleeding, which may be fatal. A few cases of cancer of the liver have been reported in women using oral contraceptives, but it is not yet known whether the drug caused them.

c. *Dangers to a developing child if oral contraceptives are used in or immediately preceding pregnancy.* Oral contraceptives should not be taken by pregnant women because they may damage the developing child. An increased risk of birth defects, including heart defects and limb defects, has been associated with the use of sex hormones, including oral contraceptives, in pregnancy. In addition, the developing female child whose mother has received DES (diethylstilbestrol), an estrogen, during pregnancy has a risk of getting cancer of the vagina or cervix in her teens or young adulthood. This risk is estimated to be about 1 to 4 in 1000 exposures. Abnormalities of the urinary and sex organs have been reported in male offspring so exposed. It is possible that other estrogens, such as the estrogens in oral contraceptives, could have the same effect in the child if the mother takes them during pregnancy.
If you stop taking oral contraceptives to become pregnant, your doctor may recommend that you use another method of contraception for a short while, for example three months. The reason for this is that there is evidence from studies in women who have had "miscarriages" soon after stopping the pill, that the lost fetuses are more likely to be abnormal. Whether there is an overall increase in "miscarriage" in women who become pregnant soon after stopping the pill as compared with women who do not use the pill is not known, but it is possible that there may be. If, however, you do become pregnant soon after stopping oral contraceptives, and do not have a miscarriage, there does not appear to be evidence that the baby has an increased risk of being abnormal.

d. *Gallbladder disease.* Women who use oral contraceptives have a greater risk than nonusers of having gallbladder disease requiring surgery. The increased risk may first appear within one year of use and may double after four or five years of use.

e. *Other side effects of oral contraceptives.* Some women using oral contraceptives experience unpleasant side effects. Some of these may be temporary. Your breasts may feel tender, nausea and vomiting may occur, you may gain or lose weight, and your ankles may swell. A spotty darkening of the skin, particularly of the face, is possible and may persist. You may notice unexpected vaginal bleeding or changes in your menstrual period. Irregular bleeding is frequently seen when using the mini-pill or combinaton oral contraceptives containing less than 50 micrograms of estrogen.
More serious side effects include worsening of migraine, asthma, epilepsy, and kidney or heart disease because of a tendency for water to be retained in the body when oral contraceptives are used. Other side effects are growth of preexisting fibroid tumors of the uterus; mental depression; and liver problems with jaundice (yellowing of the skin). Your doctor may find that levels of sugar and fatty substances in your blood are elevated; the long-term effects of these changes are not known. Some women develop high blood pressure while taking oral contraceptives, which ordinarily returns to the original levels when the oral contraceptive is stopped.
Other reactions, although not proved to be caused by oral contraceptives, are occasionally reported. These include more frequent urination and some discomfort when urinating, kidney disease, nervousness, dizziness, some loss of scalp hair, an increase in body hair, an increase or decrease in sex drive, appetite changes, cataracts, and a need for change in contact lens prescription or inability to use contact lenses.

Continued on next page

Ortho Pharm.—Cont.

After you stop using oral contraceptives there may be a delay before you are able to become pregnant or before you resume having menstrual periods. This is especially true of women who had irregular menstrual cycles prior to the use of oral contraceptives. As discussed previously, your doctor may recommend that you wait a short while after stopping the pill before you try to become pregnant. During this time, use another form of contraception. You should consult your physician before resuming use of oral contraceptives after childbirth, especially if you plan to nurse your baby. Drugs in oral contraceptives are known to appear in the milk, and the long-range effect on infants is not known at this time. Furthermore, oral contraceptives may cause a decrease in your milk supply as well as in the quality of the milk.

4. Comparison of the Risks of Oral Contraceptives and Other Contraceptive Methods.
The many studies on the risks and effectiveness of oral contraceptives and other methods of contraception have been analyzed to estimate the risk of death associated with various methods of contraception. This risk has two parts: (a) the risk of the method itself (e.g., the risk that oral contraceptives will cause death due to abnormal clotting), and (b) the risk of death due to pregnancy or abortion in the event the method fails. The results of this analysis are shown in the bar graph (Figure 1). The height of the bars is the number of deaths per 100,000 women each year. There are six sets of bars, each set referring to a specific age group of women. Within each set of bars there is a single bar for each of the different contraceptive methods. For oral contraceptives, there are two bars—one for smokers and the other for nonsmokers. The analysis is based on present knowledge and new information could, of course, alter it. The analysis shows that the risk of death from all methods of birth control is low and below that associated with childbirth, except for oral contraceptives in women over 40 who smoke. It shows that the lowest risk of death is associated with the condom or diaphragm (traditional contraception) backed up by early abortion in case of failure of the condom or diaphragm to prevent pregnancy. Also, at any age the risk of death (due to unexpected pregnancy) from the use of traditional contraception, even without a backup of abortion, is generally the same as or less than that from use of oral contraceptives.

How To Use Oral Contraceptives As Effectively As Possible, Once You Have Decided To Use Them:

1. What to Tell your Doctor.
You can make use of the pill as effectively as possible by telling your doctor if you have any of the following:

a. Conditions that mean you should not use oral contraceptives:
Clots in the legs or lungs.
Clots in the legs or lungs in the past.
A stroke, heart attack, or angina pectoris.
Known or suspected cancer of the breast or sex organs.
Unusual vaginal bleeding that has not yet been diagnosed.
Known or suspected pregnancy.

b. Conditions that your doctor will want to watch closely or which might cause him to suggest another method of contraception:
A family history of breast cancer.
Breast nodules, fibrocystic disease of the breast, or an abnormal mammogram.
Diabetes.
High blood pressure.
High cholesterol.
Cigarette smoking.
Migraine headaches.
Heart or kidney disease.
Epilepsy.
Mental depression.
Fibroid tumors of the uterus.
Gallbladder disease.

c. Once you are using oral contraceptives, you should be alert for signs of a serious adverse effect and call your doctor if they occur:
Sharp pain in the chest, coughing blood, or sudden shortness of breath (indicating possible clots in the lung).
Pain in the calf (possible clot in the leg).
Crushing chest pain or heaviness (indicating possible heart attack).
Sudden severe headache or vomiting, dizziness or fainting, disturbance of vision or speech or weakness or numbness in an arm or leg (indicating a possible stroke).
Sudden partial or complete loss of vision (indicating a possible clot in the eye).
Breast lumps (you should ask your doctor to show you how to examine your own breasts).
Severe pain in the abdomen (indicating a possible ruptured tumor of the liver).
Severe depression.
Yellowing of the skin (jaundice).

2. How to Take the Pill So That it is Most Effective.
To achieve maximum contraceptive effectiveness. ORTHO-NOVUM, MODICON and MICRONOR must be taken exactly as directed and at intervals not exceeding 24 hours.

21-Day Regimen: Counting the first day of menstrual flow as "Day 1," take one tablet daily from the 5th through the 25th day of the menstrual cycle. If the first tablet is taken later than the 5th day of the menstrual cycle or postpartum, contraceptive reliance should not be placed on ORTHO-NOVUM or MODICON until after the first seven consecutive days of administration. Take a tablet the same time each day, preferably at bedtime, for 21 days, then wait for 7 days during which time a menstrual period usually occurs. Following this 7-day waiting period, start taking a tablet each day for the next 21 days, thus using a three weeks-on, one-week off dosage regimen.

When ORTHO-NOVUM 2 mg□21 Tablets are used for the treatment of hypermenorrhea, your physician will discuss the regimen with you.

ORTHO-NOVUM 10 mg□21: In the treatment of hypermenorrhea or endometriosis, your physician will discuss the regimen with you.

28-Day Regimen: The first white or yellow tablet should be taken on the first Sunday after the menstrual period begins. If period begins on Sunday, begin taking tablets that day. Take one white or yellow tablet at the same time each day for 21 consecutive days, then take one green tablet daily for 7 days during which time your menstrual period usually occurs. During the FIRST cycle, it is important that you use another method of birth control until you have taken a white or yellow tablet daily for seven consecutive days. After 28 tablets have been taken, (last green tablet will always be taken on a Saturday) take the first tablet (white or yellow) from your next package the following day (Sunday) whether or not you are still menstruating. With the 28-day regimen, pills are taken every day of the year.

Continuous Regimen (MICRONOR): The first MICRONOR Tablet should be taken on the first day of the menstrual period.
Take one tablet at the same time each day without interruption for as long as contraceptive protection is desired.
The effectiveness of progestogen-only oral contraceptives, such as MICRONOR, is lower than that of the combination oral contraceptives containing both estrogen and progestogen. If 100 women utilized an estrogen-containing oral contraceptive for a period of one year, generally less than one pregnancy would be expected to occur, however, if MICRONOR had been utilized, approximately three pregnancies might occur.
Women who participated in the clinical studies with MICRONOR and who had not taken other oral contraceptives before starting MICRONOR had a higher pregnancy rate (four women out of 100), particularly during the first six months of therapy, and to a large extent because they did not take their tablets correctly.
Of course, if you don't take your tablets as directed, or forget to take them every day, the chance you may become pregnant is naturally greater.
MICRONOR (norethindrone) will probably cause some changes in your menstrual pattern. Your cycle, that is the time between menstrual periods, will vary. For example, you might have a 28-day cycle, followed by a 17-day cycle, followed by a 35-day cycle etc. This is common with MICRONOR.
While using MICRONOR, your period may be longer or shorter than before. If bleeding lasts more than eight days, be sure to let your doctor know.

At times there may be no menstrual period after a cycle of pills. Therefore, if you miss one menstrual period but have taken the pills *exactly as you were supposed to,* continue as usual into the next cycle. If you have not taken them correctly and miss a menstrual period, or if you are taking mini-pills and it is 45 days or more from the start of your last menstrual period, you may be pregnant and should stop taking oral contraceptives until your doctor determines whether or not you are pregnant. Until you can get to your doctor, use another form of contraception. If two consecutive menstrual periods are missed, you should stop taking pills until it is determined whether you are pregnant. If you do become pregnant while using oral contraceptives, you should discuss the risks to the developing child with your doctor.

3. Periodic Examination.
Your doctor will take a complete medical and family history before prescribing oral contraceptives. At that time and about once a year thereafter, he will generally examine your blood pressure, breasts, abdomen, and pelvic organs (including a Papanicolaou smear, i.e., test for cancer).

Summary: Oral contraceptives are the most effective method, except sterilization, for preventing pregnancy. Other methods, when used conscientiously, are also very effective and have fewer risks.
Women who use oral contraceptives should not smoke.
In addition, if you have certain conditions or have had these conditions in the past, you should not use oral contraceptives because the risk is too great. These conditions are listed in the booklet. If you do not have these conditions and decide to use the "pill," please read te booklet carefully so that you can use the "pill."

Based on his or her assessment of your medical needs, your doctor has prescribed this drug for you. Do not give the drug to anyone else.

[*Shown in Product Identification Section*]
*Trademark

SULTRIN® Triple Sulfa Cream and Vaginal Tablets ℞

Composition: SULTRIN Cream contains sulfathiazole 3.42%, sulfacetamide 2.86%, sulfabenzamide 3.7% and urea 0.64%, compounded with glyceryl monostearate, cetyl alcohol 2%, stearic acid, cholesterol, lanolin, lecithin, peanut oil, propylparaben, propylene glycol, diethylaminoethyl stearamide, phosphoric acid, methylparaben and water.

Composition: Each SULTRIN tablet contains sulfathiazole 172.5 mg, sulfacetamide 143.75 mg, and sulfabenzamide 184.0 mg, compounded with urea, lactose, guar gum, starch and magnesium stearate.

Indications: SULTRIN Cream and SULTRIN Tablets are indicated for treatment of *Haemophilus vaginalis* vaginitis. They may also be used as a deodorant for saprophytic infection following radiation therapy.
Contraindications: Sulfonamide sensitivity and kidney disease.
Dosage: SULTRIN Cream. One applicatorful intravaginally twice daily for 4 to 6 days. The dosage may then be reduced one-half to one-quarter.
SULTRIN Vaginal Tablets. 1 tablet intravaginally before retiring and again in the morning for 10 days. This course may be repeated if necessary.
Packaging: Cream — 78 g tubes with the ORTHO® Measured-Dose Applicator.
Vaginal Tablets—Package of 20 foil-wrapped tablets with vaginal applicator.

Ortho Pharmaceutical Corporation
DERMATOLOGICAL DIVISION
RARITAN, NEW JERSEY 08869
a Johnson & Johnson Company

GRIFULVIN V® (griseofulvin microsize) ℞
tablets, suspension
250 mg (500's):
VA NSN 6505-00-778-0410
500 mg (500's):
Military & VA
NSN 6505-00-782-6510

Description: Griseofulvin microsize is an antibiotic derived from a species of *Penicillium.*
Actions: GRIFULVIN V griseofulvin microsize acts systemically to inhibit the growth of Trichophyton, Microsporum, and Epidermophyton genera of fungi. Fungistatic amounts are deposited in the keratin, which is gradually exfoliated and replaced by noninfected tissue. Griseofulvin absorption from the gastrointestinal tract varies considerably among individuals, mainly because of insolubility of the drug in aqueous media of the upper G.I. tract. The peak serum level found in fasting adults given 0.5 gm. occurs at about four hours and ranges between 0.5 to 2.0 mcg./ml.
It should be noted that some individuals are consistently "poor absorbers" and tend to attain lower blood levels at all times. This may explain unsatisfactory therapeutic results in some patients. Better blood levels can probably be attained in most patients if the tablets are administered after a meal with a high fat content.
Indications: Major indications for GRIFULVIN V griseofulvin microsize are:
- Tinea capitis (ringworm of the scalp)
- Tinea corporis (ringworm of the body)
- Tinea pedis (athlete's foot)
- Tinea unguium (onychomycosis; ringworm of the nails)
- Tinea cruris (ringworm of the thigh)
- Tinea barbae (barber's itch)

GRIFULVIN V griseofulvin microsize inhibits the growth of those genera of fungi that commonly cause ringworm infections of the hair, skin, and nails, such as:
- Trichophyton rubrum
- Trichophyton tonsurans
- Trichophyton mentagrophytes
- Trichophyton interdigitalis
- Trichophyton verrucosum
- Trichophyton sulphureum
- Trichophyton schoenleini
- Microsporum audouini
- Microsporum canis
- Microsporum gypseum
- Epidermophyton floccosum
- Trichophyton megnini
- Trichophyton gallinae
- Trichophyton crateriform

Note: Prior to therapy, the type of fungi responsible for the infection should be identified. The use of the drug is not justified in minor or trivial infections which will respond to topical antifungal agents alone.
It is *not* effective in:
- Bacterial infections
- Candidiasis (Moniliasis)
- Histoplasmosis
- Actinomycosis
- Sporotrichosis
- Chromoblastomycosis
- Coccidioidomycosis
- North American Blastomycosis
- Cryptococcosis (Torulosis)
- Tinea versicolor
- Nocardiosis

Contraindications: This drug is contraindicated in patients with porphyria, hepatocellular failure, and in individuals with a history of hypersensitivity to griseofulvin.
Warnings:
Usage in Pregnancy: Safe use of GRIFULVIN V griseofulvin microsize in pregnancy has not been established.
Prophylactic Usage: Safety and efficacy of prophylactic use of this drug has not been established.
Chronic feeding of griseofulvin, at levels ranging from 0.5–2.5% of the diet, resulted in the development of liver tumors in several strains of mice, particularly in males. Smaller particle sizes result in an enhanced effect. Lower oral dosage levels have not been tested. Subcutaneous administration of relatively small doses of griseofulvin once a week during the first three weeks of life has also been reported to induce hepatomata in mice. Although studies in other animal species have not yielded evidence of tumorigenicity, these studies were not of adequate design to form a basis for conclusions in this regard.
In subacute toxicity studies, orally administered griseofulvin produced hepatocellular necrosis in mice, but this has not been seen in other species. Disturbances in prophyrin metabolism have been reported in griseofulvin-treated laboratory animals. Griseofulvin has been reported to have a colchicine-like effect on mitosis and cocarcinogenicity with methylcholanthrene in cutaneous tumor induction in laboratory animals.
Reports of animal studies in the Soviet literature state that a griseofulvin preparation was found to be embryotoxic and teratogenic on oral administration to pregnant Wistar rats. Rat reproduction studies done thus far in the U.S. and Great Britain have been inconclusive in this regard, and additional animal reproduction studies are underway. Pups with abnormalities have been reported in the litters of a few bitches treated with griseofulvin.
Suppression of spermatogenesis has been reported to occur in rats but investigation in man failed to confirm this.
Precautions: Patients on prolonged therapy with any potent medication should be under close observation. Periodic monitoring of organ system function, including renal, hepatic and hemopoietic, should be done.
Since griseofulvin is derived from species of penicillin, the possibility of cross sensitivity with penicillin exists; however, known penicillin-sensitive patients have been treated without difficulty.
Since a photosensitivity reaction is occasionally associated with griseofulvin therapy, patients should be warned to avoid exposure to intense natural or artificial sunlight. Should a photosensitivity reaction occur, lupus erythematosus may be aggravated.
Patients on warfarin-type anticoagulant therapy may require dosage adjustment of the anticoagulant during and after griseofulvin therapy. Concomitant use of barbiturates usually depresses griseofulvin activity and may necessitate raising the dosage.
Adverse Reactions: When adverse reactions occur, they are most commonly of the hypersensitivity type such as skin rashes, urticaria and rarely, angioneurotic edema, and may necessitate withdrawal of therapy and appropriate countermeasures. Paresthesias of the hands and feet have been reported rarely after extended therapy. Other side effects reported occasionally are oral thrush, nausea, vomiting, epigastric distress, diarrhea, headache, fatigue, dizziness, insomnia, mental confusion and impairment of performance of routine activities.
Proteinuria and leukopenia have been reported rarely. Administration of the drug should be discontinued if granulocytopenia occurs.
When rare, serious reactions occur with griseofulvin, they are usually associated with high dosages, long periods of therapy, or both.
Dosage and Administration: Accurate diagnosis of the infecting organism is essential. Identification should be made either by direct microscopic examination of a mounting of infected tissue in a solution of potassium hydroxide or by culture on an appropriate medium. Medication must be continued until the infecting organism is completely eradicated as indicated by appropriate clincal or laboratory examination. Representative treatment periods are tinea capitis, 4 to 6 weeks; tinea corporis, 2 to 4 weeks; tinea pedis, 4 to 8 weeks; tinea unguium—depending on rate of growth—fingernails, at least 4 months; toenails, at least 6 months.
General measures in regard to hygiene should be observed to control sources of infection or reinfection. Concomitant use of appropriate topical agents is usually required, particularly in treatment of tinea pedis since in some forms of athlete's foot, yeasts and bacteria may be involved. Griseofulvin will not eradicate the bacterial or monilial infection.
Adults: A daily dose of 500 mg. will give a satisfactory response in most patients with tinea corporis, tinea cruris, and tinea capitis. For those fungus infections more difficult to eradicate such as tinea pedis and tinea unguium, a daily dose of 1.0 gram is recommended.
Children: Approximately 5 mg. per pound of body weight per day is an effective dose for most children. On this basis the following dosage schedule for children is suggested:
Children weighing 30 to 50 pounds—125 mg. to 250 mg. daily.
Children weighing over 50 pounds—250 mg. to 500 mg daily.
How Supplied: Tablets (colored white, scored, imprinted "McNEIL") 125 mg. **NDC** 0045-0208, 250 mg. **NDC** 0045-0211, bottles of 100, and 500 mg. **NDC** 0045-0214—bottles of 50, 100 and 500. Suspension (125 mg. per 5 ml.)—bottles of 4 fl. oz. **NDC** 0045-0206-04.
U.S. Patent Nos. 2,900,304; 3,330,727

MICATIN Brand ℞
miconazole nitrate 2%

Description: MicaTin brand miconazole nitrate cream 2% and lotion 2% each contain miconazole nitrate 2%, formulated into a water miscible base consisting of pegoxol 7 stearate, peglicol 5 oleate, mineral oil, benzoic acid, and butylated hydroxyanisole.
Actions: Miconazole nitrate is a synthetic antifungal agent which inhibits the growth of the common dermatophytes, *Trichophyton rubrum, Trichophyton mentagrophytes,* and *Epidermophyton floccosum,* the yeast-like fungus, *Candida albicans,* and the organism responsible for tinea versicolor *(Malassezia furfur).*
Indications: For topical application in the treatment of tinea pedis (athlete's foot), tinea

Continued on next page

Ortho Derm.—Cont.

cruris, and tinea corporis caused by *Trichophyton rubrum, Trichophyton mentagrophytes,* and *Epidermophyton floccosum,* in the treatment of cutaneous candidiasis (moniliasis), and in the treatment of tinea versicolor.

Contraindications: MicaTin has no known contraindications.

Precautions: If a reaction suggesting sensitivity or chemical irritation should occur, use of the medication should be discontinued.

For external use only. Avoid introduction of MicaTin brand miconazole nitrate cream 2% and lotion 2% into the eyes.

Adverse Reactons: There have been isolated reports of irritation, burning, and maceration associated with application of MicaTin.

Dosage and Administration: Sufficient MicaTin cream should be applied to cover affected areas twice daily (morning and evening) in patients with tinea pedis, tinea cruris, tinea corporis, and cutaneous candidiasis and once daily in patients with tinea versicolor. It is preferable to use MicaTin lotion in intertriginous areas; if the cream is used, it should be applied sparingly and smoothed in well to avoid maceration effects.

Early relief of symptoms (2 to 3 days) is experienced by the majority of patients and clinical improvement may be seen fairly soon after treatment is begun; however, Candida infections and tinea cruris and corporis should be treated for two weeks and tinea pedis for one month in order to reduce the possibility of recurrence. If a patient shows no clinical improvement after a month of treatment, the diagnosis should be redetermined. Patients with tinea versicolor usually exhibit clinical and mycological clearing after two weeks of treatment.

How Supplied: MicaTin brand cream 2% containing miconazole nitrate at 2% strength is supplied in 3 oz., 1 oz. and 15 g. tubes. MicaTin brand lotion 2% containing miconazole nitrate at 2% w/w strength is supplied in polyethylene squeeze bottles in quantities of 30 and 12 ml.

FSN #6505-01-060-1864 (1-oz.)

PURPOSE Brand Dry Skin Cream

(See PDR For Nonprescription Drugs)

PURPOSE Brand Shampoo

(See PDR For Nonprescription Drugs)

PURPOSE Brand Soap

(See PDR For Nonprescription Drugs)

RETIN-A Brand tretinoin ℞

Description: RETIN-A Brand tretinoin acne treatment is available in gel, cream and liquid vehicles. RETIN-A Brand tretinoin Gel contains tretinoin (retinoic acid; vitamin A acid) in either of two strengths, 0.025% or 0.01% by weight, in a gel vehicle of butylated hydroxytoluene, hydroxypropyl cellulose, and alcohol 90% w/w. RETIN-A Brand tretinoin Cream contains tretinoin in either of two strengths, 0.1% or 0.05% by weight, in a hydrophilic cream vehicle of stearic acid, isopropyl myristate, polyoxyl 40 stearate, stearyl alcohol, xanthan gum, sorbic acid, and butylated hydroxytoluene. RETIN-A Brand tretinoin liquid contains tretinoin 0.05% by weight, polyethylene glycol 400, butylated hyroxytoluene, and alcohol 55%.

Indications: RETIN-A Brand tretinoin is indicated for topical application in the treatment of acne vulgaris, primarily grades I, II, and III in which comedones, papules, and pustules predominate. It is not effective in most cases of severe pustular and deep cystic nodular varieties (ance conglobata).

Contraindications: Use of the product should be discontinued if hypersensitivity to any of the ingredients is noted.

Warnings: Recent studies in hairless albino mice suggest that tretinoin may accelerate the tumorigenic potential of ultraviolet radiation. Although the significance to man is not clear, patients should avoid or minimize exposure to sun.

Concomitant topical medication should be used with caution because of possible interaction with tretinoin. Particular caution should be exercised in using preparations containing peeling agents (such as sulfur, resorcinol, benzoyl peroxide, or salicylic acid) with RETIN-A. It also is advisable to "rest" a patient's skin until the effects of peeling agents subside before use of RETIN-A is begun.

Exposure to sunlight, including sunlamps, should be minimized during the use of RETIN-A and patients with sunburn should be adivsed not to use the product until fully recovered because of heightened susceptibility to sunlight as a result of the use of tretinoin. Patients who may be required to have considerable sun exposure due to occupation and those with inherent sensitivity to the sun should exercise particular caution. Use of sunscreen products and protective clothing over treated areas may be prudent when exposure cannot be avoided. Other weather extremes, such as wind or cold, also may be irritating to patients under treatment with tretinoin. RETIN-A should be kept away from the eyes, the mouth, angles of the nose, and mucous membranes. Topical use may induce severe local erythema and peeling at the site of application. If the degree of local irritation warrants, patients should be directed to use the medication less frequently, discontinue use temporarily, or discontinue use altogether. Tretinoin has been reported to cause severe irritation on eczematous skin and should be used with utmost caution in patients with this condition.

Precautions: Medicated or abrasive soaps and cleansers, soaps and cosmetics that have a strong drying effect, and products with high concentrations of alcohol, astringents, spices, or lime should be used with caution because of possible interaction with tretinoin. If medication is applied excessively, no more rapid or better results will be obtained and marked redness, peeling, or disciomfort may occur.

Adverse Reactions: The skin of certain sensitive individuals may become excessively red, edematous, blistered, or crusted. If these effects occur, the medication should either be discontinued until the integrity of the skin is restored or the medication should be adjusted to a level the patient can tolerate. True contact allergy to topical tretinoin is rarely encountered. Temporary hyper- or hypopigmentation has been reported with repeated application of RETIN-A Brand tretinoin. Some individuals have been reported to have heightened susceptibility to sunlight while under treatment with RETIN-A. To date, all adverse effects of RETIN-A have been reversible upon discontinuance of therapy (see Dosage and Administration Section).

Dosage and Administration: RETIN-A Gel, Cream or Liquid should be applied once a day, before retiring, to the skin where acne lesions appear, using enough to cover the entire affected area lightly. Liquid: The liquid may be applied using a fingertip, gauze pad, or cotton swab. If gauze or cotton is employed, care should be taken not to oversaturate it to the extent that the liquid would run into areas where treatment is not intended. Swab: One RETIN-A swab should be applied once a day, before retiring, to the skin where acne lesions appear, using enough to cover the affected area lightly. One swab supplies enough of the preparation to treat an area the size of the face. If other sites are treated, such as the back, additional swabs should be used. Gel: Excessive application results in "pilling" of the gel, which minimizes the likelihood of overapplication by the patient.

Application may cause a transitory feeling of warmth or slight stinging. In cases where it has been necessary to temporarily discontinue therapy or to reduce the frequency of application, therapy may be resumed or frequency of application increased when the patients become able to tolerate the treatment. When it has been necessary to discontinue therapy with 0.1% cream temporarily, patients may be better able to tolerate the 0.05% strength when therapy is resumed.

It should be noted that just as some patients require less frequent applications or other dosage forms, others may respond better to more frequent applications of tretinoin. Alterations of vehicle, drug concentration, or dose frequency should be closely monitored by careful observation of the clinical therapeutic response and skin tolerance. During the early weeks of therapy, an apparent exacerbation of inflammatory lesions may occur. This is due to the action of the medication on deep, previously unseen lesions and should not be considered a reason to discontinue therapy.

Therapeutic results should be noticed after two to three weeks, but more than six weeks of therapy may be required before definite beneficial effects are seen. Once the acne lesions have responded satisfactorily, it may be possible to maintain the improvement with less frequent applicaions, or other dosage forms.

Patients treated with RETIN-A may use cosmetics, but the areas to be treated should be cleansed thoroughly before the medication is applied.

How Supplied: RETIN-A Brand tretinoin is supplied as

(1) 0.025% Gel in tubes of 15 grams and 45 grams and 0.01% gel in tubes of 15 grams and 45 grams. FSN # (0.025%) 6505-01-066-3354.

(2) 0.1% Cream in tubes of 20 grams 0.05% Cream in tubes of 20 grams and 45 grams. FSN #s (0.1%) 6505-01-044-9388, (0.05%) 6505-01-044-9389

(3) 0.05% Liquid in amber bottles containing 28 ml. FSN #6505-01-009-0266

(4) Foil-covered swabs saturated with the 0.05% liquid, in boxes of 30. FSN #6510-00-117-9010

Parke-Davis

Division Of Warner-Lambert Company
201 TABOR ROAD
MORRIS PLAINS, NJ 07950

PARCODE®
(Parke-Davis Accurate Recognition Code)

Code Number	Product Name
001-006	*Unassigned*
007	**Dilantin® Infatabs®** Each tablet contains 50 mg phenytoin, USP.
008-009	*Unassigned*
010	**Chlorpromazine Hydrochloride Tablets, USP (Promapar®)** Each tablet contains 10 mg chlorpromazine hydrochloride, USP.
011-024	*Unassigned*
025	**Chlorpromazine Hydrochloride Tablets, USP (Promapar®)** Each tablet contains 25 mg chlorpromazine hydrochloride, USP.
026-036	*Unassigned*
037	**Ferrous Sulfate Filmseals, USP (325 mg)**

Each film-coated tablet contains 325 mg (5 grains) ferrous sulfate.

038-
049 *Unassigned*

050 **Chlorpromazine Hydrochloride Tablets, USP (Promapar®)**
Each tablet contains 50 mg chlorpromazine hydrochloride, USP.

051-
054 *Unassigned*

055 **Cascara Sagrada Extract Filmseal®**
Each film-coated tablet contains 325 mg (5 grains) cascara sagrada extract.

056-
099 *Unassigned*

100 **Chlorpromazine Hydrochloride Tablets, USP (Promapar®)**
Each tablet contains 100 mg chlorpromazine hydrochloride, USP.

101-
110 *Unassigned*

111 **Ergostat® Sublingual Tablets**
Each tablet contains 2 mg ergotamine tartrate.

112-
199 *Unassigned*

200 **Chlorpromazine Hydrochloride Tablets, USP (Promapar®)**
Each tablet contains 200 mg chlorpromazine hydrochloride, USP.

201-
211 *Unassigned*

212 **Natafort® Filmseal®**
Each tablet represents vitamin A (acetate), (1.8 mg) 6,000 IU*; vitamin D (ergocalciferol), (10 mcg) 400 IU; folic acid, 1 mg; vitamin B_1 (thiamine mononitrate), 3 mg; vitamin B_2 (riboflavin), 2 mg; vitamin B_6 (pyridoxine hydrochloride), 15 mg; vitamin B_{12} (cyanocobalamin), crystalline, 6 mcg; vitamin C (ascorbic acid), 120 mg; nicotinamide (niacinamide), 20 mg; vitamin E (*dl*-alpha tocopheryl acetate), (30 mg) 30 IU; calcium,† 350 mg; magnesium,† 100 mg; iodine,† 0.15 mg; iron,† 65 mg, zinc, 25 mg; and dioctyl sodium sulfosuccinate, 50 mg.

*IU = international units
†The minerals are supplied as calcium carbonate, magnesium oxide, potassium iodide, ferrous fumarate, and zinc oxide.

213-
236 *Unassigned*

237 **Zarontin® Capsules**
Each capsule contains 250 mg ethosuximide, USP.

238-
245 *Unassigned*

246 **©Chloral Hydrate Capsules, USP**
Each capsule contains 500 mg (7½ grains) chloral hydrate.

247 **Dioctyl Sodium Sulfosuccinate Capsules, USP (D-S-S)**
Each capsule contains 100 mg dioctyl sodium sulfosuccinate.

248 **Dioctyl Sodium Sulfosuccinate with Casanthranol Capsules (D-S-S Plus)**
Each capsule contains 100 mg dioctyl sodium sulfosuccinate and 30 mg casanthranol.

249-
350 *Unassigned*

351 **Digifortis® Kapseals®, 100 mg**
Each capsule is equivalent to 1 NF digitalis unit.

352-
361 *Unassigned*

362 **Dilantin® Kapseals®**
Each Kapseal contains 100 mg phenytoin sodium, USP. The Kapseal is a No. 3 capsule with Orange band. (The Orange band on White capsule is a trademark registered in the US Patent Office.)

363 **Combex® Kapseals®**
Each Kapseal contains thiamine mononitrate, 10 mg; riboflavin, 10 mg; cyanocobalamin, 1 mcg; niacinamide, 10 mg; *dl*-panthenol, 6 mg; liver concentrate, 0.38 g. The Kapseal is a Brown No. 1 capsule with Black band.

364 *Unassigned*

365 **Dilantin® Kapseals®**
Each Kapseal contains 30 mg phenytoin sodium, USP. The Kapseal is a No. 4 capsule with Pink opaque band.

366 *Unassigned*

367 **Combex® with Vitamin C Kapseals®**
Each Kapseal contains thiamine mononitrate, 10 mg; riboflavin, 10 mg; cyanocobalamin, 1 mcg; niacinamide, 10 mg; *dl*-panthenol, 6 mg; ascorbic acid, 50 mg; liver concentrate, 0.34 g. The Kapseal is a Brown No. 1 capsule with White opaque band.

368 **Taka-Combex® Kapseals®**
Each Kapseal represents Taka-Diastase® (*Aspergillus oryzae* enzymes), 2½ grains; thiamine mononitrate, 10 mg; riboflavin, 10 mg; pyridoxine hydrochloride, 0.5 mg; cyanocobalamin, 1 mcg; niacinamide, 10 mg; *dl*-panthenol, 6 mg; ascorbic acid, 30 mg; liver concentrate, 0.34 g. The Kapseal is a Brown No. 1 capsule with Yellow opaque band.

369-
370 *Unassigned*

371 **Abdec® Kapseals®**
Each Kapseal represents vitamin A (acetate) (3 mg), 10,000 IU; ergocalciferol, (10 mcg) 400 IU; ascorbic acid, 75 mg; thiamine mononitrate, 5 mg; riboflavin, 3 mg; pyridoxine hydrochloride, 1.5 mg; cyanocobalamin, 2 mcg; niacinamide, 25 mg; *dl*-panthenol, 10 mg; *dl*-alpha tocopheryl acetate (5 mg), 5 IU. The Kapseal is a Garnet No. 3 capsule with Black band.

372 **©Carbrital® Kapseals®**
Each Kapseal contains pentobarbital sodium, 1½ grains; carbromal, 4 grains. The Kapseal is a No. 1 white capsule with Blue band. (The Blue band on White capsule is a trademark registered in the US Patent Office.)

373 **Benadryl® Kapseals®**
Each Kapseal contains 50 mg diphenhydramine hydrochloride. The Kapseal is a Pink No. 4 capsule with White opaque band. (The White band on Pink capsule is a trademark registered in the US Patent Office.)

374 **Thera-Combex® Kapseals®**
Each Kapseal contains thiamine mononitrate, 25 mg; riboflavin, 15 mg; pyridoxine hydrochloride, 1 mg; cyanocobalamin, 5 mcg; niacinamide, 100 mg; *dl*-panthenol, 20 mg; ascorbic acid, 250 mg; Taka-Diastase® (*Aspergillus oryzae* enzymes), 2½ grains. The Kapseal is a Brown No. 1 capsule with Dark Red opaque band.

375 **Dilantin® with Phenobarbital (¼ grain) Kapseals®**
Each Kapseal contains Dilantin (phenytoin sodium), 100 mg; phenobarbital, 16 mg (¼ grain). The Kapseal is a No. 3 capsule with Garnet band.

376 **©Carbrital® (Half Strength) Kapseals®**
Each Kapseal contains pentobarbital sodium, ¾ grain; carbromal, 2 grains. The Kapseal is a No. 4 capsule with Blue band. (The Blue band on White capsule is a trademark registered in the US Patent Office.)

377 *Unassigned*

378 **Benadryl® with Ephedrine Sulfate Kapseals ®**
Each Kapseal contains Benadryl (diphenhydramine hydrochloride), 50 mg; ephedrine sulfate, 25 mg. The Kapseal is a Pink No. 4 capsule with Dark Blue band.

379 **Chloromycetin® Kapseals®**
Each Kapseal contains 250 mg chloramphenicol. The Kapseal is a White opaque No. 2 capsule with Gray opaque band. (The Gray band on White capsule is a trademark registered in the US Patent Office.)

380-
381 *Unassigned*

382 **Geriplex® Kapseals®**
Each Kapseal represents vitamin A (acetate), (1.5 mg) 5,000 IU; ascorbic acid,* 50 mg; thiamine mononitrate, 5 mg; riboflavin, 5 mg; cyanocobalamin, 2 mcg; choline dihydrogen citrate, 20 mg; niacinamide, 15 mg; *dl*-alpha tocopheryl acetate, (5 mg), 5 IU; ferrous sulfate,† 30 mg; copper sulfate, 4 mg; manganese sulfate (monohydrate), 4 mg; zinc sulfate, 2 mg; calcium phosphate, dibasic (anhydrous), 200 mg. The Kapseal is a Blue No. 1 capsule with Yellow opaque band.

*Supplied as sodium ascorbate.
†Supplied as dried ferrous sulfate equivalent to the labeled amount of ferrous sulfate.

383-
388 *Unassigned*

389 **Ambodryl® Hydrochloride Kapseals®**
Each Kapseal contains 25 mg bromodiphenhydramine hydrochloride. The Kapseal is a Pink Tint No. 4 capsule with Pink band.

390 **Natabec® Kapseals®**
Each Kapseal represents: Vitamin A (acetate), 4,000 IU; vitamin D (ergocalciferol), 400 IU; vitamin C (ascorbic acid), 50 mg; thiamine HCl (as thiamine mononitrate; vitamin B_1), 3.0 mg; riboflavin (vitamin B_2), 2.0 mg; niacin (as niacinamide; nicotinic acid), 10 mg; pyridoxine (as pyridoxine HCl; vitamin B_6), 3.0 mg; vitamin B_{12} (cyanocobalamin), 5.0 mcg; calcium carbonate, 600 mg; ferrous sulfate, 150 mg.

391-
392 *Unassigned*

393 **Milontin® Kapseals®**
Each Kapseal contains 500 mg phensuximide, NF. The Kapseal is a Light Orange No. 0 capsule with Orange band.

394-
397 *Unassigned*

398 **Eldec® Kapseals®**
Each capsule represents vitamin A (acetate), (0.5 mg) 1,667 IU; vitamin C (ascorbic acid), 66.7 mg; vitamin B_1 (thiamine mononitrate nicotinamide (10 mg; vitamin B_2 (riboflavin) 0.87 mg; pyridoxine hydrochloride, 0.67 mg), niacinamide), 16.7 mg; *dl*-panthenol, 10 mg; ferrous sulfate, dried, 16.7 mg; iodine (as potassium iodide), 0.05 mg; calcium carbonate, 66.7 mg; vitamin E (*dl*-alpha tocopheryl acetate), (10 mg) 10 IU; vitamin B_{12} (cyanocobalamin), 2 mcg; folic acid, 0.33 mg. The Kapseal is a Dark Blue No. 1 capsule with Light Blue opaque band.

Continued on next page

This product information was prepared in August, 1979. On these and other Parke-Davis Products, detailed information may be obtained by addressing PARKE-DAVIS, Division of Warner-Lambert Company, Morris Plains, NJ 07950.

Parke-Davis—Cont.

399-
401 *Unassigned*
402 **Amcill® Capsules, 250 mg**
Each capsule contains ampicillin trihydrate equivalent to 250 mg ampicillin.
403 *Unassigned*
404 **Amcill® Capsules, 500 mg**
Each capsule contains ampicillin trihydrate equivalent to 500 mg ampicillin.
405-
406 *Unassigned*
407 **Tetracycline Hydrochloride Capsules, USP, 250 mg (Cyclopar®)**
Each capsule contains 250 mg tetracycline hydrochloride, USP.
408-
419 *Unassigned*
420 **Quinine Sulfate Capsules, USP**
Each capsule contains 0.325 g (5 grains) quinine sulfate.
421-
436 *Unassigned*
437 **Estrovis® Tablets**
Each tablet contains 100 mcg quinestrol.
438-
454 *Unassigned*
455 **Panteric® Capsules**
Each capsule contains 5 grains (0.325 g) pancreatin, triple strength.
456-
470 *Unassigned*
471 **Benadryl® Capsules**
Each capsule contains 25 mg diphenhydramine hydrochloride.
472-
476 *Unassigned*
477 **Chloromycetin® Capsules**
Each capsule contains 50 mg chloramphenicol, USP.
478-
479 *Unassigned*
480 **Chloromycetin® Capsules**
Each capsule contains 100 mg chloramphenicol, USP.
481-
502 *Unassigned*
503 **Panteric® Filmseals**
Each film-coated tablet contains 5 grains (0.325 g) pancreatin, triple strength.
504-
521 *Unassigned*
522 **Natabec® with Fluoride Kapeals®**
Each Kapseal represents vitamin A (acetate) (2.4 mg), 8,000 IU*; vitamin D (ergocalciferol) (10 mcg), 400 IU; vitamin E (*dl*-alpha tocopheryl acetate) (30 mg), 30 IU; vitamin C (ascorbic acid), 60 mg; folic acid, 0.8 mg; thiamine mononitrate (vitamin B_1), 1.7 mg; riboflavin (vitamin B_2), 2.0 mg; niacin (nicotinic acid)†, 20 mg; vitamin B_6 (pyridoxine hydrochloride), 2.5 mg; vitamin B_{12}, crystalline (cyanocobalamin), 8.0 mcg; calcium, 125 mg; iodine, 150 mcg; iron, 30 mg; magnesium, 100 mg; fluoride, 1.0 mg.

---

*international units
†supplied as niacinamide. The minerals are supplied as precipitated calcium carbonate, potassium iodide, dried ferrous sulfate, magnesium oxide, and sodium fluoride.

The Kapseal is a Pastel Pink No. 0 capsule with Ruby Red opaque band.

523-
524 *Unassigned*
525 **Celontin® Kapseals®**
Each Kapseal contains 300 mg methsuximide, NF. The Kapseal is a Yellow Tint No. 2 capsule with Orange band.
526 *Unassigned*
528 *Unassigned*
529 **Humatin® Capsules**
Each capsule contains paromomycin sulfate, NF, equivalent to 250 mg paromomycin.
530 *Unassigned*
531 **Dilantin® with Phenobarbital (½ grain) Kapseals®**
Each Kapseal contains Dilantin (phenytoin sodium), 100 mg; phenobarbital, 32 mg (½ grain). The Kapseal is a No. 3 capsule with Black band.
532 *Unassigned*
533 **Calcium Lactate Tablets, USP**
Each tablet contains 325 mg calcium lactate.
534-
536 *Unassigned*
537 **Celontin® (Half Strength) Kapseals®**
Each Kapseal contains 150 mg methsuximide, NF. The Kapseal is a Yellow Tint No. 4 capsule with Brown opaque band.
538-
539 *Unassigned*
540 **Ponstel® Kapseals®**
Each Kapseal contains 250 mg mefenamic acid. The Kapseal is an Ivory opaque No. 1 capsule with Light Blue opaque band. The blue band on ivory capsule combination is a Parke-Davis trademark.
541 **Natabec-F.A.® Kapseals®**
Each Kapseal represents vitamin A (acetate), (1.2 mg) 4,000 IU; ergocalciferol (10 mcg), 400 IU; ascorbic acid, 50 mg; thiamine mononitrate, 3 mg; riboflavin, 2 mg; pyridoxine hydrochloride, 3 mg; cyanocobalamin, 5 mcg; folic acid, 0.1 mg; niacinamide, 10 mg; calcium carbonate, precipitated, 600 mg; ferrous sulfate,* 150 mg.

---

*Supplied as dried ferrous sulfate equivalent to the labeled amount of ferrous sulfate.

The Kapseal is a Pink Tint opaque No. 0 capsule with White opaque band.

542-
543 *Unassigned*
544 **Geriplex-FS® Kapseals®**
Each Kapseal represents vitamin A (acetate) (1.5 mg), 5,000 IU; ascorbic acid,* 50 mg; thiamine mononitrate, 5 mg; riboflavin, 5 mg; cyanocobalamin, 2 mcg; choline dihydrogen citrate, 20 mg; niacinamide, 15 mg; *dl*-alpha tocopheryl acetate (5 mg), 5 IU; ferrous sulfate,† 30 mg; copper sulfate, 4 mg; manganese sulfate (monohydrate), 4 mg; zinc sulfate, 2 mg; calcium phosphate, dibasic (anhydrous), 200 mg; dioctyl sodium sulfosuccinate, 100 mg.

---

*Supplied as sodium ascorbate.
†Supplied as dried ferrous sulfate equivalent to the labeled amount of ferrous sulfate.

The Kapseal is a Blue No. 0 capsule with White opaque band.

545-
546 *Unassigned*
547 **Natabec ℞® Kapseals®**
Each Kapseal represents vitamin A (acetate) (1.2 mg), 4,000 IU; ergocalciferol, (10 mcg) 400 IU; ascorbic acid, 50 mg; thiamine mononitrate, 3 mg; riboflavin, 2 mg; pyridoxine hydrochloride, 3 mg; cyanocobalamin, 5 mcg; niacinamide, 10 mg; folic acid, 1 mg; calcium carbonate, precipitated, 600 mg; ferrous sulfate,* 150 mg.

---

*Supplied as dried ferrous sulfate equivalent to the labeled amount of ferrous sulfate.

The Kapseal is a Blue opaque No. 0 capsule with Pink opaque band. The banded capsule is a Parke-Davis trademark registered in the US Patent Office.

548-
549 *Unassigned*
550 **Thera-Combex H-P® Kapseals®**
Each Kapseal contains: ascorbic acid, 500 mg; thiamine mononitrate, 25 mg; riboflavin, 15 mg; pyridoxine hydrochloride, 10 mg; cyanocobalamin, 5 mcg; niacinamide, 100 mg; *dl*-panthenol, 20 mg.
The Kapseal is a Brown No. 0 capsule with Green opaque band.
551-
571 *Unassigned*
572 **Ⓒ Parest-200™ Capsules**
Each capsule contains 200 mg methaqualone hydrochloride.
573 *Unassigned*
574 **Ⓒ Parest-400™ Capsules**
Each capsule contains 400 mg methaqualone hydrochloride.
575-
600 *Unassigned*
601 **Sodium Chloride Tablets, USP**
Each tablet contains 1 g (15½ grains) sodium chloride.
602-
603 *Unassigned*
604 **Calcium Lactate Tablets, USP**
Each tablet contains 650 mg (10 grains) calcium lactate.
605 *Unassigned*
606 **Aspirin Tablets, USP (White)**
Each tablet contains 0.325 mg (5 grains) aspirin.
607 **Ⓒ Phenobarbital Tablets, USP**
Each tablet contains 65 mg (1 grain) phenobarbital.
608-
617 *Unassigned*
618 **Placebo tablet in Norlestrin [28] 1/50.**
619-
621 *Unassigned*
622 **Ferrous Fumarate Tablets**
Each tablet contains 75 mg ferrous fumarate, USP.
623 *Unassigned*
624 **Aspirin Tablets, USP (Pink)**
Each tablet contains 0.325 g (5 grains) aspirin.
625-
632 *Unassigned*
633 **Amcill® Chewable Tablets**
Each chewable tablet contains ampicillin trihydrate equivalent to 125 mg ampicillin.
634 **Acetaminophen with Codeine Phosphate, Tablets, No. 2**
Each tablet contains 300 mg acetaminophen and 15 mg (¼ grain) codeine phosphate.
635 **Acetaminophen with Codeine Phosphate Tablets, No. 3**
Each tablet contains 300 mg acetaminophen and 30 mg (½ grain) codeine phosphate.
636 **Betapar® Tablets**
Each scored, light-green tablet contains 4 mg meprednisone, NF.
637 *Unassigned*
638 **Tabron® Filmseal®**
Each film-coated tablet represents ferrous fumarate, 304.2 mg (represents 100 mg of elemental iron); ascorbic acid, 500 mg; thiamine mononitrate, 6 mg; riboflavin, 6 mg; pyridoxine hydrochloride, 5 mg; cyanocobalamin, 25 mcg; folic acid, 1 mg; niacinamide, 30 mg;

calcium pantothenate, 10 mg; *dl*-alpha tocopheryl acetate (30 mg), 30 IU; dioctyl sodium sulfosuccinate, 50 mg.

639 *Unassigned*

640 **Acetaminophen Tablets, USP (Tapar®)**
Each tablet contains 325 mg (5 grains) acetaminophen, USP.

641-
646 *Unassigned*

647 **ⒸMeprobamate Tablets, USP**
Each tablet contains 400 mg meprobamate, USP.

648 **Penicillin V Potassium Tablets, USP, 250 mg (Penapar VK®)**
Each tablet contains penicillin V potassium equivalent to 250 mg (400,000 units) penicillin V.

649-
669 *Unassigned*

670 **Oxytetracycline Hydrochloride Capsules, USP (Oxlopar®)**
Each capsule contains oxytetracycline hydrochloride, USP, equivalent to 250 mg oxytetracycline.

671 *Unassigned*

672 **Erythromycin Stearate Filmseals (Erypar®)**
Each Filmseal® contains 250 mg erythromycin stearate as erythromycin stearate.

673 **Penicillin V Potassium Tablets, USP, 500 mg (Penapar VK®)**
Each tablet contains penicillin V potassium equivalent to 500 mg (800,000 units) penicillin V.

674-
678 *Unassigned*

679 **Aspirin Compound Tablets, White**
Each tablet contains aspirin, 3½ grains; phenacetin, 2½ grains; caffeine, ½ grain.

680-
683 *Unassigned*

684 **Taka-Diastase® Tablets**
Each tablet contains 160 mg (2½ grains) Taka-Diastase (*Aspergillus oryzae* enzymes).

685-
691 *Unassigned*

692 **Propoxyphene Hydrochloride Capsules, USP**
Each capsule contains 65 mg propoxyphene hydrochloride.

693 *Unassigned*

694 **Propoxyphene Compound 65, Capsules**
Each capsule contains 65 mg propoxyphene hydrochloride, 227 mg aspirin, 162 mg phenacetin, and 32.4 mg caffeine.

695-
696 *Unassigned*

697 **Tetracycline Hydrochloride Capsules, USP, 500 mg (Cyclopar® 500)**
Each capsule contains 500 mg tetracycline hydrochloride, USP.

698 **ⒸPhenobarbital Tablets, USP**
Each tablet contains 100 mg (1½ grains) phenobarbital.

699 **ⒸPhenobarbital Tablets, USP**
Each tablet contains 15 mg (¼ grain) phenobarbital.

700 **ⒸPhenobarbital Tablets, USP**
Each tablet contains 30 mg (½ grain) phenobarbital.

701 *Unassigned*

702 **Hydrochlorothiazide Tablets, USP (Thiuretic®)**
Each tablet contains 25 mg hydrochlorothiazine.

703-
709 *Unassigned*

710 **Hydrochlorothiazide Tablets, USP (Thiuretic®)**
Each tablet contains 50 mg hydrochlorothiazide.

711-
729 *Unassigned*

730 **Amoxicillin Capsules (Utimox™) 250 mg**
Each capsule contains 250 mg amoxicillin.

731 **Amoxicillin Capsules (Utimox™) 500 mg**
Each capsule contains 500 mg amoxicillin.

732 -
746 *Unassigned*

747 **Povan® Filmseal®**
Each film-coated tablet contains pyrvinium pamoate equivalent to 50 mg pyrvinium.

748 **Paladac® with Minerals Tablets**
Each tablet represents: *Vitamins:* vitamin A (acetate), (1.2 mg) 4,000 IU; ergocalciferol, (10 mcg) 400 units; ascorbic acid,* 50 mg; thiamine mononitrate, 3 mg; riboflavin, 3 mg; pyridoxine hydrochloride, 1 mg; cyanocobalamin, 5 mcg; niacinamide, 20 mg; pantothenic acid (as the calcium salt), 5 mg; *dl*-alpha tocopheryl acetate (10 mg), 10 IU. *Minerals*†: calcium, 23 mg; iron, 5 mg; phosphorus, 17 mg; iodine, 0.05 mg; potassium, 2.5 mg; magnesium, 1 mg.

*Supplied partly as sodium ascorbate.
†Supplied as calcium phosphate dibasic, ferric phosphate, potassium iodide, potassium sulfate, and magnesium oxide.

749-
763 *Unassigned*

764 **Calcium Gluconate Tablets, USP**
Each tablet contains 1 g (15½ grains) calcium gluconate.

765-
770 *Unassigned*

771 **Niacin Tablets, NF**
Each tablet contains 50 mg niacin, NF.

772-
780 *Unassigned*

781 **Aspirin Compound Tablets, Pink**
Each tablet contains aspirin, 3½ grains; phenacetin, 2½ grains; caffeine, ½ grain.

782 *Unassigned*

783 **Vitamin C Tablets, USP**
Each tablet contains 100 mg ascorbic acid.

784-
791 *Unassigned*

792 **ⒸAspirin Compound with Codeine Phosphate Tablets, No. 2**
Each tablet contains codeine phosphate, ¼ grain; aspirin, 3½ grains; phenacetin, 2½ grains; caffeine, ½ grain.

793 **ⒸAspirin Compound with Codeine Phosphate Tablets, No. 3**
Each tablet contains codeine phosphate, ½ grain; aspirin, 3½ grains; phenacetin, 2½ grains; caffeine, ½ grain.

794 **Niacin Tablets, NF**
Each tablet contains 100 mg niacin, NF.

795-
799 *Unassigned*

800 **ⒸChlordiazepoxide Hydrochloride Capsules, USP**
Each capsule contains 5 mg chlordiazepoxide hydrochloride.

801 **ⒸChlordiazepoxide Hydrochloride Capsules, USP**
Each capsule contains 10 mg chlordiazepoxide hydrochloride.

802 **ⒸChlordiazepoxide Hydrochloride Capsules, USP**
Each capsule contains 25 mg chlordiazepoxide hydrochloride.

803-
813 *Unassigned*

814 **Vitamin C Tablets, USP**
Each tablet contains 250 mg ascorbic acid.

815-
817 *Unassigned*

818 **Thiamine Hydrochloride Tablets, USP (Vitamin B_1)**
Each tablet contains 50 mg thiamine hydrochloride.

819-
820 *Unassigned*

821 **Digitoxin Tablets, USP**
Each tablet contains 0.2 mg digitoxin.

822-
824 *Unassigned*

825 **Thiamine Hydrochloride Tablets, USP (Vitamin B_1)**
Each tablet contains 100 mg thiamine hydrochloride.

826-
835 *Unassigned*

836 **Propylthiouracil Tablets, USP**
Each tablet contains 50 mg (¾ grain) propylthiouracil.

837-
840 *Unassigned*

841 **Digitoxin Tablets, USP**
Each tablet contains 0.1 mg digitoxin.

842-
848 *Unassigned*

849 **Quinidine Sulfate Tablets, USP**
Each tablet contains 3 grains (200 mg) quinidine sulfate.

850 **Duraquin® (quinidine gluconate) Tablets, 330 mg**
Each scored, white, sustained-release tablet contains 330 mg quinidine gluconate.

851-
881 *Unassigned*

882 **Norlutin® Tablets**
Each tablet contains 5 mg norethindrone, USP.

883-
888 *Unassigned*

889 **Pitocin® Citrate, Buccal Tablets**
Each tablet contains 200 USP units oxytocin.

890 **Palaflor® Tablets**
Each tablet represents: *Vitamins:* vitamin A (acetate), (1.2 mg) 4,000 IU; ergocalciferol (10 mcg), 400 IU; ascorbic acid,* 50 mg; thiamine mononitrate, 3 mg; riboflavin, 3 mg; pyridoxine hydrochloride, 1 mg; cyanocobalamin, 5 mcg; niacinamide, 20 mg; calcium pantothenate,† 5.4 mg; *dl*-alpha tocopheryl acetate, 10 IU; *Minerals:* calcium phosphate, dibasic (anhydrous), 78 mg; potassium sulfate, 5.5 mg; ferric phosphate, 13.5 mg; magnesium oxide, 1.65 mg; sodium fluoride, 2.2 mg (provides 1 mg fluoride).

*Supplied partly as sodium ascorbate.
†Equivalent to 5 mg pantothenic acid.

891-
892 *Unassigned*

893 **Adroyd® Tablets**
Each tablet contains 5 mg oxymetholone, NF.

Continued on next page

This product information was prepared in August, 1979. On these and other Parke-Davis Products, detailed information may be obtained by addressing PARKE-DAVIS, Division of Warner-Lambert Company, Morris Plains, NJ 07950.

Parke-Davis—Cont.

894-
899 *Unassigned*
900 **Adroyd® Tablets**
Each tablet contains 10 mg oxymetholone, NF.
901 **Norlestrin® 2.5/50 Tablets**
Each tablet contains norethindrone acetate, 2.5 mg; ethinyl estradiol, 50 mcg.
902-
903 *Unassigned*
904 **Norlestrin® 1/50 Tablets**
Each tablet contains norethindrone acetate, 1 mg; ethinyl estradiol, 50 mcg.
905 *Unassigned*
906 **Vitamin C Tablets, USP**
Each tablet contains 500 mg ascorbic acid.
907-
910 *Unassigned*
911 **Digitoxin Tablets, USP (Pink)**
Each tablet contains 0.1 mg digitoxin.
912-
914 *Unassigned*
915 **Loestrin® 1/20 Tablets**
Each tablet contains norethindrone acetate, 1 mg; ethinyl estradiol, 20 mcg.
916 **Loestrin® 1.5/30 Tablets**
Each tablet contains norethindrone acetate, 1.5 mg; ethinyl estradiol, 30 mcg.
917 *Unassigned*
918 **Norlutate® Tablets**
Each tablet contains 5 mg norethindrone acetate.
919 **Erythromycin Stearate Filmseals (Erypar®)**
Each Filmseal® contains 500 mg erythromycin as erythromycin stearate.
920-
924 *Unassigned*
925 **Renoquid® Tablets**
Each tablet contains 250 mg sulfacytine.
926-
931 *Unassigned*
932 **©Meprobamate Tablets, USP**
Each tablet contains 200 mg meprobamate.
933 **Bisacodyl Tablets, USP**
Each tablet contains 5 mg bisacodyl.
934-
9999 *Unassigned*

Identification Number	Product
071	**Agoral® Plain**
072	**Agoral® Raspberry** (with phenolphthalein)
070	**Agoral® Marshmallow** (with phenolphthalein)
272	**Amitril®** (amitriptyline HCl) 10 mg
273	**Amitril®** (amitriptyline HCl) 25 mg
274	**Amitril®** (amitriptyline HCl) 50 mg
275	**Amitril®** (amitriptyline HCl) 75 mg
271	**Amitril®** (amitriptyline HCl) 100 mg
278	**Amitril®** (amitriptyline HCl) 150 mg
088	**Anusol® Suppositories**
075	**Anusol® Ointment**
089	**Anusol-HC® Suppositories**
090	**Anusol-HC® Cream**
175	**Azo-Mandelamine®**
201	**Brondecon® Elixir**
200	**Brondecon® Tablets**
215	**Choledyl® Elixir** (oxtriphylline)
217	**Choledyl Pediatric Syrup**
210	**Choledyl® Tablets** (oxtriphylline) 100 mg
211	**Choledyl® Tablets** (oxtriphylline) 200 mg
145	**Coly-Mycin® M Parenteral** 150 mg (sterile colistimethate sodium)
144	**Coly-Mycin® M Parenteral** 20 mg (sterile colistimethate sodium)
142	**Coly-Mycin® S Oral Suspension** (colistin sulfate for oral suspension)
141	**Coly-Mycin® S Otic w/Neomycin & Hydrocortisone** (colistin sulfate—neomycin sulfate— thonzonium bromide—hydrocortisone acetate otic suspension)
	Dolonil—See Pyridium® Plus
260	**Euthroid®-½** (liotrix)
261	**Euthroid®-1** (liotrix)
262	**Euthroid®-2** (liotrix)
263	**Euthroid®-3** (liotrix)
034	**Gelusil® Tablets**
036	**Gelusil® Liquid**
043	**Gelusil-II® Tablets**
042	**Gelusil-II® Liquid**
045	**Gelusil-M® Tablets**
044	**Gelusil-M® Liquid**
172	**Mandelamine®** (methenamine mandelate) 1.0 gram
171	**Mandelamine®** (methenamine mandelate) 0.5 gram
170	**Mandelamine®** (methenamine mandelate) 0.25 gram
176	**Mandelamine® Granules** (methenamine mandelate) 1.0 gram
177	**Mandelamine® Granules** (methenamine mandelate) 0.5 gram
174	**Mandelamine® Suspension Forte (methenamine mandelate)**
173	**Mandelamine® Suspension** (methenamine mandelate)
270	**Nardil®** (phenelzine sulfate)
300	**Papase®** (proteolytic enzymes extracted from *Carica papaya*)
004	**Peritrate® SA Sustained Action** 80 mg (pentaerythritol tetranitrate)
007	**Peritrate®** 10 mg (pentaerythritol tetranitrate)
001	**Peritrate®** 20 mg (pentaerythritol tetranitrate)
008	**Peritrate®** 40 mg (pentaerythritol tetranitrate)
005	**Peritrate w/Phenobarbital SA Sustained Action**
002	**Peritrate®** 10 mg **w/Phenobarbital**
003	**Peritrate®** 20 mg **w/Phenobarbital**
310	**Pre-Sate** (chlorphentermine HCl)
250	**Proloid® Tablets** (thyroglobulin ¼ grain
251	**Proloid® Tablets** (thyroglobulin) ½ grain
252	**Proloid® Tablets** (thyroglobulin) 1 grain
253	**Proloid® Tablets** (thyroglobulin) 1½ grain
257	**Proloid® Tablets** (thyroglobulin) 2 grain
254	**Proloid® Tablets** (thyroglobulin) 3 grain
180	**Pyridium®** (phenazopyridine HCl) 100 mg
181	**Pyridium®** (phenazopyridine HCl) 200 mg
182	**Pyridium® Plus**
100	**Sinubid®**
230	**Tedral®**
232	**Tedral® Anti-H**
231	**Tedral® SA Sustained Action**
242	**Tedral® Elixir**
237	**Tedral® Suspension**
238	**Tedral-25®**
239	**Tedral® Expectorant**
276	**Verstran®** (prazepam) 10 mg

Each tablet represents:		Percentages of US Recommended Daily Allowances (US RDA)
Vitamin A (acetate) (2.25 mg)	7,500 IU*	150%
Vitamin D (ergocalciferol) (10 mg)	400 IU	
Vitamin E (*dl*-alpha tocopheryl acetate, 30 mg)	30 IU	100%
Vitamin C (ascorbic acid)	180 mg	300%
Vitamin B_1 (thiamine mononitrate, 4.37 mg)	4.5 mg	300%
Vitamin B_2 (riboflavin)	5.1 mg	300%
Vitamin B_6 (pyridoxine hydrochloride, 7.3 mg)	6 mg	300%
Vitamin B_{12} crystalline (cyanocobalamin)	6 mcg	100%
Niacin (niacinamide, 59.5 mg)	60 mg$^+$	300%

*IU = International Units
$^+$Niacin (nicotinic acid) content is supplied as 59.5 mg niacinamide (nicotinamide) equivalent to 60 mg of the reference form nicotinic acid.

abdec teens™ FILMSEALS

Description: High-potency dietary vitamin supplement for teenagers
Composition:
[See table below, left].
Actions and Uses: A high-potency dietary vitamin supplement containing vitamins A, B, D, E, and C to help prevent vitamin deficiencies that may occur in growing, active teenagers.
Dosage: One tablet daily
How Supplied: N 0071-0381- Bottles of 100 and trial-size packages of 7s.

abdec teens™ with Iron

Description: High-potency vitamin supplement with iron for teenagers
Ingredients: Ascorbic acid, cellulose, niacinamide, ferrous fumarate, vitamin E acetate, hydroxypropyl methylcellulose, hydroxypropyl cellulose, gelatin, pyridoxine hydrochloride, riboflavin, thiamine mononitrate, propylene glycol, silica gel, magnesium stearate, vitamin A acetate, FD&C Red No. 3, FD&C Yellow No. 6, FD&C Blue No. 2, titanium dioxide, wax, vanillin, vitamin D_2, and vitamin B_{12}.
Composition:
Each tablet represents:

VITAMINS		Percentages of US Recommended Daily Allowances (US RDA)
Vitamin A	7,500 IU*	150%
Vitamin D	400 IU	100%
Vitamin E	30 IU	100%
Vitamin C (ascorbic acid)	180 mg	300%
Thiamine (vitamin B_1)	4.5 mg	300%
Riboflavin (vitamin B_2)	5.1 mg	300%
Niacin$^+$	60 mg	300%
Vitamin B_6	6 mg	300%
Vitamin B_{12}	6 mcg	100%
MINERALS		
Iron	18 mg	100%

*IU = International Units
$^+$ Supplied as niacinamide

Actions and Uses: A high-potency vitamin supplement with iron to help prevent vitamin

and iron deficiencies that may occur in growing, active teenagers
Dosage: One tablet daily
How Supplied: N 0071-0481- Bottles of 100 and trial-size packages of 7s

ADRENALIN® CHLORIDE SOLUTION ℞
(epinephrine injection, USP)

Description: Each milliliter contains 1 mg Adrenalin (epinephrine) as the hydrochloride dissolved in isotonic sodium chloride solution. The ampoules contain not more than 0.1% sodium bisulfite as a preservative. The Steri-Vials contain 0.5% Chloretone® (chlorobutanol) (chloroform derivative) and not more than 0.15% sodium bisulfite as preservatives. Epinephrine is the active principle of the adrenal medulla. Chemically, Adrenalin Chloride Solution is described as (—)-3,4-dihydroxy-α-([methylamino] methyl) benzyl alcohol.
Action: Adrenalin (epinephrine), a sympathomimetic drug, activates an adrenergic receptive mechanism on effector cells and imitates all actions of the sympathetic nervous system except those on the arteries of the face and sweat glands. Epinephrine acts on both alpha and beta receptors and is the most potent alpha receptor activator.
Indications: In general, the most common uses of epinephrine are to relieve respiratory distress due to bronchospasm, to provide rapid relief of hypersensitivity reactions to drugs and other allergens, and to prolong the action of infiltration anesthetics. The cardiac effects of epinephrine may be of use in restoring cardiac rhythm in cardiac arrest due to various causes, but the drug is not used in cardiac failure or in hemorrhagic, traumatic, or cardiogenic shock.
Epinephrine is used as a hemostatic agent and is also used in treating mucosal congestion of hay fever, rhinitis, and acute sinusitis; to relieve bronchial asthmatic paroxysms; in syncope due to complete heart block or carotid sinus hypersensitivity; for symptomatic relief of serum sickness, urticaria, angioneurotic edema; for resuscitation in cardiac arrest following anesthetic accidents; in simple (open angle) glaucoma; for relaxation of uterine musculature, and to inhibit uterine contractions. Epinephrine injection can be utilized to prolong the action of intraspinal and local anesthetics (see Contraindications).
Contraindications: Epinephrine is contraindicated in narrow-angle (congestive) glaucoma, shock, during general anesthesia with halogenated hydrocarbons or cyclopropane, and in individuals with organic brain damage. Epinephrine is also contraindicated with local anesthesia of certain areas, eg, fingers, toes, because of the danger of vasoconstriction producing sloughing of tissue; in labor because the drug may delay the second stage; in cardiac dilatation, and in coronary insufficiency.
Warnings: Administer with caution to elderly people; to those with cardiovascular disease, hypertension, diabetes, or hyperthyroidism; in psychoneurotic individuals; and in pregnancy.
Patients with long-standing bronchial asthma and emphysema who have developed degenerative heart disease should be administered the drug with extreme caution.
Overdosage or inadvertent intravenous injection of epinephrine may cause cerebrovascular hemorrhage resulting from the sharp rise in blood pressure.
Fatalities may also result from pulmonary edema because of the peripheral constriction and cardiac stimulation produced. Rapidly acting vasodilators, such as nitrites, or alpha-blocking agents, may counteract the marked pressor effects of epinephrine.
Use of epinephrine with excessive doses of digitalis, mercurial diuretics, or other drugs that sensitize the heart to arrhythmias is not recommended. Anginal pain may be induced when coronary insufficiency is present.
Precautions: Adrenalin (epinephrine injection) should be protected from exposure to light. Do not remove ampoules or syringes from carton until ready to use. The solution should not be used if it is brown in color, or contains a precipitate.
Epinephrine is readily destroyed by alkalies and oxidizing agents. In the latter category are oxygen, chlorine, bromine, iodine, permanganates, chromates, nitrites, and salts of easily reducible metals, especially iron.
The effects of epinephrine may be potentiated by tricyclic antidepressants; certain antihistamines, eg, diphenhydramine, tripelennamine, *d*-chlorpheniramine; and sodium *l*-thyroxine.
Adverse Reactions: Transient and minor side effects of anxiety, headache, fear, and palpitations often occur with therapeutic doses, especially in hyperthyroid individuals. Repeated local injections can result in necrosis at sites of injection from vascular constriction. "Epinephrine-fastness" can occur with prolonged use.
Dosage and Administration: Intramuscularly or subcutaneously—0.2 to 1 ml. Start with small dose and increase if required.
For bronchial asthma and certain allergic manifestations, eg, angioedema, urticaria, serum sickness, anaphylactic shock, use epinephrine subcutaneously. For bronchial asthma in pediatric patients, administer 0.01 ml/kg or 0.3 ml/m^2 to a maximum of 0.5 ml subcutaneously, repeated every four hours if required.
For cardiac resuscitation—A dose of 0.5 ml diluted to 10 ml with sodium chloride injection can be administered intravenously or intracardially to restore myocardial contractility. External cardiac massage should follow intracardial administration to permit the drug to enter coronary circulation. The drug should be used secondarily to unsuccessful attempts with physical or electromechanical methods.
Ophthalmologic use (for producing conjunctival decongestion, to control hemorrhage, produce mydriasis, and reduce intraocular pressure)—use a concentration of 1:10,000 to 1:1,000.
Intraspinal use—Ampoule 88—Usual dose is 0.2 to 0.4 ml added to anesthetic spinal fluid mixture (may prolong anesthetic action by limiting absorption). For use with local anesthetic—Epinephrine 1:100,000 to 1:20,000 is the usual concentration employed with local anesthetics.
How Supplied:
N 0071-4188-03 (Ampoule 88) Sterile solution containing 1 mg Adrenalin (epinephrine) as the hydrochloride in each 1-ml ampoule (1:1,000). For intramuscular or subcutaneous use. When diluted, the product may also be administered intracardially or intravenously, or intraspinally. Supplied in packages of 10.
N 0071-4011-13 (Steri-Vial® 11) Sterile solution containing 1 mg Adrenalin (epinephrine) as the hydrochloride (1:1,000). For intramuscular or subcutaneous use. When diluted, the drug may also be administered intracardially or intravenously. Supplied in a 30-ml Steri-Vial (rubber diaphragm-capped vial).
AHFS 12:12 **YC**

AGORAL® PLAIN
AGORAL® RASPBERRY
AGORAL® MARSHMALLOW

Description: Each tablespoonful (15 ml) of Agoral Plain (white) contains 4.2 grams mineral oil in a thoroughly homogenized emulsion with agar, tragacanth, acacia, egg albumin, glycerin and water.
Each tablespoonful (15 ml) of Agoral Raspberry (pink) or of Agoral Marshmallow (white) contains 4.2 grams mineral oil and 0.2 grams phenolphthalein in a thoroughly homogenized emulsion with agar, tragacanth, acacia, egg albumin, glycerin and water.
Actions: Agoral, containing mineral oil, facilitates defecation by lubricating the fecal mass and softening the stool. More effective than nonemulsified oil in penetrating the feces, Agoral thereby greatly reduces the possibility of oil leakage at the anal sphincter. Phenolphthalein gently stimulates motor activity of the lower intestinal tract. Agoral's combined lubricating-softening and peristaltic actions can help to restore a normal pattern of evacuation.
Indications: Relief of constipation. Agoral may be especially required when straining at stool is a hazard, as in hernia, cardiac, or hypertensive patients; during convalescence from surgery; before and after surgery for hemorrhoids or other painful anorectal disorders; for obstetrical patients; for patients confined to bed.
The management of chronic constipation should also include attention to fluid intake, diet and bowel habits.
Contraindications: Sensitivity to phenolphthalein.
Dosage and Management:

	Adults	Children over 6 years
Agoral Plain (without phenolphthalein)	1 to 2 tablespoonfuls	2 to 4 teaspoonfuls
Agoral Raspberry	½ to 1 tablespoonful	1 to 2 teaspoonfuls
Agoral Marshmallow	½ to 1 tablespoonful	1 to 2 teaspoonfuls

Take at bedtime only, unless other time is advised by physician.
Agoral may be taken alone or in milk, water or any miscible food.
Expectant or nursing mothers, bedridden or aged patients, young children or infants: use only on advice of physician.
Supplied: Agoral Plain (without phenolphthalein), plastic bottles of 16 fl oz (N 0047-0071-16). Agoral (raspberry flavor), plastic bottles of 16 fl oz (N 0047-0072-16). Agoral (marshmallow flavor), plastic bottles of 8 fl oz (N 0047-0070-08) and 16 fl oz (N 0047-0070-16).
STORE BETWEEN 59° and 86°F (15° and 30°C).

AMCILL® ℞
(ampicillin, USP) as the trihydrate
Capsules, 250 mg and 500 mg
For Oral Suspension, 125 mg/5 ml and 250 mg/5 ml

Description: Ampicillin is a semisynthetic penicillin derived from the basic penicillin nucleus, 6-aminopenicillanic acid.
Actions: Microbiology: *In vitro* studies have shown sensitivity of the following microorganisms to ampicillin:
Gram-Positive: Alpha- and beta-hemolytic streptococci, *Diplococcus pneumoniae,* staphylococci (nonpenicillinase-producing), *Bacillus anthracis, Clostridia* species, *Corynebacterium xerose,* and most strains of enterococci.
The drug does not resist destruction by penicillinase, hence is not effective against penicillin G-resistant staphylococci.
Gram-Negative: *Hemophilus influenzae, Neisseria gonorrhoeae, N meningitidis, Proteus mirabilis,* and many strains of *Salmonella* (including *S typhosa), Shigella,* and *Escherichia coli.*

Continued on next page

This product information was prepared in August, 1979. On these and other Parke-Davis Products, detailed information may be obtained by addressing PARKE-DAVIS, Division of Warner-Lambert Company, Morris Plains, NJ 07950.

Parke-Davis—Cont.

Testing for Susceptibility: The invading organism should be cultured and its sensitivity demonstrated as a guide to therapy. If the Kirby-Bauer method of disk sensitivity is used, a 10-mcg ampicillin disk should be used to determine the relative *in vitro* susceptibility.

Human Pharmacology: Ampicillin is stable in the presence of gastric acid and is well-absorbed from the gastrointestinal tract. Ampicillin diffuses readily into most body tissues and fluids. However, penetration into the cerebrospinal fluid and brain occurs only with meningeal inflammation. Ampicillin is excreted largely unchanged in the urine. Ampicillin excretion can be delayed by concurrent administration of probenecid. Ampicillin is the least-serum bound of all the penicillins, averaging 20% compared to 60 to 90% for other penicillins.

Indications: Ampicillin is indicated primarily in the treatment of infections caused by susceptible strains of the following microorganisms: *Shigella, Salmonella* (including *S typhosa), E coli, H influenzae, P mirabilis,* and *N gonorrhoeae.* Ampicillin may also be indicated in certain infections caused by susceptible gram-positive organisms: penicillin G-sensitive staphylococci, streptococci, pneumococci, and enterococci.

Bacteriology studies to determine the causative organisms and their sensitivity to ampicillin should be performed. Therapy may be initiated prior to the results of sensitivity testing.

Contraindication: Ampicillin is contraindicated in patients with a history of a hypersensitivity reaction to the penicillins.

Warning: Serious and occasionally fatal hypersensitivity (anaphylactic) reactions have been reported in patients on penicillin therapy. Although anaphylaxis is more frequent following parenteral therapy, it has occurred in patients on oral penicillins. These reactions are more apt to occur in individuals with a history of sensitivity to multiple allergens.

There have been reports of individuals with a history of penicillin hypersensitivity who experienced severe reactions when treated with cephalosporins. Before therapy with any penicillin, careful inquiry should be made concerning previous hypersensitivity reactions to penicillins, cephalosporins, or other allergens. **Serious anaphylactoid reactions require immediate emergency treatment with epinephrine. Oxygen, intravenous steroids, and airway management, including intubation, should also be administered as indicated.**

Usage in Pregnancy: Safety for use in pregnancy has not been established.

Precautions: As with any potent drug, periodic assessment of renal, hepatic, and hematopoietic functions should be made during prolonged therapy.

The possibility of superinfections with mycotic or bacterial pathogens should be kept in mind during therapy. If superinfections occur, appropriate therapy should be instituted.

Adverse Reactions: As with other penicillins, it may be expected that untoward reactions will be essentially limited to sensitivity phenomena. They are more likely to occur in individuals who have previously demonstrated hypersensitivity to penicillins and in those with a history of allergy, asthma, hay fever, or urticaria.

The following adverse reactions have been reported as associated with the use of ampicillin.

Gastrointestinal—Glossitis, stomatitis, black "hairy" tongue, nausea, vomiting, enterocolitis, pseudomembranous colitis, and diarrhea have been reported. (These reactions are usually associated with oral dosage forms.)

Hypersensitivity Reactions—Erythematous maculopapular rashes have been reported fairly frequently. Urticaria, erythema multiforme, and an occasional case of exfoliative dermatitis have been reported. Anaphylaxis is the most serious reaction experienced and has usually been associated with the parenteral dosage form.

NOTE: Urticaria, other skin rashes, and serum sickness-like reactions may be controlled with antihistamines and, if necessary, systemic corticosteroids. Whenever such reactions occur, ampicillin should be discontinued unless, in the opinion of the physician, the condition being treated is life-threatening and amenable only to ampicillin therapy. Serious anaphylactic reactions require the immediate use of epinephrine, oxygen, and intravenous steroids.

Liver—A moderate rise in serum glutamic oxaloacetic transaminase (SGOT) has been noted, particularly in infants, but the significance of this finding is unknown.

Hemic and Lymphatic Systems—Anemia, thrombocytopenia, thrombocytopenic purpura, eosinophilia, leukopenia, and agranulocytosis have been reported during therapy with the penicillins. These reactions are usually reversible on discontinuation of therapy and are believed to be hypersensitivity phenomena.

Other—Because infectious mononucleosis is viral in origin, ampicillin should not be used in the treatment. A high percentage of patients with mononucleosis who received ampicillin developed a skin rash.

Dosage and Administration:

Infections of the respiratory tract and soft tissues

Patients weighing 20 kg (44 lb) or more: 250 mg every six hours

Patients weighing less than 20 kg (44 lb): 50 mg/kg/day in equally divided doses at six- or eight-hour intervals

Infections of the gastrointestinal and genitourinary tracts

Patients weighing 20 kg (44 lb) or more: 500 mg every six hours

Patients weighing less than 20 kg (44 lb): 100 mg/kg/day in equally divided doses at six- or eight-hour intervals

In the treatment of chronic urinary tract and intestinal infections, frequent bacteriologic and clinical appraisal is necessary. Smaller doses than those recommended above should not be used. Higher doses should be used for stubborn or severe infections. In stubborn infections, therapy may be required for several weeks. It may be necessary to continue clinical and/or bacteriologic follow-up for several months after cessation of therapy.

Urethritis in males or females due to *N gonorrhoeae:*

3.5 g with 1 g probenecid, administered simultaneously.

In the treatment of complications of gonorrheal urethritis, such as prostatitis and epididymitis, prolonged and intensive therapy is recommended. Cases of gonorrhea with a suspected primary lesion of syphilis should have darkfield examinations before receiving treatment. In all other cases where concomitant syphilis is suspected, monthly serologic tests should be made for a minimum of four months.

Treatment of all infections should be continued for a minimum of 48 to 72 hours beyond the time that the patient becomes asymptomatic or evidence of bacterial eradication has been obtained. A minimum of 10 days' treatment is recommended for any infection caused by group A beta-hemolytic streptococci to help prevent the occurrence of acute rheumatic fever or acute glomerulonephritis.

Directions For Dispensing Oral Suspensions

Prepare suspension at time of dispensing. For ease in preparation, add water to the bottle in two portions, and shake well after each addition.

125 mg/5 ml

Add a total of 83 ml to the 100-ml package, 105 ml to the 150-ml package, and 165 ml to the 200-ml package. This will provide 100, 150, and 200 ml of suspension. Each 5 ml (teaspoonful) will contain ampicillin trihydrate equivalent to 125 mg ampicillin. The reconstituted suspension is stable for 14 days under refrigeration.

250 mg/5 ml

Add a total of 70 ml to the 100-ml package, 105 ml to the 150-ml package, and 140 ml to the 200-ml package. This will provide 100, 150, and 200 ml of suspension. Each 5 ml (teaspoonful) will contain ampicillin trihydrate equivalent to 250 mg ampicillin. The reconstituted suspension is stable for 14 days under refrigeration.

How Supplied:

N 0071-0402 (Capsule 402)—Amcill Capsules, 250 mg. Each capsule contains ampicillin trihydrate equivalent to 250 mg ampicillin. Bottles of 100 and 500, and unit-dose packages of 100 (10 strips of 10 capsules each). Parcode® No. 402

N 0071-0404 (Capsule 404)—Amcill Capsules, 500 mg. Each capsule contains ampicillin trihydrate equivalent to 500 mg ampicillin. Bottles of 100 and 500, and unit-dose packages of 100 (10 strips of 10 capsules each). Parcode No. 404

[*Shown in Product Identification Section*]

N 0071-2301 (No. 301)—Amcill for Oral Suspension 125 mg/5 ml. Each 5 ml of reconstituted suspension contains ampicillin trihydrate equivalent to 125 mg ampicillin. Available in 100-ml, 150-ml, and 200-ml bottles.

N 0071-2302 (No. 302)—Amcill for Oral Suspension 250 mg/5 ml. Each 5 ml of reconstituted suspension contains ampicillin trihydrate equivalent to 250 mg ampicillin. Available in 100-ml and 200-ml bottles.

AHFS 8:12.16 **YB**

Also Available:

Amcill-S® (sterile sodium ampicillin, USP) in Steri-Vials containing ampicillin sodium equivalent to 125, 250, 500 mg, or 1 g ampicillin per vial. Available in packages of 10.

N 0071-4169-01 (Steri-Vial® 169)—125-mg vial
N 0071-4170-01 (Steri-Vial 170)—250-mg vial
N 0071-4171-02 (Steri-Vial 171)—500-mg vial
N 0071-4172-03 (Steri-Vial 172)—1-g vial

AMITRIL® Tablets ℞
(amitriptyline HCl)

Caution: Federal law prohibits dispensing without prescription.

Description: Amitriptyline hydrochloride, a dibenzocycloheptadiene derivative, is a white to practically white crystalline compound that is freely soluble in water.

It is designated chemically as 1-Propanamine, 3- (10, 11-dihydro-5*H*-dibenzo [*a,d*] cyclohepten-5-ylidene) -*N, N*-dimethyl-, hydrochloride. The molecular weight is 313.87. The empirical formula is $C_{20}H_{23}N \cdot HCl$.

Actions: Amitril (amitriptyline HCl) is an antidepressant with an anxiety-reducing, sedative component. The mechanism of action in man is not known. It is not a monoamine oxidase inhibitor and it does not act primarily by stimulation of the central nervous system.

Amitril (amitriptyline HCl) inhibits the membrane pump mechanism responsible for reuptake of norepinephrine into adrenergic neurons. Pharmacologically this action may potentiate or prolong sympathetic activity, since reuptake of norepinephrine is important physiologically in terminating its transmitting actions. This interference with reuptake of norepinephrine is believed by some to underlie the antidepressant activity of amitriptyline.

Indications: For the relief of symptoms of depression. Endogenous depression is more likely to be alleviated than are other depressive states.

Contraindications: Amitril (amitriptyline HCl) is contraindicated in patients who have shown prior hypersensitivity to it.

It should not be given concomitantly with monoamine oxidase inhibitors. Hyperpyretic crises, severe convulsions, and deaths have occurred in patients receiving tricyclic antidepressant and monoamine oxidase inhibiting drugs simultaneously. When it is desired to replace a monoamine oxidase inhibitor with Amitril (amitriptyline HCl), a minimum of 14 days should be allowed to elapse after the former is discontinued. Amitril (amitriptyline HCl) should then be initiated cautiously with gradual increase in dosage until optimum response is achieved.

Amitril (amitriptyline HCl) is not recommended for use during the acute recovery phase following myocardial infarction.

Warnings: Amitril (amitriptyline HCl) may block the antihypertensive action of guanethidine or similarly acting compounds.

It should be used with caution in patients with a history of seizures and, because of its atropine-like action, in patients with a history of urinary retention, angle-closure glaucoma or increased intraocular pressure. In patients with angle-closure glaucoma, even average doses may precipitate an attack.

Patients with cardiovascular disorders should be watched closely. Tricyclic antidepressant drugs, including Amitril (amitriptyline HCl), particularly when given in high doses, have been reported to produce arrhythmias, sinus tachycardia, and prolongation of the conduction time. Myocardial infarction and stroke have been reported with drugs of this class.

Close supervision is required when Amitril (amitriptyline HCl) is given to hyperthyroid patients or those receiving thyroid medication.

This drug may impair mental and/or physical abilities required for performance of hazardous tasks, such as operating machinery or driving a motor vehicle.

Usage in Pregnancy—Safe use of Amitril (amitriptyline HCl) during pregnancy and lactation has not been established; therefore, in administering the drug to pregnant patients, nursing mothers, or women who may become pregnant, the possible benefits must be weighed against the possible hazards to mother and child.

Animal reproduction studies have been inconclusive and clinical experience has been limited.

Usage in Children—In view of the lack of experience with the use of this drug in children, it is not recommended at the present time for patients under 12 years of age.

Precautions: Schizophrenic patients may develop increased symptoms of psychosis; patients with paranoid symptomatology may have an exaggeration of such symptoms; manic depressive patients may experience a shift to the manic phase.

In these circumstances the dose of Amitril (amitriptyline HCl) may be reduced or a major tranquilizer such as perphenazine may be administered concurrently.

When Amitril (amitriptyline HCl) is given with anticholinergic agents or sympathomimetic drugs, including epinephrine combined with local anesthetics, close supervision and careful adjustment of dosages are required.

Caution is advised if patients receive large doses of ethchlorvynol concurrently. Transient delirium has been reported in patients who were treated with one gram of ethchlorvynol and 75-150 mg of amitriptyline HCl.

Amitril (amitriptyline HCl) may enhance the response to alcohol and the effects of barbiturates and other CNS depressants.

The possibility of suicide in depressed patients remains during treatment and until significant remission occurs. This type of patient should not have access to large quantities of the drug.

Concurrent administration of Amitril (amitriptyline HCl) and electroshock therapy may increase the hazards associated with such therapy. Such treatment should be limited to patients for whom it is essential.

When possible, the drug should be discontinued several days before elective surgery.

Both elevation and lowering of blood sugar levels have been reported.

Adverse Reactions:

Note: Included in the listing which follows are a few adverse reactions which have not been reported with this specific drug. However, pharmacological similarities among the tricyclic antidepressant drugs require that each of the reactions be considered when amitriptyline is administered.

Cardiovascular: Hypotension, hypertension, tachycardia, palpitation, myocardial infarction, arrhythmias, heart block, stroke.

CNS and Neuromuscular: Confusional states; disturbed concentration; disorientation; delusions, hallucinations; excitement; anxiety; restlessness, insomnia; nightmares; numbness, tingling, and paresthesias of the extremities; peripheral neuropathy; incoordination; ataxia; tremors; seizures; alteration in EEG patterns; extrapyramidal symptoms; tinnitus; syndrome of inappropriate ADH (antidiuretic hormone) secretion.

Anticholinergic: Dry mouth, blurred vision, disturbance of accommodation, constipation, paralytic ileus, urinary retention, dilatation of urinary tract.

Allergic: Skin rash, urticaria, photosensitization, edema of face and tongue.

Hematologic: Bone marrow depression, including agranulocytosis, leukopenia, eosinophilia, purpura, thrombocytopenia.

Gastrointestinal: Nausea, epigastric distress, vomiting, anorexia, stomatitis, peculiar taste, diarrhea, parotid swelling, black tongue.

Endocrine: Testicular swelling and gynecomastia in the male, breast enlargement and galactorrhea in the female, increased or decreased libido, elevation and lowering of blood sugar levels.

Other: Dizziness, weakness, fatigue, headache, weight gain or loss, increased perspiration, urinary frequency, mydriasis, drowsiness, jaundice, alopecia.

Withdrawal Symptoms: Abrupt cessation of treatment after prolonged administration may produce nausea, headache, and malaise. These are not indicative of addiction.

Dosage and Administration:

Oral Dosage

Dosage should be initiated at a low level and increased gradually, noting carefully the clinical response and any evidence of intolerance.

Initial Dosage for Adults—For outpatients 75 mg of amitriptyline HCl a day in divided doses usually is satisfactory. If necessary, this may be increased to a total of 150 mg per day. Increases are made preferably in the late afternoon and/or bedtime doses. A sedative effect may be apparent before the antidepressant effect is noted, but an adequate therapeutic effect may take as long as 30 days to develop.

An alternative method of initiating therapy in outpatients is to begin with 50 to 100 mg Amitril (amitriptyline HCl) at bedtime. This may be increased by 25 or 50 mg as necessary in the bedtime dose to a total of 150 mg per day.

Hospitalized patients may require 100 mg a day initially. This can be increased gradually to 200 mg a day if necessary. A small number of hospitalized patients may need as much as 300 mg daily.

Adolescent and Elderly Patients—In general, lower dosages are recommended for these patients. Ten mg 3 times a day with 20 mg at bedtime may be satisfactory in adolescent and elderly patients who do not tolerate higher dosages.

Maintenance—The usual maintenance dosage of Amitril (amitriptyline HCl) is 50 to 100 mg per day. In some patients 40 mg per day is sufficient. For maintenance therapy the total daily dosage may be given in a single dose preferably at bedtime. When satisfactory improvement has been reached, dosage should be reduced to the lowest amount that will maintain relief of symptoms. It is appropriate to continue maintenance therapy 3 months or longer to lessen the possibility of relapse.

Usage in Children

In view of the lack of experience with the use of this drug in children, it is not recommended at the present time for patients under 12 years of age.

Overdosage:

Manifestations—High doses may cause temporary confusion, disturbed concentration, or transient visual hallucinations. Overdosage may cause drowsiness; hypothermia; tachycardia and other arrhythmic abnormalities, such as bundle branch block; ECG evidence of impaired conduction; congestive heart failure; dilated pupils; convulsions; severe hypotension; stupor; and coma. Other symptoms may be agitation, hyperactive reflexes, muscle rigidity, vomiting, hyperpyrexia, or any of those listed under Adverse Reactions.

All patients suspected of having taken an overdosage should be admitted to a hospital as soon as possible. *Treatment* is symptomatic and supportive. Empty the stomach as quickly as possible by emesis followed by gastric lavage upon arrival at the hospital. An ECG should be taken and close monitoring of cardiac function instituted if there is any sign of abnormality. Maintain an open airway and adequate fluid intake; regulate body temperature.

The intravenous administration of 1-3 mg of physostigmine salicylate is reported to reverse the symptoms of tricyclic antidepressant poisoning. Because physostigmine is rapidly metabolized, the dosage of physostigmine should be repeated as required particularly if life-threatening signs such as arrhythmias, convulsions, and deep coma recur or persist after the initial dosage of physostigmine.

Standard measures should be used to manage circulatory shock and metabolic acidosis. Cardiac arrhythmias may be treated with neostigmine, pyridostigmine, or propranolol. Should cardiac failure occur, the use of digitalis should be considered. Close monitoring of cardiac function for not less than five days is advisable.

Anticonvulsants may be given to control convulsions. Amitriptyline increases the CNS depressant action but not the anticonvulsant action of barbiturates; therefore, an inhalation anesthetic, diazepam, or paraldehyde is recommended for control of convulsions.

Dialysis is of no value because of low plasma concentrations of the drug.

Since overdosage is often deliberate, patients may attempt suicide by other means during the recovery phase.

Deaths by deliberate or accidental overdosage have occurred with this class of drugs.

How Supplied: Amitril (amitriptyline HCl) tablets are supplied as film-coated tablets:

10 mg (tan)	in bottles of 100 (N 0047-0272-51)
10 mg (tan)	in bottles of 1000 (N 0047-0272-60)
25 mg (coral)	in bottles of 100 (N 0047-0273-51)
25 mg (coral)	in bottles of 1000 (N 0047-0273-60)
50 mg (blue/purple)	in bottles of 100 (N 0047-0274-51)
50 mg (blue/purple)	in bottles of 1000 (N 0047-0274-60)
75 mg (green)	in bottles of 100 (N 0047-0275-51)
75 mg (green)	in bottles of 1000 (N 0047-0275-60)

This product information was prepared in August, 1979. On these and other Parke-Davis Products, detailed information may be obtained by addressing PARKE-DAVIS, Division of Warner-Lambert Company, Morris Plains, NJ 07950.

Continued on next page

Parke-Davis—Cont.

100 mg (brown/mustard)	in bottles of 100 (N 0047-0271-51)
100 mg (brown/mustard)	in bottles of 1000 (N 0047-0271-60)
150 mg (orange)	in bottles of 100 (N 0047-0278-51)

Store between 59°–86° F (15°–30°C).

323 G 301 **8-78**

[*Shown in Product Identification Section*]

AMOXICILLIN ℞

(Utimox™)

Capsules—250 and 500 mg

For Oral Suspension—125 mg/5 ml and 250 mg/5 ml

Pediatric Drops—50 mg/ml

Description: Amoxicillin is a semisynthethic penicillin, an analogue of ampicillin, with a broad spectrum of bactericidal activity against many gram-positive and gram-negative microorganisms. Chemically, amoxicillin is D-(-)-α-amino-p-hydroxybenzyl penicillin trihydrate.

Actions:

Pharmacology

Amoxicillin is stable in the presence of gastric acid and may be given without regard for food. Amoxicillin is rapidly absorbed after oral administration and diffuses readily into most body tissues and fluids, with the exception of brain and spinal fluid, except when meninges are inflamed. The half-life of amoxicillin is one hour. Most of the amoxicillin is excreted unchanged in the urine and excretion can be delayed by concurrent administration of probenecid. Amoxicillin is not highly protein-bound. In blood serum, amoxicillin is approximately 20% protein-bound as compared with 60% for penicillin G.

Orally administered doses of 250 mg and 500 mg amoxicillin capsules result in average peak blood levels, one to two hours after administration, in the range of 3.5 mcg/ml to 5.0 mcg/ml, and 5.5 mcg/ml to 7.5 mcg/ml, respectively.

Orally administered doses of amoxicillin suspension, 125 mg/5 ml and 250 mg/5 ml, result in average peak blood levels, one to two hours after administration, in the range of 1.5 mcg/ml to 3.0 mcg/ml, and 3.5 mcg/ml to 5.0 mcg/ml, respectively.

Detectable serum levels are observed up to eight hours after an orally administered dose of amoxicillin. Approximately 60% of an orally administered dose of amoxicillin is excreted in the urine within six to eight hours.

Microbiology

Amoxicillin is similar to ampicillin in its bactericidal action against susceptible organisms during the stage of active multiplication. Amoxicillin acts through the inhibition of biosynthesis of cell wall mucopeptide. *In vitro* studies have demonstrated the susceptibility of most strains of the following gram-positive bacteria: alpha- and beta-hemolytic streptococci, *Diplococcus pneumoniae,* nonpenicillinase-producing staphylococci, and *Streptococcus faecalis.* Amoxicillin is active *in vitro* against many strains of *Hemophilus influenzae, Neisseria gonorrhoeae, Escherichia coli,* and *Proteus mirabilis.* Because amoxicillin does not resist destruction by penicillinase, the drug is not effective against penicillinase-producing bacteria, particularly resistant staphylococci. All strains of *Pseudomonas* and most strains of *Klebsiella* and *Enterobacter* are resistant.

Disk Susceptibility Tests

Quantitative methods that require measurement of zone diameters give the most precise estimates of antibiotic susceptibility. One such procedure has been recommended for use with disks for testing susceptibility to ampicillin-class antibiotics. Interpretations correlate diameters of the disk test with MIC values for amoxicillin. With this procedure, a report from the laboratory of "susceptible" indicates that the infecting organism is likely to respond to therapy. A report of "resistant" indicates that the infecting organism is not likely to respond to therapy. A report of "intermediate susceptibility" suggests that the organism would be susceptible if high dosage is used, or if the infection is confined to tissues and fluids (eg, urine), in which high antibiotic levels are attained.

Indications: Amoxicillin is indicated in the treatment of infections due to susceptible strains of the following.

Gram-negative organisms—*H influenzae, E coli, P mirabilis,* and *N gonorrhoeae*

Gram-positive organisms—Streptococci (including *Str faecalis), D pneumoniae,* and nonpenicillinase-producing staphylococci

Therapy may be instituted prior to obtaining results from bacteriological and susceptibility studies to determine the causative organisms and their susceptibility to amoxicillin.

Indicated surgical procedures should be performed.

Contraindication: The use of this drug is contraindicated in individuals with a history of an allergic reaction to the penicillins.

Warnings: SERIOUS AND OCCASIONALLY FATAL HYPERSENSITIVITY (ANAPHYLACTOID) REACTIONS HAVE BEEN REPORTED IN PATIENTS ON PENICILLIN THERAPY. ALTHOUGH ANAPHYLAXIS IS MORE FREQUENT FOLLOWING PARENTERAL THERAPY, IT HAS OCCURED IN PATIENTS ON ORAL PENICILLINS. THESE REACTIONS ARE MORE APT TO OCCUR IN INDIVIDUALS WITH A HISTORY OF SENSITIVITY TO MULTIPLE ALLERGENS.

THERE HAVE BEEN REPORTS OF INDIVIDUALS WITH A HISTORY OF PENICILLIN HYPERSENSITIVITY WHO HAVE EXPERIENCED SEVERE REACTIONS WHEN TREATED WITH CEPHALOSPORINS. BEFORE THERAPY WITH ANY PENICILLIN, CAREFUL INQUIRY SHOULD BE MADE CONCERNING PREVIOUS HYPERSENSITIVITY REACTIONS TO PENICILLINS, CEPHALOSPORINS, AND OTHER ALLERGENS. IF AN ALLERGIC REACTION OCCURS, APPROPRIATE THERAPY SHOULD BE INSTITUTED AND DISCONTINUANCE OF AMOXICILLIN THERAPY CONSIDERED.

SERIOUS ANAPHYLACTOID REACTIONS REQUIRE IMMEDIATE EMERGENCY TREATMENT WITH EPINEPHRINE. OXYGEN, INTRAVENOUS STEROIDS, AND AIRWAY MANAGEMENT, INCLUDING INTUBATION, SHOULD ALSO BE ADMINISTERED AS INDICATED.

Usage in Pregnancy—Safety for use in pregnancy has not been established.

Precautions: As with any potent drug, periodic assessment of renal, hepatic, and hematopoietic functions should be made during prolonged therapy.

The possibility of superinfections with mycotic or bacterial pathogens should be kept in mind during therapy. If superinfections occur (usually involving *Enterobacter, Pseudomonas,* or *Candida),* the drug should be discontinued and/or appropriate therapy instituted.

Adverse Reactions: As with other penicillins, it may be expected that untoward reactions will be essentially limited to sensitivity phenomena. They are more likely to occur in individuals who have previously demonstrated hypersensitivity to penicillins and in those with a history of allergy, asthma, hay fever, or urticaria.

The following adverse reactions have been reported as associated with the use of penicillins.

Gastrointestinal—Nausea, vomiting, and diarrhea

Hypersensitivity Reactions—Erythematous, maculopapular rashes and urticaria have been reported.

Note—Urticaria, other skin rashes, serum sickness-like reactions may be controlled with antihistamines and, if necessary, systemic corticosteroids. Whenever such reactions occur, amoxicillin should be discontinued unless, in the opinion of the physician, the condition being treated is life-threatening and amenable only to amoxicillin therapy.

Liver—A moderate rise in serum glutamic oxaloacetic transaminase (SGOT) has been noted, but the significance of this finding is unknown.

Hemic and Lymphatic Systems—Anemia, thrombocytopenia, thrombocytopenic purpura, eosinophilia, leukopenia, and agranulocytosis have been reported during therapy with the penicillins. These reactions are usually reversible on discontinuation of therapy and are believed to be hypersensitivity phenomena.

Dosage and Administration: Infections of the ear, nose, and throat due to streptococci, pneumococci, nonpenicillinase-producing staphylococci, and *H influenzae:*

Infections of the genitourinary tract due to *E coli, P mirabilis,* and *Str faecalis:*

Infections of the skin and soft tissues due to streptococci, susceptible staphylococci, and *E coli:*

Usual Dosage:

Adults: 250 mg every eight hours

Children: 20 mg/kg/day in divided doses every eight hours Children weighing 20 kg or more should be dosed according to the adult recommendations.

In severe infections or those caused by less susceptible organisms: 500 mg every eight hours for adults, and 40 mg/kg/day in divided doses every eight hours for children may be needed.

Infections of the lower respiratory tract due to streptococci, pneumococci, nonpenicillinase-producing staphylococci, and *H influenzae:*

Usual Dosage:

Adults: 500 mg every eight hours

Children: 40/kg/day in divided doses every eight hours

Children weighing 20 kg or more should be dosed according to the adult recommendations.

Gonorrhea, acute, uncomplicated anogenital and urethral infections due to *N gonorrhoeae:* (males and females) 3 g as a single, oral dose.

Cases of gonorrhea with a suspected lesion of syphilis should have darkfield examinations before receiving amoxicillin, and monthly serological tests for a minimum of four months.

Larger doses may be required for stubborn or severe infections.

The children's dosage is intended for individuals whose weight will not cause a dosage to be calculated greater than that recommended for adults.

It should be recognized that in the treatment of chronic urinary tract infections, frequent bacteriological and clinical appraisals are necessary. Smaller dosages than those recommended above should not be used. Even higher dosages may be needed at times. In stubborn infections, therapy may be required for several weeks. It may be necessary to continue clinical and/or bacteriological follow-up for several months after cessation of therapy. Except for gonorrhea, treatment should be continued for a minimum of 48 to 72 hours beyond the time that the patient becomes asymptomatic or evidence of bacterial eradication has been obtained.

It is recommended that there be at least 10 days' treatment for any infection caused by hemolytic streptococci to prevent the occurence of acute rheumatic fever or glomerulonephritis.

Dosage and Administration of Pediatric Drops:

Usual dosage for all indications except infections of the lower respiratory tract:

Under 6 kg (13 lb): 0.5 ml every eight hours
6 to 8 kg (13 to 18 lb): 1 ml every eight hours
Infections of the lower respiratory tract:
Under 6 kg (13 lb): 1 ml every eight hours
6 to 8 kg (13 to 18 lb): 2 ml every eight hours
Children weighing more than 8 kg (18 lb) should receive the appropriate dosage of the oral suspension, 125 mg/5 ml or 250 mg/5 ml. After reconstitution, the required amount of suspension should be placed directly on the child's tongue for swallowing. Alternate means of administration are to add the required amount of suspension to formula, milk, fruit juice, water, ginger ale, or cold drinks. These preparations should then be taken immediately. To be certain the child is receiving full dosage, such preparations should be consumed in their entirety.

Directions for Preparing Oral Suspension: Prepare suspension at the time of dispensing. For ease of preparation, add water to the bottle in two portions and shake well after each addition. Each teaspoonful (5 ml) will contain 125 mg or 250 mg amoxicillin.

Product	Bottle Size	Amount of Water Required for Reconstitution
125 mg/5 ml	80 ml	66 ml
	100 ml	83 ml
	150 ml	125 ml
250 mg/5 ml	80 ml	56 ml
	100 ml	70 ml
	150 ml	105 ml

Directions for Preparing Pediatric Drops: Add 10.6 ml of water to the bottle and shake vigorously. Each milliliter of suspension will contain 50 mg amoxicillin.

NOTE: SHAKE WELL BEFORE USING THE ORAL SUSPENSION AND THE PEDIATRIC DROPS.

Keep bottle tightly closed. Any unused portion of the reconstituted suspension must be discarded after 14 days. Refrigeration is preferable, but not requried.

How Supplied: N 0071-0730—Amoxicillin capsules, 250 mg. Each capsule contains amoxicillin trihydrate equivalent to 250 mg amoxicillin. Bottles of 100 and 500 and unit-dose packages of 100 (10 strips of 10 capsules each).
N 0071-0731—Amoxicillin capsules, 500 mg. Each capsule contains amoxicillin trihydrate equivalent to 500 mg amoxicillin. Bottles of 50 and 100 and unit-dose packages of 100 (10 strips of 10 capsules each).

[*Shown in Product Identification Section*]

N 0071-2500—Amoxicillin for oral suspension, 125 mg/5 ml. Each 5 ml of reconstituted suspension contains amoxicillin trihydrate equivalent to 125 mg amoxicillin. Available in 80-ml, 100-ml, and 150-ml bottles.
N 0071-2501—Amoxicillin for oral suspension, 250 mg/5 ml. Each 5 ml of reconstituted suspension contains amoxicillin trihydrate equivalent to 250 mg amoxicillin. Available in 80-ml, 100-ml, and 150-ml bottles.
N 0071-2502-11—Amoxicillin pediatric drops, 50 mg/ml. Each milliliter of reconstituted suspension contains amoxicillin trihydrate equivalent to 50 mg amoxicillin. Available in 15-ml bottles.
AHFS: 8:12.16 **YB**

ANUSOL® Suppositories/Ointment

Description:

	Anusol Suppositories each contains	Anusol Ointment each gram
Bismuth subgallate	2.25%	—
Bismuth Resorcin Compound	1.75%	—
Benzyl Benzoate	1.2 %	12 mg
Peruvian Balsam	1.8 %	18 mg
Zinc Oxide	11.0 %	110 mg
Analgine™ (pramoxine hydrochloride)	—	10 mg
	Also contains the following inactive ingredients: bismuth subiodide, calcium phosphate and certified coloring in a hydrogenated vegetable oil base.	Also contains the following inactive ingredients: calcium phosphate and kaolin in a liquid petrolatum-cocoa butter-polyethylene wax base containing glyceryl monooleate and glyceryl stearate.

Actions: Anusol Suppositories and Anusol Ointment help to relieve pain, itching and discomfort arising from irritated anorectal tissues. They have a soothing, lubricant action on mucous membranes.
Analgine (pramoxine hydrochloride) in Anusol Ointment is a rapidly acting local anesthetic for the skin and mucous membranes of the anus and rectum. Analgine is also chemically distinct from procaine, cocaine, and dibucaine and can often be used in the patient previously sensitized to other surface anesthetics. Surface analgesia lasts for several hours.

Indications: Anusol Suppositories and Anusol Ointment are adjunctive therapy for the symptomatic relief of pain and discomfort in: external and internal hemorrhoids, proctitis, papillitis, cryptitis, anal fissures, incomplete fistulas, and relief of local pain and discomfort following anorectal surgery.
Anusol Ointment is also indicated for pruritus ani.

Contraindications: Anusol Suppositories and Anusol Ointment are contraindicated in those patients with a history of hypersensitivity to any of the components of the preparations.

Precautions: Symptomatic relief should not delay definitive diagnoses or treatment.
If irritation develops, these preparations should be discontinued. These preparations are not for ophthalmic use.

Adverse Reactions: Upon application of Anusol Ointment which contains Analgine, a patient may occasionally experience burning, especially if the anoderm is not intact. Sensitivity reactions have been rare; discontinue medication if suspected.

Dosage and Administration: Anusol Suppositories—Adults: Remove foil wrapper and insert suppository into the anus. One suppository in the morning and one at bedtime, and one immediately following each evacuation.
Anusol Ointment—Adults: After gentle bathing and drying of the anal area, remove tube cap and apply freely to the exterior surface and gently rub in. For internal use, attach the plastic applicator and insert into the anus by applying gentle continuous pressure. Then squeeze the tube to deliver medication. Ointment should be applied every 3 or 4 hours, or, when necessary, every 2 hours.
NOTE: If staining from either of the above products occurs, the stain may be removed from fabric by hand or machine washing with household detergent.

How Supplied: Anusol Suppositories—boxes of 12 (N 0047-0088-12), 24 (N 0047-0088-24) and 48 (N 0047-0088-48); in silver foil strips with Anusol W/C printed in red.

[*Shown in Product Identification Section*]

Anusol Ointment—one-ounce tubes (N 0047-0075-01) with plastic applicator.
Store between 59°–86° F (15°–30° C).

ANUSOL–HC® SUPPOSITORIES ℞
Hemorrhoidal Suppositories

ANUSOL–HC® CREAM ℞
Rectal Cream
with Hydrocortisone Acetate

Caution: Federal law prohibits dispensing without prescription.

Description:

	Anusol-HC Suppositories each contains	Anusol-HC Cream each gram
Hydrocortisone Acetate	10.0 mg	5.0 mg
Bismuth Subgallate	2.25%	22.5 mg
Bismuth Resorcin Compound	1.75%	17.5 mg
Benzyl Benzoate	1.2 %	12.0 mg
Peruvian Balsam	1.8 %	18.0 mg
Zinc Oxide	11.0 %	110.0 mg
	Also contains the following inactive ingredients: dibasic calcium phosphate, and certified coloring in a hydrogenated vegetable oil base.	Also contains the following inactive ingredients: propylene glycol, propylparaben, methylparaben, polysorbate 60 and sorbitan monostearate in a water-miscible base of mineral oil, glyceryl stearate and water.

Actions: Anusol-HC Suppositories and Anusol-HC Cream help to relieve pain, itching and discomfort arising from irritated anorectal tissues. These preparations have a soothing, lubricant action on mucous membranes, and the antiinflammatory action of hydrocortisone acetate in Anusol-HC helps to reduce hyperemia and swelling.
The hydrocortisone acetate in Anusol-HC is primarily effective because of its antiinflammatory, antipruritic and vasoconstrictive actions.

Indications: Anusol-HC Suppositories and Anusol-HC Cream are adjunctive therapy for the symptomatic relief of pain and discomfort in: external and internal hemorrhoids, proctitis, papillitis, cryptitis, anal fissures, incomplete fistulas and relief of local pain and discomfort following anorectal surgery.
Anusol-HC Cream is also indicated for pruritus ani.
Anusol-HC is especially indicated when inflammation is present. After acute symptoms subside, most patients can be maintained on regular Anusol® Suppositories or Ointment.

Contraindications: Anusol-HC Suppositories and Anusol-HC Cream are contraindicated in those patients with a history of hypersensitivity to any of the components of the preparations.

Warnings: The safe use of topical steroids during pregnancy has not been fully established. Therefore, during pregnancy, they should not be used unnecessarily on extensive areas, in large amounts, or for prolonged periods of time.

Precautions: Symptomatic relief should not delay definitive diagnoses or treatment.
If irritation develops, Anusol-HC Suppositories and Anusol-HC Cream should be discontinued and appropriate therapy instituted.
In the presence of an infection the use of an appropriate antifungal or antibacterial agent should be instituted. If a favorable response does not occur promptly, the corticosteroid should be discontinued until the infection has been adequately controlled.
Care should be taken when using the corticosteroid hydrocortisone acetate in children and infants.
Anusol-HC is not for ophthalmic use.

Dosage and Administration: Anusol-HC Suppositories—Adults: Remove foil wrapper

Continued on next page

This product information was prepared in August, 1979. On these and other Parke-Davis Products, detailed information may be obtained by addressing PARKE-DAVIS, Division of Warner-Lambert Company, Morris Plains, NJ 07950.

Parke-Davis—Cont.

and insert suppository into the anus. One suppository in the morning and one at bedtime, for 3 to 6 days or until inflammation subsides. Then maintain patient comfort with regular Anusol Suppositories.
Anusol-HC Cream—Adults: After gentle bathing and drying of the anal area, remove tube cap and apply to the exterior surface and gently rub in. For internal use, attach the plastic applicator and insert into the anus by applying gentle continuous pressure. Then squeeze the tube to deliver medication. Cream should be applied 3 or 4 times a day for 3 to 6 days until inflammation subsides. Then maintain patient comfort with regular Anusol Ointment.
How Supplied: Anusol-HC Suppositories—boxes of 12 (N 0047-0089-12) and boxes of 24 (0047-0089-24); in silver foil strips with Anusol-HC W/C printed in black.
[*Shown in Product Identification Section*]
Anusol-HC Cream—one-ounce tube (N 0047-0090-01); with plastic applicator.
Store between 59°–86° F (15°–30° C).
[*Shown in Product Identification Section*]

APLISOL® ℞
(tuberculin purified protein derivative, diluted)
Stabilized Solution

For complete product information, consult Diagnostic Products Information Section.

APLITEST® ℞
(tuberculin purified protein derivative)
Multiple-Puncture Device

For complete product information, consult Diagnostic Products Information Section.

AZO-MANDELAMINE® ℞
methenamine mandelate & phenazopyridine hydrochloride

Caution: Federal law prohibits dispensing without prescription.
Description: Each tablet contains 500 mg methenamine mandelate (Mandelamine®) and 50 mg phenazopyridine hydrochloride (Pyridium®).
Actions: Azo-Mandelamine conveniently combines the urinary analgesic Pyridium (phenazopyridine hydrochloride) with the urinary antibacterial Mandelamine (methenamine mandelate). Methenamine mandelate is excreted by the kidney as mandelic acid and methenamine. In an acid urine, the excreted mandelic acid provides antibacterial action and contributes to acidification. In an acid urine, methenamine is hydrolyzed to ammonia and the bactericidal agent formaldehyde. If acidification of the urine is not attained, there will be no antibacterial effect (see Dosage and Management). The analgesic component, phenazopyridine hydrochloride, is also excreted in the urine, where it exerts a topical analgesic effect on the mucosa of the urinary tract. This action helps to relieve pain, burning, urgency and frequency. Phenazopyridine hydrochloride (Pyridium) may reduce or eliminate the need for systemic analgesics or narcotics and can help to relieve symptoms before the infection is controlled.
Indications: Azo-Mandelamine is indicated for urinary tract infections, such as cystitis, or postoperative infection, in which analgesic relief of symptoms as well as suppression or elimination of bacteriuria is required. Azo-Mandelamine should not be used for repeated or prolonged treatment without full diagnostic investigation.
Contraindications: Renal insufficiency. A yellowish tinge of the skin or sclerae may indicate accumulation due to impaired renal excretion and the need to discontinue therapy.
Precautions: Overacidification and/or higher than recommended dosage may cause symptoms of urinary tract irritation.
Adverse Reactions: Occasional gastrointestinal disturbances or generalized skin rash.
Dosage and Management: The average adult dosage is two tablets 4 times a day, after meals and at bedtime.
When symptomatic therapy is no longer required, Mandelamine (methenamine mandelate) alone should be used. Since an acid urine is essential for antibacterial activity with maximum effect at pH 5.5 or below, restriction of alkalinizing foods or medication is desirable. If testing of urine pH reveals the need, supplemental acidification should be given. When acidification is contraindicated or unattainable (as with some urea-splitting bacteria), the drug is not recommended.
Note: Patients should be told that Azo-Mandelamine produces a reddish-orange discoloration of the urine.
Supplied: Red, enteric-coated capsule-shaped tablets in bottles of 100 (N 0047-0175-51).
Store between 59° and 86°F (15° and 30°C).
[*Shown in Product Identification Section*]
367 G 123 **R-1-78**

BENADRYL® ℞
(diphenhydramine hydrochloride USP)
Kapseals®
Capsules
Elixir
Parenteral

Description: Benadryl (diphenhydramine hydrochloride) is 2-(diphenylmethoxy)-N, N-dimethylethylamine hydrochloride, occurs as a white, crystalline powder, and is freely soluble in water and alcohol.
Actions: Diphenhydramine hydrochloride is an antihistamine with anticholinergic (drying) and sedative side effects. Antihistamines appear to compete with histamine for cell receptor sites on effector cells.
Indications: *Oral:* Benadryl in the oral form is effective for the following indications.
Antihistaminic: For perennial and seasonal (hay fever) allergic rhinitis; vasomotor rhinitis, allergic conjunctivitis due to inhalant allergens and foods: mild, uncomplicated allergic skin manisfestations of urticaria and angioedema; amelioration of allergic reactions to blood or plasma, dermatographism; as therapy for anaphylactic reactions *adjunctive* to epinephrine and other standard measures after the acute manifestations have been controlled
Motion sickness: For active and prophylactic treatment of motion sickness
Antiparkinsonism: For parkinsonism (including drug-induced extrapyramidal reactions) in the elderly unable to tolerate more potent agents; mild cases of parkinsonism (including drug-induced) in other age groups; in other cases of parkinsonsim (including drug-induced) in combination with centrally acting anticholinergic agents
Parenteral: Benadryl in the injectable form is effective for the following conditions when Benadryl in the oral form is impractical.
Antihistaminic: For amelioration of allergic reactions to blood or plasma; in anaphylaxis as an adjunct to epinephrine and other standard measures after the acute symptoms have been controlled; and for other uncomplicated allergic conditions of the immediate type when oral therapy is impossible or contraindicated.
Motion Sickness: For active treatment of motion sickness
Antiparkinsonism: For use in parkinsonism when oral therapy is impossible or contraindicated, as follows: parkinsonism in the elderly who are unable to tolerate more potent agents, mild cases of parkinsonism in other age groups, and in other cases of parkinsonism in combinaton with centrally acting anticholinergic agents.
Contraindications: ***Oral and Parenteral:***
Usage in Newborn or Premature Infants: This drug should *not* be used in newborn or premature infants.
Usage in Nursing Mothers: Because of the higher risk of antihistamines for infants generally, and for newborns and prematures in particular, antihistamine therapy is contraindicated in nursing mothers.
Usage in Lower Respiratory Disease: Antihistamines *should NOT* be used to treat lower respiratory tract symptoms, including asthma.
Antihistamines are also contraindicated in the following conditions.
Hypersensitivity to diphenhydramine hydrochloride and other antihistamines of similar chemical structure
Monoamine oxidase inhibitor therapy (See Drug Interactions section.)
Warnings: ***Oral and Parenteral:*** Antihistamines should be used with considerable caution in patients with narrow-angle glaucoma, stenosing peptic ulcer, pyloroduodenal obstruction, symptomatic prostatic hypertrophy, bladder-neck obstruction.
Usage in Children: In infants and children, especially, antihistamines in *overdosage* may cause hallucinations, convulsions, or death.
As in adults, antihistamines may diminish mental alertness in children. In the young child, particularly, antihistamines may produce excitation.
Usage in Pregnancy: Experience with this drug in pregnant women is inadequate to determine whether there exists a potential for harm to the developing fetus.
Usage With CNS Depressants: Diphenhydramine hydrochloride has additive effects with alcohol and other CNS depressants (hypnotics, sedatives, tranquilizers, etc).
Usage in Activities Requiring Mental Alertness: Patients should be warned about engaging in activities requiring mental alertness, such as driving a car or operating appliances, machinery, etc.
Usage in the Elderly (approximately 60 years or older): Antihistamines are more likely to cause dizziness, sedation, and hypotension in elderly patients.
Precautions: ***Oral and Parenteral:*** Diphenhydramine hydrochloride has an atropine-like action and, therefore, should be used with caution in patients with a history of bronchial asthma, increased intraocular pressure, hyperthyroidism, cardiovascular disease, hypertension.
Drug Interactions: ***Oral and Parenteral:*** MAO inhibitors prolong and intensify the anticholinergic (drying) effects of antihistamines.
Adverse Reactions: ***Oral and Parenteral:*** The most frequent adverse reactions are underscored.

1. *General:* Urticaria, drug rash, anaphylactic shock, photosensitivity, excessive perspiration, chills, dryness of mouth, nose, and throat
2. *Cardiovascular System:* Hypotension, headache, palpitations, tachycardia, extrasystoles
3. *Hematologic System:* Hemolytic anemia, thrombocytopenia, agranulocytosis
4. *Nervous System:* Sedation, sleepiness, dizziness, disturbed coordination, fatigue, confusion, restlessness, excitation, nervousness, tremor, irritability, insomnia, euphoria, paresthesia, blurred vision, diplopia, vertigo, tinnitus, acute labyrinthitis, hysteria, neuritis, convulsions
5. *G I System:* Epigastric distress, anorexia, nausea, vomiting, diarrhea, constipation
6. *G U System:* Urinary frequency, difficult urination, urinary retention, early menses
7. *Respiratory System:* Thickening of bronchial secretions, tightness of chest and wheezing, nasal stuffiness

Overdosage: ***Oral and Parenteral:*** Antihistamine overdosage reactions may vary from central nervous system depression to stimulation. Stimulation is particularly likely in children. Atropine-like signs and symptoms—dry mouth; fixed, dilated pupils; flushing—and gastrointestinal symptoms may also occur.

Stimulants should *not* be used.

Vasopressors may be used to treat hypotension.

For antihistamines administered orally:

If vomiting has not occurred spontaneously, the patient should be induced to vomit. This is best done by having him drink a glass of water or milk, after which he should be made to gag. Precautions against aspiration must be taken, especially in infants and children.

If vomiting is unsuccessful, gastric lavage is indicated within three hours after ingestion and even later, if large amounts of milk or cream were given beforehand. Isotonic and one half isontonic saline is the lavage solution of choice.

Saline cathartics, as milk of magnesia, by osmosis, draw water into the bowel and, therefore, are valuable for their action in rapid dilution of bowel content.

Dosage and Administration: ***Oral and Parenteral:***

DOSAGE SHOULD BE INDIVIDUALIZED ACCORDING TO THE NEEDS AND THE RESPONSE OF THE PATIENT.

Oral:

A single, oral dose of diphenhydramine hydrochloride is quickly absorbed with maximum activity occurring in approximately one hour. The duration of activity following an average dose of Benadryl (diphenhydramine hydrochloride) is from four to six hours.

ADULTS: 50 mg three or four times daily

CHILDREN (over 20 lb): 12.5 to 25 mg three to four times daily. Maximum daily dosage not to exceed 300 mg. For physicians who wish to calculate the dose on the basis of body weight or surface area, the recommended dosage is 5 mg/kg/24 hours or 150 mg/m^2/24 hours.

The basis for determining the most effective dosage regimen will be the response of the patient to medication and the condition under treatment.

In motion sickness, full dosage is recommended for prophylactic use, the first dose to be given 30 minutes before exposure to motion and similar doses before meals and upon retiring for the duration of exposure.

Parenteral: Benadryl in the injectable form is indicated when the oral form is impractical.

CHILDREN: 5 mg/kg/24 hours or 150 mg/m^2/24 hours. Maximum daily dosage is 300 mg. Divide into four doses, administered intravenously or deeply intramuscularly.

ADULTS: 10 to 50 mg intravenously or deeply intramuscularly; 100 mg if required; maximum daily dosage is 400 mg.

How Supplied:

Benadryl (diphenhydramine hydrochloride) is supplied in the oral form as:

N 0071-0373-24—bottle of 100
N 0071-0373-32—bottle of 1000
N 0071-0373-40—unit-dose (ten 10s)

Each capsule contains 50 mg diphenhydramine hydrochloride.

N 0071-0471-24—bottle of 100
N 0071-0471-32—bottle of 1000
N 0071-0471-40—unit-dose (ten 10s)

Each capsule contains 25 mg diphenhydramine hydrochloride.

[*Shown in Product Identification Section*]

Benadryl is also supplied in the following forms:

N 0071-0378-24—bottle of 100

Each capsule contains 50 mg diphenhydramine hydrochloride and 25 mg ephedrine sulfate.

N 0071-2220-17—4-oz bottle
N 0071-2220-23—pt bottle
N 0071-2220-32—gal bottle

Each 5 ml of elixir contains 12.5 mg diphenhydramine hydrochloride with 14% alcohol.

WL/YA

Benadryl in parenteral form is supplied as:

N 0071-4015-10 (10-ml vial)
N 0071-4015-13 (30-ml vial)

Sterile solution for parenteral use containing 10 mg diphenhydramine hydrochloride in each milliliter of solution with 0.1 mg/ml benzethonium chloride as a germicidal agent. Supplied in multiple-dose vials (Steri-Vials).

N 0071-4402-10 1-ml ampoule

Sterile solution for parenteral use containing 50 mg diphenhydramine hydrochloride in each milliliter of solution with 0.1 mg/ml benzethonium chloride as a germicidal agent. Supplied in multiple-dose vials (Steri-Vials).

N 0071-4259-03 (Ampoule 259)

Sterile solution for parenteral use containing 50 mg diphenhydramine hydrochloride. Supplied in packages of 10.

N 0071-4259-40 Steri-Dose Disposable Syringe (individual cartons)

N 0071-4259-41 Steri-Dose Disposable Syringe (two trays of five syringes each)

Sterile solution for parenteral use containing 50 mg diphenhydramine hydrochloride in a 1-ml disposable syringe. Supplied in packages of 10.

The pH of the solutions for parenteral use have been adjusted with either sodium hydroxide or hydrochloric acid. **YC**

BENYLIN® COUGH SYRUP ℞

Each 5 ml contains:

Benadryl® (diphenhydramine hydrochloride) .... 12.5 mg
Alcohol 5%

Also contains, as inactive ingredients, sugar; water; glucose liquid; glycerin; ammonium chloride; sodium citrate; raspberry imitation flavor; sodium saccharin; citric acid; caramel; menthol; FD&C Red No. 40; and D&C Red No. 33.

Description: Diphenhydramine hydrochloride is a chemical compound, 2-(diphenylmethoxy)-N, N-dimethylethylamine hydrochloride.

Actions: Diphenhydramine hydrochloride is a potent antihistaminic agent, which also possesses an antitussive action.

Indications: Benylin Cough Syrup is indicated as an antitussive for the control of cough due to colds or allergy.

> Based on a review of this drug by the National Academy of Sciences - National Research Council and/or other information, FDA has classified this indication as follows.
>
> There is a lack of substantial evidence that this fixed combination drug has the effect purported. Final classification of the less-than-effective indication requires further investigation.

Contraindications:

Usage in Newborn or Premature Infants

This drug should not be used in newborn or premature infants.

Usage in Nursing Mothers

Because of the higher risk of antihistamines for infants generally, and for newborns and prematures in particular, antihistamine therapy is contraindicated in nursing mothers.

Usage in Lower Respiratory Disease

Antihistamines *should NOT* be used to treat lower respiratory tract symptoms, including asthma.

Antihistamines are also contraindicated in the following conditions.

Hypersensitivity to diphenhydramine hydrochloride and other antihistamines of similar chemical structure.

Monoamine oxidase inhibitor therapy (See **Drug Interactions** section.)

Warnings: Antihistamines should be used with considerable caution in patients with narrow-angle glaucoma, stenosing peptic ulcer, symptomatic prostatic hypertrophy, bladderneck obstruction, or pyloroduodenal obstruction.

Usage in Children

In infants and children, especially, antihistamines in *overdosage* may cause hallucinations, convulsions, or death.

As in adults, antihistamines may diminish mental alertness in children. In the young child, particularly, antihistamines may produce excitation.

Usage in Pregnancy

Experience with this drug in pregnant women is inadequate to determine whether there exists a potential for harm to the developing fetus.

Usage with CNS Depressants

Diphenhydramine hydrochloride has additive effects with alcohol and other CNS depressants (hypnotics, sedatives, tranquilizers, etc).

Usage in Activities Requiring Mental Alertness

Patients should be warned about engaging in activities requiring mental alertness, such as driving a car or operating appliances, machinery, etc.

Usage in the Elderly (approximately 60 years or older)

Antihistamines are more likely to cause dizziness, sedation, and hypotension in elderly patients.

Precautions: Diphenhydramine hydrochloride has an atropine-like action and, therefore, should be used with caution in patients with a history of bronchial asthma, increased intraocular pressure, hyperthyroidism, cardiovascular disease, or hypertension.

Drug Interactions: MAO inhibitors prolong and intensify the anticholinergic (drying) effects of antihistamines.

Adverse Reactions: The most frequent adverse reactions are underlined.

1. *General:* Urticaria; drug rash; anaphylactic shock; photosensitivity; excessive perspiration; chills; dryness of mouth, nose, and throat
2. *Cardiovascular System:* Hypotension, headache, palpitations, tachycardia, extrasystoles
3. *Hematologic System:* Hemolytic anemia, thrombocytopenia, agranulocytosis
4. *Nervous System:* Sedation, sleepiness, dizziness, disturbed coordination, fatigue, confusion, restlessness, excitation, nervousness, tremor, irritability, insomnia, euphoria, paresthesias, blurred vision, diplopia, vertigo, tinnitus, acute labyrinthitis, hysteria, neuritis, convulsions
5. *GI System:* Epigastric distress, anorexia, nausea, vomiting, diarrhea, constipation
6. *GU System:* Urinary frequency, difficult urination, urinary retention, early menses
7. *Respiratory System:* Thickening of bronchial secretions, tightness of chest and wheezing, nasal stuffiness

Overdosage: Antihistamine overdosage reactions may vary from central nervous system depression to stimulation. Stimulation is particularly likely in children. Atropine-like signs

Continued on next page

This product information was prepared in August, 1979. On these and other Parke-Davis Products, detailed information may be obtained by addressing PARKE-DAVIS, Division of Warner-Lambert Company, Morris Plains, NJ 07950.

Parke-Davis—Cont.

and symptoms, such as dry mouth; fixed, dilated pupils; flushing; and gastrointestinal symptoms, may also occur.

If vomiting has not occurred spontaneously, the patient should be induced to vomit. This is best done by having him drink a glass of water or milk, after which he should be made to gag. Precautions against aspiration must be taken, especially in infants and children.

If vomiting is unsuccessful, gastric lavage is indicated within three hours after ingestion and even later if large amounts of milk or cream were given beforehand. Isotonic or one half isotonic saline is the lavage solution of choice. *Saline cathartics,* such as milk of magnesia, draw water into the bowel by osmosis and, therefore, are valuable for their action in rapid dilution of bowel content.

Stimulants should *not* be used.

Vasopressors may be used to treat hypotension.

Dosage and Administration:

Usual Dosage:

Adults — Two teaspoonfuls (10 ml) every 4 hours, not to exceed eight teaspoonfuls in 24 hours

Children — 6 to under 12 years of age: one teaspoonful (5 ml) every 4 hours, not to exceed four teaspoonfuls in 24 hours

Children — 2 to under 6 years of age: one half teaspoonful (2.5 ml) every 4 hours, not to exceed two teaspoonfuls in 24 hours

Usage in children under 2 years of age is only at the discretion of the physician.

How Supplied: Benylin Cough Syrup is supplied in 4-oz, 1-pt, 1-gal bottles, and unit-dose bottles of 5 ml and 10 ml. N 0071-2195

(4 oz only: NSN 6505-00-687-4469)

AHFS 48:00 YA

BETAPAR® ℞

(meprednisone tablets, NF)

Description: Glucocorticoids are adrenocortical steroids, both naturally occurring and synthetic, which are readily absorbed from the gastrointestinal tract. The formula for meprednisone is $C_{22}H_{28}O_5$. Chemically, meprednisone is pregna-1,4-diene-3,11,20-trione,17,21-dihydroxy-16-methyl-,(16β).

Meprednisone occurs as a white to creamy white, odorless powder and has a molecular weight of 372.46. Meprednisone melts at about 200 C with decomposition. Meprednisone is very slightly soluble in water and ether; soluble in alcohol and dioxane; and freely soluble in chloroform. Each Betapar Tablet contains 4 mg of meprednisone, NF.

Actions: Naturally occurring glucocorticoids (hydrocortisone and cortisone), which also have salt-retaining properties, are used as replacement therapy in adrenocortical deficiency states. Their synthetic analogs, such as meprednisone, are primarily used for their potent anti-inflammatory effects in disorders of many organ systems.

Glucocorticoids, such as meprednisone, cause profound and varied metabolic effects. In addition, they modify the body's immune responses to diverse stimuli.

Indications:

Endocrine disorders: primary or secondary adrenocortical insufficiency (hydrocortisone or cortisone is the first choice; synthetic analogs may be used in conjunction with mineralocorticoids where applicable; in infancy, mineralocorticoid supplementation is of particular importance); congenital adrenal hyperplasia; nonsuppurative thyroiditis; hypercalcemia associated with cancer

Rheumatic disorders: as adjunctive therapy for short-term administration (to tide the patient over an acute episode or exacerbation) in psoriatic arthritis; rheumatoid arthritis, including juvenile rheumatoid arthritis (selected cases may require low-dose maintenance therapy); ankylosing spondylitis; acute and subacute bursitis; acute nonspecific tenosynovitis; acute gouty arthritis; posttraumatic osteoarthritis; synovitis of osteoarthritis; epicondylitis

Collagen diseases: during an exacerbation or as maintenance therapy in selected cases of systemic lupus erythematosus; acute rheumatic carditis

Dermatologic diseases: pemphigus; bullous dermatitis herpetiformis; severe erythema multiforme (Stevens-Johnson syndrome); exfoliative dermatitis; mycosis fungoides; severe psoriasis; severe seborrheic dermatitis

Allergic states: control of severe or incapacitating allergic conditions intractable to adequate trials of conventional treatment; seasonal or perennial allergic rhinitis; bronchial asthma; contact dermatitis; atopic dermatitis; and serum sickness; drug hypersensitivity reactions

Ophthalmic diseases: severe, acute and chronic allergic and inflammatory processes involving the eye and its adnexa, such as allergic conjunctivitis; keratitis; allergic corneal marginal ulcers; herpes zoster ophthalmicus; iritis and iridocyclitis; chorioretinitis; anterior segment inflammation; diffuse posterior uveitis and choroiditis; optic neuritis; sympathetic ophthalmia

Respiratory diseases: symptomatic sarcoidosis; Loeffler's syndrome not manageable by other means; berylliosis; fulminating or disseminated pulmonary tuberculosis when used concurrently with appropriate antituberculous chemotherapy; aspiration pneumonitis

Hematologic disorders: idiopathic thrombocytopenic in adults: secondary thrombocytopenia in adults; acquired (autoimmune) hemolytic anemia; erythroblastopenia (RBC anemia); congenital (erythroid) hypoplastic anemia

Neoplastic diseases: for palliative management of leukemias and lymphomas in adults; acute leukemia of childhood

Edematous states: to induce a diuresis or remission of proteinuria in the nephrotic syndrome, without uremia, of the idiopathic type or that due to lupus erythematosus

Gastrointestinal diseases: to tide the patient over a critical period of the disease in ulcerative colitis; regional enteritis

Miscellaneous: tuberculous meningitis with subarachnoid block or impending block when used concurrently with appropriate antituberculous chemotherapy; trichinosis with neurologic or myocardial involvement

In addition to the above indications, Betapar Tablets are indicated for systemic dermatomyositis (polymyositis).

Contraindications: Betapar (meprednisone) Tablets are contraindicated in systemic fungal infections.

Warnings: In patients on corticosteroid therapy subjected to unusual stress, increased dosage of rapidly acting corticosteroids before, during, and after the stressful situation is indicated.

Corticosteroids may mask some signs of infection, and new infections may appear during their use. There may be decreased resistance and inability to localize infection when corticosteroids are used.

Prolonged use of corticosteroids may produce posterior subcapsular cataracts, glaucoma with possible damage to the optic nerves, and may enhance the establishment of secondary ocular infections due to fungi or viruses.

Usage in pregnancy: Because adequate human reproduction studies have not been done with corticosteroids, the use of these drugs in pregnancy, nursing mothers, or women of childbearing potential requires that the possible benefits of the drug be weighed against the potential hazards to the mother and embryo or fetus. Infants born of mothers who have received substantial doses of corticosteroids during pregnancy should be carefully observed for signs of hypoadrenalism.

Average and large doses of hydrocortisone or cortisone can cause elevation of blood pressure, salt and water retention, and increased excretion of potassium. These effects are less likely to occur with the synthetic derivatives except when used in large doses. Dietary salt restriction and potassium supplementation may be necessary. All corticosteroids increase calcium excretion.

While on corticosteroid therapy, patients should not be vaccinated against smallpox. Other immunization procedures should not be undertaken in patients who are on corticosteroids, especially on high doses, because of possible hazards of neurological complications and a lack of antibody response.

The use of Betapar Tablets in active tuberculosis should be restricted to those cases of fulminating or disseminated tuberculosis in which the corticosteroid is used for the management of the disease in conjunction with an appropriate antituberculous regimen.

If corticosteroids are indicated in patients with latent tuberculosis or tuberculin reactivity, close observation is necessary as reactivation of the disease may occur. During prolonged corticosteroid therapy, these patients should receive chemoprophylaxis.

Precautions: Drug-induced secondary adrenocortical insufficiency may be minimized by gradual reduction of dosage. This type of relative insufficiency may persist for months after discontinuation of therapy; therefore, in any situation of stress occurring during that period, hormone therapy should be reinstituted. Because mineralocorticoid secretion may be impaired, salt and/or a mineralocorticoid should be administered concurrently.

There is an enhanced effect of corticosteroids on patients with hypothyroidism and in those with cirrhosis.

Corticosteroids should be used cautiously in patients with ocular herpes simplex because of possible corneal perforation.

The lowest possible dose of corticosteroid should be used to control the condition under treatment, and when reduction in dosage is possible, the reduction should be gradual.

Psychic derangements may appear when corticosteroids are used, ranging from euphoria, insomnia, mood swings, personality changes, and severe depression, to frank psychotic manifestations. Also, existing emotional instability or psychotic tendencies may be aggravated by corticosteroids.

Aspirin should be used cautiously in conjunction with corticosteroids in hypoprothrombinemia.

Steroids should be used with caution in nonspecific ulcerative colitis, if there is a probability of impending perforation, abscess, or other pyogenic infection; diverticulitis; fresh intestinal anastomoses; active or latent peptic ulcer; renal insufficiency; hypertension; osteoporosis; and myasthenia gravis.

Growth and development of infants and children on prolonged corticosteroid therapy should be carefully observed.

Adverse Reactions:

Fluid and electrolyte disturbances: sodium retention, fluid retention, congestive heart failure in susceptible patients, potassium loss, hypokalemic alkalosis, hypertension

Musculoskeletal: muscle weakness, steroid myopathy, loss of muscle mass, osteoporosis, vertebral compression fractures, aseptic necrosis of femoral and humeral heads, pathologic fracture of long bones

Gastrointestinal: peptic ulcer with possible perforation and hemorrhage, pancreatitis, abdominal distention, ulcerative esophagitis

Dermatologic: impaired wound healing, thin fragile skin, petechiae and ecchymoses, facial erythema, increased sweating, may suppress reactions to skin tests

Neurological: convulsions, increased intracranial pressure with papilledema (pseudotumor cerebri) usually after treatment, vertigo, headache
Endocrine: menstrual irregularities; development of Cushingoid state; suppression of growth in children; secondary adrenocortical and pituitary unresponsiveness, particularly in times of stress, as in trauma, surgery, or illness; decreased carbohydrate tolerance; manifestations of latent diabetes mellitus; increased requirements of insulin or oral hypoglycemic agents in diabetes
Ophthalmic: posterior subcapsular cataracts, increased intraocular pressure, glaucoma, exophthalmos
Metabolic: negative nitrogen balance due to protein catabolism
Dosage and Administration: The initial dosage of Betapar (meprednisone) may vary from 8 to 60 mg per day depending on the specific disease entity being treated. In situations of less severity, lower doses will generally suffice, while in selected patients, higher initial doses may be required. The initial dosage should be maintained or adjusted until a satisfactory response is noted. If after a reasonable period of time there is a lack of satisfactory clinical response, Betapar should be discontinued and the patient transferred to other appropriate therapy. **It should be emphasized that dosage requirements are variable and must be individualized on the basis of the disease under treatment and the response of the patient.** After a favorable response is noted, the proper maintenance dosage should be determined by decreasing the initial drug dosage in small increments at appropriate time intervals until the lowest dosage which will maintain an adequate clinical response is reached. It should be kept in mind that constant monitoring is needed in regard to drug dosage. Included in the situations which may make dosage adjustments necessary are changes in clinical status secondary to remissions or exacerbations in the disease process, the patient's individual drug responsiveness, and the effect of patient exposure to stressful situations not directly related to the disease entity under treatment; in this latter situation it may be necessary to increase the dosage of Betapar for a period of time consistent with the patient's condition. If after long-term therapy the drug is to be stopped, it is recommended that it be withdrawn gradually rather than abruptly.
How Supplied: N 0071-0636-24—Betapar (Tablet 636) is supplied as 4-mg scored tablets, in bottles of 100. Betapar is manufactured according to Parke-Davis specifications and Quality Control procedures by Schering Corporation, Kenilworth, NJ 07033. Parcode® No. 636
AHFS 68:04 **UC**

APLISOL® ℞
(tuberculin purified protein derivative, diluted)
Stabilized Solution

For complete prescribing information, consult Diagnostic Products Information Section.

APLITEST® ℞
(tuberculin, purified protein derivative)
Multiple-Puncture Device

For complete prescribing information, consult Diagnostic Products Information Section.

FLUOGEN® ℞
(influenza virus vaccine)
Immunizing Antigen, Ether Extracted Subvirion

For further information, consult alphabetical product monograph.

GAMULIN® Rh ℞
(Rh_0[D] immune globulin [human])

For complete prescribing information, consult alphabetical product monograph.

HUMAFAC® ℞
(antihemophilic factor [human])

For complete prescribing information, consult alphabetical product monograph.

IMMU-G® ℞
(immune serum globulin [human], USP)
gamma globulin (human)

For complete prescribing information, consult alphabetical product monograph.

NORMAL SERUM ALBUMIN (HUMAN) ALBUSPAN® ℞

For complete prescribing information, consult alphabetical product monograph.

POISON IVY EXTRACT ℞

Description: Poison Ivy Extract consists of the toluene-absolute, alcohol-soluble irritating principle from the leaves of *Rhus toxicodendron* (poison ivy, poison oak) dissolved in sterile almond oil. Chloretone® (chlorobutanol), 0.6%, is included as a preservative. The activity is controlled by biological assay.
How Supplied: Poison Ivy Extract is supplied as:
N 0071-4397-03 (Bio 397)—1-ml rubber diaphragm-capped vial. **AH**

TETANUS TOXOID ADSORBED ℞

Description: Tetanus Toxoid Adsorbed is prepared by detoxifying tetanus toxin, produced by growing *Clostridium tetani* in Modified Mueller's (meat-free) semisynthetic medium with formaldehyde. The toxoid is refined by ultrafiltration and 5 L_f adsorbed under controlled conditions on 2.5 mg of aluminum phosphate suspension in saline per 0.5-ml dose. Thimerosal (mercury derivative), 0.01%, is included as a preservative. This product meets all applicable standards.
How Supplied: Tetanus Toxoid Adsorbed is supplied as:
N 0071-4124-08 (Bio 2124)........................ 5 ml
(five immunizations);
N 0071-4124-40 (Bio 1377)........................ 0.5 ml
Steri-Dose® Disposable Syringe.

THROMBIN, TOPICAL ℞
(thrombin, USP)
bovine origin

For complete prescribing information, consult alphabetical product monograph.

TRIOGEN® ℞
(diphtheria and tetanus toxoids and pertussis vaccine adsorbed)

Description: Triogen (diphtheria and tetanus toxoids and pertussis vaccine adsorbed) is a combination of three antigens—diphtheria toxoid, tetanus toxoid, and pertussis vaccine—in which the diphtheria and tetanus toxoids prepared from toxin produced in semisynthetic media have been highly purified by ultrafiltration, adsorbed on preformed aluminum phosphate in saline in standardized proportions, and combined with pertussis vaccine.
How Supplied: Triogen (diphtheria and tetanus toxoids and pertussis vaccine adsorbed) is supplied as:
N 0071-4192-09 (Bio 2092)........................ 7.5 ml

* * * * *

BRONDECON® ℞
oxtriphylline and guaifenesin

Caution: Federal law prohibits dispensing without prescription.
Description: Each tablet contains 200 mg oxtriphylline and 100 mg guaifenesin. Each 5 ml teaspoonful of elixir contains 100 mg oxtriphylline and 50 mg guaifenesin; alcohol 20%.
NOTE: 100 mg oxtriphylline is equivalent to 64 mg anhydrous theophylline.
Actions: Brondecon, a bronchodilator and expectorant, helps to relieve symptoms of bronchospasm as well as obstruction caused by viscid mucus in the bronchioles.
Oxtriphylline, the choline salt of theophylline, is a xanthine bronchodilating agent. Compared to aminophylline, oxtriphylline is less irritating to the gastric mucosa, better absorbed from the gastrointestinal tract, more stable and more soluble. The expectorant component of Brondecon is guaifenesin, which tends to increase the secretion and decrease the viscosity of fluids of the respiratory tract. These physiologic fluids help to lubricate the inflamed mucous membranes of the bronchi and also help the patient to expel viscid mucus thus making cough more productive.
Indications: Brondecon is an adjunct in the management of bronchitis, bronchial asthma, asthmatic bronchitis, pulmonary emphysema, and similar chronic obstructive lung disease. It is indicated when both relaxation of bronchospasm and expectorant action are desirable.
Precautions: Concurrent use of other xanthine preparations may lead to adverse reactions, particularly CNS stimulation in children.
Adverse Reactions: Gastric distress and, occasionally, palpitation and CNS stimulation have been reported.
Dosage: Tablets—over 12 years of age: one tablet, 4 times a day.
Elixir—over 12 years of age: two teaspoonfuls, 4 times a day; from 2 to 12 years: one teaspoonful per 60 lb body weight, 4 times a day.
Above recommendations are averages. Dosage should be individualized.
Supplied: Salmon-pink tablets in bottles of 100 (N 0047-0200-51). Elixir, dark red, cherry-flavored in 237 ml (8 fl oz) (N 0047-0201-08) and 474 ml (16 fl oz) (N 0047-0201-16) bottles.
Store between 59° and 86°F (15° and 30°C).
[*Shown in Product Identification Section*]
306 G 574 R-1-78

KAPSEALS® CARBRITAL® Ⓒ ℞

Each Carbrital Kapseal contains:
Pentobarbital sodium .... 1½ grains
Carbromal .... 4 grains
Description: Pentobarbital sodium is the sodium salt of 5-ethyl-5-(1-methylbutyl) barbituric acid. Carbromal is bromdiethylacetylurea, a nonbarbiturate, brominated monoureide.
Action: Pentobarbital sodium is primarily a short-acting hypnotic with some prolonged mild sedative activity. Carbromal is primarily a sedative with some mild hypnotic activity.

INDICATIONS
Based on a review of this drug by the National Academy of Sciences—National Research Council and/or other information, FDA has classified the indications as follows.

Continued on next page

This product information was prepared in August, 1979. On these and other Parke-Davis Products, detailed information may be obtained by addressing PARKE-DAVIS, Division of Warner-Lambert Company, Morris Plains, NJ 07950.

Parke-Davis—Cont.

> "Possibly" effective:
> Carbrital is indicated as a sedative and hypnotic for insomnia.
> Final classification of the less-than-effective indications requires further investigation.

Contraindications: Carbrital is contraindicated in the following conditions: hypersensitivity to barbiturates and/or carbromal; known previous addiction to sedative-hypnotics; latent or manifest porphyria or familial history of intermittent porphyria; uncontrolled pain; history of confusion or restlessness from hypnotics; history of abnormal reaction to barbiturates; severe pulmonary insufficiency; premonitory signs of hepatic coma.

Warning: May be habit-forming

Precautions: Carbrital should be used with caution in patients with severely impaired liver function, severe anemia, congestive heart failure, fever, neuroses, hyperthyroidism, diabetes mellitus, and any condition in which respiratory depression may be characteristic.

Marked excitement, rather than depression, may occur in aged or debilitated patients, particularly those with cerebral arteriosclerosis.

Confusion or euphoria may result if dosage is not adequate to produce sleep. Symptoms of mentally ill, phobic, and emotionally disturbed patients may be accentuated. Prolonged usage may produce psychological habituation. Sudden discontinuation or radical reduction of dosage may precipitate withdrawal symptoms in patients who have taken the drug for prolonged periods; dosage should be gradually reduced to the point of complete discontinuation.

Barbiturates should be prescribed with extreme caution for persons known or suspected of routinely or periodically consuming large quantities of alcoholic beverages. Potentiation of effect, even to the extent of causing death, may result from consumption of barbiturates by patients with high serum alcohol levels.

Carbrital should be prescribed with great caution, or not at all, for persons with suicidal tendencies, a predilection for excessive use of medications, or the likelihood of becoming drug-dependent.

The effects of Carbrital may be increased by many drugs, including antihistamines, tranquilizers, corticosteroids, monoamine oxidase inhibitors, narcotic analgesics, amitriptyline, imipramine, and rauwolfia alkaloids.

Carbromal is metabolized in the body to yield free bromide ion. Accumulation of bromide as a result of prolonged use may result in the development of bromism.

Barbiturates readily cross the placental barrier and, if administered during labor, may have a depressant effect on the fetus; infants born of mothers receiving barbiturates may have difficulty breathing spontaneously. Following large doses, small amounts of barbiturates are found in the milk of nursing mothers.

Positive direct Coombs test results have been reported occasionally in patients receiving Carbrital; hemolysis has not been demonstrated or reported.

Adverse Reactions: Allergic dermatoses, undue lassitude, vertigo, nausea, vomiting, diarrhea, headache, excitement, hangover, and pain (myalgia, neuralgia, arthralgia) have been reported. Hypersensitivity reactions occur occasionally; they are more likely to appear in patients with asthma, urticaria, or angioneurotic edema. Jaundice is occasionally seen in patients who have become hypersensitive to barbiturates or who are suffering from barbiturate poisoning. Long-continued use of Carbrital could result in bromism, which is characterized by numerous toxic manifestations, such as impaired mental processes; delirium; delusions; auditory and visual hallucinations; mania; loss of memory; drowsiness; disorientation; emotional disturbances; dermatitis; coma; tremors of the hands, lips, and tongue; speech defects; and motor incoordination.

Dosage and Administration:

Adults—One or two Carbrital Kapseals

Treatment of Overdosage—In acute barbiturate toxicity, general physiologic supportive methods should be undertaken immediately. Most important of these is correction of anoxia, which may be accomplished by removal of airway obstruction, oxygen administration, artificial respiration, or analeptic therapy, or a combination of these procedures. Analeptic therapy should be avoided unless a definite need exists. Absorption of the drug should be minimized by emesis, gastric lavage, or gastric aspiration. Peritoneal dialysis or hemodialysis may be lifesaving in severe poisoning. Alkalization of the urine may increase diuresis and thereby increase the rate of urinary clearance of pentobarbital. Good nursing care is essential.

The treatment of bromide accumulation consists of supplementing the daily diet with up to 200 mEq of chloride as sodium or ammonium chloride. In serious cases, more rapid removal of the drug may be achieved by forced diuresis. Extracorporeal hemodialysis has demonstrated more rapid removal than forced diuresis.

How Supplied:

N 0071-0372 (Kapseal 372)—Carbrital Kapseals, each containing 1½ grains pentobarbital sodium and 4 grains carbromal, are available in bottles of 100 and 1,000, and unit-dose packages of 100 (10 strips of 10 capsules). Parcode® No. 372.

UF

[*Shown in Product Identification Section*]

CELONTIN® KAPSEALS® ℞
(methsuximide capsules, NF)

Description: Celontin (methsuximide) is an anticonvulsant succinimide, chemically designated as N,2-dimethyl-2-phenylsuccinimide.

Action: Methsuximide suppresses the paroxysmal three-cycle-per-second spike and wave activity associated with lapses of consciousness which is common in absence (petit mal) seizures. The frequency of epileptiform attacks is reduced, apparently by depression of the motor cortex and elevation of the threshold of the central nervous system to convulsive stimuli.

Indication: Celontin is indicated for the control of absence (petit mal) seizures that are refractory to other drugs.

Contraindication: Methsuximide should not be used in patients with a history of hypersensitivity to succinimides.

Warnings: Blood dyscrasias, including some with fatal outcome, have been reported to be associated with the use of succinimides; therefore, periodic blood counts should be performed.

It has been reported that succinimides have produced morphological and functional changes in animal liver. For this reason, methsuximide should be administered with extreme caution to patients with known liver or renal diseases. Periodic urinalysis and liver function studies are advised for all patients receiving the drug.

Cases of systemic lupus erythematosus have been reported with the use of succinimides. The physician should be alert to this possibility.

Usage in Pregnancy: The effects of Celontin in human pregnancy and nursing infants are unknown.

Recent reports suggest an association between the use of anticonvulsant drugs by women with epilepsy and an elevated incidence of birth defects in children born to these women. Data is more extensive with respect to phenytoin and phenobarbital, but these are also the most commonly prescribed anticonvulsants. Less systematic or ancecdotal reports suggest a possible similar association with the use of all known anticonvulsant drugs.

The reports suggesting an elevated incidence of birth defects in children of drug-treated epileptic women cannot be regarded as adequate to prove a definite cause-and-effect relationship. There are intrinsic methodological problems in obtaining adequate data on drug teratogenicity in humans. The possibility also exists that other factors, eg, genetic factors or the epileptic condition itself, may be more important than drug therapy in leading to birth defects. The great majority of mothers on anticonvulsant medication deliver normal infants. It is important to note that anticonvulsant drugs should not be discontinued in patients in whom the drug is administered to prevent major seizures because of the strong possibility of precipitating status epilepticus with attendant hypoxia and threat to life. In individual cases where the severity and frequency of the seizure disorder are such that the removal of medication does not pose a serious threat to the patient, discontinuation of the drug may be considered prior to and during pregnancy, although it cannot be said with any confidence that even minor seizures do not pose some hazard to the developing embryo or fetus.

The prescribing physician will wish to weigh these considerations in treating or counseling epileptic women of childbearing potential.

Hazardous Activities: Methsuximide may impair the mental and/or physical abilities required for the performance of potentially hazardous tasks, such as driving a motor vehicle or other such activity requiring alertness; therefore, the patient should be cautioned accordingly.

Precautions: It is recommended that the physician withdraw the drug slowly on the appearance of unusual depression, aggressiveness, or other behavioral alterations.

As with other anticonvulsants, it is important to proceed slowly when increasing or decreasing dosage, as well as when adding or eliminating other medication. Abrupt withdrawal of anticonvulsant medication may precipitate absence (petit mal) status.

Methsuximide, when used alone in mixed types of epilepsy, may increase the frequency of grand mal seizures in some patients.

Adverse Reactions: Gastrointestinal System: Gastrointestinal symptoms occur frequently and have included nausea or vomiting, anorexia, diarrhea, weight loss, epigastric and abdominal pain, and constipation.

Hemopoietic System: Hemopoietic complications associated with the administration of methsuximide have included eosinophilia, leukopenia, monocytosis, and pancytopenia.

Nervous System: Neurologic and sensory reactions reported during therapy with methsuximide have included drowsiness, ataxia or dizziness, irritability and nervousness, headache, blurred vision, photophobia, hiccups, and insomnia. Drowsiness, ataxia, and dizziness have been the most frequent side effects noted. Psychologic abnormalities have included confusion, instability, mental slowness, depression, hypochondriacal behavior, and aggressiveness. There have been rare reports of psychosis, suicidal behavior, and auditory hallucinations.

Integumentary System: Dermatologic manifestations which have occurred with the administration of methsuximide have included urticaria, Stevens-Johnson syndrome, and pruritic erythematous rashes.

Other: Miscellaneous reactions reported include periorbital edema and hyperemia.

Dosage and Administration: Optimum dosage of Celontin must be determined by trial. A suggested dosage schedule is 300 mg per day for the first week. If required, dosage may be increased thereafter at weekly intervals by 300 mg per day for the three weeks following to a daily dosage of 1.2 g. Because therapeutic effect and tolerance vary among patients, therapy with Celontin must be individualized according to the response of each patient. Optimal dosage is that amount of Celontin which is barely sufficient to control seizures so that side effects may be kept to a minimum. The smaller Kapseal (150 mg) facilitates administration to small children.

Celontin (methsuximide) may be administered in combination with other anticonvulsants when other forms of epilepsy coexist with absence (petit mal.)

How Supplied:

N 0071-0525-24 (Kapseal 525)—Celontin Kapseals, each containing 300 mg methsuximide; bottles of 100. Parcode® No. 525

N 0071-0537-24 (Kapseal 537)—Celontin Kapseals, Half Strength, each containing 150 mg methsuximide, bottles of 100. Parcode No. 527

WL

[*Shown in Product Identification Section*]

CHLOROMYCETIN® CREAM, 1% ℞

(chloramphenicol cream)

Description: Each gram of Chloromycetin Cream, 1%, contains 10 mg chloramphenicol with 0.1% propylparaben in a water-miscible ointment base of liquid petrolatum, cetyl alcohol, sodium lauryl sulfate, sodium phosphate buffer, and water.

Actions: Chloramphenicol, a broad-spectrum antibiotic originally isolated from *Streptomyces venezuelae*, is primarily bacteriostatic and acts by inhibition of protein synthesis by interfering with the transfer of activated amino acids from soluble RNA to ribosomes. Development of resistance to chloramphenicol can be regarded as minimal for staphylococci and many other species of bacteria.

Indications: Chloromycetin Cream, 1%, is indicated for the treatment of superficial skin infections caused by bacteria susceptible to chloramphenicol. Deeper cutaneous infections should be treated with appropriate systemic antibiotics.

Contraindication: This product is contraindicated in persons sensitive to any of its components.

Warnings: Prolonged or frequent intermittent use of topical chloramphenicol should be avoided because of the possibility of hypersensitivity reactions, including bone marrow hypoplasia.

Precautions: The prolonged use of antibiotics may occasionally result in overgrowth of nonsusceptible organisms, including fungi. If new infections appear during medication, the drug should be discontinued and appropriate measures should be taken.

In all except very superficial infections, the topical use of chloramphenicol should be supplemented by appropriate systemic medication.

Adverse Reactions: Signs of local irritation with subjective symptoms of itching or burning, angioneurotic edema, urticaria, vesicular and maculopapular dermatitis have been reported in patients sensitive to chloramphenicol and are causes for discontinuing the medication. Similar sensitivity reactions to other materials in topical preparations may also occur. Blood dyscrasias may be associated with the systemic use of chloramphenicol.

Dosage and Administration: Apply to the infected area three or four times daily after cleansing.

How Supplied:

N 0071-3166-13 (Ointment 66)

Chloromycetin Cream (chloramphenicol cream), 1%, is supplied in 1-oz tubes.

AHFS 84:04.04 SL

CHLOROMYCETIN® KAPSEALS® ℞

(chloramphenicol capsules, USP)

CHLOROMYCETIN PALMITATE

(chloramphenicol palmitate for oral suspension, USP)

ORAL SUSPENSION

WARNING

Serious and fatal blood dyscrasias (aplastic anemia, hypoplastic anemia, thrombocytopenia, and granulocytopenia) are known to occur after the administration of chloramphenicol. In addition, there have been reports of aplastic anemia attributed to chloramphenicol which later terminated in leukemia. Blood dyscrasias have occurred after both short-term and prolonged therapy with this drug. Chloramphenicol must not be used when less potentially dangerous agents will be effective, as described in the Indications section. *It must not be used in the treatment of trivial infections or where it is not indicated, as in colds, influenza, infections of the throat; or as a prophylactic agent to prevent bacterial infections.*

Precautions: It is essential that adequate blood studies be made during treatment with the drug. While blood studies may detect early peripheral blood changes, such as leukopenia, reticulocytopenia, or granulocytopenia, before they become irreversible, such studies cannot be relied on to detect bone marrow depression prior to development of aplastic anemia. To facilitate appropriate studies and observation during therapy, it is desirable that patients be hospitalized.

Description: Chloramphenicol is an antibiotic that is clinically useful for, *and should be reserved for*, serious infections caused by organisms susceptible to its antimicrobial effects when less potentially hazardous therapeutic agents are ineffective or contraindicated. Sensitivity testing is essential to determine its indicated use, but may be performed concurrently with therapy initiated on clinical impression that one of the indicated conditions exists (see Indications section).

Actions and Pharmacology: *In vitro* chloramphenicol exerts mainly a bacteriostatic effect on a wide range of gram-negative and gram-positive bacteria and is active *in vitro* against rickettsias, the lymphogranuloma-psittacosis group, and *Vibrio cholerae*. Chloramphenicol is particularly active against *Salmonella typhi* and *Hemophilus influenzae*. The mode of action is through interference or inhibition of protein synthesis in intact cells and in cell-free systems.

Chloramphenicol administered orally is absorbed rapidly from the intestinal tract. In controlled studies in adult volunteers using the recommended dosage of 50 mg/kg/day, a dosage of 1 g every six hours for eight doses was given. Using the microbiological assay method, the average peak serum level was 11.2 mcg/ml one hour after the first dose. A cumulative effect gave a peak rise to 18.4 mcg/ml after the fifth dose of 1 g. Mean serum levels ranged from 8 to 14 mcg/ml over the 48-hour period. Total urinary excretion of chloramphenicol in these studies ranged from a low of 68% to a high of 99% over a three-day period. From 8 to 12% of the antibiotic excreted is in the form of free chloramphenicol; the remainder consists of microbiologically inactive metabolites, principally the conjugate with glucuronic acid. Because the glucuronide is excreted rapidly, most chloramphenicol detected in the blood is in the microbiologically active free form. Despite the small proportion of unchanged drug excreted in the urine, the concentration of free chloramphenicol is relatively high, amounting to several hundred mcg/ml in patients receiving divided doses of 50 mg/kg/day. Small amounts of active drug are found in bile and feces. Chloramphenicol diffuses rapidly, but its distribution is not uniform. Highest concentrations are found in liver and kidney, and lowest concentrations are found in brain and cerebrospinal fluid. Chloramphenicol enters cerebrospinal fluid even in the absence of meningeal inflammation, appearing in concentrations about half of those found in the blood. Measurable levels are also detected in pleural and in ascitic fluids, saliva, milk, and in the aqueous and vitreous humors. Transport across the placental barrier occurs with somewhat lower concentration in cord blood of newborn infants than in maternal blood.

Indications: In accord with the concepts in the warning box and this indications section, chloramphenicol must be used only in those serious infections for which less potentially dangerous drugs are ineffective or contraindicated. However, chloramphenicol may be chosen to initiate antibiotic therapy on the clinical impression that one of the conditions below is believed to be present; *in vitro* sensitivity tests should be performed concurrently so that the drug may be discontinued as soon as possible if less potentially dangerous agents are indicated by such tests. The decision to continue use of chloramphenicol rather than another antibiotic when both are suggested by *in vitro* studies to be effective against a specific pathogen should be based upon severity of the infection, susceptibility of the pathogen to the various antimicrobial drugs, efficacy of the various drugs in the infection, and the important additional concepts contained in the Warning Box above:

1. Acute infections caused by *S typhi*

Chloramphenicol is a drug of choice.* It is not recommended for the routine treatment of the typhoid "carrier state."

2. Serious infections caused by susceptible strains in accordance with the concepts expressed above:

a. *Salmonella* species

b. *H influenzae*, specifically meningeal infections

c. Rickettsia

d. Lymphogranuloma-psittacosis group

e. Various gram-negative bacteria causing bacteremia, meningitis, or other serious gram-negative infections

f. Other susceptible organisms which have been demonstrated to be resistant to all other appropriate antimicrobial agents.

3. Cystic fibrosis regimens

Contraindications: Chloramphenicol is contraindicated in individuals with a history of previous hypersensitivity and/or toxic reaction to it. *It must not be used in the treatment of trivial infections or where it is not indicated, as in colds, influenza, infections of the throat; or as a prophylactic agent to prevent bacterial infections.*

---

*In the treatment of typhoid fever, some authorities recommend that chloramphenicol be administered at therapeutic levels for 8 to 10 days after the patient has become afebrile to lessen the possibility of relapse.

Precautions: 1. Baseline blood studies should be followed by periodic blood studies approximately every two days during therapy. The drug should be discontinued upon appearance of reticulocytopenia, leukopenia, thrombocyto-

Continued on next page

This product information was prepared in August, 1979. On these and other Parke-Davis Products, detailed information may be obtained by addressing PARKE-DAVIS, Division of Warner-Lambert Company, Morris Plains, NJ 07950.

Parke-Davis—Cont.

penia, anemia, or any other blood study findings attributable to chloramphenicol. However, it should be noted that such studies do not exclude the possible later appearance of the irreversible type of bone marrow depression.

2. Repeated courses of the drug should be avoided if at all possible. Treatment should not be continued longer than required to produce a cure with little or no risk of relapse of the disease.

3. Concurrent therapy with other drugs that may cause bone marrow depression should be avoided.

4. Excessive blood levels may result from administration of the recommended dose to patients with impaired liver or kidney functions, including that due to immature metabolic processes in the infant. The dosage should be adjusted accordingly or, preferably, the blood concentration should be determined at appropriate intervals.

5. There are no studies to establish the safety of this drug in pregnancy.

6. Because chloramphenicol readily crosses the placental barrier, caution in use of the drug is particularly important during pregnancy at term or during labor because of potential toxic effects on the fetus (gray syndrome).

7. Precaution should be used in therapy of premature and full-term infants to avoid gray syndrome toxicity. (See Adverse Reactions.) Serum drug levels should be carefully followed during therapy of the newborn infant.

8. Precaution should be used in therapy during lactation because of the possibility of toxic effects on the nursing infant.

9. The use of this antibiotic, as with other antibiotics, may result in an overgrowth of nonsusceptible organisms, including fungi. If infections caused by nonsusceptible organisms appear during therapy, appropriate measures should be taken.

Adverse Reactions:

1. Blood Dyscrasias

The most serious adverse effect of chloramphenicol is bone marrow depression. Serious and fatal blood dyscrasias (aplastic anemia, hypoplastic anemia, thrombocytopenia, and granulocytopenia) are known to occur after the administration of chloramphenicol. An irreversible type of marrow depression leading to aplastic anemia with a high rate of mortality is characterized by the appearance weeks or months after therapy of bone marrow aplasia or hypoplasia. Peripherally, pancytopenia is most often observed, but in a small number of cases only one or two of the three major cell types (erythrocytes, leukocytes, platelets) may be depressed.

A reversible type of bone marrow depression, which is dose-related, may occur. This type of marrow depression is characterized by vacuolization of the erythroid cells, reduction of reticulocytes, and leukopenia, and responds promptly to the withdrawal of chloramphenicol.

An exact determination of the risk of serious and fatal blood dyscrasias is not possible because of lack of accurate information regarding (1) the size of the population at risk, (2) the total number of drug-associated dyscrasias, and (3) the total number of nondrug-associated dyscrasias.

In a report to the California State Assembly by the California Medical Association and the State Department of Public Health in January 1967, the risk of fatal aplastic anemia was estimated at 1:24,200 to 1:40,500 based on two dosage levels.

There have been reports of aplastic anemia attributed to chloramphenicol which later terminated in leukemia.

Paroxysmal nocturnal hemoglobinuria has also been reported.

2. Gastrointestinal Reactions

Nausea, vomiting, glossitis and stomatitis, diarrhea, and enterocolitis may occur in low incidence.

3. Neurotoxic Reactions

Headache, mild depression, mental confusion, and delirium have been described in patients receiving chloramphenicol. Optic and peripheral neuritis have been reported, usually following long-term therapy. If this occurs, the drug should be promptly withdrawn.

4. Hypersensitivity Reactions

Fever, macular and vesicular rashes, angioedema, urticaria, and anaphylaxis may occur. Herxheimer reactions have occurred during therapy for typhoid fever.

5. "Gray Syndrome"

Toxic reactions including fatalities have occurred in the premature and newborn; the signs and symptoms associated with these reactions have been referred to as the gray syndrome. One case of gray syndrome has been reported in an infant born to a mother having received chloramphenicol during labor. One case has been reported in a 3-month-old infant. The following summarizes the clinical and laboratory studies that have been made on these patients:

(1) In most cases, therapy with chloramphenicol had been instituted within the first 48 hours of life.
(2) Symptoms first appeared after three to four days of continued treatment with high doses of chloramphenicol.
(3) The symptoms appeared in the following order:
  (a) abdominal distention with or without emesis;
  (b) progressive pallid cyanosis;
  (c) vasomotor collapse, frequently accompanied by irregular respiration;
  (d) death within a few hours of onset of these symptoms.
(4) The progression of symptoms from onset to exitus was accelerated with higher dose schedules.
(5) Preliminary blood serum level studies revealed unusually high concentrations of chloramphenicol (over 90 mcg/ml after repeated doses).
(6) Termination of therapy upon early evidence of the associated symptomatology frequently reversed the process with complete recovery.

Dosage and Administration:

DOSAGE RECOMMENDATIONS FOR ORAL CHLORAMPHENICOL PREPARATIONS

The majority of microorganisms susceptible to chloramphenicol will respond to a concentration between 5 and 20 mcg/ml. The desired concentration of active drug in blood should fall within this range over most of the treatment period. Dosage of 50 mg/kg/day divided into four doses at intervals of six hours will usually achieve and sustain levels of this magnitude.

Except in certain circumstances (eg, premature and newborn infants and individuals with impairment of hepatic or renal functions), lower doses may not achieve these concentrations. Chloramphenicol, like other potent drugs, should be prescribed at recommended doses known to have therapeutic activity. Close observation of the patient should be maintained and in the event of any adverse reactions, dosage should be reduced or the drug discontinued, if other factors in the clinical situation permit.

Adults

Adults should receive 50 mg/kg/day (approximately one 250-mg capsule per each 10 lb body weight) in divided doses at six-hour intervals. In exceptional cases, patients with infections due to moderately resistant organisms may require increased dosage up to 100 mg/kg/day to achieve blood levels inhibiting the pathogen, but these high doses should be decreased as soon as possible. Adults with impairment of hepatic or renal functions or both may have reduced ability to metabolize and excrete the drug. In instances of impaired metabolic processes, dosages should be adjusted accordingly. (See discussion under Newborn Infants.) Precise control of concentration of the drug in the blood should be carefully followed in patients with impaired metabolic processes by the available microtechniques (information available on request).

Children

Dosage of 50 mg/kg/day divided into four doses at six-hour intervals yields blood levels in the range effective against most susceptible organisms. Severe infections (eg, bacteremia or meningitis), especially when adequate cerebrospinal fluid concentrations are desired, may require dosage up to 100 mg/kg/day; however, it is recommended that dosage be reduced to 50 mg/kg/day as soon as possible. Children with impaired liver or kidney functions may retain excessive amounts of the drug.

Newborn Infants

(See section titled Gray Syndrome under Adverse Reactions.)

A total of 25 mg/kg/day in four equal doses at six-hour intervals usually produces and maintains concentrations in blood and tissues adequate to control most infections for which the drug is indicated. Increased dosage in these individuals, demanded by severe infections, should be given only to maintain the blood concentration within a therapeutically effective range. After the first two weeks of life, full-term infants ordinarily may receive up to a total of 50 mg/kg/day equally divided into four doses at six-hour intervals. *These dosage recommendations are extremely important because blood concentration in all premature infants and full-term infants under two weeks of age differs from that of other infants.* This difference is due to variations in the maturity of the metabolic functions of the liver and the kidneys.

When these functions are immature (or seriously impaired in adults), high concentrations of the drug are found which tend to increase with succeeding doses.

Infants and Children with Immature Metabolic Processes

In young infants and other children in whom immature metabolic functions are suspected, a dosage of 25 mg/kg/day will usually produce therapeutic concentrations of the drug in the blood. In this group particularly, the concentration of the drug in the blood should be carefully followed by microtechniques. (Information available on request.)

How Supplied: N 0071-0379 (Kapseal 379) Chloromycetin (chloramphenicol capsules, USP) Kapseals, each contains 250 mg chloramphenicol, supplied in packages of 16 and 100, and unit-dose packages of 10/10s. Parcode® No. 379.

[*Shown in Product Identification Section*]

The banded capsule is a Parke-Davis trademark registered in the US Patent Office.

AHFS 8:12.08 **WL**

N 0071-2310-15 Oral Suspension Chloromycetin Palmitate (chloramphenicol palmitate for oral suspension, USP). Each 5 ml contains chloramphenicol palmitate equivalent to 150 mg chloramphenicol with 0.5% sodium benzoate as preservative, in bottles of 60 ml.

Chloramphenicol Palmitate is hydrolyzed to chloramphenicol before absorption. Resulting blood concentration is similar to that produced by the oral administration of chloramphenicol.

AHFS 8:12:08 **TG**

CHLOROMYCETIN® OPHTHALMIC OINTMENT, 1% ℞

(chloramphenicol ophthalmic ointment, USP)

Description: Each gram of Chloromycetin Ophthalmic Ointment, 1%, contains 10 mg chloramphenicol in a special base of liquid petrolatum and polyethylene. The product contains no preservatives.

Actions: Chloramphenicol, a broad-spectrum antibiotic originally isolated from *Streptomyces venezuelae,* is primarily bacteriostatic and acts by inhibition of protein synthesis by interfering with the transfer of activated amino acids from soluble RNA to ribosomes. Studies have shown that chloramphenicol is not absorbed in measurable amounts by topical application to the eye. Development of resistance to chloramphenicol can be regarded as minimal for staphylococci and many other species of bacteria.

Indications: Chloromycetin Ophthalmic Ointment, 1%, is indicated for the treatment of superficial ocular infections involving the conjunctiva and/or cornea caused by chloramphenicol-susceptible organisms. Bacteriological studies should be performed to determine the causative organisms and their sensitivity to chloramphenicol.

Contraindication: This product is contraindicated in persons sensitive to any of its components.

Warnings: Prolonged or frequent intermittent use of topical chloramphenicol should be avoided because of the possibility of hypersensitivity reactions, including bone-marrow hypoplasia.

Precautions: The prolonged use of antibiotics may occasionally result in overgrowth of nonsusceptible organisms, including fungi. If new infections appear during medication, the drug should be discontinued and appropriate measures should be taken.

In all except very superficial infections, the topical use of chloramphenicol should be supplemented by appropriate systemic medication.

Adverse Reactions: Blood dyscrasias may be associated with the systemic use of chloramphenicol. Bone-marrow hypoplasia following the topical use of chloramphenicol eye drops has been reported.

Dosage and Administration: A small amount of ointment placed in the lower conjunctival sac every three hours, or more frequently if deemed advisable by the prescribing physician. Administration should be continued day and night for the first 48 hours, after which the interval between applications may be increased. Treatment should be continued for at least 48 hours after the eye appears normal.

How Supplied: N 0071-3070-07—Chloromycetin Ophthalmic Ointment, 1%, is supplied in ophthalmic ointment tubes of 3.5 g.

AHFS 52:04.04 **WC**

CHLOROMYCETIN® ℞
(chloramphenicol)
OTIC

Description: Each milliliter of Chloromycetin Otic contains 5 mg (0.5%) chloramphenicol in propylene glycol.

Actions: Chloramphenicol, a broad-spectrum antibiotic originally isolated from *Streptomyces venezuelae,* is primarily bacteriostatic and acts by inhibition of protein synthesis by interfering with the transfer of activated amino acids from soluble RNA to ribosomes. Development of resistance to chloramphenicol can be regarded as minimal for staphylococci and many other species of bacteria.

Indications: Chloromycetin (chloramphenicol) Otic is indicated for the treatment of superficial infections of the external auditory canal caused by susceptible strains of various gram-positive and gram-negative organisms including:

Staphylococcus aureus, Escherichia coli, Hemophilus influenzae, Pseudomonas aeruginosa, Aerobacter aerogenes, Klebsiella pneumoniae, and *Proteus* species.

Deeper infections should be treated with appropriate systemic antibiotics.

Contraindication: This product is contraindicated in persons sensitive to any of its components.

Warnings: Prolonged or frequent intermittent use of topical chloramphenicol should be avoided because of the possibility of hypersensitivity reactions, including bone marrow hypoplasia.

Precautions: The prolonged use of antibiotics may occasionally result in overgrowth of nonsusceptible organisms, including fungi. If new infections appear during medication, the drug should be discontinued and appropriate measures should be taken.

In all except very superficial infections, the topical use of chloramphenicol should be supplemented by appropriate systemic medication.

Adverse Reactions: Signs of local irritation, with subjective symptoms of itching or burning, angioneurotic edema, urticaria, vesicular and maculopapular dermatitis, have been reported in patients sensitive to chloramphenicol and are causes for discontinuing the medication. Similar sensitivity reactions to other materials in topical preparations may also occur. Blood dyscrasias may be associated with the systemic use of chloramphenicol.

Dosage and Administration: Instill two or three drops into the ear three times daily.

How Supplied: N 0071-3313-11—Chloromycetin (chloramphenicol) Otic is supplied in 15-ml vials with droppers.

AHFS 52:04.04 **WB**

CHLOROMYCETIN® ℞
SODIUM SUCCINATE
(chloramphenicol sodium succinate for injection, USP)
FOR INTRAVENOUS ADMINISTRATION

WARNING

Serious and fatal blood dyscrasias (aplastic anemia, hypoplastic anemia, thrombocytopenia, and granulocytopenia) are known to occur after the administration of chloramphenicol. In addition, there have been reports of aplastic anemia attributed to chloramphenicol which later terminated in leukemia. Blood dyscrasias have occurred after both short-term and prolonged therapy with this drug. Chloramphenicol must not be used when less potentially dangerous agents will be effective, as described in the Indications section. *It must not be used in the treatment of trivial infections or where it is not indicated, as in colds, influenza, infections of the throat; or as a prophylactic agent to prevent bacterial infections.*

Precautions: It is essential that adequate blood studies be made during treatment with the drug. While blood studies may detect early peripheral blood changes, such as leukopenia, reticulocytopenia, or granulocytopenia, before they become irreversible, such studies cannot be relied on to detect bone marrow depression prior to development of aplastic anemia. To facilitate appropriate studies and observation during therapy, it is desirable that patients be hospitalized.

IMPORTANT CONSIDERATIONS IN PRESCRIBING INJECTABLE CHLORAMPHENICOL SODIUM SUCCINATE

CHLORAMPHENICOL SODIUM SUCCINATE IS INTENDED FOR INTRAVENOUS USE ONLY. IT HAS BEEN DEMONSTRATED TO BE INEFFECTIVE WHEN GIVEN INTRAMUSCULARLY.

1. Chloramphenicol sodium succinate must be hydrolyzed to its microbiologically active form and there is a lag in achieving adequate blood levels compared with the base given intravenously.
2. The oral form of chloramphenicol is readily absorbed and adequate blood levels are achieved and maintained on the recommended dosage.
3. Patients started on intravenous chloramphenicol sodium succinate should be changed to the oral form as soon as practicable.

Description: Chloramphenicol is an antibiotic that is clinically useful for, *and should be reserved for,* serious infections caused by organisms susceptible to its antimicrobial effects when less potentially hazardous therapeutic agents are ineffective or contraindicated. Sensitivity testing is essential to determine its indicated use, but may be performed concurrently with therapy initiated on clinical impression that one of the indicated conditions exists (see Indications section).

Each gram (10 ml of a 10% solution) of chloramphenicol sodium succinate contains approximately 52 mg (2.25 mEq) of sodium.

Actions and Pharmacology: *In vitro* chloramphenicol exerts mainly a bacteriostatic effect on a wide range of gram-negative and gram-positive bacteria and is active *in vitro* against rickettsias, the lymphogranuloma-psittacosis group, and *Vibrio cholerae.* Chloramphenicol is particularly active against *Salmonella typhi* and *Hemophilus influenzae.* The mode of action is through interference or inhibition of protein synthesis in intact cells and in cell-free systems.

Chloramphenicol administered orally is absorbed rapidly from the intestinal tract. In controlled studies in adult volunteers using the recommended dosage of 50 mg/kg/day, a dosage of 1 g every six hours for eight doses was given. Using the microbiological assay method, the average peak serum level was 11.2 mcg/ml one hour after the first dose. A cumulative effect gave a peak rise to 18.4 mcg/ml after the fifth dose of 1 g. Mean serum levels ranged from 8 to 14 mcg/ml over the 48-hour period. Total urinary excretion of chloramphenicol in these studies ranged from a low of 68% to a high of 99% over a three-day period. From 8 to 12% of the antibiotic excreted is in the form of free chloramphenicol; the remainder consists of microbiologically inactive metabolites, principally the conjugate with glucuronic acid. Because the glucuronide is excreted rapidly, most chloramphenicol detected in the blood is in the microbiologically active free form. Despite the small proportion of unchanged drug excreted in the urine, the concentration of free chloramphenicol is relatively high, amounting to several hundred mcg/ml in patients receiving divided doses of 50 mg/kg/day. Small amounts of active drug are found in bile and feces. Chloramphenicol diffuses rapidly, but its distribution is not uniform. Highest concentrations are found in liver and kidney, and lowest concentrations are found in brain and cerebrospinal fluid. Chloramphenicol enters cerebrospinal fluid even in the absence of meningeal inflammation, appearing in concentrations about half of those found in the blood. Measurable levels are also detected in pleural and in ascitic fluids, saliva, milk, and in the aqueous and vitreous humors. Transport across the placental barrier occurs with somewhat lower concentration in cord blood of newborn infants than in maternal blood.

Indications: In accord with the concepts in the warning box and this Indications section, chloramphenicol must be used only in those serious infections for which less potentially

Continued on next page

This product information was prepared in August, 1979. On these and other Parke-Davis Products, detailed information may be obtained by addressing PARKE-DAVIS, Division of Warner-Lambert Company, Morris Plains, NJ 07950.

Parke-Davis—Cont.

dangerous drugs are ineffective or contraindicated. However, chloramphenicol may be chosen to initiate antibiotic therapy on the clinical impression that one of the conditions below is believed to be present; *in vitro* sensitivity tests should be performed concurrently so that the drug may be discontinued as soon as possible if less potentially dangerous agents are indicated by such tests. The decision to continue use of chloramphenicol rather than another antibiotic when both are suggested by *in vitro* studies to be effective against a specific pathogen should be based upon severity of the infection, susceptibility of the pathogen to the various antimicrobial drugs, efficacy of the various drugs in the infection, and the important additional concepts contained in the Warning Box above:

1. Acute infections caused by *S typhi**
It is not recommended for the routine treatment of the typhoid carrier state.

2. Serious infections caused by susceptible strains in accordance with the concepts expressed above:

a. *Salmonella* species
b. *H influenzae*, specifically meningeal infections
c. Rickettsia
d. Lymphogranuloma-psittacosis group
e. Various gram-negative bacteria causing bacteremia, meningitis, or other serious gram-negative infections
f. Other susceptible organisms which have been demonstrated to be resistant to all other appropriate antimicrobial agents.

3. Cystic fibrosis regimens

*In the treatment of typhoid fever, some authorities recommend that chloramphenicol be administered at therapeutic levels for 8 to 10 days after the patient has become afebrile to lessen the possibility of relapse.

Contraindications: Chloramphenicol is contraindicated in individuals with a history of previous hypersensitivity and/or toxic reaction to it. *It must not be used in the treatment of trivial infections or where it is not indicated, as in colds, influenza, infections of the throat; or as a prophylactic agent to prevent bacterial infection.*

Precautions:

1. Baseline blood studies should be followed by periodic blood studies approximately every two days during therapy. The drug should be discontinued upon appearance of reticulocytopenia, leukopenia, thrombocytopenia, anemia, or any other blood study findings attributable to chloramphenicol. However, it should be noted that such studies do not exclude the possible later appearance of the irreversible type of bone marrow depression.

2. Repeated courses of the drug should be avoided if at all possible. Treatment should not be continued longer than required to produce a cure with little or no risk of relapse of the disease.

3. Concurrent therapy with other drugs that may cause bone marrow depression should be avoided.

4. Excessive blood levels may result from administration of the recommended dosage to patients with impaired liver or kidney functions, including that due to immature metabolic processes in the infant. The dosage should be adjusted accordingly or, preferably, the blood concentration should be determined at appropriate intervals.

5. There are no studies to establish the safety of this drug in pregnancy.

6. Because chloramphenicol readily crosses the placental barrier, caution in use of the drug is particularly important during pregnancy at term or during labor because of potential toxic effects on the fetus (gray syndrome).

7. Precaution should be used in therapy of premature and full-term infants to avoid gray syndrome toxicity (see Adverse Reactions). Serum drug levels should be carefully followed during therapy of the newborn infant.

8. Precaution should be used in therapy during lactation because of the possibility of toxic effects on the nursing infant.

9. The use of this antibiotic, as with other antibiotics, may result in an overgrowth of nonsusceptible organisms, including fungi. If infections caused by nonsusceptible organisms appear during therapy, appropriate measures should be taken.

Adverse Reactions:

1. Blood Dyscrasias
The most serious adverse effect of chloramphenicol is bone marrow depression. Serious and fatal blood dyscrasias (aplastic anemia, hypoplastic anemia, thrombocytopenia, and granulocytopenia) are known to occur after the administration of chloramphenicol. An irreversible type of marrow depression leading to aplastic anemia with a high rate of mortality is characterized by the appearance weeks or months after therapy of bone marrow aplasia or hypoplasia. Peripherally, pancytopenia is most often observed, but in a small number of cases only one or two of the three major cell types (erythrocytes, leukocytes, platelets) may be depressed.

A reversible type of bone marrow depression, which is dose-related, may occur. This type of marrow depression is characterized by vacuolization of the erythroid cells, reduction of reticulocytes, and leukopenia, and responds promptly to the withdrawal of chloramphenicol.

An exact determination of the risk of serious and fatal blood dyscrasias is not possible because of lack of accurate information regarding (1) the size of the population at risk, (2) the total number of drug-associated dyscrasias, and (3) the total number of nondrug-associated dyscrasias.

In a report to the California State Assembly by the California Medical Association and the State Department of Public Health in January 1967, the risk of fatal aplastic anemia was estimated at 1:24,200 to 1:40,500 based on two dosage levels.

There have been reports of aplastic anemia attributed to chloramphenicol which later terminated in leukemia.

Paroxysmal nocturnal hemoglobinuria has also been reported.

2. Gastrointestinal Reactions
Nausea, vomiting, glossitis and stomatitis, diarrhea, and enterocolitis may occur in low incidence.

3. Neurotoxic Reactions
Headache, mild depression, mental confusion, and delirium have been described in patients receiving chloramphenicol. Optic and peripheral neuritis have been reported, usually following long-term therapy. If this occurs, the drug should be promptly withdrawn.

4. Hypersensitivity Reactions
Fever, macular and vesicular rashes, angioedema, urticaria, and anaphylaxis may occur. Herxheimer reactions have occurred during therapy for typhoid fever.

5. "Gray Syndrome"
Toxic reactions including fatalities have occurred in the premature and newborn; the signs and symptoms associated with these reactions have been referred to as the gray syndrome. One case of gray syndrome has been reported in an infant born to a mother having received chloramphenicol during labor. One case has been reported in a 3-month-old infant. The following summarizes the clinical and laboratory studies that have been made on these patients:

(1) In most cases, therapy with chloramphenicol had been instituted within the first 48 hours of life.
(2) Symptoms first appeared after three to four days of continued treatment with high doses of chloramphenicol.
(3) The symptoms appeared in the following order:
  (a) abdominal distention with or without emesis;
  (b) progressive pallid cyanosis;
  (c) vasomotor collapse, frequently accompanied by irregular respiration;
  (d) death within a few hours of onset of these symptoms.
(4) The progression of symptoms from onset to exitus was accelerated with higher dose schedules.
(5) Preliminary blood serum level studies revealed unusually high concentrations of chloramphenicol (over 90 mcg/ml after repeated doses).
(6) Termination of therapy upon early evidence of the associated symptomatology frequently reversed the process with complete recovery.

Administration: Chloramphenicol, like other potent drugs, should be prescribed at recommended doses known to have therapeutic activity. Administration of 50 mg/kg/day in divided doses will produce blood levels of the magnitude to which the majority of susceptible microorganisms will respond.

As soon as feasible, an oral dosage form of chloramphenicol should be substituted for the intravenous form because adequate blood levels are achieved with chloramphenicol by mouth.

The following method of administration is recommended:

Intravenously as a 10% (100 mg/ml) solution to be injected over at least a one-minute interval. This is prepared by the addition of 10 ml of an aqueous diluent, such as water for injection or 5% dextrose injection.

Dosage:

Adults
Adults should receive 50 mg/kg/day in divided doses at six-hour intervals. In exceptional cases, patients with infections due to moderately resistant organisms may require increased dosage up to 100 mg/kg/day to achieve blood levels inhibiting the pathogen, but these high doses should be decreased as soon as possible. Adults with impairment of hepatic or renal functions or both may have reduced ability to metabolize and excrete the drug. In instances of impaired metabolic processes, dosages should be adjusted accordingly. (See discussion under Newborn Infants.) Precise control of concentration of the drug in the blood should be carefully followed in patients with impaired metabolic processes by the available microtechniques (information available on request).

Children
Dosage of 50 mg/kg/day divided into four doses at six-hour intervals yields blood levels in the range effective against most susceptible organisms. Severe infections (eg, bacteremia or meningitis), especially when adequate cerebrospinal fluid concentrations are desired, may require dosage up to 100 mg/kg/day; however, it is recommended that dosage be reduced to 50 mg/kg/day as soon as possible. Children with impaired liver or kidney functions may retain excessive amounts of the drug.

Newborn Infants
(See section titled Gray Syndrome under Adverse Reactions.)
A total of 25 mg/kg/day in four equal doses at six-hour intervals usually produces and maintains concentrations in blood and tissues adequate to control most infections for which the drug is indicated. Increased dosage in these individuals, demanded by severe infections, should be given only to maintain the blood concentration within a therapeutically effective range. After the first two weeks of life, full-term infants ordinarily may receive up to a total of 50 mg/kg/day equally divided into four

doses at six-hour intervals. *These dosage recommendations are extremely important because blood concentration in all premature infants and full-term infants under two weeks of age differs from that of other infants.* This difference is due to variations in the maturity of the metabolic functions of the liver and the kidneys.

When these functions are immature (or seriously impaired in adults), high concentrations of the drug are found which tend to increase with succeeding doses.

Infants and Children with Immature Metabolic Processes

In young infants and other children in whom immature metabolic functions are suspected, a dose of 25 mg/kg/day will usually produce therapeutic concentrations of the drug in the blood. In this group particularly, the concentration of the drug in the blood should be carefully followed by microtechniques. (Information available on request.)

How Supplied: N 0071-4057-03—(Steri-Vial® No. 57) Chloromycetin (chloramphenicol) Sodium Succinate is supplied as a dried powder in Steri-Vials (rubber diaphragm-capped vials). When reconstituted as directed, each vial contains a sterile solution equivalent to 100 mg of chloramphenicol per milliliter (1 g/10 ml). Available in packages of 10 vials.

AHFS 8:12.08 **RJ**

CHLOROMYXIN™ ℞

(chloramphenicol-polymyxin ophthalmic ointment)

Description: Each gram of Chloromyxin (chloramphenicol-polymyxin ophthalmic ointment) contains 10 mg (1%) chloramphenicol and 5,000 units polymyxin B (as the sulfate) in a special base of liquid petrolatum and polyethylene.

Actions: Chloramphenicol, a broad-spectrum antibiotic originally isolated from *Streptomyces venezuelae,* is primarily bacteriostatic and acts by inhibition of protein synthesis by interfering with the transfer of activated amino acids from soluble RNA to ribosomes. Studies have shown that chloramphenicol is not absorbed in measurable amounts by topical application to the eye. Development of resistance to chloramphenicol can be regarded as minimal for staphylococci and many other species of bacteria.

Polymyxin B sulfate is one of a group of basic polypeptide antibiotics derived from *Bacillus polymyxa (B aerosporus)* and has a bactericidal action against almost all gram-negative bacilli except the *Proteus* group. Polymyxins increase the permeability of bacterial cell wall membranes. All gram-positive bacteria, fungi, and the gram-negative cocci, *Neisseria gonorrhoeae* and *N meningitidis,* are resistant.

Indications: Chloromyxin (chloramphenicol-polymyxin ophthalmic ointment) is indicated for the treatment of superficial ocular infections involving the conjunctiva and/or cornea caused by chloramphenicol- and/or polymyxin-susceptible organisms.

Contraindication: This product is contraindicated in persons sensitive to any of its components.

Warnings: Prolonged or frequent intermittent use of topical chloramphenicol should be avoided because of the possibility of hypersensitivity reactions, including bone marrow hypoplasia.

Precautions: The prolonged use of antibiotics may occasionally result in overgrowth of nonsusceptible organisms, including fungi. If new infections appear during medication, the drug should be discontinued and appropriate measures should be taken.

In all except very superficial infections, the topical use of chloramphenicol should be supplemented by appropriate systemic medication.

Adverse Reactions: Blood dyscrasias may be associated with the systemic use of chloramphenicol. Bone marrow hypoplasia following the topical use of chloramphenicol eye drops has been reported.

Dosage and Administration: A small amount of ointment placed in the lower conjunctival sac every three hours, or more frequently if deemed advisable by the prescribing physician. Administration should be continued day and night for the first 48 hours, after which the interval between applications may be increased. Treatment should be continued for at least 48 hours after the eye appears normal.

Total dosage of polymyxin, systemic and ophthalmic, exceeding 2.5 mg (25,000 units)/kg/day should be avoided.

How Supplied: N 0071-3082-07 Chloromyxin (chloramphenicol-polymyxin ophthalmic ointment) is supplied sterile in ophthalmic ointment tubes of 3.5 g.

AHFS 52:04.04 **UL**

CHOLEDYL® ℞

Tablets/Elixir
(oxtriphylline)

Caution: Federal law prohibits dispensing without prescription.

Description: Each partially enteric coated tablet contains 200 mg or 100 mg oxtriphylline. Each 5 ml teaspoonful of the elixir contains 100 mg oxtriphylline; alcohol 20%.

NOTE: 100 mg oxtriphylline is equivalent to 64 mg anhydrous theophylline.

Actions: Choledyl (oxtriphylline) is a xanthine bronchodilator—the choline salt of theophylline. Choledyl (oxtriphylline), compared to aminophylline, is less irritating to the gastric mucosa, more readily absorbed from the gastrointestinal tract, more stable and more soluble.

Like other xanthines, Choledyl (oxtriphylline) is known to increase vital capacity which has been impaired by bronchospasm and air-trapping. Development of tolerance has been reported infrequently, and therefore Choledyl is useful for long-term therapy of bronchospasm.

Indications: Choledyl (oxtriphylline) is indicated for relief of acute bronchial asthma and for reversible bronchospasm associated with chronic bronchitis and emphysema.

Warning: Use in pregnancy—animal studies revealed no evidence of teratogenic potential. Safety in human pregnancy has not been established; use during lactation or in patients who are or who may become pregnant requires that the potential benefits of the drug be weighed against its possible hazards to the mother and child.

Precautions: Concurrent use of other xanthine-containing preparations may lead to adverse reactions, particularly CNS stimulation in children.

Adverse Reactions: Gastric distress and, occasionally, palpitation and CNS stimulation have been reported.

Dosage:

Tablets—Adults: 200 mg, 4 times a day.

Elixir—Adults: 200 mg (two teaspoonfuls or 10 ml), 4 times a day; Children (2 to 12): 100 mg (one teaspoonful or 5 ml) per 60 lb body weight, 4 times a day.

Above recommendations are averages. Dosage should be individualized.

Supplied: 200 mg yellow, partially enteric coated tablets in bottles of 100 (N 0047-0211-51) and 1000 (N 0047-0211-60); Unit Dose, 10 × 10 strips (N 0047-0211-11), 100 mg red, partially enteric coated tablets in bottles of 100 (N 0047-0210-51). Elixir, cherry-flavored, bottles of 16 fl oz (1 pint) 474 ml (N 0047-0215-16).

Store between 59° and 86°F (15° and 30°C).

Toxicity:

Oxtriphylline, aminophylline and caffeine appear to be more toxic to newborn than to adult rats. No teratogenic effects have been seen.

[*Shown in Product Identification Section*]

306 G 628 **R-1-78**

CHOLEDYL® PEDIATRIC SYRUP ℞

(oxtriphylline)

Caution: Federal law prohibits dispensing without prescription.

Description: Choledyl (oxtriphylline) is a xanthine bronchodilator—the choline salt of theophylline.

Each 5 ml of Choledyl Pediatric Syrup contains 50 mg oxtriphylline (equivalent to 32 mg of anhydrous theophylline).

Clinical Pharmacology: Theophylline directly relaxes the smooth muscle of the bronchial airways and pulmonary blood vessels, thus acting mainly as a bronchodilator, pulmonary vasodilator and smooth muscle relaxant. The drug also possesses other actions typical of the xanthine derivatives: coronary vasodilator, diuretic, cardiac stimulant, cerebral stimulant and skeletal muscle stimulant. The actions of theophylline may be mediated through inhibition of phosphodiesterase and a resultant increase in intracellular cyclic AMP which could mediate smooth muscle relaxation. At concentrations higher than attained *in vivo,* theophylline also inhibits the release of histamine by mast cells.

Theophylline has been shown to react additively with beta agonists that increase intracellular cyclic AMP through the stimulation of adenyl cyclase (isoproterenol).

Apparently, the development of tolerance does not occur with chronic use of theophylline.

The half-life is shortened with cigarette smoking. The half-life is prolonged in alcoholism, reduced hepatic or renal function, congestive heart failure, and in patients receiving antibiotics such as TAO (troleandomycin), erythromycin and clindamycin. High fever for prolonged periods may decrease theophylline elimination.

Theophylline Elimination Characteristics

	Theophylline Clearance Rates (mean ± S.D.)	Half-life Average (mean ± S.D.)
Children (over 6 months of age)	1.45 ± .58 ml/kg/min	3.7 ± 1.1 hours
Adult non-smokers with uncomplicated asthma	.65 ± .19 ml/kg/min	8.7 ± 2.2 hours

Newborn infants have extremely slow clearances and half-lives exceeding 24 hours, which approach those seen for older children after about 3–6 months.

The half-life of theophylline is prolonged in patients with congestive heart failure, in those with reduced hepatic or renal function, and in alcoholism. The half-life of theophylline may also be prolonged by concurrent use of various drugs such as phenobarbital, and certain antibiotics, including troleandomycin, erythromycin, and lincomycin.

Theophylline half-life is shortened in cigarette smokers (1 to 2 packs/day) as compared to nonsmokers. The increase in theophylline clearance caused by smoking is probably the result of induction of drug metabolizing enzymes that do not readily normalize after cessation of smoking. It appears that between 3

Continued on next page

This product information was prepared in August, 1979. On these and other Parke-Davis Products, detailed information may be obtained by addressing PARKE-DAVIS, Division of Warner-Lambert Company, Morris Plains, NJ 07950.

Parke-Davis—Cont.

months and 2 years may be necessary for normalization of the effect of smoking on theophylline pharmacokinetics.

Actions: Choledyl (oxtriphylline), the choline salt of theophylline, effects significant improvement in pulmonary function parameters which have been impaired by bronchospasm. It is more soluble than either aminophylline or theophylline.

Indications: Choledyl (oxtriphylline) is indicated for relief of acute and chronic bronchial asthma and for reversible bronchospasm associated with chronic bronchitis and emphysema.

Contraindications: Choledyl is contraindicated in individuals who have shown hypersensitivity to theophylline or to Choledyl (oxtriphylline) or any of its components.

Warnings: Status asthmaticus is a medical emergency. Optimal therapy frequently requires additional medication including corticosteroids when the patient is not rapidly responsive to bronchodilators.

Excessive theophylline doses may be associated with toxicity, and serum theophylline levels are recommended to assure maximal benefit without excessive risk, incidence of toxicity increases at levels greater than 20 mcg theophylline/ml. Morphine, curare, and stilbamidine should be used with caution in patients with airflow obstruction since they stimulate histamine release and can induce asthmatic attacks. These drugs may also suppress respiration leading to respiratory failure. Alternative drugs should be chosen whenever possible.

There is an excellent correlation between high blood levels of theophylline resulting from conventional doses and associated clinical manifestations of toxicity in patients with liver dysfunction or chronic obstructive lung disease.

There is excellent correlation between high serum levels of theophylline (over 20 mcg/ml) and the clinical manifestations of toxicity. Careful reduction of dosage and monitoring of serum levels are especially important in patients manifesting a decrease in total body theophylline clearance rate, including those with generalized debility, acute hypoxia, cardiac decompensation, hepatic dysfunction, or renal failure. Dosage reduction may also be necessary in patients who are older than 55 years of age, particularly males.

Serious toxic effects may occur suddenly and are not invariably preceded by minor adverse effects such as nausea, vomiting, and restlessness. Convulsions, tachycardia, or ventricular arrhythmias may be the first sign of toxicity. Children have a marked sensitivity to the CNS stimulant action of theophylline. Serious toxic effects, including fatalities have been reported in children as well as adults.

Theophylline products may worsen pre-existing arrhythmias.

Usage in Pregnancy: Safe use of Choledyl (oxtriphylline) in pregnancy and lactation has not been established relative to possible adverse effects on fetal or neonatal development. Therefore Choledyl (oxtriphylline) should not be used in patients who are pregnant or who may become pregnant, or during lactation unless, in the judgment of the physician, the potential benefits outweigh the possible hazards.

Precautions: Mean half-life in smokers is shorter than nonsmokers. Therefore, smokers may require larger doses of theophylline. Theophylline should not be administered concurrently with other xanthine medications or with xanthine-containing beverages or foods. Use with caution in patients with severe cardiac disease, severe hypoxemia, hypertension, hyperthyroidism, acute myocardial injury, cor pulmonale, congestive heart failure, or liver disease, and in the elderly (especially males) and in neonates. Great caution should especially be used in giving theophylline to patients in congestive heart failure. Such patients have shown markedly prolonged theophylline blood level curves with theophylline persisting in serum for long periods following discontinuation of the drug.

Use theophylline cautiously in patients with a history of peptic ulcer. Theophylline may occasionally act as a local irritant to the G.I. tract although gastrointestinal symptoms are more commonly central and associated with serum theophylline concentrations over 20 mcg/ml.

Adverse Reactions: The most consistent adverse reactions are usually due to overdose and are:

1. Gastrointestinal: nausea, vomiting, epigastric pain, hematemesis, diarrhea.
2. Central nervous system: headaches, irritability, restlessness, insomnia, reflex hyperexcitability, muscle twitching, clonic and tonic generalized convulsions.
3. Cardiovascular: palpitation, tachycardia, extrasystoles, flushing, hypotension, circulatory failure, life-threatening ventricular arrhythmias.
4. Respiratory: tachypnea.
5. Renal: albuminuria, increased excretion of renal tubular cells and red blood cells, diuresis.
6. Others: hyperglycemia and inappropriate antidiuretic hormone (ADH) syndrome.

Drug Interactions: Theophylline-containing preparations have exhibited interaction with the following drugs:

Drug	Effect
Lithium carbonate	Increased excretion of lithium carbonate.
Propranolol	Antagonism of propranolol effect.
Furosemide	Increased furosemide diuresis.
Hexamethonium	Decreased hexamethonium-induced chronotropic effect.
Reserpine	Reserpine-induced tachycardia.
Chlordiazepoxide	Chlordiazepoxide-induced fatty acid mobilization.
Troleandomycin erythromycin or lincomycin	Increased theophylline plasma levels.

Dosage and Administration: Therapeutic serum levels associated with optimal likelihood of benefit and minimal risk of toxicity are considered to be between 10 mcg/ml and 20 mcg/ml. Levels above 20 mcg/ml may produce toxic effects. There is great variation from patient to patient in dosage needed in order to achieve a therapeutic blood level because of variable rates of elimination. Because of this wide variation from patient to patient and the relatively narrow therapeutic blood level range, dosage must be individualized; monitoring of theophylline serum levels is highly recommended.

Dosage should be calculated on the basis of lean (ideal) body weight-mg/kg. Theophylline does not distribute into fatty tissue.

Giving theophylline with food may prevent the rare case of stomach irritation, and although absorption may be slower, it is still complete. When rapidly absorbed products such as solutions are used, dosing to maintain "around the clock" blood levels generally requires administration every 6 hours to obtain the greatest efficacy for use in children; dosing intervals up to 8 hours may be satisfactory for adults because of their slower elimination. Children and adults requiring higher than average doses may benefit from products with slower absorption. This may allow longer dosing intervals and/or less fluctuation in serum concentration over a dosing interval during chronic therapy.

In patients receiving concurrent bronchodilator therapy, eg, beta agonists, downward adjustment of Choledyl (oxtriphylline) dosage is necessary.

[See table below].

II. *Those currently receiving theophylline products:*

Determine where possible, the time, amount, route of administration and form of the patient's last dose.

The loading dose for theophylline will be based on the principle that each 0.8 mg/kg of Choledyl (oxtriphylline) (0.5 mg/kg of theophylline) administered as a loading dose will result in a 1 mcg/ml increase in serum theophylline concentration. Ideally, then, the loading dose should be deferred if a serum theophylline concentration can be rapidly obtained. If this is not possible, the clinician must exercise his judgment in selecting a dose based on the potential for benefit and risk. When there is sufficient respiratory distress to warrant a small risk, 4 mg/kg Choledyl (oxtriphylline) (2.5 mg/kg of theophylline) is likely to increase the serum concentration when administered as a loading dose in rapidly absorbed form by only about 5 mcg/ml. If the patient is not already experiencing theophylline toxicity, this is unlikely to result in dangerous adverse effects. Following the decision regarding loading dose in this group of patients, the subsequent maintenance dosage recommendations are the same as those described above.

To achieve optimal therapeutic theophylline dosage, monitoring of serum theophylline concentrations is recommended. However, it is not always possible or practical to obtain a serum theophylline level.

CHOLEDYL (OXTRIPHYLLINE) DOSAGE FOR PATIENT POPULATION

Acute Symptoms of Asthma Requiring Rapid Theophyllinization:

I. *Not currently receiving theophylline products:*

GROUP	ORAL LOADING DOSE CHOLEDYL	MAINTENANCE DOSE FOR NEXT 12 HOURS CHOLEDYL	MAINTENANCE DOSE BEYOND 12 HOURS CHOLEDYL
1. Children 6 months to 9 years	9.4 mg/kg *(6 mg/kg)	6.2 mg/kg q4 hrs *(4 mg/kg q4 hrs)	6.2 mg/kg q6 hrs *(4 mg/kg q6 hrs)
2. Children age 9–16 and young adult smokers	9.4 mg/kg *(6 mg/kg)	4.7 mg/kg q4 hrs *(3 mg/kg q4 hrs)	4.7 mg/kg q6 hrs *(3 mg/kg q6 hrs)
3. Otherwise healthy nonsmoking adults	9.4 mg/kg *(6 mg/kg)	4.7 mg/kg q6 hrs *(3 mg/kg q6 hrs)	4.7 mg/kg q8 hrs *(3 mg/kg q8 hrs)
4. Older patients and patients with cor pulmonale	9.4 mg/kg *(6 mg/kg)	3.1 mg/kg q6 hrs *(2 mg/kg q6 hrs)	3.1 mg/kg q8 hrs *(2 mg/kg q8 hrs)
5. Patients with congestive heart failure, liver failure	9.4 mg/kg *(6 mg/kg)	3.1 mg/kg q8 hrs *(2 mg/kg q8 hrs)	1.6–3.1 mg/kg q12 hrs *(1–2 mg/kg q12 hrs)

*Anhydrous theophylline indicated in ( )

Patients should be closely monitored for signs of toxicity. The present data suggest that the above dosage recommendations will achieve therapeutic serum concentrations with minimal risk of toxicity for most patients. However, some risk of toxic serum concentration is still present.

Adverse reactions to theophylline often occur when serum theophylline levels exceed 20 mcg/ml.

Chronic Asthma

Theophyllinization is a treatment of first choice for the management of chronic asthma (to prevent symptoms and maintain patent airways). Slow clinical titration is generally preferred to assure acceptance and safety of the medication.

	Choledyl (oxtriphylline)
Initial dose:	25 mg*/kg/day or 625 mg/day (whichever is lower) in 3 to 4 divided doses at 6–8 hour intervals.
Increased dose:	The above dosage may be increased in approximately 25 percent increments at 2 to 3 day intervals so long as no intolerance is observed until the maximum, indicated below, is reached.

*25 mg Choledyl = 16 mg anhydrous theophylline

Maximum dose of Choledyl Pediatric Syrup without measurement of serum theophylline concentration:

Not to exceed the following: (WARNING: DO NOT ATTEMPT TO MAINTAIN ANY DOSE THAT IS NOT TOLERATED)

Age < 9 years	—37.5 mg/kg/day **(24 mg/kg/day)
Age 9–12 years	—31 mg/kg/day **(20 mg/kg/day)
Age 12–16 years	—28 mg/kg/day **(18 mg/kg/day)
Age > 16 years	—20 mg/kg/day or 1400 mg/day (WHICHEVER IS LESS) **(13 mg/kg/day or 900 mg/day (WHICHEVER IS LESS)

NOTE: Use ideal body weight for obese patients.

**anhydrous theophylline indicated in ()

To assist in determining dosage of Choledyl Pediatric Syrup in chronic asthma the above information has been summarized in the following table.

[See table above].

Measurement of serum theophylline concentration during chronic therapy

If the above maximum dosages are to be maintained or exceeded, serum theophylline measurement is recommended. This should be obtained at the approximate time of peak absorption (1 to 1½ hours after dosing) during chronic therapy. It is important that the patient will have missed *no* doses during the previous 48 hours and that dosing intervals will have been reasonably typical, with no added doses during that period of time.

DOSAGE ADJUSTMENT BASED ON SERUM THEOPHYLLINE MEASUREMENTS IF THE ABOVE INSTRUCTIONS HAVE NOT BEEN FOLLOWED MAY RESULT IN RISK OF TOXICITY TO THE PATIENT.

Caution should be exercised for younger children who cannot complain of minor side effects. Older adults, those with cor pulmonale, congestive heart failure, and/or liver disease, may have unusually low dosage requirements and thus may experience toxicity at the maximal dosage recommended above.

It is important that no patient be maintained on any dosage that he is not tolerating. In instructing patients to increase dosage according to the schedule above, they should be instructed to not take a subsequent dose if apparent side effects occur and to resume therapy at a lower dose once adverse effects have disappeared.

Overdosage: Serious toxic effects due to overdosage may occur suddenly and are not invariably preceded by minor adverse effects. Therefore, careful observation of the patient and prompt institution of appropriate therapeutic measures are essential in all cases of overdosage. All patients suspected of overdosage should be hospitalized.

Signs and symptoms of overdosage are related primarily to the cardiovascular, gastrointestinal, and central nervous systems.

Cardiovascular symptoms include precordial pain, tachycardia, ventricular and other arrhythmias; also varying degrees of hypotension including in extreme cases, severe shock, cardiovascular collapse and death.

Gastrointestinal symptoms include abdominal pain, nausea, persistent vomiting, and hematemesis.

Central nervous system symptoms include headache, dizziness, restlessness, irritability, tremors, hyperactivity, and agitation followed, in severe cases, by convulsions, drowsiness, coma and death.

Treatment of overdosage should be directed toward minimizing absorption and supporting vital functions.

In the alert patient emesis should be induced, followed by appropriate additional measures, as listed below. In the obtunded patient, the airway should be secured immediately by means of an endotracheal tube with cuff inflated. After the airway has been secured, lavage should be carried out, and activated charcoal slurry and a cathartic should be administered.

CNS stimulation may be controlled with diazepam, 0.1–0.3 mg/kg intravenously in children, and 10 mg intravenously in adults. Respiration should be supported by appropriate means. Hypotension and shock should be treated with appropriate fluid replacement, avoiding the use of vasopressors, if possible. Additional supportive measures should be carried out as required.

Serial serum theophylline levels are of value in following the patient's course and in guiding further management.

Forced diuresis is of no value because of the small amount of theophylline excreted unchanged by the kidney. There has been a single report of survival with the use of an activated charcoal column (hemoperfusion) in massive theophylline overdosage.

How Supplied: N 0071-2217-23—Choledyl Pediatric Syrup (oxtriphylline) is a vanilla-mint flavored syrup supplied in bottles of 16 fl oz (1 pint) 474 ml.

Store between 59°–86° F (15°–30° C).

2217G050 6-79

Approximate Choledyl Pediatric Syrup Dosage (administered every 6 hours)

Body Weight		< 9 years Initial Dose	Max. Dose	9–12 years Initial Dose	Max. Dose	12–16 years Initial Dose	Max. Dose	> 16 years Initial Dose	Max. Dose
lbs.	Kg.	6.2 mg/kg	9.4 mg/kg	6.2 mg/kg	7.8 mg/kg	6.2 mg/kg	7 mg/kg	6.2 mg/kg	5
18	8	1 tsp	1½ tsp	—	—	—	—	—	—
36	16	2 tsp	3 tsp	2 tsp	2½ tsp	—	—	—	—
54	24	3 tsp*	4½ tsp	3 tsp*	3½ tsp	3 tsp*	3½ tsp	—	—
72	32	3 tsp*	6 tsp	3 tsp*	5 tsp	3 tsp*	4½ tsp	3 tsp*	3 tsp
90	40	3 tsp*	7 tsp**	3 tsp*	6 tsp	3 tsp*	5½ tsp	3 tsp*	4 tsp
108	48	3 tsp*	7 tsp**	3 tsp*	7 tsp**	3 tsp*	6½ tsp	3 tsp*	5 tsp

NOTE: The initial dosage may be increased in approximately 25 percent increments at 2 to 3 day intervals as clinically indicated and tolerated until the maximum dosage is reached.

1 mg Choledyl (oxtriphylline) = 0.64 mg anhydrous theophylline

*Initial Dosage should not exceed 625 mg/day Choledyl (400 mg/day theophylline)

**Maximum Dosage should not exceed 1400 mg/day Choledyl (900 mg/day theophylline)

COLY-MYCIN® M PARENTERAL ℞

(sterile colistimethate sodium) for intramuscular and intravenous use

Caution: Federal law prohibits dispensing without prescription.

Coly-Mycin M Parenteral (sterile colistimethate sodium) contains the sodium salt of colistimethate. Colistimethate sodium is a polypeptide antibiotic with an approximate molecular weight of 1750; the empirical formula is $C_{58}H_{105}N_{16}Na_5O_{28}S_5$.

Actions:

Microbiology

Coly-Mycin M Parenteral has bactericidal activity against the following gram-negative bacilli: *Enterobacter aerogenes, Escherichia coli, Klebsiella pneumoniae,* and *Pseudomonas aeruginosa.*

Human Pharmacology

Typical serum and urine levels following a single 150 mg dose of Coly-Mycin M Parenteral IM or IV in normal adult subjects are shown in Figure 1.

FIGURE I: URINE AND SERUM VALUES IN ADULTS FOLLOWING PARENTERAL (IM OR IV) ADMINISTRATION OF COLY-MYCIN M PARENTERAL.

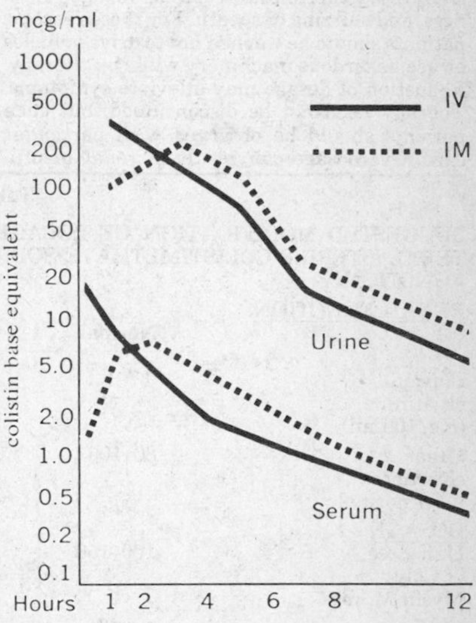

Continued on next page

This product information was prepared in August, 1979. On these and other Parke-Davis Products, detailed information may be obtained by addressing PARKE-DAVIS, Division of Warner-Lambert Company, Morris Plains, NJ 07950.

Parke-Davis—Cont.

Higher serum levels were obtained at 10 minutes following IV administration. Serum concentration declined with a half-life of 2-3 hours following either intravenous or intramuscular administration in adults and children, including premature infants.
Colistimethate sodium is transferred across the placental barrier, and blood levels of about 1 mcg/ml are obtained in the fetus following intravenous administration to the mother.
Average urine levels ranged from about 270 mcg/ml at 2 hours to about 15 mcg/ml at 8 hours after intravenous administration and from about 200 to about 25 mcg/ml during a similar period following intramuscular administration.
Indications: Coly-Mycin M Parenteral (sterile colistimethate sodium) is indicated for the treatment of acute or chronic infections due to sensitive strains of certain gram-negative bacilli. It is particularly indicated when the infection is caused by sensitive strains of ***Pseudomonas aeruginosa.*** This antibiotic is not indicated for infections due to *Proteus* or *Neisseria.* Coly-Mycin M Parenteral has proven clinically effective in treatment of infections due to the following gram-negative organisms:
Enterobacter aerogenes, Escherichia coli, Klebsiella pneumoniae, and ***Pseudomonas aeruginosa.***
Pending results of appropriate bacteriologic cultures and sensitivity tests, Coly-Mycin M Parenteral may be used to initiate therapy in serious infections that are suspected to be due to gram-negative organisms.
Contraindications: The use of Coly-Mycin M Parenteral (sterile colistimethate sodium) is contraindicated for patients with a history of sensitivity to the drug.
Warning: Maximum daily dose should not exceed 5 mg/kg/day (2.3 mg/lb) with normal renal function.
Transient neurological disturbances may occur. These include circumoral paresthesias or numbness, tingling or formication of the extremities, generalized pruritus, vertigo, dizziness, and slurring of speech. For these reasons, patients should be warned not to drive vehicles or use hazardous machinery while on therapy. Reduction of dosage may alleviate symptoms. Therapy need not be discontinued, but such patients should be observed with particular care. Overdosage can result in renal insufficiency, muscle weakness and apnea. See PRECAUTIONS for use concomitantly with curariform drugs, and DOSAGE and ADMINISTRATION Section for use in renal impairment.
Use in Pregnancy: The safety of colistimethate sodium during human pregnancy has not been established.
Precautions: Since Coly-Mycin M Parenteral (sterile colistimethate sodium) is eliminated mainly by renal excretion, it should be used with caution when the possibility of impaired renal function exists. The decline in renal function with advanced age should be considered.
When actual renal impairment is present, Coly-Mycin M Parenteral may be used, but the greatest caution should be exercised and the dosage should be reduced in proportion to the extent of the impairment. Administration of amounts of Coly-Mycin M Parenteral in excess of renal excretory capacity will lead to high serum levels and can result in further impairment of renal function, initiating a cycle which, if not recognized, can lead to acute renal insufficiency, renal shutdown and further concentration of the antibiotic to toxic levels in the body. At this point, interference of nerve transmission at neuromuscular junctions may occur and result in muscle weakness and apnea.
Easily recognized signs indicating the development of impaired renal function are diminishing urine output, rising BUN and serum creatinine. If present, therapy with Coly-Mycin M Parenteral (sterile colistimethate sodium) should be discontinued immediately.
If a life-threatening situation exists, therapy may be reinstated at a lower dosage after blood levels have fallen.
Certain other antibiotics (kanamycin, streptomycin, dihydrostreptomycin, polymyxin, neomycin) have also been reported to interfere with the nerve transmission at the neuromuscular junction. Based on this reported activity, they should not be given concomitantly with Coly-Mycin M Parenteral except with the greatest caution. The antibiotics with a gram-positive antimicrobial spectrum, e.g., penicillin, tetracycline, sodium cephalothin, have not been reported to interfere with nerve transmission and, accordingly, would not be expected to potentiate this activity of Coly-Mycin M Parenteral.
Other drugs, including curariform muscle relaxants (ether, tubocurarine, succinylcholine, gallamine, decamethonium and sodium citrate), potentiate the neuromuscular blocking effect and should be used with extreme caution in patients being treated with Coly-Mycin M Parenteral.
If apnea occurs, it may be treated with assisted respiration, oxygen, and calcium chloride injections.
Adverse Reactions: Respiratory arrest has been reported following intramuscular administration of colistimethate sodium. Impaired renal function increases the possibility of apnea and neuromuscular blockade following administration of colistimethate sodium. This has been generally due to failure to follow recommended guidelines, usually overdosage, failure to reduce dose commensurate with degree of renal impairment, and/or concomitant use of other antibiotics or drugs with neuromuscular blocking potential.
A decrease in urine output or increase in blood urea nitrogen or serum creatinine can be interpreted as signs of nephrotoxicity, which is probably a dose-dependent effect of colistimethate sodium. These manifestations of nephrotoxicity are reversible following discontinuation of the antibiotic.
Increases of blood urea nitrogen have been reported for patients receiving Coly-Mycin M Parenteral (sterile colistimethate sodium) at dose levels of 1.6-5 mg/kg per day. The BUN values returned to normal following cessation of Coly-Mycin M Parenteral administration.
Paresthesia, tingling of the extremities or tingling of the tongue and generalized itching or urticaria have been reported by patients who received Coly-Mycin M Parenteral by intravenous or intramuscular injection. In addition, the following adverse reactions have been reported for colistimethate sodium: drug fever and gastrointestinal upset, vertigo, and slurring of speech. The subjective symptoms reported by the adult may not be manifest in infants or young children, thus requiring close attention to renal function.
Dosage and Administration:
Important: Coly-Mycin M Parenteral (sterile colistimethate sodium) is supplied in vials containing colistimethate sodium equivalent to 20 mg (green cap) or 150 mg (red cap) colistin base activity per vial.
Reconstitution: The *20 mg* vial should be reconstituted with *2.2 ml* Sterile Water for Injection USP. The reconstituted solution provides colistimethate sodium at a concentration of 10 mg/ml for convenient and accurate pediatric administration. The *150 mg* vial should be reconstituted with *2.0 ml* Sterile Water for Injection USP. The reconstituted solution provides colistimethate sodium at a concentration of 75 mg/ml.
During reconstitution swirl *gently* to avoid frothing.
Dosage: *Adults and children—intravenous or intramuscular administration*—Coly-Mycin M Parenteral should be given in 2 to 4 divided doses at dose levels of 2.5 to 5 mg/kg per day for patients with normal renal function, depending on the severity of the infection.
The daily dose should be reduced in the presence of any renal impairment, which can often be anticipated from the history.
Modifications of dosage in the presence of renal impairment are presented in Table 1.
[See table at left].

Table 1

SUGGESTED MODIFICATION OF DOSAGE SCHEDULES OF COLY-MYCIN M PARENTERAL (STERILE COLISTIMETHATE SODIUM) FOR ADULTS WITH IMPAIRED RENAL FUNCTION

RENAL FUNCTION		DEGREE OF IMPAIRMENT		
	Normal	Mild	Moderate	Considerable
Plasma creatinine, (mg/100 ml)	0.7–1.2	1.3–1.5	1.6–2.5	2.6–4.0
Urea clearance, % of normal	80–100	40–70	25–40	10–25
DOSAGE				
Unit dose of Coly-Mycin M, mg	100–150	75–115	66–150	100–150
Frequency, times/day	4 to 2	2	2 or 1	every 36 hr
Total daily dose, mg	300	150–230	133–150	100
Approximate daily dose, mg/kg/day	5.0	2.5–3.8	2.5	1.5

Note: The suggested unit dose is 2.5–5 mg/kg; however, the time INTERVAL between injections should be increased in the presence of impaired renal function.

INTRAVENOUS ADMINISTRATION

1. Direct Intermittent Administration — slowly inject one-half of the total daily dose over a period of 3 to 5 minutes every 12 hours.
2. Continuous Infusion — slowly inject one-half the total daily dose over 3 to 5 minutes. Add the remaining half of the total daily dose of Coly-Mycin M Parenteral to one of the following: 0.9% NaCl; 5% dextrose in 0.9% NaCl; 5% dextrose in water; 5% dex-

trose in 0.45% NaCl; 5% dextrose in 0.225% NaCl; lactated Ringer's solution, or 10% invert sugar solution. There are not sufficient data to recommend usage of Coly-Mycin M Parenteral with other drugs or with other than the above listed infusion solutions.

Administer by slow intravenous infusion starting 1 to 2 hours after the initial dose at a rate of 5-6 mg/hr in the presence of normal renal function. In the presence of impaired renal function, reduce the infusion rate depending on the degree of renal impairment.

The choice of intravenous solution and the volume to be employed are dictated by the requirements of fluid and electrolyte management.

Any infusion solution containing colistimethate sodium should be freshly prepared and used for no longer than 24 hours.

How Supplied: Coly-Mycin M Parenteral (sterile colistimethate sodium) is supplied in vials containing colistimethate sodium (20 or 150 mg colistin base equivalent per vial) as a white to slightly yellow lyophilized cake.

STORE AT CONTROLLED ROOM TEMPERATURE (59° to 86°F) (15° to 30°C).

150 mg vial, red cap (N 0047-0145-50) 50 vials per carton or (N 0047-0145-01) one vial per carton.

STORE RECONSTITUTED SOLUTION IN REFRIGERATOR (36° to 46°F) (2° to 8°C) OR AT CONTROLLED ROOM TEMPERATURE (59° to 86°F) (15° to 30°C), and use within 7 days.

Toxicology and Animal Pharmacology:

Acute Toxicity: The intravenous LD_{50} was 41.5 mg/kg in the dog and 739 mg/kg in the mouse; intramuscular toxicity was 42 mg/kg in the dog and 267 mg/kg in the mouse.

Subacute Toxicity: In albino rabbits and beagle dogs, IV doses of 5, 10 and 20 mg/kg/day for 28 days resulted in elevated blood urea nitrogen in the dog (10 mg/kg/day dose group) and in both 20 mg/kg dose groups.

Clinical Studies: Clinically, Coly-Mycin M Parenteral (sterile colistimethate sodium) has been of particular therapeutic value in acute and chronic urinary tract infections caused by sensitive strains of *Pseudomonas aeruginosa*.

Colistimethate sodium is clinically effective in the treatment of infections due to other sensitive gram-negative pathogenic bacilli that have become resistant to broad-spectrum antibiotics.

Colistimethate sodium has been used to treat bacteriuria and overt urinary infections in pregnant women during the third trimester. However, in view of the evidence of possible embryotoxic and teratogenic effects of colistimethate sodium in pregnant rabbits, caution should be exercised in use of this drug in women of childbearing potential.

365 G 780 R-11-76

COLY-MYCIN® S ORAL SUSPENSION ℞

(colistin sulfate for oral suspension)
FOR ORAL USE ONLY

Caution: Federal law prohibits dispensing without prescription.

Coly-Mycin S Oral Suspension (colistin sulfate for oral suspension) contains the sulfate salt of colistin, a polypeptide antibiotic with a molecular weight of approximately 1170. The empirical formula of colistin is $C_{53}H_{100}N_{16}O_{13}$.

Actions: Coly-Mycin S Oral Suspension has *in vitro* bactericidal activity against most gram-negative enteric pathogens, especially enteropathogenic *E. coli* and *Shigella* (but not *Proteus*). In infants and children, it has effectively controlled acute infections of the intestinal tract due to these pathogens. Susceptible strains of *E. coli* and *Shigella in vitro* or *in vivo* rarely develop resistance to Coly-Mycin S Oral Suspension. Cross resistance to polymyxin B sulfate does exist, but cross resistance to broad spectrum antibiotics has not been encountered.

Indications: Diarrhea in infants and children, caused by susceptible strains of enteropathogenic *E. coli*.

Gastroenteritis due to *Shigella* organisms. Clinical response may vary due to the absence of tissue levels in the bowel wall.

Contraindications: Known hypersensitivity to the drug.

Warnings: Although Coly-Mycin S Oral Suspension is not absorbed systemically in measurable amounts, it is assumed that slight absorption may occur. Therefore, in the presence of azotemia or, if dosages above the recommended range are used, a potential for possible renal toxicity exists.

With prolonged usage, suppression of intestinal bacterial flora may occur. There may be a resultant overgrowth of organisms (such as *Proteus*); appropriate therapy should be initiated immediately.

Precautions: Renal function should be assessed prior to initiation of therapy.

Adverse Reactions: Within the recommended dosage range, none reported.

Preparation: Coly-Mycin S Oral Suspension (colistin sulfate for oral suspension) is a dry powder which is reconstituted with 37 ml of distilled water. To reconstitute, slowly add one half of the diluent, replace the cap and shake well. Add the remaining diluent and repeat shaking. Volume after reconstitution is 60 ml. When reconstituted, Coly-Mycin S Oral Suspension is a chocolate-flavored mixture, each 5 ml teaspoonful containing the equivalent of 25 mg of colistin base. Reconstituted Coly-Mycin S Oral Suspension is stable for two weeks when kept below 59°F (15°C).

Dosage and Administration: The usual dosage of colistin sulfate is 5–15 mg/kg/day (2.3–6.9 mg/pound/day) given in three divided doses. Higher doses may be necessary. Each 5 ml of Coly-Mycin S Oral Suspension contains the equivalent of 25 mg colistin sulfate. A 10-pound infant would require 23–69 mg of colistin sulfate or approximately ⅓ to 1 teaspoon three times a day. A 50-pound patient would require 115–340 mg colistin sulfate or approximately 1½ to 4½ teaspoons three times a day.

Supplied: Bottles containing colistin sulfate equivalent to 300 mg colistin base (N 0047-0142-53).

Before reconstitution store between 59° and 86°F (15° and 30°C).

365 G 485 R-3-77

COLY-MYCIN® S OTIC ℞

with Neomycin and Hydrocortisone (colistin sulfate—neomycin sulfate—thonzonium bromide—hydrocortisone acetate otic suspension)

Caution: Federal law prohibits dispensing without prescription.

Description: Coly-Mycin S Otic with Neomycin and Hydrocortisone (colistin sulfate-neomycin sulfate-thonzonium bromide-hydrocortisone acetate otic suspension) is a sterile aqueous suspension containing in each ml: Colistin base activity, 3 mg (as the sulfate); Neomycin base activity, 3.3 mg (as the sulfate); Hydrocortisone acetate, 10 mg (1%); Thonzonium bromide, 0.5 mg (0.05%); Polysorbate 80, acetic acid, and sodium acetate in a buffered aqueous vehicle. Thimerosal, 0.002%, added as a preservative. It is a non-viscous liquid, buffered at pH 5, for instillation into the canal of the external ear or direct application to the affected aural skin.

Actions:

1. Colistin sulfate—an antibiotic with bactericidal action against most gram-negative organisms, notably *Pseudomonas aeruginosa*, *E. coli.*, and *Klebsiella-Aerobacter*.
2. Neomycin sulfate—a broad-spectrum antibiotic, bactericidal to many pathogens, notably *Staph. aureus* and *Proteus* sp.
3. Hydrocortisone acetate—a corticosteroid that controls inflammation, edema, pruritus and other dermal reactions.
4. Thonzonium bromide—a surface-active agent that promotes tissue contact by dispersion and penetration of the cellular debris and exudate.

Indications: For the treatment of superficial bacterial infections of the external auditory canal, caused by organisms susceptible to the action of the antibiotics; and for the treatment of infections of mastoidectomy and fenestration cavities, caused by organisms susceptible to the antibiotics.

Contraindications: This product is contraindicated in those individuals who have shown hypersensitivity to any of its components, and in herpes simplex, vaccinia and varicella.

Warnings: As with other antibiotic preparations, prolonged treatment may result in overgrowth of nonsusceptible organisms and fungi. If the infection is not improved after one week, cultures and susceptibility tests should be repeated to verify the identity of the organism and to determine whether therapy should be changed.

Patients who prefer to warm the medication before using should be cautioned against heating the solution above body temperature, in order to avoid loss of potency.

Precautions: If sensitization or irritation occurs, medication should be discontinued promptly.

This drug should be used with care in cases of perforated eardrum and in long-standing cases of chronic otitis media because of the possibility of ototoxicity caused by neomycin.

Treatment should not be continued for longer than ten days.

Allergic cross-reactions may occur which could prevent the use of any or all of the following antibiotics for the treatment of future infections: kanamycin, paromomycin, streptomycin, and possibly gentamicin.

Adverse Reactions: Neomycin is a not uncommon cutaneous sensitizer. There are articles in the current literature that indicate an increase in the prevalence of persons sensitive to neomycin.

Dosage and Administration: The external auditory canal should be thoroughly cleansed and dried with a sterile cotton applicator.

For adults, 4 drops of the suspension should be instilled into the affected ear 3 or 4 times daily. For infants and children, 3 drops are suggested because of the smaller capacity of the ear canal.

The patient should lie with the affected ear upward and then the drops should be instilled. This position should be maintained for 5 minutes to facilitate penetration of the drops into the ear canal. Repeat, if necessary, for the opposite ear.

If preferred, a cotton wick may be inserted into the canal and then the cotton may be saturated with the solution. This wick should be kept moist by adding further solution every 4 hours. The wick should be replaced at least once every 24 hours.

Continued on next page

This product information was prepared in August, 1979. On these and other Parke-Davis Products, detailed information may be obtained by addressing PARKE-DAVIS, Division of Warner-Lambert Company, Morris Plains, NJ 07950.

Parke-Davis—Cont.

How Supplied: In bottles containing 5 ml (N 0047-0141-05) or 10 ml (N 0047-0141-10). Each package contains a sterile dropper calibrated at 4 drops.

SHAKE WELL BEFORE USING.

Store at controlled room temperature (59° - 86° F) (15° - 30° C). Stable for 18 months at room temperature; prolonged exposure to higher temperatures should be avoided.

365 G 840 **R-12-77**

DILANTIN® KAPSEALS® ℞
(phenytoin sodium capsules, USP)

Parenteral
DILANTIN ℞
(phenytoin sodium injection)

> **IMPORTANT NOTE**
> **This drug must be administered slowly.**
> **Do not exceed 50 mg per minute intravenously.**

Description:

Oral:

Dilantin (phenytoin sodium) is related to the barbiturates in chemical structure, but has a five-membered ring. The chemical name is sodium 5,5-diphenyl-2,4-imidazolidinedione.

Parenteral:

Ampoule Dilantin (phenytoin sodium injection) is a ready-mixed solution of phenytoin sodium in a vehicle containing 40% propylene glycol and 10% alcohol in water for injection, adjusted to pH 12 with sodium hydroxide. Phenytoin sodium is related to the barbiturates in chemical structure, but has a five-membered ring. The chemical name is 5,5-diphenyl-2,4-imidazolidinedione.

Clinical Pharmacology:

Oral:

Phenytoin is an anticonvulsant drug which can be useful in the treatment of epilepsy.

Parenteral:

Phenytoin is an anticonvulsant which may be useful in the treatment of status epilepticus of the grand mal type.

Oral and Parenteral:

The primary site of action appears to be the motor cortex where spread of seizure activity is inhibited. Possibly by promoting sodium efflux from neurons, phenytoin tends to stabilize the threshold against hyperexcitability caused by excessive stimulation or environmental changes capable of reducing membrane sodium gradient. This includes the reduction of posttetanic potentiation at synapses. Loss of posttetanic potentiation prevents cortical seizure foci from detonating adjacent cortical areas. Phenytoin reduces the maximal activity of brain stem centers responsible for the tonic phase of grand mal seizures.

Oral:

The plasma half-life in man after oral administration of phenytoin averages 22 hours, with a range of 7 to 42 hours. Steady-state therapeutic levels are achieved 7 to 10 days after initiation of therapy with recommended dosage of 300 mg/day. The clinically effective serum level is usually 10 to 20 mcg/ml.

The majority of phenytoin is excreted in the bile as inactive metabolites, which are then reabsorbed from the intestinal tract and excreted in the urine. Urinary excretion of phenytoin and its metabolites occurs partly through glomerular filtration but, more importantly, by tubular secretion.

In most patients maintained at a steady dosage, a stable phenytoin blood level is achieved. Some patients manifest a large variation in plasma levels despite equivalent dosages. Patients with unusually low plasma levels may not be absorbing phenytoin, may be noncompliant, or are hypermetabolizers of phenytoin. Unusually high plasma levels result from liver disease, congenital enzyme deficiency, or drug interactions which result in metabolic interference. The patient with large variations in phenytoin plasma levels, despite standard dosage, presents a difficult clinical problem and may benefit from serum level determinations.

Clinical studies with this drug have indicated that both single and divided dosage schedules demonstrate similar rates of absorption and equilibrium levels. This means that a patient stabilized with a dosage of a 100-mg dose three times daily may respond to the more convenient, single, daily dose of 300 mg. After the divided dosage of 300 mg daily has adequately controlled the seizures, changeover to a single, daily dose of 300 mg can be considered.

There has been no reported evidence of increased drug toxicity when single, daily doses of 300 mg have been administered to patients previously receiving the same quantity in divided doses.

Parenteral:

A fall in plasma levels may occur when patients are changed from oral to intramuscular administration. The drop is caused by slower absorption, as compared to oral administration, due to the poor water solubility of phenytoin. Intravenous administration is the preferred route for producing rapid therapeutic serum levels.

There are occasions when intramuscular administration may be required: ie, postoperatively, in comatose patients, for GI upsets. During these periods, a sufficient dose must be administered intramuscularly to maintain the plasma level within the therapeutic range. Where oral dosage is resumed following intramuscular usage, the oral dosage should be properly adjusted to compensate for the slow, continuing IM absorption to avoid toxic symptoms.

Patients stabilized on a daily oral regimen of Dilantin (phenytoin sodium) experience a drop in peak blood levels to 50 to 60% of stable levels if crossed over to an equal dose administered intramuscularly. However, the intramuscular depot of poorly soluble material is eventually absorbed, as determined by urinary excretion of 5-(p-hydroxyphenyl)-5-phenylhydantoin (HPPH), the principal metabolite, as well as the total amount of drug eventually appearing in the blood.

A short-term (one week) study indicates that patients do not experience the expected drop in blood levels when crossed over to the intramuscular route, if the Dilantin IM dosage is increased by 50% over the previously established oral dosage. To avoid drug cumulation due to absorption from the muscle depots, it is recommended that for the first week back on oral Dilantin, the dosage be reduced to one half of the original oral dosage (one third of the IM dosage). Experience for periods greater than one week are lacking and blood level monitoring is recommended. For administration of Dilantin in patients who cannot take oral medication for periods greater than a week, gastric intubation may be considered.

Indications:

Oral:

Dilantin is indicated for the control of grand mal and psychomotor seizures.

Parenteral:

Parenteral Dilantin is indicated for the control of status epilepticus of the grand mal type, and for prevention and treatment of seizures occurring during neurosurgery.

Contraindications:

Oral and Parenteral:

Phenytoin is contraindicated in those patients with a history of hypersensitivity to hydantoin products.

Parenteral:

Because of its effect on ventricular automaticity, phenytoin is contraindicated in sinus bradycardia, sino-artrial block, second- and third-degree A-V block, and patients with Adams-Stokes syndrome.

Warnings:

Oral

Abrupt withdrawal of phenytoin in epileptic patients may precipitate status epilepticus. When, in the judgment of the clinician, the need for dosage reduction, discontinuation, or substitution of other anticonvulsant medication arises, this should be done gradually. In the event of an allergic or hypersensitivity reaction, more rapid substitution of alternative therapy may be necessary. In this case, alternative therapy should be an anticonvulsant not belonging to the hydantoin chemical class.

Parenteral:

Intravenous administration should not exceed 50 mg per minute.

Oral and Parenteral:

Phenytoin and phenytoin sodium injection are not indicated in seizures due to hypoglycemia or other causes which may be immediately identified and corrected. Appropriate diagnostic procedures should be performed as indicated.

Phenytoin metabolism may be significantly altered by the concomitant use of other drugs, such as the following.

Oral:

1. Barbiturates may enhance the rate of metabolism of phenytoin. This effect, however, is variable and unpredictable.
2. Coumarin anticoagulants, disulfiram, phenylbutazone, and sulfaphenazole may inhibit the metabolism of phenytoin, resulting in increased serum levels of the drug. This may lead to an increased incidence of nystagmus, ataxia, or other toxic signs. The effect of dicumarol in inhibiting the metabolism of phenytoin in the liver has been well-documented.
3. Isoniazid inhibits the metabolism of phenytoin so that, with combined therapy, patients who are slow acetylators may suffer from phenytoin intoxication.
4. Tricyclic antidepressants in high doses may precipitate seizures, and the dosage of phenytoin may have to be adjusted accordingly.

Phenytoin may interfere with the metyrapone and the 1-mg dexamethasone tests. It may also suppress the protein-bound iodine. However, this has not been associated with any clinical signs of hypothyroidism; the T3 is normal.

Parenteral:

1. Barbiturates may enhance the rate of metabolism of phenytoin. This effect, however, is variable and unpredictable. It has been reported that, in some cases, the concomitant administration of carbamazepine resulted in an increased rate of phenytoin metabolism.
2. Coumarin anticoagulants, disulfiram, phenylbutazone, and sulfaphenazole may inhibit the metabolism of phenytoin, resulting in signs of phenytoin toxicity. The effect of dicumarol in inhibiting the metabolism of phenytoin in the liver has been well-documented.
3. Isoniazid inhibits the metabolism of phenytoin so that, with combined therapy, patients who are slow acetylators may suffer from phenytoin intoxication.
4. Tricyclic antidepressants in high doses may precipitate seizures, and the dosage of phenytoin may have to be adjusted.

The results of certain clinical laboratory tests, eg, metyrapone, 1-mg dexamethasone, and protein-bound iodine, may be altered if the patient has been receiving phenytoin.

Phenytoin should be used with caution in patients with hypotension and severe myocardial insufficiency.

The intramuscular route is not recommended for the treatment of status epilepticus because blood levels of phenytoin in the therapeutic range cannot be readily achieved with doses and methods of administration ordinarily employed.

Oral and Parenteral:

Usage in Pregnancy: The effects of Dilantin (phenytoin sodium) in human pregnancy and nursing infants are unknown.

Recent reports suggest an association between the use of anticonvulsant drugs by women with epilepsy and an elevated incidence of birth defects in children born to these women. Data is more extensive with respect to phenytoin and phenobarbital, but these are also the most commonly prescribed anticonvulsants; less systematic or anecdotal reports suggest a possible similar association with the use of all known anticonvulsant drugs.

The reports suggesting an elevated incidence of birth defects in children of drug-treated epileptic women cannot be regarded as adequate to prove a definite cause and effect relationship. There are intrinsic methodologic problems in obtaining adequate data on drug teratogenicity in humans; the possibility also exists that other factors, eg, genetic factors or the epileptic condition itself, may be more important than drug therapy in leading to birth defects. The great majority of mothers on anticonvulsant medication deliver normal infants. It is important to note that anticonvulsant drugs should not be discontinued in patients in whom the drug is administered to prevent major seizures because of the strong possibility of precipitating status epilepticus with attendant hypoxia and threat to life. In individual cases where the severity and frequency of the seizure disorder are such that the removal of medication does not pose a serious threat to the patient, discontinuation of the drug may be considered prior to and during pregnancy, although it cannot be said with any confidence that even minor seizures do not pose some hazard to the developing embryo or fetus.

The prescribing physician will wish to weigh these considerations in treating or counseling epileptic women of childbearing potential.

Precautions:

Parenteral:

The addition of Dilantin solution to intravenous infusion is not recommended due to lack of solubility and resultant precipitation.

Oral and Parenteral:

The liver is the chief site of biotransformation of phenytoin: patients with impaired liver function may show early signs of toxicity. Elderly patients or those who are gravely ill may show early signs of toxicity.

A small percentage of individuals who have been treated with phenytoin have been shown to metabolize the drug slowly. Slow metabolism may be due to limited enzyme availability and lack of induction and appears to be genetically determined.

Oral:

Phenytoin has been associated with reversible lymph node hyperplasia. If lymph node enlargement occurs in patients on phenytoin, every effort should be made to substitute another anticonvulsant drug or drug combination.

Oral and Parenteral:

Drugs that control grand mal are not effective against absence (petit mal) seizures. Therefore, if both conditions are present, combined drug therapy is needed.

Oral:

The drug should be discontinued if a skin rash appears (See Warnings section regarding drug discontinuation). If the rash is exfoliative, purpuric, or bullous, use of the drug should not be resumed. If the rash is a milder type (measles-like or scarlatiniform), therapy may be resumed after the rash has completely disappeared. If the rash recurs upon reinstitution of therapy, further phenytoin sodium administration is contraindicated.

Osteomalacia has been associated with anticonvulsant therapy, including phenytoin.

Parenteral:

Each injection of intravenous Dilantin (phenytoin sodium injection) should be followed by an injection of sterile saline through the same needle or intravenous catheter to avoid local venous irritation due to the alkalinity of the solution. Continuous infusion should be avoided.

Oral and Parenteral:

Hyperglycemia, resulting from the drug's inhibitory effect on insulin release, has been reported. Phenytoin may also raise the blood sugar level in persons already suffering from hyperglycemia.

Adverse Reactions:

Oral:

Central Nervous System: The most common manifestations encountered with phenytoin therapy are referable to this system. These include nystagmus, ataxia, slurred speech, and mental confusion. Dizziness, insomnia, transient nervousness, motor twitchings, and headache have also been observed. These side effects may disappear with continuing therapy at a reduced dosage level.

Gastrointestinal System: Phenytoin may cause nausea, vomiting, and constipation. Administration of the drug with or immediately after meals may help prevent gastrointestinal discomfort.

Integumentary System: Dermatological manifestations sometimes accompanied by fever have included scarlatiniform or morbilliform rashes. A morbilliform rash (measles-like) is the most common; other types of dermatitis are seen more rarely. Rashes are more frequent in children and young adults. Other, more serious forms which may be fatal have included bullous, exfoliative, or purpuric dermatitis, lupus erythematosus, and Stevens-Johnson syndrome.

Hemopoietic System: Hemopoietic complications, some fatal, have occasionally been reported in association with administration of phenytoin. These have included thrombocytopenia, leukopenia, granulocytopenia, agranulocytosis, and pancytopenia. While marcrocytosis and megaloblastic anemia have occurred, these conditions usually respond to folic acid therapy. The occasional occurrence of lymphadenopathy indicates the need to differentiate such a condition from other lymph gland pathology.

Other: Gingival hyperplasia occurs frequently; the incidence may be reduced by good oral hygiene including gum massage, frequent brushing, and appropriate dental care. Polyarthropathy and hirsutism occur occasionally. Hyperglycemia has been reported. Toxic hepatitis, liver damage, and periarteritis nodosa may occur and can be fatal.

Parenteral:

The most notable signs of toxicity associated with the intravenous use of this drug are cardiovascular collapse and/or central nervous system depression. Hyptension does occur when the drug is administered rapidly by the intravenous route. The <u>rate</u> of administration is very important; it should not exceed 50 mg per minute. At this rate, toxicity should be minimized.

Severe cardiotoxic reactions and fatalities have been reported with atrial and ventricular conduction depression and ventricular fibrillation. Severe complications are most commonly encountered in elderly or gravely ill patients. Parenteral Dilantin (phenytoin sodium parenteral) sometimes causes drowsiness, nystagmus, circumoral tingling, vertigo, nausea, and, rarely, vomiting. When these effects are observed, the plasma concentration is usually above 20 mcg/ml, which is just above the usual therapeutic plasma concentration.

Administration of this drug has produced an elevation in plasma glucose concentration.

Dosage and Administration:

Oral:

Dosage should be individualized to provide maximum benefit. In some cases, serum blood level determinations may be necessary for optimal dosage adjustments—the clinically effective serum level is usually in the range of 10 to 20 mcg/ml. With recommended dosage, a period of 7 to 10 days may be required to achieve therapeutic blood levels with Dilantin (phenytoin sodium).

Adult Dosage: Patients who have received no previous treatment may be started on one 100-mg Dilantin Kapseal three times daily, and the dosage then adjusted to suit individual requirements. For most adults, the satisfactory maintenance dosage will be three to four Kapseals daily. An increase to six Kapseals daily may be made, if necessary.

Pediatric Dosage: Initially, 5 mg/kg/day in two or three equally divided doses, with subsequent dosage individualized to a maximum of 300 mg daily. A recommended daily maintenance dosage is usually in the range of 4 to 8 mg/kg. Children over 6 years old may require the minimal adult dosage (300 mg/day). Pediatric dosage forms available include a 30-mg Kapseal, a palatably flavored 50-mg Infatab, or an oral suspension form containing 30 mg of Dilantin in each 5 ml.

Alternative Dosage: Once-a-day dosage for adults with 300 mg of Dilantin may be considered if seizure control is established with divided doses of three 100-mg Kapseals daily. Studies comparing divided doses of 100 mg three times daily with a single, daily dose of 300 mg indicated that absorption, peak plasma levels, biologic half-life, difference between peak and minimum values, and urinary recovery were equivalent. Once-a-day dosage offers a convenience to the individual patient or to nursing personnel for institutionalized patients, and is intended to be used only for patients requiring this amount of drug daily. A major problem in motivating noncompliant patients may be lessened also when the patient can take all of the medication once a day. However, patients should be cautioned not to miss a dose inadvertently.

Parenteral:

The addition of Dilantin (phenytoin sodium) solution to intravenous infusion is not recommended due to lack of solubility and resultant precipitation.

Not to exceed 50 mg per minute, intravenously. There is a relatively small margin between full therapeutic effect and minimally toxic doses of this drug.

The solution is suitable for use as long as it remains free of haziness and precipitate. Upon refrigeration or freezing, a precipitate might form; this will dissolve again after the solution is allowed to stand at room temperature. The product is still suitable for use. Only a clear solution should be used. A faint yellow coloration may develop; however, this has no effect on the potency of the solution.

In the treatment of status epilepticus, the intravenous route is preferred because of the delay in absorption of phenytoin when administered intramuscularly.

Status Epilepticus:

Intravenously: 150 to 250 mg administered slowly, then 100 to 150 mg 30 minutes later if necessary. Higher doses may be required to control seizures. Dosage for children is usually determined according to weight in proportion

Continued on next page

This product information was prepared in August, 1979. On these and other Parke-Davis Products, detailed information may be obtained by addressing PARKE-DAVIS, Division of Warner-Lambert Company, Morris Plains, NJ 07950.

Parke-Davis—Cont.

to the dosage for a 150-lb adult. Pediatric dosage may also be calculated on the basis of 250 mg per square meter of body surface.
If the state of the patient is such that immobilization of an extremity is impossible due to convulsions, or veins are inaccessible, medication can be given intramuscularly during the attack.
If administration of phenytoin does not terminate the seizure, the clinician may consider the use of other anticonvulsants, intravenous barbiturates, general anesthesia, or other measures.

Neurosurgery:
Prophylactic dosage—100 to 200 mg (2 to 4 ml) intramuscularly at approximately four-hour intervals during surgery and continued during the postoperative period.
When intramuscular administration is required for a patient previously stabilized orally, compensating dosage adjustments are necessary to maintain therapeutic plasma levels. An intramuscular dose 50% greater than the oral dosage is necessary to maintain these levels. When returned to oral administration, the dosage should be reduced by 50% of the original oral dosage for one week to prevent excessive plasma levels due to sustained release from intramuscular tissue sites.
If the patient requires more than a week of IM Dilantin, alternative routes should be explored, such as gastric intubation. For time periods less than one week, the patient shifted back from IM administration should receive one half the original oral dosage for the same period of time the patient received IM Dilantin (phenytoin sodium injection). Monitoring plasma levels would help prevent a fall into the subtherapeutic range.

Management of Overdosage:
Oral and Parenteral:
The mean lethal dose in adults is estimated to be 2 to 5 g. The cardinal initial symptoms are nystagmus, ataxia, and dysarthria. The patient then becomes comatose, the pupils are unresponsive, and hypotension occurs. Death is due to respiratory depression and apnea. Treatment is nonspecific because there is no known antidote. First, the stomach should be emptied. If the gag reflex is absent, the airway should be supported. Oxygen, vasopressors, and assisted ventilation may be necessary for central nervous system, respiratory, and cardiovascular depression.
Finally, hemodialysis can be considered because phenytoin is not completely bound to plasma proteins. Total exchange transfusion has been utilized in the treatment of severe intoxication in children.

How Supplied:
Oral
N 0071-0362 (Kapseal 362) Dilantin (phenytoin sodium), 100 mg; in 100s, 1,000s, and unit-dose 100s. Parcode® No. 362
N 0071-0365 (Kapseal 365) Dilantin (phenytoin sodium), 30 mg; in 100s, 1,000s, and unit-dose 100s. Parcode No. 365
[*Shown in Product Identification Section*]
Also available as:
N 0071-2214-20 Dilantin-125® Suspension (phenytoin oral suspension), 125 mg phenytoin/5 ml; 8-oz bottles
N 0071-2315-20 Pediatric Dilantin-30® Suspension (phenytoin oral suspension), 30 mg phenytoin/5 ml; 8-oz bottles
N 0071-0375 (Kapseal 375) Dilantin with Phenobarbital: each contains 100 mg phenytoin sodium with 16 mg (1/4 grain) phenobarbital; in 100s and 1,000s. Parcode No. 375
[*Shown in Product Identification Section*]
N 0071-0531 (Kapseal 531) Dilantin with Phenobarbital: each contains 100 mg phenytoin sodium with 32 mg (1/2 grain) phenobarbital; in 100s, 1,000s, and unit-dose 100s. Parcode No. 531
[*Shown in Product Identification Section*]
N 0071-0007 (Tablet 7) Dilantin Infatabs® (phenytoin tablets, USP); each contains 50 mg phenytoin; 100s and unit-dose 100s. Parcode No. 7
[*Shown in Product Identification Section*]
N 0071-1801-13 Dilantin (phenytoin sodium) powder; 1-oz bottles **WL**

Parenteral:
N 0071-4488-05 (Ampoule 1488) Dilantin ready-mixed solution containing 50 mg phenytoin sodium per milliliter is supplied in 2-ml ampoules. Packages of 10.
N 0071-4488-41 (Steri-Dose® 4488) Dilantin ready-mixed solution containing 50 mg phenytoin sodium per milliliter is supplied in a 2-ml sterile disposable syringe (22-gauge x 1 1/4-inch needle). Packages of 10.
N 0071-4475-35 (Ampoule 1475) Dilantin ready-mixed solution containing 50 mg phenytoin sodium per milliliter is supplied in 5-ml ampoules with one 6-ml sterile disposable syringe (22-gauge x 1 1/4-inch needle). Packages of 10.
N 0071-4475-08 (Ampoule 1475) Dilantin ready-mixed solution containing 50 mg phenytoin sodium per milliliter is supplied in packages of ten 5-ml ampoules without syringes.
YC

DURAQUIN® ℞
(quinidine gluconate tablets)
SUSTAINED RELEASE

Description: Quinidine gluconate is the gluconate of an alkaloid which may be obtained from various species of Cinchona and their hybrids, from Remijia pedunculata Fluckiger (Fam. Rubiaceae), or prepared from quinine. Quinidine gluconate contains, on the dry basis, not less than 99% of $C_{20}H_{24}N_2O_2 \cdot C_6H_{12}O_7$ (520.58). Quinidine is chemically described as 6-methoxy-alpha- (5-vinyl-2 quinuclidinyl) -4 quinolinemethanol and is the dextrorotatory isomer of quinine. Each 330-mg sustained-release tablet, representing 206 mg of quinidine base, is equivalent to 248 mg of quinidine sulfate.
Actions: The antiarrhythmic activity consists of two actions: (a) prolongation of effective refractory period of the atrial or ventricular muscle which leads to termination of arrhythymia; (b) decrease in excitability of ectopic foci of the heart. In addition, quinidine blocks vagal innervation and facilitates conduction in the atrial-ventricular junction.
Clinical Pharmacology: In clinical studies, single doses of Duraquin produced a mean maximum plasma level at 2 hours which was maintained for 12 hours. This broad plateau indicates slow, continuous absorption from the gastrointestinal tract.
In multiple dose studies, administration of Duraquin tablets, 660 mg every 12 hours, produced steady state (equilibrium) plasma levels shortly after 24 hours. The average quinidine plasma levels (Cramer and Isaksson assay[1]) were 0.81 mcg/ml and the mean peak levels were 1.16 mcg/ml in a group of normal male subjects weighing 75 Kg. Following the last dose at steady state, quinidine plasma levels decreased at an approximate rate of 50% in 10 hours. This compares to the expected plasma half-life of 6.3 hours for quinidine sulfate tablets, USP.
Therapeutic and toxic effects coordinate better with plasma levels than with dosage. While therapeutic levels of 3 to 6 mcg/ml with a range of 1.5 to 9 mcg/ml have been reported, these values are based on peak plasma levels determined by the less specific Edgar and Sokolow assay.[2] This procedure yields quinidine levels averaging 22% higher than the Cramer and Isaksson assay. Plasma levels vary considerably in patients receiving identical doses. Therefore, it is advisable to adjust the dosage by monitoring plasma quinidine levels.
Indications: Duraquin tablets are indicated for the prevention of premature atrial, nodal, or ventricular contractions. They are also indicated for the maintenance of normal sinus rhythm following spontaneous reversion or electrical conversion of atrial, nodal, or ventricular tachycardia, atrial flutter and fibrillation (either paroxysmal or chronic).
Contraindications:
1. History of hypersensitivity to quinidine manifested by thrombocytopenia, skin eruption, febrile reactions, etc.
2. Complete A-V block
3. Complete bundle branch block or other severe intraventricular conduction defects exhibiting marked QRS widening or bizarre complexes
4. Myasthenia gravis
5. Arrhythmias associated with digitalis toxicity

Warnings:
1. (a) In the treatment of atrial fibrillation with rapid ventricular response, ventricular rate should be controlled with digitalis glycosides *prior* to administration of quinidine.
(b) In the treatment of atrial flutter with quinidine, reversion to sinus rhythm may be preceded by progressive reduction in the degree of A-V block to a 1:1 ratio resulting in an extremely high ventricular rate. This potential hazard may be reduced by digitalization prior to administration of quinidine.

Recent reports have described increased, potentially toxic, digoxin plasma levels when quinidine is administered concurrently. When concurrent use is necessary, digoxin dosage should be reduced and plasma concentration should be monitored and patients observed closely for digitalis intoxication.

2. Quinidine cardiotoxicity may be manifested by increased PR and QT intervals, 50% widening of QRS, and/or ventricular ectopic beats or tachycardia. Appearance of these toxic signs during quinidine administration mandates immediate discontinuation of the drug, and/or close clinical and electrocardiographic monitoring. Note: Quinidine effect is enhanced by potassium and reduced in the presence of hypokalemia.
3. "Quinidine Syncope" may occur as a complication of long-term therapy. It is manifested by sudden loss of consciousness and ventricular arrhythmias with bizarre QRS complexes. This syndrome does not appear to be related to dose or plasma levels but occurs more often with prolonged QT intervals.
4. Because quinidine antagonizes the effect of vagal excitation upon the atrium and the A-V node, the administration of parasympathomimetic drugs (choline esters) or the use of any other procedure to enhance vagal activity may fail to terminate paroxysmal supraventricular tachycardia in patients receiving quinidine.
5. Quinidine should be used with extreme caution in: a) the presence of incomplete A-V block, since a complete block and asystole may result. Quinidine may cause unpredictable abnormalities of rhythm in digitalized hearts. Therefore, it should be used with caution in the presence of digitalis intoxication. (See 1.(b) above).
b) Partial bundle branch block.
c) Severe congestive heart failure and hypotensive states due to the depressant effects of quinidine on myocardial contractility and arterial pressure.
d) Poor renal function, especially renal tubular acidosis, because of the potential accumulation of quinidine in plasma leading to toxic concentrations.

Precautions:
1. Test Dose
A preliminary test dose of a single tablet of quinidine *sulfate* should be administered prior to the initiation of the sustained release gluconate to determine whether the patient has an idiosyncrasy to the quinidine molecule.
2. Hypersensitivity
During the first weeks of therapy; hypersensitivity to quinidine, although rare, should be considered (eg, angioedema, purpura, acute asthmatic episode, vascular collapse).
3. Long-Term Therapy
Periodic blood counts and liver and kidney function tests should be performed during long-term therapy and the drug should be discontinued if blood dyscrasias or signs of hepatic or renal disorders occur.
4. Large Doses
ECG monitoring and determination of plasma quinidine levels are recommended when doses greater than 2.5 g/day are administered.
5. Usage in Pregnancy
The use of quinidine, in pregnancy, should be reserved only for those cases where the benefits outweigh the possible hazards to the patient and fetus.
6. Nursing Mothers
The drug should be used with extreme caution in nursing mothers because the drug is excreted in breast milk.
7. General
In patients exhibiting asthma, muscle weakness, and infection with fever *prior* to quinidine administration, hypersensitivity reactions to the drug may be masked.

Drug Interactions:
1. Caution should be used when quinidine and its analogs are administered concurrently with coumarin anticoagulants. This combination may reduce prothrombin levels and cause bleeding.
2. Quinidine, a weak base, may have its half-life prolonged in patients who are concurrently taking drugs that can alkalize the urine, such as thiazide diuretics, sodium bicarbonate, and carbonic anhydrase inhibitors. Quinidine and drugs which alkalize the urine should be used together cautiously.
3. Quinidine exhibits a distinct anticholinergic activity in the myocardial tissues. An additive vagolytic effect may be seen when quinidine and drugs having anticholinergic blocking activity are used together. Drugs having cholinergic activity may be antagonized by quinidine.
4. Quinidine and other antiarrhythmic agents may produce additive cardiac depressant effects when administered together.
5. Quinidine interaction with cardiac glycosides (digoxin); See WARNINGS.
6. Antacids may delay absorption of quinidine but appear unlikely to cause incomplete absorption.
7. Phenobarbital and phenytoin may reduce plasma $t_{1/2}$ of quinidine by 50%.
8. Quinidine may potentiate the neuromuscular blocking effect in ventilatory depression of patients receiving decamethonium, tubocurare, or succinylcholine.

Adverse Reactions: Symptoms of cinchonism (ringing in the ears, headache, disturbed vision) may appear in sensitive patients after a single dose of the drug.
Gastrointestinal: The most common side effects encountered with quinidine are referable to this system. Diarrhea frequently occurs, but it rarely necessitates withdrawal of the drug. Nausea, vomiting, and abdominal pain also occur. Some of these effects may be minimized by administering the drug with meals.
Cardiovascular: Widening of QRS complex, cardiac asystole, ventricular ectopic beats, idioventricular rhythms including ventricular tachycardias and fibrillation; paradoxical tachycardia, arterial embolism and hypotension.
Hematologic: acute hemolytic anemia, hypoprothrombinemia, thrombocytopenic purpura, agranulocytosis.
CNS: headache, fever, vertigo, apprehension, excitement, confusion, delirium and syncope, disturbed hearing (tinnitus, decreased auditory acuity), disturbed vision (mydriasis, blurred vision, disturbed color perception, photophobia, diplopia, night blindness, scotomata); optic neuritis.
Dermatologic: cutaneous flushing with intense pruritus.
Hypersensitivity reactions: angioedema, acute asthmatic episode, vascular collapse, respiratory arrest.

Dosage and Administration: **Dosage should be titrated to give the desired clinical effect, e.g., elimination of paroxysmal rhythm or reduction in premature contractions (See CLINICAL PHARMACOLOGY). This will often require prolonged ambulatory ECG monitoring, as hour-to-hour variability renders brief ECG recordings unreliable. When doses larger than 2.5g/day are used, quinidine blood levels should be monitored, if possible, and serial ECGs should be followed (See WARNINGS and PRECAUTIONS).**
For prevention of premature contractions and maintenance of normal sinus rhythm following spontaneous reversion or electrical conversion, the usual dosage is from 330 mg to 660 mg every eight hours, most patients requiring the higher dose.
In elderly patients, and in patients in the lower end of the normal weight range, plasma quinidine determinations should be considered. Dosage adjustments may be required.

Overdosage: Cardiotoxic effects of quinidine may be reversed in part by molar sodium lactate; the hypotension may be reversed by vasoconstrictors and by catecholamines (since the vasodilation is partly due to alpha-adrenergic blockade).

How Supplied: N 0071-0850 (P-D 850) Duraquin (quinidine gluconate tablets) 330-mg tablets are supplied in bottles of 100 tablets.

YD

[1] Cramer, G. and Isaksson, B. Quantitative Determination of Quinidine in Plasma, Scandinavian J. Clin. & Lab Investigation 15, 553, 1963.
[2] Edgar, A.L. and Sokolow, M. Experiences with the Photofluorometric Determination of Quinidine in Blood J. Lab Clin. Med. 36, 478, 1950.

ELASE® ℞
(fibrinolysin and desoxyribonuclease, combined [bovine])

ELASE OINTMENT ℞
(fibrinolysin and desoxyribonuclease, combined [bovine], ointment)

ELASE–CHLOROMYCETIN® OINTMENT ℞
(fibrinolysin and desoxyribonuclease, combined [bovine], with chloramphenicol ointment)

Description: Elase is a combination of two lytic enzymes, fibrinolysin and desoxyribonuclease, supplied as a lyophilized powder and in an ointment base of liquid petrolatum and polyethylene. Elase-Chloromycetin Ointment contains fibrinolysin and desoxyribonuclease combined with chloramphenicol in an ointment base. The fibrinolysin component is derived from bovine plasma and the desoxyribonuclease is isolated in a purified form from bovine pancreas. The fibrinolysin used in the combination is activated by chloroform.
Chloramphenicol, a broad-spectrum antibiotic originally isolated from *Streptomyces venezuelae*, is therapeutically active against a wide variety of susceptible organisms, both gram-positive and gram-negative. Chemically, chloramphenicol may be identified as D(-)- *threo*-1-*p*-nitrophenyl -2 -dichloroacetamido- 1, 3-propanediol.

Action: Combination of these two enzymes is based on the observation that purulent exudates consist largely of fibrinous material and nucleoprotein. Desoxyribonuclease attacks the desoxyribonucleic acid (DNA) and fibrinolysin attacks principally fibrin of blood clots and fibrinous exudates.
The activity of desoxyribonuclease is limited principally to the production of large polynucleotides, which are less likely to be absorbed than the more diffusible protein fractions liberated by certain enzyme preparations obtained from bacteria. The fibrinolytic action of Elase and of the enzymes in Elase Ointment and Elase-Chloromycetin Ointment is directed mainly against denatured proteins, such as those found in devitalized tissue, while protein elements of living cells remain relatively unaffected.
Elase, Elase Ointment, and Elase-Chloromycetin Ointment are combinations of active enzymes. This is an important consideration in treating patients suffering from lesions resulting from impaired circulation.
The enzymatic action of Elase helps to produce clean surfaces and thus supports healing in a variety of exudative lesions.
Chloramphenicol is a broad-spectrum antibiotic that is primarily bacteriostatic and acts by inhibition of protein synthesis by interfering with the transfer of activated amino acids from soluble RNA to ribosomes. Development of resistance to chloramphenicol can be regarded as minimal for staphylococci and many other species of bacteria.
The action of Elase-Chloromycetin helps to produce clean surfaces and thus supports healing in a variety of exudative lesions.

Indications: Elase and Elase Ointment are indicated for topical use as debriding agents in a variety of inflammatory and infected lesions. These include: (1) general surgical wounds; (2) ulcerative lesions—trophic, decubitus, stasis, arteriosclerotic; (3) second- and third-degree burns; (4) circumcision and episiotomy. Elase and Elase Ointment are used intravaginally in: (1) cervicitis—benign, postpartum, and postconization, and (2) vaginitis. Elase is used as an irrigating agent in the following conditions: (1) infected wounds—abscesses, fistulae, and sinus tracts; (2) otorhinolaryngologic wounds; (3) superficial hematomas (except when the hematoma is adjacent to or within adipose tissue).
Elase-Chloromycetin Ointment is indicated for use in the treatment of infected lesions, such as burns, ulcers, and wounds where the actions of both a debriding agent and a topical antibiotic are desired. This dual-purpose approach is especially useful in the treatment of infections caused by organisms that utilize a process of fibrin deposition as protective device (ie, coagulase-producing staphylococci). Appropriate measures should be taken to determine the susceptibility of the pathogen to chloramphenicol.

Contraindications: These products (Elase, Elase Ointment, Elase-Chloromycetin Ointment) are contraindicated in individuals with a history of hypersensitivity reactions to any of their components. Elase is not recommended for parenteral use because the bovine fibrinolysin may be antigenic.

Warnings: Elase-Chloromycetin Ointment—Prolonged or frequent intermittent use of topical chloramphenicol should be avoided because

Continued on next page

This product information was prepared in August, 1979. On these and other Parke-Davis Products, detailed information may be obtained by addressing PARKE-DAVIS, Division of Warner-Lambert Company, Morris Plains, NJ 07950.

Parke-Davis—Cont.

of the possibility of hypersensitivity reactions, including bone marrow hypoplasia.

Precautions: Elase-Chloromycetin Ointment—The prolonged use of antibiotics may occasionally result in overgrowth of nonsusceptible organisms, including fungi. If new infections appear during medication, the drug should be discontinued and appropriate measures should be taken.

In all except very superficial infections, the topical use of chloramphenicol should be supplemented by appropriate systemic medication.

Elase, Elase Ointment, Elase-Chloromycetin Ointment—The usual precautions against allergic reactions should be observed, particularly in persons with a history of sensitivity to materials of bovine origin or to mercury compounds.

Elase—To be maximally effective, Elase solutions must be freshly prepared before use. The loss in activity is reduced by refrigeration; however, even when stored in a refrigerator, the solution should not be used 24 hours or more after reconstitution.

Adverse Reactions: Side effects attributable to the enzymes have not been a problem at the dose and for the indications recommended herein. With higher concentrations, side effects have been minimal, consisting of local hyperemia.

Chills and fever attributable to antigenic action of profibrinolysin activators of bacterial origin are not a problem with Elase, Elase Ointment, or Elase-Chloromycetin Ointment.

Elase-Chloromycetin Ointment—Signs of local irritation, with subjective symptoms of itching or burning, angioneurotic edema, urticaria, vesicular and maculopapular dermatitis have been reported in patients sensitive to chloramphenicol and are causes for discontinuing the medication. Similar sensitivity reactions to other materials in topical preparations may also occur. Blood dyscrasias may be associated with the systemic use of chloramphenicol.

Preparation of Elase Solution: The contents of each vial may be reconstituted with 10 ml of isotonic sodium chloride solution. Higher or lower concentrations can be prepared if desired by varying the amount of the diluent.

Dosage and Administration: Because the conditions for which Elase and Elase Ointment (fibrinolysin and desoxyribonuclease, combined [bovine]), and Elase-Chloromycetin Ointment (fibrinolysin and desoxyribonuclease, combined [bovine], with chloramphenicol ointment) are helpful vary considerably in severity, dosage must be adjusted to the individual case; however, the following general recommendations can be made.

Successful use of enzymatic debridement depends on several factors: (1) dense, dry eschar, if present, should be removed surgically before enzymatic debridement is attempted; (2) the enzyme must be in constant contact with the substrate; (3) accumulated necrotic debris must be periodically removed; (4) the enzyme must be replenished at least once daily; and (5) secondary closure or skin grafting must be employed as soon as possible after optimal debridement has been attained. It is further essential that wound-dressing techniques be performed carefully under aseptic conditions and that appropriate systemically acting antibiotics be administered concomitantly if, in the opinion of the physician, they are indicated.

General Topical Uses: Selection of the product form and the duration of treatment must to a great extent be left to the discretion of the physician. Local application of the appropriate product should be repeated at intervals for as long as enzyme action is desired. A recommended procedure for the application of Elase Ointment is:

1) Clean the wound with water, peroxide, or normal saline and dry area gently. If there is a dense, dry eschar present, it should be removed surgically before applying Elase Ointment;
2) Apply a <u>thin</u> layer of Elase Ointment;
3) Cover with petrolatum gauze or another type of nonadhering dressing;
4) Change the dressing at least ONCE a day, preferably two or three times daily. Frequency of application is more important than the amount of Elase Ointment used. Flush away the necrotic debris and fibrinous exudates with saline, peroxide, or warm water so that newly applied ointment can be in direct contact with the substrate.

Elase solution may be applied topically as a liquid, spray, or wet dressing. Application of a gentle spray of the solution can be accomplished by using a conventional atomizer. A recommended procedure for the application of Elase solution is as follows.

1) Mix one vial of Elase powder with 10 to 50 ml of saline and saturate strips of fine-mesh gauze or an unfolded sterile gauze sponge with the Elase solution.
2) Pack ulcerated area with the Elase-saturated gauze, making sure the gauze remains in contact with the necrotic substrate. (If the lesion is covered with a heavy eschar, it must be removed surgically before wet-to-dry debridement is begun.)
3) ALLOW GAUZE TO DRY IN CONTACT WITH THE ULCERATED LESION (approximately six to eight hours). As the gauze dries, the necrotic tissues slough and become enmeshed in the gauze.
4) Remove dried gauze. This mechanically debrides the area. Repeat wet-to-dry procedure three or four times daily because frequent dressing changes greatly enhance results. After two, three, or four days, the area becomes clean and starts to fill in with granulation tissue.

After application, Elase, especially in solution, becomes rapidly and progressively less active and is probably exhausted for practical purposes at the end of 24 hours. The dry material for solution and the ointments are stable at room temperature through the expiration date printed on each package.

Intravaginal Use: In mild to moderate vaginitis and cervicitis, 5 ml of Elase Ointment should be deposited deep in the vagina once nightly at bedtime for approximately five applications, or until the entire contents of one 30-g tube of Elase Ointment has been used. The patient should be checked by her physician to determine possible need for further therapy. In more severe cervicitis and vaginitis, some physicians prefer initially to instill 10 ml of Elase solution intravaginally, wait one or two minutes for the enzyme to disperse, and then insert a cotton tampon in the vaginal canal. The tampon should be removed the next day, followed by as many applications of Elase Ointment as necessary.

Abscesses, empyema cavities, fistulae, sinus tracts, or subcutaneous hematomas: Despite the contraindication against parenteral use, Elase has been used in irrigating these specific conditions. The Elase solution should be drained and replaced at intervals of 6 to 10 hours to reduce the amount of by-product accumulation and minimize loss of enzyme activity. Traces of blood in the discharge usually indicate active filling in of the cavity.

How Supplied:

ELASE (fibrinolysin and desoxyribonuclease, combined [bovine])

N 0071-4256-01 Elase is supplied dried in rubber diaphragm-capped vials of 30-ml capacity containing 25 units (Loomis) of fibrinolysin and 15,000 units (modified Christensen method) of desoxyribonuclease with 0.1 mg thimerosal (mercury derivative).

AHFS 84:36

ELASE OINTMENT (fibrinolysin and desoxyribonuclease, combined [bovine], ointment)

N 0071-4279-13 Elase Ointment, 30 g.

The 30-g tube contains 30 units of fibrinolysin and 20,000 units of desoxyribonuclease with 0.12 mg thimerosal (mercury derivative) in a special ointment base of liquid petrolatum and polyethylene. For gynecologic use, six disposable vaginal applicators (V-Applicator™ —N 0071-1859-04) as a separate package are available for this tube when required to facilitate administration of the proper dose.

NSN 6505-00-958-8975A

AHFS 84:36

N 0071-4279-10 Elase Ointment, 10 g.

The 10-g tube contains 10 units of fibrinolysin and 6,666 units of desoxyribonuclease with 0.04 mg thimerosal (mercury derivative) in a special ointment base of liquid petrolatum and polyethylene.

These product forms contain sodium chloride and sucrose as incidental ingredients.

AHFS 84:36

ELASE-CHLOROMYCETIN OINTMENT (fibrinolysin and desoxyribonuclease, combined [bovine], with chloramphenicol ointment)

Elase-Chloromycetin is supplied in 30-g and 10-g ointment tubes. The 10-g tubes have an elongated nozzle to facilitate the application to surface lesions.

N 0071-4281-13 Elase-Chloromycetin Ointment, 30 g.

The 30-g tubes contain 30 units of fibrinolysin (bovine), 20,000 units of desoxyribonuclease with 0.12 mg thimerosal (mercury derivative) (as a preservative), and 0.3 g* chloramphenicol in a special ointment base of liquid petrolatum and polyethylene.

N 0071-4281-10 Elase-Chloromycetin Ointment, 10 g.

The 10-g tubes contain 10 units of fibrinolysin (bovine) and 6,666 units of desoxyribonuclease with 0.04 mg thimerosal (mercury derivative) (as a preservative) and 0.1 g* chloramphenicol in a special ointment base of liquid petrolatum and polyethylene.

This ointment also contains sodium chloride and sucrose used in its manufacture.

AHFS 84:04.04 **MD-MF**

*10 mg chloramphenicol per gram, or 1%

ELDEC® KAPSEALS® ℞

Composition: Each capsule contains vitamin A (acetate), 1,667 IU; vitamin C (ascorbic acid), 66.7 mg; vitamin B_1 (thiamine mononitrate), 10 mg; vitamin B_2 (riboflavin), 0.87 mg; vitamin B_6 (pyridoxine hydrochloride), 0.67 mg; nicotinamide (niacinamide), 16.7 mg; *dl*-panthenol, 10 mg; ferrous sulfate, dried, 16.7 mg; iodine (as potassium iodide), 0.05 mg; calcium carbonate, precipitated, 66.7 mg; vitamin E (*dl*-alpha tocopheryl acetate), (10 mg) 10 IU; vitamin B_{12} (cyanocobalamin), 2 mcg; folic acid, 0.33 mg.

Action and Uses: For certain vitamin and mineral deficiencies

Dosage: The usual dosage of Eldec is one capsule three times a day.

How Supplied: N 0071-0398-24 Eldec (Kapseal 398), bottles of 100. Parcode® No. 398.

[*Shown in Product Identification Section*]

ERGOSTAT® ℞

(ergotamine tartrate tablets)
Sublingual Tablets

Description: Each sublingual tablet contains 2 mg ergotamine tartrate.

Action: Ergotamine is an alpha-adrenergic blocking agent with a direct stimulating effect on the smooth muscle of peripheral and cranial blood vessels and produces depression of central vasomotor centers. Ergostat also has the properties of a serotonin antagonist.

Ergostat (ergotamine tartrate tablets) exerts a direct effect on cranial blood vessels, causing vasoconstriction, with concomitant decrease in the pulsations probably responsible for migraine and other vascular headache symptoms. Ergostat is thus generally considered to be a specific agent for therapy in this condition.
Because ergotamine is a nonnarcotic, it avoids the dangers inherent with repeated use of narcotics in the treatment of frequent migraine attacks.
Indications: Vascular headaches, such as migraine and cluster headache (histaminic cephalalgia)
Precautions: Avoid prolonged administration or dosage in excess of that recommended because of the danger of ergotism and gangrene.
Contraindications: Contraindicated in sepsis, occlusive vascular disease (thromboangiitis obliterans, luetic arteritis, severe arteriosclerosis, coronary artery disease, thrombophlebitis, Raynaud's disease), hepatic disease, renal disease, severe pruritis, hypertension, and pregnancy; hypersensitivity to ergot alkaloids
Adverse Reactions: When prescribed in correct dosage, in the absence of contraindications, ergotamine is a safe and useful drug; few serious complications have been reported from its use in the migraine syndrome. Unpleasant side effects which may occur include nausea and vomiting, diarrhea, weakness in the legs, muscle pains in the extremities, numbness and tingling of fingers and toes, precordial distress and pain, and transient tachycardia or bradycardia. Localized edema and itching may occur in the rare sensitive patient. Side effects are usually not such as to necessitate interruption of therapy.
Dosage and Administration: All efforts should be made to initiate therapy as soon as possible after the first symptoms of the attack are noted, because success is proportional to rapidity of treatment, and lower dosages will be effective. At the first sign of an attack, or to relieve the symptoms of the full-blown attack, one sublingual tablet (2 mg) is placed under the tongue. Another sublingual tablet (2 mg) should be placed under the tongue at half-hour intervals thereafter, if necessary, for a total of three tablets (6 mg). Dosage must not exceed three tablets (6 mg) in any 24-hour period. Limit dosage to not more than five tablets (10 mg) in any one week.
How Supplied: N 0071-0111-13 — Ergostat (ergotamine tartrate tablets) Sublingual Tablets, 2 mg, each in an individual foil pouch with two strips of 12 pouches packaged in a plastic vial
AHFS 12:16 **YB**
[*Shown in Product Identification Section*]

ERYTHROMYCIN STEARATE TABLETS, USP ℞
(Erypar®)

Description: Erythromycin, produced by a strain of *Streptomyces erythraeus,* belongs to the macrolide group of antibiotics. Erythromycin is basic and readily forms salts with acids. The base, the stearate salt, and the esters are poorly soluble in water, and are suitable for oral administration.
Film-coated tablets contain 250 mg or 500 mg of erythromycin as erythromycin stearate, USP. Each tablet is buffered with sodium citrate.
Actions: The mode of action of erythromycin is by inhibition of protein synthesis without affecting nucleic acid synthesis. Resistance to erythromycin of some strains of *Hemophilus influenzae* and staphylococci has been demonstrated. Culture and susceptibility testing should be done. If the Kirby-Bauer method of disk susceptibility is used, a 15-mcg erythromycin disk should give a zone diameter of at least 18 mm when tested against an erythromycin-susceptible organism.
Orally administered erythromycin is readily absorbed by most patients, especially on an empty stomach, but patient variation is observed.
After absorption, erythromycin diffuses readily into most body fluids. In the absence of meningeal inflammation, low concentrations are normally achieved in the spinal fluid, but passage of the drug across the blood-brain barrier increases in meningitis. In the presence of normal hepatic function, erythromycin is concentrated in the liver and excreted in the bile; the effect of hepatic dysfunction on excretion of erythromycin by the liver into the bile is not known. After oral administration, less than 5% of the activity of the administered dose can be recovered in the urine.
Erythromycin crosses the placental barrier but fetal plasma levels are generally low.
Indications: *Streptococcus pyogenes* (group A beta-hemolytic *Streptococcus*): Upper and lower respiratory tract, skin, and soft-tissue infections of mild to moderate severity
Injectable benzathine penicillin G is considered by the American Heart Association to be the drug of choice in the treatment and prevention of streptococcal pharyngitis and in long-term prophylaxis of rheumatic fever.
When oral medication is preferred for treatment of streptococcal pharyngitis, penicillin G, V, or erythromycin are alternate drugs of choice.
When oral medication is given, the importance of strict adherence by the patient to the prescribed dosage regimen must be stressed. A therapeutic dosage should be administered for at least 10 days.
Alpha-hemolytic streptococci (viridans group): Short-term prophylaxis of bacterial endocarditis prior to dental or other operative procedures in patients with a history of rheumatic fever or congenital heart disease who are hypersensitive to penicillin. (Erythromycin is not suitable prior to genitourinary surgery where the organisms likely to lead to bacteremia are gram-negative bacilli or the *Enterococcus* group of streptococci.)
Staphylococcus aureus: Acute infections of skin and soft tissue of mild to moderate severity. Resistant organisms may emerge during treatment.
Diplococcus pneumoniae: Upper respiratory tract infections (eg, otitis media, pharyngitis) and lower respiratory tract infections (eg, pneumonia) of mild to moderate degree
Mycoplasma pneumoniae (Eaton agent, PPLO): In the treatment of primary atypical pneumonia, when due to this organism
Treponema pallidum: Erythromycin is an alternate choice of treatment for primary syphilis in patients allergic to the penicillins. In treatment of primary syphilis, spinal fluid examinations should be done before treatment and as part of follow-up after therapy.
Corynebacterium diphtheriae and C minutissimum: As an adjunct to antitoxin, to prevent establishment of carriers, and to eradicate the organism in carriers
In the treatment of erythrasma
Entamoeba histolytica: In the treatment of intestinal amebiasis only
Extra-enteric amebiasis requires treatment with other agents.
Listeria monocytogenes: Infections due to this organism
Legionnaires' Disease: Although no controlled clinical efficacy studies have been conducted, *in vitro* and liimited preliminary clinical data suggests that erythromycin may be effective in treating Legionnaires' Disease.
Contraindication: Erythromycin is contraindicated in patients with known hypersensitivity to this antibiotic.
Warning: Usage in pregnancy: Safety for use in pregnancy has not been established.
Precautions: Erythromycin is principally excreted by the liver. Caution should be exercised in administering the antibiotic to patients with impaired hepatic function. There have been reports of hepatic dysfunction, with or without jaundice, occurring in patients receiving oral erythromycin products.
Recent data from studies of erythromycin reveal that its use in patients who are receiving high doses of theophylline may be associated with an increase of serum theophylline levels and potential theophylline toxicity. In case of theophylline toxicity and/or elevated serum theophylline levels, the dose of theophylline should be reduced while the patient is receiving concomitant erythromycin therapy.
Surgical procedures should be performed when indicated.
Adverse Reactions: The most frequent side effects of oral erythromycin preparations are gastrointestinal, such as abdominal cramping and discomfort, and are dose-related. Nausea, vomiting, and diarrhea occur infrequently with usual oral doses.
During prolonged or repeated therapy, there is a possibility of overgrowth of nonsusceptible bacteria or fungi. If such infections occur, the drug should be discontinued and appropriate therapy instituted.
Mild allergic reactions, such as urticaria and other skin rashes, have occurred. Serious allergic reactions, including anaphylaxis, have been reported.
Dosage and Administration: Optimum blood levels are obtained when doses are given on an empty stomach.
Adults: 250 mg every 6 hours is the usual dosage; or 500 mg every 12 hours, one hour before meals. Dosage may be increased up to 4 g or more per day according to the severity of the infection.
Children: Age, weight, and severity of the infection are important factors in determining the proper dosage: 30 to 50 mg/kg/day, in divided doses, is the usual dosage. For more severe infections, this dosage may be doubled.
If dosage is desired on a twice-a-day schedule in either adults or children, one half of the total daily dosage may be given every 12 hours, one hour before meals.
In the treatment of streptococcal infections, a therapeutic dosage of erythromycin should be administered for at least 10 days. In continuous *prophylaxis* of streptococcal infections in persons with a history of rheumatic heart disease, the dosage is 250 mg twice a day.
When used prior to surgery to prevent endocarditis (see alpha-hemolytic streptococci), a recommended schedule for adults is 500 mg before the procedure and 250 mg every six hours for four doses after the procedure. For small children: 30 to 50 mg/kg/day divided into three or four evenly spaced doses.
For treatment of primary syphilis: 30 to 40 g given in divided doses over a period of 10 to 15 days.
For dysenteric amebiasis: Adults: 250 mg four times daily for 10 to 14 days. Children: 30 to 50 mg/kg/day in divided doses for 10 to 14 days.
For treatment of Legionnaires' Disease: Although optimal dosage has not been established, doses utilized in reported clinical data were those recommended above (1 to 4 g erythromycin stearate daily in divided doses).
How Supplied:
N 0071-0672 (Tablet 672). Each Filmseal® (film-coated tablet) contains 250 mg erythromycin as erythromycin stearate; in bottles of 100 and 500, and unit-dose packages of 100 (10 strips of 10 tablets). Parcode® No. 672

Continued on next page

This product information was prepared in August, 1979. On these and other Parke-Davis Products, detailed information may be obtained by addressing PARKE-DAVIS, Division of Warner-Lambert Company, Morris Plains, NJ 07950.

Parke-Davis—Cont.

N 0071-0919-24 (Tablet 919). Film-coated tablets, each containing 500 mg erythromycin as erythromycin stearate, in bottles of 100. Parcode No. 919
AHFS 8:12.12 **WH**
[*Shown in Product Identification Section*]

ESTROVIS® ℞
(Quinestrol)

Caution: Federal law prohibits dispensing without prescription.

Warning:

1. Estrogens Have Been Reported to Increase the Risk of Endometrial Carcinoma.

Three independent case control studies have shown an increased risk of endometrial cancer in postmenopausal women exposed to exogenous estrogens for prolonged periods.[1–3] This risk was independent of the other known risk factors for endometrial cancer. These studies are further supported by the finding that incidence rates of endometrial cancer have increased sharply since 1969 in eight different areas of the United States with population-based cancer reporting systems, an increase which may be related to the rapidly expanding use of estrogens during the last decade.[4]

The three case control studies reported that the risk of endometrial cancer in estrogen users was about 4.5 to 13.9 times greater than in nonusers. The risk appears to depend on both duration of treatment[1] and on estrogen dose.[3] In view of these findings, when estrogens are used for the treatment of menopausal symptoms, the lowest dose that will control symptoms should be utilized and medication should be discontinued as soon as possible. When prolonged treatment is medically indicated, the patient should be reassessed on at least a semiannual basis to determine the need for continued therapy. Although the evidence must be considered preliminary, one study suggests that cyclic administration of low doses of estrogen may carry less risk than continuous administration,[3] it, therefore, appears prudent to utilize such a regimen.

Close clinical surveillance of all women taking estrogens is important. In all cases of undiagnosed persistent or recurring abnormal vaginal bleeding, adequate diagnostic measures should be undertaken to rule out malignancy. There in no evidence at present that "natural" estrogens are more or less hazardous than "synthetic" estrogens at equiestrogenic doses.

2. Estrogens Should not be Used During Pregnancy.

The use of female sex hormones, both estrogens and progestogens, during early pregnancy may seriously damage the offspring. It has been shown that females exposed *in utero* to diethylstilbestrol, a nonsteroidal estrogen, have an increased risk of developing in later life a form of vaginal or cervical cancer that is ordinarily extremely rare.[5–6] This risk has been estimated as not greater than 4 per 1,000 exposures.[7] Furthermore, a high percentage of such exposed women (from 30 to 90 percent) have been found to have vaginal adenosis,[8–12] epithelial changes of the vagina and cervix. Although these changes are histologically benign, it is not known whether they are precursors of malignancy. Although similar data are not available with the use of other estrogens, it cannot be presumed they would not induce similar changes. Several reports suggest an association between intrauterine exposure to female sex hormones and congenital anomalies, including congenital heart defects and limb-reduction defects.[13–16] One case control study[16] estimated a 4.7-fold increased risk of limb-reduction defects in infants exposed *in utero* to sex hormones (oral contraceptives, hormone withdrawal tests for pregnancy, or attempted treatment for threatened abortion). Some of these exposures were very short and involved only a few days of treatment. The data suggest that the risk of limb-reduction defects in exposed fetuses is somewhat less than 1 per 1,000.

In the past, female sex hormones have been used during pregnancy in an attempt to treat threatened or habitual abortion. There is considerable evidence that estrogens are ineffective for these indications, and there is no evidence from well-controlled studies that progestogens are effective for these uses.

If Estrovis (quinestrol) is used during pregnancy, or if the patient becomes pregnant while taking this drug, she should be apprised of the potential risks to the fetus, and the advisability of pregnancy continuation.

Description: Estrovis (quinestrol) is available as a 100-mcg oral tablet. It is an estrogen. Estrovis (quinestrol) is the 3-cyclopentylether of ethinyl estradiol. The chemical name is 3-cyclopentyloxy-17α-ethynylestra-1, 3, 5 (10)-trien-17β-ol.

It is a white, essentially odorless powder, insoluble in water and soluble in alcohol, chloroform, and ether.

Clinical Pharmacology: Estrovis (quinestrol) is an orally effective estrogen as judged by conventional assay procedures employing vagina and uterine end-points in mice, rats and rabbits.

The estrogenic effects of Estrovis have been demonstrated in clinical studies by its effects on the endometrium, maturation of the vaginal epithelium, thinning of cervical mucus, suppression of pituitary gonadotropin, inhibition of ovulation, and prevention of postpartum breast discomfort.

Indications: Estrovis (quinestrol) is indicated in the treatment of:

1. Moderate to severe vasomotor symptoms associated with the menopause. (There is no evidence that estrogens are effective for nervous symptoms or depression which might occur during menopause, and they should not be used to treat these conditions.)
2. Atrophic vaginitis
3. Kraurosis vulvae
4. Female hypogonadism
5. Female castration
6. Primary ovarian failure

Estrovis (Quinestrol) Has Not Been Shown to be Effective for any Purpose during Pregnancy and Its Use May Cause Severe Harm to the Fetus (See Boxed Warning).

Contraindications: Estrogens should not be used in women (or men) with any of the following conditions:

1. Known or suspected cancer of the breast except in appropriately selected patients being treated for metastatic disease
2. Known or suspected estrogen-dependent neoplasia
3. Known or suspected pregnancy (See Boxed Warning)
4. Undiagnosed abnormal genital bleeding
5. Active thrombophlebitis or thromboembolic disorders
6. A past history of thrombophlebitis, thrombosis, or thromboembolic disorders associated with previous estrogen use (except when used in treatment of breast or prostatic malignancy)

Warnings:

1. *Induction of malignant neoplasms.* Long-term continuous administration of natural and synthetic estrogens in certain animal species increases the frequency of carcinomas of the breast, cervix, vagina, and liver. There is now evidence that estrogens increase the risk of carcinoma of the endometrium in humans. (See Boxed Warning.)

At the present time there is no satisfactory evidence that estrogens given to postmenopausal women increase the risk of cancer of the breast,[18] although a recent long-term follow up of a single physician's practice has raised this possibility.[18a] Because of the animal data, there is a need for caution in prescribing estrogens for women with a strong family history of breast cancer or who have breast nodules, fibrocystic disease, or abnormal mammograms.

2. *Gallbladder disease.* A recent study has reported a 2- to 3-fold increase in the risk of surgically confirmed gallbladder disease in women receiving postmenopausal estrogens,[18] similar to the 2-fold increase previously noted in users of oral contraceptives.[19–24] In the case of oral contraceptives the increased risk appeared after two years of use.[24]

3. *Effects similar to those caused by estrogen-progestogen oral contraceptives.* There are several serious adverse effects of oral contraceptives, most of which have not, up to now, been documented as consequences of postmenopausal estrogen therapy. This may reflect the comparatively low doses of estrogen used in postmenopausal women. It would be expected that the larger doses of estrogen used to treat prostatic or breast cancer or postpartum breast engorgement are more likely to result in these adverse effects, and, in fact, it has been shown that there is an increased risk of thrombosis in men receiving estrogens for prostatic cancer and women for postpartum breast engorgement.[20–23]

a. *Thromboembolic disease.* It is now well established that users of oral contraceptives have an increased risk of various thromboembolic and thrombotic vascular diseases, such as thrombophlebitis, pulmonary embolism, stroke, and myocardial infarction.[24–31] Cases of retinal thrombosis, mesenteric thrombosis, and optic neuritis have been reported in oral contraceptive users. There is evidence that the risk of several of these adverse reactions is related to the dose of the drug.[32,33] An increased risk of postsurgery thromboembolic complications has also been reported in users of oral contraceptives.[34,35] If feasible, estrogen should be discontinued at least 4 weeks before surgery of the type associated with an increased risk of thromboembolism, or during periods of prolonged immobilization.

While an increased rate of thromboembolic and thrombotic disease in postmenopausal users of estrogens has not been found,[18,36] this does not rule out the possibility that such an increase may be present or that subgroups of women who have underlying risk factors or who are receiving relatively large doses of estrogens may have increased risk. Therefore, estrogens should not be used in persons with active thrombophlebitis or thromboembolic disorders, and they should not be used (except in treatment of malignancy) in persons with a history of such disorders in association with estrogen use. They should be used with caution in patients with cerebral vascular or coronary artery disease and only for those in whom estrogens are clearly needed.

Large doses of estrogen (5 mg conjugated estrogens per day), comparable to those used to treat cancer of the prostate and breast, have been shown in a large prospective clinical trial in men[37] to increase the risk of nonfatal myocardial infarction, pulmonary embolism and thrombophlebitis. When estrogen doses of this size are used, any of the thromboembolic and thrombotic adverse effects associated with oral contraceptive use should be considered a clear risk.

b. *Hepatic adenoma.* Benign hepatic adenomas appear to be associated with the use of oral contraceptives.[38–40] Although benign, and rare, these may rupture and may cause death through intra-abdominal hemorrhage. Such lesions have not yet been reported in association with other estrogen or progestogen preparations but should be considered in estrogen users having abdominal pain and tenderness, abdominal mass, or hypovolemic shock. Hepatocellular carcinoma has also been reported in women taking estrogen-containing oral contraceptives.[39] The relationship of this malignancy to these drugs is not known at this time.

c. *Elevated blood pressure.* Increased blood pressure is not uncommon in women using oral contraceptives. There is now a report that this may occur with use of estrogens in the menopause[11] and blood pressure should be monitored with estrogen use, especially if high doses are used.

d. *Glucose tolerance.* A worsening of glucose tolerance has been observed in a significant percentage of patients on estrogen-containing oral contraceptives. For this reason, diabetic patients should be carefully observed while receiving estrogen.

4. *Hypercalcemia.* Administration of estrogens may lead to severe hypercalcemia in patients with breast cancer and bone metastases. If this occurs, the drug should be stopped and appropriate measures taken to reduce the serum calcium level.

Precautions:

A. General Precautions

1. A complete medical and family history should be taken prior to the initiation of any estrogen therapy. The pretreatment and periodic physical examinations should include special reference to blood pressure, abdomen, and pelvic organs, and should include a Papanicolau smear. As a general rule, estrogen should not be prescribed for longer than one year without another physical examination being performed.
2. Fluid retention—Because estrogens may cause some degree of fluid retention, conditions which might be influenced by this factor, such as epilepsy, migraine, and cardiac or renal dysfunction, require careful observation.
3. Certain patients may develop undesirable manifestations or excessive estrogenic stimulation, such as abnormal or excessive uterine bleeding, mastodynia, etc.
4. Oral contraceptives appear to be associated with an increased incidence of mental depression.[24] Although it is not clear whether this is due to the estrogenic or progestogenic component of the contraceptive, patients with a history of depression should be carefully observed.
5. Preexisting uterine leiomyomata may increase in size during estrogen use.
6. The pathologist should be advised of estrogen therapy when relevant specimens are submitted.
7. Patients with a past history of jaundice during pregnancy have an increased risk of recurrence of jaundice while receiving estrogen-containing oral contraceptive therapy. If jaundice develops in any patient receiving estrogen, the medication should be discontinued while the cause is investigated.
8. Estrogens may be poorly metabolized in patients with impaired liver function and they should be administered with caution in such patients.
9. Because estrogens influence the metabolism of calcium and phosphorus, they should be used with caution in patients with metabolic bone diseases that are associated with hypercalcemia or in patients with renal insufficiency.
10. Because of the effects of estrogens on epiphyseal closure, they should be used judiciously in young patients in whom bone growth is not complete.
11. Certain endocrine and liver function tests may be affected by estrogen-containing oral contraceptives. The following similar changes may be expected with larger doses of estrogen:

a. Increased sulfobromophthalein retention.
b. Increased prothrombin and factors VII, VIII, IX, and X; decreased antithrombin 3; increased norepinephrine-induced platelet aggregability.
c. Increased thyroid binding globulin (TBG) leading to increased circulating total thyroid hormone, as measured by PHI, T4 by column, or T4 by radioimmunoassay. Free T3 resin uptake is decreased, reflecting the elevated TBG; free T4 concentration is unaltered.
d. Impaired glucose tolerance.
e. Decreased pregnanediol excretion.
f. Reduced response to metyrapone test.
g. Reduced serum folate concentration.
h. Increased serum triglyceride and phospholipid concentration.

B. Information for the patient. See text of Patient Package Insert.

C. Pregnancy. See Contraindications and Boxed Warning.

D. Nursing Mothers. As a general principle, the administration of any drug to nursing mothers should be done only when clearly necessary because many drugs are excreted in human milk.

Adverse Reactions: (See Warnings regarding induction of neoplasia, adverse effects on the fetus, increased incidence of gallbladder disease, and adverse effects similar to those of oral contraceptives, including thromboembolism.) The following additional adverse reactions have been reported with estrogenic therapy, including oral contraceptives:

1. *Genitourinary system.*
Breakthrough bleeding, spotting, change in menstrual flow
Dysmenorrhea
Premenstrual-like syndrome
Amenorrhea during and after treatment
Increase in size of uterine fibromyomata
Vaginal candidiasis
Change in cervical eversion and in degree of cervical secretion
Cystitis-like syndrome

2. *Breasts.*
Tenderness, enlargement, secretion

3. *Gastrointestinal.*
Nausea, vomiting
Abdominal cramps, bloating
Cholestatic jaundice

4. *Skin.*
Chloasma or melasma which may persist when drug is discontinued
Erythema multiforme
Erythema nodosum
Hemorrhagic eruption
Loss of scalp hair
Hirsutism

5. *Eyes.*
Steepening of corneal curvature
Intolerance to contact lenses

6. *CNS.*
Headache, migraine, dizziness
Mental depression
Chorea

7. *Miscellaneous.*
Increase or decrease in weight
Reduced carbohydrate tolerance
Aggravation of porphyria
Edema
Changes in libido

Acute Overdosage: Numerous reports of ingestion of large doses of estrogen-containing oral contraceptives by young children indicate that serious ill effects do not occur. Overdosage of estrogen may cause nausea, and withdrawal bleeding may occur in females.

Dosage and Administration: For treatment of moderate to severe vasomotor symptoms associated with the menopause, and for atrophic vaginitis, kraurosis vulvae, female hypogonadism, female castration and primary ovarian failure.

One Estrovis (quinestrol) 100-mcg tablet once daily for seven days, followed by one 100-mcg tablet weekly as a maintenance schedule, commencing two weeks after inception of treatment. The dosage may be increased to 200 mcg weekly if the therapeutic response is not that which may be desirable or considered optimal. The lowest maintenance dose that will control symptoms should be chosen and medication should be discontinued as promptly as possible. Attempts to discontinue or taper medication should be made at three- to six-month intervals.

Treated patients with an intact uterus should be monitored closely for signs of endometrial cancer and appropriate diagnostic measures should be taken to rule out malignancy in the event of persistent or recurring abnormal vaginal bleeding.

How Supplied: N 0071-0437 (P-D 437) Estrovis (quinestrol) 100-mcg tablets are supplied in bottles of 100. **YD**

Physician References:

1. Ziel, H.K. and W.D. Finkle, "Increased Risk of Endometrial Carcinoma Among Users of Conjugated Estrogens." *New England Journal of Medicine,* 293:1167–1170, 1975.
2. Smith, D.C., R. Prentic, D.J. Thompson, and W.L. Hermann, "Association of Exogenous Estrogen and Endometrial Carcinoma." *New England Journal of Medicine,* 293:1164–1167, 1975.
3. Mack, T.M., M.C. Pike, B.E. Henderson, R.I. Pfeffer, V.R. Gerkins, M. Arthur, and S.E. Brown, "Estrogens and Endometrial Cancer in a Retirement Community." *New England Journal of Medicine,* 294:1262–1267, 1976.
4. Weiss, N.D., D.R. Szekely and D.F. Austin, "Increasing Incidence of Endometrial Cancer in the United States." *New England Journal of Medicine,* 294:1259–1262, 1976.
5. Herbst, A.L., H. Ulfelder and D.C. Poskanzer, "Adenocarcinoma of Vagina." *New England Journal of Medicine,* 284:878–881, 1971.
6. Greenwald, P., J. Barlow, P. Nasca, and W. Burnett, "Vaginal Cancer after Maternal Treatment with Synthetic Estrogens." *New England Journal of Medicine,* 285:390–392, 1971.
7. Lanier, A., K. Noller, D. Decker, L. Elveback, and L. Kurland, "Cancer and Stilbestrol, A Follow-Up of 1719 Persons Exposed to Estrogens in *Utero* and Born 1943–1959." *Mayo Clinic Proceedings,* 48:793–799, 1973.
8. Herbst, A., R. Kurman, and R. Scully, "Vaginal and Cervical Abnormalities After Exposure to Stilbestrol in Utero." *Obstetrics and Gynecology,* 40:287–298, 1972.
9. Herbst, A., S. Robboy, G. Macdonald, and R. Scully, "The Effects of Local Progesterone on Stilbestrol-Associated Vaginal Adenosis." *American Journal of Obstetrics and Gynecology,* 118:607–615, 1974.
10. Herbst, A., D. Poskanzer, S. Robboy, L. Friedlander, and R. Scully, "Prenatal Exposure to Stilbestrol, A Prospective Comparison of Exposed Female Offspring with Unexpected Controls." *New England Journal of Medicine,* 292:334–339, 1975.
11. Stafl, A., R. Mattingly, D. Foley, and W. Fetherston, "Clinical Diagnosis of Vaginal Adenosis." *Obstetrics and Gynecology,* 43:118–128, 1974.

Continued on next page

This product information was prepared in August, 1979. On these and other Parke-Davis Products, detailed information may be obtained by addressing PARKE-DAVIS, Division of Warner-Lambert Company, Morris Plains, NJ 07950.

Parke-Davis—Cont.

12. Sherman, A.I., M. Goldrath, A. Berlin, V. Vakhariya, F. Banooni, W. Michaels, P. Goodman, S. Brown, "Cervical-Vaginal Adenosis After *In Utero* Exposure to Synthetic Estrogens," *Obstetrics and Gynecology,* 44:531–545, 1974.
13. Gal, I., B. Kirman, and J. Stern, "Hormone Pregnancy Tests and Congenital Malformation," *Nature,* 216:83, 1967.
14. Levy, E.P., A. Cohen, and F.C. Fraser, "Hormone Treatment During Pregnancy and Congenital Heart Defects," *Lancet,* 1:611, 1973.
15. Nora, J. and A. Nora, "Birth Defects and Oral Contraceptives," *Lancet,* 1:941–942, 1973.
16. Janerich, D.T., J.M. Piper, and D.M. Glebatis, "Oral Contraceptives and Congenital Limb-Reduction Defects," *New England Journal of Medicine,* 291:697–700, 1974.
17. "Estrogens for Oral or Parenteral Use," *Federal Register,* 40:8212, 1975.
18. Boston Collaborative Drug Surveillance Program "Surgically Confirmed Gallbladder Disease, Venous Thromboembolism and Breast Tumors in Relation to Post-Menopausal Estrogen Therapy," *New England Journal of Medicine,* 210:15–19, 1974.
18a. Hoover, R., L.A. Gray, Sr., P. Cole, and B. MacMahon, "Menopausal Estrogens and Breast Cancer." *New England Journal of Medicine,* 295:401–405, 1976.
19. Boston Collaborative Drug Surveillance Program, "Oral Contraceptives and Venous Thromboembolic Disease, Surgically Confirmed Gallbladder Disease, and Breast Tumors," *Lancet,* 1:1399–1404, 1973.
20. Daniel, D.G., H. Campbell, and A.C. Turnbull, "Puerperal Thromboembolism and Suppression of Lactation." *Lancet,* 2:287–289, 1967.
21. The Veterans Administration Cooperative Urological Research Group, "Carcinoma of the Prostate: Treatment Comparisons," *Journal of Urology,* 98:516–522, 1967.
22. Ballar, J.C., "Thromboembolism and Oestrogen Therapy," *Lancet,* 2, 560. 1967.
23. Blackard, C., R. Doe, G. Mellinger, and D. Byar, "Incidence of Cardiovascular Disease and Death in Patients Receiving Diethylstilbestrol for Carcinoma of the Prostate," *Cancer,* 26:249–256, 1970.
24. Royal College of General Practitioners, "Oral Contraception and Thromboembolic Disease," *Journal of the Royal College of General Practitioners,* 13, 267–279, 1967.
25. Inman, W.H.W. and M.P. Vessey, "Investigation of Deaths from Pulmonary, Coronary, and Cerebral Thrombosis and Embolism in Women of Child-Bearing Age." *British Medical Journal,* 2:193–199, 1968.
26. Vessey, M.P. and R. Doll, "Investigation of Relation Between Use of Oral Contraceptives and Thromboembolic Disease, A Further Report," *British Medical Journal,* 2:651–657, 1969.
27. Sartwell, P.E., A.T. Masi, F.G. Arthes, G.R. Greene and H.E. Smith, "Thromboembolism and Oral Contraceptives: An Epidemiological Case Control Study." *American Journal of Epidemology,* 90:365–380, 1969.
28. Collaborative Group for the Study of Stroke in Young Women, "Oral Contraception and Increased Risk of Cerebral Ischemia or Thrombosis," *New England Journal of Medicine,* 288:871–878, 1973.
29. Collaborative Group for the Study of Stroke in Young Women: "Oral Contraceptives and Stroke in Young Women: Associated Risk Factors," 231:718–722, 1975. *Journal of the American Medical Assoc.* 231:718–722, 1975.
30. Mann, J.I. and W.H.W. Inman, "Oral Contraceptives and Death from Myocardial Infarction," *British Medical Journal,* 2:245–248, 1975.
31. Mann, J.I., M.P. Vessey, M. Thorogood, and R. Doll, "Myocardial Infarction in Young Women with Special Reference to Oral Contraceptive Practice," *British Medical Journal,* 2:241–245, 1975.
32. Inman, W.H.W., M.P. Vessey, B. Westerholm, and A. Engelund. "Thromboembolic Disease and the Steroidal Content of Oral Contraceptives," *British Medical Journal,* 2:203–209, 1970.
33. Stolley, P.D., J.A. Tonascia, M.S. Tockman, P.E. Sartwell, A.H. Rutledge, and M.P. Jacobs, "Thrombosis with Low-Estrogen Oral Contraceptives," *American Journal of Epidemology,* 102:197–208, 1975.
34. Vessey, M.P., R. Doll, A.S. Fairbairn, and G. Glober, "Post-Operative Thromboembolism and the use of the Oral Contraceptives," *British Medical Journal,* 3:123–126, 1970.
35. Greene, G.R. and P.E. Sartwell, "Oral Contraceptive Use in Patients with Thromboembolism Following Surgery, Trauma or Infection," *American Journal of Public Health,* 62:680–685, 1972.
36. Rosenberg, L., M.B. Armstrong and H. Jick "Myocardial Infarction and Estrogen Therapy in Post-menopausal Women," *New England Journal of Medicine,* 294:1256–1259, 1976.
37. Coronary Drug Project Research Group, "The Coronary Drug Project: Initial Findings Leading to Modifications of Its Research Protocol," *Journal of the American Medical Association,* 214:1303–1313, 1970.
38. Baum, J., F. Holtz, J.J. Bookstein, and E.W. Klein, "Possible Association between Benign Hepatomas and Oral Contraceptives," *Lancet,* 2:926–928, 1973.
39. Mays, E.T., W.M. Christopherson, M.M. Mahr, and H.C. Williams, "Hepatic Changes in Young Women Ingesting Contraceptive Steroids, Hepatic Hemorrhage and Primary Hepatic Tumors," *Journal of the American Medical Association,* 235:780–782, 1976.
40. Edmondson, H.A., B. Henderson, and B. Benton, "Liver Cell Adenomas Association with the Use of Oral Contraceptives," *New England Journal of Medicine,* 294:470–472, 1976.
41. Pfeffer, A.I. and S. Van Den Noore, "Estrogen use and Stroke Risk in Post-menopausal Women," *American Journal of Epidemiology,* 103:545–546, 1976.

EUTHROID® ℞
(liotrix)

Caution: Federal law prohibits dispensing without prescription.

Description: Euthroid is synthetic microcrystalline levothyroxine sodium (T_4) USP and synthetic microcrystalline liothyronine sodium (T_3) USP combined in a constant 4:1 ratio.

Actions: Euthroid provides replacement therapy for the thyroactive material normally supplied by the human thyroid. The normal thyroid gland produces and stores thyroglobulin, the active components of which are two metabolically active hormones: levothyroxine and liothyronine. Euthroid (liotrix) provides a combination of these hormones in purified, synthetic form, supplied in a constant 4:1 ratio in order to simulate as closely as possible the physiologic and metabolic effects of normal endogenous thyroid secretions.

In contrast with the individual synthetic, metabolically active hormones, Euthroid will usually produce normal results for PBI, T_3, and other thyroid function tests—consistent with clinical progress—when persons with endogenous thyroid deficiencies are made euthyroid. Liothyronine sodium (T_3) acts more rapidly and for a shorter period of time than preparations of biological origin. Customarily, its use as a single agent produces inappropriately decreased PBI values. Levothyroxine sodium (T_4), on the other hand, is more tightly bound by plasma protein fractions and is somewhat slower acting than liothyronine sodium (T_3); its use as a single agent tends to produce inappropriately elevated PBI values. Euthroid, with its unvarying 4:1 ratio of T_4/T_3, permits interpretation of appropriate laboratory tests consistent with the total clinical status of the patient.

Indications: Euthroid (liotrix) provides thyroid replacement therapy in all conditions of inadequate production of thyroid hormones, namely:

1) Hypothyroidism, including cretinism and myxedema.
2) Simple (nontoxic) goiter.
3) Subacute or chronic thyroiditis including Hashimoto's disease.
4) Prevention of goiter in hyperthyroid patients undergoing treatment with thiouracil derivatives.
5) Usage in patients who may manifest intolerance to thyroid products of animal origin.

Contraindications: Acute myocardial infarction, adrenal insufficiency, hypersensitivity to any component of this drug.

Warnings:

> Drugs with thyroid hormone activity, alone or together with other therapeutic agents, have been used for the treatment of obesity. In euthyroid patients, doses within the range of daily hormonal requirements are ineffective for weight reduction. Larger doses may produce serious or even life-threatening manifestations of toxicity, particularly when given in association with sympathomimetic amines such as those used for their anorectic effects.

Liotrix should not be used in the presence of cardiovascular disease unless thyroid replacement therapy is clearly indicated. If the latter exists, low doses should be instituted (Euthroid-½ or Euthroid-1) and increased by the same amount in increments at 2-week intervals. This demands careful clinical judgment. Morphologic hypogonadism and nephroses should be ruled out and adrenal deficiency due to hypopituitarism corrected before liotrix therapy is started.

If hypothyroidism and adrenal insufficiency exist concomitantly, cortisone or similar steroids should be given at dose levels sufficient to correct the adrenal insufficiency before attempting replacement therapy with thyroid hormones.

Likewise, the possibility of alterations in the prothrombin time must be considered and closely monitored in patients on anticoagulant therapy.

Myxedematous patients are very sensitive to thyroid hormones, and dosage should be started at a very low level and increased gradually.

Surgery: Euthroid-treated patients with coronary artery disease should be carefully observed during surgery, since the possibility of precipitating cardiac arrhythmias may be greater in patients treated with thyroid hormones.

Precautions: Hypothyroid patients are especially sensitive to thyroid preparations, and those with severe hypothyroidism may be unusually so.

Initiation of thyroid replacement therapy in patients with diabetes must be carefully monitored because of potential fluctuation in daily insulin or oral hypoglycemic requirements.

As with all thyroid preparations, this drug will alter the results of thyroid function tests.

Adverse Reactions: Overdosage or too rapid increase in dosage of thyroid preparations can produce signs and symptoms of hyperthyroidism, such as menstrual irregularities, nervousness, cardiac arrhythmias, and angina pectoris.

Drug Interactions: The possibility of alterations in the prothrombin time must be considered and closely monitored in patients on anticoagulant therapy.

Dosage and Administration: Initial dosage should be low and gradually increased at 2-week intervals until the desired clinical response is obtained.

Laboratory criteria of euthyroidism include a PBI of 3.5 to 8 mcg; T_3, T_4, and BEI tests are useful.

For most patients, a single daily dose of Euthroid-1, -2, or -3 will maintain euthyroidism. Transfer of a patient from a maintenance dose of another thyroid preparation to Euthroid can usually be effected smoothly. See table for initiating therapy or converting from other thyroid preparations.

[See table above].

Dosage for cretinism or severe hypothyroidism in children is the same as for adults with myxedema. Eventual maintenance dosage in the growing child may be higher than in the adult.

Overdosage:

Symptoms: Headache, instability, nervousness, sweating, tachycardia, and unusual bowel motility. Angina pectoris or congestive heart failure may be induced or aggravated. Shock may develop. Massive overdosage may result in symptoms resembling thyroid storm; chronic excessive dosage will produce the signs and symptoms of hyperthyroidism.

Treatment: Shock—Supportive measures should be utilized. Treatment of unrecognized adrenal insufficiency should be considered.

Supplied: Square W/C monogrammed tablets of four potencies, each identified by a different color (see accompanying table).

Euthroid is supplied in ½ grain, pale orange tablets in bottles of 100 (N 0470-0260-51) and 1000 (N 0470-0260-60); 1 grain, light brown tablets in bottles of 100 (N 0470-0261-51) and 1000 (N 0470-0261-60); 2 grain, violet tablets in bottles of 100 (N 0470-0262-51) and 3 grain, gray tablets in bottles of 100 (N 0470-0263-51).

STORE BETWEEN 59° and 86°F (15° and 30°C).

Licensed under U.S. Patent 2,823,164

[Shown in Product Identification Section]

339 G 600 **R-2-79**

Euthroid (liotrix)			Approximate Equivalents		
			Natural	Synthetic	
Tablet	T_4*/T_3**	Color	Thyroid USP	T_4*	T_3**
	mcg				
Euthroid-½	(30/7.5)	pale orange	½ grain	.05 mg	12.5 mcg
Euthroid-1	(60/15)	light brown	1 grain	.1 mg	25.0 mcg
Euthroid-2	(120/30)	violet	2 grains	.2 mg	50.0 mcg
Euthroid-3	(180/45)	gray	3 grains	.3 mg	75.0 mcg

*T_4 = levothyroxine sodium (*l*-thyroxine)

**T_3 = liothyronine sodium (*l*-triiodothyronine)

FLUOGEN® ℞
(influenza virus vaccine)

The formulation of influenza virus vaccine for use during each season is established by the Bureau of Biologics, Food and Drug Administration, Public Health Service. For information regarding the current formulation, please refer to the product package insert, contact your Parke-Davis representative, or call (201) 540-2000.

GAMULIN® Rh ℞
Rh_o (D) immune globulin (human)

Description: Gamulin Rh (Rh_o [D] immune globulin [human]) is a sterile gamma globulin solution containing Rh_o(D) antibodies. It is obtained by alcohol fractionation of plasma from human blood donors, concentrated and standardized to give a total globulin content of 11.5 ± 1.5%. All lots are assayed for Rh_o(D) antibody content by the radioimmune technique. The Rh_o(D) antibody level in each vial of Gamulin Rh is equal to or greater than that of the Bureau of Biologics Reference Rh_o(D) Immune Globulin (Human). This dose has been shown to effectively inhibit the immunizing potential of up to 15 ml of Rh-positive packed red blood cells. All plasma used in the production of Gamulin Rh has been tested and found nonreactive for hepatitis B surface antigen (HB_s Ag). The final product contains 0.3 *M* glycine as a stabilizer and 0.01% thimerosal (mercury derivative) as a preservative.

Action: Gamulin Rh effectively suppresses the immune response of nonsensitized Rh_o(D) negative, D^u negative individuals who receive Rh_o(D) positive or D^u positive blood as the result of a fetomaternal hemorrhage or a transfusion accident.

Indications: *Full Term Delivery.* Gamulin Rh is used to prevent sensitization to the Rh_o(D) factor and thus to prevent hemolytic disease of the newborn (erythroblastosis fetalis) in a pregnancy that follows the injection of Gamulin Rh. It effectively suppresses the immune response of nonsensitized Rh-negative mothers after delivery of an Rh-positive infant.

Criteria for an Rh-incompatible pregnancy requiring administration of Gamulin Rh are:

1. The mother must be Rh_o(D) negative and D^u negative.
2. The mother should not have been previously sensitized to the Rh_o(D) factor.
3. The infant must be Rh_o(D) positive or D^u positive and direct Coombs negative. A positive direct Coombs test may be due to antibodies other than Rh_o(D). These antibodies should be investigated. If the positive Coombs test is due to Rh_o(D) antibodies, Gamulin Rh should not be given to the mother.

ABO incompatibility between mother and infant provides some protection against Rh isoimmunization but this protection is incomplete. In cases meeting the Rh-incompatibility criteria, Gamulin Rh should be used regardless of ABO incompatibility.

Incomplete Pregnancy. Gamulin Rh should be administered to all nonsensitized Rh-negative women after spontaneous or induced abortions, after ruptured tubal pregnancies, or any occurrence of transplacental hemorrhage unless the blood type of the fetus has been determined to be Rh_o(D) negative and D^u negative.

Note: In a case of abortion or ectopic pregnancy when Rh typing of the fetus is not possible, the fetus must be assumed to be Rh_o(D) positive or D^u positive. In such an instance, the patient should be considered a candidate for administration of Gamulin Rh.

If the father can be determined to be Rh_o(D) negative and D^u negative, Gamulin Rh need not be given.

Gamulin Rh should be given within 72 hours following an Rh-incompatible delivery, miscarriage, or abortion.

Transfusions. Gamulin Rh can be used to prevent Rh_o(D) sensitization in Rh_o(D) negative patients accidentally transfused with Rh_o(D) positive blood.

Gamulin Rh should be administered within 72 hours following an Rh-incompatible transfusion.

Contraindications: Gamulin Rh should not be given to the following.

1. The infant
2. An Rh_o(D) positive or D^u positive individual
3. An Rh_o(D) negative and D^u negative individual previously sensitized to the Rh_o(D) or D^u antigen

Note: Although there is no need to administer Gamulin Rh to a woman who is already sensitized to the Rh factor, there is no more risk than when it is given to a woman who is not sensitized. When there is doubt, Gamulin Rh should be given.

Warnings: Gamulin Rh must not be given to the infant. Do not give intravenously.

Precautions: Before administering Gamulin Rh, it is desirable that all diagnostic laboratory criteria be met, as outlined in the **PREADMINISTRATION LABORATORY PROCEDURES** section.

Adverse Reactions: Because Gamulin Rh is an Rh_o(D) immune globulin derived from homologous human serum proteins, allergic reactions are not expected but the possibility cannot be ruled out. Such reactions have been reported following extensive use of immune serum globulin (gamma globulin) in hypogammaglobulinemic patients.

On occasion, a patient has shown a systemic reaction manifested by a low-grade fever but, generally, reactions have been mild, infrequent, and confined to the site of injection.

Rh_o(D) negative patients inadvertently transfused with Rh_o(D) positive blood have received from 15 to 33 vials of Gamulin Rh with no adverse reaction other than soreness at the injection site. A 1 F temperature elevation in one patient, which could have been due to the underlying illness, has been reported.

PREADMINISTRATION LABORATORY PROCEDURE: *Infant.* Immediately post partum, determine the infant's blood type (ABO, Rh_o[D], and D^u) and perform a direct Coombs test. Umbilical cord, venous, or capillary blood may be used.

Gamulin Rh and Crossmatch Solution: Verify that the lot numbers are the same for the crossmatch solution and the Gamulin Rh to be administered.

Mother. Confirm that the mother is Rh_o(D) negative and D^u negative by crossmatching the mother's blood with the crossmatch solution provided in a separate vial. This solution is a 1:1,000 dilution of an aliquot from the same lot of Gamulin Rh. Perform a minor crossmatch test according to an established procedure by using one drop of a 5% suspension of the mother's red blood cells, freshly drawn, in physiological saline and two drops of the crossmatch solution.

An incompatible crossmatch may indicate that:

1. The patient has been incorrectly typed, in which case typing should be repeated.
2. The crossmatch solution is reacting with fetal red blood cells which entered the mother's blood after a profuse transplacental (fetomaternal) bleeding.
3. Rh-incompatible blood has recently been transfused and the crossmatch solution is reacting with the donor's red blood cells.

If it can be established that the patient is Rh_o(D) negative and D^u negative, Gamulin Rh may be administered regardless of the results of crossmatching.

Continued on next page

This product information was prepared in August, 1979. On these and other Parke-Davis Products, detailed information may be obtained by addressing PARKE-DAVIS, Division of Warner-Lambert Company, Morris Plains, NJ 07950.

Parke-Davis—Cont.

Dosage: *Obstetrical Usage:* One vial of Gamulin Rh is sufficient to prevent maternal sensitization to the Rh factor if the fetal packed red blood cell volume, which entered the mother's blood due to fetomaternal hemorrhage, is less than 15 ml (30 ml of whole blood). When the fetomaternal hemorrhage exceeds 15 ml of packed cells or 30 ml of whole blood, more than one vial of Gamulin Rh should be administered.
To determine the number of vials required, the volume of packed fetal red blood cells must be determined by an approved laboratory assay, such as the Kleihauer-Betke Acid Elution Technic or the Clayton Modification.
The volume of fetomaternal hemorrhage divided by two gives the volume of packed fetal red blood cells in the maternal blood. The number of vials of Gamulin Rh to be administered is determined by dividing the volume (ml) of packed red blood cells by 15.

Procedure for the Kleihauer-Betke Acid Elution Technic:

Reagents:
1. Buffer: 1.46 g citric acid monohydrate and 0.86 g Na_2HPO_4
(Dissolve and qs to 100 ml with distilled water. Final pH 3.5)

Note: Buffer must be fresh. Prepare just prior to use.

2. Stain: Erythrosin B (0.5% in water)
3. Fixative: 80% ethyl alcohol

Controls:
1. Positive:
a) Mixture of 10 parts of adult blood with one part of cord blood (ABO compatible)
b) Cord blood
2. Negative: Adult blood (preferably from a male)

PROCEDURE:
1. Collect blood using EDTA or oxalate as anticoagulant.
2. Dilute blood with equal volume of 0.9% sodium chloride.
3. Prepare thin smears and fix in 80% ethyl alcohol for five minutes.
4. Wash smears with distilled water and airdry.
5. Immerse smears in citric phosphate buffer (pH 3.5) at 37 C for 10 minutes.
6. Wash smears with distilled water.
7. Immerse smears in Erythrosin B for five minutes.
8. Wash smears in running tap water for one minute. (Smears may be counterstained with acid hematoxylin if desired. To do this, after rinsing smears, immerse them in acid hematoxylin for five minutes. Rinse again in running tap water for one minute.)
9. Air-dry smears.
10. Observe under a microscope using 40x magnification. An ocular grid facilitates the counting of cells.

Interpretation:
Normal adult red blood cells appear as pale gray-pink bodies.
Fetal red blood cells appear as bright pink refractile bodies.

Calculation of volume of fetomaternal hemorrhage:
[See table below].

Transfusion Accidents: The number of vials of Gamulin Rh to be administered is dependent on the volume of packed red cells or whole blood transfused. The method to determine the number of vials of Gamulin Rh required to prevent sensitization is outlined below. If the dose calculation results in a fraction, administer the next whole number of vials of Gamulin Rh.

Procedure:
a) Multiply the volume (in ml) of Rh-positive whole blood administered by the hematocrit of the donor unit. This value equals the volume of packed red blood cells transfused.
b) Divide the volume (in ml) of packed red blood cells by 15 to obtain the number of vials of Gamulin Rh (human) to be administered.

ADMINISTRATION:
One-vial dose. Using the sterile disposable syringe provided, withdraw and inject intramuscularly the entire contents of the vial of Gamulin Rh.
Two or more vials dose. Using sterile 5- or 10-ml syringe(s), withdraw the contents from the vials to be administered at one time and inject intramuscularly. The contents of the total number of vials may be injected as a divided dose at different injection sites at the same time, or the total dosage may be divided and injected at intervals provided the total dosage to be given is injected within 72 hours post partum or after a transfusion accident.
This product should be administered within 72 hours after Rh-incompatible delivery or transfusion.
Do not inject intravenously.
Do not inject infant.
For convenience of record keeping, a special form is provided with this product. The form should be carefully filled out and attached to the patient's hospital records. If the form is not used, the following information should be included in the patient's records.
1. Patient's complete identification
2. Patient's ABO and Rh type, and date determined
3. Crossmatch results and date
4. Result of test for prior Rh sensitization
5. Infant's ABO and Rh type, when known, and result of direct Coombs test, or in the case of a transfusion accident, the ABO and Rh types of the donor blood and the volume transfused
6. Notification to patient concerning nature of medication, date, and reason for giving it
7. Lot number of Gamulin Rh and date and time of injection, and the number of vials injected
8. Adequate documentation, if medication is refused by the patient

Caution: Federal law prohibits dispensing without prescription.
How Supplied: Gamulin Rh is supplied in individual packages containing the following.
1. One single-dose vial of Gamulin Rh (N 0071-4002-35)
2. One vial of crossmatch material (1:1,000 dilution of an aliquot from the same lot of Gamulin Rh)
3. A sterile, disposable, 3-ml syringe with 22-gauge, 1 ¼-inch needle
4. Patient identification card
5. Laboratory data sheets
6. Directions for use

Keep refrigerated at 2 to 8 C (35 to 46 F). Do not freeze. **WC**

Total volume of maternal blood in ml*	×	Number of fetal cells / Number of maternal cells	=	Volume of fetomaternal hemorrhage

*Estimated maternal blood volume (5,000 ml: Kleihauer formula) or from normal Tables.

GELUSIL®
Antacid-Antiflatulent
Liquid/Tablets

Each teaspoonful (5 ml) or tablet contains:
200 mg aluminum hydroxide
200 mg magnesium hydroxide
25 mg simethicone

Advantages:
- High acid-neutralizing capacity
- Low sodium content
- Simethicone for antiflatulent activity
- Good taste for better patient compliance
- Fast dissolution of chewed tablets for prompt relief

Indications: Gelusil, a carefully balanced combination of two widely used antacids and the antiflatulent simethicone, is effective for the relief of symptoms associated with heartburn, sour stomach and acid indigestion. Gelusil also provides symptomatic relief of hyperacidity associated with the diagnosis of peptic ulcer, gastritis, peptic esophagitis, gastric hyperacidity and hiatal hernia. Gelusil is also indicated to alleviate or relieve the symptoms of gas, postoperative gas pain or for use in endoscopic examination.
Actions and Uses: The proven neutralizing power of aluminum hydroxide and of magnesium hydroxide combine to give Gelusil dependable antacid action without the acid rebound sometimes associated with calcium carbonate.
The pleasant peppermint-flavored taste of Gelusil Liquid and Tablets encourages patient acceptance of, and compliance with, recommended antacid regimens.
Gelusil Tablets are easy to chew and are specifically formulated to dissolve readily, providing prompt onset of action and reliable relief of symptoms.
Gelusil is appropriate whenever there is a need for well-accepted, effective antacid-antiflatulent therapy.
Dosage and Administration: Two or more teaspoonfuls or tablets one hour after meals and at bedtime, or as directed by a physician. Tablets should be chewed.
The following information is provided to facilitate treatment:

Gelusil	LIQUID	TABLETS
Acid-neutralizing capacity	24 mEq/ 10 ml	22 mEq/ 2 tabs
Sodium	0.7 mg/ 5 ml	0.8 mg/ tab
Lactose	0	0

Warnings: Do not take more than 12 tablets or teaspoonfuls in a 24-hour period, or use this maximum dosage for more than 2 weeks, or use this product if you have kidney disease, except under the advice and supervision of a physician.
Keep this and all drugs out of the reach of children.
Drug Interaction Precaution: Do not take this product if you are presently taking a prescription antibiotic drug containing any form of tetracycline. As with all aluminum-containing antacids, Gelusil may prevent proper absorption of the tetracycline.
How Supplied:
Liquid—In plastic bottles of 6 fl oz (N 0047-0036-06) and 12 fl oz (N 0047-0036-12).
Tablets—White, embossed W/C Gelusil 034—individual strips of 10 in boxes of 50 (N 0047-0034-50), 100 (N 0047-0034-51) and 1000 (N 0047-0034-60); 165 tablets loose-packed in plastic bottles (N 0047-0034-32).
Store between 59° - 86° F (15° - 30° C).
[*Shown in Product Identification Section*]

GELUSIL-M®
Antacid-Antiflatulent
Liquid/Tablets

Each teaspoonful (5 ml) or tablet contains:
300 mg aluminum hydroxide
200 mg magnesium hydroxide
25 mg simethicone

Advantages:
- High acid-neutralizing capacity
- Low sodium content
- Simethicone for antiflatulent activity
- Good taste for better patient compliance
- Fast dissolution of chewed tablets for prompt relief

• Especially useful for those whose bowel functions are adversely effected by magnesium hydroxide.

Indications: Gelusil-M, a carefully balanced combination of two widely used antacids and the antiflatulent simethicone, is effective for the relief of symptoms associated with heartburn, sour stomach, and acid indigestion. Gelusil-M also provides symptomatic relief of hyperacidity associated with the diagnosis of peptic ulcer, gastritis, peptic esophagitis, gastric hyperacidity and hiatal hernia. Gelusil-M is also indicated to alleviate or relieve the symptoms of gas, postoperative gas pain or for use in endoscopic examination.

Actions and Uses: The proven neutralizing power of aluminum hydroxide and magnesium hydroxide combine to give Gelusil-M dependable antacid action without the acid rebound sometimes associated with calcium carbonate. The pleasant spearmint-flavored taste of Gelusil-M Liquid and Tablets encourages patient acceptance of, and compliance with, recommended antacid regimens.

Gelusil-M Tablets are easy to chew and are specifically formulated to dissolve readily providing prompt onset of action and reliable relief of symptoms.

Gelusil-M is appropriate whenever there is a need for well-accepted, effective antacid-antiflatulent therapy.

Dosage and Administration: Two or more teaspoonfuls or tablets one hour after meals and at bedtime, or as directed by a physician. Tablets should be chewed.

The following information is provided to facilitate treatment:

Gelusil-M	LIQUID	TABLETS
Acid-neutralizing capacity	30 mEq/ 10 ml	25 mEq/ 2 tabs
Sodium	1.2 mg/ 5 ml	1.3 mg/ tab
Lactose	0	0

Warnings: Do not take more than 10 teaspoonfuls or tablets in a 24-hour period, or use this maximum dosage for more than 2 weeks, or use this product if you have kidney disease, except under the advice and supervision of a physician.

Keep this and all drugs out of the reach of children.

Drug Interaction Precaution: Do not take this product if you are presently taking a prescription antibiotic drug containing any form of tetracycline. As with all aluminum-containing antacids, Gelusil-M may prevent proper absorption of the tetracycline.

How Supplied:

Liquid—In plastic bottles of 12 fl oz (N 0047-0044-12).

Tablets—White, embossed W/C 045—individual strips of 10 in boxes of 100 (N 0047-0045-51).

Store between 59° - 86°F (15° - 30°C).

GELUSIL-II®

Antacid-Antiflatulent
Liquid/Tablets
High Potency

Each teaspoonful (5 ml) or tablet contains:
400 mg aluminum hydroxide
400 mg magnesium hydroxide
30 mg simethicone

Advantages:
- High acid-neutralizing capacity
- Low sodium content
- Simethicone for antiflatulent activity
- Good taste for better patient compliance
- Fast dissolution of chewed tablets for prompt relief
- Double strength antacid

Indications: Gelusil-II, a carefully balanced high-potency combination of two widely used antacids and the antiflatulent simethicone, is effective for the relief of symptoms associated with heartburn, sour stomach and acid indigestion. Gelusil-II also provides symptomatic relief of hyperacidity associated with the diagnosis of peptic ulcer, gastritis, peptic esophagitis, gastric hyperacidity and hiatal hernia. Gelusil-II may be used concomitantly for relief of pain. Gelusil-II is also indicated to alleviate or relieve the symptoms of gas, postoperative gas pain or for use in endoscopic examination.

Actions and Uses: The proven neutralizing power of aluminum hydroxide and magnesium hydroxide combine to give Gelusil-II dependable antacid action without the acid rebound sometimes associated with calcium carbonate. The higher potency of Gelusil-II is achieved by greater concentration of antacid ingredients per dosage unit.

The pleasant taste of Gelusil-II Liquid (citrus-flavored) and Tablets (orange-flavored) encourages patient acceptance of, and compliance with, recommended antacid regimens.

Gelusil-II Tablets are easy to chew and are specifically formulated to dissolve readily, providing prompt onset of action and reliable relief of symptoms.

Gelusil-II is appropriate whenever there is a need for well-accepted, effective antacid-antiflatulent therapy.

Dosage and Administration: Two or more teaspoonfuls or tablets one hour after meals and at bedtime, or as directed by a physician. Tablets should be chewed.

The following information is provided to facilitate treatment:

Gelusil–II	LIQUID	TABLETS
Acid-neutralizing capacity	48 mEq/ 10 ml	42 mEq/ 2 tabs
Sodium	1.3 mg/ 5 ml	2.1 mg/ tab
Lactose	0	0

Warnings: Do not take more than 8 tablets or teaspoonfuls in a 24-hour period, or use this maximum dosage for more than 2 weeks, or use this product if you have kidney disease, except under the advice and supervision of a physician.

Keep this and all drugs out of the reach of children.

Drug Interaction Precaution: Do not take this product if you are presently taking a prescription antibiotic containing any form of tetracycline. As with all aluminum-containing antacids, Gelusil-II may prevent proper absorption of the tetracycline.

How Supplied:

Liquid —In plastic bottles of 12 fl oz (N-0047-0042-12).

Tablets —Double-layered white/orange, embossed W/C 043 - individual strips of 10 in boxes of 80 (N 0047-0043-80).

Store between 59° - 86°F (15° - 30°C).

[*Shown in Product Identification Section*]

GENERICS

The following is a list of the generic names of all Parke-Davis solid-oral product forms which are marketed under the generic name or a trade name.

25-634-		**Acetaminophen with Codeine Phosphate Tablets, No. 22**
25-635-		**Acetaminophen with Codeine Phosphate Tablets, No. 3**
25-640-		**Acetaminophen Tablets, USP (Tapar®), 325 mg**
6-402-		**Ampicillin Capsules, USP (Amcill® Capsules), 250 mg**
6-404-		**Ampicillin Capsules, USP (Amcill® Capsules), 500 mg**
6–730–		**Amoxicillin (Utimox™) Capsules, 250 mg**
6–731–		**Amoxicillin (Utimox™) Capsules, 500 mg**
25-906-		**Ascorbic Acid Tablets, USP (Vitamin C Tablets), 500 mg**
25-606-		**Aspirin Tablets, USP, 325 mg**
25-624-		**Aspirin Tablets, USP, 325 mg, Pink**
25-679-		**Aspirin Compound Tablets**
25-781-		**Aspirin Compound Tablets, Pink**
25-792-	©III	**Aspirin Compound with Codeine Phosphate Tablets No. 2**
25-793-	©III	**Aspirin Compound with Codeine Phosphate Tablets No. 3**
15-389-		**Bromodiphenhydramine Hydrochloride Capsules, NF (Ambodryl® Kapseals®), 25 mg**
25-764-		**Calcium Gluconate Tablets, USP, 1 g**
25-533-		**Calcium Lactate Tablets, USP, 325 mg**
25-604-		**Calcium Lactate Tablets, USP, 650 mg**
25-55-		**Cascara Tablets, NF (Cascara Sagrada Extract Filmseal®), 325 mg**
7-246-	©IV	**Chloral Hydrate Capsules, USP, 500 mg**
15-379-		**Chloramphenicol Capsules, USP (Chloromycetin Kapseals), 250 mg**
6-800-	©IV	**Chlordiazepoxide Hydrochloride Capsules, USP, 5 mg**
6-801-		**Chlordiazepoxide Hydrochloride Capsules, USP, 10 mg**
6-802-		**Chlordiazepoxide Hydrochloride Capsules, USP, 25 mg**
25-10-		**Chlorpromazine Hydrochloride Tablets, USP (Promapar®), 10 mg**
25-25-		**Chlorpromazine Hydrochloride Tablets, USP, 25 mg**
25-50-		**Chlorpromazine Hydrochloride Tablets, USP, 50 mg**
25-100-		**Chlorpromazine Hydrochloride Tablets, USP, 100 mg**
25-200-		**Chlorpromazine Hydrochloride Tablets, USP, 200 mg**
15-351-		**Digitalis Capsules, NF (Digifortis® Kapseals), 100 mg**
6-471-		**Diphenhydramine Hydrochloride Capsules, USP (Benadryl®), 25 mg**
15-373-		**Diphenhydramine Hydrochloride Capsules, USP (Benadryl Kapseals), 50 mg**
7-247-		**Dioctyl Sodium Sulfosuccinate Capsules, (D-D-S Capsules), 100 mg**
7-248-		**Dioctyl Sodium Sulfosuccinate with Casanthranol Capsules (D-S-S Plus Capsules)**
27-111-		**Ergotamine Tartrate Tablets (Ergostat® Sublingual Tablets), 2 mg**
25-672-		**Erythromycin Stearate Tablets, USP (Erypar® Filmseal), 250 mg**
25-919-		**Erythromycin Stearate Tablets, USP (Erypar® Filmseal), 500 mg**
7-237-		**Ethosuximide Capsules, USP (Zarontin® Capsules), 250 mg**
25-37-		**Ferrous Sulfate Filmseal, 325 mg**
25-702-		**Hydrochlorothiazide Tablets, USP (Thiuretic®), 25 mg**

Continued on next page

This product information was prepared in August, 1979. On these and other Parke-Davis Products, detailed information may be obtained by addressing PARKE-DAVIS, Division of Warner-Lambert Company, Morris Plains, NJ 07950.

Parke-Davis—Cont.

25-710- Hydrochlorothiazide Tablets, USP (Thiuretic®), 50 mg
15-540- Mefenamic Acid (Ponstel® Kapseals), 250 mg
25-636- Meprednisone Tablets, NF (Betapar® Tablets), 4 mg
25-932- Ⓒ Meprobamate Tablets, USP, 200 mg
25-647- Meprobamate Tablets, USP, 400 mg
6-574- Ⓒ Methaqualone Hydrochloride Capsules, NF (Parest-400™), 400 mg
15-525- Methsuximide Capsules, NF (Celontin® Kapseals), 300 mg
15-537- Methsuximide Capsules, NF (Celontin Kapseals), 150 mg
25-771- Niacin Tablets, NF (Nicotinic Acid Tablets), 50 mg
25-794- Niacin Tablets, NF (Nicotinic Acid Tablets), 100 mg
27-1460- Nitroglycerin Tablets, USP (Nitrostat® Sublingual Tablets), 0.15 mg
27-1469- Nitroglycerin Tablets, USP (Nitrostat Sublingual Tablets), 0.3 mg
27-1470- Nitroglycerin Tablets, USP (Nitrostat Sublingual Tablets), 0.4 mg
27-1471- Nitroglycerin Tablets, USP (Nitrostat Sublingual Tablets), 0.6 mg
25-882- Norethindrone Tablets, USP (Norlutin® Tablets), 5 mg
25-918- Norethindrone Acetate Tablets, NF (Norlutate® Tablets), 5 mg
6-670- Oxytetracycline Hydrochloride Capsules, USP (Oxlopar®), 250 mg
25-889- Oxytocin Citrate, Buccal Tablets (Pitocin® Citrate, Buccal Tablets), 200 units
6-455- Pancreatin Capsules, NF (Panteric® Capsules), 325 mg
25-503- Pancreatin Tablets, NF (Panteric Filmseal), 325 mg
6-529- Paromomycin Sulfate Capsules, NF (Humatin® Kapseals), 250 mg
25-676- Penicillin G Potassium Tablets, USP, 400,000 units
25-648- Penicillin V Potassium Tablets, USP (Penapar VK®), 250 mg
25-673- Penicillin V Potassium Tablets, USP (Penapar VK), 500 mg
25-699- Ⓒ Phenobarbital Tablets, USP, 15 mg
25-700- Phenobarbital Tablets, USP, 30 mg
25-607- Phenobarbital Tablets, USP, 60 mg
25-698- Phenobarbital Tablets, USP, 100 mg
15-393- Phensuximide Capsules, NF (Milontin® Kapseals), 500 mg
36-7- Phenytoin Tablets, USP (Dilantin® Infatabs®), 50 mg
15-362- Phenytoin Sodium Capsules, USP (Dilantin Kapseals), 100 mg
15-365- Phenytoin Sodium Capsules, USP (Dilantin Kapseals), 30 mg
6-692- Ⓒ Propoxyphene Hydrochloride Capsules, USP, 65 mg
6-694- Ⓒ Propoxyphene Compound 65, Capsules
25-836- Propylthiouracil Tablets, USP, 50 mg
25-747- Pyrvinium Pamoate Tablets, USP (Povan® Filmseal), 50 mg
25-437 Quinestrol tablets (Estrovis® Tablets), 100 mcg
25-850- Quinidine Gluconate Tablets (Duraquin® Tablets), 330 mg
25-849- Quinidine Sulfate Tablets, USP, 200 mg
6-420- Quinine Sulfate Capsules, USP, 325 mg
25-601- Sodium Chloride Tablets, USP, 1 g
25-925- Sulfacytine Tablets (Renoquid® Tablets), 250 mg
6-407- Tetracycline Hydrochloride Capsules, USP (Cyclopar®), 250 mg
6-697- Tetracycline Hydrochloride Capsules, USP (Cyclopar 500), 500 mg
25-818- Thiamine Hydrochloride Tablets, USP, 50 mg
25-825- Thiamine Hydrochloride Tablets, USP, 100 mg
7-685- Vitamin E Synthetic Capsules, 400 IU
7-1574- Vitamin E Natural Capsules, 400 IU

GERIPLEX®
Geriatric Vitamin-Mineral Formula

Composition: Each Kapseal represents:
Vitamins:
Vitamin A (acetate) ....(1.5 mg) 5,000 IU*
Vitamin C (ascorbic acid)† .... 50 mg
Vitamin B_1 (thiamine mononitrate) .... 5 mg
Vitamin B_2(G) (riboflavin) .... 5 mg
Vitamin B_{12}, crystalline (cyanocobalamin) .... 2 mcg
Choline dihydrogen citrate .... 20 mg
Nicotinamide (niacinamide) .... 15 mg
Vitamin E (*dl*-alpha tocopheryl acetate) .... (5 mg) 5 IU*
Minerals and Enzymes:
Ferrous sulfate‡ .... 30 mg
Copper sulfate .... 4 mg
Manganese sulfate (monohydrate) .... 4 mg
Zinc sulfate .... 2 mg
Calcium phosphate, dibasic (anhydrous) .... 200 mg
Taka-Diastase® (aspergillus oryzae enzymes) .... 2½ gr

* International Units
†Supplied as sodium ascorbate
‡Supplied as dried ferrous sulfate equivalent to the labeled amount of ferrous sulfate

Action and Uses: A preparation containing vitamins and minerals for middle-aged and older individuals.
Administration and Dosage: USUAL DOSAGE—one Kapseal daily, with or immediately after a meal.
How Supplied: N 0071-0382—Bottles of 100. Parcode® No. 382.

GERIPLEX-FS® KAPSEALS®

Composition: Each Kapseal represents:
Vitamin A (acetate) ....(1.5 mg) 5,000 IU*
Vitamin C (ascorbic acid)† .... 50 mg
Vitamin B_1 (thiamine mononitrate) .... 5 mg
Vitamin B_2 (riboflavin) .... 5 mg
Vitamin B_{12}, crystalline (cyanocobalamin) .... 2 mcg
Choline dihydrogen citrate .... 20 mg
Nicotinamide (niacinamide) .... 15 mg
Vitamin E (*dl*-alpha tocopheryl acetate) .... (5 mg) 5 IU*
Ferrous sulfate‡ .... 30 mg
Copper sulfate .... 4 mg
Manganese sulfate (monohydrate) .... 4 mg
Zinc sulfate .... 2 mg
Calcium phosphate, dibasic (anhydrous) .... 200 mg
Taka-Diastase® (aspergillus oryzae enzymes) .... 2½ gr
Dioctyl sodium sulfosuccinate .... 100 mg

* International Units
†Supplied as sodium ascorbate
‡Supplied as dried ferrous sulfate equivalent to the labeled amount of ferrous sulfate

Action and Uses: A preparation containing vitamins, minerals, and a fecal softener for middle-aged and older individuals. The fecal softening agent, dioctyl sodium sulfosuccinate, acts to soften stools and make bowel movements easier.
Administration and Dosage: USUAL DOSAGE—One Kapseal daily, with or immediately after a meal.
How Supplied: N 0071-0544—Bottles of 100 and in unit-dose packages of 100 (10 strips of 10). Parcode® No. 544.
[*Shown in Product Identification Section*]

GERIPLEX-FS® LIQUID
Geriatric Vitamin Formula with Iron and a Fecal Softener

Composition: Each 30 ml represents vitamin B_1 (thiamine hydrochloride), 1.2 mg; vitamin B_2 (as riboflavin-5'-phosphate sodium), 1.7 mg; vitamin B_6 (pyridoxine hydrochloride), 1 mg; vitamin B_{12} (cyanocobalamin) crystalline, 5 mcg; niacinamide, 15 mg; iron (as ferric ammonium citrate, green), 15 mg; Pluronic® F-68,* 200 mg; alcohol, 18%.
Administration and Dosage: USUAL ADULT DOSAGE—Two tablespoonfuls (30 ml) daily or as recommended by the physician.
How Supplied: N 0071-2454-23—Bottles of 16 oz (1 pt).

*Pluronic is a registered trademark of BASF Wyandotte Corporation for polymers of ethylene oxide and propylene oxide.

HISTOPLASMIN, DILUTED ℞

For complete product information, consult Diagnostic Products Information Section.

HUMAFAC® ℞
(antihemophilic factor [human])
Factor VIII

Description: Humafac is a lyophilized preparation of human antihemophilic factor (factor VIII, AHF, AHG) prepared from frozen venous plasma that was found nonreactive when individual units were tested for hepatitis B surface antigen by the radioimmunoassay (RIA) method. The freeze-dried concentrate of antihemophilic factor is prepared from the factor VIII-rich cryoprotein of plasma by a modification of the method described by Hershgold, Pool, and Pappenhagen.
Each lot of Humafac is assayed and labeled according to its factor VIII content, making both estimation of dose and prediction of effects possible. Humafac reconstitutes relatively rapidly and easily. A few proteinic particles may become coated with microscopic-sized air bubbles which may prolong solubilization time. This formation of foam or bubbles should also be avoided due to the potential inactivation of AHF. (See **Reconstitution.**) Humafac can be administered rapidly by direct syringe intravenous injection, which takes less than two minutes per single dose.
Because each vial of Humafac can be reconstituted with 6 ml of diluent, sufficient material

for an average dose can be administered with a relatively small total volume. Increased amounts of AHF necessary to overcome inhibitors can also be safely and conveniently given. The total amount of diluent provided, 10 ml, may be used if a less viscous solution is desired. A 10-ml vial of Sterile Water for Injection, USP, is enclosed to be used as the diluent. Sterile Water for Injection, USP, is water for injection sterilized. It is not suitable for intravascular injection by itself.

Action: Antihemophilic factor (human) accelerates the abnormally slow clotting time of hemophiliacs, which is due to a deficiency of factor VIII.

Indication: Antihemophilic factor (human) is intended for use in the therapy of classical hemophilia (hemophilia A), a congenital deficiency characterized by a life-long tendency to prolonged hemorrhage. Classical hemophilia appears to be due to a deficiency of a specific plasma protein, antihemophilic factor. The abnormality is attributable to a sex-linked, recessive, mutant gene, so the disease occurs almost exclusively in males. However, homozygous females, very rarely encountered, may have typical manifestations of the disease. An adequate supply of AHF concentrate should be available to maintain known hemophiliacs free of hemorrhagic episodes and for control of nonanticipated major hemorrhagic episodes and emergency and elective surgery.

Antihemophilic factor (human) is not indicated for the management of bleeding in patients with von Willebrand's disease.

Warning: Humafac (antihemophilic factor, [human]) is prepared from human plasma and, consequently, the risk of transmitting hepatitis is present. However, both the individual units of plasma used in the preparation of Humafac and each lot of final product have been found nonreactive when tested for hepatitis B surface antigen using the radioimmunoassay method. Because presently available testing methods are not sensitive enough to detect all potentially infectious antigen, the risk of transmitting hepatitis still exists.

Precautions: Humafac is for intravenous use only.

A separate, sterile, disposable syringe should be used for each injection to avoid possible contamination of the syringes with blood containing the virus of homologous serum hepatitis. The use of a plastic syringe is recommended because solutions of Humafac may cause binding of ground-glass surfaces.

Identification of the deficiency as one of factor VIII in classical hemophilia is imperative before administration of this highly concentrated factor. No benefit can be expected from this product in treating deficiencies other than that described in the **Indication** section.

This preparation contains groups A and B isoagglutinins. When large volumes are given to individuals of blood groups A, B, or AB, the physician should watch for symptoms of intravascular hemolysis.

Adverse Reactions: In clinical trials, one child developed abnormal laboratory tests consistent with hepatitis several months after administration; the child was asymptomatic and laboratory values subsequently returned to normal.

Acute reactions, such as erythema, hives, fever, and backache, may occur infrequently and ordinarily will disappear within 15 to 20 minutes.

Reconstitution:

1. Warm the Humafac vial and the diluent vial to between 30 and 37 C (86 and 99 F) just prior to use. Use of a water bath will facilitate temperature adjustment. Reconstitution of the Humafac with cold diluent or reconstitution of a Humafac vial at refrigerator temperature will markedly prolong the time necessary for complete reconstitution.
2. Remove perforated center from product vial cap and plastic protective cover from diluent. Cleanse stoppers with suitable antiseptic.
3. Attach filter needle to syringe (use plastic syringe) and solubilize the contents of the Humafac (antihemophilic factor [human]) vial by aseptically transferring 6 or 10 ml of the warmed diluent. Attention should be given to puncturing the rubber stopper through the slot, at an angle, to deliver the diluent down the inside walls of the product vial, *slowly,* so that foam does not form. Care should be taken so that the vacuum inside the vial does not cause the diluent to rush into the vial causing the formation of foam, thereby prolonging the time necessary for complete solubilization. *Do not* shake the product vial during this transfer. Thereafter, withdraw 5 to 10 ml of air from the vial by means of the syringe and filter needle, leaving the vial under a slight vacuum. Remove the filter needle and syringe from the vial without agitating the contents, leave filter needle on syringe, and protect needle from contamination.
4. Allow the contents to sit for one to two minutes without motion so that the contents become thoroughly wetted. Then swirl the product vial with a *gentle* rotary motion until the contents are completely dissolved.
5. Reinsert filter needle (on syringe) through vial stopper and withdraw reconstituted AHF into syringe.
6. Remove filter needle from syringe and discard, attach the 23-gauge x 1-inch vein needle, and administer promptly. The solution should be administered within two hours after reconstitution because no preservative has been added. The reconstituted material should not be refrigerated because precipitation of some active material may result.

Note: Entrapment of powder particles within foam greatly prolongs reconstitution time. Avoid foam formation. Normal reconstitution time is less than 10 minutes, averaging about 8 minutes. Expect to see a homogeneous, opalescent, somewhat viscous solution, slightly tannish colored.

Dosage and Administration: Each vial of Humafac (antihemophilic factor [human]) is labeled with the number of AHF units it contains. One AHF unit is defined as the equivalent of the activity present in 1 ml plasma pooled from at least 10 donors and tested within three hours of collection of the first unit represented in the pool.

Dosage must be individualized according to the weight of the patient, the severity of the bleeding, the severity of the blood condition, the source of the bleeding, the presence of inhibitors, and other factors as determined by the physician.

The following dosage schedules for various clinical conditions are suggested.

1. *Joint and muscle hemorrhages*—Joint and muscle hemorrhages should be treated with 25 units/kg once daily, with repeated daily administration if the patient does not respond. A partial thromboplastin time assay obtained after infusion of AHF should demonstrate significant improvement; otherwise the presence of factor VIII antibodies should be suspected, necessitating additional doses.
2. *Overt bleeding*(cut lips, tongue, cheeks; various cuts and wounds)—Initially, 20 units/kg, followed by 10 units/kg every 6 to 8 hours for 24 hours, then every 12 hours for three to four days.
3. *Massive wounds*—Infusion should be maintained until bleeding is stopped. The partial thromboplastin time results should approach the normal control value.
4. *Surgery*—Levels of 40% AHF or more are required. Thirty to 40 units per kilogram body weight are needed prior to surgery, followed by 20 units/kg every eight hours after surgery. This should be done with laboratory control and the dosage should be increased if the AHF level is less than 30% just prior to the next infusion. The postinfusion level should be around 60% AHF (McMillan et al have suggested that the AHF level be raised to 30 to 60% of normal initially and then maintained at 15 to 30% for at least 10 days postoperatively).

For each unit of antihemophilic factor administered per kilogram of body weight, a 2% rise in factor VIII activity was observed by Abildgaard et al. This linear dose-response relationship can be shown by the following formula.

$$\text{Exp. AHF increase (in \% of "normal")} = \frac{2 \times \text{units administered}}{\text{body weight (in kg)}}$$

The clinical effect on the patient is the most important factor in the evaluation of adequacy of therapy. It may, therefore, be necessary to administer more Humafac than would be estimated to obtain the desired result. The dosage requirements of AHF, when inhibitors are present, are extremely variable, and the dosage can only be determined by clinical response.

Laboratory Control: Whenever possible, clinical observations should be supplemented by appropriate laboratory tests to assure that adequate AHF levels have been reached and are maintained. Factor VIII-deficient plasma exhibits a prolonged, partial thromboplastin time and the PTT assay may be used as a crude means of measuring the patient's response. Approximately 25 to 30% AHF is necessary for a normal value. A complete set of reagents, including reference plasma, is commercially available for determination of AHF level by the PTT assay. Other laboratory findings in severe cases are a prolonged clotting time and a high level of residual prothrombin in the serum. Bleeding time and prothrombin time are normal.

If the AHF level fails to reach expected levels or if bleeding is not controlled after apparently adequate dosage, the presence of AHF inhibitors should be suspected. After sufficient dosage to neutralize inhibitors, additional dosage produces predicted clinical response. When inhibitors are present, measurement of Lee-White clotting time may be a better indicator of dosage adequacy than measurement of circulating AHF.

Storage: Humafac (antihemophilic factor [human]) should be stored under refrigeration between 2 and 8 C. If refrigeration is not available, Humafac may be stored at room temperature for up to six months. Although not harmful to the unreconstituted AHF, freezing may cause damage to the diluent bottle.

Reconstituted Humafac should not be refrigerated.

How Supplied: Humafac is supplied as a lyophilized powder in single-dose vials with 10 ml Sterile Water for Injection, USP, one 23-gauge x 1-inch thin-wall needle, and one filter needle. The number of AHF units per vial is stated on the label and on the carton. YF

HYDROCHLOROTHIAZIDE TABLETS, USP ℞
(Thiuretic®)

Description: Hydrochlorothiazide is a member of the benzothiadiazine (thiazide) family of drugs. It is closely related to chlorothiazide. Clinically, hydrochlorothiazide is an orally active diuretic-antihypertensive agent.

Actions: The diuretic and saluretic effects of hydrochlorothiazide result from a drug-induced inhibition of the renal tubular reabsorp-

Continued on next page

This product information was prepared in August, 1979. On these and other Parke-Davis Products, detailed information may be obtained by addressing PARKE-DAVIS, Division of Warner-Lambert Company, Morris Plains, NJ 07950.

Parke-Davis—Cont.

tion of electrolytes. The excretion of sodium and chloride is greatly enhanced. Potassium excretion is enhanced also to a variable degree, as it is with other thiazides. Although urinary excretion of bicarbonate is increased slightly, there is usually no significant change in urinary pH. Hydrochlorothiazide has a per milligram natriuretic activity approximately 10 times that of the prototype thiazide, chlorothiazide. At maximal therapeutic dosages, all thiazides are approximately equal in their diuretic/natriuretic effects.

There is significant natriuresis and diuresis within two hours after administration of a single, oral dose of hydrochlorothiazide. These effects reach a peak in about 6 hours and persist for about 12 hours following oral administration of a single dose.

Like other benzothiadiazines, hydrochlorothiazide also has antihypertensive properties, and may be used for this purpose either alone or to enhance the antihypertensive action of other drugs. The mechanism by which the benzothiadiazines, including hydrochlorothiazide, produce a reduction of elevated blood pressure is not known. However, sodium depletion appears to be involved.

Hydrochlorothiazide is readily absorbed from the gastrointestinal tract and is excreted unchanged by the kidneys.

Indications: Hydrochlorothiazide is indicated in the management of hypertension either as the sole therapeutic agent or to enhance the effect of other antihypertensive drugs in the more severe forms of hypertension.

Hydrochlorothiazide is indicated as adjunctive therapy in edema associated with congestive heart failure, hepatic cirrhosis, and corticosteroid and estrogen therapy.

Hydrochlorothiazide has been found useful also in edema due to various forms of renal dysfunction, such as the nephrotic syndrome, acute glomerulonephritis, and chronic renal failure.

Usage in Pregnancy: The routine use of diuretics in an otherwise healthy pregnant woman is inappropriate and exposes mother and fetus to unnecessary hazard. Diuretics do not prevent development of toxemia of pregnancy, and there is no satisfactory evidence that they are useful in the treatment of developed toxemia.

Edema during pregnancy may arise from pathological causes or from the physiological and mechanical consequences of pregnancy. Thiazides are indicated in pregnancy when edema is due to pathological causes, just as the drugs are in the absence of pregnancy (however, see Warnings). Dependent edema in pregnancy, resulting from restriction of venous return by the expanded uterus, is properly treated through elevation of the lower extremities and use of support hose; use of diuretics to lower intravascular volume in this case is illogical and unnecessary. There is hypervolemia during normal pregnancy which is harmful to neither the fetus nor the mother (in the absence of cardiovascular disease), but which is associated with edema, including generalized edema, in the majority of pregnant women. If this edema produces discomfort, increased recumbency will often provide relief. In rare instances, this edema may cause extreme discomfort which is not relieved by rest. In these cases, a short course of diuretics may provide relief and may be appropriate.

Contraindications:

Renal decompensation

Hypersensitivity to this or other sulfonamide-derived drugs

Warnings: Hydrochlorothiazide shares with other thiazides the propensity to deplete potassium reserves to an unpredictable degree.

Thiazides should be used with caution in patients with renal disease or significant impairment of renal function, because azotemia may be precipitated and cumulative drug effects may occur.

Thiazides should be used with caution in patients with impaired hepatic function or progressive liver disease, because minor alterations of fluid and electrolyte balance may precipitate hepatic coma.

Thiazides may be additive or potentiative of the action of other antihypertensive drugs. Potentiation occurs with ganglionic or peripheral adrenergic blocking drugs.

Sensitivity reactions may occur in patients with a history of allergy or bronchial asthma. The possibility of exacerbation or activation of systemic lupus erythematosus has been reported.

Usage in Pregnancy: Thiazides cross the placental barrier and appear in cord blood. The use of thiazides in pregnant women requires that the anticipated benefit be weighed against possible hazards to the fetus. These hazards include fetal or neonatal jaundice, thrombocytopenia, and possible other adverse reactions that have occurred in the adult.

Nursing Mothers: Thiazides appear in breast milk. If use of the drug is deemed essential, the patient should stop nursing.

Precautions: Periodic determinations of serum electrolytes should be performed at appropriate intervals for the purpose of detecting possible electrolyte imbalances, such as hyponatremia, hypochloremic alkalosis, and hypokalemia. Serum and urine electrolyte determinations are particularly important when a patient is vomiting excessively or receiving parenteral fluids. All patients should be observed for other clinical signs of electrolyte imbalances, such as dryness of mouth, thirst, weakness, lethargy, drowsiness, restlessness, muscle pains or cramps, muscular fatigue, hypotension, oliguria, tachycardia, and gastrointestinal disturbances, such as nausea and vomiting.

Hypokalemia may develop with thiazides as with any other potent diuretic, especially when brisk diuresis occurs, severe cirrhosis is present, or corticosteroids or ACTH are given concomitantly. Interference with the adequate oral intake of electrolytes will also contribute to the possible development of hypokalemia. Potassium depletion, even of a mild degree, resulting from thiazide use, may sensitize a patient to the effects of cardiac glycosides, such as digitalis.

Any chloride deficit is generally mild and usually does not require specific treatment except under extraordinary circumstances (as in liver disease or renal disease). Dilutional hyponatremia may occur in edematous patients in hot weather; appropriate therapy is water restriction, rather than administration of salt, except in rare instances when the hyponatremia is life-threatening.

In actual salt depletion, appropriate replacement is the therapy of choice.

Hyperuricemia may occur or frank gout may be precipitated in certain patients receiving thiazide therapy.

Insulin requirements in diabetic patients may be increased, decreased, or unchanged. Latent diabetes mellitus may become manifest during thiazide administration.

Thiazide drugs may increase the responsiveness to tubocurarine.

The antihypertensive effects of the drug may be enhanced in the postsympathectomy patient.

Thiazides may decrease arterial responsiveness to norepinephrine. This diminution is not sufficient to preclude effectiveness of the pressor agent for therapeutic use.

If progressive renal impairment becomes evident as indicated by a rising-nonprotein nitrogen or blood urea nitrogen, a careful reappraisal of therapy is necessary, with consideration given to withholding or discontinuing diuretic therapy.

Thiazides may decrease serum PBI levels without signs of thyroid disturbance.

Thiazides have been reported, on rare occasions, to have elevated serum calcium to hypercalcemic levels. The serum calcium levels have returned to normal when the medication has been stopped. This phenomenon may be related to the ability of the thiazide diuretics to lower the amount of calcium excreted in the urine.

Adverse Reactions: Gastrointestinal system reactions—anorexia, gastric irritation, nausea, vomiting, cramping, diarrhea, constipation, jaundice, (intrahepatic cholestatic jaundice), pancreatitis

Central nervous system reactions—dizziness, vertigo, paresthesias, headache, xanthopsia

Hematologic reactions—leukopenia, agranulocytosis, thrombocytopenia, aplastic anemia

Dermatologic—hypersensitivity reactions: purpura, photosensitivity, rash, urticaria, necrotizing angiitis (vasculitis) (cutaneous vasculitis)

Cardiovascular reaction—orthostatic hypotension may occur and may be aggravated by alcohol, barbiturates, or narcotics.

Other—hyperglycemia, glycosuria, hypercalcemia, hyperuricemia, muscle spasm, weakness, restlessness

There have been isolated reports that certain nonedematous individuals developed severe fluid and electrolyte derangements after only brief exposure to normal doses of thiazide and nonthiazide diuretics. The condition is usually manifested as severe dilutional hyponatremia, hypokalemia, and hypochloremia. This syndrome has been reported to be due to inappropriately increased ADH secretion and appears to be idiosyncratic. Potassium replacement is apparently the most important therapy in the treatment of this syndrome along with removal of the offending drug.

Whenever adverse reactions are severe, treatment should be discontinued.

Dosage and Administration: Hydrochlorothiazide is administered orally. Therapy should be individualized according to patient response. This therapy should be titrated to gain maximal therapeutic response as well as the minimal dosage possible to maintain that therapeutic response.

For the management of edema, the adult dosage ranges from 25 to 200 mg daily and may be given in single or divided doses. Usually, 75 to 100 mg will produce the desired diuretic effect.

For the management of hypertension, the usual initial adult dosage is 25 to 50 mg two times daily. The dosage may be increased if necessary to a maximum of 100 mg twice daily.

When therapy is prolonged or large dosages are given, particular attention should be given to the patient's electrolyte status. Supplemental potassium may be required.

In the treatment of hypertension, hydrochlorothiazide may be employed either alone or concurrently with other antihypertensive drugs. Combined therapy may provide adequate control of hypertension with lower dosage of the component drugs and fewer or less severe side effects.

For treatment of moderately severe or severe hypertension, supplemental use of other potent antihypertensive agents may be indicated. When other antihypertensive agents are to be added to the regimen, this should be accomplished gradually. Additional potent antihypertensive agents should be given at only half the usual dosage because their effect is potentiated by pretreatment with hydrochlorothiazide.

Overdosage: Symptoms of overdosage include electrolyte imbalance and signs of potassium deficiency, such as confusion, dizziness, muscular weakness, and gastrointestinal disturbances. General supportive measures including replacement of fluids and electrolytes may be indicated in the treatment of overdosage.

How Supplied:
N 0071-0702 (Tablet 702)—Hydrochlorothiazide, 25 mg; in 100s and unit-dose 100s. Parcode® No. 702
N 0071-0710 (Tablet 710)—Hydrochlorothiazide, 50 mg; in 100s, 1,000s, and unit-dose 100s. Parcode No. 710
Manufactured by Abbott Laboratories, North Chicago, IL, 60064, for distribution by Parke-Davis, Division of Warner-Lambert Company, Morris Plains, NJ 07950. **WK**

IMMU-G® ℞

(immune serum globulin [human], USP)
gamma globulin (human)

Description: Immu-G is a sterile, concentrated solution of antibodies found in normal human blood. The product is prepared from large pools of adult human blood of venous and placental origin by a special fractionation process involving a series of controlled precipitations with cold alcohol (Cohn process). Each unit of venous plasma used in this product has been shown to be nonreactive when tested for hepatitis B surface antigen (HB_sAg). The placental plasma used is obtained from hospital maternity populations whose patient sera have been screened to meet accepted criteria for hepatitis B surface antigen (HB_sAg). The active component is highly refined gamma globulin (approximately 165 mg/ml) dissolved in a 2.25% solution of aminoacetic acid (glycine) and containing approximately 0.2% sodium chloride, preserved with 0.01% thimerosal (mercury derivative) and adjusted to pH 6.8 with sodium acetate buffer. The color normally varies from clear amber to dark reddish-brown but these variations in no way affect potency or stability of the product.
The presence of several marker antibodies is demonstrated by immunological tests in laboratory animals and tissue cultures. Specifically, the antibody content meets or exceeds the potency requirement for Measles Immune Globulin (Human) and meets the potency requirement for Poliomyelitis Globulin (Human). In addition, the diphtheria antitoxin content is titrated in each lot.

Indications: Solutions of human immune serum globulin offer highly effective protection against the clinical manifestations of hepatitis A (formerly infectious hepatitis). Immune serum globulin is also effective in the prevention or modification of measles (rubeola) and the treatment of antibody-deficiency disease. In addition, immune serum globulin has been reported effective in various degrees for the prevention or modification of German measles (rubella) in the first trimester of pregnancy, the prevention or modification of varicella in certain high-risk patients, and as an adjunct in the treatment of various bacterial infections that do not respond well to antibiotic therapy alone.

Adverse Reactions: Reactions following intramuscular injections of Immu-G, as with any gamma globulin product, are infrequent, usually of a mild nature, and confined to the area of injection. An occasional patient may react more strongly with localized tenderness, erythema, or low-grade fever. Repeated injections may possibly sensitize an individual to the protein content and, rarely, spontaneous hypersensitivity may exist. However, because of the extreme rarity of patient hypersensitivity and the high incidence of local irritation to intradermal injection, which could be mistaken for a positive reaction, it is recommended that a sensitivity test should not be made. A decision based on a false-positive reaction could deny the patient the benefit of this product.

Dosage and Administration:
Do Not Inject Intravenously
Immu-G should be administered intramuscularly; it should not be injected intravenously as untoward reactions may result. A separate, sterile syringe and needle should be used for each individual injection to avoid possible contamination of the syringe with blood containing the virus of hepatitis B; immune globulin (human) itself has been reported to be free of the hepatitis B virus. To facilitate injection, a large bore needle (18 or 20 gauge) is recommended. The rate of injection should be slow in order to accommodate the relatively large volume which is sometimes administered and to minimize the discomfort of the patient. Further, for doses over 10 ml, multiple injection sites are suggested.

Hepatitis A (formerly infectious hepatitis) is thought to be caused by a virus transmitted principally by the fecal-oral route under conditions of poor sanitation and close contact with infected persons. Numerous field studies during the past two decades have documented the protection against hepatitis A conferred by immune serum globulin administered before exposure or during the incubation period. The relative effectiveness of immune serum globulin depends on timing and dose. When administered before or within one to two weeks after exposure to hepatitis A in the appropriate dose, immune serum globulin prevents illness in 80 to 90% of those exposed. However, because immune serum globulin may not suppress inapparent infection, long-lasting, natural immunity may result.
Immune serum globulin should be given as soon as possible after a known exposure. The prophylactic value of immune serum globulin is greatest when given early in the incubation period and decreases with time after exposure. The use of immune serum globulin more than six weeks after exposure or after onset of clinical illness is not indicated.
The dosage patterns of immune serum globulin in common use were derived primarily from field and clinical observations. Under most conditions of exposure, protection is afforded by intramuscular injection of 0.02 ml/kg (0.01 ml/lb) of body weight (see Table 1).

Table 1

Person's Weight (lb)	Immune Serum Globulin Dose (ml)*
up to 50	0.5
50 to 100	1.0
over 100	2.0

*Within limits, larger doses of immune serum globulin provide longer-lasting but not necessarily more protection. Higher doses are, therefore, used under certain circumstances.

For high-risk situations—Where hepatitis A exists endemically, particularly in very large institutions with high rates of admission and discharge, residents and staff personnel may be subject to frequent and continuing exposure. Under these conditions, use of immune serum globulin has not resulted in eradication of hepatitis. However, immune serum globulin has been shown to provide temporary protection when administered in doses of 0.05 to 0.1 ml/kg (0.02 to 0.05 ml/lb) of body weight at the time of admission or employment. It may be necessary to re-administer immune serum globulin in the same dose after six months if the risk is felt to persist.
The risk of acquiring hepatitis A for United States residents traveling abroad appears to be small; it varies with living conditions, prevalence of hepatitis A in the area visited, and, particularly the length of stay.
Travelers to foreign countries may be at no greater risk than in the United States when their travel involves ordinary tourist routes and is for less than three months. Travelers to tropical areas or developing countries planning to stay three months or less, and who bypass ordinary tourist routes, are at greater risk of acquiring hepatitis A. The recommended dose of immune serum globulin is shown in Table 2 (length of stay less than three months).
Travelers planning to stay three or more months in tropical areas or developing countries, where hepatitis A is more common, and where they may be exposed to infected persons and contaminated food and water, are also at greater risk of acquiring hepatitis A. The dosage of immune serum globulin shown in Table 2 (length of stay three months or more) is recommended for them.
For persons residing abroad in tropical areas or developing countries, the risk of hepatitis appears to persist. Experience has shown that regular administration of immune serum globulin offers at least partial protection against hepatitis. It is recommended that prophylactic immune serum globulin be repeated every four to six months at the higher doses (length of stay three months or more) shown in Table 2. [See table above].

Table 2
Immune Serum Globulin for Protection Against Hepatitis A for US Residents Traveling or Living in Foreign Countries

Length of Stay	Body Weight kg	lb	Immune Serum Globulin Dose ml
Short-term travel (less than three months)	up to 23	50	0.5
	23–45	50–100	1.0
	over 45	100	2.0
Long-term travel (more than three months)	up to 23	50	1.0
	23–45	50–100	2.5
	over 45	100	5.0

Measles (rubeola)—Immu-G may be used for either modification or prevention of measles.
Preventive dose: 0.25 ml/kg (0.1 ml/lb) of body weight. For maximum effect, it is recommended that the dose be administered as soon as possible within four days after exposure.
Modification dose: 0.05 ml/kg (0.02 ml/lb) of body weight. The dose should be administered within the six days following exposure.
Clinical response in measles prophylaxis is best in persons who receive immune globulin soon after exposure to the disease. When given late in the incubation period, results are more variable and attempts at complete prevention are seldom successful.
Modification of measles is preferred to prevention because the immunity acquired from modified measles is, in most cases, sufficient to protect against any future exposures. Preventive treatment is generally limited to all children under 2 or 3 years of age and to individuals where measles infection would constitute a

Continued on next page

This product information was prepared in August, 1979. On these and other Parke-Davis Products, detailed information may be obtained by addressing PARKE-DAVIS, Division of Warner-Lambert Company, Morris Plains, NJ 07950.

Parke-Davis—Cont.

definite hazard to themselves or members of their families or associates, such as in a hospital or other institution. In such instances, another protective dose may be necessary should exposure to measles recur after the passive immunity conferred by the initial dosage has waned. The passive immunity acquired from an effective dose usually persists for about four weeks.

Antibody-deficiency disease—Antibody-deficiency states, leading to an increased susceptibility to disease, may be responsive to immune serum globulin therapy. Only deficiency states proved to involve IgG should be treated with immune serum globulin replacement therapy. The usual dosage consists of an initial dose of 1.2 ml/kg (0.6 ml/lb) followed in three or four weeks by 0.66 ml/kg (0.3 ml/lb) to be given every three or four weeks. The response of the individual patient may determine the need for more frequent injections of immune serum globulin.

German measles (rubella)—The use of immune serum globulin for the prevention of rubella in pregnant women has been controversial for many years. Available evidence indicates that immune serum globulin may modify or suppress the clinical manifestations without preventing viremia. Some studies suggest that the use of immune serum globulin in exposed, susceptible women can lessen the likelihood of infection and fetal damage. Therefore, the use of immune serum globulin in women in the first trimester of pregnancy, in a dose of 20 ml, may be considered for those who would not consider a therapeutic abortion.

Chickenpox (varicella)—Immune serum globulin may be of value for the modification, and possibly the prevention, of varicella-zoster viral infections in the high-risk patient. The dose for patients in this increased-risk group is 0.6 to 1.2 ml/kg (0.3 to 0.6 ml/lb) of body weight given as soon as possible after exposure to the disease.

Bacterial infections—Kabat has reviewed the various reports of the use of human gamma globulin prepared from random pools of normal blood in the treatment of resistant bacterial infections. These included those which cause particular problems in therapy—staphylococci, *Pseudomonas aeruginosa*, and *Proteus* species. In general, very large doses were used, ranging from 0.25 to 1.5 ml/lb (0.55 to 3.3 ml/kg) of body weight. Doses were sometimes repeated for several weeks to prevent recurrence. In burns, the use of gamma globulin, again in large doses, was cited as a valuable adjunct to antibiotic therapy in reducing the incidence of septicemia and late deaths.

How Supplied: Immu-G is supplied as:
N 0071-4618-10 (Bio 619)—10-ml rubber diaphragm-capped vial

TG

KETALAR® ℞
(ketamine hydrochloride injection, NF)

SPECIAL NOTE

EMERGENCE REACTIONS HAVE OCCURRED IN APPROXIMATELY 12% OF PATIENTS.

THE PSYCHOLOGICAL MANIFESTATIONS VARY IN SEVERITY BETWEEN PLEASANT DREAMLIKE STATES, VIVID IMAGERY, HALLUCINATIONS, AND EMERGENCE DELIRIUM. IN SOME CASES, THESE STATES HAVE BEEN ACCOMPANIED BY CONFUSION, EXCITEMENT, AND IRRATIONAL BEHAVIOR WHICH A FEW PATIENTS RECALL AS AN UNPLEASANT EXPERIENCE. THE DURATION ORDINARILY LASTS NO MORE THAN A FEW HOURS; IN A FEW CASES, HOWEVER, RECURRENCES HAVE TAKEN PLACE UP TO 24 HOURS POSTOPERATIVELY. NO RESIDUAL PSYCHOLOGICAL EFFECTS ARE KNOWN TO HAVE RESULTED FROM USE OF KETALAR.

THE INCIDENCE OF THESE EMERGENCE PHENOMENA IS LEAST IN THE YOUNG (15 YEARS OF AGE OR LESS) AND ELDERLY (OVER 65 YEARS OF AGE) PATIENT. ALSO, THEY ARE LESS FREQUENT WHEN THE DRUG IS GIVEN INTRAMUSCULARLY.

THESE REACTIONS MAY BE REDUCED IF VERBAL, TACTILE, AND VISUAL STIMULATION OF THE PATIENT IS MINIMIZED DURING THE RECOVERY PERIOD. THIS DOES NOT PRECLUDE THE MONITORING OF VITAL SIGNS. IN ADDITION, THE USE OF A SMALL HYPNOTIC DOSE OF A SHORT-ACTING OR ULTRASHORT-ACTING BARBITURATE MAY BE REQUIRED TO TERMINATE A SEVERE EMERGENCE REACTION. THE INCIDENCE OF EMERGENCE REACTIONS IS REDUCED AS EXPERIENCE WITH THE DRUG IS GAINED.

WHEN KETALAR IS USED ON AN OUTPATIENT BASIS, THE PATIENT SHOULD NOT BE RELEASED UNTIL RECOVERY FROM ANESTHESIA IS COMPLETE AND THEN SHOULD BE ACCOMPANIED BY A RESPONSIBLE ADULT.

Description: Ketalar is a nonbarbiturate anesthetic chemically designated *dl* 2-(o-chlorophenyl)-2-(methylamino) cyclohexanone hydrochloride. It is formulated as a slightly acid (pH 3.5 to 5.5) solution for intravenous or intramuscular injection in concentrations containing the equivalent of either 10, 50, or 100 mg ketamine base per milliliter and contains 0.1 mg/ml Phemerol® (benzethonium chloride) as a preservative. The 10 mg/ml solution has been made isotonic with sodium chloride.

Action: Ketalar is a rapid-acting general anesthetic producing an anesthetic state characterized by profound analgesia, normal pharyngeal-laryngeal reflexes, normal or slightly enhanced skeletal muscle tone, cardiovascular and respiratory stimulation, and occasionally a transient and minimal respiratory depression.

A patent airway is maintained partly by virtue of unimpaired pharyngeal and laryngeal reflexes. (See Warnings and Precautions.)

The anesthetic state produced by Ketalar (ketamine hydrochloride) has been termed "dissociative anesthesia" in that it appears to selectively interrupt association pathways of the brain before producing somesthetic sensory blockade. Ketalar may selectively depress the thalamoneocortical system before significantly obtunding the more ancient cerebral centers and pathways (reticular-activating and limbic systems).

Elevation of blood pressure begins shortly after injection, reaches a maximum within a few minutes and usually returns to preanesthetic values within 15 minutes after injection. The median peak rise has ranged from 20 to 25% of preanesthetic values.

Ketamine has a wide margin of safety; several instances of unintentional administration of overdoses of Ketalar (up to 10 times that usually required) have been followed by prolonged but complete recovery.

Indications:

Ketalar is recommended:

1. as the sole anesthetic agent for diagnostic and surgical procedures that do not require skeletal muscle relaxation. Ketalar is best suited for short procedures but it can be used, with additional doses, for longer procedures;
2. for the induction of anesthesia prior to the administration of other general anesthetic agents;
3. to supplement low-potency agents, such as nitrous oxide.

Specific areas of application are described in the section Clinical Studies.

Contraindications: Ketamine hydrochloride is contraindicated in those in whom a significant elevation of blood pressure would constitute a serious hazard and those who have shown hypersensitivity to the drug.

Warnings:

1. Ketalar should be used by or under the direction of physicians experienced in administering general anesthetics and in maintenance of an airway and in the control of respiration.
2. Cardiac function should be continually monitored during the procedure in patients found to have hypertension or cardiac decompensation.
3. Barbiturates and Ketalar, being chemically incompatible because of precipitate formation, *should not* be injected from the same syringe.
4. Prolonged recovery time may occur if barbiturates and/or narcotics are used concurrently with Ketalar.
5. Postoperative confusional states may occur during the recovery period.
6. Respiratory depression may occur with overdosage or too rapid a rate of administration of Ketalar, in which case supportive ventilation should be employed. Mechanical support of respiration is preferred to administration of analeptics.

Usage in Pregnancy:

Because the safe use in pregnancy, including obstetrics (either vaginal or abdominal delivery), has not been established, such use is not recommended (see Animal Pharmacology).

Precautions:

1. Because pharyngeal and laryngeal reflexes are usually active, Ketalar should not be used alone in surgery or diagnostic procedures of the pharynx, larynx, or bronchial tree. Mechanical stimulation of the pharynx should be avoided, whenever possible, if Ketalar (ketamine hydrochloride) is used alone. Muscle relaxants, with proper attention to respiration, may be required in both of these instances.
2. Resuscitative equipment should be ready for use.
3. ***The incidence of emergence reactions may be reduced*** if verbal and tactile stimulation of the patient is minimized during the recovery period. This does not preclude the monitoring of vital signs (see SPECIAL NOTE).
4. The intravenous dose should be administered over a period of 60 seconds. More rapid administration may result in respiratory depression or apnea and enhanced pressor response.
5. In surgical procedures involving visceral pain pathways, Ketalar should be supplemented with an agent which obtunds visceral pain.
6. Use with caution in the chronic alcoholic and the acutely alcohol-intoxicated patient.
7. An increase in cerebrospinal fluid pressure has been reported following administration of ketamine hydrochloride. Use with extreme caution in patients with preanesthetic elevated cerebrospinal fluid pressure.

Adverse Reactions:

Cardiovascular: Blood pressure and pulse rate are frequently elevated following administration of Ketalar. However, hypotension and bradycardia have been observed. Arrhythmia has also occurred.

Respiration: Although respiration is frequently stimulated, severe depression of respiration or apnea may occur following rapid intravenous administration of high doses of Ketalar. Laryngospasms and other forms of airway obstruction have occurred during Ketalar anesthesia.

Eye: Diplopia and nystagmus have been noted following Ketalar (ketamine hydrochloride) administration. Ketalar also may cause a

slight elevation in intraocular pressure measurement.
Psychological: (See SPECIAL NOTE.)
Neurological: In some patients, enhanced skeletal muscle tone may be manifested by tonic and clonic movements sometimes resembling seizures (see Dosage and Administration).
Gastrointestinal: Anorexia, nausea, and vomiting have been observed; however, this is not usually severe and allows the great majority of patients to take liquids by mouth shortly after regaining consciousness (see Dosage and Administration).
General: Local pain and exanthema at the injection site have infrequently been reported. Transient erythema and/or morbilliform rash have also been reported.

Dosage and Administration:

Preoperative Preparations:

1. While vomiting has been reported following Ketalar administration, airway protection is usually afforded because of active laryngeal-pharyngeal reflexes. However, because these reflexes may also be diminished by supplementary anesthetics or muscle relaxants, the possibility of aspiration must be considered. Ketalar is recommended for use in the patient whose stomach is not empty when, in the judgment of the practitioner, the benefits of the drug outweigh the possible risks.
2. Atropine, scopolamine, or other drying agents should be given at an appropriate interval prior to induction.

Dosage:
As with other general anesthetic agents, the individual response to Ketalar is somewhat varied depending on the dose, route of administration, and age of patient, so that dosage recommendation cannot be absolutely fixed. The drug should be titrated against the patient's requirements.

Onset and Duration:
Because of rapid induction following the initial intravenous injection, the patient should be in a supported position during administration.
The onset of action of Ketalar is rapid; an intravenous dose of 2 mg/kg (1 mg/lb) of body weight usually produces surgical anesthesia within 30 seconds after injection, with the anesthetic effect usually lasting 5 to 10 minutes. If a longer effect is desired, additional increments can be administered intravenously or intramuscularly to maintain anesthesia without producing significant cumulative effects.
Intramuscular doses, from experience primarily in children, in a range of 9 to 13 mg/kg (4 to 6 mg/lb) usually produce surgical anesthesia within three to four minutes following injection, with the anesthetic effect usually lasting 12 to 25 minutes.

Induction:
Intravenous Route: The initial dose of Ketalar (ketamine hydrochloride) administered intravenously may range from 1 mg/kg to 4.5 mg/kg (0.5 to 2 mg/lb). The average amount required to produce 5 to 10 minutes of surgical anesthesia has been 2 mg/kg (1 mg/lb).
NOTE: The 100 mg/ml concentration (Steri-Vial® 1585) of Ketalar, *should not* be injected intravenously without proper dilution. It is recommended the drug be diluted with an equal volume of either Sterile Water for Injection, USP, Normal Saline, or 5% Dextrose in Water.
Rate of Administration: It is recommended that Ketalar be administered slowly (over a period of 60 seconds). More rapid administration may result in respiratory depression and enhanced pressor response.
Intramuscular Route: The initial dose of Ketalar administered intramuscularly may range from 6.5 to 13 mg/kg (3 to 6 mg/lb). A dose of 10 mg/kg (5 mg/lb) will usually produce 12 to 25 minutes of surgical anesthesia.

Maintenance of Anesthesia:
Increments of one half to the full induction dose may be repeated as needed for maintenance of anesthesia. However, it should be noted that purposeless and tonic-clonic movements of extremities may occur during the course of anesthesia. These movements do not imply a light plane and are not indicative of the need for additional doses of the anesthetic. It should be recognized that the larger the total dose of Ketalar administered, the longer will be the time to complete recovery.

Supplementary Agents:
Ketalar is clinically compatible with the commonly used general and local anesthetic agents when an adequate respiratory exchange is maintained.

How Supplied:
Ketalar (ketamine hydrochloride) is supplied as the hydrochloride in concentrations equivalent to ketamine base.
N 0071-4581-15—Each 50-ml vial contains 10 mg/ml. Supplied in cartons of 10.
NSN 6505-00-151-6366
N 0071-4581-12—Each 20-ml vial contains 10 mg/ml. Supplied in cartons of 10.
NSN 6505-00-079-9736
N 0071-4582-10—Each 10-ml vial contains 50 mg/ml. Supplied in cartons of 10.
NSN 6505-00-432-7047
N 0071-4585-08—Each 5-ml vial contains 100 mg/ml. Supplied in cartons of 10.
NSN 6505-00-079-9846

Animal Pharmacology and Toxicology:
Toxicity: The acute toxicity of Ketalar (ketamine hydrochloride) has been studied in several species. In mature mice and rats, the intraperitoneal LD_{50} values are approximately 100 times the average human intravenous dose and approximately 20 times the average human intramuscular dose. A slightly higher acute toxicity observed in neonatal rats was not sufficiently elevated to suggest an increased hazard when used in children. Daily intravenous injections in rats of five times the average human intravenous dose and intramuscular injections in dogs at four times the average human intramuscular dose demonstrated excellent tolerance for as long as six weeks. Similarly, twice-weekly anesthetic sessions of one, three, or six hours' duration in monkeys over a four- to six-week period were well-tolerated.
Interaction With Other Drugs Commonly Used For Preanesthetic Medication: Large doses (three or more times the equivalent effective human dose) of morphine, meperidine, and atropine increased the depth and prolonged the duration of anesthesia produced by a standard anesthetizing dose of Ketalar in *Rhesus* monkeys. The prolonged duration was not of sufficient magnitude to contraindicate the use of these drugs for preanesthetic medication in human clinical trials.
Blood Pressure: Blood pressure responses to Ketalar vary with the laboratory species and experimental conditions. Blood pressure is increased in normotensive and renal hypertensive rats with and without adrenalectomy and under pentobarbital anesthesia.
Intravenous Ketalar produces a fall in arterial blood pressure in the *Rhesus* monkey and a rise in arterial blood pressure in the dog. In this respect, the response in the dog mimics the cardiovascular effect observed in man. The pressor response to Ketalar injected into intact, unanesthetized dogs is accompanied by a tachycardia, rise in cardiac output, and a fall in total peripheral resistance. Ketalar causes a fall in perfusion pressure following a large dose injected into an artificially perfused vascular bed (dog hindquarters), and has little or no potentiating effect upon vasoconstriction responses of epinephrine or norepinephrine. The pressor response to Ketalar is reduced or blocked by chlorpromazine (central depressant and peripheral α-adrenergic blockade), by β-adrenergic blockade, and by ganglionic blockade. The tachycardia and increase in myocardial contractile force seen in intact animals do not appear in isolated hearts (Langendorff) at a concentration of 0.1 mg of Ketalar nor in Starling dog heart-lung preparations at a Ketalar concentration of 50 mg/kg of HLP. These observations support the hypothesis that the hypertension produced by Ketalar is due to selective activation of central cardiac stimulating mechanisms leading to an increase in cardiac output. The dog myocardium is not sensitized to epinephrine and Ketalar appears to have a weak antiarrhythmic activity.
Metabolic Disposition: Ketalar (ketamine hydrochloride) is rapidly absorbed following parenteral administration. Animal experiments indicated that Ketalar was rapidly distributed into body tissues, with relatively high concentrations appearing in body fat, liver, lung, and brain; lower concentrations were found in the heart, skeletal muscle, and blood plasma. Placental transfer of the drug was found to occur in pregnant dogs and monkeys. No significant degree of binding to serum albumin was found with Ketalar.
Balance studies in rats, dogs, and monkeys resulted in the recovery of 85 to 95% of the dose in the urine, mainly in the form of degradation products. Small amounts of drug were also excreted in the bile and feces. Balance studies with tritium-labeled Ketalar in human subjects (1 mg/lb given intravenously) resulted in the mean recovery of 91% of the dose in the urine and 3% in the feces. Peak plasma levels averaged about 0.75 mcg/ml, and CSF levels were about 0.2 mcg/ml, one hour after dosing.
Ketalar undergoes N-demethylation and hydroxylation of the cyclohexanone ring, with the formation of water-soluble conjugates which are excreted in the urine. Further oxidation also occurs with the formation of a cyclohexenone derivative. The unconjugated N-demethylated metabolite was found to be less than one sixth as potent as Ketalar. The unconjugated demethyl cyclohexenone derivative was found to be less than one tenth as potent as Ketalar (ketamine hydrochloride). Repeated doses of Ketalar administered to animals did not produce any detectable increase in microsomal enzyme activity.
Reproduction: Male and female rats, when given five times the average human intravenous dose of Ketalar for three consecutive days about one week before mating had a reproductive performance equivalent to that of saline-injected controls. When given to pregnant rats and rabbits intramuscularly at twice the average human intramuscular dose during the respective periods of organogenesis, the litter characteristics were equivalent to those of saline-injected controls. A small group of rabbits was given a single, large dose (six times the average human dose) of Ketalar on Day 6 of pregnancy to simulate the effect of an excessive clinical dose around the period of nidation. The outcome of pregnancy was equivalent in control and treated groups.
To determine the effect of Ketalar on the perinatal and postnatal period, pregnant rats were given twice the average human intramuscular dose during Days 18 to 21 of pregnancy. Litter characteristics at birth and through the weaning period were equivalent to those of the control animals. There was a slight increase in incidence of delayed parturition by one day in treated dams of this group. Three groups each of mated beagle bitches were given 2.5 times the average human intramuscular dose twice weekly for the three weeks of the first, second, and third trimesters of pregnancy, respec-

Continued on next page

This product information was prepared in August, 1979. On these and other Parke-Davis Products, detailed information may be obtained by addressing PARKE-DAVIS, Division of Warner-Lambert Company, Morris Plains, NJ 07950.

Parke-Davis—Cont.

tively, without the development of adverse effects in the pups.

Clinical Studies: Ketalar (ketamine hydrochloride) has been studied in over 12,000 operative and diagnostic procedures, involving over 10,000 patients from 105 separate studies. During the course of these studies, Ketalar was administered as the sole agent, as induction for other general agents, or to supplement low-potency agents. Specific areas of application have included the following:

1. debridement, painful dressings, and skin grafting in burn patients, as well as other superficial surgical procedures;
2. neurodiagnostic procedures, such as pneumoencephalograms, ventriculograms, myelograms, and lumbar punctures;
3. diagnostic and operative procedures of the eye, ear, nose, and mouth, including dental extractions;
4. diagnostic and operative procedures of the pharynx, larynx, or bronchial tree; NOTE: Muscle relaxants, with proper attention to respiration, may be required (see Precautions).
5. sigmoidoscopy and minor surgery of the anus and rectum, and circumcision;
6. extraperitoneal procedures used in gynecology, such as dilatation and curettage;
7. orthopedic procedures, such as closed reductions, manipulations, femoral pinning, amputations, and biopsies;
8. as an anesthetic in poor-risk patients with depression of vital functions;
9. in procedures where the intramuscular route of administration is preferred;
10. in cardiac catheterization procedures.

In these studies, the anesthesia was rated either "excellent" or "good" by the anesthesiologist and the surgeon at 90 and 93%, respectively; rated "fair" at 6 and 4%, respectively; and rated "poor" at 4 and 3%, respectively. In a second method of evaluation, the anesthesia was rated "adequate" in at least 90%, and "inadequate" in 10% or less of the procedures.

SG

LOESTRIN® [21] 1/20 ℞
LOESTRIN [Fe] 1/20
LOESTRIN [21] 1.5/30
LOESTRIN [Fe] 1.5/30
NORLESTRIN® [21] 1/50
NORLESTRIN [28] 1/50
NORLESTRIN [Fe] 1/50
NORLESTRIN [21] 2.5/50
NORLESTRIN [Fe] 2.5/50
(norethindrone acetate and ethinyl estradiol tablets, USP)

Loestrin and Norlestrin are products of Parke Davis Laboratories, Fajardo, PR 00648.

Loestrin [21] 1/20
Each white tablet contains: norethindrone acetate (17 alpha-ethinyl-19-nortestosterone acetate), 1 mg; ethinyl estradiol (17 alpha-ethinyl-1, 3, 5(10)-estratriene-3, 17 beta-diol), 20 mcg.

Loestrin [Fe] 1/20
Each white tablet contains: norethindrone acetate, 1 mg; ethinyl estradiol, 20 mcg.
Each brown tablet contains 75 mg ferrous fumarate, USP.

Loestrin [21] 1.5/30
Each green tablet contains: norethindrone acetate, 1.5 mg; ethinyl estradiol, 30 mcg.

Loestrin [Fe] 1.5/30
Each green tablet contains norethindrone acetate, 1.5 mg; ethinyl estradiol, 30 mcg.
Each brown tablet contains 75 mg ferrous fumarate, USP.

Norlestrin [21] 1/50
Each yellow tablet contains: norethindrone acetate (17 alpha-ethinyl-19-nortestosterone acetate), 1 mg; ethinyl estradiol (17 alpha-ethinyl-1,3,5(10)-estratriene-3, 17 beta-diol), 50 mcg.

Nausea and/or vomiting, [28] 1/50 reactions,
Each yellow tablet contains: norethindrone acetate, 1 mg; ethinyl estradiol, 50 mcg. Each compact contains 21 yellow tablets and 7 white inert tablets.

Norlestrin [Fe] 1/50
Each yellow tablet contains: norethindrone acetate, 1 mg; ethinyl estradiol, 50 mcg. Each brown tablet contains 75 mg ferrous fumarate.

Norlestrin [21] 2.5/50
Each pink tablet contains: norethindrone acetate, 2.5 mg; ethinyl estradiol, 50 mcg.

Norlestrin [Fe] 2.5/50
Each pink tablet contains: norethindrone acetate, 2.5 mg; ethinyl estradiol, 50 mcg. Each brown tablet contains 75 mg ferrous fumarate.

Description: Loestrin [21] 1/20, Loestrin [21] 1.5/30, Norlestrin [21] 1/50, and Norlestrin [21] 2.5/50 are progestogen-estrogen combinations.

Loestrin [Fe] 1/20, Loestrin [Fe] 1.5/30, Norlestrin [Fe] 1/50, and Norlestrin [Fe] 2.5/50
Loestrin 1/20, Loestrin 1.5/30, Norlestrin 1/50, and Norlestrin 2.5/50 are progestogen-estrogen combinations.
Loestrin [Fe] 1/20, Loestrin [Fe] 1.5/30, Norlestrin [Fe] 1/50, and Norlestrin [Fe] 2.5/50 provide a continuous dosage regimen consisting of 21 oral contraceptive tablets and seven ferrous fumarate tablets. The ferrous fumarate tablets are present to facilitate ease of drug administration via a 28-day regimen and are not intended to serve any therapeutic purpose.
Norelstrin [28] 1/50 provides a continuous dosage regimen consisting of 21 oral contraceptive tablets and 7 inert tablets.

Clinical Pharmacology: Combination oral contraceptives act primarily through the mechanism of gonadotropin suppression due to the estrogenic and progestational activity of the ingredients. Although the primary mechanism of action is inhibition of ovulation, alterations in the genital tract, including changes in the cervical mucus (which increases the difficulty of sperm penetration) and in the endometrium (which reduces the likelihood of implantation), may also contribute to the contraceptive effectiveness.

Indications and Usage: Loestrin Products and Norlestrin Products are indicated for the prevention of pregnancy in women who elect to use oral contraceptives as a method of contraception.

Oral contraceptives are highly effective. The pregnancy rate in women using conventional combination oral contraceptives (containing 35 mcg or more of ethinyl estradiol or 50 mcg or more of mestranol) is generally reported as less than one pregnancy per 100 women years of use. Slightly higher rates (somewhat more than one pregnancy per 100 women years of use) are reported for some combination products containing 35 mcg or less of ethinyl estradiol, and rates on the order of three pregnancies per 100 women years are reported for the progestogen-only contraceptives.

These rates are derived from separate studies conducted by different investigators in several population groups and cannot be compared precisely. Furthermore, pregnancy rates tend to be lower as clinical studies are continued, possibly due to selective retention in the longer studies of those patients who accept the treatment regimen and do not discontinue as a result of adverse reactions, pregnancy, or other reasons.

Loestrin [21] 1/20 and Loestrin [Fe] 1/20
In clinical trials with Loestrin 1/20, 1,431 patients completed 15,899 cycles and a total of 10 pregnancies was reported. This represents a pregnancy rate of 0.75 per 100 women years based upon data that includes the cases where patients failed to comply with the dosage regimen. The pregnancy rate in patients who adhered to the dosage regimen was 0.30 per 100 women years (four pregnancies in these trials).

Loestrin [21] 1.5/30 and Loestrin [Fe] 1.5/30
In clinical trials with Loestrin 1.5/30, 1,289 patients completed 17,139 cycles and a total of seven pregnancies was reported. This represents a pregnancy rate of 0.49 per 100 women-years based upon data that includes the cases where patients failed to comply with the dosage regimen. The pregnancy rate in patients who adhered to the dosage regimen was 0.07 per 100 women-years (one pregnancy in these trials).

Norlestrin [21] 1/50, Norlestrin [28] 1/50, and Norlestrin [Fe] 1/50
In clinical trials with Norlestrin 1/50, 1,156 patients completed 25,983 cycles and a total of one pregnancy was reported. This represents a pregnancy rate of 0.05 per 100 women-years.

Norlestrin [21] 2.5/50 and Norlestrin [Fe] 2.5/50
In clinical trials with Norlestrin 2.5/50, 3,829 patients completed 96,388 cycles and a total of 18 pregnancies was reported. This represents a pregnancy rate of 0.22 per 100 women-years based upon data that includes the cases where patients failed to comply with the dosage regimen. The pregnancy rate in patients who adhered to the dosage regimen was 0.02 per 100 women-years (two pregnancies in these trials).

Table 1 gives ranges of pregnancy rates reported in the literature[1] for other means of contraception. The efficacy of these means of contraception (except the IUD) depends upon the degree of adherence to the method.

Table 1: Pregnancies Per 100 Women Years:
IUD, less than 1–6
Diaphragm with spermicidal product (creams or jellies), 2–20
Condom, 3–36
Aerosol foams, 2–29
Jellies and creams, 4–36
Periodic abstinence (rhythm) all types, less than 1–47
1. Calendar method, 14–47
2. Temperature method, 1–20
3. Temperature method—intercourse in postovulatory phase only, less than 1–7
4. Mucus method, 1–25
No contraception, 60–80

Dose-Related Risk of Thromboembolism From Oral Contraceptives
Two studies have shown a positive association between the dose of estrogens in oral contraceptives and the risk of thromboembolism.[2,3] For this reason, it is prudent and in keeping with good principles of therapeutics to minimize exposure to estrogen. The oral contraceptive product prescribed for any given patient should be that product which contains the least amount of estrogen that is compatible with an acceptable pregnancy rate and patient acceptance. It is recommended that new acceptors of oral contraceptives should be started on preparations containing 0.05 mg or less of estrogen.

Contraindications: Oral contraceptives should not be used in women with any of the following conditions.
1. Thrombophlebitis or thromboembolic disorders
2. A past history of deep-vein thrombophlebitis or thromboembolic disorders
3. Cerebral vascular or coronary artery disease
4. Known or suspected carcinoma of the breast
5. Known or suspected estrogen-dependent neoplasia
6. Undiagnosed abnormal genital bleeding
7. Known or suspected pregnancy (See Warning No. 5.)

Warnings:

Cigarette smoking increases the risk of serious cardiovascular side effects from oral contraceptive use. This risk increases with age and with heavy smoking (15 or more cigarettes per day) and is quite marked in women over 35 years of age.

Women who use oral contraceptives should be strongly advised not to smoke. The use of oral contraceptives is associated with increased risk of several serious conditions including thromboembolism, stroke, myocardial infarction, hepatic adenoma, gall bladder disease, hypertension. Practitioners prescribing oral contraceptives should be familiar with the following information relating to these risks.

1. *Thromboembolic Disorders and Other Vascular Problems:* An increased risk of thromboembolic and thrombotic disease associated with the use of oral contraceptives is well-established. Three principal studies in Great Britain[4–6] and three in the United States[7–10] have demonstrated an increased risk of fatal and nonfatal venous thromboembolism and stroke, both hemorrhagic and thrombotic. These studies estimate that users of oral contraceptives are 4 to 11 times more likely (Table 2) than nonusers to develop these diseases without evident cause.

Cerebrovascular Disorders

In a collaborative American study[9,10] of cerebrovascular disorders in women with and without predisposing causes, it was estimated that the risk of hemorrhagic stroke was 2.0 times greater in users than nonusers, and the risk of thrombotic stroke was 4.0 to 9.5 times greater in users than in nonusers (Table 2).

Table 2

Summary of relative risk of thromboembolic disorders and other vascular problems in oral contraceptive users compared to nonusers

	Relative risk, times greater
Idiopathic thromboembolic disease	4 to 11
Postsurgery thromboembolic complications	4 to 6
Thrombotic stroke	4 to 9.5
Hemorrhagic stroke	2
Myocardial infarction	2 to 12

Myocardial Infarction

An increased risk of myocardial infarction associated with the use of oral contraceptives has been reported,[11–13] confirming a previously suspected association. These studies, conducted in the United Kingdom, found, as expected, that the greater the number of underlying risk factors for coronary artery disease (cigarette smoking, hypertension, hypercholesterolemia, obesity, diabetes, history of preeclamptic toxemia) the higher the risk of developing myocardial infarction, regardless of whether the patient was an oral contraceptive user or not. Oral contraceptives, however, were found to be a clear additional risk factor.

In terms of relative risk, it has been estimated[52] that oral contraceptive users who do not smoke (smoking is considered a major predisposing condition to myocardial infarction) are about twice as likely to have a fatal myocardial infarction as nonusers who do not smoke. Oral contraceptive users who are also smokers have about a fourfold increased risk of fatal infarction compared to users who do not smoke, but about a tenfold to twelvefold increased risk compared to nonusers who do not smoke. Furthermore, the amount of smoking is also an important factor. In determining the importance of these relative risks, however, the baseline rates for various age groups, as shown in Table 3, must be given serious consideration. The importance of other predisposing conditions mentioned above in determining relative and absolute risks has not as yet been quantified; it is quite likely that the same synergistic action exists, but perhaps to a lesser extent.

Table 3

Estimated annual mortality rate per 100,000 women from myocardial infarction by use of oral contraceptives, smoking habits, and age (in years)

	Myocardial Infarction			
	Women aged 30–39		Women aged 40–44	
Smoking habits	Users	Non-users	Users	Non-users
All smokers	10.2	2.6	62.0	15.9
Heavy*	13.0	5.1	78.7	31.3
Light	4.7	0.9	28.6	5.7
Nonsmokers	1.8	1.2	10.7	7.4
Smokers and nonsmokers	5.4	1.9	32.8	11.7

*Heavy smoker: 15 or more cigarettes per day. From Jain, A.K., *Studies in Family Planning,* **8**:50, 1977.

Risk of Dose

In an analysis of data derived from several national adverse reaction reporting systems,[2] British investigators concluded that the risk of thromboembolism, including coronary thrombosis, is directly related to the dose of estrogen used in oral contraceptives. Preparations containing 100 mcg or more of estrogen were associated with a higher risk of thromboembolism than those containing 50 to 80 mcg of estrogen. Their analysis did suggest, however, that the quantity of estrogen may not be the sole factor involved. This finding has been confirmed in the United States.[3] Careful epidemiological studies to determine the degree of thromboembolic risk associated with progestogen-only oral contraceptives have not been performed. Cases of thromboembolic disease have been reported in women using these products, and they should not be presumed to be free of excess risk.

Estimate of Excess Mortality From Circulatory Diseases

A large prospective study[53] carried out in the U.K. estimated the mortality rate per 100,000 women per year from diseases of the circulatory system for users and nonusers of oral contraceptives according to age, smoking habits, and duration of use. The overall excess death rate annually from circulatory diseases for oral contraceptive users was estimated to be 20 per 100,000 (ages 15 to 34—5/100,000; ages 35 to 44—33/100,000; ages 45 to 49—140/100,000), the risk being concentrated in older women, in those with a long duration of use, and in cigarette smokers. It was not possible, however, to examine the interrelationships of age, smoking, and duration of use, nor to compare the effects of continuous versus intermittent use. Although the study showed a tenfold increase in death due to circulatory diseases in users for five or more years, all of these deaths occurred in women 35 or older. Until larger numbers of women under 35 with continuous use for five or more years are available, it is not possible to assess the magnitude of the relative risk for this younger age group.

The available data from a variety of sources has been analyzed[14] to estimate the risk of death associated with various methods of contraception. The estimates of risk of death for each method include the combined risk of the contraceptive method (eg, thromboembolic and thrombotic disease in the case of oral contraceptives) plus the risk attributable to pregnancy or abortion in the event of method failure. This latter risk varies with the effectiveness of the contraceptive method. The findings of this analysis are shown in Figure 1.[14] The study concluded that the mortality associated with all methods of birth control is low and below that associated with childbirth, with the exception of oral contraceptives in women over 40 who smoke. (The rates given for Pill/only smokers for each age group are for smokers as a class. For "heavy" smokers [more than 15 cigarettes a day], the rates given would be about double; for "light" smokers [less than 15 cigarettes a day], about 50%). The lowest mortality is associated with the condom or diaphragm backed up by early abortion.

(See Figure 1 next page)

The risk of thromboembolic and thrombotic disease associated with oral contraceptives increases with age after approximately age 30 and, for myocardial infarction, is further increased by hypertension, hypercholesterolemia, obesity, diabetes, or history of preeclamptic toxemia, and especially by cigarette smoking.

Based on the data currently available, the following chart gives a gross estimate of the risk of death from circulatory disorders associated with the use of oral contraceptives:

SMOKING HABITS AND OTHER PREDISPOSING CONDITIONS—RISK ASSOCIATED WITH USE OF ORAL CONTRACEPTIVES

Age	Below 30	30–39	40+
Heavy smokers	C	B	A
Light smokers	D	C	B
Nonsmokers (no predisposing conditions)	D	C, D	C
Nonsmokers (other predisposing conditions)	C	C, B	B, A

A—Use associated with very high risk
B—Use associated with high risk
C—Use associated with moderate risk
D—Use associated with low risk

The physician and the patient should be alert to the earliest manifestations of thromboembolic and thrombotic disorders (eg, thrombophlebitis, pulmonary embolism, cerebrovascular insufficiency, coronary occlusion, retinal thrombosis, and mesenteric thrombosis). Should any of these occur or be suspected, the drug should be discontinued immediately.

A fourfold to sixfold increased risk of postsurgery thromboembolic complications has been reported in oral contraceptive users.[15,16] If feasible, oral contraceptives should be discontinued at least four weeks before surgery of a type associated with an increased risk of thromboembolism or prolonged immobilization.

2. *Ocular lesions.* There have been reports of neuro-ocular lesions, such as optic neuritis or retinal thrombosis, associated with the use of oral contraceptives. Discontinue oral contraceptive medication if there is unexplained sudden or gradual, partial or complete loss of vision; sudden onset of proptosis or diplopia; papilledema; or retinal vascular lesions, and institute appropriate diagnostic and therapeutic measures.

3. *Carcinoma.* Long-term continuous administration of either natural or synthetic estrogen in certain animal species increases the frequency of carcinoma of the breast, cervix, vagina, and liver. Certain synthetic progestogens, none currently contained in oral contraceptives, have been noted to increase the incidence of mammary nodules, benign and malignant, in dogs.

In humans, three case-control studies have reported an increased risk of endometrial carcinoma associated with the prolonged use of exogenous estrogen in postmenopausal women.[17–19] One publication[20] reported on the first 21 cases submitted by physicians to a reg-

Continued on next page

This product information was prepared in August, 1979. On these and other Parke-Davis Products, detailed information may be obtained by addressing PARKE-DAVIS, Division of Warner-Lambert Company, Morris Plains, NJ 07950.

Parke-Davis—Cont.

istry of cases of adenocarcinoma of the endometrium in women under 40 on oral contraceptives. Of the cases found in women without predisposing risk factors for adenocarcinoma of the endometrium (eg, irregular bleeding at the time oral contraceptives were first given, polycystic ovaries), nearly all occurred in women who had used a sequential oral contraceptive. These products are no longer marketed. No evidence has been reported suggesting an increased risk of endometrial cancer in users of conventional combination or progestogen-only oral contraceptives.

Several studies[8,21–24] have found no increase in breast cancer in women taking oral contraceptives or estrogens. One study,[25] however, while also noting no overall increased risk of breast cancer in women treated with oral contraceptives, found an excess risk in the subgroups of oral contraceptive users with documented benign breast disease. A reduced occurrence of benign breast tumors in users of oral contraceptives has been well-documented.[8,21,25–27]

In summary, there is at present no confirmed evidence from human studies of an increased risk of cancer associated with oral contraceptives. Close clinical surveillance of all women taking oral contraceptives is, nevertheless, essential. In all cases of undiagnosed persistent or recurrent abnormal vaginal bleeding, appropriate diagnostic measures should be taken to rule out malignancy. Women with a strong family history of breast cancer or who have breast nodules, fibrocystic disease, or abnormal mammograms, should be monitored with particular care if they elect to use oral contraceptives instead of other methods of contraception.

4. *Hepatic Tumors.* Benign hepatic adenomas have been found to be associated with the use of oral contraceptives.[28–30,46] One study[46] showed that oral contraceptive formulations with high hormonal potency were associated with a higher risk than lower potency formulations. Although benign, hepatic adenomas may rupture and may cause death through intra-abdominal hemorrhage. This has been reported in short-term as well as long-term users of oral contraceptives. Two studies relate risk with duration of use of contraceptive, the risk being much greater after four or more years of oral contraceptive use.[30,46] While hepatic adenoma is a rare lesion, it should be considered in women presenting abdominal pain and tenderness, abdominal mass, or shock.

A few cases of hepatocellular carcinoma have been reported in women taking oral contraceptives. The relationship of these drugs to this type of malignancy is not known at this time.

5. *Usage in or Immediately Preceding Pregnancy; Birth Defects in Offspring, and Malignancy in Female Offspring.* The use of female sex hormones—both estrogenic and progestational agents—during early pregnancy may seriously damage the offspring. It has been shown that females exposed *in utero* to diethylstilbestrol, a nonsteroidal estrogen, have an increased risk of developing in later life a form of vaginal or cervical cancer that is ordinarily extremely rare.[31,32] This risk has been estimated to be of the order of 1 in 1,000 exposures or less[33,47] Although there is no evidence at the present time that oral contraceptives further enhance the risk of developing this type of malignancy, such patients should be monitored with particular care if they elect to use oral contraceptives instead of other methods of contraception. Furthermore, a high percentage of such exposed women (from 30 to 90%) have been found to have epithelial changes of the vagina and cervix.[34–38]

Although these changes are histologically benign, it is not known whether this condition is a precursor of vaginal malignancy. Male children so exposed may develop abnormalities of the urogenital tract.[48–50] Although similar data is not available with the use of other estrogens, it cannot be presumed that they would not induce similar changes.

An increased risk of congenital anomalies, including heart defects and limb defects, has been reported with the use of sex hormones, including oral contraceptives, in pregnancy.[39–42,51] One case-control study[42] has estimated a 4.7-fold increase in risk of limb-reduction defects in infants exposed *in utero* to sex hormones (oral contraceptives, hormonal withdrawal tests for pregnancy, or attempted treatment for threatened abortion). Some of these exposures were very short and involved only a few days of treatment. The data suggests that the risk of limb-reduction defects in exposed fetuses is somewhat less than 1 in 1,000 live births.

In the past, female sex hormones have been used during pregnancy in an attempt to treat threatened or habitual abortion. There is considerable evidence that estrogens are ineffective for these indications, and there is no evidence from well-controlled studies that progestogens are effective for these uses.

There is some evidence that triploidy and possibly other types of polyploidy are increased among abortuses from women who become pregnant soon after ceasing oral contraceptives.[43] Embryos with these anomalies are virtually always aborted spontaneously. Whether there is an overall increase in spontaneous abortion of pregnancies conceived soon after stopping oral contraceptives is unknown.

It is recommended that for any patient who has missed two consecutive periods, pregnancy should be ruled out before continuing the contraceptive regimen. If the patient has not adhered to the prescribed schedule, the possibility of pregnancy should be considered at the time of the first missed period, and further use of oral contraceptives should be withheld until pregnancy has been ruled out. If pregnancy is confirmed, the patient should be apprised of the potential risks to the fetus and the advisability of continuation of the pregnancy should be discussed in the light of these risks.

It is also recommended that women who discontinue oral contraceptives with the intent of becoming pregnant use an alternate form of contraception for a period of time before attempting to conceive. Many clinicians recommend three months, although no precise information is available on which to base this recommendation.

The administration of progestogen-only or progestogen-estrogen combinations to induce withdrawal bleeding should not be used as a test of pregnancy.

6. *Gallbladder Disease.* Studies[8,23,26] report an increased risk of surgically confirmed gallbladder disease in users of oral contraceptives or estrogens. In one study, an increased risk appeared after two years of use and doubled after four or five years of use. In one of the other studies, an increased risk was apparent between 6 and 12 months of use.

7. *Carbohydrate and Lipid Metabolic Effects.* A decrease in glucose tolerance has been observed in a significant percentage of patients on oral contraceptives. For this reason, prediabetic and diabetic patients should be carefully observed while receiving oral contraceptives.

Figure 1. Estimated annual number of deaths associated with control of fertility and no control per 100,000 nonsterile women, by regimen of control and age of woman.

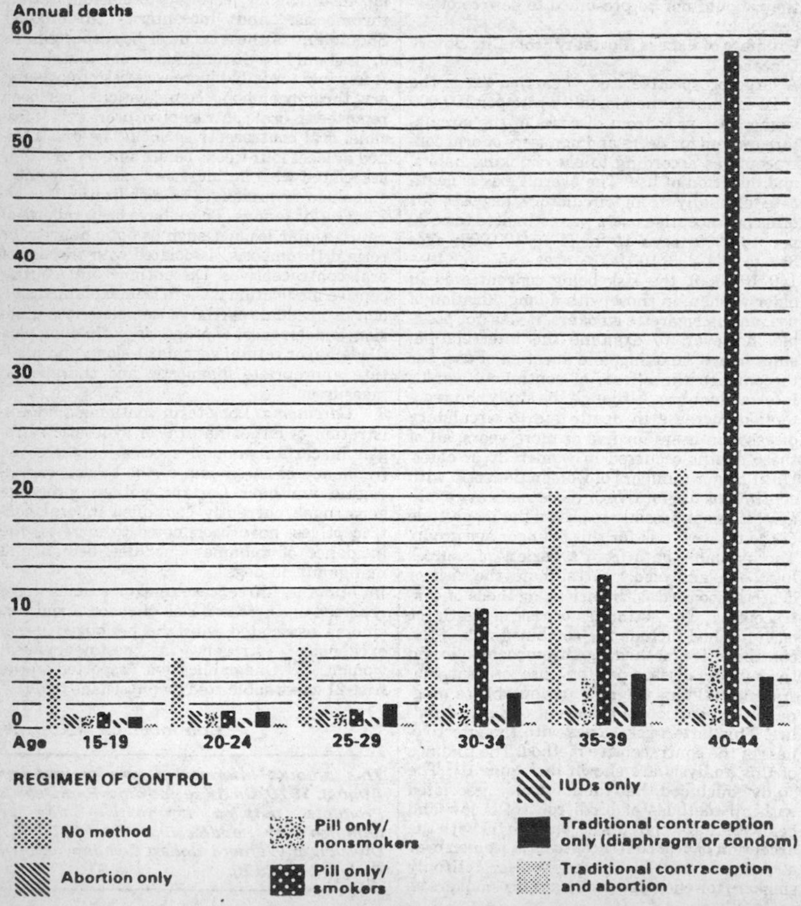

An increase in triglycerides and total phospholipids has been observed in patients receiving oral contraceptives.[44] The clinical significance of this finding remains to be defined.

8. *Elevated Blood Pressure.* An increase in blood pressure has been reported in patients receiving oral contraceptives[26]. In some women, hypertension may occur within a few months of beginning oral contraceptive use. In the first year of use, the prevalence of women with hypertension is low in users and may be no higher than that of a comparable group of nonusers. The prevalence in users increases, however, with longer exposure, and in the fifth year of use, is two and a half to three times the reported prevalence in the first year. Age is also strongly correlated with the development of hypertension in oral contraceptive users. Women who previously have had hypertension during pregnancy may be more likely to develop elevation of blood pressure when given oral contraceptives. Hypertension that develops as a result of taking oral contraceptives usually returns to normal after discontinuing the drug.

9. *Headache.* The onset or exacerbation of migraine or development of headache of a new pattern which is recurrent, persistent, or severe, requires discontinuation of oral contraceptives and evaluation of the cause.

10. *Bleeding Irregularities.* Breakthrough bleeding, spotting, and amenorrhea are frequent reasons for patients discontinuing oral contraceptives. In breakthrough bleeding, as in all cases of irregular bleeding from the vagina, nonfunctional causes should be borne in mind. In undiagnosed persistent or recurrent abnormal bleeding from the vagina, adequate diagnostic measures are indicated to rule out pregnancy or malignancy. If pathology has been excluded, time or a change to another formulation may solve the problem. Changing to an oral contraceptive with a higher estrogen content, while potentially useful in minimizing menstrual irregularity, should be done only if necessary, because this may increase the risk of thromboembolic disease.

Women with a past history of oligomenorrhea or secondary amenorrhea or young women without regular cycles may have a tendency to remain anovulatory or to become amenorrheic after discontinuation of oral contraceptives. Women with these preexisting problems should be advised of this possibility and encouraged to use other contraceptive methods. Postuse anovulation, possibly prolonged, may also occur in women without previous irregularities.

11. *Ectopic Pregnancy.* Ectopic as well as intrauterine pregnancy may occur in contraceptive failures. However, in progestogen-only oral contraceptive failures, the ratio of ectopic to intrauterine pregnancies is higher than in women who are not receiving oral contraceptives because the drugs are more effective in preventing intrauterine than ectopic pregnancies.

12. *Breast Feeding.* Oral contraceptives given in the postpartum period may interfere with lactation. There may be a decrease in the quantity and quality of breast milk. Furthermore, a small fraction of the hormonal agents in oral contraceptives has been identified in the milk of mothers receiving these drugs.[45] The effects, if any, on the breast-fed child have not been determined. If feasible, the use of oral contraceptives should be deferred until the infant has been weaned.

Precautions:

General

1. A complete medical and family history should be taken prior to the initiation of oral contraceptives. The pretreatment and periodic physical examinations should include special reference to blood pressure, breasts, abdomen, and pelvic organs, including Papanicolaou smear and relevant laboratory tests. As a general rule, oral contraceptives should not be prescribed for longer than one year without another physical examination being performed.

2. Under the influence of estrogen-progestogen preparations, preexisting uterine leiomyomata may increase in size.

3. Patients with a history of psychic depression should be carefully observed and the drug discontinued if depression recurs to a serious degree. Patients becoming significantly depressed while taking oral contraceptives should stop the medication and use an alternate method of contraception in an attempt to determine whether the symptom is drug-related.

4. Oral contraceptives may cause some degree of fluid retention. They should be prescribed with caution, and only with careful monitoring, in patients with conditions which might be aggravated by fluid retention, such as convulsive disorders, migraine syndrome, asthma, or cardiac or renal insufficiency.

5. Patients with a past history of jaundice during pregnancy have an increased risk of recurrence of jaundice while receiving oral contraceptive therapy. If jaundice develops in any patient receiving such drugs, the medication should be discontinued.

6. Steroid hormones may be poorly metabolized in patients with impaired liver function, and should be administered with caution in such patients.

7. Oral contraceptive users may have disturbances in normal tryptophan metabolism which may result in a relative pyridoxine deficiency. The clinical significance of this is yet to be determined.

8. Serum folate levels may be depressed by oral contraceptive therapy. Because the pregnant woman is predisposed to the development of folate deficiency and the incidence of folate deficiency increases with increasing gestation, it is possible that if a woman becomes pregnant shortly after stopping oral contraceptives, she may have a greater chance of developing folate deficiency and complications attributed to this deficiency.

9. The pathologist should be advised of oral contraceptive therapy when relevant specimens are submitted.

10. Certain endocrine and liver function tests and blood components may be affected by estrogen-containing oral contraceptives.

a) Increased sulfobromophthalein retention
b) Increased prothrombin and factors VII, VIII, IX, and X; decreased antithrombin 3; increased norepinephrine-induced platelet aggregability
c) Increased thyroid-binding globulin (TBG) leading to increased circulating total thyroid hormone, as measured by protein-bound iodine (PBI), T4 by column, or T4 by radioimmunoassay. Free T3 resin uptake is decreased, reflecting the elevated TBG; free T4 concentration is unaltered
d) Decreased pregnanediol excretion
e) Reduced response to metyrapone test

Information For The Patient: See Patient Labeling printed following **REFERENCES** section.

Drug Interactions: Reduced efficacy and increased incidence of breakthrough bleeding have been associated with concomitant use of rifampin. A similar association has been suggested with barbiturates, phenylbutazone, phenytoin sodium, and ampicillin.

Carcinogenesis: See **WARNINGS** section for information on the carcinogenic potential of oral contraceptives.

Pregnancy: Pregnancy category X. See **CONTRAINDICATIONS** and **WARNINGS.**

Nursing Mothers: See **WARNINGS.**

Adverse Reactions: An increased risk of the following serious adverse reactions has been associated with the use of oral contraceptives (see **WARNINGS**).

Thrombophlebitis
Pulmonary embolism
Coronary thrombosis
Cerebral thrombosis
Cerebral hemorrhage
Hypertension
Gallbladder disease
Benign hepatomas
Congenital anomalies

There is evidence of an association between the following conditions and the use of oral contraceptives, although additional confirmatory studies are needed.

Mesenteric thrombosis
Neuro-ocular lesions, eg, retinal thrombosis and optic neuritis

The following adverse reactions have been reported in patients receiving oral contraceptives and are believed to be drug-related.

Nausea and/or vomiting, usually the most common adverse reactions, occur in approximately 10% or less of patients during the first cycle. Other reactions, as a general rule, are seen much less frequently or only occasionally.
Gastrointestinal symptoms (such as abdominal cramps and bloating)
Breakthrough bleeding
Spotting
Change in menstrual flow
Dysmenorrhea
Amenorrhea during and after treatment
Temporary infertility after discontinuance of treatment
Edema
Chloasma or melasma which may persist
Breast changes: tenderness, enlargement, and secretion
Change in weight (increase or decrease)
Change in cervical erosion and cervical secretion
Possible diminution in lactation when given immediately post partum
Cholestatic jaundice
Migraine
Increase in size of uterine leiomyomata
Rash (allergic)
Mental depression
Reduced tolerance to carbohydrates
Vaginal candidiasis
Change in corneal curvature (steepening).
Intolerance to contact lenses

The following adverse reactions have been reported in users of oral contraceptives, and the association has been neither confirmed nor refuted.

Premenstrual-like syndrome
Cataracts
Changes in libido
Chorea
Changes in appetite
Cystitis-like syndrome
Headache
Nervousness
Dizziness
Hirsutism
Loss of scalp hair
Erythema multiforme
Erythema nodosum
Hemorrhagic eruption
Vaginitis
Porphyria

Acute Overdose: Serious ill effects have not been reported following acute ingestion of large doses of oral contraceptives by young children. Overdosage may cause nausea, and withdrawal bleeding may occur in females.

Continued on next page

This product information was prepared in August, 1979. On these and other Parke-Davis Products, detailed information may be obtained by addressing PARKE-DAVIS, Division of Warner-Lambert Company, Morris Plains, NJ 07950.

Parke-Davis—Cont.

Dosage and Administration:

Loestrin [21] 1/20 (norethindrone acetate and ethinyl estradiol tablets, USP)

To achieve maximum contraceptive effectiveness, Loestrin [21] 1/20 must be taken exactly as directed and at intervals not exceeding 24 hours. Loestrin [21] 1/20 provides the patient with a convenient tablet schedule of "three weeks on — one week off."

The first day of menstrual flow is considered Day 1. Initially, the patient begins taking tablets on Day 5 and takes one tablet daily for 21 days. She then takes no tablets for seven days. After the 7 days during which no tablets are taken, the patient begins a new course of one tablet daily for 21 days. Each course of tablets will begin on the same day of the week as the first course. Likewise, the interval of no tablets will always start on the same day of the week.

Tablets should be taken regularly with a meal or at bedtime. It should be stressed that efficacy of medication depends on strict adherence to the dosage schedule.

Special Notes on Administration

Menstruation usually begins two or three days, but may begin as late as the fourth or fifth day, after discontinuing medication. Because of the relatively low estrogenic content, Loestrin [21] 1/20 is not a good cyclic regulator. There are patients whose inherent hormone balance will require larger amounts of estrogen to achieve cyclic regularity than that contained in Loestrin [21] 1/20. These patients experience altered bleeding patterns, which do not conform to treatment schedules, while taking Loestrin [21] 1/20 Tablets. However, it is important that patients adhere to the dosage schedule regardless of when bleeding occurs.

The occurrence of altered bleeding is highest in Cycle 1. The majority of patients will have seven days or less of total bleeding during the 28-day cycle (including both withdrawal bleeding and breakthrough bleeding and spotting). Should irregular bleeding occur, patients should be reassured and instructed to continue taking the tablets as directed. If by the third cycle the irregular patterns are unacceptable, consideration should be given to changing the medication to a product with higher estrogen content (Norlestrin* 1/50 or Norlestrin 2.5/50). The physician should be alert to the fact that the irregular bleeding patterns could mask bleeding from organic causes, and appropriate diagnostic measures should be taken if the bleeding persists or continues after changing to a higher estrogen-content product.

If a patient forgets to take one or more tablets, the following is suggested. If one tablet is missed, take it as soon as remembered, or take two tablets the next day. If two consecutive tablets are missed, take two tablets daily for the next two days, then resume the regular schedule. However, an additional means of contraception should be used for seven consecutive days. If three consecutive tablets are missed, begin a new compact of tablets, starting seven days after the last tablet was taken. The patient should use an alternative means of contraception (other than oral tablets) until the start of the next menstrual period.

The possibility of ovulation occurring increases with each successive day that scheduled tablets are missed. While there is little likelihood of ovulation occurring if only one tablet is missed, the possibility of spotting or bleeding is increased. This is particularly likely to occur if two or more consecutive tablets are missed.

*Norlestrin (norethindrone acetate and ethinyl estradiol tablets, USP)

Loestrin [Fe] 1/20 (norethindrone acetate and ethinyl estradiol tablets, USP)

To achieve maximum contraceptive effectiveness, Loestrin [Fe] 1/20 must be taken exactly as directed and at intervals not exceeding 24 hours.

Loestrin [Fe] 1/20 provides a continuous administration regimen consisting of 21 *white* tablets of Loestrin 1/20 and *seven* brown tablets of ferrous fumarate. There is no need for the patient to count days between cycles because there are no "off-tablet days."

The dosage schedule is one *white* tablet daily for 21 days, starting initially on Day 5 of the menstrual cycle, followed without interruption by one *brown* tablet daily for 7 days. The first day of menstrual flow is considered Day 1. Upon completion of this first course of tablets, a second course of tablets is started without interruption. All subsequent courses are also taken without interruption.

Tablets should be taken regularly with a meal or at bedtime. It should be stressed that efficacy of medication depends on strict adherence to the dosage schedules.

Special Notes on Administration

Menstruation usually begins two or three days, but may begin as late as the fourth or fifth day, after the *brown* tablets have been started. Because of the relatively low estrogenic content, Loestrin [Fe] 1/20 is not a good cyclic regulator. There are patients whose inherent hormone balance will require larger amounts of estrogen to achieve cyclic regularity than that contained in Loestrin [Fe] 1/20. These patients experience altered bleeding patterns, which do not conform to treatment schedules, while taking the *white* Loestrin [Fe] 1/20 Tablets. However, it is important that patients adhere to the dosage schedule regardless of when bleeding occurs.

The occurrence of altered bleeding is highest in Cycle 1. The majority of patients will have seven days or less of total bleeding during the 28-day cycle (including both withdrawal bleeding and breakthrough bleeding and spotting). Should irregular bleeding occur, patients should be reassured and instructed to continue taking the tablets as directed. If by the third cycle the irregular patterns are unacceptable, consideration should be given to changing the medication to a product with higher estrogen content (Norlestrin* 1/50 or Norlestrin 2.5/50). The physician should be alert to the fact that the irregular bleeding patterns could mask bleeding from organic causes, and appropriate diagnostic measures should be taken if the bleeding persists or continues after changing to a higher estrogen-content product.

If a patient forgets to take one or more *white* tablets, the following is suggested. If one *white* tablet is missed, take it as soon as remembered, or take two *white* tablets the next day. If two consecutive *white* tablets are missed, take two *white* tablets daily for the next two days, then resume the regular schedule. However, an additional means of contraception should be used for seven consecutive days. If three consecutive *white* tablets are missed, begin a new compact of tablets, starting seven days after the last tablet was taken. The patient should use an alternative means of contraception (other than oral tablets) until the start of the next menstrual period.

*Norlestrin (norethindrone acetate and ethinyl estradiol tablets, USP)

The possibility of ovulation occurring increases with each successive day that scheduled *white* tablets are missed. While there is little likelihood of ovulation occurring if only one *white* tablet is missed, the possibility of spotting or bleeding is increased. This is particularly likely to occur if two or more consecutive *white* tablets are missed.

If one or more *brown* tablets are missed, the *white* tablets should be started no later than the eighth day after the last *white* tablet was taken. The possibility of conception occurring is not increased if *brown* tablets are missed.

Loestrin [21] 1.5/30 (norethindrone acetate and ethinyl estradiol tablets, USP)

To achieve maximum contraceptive effectiveness, Loestrin [21] 1.5/30 must be taken exactly as directed and at intervals not exceeding 24 hours. Loestrin [21] 1.5/30 provides the patient with a convenient tablet schedule of "three weeks on — one week off."

The first day of menstrual flow is considered Day 1. Initially, the patient begins taking a *green* tablet on Day 5 and takes one tablet daily for 21 days. She then takes no tablets for seven days.

After the seven days during which no tablets are taken, the patient begins a new course of one *green* tablet daily for 21 days. Each course of tablets will begin on the same day of the week as the first course. Likewise, the interval of no tablets will always start on the same day of the week.

Tablets should be taken regularly with a meal or at bedtime. It should be stressed that efficacy of medication depends on strict adherence to the dosage schedule.

Special Notes on Administration

Menstruation usually begins two or three days, but may begin as late as the fourth or fifth day, after discontinuing medication. Because of the relatively low estrogenic content, Loestrin [21] 1.5/30 is not a good cyclic regulator. There are patients whose inherent hormone balance will require larger amounts of estrogen to achieve cyclic regularity than that contained in Loestrin [21] 1.5/30. These patients experience altered bleeding patterns, which do not conform to treatment schedules, while taking Loestrin [21] 1.5/30 Tablets. However, it is important that patients adhere to the dosage schedule regardless of when bleeding occurs.

The occurrence of altered bleeding is highest in Cycle 1. The majority of patients will have seven days or less of total bleeding during the 28-day cycle (including both withdrawal bleeding and breakthrough bleeding and spotting). Should irregular bleeding occur, patients should be reassured and instructed to continue taking the tablets as directed. If by the third cycle the irregular patterns are unacceptable, consideration should be given to changing the medication to a product with higher estrogen content (Norlestrin* 1/50 or Norlestrin 2.5/50). The physician should be alert to the fact that the irregular bleeding patterns could mask bleeding from organic causes, and appropriate diagnostic measures should be taken if the bleeding persists or continues after changing to a higher estrogen-content product.

*Norlestrin (norethindrone acetate and ethinyl estradiol tablets, USP)

If a patient forgets to take one or more tablets, the following is suggested. If one tablet is missed, take it as soon as remembered, or take two tablets the next day. If two consecutive tablets are missed, take two tablets daily for the next two days, then resume the regular schedule. If three consecutive tablets are missed, begin a new compact of tablets, starting seven days after the last tablet was taken. The patient should use an alternative means of contraception (other than oral tablets) until the start of the next menstrual period.

The possibility of ovulation occurring increases with each successive day that scheduled tablets are missed. While there is little likelihood of ovulation occurring if only one tablet is missed, the possibility of spotting or bleeding is increased. This is particularly likely to occur if two or more consecutive tablets are missed.

Loestrin [Fe] 1.5/30 (norethindrone acetate and ethinyl estradiol tablets, USP)

To achieve maximum contraceptive effectiveness, Loestrin [Fe] 1.5/30 must be taken exactly as directed and at intervals not exceeding 24 hours.

Loestrin Fe 1.5/30 provides a continuous administration regimen consisting of 21 *green* tablets of Loestrin 1.5/30 and *seven* brown tablets of ferrous fumarate. There is no need for the patient to count days between cycles because there are no "off-tablet days."

The dosage schedule is one *green* tablet daily for 21 days, starting initially on Day 5 of the menstrual cycle, followed without interruption by one *brown* tablet daily for 7 days. The first day of menstrual flow is considered Day 1. Upon completion of this first course of tablets, a second course of tablets is started without interruption. All subsequent courses are also taken without interruption.

Tablets should be taken regularly with a meal or at bedtime. It should be stressed that efficacy of medication depends on strict adherence to the dosage schedule.

Special Notes on Administration

Menstruation usually begins two or three days, but may begin as late as the fourth or fifth day, after the *brown* tablets have been started. Because of the relatively low estrogenic content, Loestrin Fe 1.5/30 is not a good cyclic regulator. There are patients whose inherent hormone balance will require larger amounts of estrogen to achieve cyclic regularity than that contained in Loestrin Fe 1.5/30. These patients experience altered bleeding patterns, which do not conform to treatment schedules, while taking the green Loestrin Fe 1.5/30 Tablets. However, it is important that patients adhere to the dosage schedule regardless of when bleeding occurs.

The occurrence of altered bleeding is highest in Cycle 1. The majority of patients will have seven days or less of total bleeding during the 28-day cycle (including both withdrawal bleeding and breakthrough bleeding and spotting). Should irregular bleeding occur, patients should be reassured and instructed to continue taking the tablets as directed. If by the third cycle the irregular patterns are unacceptable, consideration should be given to changing the medication to a product with higher estrogen content (Norlestrin* 1/50 or Norlestrin 2.5/50). The physician should be alert to the fact that the irregular bleeding patterns could mask bleeding from organic causes, and appropriate diagnostic measures should be taken if the bleeding persists or continues after changing to a higher estrogen-content product.

*Norlestrin (norethindrone acetate and ethinyl estradiol tablets, USP)

If a patient forgets to take one or more *green* tablets, the following is suggested. If one *green* tablet is missed, take it as soon as remembered, or take two *green* tablets the next day. If two consecutive *green* tablets are missed, take two *green* tablets daily for the next two days, then resume the regular schedule. If three consecutive *green* tablets are missed, begin a new compact of tablets, starting seven days after the last tablet was taken. The patient should use an alternative means of contraception (other than oral tablets) until the start of the next menstrual period.

The possibility of ovulation occurring increases with each successive day that scheduled *green* tablets are missed. While there is little likelihood of ovulation occurring if only one *green* tablet is missed, the possibility of spotting or bleeding is increased. This is particularly likely to occur if two or more consecutive *green* tablets are missed.

If one or more *brown* tablets are missed, the *green* tablets should be started no later than the eighth day after the last *green* tablet was taken. The possibility of conception occurring is not increased if *brown* tablets are missed.

Norlestrin 21 1/50 (norethindrone acetate and ethinyl estradiol tablets, USP)

To achieve maximum contraceptive effectiveness, Norlestrin 21 1/50 must be taken exactly as directed and at intervals not exceeding 24 hours. Norlestrin 21 1/50 provides the patient with a convenient tablet schedule of "three weeks on — one week off."

The first day of menstrual flow is considered Day 1. Initially, the patient takes a tablet on Day 5 and takes one tablet daily for 21 days. She then takes no tablets for seven days.

After the seven days during which no tablets are taken, the patient begins a new course of one tablet daily for 21 days. Each course of tablets will begin on the same day of the week as the first course. Likewise, the interval of no tablets will always start on the same day of the week.

Tablets should be taken regularly with a meal or at bedtime. It should be stressed that efficacy of medication depends on strict adherence to the dosage schedule.

Special Notes on Administration

Menstruation usually begins two or three days, but may begin as late as the fourth or fifth day, after discontinuing medication.

If spotting occurs while on the usual regimen of one tablet daily, the patient should continue medication without interruption.

If a patient forgets to take one or more tablets, the following is suggested. If one tablet is missed, take it as soon as remembered, or take two tablets the next day. If two consecutive tablets are missed, take two tablets daily for the next two days, then resume the regular schedule. If three consecutive tablets are missed, begin a new compact of tablets, starting seven days after the last tablet was taken. The possibility of ovulation occurring increases with each successive day that scheduled tablets are missed. When three consecutive tablets are missed, the patient should use an alternative means of contraception (other than oral tablets) until the start of the next menstrual period.

While there is little likelihood of ovulation occurring if only one tablet is missed, the possibility of spotting or bleeding is increased. This is particularly likely to occur if two or more consecutive tablets are missed.

In the rare case of bleeding which resembles menstruation, the patient should be advised to discontinue medication and then begin taking tablets from a new compact on the fifth day (Day 5). Persistent bleeding which is not controlled by this method indicates the need for reexamination of the patient, at which time nonfunctional causes should be borne in mind.

Norlestrin 28 1/50 (norethindrone acetate and ethinyl estradiol tablets, USP)

To achieve maximum contraceptive effectiveness, Norlestrin 28 1/50 must be taken exactly as directed and at intervals not exceeding 24 hours.

Norlestrin 28 1/50 provides a continuous administration regimen consisting of 21 *yellow* tablets of Norlestrin 1/50 and 7 *white* inert tablets. There is no need for the patient to count days between cycles because there are no "off-tablet days."

The dosage schedule is one *yellow* tablet daily for 21 days, starting initially on Day 5 of the menstrual cycle, followed without interruption by one *white* inert tablet daily for 7 days. The first day of menstrual flow is considered Day 1. Upon completion of this first course of tablets, a second course of tablets is started without interruption. All subsequent courses are also taken without interruption.

Tablets should be taken regularly with a meal or at bedtime. It should be stressed that efficacy of medication depends on strict adherence to the dosage schedule.

Special Notes on Administration

Menstruation usually begins two or three days, but may begin as late as the fourth or fifth day, after the *white* tablets have been started. In any event, the next course of tablets should be started without interruption. There should never be a day when the patient is not taking a tablet.

If spotting occurs while the patient is taking *yellow* tablets, continue medication without interruption.

If a patient forgets to take one or more *yellow* tablets, the following is suggested. If one *yellow* tablet is missed, take it as soon as remembered, or take two *yellow* tablets the next day. If two consecutive *yellow* tablets are missed, take two *yellow* tablets daily for the next two days, then resume the regular schedule. If three consecutive *yellow* tablets are missed, begin a new compact of tablets, starting seven days after the last tablet was taken.

The possibility of ovulation occurring increases with each successive day that scheduled *yellow* tablets are missed. When three consecutive *yellow* tablets are missed, the patient should use an alternative means of contraception (other than oral tablets) until the start of the next menstrual period).

While there is little likelihood of ovulation occurring if only one *yellow* tablet is missed, the possibility of spotting or bleeding is increased. This is particularly likely to occur if two or more consecutive *yellow* tablets are missed.

If one or more *white* tablets are missed, the *yellow* tablets should be started no later than the eighth day after the last *yellow* tablet was taken. The possibility of conception occurring is not increased if *white* tablets are missed.

In the rare case of bleeding which resembles menstruation, the patient should be advised to discontinue medication and then begin taking tablets from a new compact on the fifth day (Day 5). Persistent bleeding which is not controlled by this method indicates the need for reexamination of the patient, at which time nonfunctional causes should be borne in mind.

Norlestrin Fe 1/50 (norethindrone acetate and ethinyl estradiol tablets, USP)

To achieve maximum contraceptive effectiveness, Norlestrin Fe 1/50 must be taken exactly as directed and at intervals not exceeding 24 hours. Norlestrin Fe 1/50 provides a continuous administration regimen consisting of 21 *yellow* tablets of Norlestrin 1/50 and 7 *brown* tablets of ferrous fumarate. There is no need for the patient to count days between cycles because there are no "off-tablet days."

The dosage schedule is one *yellow* tablet daily for 21 days, starting initially on Day 5 of the menstrual cycle, followed without interruption by one *brown* tablet daily for 7 days. The first day of menstrual flow is considered Day 1. Upon completion of this first course of tablets, a second course of tablets is started without interruption. All subsequent courses are also taken without interruption.

Tablets should be taken regularly with a meal or at bedtime. It should be stressed that efficacy of medication depends on strict adherence to the dosage schedule.

Special Notes on Administration

Menstruation usually begins two or three days, but may begin as late as the fourth or fifth day, after the *brown* tablets have been started. In any event, the next course of tablets should be started without interruption. There should never be a day when the patient is not taking a tablet.

If spotting occurs while the patient is taking *yellow* tablets, continue medication without interruption.

If a patient forgets to take one or more *yellow* tablets, the following is suggested. If one *yellow* tablet is missed, take it as soon as remembered,

Continued on next page

This product information was prepared in August, 1979. On these and other Parke-Davis Products, detailed information may be obtained by addressing PARKE-DAVIS, Division of Warner-Lambert Company, Morris Plains, NJ 07950.

Parke-Davis—Cont.

or take two *yellow* tablets the next day. If two consecutive *yellow* tablets are missed, take two *yellow* tablets daily for the next two days, then resume the regular schedule. If three consecutive *yellow* tablets are missed, begin a new compact of tablets, starting seven days after the last tablet was taken.

The possibility of ovulation occurring increases with each successive day that scheduled *yellow* tablets are missed. When three consecutive *yellow* tablets are missed, the patient should use an alternative means of contraception (other than oral tablets) until the start of the next menstrual period.

While there is little likelihood of ovulation occurring if only one *yellow* tablet is missed, the possibility of spotting or bleeding is increased. This is particularly likely to occur if two or more consecutive *yellow* tablets are missed.

If one or more *brown* tablets are missed, the *yellow* tablets should be started no later than the eighth day after the last *yellow* tablet was taken. The possibility of conception occurring is not increased if *brown* tablets are missed.

In the rare case of bleeding which resembles menstruation, the patient should be advised to discontinue medication and then begin taking tablets from a new compact on the fifth day (Day 5). Persistent bleeding which is not controlled by this method indicates the need for reexamination of the patient, at which time nonfunctional causes should be borne in mind.

Norlestrin 21 2.5/50 (norethindrone acetate and ethinyl estradiol tablets, USP)

To achieve maximum contraceptive effectiveness, Norlestrin 21 2.5/50 must be taken exactly as directed and at intervals not exceeding 24 hours. Norlestrin 21 2.5/50 provides the patient with a convenient tablet schedule of "three weeks on — one week off."

The first day of menstrual flow is considered Day 1. Initially, the patient takes a tablet on Day 5 and takes one tablet daily for 21 days. She then takes no tablets for seven days.

After the seven days during which no tablets are taken, the patient begins a new course of one tablet daily for 21 days. Each course of tablets will begin on the same day of the week as the first course. Likewise, the interval of no tablets will always start on the same day of the week.

Tablets should be taken regularly with a meal or at bedtime. It should be stressed that efficacy of medication depends on strict adherence to the dosage schedule.

Special Notes on Administration

Menstruation usually begins two or three days, but may begin as late as the fourth or fifth day, after discontinuing medication.

If spotting occurs while on the usual regimen of one tablet daily, the patient should continue medication without interruption.

If a patient forgets to take one or more tablets, the following is suggested. If one tablet is missed, take it as soon as remembered, or take two tablets the next day. If two consecutive tablets are missed, take two tablets daily for the next two days, then resume the regular schedule. If three consecutive tablets are missed, begin a new compact of tablets, starting seven days after the last tablet was taken.

The possibility of ovulation occurring increases with each successive day that scheduled tablets are missed. When three consecutive tablets are missed, the patient should use an alternative means of contraception (other than oral tablets) until the start of the next menstrual period.

While there is little likelihood of ovulation occurring if only one tablet is missed, the possibility of spotting or bleeding is increased. This is particularly likely to occur if two or more consecutive tablets are missed.

In the rare case of bleeding which resembles menstruation, the patient should be advised to discontinue medication and then begin taking tablets from a new compact on the fifth day (Day 5). Persistent bleeding which is not controlled by this method indicates the need for reexamination of the patient, at which time nonfunctional causes should be borne in mind.

Norlestrin Fe 2.5/50 (norethindrone acetate and ethinyl estradiol tablets, USP)

To achieve maximum contraceptive effectiveness, Norlestrin Fe 2.5/50 must be taken exactly as directed and at intervals not exceeding 24 hours. Norlestrin Fe 2.5/50 provides a continuous administration regimen consisting of 21 *pink* tablets of Norlestrin 2.5/50 and 7 *brown* tablets of ferrous fumarate. There is no need for the patient to count days between cycles because there are no "off-tablet days."

The dosage schedule is one *pink* tablet daily for 21 days, starting initially on Day 5 of the menstrual cycle, followed without interruption by one *brown* tablet daily for 7 days. The first day of menstrual flow is considered Day 1. Upon completion of this first course of tablets, a second course of tablets is started without interruption. All subsequent courses are also taken without interruption.

Tablets should be taken regularly with a meal or at bedtime. It should be stressed that efficacy of medication depends on strict adherence to the dosage schedule.

Special Notes on Administration

Menstruation usually begins two or three days, but may begin as late as the fourth or fifth day, after the *brown* tablets have been started. In any event, the next course of tablets should be started without interruption. There should never be a day when the patient is not taking a tablet.

If spotting occurs while the patient is taking *pink* tablets, continue medication without interruption.

If a patient forgets to take one or more *pink* tablets, the following is suggested. If one *pink* tablet is missed, take it as soon as remembered, or take two *pink* tablets the next day. If two consecutive *pink* tablets are missed, take two *pink* tablets daily for the next two days, then resume the regular schedule. If three consecutive *pink* tablets are missed, begin a new compact of tablets, starting seven days after the last tablet was taken.

The possibility of ovulation occurring increases with each successive day that scheduled *pink* tablets are missed. When three consecutive *pink* tablets are missed, the patient should use an alternative means of contraception (other than oral tablets) until the start of the next menstrual period.

While there is little likelihood of ovulation occurring if only one *pink* tablet is missed, the possibility of spotting or bleeding is increased. This is particularly likely to occur if two or more consecutive *pink* tablets are missed.

If one or more *brown* tablets are missed, the *pink* tablets should be started no later than the eighth day after the last *pink* tablet was taken. The possibility of conception occurring is not increased if *brown* tablets are missed.

In the rare case of bleeding which resembles menstruation, the patient should be advised to discontinue medication and then begin taking tablets from a new compact on the fifth day (Day 5). Persistent bleeding which is not controlled by this method indicates the need for reexamination of the patient, at which time nonfunctional causes should be borne in mind.

Loestrin and Norlestrin Products

Use of oral contraceptives in the event of a missed menstrual period:

1. If the patient has not adhered to the prescribed dosage regimen, the possibility of pregnancy should be considered after the first missed period and oral contraceptives should be withheld until pregnancy has been ruled out.
2. If the patient has adhered to the prescribed regimen and misses two consecutive periods, pregnancy should be ruled out before continuing the contraceptive regimen.

After several months on treatment, bleeding may be reduced to a point of virtual absence. This reduced flow may occur as a result of medication, in which event it is not indicative of pregnancy.

How Supplied:

Loestrin 21 1/20 (norethindrone acetate and ethinyl estradiol tablets, USP) is available in compacts each containing 21 white tablets (Parcode® No. 915). Each white tablet contains 1 mg of norethindrone acetate and 20 mcg of ethinyl estradiol. Available in packages of five compacts (N 0710-0915-46) and packages of five refills (N 0710-0915-47).

Loestrin Fe 1/20 is available in compacts, each containing 21 white tablets (Parcode No. 915) and 7 brown tablets (Parcode No. 622). Each white tablet contains 1 mg of norethindrone acetate and 20 mcg of ethinyl estradiol. Each brown tablet contains 75 mg of ferrous fumarate. Available in packages of five minicompacts (N 0710-0913-46) and packages of five refills (N 0710-0913-47).

Loestrin 21 1.5/30 is available in packages each containing 21 green tablets (Parcode No. 916). Each green tablet contains 1.5 mg of norethindrone acetate and 30 mcg ethinyl estradiol. Available in packages of five minicompacts (N 0710-0916-46) and packages of five refills (N 0710-0916-47).

Loestrin Fe 1.5/30 is available in compacts, each containing 21 green tablets (Parcode No. 916) and 7 brown tablets (Parcode No. 622). Each green tablet contains 1.5 mg of norethindrone acetate and 30 mcg ethinyl estradiol. Each brown tablet contains 75 mg ferrous fumarate. Available in packages of five minicompacts (N 0710-0917-46) and packages of five refills (N 0710-0917-47).

Norlestrin 21 1/50 is available in compacts, each containing 21 yellow tablets (Parcode No. 904). Each yellow tablet contains 1 mg of norethindrone acetate and 50 mcg ethinyl estradiol. Available in packages of five minicompacts (N 0710-0904-46) and packages of five refills (N 0710-0904-47).

Norlestrin 28 1/50 is available in compacts, each containing 21 yellow tablets (Parcode No. 904) and 7 white inert tablets (Parcode No. 618). Each yellow tablet contains 1 mg norethindrone acetate and 50 mcg ethinyl estradiol. Available in packages of five minicompacts (N 0710-0903-46) and packages of five refills (N 0710-0903-47).

Norlestrin Fe 1/50 is available in compacts, each containing 21 yellow tablets (Parcode No. 904) and 7 brown tablets (Parcode No. 622). Each yellow tablet contains 1 mg norethindrone acetate and 50 mcg ethinyl estradiol. Each brown tablet contains 75 mg ferrous fumarate. Available in packages of five minicompacts (N 0710-0905-46) and packages of five refills (N 0710-0905-47).

Norlestrin 21 2.5/50 is available in compacts, each containing 21 pink tablets (Parcode No. 901). Each pink tablet contains 2.5 mg norethindrone acetate and 50 mcg ethinyl estradiol. Available in packages of five minicompacts (N 0710-901-46) and packages of five refills (N 0710-0901-47).

Norlestrin Fe 2.5/50 is available in compacts, each containing 21 pink tablets (Parcode No. 901) and 7 brown tablets (Parcode No. 622). Each pink tablet contains 2.5 mg norethindrone acetate and 50 mcg ethinyl estradiol. Each brown tablet contains 75 mg ferrous fumarate. Available in packages of five minicompacts (N 0710-0907-46) and packages of five refills (N 0710-0907-47).

References:

1. Population Reports, Series H, No. 2, May 1974; Series I, No. 1, June 1974; Series B, No. 2, January 1975; Series H, No. 3, 1975; Series H, No. 4, January 1976. Pop-

ulation Information Program, The George Washington University Medical Center, Washington, DC.
2. Inman WHW, et al: Thromboembolic disease and the steroidal content of oral contraceptives, A report to the Committee on Safety of Drugs. *Brit Med J* **2**:203–209, 1970.
3. Stolley PD, et al: Thrombosis with low-estrogen oral contraceptives. *Am J Epidemiol* **102**:197–208, 1975.
4. Oral contraception and thromboembolic disease, Royal College of General Practitioners. *J Coll Gen Pract* **13**:267–279, 1967.
5. Inman WHW, Vessey MP: Investigation of deaths from pulmonary, coronary and cerebral thrombosis and embolism in women of childbearing age. *Brit Med J* **2**:193–199, 1968.
6. Vessey MP, Doll R: Investigation of relation between use of oral contraception and thromboembolic disease. A further report. *Brit Med J* **2**:651–657, 1969.
7. Sartwell PE, et al: Thromboembolism and oral contraceptives: an epidemiological case control study. *Am J Epidemiol* **90**:365–380, 1969.
8. Oral contraceptives and venous thromboembolic disease, surgically confirmed gallbladder disease and breast tumors, Boston Collaborative Drug Surveillance Program. *Lancet* **1**:1399–1404, 1973.
9. Oral contraception and increased risk of cerebral ischemia or thrombosis, Collaborative Group for the Study of Stroke in Young Women. *N Engl J Med* **288**:871–878, 1973.
10. Oral contraceptives and stroke in young women: associated risk factors, Collaborative Group for the Study of Stroke in Young Women. *JAMA* **231**:718–722, 1975.
11. Mann JI, Inman WHW: Oral contraceptives and death from myocardial infarction. *Brit Med J* **2**:245–248, 1975.
12. Mann JI, et al: Oral contraceptive use in older women and fatal myocardial infarction. *Brit Med J* **2**:445–447, 1976.
13. Mann JI, et al: Myocardial infarction in young women with special reference to oral contraceptive practice. *Brit Med J* **2**:241–245, 1975.
14. Tietze C: New Estimates of Mortality Associated with Fertility Control. *Family Planning Perspectives* **9**:74–76, 1977.
15. Vessey MP, et al: Post-operative thromboembolism following the use of oral contraceptives. *Brit Med J* **3**:123–126, 1970.
16. Greene RG, Sartwell PE: Oral contraceptive use in patients with thromboembolism following surgery, trauma or infection. *Am J Pub Health* **62**:680–685, 1972.
17. Smith DC, et al: Association of exogenous estrogen and endometrial carcinoma. *N Engl J Med* **293**:1164–1167, 1975.
18. Ziel HK, Finkle WD: Increased risk of endometrial carcinoma among users of conjugated estrogens. *N Engl J Med* **293**:1167–1170, 1975.
19. Mack TN, et al: Estrogens and endometrial cancer in a retirement community. *N Engl J Med* **294**:1262–1267, 1976.
20. Silverberg SG, Makowski EL: Endometrial carcinoma in young women taking oral contraceptive agents. *Obstet Gynecol* **46**:503–506, 1975.
21. Vessey MP, et al: Oral contraceptives and breast neoplasia: a retrospective study. *Brit Med J* **3**:719–724, 1972.
22. Vessey MP, et al: Oral contraceptives and breast cancer. Progress report of an epidemiological study. *Lancet* **1**:941–943, 1975.
23. Surgically confirmed gallbladder disease, venous thromboembolism and breast tumors in relation to postmenopausal estrogen therapy, Boston Collaborative Drug Surveillance Program. *N Engl J Med* **290**:15–19, 1974.
24. Arthes FG, et al: The pill, estrogens, and the breast. Epidemiologic aspects. *Cancer* **28**:1391–1394, 1971.
25. Fasal E, Paffenbarger RS: Oral contraceptives as related to cancer and benign lesions of the breast. *J Natl Cancer Inst* **55**:767–773, 1975.
26. *Oral Contraceptives and Health.* Royal College of General Practitioners, London, Pitman, 1974.
27. Ory H, et al: Oral contraceptives and reduced risk of benign breast diseases. *N Engl J Med* **294**:419–422, 1976.
28. Baum J, et al: Possible association between benign hepatomas and oral contraceptives. *Lancet* **2**:926–928, 1973.
29. Mays ET, et al: Hepatic changes in young women ingesting contraceptive steroids. Hepatic hemorrhage and primary hepatic tumors. *JAMA* **235**:730–732, 1976.
30. Edmondson HA, et al: Liver-cell adenomas associated with use of oral contraceptives. *N Engl J Med* **294**:470–472, 1976.
31. Herbst AL, et al: Adenocarcinoma of the vagina. *N Engl J Med* **284**:878–881, 1971.
32. Greenwald P, et al: Vaginal cancer after maternal treatment with synthetic estrogens. *N Engl J Med* **285**:390–392, 1971.
33. Lanier AP, et al: Cancer and stilbestrol. A follow-up of 1719 persons exposed to estrogens in utero and born 1943-1959. *Mayo Clin Pro* **48**:793–799, 1973.
34. Herbst AL, et al.: Vaginal and cervical abnormalities after exposure to stilbestrol in utero. *Obstet Gynecol* **40**:287–298, 1972.
35. Herbst AL, et al.: The effects of local progesterone on stilbestrol-associated vaginal adenosis. *Am J Obstet Gynecol* **118**:607–615, 1974.
36. Herbst AL, et al: Prenatal exposure to stilbestrol: a prospective comparison of exposed female offspring with unexposed controls. *N Engl J Med* **292**:334–339, 1975.
37. Stafl A, et al: Clinical diagnosis of vaginal adenosis. *Obstet Gynecol* **43**:118–128, 1974.
38. Sherman AI, et al: Cervical-vaginal adenosis after in utero exposure to synthetic estrogens. *Obstet Gynecol* **44**:531–545, 1974.
39. Gal I, et al: Hormone pregnancy tests and congenital malformation. *Nature* **216**:83, 1967.
40. Levy EP, et al: Hormone treatment during pregnancy and congenital heart defects. *Lancet* **1**:611, 1973.
41. Nora JJ, Nora AH: Birth defects and oral contraceptives. *Lancet* **1**:941–942, 1973.
42. Janerich DT, et al: Oral contraceptives and congenital limb-reduction defects. *N Engl J Med* **291**:697–700, 1974.
43. Carr DH: Chromosome studies in selected spontaneous abortions: I. Conception after oral contraceptives. *Canad Med Assoc J* **103**:343–348, 1970.
44. Wynn V, et al: Some effects of oral contraceptives on serum-lipid and lipoprotein levels. *Lancet* **2**:720–723, 1966.
45. Laumas KR, et al: Radioactivity in the breast milk of lactating women after oral administration of 3 H-norethynodrel. *Am J Obstet Gynecol* **98**:411–413, 1967.
46. Increased risk of hepatocellular adenoma in women with long-term use of oral contraceptives. *Morbidity Mortality Weekly Rep* **26**:293–294, Center for Disease Control, 1977.
47. Herbst AL, et al: Age-incidence and risk of diethylstilbestrol-related clear cell adenocarcinoma of the vagina and cervix. *Am J Obstet Gynecol* **128**:43–50, 1977.
48. Bibbo M, et al: Follow-up study of male and female offspring of DES-treated mothers. A Preliminary Report. *J Repro Med* **15**:29–32, 1975.
49. Gill, WB, et al: Structural and functional abnormalities in the sex organs of male offspring of mothers treated with diethylstilbestrol (DES). *J Repro Med* **16**:147–153, 1976.
50. Henderson BE, et al: Urogenital tract abnormalities in sons of women treated with diethylstilbestrol. *Pediatrics* **58**:505–507, 1976.
51. Heinonen OP, et al: Cardiovascular birth defects and antenatal exposure to female sex hormones. *N Engl J Med* **296**:67–70, 1977.
52. Jain AK: Mortality risk associated with the use of oral contraceptives. *Studies in Family Planning* **8**:50–54, 1977.
53. Beral V: Mortality among oral contraceptive users, *Lancet* **2**:727–731, 1977.

The patient labeling for oral contraceptive drug products is set forth below.

Brief Summary Patient Package Insert:

Cigarette smoking increases the risk of serious adverse effects on the heart and blood vessels from oral contraceptive use. This risk increases with age and with heavy smoking (15 or more cigarettes per day) and is quite marked in women over 35 years of age. Women who use oral contraceptives should not smoke.

Oral contraceptives taken as directed are about 99% effective in preventing pregnancy. (The minipill, however, is somewhat less effective.) Forgetting to take your pills increases the chance of pregnancy.

Women who have or have had clotting disorders, cancer of the breast or sex organs, unexplained vaginal bleeding, a stroke, heart attack, angina pectoris, or who suspect they may be pregnant should not use oral contraceptives.

Most side effects of the Pill are not serious. The most common side effects are nausea, vomiting, bleeding between menstrual periods, weight gain, and breast tenderness. However, proper use of oral contraceptives requires that they be taken under your doctor's continuous supervision because they can be associated with serious side effects which may be fatal. Fortunately, these occur very infrequently. The serious side effects are:

1. Blood clots in the legs, lungs, brain, heart, or other organs and hemorrhage into the brain due to bursting of a blood vessel;
2. Liver tumors, which may rupture and cause severe bleeding;
3. Birth defects, if the Pill is taken while you are pregnant;
4. High blood pressure;
5. Gallbladder disease.

The symptoms associated with these serious side effects are discussed in the detailed leaflet given you with your supply of pills. Notify your doctor if you notice any unusual physical disturbance while taking the Pill.

The estrogen in oral contraceptives has been found to cause breast cancer and other cancers in certain animals. These findings suggest that oral contraceptives may also cause cancer in humans. However, studies to date in women taking currently marketed oral contraceptives have not confirmed that oral contraceptives cause cancer in humans.

The detailed leaflet describes more completely the benefits and risks of oral contraceptives. It

Continued on next page

This product information was prepared in August, 1979. On these and other Parke-Davis Products, detailed information may be obtained by addressing PARKE-DAVIS, Division of Warner-Lambert Company, Morris Plains, NJ 07950.

Parke-Davis—Cont.

also provides information on other forms of contraception. Read it carefully. If you have any questions, consult your doctor.

Caution. Oral contraceptives are of no value in the prevention or treatment of venereal disease.

Detailed Patient Labeling:

What You Should Know About Oral Contraceptives

Oral contraceptives ("the Pill") are the most effective way (except for sterilization) to prevent pregnancy. They are also convenient and, for most women, free of serious or unpleasant side effects. Oral contraceptives must always be taken under the continuous supervision of a physician.

It is important that any woman who considers using an oral contraceptive understands the risks involved. Although the oral contraceptives have important advantages over other methods of contraception, they have certain risks that no other method has. Only you can decide whether the advantages are worth these risks. This leaflet will tell you about the most important risks. It will explain how you can help your doctor prescribe the Pill as safely as possible by telling him about yourself and being alert for the earliest signs of trouble. And, it will tell you how to use the Pill properly, so that it will be as effective as possible. There is more detailed information available in the leaflet prepared for doctors. Your pharmacist can show you a copy; you may need your doctor's help in understanding parts of it.

Who Should Not Use Oral Contraceptives

A. If you have any of the following conditions you should not use the Pill.
   1. Clots in the legs or lungs
   2. Angina pectoris
   3. Known or suspected cancer of the breast or sex organs
   4. Unusual vaginal bleeding that has not yet been diagnosed
   5. Known or suspected pregnancy

B. If you have had any of the following conditions, you should not use the Pill.
   1. Heart attack or stroke
   2. Clots in the legs or lungs

C. Cigarette smoking increases the risk of serious adverse effects on the heart and blood vessels from oral contraceptive use. This risk increases with age and with heavy smoking (15 or more cigarettes per day) and is quite marked in women over 35 years of age. Women who use oral contraceptives should not smoke.

D. If you have scanty or irregular periods or are a young woman without a regular cycle, you should use another method of contraception because, if you use the Pill, you may have difficulty becoming pregnant or may fail to have menstrual periods after discontinuing the Pill.

Deciding To Use Oral Contraceptives

If you do not have any of the conditions listed above and are thinking about using oral contraceptives, to help you decide, you need information about the advantages and risks of oral contraceptives and of other contraceptive methods as well. This leaflet describes the advantages and risks of oral contraceptives. Except for sterilization, the IUD and abortion, which have their own exclusive risks, the only risks of other methods of contraception are those due to pregnancy should the method fail. Your doctor can answer questions you may have with respect to other methods of contraception. He can also answer any questions you may have after reading this leaflet on oral contraceptives.

1. What Oral Contraceptives Are and How They Work. Oral contraceptives are of two types. The most common, often simply called the Pill, is a combination of an estrogen and a progestogen, two kinds of female hormones. The amount of estrogen and progestogen can vary, but the amount of estrogen is most important because both the effectiveness and some of the dangers of oral contraceptives are related to the amount of estrogen. This kind of oral contraceptive works principally by preventing release of an egg from the ovary. When the amount of estrogen is 50 micrograms or more, and the Pill is taken as directed, oral contraceptives are more than 99% effective (ie, there would be less than one pregnancy if 100 women used the Pill for one year). Pills that contain 20 to 35 micrograms of estrogen vary slightly in effectiveness, ranging from 98% to more than 99% effective. Loestrin 1/20, Loestrin 1.5/30, Norlestrin 1/50, and Norlestrin 2.5/50 were shown, in clinical trials, to be more than 99% effective.

The second type of oral contraceptive, often called the "minipill," contains only a progestogen. It works in part by preventing release of an egg from the ovary but also by keeping sperm from reaching the egg and by making the uterus (womb) less receptive to any fertilized egg that reaches it. The minipill is less effective than the combination oral contraceptive, about 97% effective.

In addition, the progestogen-only pill has a tendency to cause irregular bleeding which may be quite inconvenient, or cessation of bleeding entirely. The progestogen-only pill is used despite its lower effectiveness in the hope that it will prove not to have some of the serious side effects of the estrogen-containing pill (see below) but it is not yet certain that the minipill does in fact have fewer serious side effects. The discussion below, while based mainly on information about the combination pills, should be considered to apply as well to the minipill.

2. Other Nonsurgical Ways to Prevent Pregnancy. As this leaflet will explain, oral contraceptives have several serious risks. Other methods of contraception have lesser risks or none at all. They are also less effective than oral contraceptives, but, used properly, may be effective enough for many women. The following Table gives reported pregnancy rates (the number of women out of 100 who would become pregnant in one year) for these methods.

Pregnancies Per 100 Women Per Year

Intrauterine device (IUD), less than 1–6
Diaphragm with spermicidal products (creams or jellies), 2–20
Condom (rubber), 3–36
Aerosol foams, 2–29
Jellies and creams, 4–36
Periodic abstinence (rhythm) types, less than 1–47
1. Calendar method, 14–47
2. Temperature method, 1–20
3. Temperature method—intercourse in postovulatory phase only, less than 1–7
4. Mucus method, 1–25
No contraception, 60–80

The figures (except for the IUD) vary widely because people differ in how well they use each method. Very faithful users of the various methods obtain very good results except for users of the calendar method of periodic abstinence (rhythm). Except for the IUD, effective use of these methods requires somewhat more effort than simply taking a single Pill every morning, but it is an effort that many couples undertake successfully. Your doctor can tell you a great deal more about these methods of contraception.

3. The Dangers of Oral Contraceptives

a) *Circulatory disorders (abnormal blood clotting and stroke due to hemorrhage).* Blood clots (in various blood vessels of the body) are the most common of the serious side effects of oral contraceptives. A clot can result in a stroke (if the clot is in the brain), a heart attack (if the clot is in a blood vessel of the heart), or a pulmonary embolus (a clot which forms in the legs or pelvis, then breaks off, and travels to the lungs). Any of these can be fatal. Clots also occur rarely in the blood vessels of the eye, resulting in blindness or impairment of vision in that eye. There is evidence that the risk of clotting increases with higher estrogen dosages. It is, therefore, important to keep the dosage of estrogen as low as possible, so long as the oral contraceptive used has an acceptable pregnancy rate and doesn't cause unacceptable changes in the menstrual pattern.

Furthermore, cigarette smoking by oral contraceptive users increases the risk of serious adverse effects on the heart and blood vessels. This risk increases with age and with heavy smoking (15 or more cigarettes per day) and begins to become quite marked in women over 35 years of age. For this reason, women who use oral contraceptives should not smoke.

The risk of abnormal clotting increases with age in both users and nonusers of oral contraceptives, but the increased risk from the contraceptive appears to be present at all ages. For oral contraceptive users in general, it has been estimated that in women between the ages of 15 and 34 the risk of death due to a circulatory disorder is about 1 in 12,000 per year, whereas for nonusers the rate is about 1 in 50,000 per year. In the age group 35 to 44, the risk is estimated to be about 1 in 2,500 per year for oral contraceptive users and about 1 in 10,000 per year for nonusers.

Even without the Pill, the risk of having a heart attack increases with age and is also increased by such heart attack risk factors as high blood pressure, high cholesterol, obesity, diabetes, and cigarette smoking. Without any risk factors present, the use of oral contraceptives alone may double the risk of heart attack. However, the combination of cigarette smoking, especially heavy smoking, and oral contraceptive use greatly increases the risk of heart attack. Oral contraceptive users who smoke are about 5 times more likely to have a heart attack than users who do not smoke and about 10 times more likely to have a heart attack than nonusers who do not smoke. It has been estimated that users between the ages of 30 and 39 who smoke have about a 1 in 10,000 chance each year of having a fatal heart attack compared to about a 1 in 50,000 chance in users who do not smoke, and about a 1 in 100,000 chance in nonusers who do not smoke. In the age group 40 to 44, the risk is about 1 in 1,700 per year for users who smoke compared to about 1 in 10,000 for users who do not smoke and to about 1 in 14,000 per year for nonusers who do not smoke. Heavy smoking (about 15 cigarettes or more a day) further increases the risk. If you do not smoke and have none of the other heart attack risk factors described above, you will have a smaller risk than listed. If you have several heart attack risk factors, the risk may be considerably greater than listed.

In addition to blood-clotting disorders, it has been estimated that women taking oral contraceptives are twice as likely as nonusers to have a stroke due to rupture of a blood vessel in the brain.

b) *Formation of tumors.* Studies have found that when certain animals are given the female sex hormone estrogen, which is an ingredient of oral contraceptives, continuously for long periods, cancers may develop in the breast, cervix, vagina, and liver.

These findings suggest that oral contraceptives may cause cancer in humans. However, studies to date in women taking currently marketed oral contraceptives have not confirmed that oral contraceptives cause cancer in humans. Several studies have found no increase in breast cancerin users, although one study suggested oral contraceptives might cause an increase in breast cancer in women who already have benign breast disease (eg, cysts).

Women with a strong family history of breast cancer or who have breast nodules, fibrocystic disease, or abnormal mammograms, or who were exposed to DES (diethylstebestrol), an estrogen, during their mothers' pregnancies must be followed very closely by their doctors if they choose to use oral contraceptives instead of another method of contraception. Many studies have shown that women taking oral contraceptives have less risk of getting benign breast disease than those who have not used oral contraceptives. Recently, strong evidence has emerged that estrogens (one component of oral contraceptives) when given for periods of more than one year to women after the menopause, increase the risk of cancer of the uterus (womb). There is also some evidence that a kind of oral contraceptive which is no longer marketed, the sequential oral contraceptive, may increase the risk of cancer of the uterus. There remains no evidence, however, that the oral contraceptives now available increase the risk of this cancer.

Oral contraceptives do cause, although rarely, a benign (nonmalignant) tumor of the liver. These tumors do not spread, but they may rupture and cause internal bleeding, which may be fatal. A few cases of cancer of the liver have been reported in women using oral contraceptives, but it is not yet known whether the drug caused them.

c) *Dangers to a developing child if oral contraceptives are used in or immediately following pregnancy.* Oral contraceptives should not be taken by pregnant women because they may damage the developing child. An increased risk of birth defects, including heart defects and limb defects, has been associated with the use of sex hormones, including oral contraceptives, in pregnancy. In addition, the developing female child whose mother has received DES (diethylstilbestrol), an estrogen, during pregnancy has a risk of getting cancer of the vagina or cervix in her teens or young adulthood. This risk is estimated to be about 1 in 1,000 exposures or less. Abnormalities of the urinary and sex organs have been reported in male offspring so exposed. It is possible that other estrogens, such as the estrogens in oral contraceptives, could have the same effect in the child if the mother takes them during pregnancy.

If you stop taking oral contraceptives to become pregnant, your doctor may recommend that you use another method of contraception for a short while. The reason for this is that there is evidence from studies in women who have had "miscarriages" soon after stopping the Pill, that the lost fetuses are more likely to be abnormal. Whether there is an overall increase in miscarriage in women who become pregnant soon after stopping the Pill, as compared with women who do not use the Pill, is not known, but it is possible that there may be. If, however, you do become pregnant soon after stopping oral contraceptives, and do not have a miscarriage, there is no evidence that the baby has an increased risk of being abnormal.

d) *Gallbladder disease.* Women who use oral contraceptives have a greater risk than nonusers of having gallbladder disease requiring surgery. The increased risk may first appear within one year of use and may double after four or five years of use.

e) *Other side effects of oral contraceptives.* Some women using oral contraceptives experience unpleasant side effects that are not dangerous and are not likely to damage their health. Some of these may be temporary. Your breasts may feel tender, nausea and vomiting may occur, you may gain or lose weight, and your ankles may swell. A spotty darkening of the skin, particularly of the face, is possible and may persist. You may notice unexpected vaginal bleeding or changes in your menstrual period. Irregular bleeding is frequently seen when using the minipill or combination oral contraceptives containing less than 50 micrograms of estrogen.

More serious side effects include worsening of migraine, asthma, epilepsy, and kidney or heart disease because of a tendency for water to be retained in the body when oral contraceptives are used. Other side effects are growth of preexisting fibroid tumors of the uterus, mental depression, and liver problems with jaundice (yellowing of the skin). Your doctor may find that levels of sugar and fatty substances in your blood are elevated; the long-term effects of these changes are not known. Some women develop high blood pressure while taking oral contraceptives, which ordinarily returns to the original levels when the oral contraceptive is stopped.

Other reactions, although not proved to be caused by oral contraceptives, are occasionally reported. These include more frequent urination and some discomfort when urinating, nervousness, dizziness, some loss of scalp hair, an increase in body hair, an increase or decrease in sex drive, appetite changes, cataracts, and a need for a change in contact lens prescription or inability to use contact lenses.

After you stop using oral contraceptives, there may be a delay before you are able to become pregnant or before you resume having menstrual periods. This is especially true of women who had irregular menstrual cycles prior to the use of oral contraceptives. As discussed previously, you should wait a short while after stopping the Pill before you try to become pregnant. During this time, use another form of contraception. You should consult your physician before resuming use of oral contraceptives after childbirth, especially if you plan to nurse your baby. Drugs in oral contraceptives are known to appear in the milk, and the long-range effect on infants is not known at this time. Furthermore, oral contraceptives may cause a decrease in your milk supply as well as in the quality of the milk.

Figure 1. Estimated annual number of deaths associated with control of fertility and no control per 100,000 nonsterile women, by regimen of control and age of woman.

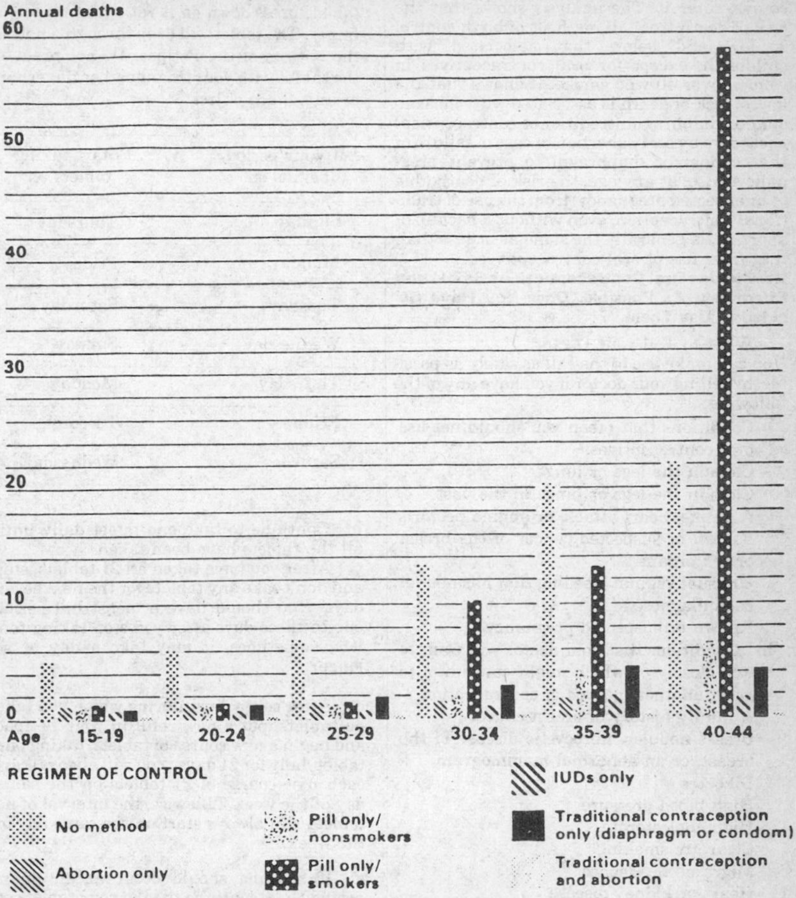

4. Comparison of the Risks of Oral Contraceptives and Other Contraceptive Methods. The many studies on the risks and effectiveness of oral contraceptives and other methods of contraception have been analyzed to estimate the risk of death associated with various methods of contraception. This risk has two parts: (1) the risk of the method itself (eg, the risk that oral contraceptives will cause death due to abnormal clotting); and (2) the risk of death due to pregnancy or abortion in the event the method fails. The results of this analysis are shown in the bar graph (Fig. 1). The height of the bars is the number of deaths per 100,000 women each year. There are six sets of bars, each set referring to a specific age group of women. Within each set of bars, there is a single bar for each of the different contraceptive methods. For oral contraceptives, there are two bars—one for smokers and the other for nonsmokers. The analysis is based on present

Continued on next page

This product information was prepared in August, 1979. On these and other Parke-Davis Products, detailed information may be obtained by addressing PARKE-DAVIS, Division of Warner-Lambert Company, Morris Plains, NJ 07950.

Parke-Davis—Cont.

knowledge and new information could, of course, alter it. The analysis shows that the risk of death from all methods of birth control is low and below that associated with childbirth, except for oral contraceptives in women over 40 who smoke. It shows that the lowest risk of death is associated with the condom or diaphragm (traditional contraception) backed up by early abortion in case of failure of the condom or diaphragm to prevent pregnancy. Also, at any age, the risk of death (due to unexpected pregnancy) from the use of traditional contraception, even without a backup of abortion, is generally the same as or less than that from use of oral contraceptives.

How to Use Oral Contraceptives As Safely and Effectively As Possible, Once You Have Decided to Use Them

1. What to Tell your Doctor.
You can make use of the Pill as safely as possible, by telling your doctor if you have any of the following.

a) Conditions that mean you should not use oral contraceptives:
Clots in the legs or lungs
Clots in the legs or lungs in the past
A stroke, heart attack, or angina pectoris
Known or suspected cancer of the breast or sex organs
Unusual vaginal bleeding that has not yet been diagnosed
Known or suspected pregnancy

b) Conditions that your doctor will want to watch closely or which might cause him to suggest another method of contraception.
A family history of breast cancer
Breast nodules, fibrocystic disease of the breast, or an abnormal mammogram
Diabetes
High blood pressure
High cholesterol
Cigarette smoking
Migraine headaches
Heart or kidney disease
Epilepsy
Mental depression
Fibroid tumors of the uterus
Gallbladder disease

c) Once you are using oral contraceptives, you should be alert for signs of serious adverse effects and call your doctor if they occur.
Sharp pain in the chest, coughing blood, or sudden shortness of breath (indicating possible clots in the lungs)
Pain in the calf (possible clot in the leg)
Crushing chest pain or heaviness (indicating possible heart attack)
Sudden severe headache or vomiting, dizziness or fainting, disturbance of vision or speech, or weakness or numbness in an arm or leg (indicating a possible stroke)
Sudden partial or complete loss of vision (indicating a possible clot in the eye)
Breast lumps (you should ask your doctor to show you how to examine your own breasts)
Severe pain in the abdomen (indicating a possible ruptured tumor of the liver)
Severe depression
Yellowing of the skin (jaundice)

2. How to take the Pill So That it is Most Effective

Directions

Loestrin [21] 1/20

a) The first day of your period is Day 1. On the fifth day (Day 5), start taking a tablet daily, beginning with the tablet in the upper left corner of the Petipac®. In the space provided, write the day you start. To remove the tablet, press down on it with your thumb or finger. The tablet will drop through a hole in the bottom of the Petipac. Do not press on the tablet with your thumbnail or fingernail, or any sharp object.

If your period begins on:	Start taking tablets on:
Sunday	Thursday
Monday	Friday
Tuesday	Saturday
Wednesday	Sunday
Thursday	Monday
Friday	Tuesday
Saturday	Wednesday

b) Continue to take one tablet daily until all the tablets have been taken.

c) After you have taken all 21 tablets, stop and don't take any tablets for the next seven days. You should have a menstrual period one to three days after you stop taking tablets; sometimes, it may take a day or so longer.

d) After seven days, during which you take no tablets, put a new refill in your Petipac and begin a new course of tablets, taking one tablet daily for 21 days. You will always start each new course of 21 tablets on the same day of the week. Likewise, the interval of no tablets will always start on the same day of the week.

e) If spotting should occur at an unexpected time, continue to take your tablets as directed. Spotting is usually temporary and without significance. However, if bleeding should occur at an unexpected time, consult your physician. Call your physician regarding any problem or change in your general health that may concern you.

f) If you forget to take a tablet, take it as soon as you remember, even if it is the next day. Then, take the next scheduled tablet at the usual time. If you miss two consecutive tablets, take two tablets daily for the next two days. Then, resume the regular schedule. However, you should use an additional means of contraception for seven consecutive days. If you miss three consecutive tablets, discard any tablets remaining, and begin a new course of tablets, starting seven days after the last tablet was taken, even if you are still menstruating. You should use an alternate means of contraception, other than oral tablets, until the start of your next menstrual period.

Loestrin [Fe] 1/20

a) The first day of your period is Day 1. On the fifth day (Day 5), start taking one *white* tablet daily, beginning with the tablet in the upper left corner of the Petipac. In the space provided, write the day you start. To remove the tablet, press down on it with your thumb or finger. The tablet will drop through a hole in the bottom of the Petipac. Do not press on the tablet with your thumbnail or fingernail, or any other sharp object.

If your period begins on:	Start taking tablets on:
Sunday	Thursday
Monday	Friday
Tuesday	Saturday
Wednesday	Sunday
Thursday	Monday
Friday	Tuesday
Saturday	Wednesday

b) On the day after taking the last *white* tablet, begin taking one *brown* tablet daily until all the tablets have been taken.

c) When the last tablet has been taken, put a new refill in your Petipac and, without interruption, begin a new course of tablets by taking the *white* tablets first, followed by the *brown* tablets. There should never be a day when you are not taking a tablet.

d) Continue taking *white* tablets without interruption whether or not your period has occurred or is still in progress. Your period will usually occur during the time you are taking *brown* tablets.

e) If spotting should occur at an unexpected time, continue to take your tablets as directed. Spotting is usually temporary and without significance. However, if bleeding should occur at an unexpected time, consult your physician. Call your physician regarding any problem or change in your general health that may concern you.

f) If you forget to take a *white* tablet, take it as soon as you remember, even if it is the next day. Then, take the next scheduled tablet at the usual time. If you miss two consecutive *white* tablets, take two tablets daily for the next two days. Then, resume the regular schedule. However, you should use an additional means of contraception for seven consecutive days. If you miss three consecutive *white* tablets, discard any tablets remaining, and begin a new course of tablets, starting seven days after the last tablet was taken, even if you are still menstruating. You should use an alternate means of contraception, other than oral tablets, until the start of your next menstrual period.

g) If you miss one or more *brown* tablets, discard the remainder and begin a new course of tablets no later than the eighth day after you took the last *white* tablet. Under no circumstances should you substitute a *brown* tablet for a *white* one, or take any *brown* tablets before you have taken all the *white* tablets, unless your physician advises you to do so.

Loestrin [21] 1.5/30

a) The first day of your period is Day 1. One the fifth day (Day 5), start taking a tablet daily, beginning with the tablet in the upper left corner of the Petipac. In the space provided, write the day you start. To remove the tablet, press down on it with your thumb or finger. The tablet will drop through a hole in the bottom of the Petipac. Do not press on the tablet with your thumbnail or fingernail, or any other sharp object.

If your period begins on:	Start taking tablets on:
Sunday	Thursday
Monday	Friday
Tuesday	Saturday
Wednesday	Sunday
Thursday	Monday
Friday	Tuesday
Saturday	Wednesday

b) Continue to take one tablet daily until all the tablets have been taken.
c) After you have taken all 21 tablets, stop and don't take any tablets for the next seven days. You should have a menstrual period one to three days after you stop taking tablets; sometimes, it may take a day or so longer.
d) After seven days, during which you take no tablets, put a new refill in your Petipac and begin a new course of tablets, taking one tablet daily for 21 days. You will always start each new course of 21 tablets on the same day of the week. Likewise, the interval of no tablets will always start on the same day of the week.
e) If spotting should occur at an unexpected time, continue to take your tablets as directed. Spotting is usually temporary and without significance. However, if bleeding should occur at an unexpected time, consult your physician. Call your physician regarding any problem or change in your general health that may concern you.
f) If you forget to take a tablet, take it as soon as you remember, even if it is the next day. Then, take the next scheduled tablet at the usual time. If you miss two consecutive tablets, take two tablets daily for the next two days. Then, resume the regular schedule. While there is little likelihood of pregnancy occurring if you miss only one or two tablets, the possibility of pregnancy increases with each successive day that tablets are missed. If you miss three consecutive tablets, discard any tablets remaining, and begin a new course of tablets, starting seven days after the last tablet was taken, even if you are still menstruating. You should use an alternate means of contraception, other than oral tablets, until the start of your next menstrual period.

Loestrin Fe 1.5/30

a) The first day of your period is Day 1. On the fifth day (Day 5), start taking one *green* tablet daily, beginning with the tablet in the upper left corner of the Petipac. In the space provided, write the day you start. To remove the tablet, press down on it with your thumb or finger. The tablet will drop through a hole in the bottom of the Petipac. Do not press on the tablet with your thumbnail or fingernail, or any other sharp object.

If your period begins on:	Start taking tablets on:
Sunday	Thursday
Monday	Friday
Tuesday	Saturday
Wednesday	Sunday
Thursday	Monday
Friday	Tuesday
Saturday	Wednesday

b) On the day after taking the last *green* tablet, begin taking one *brown* tablet daily until all the tablets have been taken.
c) When the last tablet has been taken, put a new refill in your Petipac and, without interruption, begin a new course of tablets by taking the *green* tablets first, followed by the *brown* tablets. There should never be a day when you are not taking a tablet.
d) Continue taking *green* tablets without interruption whether or not your period has occurred or is still in progress. Your period will usually occur during the time you are taking *brown* tablets.
e) If spotting should occur at an unexpected time, continue to take your tablets as directed. Spotting is usually temporary and without significance. However, if bleeding should occur at an unexpected time, consult your physician. Call your physician regarding any problem or change in your general health that may concern you.
f) If you forget to take a *green* tablet, take it as soon as you remember, even if it is the next day. Then, take the next scheduled tablet at the usual time. If you miss two consecutive *green* tablets, take two tablets daily for the next two days. Then, resume the regular schedule. While there is little likelihood of pregnancy occurring if you miss only one or two *green* tablets, the possibility of pregnancy increases with each successive day that scheduled tablets are missed. If you miss three consecutive *green* tablets, discard any tablets remaining, and begin a new course of tablets, starting seven days after the last tablet was taken, even if you are still menstruating. You should use an alternate means of contraception, other than oral tablets, until the start of your next menstrual period.
g) If you miss one or more *brown* tablets, discard the remainder and begin a new course of tablets no later than the eighth day after you took the last *green* tablet. Under no circumstances should you substitute a *brown* tablet for a *green* one, or take any *brown* tablets before you have taken all the *green* tablets, unless your physician advises you to do so.

Norlestrin 21 1/50

a) The first day of your period is Day 1. On the fifth day (Day 5), start taking a tablet daily, beginning with the tablet in the upper left corner of the Petipac. In the space provided, write the day you start. To remove the tablet, press down on it with your thumb or finger. The tablet will drop through a hole in the bottom of the Petipac. Do not press on the tablet with your thumbnail or fingernail, or any other sharp object.

If your period begins on:	Start taking tablets on:
Sunday	Thursday
Monday	Friday
Tuesday	Saturday
Wednesday	Sunday
Thursday	Monday
Friday	Tuesday
Saturday	Wednesday

b) Continue to take one tablet daily until all the tablets have been taken.
c) After you have taken all 21 tablets, stop and don't take any tablets for the next seven days. You should have a menstrual period one to three days after you stop taking tablets; sometimes, it may take a day or so longer.
d) After seven days, during which you take no tablets, put a new refill in your Petipac and begin a new course of tablets, taking one tablet daily for 21 days. You will always start each new course of 21 tablets on the same day of the week. Likewise, the interval of no tablets will always start on the same day of the week.
e) If spotting should occur at an unexpected time, continue to take your tablets as directed. Spotting is usually temporary and without significance. However, if bleeding should occur at an unexpected time, consult your physician. Call your physician regarding any problem or change in your general health that may concern you.
f) If you forget to take a tablet, take it as soon as you remember, even if it is the next day. Then, take the next scheduled tablet at the usual time. If you miss two consecutive tablets, take two tablets daily for the next two days. Then, resume the regular schedule. While there is little likelihood of pregnancy occurring if you miss only one or two tablets, the possibility of pregnancy increases with each successive day that tablets are missed. If you miss three consecutive tablets, discard any tablets remaining, and begin a new course of tablets, starting seven days after the last tablet was taken, even if you are still menstruating. You should use an alternate means of contraception, other than oral tablets, until the start of your next menstrual period.

Norlestrin 28 1/50

a) The first day of your period is Day 1. On the fifth day (Day 5), start taking one *yellow* tablet daily, beginning with the tablet in the upper left corner of the Petipac. In the space provided, write the day you start. To remove the tablet, press down on it with your thumb or finger. The tablet will drop through a hole in the bottom of the Petipac. Do not press on the tablet with your thumbnail or fingernail, or any other sharp object.

If your period begins on:	Start taking tablets on:
Sunday	Thursday
Monday	Friday
Tuesday	Saturday
Wednesday	Sunday
Thursday	Monday
Friday	Tuesday
Saturday	Wednesday

b) On the day after taking the last *yellow* tablet, begin taking one *white* tablet daily until all the tablets have been taken.
c) When the last tablet has been taken, put a new refill in your Petipac and, without interruption, begin a new course of tablets by taking the *yellow* tablets first, followed by the *white* tablets. There should never be a day when you are not taking a tablet.
d) Continue taking *yellow* tablets without interruption whether or not your period has occurred or is still in progress. Your period will usually occur during the time you are taking *white* tablets.
e) If spotting should occur at an unexpected time, continue to take your tablets as directed. Spotting is usually temporary and without significance. However, if bleeding

Continued on next page

This product information was prepared in August, 1979. On these and other Parke-Davis Products, detailed information may be obtained by addressing PARKE-DAVIS, Division of Warner-Lambert Company, Morris Plains, NJ 07950.

Parke-Davis—Cont.

should occur at an unexpected time, consult your physician. Call your physician regarding any problem or change in your general health that may concern you.

f) If you forget to take a *yellow* tablet, take it as soon as you remember, even if it is the next day. Then, take the next scheduled tablet at the usual time. If you miss two consecutive *yellow* tablets, take two tablets daily for the next two days. Then, resume the regular schedule. While there is little likelihood of pregnancy occurring if you miss only one or two *yellow* tablets, the possibility of pregnancy increases with each successive day that scheduled tablets are missed. If you miss three consecutive *yellow* tablets, discard any tablets remaining, and begin a new course of tablets, starting seven days after the last tablet was taken, even if you are still menstruating. You should use an alternate means of contraception, other than oral tablets, until the start of your next menstrual period.

g) If you miss one or more *white* tablets, discard the remainder and begin a new course of tablets no later than the eighth day after you took the last *yellow* tablet. Under no circumstances should you substitute a *white* tablet for a *yellow* one, or take any *white* tablets before you have taken all the *yellow* tablets, unless your physician advises you to do so.

Norlestrin Fe 1/50

a) The first day of your period is Day 1. On the fifth day (Day 5), start taking one *yellow* tablet daily, beginning with the tablet in the upper left corner of the Petipac. In the space provided, write the day you start. To remove the tablet, press down on it with your thumb or finger. The tablet will drop through a hole in the bottom of the Petipac. Do not press on the tablet with your thumbnail or fingernail, or any other sharp object.

If your period begins on:	Start taking tablets on:
Sunday	Thursday
Monday	Friday
Tuesday	Saturday
Wednesday	Sunday
Thursday	Monday
Friday	Tuesday
Saturday	Wednesday

b) On the day after taking the last *yellow* tablet, begin taking one *brown* tablet daily until all the tablets have been taken.

c) When the last tablet has been taken, put a new refill in your Petipac and, without interruption, begin a new course of tablets by taking the *yellow* tablets first, followed by the *brown* tablets. There should never be a day when you are not taking a tablet.

d) Continue taking *yellow* tablets without interruption whether or not your period has occurred or is still in progress. Your period will usually occur during the time you are taking *brown* tablets.

e) If spotting should occur at an unexpected time, continue to take your tablets as directed. Spotting is usually temporary and without significance. However, if bleeding should occur at an unexpected time, consult your physician. Call your physician regarding any problem or change in your general health that may concern you.

f) If you forget to take a *yellow* tablet, take it as soon as you remember, even if it is the next day. Then, take the next scheduled tablet at the usual time. If you miss two consecutive *yellow* tablets, take two tablets daily for the next two days. Then, resume the regular schedule. While there is little likelihood of pregnancy occurring if you miss only one or two *yellow* tablets, the possibility of pregnancy increases with each successive day that scheduled tablets are missed. If you miss three consecutive *yellow* tablets, discard any tablets remaining, and begin a new course of tablets, starting seven days after the last tablet was taken, even if you are still menstruating. You should use an alternate means of contraception, other than oral tablets, until the start of your next menstrual period.

g) If you miss one or more *brown* tablets, discard the remainder and begin a new course of tablets no later than the eighth day after you took the last *yellow* tablet. Under no circumstances should you substitute a *brown* tablet for a *yellow* one, or take any *brown* tablets before you have taken all the *yellow* tablets, unless your physician advises you to do so.

Norlestrin 21 2.5/50

a) The first day of your period is Day 1. On the fifth day (Day 5), start taking a tablet daily, beginning with the tablet in the upper left corner of the Petipac. In the space provided, write the day you start. To remove the tablet, press down on it with your thumb or finger. The tablet will drop through a hole in the bottom of the Petipac. Do not press on the tablet with your thumbnail or fingernail, or any other sharp object.

If your period begins on:	Start taking tablets on:
Sunday	Thursday
Monday	Friday
Tuesday	Saturday
Wednesday	Sunday
Thursday	Monday
Friday	Tuesday
Saturday	Wednesday

b) Continue to take one tablet daily until all the tablets have been taken.

c) After you have taken all 21 tablets, stop and don't take any tablets for the next seven days. You should have a menstrual period one to three days after you stop taking tablets; sometimes, it may take a day or so longer.

d) After 7 days, during which you take no tablets, put a new refill in your Petipac and begin a new course of tablets, taking one tablet daily for 21 days. You will always start each new course of 21 tablets on the same day of the week. Likewise, the interval of no tablets will always start on the same day of the week.

e) If spotting should occur at an unexpected time, continue to take your tablets as directed. Spotting is usually temporary and without significance. However, if bleeding should occur at an unexpected time, consult your physician. Call your physician regarding any problem or change in your general health that may concern you.

f) If you forget to take a tablet, take it as soon as you remember, even if it is the next day. Then, take the next scheduled tablet at the usual time. If you miss two consecutive tablets, take two tablets daily for the next two days. Then, resume the regular schedule. While there is little likelihood of pregnancy occurring if you miss only one or two tablets, the possibility of pregnancy increases with each successive day that tablets are missed. If you miss three consecutive tablets, discard any tablets remaining, and begin a new course of tablets, starting seven days after the last tablet was taken, even if you are still menstruating. You should use an alternate means of contraception, other than oral tablets, until the start of your next menstrual period.

Norlestrin Fe 2.5/50

a) The first day of your period is Day 1. On the fifth day (Day 5), start taking one *pink* tablet daily, beginning with the tablet in the upper left corner of the Petipac. In the space provided, write the day you start. To remove the tablet, press down on it with your thumb or finger. The tablet will drop through a hole in the bottom of the Petipac. Do not press on the tablet with your thumbnail or fingernail, or any other sharp object.

If your period begins on:	Start taking tablets on:
Sunday	Thursday
Monday	Friday
Tuesday	Saturday
Wednesday	Sunday
Thursday	Monday
Friday	Tuesday
Saturday	Wednesday

b) On the day after taking the last *pink* tablet, begin taking one *brown* tablet daily until all the tablets have been taken.

c) When the last tablet has been taken, put a new refill in your Petipac and, without interruption, begin a new course of tablets by taking the *pink* tablets first, followed by the *brown* tablets. There should never be a day when you are not taking a tablet.

d) Continue taking *pink* tablets without interruption whether or not your period has occurred or is still in progress. Your period will usually occur during the time you are taking *brown* tablets.

e) If spotting should occur at an unexpected time, continue to take your tablets as directed. Spotting is usually temporary and without significance. However, if bleeding should occur at an unexpected time, consult your physician. Call your physician regarding any problem or change in your general health that may concern you.

f) If you forget to take a *pink* tablet, take it as soon as you remember, even if it is the next day. Then, take the next scheduled tablet at the usual time. If you miss two consecutive *pink* tablets, take two tablets daily for the next two days. Then, resume the regular schedule. While there is little likelihood of pregnancy occurring if you miss only one or two *pink* tablets, the possibility of pregnancy increases with each successive day that scheduled tablets are missed. If you miss three consecutive *pink* tablets, discard any tablets remaining, and begin a new course of tablets, starting seven days after the last tablet was taken, even if you are still menstruating. You should use an alternate means of contraception, other than oral tablets, until the start of your next menstrual period.

g) If you miss one or more *brown* tablets, discard the remainder and begin a new course of tablets no later than the eighth day after you took the last *pink* tablet. Under no circumstances should you substitute a *brown* tablet for a *pink* one, or take any *brown* tablets before you have taken all the *pink* tablets, unless your physician advises you to do so.

Loestrin and Norlestrin Products

At times, there may be no menstrual period after a cycle of pills. Therefore, if you miss one menstrual period, but have taken the pills *exactly as you were supposed to,* continue as usual into the next cycle. If you have not taken the pills correctly and miss a menstrual period, *you may be pregnant* and should stop taking oral contraceptives until your doctor determines whether or not you are pregnant. Until you can get to your doctor, use another form of contraception. If two consecutive menstrual periods are missed, you should stop taking pills until it is determined whether you are pregnant. If you do become pregnant while using oral contraceptives, you should discuss the risks to the developing child with your doctor.

3. Periodic Examination.

Your doctor will take a complete medical and family history before prescribing oral contraceptives. At that time and about once a year thereafter, he will generally examine your blood pressure, breasts, abdomen, and pelvic organs (including a Papanicolaou smear, ie, test for cancer).

Summary: Oral contraceptives are the most effective method, except sterilization, for preventing pregnancy. Other methods, when used conscientiously, are also very effective and have fewer risks. The serious risks of oral contraceptives are uncommon and the Pill is a very convenient method of preventing pregnancy.

If you have certain conditions or have had these conditions in the past, you should not use oral contraceptives because the risk is too great. These conditions are listed in this leaflet. If you do not have these conditions, and decide to use the Pill, please read this leaflet carefully so that you can use the Pill most safely and effectively.

Based on his or her assessment of your medical needs, your doctor has prescribed this drug for you. Do not give this drug to anyone else.

WC

[*Shown in Product Identification Section*]

MANDELAMINE® ℞
(methenamine mandelate)

Caution: Federal law prohibits dispensing without prescription.
[See table above].

DOSAGES
Mandelamine (methenamine mandelate)

	Dosage: Adults	Dosage: Children	Supplied
Tablets and Granules			
1.0 gram	1 tablet q.i.d.	—	Tablets W/C 172: purple, enteric coated in bottles of 100 (N 0047-0172-51) and 1000 (N 0047-0172-60); also unit dose in 10 x 10 strips (N 0047-0172-11)
	1 packet* q.i.d.	—	Granules:* orange-flavored individual packets; cartons of 56 (N 0047-0176-11)
0.5 gram	2 tablets q.i.d.	(Ages 6–12) 1 tablet q.i.d.	Tablets W/C 171: brown, enteric coated in bottles of 100 (N 0047-0171-51) and 1000 (N 0047-0171-60); unit dose in 10 x 10 strips (N 0047-0171-11)
	—	(Ages 6–12) 1 packet* q.i.d.	Granules:* orange-flavored individual packets; cartons of 56 (N 0047-0177-11)
0.25 gram	—	(Age under 6) 1 tablet per 30 lb body weight q.i.d.	Tablets W/C 170: brown, enteric coated in bottles of 100 (N 0047-0170-51) and 1000 (N 0047-0170-60)
Suspension Forte 500 mg/5 ml teaspoonful	2 teaspoonfuls (10 ml) q.i.d.	(Ages 6–12) 1 teaspoonful (5 ml) q.i.d.	Suspension Forte†: pink, cherry-flavored in bottles of 8 fl oz (N 0047-0174-08) and 16 fl oz (N 0047-0174-16). U.S. Patent No. 3,077,438
Suspension 250 mg/5 ml teaspoonful	—	(Age under 6) 1 teaspoonful (5 ml) per 30 lb body weight q.i.d.	Suspension†: cream-colored, coconut-flavored in bottles of 16 fl oz (N 0047-0173-16)

*Contents of packet to be dissolved in 2–4 oz water immediately before using.
†Suspensions are in vegetable oil. Shake well before using.

Description: Mandelamine, a urinary antibacterial agent, is the chemical combination of mandelic acid with methenamine.

Actions: Mandelamine is readily absorbed but remains essentially inactive until it is excreted by the kidney and concentrated in the urine. An acid urine is essential for antibacterial action with maximum efficacy occurring at pH 5.5 or less. In an acid urine, mandelic acid exerts its antibacterial action and also contributes to the acidification of the urine. Mandelic acid is excreted by both glomerular filtration and tubular excretion. The methenamine component, in an acid urine, is hydrolyzed to ammonia and to the bactericidal agent formaldehyde. There is equally effective antibacterial activity against both gram-positive and gram-negative organisms, since the antibacterial action of mandelic acid and formaldehyde is nonspecific. There are reports that Mandelamine is ineffective in some infections with *Proteus vulgaris* and urea-splitting strains of *Pseudomonas aeruginosa* and *A. aerogenes.* Since urea-splitting strains may raise the pH of the urine, particular attention to supplementary acidification is required. However, results in any single case will depend to a large extent on the underlying pathology and the overall management.

Rationale: *Prophylactic use*—Urine is a good culture medium for many urinary pathogens. Inoculation by a few organisms (relapse or reinfection) may lead to bacteriuria in susceptible individuals. Thus, the rationale of management in recurring urinary tract infection (bacteriuria) is to change the urine from a growth-supporting to a growth-inhibiting medium. There is a growing body of evidence that long-term administration of Mandelamine can prevent the recurrence of bacteriuria in patients with chronic pyelonephritis.

Therapeutic use—Mandelamine helps to sterilize the urine and, in some situations in which underlying pathologic conditions prevent sterilization by any means, it can help to suppress the bacteriuria. Mandelamine should not be used alone for acute infections with parenchymal involvement causing systemic symptoms such as chills and fever. A thorough diagnostic investigation as a part of the overall management of the urinary tract infection should accompany the use of Mandelamine.

Indications: Mandelamine (methenamine mandelate) is indicated for the suppression or elimination of bacteriuria associated with pyelonephritis, cystitis, and other chronic urinary tract infections; also for infected residual urine sometimes accompanying neurologic diseases.

When used as recommended, Mandelamine is particularly suitable for long-term therapy because of its safety and because resistance to the nonspecific bactericidal action of formaldehyde does not develop. Pathogens resistant to other antibacterial agents may respond to Mandelamine because of the nonspecific effect of formaldehyde formed in an acid urine.

Contraindication: Renal insufficiency.

Precautions: Dysuria may occur (usually at higher than recommended dosage). This can be controlled by reducing the dosage and the acidification. When urine acidification is contraindicated or unattainable (as with some urea-splitting bacteria), the drug is not recommended.

Continued on next page

This product information was prepared in August, 1979. On these and other Parke-Davis Products, detailed information may be obtained by addressing PARKE-DAVIS, Division of Warner-Lambert Company, Morris Plains, NJ 07950.

Parke-Davis—Cont.

To avoid inducing lipid pneumonia, administer Mandelamine Suspension Forte and Mandelamine Suspension with care to elderly, debilitated or otherwise susceptible patients.
Adverse Reactions: An occasional patient may experience gastrointestinal disturbance or a generalized skin rash.
Dosage and Management: The average adult dosage is 4 grams daily given as 1.0 gram after each meal and at bedtime. Children 6 to 12 should receive half the adult dose and children under 6 years of age should receive 250 mg per 30 lb body weight, four times daily. [See accompanying Chart on preceding page]
Since an acid urine is essential for antibacterial activity with maximum efficacy occurring at pH 5.5 or below, restriction of alkalinizing foods and medication is thus desirable. If testing of urine pH reveals the need, supplemental acidification should be given.
STORE BETWEEN 59°–86°F (15°–30°C).
[*Shown in Product Identification Section*]
308 G 903 **9-77**

METED® /METED® 2
antidandruff
Lotion Shampoos

Description: Meted is for oily dandruff and scalp and hair problems. Meted 2 is for dry scaly dandruff.

	Meted	Meted 2
Sulfur	3%	—
Colloidal sulfur	—	2.3%
Salicylic Acid	2%	1%

These shampoos also contain polyethylene glycol 400, sodium lauryl sulfate, polyoxyethylene lauryl ether, magnesium aluminum silicate, synthetic perfume and purified water. Meted 2 also contains methylparaben.
Actions: Meted lotion shampoo helps control symptoms of seborrheic dermatitis and other seborrheic problems through the actiion of sulfur and salicylic acid combined with a concentrated degergent system. In Meted, the combination of sulfur and salicylic acid with a highly concentrated degreasing system for oily hair and scalp helps control the scaling, oiliness and pruritus associated with oily dandruff. Meted can also be used as an oily skin cleanser.
Meted 2 lotion shampoo helps control symptoms of pityriasis sicca through the actions of colloidal sulfur, salicylic acid and a detergent system for dry hair and scalp. The antiseborrheic and keratolytic/keratoplastic properties of sulfur and salicylic acid incorporated into Meted and Meted 2 have long been recognized as effective controls for symptoms of seborrhea capitis.
Advantages: Meted and Meted 2 are effective, easy to use, and pleasantly scented. After being rinsed, hair, scalp and skin areas feel clean. Meted and Meted 2 contain a special conditioning agent to leave the hair easy to manage, soft and glossy.
Contraindications: Hypersentitivity to any components of these preparations.
Precautions and Adverse Reactions: Avoid contact with eyes. If lather gets into eyes, flush well with water. If undue skin irritation develops or increases, discontinue use. Keep this and all medications out of reach of children.
Directions: SHAKE WELL BEFORE USING.
Meted:
Apply to wet hair and scalp, rub into scalp, adding water liberally to produce lather. Rinse and repeat. For simple oily scalp, allow lather to remain 2–3 minutes; for extremely oily conditions, allow second lather to remain up to 10 minutes. Most patients find one or two shampoos per week sufficient; those with extremely oily conditions may use Meted more frequently until the condition is controlled.
As an oily skin cleanser: Apply to moistened skin. Massage to lather. Leave on skin 2–5 minutes. Rinse.
Meted 2: Apply liberally to wet hair and scalp; rub into scalp to produce lather. Rise and repeat. Most patients will find two shampoos per week to be sufficient.
How Supplied: Meted Lotion Shampoo–4-oz plastic bottles (N 0064-3910-04).
Meted 2 Lotion Shampoo—4-oz plastic bottles (N 0064-3913-04).

MILONTIN® ℞
(phensuximide, NF)

Description: Milontin (phensuximide) is an anticonvulsant succinimide, chemically designated as N-methyl-2-phenylsuccinimide.
Action: Phensuximide suppresses the paroxysmal three-cycle-per-second spike and wave activity associated with lapses of consciousness which is common in absence (petit mal) seizures. The frequency of epileptiform attacks is reduced, apparently by depression of the motor cortex and elevation of the threshold of the central nervous system to convulsive stimuli.
Indication: Milontin is indicated for the control of absence (petit mal) seizures.
Contraindication: Phensuximide should not be used in patients with a history of hypersensitivity to succinimides.
Warnings: Blood dyscrasias, including some with fatal outcome, have been reported to be associated with the use of succinimides; therefore, periodic blood counts should be performed.
It has been reported that succinimides have produced morphological and functional changes in animal liver. For this reason, phensuximide should be administered with extreme caution to patients with known liver or renal diseases. Periodic urinalysis and liver function studies are advised for all patients receiving the drug.
Cases of systemic lupus erythematosus have been reported with the use of succinimides. The physician should be alert to this possibility.
Usage in pregnancy: The effects of Milontin in human pregnancy and nursing infants are unknown.
Recent reports suggest an association between the use of anticonvulsant drugs by women with epilepsy and an elevated incidence of birth defects in children born to these women. Data is more extensive with respect to phenytoin and phenobarbital, but these are also the most commonly prescribed anticonvulsants; less systematic or anecdotal reports suggest a possible similar association with the use of all known anticonvulsant drugs.
The reports suggesting an elevated incidence of birth defects in children of drug-treated epileptic women cannot be regarded as adequate to prove a definite cause-and-effect relationship. There are intrinsic methodologic problems in obtaining adequate data on drug teratogenicity in humans; the possibility also exists that other factors, eg, genetic factors or the epileptic condition itself, may be more important than drug therapy in leading to birth defects. The great majority of mothers on anticonvulsant medication deliver normal infants. It is important to note that anticonvulsant drugs should not be discontinued in patients in whom the drug is administered to prevent major seizures because of the strong possibility of precipitating status epilepticus with attendant hypoxia and threat to life. In individual cases where the severity and frequency of the seizure disorder are such that the removal of medication does not pose a serious threat to the patient, discontinuation of the drug may be considered prior to and during pregnancy, although it cannot be said with any confidence that even minor seizures do not pose some hazard to the developing embryo or fetus.
The prescribing physician will wish to weigh these considerations in treating or counseling epileptic women of childbearing potential.
Hazardous activities: Phensuximide may impair the mental and/or physical abilities required for the performance of potentially hazardous tasks, such as driving a motor vehicle or other such activity requiring alertness; therefore, the patient should be cautioned accordingly.
Precautions: Phensuximide, when used alone in mixed types of epilepsy, may increase the frequency of grand mal seizures in some patients.
As with other anticonvulsants, it is important to proceed slowly when increasing or decreasing dosage, as well as when adding or eliminating other medication. Abrupt withdrawal of anticonvulsant medication may precipitate absence (petit mal) status.
Adverse Reactions:
Gastrointestinal System: Gastrointestinal symptoms, such as nausea, vomiting, and anorexia, occur frequently, but may be the result of overdosage.
Nervous System: Neurologic and sensory reactions reported during therapy with phensuximide have included drowsiness, dizziness, ataxia, headache, dreamlike state, and lethargy. Side effects, such as drowsiness and dizziness, may be relieved by a reduction in total dosage.
Integumentary System: Dermatologic manifestations reported to be associated with the administration of phensuximide have included pruritus, skin eruptions, erythema multiforme, and erythematous rashes.
Genitourinary System: Genitourinary complications which have been reported include urinary frequency, renal damage, and hematuria.
Hemopoietic System: Hemopoietic complications associated with the administration of phensuximide include granulocytopenia, transient leukopenia, and pancytopenia.
Other: Miscellaneous reactions reported have been alopecia and muscular weakness.
Dosage and Administration: Milontin (phensuximide, NF) is administered by the oral route in doses of 500 mg to 1 g two or three times daily. As with other anticonvulsant medication, the dosage should be adjusted to suit individual requirements. The total dosage, irrespective of age, may, therefore, vary between 1 and 3 g per day, the average being 1.5 g. For pediatric administration, phensuximide is available as a pleasant-flavored liquid. Because each 5 ml of the oral suspension contains 300 mg of the drug, the usual dose may vary from 2 to 4 teaspoonfuls two or three times daily.
Milontin may be administered in combination with other anticonvulsants when other forms of epilepsy coexist with absence (petit mal).
How Supplied:
N 0071-0393-24 (Kapseal 393)—Milontin Kapseals, each containing 500 mg phensuximide; bottles of 100. Parcode® No. 393
N 0071-2321-23—Milontin Suspension, each 5 ml contains 300 mg phensuximide; in 16-oz bottles.
YA

MYADEC®

Each tablet represents:		% of US Recommended Daily Allowances (US RDA)
Vitamins		
Vitamin A	10,000 IU*	200%
Vitamin D	400 IU	100%
Vitamin E	30 IU	100%
Vitamin C	250 mg	417%
Folic Acid	0.4 mg	100%
Thiamine	10 mg	667%
Riboflavin	10 mg	588%
Niacin†	100 mg	500%

Vitamin B_6	5 mg	250%
Vitamin B_{12}	6 mcg	100%
Pantothenic Acid	20 mg	200%
Minerals		
Iodine	150 mcg	100%
Iron	20 mg	111%
Magnesium	100 mg	25%
Copper	2 mg	100%
Zinc	20 mg	133%
Manganese	1.25 mg	‡

Ingredients: Sodium ascorbate, magnesium oxide, microcrystalline cellulose, niacinamide, ferrous fumarate, ascorbic acid, zinc sulfate monohydrate, gelatin, vitamin E acetate, polyvinylpyrrolidone, calcium pantothenate, hydroxypropyl methylcellulose, silicon dioxide, riboflavin, thiamine mononitrate, magnesium stearate, pyridoxine hydrochloride, propylene glycol, cupric sulfate anhydrous, sugar, manganese sulfate monohydrate, vitamin A acetate, ethylcellulose, citric acid anhydrous, polysorbate 80, folic acid, wax, potassium iodide vitamin D_2, titanium dioxide, vanillin, FD&C Yellow No. 6, FD&D Blue No. 2, FD&C Red No. 3, and vitamin B_{12}.

* International Units
† Supplied as niacinamide
‡ No US Recommended Daily Allowance (US RDA) has been established for this nutrient.

Actions and Uses: For prevention of certain vitamin deficiencies. Also supplies various minerals normally present in body tissues.
Dosage: One tablet daily
How Supplied: N 0071-0335. In bottles of 130 and 250.

NARDIL® ℞
(phenelzine sulfate)

Caution: Federal law prohibits dispensing without prescription.
Description: Nardil (phenelzine sulfate) is a potent inhibitor of monoamine oxidase (MAO). Chemically, it is a hydrazine derivative, phenethylhydrazine sulfate.
Actions: Monoamine oxidase is a complex enzyme system, widely distributed throughout the body. Drugs that inhibit monoamine oxidase in the laboratory are associated with a number of clinical effects. Thus, it is unknown whether MAO inhibition *per se*, other pharmacologic actions, or an interaction of both is responsible for the clinical effects observed. Therefore, the physician should become familiar with all the effects produced by drugs of this class.
Indications: Nardil (phenelzine sulfate) has been found to be effective in depressed patients clinically characterized as "atypical," "nonendogenous," or "neurotic." These patients often have mixed anxiety and depression and phobic or hypochondriacal features. There is less conclusive evidence of its usefulness with severely depressed patients with endogenous features.
Nardil should rarely be the first antidepressant drug used. Rather, it is more suitable for use with patients who have failed to respond to the drugs more commonly used for these conditions.
Nardil has had considerable use in combination with dibenzazepine derivatives in treatment-resistant patients without a significant incidence of serious side effects.
Contraindications: Nardil (phenelzine sulfate) is contraindicated in patients with known sensitivity to the drug, pheochromocytoma, congestive heart failure, a history of liver disease, or abnormal liver function tests. (See WARNINGS for other conditions.)
The potentiation of sympathomimetic substances by MAO inhibitors may result in hypertensive crises (See WARNINGS); therefore, patients taking Nardil (phenelzine sulfate) should not be given **sympathomimetic drugs** (including methyl dopa, L-dopa, dopamine, and tryptamine-containing substances as well as epinephrine and norepinephrine); or foods with a high concentration of tryptamine-containing substances or **tyramine** (pods of broad beans, aged cheeses, beer, wines, pickled herring, chicken liver, yeast extract). Excessive amounts of caffeine and chocolate can also cause hypertensive reactions.
Nardil (phenelzine sulfate) should not be used in combination with some CNS depressants such as alcohol and narcotics (e.g., meperidine); death has been reported in patients who have received meperidine and Nardil (phenelzine sulfate) concomitantly. Nardil (phenelzine sulfate) should not be administered together with or in rapid succession to other MAO inhibitors because HYPERTENSIVE CRISES and convulsive seizures, fever, marked sweating, excitation, delirium, tremor, coma, and circulatory collapse may occur.

List of MAO Inhibitors

Generic Name	Trademark
pargyline hydrochloride	Eutonyl® (Abbott Laboratories)
pargyline hydrochloride and methylclothiazide	Eutron® (Abbott Laboratories)
furazolidone	Furoxone® (Eaton Laboratories)
isocarboxazid	Marplan® (Roche Laboratories)
nialamide	Niamid® (Pfizer Laboratories)
tranylcypromine	Parnate® (Smith Kline & French Laboratories)

Patients taking Nardil (phenelzine sulfate) should not undergo elective surgery requiring general anesthesia. Also, they should not be given cocaine or local anesthesia containing sympathomimetic vasoconstrictors. The possible combined hypotensive effects of Nardil (phenelzine sulfate) and spinal anesthesia should be kept in mind. Nardil (phenelzine sulfate) should be discontinued at least 10 days prior to elective surgery.
IMPORTANT
Warnings: The most serious reactions to Nardil (phenelzine sulfate) involve changes in blood pressure.
Hypertensive Crises: The most important reaction associated with Nardil (phenelzine sulfate) administration is the occurrence of hypertensive crises, which have sometimes been fatal.
These crises are characterized by some or all of the following symptoms: occipital headache which may radiate frontally, palpitation, neck stiffness or soreness, nausea, vomiting, sweating (sometimes with fever and sometimes with cold, clammy skin), dilated pupils, and photophobia. Either tachycardia or bradycardia may be present and can be associated with constricting chest pain.
NOTE: Intracranial bleeding has been reported in association with the increase in blood pressure.
Blood pressure should be observed frequently to detect evidence of any pressor response in all patients receiving Nardil (phenelzine sulfate). Therapy should be discontinued immediately upon the occurrence of palpitation or frequent headaches during therapy.
Recommended treatment in hypertensive crisis: If a hypertensive crisis occurs, Nardil (phenelzine sulfate) should be discontinued immediately and therapy to lower blood pressure should be instituted immediately. On the basis of present evidence, phentolamine is recommended. (The dosage reported for phentolamine is 5 mg intravenously.) Care should be taken to administer this drug slowly in order to avoid producing an excessive hypotensive effect. Fever should be managed by means of external cooling.
Warning to the patient: All patients should be warned against eating foods with high tyramine content (aged cheeses, wines, beer, pickled herring, broad bean pods, chicken liver, yeast extract); any high protein food that is aged or has undergone breakdown by putrefaction process to improve flavor is suspect of being able to produce a hypertensive crisis in patients taking MAO inhibitors; against drinking alcoholic beverages and against self-medication with certain proprietary agents such as cold, hay fever or reducing preparations while undergoing Nardil (phenelzine sulfate) therapy. Beverages containing caffeine may be used in moderation.
Patients should be instructed to report promptly the occurrence of headache or other unusual symptoms.
Concomitant Use with Tricyclic (Dibenzazepine) Derivatives
If the decision is made to administer Nardil concurrently with other antidepressant drugs, or within less than 10 days after discontinuation of antidepressant therapy, the patient should be cautioned by the physician regarding the possibility of adverse drug interaction.

List of Tricyclic (dibenzazepine derivative) Drugs

Generic Name	Trademark
nortriptyline hydrochloride	Aventyl® (Eli Lilly & Co.)
amitriptyline hydrochloride	Amitril® (Parke-Davis)
amitriptyline hydrochloride	Elavil® (Merck Sharp & Dohme)
amitriptyline hydrochloride	Endep® (Roche Laboratories)
perphenazine & amitriptyline hydrochloride	Etrafon® (Schering Corporation)
perphenazine & amitriptyline hydrochloride	Triavil® (Merck Sharp & Dohme)
desipramine hydrochloride	Norpramin® (Merrell-National)
desipramine hydrochloride	Pertofrane® (USV)
imipramine hydrochloride	Tofranil® (Geigy)

Nardil (phenelzine sulfate) should be used with caution in combination with antihypertensive drugs, including thiazide diuretics, since hypotension may result. MAO inhibitors including Nardil (phenelzine sulfate) are contraindicated in patients receiving guanethidine.
Use in Pregnancy: The safe use of Nardil (phenelzine sulfate) during pregnancy or lactation has not been established. The potential benefit of this drug, if used during pregnancy, lactation, or in women of childbearing age, should be weighed against the possible hazard to the mother or fetus.
Doses of Nardil (phenelzine sulfate) in pregnant mice well exceeding the maximum recommended human dose have caused a significant decrease in the number of viable offspring per mouse. In addition, the growth of young dogs and rats has been retarded by doses exceeding the maximum human dose.
Use in Children: Nardil (phenelzine sulfate) is not recommended for patients under 16 years of age since there are no controlled studies of safety in this age group.
Nardil (phenelzine sulfate), as with other hydrazine derivatives, has been reported to induce pulmonary and vascular tumors in an uncontrolled lifetime study in mice.
Precautions: In depressed patients, the possibility of suicide should always be considered and adequate precautions taken. It is recom-

Continued on next page

This product information was prepared in August, 1979. On these and other Parke-Davis Products, detailed information may be obtained by addressing PARKE-DAVIS, Division of Warner-Lambert Company, Morris Plains, NJ 07950.

Parke-Davis—Cont.

mended that careful observations of patients undergoing Nardil (phenelzine sulfate) treatment be maintained until control of depression is achieved. If necessary, additional measures (ECT, hospitalization, etc.) should be instituted.
All patients undergoing treatment with Nardil (phenelzine sulfate) should be closely followed for symptoms of postural hypotension. Hypotensive side effects have occurred in hypertensive as well as normal and hypotensive patients. Blood pressure usually returns to pretreatment levels rapidly when the drug is discontinued or the dosage is reduced.
Because the effect of Nardil (phenelzine sulfate) on the convulsive threshold may be variable, adequate precautions should be taken when treating epileptic patients.
Of the more severe side effects that have been reported with any consistency, hypomania has been the most common. This reaction has been largely limited to patients in whom disorders characterized by hyperkinetic symptoms coexist with, but are obscured by, depressive affect; hypomania usually appeared as depression improved. If agitation is present, it may be increased with Nardil (phenelzine sulfate). Hypomania and agitation have also been reported at higher than recommended doses, or following long-term therapy.
Nardil (phenelzine sulfate) may cause excessive stimulation in schizophrenic patients; in manic-depressive states it may result in a swing from a depressive to a manic phase.
MAO inhibitors, including Nardil (phenelzine sulfate), potentiate hexobarbital hypnosis in animals. Therefore, barbiturates should be given at a reduced dose with Nardil (phenelzine sulfate).
MAO inhibitors inhibit the destruction of serotonin and norepinephrine, which are believed to be released from tissue stores by rauwolfia alkaloids. Accordingly, caution should be exercised when rauwolfia is used concomitantly with an MAO inhibitor, including Nardil (phenelzine sulfate).
There is conflicting evidence as to whether or not MAO inhibitors affect glucose metabolism or potentiate hypoglycemic agents. This should be kept in mind if Nardil (phenelzine sulfate) is administered in diabetics.
Adverse Reactions: Nardil (phenelzine sulfate) is a potent inhibitor of monoamine oxidase. Because this enzyme is widely distributed throughout the body, diverse pharmacologic effects can be expected to occur. When they occur, such effects tend to be mild or moderate in severity (see below), often subside as treatment continues, and can be minimized by adjusting dosage; rarely is it necessary to institute counteracting measures or to discontinue Nardil (phenelzine sulfate). Common side effects include dizziness, constipation, dry mouth, postural hypotension, drowsiness, weakness and fatigue, edema, gastrointestinal disturbances, tremors, twitching, and hyperreflexia.
Less common mild to moderate side effects, some of which have been reported in a single patient or by a single physician, include blurred vision, glaucoma, sweating, skin rash, jitteriness, palilalia, urinary retention, euphoria, nystagmus, sexual disturbances and hypernatremia.
Although reported less frequently, and sometimes only once, additional severe side effects have included ataxia, shock-like coma, edema of the glottis, transient respiratory and cardiovascular depression following ECT, leukopenia, toxic delirium, reversible jaundice, manic reaction, convulsions, acute anxiety reaction and precipitation of schizophrenia. To date, fatal progressive necrotizing hepatocellular damage has been reported in a very few patients.
Dosage and Administration: *Initial dose*—the usual starting dose of Nardil (phenelzine sulfate) is one tablet (15 mg) three times a day.
Early phase treatment: dosage should be increased to at least 60 mg per day at a fairly rapid pace consistent with patient tolerance. It may be necessary to increase dosage up to 90 mg per day to obtain sufficient MAO inhibition. Many patients do not show a clinical response until treatment at 60 mg has been continued for at least 4 weeks.
Maintenance dose—after maximum benefit from Nardil (phenelzine sulfate) is achieved, dosage should be reduced slowly over several weeks. Maintenance dose may be as low as 1 tablet, 15 mg, a day or every other day, and should be continued for as long as is required.
Overdosage: Accidental or intentional overdosage with any medication is possible and may be somewhat more common in patients who are depressed. Mild overdoses of Nardil (phenelzine sulfate) are characterized by the appearance of drowsiness, followed by dizziness, ataxia, and irritability. With the usual supportive measures and no specific treatment, complete recovery from mild overdoses usually occurs within 3 to 4 days.
There are no data on the average lethal dose in man.
In severe overdosage of Nardil (phenelzine sulfate) the initial manifestation is faintness, with hypotension and, occasionally, precordial pain and intense headache. Should hypotension require the use of vasopressors it should be remembered that they are potentiated by Nardil (phenelzine sulfate). Hyperactivity and marked agitation may occur. The skin may be cool and clammy with profuse perspiration; coma, seizures, and signs of peripheral circulatory collapse may also occur. In some cases trismus and opisthotonos may be observed, the pulse may become fast and irregular, and respiration may become shallow. Treatment is largely symptomatic and may vary from patient to patient. Measures generally recommended to counteract overdosage of MAO inhibitors should be followed; mainly, these include bed rest, maintenance of hydration and electrolyte balance, avoidance of CNS stimulants, and, when necessary, use of an intravenous phenothiazine.
How Supplied: Tablets—each orange-coated tablet bears the W/C 270 monogram and contains phenelzine sulfate equivalent to 15 mg of phenelzine base; bottles of 100 (N 0047-0270-51).
Store Between 59° and 86°F (15° and 30°C).
[*Shown in Product Identification Section*]
323 G 440 **4-78**

NATABEC® KAPSEALS®

Each capsule represents:

Vitamins	
Vitamin A	4,000 IU*
Vitamin D	400 IU
Vitamin C (ascorbic acid)	50 mg
Thiamine (vitamin B_1)	3 mg
Riboflavin (vitamin B_2)	2.0 mg
Niacin	20 mg⁺
Vitamin B_6	3 mg
Vitamin B_{12}	5 mcg
Minerals	
Calcium Carbonate	600 mg
Ferrous Sulfate	150 mg
Iron	30 mg

*IU = International Units
⁺Supplied as niacinamide

Action and Uses: A multivitamin and multimineral supplement for use during pregnancy and lactation
Dosage: One Kapseal daily, or as directed by physician
How Supplied: N 0071-0390. In bottles of 100 and 1,000. Parcode® 390
The color combination of the banded capsule is a Parke-Davis trademark registered in the US Patent Office.
[*Shown in Product Identification Section*]

NATABEC Rx® KAPSEALS® ℞

Vitamin and Mineral Formula Containing 1 mg of Folic Acid

Each Kapseal Represents: Vitamin A (acetate) (1.2 mg), 4,000 units; vitamin D (ergocalciferol) (10 mcg), 400 units; vitamin C (ascorbic acid), 50 mg; vitamin B_1 (thiamine mononitrate), 3 mg; vitamin B_2 (riboflavin), 2 mg; vitamin B_6 (pyridoxine hydrochloride), 3 mg; vitamin B_{12} crystalline (cyanocobalamin), 5 mcg; nicotinamide (niacinamide), 10 mg; folic acid, 1 mg; calcium carbonate precipitated, 600 mg; ferrous sulfate,* 150 mg.

*Supplied as dried ferrous sulfate equivalent to the labeled amount of ferrous sulfate.

Actions and Uses: Vitamin and mineral formula for use during pregnancy and lactation containing 1 mg of folic acid to help prevent megaloblastic anemia of pregnancy
Caution: Federal law prohibits dispensing without prescription.
Dosage: One capsule daily or as directed by the physician
Precautions: **Caution**—Folic acid may obscure pernicious anemia; the peripheral blood picture may revert to normal while neurological manifestations remain progressive.
How Supplied: N 0071-0547-04. Supplied in bottles of 100
The pink band on blue capsule is a Parke-Davis trademark registered in the US Patent Office.
[*Shown in Product Identification Section*]

NATAFORT® FILMSEAL® ℞

Each tablet represents:

Vitamin A	6,000 IU*
Vitamin D	400 IU
Vitamin C	120 mg
Thiamine (vitamin B_1)	3 mg
Riboflavin (vitamin B_2)	2 mg
Vitamin B_6	15 mg
Vitamin B_{12}	6 mcg
Folic acid	1 mg
Nicotinamide	20 mg
Vitamin E	30 IU
Calcium†	350 mg
Iodine†	0.15 mg
Magnesium†	100 mg
Zinc†	25 mg
Dioctyl sodium succinate	50 mg

*IU = International Units
†The minerals are supplied as calcium carbonate, magnesium oxide, potassium iodide, ferrous fumarate, and zinc oxide.
Indication: Comprehensive prenatal vitamin and mineral formula including 1 mg of folic acid to help prevent megaloblastic anemia of pregnancy
Caution: Folic acid may obscure pernicious anemia; the peripheral blood picture may revert to normal while neurological manifestations remain progressive.
Usual Dosage: One tablet daily
How Supplied: Bottles of 100 tablets each. N 0071-0212-24
[*Shown in Product Identification Section*]

NITROSTAT® ℞

(nitroglycerin tablets, USP)
Sublingual Tablets
Stabilized Formula

Description: Nitrostat is a stabilized nitroglycerin tablet manufactured by a unique process for which a patent has been granted, and is superior to conventional molded sublingual tablets in terms of stability and product uniformity.

Action: Nitroglycerin relaxes smooth muscles, principally in the smaller blood vessels, and dilates the arterioles and capillaries, especially in the coronary circulation. In therapeutic doses, this allows increased blood supply to the myocardium, tending to relieve myocardial ischemia, which has been suggested as the basis for the pain of angina pectoris.

Indications: Nitrostat is indicated for the treatment of acute angina pectoris episodes and for the management of angina pectoris associated with or resulting from coronary insufficiency, coronary artery disease, coronary occlusion, or subacute myocardial infarction.

Contraindications: Sublingual nitroglycerin therapy is contraindicated in patients with early myocardial infarction, severe anemia, increased intracranial pressure, and those with a known hypersensitivity to nitroglycerin.

Precautions: Only the smallest dose required for effective relief of the acute anginal attack should be used. Excessive use may lead to the development of tolerance. The tablets are intended for sublingual or buccal administration and should not be swallowed. The drug should be discontinued if blurring of vision or drying of the mouth occur. Excessive dosage may produce violent headache.

Adverse Reactions: Transient headache may occur immediately after use. Vertigo, weakness, palpitation, and other manifestations of postural hypotension may develop occasionally, particularly in erect, immobile patients. Syncope due to nitrate vasodilation, though rare, has been reported.

Method of Administration: One tablet should be dissolved under the tongue or in the buccal pouch immediately upon indication of an acute anginal attack. The dose may be repeated as needed until relief is obtained. Nitrostat may be used prophylactically prior to engaging in activities known to precipitate an acute attack.

How Supplied: Nitrostat is supplied in four strengths in bottles, containing 100 tablets each, with color-coded labels, and in color-coded Patient Convenience Packages of four bottles of 25 tablets each.

0.15 mg (1/400 grain):
N 0071-0568-24—Bottles of 100
N 0071-0568-13—Convenience Package
0.3 mg (1/200 grain):
N 0071-0569-24—Bottles of 100
N 0071-0569-13—Convenience Package
0.4 mg (1/150 grain):
N 0071-0570-24—Bottles of 100
N 0071-0570-13—Convenience Package
0.6 mg (1/100 grain):
N 0071-0571-24—Bottles of 100
N 0071-0571-13—Convenience Package
AHFS 24:12
[*Shown in Product Identification Section*]

NORLUTIN® ℞
(norethindrone tablets, USP)
NORLUTATE® ℞
(norethindrone acetate tablets, NF)

WARNING
The use of progestational agents during the first four months of pregnancy is not recommended.
Progestational agents have been used beginning with the first trimester of pregnancy in an attempt to prevent habitual abortion or to treat threatened abortion. There is no adequate evidence that such use is effective and there is evidence of potential harm to the fetus when such drugs are given during the first four months of pregnancy. Furthermore, in the vast majority of women, the cause of abortion is a defective ovum, which progestational agents could not be expected to influence. In addition, the use of progestational agents, with their uterine-relaxant properties, in patients with fertilized defective ova may cause a delay in spontaneous abortion. Therefore, the use of such drugs during the first four months of pregnancy is not recommended.
Several reports suggest an association between intrauterine exposure to female sex hormones and congenital anomalies, including congenital heart defects and limb reduction defects. One study estimated a 4.7 fold increased risk of limb reduction defects in infants exposed *in utero* to sex hormones (oral contraceptives, hormone withdrawal test for pregnancy, or attempted treatment for threatened abortion). Some of these exposures were very short and involved only a few days of treatment. The data suggests that the risk of limb reduction defects in exposed fetuses is somewhat less than 1 in 1,000.
If the patient is exposed to Norlutin or Norlutate during the first four months of pregnancy or if she becomes pregnant while taking either of these drugs, she should be apprised of the potential risk to the fetus.

Description: Norlutin is the 17 alpha-ethinyl derivative of 19-nortestosterone. It is a purified crystalline compound that provides orally potent progestational action. The use of norethindrone is indicated in those clinical conditions associated with a deficiency in the secretion of progesterone.
Norlutate is the acetic acid ester of norethindrone, which is the 17 alpha-ethinyl derivative of 19-nortestosterone. The use of norethindrone acetate is indicated in those clinical conditions associated with a deficiency in the secretion of progesterone.
Norethindrone acetate differs from norethindrone only in potency; the acetate is approximately twice as potent.

Actions: Transforms proliferative endometrium into secretory endometrium
Inhibits (at the usual dosage range) the secretion of pituitary gonadotropins, which in turn prevents follicular maturation and ovulation
May also demonstrate some estrogenic, anabolic, or androgenic activity but should not be relied upon

Indications: Norlutin (norethindrone tablets, USP) and Norlutate (norethindrone acetate tablets, NF) are indicated in amenorrhea; in abnormal uterine bleeding due to hormonal imbalance in the absence of organic pathology, such as submucous fibroids or uterine cancer; and in endometriosis.

Contraindications:
1. Thrombophlebitis, thromboembolic disorders, cerebral apoplexy, or patients with a past history of these conditions
2. Markedly impaired liver function or disease
3. Known or suspected carcinoma of the breast
4. Undiagnosed vaginal bleeding
5. Missed abortion
6. As a diagnostic test for pregnancy

Warnings:
1. Discontinue medication pending examination if there is a sudden partial or complete loss of vision, or if there is sudden onset of proptosis, diplopia, or migraine. If examination reveals papilledema or retinal vascular lesions, medication should be withdrawn.
2. Detectable amounts of progestogens have been identified in the milk of mothers receiving them. The effect of this on the nursing infant has not been determined.
3. Because of the occasional occurrence of thrombophlebitis and pulmonary embolism in patients taking progestogens, the physician should be alert to the earliest manifestations of the disease.
4. Masculinization of the female fetus has occurred when progestogens have been used in pregnant women.
5. Some beagle dogs treated with medroxyprogesterone acetate developed mammary nodules. Although nodules occasionally appeared in control animals, they were intermittent in nature, whereas nodules in treated animals were larger and more numerous, and persisted. There is no general agreement as to whether the nodules are benign or malignant. Their significance with respect to humans has not been established.

Precautions:
1. The pretreatment physical examination should include special reference to breasts and pelvic organs, as well as a Papanicolaou smear.
2. Because this drug may cause some degree of fluid retention, conditions which might be influenced by this factor, such as epilepsy, migraine, asthma, cardiac or renal dysfunctions, require careful observation.
3. In cases of breakthrough bleeding, as in all cases of irregular bleeding per vaginam, nonfunctional causes should be borne in mind. In cases of undiagnosed vaginal bleeding, adequate diagnostic measures are indicated.
4. Patients who have a history of psychic depression should be carefully observed and the drug discontinued if the depression recurs to a serious degree.
5. Any possible influence of prolonged progestogen therapy on pituitary, ovarian, adrenal, hepatic, or uterine functions awaits further study.
6. A decrease in glucose tolerance has been observed in a small percentage of patients on estrogen-progestogen combination drugs. The mechanism of this decrease is obscure. For this reason, diabetic patients should be carefully observed while receiving progestogen therapy.
7. The age of the patient constitutes no absolute limiting factor, although treatment with progestogens may mask the onset of the climacteric.
8. The pathologist should be advised of progestogen therapy when relevant specimens are submitted.

Adverse Reactions: The following adverse reactions have been observed in women taking progestogens.
1. Breakthrough bleeding
2. Spotting
3. Change in menstrual flow
4. Amenorrhea
5. Edema
6. Changes in weight (increase or decrease)
7. Changes in cervical erosion and cervical secretions
8. Cholestatic jaundice
9. Rash (allergic) with and without pruritus
10. Melasma or chloasma
11. Mental depression

The following laboratory result may be altered by the use of progestogens: pregnanediol determination.
In addition, the following laboratory results may be altered by the concomitant use of estrogens with progestogens.

Continued on next page

This product information was prepared in August, 1979. On these and other Parke-Davis Products, detailed information may be obtained by addressing PARKE-DAVIS, Division of Warner-Lambert Company, Morris Plains, NJ 07950.

Parke-Davis—Cont.

1. Hepatic function
2. Coagulation tests: increase in prothrombin, factors VII, VIII, IX, and X
3. Increase in PBI, BEI, and a decrease in T3 uptake
4. Metyrapone test

A statistically significant association has been demonstrated between use of estrogen-progestogen combination drugs and the following serious adverse reactions: thrombophlebitis; pulmonary embolism, and cerebral thrombosis and embolism. For this reason, patients on progestogen therapy should be carefully observed.
Although available evidence is suggestive of an association, such a relationship has been neither confirmed nor refuted for the following serious adverse reactions:
Neuro-ocular lesions, eg, retinal thrombosis and optic neuritis.
The following adverse reactions have been observed in patients receiving estrogen-progestogen combination drugs.

1. Rise in blood pressure in susceptible individuals
2. Premenstrual-like syndrome
3. Changes in libido
4. Changes in appetite
5. Cystitis-like syndrome
6. Headache
7. Nervousness
8. Dizziness
9. Fatigue
10. Backache
11. Hirsutism
12. Loss of scalp hair
13. Erythema multiforme
14. Erythema nodosum
15. Hemorrhagic eruption
16. Itching

In view of these observations, patients on progestogen therapy should be carefully observed.
Dosage and Administration: Norlutin (norethindrone tablets, USP): *Therapy with Norlutin must be adapted to the specific indications and therapeutic response of the individual patient.*
This dosage schedule assumes the interval between menses to be 28 days.
Amenorrhea, abnormal uterine bleeding due to hormonal imbalance in the absence of organic pathology: 5 to 20 mg Norlutin starting with the fifth day of the menstrual cycle and ending on the 25th day.
Endometriosis: Initial daily dosage of 10 mg Norlutin for two weeks with increments of 5 mg per day of Norlutin every two weeks until 30 mg per day of Norlutin is reached. Therapy may be held at this level for from six to nine months or until annoying breakthrough bleeding demands temporary termination.
Norlutate (norethindrone acetate tablets, NF): *Therapy with Norlutate must be adapted to the specific indications and therapeutic response of the individual patient.*
This dosage schedule assumes the interval between menses to be 28 days.
Amenorrhea, abnormal uterine bleeding due to hormonal imbalance in the absence of organic pathology: 2.5 to 10 mg Norlutate starting with the fifth day of the menstrual cycle and ending on the 25th day.
Endometriosis: Initial daily dosage of 5 mg Norlutate for two weeks, with increments of 2.5 mg per day of Norlutate every two weeks until 15 mg per day of Norlutate is reached. Therapy may be held at this level for from six to nine months or until annoying breakthrough bleeding demands temporary termination.
How Supplied: N 0071-0882-19 (Tablet 882)—Norlutin (norethindrone) is supplied as 5-mg scored tablets in bottles of 50. Parcode® No. 882
[*Shown in Product Identification Section*]
N 0710-0918-19 (Tablet 918)—Norlutate (norethindrone acetate) is supplied as 5-mg scored tablets in bottles of 50. Parcode® 918
Norlutin and Norlutate are manufactured by Parke Davis Laboratories, Fajardo, Puerto Rico and are distributed by Parke-Davis, Division of Warner-Lambert Company, Morris Plains, NJ 07950.
AHFS 68:32
[*Shown in Product Identification Section*]

PATIENT LABELING FOR PROGESTOGENS
WARNING FOR WOMEN
There is an increased risk of birth defects in children whose mothers take this drug during the first four months of pregnancy.
Norlutin and Norlutate are similar to the progesterone hormones naturally produced by the body. Progesterone and progesterone-like drugs are used to treat menstrual disorders, to test if the body is producing certain hormones, and to treat some forms of cancer in women. These drugs have been used as a test for pregnancy but such use is no longer considered safe because of possible damage to a developing baby. Also, more rapid methods for testing for pregnancy are now available.
These drugs have also been used to prevent miscarriage in the first few months of pregnancy. No adeuate evidence is available to show that they are effective for this purpose and there is evidence of an increased risk of birth defects, such as heart or limb defects, if these drugs are taken during during the first four months of pregnancy. Furthermore, most cases of early miscarriage are due to causes which could not be helped by these drugs.
The exact risk of taking these drugs early in pregnancy and having a baby with a birth defect is not known. However, one study found that babies born to women who had taken sex hormones (such as progesterone-like drugs) during the first three months of pregnancy were 4 to 5 times more likely to have abnormalities of the arms or legs than if their mothers had not taken such drugs. Some of these women had taken these drugs for only a few days. The chance that an infant whose mother had taken this drug will have this type of defect is about 1 in 1,000.
If you take Norlutin or Norlutate and later find you were pregnant when you took it, be sure to discuss this with your doctor as soon as possible.

WK

NORMAL SERUM ALBUMIN (HUMAN), USP ℞
Albuspan®

Description: Albuspan (normal serum albumin [human]) is supplied in two different strengths of solution: 5% and 25%. The 5% product is a sterile, pyrogen-free, aqueous solution of serum albumin isotonic and iso-osmotic with pooled whole human plasma. The 25% product is a salt-poor, aqueous solution approximately isoviscous with whole blood and osmotically equivalent to five times its volume of pooled whole blood plasma. Albuspan is prepared from venous and placental plasma by a special fractionation process involving a series of controlled precipitations with cold alcohol according to the Cohn process and pasteurized in the final container at 60 C for 10 hours. Each unit of venous plasma used in this product has been shown to be nonreactive when tested for hepatitis B surface antigen (HB_sAg). The placental plasma used is obtained from hospitalized maternity populations whose patient sera have been screened to meet accepted criteria for hepatitis B surface antigen (HB_sAg). Both the 5% and 25% products are stabilized with 0.08 millimole of sodium acetyltryptophanate and 0.08 millimole of sodium caprylate per gram of albumin. The 5% solution is prepared in 0.15 *M* sodium chloride and contains not more than 32.5 mEq of sodium per 250 ml of solution and 65 to 80 mEq of sodium per 500 ml of solution. The 25% solution contains 8 mEq of sodium per 50 ml (130 to 160 mEq per liter) of solution. The solutions may have had sodium bicarbonate or acetic acid added to adjust pH. Neither strength includes an antimicrobial preservative. Both concentrations meet all requirements of the Food and Drug Administration and the USP for this product.
Action: Highly active osmotically, serum albumin is an important factor in the regulation of the volume of circulating blood. The albumin component normally constitutes approximately 60% of plasma protein and, because of its relatively low molecular weight, exerts 80% of the colloidal osmotic pressure of the blood.
Fluid shifts rapidly from the interstitial spaces into the circulation during intravenous injection of concentrated serum albumin. A slight increase, therefore, occurs in the concentration of plasma protein. The degree of volume expansion is determined by the initial blood volume. When concentrated albumin solution is administered to an individual with normal blood volume, the excess fluid and protein are lost from the circulation within a few hours. When albumin is administered to a patient with diminished blood volume, the gain tends to be sustained.
In addition to its osmotic function, albumin serves as a carrier of intermediate metabolites, and is thus important to the transport and exchange of tissue products.
Unlike whole blood and plasma, albumin is free of the danger of homologous serum hepatitis B. Albumin, stable at room temperature (37 C or less) and quite soluble, is ready for immediate use, with no reconstitution or cross matching necessary. In concentrated form, albumin is compact, requires no refrigeration, and makes possible more rapid therapeutic infusion.
Indications: Albuspan is useful in the following clinical conditions.
Shock
Shock, due to burns, trauma, crushing injuries, abdominal emergencies, or other similar conditions, is manifested in the circulatory system by a sudden and severe drop in blood pressure. This is due to loss of fluid from the circulating blood and a greatly expanded volume of the peripheral vascular bed. There is thus created an urgent need for expansion of the volume of circulating blood, and this can be brought about by the osmotic pull of serum albumin administered intravenously. In cases in which there has been a considerable loss of red blood cells, transfusion with whole blood (human) or red blood cells (human) is indicated.
Hypoproteinemia
Hypoproteinemia, as in the nephrotic syndrome, hepatic cirrhosis, and toxemia of pregnancy; also in postoperative patients, tuberculous patients, and premature infants—
These various clinical situations are characterized by a low concentration of plasma protein and, consequently, a reduced volume of circulating blood.
Unless the condition responsible for the hypoproteinemia can be corrected, albumin will provide only supportive relief.
Hyperbilirubinemia and erythroblastosis fetalis
Albumin can be a useful adjunct in exchange transfusions for these two conditions because it reduces the necessity for reexchange and increases the amount of bilirubin removed with each transfusion.
Contraindications: Albuspan is contraindicated in patients with severe anemia or cardiac failure.
Precautions: Do not administer more than 250 g in 48 hours. Patients who require more than this amount probably need whole blood or plasma. Normal serum albumin should be ad-

ministered with caution to patients with low cardiac reserve or with no albumin deficiency because a rapid increase in plasma volume may cause circulatory embarrassment or pulmonary edema.

Do not use any solution of normal serum albumin (human) if it appears turbid or if there is sediment in the bottle. **Do not use if more than four hours elapse after entering the container.** Normal serum albumin contains no preservative and, therefore, should be used promptly after opening the bottle.

Patients with marked dehydration require administration of additional fluids, because drawing additional fluids from the tissues of a dehydrated patient is undesirable. The fluid may be given by any route, including oral.

Infusion of this product may result in an elevated level of alkaline phosphatase. While not detrimental, the possibility of an increased level following administration may result in confusion over the patient's true endogenous level of this enzyme.

Adverse Reactions: Adverse reactions have been associated with the administration of normal serum albumin (human). These are infrequent, and may be due to allergy or to protein overload resulting from high dosage or repeated administration. Side effects include chills and fever, urticaria, and effect on blood pressure, pulse, and respiration. Antihistamines may be of value in prevention and treatment of allergic symptoms.

Dosage and Administration:

Dilution

Albuspan, 5%, is administered without further dilution.

Albuspan, 25%, may be diluted with sodium chloride injection or other suitable fluids, in conditions *other than nephrosis.* The undiluted solution should be used in treating patients with nephrosis. A solution approximately isotonic with citrated plasma can be prepared by adding one volume of Albuspan, 25%, to four volumes of sodium chloride injection or 5% dextrose injection. Dilution with dextrose injection is preferable for use in edematous conditions. The 25% concentration may be administered cautiously without dilution provided the rate of infusion is slow enough to prevent too rapid expansion of plasma volume.

Shock

For treatment of adults and for emergencies in children, an initial dose of 25 g is suggested. Some patients will require twice this amount. Therapy should be guided by the degree of venous and pulmonary congestion, and hemoglobin or hematocrit measurements.

In the treatment of patients with greatly reduced blood volume, Albuspan, 5%, or 25%, may be administered as rapidly as desired. A repeat dose may be given in 15 to 30 minutes if the initial dose proves inadequate. The rate of administration in patients with relatively normal blood volume, however, should not exceed 1 ml per minute for Albuspan, 25%, or 2 to 4 ml per minute with the 5% concentration.

In burns, the dosage will depend on the extent of the injury. Initially, electrolyte solutions are usually given to keep the patient hemodynamically stable. There is little evidence that albumin is therapeutically useful during the first 24 hours after severe burns. Thereafter, the ratio of albumin to electrolyte solution administered may be increased. An optimal therapeutic regimen for the use of colloids, crystalloids, and fluids has not been established. The dosage must be sufficient to correct the decreased plasma volume and hemoconcentration.

Hypoproteinemia

Hypoproteinemia is caused by a wide variety of conditions: (1) inadequate protein intake, (2) impaired protein synthesis, or (3) sudden or excessive loss of albumin. Albumin is particularly advantageous in the treatment of many of these conditions because 100 ml of normal serum albumin (human), 25%, provides about as much plasma protein as does 500 ml of plasma or 2 pints of whole blood. Administration of serum albumin intravenously will restore plasma proteins and relieve edema, but it must be kept in mind that this is an interim measure. The underlying cause of the condition must be corrected for permanent restoration of the plasma protein level. Prophylactic administration of the 25% concentration of serum albumin, in doses of 3 to 4 ml/lb body weight (6.6 to 8 ml/kg), has been found advantageous in premature infants with low serum protein levels.

Dosage in nonemergency treatment of children is regulated by the age of the child and the type of condition being treated. A dose one quarter to one half the adult dose may be administered; or dosage may be calculated on the basis of 1 ml Albuspan, 25%, per lb body weight (2.2 ml/kg).

1. ***Hepatic Cirrhosis***

The liver is the site of production of plasma albumin and the rate of synthesis may be decreased in cirrhosis. Normal serum albumin may be effective in temporarily restoring plasma protein levels in the absence of ascites. If ascites is present, albumin may be of value after the removal of a large volume of fluid (eg, more than 1,500 ml of ascitic fluid during a single paracentesis). Otherwise, there is little evidence that albumin is effective in the management of the hypoproteinemia of cirrhosis.

2. ***Nephrosis***

The nephrosis accompanying chronic glomerulonephritis is characterized by albuminuria, hypoalbuminemia, and hypercholesteremia. The administration of concentrated human serum albumin raises the osmotic pressure of the blood, increases the circulating volume while removing edema fluid, and stimulates salt excretion. The initial dose of 100 to 200 ml of Albuspan, 25%, may be repeated at intervals of one or two days. Because of rapid loss of albumin from the circulation, the effects in most cases are not sustained after discontinuation of therapy.

Hyperbilirubinemia and erythroblastosis fetalis

The use of albumin in exchange transfusions for hyperbilirubinemia or erythroblastosis fetalis has been shown in numerous studies to reduce the necessity for reexchange and to increase the amount of bilirubin removed with each exchange transfusion. Normal serum albumin is generally administered at a dosage of 1 g/kg of body weight one to two hours before transfusion of blood. In some cases, albumin has been administered as part of the transfusion by substituting 50 ml (12.5 g) normal serum albumin (25% concentration) for 50 ml of plasma in the blood to be transfused.

How Supplied: Albuspan (normal serum albumin [human]) is a brownish-to-amber-colored, clear, sterile, moderately viscous fluid.

The 5% concentration is supplied in packages as:

N 0071-4698-35 (Bio 698)—containing one 250-ml bottle of 12.5 g normal serum albumin (human) and one sterilized, pyrogen-free, disposable intravenous injection set.

N 0071-4698-36 (Bio 699)—containing one 500-ml bottle of 25 g normal serum albumin (human) and one sterilized, pyrogen-free, disposable intravenous injection set.

The 25% concentration is supplied in packages as:

N 0071-4864-35 (Bio 864)—containing one 50-ml bottle of 12.5 normal serum albumin (human) and one sterilized, pyrogen-free, disposable intravenous injection set.

AHFS 16:00 **UH**

OPHTHOCHLOR® ℞

(chloramphenicol ophthalmic solution, USP) 0.5%

Description: Ophthochlor Ophthalmic Solution, 0.5%, is a sterile, buffered solution containing 0.5% (5 mg/ml) of chloramphenicol. Ophthochlor contains no preservatives.

Actions: Chloramphenicol, a broad-spectrum antibiotic originally isolated from *Streptomyces venezuelae,* is primarily bacteriostatic and acts by inhibition of protein synthesis by interfering with the transfer of activated amino acids from soluble RNA to ribosomes. Studies have shown that chloramphenicol is not absorbed in measurable amounts by topical application to the eye. Development of resistance to chloramphenicol can be regarded as minimal for staphylococci and many other species of bacteria.

Indications: Ophthochlor Ophthalmic Solution, 0.5%, is indicated for the treatment of superficial ocular infections involving the conjunctiva and/or cornea caused by chloramphenicol-susceptible organisms. Bacteriological studies should be performed to determine the causative organisms and their sensitivity to chloramphenicol.

Contraindication: This product is contraindicated in persons sensitive to any of its components.

Warnings: Prolonged or frequent intermittent use of topical chloramphenicol should be avoided because of the possibility of hypersensitivity reactions, including bone marrow hypoplasia.

Precautions: The prolonged use of antibiotics may occasionally result in overgrowth of nonsusceptible organisms, including fungi. If new infections appear during medication, the drug should be discontinued and appropriate measures should be taken.

In all except very superficial infections, the topical use of chloramphenicol should be supplemented by appropriate systemic medication.

Adverse Reactions: Blood dyscrasias may be associated with the systemic use of chloramphenicol. Bone marrow hypoplasia following topical use of chloramphenicol eye drops has been reported.

Dosage and Administration: Two drops applied to the affected eye every three hours, or more frequently if deemed advisable by the prescribing physician. Administration should be continued day and night for the first 48 hours, after which the interval between applications may be increased. Treatment should be continued for at least 48 hours after the eye appears normal.

How Supplied: N 0071-3395-11—15-ml bottles—Ophthochlor Ophthalmic Solution, 0.5%, is supplied in plastic dropper bottles and contains no preservatives. Each milliliter contains 5 mg chloramphenicol in a boric acid-sodium borate buffer solution. Sodium hydroxide may have been added for adjustment of pH. To protect it from light, the solution should be dispensed in the carton. This product should be stored in a refrigerator until dispensed. Discard solution within 21 days from date dispensed.

NSN 6505-00-126-2037

AHFS 52:04.04 **WA**

[*Shown in Product Identification Section*]

PAPASE® ℞

(proteolytic enzymes extracted from *Carica papaya*)

Caution: Federal law prohibits dispensing without prescription.

Description: Each tablet of Papase contains proteolytic enzymes extracted from *Carica papaya;* the tablet is standardized to 10,000

Continued on next page

This product information was prepared in August, 1979. On these and other Parke-Davis Products, detailed information may be obtained by addressing PARKE-DAVIS, Division of Warner-Lambert Company, Morris Plains, NJ 07950.

Parke-Davis—Cont.

Warner/Chilcott Units of enzyme activity. Tablets may be administered orally or buccally.

Actions: Papase contains an extract of proteolytic enzymes of *Carica papaya*. Each tablet furnishes enzymatic activity equal to 10,000 Warner/Chilcott Units, thereby providing optimal therapeutic activity.

Indications
Based on a review of this drug by the National Academy of Sciences—National Research Council and/or other information, FDA has classified the indications as follows:
"Possibly" effective for relieving symptomatology related to episiotomy.
Final classification of the less-than-effective indications requires further investigation.

Contraindications: Concomitant use with anticoagulants is the only known contraindication. However, it is not recommended in generalized or systemic infections, or in severe disorders of blood clotting, or in patients with a prior allergic reaction to Papase (proteolytic enzymes extracted from *Carica papaya*) or papain.

Warning—Use in Pregnancy: Safe use of this drug in pregnancy has not been established.

Precautions: This drug should be used with caution in patients with severe renal or hepatic disease.

Adverse Reactions: The incidence of side effects is low. The following reactions have been described: nausea, vomiting, diarrhea, dizziness, pruritis, rash, and urticaria. To date, buccal ulceration has not been observed in patients, even those receiving Papase (proteolytic enzymes extracted from *Carica papaya*) for prolonged periods. An occasional patient, however, has experienced a mild, local tingling at the site of buccal absorption; this sensation usually subsided when the tablet was moved.

Dosage and Administration: Prophylactic Dosage—Two tablets, 1 or 2 hours before episiotomy.
Therapeutic Dosage—Two tablets 4 times a day for at least five days.
Tablets may be administered buccally or orally, swallowed with water, or chewed.

Supplied: Green peppermint-flavored tablets (with desiccant) in bottles of 100 (N 0047-0300-51) and 1000 (N 0047-0300-60).

Standardization — Since antiinflammatory action is related to enzymatic activity, Papase (proteolytic enzymes extracted from *Carica papaya*) has been specially prepared and carefully standardized on this basis. The method used is a milk-clotting assay,[1] the results of which are expressed in Warner/Chilcott Units. One Warner/Chilcott Unit is that quantity of proteolytic enzymes extracted from *Carica papaya* which, under the conditions specified in the method of assay, will clot 2.64 microliters of milk substrate in 2 minutes at 40° C.
Store between 59° and 86°F (15° and 30°C).

Reference: 1. Hinkle ET Jr, Alford, AC: *Ann. New York Acad. Sc. 54*(2):208, 1951.

[*Shown in Product Identification Section*]

342 G 270 **R-1-77**

PAREST® Ⓒ ℞
(methaqualone hydrochloride capsules, NF)

PAREST-400*

Each Parest-400 capsule contains:
Methaqualone HCl .... 400 mg
(Equivalent to 350 mg methaqualone base)

Description: Methaqualone is chemically 2-methyl-3- (2-methylphenyl) -4(3H)-quinazolinone. Methaqualone occurs as a white, crystalline powder with a bitter taste and is very slightly soluble in water and freely soluble in alcohol. The drug is highly lipid soluble.
The hydrochloride salt of methaqualone occurs as a white, crystalline powder and is sparingly soluble in water and in alcohol.

Clinical Pharmacology: Methaqualone and methaqualone hydrochloride are rapidly absorbed from the G.I. tract. The onset of action of the drug is rapid; sleep is usually induced within 30 minutes and lasts 5 to 8 hours following usual hypnotic doses.
The decline of serum levels of methaqualone is biphasic. The half-life for the first (distribution) phase is 1 to 4 hours and the half-life for the second (elimination) phase has been reported to be 19 to 40 hours. There is extensive tissue localization of the drug, particularly in adipose tissue. Steady-state equilibrium is achieved in less than one week.
Although the metabolic fate of methaqualone has not been completely elucidated, there is considerable evidence that therapeutic doses of methaqualone are almost completely metabolized in the liver by hydroxylation. In doses of up to 300 mg in man, very little unchanged drug is found in the urine.

Indications: Methaqualone and methaqualone hydrochloride are hypnotics for the treatment of simple insomnia. The prolonged administration of Parest is *not* recommended since it has not been shown to be effective for more than 14 days. Attempts should be made to find alternative nondrug therapy in chronic insomnia.

Contraindications: Parest is contraindicated in patients with known hypersensitivity to methaqualone and in women who are or may become pregnant. Reproduction studies in the rat revealed minor but clear-cut skeletal abnormalities in the young.

Warnings: The hypnotic dose should be taken only at bedtime, immediately before the patient retires, since methaqualone may produce drowsiness within 10 to 20 minutes.
The patient on Parest must be warned against driving a car or operating dangerous machinery while on the drug, because methaqualone may impair the ability to perform hazardous activities requiring mental alertness or physical coordination.
The patient should be warned about the possible additive effects when methaqualone is taken concomitantly with other central nervous system depressants such as alcohol or barbiturates.

Usage in children:
Methaqualone is *not* recommended for use in children, because its safety and effectiveness in the pediatric age group have not been established.

Physical and psychological dependence:
Psychological and physical dependence with methaqualone have been reported. Excessive use of the drug or abuse of the drug for nontherapeutic purposes may lead to severe psychological or physical dependence.
Because methaqualone is known to have value on the illicit drug market, caution must be exercised in prescribing methaqualone to individuals whose history suggests they may increase the dosage on their own initiative. Ordinarily, an amount adequate for one week is sufficient. The patient should be reevaluated before represcribing.

Precautions: The possibility of the use of hypnotic drugs in suicide attempts should be kept in mind and the drugs prescribed in small quantities.
Because methaqualone is metabolized in the liver, it should be given in reduced doses, if at all, to those with impaired hepatic function.

Adverse Reactions:
Neuropsychiatric: headache, hangover, fatigue, dizziness, torpor, transient paresthesia of the extremities. Peripheral neuropathy has been reported. Restlessness or anxiety occurs occasionally.
Hematologic: aplastic anemia possibly related to methaqualone has been reported.
Gastrointestinal: dry mouth, anorexia, nausea, emesis, epigastric discomfort, diarrhea.
Dermatologic: diaphoresis, bromhidrosis, exanthema. Urticaria has been particularly well documented.

Dosage and Administration:
Usual Adult Dosage—The usual adult hypnotic dose of methaqualone hydrochloride is 200 to 400 mg at bedtime.
Geriatric Dosage—Dosage for aged, debilitated, or highly agitated patients should be individualized in accordance with the judgment of the physician. The principle to be followed is to observe the response to small doses and determine the desirability of adjusting the dose.

Overdosage: Acute overdosage may result in delirium and coma, with restlessness and hypertonia, progressing to convulsions. Pupillary dilatation, tachycardia, and hyperreflexia may also occur. Spontaneous vomiting and increased secretions are common and may lead to aspiration pneumonitis or respiratory obstruction. Large overdoses have been accompanied by cutaneous edema, pulmonary edema, hepatic damage, renal insufficiency, and bleeding. Shock and respiratory arrest may occasionally occur. Coma has occurred with acute overdoses averaging 2.4 grams. Death has occurred following ingestion of 8 grams of methaqualone.
Recommended management includes prompt evacuation of gastric contents, maintenance of adequate ventilation, support of blood pressure if necessary, and the usual supportive measures for the unconscious patient. Dialysis may be helpful. Analeptics are contraindicated.
Sudden discontinuation of methaqualone in physically dependent patients may produce severe withdrawal symptoms including nausea, vomiting, nervousness, tremulousness, headache, anxiety, confusion, weakness, abdominal cramps, insomnia, nightmares, hallucinations and convulsions. Treatment of methaqualone physical dependence consists of cautious and gradual withdrawal of the drug. Patients being withdrawn from methaqualone should be closely monitored, preferably hospitalized, and general supportive therapy given as needed.

How Supplied:
N 0071-0574-24 (Stock 6-574-4)—Parest-400 capsules, each containing 400 mg methaqualone HCl, are available in bottles of 100 capsules.
AHFS Category 28:24 **WK**

[*Shown in Product Identification Section*]

PENICILLIN V POTASSIUM ℞
(Penapar VK®)

Description: Penicillin V is the phenoxymethyl analogue of penicillin G.

Action and Pharmacology: Penicillin V exerts a bactericidal action against penicillin-sensitive microorganisms during the stage of active multiplication and acts through the inhibition of biosynthesis of cell wall mucopeptide. Penicillin V Potassium is not active against the penicillinase-producing bacteria, which includes many strains of staphylococci. The drug exerts high *in vitro* activity against staphylococci (except penicillinase-producing strains), streptococci (groups A, C, G, H, L, and M), and pneumococci. Other organisms sensitive *in vitro* to penicillin V are *Corynebacterium diphtheriae, Bacillus anthracis, Clostridia, Actinomyces bovis, Streptobacillus moniliformis, Listeria monocytogenes, Leptospira,* and *Neisseria gonorrhoeae. Treponema pallidum* is extremely sensitive.
Penicillin V has the distinct advantage over penicillin G in resistance to inactivation by gastric acid and may be given with meals; however, blood levels are slightly higher when the drug is given on an empty stomach. Average

blood levels are two to five times higher than the levels following the same dose of oral penicillin G and also show much less individual variation.

Once absorbed, penicillin V is about 80% bound to serum protein. Tissue levels are highest in the kidneys, with lesser amounts in the liver, skin, and intestines. Small amounts are found in all other body tissues and the cerebrospinal fluid. The drug is excreted as rapidly as it is absorbed in individuals with normal kidney function; however, recovery of the drug from the urine indicates that only about 25% of the dose given is absorbed. In neonates, young infants, and individuals with impaired kidney function, excretion is considerably delayed.

Indications: Penicillin V is indicated in the treatment of mild to moderately severe infections due to penicillin G-sensitive microorganisms that are sensitive to the low serum levels common to this particular dosage form. Therapy should be guided by bacteriologic studies (including sensitivity tests) and by clinical response.

NOTE: Severe pneumonia, empyema, bacteremia, pericarditis, meningitis, and arthritis should not be treated with penicillin V during the acute stage.

Indicated surgical procedures should be performed.

The following infections will usually respond to adequate dosage of penicillin V.

Streptococcal infections (without bacteremia); mild to moderate infections of the upper respiratory tract, scarlet fever, and mild erysipelas

NOTE: Streptococci in groups A, C, G, H, L, and M are very sensitive to penicillin. Other groups, including group D *(Enterococcus)*, are resistant.

Pneumococcal infections; mild to moderately severe infections of the respiratory tract

Staphylococcal infections—penicillin G-sensitive; mild infections of the skin and soft tissues.

NOTE: Reports indicate an increasing number of strains of staphylococci resistant to penicillin G, emphasizing the need for culture and sensitivity studies in treating suspected staphylococcal infections.

Fusospirochetosis (Vincent's gingivitis and pharyngitis); mild to moderately severe infections of the oropharynx usually respond to therapy with oral penicillin.

NOTE: Necessary dental care should be accomplished in infections involving the gum tissue.

Medical conditions in which oral penicillin therapy is indicated as prophylaxis:

For the prevention of recurrence following rheumatic fever and/or chorea: prophylaxis with oral penicillin on a continuing basis has proved effective in preventing recurrence of these conditions.

To prevent bacterial endocarditis in patients with congenital and/or rheumatic heart lesions who are to undergo dental procedures or minor upper respiratory tract surgery or instrumentation; prophylaxis should be instituted the day of the procedure and for two or more days following. Patients who have a past history of rheumatic fever and are receiving continuous prophylaxis may harbor increased numbers of penicillin-resistant organisms; use of another prophylaxis anti-infective agent should be considered. If penicillin is to be used in these patients at surgery, the regular rheumatic fever program should be interrupted one week prior to the contemplated surgery. At the time of surgery, penicillin may be reinstituted as a prophylactic measure against the hazards of surgically induced bacteremia.

NOTE: Oral penicillin should not be used as adjunctive prophylaxis for genitourinary instrumentation or surgery, lower intestinal tract surgery, sigmoidoscopy, and childbirth.

Contraindication: A previous hypersensitivity reaction to any penicillin is a contraindication.

Warnings: Serious and occasionally fatal hypersensitivity (anaphylactoid) reactions have been reported in patients on penicillin therapy. Although anaphylaxis is more frequent following parenteral therapy, it has occurred in patients on oral penicillins. These reactions are more apt to occur in individuals with a history of sensitivity to multiple allergens.

There have been well-documented reports of individuals with a history of penicillin hypersensitivity reactions who have experienced severe hypersensitivity reactions when treated with a cephalosporin. Before therapy with a penicillin, careful inquiry should be made concerning previous hypersensitivity reactions to penicillins, cephalosporins, and other allergens. If an allergic reaction occurs, the drug should be discontinued and the patient should be treated with the usual agents, eg, pressor amines, antihistamines, and corticosteroids.

Precautions: Penicillin should be used with caution in individuals with histories of significant allergies and/or asthma.

The oral route of administration should not be relied upon in patients with severe illness, or with nausea, vomiting, gastric dilatation, cardiospasm, or intestinal hypermotility.

Occasional patients will not absorb therapeutic amounts of orally administered penicillin.

In streptococcal infections, therapy must be sufficient to eliminate the organism (minimum, 10 days); otherwise, the sequelae of streptococcal disease may occur. Cultures should be taken following completion of treatment to determine whether streptococci have been eradicated.

Prolonged use of antibiotics may promote the overgrowth of nonsusceptible organisms, including fungi. Should superinfection occur, appropriate measures should be taken.

Adverse Reactions: Although the incidence of reactions to oral penicillins has been reported with much less frequency than following parenteral therapy, it should be remembered that all degrees of hypersensitivity, including fatal anaphylaxis, have been reported with oral penicillin.

The most common reactions to oral penicillin are nausea, vomiting, epigastric distress, diarrhea, and black, hairy tongue. The hypersensitivity reactions reported are skin eruptions (maculopapular to exfoliative dermatitis), urticaria and other serum sickness reactions, laryngeal edema, and anaphylaxis. Fever and eosinophilia may frequently be the only reaction observed. Hemolytic anemia, leukopenia, thrombocytopenia, neuropathy, and nephropathy are infrequent reactions and are usually associated with high doses of parenteral penicillin.

Dosage and Administration: The dosage of penicillin V should be determined according to the sensitivity of the causative microorganisms and the severity of the infection, and adjusted to the clinical response of the patient.

The usual dosage recommendations for adults and children 12 years and over are as follows.

Streptococcal infections—mild to moderately severe—of the upper respiratory tract and including scarlet fever and erysipelas: 200,000 to 500,000 units every six to eight hours for 10 days

Pneumococcal infections—mild to moderately severe—of the respiratory tract, including otitis media: 400,000 to 500,000 units every six hours until the patient has been afebrile for at least two days

Staphylococcal infections—mild infections of skin and soft tissue (culture and sensitivity tests should be performed): 400,000 to 500,000 units every six to eight hours

Fusospirochetosis (Vincent's infection) of the oropharynx—mild to moderately severe infections: 400,000 to 500,000 units every six to eight hours

For the prevention of recurrence following rheumatic fever and/or chorea: 200,000 to 250,000 units twice daily on a continuing basis.

To prevent bacterial endocarditis in patients with rheumatic or congenital heart lesions who are to undergo dental or upper respiratory tract surgery or instrumentation: 500,000 units given the day of the procedure, 500,000 units of aqueous penicillin G intramuscularly one hour before the procedure, and 500,000 units every six hours for two days following the procedure.

NOTE: Therapy for children under 12 years of age is calculated on the basis of body weight. For infants and small children, the suggested dosage is 25,000 to 90,000 units per kg per day in three to six divided doses.

How Supplied: Penicillin V Potassium is supplied as:

Tablet 648 (N 0071-0648)—250 mg

Each tablet contains penicillin V potassium equivalent to 250 mg (400,000 units) penicillin V, bottles of 100, 1,000, and unit-dose packages of 100 (10 strips of 10). Parcode® No. 648

Tablet 673 (N 0071-0673-24)—500 mg

Each tablet contains penicillin V potassium equivalent to 500 mg (800,000 units) penicillin V, bottles of 100. Parcode No. 673

[*Shown in Product Identification Section*]

N 0071-2449—For Oral Solution, 125 mg/5 ml

When reconstituted according to directions, each 5 ml contains penicillin V potassium equivalent to 125 mg (200,000 units) penicillin V per 5 ml, 100- and 200-ml bottles, and 10-ml unit-dose bottles.

N 0071-2506—For Oral Solution, 250 mg/5 ml

When reconstituted according to directions, each 5 ml contains penicillin V potassium equivalent to 250 mg (400,000 units) penicillin V per 5 ml, 100- and 200-ml bottles.

AHFS 8:12.16 **YB**

PENTRAX® TAR SHAMPOO

Description: Pentrax Tar Shampoo contains 8.75% Fractar® (which is equivalent to 4.3% crude coal tar), a patented standardized extract of coal tar; a blend of highly-concentrated detergents; and a conditioning agent. Fractar contains the major homologues of benzene, such as anthracene, phenanthrene, naphthalene and other aromatic hydrocarbons found in crude coal tar. Spectrophotometric standardization, based on hydrocarbon analysis, assures uniform tar content from batch to batch. Pentrax Tar Shampoo does not contain hexachlorophene, parabens or other preservatives.

Action: Coal tar helps correct abnormalities of keratinization by decreasing epidermal proliferation and dermal infiltration.

Indications: For the adjunctive, topical management of seborrhea, psoriasis and subacute and chronic eczematous dermatoses of the scalp.

Contraindications: Pentrax Tar Shampoo is contraindicated in patients with a history or hypersensitivity to tar and other components of the formulation.

Precautions: Not for ophthalmic use. Minor dermatologic side effects have been reported from use of topical tar preparations. These include primary irritation, folliculitis from long-term use, allergic contact dermatitis and phototoxicity. May stain hair and fabrics. Keep out of reach of children.

Continued on next page

This product information was prepared in August, 1979. On these and other Parke-Davis Products, detailed information may be obtained by addressing PARKE-DAVIS, Division of Warner-Lambert Company, Morris Plains, NJ 07950.

Parke-Davis—Cont.

Directions: Apply Pentrax Tar Shampoo to wet hair; massage, adding water liberally to produce lather. Rinse. Re-apply. Second lather may be allowed to remain up to 10 minutes. Rinse. Shampoo twice weekly.
Packaging: 4-oz plastic bottles (N 0064-3916-04).

PERITRATE® SA ℞
Sustained Action
(pentaerythritol tetranitrate) 80 mg

Caution: Federal law prohibits dispensing without prescription.

PERITRATE® ℞
(pentaerythritol tetranitrate) 40 mg

Caution: Federal law prohibits dispensing without prescription.

PERITRATE® ℞
(pentaerythritol tetranitrate) 20 mg

Caution: Federal law prohibits dispensing without prescription.

PERITRATE® ℞
(pentaerythritol tetranitrate) 10 mg

Caution: Federal law prohibits dispensing without prescription.

Peritrate SA Sustained Action 80 mg: each tablet contains pentaerythritol tetranitrate 80 mg (20 mg in the immediate release layer and 60 mg in sustained release base).
Peritrate 40 mg: each tablet contains pentaerythritol tetranitrate 40 mg.
Peritrate 20 mg: each tablet contains pentaerythritol tetranitrate 20 mg.
Peritrate 10 mg: each tablet contains pentaerythritol tetranitrate 10 mg.
Peritrate (pentaerythritol tetranitrate) is a nitric acid ester of a tetrahydric alcohol (pentaerythritol).
Actions: The exact cause of angina pectoris (that is, the pain associated with coronary artery disease) remains obscure, despite the numerous and often conflicting hypotheses concerning its pathophysiology. Therapy at the present time, therefore, remains essentially empirical. Customarily, clinical improvement has been measured by: reduction in (1) number, intensity and duration of angina pectoris attacks and (2) necessity for glyceryl trinitrate intake for prevention or relief of anginal attacks. Peritrate SA Sustained Action (pentaerythritol tetranitrate) 80 mg and Peritrate (pentaerythritol tetranitrate) have been reported in clinical usage to reduce in number and severity the incidence of angina pectoris attacks, with concomitant reduction in glyceryl trinitrate intake.
In the evaluation of Peritrate (pentaerythritol tetranitrate) and Peritrate SA Sustained Action (pentaerythritol tetranitrate) 80 mg in angina pectoris, clinical improvement has been customarily measured subjectively by: reduction in number and severity of attacks and necessity for glyceryl trinitrate intake for prevention or abortion of anginal attacks. Individual patterns of angina pectoris differ widely as does the symptomatic response to antianginal agents such as pentaerythritol tetranitrate. The published literature contains both favorable and unfavorable clinical reports. In conjunction with total management of the patient with angina pectoris, Peritrate (pentaerythritol tetranitrate) and Peritrate SA Sustained Action 80 mg have been accepted as safe for prolonged administration and widely regarded as useful.

Indications
Based on a review of this drug by the National Academy of Sciences—National Research Council and/or other information, FDA has classified the indications as follows:
"Possibly" effective: Peritrate (pentaerythritol tetranitrate) is indicated for the relief of angina pectoris (pain associated with coronary artery disease). It is not intended to abort the acute anginal episode but is widely regarded as useful in the prophylactic treatment of angina pectoris.
Final classification of the less-than-effective indications requires further investigation.

Contraindications: Peritrate SA Sustained Action (pentaerythritol tetranitrate) 80 mg and Peritrate (pentaerythritol tetranitrate) are contraindicated in patients who have a history of sensitivity to the drug.
Warnings: Data supporting the use of Peritrate (pentaerythritol tetranitrate) during the early days of the acute phase of myocardial infarction (the period during which clinical and laboratory findings are unstable) are insufficient to establish safety.
This drug can act as a physiological antagonist to norepinephrine, acetylcholine, histamine, and many other agents.
Precautions: Should be used with caution in patients who have glaucoma. Tolerance to this drug and cross-tolerance to other nitrites and nitrates may occur.
Adverse Reactions: Side effects reported to date have been predominantly related to rash (which requires discontinuation of medication) and headache and gastrointestinal distress, which are usually mild and transient with continuation of medication. In some cases severe persistent headaches may occur. In addition, the following adverse reactions to nitrates such as pentaerythritol tetranitrate have been reported in the literature:
(a) Cutaneous vasodilatation with flushing.
(b) Transient episodes of dizziness and weakness, as well as other signs of cerebral ischemia associated with postural hypotension, may occasionally develop.
(c) An occasional individual exhibits marked sensitivity to the hypotensive effects of nitrite and severe responses (nausea, vomiting, weakness, restlessness, pallor, perspiration and collapse) can occur, even with the usual therapeutic doses. Alcohol may enhance this effect.

Dosage: Peritrate (pentaerythritol tetranitrate) may be administered in individualized doses up to 160 mg a day. Dosage can be initiated at one 10 mg or 20 mg tablet q.i.d. and titrated upward to 40 mg (two 20 mg tablets or one 40 mg tablet) q.i.d. one-half hour before or one hour after meals and at bedtime. Alternatively, Peritrate Sustained Action 80 mg can be administered on a convenient b.i.d. dosage schedule. One tablet immediately on arising and 1 tablet 12 hours later (on an empty stomach). Tablets should not be chewed.
Supplied:
Peritrate SA Sustained Action 80 mg—double layer, biconvex, dark green/light green tablets in bottles of 100 (N 0740-0004-51) and 1000 (N 0740-0004-60).
[Shown in Product Identification Section]
Also Unit Dose in package of 10 × 10 strips (N 0740-0004-11).
Peritrate 40 mg—coral scored tablets in bottles of 100 (N 0470-0008-51).
[Shown in Product Identification Section]
Peritrate 20 mg—light green, scored tablets in bottles of 100 (N 0470-0001-51) and 1000 (N 0470-0001-60).
[Shown in Product Identification Section]
Also Unit Dose in package of 10 × 10 strips (N 0470-0001-11).
Peritrate 10 mg—light green, unscored tablets in bottles of 100 (N 0470-0007-51).
STORE BETWEEN 59° and 86°F (15° and 30°C).
Animal Pharmacology: In a series of carefully designed studies in pigs, Peritrate (pentaerythritol tetranitrate) was administered for 48 hours before an artificially induced occlusion of a major coronary artery and for seven days thereafter. The pigs were sacrificed at various intervals for periods up to six weeks. The result showed a significantly larger number of survivors in the drug-treated group. Damage to myocardial tissue in the drug-treated survivors was less extensive than in the untreated group. Studies in dogs subjected to oligemic shock through progressive bleeding have demonstrated that Peritrate (pentaerythritol tetranitrate) is vasoactive at the postarteriolar level, producing increased blood flow and better tissue perfusion. These animal experiments cannot be translated to the drug's actions in humans.
303 G 720 **R-SA-2-79**

PERITRATE® ℞
with Phenobarbital SA Sustained Action
PERITRATE® 20 mg with Phenobarbital
PERITRATE® 10 mg with Phenobarbital

Caution: Federal law prohibits dispensing without prescription.
Peritrate with Phenobarbital SA Sustained Action: each tablet contains pentaerythritol tetranitrate 80 mg and phenobarbital 45 mg. The immediate release layer contains 20 mg pentaerythritol tetranitrate and 10 mg phenobarbital; the sustained release base contains 60 mg pentaerythritol tetranitrate and 35 mg phenobarbital.
Peritrate 20 mg with Phenobarbital: each tablet contains pentaerythritol tetranitrate 20 mg and phenobarbital 15 mg.
Peritrate 10 mg with Phenobarbital: each tablet contains pentaerythritol tetranitrate 10 mg and phenobarbital 15 mg.
Peritrate (pentaerythritol tetranitrate) is a nitric acid ester of a tetrahydric alcohol (pentaerythritol).
DOSAGE FORMS CONTAINING PHENOBARBITAL MAY BE HABIT-FORMING.
Actions: The exact cause of angina pectoris (that is, the pain associated with coronary artery disease) remains obscure, despite the numerous and often conflicting hypotheses concerning its pathophysiology. Therapy at the present time, therefore, remains essentially empirical. Customarily, clinical improvement has been measured by: reduction in (1) number, intensity and duration of angina pectoris attacks and (2) reduction in necessity for glyceryl trinitrate intake for prevention or relief of anginal attacks. Peritrate (pentaerythritol tetranitrate) has been reported in clinical usage to reduce in number and severity the incidence of angina pectoris attacks, with concomitant reduction in glyceryl trinitrate intake.
In the evaluation of Peritrate (pentaerythritol tetranitrate) in angina pectoris, clinical improvement has been customarily measured subjectively by: reduction in number and severity of attacks and necessity for glyceryl trinitrate intake for prevention or abortion of anginal attacks. Individual patterns of angina pectoris differ widely as does the symptomatic response to antianginal agents such as pentaerythritol tetranitrate. The published literature contains both favorable and unfavorable clinical reports. In conjunction with total management of the patient with angina pectoris, Peritrate (pentaerythritol tetranitrate) has been accepted as safe for prolonged administration and widely regarded as useful.

Indications
Based on a review of this drug by the National Academy of Sciences-National Research Council and/or other information, FDA has classified the indications as follows:

"Possibly" effective: Peritrate (pentaerythritol tetranitrate), alone or in combination forms, is indicated for the relief of angina pectoris (pain associated with coronary artery disease). It is not intended to abort the acute anginal episode but is widely regarded as useful in the prophylactic treatment of angina pectoris.
The dosage forms containing phenobarbital are especially indicated for the relief of angina pectoris precipitated or complicated by emotional tension, anxiety, and physical agitation.
Final classification of the less-than-effective indications requires further investigation.

Contraindications: Peritrate (pentaerythritol tetranitrate), alone or in combination forms, is contraindicated in patients who have a history of sensitivity to the component drugs. Phenobarbital is contraindicated in patients who have porphyria.

Warnings: Data supporting the use of Peritrate (pentaerythritol tetranitrate) during the early days of the acute phase of myocardial infarction (the period during which clinical and laboratory findings are unstable) are insufficient to establish safety.
This drug can act as a physiological antagonist to norepinephrine, acetylcholine, histamine, and many other agents.
PHENOBARBITAL MAY BE HABIT-FORMING.

Precautions: Should be used with caution in patients who have glaucoma. Tolerance to this drug and cross-tolerance to other nitrites and nitrates may occur.

Adverse Reactions: Side effects reported to date have been predominantly related to rash (which requires discontinuation of medication) and headache and gastrointestinal distress, which are usually mild and transient with continuation of medication. In some cases severe persistent headaches may occur.
In addition, the following adverse reactions to nitrates such as pentaerythritol tetranitrate have been reported in the literature:
(a) Cutaneous vasodilatation with flushing.
(b) Transient episodes of dizziness and weakness, as well as other signs of cerebral ischemia associated with postural hypotension, may occasionally develop.
(c) An occasional individual exhibits marked sensitivity to the hypotensive effects of nitrite, and severe responses (nausea, vomiting, weakness, restlessness, pallor, perspiration and collapse) can occur, even with the usual therapeutic doses. Alcohol may enhance this effect.

Dosage: Peritrate with Phenobarbital SA Sustained Action (b.i.d. on an empty stomach): 1 tablet immediately on arising and 1 tablet 12 hours later. Tablets should not be chewed.
Peritrate 20 mg with Phenobarbital: (q.i.d. on an empty stomach); 1 tablet at least ½ hour before or 1 hour after meals and at bedtime. Dosage can be initiated at 10 mg q.i.d. and should be individualized.
Peritrate 10 mg with Phenobarbital (q.i.d. on an empty stomach); 1 or 2 tablets at least ½ hour before or 1 hour after meals and at bedtime.

Supplied:
Peritrate with Phenobarbital SA Sustained Action (pentaerythritol tetranitrate 80 mg with phenobarbital 45 mg)—double-layer, biconvex, dark yellow/light yellow tablets in bottles of 100 (N 0740-0005-51) and 1000 (N 0470-0005-60).
[*Shown in Product Identification Section*]
Peritrate 20 mg with Phenobarbital—yellow, scored tablets in bottles of 100 (N 0470-0003-51) and 1000 (N 0470-0003-60).
[*Shown in Product Identification Section*]
Peritrate 10 mg with Phenobarbital—yellow, scored tablets in bottles of 100 (N 0470-0002-51) and 1000 (N 0470-0002-60).

Animal Pharmacology: In a series of carefully designed studies in pigs, Peritrate (pentaerythritol tetranitrate) was administered for 48 hours before an artificially induced occlusion of a major coronary artery and for seven days thereafter. The pigs were sacrificed at various intervals for periods up to six weeks. The result showed a significantly larger number of survivors in the drug-treated group. Damage to myocardial tissue in the drug-treated survivors was less extensive than in the untreated group. Studies in dogs subjected to oligemic shock through progressive bleeding have demonstrated that Peritrate (pentaerythritol tetranitrate) is vasoactive at the postarteriolar level, producing increased blood flow and better tissue perfusion.
These animal experiments cannot be translated to the drug's actions in humans.
STORE BETWEEN 59°-86°F (15°-30°C).
315 G 750 **R-2-79**

PITOCIN® ℞
(oxytocin injection, USP) synthetic

IMPORTANT NOTICE
Pitocin is not indicated for the elective induction of labor because available data and information are inadequate to define the benefits-to-risks considerations in the use of the drug product. Elective induction of labor is defined as the initiation of labor in an individual with a term pregnancy who is free of medical indications for the initiation of labor.

Description: Pitocin (oxytocin injection, USP) is a sterile, aqueous solution of synthetic oxytocic hormone standardized to contain 10 units/ml and containing 0.5% Chloretone® (chlorobutanol, USP) (chloral derivative) as a preservative, with the acidity adjusted with acetic acid. The drug is prepared synthetically to avoid possible contamination with vasopressin (ADH) and its antidiuretic and cardiovascular effects. However, the physician should be cognizant of the fact that even highly purified synthetic oxytocin contains inherent pressor-antidiuretic properties which may become manifest following administration of large doses (see Precautions).

Action: Uterine motility is controlled by a variety of biochemical and regulatory processes. Oxytocin appears to act primarily on uterine myofibril activity by increasing the permeability of the cell membranes to sodium ions, thus augmenting the number of contracting myofibrils, and thereby enabling the uterus to produce the necessary number of contractions. The effect depends on the uterine threshold of excitability. The sensitivity of the uterus to oxytocin increases gradually during gestation; then increases sharply before parturition.

Indications: **Ante partum:** Pitocin is indicated for the initiation or improvement of uterine contractions, where this is desirable and considered suitable, for the following purposes: induction of labor in patients with a medical indication for the initiation of labor, such as mild preeclampsia at or near term, when delivery is in the best interest of mother and fetus or when membranes are prematurely ruptured and delivery is indicated; stimulation or reinforcement of labor, as in selected cases of uterine inertia; management of inevitable, incomplete, or missed abortion.
Post partum: Pitocin is indicated to produce uterine contractions during the third stage of labor and to control postpartum bleeding or hemorrhage.

Contraindications: Pitocin is contraindicated in any of the following conditions: significant cephalopelvic disproportion; unfavorable fetal positions or presentations which are undeliverable without conversion prior to delivery (as, for example, transverse lies); in obstetrical emergencies where the benefit-to-risk ratio for either the fetus or the mother favors surgical intervention; in cases of fetal distress where delivery is not imminent; prolonged use in uterine inertia or severe toxemia; hypertonic uterine patterns; patients with hypersensitivity to the drug; induction or augmentation of labor in those cases where vaginal delivery is contraindicated, such as cervical carcinoma, cord presentation or prolapse, total placentia previa, and vasa previa.

Warnings: **Pitocin, when given for induction or stimulation of labor, must be administered only by the intravenous route and with adequate medical supervision in a hospital.**
Oxytocin should not be used simultaneously by more than one route, such as transbuccally and parenterally at the same time. Such use would complicate the problem of controlling dosage; however, clinical trials have shown that oxytocin by intravenous infusion may be used successfully after an unsuccessful trial of oxytocin by the buccal route. Conversely, buccal oxytocin could be employed in a patient who had previously received the drug intravenously.

Precautions:
1. All patients receiving intravenous oxytocin must be under continuous observation by trained personnel with a thorough knowledge of the drug and qualified to identify complications. A physician qualified to manage any complications should be immediately available.
2. When properly administered, oxytocin should stimulate uterine contractions comparable to those seen in normal labor. Overstimulation of the uterus by improper administration can be hazardous to both mother and fetus. Even with proper administration and adequate supervision, hypertonic contractions can occur in patients whose uteri are hypersensitive to oxytocin. This fact must be considered by the physician in exercising his judgment regarding patient selection.
3. Except in unusual circumstances, oxytocin should not be administered in the following conditions: fetal distress, partial placenta previa, prematurity, borderline cephalopelvic disproportion, and in any conditions where there is a predisposition for uterine rupture, such as previous major surgery on the cervix or uterus including cesarean section, overdistention of the uterus, grand multiparity, or past history of uterine sepsis or of traumatic delivery. Because of the variability of the combinations of factors which may be present in the conditions listed above, the definition of "unusual circumstances" must be left to the judgment of the physician. The decision can only be made by carefully weighing the potential benefits which oxytocin can provide in a given case against rare but definite potential for the drug to produce hypertonicity or tetanic spasm.
4. Maternal deaths due to hypertensive episodes, subarachnoid hemorrhage, rupture of the uterus, and fetal deaths due to various causes have been reported associated with the use of parenteral oxytocic drugs for induction of labor or for augmentation in the first and second stages of labor.
5. Oxytocin has been shown to have an intrinsic antidiuretic effect, acting to increase water reabsorption from the glomerular filtrate. Consideration should, therefore, be given to the

Continued on next page

This product information was prepared in August, 1979. On these and other Parke-Davis Products, detailed information may be obtained by addressing PARKE-DAVIS, Division of Warner-Lambert Company, Morris Plains, NJ 07950.

Parke-Davis—Cont.

possibility of water intoxication, particularly when oxytocin is administered continuously by infusion and the patient is receiving fluids by mouth.

6. When oxytocin is used for induction or reinforcement of already existent labor, patients should be carefully selected. Pelvic adequacy must be considered and maternal and fetal conditions evaluated before use of the drug.

Adverse Reactions: Fetal bradycardia, anaphylactic reaction, postpartum hemorrhage, cardiac arrhythmia, and pelvic hematoma have been reported.

Excessive dosage or hypersensitivity to the drug may result in uterine hypertonicity, spasm, tetanic contraction, or rupture.

Side effects that may also occur during spontaneous labor, such as nausea, vomiting, and premature ventricular contractions, have been noted occasionally with oxytocin.

A fatality due to afibrinogenemia has been reported, naming oxytocin injection as a possible cause. The possibility of increased blood loss and afibrinogenemia should be kept in mind when administering the drug.

Severe water intoxication with convulsions and coma has occurred, associated with a slow oxytocin infusion over a 24-hour period. Maternal death due to oxytocin-induced water intoxication has been reported.

Dosage and Administration: Dosage of oxytocin is determined by uterine response. The following dosage information is based upon the various regimens and indications in general use.

A. Induction or Stimulation of Labor

Intravenous infusion (drip method) is the only acceptable method of parenteral administration for the induction or stimulation of labor. Accurate control of the rate of infusion flow is essential. An infusion pump or other such device and at least external electronic monitoring are necessary for the safe administration of oxytocin for the induction or stimulation of labor. If uterine contractions become too powerful, the infusion can be abruptly stopped, and oxytocic stimulation of the uterine musculature will soon wane.

1. An intravenous infusion of non-oxytocin containing solution should be started. (Physiologic electrolyte solution should be used.)
2. To prepare the standard solution for infusion the contents of one 1-ml ampoule is combined aseptically with 1,000 ml of 0.9% aqueous sodium chloride solution or other nonhydrating diluent. The combined solution (1 ml = 10 milliunits) is rotated in the infusion bottle to insure thorough mixing. Add the container with dilute oxytocic solution to the system through use of a constant infusion pump.
3. The initial dose should be 1–2 mU/minute. At 15–30 minute intervals, the dose should be gradually increased in increments of 1 to 2 mU/minute until the desired contraction pattern has been established, which should be comparable to that seen in normal labor.
4. The fetal heart rate, resting uterine tone, and the frequency, duration, and force of contractions should be monitored.
5. The oxytocin infusion should be discontinued immediately in the event of uterine hyperactivity or fetal distress. Oxygen should be administered to the mother. The mother and the fetus must be evaluated by the responsible physician.

B. Control of Postpartum Uterine Bleeding

1. Intravenous Infusion (Drip Method)

To control postpartum bleeding, 10 to 40 units of oxytocin may be added to 1,000 ml of 5% dextrose injection and run at a rate necessary to control uterine atony.

Intramuscular Administration

1 ml (10 units) of oxytocin can be given after delivery of the placenta.

How Supplied: N 0071-4160-02 (Ampoule 163)
Contains 5 units in a 0.5-ml ampoule, packages of 10
N 0071-4160-03 (Ampoule 160)
Contains 10 units in a 1-ml ampoule, packages of 10
N 0071-4160-10 (Steri-Vial® 1541) contains 10 units per milliliter in a 10-ml Steri-Vial (rubber diaphragm-capped vial)
N 0071-4160-40 (Steri-Dose® syringe 1489)
Contains 10 units in a 1-ml sterile disposable syringe, packages of 10
AHFS 76:00 **WM**
Ampoule 160
NSN 6505-00-116-1376 (20s)
NSN 6505-00-965-2512 (100s)

PITOCIN® Citrate, Buccal ℞
(oxytocin citrate, buccal tablets)

> **IMPORTANT NOTE**
> Patients must be carefully selected: before the use of this drug, pelvic adequacy must be considered, and maternal and fetal conditions evaluated. Erroneous assumption of fetal maturity is one of the most serious dangers in elective induction.

Description: Pitocin Citrate, Buccal (oxytocin citrate, buccal tablets), is a preparation of synthetic oxytocin for buccal administration. Each tablet possesses an oxytocic activity equivalent to 200 USP units of oxytocin.

Action: The buccal tablets are designed to release oxytocin at a regular rate and, with the exception of the first few minutes, the rate of absorption is restricted by local mucosal vasoconstriction, but remains relatively steady until the tablet dissolves completely. This vasoconstriction is strictly a local effect and does not extend to systemic vessels. Oxytocin is not a vasopressor. Dosage is regulated until firm and regular contractions are produced. (See Dosage and Administration.)

Uterine motility is controlled by a variety of biochemical and regulatory processes. Oxytocin appears to act primarily on uterine myofibril activity by increasing the permeability of the cell membranes to sodium ions, thus augmenting the number of contracting myofibrils, and thereby enabling the uterus to produce the necessary number of contractions. The effect depends on the uterine threshold of excitability. The sensitivity of the uterus to oxytocin increases gradually during gestation; then increases sharply before parturition.

Indications: Pitocin Buccal is indicated for the initiation or improvement of uterine contractions where this is desirable and considered suitable as in the following.

1. To achieve gradual effacement in a responsive cervix when early vaginal delivery (36 weeks or more) for fetal reasons is indicated but not immediately necessary (eg, Rh problems, maternal diabetes)
2. Induction of labor in patients with mild preeclampsia at or near term, when delivery is in the best interest of mother and fetus
3. Induction of labor when membranes are prematurely ruptured and delivery is indicated
4. Elective induction when presentation is normal and other conditions favorable
5. Stimulation or reinforcement of labor, as in selected cases of uterine inertia

Contraindications: Pitocin Citrate, Buccal, is contraindicated in any of the following conditions: significant cephalopelvic disproportion; unfavorable fetal positions or presentations which are undeliverable without conversion prior to delivery (as, for example, transverse lies); in obstetrical emergencies where the benefit-to-risk ratio for either the fetus or the mother favors surgical intervention; in cases of fetal distress where delivery is not imminent; prolonged use in uterine inertia or severe toxemia; hypertonic uterine patterns; patients with hypersensitivity to the drug; or in an unconscious patient.

Pitocin Buccal is contraindicated for management and control of the third stage, to expel the placenta; control of postpartum bleeding and hemorrhage; and management of inevitable, incomplete, or missed abortion.

Warnings: *Pitocin Buccal is for hospital use only and must be administered with adequate medical supervision.*

Oxytocin *should not* be used simultaneously by more than one route, such as transbuccally and parenterally at the same time. Such use would complicate the problem of controlling dosage; however, clinical trials have shown that oxytocin by intravenous infusion may be used successfully after an unsuccessful trial of oxytocin by the buccal route. Conversely, buccal oxytocin could be employed in a patient who had previously received the drug intravenously.

Precautions: Administration of oxytocin by the buccal route in the first and second stages of labor should be supervised by persons having a thorough knowledge of the drug and qualified to identify complications. A qualified physician should be available at all times to manage any complications. Because of the variability in individual sensitivity to oxytocin and the response which is often accentuated in the second stage of labor, administration by untrained medical personnel is dangerous. When properly administered, oxytocin should stimulate uterine contractions identical to those seen in normal labor. Overstimulation of the uterus by improper administration can be hazardous to both the mother and fetus. Even with proper administration and adequate supervision, hypertonic contractions can occur in patients whose uteri are hypersensitive to oxytocin. Therefore, the physician must exercise careful judgment in his patient-selection criteria. Except in unusual circumstances, Pitocin Citrate, Buccal (oxytocin citrate, buccal tablets), should not be administered in the following conditions: fetal distress, prematurity, placenta praevia, abruptio placentae, borderline cephalopelvic disproportion, and in any condition where there is a predisposition for uterine rupture, such as previous major surgery on the cervix or uterus including cesarean section; overdistention of the uterus; grand multiparity; or past history of uterine sepsis or of traumatic delivery. Because of the variability of the combinations of factors which may be present in the conditions listed above, the definition of "unusual circumstances" must be left to the judgment of the physician. The decision can only be made by carefully weighing the potential benefits which oxytocin can provide in a given case against the rare but definite potential for the drug to produce hypertonicity or tetanic spasm.

Maternal deaths due to hypertensive episodes, subarachnoid hemorrhage, rupture of the uterus, and fetal deaths due to various causes have been reported associated with the use of parenteral oxytocic drugs for induction of labor or for augmentation in the first and second stages of labor.

Adverse Reactions: Fetal bradycardia, anaphylactic reactions, postpartum hemorrhage, cardiac arrhythmia, and pelvic hematoma have been reported.

Excessive dosage or hypersensitivity to the drug may result in uterine hypertonicity, spasm, tetanic contraction, or rupture.

Side effects that may also occur during spontaneous labor, such as nausea, vomiting, and premature ventricular contractions, have been noted occasionally with oxytocin.

A fatality due to afibrinogenemia has been reported, naming oxytocin injection as a possible cause. The possibility of increased blood loss and afibrinogenemia should be kept in mind when administering the drug.

Severe water intoxication with convulsions and coma has occurred, due to a slow oxytocin infusion over a 24-hour period. This suggests that oxytocin possesses some intrinsic antidiuretic action similar to that of vasopressin (ADH) and may thus affect fluid balance.

Dosage and Administration: Buccal administration of oxytocin must be adapted to the patient's response, and used only for induction or stimulation of labor.

The patient should be instructed to avoid disturbing the tablets after they are placed in the parabuccal space. Leaving the tablets undisturbed favors better absorption. Accidental swallowing of a tablet does not harm the patient; however, because oxytocin is inactivated by chymotrypsin, the oxytocic action of that tablet is destroyed in the digestive tract. If the mucous membranes become dry during the induction period, the patient may be allowed to rinse her mouth with cold water before replacing the tablets or receiving the next dose.

The initial dose is limited to one tablet to avoid the possibility of excessive absorption which may occur before local vasoconstriction has occurred. The tablets are then placed in alternate cheek pouches every 30 minutes until a dosage is found that produces the desired response. To find this dosage, give tablets according to the following schedule.

First hour:

One tablet (200 units) to start, repeat one tablet 30 minutes later.

If the desired response is obtained during the first hour, maintain the same number of tablets in the parabuccal spaces until delivery, or until a total of 15 tablets has been given (over a 24-hour period).

Second hour:

If no response, increase dosage to two tablets; repeat two tablets 30 minutes later.

If the desired response is obtained during the second hour, maintain the same number of tablets in the parabuccal spaces until delivery, or until a total of 15 tablets has been given (over a 24-hour period).

Third hour and until delivery:

If no response, increase dosage to three tablets; repeat three tablets every 30 minutes.

If the desired response is obtained during the third hour, maintain the same number of tablets in the parabuccal spaces until delivery, or until a total of 15 tablets has been given (over a 24-hour period).

This schedule, which increases dosage in increments of whole tablets at half-hour intervals, is continued until the desired response, ie, firm and regular uterine contractions not exceeding 40 to 60 seconds' duration and not occurring more frequently than every three minutes, is produced. Subject to the judgment of the physician, and provided effective autonomous labor has not been established, buccal dosage should then be maintained at the dosage level which has provided firm and regular uterine contractions. This buccal dosage should be maintained until a total of 15 tablets (3,000 units) has been given over a 24-hour period or until delivery is imminent or anesthesia is contemplated. If, for example, four tablets are required in the parabuccal spaces at one time to establish labor, the same number of tablets should be maintained parabuccally to sustain nonautonomous labor.

The average dosage required to complete labor in the original clinical work on Pitocin Citrate, Buccal, was approximately 1,700 units (between eight and nine tablets).

The technique for stimulation of labor is the same as that for induction, but the total dosage for stimulation may be less than that required for induction.

How Supplied: N 0071-0889-06 (Parcode® No. 889)

Pitocin Citrate, Buccal (oxytocin citrate, buccal tablets) is supplied as white rectangular tablets, wrapped individually in foil, each containing 200 USP units of oxytocin, packages of 10.

AHFS 76:00 **SA**

PITRESSIN® ℞
(vasopressin injection, USP)
synthetic

Description: Pitressin (vasopressin injection) is a sterile, aqueous solution of synthetic vasopressin (8-arginine vasopressin) of the posterior pituitary gland, is substantially free from the oxytocic principle, and is standardized to contain 20 pressor units/ml. The solution contains 0.5% Chloretone® (chlorobutanol) (chloroform derivative) as a preservative. The acidity of the solution is adjusted with acetic acid.

Action: The antidiuretic action of vasopressin is ascribed to increasing reabsorption of water by the renal tubules.

Vasopressin can cause contraction of smooth muscle of the gastrointestinal tract and of all parts of the vascular bed, especially the capillaries, small arterioles, and venules, with less effect on the smooth musculature of the large veins. The direct effect on the contractile elements is neither antagonized by adrenergic blocking agents nor prevented by vascular denervation.

Contraindication: Anaphylaxis or hypersensitivity to the drug or its components.

Indications: Pitressin is indicated for prevention and treatment of postoperative abdominal distention, in abdominal roentgenography to dispel interfering gas shadows, and in diabetes insipidus.

Warnings: This drug should not be used in patients with vascular disease, especially disease of the coronary arteries, except with extreme caution. In such patients, even small doses may precipitate anginal pain, and with larger doses, the possibility of myocardial infarction should be considered.

Vasopressin may produce water intoxication. The early signs of drowsiness, listlessness, and headaches should be recognized to prevent terminal coma and convulsions.

Precautions: Vasopressin should be used cautiously in the presence of epilepsy, migraine, asthma, heart failure, or any state in which a rapid addition to extracellular water may produce hazard for an already overburdened system.

Chronic nephritis with nitrogen retention contraindicates the use of vasopressin until reasonable nitrogen blood levels have been attained.

Adverse Reactions: Local or systemic allergic reactions may occur in hypersensitive individuals. The following side effects have been reported following the administration of vasopressin: tremor, sweating, vertigo, circumoral pallor, "pounding" in head, abdominal cramps, passage of gas, nausea, vomiting, urticaria, bronchial constriction. Anaphylaxis (cardiac arrest and/or shock) has been observed shortly after injection of vasopressin.

Dosage and Administration: Pitressin (vasopressin injection, USP) may be administered subcutaneously or intramuscularly.

Ten units of Pitressin (0.5 ml) will usually elicit full physiologic response in adult patients; 5 units will be adequate in many cases. Pitressin should be given intramuscularly at three- or four-hour intervals as needed. The dosage should be proportionately reduced for children. (For an additional discussion of dosage, consult the following sections.)

When determining the dose of Pitressin for a given case, the following should be kept in mind.

It is particularly desirable to give a dose not much larger than is just sufficient to elicit the desired physiologic response. Excessive dosage may cause undesirable side actions—blanching of the skin, abdominal cramps, nausea—which, though not serious, may be alarming to the patient. Spontaneous recovery from such side actions occurs in a few minutes. It has been found that one or two glasses of water given at the time Pitressin is administered reduces such symptoms.

Abdominal Distention: In the average postoperative adult patient, give 5 units (0.25 ml) initially; increase to 10 units (0.5 ml) at subsequent injections if necessary. It is recommended that Pitressin be given intramuscularly and that injections be repeated at three- or four-hour intervals as required. Dosage to be reduced proportionately for children.

Pitressin used in this manner will frequently prevent, or relieve, postoperative distention. These recommendations apply also to distention complicating pneumonia or other acute toxemias.

Abdominal Roentgenography: For the average case, two injections of 10 units each (0.5 ml) are suggested. These should be given two hours and one half hour, respectively, before films are exposed. Many roentgenologists advise giving an enema prior to the first dose of Pitressin.

Diabetes Insipidus: Pitressin may be given by injection or administered intranasally on cotton pledgets, by nasal spray, or by dropper. The dosage by injection is 5 to 10 units (0.25 to 0.5 ml) repeated two or three times daily as needed. When Pitressin is administered intranasally by spray or on pledgets, the dosage and interval between treatments must be determined for each patient.

How Supplied: *Pitressin (vasopressin injection, USP) synthetic is supplied in ampoules as follows.*

N 0071-4200-02
0.5 ml (10 pressor units). Packages of 10
N 0071-4200-03
1 ml (20 pressor units). Packages of 10

Note: When ordering Pitressin Ampoules, Synthetic, be sure to state whether the 10- or 20-unit is desired. **UM**

PITRESSIN® TANNATE IN OIL ℞
(vasopressin tannate)

Description: Pitressin Tannate (vasopressin tannate) is a water-insoluble chemical compound of vasopressin, the pressor fraction of the posterior lobe of the pituitary gland, and tannic acid.

Action: The antidiuretic action of vasopressin tannate is ascribed to increasing reabsorption of water by the renal tubules.

Vasopressin can cause contraction of smooth muscle of the gastrointestinal tract and of all parts of the vascular bed, especially the capillaries, small arterioles, and venules, with less effect on the smooth musculature of the large veins. These effects are ordinarily not seen to a significant degree with recommended antidiuretic doses of vasopressin tannate. The direct effect on the contractile elements is neither antagonized by adrenergic blocking agents nor prevented by vascular denervation.

Indications: Pitressin Tannate in Oil is indicated for the control or prevention of the symptoms and complications of diabetes insipidus due to a deficiency of endogenous posterior pituitary antidiuretic hormone.

Contraindication: Anaphylaxis or hypersensitivity to the drug or its components.

Continued on next page

This product information was prepared in August, 1979. On these and other Parke-Davis Products, detailed information may be obtained by addressing PARKE-DAVIS, Division of Warner-Lambert Company, Morris Plains, NJ 07950.

Parke-Davis—Cont.

Warnings:
This preparation should never be administered intravenously.
This drug should not be used in patients with vascular disease, especially disease of the coronary arteries, except with extreme caution. In such patients, even small doses may precipitate anginal pain.
Vasopressin may produce water intoxication. The early signs of drowsiness, listlessness, and headaches should be recognized to prevent terminal coma and convulsions.
Precautions: Vasopressin should be used cautiously in the presence of epilepsy, migraine, asthma, heart failure, or any state in which a rapid addition to extracellular water may produce hazard for an already overburdened system.
Chronic nephritis with nitrogen retention contraindicates the use of vasopressin until reasonable nitrogen blood levels have been attained.
Adverse Reactions: Local or systemic allergic reactions may occur in hypersensitive individuals. The following side effects have been reported following the administration of vasopressin: tremor, sweating, vertigo, circumoral pallor, "pounding" in head, abdominal cramps, passage of gas, nausea, vomiting, urticaria, bronchial constriction, anaphylaxis, cardiac arrest.
Dosage and Administration: Intramuscular —0.3 to 1 ml repeated as required. The duration of action varies with the patient and his condition, and may be as prolonged as 48 to 96 hours.
How Supplied:
N 0071-4302-03 (Ampoule 302)
Pitressin Tannate in Oil (vasopressin tannate) is supplied as a suspension containing 5 pressor units per milliliter in peanut oil, in 1-ml ampoules, packages of 10.
AHFS 68:28 **YC**

PONSTEL® ℞
(mefenamic acid)

Description: Ponstel is an analgetic agent, chemically designated N-(2,3-xylyl)-anthranilic acid, supplied in Kapseals® containing 250 mg mefenamic acid.
Action: The analgetic activity of Ponstel has been demonstrated in clinical trials. In pharmacologic studies conducted in animals, analgetic, antipyretic, and anti-inflammatory activities have been demonstrated. Pharmacologic studies in monkeys showed Ponstel to be devoid of any capacity to relieve morphine-abstinence signs in abstinent, morphine-habituated monkeys.
Metabolic studies show that Ponstel is excreted in urine and feces both as free drug and as metabolites.
Indications: Ponstel is indicated for the relief of mild to moderate pain when therapy will not exceed one week.
Contraindications: Ponstel is contraindicated in patients with ulceration or chronic inflammation of either the upper or lower gastrointestinal tract.
Ponstel should not be given to children under 14 years of age, because safe and effective use in this age group has not been established.
This drug is contraindicated in patients known to be hypersensitive to mefenamic acid.
Warnings: Administration of Ponstel (mefenamic acid) for periods exceeding one week is not recommended. If diarrhea occurs, the drug should be promptly discontinued. The patient so affected is usually unable to tolerate mefenamic acid thereafter.
Ponstel should be used with caution in patients with a history of kidney or liver disease. BUN values may rise during therapy. Microscopic examination in dogs given 100 or 200 mg per kg revealed slight centrolobular hepatocellular vacuolation. There was some evidence of edema and blunting of renal papilla in dogs administered 200 mg/kg. Rats given 100 mg/kg also showed microscopic evidence of renal papillary necrosis with epithelial cell degeneration.
Usage in Pregnancy—Reproduction studies in rats have shown a decreased rate of survival to weaning (possibly due to maternal neglect), delay in parturition, and decrease in fertility. In rabbits, an increase in the number of resorptions was noted. There were no fetal anomalies induced in mice, rats, rabbits, or dogs. Because there is no data on use of this drug in pregnant women, safety in pregnancy has not been established.
Precautions: The drug should be administered with caution to patients with inflammatory disease of the gastrointestinal tract. In animal toxicity studies, rats given 100 mg/kg of the drug have been known to develop small intestinal mucosal erosions and ulcers.
If rash occurs, the drug should be promptly withdrawn.
Ponstel may prolong prothrombin time. Therefore, when the drug is administered to patients receiving oral anticoagulant drugs, frequent monitoring of prothrombin time is necessary.
Ponstel should be used with caution in asthmatics, because the drug may cause an acute exacerbation of their condition.
A false-positive reaction for urinary bile, using the diazo tablet test, may result after mefenamic acid administration. If biliuria is suspected, other diagnostic procedures, such as the Harrison test, should be performed.
Adverse Reactions: Gastrointestinal: Nausea, gastrointestinal discomfort, vomiting, gas, and diarrhea, which may be severe and at times associated with inflammation of the bowel or hemorrhage, may occur in patients taking mefenamic acid.
Hematopoietic: Severe autoimmune hemolytic anemia may occur in patients given this drug for prolonged periods of time. Leukopenia, eosinophilia, thrombocytopenic purpura, agranulocytosis, pancytopenia, and bone marrow hypoplasia have also been reported in association with mefenamic acid therapy.
Nervous System: Drowsiness, dizziness, nervousness, headache, blurred vision, and insomnia have occurred.
Dermatologic: Urticaria, rash, and facial edema have been reported.
Renal: Mild renal toxicity, dysuria, and hematuria have occurred.
Other: Eye irritation, ear pain, perspiration, mild hepatic toxicity, and increased need for insulin in a diabetic have been reported. There have been rare reports of palpitation, dyspnea, and reversible loss of color vision.
Dosage and Administration: Administration is by the oral route, preferably with food. The recommended regimen for adults and children over 14 years of age is 500 mg Ponstel as an initial dose, followed by 250 mg every six hours as needed. Ponstel is indicated for short-term administration not exceeding one week of therapy. The margin of safety is reduced at higher doses and for longer administration.
How Supplied: N 0071-0540-24—Ponstel is available in Kapseals of 250 mg, bottles of 100. Parcode® No. 540
AHFS 28:08 **WL**
[Shown in Product Identification Section]

POVAN® FILMSEAL® ℞
(pyrvinium pamoate tablets, USP)
POVAN SUSPENSION ℞
(pyrvinium pamoate oral suspension, USP)

Description: Pyrvinium pamoate, a cyanine dye, is 6-dimethylamino-2-(2-[2, 5-dimethyl-1-phenyl-3-pyrrolyl] - vinyl) -1- methylquinolinium as the pamoate. It is a deep red crystalline powder which is stable to heat, light, and air, and is practically insoluble in water.
Actions: Pyrvinium pamoate appears to exert its anthelmintic effect by preventing the parasite from using exogenous carbohydrates. The parasite's endogenous reserves are depleted, and it dies. Povan is not appreciably absorbed from the gastrointestinal tract.
Indication: Povan is indicated for the treatment of enterobiasis.
Warnings: No animal or human reproduction studies have been performed. Therefore, the use of this drug during pregnancy requires that the potential benefits be weighed against its possible hazards to the mother and fetus.
Precautions: To forestall undue concern and help avoid accidental staining, patients and parents should be advised of the staining properties of Povan. Care should be exercised not to spill the suspension because it will stain most materials. Parents and patients should be informed that pyrvinium pamoate will color the stool a bright red. This is not harmful to the patient. If emesis occurs, the vomitus will probably be colored red and will stain most materials.
Adverse Reactions: Nausea, vomiting, cramping, diarrhea, and hypersensitivity reactions (photosensitization and other allergic reactions) have been reported. The gastrointestinal reactions occur more often in older children and adults who have received large doses. Emesis is more frequently seen with Povan Suspension than with Povan Filmseals.
Dosage and Administration: For control of pinworm infections in children and adults, Povan is administered orally in a single dose of 5 mg pyrvinium per kilogram body weight. If necessary, the dose may be repeated in two or three weeks. For convenience, a 5-ml teaspoonful of suspension per 10 kg (22 lb) body weight is recommended.
Pinworm infection can pass easily from person to person by transfer of eggs through direct contact, handling contaminated objects, and breathing airborne eggs in dust. Therefore, if an infection is detected in any member of a family or institution group, treatment of all members should be considered for complete parasite eradication.
Dosage may be conveniently determined by referring to the Table.
[See table on next page].
How Supplied:
N 0710-0747-19 (Tablet 747)—Povan film-coated tablets, each containing pyrvinium pamoate equivalent to 50 mg pyrvinium, are supplied in bottles of 50; Parcode® No. 747.
Povan Filmseal is a product of Parke Davis Laboratories, Fajardo, PR 00648.
[Shown in Product Identification Section]
N 0071-2253-53 (Suspension 253)—Povan Suspension, a pleasant-tasting strawberry-flavored preparation containing pyrvinium pamoate equivalent to 10 mg pyrvinium per milliliter, is supplied in 2-oz bottles.
NSN: 6505-00-890-1093
AHFS 8:08 **YE**

PRE-SATE® Ⓒ ℞
(chlorphentermine hydrochloride)

Caution: Federal law prohibits dispensing without prescription.
Description: Pre-Sate (chlorphentermine hydrochloride) is 4-Chloro-α α-dimethylphenethylamine hydrochloride.
Actions: Pre-Sate (chlorphentermine hydrochloride) is a sympathomimetic amine with some pharmacologic activities similar to and some activities differing from the prototype drugs used in obesity, the amphetamines. Tolerance has been demonstrated with all drugs of this class in which this phenomenon has been looked for.
Drugs of this class used in obesity are commonly known as "anorectics" or "anorexigenics." It has not been established, however, that the action of such drugs in treating obesity is primarily one of appetite suppression. Other

central nervous system actions or metabolic effects may be involved.

Adult obese subjects instructed in dietary management and treated with "anorectic" drugs lose more weight on the average than those treated with placebo and diet, as determined in relatively short-term clinical trials. The magnitude of increased weight loss by drug-treated patients over placebo-treated patients—in various study designs—is statistically significant at a fraction of a pound a week. The rate of weight loss is greatest in the first weeks of therapy for both drug and placebo subjects and tends to decrease in succeeding weeks. The possible origins of the increased weight loss due to the various drug effects are not established. The amount of weight loss associated with the use of an "anorectic" drug varies from trial to trial, and the increased weight loss appears to be related in part to variables other than the drugs prescribed, such as the physician-investigator, the population treated, and the diet prescribed. Studies do not permit conclusions as to the relative importance of the drug and non-drug factors on weight loss.

The natural history of obesity is measured in years, whereas the studies cited are restricted to a few weeks' duration; thus, the total impact of drug-induced weight loss over that of diet alone must be considered clinically limited.

Indications: Pre-Sate (chlorphentermine hydrochloride) is indicated in the management of exogenous obesity as a short term (a few weeks) adjunct in a regimen of weight reduction based on caloric restriction. The limited usefulness of agents of this class (see Actions) should be measured against possible risk factors inherent in their use such as those described below.

Contraindications: Glaucoma, advanced arteriosclerosis, hypersensitive response to chlorphentermine or other sympathomimetic amines, severe hypertension, hyperthyroidism.

Patients with a history of drug abuse, agitated states. Administration during or within 14 days following the administration of monoamine oxidase inhibitors, since hypertensive crises may result.

Warnings: Tolerance to the anorectic effect often develops within a few weeks. When this occurs, the recommended dose should not be exceeded in an attempt to increase the effect; rather, the drug should be discontinued.

Pre-Sate (chlorphentermine hydrochloride) may impair the ability of the patient to engage in potentially hazardous activities such as operating machinery or driving a motor vehicle; the patient should therefore be cautioned accordingly.

There have been reports of pulmonary hypertension in patients who received related drugs.

Drug Dependence: Chlorphentermine hydrochloride is related chemically and to some extent pharmacologically to the amphetamines. Amphetamines and related stimulant drugs have been extensively abused. Clinical use of Pre-Sate (chlorphentermine hydrochloride) over a number of years has not demonstrated clear-cut abuse potential; but the possibility of abuse should be kept in mind when evaluating the desirability of including this or any other anorectic drug as part of a weight reduction program. Abuse of amphetamines and some related drugs may be associated with intense psychological dependence, severe social dysfunction, and changes in sleep EEG, although not reported with Pre-Sate (chlorphentermine hydrochloride). Manifestations of chronic intoxication with amphetamines and some related drugs include severe dermatoses, marked insomnia, irritability, hyperactivity, and personality changes. The most severe manifestation of chronic intoxications with amphetamines and some related drugs is psychosis, often clinically indistinguishable from schizophrenia.

BODY WEIGHT		DOSAGE	DOSAGE
lb	kg	(Number of Teaspoonfuls)	(Number of Tablets)
154*	70	7 (35 ml)	7
143	65	6½ (32.5 ml)	7
132	60	6 (30 ml)	6
121	55	5½ (27.5 ml)	6
110	50	5 (25 ml)	5
99	45	4½ (22.5 ml)	5
88	40	4 (20 ml)	4
77	35	3½ (17.5 ml)	4
66	30	3 (15 ml)	3
55	25	2½ (12.5 ml)	3
44	20	2 (10 ml)	2
33	15	1½ (7.5 ml)	2

*Because the gastrointestinal tract of adults does not appreciably increase in size with increased weight gain, the dosage for adults need not exceed that recommended for a patient weighing 154 lb. A single dose of seven tablets or teaspoonfuls should be adequate for patients who weigh more than 154 lb.

Usage in Pregnancy: Mammalian reproductive and teratogenic studies with high multiples of the human dose have been negative. There have been no reports of adverse reproductive or teratogenic effects in humans. Use of Pre-Sate (chlorphentermine hydrochloride) by women who are or may become pregnant requires that the potential benefit be weighed against possible hazards to mother and infant.

Usage in Children: Pre-Sate (chlorphentermine hydrochloride) is not recommended for use in children under 12 years of age.

Precautions: Use only with caution in hypertension, with monitoring of blood pressure, since evidence is insufficient to rule out a possible adverse effect on blood pressure in some hypertensive patients. The drug is not recommended for patients with symptomatic cardiovascular disease, including arrhythmias.

Insulin requirements in diabetes mellitus may be altered in association with the use of chlorphentermine hydrochloride and a concomitant dietary regimen.

The least amount feasible of chlorphentermine hydrochloride should be prescribed or dispensed at one time in order to minimize the possibility of overdosage.

Adverse Reactions: *Cardiovascular:* Palpitation, tachycardia, elevation of blood pressure is rare and usually not serious.

Central Nervous System: Sedation, drowsiness, overstimulation, restlessness, dizziness, insomnia, euphoria, dysphoria, tremor, headache; rarely, psychotic episodes at recommended doses.

Gastrointestinal: Dryness of the mouth, unpleasant taste, diarrhea, constipation, other gastrointestinal disturbances.

Allergic: Urticaria.

Endocrine: Impotence, changes in libido.

Also: Mydriasis, diuresis and rarely, difficulty in initiating micturition.

Dosage and Administration: The recommended adult daily dose of Pre-Sate (chlorphentermine hydrochloride) is one tablet (equivalent to 65 mg chlorphentermine base) taken after the first meal of the day. Use in children under 12 is not recommended.

Overdosage: *Manifestations:* Restlessness, confusion, assaultiveness, hallucinations, panic states, and hyperpyrexia may be manifestations of acute intoxication with anorectic agents. Fatigue and depression usually follow the central stimulation.

Cardiovascular effects include arrhythmias, hypertension, or hypotension and circulatory collapse. Gastrointestinal symptoms include nausea, vomiting, diarrhea, and abdominal cramps. Fatal poisoning usually terminates in convulsions and coma.

Management: Management of acute intoxication with sympathomimetic amines is largely symptomatic and supportive and often includes sedation with a barbiturate. If hypertension is marked, the use of a nitrate or rapidly acting alpha-receptor blocking agent should be considered. Experience with hemodialysis or peritoneal dialysis is inadequate to permit recommendations.

How Supplied: Each Pre-Sate (chlorphentermine hydrochloride) tablet contains the equivalent of 65 mg chlorphentermine base; bottles of 100 (N 0047-0310-51).

STORE BETWEEN 59° and 86°F (15° and 30°C).

[*Shown in Product Identification Section*]

326 G 231 **4-78**

PROLOID® TABLETS ℞
(thyroglobulin)

Caution: Federal law prohibits dispensing without prescription.

Description: Proloid (thyroglobulin) is obtained from a purified extract of hog thyroid. It contains the known calorigenically active components, levothyroxine (T_4) and liothyronine (T_3). Proloid (thyroglobulin) conforms to the primary USP specifications for desiccated thyroid — for iodine based on chemical assay — and is also biologically assayed and standardized in animals.

Chromatographic analysis to standardize the levothyroxine and liothyronine content of Proloid (thyroglobulin) is routinely employed.

Proloid (thyroglobulin) is stable when stored at room temperature.

Actions: The actions of the thyroid hormone(s) involve the maturation and proper function of such organ systems as the endocrine, nervous, skeletal, reproductive, and gastrointestinal. The calorigenic and other actions of thyroid hormone(s) are instrumental in maintaining the normal functional capacity of tissues in organ systems throughout the body.

Indications: Proloid (thyroglobulin) is thyroid replacement therapy for conditions of inadequate endogenous thyroid production: e.g., cretinism and myxedema. Replacement therapy will be effective only in manifestations of hypothyroidism.

In simple (nontoxic) goiter, Proloid (thyroglobulin) may be tried therapeutically, in nonemergency situations, in an attempt to reduce the size of such goiters.

Contraindication: Thyroid preparations are contraindicated in the presence of uncorrected adrenal insufficiency.

Continued on next page

This product information was prepared in August, 1979. On these and other Parke-Davis Products, detailed information may be obtained by addressing PARKE-DAVIS, Division of Warner-Lambert Company, Morris Plains, NJ 07950.

Parke-Davis—Cont.

Warnings:

> Drugs with thyroid hormone activity, alone or together with other therapeutic agents, have been used for the treatment of obesity. In euthyroid patients, doses within the range of daily hormonal requirements are ineffective for weight reduction. Larger doses may produce serious or even life-threatening manifestations of toxicity, particularly when given in association with sympathomimetic amines such as those used for their anorectic effects.

Thyroglobulin should not be used in the presence of cardiovascular disease unless thyroid-replacement therapy is clearly indicated. If the latter exists, low doses should be instituted beginning at 0.5 to 1.0 grain (approximately 32 to 65 mg) and increased by the same amount in increments at two-week intervals. This demands careful clinical judgment.

Morphologic hypogonadism and nephroses should be ruled out before the drug is administered. If hypopituitarism is present, the adrenal deficiency must be corrected prior to starting the drug.

Myxedematous patients are very sensitive to thyroid and dosage should be started at a very low level and increased gradually.

Precaution: As with all thyroid preparations this drug will alter results of thyroid function tests.

Adverse Reactions: Overdosage or too rapid increase in dosage may result in signs and symptoms of hyperthyroidism, such as menstrual irregularities, nervousness, cardiac arrhythmias, and angina pectoris.

Dosage and Administration: Optimal dosage is usually determined by the patient's clinical response. Confirmatory tests include BMR, $T_3{}^{131}I$ resin sponge uptake, $T_3{}^{131}I$ red cell uptake, Thyro Binding Index (TBI), and Achilles Tendon Reflex Test. Clinical experience has shown that a normal PBI (3.5-8 mcg/100 ml) will be obtained in patients made clinically euthyroid when the content of T_4 and T_3 is adequate. Dosage should be started in small amounts and increased gradually with increments at intervals of one to two weeks. Usual maintenance dose is 0.5 to 3.0 grains (approximately 32 to 200 mg) daily.

Instructions for Use: The following conversion table lists the approximate equivalents of other thyroid preparations to Proloid (thyroglobulin) when changing medication from desiccated thyroid, T_4 (levothyroxine sodium), T_3 (liothyronine sodium), or T_4/T_3 (liotrix).

[See accompanying table below].

In changing from Thyroid USP to Proloid (thyroglobulin), substitute the equivalent dose of Proloid (thyroglobulin). Each patient may still require fine adjustment of dosage because the equivalents are only estimates.

Overdosage Symptoms: Headache, instability, nervousness, sweating, tachycardia, with unusual bowel motility. Angina pectoris or congestive heart failure may be induced or aggravated. Shock may develop. Massive overdosage may result in symptoms resembling thyroid storm. Chronic excessive dosage will produce the signs and symptoms of hyperthyroidism.

(Treatment: In shock, supportive measures should be utilized. Treatment of unrecognized adrenal insufficiency should be considered.)

Supplied: ½ grain (32 mg) tablets in bottles of 100 (N 0047-0251-51) and 1000 (N 0047-0251-60); scored 1 grain (65 mg) tablets in bottles of 100 (N 0047-0252-51) and 1000 (N 0047-0252-60); 1½ grain (100 mg) tablets in bottles of 100 (N 0047-0253-51) and 1000 (N 0047-0253-60); scored 2 grain (130 mg) tablets in bottles of 100 (N 0047-0257-51); 3 grain (200 mg) tablets in bottles of 100 (N 0047-0254-51) and 1000 (N 0047-0254-60).

STORE BETWEEN 59° and 86° F (15° and 30° C).

[*Shown in Product Identification Section*]

378 G 184 **R-6-78**

Conversion Table

Dose of Proloid (thyroglobulin) grain	mg	Dose of Desiccated Thyroid grain	Dose of T_4 (levothyroxine sodium) mg	Dose of T_3 (liothyronine sodium) mcg	Dose of liotrix (T_4/T_3)
1	(65)	1	0.1	25	#1 (60 mcg/15 mcg)
2	(130)	2	0.2	50	#2 (120 mcg/30 mcg)
3	(200)	3	0.3	75	#3 (180 mcg/45 mcg)
4	(260)	4	0.4	100	

PYRIDIUM® ℞
(phenazopyridine HCl)

Caution: Federal law prohibits dispensing without prescription.

Description: 200 mg—Each tablet contains 0.2 gram Pyridium (phenazopyridine HCl) and bears the inscription W/C 181. 100 mg—Each tablet contains 0.1 gram Pyridium (phenazopyridine HCl) and bears the inscription W/C 180.

Actions: Pyridium (phenazopyridine HCl) is excreted in the urine where it exerts a topical analgesic effect on the mucosa of the urinary tract. This action helps to relieve pain, burning, urgency and frequency. Since Pyridium (phenazopyridine HCl) is an analgesic, it should be used only for relief of symptoms. It is, however, compatible with antibacterial therapy and can help to relieve pain and discomfort during the interval before antibacterial therapy controls the infection.

Indications: Symptomatic relief of pain, burning, urgency, frequency, and other discomforts arising from irritation of the lower urinary tract mucosa. These symptoms may result from infection, trauma, surgery, endoscopic procedures, or passage of sounds or catheters. Its topical, analgesic action may reduce or eliminate the need for systemic analgesics or narcotics. The use of Pyridium (phenazopyridine HCl) for symptomatic relief should not delay definitive diagnosis and treatment.

Contraindications: Renal insufficiency. A yellowish tinge of the skin or sclerae may indicate accumulation due to impaired renal excretion and the need to discontinue therapy.

Adverse Reactions: Occasional gastrointestinal disturbance. Methemoglobinemia, hemolytic anemia, renal and hepatic toxicity have been described, usually at overdose levels (see Overdosage section).

Dosage and Management: 200 mg tablets: Average adult dosage is one tablet 3 times a day after meals. 100 mg tablets: Average adult dosage is two tablets 3 times a day after meals. Note: Patients should be told that Pyridium (phenazopyridine HCl) produces a reddish-orange discoloration of the urine.

Overdosage: Exceeding the recommended dose in patients with good renal function or administering the usual dose to patients with impaired renal function (common in elderly patients), may lead to increased serum levels and toxic reactions. Methemoglobinemia generally follows a massive, acute overdose. Methylene blue, 1 to 2 mg/kg body weight intravenously, or ascorbic acid 100 to 200 mg given orally should cause prompt reduction of the methemoglobinemia and disappearance of the cyanosis which is an aid in diagnosis. Oxidative Heinz body hemolytic anemia may also occur, and "bite cells" (degmacytes) may be present in a chronic overdosage situation. Red blood cell G-6-PD deficiency may predispose to hemolysis. Renal and hepatic impairment and occasional failure, usually due to hypersensitivity, may also occur.

Supplied: The 200 mg dark maroon, coated tablets are supplied in bottles of 100 (N 0047-0181-51) and 1000 (N 0047-0181-60). Also in unit dose—package of 10 × 10 strips (N 0047-0181-11).

The 100 mg dark maroon, coated tablets are supplied in bottles of 100 (N 0047-0180-51) and 1000 (N 0047-0180-60). Also in unit dose—package of 10 × 10 strips (N 0047-0180-11).

STORE BETWEEN 59° and 86°F (15° and 30°C).

[*Shown in Product Identification Section*]

304 G 822 **R-4-78**

PYRIDIUM® PLUS ℞
(formerly Dolonil®)

Caution: Federal law prohibits dispensing without prescription.

Description: Each tablet contains 150 mg phenazopyridine hydrochloride (Pyridium®); 0.3 mg hyoscyamine hydrobromide; 15 mg butabarbital.

Actions: Relieves lower urinary symptoms of pain, frequency, urgency, burning and dysuria arising from inflammation of the urothelium, the mucosal lining of the lower urinary tract. Lower urinary tract pain can cause reflex spasm of the detrusor. Pain and spasm are often aggravated by apprehension to promote a pain-spasm-apprehension cycle. The three pharmacologic components of Pyridium Plus act against each phase of this cycle.

Phenazopyridine hydrochloride (Pyridium), excreted in the urine, is a topical analgesic, to relieve pain and discomfort.

Hyoscyamine hydrobromide, a parasympatholytic, acts to relieve detrusor muscle spasm.

Butabarbital, a short-to-intermediate-acting sedative, helps to allay associated anxiety and apprehension.

Indications: Pyridium Plus is indicated for the symptomatic relief of pain, burning, frequency, urgency, and dysuria, particularly when accompanied by detrusor muscle spasm and apprehension. These symptoms may arise from infection, trauma, surgery, endoscopic procedures, or passage of sounds or catheters. Pyridium Plus therapy does not interfere with antibacterial therapy and can help to relieve symptoms of pain and discomfort before definitive treatment is effective. The use of Pyridium Plus for symptomatic relief should not delay definitive diagnosis and treatment. In the absence of infection, Pyridium Plus may be the only medication required.

Contraindications: Renal or hepatic insufficiency; glaucoma; porphyria; sensitivity to any component. A yellowish tinge of the skin or sclerae may indicate accumulation due to impaired renal excretion and the need to discontinue therapy.

Warning: Butabarbital may be habit-forming.

Precautions: Not recommended for patients with bladder-neck obstruction.

Adverse Reactions: Dry mouth, drowsiness or dizziness is noted in more than one-third of patients (and may occur in half of the patients of older age groups). These symptoms seldom require discontinuation of medication. Other atropine-like effects such as blurred vision may also occur. There may be occasional gastrointestinal disturbances.

Dosage: Average adult dosage: one tablet 4 times a day (after meals and at bedtime).

Note: Patients should be told that Pyridium Plus produces a reddish-orange discoloration of the urine.
Supplied: Dark maroon, square tablets in bottles of 100 (N 0740-0182-24).
STORE BETWEEN 59° and 86°F (15° and 30°C).
[*Shown in Product Identification Section*]
0182 G 010 **9-79**

RENOQUID® ℞
(sulfacytine)
250-mg Tablets

Description: Sulfacytine, a short-acting sulfonamide, is a white, crystalline solid with a melting point in the range of 168.5 to 170 C. It is slightly soluble in pH 5 buffer (109 mg/100 ml). It can be dissolved in human urine to 500 mg/100 ml at pH 6. One gram in 5 ml hot 70% aqueous methanol makes a clear solution. Chemically, sulfacytine is 1-ethyl-N-sulfanilylcytosine.
Actions: The systemic sulfonamides are bacteriostatic agents having a similar spectrum of activity. Sulfonamides competitively inhibit bacterial synthesis of folic acid (pteroylglutamic acid) from aminobenzoic acid. Resistant strains are capable of utilizing folic acid precursors or preformed folic acid.
Indications: Sulfacytine is indicated for the treatment of acute urinary tract infections only (primarily pyelonephritis, pyelitis, and cystitis), in the absence of obstructive uropathy or foreign bodies, when due to susceptible strains of the following microorganisms: *Escherichia coli, Klebsiella-Enterobacter, Staphylococcus aureus, Proteus mirabilis,* and *P vulgaris.*
Important Note: *In vitro* sulfonamide sensitivity tests are not always reliable. The test must be carefully coordinated with bacteriologic and clinical response. When the patient is already taking sulfonamides, follow-up cultures should have aminobenzoic acid added to the culture media.
Currently, the increasing frequency of resistant microorganisms is a limitation of the usefulness of antibacterial agents including the sulfonamides.
Contraindications: Hypersensitivity to sulfonamides. Infants less than 2 months of age. Pregnancy at term and during the nursing period because sulfonamides cross the placenta and are excreted in breast milk and may cause kernicterus.
Warnings: Deaths associated with the administration of sulfonamides have been reported from hypersensitivity reactions, agranulocytosis, aplastic anemia, and other blood dyscrasias. The presence of clinical signs, such as sore throat, fever, pallor, purpura, or jaundice, may be early indications of serious blood disorders.
Complete blood counts should be done frequently in patients receiving sulfonamides.
The frequency of renal complications is considerably lower in patients receiving the more soluble sulfonamides. Urinalysis with careful microscopic examination should be performed frequently for patients receiving sulfonamides.
Due to lack of clinical experience in the pediatric age group, sulfacytine is not recommended for use in children under age 14.
Precautions: Sulfonamides should be given with caution to patients with impaired renal or hepatic functions and to those with severe allergies or bronchial asthma.
Adequate fluid intake must be maintained in order to prevent crystalluria and formation of calculi.
In glucose-6-phosphate dehydrogenase-deficient individuals, hemolysis may occur. This reaction is frequently dose-related.
Usage in Pregnancy: Reproduction studies have been performed in rats and rabbits and have revealed no evidence of impaired fertility or harm to the fetus due to sulfacytine. There are no well-controlled studies in pregnant women. Therefore, sulfacytine should be used in pregnant women only when clearly needed.
Adverse Reactions: The most common adverse reactions associated with sulfacytine are headache, gastrointestinal disturbances, and allergic reactions (rash).
The following reactions have been associated with sulfonamide therapy.
Blood dyscrasias: agranulocytosis, aplastic anemia, thrombocytopenia, leukopenia, hemolytic anemia, purpura, hypoprothrombinemia, methemoglobinemia
Allergic reactions: erythema multiforme (including Stevens-Johnson syndrome), generalized skin eruptions, epidermal necrolysis, urticaria, serum sickness, pruritus, exfoliative dermatitis, anaphylactoid reactions, periorbital edema, conjunctival and scleral injection, photosensitization, arthralgia, and allergic myocarditis
Gastrointestinal reactions: nausea, emesis, abdominal pains, hepatitis, diarrhea, anorexia, pancreatitis, and stomatitis
CNS reactions: headache, peripheral neuritis, mental depression, convulsions, ataxia, hallucinations, tinnitus, vertigo, and insomnia
Miscellaneous reactions: drug fever, chills, and toxic nephrosis with oliguria and anuria. Periarteritis nodosa and lupus erythematosus phenomena have occurred.
The sulfonamides bear certain chemical similarities to some goitrogens, diuretics (acetazolamide and the thiazides), and oral hypoglycemia agents. Goiter production, diuresis, and hypoglycemia have occurred rarely in patients receiving sulfonamides. Cross-sensitivity may exist with these agents.
Rats appear to be especially susceptible to the goitrogenic effects of sulfonamides, and long-term administration has produced thyroid malignancies in the species.

Dosage and Administration: The usual adult dosage is 500 mg initially as a loading dose, then 250 mg four times daily for 10 days. Due to lack of clinical experience in the pediatric age group, sulfacytine is not recommended for use in children under age 14.

How Supplied: N 0071-0925-Renoquid (sulfacytine) Tablets, 250 mg, are supplied in bottles of 100, and in a Therapy Pack containing 41 tablets (10-day dosage regimen). Parcode® No. 925

Clinical Pharmacology: Sulfacytine is rapidly absorbed following single, oral doses of 0.5, 1.0, 2.0, and 4.0 g. Peak blood levels occur within two to three hours. The area under the blood level curve indicates essentially complete oral absorption. The plasma half-life is four hours.
A sulfacytine dosage of 250 mg four times daily for seven days will produce a mean total sulfonamide plasma level of 16.8 mcg/ml, mean free plasma level of 16.5 mcg/ml for Days 2 to 7.
Protein-binding studies indicate that the unbound fraction of sulfacytine is 14%. The binding is readily reversible. Dialysis equilibrium studies with human plasma yielded a dissociation constant of $5 \times 10^{-5} M$ for sulfacytine.
Sulfacytine is rapidly excreted by the kidneys. Following a single, oral dose of 500 mg, 88% was recovered in the urine at the end of 24 hours, 95% at the end of five days. Following a dosage of 250 mg four times daily for seven days, chromatographic analysis of the urine on the final day showed the following distribution: 79% free drug, 11% N-glucuronides, and 10% acetylated metabolite (inactive). The "free" form is considered to be the therapeutically active form.
Following administration of 500 mg initially, then 250 mg four times daily for seven days, the mean urinary concentration of free sulfacytine for all sampling periods was 419 mcg/ml. This is over 10 times the highest minimal inhibitory concentration (MIC) for sensitive strains of *E coli, Enterobacter,* and *Proteus* (31 mcg/ml).
WL
[*Shown in Product Identification Section*]

SAF TIP® PHOSPHATE ENEMA
Saline Laxative

Composition: Active ingredients: Each 120 ml (4 fl oz) contains 19 g of sodium biphosphate and 7 g of sodium phosphate. Sodium content is 4.4 g per 120 ml.
Action: Saf Tip Phosphate Enema (a saline laxative) increases water in the intestine, thereby promoting bowel movement.
Indication: For short-term relief of constipation
Warnings: Do not use this product when abdominal pain, nausea, or vomiting are present.
If you have noticed a sudden change in bowel habits that persists over a period of two weeks, consult a physician before using a laxative.
For occasional use only. Serious side effects from prolonged use or overdosage may occur.
Except on the advice and under the supervision of a physician,
do not give to children under 2 years of age;
do not use this product for a period of longer than one week;
do not use this product if you have kidney disease;
do not use this product if you are on a low-salt diet.
Dosage: Adults, 120 ml (4 fl oz) (delivered dose) daily, as a single, rectal dose; children over 2 years of age, 60 ml (2 fl oz) daily as a single, rectal dose. Do not exceed the recommended dosage except on the advice and under the supervision of a physician.
How Supplied: N 0071-1396-18. 4½-oz squeeze bottles.
WD

SINUBID® ℞
Caution: Federal law prohibits dispensing without prescription.
Description: Each Sinubid tablet contains:

acetaminophen	300 mg
phenacetin	300 mg
phenylpropanolamine hydrochloride	100 mg
phenyltoloxamine citrate	66 mg

Actions: Sinubid is designed to provide symptomatic relief of coryza and nasal congestion when given twice a day (every 12 hours). Sinubid can provide symptomatic relief of headache, fever, and other symptoms associated with mucosal congestion (nasopharyngeal), general malaise, and irritability associated with the common cold, allergic and vasomotor disorders, sinusitis, and rhinitis.
Sinubid contains two analgesic-antipyretics (acetaminophen and phenacetin) to relieve the pain of sinus headache and nasal congestion. These analgesic-antipyretics are rapidly absorbed and as effective as aspirin in raising the pain threshold but have the advantage of causing little or no gastric irritation. Sinubid, because it contains no salicylates, can be used by patients who are allergic to aspirin.
Decongestion of the nasopharyngeal mucosa is provided by phenylpropanolamine hydrochloride, a sympathomimetic amine which provides symptomatic relief. Because its vasoconstrictor activity is similar to that of ephedrine, but less likely to cause CNS stimulation, Sinubid may eliminate the need for topical decongestants.

Continued on next page

This product information was prepared in August, 1979. On these and other Parke-Davis Products, detailed information may be obtained by addressing PARKE-DAVIS, Division of Warner-Lambert Company, Morris Plains, NJ 07950.

Parke-Davis—Cont.

Phenyltoloxamine citrate is a mild antihistamine which may provide symptomatic relief of seasonal and perennial allergic rhinitis, vasomotor rhinitis, nasal and sinus symptoms of sinusitis, and adjunctive therapy for bacterial sinusitis in uncomplicated upper respiratory infections.
Indications: Sinubid is indicated for the rapid, prolonged, symptomatic relief of nasal congestion in sinus or other frontal headache; allergic and vasomotor manifestations of upper respiratory disorders such as sinusitis, allergic rhinitis, vasomotor rhinitis, coryza; facial pain and "pressure" of acute and chronic sinusitis; and for the relief of accompanying fever. Sinubid is indicated only for intermittent treatment of the above noted acute symptoms.
Contraindications: This compound should not be used in patients whose oversensitivity to small doses of sympathomimetic amines produces sleeplessness, dizziness, lightheadedness, weakness, tremulousness, or cardiac arrhythmias. The drug is contraindicated in any patient hypersensitive to any of the ingredients of the formulation.
Warnings: Instruct patients not to drive or operate machinery if drowsiness occurs. Individuals should not ingest alcoholic beverages, monoamine oxidase inhibitors, or barbiturates while taking this medication.
Precautions: Individuals with high blood pressure, heart disease, diabetes mellitus, chronic renal disease, or thyroid disease should use only as directed by a physician. Excessive or prolonged use of phenacetin-containing products should be avoided.
Usage in Pregnancy: Since there is no adequate experience in pregnant women who have received this drug, safety in pregnancy has not been established. This drug should not be used in nursing mothers.
Adverse Reactions: The following adverse reactions have been reported for each of the individual or combinations of ingredients: *Acetaminophen*—urticaria, epigastric distress, dizziness, and palpitation. *Phenacetin*—cyanosis with methemoglobinemia, hemolytic anemia, dyspnea, headache, vascular collapse, and kidney damage from prolonged use. *Phenylpropanolamine HCl*—anxiety, restlessness, tension, insomnia, tremor, weakness, headache, vertigo, sweating, arrhythmia, nausea, and vomiting. *Phenyltoloxamine Citrate*—urticaria, drowsiness, disturbed coordination, inability to concentrate, dizziness, insomnia, tremors, nervousness, palpitation, convulsions, muscular weakness, gastric distress, diarrhea, intestinal cramps, blurred vision, hypotension, urinary retention, dryness of mouth, throat and nose.
Dosage:
Adults: One tablet twice daily (every 12 hours). Children (6-12 years of age): One-half tablet twice daily (every 12 hours).
Tablets should not be chewed.
Supplied: Sinubid is an ellipsoid, bi-layered (light pink/pink), scored tablet, bearing the Warner/Chilcott monogram. Bottles of 100 (N 0047-0100-51).
STORE BETWEEN 59° and 86°F (15° and 30°C).
[*Shown in Product Identification Section*]
364 G 396 **R-10-78**

SURITAL® Ⓒ
(thiamylal sodium for injection, NF)

Description: Surital (thiamylal sodium for injection, NF) is sodium-5-allyl-5-(1-methylbutyl)-2-thiobarbiturate.
Actions: Thiamylal sodium is a rapid, ultrashort-acting barbiturate, intravenous, anesthetic agent.
Indications: Surital is indicated for induction of anesthesia, for supplementing other anesthetic agents, as intravenous anesthesia for short surgical procedures with minimal painful stimuli, or as an agent for inducing a hypnotic state.
Contraindications: Thiamylal sodium is contraindicated when general anesthesia is contraindicated, in patients with latent or manifest porphyria, or in patients with a known hypersensitivity to barbiturates.
Warnings: RESUSCITATIVE EQUIPMENT AND DRUGS SHOULD BE IMMEDIATELY AVAILABLE. This drug should be administered by persons qualified in the use of intravenous anesthetics.
Repeated and continuous infusion may cause cumulative effects resulting in prolonged somnolence, and respiratory and circulatory depression.
Usage in pregnancy: Safe use of thiamylal sodium has not been established with respect to adverse effects upon fetal development. Therefore, thiamylal sodium should not be used in women of childbearing potential, and particularly during early pregnancy, unless, in the judgment of the physician, the expected benefits outweigh the potential hazards.
Precautions: Respiratory depression, apnea, or hypotension may occur due to variations in tolerance from individual to individual or to physical status of patient. Caution should be exercised in debilitated patients, or those with impaired function of respiratory, circulatory, renal, hepatic, and endocrine systems.
Thiamylal sodium should be used with extreme caution in patients in status asthmaticus.
Extravascular injection may cause pain, swelling, ulceration, and necrosis. Intra-arterial injection is dangerous and may produce gangrene of an extremity.
Adverse Reactions: The following adverse reactions have been reported: circulatory depression, thrombophlebitis, pain at injection site, and respiratory depression, including apnea, laryngospasm, bronchospasm, salivation, hiccups, emergence delirium, headache, injury to nerves adjacent to injection site, skin rashes, urticaria, nausea, and emesis.
Dosage and Administration: The dosage is individualized according to the patient's response.
A 2.5% solution is recommended for induction of anesthesia as well as for maintenance by intermittent intravenous injection. A dilute solution (0.3%) may be used by continuous drip for maintenance. The rate of injection during induction should be approximately 1 ml of 2.5% solution every five seconds; an initial injection of 3 to 6 ml of 2.5% solution is generally sufficient to produce short periods of surgical anesthesia.
Sterile water for injection is the preferred solvent for preparing Surital (thiamylal sodium for injection, NF) solutions. Initially, Surital solutions are clear, but they may become cloudy on aging. Thiamylal sodium cannot be reconstituted with Ringer's Solution or solutions containing bacteriostatic or buffer agents, because they may tend to cause precipitation. In preparing dilute solutions for continuous drip maintenance, either 5% dextrose or isotonic sodium chloride should be used instead of sterile water for injection to avoid extreme hypotonicity. Dextrose solutions are occasionally sufficiently acid, however, to cause precipitation. Injection of air into the solution should be avoided because this may hasten the development of cloudiness.
Solutions of atropine sulfate, *d*-tubocurarine, or succinylcholine may be given concurrently with Surital, but they should not be mixed prior to administration.
Thiamylal sodium solutions should be prepared under aseptic conditions. Solutions cannot be heated for sterilization. The solutions should be stored in a refrigerator and used within six days. If kept at room temperature, the solution should be used within 24 hours. Only clear solutions should be used; discard if cloudiness or precipitate form. Refrigeration of the reconstituted Surital contributes to the maintenance of a clear solution.
[See table below].

TABLE FOR PREPARING SOLUTIONS

Surital (g)	Amount of solvent required (in ml) for percentage solutions shown								
	0.2%	0.3%	0.4%	2%	2.5%	3%	4%	5%	10%
1	500	333	250	50	40	33.3	25	20	10
5	2,500	1,670	1,250	250	200	167	125	100	50
10	5,000	3,333	2,500	500	400	333	250	200	100

How Supplied: Surital is supplied as follows.
1 g, in packages of 25 (Steri-Vial® 64)
N 0071-4064-03 (35-64-25)
5 g, packaged individually and in packages of 25 (Ampoule 265)
N 0071-4265-08 (3-265-1)
5 g, in packages of 10 (Steri-Vial 122)
N 0071-4122-08 (35-122-10)
10 g, in packages of 10 (Steri-Vial 123)
N 0071-4123-10 (35-123-10)
UC

TABRON® FILMSEAL® ℞

Each tablet represents:

Ferrous fumarate	304.2 mg
(represents 100 mg of elemental iron)	
Vitamin C (ascorbic acid)	500 mg
Vitamin B_1 (thiamine mononitrate)	6 mg
Vitamin B_2 (riboflavin)	6 mg
Vitamin B_6 (pyridoxine hydrochloride)	5 mg
Vitamin B_{12} (cyanocobalamin), crystalline	25 mcg
Folic acid	1 mg
Nicotinamide (niacinamide)	30 mg
Calcium pantothenate	10 mg
Vitamin E (*dl*-alpha tocopheryl acetate)	(30 mg) 30 IU
Dioctyl sodium sulfosuccinate	50 mg

Caution: Folic acid may obscure pernicious anemia; the peripheral blood picture may revert to normal while neurological manifestations remain progressive.
Indications: Tabron is a hematinic for the treatment of iron-deficiency anemia and folate deficiency.
Dosage: Usual adult dose: One tablet per day.
How Supplied: N 0071-0638—Bottles of 100 and unit-dose packages of 100 (ten 10s). Parcode® No. 638
[*Shown in Product Identification Section*]

TEDRAL®
TEDRAL® SA ℞
Sustained Action
TEDRAL-25® ℞
TEDRAL® EXPECTORANT ℞
TEDRAL® SUSPENSION
TEDRAL® ELIXIR

Caution: Federal law prohibits dispensing Tedral SA, Tedral-25, or Tedral Expectorant without prescription.

Description:

Tedral: each tablet contains 130 mg theophylline, 24 mg ephedrine hydrochloride, and 8 mg phenobarbital.

Tedral SA: each tablet contains 180 mg anhydrous theophylline (90 mg in the immediate release layer and 90 mg in the sustained release layer); 48 mg ephedrine hydrochloride (16 mg in the immediate release layer and 32 mg in the sustained release layer); 25 mg phenobarbital in the immediate release layer.

Tedral-25: each tablet contains 130 mg theophylline, 24 mg ephedrine hydrochloride, and 25 mg butabarbital.

Tedral Expectorant: each tablet contains 130 mg theophylline, 24 mg ephedrine hydrochloride, 8 mg phenobarbital, and 100 mg guaifenesin.

Tedral Suspension: each 5 ml teaspoonful of suspension contains 65 mg theophylline, 12 mg ephedrine hydrochloride, and 4 mg phenobarbital.

Tedral Elixir: each 5 ml teaspoonful contains 32.5 mg theophylline, 6 mg ephedrine hydrochloride, and 2 mg phenobarbital; the alcohol content is 15%.

Actions: The Tedral formulations combine theophylline and ephedrine—widely accepted oral bronchodilators, with differing modes of action—with a sedative (phenobarbital or butabarbital).

From experimental evidence,[1] it appears that a combination of a sympathomimetic and methylxanthine is more effective than either drug alone in inhibiting the release of bronchoconstricting mediators (histamine and slow-reacting substance of anaphylaxis) produced by antigen-antibody (IgE) interaction on sensitive cells. The β-adrenergic stimulation by the sympathomimetics produces cyclic 3′5′-adenosine monophosphate (cAMP), and the degradation of cAMP by the specific enzyme phosphodiesterase is inhibited by methylxanthines. Thus, at present, the principal action of the Tedral formulations in the relief or prevention of bronchoconstriction appears to be involved with the cAMP system.

Phenobarbital is incorporated to counteract possible stimulation by ephedrine and to provide a mild, long-acting sedative for the apprehensive asthmatic patient.

Tedral SA provides sustained as well as immediate bronchodilatation for the asthmatic patient, with the convenience of b.i.d. dosage.

The nervous or apprehensive asthmatic patient can benefit from butabarbital in **Tedral-25**. This formulation can also be useful in the occasional patient who is unduly sensitive to ephedrine.

Tedral Expectorant combines Tedral with guaifenesin which helps to increase the volume and decrease the viscosity of fluids of the respiratory tract. By aiding lubrication of the mucous membranes of the bronchi, Tedral Expectorant helps the patient to cough up viscid mucus.

Tedral Suspension and **Tedral Elixir** are convenient formulations for children and other persons who may have difficulty in swallowing tablets.

Indications: Tedral, Tedral SA, Tedral-25, Tedral Expectorant, Tedral Suspension and **Tedral Elixir** are indicated for the symptomatic relief of bronchial asthma, asthmatic bronchitis, and other bronchospastic disorders. They may also be used prophylactically to abort or minimize asthmatic attacks and are of value in managing occasional, seasonal or perennial asthma.

Tedral SA provides sustained as well as immediate bronchodilatation for the asthmatic patient, with the convenience of b.i.d. dosage.

Tedral-25 is indicated when there is excessive nervousness, apprehension or sensitivity to ephedrine.

Tedral Expectorant is indicated only when both relaxation of bronchospasm and expectoration are desired.

Tedral Suspension and **Tedral Elixir** are convenient for persons who may have difficulty in swallowing tablets.

These Tedral formulations are adjuncts in the total management of the asthmatic patient. Acute or severe asthmatic attacks may necessitate supplemental therapy with other drugs by inhalation or other parenteral routes.

Contraindications: Sensitivity to any of the ingredients; porphyria.

Warnings: Drowsiness may occur. PHENOBARBITAL AND BUTABARBITAL MAY BE HABIT-FORMING.

Precautions: Use with caution in the presence of cardiovascular disease, severe hypertension, hyperthyroidism, prostatic hypertrophy, or glaucoma.

Adverse Reactions: Mild epigastric distress, palpitation, tremulousness, insomnia, difficulty of micturition, and CNS stimulation have been reported.

Average Dosage: *Prophylactic or Therapeutic*

Tedral

Adults—One or two tablets every 4 hours.
Children—(Over 60 lb) one-half the adult dose.

Tedral SA

Adults—One tablet on arising and one tablet 12 hours later. Tablets should not be chewed.
Children—Not established for children under 12.

Tedral-25

Adults—One tablet every 4 hours.
Children—(6–12) one-half the adult dose.

Tedral Expectorant

Adults—One or two tablets q.i.d.
Children—Not established for children under 12.

Tedral Suspension

Note: One teaspoonful is equivalent to *one-half* a Tedral tablet.
Adults—Two to four teaspoonfuls every 4 hours.
Children—One teaspoonful per 60 lb body weight, every 4–6 hours, unless prescribed otherwise by physician. Should be given to children under 2 years of age only with extreme caution.
SHAKE BOTTLE WELL.

Tedral Elixir

Note: One teaspoonful is equivalent to *one-quarter* Tedral tablet.
Children—One teaspoonful per 30 lb body weight, every 4–6 hours, unless prescribed otherwise by physician. Should be given to children under 2 years of age only with extreme caution.
Adults—One to two tablespoonfuls every four hours.

Supplied:

Tedral

White, uncoated scored tablets in bottles of 24 (N 0047-0230-24), 100 (N 0047-0230-51) and 1000 (N 0047-0230-60). Also in Unit Dose—package of 10 × 10 strips (N 0047-0230-11).

Tedral SA

Double-layered, uncoated, coral/mottled white tablets in bottles of 100 (N 0047-0231-51) and 1000 (N 0047-0231-60). Also in Unit Dose—package of 10 × 10 strips (N 0047-0231-11).

Tedral-25

Light orange, uncoated, scored tablets in bottles of 100 (N 0047-0238-51).

Tedral Expectorant

White tablets in bottles of 100 (N 0047-0239-51).

Tedral Suspension

Yellow, licorice-flavored suspension in bottles of 237 ml (8 fl oz) (N 0047-0237-08) and 474 ml (16 fl oz) (N 0047-0237-16).

Tedral Elixir

Dark red, cherry-flavored in 474 ml (16 fl oz) bottles (N 0047-0242-16).
STORE BETWEEN 59°–86° F (15°–30° C).

Reference:

1. Koopman WJ, Orange RP, Austen KF: *J. Immunol.* 105: 1096, November 1970.

[*Shown in Product Identification Section*]

958 G 040 **R-7-77**

TETRACYCLINE HYDROCHLORIDE CAPSULES, USP ℞
(Cyclopar® 500—500-mg Capsules)
(Cyclopar—250-mg Capsules)

Description: Cyclopar 500 Capsules: each contains 500 mg of the broad-spectrum antibiotic, tetracycline hydrochloride. Each Cyclopar Capsule contains 250 mg tetracycline hydrochloride. Tetracycline hydrochloride is a yellow, odorless, crystalline powder with the chemical formula $C_{22}H_{24}N_2O_8 \cdot HCl$.

Actions: The tetracyclines are primarily bacteriostatic and are thought to exert their antimicrobial effect by the inhibition of protein synthesis. Tetracyclines are active against a wide range of gram-negative and gram-positive organisms.

The drugs in the tetracycline class have closely similar antimicrobial spectra, and cross-resistance among them is common. Microorganisms may be considered susceptible if the MIC (minimum inhibitory concentration) is not more than 4.0 mcg/ml, and intermediate if the MIC is 4.0 to 12.5 mcg/ml.

Susceptibility plate testing: A tetracycline disk may be used to determine microbial susceptibility to drugs in the tetracycline class. If the Kirby-Bauer method of disk susceptibility testing is used, a 30-mcg tetracycline disk should give a zone of at least 19 mm when tested against a tetracycline-susceptible bacterial strain.

Tetracyclines are readily absorbed and are bound to plasma proteins in varying degree. Tetracyclines are concentrated by the liver in the bile and excreted in the urine and feces at high concentrations and in a biologically active form.

Indications: Tetracycline is indicated in infections caused by the following microorganisms.

- Rickettsiae (Rocky Mountain spotted fever, typhus fever and the typhus group, Q fever, rickettsialpox, and tick fevers)
- *Mycoplasma pneumoniae* (PPLO, Eaton agent)
- Agents of psittacosis and ornithosis
- Agents of lymphogranuloma venereum and granuloma inguinale
- The spirochetal agent of relapsing fever *(Borrelia recurrentis)*
- The following gram-negative microorganisms:
  - *Hemophilus ducreyi* (chancroid)
  - *Pasteurella pestis* and *P tularensis*
  - *Bartonella bacilliformis*
  - *Bacteroides* species
  - *Vibrio comma* and *V fetus*
  - *Brucella* species (in conjunction with streptomycin)

Because many strains of the following groups of microorganisms have been shown to be resis-

Continued on next page

This product information was prepared in August, 1979. On these and other Parke-Davis Products, detailed information may be obtained by addressing PARKE-DAVIS, Division of Warner-Lambert Company, Morris Plains, NJ 07950.

Parke-Davis—Cont.

tant to tetracyclines, culture and susceptibility testing are recommended.
Tetracycline is indicated for treatment of infections caused by the following gram-negative microorganisms when bacteriologic testing indicates appropriate susceptibility to the drug.

Escherichia coli
Enterobacter aerogenes (formerly *Aerobacter aerogenes)*
Shigella species
Mima species and *Herellea* species
H influenzae (respiratory infections)
Klebsiella species (respiratory and urinary infections)

Tetracycline is indicated for treatment of infections caused by the following gram-positive microorganisms when bacteriologic testing indicates appropriate susceptibility to the drug.

Streptococcus species:
Up to 44% of strains of *Str pyogenes* and 74% of *Str faecalis* have been found to be resistant to tetracycline drugs. Therefore, tetracyclines should not be used for streptococcal disease unless the organism has been demonstrated to be sensitive.
For upper respiratory infections due to group A beta-hemolytic streptococci, penicillin is the usual drug of choice, including prophylaxis of rheumatic fever.

Diplococcus pneumoniae
Staphylococcus aureus
Skin and soft-tissue infections. Tetracyclines are not the drugs of choice in the treatment of any type of staphylococcal infection.

When penicillin is contraindicated, tetracyclines are alternative drugs in the treatment of infections due to:

Neisseria gonorrhoeae,
Treponema pallidum and *T pertenue* (syphilis and yaws),
Listeria monocytogenes,
Clostridium species,
Bacillus anthracis,
Fusobacterium fusiforme (Vincent's infection),
Actinomyces species.

In acute intestinal amebiasis, the tetracyclines may be a useful adjunct to amebicides.
In severe acne, the tetracyclines may be useful adjunctive therapy.
Tetracyclines are indicated in the treatment of trachoma, although the infectious agent is not always eliminated, as judged by immunofluorescence.
Inclusion conjunctivitis may be treated with oral tetracyclines or with a combination of oral and topical agents.
Contraindication: This drug is contraindicated in persons who have shown hypersensitivity to any of the tetracyclines.
Warnings: THE USE OF DRUGS OF THE TETRACYCLINE CLASS DURING TOOTH DEVELOPMENT (LAST HALF OF PRENANCY, INFANCY, AND CHILDHOOD TO THE AGE OF 8 YEARS) MAY CAUSE PERMANENT DISCOLORATION OF THE TEETH (YELLOW-GRAY-BROWN). This adverse reaction is more common during long-term use of the drugs but has been observed following repeated short-term courses. Enamel hypoplasia has also been reported. TETRACYCLINE DRUGS, THEREFORE, SHOULD NOT BE USED IN THIS AGE GROUP UNLESS OTHER DRUGS ARE NOT LIKELY TO BE EFFECTIVE OR ARE CONTRAINDICATED.
If renal impairment exists, even usual oral or parenteral doses may lead to excessive systemic accumulation of the drug and possible liver toxicity. Under such conditions, lower than usual total doses are indicated and, if therapy is prolonged, serum level determinations of the drug may be advisable.
Photosensitivity manifested by an exaggerated sunburn reaction has been observed in some individuals taking tetracyclines. Patients apt to be exposed to direct sunlight or ultraviolet light should be advised that this reaction can occur with tetracycline drugs, and treatment should be discontinued at the first evidence of skin erythema.
The antianabolic action of the tetracyclines may cause an increase in BUN. While this is not a problem in those with normal renal function, in patients with significantly impaired function, higher serum levels of tetracycline may lead to azotemia, hyperphosphatemia, and acidosis.
Usage in pregnancy. (See above Warnings about use during tooth development).
Results of animal studies indicate that tetracyclines cross the placenta, are found in fetal tissues, and can have toxic effects on the developing fetus (often related to retardation of skeletal development.) Evidence of embryotoxicity has also been noted in animals treated early in pregnancy.
Usage in newborns, infants, and children. (See above Warnings about use during tooth development.)
All tetracyclines form a stable calcium complex in any bone-forming tissue. A decrease in the fibula growth rate has been observed in prematures given oral tetracycline in doses of 25 mg/kg every six hours. This reaction was shown to be reversible when the drug was discontinued.
Tetracyclines are present in the milk of lactating women who are taking a drug in this class.
Precautions: As with other antibiotic preparations, use of this drug may result in overgrowth of nonsusceptible organisms, including fungi. If superinfection occurs, the antibiotic should be discontinued and appropriate therapy instituted.
In venereal diseases when coexistent syphilis is suspected, darkfield examination should be done before treatment is started and the blood serology repeated monthly for at least four months.
Because tetracyclines have been shown to depress plasma prothrombin activity, patients who are on anticoagulant therapy may require downward adjustment of their anticoagulant dosage.
In long-term therapy, periodic laboratory evaluation of organ systems, including hematopoietic, renal, and hepatic studies, should be performed.
All infections due to group A beta-hemolytic streptococci should be treated for at least 10 days.
Because bacteriostatic drugs may interfere with the bactericidal action of penicillin, it is advisable to avoid giving tetracycline in conjunction with penicillin.
Adverse Reactions: Gastrointestinal: anorexia, nausea, vomiting, diarrhea, glossitis, dysphagia, enterocolitis, and inflammatory lesions (with monilial overgrowth) in the anogenital region. These reactions have been caused by both the oral and parenteral administration of tetracyclines.
Skin: maculopapular and erythematous rashes. Exfoliative dermatitis has been reported but is uncommon. Photosensitivity is discussed above. (See Warnings.)
Renal toxicity: rise in BUN has been reported and is apparently dose-related. (See Warnings.)
Hypersensitivity reactions: urticaria, angioneurotic edema, anaphylaxis, anaphylactoid purpura, pericarditis, and exacerbation of systemic lupus erythematosus
Bulging fontanels have been reported in young infants following full therapeutic dosage. This sign disappeared rapidly when the drug was discontinued.
Blood: hemolytic anemia, thrombocytopenia, neutropenia, and eosinophilia have been reported.
When given over prolonged periods, tetracyclines have been reported to produce brown-black microscopic discoloration of thyroid glands. No abnormalities of thyroid function studies are known to occur.
Dosage and Administration: Therapy should be continued for at least 24 to 48 hours after symptoms and fever have subsided.
Concomitant therapy: Antacids containing aluminum, calcium, or magnesium impair absorption and should not be given to patients taking oral tetracycline.
Food and some dairy products also interfere with absorption. Oral forms of tetracycline should be given one hour before or two hours after meals. Pediatric oral dosage forms should not be given with milk formulas and should be given at least one hour prior to feeding.
In patients with renal impairment: (See Warnings.) Total dosage should be decreased by reduction of recommended individual doses and/or by extending time intervals between doses.
In the treatment of streptococcal infections, a therapeutic dosage of tetracycline should be administered for at least 10 days.
Adults: Usual daily dosage, 1 to 2 g divided in two or four equal doses, depending on the severity of the infection.
For children above 8 years of age: Usual daily dosage, 10 to 20 mg (25 to 50 mg/kg) per pound of body weight divided in four equal doses.
For treatment of brucellosis, 500 mg tetracycline four times daily for three weeks should be accompanied by streptomycin, 1 g, intramuscularly twice daily the first week and once daily the second week.
For treatment of syphilis, a total of 30 to 40 g in equally divided doses over a period of 10 to 15 days should be given. Close follow-up, including laboratory tests, is recommended.
For the treatment of acute gonococcal urethritis, a single, initial dose of 1.5 g followed by 0.5 g every four to six hours for four to six days should be given. Female patients may require more prolonged therapy.
How Supplied: Tetracycline hydrochloride capsules, USP, 500 mg (Cyclopar 500)—each capsule contains 500 mg tetracycline hydrochloride. Tetracycline hydrochloride capsules, USP, 250 mg (Cyclopar)—each capsule contains 250 mg tetracycline hydrochloride.
N 0071-0697—Cyclopar 500—Bottles of 100. Parcode® No. 697
N 0071-0407—Cyclopar—Bottles of 100 and 1,000. Parcode No. 407
AHFS 8:12.24 **WL**
[Shown in Product Identification Section]

TEXACORT® SCALP LOTION ℞

Description: Texacort Scalp Lotion contains hydrocortisone in a concentration of 1% (10 mg/g). Hydrocortisone (cortisol) has the chemical formula of 11β,17,21-trihydroxypregn-4-ene-3,20 dione. The vehicle contains: 33% alcohol, propylene glycol, polysorbate 20, benzalkonium chloride, and purified water. Texacort Scalp Lotion is lipid-free and paraben-free.
Actions: Topical steroids are primarily effective because of their antiinflammatory, antipruritic, and vasoconstrictive actions.
Indications: For relief of the inflammatory manifestations of corticosteroid-responsive dermatoses.
Contraindications: Topical steroids are contraindicated in those patients with a history of hypersensitivity to any components of the preparation. Topical steroids should not be used when circulation is markedly impaired. Not for ophthalmic use.
Warnings: Usage in Pregnancy: Although topical steroids have not been reported to have an adverse effect on human pregnancy, the safety of their use in pregnant women has not

been absolutely established. In laboratory animals, increases in incidence of fetal abnormalities have been associated with exposure of gestating females to topical corticosteroids, in some cases at rather low dosage levels. Therefore, drugs of this class should not be used extensively on pregnant patients, in large amounts, or for prolonged periods of time.
Precautions: If irritation develops, Texacort Scalp Lotion should be discontinued and appropriate therapy instituted.
In the presence of an infection the use of an appropriate antifungal or antibacterial agent should be instituted. If a favorable response does not occur promptly, the corticosteroid should be discontinued until the infection has been adequately controlled.
If extensive areas are treated or if the occlusive technique is used there will be increased systemic absorption of the corticosteroid and suitable precautions should be taken, particularly in children and infants.
Adverse Reactions: The following local adverse reactions have been reported with topical corticosteroids, especially under occlusive dressings: burning, itching, irritation, dryness, folliculitis, hypertrichosis, acneform eruptions, hypopigmentation, perioral dermatitis, allergic contact dermatitis, maceration of the skin, secondary infection, skin atrophy, striae and miliaria.
Dosage and Administration: Apply to affected areas 3 or 4 times daily. When a favorable response is obtained, gradually reduce dosage and eventually discontinue.
How Supplied: Texacort Scalp Lotion is supplied in 1-oz bottles with dropper (N 0064-3912-01).

THERA-COMBEX H-P®
High-Potency Vitamin B Complex with 500 mg Vitamin C

Composition: Each Kapseal contains:

Ascorbic acid (vitamin C)	500 mg
Thiamine (vitamin B_1) mononitrate	25 mg
Riboflavin (vitamin B_2)	15 mg
Pyridoxine hydrochloride (vitamin B_6)	10 mg
Vitamin B_{12} (cyanocobalamin)	5 mcg
Nicotinamide (niacinamide)	100 mg
dl-Panthenol	20 mg

Uses: For the prevention or treatment of vitamin B complex and vitamin C deficiencies.
Dosage: One or two capsules daily
How Supplied: N 0071-0550—Bottles of 30, 100, and 1,000; also unit-dose packages of ten 10s; Parcode® No. 550
[*Shown in Product Identification Section*]

THERAPADS®
Composition: Nonwoven, textured pads saturated with a solution containing salicylic acid, 1.5%, and ethyl alcohol, 50%.
Action and Uses: As a therapeutic wipe in acne and other oily skin conditions to cleanse away sebaceous film and exert a mild, drying, keratolytic action.
Warning: Flammable. For external use only.
Precaution: Avoid contact with eyes.
Side Effects: Reduce frequency or discontinue use if excessive drying of skin occurs.
Administration: Wipe affected skin areas thoroughly two or three times daily or as indicated by severity of condition or response to therapy.
How Supplied: Jars of 40 and 100 with resealable, plastic pouch. N 0071-1705

THERAPADS® PLUS
Composition: Mildly abrasive, nonwoven wipes saturated with solution of ethyl alcohol, 70%; salicylic acid, 1.5%; and sodium alkyl aryl polyether sulfonate, 0.1%.
Action and Uses: For use as a therapeutic cleansing wipe in acne and other excessively oily skin conditions where a drying, keratolytic effect is indicated.
Warning: Flammable. For external use only.
Precaution: Avoid contact with eyes.
Side Effect: Reduce frequency or discontinue use if excessive drying of skin occurs.
Dosage and Administration: Wipe affected area two or three times daily (as indicated by condition).
How Supplied: Individually foil-wrapped wipes, packed 30 in a carton. N 0071-1706-11

THROMBIN, TOPICAL ℞
(bovine origin)

Thrombin, Topical, Must Not Be Injected! Apply On The Surface Of Bleeding Tissue As A Solution Or Powder.
Description: Thrombin, Topical, is a protein substance produced through a conversion reaction in which prothrombin is activated by tissue thromboplastin in the presence of calcium chloride. Thrombin, Topical, is supplied as a sterile powder that has been freeze-dried in the final container. Also contained in this preparation are calcium chloride, sodium chloride, aminoacetic acid (glycine), and Phemerol® (benzethonium chloride). Glycine is included to make the dried product friable and more readily soluble, and benzethonium chloride as a preservative as follows: 0.4 mg per 1,000-unit vial, 0.1 mg per 5,000-unit vial, and 0.2 mg per 10,000-unit vial.
A 5-ml vial of Isotonic Saline is enclosed to be used as a diluent with the 5-ml, 5,000 US (NIH) unit vial of Thrombin.
Isotonic Saline is a sterile, isotonic solution of sodium chloride in Water for Injection, USP. It contains Phemerol® (benzethonium chloride), 0.02 mg/ml, as a preservative. (See Dosage and Administration for additional information on diluents which may be used.)
This product is prepared under rigid assay control. A United States National Institutes of Health unit is defined as the amount required to clot 1 ml of standardized fibrinogen solution in 15 seconds. Approximately 2 US (NIH) units are required to clot 1 ml of oxalated human plasma in the same period of time.
Action: Thrombin, Topical, requires no intermediate physiological agent for its action. Thrombin, Topical, clots the fibrinogen of the blood directly. **Failure to clot blood occurs in the rare case where the primary clotting defect is the absence of fibrinogen itself.** The speed with which thrombin clots blood is dependent upon its concentration. For example, the contents of a 5,000 US (NIH) unit vial of Thrombin, Topical, dissolved in 5 ml of saline diluent is capable of clotting an equal volume of blood in less than a second, or 1,000 ml in less than a minute.
Indications: Thrombin is indicated as an aid in hemostasis wherever oozing blood from capillaries and venules is accessible.
In various types of surgery, solutions of Thrombin, Topical, may be used in conjunction with absorbable gelatin sponge, USP, for hemostasis.
Precaution: Consult the absorbable gelatin sponge product labeling for complete information prior to utilizing the thrombin-saturated sponge procedure.
Contraindication: Thrombin, Topical, is contraindicated in persons known to be sensitive to any of its components and/or to material of bovine origin.
Warning: Because of its action in the clotting mechanism, Thrombin, Topical, must not be injected or otherwise allowed to enter large blood vessels. Extensive intravascular clotting and even death may result. Thrombin is an antigenic substance and has caused sensitivity and allergic reactions when injected into animals.
Adverse Reactions: An allergic-type reaction following the use of thrombin for treatment of epistaxis has been reported. Febrile reactions have also been observed following the use of thrombin in certain surgical procedures but no cause-effect relationship has been established.
Dosage and Administration: Solutions of Thrombin, Topical, may be prepared in Sterile Distilled Water or isotonic saline. The intended use determines the strength of the solution to prepare.
For general use in plastic surgery, dental extractions, skin grafting, neurosurgery, etc, solutions containing approximately 100 units/ml are frequently used. For this, 10 ml of diluent added to the 1,000-unit package (Bio 2077) is suitable.
Where bleeding is profuse, as from cut surfaces of liver and spleen, concentrations as high as 1,000 to 2,000 units per milliliter may be required. For this, the 5,000-unit vial (Bio 2073) dissolved in 5 ml or 2.5 ml, respectively, of the diluent supplied in the package is convenient. Intermediate strengths to suit the needs of the case may be prepared by selecting the proper strength package and dissolving the contents in an appropriate volume of diluent.
In many situations, it may be advantageous to use Thrombin, Topical, in dry form on oozing surfaces.
Caution: Solutions should be used the day they are prepared. If several hours are to elapse, the solution should be refrigerated, preferably frozen, and not used after 48 hours. Dilute acid, alkalies, salts of heavy metals, and heat are detrimental to thrombin activity; therefore, stomach acids must be neutralized prior to oral administration of Thrombin, Topical.
The following techniques are suggested for the topical application of thrombin.
1. The recipient surface should be sponged (not wiped) free of blood before Thrombin, Topical, is applied.
2. A spray may be used or the surface may be flooded using a sterile syringe and small-gauge needle. The most effective hemostasis results when Thrombin, Topical, mixes freely with the blood as soon as it reaches the surface.
3. In instances where thrombin in dry form is needed, the vial is opened by removing the metal ring by grasping the edge where it is scored, and tearing, using sterile pliers. The rubber-diaphragm cap may be easily removed and the dried thrombin is then broken up into a powder by means of a sterile glass rod or other suitable sterile instrument.
4. Sponging of treated surfaces should be avoided in order that the clot remain securely in place.
Thrombin, Topical, may be used in conjunction with absorbable gelatin sponge, USP, as follows.
1. Prepare thrombin solution of the desired strength.
2. Immerse sponge strips of the desired size in the thrombin solution. Knead the sponge strips vigorously with moistened gloved fingers to remove trapped air, thereby facilitating saturation of the sponge.
3. Apply saturated sponge to bleeding area. Hold in place for 10 to 15 seconds with a pledget of cotton, or a small gauze sponge.
How Supplied: Thrombin, Topical, is supplied as follows.
N 0071-4173-35 (Bio 2073)—Package contains one 5,000 US (NIH) unit vial of Thrombin, Top-

Continued on next page

This product information was prepared in August, 1979. On these and other Parke-Davis Products, detailed information may be obtained by addressing PARKE-DAVIS, Division of Warner-Lambert Company, Morris Plains, NJ 07950.

Parke-Davis—Cont.

ical, and one 5-ml vial of isotonic saline diluent with Phemerol, 0.02 mg/ml, as a preservative.
NSN 6505-00-161-2950
N 0071-4176-01 (Bio 2076)—Package contains one 10,000 US (NIH) unit vial of Thrombin, Topical.
N 0071-4177-01 (Bio 2077)—Package contains one 1,000 US (NIH) unit vial of Thrombin, Topical.
AHFS 20:12.16 **YF**

TUCKS®
Premoistened Pads

Composition: Premoistened pads saturated with a solution containing witch hazel, 50%; glycerin, USP, 10%; purified water, USP, deionized, qs; buffered to approximately pH 4.6; methylparaben, USP, 0.1%, and benzalkonium chloride, USP, 0.003%, added as preservatives
Action and Uses: *Prophylactically,* as an after-stool wipe to remove most causes of local irritation; temporarily helps prevent pruritus ani and vulvae, and similar perianal or perineal irritations
As soothing, *cleansing* pad during menstruation, and in the temporary management of vulvitis, pruritus ani and vulvae
As a *compress,* to temporarily help relieve the discomfort of simple hemorrhoids, anorectal surgical wounds, episiotomies
Warning: In case of continued irritation or rectal bleeding, discontinue use.
Dosage and Administration: Use in addition to toilet tissue. For further temporary relief, apply Tucks to affected areas for 15 to 30 minutes as needed.
How Supplied: Jars of 40 and 100. Also available as Tucks Take-Alongs®, individual, foil-wrapped, nonwoven wipes, 12 packets per box
Tucks—N 0071-1703
Tucks Take-Alongs—N 0071-1704-01

TUCKS® OINTMENT, CREAM

Composition: Tucks Ointment and Cream contain a specially formulated aqueous phase of 50% witch hazel (hamamelis water). Both have an acid pH, pleasant odor, and are nonstaining.
Action and Uses: Tucks Ointment and Tucks Cream exert a temporary, soothing, mildly astringent effect on such superficial irritations as hemorrhoids, pruritus ani and vulvae, postpartum discomfort, anorectal wounds. Tucks Cream is excellent for nipple care by nursing mothers.
Warning: In case of continued irritation or rectal bleeding, discontinue use.
Dosage and Administration: Apply locally three or four times daily. Applicator provided for rectal instillation.
How Supplied: Tucks Ointment and Tucks Cream (water-washable) in 40-g tubes with rectal applicators
Tucks Ointment—N 0071-3021-14
Tucks Cream—N 0071-3022-14 **UH**

UTICORT® ℞
(betamethasone benzoate, USP)
Cream, 0.025%
Gel, 0.025%
For External Use Only

Description: Uticort Gel and Uticort Cream contain the active fluorinated steroid compound, betamethasone benzoate, the 17-benzoate ester of betamethasone, having the chemical formula of 9-fluoro-11β,17,21-trihydroxy-16 β-methylpregna-1, 4-diene-3, 20-dione 17-benzoate.
Each gram of Uticort Cream contains 0.25 mg of betamethasone benzoate in a water-washable, emollient cream base consisting of cetyl alcohol, glyceryl stearate, light mineral oil, propylene glycol, disodium monooleamidosulfosuccinate, citric acid, and purified water.
Each gram of Uticort Gel, 0.025%, contains 0.25 mg of betamethasone benzoate in a specially formulated gel base consisting of 13.8% (w/w) alcohol, carboxy-vinyl polymer, propylene glycol, disodium edetate, diisopropanolamine, and purified water. The gel is self-liquefying, clear, greaseless, and nonstaining. The active ingredient is completely solubilized and remains in the clear film without crystallization after evaporation of volatile substances.
Actions: Uticort Cream and Gel are primarily effective because of its anti-inflammatory, antipruritic, and vasoconstrictive actions.
Indications: Uticort Cream and Gel are intended for relief of the inflammatory manifestations of corticosteroid-responsive dermatoses.
Contraindications: Topical steroids are contraindicated in those patients with a history of sensitivity to any components of the preparation.
Precautions: If irritation develops, the Uticort Cream or Gel should be discontinued and appropriate therapy instituted.
In the presence of an infection, the use of appropriate antifungal or antibacterial agents should be instituted. If a favorable response does not occur promptly, the corticosteroid should be discontinued until the infection has been adequately controlled.
If extensive areas are treated, or if the occlusive technique is used, there will be increased systemic absorption of the corticosteroid, and suitable precautions should be taken, particularly in infants and children.
Although topical steroids have not been reported to have an adverse effect on human pregnancy, the safety of their use in pregnant women has not been established absolutely.
In laboratory animals, increases in incidence of fetal abnormalities have been associated with exposure of gestating females to topical corticosteroids, in some cases at rather low dosage levels. Therefore, drugs of this class should not be used extensively on pregnant patients, in large amounts, or for prolonged periods of time.
Due to the alcohol content of the vehicle, Uticort Gel (betamethasone benzoate gel, USP) may cause mild, transient stinging without irritation if used on excoriated skin.
Uticort Cream and Gel are not for ophthalmic use.
Adverse Reactions: The following local adverse reactions have been reported with topical corticosteroids, especially under occlusive dressings: burning, itching, irritation, dryness, folliculitis, hypertrichosis, acneiform eruptions, hypopigmentation, perioral dermatitis, allergic contact dermatitis, maceration of the skin, secondary infection, skin atrophy, striae, and miliaria.
Dosage and Administration: Apply to affected areas two to four times daily as needed.
How Supplied: N 0071-3027 Uticort Cream, 0.025%, is supplied in 15-g and 60-g tubes. N 0071-3025 Uticort Gel, 0.025%, is supplied in 15-g and 60-g tubes.
US Patent Nos. 3,529,060 and 3,749,773 **WK**
[*Shown in Product Identification Section*]

VERSTRAN® Ⓒ
(prazepam)

Caution: Federal law prohibits dispensing without prescription.
Description: Verstran (prazepam), a benzodiazepine derivative, is identified chemically as 7-chloro-1-(cyclopropylmethyl)-1, 3-dihydro-5-phenyl-2H-1, 4-benzodiazepin-2-one. The molecular weight is 324.8.
Clinical Pharmacology: Studies in normal subjects have shown that Verstran (prazepam) has depressant effects on the central nervous system. Oral administration of single doses as high as 60 mg and divided doses up to 100 mg t.i.d. (300 mg total daily dose) were without toxic effects.
Single oral doses of Verstran in normal subjects produced average peak blood levels of the major metabolite norprazepam at 6 hours post-administration, with significant amounts still present after 48 hours. Verstran was slowly absorbed over a prolonged period, rather constant blood levels were maintained, and excretion was prolonged. The mean half-life of prazepam measured in subjects given 10 mg t.i.d. for one week was 63 ($\pm$15 s.d.) hours before and 70 ($\pm$10 s.d.) hours after multiple dosing—a nonsignificant difference. Human metabolism studies showed that prior to elimination from the body, prazepam is metabolized in large part to 3-hydroxyprazepam and oxazepam.
Indications: Verstran (prazepam) is indicated for the symptomatic relief of anxiety associated with anxiety neurosis, in other psychoneuroses in which anxiety symptoms are prominent features, and as an adjunct in disease states in which anxiety is manifested. The effectiveness of Verstran (prazepam) in long-term use, that is, more than 4 months, has not been assessed by systematic clinical studies. The physician should reassess periodically the usefulness of the drug for the individual patient.
Contraindications: Verstran (prazepam) is contraindicated in patients with a known sensitivity to the drug and in those with acute narrow-angle glaucoma.
Warnings: Verstran (prazepam) is not recommended in psychotic states and in those psychiatric disorders in which anxiety is not a prominent feature.
Patients taking Verstran should be cautioned against engaging in hazardous occupations requiring mental alertness, such as operating dangerous machinery, including motor vehicles.
Because Verstran has a central nervous system depressant effect, patients should be advised against the simultaneous use of other CNS-depressant drugs, including phenothiazines, narcotics, barbiturates, MAO inhibitors, and other antidepressants. The effects of alcohol may also be increased.
Physical and Psychological Dependence: Withdrawal symptoms similar in character to those noted with barbiturates and alcohol have occurred following abrupt discontinuance of benzodiazepine drugs. These symptoms include convulsions, tremor, abdominal and muscle cramps, vomiting and sweating. Addiction-prone individuals, such as drug addicts and alcoholics, should be under careful surveillance when receiving benzodiazepines because of the predisposition of such patients to habituation and dependence.
Precautions:
Use in Pregnancy and Lactation: *An increased risk of congenital malformations associated with the use of minor tranquilizers (chlordiazepoxide, diazepam, and meprobamate) during the first trimester of pregnancy has been suggested in several studies. Verstran (prazepam), a benzodiazepine derivative, has not been studied adequately to determine whether it, too, may be associated with an increased risk of fetal abnormality. Because use of these drugs is rarely a matter of urgency, their use during this period should almost always be avoided. The possibility that a woman of childbearing potential may be pregnant at the time of institution of therapy should be considered. Patients should be advised that if they become pregnant during therapy or intend to become pregnant they should communicate with their physician about the desirability of discontinuing the drug. In view of their molecular size, Verstran and its metabolites are probably excreted in human milk. Therefore, this drug should not be given to nursing mothers.*

In those patients in whom a degree of depression accompanies the anxiety, suicidal tendencies may be present, and protective measures may be required. The least amount of drug that is feasible should be available to the patient at any one time.
Patients taking Verstran for prolonged periods should have blood counts and liver function tests periodically. The usual precautions in treating patients with impaired renal or hepatic function should also be observed. Hepatomegaly and cholestasis were observed in chronic toxicity studies in rats and dogs.
In elderly or debilitated patients, the initial dose should be small, and increments should be made gradually, in accordance with the response of the patient, to preclude ataxia or excessive sedation.

Pediatric Use: Safety and effectiveness in patients below the age of 18 have not been established.

Adverse Reactions: The side effects most frequently reported during double-blind placebo-controlled trials employing a typical 30 mg divided total daily dose and the percent incidence in the Verstran (prazepam) group were: fatigue (11.6%), dizziness (8.7%), weakness (7.7%), drowsiness (6.8%), lightheadedness (6.8%), and ataxia (5.0%). Less frequently reported were: headache, confusion, tremor, vivid dreams, slurred speech, palpitation, stimulation, dry mouth, diaphoresis, and various gastrointestinal complaints. Other side effects included: pruritus, transient skin rashes, swelling of feet, joint pains, various genitourinary complaints, blurred vision, and syncope.
Single nightly dose, controlled trials of variable dosages showed a dose-related incidence of these same side effects. Transient and reversible aberrations of liver function tests have been reported, as have been slight decreases in blood pressure and increases in body weight. These findings are characteristic of benzodiazepine drugs.

Overdosage: As in the management of overdosage with any drug, it should be borne in mind that multiple agents may have been taken.
If vomiting has not occurred spontaneously, it should be induced. Immediate gastric lavage is also recommended. General supportive care, including frequent monitoring of the vital signs and close observation of the patient, is indicated. Hypotension, though unlikely, may be controlled with Levophed® (levarterenol bitartrate) or Aramine® (metaraminol bitartrate). Caffeine and Sodium Benzoate Injection, USP, may be used to counteract central nervous system depressant effects.

Dosage and Administration: Verstran (prazepam) is administered orally in divided doses. The usual daily dose is 30 mg. The dose should be adjusted gradually within the range of 20 to 60 mg daily in accordance with the response of the patient. In elderly or debilitated patients it is advisable to initiate treatment at a divided daily dose of 10 to 15 mg. (See Precautions.)
Prazepam may also be administered as a single dose daily at bedtime. The recommended starting nightly dose is 20 mg. The response of the patient to several days' treatment will permit the physician to adjust the dose upward or, occasionally, downward to maximize antianxiety effect with a minimum of daytime drowsiness. The optimum dosage will usually range from 20 to 40 mg.

Drug Interactions: If Verstran (prazepam) is to be combined with other drugs acting on the central nervous system, careful consideration should be given to the pharmacology of the agents to be employed. The actions of the benzodiazepines may be potentiated by barbiturates, narcotics, phenothiazines, monoamine oxidase inhibitors or other antidepressants.
If Verstran is used to treat anxiety associated with somatic disease states, careful attention must be paid to possible drug interaction with concomitant medication.

How Supplied: Verstran (prazepam) 10 mg light blue, scored tablets in bottles of 100 (N 0047-0276-51) and 1000 (N 0047-0276-60). Unit dose 10 × 10 strips (N 0047-0276-11).
STORE BETWEEN 59°–86° F (15°–30°C).
Licensed under U.S. Patents 3192199, 3192200.
[*Shown in Product Identification Section*]
319 G 511 **6-79**

VIRA-A® ℞
(vidarabine for infusion)

Description: Vira-A for infusion (ara-A, vidarabine, adenine arabinoside) is a sterile antiviral drug for intravenous administration only. Vira-A is a purine nucleoside obtained from fermentation cultures of *Streptomyces antibioticus*. Each milliliter of suspension contains 200 mg of vidarabine monohydrate equivalent to 187.4 mg of vidarabine. Each milliliter contains 0.1 mg Phemerol® (benzethonium chloride) as a preservative; sodium phosphate dibasic, 0.957 mg, and sodium phosphate monobasic, 4.138 mg, as buffering agents. Hydrochloric acid may have been added to adjust pH.
Vira-A is a white, crystalline solid with this empirical formula: $C_{10}H_{13}N_5O_4 \cdot H_2O$. The molecular weight is 285.2; the solubility is 0.45 mg/ml at 25 C; and the melting point ranges from 260 to 270 C. The chemical name is 9-β-D-arabinofuranosyladenine monohydrate.

Clinical Pharmacology: Following intravenous administration, Vira-A is rapidly deaminated into arabinosylhypoxanthine (Ara-Hx), the principal metabolite, which is promptly distributed into the tissues. Peak Ara-Hx and Ara-A plasma levels ranging from 3 to 6 μg/ml and 0.2 to 0.4 μg/ml, respectively, are attained after slow intravenous infusion of Vira-A doses of 10 mg/kg of body weight. These levels reflect the rate of infusion and show no accumulation across time. The mean half-life of Ara-Hx is 3.3 hours. Ara-Hx penetrates into the cerebrospinal fluid (CSF) to give a CSF/plasma ratio of approximately 1:3.
Excretion of Vira-A is principally via the kidneys. Urinary excretion is constant over 24 hours. Forty-one to 53% of the daily dose is recovered in the urine as Ara-Hx with 1 to 3% appearing as the parent compound. There is no evidence of fecal excretion of drug or metabolites. In patients with impaired renal function Ara-Hx may accumulate in the plasma and reach levels several-fold higher than those described above.

Microbiology: Vira-A possesses *in vitro* and *in vivo* antiviral activity against *Herpesvirus* simplex (Herpes simplex virus) types 1 and 2. The antiviral mechanism of action has not yet been established. The drug is converted into nucleotides which appear to be involved with the inhibition of viral replication. In KB cells infected with Herpes simplex virus type 1, Vira-A inhibits viral DNA synthesis. Vira-A is rapidly deaminated to Ara-Hx, the principal metabolite, in cell cultures, laboratory animals, and humans.
Ara-Hx also possesses *in vitro* antiviral activity but this activity is significantly less than the activity of Vira-A.

Indications and Usage: Vira-A is indicated in the treatment of Herpes simplex virus encephalitis. Controlled studies indicate that Vira-A therapy will reduce the mortality caused by Herpes simplex virus encephalitis from 70 to 28%. Vira-A therapy does not appear to alter morbidity and resulting serious neurological sequelae in the comatose patient. Therefore, early diagnosis and treatment are essential.
Herpes simplex virus encephalitis should be suspected in patients with a history of an acute febrile encephalopathy associated with disordered mentation, altered level of consciousness and focal cerebral signs.
Studies which may support the suspected diagnosis include examination of cerebrospinal fluid and localization of an intra-cerebral lesion by brain scan, electroencephalography or computerized axial tomography (CAT).
Brain biopsy is required in order to confirm the etiological diagnosis by means of viral isolation in cell cultures.
Detection of Herpes simplex-virus in the biopsied brain tissue can also be reliably done by specific fluorescent antibody techniques. Detection of Herpes virus-like particles by electron microscopy or detection of intranuclear inclusions by histopathologic techniques only provides a presumptive diagnosis.
There are no reports available to indicate that Vira-A for infusion is effective in the management of encephalitis due to varicella-zoster or vaccinia viruses. Vira-A is not effective against infections caused by adenovirus or RNA viruses. It is also not effective against bacterial or fungal infections. There are no data to support efficacy of Vira-A against cytomegalovirus, vaccinia virus, or smallpox virus.

Contraindications: Vira-A is contraindicated in patients who develop hypersensitivity reactions to it.

Warnings: Vira-A should not be administered by the intramuscular or subcutaneous route because of its low solubility and poor absorption.

Precautions: Treatment should be discontinued in the patient with a brain biopsy negative for Herpes simplex virus in cell culture.
Special care should be exercised when administering Vira-A to patients susceptible to fluid overloading or cerebral edema. Examples are patients with CNS infections and impaired renal function.
Patients with impaired renal function, such as post-operative renal transplant recipients, may have a slower rate of renal excretion of Ara-Hx. Therefore, the dose of Vira-A may need to be adjusted according to the severity of impairment. These patients should be carefully monitored.
Patients with impaired liver function should also be observed for possible adverse effects.
Appropriate hematologic tests are recommended during Vira-A administration since hemoglobin, hematocrit, white blood cells, and platelets may be depressed during therapy.
Some degree of immunocompetence must be present in order for Vira-A to achieve clinical response.

Usage in Pregnancy. Vira-A given parenterally is teratogenic in rats and rabbits. Doses of 5 mg/kg or higher given intramuscularly to pregnant rabbits during organogenesis induced fetal abnormalities. Doses of 3 mg/kg or less did not induce teratogenic changes in pregnant rabbits. Vira-A doses ranging from 30 to 250 mg/kg were given intramuscularly to pregnant rats during organogenesis; signs of maternal toxicity were induced at doses of 100 mg/kg or higher and frank fetal anomalies were found at doses of 150 to 250 mg/kg.
A safe dose for the human embryo or fetus has not been established.
Consequently, the use of Vira-A in pregnant patients should be limited to life-threatening illnesses where the possible benefits outweigh the potential risks involved.
It is not known whether Vira-A is excreted in human milk. As a general rule, nursing should not be undertaken while a patient is under treatment since many drugs are excreted in

Continued on next page

This product information was prepared in August, 1979. On these and other Parke-Davis Products, detailed information may be obtained by addressing PARKE-DAVIS, Division of Warner-Lambert Company, Morris Plains, NJ 07950.

Parke-Davis—Cont.

human milk. However, Vira-A is rapidly deaminated in the gastrointestinal tract.

Adverse Reactions: The principal adverse reactions involve the gastrointestinal tract and are anorexia, nausea, vomiting, and diarrhea. These reactions are mild to moderate, and seldom require termination of Vira-A therapy.

CNS disturbances have been occasionally reported at therapeutic doses. These are tremor, dizziness, hallucinations, confusion, psychosis, and ataxia.

Hematologic clinical laboratory changes noted in controlled and uncontrolled studies were a decrease in hemoglobin or hematocrit, white blood cell count, and platelet count. SGOT elevations were also observed. Other changes occasionally observed were decreases in reticulocyte count and elevated total bilirubin.

Other symptoms which have been reported are weight loss, malaise, pruritus, rash, hematemesis, and pain at the injection site.

Overdosage: Acute massive overdose of the intravenous form has been reported without any serious evidence of adverse effect. Acute water overloading would pose a greater threat to the patient than Vira-A, due to its low solubility. Doses of Vira-A over 20 mg/kg/day can produce bone marrow depression with concomitant thrombocytopenia and leukopenia. If a massive overdose of the intravenous form occurs, hematologic, liver, and renal functions should be carefully monitored.

Acute massive oral ingestion is not expected to be toxic because drug absorption from the gastrointestinal tract is minimal. The oral LD_{50} for Vira-A is greater than 5,020 mg/kg in mice and rats.

Dosage and Administration: CAUTION—THE CONTENTS OF THE VIAL MUST BE DILUTED IN AN APPROPRIATE INTRAVENOUS SOLUTION PRIOR TO ADMINISTRATION. RAPID OR BOLUS INJECTION MUST BE AVOIDED.

Dosage. Herpes simplex virus encephalitis—15 mg/kg/day for 10 days.

Method of Preparation. Each vial contains 200 mg of Vira-A per ml of suspension. The solubility of Vira-A in intravenous infusion fluids is limited. Each 1 mg of Vira-A requires 2.22 ml of intravenous infusion fluid for complete solubilization. Therefore, each 1 liter of intravenous infusion fluid will solubilize a maximum of 450 mg of Vira-A.

Any appropriate intravenous solution is suitable for use as a diluent *EXCEPT* biologic or colloidal fluids (eg, blood products, protein solutions, etc.).

Shake the Vira-A vial well to obtain a homogeneous suspension before measuring and transferring.

Prepare the Vira-A solution for intravenous administration by aseptically transferring the proper dose of Vira-A into an appropriate intravenous infusion fluid. The intravenous infusion fluid used to prepare the Vira-A solution may be prewarmed to 35 to 40 C (95 to 100 F) to facilitate solution of the drug following its transference. Depending on the dose to be given, more than one liter of intravenous infusion fluid may be required. Thoroughly agitate the prepared admixture until *completely* clear. Complete solubilization of the drug, as indicated by a completely clear solution, is ascertained by careful visual inspection. Final filtration with an in-line membrane filter (0.45 μ pore size or smaller) is necessary.

Once in solution, the drug has been found to be chemically stable at room temperature (below 86 F) for at least two weeks. Dilution should be made just prior to administration and used at least within 48 hours. Subsequent agitation, shaking, or inversion of the bottle is unnecessary once the drug is completely in solution.

Administration. Using aseptic technique, slowly infuse the total daily dose by intravenous infusion (prepared as discussed above) at a constant rate over a 12- to 24-hour period.

How Supplied: N 0071-4150-08 (Steri-Vial® 4150) Vira-A (Vidarabine for Infusion), a sterile suspension containing 200 mg/ml, is supplied in 5-ml Steri-Vials; packages of 10.

WK

Animal Pharmacology and Toxicity: Acute Toxicity: The intraperitoneal LD_{50} for Vira-A ranged from 3,890 to 4,500 mg/kg in mice, and from 2,239 to 2,512 mg/kg in rats, suggesting a low order of toxicity to a single parenteral dose. Hepatic megalocytosis was observed in rats after single, intraperitoneal injections at doses near and exceeding the LD_{50} value. The hepatic megalocytosis appeared to regress completely over several months. Acute intravenous LD_{50} values could not be obtained because of the limited solubility of Vira-A.

Subacute Toxicity. Rats, dogs, and monkeys have been given daily intramuscular injections of Vira-A as a 20% suspension for 28 days. These animal species showed dose related decreases in hemoglobin, hematocrit, and lymphocytes. Bone marrow depression was also observed in monkeys. Except for localized, injection-site injury and weight gain inhibition or loss, rats tolerated daily doses up to 150 mg/kg, and dogs tolerated daily doses up to 50 mg/kg. Megalocytosis was not seen in the rats dosed by the intramuscular route for 28 days. Rhesus monkeys were particularly sensitive to Vira-A. Daily intramuscular doses of 15 mg/kg were tolerable, but doses of 25 mg/kg or higher induced progressively severe clinical signs of CNS toxicity. Three monkeys given slow intravenous infusions of Vira-A in solution at a dose of 15 mg/kg daily for 28 days had no significant adverse reactions.

Tumorigenicity. Chronic parenteral (IM) studies of vidarabine have been conducted in mice and rats.

In the mouse study, there was a statistically significant increase in liver tumor incidence among the vidarabine-treated females. In the same study, some vidarabine-treated male mice developed kidney neoplasia. No renal tumors were found in the vehicle-treated control mice or the vidarabine-treated female mice.

In the rat study, intestinal, testicular, and thyroid neoplasia occurred with greater frequency among the vidarabine-treated animals then in the vehicle-treated controls. The increases in thyroid adenoma incidence in the high-dose (50 mg/kg) males and the low-dose (30 mg/kg) females were statistically significant.

Hepatic megalocytosis, associated with vidarabine treatment, has been found in short- and long-term rodent (rat and mouse) studies. It is not clear whether or not this represents a preneoplastic change.

Mutagenicity. Results of *in vitro* experiments indicate that vidarabine can be incorporated into mammalian DNA and can induce mutation in mammalian cells (mouse L5178Y cell line). Thus far, *in vivo* studies have not been as conclusive, but there is some evidence (dominant lethal assay in mice) that vidarabine may be capable of producing mutagenic effects in male germ cells.

It has also been reported that vidarabine causes chromosome breaks and gaps when added to human leukocytes *in vitro*. While the significance of these effects in terms of mutagenicity is not fully understood, there is a well-known correlation between the ability of various agents to produce such effects and their ability to produce heritable genetic damage.

VIRA-A® ℞
(vidarabine ophthalmic ointment), 3%

Description: Vira-A (vidarabine, adenine arabinoside, or Ara-A) is an antiviral drug for topical ophthalmic administration. The chemical name is 9-β-D-arabinofuranosyladenine. Each gram of the ophthalmic ointment contains 30 mg of vidarabine monohydrate equivalent to 28.11 mg of vidarabine in a sterile, inert, petroleum base.

Clinical Pharmacology: Vira-A is a purine nucleoside obtained from fermentation cultures of *Streptomyces antibioticus*. Vira-A possesses *in vitro* and *in vivo* antiviral activity against Herpes simplex types 1 and 2, Varicella-Zoster, and Vaccinia viruses. Except for Rhabdovirus and Oncornavirus, Vira-A does not display *in vitro* antiviral activity against the other RNA or DNA viruses, including Adenovirus.

The antiviral mechanism of action has not been established. Vira-A appears to interfere with the early steps of viral DNA synthesis. Vira-A is rapidly deaminated to arabinosylhypoxanthine (Ara-Hx), the principal metabolite. Ara-Hx also possesses *in vitro* antiviral activity but this activity is less than that of Vira-A. Because of the low solubility of Vira-A, trace amounts of both Vira-A and Ara-Hx can be detected in the aqueous humor only if there is an epithelial defect in the cornea. If the cornea is normal, only trace amounts of Ara-Hx can be recovered from the aqueous humor.

Systemic absorption of Vira-A should not be expected to occur following ocular administration and swallowing lacrimal secretions. In laboratory animals, Vira-A is rapidly deaminated in the gastrointestinal tract to Ara-Hx. In contrast to topical idoxuridine, Vira-A demonstrated less cellular toxicity in the regenerating corneal epithelium in the rabbit.

Indications and Usage: Vira-A Ophthalmic Ointment, 3%, is indicated for the treatment of acute keratoconjunctivitis and recurrent epithelial keratitis due to Herpes simplex virus types 1 and 2. Vira-A is also effective in superficial keratitis caused by Herpes simplex virus which has not responded to topical idoxuridine or when toxic or hypersensitivity reactions to idoxuridine have occurred. The effectiveness of Vira-A Ophthalmic Ointment, 3%, against stromal keratitis and uveitis due to Herpes simplex virus has not been established.

The clinical diagnosis of keratitis caused by Herpes simplex virus is usually established by the presence of typical dendritic or geographic lesions on slit-lamp examination.

In controlled and uncontrolled clinical trials, an average of seven and nine days of continuous Vira-A Ophthalmic Ointment, 3%, therapy was required to achieve corneal re-epithelialization. In the controlled trials, 70 of 81 subjects (86%) re-epithelialized at the end of three weeks of therapy. In the uncontrolled trials, 101 of 142 subjects (71%) re-epithelialized at the end of three weeks. Seventy-five percent of the subjects in these uncontrolled trials had either not healed previously or had developed hypersensitivity to topical idoxuridine therapy.

The following topical antibiotics: gentamicin, erythromycin, and chloramphenicol; or topical steroids: prednisolone or dexamethasone, have been administered concurrently with Vira-A Ophthalmic Ointment, 3%, without an increase in adverse reactions.

Normally, corticosteroids alone are contraindicated in Herpes simplex virus infections of the eye. If Vira-A Ophthalmic Ointment, 3%, is administered concurrently with topical corticosteroid therapy, corticosteroid-induced ocular side effects must be considered. These include corticosteroid-induced glaucoma or cataract formation and progression of a bacterial or viral infection.

Vira-A (vidarabine ophthalmic ointment) is not effective against RNA virus or adenoviral ocular infections. Vira-A is also not effective against bacterial, fungal, or chlamydial infections of the cornea or nonviral trophic ulcers.

Contraindication: Vira-A Ophthalmic Ointment, 3%, is contraindicated in patients who develop hypersensitivity reactions to it.

Warnings:

Usage in Pregnancy

Vira-A parenterally is teratogenic in rats and rabbits. Ten percent Vira-A Ointment applied to 10% of the body surface during organogenesis induced fetal abnormalities in rabbits. When 10% Vira-A Ointment was applied to 2 to 3% of the body surface of rabbits, no fetal abnormalities were found. This dose greatly exceeds the total ophthalmic dose in humans. The possibility of embryonic or fetal damage in pregnant women receiving Vira-A Ophthalmic Ointment, 3%, is remote. The topical ophthalmic dose is small, and the drug relatively insoluble. Its ocular penetration is very low. However, a safe dose for a human embryo or fetus has not been established. Consequently, Vira-A should be used only when clearly indicated.

It is not known whether Vira-A is excreted in human milk. As a general rule, because many drugs are excreted in human milk, nursing should not be undertaken while a patient is under treatment. However, excretion of vidarabine in breast milk is unlikely because Vira-A is rapidly deaminated in the gastrointestinal tract.

Mutagenic Potential

Results of *in vitro* experiments indicate that vidarabine can be incorporated into mammalian DNA and can induce mutation in mammalian cells (mouse L5178Y cell line). Thus far, *in vivo* studies have not been as conclusive, but there is some evidence (dominant lethal assay in mice) that vidarabine may be capable of producing mutagenic effects in male germ cells.

It has also been reported that vidarabine causes chromosome breaks and gaps when added to human leukocytes *in vitro*. While the significance of these effects in terms of mutagenicity is not fully understood, there is a well-known correlation between the ability of various agents to produce such effects and their ability to produce heritable genetic damage.

Oncogenic Potential

Chronic parenteral (IM) studies of vidarabine have been conducted in mice and rats.

In the mouse study, there was a statistically significant increase in liver tumor incidence among the vidarabine-treated females. In the same study, some vidarabine-treated male mice developed kidney neoplasia. No renal tumors were found in the vehicle-treated control mice or in the vidarabine-treated female mice.

In the rat study, intestinal, testicular, and thyroid neoplasia occurred with greater frequency among the vidarabine-treated animals than in the vehicle-treated controls. The increases in thyroid adenoma incidence in the high-dose (50 mg/kg) males and the low-dose (30 mg/kg) females were statistically significant.

Hepatic megalocytosis, associated with vidarabine treatment, has been found in short- and long-term rodent (rats and mice) studies. It is not clear whether or not this represents a preneoplastic change.

The recommended frequency and duration of administration should not be exceeded (see Dosage and Administration).

Precautions: The diagnosis of keratoconjunctivitis due to Herpes simplex virus should be established clinically prior to prescribing Vira-A (vidarabine ophthalmic ointment), 3%.

Patients should be forewarned that Vira-A Ointment, 3%, like any ophthalmic ointment, may produce a temporary visual haze.

Although viral resistance to Vira-A has not been observed, this possibility may exist.

Adverse Reactions: Lacrimation, foreign-body sensation, conjunctival injection, burning, irritation, superficial punctate keratitis, pain, photophobia, punctal occlusion, and sensitivity has been reported with Vira-A Ophthalmic Ointment, 3%. The following have been reported also but appear disease-related: uveitis, stromal edema, secondary glaucoma, trophic defects, corneal vascularization, and hyphema.

Overdosage: Acute massive overdosage by oral ingestion of the ophthalmic ointment has not occurred. However, the rapid deamination to arabinosylhypoxanthine should preclude any difficulty. The oral LD_{50} for vidarabine is greater than 5,020 mg/kg in mice and rats. No untoward effects should result from ingestion of the entire contents of a tube.

Overdosage by ocular administration is unlikely because any excess should be expelled quickly from the conjunctival sac. Too frequent administration should be avoided.

Dosage and Administration: Administer approximately one half inch of Vira-A Ophthalmic Ointment, 3%, into the lower conjunctival sac five times daily at three-hour intervals.

If there are no signs of improvement after 7 days, or complete re-epithelialization has not occurred by 21 days, other forms of therapy should be considered. Some severe cases may require longer treatment.

After re-epithelialization has occurred, treatment for an additional seven days at a reduced dosage (such as twice daily) is recommended in order to prevent recurrence.

How Supplied:

N 0071-3677-07

Vira-A Ophthalmic Ointment, 3%, is supplied sterile in ophthalmic ointment tubes of 3.5 g. The base is a 60:40 mixture of solid and liquid petrolatum. **UK**

[*Shown in Product Identification Section*]

ZARONTIN® ℞

(ethosuximide, USP)
Capsules
Syrup

Description: Zarontin (ethosuximide) is an anticonvulsant succinimide, chemically designated as alpha-ethyl-alpha-methyl-succinimide.

Action: Ethosuximide suppresses the paroxysmal three-cycle-per-second spike and wave activity associated with lapses of consciousness which is common in absence (petit mal) seizures. The frequency of epileptiform attacks is reduced, apparently by depression of the motor cortex and elevation of the threshold of the central nervous system to convulsive stimuli.

Indication: Zarontin is indicated for the control of absence (peti mal) epilepsy.

Contraindication: Ethosuximide should not be used in patients with a history of hypersensitivity to succinimides.

Warnings: Blood dyscrasias, including some with fatal outcome, have been reported to be associated with the use of ethosuximide; therefore, periodic blood counts should be performed.

Ethosuximide is capable of producing morphological and functional changes in the animal liver. In humans, abnormal liver and renal function studies have been reported.

Ethosuximide should be administered with extreme caution to patients with known liver or renal diseases. Periodic urinalysis and liver function studies are advised for all patients receiving the drug.

Cases of systemic lupus erythematosus have been reported with the use of ethosuximide. The physician should be alert to this possibility.

Usage in Pregnancy: The effects of Zarontin in human pregnancy and nursing infants is unknown.

Recent reports suggest an association between the use of anticonvulsant drugs by women with epilepsy and an elevated incidence of birth defects in children born to these women. Data is more extensive with respect to phenytoin and phenobarbital, but these are also the most commonly prescribed anticonvulsants. Less systematic or anecdotal reports suggest a possible similar association with the use of all known anticonvulsant drugs.

The reports suggesting an elevated incidence of birth defects in children of drug-treated epileptic women cannot be regarded as adequate to prove a definite cause-and-effect relationship. There are intrinsic methodological problems in obtaining adequate data on drug teratogenicity in humans. The possibility also exists that other factors, eg, genetic factors or the epileptic condition itself, may be more important than drug therapy in leading to birth defects. The great majority of mothers on anticonvulsant medication deliver normal infants. It is important to note that anticonvulsant drugs should not be discontinued in patients in whom the drug is administered to prevent major seizures because of the strong possibility of precipitating status epilepticus with attendant hypoxia and threat to life. In individual cases where the severity and frequency of the seizure disorder are such that the removal of medication does not pose a serious threat to the patient, discontinuation of the drug may be considered prior to and during pregnancy, although it cannot be said with any confidence that even minor seizures do not pose some hazard to the developing embryo or fetus.

The prescribing physician will wish to weigh these considerations in treating or counseling epileptic women of childbearing potential.

Hazardous Activities: Ethosuximide may impair the mental and/or physical abilities required for the performance of potentially hazardous tasks, such as driving a motor vehicle or other such activity requiring alertness; therefore, the patient should be cautioned accordingly.

Precautions: Ethosuximide, when used alone in mixed types of epilepsy, may increase the frequency of grand mal seizures in some patients.

As with other anticonvulsants, it is important to proceed slowly when increasing or decreasing dosage, as well as when adding or eliminating other medication. Abrupt withdrawal of anticonvulsant medication may precipitate absence (petit mal) status.

Adverse Reactions:

Gastrointestinal System: Gastrointestinal symptoms occur frequently and include anorexia, vague gastric upset, nausea and vomiting, cramps, epigastric and abdominal pain, weight loss, and diarrhea.

Hemopoietic System: Hemopoietic complications associated with the administration of ethosuximide have included leukopenia, agranulocytosis, pancytopenia, aplastic anemia, and eosinophilia.

Nervous System: Neurologic and sensory reactions reported during therapy with ethosuximide have included drowsiness, headache, dizziness, euphoria, hiccups, irritability, hyperactivity, lethargy, fatigue, and ataxia. Psychiatric or psychological aberrations associated with ethosuximide administration have included disturbances of sleep, night terrors, inability to concentrate, and aggressiveness. These effects may be noted particularly in patients who have previously exhibited psychological abnormalities. There have been rare reports of paranoid psychosis, increased libido, and increased state of depression with overt suicidal intentions.

Integumentary System: Dermatologic manifestations which have occurred with the administration of ethosuximide have included

Continued on next page

This product information was prepared in August, 1979. On these and other Parke-Davis Products, detailed information may be obtained by addressing PARKE-DAVIS, Division of Warner-Lambert Company, Morris Plains, NJ 07950.

Parke-Davis—Cont.

urticaria, Stevens-Johnson syndrome, systemic lupus erythematosus, and pruritic erythematous rashes.

Miscellaneous: Other reactions reported have included myopia, vaginal bleeding, swelling of the tongue, gum hypertrophy, and hirsutism.

Dosage and Administration:

Zarontin Capsules (ethosuximide capsules, USP): Zarontin is administered by the oral route. The initial dosage for patients 3 to 6 years of age is one capsule (250 mg) per day; for patients 6 years of age and older, 2 capsules (500 mg) per day. The dosage thereafter must be individualized according to the patient's response. Dosage should be increased by small increments. One useful method is to increase the daily dosage by 250 mg every four to seven days until control is achieved with minimal side effects. Dosages exceeding 1.5 g daily, in divided doses, should be administered only under the strictest supervision of the physician.

The *optimal* dosage for most children is 20 mg/kg/day. This dose has given average plasma levels within the accepted therapeutic range of 40 to 100 mcg/ml. Subsequent dosage schedules can be based on effectiveness and plasma level determinations.

Zarontin Syrup: Zarontin is administered by the oral route. The initial dosage for patients 3 to 6 years of age is one teaspoonful (250 mg) per day; for patients 6 years of age and older, 2 teaspoonsful (500 mg) per day. The dosage thereafter must be individualized according to the patient's response. Dosage should be increased by small increments. One useful method is to increase the daily dosage by 250 mg every four to seven days until control is achieved with minimal side effects. Dosages exceeding 1.5 g daily, in divided doses, should be administered only under the strictest supervision of the physician.

The *optimal* dosage for most children is 20 mg/kg/day.

Zarontin Capsules and Syrup:
Zarontin may be administered in combination with other anticonvulsants when other forms of epilepsy coexist with absence (petit mal).

The *optimal* dosage for most children is 20 mg/kg/day.

How Supplied:

N 0071-0237-24 (Capsule 237)—Each capsule contains 250 mg ethosuximide, supplied in bottles of 100. Parcode® No. 237

[*Shown in Product Identification Section*]

N 0071-2418-24—Zarontin Syrup, each 5 ml contains 250 mg ethosuximide in a raspberry-flavored base; in 16-oz bottles.

YC

Pennwalt
Rx DIVISION
Pennwalt Corporation
ROCHESTER, NEW YORK 14623

ADAPIN® ℞
(doxepin HCl)

Description: Adapin (doxepin HCl) is an isomeric mixture of N,N-dimethyl-dibenz(b,e) oxepin-$\Delta^{11(6H)}$,γpropylamine hydrochloride.

Actions: Adapin has a variety of pharmacological actions with its predominant action on the central nervous system. While its mechanism of action is not known, studies have demonstrated that it is neither a monoamine oxidase inhibitor nor a primary stimulant of the central nervous system.

In a large series of patients systematically observed for withdrawal symptoms, none were reported—a finding which is consistent with the virtual absence of euphoria as a side effect and the lack of addictive potential characteristic of this type of chemical compound.

Indications: In controlled clinical evaluations, Adapin has shown marked antianxiety and significant antidepressant effects. Adapin has been found to be well tolerated even in elderly patients.

Adapin is indicated for the treatment of patients with:

1. Psychoneurotic anxiety and/or depressive reactions.
2. Mixed symptoms of anxiety and depression.
3. Anxiety and/or depression associated with alcoholism.
4. Anxiety associated with organic disease.
5. Psychotic depressive disorders including involutional depression and manic-depressive reactions.

Target symptoms of psychoneurosis that respond particularly well to Adapin include: anxiety, tension, depression, somatic symptoms and concerns, insomnia, guilt, lack of energy, fear, apprehension and worry.

Because Adapin provides antidepressant as well as antianxiety effects, it is of particular value in patients in whom anxiety masks depression. Patients who have not responded to other antianxiety or antidepressant drugs may benefit from Adapin.

Contraindications: Because Adapin has an anticholinergic effect, it is contraindicated in patients with glaucoma or a tendency toward urinary retention.

Use of Adapin is contraindicated in patients who have been found hypersensitive to it.

Warnings: *Usage in Pregnancy:* Adapin has not been evaluated in pregnant patients. Therefore, it should not be used during pregnancy unless, in the judgment of the physician, it is essential to the welfare of the patient.

In animal reproduction studies of Adapin, gross and microscopic examination of the offspring gave no evidence of drug-related teratogenic effect. Following doses of up to 25 mg./kg./day for 8 to 9 months, no changes were observed in the number of live births, litter size, or lactation. A decreased rate of conception was observed when male rats were given 25 mg./kg./day for prolonged periods—an effect which has occurred with other psychotropic drugs and has been attributed to drug effect on the central and/or autonomic nervous systems.

Usage in Children: The use of Adapin in children under 12 years of age is not recommended, because safe conditions for its use have not been established.

MAO Inhibitors: Serious side effects and even death have been reported following the concomitant use of certain drugs with MAO inhibitors. Therefore, MAO inhibitors should be discontinued at least two weeks prior to the cautious initiation of therapy with Adapin (doxepin HCl). The exact length of time may vary and is dependent upon the particular MAO inhibitor being used, the length of time it has been administered, and the dosage involved.

Alcohol: In patients who may use alcohol excessively, it should be borne in mind that the potentiation may increase the danger inherent in any suicide attempt or overdosage.

Precautions: Drowsiness may occur with Adapin (doxepin HCl); therefore, patients should be warned of its possible occurrence and cautioned against driving a motor vehicle or operating hazardous machinery while taking the drug.

Patients should also be cautioned that the effects of alcoholic beverages may be increased. Since suicide is an inherent risk in depressed patients and remains a risk through the initial phases of improvement, depressed patients should be closely supervised.

Although Adapin has shown effective tranquilizing activity, the possibility of activating or unmasking latent psychotic symptoms should be kept in mind.

Compounds structurally related to Adapin can block the effects of guanethidine and similarly acting compounds. However, at the usual clinical dosages, 75 mg. to 150 mg. per day, Adapin has been given concomitantly with guanethidine without blocking its antihypertensive effect. But at dosages of 300 mg. per day or higher, Adapin has exerted a significant blocking effect.

Adapin, like other structurally related psychotropic drugs, potentiates norepinephrine response in animals. But this effect has not been observed with Adapin in humans, which is in accord with the low incidence of tachycardia reported clinically.

Adverse Reactions: *Anticholinergic Effects:* Dry mouth, blurred vision and constipation have been reported. These are usually mild, and often subside as therapy is continued or dosage reduced.

Central Nervous System Effects: Drowsiness has been observed. It usually occurs early in the course of therapy and tends to subside as therapy continues. (See Dosage and Administration section.)

Cardiovascular Effects: Tachycardia and hypotension have been reported infrequently.

Other infrequently reported adverse effects include extrapyramidal symptoms, gastrointestinal reactions, secretory effects (such as increased sweating), weakness, dizziness, fatigue, weight gain, edema, paresthesias, flushing, chills, tinnitus, photophobia, decreased libido, rash, and pruritus.

Dosage and Administration: *In most patients with mild to moderate anxiety and/or depression:* A starting dose of 25 mg. t.i.d. is recommended. Decrease or increase the dosage at appropriate intervals according to individual response. Usual optimum dosage is 75 mg. to 150 mg. per day. As an alternate regimen the total daily dosage, up to 150 mg., may be given at bedtime without loss of effectiveness. In some patients with mild symptomatology or emotional symptoms accompanying organic disease, dosage as low as 25 mg. to 50 mg. per day has provided effective control.

In more severe anxiety and/or depression: 50 mg. t.i.d. may be required to start—if necessary, gradually increase to 300 mg. per day. Additional effectiveness is rarely obtained by exceeding 300 mg. per day.

Although optimal antidepressant response may not be evident for two to three weeks, antianxiety activity is rapidly apparent.

Overdosage: Symptoms—An increase of any of the reported adverse reactions, primarily excessive sedation and anticholinergic effects such as blurred vision and dry mouth. Other effects may be: pronounced tachycardia, hypotension and extrapyramidal symptoms. Treatment—Essentially symptomatic; supportive therapy in the case of hypotension and excessive sedation.

How Supplied: Each capsule contains doxepin, as the hydrochloride, 10 mg. (NDC 0018-0356), 25 mg. (NDC 0018-0357), 50 mg. (NDC 0018-0358) and 100 mg (NDC 0018-0359) capsules in bottles of 100, and 1000.

Rev 12/77

[*Shown in Product Identification Section*]

IONAMIN® ©
(phentermine resin)

Description: Ionamin '15' and Ionamin '30' contain 15 mg. and 30 mg. respectively of phentermine as the cationic exchange resin complex. Phentermine is α, α-dimethyl phenylethylamine (phenyl-tertiary-butylamine).

Actions: Ionamin is a sympathomimetic amine with pharmacologic activity similar to the prototype drug of this class used in obesity, amphetamine (d- and *dl*-amphetamine). Actions include central nervous system stimula-

tion and elevation of blood pressure. Tachyphylaxis and tolerance have been demonstrated with all drugs of this class in which these phenomena have been looked for.
Drugs of this class used in obesity are commonly known as "anorectics" or "anorexigenics." It has not been established, however, that the action of such drugs in treating obesity is primarily one of appetite suppression. Other central nervous system actions, or metabolic effects may be involved.
Adult obese subjects instructed in dietary management and treated with "anorectic" drugs, lose more weight on the average than those treated with placebo and diet, as determined in relatively short-term clinical trials.
The magnitude of increased weight loss of drug-treated patients over placebo-treated patients is only a fraction of a pound a week. The rate of weight loss is greatest in the first weeks of therapy for both drug and placebo subjects and tends to decrease in succeeding weeks. The possible origins of the increased weight loss due to the various drug effects are not established. The amount of weight loss associated with the use of an "anorectic" drug varies from trial to trial, and the increased weight loss appears to be related in part to variables other than the drugs prescribed, such as the physician-investigator, the population treated, and the diet prescribed. Studies do not permit conclusions as to the relative importance of the drug and non-drug factors on weight loss.
The natural history of obesity is measured in years, whereas the studies cited are restricted to a few weeks or months duration; thus, the total impact of drug-induced weight loss over that of diet alone must be considered clinically limited.
The bioavailability of Ionamin has been studied in humans in which blood levels of phentermine were measured by a gas-chromatography method. Blood levels obtained with the 15 mg. and 30 mg. resin complex formulations indicated slower absorption with a reduced but prolonged peak concentration and without a significant difference in prolongation of blood levels when compared with the same doses of phentermine hydrochloride. The clinical significance of these differences is not known. In clinical trials establishing the efficacy of Ionamin, a single daily dose produced an effect comparable to that produced by other regimens of "anorectic" drug therapy.
Indication: Ionamin is indicated in the management of exogenous obesity as a short-term (a few weeks) adjunct in a regimen of weight reduction based on caloric restriction. The limited usefulness of agents of this class (see ACTIONS) should be measured against possible risk factors inherent in their use such as those described below.
Contraindications: Advanced arterlosclerosis, symptomatic cardiovascular disease, moderate to severe hypertension, hyperthyroidism, known hypersensitivity, or idiosyncrasy to the sympathomimetic amines, glaucoma.
Agitated states.
Patients with a history of drug abuse.
During or within 14 days following the administration of monoamine oxidase inhibitors (hypertensive crises may result).
Warnings: If tolerance to the "anorectic" effect develops, the recommended dose should not be exceeded in an attempt to increase the effect: rather, the drug should be discontinued. Ionamin may impair the ability of the patient to engage in potentially hazardous activities such as operating machinery or driving a motor vehicle; the patient should therefore be cautioned accordingly.
Drug Dependence: Ionamin is related chemically and pharmacologically to amphetamine (d- and d*l*- amphetamine) and other stimulant drugs that have been extensively abused. The possibility of abuse of Ionamin should be kept in mind when evaluating the desirability of including a drug as part of a weight reduction program. Abuse of amphetamine (d- and d*l*-amphetamine) and related drugs may be associated with intense psychological dependence and severe social dysfunction. There are reports of patients who have increased the dosage of some of these drugs to many times that recommended. Abrupt cessation following prolonged high dosage administration results in extreme fatigue and mental depression; changes are also noted on the sleep EEG. Manifestations of chronic intoxication with anorectic drugs include severe dermatoses, marked insomnia, irritability, hyperactivity, and personality changes. The most severe manifestation of chronic intoxications is psychosis, often clinically indistinguishable from schizophrenia.
Usage in Pregnancy: Safe use in pregnancy has not been established. Use of Ionamin by women who are or may become pregnant requires that the potential benefit be weighed against the possible hazard to mother and infant.
Usage in Children: Ionamin is not recommended for use in children under 12 years of age.
Precautions: Caution is to be exercised in prescribing Ionamin for patients with even mild hypertension. Insulin requirements in diabetes mellitus may be altered in association with the use of Ionamin and the concomitant dietary regimen.
Ionamin may decrease the hypotensive effect of guanethidine.
The least amount feasible should be prescribed or dispensed at one time in order to minimize the possibility of overdosage.
Adverse Reactions:
Cardiovascular: Palpitation, tachycardia, elevation of blood pressure.
Central Nervous System: Overstimulation, restlessness, dizziness, insomnia, euphoria, dysphoria, tremor, headache; rarely psychotic episodes at recommended doses with some drugs in this class.
Gastrointestinal: Dryness of the mouth, unpleasant taste, diarrhea, constipation, other gastrointestinal disturbances.
Allergic: Urticaria.
Endocrine: Impotence, changes in libido.
Dosage and Administration: One capsule daily, before breakfast or 10–14 hours before retiring. For individuals exhibiting greater drug responsiveness, Ionamin '15' will usually suffice. Ionamin '30' is recommended for less responsive patients. Ionamin is not recommended for use in children under 12 years of age.
Overdosage: Manifestations of acute overdosage may include restlessness, tremor, hyperreflexia, rapid respiration, confusion, assaultiveness, hallucinations, panic states.
Fatigue and depression usually follow the central stimulation.
Cardiovascular effects include arrhythmias, hypertension, or hypotension and circulatory collapse. Gastrointestinal symptoms include nausea, vomiting, diarrhea, and abdominal cramps. Overdosage of pharmacologically similar compounds has resulted in fatal poisoning, usually terminating in convulsions and coma.
Management of acute Ionamin intoxication is largely symptomatic and includes lavage and sedation with a barbiturate. Experience with hemodialysis or peritoneal dialysis is inadequate to permit recommendation in this regard. Intravenous phentolamine (Regitine) has been suggested on pharmacologic grounds for possible acute, severe hypertension, if this complicates overdosage.
How Supplied: Two strengths: Ionamin (phentermine resin) 15 mg. (NDC 0018-0903) yellow and gray capsules; Ionamin (phentermine resin) 30 mg. (NDC 0018-0904) yellow capsules. Available on prescription only. Stock bottles of 100 and 400. Rev 4/78
[Shown in Product Identification Section]

KOLYUM® LIQUID/KOLYUM® POWDER ℞

Description: Each tablespoonful (15 ml.) of Kolyum Liquid or 5 g. packet of Kolyum Powder provides 20 mEq. of potassium ion and 3.4 mEq. of chloride ion in a sugar-free, cherry-flavored vehicle. These mEq. quantities are derived from the presence of potassium gluconate 3.9 g. and potassium chloride 0.25 g. The blandness of the potassium gluconate and the presence of sorbitol in the formulation permit a high level of gastrointestinal tolerance. Both adults and children find Kolyum palatable.
Indications: Prevention and treatment of hypokalemia which may occur secondary to diuretic or corticosteroid administration. May be used in the treatment of cardiac arrhythmias due to digitalis intoxication. In hypokalemic states, especially in patients on salt-free diets, hypochloremic alkalosis may occur; treatment may then require chloride in addition to potassium supplementation. Kolyum provides 3.4 mEq. of chloride per dose as an adjunct to the treatment of hypochloremic alkalosis.
Contraindications: Severe renal impairment with oliguria or azotemia, untreated Addison's disease, adynamia episodica hereditaria (periodic paralysis; hyperkalemic type), acute dehydration, heat cramps and hyperkalemia from any causes.
Precautions: In response to a rise in the concentration of potassium, renal excretion of the ion is increased. With normal kidney function it is difficult to produce potassium intoxication by oral administration. Nevertheless, potassium supplements must be administered with caution, since the amount of the deficiency and the daily intake are not accurately known. Other medications, such as potassium penicillins, may contain appreciable potassium.
The clinical status of the patient should be assessed frequently. Periodic ECG tracings should be performed, and serum potassium levels should be determined at frequent intervals. High serum concentrations of potassium ion may cause death as a result of cardiac depression, arrhythmias or arrest. This drug should be used with caution in the presence of heart disease.
Extreme caution should be exercised in patients receiving aldosterone antagonists or potassium sparing diuretics. In both instances potassium intoxication may occur.
Adverse Reactions: Nausea, vomiting, diarrhea and abdominal discomfort have been reported. The symptoms and signs of potassium intoxication include paresthesias and weakness of the extremities, flaccid paralysis, listlessness, mental confusion, hypotension, cardiac arrhythmias and heart block.
The following ECG abnormalities may be present in hyperkalemia: disappearance of the P wave, widening and slurring of the QRS complex, changes of the ST segment, and tall, peaked T waves, particularly in the right precordial leads.
Dosage: The usual adult dose of Kolyum Liquid is one tablespoonful (15 ml.) in 30 ml. (one fluid ounce) or more of water twice daily. The usual adult dose of Kolyum Powder is one packet (5 g.) dissolved in 3-4 fluid ounces of cool water twice daily.
This daily dose of Kolyum Liquid or Kolyum Powder supplies 40 mEq. of potassium ion, the approximate daily requirement, as well as 6.7 mEq. of chloride ion. Deviations from this recommendation may be indicated; as no average total daily dose can be defined, the response of the patient to the dose of the drug must be assessed clinically. Larger doses may be required, but should be administered under close supervision because of the possibility of potassium intoxication.

Continued on next page

Pennwalt—Cont.

Overdosage: Potassium intoxication may result from overdose of potassium or from ordinary therapeutic doses in conditions stated in the section on "Contraindications". Hyperkalemia, when detected, must be treated immediately because lethal levels can be reached in a few hours.

Treatment of Hyperkalemia:

1. Dextrose solution, 10% or 25%, containing 10 units of crystalline insulin per 20 g. dextrose, given I.V. in a dose of 300-500 ml. in one hour.
2. Absorption and exchange of potassium using sodium or ammonium cycle cation exchange resin, orally and as retention enema. (Caution: Ammonium compounds should not be used in patients with hepatic cirrhosis).
3. Hemodialysis and peritoneal dialysis.
4. Ingestion of potassium-containing foods and medication should be stopped.
5. Transition from the hyperkalemic state to one of hypokalemia should be guarded against, especially in patients taking digitalis, as hypokalemia increases sensitivity to digitalis.

How Supplied: Available on prescription only.

Kolyum Liquid
Stock bottles of 1 gallon, 1 pint (NDC-0018-0858). Dispense in amber glass bottles. Store at room temperature.

Kolyum Powder
Cartons containing 30, 5 g. packets (NDC-0018-0604). Dispense in original packet to keep product moisture-free. Store at room temperature.

Rev 3/30/77

NESACAINE® ℞
(Chloroprocaine Hydrochloride)
FOR INFILTRATION AND REGIONAL ANESTHESIA
NESACAINE®–CE
(Chloroprocaine Hydrochloride)
FOR CAUDAL AND EPIDURAL ANESTHESIA

Description: NESACAINE and NESACAINE-CE (Chloroprocaine Hydrochloride) is β - diethylaminoethyl 2-chloro-4-aminobenzoate hydrochloride.

Chloroprocaine Hydrochloride is an amorphous white powder or a colorless crystalline substance which is water-soluble, melts at 173° to 176° C., and has a molecular weight of 307.2. It is incompatible with caustic alkalis and their carbonates, soaps, silver salts, iodine, and iodides.

NESACAINE (Chloroprocaine Hydrochloride), multidose vials, should not be used for caudal or epidural anesthesia since it contains a preservative.

NESACAINE-CE (Chloroprocaine Hydrochloride), single dose vials, for caudal and epidural anesthesia contains no preservative and any unused portion should be discarded.

NESACAINE and NESACAINE-CE (Chloroprocaine Hydrochloride) solutions are sterile so that autoclaving is unnecessary. Since hydrolysis resulting in impairment of potency is accelerated at the temperature of steam sterilization, these solutions should not be autoclaved.

As with other anesthetics having a free aromatic amino group, NESACAINE and NESACAINE-CE (Chloroprocaine Hydrochloride) solutions are slightly photosensitive and may become discolored after prolonged exposure to light. It is recommended that these vials be stored in the original outer containers, protected from direct sunlight. Discolored solutions should not be administered. If stored at low temperatures, NESACAINE and NESACAINE-CE (Chloroprocaine Hydrochloride) may deposit crystals which, when returned to room temperature, will redissolve.

Actions: The parenteral administration of NESACAINE and NESACAINE-CE (Chloroprocaine Hydrochloride) stabilizes the neuronal membrane and prevents the initiation and transmission of nerve impulses, thereby effecting local anesthetic action.

The onset of action of NESACAINE (Chloroprocaine Hydrochloride) is from 6 to 12 minutes and the duration of anesthesia is from 30 to 60 minutes depending upon the amount used.

NESACAINE and NESACAINE-CE (Chloroprocaine Hydrochloride) is hydrolyzed in plasma by pseudocholinesterase. The hydrolysis of 2-chloroprocaine results in the production of 2-chloro-4-aminobenzoic acid and β-diethylaminoethanol.

Solutions of NESACAINE and NESACAINE-CE (Chloroprocaine Hydrochloride) do not injure nervous tissue and are not irritating to other tissues in the concentrations employed for infiltration, regional, caudal and epidural anesthesia.

Indications: NESACAINE in multiple dose vials and NESACAINE-CE in *single dose* vials without preservatives are indicated for production of local anesthesia by infiltration injection and nerve block.*

NESACAINE-CE in *single dose* vials without preservatives is also indicated for production of local anesthesia by caudal or other epidural block.*

*NESACAINE in multiple dose vials with preservatives is not to be used for caudal or epidural anesthesia. NESACAINE-CE contains no preservatives and the unused portion must be discarded after initial use.

Contraindications: NESACAINE and NESACAINE-CE (Chloroprocaine Hydrochloride) are contraindicated in patients hypersensitive (allergic) to drugs of the PABA ester group.

Although central nervous system disease is generally considered a contraindication to caudal or epidural nerve block, it is not a contraindication to peripheral nerve block. Pathologic changes of the vertebral column may make epidural puncture impossible or inadvisable.

Warnings: RESUSCITATIVE EQUIPMENT AND DRUGS SHOULD BE IMMEDIATELY AVAILABLE WHEN ANY LOCAL ANESTHETIC IS USED. NESACAINE (Chloroprocaine Hydrochloride) contains a preservative and should not be used for caudal or epidural anesthesia. As NESACAINE-CE (Chloroprocaine Hydrochloride) contains no preservative, discard unused drug remaining in vial after initial use. Equipment and drugs necessary for the treatment of inadvertent intravascular injection, intrathecal injection, or excessive dosage should be immediately available.

Usage in Pregnancy: Safe use of chloroprocaine hydrochloride has not been established with respect to adverse effects upon fetal development. Therefore, it should not be used in women of childbearing potential unless in the judgment of the physician the potential benefits outweigh the unknown hazards.

In obstetrics, if vasoconstrictor drugs are used either to correct hypotension or are added to the local anesthetic solution, the obstetrician should be warned that some oxytocic drugs may cause severe persistent hypertension and even rupture of a cerebral blood vessel may occur during the post partum period.

Solutions containing vasoconstrictors, particularly epinephrine and norepinephrine, should be used with extreme caution in patients receiving certain antidepressants such as MAO inhibitors, and tricyclic compounds since a severe prolonged hypertension may occur.

Precautions: The safety and effectiveness of chloroprocaine hydrochloride depends upon proper dosage, correct technique, adequate precautions and readiness for emergencies.

The lowest dosage that results in effective anesthesia should be used to avoid high plasma levels and serious undesirable systemic side effects. Tolerance varies with the status of the patient. Debilitated patients, elderly patients, acutely ill patients, and children should be given reduced doses commensurate with their age and physical status.

Solutions containing vasoconstrictors should be used cautiously in the presence of disease which may adversely affect the patient's cardiovascular system.

Chloroprocaine hydrochloride should be employed cautiously in persons with known drug allergies or sensitivities.

The decision whether or not to use local anesthesia in the following conditions depends on the physician's appraisal of the advantages as opposed to the risk:

Paracervical block when fetal distress is anticipated or when predisposing factors causative of fetal distress are present (i.e. toxemia, prematurity, diabetes, etc.)

Injection of solutions containing epinephrine in areas where the blood supply is limited (i.e. ears, nose, digits, etc.) or when peripheral vascular disease is present.

Serious cardiac arrhythmias may occur if preparations containing a vasopressor are employed in patients during or following the administration of chloroform, halothane, cyclopropane, trichloroethylene, or other related agents.

Adverse Reactions: Adverse reactions result from high plasma levels due to rapid absorption, inadvertent intravascular injection or excessive dosage. Hypersensitivity, idiosyncrasy, or diminished tolerance are other causes of reactions. Reactions due to overdosage (high plasma levels) are systemic and involve the central nervous system and the cardiovascular system.

Reactions involving the central nervous system are characterized by excitation and/or depression. Nervousness, dizziness, blurred vision or tremors may occur followed by drowsiness, convulsions, unconsciousness and possibly respiratory arrest. Since excitement may be transient or absent, the first manifestations may be drowsiness merging into unconsciousness and respiratory arrest.

Reactions involving the cardiovascular system include depression of the myocardium, hypotension, bradycardia and even cardiac arrest.

Treatment of a patient with toxic manifestations consists of maintaining an airway, and supporting ventilation using oxygen and assisted or controlled respiration as required. Supportive treatment of the cardiovascular system consists of using vasopressors, preferably those that stimulate the myocardium (e.g. ephedrine), and intravenous fluids. Convulsions may be controlled by the intravenous administration in small increments of an ultrashort acting barbiturate (i.e. thiopental, thiamylal) or a short acting barbiturate if these are not available (secobarbital, pentobarbital) or a short acting muscle relaxant (succinylcholine), together with oxygen. Muscle relaxants and intravenous barbiturates should be used only by those familiar with their use.

Allergic reactions are characterized by cutaneous lesions, urticaria, edema and other manifestations of allergy. The detection of sensitivity by skin testing is of doubtful value.

Dosage and Administration: As with all local anesthetics the dosage varies and depends upon the area to be anesthetized, vascularity of the tissues, number of neuronal segments to be blocked, individual tolerance and the technique of anesthesia. The lowest dosage needed to provide effective anesthesia should be administered. For specific techniques and procedures refer to standard textbooks.

The maximum single recommended doses of chloroprocaine hydrochloride with and without epinephrine (1:200,000) are 1000 mg. and 800 mg. respectively.

1. Infiltration and Nerve Block
A guide to the volume and concentration of NESACAINE (Chloroprocaine Hydrochloride) for regional nerve blocks is given below:
(See table at right)
2. Caudal and Epidural Block
For Caudal anesthesia the initial dose is 15 to 25 ml. of a 2 percent or 3 percent solution. Repeated doses may be given at 40 to 60 minute intervals.
For Epidural anesthesia in the cervical or thoracic region, 1.5 to 2.0 ml. for each segment can be used. In the lumbar and sacral regions 2.0 to 2.5 ml. per segment can be used. The usual total volume of NESACAINE-CE (Chloroprocaine Hydrochloride) is from 15 to 25 ml.
Repeated doses 2 to 6 ml. less than the original dose may be given at 40 to 50 minute intervals.
Preparation of Epinephrine Solutions—To prepare a 1 to 200,000 epinephrine-chloroprocaine hydrochloride solution add 0.15 milliliters of a 1 to 1,000 epinephrine injection U.S.P. solution per 30 milliliters of NESACAINE-CE (Chloroprocaine Hydrochloride).
How Supplied: NESACAINE (Chloroprocaine Hydrochloride) is supplied as follows:
1 percent solution (10 mg/ml) in 30 ml. multiple-dose vials, 12 vials per carton.
2 percent solution (20 mg/ml) in 30 ml. multiple-dose vials, 12 vials per carton.
NESACAINE-CE (Chloroprocaine Hydrochloride) is supplied as follows:
2 percent solution (20 mg/ml) in 30 ml. single-dose vials, packaged 12 vials per carton.
3 percent solution (30 mg/ml) in 30 ml. single-dose vials, packaged 12 vials per carton.
7/77

Type of Block	Volume	Concentration
Occipital	3–5 ml.	1%–2%
Mandibular	2–3 ml.	2%
Maxillary	2–3 ml.	2%
Infra-orbital	0.5–1 ml.	2%
Cervical	3–4 ml. (for each segment)	1%–2%
Brachial plexus	30–40 ml.	2%
Ulnar nerve	3–5 ml.	2%
Paravertebral	3–5 ml.	2%
Intercostal	3 ml.	1%–2%
Sciatic nerve	10–15 ml.	2%
Stellate ganglion	5–10 ml.	1%–2%
Lumbar sympathetic (1 needle technic)	15–20 ml.	1%–2%
Interdigital	3–4 ml. (without epinephrine)	1%–2%

Fractional doses, up to 300 to 600 mg., may be given at 50 minute intervals.

Antitussive
TUSSIONEX® Ⓒ
(Resin Complexes of Hydrocodone and Phenyltoloxamine)

TUSSIONEX® Capsules, Suspension and Tablets
Composition: Each capsule, teaspoonful (5 ml.) or tablet contains 5 mg. hydrocodone (*Warning:* may be habit-forming), and 10 mg. phenyltoloxamine as cationic resin complexes.
Effects: An effective antitussive which acts for approximately 12 hours.
Dosage: *Adults:* 1 teaspoonful (5 ml.), capsule or tablet every 8-12 hours. May be adjusted to individual requirements. *Children:*
Under 1 year: ¼ teaspoonful every 12 hours.
From 1-5 years: ½ teaspoonful every 12 hours.
Over 5 years: 1 teaspoonful every 12 hours.
Side Effects: Negligible, but when encountered may include mild constipation, nausea, facial pruritus, drowsiness, which disappear with adjustment of dose or discontinuance of treatment.
Precaution: In young children the respiratory center is especially susceptible to the depressant action of narcotic cough suppressants. Benefit to risk ratio should be carefully considered especially in children with respiratory embarrassment. Estimation of dosage relative to the age and weight of the child is of great importance.
Overdosage: Immediately evacuate the stomach. Respiratory depression, if any, can be counteracted by respiratory stimulants. Convulsions, sometimes seen in children, can be controlled by intravenous administration of short-acting barbiturates. Hypothermia can be controlled by the usual supportive methods.
How Supplied: Tussionex Suspension, neutral in taste, golden color; 16 oz. and 900 ml. bottles. Tussionex Tablets, light brown, scored; bottles of 100. Tussionex Capsules, green and white; bottles of 50. A prescription for 2 oz. of the Suspension, or 12 Capsules or Tablets, constitutes a 6 day supply in the average case.
Rev 11/79

Diuretic, Antihypertensive
ZAROXOLYN® ℞
(Metolazone)

Each ZAROXOLYN Tablet contains 2½, 5, or 10 mg of metolazone.
Description: ZAROXOLYN (metolazone) has the molecular formula $C_{16}H_{16}ClN_3O_3S$ and a molecular weight of 365.84 and its chemical name is 7-chloro-1,2,3,4-tetrahydro-2-methyl-4-oxo-3-o-tolyl-6-quinazolinesulfonamide.
Metolazone is only sparingly soluble in water, but more soluble in plasma, blood, alkali, and organic solvents.
Actions: ZAROXOLYN (metolazone) is a diuretic/saluretic/antihypertensive drug. The action of ZAROXOLYN results in an interference with the renal tubular mechanism of electrolyte reabsorption. The mechanism of this action is unknown. ZAROXOLYN acts primarily to inhibit sodium reabsorption at the cortical diluting site and in the proximal convoluted tubule. Sodium and chloride ions are excreted in approximately equivalent amounts. The increased delivery of sodium to the distal tubular exchange site may result in increased potassium excretion.
DRUG INTERACTION STUDIES: In animals pretreated with ZAROXOLYN, the drug did not alter the characteristic effect of heparin on clotting time nor protamine antagonism; dicumarol on prothrombin time nor Vitamin K antagonism; the response of guanethidine, reserpine and hydralazine to cardiovascular parameters nor the pressor response of the subsequent dose of norepinephrine.
ZAROXOLYN and furosemide, administered concurrently have produced marked diuresis in some patients where edema or ascites was refractory to treatment with maximum recommended doses of these or other diuretics administered alone. The mechanism of this interaction is not known.
In clinical usage, ZAROXOLYN does not inhibit carbonic anhydrase. Its proximal action has been evidenced in humans by increased excretion of phosphate and magnesium ions, by markedly increased fractional excretion of sodium in patients with severely compromised glomerular filtration, and in animals by the results of micropuncture studies. Decrease in calcium ion excretion has not been noted.
At maximum therapeutic dosage ZAROXOLYN is approximately equal to thiazide diuretics in its diuretic potency. However, ZAROXOLYN may produce diuresis in patients with glomerular filtration rates below 20 ml/min.
When ZAROXOLYN is given, diuresis and saluresis usually begin within one hour and persist for 12 to 24 hours depending on dosage. Maximum effect occurs about two hours after administration. At the higher recommended dosages, effect may be prolonged beyond 24 hours. *A single daily dose is recommended.* For most patients the duration of effect can be varied by adjusting the daily dose.
The prolonged duration of action of ZAROXOLYN is attributed to protein-binding and enterohepatic recycling. A small amount of ZAROXOLYN is metabolized and the fraction so changed is nontoxic. The primary route of excretion is renal.
The mechanism whereby diuretics function in the control of hypertension is unknown; both renal and extra-renal actions may be involved. An antihypertensive effect may be seen as early as three to four days after ZAROXOLYN has been started. Administration for three to four weeks, however, is usually required for optimum antihypertensive effect.
Indications: ZAROXOLYN (metolazone) is indicated in the management of hypertension either as the sole therapeutic agent or to enhance the effectiveness of other antihypertensive drugs in the more severe forms of hypertension.
ZAROXOLYN (metolazone) is indicated for the treatment of salt and water retention including
—edema accompanying congestive heart failure
—edema accompanying renal diseases, including the nephrotic syndrome, and states of diminished renal function

Usage in Pregnancy
The routine use of diuretics in an otherwise healthy woman is inappropriate and exposes mother and fetus to unnecessary hazard. Diuretics do not prevent development of toxemia of pregnancy, and there is no satisfactory evidence that they are useful in the treatment of developed toxemia.
Edema during pregnancy may arise from pathological causes or from the physiologic and mechanical consequences of pregnancy. ZAROXOLYN is indicated in pregnancy when edema is due to pathologic causes, just as it is in the absence of pregnancy (however, see Warnings, below). Dependent edema in pregnancy, resulting from restriction of venous return by the expanded uterus, is properly treated through elevation of the lower extremities and use of support hose; use of diuretics to lower intravascular volume in this case is illogical and unnecessary. There is hypervolemia during normal pregnancy which is harmful to neither the fetus nor the mother (in the absence of cardiovascular disease), but which is associated with edema, including generalized edema, in the majority of pregnant women. If this edema produces discomfort, increased recumbency will often provide relief. In rare instances, this edema may cause extreme discomfort which is not relieved by rest. In these cases, a short course of diuretics may provide relief and may be appropriate.
Contraindications: Anuria.
Hepatic coma or pre-coma; known allergy or hypersensitivity to ZAROXOLYN (metolazone).

Continued on next page

Pennwalt—Cont.

Warnings: While not reported to date, cross-allergy theoretically may occur when ZAROXOLYN (metolazone) is given to patients known to be allergic to sulfonamide-derived drugs, thiazides, or quinethazone.
Hypokalemia may occur, with consequent weakness, cramps, and cardiac dysrhythmias. Hypokalemia is a particular hazard in digitalized patients; dangerous or fatal arrhythmias may be precipitated.
Azotemia and hyperuricemia may be noted or precipitated during the administration of ZAROXOLYN. (Infrequently, gouty attacks have been reported in persons with history of gout.)
If azotemia and oliguria worsen during treatment of patients with severe renal disease, ZAROXOLYN should be discontinued.
Until additional data have been obtained, ZAROXOLYN is not recommended for patients in the pediatric age group.
Unusually large or prolonged effects on volume and electrolytes may result when ZAROXOLYN and furosemide are administered concurrently. It is recommended that concurrent administration of these diuretics for treatment of resistant edema be started under hospital conditions in order to provide for adequate monitoring.
When ZAROXOLYN is used with other antihypertensive drugs, particular care must be taken, especially during initial therapy. Dosage of other antihypertensive agents, especially the ganglionic blockers, should be reduced.
ZAROXOLYN may be given with a potassium-sparing diuretic when indicated. In this circumstance, diuresis may be potentiated and dosages should be reduced. Potassium retention and hyperkalemia may result; the serum potassium should be determined frequently. Potassium supplementation is contraindicated when a potassium-sparing diuretic is given.

Usage in Pregnancy
ZAROXOLYN crosses the placental barrier and appears in cord blood. The use of ZAROXOLYN in pregnant women requires that the anticipated benefit be weighed against possible hazards to the fetus. These hazards include fetal or neonatal jaundice, thrombocytopenia, and possibly other adverse reactions which have occurred in the adult.

Nursing Mothers
ZAROXOLYN appears in breast milk. If use of the drug is deemed essential, the patient should stop nursing.

Precautions: Periodic determination of serum electrolytes to detect possible electrolyte imbalance should be performed at appropriate intervals. Blood urea nitrogen, uric acid, and glucose levels should be assessed at intervals during diuretic therapy.
All patients receiving ZAROXOLYN (metolazone) therapy should be observed for clinical signs of fluid and/or electrolyte imbalance; namely, hyponatremia, hypochloremic alkalosis, and hypokalemia. Serum and urine electrolyte determinations are particularly important when the patient is vomiting excessively or receiving parenteral fluids. Medication such as digitalis may also influence serum electrolytes. Warning signs, irrespective of cause, are: dryness of mouth, thirst, weakness, lethargy, drowsiness, restlessness, muscle pains or cramps, muscular fatigue, hypotension, oliguria, tachycardia, and gastrointestinal disturbances such as nausea and vomiting.
The serum potassium should be determined at regular intervals, and potassium supplementation instituted whenever indicated. Hypokalemia will be more common in association with intensive or prolonged diuretic therapy, with concomitant steroid or ACTH therapy, and with inadequate electrolyte intake.
While not reported to date for ZAROXOLYN, related diuretics have increased responsiveness to tubocurarine and decreased arterial responsiveness to norepinephrine. Accordingly, it may be advisable to discontinue ZAROXOLYN three days before elective surgery.
Caution should be observed when administering ZAROXOLYN to hyperuricemic or gouty patients. ZAROXOLYN exerts minimal effects on glucose metabolism; insulin requirements may be affected in diabetics, and hyperglycemia and glycosuria may occur in patients with latent diabetes.
Chloride deficit and hypochloremic alkalosis may occur. In patients with severe edema accompanying cardiac failure or renal disease, a low-salt syndrome may be produced; hot weather and a low-salt diet will contribute.
Caution should be observed when administering ZAROXOLYN to patients with severely impaired renal function. As most of the drug is excreted by the renal route, cumulative effects may be seen in this circumstance.
Orthostatic hypotension may occur, this may be potentiated by alcohol, barbiturates, narcotics, or concurrent therapy with other antihypertensive drugs.
While not reported for ZAROXOLYN, use of other diuretics has been associated on rare occasions with pathological changes in the parathyroid glands, with hypercalcemia and hypophosphatemia. This possibility should be kept in mind with clinical use of ZAROXOLYN.

Adverse Reactions: Adverse reactions encountered during therapy with potent medications should be considered in two groups: those that represent extensions of the expected pharmacologic actions of the drug, and those which are pharmacologically unexpected, idiosyncratic, specially toxic, due to allergy or hypersensitivity, or due to unexplained causes.
For ZAROXOLYN (metolazone), adverse reactions constituting extensions of the expected pharmacologic actions of this potent diuretic/saluretic/antihypertensive drug may include:
Gastrointestinal reactions: constipation.
Central nervous system reactions: syncope, dizziness, drowsiness.
Cardiovascular reactions: orthostatic hypotension, excessive volume depletion, hemoconcentration, venous thrombosis.
Other reactions: dryness of the mouth, symptomatic and asymptomatic hypokalemia, hyponatremia, hypochloremia; hypochloremic alkalosis, hyperuricemia, hyperglycemia, glycosuria, increase in BUN or creatinine, fatigue, muscle cramps or spasm, weakness, restlessness.
In the second classification, adverse reactions to ZAROXOLYN may include:
Gastrointestinal reactions: nausea, vomiting, anorexia, diarrhea, abdominal bloating, epigastric distress, intrahepatic cholestatic jaundice, hepatitis.
Central nervous system reactions: vertigo, headache.
Hematologic reactions: leukopenia.
Dermatologic-hypersensitivity reactions: urticaria and other skin rashes.
Cardiovascular reactions: palpitation, chest pain.
Other reactions: chills, acute gouty attacks.
Adverse reactions which have occurred with other diuretics, but which have not been reported to date for ZAROXOLYN (metolazone), include:
pancreatitis, paresthesias, xanthopsia, agranulocytosis, thrombocytopenia, aplastic anemia, purpura, photosensitivity, and necrotizing angiitis (cutaneous vasculitis). These reactions should be considered as possible occurrences with clinical usage of ZAROXOLYN.
Whenever adverse reactions are moderate or severe, ZAROXOLYN dosage should be reduced or therapy withdrawn.

Dosage and Administration: Therapy should be individualized according to patient response. Programs of therapy with ZAROXOLYN (metolazone) should be titrated to gain a maximal initial therapeutic response, and to determine the minimal dose possible to maintain that therapeutic response.
ZAROXOLYN is a potent drug with a prolonged, 12-to-24-hour duration of action. When an initially-desired therapeutic effect has been obtained, it is ordinarily advisable to reduce the dosage of ZAROXOLYN to a lower maintenance level. The time interval required for the initial higher-dosage regimen may vary from days in edematous states to three or four weeks in the treatment of elevated blood pressure.
The daily dosage depends on the severity of each patient's condition, his sodium intake, and his responsiveness. Therefore, dosage adjustment is usually necessary during the course of therapy. A decision to reduce the daily dosage of ZAROXOLYN from a higher induction level to a lower maintenance level should be based on the results of thorough clinical and laboratory evaluations. If antihypertensive drugs or diuretics are given concurrently with ZAROXOLYN, careful dosage adjustment may be necessary.

Usual single daily dosage schedules
Suitable initial dosages will usually fall in the ranges given:
Edema of cardiac failure: ZAROXOLYN 5–10 mg. once daily
Edema of renal disease: ZAROXOLYN 5–20 mg. once daily
Mild to moderate essential hypertension:
ZAROXOLYN 2½–5 mg. once daily
For patients with congestive cardiac failure who tend to experience paroxysmal nocturnal dyspnea, it is usually advisable to employ a dosage near the upper end of the range, to ensure prolongation of diuresis and saluresis for a full 24-hour period.

How Supplied: ZAROXOLYN (metolazone) is provided as: pink 2½ mg tablets, blue 5 mg tablets, and yellow 10 mg tablets; in package sizes of 100, 500, 1000 and unit-dose strip packages of 100 (10 × 10's).

Rev 5/14/79

[*Shown in Product Identification Section*]

Persōn & Covey, Inc.
616 ALLEN AVENUE
Glendale, CA 91201

A.C.N.® OTC
Water-miscible Vitamin A, C, and Niacinamide Tablets

Description:

Each tablet contains:		% of U.S. RDA*
Vitamin A	25,000 I.U.	500
Ascorbic Acid	250 mg	417
Niacinamide	25 mg	125

*Percentage of U.S. Recommended Daily Allowance.

Indication: For use as a dietary supplement.
Dosage: One tablet daily as a dietary supplement. For adults and children 4 or more years of age.
Warnings: Keep all medication out of the reach of children. Store in a dry place at room temperature. Avoid heat.
How Supplied: In bottles of 100 tablets.
NDC 0096-0014-11

DHS* Shampoo OTC
Dermatological Hair and Scalp Shampoo

DHS* Shampoo contains: distilled water, TEA-lauryl sulfate, sodium chloride, PEG-8 distearate, cocamide DEA, cocamide MEA, fragrance and FD&C yellow #6.
DHS* contains a unique blend of special cleansing agents that provide a luxurious lather which cleans the hair and scalp.

DHS* conditioners reduce the need for after rinses and leave the hair lustrously clean.
DHS* is especially formulated for pH balance.
DHS* may be used daily.
Directions: (1) Wet hair thoroughly; apply DHS*, lather and rinse. (2) Reapply DHS, lather and rinse again. Repeat as necessary or as directed by your physician.
Caution: For external use only. Keep out of the reach of children. Avoid contact with the eyes.
How Supplied: 8 fluid ounce plastic bottles with easy to use dispenser.
*T.M.

DHS* Tar Shampoo OTC
Dermatological Hair and Scalp Shampoo

DHS* Tar Shampoo contains: Tar, equivalent to 0.5% Coal Tar, U.S.P., TEA-lauryl sulfate, distilled water, sodium chloride, PEG-8 distearate, cocamide DEA, cocamide MEA.
DHS* Tar Shampoo aids in the control of the scaling of seborrhea (dandruff) and psoriasis of the scalp.
Directions: (1) Wet hair thoroughly; apply a liberal quantity of DHS* Tar Shampoo and massage into a lather. (2) Rinse thoroughly and repeat application. (3) Allow lather to remain on scalp for about 5 minutes. (4) Use DHS Tar Shampoo once or twice weekly or as directed by your physician.
Caution: Avoid contact with the eyes. In case of contact, wash out with water. If irritation occurs, discontinue use and consult physician.
Warning: KEEP OUT OF THE REACH OF CHILDREN. FOR EXTERNAL USE ONLY.
How Supplied: 4 and 8 fluid ounce plastic bottles with easy to use dispenser.
NDC 0096-0728-04
NDC 0096-0728-08
*T.M.

DRYSOL™ ℞

A Solution of:
Aluminum Chloride (Hexahydrate) 20% w/v in Anhydrous Ethyl Alcohol (S.D. Alcohol 40) 93% v/v.
Indication: An aid in the management of hyperhidrosis.
Directions: Apply Drysol™ to the affected area once a day, only at bedtime. To help prevent irritation, the area should be completely dry prior to application. Do not apply Drysol to broken, irritated or recently shaved skin.
For Maximum Effect: Your doctor may instruct you to cover the treated area with saran wrap held in place by a snug fitting "T" or body shirt, mitten or sock. (Never hold saran in place with tape.) Wash the treated area the following morning. Excessive sweating may be stopped after two or more treatments. Thereafter, apply Drysol™ once or twice weekly or as needed.
Notice: Drysol™ will probably produce a burning or prickling sensation. Keep cap tightly closed when not in use to prevent evaporation.
Warning: For external use only. Keep out of the reach of children. Avoid contact with the eyes. If irritation or sensitization occurs, discontinue use or consult with a physician. Drysol™ may be harmful to certain fabrics.
Package: 37.5 cc polyethylene bottle. NDC 0096-0707-37.
30 cc bottle with convenient Dab-O-Matic™ applicator head. NDC 0096-0707-30.
Patient instruction sheets are available upon request.

ENISYL* Tablets OTC
L-Lysine Monohydrochloride

Composition: Each tablet contains L-Lysine 334 mg (from the hydrochloride).
Indication: For use as a dietary supplement.
Dosage: Adults: one to three tablets daily as a dietary supplement.
Actions: Improves utilization of vegetable proteins such as rice, wheat, corn, etc.
Warning: Keep out of the reach of children. Store in a dry place at room temperature. Avoid heat.
How Supplied: In bottles of 100 tablets.
NDC 0096-0777-11
*TM

SOLBAR® OTC
Dioxybenzone and Oxybenzone Cream, U.S.P.

Composition:
Dioxybenzone, U.S.P. 3%
Oxybenzone, U.S.P. 3%
Action and Uses: When properly applied, Solbar® protects the skin from sunburning and aids in the prevention of visible changes in the skin such as wrinkling, drying and freckling due to overexposure to sun.
Directions: Smooth Solbar® gently and evenly on exposed skin areas. Do not rub. Allow to dry. Solbar will leave a transparent film containing the sun protectant, which is colorless, odorless, tasteless, non-staining, and cosmetically acceptable for men or women. Apply Solbar before exposure to sun. Reapply after swimming, bathing or prolonged exposure.
Caution: If irritation or sensitization occurs, discontinue use and consult a physician. Avoid contact with eyes.
Protect from freezing.
Keep out of the reach of children.
How Supplied: Packaged in 2½ oz. polyethylene plastic tubes. NDC 0096-0680-75

XERAC® OTC
(alcohol gel)

Composition: Isopropyl Alcohol 44%
Microcrystalline Sulfur 4%
Effects: A medicated antiseptic gel to promote drying and peeling of the skin. An aid in the management of acne. Invisible when applied to the skin.
Directions: Apply a thin film to affected areas one to three times daily, or as directed by physician.
Precautions: Avoid overuse. If undue skin irritation develops or becomes excessive, discontinue use and consult physician. Avoid contact with eyes. Keep this and all medication out of the reach of children. For external use only.
How Supplied: 45 g (1-½ oz.) plastic tube.
NDC 0096-0787-45

XERAC A C™ ℞
Aluminum Chloride Hexahydrate in Anhydrous Ethanol
Anhidrotic/Antibacterial

Description: A solution of Aluminum Chloride (Hexahydrate) 6.25% (w/v) in Anhydrous Ethyl Alcohol (S. D. Alcohol 40) 96% (v/v).
Indication: For topical application as an anhidrotic and antibacterial.
Actions: The unique action of XERAC A C™ derives from its combined anhidrotic and antibacterial effects on the skin. Its action is sustained by the substantive retention of the aluminum ion in the stratum corneum.
Directions: Apply to affected areas at bedtime. Additional applications during the day may benefit certain patients. Do not apply immediately after washing. Apply only to skin which is completely dry. Treatment of large areas is facilitated by the special swab applicator head of the XERAC A C™ dispenser. For small areas, particularly near the eyes and lips, XERAC A C™ may be applied more precisely with the fingertips which have been moistened with the solution. Contact with the eyes should be avoided.
Contraindication—Precautions: Do not use on acutely irritated erythematous skin. If irritation develops, the formulation should be discontinued.
Adverse Reactions: Transient stinging or itching may occur. It is not evidence of contact sensitivity and may be prevented or reduced by applying XERAC A C™ only to skin which is completely dry or by removing the solution with soap and water. Rarely, the skin may become irritated. This can be alleviated when application of the product is stopped.
Warning: Keep this and all medication out of the reach of children. For external use only. Avoid contact with the eyes. This product may be harmful to certain fabrics. Keep the container tightly closed.
How Supplied: 30 cc bottle with special swab applicator head.
Xerac AC™ 30 cc bottle—NDC 0096-0709-30

XERAC BP5™ ℞
XERAC BP10™ ℞
(benzoyl peroxide hydrogel*)

Composition: Xerac BP5™ contains 5% Benzoyl Peroxide, Laureth-4, Carbomer-934, Triethanolamine, Disodium EDTA and Distilled Water.
Xerac BP10™ contains 10% Benzoyl Peroxide, Laureth-4, Carbomer-934, Triethanolamine, Disodium EDTA and Distilled Water.
Indication: A topical aid in the management of acne.
Actions: Provides the drying and desquamation necessary in the topical treatment of acne.
Administration and Dosage: After washing affected area, rub Xerac BP™ into affected area once or twice daily. The desired degree of drying and peeling may be regulated by increasing or decreasing the dosage schedule.
Contraindication: Should not be used by individuals known to be sensitive to any ingredient of Xerac BP™.
Precautions: For external use only. Avoid contact with the eyes, eyelids and mucous membranes. Keep all medication out of the reach of children. May bleach colored fabrics. If excessive irritation develops, discontinue use and consult physician.
How Supplied: 45 g (1.5 oz.) and 90 g (3 oz.) plastic tubes.
45 g tubes
Xerac BP5™ - NDC 0096-0790-45
Xerac BP10™ - NDC 0096-0791-45
90 g tubes
Xerac BP5™ - NDC 0096-0790-90
Xerac BP10™ - NDC 0096-0791-90
*TM

Z-PRO-C™ ℞
Zinc Sulfate and Ascorbic Acid

Composition: Each Z-PRO-C™ tablet contains 45 mg of elemental Zinc (from Zinc Sulfate Monohydrate, equivalent in Zinc content to 200 mg Zinc Sulfate, U.S.P.) and 100 mg Ascorbic Acid, U.S.P.
Indications: For use in Zinc and Ascorbic Acid deficiency.
Dosage: One tablet as prescribed by physician. Take with a meal to help avoid gastric irritation, but not with dairy products or bran products, including brown bread, as this will decrease the absorption of Zinc.
Concomitant Therapy: Zinc will impair the absorption of tetracycline hydrochloride. If a patient is taking tetracycline, the physician should be consulted for dosage directions for Z-PRO-C™.
Warnings: Do not exceed recommended dosage. A single dose of 10 tablets may have an emetic effect. Overdose may cause severe vomiting, dehydration or restlessness. Keep all medication out of the reach of children. Store

Continued on next page

Persōn & Covey—Cont.

in a dry place at room temperature. Avoid heat.

How Supplied: 100's.
NDC 0096-0099-11

Pfipharmecs Division
PFIZER INC.
235 EAST 42ND STREET
NEW YORK, NEW YORK 10017

Pfipharmecs is a division of Pfizer Inc. which provides economical distribution of a line of time honored antibiotics and certain over-the-counter products to retail and hospital pharmacists. These products include those listed here. Full color identification photographs of the solid oral dosage forms of the prescription products listed here can be found in the Product Identification Section.

PRODUCT IDENTIFICATION CODES

To provide quick and positive identification of Pfipharmecs Division products, we have imprinted the product identification number of the National Drug Code on tablets and capsules.

In order that you may quickly identify a product by its code number, we have compiled below a numerical list of code numbers of prescription products with their corresponding product names.

Product Identification Code	NUMERICAL PRODUCT INDEX Product
015	Tetracyn (tetracycline HCl) 250 mg capsules
016	Tetracyn (tetracycline HCl) 500 mg capsules
024	Pfizer-E (erythromycin stearate) 250 mg tablets
028	Pfizer-E (erythromycin stearate) 500 mg tablets
029	Tetrastatin (tetracycline HCl & nystatin) 250 mg capsules
041	Neobiotic (neomycin sulfate) 500 mg tablets
046	Pfizerpen G (penicillin G potassium) 200,000 units tablets
047	Pfizerpen G (penicillin G potassium) 250,000 units tablets
048	Pfizerpen G (penicillin G potassium) 400,000 units tablets
104	Pfizerpen G (penicillin G potassium) 800,000 units tablets
105	Pfizerpen VK (penicillin V potassium) 250 mg tablets
106	Pfizerpen VK (penicillin V potassium) 500 mg tablets
166	Tetracyn (tetracycline HCl) 250 mg capsules
172	Tetracyn 500 (tetracycline HCl) 500 mg capsules
175	Tetracyn (tetracycline HCl) 250 mg capsules
300	Pen-A (ampicillin) 250 mg capsules
310	Pen-A (ampicillin) 500 mg capsules
335	Sterane (prednisolone) 5 mg tablets

BACITRACIN TOPICAL OINTMENT

How Supplied: Each gram contains 500 units of Bacitracin. Available in ½ ounce tubes sold in cartons of twelve. A prescription is not required.

BONINE
(meclizine) HCl

For motion sickness. Available in convenient OTC packet of 8 chewable tablets of 25 mg meclizine HCl. No prescription required.

CORTRIL® ℞
(hydrocortisone)
Topical Ointment

How Supplied: Topical Ointment 1.0%: ½ oz. (14.2 Gm.) tube containing 10 mg./Gm. of hydrocortisone.

CORYBAN®-D CAPSULES
Decongestant Cold Capsules

Composition: Each capsule contains:
Caffeine U.S.P. ....30 mg.
Chlorpheniramine maleate U.S.P. ....2 mg.
Phenylpropanolamine HCl ....25 mg.

Indications: Coryban-D is a combination of ingredients designed to relieve nasal/sinus congestion, runny nose and watery eyes.

Administration and Dosage: Adults—two capsules 3 times a day, not to exceed six capsules in 24 hours. Children 6 to 12—one capsule three times a day, not to exceed three capsules in 24 hours. A physician should be consulted if symptoms persist. For children under 6 years, as directed by a physician.

Warning: Drowsiness may appear in some cases. If this occurs, the operation of vehicles or machinery should be avoided. Individuals with high blood pressure, heart disease, diabetes or thyroid disease should use only as directed by a physician. Coryban-D should be kept out of the reach of children.

How Supplied: In bottles of 24 or packs of 12, light and dark blue capsules.

CORYBAN®-D COUGH SYRUP
With Decongestant

Composition: Each 5 ml (1 teaspoonful) contains:
Dextromethorphan HBr U.S.P. ....7.5 mg.
Guaifenesin ....50 mg.
Phenylephrine HCl ....5 mg.
Acetaminophen ....120 mg.
Alcohol* 7.5%
* Small loss unavoidable

Description: Coryban-D cough syrup is a non-narcotic, cough suppressant containing a combination of ingredients which act to provide relief of common symptoms associated with coughs due to colds or allergy.

Indications:
Coryban-D provides effective relief from
- irritating coughs due to colds, flu or allergy yet non-narcotic.
- stuffy nose due to the common cold, hay fever and other allergies.
- chest congestion by liquefying and loosening bronchial mucus.
- aches and pains accompanying a cold.

Administration and Dosage: Adults—two teaspoonfuls every four hours not to exceed 8 teaspoonfuls in a 24 hour period. Children 6 to 12 years—one-half adult dosage. Children 3 to 6 years—one half teaspoonful every four hours not to exceed three teaspoonfuls in a 24 hour period.

Warning: Unless directed by a physician, the recommended dosage should not be exceeded. Coryban-D Cough Syrup should not be used longer than ten days, or given to children under 6 years of age. Because drowsiness may occur, patients should not drive or operate machinery. If high fever or persistent coughs are observed, a serious condition may be present and Coryban-D Cough Syrup should be used only with the physician's approval. Individuals with high blood pressure, heart disease, diabetes, or thyroid disease should use only as directed by the physician. Keep out of the reach of children.

How Supplied: Coryban-D Cough Syrup is available in 4-ounce dripless spout bottles. Sorbitol, which is contained in this product, is a nutritive, carbohydrate sweetening agent which is metabolized more slowly than sugar.

Recommended Storage: Store below 77°F. (25°C.)
Do not refrigerate.

NEOBIOTIC® TABLETS ℞
(neomycin sulfate)

How Supplied: Available in 500 mg. white tablets, in bottles of 100. Identification code #041.

[*Shown in Product Identification Section*]

OBRON—6® TABLETS OTC
Prenatal Vitamins

Each tablet provides the listed vitamins and minerals:

VITAMINS	AMOUNT	% US RDA*
Vitamin A	5,000 IU	62.5
Vitamin D	400 IU	100
Vitamin C	50 mg	83
Vitamin B_1	3 mg	176
Vitamin B_2	2 mg	100
Niacin	20 mg	100
Vitamin B_6	8.2 mg	328
Vitamin B_{12}	2 mcg	25
Pantothenic Acid	0.92 mg	9
MINERALS		
Calcium	243 mg	18.7
Iron	33 mg	183
Magnesium	1 mg	0.2
Zinc	0.4 mg	2.7
Manganese	0.33 mg	**
Potassium	1.7 mg	**

Recommended Dosage: One tablet daily, or as directed by physician.

How Supplied: In bottles of 100 pink sugar free tablets

*Percentage of U.S. Recommended Daily Allowance (RDA) for pregnant or lactating women.

**Manganese and potassium are recognized as essential in human nutrition, but no U.S. RDA has been established.

PEN A® ℞
(ampicillin)
CAPSULES AND POWDER FOR ORAL SUSPENSION

Indications: Pen A (ampicillin) is indicated in the treatment of infections due to susceptible strains of the following:

gram-negative organisms—Shigellae, Salmonellae (including *S. typhosa), H. influenzae, E. coli* and *P. mirabilis, N. gonorrhoeae,* and *N. meningitidis;*

gram-positive organisms—Streptococci, *D. pneumoniae,* and nonpenicillinase-producing staphylococci.

Because of its wide spectrum and bactericidal action, it may be useful in instituting therapy; however, bacteriological studies to determine the causative organisms and their sensitivity to ampicillin should be performed.

Indicated surgical procedures should be performed.

Contraindications: A history of allergic reaction to any of the penicillins is a contraindication.

Warnings: SERIOUS AND OCCASIONALLY FATAL HYPERSENSITIVITY (ANAPHYLACTOID) REACTIONS HAVE BEEN REPORTED IN PATIENTS ON PENICILLIN THERAPY. ALTHOUGH ANAPHYLAXIS IS MORE FREQUENT FOLLOWING PARENTERAL THERAPY, IT HAS OCCURRED IN PATIENTS ON ORAL PENICILLINS. THESE REACTIONS ARE MORE APT TO OCCUR IN INDIVIDUALS WITH A HISTORY OF PENICILLIN HYPERSENSITIVITY AND/OR HYPERSENSITIVITY REACTIONS TO MULTI-

PLE ALLERGENS. THERE HAVE BEEN REPORTS OF INDIVIDUALS WITH A HISTORY OF PENICILLIN HYPERSENSITIVITY WHO HAVE EXPERIENCED SEVERE REACTIONS WHEN TREATED WITH CEPHALOSPORINS. BEFORE THERAPY WITH A PENICILLIN, CAREFUL INQUIRY SHOULD BE MADE CONCERNING PREVIOUS HYPERSENSITIVITY REACTIONS TO PENICILLINS, CEPHALOSPORINS, AND OTHER ALLERGENS. IF AN ALLERGIC REACTION OCCURS, THE DRUG SHOULD BE DISCONTINUED AND THE APPROPRIATE THERAPY INSTITUTED.

SERIOUS ANAPHYLACTOID REACTIONS REQUIRE IMMEDIATE EMERGENCY TREATMENT WITH EPINEPHRINE. OXYGEN, INTRAVENOUS STEROIDS, AND AIRWAY MANAGEMENT, INCLUDING INTUBATION, SHOULD ALSO BE ADMINISTERED AS INDICATED.

USAGE IN PREGNANCY: Safety for use in pregnancy has not been established.

Precautions: As with any antibiotic preparation, constant observations for signs of overgrowth of nonsusceptible organisms, including fungi, are essential. Should superinfection occur (usually involving Aerobacter, Pseudomonas, or Candida), the drug should be discontinued and/or appropriate therapy instituted. As with any potent agent, it is advisable to check periodically for organ system dysfunction during prolonged therapy; this includes renal, hepatic, and hematopoietic systems. This is particularly important in prematures, neonates and other infants.

Adverse Reactions: As with other penicillins, it may be expected that untoward reactions will be essentially limited to sensitivity phenomena. They are more likely to occur in individuals who have previously demonstrated hypersensitivity to penicillins and in those with a history of allergy, asthma, hay fever, or urticaria. The following adverse reactions have been reported as associated with the use of ampicillin:

Gastrointestinal—glossitis, stomatitis, black "hairy" tongue, nausea, vomiting, enterocolitis, pseudomembranous colitis and diarrhea. (These reactions are usually associated with oral dosage forms.)

Hypersensitivity reactions—An erythematous maculopapular rash has been reported fairly frequently. Urticaria and erythema multiforme have been reported occasionally. A few cases of exfoliative dermatitis have been reported. Anaphylaxis is the most serious reaction experienced and has usually been associated with the parenteral dosage form.

Note: Urticaria, other skin rashes, and serum sickness-like reactions may be controlled with antihistamines, and if necessary, systemic corticosteroids. Whenever such reactions occur, ampicillin should be discontinued, unless, in the opinion of the physician, the condition being treated is life-threatening and amenable only to ampicillin therapy.

Liver—A moderate rise in serum glutamic oxaloacetic transaminase (SGOT) has been noted, particularly in infants, but the significance of this finding is unknown.

Hemic and Lymphatic Systems—Anemia, thrombocytopenia, thrombocytopenic purpura, eosinophilia, leukopenia, and agranulocytosis have been reported during therapy with the penicillins. These reactions are usually reversible on discontinuation of therapy and are believed to be sensitivity reactions.

Dosage: *Infections of the ear, nose, throat, and lower respiratory tract* due to streptococci, pneumococci, and nonpenicillinase-producing staphylococci, and also those infections of *the upper and lower respiratory tract due to H. influenzae:*

Adults— 250 mg every 6 hours.
Children— 50 mg/kg/day in divided doses every 6 or 8 hours.

Infections of the genitourinary tract caused by sensitive gram-negative and gram-positive bacteria:

Adults— 500 mg every 6 hours. Larger doses may be required for severe infections.
Children— 100 mg/kg/day in divided doses every 6 hours.

Uncomplicated urethritis due to N. gonorrhoeae:
Adult males and females—3.5 grams single oral dose administered simultaneously with 1.0 gram of probenecid.

Cases of gonorrhea with a suspected lesion of syphilis should have dark field examinations before receiving ampicillin, and monthly serological tests for a minimum of 4 months.

Infections of the gastrointestinal tract:
Adults— 500 mg every 6 hours.
Children— 100 mg/kg/day in divided doses every 6 hours.

Larger doses may be required for stubborn or severe infections. The children's dosage is intended for individuals whose weight will not cause a dosage to be calculated greater than that recommended for adults. Children weighing more than 20 kg should be dosed according to the adult recommendations.

It should be recognized that in the treatment of chronic urinary tract and intestinal infections, frequent bacteriological and clinical appraisals are necessary. Smaller doses than those recommended above should not be used. Even higher doses may be needed at times. In stubborn infections, therapy may be required for several weeks. It may be necessary to continue clinical and/or bacteriological follow-up for several months after cessation of therapy.

Treatment should be continued for a minimum of 48 to 72 hours beyond the time that the patient becomes asymptomatic or evidence of bacterial eradication has been obtained. It is recommended that there be at least 10 days' treatment for any infection caused by hemolytic streptococci, to help prevent the occurrence of acute rheumatic fever or glomerulonephritis.

Directions For Mixing Oral Suspensions: Prepare suspension at time of dispensing as follows: Add 66 ml of water to the 100 ml package and 132 ml of water to the 200 ml package. Shake vigorously. This will provide 100 and 200 ml of suspension, respectively. Each teaspoonful (5 ml) will contain 125 mg or 250 mg ampicillin. SHAKE WELL BEFORE USING. Keep bottle tightly closed. Any unused portion of the reconstituted suspension must be discarded after 7 days at room temperature or 14 days under refrigeration.

How Supplied: Pen A (ampicillin) Capsules: Ampicillin trihydrate equivalent to 250 mg or 500 mg ampicillin per capsule.
250 mg: bottles of 100 and 500.
500 mg: bottles of 100.
[*Shown in Product Identification Section*]
Pen A (ampicillin) for Oral Suspension: Each 5 ml of reconstituted suspension contains ampicillin trihydrate equivalent to 125 mg or 250 mg ampicillin.
125 mg/5 ml: bottles of 100 ml and 200 ml.
250 mg/5 ml: bottles of 100 ml and 200 ml.

PFIZER-E® ℞
(erythromycin stearate)
Film Coated Tablets

Indications: *Streptococcus pyogenes* (Group A beta hemolytic streptococcus): Upper and lower respiratory tract, skin, and soft tissue infections of mild to moderate severity.

Injectable benzathine penicillin G is considered by the American Heart Association to be the drug of choice in the treatment and prevention of streptococcal pharyngitis and in long term prophylaxis of rheumatic fever.

When oral medication is preferred for treatment of the above conditions, penicillin G, V, or erythromycin are alternate drugs of choice. When oral medication is given, the importance of strict adherence by the patient to the prescribed dosage regimen must be stressed. A therapeutic dose should be administered for at least 10 days.

Alpha-hemolytic streptococci (viridans group): Short term prophylaxis of bacterial endocarditis prior to dental or other operative procedures in patients with a history of rheumatic fever or congenital heart disease who are hypersensitive to penicillin. (Erythromycin is not suitable prior to genitourinary surgery where the organisms likely to lead to bacteremia are gram-negative bacilli or the enterococcus group of streptococci.)

Staphylococcus aureus: Acute infections of skin and soft tissue of mild to moderate severity. Resistant organisms may emerge during treatment.

Diplococcus pneumoniae: Upper respiratory tract infections (e.g. otitis media, pharyngitis) and lower respiratory tract infections (e.g. pneumonia) of mild to moderate degree.

Mycoplasma pneumoniae (Eaton agent, PPLO): For respiratory infections due to this organism.

Hemophilus influenzae: For upper respiratory tract infections of mild to moderate severity when used concomitantly with adequate doses of sulfonamides. Not all strains of this organism are susceptible at the erythromycin concentrations ordinarily achieved. (See appropriate sulfonamide labeling for prescribing information.)

Treponema pallidum: Erythromycin is an alternate choice of treatment for primary syphilis in patients allergic to the penicillins. In treatment of primary syphilis, spinal fluid examinations should be done before treatment and as part of follow-up after therapy.

Corynebacterium diphtheriae and *C. minutissimum:* As an adjunct to antitoxin, to prevent establishment of carriers, and to eradicate the organism in carriers.

In the treatment of erythrasma.

Entamoeba histolytica: In the treatment of intestinal amebiasis only. Extra-enteric amebiasis requires treatment with other agents.

Listeria monocytogenes: Infections due to this organism.

Neisseria gonorrhoeae: Erythromycin lactobionate for injection-I.V. in conjunction with erythromycin stearate orally, as an alternative drug in treatment of acute pelvic inflammatory disease caused by *N. gonorrhoeae* in female patients with a history of sensitivity to penicillin. Before treatment of gonorrhea, patients who are suspected of also having syphilis should have a microscopic examination for *T. pallidum* (by immunofluorescence or dark field) before receiving erythromycin, and monthly serologic tests for a minimum of 4 months.

Legionnaires' Disease: Although no controlled clinical efficacy studies have been conducted, *in vitro* and limited preliminary clinical data suggest that erythromycin may be effective in treating Legionnaires' Disease.

Contraindications: Erythromycin is contraindicated in patients with known hypersensitivity to this antibiotic.

Warnings: Usage in pregnancy: Safety for use in pregnancy has not been established.

Precautions: Erythromycin is principally excreted by the liver. Caution should be exercised in administering the antibiotic to patients with impaired hepatic function. There have been reports of hepatic dysfunction, with or without jaundice, occurring in patients receiving oral erythromycin products.

Recent data from studies of erythromycin reveal that its use in patients who are receiving high doses of theophylline may be associated with an increase of serum theophylline levels and potential theophylline toxicity. In case of

Continued on next page

Pfipharmecs—Cont.

theophylline toxicity and/or elevated serum theophylline levels, the dose of theophylline should be reduced while the patient is receiving concomitant erythromycin therapy.
Surgical procedures should be performed when indicated.
Adverse Reactions: The most frequent side effects of oral erythromycin preparations are gastrointestinal, such as abdominal cramping and discomfort, and are dose-related. Nausea, vomiting, and diarrhea occur infrequently with usual oral doses.
During prolonged or repeated therapy, there is a possibility of overgrowth of nosusceptible bacteria or fungi. If such infections occur, the drug should be discontinued and appropriate therapy instituted.
Mild allergic reactions such as urticaria and other skin rashes have occurred. Serious allergic reactions, including anaphylaxis, have been reported.
Dosage and Administration: Optimum blood levels are obtained when doses are given on an empty stomach.
Adults: 250 mg every six hours is the usual dose; or 500 mg every 12 hours one hour before meals. Dosage may be increased up to 4 or more grams per day according to the severity of the infection.
Children: Age, weight, and severity of the infection are important factors in determining the proper dosage. 30–50 mg/kg/day, in divided doses, is the usual dose. For more severe infections this dose may be doubled.
When dosage is desired on a twice-a-day schedule in either adults or children, one-half of the total daily dose may be given every 12 hours, one hour before meals.
In the treatment of streptococcal infections, a therapeutic dosage of erythromycin should be administered for at least 10 days. In continuous *prophylaxis* of streptococcal infections in persons with a history of rheumatic heart disease, the dose is 250 mg twice a day.
When used prior to surgery to prevent endocarditis (see *Alpha-hemolytic streptococci*), a recommended schedule for adults is: 500 mg before the procedure and 250 mg every 6 hours for 4 doses after the procedure. For small children: 30 to 50 mg/kg/day divided into three or four evenly spaced doses.
For treatment of primary syphilis: 30–40 grams given in divided doses over a period of 10–15 days.
For treatment of acute pelvic inflammatory disease caused by *N. gonorrhoeae:* 500 mg erythromycin lactobionate for injection-I.V. every 6 hours for 3 days, followed by 250 mg erythromycin stearate every 6 hours for 7 days.
For intestinal amebiasis: Adults: 250 mg four times daily for 10 to 14 days. Children: 30–50 mg/kg/day in divided doses for 10 to 14 days.
For treatment of Legionnaires' Disease: Although optimal doses have not been established, daily doses of erythromycin stearate utilized in reported clinical data were 1 to 4 grams in divided doses.
How Supplied: Pfizer-E (erythromycin stearate) Film Coated Tablets, 250 mg. Each tablet contains erythromycin stearate equivalent to 250 mg erythromycin.
Bottles of 100's and 500's.
Unit Dose package of 100's.
Pfizer-E (erythromycin stearate) Film Coated Tablets, 500 mg. Each tablet contains erythromycin stearate equivalent to 500 mg erythromycin.
Bottles of 100's.
Unit Dose package of 100's.
[*Shown in Product Identification Section*]

PFIZERPEN G® ℞
(penicillin G potassium)
POWDER FOR SYRUP/TABLETS
BUFFERED
FOR ORAL ADMINISTRATION

Indications: Oral penicillin G is indicated in the treatment of mild to moderately severe infections due to penicillin G-sensitive microorganisms that are sensitive to the low serum levels common to this particular dosage form. Therapy should be guided by bacteriological studies (including sensitivity tests) and by clinical response.
NOTE: Severe pneumonia, empyema, bacteremia, pericarditis, meningitis, and purulent or septic arthritis should not be treated with oral penicillin during the acute stage.
Indicated surgical procedures should be performed.
The following infections will usually respond to adequate dosage of oral penicillin G.
1. *Streptococcal infections* (Group A) (without bacteremia). Mild to moderate infections of the upper respiratory tract (including middle ear infections—otitis media), skin and soft tissue infections, scarlet fever, and mild erysipelas.
NOTE: Streptococci in groups A, C, H, G, L, and M are very sensitive to penicillin G. Other groups, including group D (enterococcus) are resistant.
2. *Pneumococcal infections.* Mild to moderately severe infections of the respiratory tract (including middle ear infections—otitis media).
3. *Staphylococcal infections.* Penicillin G sensitive. Mild infections of the skin and soft tissues.
NOTE: Reports indicate an increasing number of strains of staphylococci resistant to penicillin G, emphasizing the need for culture and sensitivity studies in treating suspected staphylococcal infections.
4. *Fusospirochetosis* (Vincent's gingivitis and pharyngitis)—Mild to moderately severe infections of the oropharynx usually respond to therapy with oral penicillin G.
NOTE: Necessary dental care should be accomplished in infections involving the gum tissue.
5. *Oral penicillin G therapy is indicated as prophylaxis for the prevention of recurrence following rheumatic fever and/or chorea.* Prophylaxis with oral penicillin G on a continuing basis has proven effective in preventing recurrence of these conditions.
Contraindications: A previous hypersensitivity reaction to any penicillin is a contraindication.
Warnings: Serious and occasionally fatal hypersensitivity (anaphylactoid) reactions have been reported in patients on penicillin therapy. Although anaphylaxis is more frequent following parenteral therapy it has occurred in patients on oral penicillins. These reactions are more apt to occur in individuals with a history of sensitivity to multiple allergens.
There have been well documented reports of individuals with a history of penicillin hypersensitivity reactions who have experienced severe hypersensitivity reactions when treated with a cephalosporin. Before therapy with a penicillin, careful inquiry should be made concerning previous hypersensitivity reactions to penicillins, cephalosporins, and other allergens. If an allergic reaction occurs, the drug should be discontinued and the patient treated with the usual agents e.g., pressor amines, antihistamines and corticosteroids.
Precautions: Penicillin should be used with caution in individuals with histories of significant allergies and/or asthma.
The oral route of administration should not be relied upon in patients with severe illness, or with nausea, vomiting, gastric dilatation, cardiospasm or intestinal hypermotility.
Occasional patients will not absorb therapeutic amounts of orally administered penicillin.
In streptococcal infections, therapy must be sufficient to eliminate the organism (10 days minimum); otherwise the sequelae of streptococcal disease may occur. Cultures should be taken following completion of treatment to determine whether streptococci have been eradicated.
Prolonged use of antibiotics may promote the overgrowth of nonsusceptible organisms, including fungi. Should superinfection occur, appropriate measures should be taken.
Adverse Reactions: Although the incidence of reactions to oral penicillins has been reported with much less frequency than following parenteral therapy, it should be remembered that all degrees of hypersensitivity including fatal anaphylaxis, have been reported with oral penicillin.
The most common reactions to oral penicillin are nausea, vomiting, epigastric distress, diarrhea, and black hairy tongue. The hypersensitivity reactions reported are skin eruptions (maculopapular to exfoliative dermatitis), urticaria and other serum sickness reactions, laryngeal edema and anaphylaxis. Fever and eosinophilia may frequently be the only reaction observed. Hemolytic anemia, leukopenia, thrombocytopenia, neuropathy, and nephropathy are infrequent reactions and usually associated with high doses of parenteral penicillin.
Dosage and Administration: The dosage of penicillin G (oral) should be determined according to the sensitivity of the causative microorganism and the severity of infection, and adjusted to the clinical response of the patient.
Oral penicillin G should be given at least 1 hour before or 2 hours after meals.
The usual dosage recommendation for adults and children 12 years and over is as follows:
Streptococcal infections—Mild to moderately severe—of the upper respiratory tract and including scarlet fever and mild erysipelas.
200,000–250,000 units q. 6–8 hours for 10 days for mild infections.
400,000–500,000 units q. 8 hours for 10 days for moderately severe infections; alternatively, 500 mg (800,000 units) may be given b.i.d.
Pneumococcal infections—Mild to moderately severe—of the respiratory tract, including otitis media.
400,000–500,000 units q. 6 hours until the patient has been afebrile for at least 2 days.
Staphylococcal infections—Mild infections of skin and soft tissue (culture and sensitivity tests should be performed).
200,000–500,000 units q. 6–8 hours until infection is cured.
Fusospirochetosis (Vincent's infection) of the oropharynx—Mild to moderately severe infections.
400,000–500,000 units q. 6–8 hours.
For the prevention of recurrence following rheumatic fever and/or chorea:
200,000–250,000 units twice daily on a continuing basis.
NOTE: Therapy for children under 12 years of age is calculated on the basis of body weight. For infants and small children the suggested dose is 25,000 to 90,000 units per kg per day in 3 to 6 divided doses.
How Supplied: Pfizerpen G (penicillin G potassium) Powder for Syrup buffered, for oral administration when reconstituted as directed, is available in the following form:
400,000 units per 5 ml—bottles of 100 ml and 200 ml.
Pfizerpen G (penicillin G potassium) Tablets, buffered with calcium carbonate, for oral administration are available in the following forms and quantities:
200,000 units—bottles of 100 and 500 tablets.
250,000 units—bottles of 100 tablets.
400,000 units—bottles of 100 and 1000 tablets.
800,000 units—bottles of 100 tablets.
Tablets are white, and are scored for easy calibration of dosage.
[*Shown in Product Identification Section*]

PFIZERPEN VK® ℞
(penicillin V potassium)
Tablets and Powder For Oral Solution

Indications: Penicillin V potassium is indicated in the treatment of mild to moderately severe infections due to penicillin G-sensitive microorganisms that are sensitive to the low serum levels common to this particular dosage form. Therapy should be guided by bacteriological studies (including sensitivity tests) and by clinical response.
NOTE: Severe pneumonia, empyema, bacteremia, pericarditis, meningitis, and arthritis should not be treated with penicillin V during the acute stage.
Indicated surgical procedures should be performed.
The following infections will usually respond to adequate dosage of penicillin V:
Streptococcal infections (without bacteremia). Mild to moderate infections of the upper respiratory tract, scarlet fever, and mild erysipelas.
NOTE: Streptococci in groups A, C, G, H, L, and M are very sensitive to penicillin. Other groups, including group D (enterococcus) are resistant.
Pneumococcal infections. Mild to moderately severe infections of the respiratory tract.
Staphylococcal infections—penicillin G-sensitive. Mild infections of the skin and soft tissues.
NOTE: Reports indicate an increasing number of strains of staphylococci resistant to penicillin G, emphasizing the need for culture and sensitivity studies in treating suspected staphylococcal infections.
Fusospirochetosis (Vincent's gingivitis and pharyngitis). Mild to moderately severe infections of the oropharynx usually respond to therapy with oral penicillin.
NOTE: Necessary dental care should be accomplished in infections involving the gum tissue.
Medical conditions in which oral penicillin therapy is indicated as prophylaxis:
For the prevention of recurrence following rheumatic fever and/or chorea. Prophylaxis with oral penicillin on a continuing basis has proven effective in preventing recurrence of these conditions.
To prevent bacterial endocarditis in patients with congenital and/or rheumatic heart lesions in patients to undergo dental procedures or minor upper respiratory tract surgery or instrumentation. Prophylaxis should be instituted the day of the procedure and for 2 or more days following. Patients who have a past history of rheumatic fever and are receiving continuous prophylaxis may harbor increased numbers of penicillin-resistant organisms; use of another prophylactic anti-infective agent should be considered. If penicillin is to be used in these patients at surgery, the regular rheumatic fever program should be interrupted 1 week prior to the contemplated surgery. At the time of surgery, penicillin may be reinstituted as a prophylactic measure against the hazards of surgically induced bacteremia.
NOTE: Oral penicillin should not be used as adjunctive prophylaxis for genitourinary instrumentation or surgery, lower intestinal tract surgery, sigmoidoscopy, and childbirth.
Contraindications: A previous hypersensitivity reaction to any penicillin is a contraindication.
Warnings: Serious and occasionally fatal hypersensitivity (anaphylactoid) reactions have been reported in patients on penicillin therapy. Although anaphylaxis is more frequent following parenteral therapy it has occurred in patients on oral penicillins. These reactions are more apt to occur in individuals with a history of sensitivity to multiple allergens.
There have been well documented reports of individuals with a history of penicillin hypersensitivity reactions who have experienced severe hypersensitivity reactions when treated with a cephalosporin. Before therapy with a penicillin, careful inquiry should be made concerning previous hypersensitivity reactions to penicillins, cephalosporins, and other allergens. If an allergic reaction occurs, the drug should be discontinued and the patient treated with the usual agents e.g., pressor amines, antihistamines, and corticosteroids.
Precautions: Penicillin should be used with caution in individuals with histories of significant allergies and/or asthma.
The oral route of administration should not be relied upon in patients with severe illness, or with nausea, vomiting, gastric dilatation, cardiospasm, or intestinal hypermotility.
Occasional patients will not absorb therapeutic amounts of orally administered penicillin.
In streptococcal infections, therapy must be sufficient to eliminate the organism (10 days minimum); otherwise the sequelae of streptococcal disease may occur. Cultures should be taken following completion of treatment to determine whether streptococci have been eradicated.
Prolonged use of antibiotics may promote the overgrowth of nonsusceptible organisms, including fungi. Should superinfection occur, appropriate measures should be taken.
Adverse Reactions: Although the incidence of reactions to oral penicillins has been reported with much less frequency than following parenteral therapy, it should be remembered that all degrees of hypersensitivity including fatal anaphylaxis, have been reported with oral penicillin.
The most common reactions to oral penicillin are nausea, vomiting, epigastric distress, diarrhea, and black hairy tongue. The hypersensitivity reactions reported are skin eruptions (maculopapular to exfoliative dermatitis), urticaria and other serum sickness reactions, laryngeal edema, and anaphylaxis. Fever and eosinophilia may frequently be the only reaction observed. Hemolytic anemia, leukopenia, thrombocytopenia, neuropathy, and nephropathy are infrequent reactions and usually associated with high doses of parenteral penicillin.
Administration and Dosage: The dosage of penicillin V should be determined according to the sensitivity of the causative microorganisms and the severity of infection, and adjusted to the clinical response of the patient.
The usual dosage recommendations for adults and children 12 years and over are as follows:
Streptococcal infections—mild to moderately severe—of the upper respiratory tract and including scarlet fever and erysipelas: 200,000 to 500,000 units every 6 to 8 hours for 10 days.
Pneumococcal infections—mild to moderately severe—of the respiratory tract, including otitis media; 400,000 to 500,000 units every 6 hours until the patient has been afebrile for at least 2 days.
Staphylococcal infections—mild infections of skin and soft tissue (culture and sensitivity tests should be performed): 400,000 to 500,000 units every 6 to 8 hours.
Fusospirochetosis (Vincent's infection) of the oropharynx—mild to moderately severe infections: 400,000 to 500,000 units every 6 to 8 hours.
For the prevention of recurrence following rheumatic fever and/or chorea: 200,000 to 250,000 units twice daily on a continuing basis.
To prevent bacterial endocarditis in patients with rheumatic or congenital heart lesions who are to undergo dental or upper respiratory tract surgery or instrumentation: 500,000 units given the day of the procedure, 500,000 aqueous penicillin G I.M. units 1 hour before the procedure, and 500,000 units every 6 hours for 2 days.
NOTE: Therapy for children under 12 years of age is calculated on the basis of body weight. For infants and small children the suggested dose is 25,000 to 90,000 units per kg. per day in three to six divided doses.
How Supplied: Pfizerpen VK (penicillin V potassium) for Oral Solution. Each 5 ml of reconstituted solution contains penicillin V potassium equivalent to 125 or 250 mg penicillin V.
125 mg (200,000 units): bottles of 100 ml, 150 ml, and 200 ml
250 mg (400,000 units): bottles of 100 ml, 150 ml, and 200 ml
Pfizerpen VK (penicillin V potassium) tablets. Each tablet contains penicillin V potassium equivalent to 250 mg (400,000 units) or 500 mg (800,000 units) penicillin V.
250 mg (400,000 units): bottles of 100 and 1000.
500 mg (800,000 units): bottles of 100.
[*Shown in Product Identification Section*]
Directions for Reconstituting Oral Solutions: Prepare the formulation at the time of dispensing. For ease in preparation, tap bottle lightly to loosen powder, add water to the bottle in two portions and shake well after each addition. The reconstituted solutions are stable for 14 days under refrigeration.

125 mg/5 ml

Add 60 ml water to the 100 ml package, 90 ml water to the 150 ml package, and 120 ml water to the 200 ml package. This will provide 100 ml, 150 ml, and 200 ml of solution respectively. Each 5 ml (teaspoonful) will contain penicillin V potassium equivalent to 125 mg of penicillin V.

250 mg/5 ml

Add 60 ml water to the 100 ml package, 90 ml water to the 150 ml package, and 120 ml water to the 200 ml package. This will provide 100 ml, 150 ml, and 200 ml of solution respectively. Each 5 ml (teaspoonful) will contain penicillin V potassium equivalent to 250 mg of penicillin V.

RID™
Liquid Pediculicide

Description: Rid is a liquid pediculicide whose active ingredients are: pyrethrins 0.3%, piperonyl butoxide, technical 3.00%, equivalent to 2.4% (butylcarbityl) (6-propylpiperonyl) ether and to 0.6% related compounds, petroleum distillate 1.20% and benzyl alcohol 2.4%. Inert ingredients 93.1%.
Actions: RID kills head lice (Pediculus humanus capitis), body lice (Pediculus humanus humanus), and pubic or crab lice (Phthirus pubis), and their eggs on contact.
The pyrethrins act as a contact poison and affect the parasite's nervous system, resulting in paralysis and death. The efficacy of the pyrethrins is enhanced by the synergist, piperonyl butoxide.
Indications: RID is indicated for the treatment of infestations of head lice, body lice and pubic (crab) lice and their eggs.
Warning: RID should not be used by ragweed sensitized persons.
Precautions: This product is for external use only. It is harmful if swallowed. It should not be inhaled. It should be kept out of the eyes and contact with mucous membranes should be avoided. If accidental contact with eyes occurs, flush immediately with water. In case of infection or skin irritation, discontinue use and consult a physician. Consult a physician if infestation of eyebrows or eyelashes occurs. Avoid contamination of feed or foodstuffs. Do not reuse container. Destroy when empty.
Do not transport or store below 32°F (0°C).
Dosage and Administration: (1) Apply RID undiluted to hair and scalp or to any other infested area until entirely wet. Do not use on eyelashes or eyebrows. (2) Allow RID to remain on area for 10 minutes but no longer. (3) Wash thoroughly with warm water and soap or shampoo. (4) Dead lice and eggs may require removal with fine-toothed comb provided. A second application is seldom needed. If necessary, treatment may be repeated but do not

Continued on next page

Pfipharmecs—Cont.

exceed two consecutive applications within 24 hours.
Since lice infestations are spread by contact, each family member should be examined carefully. If infested, he or she should be treated promptly to avoid spread or reinfestation of previously treated individuals. Contaminated clothing and other articles, such as hats, etc. should be dry cleaned, boiled or otherwise treated until decontaminated to prevent reinfestation or spread.
How Supplied: In 2 and 4 fl. oz. bottles. Fine-toothed comb to aid in removal of dead lice and nits and patient instruction booklet are included in each package of RID.

ROERIBEC® TABLETS
High Potency B Complex with 500 mg. of Vitamin C

Composition: Each tablet contains:

		%RDA
Vitamin C (L-Ascorbic Acid)	500 mg	833
Vitamin B_1 (Thiamine Mononitrate)	10 mg	666
Vitamin B_2 (Riboflavin)	10 mg	590
Niacin (Niacinamide)	100 mg	500
Vitamin B_6 (Pyridoxine Hydrochloride)	8.2 mg	410
Vitamin B_{12} (Cyanocobalamin)	4 mcg	67
Pantothenic Acid (Calcium Pantothenate)	18 mg	180

Dosage: One tablet daily or as directed by the physician.
How Supplied: RoeriBeC is supplied in bottles of 100 red, easy-to-swallow film coated (sugar free) tablets.

STERANE® TABLETS ℞
(prednisolone)
For Oral Administration

Indications:
1. Endocrine Disorders:
Primary or secondary adrenocortical insufficiency (hydrocortisone or cortisone is the first choice; synthetic analogs may be used in conjunction with mineralocorticoids where applicable; in infancy mineralocorticoid supplementation is of particular importance).
Congenital adrenal hyperplasia.
Nonsuppurative thyroiditis.
Hypercalcemia associated with cancer.
2. Rheumatic Disorders:
As adjunctive therapy for short term administration (to tide the patient over an acute episode or exacerbation) in:
Psoriatic arthritis.
Rhemuatoid arthritis including juvenile rheumatoid arthritis (selected cases may require low-dose maintenance therapy).
Ankylosing spondylitis.
Acute and subacute bursitis.
Acute nonspecific tenosynovitis.
Acute gouty arthritis.
Post-traumatic osteoarthritis.
Synovitis of osteoarthritis.
Epicondylitis.
3. Collagen Diseases:
During an exacerbation or as maintenance therapy in selected cases of—
Systemic lupus erythematosus.
Systemic Dermatomyositis (polymyositis)
Acute rheumatic carditis.
4. Dermatologic Diseases:
Pemphigus.
Bullous dermatitis herpetiformis.
Severe erythema multiforme (Stevens-Johnson syndrome)
Exfoliative dermatitis.
Mycosis fungoides.
Severe psoriasis.
Severe seborrheic dermatitis.
5. Allergic States:
Control of severe or incapacitating allergic conditions intractable to adequate trials of conventional treatment:
Seasonal or perennial allergic rhinitis.
Bronchial asthma.
Contact dermatitis.
Atopic dermatitis.
Serum sickness.
Drug hypersensitivity reactions.
6. Ophthalmic Diseases:
Severe acute and chronic allergic and inflammatory processes involving the eye and its adnexa such as—
Allergic conjunctivitis.
Keratitis.
Allergic corneal marginal ulcers.
Herpes zoster ophthalmicus.
Iritis and iridocyclitis.
Chorioretinitis.
Anterior segment inflammation.
Diffuse posterior uveitis and choroiditis.
Optic neuritis.
Sympathetic ophthalmia.
7. Respiratory Diseases:
Symptomatic sarcoidosis.
Loeffler's syndrome not manageable by other means.
Fulminating or disseminated pulmonary tuberculosis when used concurrently with appropriate antituberculous chemotherapy.
Aspiration pneumonitis.
Berylliosis.
8. Hematologic Disorders:
Idiopathic thrombocytopenic purpura in adults.
Secondary thrombocytopenia in adults.
Acquired (autoimmune) hemolytic anemia.
Erythroblastopenia (RBC anemia).
Congenital (erythroid) hypoplastic anemia.
9. Neoplastic Diseases:
For palliative management of:
Leukemias and lymphomas in adults.
Acute leukemia of childhood.
10. Edematous States:
To induce a diuresis or remission of proteinuria in the nephrotic syndrome, without uremia, of the idiopathic type or that due to lupus erythematosus.
11. Gastrointestinal Diseases:
To tide the patient over a critical period of the disease in:
Ulcerative colitis.
Regional enteritis.
12. Miscellaneous:
Tuberculous meningitis with subarachnoid block or impending block when used concurrently with appropriate antituberculous chemotherapy.
Trichinosis with neurologic or myocardial involvement.
Contraindications: Systemic fungal infections.
Warnings: In patients on corticosteroid therapy subjected to unusual stress, increased dosage of rapidly acting corticosteroids before, during, and after the stressful situation is indicated.
Corticosteroids may mask some signs of infection, and new infections may appear during their use. There may be decreased resistance and inability to localize infection when corticosteroids are used.
Prolonged use of corticosteroids may produce posterior subcapsular cataracts, glaucoma with possible damage to the optic nerves, and may enhance the establishment of secondary ocular infections due to fungi or viruses.
Usage in pregnancy: Since adequate human reproduction studies have not been done with corticosteroids, the use of these drugs in pregnancy, nursing mothers or women of childbearing potential requires that the possible benefits of the drug be weighed against the potential hazards to the mother and embryo or fetus. Infants born of mothers who have received substantial doses of corticosteroids during pregnancy, should be carefully observed for signs of hypoadrenalism.
Average and large doses of hydrocortisone or cortisone can cause elevation of blood pressure, salt and water retention, and increased excretion of potassium. These effects are less likely to occur with the synthetic derivatives except when used in large doses. Dietary salt restriction and potassium supplementation may be necessary. All corticosteroids increase calcium excretion.
While on Corticosteroid Therapy Patients Should Not Be Vaccinated Against Smallpox. Other Immunization Procedures Should Not Be Undertaken in Patients Who Are on Corticosteroids, Especially on High Dose, Because of Possible Hazards of Neurological Complications and a Lack of Antibody Response.
The use of Sterane in active tuberculosis should be restricted to those cases of fulminating or disseminated tuberculosis in which the corticosteroid is used for the management of the disease in conjunction with an appropriate antituberculous regimen.
If corticosteroids are indicated in patients with latent tuberculosis or tuberculin reactivity, close observation is necessary as reactivation of the disease may occur. During prolonged corticosteroid therapy, these patients should receive chemoprophylaxis.
Precautions: Drug-induced secondary adrenocortical insufficiency may be minimized by gradual reduction of dosage. This type of relative insufficiency may persist for months after discontinuation of therapy; therefore, in any situation of stress occurring during that period, hormone therapy should be reinstituted. Since mineralocorticoid secretion may be impaired, salt and/or a mineralocorticoid should be administered concurrently.
There is an enhanced effect of corticosteroids on patients with hypothyroidism and in those with cirrhosis.
Corticosteroids should be used cautiously in patients with ocular herpes simplex because of possible corneal perforation.
The lowest possible dose of corticosteroid should be used to control the condition under treatment, and when reduction in dosage is possible, the reduction should be gradual.
Psychic derangements may appear when corticosteroids are used, ranging from euphoria, insomnia, mood swings, personality changes, and severe depression, to frank psychotic manifestations. Also, existing emotional instability or psychotic tendencies may be aggravated by corticosteroids.
Aspirin should be used cautiously in conjunction with corticosteroids in hypoprothrombinemia.
Steroids should be used with caution in nonspecific ulcerative colitis, if there is a probability of impending perforation, abscess or other pyogenic infection; diverticulitis; fresh intestinal anastomoses; active or latent peptic ulcer; renal insufficiency; hypertension; osteoporosis; and myasthenia gravis.
Growth and development of infants and children on prolonged corticosteroid therapy should be carefully observed.
Adverse Reactions:
Fluid and Electrolyte Disturbances.
Sodium retention.
Fluid retention.
Congestive heart failure in susceptible patients.
Potassium loss.
Hypokalemic alkalosis.
Hypertension.
Musculoskeletal.
Muscle weakness.
Steroid myopathy.
Loss of muscle mass.

Osteoporosis.
Vertebral compression fractures.
Aseptic necrosis of femoral and humeral heads.
Pathologic fracture of long bones.

Gastrointestinal.
Peptic ulcer with possible perforation and hemorrhage.
Pancreatitis.
Abdominal distention.
Ulcerative esophagitis.

Dermatologic.
Mild hirsutism.
Impaired wound healing.
Thin fragile skin.
Petechiae and ecchymoses.
Facial erythema.
Increased sweating.
May suppress reactions to skin tests.

Neurological.
Convulsions.
Increased intracranial pressure with papilledema (pseudo-tumor cerebri) usually after treatment.
Vertigo.
Headache.

Endocrine.
Menstrual irregularities.
Development of Cushingoid state.
Suppression of growth in children.
Secondary adrenocortical and pituitary unresponsiveness, particularly in times of stress, as in trauma, surgery or illness.
Decreased carbohydrate tolerance.
Manifestations of latent diabetes mellitus.
Increased requirements for insulin or oral hypoglycemic agents in diabetics.

Ophthalmic.
Posterior subcapsular cataracts.
Increased intraocular pressure.
Glaucoma.
Exophthalmos.

Metabolic.
Negative nitrogen balance due to protein catabolism.

Dosage and Administration: The initial dosage of Sterane (prednisolone) may vary from 5 mg to 60 mg per day depending on the specific disease entity being treated. In situations of less severity lower doses will generally suffice while in selected patients higher initial doses may be required. The initial dosage should be maintained or adjusted until a satisfactory response is noted. If after a reasonable period of time there is a lack of satisfactory clinical response, Sterane should be discontinued and the patient transferred to other appropriate therapy. *IT SHOULD BE EMPHASIZED THAT DOSAGE REQUIREMENTS ARE VARIABLE AND MUST BE INDIVIDUALIZED ON THE BASIS OF THE DISEASE UNDER TREATMENT AND THE RESPONSE OF THE PATIENT.* After a favorable response is noted, the proper maintenance dosage should be determined by decreasing the initial drug dosage in small increments at appropriate time intervals until the lowest dosage which will maintain an adequate clinical response is reached. It should be kept in mind that constant monitoring is needed in regard to drug dosage. Included in the situations which may make dosage adjustments necessary are changes in clinical status secondary to remissions or exacerbations in the disease process, the patient's individual drug responsiveness, and the effect of patient exposure to stressful situations not directly related to the disease entity under treatment; in this latter situation it may be necessary to increase the dosage of Sterane for a period of time consistent with the patient's condition. If after long term therapy the drug is to be stopped, it is recommended that it be withdrawn gradually rather than abruptly.

How Supplied: Sterane (prednisolone) is supplied in 5 mg tablets, bottles of 100 and 1000.

[*Shown in Product Identification Section*]

TERRAMYCIN® OINTMENT
(oxytetracycline hydrochloride topical ointment with polymyxin B sulfate)

How Supplied: Each gram contains oxytetracycline hydrochloride equivalent to 30 mg. of oxytetracycline; and also 10,000 units of polymyxin B sulfate.
Available in ½ ounce and one ounce tubes, both sizes sold in cartons of twelve. A prescription is *not* required.

TETRACYN® ℞
(tetracycline)
(tetracycline hydrochloride)
CAPSULES AND SYRUP

Indications: Tetracycline is indicated in infections caused by the following microorganisms:
Rickettsiae: Rocky Mountain spotted fever, typhus fever and the typhus group, Q fever, rickettsialpox and tick fevers.
Mycoplasma pneumoniae (PPLO, Eaton agent),
Agents of psittacosis and ornithosis,
Agents of lymphogranuloma venereum and granuloma inguinale,
The spirochetal agent of relapsing fever *(Borrelia recurrentis).*
The following gram-negative microorganisms:
Haemophilus ducreyi (chancroid),
Pasteurella pestis and *Pasteurella tularensis,*
Bartonella bacilliformis,
Bacteroides species,
Vibrio comma and *Vibrio fetus,*
Brucella species (in conjunction with streptomycin).
Because many strains of the following groups of microorganisms have been shown to be resistant to tetracyclines, culture and susceptibility testing are recommended.
Tetracycline is indicated for treatment of infections caused by the following gram-negative microorganisms, when bacteriologic testing indicates appropriate susceptibility to the drug.
Escherichia coli,
Enterobacter aerogenes (formerly *Aerobacter aerogenes*),
Shigella species,
Mima species and *Herellea* species,
Haemophilus influenzae (respiratory infections),
Klebsiella species (respiratory and urinary infections).
Tetracycline is indicated for treatment of infections caused by the following gram-positive microorganisms when bacteriologic testing indicates appropriate susceptibility to the drug:
Streptococcus species:
Up to 44 percent of strains of *Streptococcus pyogenes* and 74 percent of *Streptococcus faecalis* have been found to be resistant to tetracycline drugs. Therefore, tetracyclines should not be used for streptococcal disease unless the organism has been demonstrated to be sensitive.
For upper respiratory infections due to Group A beta-hemolytic streptococci, penicillin is the usual drug of choice, including prophylaxis of rheumatic fever.
Diplococcus pneumoniae,
Staphylococcus aureus, skin and soft tissue infections. Tetracyclines are not the drugs of choice in the treatment of any type of staphylococcal infections.
When penicillin is contraindicated, tetracyclines are alternative drugs in the treatment of infections due to:
Neisseria gonorrhoeae,
Treponema pallidum and *Treponema pertenue* (syphilis and yaws),
Listeria monocytogenes,
Clostridium species,
Bacillus anthracis,
Fusobacterium fusiforme (Vincent's infection),
Actinomyces species.
In acute intestinal amebiasis, the tetracyclines may be a useful adjunct to amebicides.
In severe acne, the tetracyclines may be useful adjunctive therapy.
Tetracyclines are indicated in the treatment of trachoma, although the infectious agent is not always eliminated, as judged by immunofluorescence.
Inclusion conjunctivitis may be treated with oral tetracyclines or with a combination of oral and topical agents.

Contraindications: This drug is contraindicated in persons who have shown hypersensitivity to any of the tetracyclines.

Warnings: THE USE OF DRUGS OF THE TETRACYCLINE CLASS DURING TOOTH DEVELOPMENT (LAST HALF OF PREGNANCY, INFANCY, AND CHILDHOOD TO THE AGE OF 8 YEARS) MAY CAUSE PERMANENT DISCOLORATION OF THE TEETH (YELLOW-GRAY-BROWN). This adverse reaction is more common during long term use of the drugs but has been observed following repeated short term courses. Enamel hypoplasia has also been reported. *TETRACYCLINE DRUGS, THEREFORE, SHOULD NOT BE USED IN THIS AGE GROUP UNLESS OTHER DRUGS ARE NOT LIKELY TO BE EFFECTIVE OR ARE CONTRAINDICATED.*
If renal impairment exists, even usual oral or parenteral doses may lead to excessive systemic accumulation of the drug and possible liver toxicity. Under such conditions, lower than usual total doses are indicated and, if therapy is prolonged, serum level determinations of the drug may be advisable.
Photosensitivity manifested by an exaggerated sunburn reaction has been observed in some individuals taking tetracyclines. Patients apt to be exposed to direct sunlight or ultraviolet light should be advised that this reaction can occur with tetracycline drugs, and treatment should be discontinued at the first evidence of skin erythema.
The antianabolic action of the tetracyclines may cause an increase in BUN. While this is not a problem in those with normal renal function, in patients with significantly impaired function, higher serum levels of tetracycline may lead to azotemia, hyperphosphatemia, and acidosis.
Usage in pregnancy. (See above "Warnings" about use during tooth development.)
Results of animal studies indicate that tetracyclines cross the placenta, are found in fetal tissues and can have toxic effects on the developing fetus (often related to retardation of skeletal development). Evidence of embryotoxicity has also been noted in animals treated early in pregnancy.
Usage in newborns, infants, and children. (See above "Warnings" about use during tooth development.)
All tetracyclines form a stable calcium complex in any bone-forming tissue. A decrease in the fibula growth rate has been observed in prematures given oral tetracycline in doses of 25 mg/kg every 6 hours. This reaction was shown to be reversible when the drug was discontinued.
Tetracyclines are present in the milk of lactating women who are taking a drug in this class.

Precautions: As with other antibiotic preparations, use of this drug may result in overgrowth of nonsusceptible organisms, including fungi. If superinfection occurs, the antibiotic should be discontinued and appropriate therapy instituted.

Continued on next page

Pfipharmecs—Cont.

In venereal diseases when coexistent syphilis is suspected, a dark field examination should be done before treatment is started and the blood serology repeated monthly for at least 4 months.
Because tetracyclines have been shown to depress plasma prothrombin activity, patients who are on anticoagulant therapy may require downward adjustment of their anticoagulant dosage.
In long term therapy, periodic laboratory evaluation of organ systems, including hematopoietic, renal and hepatic studies should be performed.
All infections due to Group A beta-hemolytic streptococci should be treated for at least 10 days.
Since bacteriostatic drugs may interfere with the bactericidal action of penicillin, it is advisable to avoid giving tetracycline in conjunction with penicillin.
Adverse Reactions: Gastrointestinal: Anorexia, nausea, vomiting, diarrhea, glossitis, dysphagia, enterocolitis, and inflammatory lesions (with monilial overgrowth) in the anogenital region. These reactions have been caused by both the oral and parenteral administration of tetracyclines.
Skin: maculopapular and erythematous rashes. Exfoliative dermatitis has been reported but is uncommon. Photosensitivity is discussed above. (See "Warnings").
Renal toxicity: Rise in BUN has been reported and is apparently dose related. (See "Warnings").
Hypersensitivity reactions: urticaria, angioneurotic edema, anaphylaxis, anaphylactoid purpura, pericarditis, and exacerbation of systemic lupus erythematosus.
Bulging fontanels in infants and benign intracranial hypertension in adults have been reported in individuals receiving full therapeutic dosages. These conditions disappeared rapidly when the drug was discontinued.
Blood: Hemolytic anemia, thrombocytopenia, neutropenia, and eosinophilia have been reported.
When given over prolonged periods, tetracyclines have been reported to produce brown-black microscopic discoloration of thyroid glands. No abnormalities of thyroid function studies are known to occur.
Dosage and Administration: Therapy should be continued for at least 24–48 hours after symptoms and fever have subsided.
Concomitant therapy: Antacids containing aluminum, calcium, or magnesium impair absorption and should not be given to patients taking oral tetracycline. Food and some dairy products also interfere with absorption. Oral forms of tetracycline should be given one hour before or two hours after meals. Pediatric oral dosage forms should not be given with milk formulas and should be given at least one hour prior to feeding.
In patients with renal impairment (See "Warnings") total dosage should be decreased by reduction of recommended individual doses and/or by extending time intervals between doses.
In the treatment of streptococcal infections, a therapeutic dose of tetracycline should be administered for at least 10 days. The dosage required to produce optimum therapeutic response will vary from one patient to another depending upon the severity of the infection, the degree of susceptibility of the organism, and the response of the individual.
The suggested minimum adult dosage for tetracycline is 1 gram daily in divided doses given as 500 mg twice a day or 250 mg four times a day. Higher doses, such as 500 mg four times daily, may be required for severe infections or for those infections which do not respond to the smaller dose.
For children above eight years of age: Usual daily dose, 10–20 mg per pound (25–50 mg/kg) of body weight divided in four equal doses.
A gram a day in two divided doses of 500 mg each, has been found effective in certain types of skin infections.
For treatment of brucellosis, 500 mg tetracycline four times daily for three weeks should be accompanied by streptomycin, one gram intramuscularly twice daily the first week and once daily the second week.
For treatment of uncomplicated gonorrhea, when penicillin is contraindicated, tetracycline may be used for the treatment of both males and females in the following divided dosage schedule: 1.5 grams initially, followed by 0.5 gram q.i.d. for a total of 9.0 grams.
For treatment of syphilis, a total of 30 to 40 grams in equally divided doses over a period of 10–15 days should be given. Close follow-up, including laboratory tests, is recommended.
How Supplied: Tetracyn (tetracycline HCl) Capsules, available in opaque, black and white, hard gelatin capsules contain 250 mg of tetracycline HCl: bottles of 100, 1000.
Tetracyn® 500 (tetracycline HCl) Capsules, available in opaque, black and blue, hard gelatin capsules contain 500 mg of tetracycline HCl: bottles of 100.
[*Shown in Product Identification Section*]
Tetracyn (tetracycline) Syrup, available as a preconstituted, cherry-flavored aqueous suspension, contains in each teaspoonful (5 ml) tetracycline equivalent to 125 mg of tetracycline HCl: 1 pint bottle.

TETRASTATIN® ℞
tetracycline HCl 250 mg.
nystatin 250,000 units
CAPSULES

Actions: Tetracyn® (tetracycline HCl) is a crystalline antibiotic which possesses potent antimicrobial activity. It is well tolerated and effective in the treatment of many diseases caused by gram-positive or gram-negative bacteria.
Nystatin is an antibiotic with activity against a number of fungi, including *Candida albicans* (Monilia). It adds significant prophylaxis against overgrowth or superinfection by such fungi.

Indications:
Based on a review of this drug by the National Academy of Sciences-National Research Council and/or other information, FDA has classified the indications as follows:
"Lacking substantial evidence of effectiveness as a fixed combination":
Tetrastatin is indicated in a wide variety of infections caused by susceptible bacteria. Tetracyn (tetracycline HCl) is very rapidly absorbed, diffuses readily into tissues to combat infection, and is well tolerated. Nystatin, the first available antifungal antibiotic, has been used successfully as a prophylactic agent for the suppression of *Candida albicans* and as a therapeutic agent in the management of active monilial infections.
The following have been clinically established as indications for the use of Tetracyn (tetracycline HCl):
RESPIRATORY TRACT INFECTIONS: Pneumococcal pneumonia; other types of bacterial pneumonia; bronchopneumonia; pertussis; follicular tonsillitis; acute bronchitis; otitis media; mastoiditis, and a number of upper respiratory infections.
GENITOURINARY INFECTIONS: Acute and chronic urinary infections such as cystitis; urethritis; pyelonephritis; ureteritis; and prostatitis; caused by susceptible staphylococci, streptococci, A. aerogenes, E. coli, and some mixed infections; gonorrhea.
INFECTIONS OF THE NERVOUS SYSTEM: Bacterial meningitis caused by the meningococcus, H. influenzae and other susceptible organisms, as well as bacterial infections localized elsewhere in the nervous system.
SURGICAL INFECTIONS: Peritonitis, acute bacterial cholecystitis, infected wounds and incisions, serious soft tissue infections, and osteomyelitis.
In the treatment of staphylococcal infections, indicated surgical procedures should be carried out in all cases.
INFECTIONS IN OBSTETRICS AND GYNECOLOGY: Puerperal infection, salpingo-oophoritis, pelvic inflammatory disease, and infection resulting from incomplete abortion.
OTHER INFECTIONS: Eye infections, gastrointestinal infections, and skin infections caused by susceptible bacteria; rickettsial infections such as Rocky Mountain spotted fever and epidemic typhus; certain infections with large viruses such as lymphogranuloma venereum and psittacosis; brucellosis and bartonellosis; bacillary dysentery; acute intestinal amebic infections; septicemia, and subacute bacterial endocarditis due to susceptible organisms. It is usually not possible to predict with certainty which patients may develop clinical moniliasis as a result of broad-spectrum antibiotic therapy. However, the added protection afforded by Tetrastatin against monilial superinfection of intestinal origin is especially important for patients who are most likely to be susceptible to the overgrowth of *Candida albicans.* Among such patients are those requiring high or prolonged antibiotic dosage; debilitated or elderly patients; diabetics; infants; patients receiving concomitant cortisone or related steroid therapy; patients who have developed a monilial complication on previous broad-spectrum therapy; and women particularly during pregnancy.
Final classification of the less than effective indications require further investigation. Clinical studies to substantiate the efficacy of Tetrastatin are ongoing. Completion of these ongoing studies will provide data for final classification of these indications.

Contraindications: This drug is contraindicated in individuals who have shown hypersensitivity to any of its components.
Warnings: Tetracycline may form a stable calcium complex in any bone forming tissue with no serious harmful effects reported thus far in humans. However, use of tetracycline during tooth development (last trimester of pregnancy, neonatal period and early childhood) may cause discoloration of the teeth (yellow-grey-brownish). This effect occurs mostly during long-term use of the drug but it has also been observed in usual short treatment courses.
If renal impairment exists even usual doses may lead to excessive accumulation of the drug and possible liver toxicity. Under such conditions, lower than usual doses are indicated and if therapy is prolonged, tetracycline serum level determinations may be advisable.
Certain hypersensitive individuals may develop a photodynamic reaction precipitated by a direct exposure to natural or artificial sunlight during the use of this drug. This reaction is usually of the photoallergic type which may also be produced by other tetracycline derivatives. Individuals with a history of photosensitivity reactions should be instructed to avoid direct exposure to natural or artificial sunlight

while under treatment with this or other tetracycline drugs, and treatment should be discontinued at first evidence of skin discomfort.
NOTE: Tetracyn (tetracycline HCl) has been rarely implicated as the causative agent of photosensitivity.
Precautions: If a superimposed infection which may be caused by resistant organisms is observed, the antibiotic should be discontinued and a therapeutic trial of other antibiotics as indicated by susceptibility testing may be indicated.
Increased intracranial pressure with bulging fontanelles has been observed occasionally in infants receiving therapeutic doses of tetracycline. Although the mechanism for this phenomenon is unknown, the signs and symptoms have disappeared rapidly upon cessation of treatment with no sequelae.
In long term therapy with this as with other potent drugs, periodic laboratory evaluation of organ systems, including hematopoietic, renal and hepatic studies should be accomplished.
When treating gonorrhea in which lesions of primary or seconary syphilis are suspected, proper diagnostic procedures including darkfield examinations, should be followed. In other cases in which concomitant syphilis is suspected, monthly serological tests should be made for at least four months.
Adverse Reactions: Glossitis, stomatitis, proctitis, nausea, diarrhea, vaginitis, and dermatitis as well as reactions of an allergic nature may occur but are rare. If adverse reactions occur or individual idiosyncrasy or allergy occurs, discontinue medication.
With tetracycline therapy bulging fontanels in infants and benign intracranial hypertension in adults have been reported in individuals receiving full therapeutic dosages. These conditions disappeared rapidly when the drug was discontinued.
Elevation of SGOT or SGPT values or elevated BUN have been reported with the use of tetracyclines, the significance of which is not known at this time. Anemia, neutropenia, and eosinophilia have been reported with the use of tetracyclines.
Dosage: The dosage of Tetrastatin required to produce optimum therapeutic response will vary from one patient to another depending upon the severity of the infection, the degree of susceptibility of the organism, and the response of the individual to treatment. In the average adult the suggested daily dose should be 1 to 2 g of tetracycline HCl divided into four equal parts (250 mg to 500 mg q.i.d. or 1 to 2 capsules of Tetrastatin q.i.d.). Higher daily doses may be required for severe infections or for those patients who do not respond rapidly to lower dosage. Therapy should continue for at least 24 to 48 hours after symptoms and fever have subsided. When used in streptococcal infections therapy should continue for ten days to prevent the possible development of rheumatic fever or glomerulonephritis.
In subacute bacterial endocarditis, therapy for 6 to 8 weeks should be maintained. A rest period may be given at the end of these periods of treatment and therapy again begun if the specific infectious agent can still be demonstrated.
When using Tetracyn (tetracycline HCl) in the treatment of brucellosis, the course of therapy should be three weeks and supplemented with intramuscular injections of streptomycin in a dosage of 1 g twice daily the first week, and 1 g daily the second and third weeks.
The recommended dosage of Tetrastatin as indicated above is the same as that for Tetracyn (tetracycline HCl). Because of the diminished possibility of fungal overgrowth it may be anticipated that gastrointestinal disturbances should be minimized.
To aid absorption of the drug, it should be given at least one hour before or two hours after eating. Tetracycline should not be given with milk formulas or calcium-containing foods. Aluminum hydroxide gel and similar substances when given with antibiotics have been shown to decrease absorption and are contraindicated.
How Supplied: Tetrastatin Capsules are available in opaque, black and pink, hard gelatin capsules; each capsule contains 250 mg of tetracycline HCl and 250,000 units of nystatin: bottles of 100.
[*Shown in Product Identification Section*]

VITERRA C

How Supplied: Available as 250 mg and 500 mg tablets, in bottles of 100.

VITERRA E

How Supplied: Available as capsules of 100 I.U., 200 I.U., 400 I.U. and 600 I.U., in bottles of 100.

VITERRA® ORIGINAL FORMULA TABLETS

Vitamins and Minerals

Composition: Each tablet contains:

Vitamins	Amount	% U.S. RDA*
Vitamin A (Vitamin A Acetate)	5,000 IU	100
Vitamin D (Ergocalciferol)	400 IU	100
Vitamin E (dl-Alpha Tocopheryl Acetate)	3.7 IU	12
Vitamin C (L-Ascorbic Acid)	50 mg	83
Vitamin B_1 (Thiamine Mononitrate)	3 mg	200
Vitamin B_2 (Riboflavin)	3 mg	176
Niacin (Niacinamide)	25 mg	125
Vitamin B_6 (Pyridoxine Hydrochloride)	0.82 mg	41
Vitamin B_{12} (Cyanocobalamin)	2 mcg	33
Pantothenic Acid (D-Calcium Pantothenate)	4.6 mg	46
Minerals		
Calcium (Calcium Carbonate and Dibasic Calcium Phosphate)	140 mg	14
Phosphorous (Dibasic Calcium Phosphate)	70 mg	7
Iodine (Potassium Iodide)	150 mcg	100
Iron (Ferrous Fumarate)	10 mg	55
Magnesium (Magnesium Sulfate)	5 mg	1.25
Copper (Cupric Sulfate)	1 mg	50
Zinc (Zinc Sulfate)	1.2 mg	8
Manganese (Manganese Sulfate)	1 mg	**

* Percentage of U.S. Recommended Daily Allowance (RDA) for adults and children 4 or more years of age.
** Manganese is recognized as essential in human nutrition but no U.S. RDA has been established.

Description: An original formula containing vitamins plus minerals.
Administration and Dosage: One tablet daily, or as directed by the physician.
How Supplied: In bottles of 100 yellow film coated (sugar free) tablets.

VITERRA® HIGH POTENCY TABLETS

Vitamins and Minerals

Composition: Each tablet contains:

Vitamins	Amount	% U.S. RDA*
Vitamin A (Vitamin A Acetate)	10,000 IU	200
Vitamin D-(Ergocalciferol)	400 IU	100
Vitamin E (dl Alpha Tocopheryl Acetate)	5 IU	16.7
Vitamin C (L-Ascorbic Acid)	150 mg	250
Vitamin B_1 (Thiamine Mononitrate)	10 mg	666
Vitamin B_2 (Riboflavin)	10 mg	590
Niacin (Niacinamide)	100 mg	500
Vitamin B_6 (Pyridoxine Hydrochloride)	1.6 mg	80
Vitamin B_{12} (Cyanocobalamin)	5 mcg	83
Pantothenic Acid (Calcium Pantothenate)	4.6 mg	46
Minerals		
Calcium (Calcium Carbonate)	0.05 g	5
Iodine (Potassium Iodide)	150 mcg	100
Iron (Ferrous Fumarate)	10 mg	55
Magnesium (Magnesium Sulfate)	5 mg	1.25
Copper (Cupric Sulfate)	1 mg	50
Zinc (Zinc Sulfate)	1.2 mg	8
Manganese (Manganese Sulfate)	1 mg	**

* Percentage of U.S. Recommended Daily Allowance (RDA) for adults and children 4 or more years of age.
** Manganese is recognized as essential in human nutrition but no U.S. RDA has been established.

Description: A higher potency formula containing vitamins plus minerals.
Administration and Dosage: One tablet daily, or as directed by the physician.
How Supplied: In bottles of 100 salmon-red film coated (sugar free) tablets.

Pfizer Laboratories Division

PFIZER INC.
235 EAST 42ND STREET
NEW YORK, NEW YORK 10017

Full prescribing information for all Pfizer Laboratories products is available from your Pfizer Laboratories representative.

Product Identification Codes

To provide quick and positive identification of Pfizer Laboratories Division products, we have imprinted the product identification number of the National Drug Code on most tablets and capsules.
In order that you may quickly identify a product by its code number, we have compiled below a numerical list of code numbers with their corresponding product names. We are also listing the code numbers by alphabetical order of products.

NUMERICAL PRODUCT INDEX

Product Identification Code	Product
072	Terramycin® (Oxytetracycline HCl) Capsules 125 mg.
073	Terramycin® (Oxytetracycline HCl) Capsules 250 mg.
084	Terramycin® (Oxytetracycline) Tablets (film coated) 250 mg.
087	Terramycin® (Oxytetracycline HCl) Vaginal Tablets with Polymyxin B Sulfate
088	Terrastatin® (Oxytetracycline with Nystatin) Capsules 250 mg.
094	Vibramycin® Hyclate (Doxycycline Hyclate) Capsules 50 mg.
095	Vibramycin® Hyclate (Doxycycline Hyclate) Capsules 100 mg.
180	Vistrax® 5 (Oxyphencyclimine HCl 5 mg. and Hydroxyzine HCl 25 mg.) Tablets
181	Vistrax® 10 (Oxyphencyclimine HCl 10 mg. and Hydroxyzine HCl 25 mg.) Tablets
201	Bonine® (Meclizine HCl) Chewable Tablets 25 mg.
320	Ataraxoid® (Prednisolone 2.5 mg. and Hydroxyzine HCl 10 mg.) Tablets 2.5 mg.

Continued on next page

Pfizer—Cont.

321	Ataraxoid® (Prednisolone 5.0 mg. and Hydroxyzine HCl 10 mg.) Tablets 5.0 mg.
375	Renese® (Polythiazide) Tablets 1 mg.
376	Renese® (Polythiazide) Tablets 2 mg.
377	Renese® (Polythiazide) Tablets 4 mg.
393	Diabinese® (Chlorpropamide) Tablets 100 mg.
394	Diabinese® (Chlorpropamide) Tablets 250 mg.
431	Minipress® (Prazosin HCl) Capsules 1 mg.
437	Minipress® (Prazosin HCl) Capsules 2 mg.
438	Minipress® (Prazosin HCl) Capsules 5 mg.
441	Moderil® (Rescinnamine) Tablets 0.25 mg.
442	Moderil® (Rescinnamine) Tablets 0.5 mg.
446	Renese®-R (Polythiazide 2.0 mg. and Reserpine 0.25 mg.) Tablets
534	Sinequan® (Doxepin HCl) Capsules 10 mg.
535	Sinequan® (Doxepin HCl) Capsules 25 mg.
536	Sinequan® (Doxepin HCl) Capsules 50 mg.
537	Sinequan® (Doxepin HCl) Capsules 150 mg.
538	Sinequan® (Doxepin HCl) Capsules 100 mg.
539	Sinequan® (Doxepin HCl) Capsules 75 mg.
541	Vistaril® (Hydroxyzine Pamoate) Capsules 25 mg.
542	Vistaril® (Hydroxyzine Pamoate) Capsules 50 mg.
543	Vistaril® (Hydroxyzine Pamoate) Capsules 100 mg.

ALPHABETICAL PRODUCT INDEX

Product	Product Identification Code
Ataraxoid® (Prednisolone 2.5 mg. and Hydroxyzine HCl 10 mg.) Tablets 2.5 mg.	320
Ataraxoid® (Prednisolone 5.0 mg. and Hydroxyzine HCl 10 mg.) Tablets 5.0 mg.	321
Bonine® (Meclizine HCl) Chewable Tablets 25 mg.	201
Diabinese® (Chlorpropamide) Tablets 100 mg.	393
Diabinese® (Chlorpropamide) Tablets 250 mg.	394
Minipress® (Prazosin HCl) Capsules 1 mg.	431
Minipress® (Prazosin HCl) Capsules 2 mg.	437
Minipress® (Prazosin HCl) Capsules 5 mg.	438
Moderil® (Rescinnamine) Tablets 0.25 mg.	441
Moderil® (Rescinnamine) Tablets 0.5 mg.	442
Renese® (Polythiazide) Tablets 1 mg.	375
Renese® (Polythiazide) Tablets 2 mg.	376
Renese® (Polythiazide) Tablets 4 mg.	377
Renese®-R (Polythiazide 2.0 mg. and Reserpine 0.25 mg.) Tablets	446
Sinequan® (Doxepin HCl) Capsules 10 mg.	534
Sinequan® (Doxepin HCl) Capsules 25 mg.	535
Sinequan® (Doxepin HCl) Capsules 50 mg.	536
Sinequan® (Doxepin HCl) Capsules 75 mg.	539
Sinequan® (Doxepin HCl) Capsules 100 mg.	538
Sinequan® (Doxepin HCl) Capsules 150 mg.	537
Terramycin® (Oxytetracycline HCl) Capsules 125 mg.	072
Terramycin® (Oxytetracycline HCl) Capsules 250 mg.	073
Terramycin® (Oxytetracycline) Tablets (film coated) 250 mg.	084
Terramycin® (Oxytetracycline HCl) Vaginal Tablets with Polymyxin B Sulfate	087
Terrastatin® (Oxytetracycline with Nystatin) Capsules 250 mg.	088
Vibramycin® Hyclate (Doxycycline Hyclate) Capsules 50 mg.	094
Vibramycin® Hyclate (Doxycycline Hyclate) Capsules 100 mg.	095
Vistaril® (Hydroxyzine Pamoate) Capsules 25 mg.	541
Vistaril® (Hydroxyzine Pamoate) Capsules 50 mg.	542
Vistaril® (Hydroxyzine Pamoate) Capsules 100 mg.	543
Vistrax® 5 (Oxyphencyclimine HCl 5 mg. and Hydroxyzine HCl 25 mg.) Tablets	180
Vistrax® 10 (Oxyphencyclimine HCl 10 mg. and Hydroxyzine HCl 25 mg.) Tablets	181

BONINE® OTC
(meclizine hydrochloride)
Chewable Tablets

Actions: BONINE is an antihistamine which shows marked protective activity against nebulized histamine and lethal doses of intravenously injected histamine in guinea pigs. It has a marked effect in blocking the vasodepressor response to histamine, but only a slight blocking action against acetylcholine. Its activity is relatively weak in inhibiting the spasmogenic action of histamine on isolated guinea pig ileum.
Antihistamines have been observed to have both stimulant and depressant effects on the CNS, but no clear explanation exists in regard to their diverse central actions. The site and mode of their central action is unknown.
Indications: BONINE is effective in the management of nausea, vomiting and dizziness associated with motion sickness.
Contraindications: Administration of BONINE during pregnancy or to women who may become pregnant is contraindicated in view of the teratogenic effect of the drug in rats.
The administration of meclizine to pregnant rats during the 12th-15th day of gestation has produced cleft palate in the offspring. Limited studies using doses of over 100 mg./kg./day in rabbits and 10 mg./kg./day in pigs and monkeys did not show cleft palate. Congeners of meclizine have caused cleft palate in species other than the rat.
Meclizine HCl is contraindicated in individuals who have shown a previous hypersensitivity to it.
Warnings: Since drowsiness may occur with the use of this drug, patients should be warned of this possibility and cautioned against driving a car or operating dangerous machinery.
Usage in Children:
Clinical studies establishing safety and effectiveness in children have not been done; therefore, usage is not recommended in the pediatric age group.
Usage in Pregnancy:
See "Contraindications".
Adverse Reactions: Drowsiness, dry mouth, and on rare occasions, blurred vision have been reported.
Dosage and Administration: The initial dose of 25-50 mg. of BONINE should be taken one hour prior to embarkation against motion sickness. Thereafter, the dose may be repeated every 24 hours for the duration of the journey.
How Supplied: BONINE (meclizine HCl) is supplied as 25 mg. scored chewable tablets (imprinted with code number 201) (bottles of 100 and 500). (60-1464-00-5)
Literature Available: Yes.

DIABINESE® ℞
(chlorpropamide)
Tablets

Actions: DIABINESE (chlorpropamide) IS AN ORAL HYPOGLYCEMIC AGENT. IT IS NOT AN ORAL INSULIN, THOUGH THE PRECISE MECHANISM OF ACTION IS NOT COMPLETELY UNDERSTOOD.
DIABINESE was discovered and synthesized by researchers of Pfizer Inc. It was evaluated thoroughly in a broad clinical program, and these studies have shown it to be a potent, active, oral hypoglycemic agent, valuable in the treatment of selected diabetic patients. It is generally used alone to control the mild to moderately severe maturity-onset, stable diabetic. While chlorpropamide is a sulfonamide derivative, it is devoid of antibacterial activity. A method developed by chemists at Pfizer Inc. (description available on request) permits the easy measurement of the drug in blood. Chlorpropamide does not interfere with the usual tests to detect albumin in the urine.
DIABINESE is absorbed rapidly from the gastrointestinal tract. Within one hour after a single oral dose, it is readily detectable in the blood, and the level reaches a maximum within two to four hours. It is not significantly metabolized or deactivated. It is slowly excreted in the urine, for the most part as unchanged chlorpropamide. The biological half-life of chlorpropamide averages about 36 hours. Within 96 hours, 80–90% of a single oral dose is excreted in the urine. However, long-term administration of therapeutic doses does not result in undue accumulation in the blood, since absorption and excretion rates become stabilized in about 5 to 7 days after the initiation of therapy.
DIABINESE exerts a hypoglycemic effect in normal humans within one hour, becoming maximal at 3 to 6 hours and persisting for at least 24 hours. The potency of chlorpropamide is approximately six times that of tolbutamide. Some experimental results suggest that its increased effectiveness may be the result of slower excretion and absence of significant deactivation.
The mode of action of chlorpropamide is believed to be that of stimulation of synthesis and release of endogenous insulin.
There is now evidence that improvement in pancreatic beta cell function, with consequent improvement in glucose tolerance, may occur with prolonged administration of chlorpropamide. Accordingly, in individuals with asymptomatic diabetes mellitus, principally manifested by an abnormal glucose tolerance, continuous use of chlorpropamide may result in "normalization" of their tolerance to glucose.
Indications: DIABINESE is indicated in uncomplicated diabetes mellitus of the stable, mild or moderately severe, non-ketotic, maturity-onset type, which cannot be completely controlled by diet alone. It can often be used in patients of this type in place of insulin. It may also prove effective in controlling certain patients who have shown an inadequate response or true primary or secondary failure to other sulfonylurea agents. In patients requiring high doses or frequent administration of another oral agent, control may be facilitated through its use.
Patient selection: The most likely patient for therapy is one in whom diabetes is of the maturity-onset (adult) type, stable, and not controllable by dietary regulation alone. A past history of diabetic coma does not necessarily preclude successful therapeutic control with DIABINESE. A trial period may be indicated in certain patients who might be expected to respond to this type of medication, but failed in initial trials with tolbutamide or subsequently after having been on other sulfonylureas for variable periods of time, or in patients whose diabetic control with tolbutamide is not as good as the physician would think best

for his patient. DIABINESE may provide effective and improved control of the diabetes. The final evaluation of response in patients who qualify as candidates for DIABINESE is a therapeutic trial for a period of at least seven days. During the trial period, the absence of ketonuria together with a satisfactory reduction of glycosuria and hyperglycemia, or maintenance of previously satisfactory control, indicates that the patient is responsive and amenable to control with the drug. However, the development of ketonuria within 24 hours after withdrawal of insulin usually will be indicative of a poor response. The patient is considered nonresponsive if he fails to achieve satisfactory lowering of blood sugar levels or fails to obtain objective or subjective clinical improvement and if he develops ketonuria or glycosuria. Insulin is indicated for the therapy of such patients.

Contraindications: Use of DIABINESE is not indicated in patients having:

1. Juvenile or growth-onset diabetes mellitus.
2. Severe or unstable "brittle" diabetes.
3. Diabetes complicated by ketosis and acidosis, diabetic coma, major surgery, severe infection, or severe trauma.

DIABINESE is contraindicated during pregnancy. Safe conditions for the use of DIABINESE in pregnancy have not been established, and serious consideration should be given to the potential hazard of its use in women of the childbearing age who may become pregnant.

DIABINESE is contraindicated in patients with serious impairment of hepatic, renal, or thyroid function. Pseudo-diabetes with azotemia due to chronic renal disease has been misdiagnosed as diabetes mellitus.

Precautions: Since animal studies suggest that the action of barbiturates may be prolonged by therapy with chlorpropamide, barbiturates should be employed with caution. Similarly, studies showing an exaggerated hypoglycemic effect of chlorpropamide in adrenalectomized animals suggest cautious use in patients with Addison's disease. In some patients, a disulfiram-like reaction may be produced by the ingestion of alcohol.

Caution should be exercised when antibacterial sulfonamides, phenylbutazone, salicylates, probenecid, dicoumarol, or MAO inhibitors are administered concomitantly with chlorpropamide as hypoglycemia resultant from either potentiation or accumulation of sulfonylureas has been reported.

During the first six weeks of therapy, the physician should be in contact with the patient at least once a week. During this initial period, the patient must be observed for evidence of occasional drug reactions as described in the ADVERSE REACTIONS section. Because of the possibility of the following manifestations of hypersensitivity the patient should be instructed to report immediately to his physician if he does not feel as well as usual, or notes any pruritus, rash, jaundice, dark urine, light colored stools, low-grade fever, sore throat or diarrhea. As with all drugs, careful attention must be given to weigh the therapeutic advantages against the nature and incidence of side effects.

During the period of transition to DIABINESE (chlorpropamide), the patient's urine should be tested for sugar and acetone at least three times daily and the results reviewed by the physician at least once a week. Frequent laboratory determinations of liver function should also be seriously considered. Although transient minor alterations, particularly of cephalin flocculation, thymol turbidity, and serum alkaline phosphatase levels are not unusual and are probably of no clinical significance, a progressive rise in the alkaline phosphatase value should alert the physician to the possibility of incipient biliary stasis and jaundice, and chlorpropamide therapy should be promptly discontinued. After the initial six weeks of therapy, subsequent patient-physician contacts may be at less frequent intervals, the exact frequency dependent on the judgment of the physician.

The drug should be used as an adjunct to, not a substitute for, dietary regulation, for this remains the primary consideration of diabetic management. It does not alter the need to educate the patient to such standard prophylactic and therapeutic measures as weight and exercise control, proper hygiene, and prompt care of intercurrent infection.

Alcohol and decreased diet may lead to hypoglycemia, ketosis, coma and death. Thiazides, on the other hand, have been shown to suppress insulin secretion, and therefore will contribute to hyperglycemia.

Warnings: DIABINESE SHOULD NOT BE USED IN JUVENILE DIABETES OR IN DIABETES COMPLICATED BY ACIDOSIS, COMA, SEVERE INFECTION, MAJOR SURGICAL PROCEDURES, OR SEVERE TRAUMA. HERE, INSULIN IS INDISPENSABLE.

Although DIABINESE given alone has controlled some patients with mild maturity-onset diabetes of the stable type during the stress of mild infection or minor surgery, insulin therapy is generally essential during intercurrent complications (for example, ketoacidosis, severe trauma, major surgical procedures, severe infections, severe diarrhea, nausea and vomiting, etc.). The severity of the diabetes, the nature of the complication, and availability of laboratory facilities determine whether therapy with chlorpropamide can be continued or should be withdrawn while insulin is being used.

IN CASES OF ACCIDENTAL INGESTION BY CHILDREN, DUE NOTE SHOULD BE TAKEN OF THE FACT THAT 3–5 DAYS ARE REQUIRED FOR COMPLETE ELIMINATION OF CHLORPROPAMIDE FROM THE BODY, AND THE PATIENT SHOULD BE KEPT UNDER CLOSE OBSERVATION FOR THIS PERIOD OF TIME DESPITE APPARENT RECOVERY.

Since insulin still remains the standard therapy for patients during periods of stress or complication, the patient on chlorpropamide must be instructed in the use of insulin. The patient must also be alerted to the early detection and prompt treatment of hypoglycemia since this complication although less frequent, may develop on sulfonylurea therapy as well as on insulin therapy. HYPOGLYCEMIA IF IT OCCURS, MAY BE PROLONGED. (See section on ADVERSE REACTIONS.)

During the initial period of therapy with chlorpropamide, hypoglycemic reactions may occasionally occur, particularly during the transition from insulin to the oral drug. Hypoglycemia within 24 hours after withdrawal of the intermediate or long-acting types of insulin will usually prove to be the result of insulin carry-over and not primarily due to the effect of chlorpropamide.

Adverse Reactions: The majority of the side effects have been dose-related, transient, and have responded to dose reduction or withdrawal of the medication. However, clinical experience thus far has shown that, as with other sulfonylureas, some side effects associated with hypersensitivity may be severe and deaths have been reported in some instances. Chlorpropamide has a somewhat higher reported incidence of side effects than tolbutamide.

Certain untoward reactions associated with idiosyncrasy or hypersensitivity have occurred, including jaundice, skin eruptions rarely progressing to erythema multiforme and exfoliative dermatitis, and probably depression of formed elements of the blood, and show no direct relationship to the size of the dose. They occur characteristically during the first six weeks of therapy. With a few exceptions, these manifestations have been mild and readily reversible on the withdrawal of the drug.

The more severe manifestations may require other therapeutic measures, including corticosteroid therapy. DIABINESE (chlorpropamide) should be discontinued promptly when the development of sensitivity is suspected.

Jaundice has been reported, and is usually promptly reversible on discontinuance of therapy. On the basis of considerable histopathologic evidence, the jaundice is cholangiolitic and results primarily from intracanalicular biliary stasis rather than hepatocellular degeneration. The alkaline phosphatase which frequently shows serial and progressive elevation in these patients is of particular diagnostic value. THE OCCURRENCE OF PROGRESSIVE ELEVATION SHOULD SUGGEST THE POSSIBILITY OF INCIPIENT JAUNDICE AND CONSTITUTES AN INDICATION FOR WITHDRAWAL OF THE DRUG.

In contrast, transient alterations of certain liver function tests seen occasionally following institution of sulfonylurea therapy, appear to be of no clinical significance.

Skin rash may be either the only manifestation of sensitivity, or occur in association with jaundice, frequently preceding it. Low grade fever and eosinophilia may also occur in association with, or preceding the development of, clinical jaundice. Rarely, severe diarrhea, sometimes accompanied by bleeding into the lower bowel and due to nonspecific proctocolitis, has been associated with other hypersensitivity manifestations, particularly jaundice, skin rash, or both. The occurrence, singly or together, of any of these hypersensitivity manifestations, should constitute an indication for prompt termination of the drug, and such other therapeutic measures as are dictated by the circumstances should be instituted.

Leukopenia, thrombocytopenia and mild anemia, which occur occasionally, are generally benign and revert to normal, following cessation of the drug. Leukopenia of mild degree, and not associated with a shift in the differential count, may be transient and frequently reverts to normal even while the drug is continued.

Cases of aplastic anemia and agranulocytosis, generally similar to blood dyscrasias associated with other sulfonylureas have been reported. Lymphocytosis appears to be of no clinical significance.

Dose-related side effects previously mentioned are generally transient and not of a serious nature and would include anorexia, nausea, vomiting, and epigastric discomfort as evidence of gastrointestinal intolerance, and various vague neurologic symptoms, particularly weakness and paresthesias. These manifestations are generally a direct function of dosage and were reported much more frequently during the early clinical history of the drug when some clinicians employed relatively high doses. These side effects are reversible on reduction of the daily dosage, or if necessary, by withdrawal of the medication.

Administration of the total daily drug requirement in two doses rather than one is sometimes an effective measure for alleviating symptoms of gastrointestinal intolerance.

Hypoglycemia, although not a true side effect, but rather an exaggeration of the expected therapeutic action, may be the result of dosage in excess of the patient's immediate requirements, as in the case with any hypoglycemic agent. Since the development of hypoglycemia is a function of many factors including diet, this effect is at times seen in patients on the usual recommended dosage. It is readily controlled by administration of glucose. Its occurrence is an obvious indication for immediate

Continued on next page

Pfizer—Cont.

re-evaluation and adjustment of the insulin or chlorpropamide dosage.
BECAUSE OF THE PROLONGED HYPOGLYCEMIC ACTION OF DIABINESE, PATIENTS WHO BECOME HYPOGLYCEMIC DURING THERAPY WITH THIS DRUG REQUIRE CLOSE SUPERVISION FOR A MINIMUM PERIOD OF 3 TO 5 DAYS, during which time frequent feedings or glucose administration are essential. The anorectic patient or the profoundly hypoglycemic patient should be hospitalized.
Rare cases of phototoxic reactions have been reported.
Edema associated with hyponatremia has been infrequently reported with DIABINESE therapy. This is thought to occur by potentiation of available ADH with subsequent water retention. The condition is usually readily reversible upon discontinuation of medication.
Dosage: The total daily dosage is generally taken at a single time each morning with breakfast. Occasionally cases of gastrointestinal intolerance may be relieved by dividing the daily dosage. A LOADING OR PRIMING DOSE IS NOT NECESSARY AND SHOULD NOT BE USED.
Initial Therapy: 1. The mild to moderately severe, middle-aged, stable diabetic patient should be started on 250 mg daily. Because the geriatric diabetic patient appears to be more sensitive to the hypoglycemic effect of sulfonylurea drugs, older patients should be started on smaller amounts of DIABINESE, in the range of 100 to 125 mg daily.
2. No transition period is necessary when transferring patients from other oral hypoglycemic agents to DIABINESE. The other agent may be discontinued abruptly and chlorpropamide started at once. In prescribing chlorpropamide, due consideration must be given to its greater potency.
3. The large majority of mild to moderately severe middle-aged, stable diabetic patients receiving insulin can be placed directly on the oral drug and their insulin abruptly discontinued. For patients requiring more than 40 units of insulin daily, therapy with DIABINESE may be initiated with a 50 per cent reduction in insulin for the first few days, with subsequent further reductions dependent upon the response.
During the insulin withdrawal period, the patient should test his urine for sugar and ketone bodies at least three times daily and report the results frequently to his physician. If they are abnormal, the physician should be notified immediately. In some cases, it may be advisable to consider hospitalization during the transition period.
Five to seven days after the initial therapy, the blood level of chlorpropamide reaches a plateau. Dosage may subsequently be adjusted upward or downward by increments of not more than 50 to 125 mg at intervals of three to five days to obtain optimal control. More frequent adjustments are usually undesirable.
Maintenance Therapy: Most moderately severe, middle-aged stable diabetic patients are controlled by approximately 250 mg daily. Many investigators have found that some milder diabetics do well on daily doses of 100 mg or less. Many of the more severe diabetics may require 500 mg daily for adequate control. PATIENTS WHO DO NOT RESPOND COMPLETELY TO 500 MG DAILY WILL USUALLY NOT RESPOND TO HIGHER DOSES. Maintenance doses above 750 mg daily should be avoided.
Supply: DIABINESE (chlorpropamide) Tablets:
250 mg: Blue "D"-shaped, scored tablets (imprinted with code #394)—bottles of 100's, 250's, 1000's, and Unit-Dose packages of 100.
100 mg: Blue "D"-shaped, scored tablets (imprinted with code #393)—bottles of 100's, 500's, and Unit-Dose packages of 100.
(60-2141-37-3)
Literature Available: Yes.
[Shown in Product Identification Section]

MINIPRESS® CAPSULES ℞
(prazosin hydrochloride)
For Oral Use

Description: MINIPRESS (prazosin hydrochloride), a quinazoline derivative, is the first of a new chemical class of antihypertensives. It is the hydrochloride salt of 1-(4-amino-6,7-dimethoxy-2-quinazolinyl)-4-(2-furoyl) piperazine.
It is a white, crystalline substance, slightly soluble in water and isotonic saline and has a molecular weight of 419.87. Each 1 mg capsule of MINIPRESS (prazosin hydrochloride) contains drug equivalent to 1 mg free base.
Actions: The exact mechanism of the hypotensive action of prazosin is unknown. Prazosin causes a decrease in total peripheral resistance and was originally thought to have a direct relaxant action on vascular smooth muscle. Recent animal studies, however, have suggested that the vasodilator effect of prazosin is also related to blockade of postsynaptic *alpha*-adrenoceptors. The results of dog forelimb experiments demonstrate that the peripheral vasodilator effect of prazosin is confined mainly to the level of the resistance vessels (arterioles). Unlike conventional *alpha*-blockers, the antihypertensive action of prazosin is usually not accompanied by a reflex tachycardia. Tolerance has not been observed to develop in long term therapy.
Hemodynamic studies have been carried out in man following acute single dose administration and during the course of long term maintenance therapy. The results confirm that the therapeutic effect is a fall in blood pressure unaccompanied by a clinically significant change in cardiac output, heart rate, renal blood flow and glomerular filtration rate. There is no measurable negative chronotropic effect.
In clinical studies to date, MINIPRESS (prazosin hydrochloride) has not increased plasma renin activity.
In man, blood pressure is lowered in both the supine and standing positions. This effect is most pronounced on the diastolic blood pressure.
Following oral administration, human plasma concentrations reach a peak at about three hours with a plasma half-life of two to three hours. The drug is highly bound to plasma protein. Bioavailability studies have demonstrated that the total absorption relative to the drug in a 20% alcoholic solution is 90%, resulting in peak levels approximately 65% of that of the drug in solution. Animal studies indicate that MINIPRESS (prazosin hydrochloride) is extensively metabolized, primarily by demethylation and conjugation, and excreted mainly via bile and feces. Less extensive human studies suggest similar metabolism and excretion in man.
MINIPRESS (prazosin hydrochloride) has been administered without any adverse drug interaction in limited clinical experience to date with the following: (1) cardiac glycosides—digitalis and digoxin; (2) hypoglycemics—insulin, chlorpropamide, phenformin, tolazamide, and tolbutamide; (3) tranquilizers and sedatives—chlordiazepoxide, diazepam, and phenobarbital; (4) antigout—allopurinol, colchicine, and probenecid; (5) antiarrhythmics—procainamide, propranolol (see WARNINGS however), and quinidine; and (6) analgesics, antipyretics and anti-inflammatories—propoxyphene, aspirin, indomethacin, and phenylbutazone.
Indications: MINIPRESS (prazosin hydrochloride) is indicated in the treatment of hypertension. As an antihypertensive drug, it is mild to moderate in activity. It can be used as the initial agent or it may be employed in a general treatment program in conjunction with a diuretic and/or other antihypertensive drugs as needed for proper patient response.
Warnings: MINIPRESS (prazosin hydrochloride) may cause syncope with sudden loss of consciousness. In most cases this is believed to be due to an excessive postural hypotensive effect, although occasionally the syncopal episode has been preceded by a bout of severe tachycardia with heart rates of 120–160 beats per minute. Syncopal episodes have usally occurred within 30 to 90 minutes of the initial dose of the drug; occasionally they have been reported in association with rapid dosage increases or the introduction of another antihypertensive drug into the regimen of a patient taking high doses of MINIPRESS (prazosin hydrochloride). The incidence of syncopal episodes is approximately 1% in patients given an initial dose of 2 mg or greater. Clinical trials conducted during the investigational phase of this drug suggest that syncopal episodes can be minimized by limiting the initial dose of the drug to 1 mg, by subsequently increasing the dosage slowly, and by introducing any additional antihypertensive drugs into the patient's regimen with caution (see DOSAGE AND ADMINISTRATION). Hypotension may develop in patients given MINIPRESS who are also receiving a beta-blocker such as propranolol.
If syncope occurs, the patient should be placed in the recumbent position and treated supportively as necessary. This adverse effect is self-limiting and in most cases does not recur after the initial period of therapy or during subsequent dose titration.
Patients should always be started on the 1 mg capsules of MINIPRESS (prazosin hydrochloride). The 2 and 5 mg capsules are not indicated for initial therapy.
More common than loss of consciousness are the symptoms often associated with lowering of the blood pressure, namely, dizziness and lightheadedness. The patient should be cautioned about these possible adverse effects and advised what measures to take should they develop. The patient should also be cautioned to avoid situations where injury could result should syncope occur during the initiation of MINIPRESS (prazosin hydrochloride) therapy.
Usage in Pregnancy:
Although no teratogenic effects were seen in animal testing, the safety of MINIPRESS (prazosin hydrochloride) in pregnancy has not been established. MINIPRESS (prazosin hydrochloride) is not recommended in pregnant women unless the potential benefit outweighs potential risk to mother and fetus.
Usage in Children:
No clinical experience is available with the use of MINIPRESS (prazosin hydrochloride) in children.
Adverse Reactions: The most common reactions associated with MINIPRESS (prazosin hydrochloride) therapy are: dizziness 10.3%, headache 7.8%, drowsiness 7.6%, lack of energy 6.9%, weakness 6.5%, palpitations 5.3%, and nausea 4.9%. In most instances side effects have disappeared with continued therapy or have been tolerated with no decrease in dose of drug.
The following reactions have been associated with MINIPRESS (prazosin hydrochloride), some of them rarely. (In some instances exact causal relationships have not been established).
Gastrointestinal: vomiting, diarrhea, constipation, abdominal discomfort and/or pain.
Cardiovascular: edema, dyspnea, syncope, tachycardia.
Central Nervous System: nervousness, vertigo, depression, paresthesia.

Dermatologic: rash, pruritus.
Genitourinary: urinary frequency, incontinence, impotence.
EENT: blurred vision, reddened sclera, epistaxis, tinnitus, dry mouth, nasal congestion.
Other: diaphoresis.
Single reports of pigmentary mottling and serous retinopathy, and a few reports of cataract development or disappearance have been reported. In these instances, the exact causal relationship has not been established because the baseline observations were frequently inadequate.
In more specific slit-lamp and funduscopic studies, which included adequate baseline examinations, no drug-related abnormal ophthalmological findings have been reported.
Dosage and Administration: The dose of MINIPRESS (prazosin hydrochloride) should be adjusted according to the patient's individual blood pressure response. The following is a guide to its administration:
Initial Dose:
1 mg two or three times a day. (See Warnings)
Maintenance Dose:
Dosage may be slowly increased to a total daily dose of 20 mg given in divided doses. The therapeutic dosages most commonly employed have ranged from 6 mg to 15 mg daily given in divided doses. Doses higher than 20 mg usually do not increase efficacy, however a few patients may benefit from further increases up to a daily dose of 40 mg given in divided doses. After initial titration some patients can be maintained adequately on a twice daily dosage regimen.
Use With Other Drugs:
When adding a diuretic or other antihypertensive agent, the dose of MINIPRESS (prazosin hydrochloride) should be reduced to 1 mg or 2 mg three times a day and retitration then carried out.
Overdosage: Accidental ingestion of at least 50 mg of MINIPRESS (prazosin hydrochloride) in a two year old child resulted in profound drowsiness and depressed reflexes. No decrease in blood pressure was noted. Recovery was uneventful.
Should overdosage lead to hypotension, support of the cardiovascular system is of first importance. Restoration of blood pressure and normalization of heart rate may be accomplished by keeping the patient in the supine position. If this measure is inadequate, shock should first be treated with volume expanders. If necessary, vasopressors should then be used. Renal function should be monitored and supported as needed. Laboratory data indicate MINIPRESS (prazosin hydrochloride) is not dialysable because it is protein bound.
Toxicology: Testicular changes, necrosis and atrophy have occurred at 25 mg/kg/day (60 times the usual maximum recommended dose of 20 mg per day in humans) in long term (one year or more) studies in rats and dogs. No testicular changes were seen in rats or dogs at the 10 mg/kg/day level (24 times the usual maximum recommended dose of 20 mg per day in humans). In view of the testicular changes observed in animals, 105 patients on long term MINIPRESS (prazosin hydrochloride) therapy were monitored for 17-ketosteroid excretion and no changes indicating a drug effect were observed. In addition, 27 males on MINIPRESS (prazosin hydrochloride) alone for up to 51 months did not demonstrate changes in sperm morphology suggestive of drug effect.
How Supplied: MINIPRESS (prazosin hydrochloride) is available in 1 mg (white #431), 2 mg (pink and white #437) capsules in bottles of 250, 1000, and unit dose institutional packages of 100 (10 × 10's); and 5 mg (blue and white #438) capsules in bottles of 250, 500 and unit dose institutional packages of 100 (10 × 10's).
60-2318-00-5
Literature Available—Yes.
[*Shown in Product Identification Section*]

MODERIL® ℞
(rescinnamine)
TABLETS

Description: Rescinnamine is a pure crystalline alkaloid that has been identified chemically as the 3,4,5-trimethoxycinnamic acid ester of methyl reserpate. Pure rescinnamine occurs as white, needle-shaped crystals that are readily absorbed when ingested.
Moderil is available as oval, scored salmon tablets providing 0.5 mg. of crystalline rescinnamine or as oval, scored yellow tablets providing 0.25 mg. of crystalline rescinnamine.
Actions: Rescinnamine probably produces its antihypertensive effects through depletion of tissue stores of catecholamines (epinephrine and norepinephrine) from peripheral sites. By contrast, its sedative and tranquilizing properties are thought to be related to depletion of 5-hydroxytryptamine from the brain.
Rescinnamine is characterized by slow onset of action and sustained effect. Both its cardiovascular and central nervous system effects may persist following withdrawal of the drug.
Indications: Indicated in the treatment of mild essential hypertension.
Contraindications: Do not use in patients with known hypersensitivity, mental depression—especially with suicidal tendencies, active peptic ulcer, and ulcerative colitis. It is also contraindicated in patients receiving electroconvulsive therapy.
Warnings: Extreme caution should be exercised in treating patients with a history of mental depression. Discontinue the drug at the first sign of despondency, early morning insomnia, loss of appetite, impotence, or self-depreciation. Drug-induced depression may persist for several months after drug withdrawal and may be severe enough to result in suicide.
Usage in pregnancy: The safety of rescinnamine for use during pregnancy or lactation has not been established. Therefore, the drug should be used in pregnant patients or in women of child-bearing potential only when, in the judgment of the physician, its use is deemed essential to the welfare of the patient. Increased respiratory secretions, nasal congestion, cyanosis, and anorexia may occur in infants born to rescinnamine-treated mothers, since this preparation is known to cross the placental barrier, appearing in cord blood and breast milk.
Precautions: Because Rauwolfia preparations increase gastrointestinal motility and secretion, this drug should be used cautiously in patients with a history of peptic ulcer, ulcerative colitis, or gallstones where biliary colic may be precipitated.
Caution should be exercised when treating hypertensive patients with renal insufficiency since they adjust poorly to lowered blood pressure levels.
Use rescinnamine cautiously with digitalis and quinidine since cardiac arrhythmias have occurred with Rauwolfia preparations.
Preoperative withdrawal of rescinnamine does not assure that circulatory instability will not occur. It is important that the anesthesiologist be aware of the patient's drug intake and consider this in the over-all management, since hypotension has occurred in patients receiving Rauwolfia preparations. Anticholinergic and/or adrenergic drugs (metaraminol, norepinephrine) have been employed to treat adverse vagocirculatory effects.
Adverse Reactions: Rauwolfia preparations have caused gastrointestinal reactions including hypersecretion, nausea and vomiting, anorexia, and diarrhea; cardiovascular reactions including angina-like symptoms, arrhythmias particularly when used concurrently with digitalis or quinidine, and bradycardia; and central nervous system reactions including drowsiness, depression, nervousness, paradoxical anxiety, nightmares, rare parkinsonian syndrome, C.N.S. sensitization manifested by dull sensorium, deafness, glaucoma, uveitis, and optic atrophy. Nasal congestion is a frequent complaint; and pruritus, rash, dryness of mouth, dizziness, headache, dyspnea, purpura, impotence or decreased libido, dysuria, muscular aches, conjunctival injection, and weight gain have been reported. Extrapyramidal tract symptoms have also occurred. These reactions are usually reversible and disappear when the drug is discontinued.
Water retention with edema in patients with hypertensive vascular disease may occur rarely, but the condition generally clears with cessation of therapy, or with the administration of a diuretic agent.
Dosage and Administration: For adults the average initial dose is 0.5 mg. orally, twice daily. Increase dosage gradually, if necessary. Maintenance doses may vary from 0.25 mg. to 0.5 mg. daily. Higher doses should be used cautiously because serious mental depression and other side effects may be increased considerably.
Concomitant use of rescinnamine and ganglionic blocking agents, guanethidine, veratrum, hydralazine, methyldopa, chlorthalidone, or thiazides necessitates careful titration of dosage with each agent.
Supply:
0.25 mg. tablets, oval, scored, yellow (imprinted with code number 441): bottles of 100
0.5 mg. tablets, oval, scored, salmon (imprinted with code number 442): bottles of 100
(60-0695-00-7)
[*Shown in Product Identification Section*]

Buffered ℞
PFIZERPEN® for Injection
(penicillin G potassium)

Description: Buffered Pfizerpen (penicillin G potassium) for Injection is a sterile, pyrogen-free powder which is stable for 36 months when stored at room temperature.
Each million units contains approximately 6.8 milligrams of sodium (0.3 mEq.) and 65.6 milligrams of potassium (1.68 mEq.).
Actions and Pharmacology: Penicillin G exerts a bactericidal action against penicillin-sensitive microorganisms during the stage of active multiplication. It acts through the inhibition of biosynthesis of cell wall mucopeptide. It is not active against the penicillinase-producing bacteria, which include many strains of staphylococci. Penicillin G exerts high in vitro activity against staphylococci (except penicillinase-producing strains), streptococci (groups A, C, G, H, L, and M) and pneumococci. Other organisms sensitive to penicillin G are *N. gonorrhoeae, Corynebacterium diphtheriae, Bacillus anthracis,* Clostridia, *Actinomyces bovis, Streptobacillus moniliformis, Listeria monocytogenes* and Leptospira. *Treponema pallidum* is extremely sensitive to the bactericidal action of penicillin G. Some species of gram-negative bacilli are sensitive to moderate to high concentrations of the drug obtained with intravenous administration. These include most strains of *Escherichia coli,* all strains of *Proteus mirabilis,* Salmonella and Shigella and some strains of *Aerobacter aerogenes* and *Alcaligenes fecalis.*
Sensitivity Plate Testing: If the Kirby-Bauer method of disc sensitivity is used, a 10 unit penicillin disc should give a zone greater than 28 mm. when tested againt a penicillin-sensitive bacterial strain.
Aqueous penicillin G is rapidly absorbed following both intramuscular and subcutaneous injection. Approximately 60 percent of the total dose of 300,000 units is excreted in the urine within this 5-hour period. For this reason high and frequent doses are required to maintain the elevated serum levels desirable in treating certain severe infections in individu-

Continued on next page

Pfizer—Cont.

als with normal kidney function. In neonates and young infants and in individuals with impaired kidney function, excretion is considerably delayed.

Indications: Aqueous penicillin G (parenteral) is indicated in the therapy of severe infections caused by penicillin G sensitive microorganisms when rapid and high penicillinemia is required. Therapy should be guided by bacteriological studies (including sensitivity tests) and by clinical response.

The following infections will usually respond to adequate dosage of aqueous penicillin G (parenteral):

Streptococcal infections.

NOTE: Streptococci in groups A, C, H, G, L, and M are very sensitive to penicillin G. Some group D organisms are sensitive to the high serum levels obtained with aqueous penicillin G.

Aqueous penicillin (parenteral) is the penicillin dosage form of choice for bacteremia, empyema, severe pneumonia, pericarditis, endocarditis, meningitis and other severe infections caused by sensitive strains of the gram-positive species listed above.

Pneumococcal infections.

Staphylococcal infections—penicillin G sensitive.

Other infections:

Anthrax.

Actinomycosis.

Clostridial infections (including tetanus).

Diphtheria (to prevent carrier state).

Erysipeloid (Erysipelothrix insidiosa) endocarditis.

Fusospirochetal infections-severe infections of the oropharynx (Vincent's), lower respiratory tract and genital area due to *Fusobacterium fusiformisans* spirochetes.

Gram-negative bacillary infections (bacteremias)—*(E. coli, A. aerogenes, A. faecalis,* Salmonella, Shigella and *P. mirabilis)*

Listeria infections *(Listeria monocytogenes).*

Meningitis and endocarditis.

Pasteurella infections *(pasteurella multocida).*

Bacteremia and meningitis.

Rat-bite fever *(Spirillum minus* or *Streptobacillus moniliformis*

Gonorrheal endocarditis and arthritis *(N. gonorrhoeae).*

Syphilis *(T. pallidum)* including congenital syphilis.

Meningococcic meningitis.

Prophylaxis against bacterial endocarditis in patients with rheumatic or congenital heart disease when undergoing dental or upper respiratory tract surgery or instrumentation, surgery of the lower intestinal tract, childbirth, and instrumentation of the genitourinary tract.

NOTE: Because patients who have a past history of rheumatic fever and are receiving continuous prophylaxis may harbor increased numbers of penicillin-resistant organisms, use of another prophylactic antiinfective agent should be considered. If penicillin is to be used in these patients at surgery, the regular rheumatic fever program should be interrupted 1 week prior to the contemplated surgery. At the time of surgery, penicillin may be reinstituted as a prophylactic measure against the hazards of surgically induced bacteremia.

Contraindications: A history of a previous hypersensitivity reaction to any of the penicillins is a contraindication.

Warning: Serious and occasionally fatal hypersensitivity (anaphylactoid) reactions have been reported in patients on penicillin therapy. Although anaphylaxis is more frequent following parenteral therapy it has occurred in patients on oral penicillins. These reactions are more apt to occur in individuals with a history of sensitivity to multiple allergens.

There have been well documented reports of individuals with a history of penicillin hypersensitivity reactions who have experienced severe hypersensitivity reactions when treated with a cephalosporin. Before therapy with a penicillin, careful inquiry should be made concerning previous hypersensitivity reactions to penicillins, cephalosporins, and other allergens. If an allergic reaction occurs, the drug should be discontinued and the patient treated with the usual agents e.g., pressor amines, antihistamines and corticosteroids.

Precautions: Penicillin should be used with caution in individuals with histories of significant allergies and/or asthma.

In streptococcal infections, therapy must be sufficient to eliminate the organism (10 days minimum) otherwise the sequelae of streptococcal disease may occur. Cultures should be taken following the completion of treatment to determine whether streptococci have been eradicated.

Aqueous penicillin G by the intravenous route in high doses (above 10 million units), should be administered slowly because of the adverse effects of electrolyte imbalance from either the potassium or sodium content of the penicillin. The patient's renal, cardiac and vascular status should be evaluated and if impairment of function is suspected or known to exist a reduction in the total dosage should be considered. Frequent evaluation of electrolyte balance, renal and hematopoietic function is recommended during therapy when high doses of intravenous aqueous penicillin G are used.

Prolonged use of antibiotics may promote overgrowth of nonsusceptible organisms, including fungi. Should superinfection occur, appropriate measures should be taken. Indwelling intravenous catheters encourage superinfections and should be avoided whenever possible.

Therapy of susceptible infections should be accompanied by any indicated surgical procedures.

Adverse Reactions: Penicillin is a substance of low toxicity but does have a significant index of sensitization. The following hypersensitivity reactions have been reported: skin rashes ranging from maculopapular eruptions to exfoliative dermatitis: urticaria and reactions resembling serum sickness, including chills, fever, edema, arthralgia and prostration. Severe and occasionally fatal anaphylaxis has occurred (see Warnings).

Hemolytic anemia, leucopenia, thrombocytopenia, nephropathy, and neuropathy are rarely observed adverse reactions and are usually associated with high intravenous dosage. Patients given continuous intravenous therapy with penicillin G potassium in high dosage (10 million to 100 million units daily) may suffer severe or even fatal potassium poisoning, particularly if renal insufficiency is present. Hyperreflexia, convulsions and coma may be indicative of this syndrome.

Cardiac arrhythmias and cardiac arrest may also occur. (High dosage of penicillin G sodium may result in congestive heart failure due to high sodium intake.)

The Jarisch-Herxheimer reaction has been reported in patients treated for syphilis.

Administration and Dosage: *Severe infections due to Susceptible Strains of Streptococci, Pneumococci and Staphylococci*—bacteremia, pneumonia, endocarditis, pericarditis, empyema, meningitis and other severe infections—a minimum of 5 million units daily.

Syphilis—Aqueous penicillin G may be used in the treatment of acquired and congenital syphilis, but because of the necessity of frequent dosage, hospitalization is recommended. Dosage and duration of therapy will be determined by age of patient and stage of the disease.

Gonorrheal Endocarditis—a minimum of 5 million units daily.

Meningococcic meningitis—1-2 million units intramuscularly every 2 hours, or continuous I.V. drip of 20-30 million units/day.

Actinomycosis—1-6 million units/day for cervico-facial cases; 10-20 million units/day for thoracic and abdominal disease.

Clostridial infections—20 million units/day; penicillin is adjunctive therapy to antitoxin.

Fusospirochetal infections—severe infections of oropharynx, lower respiratory tract and genital area—5-10 million units/day.

Rat-bite Fever (Spirillum minus or streptobacillus moniliformis)—12-15 million units/day for 3-4 weeks.

Listeria infections (Listeria monocytogenes).

Neonates—500,000 to 1 million units/day.

Adults with meningitis—15-20 million units/day for 2 weeks.

Adults with endocarditis—15-20 million units/day for 4 weeks.

Pasteurella infections (Pasteurella multocida).

Bacteremia and meningitis—4-6 million units/day for 2 weeks.

Erysipeloid (Erysipelothrix insidiosa).

Endocarditis 2-20 million units/day for 4-6 weeks.

Gram-negative bacillary infections (E. coli, A. aerogenes, A. faecalis, Salmonella, Shigella and *Proteus mirabilis).*

Bacteremia—20-80 million units/day.

Diphtheria (carrier state).

300,000—400,000 unts of penicillin/day in divided doses for 10-12 days.

Anthrax—

A minimum of 5 million units of penicillin/day in divided doses until cure is effected.

Prophylaxis *Against Bacterial Endocarditis* in patients with rheumatic or congenital heart disease when undergoing dental or other operative procedures.

600,000 units of penicillin G procaine the day of operation.

600,000 units of aqueous penicillin G (K or Na) 1-2 hours before operation.

600,000 units of penicillin G procaine daily for 2 days following operation.

The following table shows the amount of solvent required for solution of various concentrations.

[See table at left].

Desired Concentration (units/ml)	Approx. Volume (ml) 1,000,000 units	Solvent for Vial of 5,000,000 units	Infusion Only 20,000,000 units
50,000	19.6	...	...
100,000	9.6	...	...
250,000	3.6	18.2	74.2
500,000	1.6	8.2	32.4
750,000	...	4.8	...
1,000,000	...	3.2	11.5

When the required volume of solvent is greater than the capacity of the vial, the penicillin can be dissolved by first injecting only a portion of the solvent into the vial, then withdrawing the resultant solution and combining it with the remainder of the solvent in a larger sterile container.

Buffered Pfizerpen (penicillin G potassium) for Injection is highly water soluble. It may be dissolved in small amounts of Water for Injection, or Sterile Isotonic Sodium Chloride solution for Parenteral Use. All solutions should be stored in a refrigerator. When refrigerated, penicillin solutions may be stored for seven days without significant loss of potency.

Buffered Pfizerpen (penicillin G potassium) for Injection may be given intramuscularly or by continuous intravenous drip for dosages of 500,000, 1,000,000, or 5,000,000 units. It is also suitable for intrapleural, intraarticular, and other local instillations.

THE 20,000,000 UNIT DOSAGE MAY BE ADMINISTERED BY INTRAVENOUS INFUSION ONLY.

(1) Intramuscular Injection: Keep total volume of injection small. The intramuscular route is the preferred route of administration. Solutions containing up to 100,000 units of penicillin per ml of diluent may be used with a minimum of discomfort. Greater concentration of penicillin G per ml is physically possible and may be employed where therapy demands. When large dosages are required, it may be advisable to administer aqueous solutions of penicillin by means of continuous intravenous drip.

(2) Continuous Intravenous Drip: Determine the volume of fluid and rate of its administration required by the patient in a 24-hour period in the usual manner for fluid therapy, and add the appropriate daily dosage of penicillin to this fluid. For example, if an adult patient requires 2 liters of fluid in 24 hours and a daily dosage of 10 million units of penicillin, add 5 million units to 1 liter and adjust the rate of flow so that the liter will be infused in 12 hours.

(3) Intrapleural or Other Local Infusion: If fluid is aspirated, give infusion in a volume equal to ¼ or ½ the amount of fluid aspirated; otherwise, prepare as for intramuscular injection.

(4) Intrathecal Use: The intrathecal use of penicillin in meningitis must be highly individualized. It should be employed only with full consideration of the possible irritating effects of penicillin when used by this route. The preferred route of therapy in bacterial meningitides is intravenous, supplemented by intramuscular injection.

How Supplied: Buffered Pfizerpen (penicillin G potassium) for Injection is available in vials containing respectively 1,000,000, 5,000,000, and 20,000,000 units of dry powder for reconstitution; buffered with sodium citrate and citric acid to an optimum pH.

Each million units contain approximately 6.8 milligrams of sodium (0.3 mEq.) and 65.6 milligrams of potassium (1.68 mEq.).

60-0077-00-3

RENESE® ℞
(polythiazide)
TABLETS
for Oral Administration

Description: Renese is designated generically as polythiazide, and chemically as 2-methyl-3, 4-dihydro-3-(2,2,2-trifluoroethylthiomethyl)-6-chloro-7-sulfamyl 1,2,4-benzothiadiazine 1,1 dioxide. It is a white crystalline substance, insoluble in water but readily soluble in alkaline solution.

Action: The mechanism of action results in an interference with the renal tubular mechanism of electrolyte reabsorption. At maximal therapeutic dosage all thiazides are approximately equal in their diuretic potency. The mechanism whereby thiazides function in the control of hypertension is unknown.

Indications: Renese is indicated as adjunctive therapy in edema associated with congestive heart failure, hepatic cirrhosis, and corticosteroid and estrogen therapy.

Renese has also been found useful in edema due to various forms of renal dysfunction as: Nephrotic syndrome; Acute glomerulonephritis; and Chronic renal failure.

Renese is indicated in the management of hypertension either as the sole therapeutic agent or to enhance the effectiveness of other antihypertensive drugs in the more severe forms of hypertension.

Usage in Pregnancy: The routine use of diuretics in an otherwise healthy woman is inappropriate and exposes mother and fetus to unnecessary hazard. Diuretics do not prevent development of toxemia of pregnancy, and there is no satisfactory evidence that they are useful in the treatment of developed toxemia. Edema during pregnancy may arise from pathological causes or from the physiologic and mechanical consequences of pregnancy. Thiazides are indicated in pregnancy when edema is due to pathologic causes, just as they are in the absence of pregnancy (however, see Warnings, below). Dependent edema in pregnancy, resulting from restriction of venous return by the expanded uterus, is properly treated through elevation of the lower extremities and use of support hose; use of diuretics to lower intravascular volume in this case is illogical and unnecessary. There is hypervolemia during normal pregnancy which is harmful to neither the fetus nor the mother (in the absence of cardiovascular disease), but which is associated with edema, including generalized edema, in the majority of pregnant women. If this edema produces discomfort, increased recumbency will often provide relief. In rare instances, this edema may cause extreme discomfort which is not relieved by rest. In these cases, a short course of diuretics may provide relief and may be appropriate.

Contraindications: Anuria. Hypersensitivity to this or other sulfonamide derived drugs.

Warnings: Thiazides should be used with caution in severe renal disease. In patients with renal disease, thiazides may precipitate azotemia. Cumulative effects of the drug may develop in patients with impaired renal function. Thiazides should be used with caution in patients with impaired hepatic function or progressive liver disease, since minor alterations of fluid and electrolyte balance may precipitate hepatic coma.

Thiazides may add to or potentiate the action of other antihypertensive drugs. Potentiation occurs with ganglionic or peripheral adrenergic blocking drugs.

Sensitivity reactions may occur in patients with a history of allergy or bronchial asthma. The possibility of exacerbation or activation of systemic lupus erythematosus has been reported.

Usage in pregnancy. Thiazides cross the placental barrier and appear in cord blood. The use of thiazides in pregnant women requires that the anticipated benefit be weighed against possible hazards to the fetus. These hazards include fetal or neonatal jaundice, thrombocytopenia, and possibly other adverse reactions which have occurred in the adult.

Nursing Mothers. Thiazides appear in breast milk. If use of the drug is deemed essential, the patient should stop nursing.

Precautions: Periodic determination of serum electrolytes to detect possible electrolyte imbalance should be performed at appropriate intervals.

All patients receiving thiazide therapy should be observed for clinical signs of fluid or electrolyte imbalance; namely, hyponatremia, hypochloremic alkalosis, and hypokalemia. Serum and urine electrolyte determinations are particularly important when the patient is vomiting excessively or receiving parenteral fluids. Medication such as digitalis may also influence serum electrolytes. Warning signs, irrespective of cause, are: dryness of mouth, thirst, weakness, lethargy, drowsiness, restlessness, muscle pains or cramps, muscular fatigue, hypotension, oliguria, tachycardia, and gastrointestinal disturbances such as nausea and vomiting.

Hypokalemia may develop with thiazides as with any other potent diuretic, especially with brisk diuresis, when severe cirrhosis is present, or during concomitant use of corticosteroids or ACTH.

Interference with adequate oral electrolyte intake will also contribute to hypokalemia. Digitalis therapy may exaggerate metabolic effects of hypokalemia especially with reference to myocardial activity.

Any chloride deficit is generally mild and usually does not require specific treatment except under extraordinary circumstances (as in liver disease or renal disease). Dilutional hyponatremia may occur in edematous patients in hot weather; appropriate therapy is water restriction, rather than administration of salt except in rare instances when the hyponatremia is life threatening. In actual salt depletion, appropriate replacement is the therapy of choice.

Hyperuricemia may occur or frank gout may be precipitated in certain patients receiving thiazide therapy.

Insulin requirements in diabetic patients may be increased, decreased, or unchanged. Latent diabetes mellitus may become manifest during thiazide administration.

Thiazide drugs may increase the responsiveness to tubocurarine.

The antihypertensive effects of the drug may be enhanced in the postsympathectomy patient.

Thiazides may decrease arterial responsiveness to norepinephrine. This diminution is not sufficient to preclude effectiveness of the pressor agent for therapeutic use.

If progressive renal impairment becomes evident, as indicated by a rising nonprotein nitrogen or blood urea nitrogen, a careful reappraisal of therapy is necessary with consideration given to withholding or discontinuing diuretic therapy.

Thiazides may decrease serum PBI levels without signs of thyroid disturbance.

Adverse Reactions:

A. GASTROINTESTINAL SYSTEM REACTIONS

1. anorexia	6. diarrhea
2. gastric irritation	7. constipation
3. nausea	8. jaundice (intrahepatic cholestatic jaundice)
4. vomiting	9. pancreatitis
5. cramping	

B. CENTRAL NERVOUS SYSTEM REACTIONS

1. dizziness	4. headache
2. vertigo	5. xanthopsia
3. paresthesias	

C. HEMATOLOGIC REACTIONS

1. leukopenia	3. thrombocytopenia
2. agranulocytosis	4. aplastic anemia

D. DERMATOLOGIC–HYPERSENSITIVITY REACTIONS

1. purpura	5. necrotizing angiitis (vasculitis) (cutaneous vasculitis)
2. photosensitivity	
3. rash	
4. urticaria	

E. CARDIOVASCULAR REACTION

Orthostatic hypotension may occur and may be aggravated by alcohol, barbiturates or narcotics.

F. OTHER

1. hyperglycemia	4. muscle spasm
2. glycosuria	5. weakness
3. hyperuricemia	6. restlessness

Whenever adverse reactions are moderate or severe, thiazide dosage should be reduced or therapy withdrawn.

Dosage and Administration: Therapy should be individualized according to patient response. This therapy should be titrated to gain maximal therapeutic response as well as the minimal dose possible to maintain that therapeutic response. The usual dosage of Renese tablets for diuretic therapy is 1 to 4 mg daily, and for antihypertensive therapy is 2 to 4 mg daily.

How Supplied: RENESE (polythiazide) Tablets are available as:

1 mg white, scored tablets (imprinted with code number 375) in bottles of 100 and 1000.

2 mg yellow, scored tablets (imprinted with code number 376) in bottles of 100 and 1000.

Continued on next page

Pfizer—Cont.

4 mg white, scored tablets (imprinted with code number 377) in bottles of 100 and 1000.
(60-1116-00-2)

Literature Available: Yes.
[*Shown in Product Identification Section*]

RENESE®-R ℞

> **Warning**
> This fixed combination drug is not indicated for initial therapy of hypertension. Hypertension requires therapy titrated to the individual patient. If the fixed combination represents the dosage so determined, its use may be more convenient in patient management. The treatment of hypertension is not static, but must be reevaluated as conditions in each patient warrant.

RENESE-R tablets combine polythiazide and reserpine, two antihypertensive agents with complementary properties. Each blue, scored tablet of RENESE-R provides:
Renese (polythiazide) .... 2.0 mg
Reserpine .... 0.25 mg

Actions: RENESE (polythiazide) is a member of the benzothiadiazine (thiazide) family of diuretic/antihypertensive agents. RENESE (polythiazide) alone has demonstrated clinical effectiveness in lowering elevated blood pressure in patients without visible edema as well as in edematous hypertensive patients. This antihypertensive action probably comes about through depletion of sodium and fluid accumulation in the blood vessel wall.

RENESE (polythiazide) is 2-methyl-3,4-dihydro-3 (2,2,2-trifluoroethylthiomethyl)-6-chloro-7-sulfamyl 1,2,4-benzothiadiazine 1,1 dioxide.

Reserpine, an alkaloid of Rauwolfia serpentina has several complementary actions of benefit to the hypertensive patient, including a calming effect and a slowing of the pulse rate. Its ultimate effect in lowering blood pressure is thought to be due to vasodilatation unaccompanied by reduction in cardiac performance, probably as a result of depletion of norepinephrine from tissue receptor sites.

Since polythiazide reduces or eliminates the sodium and fluid retention frequently associated with hypertension, it enhances the efficacy of reserpine in lowering elevated blood pressure. RENESE-R often has been found to be more effective than equivalent doses of either agent alone. Both the cardiovascular and central nervous system effects may persist following withdrawal of the drug.

Indications: Hypertension (see box warning).

Contraindications:

A. Related to polythiazide:
1. Advanced renal or hepatic failure.
2. Hypersensitivity to this or other sulfonamide derivatives.

B. Related to reserpine:
1. Demonstrated hypersensitivity.
2. Mental depression.
3. Demonstrated peptic ulcer or ulcerative colitis.

Warnings: Serum electrolyte determinations are especially indicated for patients with severe derangement of metabolic processes, e.g., surgery, vomiting, or parenteral fluid therapy. Electrolyte imbalance may be caused by certain diseases such as cirrhosis, or it may result from drug therapy, such as therapy with corticosteroids. Patients with cirrhosis who are continually receiving RENESE-R should be observed carefully for the development of hepatic precoma or coma. Indications of impending hepatic failure are tremor, confusion, drowsiness, and hepatic fetor.

Thiazides may precipitate kidney failure and uremia in patients with pre-existing renal pathology and impaired renal function.

Available information tends to implicate all oral dosage forms of potassium salts ingested in solid form with or without thiazides in the etiology of nonspecific, small bowel lesions consisting of ulceration with or without stenosis, causing obstruction, hemorrhage and perforation, and frequently requiring surgery. Deaths due to these complications have been reported. All oral dosage forms of potassium salts ingested in solid form should be used only when adequate dietary supplementation is not practical and should be discontinued immediately if abdominal pain, distention, nausea, vomiting or gastrointestinal bleeding occur.

RENESE-R does not itself contain enteric-coated potassium.

Electroshock therapy should not be given within one week of cessation of reserpine.

Usage in Pregnancy and the Childbearing Age. Since thiazides appear in breast milk, the usage of polythiazide is contraindicated in nursing mothers. Thiazides cross the placental barrier and appear in cord blood. The safety of reserpine for use during pregnancy or lactation has not been established. When polythiazide and reserpine are used in women of childbearing age, the potential benefits of this drug combination should be weighed against the possible hazards to the fetus. The hazards include fetal or neonatal jaundice, thrombocytopenia, and possibly other adverse reactions which have occurred in the adult.

Precautions: Since all diuretic agents may reduce serum levels of sodium, chloride, and potassium, especially with brisk diuresis or when used concurrently with steroids, patients should be observed regularly for early signs of fluid or electrolyte imbalance and serum electrolyte studies should be performed periodically. Warning signs of possible electrolyte imbalance irrespective of cause include fatigue, muscle cramps, gastrointestinal disturbances, lethargy, oliguria, and tachycardia. In extreme cases, hypotension, shock, and coma may develop. Frequently, serum electrolyte levels do not correlate with signs or symptoms of electrolyte imbalance. Unduly restricted salt intake as well as concurrent administration of digitalis may exaggerate metabolic effects of hypokalemia. A favorable ratio of potassium to sodium excretion lessens the possibility of hypokalemia. However, should this occur or be suspected, foods with a high potassium content (bananas, apricots, citrus fruits, prune juice, etc.) should be given. When necessary, oral potassium supplements may be administered. If other antihypertensive agents are used concurrently, lower than usual doses of RENESE-R and of the other agents should be considered.

Like other thiazide diuretics, polythiazide may cause a rise in serum uric acid levels with or without overt symptoms of gout. Thiazides are known to disturb glucose tolerance in some individuals, even when there is no history of glucose intolerance or diabetes in the individual or his family. Likewise, thiazides may decrease PBI levels without signs of thyroid disturbances.

Thiazide drugs may augment the paralyzing actions of tubocurarine, and may decrease the arterial responsiveness to norepinephrine. Extra precautions may be necessary in patients who may require these drugs or their derivatives, as in surgery. The antihypertensive effects of the drug may be enhanced in the postsympathectomy patient.

Reserpine: Since reserpine may increase gastric acid secretion, it should be used cautiously in patients with a history of peptic ulcer or ulcerative colitis. Extreme caution is needed in patients with a history of mental depression, and reserpine should be discontinued at the first sign of depressive symptoms. Parkinsonism and confusion have been encountered, particularly in psychiatric patients, and constitute an indication for withdrawal of the drug. Caution should be exercised when treating patients with impairment of renal function, as lowered blood pressure may result in further decompensation and embarrassment of function. Reserpine should be used cautiously with digitalis or quinidine as the concurrent use may enhance the appearance of arrhythmias. Discontinue the drug one to two weeks prior to elective surgery since an unexpected degree of hypotension and bradycardia have been reported in patients receiving anesthetic agents concurrently with reserpine, probably due to a reduced responsiveness to norepinephrine. For emergency surgical procedures vagal blocking agents may be given parenterally to prevent or reverse hypotension and/or bradycardia. Reserpine may cause increased appetite and weight gain in some patients.

Adverse Reactions: **Polythiazide:** Side effects such as nausea, vertigo, weakness, paresthesias, and fatigue occur but seldom require cessation of therapy. Most of these can be overcome by reducing the dose or taking measures to improve electrolyte imbalance. Maculopapular skin rash has been reported, as has reversible cholestatic jaundice. Leukopenia (neutropenia) and purpura, with or without thrombocytopenia, have been reported rarely, and agranulocytosis and aplastic anemia have been reported with the older thiazides but not as yet with the newer compounds such as polythiazide. Pancreatitis, photosensitivity reactions, gastrointestinal disturbances, headache, xanthopsia, necrotizing angiitis, orthostatic hypotension, and dizziness have all been reported following the use of the benzothiadiazine class of diuretics.

Reserpine: Gastrointestinal reactions include hypersecretion, nausea and vomiting, anorexia, and diarrhea. Cardiovascular reactions reported include angina-like symptoms, arrhythmias—particularly when used concurrently with digitalis or quinidine, flushing of the skin, and bradycardia. Central nervous system reactions range from drowsiness, depression, nervousness, paradoxical anxiety, nightmares, and a rare Parkinsonian syndrome to C.N.S. sensitization manifested by deafness, glaucoma, uveitis, and optic atrophy. Nasal congestion is a frequent complaint, and pruritus, rash, dryness of mouth, dizziness, headache, purpura, impotence or decreased libido, and miosis have been reported with use of this drug. These reactions are usually reversible and disappear when the drug is discontinued.

Dosage: As determined by individual titration (see box warning).

Initial dosages of the combination should conform to those dosages of the individual components established during titration.

Maintenance dosages range from ½ tablet to 2 tablets daily. Dosage of other antihypertensive agents, particularly ganglionic blockers, that are used concomitantly should be reduced.

Supply: RENESE-R tablets (2 mg polythiazide-0.25 mg reserpine) are available as blue, scored tablets (imprinted with code number 446) in bottles of 100 and 1,000.

Literature Available: Yes. (60-1200-00-7)
[*Shown in Product Identification Section*]

SINEQUAN® ℞
(doxepin HCl)
Capsules
Oral Concentrate

Description: SINEQUAN (doxepin hydrochloride) is one of a class of psychotherapeutic agents known as dibenzoxepin tricyclic compounds. The molecular formula of the compound is $C_{19}H_{21}NO \cdot HCl$ having a molecular weight of 316. It is a white crystalline solid readily soluble in water, lower alcohols and chloroform.

Chemistry: SINEQUAN (doxepin HCl) is a dibenzoxepin derivative and is the first of a family of tricyclic psychotherapeutic agents. Specifically, it is an isomeric mixture of N, N-dimethyl-dibenz (b,e) oxepin-$\Delta^{11(6H)}$, γ-propylamine hydrochloride.

Actions: The mechanism of action of SINEQUAN (doxepin HCl) is not definitely known. It is not a central nervous system stimulant nor a monoamine oxidase inhibitor. The current hypothesis is that the clinical effects are due, at least in part, to influences on the adrenergic activity at the synapses so that deactivation of norepinephrine by reuptake into the nerve terminals is prevented. Animal studies suggest that doxepin HCl does not appreciably antagonize the antihypertensive action of guanethidine. In animal studies anticholinergic, antiserotonin and antihistamine effects on smooth muscle have been demonstrated. At higher than usual clinical doses, norepinephrine response was potentiated in animals. This effect was not demonstrated in humans.

At clinical dosages up to 150 mg per day, SINEQUAN can be given to man concomitantly with guanethidine and related compounds without blocking the antihypertensive effect. At dosages above 150 mg per day blocking of the antihypertensive effect of these compounds has been reported.

There have been no reports of physical dependency or withdrawal symptoms associated with SINEQUAN therapy. This is consistent with the virtual absence of euphoria as a side effect and the lack of addiction potential characteristic of this type of chemical compound.

Indications: SINEQUAN is recommended for the treatment of:

1. Psychoneurotic patients with depression and/or anxiety.
2. Depression and/or anxiety associated with alcoholism (not to be taken concomitantly with alcohol).
3. Depression and/or anxiety associated with organic disease (the possibility of drug interaction should be considered if the patient is receiving other drugs concomitantly).
4. Psychotic depressive disorders with associated anxiety including involutional depression and manic-depressive disorders.

The target symptoms of psychoneurosis that respond particularly well to SINEQUAN include anxiety, tension, depression, somatic symptoms and concerns, sleep disturbances, guilt, lack of energy, fear, apprehension and worry.

Clinical experience has shown that SINEQUAN is safe and well-tolerated even in the elderly patient. Owing to lack of clinical experience in the pediatric population, SINEQUAN is not recommended for use in children under 12 years of age.

Contraindications: SINEQUAN is contraindicated in individuals who have shown hypersensitivity to the drug. Possibility of cross sensitivity with other dibenzoxepines should be kept in mind.

SINEQUAN is contraindicated in patients with glaucoma or a tendency to urinary retention. These disorders should be ruled out, particularly in older patients.

Warnings: The once-a-day dosage regimen of SINEQUAN in patients with intercurrent illness or patients taking other medications should be carefully adjusted. This is especially important in patients receiving other medications with anticholinergic effects.

Usage in Geriatrics

The use of SINEQUAN on a once-a-day dosage regimen in geriatric patients should be adjusted carefully based on the patient's condition.

Usage in Pregnancy

Reproduction studies have been performed in rats, rabbits, monkeys and dogs and there was no evidence of harm to the animal fetus. The relevance to humans is not known. Since there is no experience in pregnant women who have received this drug, safety in pregnancy has not been established. There are no data with respect to the secretion of the drug in human milk and its effect on the nursing infant.

Usage in Children

The use of SINEQUAN in children under 12 years of age is not recommended because safe conditions for its use have not been established.

MAO Inhibitors

Serious side effects and even death have been reported following the concomitant use of certain drugs with MAO inhibitors. Therefore, MAO inhibitors should be discontinued at least two weeks prior to the cautious initiation of therapy with SINEQUAN. The exact length of time may vary and is dependent upon the particular MAO inhibitor being used, the length of time it has been administered, and the dosage involved.

Usage with Alcohol

It should be borne in mind that alcohol ingestion may increase the danger inherent in any intentional or unintentional SINEQUAN overdosage. This is especially important in patients who may use alcohol excessively.

Precautions: Since drowsiness may occur with the use of this drug, patients should be warned of the possibility and cautioned against driving a car or operating dangerous machinery while taking the drug. Patients should also be cautioned that their response to alcohol may be potentiated.

Since suicide is an inherent risk in any depressed patient and may remain so until significant improvement has occurred, patients should be closely supervised during the early course of therapy. Prescriptions should be written for the smallest feasible amount.

Should increased symptoms of psychosis or shift to manic symptomatology occur, it may be necessary to reduce dosage or add a major tranquilizer to the dosage regimen.

Adverse Reactions:

NOTE: Some of the adverse reactions noted below have not been specifically reported with SINEQUAN use. However, due to the close pharmacological similarities among the tricyclics, the reactions should be considered when prescribing SINEQUAN (doxepin HCl).

Anticholinergic Effects: Dry mouth, blurred vision, constipation, and urinary retention have been reported. If they do not subside with continued therapy, or become severe, it may be necessary to reduce the dosage.

Central Nervous System Effects: Drowsiness is the most commonly noticed side effect. This tends to disappear as therapy is continued. Other infrequently reported CNS side effects are confusion, disorientation, hallucinations, numbness, paresthesias, ataxia, and extrapyramidal symptoms and seizures.

Cardiovascular: Cardiovascular effects including hypotension and tachycardia have been reported occasionally.

Allergic: Skin rash, edema, photosensitization, and pruritus have occasionally occurred.

Hematologic: Eosinophilia has been reported in a few patients. There have been occasional reports of bone marrow depression manifesting as agranulocytosis, leukopenia, thrombocytopenia, and purpura.

Gastrointestinal: Nausea, vomiting, indigestion, taste disturbances, diarrhea, anorexia, and aphthous stomatitis have been reported. (See anticholinergic effects.)

Endocrine: Raised or lowered libido, testicular swelling, gynecomastia in males, enlargement of breasts and galactorrhea in the female, raising or lowering of blood sugar levels have been reported with tricyclic administration.

Other: Dizziness, tinnitus, weight gain, sweating, chills, fatigue, weakness, flushing, jaundice, alopecia, and headache have been occasionally observed as adverse effects.

Dosage and Administration: For most patients with illness of mild to moderate severity, a starting daily dose of 75 mg is recommended. Dosage may subsequently be increased or decreased at appropriate intervals and according to individual response. The usual optimum dose range is 75 mg/day to 150 mg/day.

In more severely ill patients higher doses may be required with subsequent gradual increase to 300 mg/day if necessary. Additional therapeutic effect is rarely to be obtained by exceeding a dose of 300 mg/day.

In patients with very mild symptomatology or emotional symptoms accompanying organic disease, lower doses may suffice. Some of these patients have been controlled on doses as low as 25-50 mg/day.

The total daily dosage of SINEQUAN may be given on a divided or once-a-day dosage schedule. If the once-a-day schedule is employed the maximum recommended dose is 150 mg/day. This dose may be given at bedtime. **The 150 mg capsule strength is intended for maintenance therapy only and is not recommended for initiation of treatment.**

Anti-anxiety effect is apparent before the antidepressant effect. Optimal antidepressant effect may not be evident for two to three weeks.

Overdosage:

A. Signs and Symptoms
   1. Mild: Drowsiness, stupor, blurred vision, excessive dryness of mouth.
   2. Severe: Respiratory depression, hypotension, coma, convulsions, cardiac arrhythmias and tachycardias.

   Also: urinary retention (bladder atony), decreased gastrointestinal motility (paralytic ileus), hyperthermia (or hypothermia), hypertension, dilated pupils, hyperactive reflexes.

B. Management and Treatment
   1. Mild: Observation and supportive therapy is all that is usually necessary.
   2. Severe: Medical management of severe SINEQUAN overdosage consists of aggressive supportive therapy. If the patient is conscious, gastric lavage, with appropriate precautions to prevent pulmonary aspiration, should be performed even though SINEQUAN is rapidly absorbed. The use of activated charcoal has been recommended, as has been continuous gastric lavage with saline for 24 hours or more. An adequate airway should be established in comatose patients and assisted ventilation used if necessary. EKG monitoring may be required for several days, since relapse after apparent recovery has been reported. Arrhythmias should be treated with the appropriate antiarrhythmic agent. It has been reported that many of the cardiovascular and CNS symptoms of tricyclic antidepressant poisoning in adults may be reversed by the slow intravenous administration of 1 mg to 3 mg of physostigmine salicylate. Because physostigmine is rapidly metabolized, the dosage should be repeated as required. Convulsions may respond to standard anticonvulsant therapy, however, barbiturates may potentiate any respiratory depression. Dialysis and forced diuresis generally are not of value in the management of overdosage due to high tissue and protein binding of SINEQUAN.

Supply:

SINEQUAN is available as capsules containing doxepin HCl equivalent to: 10 mg (imprinted with code #534), 75 mg (imprinted with code #539), and 100 mg (imprinted with code #538) doxepin; bottles of 100, 1000, and unit-dose packages of 100 (10 × 10's).

25 mg (imprinted with code #535) and 50 mg (imprinted with code #536) doxepin: bottles

Continued on next page

Pfizer—Cont.

of 100, 1000, 5000, and unit-dose packages of 100 (10 × 10's).
150 mg (imprinted with code #537) doxepin: bottles of 50, 500, and unit-dose packages of 100 (10 × 10's).

SINEQUAN Oral Concentrate is available in 120 ml bottles with an accompanying dropper calibrated at 5 mg, 10 mg, 15 mg, 20 mg, and 25 mg. Each ml contains doxepin HCl equivalent to 10 mg doxepin. Just prior to administration, SINEQUAN Oral Concentrate should be diluted with approximately 120 ml of water, whole or skimmed milk, or orange, grapefruit, tomato, prune or pineapple juice. SINEQUAN Oral Concentrate is not physically compatible with a number of carbonated beverages. For those patients requiring antidepressant therapy who are on methadone maintenance, SINEQUAN Oral Concentrate and methadone syrup can be mixed together with Gatorade®, lemonade, orange juice, sugar water, Tang®, or water; but not with grape juice. Preparation and storage of bulk dilutions is not recommended.

(67-2135-37-9)

Literature Available: Yes.
[*Shown in Product Identification Section*]

TERRA-CORTRIL® ℞
Terramycin® (oxytetracycline HCl)—
Cortril® (hydrocortisone acetate)
OPHTHALMIC SUSPENSION
Each ml contains:

Terramycin (oxytetracycline HCl) equivalent to 5 mg of oxytetracycline, and 15 mg of Cortril (hydrocortisone acetate) incorporated in mineral oil with aluminum tristearate.

For Ophthalmic Use Only

How Supplied: Terra-Cortril Ophthalmic Suspension is supplied in 5 ml vials with separate sterile dropper.

TERRA-CORTRIL® SPRAY ℞
with POLYMYXIN B SULFATE
Each 85 Gm. can contains:
TERRAMYCIN® (oxytetracycline HCl equivalent to 300 mg. of oxytetracycline)
CORTRIL® (hydrocortisone) 100 mg.
Polymyxin B as the sulfate 100,000 units

For external use only. Do not spray into eyes.

How Supplied: Terra-Cortril Spray with Polymyxin B Sulfate is available in 85 Gm. seamless, pressurized cans requiring approximately 120 seconds of spraying time to empty contents. Each second of spraying time covers approximately 4 square inches in area.
The active ingredients are incorporated in an isopropyl myristate, lecithin, and sorbitan trioleate vehicle with propellants.

TERRA-CORTRIL® ℞
Terramycin® (oxytetracycline HCl)—
Cortril® (hydrocortisone)
TOPICAL OINTMENT

Contains Terramycin (oxytetracycline HCl) equivalent to 30 mg of oxytetracycline, and 10 mg of Cortril (hydrocortisone) in each gram of petrolatum base.

Not for Ophthalmic Use

How Supplied: Terra-Cortril Topical Ointment is supplied in ½ oz (14.2 Gm) tubes. The active ingredients are incorporated in mineral oil and petrolatum.

TERRAMYCIN® ℞
Capsules
(oxytetracycline HCl)
Syrup
(calcium oxytetracycline)
Film-coated Tablets
(oxytetracycline)

TERRAMYCIN® Intramuscular Solution ℞
(oxytetracycline)
TERRAMYCIN® Intravenous ℞
(oxytetracycline HCl)

Description: Oxytetracycline is a product of the metabolism of *Streptomyces rimosus* and is one of the family of tetracycline antibiotics.
Oxytetracycline diffuses readily through the placenta into the fetal circulation, into the pleural fluid and, under some circumstances, into the cerebrospinal fluid. It appears to be concentrated in the hepatic system and excreted in the bile, so that it appears in the feces, as well as in the urine, in a biologically active form.
Oral only: A 1 percent solution in water is acidic (pH about 2.5). Its potency is affected in solutions more acid than pH 2 and it is rapidly destroyed by alkali hydroxides.
Intravenous only: Terramycin (oxytetracycline HCl) Intravenous is a sterile, pyrogen-free dry mixture of crystalline oxytetracycline hydrochloride, buffered with ascorbic acid. When dissolved in water, a clear, yellow solution results. Such solutions should be stored at refrigerator temperature, and will maintain their potencies for at least 48 hours.
Actions: Oxytetracycline is primarily bacteriostatic and is thought to exert its antimicrobial effect by the inhibition of protein synthesis. Oxytetracycline is active against a wide range of gram-negative and gram-positive organisms. The drugs in the tetracycline class have closely similar antimicrobial spectra, and cross-resistance among them is common. Microorganisms may be considered susceptible if the M.I.C. (minimum inhibitory concentration) is not more than 4.0 mcg/ml and intermediate if the M.I.C. is 4.0 to 12.5 mcg/ml.
Susceptibility plate testing: A tetracycline disc may be used to determine microbial susceptibility to drugs in the tetracycline class. If the Kirby-Bauer method of disc susceptibility testing is used, a 30 mcg tetracycline disc should give a zone of at least 19 mm when tested against a tetracycline-susceptible bacterial strain.
Tetracyclines are readily absorbed and are bound to plasma proteins in varying degree. They are concentrated by the liver in the bile and excreted in the urine and feces at high concentrations and in a biologically active form.
Indications: Oxytetracycline is indicated in infections caused by the following microorganisms:
Rickettsiae (Rocky Mountain spotted fever, typhus fever and the typhus group, Q fever, rickettsialpox and tick fevers),
Mycoplasma pneumoniae (PPLO, Eaton Agent),
Agents of psittacosis and ornithosis,
Agents of lymphogranuloma venereum and granuloma inguinale,
The spirochetal agent of relapsing fever (*Borrelia recurrentis*).
The following gram-negative microorganisms:
Haemophilus ducreyi (chancroid),
Pasteurella pestis and *Pasteurella tularensis*,
Bartonella bacilliformis,
Bacteroides species,
Vibrio comma and *Vibrio fetus*,
Brucella species (in conjunction with streptomycin).
Because many strains of the following groups of microorganisms have been shown to be resistant to tetracyclines, culture and susceptibility testing are recommended.
Oxytetracycline is indicated for treatment of infections caused by the following gram-negative microorganisms, when bacteriologic testing indicates appropriate susceptibility to the drug:
Escherichia coli,
Enterobacter aerogenes (formerly *Aerobacter aerogenes*),
Shigella species,
Mima species and *Herellea* species,
Haemophilus influenzae (respiratory infections),
Klebsiella species (respiratory and urinary infections).
Oxytetracycline is indicated for treatment of infections caused by the following gram-positive microorganisms when bacteriologic testing indicates appropriate susceptibility to the drug:
Streptococcus species:
Up to 44 percent of strains of *Streptococcus pyogenes* and 74 percent of *Streptococcus faecalis* have been found to be resistant to tetracycline drugs. Therefore, tetracyclines should not be used for streptococcal disease unless the organism has been demonstrated to be sensitive.
For upper respiratory infections due to Group A beta-hemolytic streptococci, penicillin is the usual drug of choice, including prophylaxis of rheumatic fever.
Diplococcus pneumoniae,
Staphylococcus aureus, skin and soft tissue infections. Oxytetracycline is not the drug of choice in the treatment of any type of staphylococcal infections.
When penicillin is contraindicated, tetracyclines are alternative drugs in the treatment of infections due to:
Neisseria gonorrhoeae
Intravenous only: *Neisseria meningitidis*
Treponema pallidum and *Treponema pertenue* (syphilis and yaws),
Listeria monocytogenes,
Clostridium species,
Bacillus anthracis,
Fusobacterium fusiforme (Vincent's infection),
Actinomyces species.
In acute intestinal amebiasis, the tetracyclines may be a useful adjunct to amebicides.
In severe acne, the tetracyclines may be useful adjunctive therapy. (This indication is for the oral use only, not for I.M. or I.V.)
Tetracyclines are indicated in the treatment of trachoma, although the infectious agent is not always eliminated, as judged by immunofluorescence.
Inclusion conjunctivitis may be treated with oral tetracyclines or with a combination of oral and topical agents.
Contraindications: This drug is contraindicated in persons who have shown hypersensitivity to any of the tetracyclines.
Warnings: In the presence of renal dysfunction, particularly in pregnancy, intravenous tetracycline therapy in daily doses exceeding 2 grams has been associated with deaths through liver failure.
When the need for intensive treatment outweighs its potential dangers (mostly during pregnancy or in individuals with known or suspected renal or liver impairment), it is advisable to perform renal and liver function tests before and during therapy. Also, tetracycline serum concentrations should be followed.
If renal impairment exists, even usual oral or parenteral doses may lead to excessive systemic accumulation of the drug and possible liver toxicity. Under such conditions, lower than usual total doses are indicated, and if therapy is prolonged, serum level determinations of the drug may be advisable. This hazard is of particular importance in the parenteral administration of tetracyclines to pregnant or postpartum patients with pyelonephritis. When used under these circumstances, the blood level should not exceed 15 mcg/ml and liver function tests should be made at frequent intervals. Other potentially hepatotoxic drugs should not be prescribed concomitantly.
THE USE OF DRUGS OF THE TETRACYCLINE CLASS DURING TOOTH DEVELOP-

MENT (LAST HALF OF PREGNANCY, INFANCY, AND CHILDHOOD TO THE AGE OF 8 YEARS) MAY CAUSE PERMANENT DISCOLORATION OF THE TEETH (YELLOW-GRAY-BROWN). This adverse reaction is more common during long term use of the drugs but has been observed following repeated short term courses. Enamel hypoplasia has also been reported. *TETRACYCLINE DRUGS, THEREFORE, SHOULD NOT BE USED IN THIS AGE GROUP UNLESS OTHER DRUGS ARE NOT LIKELY TO BE EFFECTIVE OR ARE CONTRAINDICATED.*
Photosensitivity manifested by an exaggerated sunburn reaction has been observed in some individuals taking tetracyclines. Patients apt to be exposed to direct sunlight or ultraviolet light should be advised that this reaction can occur with tetracycline drugs, and treatment should be discontinued at the first evidence of skin erythema.

Precautions: As with other antibiotic preparations, use of this drug may result in overgrowth of nonsusceptible organisms, including fungi. If superinfection occurs, the antibiotic should be discontinued and appropriate therapy instituted.
In venereal diseases when coexistent syphilis is suspected, a dark field examination should be done before treatment is started and the blood serology repeated monthly for at least 4 months.
Because tetracyclines have been shown to depress plasma prothrombin activity, patients who are on anticoagulant therapy may require downward adjustment of their anticoagulant dosage.
In long term therapy, periodic laboratory evaluation of organ systems, including hematopoietic, renal and hepatic studies should be performed.
All infections due to Group A beta-hemolytic streptococci should be treated for at least 10 days.
Since bacteriostatic drugs may interfere with the bactericidal action of penicillin, it is advisable to avoid giving tetracycline in conjunction with penicillin.
As with all intramuscular preparations, Terramycin (oxytetracycline) Intramuscular Solution should be injected well within the body of a relatively large muscle. ADULTS: The preferred sites are the upper outer quadrant of the buttock, (i.e., gluteus maximus), and the midlateral thigh. CHILDREN: It is recommended that intramuscular injections be given preferably in the mid-lateral muscles of the thigh. In infants and small children the periphery of the upper outer quadrant of the gluteal region should be used only when necessary, such as in burn patients, in order to minimize the possibility of damage to the sciatic nerve.
The deltoid area should be used only if well developed such as in certain adults and older children, and then only with caution to avoid radial nerve injury. Intramuscular injections should not be made into the lower and mid-thirds of the upper arm. As with all intramuscular injections, aspiration is necessary to help avoid inadvertent injection into a blood vessel.

Adverse Reactions: Local irritation may be present after intramuscular injection. The injection should be deep, with care taken not to injure the sciatic nerve nor inject intravascularly.
Gastrointestinal: anorexia, nausea, vomiting, diarrhea, glossitis, dysphagia, enterocolitis, and inflammatory lesions (with monilial overgrowth) in the anogenital region. These reactions have been caused by both the oral and parenteral administration of tetracyclines.
Skin: maculopapular and erythematous rashes. Exfoliative dermatitis has been reported but is uncommon. Photosensitivity is discussed above. (See "Warnings.")
Renal toxicity: Rise in BUN has been reported and is apparently dose related. (See "Warnings.")

contents per ml (w/v)

Ingredient	2 ml Single Dose Ampules and Isoject 100 mg/2 ml	2 ml Single Dose Ampules and Isoject 250 mg/2 ml	10 ml Vial Multidose 50 mg/ml 10 ml (5 × 2 ml Doses)
oxytetracycline	50 mg	125 mg	50 mg
lidocaine	2.0%	2.0%	2.0%
magnesium chloride hexahydrate	2.5%	6.0%	2.5%
sodium formaldehyde sulfoxylate	0.5%	0.5%	0.3%
α-monothioglycerol	—	—	1.0%
monoethanolamine	approx. 1.7%	approx. 4.2%	approx. 2.6%
citric acid	—	—	1.0%
propyl gallate	—	—	0.02%
propylene glycol	75.2%	67.0%	74.1%
water	18.8%	16.8%	18.5%

Hypersensitivity reactions: Urticaria, angioneurotic edema, anaphylaxis, anaphylactoid purpura, pericarditis and exacerbation of systemic lupus erythematosus.
Bulging fontanels in infants and benign intracranial hypertension in adults have been reported in individuals receiving full therapeutic dosages. These conditions disappeared rapidly when the drug was discontinued.
Blood: Hemolytic anemia, thrombocytopenia, neutropenia and eosinophilia have been reported.
When given over prolonged periods, tetracyclines have been reported to produce brown-black microscopic discoloration of thyroid glands. No abnormalities of thyroid function studies are known to occur.

Dosage and Administration:

Oral: Capsules and Syrup only:
Adults: Usual daily dose, 1-2 g divided in four equal doses, depending on the severity of the infection.

Film-coated Tablets only:
Adults: A dosage schedule providing 2 tablets initially, then 1 tablet every six hours is the usual average dose. In severe infections a larger dose (2 to 4 grams daily) may be indicated.
The total daily dose should be administered in four equal portions given at six hour intervals.

All Oral Forms:
For children above eight years of age: Usual daily dose, 10-20 mg per pound (25-50) mg/kg) of body weight divided in four equal doses.
Therapy should be continued for at least 24-48 hours after symptoms and fever have subsided.
For treatment of brucellosis, 500 mg oxytetracycline four times daily for 3 weeks should be accompanied by streptomycin, 1 gram intramuscularly twice daily the first week, and once daily the second week.
For treatment of uncomplicated gonorrhea, when penicillin is contraindicated, tetracycline may be used for the treatment of both males and females in the following divided dosage schedule: 1.5 grams initially followed by 0.5 gram q.i.d. for a total of 9.0 grams.
For treatment of syphilis, a total of 30-40 grams in equally divided doses over a period of 10-15 days should be given. Close follow-up, including laboratory tests, is recommended.
Concomitant therapy: Antacids containing aluminum, calcium, or magnesium impair absorption and should not be given to patients taking oral tetracyclines.
Food and some dairy products also interfere with absorption. Oral forms of tetracyclines should be given 1 hour before or 2 hours after meals. Pediatric oral dosage forms should not be given with milk formulas and should be given at least 1 hour prior to feeding.
In patients with renal impairment: (See "Warnings.") Total dosage should be decreased by reduction of recommended individual doses and/or by extending time intervals between doses.
In the treatment of streptococcal infections, a therapeutic dose of oxytetracycline should be administered for at least 10 days.

Intramuscular Administration:
Adults: The usual daily dose is 250 mg administered once every 24 hours or 300 mg given in divided doses at 8 to 12 hour intervals.
For children above eight years of age: 15-25 mg/kg body weight up to a maximum of 250 mg per single daily injection. Dosage may be divided and given at 8 to 12 hour intervals.
Intramuscular therapy should be reserved for situations in which oral therapy is not feasible.
The intramuscular administration of oxytetracycline produces lower blood levels than oral administration in the recommended dosages.
Patients placed on intramuscular oxytetracycline should be changed to the oral dosage form as soon as possible. If rapid, high blood levels are needed, oxytetracycline should be administered intravenously.
In patients with renal impairment: (See "Warnings.") Total dosage should be decreased by reduction of recommended individual doses and/or by extending time intervals between doses.

Intravenous Administration:
NOTE: Rapid administration is to be avoided. Parenteral therapy is indicated only when oral therapy is not adequate or tolerated. Oral therapy should be instituted as soon as possible. If intravenous therapy is given over prolonged periods of time, thrombophlebitis may result.
Adults: If in powder form, dissolve oxytetracycline powder in 10 ml Sterile Water for Injection U.S.P., or 5 percent Dextrose Injection U.S.P. Then redilute, to make at least 100 ml Dextrose 5 percent in water. Isotonic Sodium Chloride Solution or Ringer's solution may be used. The usual adult dose is 250 to 500 mg every 12 hours and should not exceed 500 mg every 6 hours.
For children above eight years of age: The usual dose is 12 mg/kg/day, divided into two doses, but from 10 to 20 mg/kg/day may be given, depending on the severity of the infection.
In patients with renal impairment: (See "Warnings.") Total dosage should be decreased by reduction of recommended individual doses and/or by extending time intervals between doses.
Intravenous solutions should be injected directly into the vein: they should not be injected intramuscularly or subcutaneously. Caution should be taken to avoid the inadvertent introduction of the intravenous solution into the adjacent soft tissue.

Continued on next page

Pfizer—Cont.

How Supplied:
Oral: Terramycin (oxytetracycline HCl) Capsules are available as opaque, yellow, hard gelatin capsules which contain either oxytetracycline HCl equivalent to 250 mg of oxytetracycline, and glucosamine hydrochloride (imprinted with code number 073): bottles of 16, 100, and 500; or oxytetracycline HCl equivalent to 125 mg of oxytetracycline, and glucosamine hydrochloride (imprinted with code number 072): bottles of 100.
Terramycin (calcium oxytetracycline) Syrup is available as a preconstituted fruit-flavored aqueous suspension. Each teaspoonful (5 ml) contains calcium oxytetracycline equivalent to 125 mg of oxytetracycline, and N-acetylglucosamine: bottles of 2 oz. and 1 pint.
Terramycin (oxytetracycline) Tablets are available as:
250 mg film-coated tablets (imprinted with code number 084): bottles of 100.
Intramuscular: Terramycin (oxytetracycline) Intramuscular Solution is available as follows:

Potency of 250 mg/2 ml—
- in 2 ml pre-scored glass ampules, packages of 5 and 100.
- 2 ml Isoject® disposable syringe, packages of 10.

Potency of 100 mg/2 ml—
- in 2 ml pre-scored glass ampules, packages of 5 and 100.
- 2 ml Isoject® disposable syringe, packages of 10.

Potency of 50 mg/ml—
- in 10 ml multiple dose vials, packages of 5.

*U.S. Pat. Nos. 3,017,323 and 3,026,248.
Composition:
Intramuscular only:
(See table on preceding page)
Intravenous: Terramycin (oxytetracycline HCl) Intravenous is available in two convenient sizes for intravenous administration: 250 mg vials buffered with 1.0 gram ascorbic acid, packages of 5, and 500 mg vials buffered with 2.0 grams ascorbic acid, packages of 5 and 100.

[*Capsules Shown in Product Identification Section*]

(I.M.)	60-1051-00-0
(Capsules & Syrup)	60-0755-00-3
(Film-coated Tablets)	23-1127-00-1
(I.V.)	60-0137-00-4

TERRAMYCIN® ℞
oxytetracycline HCl
with POLYMYXIN B SULFATE
OPHTHALMIC OINTMENT
Sterile

Each gram of sterile ointment contains oxytetracycline HCl equivalent to 5 mg oxytetracycline, 10,000 units of polymyxin B sulfate, white petrolatum, and liquid petrolatum.
How Supplied: Terramycin with Polymyxin B Sulfate Ophthalmic Ointment is supplied in ⅛ oz (3.5 g) tubes.

TERRAMYCIN® ℞
oxytetracycline HCl
with POLYMYXIN B SULFATE
OTIC OINTMENT
Sterile

Each gram of sterile ointment contains oxytetracycline HCl equivalent to 5 mg oxytetracycline, 10,000 units of polymyxin B sulfate, white petrolatum, and liquid petrolatum.
How Supplied: Terramycin with Polymyxin B Sulfate Otic Ointment is supplied in ⅛ oz (3.5 g) tubes.

TERRAMYCIN® ℞
oxytetracycline hydrochloride
VAGINAL TABLETS
with POLYMYXIN B SULFATE

Contains: oxytetracycline HCl equivalent to 100 mg of oxytetracycline, and 100,000 units of Polymyxin B Sulfate (equivalent to 10 mg Polymyxin B Standard), and starch, sodium carboxymethylcellulose, lactose, magnesium stearate; as preservatives: 0.3% methylparaben, and 0.07% propylparaben.
How Supplied: The tablets are packaged in foil strips of ten, each strip to be contained in an individual printed carton.
[*Shown in Product Identification Section*]

TERRASTATIN® ℞
oxytetracycline....................250 mg
nystatin....................250,000 units
glucosamine hydrochloride

How Supplied: Terrastatin Capsules are available as:
opaque, pink and yellow hard gelatin capsules (imprinted with code number 008); bottles of 50. (60-1060-00-3)
[*Shown in Product Identification Section*]

VIBRAMYCIN® Hyclate ℞
(doxycycline hyclate)
CAPSULES
VIBRAMYCIN® Calcium
(doxycycline calcium oral suspension)
SYRUP
VIBRAMYCIN® Monohydrate
(doxycycline monohydrate)
For ORAL SUSPENSION

Description: Vibramycin is a broad-spectrum antibiotic synthetically derived from oxytetracycline, and is available as Vibramycin Monohydrate (doxycycline monohydrate), Vibramycin Hyclate (doxycycline hydrochloride hemiethanolate hemihydrate), and Vibramycin Calcium (doxycycline calcium). The chemical designation of this light-yellow crystalline powder is alpha-6-deoxy-5-oxytetracycline. Doxycycline has a high degree of lipoid solubility and a low affinity for calcium binding. It is highly stable in normal human serum. Doxycycline will not degrade into an epianhydro form.
Actions: Doxycycline is primarily bacteriostatic and is thought to exert its antimicrobial effect by the inhibition of protein synthesis. Doxycycline is active against a wide range of gram-positive and gram-negative organisms.
The drugs in the tetracycline class have closely similar antimicrobial spectra, and cross resistance among them is common. Microorganisms may be considered susceptible if the M.I.C. (minimum inhibitory concentration) is less than 4.0 mcg/ml and intermediate if the M.I.C. is 4.0 to 12.5 mcg/ml.
Susceptibility plate testing: If the Kirby-Bauer method of disc susceptibility testing is used, a 30 mcg doxycycline disc should give a zone of at least 16 mm when tested against a doxycycline-susceptible bacterial strain. A tetracycline disc may be used to determine microbial susceptibility. If the Kirby-Bauer method of disc susceptibility testing is used, a 30 mcg tetracycline disc should give a zone of at least 19 mm when tested against a tetracycline-susceptible bacterial strain.
Tetracyclines are readily absorbed and are bound to plasma proteins in varying degree. They are concentrated by the liver in the bile, and excreted in the urine and feces at high concentrations and in a biologically active form.
Doxycycline is virtually completely absorbed after oral administration.
Following a 200 mg dose, normal adult volunteers averaged peak serum levels of 2.6 mcg/ml of doxycycline at 2 hours decreasing to 1.45 mcg/ml at 24 hours. Excretion of doxycycline by the kidney is about 40%/72 hours in individuals with normal function (creatinine clearance about 75 ml/min.). This percentage excretion may fall as low as 1-5%/72 hours in individuals with severe renal insufficiency (creatinine clearance below 10 ml/min.). Studies have shown no significant difference in serum half-life of doxycycline (range 18-22 hours) in individuals with normal and severely impaired renal function.
Hemodialysis does not alter serum half-life.
Indications: Doxycycline is indicated in infections caused by the following microorganisms:
- Rickettsiae: Rocky Mountain spotted fever, typhus fever and the typhus group, Q. fever, rickettsialpox, and tick fevers.
- *Mycoplasma pneumoniae* (PPLO, Eaton agent),
- Agents of psittacosis and ornithosis,
- Agents of lymphogranuloma venereum and granuloma inguinale,
- The spirochetal agent of relapsing fever *(Borrelia recurrentis).*

The following gram-negative microorganisms:
- *Haemophilus ducreyi* (chancroid),
- *Pasteurella pestis,* and *Pasteurella tularensis,*
- *Bartonella bacilliformis,*
- *Bacteroides* species,
- *Vibrio comma* and *Vibrio fetus,*
- *Brucella* species (in conjunction with streptomycin).

Because many strains of the following groups of microorganisms have been shown to be resistant to tetracyclines, culture and susceptibility testing are recommended.
Doxycycline is indicated for treatment of infections caused by the following gram-negative microorganisms, when bacteriologic testing indicates appropriate susceptibility to the drug:
- *Escherichia coli,*
- *Enterobacter aerogenes* (formerly *Aerobacter aerogenes),*
- *Shigella* species,
- *Mima* species and *Herellea* species,
- *Haemophilus influenzae* (respiratory infections),
- *Klebsiella* species (respiratory and urinary infections).

Doxycycline is indicated for treatment of infections caused by the following gram-positive microorganisms when bacteriologic testing indicates appropriate susceptibility to the drug:
Streptococcus species:
Up to 44 percent of strains of *Streptococcus pyogenes* and 74 percent of *Streptococcus faecalis* have been found to be resistant to tetracycline drugs. Therefore, tetracyclines should not be used for streptococcal disease unless the organism has been demonstrated to be sensitive.
For upper respiratory infections due to group A beta-hemolytic streptococci, penicillin is the usual drug of choice, including prophylaxis of rheumatic fever.
- *Diplococcus pneumoniae,*
- *Staphylococcus aureus,* respiratory, skin and soft-tissue infections. Tetracyclines are not the drug of choice in the treatment of any type of staphylococcal infection.

When penicillin is contraindicated, doxycycline is an alternative drug in the treatment of infections due to:
- *Neisseria gonorrhoeae,*
- *Treponema pallidum* and *Treponema pertenue* (syphilis and yaws),
- *Listeria monocytogenes,*
- *Clostridium* species,
- *Bacillus anthracis,*
- *Fusobacterium fusiforme* (Vincent's infection),
- *Actinomyces* species.

In acute intestinal amebiasis doxycycline may be a useful adjunct to amebicides.
In severe acne doxycycline may be useful adjunctive therapy.
Doxycycline is indicated in the treatment of trachoma, although the infectious agent is not

always eliminated, as judged by immunofluorescence.
Inclusion conjunctivitis may be treated with oral doxycycline alone, or with a combination of topical agents.
Contraindications: This drug is contraindicated in persons who have shown hypersensitivity to any of the tetracyclines.
Warnings: THE USE OF DRUGS OF THE TETRACYCLINE CLASS DURING TOOTH DEVELOPMENT (LAST HALF OF PREGNANCY, INFANCY AND CHILDHOOD TO THE AGE OF 8 YEARS) MAY CAUSE PERMANENT DISCOLORATION OF THE TEETH (YELLOW-GRAY-BROWN). This adverse reaction is more common during long term use of the drugs but has been observed following repeated short term courses. Enamel hypoplasia has also been reported. *TETRACYCLINE DRUGS, THEREFORE, SHOULD NOT BE USED IN THIS AGE GROUP UNLESS OTHER DRUGS ARE NOT LIKELY TO BE EFFECTIVE OR ARE CONTRAINDICATED.*
Photosensitivity manifested by an exaggerated sunburn reaction has been observed in some individuals taking tetracyclines. Patients apt to be exposed to direct sunlight or ultraviolet light should be advised that this reaction can occur with tetracycline drugs, and treatment should be discontinued at the first evidence of skin erythema.
The antianabolic action of the tetracyclines may cause an increase in BUN. Studies to date indicate that this does not occur with the use of doxycycline in patients with impaired renal function.
Usage in Pregnancy: (See above "Warnings" about use during tooth development.)
Results of animal studies indicate that tetracyclines cross the placenta, are found in fetal tissues, and can have toxic effects on the developing fetus (often related to retardation of skeletal development). Evidence of embryo-toxicity has also been noted in animals treated early in pregnancy.
Usage in Newborns, Infants, and Children: (See above "Warnings" about use during tooth development.)
As with other tetracyclines, doxycycline forms a stable calcium complex in any bone-forming tissue. A decrease in the fibula growth rate has been observed in prematures given oral tetracycline in doses of 25 mg/kg every six hours. This reaction was shown to be reversible when the drug was discontinued.
Tetracyclines are present in the milk of lactating women who are taking a drug in this class.
Precautions: As with other antibiotic preparations, use of this drug may result in overgrowth of nonsusceptible organisms, including fungi. If superinfection occurs, the antibiotic should be discontinued and appropriate therapy should be instituted.
In venereal disease when coexistent syphilis is suspected, a dark field examination should be done before treatment is started and the blood serology repeated monthly for at least four months.
Because the tetracyclines have been shown to depress plasma prothrombin activity, patients who are on anticoagulant therapy may require downward adjustment of their anticoagulant dosage.
In long term therapy, periodic laboratory evaluation of organ systems, including hematopoietic, renal, and hepatic studies should be performed.
All infections due to group A beta-hemolytic streptococci should be treated for at least 10 days.
Since bacteriostatic drugs may interfere with the bactericidal action of penicillin, it is advisable to avoid giving tetracycline in conjunction with penicillin.
Adverse Reactions: Due to Vibramycin's (doxycycline) virtually complete absorption, side effects of the lower bowel, particularly diarrhea, have been infrequent. The following adverse reactions have been observed in patients receiving tetracyclines:
Gastrointestinal: anorexia, nausea, vomiting, diarrhea, glossitis, dysphagia, enterocolitis, and inflammatory lesions (with monilial overgrowth) in the anogenital region. These reactions have been caused by both the oral and parenteral administration of tetracyclines.
Skin: maculopapular and erythematous rashes. Exfoliative dermatitis has been reported but is uncommon. Photosensitivity is discussed above (see "Warnings").
Renal toxicity: Rise in BUN has been reported and is apparently dose related. (See "Warnings".)
Hypersensitivity reactions: urticaria, angioneurotic edema, anaphylaxis, anaphylactoid purpura, pericarditis, and exacerbation of systemic lupus erythematosus.
Bulging fontanels in infants and benign intracranial hypertension in adults have been reported in individuals receiving full therapeutic dosages. These conditions disappeared rapidly when the drug was discontinued.
Blood: Hemolytic anemia, thrombocytopenia, neutropenia, and eosinophilia have been reported with tetracyclines.
When given over prolonged periods, tetracyclines have been reported to produce brown-black microscopic discoloration of thyroid glands. No abnormalities of thyroid function studies are known to occur.
Dosage and Administration: THE USUAL DOSAGE AND FREQUENCY OF ADMINISTRATION OF DOXYCYCLINE DIFFERS FROM THAT OF THE OTHER TETRACYCLINES. EXCEEDING THE RECOMMENDED DOSAGE MAY RESULT IN AN INCREASED INCIDENCE OF SIDE EFFECTS.
Adults: The usual dose of Vibramycin is 200 mg on the first day of treatment (administered 100 mg every 12 hours) followed by a maintenance dose of 100 mg/day. The maintenance dose may be administered as a single dose or as 50 mg every 12 hours. In the management of more severe infections (particularly chronic infections of the urinary tract), 100 mg every 12 hours is recommended.
For children above eight years of age: The recommended dosage schedule for children weighing 100 pounds or less is 2 mg/lb. of body weight divided into two doses on the first day of treatment, followed by 1 mg/lb. of body weight given as a single daily dose or divided into two doses, on subsequent days. For more severe infections up to 2 mg/lb. of body weight may be used. For children over 100 lbs. the usual adult dose should be used.
Acute gonococcal infections: 200 mg stat, and 100 mg at bedtime, the first day, followed by 100 mg b.i.d. for 3 days.
As an alternate single visit dose, administer 300 mg stat followed in one hour by a second 300 mg dose. The dose may be administered with food, including milk or carbonated beverage, as required.
Primary and secondary syphilis: 300 mg a day in divided doses for at least 10 days.
The therapeutic antibacterial serum activity will usually persist for 24 hours following recommended dosage.
When used in streptococcal infections, therapy should be continued for 10 days.
If gastric irritation occurs, it is recommended that doxycycline be given with food or milk. The absorption of doxycycline is not markedly influenced by simultaneous ingestion of food or milk.
Concomitant therapy: Antacids containing aluminum, calcium, or magnesium impair absorption and should not be given to patients taking oral doxycycline.
Studies to date have indicated that administration of Vibramycin at the usual recommended doses does not lead to excessive accumulation of the antibiotic in patients with renal impairment.
How Supplied: Vibramycin Hyclate (doxycycline hyclate) is available in capsules containing doxycycline hyclate equivalent to:
50 mg doxycycline (imprinted with code number 094)
bottles of 50
unit-dose pack of 100 (10 x 10's)
X-pack of 50 (5 x 10's)
100 mg doxycycline (imprinted with code number 095)
bottles of 50 and 500
unit-dose pack of 100 (10 x 10's)
V-pack of 25 (5 x 5's)
Nine-Paks (10 x 9's)
Vibramycin Calcium Syrup (doxycycline calcium oral suspension) is available as a raspberry-apple flavored oral suspension. Each teaspoonful (5 ml) contains doxycycline calcium equivalent to 50 mg of doxycycline: bottles of 1 oz. (30 ml) and 1 Pint (473 ml).
Vibramycin Monohydrate (doxycycline monohydrate) for Oral Suspension is available as a pleasant tasting, raspberry flavored, dry powder for oral suspension. When reconstituted, each teaspoonful (5 ml) contains doxycycline monohydrate equivalent to 25 mg of doxycycline: 2 oz. (60 ml) bottles.
(60-1680-00-0)
Literature Available: Yes.
[*Shown in Product Identification Section*]

VIBRAMYCIN® Hyclate ℞
(doxycycline hyclate for injection)
INTRAVENOUS
For Intravenous Use Only

Description: Vibramycin (doxycycline hyclate for injection) Intravenous is a broad-spectrum antibiotic synthetically derived from oxytetracycline, and is available as Vibramycin Hyclate (doxycycline hydrochloride hemiethanolate hemihydrate). The chemical designation of this light-yellow crystalline powder is alpha-6-deoxy-5-oxytetracycline. Doxycycline has a high degree of lipoid solubility and a low affinity for calcium binding. It is highly stable in normal human serum.
Actions: Doxycycline is primarily bacteriostatic and thought to exert its antimicrobial effect by the inhibition of protein synthesis. Doxycycline is active against a wide range of gram-positive and gram-negative organisms.
The drugs in the tetracycline class have closely similar antimicrobial spectra and cross resistance among them is common. Microorganisms may be considered susceptible to doxycycline (likely to respond to doxycycline therapy) if the minimum inhibitory concentration (M.I.C.) is not more than 4.0 mcg/ml. Microorganisms may be considered intermediate (harboring partial resistance) if the M.I.C. is 4.0 to 12.5 mcg/ml and resistant (not likely to respond to therapy) if the M.I.C. is greater than 12.5 mcg/ml.
Susceptibility plate testing: If the Kirby-Bauer method of disc susceptibility testing is used, a 30 mcg doxycycline disc should give a zone of at least 16 mm when tested against a doxycycline-susceptible bacterial strain. A tetracycline disc may be used to determine microbial susceptibility. If the Kirby-Bauer method of disc susceptibility testing is used, a 30 mcg tetracycline disc should give a zone of at least 19 mm when tested against a tetracycline-susceptible bacterial strain.
Tetracyclines are readily absorbed and are bound to plasma proteins in varying degree. They are concentrated by the liver in the bile, and excreted in the urine and feces at high concentrations and in a biologically active form.
Following a single 100 mg dose administered in a concentration of 0.4 mg/ml in a one-hour infusion, normal adult volunteers average a peak of 2.5 mcg/ml, while 200 mg of a concen-

Continued on next page

Pfizer—Cont.

tration of 0.4 mg/ml administered over two hours averaged a peak of 3.6 mcg/ml.
Excretion of doxycycline by the kidney is about 40 percent/72 hours in individuals with normal function (creatinine clearance about 75 ml/min.). This percentage excretion may fall as low as 1-5 percent/72 hours in individuals with severe renal insufficiency (creatinine clearance below 10 ml/min.). Studies have shown no significant difference in serum half-life of doxycycline (range 18-22 hours) in individuals with normal and severely impaired renal function.
Hemodialysis does not alter this serum half-life of doxycycline.
Indications: Doxycycline is indicated in infections caused by the following microorganisms:
Rickettsiae (Rocky Mountain spotted fever, typhus fever, and the typhus group, Q fever, rickettsialpox and tick fevers).
Mycoplasma pneumoniae (PPLO, Eaton Agent).
Agents of psittacosis and ornithosis.
Agents of lymphogranuloma venereum and granuloma inguinale.
The spirochetal agent of relapsing fever *(Borrelia recurrentis).*
The following gram-negative microorganisms:
Haemophilus ducreyi (chancroid),
Pasteurella pestis and *Pasteurella tularensis,*
Bartonella bacilliformis,
Bacteroides species,
Vibrio comma and *Vibrio fetus,*
Brucella species (in conjunction with streptomycin).
Because many strains of the following groups of microorganisms have been shown to be resistant to tetracyclines, culture and susceptibility testing are recommended.
Doxycycline is indicated for treatment of infections caused by the following gram-negative microorganisms when bacteriologic testing indicates appropriate susceptibility to the drug:
Escherichia coli,
Enterobacter aerogenes (formerly *Aerobacter aerogenes),*
Shigella species,
Mima species and *Herellea* species,
Haemophilus influenzae (respiratory infections),
Klebsiella species (respiratory and urinary infections).
Doxycycline is indicated for treatment of infections caused by the following gram-positive microorganisms when bacteriologic testing indicates appropriate susceptibility to the drug:
Streptococcus species:
Up to 44 percent of strains of *Streptococcus pyogenes* and 74 percent of *Streptococcus faecalis* have been found to be resistant to tetracycline drugs. Therefore, tetracyclines should not be used for streptococcal disease unless the organism has been demonstrated to be sensitive.
For upper respiratory infections due to group A beta-hemolytic streptococci, penicillin is the usual drug of choice, including prophylaxis of rheumatic fever.
Diplococcus pneumoniae,
Staphylococcus aureus, respiratory, skin and soft tissue infections. Tetracyclines are not the drugs of choice in the treatment of any type of staphylococcal infections.
When penicillin is contraindicated, doxycycline is an alternative drug in the treatment of infections due to:
Neisseria gonorrhoeae and *N. meningitidis,*
Treponema pallidum and *Treponema pertenue* (syphilis and yaws),
Listeria monocytogenes,
Clostridium species,
Bacillus anthracis,
Fusobacterium fusiforme (Vincent's infection),
Actinomyces species.
In acute intestinal amebiasis, doxycycline may be a useful adjunct to amebicides.
Doxycycline is indicated in the treatment of trachoma, although the infectious agent is not always eliminated, as judged by immunofluorescence.
Contraindications: This drug is contraindicated in persons who have shown hypersensitivity to any of the tetracyclines.
Warnings: THE USE OF DRUGS OF THE TETRACYCLINE CLASS DURING TOOTH DEVELOPMENT (LAST HALF OF PREGNANCY, INFANCY AND CHILDHOOD TO THE AGE OF 8 YEARS) MAY CAUSE PERMANENT DISCOLORATION OF THE TEETH (YELLOW-GRAY-BROWN). This adverse reaction is more common during long-term use of the drugs but has been observed following repeated short-term courses. Enamel hypoplasia has also been reported. *TETRACYCLINE DRUGS, THEREFORE, SHOULD NOT BE USED IN THIS AGE GROUP UNLESS OTHER DRUGS ARE NOT LIKELY TO BE EFFECTIVE OR ARE CONTRAINDICATED.*
Photosensitivity manifested by an exaggerated sunburn reaction has been observed in some individuals taking tetracyclines. Patients apt to be exposed to direct sunlight or ultraviolet light should be advised that this reaction can occur with tetracycline drugs, and treatment should be discontinued at the first evidence of skin erythema.
The antianabolic action of the tetracyclines may cause an increase in BUN. Studies to date indicate that this does not occur with the use of doxycycline in patients with impaired renal function.

Usage in Pregnancy
(See above "Warnings" about use during tooth development.)
Vibramycin (doxycycline hyclate for injection) Intravenous has not been studied in pregnant patients. It should not be used in pregnant women unless, in the judgement of the physician, it is essential for the welfare of the patient.
Results of animal studies indicate that tetracyclines cross the placenta, are found in fetal tissues and can have toxic effects on the developing fetus (often related to retardation of skeletal development). Evidence of embryotoxicity has also been noted in animals treated early in pregnancy.

Usage in Children
The use of Vibramycin Intravenous in children under 8 years is not recommended because safe conditions for its use have not been established.
(See above "Warnings" about use during tooth development.)
As with other tetracyclines, doxycycline forms a stable calcium complex in any bone-forming tissue. A decrease in the fibula growth rate has been observed in prematures given oral tetracycline in doses of 25 mg/kg every 6 hours. This reaction was shown to be reversible when the drug was discontinued.
Tetracyclines are present in the milk of lactating women who are taking a drug in this class.
Precautions: As with other antibiotic preparations, use of this drug may result in overgrowth of nonsusceptible organisms, including fungi. If superinfection occurs, the antibiotic should be discontinued and appropriate therapy instituted.
In venereal diseases when coexistent syphilis is suspected, a dark field examination should be done before treatment is started and the blood serology repeated monthly for at least 4 months.
Because tetracyclines have been shown to depress plasma prothrombin activity, patients who are on anticoagulant therapy may require downward adjustment of their anticoagulant dosage.
In long-term therapy, periodic laboratory evaluation of organ systems, including hematopoietic, renal, and hepatic studies should be performed.
All infections due to group A beta-hemolytic streptococci should be treated for at least 10 days.
Since bacteriostatic drugs may interfere with the bactericidal action of penicillin, it is advisable to avoid giving tetracycline in conjunction with penicillin.
Adverse Reactions: Gastrointestinal: anorexia, nausea, vomiting, diarrhea, glossitis, dysphagia, enterocolitis, and inflammatory lesions (with monilial overgrowth) in the anogenital region. These reactions have been caused by both the oral and parenteral administration of tetracyclines.
Skin: maculopapular and erythematous rashes. Exfoliative dermatitis has been reported but is uncommon. Photosensitivity is discussed above. (See "Warnings.")
Renal toxicity: Rise in BUN has been reported and is apparently dose related. (See "Warnings.")
Hypersensitivity reactions: urticaria, angioneurotic edema, anaphylaxis, anaphylactoid purpura, pericarditis and exacerbation of systemic lupus erythematosus.
Bulging fontanels in infants and benign intracranial hypertension in adults have been reported in individuals receiving full therapeutic dosages. These conditions disappeared rapidly when the drug was discontinued.
Blood: Hemolytic anemia, thrombocytopenia, neutropenia and eosinophilia have been reported.
When given over prolonged periods, tetracyclines have been reported to produce brown-black microscopic discoloration of thyroid glands. No abnormalities of thyroid function studies are known to occur.
Dosage and Administration: Note: Rapid administration is to be avoided. Parenteral therapy is indicated only when oral therapy is not indicated. Oral therapy should be instituted as soon as possible. If intravenous therapy is given over prolonged periods of time, thrombophlebitis may result.
THE USUAL DOSAGE AND FREQUENCY OF ADMINISTRATION OF VIBRAMYCIN I.V. (100-200 MG/DAY) DIFFERS FROM THAT OF THE OTHER TETRACYCLINES (1-2 G/DAY). EXCEEDING THE RECOMMENDED DOSAGE MAY RESULT IN AN INCREASED INCIDENCE OF SIDE EFFECTS.
Studies to date have indicated that Vibramycin at the usual recommended doses does not lead to excessive accumulation of the antibiotic in patients with renal impairment.
Adults: The usual dosage of Vibramycin (doxycycline hyclate for injection) I.V. is 200 mg on the first day of treatment administered in one or two infusions. Subsequent daily dosage is 100 to 200 mg depending upon the severity of infection, with 200 mg administered in one or two infusions.
In the treatment of primary and secondary syphilis, the recommended dosage is 300 mg daily for at least 10 days.
For children above eight years of age: The recommended dosage schedule for children weighing 100 pounds or less is 2 mg/lb. of body weight on the first day of treatment, administered in one or two infusions. Subsequent daily dosage is 1 to 2 mg/lb. of body weight given as one or two infusions, depending on the severity of the infection. For children over 100 pounds the usual adult dose should be used. (See "Warning" Section for Usage in Children.)
General: The duration of infusion may vary with the dose (100 to 200 mg per day), but is

usually one to four hours. A recommended minimum infusion time for 100 mg of a 0.5 mg/ml solution is one hour. Therapy should be continued for at least 24-48 hours after symptoms and fever have subsided. The therapeutic antibacterial serum activity will usually persist for 24 hours following recommended dosage.
Intravenous solutions should not be injected intramuscularly or subcutaneously. Caution should be taken to avoid the inadvertent introduction of the intravenous solution into the adjacent soft tissue.

Preparation of Solution: To prepare a solution containing 10 mg/ml, the contents of the vial should be reconstituted with 10 ml (for the 100 mg/vial container) or 20 ml (for the 200 mg/vial container) of Sterile Water for Injection or any of the ten intravenous infusion solutions listed below. Each 100 mg of Vibramycin (i.e., withdraw entire solution from the 100 mg vial) is further diluted with 100 ml to 1000 ml of the intravenous solutions listed below. Each 200 mg of Vibramycin (i.e., withdraw entire solution from the 200 mg vial) is further diluted with 200 ml to 2000 ml of the following intravenous solutions:

1. Sodium Chloride Injection, USP
2. 5% Dextrose Injection, USP
3. Ringer's Injection, USP
4. Invert Sugar, 10% in Water
5. Lactated Ringer's Injection, USP
6. Dextrose 5% in Lactated Ringer's
7. Normosol-M® in D5-W (Abbott)
8. Normosol-R® D5-W (Abbott)
9. Plasma-Lyte® 56 in 5% Dextrose (Travenol)
10. Plasma-Lyte® 148 in 5% Dextrose (Travenol)

This will result in desired concentrations of 0.1 to 1.0 mg/ml. Concentrations lower than 0.1 mg/ml or higher than 1.0 mg/ml are not recommended.

Stability:
When diluted with Sodium Chloride Injection, USP, or 5% Dextrose Injection, USP, or Ringer's Injection, USP, or Invert Sugar, 10% in Water, or Normosol-M® in D5-W (Abbott), or Normosol-R® in D5-W (Abbott), or Plasma-Lyte® 56 in 5% Dextrose (Travenol), or Plasma-Lyte® 148 in 5% Dextrose (Travenol), infusion of the solution (ca. 1.0 mg/ml) or lower concentrations (not less than 0.1 mg/ml) must be completed within 12 hours after reconstitution to ensure adequate stability. During infusion, the solution must be protected from direct sunlight. Reconstituted solutions (1.0 to 0.1 mg/ml) may also be stored up to 72 hours prior to start of infusion, if refrigerated and protected from sunlight and artificial light. Again, infusion must then be completed within 12 hours. Solutions must be used within these time periods or discarded.
When diluted with Lactated Ringer's Injection, USP, or Dextrose 5% in Lactated Ringer's, infusion of the solution (ca. 1.0 mg/ml) or lower concentrations (not less than 0.1 mg/ml) must be completed within six hours after reconstitution to ensure adequate stability. During infusion, the solution must be protected from direct sunlight. Solutions must be used within this time period or discarded.
Solutions of Vibramycin (doxycycline hyclate for injection) at a concentration of 10 mg/ml in Sterile Water for Injection, when frozen immediately after reconstitution are stable for 8 weeks when stored at −20°C. If the product is warmed, care should be taken to avoid heating it after the thawing is complete. Once thawed the solution should not be refrozen.

How Supplied: Vibramycin (doxycycline hyclate for injection) Intravenous is available as a sterile powder in a vial containing doxycycline hyclate equivalent to 100 mg of doxycycline with 480 mg of ascorbic acid, packages of 5; and in individually packaged vials containing doxycycline hyclate equivalent to 200 mg of doxycycline with 960 mg of ascorbic acid.
(60-1940-00-8)

Literature Available: Yes.

VISTARIL® ℞
(hydroxyzine pamoate)
Capsules and Oral Suspension

Description: Hydroxyzine pamoate is designated chemically as 1-(p-chlorobenzhydryl) 4-[2-(2-hydroxyethoxy) ethyl] diethylenediamine salt of 1,1′- methylene bis (2 hydroxy-3-naphthalene carboxylic acid).

Clinical Pharmacology: Vistaril (hydroxyzine pamoate) is unrelated chemically to the phenothiazines, reserpine, meprobamate, or the benzodiazepines.
Vistaril is not a cortical depressant, but its action may be due to a suppression of activity in certain key regions of the subcortical area of the central nervous system. Primary skeletal muscle relaxation has been demonstrated experimentally. Bronchodilator activity, and antihistaminic and analgesic effects have been demonstrated experimentally and confirmed clinically. An antiemetic effect, both by the apomorphine test and the veriloid test, has been demonstrated. Pharmacological and clinical studies indicate that hydroxyzine in therapeutic dosage does not increase gastric secretion or acidity and in most cases has mild antisecretory activity. Hydroxyzine is rapidly absorbed from the gastrointestinal tract and Vistaril's clinical effects are usually noted within 15 to 30 minutes after oral administration.

Indications: For symptomatic relief of anxiety and tension associated with psychoneurosis and as an adjunct in organic disease states in which anxiety is manifested.
Useful in the management of pruritus due to allergic conditions such as chronic urticaria and atopic and contact dermatoses, and in histamine-mediated pruritus.
As a sedative when used as premedication and following general anesthesia, **Hydroxyzine may potentiate meperidine (Demerol®) and barbiturates,** so their use in pre-anesthetic adjunctive therapy should be modified on an individual basis. Atropine and other belladonna alkaloids are not affected by the drug. Hydroxyzine is not known to interfere with the action of digitalis in any way and it may be used concurrently with this agent.
The effectiveness of hydroxyzine as an antianxiety agent for long term use, that is more than 4 months, has not been assessed by systematic clinical studies. The physician should reassess periodically the usefulness of the drug for the individual patient.

Contraindications: Hydroxyzine, when administered to the pregnant mouse, rat, and rabbit, induced fetal abnormalities in the rat and mouse at doses substantially above the human therapeutic range. Clinical data in human beings are inadequate to establish safety in early pregnancy. Until such data are available, hydroxyzine is contraindicated in early pregnancy.
Hydroxyzine pamoate is contraindicated for patients who have shown a previous hypersensitivity to it.

Warnings: **Nursing Mothers:** It is not known whether this drug is excreted in human milk. Since many drugs are so excreted, hydroxyzine should not be given to nursing mothers.

Precautions: THE POTENTIATING ACTION OF HYDROXYZINE MUST BE CONSIDERED WHEN THE DRUG IS USED IN CONJUNCTION WITH CENTRAL NERVOUS SYSTEM DEPRESSANTS SUCH AS NARCOTICS, NON-NARCOTIC ANALGESICS AND BARBITURATES. Therefore, when central nervous system depressants are administered concomitantly with hydroxyzine their dosage should be reduced. Since drowsiness may occur with use of the drug, patients should be warned of this possibility and cautioned against driving a car or operating dangerous machinery while taking Vistaril (hydroxyzine pamoate). Patients should be advised against the simultaneous use of other CNS depressant drugs, and cautioned that the effect of alcohol may be increased.

Adverse Reactions: Side effects reported with the administration of Vistaril are usually mild and transitory in nature.
Anticholinergic: Dry mouth.
Central Nervous System: Drowsiness is usually transitory and may disappear in a few days of continued therapy or upon reduction of the dose. Involuntary motor activity including rare instances of tremor and convulsions has been reported, usually with doses considerably higher than those recommended. Clinically significant respiratory depression has not been reported at recommended doses.

Overdosage: The most common manifestation of overdosage of Vistaril is hypersedation. As in the management of overdosage with any drug, it should be borne in mind that multiple agents may have been taken.
If vomiting has not occurred spontaneously, it should be induced. Immediate gastric lavage is also recommended. General supportive care, including frequent monitoring of the vital signs and close observation of the patient, is indicated. Hypotension, though unlikely, may be controlled with intravenous fluids and Levophed® (levarterenol) or Aramine® (metaraminol). Do not use epinephrine as Vistaril counteracts its pressor action. Caffeine and Sodium Benzoate Injection, U.S.P., may be used to counteract central nervous system depressant effects.
There is no specific antidote. It is doubtful that hemodialysis would be of any value in the treatment of overdosage with hydroxyzine. However, if other agents such as barbiturates have been ingested concomitantly, hemodialysis may be indicated. There is no practical method to quantitate hydroxyzine in body fluids or tissue after its ingestion or administration.

Dosage: For symptomatic relief of anxiety and tension associated with psychoneurosis and as an adjunct in organic disease states in which anxiety is manifested: in adults, 50–100 mg q.i.d.; children under 6 years, 50 mg daily in divided doses and over 6 years, 50–100 mg daily in divided doses.
For use in the management of pruritus due to allergic conditions such as chronic urticaria and atopic and contact dermatoses, and in histamine-mediated pruritus: in adults, 25 mg t.i.d. or q.i.d.; children under 6 years, 50 mg daily in divided doses and over 6 years, 50–100 mg daily in divided doses.
As a sedative when used as a premedication and following general anesthesia: 50–100 mg in adults, and 0.6 mg/kg in children.
When treatment is initiated by the intramuscular route of administration, subsequent doses may be administered orally.
As with all medications, the dosage should be adjusted according to the patient's response to therapy.

Supply:
Vistaril Capsules (hydroxyzine pamoate equivalent to hydroxyzine hydrochloride)
25 mg: 100's and 500's and unit dose (10 × 10's)—two-tone green capsules (imprinted with code number 541).
50 mg: 100's and 500's and unit dose 10 × 10's)—green and white capsules (imprinted with code number 542).
100 mg: 100's and 500's and unit dose (10 × 10's)—green and gray capsules (imprinted with code number 543).
Vistaril Oral Suspension (hydroxyzine pamoate equivalent to 25 mg hydroxyzine hydro-

Continued on next page

Pfizer—Cont.

chloride per teaspoonful-5 ml): 1 pint bottles and 4 ounce (120 ml) bottles in packages of 4.
Bibliography: Available on request.
(60-0846-00-9)
[*Shown in Product Identification Section*]

VISTARIL® ℞
(hydroxyzine hydrochloride)
Intramuscular Solution
For Intramuscular Use Only

Chemistry: Hydroxyzine hydrochloride is designated chemically as 1-(p-chlorobenzhydryl) 4-[2-(2-hydroxyethoxy) ethyl] piperazine dihydrochloride.
Actions: VISTARIL (hydroxyzine hydrochloride) is unrelated chemically to phenothiazine, reserpine, and meprobamate. Hydroxyzine has demonstrated its clinical effectiveness in the chemotherapeutic aspect of the total management of neuroses and emotional disturbances manifested by anxiety, tension, agitation, apprehension or confusion.
Hydroxyzine has been shown clinically to be a rapid-acting true ataraxic with a wide margin of safety. It induces a calming effect in anxious, tense, psychoneurotic adults and also in anxious, hyperkinetic children without impairing mental alertness. It is not a cortical depressant, but its action may be due to a suppression of activity in certain key regions of the subcortical area of the central nervous system.
Primary skeletal muscle relaxation has been demonstrated experimentally.
Hydroxyzine has been shown experimentally to have antispasmodic properties, apparently mediated through interference with the mechanism that responds to spasmogenic agents such as serotonin, acetylcholine, and histamine.
Antihistaminic effects have been demonstrated experimentally and confirmed clinically.
An antiemetic effect, both by the apomorphine test and the veriloid test, has been demonstrated. Pharmacological and clinical studies indicate that hydroxyzine in therapeutic dosage does not increase gastric secretion or acidity and in most cases provides mild antisecretory benefits.
Indications: The total management of anxiety, tension, and psychomotor agitation in conditions of emotional stress requires in most instances a combined approach of psychotherapy and chemotherapy. Hydroxyzine has been found to be particularly useful for this latter phase of therapy in its ability to render the disturbed patient more amenable to psychotherapy in long term treatment of the psychoneurotic and the psychotic, although it should not be used as the sole treatment of psychosis or of clearly demonstrated cases of depression.
Hydroxyzine is also useful in alleviating the manifestations of anxiety and tension as in the preparation for dental procedures and in acute emotional problems. It has also been recommended for the management of anxiety associated with organic disturbances and as adjunctive therapy in alcoholism and allergic conditions with strong emotional overlay, such as in asthma, chronic urticaria, and pruritus.
VISTARIL (hydroxyzine hydrochloride) Intramuscular Solution is useful in treating the following types of patients when intramuscular administration is indicated:

1. The acutely disturbed or hysterical patient.
2. The acute or chronic alcoholic with anxiety withdrawal symptoms or delirium tremens.
3. As pre- and postoperative and pre- and postpartum adjunctive medication to permit reduction in narcotic dosage, allay anxiety, and control emesis.

VISTARIL (hydroxyzine hydrochloride) has also demonstrated effectiveness in controlling nausea and vomiting, excluding nausea and vomiting of pregnancy. (See Contraindications.)
In prepartum states, the reduction in narcotic requirement effected by hydroxyzine is of particular benefit to both mother and neonate.
Hydroxyzine benefits the cardiac patient by its ability to allay the associated anxiety and apprehension attendant to certain types of heart disease. Hydroxyzine is not known to interfere with the action of digitalis in any way and may be used concurrently with this agent.
The effectiveness of hydroxyzine in long-term use, that is, more than 4 months, has not been assessed by systematic clinical studies. The physician should reassess periodically the usefulness of the drug for the individual patient.
Contraindications: Hydroxyzine hydrochloride intramuscular solution is intended only for intramuscular administration and should not, under any circumstances, be injected subcutaneously, intraarterially or intravenously.
This drug is contraindicated for patients who have shown a previous hypersensitivity to it.
Hydroxyzine, when administered to the pregnant mouse, rat, and rabbit, induced fetal abnormalities in the rat at doses substantially above the human therapeutic range. Clinical data in human beings are inadequate to establish safety in early pregnancy. Until such data are available, hydroxyzine is contraindicated in early pregnancy.
Precautions: THE POTENTIATING ACTION OF HYDROXYZINE MUST BE CONSIDERED WHEN THE DRUG IS USED IN CONJUNCTION WITH CENTRAL NERVOUS SYSTEM DEPRESSANTS SUCH AS NARCOTICS AND BARBITURATES. Therefore when central nervous system depressants are administered concomitantly with hydroxyzine their dosage should be reduced up to 50 per cent. The efficacy of hydroxyzine as adjunctive pre- and postoperative sedative medication has also been well established, especially as regards its ability to allay anxiety, control emesis, and reduce the amount of narcotic required.
HYDROXYZINE MAY POTENTIATE NARCOTICS AND BARBITURATES, so their use in preanesthetic adjunctive therapy should be modified on an individual basis. Atropine and other belladonna alkaloids are not affected by the drug.
When hydroxyzine is used preoperatively or prepartum, narcotic requirements may be reduced as much as 50 per cent. Thus, when 50 mg of VISTARIL (hydroxyzine hydrochloride) Intramuscular Solution is employed, meperidine dosage may be reduced from 100 mg to 50 mg.
Since drowsiness may occur with use of this drug, patients should be warned of this possibility and cautioned against driving a car or operating dangerous machinery while taking this drug.
As with all intramuscular preparations, VISTARIL Intramuscular Solution should be injected well within the body of a relatively large muscle. Inadvertent subcutaneous injection may result in significant tissue damage.
ADULTS: The preferred site is the upper outer quadrant of the buttock (i.e., gluteus maximus), or the mid-lateral thigh.
CHILDREN: It is recommended that intramuscular injections be given preferably in the mid-lateral muscles of the thigh. In infants and small children the periphery of the upper outer quadrant of the gluteal region should be used only when necessary, such as in burn patients, in order to minimize the possibility of damage to the sciatic nerve.
The deltoid area should be used only if well developed such as in certain adults and older children, and then only with caution to avoid radial nerve injury. Intramuscular injections should not be made into the lower and mid-third of the upper arm. As with all intramuscular injections, aspiration is necessary to help avoid inadvertent injection into a blood vessel.
Adverse Reactions: Therapeutic doses of hydroxyzine seldom produce impairment of mental alertness. However, drowsiness may occur; if so, it is usually transitory and may disappear in a few days of continued therapy or upon reduction of the dose. Dryness of the mouth may be encountered at higher doses. Extensive clinical use has substantiated the absence of toxic effects on the liver or bone marrow when administered in the recommended doses for over four years of uninterrupted therapy. The absence of adverse effects has been further demonstrated in experimental studies in which excessively high doses were administered.
Involuntary motor activity, including rare instances of tremor and convulsions, has been reported, usually with doses considerably higher than those recommended. Continuous therapy with over one gram per day has been employed in some patients without these effects having been encountered.
Dosage and Administration: The recommended dosages for VISTARIL (hydroxyzine hydrochloride) Intramuscular Solution are:
For adult psychiatric and emotional emergencies, including acute alcoholism.
I.M.: 50–100 mg stat., and q. 4–6h., p.r.n.
Nausea and vomiting excluding nausea and vomiting of pregnancy.
Adults: 25–100 mg I.M. Children: 0.5 mg/lb. body weight I.M.
Pre- and postoperative adjunctive medication.
Adults: 25–100 mg I.M. Children: 0.5 mg/lb. body weight I.M.
Pre- and postpartum adjunctive therapy.
25–100 mg I.M.
As with all potent medications, the dosage should be adjusted according to the patient's response to therapy.
FOR ADDITIONAL INFORMATION OF THE ADMINISTRATION AND SITE OF SELECTION SEE PRECAUTIONS SECTION. NOTE: VISTARIL (hydroxyzine hydrochloride) Intramuscular Solution may be administered without further dilution.
Patients may be started on intramuscular therapy when indicated. They should be maintained on oral therapy whenever this route is practicable.
Supply:
VISTARIL (hydroxyzine hydrochloride) Intramuscular Solution
25 mg/ml: 10 ml vials
50 mg/ml: 10 ml vials
100 mg/2 ml: 2 ml vials, packages of 10 vials
Isoject®
25 mg/ml—1 ml fill: packages of 10 Isojects
50 mg/ml—1 ml fill: packages of 10 Isojects
100 mg/2 ml—2 ml fill: packages of 10 Isojects
Formula:

Each ml contains:	25 mg/ml	50 mg/ml 100 mg/2 ml
Hydroxyzine hydrochloride	25 mg	50 mg
Benzyl Alcohol	0.9%	0.9%
Sodium hydroxide	to adjust to optimum pH	

Bibliography: Available on request.
(60-0843-00-0)

VISTRAX® TABLETS ℞
(oxyphencyclimine HCl and hydroxyzine HCl)

Composition: Each Vistrax 5 tablet contains:
oxyphencyclimine HCl ....5 mg
hydroxyzine HCl..25 mg
Each Vistrax 10 tablet contains:
oxyphencyclimine HCl ....10 mg
hydroxyzine HCl..25 mg
Description: Vistrax is a combination of oxyphencyclimine HCl and hydroxyzine HCl. Oxyphencyclimine HCl is a crystalline sub-

stance designated chemically as: (1,4,5,6-tetrahydro-1-methyl-2-pyrimidinyl) methyl alpha-phenylcyclohexaneglycolate monohydrochloride.
Hydroxyzine HCl is designated chemically as: 2-[2- [4- (p-chloro-alpha-phenylbenzyl) -1-piperazinyl] ethoxy] ethanol dihydrochloride.
Actions: Oxyphencyclimine HCl provides long acting suppression of gastric secretion through its anticholinergic action. The mechanism of this action is the inhibition of acetylcholine at postganglionic cholinergic sites in structures innervated by postganglionic parasympathetic nerves and on smooth muscle not so innervated but responsive to acetylcholine.
Hydroxyzine HCl has been shown clinically to be an effective antianxiety agent. It induces a calming effect in anxious, tense individuals without impairing mental alertness. It is not a cortical depressant, but its action may be due to a suppression of activity in certain key regions of the subcortical area of the central nervous system.

Indications
Based on a review of this drug by the National Academy of Sciences—National Research Council and/or other information, FDA has classified the indications as follows:
Possibly Effective: As adjunctive therapy in peptic ulcer; irritable bowel syndrome (irritable colon, spastic colon, mucous colitis, functional gastrointestinal disorders); functional diarrhea; drug induced diarrhea; ulcerative colitis, and urinary bladder spasm and ureteral spasm (i.e., smooth muscle spasm).
Final classification of these less than effective indications requires further investigation.

Contraindications: Because of its anticholinergic activity, Vistrax is contraindicated in the presence of glaucoma, obstructive uropathy (i.e. bladder neck obstruction due to prostatic hypertrophy), obstructive disease of the gastrointestinal tract (as in achalasia, pyloroduodenal stenosis, etc.); paralytic ileus; intestinal atony of the elderly or debilitated patient; unstable cardiovascular status in acute hemorrhage; severe ulcerative colitis; toxic megacolon complicating ulcerative colitis; myasthenia gravis.
Warnings: Hydroxyzine, when administered to the pregnant mouse, rat, and rabbit, induced fetal abnormalities in the rat at doses substantially above the human therapeutic range. Clinical data in human beings are inadequate to establish safety in early pregnancy. Until such data are available, hydroxyzine-containing drugs are not advised in early pregnancy.
In the presence of a high environmental temperature, heat prostration can occur with drug use (fever and heatstroke due to decreased sweating).
Diarrhea may be an early symptom of incomplete intestinal obstruction, especially in patients with ileostomy or colostomy. In this instance treatment with this drug would be inappropriate and possibly harmful.
Vistrax may produce drowsiness or blurred vision. In this event, the patient should be warned not to engage in activities requiring mental alertness such as operating a motor vehicle or other machinery, or perform hazardous work while taking this drug.
Precautions: Anticholinergics should be used with caution in patients with:
autonomic neuropathy,
hepatic or renal disease,
ulcerative colitis—(Large doses may suppress intestinal motility to the point of producing a paralytic ileus and the use of this drug may precipitate or aggravate the serious complication of toxic megacolon.),
hyperthyroidism, coronary heart disease, congestive heart failure, cardiac arrhythmias, hypertension and nonobstructing prostatic hypertrophy; hiatal hernia associated with reflux esophagitis, since anticholinergic drugs may aggravate this condition.
It should be noted that the use of anticholinergic drugs in the treatment of gastric ulcer may produce a delay in gastric emptying time and may complicate such therapy (antral stasis).
The use of this drug in the presence of complication of biliary tract disease should not be relied upon.
Tachycardia should be thoroughly investigated before giving anticholinergic (atropine-like) drugs since they may increase the heart rate.
With overdosage, a curare-like action may occur.
Adverse Reactions: As with other anticholinergics, oxyphencyclimine HCl produces certain effects which may be physiologic or toxic depending upon the individual patient's response. The physician must delineate these.
Adverse reactions may include xerostomia; urinary hesitancy and retention; blurred vision and tachycardia; palpitations; mydriasis; dilatation of the pupil; cycloplegia, increased ocular tension; loss of taste; headaches; nervousness; drowsiness; weakness; dizziness; insomnia; nausea; vomiting; impotence; suppression of lactation; constipation; bloated feeling; severe allergic reaction or drug idiosyncrasies including anaphylaxis, urticaria and other dermal manifestation; some degree of mental confusion and/or excitement especially in elderly persons.
Decreased sweating is another adverse reaction that may occur. It should be noted that adrenergic innervation of the eccrine sweat glands on the palms and soles make complete control of sweating impossible. An end point of complete anhidrosis cannot occur because large doses of drug would be required, and this would produce severe side effects from parasympathetic paralysis.
Side effects which occasionally occur with hydroxyzine HCl are drowsiness, xerostomia, and, at extremely high doses, involuntary motor activity, all of which may be controlled by reduction of the dosage or discontinuation of the medication.
Dosage and Administration: The recommended adult dose is usually one Vistrax 5 or one Vistrax 10 tablet two times a day or three times a day, depending on individual response. Proper diet and antacids should be used where indicated as concomitant therapy. The safe use of Vistrax in children has not been established; therefore, the drug should not be used in children.
Drug Interactions: The potentiating action of hydroxyzine must be considered when the drug is used in combination with central nervous system depressants.
How Supplied: Vistrax 5 is available as white scored tablets (imprinted with code number 180) in bottles of 100. Vistrax 10 is available as black and white scored tablets (imprinted with code number 181) in bottles of 100. (60-2258-00-1)
Literature Available: Yes.
[*Shown in Product Identification Section*]

Products are cross-indexed by
generic and chemical names
in the
YELLOW SECTION

Pharmacia Laboratories

Division of Pharmacia Inc.
800 CENTENNIAL AVENUE
PISCATAWAY, NJ 08854

AZULFIDINE® ℞
(sulfasalazine, N.F.)
Tablets

Description: AZULFIDINE Tablets contain sulfasalazine N.F. which is synthesized by the diazotization of sulfapyridine and the coupling of the diazonium salt with salicylic acid. Further processing results in a bright orange-colored substance that chemically is designated: 5-[[p-(2-Pyridylsulfamoyl) phenyl]azo] salicylic acid. Reductive splitting of the azo linkage yields sulfapyridine and 5-aminosalicylic acid.
Actions: After oral administration, AZULFIDINE is partially absorbed and extensively metabolized, as described below.
About one-third of a given dose of sulfasalazine (SS) is absorbed from the small intestine. The remaining two-thirds pass to the colon where the compound is split (presumably by intestinal bacteria) into its components, 5-aminosalicylic acid (5-ASA) and sulfapyridine (SP). Most of the SP thus liberated is absorbed, whereas only about one-third of the 5-ASA is absorbed, the remainder being excreted in the feces. The distribution, metabolism and excretion of SS and its two components are as follows:
Sulfasalazine (SS)—Detectable serum concentrations of SS have been found in healthy subjects within 90 minutes after the ingestion of a single 2 g dose of AZULFIDINE Tablets. Maximum concentrations of SS occur between 1.5 and 6 hours, with the mean peak concentration (14 mcg/ml) occurring at 3 hours. Small amounts of SS are excreted unchanged in the urine.
Sulfapyridine (SP)—Following absorption and distribution, SP is acetylated and hydroxylated in the liver, and then conjugated with glucuronic acid. After ingestion of a single 2 g dose of AZULFIDINE Tablets by healthy subjects, SP and its various metabolites appear in the serum within 3 to 6 hours. Maximum concentrations of total SP occur between 6 and 24 hours, with the mean peak concentration (21 mcg/ml) occurring at 12 hours. The total recovery of SS and its SP metabolites from the urine of healthy subjects 3 days after the administration of a single 2 g dose of AZULFIDINE Tablets averaged 91%.
Mean serum concentrations of total SP, i.e., SP + its metabolites, tend to be significantly greater in patients with a slow acetylator phenotype than in those with a fast acetylator phenotype. SP serum concentrations greater than 50 mcg/ml appear to be associated with adverse reactions.
5-Aminosalicylic Acid (5-ASA)—The serum concentration of 5-ASA in patients with ulcerative colitis was found to range from 0 to 4 mcg/ml, and to exist mainly in the form of free 5-ASA. The urinary recovery of this compound was mostly in the acetylated form.
The mode of action of AZULFIDINE is still under investigation. It may be related to the immunosuppressant properties that have been observed in animal and *in vitro* models, to its affinity for connective tissue, and/or to the relatively high concentration it reaches in serous fluids, the liver and intestinal wall, as demonstrated in autoradiographic studies in animals. AZULFIDINE has also been described as a highly efficient vehicle for carrying its principal metabolites, SP and 5-ASA, to the colon, where a local action for both of them has been postulated.

Continued on next page

Pharmacia—Cont.

Indications: AZULFIDINE is indicated in the treatment of mild to moderate ulcerative colitis, and as adjunctive therapy in severe ulcerative colitis.

Contraindications: Hypersensitivity to sulfonamides or salicylates. In infants under 2 years. Intestinal and urinary obstruction. Pregnancy at term and during nursing because sulfonamides are excreted in the milk. In the newborn, they compete with bilirubin for binding sites on the plasma proteins and may thus cause kernicterus. Patients with porphyria should not receive sulfonamides, as these drugs have been reported to precipitate an acute attack.

Warnings:

Use in Pregnancy—The safe use of sulfonamides in pregnancy has not been established. The benefit to risk ratio must be carefully evaluated when sulfonamides are given during pregnancy, especially at term since kernicterus may be produced in the newborn. The teratogenic potential of most sulfonamides has not been thoroughly investigated in either animals or humans. However, a significant increase in the incidence of cleft palate and other bony abnormalities of offspring has been observed when certain sulfonamides of the short-, intermediate- and long-acting types were given to pregnant rats and mice at high oral doses (7 to 25 times the human therapeutic dose).

Other Warnings—Only after critical appraisal should AZULFIDINE be used in patients with hepatic or renal damage or blood dyscrasias. Deaths associated with the administration of AZULFIDINE have been reported from hypersensitivity reactions, agranulocytosis, aplastic anemia, other blood dyscrasias, renal and liver damage, irreversible neuromuscular and CNS changes, and fibrosing alveolitis. The presence of clinical signs such as sore throat, fever, pallor, purpura, or jaundice may be indications of serious blood disorders. Complete blood counts as well as urinalysis with careful microscopic examination should be done frequently in patients receiving AZULFIDINE.

Precautions: AZULFIDINE should be given with caution to patients with severe allergy or bronchial asthma. Adequate fluid intake must be maintained in order to prevent crystalluria and stone formation. Patients with glucose-6-phosphate dehydrogenase deficiency should be observed closely for signs of hemolytic anemia. This reaction is frequently dose related. If toxic or hypersensitivity reactions occur, the drug should be discontinued immediately.

Adverse Reactions: Adverse reactions have been observed in 5 to 55% of patients included in clinical studies reported in the literature. Experience suggests that with daily dosages of 4 g or more, adverse reactions tend to increase. The most common adverse reactions associated with AZULFIDINE therapy are anorexia, nausea, vomiting, and gastric distress. The following adverse reactions have been reported to occur during therapy with AZULFIDINE.

Blood dyscrasias: Agranulocytosis, aplastic anemia, thrombocytopenia, leukopenia, hemolytic anemia, Heinz Body anemia, purpura, hypoprothrombinemia, "cyanosis", and methemoglobinemia.

Hypersensitivity reactions: Generalized skin eruptions, erythema multiforme (Stevens-Johnson syndrome), parapsoriasis varioliformis acuta (Mucha-Haberman syndrome), exfoliative dermatitis, epidermal necrolysis (Lyell's syndrome) with corneal damage, pruritus, urticaria, photosensitization, anaphylaxis, serum sickness syndrome, chills, drug fever, periorbital edema, conjunctival and scleral injection, arthralgia, transient pulmonary changes with eosinophilia and decreased pulmonary function, allergic myocarditis, polyarteritis nodosa, L. E. phenomenon, and hepatitis with immune complexes.

Gastrointestinal reactions: Anorexia, nausea, emesis, abdominal pains, diarrhea, bloody diarrhea, impaired folic acid and digoxin absorption, stomatitis, pancreatitis, and hepatitis.

CNS reactions: Headache, vertigo, tinnitus, hearing loss, peripheral neuropathy, transient lesions of posterior spinal column, transverse myelitis, ataxia, convulsions, insomnia, mental depression, hallucinations and drowsiness.

Renal reactions: Crystalluria, hematuria, proteinuria, and nephrotic syndrome. Toxic nephrosis with oliguria and anuria.

Incidents of alopecia and reduction in sperm count and viability have also been reported.

The sulfonamides bear certain chemical similarities to some goitrogens, diuretics (acetazolamide and the thiazides), and oral hypoglycemic agents. Goiter production, diuresis, and hypoglycemia have occurred rarely in patients receiving sulfonamides. Cross sensitivity may exist with these agents.

Rats appear to be especially susceptible to the goitrogenic effects of sulfonamides and long-term administration has produced thyroid malignancies in the species.

AZULFIDINE produces an orange-yellow color when the urine is alkaline. Similar discoloration of the skin has also been reported.

Treatment of Overdosage and Sensitivity Reactions:

Overdosage—Gastric lavage or emesis plus catharsis as indicated. Alkalinize urine. If kidney function is normal, force fluids. If anuria is present, restrict fluids and salt, and treat for renal failure. Catheterization of the ureters may be indicated for complete renal blockage by crystals. For agranulocytosis discontinue the drug immediately, hospitalize the patient and institute appropriate therapy.

Sensitivity reactions—Discontinue treatment immediately. Urticaria, other skin rashes, and serum sickness-like reactions may be controlled with antihistamines and, if necessary, systemic corticosteroids.

Dosage and Administration: Dosage should be adjusted to each individual's response and tolerance. The drug should be given in evenly divided doses over each 24-hour period, intervals between nighttime doses should not exceed 8 hours, with administration after meals recommended when feasible. Experience suggests that with daily dosages of 4 g or more adverse reactions tend to increase, hence patients receiving these dosages should be carefully observed for the appearance of adverse effects.

Usual Dosage:

Initial Therapy:

Adults: 3–4 g (6–8 tablets) daily in evenly divided doses. In some cases it is advisable to initiate therapy with a smaller dosage, e.g., 1–2 g (2–4 tablets) daily, to lessen adverse gastrointestinal effects. If daily doses up to 8 g (16 tablets) are required to achieve desired effects, the increased risk of toxicity should be kept in mind.

Children: 40–60 mg per kg body weight in each 24-hour period, divided into 3–6 doses.

Maintenance Therapy:

Adults: 2 g daily (1 tablet q.i.d.).

Children: 30 mg per kg body weight in each 24-hour period, divided into 4 doses.

Response to therapy and adjustment of dosage should be determined by periodic examination. It is often necessary to continue medication, even when clinical symptoms, including diarrhea, have been controlled. When endoscopic examination confirms satisfactory improvement dosage is reduced to a maintenance level. If diarrhea recurs, dosage should be increased to previous effective levels.

If symptoms of gastric intolerance (anorexia, nausea, vomiting, etc.) occur after the first few doses of AZULFIDINE, they are probably due to mucosal irritation, and may be alleviated by distributing the total daily dose more evenly over the day or by giving enteric coated EN-tabs. If such symptoms occur after the first few days of treatment with AZULFIDINE, they are probably due to increased serum levels of total sulfapyridine, and may be alleviated by halving the dose and subsequently increasing it gradually over several days. If symptoms continue, the drug should be stopped for five to seven days, then reinstituted at a lower daily dose.

How Supplied:

AZULFIDINE Tablets 500 mg 100's
NDC No. 0016-0101-01

AZULFIDINE Tablets 500 mg 500's
NDC No. 0016-0101-05

AZULFIDINE Tablets 500 mg Unit Dose 100's
NDC No. 0016-0101-11

AZULFIDINE Tablets 500 mg Unit Dose 10 × 100 (1000's)
NDC No. 0016-0101-10

Also available as

AZULFIDINE EN-tabs 500 mg 100's
NDC No. 0016-0102-01

AZULFIDINE EN-tabs 500 mg 500's
NDC No. 0016-0102-05

[*Shown in Product Identification Section*]

AZULFIDINE ℞

(sulfasalazine, N.F.)
EN-tabs®

Description: AZULFIDINE enteric-coated EN-tabs contain sulfasalazine N.F. which is synthesized by the diazotization of sulfapyridine and the coupling of the diazonium salt with salicylic acid. Further processing results in a bright orange-colored substance that chemically is designated: 5-[[p-(2-Pyridylsulfamoyl)phenyl]azo] salicylic acid. Reductive splitting of the azo linkage yields sulfapyridine and 5- aminosalicylic acid.

AZULFIDINE EN-tabs are film coated with cellulose acetate phthalate to prevent disintegration of the tablet in the stomach and thus to reduce possible irritation of the gastric mucosa. Cellulose acetate phthalate coatings disintegrate due to the hydrolytic effect of the intestinal esterases, even when the intestinal contents are acid.

Actions: After oral administration, AZULFIDINE is partially absorbed and extensively metabolized, as described below.

About one-third of a given dose of sulfasalazine (SS) is absorbed from the small intestine. The remaining two-thirds pass to the colon where the compound is split (presumably by intestinal bacteria) into its components, 5-aminosalicylic acid (5-ASA) and sulfapyridine (SP). Most of the SP thus liberated is absorbed, whereas only about one-third of the 5-ASA is absorbed, the remainder being excreted in the feces. The distribution, metabolism and excretion of SS and its two components are as follows:

Sulfasalazine (SS)—Detectable serum concentrations of SS have been found in healthy subjects within 90 minutes after the ingestion of a single 2 g dose of AZULFIDINE EN-tabs. Maximum concentrations of SS occur between 3 and 12 hours, with the mean peak concentrations (6 mcg/ml) occurring at 6 hours. Small amounts of SS are excreted unchanged in the urine.

Sulfapyridine (SP)—Following absorption and distribution, SP is acetylated and hydroxylated in the liver, and then conjugated with glucuronic acid. After ingestion of a single 2 g dose of AZULFIDINE EN-tabs by healthy subjects, peak concentrations of SP and its various metabolites appear in the serum between 12 and 24 hours, with the peak concentration (13 mcg/ml) occurring at 12 and lasting until 24 hours. The total recovery of SS and its SP metabolites from the urine of healthy subjects 3 days after the administration of a single 2 g dose of AZULFIDINE EN-tabs averaged 81%.

Mean serum concentrations of total SP, i.e., SP + its metabolites, tend to be significantly greater in patients with a slow acetylator phenotype than in those with a fast acetylator phenotype. SP serum concentrations greater than 50 mcg/ml appear to be associated with adverse reactions.

5-Aminosalicylic Acid (5-ASA)—The serum concentration of 5-ASA in patients with ulcerative colitis was found to range from 0 to 4 mcg/ml, and to exist mainly in the form of free 5-ASA. The urinary recovery of this compound was mostly in the acetylated form.

The mode of action of AZULFIDINE is still under investigation. It may be related to the immunosuppressant properties that have been observed in animal and *in vitro* models, to its affinity for connective tissue, and/or to the relatively high concentration it reaches in serous fluids, the liver and intestinal wall, as demonstrated in autoradiographic studies in animals. AZULFIDINE has also been described as a highly efficient vehicle for carrying its principal metabolites, SP and 5-ASA, to the colon, where a local action for both of them has been postulated.

Indications: AZULFIDINE is indicated in the treatment of mild to moderate ulcerative colitis, and as adjunctive therapy in severe ulcerative colitis.

AZULFIDINE EN-tabs are particularly indicated in patients who cannot take the regular AZULFIDINE tablet because of gastrointestinal intolerance, and in whom there is evidence that this intolerance is not primarily due to high blood levels of sulfapyridine and its metabolites, e.g. patients experiencing nausea, vomiting, etc., when taking the first few doses of the drug, or patients in whom a reduction in dosage does not alleviate the gastrointestinal side effects.

Contraindications: Hypersensitivity to sulfonamides or salicylates. In infants under 2 years. Intestinal and urinary obstruction. Pregnancy at term and during nursing because sulfonamides are excreted in the milk. In the newborn, they compete with bilirubin for binding sites on the plasma proteins and may thus cause kernicterus. Patients with porphyria should not receive sulfonamides, as these drugs have been reported to precipitate an acute attack.

Warnings:

Use in Pregnancy—The safe use of sulfonamides in pregnancy has not been established. The benefit to risk ratio must be carefully evaluated when sulfonamides are given during pregnancy, especially at term since kernicterus may be produced in the newborn. The teratogenic potential of most sulfonamides has not been thoroughly investigated in either animals or humans. However, a significant increase in the incidence of cleft palate and other bony abnormalities of offspring has been observed when certain sulfonamides of the short-, intermediate- and long-acting types were given to pregnant rats and mice at high oral doses (7 to 25 times the human therapeutic dose).

Other Warnings—Only after critical appraisal should AZULFIDINE EN-tabs be used in patients with hepatic or renal damage or blood dyscrasias. Deaths associated with the administration of AZULFIDINE have been reported from hypersensitivity reactions, agranulocytosis, aplastic anemia, other blood dyscrasias, renal and liver damage, irreversible neuromuscular and CNS changes, and fibrosing alveolitis. The presence of clinical signs such as sore throat, fever, pallor, purpura, or jaundice may be indications of serious blood disorders. Complete blood counts as well as urinalysis with careful microscopic examination should be done frequently in patients receiving AZULFIDINE.

Precautions: AZULFIDINE EN-tabs should be given with caution to patients with severe allergy or bronchial asthma. Adequate fluid intake must be maintained in order to prevent crystalluria and stone formation. Patients with glucose-6-phosphate dehydrogenase deficiency should be observed closely for signs of hemolytic anemia. This reaction is frequently dose related. If toxic or hypersensitivity reactions occur, the drug should be discontinued immediately. Isolated instances have been reported when AZULFIDINE EN-tabs have passed undisintegrated. This may be due to a lack of intestinal esterases in these patients (see description). If this is observed, the administration of AZULFIDINE EN-tabs should be discontinued immediately.

Adverse Reactions: Adverse reactions have been observed in 5 to 55% of patients included in clinical studies reported in the literature. Experience suggests that with daily dosages of 4 g or more, adverse reactions tend to increase. The most common adverse reactions associated with AZULFIDINE therapy are anorexia, nausea, vomiting, and gastric distress. The following adverse reactions have been reported to occur during therapy with AZULFIDINE.

Blood dyscrasias: Agranulocytosis, aplastic anemia, thrombocytopenia, leukopenia, hemolytic anemia, Heinz Body anemia, purpura, hypoprothrombinemia, "cyanosis", and methemoglobinemia.

Hypersensitivity reactions: Generalized skin eruptions, erythema multiforme (Stevens-Johnson syndrome), parapsoriasis varioliformis acuta (Mucha-Haberman syndrome), exfoliative dermatitis, epidermal necrolysis (Lyell's syndrome) with corneal damage, pruritus, urticaria, photosensitization, anaphylaxis, serum sickness syndrome, chills, drug fever, periorbital edema, conjunctival and scleral injection, arthralgia, transient pulmonary changes with eosinophilia and decreased pulmonary function, allergic myocarditis, polyarteritis nodosa, L. E. phenomenon, and hepatitis with immune complexes.

Gastrointestinal reactions: Anorexia, nausea, emesis, abdominal pains, diarrhea, bloody diarrhea, impaired folic acid and digoxin absorption, stomatitis, pancreatitis, and hepatitis.

CNS reactions: Headache, vertigo, tinnitus, hearing loss, peripheral neuropathy, transient lesions of posterior spinal column, transverse myelitis, ataxia, convulsions, insomnia, mental depression, hallucinations and drowsiness.

Renal reactions: Crystalluria, hematuria, proteinuria, and nephrotic syndrome. Toxic nephrosis with oliguria and anuria.

Incidents of alopecia and reduction in sperm count and viability have also been reported.

The sulfonamides bear certain chemical similarities to some goitrogens, diuretics (acetazolamide and the thiazides), and oral hypoglycemic agents. Goiter production, diuresis, and hypoglycemia have occurred rarely in patients receiving sulfonamides. Cross sensitivity may exist with these agents.

Rats appear to be especially susceptible to the goitrogenic effects of sulfonamides and long-term administration has produced thyroid malignancies in the species.

AZULFIDINE EN-tabs produce an orange-yellow color when the urine is alkaline. Similar discoloration of the skin has also been reported.

Treatment of Overdosage and Sensitivity Reactions:

Overdosage—Gastric lavage or emesis plus catharsis as indicated. Alkalinize urine. If kidney function is normal, force fluids. If anuria is present, restrict fluids and salt, and treat for renal failure. Catheterization of the ureters may be indicated for complete renal blockage by crystals. For agranulocytosis discontinue the drug immediately, hospitalize the patient and institute appropriate therapy.

Sensitivity reactions—Discontinue treatment immediately. Urticaria, other skin rashes, and serum sickness-like reactions may be controlled with antihistamines and, if necessary, systemic corticosteroids.

Dosage and Administration: Dosage should be adjusted to each individual's response and tolerance. The drug should be given in evenly divided doses over each 24-hour period, intervals between nighttime doses should not exceed 8 hours, with administration after meals recommended when feasible. Experience suggests that with daily dosages of 4 g or more adverse reactions tend to increase, hence patients receiving these dosages should be carefully observed for the appearance of adverse effects.

Usual Dosage:

Initial Therapy:

Adults: 3–4 g (6–8 EN-tabs) daily in evenly divided doses. In some cases it is advisable to initiate therapy with a smaller dosage, e.g., 1–2 g (2–4 EN-tabs) daily, to lessen adverse gastrointestinal effects. If daily doses up to 8 g (16 EN-tabs) are required to achieve desired effects, the increased risk of toxicity should be kept in mind.

Children: 40–60 mg per kg body weight in each 24-hour period, divided into 3–6 doses.

Maintenance Therapy:

Adults: 2 g daily (1 EN-tab q.i.d.).

Children: 30 mg per kg body weight in each 24-hour period, divided into 4 doses.

Response to therapy and adjustment of dosage should be determined by periodic examination. It is often necessary to continue medication, even when clinical symptoms, including diarrhea, have been controlled. When endoscopic examination confirms satisfactory improvement, dosage is reduced to a maintenance level. If diarrhea recurs, dosage should be increased to previous effective levels.

If symptoms of gastric intolerance (anorexia, nausea, vomiting, etc.) occur after the first few days of treatment with AZULFIDINE EN-tabs, they are probably due to increased serum levels of total sulfapyridine, and may be alleviated by halving the dose and subsequently increasing it gradually over several days. If symptoms continue, the drug should be stopped for five to seven days, then reinstituted at a lower daily dose.

How Supplied:

AZULFIDINE EN-tabs 500 mg 100's
NDC No. 0016-0102-01

AZULFIDINE EN-tabs 500 mg 500's
NDC No. 0016-0102-05

Also available as

AZULFIDINE Tablets 500 mg 100's
NDC No. 0016-0101-01

AZULFIDINE Tablets 500 mg 500's
NDC No. 0016-0101-05

AZULFIDINE Tablets 500 mg. Unit Dose 100's
NDC No. 0016-0101-11

AZULFIDINE Tablets 500 mg. Unit Dose 10 × 100's (1000's)
NDC No. 0016-0101-10

[*Shown in Product Identification Section*]

DEBRISAN® ℞
(dextranomer)

Description: DEBRISAN® consists of spherical hydrophilic beads of dextranomer, 0.1–0.3 mm in diameter. The beads are composed of a three dimensional network of macromolecular chains of cross-linked dextran which is large enough to allow substances with a molecular weight of less than 1000 to enter freely. Substances with a molecular weight of 1000–5000 enter the beads less freely, while those with a molecular weight greater than 5000 remain in the interspaces between the beads.

Continued on next page

Pharmacia—Cont.

Characteristics: Because of its hydrophilic properties, each gram of DEBRISAN beads absorbs approximately 4 ml of fluid. This action, which is continuous as long as unsaturated beads are in proximity to the lesion, allows DEBRISAN to generate suction forces up to 200 mm Hg.
When DEBRISAN is applied to the surface of exuding lesions, its suction forces immediately begin removing various exudates and particles that tend to impede tissue repair. For example, low molecular weight components of wound exudates are drawn-up within the DEBRISAN beads, while higher molecular weight components, such as plasma proteins, fibrinogen and its high molecular weight split products, are found between the swollen beads. Removal of these latter components, particularly fibrin and fibrinogen split products, retards eschar formation and keeps the lesion soft and pliable. The ability of DEBRISAN to remove exudates rapidly and continuously from the surface of the wound results in a concomitant reduction of inflammation, edema and pain. Additionally, there is in vitro evidence that the suction forces created by DEBRISAN may also remove bacteria and bacterial toxins from the surface of the wound. This overall wound cleansing action of DEBRISAN appears to speed-up the formation of granulation tissue and to reduce the time necessary for wound healing or skin grafting.
Indications: DEBRISAN is indicated for use in cleansing exuding lesions such as venous stasis ulcers, decubitus ulcers, infected traumatic and surgical wounds, and infected burns.
Precautions: To minimize the possibility of cross-contamination, contents of a DEBRISAN container should be limited to use in one patient.
When treating cratered decubitus ulcers, do not pack the wound tightly. Allow for expansion of the beads.
Maceration of surrounding skin may result if occlusive dressings are used.
Once the beads are saturated they should be removed, thereby avoiding encrustation which makes removal more difficult.
Wounds may appear larger during the first few days of treatment due to the reduction of edema.
DEBRISAN is not effective in cleansing non-secreting lesions.
Not all lesions require treatment with DEBRISAN to complete healing. When the wound is no longer exuding and a healthy granulation base has been established, DEBRISAN should be discontinued. At this point, the continued natural healing process usually leads to complete closure of the lesion.
Treatment of the underlying condition (venous or arterial flow, pressure, etc.) should proceed concurrently with the use of DEBRISAN.
Adverse Reactions: Upon application and/or removal of beads, transitory pain, bleeding, blistering and erythema have been reported in isolated cases.
Application: Clean the lesion using sterile water, saline or another appropriate cleansing solution. Leave the cleansed area moist. Pour on a sufficient amount of DEBRISAN to cover the area being treated to a thickness of 3 mm (1/8"–1/4"). A wound or ulcer 1½" × 1½" covered to the proper thickness should require approximately 4 g of DEBRISAN. Lightly bandage to hold the DEBRISAN in place. No special bandaging technique is required because the performance of DEBRISAN does not depend on the type of bandage or final dressing. When DEBRISAN is saturated it becomes greyish-yellow, indicating that it should be removed. Removal should be as complete as possible and is best achieved by irrigating with sterile water, saline, or another cleansing solution. Occasionally vigorous irrigation may be required to remove patches of DEBRISAN beads that adhere to the lesion surface.
DEBRISAN dressings usually require changing once or twice a day. If the lesion is draining profusely, 3 or 4 dressing changes a day may be required. The degree of secretion from the lesion will determine how often DEBRISAN® must be changed. It is advisable to change DEBRISAN before it becomes fully saturated to prevent drying and make removal easier.
For further information, see the directions for use which accompany each package.
How Supplied: DEBRISAN is supplied sterile, in containers of 60 and 120 g and in packages containing seven or fourteen 4 g packets.
Keep dry and store in a well closed container.
Avoid contact with eyes.
For external use only.
Keep out of reach of children.
Avoid spilling beads onto floor, as this will result in a slippery surface.
See accompanying directions for use.
Caution: Federal law restricts this device to sale by or on the order of a physician.

HYSKON® Hysteroscopy Fluid ℞
32% (W/V) dextran 70 in dextrose

Description: HYSKON Hysteroscopy Fluid is a clear, viscid, sterile, non-pyrogenic solution of dextran 70 (32% W/V) in dextrose (10% W/V). Dextran 70 is that fraction of dextran, a branched polysaccharide composed of glucose units, having a weight average molecular weight of 70,000. The fluid is electrolyte-free and non-conductive. At room temperature HYSKON Hysteroscopy Fluid has a viscosity of 220 cSt.
HYSKON has a tendency to crystalize when subjected to temperature variations or when stored for long periods. If flakes of dextran are present, heat at 100°–110° C until complete dissolution is achieved.
Indications: HYSKON Hysteroscopy Fluid is indicated for use with the hysteroscope as an aid in distending the uterine cavity and in irrigating and visualizing its surfaces.
Contraindications: HYSKON Hysteroscopy Fluid should not be instilled in patients known to be hypersensitive to dextran. All other contraindications are those relative to the hysteroscopic procedure itself, such as pregnancy, endometrial carcinoma, etc.
Warnings: It is not known to what extent systemic absorption of dextran 70 occurs from the uterine and peritoneal cavities. Because of the possibility that absorption can occur, the physician should familiarize himself with the systemic effects of this drug. The most alarming are severe, sometimes fatal anaphylactoid reactions, which are quite rare. Other noteworthy effects include plasma volume expansion and transient prolongation of bleeding time.
Adverse Reactions: The physician should be mindful of the fact that adverse reactions are known to occur with the administration of dextran 70. Such reactions, some of which have also been reported with the use of HYSKON, have included: allergic phenomena (generalized itching, macular rash, anaphylactoid reactions, urticaria, nasal congestion, wheezing, tightness of chest and mild hypotension), nausea, vomiting, fever and joint pains.
Dosage and Administration: The amount of HYSKON Hysteroscopy Fluid required per patient depends on a number of factors, such as the type and length of the diagnostic procedure, whether or not manipulation or surgery is performed, etc. Most often, however, the amount of HYSKON instilled into the uterus will be between 50 and 100 milliliters.
HYSKON should be introduced into the uterine cavity through the cannula of a hysteroscope under low pressure (approximately 100 mm Hg) until the uterus is sufficiently distended to permit adequate visualization. During the hysteroscopic examination, HYSKON should be infused at a rate that keeps the cavity suitably distended. To avoid injection of the fluid into the tissues of the uterus and parametria and to avoid having unnecessary amounts of the fluid pass into the peritoneal cavity and backwards along the side of the hysteroscope, infusion pressures greater than 150 mm Hg should not be used.
How Supplied: HYSKON Hysteroscopy Fluid (32% W/V dextran 70 in 10% W/V dextrose) is available as a sterile, nonpyrogenic solution in 100 ml bottles packed 12 to a carton. ....**NDC** No. 0016-0231-61.
Keep from cold during transportation.
Caution: Federal law prohibits dispensing without prescription.

MACRODEX® ℞
(Plasma Volume Expander)

6% Dextran 70 in 5% Dextrose Injection. 500 ml.
6% Dextran 70 in 0.9% Sodium Chloride Injection. 500 ml.

RECTOID® ℞
(hydrocortisone retention enema)

Description: RECTOID enema is a convenient, disposable, single-dose hydrocortisone enema designed for easy self-administration. Each single dose bottle (60 ml.) contains 100 mg of hydrocortisone in aqueous isotonic saline with methylcellulose, carboxypolymethylene, polysorbate 80, disodium edetate, methylparaben and propylparaben. Hydrocortisone is a naturally occurring glucocorticoid (adrenal corticosteroid).
Actions: RECTOID enema provides the potent anti-inflammatory effect of hydrocortisone by means of rectal administration. Data from pharmacokinetic studies in healthy humans indicate that up to 94% of the rectally administered dose of hydrocortisone may be absorbed and cause relatively prolonged plasma hydrocortisone levels. Although rectally administered hydrocortisone has a low incidence of reported adverse reactions, prolonged use can cause systemic reactions similar to those associated with oral dosage forms.
Indications: RECTOID enema is indicated as adjunctive therapy in the treatment of ulcerative colitis.
Contraindications: Systemic fungal infections. Ileocolostomy during the immediate or early postoperative period.
Warnings: In severe ulcerative colitis, it is hazardous to delay needed surgery while awaiting response to medical treatment.
Damage to the rectal wall can result from careless or improper insertion of an enema tip.
In patients on corticosteroid therapy who are subjected to unusual stress, an increased dosage of rapidly acting corticosteroids before, during, and after the stressful situation is indicated.
Corticosteroids may mask some signs of infection, and new infections may appear during their use. There may be decreased resistance and inability to localize infection when corticosteroids are used.
Prolonged use of corticosteroids may produce posterior subcapsular cataracts, glaucoma with possible damage to the optic nerves, and may enhance the establishment of secondary ocular infections due to fungi or viruses.
Usage in pregnancy: Since adequate human reproduction studies have not been done with corticosteroids, the use of these drugs in pregnancy, nursing mothers or women of childbearing potential requires that the possible benefits of the drug be weighed against the potential hazards to the mother and embryo or fetus. Infants born of mothers who have received substantial doses of corticosteroids during pregnancy, should be carefully observed for signs of hypoadrenalism.

Average and large doses of hydrocortisone or cortisone can cause elevation of blood pressure, salt and water retention, and increased excretion of potassium. These effects are less likely to occur with the synthetic derivatives except when used in large doses. Dietary salt restriction and potassium supplementation may be necessary. All corticosteroids increase calcium excretion.
While on corticosteroid therapy patients should not be vaccinated against smallpox. Other immunization procedures should not be undertaken in patients who are on corticosteroids, especially on high dose, because of possible hazards of neurological complications and lack of antibody response. If corticosteroids are indicated in patients with latent tuberculosis or tuberculin reactivity, close observation is necessary as reactivation of the disease may occur. During prolonged corticosteroid therapy, these patients should receive chemoprophylaxis.
Precautions: RECTOID enema should be used with caution where there is a probability of impending perforation, abscess or other pyogenic infection; fresh intestinal anastomoses; obstruction; or extensive fistulas. Use with caution in the presence of active or latent peptic ulcer; diverticulitis; renal insufficiency; hypertension; osteoporosis; or myasthenia gravis.
Steroid therapy might impair prognosis in surgery by increasing the hazard of infection. If infection is suspected, appropriate antibiotic therapy must be administered, usually in larger than ordinary doses.
Drug-induced secondary adrenocortical insufficiency may occur with prolonged RECTOID enema therapy. This is minimized by gradual reduction of dosage. This type of relative insufficiency may persist for months after discontinuation of therapy; therefore, in any situation of stress occurring during that period, hormone therapy should be reinstituted. Since mineralocorticoid secretion may be impaired, salt and/or a mineralocorticoid should be administered concurrently. There is an enhanced effect of corticosteroids on patients with hypothydroidism and in those with cirrhosis. Corticosteroids should be used cautiously in patients with ocular herpes simplex because of possible corneal perforation.
The lowest possible dose of corticosteroid should be used to control the condition under treatment, and when reduction in dosage is possible, the reduction should be gradual.
Psychic derangement may appear when corticosteroids are used, ranging from euphoria, insomnia, mood swings, personality changes, and severe depression, to frank psychotic manifestations. Also, existing emotional instability or psychotic tendencies may be aggravated by corticosteroids.
Aspirin should be used cautiously in conjunction with corticosteroids in hypoprothrombinemia.
Growth and development of infants and children on prolonged corticosteroid therapy should be carefully observed.
Adverse Reactions: Local pain or burning, rectal bleeding, and apparent exacerbations of the disease or sensitivity reactions may occur in rare instances. The following adverse reactions should be kept in mind whenever corticosteroids are given.
Fluid and Electrolyte Disturbances: Sodium retention; fluid retention; congestive heart failure in susceptible patients; potassium loss; hypokalemic alkalosis; hypertension. *Musculoskeletal:* Muscle Weakness; steroid myopathy; loss of muscle mass; osteoporosis; vertebral compression fractures; aseptic necrosis of femoral and humeral heads; pathologic fracture of long bones. *Gastrointestinal:* Peptic ulcer with possible perforation and hemorrhage; pancreatitis; abdominal distention; ulcerative esophagitis. *Dermatologic:* Impaired wound healing; thin fragile skin; petechiae and ecchymoses; facial erythema; increased sweating; may suppress reactions to skin tests. *Neurological:* Convulsions; increased intracranial pressure with papilledema (pseudo-tumor cerebri) usually after treatment; vertigo; headache. *Endocrine:* Menstrual irregularities; development of Cushingoid state; suppression of growth in children; secondary adrenocortical and pituitary unresponsiveness, particularly in times of stress, as in trauma, surgery or illness; decreased carbohydrate tolerance; manifestations of latent diabetes mellitus; increased requirements for insulin or oral hypoglycemic agents in diabetics. *Ophthalmic:* Posterior subcapsular cataracts; increased intraocular pressure; glaucoma; exophthalmos. *Metabolic:* Negative nitrogen balance due to protein catabolism.
Dosage and Administration: The use of RECTOID enema should complement the concomitant use of other measures such as dietary control, sedatives, anti-diarrheal agents, antibacterial therapy, blood replacement, etc.
The usual course of therapy is one RECTOID enema nightly for 21 days, or until clinical and proctological remission is obtained.
Clinical symptoms usually subside promptly within 3 to 5 days. Improvement in the appearance of the mucosa, as seen by sigmoidoscopic examination, may lag somewhat behind clinical improvement. Difficult cases may require as long as 2 or 3 months of RECTOID enema treatment. Where the course of therapy extends beyond 21 days, RECTOID enema should be discontinued gradually by reducing administration to every other night for 2 or 3 weeks. If clinical or proctologic improvement fails to occur within 2 or 3 weeks after starting RECTOID enema, discontinue its use.
Symptomatic improvement, evidenced by decreased diarrhea and bleeding; weight gain; improved appetite; lessened fever; and decrease in leukocytosis, may be misleading and should not be used as the sole criterion in judging efficacy. Sigmoidoscopic examination and X-ray visualization are essential for adequate monitoring.
Patient instructions for administering RECTOID enema are enclosed in each package. It is recommended that the patient lie on his left side during administration and for 30 minutes thereafter, so that the fluid will distribute throughout the left colon. Every effort should be made to retain the enema for at least an hour and, preferably, all night. This may be facilitated by prior sedation and/or antidiarrheal medication, especially early in therapy, when the urge to evacuate is great.
How Supplied: RECTOID enema is a Retention Enema containing hydrocortisone 100 mg and is supplied in boxes of seven 60 ml disposable single-dose bottles with lubricated rectal applicator tips. Also available as a unit-dose preparation, thirty 60 ml disposable single-dose bottles with lubricated rectal applicator tips.
NDC No. 0016-0110-07. (7's)
NDC No. 0016-0110-30. (30's)
Shake Well Before Use.
Store at Room Temperature (20–25°C)—Avoid Excessive Heat.
Caution: Federal law prohibits dispensing without prescription.

RHEOMACRODEX® ℞
(low molecular weight dextran)

10% Dextran 40 in 5% Dextrose Injection. 500 ml.
10% Dextran 40 in 0.9% Sodium Chloride Injection. 500 ml.

Pharmacraft Consumer Products

PHARMACEUTICAL DIVISION
PENNWALT CORPORATION
755 JEFFERSON ROAD
ROCHESTER, N.Y. 14623

ALLEREST® Tablets
(See PDR For Nonprescription Drugs)

ALLEREST® Timed Release Allergy Capsules
(See PDR For Nonprescription Drugs)

CALDESENE® MEDICATED OINTMENT
(See PDR For Nonprescription Drugs)

CALDESENE® MEDICATED POWDER
(See PDR For Nonprescription Drugs)

CRUEX®
Medicated Cream
(See PDR For Nonprescription Drugs)

CRUEX®
MEDICATED POWDER
(See PDR For Nonprescription Drugs)

DESENEX®
(See PDR For Nonprescription Drugs)

DESENEX® Spray-On Foot Powder
(See PDR For Nonprescription Drugs)

SINAREST® Tablets
(See PDR For Nonprescription Drugs)

Philips Roxane Laboratories, Inc.

P.O. 16532
COLUMBUS, OH 43216

HOSPITAL UNIT DOSE

Hospital Unit Dose—Philips Roxane, was developed to aid in improved drug distribution and administration. With Hospital Unit Dose, each single unit of medication moves from our quality controlled production lines to the patient's bedside in tamper proof containers, labeled for positive identification, thus protecting dosage integrity to the point of administration.
The following products are currently available in Hospital Unit Dose:
Acetaminophen Elixir USP 120mg/5ml, 325mg/12.5ml, 650mg/25ml
Acetaminophen Suppositories 120mg, 650mg
Acetaminophen Tablets USP 325mg, 650mg
Acetaminophen 300 mg with Codeine Phosphate 15 mg tablets
Acetaminophen 300 mg with Codeine Phosphate 30 mg tablets
Acetaminophen 300 mg with Codeine Phosphate 60 mg tablets
Aluminum Hydroxide Gel USP (Flavored) 30ml
Aminophylline Suppositories USP 500mg
Amitriptyline Hydrochloride Tablets USP 10mg, 25mg, 50mg, 75mg, 100mg, 150mg
Aromatic Cascara Fluidextract USP 5ml
Ascorbic Acid Tablets USP 250mg, 500mg
Aspirin Suppositories USP 125mg, 300mg, 600mg

Continued on next page

Philips Roxane—Cont.

Barium Enema Prep Kit
Bisacodyl Suppositories USP 10mg
Bisacodyl Tablets USP 5mg
Bisacodyl Patient Pack
Calcium Gluconate Tablets USP
Castor Oil USP 30ml, 60ml
Castor Oil Flavored 30ml, 60ml
Chloral Hydrate Syrup USP 500mg/10ml, 1g/10ml
Chloral Hydrate Capsules USP 500mg
Chlordiazepoxide Hydrochloride Capsules USP 10mg, 25mg
Chlorpromazine Hydrochloride Tablets USP 10mg, 25mg, 50mg, 100mg, 200mg
Dexamethasone Tablets USP 0.5 mg, 0.75mg, 1.5mg, 4mg
Digoxin Tablets USP 0.25mg
Dihydrotachysterol Tablets USP 0.125mg, 0.2mg
Dioctyl Sodium Sulfosuccinate Capsules USP 50mg, 100mg, 250mg
Dioctyl Sodium Sulfosuccinate Syrup NF 50mg/15ml, 100mg/30ml
Dioctyl Sodium Sulfosuccinate 100mg with Casanthranol 30mg Capsules
Diphenhydramine Hydrochloride Elixir USP 25mg/10ml
Diphenhydramine Hydrochloride Capsules USP 50mg
Diphenoxylate Hydrochloride 2.5mg and Atropine Sulfate 0.025mg Tablets USP
Ferrous Sulfate Liquid 300mg/5ml
Ferrous Sulfate Tablets USP 300mg
Glycerin Oral Solution USP 180 ml
Guaifenesin Syrup NF 100mg/5ml, 200mg/10ml, 300mg/15ml
Hemorrhoidal Suppositories with Hydrocortisone Acetate
Hydrochlorothiazide Tablets USP 25mg, 50mg
Imipramine Hydrochloride Tablets USP 10mg, 25mg, 50mg
Ipecac Syrup USP 15ml, 30ml
Kaolin-Pectin Suspension 30ml
Lithium Carbonate Capsules USP 300mg
Magnesia and Alumina Oral Suspension USP 30ml
Meprobamate Tablets USP 200mg, 400mg
Milk of Magnesia USP 15ml, 30ml
Milk of Magnesia Concentrated Flavored 10ml, 15ml, 20ml
Milk of Magnesia—Cascara Suspension 30ml
Milk of Magnesia—Mineral Oil Emulsion 30ml
Milk of Magnesia—Mineral Oil Emulsion (Flavored) 30ml
Mineral Oil-Light Sterile 10ml, 30ml
Mineral Oil USP 30ml
Neomycin Sulfate Tablets USP 500 mg
Niacin Tablets NF 50mg, 100mg
Papaverine Hydrochloride Prolonged Release Capsules 150mg
Paregoric USP 5ml
Phenobarbital Elixir USP 20mg/5ml
Phenobarbital Tablets USP 15mg, 30mg, 60mg, 100mg
Potassium Chloride Oral Solution USP 5% (20mEq/30ml)
Potassium Chloride Oral Solution USP 10% (15mEq/11.25ml)
Potassium Chloride Oral Solution USP 10% (20mEq/15ml)
Potassium Chloride Oral Solution USP 10% (30mEq/22.5ml)
Potassium Chloride Oral Solution USP 10% (40mEq/30ml)
Potassium Chloride Oral Solution USP 20% (80mEq/30ml)
Potassium Chloride for Oral Solution USP 20mEq/4g
Potassium Chloride USP Powder Unflavored 20mEq/1.5g
Potassium Gluconate Elixir NF 20mEq/15ml
Potassium Iodide Liquid 500mg/15ml
Prednisolone Tablets USP 5mg
Prednisone Tablets USP 5mg, 10mg, 20mg, 50mg
Propantheline Bromide Tablets USP 15mg
Propoxyphene Hydrochloride Capsules USP 65 mg
Propoxyphene Hydrochloride 65 mg and APC Capsules USP
Quinidine Sulfate Tablets USP 200mg, 300mg
Reserpine Tablets USP 0.25mg
SSKI 1g/ml
Sodium Phosphate and Biphosphate Oral Solution USP 30ml
Sulfisoxazole Tablets USP 500mg
Terpin Hydrate and Codeine Elixir NF 5ml
Theophylline Elixir 80mg/15ml, 160mg/30ml

As research continues, new Philips Roxane Laboratories' products will be available in Hospital Unit Dose packages.

DIHYDROTACHYSTEROL TABLETS USP ℞

Description: Each tablet contains:
Dihydrotachysterol...... 0.125mg, 0.2mg, or 0.4 mg
Dihydrotachysterol is a synthetic reduction product of tachysterol, a close isomer of vitamin D.

Actions: Dihydrotachysterol is hydroxylated in the liver to 25-hydroxydihydrotachysterol, which is the major circulating active form of the drug. It does not undergo further hydroxylation by the kidney and therefore is the analogue of 1,25-dihydroxyvitamin D. Dihydrotachysterol is effective in the elevation of serum calcium by stimulating intestinal calcium absorption and mobilizing bone calcium in the absence of parathyroid hormone and of functioning renal tissue. Dihydrotachysterol also increases renal phosphate excretion. In contrast to parathyroid extract, Dihydrotachysterol is active when taken orally, exerts a slow but persistent effect, and may be used for long periods without increasing the dosage or causing tolerance. Dihydrotachysterol is faster-acting than pharmacologic doses of vitamin D and is less persistent after cessation of treatment, thus decreasing the risk of accumulation and of hypercalcemia.

Indications: Dihydrotachysterol is indicated for the treatment of acute, chronic, and latent forms of postoperative tetany, idiopathic tetany, and hypoparathyroidism.

Contraindications: Contraindicated in patients with hypercalcemia, abnormal sensitivity to the effects of vitamin D, and hypervitaminosis D.

Warning: **Usage in Pregnancy.** The safety of dihydrotachysterol during pregnancy has not been established. Animal reproduction studies have shown fetal abnormalities in several species associated with hypervitaminosis D. These are similar to the supravalvular aortic stenosis syndrome described in infants by Black in England (1963). This syndrome was characterized by supravalvular aortic stenosis, elfin facies, and mental retardation. For the protection of the fetus, therefore, the use of Dihydrotachysterol during normal pregnancy should be avoided unless, in the judgment of the physician, the potential benefits outweigh the possible hazards.

Precautions: To prevent hypercalcemia, treatment should always be controlled by regular determinations of blood calcium level, which should be maintained within the normal range. The difference between therapeutic dose and intoxicating dose may be small in any patient and therefore dosage must be individualized and periodically reevaluated.
Because of its effect on serum calcium, Dihydrotachysterol should be administered to pregnant patients or to patients with renal stones only when, in the judgment of the physician, the potential benefits outweigh the possible hazards.
In patients with renal osteodystrophy accompanied by hyperphosphatemia, maintenance of a normal serum phosphorus level by dietary phosphate restriction and/or administration of aluminum gels as intestinal phosphate binders is essential to prevent metastatic calcification. Administration of thiazide diuretics to hypoparthyroid patients who are concurrently being treated with Dihydrotachysterol may cause hypercalcemia.

Dosage and Administration: The dosage depends on the nature and seriousness of the disorder and should be adapted to each individual patient. Serum calcium levels should be maintained between 9 to 10 mg per 100 ml. The following dosage schedule will serve as a guide: *Initial dose:* 0.8 mg to 2.4 mg daily for several days. *Maintenance dose:* 0.2 mg to 1.0 mg daily as required for normal serum calcium levels. The average maintenance dose is 0.6 mg daily. This dose may be supplemented with 10 to 15 grams of calcium lactate or gluconate by mouth daily.

Overdosage: The effects of Dihydrotachysterol can persist for up to one month after cessation of treatment.
Manifestations: Toxicity associated with dihydrotachysterol is similar to that seen with large doses of vitamin D. Overdosage is manifested by symptoms of hypercalcemia, i.e., weakness, headache, anorexia, nausea, vomiting, abdominal cramps, diarrhea, constipation, vertigo, tinnitus, ataxia, hypotonia, lethargy, depression, amnesia, disorientation, hallucinations, syncope, and coma. Impairment of renal function may result in polyuria, polydipsia, and albuminuria. Widespread calcification of soft tissues, including heart, blood vessels, kidneys, and lungs can occur. Death can result from cardiovascular or renal failure.
Treatment: Treatment of overdosage consists of withdrawal of Dihydrotachysterol, bed rest, liberal intake of fluids, a low-calcium diet, and administration of a laxative. Hypercalcemic crisis with dehydration, stupor, coma, and azotemia requires more vigorous treatment. The first step should be hydration of the patient. Intravenous saline may quickly and significantly increase urinary calcium excretion. A loop diuretic (furosemide or ethacrynic acid) may be given with the saline infusion to further increase renal calcium excretion. Other reported therapeutic measures include dialysis or the administration of citrates, sulfates, phosphates, corticosteroids, EDTA (ethylenediaminetetraacetic acids), and mithramycin via appropriate regimens.

How Supplied:
0.125 mg white tablets.
NDC 0054-8172-25: Unit dose, 10 tablets per strip, 10 strips per shelf pack, 10 shelf packs per shipper.
NDC 0054-4190-19: Bottles of 50 tablets.
0.2 mg pink tablets.
NDC 0054-8182-25: Unit dose, 10 tablets per strip, 10 strips per shelf pack, 10 shelf packs per shipper.
NDC 0054-4189-25: Bottles of 100 tablets.
0.4 mg white tablets.
NDC 0054-4191-19: Bottles of 50 tablets.

IMIPRAMINE HYDROCHLORIDE TABLETS USP ℞

How Supplied:
10 mg Film Coated tablets.
NDC 0054-8418-25: Unit dose, 10 tablets per strip, 10 strips per shelf pack, 10 shelf packs per shipper.
NDC 0054-4418-25: Bottles of 100 tablets.
NDC 0054-4418-31: Bottles of 1000 tablets.
25 mg Film Coated tablets.
NDC 0054-8419-25: Unit dose, 10 tablets per strip, 10 strips per shelf pack, 10 shelf packs per shipper.

NDC 0054-4419-31: Bottles of 1000 tablets.
50 mg Film Coated tablets.
NDC 0054-8420-25: Unit dose, 10 tablets per strip, 10 strips per shelf pack, 10 shelf packs per shipper.
NDC 0054-4420-31: Bottles of 1000 tablets.

LITHIUM CARBONATE ℞ CAPSULES AND TABLETS USP, 300 mg

For Control of Manic Episodes in Manic-Depressive Psychosis

WARNING
Lithium toxicity is closely related to serum lithium levels, and can occur at doses close to therapeutic levels. Facilities for prompt and accurate serum lithium determinations should be available before initiating therapy.

Description: Lithium carbonate is a white, light, alkaline powder with molecular formula Li_2CO_3 and molecular weight 73.89. Lithium is an element of the alkali-metal group with atomic number 3, atomic weight 6.94 and an emission line at 671 on the flame photometer.

Actions: Preclinical studies have shown that lithium alters sodium transport in nerve and muscle cells and effects a shift toward intraneuronal metabolism of catecholamines, but the specific biochemical mechanism of lithium action in mania is unknown.

Indications: Lithium carbonate is indicated in the treatment of manic episodes of manic depressive illness. Maintenance therapy prevents or diminishes the intensity of subsequent episodes in those manic-depressive patients with a history of mania.

Typical symptoms of mania include pressure of speech, motor hyperactivity, reduced need for sleep, flight of ideas, grandiosity, elation, poor judgment, aggressiveness, and possibly hostility. When given to a patient experiencing a manic episode, lithium may produce a normalization of symptomatology within 1 to 3 weeks.

Warnings: Lithium should generally not be given to patients with significant renal or cardiovascular disease, severe debilitation or dehydration, or sodium depletion, and to patients receiving diuretics, since the risk of lithium toxicity is very high in such patients. If the psychiatric indication is life-threatening, and if such a patient fails to respond to other measures, lithium treatment may be undertaken with extreme caution, including daily serum lithium determinations and adjustment to the usually low doses ordinarily tolerated by these individuals. In such instances, hospitalization is a necessity.

Lithium therapy has been reported in some cases to be associated with morphologic changes in the kidneys. The relationship between such changes and renal function has not been established.

Lithium toxicity is closely related to serum lithium levels, and can occur at doses close to therapeutic levels (see DOSAGE AND ADMINISTRATION).

Outpatients and their families should be warned that the patient must discontinue lithium carbonate therapy and contact his physician if such clinical signs of lithium toxicity as diarrhea, vomiting, tremor, mild ataxia, drowsiness, or muscular weakness occur.

Combined use of haloperidol and lithium: An encephalopathic syndrome (characterized by weakness, lethargy, fever, tremulousness and confusion, extrapyramidal symptoms, leucocytosis, elevated serum enzymes, BUN and FBS) followed by irreversible brain damage has occurred in a few patients treated with lithium plus haloperidol. A causal relationship between these events and the concomitant administration of lithium and haloperidol has not been established; however, patients receiving such combined therapy should be monitored closely for early evidence of neurological toxicity and treatment discontinued promptly if such signs appear.

Usage in Pregnancy: Adverse effects on nidation in rats, embryo viability in mice, and metabolism in-vitro of rat testis and human spermatozoa have been attributed to lithium, as have teratogenicity in submammalian species and cleft palates in mice. Studies in rats, rabbits and monkeys have shown no evidence of lithium-induced teratology.

There are lithium birth registries in the United States and elsewhere; however there are at the present time insufficient data to determine the effects of lithium carbonate on human fetuses. Therefore, at this point, lithium should not be used in pregnancy, especially the first trimester, unless in the opinion of the physician, the potential benefits outweigh the possible hazards.

Usage in Children: Since information regarding the safety and effectiveness of lithium carbonate in children under 12 years of age is not available, its use in such patients is not recommended at this time.

Precautions: The ability to tolerate lithium is greater during the acute manic phase and decreases when manic symptoms subside (see DOSAGE AND ADMINISTRATION).

The distribution space of lithium approximates that of total body water. Lithium is primarily excreted in urine with insignificant excretion in feces. Renal excretion of lithium is proportional to its plasma concentration. The half-elimination time of lithium is approximately 24 hours. Lithium decreases sodium reabsorption by the renal tubules which could lead to sodium depletion. Therefore, it is essential for the patient to maintain a normal diet, including salt, and an adequate fluid intake (2500–3000 ml) at least during the initial stabilization period. Decreased tolerance to lithium has been reported to ensue from protracted sweating or diarrhea and, if such occur, supplemental fluid and salt should be administered.

In addition to sweating and diarrhea, concomitant infection with elevated temperatures may also necessitate a temporary reduction or cessation of medication.

The possibility of adverse interaction with antipsychotic medications exists.

Adverse Reactions: Adverse reactions are seldom encountered at serum lithium levels below 1.5 mEq/1, except in the occasional patient sensitive to lithium. Mild to moderate toxic reactions may occur at levels from 1.5–2.5 mEq/1, and moderate to severe reactions may be seen at levels from 2.0–2.5 mEq/1 depending upon individual response to the drug.

Fine hand tremor, polyuria and mild thirst may occur during initial therapy for the acute manic phase, and may persist throughout treatment. Transient and mild nausea and general discomfort may also appear during the first few days of lithium administration.

These side effects are an inconvenience rather than a disabling condition, and usually subside with continued treatment or a temporary reduction or cessation of dosage. If persistent, a cessation of dosage is indicated.

Diarrhea, vomiting, drowsiness, muscular weakness and lack of coordination may be early signs of lithium intoxication, and can occur at lithium levels below 2.0 mEq/1. At higher levels, giddiness, ataxia, blurred vision, tinnitus and a large output of dilute urine may be seen. Serum lithium levels above 3.0 mEq/1 may produce a complex clinical picture involving multiple organs and organ systems. Serum lithium levels should not be permitted to exceed 2.0 mEq/1 during the acute treatment phase.

The following toxic reactions have been reported and appear to be related to serum lithium levels:

Neuromuscular: tremor, muscle hyperirritability (fasciculations, twitching, clonic movements of whole limbs), ataxia, choreo-athetotic movements, hyperactive deep tendon reflexes.

Central Nervous System: blackout spells, epileptiform seizures, slurred speech, dizziness, vertigo, incontinence of urine or feces, somnolence, psychomotor retardation, restlessness, confusion, stupor, coma.

Cardiovascular: cardiac arrhythmia, hypotension, peripheral circulatory collapse.

Gastrointestinal: anorexia, nausea, vomiting, diarrhea.

Genitourinary: albuminuria, oliguria, polyuria, glycosuria.

Dermatologic: drying and thinning of hair, anesthesia of skin, chronic folliculitis, xerosis cutis.

Autonomic Nervous System: blurred vision, dry mouth.

Miscellaneous: fatigue, lethargy, tendency to sleep, dehydration, weight loss, transient scotomata.

Thyroid Abnormalities: Euthyroid goiter and/or hypothyroidism (including myxedema) accompanied by lower T_3 and T_4. I_{131} iodine uptake may be elevated. Underlying thyroid disorders do not constitute a contraindication to lithium treatment; careful monitoring of thyroid function during lithium stabilization and maintenance allows for correction of changing thyroid parameters, if any. They can be treated by prescribing thyroid in these cases.

EEG Changes: diffuse slowing, widening of frequency spectrum, potentiation and disorganization of background rhythm.

EKG Changes: reversible flattening, isoelectricity or inversion of T-waves.

Miscellaneous reactions unrelated to dosage are: transient electroencephalographic and electrocardiographic changes, leucocytosis, headache, diffuse nontoxic goiter with or without hypothyroidism, transient hyperglycemia, generalized pruritis with or without rash, cutaneous ulcers, albuminuria, worsening of organic brain syndromes, excessive weight gain, edematous swelling of ankles or wrists, and thirst or polyuria, sometimes resembling diabetes insipidus.

A single report has been received of the development of painful discoloration of fingers and toes and coldness of the extremities within one day of the starting of treatment of lithium. The mechanism through which these symptoms (resembling Reynaud's Syndrome) developed is not known. Recovery followed discontinuance.

Dosage and Administration:

Acute Mania: Optimal patient response to lithium carbonate usually can be established and maintained with 600 mg t.i.d. Such doses will normally produce an effective serum lithium level ranging between 1.0 and 1.5 mEq/1. Dosage must be individualized according to serum levels and clinical response. Regular monitoring of the patient's clinical state and of serum lithium levels is necessary. Serum levels should be determined twice per week during the acute phase, and until the serum level and clinical condition of the patient have been stabilzed.

Long-term Control: The desirable lithium levels are 0.6 to 1.2 mEq/1. Dosage will vary from one individual to another, but usually 300 mg t.i.d. or q.i.d. will maintain this level. Serum lithium levels in uncomplicated cases receiving maintenance therapy during remission should be monitored at least every two months.

Patients abnormally sensitive to lithium may exhibit toxic signs at serum levels of 1.0 to 1.5 mEq/1. Elderly patients often respond to reduced dosage, and may exhibit signs of toxicity at serum levels ordinarily tolerated by other patients.

N. B.: Blood samples for serum lithium determination are drawn 8–12 hours after the previ-

Continued on next page

Philips Roxane—Cont.

ous dose when lithium concentrations are relatively stable. Total reliance must not be placed on serum levels alone. Accurate patient evaluation requires both clinical and laboratory analysis.

Overdosage: The toxic levels for lithium are close to the therapeutic levels. It is therefore important that patients and their families be cautioned to watch for early toxic symptoms and to discontinue the drug and inform the physician should they occur. Toxic symptoms are listed in detail under ADVERSE REACTIONS.

Treatment: No specific antidote for lithium poisoning is known. Early symptoms of lithium toxicity can usually be treated by reduction or cessation of dosage of the drug and resumption of the treatment at a lower dose after 24 to 48 hours. In severe cases of lithium poisoning, the first and foremost goal of treatment consists of elimination of this ion from the organism.

Treatment is essentially the same as that used in barbiturate poisoning: 1) lavage, 2) correction of fluid and electrolyte imbalance and 3) regulation of kidney functioning. Urea, mannitol, and aminophylline all produce significant increases in lithium excretion. Infection prophylaxis, regular chest X-rays, and preservation of adequate respiration are essential.

How Supplied:

300 mg flesh-colored capsules.

NDC 0054-8527-25: Unit dose, 10 capsules per strip, 10 strips per shelf pack, 10 shelf packs per shipper.

NDC 0054-2527-25: Bottles of 100 capsules.

NDC 0054-2527-31: Bottles of 1000 capsules.

300 mg white, scored tablets.

NDC 0054-4527-25: Bottles of 100 tablets.

NDC 0054-4527-31: Bottles of 1000 tablets.

LITHIUM CITRATE SYRUP ℞

8 mEq of Lithium per 5 ml
SUGAR FREE
FOR ORAL ADMINISTRATION ONLY
For Control of Manic Episodes in Manic-Depressive Psychosis

> WARNING
> **Lithium toxicity is closely related to serum lithium levels, and can occur at doses close to therapeutic levels. Facilities for prompt and accurate serum lithium determinations should be available before initiating therapy.**

Description: Lithium Citrate Syrup is a palatable oral dosage form of lithium ion. Lithium citrate is prepared in solution from lithium hydroxide and citric acid in a ratio approximating di-lithium citrate:

Each 5 ml of Lithium Citrate Syrup contains 8 mEq of lithium ion (Li+), equivalent to the amount of lithium in 300 mg of lithium carbonate. Lithium is an element of the alkali-metal group with atomic number 3, atomic weight 6.94, and an emission line at 671nm on the flame photometer.

Actions: Preclinical studies have shown that lithium alters sodium transport in nerve and muscle cells and effects a shift toward intraneuronal metabolism of catecholamines, but the specific biochemical mechanism of lithium action in mania is unknown.

Indications: Lithium Citrate Syrup is indicated in the treatment of manic episodes of manic depressive illness. Maintenance therapy prevents or diminishes the intensity of subsequent episodes in those manic-depressive patients with a history of mania.

Typical symptoms of mania include pressure of speech, motor hyperactivity, reduced need for sleep, flight of ideas, grandiosity, elation, poor judgment, aggressiveness, and possibly hostility. When given to a patient experiencing a manic episode, lithium may produce a normalization of symptomatology within 1 to 3 weeks.

Warnings: Lithium should generally not be given to patients with significant renal or cardiovascular disease, severe debilitation or dehydration, or sodium depletion, and to patients receiving diuretics, since the risk of lithium toxicity is very high in such patients. If the psychiatric indication is life-threatening, and if such a patient fails to respond to other measures, lithium treatment may be undertaken with extreme caution, including daily serum lithium determinations and adjustment to the usually low doses ordinarily tolerated by these individuals. In such instances, hospitalization is a necessity.

Lithium therapy has been reported in some cases to be associated with morphologic changes in the kidneys. The relationship between such changes and renal function has not been established.

Lithium toxicity is closely related to serum lithium levels, and can occur at dose close to therapeutic levels (see DOSAGE AND ADMINISTRATION).

Outpatients and their families should be warned that the patient must discontinue lithium therapy and contact his physician if such clinical signs of lithium toxicity as diarrhea, vomiting, tremor, mild ataxia, drowsiness, or muscular weakness occur.

Combined use of haloperidol and lithium: An encephalopathic syndrome (characterized by weakness, lethargy, fever, tremulousness and confusion, extrapyramidal symptoms, leucocytosis, elevated serum enzymes, BUN and FBS) followed by irreversible brain damage has occurred in a few patients treated with lithium plus haloperidol. A causal relationship between these events and the concomitant administration of lithium and haloperidol has not been established; however, patients receiving such combined therapy should be monitored closely for early evidence of neurological toxicity and treatment discontinued promptly if such signs appear.

Usage in Pregnancy: Adverse effects on nidation in rats, embryo viability in mice, and metabolism in-vitro of rat tests and human spermatozoa have been attributed to lithium, as have teratogenicity in submammalian species and cleft palates in mice. Studies in rats, rabbits and monkeys have shown no evidence of lithium-induced teratology.

There are lithium birth registries in the United States and elsewhere; however there are at the present time insufficient data to determine the effects of lithium on human fetuses.

Therefore, at this point, lithium should not be used in pregnancy, especially the first trimester, unless in the opinion of the physician, the potential benefits outweigh the possible hazards.

Usage in Children: Since information regarding the safety and effectiveness of lithium in children under 12 years of age is not available, its use in such patients is not recommended at this time.

Precautions: The ability to tolerate lithium is greater during the acute manic phase and decreases when manic symptoms subside (see DOSAGE AND ADMINISTRATION).

The distribution space of lithium approximates that of total body water. Lithium is primarily excreted in urine with insignificant excretion in feces. Renal excretion of lithium is proportional to its plasma concentration. The half-elimination time of lithium is approximately 24 hours. Lithium decreases sodium reabsorption by the renal tubules which could lead to sodium depletion. Therefore, it is essential for the patient to maintain a normal diet, including salt, and an adequate fluid intake (2500–3000 ml) at least during the initial stabilization period. Decreased tolerance to lithium has been reported to ensue from protracted sweating or diarrhea and, if such occur, supplemental fluid and salt should be administered.

In addition to sweating and diarrhea, concomitant infection with elevated temperatures may also necessitate a temporary reduction or cessation of medication.

The possibility of adverse interaction with antipsychotic medications exists.

Adverse Reactions: Adverse reactions are seldom encountered at serum lithium levels below 1.5 mEq/l except in the occasional patient sensitive to lithium. Mild to moderate toxic reactions may occur at levels from 1.5–2.5 mEq/1, and moderate to severe reactions may be seen at levels from 2.0–2.5 mEq/1, depending upon individual response to the drug.

Fine hand tremor, polyuria and mild thirst may occur during initial therapy for the acute manic phase, and may persist throughout treatment. Transient and mild nausea and general discomfort may also appear during the first few days of lithium administration.

These side effects are an inconvenience rather than a disabling condition, and usually subside with continued treatment or a temporary reduction or cessation of dosage. If persistent, a cessation of dosage is indicated.

Diarrhea, vomiting, drowsiness, muscular weakness and lack of coordination may be early signs of lithium intoxication, and can occur at lithium levels below 2.0 mEq/l. At higher levels, giddiness, ataxia, blurred vision, tinnitus and a large output of dilute urine may be seen. Serum lithium levels above 3.0 mEq/l may produce a complex clinical picture involving multiple organs and organ systems. Serum lithium levels should not be permitted to exceed 2.0 mEq/l during the acute treatment phase.

The following toxic reactions have been reported and appear to be related to serum lithium levels:

Neuromuscular: tremor, muscle hyperirritability (fasciculations, twitching, clonic movements of whole limbs), ataxia, choreoathetotic movements, hyperactive deep tendon reflexes.

Central Nervous System: blackout spells, epileptiform seizures, slurred speech, dizziness, vertigo, incontinence of urine or feces, somnolence, psychomotor retardation, restlessness, confusion, stupor, coma.

Cardiovascular: cardiac arrhythmia, hypotension, peripheral circulatory collapse.

Gastrointestinal: anorexia, nausea, vomiting, diarrhea.

Genitourinary: Albuminuria, oliguria, polyuria, glycosuria.

Dermatologic: drying and thinning of hair, anesthesia of skin, chronic folliculitis, xerosis cutis.

Autonomic Nervous System: blurred vision, dry mouth.

Miscellaneous: fatigue, lethargy, tendency to sleep, dehydration, weight loss, transient scotomata.

Thyroid Abnormalities: Euthyroid goiter and/or hypothyroidism (including myxedema) accompanied by lower T_3 and T_4. Iodine 131 uptake may be elevated. Underlying thyroid disorders do not constitute a contraindication to lithium treatment; careful monitoring of thyroid function during lithium stabilization and maintenance allows for correction of changing thyroid parameters, if any. They can be treated by prescribing thyroid in these cases.

EEG Changes: diffuse slowing, widening of frequency spectrum, potentiation and disorganization of background rhythm.

EKG Changes: reversible flattening, isoelectricity or inversion of T-waves.

Miscellaneous reactions unrelated to dosage are: transient electroencephalographic and electrocardiographic changes, leucocytosis, headache, diffuse nontoxic goiter with or without hypothyroidism, transient hyperglycemia, generalized pruritis with or without rash, cutaneous ulcers, albuminuria, worsening of organic brain syndromes, excessive weight gain, edematous swelling of ankles or wrists, and thirst or polyuria, sometimes resembling diabetes insipidus.

A single report has been received of the development of painful discoloration of fingers and toes and coldness of the extremities within one day of the starting of treatment of lithium. The mechanism through which these symptoms (resembling Raynaud's Syndrome) developed is not known. Recovery followed discontinuance.

Dosage and Administration:

Acute Mania: Optimal patient response to Lithium Citrate Syrup usually can be established and maintained with 10 ml (2 teaspoons) (16 mEq of lithium) t.i.d. Such doses will normally produce an effective serum lithium level ranging between 1.0 and 1.5 mEq/l. Dosage must be individualized according to serum levels and clinical response. Regular monitoring of the patient's clinical state and of serum lithium levels is necessary. Serum levels should be determined twice per week during the acute phase, and until the serum level and clinical condition of the patient have been stabilized.

Long-term Control: The desirable serum lithium levels are 0.6 to 1.2 mEq/l. Dosage will vary from one individual to another, but usually 5 ml (1 teaspoon) (8 mEq of lithium) t.i.d. or q.i.d. will maintain this level. Serum lithium levels in uncomplicated cases receiving maintenance therapy during remission should be monitored at least every two months.

Patients abnormally sensitive to lithium may exhibit toxic signs at serum levels of 1.0 to 1.5 mEq/l. Elderly patients often respond to reduced dosage, and may exhibit signs of toxicity at serum levels ordinarily tolerated by other patients.

N.B.: Blood samples for serum lithium determinations are drawn 8–12 hours after the previous dose when lithium concentrations are relatively stable. Total reliance must not be placed on serum levels alone. Accurate patient evaluation requires both clinical and laboratory analysis.

Overdosage: The toxic levels for lithium are close to the therapeutic levels. It is therefore important that patients and their families be cautioned to watch for early symptoms and to discontinue the drug and inform the physician should they occur. Toxic symptoms are listed in detail under ADVERSE REACTIONS.

Treatment: No specific antidote for lithium poisoning is known. Early symptoms of lithium toxicity can usually be treated by reduction or cessation of dosage of the drug and resumption of the treatment at a lower dose after 24 to 48 hours. In severe cases of lithium poisoning, the first and foremost goal of treatment consists of elimination of this ion from the organism.

Treatment is essentially the same as that used in barbiturate poisoning: 1) lavage, 2) correction of fluid and electrolyte imbalance and 3) regulation of kidney functioning. Urea, mannitol, and aminophylline all produce significant increases in lithium excretion. Infection prophylaxis, regular chest X-rays, and preservation of adequate respiration are essential.

How Supplied:

Lithium Citrate Syrup, 8 mEq per 5 ml

NDC 0054-3527-62: Bottles of 480 ml.

Caution: Federal law prohibits dispensing without prescription.

POTASSIUM CHLORIDE ORAL SOLUTION USP, POTASSIUM CHLORIDE POWDER USP, and POTASSIUM CHLORIDE for ORAL SOLUTION USP ℞

Description: Potassium chloride is usually the salt of choice in the treatment of hypopotassemia since chloride and potassium deficiencies are likely to be associated with each other.

Indications: Potassium chloride is used in the treatment of conditions characterized by hypopotassemia. Diarrhea and vomiting may give rise to potassium deficiency since the gastric secretion contains approximately ten times as much potassium as does the serum and the intestinal secretions contain about twice as much potassium as does the serum. Other factors which tend to decrease serum potassium levels include decreased potassium intake; increased renal excretion of potassium, which may occur in diuresis, acidosis, or adrenal cortical hyperactivity; injection of potassium-free fluids which increase extracellular fluid volume; and increased glucose uptake by the cells such as occurs in diabetic acidosis treated with insulin.

The use of potassium salts is indicated in the treatment of diabetic acidosis; diarrhea and vomiting; in surgical conditions accompanied by nitrogen loss, vomiting, suction drainage, diarrhea, and increased urinary excretion of potassium; in certain cases of uremia in which large amounts of potassium are excreted in the urine; when high excretion of potassium takes place as in hyperadrenalism; after over-doses of desoxycorticosterone or following cortisone or ACTH therapy; in starvation and debilitation; in severe or persistent alkalosis; in familial periodic paralysis; and in cardiac arrhythmias due to digitalis intoxication.

Contraindications: Severe renal impairment with oliguria or azotemia, untreated Addison's disease, adynamia episodica hereditaria, acute dehydration, heat cramps and hyperkalemia from any cause.

Precautions: In response to a rise in the concentration of body potassium, renal excretion of the ion is increased. With normal kidney function, it is difficult, therefore, to produce potassium intoxication by oral administration. However, potassium supplements must be administered with caution, since the amount of the dietary or daily dosage is not accurately known. Frequent checks of the clinical status of the patient, and periodic ECG and/or serum potassium levels should be made. High serum concentrations of potassium ion may cause death through cardiac depression, arrhythmias, or arrest. This drug should be used with caution in the presence of cardiac disease. It should be borne in mind that there is a hazard in prescribing potassium in digitalis intoxication manifested by digitalis-induced atrio-ventricular (A-V) conduction disturbance.

Adverse Reactions: Adverse reactions reported with the use of potassium-containing drugs include vomiting, diarrhea, nausea, and abdominal discomfort.

The symptoms and signs of potassium intoxication include paresthesias of the extremities, flaccid paralysis, listlessness, mental confusion, weakness and heaviness of the legs, fall in blood pressure, cardiac arrhythmias and heart block. Hyperkalemia may exhibit the following electrocardiographic abnormalities (disappearance of the P wave, widening and slurring of QRS complex, changes of the S-T segment, tall peaked T waves, etc.).

Toxicity: Potassium intoxication may result from overdosage of potassium chloride or from therapeutic dosage in conditions stated under "Contraindication". Hyperkalemia, when detected, must be treated immediately because lethal levels can be reached in a few hours.

Overdosage: Overdosage may lead to a clinical syndrome of listlessness, mental confusion, numbness and tingling of the extremities; weakness and heaviness of the legs; pallor; bradycardia; arrhythmia; peripheral vascular collapse; rapidly ascending flaccid paralysis; and cardiac arrest.

Dosage and Administration: The usual daily dose is up to 6 grams (approximately 80 mEq) per 24 hours for adults. Deviations from this recommendation may be indicated, since no average total daily dose can be defined, but must be governed by close observation for clinical effects. However, potassium intoxication may result from any therapeutic dosage. See under "Toxicity" and "Precautions".

Important: To assure against gastrointestinal injury and to minimize the possibility of a saline laxative effect, both of which have been associated with the oral ingestion of concentrated potassium salt preparations, it is recommended that these preparations be given with a full glass of water or fruit juice.

Treatment of Hyperkalemia:

1. Dextrose solution, 10% or 25%, containing 10 units of crystalline insulin per 20 g dextrose, given I.V. in a dose of 300 to 500 ml in an hour.
2. Absorption and exchange of potassium using sodium or ammonium cycle cation exchange resin, orally and as retention enema.
3. Hemodialysis and peritoneal dialysis. The use of potassium-containing foods or medicaments must be eliminated. However, in cases of digitalization too rapid a lowering of plasma potassium concentration can cause digitalis toxicity.

How Supplied:

POTASSIUM CHLORIDE ORAL SOLUTION USP, 5%

20 mEq of potassium per 30 ml

NDC 0054-8715-04: Unit dose Patient Cups™ filled to deliver 30 ml, ten 30 ml Patient Cups™ per shelf pack, ten shelf packs per shipper.

NDC 0054-3715-63: Bottles of 500 ml.

NDC 0054-3715-75: Bottles of 5 liter.

POTASSIUM CHLORIDE ORAL SOLUTION USP, 10%

15 mEq of potassium per 11.25 ml

NDC 0054-8711-04: Unit dose Patient Cups™ filled to deliver 11.25 ml, ten 11.25 ml Patient Cups™ per shelf pack, ten shelf packs per shipper.

20 mEq of potassium per 15 ml

NDC 0054-8714-04: Unit dose Patient Cups™ filled to deliver 15ml, ten 15ml Patient Cups™ per shelf pack, ten shelf packs per shipper.

30 mEq of potassium per 22.5 ml

NDC 0054-8712-04: Unit dose Patient Cups™ filled to deliver 22.5 ml, ten 22.5 ml Patient Cups™ per shelf pack, ten shelf packs per shipper.

40 mEq potassium per 30 ml

NDC 0054-8713-04: Unit dose Patient Cups™ filled to deliver 30ml, ten 30ml Patient Cups™ per shelf pack, ten shelf packs per shipper.

NDC 0054-3716-54: Bottles of 180 ml.

NDC 0054-3716-63: Bottles of 500 ml.

NDC 0054-3716-68: Bottles of 1 liter.

NDC 0054-3716-75: Bottles of 5 liter.

POTASSIUM CHLORIDE ORAL SOLUTION USP, 20%

80 mEq of potassium per 30 ml

NDC 0054-3714-54: Bottles of 180 ml.

NDC 0054-3714-63: Bottles of 500 ml.

NDC 0054-3714-68: Bottles of 1 liter.

NDC 0054-3714-75: Bottles of 5 liter.

POTASSIUM CHLORIDE POWDER USP

20 mEq of potassium per 1.5 g (unflavored)

NDC 0054-8490-13: Unit dose, 1.5 g packets, 30 packets per carton.

NDC 0054-8490-25: Unit dose, 1.5 g packets, 100 packets per carton.

POTASSIUM CHLORIDE for ORAL SOLUTION USP

20 mEq of potassium per 4 g (cherry flavored)

NDC 0054-8716-13: Unit dose, 4 g packets, 30 packets per carton.

NDC 0054-8716-25: Unit dose, 4 g packets 100 packets per carton.

Continued on next page

Philips Roxane—Cont.

PREDNISONE TABLETS USP ℞
5 mg, 10 mg, 20 mg, or 50 mg

Description: Each tablet contains:
Prednisone.... 5 mg, 10 mg, 20 mg, or 50 mg
Glucocorticoids are adrenocortical steroids, both naturally occurring and synthetic, which are readily absorbed from the gastrointestinal tract.
Prednisone chemically is 17,21-Dihydroxy-pregna-1,4-diene-3,11,20-trione. A synthetic deriviative of cortisone, it is a white to practically white, odorless, crystalline powder. It is very slightly soluble in water, and slightly soluble in alcohol, in chloroform, in dioxane, and in methanol.
Actions: Naturally occurring glucocorticoids (hydrocortisone and cortisone), which also have salt-retaining properties, are used as replacement therapy in adrenocortical deficiency states. Their synthetic analogs are primarily used for their potent anti-inflammatory effects in disorders of many organ systems.
Glucocorticoids cause profound and varied metabolic effects. In addition, they modify the body's immune responses to diverse stimuli.
Indications:
1. *Endocrine disorders:*
   Primary or secondary adrenocortical insufficiency (hydrocortisone or cortisone is the first choice; synthetic analogs may be used in conjunction with mineralocorticoids where applicable; in infancy mineralocorticoid supplementation is of particular importance).
   Congenital adrenal hyperplasia
   Nonsuppurative thyroiditis
   Hypercalcemia associated with cancer
2. *Rheumatic disorders:* As adjunctive therapy for short-term administration (to tide the patient over an acute episode or exacerbation) in:
   Psoriatic arthritis
   Rheumatoid arthritis, including juvenile rheumatoid arthritis (selected cases may require low-dose maintenance therapy)
   Ankylosing spondylitis
   Acute and subacute bursitis
   Acute nonspecific tenosynovitis
   Acute gouty arthritis
   Post-traumatic osteoarthritis
   Synovitis of osteoarthritis
   Epicondylitis
3. *Collagen diseases:* During an exacerbation or as maintenance therapy in selected cases of:
   Systemic lupus erythematosus
   Acute rheumatic carditis
   Systemic dermatomyositis (polymyositis)
4. *Dermatologic diseases:*
   Pemphigus
   Bullous dermatitis herpetiformis
   Severe erythema multiforme (Stevens-Johnson syndrome)
   Exfoliative dermatitis
   Mycosis fungoides
   Severe psoriasis
   Severe seborrheic dermatitis
5. *Allergic states:* Control of severe or incapacitating allergic conditions intractable to adequate trials of conventional treatment:
   Seasonal or perennial allergic rhinitis
   Bronchial asthma
   Contact dermatitis
   Atopic dermatitis
   Serum sickness
   Drug hypersensitivity reactions
6. *Ophthalmic diseases:* Severe acute and chronic allergic and inflammatory processes involving the eye and its adnexa such as:
   Allergic conjunctivitis
   Keratitis
   Allergic corneal marginal ulcers
   Herpes zoster ophthalmicus
   Iritis and iridocyclitis
   Chorioretinitis
   Anterior segment inflammation
   Diffuse posterior uveitis and choroiditis
   Optic neuritis
   Sympathetic ophthalmia
7. *Respiratory Diseases:*
   Symptomatic sarcoidosis
   Loeffler's syndrome not manageable by other means
   Berylliosis
   Fulminating or disseminated pulmonary tuberculosis when used concurrently with appropriate antituberculus chemotherapy.
   Aspiration pneumonitis
8. *Hematologic disorders:*
   Idiopathic thrombocytopenic purpura in adults
   Secondary thrombocytopenia in adults
   Acquired (autoimmune) hemolytic anemia
   Erythroblastopenia (RBC anemia)
   Congenital (erythroid) hypoplastic anemia
9. *Neoplastic diseases:* For palliative management of:
   Leukemias and lymphomas in adults
   Acute leukemia of childhood
10. *Edematous states:* To induce a diuresis or remission of proteinuria in the nephrotic syndrome, without uremia, of the idiopathic type or that due to lupus erythematosus.
11. *Gastrointestinal diseases:* To tide the patient over a critical period of the disease in:
    Ulcerative colitis
    Regional enteritis
12. *Nervous System:*
    Acute exacerbations of multiple sclerosis.
13. *Miscellaneous:*
    Tuberculous meningitis with subarachnoid block or impending block when used concurrently with appropriate antituberculous chemotherapy.
    Trichinosis with neurologic or myocardial involvement.

Contraindications: Systemic fungal infections.
Warnings: In patients on corticosteroid therapy subjected to unusual stress, increased dosage of rapidly acting corticosteroids before, during, and after the stressful situation is indicated.
Corticosteroids may mask some signs of infection, and new infections may appear during their use. There may be decreased resistance and inability to localize infection when corticosteroids are used.
Prolonged use of corticosteroids may produce posterior subcapsular cataracts, glaucoma with possible damage to the optic nerves, and may enhance the establishment of secondary ocular infections due to fungi or viruses.
USAGE IN PREGNANCY: Since adequate human reproduction studies have not been done with corticosteroids, the use of these drugs in pregnancy, nursing mothers or women of childbearing potential requires that the possible benefits of the drug be weighed against the potential hazards to the mother and embryo or fetus. Infants born of mothers who have received substantial doses of corticosteroids during pregnancy should be carefully observed for signs of hypoadrenalism.
Average and large doses of hydrocortisone or cortisone can cause elevation of blood pressure, salt and water retention, and increased excretion of potassium. These effects are less likely to occur with prednisone except when used in large doses. Dietary salt restriction and potassium supplementation may be necessary. All corticosteroids increase calcium excretion.
While on Corticosteroid Therapy Patients Should Not Be Vaccinated Against Smallpox. Other Immunization Procedures Should Not Be Undertaken in Patients Who are on Corticosteroids, Especially on High Dose, Because of Possible Hazards of Neurological Complications and a Lack of Antibody Response.
The use of prednisone in active tuberculosis should be restricted to those cases of fulminating or disseminated tuberculosis in which the corticosteroid is used for the management of the disease in conjunction with an appropriate antituberculous regimen.
If corticosteroids are indicated in patients with latent tuberculosis or tuberculin reactivity, close observation is necessary as reactivation of the disease may occur. During prolonged corticosteroid therapy, these patients should receive chemoprophylaxis.
Precautions: Drug-induced secondary adrenocortical insufficiency may be minimized by gradual reduction of dosage. This type of relative insufficiency may persist for months after discontinuation of therapy; therefore, in any situation of stress occurring during that period, hormone therapy should be reinstituted. Since mineralocorticoid secretion may be impaired, salt and/or a mineralocorticoid should be administered concurrently.
There is an enhanced effect on corticosteroids on patients with hypothyroidism and in those with cirrhosis.
Corticosteroids should be used cautiously in patients with ocular herpes simplex because of possible corneal perforation.
The lowest possible dose of corticosteroid should be used to control the condition under treatment, and when reduction in dosage is possible, the reduction should be gradual.
Psychic derangements may appear when corticosteroids are used, ranging from euphoria, insomnia, mood swings, personality changes, and severe depression, to frank psychotic manifestations. Also, existing emotional instability or psychotic tendencies may be aggravated by corticosteroids.
Aspirin should be used cautiously in conjunction with corticosteroids in hypoprothrombinemia.
Steroids should be used with caution in nonspecific ulcerative colitis, if there is a probability of impending perforation, abscess or other pyogenic infection; diverticulitis; fresh intestinal anastomoses; active or latent peptic ulcer; renal insufficiency; hypertension; osteoporosis; and myasthenia gravis.
Growth and development of infants and children on prolonged corticosteroid therapy should be carefully observed.
Although controlled clinical trials have shown corticosteroids to be effective in speeding the resolution of acute exacerbations of multiple sclerosis they do not show that they affect the ultimate outcome or natural history of the disease. The studies do show that relatively high doses of corticosteroids are necessary to demonstrate a significant effect. (See DOSAGE AND ADMINISTRATION Section).
Since complications of treatment with glucocorticoids are dependent on the size of the dose and the duration of treatment a risk/benefit decision must be made in each individual case as to dose and duration of treatment and as to whether daily or intermittent therapy should be used.
Adverse Reactions:
Fluid and Electrolyte Disturbances.
Sodium retention.
Fluid retention.
Congestive heart failure in susceptible patients.
Potassium loss.
Hypokalemic alkalosis.
Hypertension.
Musculoskeletal.
Muscle weakness.
Steroid myopathy.
Loss of muscle mass.
Osteoporosis.
Vertebral compression fractures.
Aseptic necrosis of femoral and humeral heads.

Pathologic fracture of long bones.
Gastrointestinal.
Peptic ulcer with possible perforation and hemorrhage.
Pancreatitis.
Abdominal distention.
Ulcerative esophagitis.
Dermatologic.
Impaired wound healing.
Thin fragile skin.
Petechiae and ecchymoses.
Facial erythema.
Increased sweating.
May suppress reactions to skin tests.
Neurological.
Convulsions.
Increased intracranial pressure with papilledema (pseudo-tumor cerebri) usually after treatment.
Vertigo.
Headache.
Endocrine.
Menstrual irregularities.
Development of Cushingoid state.
Suppression of growth in children.
Secondary adrenocortical and pituitary unresponsiveness, particularly in times of stress, as in trauma, surgery or illness.
Decreased carbohydrate tolerance.
Manifestations of latent diabetes mellitus.
Increased requirements for insulin or oral hypoglycemic agents in diabetics.
Ophthalmic.
Posterior subcapsular cataracts.
Increased intraocular pressure.
Glaucoma.
Exophthalmos.
Metabolic.
Negative nitrogen balance due to protein catabolism.

Dosage and Administration:
1. Dosage should be individualized according to the severity of the disease and the response of the patient. For infants and children, the recommended dosage should be governed by the same considerations rather than by strict adherence to the ratio indicated by age or body weight.
2. Hormone therapy is an adjunct to, and not a replacement for, conventional therapy.
3. Dosage should be decreased or discontinued gradually when the drug has been administered for more than a few days.
4. The severity, prognosis and expected duration of the disease and the reaction of the patient to medication are primary factors in determining dosage.
5. If a period of spontaneous remission occurs in a chronic condition, treatment should be discontinued.
6. Blood pressure, body weight, routine laboratory studies, including 2-hour post-prandial blood glucose and serum potassium, and a chest X-ray should be obtained at regular intervals during prolonged therapy. Upper GI X-rays are desirable in patients with known or suspected peptic ulcer disease.

Dosage Recommendations: The initial dosage of Prednisone may vary from 5 mg to 60 mg per day depending on the specific disease entity being treated. In situations of less severity lower doses will generally suffice, while in selected patients higher initial doses may be required. The initial dosage should be maintained or adjusted until a satisfactory response is noted. If after a reasonable period of time there is a lack of satisfactory clinical response, Prednisone should be discontinued and the patient transferred to other appropriate therapy.
In the treatment of acute exacerbations of multiple sclerosis daily doses of 200 mg of prednisolone for a week followed by 80 mg. every other day or 4–8 mg. dexamethasone every other day for 1 month have been shown to be effective.
For the purpose of comparison, the following is the *equivalent milligram dosage* of the various glucocorticoids: *cortisone, 25; hydrocortisone, 20; prednisolone, 5; prednisone, 5; methylprednisolone, 4; triamicinolone, 4; paramethasone, 2; betamethasone, 0.75; dexamethasone 0.75.* These dose relationships apply only to oral or intravenous administration of these compounds. When these substances or their derivatives are injected intramuscularly or into joint spaces, their relative properties may be greatly altered.
IT SHOULD BE EMPHASIZED THAT DOSAGE REQUIREMENTS ARE VARIABLE AND MUST BE INDIVIDUALIZED ON THE BASIS OF THE DISEASE UNDER TREATMENT AND THE RESPONSE OF THE PATIENT.
After a favorable response is noted, the proper maintenance dosage should be determined by decreasing the initial drug dosage in small increments at appropriate time intervals until the lowest dosage which will maintain an adequate clinical response is reached. It should be kept in mind that constant monitoring is needed in regard to drug dosage. Included in the situations which may make dosage adjustments necessary are changes in clinical status secondary to remissions or exacerbations in the disease process, the patient's individual drug responsiveness, and the effect of patient exposure to stressful situations not directly related to the disease entity under treatment; in this latter situation it may be necessary to increase the dosage of Prednisone for a period of time consistent with the patient's condition. If after long-term therapy the drug is to be stopped, it is recommended that it be withdrawn gradually rather than abruptly.

How Supplied:
5 mg white, scored tablets.
NDC 0054-8724-25: Unit dose, 10 tablets per strip, 10 strips per shelf pack, ten shelf packs per shipper.
NDC 0054-4728-25: Bottles of 100 tablets.
NDC 0054-4728-31: Bottles of 1000 tablets.
10 mg white, scored tablets.
NDC 0054-8725-25: Unit dose, 10 tablets per strip, 10 strips per shelf pack, 10 shelf packs per shipper.
NDC 0054-4730-25: Bottles of 100 tablets.
NDC 0054-4730-29: Bottles of 500 tablets.
20 mg white, scored tablets.
NDC 0054-8726-25: Unit dose, 10 tablets per strip, 10 strips per shelf pack, 10 shelf packs per shipper.
NDC 0054-4729-25: Bottles of 100 tablets.
NDC 0054-4729-29: Bottles of 500 tablets.
50 mg white, scored tablets.
NDC 0054-8729-25: Unit dose, 10 tablets per strip, 10 strips per shelf pack, 10 shelf packs per shipper.
NDC 0054-4733-25: Bottles of 100 tablets.

Poythress & Co., Wm. P., Incorporated

16 N. 22nd ST.
POST OFFICE BOX 26946
RICHMOND, VA 23261

ANTROCOL® ℞
TABLETS AND CAPSULES

Composition: Each tablet or capsule contains atropine sulfate, 0.195 mg.; phenobarbital, 16 mg. (Warning: may be habit-forming); blended for even absorption.
Action and Uses: Antrocol provides the prompt and predictable antispasmodic and antisecretory actions of atropine, blended for mild sedation. In peptic ulcer the ratio of stronger than usual parasympatholytic to sedative activity in Antrocol permits effective lowering of the gastric acid titer without exceeding optimal mild continuous sedation. In addition to the treatment of peptic ulcer, Antrocol is useful in correcting many digestive disturbances and is also effective in preventing recurrence of ulcer.
Dosage: 2 to 8 tablets or capsules per day as indicated. Functional gastro-intestinal spasms: One tablet or capsule after each meal. Peptic Ulcer: To obtain the desired antisecretory effect, dosage up to 8 tablets or capsules per day. Prophylactic: One tablet or capsule after the morning and evening meal is usually sufficient to help prevent recurrence of ulcer.
Side Effects: Toxic levels of atropine may produce flushing, dryness of mouth, cycloplegia, tachycardia and urinary retention.
Precautions: Use cautiously in prostatic hypertrophy. Do not use in glaucoma.
How Supplid: Tablets in bottles of 100, 500. Capsules in bottles of 100, 500.
[*Shown in Product Identification Section*]

ANTROCOL® ELIXIR ℞
A Sugar-free Antisecretory—Sedative

Composition: Each 1 cc contains atropine sulate 0.039 mg., phenobarbital (Warning: may be habit-forming) 3 mg., and 20% alcohol (v/v) in a citrus flavored—artifically colored elixir.
Caution: Federal law prohibits dispensing without prescription.
Actions and Uses: Antrocol Elixir provides the prompt and predictable antispasmodic and antisecretory action of the belladonna alkaloid, atropine, in a stronger than usual ratio with phenobarbital, permitting effective spasmolysis without exceeding optimal mild sedation. Antrocol Elixir is indicated for the symptomatic relief of colic, pylorospasm and a wide range of functional gastrointestinal disturbances. In peptic ulcer the ratio of stronger than usual parasympatholytic to sedative activity in Antrocol permits effective lowering of the gastric acid titer without exceeding optimal mild continuous sedation.
Contraindicated in glaucoma.
Dosage (average): 0.5 cc for each 15 lbs of body weight. 5 cc (1 teaspoonful) is the average adult dose. May be repeated 3 to 4 times daily.
Suggested Average Pediatric Dosage:
(Clark's Rule)

Weight of Child	Dosage
15 lbs.	0.5 cc (10 drops)
30 lbs.	1 cc (20 drops)
45 lbs.	1.5 cc (30 drops)
60 lbs.	2 cc
90 lbs.	3 cc

Side Effects: Toxic levels of atropine may produce flushing, dryness of the mouth, cycloplegia, tachycardia and urinary retention.
Precautions: Use cautiously in prostatic hypertrophy. Do not use in glaucoma.
How Supplied: 1 pint and 1 fl. oz. (30 cc) dropper bottles in individual printed cartons with individually wrapped droppers calibrated from 0.5 cc to 1 cc.

BENSULFOID® ℞

Composition: Issued in 130 mg. tablets and in powder form, Bensulfoid is a fusion, 33% by weight, of a highly reactive sulfur onto colloidal bentonite. The particles of Bensulfoid (300 mesh) consist of tiny disks of bentonite on which sulfur is adsorbed on the laminar structure. The distinctive manufacturing process of Bensulfoid produces a finely-divided physical complex, colloidal in nature, which possesses the gelforming and adsorbing properties of bentonite. This is accomplished by fusing one part of precipitated sulfur, U.S.P., with two parts of bentonite, U.S.P., in an electrically heated blending reactor. The resulting sulfur-coated bentonite particles are as finely divided as bentonite, and they retain all of the physical properties of bentonite. In addition, the chemical reactivity of the sulfur is increased many times. In contrast to bentonite, which has a pH

Continued on next page

Poythress—Cont.

of 9, the pH of Bensulfoid is close to neutral, and its adsorption is based on its finely divided state rather than on ion exchange.
Action and Uses: Bensulfoid has many physical properties that are useful in prescription compounding. When combined with oral medications Bensulfoid acts as a dispersing agent and carrier for the active drugs. Its affinity for neutral drug molecules in aqueous mixtures is greater than that of bentonite, but it readily releases these drugs to physiologically absorbing surfaces. This promotes more even drug absorption. When taken orally the sulfur exerts practically no pharmacological effect in the recommended dosage. It is absorbed as sulfide and oxidized to sulfate. Topically Bensulfoid is very effective as a skin fungicide and keratolytic agent. Its sulfur is converted into soluble sulfides 40 times faster than precipitated sulfur. Topical prescriptions should not contain more than 8.5% Bensulfoid and its use should be discontinued if skin irritation develops.
How Supplied: Powder, 1-ounce bottles. Tablets, bottles of 100. Each tablet contains 130 mg. of Bensulfoid .

BENSULFOID® LOTION

(See PDR For Nonprescription Drugs)

MUDRANE® Tablets ℞

Composition: Each tablet contains potassium iodide, 195 mg.; aminophylline (anhydrous), 130 mg.; phenobarbital, 8 mg. (Warning: may be habit-forming); ephedrine HCl, 16 mg.
Indications: A bronchodilator-mucolytic, Mudrane gives prompt symptomatic relief in bronchial asthma, emphysema and asthmatic bronchitis. Mudrane dilates the bronchi, liquefies the mucus plugs. The stability of Mudrane has been achieved without coating the potassium iodide; thus all the components in the fast-disintegrating tablet begin their actions promptly. The phenobarbital in slight excess of ephederine minimizes the side-effect of nervousness. Mudrane is buffered for gastric tolerance.
Contraindications: *Aminophylline/theopylline* is contraindicated in the presence of severe cardiac arrhythmias in patients with massive myocardial damage. *Ephedrine* is contraindicated in the presence of severe heart disease, severe hypertension and in hyperthyroidism. *Phenobarbital* is contraindicated in porphyria and in patients with known phenobarbital sensitivity. *Potassium iodide* is contraindicated in pregnancy (to protect the fetus against possible iodide-induced depression of thyroid activity), in tuberculosis (produces gumma dissolution), and in acne; also, in the presence of known iodide sensitivity.
Precautions: *Aminophylline/theophylline* should be avoided in patients with massive myocardial damage and/or severe cardiac arrhythmias, and severe agitation. *Ephedrine* should be used with caution in the presence of severe cardiac disease, particularly arrhythmias and angina pectoris, it should be avoided in hyperthyroidism and severe hypertension. *Phenobarbial* may be habit-forming. Avoid overdosage. *Potassium iodide:* Discontinue in the presence of skin rash, swelling of the eyelids, or severe frontal headache. Long use may cause goiter.
Adverse Reactions: *Aminophylline/theophylline* may cause cardiac arrhythmias and aggravate severe myocardial disease; may cause headaches and tachycardia; vomiting and dizziness are not uncommon. *Ephedrine* may cause nervousness, tachycardia, extrasystole and ventricular arrhythmias in patients hypersensitive to CNS stimulation. Also, ephedrine may cause urinary retention, especially in the presence of partial prostatic obstruction. Psychoneurosis may be aggravated. Pre-existing anginal pain will be aggravated. *Phenobarbital* may produce severe skin rash; avoid overdosage; may be habit-forming. *Potassium iodide* may cause nausea; over very long period of use, iodides may cause goiter. Discontinue if patient developes skin rash, eye irritation, eyelid swelling or severe frontal headache.
Dosage: One tablet witn full glass of water, 3 or 4 times daily, as required. Divide tablet for child's dose.
How Supplied: Mudrane Yellow scored tablets in bottles or 100 and 1,000.
[*Shown in Product Identification Section*]

MUDRANE®-2 TABLETS ℞

Composition: Each tablet contains potassium iodide 195 mg. aminophylline (anhydrous) 130 mg.
Indications: When ephedrine is too exciting or contraindicated, Mudrane-2 gives prompt symptomatic relief in asthma, emphysema and asthmatic bronchitis through its bronchodilator-mucolytic actions. The stability of Mudrane-2 has been achieved without coating the potassium iodide; thus the components in the fast disintegrating tablet begin their actions promptly.
Contraindications: Precautions: Adverse Reactions: See under Mudrane tablets above, as listed for aminophylline/theophylline and potassium iodide.
Dosage: One tablet with full glass of water, 3 or 4 times daily.
How Supplied: White scored tablets in bottles of 100.
[*Shown in Product Identification Section*]

MUDRANE® GG TABLETS ℞

Composition: Each tablet contains aminophylline (anhydrous), 130 mg.; ephedrine HCl, 16 mg.; phenobarbital, 8 mg. (Warning: may be habit-forming); Guaifenesin, 100 mg.
Indications: Same as Mudrane, EXCEPT Guaifenesin, 100 mg. replaces potassium iodide as a mucolytic-expectorant. Mudrane GG should be prescribed when acne or tuberculosis co-exist, during pregnancy, or when iodide intolerance is present. In emphysema, requiring constant Mudrane therapy, Mudrane GG may be substituted every fourth week to reduce the possibility of iodide sensitivity.
Contraindications: Precautions: Adverse Reactions: See under Mudrane tablets above, as listed for aminophylline/theophylline, ephedrine HCl, and phenobarbital.
Dosage: One tablet with full glass of water, 3 or 4 times daily.
How Supplied: Yellow, mottled, GG embossed tablets in bottles of 100 and 1,000.
[*Shown in Product Identification Section*]

MUDRANE® GG-2 TABLETS ℞

Composition: Each tablet contains aminophylline (anhydrous), 130 mg.; Guaifenesin, 100 mg.
Indications: When ephedrine is too exciting or contraindicated, Mudrane GG-2 gives prompt symptomatic relief in asthma, emphysema and asthmatic bronchitis through its bronchodilator-mucolytic actions.
Contraindications: Precautions: Adverse Reactions: See under Mudrane tablets above, as listed for aminophylline/theophylline.
Dosage: One tablet with full glass of water, 3 or 4 times daily.
How Supplied: Green, mottled, GG embossed tablets in bottles of 100.
[*Shown in Product Identification Section*]

MUDRANE® GG ELIXIR ℞

Composition: Each 5 ml teaspoonful contains theophylline, 20 mg.; ephedrine HCl, 4 mg.; phenobarbital 2.5 mg. (Warning: may be habit-forming); Guaifenesin, 26 mg. The theophylline in the Elixir is in solution. (The theophylline in the tablet is supplied by aminophylline for prompt solubility from the rapid-disintegrating, uncoated tablet). Preserved with 0.1% paraben. Contains 20% alcohol.
Indications: Mudrane GG Elixir is a sugar-free bronchodilator-mucolytic especially formulated for pediatric use. Mudrane GG Elixir supplies the active ingredients of Mudrane GG tablets for the relief of asthma and asthmatic bronchitis.
Contraindications: Precautions: Adverse Reactions: See under Mudrane tablets above, as listed for aminophylline/theophylline, ephedrine HCl, and phenobarbital.
Dosage: Children, 1 ml for each 10 lbs. of body weight; one teaspoonful for 50 lb. child. May be repeated 3 or 4 times daily. Adult, one tablespoonful, 3 or 4 times daily. All doses should be followed with water.
How Supplied: A red liquid in pints and one-half gallon bottles.

PANALGESIC

Composition: Methyl salicylate, 50%; aspirin, 8%; menthol and camphor, 4%; emollient oils, 20%; alcohol, 18% by weight.
Action and Uses: Panalgesic, an external application for relief of superficial aches and pains, supplies salicylates in the proper environment for maximum skin absorption, producing counterirritation, analgesia,local anesthesia, and asepsis. Panalgesic lessens the discomfort of muscular fatigue, and of trauma, and increases the blood level of salicylate by dermal absorption.
Method of Application: Apply externally to affected area with a gentle massage 3 or 4 times daily.
Warning: Do not use otherwise than as directed. Keep out of reach of children to avoid accidental poisoning. Discontinue use if excessive irritation of the skin develops. Avoid getting into eyes or on mucous membrane.
How Supplied: 4-ounce; 1-pint; one-half gallon bottles.

SOLFOTON® TABLETS, CAPSULES, AND S/C (SUGAR-COATED) TABLETS ©

Composition: Each tablet or capsule contains phenobarbital, 16 mg. (Warning: may be habit-forming). Blended for even absorption.
Action and Uses: Solfoton is safe for maintaining mild continuous sedation over long periods. No bizarre physical or psychic states nor reduced effectiveness have been noted following prolonged use. The mild continuous sedation of Solfoton therapy will help in creating empathy with the patient preparatory to outlining a health plan. Solfoton is the ideal clinical approach to frequently encountered mild chronic anxiety states—it subtly blunts and normalizes the hyper-reactive CNS to environmental stimuli.
Administration and Dosage: One tablet or capsule at 6-hour intervals will usually maintain sedation at the threshold of calmness.
Side Effects: Identical to those of 16 mg. phenobarbital.
How Supplied: Uncoated tablets: bottles of 100, 500, 5,000. Tablets S./C: bottles 100, 500. Capsules: bottles 100, 500.
[*Shown in Product Identification Section*]

TROCINATE ℞
(Thiphenamil hydrochloride)

Description: Trocinate, chemically, is 2-diethylaminoethyldiphenylthioacetate hydrochloride. Trocinate may be dispensed only upon the prescription of a physician. Trocinate is manufactured by Wm. P. Poythress and Company, Incorporated, Richmond, Virginia, and has been marketed since 1950.

Actions: Trocinate is a potent antispasmodic and smooth muscle relaxant that acts like papaverine on smooth muscle. Trocinate exerts a strong local anesthetic effect on contact with mucous membranes.

INDICATIONS
Trocinate is indicated for relief of smooth muscle spasm.
In Gastroenterology: for relief of pain and discomfort due to smooth muscle spasm associated with spastic colitis, irritable colon, mucous colitis, acute enterocolitis, and functional gastrointestinal disorders.
LIMITATIONS OF EFFECTIVENESS
On the basis of the opinions of the National Academy of Science and National Research Council Committees and other information, the Food and Drug Administration considers this drug to be limited in its effectiveness, as follows:
Probably effective, as follows: May be useful in the irritable bowel syndrome (irritable colon, spastic colon, mucous colitis, acute enterocolitis, and functional gastrointestinal disorders); and in neurogenic bowel disturbances (including the splenic flexure syndrome and neurogenic colon).
To be effective the dosage must be titrated to the individual patient's needs.

Contraindications: Trocinate is contraindicated in obstructive uropathy (for example, bladder neck obstruction due to prostatic hypertrophy); obstructive disease of the gastrointestinal tract (as in achalasia, paralytic ileus, pyloroduodenal stenosis, etc.); intestinal atony of elderly or debilitated patient; severe ulcerative colitis; toxic megacolon complicating ulcerative colitis; myasthenia gravis.
Warnings: Use in Pregnancy—The safety of the use of Trocinate during pregnancy has not been established.
Diarrhea may be an early symptom of incomplete intestinal obstruction, especially in patients with ileostomy or colostomy. In this instance treatment with this drug may be inappropriate and possibly harmful.
Dosage and Administration: Adult: Initially, 400 milligrams. May be repeated four hours later. Trocinate acts very promptly and, when effective, relieves discomfort with two to four doses. Relief may usually be maintained with reduced frequency of dosage.
The safety and efficacy of Trocinate in children has not been determined, and Trocinate should not be administered to children.
Management of Overdosage: In twenty years of usage of Trocinate, side-effects have been so very infrequent that no typical symptoms and physical signs of overdosage have become known. Skin rash, mild hypotension and colicky abdominal pain when observed have rapidly disappeared with stoppage of the drug.
How Supplied:
400 mg. branded, pink sugar-coated tablets
Bottles of 25's..........NDC 95-0029-26
Bottles of 100's..........NDC 95-0029-01
100 mg. branded, pink sugar-coated tablets
Bottles of 100's..........NDC 95-0028-01
Bottles of 500's..........NDC 95-0028-05
[*Shown in Product Identification Section*]

URO-PHOSPHATE TABLETS ℞
(Methenamine, sodium acid phosphate)

Protect from Heat. Store at room temperature 60°–75°F

Description: Uro-Phosphate, a urinary antibacterial agent, is the combination of methenamine 300 mg. and sodium acid phosphate 500 mg. supplied in a white sugar-coated tablet.
Actions: Methenamine is readily absorbed from the gastrointestinal tract but remains essentially inactive until concentrated and excreted by the kidney in an acid urine where hydrolysation produces antibacterial formaldehyde. An acid urine is essential for the conversion of methenamine to antibacterial formaldehyde with the maximum efficacy occurring at pH 5.5 or less. Methenamine alone may be ineffective in some infections with Proteus vulgaris and urea-splitting strains of Pseudomonas aeruginosa and A. aerogenes as they may raise the pH of the urine inhibiting formaldehyde formation. Sodium acid phosphate, a natural urine acidifier, generally provides urine pH at an acid level conducive to formaldehyde production. Results in any individual case will depend on dosage, underlying pathology and overall management.
Indications: Uro-Phosphate (methenamine and sodium acid phosphate) is indicated for suppressive or prophylactic treatment of chronic bacteriuria associated with pyelonephritis, cystitis, significant residual urine accompanying some neurological diseases and with prolonged bladder catheterization. The safety and nonspecific bacteriacidal effect of formaldehyde does not lead to bacterial resistance to Uro-Phosphate.
Contraindications: Renal insufficiency, severe dehydration or acidosis. Methenamine preparations should not be given patients taking sulfonamides since formaldehyde may form an insoluble precipitate with some sulfonamides in urine.
Warning: Safe use in pregnancy is not established.
Precautions: Large doses of methenamine (8 grams daily for 3 to 4 weeks) have caused bladder irritation, painful and frequent micturition, albuminures and gross hematuria. Care should be taken to maintain an acid pH of the urine especially when treating infections due to urea-splitting pathogens such as Proteus and strains of Pseudomonas.
Adverse Reactions: Minor adverse reactions have been reported in fewer than 3.5% of patients treated. These reactions have included nausea, upset stomach, dysuria and rash.
Dosage and Administration: 1 or 2 tablets at 4 to 6 hour intervals is usually sufficient to maintain proper urine acidity. Two tablets on retiring will maintain comfort and lessen frequency when residual urine is present.
How Supplied: White sugar-coated tablets:
Bottles of 100's NDC 0095-0031-01
Bottles of 1000's NDC 0095-0031-10
Mfd. for Wm. P. Poythress Co., Inc., Richmond, Virginia 23261 by ICN Pharmaceuticals, Inc., Cincinnati, Ohio 45213
[*Shown in Product Identification Section*]

Premo Pharmaceutical Laboratories, Inc.

111 LEUNING STREET
SOUTH HACKENSACK, NJ 07606

NDC 0331	Product
0979	**ACTI-PREM TABLETS** ℞ (Triprolidine HCl & Pseudoephedrine HCl)
0621	**ALGEMOL VELVETABS** OTC
	ALLOPURINOL TABLETS ℞
0453	100 mg.
0455	300 mg.
	AMOXICILLIN CAPSULES ℞
0613	250 mg.
0615	500 mg.
	AMPICILLIN TRIHYDRATE CAPSULES ℞
0765	250 mg.
0767	500 mg.
0673	**BETA-VAL CREAM** ℞ (Betamethasone Valerate Cream, 0.1%)
	CEPHALEXIN MONOHYDRATE CAPSULES ℞
0541	250 mg. Green/white, Hard Shell Capsule
0543	500 mg. Two-tone Green, Hard Shell Capsule
	CHLORDIAZEPOXIDE HCl CAPSULES Ⓒ
0053	5 mg.
0055	10 mg.
0057	25 mg.
0617	**CHLORDINIUM SEALETS** ℞ (Chlordiazepoxide HCl & Clidinium Bromide)
0545	**CHLORZOXAZONE with APAP TABLETS** ℞
	CHLOROTHIAZIDE TABLETS ℞
0049	250 mg.
0051	500 mg.
	CYCLANDELATE CAPSULES ℞
0919	200 mg.
0977	400 mg.
0471	**DECON-AID T R CAPSULES** ℞ (Chlorpheniramine Maleate, Phenylpropanolamine HCl, Isopropamide Iodide)
0477	**DECON-TUSS T R CAPSULES** ℞ (Caramiphen Edisylate, Chlorpheniramine Maleate, Phenylpropanolmine, Isopropamide Iodide)
	DIPHENHYDRAMINE HCl CAPSULES ℞
0245	25 mg.
0247	50 mg.
0027	**DIPYRIDAMOLE TABLETS** ℞ 25 mg.
0597	**DOXINE TABLETS** ℞ (Doxylamine Succinate & Pyridoxine HCl)
0981	**DYNOHIST S. A. TABLETS** ℞ (D-Isoephedrine Sulfate & Brompheniramine Maleate)
0775	**ERYTHROMYCIN STEARATE TABLETS** ℞ 250 mg.
	FLUOCIN CREAM ℞ (Fluocinolone Cream)
0665	0.025%
0663	0.1%
0843	**FOLIC ACID TABLETS** ℞ 1 mg.
	HYDRALAZINE HCl TABLETS ℞
0945	25 mg.
0947	50 mg.
0887	**HYDRAP-ES TABLETS** ℞ (Hydralazine HCl, Hydrochlorothiazide & Reserpine)
	HYDERGOT SUBLINGUAL TABLETS ℞ (Hydrogenated Ergot Alkaloids)
0967	0.5 mg.
0969	1.0 mg.
	HYDROCHLOROTHIAZIDE ℞
0777	25 mg.
0779	50 mg.
0329	**HYDROCORTISONE TABLETS** ℞ 20 mg.
	HYDRO-SERP TABLETS ℞
0923	"25"
0921	"50"
	HYDROXYZINE HCl TABLETS ℞
0019	10 mg.
0021	25 mg.
0023	50 mg.
	HY-PAM CAPSULES ℞ (Hydroxyzine Pamoate)
0033	25 mg.
0035	50 mg.
0037	100 mg.
	IMIPRAMINE HCl TABLETS ℞
0925	10 mg.
0927	25 mg.
0929	50 mg.
0013	**INSULASE™ TABLETS** ℞ (Chlorpropamide) 250 mg.

Continued on next page

Premo—Cont.

0469 **ISO-PERAZINE T R CAPSULES** ℞
(Isopropamide Iodide, Prochlorperazine Maleate)
ISOXSUPRINE HCl TABLETS ℞
0911 10 mg.
0913 20 mg.
MECLIZINE HCl TABLETS OTC
0579 12.5 mg.
0581 25 mg.
MEPROBAMATE TABLETS Ⓒ
0365 200 mg.
0367 400 mg.
0539 **MEPROGESIC TABLETS** Ⓒ
(Meprobamate, Aspirin & Ethoheptazine Citrate)
MEPRO-HEX TABLETS ℞
(Tridihexethyl Chloride & Meprobamate)
0609 "200"
0611 "400"
0941 **MYCO TRIACET CREAM** ℞
(Nystatin-Neomycin Sulfate-Gramicidin-Triamcinolone Acetonide Cream)
0677 **MYCO TRIACET OINTMENT**
(Nystatin-Neomycin Sulfate-Gramicidin-Triamcinolone Acetonide Ointment)
NITROFURANTOIN TABLETS ℞
0683 50 mg.
0685 100 mg.
NYLIDRIN HCl TABLETS ℞
0963 6 mg.
0965 12 mg.
0955 **NYSTATIN CREAM** ℞
0983 **NYSTATIN ORAL TABLETS** ℞
500,000 Units
0943 **NYSTATIN VAGINAL TABLETS** ℞
100,000 Units
0949 **OXYTETRACYCLINE HCl CAPSULES** ℞
250 mg.
0727 **PAPAVERINE HCl T R CAPSULES** ℞
150 mg.
0901 **PHENATAPP EXTEND TABLETS** ℞
(Phenylephrine, Phenylpropanolamine & Brompheniramine Maleate)
0499 **PHENTERMINE HCl CAPSULES** ℞
30 mg.
0523 **PHENTERMINE RESIN CAPSULES** ℞
30 mg.
0989 **PHENYLBUTAZONE ALKA CAPSULES** ℞
(Phenylbutazone, Dried Aluminum Hydroxide Gel & Magnesium Trisilicate)
0857 **PHENYTOIN SODIUM CAPSULES** ℞
100 mg.
0507 **PREDNISOLONE TABLETS** ℞
5 mg.
0509 **PREDNISONE TABLETS** ℞
5 mg.
0783 **PROPOXYPHENE COMPOUND-65 CAPSULES** Ⓒ
(Propoxyphene HCl & A.P.C.)
PROPOXYPHENE HCl CAPSULES Ⓒ
0047 32 mg.
0741 65 mg.
0917 **PSEUDOEPHEDRINE HCl TABLETS** ℞
60 mg.
0401 **TETRACYCLINE HCl CAPSULES** ℞
250 mg.
0549 **THEOPHEDRIZINE TABLETS** ℞
(Theophylline, Ephedrine Sulfate & Hydroxyzine HCl)
THIORIDAZINE HCl TABLETS ℞
0567 25 mg.
0569 50 mg.
0571 100 mg.
0759 **TOLBUTAMIDE TABLETS 0.5 g.** ℞
TRIACET CREAM ℞
(Triamcinolone Acetonide Cream)
0935 0.025%
0937 0.1%
0939 0.5%
0503 **TRIAMTERENE WITH HYDROCHLOROTHIAZIDE** ℞
TRIFLUOPERAZINE TABLETS ℞
0641 2 mg.
0643 5 mg.

Procter & Gamble

P. O. BOX 171
CINCINNATI, OHIO 45201

DIDRONEL® ℞
(etidronate disodium)

Description: DIDRONEL (etidronate disodium) is the disodium salt of (1-Hydroxyethylidene) diphosphonic acid. The compound, often referred to in the literature as EHDP or Na_2 EHDP, is a white powder, highly soluble in water, with a molecular weight of 250. DIDRONEL is supplied in rectangular white tablets containing 200 mg of etidronate disodium for oral administration.

Clinical Pharmacology:
DIDRONEL acts primarily on bone. It can modify the crystal growth of calcium hydroxyapatite by chemisorption onto the crystal surface. Depending on concentration, the drug may either inhibit crystal resorption or crystal growth.

Serum phosphate elevations have been observed when DIDRONEL is administered at daily doses of 10 mg/kg body weight/day or above and occasionally at 5 mg/kg/day. This has not been found to be an indication for discontinuing therapy. This drug-related elevation appears to be the result of increased tubular reabsorption of phosphate by the kidney, and serum values in excess of 7 mg% have been observed with high doses. No adverse effects of DIDRONEL-induced hyperphosphatemia have been found. Serum phosphate levels generally return to normal 2–4 weeks after stopping medication. DIDRONEL therapy is not accompanied by clinically significant changes in serum parathyroid hormone or serum calcium levels.

DIDRONEL is not metabolized. Patients absorb an average of about 1% of an oral dose of 5 mg/kg body weight/day. The absorption increases with dose level to about 2.5% at 10 mg/kg/day and 6% at 20 mg/kg/day. Most of the absorbed drug is cleared from the blood within six hours. Within 24 hours about one-half of the absorbed dose is excreted in the urine. The remainder is chemically adsorbed on the bone and is slowly eliminated. Unabsorbed drug is excreted in the feces.

Paget's Disease
Paget's disease is an idiopathic bone disorder characterized by abnormal and accelerated bone resorption and formation in one or more bones. The extent and severity of the disease is highly variable. Characteristic symptoms may be bone pain, varying degrees of bone deformity, neurologic disorders, and less frequently, vascular disorders, including abnormally elevated cardiac output secondary to the increased vascularity associated with Paget's disease. Increased bone resorption results in increased urinary excretion of hydroxyproline and increased bone formation is reflected by increased levels of serum alkaline phosphatase.

DIDRONEL slows the rate of bone turnover (bone resorption and new bone accretion) in Pagetic bone lesions and in the normal remodeling process.

Histologic examination of bone from Pagetic patients on DIDRONEL therapy shows a reduction in the excessive cellular activity accompanied by a suppression of bone resorption and accretion and a return towards normal of the histologic patterns. Accumulation of unmineralized osteoid has been frequently observed in patients treated with a dose of 20 mg/kg/day and in some patients after six months of therapy at lower doses (see Precautions—"Paget's Disease").

DIDRONEL therapy affects several clinical abnormalities seen in patients with Paget's disease: lowering elevated urinary hydroxyproline excretion, lowering elevated serum alkaline phosphatase, and reducing the uptake of radionuclide bone imaging agents at active Pagetic bone sites. These changes are consistent with a reduction in bone turnover rate which has been demonstrated in man by calcium kinetic and balance studies and by morphometric studies of bone. In addition, DIDRONEL therapy reduces vascularity of Pagetic bone, reduces abnormally elevated cardiac output associated with active Paget's disease, and lowers the temperature over superficially located Pagetic lesions. These actions may be accompanied by symptomatic improvement, including reduced bone pain. The first evidence of therapeutic response to DIDRONEL in Paget's disease, reduction of urinary hydroxyproline excretion, usually occurs after one to three months of medication.

Heterotopic Ossification due to Spinal Cord Injury
Heterotopic ossification following spinal cord injury commonly occurs in about 40% of patients. Although a complete understanding of the sequence and nature of events which lead to heterotopic bone masses in soft tissue is unknown, the formation is the result of metaplastic osteogenesis and mineralization. Heterotopic ossification appears to be most active during the period immediately following injury.

DIDRONEL chemisorbs to calcium hydroxyapatite crystals, blocking further crystal growth and mineralization. This is thought to be the mechanism of action which prevents or retards heterotopic bone formation during the active stage.

Indications and Usage:
Paget's Disease
DIDRONEL is indicated for the treatment of symptomatic Paget's disease of bone (osteitis deformans). Effectiveness has been demonstrated primarily in patients with polyostotic Paget's disease with symptoms of pain and with clinically significant elevations of urinary hydroxyproline and serum alkaline phosphatase. In patients treated with DIDRONEL at the dose of 5 mg/kg/day, the elevated urinary hydroxyproline and serum alkaline phosphatase decreased by 30% or more in about 4 out of 5 patients. Hydroxyproline either returned to normal or was decreased by at least 50% in about 3 out of 5 patients and alkaline phosphatase in about one-half of the patients.

In controlled studies, approximately 3 out of 5 patients experienced decreased pain and/or improved mobility. About 2 out of 5 patients in the placebo group showed similar subjective improvement. Objective measurements in DIDRONEL-treated patients have shown reductions of elevated cardiac output in about 2 out of 3 patients. Reductions in elevated skin temperature over Pagetic lesions have also been measured. The number of treated patients in these categories is still too small to predict with certainty how likely such a result will be in any given patient. Objective evidence of hearing improvement has not been demonstrated.

The majority of patients with localized, especially monostotic disease, do not develop symptoms and most patients with mild symptoms can be managed by analgesics. There is no evidence that the prophylactic use of DIDRONEL is beneficial in asymptomatic patients although treatment may be considered in exceptional circumstances in which there is extensive involvement of the skull or the spinal cord with the prospect of irreversible neurologic damage. In these instances, treatment would be based on the demonstrated effect of DIDRONEL on Pagetic bone rather than on clinical studies in that patient population.

Heterotopic Ossification

DIDRONEL is indicated in the prevention and treatment of heterotopic ossification due to spinal cord injury.

In placebo-controlled studies among spinal cord injured patients, DIDRONEL therapy resulted in significant reduction in the incidence of heterotopic bone; 4 out of 69 (6%) DIDRONEL-treated patients developed heterotopic ossification versus 17 out of 63 (27%) placebo-treated patients.

In those patients with radiographic evidence of early heterotopic ossification or who developed masses while on therapy, DIDRONEL was effective in retarding the progression of these immature masses. Progression was observed in 6 out of 81 (7%) DIDRONEL-treated patients versus 26 out of 76 (34%) placebo-treated patients.

DIDRONEL has been shown to reduce significantly the severity of clinically important heterotopic ossification masses, i.e., masses of sufficient size to restrict range of motion, require surgical removal or be of other clinical significance.

Follow-up data from controlled studies are inadequate to define the post-treatment benefits of the drug.

Contraindications:

At present, clinical trials have demonstrated no absolute contraindications to DIDRONEL.

Warnings:

The physician should adhere to the recommended dose regimen in order to avoid overtreatment with DIDRONEL (see Precautions and Adverse Reactions).

Paget's Disease

The response to therapy may be of slow onset and may continue even for months after treatment with the drug has been discontinued. Dosage should not be increased prematurely nor should treatment be resumed before there is clear evidence of reactivation of the disease process. Retreatment should not be initiated until the patient has had at least a three month drug-free interval.

The incidence of osteogenic sarcoma is known to be increased in Paget's disease. Pagetic lesions, with or without therapy, may appear by x-ray to progress markedly, possibly with some loss of definition of periosteal margins. Such lesions should be evaluated carefully to differentiate these from osteogenic sarcoma.

Heterotopic Ossification

There are no warnings specific to patients with spinal cord injury.

Precautions:

1. General

Patients should maintain an adequate nutritional status, and particularly, an adequate intake of calcium and vitamin D. Patients with restricted vitamin D and calcium intake may be particularly sensitive to drugs that affect calcium homeostasis and should be closely followed while under treatment with DIDRONEL.

DIDRONEL therapy has been withheld from patients with enterocolitis because increased frequency of bowel movements and diarrhea are seen in some patients when DIDRONEL is administered at a dose of 20 mg/kg/day and may be increased occasionally at lower doses.

DIDRONEL is not metabolized and is excreted intact via the kidney; therefore, treatment of patients with impaired renal function should be approached very cautiously, if at all.

Paget's Disease

When administered at doses of 20 mg/kg/day, DIDRONEL suppresses bone turnover and essentially stops mineralization of new bone in Pagetic lesions and, to a lesser extent, in the uninvolved skeleton. Mineralization of Pagetic lesions has been demonstrated to occur normally after discontinuation of the drug.

DIDRONEL retards mineralization of osteoid laid down during the bone accretion process. This effect is dose and time dependent. There may be an overlap of beneficial and mineralization inhibition effects in some patients at higher doses. Extended periods of medication should be approached cautiously.

Heterotopic Ossification

Concomitant fractures are common in patients with spinal cord injury. In controlled studies, no problems of fracture healing or stabilization of the spine were encountered. In cases with multiple long bone fractures, it may be advisable to delay therapy for a short time until callus formation is evidenced.

2. Pregnancy

Reproduction studies have been performed in rats and rabbits. In some of these studies there was a decrease in the number of live born fetuses. There were no teratogenic effects. Because DIDRONEL does not cross the placental barrier in these species, the decrease in number of live fetuses may have been due to a metabolic effect of DIDRONEL in the mother. There is no experience in pregnant women given DIDRONEL. DIDRONEL should be used only when clearly needed in women who are or may become pregnant.

3. Nursing Mothers

It is not known whether this drug is excreted in human milk. As a general rule, nursing should not be undertaken while the patient is on a drug since many drugs are excreted in human milk.

4. Pediatric Use

Paget's Disease

Disorders of bone in children, referred to as juvenile Paget's disease, have been reported rarely. The relationship to adult Paget's disease has not been established. No data support the use of DIDRONEL in children.

Heterotopic Ossification

There are no data to support the use of DIDRONEL for this condition in children.

Adverse Reactions:

Gastrointestinal complaints such as diarrhea, loose bowel movement, and nausea are increased in some patients when DIDRONEL is administered at doses greater than 5 mg/kg/day. The incidence is about 1 out of 15 in both placebo-treated patients and in patients on DIDRONEL, 5 mg/kg/day. The incidence rises to approximately 2 out of 10 in patients treated with DIDRONEL at the dose of 20 mg/kg/day.

Paget's Disease

Increased or recurrent bone pain at existing Pagetic sites and/or the appearance of pain at sites previously asymptomatic has been reported. At the recommended dose (5 mg/kg/day) 1 out of 10 patients reported the phenomena; at higher doses the figure rose to 2 out of 10. In placebo-treated patients, the occurrence was 1 out of 15. In DIDRONEL-treated patients, the pain resolved while therapy was continued in some patients but persisted for several months in others.

Fractures are recognized as a common feature in patients with Paget's disease. The risk of fracture may be increased when DIDRONEL is taken at a dose level of 20 mg/kg/day in excess of 3 months. This risk may be greater in patients with extensive and severe disease, a history of multiple fractures, and/or rapidly advancing osteolytic lesions. It is recommended that the drug be discontinued when fractures occur and that therapy not be reinstated until fracture healing is complete.

Heterotopic Ossification

There are no adverse reactions peculiar to patients with spinal cord injury.

Overdosage:

While there is no experience with acute overdosage, it is theoretically possible that enough DIDRONEL could be taken to result in hypocalcemia.

Dosage and Administration:

DIDRONEL should be administered as a single, oral dose, two hours before meals. It may be given with fruit juice or water. Food, particularly materials high in calcium content such as milk, in the stomach or upper portion of the small intestine may reduce absorption. Therefore, eating should be avoided for two hours before and after drug administration.

Paget's Disease

Initial Treatment Guidelines: The recommended initial dose of DIDRONEL for most patients is 5 mg/kg body weight/day, not to exceed a period of six months. Doses above 10 mg/kg should be reserved for use when there is an overriding requirement for suppression of increased bone turnover associated with Paget's disease or when the patient requires more prompt reduction of elevated cardiac output. Treatment with doses above 10 mg/kg/day should be approached cautiously and should not exceed three months duration. Doses in excess of 20 mg/kg/day are not recommended. Urinary hydroxyproline excretion and/or serum alkaline phosphatase levels should be monitored periodically during the course of DIDRONEL therapy.

Retreatment Guidelines: Retreatment should be undertaken only after a drug-free period of at least three months and after it is evident that reactivation of the disease has occurred and biochemical indices of the disease have become substantially re-elevated or approach pretreatment values (approximately twice the upper limit of normal or 75% of pretreatment value). In no case should duration of retreatment exceed the maximum duration of the initial treatment. Premature retreatment should be avoided. In clinical trials the biochemical improvements obtained during drug therapy have generally persisted for a period of three months to, in some cases, almost a year after drug withdrawal.

Heterotopic Ossification due to Spinal Cord Injury

The recommended dose is 20 mg/kg/day for 2 weeks followed by 10 mg/kg/day for 10 weeks. The total treatment period is 12 weeks.

This recommended dosing regimen should be instituted as soon as is medically feasible following the injury, preferably prior to any radiographic evidence of heterotopic ossification. Retreatment has not been studied since the heterotopic ossification process is most active during the period immediately following injury. There is no evidence that DIDRONEL therapy will affect mature heterotopic bone.

How Supplied:

DIDRONEL is supplied as a rectangular white tablet containing 200 mg of etidronate disodium. The tablets are packaged in bottles of 60.

NDC 37000-402

Made in U.S.A. for PROCTER & GAMBLE, Cincinnati, Ohio 45202 by Chase Chemical Co. Newark, N.J. 07105.

[*Shown in Product Identification Section*]

HEAD & SHOULDERS®
Antidandruff Shampoo

(See PDR For Nonprescription Drugs)

TOPICYCLINE® ℞
(tetracycline hydrochloride for topical solution)

Description: TOPICYCLINE is a topical preparation containing 2.2 mg of tetracycline

Continued on next page

Procter & Gamble—Cont.

hydrochloride per ml as the active ingredient, as well as 4-epitetracycline hydrochloride and sodium bisulfite in a base of 40% ethanol, n-decyl methyl sulfoxide and sucrose esters.
Each package supplies the patient with 70 ml of the medication containing 154 mg of tetracycline hydrochloride. In order to maintain an effective concentration of tetracycline hydrochloride, TOPICYCLINE contains sufficient 4-epitetracycline hydrochloride to maintain an equilibrium mixture of the two. Sodium bisulfite is included as a color stabilizer.

Actions (Clinical Pharmacology): TOPICYCLINE delivers tetracycline to the pilosebaceous apparatus and the adjacent tissues.
In clinical studies, use of TOPICYCLINE on the face and neck twice daily delivered to the skin an average dose of 2.9 mg of tetracycline hydrochloride per day. Patients who used the medication twice daily on other acne-involved areas in addition to the face and neck applied an average dose of 4.8 mg of tetracycline hydrochloride per day.
The serum level of tetracycline resulting from continuing twice-daily use of TOPICYCLINE is 0.1 µg/ml or less; this is the lower limit of detection of the analytical method. By comparison, an orally-administered divided dose of 500 mg of tetracycline hydrochloride per day results in a serum level of approximately 1.5 µg/ml.

Indications: TOPICYCLINE is indicated in the treatment of *acne vulgaris*. In 12-week controlled clinical studies employing a total of 256 patients, the following reductions in acne severity were determined: TOPICYCLINE 37%; oral tetracycline (500 mg/day) 44%; placebo 17%.

Contraindications: TOPICYCLINE is contraindicated in persons who have shown hypersensitivity to any of its ingredients or to any of the other tetracyclines.

Warnings: Because the serum level of tetracycline resulting from the use of TOPICYCLINE (less than 0.1 µg/ml) is less than 7% of that associated with a therapeutic dose of 500 mg/day of tetracycline administered orally, liver damage from the use of TOPICYCLINE is highly unlikely, even in patients with renal impairment. Nevertheless, the warnings associated with the use of tetracycline orally should be considered before prescribing TOPICYCLINE for patients with renal impairment.
Reproduction studies in rats and rabbits have revealed no evidence of impaired fertility or harm to the fetus from TOPICYCLINE. There are no data, however, on use of this drug in pregnant women.
It is not known whether tetracycline or any other component of TOPICYCLINE, administered in this topical form, is secreted in human milk. As a general rule, nursing should not be undertaken while a patient is receiving any drug treatment because many drugs are excreted in human milk.

Precautions: This drug is for external use only, and care should be taken to keep it out of the eyes, nose, and mouth.

Adverse Reactions: Among the 733 patients treated with TOPICYCLINE under normal usage conditions during clinical evaluation, there was one instance of severe dermatitis requiring systemic steroid therapy.
About one-third of patients are likely to experience a stinging or burning sensation upon application of TOPICYCLINE. The sensation ordinarily lasts no more than a few minutes, and does not occur at every application. There has been no indication that patients experience sufficient discomfort to reduce the frequency of use or to discontinue use of the product.
A slight yellowing of the skin in the areas of application can be noticed by most users of TOPICYCLINE, particularly by those with light complexions. This condition is superficial, and the color can be eliminated by washing. Treated areas of skin will also fluoresce under an ultraviolet light source.
The kinds of side effects often associated with oral or parenteral administration of tetracyclines (e.g., various gastrointestinal complaints, vaginitis, hematologic abnormalities, manifestations of systemic hypersensitivity reactions, and dental and skeletal disorders) have not been observed with TOPICYCLINE. Because of TOPICYCLINE's topical form of administration and its resultant low serum levels, it is highly unlikely that such side effects will occur from its use.

Dosage and Administration: It is recommended that TOPICYCLINE be applied to the affected areas twice daily, morning and evening. The medication should be applied generously until the skin is thoroughly wet.
The medication is applied by tilting the bottle and rubbing the applicator top over the skin while gently applying pressure. The rate of flow may be controlled by increasing or decreasing the pressure against the skin. Instructions to the patient for proper application are provided on the TOPICYCLINE bottle label.
The average amount of TOPICYCLINE delivered to the skin by application to the face and neck twice daily is approximately 1.3 ml/day. This quantity of the medication contains 2.9 mg of tetracycline hydrochloride. Twice-daily use of TOPICYCLINE on other acne-involved areas in addition to the face and neck results in the application of about 2.2 ml/day, or 4.8 mg of tetracycline hydrochloride.
Patients may continue their normal use of cosmetics.

How Supplied: TOPICYCLINE is supplied in a single carton containing a powder and a liquid which must be mixed together by the pharmacist or physician prior to dispensing.
The liquid is a solution of n-decyl methyl sulfoxide and sucrose esters in 40% aqueous ethanol. It is contained in an amber glass bottle.
The powder is a premeasured mixture of tetracycline hydrochloride, 4-epitetracycline hydrochloride, and sodium bisulfite. The powder is contained in a plastic unit which, when inserted into the bottle, also acts as the applicator. At the time of dispensing, the applicator containing the powder is inserted into the bottle, and its powder contents are released into the liquid by pressing firmly on the center of the applicator top. Complete instructions for mixing are contained in the package.
The TOPICYCLINE bottle contains 70 ml of medication as dispensed. This constitutes about an eight-week supply for patients treating the face and neck, and about a four-week supply for patients treating other acne-involved areas in addition to the face and neck. Differences in individual usage habits will result in variation from these averages.
TOPICYCLINE should be kept at controlled room temperature or below, away from excessive heat.
TOPICYCLINE should be dispensed prior to the date marked on the bottle's back label. After dispensing, the medication should be used by the patient within 2 months.

Caution: Federal law prohibits dispensing without prescription.

NDC 37000-401-01

Made in U.S.A. for PROCTER & GAMBLE, Cincinnati, Ohio 45202 by Taylor Pharmacal, Decatur, Ill. 62525. A product of Procter & Gamble research.
U.S. Patents 3527864, 3896238, 3952099.

[*Shown in Product Identification Section*]

Purdue Frederick Company, The
50 WASHINGTON STREET
NORWALK, CT 06856

ARTHROPAN® Liquid
(choline salicylate)
Analgesic, Anti-inflammatory, Antipyretic

Composition: ARTHROPAN Liquid is an aqueous mint-flavored solution, each teaspoonful containing choline salicylate equivalent in salicylate content to 10 grains of aspirin.

Action: ARTHROPAN Liquid is an analgesic, anti-inflammatory, antipyretic agent, providing therapeutic effectiveness in salicylate therapy equal to that of aspirin, but with more rapid absorption and greater gastric tolerance. When taken on an empty stomach, ARTHROPAN Liquid is absorbed 5 times as rapidly as aspirin and reaches peak blood levels 12 times as rapidly as aspirin. In rheumatoid arthritis, beneficial results, such as relief of pain, have been demonstrated with ARTHROPAN Liquid in therapeutic doses. **Clinical studies show that ARTHROPAN Liquid is less irritating to the stomach than salicylates in common use. Radioactive chromium tagging of red blood cells demonstrated that administration of ARTHROPAN Liquid is associated with minimal incidence of intestinal bleeding no greater than in healthy volunteers.**

Indications: As a well-tolerated salicylate, ARTHROPAN Liquid is indicated as base therapy and long-term therapy as an analgesic and anti-inflammatory for the temporary relief of pain of rheumatoid arthritis, rheumatic fever, osteoarthritis, and other conditions for which oral salicylates are recommended. In addition, ARTHROPAN Liquid may be indicated for geriatric and other adult patients who have difficulty in swallowing tablets or capsules; for many patients who experience gastric distress after taking aspirin; in conditions where higher doses of salicylates may be desirable, yet there is difficulty in administering such doses in tablet form; and for patients who should avoid the use of sodium-containing salicylates.

Precautions and Adverse Reactions: Administration of ARTHROPAN Liquid is associated with a minimal incidence of gastrointestinal blood loss, and many patients can tolerate ARTHROPAN Liquid in larger doses than ordinary salicylates. Overdosage may lead to salicylism which should be treated in the established manner.

Dosage and Administration: Recommended dosage for adults and children over 12 years is 1 (one) teaspoonful; may be mixed with fruit juices, carbonated beverages, or water. Dosage may be repeated every 3 or 4 hours, if necessary, but not more than 6 times in one day. Patients with rheumatoid arthritis may start on 1 to 2 teaspoonfuls up to 4 times daily.

Supplied: Bottles of 8 and 16 fluid ounces (1 pint).

BETADINE® HĒLAFOAM™ SOLUTION
(povidone-iodine)
Topical Antiseptic Microbicide

Description: BETADINE Hēlafoam Solution is a unique, broad-spectrum microbicidal foam which helps prevent infection in burns and wounds. The light, protective foam may be applied directly from canister to burn site. BETADINE Hēlafoam Solution adheres to the site of the burn wound with virtually no runoff.

Action and Uses: For use as a microbicide of choice for disinfection of wounds and for antiseptic treatment of lacerations, abrasions, and first-, second- and third-degree burns. For use as a prophylactic anti-infective agent in hospital and office procedures, including postopera-

tive application to incisions to protect against possible infection. BETADINE Hēlafoam Solution may be bandaged or covered with gauze. By helping to control bacterial proliferation, BETADINE Hēlafoam Solution aids in prevention of partial-thickness burns progressing to full-thickness burns. A lower incidence of burn wound sepsis may help reduce the need for grafting or permit earlier grafting and shorten hospital stay.
Dosage and Administration: Shake well. Hold can upright and firmly press release button on top of can. Apply directly to treatment site, spreading gently with sterile-gloved hand or with sterile tongue-depressor. Alternative methods of application are to dispense directly onto sterile-gloved hand and apply gently over the treatment site; or onto sterile gauze and cover the wound thoroughly with the impregnated gauze. Apply BETADINE Hēlafoam Solution liberally, as needed.
Warning: Contents under pressure. Do not puncture or incinerate. Do not expose to temperatures above 120° Fahrenheit. Store at controlled room temperature (59°–86°F).
Supplied: Aerosol, 9 oz. (250 gm.) canister.

BETADINE® SOLUTION
(povidone-iodine)
Antiseptic, germicide

Action and Uses: For preoperative prepping of operative site, including the vagina, and as a general topical microbicide for: disinfection of wounds; emergency treatment of lacerations and abrasions; second– and third–degree burns; as a prophylactic anti-infective agent in hospital and office procedures, including postoperative application to incisions to help prevent infection; trichomonal, monilial, and nonspecific infectious vaginitis; oral moniliasis (thrush); bacterial and mycotic skin infections; decubitus and stasis ulcers; preoperatively, in the mouth and throat, as a swab. BETADINE Solution is microbicidal, and not merely bacteriostatic. It *kills* gram-positive and gram-negative bacteria (including antibiotic-resistant strains), fungi, viruses, protozoa and yeasts.
Administration: Apply full strength as often as needed as a paint, spray, or wet soak. May be bandaged.
How Supplied: ½ oz., 8 oz., 16 oz. (1 pt.), 32 oz. (1 qt.) and 1 gal. plastic bottles and 1 oz. packettes.
Also Available: BETADINE SOLUTION SWAB AIDS for degerming small areas of skin or mucous membranes prior to injections, aspirations, catheterization and surgery; boxes of 100 packettes. Also: disposable BETADINE SOLUTION SWABSTICKS, in packettes of 1's and 3's.

BETADINE® AEROSOL SPRAY
(povidone-iodine)
Antiseptic, germicide

The nitrogen pressurized spray is easy to apply over large areas, eliminates the use of a contact applicator on the tender site. Also used for pre- and postoperative prepping of operative site, treatment of burns, including third-degree burns, decubitus and stasis ulcers, as a spray on the skin to be covered with a cast, and as a general topical microbicide.
BETADINE Aerosol Spray is film-forming and may be applied with or without bandages.
Administration: Spray the affected area thoroughly as needed. The improved actuator permits spraying from any angle.
How Supplied: Aerosol, nitrogen propelled, 3 fl. oz. bottle.

BETADINE® SURGICAL SCRUB
(povidone-iodine)

Action and Uses: An antiseptic, germicidal, sudsing skin cleanser for pre- and postoperative scrubbing or washing by hospital operating room personnel; for preoperative use on patients; and general use as an antiseptic germicide in physician's office. Forms rich, golden lather, virtually nonirritating; nonstaining to skin and natural fabrics.
Caution: In rare instance of local irritation or sensitivity, discontinue use by individual.
Directions for Use:
A. For Preoperative Washing by Operating Personnel
1. Wet hands and forearms with water. Pour about 5 cc. (1 teaspoonful) of BETADINE Surgical Scrub on the palm of the hand and spread over both hands and forearms. Without adding more water, rub the Scrub thoroughly over all areas for about five minutes. Use a brush if desired. Clean thoroughly under fingernails. Add a little water and develop copious suds. Rinse thoroughly under running water.
2. Complete the wash by scrubbing with another 5 cc. of BETADINE Surgical Scrub in the same way.

B. For Preoperative Use on Patients
After the skin area is shaved, wet it with water. Apply BETADINE Surgical Scrub (1 cc. is sufficient to cover an area of 20-30 square inches), develop lather and scrub thoroughly for about five minutes. Rinse off by aid of sterile gauze saturated with water. The area may then be painted with BETADINE Solution or sprayed with BETADINE Aerosol Spray and allowed to dry.
C. For use in the Physician's Office
Use for washing whenever a germicidal detergent is required. For maximum degerming of the hands proceed as under (A). To prepare the patient's skin proceed as under (B).
Note: Blue stains on starched linen will wash off with soap and water.
Supplied: 16 oz. (1 pint) plastic bottle with and without pump, 32 oz. (1 quart) and 1 gal. plastic bottles, and ½ oz. packettes.

BETADINE® DOUCHE
(povidone-iodine)

A pleasantly scented solution, clinically effective in nonspecific infectious vaginitis and against vaginal moniliasis and *Trichomonas vaginalis* vaginitis. Also effective as a cleansing douche.
Advantages: Low surface tension, with uniform wetting action to assist penetration into vaginal crypts and crevices. Active in the presence of blood, pus, or vaginal secretions. Virtually nonirritating to vaginal mucosa. Will not stain skin or natural fabrics.
Directions for Use: As a Therapeutic Douche: Two (2) tablespoonfuls to a quart of lukewarm water once daily. As a Routine Cleansing Douche: One (1) tablespoonful to a quart of lukewarm water once or twice per week.
How Supplied: 1 oz., 8 oz., 1 gallon plastic bottles. Disposable ½ oz. (1 tablespoonful) packettes.
Also Available: BETADINE DOUCHE KIT.

BETADINE® VAGINAL GEL ℞
(povidone-iodine)

Action and Uses: For use in the treatment of *Trichomonas vaginalis* vaginitis, monilial vaginitis and nonspecific vaginitis.

> Based on a review of this drug by the National Academy of Sciences—National Research Council and/or other information, FDA has classified the indications as follows: possibly effective for use in the management of trichomonas vaginalis vaginitis, monilial vaginitis and nonspecific vaginitis. Final classification of the less-than-effective indications requires further investigation.

BETADINE Vaginal Gel (povidone-iodine) makes available elemental iodine in a form that maintains iodine's microbicidal activity, yet is virtually nonirritating, nontoxic and is nonstaining to skin and natural fabrics. It kills trichomonas, monilia and other iodine-susceptible vaginal organisms responsible for specific and nonspecific vaginal infections. Active in the presence of blood, pus or vaginal secretions, virtually nonirritating to vaginal mucosa, nonstaining to skin, linen or clothing of natural fabrics; color can be washed off with water.
Recommended Regimen: In the office, swab the cervix and vulvovaginal area with BETADINE Solution. Prescribe BETADINE Vaginal Gel (povidone-iodine) as follows: Insert one (1) applicatorful each night, followed the next morning by BETADINE Douche in its therapeutic concentration (2 tablespoonfuls to a quart of lukewarm water). This regimen is to be followed through the entire menstrual cycle, including days of menses. If further therapy is warranted, the regimen should be continued through the next two cycles. The patient may be instructed to return for an office visit following two weeks of therapy.
Precaution: If irritation, redness or swelling develop, discontinue use. The rare individual with history of iodine sensitization should not use this product, pending further investigation.
Recommended Dosage: One applicatorful (5 Gm). Each five grams (one applicatorful) is equivalent to fifty milligrams of available iodine.
Supplied: 18 Gm. and 3 oz. tubes with applicator. Only on prescription.
[*Shown in Product Identification Section*]

BETADINE® SKIN CLEANSER
(povidone-iodine)

BETADINE Skin Cleanser is a sudsing antiseptic liquid cleanser. It essentially retains the nonselective microbicidal action of iodine, yet virtually without the undesirable features associated with iodine. BETADINE Skin Cleanser kills gram-positive and gram-negative bacteria (including antibiotic-resistant strains), fungi, viruses, protozoa and yeasts. It forms rich golden lather, virtually nonirritating; nonstaining to skin and natural fabrics.
Indications: BETADINE Skin Cleanser aids in degerming the skin of patients with common pathogens, including Staphylococcus aureus. To help prevent the recurrence of acute inflammatory skin infections caused by iodine-susceptible pyogenic bacteria. In pyodermas, as a topical adjunct to systemic antimicrobial therapy. To help prevent spread of infection in acne pimples.
Directions for Use: Wet the skin and apply a sufficient amount of Skin Cleanser to work up a rich golden lather. Allow lather to remain about 3 minutes. Then rinse. Repeat 2-3 times a day or as needed.
Caution: In rare instances of local sensitivity, discontinue use by the individual.
How Supplied: 1 fl. oz. and 4 fl. oz. plastic bottles.
Note: Blue stains on starched linen will wash off with soap and water.

BETADINE® OINTMENT
(povidone-iodine)

Action and Uses: To help prevent infection in burns, lacerations and abrasions. Infected stasis ulcers. Common skin infections. For degerming skin in hyperalimentation, catheter care, the umbilical area or circumcision.
BETADINE Ointment, in a water-soluble base, is a topical agent active against organisms commonly encountered in skin and wound infections. The active ingredient substantially

Continued on next page

Purdue Frederick—Cont.

retains the broad-spectrum germicidal activity of iodine without the undesirable features or disadvantages of iodine. BETADINE Ointment is virtually nonirritating, does not block air from reaching the site of application, and washes easily off skin and natural fabrics. The site to which BETADINE Ointment is applied can be bandaged.
Administration: Apply directly to affected area as needed. May be bandaged.
Supplied: 1/32 oz. and 1/8 oz. packettes; 1 oz. tubes; 16 oz. (1 lb.) (av.) jars .

BETADINE® Mouthwash/Gargle
(povidone-iodine)

Description: BETADINE Mouthwash/Gargle is a flavored solution of povidone-iodine. It contains alcohol 8% by volume.
Action and Uses: An aromatic mouth freshener to help provide soothing temporary relief of dryness and minor irritations of the mouth and throat. May also be used as an aid to the daily care of the mouth and as a refreshing mouth rinse to cause the mouth to feel clean.
Directions for Use: Can be diluted with 2 parts of water or used full strength as a mouthwash, gargle, or rinse.
How Supplied: 6 oz. and 12 oz. bottles.

BETADINE® Viscous Formula Antiseptic Gauze Pad
(povidone-iodine)

Description: BETADINE Viscous Formula Antiseptic Gauze Pad is a 3″ × 9″ regular mesh gauze pad impregnated with BETADINE Solution (povidone-iodine) in a viscous base that is formulated to remain moist for an extended period of time.
Actions: The active ingredient in BETADINE Viscous Formula Antiseptic Gauze Pad kills both gram-positive and gram-negative bacteria (including antibiotic-resistant strains), viruses, fungi, protozoa and yeasts. It is rapidly effective against *Staphylococcus aureus.* It is microbicidal, not merely bacteriostatic. . . and maintains its activity in the presence of blood, pus and serum.
Uses: AS A TOPICAL MICROBICIDAL DRESSING
To help prevent topical infection; for disinfection of wounds; for antiseptic treatment of lacerations, abrasions and first-, second- and third-degree burns; for use as a prophylactic anti-infective agent in hospital and office procedures; for postoperative application to incisions to help protect against possible infection; for antiseptic treatment of cutaneous ulcers.
Directions for use: To open, separate seam in either corner of packette and peel down. Remove the gauze pad and apply directly to affected area. Gauze pad may be bandaged.
Supplied: Boxes of 12 and 50.
Also Available: BETADINE® Antiseptic Gauze Pad, impregnated with BETADINE SOLUTION in a water-soluble base of propylene glycol.

CARDIOQUIN® TABLETS ℞
(quinidine polygalacturonate)

Composition: Each CARDIOQUIN Tablet (quinidine polygalacturonate 275 mg.) is equivalent in quinidine content to 3 grains (200 mg.) of quinidine sulfate.
Action: CARDIOQUIN Tablets possess full cardiodynamic quinidine effects in arrhythmias, with significantly lower incidence of local gastrointestinal irritation than with quinidine sulfate.
Indications: CARDIOQUIN Tablets (quinidine polygalacturonate) are indicated in the treatment of: premature atrial and ventricular contractions; paroxysmal atrial tachycardia; paroxysmal AV junctional rhythm; atrial flutter; paroxysmal atrial fibrillation; established atrial fibrillation when therapy is appropriate; paroxysmal ventricular tachycardia when not associated with complete heartblock; maintenance therapy after electrical conversion of atrial fibrillation and/or flutter.
Contraindications: Aberrant impulses and abnormal rhythms due to escape mechanisms should not be treated with quinidine.
Warning: In the treatment of atrial flutter reversion to sinus rhythm may be preceded by a progressive reduction in the degree of AV block to a 1:1 ratio and resulting extremely rapid ventricular rate.
Administration and Dosage: Dosage must be adjusted to individual patient's needs, both for conversion and maintenance. An initial dose of 1 to 3 tablets may be used to terminate arrhythmia, and may be repeated in 3-4 hours. If normal sinus rhythm is not restored after 3 or 4 equal doses, the dose may be increased by 1/2 to 1 tablet (137.5 to 275 mg.) and administered three to four times before any further dosage increase. For maintenance, one tablet may be used two or three times a day; generally, one tablet morning and night will be adequate.
How Supplied: Uncoated, scored tablets in bottles of 100 and 500.
[*Shown in Product Identification Section*]

CERUMENEX® DROPS ℞
(triethanolamine polypeptide oleate-condensate)

A UNIQUE CERUMENOLYTIC AGENT FOR EFFECTIVE AND EASY REMOVAL OF EARWAX
Composition: CERUMENEX Drops contain (10%) Triethanolamine polypeptide oleate-condensate in propylene glycol with chlorbutanol (0.5%), for effective, convenient cerumenolytic action and easy removal of earwax.
Among its properties are:
1. Aqueous-miscible solution—low surface tension and optimal viscosity.
2. Slightly acid pH range to approximate surface of normal ear canal.
3. Hygroscopic—helps absorb aqueous transudates.
4. Antiseptic protection against contamination.

Advantages:
- USUALLY EFFECTIVE WITH A SINGLE 15-30 MINUTE TREATMENT.
- EXCELLENT RESULTS REPORTED IN OVER 90% OF ABOUT 2,700 ADULT AND PEDIATRIC PATIENTS.
- HELPS AVOID PAINFUL INSTRUMENTATION.
- SIMPLE AND EASY TO ADMINISTER.

Action: CERUMENEX Drops are specifically designed as a cerumenolytic agent, to emulsify and disperse excess or impacted earwax for easier removal without painful instrumentation. They are usually effective with a single 15-30 minute treatment, and are simple and easy to administer (See Dosage and Administration).
Indications:
- REMOVAL OF CERUMEN.
- REMOVAL OF IMPACTED CERUMEN PRIOR TO EAR EXAMINATION.
- REMOVAL OF IMPACTED CERUMEN PRIOR TO OTOLOGIC THERAPY.
- REMOVAL OF IMPACTED CERUMEN PRIOR TO AUDIOMETRY.

Contraindications:
- A history of a previous untoward reaction to CERUMENEX Drops.
- A positive patch test (see "Precautions").
- Knowledge or suspicion of a perforated eardrum or otitis media may be considered as a relative contraindication.

Precautions:
It is recommended that the following precautions be observed in prescribing and administration of this agent:
1. Extreme caution is indicated in patients with demonstrable dermatologic idiosyncrasies or with history of allergic reactions in general.
2. In case of doubt, a patch test should be performed by placing a drop of CERUMENEX Drops on the flexor surface of the arm or forearm and covering it with a small Band-Aid strip. The results are read and interpreted after 24 hours. Positive reaction indicates the probability of an allergic reaction following instillation in the ear.
3. Exposure of the ear canal to the CERUMENEX Drops should be limited to 15-30 minutes.
4. Patients must be instructed not to exceed the time of exposure, nor to use the medication more frequently than directed by the physician.
5. When administering CERUMENEX Drops, care must be taken to avoid undue exposure of the periaural skin during the instillation and the flushing out of the medication. If the medication comes in contact with the skin, the area should be washed with soap and water. Use of proper technique (see Dosage and Administration) will help avoid such undue exposure.
6. Although introduction of CERUMENEX Drops (triethanolamine polypeptide oleate-condensate) into the middle ear of animals with surgically perforated drums or into patients with ruptured drums has been accomplished without untoward reactions, the use of this medication should be avoided in the presence of underlying disease in the middle ear (otitis media, perforated drum) and it should be used only with caution in certain types of external otitis.
7. Patients should be advised to discontinue the use of the medication in case of a possible reaction and to consult their physician promptly.

Adverse Reactions:
Clinical Reactions of Possible Allergic Origin
Localized dermatitis reactions were reported in about 1% of 2,700 patients treated, ranging from a very mild erythema and pruritus of the external canal to a severe eczematoid reaction involving the external ear and periauricular tissue, generally with duration of 2-10 days. In all cases, complete and uneventful resolution occurred without residual sequelae, sometimes without supplemental therapy. Such therapy may consist of only symptomatic relief in mild cases and may include anti-inflammatory agents when indicated. Thus, while reactions of a possible allergic origin may occur, their incidence is minimal and usually not disproportionate to other commonly used dermatologic agents.
Dosage and Administration:
1. Fill ear canal with CERUMENEX Drops with the patient's head tilted at a 45° angle.
2. Insert cotton plug and allow to remain 15-30 minutes.
3. Then gently flush ear with lukewarm water, using soft rubber syringe (avoid excessive pressure). Avoid undue exposure of large skin areas to the drug. If a second application is necessary in unusually hard impactions, the procedure may be repeated.

How Supplied: 8 cc. and 15 cc. bottles with cellophane wrapped blunt-end dropper.
[*Shown in Product Identification Section*]

SENOKOT® SYRUP
(standardized extract of senna fruit)

Action and Uses: For relief of functional constipation and whenever gentle laxation is indicated. A deliciously flavored liquid laxative, predictably and reliably effective.
Contraindications: Acute surgical abdomen.
Administration and Dosage: Preferably at bedtime. Adults: 2 to 3 tsp. (maximum—3 tsp. b.i.d.). For older, debilitated, and OB/GYN patients, the physician may consider prescribing ½ the initial adult dose. Children 5-15 years: 1 to 2 tsp. (maximum—2 tsp. b.i.d.). 1-5 years: ½ to 1 tsp. (maximum—1 tsp. b.i.d.). 1 month to 1 year: ¼ to ½ tsp. (maximum—½ tsp. b.i.d.). If comfortable evacuation is not achieved by the second day, decrease or increase daily dosage (up to maximum) by one half the starting dose until optimum dose for evacuation is established.
How Supplied: Bottles of 2 and 8 fl. oz.

SENOKOT® TABLETS/GRANULES
(standardized senna concentrate)

Action and Uses: Indicated for relief of functional constipation (chronic or occasional). SENOKOT Tablets/Granules contain a natural vegetable derivative, purified and standardized for uniform action. The current theory of the mechanism of action is that glycosides are transported to the colon, where they are changed to aglycones that stimulate Auerbach's plexus to induce peristalsis. This virtually colon-specific action is gentle, effective and predictable, usually inducing comfortable evacuation of well-formed stool within 8-10 hours. Found effective even in many previously intractable cases of functional constipation, SENOKOT preparations may aid in rehabilitation of the constipated patient by facilitating regular elimination. At proper dosage levels, SENOKOT preparations are virtually free of adverse reactions (such as loose stools or abdominal discomfort) and enjoy high patient acceptance. Numerous and extensive clinical studies show their high degree of effectiveness in varieties of functional constipation: chronic, geriatric, antepartum and postpartum, drug-induced, pediatric, as well as in functional constipation concurrent with heart disease or anorectal surgery.
Contraindications: Acute surgical abdomen.
Administration and Dosage: Preferably at bedtime. GRANULES (deliciously cocoa-flavored): Adults: 1 level tsp. (maximum—2 level tsp. b.i.d.). For older, debilitated, and OB/GYN patients, the physician may consider prescribing ½ the initial adult dose. Children above 60 lb.: ½ level tsp. (maximum—1 level tsp. b.i.d.). TABLETS: Adults: 2 tablets (maximum—4 tablets b.i.d.). For older, debilitated, and OB/-GYN patients, the physician may consider prescribing ½ the initial dose. Children above 60 lb.: 1 tablet (maximum—2 tablets b.i.d.). To meet individual requirements, if comfortable bowel movement is not achieved by the second day, decrease or increase daily by ½ level tsp. or 1 tablet (up to maximum) until optimal dose for evacuation is established.
How Supplied: Granules: 2, 6, and 12 oz. plastic canisters. Tablets: Box of 20, bottles of 50 and 100.
SENOKOT Tablets Unit Strip Packs in boxes of 100 tablets; each tablet individually sealed in see-through pockets.

SENOKOT®-S Tablets
(standardized senna concentrate and dioctyl sodium sulfosuccinate)
Natural Laxative/Stool Softener Combination

Action and Uses: SENOKOT-S Tablets are designed to relieve both aspects of functional constipation—bowel inertia and hard, dry stools. They provide a natural neuroperistaltic stimulant combined with a classic stool softener: standardized senna concentrate gently stimulates Auerbach's plexus in the colonic wall, while DSS softens the stool for smoother and easier evacuation. This coordinated dual action of the two ingredients results in colon-specific, predictable laxative effect, usually in 8–10 hours. Administering the tablets at bedtime allows the patient an uninterrupted night's sleep, with a comfortable evacuation in the morning. Flexibility of dosage permits fine adjustment to individual requirements. At proper dosage levels, SENOKOT-S Tablets are virtually free from side effects. SENOKOT-S Tablets are highly suitable for relief of postsurgical and postpartum constipation, and effectively counteract drug-induced constipation. They facilitate regular elimination in impaction-prone and elderly patients, and are indicated in the presence of cardiovascular disease where straining must be avoided, as well as in the presence of hemorrhoids and anorectal disease.
Contraindications: Acute surgical abdomen.
Administration and Dosage: (preferably at bedtime) Recommended Initial Dosage: ADULTS—2 tablets (maximum dosage—4 tablets b.i.d.); CHILDREN (above 60 lbs.)—1 tablet (maximum dosage—2 tablets b.i.d.). For older or debilitated patients, the physician may consider prescribing half the initial adult dose. To meet individual requirements, if comfortable bowel movement is not achieved by the second day, dosage may be decreased or increased by 1 tablet, up to maximum, until the most effective dose is established.
Supplied: Bottles of 30 and 60 Tablets.

TRILISATE® Tablets ℞
(choline magnesium trisalicylate)
500 mg*
***present as 293 mg of choline salicylate combined with 362 mg of magnesium salicylate to provide 500 mg salicylate content.**

Description: TRILISATE Tablets contain a combination of choline salicylate and magnesium salicylate, which is freely soluble in water (greater than 100 mg/ml salicylate equivalent). TRILISATE Tablets are pale pink, capsule-shaped, and scored to permit flexible dosage. Each 500 mg tablet contains 293 mg of choline salicylate and 362 mg of magnesium salicylate to provide 500 mg. of salicylate content.
Clinical Pharmacology: TRILISATE Tablets are a non-steroidal, anti-inflammatory agent, with analgesic and anti-pyretic activity. In patients with rheumatoid arthritis, the anti-inflammatory action has been shown by a reduction in joint swelling, a reduction in pain, a reduction in duration of morning stiffness, and a reduction in disease activity as assessed by both the investigator and patient. As with other non-steroidal, anti-inflammatory drugs (including the salicylates), the mode of action is not known.
When TRILISATE Tablets are administered, the salicylate is absorbed rapidly and reaches peak blood levels within two hours. The primary route of excretion is through the kidneys, the excretion products being chiefly the glycine and glucuronide conjugates. At recommended doses, the therapeutic range of 5 to 30 mg/100 ml is achieved, and a steady-state condition is normally reached after 4–5 doses. The half-life of this drug is 9 to 17 hours. This permits a b.i.d. dosage schedule with maintenance of adequate blood levels throughout the 12-hour interval.
Utilizing radioactive chromium tagging of red blood cells to measure occult blood loss in feces, a double-blind comparative study of 14 days duration, involving 10 normal volunteers in each group, showed that TRILISATE Tablets did not induce a significant increase in blood loss over that observed during a 7-day drug-free control period. In the same study, aspirin produced a significantly greater blood loss than occurred during the drug-free control period, and a significantly greater blood loss than that observed in the group treated with TRILISATE Tablets.
Unlike aspirin and other non-steroidal, anti-inflammatory arylpropionic acid derivatives and arylacetic acid derivatives, TRILISATE Tablets, at therapeutic dosage levels, do not affect platelet aggregation, as shown by *in vitro* and *in vivo* studies.
In a double-blind, controlled crossover clinical trial in patients suffering from rheumatoid arthritis, TRILISATE Tablets did not cause the high incidence of gastric mucosal erosion endoscopically observed with aspirin, which produced the typical hyperemic and early ulcerative changes, such as have been reported in the literature. After aspirin tablets, 18 of 20 patients revealed marked gastric hyperemic mucosa and hemorrhagic erosions. After TRILISATE Tablets, gastric mucosal erosion was seen in only one of the 20 patients.
Indications and Usage: TRILISATE Tablets are indicated for relief of the signs and symptoms of rheumatoid arthritis, osteoarthritis and other arthritides. TRILISATE Tablets are indicated in the treatment of acute flare and in the long-term management of the disease.
TRILISATE Tablets are generally well tolerated, and since salicylates are considered the therapy of choice in the arthritides, TRILISATE Tablets may be regarded as a logical choice whenever salicylate therapy is indicated. TRILISATE Tablets are particularly to be chosen when b.i.d. dosage regimen is of importance for patient compliance with the dosage schedule; when gastrointestinal intolerance to aspirin is encountered; when gastrointestinal microbleeding or hematologic effects of aspirin are considered a patient hazard; and when interference (or the risk of interference) with normal platelet function by aspirin or by propionic acid derivatives is considered to be clinically undesirable.
In those rheumatoid arthritis patients who are designated by the American Rheumatism Association as Functional Class IV (incapacitated, largely or wholly bedridden or confined to a wheelchair, with little or no self-care), the safety and efficacy of TRILISATE Tablets have not been established.
In double-blind clinical trials, in patients treated with TRILISATE Tablets (on a b.i.d. schedule) for rheumatoid arthritis, the anti-inflammatory and analgesic action has been demonstrated by broad-spectrum improvement within one week of therapy in the major parameters of measurement of this disease's processes. Among these parameters are clinically and statistically significant ($P < 0.001$) reduction in the number of swollen joints and in the number of painful joints; clinically and statistically significant ($P < 0.001$) reduction in the swelling index and in the articular index; and a reduction in disease activity as assessed by both the investigator and patient. In rheumatoid arthritis patients, there was a clinically and statistically significant ($P < 0.001$) reduction in the duration of morning stiffness.
In double-blind clinical trials comparing TRILISATE Tablets with aspirin and ibuprofen in rheumatoid arthritis, and with indomethacin in osteoarthritis, TRILISATE Tablets were demonstrated to be a significantly effective non-steroidal antiarthritic agent.
TRILISATE Tablets may be used in combination with gold salts.
Effectiveness and excellent patient tolerance (especially by the gastrointestinal system) establish TRILISATE Tablets as an agent of choice in the treatment of the arthritides. This consideration is especially pertinent for pa-

Continued on next page

Purdue Frederick—Cont.

tients with demonstrated gastrointestinal intolerance to aspirin.
Contraindication: Patients who are hypersensitive to salicylates should not take TRILISATE Tablets.
Precautions: As with other salicylates, TRILISATE Tablets should be used with caution in patients with chronic renal insufficiency, or with active erosive gastritis or peptic ulcer.
Reports indicate that when salicylates are given with steroids, the butazones, or alcohol, the risk of gastrointestinal ulceration is increased. Caution should also be exercised in patients requiring coumarin or indandione anticoagulants, or heparin.
While salicylates are not known to be associated with teratogenic potential in man, the usual care should be exercised in the administration of any drug during pregnancy. Because of the possible inhibition of prostaglandin with high doses of salicylates, the use of TRILISATE Tablets is not recommended prior to parturition. TRILISATE Tablets are at present not recommended in children under twelve years.
Adverse Reactions: TRILISATE Tablets are generally well tolerated at recommended dosage ranges and have been shown to be particularly well tolerated by the gastrointestinal system. Since they are a salicylate, in large doses or extended therapy, salicylism and/or salicylate intoxication may occur.
Tinnitus may be regarded as a therapeutic guide. Should it develop, it is recommended that dosage be reduced.
Dosage: The recommended dosage of TRILISATE Tablets is two to three 500 mg tablets b.i.d. (q. 12 h.) for rheumatoid arthritis, for osteoarthritis and for the more severe arthritides.
One to two tablets b.i.d. (q. 12 h.) is the recommended dosage for mild to moderate arthritides. Each TRILISATE Tablet is equivalent in salicylate content to 10 gr of aspirin.
If the physician prefers, one to two tablets t.i.d. may be administered.
Therapeutic blood levels of 5 to 30 mg/100 ml are usually achieved and sustained by any of the above recommended dosage schedules.
As with other therapeutic agents, individual dose titration is advisable, and some patients may require higher or lower dosage than the recommended schedules. Some patients may require 2–3 weeks therapy for optimal effect.
Caution: Federal law prohibits dispensing without prescription.
How Supplied: TRILISATE Tablets are supplied in bottles of 100 Tablets.
U.S. Patent Nos. 3069321, 3759980 and 4067974.
[*Shown in Product Identification Section*]

IDENTIFICATION PROBLEM?

Consult PDR's

Product Identification Section

where you'll find over 900

products pictured actual size

and in full color.

Purepac Pharmaceutical Co.

200 ELMORA AVENUE
ELIZABETH, NEW JERSEY 07207

ACETAMINOPHEN TABLETS, USP
5 gr. (White scored)
ACETAMINOPHEN ELIXIR, USP
ACETAMINOPHEN W/CODEINE TABLETS ℞ Ⓒ
½ gr. No. 3 (White scored)
1 gr. No. 4 (White scored)
AMINOPHYLLINE SUPPOSITORIES, USP ℞
7½ gr. (Foil wrapped)
AMINOPHYLLINE TABLETS, USP ℞
3 gr., 1½ gr. (White)
AMITRIPTYLINE HCl TABLETS, USP ℞
10 mg. (FC Blue)
25 mg. (FC Yellow)
50 mg. (FC Tan)
75 mg. (FC Orange)
100 mg. (FC Pink)
AMPICILLIN FOR ORAL SUSPENSION, USP ℞
125 mg./5cc, 250 mg./5cc
AMPICILLIN TRIHYDRATE CAPSULES, USP ℞
250 mg., 500 mg. (Gray-Maroon)
A.P.C. TABLETS
(White)
A.P.C. W/BUTALBITAL TABLETS ℞ Ⓒ
(White)
A.P.C. W/CODEINE PHOSPHATE TABLETS ℞ Ⓒ
½ gr. No. 3, 1 gr. No. 4 (White Scored)
ASPIRIN SUPPOSITORIES, USP
2 gr., 5 gr., 10 gr. (Foil wrapped)
ASPIRIN TABLETS, USP
5 gr. (White)
AZMA-AID TABLETS
(White scored)
BELLADONNA ALKALOIDS with PHENOBARBITOL TABLETS ℞
(White scored)
BELLADONNA ALKALOIDS with PHENOBARBITAL ELIXIR ℞
(Green)
BELLADONNA TINCTURE USP ℞
Pint
BISACODYL SUPPOSITORIES, USP
10 mg.
BISACODYL TABLETS, USP
5 mg. (EC Orange)
PURETANE TABLETS ℞
(Brompheniramine Maleate)
4 mg. (SC Lt. Orange Scored) NF
12 mg. (SC Peach) Time Release
PURETAPP PA TABLETS ℞
(Brompheniramine Maleate with Phenylephrine HCl & Phenylpropanolamine HCl)
12 mg. (SC Lt. Blue)
PURETAPP ELIXIR ℞
(Brompheniramine Maleate with Phenylephrine HCl, Phenylpropanolamine HCl & Alcohol)
4 mg/5ml
PURETANE EXPECTORANT ℞
(Brompheniramine Maleate Expectorant)
PURETANE DC EXPECTORANT ℞ Ⓒ
(Brompheniramine Maleate DC Expectorant)
BUTABARBITAL SODIUM TABS., NF ℞ Ⓒ
¼ gr. (Lavender Scored)
½ gr. (Lt. Green Scored)
BUTABARBITAL SODIUM ELIXIR, NF Ⓒ
(Green Peppermint Fl.)
CALCIUM LACTATE TABLETS, USP
5 gr., 10 gr. (White)
CHLORAL HYDRATE CAPSULES, USP ℞ Ⓒ
500 mg. (7½ gr.) Red
500 mg. (7½ gr.) Green
250 mg. (3–¾ gr.) Green
CHLORAL HYDRATE SYRUP, USP Ⓒ
CHLORDIAZEPOXIDE HCl CAPSULES, USP ℞ Ⓒ
5 mg. (Green-Yellow)
10 mg. (Black-Green)
25 mg. (White-Green)
CHLOROTHIAZIDE TABLETS, USP ℞
250 mg., 500 mg. (White scored)
CHLORPHENIRAMINE MALEATE CAPSULES, USP TIME RELEASE ℞
8 mg., 12 mg. (Clear-Green)
CHLORPHENIRAMINE MALEATE TABLETS, USP ℞
4 mg. (Yellow)
CHLORPROMAZINE HCl TABLETS, USP ℞
10 mg., 25 mg., 50 mg., 100 mg., 200 mg. (SC Tan)
COLCHICINE TABLETS, USP ℞
1/100 gr. (White)
CONJUGATED ESTROGENS TABLETS, USP ℞
0.625 mg. (SC Maroon)
1.25 mg. (SC Yellow)
CORTISONE ACETATE TABLETS, USP ℞
25 mg. (White Scored)
CYCLANDELATE CAPSULES ℞
200 mg. (Blue)
400 mg. (Red-Blue)
DEXAMETHASONE TABLETS, USP ℞
0.75 mg. (Lt. Blue Scored, Pentagon)
DIGITOXIN TABLETS, USP ℞
0.1 mg. (Pink)
0.2 mg. (White)
DIGOXIN TABLETS, USP ℞
0.25 mg. (White scored)
DIMENHYDRINATE TABLETS, USP
50 mg. (Yellow)
DOCTASE
(Dioctyl Sodium Sulfosuccinate Capsules, 100 mg. w/Casanthranol)
30 mg. (Brown)
DIOCTO
(Dioctyl Sodium Sulfosuccinate Capsules, USP)
100 mg., 250 mg. (Red)
DIPHENYDRAMINE HCl CAPS., USP ℞
25 mg. (Clear-Pink)
50 mg. (Pink-Pink)
DIPHENHYDRAMINE HCl ELIXIR ℞
DIPHENHYDRAMINE HCl EXPECTORANT ℞
DIPHENOXYLATE HCl & ATROPINE SULFATE TABLETS ℞ Ⓒ
2.5 mg. (White)
DIPHENOXYLATE HCl & ATROPINE SULFATE LIQUID ℞ Ⓒ
DOXYCYCLINE HYCLATE CAPS., USP ℞
50 mg. (White-Blue)
100 mg. (Lt. Blue)
ERGONOVINE MALEATE TABLETS, NF ℞
0.2 mg.
ERGOTAMINE TARTRATE AND CAFFEINE TABLETS, NF ℞
ERYTHROMYCIN STEARATE TABS., USP ℞
250 mg. (FC Pink)
ESTROGENIC AQUEOUS INJECTABLE ℞
2 mg.
ESTROGENIC OIL INJECTABLE ℞
2 mg.
ESTRONE AQUEOUS SUSPENSION INJECTABLE ℞
5 mg.
FERROUS FUMURATE TABLETS, USP
5 gr. (SC Red)
FERROUS GLUCONATE TABLETS
5 gr. (SC Green)
FERROUS SULFATE CAPSULES, TIME RELEASE
250 mg. (Time Release) Clear-Red
FERROUS SULFATE TABLETS, USP
5 gr. SC (Green)
5 gr. SC (Red)
FOLIC ACID TABLETS, USP ℞
1 mg. (Yellow Scored)
GLUTETHIMIDE TABLETS, NF ℞ Ⓒ
500 mg. (White Scored)
HYDRALAZINE HCl TABLETS ℞
25 mg. (Blue)
50 mg. (Pink)
HYDROCHLOROTHIAZIDE TABLETS ℞
25 mg., 50 mg.
HYDROCHLOROTHIAZIDE 50 mg. with RESERPINE 0.125 mg. Tablets, ℞

HYDROCHLOROTHIAZIDE with RESERPINE AND HYDRALAZINE TABLETS ℞

HYDROCORTISONE TABLETS, USP ℞
10 mg., 20 mg. (White Scored)

HYDROCORTISONE ACETATE ℞
Cream
½%, 1%
Lotion
0.5%
Powder

IMIPRAMINE HCl TABLETS, USP ℞
10 mg., 25 mg., 50 mg. (SC Orange)

IODINE SOLUTION STRONG USP ℞
(Lugols)

ISONIAZID TABLETS, USP ℞
100 mg. (White Scored)

ISOSORBIDE DINITRATE TABLETS, USP ℞
10 mg. (White Scored) (Oral)
5 mg. (Pink) (Sublingual)

ISOSORBIDE DINITRATE TD TABLETS ℞
40 mg. (Yellow-Green Scored)

MECLIZINE TABLETS, USP CHEWABLE ℞
25 mg. (Pink)

MECLIZINE MULTI-LAYERED TABLETS, USP ℞
12.5 mg. (White-Yellow Scored)
25 mg. (White-Yellow Scored)

MEPROBAMATE TABLETS, USP ℞ Ⓒ
200 mg., 400 mg. (White Scored)

METHENAMINE MANDELATE TABLETS, USP ℞
500 mg. (EC Brown)
1 gm.

METHOCARBAMOL TABLETS ℞
500 mg., 750 mg. (White Scored)

METHYLTESTOSTERONE TABLETS, USP ℞
10 mg. (Buccal, Yellow Scored)
25 mg. (Yellow Scored)

NITROFURANTOIN TABLETS, USP ℞
50 mg., 100 mg. (Yellow Scored)

NITROGLYCERIN CAPSULES, TIME RELEASED ℞
2.5 mg. (Clear-Purple)
6.5 mg. (Yellow-Purple)

OXYTETRACYCLINE HCl CAPS., USP ℞
250 mg. (Yellow Opaque)

PAPAVERINE HYDROCHLORIDE CAPSULES, TR ℞
150 mg. (Brown-Clear)

PAPAVERINE HYDROCHLORIDE TABLETS, NF ℞
1½ gr. (White Scored)

PAREGORIC, USP ℞ Ⓒ

PENICILLIN G TABLETS, BUFFERED, USP ℞
200 MU, 250 MU, 400 MU (White Scored)

PENICILLIN G POTASSIUM POWDERED, USP ℞
(For Oral Suspension)
250 MU 5cc, 400 MU 5cc

PENICILLIN V POTASSIUM TABS., USP ℞
125 mg. 200 MU, 250 mg. 400 MU, 500 mg. 800 MU (White scored)

PENICILLIN V (BUFFERED POTASSIUM PENICILLIN V POWDER) ℞
(For Oral Suspension)
125 mg. 200 MU 5cc, 250 mg. 400 MU 5cc

PENTAERYTHRITOL TETRANITRATE TABLETS, NF ℞
10 mg., 20 mg. (Green)

PENTAERYTHRITOL TETRANITRATE CAPSULES, TIME RELEASE ℞
80 mg. Clear-White

PENTOBARBITAL SODIUM CAPSULES, USP ℞ Ⓒ
100 mg. (1½ gr.) (Yellow)

PHENOBARBITAL TABLETS, USP ℞ Ⓒ
¼ gr., ½ gr., 1½ gr. (White Scored)

PHENOBARBITAL ELIXIR, USP ℞ Ⓒ

PHENYTOIN SODIUM CAPSULES, USP ℞
100 mg. (Clear)

POTASSIUM CHLORIDE ORAL SOLUTION, 10% (Sugar Free) ℞

POTASSIUM CHLORIDE ORAL SOLUTION, 20% (Sugar Free) ℞

PREDNISOLONE TABLETS, USP ℞
5 mg. (Orange Scored)

PREDNISOLONE INJECTABLE ℞
25 mg.

PREDNISONE TABLETS, USP ℞
2.5 mg. (White)
5 mg. (White Scored)
10 mg. (Blue Scored)
20 mg. (Lt. Orange Scored)

PROBENECID and COLCHICINE TABLETS ℞
250 mg., 500 mg. (Yellow)

PROCAINAMIDE HCl CAPSULES, USP ℞
250 mg. (Yellow)

PROGESTERONE IN OIL INJECTABLE ℞
100 mg.

PROMETHAZINE HCl TABLETS, USP ℞
25 mg. (White Scored)
50 mg. (Pink)

PROMETHAZINE EXPECTORANT VC W/CODEINE ℞ Ⓒ

PROMETHAZINE HYDROCHLORIDE EXPECTORANT W/CODEINE, USP ℞ Ⓒ

PROMETHAZINE HYDROCHLORIDE EXPECTORANT ℞

PROPANTHELINE BROMIDE TABS., USP ℞
15 mg. (SC Beige)

PROPOXYPHENE HCl CAPSULES, USP ℞ Ⓒ
65 mg. (Pink)

PROPOXYPHENE COMPOUND 65 ℞ Ⓒ
(Red-Gray)

PROPOXYPHENE HCl & APAP TABLETS ℞ Ⓒ
(FC Lt. Red)

PROPYLTHIOURACIL TABLETS, USP ℞
50 mg. (White Scored)

PYRIDOXINE HCl INJECTABLE ℞
100 mg.

QUINIDINE SULFATE TABLETS, USP ℞
200 mg. (3 gr.) (White Scored)

QUININE SULFATE CAPSULES, USP
3 gr. (Clear)

QUININE SULFATE CAPSULES, USP
5 gr. (Clear)

RAUWOLFIA SERPENTINA TABLETS, NF ℞
50 mg., 100 mg. (SC Red)

RESERPINE TABLETS, USP ℞
0.1 mg., 0.25 mg. (White Scored)

SECOBARBITAL SODIUM CAPSULES, USP ℞ Ⓒ
100 mg. (1½ gr.) (Red-Orange)

SPIRONOLACTONE TABLETS ℞
25 mg.

SPIRONOLACTONE 25 mg. W/HYDROCHLOROTHIAZIDE 25 mg. ℞

SULFAMETHOXAZOLE TABLETS, NF ℞
500 mg.

SULFISOXAZOLE TABLETS, USP ℞
0.5 gm. (White Scored)

TESTOSTERONE AQUEOUS SUSPENSION INJECTABLE ℞
25 mg., 50 mg., 100 mg.

TESTOSTERONE PROPIONATE IN OIL INJECTABLE ℞
100 mg.

TETRACYCLINE HCl CAPSULES, USP ℞
250 mg. (Yellow-Orange)
500 mg. (Yellow-Black)

TETRACYCLINE SYRUP ℞
125 mg./5cc

THYROID TABLETS, USP ℞
¼ gr., ½ gr., 1 gr., 2 gr. (Tan)

TOLBUTAMIDE 0.5 gm TABLETS USP ℞

TRIAMCINOLONE TABLETS ℞
4 mg. (White Scored)

TRIDIHEXETHYL CHLORIDE W/MEPROBAMATE TABLETS ℞
200 mg. (SC Yellow)
400 mg. (Lt. Yellow)

TRIPLE ANTIBIOTIC OINTMENT
(Bacitracin, Polymixin, Neomycin)

TRIPROLIDINE HCl 2.5 MG. W/PSEUDOEPHEDRINE HCl 60 MG. TABLETS ℞
(White Scored)

TRIPROLIDINE HCl 1.25 MG. W/PSEUDOEPHEDRINE HCl 30 MG. SYRUP ℞

Reed & Carnrick
30 BORIGHT AVE.
KENILWORTH, NJ 07033

ALPHOSYL®
Lotion, Cream

Description: Special crude coal tar extract 5.0% and allantoin 1.7% in combination in a greaseless, stainless vanishing cream base.

Actions: In the treatment of psoriasis and other chronic dermatoses with itching, scaling and erythema.

Precautions: Alphosyl is safe for use as directed. However, if irritation and/or redness occurs, discontinue use and consult physician. Alphosyl is for external use only; avoid contact with the eyes.

Directions for use: SHAKE WELL BEFORE USING.

1.) Apply Alphosyl Lotion to affected areas two to four times daily, morning and night, massaging thoroughly into the lesions.

2.) For persistent, long term cases, with heavy scaling and crusting, a hot daily bath is recommended to soften and facilitate removal of scales, prior to applying Alphosyl Lotion.

3.) MAINTENANCE THERAPY: Once the condition is under control, Alphosyl Lotion should be applied 2 to 3 times weekly to help prevent recurrence. Treatments may be repeated as directed by physician.

How Supplied: ALPHOSYL Lotion 8 fl. oz.; ALPHOSYL Cream 2 oz. tube.

ALSO AVAILABLE as ALPHOSYL-HC Lotion (0.5% hydrocortisone) in 4 oz. bottles and ALPHOSYL-HC Cream (0.5% hydrocortisone) in 30 gm. tubes, on prescription.

CORTIFOAM® ℞
(hydrocortisone acetate 10%)

Description: Contains hydrocortisone acetate 10% as the sole active ingredient in 20 Gms. of a foam containing propylene glycol, ethoxylated stearyl alcohol, polyoxyethylene-10-stearyl ether, cetyl alcohol, methyl and propyl parabens, triethanolamine, water and inert propellants, dichlorodifluoromethane and dichlorotetrafluoroethane.

Each application delivers approximately 900 mg. of foam containing 80 mg. of hydrocortisone (90 mg. of hydrocortisone acetate).

Clinical Pharmacology: CORTIFOAM provides effective topical administration of an anti-inflammatory corticosteroid as adjunctive therapy of ulcerative proctitis.

Indications: CORTIFOAM is indicated as adjunctive therapy in the topical treatment of ulcerative proctitis of the distal portion of the rectum. It is especially useful in patients who cannot retain hydrocortisone or other corticosteroid enemas. Direct observations of methylene blue-containing foam have shown staining about 10 centimeters into the rectum.

Contraindications: Local contraindications to the use of intrarectal steroids include obstruction, abscess, perforation, peritonitis, fresh intestinal anastomoses, extensive fistulas and sinus tracts. Tuberculosis (active, latent or questionably healed), ocular herpes simplex and acute psychosis are usually considered absolute contraindications to the use of corticosteroids. Relative contraindications include active peptic ulcer, acute glomerulonephritis, myasthenia gravis, osteoporosis, diverticulitis, thrombophlebitis, psychic disturbances, pregnancy, diabetes, hyperthyroidism, acute coronary disease, hypertension, limited cardiac reserve and local or systemic infections, including fungal or exanthematous diseases. Where these conditions exist, the expected benefits from steroid therapy must be weighed against the risks involved in its use. Pregnancy is a relative contraindication to

Continued on next page

Reed & Carrnick—Cont.

corticosteroids, particularly during third trimester. If corticosteroids must be administered in pregnancy, watch newborn infant closely for signs of hypoadrenalism, and administer appropriate therapy if needed.
Warning: Do not insert any part of the aerosol container into the anus. Contents of the container are under pressure, but not flammable. Do not burn or puncture the aerosol container. Store at room temperature—not over 120° F. Because CORTIFOAM is not expelled systemic hydrocortisone absorption may be greater from CORTIFOAM than from corticosteroid enema formulations. If there is no evidence of clinical or proctologic improvement within two or three weeks after starting CORTIFOAM therapy, or if the patient's condition worsens, discontinue the drug.
Precautions: Steroid therapy should be administered with caution in patients with severe ulcerative disease because these patients are predisposed to perforation of the bowel wall. Where surgery is imminent, it is hazardous to wait more than a few days for a satisfactory response to medical treatment. General precautions common to all corticosteroid therapy should be observed during treatment with CORTIFOAM. These include gradual withdrawal of therapy to allow for possible adrenal insufficiency and awareness to possible growth suppression in children. Patients should be kept under close observation, for, as with all drugs, rare individuals may react unfavorably under certain conditions. If severe reactions or idiosyncrasies occur, steroids should be discontinued immediately and appropriate measures instituted. Do not employ in immediate or early postoperative period following ileorectostomy.
Adverse Reactions: Corticosteroid therapy may produce side effects which include moon face, fluid retention, excessive appetite and weight gain, abnormal fat deposits, mental symptoms, hypertrichosis, acne, ecchymosis, increased sweating, pigmentation, dry scaly skin, thinning scalp hair, thrombophlebitis, decreased resistance to infection, negative nitrogen balance with delayed bone and wound healing, menstrual disorders, neuropathy, peptic ulcer, decreased glucose tolerance, hypopotassemia, adrenal insufficiency, necrotizing angiitis, hypertension, pancreatitis and increased intraocular pressure. In children, suppression of growth may occur. Increased intercranial pressure may occur and possibly account for headache, insomnia and fatigue. Supcapsular cataracts may result from prolonged usage. Long-term use of all corticosteroids results in catabolic effects characterized by negative protein and calcium balance. Osteoporosis, spontaneous fractures and aseptic necrosis of the hip and humerus may occur as part of this catabolic phenomenon. Where hypopotassemia and other symptoms associated with fluid and electrolyte imbalance call for potassium supplementation and salt poor or salt-free diets, these may be instituted and are compatible with diet requirements for ulcerative proctitis.
Administration and Dosage: Usual dose is one applicatorful once or twice daily for two or three weeks, and every second day thereafter, administered rectally. The patient direction package with the applicator describes how to use the aerosol container and applicator. Satisfactory response usually occurs within five to seven days marked by a decrease in symptoms. Symptomatic improvement in ulcerative proctitis should not be used as the sole criterion for evaluating efficacy. Sigmoidoscopy is also recommended to judge dosage adjustment, duration of therapy and rate of improvement. Directions For Use: 1) Shake foam container vigorously before use. Hold container upright and insert into opening of the tip of the applicator. Be sure applicator plunger is drawn all the way out. Container must be held upright to obtain proper flow of medication 2) To fill, press down slowly on container cap. When foam reaches fill line in the applicator, it is ready for use. Caution: The aerosol container should never be inserted directly into the anus. 3) Remove applicator from container. Allow some foam to remain on the applicator tip. Hold applicator by barrel and gently insert tip into the anus. With applicator in place, push plunger in order to expel foam, then withdraw applicator. (Applicator parts should be pulled apart for thorough cleaning with warm water.)
How Supplied: CORTIFOAM is supplied in an aerosol container with a special rectal applicator. Each applicator delivers approximately 900 mg. of foam containing approximately 80 mg. of hydrocortisone as 90 mg. of hydrocortisone acetate. The aerosol container will deliver a minimum of 14 applications.
Literature Available: Patient information and instruction pads available on request.
[*Shown in Product Identification Section*]

DILATRATE-™ SR ℞
[isosorbide dinitrate]
Sustained Release Capsules 40 mg.

Description: Dilatrate-SR (isosorbide dinitrate) provides up to 12 hours of continuous vasodilatation.
Actions: The basic action is that of all nitrates, the relaxation of smooth muscle. How this relates to its clinical usefulness in the treatment of angina pectoris (pain of coronary artery disease) is not clear, since the exact cause of this pain is also obscure.
The objective of therapy is a decrease in the frequency and severity of attacks of angina pectoris and a decrease in the need to use nitroglycerin. This is the only practical way to judge the effects of therapy, especially since there is a wide variation in symptomatic response to treatment.

Indications:
Based on a review of this drug by the National Academy of Sciences-National Research Council and/or other information, FDA has classified the indications as follows:
"Possibly" effective: When taken by the oral route, is indicated for the relief of angina pectoris (pain of coronary artery disease). It is not intended to abort the acute anginal episode, but is widely regarded in the prophylactic treatment of angina pectoris.
Final classification of the less-than-effective indication requires further investigation.

Contraindications: Idiosyncracy to this drug.
Warnings: Data supporting the use of nitrates and nitrites during the early days of the acute phase of myocardial infarction (the period during which clinical and laboratory findings are unstable) are insufficient to establish safety.
Precautions:
1. Tolerance to this drug, and cross-tolerance to other nitrates or nitrites may occur.
2. In patients with functional or organic gastrointestinal hypermotility or malabsorption syndrome it is suggested that either the 5 mg. or 10 mg. oral tablets or 2.5 mg. or 5 mg. sublingual tablets be the preferred therapy.

Adverse Reactions:
1. Cutaneous vasodilation with flushing.
2. Headache is common and may be severe and persistent.
3. Transient episodes of dizziness and weakness, as well as other signs of cerebral ischemia associated with postural hypotension, may occasionally develop.
4. This drug can act as a physiological antagonist to norepinephrine, acetylcholine, histamine, and many other agents.
5. An occasional individual exhibits marked sensitivity to the hypotensive effects of nitrite, and severe responses (nausea, vomiting, weakness, restlessness, pallor, perspiration and collapse) can occur even with the usual therapeutic dose. Alcohol may enhance this effect.
6. Drug rash and/or exfoliative dermatitis may occasionally occur.

Dosage and Administration:
Initiating Therapy: In starting patients on isosorbide dinitrate, it is necessary to adjust the dosage until the smallest effective dose is determined.
Occasionally, severe hypotensive responses may occur with this dosage form, even with doses as low as 5 mg.
Dilatrate-SR 40 mg. sustained release capsules: Average dose is one capsule orally, every 10 to 12 hrs. according to need.
It is recommended that Dilatrate-SR be taken on an empty stomach. If vascular headache cannot be effectively controlled by ordinary measures, dosages may be taken with meals to minimize this side effect.
How Supplied: Bottles of 100 (opaque pink cap and colorless body).
Storage: Keep bottle tightly closed. Protect from light, heat and moisture.
Warning: Keep out of reach of children.
Caution: Federal law prohibits dispensing without prescription.

EPIFOAM™ ℞
(hydrocortisone acetate 1%)

Description: A topical steroid foam containing hydrocortisone acetate 1%
Inactive ingredients: Pramoxine HCl, propylene glycol, cetyl alcohol, PEG-100 stearate, glyceryl stearate, laureth-23, polyoxyl-40 stearate, methylparaben, propylparaben, triethanolamine or hydrochloric acid to adjust pH, purified water, propellant (inert), butane and propane.
Actions: Topical steroids are primarily effective because of their anti-inflammatory, antipruritic and vasoconstrictive actions.
Indications: For relief of the inflammatory manifestations of corticosteroid-responsive dermatoses.
Contraindications: Topical steroids are contraindicated in those patients with a history of hypersensitivity to any of the components of the preparation.
Precautions: If irritation develops, the product should be discontinued and appropriate therapy instituted.
In the presence of an infection, the use of appropriate antifungal or antibacterial agents should be instituted. If a favorable response does not occur promptly, the corticosteroid should be discontinued until the infection has been adequately controlled.
If extensive areas are treated or if the occlusive technique is used, the possibility exists of increased systemic absorption of the corticosteroid and suitable precautions should be taken, particularly in children and infants. Although topical steroids have not been reported to have any adverse effect on human pregnancy, the safety of their use in pregnant women has not absolutely been established. In laboratory animals, increases in incidence of fetal abnormalities have been associated with exposure of gestating females to topical corticosteroids, in some cases at rather low dosage levels. Therefore, drugs of this class should not be used extensively on pregnant patients, in large amounts, or for prolonged periods of time.
The product is not for ophthalmic use.
Adverse Reactions: The following local adverse reactions have been reported with topi-

cal corticosteroids: Burning, itching, irritation, dryness, folliculitis, hypertrichosis, acneiform eruptions, hypopigmentation, allergic contact dermatitis, maceration of the skin, secondary infection, skin atrophy, striae and miliaria.
Dosage and Administration: Apply to affected areas 3 or 4 times daily. Transfer the medication to a pad and apply gently, or apply the foam directly. Refer to the enclosed "Directions for Use"
How Supplied: Available in 10 gram pressurized cans.

KWELL® Cream ℞
LINDANE (gamma benzene hexachloride Cream) USP 1%

KWELL CREAM (gamma benzene hexachloride, Cream, USP 1%)
Description: Active ingredient lindane (gamma benzene hexachloride, USP) 1%, Inert ingredients: 99% in a pleasantly scented water dispersible cream, containing stearic acid, lanolin, glycerin, 2-amino-2-methyl-1-propanol, perfume and purified water.
Actions: KWELL CREAM is an ectoparasiticide for Sarcoptes scabiei (scabies), Pediculus capitis (head lice), Phthirus pubis (crab lice), and their ova.
Indications: KWELL CREAM is indicated for the treatment of patients with Sarcoptes scabiei (scabies), as well as infestations of Pediculus capitis (head lice), Phthirus pubis (crab lice), and their ova.
Contraindications: KWELL CREAM is contraindicated for individuals with known sensitivity to the product or to any of its components.
Warning: KWELL SHOULD BE USED WITH CAUTION, ESPECIALLY ON INFANTS, CHILDREN AND ON PREGNANT WOMEN. GAMMA BENZENE HEXACHLORIDE PENETRATES HUMAN SKIN AND HAS THE POTENTIAL FOR CNS TOXICITY. STUDIES INDICATE THAT POTENTIAL TOXIC EFFECTS OF TOPICALLY APPLIED LINDANE ARE GREATER IN THE YOUNG. Seizures have been reported after the use of gamma benzene hexachloride, but a cause and effect relationship has not been established.
Simultaneous application of creams, ointments or oils may enhance the percutaneous absorption of gamma benzene hexachloride.
Precautions: If accidental ingestion occurs, prompt gastric lavage will rid the body of large amounts of the toxicant. However, since oils favor absorption, saline cathartics for intestinal evacuation should be given rather than oil laxatives. If central nervous system manifestations occur, they can be antagonized by the administration of pentobarbital or phenobarbital.
If accidental contact with the eyes occurs, flush with water. If irritation or sensitization occurs, discontinue use and contact a physician.
Adverse Reactions: Eczematous eruptions due to irritation from this product have been reported.

ADMINISTRATION
CAUTION: USE ONLY AS DIRECTED. DO NOT EXCEED RECOMMENDED DOSAGE.
NOTE: PLEASE READ CAREFULLY.

Directions for Use:
Pediculosis capitis (head lice)—Kwell Shampoo is the most convenient dosage form but the lotion and cream are also effective.
Apply a quantity sufficient to cover only the affected and adjacent hairy areas. The cream should be rubbed into scalp and hair and left in place for 12 hours followed by thorough washing.
Retreatment is usually not necessary. Demonstrable living lice after 7 days indicates that retreatment is necessary.
Pediculosis pubis (crab lice)—Apply a sufficient quantity only to cover thinly the hair and skin of the pubic area, and if infested the thighs, trunk, and axillary regions. The material should be rubbed into the skin and hair, and left in place for 12 hours followed by a thorough washing.
Retreatment is usually not necessary. Demonstrable living lice after 7 days indicates that retreatment is necessary. Sexual contacts should be treated simultaneously.
Scabies (Sarcoptes scabiei)—The cream should be applied to dry skin in a thin layer and rubbed in thoroughly. If crusted lesions are present, a warm bath preceding the medication is helpful. If a warm bath is used, allow the skin to dry and cool before applying the cream. Usually one ounce is sufficient for an adult. A total body application should be made from the neck down. Scabies rarely affects the head of children or adults but may occur in infants. The cream should be left on 8–12 hours and should then be removed by thorough washing. ONE APPLICATION IS USUALLY CURATIVE.
Many patients exhibit persistent pruritus after treatment; this is rarely a sign of treatment failure and is not an indication for retreatment, unless living mites can be demonstrated.
CAUTION: Federal law prohibits dispensing without prescription.
How Supplied: KWELL CREAM in tubes of 2 oz (57G) and jars of 16 oz (454G).
Literature Available: Patient information and instruction pads with directions for use available on request.

KWELL® Lotion ℞
LINDANE (gamma benzene hexachloride Lotion) USP 1%

KWELL LOTION (gamma benzene hexachloride, Lotion, USP 1%)
Description: Active ingredient lindane (gamma benzene hexachloride, USP) 1%. Inert ingredients: 99% in a non-greasy, pleasantly scented base, containing glyceryl monostearate, cetyl alcohol, stearic acid, triethanolamine, 2-amino-2-methyl-1-propanol, butyl p-hydroxybenzoate, methyl p-hydroxybenzoate, Irish moss extract, perfume and purified water.
Actions: KWELL LOTION is an ectoparasiticide for Sarcoptes scabiei (scabies), Pediculus capitis (head lice), Phthirus pubis (crab lice), and their ova.
Indications: KWELL LOTION is indicated for the treatment of patients with Sarcoptes scabiei (scabies), as well as infestations of Pediculus capitis (head lice), Phthirus pubis (crab lice), and their ova.
Contraindications: KWELL LOTION is contraindicated for individuals with known sensitivity to the product or to any of its components.
Warning: KWELL SHOULD BE USED WITH CAUTION, ESPECIALLY ON INFANTS, CHILDREN AND ON PREGNANT WOMEN. GAMMA BENZENE HEXACHLORIDE PENETRATES HUMAN SKIN AND HAS THE POTENTIAL FOR CNS TOXICITY. STUDIES INDICATE THAT POTENTIAL TOXIC EFFECTS OF TOPICALLY APPLIED LINDANE ARE GREATER IN THE YOUNG. Seizures have been reported after the use of gamma benzene hexachloride, but a cause and effect relationship has not been established.
Simultaneous application of creams, ointments or oils may enhance the percutaneous absorption of gamma benzene hexachloride.
Precautions: If accidental ingestion occurs, prompt gastric lavage will rid the body of large amounts of the toxicant. However, since oils favor absorption, saline cathartics for intestinal evacuation should be given rather than oil laxatives. If central nervous system manifestations occur, they can be antagonized by the administration of pentobarbital or phenobarbital.
If accidental contact with the eyes occurs, flush with water. If irritation or sensitization occurs discontinue use and contact a physician.
Adverse Reactions: Eczematous eruptions due to irritation from this product have been reported.

ADMINISTRATION
CAUTION: USE ONLY AS DIRECTED. DO NOT EXCEED RECOMMENDED DOSAGE.
NOTE: PLEASE READ CAREFULLY.

Directions For Use:
Pediculosis capitis (head lice)—Kwell Shampoo is the most convenient dosage form but the lotion and cream are also effective.
Apply a quantity sufficient to cover only the affected and adjacent hairy areas. The lotion should be rubbed into scalp and hair and left in place for 12 hours followed by thorough washing.
Retreatment is usually not necessary. Demonstrable living lice after 7 days indicates that retreatment is necessary.
Pediculosis pubis (crab lice)—Apply a sufficient quantity only to cover thinly the hair and skin of the pubic area, and if infested, the thighs, trunk, and axillary regions. The material should be rubbed into the skin and hair and left in place for 12 hours followed by a thorough washing.
Retreatment is usually not necessary. Demonstrable living lice after 7 days indicates that retreatment is necessary. Sexual contacts should be treated simultaneously.
Scabies (Sarcoptes scabiei)—The lotion should be applied to dry skin in a thin layer and rubbed in thoroughly. If crusted lesions are present, a warm bath preceding the medication is helpful. If a warm bath is used, allow the skin to dry and cool before applying the lotion. Usually one ounce is sufficient for an adult. A total body application should be made from the neck down. Scabies rarely affects the head of children or adults but may occur in infants. The lotion should be left on for 8–12 hours and should then be removed by thorough washing. ONE APPLICATION IS USUALLY CURATIVE.
Many patients exhibit persistent pruritus after treatment; this is rarely a sign of treatment failure and is not an indication for retreatment, unless living mites can be demonstrated.
Caution: Federal law prohibits dispensing without prescription.
How Supplied: KWELL LOTION in bottles of 2 oz (59ml), 16 oz (472ml) and 1 gallon (3.8 L).
Literature Available: Patient information and instruction pads with directions for use available on request.

KWELL® Shampoo ℞
LINDANE (gamma benzene hexachloride, USP) Shampoo, 1%

KWELL SHAMPOO (gamma benzene hexachloride, shampoo 1%)
Description: Active ingredient lindane (gamma benzene hexachloride, USP) 1%. Inert ingredients: 99% in a cosmetically pleasant shampoo base, containing polyoxyethylene sorbitan monostearate, triethanolamine lauryl sulfate, acetone and purified water.
Actions: KWELL SHAMPOO is an ectoparasiticide and ovicide toxic to the parasites, Pediculus capitis (head lice), Phthirus pubis (crab lice), and their ova.
Indications: KWELL SHAMPOO is indicated for the treatment of patients with Pediculus capitis (head lice), Phthirus pubis (crab lice), and their ova.
Contraindications: KWELL SHAMPOO is contraindicated for individuals with known sensitivity to the product or to any of its components.
Warning: KWELL SHAMPOO SHOULD BE USED WITH CAUTION, ESPECIALLY ON INFANTS, CHILDREN AND ON PREGNANT WOMEN. GAMMA BENZENE HEXACHLORIDE PENETRATES HUMAN SKIN AND HAS THE POTENTIAL FOR CNS TOX-

Continued on next page

Reed & Carnrick—Cont.

ICITY. STUDIES INDICATE THAT POTENTIAL TOXIC EFFECTS OF TOPICALLY APPLIED LINDANE ARE GREATER IN THE YOUNG. Seizures have been reported after the use of gamma benzene hexachloride, but a cause and effect relationship has not been established.
Simultaneous application of creams, ointments or oils may enhance the percutaneous absorption of gamma benzene hexachloride.
Precautions: If accidental ingestion occurs, prompt gastric lavage will rid the body of large amounts of the toxicant. However, since oils favor absorption, saline cathartics for intestinal evacuation should be given rather than oil laxatives. If central nervous system manifestations occur, they can be antagonized by the administration of pentobarbital, or phenobarbital.
If accidental contact with the eyes, occurs flush with water. If irritation or sensitization occurs discontinue use and contact a physician.
Adverse Reactions: Eczematous eruptions due to irritation from this product have been reported.

ADMINISTRATION
CAUTION: USE ONLY AS DIRECTED. DO NOT EXCEED RECOMMENDED DOSAGE.
NOTE: PLEASE READ CAREFULLY

Directions For Use:
Pediculosis capitis (head lice)—1) Apply a sufficient quantity of the shampoo to thoroughly wet the hair and skin of the infested and adjacent, hairy areas. 2) When the hair and skin are thoroughly wetted with the shampoo, add small quantities of water at a time working the shampoo into the hair and skin until a good lather forms. 3) Continue shampooing for four minutes. 4) Rinse thoroughly. Towel briskly. When the hair is dry, any remaining nits or nit shells may be removed by fine-tooth combing or with tweezers.
Retreatment is usually not necessary. Demonstrable living lice after 7 days indicates that retreatment is necessary.
Pediculosis pubis (crab lice)—1) Apply a sufficient quantity of the shampoo to thoroughly wet the hair and skin of the infested and adjacent, hairy areas. 2) When the hair and skin are thoroughly wetted with the shampoo, add small quantities of water at a time working the shampoo into the hair and skin until a good lather forms. 3) Continue shampooing for four minutes. 4) Rinse thoroughly. Towel briskly. Retreatment is usually not necessary. Demonstrable living lice after 7 days indicates that retreatment is required. Sexual contacts should be treated simultaneously.
NOTE: Kwell Shampoo is intended only for head lice and crab lice infestations and should not be used as a routine shampoo. For other ectoparasitic infestions, such as scabies, the use of Kwell Cream or Kwell Lotion is recommended.
Caution: Federal law prohibits dispensing without prescription.
How Supplied: Kwell Shampoo in bottles of 2 fl. oz (59ml), 16 fl. oz (472ml) and 1 gallon (3.8L).
Literature Available: Patient information and instruction pads with directions for use available on request.

PHAZYME® Tablets

Description: A pink coated two-phase tablet. The outer layer releases in the stomach: simethicone, NF, specially activated 20 mg. The enteric coated core releases in the small intestine: pancreatic enzymes (protease 3,000 NF units, lipase 240 NF units, amylase 2,000 NF units), and simethicone, NF, specially activated 40 mg.
Actions: Phazyme is the only dual approach to the problem of gastrointestinal gas. Simethicone, the gas releasing agent, minimizes gas formation and relieves gas entrapment in both the stomach and the lower G.I. tract. This action combats pain, due to gastrointestinal gas. Pancreatic enzymes enhance the normal digestive process and help to reduce gas formation. Also, for relief of gas distress associated with other functional or organic conditions such as: diverticulitis, spastic colitis, hyperacidity, post-cholecystectomy syndrome and chronic cholecystitis.
Indications: Phazyme is indicated for the relief of occasional or chronic pain caused by gas entrapped in the stomach or in the lower gastrointestinal tract—resulting from aerophagia, postoperative distention, dyspepsia and food intolerance.
Contraindications: A known sensitivity to an ingredient.
Dosage: One or two tablets with meals and upon retiring or as required.
How Supplied: Pink coated two-phase tablet in bottles of 50, 100, and 1,000.
[*Shown in Product Identification Section*]

PHAZYME®-95 Tablets

Description: A red coated two phase tablet with the highest dose of simethicone available in a single tablet. The outer layer releases in the stomach: simethicone, NF, specially activated 25 mg. The enteric coated core releases in the small intestine: pancreatic enzymes (protease 6,000 NF units, lipase 480 NF units, amylase 4,000 NF units), and simethicone, NF, specially activated 70 mg.
Actions: Phazyme®-95 is the only dual approach to the problem of gastrointestinal gas. Simethicone, the gas releasing agent, minimizes gas formation and relieves gas entrapment in both the stomach and the lower G.I. tract. This action combats pain due to gastrointestinal gas. Pancreatic enzymes enhance the normal digestive process and help to reduce gas formation. Also, for relief of gas distress associated with other functional or organic conditions such as: diverticulitis, spastic colitis, hyperacidity, post-cholecystectomy syndrome and chronic cholecystitis.
Indications: Phazyme®-95 is indicated for the relief of acute severe lower intestinal pain due to gas—resulting from aerophagia, postoperative distention, dyspepsia and food intolerance.
Contraindications: A known sensitivity to any ingredient.
Dosage: One tablet with meals and at bedtime, or as required.
How Supplied: Red coated two-phase tablets, in bottles of 100.
[*Shown in Product Identification Section*]

PHAZYME®-PB Tablets ℭ ℞

Description: A yellow coated two-phase tablet. The outer layer releases in the stomach: simethicone, NF, specially activated 20 mg. and phenobarbital 15 mg., (WARNING: MAY BE HABIT FORMING). The enteric coated core releases in the small intestine: pancreatic enzymes (protease 3,000 NF units, lipase 240 NF units, amylase 2,000 NF units), and simethicone, NF, specially activated 40 mg.
Actions: Phazyme®-PB provides the same advantages of the Phazyme formula (minimizes gas formation, relieves gas entrapment) and in addition, supplies the calming benefits of phenobarbital to control the emotional component of gastrointestinal gas pain. Also, for relief of gas distress associated with other functional or organic conditions such as: diverticulitis, spastic colitis, hyperacidity, post-cholecystectomy syndrome and chronic cholecystitis.
Indications: Phazyme®-PB is indicated for gas pain associated with anxiety-resulting in aerophagia, post-operative distention, dyspepsia and food intolerance.
Contraindications: Sensitivity to barbiturates or known allergy to an ingredient.
Warning: May be habit forming.
Precautions: Excessive use may produce drowsiness.
Dosage: One or two tablets with meals and at bedtime or as required.
How Supplied: Yellow coated two-phase tablets in bottles of 100 and 1000.
[*Shown in Product Identification Section*]

proctoFoam®/non-steroid
(Pramoxine HCl 1%)

Description: proctoFoam is a foam for anal and perianal use containing pramoxine hydrochloride 1%, in a water-miscible mucoadhesive foam base of mineral oil, cetyl alcohol, ethoxylated stearyl alcohol, sorbitan sesquioleate, polysorbate 60, propyl and methyl parabens and water.
Actions: proctoFoam is an anesthetic mucoadhesive foam which medicates the anorectal mucosa, and provides prompt temporary relief from itching and pain. Its lubricating action helps make bowel evacuations more comfortable.
Indications: Prompt, temporary relief of anorectal inflammation, pruritus and pain associated with hemorrhoids, proctitis, cryptitis, fissures, postoperative pain and pruritus ani.
Contraindications: Contraindicated in persons hypersensitive to any of the ingredients.
Warning: Not for prolonged use. Do not use more than four consecutive weeks. If redness, pain, irritation or swelling persists or rectal bleeding occurs, discontinue use. Keep this and all medicines out of the reach of children.
Caution: Do not insert any part of the aerosol container into the anus. Contents of the container are under pressure, but not flammable. Do not burn or puncture the aerosol container. Store at room temperature, not over 120° F.
Dosage and Administration:

1. To fill—Shake foam container vigorously before use. Hold container upright and insert into opening of applicator tip. With plunger of applicator drawn out to mechanical stop, press down on container cap. When foam reaches fill line in the applicator, it is ready to use.
2. To administer—Separate applicator from container. Hold applicator by barrel and gently insert into the anus. With applicator in place, push plunger in order to expel foam, then withdraw applicator. (Applicator parts should be pulled apart for thorough cleaning with warm water.)

Note: To relieve itching place some foam on a tissue and apply externally.
Dosage: One application two or three times daily and after bowel evacuation.
How Supplied: Available in 15 gm. aerosol container, with special plastic applicator. The aerosol supplies approximately 18 applications.
Literature Available: Instruction pads with directions for use available upon request.
[*Shown in Product Identification Section*]

PROCTOFOAM®-HC ℞
(hydrocortisone acetate 1%)

Description: PROCTOFOAM-HC contains as active ingredient: Hydrocortisone acetate 1% in a hydrophilic base containing: pramoxine hydrochloride, propylene glycol, ethoxylated cetyl and stearyl alcohol, polyoxyethylene 10 stearyl ether, cetyl alcohol, methyl paraben, propyl paraben, triethanolamine, purified water; propellant (inert) dichlorodifluoromethane and dichlorotetrafluoroethane.
Actions: Topical steroids are primarily effective because of their anti-inflammatory, antipruritic and vasoconstrictive actions.

Indications: For relief of the inflammatory manifestations of corticosteroid-responsive dermatoses of the anogenital area.
Contraindications: Topical steroids are contraindicated in those patients with a history of sensitivity to any of the components of the preparation.
Precautions: If irritation develops, the product should be discontinued and appropriate therapy instituted.
In the presence of an infection, the use of appropriate antifungal or antibacterial agents should be instituted. If a favorable response does not occur promptly, the corticosteroid should be discontinued until the infection has been adequately controlled.
If extensive areas are treated or if the occlusive technique is used, the possibility exists of increased systemic absorption of the corticosteroid and suitable precautions should be taken particularly in children and infants.
Although topical steroids have not been reported to have an adverse effect on human pregnancy, the safety of their use in pregnant women has not absolutely been established. In laboratory animals, increases in incidence of fetal abnormalities have been associated with exposure of gestating females to topical corticosteroids, in some cases at rather low dosage levels. Therefore, drugs of this class should not be used extensively on pregnant patients, in large amounts, or for prolonged periods of time.
This product is not for ophthalmic use.
Adverse Reactions: The following local adverse reactions have been reported with topical corticosteroids, especially under occlusive dressings: burning, itching, irritation, dryness, folliculitis, hypertrichosis, acneiform eruptions, hypopigmentation, allergic contact dermatitis, maceration of the skin, secondary infection, skin atrophy, striae, and miliaria.
Dosage and Administration: Apply to affected areas 3 or 4 times daily. Use the applicator supplied for rectal application. For perianal use, transfer a small quantity to a tissue and rub in gently.
1.) Shake foam container vigorously before use. Hold container upright and insert into opening of the tip of the applicator. Be sure applicator plunger is drawn all the way out. Container must be held upright to obtain proper flow of medication.
2.) To fill, press down slowly on container cap. When foam reaches fill line in the applicator, it is ready for use. Caution: The aerosol contrainer should never be inserted directly into the anus.
3.) Remove applicator from container. Allow some foam to remain on the applicator tip. Hold applicator by barrel and gently insert tip into the anus. With applicator in place, push plunger in order to expel foam, then withdraw applicator. (Applicator parts should be pulled apart for thorough cleaning with warm water.) (See accompanying illustration)

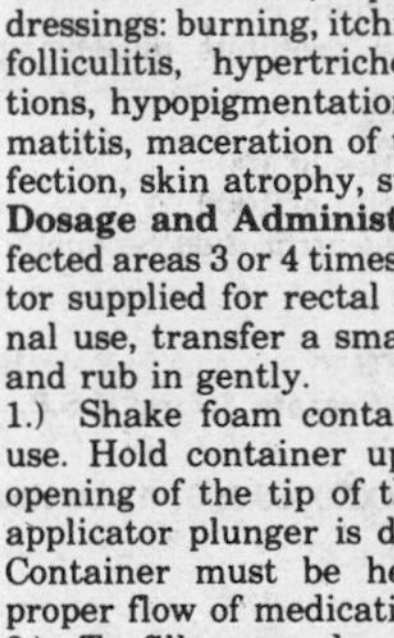

Caution: Federal law prohibits dispensing without a prescription.

How Supplied: In aerosol container containing 10 Gms., with special rectal applicator. The aerosol supplies approximately 24 applications.
Literature Available: Instruction pads with directions for use available upon request.
[*Shown in Product Identification Section*]

PROXIGEL®
(carbamide peroxide 11%)

Description: Proxigel is an antiseptic, cleansing and healing aid for minor oral inflammations. Active ingredient: Carbamide peroxide 11% in a water free gel base.
Actions: Proxigel releases oxygen on contact with mouth tissues to provide cleansing effects. Unlike liquid preparations, Proxigel's unique viscous base adheres to affected areas for longer oxygenating action or debriding action.
Indications: Proxigel is recommended for recurrent aphthous ulcerations (canker sores) and relief of minor inflammation of gums and other surfaces of the mouth and lips. Proxigel is also useful as adjunctive therapy in gingivitis, periodontitis, stomatitis, Vincent's infection and denture irritation. It is bactericidal against pathogens and other microorganisms which may be found in the oral cavity. Proxigel helps to inhibit odor causing bacteria, helps soothe the painful tissues and thus aids in healing.
Precautions: If condition persists or worsens, or irritation develops, discontinue use.
Dosage and Administration: Do not dilute. Use 4 times a day, or as directed. Apply directly with or without nozzle. Gently massage medication with finger or swab on affected area. Do not drink or rinse for 5 minutes. Always replace cap on nozzle after use. Store in cool place between 46° and 59°F (8° and 15 °C) or in a refrigerator.
How Supplied: Plastic tubes 1.2 oz. with special applicator top and guard cap.

R&C® SPRAY Insecticide

Description: Active ingredients: 3-Phenoxybenzyl d-cis and trans 2,2-dimethyl-3-(2-methylpropenyl)

cyclopropanecarboxylate	0.382%
Other Isomers	0.018%
Petroleum Distillates	4.255%
Inert Ingredients:	95.345%
	100.000%

Actions: R&C Spray is specially formulated to kill lice and their nits on inanimate objects.
Indications: R&C Spray is recommended for use only on bedding, mattresses, furniture and other objects infested or possibly infested with lice which cannot be laundered or dry cleaned.
Warnings: Contents under pressure. Do not use or store near heat or open flame. Do not puncture or incinerate container. Exposure to temperatures above 130°F may cause bursting. It is a violation of Federal law to use this product in a manner inconsistent with its labeling. NOT FOR USE ON HUMANS OR ANIMALS.
Caution: Avoid spraying in eyes. Avoid breathing spray mist. Avoid contact with the skin. May be absorbed through the skin: In case of contact, wash immediately with soap and water. Harmful if swallowed. Vacate room after treatment and ventilate before reoccupying. Avoid contamination of feed and foodstuffs.
Remove pets, birds and cover fish aquariums before spraying.
Directions: SHAKE WELL BEFORE AND OCCASIONALLY DURING USE. Spray on an inconspicuous area to test for possible staining or discoloration. Inspect after drying, then proceed to spray entire area to be treated.
Hold container upright with nozzle away from you. Depress valve and spray from a distance of 8 to 10 inches.
Spray each square foot for about three seconds. For mattresses, furniture, or similar objects (that cannot be laundered or dry cleaned): Spray thoroughly. Do not use article until spray is dry. Repeat treatment as necessary. Do not use in commercial food processing, preparation, storage or serving areas.
How Supplied: In 5 oz. aerosol container.

SIDONNA® Tablets ℞

Description: Each tablet contains:

Simethicone, NF, specially activated	25 mg.
Sodium butabarbital, NF	16 mg.
(Warning: May Be Habit Forming)	
Hyoscyamine sulfate, NF	0.1037 mg.
Atropine sulfate, USP	0.0194 mg.
Scopolamine hydrobromide, USP	0.0065 mg.

Actions: This drug combination provides natural belladonna alkaloids in a specific, fixed ratio combined with butabarbital to provide anticholinergic/antispasmodic action and mild sedation. In addition, simethicone disperses gastrointestinal gas to combat gas pain, flatulence, and distention.

Indications: Based on a review of this drug by the national Academy of Sciences—National Research Council and/or other information, FDA has classified the indications as "possibly" effective.
For use as adjunctive therapy in the treatment of patients with irritable bowel syndrome (irritable colon, spastic colon, mucous colitis), and acute enterocolitis.
Final classification of the less-than effective indications requires further investigation.

Contraindications: Glaucoma, obstructive uropathy (for example, bladder neck obstruction due to prostatic hypertrophy); obstructive disease of the gastrointestinal tract (as in achalasia, pyloroduodenal stenosis, etc.); paralytic ileus, intestinal atony of the elderly or debilitated patient, unstable cardiovascular status in acute hemorrhage; severe ulcerative colitis especially if complicated by toxic megacolon; myasthenia gravis; hiatal hernia associated with reflex esophagitis.
Butabarbital is contraindicated in acute intermittent porphyria. A sensitivity to butabarbital contraindicates the use of belladonna alkaloids with butabarbital and in those patients in whom butabarbital produces restlessness and/or excitement.
Warnings: Belladonna alkaloids with butabarbital should be used in pregnancy, lactation, or in women of childbearing age only, when in the judgment of the physician, the expected benefits outweight the potential hazards to the mother and child.
In the presence of a high environmental temperature, heat prostration can occur with the drug use (fever and heatstroke due to decreased sweating).
Diarrhea may be an early symptom of incomplete intestinal obstruction, especially in patients with ileostomy or colostomy. In this instance treatment with this drug would be inappropriate and possibly harmful.
Belladonna alkaloids with butabarbital may produce drowsiness or blurred vision. In this event, the patient should be warned not to engage in activities requiring mental alertness such as operating a motor vehicle or other machinery, or perform hazardous work while taking this drug.
Butabarbital in patients taking anticoagulants may decrease the effect of the anticoagulant and thus require larger doses of the anticoagulant for optimal effect. When the butabarbital is discontinued, the dose of the anticoagulant

Continued on next page

Reed & Carnrick—Cont.

may have to be decreased. Barbiturates may thus decrease the action of anticoagulant drugs.
Butabarbital may be habit forming and should not be administered to individuals known to be addiction prone or to those with a history of physical and/or psychological dependence upon habit forming drugs. Since barbiturates are metabolized in the liver, use with initial small doses and caution in patients with hepatic dysfunction.
Precautions: Use with caution in patients with:
Autonomic neuropathy.
Hepatic or renal disease.
Hyperthyroidism, coronary heart disease, congestive heart failure, cardiac arrhythmias, and hypertension.
It should be noted that the use of anticholinergic/antispasmodic drugs in the treatment of gastric ulcer may produce a delay in gastric emptying time and may complicate such therapy (antral stasis).
Do not rely on the use of the drug in the presence of complication of biliary tract disease.
Investigate any tachycardia before giving anticholinergic (atropine-like) drugs since they may increase the heart rate.
With overdosage, a curare-like action may occur.
Adverse Reactions: Adverse reactions may include xerostomia; urinary hesitancy and retention; blurred vision and tachycardia; palpitation; mycriasis; cycloplegia; increased ocular tension; loss of taste sense; headache; nervousness; drowsiness; weakness; dizziness; insomnia; nausea; vomiting; impotence; suppression of lactation; constipation; bloated feeling; severe allergic reaction or drug idiosyncrasies including anaphylaxis; urticaria and other dermal manifestations; and decreased sweating. Elderly patients may react with symptoms of excitement, agitation, drowsiness, and other untoward manifestations to even small doses of the drug.
Butabarbital may produce excitement in some patients rather than a sedative effect. An occasional patient may experience musculoskeletal pain. Some patients may acquire a sensitivity to barbiturates and experience allergic phenomena and/or dermatologic response.
In patients habituated to barbiturates, abrupt withdrawal may produce delerium or convulsions.
Dosage and Administration: The dosage should be adjusted to the needs of the individual patient to assure symptomatic control with a minimum of adverse effects.
Belladonna Alkaloids with Butabarbital Tablets
Adults: One or two tablets three or four times a day preferably before meals and at bedtime according to condition and severity of symptoms.
Management of Overdosage: The signs and symptoms of overdose are headache, nausea, vomiting, blurred vision, dilated pupils, hot dry skin, dizziness, dryness of the mouth, difficulty in swallowing, CNS stimulation. Treatment should consist of gastric lavage, emetics, and activated charcoal. If indicated, parenteral cholinergic agents such as bethanechol chloride USP should be used.
Caution: Federal law prohibits dispensing without a prescription.
How Supplied: Bottles of 100 scored tablets.

TRICHOTINE® Powder, Vaginal Douche

Description: A detergent, mucolytic, vaginal douche containing sodium lauryl sulfate, USP, in combination with sodium perborate, sodium chloride, and aromatics.
Actions: Low surface tension enables TRICHOTINE to penetrate the rugal folds, remove mucous, debris, and vaginal discharge thereby making treatment of vaginitis more effective. TRICHOTINE deodorizes and affords prompt relief from itching and burning.
Indications: TRICHOTINE helps to establish a normal healthy mucosa in postmenstrual, postcoital or routine vaginal cleansing, and as an adjunct in therapy of vaginitis.
Contraindications: None reported.
Warning: For routine use, do not use more than twice weekly. May be used more frequently in concomitant use for treatment of vaginitis.
Precautions: Use only in fresh solution—never use dry.
Side Effects: None reported.
Directions For Use: Dissolve one tablespoonful to each quart of warm water and mix thoroughly.
How Supplied: 5 oz., 12 oz., and 20 oz.
Literature Available: Instructions for the use of TRICHOTINE available in pads of 50 sheets.

TRICHOTINE® Liquid Vaginal Douche

Description: A detergent, mucolytic, vaginal douche containing sodium lauryl sulfate, USP; sodium borate, USP; alcohol (SDA 23A) 8% and aromatics.
Actions: (See TRICHOTINE Powder above).
Indications: (See TRICHOTINE powder above).
Contraindications: None reported.
Warning: For routine use, do not use more than twice weekly. May be used more frequently in concomitant use for treatment of vaginitis.
Precautions: Use only fresh solution. Do not use full strength.
Side Effects: None reported.
Directions For Use: Two capfuls mixed well to each quart of warm water.
How Supplied: 4 and 8 fl. oz. plastic bottles.
Literature Available: Instructions for the use of Trichotine are available in pads of 50 sheets.

TRICHOTINE®-D Disposable Vaginal Douche

Description: A detergent, mucolytic, vaginal douche containing sodium chloride, sodium lauryl sulfate, USP, and tetrasodium EDTA, premeasured in a disposable bag. Designed to be used once and thrown away to avoid the risk of infection from an improperly cleaned nozzle or syringe.
Actions: (See Trichotine Powder above)
Indications: (See Trichotine Powder above)
Contraindications: None reported.
Warning: For routine use, do not use more than twice weekly. May be used more frequently in concomitant use for treatment of vaginitis. Discontinue use if irritation develops.
Precautions: For one time use only, do not refill.
Side Effects: None reported.
Directions for Use: Hold bag in an upright position to avoid loss of premeasured powder, and remove foil cover from neck of bag. Fill with water up to the "Fill Line" (12 oz.). Screw the nozzle on the neck of the bag until locked tightly into position. Dispose of unit after use.
How Supplied: Twin Pack - Consisting of two disposable douche units, each containing premeasured powder which holds 12 oz. when filled with water. Each unit is individually sealed in a sanitary wrapper.
Literature Available: Instructions for the use of Trichotine-D are available in pads of 50 sheets.

Reid-Provident Laboratories Inc.

Executive Offices
640 TENTH STREET, N.W.
ATLANTA, GA 30318
Scientific Affairs and Manufacturing
25 FIFTH ST., N.W.
ATLANTA, GA 30308

CALINATE®-FA ℞

Prenatal dietary supplement containing:
Ascorbic Acid (As Sodium Ascorbate)...50 mg.
Niacinamide ....20 mg.
d-panthenol ....1 mg.
Iron (From Ferrous Fumarate) ....60 mg.
Iodine (From Potassium Iodide) ....0.02 mg.
Manganese (From Manganese Oxide) 0.2 mg.
Magnesium (From Magnesium Oxide) 0.2 mg.
Zinc (From Zinc Oxide) ....0.1 mg.
Copper (From Cupric Oxide) ....0.15 mg.
Calcium (Calcium Carbonate 625 mg.) 250 mg.
Vitamin A (Palmitate)....4000 USP Units
Vitamin D_2 (Calciferol) ....400 USP Units
Thiamine Mononitrate (Vitamin B_1) ....3 mg.
Riboflavin (Vitamin B_2) ....3 mg.
Pyridoxine HCl (Vitamin B_6) ....5 mg.
Cyanocobalamin (Vitamin B_{12}) ....1 mcg.
Folic Acid ....1 mg.
Indications: Prenatal dietary supplement.
Precautions: Folic acid may obscure pernicious anemia in that the peripheral blood picture may revert to normal while neurological manifestations remain progressive.
Usual Dosage: One tablet daily before a meal, or as directed by physician.
Caution: Federal law prohibits dispensing without prescription.
Supplied:
NDC 0063-1139-06 bottles of 100
NDC 0063-1139-09 bottles of 1000
[Shown in Product Identification Section]

CURRETAB TABLETS ℞
Medroxyprogesterone Acetate 10 mg U.S.P.

How Supplied:
White scored tablet NDC 0063-1007-42 bottles of 50

ESTRATAB® ℞
Esterified Estrogens
0.625 mg. 1.25 mg. 2.5 mg.

How Supplied:

NDC	063-1022-06	0.625 mg.	Bottles of 100
NDC	063-1022-09	0.625 mg.	Bottles of 1000
NDC	063-1024-06	1.25 mg.	Bottles of 100
NDC	063-1024-09	1.25 mg.	Bottles of 1000
NDC	063-1025-06	2.5 mg.	Bottles of 100
NDC	063-1025-09	2.5 mg.	Bottles of 1000

[Shown in Product Identification Section]

ESTRATEST® ℞
ESTRATEST® H.S. (Half-Strength) ℞
Androgen-Estrogen Therapy

Description:
ESTRATEST® Oral Tablets
Each dark green tablet contains:
Esterified Estrogens, U.S.P. ....1.25 mg
Methyltestosterone, U.S.P. ....2.5 mg
ESTRATEST® H.S. (Half-Strength) Oral Tablets
Each light green tablet contains:
Esterified Estrogens, U.S.P. ....0.625 mg
Methyltestosterone, U.S.P. ....1.25 mg
How Supplied:
Estratest® NDC 0063-1026-06 bottles of 100
NDC 0063-1026-09 bottles of 1000
Estratest® H.S. NDC 0063-1023-06 bottles of 100
[Shown in Product Identificaion Section]

HISTALET® Syrup ℞
HISTALET® DM Syrup
HISTALET® X Syrup
HISTALET® X Tablets
HISTALET® FORTE Tablets
for oral use only

Formula:
(See table at right)

Formula:	Per 5 ml: Histalet® Syrup	Histalet® DM Syrup	Histalet® X Syrup	Per tab Histalet® X Tablets
Pseudoephedrine HCl	45 mg	45 mg	45 mg	120 mg
Chlorpheniramine Maleate	3 mg	3 mg	3 mg	8 mg
Dextromethorphan HBr		15 mg		
Guaifenesin			200 mg	200 mg

Histalet® Forte Tablets:
Each tablet contains:
Phenylephrine HCl ....10 mg.
Phenylpropanolamine HCl ....50 mg.
Pyrilamine Maleate ....25 mg.
Chlorpheniramine Maleate ....4 mg.
Histalet® X Tablets and Histalet® Forte Tablets Are Prepared In A Special Base Which Provides For Prolonged Therapeutic Effect.
Do Not Exceed Recommended Dosage.
Indications: The Histalets® are indicated for the Common Cold, Nasal Congestion, Acute Upper Respiratory Infections, Sinusitis, Hay Fever or Upper Respiratory Allergies, Seasonal and Perennial Allergic Rhinitis, Vasomotor Rhinitis, Rhinorrhea, Allergic Asthma, Non Productive and Productive Cough, Acute Bronchitis, Croup, Emphysema, Trachebronchitis and Influenza. Decongestants have been used for many years to relieve eustachian tube congestion associated with acute eustachian salpingitis, aerotitis media, acute otitis media and serous otitis media.
Contraindications: Contraindicated in patients with severe hypertension, severe coronary artery disease, hyperthyroidism, and in patients on MAO inhibitor therapy. Patient idiosyncrasy to adrenergic agents may be manifested by insomnia, dizziness, weakness, tremor or arrhythmias.
Nursing Mothers: Pseudoephedrine is contraindicated in nursing mothers because of the higher than usual risk for infants from sympathomimetic amines.
Hypersensitivity: This drug is contraindicated in patients with hypersensitivity or idiosyncrasy to sympathomimetic amines or antihistamines & dextromethorphan.
Precautions: Pseudoephedrine should be used with caution in patients with diabetes, hypertension, cardiovascular disease and hyper-reactivity to ephedrine. The antihistaminic agent may cause drowsiness and ambulatory patients who operate machinery or motor vehicles should be cautioned accordingly.
Warnings: Should be used judiciously and sparingly in patients with hypertension, diabetes mellitus, ischemic heart disease, increased intraocular pressure, and prostatic hypertrophy, See, however, **Contraindications.** Sympathomimetics may produce central nervous stimulation with convulsions or cardiovascular collapse with accompanying hypotension.
Do not exceed recommended dosage.
Usage in Pregnancy: The safety of pseudoephedrine for use during pregnancy has not been established.
Use in Elderly: The elderly (60 years and older) are more likely to have adverse reactions to sympathomimetics. Overdosage of sympathomimetics in this age group may cause hallucinations, convulsions, CNS depression, and death.
Dosage: Histalet® Syrup, Histalet® DM Syrup and Histalet® X Syrup—ADULTS—2 teaspoonfuls 4 times daily, CHILDREN (6-12)—1 teaspoonful 4 times daily, CHILDREN (2-6)—½ teaspoonful 4 times daily, CHILDREN (under 2)—only as directed by physician.
DO NOT EXCEED 4 DOSES IN 24 HOUR PERIOD
Histalet® X Tablets—ADULTS—1 tablet, 2-3 times daily, CHILDREN (6—12)—½ tablet 2-3 times daily, CHILDREN (under 6)—only as directed by physician.
Histalet® Forte Tablets—1 tablet 2-3 times daily or as directed by physician.
Do not exceed recommended dosage.
How Supplied:
Histalet® Syrup NDC 0063-1035-12, pint bottles
Histalet® DM Syrup NDC 0063-1037-12, pint bottles
Histalet® X Syrup NDC 0063-1045-12, pint bottles
Histalet® X Tablets NDC 0063-1046-06, bottles of 100 tablets
Histalet® Forte Tablets NDC 0063-1039-06 bottles of 100 tablets
NDC 0063-1039-07 bottles of 250 tablets
[Shown in Product Identification Section]

MELFIAT® Ⓒ
Phendimetrazine Tartrate 35 mg tablets

How Supplied:
NDC 0063-1079-06 Bottles of 100
NDC 0063-1079-09 Bottles of 1000
[Shown in Product Identification Section]

P-V-TUSSIN® SYRUP Ⓒ
P-V-TUSSIN® TABLETS
Antitussive-Antihistamine-Expectorant Liquid and Tablets

Description: Each teaspoonful (5 ml) of P-V-TUSSIN® Syrup contains: Hydrocodone Bitartrate 2.5 mg (WARNING: May be habit forming), Phenylephrine HCl 5 mg, Pyrilamine Maleate 6 mg, Chlorpheniramine Maleate 2 mg, Phenindamine Tartrate 5 mg, Ammonium Chloride 50 mg; Alcohol 5%
Each Scored P-V-TUSSIN® Tablet contains: Hydrocodone Bitartrate 5 mg (WARNING: May be habit forming), Phenindamine Tartrate 25 mg, Guaifenesin 200 mg.
Indications: For the symptomatic relief of cough and nasal congestion due to common cold, upper respiratory tract congestion associated with the common cold, influenza, bronchitis and sinusitis.
Precautions: The patient should be advised not to drive a car or operate dangerous machinery if drowsiness occurs. Use with caution in the presence of hypertension, cardiovascular disease, hyperthyroidism or diabetes.
Warning: Hydrocodone should be prescribed and administered with the same degree of caution as all oral medications containing a narcotic analgesic.
Adverse Reactions: Adverse reactions, when they occur, include sedation, nausea, vomiting and constipation.
Drug Interactions: Hydrocodone may potentiate the effects of other narcotics, general anesthetics, tranquilizers, sedatives and hypnotics, tricyclic antidepressants, MAO inhibitors, alcohol and other CNS depressants.
Dosage and Administration:
P-V-Tussin® Syrup:
Adults, 2 teaspoonfuls every 4 to 6 hours
Children 6 to 12, 1 teaspoonful every 4 to 6 hours
Children 1 to 6, ½ teaspoonful every 4 to 6 hours
Dose for children should not be repeated more than 4 times in a 24 hour period.
P-V-Tussin® Tablets:
Adults and children over 12, 1 tablet 4 times daily or as directed by physician. Should be taken after meals and at bedtime, not less than 4 hours apart. Do not exceed the recommended dosage.
Caution: Federal law prohibits dispensing without prescription.
How Supplied:
P-V-Tussin® Syrup
NDC 0063-1087-12, pint bottles
NDC 0063-1087-13, gallon bottles
P-V-Tussin® Tablets
NDC 0063-1088-06, bottles of 100 tablets
[Shown in Product Identification Section]

UNIPRES® ℞

Formula: Each tablet contains:
Hydralazine Hydrochloride....................25 mg.
Hydrochlorothiazide....................15 mg.
Reserpine....................0.1 mg.
How Supplied:
NDC 0063-1132-06 Bottles of 100
NDC 0063-1132-09 Bottles of 1000
[Shown in Product Identification Section]

Research Industries Corporation

Pharmaceutical Division
1847 WEST 2300 SOUTH
SALT LAKE CITY, UTAH 84119

RIMSO®-50 ℞
(brand of dimethyl sulfoxide)

Description:
Rimso®-50, brand of dimethyl sulfoxide (DMSO)
50% w/w Aqueous Solution for intravesical instillation
Each ml contains 0.54 gm dimethyl sulfoxide
STERILE AND PYROGEN-FREE
Intravesical instillation for the treatment of interstitial cystitis
NOT FOR I.M. OR I.V. INJECTION
Caution: Federal law prohibits dispensing without a prescription
The active component of RIMSO®-50 is dimethyl sulfoxide which has the empirical formula C_2H_6OS.
Dimethyl sulfoxide is a clear, colorless and essentially odorless liquid which is miscible with water and most organic solvents. Other physical characteristics include: molecular weight 78.13, melting point 18.4°C, and a specific gravity of 1.100.
Clinical Pharmacology: Dimethyl sulfoxide is metabolized in man by oxidation to dimethyl sulfone or by reduction to dimethyl sulfide. Dimethyl sulfoxide and dimethyl sulfone are excreted in the urine and feces. Dimethyl sulfide is eliminated through the breath and skin and is responsible for the characteristic odor from patients on dimethyl sulfoxide medication. Dimethyl sulfone can persist in serum for longer than two weeks after a single intravesical instillation. No residual accumulation of dimethyl sulfoxide has occurred in man or lower animals who have received treatment for protracted periods of time. Following topical application, dimethyl sulfoxide is absorbed and generally distributed in the tissues and body fluids.
The pharmacological mode of action is unknown at this time. Dimethyl sulfoxide has a wide spectrum of primary pharmacological activity including:

Continued on next page

Research Industries—Cont.

a) membrane penetrant
b) solute "carrier" across membranes
c) anti-inflammatory agent
d) analgesic
e) bacteriostatic
f) diuretic
g) inhibitor of cholinesterase
h) muscle relaxant
i) vasodilator
j) penetrant of blood brain barrier

Indications and Usage: RIMSO®-50 (dimethyl sulfoxide) is indicated for the symptomatic relief of patients with interstitial cystitis. RIMSO®-50 has not been approved as being safe and effective for any other indication. There is no clinical evidence of effectiveness of dimethyl sulfoxide in the treatment of bacterial infections of the urinary tract.

Contraindications: None known.

Warnings: DIMETHYL SULFOXIDE CAN INITIATE THE LIBERATION OF HISTAMINE AND THERE HAS BEEN OCCASIONAL HYPERSENSITIVITY REACTION WITH TOPICAL ADMINISTRATION OF DIMETHYL SULFOXIDE. THIS HYPERSENSITIVITY HAS NOT OCCURRED IN PATIENTS RECEIVING INTRAVESICAL RIMSO®-50: HOWEVER, THE PHYSICIAN SHOULD BE COGNIZANT OF THIS POSSIBILITY IN PRESCRIBING RIMSO®-50. IF ANAPHALACTOID SYMPTOMS DEVELOP, APPROPRIATE THERAPY SHOULD BE INSTITUTED.

Precautions: Changes in the refractive index have been seen in monkeys, dogs and rats given dimethyl sulfoxide chronically. No ophthalmic changes attributable to intravesical instillation of dimethyl sulfoxide have been reported in patients carefully followed for up to 17 months; nevertheless, full eye evaluations, including slit lamp examinations, are recommended prior to and periodically during treatment.

Approximately every six months patients receiving dimethyl sulfoxide should have a biochemical screening, particularly liver and renal function tests, and complete blood count.

Intravesical instillation of RIMSO®-50 may be harmful to patients with urinary tract malignancy because of dimethyl sulfoxide-induced vasodilation.

Some data indicates that dimethyl sulfoxide potentiates other concomitantly administered medications.

Pregnancy Catagory C. Dimethyl sulfoxide caused teratogenic responses in hamsters, rats and mice when administered intraperitoneally at high doses (5–12 gm/kg). Oral or topical doses of dimethyl sulfoxide did not cause problems of reproduction in rats, mice and hamsters. Topical doses (5 gm/kg first two days, then 2.5 gm/kg—last eight days) produced terata in rabbits, but in another study, topical doses of 1.1 gm/kg days 3 through 16 of gestation failed to produce any abnormalities. There are no adequate and well controlled studies in pregnant women. Dimethyl sulfoxide should be used during pregnancy only if the potential benefit justifies the potential risk to the fetus. It is not known whether this drug is excreted in human milk. Because many drugs are excreted in human milk, caution should be exercised when dimethyl sulfoxide is administered to a nursing woman.

Safety and effectiveness in children have not been established.

Information available to be given to the patient is reprinted at the end of this text.

Adverse Reactions: A garlic-like taste may be noted by the patient within a few minutes after instillation of RIMSO®-50 (dimethyl sulfoxide). This taste may last several hours and because of the presence of metabolites an odor on the breath and skin may remain for 72 hours.

Transient chemical cystitis has been noted following instillation of 100% dimethyl sulfoxide.

The patient may experience moderately severe discomfort on administration. Usually this becomes less prominent with repeated administration.

Drug Abuse and Dependence: None known.

Overdosage: The oral LD_{50} of dimethyl sulfoxide in the dog is greater than 10 mg/kg. It is most improbable that this dosage level could be obtained with intravesical instillation of RIMSO®-50 in the patient.

Dosage and Administration: Instillation of 50 ml of RIMSO®-50 (dimethyl sulfoxide) directly into the bladder may be accomplished by catheter or asepto syringe and allowed to remain for 15 minutes. Application of an analgesic lubricant gel such as lidocaine jelly to the urethra is suggested prior to insertion of the catheter to avoid spasm. The medication is expelled by spontaneous voiding. It is recommended that the treatment be repeated every two weeks until maximum symptomatic relief is obtained. Thereafter, time intervals between therapy may be increased appropriately.

In selected cases where symptomatic relief is not complete, the bladder may be gently distended by gravity instillation with up to 500 ml of a dimethyl sulfoxide solution (one part RIMSO®-50 and one part sterile water) prepared in a glass delivery container immediately prior to the procedure. After retention of the solution it is expelled by spontaneous voiding. Discard any remaining solution. A standard dose of 50 ml of RIMSO®-50 should then be instilled for an additional 15 minutes, followed again by spontaneous voiding.

Administration of oral analgesic medication or suppositories containing belladonna and opium prior to the instillation of RIMSO®-50 can reduce bladder spasm.

In patients with severe interstitial cystitis with very sensitive bladders, the initial treatment, and possibly the second and third (depending on patient response) should be done under anesthesia. (Saddle block has been suggested.)

How Supplied:

Bottles contain 50 ml of sterile and pyrogen-free RIMSO®-50 (50% w/w dimethyl sulfoxide aqueous solution).

Dimethyl sulfoxide is clear and colorless.
Protect from strong light.
Store at room temperature (59° to 86°F).
Do not autoclave.
NDC #0433-0433-05

For additional information concerning RIMSO®-50, contact the Pharmaceutical Division, Research Industries Corporation, Salt Lake City, Utah.

RIMSO®-50 is manufactured by Tera Pharmaceuticals, Inc., Buena Park, California, for the Pharmaceutical Division, Research Industries Corp., Salt Lake City, Utah.

Clinical Studies:

References

1. *Stewart, B.H., et al., J. Urol., 107: 377, 1972.*
2. *Kligman, A.M., J.A.M.A., 193:923, 1965.*
3. *Weisman, G., et al., Ann. N.Y. Acad. Sci., 141:326, 1967.*
4. *Shealy, C.N., Headache, 6:101, 1966.*
5. *Jacob, S.W., et al., Curr. Ther. Res., 6:134, 1964.*
6. *Formanek, K., and Sucket, R., "Diuretische wirkung von DMSO," in DMSO Symposium, 1966, Saladruck, Berlin, 1966, p. 21.*
7. *Engel, M.F., Ann. N.Y. Acad. Sci., 141:638, 1967.*
8. *Adamson, J.E., et al., Plast. Reconstr. Surg., 37:105, 1967.*
9. *Caujolle, F.M.E., et al., Ann. N.Y. Acad. Sci., 141:110, 1967.*
10. *Sawada, Y., and Chang, M. C., Fertil, and Steril., 15:222, 1964.*
11. *Wilmut, I., and Rowson, L.E.A., The Vt. Rec., 92:686, 1973.*
12. *Whittingham, D.G., et al., Science, 1978:411, 1972.*
13. *Demos, C.H., et al., Ann. N.Y. Acad. Sci., 141:517, 1967.*
14. *DMSO as a therapeutic agent, Report of the Ad Hoc Committee, Nat. Acad. Sci.— Nat. Res. Cov., prepared for the FDA, Aug., 1973 (PB-224574).*
15. *John, H., and Laudahn, G., Ann. N.Y. Acad. Sci., 141:506, 1967.*
16. *Stewart, B.H., et al., J. Urol., 36:116, 1976.*
17. *Shirley, S.W., et al., Urol., Vol. XI, # 3, 215, 1978.*

INFORMATION FOR PATIENTS

RIMSO®-50 is a 50% water solution of dimethyl sulfoxide (DMSO) that has been approved by the U.S. Food and Drug Administration for use in the symptomatic relief of patients with interstitial cystitis.

RIMSO®-50 will be instilled in the bladder on an in-patient or out-patient basis, which will be determined by your physician.

Some data indicates that dimethyl sulfoxide could change the effectiveness of any medication(s) that you may be presently receiving. Be sure to mention the names and dosage of all medications you are taking to your physician before a RIMSO®-50 instillation.

A garlic-like taste may be noted by the patient within a few minutes after instillation of RIMSO®-50 (dimethyl sulfoxide). This taste may last several hours. An odor on the breath and skin may be present and remain for up to 72 hours.

Some patients may experience discomfort on administration of the drug. Usually this becomes less prominent with repeated administration.

If you are pregnant or nursing, ask your physician about the advisability of using RIMSO®-50.

Rexall Drug Company

3901 NO. KINGSHIGHWAY BLVD.
ST. LOUIS, MO 63115

NDC-0122	Product		
	AMPICILLIN Capsules, USP Red and Gray		℞
0356-01	250 mg.	100's	
0356-05	250 mg.	500's	
0357-01	500 mg.	100's	
0357-05	500 mg.	500's	
	AMPICILLIN Powder For Oral Suspension		℞
0358-37	125 mg./5 ml.	100 cc.	
0358-39	125 mg./5 ml.	200 cc.	
0359-37	250 mg./5 ml.	100 cc.	
0359-39	250 mg./5 ml.	200 cc.	
	CHLORAL HYDRATE Capsules, USP		C
0005-01	500 mg.	100's	
	ERYTHROMYCIN STEARATE Tablets, USP Pink		℞
0153-01	250 mg.	100's	
0153-05	250 mg.	500's	
0409-01	500 mg.	100's	
	HYDROCHLOROTHIAZIDE Tablets, USP		℞
0411-10	25 mg.	1,000's	
0412-10	50 mg.	1,000's	
	MEPROBAMATE Tablets, USP Bisected, White		C
0012-10	400 mg.	1,000's	
	MONACET® (APC) w/CODEINE, Tablets White		C
0014-24	2 mg. (1/30) gr.	24's	

	PABIZOL® WITH PAREGORIC	Ⓒ
0043-04	4 oz.	
0043-08	8 oz.	
0043-16	16 oz.	
	PAPAVERINE HYDROCHLORIDE TIMED RELEASE Capsules	℞
0360-01	150 mg. 100's	
0360-10	150 mg. 1,000's	
	PAREGORIC, USP	Ⓒ
0044-16	16 oz.	
0044-28	1 gal.	
	PENICILLIN G. POTASSIUM Tablets, USP	℞
0016-10	200,000 Units 1,000's	
0018-01	400,000 Units 100's	
0018-10	400,000 Units 1,000's	
	PENICILLIN V. POTASSIUM For Oral Suspension	℞
0377-37	200,000 Units per 5 ml. (125 mg. per 100 ml.)	
0378-37	400,000 Units per 5 ml. (250 mg. per 100 ml.)	
0377-39	200,000 Units per 5 ml. (125 mg. per 200 ml.)	
0378-39	400,000 Units per 5 ml. (250 mg. per 200 ml.)	
	PENICILLIN V. POTASSIUM Tablets, USP	℞
0138-01	400,000 Units 100's 250 mg.	
0138-10	400,000 Units 1,000's 250 mg.	
432-01	800,000 Units 100's 500 mg.	
	PHENOBARBITAL ELIXIR, USP	Ⓒ
0045-28	1 gal.	
	PHENOBARBITAL Tablets, USP	Ⓒ
0021-51	¼ gr. 5,000's	
0022-51	½ gr. 5,000's	
0023-10	1 gr. 1,000's	
	PREDNISOLONE Tablets, USP	℞
0025-10	5 mg. 1,000's	
	PREDNISONE Tablets, USP	℞
0026-10	5 mg. 1,000's	
	PROPOXYPHENE HYDROCHLORIDE Capsules, USP	Ⓒ
0361-05	65 mg. 500's	
	PROPOXYPHENE HYDROCHLORIDE w/A.P.C. Capsules	Ⓒ
0362-05	65 mg. 500's	
	QUINIDINE SULFATE Tablets, USP	℞
0028-10	200 mg. 1,000's	
	RESERPINE Tablets, USP White	℞
0031-10	0.25 mg. 1,000's	
	TERPIN HYDRATE & CODEINE ELIXIR, NF	Ⓒ
0050-02	2 oz.	
0050-04	4 oz.	
0050-28	1 gal.	
	TETRACYCLINE HYDROCHLORIDE Capsules, USP	℞
0032-01	(Orange-Yellow) 250 mg. 100's	
0032-10	(Orange-Yellow) 250 mg. 1,000's	
0408-01	(Black-Yellow) 500 mg. 100's	
0408-10	(Black-Yellow) 500 mg. 1,000's	
	TETRACYCLINE SYRUP (125 mg. per 5 cc)	℞
0140-16	16 oz.	
	THYROID Tablets, USP	℞
0036-10	1 gr. 1,000's	
0037-05	2 gr. 500's	

QUINIDINE SULFATE TABLETS, USP ℞

200 mg. (3 gr.)

Description: Quinidine sulfate is the sulfate of an alkaloid obtained from various species of Cinchona and their hybrids and from Remijia pedunculata Flückiger (Fam. Rubiaceae), or prepared from quinine. Quinidine is a dextrorotatory stereoisomer of quinine. Quinidine sulfate occurs as fine, needlelike, white crystals, frequently cohering in masses, or fine, white powder. It is odorless, has a very bitter taste, and darkens on exposure to light. Its solutions are neutral or alkaline to litmus. It is slightly soluble in water; soluble in alcohol and in chloroform; insoluble in ether. Chemically, it is $(C_{20}H_{24}N_2O_2)_2 \cdot H_2SO_4 \cdot 2H_2O$.

Actions: Quinidine is generally regarded as a myocardial depressant drug because it depresses excitability, conduction velocity and contractility of the myocardium. Besides these direct effects quinidine exerts some indirect effects on the heart through an anticholinergic action. Large oral doses may reduce the arterial pressure due to peripheral vasodilatation. Hypotension of a serious degree is more likely with the parenteral use of the drug.

Quinidine is essentially completely absorbed after oral administration; maximal effects occur within 1 to 3 hours, and persist for 6 to 8 or more hours. Blood levels of quinidine can be measured; the average therapeutic range is between 3 and 6 mg. per liter of plasma. Toxic reactions are almost certain to appear at levels above 8 mg. per liter.

Indications: Quinidine sulfate is indicated in the treatment of:

Premature atrial and ventricular contractions.
Paroxysmal atrial tachycardia.
Paroxysmal A-V junctional rhythm.
Atrial flutter.
Paroxysmal atrial fibrillation.
Established atrial fibrillation when therapy is appropriate.
Paroxysmal ventricular tachycardia when not associated with complete heartblock.
Maintenance therapy after electrical conversion of atrial fibrillation and/or flutter.

Contraindications: Hypersensitivity or idiosyncrasy to the drug. History of thrombocytopenic purpura associated with previous quinidine administration. Digitalis intoxication manifested by A-V conduction disorders. Complete A-V block with an A-V nodal or idioventricular pacemaker. Ectopic impulses and rhythms due to escape mechanisms.

Warnings: In the treatment of atrial flutter, reversion to sinus rhythm may be preceded by a progressive reduction in the degree of A-V block to a 1=1 ratio resulting in extremely rapid ventricular rate. This possible hazard may be decreased by digitalization prior to giving quinidine. Evidence of quinidine cardiotoxicty (50% widening of QRS, frequent ventricular ectopic beats) mandates immediate discontinuation of the drug followed with close observation (ECG—monitoring) of the patient.

Usage in Pregnancy: The use of quinidine in pregnancy should be reserved only for those cases where the benefits outweigh the possible hazards to patient and fetus.

Precautions: Use quinidine with extreme caution in the presence of incomplete A-V block since complete block and asystole may result. Quinidine may cause unpredictable abnormalities of rhythm in digitalized hearts and it should be used with special caution in the presence of digitalis intoxication.

Note: Quinidine effect is enhanced by potassium and reduced in presence of hypokalemia. The depressant actions of quinidine on cardiac contractility and arterial blood pressure limit its use in congestive heart failure and in hypotensive states unless these conditions are due to or aggravated by the arrhythmia. The potential disadvantages and benefits must be weighed.

Continuous ECG-monitoring and determination of plasma quinidine levels are indicated when large doses, more than 2 g./day, are used.

Adverse Reactions: *Symptoms of cinchonism* (ringing in the ears, headache, nausea, disturbed vision) may appear (in sensitive patients) after a single dose of the drug.

Cardiovascular: Widening of QRS-complex, cardiac asystole, ventricular ectopic beats, idioventricular rhythms including ventricular tachycardia and fibrillation, paradoxical tachycardia, arterial embolism.

Gastrointestinal: Nausea, vomiting, abdominal pain, diarrhea.

Hematologic: Acute hemolytic anemia, hypoprothrombinemia, thrombocytopenic purpura, agranulocytosis.

CNS: Headache, fever, vertigo, apprehension, excitement, confusion, delirium and syncope, disturbed hearing (tinnitus, decreased auditory acuity), disturbed vision (mydriasis, blurred vision, disturbed color perception, photophobia, diplopia, night blindness, scotomata), optic neuritis.

Dermatologic: Cutaneous flushing with intense pruritus.

Hypersensitivity reactions: Angioedema, acute asthmatic episode, vascular collapse, respiratory arrest.

Dosage and Administration: A preliminary test dose of a single tablet of quinidine sulfate should be administered to determine whether the patient has an idiosyncrasy to it. Continuous ECG-monitoring is recommended in all cases where quinidine is used in large doses.

Usual Adult Dose:

Premature atrial and ventricular contractions: 0.2–0.3 g. 3 or 4 times daily.

Paroxysmal supraventricular tachycardias: 0.4 to 0.6 g. in every 2 or 3 hours until the paroxysm is terminated.

Atrial flutter: Quinidine should be administered after digitalization for this indication. Dosage is to be individualized.

Conversion of atrial fibrillations: Various schedules of quinidine administration have been in clinical use. A widely used technique is the administration of 0.2 g. of quinidine orally in every 2 or 3 hours for 5 to 8 doses, with subsequent daily increase of the individual dose until sinus rhythm is restored or toxic effects occur. The total daily dose should not exceed 3 to 4 g. given by any schedule. Prior to quinidine administration the ventricular rate and congestive failure (if present) should be brought under control by digitalis therapy.

Maintenance therapy: 0.2 to 0.3 g. three or four times daily.

Overdosage: Cardiotoxic effects of quinidine may be reversed in part by molar sodium lactate; the hypotension by vasoconstrictors and by catecholamines (since the vasodilation is partly due to adrenergic blockade).

How Supplied: Quinidine Sulfate Tablets, 200 mg. (3 gr.) bisected are supplied in bottles of 100 tablets and bottles of 1000 tablets.

SUPER PLENAMINS® MULTIPLE VITAMINS with MINERALS

Composition: Each sugar-coated, red, oval-shaped tablet contains:

Vitamin A (Acetate) (8000 I.U.)	2.4 mg.
Vitamin D_2 (Ergocalciferol) (400 I.U.)	10 mcg.
Vitamin B_1	2.5 mg.
Vitamin B_2	2.5 mg.
Vitamin C	75 mg.
Niacinamide	20 mg.
Vitamin B_6	1.0 mg.
Vitamin B_{12}	3.0 mcg.
Biotin	20 mcg.
Vitamin E (dl-Alpha Tocopheryl Acetate) (1.0 I.U.)	1.0 mg.
Pantothenic Acid	3.0 mg.
Liver Concentrate	100 mg.
Iron (from $FeSO_4$)	30 mg.
Calcium (from $CaHPO_4$)	75 mg.
Phosphorus (from $CaHPO_4$)	58 mg.
Iodine (from KI)	0.15 mg.
Copper (from $CuSO_4$)	0.75 mg.
Manganese (from $MnSO_4$)	1.25 mg.
Magnesium (from $MgSO_4$)	10.0 mg.

Continued on next page

Rexall—Cont.

Zinc (from $ZnSO_4$) ....1.0 mg.
Action and Uses: A dietary supplement.
Administration and Dosage: Adults and children 12 years and older, 1 tablet daily. Children under 12, only as physician directs.
How Supplied: Super Plenamins in bottles of 36, 72, 144, 288 and 365. NDC 122-66.
Available at Rexall pharmacies.

Riker Laboratories, Inc.
NORTHRIDGE, CA 91324

[See table below].

CALCIUM DISODIUM VERSENATE* ℞
(calcium disodium edetate injection, U.S.P.)
Injection

WARNING
Calcium Disodium Edetate is capable of producing toxic and potentially fatal effects. The dosage schedule should be followed and at no time should the recommended daily dose be exceeded. In lead encephalopathy avoid rapid infusion; intramuscular route is preferred.

Description: Calcium Disodium Versenate Injection (Calcium Disodium Edetate Injection, U.S.P.) is a sterile concentrated solution (20%) containing 200 mg. of calcium disodium edetate per ml. for intravenous infusion or intramuscular injection.
Actions: The calcium in calcium disodium edetate is readily displaced by heavy metals, such as lead, to form stable complexes. Following parenteral injection, the chelate formed is excreted in the urine, with 50 percent appearing in the first hour after administration.
Indications: Calcium disodium edetate is indicated for the reduction of blood levels and depot stores of lead in lead poisoning (acute and chronic) and lead encephalopathy.
Contraindications: Calcium disodium edetate should not be given during periods of anuria.
Warnings: See box warning above.
Usage in pregnancy: The safe use of calcium disodium edetate has not been established with respect to possible adverse effects upon fetal development. Therefore, it should not be used in women of child-bearing potential and particularly during early pregnancy unless, in the judgment of the physician, the potential benefits outweigh the possible hazards.
Precautions: Severe acute lead poisoning by itself may cause proteinuria and microscopic hematuria. Calcium disodium edetate may produce the same signs of renal damage. Routine urinalysis should be done daily during each course of therapy to determine whether the proteinuria and hematuria is improving or the evidence of renal tubular injury is getting worse. The presence of large renal epithelial cells or increasing numbers of red blood cells in the urinary sediment or greater proteinuria call for immediate stopping of calcium disodium edetate administration. Evidence of renal impairment should be looked for by periodic blood urea nitrogen determinations before and during each course of therapy. The patient should also be monitored for irregularities of cardiac rhythm.
Adverse Reactions: The principal toxic effect is renal tubular necrosis.
Dosage and Administration: Calcium disodium edetate is equally effective whether administered intravenously, subcutaneously or intramuscularly. Because of convenience in administration and greater safety in treating symptomatic children, many physicians experienced in the treatment of lead poisoning prefer the intramuscular route which is recommended in patients with either overt or incipient lead encephalopathy. Rapid intravenous infusions may be lethal by suddenly increasing intracranial pressure in this group of patients with cerebral edema.
Note: In patients with lead encephalopathy and increased intracranial pressure, excess fluids must be avoided. In such case a 20 percent solution of calcium disodium edetate is mixed with procaine to give a final concentration of 0.5 percent of procaine in the mixture which is administered intramuscularly.
Acutely ill individuals may be dehydrated from vomiting. Since calcium disodium edetate is excreted almost exclusively in the urine, it is very important to establish urine flow by intravenous infusion before the first dose of the chelating agent is given. Once urine flow is established further intravenous fluid is restricted to basal water and electrolyte requirements. Administration of calcium disodium edetate should be stopped whenever there is cessation of urine flow in order to avoid unduly high tissue levels of the drug.
Intravenous Administration: Dilute the 5 ml. (1 gram, 20% solution) from an ampule with 250-500 ml. of Solution Isotonic Sodium Chloride, USP, or sterile 5% dextrose solution in water. In asymptomatic adults, administer this diluted solution over a period of at least one hour. Such doses may be administered twice daily for periods up to 5 days. The therapy should then be interrupted for 2 days and followed by an additional 5 days of treatment, if indicated.
In mildly affected or asymptomatic individuals the dosage of 50 mg./kg. per day should not be exceeded.
In symptomatic adults, fluids should be kept to basal levels and the time of administration increased to two hours. A second daily infusion is to be given six or more hours after the first.
Intramuscular Administration: This is the route of choice for children.[1-8] The dosage should not exceed 0.5 gram per 30 pounds of body weight twice daily (total, 1.0 gram/30 lbs./day). This is equivalent to 35 mg./kg. twice daily (total, approx. 75 mg./kg./day). In mild cases a dose of 50 mg./kg. per day should not be exceeded. For young children the total daily dose may be given in divided doses every 8 or 12 hours for 3 to 5 days. A second course may be given after a rest period of 4 or more days. Procaine to produce a concentration of 0.5% should be added to minimize pain at injection site. (1 ml. of 1% procaine solution for each ml. of concentrated Calcium Disodium Versenate solution, or crystalline procaine may be used to reduce volume.)
Regardless of method of administration, doses larger than those recommended should not be undertaken.
Lead Encephalopathy: This condition is relatively rare in adults but is quite common in children in whom the mortality rate has been high. Recent reports by Chisolm[3,4] and by Coffin et al, who employed a combination of BAL and calcium disodium edetate, suggest that this may be the preferred treatment, although calcium disodium edetate alone has been used over a longer period of time. Each group administered calcium disodium edetate intramuscularly concurrently with BAL in separate deep I.M. sites. Procaine was added to the 20% solution of calcium disodium edetate to give a procaine concentration of 0.5%. In the studies of Coffin and Chisolm, 125 children with acute lead encephalopathy have been treated with this combined therapy with only one death. Since these instructions are concerned only with Calcium Disodium Versenate, information on dosage of combined therapy will be found in references 3-8.
How Supplied: Calcium Disodium Versenate Injection, 5 ml. ampules containing 200 mg. of calcium disodium edetate per ml., boxes containing 6 ampules. (NDC **0089-0510-06**).
Bibliography:

1. Shrand, H.: Treatment of Lead Poisoning with Intramuscular Edathamil Calcium-Disodium, Lancet, p 310, February 11, 1961.
2. Statement on Diagnosis and Treatment of Lead Poisoning in Childhood, Pediatrics, *27*:676, 1961.
3. Chisolm, J. J., Jr.: Treatment of Lead Poisoning, Modern Treatment, *4*:710, 1967.

The following Riker products are available in Military and Veterans Administration depots:

Military Depot Items	National Stock Number
Circanol® Tablets 1 mg. 100's	6505-01-017-1626
Duo-Medihaler® (aerosol) w/adapter 22.5 ml.	6505-00-071-7861
Lipo-Hepin® (heparin sodium injection, U.S.P. aqueous)	
1,000 U/ml. 10 ml. vial	6505-00-153-9740
10,000 U/ml. 5 ml. vial	6505-00-584-2914
20,000 U/ml. 2 ml. vial	6505-00-579-8432
Medihaler-Iso® (aerosol) w/adapter 15 ml.	6505-00-023-6481
Medihaler-Iso® (aerosol) w/adapter 22.5 ml.	6505-00-014-8486
Norflex® Tablets 100's	6505-00-138-8462
Norgesic® Tablets 500's	6505-00-952-6762
Norgesic® Forte Tablets 500's	6505-01-029-9116
Tepanil® Ten-tab® (controlled-release tablet) 75 mg. 100's	6505-00-082-2684
Titralac® Tablets 500's	6505-00-890-1658
Titralac® Tablets 100's strip pack	6505-01-044-3763
Urex® Tablets 100's	6505-00-126-3207

Veterans Administration Depot Items	National Stock Number
Alu-Cap® Capsules 100's	6505-00-166-7844
Duo-Medihaler® (aerosol) w/adapter 22.5 ml.	6505-00-071-7861A
Lipo Hepin®/BL (heparin sodium injection, U.S.P. aqueous) (Derived from beef lung)	
1000 U/ml. 10 ml. vial	6505-00-088-6747
1000 U/ml. 30 ml. vial	6505-01-030-3253
10,000 U/ml. 4 ml. vial	6505-00-584-2916
Medihaler-Iso® (aerosol) w/adapter 22.5 ml.	6505-00-014-8486A
Norflex® Tablets 100's	6505-00-550-4903A
Norgesic® Tablets 500's	6505-00-952-6762A
Norgesic® Forte Tablets 500's	6505-01-032-1442A
Theolair™ Tablets 125 mg. 250's	6505-01-075-8307A
Theolair™ Tablets 250 mg. 250's	6505-01-075-8308A
Titralac® Tablets 1000's	6505-00-065-4249
Urex® Tablets 500's	6505-00-443-4501

4. Chisolm, J. J., Jr.: The Use of Chelating Agents in the Treatment of Acute and Chronic Lead Intoxication in Childhood. Jour. Pediatrics, *73*:1, 1968.
5. Coffin, R., Phillips, J. L., Staples, W. I., and Spector, S.: Treatment of Lead Encephalopathy in Children, Jour. Pediatrics, *69*:198, 1966.
6. Chisolm, J. J., Jr. and Harrison, H. E.: Lead Intoxication, in Current Pediatric Therapy 3, Edited by Gellis and Kagan, Saunders, Philadelphia, 1968, p 918.
7. Silver, W. and Rodrigues-Torres, R.: Lead Intoxication, Pediatric Therapy 4. Edited by Gellis and Kagan, Saunders, Philadelphia, 1970, p 958.
8. Sachs, H. K., et al: Ambulatory Treatment of Lead Poisoning: Report of 1,155 Cases. Pediatrics *46*:389, 1970.

*Registered trademark of the Dow Chemical Company

CALCIUM DISODIUM VERSENATE* ℞
(calcium disodium edetate)
Tablets

> **WARNING:**
> Calcium Disodium Edetate is capable of producing toxic and potentially fatal effects. The dosage schedule should be followed and at no time should the recommended daily dose be exceeded.

Description: Calcium Disodium Versenate (Calcium Disodium Edetate) Tablets contain 500 mg. of calcium disodium edetate per tablet.
Actions: The calcium in calcium disodium edetate is readily displaced by heavy metals, such as lead, to form stable complexes. The drug is poorly absorbed from the gastrointestinal tract. About 5 to 10% of oral calcium disodium edetate is absorbed in man. Orally administered calcium disodium edetate may enhance the absorption of lead and promote its excretion in the urine. Oral Versenate appears less effective in promoting the excretion of nonionized organic lead compounds, such as tetra-ethyl lead, than it is in promoting the excretion of ionized inorganic lead compounds. With the increased excretion of lead in urine there is a concomitant decrease in blood lead levels and in urine coproporphyrin.
Indication: To promote the continued excretion of lead following treatment of lead poisoning and lead encephalopathy by more vigorous means, such as use of calcium disodium versenate by injection.
Contraindications: Calcium Disodium Versenate Tablets should not be given to patients with severe renal disease.
Warnings: See box above.
Chronic oral use of Versenate should not be used as a substitute for adequate measures to avoid undue exposure to lead. Because Versenate chelates other metals, e.g. zinc, copper, etc., the possibility of depletion of such metals in persons taking Versenate on a long-term basis should be considered, and steps taken to avoid such deficiencies. Although urinary excretion of lead usually does increase following administration of Versenate, there is the possibility that, in some cases, a concomitant decrease in fecal excretion occurs. If this were to happen, the total amount of lead excreted might appear greater than is actually the case.
Usage in pregnancy: The safe use of calcium disodium edetate has not been established with respect to possible adverse effects upon fetal development. Therefore, it should not be used in women of child-bearing potential and particularly during early pregnancy unless, in the judgment of the physician, the potential benefits outweigh the possible hazards.
Precautions: The drug should be used with caution in tuberculosis, active or healed, and in the presence of renal disease. There have been reports of increased absorption of lead from the gut following the use of oral Versenate.
Adverse Reactions: Calcium Disodium Versenate when administered orally may act as a gastrointestinal irritant in some patients, producing diarrhea, abdominal cramps, and vomiting. Such symptoms are more likely to occur when the daily dose exceeds 3 gms. Other side actions reported in a relatively small percentage of patients were leg and other muscle cramps, weakness, malaise, and albumin or red cells in the urine. Excessive doses may result in renal toxicity.
Dosage and Administration: Adults: The average daily dosage is 8 tablets (4 gm.) in divided doses.
Children: Two tablets (1 gm.) daily per 35 pounds of body weight in divided doses.
How Supplied: Calcium Disodium Versenate Tablets, bottles of 250 tablets containing 500 mg. of calcium disodium edetate per tablet. (NDC **0089-0115-25**)
*Registered trademark of The Dow Chemical Company.

CIRCANOL® ℞
(hydrogenated ergot alkaloids)
TABLETS FOR SUBLINGUAL ADMINISTRATION

Description: Each white, round, sublingual 0.5 mg tablet contains dihydroergocornine 0.167 mg, dihydroergocristine 0.167 mg and dihydroergocryptine 0.167 mg. (dihydro-alpha-ergocryptine and dihydro-beta-ergocryptine in the proportion of 2:1) as the methanesulfonates (mesylates), representing a total of 0.5 mg.
Each white, oval, sublingual 1.0 mg tablet contains dihydroergocornine 0.333 mg, dihydroergocristine 0.333 mg and dihydroergocryptine 0.333 mg. (dihydro-alpha-ergocryptine and dihydro-beta-ergocryptine in the proportion of 2:1) as the methanesulfonates (mesylates), representing a total of 1.0 mg.
Action: There is no specific evidence which clearly establishes the mechanism by which hydrogenated ergot alkaloids produces its mental effects, nor is there conclusive evidence that it particularly affects cerebral arteriosclerosis or cerebrovascular insufficiency.
Indications: Circanol is indicated for the treatment of selected symptoms in elderly patients. Short-term clinical studies have demonstrated modest improvement in levels of performance of self care and such symptoms as mood-depression, confusion, unsociability, and dizziness. These symptoms are of unknown etiology and are not specific to any age group or disease. However, to date only short-term studies conducted with elderly patients have been reported.
Contraindications: Hydrogenated ergot alkaloids is contraindicated in individuals who have previously shown hypersensitivity to the drug.
Precautions: Practitioners are advised that because the target symptoms are of unknown etiology careful diagnosis should be attempted before prescribing Circanol (hydrogenated ergot alkaloids).
Adverse Reactions: Circanol (hydrogenated ergot alkaloids) sublingual tablets have not been found to produce serious side effects. Some sublingual irritation, transient nausea, and gastric disturbances have been reported. Circanol does not possess the vasoconstrictor properties of the natural ergot alkaloids.
Dosage and Administration: 0.5 mg tablets: two sublingual tablets three times daily; 1.0 mg tablets: one sublingual tablet three times daily. Alleviation of symptoms is usually gradual and results may not be observed for 3 to 4 weeks.
How Supplied: Circanol (hydrogenated ergot alkaloids) sublingual tablets are supplied as 0.5 mg white round tablets in bottles of 100 (NDC **0089-0121-10**) and 1,000 (NDC **0089-0121-80**) and 1.0 mg white oval tablets in bottles of 1,000 (NDC **0089-0123-80**) and 100 (NDC **0089-0123-10**).
[Shown in Product Identification Section]

DEANER® and DEANER®-250 ℞
(deanol acetamidobenzoate)

Description: Each tablet contains 250 mg., 100 mg. or 25 mg. of deanol (2-dimethylaminoethanol) as the para-acetamidobenzoic acid salt.
Pharmacology: The concept that deanol is a precursor of acetylcholine which affects the central nervous system is supported by evidence derived from biochemical and pharmacologic studies. Studies with Carbon 14-labeled deanol indicate that it crosses the blood-brain barrier and probably is converted intracellularly to acetylcholine. It does not depress the appetite or cause jitteriness, as does amphetamine. Deanol does not affect the BMR, blood pressure, or pulse rate, and is not an MAO inhibitor.
The toxicity of deanol is very low. Laboratory tests and clinical, pathological and histopathological examinations have disclosed no harmful changes attributable to the drug.

> **Indications:**
> Based on a review of this drug by the National Academy of Sciences—National Research Council and/or other information, FDA has classified the indications as follows:
> "Possibly" effective:
> 1. Learning problems—learning in deficit of that usually associated with apparent level of intelligence, including I.Q. Reading difficulties. Shortened attention span.
> 2. Behavior problems—hyperkinetic behavior problem syndrome characterized by distractibility, motor disinhibition, dissociation and perseveration.
> 3. Or, as more frequently encountered, hyperkinetic behavior and learning disorders incorporating varying combinations of both of the above. Under-achievers, Reading, and speech difficulties. Impaired motor coordination. Hyperactive, impulsive/compulsive behavior, often described as asocial, antisocial, delinquent, stimulus-governed.
> Final classification of the less than effective indications requires further investigation.

Contraindications: No absolute contraindications are known. Grand mal epilepsy and mixed epilepsy with a grand mal component are relative contraindications.
Side Actions: Neither sensitization nor serious side effects have been reported with DEANER (deanol acetamidobenzoate). Mild overstimulation and the following minor side actions, if encountered, usually disappear with continued treatment or with reduction in dosage: dull occipital headache early in therapy; constipation; tenseness in neck, masseter and quadriceps muscles; insomnia; pruritus; transient rash. Rarely postural hypotension occurs.
Administration and Dosage: Starting dose: 500 mg. daily. If satisfactory improvement occurs, the maintenance dosage will vary from 250 to 500 mg. daily. The maintenance dosage should be adjusted to the needs of the individual patient.
How Supplied: Deaner-250: 250 mg. scored, white, capsule shaped, film coated tablets in bottles of 50 (NDC **0089-0135-05**); Deaner: 100 mg. scored, pink, round tablets in bottles of 50 (NDC **0089-0137-05**) and 25 mg. scored, white, round tablets in bottles of 100 (NDC **0089-0131-10**) and 500 (NDC **0089-0131-50**).
[Shown in Product Identification Section]

Continued on next page

Riker—Cont.

DISALCID® ℞
(salsalate)
Tablets and Capsules

Description: Each round, aqua, film coated Disalcid tablet contains 500 mg salsalate (salicylsalicylic acid). Each aqua and white Disalcid capsule contains 500 mg salsalate (salicylsalicylic acid).
Action: Disalcid is a non-steroidal anti-inflammatory agent with analgesic and antipyretic activity.
The mode of action of non-steroidal anti-inflammatory agents (including salicylates) has not been conclusively determined. However, the mode of action of Disalcid is thought to be similar to that of other non-acetylated salicylates.
In studies utilizing radioactive chromium tagging of red blood cells, Disalcid, unlike aspirin, has been shown not to be associated with gastrointestinal hemorrhage. In addition, other studies indicate that the incidence of gastric erosion is not significant with the use of Disalcid. Like other non-acetylated salicylates, Disalcid is not believed to inhibit platelet aggregation.
Clinical Pharmacology: Salsalate is insoluble in gastric acid medium, and upon absorption in the small intestine each ester molecule of salsalate is hydrolized into two free salicylic acid molecules.
It has been shown that after three days of continuous administration at the recommended dosage, blood salicylate levels are maintained within the therapeutic range for at least 16 hours after discontinuation of treatment.
Indications: Disalcid is indicated for the relief of the signs and symptoms of rheumatoid arthritis, osteoarthritis and other related rheumatic disorders.
Precautions: As with all salicylates, caution should be exercised in the use of Disalcid in chronic renal insufficiency and peptic ulcer.
Salicylates, in large doses, displace oral anticoagulants from protein binding sites, raising the possibility of systemic hemorrhage. Caution, therefore, should be observed with the concomitant use of anticoagulants and Disalcid.
As with all drugs, usual precautions should be followed during pregnancy.
Contraindications: Disalcid is contraindicated in patients hypersensitive to salicylates.
Adverse Reactions: Mild reactions to salicylates (nausea, dyspepsia, heartburn) may occur occasionally.
Salsalate has not been associated with reactions causing asthmatic attacks in susceptible individuals.
Dosage and Administration:
Adults: The usual dosage is 6 tablets or capsules daily, given as 2 tablets or capsules three times daily or 3 tablets or capsules twice daily. As with other salicylates, dosage should be titrated depending on individual response. It is recommended that the last daily dose be taken at bedtime.
Children: Disalcid has not been evaluated in children. No dosage recommendations can, therefore, be made for children under 12 years of age.
Overdosage:
Symptoms: Overdosage with Disalcid produces the usual symptoms of salicylism: tinnitus, vertigo, headache, confusion, drowsiness, sweating, hyperventilation, vomiting or diarrhea.
Treatment: Further absorption of salicylate from the G.I. tract should be prevented by emesis (syrup of ipecac) and, if necessary, by gastric lavage. Fluid and electrolyte imbalance should be corrected by the administration of appropriate I.V. therapy. Adequate renal function should be maintained. Hemo or peritoneal dialysis may be required in extreme cases.
How Supplied: 500 mg tablets, in bottles of 100 (**NDC 0089-0149-10**) and 500 mg capsules, in bottles of 100 (**NDC 0089-0148-10**).
[Shown in Product Identification Section]

DISIPAL® ℞
(orphenadrine hydrochloride) Tablets

Description: Each tablet contains 50 mg. orphenadrine hydrochloride (2-dimethylaminoethyl 2-methylbenzhydryl ether hydrochloride).
Actions: In the laboratory, DISIPAL (orphenadrine hydrochloride) demonstrates parasympatholytic and antitremor activity, as well as clinically unimportant degrees of antihistaminic and local anesthetic actions. The drug acts centrally, producing effective relaxation of muscle spasm. DISIPAL (orphenadrine hydrochloride) has greater parasympatholytic and antitremor activity than its chemical relative, diphenhydramine. An outstanding difference between orphenadrine and diphenhydramine is the absence of a soporific action.
Chronic toxicity studies, in rats and dogs, have shown no gross or microscopic evidence of drug induced pathology. The daily oral dosage was 20 milligrams per kilogram for the dog and 75 milligrams per kilogram for the rats. No abnormalities of the blood or urine were produced during a six month period of continuous medication.
Indications: DISIPAL (orphenadrine hydrochloride) is effective for use as an adjunct in the therapy of all forms of parkinsonism (postencephalitic, arteriosclerotic, idiopathic).
Contraindications: Contraindications are due to the anticholinergic action of orphenadrine. DISIPAL (orphenadrine hydrochloride) should not be used in patients with glaucoma, pyloric or duodenal obstruction, stenosing peptic ulcers, prostatic hypertrophy or obstructions at the bladder neck, achalasia (megaesophagus) and myasthenia gravis. DISIPAL (orphenadrine hydrochloride) should be used with caution in patients with tachycardia.
Since mental confusion, anxiety and tremors have been reported in patients receiving orphenadrine and propoxyphene concurrently, it is recommended that DISIPAL not be given in combination with propoxyphene (Darvon®).
Warning: Use in pregnancy: Since safety of the use of this preparation in pregnancy, during lactation, or in the child-bearing age has not been established, use of the drug in such patients requires that the potential benefits of the drug be weighed against its possible hazard to the mother and child.
Adverse Reactions: Side effects of DISIPAL (orphenadrine hydrochloride) are mainly due to the mild anticholinergic action of orphenadrine and are usually associated with higher dosage. Dryness of the mouth is the first side effect to appear. When the daily dose is increased, possible side actions include: tachycardia, palpitation, urinary hesitancy or retention, blurred vision, dilatation of the pupil, increased ocular tension, weakness, nausea, vomiting, headache, dizziness, constipation and drowsiness and rarely, urticaria and other dermatoses. Infrequently, an elderly patient may experience some degree of mental confusion. These mild side effects can usually be eliminated by reduction in dosage. Two cases of aplastic anemia associated with orphenadrine citrate have been reported. No causal relationship has been established, and no reports were received in connection with the use of DISIPAL.
Dosage and Administration: Usual dosage, one tablet (50 mg.) three times daily. In combination with other agents and in the treatment of Parkinson's syndrome, smaller doses often suffice. Doses up to 250 mg. daily have been used without the occurrence of disagreeable side effects.
How Supplied: Bottles of 100 (NDC **0089-0161-10**).
[Shown in Product Identification Section]

DORBANE®
(brand of danthron)
Laxative

Composition: Each tablet contains: Danthron 75 mg.
Dorbane promotes colonic peristalsis and is a superior laxative in the management and treatment of constipation.
Dosage: 1 or 2 tablets once daily, 1 hour after the evening meal. As treatment progresses, dosage may be gradually decreased. May cause harmless discoloration of the urine.
Warning: Do not use when abdominal pain, nausea, or vomiting are present. Frequent or prolonged use of this preparation may result in dependence on laxatives.
Keep this and all medications out of the reach of children.
NOTE: Variation in color may occur from lot to lot, but this has no effect on the laxative action of the tablets.
Availability: Bottles of 100 (NDC **0089-0173-10**), 500 (NDC **0089-0173-50**) and 1000 (NDC **0089-0173-80**) orange, scored tablets.
[Shown in Product Identification Section]

DORBANTYL® Laxative
Stool Softener

For relief of occasional constipation. May cause harmless discoloration of urine.
Composition: Each capsule contains: Danthron, 25 mg.; docusate sodium, 50 mg.
Dosage: ADULTS: 2 capsules at bedtime; repeat if needed to cause bowel movement. CHILDREN: 6 to 12 years of age: 1 capsule taken as above. Under 6 years of age: use only on advice of physician.
Warning: Do not use when abdominal pain, nausea, or vomiting are present. Frequent or prolonged use of this preparation may result in dependence on laxatives.
Keep this and all medications out of the reach of children. Professional literature available to physicians on request.
Availability: Bottles of 30 NDC **0089-0174-03** 100 NDC **0089-0174-10** and 250 orange NDC **0089-0174-25** and black capsules.
[Shown in Product Identification Section]

DORBANTYL® FORTE Laxative
Stool Softener

For relief of occasional constipation. May cause harmless discoloration of urine.
Composition: Each capsule contains: Danthron, 50 mg.; docusate sodium, 100 mg.
Dosage: ADULTS: 1 capsule at bedtime; repeat if needed to cause bowel movement. CHILDREN: Use regular Dorbantyl.
Warning: Do not use when abdominal pain, nausea, or vomiting are present. Frequent or prolonged use of this preparation may result in dependence on laxatives.
Keep this and all medication out of the reach of children.
Note: 1 Dorbantyl **Forte** capsule is equivalent to 2 regular Dorbantyl capsules.
Professional literature available to physicians on request.
Availability: Bottles of 30 (NDC **0089-0178-03**), 100 (NDC **0089-0178-10**) and 250 (NDC **0089-0178-25**) orange and grey capsules.
[Shown in Product Identification Section]

LIPO-HEPIN® ℞
(heparin sodium injection, U.S.P.) Aqueous
DERIVED FROM PORCINE INTESTINAL MUCOSA
LIPO-HEPIN®/BL ℞
(heparin sodium injection, U.S.P.) Aqueous
DERIVED FROM BEEF LUNG

Description: Heparin Sodium Injection, USP is a sterile solution of heparin sodium derived from animal tissues (i.e. porcine intestinal mucosa, or bovine lung tissue) standardized for use as an anticoagulant, in water for injection with 0.9% benzyl alcohol as a preservative and sodium chloride to make solutions under 10,000 U/ml isotonic. The potency is determined by biological assay using a USP reference standard based upon units of heparin activity per milligram.
Actions: Heparin inhibits reactions which lead to the clotting of blood and the formation of fibrin clots both **in vitro** and **in vivo**. Heparin acts at multiple sites in the normal coagulation system. Small amounts of heparin in combination with antithrombin III (heparin co-factor) can prevent the development of a hypercoagulable state by inactivating activated Factor X, preventing the conversion of prothrombin to thrombin. Once a hypercoagulable state exists, larger amounts of heparin in combination with antithrombin III can inhibit the coagulation process by inactivating thrombin and earlier clotting intermediates, thus preventing the conversion of fibrinogen to fibrin. Heparin also prevents the formation of a stable fibrin clot by inhibiting the activation of the fibrin stabilizing factor.
Bleeding time is usually unaffected by heparin. Clotting time is prolonged by full therapeutic doses of heparin; in most cases it is not measurably affected by low doses of heparin.
Heparin does not have fibrinolytic activity; therefore, it will not lyse existing clots.
Indications: Heparin sodium injection is indicated for anticoagulant therapy in prophylaxis and treatment of venous thrombosis and its extension; in low-dose regimen for prevention of postoperative deep venous thrombosis and pulmonary embolism in patients undergoing major abdomino-thoracic surgery who are at risk of developing thromboembolic disease (see DOSAGE AND ADMINISTRATION section); for prophylaxis and treatment of pulmonary embolism; in atrial fibrillation with embolization; for diagnosis and treatment of acute and chronic consumptive coagulopathies (disseminated intravascular coagulation); for prevention of clotting in arterial and cardiac surgery; and for prevention of cerebral thrombosis in evolving stroke.
Heparin is indicated as an adjunct in treatment of coronary occlusion with acute myocardial infarction, and in prophylaxis and treatment of peripheral arterial embolism.
Heparin may also be employed as an anticoagulant in blood transfusions, extracorporeal circulation, dialysis procedures, and in blood samples for laboratory purposes.
Contraindications: Hypersensitivity to heparin.
Inability to perform suitable blood coagulation tests, e.g. the whole blood clotting time, partial thromboplastin time, etc., at required intervals. There is usually no need to monitor the effect of low-dose heparin in patients with normal coagulation parameters.
Uncontrollable bleeding.
Warnings:

> Heparin sodium should be used with extreme caution in disease states in which there is an increased danger of hemorrhage.

Administration of Heparin Sodium Injection, USP, when used in therapeutic dosage, should be regulated by frequent blood coagulation tests. If these are unduly prolonged or if hemorrhage occurs, heparin sodium should be promptly discontinued. See **OVERDOSAGE** section.
Some of the conditions in which increased danger of hemorrhage exists are:

Cardiovascular	subacute bacterial endocarditis; arterial sclerosis; increased capillary permeability; during and immediately following a) spinal tap or spinal anesthesia, b) major surgery, especially involving the brain, spinal cord, or eye.
Hematologic	conditions associated with increased bleeding tendencies such as hemophilia, some purpuras, and thrombocytopenia.
Gastrointestinal	inaccessible ulcerative lesions and continuous tube drainage of the stomach or small intestine.

Heparin sodium may prolong the one-stage prothrombin time. Accordingly, when heparin sodium is given with dicumarol or warfarin sodium, a period of at least 5 hours after the last intravenous dose and 24 hours after the last subcutaneous (intrafat) dose of heparin sodium should elapse before blood is drawn, if a valid prothrombin time is to be obtained.
Drugs (such as acetylsalicylic acid, dextran, phenylbutazone, ibuprofen, indomethacin, dipyridamole and hydroxychloroquine) which interfere with platelet aggregation reactions (the main hemostatic defense of heparinized patients) may induce bleeding and should be used with caution in patients on heparin therapy.
While there is experimental evidence that heparin may antagonize the action of ACTH, insulin, or corticoids, this effect has not been clearly defined.
There is also evidence in animal experiments that heparin may modify or inhibit allergic reactions. However, the application of these findings to human patients has not been fully defined.
Larger doses of heparin may be necessary in the febrile state.
The use of digitalis, tetracyclines, nicotine, or antihistamines may partially counteract the anticoagulant action of heparin. An increased resistance to heparin is frequently encountered in cases of thrombosis, thrombophlebitis, infections with thrombosing tendency, myocardial infarction, cancer, and in the postoperative patient.
Use in Pregnancy: Heparin sodium injection should be used with caution during pregnancy, especially during the last trimester and in the immediate post partum period.
There is no adequate information as to whether heparin may affect human fertility, or have a teratogenic potential or other adverse effects to the fetus.
Heparin does not cross the placental barrier; it is not excreted in human milk.
Precautions: Because heparin sodium injection is derived from animal tissue, it should be used with caution in patients with a history of allergy. Before a therapeutic dose is given to such a patient, a trial dose of 1,000 units may be advisable.
Heparin sodium should also be used with caution in the presence of hepatic or renal disease, hypertension, during menstruation, or in patients with indwelling catheters.
A higher incidence of bleeding may be seen in women over 60 years of age.
Caution should be exercised when administering ACD-converted blood (i.e. blood collected in heparin sodium and later converted to ACD blood), since the anticoagulant activity of its heparin sodium content persists without loss for 22 days. ACD- converted blood may alter the coagulation system of the recipient, especially if it is given in multiple transfusions.
Adverse Reactions: Hemorrhage is the chief complication that may result from heparin therapy. An overly prolonged clotting time or minor bleeding during therapy can usually be controlled by withdrawing the drug. See **OVERDOSAGE** section.
The occurrence of significant gastrointestinal or urinary tract bleeding during anticoagulant therapy may indicate the presence of an underlying occult lesion.
Adrenal hemorrhage with resultant acute adrenal insufficiency has occurred during anticoagulant therapy. Therefore such treatment should be discontinued in patients who develop signs and symptoms compatible with acute adrenal hemorrhage and insufficiency. Plasma cortisol levels should be measured immediately, and vigorous therapy with intravenous corticosteroids should be instituted promptly. Initiation of therapy should not depend upon laboratory confirmation of the diagnosis, since any delay in an acute situation may result in the patient's death.
Intramuscular injection of heparin sodium frequently causes local irritation, mild pain, or hematoma, and for these reasons should be avoided. These effects are less often seen following deep subcutaneous (intrafat) injection. Histamine-like reactions have also been observed at the site of injection.
Hypersensitivity reactions have been reported with chills, fever, and urticaria as the most usual manifestations. Asthma, rhinitis, lacrimation, and anaphylactoid reactions have also been reported. Vasospastic reactions may develop independent of the origin of heparin 6 to 10 days after the initiation of therapy and last for 4 to 6 hours. The affected limb is painful, ischemic and cyanosed. An artery to this limb may have been recently catheterized. After repeat injections, the reaction may gradually increase, to include generalized vasospasm, with cyanosis, tachypnea, feeling of oppression, and headache. Protamine sulfate treatment has no marked therapeutic effect. Itching and burning, especially on the plantar side of the feet, is possibly based on a similar allergic vasospastic reaction. Chest pain, elevated blood pressure, arthralgias, and/or headache have also been reported in the absence of definite peripheral vasospasm. Anaphylactic shock has been reported rarely following the intravenous administration of heparin sodium.
Acute reversible thrombocytopenia following the intravenous administration of heparin sodium has been reported. Osteoporosis, and suppression of renal function following long-term, high-dose administration, suppression of aldosterone synthesis, delayed transient alopecia, priapism, and rebound hyperlipemia following discontinuation of heparin sodium, have also been reported.
Dosage and Administration: Heparin sodium is not effective by oral administration and should be given by deep subcutaneous (intrafat, i.e., above iliac crest or into the abdominal fat layer) injection, by intermittent intravenous injection, or intravenous infusion. The intramuscular route of administration should be avoided because of the frequent occurrence of hematoma at the injection site.
The dosage of heparin sodium should be adjusted according to the patient's coagulation test results, which during the first day of treatment should be determined just prior to each injection. There is usually no need to monitor the effect of low-dose heparin in patients with normal coagulation parameters. Dosage is considered adequate when the whole blood clotting time is elevated approximately 2.5 to 3 times the control value.
When heparin sodium is administered by continuous intravenous infusion, coagulation tests

Continued on next page

Riker—Cont.

should be performed approximately every 4 hours during the early stages of therapy. When it is administered intermittently by intravenous, or deep subcutaneous (intrafat) injection, coagulation tests should be performed before each injection during the early stages of treatment, and daily thereafter.

When an oral anticoagulant of the coumadin or similar type is administered with heparin sodium, coagulation tests and prothrombin activity should be determined at the start of therapy. For immediate anticoagulant effect, administer heparin sodium in the usual therapeutic dosage. When the results of the initial prothrombin determination are known, administer the first dose of an oral anticoagulant in the usual initial amount. Thereafter, perform a coagulation test and determine the prothrombin activity at appropriate intervals. A period of at least 5 hours after the last intravenous dose and 24 hours after the last subcutaneous (intrafat) dose of heparin sodium should elapse before blood is drawn, if a valid prothrombin time is to be obtained. When the oral anticoagulant shows full effect and prothrombin activity is in the desired therapeutic range, heparin sodium may be discontinued and therapy continued with the oral anticoagulant.

Therapeutic Anticoagulant Effect with Full-Dose Heparin

Although dosage must be adjusted for the individual patient according to the results of suitable laboratory tests, the following dosage schedules may be used as guidelines:

[See table below].

1. By deep subcutaneous (intrafat) injection. After an initial I.V. injection of 5,000 units, inject 10,000 to 20,000 units of a concentrated heparin sodium solution subcutaneously, followed by 8,000 to 10,000 units of a concentrated solution subcutaneously every eight hours, or 15,000 to 20,000 units of a concentrated solution every twelve hours. A different site should be used for each injection to prevent the development of a massive hematoma.

2. By intermittent intravenous injection. 10,000 units initially, then 5,000 to 10,000 units every four to six hours. These amounts may be given either undiluted or diluted with 50 to 100 ml of isotonic sodium chloride injection.

3. By continuous intravenous infusion. After an initial I.V. injection of 5,000 units of heparin sodium, add 20,000 to 40,000 units to 1,000 ml of isotonic sodium chloride solution for infusion. For most patients, the rate of flow should be adjusted to deliver approximately 20,000 to 40,000 units in 24 hours.

Surgery of the Heart and Blood Vessels: Patients undergoing total body perfusion for open heart surgery should receive an initial dose of not less than 150 units of heparin sodium per kilogram of body weight. Frequently a dose of 300 units of heparin sodium per kilogram of body weight is used for procedures estimated to last less than 60 minutes; or 400 units per kilogram for those estimated to last longer than 60 minutes.

Low-Dose Prophylaxis of Postoperative Thromboembolism: A number of well-controlled clinical trials have demonstrated that low-dose heparin prophylaxis, given just prior to and after surgery, will reduce the incidence of post-operative deep vein thrombosis in the legs, as measured by the I-125 fibrinogen technique and venography, and of clinical pulmonary embolism. The most widely used dosage has been 5,000 units 2 hours before surgery and 5,000 units every 8 to 12 hours thereafter for 7 days or until the patient is fully ambulatory, whichever is longer. The heparin is given by deep subcutaneous injection in the arm or abdomen with a fine needle (25-26 gauge) to minimize tissue trauma. A concentrated solution of heparin sodium is recommended. Such prophylaxis should be reserved for patients over 40 undergoing major surgery. Patients with bleeding disorders, those having neurosurgery, spinal anesthesia, eye surgery, or potentially sanguinous operations should be excluded, as well as patients receiving oral anticoagulants or platelet-active drugs (see WARNINGS). The value of such prophylaxis in hip surgery has not been established. The possibility of increased bleeding during surgery or postoperatively should be borne in mind. If such bleeding occurs, discontinuance of heparin and neutralization with protamine sulfate is advisable. If clinical evidence of thromboembolism develops despite low-dose prophylaxis, full therapeutic doses of anticoagulants should be given unless contraindicated. All patients should be screened prior to heparinization to rule out bleeding disorders, and monitoring should be performed with appropriate coagulation tests just prior to surgery. Coagulation test values should be normal or only slightly elevated. There is usually no need for daily monitoring of the effect of low-dose heparin in patients with normal coagulation parameters.

Extracorporeal Dialysis Use: Follow equipment manufacturer's operating directions carefully.

Blood Transfusion: Addition of 400 to 600 USP units per 100 ml of whole blood. Usually, 7,500 USP units of heparin sodium are added to 100 ml of Sterile Sodium Chloride Injection (or 75,000 USP units per 1,000 ml of Sterile Sodium Chloride Injection) and mixed, and from this sterile solution, 6 to 8 ml is added per 100 ml of whole blood. Leukocyte counts should be performed on heparinized blood within two hours after addition of the heparin. Heparinized blood should not be used for isoagglutinin, complement erythrocyte fragility tests, or platelet counts.

Laboratory Samples: Addition of 70 to 150 units of heparin sodium per 10 to 20 ml sample of whole blood is usually employed to prevent coagulation of the sample. See comments under "Blood Transfusion."

Overdosage: Protamine sulfate (1% solution) by slow infusion will neutralize heparin. No more than 50 mg should be given very slowly in any 10 minute period. Each mg of protamine sulfate neutralizes approximately 100 USP units of heparin (or 1.0 to 1.5 mg neutralizes approximately 1.0 mg of heparin). Heparins derived from various animal sources require different amounts of protamine sulfate for neutralization. This fact is of most importance during procedures of regional heparinization, including dialysis.

Decreasing amounts of protamine are required as time from last heparin injection increases. Thirty minutes after a dose of heparin approximately 0.5 mg of protamine is sufficient to neutralize each 100 units of administered heparin. Blood or plasma transfusions may be necessary; these dilute but do not neutralize heparin.

How Supplied: Lipo-Hepin® (heparin sodium injection, U.S.P.) derived from porcine intestinal mucosa is available in single-dose ampules, vials, and disposable syringes, and in multiple-dose vials for subcutaneous or intravenous injection.

[See table on next page].

How Supplied: Lipo-Hepin® /BL (heparin sodium injection, U.S.P.) derived from beef lung, is available in disposable syringes and in multiple-dose vials for subcutaneous or intravenous injection.

1,000 Units per ml—in 10 ml multiple dose vials (NDC 0089-0480-01).
1,000 Units per ml—in 30 ml vials for dialysis, box of 25 (NDC 0089-0483-25).
5000 u/ml in 1 ml vial (NDC 0089-0485-25)
5,000 u/ml in 10 ml vial (NDC 0089-0486-01)
10,000 u/ml in 1 ml vial (NDC 0089-0490-25)
10,000 Units per ml—in 4 ml multiple dose vials (NDC 0089-0491-01).
10,000 u/ml in 5 ml vial (NDC 0089-0492-01)
Unit Dose Syringe—to deliver 0.5 ml containing 5,000 units per 0.5 ml (NDC 0089-0495-10).

Preservative: Benzyl alcohol 0.9%. Sodium chloride added to 1,000 and 5,000 units per ml. concentrations to make solutions isotonic.

METHOD OF ADMINISTRATION	FREQUENCY	RECOMMENDED DOSE [based on 150 lb (68 kg) patient]
Deep Subcutaneous (Intrafat) Injection	Initial Dose	5,000 units by I.V. injection followed by 10,000–20,000 units of a concentrated solution, subcutaneously
	Every 8 hours	8,000–10,000 units of a concentrated solution
	(or) Every 12 hours	15,000–20,000 units of a concentrated solution
Intermittent Intravenous Injection	Initial Dose	10,000 units, either undiluted or in 50–100 ml isotonic sodium chloride injection
	Every 4 to 6 hours	5,000–10,000 units, either undiluted or in 50–100 ml isotonic sodium chloride injection
Intravenous Infusion	Initial Dose	5,000 units by I.V. injection
	Continuous	20,000–40,000 units in 1,000 ml of isotonic sodium chloride solution for infusion/day

DUO-MEDIHALER® ℞

(isoproterenol hydrochloride, phenylephrine bitartrate)

Description: Duo-Medihaler® (isoproterenol hydrochloride and phenylephrine bitartrate) is an aerosol device which delivers micronized particles of isoproterenol hydrochloride and phenylephrine bitartrate suspended in an inert mixture of sorbitan trioleate, cetylpyridinium chloride with fluorochlorohydrocarbons as propellants. This drug-propellant system is contained in a hermetically sealed metal vial. Each valve actuation releases a uniform aerosolized dose of 0.16 mg isoproterenol hydrochloride (equivalent to 0.137 mg of isoproterenol base) and 0.24 mg phenylephrine bitartrate (equivalent to 0.126 mg of phenylephrine base).

Actions: Duo-Medihaler provides rapid and prolonged symptomatic relief of dyspnea resulting from bronchospasm and congestion and edema of the respiratory mucosa. Isoproterenol acts almost exclusively by stimulating beta adrenergic receptors within the tracheobronchial tree. The main action of isoproterenol is to prevent and relieve bronchoconstriction. Phenylephrine is a powerful alpha-receptor stimulant and as such produces vaso-constriction which is of considerable value in reducing edema and congestion of the bronchiolar vascular beds. It is believed that phenylephrine is synergistic with isoproterenol through its vasoconstricting and mild bronchodilatory actions. This reduces bronchiolar blood flow, thereby decreasing the engorgement of the bronchiolar tree and slowing the systemic absorption of the isoproterenol, as well as adding further bronchodilatation.

Indications: For the treatment of bronchospasm associated with acute and chronic bronchial asthma, pulmonary emphysema, bronchitis, and bronchiectasis.

Contraindications: Known hypersensitivity to either agent constitutes a contraindication to the use of this drug. Isoproterenol preparations are generally contraindicated in patients with pre-existing cardiac arrhythmias associated with tachycardia because the cardiac stimulant effect of the drug may aggravate such disorders.

Warnings: Excessive use of an adrenergic aerosol should be discouraged, as it may lose its effectiveness. Occasional patients have been reported to develop severe paradoxical airway resistance with repeated, excessive use of isoproterenol inhalation preparations. The cause of this refractory state is unknown. It is advisable that in such instances the use of this preparation be discontinued immediately and alternative therapy instituted, since in the reported cases the patients did not respond to other forms of therapy until the drug was withdrawn.

Deaths have been reported following excessive use of isoproterenol inhalation preparations and the exact cause is unknown. Cardiac arrest was noted in several instances.

Precautions: Isoproterenol should not be administered with epinephrine, since both drugs are direct cardiac stimulants and their combined effects may produce serious arrhythmias. If desired, these drugs may be alternated, provided an interval of at least four hours has elapsed.

Although there has been no evidence of teratogenic effects with these drugs, use of any drug in pregnancy, lactation, or in women of childbearing age requires that the potential benefit of the drug be weighed against its possible hazard to the mother and child.

Duo-Medihaler should be used with caution in patients with cardiovascular disorders including coronary insufficiency, diabetes, or hyperthyroidism, and in persons sensitive to sympathomimetic amines.

Adverse Reactions: Overdosage with isoproterenol can produce palpitation, tachycardia, tremulousness, flushing, anginal-type pain, nausea, dizziness, weakness and sweating, while overdosage with phenylephrine can induce cardiac irregularities, central nervous system disturbances and reflex bradycardia.

The individual patient's sensitivity to either drug would dictate the overdosage signs. However, there is reason to believe the overdosage effects of either drug are antagonized by the other drug in the mixture.

Dosage and Administration: The recommended dose for the relief of dyspnea in the acute episode is 1 to 2 inhalations. Start with one inhalation. If no relief is evident after 2 to 5 minutes, a second inhalation may be taken. For daily maintenance, use 1 to 2 inhalations 4 to 6 times daily or as directed by the physician. No more than two inhalations should be taken at any one time, or more than 6 inhalations in any one hour during a 24-hour period, unless advised by physician.

INTESTINAL PORCINE MUCOSAL HEPARIN 1 ml AMPULES

NATIONAL DRUG CODE NO.		POTENCY: U.S.P. UNITS PER ML.
0089-0 402-50	BOX OF 50	10,000

1 ml UNIT-DOSE VIALS

NATIONAL DRUG CODE NO.		POTENCY: U.S.P. UNITS PER ML.
0089-0 414-25	BOX OF 25	5,000
0089-0 419-25	BOX OF 25	10,000
0089-0 430-25	BOX OF 25	20,000

MULTIPLE-DOSE VIALS

NATIONAL DRUG CODE NO.	VIAL CONTENT	POTENCY: U.S.P. UNITS PER ML.
0089-0 410-01	10 ml	1,000
0089-0 415-01	10 ml	5,000
0089-0 421-01	4 ml	10,000
0089-0 425-01	5 ml	10,000
0089-0 432-01	2 ml	20,000
0089-0 435-01	5 ml	20,000
0089-0 438-01	10 ml	20,000
0089-0 442-01	2 ml	40,000
0089-0 445-01	5 ml	40,000
0089-0 413-25	BOX OF 25 30 ml DIALYSIS VIAL	1,000

SYRINGES

NATIONAL DRUG CODE NO.	SYRINGES TO DELIVER	POTENCY: U.S.P. Units Per 0.5 ML.
0089-0 462-10	0.5 ml	1,000
0089-0 464-10	0.5 ml	5,000
0089-0 465-10	0.5 ml	7,500
0089-0 466-10	0.5 ml	10,000
0089-0 467-10	0.5 ml	15,000
0089-0 469-10	0.5 ml	20,000

Preservative: Benzyl alcohol 0.9%. Sodium chloride added to 1,000, 2,000 and 5,000 units per ml. concentrations to make solutions isotonic.

How Supplied:
For long-term use:
Initial Rx: Duo-Medihaler with adapter (450-doses, 22.5 ml.) NDC **0089-0732-21.**
Refill: Duo-Medihaler refill vial (450-doses, 22.5 ml.) NDC **0089-0732-11.**
For patients with less frequent need:
Initial Rx: Duo-Medihaler with adapter (300 doses, 15 ml.) NDC **0089-0735-21.**
Refill: Duo-Medihaler refill (300 doses, 15 ml.) NDC **0089-0735-11.**

MEDIHALER-EPI®
(epinephrine bitartrate)

Description: Each ml. contains 7.0 mg. epinephrine bitartrate, suspended in an inert, non-toxic aerosol vehicle. Each automatically-measured dose delivers 0.3 mg. epinephrine bitartrate, equivalent to 0.16 mg. epinephrine base.

For speed of relief and convenience, MEDIHALER oral inhaler comes ready-to-use, with a metal vial containing the medication, and a single-dose valve, which fits into the oral adapter (plastic mouthpiece). The vial can be used only with the MEDIHALER oral adapter.

Actions: Epinephrine is a short acting sympathomimetic drug, having bronchodilator, vasoconstrictor, pressor, tachycardic and central stimulating action. The value of epinephrine as an anti-allergic agent is well established. Epinephrine does not significantly alter blood pressure when given in nebulized form at recommended dosage. With increased dosage, it can cause tremulousness and tachycardia, tremulousness being seen more frequently. Epinephrine is a highly effective bronchodilator.

Indications: MEDIHALER-EPI is a dependable aerosol medication for temporary relief from acute or chronic paroxysms of bronchial asthma, drug sensitivity reactions, injected allergens, urticaria and other allergic manifestations.

Dosage: Start with one inhalation. Allow at least two minutes to elapse between inhalations. The least number of inhalations which produces relief should be used on subsequent occasions. Rarely will more than two inhalations be required.

Precautions: As with all sympathomimetic drugs, epinephrine should be used with great caution in the presence of hyperthyroidism, diabetes, cardiovascular disorders including coronary insufficiency, tuberculosis, or when there is a sensitivity to sympathomimetic amines.

Isoproterenol and epinephrine may be used interchangeably if the patient becomes unresponsive to one or the other but should not be used concurrently; an interval of 4 hours should elapse before changing from one to the other compound.

Availability: MEDIHALER-EPI with oral adapter (15 ml.) NDC **0089-0755-21.**
MEDIHALER-EPI refill vial only (15 ml.) NDC **0089-0755-11.**

Continued on next page

Riker—Cont.

MEDIHALER-ISO® ℞
(isoproterenol sulfate)

Description: Medihaler-Iso® (isoproterenol sulfate) is an aerosol device which contains a fine-particle suspension of 2.0 mg. per ml. isoproterenol sulfate in an inert propellant consisting of sorbitan trioleate and fluorochlorohydrocarbons. Each depression of the valve delivers a measured dose of 0.075 mg. to the patient.
Actions: Isoproterenol is a short-acting sympathomimetic drug. It produces pharmacologic response in the cardiovascular system and on the smooth muscles of the bronchial tree. The drug will prevent or overcome histamine-induced asthma in both experimental animals and man, and is effective when used prophylactically. It is one of the most potent bronchodilators known and can be used in patients who do not respond to the bronchodilating action of epinephrine. Isoproterenol has a cardio-accelerating effect, but its vasoconstricting action is less pronounced than that of epinephrine. Therapeutic doses may produce a slight increase in systolic blood pressure, but a slight decrease in diastolic. Larger doses may cause peripheral vasodilatation in the renal, mesenteric and femoral beds and some patients respond with a decrease in diastolic, but no change in systolic pressure. Such effects are usually of very short duration.
Indications: For the treatment of bronchospasm associated with acute and chronic bronchial asthma, pulmonary emphysema, bronchitis, and bronchiectasis.
Contraindications: Use of isoproterenol in patients with pre-existing cardiac arrhythmias associated with tachycardia is contraindicated because the cardiac stimulant effects of the drug may aggravate such disorders.
Warnings: Excessive use of an adrenergic aerosol should be discouraged, as it may lose its effectiveness. Occasional patients have been reported to develop severe paradoxical airway resistance with repeated, excessive use of isoproterenol inhalation preparations. The cause of this refractory state is unknown. It is advisable that in such instances the use of this preparation be discontinued immediately and alternative therapy instituted, since in the reported cases the patients did not respond to other forms of therapy until the drug was withdrawn.
Deaths have been reported following excessive use of isoproterenol inhalation preparations and the exact cause is unknown. Cardiac arrest was noted in several instances.
Precautions: Isoproterenol and epinephrine may be used interchangeably if the patient becomes unresponsive to one or the other but should not be used concurrently. If desired, these drugs may be alternated, provided an interval of at least four hours has elapsed.
As with all sympathomimetic drugs, isoproterenol should be used with great caution in the presence of cardiovascular disorders, including coronary insufficiency, hypertension, hyperthyroidism and diabetes, or when there is a sensitivity to sympathomimetic amines.
Although there has been no evidence of teratogenic effects with this drug, use of any drug in pregnancy, lactation, or in women of childbearing age requires that the potential benefit of the drug be weighed against its possible hazard to the mother and child.
Adverse Reactions: Only a small percentage of patients experience any side effects following oral inhalation of aerosolized isoproterenol. Overdosage may produce tachycardia with resultant coronary insufficiency, palpitations, vertigo, nausea, tremors, headache, insomnia, central excitation, and blood pressure changes. These reactions are similar to those produced by other sympathomimetic agents.
Dosage and Administration:
Dosage: The usual dose for the relief of dyspnea in the acute episode is 1 to 2 inhalations. Start with one inhalation. If no relief is evident after 2 to 5 minutes, a second inhalation may be taken. For daily maintenance, use 1 to 2 inhalations 4 to 6 times daily or as directed by the physician. The physician should be careful to instruct the patient in the proper technique of administration so that the number of inhalations per treatment and the frequency of retreatment may be titrated to the patient's response.
No more than two inhalations should be taken at any one time, or more than 6 inhalations in any one hour during a 24 hour period, unless advised by physician.
How Supplied:
Medihaler-Iso (isoproterenol sulfate) with oral adapter (15 ml.) NDC **0089-0785-21.**
Medihaler-Iso (isoproterenol sulfate) refill vial only (15 ml.) NDC **0089-0785-11.**
Medihaler-Iso (isoproterenol sulfate) with oral adapter (22.5 ml) NDC **0089-0782-21.**
Medihaler-Iso (isoproterenol sulfate) refill vial only (22.5 ml.) NDC **0089-0782-11.**

NORFLEX® ℞
(orphenadrine citrate)
Tablets and Injectable

Description: Orphenadrine citrate is the citrate salt of orphenadrine (2-dimethylaminoethyl 2-methylbenzhydryl ether citrate). It occurs as a white, crystalline powder having a bitter taste. It is practically odorless; sparingly soluble in water, slightly soluble in alcohol.
Actions: The mode of therapeutic action has not been clearly identified, but may be related to its analgesic properties. Orphenadrine citrate also possesses anti-cholinergic actions.
Indications: Orphenadrine citrate is indicated as an adjunct to rest, physical therapy, and other measures for the relief of discomfort associated with acute painful musculo skeletal conditions. The mode of action of the drug has not been clearly identified, but may be related to its analgesic properties. Orphenadrine citrate does not directly relax tense skeletal muscles in man.
Contraindications: Contraindicated in patients with glaucoma, pyloric or duodenal obstruction, stenosing peptic ulcers, prostatic hypertrophy or obstruction of the bladder neck, cardio-spasm (megaesophagus) and myasthenia gravis.
Contraindicated in patients who have demonstrated a previous hypersensitivity to the drug.
Warnings: Some patients may experience transient episodes of lightheadedness, dizziness or syncope. Norflex may impair the ability of the patient to engage in potentially hazardous activities such as operating machinery or driving a motor vehicle; ambulatory patients should therefore be cautioned accordingly.
Usage in Pregnancy: Safe use of orphenadrine has not been established with respect to adverse effects upon fetal development. Therefore, Norflex should be used in women of childbearing potential and particularly during early pregnancy only when in the judgment of the physician the potential benefits outweigh the possible hazards.
Usage in Children: Safety and effectiveness in children have not been established; therefore, this drug is not recommended for use in the pediatric age group.
Precautions: Confusion, anxiety and tremors have been reported in few patients receiving propoxyphene and orphenadrine concomitantly. As these symptoms may be simply due to an additive effect, reduction of dosage and/or discontinuation of one or both agents is recommended in such cases.
Orphenadrine citrate should be used with caution in patients with tachycardia, cardiac decompensation, coronary insufficiency, cardiac arrhythmias.
Safety of continuous long-term therapy with orphenadrine has not been established. Therefore, if orphenadrine is prescribed for prolonged use, periodic monitoring of blood, urine and liver function values is recommended.
Adverse Reactions: Adverse effects of orphenadrine are mainly due to the mild anticholinergic action of orphenadrine, and are usually associated with higher dosage. Dryness of the mouth is usually the first adverse effect to appear. When the daily dose is increased, possible adverse effects include: tachycardia, palpitation, urinary hesitancy or retention, blurred vision, dilatation of pupils, increased ocular tension, weakness, nausea, vomiting, headache, dizziness, constipation, drowsiness, hypersensitivity reactions, pruritus, hallucinations, agitation, tremor, gastric irritation, and rarely urticaria and other dermatoses. Infrequently, an elderly patient may experience some degree of mental confusion. These adverse reactions can usually be eliminated by reduction in dosage. Very rare cases of aplastic anemia associated with the use of orphenadrine tablets have been reported. No causal relationship has been established.
Rare instances of anaphylactic reaction have been reported associated with the intramuscular injection of Norflex injectable.
Dosage and Administration:
TABLETS: Adults—Two tablets per day; one in the morning and one in the evening.
INJECTABLE: Adults—One 2 ml. ampul (60 mg.) intravenously or intramuscularly; may be repeated every 12 hours. Relief may be maintained by 1 Norflex Tablet twice daily.
How Supplied:
TABLETS: Bottles of 100 (NDC **0089-0221-10**) and 500 (NDC **0089-0221-50**), each tablet containing 100 mg. of orphenadrine citrate.
INJECTABLE: Boxes of 6 (NDC **0089-0540-06**) and 50 (NDC **0089-0540-50**) 2 ml. ampuls, each ampul containing 60 mg. of orphenadrine citrate in aqueous solution, made isotonic with sodium chloride.
[100 mg. Tablet Shown in Product Identification Section]

NORGESIC® and NORGESIC® FORTE ℞

Actions: Orphenadrine citrate is a centrally acting (brain stem) compound which in animals selectively blocks facilitatory functions of the reticular formation. Orphenadrine does not produce myoneural block, nor does it affect crossed extensor reflexes. Orphenadrine prevents nicotine-induced convulsions but not those produced by strychnine.
Chronic administration of Norgesic to dogs and rats has revealed no drug-related toxicity. No blood or urine changes were observed, nor were there any macroscopic or microscopic pathological changes detected. Extensive experience with combinations containing aspirin, phenacetin and caffeine has established them as safe agents. The addition of orphenadrine citrate does not alter the toxicity of APC.
The mode of therapeutic action of orphenadrine has not been clearly identified, but may be related to its analgesic properties. Orphenadrine citrate also possesses anti-cholinergic actions.
Indications:
1. Symptomatic relief of mild to moderate pain of acute musculo-skeletal disorders.
2. The orphenadrine component is indicated as an adjunct to rest, physical therapy, and other measures for the relief of discomfort associated with acute painful musculoskeletal conditions.
   The mode of action of orphenadrine has not been clearly identified, but may be related to its analgesic and sedative properties.

Norgesic and Norgesic Forte do not directly relax tense skeletal muscles in man.

Contraindications: Because of the mild anticholinergic effect of orphenadrine, Norgesic or Norgesic Forte should not be used in patients with glaucoma, pyloric or duodenal obstruction, achalasia, prostatic hypertrophy or obstructions at the bladder neck. Norgesic or Norgesic Forte is also contraindicated in patients with myasthenia gravis and in patients known to be sensitive to aspirin, phenacetin or caffeine.

The drug is contraindicated in patients who have demonstrated a previous hypersensitivity to the drug.

Warnings: Norgesic Forte may impair the ability of the patient to engage in potentially hazardous activities such as operating machinery or driving a motor vehicle; ambulatory patients should therefore be cautioned accordingly.

Salicylates should be used with extreme caution in the presence of peptic ulcers and coagulation abnormalities.

USAGE IN PREGNANCY: Since safety of the use of this preparation in pregnancy, during lactation, or in the childbearing age has not been established, use of the drug in such patients requires that the potential benefits of the drug be weighed against its possible hazard to the mother and child.

USAGE IN CHILDREN: The safe and effective use of this drug in children has not been established. Usage of this drug in children under 12 years of age is not recommended.

Precautions: Usage of phenacetin in large amounts or for long periods of time may result in gastrointestinal disturbances, anemia, methemoglobinemia and renal damage. Caution, therefore, should be exercised when Norgesic or Norgesic Forte is administered to patients with renal disorders. It should also be used with caution in patients with tachycardia.

Confusion, anxiety and tremors have been reported in few patients receiving propoxyphene and orphenadrine concomitantly. As these symptoms may be simply due to an additive effect, reduction of dosage and/or discontinuation of one or both agents is recommended in such cases.

Safety of continuous long term therapy with Norgesic Forte has not been established; therefore, if Norgesic Forte is prescribed for prolonged use, periodic monitoring of blood, urine and liver function values is recommended.

Adverse Reactions: Side effects of Norgesic or Norgesic Forte are those seen with APC or those usually associated with mild anticholinergic agents. These may include tachycardia, palpitation, urinary hesitancy or retention, dry mouth, blurred vision, dilatation of the pupil, increased intraocular tension, weakness, nausea, vomiting, headache, dizziness, constipation, drowsiness, and rarely, urticaria and other dermatoses. Infrequently an elderly patient may experience some degree of confusion. Mild central excitation and occasional hallucinations may be observed. These mild side effects can usually be eliminated by reduction in dosage. One case of aplastic anemia associated with the use of Norgesic has been reported. No causal relationship has been established. Rare G.I. hemorrhage due to the aspirin content may be associated with the administration of Norgesic or Norgesic Forte. Some patients may experience transient episodes of light-headedness, dizziness or syncope.

Dosage and Administration:

Norgesic: Adults 1 to 2 tablets 3 to 4 times daily.

Norgesic Forte: Adults ½ to 1 tablet 3 to 4 times daily.

How Supplied: Norgesic tablets can be identified by their three layers colored light green, white and yellow. Each round tablet contains orphenadrine citrate (2-dimethylaminoethyl 2-methylbenzhydryl ether citrate) 25 mg., aspirin 225 mg., phenacetin 160 mg. and caffeine 30 mg.

Norgesic Forte tablets are exactly twice the strength of Norgesic. They are identified by their scored capsule shape and by their three layers colored light green, white and yellow. Each capsule shaped tablet contains orphenadrine citrate 50 mg., aspirin 450 mg., phenacetin 320 mg., and caffeine 60 mg.

Norgesic: Bottles of 100 (NDC **0089-0235-10**) and 500 tablets (NDC **0089-0235-50**).

Norgesic Forte: Bottles of 100 tablets (NDC **0089-0237-10**) and 500 tablets (NDC **0089-0237-50**).

[Shown in Product Identification Section]

TEPANIL® Ⓒ ℞
(diethylpropion hydrochloride, N.F.)
TEPANIL® TEN-TAB® Ⓒ ℞
(controlled release tablet)

Description: Diethylpropion hydrochloride, a sympathomimetic agent, is 1-phenyl-2-diethylamino-1-propanone hydrochloride.

In Tepanil Ten-tab tablets, diethylpropion hydrochloride is dispersed in a hydrophilic matrix. On exposure to water the diethylpropion hydrochloride is released at a relatively uniform rate as a result of slow hydration of the matrix. The result is controlled release of the anorexic agent.

Actions: Tepanil is a sympathomimetic amine with some pharmacologic activity similar to that of the prototype drugs of this class used in obesity, the amphetamines. Actions include some central nervous system stimulation and elevation of blood pressure. Tolerance has been demonstrated with all drugs of this class in which these phenomena have been looked for.

Drugs of this class used in obesity are commonly known as "anorectics" or "anorexigenics." It has not been established, however, that the action of such drugs in treating obesity is primarily one of appetite suppression. Other central nervous system actions, or metabolic effects may be involved, for example.

Adult obese subjects instructed in dietary management and treated with "anorectic" drugs lose more weight on the average than those treated with placebo and diet, as determined in relatively short-term clinical trials. The magnitude of increased weight loss of drug-treated patients over placebo-treated patients is some fraction of a pound a week. However, some patients lose more weight than this and some lose less. The rate of weight loss is greatest in the first weeks of therapy for both drug and placebo subjects and tends to decrease in succeeding weeks. The possible origins of the increased weight loss due to the various drug effects are not established. The amount of weight loss associated with the use of an "anorectic" drug varies from trial to trial, and the increased weight loss appears to be related in part to variables other than the drug prescribed, such as the physician-investigator, the population treated, and the diet prescribed. Studies do not permit conclusions as to the relative importance of the drug and non-drug factors on weight loss.

The natural history of obesity is measured in years, whereas most studies cited are restricted to a few weeks duration; thus, the total impact of drug-induced weight loss over that of diet alone must be considered clinically limited.

The controlled-release characteristics of Tepanil Ten-tab have been demonstrated by studies in humans in which plasma levels of diethylpropion-related material were measured by phosphorescence analysis. Plasma levels obtained with the 75 mg. Ten-tab formulation administered once daily indicated a more gradual release than the standard formulation. The formulation has not been shown superior in effectiveness to the same dosage of the standard, noncontrolled-release formulation.

Indication: Tepanil and Tepanil Ten-tab are indicated in the management of exogenous obesity as a short-term adjunct (a few weeks) in a regimen of weight reduction based on caloric restriction. The limited usefulness of agents of this class (see ACTIONS) should be measured against possible risk factors inherent in their use such as those described below.

Contraindications: Advanced arteriosclerosis, hyperthyroidism, known hypersensitivity, or idiosyncrasy to the sympathomimetic amines, glaucoma.

Agitated states.

Patients with a history of drug abuse.

During or within 14 days following the administration of monoamine oxidase inhibitors, hypertensive crises may result.

Warnings: If tolerance develops, the recommended dose should not be exceeded in an attempt to increase the effect; rather, the drug should be discontinued. Tepanil may impair the ability of the patient to engage in potentially hazardous activities such as operating machinery or driving a motor vehicle; the patient should therefore be cautioned accordingly.

Drug Dependence: Tepanil has some chemical and pharmacologic similarities to the amphetamines and other related stimulant drugs that have been extensively abused. There are occasional reports of subjects dependent on amphetamine later chronically abusing diethylpropion. The possibility of abuse should be kept in mind when evaluating the desirability of including a drug as part of a weight reduction program. Abuse of amphetamines and related drugs may be associated with varying degrees of psychologic dependence and social dysfunction which, in the case of certain drugs, may be severe. There are reports of patients who have increased the dosage to many times that recommended.

Abrupt cessation following prolonged high dosage administration results in extreme fatigue and mental depression; changes are also noted on the sleep EEG. Manifestations of chronic intoxication with anorectic drugs include severe dermatoses, marked insomnia, irritability, hyperactivity, and personality changes. The most severe manifestation of chronic intoxications is psychosis, often clinically indistinguishable from schizophrenia.

Use in Pregnancy: Although rat and human reproductive studies have not indicated adverse effects, the use of Tepanil by women who are pregnant or may become pregnant requires that the potential benefits be weighed against the potential risks.

Use in Children: Tepanil is not recommended for use in children under 12 years of age.

Precautions: Caution is to be exercised in prescribing Tepanil for patients with hypertension or with symptomatic cardiovascular disease, including arrhythmias. Tepanil should not be administered to patients with severe hypertension. Insulin requirements in diabetes mellitus may be altered in association with the use of Tepanil and the concomitant dietary regimen.

Tepanil may decrease the hypotensive effect of guanethidine.

The least amount feasible should be prescribed or dispensed at one time in order to minimize the possibility of overdosage.

Reports suggest that Tepanil may increase convulsions in some epileptics. Therefore, epileptics receiving Tepanil should be carefully monitored. Titration of dose or discontinuance of Tepanil may be necessary.

Adverse Reactions: Cardiovascular; Palpitation, tachycardia, elevation of blood pressure, precordial pain, arrhythmia. One published report described T-wave changes in the ECG of a healthy young male after ingestion of diethylpropion hydrochloride.

Continued on next page

Riker—Cont.

Central Nervous System: Overstimulation, nervousness, restlessness, dizziness, jitteriness, insomnia, anxiety euphoria, depression, dysphoria, tremor, headache; rarely psychotic episodes at recommended doses. In a few epileptics an increase in convulsive episodes has been reported.
Gastrointestinal: Dryness of the mouth, unpleasant taste, nausea, vomiting, abdominal discomfort, diarrhea, constipation, other gastrointestinal disturbances.
Allergic: Urticaria, rash, ecchymosis, erythema.
Endocrine: Impotence, changes in libido, menstrual upset.
Hematopoietic System: Bone marrow depression, agranulocytosis, leukopenia.
Miscellaneous: A variety of miscellaneous adverse reactions has been reported by physicians. These include complaints such as dyspnea, hair loss, muscle pain, dysuria, and polyuria.
Dosage and Administration: Tepanil (diethylpropion hydrochloride):
One 25 mg. tablet three times daily, one hour before meals, and in midevening if desired to overcome night hunger.
Tepanil Ten-tab (diethylpropion hydrochloride) controlled-release:
One 75 mg. tablet daily, swallowed whole, in midmorning.
Tepanil is not recommended for use in children under 12 years of age.
Overdosage: Manifestations of acute overdosage include restlessness, tremor, hyperreflexia, rapid respiration, confusion, assaultiveness, hallucinations, panic states. Fatigue and depression usually follow the central stimulation.
Cardiovascular effects include arrhythmias, hypertension or hypotension and circulatory collapse. Gastrointestinal symptoms include nausea, vomiting, diarrhea, and abdominal cramps. Overdose of pharmacologically similar compounds has resulted in fatal poisoning, usually terminating in convulsions and coma.
Management of acute Tepanil intoxication is largely symptomatic and includes lavage and sedation with a barbiturate. Experience with hemodialysis of peritoneal dialysis is inadequate to permit recommendation in this regard. Intravenous phentolamine (Regitine®) has been suggested on pharmacologic grounds for possible acute, severe hypertension, if this complicates Tepanil overdosage.
How Supplied: Tepanil 25 mg.: bottles of 100 (NDC **0089-0351-10**) and 1000 (NDC **0089-0351-80**) white tablets. Tepanil Ten-tab 75 mg.: bottles of 30 (NDC **0089-0353-03**), 100 (NDC **0089-0353-10**), and 250 (NDC **0089-0353-25**) white tablets.
[Shown in Product Identification Section]

THEOLAIR™ ℞
(theophylline)
Tablets
THEOLAIR™ ℞
Liquid
THEOLAIR™-SR ℞
Tablets

Description: Theophylline tablets contain not less than 94.0 percent and not more than 106.0 percent of the labeled amount of $C_7H_8N_4O_2H_2O$. Theophylline, a xanthine compound, is a white, odorless, crystalline powder, having a bitter taste. It contains one molecule of water of hydration or is anhydrous.
125 mg. Tablet: Each round, white, scored tablet contains 125 mg. theophylline U.S.P., anhydrous.
250 mg. Tablet: Each capsule shaped, white, scored tablet with "THEOLAIR 250" imprint contains 250 mg. theophylline U.S.P., anhydrous.
THEOLAIR (theophylline) Tablets provide therapeutic levels of theophylline as rapidly as do hydroalcoholic solutions of theophylline. The reliable and predictable blood levels are due to the rapid dissolution and absorption characteristics of theophylline crystals of microfine size. This is achieved without the use of highly alkaline salts such as ethylenediamine or choline or the use of hydroalcoholic media.
THEOLAIR Liquid contains 80 mg. of theophylline U.S.P., anhydrous per 15 ml. (tablespoonful) in a nonalcoholic solution.
THEOLAIR-SR 250 mg: Each round, white, scored tablet with "SR 250" imprint contains 250 mg of theophylline, USP anhydrous in a slow release formulation.
THEOLAIR-SR 500 mg: Each capsule shaped, white, scored tablet with "SR 500" imprint contains 500 mg of theophylline, USP anhydrous in a slow release formulation.
Clinical Pharmacology: Theophylline directly relaxes the smooth muscle of the bronchial airways and pulmonary blood vessels, thus acting mainly as a bronchodilator, pulmonary vasodilator and smooth muscle relaxant. The drug also possesses other actions typical of the xanthine derivatives: coronary vasodilator, diuretic, cardiac stimulant, cerebral stimulant and skeletal muscle stimulant. The actions of theophylline may be mediated through inhibition of phosphodiesterase and a resultant increase in intracellular cyclic AMP which could mediate smooth muscle relaxation. At concentrations higher than attained **in vivo**, theophylline also inhibits the release of histamine by mast cells.
In vitro, theophylline has been shown to react synergistically with beta agonists that increase intracellular cyclic AMP through the stimulation of adenyl cyclase (isoproterenol), but synergism has not been demonstrated in patient studies and more data is needed to determine if theophylline and beta agonists have clinically important additive effect **in vivo**.
Apparently, no development of tolerance occurs with chronic use of theophylline.
The half-life is shortened with cigarette smoking. The half-life is prolonged in alcoholism, reduced hepatic or renal function, congestive heart failure, and in patients receiving antibiotics such as TAO (troleandomycin), erythromycin and clindamycin. High fever for prolonged periods may decrease theophylline elimination.
[See table below].
Newborn infants have extremely slow clearances and half-lives exceeding 24 hours which approach those seen for older children after about 3–6 months.
Older adults with chronic obstructive pulmonary disease, any patients with cor pulmonale or other causes of heart failure, and patients with liver pathology may have much lower clearances with half-lives that may exceed 24 hours.
The half-life of theophylline in smokers (1 to 2 packs/day) averaged 4–5 hours among various studies, much shorter than the half-life in nonsmokers who averaged about 7–9 hours. The increase in theophylline clearance caused by smoking is probably the result of induction of drug-metabolizing enzymes that do not readily normalize after cessation of smoking. It appears that between 3 months and 2 years may be necessary for normalization of the effect of smoking on theophylline pharmacokinetics.
THEOLAIR-SR has an apparent half life of 10.7 hours. Blood levels of theophylline peak between 4 and 6 and the formulation is completely absorbed.
Indications: For relief of acute bronchial asthma and for reversible bronchospasm associated with chronic bronchitis and emphysema.
Contraindications: In individuals who have shown hypersensitivity to any of its components.
Warnings: Status asthmaticus is a medical emergency. Optimal therapy frequently requires additional medication including corticosteroids when the patient is not rapidly responsive to bronchodilators.
Excessive theophylline doses may be associated with toxicity and serum theophylline levels are recommended to assure maximal benefit without excessive risk. Incidence of toxicity increases at levels greater than 20 mcg/ml.
Morphine, curare, and stilbamidine should be used with caution in patients with airflow obstruction since they stimulate histamine release and can induce asthmatic attacks. They may also suppress respiration leading to respiratory failure. Alternative drugs should be chosen whenever possible.
There is an excellent correlation between high blood levels of theophylline resulting from conventional doses and associated clinical manifestations of toxicity in (1) patients with lowered body plasma clearances (due to transient cardiac decomposition), (2) patients with liver dysfunction or chronic obstructive lung disease, (3) patients who are older than 55 years of age, particularly males.
There are often no early signs of less serious theophylline toxicity such as nausea and restlessness, which may appear in up to 50 percent of patients prior to onset of convulsions. Ventricular arrhythmias or seizures may be the first signs of toxicity.
Many patients who have higher theophylline serum levels exhibit a tachycardia.
Theophylline products may worsen pre-existing arrhythmias.
Usage in Pregnancy: Safe use in pregnancy has not been established relative to possible adverse effects on fetal development, but neither have adverse effects on fetal development been established. This is unfortunately true for most antiasthmatic medications. Therefore, use of theophylline in pregnant women should be balanced against the risk of uncontrolled asthma.
Precautions: Mean half-life in smokers is shorter than non-smokers; therefore smokers may require larger doses of theophylline. Theophylline should not be administered concurrently with other xanthine medications. Use with caution in patients with severe cardiac disease, severe hypoxemia, hypertension, hyperthyroidism, acute myocardial injury, cor pulmonale, congestive heart failure, liver disease, and in the elderly (especially males) and in neonates. Great caution should especially be used in giving theophylline to patients with congestive heart failure. Such patients have shown markedly prolonged theophylline blood level curves with theophylline persisting in serum for long periods following discontinuation of the drug.
Use theophylline cautiously in patients with history of peptic ulcer.
Theophylline may occasionally act as a local irritant to G.I. tract although gastrointestinal symptoms are more commonly central and associated with serum concentrations over 20 mcg/ml.
Adverse Reactions: The most consistent adverse reactions are usually due to overdose and are:

Theophylline Elimination Characteristics

	Theophylline Clearance Rates (mean ± S.D.)	Half-life Average (mean ± S.D.)
Children (over 6 months of age):	1.45 ± 0.58 ml/kg/min	3.7 ± 1.1 hours
Adult nonsmokers with uncomplicated asthma	0.65 ± 0.19 ml/kg/min	8.7 ± 2.2 hours

1. Gastrointestinal: nausea, vomiting, epigastric pain, hematemesis, diarrhea.
2. Central nervous system: headaches, irritability, restlessness, insomnia, reflex hyperexcitability, muscle twitching, clonic and tonic generalized convulsions.
3. Cardiovascular: palpitation, tachycardia, extra systoles, flushing, hypotension, circulatory failure, life threatening ventricular arrhythmias.
4. Respiratory: tachypnea.
5. Renal: albuminuria, increased excretion of renal tubular potentiation or diuresis, and red blood cells.
6. Others: hyperglycemia and inappropriate ADH syndrome.

Drug Interactions: Toxic synergism with ephedrine has been documented and may occur with some other sympathomimetic bronchodilators.
[See table above].

Drug	Effect
Aminophylline with Lithium Carbonate	Increased excretion of Lithium Carbonate
Aminophylline with Propranolol	Antagonism of Propranolol effect
Theophylline with Furosemide	Increased diuresis of Furosemide
Theophylline with Hexamethonium	Decreased Hexamethonium—induced chromatropic effect
Theophylline with Reserpine	Reserpine-induced tachycardia
Theophylline with Chlordiazepoxide	Chlordiazepoxide-induced fatty acid mobilization
Theophylline with Cyclamycin (TAO = Triacetyloleandomycin): erythromycin, lincomycin	Increased Theophyllin plasma levels

Overdosage: Management:

A. If potential oral overdose is established and seizure has not occurred:
   1) Induce vomiting.
   2) Administer a cathartic (this is particularly important if sustained release preparations have been taken).
   3) Administer activated charcoal.

B. If patient is having a seizure:
   1) Establish an airway.
   2) Administer O_2.
   3) Treat the seizure with intravenous diazepam, 0.1 to 0.3 mg/kg up to 10 mg.
   4) Monitor vital signs, maintain blood pressure and provide adequate hydration.

C. Post-Seizure Coma:
   1) Maintain airway and oxygenation.
   2) If a result of oral medication, follow above recommendations to prevent absorption of drug, but intubation and lavage will have to be performed instead of inducing emesis, and the cathartic and charcoal will need to be introduced via a large bore gastric lavage tube.
   3) Continue to provide full supportive care and adequate hydration while waiting for drug to be metabolized. In general, the drug is metabolized sufficiently rapidly so as to not warrant consideration of dialysis.

D. Animal studies suggest that phenobarbital may decrease theophylline toxicity. There is as yet, however, insufficient data to recommend pre-treatment of an overdosage with phenobarbital.

Dosage and Administration: Therapeutic serum levels associated with optimal likelihood for benefit and minimal risk of toxicity are considered to be between 10 mcg/ml and 20 mcg/ml. Levels above 20 mcg/ml may produce toxic effects. There is great variation from patient to patient in dosage needed in order to achieve a therapeutic blood level because of variable rates of elimination. Because of this wide variation from patient to patient, and the relatively narrow therapeutic blood level range, dosage must be individualized and monitoring of theophylline serum levels is highly recommended.

Dosage should be calculated on the basis of lean (ideal) body weight where mg/kg doses are stated. Theophylline does not distribute into fatty tissue.

Giving theophylline with food may prevent the rare case of stomach irritation, and though absorption may be slower, it is still complete.

When rapidly absorbed products such as solutions and uncoated tablets with rapid dissolution are used, dosing to maintain "around the clock" blood levels generally requires administration every 6 hours to obtain the greatest efficacy for clinical use in children; dosing intervals up to 8 hours may be satisfactory for adults because of their slower elimination. Children, and adults requiring higher than average doses, may benefit from products with slower absorption which may allow longer dosing intervals and/or less fluctuation in serum concentration over a dosing interval during chronic therapy.
[See table below].

The loading dose for theophylline will be based on the principle that each 0.5 mg/kg of theophylline administered as a loading dose will result in a 1 mcg/ml increase in serum theophylline concentration. Ideally, then, the loading dose should be deferred if a serum theophylline concentration can be rapidly obtained. If this is not possible, the clinician must exercise his judgment in selecting a dose based on the potential for benefit and risk. When there is sufficient respiratory distress to warrant a small risk, 2.5 mg/kg of theophylline is likely to increase the serum concentration when administered as a loading dose in rapidly absorbed form by only about 5 mcg/ml. If the patient is not already experiencing theophylline toxicity, this is unlikely to result in dangerous adverse effects.

Subsequent to the modified decision regarding loading dose in this group of patients, the subsequent maintenance dosage recommendations are the same as those described above.

Comments: To achieve optimal therapeutic theophylline dosage, it is recommended to monitor serum theophylline concentrations. However, it is not always possible or practical to obtain a serum theophylline level.

Patients should be closely monitored for signs of toxicity. The present data suggest that the above dosage recommendations will achieve therapeutic serum concentrations with minimal risk of toxicity for most patients. However, some risk of toxic serum concentrations is still present.

Adverse reactions to theophylline often occur when serum theophylline levels exceed 20 mcg/ml.

Chronic Asthma:

Theophyllinization is a treatment of first choice for the management of chronic asthma (to prevent symptoms and maintain patent airways). Slow clinical titration is generally preferred to assure acceptance and safety of the medication.

Initial dose: 16 mg/kg/day or 400 mg/day (whichever is lower) in 3–4 divided doses at 6–8 hour intervals.

Increased dose: The above dosage may be increased in approximately 25 percent increments at 2–3 day intervals so long as no intolerance is observed, until the maximum indicated below is reached.

Maximum dose without measurement of serum concentration:

Not to exceed the following: (WARNING: DO NOT ATTEMPT TO MAINTAIN ANY DOSE THAT IS NOT TOLERATED)

Age <9 years — 24 mg/kg/day
Age 9–12 years — 20 mg/kg/day
Age 12–16 years — 18 mg/kg/day
Age >16 years — 13 mg/kg/day or 900 mg/day (WHICHEVER IS LESS)

NOTE: Use ideal body weight for obese patients.

Measurement of serum theophylline concentration during chronic therapy:

If the above maximum doses are to be maintained or exceeded, serum theophylline measurement is recommended. This should be obtained at the approximate time of peak absorption during chronic therapy for the product used (1–2 hours for liquids and plain uncoated tablets that undergo rapid dissolution, 3–5 hours for sustained release preparations). It is important that the patient will have missed no doses during the previous 48 hours and that dosing intervals will have been reasonably typical with no added doses during that period of time.

DOSAGE ADJUSTMENT BASED ON SERUM THEOPHYLLINE MEASUREMENTS WHEN THESE INSTRUCTIONS HAVE NOT BEEN FOLLOWED MAY RESULT IN RECOMMENDATIONS THAT PRESENT RISK OF TOXICITY TO THE PATIENT.

How Supplied:

THEOLAIR TABLETS—125 mg. tablets: Bottles of 100 (NDC **0089-0342-10**) and boxes of 250 unit dose aluminum foil, non child-resistant strips (NDC **0089-0342-26**). 250 mg tablets: Bottles of 100 (NDC **0089-0344-10**) and boxes of 250 unit dose aluminum foil, non child-resistant strips (NDC **0089-0344-26**).

THEOLAIR LIQUID—1 pint (NDC **0089-0960-16**), and 1 gallon (NDC **0089-0960-28**).

THEOLAIR-SR TABLETS—250 mg. slow release tablets: Bottles of 100 (NDC **0089-0345-10**). 500 mg. slow release tablets: Bottles of 100 (NDC **0089-0347-10**).

[Shown in Product Identification Section]

Dosage For Patient Population

ACUTE SYMPTOMS OF ASTHMA REQUIRING RAPID THEOPHYLLINIZATION:

I. Not currently receiving theophylline products.

GROUP	ORAL LOADING DOSE (THEOPHYLLINE)	MAINTENANCE DOSE FOR NEXT 12 HOURS (THEOPHYLLINE)	MAINTENANCE DOSE BEYOND 12 HOURS (THEOPHYLLINE)
1. Children 6 months to 9 years	6 mg/kg	4 mg/kg q4hrs	4 mg/kg q6hrs
2. Children age 9–16 and young adult smokers	6 mg/kg	3 mg/kg q4h	3 mg/kg q6h
3. Otherwise healthy nonsmoking adults	6 mg/kg	3 mg/kg q6h	3 mg/kg q8h
4. Older patients and patients with cor pulmonale	6 mg/kg	2 mg/kg q6h	2 mg/kg q8h
5. Patients with congestive heart failure, liver failure	6 mg/kg	2 mg/kg q8h	1–2 mg/kg q12h

II. Those currently receiving theophylline products: determine, where possible, the time, amount, route of administration and form of the patient's last dose.

Continued on next page

Riker—Cont.

TITRALAC®
Tablets and Liquid

Description:
Liquid: Each teaspoonful (5 ml.) of white, spearmint-flavored liquid contains calcium carbonate 1.00 gm. and glycine for a smooth, pleasant taste. One teaspoonful of liquid approximates two tablets.
Tablets: Each white, spearmint-flavored tablet contains calcium carbonate 0.42 gm. and glycine for a smooth, pleasant taste.
Indications: As an antacid for the relief of heartburn, sour stomach and/or acid indigestion and symptomatic relief of hyperacidity associated with the diagnosis of peptic ulcer, gastritis, peptic esophagitis, gastric hyperacidity, and hiatal hernia.
Dosage: One teaspoonful, or two tablets, taken one hour after meals or as directed by a physician. Tablets can be chewed, swallowed, or allowed to melt in the mouth.
Warnings: Do not take more than 19 tablets or 8 teaspoons in a 24 hour period, or use the maximum dose of this product for more than two weeks except under the advice and supervision of a physician.
Neutralizing Capacity:
Titralac Liquid: 19 milliequivalents per 5 ml.
Titralac Tablets: 15 milliequivalents per 2 tablets.
These neutralization equivalents are expressed as milliequivalents of acid neutralized in 15 minutes when tested in accordance with USP antacid effectiveness test as prescribed in the code of Federal Regulations for OTC antacid products.
Availability: *Tablets:* bottles of 40 (NDC **0089-0355-04**), 100 (NDC **0089-0355-10**), 500 (NDC **0089-0355-50**) and 1000 (NDC **0089-0355-80**) white, spearmint-flavored tablets and boxes containing 60 individually sealed tablets. *Liquid,* bottles of 12 fl. oz. (NDC **0089-0355-12**), spearmint-flavored Liquid. No prescription required.
[*Tablets Shown in Product Identification Section*]

UREX® ℞
(methenamine hippurate)

Description: Urex (methenamine hippurate) is the hippuric acid salt of methenamine (hexamethylenetetramine).
Actions: Urex (methenamine hippurate) is active against a broad spectrum of both gram-positive and gram-negative urinary tract pathogens. It is readily absorbed and excreted. It exerts its antibacterial activity when excreted by the kidney and concentrated in the urine where it dissociates to hippuric acid and methenamine. In an acid urine some of the methenamine component is hydrolyzed to ammonia and the bactericidal agent formaldehyde.
Indications: Urex is indicated for the suppression or elimination of bacteriuria associated with acute, chronic and recurrent infections of the urinary tract, especially when long term therapy is indicated.
Contraindications: Urex (methenamine hippurate) is contraindicated in patients with renal insufficiency, severe hepatic insufficiency or severe dehydration. It also is contraindicated as the sole therapeutic agent in acute parenchymal infections causing systemic symptoms.
Warning: Use in pregnancy: In early pregnancy the safe use of "Urex" is not established. In the last trimester, safety is suggested, but not definitely proven.
Precautions:
1. Large doses of methenamine (8 grams daily for 3 to 4 weeks) have caused bladder irritation, painful and frequent micturition, albuminuria and gross hematuria.
2. Care should be taken to maintain an acid pH of the urine especially when treating infections due to urea-splitting organisms such as Proteus and strains of Pseudomonas.
3. In a few instances in one study, the serum transaminase levels showed a mild elevation during treatment which returned to normal while the patients were still receiving Urex. Because of this one report, it is recommended that liver function studies be performed periodically on patients receiving the drug, especially those with liver dysfunction.

Adverse Reactions: Minor adverse reactions have been reported in fewer than 3.5% of patients treated. These reactions have included: nausea, "upset stomach," dysuria and rash.
Dosage and Administration: One tablet (1.0 Gm.) twice daily for adults and children over 12 years of age. One-half to one tablet (0.5 to 1.0 Gm.) twice daily for children 6-12 years of age.
The antibacterial activity of Urex is greater in acid urine. Therefore, restriction of alkalinizing foods and medications is desirable. If necessary, as indicated by urinary pH and clinical response, supplemental acidification of the urine may be instituted. As is the case with all urinary tract infections, the efficacy of therapy should be monitored by repeated urine cultures.
How Supplied: One gram scored, white tablets, bottles of 100 (NDC **0089-0371-10**) and 500 (NDC **0089-0371-50**).
Animal Pharmacology and Toxicology: Up to 600 mg./kg. of Urex in a single dose were administered intravenously to dogs and rats without toxic effects being observed. Chronic oral administration of 50-200 mg./kg./day to dogs and 800-6400 mg./kg./day to rats produced gastric and bladder irritation with some hemorrhagic sites and ulceration observed at autopsy.
Urex was administered to rats at a dose of 800 mg./kg./day as part of a study of teratogenicity. Urex did not prevent conception, increase fetal death rate or produce teratogenesis. Studies in rabbits at dosage levels producing no toxicity in the parent animals (100-113 mg./kg./day) revealed no prevention of conception, no increase in fetal death rate, no embryopathy and no teratogenicity. At a higher dose of 800 mg./kg./day (20 times the recommended human dose) most of the pregnant rabbits died. However, the two that survived bore viable normal young.
Amounts of Urex equivalent to twice the recommended human dose were administered to rats for twelve months and monkeys for six months without producing any adverse effects.
Clinical Studies: Within one-half hour after ingestion of a single one gram dose of Urex, antibacterial activity is demonstrable in the urine. Urine shows continuous antibacterial activity when Urex is administered at the recommended dosage schedule of one gram twice daily. Over 90% of methenamine moiety is excreted in the urine within 24 hours after administration of a single one gram dose. Similarly, the hippurate moiety is rapidly absorbed and excreted, and it reaches the urine by both tubular secretion and glomerular filtration. This may be of importance in older patients or those with some degree of renal impairment.
Urex is effective clinically against most common urinary tract pathogens. It has demonstrable antibacterial activity in vitro against Escherichia coli, Micrococcus pyogenes, Enterobacter aerogenes, Pseudomonas aeruginosa, and Proteus vulgaris at pH 5.0-6.8. The minimal inhibitory concentrations are significantly lower in more acidic media; therefore, the efficacy of Urex can be increased by acidification of urine.
Using the gradient plate technique of Szybalski no resistant bacterial strains were found to have developed when Urex was tested against both gram-positive and gram-negative pathogens, including Streptococcus fecalis, Proteus vulgaris, Micrococcus pyogenes, Aerobacter aerogenes and Escherichia coli.
The efficacy of Urex at the recommended dose has been established in clinical trials involving approximately 400 patients. Objective measurement of efficacy (reversal of positive cultures) has demonstrated the therapeutic effectiveness of Urex in a wide variety of urinary tract infections. Symptomatic relief was usually reported within 24-72 hours followed by culture reversal in the majority of patients monitored. Studies in children 6-12 years of age have shown similar results. Of 50 children monitored with serial urine cultures, eradication of the infecting organism was achieved in 34 (68%).
Hematologic studies were carried out in over 20% of all patients involved in the clinical trials. There was no instance of significant drug-related alteration of hemograms, blood urea nitrogen, serum creatinine, serum transaminase levels or liver profiles. Gastroscopic examination of 20 patients who received a single one gram dose of Urex revealed no mucosal irritation attributable to the drug.
[*Shown in Product Identification Section*]

Robins Company, A. H.
1407 CUMMINGS DRIVE
RICHMOND, VA 23220

ADABEE® TABLETS
ADABEE® WITH MINERALS TABLETS

Composition: **Adabee.** Each capsule-shaped tablet contains: Vitamin A, USP 10,000 USP units; Ascorbic Acid (Vit. C) (as Sodium Ascorbate, USP) 250 mg; Thiamine Mononitrate, USP (B_1) 15 mg; Riboflavin, USP (B_2) 10 mg; Pyridoxine Hydrochloride, USP (B_6) 5 mg; Niacinamide, USP 50 mg.
Adabee with Minerals. In addition to the vitamins in the Adabee formula, each capsule-shaped tablet contains the following minerals: Iron (as Dried Ferrous Sulfate, USP) 15 mg; Calcium (as Dibasic Calcium Phosphate, NF) 103 mg; Phosphorous (as Dibasic Calcium Phosphate, NF) 80 mg.
Indications: For the prevention and treatment of dietary deficiencies of Vitamins A, B and C (Adabee) and certain minerals (Adabee with Minerals).
Precautions: Do not take Adabee with minerals within two hours of oral tetracycline antibiotics, since oral iron products interfere with absorption of tetracycline. Hypervitaminosis A has been known to appear in children after excessive quantities (50,000 to 500,000 units) of Vitamin A were ingested daily for six months or longer.
Adverse Reactions: Iron-containing medications may occasionally cause gastrointestinal discomfort (such as nausea) or bowel effects (such as constipation or diarrhea).
Dosage and Administraton: One tablet daily, preferably with meals; dosage may be increased, depending on the needs of the patient.
How Supplied: Adabee—yellow, coated, capsule-shaped tablet (NDC 0031-0224); Adabee with Minerals—green, coated, capsule-shaped tablet (NDC 0031-0274). Both in 100s.

ALLBEE® WITH C CAPSULES

One capsule daily provides:

	Percentage of U.S. Recommended Daily Allowance (U.S. RDA)	
Vitamin C	500	300.0 mg
Thiamine (Vitamine B_1)	1000	15.0 mg
Riboflavin (Vitamin B_2)	600	10.2 mg

Niacin	250	50.0 mg
Vitamin B_6	250	5.0 mg
Pantothenic Acid	100	10.0 mg

Ingredients: Ascorbic Acid; Gelatin; Niacinamide; Lactose; Corn Starch; Thiamine Mononitrate; Calcium Pantothenate; Riboflavin; Magnesium Stearate; Pyridoxine Hydrochloride; Light Mineral Oil; Artificial Color; Vanillin.

Action and Uses: Allbee with C is a high potency formulation of B and C vitamins. Its components have important roles in general nutrition, healing of wounds, and prevention of hemorrhage. It is recommended for deficiencies of B-vitamins and ascorbic acid in conditions such as febrile diseases, chronic or acute infections, burns, fractures, surgery, toxic conditions, physiologic stress, alcoholism, prolonged exposure to high temperature, geriatrics, gastritis, peptic ulcer, and colitis; and in conditions involving special diets and weight-reduction diets.

In dentistry, Allbee with C is recommended for deficiencies of B-vitamins and ascorbic acid in conditions such as herpetic stomatitis, aphthous stomatitis, cheilosis, herpangina, gingivitis.

Dosage: The recommended OTC dosage for adults and children twelve or more years of age, other than pregnant or lactating women, is one capsule daily. Under the direction and supervision of a physician, the dose and frequency of administration may be increased in accordance with the patient's requirements.

How Supplied: Yellow and green capsules, monogrammed AHR, in bottles of 30, 100, 1,000 capsules and in Dis-Co® Unit Dose Packs of 500. (NDC 0031-0674)

[Shown in Product Identification Section]

ALLBEE-T® TABLETS

One tablet daily provides:

	Percentage of U.S. Recommended Daily Allowance (U.S. RDA)	
Vitamin C	833	500.0 mg
Thiamine (Vitamin B_1)	1033	15.5 mg
Riboflavin (Vitamin B_2)	588	10.0 mg
Niacin	500	100.0 mg
Vitamin B_6	410	8.2 mg
Vitamin B_{12}	83	5.0 mcg
Pantothenic Acid	230	23.0 mg

Ingredients: Sodium Ascorbate; Desiccated Liver; Lactose; Niacinamide; Hydroxypropyl Methylcellulose; Calcium Pantothenate; Stearic Acid; Povidone; Thiamine Mononitrate; Artificial Color; Propylene Glycol; Riboflavin; Pyridoxine Hydrochloride; Vanillin; Gelatin; Cyanocobalamin.

Actions and Uses: Allbee-T is a high potency, therapeutic formulation of the important B-complex vitamins with Vitamin C.

Allbee-T is indicated for the management of vitamin deficiency states involving one or more B-vitamins or Vitamin C, as in the following:

1. Conditions characterized by an increased requirement for B-complex vitamins and vitamin C, such as severe burns, fractures, surgical procedures, febrile illnesses, hyperthyroidism, acute and chronic infections and alcoholism.
2. Conditions in which the intake and/or absorption of the water-soluble vitamins may be impaired, such as gastritis, colitis, peptic ulcer disease, malabsorption syndromes, weight reduction and other therapeutic diets.
3. Conditions characterized by oral lesions such as cheilosis, gingivitis, and stomatitis where deficiencies of water-soluble vitamins may exist.

Precaution: Not intended for the treatment of pernicious anemia.

Dosage: The recommended OTC dosage for adults and children twelve or more years of age, other than pregnant or lactating women, is one tablet daily. Under the direction and supervision of a physician, the dose and frequency of administration may be increased in accordance with the patient's requirements.

How Supplied: Orange, capsule-shaped, film-coated tablets engraved AHR in bottles of 100 and 500 (NDC 0031-0688).

[Shown in Product Identification Section]

ARTHRALGEN® TABLETS

Composition: Each Arthralgen tablet contains:

Salicylamide........250 mg.
Acetaminophen, USP........250 mg.

Action and Uses: Arthralgen is indicated for the relief of pain associated with a variety of arthritic conditions, colds, flu and myalgias.

Contraindications: Hypersensitivity to any ingredient.

Adverse Reaction: Therapy with Arthralgen may rarely produce nausea or G-I upset. Occasionally mild salicylism may occur, requiring adjustment in dosage.

Administration and Dosage: One or two tablets four times daily.

How Supplied: Arthralgen (white, scored) tablets are available in bottles of 100 and 500. (NDC 0031-1462)

DIMACOL® CAPSULES DIMACOL® LIQUID

Composition: Each capsule or 5 ml (one teaspoonful) contains:

Guaifenesin, NF........100 mg
Pseudoephedrine Hydrochloride, NF........30 mg
Dextromethorphan Hydrobromide, NF........15 mg
Liquid: Alcohol........4.75%

Actions: Dimacol helps reduce nasal congestion and suppresses cough associated with the common cold and other upper respiratory disorders.

Guaifenesin enhances the output of lower respiratory tract fluid. The enhanced flow of less viscid secretions promotes ciliary action, and facilitates the removal of inspissated mucus. As a result, dry unproductive coughs become more productive and less frequent. *Pseudoephedrine hydrochloride* is an orally effective nasal decongestant. Through its vasoconstrictor action, pseudoephedrine gently but promptly reduces edema and congestion of nasal passages. *Dextromethorphan hydrobromide* is a synthetic, non-narcotic cough suppressant. The antitussive effectiveness of dextromethorphan has been demonstrated in both animal and clinical studies, and the incidence of toxic effects has been remarkably low.

Indications: Dimacol is indicated for the management of cough accompanied by nasal mucosal congestion and edema, and nasal hypersecretion, associated with the common cold, upper respiratory infection and sinusitis.

Contraindications: Hypersensitivity to any of the ingredients. Dimacol should not be administered to patients receiving MAO inhibitors.

Precautions: Administer with caution in the presence of hypertension, heart disease, peripheral vascular disease, diabetes or hyperthyroidism. As with all products containing sympathomimetic amines, use with caution in patients with prostatic hypertrophy or glaucoma.

Note: Guaifenesin has been shown to produce a color interference with certain clinical laboratory determinations of 5-hydroxyindoleacetic acid (5-HIAA) and vanilmandelic acid (VMA).

Adverse Reactions: The following adverse reactions may possibly occur: nausea, vomiting, dry mouth, nervousness, insomnia.

Dosage and Administration: Adults and children over 12 years of age, one capsule or one teaspoonful (5 ml) three times a day. Children 6 to 12 years, ½ teaspoonful 3 times a day. Children under 6 years of age, as directed by a physician.

How Supplied: Orange and green capsules in bottles of 100 and 500 and consumer packages of 12 and 24 (individually packaged). (NDC 0031-1650). Orange colored, chocolate flavored liquid in bottles of one pint. (NDC 0031-1660).

[Shown in Product Identification Section]

DIMETANE EXTENTABS® ℞

brand of Brompheniramine Maleate, NF
8 mg and 12 mg

Actions: Brompheniramine maleate is an antihistamine, with anticholinergic (drying) and sedative side effects. Antihistamines appear to compete with histamine for cell receptor sites on effector cells.

Indications: Perennial and seasonal allergic rhinitis; vasomotor rhinitis; allergic conjunctivitis due to inhalant allergens and foods; mild, uncomplicated allergic skin manifestations of urticaria and angioedema; amelioration of allergic reactions to blood or plasma; dermatographism; as therapy for anaphylactic reactions ***adjunctive*** to epinephrine and other standard measures after the acute manifestations have been controlled.

Contraindications: Use in children six years of age and under. This drug should not be used in children six years of age and under.

Use in Nursing Mothers. Because of the higher risk of antihistamines for infants generally and for newborns and prematures in particular, antihistamine therapy is contraindicated in nursing mothers.

Use in Lower Respiratory Disease. Antihistamines **should NOT** be used to treat lower respiratory tract symptoms including asthma.

Antihistamines are also contraindicated in the following conditions: hypersensitivity to brompheniramine maleate and other antihistamines of similar chemical structure; monoamine oxidase inhibitor therapy (see Drug Interaction section).

Warnings: Antihistamines should be used with considerable caution in patients with: narrow angle glaucoma; stenosing peptic ulcer; pyloroduodenal obstruction; symptomatic prostatic hypertrophy; bladder neck obstruction.

Use in Children. In infants and children, especially, antihistamines in **overdosage** may cause hallucinations, convulsions, or death.

As in adults, antihistamines may diminish mental alertness in children. In the young child, particularly, they may produce excitation.

Use in Pregnancy. Experience with this drug in pregnant women is inadequate to determine whether there exists a potential for harm to the developing fetus.

Use with CNS Depressants. Dimetane has additive effects with alcohol and other CNS depressants (hypnotics, sedatives, tranquilizers, etc.)

Use in Activities Requiring Mental Alertness. Patients should be warned about engaging in activities requiring mental alertness, such as driving a car or operating appliances, machinery, etc.

Use in the Elderly (approximately 60 years or older). Antihistamines are more likely to

Continued on next page

Prescribing information on A. H. Robins products listed here is based on official labeling in effect August 1, 1979, with Indications, Contraindications, Warnings, Precautions, Adverse Reactions, and Dosage stated in full.

Robins—Cont.

cause dizziness, sedation, and hypotension in elderly patients.

Precautions: As with other antihistamines, Dimetane has an atropine-like action, and, therefore, should be used with caution in patients with: history of bronchial asthma; increased intraocular pressure; hyperthyroidism; cardiovascular disease; hypertension.

Drug Interactions: MAO inhibitors prolong and intensify the anticholinergic (drying) effects of antihistamines.

Adverse Reactions: The most frequent adverse reactions are italicized:

General: Urticaria, drug rash, anaphylactic shock, photosensitivity, excessive perspiration, chills, dryness of mouth, nose, and throat.

Cardiovascular System: Hypotension, headache, palpitations, tachycardia, extrasystoles.

Hematologic System: Hemolytic anemia, thrombocytopenia, agranulocytosis.

Nervous System: ***Sedation, sleepiness, dizziness, disturbed coordination,*** fatigue, confusion, restlessness, excitation, nervousness, tremor, irritability, insomnia, euphoria, paresthesias, blurred vision, diplopia, vertigo, tinnitus, acute labyrinthitis, hysteria, neuritis, convulsions.

G.I. System: ***Epigastric distress,*** anorexia, nausea, vomiting, diarrhea, constipation.

G.U. System: Urinary frequency, difficult urination, urinary retention, early menses.

Respiratory System: ***Thickening of bronchial secretions,*** tightness of chest and wheezing, nasal stuffiness.

Overdosage: Antihistamine overdosage reactions may vary from central nervous system depression to stimulation. Stimulation is particularly likely in children. Atropine-like signs and symptoms—dry mouth; fixed, dilated pupils; flushing; and gastrointestinal symptoms may also occur.

If vomiting has not occurred spotaneously, the patient should be induced to vomit. This is best done by having him drink a glass of water or milk after which he should be made to gag. Precautions against aspiration must be taken, especially in infants and children.

If vomiting is unsuccessful, gastric lavage is indicated within 3 hours after ingestion and even later if large amounts of milk or cream were given beforehand. Isotonic and ½ isotonic saline is the lavage solution of choice.

NOTE: Extentabs will not be dissolved during the process of lavage, and the tubes ordinarily employed in lavage are not large enough in diameter to remove Extentabs.

Saline cathartics, as milk of magnesia, by osmosis draw water into the bowel and therefore, are valuable for their action in rapid dilution of bowel content.

Stimulants should **not** be used.

Vasopressors may be used to treat hypotension.

Dosage and Administration: DOSAGE SHOULD BE INDIVIDUALIZED ACCORDING TO THE NEEDS AND THE RESPONSE OF THE PATIENTS.

Adults: One Extentab (8 or 12 mg) every eight to twelve hours or twice daily.

Children over six. One Extentab (8 or 12 mg) every twelve hours.

How Supplied:

Extentabs, 8 mg are available as Persian rose-colored, coated tablets, in bottles of 100 and 500 (NDC 0031-1868).

Extentabs, 12 mg are available as peach-colored, coated tablets, in bottles of 100 and 500 (NDC 0031-1843).

[*Shown in Product Identification Section*]

DIMETANE®

brand of Brompheniramine Maleate, NF
Tablets—4 mg
Elixir—2 mg/5 ml
Alcohol, 3%

Actions: Brompheniramine maleate is an antihistamine, with anticholinergic (drying) and sedative side effects. Antihistamines appear to compete with histamine for cell receptor sites on effector cells.

Indications: For effective, temporary relief of hay fever/upper respiratory allergy symptoms: itchy, watery eyes; sneezing; itching nose or throat.

Contraindications: *Use in Newborn or Premature Infants.* This drug should **not** be used in newborn or premature infants.

Use in Nursing Mothers. Because of the higher risk of antihistamines for infants generally and for newborns and prematures in particular, antihistamine therapy is contraindicated in nursing mothers.

Use in Lower Respiratory Disease. Antihistamines **should NOT** be used to treat lower respiratory tract symptoms including asthma.

This drug is also contraindicated in the following conditions: hypersensitivity to brompheniramine maleate and other antihistamines of similar chemical structure; monoamine oxidase inhibitor therapy (see Drug Interaction section).

Warnings: Antihistamines should be used with considerable caution in patients with: narrow angle glaucoma; stenosing peptic ulcer; pyloroduodenal obstruction; symptomatic prostatic hypertrophy; bladder neck obstruction.

Use in Children. In infants and children, especially, antihistamines in **overdosage** may cause hallucinations, convulsions, or death.

As in adults, antihistamines may diminish mental alertness in children. In the young child, particularly, they may produce excitation.

Use in Pregnancy. Experience with this drug in pregnant women is inadequate to determine whether there exists a potential for harm to the developing fetus.

Use with CNS Depressants. Dimetane has additive effects with alcohol and other CNS depressants (hypnotics, sedatives, tranquilizers, etc.).

Use in Activities Requiring Mental Alertness. Patients should be warned about engaging in activities requiring mental alertness, such as driving a car or operating appliances, machinery, etc.

Use in the Elderly (approximately 60 years or older). Antihistamines are more likely to cause dizziness, sedation, and hypotension in elderly patients.

Precautions: As with other antihistamines, Dimetane has an atropine-like action and, therefore, should be used with caution in patients with: history of bronchial asthma; increased intraocular pressure; hyperthyroidism; cardiovascular disease; hypertension.

Drug Interactions: MAO inhibitors prolong and intensify the anticholinergic (drying) effects of antihistamines.

Adverse Reactions: The most frequent adverse reactions are italicized:

General: Urticaria, drug rash, anaphylactic shock, photosensitivity, excessive perspiration, chills, dryness of mouth, nose, and throat.

Cardiovascular System: Hypotension, headache, palpitations, tachycardia, extrasystoles.

Hematologic System: Hemolytic anemia, thrombocytopenia, agranulocytosis.

Nervous System: ***Sedation, sleepiness, dizziness, disturbed coordination,*** fatigue, confusion, restlessness, excitation, nervousness, tremor, irritability, insomnia, euphoria, paresthesias, blurred vision, diplopia, vertigo, tinnitus, acute labyrinthitis, hysteria, neuritis, convulsions.

G.I. System: ***Epigastric distress,*** anorexia, nausea, vomiting, diarrhea, constipation.

G.U. System: Urinary frequency, difficult urination, urinary retention, early menses.

Respiratory System: ***Thickening of bronchial secretions,*** tightness of chest and wheezing, nasal stuffiness.

Overdosage: Antihistamine overdosage reactions may vary from central nervous system depression to stimulation. Stimulation is particularly likely in children. Atropine-like signs and symptoms—dry mouth; fixed, dilated pupils; flushing; and gastrointestinal symptoms may also occur.

If vomiting has not occurred spontaneously, the patient should be induced to vomit. This is best done by having him drink a glass of water or milk after which he should be made to gag. Precautions against aspiration must be taken, especially in infants and children.

If vomiting is unsuccessful, gastric lavage is indicated within 3 hours after ingestion and even later if large amounts of milk or cream were given beforehand. Isotonic and ½ isotonic saline is the lavage solution of choice.

Saline cathartics, such as milk of magnesia, by osmosis draw water into the bowel and therefore, are valuable for their action in rapid dilution of bowel content.

Stimulants should **not** be used.

Vasopressors may be used to treat hypotension.

Dosage and Administration: The recommended OTC dosage is:

Adults and children 12 years of age and over: 1 tablet or 2 teaspoonfuls every four to six hours, not to exceed 6 tablets or 12 teaspoonfuls in 24 hours.

Children 6 to under 12 years: ½ tablet or 1 teaspoonful every four to six hours, not to exceed 3 tablets or 6 teaspoonfuls in 24 hours.

Children under 6 years: use as directed by a physician.

Under physician supervision, children 2 to under 6 years: ½ teaspoonful every four to six hours, not to exceed 3 teaspoonfuls in 24 hours.

How Supplied: 4 mg tablets are available as peach-colored, compressed, scored tablets in cartons of 24 individually packaged blister units, and in bottles of 100 and 500 (NDC 0031-1857). 2 mg per 5 ml peach-colored liquid is available in bottles of 4 fl. oz., 1 pint and 1 gallon (NDC 0031-1807).

[*Shown in Product Identification Section*]

DIMETANE®-TEN INJECTABLE ℞

brand of Brompheniramine
Maleate Injection, NF

Description: **Dimetane®-Ten Injectable,** for intramuscular, intravenous, or subcutaneous injection.

Each 1 ml contains:
Brompheniramine Maleate, NF ....10 mg
Water for Injection, USP ....q.s.
pH adjusted to 6.8–7.0
with sodium hydroxide

Actions: Brompheniramine maleate is an antihistamine, with anticholinergic (drying) and sedative side effects. Antihistamines appear to compete with histamine for cell receptor sites on effector cells.

Indications: For the following conditions when use of the oral form of the drug is impractical:

Amelioration of allergic reactions to blood or plasma.

In anaphylaxis as an adjunct to epinephrine and other standard measures after the acute symptoms have been controlled.

For other uncomplicated allergic conditions of the immediate type when oral therapy is impossible or contraindicated.

Contraindications: *Use in Newborn or Premature Infants.* This drug should **not** be used in newborn or premature infants.

Use in Nursing Mothers. Because of the higher risk of antihistamines for infants generally

and for newborns and prematures in particular, antihistamine therapy is contraindicated in nursing mothers.
Use in Lower Respiratory Disease. Antihistamines **should NOT** be used to treat lower respiratory tract symptoms including asthma.
This drug is also contraindicated in the following conditions: hypersensitivity to brompheniramine maleate and other antihistamines of similar chemical structure; monoamine oxidase inhibitor therapy (see Drug Interaction section).
Warnings: Antihistamines should be used with considerable caution in patients with: narrow angle glaucoma; stenosing peptic ulcer; pyloroduodenal obstruction; symptomatic prostatic hypertrophy; bladder neck obstruction.
Use in Children. In infants and children, especially, antihistamines in **overdosage** may cause hallucinations, convulsions, or death.
As in adults, antihistamines may diminish mental alertness in children. In the young child, particularly, they may produce excitation.
Use in Pregnancy. Experience with this drug in pregnant women is inadequate to determine whether there exists a potential for harm to the developing fetus.
Use With CNS Depressants. Dimetane has additive effects with alcohol and other CNS depressants (hypnotics, sedatives, tranquilizers, etc.).
Use In Activities Requiring Mental Alertness. Patients should be warned about engaging in activities requiring mental alertness as driving a car or operating appliances, machinery, etc.
Use in the Elderly (approximately 60 years or older). Antihistamines are more likely to cause dizziness, sedation, and hypotension in elderly patients.
Precautions: As with other antihistamines, Dimetane has an atropine-like action and, therefore, should be used with caution in patients with: history of bronchial asthma; increased intraocular pressure; hyperthyroidism; cardiovascular disease; hypertension.
Drug Interactions: MAO inhibitors prolong and intensify the anticholinergic (drying) effects of antihistamines.
Adverse Reactions: The most frequent adverse reactions are italicized:
1. ***General:*** Urticaria, drug rash, anaphylactic shock, photosensitivity, excessive perspiration, chills, dryness of mouth, nose, and throat.
2. ***Cardiovascular System:*** Hypotension, headache, palpitations, tachycardia, extrasystoles.
3. ***Hematologic System:*** Hemolytic anemia, thrombocytopenia, agranulocytosis.
4. ***Nervous System: Sedation, sleepiness, dizziness, disturbed coordination,*** fatigue, confusion, restlessness, excitation, nervousness, tremor, irritability, insomnia, euphoria, paresthesias, blurred vision, diplopia, vertigo, tinnitus, acute labyrinthitis, hysteria, neuritis, convulsions.
5. ***G.I. System: Epigastric distress,*** anorexia, nausea, vomiting, diarrhea, constipation.
6. ***G.U. System:*** Urinary frequency, difficult urination, urinary retention, early menses.
7. ***Respiratory System: Thickening of bronchial secretions,*** tightness of chest and wheezing, nasal stuffiness.
Overdosage: Antihistamine overdosage reactions may vary from central nervous system depression to stimulation. Stimulation is particularly likely in children. Atropine-like signs and symptoms—dry mouth; fixed, dilated pupils; flushing; and gastrointestinal symptoms may also occur.
Specific Therapy: There is no specific therapy or known antidote.
Management of Overdosage: ***Stimulants*** should ***not*** be used. Vasopressors may be used to treat hypotension.
Dosage and Administration: DOSAGE SHOULD BE INDIVIDUALIZED ACCORDING TO THE NEEDS AND THE RESPONSE OF THE PATIENTS.
Adults: The usual dose is 10 mg. The dosage range is 5 mg to 20 mg. The period of protection is three to twelve hours, and twice daily administration is usually all that is necessary. The maximum recommended dose for 24 hours is 40 mg.
Children under 12 years: 0.5 mg per kg per 24 hours, or 15 mg per M^2 per 24 hours, divided into 3–4 doses.
NOTE: Dimetane-Ten Injectable (10 mg brompheniramine maleate per ml) may be administered without further dilution intramuscularly or subcutaneously. It may also be administered intravenously either undiluted or diluted 1 to 10 with sterile saline for injection. If given intravenously, the drug should be given slowly, preferably with the patient in a recumbent position. If desired, Dimetane-Ten Injectable may be added to normal saline or 5% glucose or whole blood for intravenous administration.
How Supplied: Dimetane-Ten Injectable is supplied as 1 ml ampuls, in cartons of 6 and 100 (NDC 0031-1881), each ampul containing 10 mg brompheniramine maleate.
Caution: To protect from light, Dimetane-Ten Injectable should be stored in carton until used. Cooling below 32°F may produce brompheniramine crystals; if present, dissolve by warming to 85°F before using.

DIMETANE® EXPECTORANT ℞
DIMETANE® EXPECTORANT-DC ℞ Ⓒ

Composition: *Dimetane Expectorant:* Each 5 ml (1 teaspoonful) contains Brompheniramine Maleate, NF 2 mg., Guaifenesin, NF 100 mg., Phenylephrine Hydrochloride, USP 5 mg., Phenylpropanolamine Hydrochloride, NF 5 mg., Alcohol 3.5 per cent.
Dimetane Expectorant-DC: Same as Dimetane Expectorant, plus Codeine Phosphate, USP per 5 ml teaspoonful 10 mg. (Warning: May be habit forming.)
Actions: Dimetane Expectorant combines widely used ingredients designed for the temporary relief of coughing and the complications of allergic states including manifestations such as perennial and seasonal allergic rhinitis. Brompheniramine maleate (Dimetane®) has the clinical ability to alleviate allergic conditions. The sympathomimetic amines, phenylephrine hydrochloride and phenylpropanolamine hydrochloride, are indicated for the temporary relief of nasal congestion. Guaifenesin is present as an expectorant.
Dimetane Expectorant-DC contains codeine phosphate for greater suppression of cough, in addition to the Dimetane Expectorant ingredients.

Indications
Based on a review of these drugs by the National Academy of Sciences—National Research Council and/or other information, FDA has classified these products as lacking substantial evidence of effectiveness as fixed combinations for the following indications:
Dimetane Expectorant is indicated for relief of coughing and for symptomatic relief of many manifestations of allergic states in which expectorant action is desired. Dimetane Expectorant-DC is indicated in the same disorders as Dimetane Expectorant when the antitussive properties of codeine are desired.

Contraindications: Hypersensitivity to brompheniramine maleate and other antihistamines of similar chemical structure; hypersensitivity to any of the other active ingredients; use in pregnancy; monamine oxidase inhibitor therapy (see Drug Interaction section).
Use in Newborn or Premature Infants: Dimetane Expectorant and Dimetane Expectorant-DC should not be used in newborn or premature infants.
Use in Nursing Mothers: Because of the higher risk of antihistamines for infants generally and for newborns and prematures in particular, Dimetane Expectorant and Dimetane Expectorant-DC are contraindicated in nursing mothers.
Use in Lower Respiratory Disease: Antihistamines **should NOT** be used to treat lower respiratory tract symptoms including asthma.
Warnings: Antihistamines should be used with considerable caution in patients with: narrow angle glaucoma; stenosing peptic ulcer; pyloroduodenal obstruction; symptomatic prostatic hypertrophy; bladder neck obstruction. Codeine can produce drug dependence of the morphine type, and therefore, has the potential for being abused.
Use in Children: In infants and children, especially, antihistamines in **overdosage** may cause hallucinations, convulsions, or death.
As in adults, antihistamines may diminish mental alertness in children. In the young child, particularly, they may produce excitation.
Use in Pregnancy: Experience with brompheniramine maleate in pregnant women is inadequate to determine whether there exists a potential for harm to the developing fetus.
Use with CNS Depressants: Brompheniramine maleate and codeine phosphate have additive effects with alcohol and other CNS depressants (hypnotics, sedatives, tranquilizers, etc.).
Use in Activities Requiring Mental Alertness: Patients should be warned about engaging in activities requiring mental alertness, such as driving a car or operating appliances, machinery, etc.
Use in the Elderly (approximately 60 years or older): Antihistamines are more likely to cause dizziness, sedation, and hypotension in elderly patients.
Precautions: As with other antihistamines, brompheniramine maleate has an atropinelike action and, therefore, should be used with caution in patients with: history of bronchial asthma; increased intraocular pressure; hyperthyroidism; cardiovascular disease; hypertension. As with all preparations containing sympathomimetic amines, administer with caution to patients with cardiac or peripheral vascular diseases and hypertension.
Drug Interactions: MAO inhibitors prolong and intensify the anticholinergic (drying) effects of antihistamines. The CNS depressant effect of brompheniramine maleate and codeine phosphate may be additive with that of other CNS depressants.
Adverse Reactions: *General.* Urticaria, drug rash, anaphylactic shock, photosensitivity, excessive perspiration, chills, dryness of mouth, nose and throat.
Cardiovascular System. Hypotension, hypertension, headache, palpitations, tachycardia, extrasystoles.
Hematologic System. Hemolytic anemia, thrombocytopenia, agranulocytosis.
Nervous System. Sedation, sleepiness, dizziness, disturbed coordination, fatigue, confusion, restlessness, excitation, nervousness, tremor, irritability, insomnia, euphoria, paresthesias, blurred vision, diplopia, vertigo, tinni-

Continued on next page

Prescribing information on A. H. Robins products listed here is based on official labeling in effect August 1, 1979, with Indications, Contraindications, Warnings, Precautions, Adverse Reactions, and Dosage stated in full.

Robins—Cont.

tus, acute labyrinthitis, hysteria, neuritis, convulsions.
G.I. System. Epigastric distress, anorexia, nausea, vomiting, diarrhea, constipation.
G.U. System. Urinary frequency, difficult urination, urinary retention, early menses.
Respiratory System. Thickening of bronchial secretions, tightness of chest and wheezing, nasal stuffiness.
Note: Guaifenesin has been shown to produce a color interference with certain clinical laboratory determinations of 5-hydroxyindoleacetic acid (5-HIAA) and vanillylmandelic acid (VMA).
Overdosage: Overdosage reactions may vary from central nervous system depression to stimulation. Stimulation is particularly likely in children as a result of antihistamine overdosage. Atropine-like signs and symptoms—dry mouth; fixed, dilated pupils; flushing; and gastrointestinal symptoms—may also occur.
If vomiting has not occurred spontaneously, the patient should be induced to vomit. This is best done by having him drink a glass of water or milk after which he should be made to gag. Precautions against aspiration must be taken, especially in infants and children.
If vomiting is unsuccessful, gastric lavage is indicated within three hours after ingestion and even later if large amounts of milk or cream were given beforehand. Isotonic and one-half isotonic saline is the lavage solution of choice.
Saline cathartics, as milk of magnesia, by osmosis draw water into the bowel and therefore, are valuable for their action in rapid dilution of bowel content.
Stimulants should **not** be used.
Vasopressors may be used to treat hypotension. Naloxone may be used to treat codeine toxicity.
Suggested Dosage: Adults. 1 to 2 teaspoonfuls four times a day.
Children. ½ to 1 teaspoonful three or four times a day.
How Supplied: Dimetane Expectorant—bottles of one pint and one gallon (NDC 0031-1818).
Dimetane Expectorant-DC—bottles of one pint and one gallon (NDC 0031-1831).

DIMETAPP® ELIXIR ℞

Each 5 ml (1 teaspoonful) contains:
Brompheniramine Maleate, NF................4 mg
Phenylephrine Hydrochloride, USP.........5 mg
Phenylpropanolamine
Hydrochloride, NF..................................5 mg
Alcohol, 2.3%
Actions: Dimetapp effectively reduces excessive nasopharyngeal secretions and diminishes inflammatory mucosal edema and congestion in the upper respiratory tract.
The antihistaminic action of brompheniramine maleate reduces or abolishes the allergic response of nasal tissue. It is complemented by the mild vasoconstrictor action of phenylephrine hydrochloride and phenylpropanolamine hydrochloride which provide a nasal decongestant effect.

Indications
Based on a review of this drug by the National Academy of Sciences—National Research Council and/or other information, FDA has classified the following indications as "probably effective" for Dimetapp Elixir: The symptomatic treatment of seasonal and perennial allergic rhinitis and vasomotor rhinitis; and "lacking substantial evidence of effectiveness as a fixed combination" for the following indications: Symptomatic relief of allergic manifestations of upper respiratory illnesses, acute sinusitis, nasal congestion, and otitis.
Final classification of the less-than-effective indications requires further investigation.

Contraindications: Hypersensitivity to antihistamines of the same chemical class. Dimetapp is contraindicated during pregnancy and in concurrent MAO inhibitor therapy. Because of its drying and thickening effect on the lower respiratory secretions, Dimetapp is not recommended in the treatment of bronchial asthma.
Warnings: ***Use in children.*** In infants and children particularly, antihistamines in overdosage may produce convulsions and death.
Precautions: Administer with care to patients with cardiac or peripheral vascular diseases or hypertension. Until the patient's response has been determined, he should be cautioned against engaging in operations requiring alertness such as driving an automobile, operating machinery, etc. Patients receiving antihistamines should be warned against possible additive effects with CNS depressants such as alcohol, hypnotics, sedatives, tranquilizers, etc.
Adverse Reactions: Adverse reactions to Dimetapp may include hypersensitivity reactions such as rash, urticaria, leukopenia, agranulocytosis and thrombocytopenia; drowsiness, lassitude, giddiness, dryness of the mucous membranes, tightness of the chest, thickening of bronchial secretions, urinary frequency and dysuria, palpitation, hypotension/hypertension, headache, faintness, dizziness, tinnitus, incoordination, visual disturbances, mydriasis, CNS depressant and (less often) stimulant effect, increased irritability or excitement, anorexia, nausea, vomiting, diarrhea, constipation, and epigastric distress.
Dosage and Administration: Adults—1 to 2 teaspoonfuls 3 or 4 times daily.
Children (4 to 12 years)—1 teaspoonful 3 or 4 times daily; (2 to 4 years)—¾ teaspoonful 3 or 4 times daily; (7 months to 2 years)—½ teaspoonful 3 or 4 times daily; (1 to 6 months)—¼ teaspoonful 3 or 4 times daily.
How Supplied: Grape flavored Elixir in 4 fl. oz., pints and gallons, and 5 ml Dis-Co® Unit Dose Packs (4 × 25s) (NDC 0031-2224).

DIMETAPP EXTENTABS® ℞

Each Extentab contains:
Brompheniramine Maleate, NF.............12 mg
Phenylephrine Hydrochloride, USP.......15 mg
Phenylpropanolamine
Hydrochloride, NF...............................15 mg
Extentabs provide a continuous release of medication which affords effects for ten to twelve hours.
Actions: Dimetapp Extentabs effectively reduce excessive nasopharyngeal secretions and diminish inflammatory mucosal edema and congestion in the upper respiratory tract.
The antihistaminic action of brompheniramine maleate reduces or abolishes the allergic response of nasal tissue. It is complemented by the mild vasoconstrictor action of phenylephrine hydrochloride and phenylpropanolamine hydrochloride which provide a nasal decongestant effect.

Indications
Based on a review of this drug by the National Academy of Sciences—National Research Council and/or other information, FDA has classified the following indications as "lacking substantial evidence of effectiveness as a fixed combination" for Dimetapp Extentabs: For the symptomatic treatment of seasonal and perennial allergic rhinitis and vasomotor rhinitis, allergic manifestations of upper respiratory illnesses, acute sinusitis, nasal congestion, and otitis.
Final classification of the less-than-effective indications requires further investigation.

Contraindications: Hypersensitivity to antihistamines of the same chemical class. Dimetapp Extentabs are contraindicated during pregnancy and in children under 12 years of age. Because of its drying and thickening effect on the lower respiratory secretions, Dimetapp is not recommended in the treatment of bronchial asthma. Also, Dimetapp Extentabs are contraindicated in concurrent MAO inhibitor therapy.
Warnings: ***Use in Children.*** In infants and children particularly, antihistamines in overdosage may produce convulsions and death.
Precautions: Administer with care to patients with cardiac or peripheral vascular diseases or hypertension. Until the patient's response has been determined, he should be cautioned against engaging in operations requiring alertness such as driving an automobile, operating machinery, etc. Patients receiving antihistamines should be warned against possible additive effects with CNS depressants such as alcohol, hypnotics, sedatives, tranquilizers, etc.
Adverse Reactions: Adverse reactions to Dimetapp Extentabs may include hypersensitivity reactions such as rash, urticaria, leukopenia, agranulocytosis and thrombocytopenia; drowsiness, lassitude, giddiness, dryness of the mucous membranes, tightness of the chest, thickening of bronchial secretions, urinary frequency and dysuria, palpitation, hypotension/hypertension, headache, faintness, dizziness, tinnitus, incoordination, visual disturbances, mydriasis, CNS depressant and (less often) stimulant effect, increased irritability or excitement, anorexia, nausea, vomiting, diarrhea, constipation, and epigastric distress.
Dosage and Administration: Adults and Children 12 years and over. One Extentab morning and evening. If indicated, one Extentab every 8 hours may be given.
How Supplied: Light blue Extentabs in bottles of 100 and 500 and Dis-Co® Unit Dose Packs of 100. (NDC 0031-2274).
[*Shown in Product Identification Section*]

DONNAGEL®
DONNAGEL®-PG Ⓒ

Composition: *Donnagel:* Each 30 ml (one fluid ounce) contains kaolin (90 gr.) 6.0 g., pectin (2 gr.) 142.8 mg., hyoscyamine sulfate 0.1037 mg., atropine sulfate 0.0194 mg., hyoscine hydrobromide 0.0065 mg., sodium benzoate (preservative) 60 mg., alcohol 3.8 per cent.
Donnagel-PG: Each 30 ml (one fluid ounce) contains the basic Donnagel formula plus powdered opium, USP (equivalent to paregoric 6 ml.) 24 mg. (Warning: may be habit forming), alcohol 5.0 per cent.
Action and Uses: *Donnagel* combines the adsorbent and detoxifying effects of kaolin (which functions principally in the stomach and small intestine) and pectin (which exerts its effects mainly in the large intestine) with the antispasmodic efficacy of the natural belladonna alkaloids. The latter help control hypermotility and hypersecretion in the gastrointestinal tract.
The actions of Donnagel are adsorbent, detoxicant, demulcent, spasmolytic, and anticholinergic. Donnagel is specifically indicated for antidiarrheal use. It is also effective in gastritis, enteritis, colitis, and acute gastrointestinal upsets, and nausea which may accompany any of these conditions.
Donnagel-PG is indicated for symptomatic control of acute, non-specific diarrheas. The powdered opium content of two tablespoonfuls is equivalent to 6 ml. of paregoric. The addition of a paregoric equivalent to the Donnagel formula provides a more complete approach for

stopping diarrhea and relieving tenesmus and pain. The belladonna alkaloids partly antagonize the occasional cramping effect of opium on the colon.

Contraindications: Glaucoma, advanced renal or hepatic disease or hypersensitivity to any of the ingredients.

Precautions: As with all preparations containing belladonna alkaloids, the Donnagel formulations must be administered with care to patients with incipient glaucoma or urinary bladder neck obstruction as in prostatic hypertrophy.

Adverse Reactions: Blurring of vision, dry mouth, difficult urination, or flushing and dryness of skin may occur in a small number of patients on increased dosage, rarely at the usual dosage.

Administration and Dosage: *Donnagel: Adults*—for diarrhea, 2 tablespoonfuls at once and 1 or 2 tablespoonfuls after each stool; for other conditions, 1 tablespoonful every 3 hrs. as necessary.

Donnagel-PG: Adults—2 tablespoonfuls every 3 hours, or as needed.

Donnagel and Donnagel-PG-Pediatric Dosage Recommendations: Body Weight: 10 lb.-30 mins or ½ teaspoonful; 20 lb.-1 teaspoonful; 30 lb. and over-1-2 teaspoonfuls.

How Supplied: Donnagel is a pale green aromatized suspension packaged in 4 fl. oz. plastic bottles, and 16 fl. oz. glass bottles (NDC 0031-3016).

Donnagel-PG is a pale yellow, banana flavored suspension in 6 fl. oz. and 16 fl. oz. bottles (NDC 0031-3083).

DONNATAL® TABLETS ℞
DONNATAL® CAPSULES ℞
DONNATAL® ELIXIR ℞
DONNATAL® NO. 2 TABLETS ℞

Description: Each Donnatal tablet, capsule or 5 ml (teaspoonful) of elixir (23% alcohol) contains:

Phenobarbital (¼ gr)	16.2 mg
(Warning: May be habit forming)	
Hyoscyamine Sulfate	0.1037 mg
Atropine Sulfate	0.0194 mg
Hyoscine Hydrobromide	0.0065 mg

Each Donnatal No. 2 tablet contains the belladonna alkaloids as in Donnatal, with 32.4 mg phenobarbital (Warning: May be habit forming).

Actions: Donnatal provides natural belladonna alkaloids in a specific, fixed ratio combined with phenobarbital to provide peripheral anticholinergic/antispasmodic action and mild sedation.

Indications

Based on a review of this drug by the National Academy of Sciences—National Research Council and/or other information, FDA has classified the following indications as possibly effective: adjunctive therapy in the treatment of peptic ulcer; the treatment of the irritable bowel syndrome (irritable colon, spastic colon, mucous colitis) and acute enterocolitis.

Final classification of the less-than-effective indications requires further investigation.

Contraindications: Donnatal is contraindicated in patients with glaucoma, renal or hepatic disease, obstructive uropathy (for example, bladder neck obstruction due to prostatic hypertrophy) or a hypersensitivity to any of the ingredients.

Adverse Reactions: Blurred vision, dry mouth, difficult urination, and flushing or dryness of the skin may occur at higher dosage levels, rarely at the usual dosage.

Dosage and Administration: The dosage of Donnatal should be adjusted to the needs of the individual patient to assure symptomatic control with a minimum of adverse effects.

Donnatal Tablets or Capsules. Adults: One or two Donnatal tablets or capsules three or four times a day according to condition and severity of symptoms.

Donnatal Elixir. Adults: One or two teaspoonfuls of elixir three or four times a day according to conditions and severity of symptoms.

Children (Elixir):

Body Weight	Starting Dosage
10 lb	0.5 ml to 0.75 ml
20 lb	1.25 ml (¼ tsp) to 2.0 ml
30 lb	2.5 ml (½ tsp)
50 lb	¾ tsp to 1 tsp
75–80 lb	1 tsp to 1½ tsp

Doses may be repeated every 4 to 6 hours as needed; dosage adjustment may be necessary.

Donnatal No. 2 Tablets. Adults: One or two tablets three times a day according to condition and severity of symptoms.

How Supplied: *Donnatal Tablets.* White, compressed, scored and embossed "R"; in bottles of 100 and 1000 and Dis-Co® unit dose packs (10 × 100s) (NDC 0031-4250).

Donnatal Capsules. Green and white, monogrammed "AHR"; in bottles of 100 and 1000 (NDC 0031-4207).

Donnatal Elixir. Green, citrus flavored, in 4 fl. oz., pints and gallons, and 5 ml Dis-Co® unit dose packs (4 × 25s) (NDC 0031-4221).

Donnatal No. 2 Tablets. Pale green, compressed, scored and embossed "R"; in bottles of 100 and 1000 (NDC 0031-4264).

[*Shown in Product Identification Section*]

DONNATAL EXTENTABS® ℞

Description: Each Donnatal Extentab contains:

Phenobarbital (¾gr)	48.6 mg
(Warning: May be habit forming)	
Hyoscyamine Sulfate	0.3111 mg
Atropine Sulfate	0.0582 mg
Hyoscine Hydrobromide	0.0195 mg

Each Donnatal Extentab contains the equivalent of three Donnatal tablets. The Extentab is designed to release the ingredients gradually to provide effects for up to twelve (12) hours.

Actions: Donnatal provides natural belladonna alkaloids in a specific, fixed ratio combined with phenobarbital to provide peripheral anticholinergic/antispasmodic action and mild sedation.

INDICATIONS

Based on a review of this drug by the National Academy of Sciences—National Research Council and/or other information, FDA has classified the following indications as possibly effective: adjunctive therapy in the treatment of peptic ulcer; the treatment of the irritable bowel syndrome (irritable colon, spastic colon, mucous colitis) and acute enterocolitis.

Final classification of the less-than-effective indications requires further investigation.

Contraindications: Donnatal is contraindicated in patients with glaucoma, renal or hepatic disease, obstructive uropathy (for example, bladder neck obstruction due to prostatic hypertrophy) or a hypersensitivity to any of the ingredients.

Adverse Reactions: Blurred vision, dry mouth, difficult urination, and flushing or dryness of the skin may occur at higher dosage levels, rarely at the usual dosage.

Dosage and Administration: The dosage of Donnatal Extentabs should be adjusted to the needs of the individual patient to assure symptomatic control with a minimum of adverse reactions. The usual dose is one Extentab every twelve (12) hours. If indicated, one Extentab every eight (8) hours may be given.

How Supplied: Pale green, coated tablets, monogrammed "R" in bottles of 100 and 500 and Dis-Co® Unit Dose Packs of 100. (NDC 0031-4235).

[*Shown in Product Identification Section*]

DONNAZYME® TABLETS ℞

Composition: Each tablet contains:

Pancreatin, NF equivalent	300 mg
Pepsin	150 mg
Bile salts	150 mg
Hyoscyamine sulfate	0.0518 mg
Atropine sulfate	0.0097 mg
Hyoscine hydrobromide	0.0033 mg
Phenobarbital (⅛ gr)	8.1 mg
(Warning: May be habit forming)	

Action and Uses: Donnazyme tablets provide a logical combination of time-tested and proven agents for the comprehensive symptomatic control of the many-sided problem of "nervous indigestion." Donnazyme is a combination of belladonna alkaloids and phenobarbital with the natural digestive enzymes plus bile salts.

The outer layer of Donnazyme tablets is gastric-soluble and contains belladonna alkaloids, phenobarbital and pepsin. These ingredients become rapidly available for absorption as the tablet begins disintegrating in the stomach. The pepsin supplements the stomach's digestive secretions by aiding the breakdown of proteins into proteoses and peptones. Spasmolysis and sedation are produced as the belladonna alkaloids and phenobarbital are absorbed.

The core of the tablet containing pancreatin and bile salts is designed to break down only in an alkaline medium and therefore does not release its components until it reaches the duodenum. The pancreatin with its trypsin, amylase and lipase components is therefore released in this area in an enzymatically active state, along with the bile salts. Trypsin breaks down larger protein fractions into peptides; amylase converts starch into maltose; lipase splits fat into fatty acids and glycerin; and bile salts not only enhance the fat-splitting action of the lipase but also aid the emulsification of fats and the absorption of fatty acids.

Donnazyme is particularly useful for symptomatic relief of G-I disorders that prove purely functional and are devoid of organic pathology. It is especially recommended for the multitude of symptoms attending "nervous indigestion."

In patients over 40 years old with visceral complaints, decreased digestive enzyme secretory activity is frequently suspect, and in these patients Donnazyme may prove especially useful. It is also indicated for symptomatic relief of chronic pancreatitis, chronic gastritis, postcholecystectomy syndrome, and chronic biliary disorders.

Contraindications: Acute glaucoma, advanced renal or hepatic disease, biliary tract obstruction or a hypersensitivity to any of the ingredients.

Precautions: Administer with caution to patients with incipient glaucoma or prostatic hypertrophy. Phenobarbital in prolonged and excessive dosage may be habit forming.

Adverse Reactions: Blurring of vision, dry mouth, and difficult urination may occur at higher dosage levels, rarely on usual dosage.

Dosage: Adult dosage: two tablets after each meal.

Continued on next page

Prescribing information on A. H. Robins products listed here is based on official labeling in effect August 1, 1979, with Indications, Contraindications, Warnings, Precautions, Adverse Reactions, and Dosage stated in full.

Robins—Cont.

How Supplied: Donnazyme®—Kelly green tablets in bottles of 100 and 500 (NDC 0031-4649).

[*Shown in Product Identification Section*]

DOPRAM® INJECTABLE ℞

brand of Doxapram Hydrochloride Injection, NF

Composition: Each 1 ml contains:
Doxapram Hydrochloride, NF..............20 mg.
Water for Injection, USP ....q.s.
Chlorobutanol, USP (as preservative)......0.5%

Actions: Doxapram hydrochloride produces respiratory stimulation mediated through the peripheral carotid chemoreceptors. As the dosage level is increased, the central respiratory centers in the medulla are stimulated with progressive stimulation of other parts of the brain and spinal cord.

The onset of respiratory stimulation following the recommended single intravenous injection of doxapram hydrochloride usually occurs in 20–40 seconds with peak effect at 1–2 minutes. The duration of effect may vary from 5–12 minutes.

The respiratory stimulant action is manifested by an increase in tidal volume associated with a slight increase in respiratory rate.

A pressor response may result following doxapram administration. Provided there is no impairment of cardiac function, the pressor effect is more marked in hypovolemic than in normovolemic states. The pressor response is due to the improved cardiac output rather than peripheral vasoconstriction. Following doxapram administration an increased release of catecholamines has been noted.

Although opiate induced respiratory depression is antagonized by doxapram, the analgesic effect is not affected.

Indications:

1. ***Post-anesthesia.***
 a. When the possibility of airway obstruction and/or hypoxia have been eliminated, doxapram may be used to stimulate respiration in patients with drug-induced postanesthesia respiratory depression or apnea other than that due to muscle relaxant drugs.
 b. To pharmacologically stimulate deep breathing in the so-called "stir-up" regimen in the postoperative patient. (Simultaneous administration of oxygen is desirable.)
2. ***Drug-induced central nervous system depression.***
 Exercising care to prevent vomiting and aspiration, doxapram may be used to stimulate respiration, hasten arousal, and to encourage the return of laryngopharyngeal reflexes in patients with mild to moderate respiratory and CNS depression due to drug overdosage.
3. ***Chronic pulmonary disease associated with acute hypercapnia.***
 Doxaram is indicated as a temporary measure in hospitalized patients with acute respiratory insufficiency superimposed on chronic obstructive pulmonary disease. Its use should be for a short period of time (approximately 2 hours) as an aid in the prevention of elevation of arterial CO_2 tension during the administration of oxygen. It should not be used in conjuction with mechanical ventilation. The adequacy of ventilation MUST be assessed by measurements of arterial blood gases as well as careful monitoring of the cardiovascular indices.

Contraindications:

1. ***General Contraindications.***
 Doxapram is not recommended in the following conditions: epilepsy and other convulsive states; incompetence of the ventilatory mechanism due to muscle paresis, flail chest, pneumothorax, airway obstruction, and extreme dyspnea; severe hypertension and cerebrovascular accidents; hypersensitivity to doxapram; evidence of head injury.
2. ***Contraindications in pulmonary disease.***
 Doxapram is not recommended in the following conditions: strongly suspected or confirmed pulmonary embolism, pneumothorax, acute bronchial asthma, respiratory failure due to neuromuscular disorders, and in restrictive respiratory diseases such as pulmonary fibrosis.
3. ***Contraindications in cardiovascular disease.***
 Doxapram is not recommended in the following conditions: coronary artery disease, frank uncompensated heart failure.

Warnings:

1. ***Warning in post-anesthetic use.***
 a. Doxapram is neither an antagonist to muscle relaxant drugs nor a specific narcotic antagonist. Adequacy of airway and oxygenation must be assured prior to doxapram administration.
 b. Doxapram should be administered with great care and only under close supervision to patients with cerebral edema, history of bronchial asthma, severe tachycardia, cardiac arrhythmia, cardiac disease, hyperthyroidism, or pheochromocytoma.
 c. Since narcosis may recur after stimulation with doxapram, care should be taken to maintain close observation until the patient has been fully alert for ½ to 1 hour.
2. ***Warning in drug-induced CNS and respiratory depression.***
 Doxapram alone may not stimulate adequate spontaneous breathing or provide sufficient arousal in patients who are ***severely*** depressed either due to respiratory failure or to CNS depressant drugs, but should be used as an adjunct to establish supportive measures and resuscitative techniques.
3. ***Warning in chronic obstructive pulmonary disease.***
 a. In an attempt to lower pCO_2, the rate of infusion of doxapram should not be increased in severely ill patients because of the associated increased work in breathing.
 b. Doxapram should not be used in conjunction with mechanical ventilation.
4. ***Warning in pregnancy.***
 Clinically the safe use of doxapram in pregnancy has not been established. The physician must weigh the need against possible risks in using the drug in pregnant patients or in women of childbearing potential.
5. ***Warning in children 12 years of age and under.***
 Doxapram is not recommended for use in patients 12 years of age or under because studies to adequately evaluate its safety and efficacy have not been performed.

Precautions:

1. ***General precautions.***
 a. An adequate airway is essential.
 b. Recommended dosages of doxapram should be employed and maximum total dosages should not be exceeded. In order to avoid side effects, it is advisable to use the minimum effective dosage.
 c. Monitoring of the blood pressure and deep tendon reflexes is recommended to prevent overdosage.
 d. Vascular extravasation or use of a single injection site over an extended period should be avoided since either may lead to thrombophlebitis or local skin irritation.
 e. Rapid infusion may result in hemolysis.
 f. Lowered pCO_2 induced by hyperventilation produces cerebral vasoconstriction and slowing of the cerebral circulation. This should be taken into consideration on an individual basis.
 g. Intravenous short-acting barbiturates, oxygen and resuscitative equipment should be readily available to manage overdosage manifested by excessive central nervous system stimulation. Slow administration of the drug, careful observation of the patient during administration and for some time subsequently, are advisable. These precautions are to assure that the protective reflexes have been restored and to prevent possible posthyperventilation hypoventilation.
 h. Doxapram should be administered cautiously to patients receiving sympathomimetic or monoamine oxidase inhibiting drugs, since an additive pressor effect may occur.
 i. Blood pressure increases are generally modest but significant increases have been noted in some patients. Because of this doxapram is not recommended for use in severe hypertension (see Contraindications).
 j. If sudden hypotension or dyspnea develops, doxapram should be stopped.
2. ***Precautions in post-anesthetic use.***
 a. In patients who have received muscle relaxants, doxapram may temporarily mask the residual effects of muscle relaxant drugs.
 b. Since an increase in epinephrine release has been noted with doxapram, it is recommended that initiation of therapy be delayed for at least 10 minutes following the discontinuance of anesthetics known to sensitize the myocardium to catecholamines, such as halothane, cyclopropane and enflurane.
 c. The same consideration to pre-existing disease states should be exercised as in non-anesthetized individuals. See Contraindications and Warnings covering use in hypertension, asthma, disturbances of respiratory mechanics including airway obstruction, CNS disorders including increased cerebrospinal fluid pressure, convulsive disorders, acute agitation, and profound metabolic disorders.
3. ***Precautions in chronic obstructive pulmonary disease.***
 a. Arrhythmias seen in some patients in acute respiratory failure secondary to chronic obstructive pulmonary disease are probably the result of hypoxia. Doxapram should be used with caution in these patients.
 b. Arterial blood gases should be drawn prior to the initiation of doxapram infusion and oxygen administration, then at least every ½ hour. Doxapram administration does not diminish the need for careful monitoring of the patient or the need for supplemental oxygen in patients with acute respiratory failure. Doxapram should be stopped if the arterial blood gases deteriorate, and mechanical ventilation initiated.

Adverse Reactions: The following adverse reactions have been reported:

1. ***Central and autonomic nervous systems.***
 Headache, dizziness, apprehension, disorientation, pupillary dilatation, hyperactivity, involuntary movements, convulsions, muscle spasticity, increased deep tendon reflexes, clonus, bilateral Babinski; pyrexia, flushing, sweating; pruritus and paresthesia such as a feeling of warmth, burning, or hot sensation especially in the area of genitalia and perineum.
2. ***Respiratory***
 Cough, dyspnea, tachypnea, laryngospasm, bronchospasm, hiccough, and rebound hypoventilation.
3. ***Cardiovascular.***
 Phlebitis, variations in heart rate, lowered T-waves, arrhythmias, chest pain, tightness in chest. A mild to moderate increase in blood pressure is commonly noted. The elevation in blood pressure may be of concern only in hypertensive patients. (See Contraindications.)

4. ***Gastrointestinal.***
Nausea, vomiting, diarrhea, desire to defecate.
5. ***Genitourinary.***
Urinary retention, stimulation of urinary bladder with spontaneous voiding.
6. ***Laboratory determinations.***
A decrease in hemoglobin, hematocrit, or red blood cell count has been observed in postoperative patients. In the presence of preexisting leukopenia, a further decrease in WBC has been observed following anesthesia and treatment with doxapram hydrochloride. Elevation of BUN and albuminuria have also been observed. As some of the patients cited above had received multiple drugs concomitantly, a cause and effect relationship could not be determined.

Dosage and Administration:

1. Doxapram hydrochloride is compatible with 5% and 10% dextrose in water or normal saline. ADMIXTURE OF DOXAPRAM WITH ALKALINE SOLUTIONS SUCH AS 2.5% THIOPENTAL SODIUM OR BICARBONATE WILL RESULT IN PRECIPITATION.
2. ***In post-anesthetic use.***
a. By i.v. injection (see Table I. Dosage for post-anesthetic use—I.V.)
b. By infusion. The solution is prepared by adding 250 mg of doxapram (12.5 ml) to 250 ml of dextrose or saline solution. The infusion is initiated at a rate of approximately 5 mg/minute until a satisfactory respiratory response is observed, and maintained at a rate of 1–3 mg/minute. The rate of infusion should be adjusted to sustain the desired level of respiratory stimulation with a minimum of side effects. The recommended total dosage by infusion is 4 mg/kg (2.0 mg/lb), not to exceed 3 grams.
3. ***In the management of drug-induced CNS depression.***
(See Table II. Dosage for drug-induced CNS depression.)

METHOD ONE

Using Single and/or Repeat Single I.V. ***Injections.***

a. Give priming dose of 1.0 mg/lb (2.0 mg/kg) body weight and repeat in 5 minutes.
b. Repeat same dose q1–2h until patient wakens. Watch for relapse into unconsciousness or development of respiratory depression, since Dopram does not affect the metabolism of CNS-depressant drugs.
c. If relapse occurs, resume 1–2 hourly injections until arousal is sustained, or total maximum daily dose (3 grams) is given. Allow patient to sleep until 24 hours have elapsed from first injection of Dopram, using assisted or automatic respiration if necessary.
d. Repeat procedure until patient breathes spontaneously and sustains desired level of consciousness, or until maximum dosage (3 grams) is given.
e. Repetitive doses should be administered only to patients who have shown response to the initial dose.
f. Failure to respond appropriately indicates the need for neurologic evaluation for a possible central nervous system source of sustained coma.

Table I. Dosage for post-anesthetic use—I.V.

I.V. Administration	Recommended dosage mg/kg	mg/lb	Maximum dose per single injection mg/kg	mg/lb	Maximum total dose mg/kg	mg/lb
Single Injection	0.5–1.0	0.25–0.5	1.5	0.70	1.5	0.70
Repeat Injections (5 min. intervals)	0.5–1.0	0.25–0.5	1.5	0.70	2.0	1.0
Infusion	0.5–1.0	0.25–0.5	—	—	4.0	2.0

METHOD TWO

By Intermittent I.V. ***Infusion.***

a. Give priming dose as in Method One.
b. If patient wakens, watch for relapse; if no response, continue general supportive treatment for 1–2 hours and repeat Dopram. If some respiratory stimulation occurs, prepare I.V. infusion by adding 250 mg of Dopram (12.5 ml) to 250 ml of saline or dextrose solution. Deliver at rate of 1–3 mg/min (60–180 ml/hr) according to size of patient and depth of coma. Discontinue Dopram if patient begins to waken or at end of 2 hours.
c. Continue supportive treatment for ½ to 2 hours and repeat Step b.
d. Do not exceed 3 grams.

4. ***Chronic obstructive pulmonary disease associated with acute hypercapnia.***
a. One vial of doxapram (400 mg) should be mixed with 180 ml of the intravenous solution (concentration of 2.0 mg/ml). The infusion should be started at 1–2 mg/minute (½–1 ml/minute); if indicated, increase to a maximum of 3 mg/minute. Arterial blood gases should be determined prior to the onset of doxapram's administration and at least every half hour during the two hours of infusion to insure against the insidious development of CO_2-RETENTION AND ACIDOSIS. Alteration of oxygen concentration or flow rate may necessitate adjustment in the rate of doxapram infusion.
b. Predictable blood gas patterns are more readily established with a continuous infusion of doxapram. If the blood gases show evidence of deterioration, the infusion of doxapram should be discontinued.
c. ADDITIONAL INFUSIONS BEYOND THE SINGLE MAXIMUM TWO HOUR ADMINISTRATION PERIOD ARE NOT RECOMMENDED.

Overdosage: Excessive pressor effect, tachycardia, skeletal muscle hyperactivity, and enhanced deep tendon reflexes may be early signs of overdosage. Therefore, the blood pressure, pulse rate, and deep tendon reflexes should be evaluated periodically and the dosage or infusion rate adjusted accordingly. Convulsive seizures are unlikely at recommended dosages, but intravenous anticonvulsants, oxygen, and resuscitative equipment should be available.

How Supplied: Dopram Injectable (doxapram hydrochloride injection) is available in 20 ml multiple dose vials containing 20 mg of doxapram hydrochloride per ml, 20 mg/ml, with chlorobutanol 0.5% as the preservative (NDC 0031-4849).
Additional literature available upon request.

Table II. Dosage for drug-induced CNS depression.

Level of Depression	METHOD ONE Priming dose single/repeat i.v. injection mg/kg	mg/lb	METHOD TWO Rate of intermittent i.v. infusion mg/kg/hr	mg/lb/hr
Mild*	1.0	0.5	1.0–2.0	0.5–1.0
Moderate†	2.0	1.0	2.0–3.0	1.0–1.5

*Mild Depression
Class 0: Asleep, but can be aroused and can answer questions.
Class 1: Comatose, will withdraw from painful stimuli, reflexes intact.

†Moderate Depression
Class 2: Comatose, will not withdraw from painful stimuli, reflexes intact.
Class 3: Comatose, reflexes absent, no depression of circulation or respiration.

ENTOZYME® TABLETS ℞

Composition: Each tablet contains:

Pancreatin, NF equivalent	300 mg
Pepsin	250 mg
Bile salts	150 mg

Action and Uses: Entozyme should be considered a form of nutritional therapy as it is made up of naturally occurring digestive enzymes. Entozyme enhances proteolysis by its peptic and tryptic activity, carbohydrate digestion by amylolytic activity, and fat emulsification and transport by lipolytic activity and the action of the bile salts. The components of six Entozyme tablets will digest 60 grams of fat, 48 grams of protein, and 48 grams of carbohydrate, amounts of food principles that yield nearly 1,000 calories (one-third to one-half of many daily caloric intakes).

By effectively supplementing the patient's secretion of digestive enzymes, Entozyme promotes more complete digestion of carbohydrates, proteins, and fats.

Entozyme is primarily indicated for the management of gastrointestinal disturbances associated with a diminished secretion of pancreatic enzymes, such as pancreatitis, pancreatic fibrosis, and the postpancreatectomy state. It is also recommended for the relief of steatorrhea and such symptoms as pyrosis, flatulence, or belching associated with conditions such as cholecystitis, postcholecystectomy syndrome, subtotal gastrectomy and miscellaneous vague digestive complaints of patients with no evidence of specific disease entity. Digestive enzyme secretion is frequently diminished in older persons, and Entozyme may therefore be useful in maintaining adequate nutrition for geriatric patients. "Since protein malnutrition may be the most significant factor in the etiol-

Continued on next page

Prescribing information on A. H. Robins products listed here is based on official labeling in effect August 1, 1979, with Indications, Contraindications, Warnings, Precautions, Adverse Reactions, and Dosage stated in full.

Robins—Cont.

ogy of many chronic diseases, it seems to be logical to provide an adquate and qualitatively well-balanced protein diet, as well as the enzymes for its proper digestion."

Construction: Entozyme is a specially constructed tablet with an outer layer that dissolves quickly in the stomach and releases pepsin, and an "inner tablet" protected by an enteric coating that disintegrates in the alkaline medium of the small intestine and releases pancreatin and bile salts. This enables the pancreatin to pass safely through the stomach and arrive in the small intestine without losing its digestive potency.

Contraindications: Biliary tract obstruction. Hypersensitivity to any of the ingredients.

Adverse Reactions: Rash may occur in patients hypersensitive to any of the ingredients.

Dosage: Two tablets after each meal, or as directed. Entozyme tablets should not be crushed or chewed, but swallowed whole.

How Supplied: White, coated tablets, monogrammed "AHR," in bottles of 100 and 500 (NDC 0031-5049).

[*Shown in Product Identification Section*]

EXNA® TABLETS ℞

brand of Benzthiazide Tablets, NF

Description: Each round, yellow scored Exna tablet contains benzthiazide 50 mg.

Action: The mechanism of action results in an interference with the renal tubular mechanism of electrolyte reabsorption. At maximal therapeutic dosage all thiazides are approximately equal in their diuretic potency. The mechanism whereby thiazides function in the control of hypertension is unknown.

Indications: Exna (benzthiazide) is indicated as adjunctive therapy in edema associated with congestive heart failure, hepatic cirrhosis and corticosteroid and estrogen therapy.

Exna has also been found useful in edema due to various forms of renal dysfunction as: nephrotic syndrome; acute glomerulonephritis; and chronic renal failure.

Exna is indicated in the management of hypertension either as the sole therapeutic agent or to enhance the effectiveness of other antihypertensive drugs in the more severe forms of hypertension.

Usage in Pregnancy. The routine use of diuretics in an otherwise healthy woman is inappropriate and exposes mother and fetus to unnecessary hazard. Diuretics do not prevent development of toxemia of pregnancy, and there is no satisfactory evidence that they are useful in the treatment of developed toxemia.

Edema during pregnancy may arise from pathological causes or from the physiologic and mechanical consequences of pregnancy. Thiazides are indicated in pregnancy when edema is due to pathologic causes, just as they are in the absence of pregnancy (however, see Warnings). Dependent edema in pregnancy, resulting from restriction of venous return by the expanded uterus, is properly treated through elevation of the lower extremities and use of support hose; use of diuretics to lower intravascular volume in this case is illogical and unnecessary. There is hypervolemia during normal pregnancy which is harmful to neither the fetus nor the mother (in the absence of cardiovascular disease), but which is associated with edema, including generalized edema, in the majority of pregnant women. If this edema produces discomfort, increased recumbency will often provide relief. In rare instances, this edema may cause extreme discomfort which is not relieved by rest. In these cases, a short course of diuretics may provide relief and may be appropriate.

Contraindications: Anuria. Hypersensitivity to this or other sulfonamide derived drugs.

Warnings: Thiazides should be used with caution in severe renal disease. In patients with renal disease, thiazides may precipitate azotemia. Cumulative effects of the drug may develop in patients with impaired renal function. Thiazides should be used with caution in patients with impaired hepatic function or progressive liver disease, since minor alterations of fluid and electrolyte balance may precipitate hepatic coma.

Thiazides may add to or potentiate the action of other antihypertensive drugs. Potentiation occurs with ganglionic or peripheral adrenergic blocking drugs.

Sensitivity reactions may occur in patients with a history of allergy or bronchial asthma. The possibility of exacerbation or activation of systemic lupus erythematosus has been reported.

Usage in Pregnancy: Thiazides cross the placental barrier and appear in cord blood. The use of thiazides in pregnant women requires that the anticipated benefit be weighed against possible hazards to the fetus. These hazards include fetal or neonatal jaundice, thrombocytopenia, and possibly other adverse reactions which have occurred in the adult.

Nursing Mothers. Thiazides appear in breast milk. If use of the drug is deemed essential, the patient should stop nursing.

Precautions: Periodic determination of serum electrolytes to detect possible electrolyte imbalance should be performed at appropriate intervals.

All patients receiving thiazide therapy should be observed for clinical signs of fluid or electrolyte imbalance; namely, hyponatremia, hypochloremic alkalosis, and hypokalemia. Serum and urine electrolyte determinations are particularly important when the patient is vomiting excessively or receiving parenteral fluids. Medication such as digitalis may also influence serum electrolytes. Warning signs, irrespective of cause, are: dryness of mouth, thirst, weakness, lethargy, drowsiness, restlessness, muscle pains or cramps, muscular fatigue, hypotension, oliguria, tachycardia, and gastrointestinal disturbances such as nausea and vomiting.

Hypokalemia may develop with thiazides as with any other potent diuretic especially with brisk diuresis, when severe cirrhosis is present or during concomitant use of corticosteroids or ACTH.

Interference with adequate oral electrolyte intake will also contribute to hypokalemia. Digitalis therapy may exaggerate metabolic effects of hypokalemia especially with reference to myocardial activity.

Any chloride deficit is generally mild and usually does not require specific treatment except under extraordinary circumstances (as in liver disease or renal disease). Dilutional hyponatremia may occur in edematous patients in hot weather; appropriate therapy is water restriction, rather than administration of salt except in rare instances when the hyponatremia is life threatening. In actual salt depletion, appropriate replacement is the therapy of choice.

Hyperuricemia may occur or frank gout may be precipitated in certain patients receiving thiazide therapy.

Insulin requirements in diabetic patients may be increased, decreased, or unchanged. Latent diabetes mellitus may become manifest during thiazide administration.

Thiazide drugs may increase the responsiveness to tubocurarine.

The antihypertensive effects of the drug may be enhanced in the postsympathectomy patient.

Thiazides may decrease arterial responsiveness to norepinephrine. This diminution is not sufficient to preclude effectiveness of the pressor agent for therapeutic use.

If progressive renal impairment becomes evident, as indicated by a rising nonprotein nitrogen or blood urea nitrogen, a careful reappraisal of therapy is necessary with consideration given to withholding or discontinuing diuretic therapy.

Thiazides may decrease serum PBI levels without signs of thyroid disturbance.

Adverse Reactions: ***Gastrointestinal System Reaction:*** anorexia; gastric irritation; nausea; vomiting, cramping; diarrhea; constipation; jaundice (intrahepatic cholestatic jaundice); pancreatitis.

Central Nervous System Reactions: dizziness; vertigo; parasthesias; headache; xanthopsia.

Hematologic Reactions: leukopenia, agranulocytosis; thrombocytopenia; aplastic anemia.

Dermatologic-Hypersensitivity Reactions: purpura; photosensitivity; rash; urticaria; necrotizing angiitis (vasculitis) (cutaneous vasculitis).

Cardiovascular Reaction: Orthostatic hypotension may occur and may be aggravated by alcohol, barbiturates or narcotics.

Other: hyperglycemia; glycosuria; hyperuricemia; muscle spasm; weakness; restlessness.

Whenever adverse reactions are moderate or severe, thiazide dosage should be reduced or therapy withdrawn.

Dosage and Administration: Therapy should be individualized according to patient response. This therapy should be titrated to gain maximal therapeutic response as well as the minimal dose possible to maintain that therapeutic response.

	Diuretic	Antihypertensive
Benzthiazide	50 to 200 mg	50 to 200 mg

Edema: ***Initiation of diuresis:*** 50 to 200 mg daily should be used for several days, or until dry weight is attained. With 100 mg or more daily, it is generally preferable to administer benzthiazide in two doses, following morning and evening meals.

Maintenance of diuresis: 50 to 150 mg daily depending upon the patient's response. To maintain effectiveness, reduction to minimal effective dosage should be gradual.

Hypertension: *Initiation of antihypertensive therapy:* 50 to 100 mg daily is the average dose. It may be given in two doses of 25 mg or 50 mg each after breakfast and after lunch. This dosage may be continued until a therapeutic drop in blood pressure occurs.

Maintenance of antihypertensive therapy: Dosage should be adjusted according to the patient response, either upward to as much as 50 mg q.i.d., or downward to the minimal effective dosage level.

How Supplied: Exna (benzthiazide) is supplied in 50 mg yellow, scored tablets, packaged in bottles of 100 and 500. (NDC 0031-5449).

[*Shown in Product Identification Section*]

EXNA®-R TABLETS ℞

Composition: Each white, flat, scored tablet contains:

Benzthiazide, NF....................................50 mg.
Reserpine, USP ....0.125 mg.

Action: The mechanisms of action for Exna-R are presumably those currently postulated for the thiazide derivatives and reserpine, namely, the interference with arterial pressor mechanisms and reduction of extracellular fluid and plasma volume caused by thiazides plus the concurrent loss of catecholamines at adrenergic nerve endings induced by reserpine. The central action of reserpine in decreasing sympathetic outflow from the medullary centers, either by depressing the reticular activating system or by producing a parasympathetic dominance through effects on the hypothalamus, is similarly pertinent. While numerous and complex pharmacological effects have been recorded, the precise mechanisms whereby thiazides and reserpine function in the control of hypertension are unknown.

Indications: Based upon a review of thiazide-reserpine combination drugs by the National Academy of Sciences—National Research Council and/or other information, the FDA has classified Exna-R "Effective" for: Hypertension (See box warning).

> **Warning**
> This fixed combination drug is not indicated for initial therapy of hypertension. Hypertension requires therapy titrated to the individual patient. If the fixed combination represents the dosage so determined, its use may be more convenient in patient management. The treatment of hypertension is not static, but must be reevaluated as conditions in each patient warrant.

Contraindications:
Anuria.
Hypersensitivity to derivatives of any sulfonamide drugs or rauwolfia alkaloids; severe mental depression; active peptic ulcer or ulcerative colitis.
Electroshock therapy should not be given to patients who are receiving reserpine; severe or fatal reactions may occur. This drug should be withdrawn at least one week prior to electroshock therapy.
Progressive renal and progressive hepatic disease constitute relative contraindications to use of this drug.

Warnings: Reserpine should be avoided or administered with care in the presence of peptic ulcer disease.
Severe hypotension and bradycardia may develop during anesthesia in patients who have received reserpine therapy, and the thiazides may decrease arterial responsiveness to norepinephrine. Therefore, Exna-R should be withdrawn two weeks prior to elective surgery. If emergency surgery is indicated, pre-anesthetic and anesthetic agents should be administered in reduced dosage, especially in chronically ill or debilitated patients. When possible, the administration of opiates should be avoided.
In patients with renal disease the thiazide may precipitate or increase azotemia. Caution should be observed to avoid cumulative effects of the drug in patients with impaired renal function. In patients with severe hepatic disease, particularly those with a history of hepatic coma, electrolyte imbalance which may result from thiazide administration may precipitate hepatic coma.
Exna-R may be additive or potentiative of the action of other antihypertensive drugs. Potentiation occurs with ganglionic or peripheral adrenergic blocking drugs.
Sensitivity reactions due to thiazide may occur in patients with a history of allergy or bronchial asthma.
The possibility of exacerbation or activation of systemic lupus erythematosus has been reported with thiazides.

Usage in pregnancy: Usage of Exna-R in women of childbearing age requires that the potential benefits of the drug be weighed against its possible hazards to the fetus. The hazards of thiazides administered to pregnant patients include fetal or neonatal jaundice, thrombocytopenia, and possibly other adverse reactions which have occurred in the adult. Reserpine administered in late pregnancy may produce nasal congestion in the newborn which can cause serious respiratory difficulties.

Nursing mothers: Thiazides cross the placental barrier and appear in cord blood and breast milk. The safety of reserpine during lactation has not been established.

Precautions: The following laboratory determinations should be performed prior to and at appropriate intervals during therapy with Exna-R: serum electrolytes, BUN, uric acid, and blood sugar.
All patients receiving thiazide therapy should be observed for clinical signs of fluid or electrolyte imbalance; namely, hyponatremia, hypochloremic alkalosis, and hypokalemia. Serum and urine electrolyte determinations are particularly important when the patient is vomiting excessively or receiving parenteral fluids. Medication such as digitalis may also influence serum electrolytes. Warning signs, irrespective of cause, are: dryness of mouth, thirst, weakness, lethargy, drowsiness, restlessness, muscle pains or cramps, muscular fatigue, hypotension, oliguria, tachycardia, and gastrointestinal disturbances such as nausea and vomiting.
Hypokalemia may develop with thiazides as with any other potent diuretic, especially with brisk diuresis, when severe cirrhosis is present or during concomitant use of corticosteroids or ACTH. Caution should be exercised in the concomitant administration of digitalis and thiazide-reserpine combinations, since hypokalemia and reserpine may enhance the toxic effects of digitalis. Supplemental potassium may be indicated if the serum potassium is 4.0 mEq/liter or less, or if the patient is on digitalis.
Interference with adequate oral electrolyte intake will also contribute to hypokalemia. Digitalis therapy may exaggerate metabolic effects of hypokalemia especially with reference to myocardial activity.
Any chloride deficit induced by thiazides is generally mild and usually does not require specific treatment except under extraordinary circumstances (as in liver disease or renal disease). Dilutional hyponatremia may occur in edematous patients in hot weather; appropriate therapy is water restriction, rather than administration of salt except in rare instances when the hyponatremia is life threatening. In actual salt depletion, appropriate replacement is the therapy of choice.
Hyperuricemia may occur or frank gout may be precipitated in certain patients receiving thiazide therapy.
Insulin requirements in diabetic patients may be increased, decreased, or unchanged. Latent diabetes mellitus may become manifest during thiazide administration.
Thiazide drugs may increase the responsiveness to tubocurarine.
The antihypertensive effects of the drug may be enhanced in the postsympathectomy patient.
Thiazides may decrease arterial responsiveness to norepinephrine. This diminution is not sufficient to preclude effectiveness of the pressor agent for therapeutic use.
If progressive renal impairment becomes evident, as indicated by a rising nonprotein nitrogen or blood urea nitrogen, a careful reappraisal of therapy is necessary with consideration given to withholding or discontinuing thiazide therapy.
Thiazides may decrease serum PBI levels without signs of thyroid disturbance.
Reserpine should be used with great caution in patients with mild depression or a history of depression. The drug should be discontinued at the first sign of a developing depression or augmentation of a pre-existing one.
Reserpine may precipitate bronchial asthma in susceptible individuals or biliary colic in patients with gallstones.

Adverse Reactions: Adverse reactions reported in association with **thiazide therapy** include the following:
Gastrointestinal System Reactions: anorexia; gastric irritation; nausea; vomiting; cramping; diarrhea; constipation; jaundice (intrahepatic cholestatic jaundice); pancreatitis.
Central Nervous System Reactions: dizziness; vertigo; parasthesias; headache; xanthopsia.
Hematologic Reactions: leukopenia; agranulocytosis; thrombocytopenia; aplastic anemia.
Dermatologic - Hypersensitivity Reactions: purpura; photosensitivity; rash; urticaria; necrotizing angiitis (vasculitis) (cutaneous vasculitis).
Cardiovascular Reaction: Orthostatic hypotension may occur and may be aggravated by alcohol, barbiturates or narcotics.
Other: hyperglycemia; glycosuria; hyperuricemia; muscle spasm; weakness; restlessness.
Adverse reactions reported in association with **reserpine therapy** include the following:
Gastrointestinal System Reactions: gastrointestinal irritation; cramping; diarrhea (increased intestinal motility); gastrointestinal ulceration and hemorrhage, possibly secondary to increased gastric secretion; increased appetite and weight gain.
Central Nervous System Reactions: nightmares; psychic depression, sometimes severe; drowsiness; dizziness; headache; nystagmus; staggering gait; syncope; blurring of vision; CNS sensitization manifested by dull sensorium, deafness, glaucoma, uveitis and optic atrophy; anxiety.
Cardiovascular System Reactions: bradycardia; cardiac arrhythmias; angina-like syndrome; flushing.
Other: nasal stuffiness and/or epistaxis; conjunctival hyperemia; extrapyramidal disturbances, including parkinsonism; menstrual irregularities; galactorrhea; muscular weakness and aching; depression of libido or impotence; gynecomastia; dyspnea; fluid retention; dysuria; xerostomia or increased salivation; skin rashes and/or pruritus.
Whenever adverse reactions are moderate or severe, Exna-R dosage should be reduced or therapy withdrawn.

Dosage and Administration: As determined by titration of individual ingredients (see box warning).

How Supplied: Exna-R is supplied as white, flat, scored tablets containing 50 mg of benzthiazide and 0.125 mg of reserpine. Bottles of 100 and 500. (NDC 0031-5460).

[Shown in Product Identification Section]

HEPARIN SODIUM INJECTION, USP ℞

Description: Heparin Sodium Injection, USP is a sterile solution of heparin sodium derived from porcine intestines, standardized for use as an anticoagulant, in Water for Injection with sodium chloride, if needed for isotonicity, and may contain 1% benzyl alcohol as a preservative. See carton label for exact formula. The potency is determined by biological assay using a USP reference standard based on units of heparin activity per milligram.
Slight variations in the color of heparin sodium solutions do not affect the therapeutic efficacy.

Actions: Heparin inhibits reactions which lead to the clotting of blood and the formation of fibrin clots both *in vitro* and *in vivo*. Heparin acts at multiple sites in the normal coagulation system. Small amounts of heparin in combination with antithrombin III (heparin co-factor) can prevent the development of a hypercoagulable state by inactivating activated Factor X, preventing the conversion of prothrombin to thrombin. Once a hypercoagulable state exists, larger amounts of heparin in combination with antithrombin III can inhibit the coagulation process by inactivating thrombin and earlier clotting intermediates, thus preventing the conversion of fibrinogen to fibrin. Heparin also prevents the formation of a stable fibrin clot by

Continued on next page

Prescribing information on A. H. Robins products listed here is based on official labeling in effect August 1, 1979, with Indications, Contraindications, Warnings, Precautions, Adverse Reactions, and Dosage stated in full.

Robins—Cont.

inhibiting the activation of the fibrin stabilizing factor.
Bleeding time is usually unaffected by heparin. Clotting time is prolonged by full therapeutic doses of heparin; in most cases it is not measurably affected by low doses of heparin.
Heparin does not have fibrinolytic activity; therefore, it will not lyse existing clots.
Indications: Heparin Sodium Injection is indicated for anticoagulant therapy in prophylaxis and treatment of venous thrombosis and its extension; in low-dose regimen, for prevention of postoperative deep venous thrombosis and pulmonary embolism in patients undergoing major abdominothoracic surgery who are at risk of developing thromboembolic disease (see DOSAGE AND ADMINISTRATION section); for prophylaxis and treatment of pulmonary embolism; in atrial fibrillation with embolization; for diagnosis and treatment of acute and chronic consumptive coagulopathies (disseminated intravascular coagulation); for prevention of clotting in arterial and cardiac surgery; and for prevention of cerebral thrombosis in evolving stroke.
Heparin is indicated as an adjunct in treatment of coronary occlusion with acute myocardial infarction, and in prophylaxis and treatment of peripheral arterial embolism.
Heparin may also be employed as an anticoagulant in blood transfusions, extracorporeal circulation, dialysis procedures, and in blood samples for laboratory purposes.
Contraindications: Hypersensitivity to heparin.
Inability to perform suitable blood coagulation tests; e.g., the whole blood clotting time, partial thromboplastin time, etc., at required intervals. There is usually no need to monitor the effect of low-dose heparin in patients with normal coagulation parameters.
Uncontrollable bleeding.
WARNINGS

Heparin sodium should be used with extreme caution in disease states in which there is an increased danger of hemorrhage.

Administration of Heparin Sodium Injection, USP, when used in therapeutic dosage, should be regulated by frequent blood coagulation tests. If these are unduly prolonged or if hemorrhage occurs, heparin sodium should be promptly discontinued. See ***Overdosage*** section.
Some of the conditions in which increased danger of hemorrhage exists are:

Cardiovascular—subacute bacterial endocarditis; arterial sclerosis; increased capillary permeability; during and immediately following a) spinal tap or spinal anesthesia, b) major surgery, especially involving the brain, spinal cord, or eye.

Hematologic—conditions associated with increased bleeding tendencies such as hemophilia, some purpuras, and thrombocytopenia.

Gastrointestinal—inaccessible ulcerative lesions and continuous tube drainage of the stomach or small intestine.

Heparin sodium may prolong the one-stage prothrombin time. Accordingly, when heparin sodium is given with dicumarol or warfarin sodium, a period of at least 5 hours after the last intravenous dose and 24 hours after the last subcutaneous (intrafat) dose of heparin sodium should elapse before blood is drawn, if a valid prothrombin time is to be obtained.
Drugs (such as acetylsalicylic acid, dextran, phenylbutazone, ibuprofen, indomethacin, dipyridamole and hydroxychloroquine) which interfere with platelet aggregation reactions (the main hemostatic defense of heparinized patients) may induce bleeding and should be used with caution in patients on heparin therapy.
While there is experimental evidence that heparin may antagonize the action of ACTH, insulin, or corticoids, this effect has not been clearly defined.
There is also evidence in animal experiments that heparin may modify or inhibit allergic reactions. However, the application of these findings to human patients has not been fully defined.
Larger doses of heparin may be necessary in the febrile state.
The use of digitalis, tetracyclines, nicotine, or antihistamines may partially counteract the anticoagulant action of heparin. An increased resistance to heparin is frequently encountered in cases of thrombosis, thrombophelebitis, infections with thrombosing tendency, myocardial infarction, cancer, and in the postoperative patient.
Usage in Pregnancy: Heparin Sodium Injection should be used with caution during pregnancy, especially during the last trimester and in the immediate post partum period.
There is no adequate information as to whether heparin may affect human fertility, or have a teratogenic potential or other adverse effects to the fetus.
Heparin does not cross the placental barrier; it is not excreted in human milk.
Precautions: Because Heparin Sodium Injection is derived from animal tissue (porcine intestines), it should be used with caution in patients with a history of allergy. Before a therapeutic dose is given to such a patient, a trial dose of 1000 units may be advisable.
Heparin sodium should also be used with caution in the presence of hepatic or renal disease, hypertension, during menstruation, or in patients with indwelling catheters.
A higher incidence of bleeding may be seen in women over 60 years of age.
Caution should be exercised when administering ACD-converted blood (i.e., blood collected in heparin sodium and later converted to ACD blood), since the anticoagulant activity of its heparin sodium content persists without loss for 22 days. ACD-converted blood may alter the coagulation system of the recipient, especially if it is given in multiple transfusions.
Adverse Reactions: Hemorrhage is the chief complication that may result from heparin therapy. An overly prolonged clotting time or minor bleeding during therapy can usually be controlled by withdrawing the drug. See ***Overdosage*** section.
The occurrence of signficant gastrointestinal or urinary tract bleeding during anticoagulant therapy may indicate the presence of an underlying occult lesion.
Adrenal hemorrhage with resultant acute adrenal insufficiency has occurred during anticoagulant therapy. Therefore, such treatment should be discontinued in patients who develop signs and symptoms compatible with acute adrenal hemorrhage and insufficiency. Plasma cortisol levels should be measured immediately, and vigorous therapy with intravenous corticosteroids should be instituted promptly. Initiation of therapy should not depend upon laboratory confirmation of the diagnosis, since any delay in an acute situation may result in the patient's death.
Intramuscular injection of heparin sodium frequently causes local irritation, mild pain, or hematoma, and for these reasons should be avoided. These effects are less often seen following deep subcutaneous (intrafat) injection.
Histamine-like reactions have also been observed at the site of injection.
Hypersensitivity reactions have been reported, with chills, fever, and urticaria as the most usual manifestations. Asthma, rhinitis, lacrimation, and anaphylactoid reactions have also been reported. Vasospastic reactions may develop independent of the origin of heparin, 6 to 10 days after the initiation of therapy and last for 4 to 6 hours. The affected limb is painful, ischemic and cyanosed. An artery to this limb may have been recently catheterized. After repeat injections, the reaction may gradually increase to include generalized vasospasm with cyanosis, tachypnea, feeling of oppression, and headache. Protamine sulfate treatment has no marked therapeutic effect. Itching and burning, especially on the plantar side of the feet, is possibly based on a similar allergic vasospastic reaction. Chest pain, elevated blood pressure, arthralgias, and/or headache have also been reported in the absence of definite peripheral vasospasm. Anaphylactic shock has been reported, rarely following the intravenous administration of heparin sodium. Acute reversible thrombocytopenia following the intravenous administration of heparin sodium has been reported. Osteoporosis and suppression of renal function following long-term, high-dose administration of heparin sodium, and suppression of aldosterone synthesis, delayed transient alopecia, priapism, and rebound hyperlipemia following discontinuation of heparin sodium, have also been reported.
Dosage and Administration: Heparin sodium is not effective by oral administration and should be given by deep subcutaneous (intrafat, i.e., above iliac crest or into the abdominal fat layer) injection, by intermittent intravenous injection, or intravenous infusion. The intramuscular route of administration should be avoided because of the frequent occurrence of hematoma at the injection site.
The dosage of heparin sodium should be adjusted according to the patient's coagulation test results, which during the first day of treatment should be determined just prior to each injection. There is usually no need to monitor the effect of low-dose heparin in patients with normal coagulation parameters. Dosage is considered adequate when the whole blood clotting time is elevated approximately 2.5 to 3 times the control value.
When heparin sodium is administered by continuous intravenous infusion, coagulation tests should be performed approximately every 4 hours during the early stages of therapy. When it is administered intermittently by intravenous or deep subcutaneous (intrafat) injection, coagulation tests should be performed before each injection during the early stages of treatment, and daily thereafter.
When an oral anticoagulant of the coumadin or similar type is administered with heparin sodium, coagulation tests and prothrombin activity should be determined at the start of therapy. For immediate anticoagulant effect, administer heparin sodium in the usual therapeutic dosage. When the results of the initial prothrombin determination are known, administer the first dose of an oral anticoagulant in the usual initial amount. Thereafter, perform a coagulation test and determine the prothrombin activity of appropriate intervals. A period of at least 5 hours after the last intravenous dose and 24 hours after the last subcutaneous (intrafat) dose of heparin sodium should elapse before blood is drawn, if a valid prothrombin time is to be obtained. When the oral anticoagulant shows full effect and prothrombin activity is in the desired therapeutic range, heparin sodium may be discontinued and therapy continued with the oral anticoagulant.
Therapeutic Anticoagulant Effect with Full-Dose Heparin: Although dosage must be adjusted for the individual patient according to the results of suitable laboratory tests, the following dosage schedules may be used as guidelines:
[See table on next page].
1. ***By deep subcutaneous (Intrafat) Injection.***-
After an initial I.V. injection of 5,000 units, inject 10,000 to 20,000 units of a concentrated heparin sodium solution subcutaneously, followed by 8,000 to 10,000 units of a concen-

trated solution every eight hours, or 15,000 to 20,000 units of a concentrated solution every twelve hours. A different site should be used for each injection to prevent the development of a massive hematoma.

2. ***By intermittent intravenous Injection.*** 10,000 units initially, then 5,000 to 10,000 units every four to six hours. These amounts may be given either undiluted or diluted with 50 to 100 ml of isotonic sodium chloride injection.

3. ***By continuous Intravenous Infusion.*** After an initial I.V. injection of 5,000 units of heparin sodium, add 20,000 to 40,000 units to 1,000 ml of isotonic sodium chloride solution for infusion. For most patients, the rate of flow should be adjusted to deliver approximately 20,000 to 40,000 units in 24 hours.

Surgery of the Heart and Blood Vessels: Patients undergoing total body perfusion for open heart surgery should receive an initial dose of not less than 150 units of heparin sodium per kilogram of body weight. Frequently a dose of 300 units of heparin sodium per kilogram of body weight is used for procedures estimated to last less than 60 minutes; or 400 units per kilogram for those estimated to last longer than 60 minutes.

Low-Dose Prophylaxis of Postoperative Thromboembolism: A number of well-controlled clinical trials have demonstrated that low-dose heparin prophylaxis, given just prior to and after surgery, will reduce the incidence of postoperative deep vein thrombosis in the legs, as measured by the I-125 fibrinogen technique and venography, and clinical pulmonary embolism. The most widely used dosage has been 5,000 units 2 hours before surgery and 5,000 units every 8 to 12 hours thereafter for 7 days or until the patient is fully ambulatory, whichever is longer. The heparin is given by deep subcutaneous injection in the arm or abdomen with a fine needle (25-26 gauge) to minimize tissue trauma. A concentrated solution of heparin sodium is recommended. Such prophylaxis should be reserved for patients over 40 undergoing major surgery. Patients with bleeding disorders and those having neurosurgery, spinal anesthesia, eye surgery, or potentially sanguinous operations should be excluded, as well as patients receiving oral anticoagulants or platelet-active drugs (see ***Warnings***). The value of such prophylaxis in hip surgery has not been established. The possibility of increased bleeding during surgery or postoperatively should be borne in mind. If such bleeding occurs, discontinuance of heparin and neutralization with protamine sulfate is advisable. If clinical evidence of thrombo-embolism develops despite low-dose prophylaxis, full therapeutic doses of anticoagulants should be given unless contraindicated. All patients should be screened prior to heparinization to rule out bleeding disorders, and monitoring should be performed with appropriate coagulation tests just prior to surgery. Coagulation test values should be normal or only slightly elevated. There is usually no need for daily monitoring of the effect of low-dose heparin in patients with normal coagulation parameters.

Extracorporeal Dialysis Use: Follow equipment manufacturer's operating directions carefully.

Blood Transfusion: Add 400 to 600 USP units per 100 ml of whole blood. Usually, 7,500 USP units of heparin sodium are added to 100 ml of Sterile Sodium Chloride Injection (or 75,000 USP units per 1,000 ml of Sterile Sodium Chloride Injection) and mixed, and from this sterile solution, 6 to 8 ml is added per 100 ml of whole blood. Leukocyte counts should be performed on heparinized blood within two hours after addition of the heparin. Heparinized blood should not be used for isoagglutinin complement, erythrocyte fragility tests, or platelet counts.

Laboratory Samples: Addition of 70 to 150 units of heparin sodium per 10 to 20 ml sample

Method of Administration	Frequency	Recommended Dose [based on 150 lb (68 kg) patient]
Deep Subcutaneous (Intrafat) Injection	Initial Dose	5,000 units by I.V. injection followed by 10,000-20,000 units of a concentrated solution, subcutaneously
	Every 8 hours	8,000-10,000 units of a concentrated solution
	(or) Every 12 hours	15,000-20,000 units of a concentrated solution
Intermittent Intravenous Injection	Initial Dose	10,000 units, either undiluted or in 50-100 ml isotonic sodium chloride injection
	Every 4 to 6 hours	5,000-10,000 units, either undiluted or in 50-100 ml isotonic sodium chloride injection
Intravenous Infusion	Initial Dose	5,000 units by I.V. injection
	Continuous	20,000-40,000 units in 1,000 ml of isotonic sodium chloride solution for infusion/day

of whole blood is usually employed to prevent coagulation of the sample. See comments under "***Blood Transfusion.***"

Overdosage: Protamine sulfate (1% solution) by slow infusion will neutralize heparin. No more than 50 mg should be given very slowly, in any 10 minute period. Each mg of protamine sulfate neutralizes approximately 100 USP units of heparin (or 1.0 to 1.5 mg neutralize approximately 1.0 mg of heparin). Heparin derived from various animal sources requires different amounts of protamine sulfate for neutralization. This fact is of utmost importance during procedures of regional heparinization, including dialysis.

Decreasing amounts of protamine are required as time from last heparin injection increases. Thirty minutes after a dose of heparin, approximately 0.5 mg of protamine sulfate is sufficient to neutralize each 100 units of administered heparin. Blood or plasma transfusions may be necessary; these dilute but do not neutralize heparin.

How Supplied: 1000 USP units per ml—1ml single dose vials, 10 ml multiple dose vials, 30 ml multiple dose vials (NDC 0031-5501).
5000 USP units per ml—1 ml single dose vials, 10 ml multiple dose vials (NDC 0031-5502).
10,000 USP units per ml—1 ml single dose vials, 4 ml multiple dose vials (NDC 0031-5503).

Also Available: Heparin Lock Flush Solution, 100 USP units per ml, 2 ml single dose vials (NDC 0031-5506).

IMAVATE® TABLETS ℞

brand of Imipramine Hydrochloride Tablets, USP

Tablet Strengths: 25 and 50 mg

Description: Imipramine hydrochloride is a member of the dibenzazepine group of compounds. It is designated 5-[3-(Dimethyl-amino)-propyl]-10, 11-dihydro-5 H-dibenz [b,f] azepine Monohydrochloride. Its molecular weight is 316.9 and its empirical formula is $C_{19}H_{24}N_2 \cdot HCl$.

Imipramine hydrochloride is a white, crystalline substance that turns yellowish or reddish on long exposure to light. It is easily soluble in water, fairly soluble in acetone or alcohol, but almost insoluble in ether. It melts at 170–174°C.

Actions: The mechanism of action of imipramine hydrochloride is not definitely known. It does not appear to act primarily by stimulation of the central nervous system. The clinical effect is thought to be due to potentiation of adrenergic synapses by blocking uptake of norepinephrine at nerve endings.

Indications: For the relief of symptoms of depression. Endogenous depression is more likely to be alleviated than other depressive states.

Contraindications: The concomitant use of monoamine oxidase inhibiting compounds is contraindicated. Hyperpyretic crises or severe convulsive seizures may occur in patients receiving such combinations. The potentiation of adverse effects can be serious or even fatal. When it is desired to substitute imipramine hydrochloride, in patients receiving a monoamine oxidase inhibitor, as long an interval should elapse as the clinical situation will allow, with a minimum of 14 days. Initial dosage should be low and increases should be gradual and cautiously prescribed.

The drug is contraindicated during the acute recovery period after a myocardial infarction. Patients with a known hypersensitivity to this compound should not be given the drug. The possibility of cross-sensitivity to other dibenzazepine compounds should be kept in mind.

Warnings: ***Usage in Pregnancy:*** Safe use of imipramine hydrochloride during pregnancy and lactation has not been established; therefore, this drug should be administered to women who are or who might become pregnant, or to nursing mothers, only when the potential benefits clearly outweigh possible hazards. There have been clinical reports of congenital malformation associated with the use of this drug, but a causal relationship has not been confirmed. Animal reproduction studies with imipramine HCl have yielded inconclusive results. Oral studies in rats and mice at doses up to 2½ times, and in rabbits at doses up to 25 times the maximum human dose, showed no clear evidence of teratogenic potential, but subcutaneous studies showed a teratogenic effect in rabbits and equivocal teratogenicity in mice at respective doses up to 5 and

Continued on next page

Prescribing information on A. H. Robins products listed here is based on official labeling in effect August 1, 1979, with Indications, Contraindications, Warnings, Precautions, Adverse Reactions, and Dosage stated in full.

Robins—Cont.

6½ times the maximum human dose. Increased resorptions and stillbirths and decreased neonatal weights were seen in the oral as well as subcutaneous studies.
Extreme caution should be used when this drug is given to:
- patients with cardiovascular disease because of the possibility of conduction defects, arrhythmias, myocardial infarction, strokes and tachycardia;
- patients with increased intraocular pressure, history of urinary retention, or history of narrow-angle glaucoma because of the drug's anticholinergic properties;
- hyperthyroid patients or those on thyroid medication because of the possibility of cardiovascular toxicity;
- patients with a history of seizure disorder because this drug has been shown to lower the seizure threshold;
- patients receiving guanethidine or similar agents since imipramine hydrochloride may block the pharmacologic effects of these drugs.

Usage in Children: Pending evaluation of results from clinical trials in children, this drug is not recommended for use in patients under twelve years of age.
Since this drug may impair the mental and/or physical abilities required for the performance of tasks such as operation of an automobile or hazardous machinery, the patient should be cautioned accordingly.
Precautions: It should be kept in mind that the possibility of suicide in seriously depressed patients is inherent in the illness and may persist until significant remission occurs. Such patients should be carefully supervised during the early phase of treatment with imipramine hydrochloride and may require hospitalization. Prescriptions should be written for the smallest amount feasible.
Hypomanic or manic episodes may occur, particularly in patients with cyclic disorders. Such reactions may necessitate discontinuation of the drug. If needed, imipramine hydrochloride may be resumed in lower dosage when these episodes are relieved. Administration of a tranquilizer may be useful in controlling such episodes.
Prior to elective surgery, imipramine hydrochloride should be discontinued for as long as the clinical situation will allow.
An activation of the psychosis may occasionally be observed in schizophrenic patients and may require reduction of dosage and the addition of a phenothiazine.
In occasional susceptible patients or in those receiving anticholinergic drugs (including antiparkinsonism agents) in addition, the atropine-like effects may become more pronounced (e.g. paralytic ileus). Close supervision and careful adjustment of dosage is required when this drug is administered concomitantly with anticholinergic or sympathomimetic drugs.
Avoid the use of preparations, such as decongestants and local anesthetics, which contain any sympathomimetic amine (e.g., adrenalin, noradrenalin), since it has been reported that tricyclic antidepressants can potentiate the effects of catecholamines.
Patients should be warned that the concomitant use of alcoholic beverages may be associated with exaggerated effects.
Both elevation and lowering of blood sugar levels have been reported.
Concurrent administration of imipramine hydrochloride with electroshock therapy may increase the hazards; such treatment should be limited to those patients for whom it is essential, since there is limited clinical experience.
Adverse Reactions: Note: Although the listing which follows includes a few adverse reactions which have not been reported with this specific drug, the pharmacological similarities among the tricyclic antidepressant drugs require that each of the reactions be considered when imipramine hydrochloride is administered.
Cardiovascular: Hypotension, hypertension, tachycardia, palpitation, myocardial infarction, arrhythmias, heart block, stroke, falls.
Psychiatric: Confusional states (especially in the elderly) with hallucinations, disorientation, delusions; anxiety, restlessness, agitation; insomnia and nightmares; hypomania; exacerbation of psychosis.
Neurological: Numbness, tingling, paresthesias of extremities; incoordination, ataxia, tremors; peripheral neuropathy; extrapyramidal symptoms; seizures, alterations in EEG patterns; tinnitus.
Anticholinergic: Dry mouth, and, rarely, associated sublingual adenitis; blurred vision, disturbances of accommodation, mydriasis; constipation, paralytic ileus; urinary retention, delayed micturition, dilation of the urinary tract.
Allergic: Skin rash, petechiae, urticaria, itching, photosensitization (avoid excessive exposure to sunlight); edema (general or of face and tongue); drug fever; cross-sensitivity with desipramine.
Hematologic: Bone marrow depression including agranulocytosis; eosinophilia; purpura; thrombocytopenia. Leukocyte and differential counts should be performed in any patient who develops fever or sore throat during therapy; the drug should be discontinued if there is evidence of pathological neutrophil depression.
Gastrointestinal: Nausea and vomiting, anorexia, epigastric distress, diarrhea; peculiar taste, stomatitis, abdominal cramps, black tongue.
Endocrine: Gynecomastia in the male; breast enlargement and galactorrhea in the female; increased or decreased libido, impotence; testicular swelling; elevation or depression of blood sugar levels.
Other: Jaundice (simulating obstructive); altered liver function; weight gain or loss, perspiration; flushing; urinary frequency; drowsiness, dizziness, weakness and fatigue; headache; parotid swelling; alopecia.
Withdrawal Symptoms: Though not indicative of addiction, abrupt cessation of treatment after prolonged therapy may produce nausea, headache and malaise.
Dosage and Administration: Lower dosages are recommended for elderly patients and adolescents. Lower dosages are also recommended for outpatients as compared to hospitalized patients who will be under close supervision. Dosage should be initiated at a low level and increased gradually, noting carefully the clinical response and any evidence of intolerance. Following remission, maintenance medication may be required for a longer period of time, at the lowest dose that will maintain remission.
Usual Oral Adult Dose: Hospitalized patients—Initially, 100 mg/day in divided doses gradually increased to 200 mg/day as required. If no response after two weeks, increase to 250–300 mg/day.
Outpatients—Initially, 75 mg/day increased to 150 mg/day. Dosages over 200 mg/day are not recommended. Maintenance, 50–150 mg/day.
Adolescent and geriatric patients—Initially, 30–40 mg/day; it is generally not necessary to exceed 100 mg/day.
Overdosage: *Signs and Symptoms:* These may vary in severity depending on several factors, including the amount absorbed, age, interval between ingestion and start of treatment, etc. In infants and young children, especially, acute overdosage in any amount must be considered serious and potentially fatal.
CNS abnormalities may include drowsiness, stupor, coma, ataxia, restlessness, agitation, hyperactive reflexes, muscle rigidity, athetoid and choreiform movements, and convulsions. Cardiac abnormalities may include arrhythmia, tachycardia, ECG evidence of impaired conduction, and signs of congestive failure. Respiratory depression, cyanosis, hypotension, shock, vomiting, hyperpyrexia, mydriasis, and diaphoresis may also be present.
Treatment: Because CNS involvement, respiratory depression and cardiac arrhythmia can occur suddenly, hospitalization and close observation are necessary, even when the amount ingested is thought to be small or the initial degree of intoxication appears slight or moderate. All patients with ECG abnormalities should have continuous cardiac monitoring for at least 72 hours and be closely observed until well after cardiac status has returned to normal; relapses may occur after apparent recovery.
The ***slow*** intravenous administration of physostigmine salicylate has been reported to reverse most of the cardiovascular and CNS effects of overdosage with tricyclic antidepressants. In adults, 1 to 3 mg has been reported to be effective. In children, start with 0.5 mg and repeat at 5 minute intervals to determine the minimum effective dose; do not exceed 2 mg. Because of the short duration of action of physostigmine, repeat the effective dose at 30 to 60 minute intervals, as necessary. Avoid rapid injection to reduce the possibility of physostigmine-induced convulsions.
In the alert patient, empty the stomach promptly by induced emesis followed by lavage. In the obtunded patient, secure the airway with a cuffed endotracheal tube before beginning lavage (do not induce emesis). Continue lavage for 24 hours or longer, depending on the apparent severity of intoxication. Use normal or half-normal saline to avoid water intoxication, especially in children. Installation of activated charcoal slurry may help reduce absorption of imipramine.
Minimize external stimulation to reduce the tendency to convulsions. If anticonvulsants are necessary, diazepam, short-acting barbiturates, paraldehyde or methocarbamol may be useful. Do not use barbiturates if MAO inhibitors have been taken recently.
Maintain adequate respiratory exchange. Do not use respiratory stimulants.
Shock should be treated with supportive measures, such as intravenous fluids, oxygen and corticosteroids. Digitalis may increase conduction abnormalities and further irritate an already sensitized myocardium. If congestive heart failure necessitates rapid digitalization, particular care must be exercised.
Hyperpyrexia should be controlled by whatever external means are available, including ice packs and cooling sponge baths, if necessary.
Hemodialysis, peritoneal dialysis, exchange transfusions and forced diuresis have been generally reported as ineffective because of the rapid fixation of imipramine in tissues. Blood imipramine levels may not correlate with the degree of intoxication, and are unreliable indicators in the clinical management of the patient.
How Supplied: Imavate Tablets, brand of Imipramine Hydrochloride Tablets, USP (film-coated), 25 mg (coral) in bottles of 100 (NDC 0031-5625); and 50 mg (fuchsia) in bottles of 100 (NDC 0031-5650).

PABALATE® TABLETS
PABALATE®-SF TABLETS ℞

Composition: Each Pabalate tablet contains Sodium Salicylate, NF 0.3 g. Sodium Aminobenzoate 0.3 g.
Each Pabalate-SF (Sodium Free) tablet contains Potassium Salicylate 0.3 g. Potassium Aminobenzoate 0.3 g.
Actions and Uses: Pabalate tablets are indicated for the temporary relief of pain and in-

flammation associated with arthritis and rheumatism. Pabalate-SF tablets are indicated for the temporary relief of pain and inflammation associated with arthritis and rheumatism, complicated by conditions in which the restriction of sodium intake may be desirable, such as: congestive heart failure, essential hypertension, glomerulonephritis, and pregnancy.

Contraindications: Hypersensitivity to any of the ingredients. Presence of an active ulcer.

Warnings: Pabalate-SF—There have been several reports, published and unpublished, concerning non-specific small bowel lesions consisting of stenosis with or without ulceration, associated with the administration of enteric-coated thiazides with potassium salts. These lesions may occur with enteric-coated potassium tablets alone or when they are used with nonenteric-coated thiazides, or certain other oral diuretics.

These small bowel lesions have caused obstruction, hemorrhage and perforation. Surgery was frequently required and deaths have occurred.

Based on a large survey of physicians and hospitals, both American and foreign, the incidence of these lesions is low, and a causal relationship in man has not been definitely established.

Available information tends to implicate enteric-coated potassium salts although lesions of this type also occur spontaneously. Therefore, coated potassium-containing formulations should be administered only when indicated, and should be discontinued immediately if abdominal pain, distention, nausea, vomiting or gastrointestinal bleeding occur.

When prescribing Pabalate-SF for patients who are receiving concurrent potassium supplementation (e.g., to replace potassium excreted during thiazide therapy), it should be kept in mind that Pabalate-SF also contains potassium. A decrease in supplemental potassium dosage should be considered in order to help avoid hyperkalemia.

Precautions: When administered concurrently, aminobenzoic acid (PABA) inhibits the bacteriostatic action of sulfonamides. Hypoprothrombinemia has been observed during prolonged and intensive therapy with salicylates. If patients receiving such dosages are to undergo surgery, the prothrombin time should be determined. Pabalate is not recommended for persons on a sodium restricted diet.

Adverse Reactions: Nausea and gastrointestinal upset, fine rash with or without pruritus, and urticaria. The occasional occurrence of mild salicylism may require adjustment in dosage.

Dosage and Administration: The average adult dose of Pabalate and Pabalate-SF is two tablets four times daily. In acute exacerbations, the dose may be increased as required. Tablets should not be taken within one hour of ingesting milk or antacids, such as sodium bicarbonate.

How Supplied: Pabalate (yellow), (NDC 0031-5816) Pabalate-SF (Persian Rose), (NDC 0031-5883) enteric coated tablets, monogrammed AHR, in bottles of 100 and 500.

[*Shown in Product Identification Section*]

PHENAPHEN® WITH CODEINE NO. 2 ℞ Ⓒ

Codeine Phosphate, USP ....15 mg
(Warning: May be habit forming)
Acetaminophen, USP ....325 mg

PHENAPHEN® WITH CODEINE NO. 3 ℞ Ⓒ

Codeine Phosphate, USP ....30 mg
(Warning: May be habit forming)
Acetaminophen, USP ....325 mg

PHENAPHEN® WITH CODEINE NO. 4 ℞ Ⓒ

Codeine Phosphate, USP ....60 mg
(Warning: May be habit forming)
Acetaminophen, USP ....325 mg

Description: Acetaminophen, a non-salicylate, occurs as a white, odorless, crystalline powder which possesses a slightly bitter taste. Codeine is an alkaloid obtained from opium or prepared from morphine by methylation and occurs as colorless or white crystals. Codeine effloresces slowly in dry air and is affected by light.

Actions: Acetaminophen is an analgesic and antipyretic; codeine an analgesic and antitussive.

Indications: Phenaphen with Codeine No. 2 and Phenaphen with Codeine No. 3 are indicated for the relief of mild to moderate pain. Phenaphen with Codeine No. 4 is indicated for the relief of moderate to severe pain.

Contraindications: Hypersensitivity to acetaminophen or codeine.

Warnings: ***Drug dependence.*** Codeine can produce drug dependence of the morphine type, and therefore, has the potential for being abused. Psychic dependence, physical dependence and tolerance may develop upon repeated administration of this drug and it should be prescribed and administered with the same degree of caution appropriate to the user of other oral narcotic-containing medications. Like other narcotic-containing medications, the drug is subject to the Federal Controlled Substances Act.

Usage in ambulatory patients. Acetaminophen and codeine may impair the mental and/or physical abilities required for the performance of potentially hazardous tasks such as driving a car or operating machinery. The patient using this drug should be cautioned accordingly.

Interaction with other central nervous system depressants. Patients receiving other narcotic analgesics, general anesthetics, phenothiazines, tranquilizers, sedative-hypnotics or other CNS depressants (including alcohol) concomitantly with acetaminophen and codeine may exhibit an additive CNS depression. When such combined therapy is contemplated, the dose of one or both agents should be reduced.

Usage in Pregnancy. Safe use in pregnancy has not been established relative to possible adverse effects on fetal development. Therefore, acetaminophen and codeine should not be used in pregnant women unless, in the judgment of the physician, the potential benefits outweigh the possible hazards.

Precautions: ***Head injury and increased intracranial pressure.*** The respiratory depressant effects of narcotics and their capacity to elevate cerebrospinal fluid pressure may be markedly exaggerated in the presence of head injury, other intracranial lesions or a pre-existing increase in intracranial pressure. Furthermore, narcotics produce adverse reactions which may obscure the clinical course of patients with head injuries.

Acute abdominal condition. The administration of acetaminophen and codeine or other narcotics may obscure the diagnosis or clinical course in patients with acute abdominal conditions.

Special risk patients. Acetaminophen and codeine should be given with caution to certain patients such as the elderly or debilitated, and those with severe impairment of hepatic or renal function, hypothyroidism, Addison's disease, and prostatic hypertrophy or urethral stricture.

Adverse Reactions: The most frequently observed adverse reactions include lightheadedness, dizziness, sedation; nausea and vomiting. These effects seem to be more prominent in ambulatory than in nonambulatory patients, and some of these adverse reactions may be alleviated if the patient lies down.

Other adverse reactions include euphoria, dysphoria, constipation and pruritus.

Dosage and Administration: Dosage should be adjusted according to the severity of the pain and the response of the patient. It may occasionally be necessary to exceed the usual dosage recommended below in cases of more severe pain or in those patients who have become tolerant to the analgesic effect of narcotics. Phenaphen with codeine is given orally. The usual adult dose for Phenaphen with Codeine No. 2 and Phenaphen with Codeine No. 3 is one or two capsules every 4 hours as required. The usual adult dose for Phenaphen with Codeine No. 4 is one capsule every 4 hours as required.

Drug Interactions: The CNS depressant effect of acetaminophen and codeine may be additive with that of other CNS depressants. See WARNINGS.

Management of Overdosage: ***Signs and Symptoms.*** Serious overdose with acetaminophen and codeine is characterized by respiratory depression (a decrease in respiratory rate and/or tidal volume, Cheyne-Stokes respiration, cyanosis), extreme somnolence progressing to stupor or coma, skeletal muscle flaccidity, cold and clammy skin, and sometimes bradycardia and hypotension. In severe overdosage, apnea, circulatory collapse, cardiac arrest and death may occur. The ingestion of very large amounts of this drug may, in addition, result in acute hepatic toxicity.

Treatment. Primary attention should be given to the reestablishment of adequate respiratory exchange through provision of a patent airway and the institution of assisted or controlled ventilation. The narcotic antagonist, naloxone, is a specific antidote against respiratory depression which may result from overdosage or unusual sensitivity to narcotics, including codeine. Therefore, an appropriate dose of naloxone (usual initial adult dose: 0.4 mg) should be administered, preferably by the intravenous route, and simultaneously with efforts at respiratory resuscitation. Since the duration of action of codeine may exceed that of the antagonist, the patient should be kept under continued surveillance and repeated doses of the antagonist should be administered as needed to maintain adequate respiration.

An antagonist should not be administered in the absence of clinically significant respiratory or cardiovascular depression.

Oxygen, intravenous fluids, vasopressors and other supportive measures should be employed as indicated.

Gastric emptying may be useful in removing unabsorbed drug.

Acetaminophen in massive overdosage may cause hepatotoxicity in some patients. Clinical and laboratory evidence of hepatotoxicity may be delayed for up to one week. Close clinical monitoring and serial hepatic enzyme determinations are therefore recommended.

Treatment of acute acetaminophen overdosage is purely symptomatic.

How Supplied: ***Phenaphen with Codeine No. 2,*** black and yellow capsules (NDC 0031-6242) in bottles of 100 and 500 and Dis-Co® unit dose packs of 100 capsules (4 × 25).

Phenaphen with Codeine No. 3, black and green capsules (NDC 0031-6257), in bottles of 100 and 500 and Dis-Co® unit dose packs of 100 capsules (4 × 25).

Phenaphen with Codeine No. 4, green and white capsules (NDC 0031-6274), in bottles of 100 and 500 and Dis-Co® unit dose packs of 100 capsules (4 × 25).

Continued on next page

Prescribing information on A. H. Robins products listed here is based on official labeling in effect August 1, 1979, with Indications, Contraindications, Warnings, Precautions, Adverse Reactions, and Dosage stated in full.

Robins—Cont.

Also available without codeine as Phenaphen® Capsules and Tablets, each containing 325 mg of acetaminophen.
[*Shown in Product Identification Section*]

PHENAPHEN®-650 WITH CODEINE TABLETS ℞ ©

Each tablet contains:
Codeine Phosphate, USP .... 30 mg
(Warning: May be habit forming)
Acetaminophen, USP ....650 mg

Description: Acetaminophen, a non-salicylate, occurs as a white, odorless, crystalline powder which possesses a slightly bitter taste. Codeine is an alkaloid obtained from opium or prepared from morphine by methylation and occurs as colorless or white crystals. Codeine effloresces slowly in dry air and is affected by light.

Actions: Acetaminophen is an analgesic and antipyretic; codeine an analgesic and antitussive.

Indications: Phenaphen-650 with Codeine is indicated for the relief of mild to moderate pain.

Contraindications: Hypersensitivity to acetaminophen or codeine.

Warnings: ***Drug dependence.*** Codeine can produce drug dependence of the morphine type, and therefore, has the potential for being abused. Psychic dependence, physical dependence and tolerance may develop upon repeated administration of this drug and it should be prescribed and administered with the same degree of caution appropriate to the use of other oral narcotic-containing medications. Like other narcotic-containing medications, the drug is subject to the Federal Controlled Substances Act.

Usage in ambulatory patients. Acetaminophen and codeine may impair the mental and/or physical abilities required for the performance of potentially hazardous tasks such as driving a car or operating machinery. The patient using this drug should be cautioned accordingly.

Interaction with other central nervous system depressants. Patients receiving other narcotic analgesics, general anesthetics, phenothiazines, tranquilizers, sedative-hypnotics or other CNS depressants (including alcohol) concomitantly with acetaminophen and codeine may exhibit an additive CNS depression. When such combined therapy is contemplated, the dose of one or both agents should be reduced.

Usage in Pregnancy. Safe use in pregnancy has not been established relative to possible adverse effects on fetal development. Therefore, acetaminophen and codeine should not be used in pregnant women unless, in the judgment of the physician, the potential benefits outweigh the possible hazards.

Precautions: ***Head injury and increased intracranial pressure.*** The respiratory depressant effects of narcotics and their capacity to elevate cerebrospinal fluid pressure may be markedly exaggerated in the presence of head injury, other intracranial lesions or a pre-existing increase in intracranial pressure. Furthermore, narcotics produce adverse reactions which may obscure the clinical course of patients with head injuries.

Acute abdominal condition. The administration of acetaminophen and codeine or other narcotics may obscure the diagnosis or clinical course in patients with acute abdominal conditions.

Special risk patients. Acetaminophen and codeine should be given with caution to certain patients such as the elderly or debilitated, and those with severe impairment of hepatic or renal function, hypothyroidism. Addison's disease, and prostatic hypertrophy or urethral stricture.

Adverse Reactions: The most frequently observed adverse reactions include lightheadedness, dizziness, sedation; nausea and vomiting. These effects seem to be more prominent in ambulatory than in nonambulatory patients, and some of these adverse reactions may be alleviated if the patient lies down.
Other adverse reactions include euphoria, dysphoria, constipation and pruritus.

Dosage and Administration: Dosage should be adjusted according to the severity of the pain and the response of the patient. It may occasionally be necessary to exceed the usual dosage recommended below in cases of more severe pain or in those patients who have become tolerant to the analgesic effect of narcotics. Phenaphen-650 with Codeine is given orally. The usual adult dose for Phenaphen-650 with Codeine is one tablet every four hours as required.

Drug Interactions: The CNS depressant effect of acetaminophen and codeine may be additive with that of other CNS depressants. See WARNINGS.

Management of Overdosage: ***Signs and Symptoms.*** Serious overdose with acetaminophen and codeine is characterized by respiratory depression (a decrease in respiratory rate and/or tidal volume, Cheyne-Stokes respiration, cyanosis), extreme somnolence progressing to stupor or coma, skeletal muscle flaccidity, cold and clammy skin, and sometimes bradycardia and hypotension. In severe overdosage, apnea, circulatory collapse, cardiac arrest and death may occur. The ingestion of very large amounts of this drug may, in addition, result in acute hepatic toxicity.

Treatment. Primary attention should be given to the reestablishment of adequate respiratory exchange through provision of a patent airway and the institution of assisted or controlled ventilation. The narcotic antagonist, naloxone, is a specific antidote against respiratory depression which may result from overdosage or unusual sensitivity to narcotics, including codeine. Therefore, an appropriate dose of naloxone (usual initial adult dose: 0.4 mg) should be administered, preferably by the intravenous route, and simultaneously with efforts at respiratory resuscitation. Since the duration of action of codeine may exceed that of the antagonist, the patient should be kept under continued surveillance and repeated doses of the antagonist should be administered as needed to maintain adequate respiration.
An antagonist should not be administered in the absence of clinically significant respiratory or cardiovascular depression.
Oxygen, intravenous fluids, vasopressors and other supportive measures should be employed as indicated.
Gastric emptying may be useful in removing unabsorbed drug.
Acetaminophen in massive overdosage may cause hepatotoxicity in some patients. Clinical and laboratory evidence of hepatotoxicity may be delayed for up to one week. Close clinical monitoring and serial hepatic enzyme determinations are therefore recommended.
Treatment of acute acetaminophen overdosage is purely symptomatic.

How Supplied: Phenaphen-650 with Codeine is available as a scored, white, capsule-shaped compressed tablet, engraved AHR and 6251 (NDC 0031-6251), in bottles of 50.
[*Shown in Product Identification Section*]

PONDIMIN® TABLETS ℞ ©
brand of fenfluramine hydrochloride
Tablets—20 mg

Actions: Fenfluramine is a sympathomimetic amine the pharmacologic activity of which differs somewhat from that of the prototype drugs of this class used in obesity, the amphetamines, in appearing to produce more central nervous system depression than stimulation.
Tolerance has been demonstrated with all drugs of this class in which this phenomenon has been looked for.
Drugs of this class used in obesity are commonly known as "anorectics" or "anorexigenics." It has not been established, however, that the action of such drugs in treating obesity is primarily one of appetite suppression. Other central nervous system actions, or metabolic effects may be involved, for example.
Adult obese subjects instructed in dietary management and treated with "anorectic" drugs, lose more weight on the average than those treated with placebo and diet, as determined in relatively short-term trials.
The average magnitude of increased weight loss of drug-treated patients over placebo-treated is only a fraction of a pound a week. The rate of weight loss is greatest in the first weeks of therapy for both drug and placebo subjects and tends to decrease in succeeding weeks. The possible origins of the increased weight loss due to the various drug effects are not established. The average amount of weight loss associated with the use of an "anorectic" drug varies from trial to trial, and the increased weight loss appears to be related in part to variables other than the drug prescribed, such as the physician-investigator, the population treated and the diet prescribed. Studies do not permit conclusions as to the relative importance of the drug and non-drug factors on weight loss.
The natural history of obesity is measured in years, whereas the studies cited are restricted to a few weeks duration; thus, the total impact of drug-induced weight loss over that of diet alone must be considered clinically limited.

Indication: Pondimin is indicated in the management of exogenous obesity as a short-term (a few weeks) adjunct in a regimen of weight reduction based on caloric restriction. The limited usefulness of agents of this class (see "Actions") should be measured against possible risk factors inherent in their use such as those described below.

Contraindications: Glaucoma, hypersensitivity to fenfluramine or other sympathomimetic amines. During or within 14 days following the administration of monoamine oxidase inhibitors, since hypertensive crises may result. Patients with a history of drug abuse.
Do not administer fenfluramine to patients with alcoholism since psychiatric symptoms (paranoia, depression, psychosis) have been reported in a few such patients who had been administered this drug.

Warnings: When tolerance to the "anorectic" effect develops, the maximum recommended dose should not be exceeded in an attempt to increase the effect; rather, the drug should be discontinued.
Fenfluramine may impair the ability of the patient to engage in potentially hazardous activities such as operating machinery or driving a motor vehicle (see "Adverse Reactions"); the patient should be cautioned accordingly.
A fatal cardiac arrest has been reported shortly after the induction of anesthesia in a patient who had been taking fenfluramine prior to surgery. Fenfluramine may have a catecholamine-depleting effect when administered for prolonged periods of time; therefore, potent anesthetic agents should be administered with caution to patients taking fenfluramine. If general anesthesia cannot be avoided, full cardiac monitoring, and facilities for instant resuscitative measure are a minimum necessity.

Drug Dependence: Fenfluramine is related chemically to the amphetamines, although it differs somewhat pharmacologically. The amphetamines and related stimulant drugs have been extensively abused and can produce tolerance and severe psychological dependence, as well as other adverse organic and mental changes. In this regard, there has been a recent report of abuse of fenfluramine by subjects with a history of abuse of other drugs. Abuse of 80 to 400 milligrams of the drug has been reported to be associated with euphoria, derealization and perceptual changes. Fenfluramine did not produce signs of dependence in animals and appears to produce sedation more often than CNS stimulation at therapeutic doses. Its abuse potential appears qualitatively different from that of amphetamines. The possibility that fenfluramine may induce dependence should be kept in mind when evaluating the desirability of including the drug in the weight reduction programs of individual patients.

Usage in Pregnancy: Safe use in pregnancy has not been established. Reproduction studies in rats suggested an embryotoxic potential. However, additional reproduction studies in rabbits, mice and monkeys yielded negative results. Use of fenfluramine in women who are or may become pregnant requires that the potential benefit be weighed against the possible hazard to mother and infant.

Usage in Children: The safety and efficacy of fenfluramine in children under 12 years of age have not been established.

Precautions: Fenfluramine differs in its pharmacologic profile from other "anorectic" drugs with which the prescribing practitioner may be familiar. Correspondingly, there are possible adverse effects not associated with other "anorectics"; such effects include those of diarrhea, sedation, and depression. The possibility of these effects should be weighed against the possible advantage of decreased central nervous system stimulation and/or abuse potential.

Other CNS depressant drugs should be used with caution in patients taking fenfluramine, since the effects may be additive.

Use only with caution in hypertension, with monitoring of blood pressure, since evidence is insufficient to rule out a possible adverse effect on blood pressure in some hypertensive patients. The drug is not recommended in severely hypertensive patients. The drug is not recommended for patients with symptomatic cardiovascular disease including arrhythmias.

Fenfluramine may increase slightly the effect of antihypertensive drugs, e.g., guanethidine, methyldopa, reserpine.

Caution should be exercised in prescribing fenfluramine for patients with a history of mental depression. Further depression of mood may become evident while the patient is on fenfluramine or following withdrawal of fenfluramine.

Administer with caution to patients with alcoholism since psychiatric symptoms (paranoia, depression, psychosis) have been reported in a few such patients following the administration of fenfluramine.

Adverse Reactions: The most common secondary effects or adverse reactions of fenfluramine are drowsiness, diarrhea, and dry mouth. Less frequent adverse reactions reported in association with fenfluramine are:

Central Nervous System: Dizziness; confusion; incoordination; headache; elevated mood; depression; anxiety, nervousness, or tension; insomnia; weakness or fatigue; increased or decreased libido; agitation, dysarthria;

Gastrointestinal: Constipation, abdominal pain; nausea;

Autonomic: Sweating; chills; blurred vision;

Genitourinary: Dysuria; urinary frequency;

Cardiovascular: Palpitation; hypotension; hypertension; fainting;

Skin: Rash; urticaria; burning sensation;

Miscellaneous: Eye irritation; myalgia; fever; chest pain; bad taste.

Dosage and Administration: Therapy with fenfluramine should be initiated at a dosage of one 20 mg tablet three times daily before meals, but thereafter the dosage should be adjusted to the need and response of the patient. Depending on the degree of effectiveness and side effects, the dosage may be increased at weekly intervals by one tablet daily until a maximum dosage of two tablets three times daily is attained. In patients in whom the initial dosage is not well tolerated, dosage may be reduced to two tablets daily and thereafter gradually increased in order to minimize the chance of side effects.

Overdosage: Only limited data are available concerning clinical effects and management of fenfluramine overdosage. Reported single overdoses have ranged from 300 to 2000 mg; the lowest reported fatal dose was a few hundred mg in a small child and the highest reported non-fatal dose was 1800 mg in an adult. Agitation and drowsiness, confusion, flushing, tremor (or shivering), fever, sweating, abdominal pain, hyperventilation, and dilated nonreactive pupils seem frequent in fenfluramine overdosage. Reflexes may be either exaggerated or depressed and some patients may have rotary nystagmus. Tachycardia may be present, but blood pressure may be normal or only slightly elevated. Convulsions, coma and ventricular extrasystoles, culminating in ventricular fibrillation, may occur at higher dosage. Treatment consists of supportive measures, if possible with cardiac monitoring. However, in the more severe cases, forced diuresis with acidification of the urine may be beneficial to hasten excretion. Efficacy of peritoneal dialysis or extra-corporeal hemodialysis has not been established. Although hypertension has not been a feature of reported cases of overdosage, if it should occur, the use of intravenous phentolamine (Regitine) has been suggested on pharmacologic grounds.

How Supplied: Pondimin is available in 20 mg orange, scored compressed tablets monogrammed AHR, in bottles of 100 and 500 (NDC 0031-6447).

[*Shown in Product Identification Section*]

QUINIDEX EXTENTABS® ℞

brand of Quinidine Sulfate, USP

Composition: Each Extentab (extended action tablet) contains 300 mg. Quinidine Sulfate, USP.

Description: Quinidex Extentabs (quinidine sulfate) are constructed to release one-third of their alkaloidal salt, quinidine sulfate (100 mg), on reaching the stomach, to begin absorption in the upper intestinal tract. The remaining two-thirds of the active drug (200 mg) is evenly distributed throughout a homogeneous core which slowly dissolves as it moves along the intestinal tract, releasing the quinidine sulfate for continuous absorption over an 8-12 hour period.

Action: The action of quinidine in preventing aberrant cardiac rhythms of atrial and ventricular origin resides in its ability to (a) depress excitability of cardiac muscle, (b) slow the rate of spontaneous rhythm, (c) decrease vagal tone, and (d) prolong conduction and effective refractory period.

Indications: Quinidex Extentabs are indicated in the treatment of:

Premature atrial and ventricular contractions.
Paroxysmal atrial tachycardia.
Paroxysmal A-V junctional rhythm.
Atrial flutter.
Paroxysmal atrial fibrillation.
Established atrial fibrillation when therapy is appropriate.
Paroxysmal ventricular tachycardia when not associated with complete heartblock.
Maintenance therapy after electrical conversion of atrial fibrillation and/or flutter.

Contraindications: Intraventricular conduction defects. A-V block. Idiosyncrasy or hypersensitivity.

Aberrant impulses and abnormal rhythms due to escape mechanisms should not be treated with quinidine.

Warning: In the treatment of atrial flutter, reversion to sinus rhythm may be preceded by a progressive reduction in the degree of A-V block to a 1:1 ratio and resulting extremely rapid ventricular rate.

Precautions: All the precautions applying to regular quinidine therapy apply to the Extentab form. Use with care in patients with severe congestive failure, renal insufficiency or with digitalis intoxication.

Patients should be carefully observed for signs of toxicity: e.g., (1) allergy or idiosyncrasy, such as febrile reactions, skin eruptions, and thrombocytopenia (extremely rare); (2) "cinchonism," such as tinnitus, blurred vision, dizziness, lightheadedness, and tremor, (3) G-I symptoms (nausea, vomiting, diarrhea, and colic); (4) cardiotoxic effects such as ventricular extrasystoles occurring at a rate of one or more every 6 normal beats, an increase of the QRS complex of 50% or more, a complete A-V block, or ventricular tachycardia.

NOTE: The development of "cinchonism" is not usually sufficient reason for terminating quinidine therapy. G-I symptoms can also be minimized by giving the drug with food.

Adverse Reactions: Cases of quinidine-induced hypoprothrombinemic hemorrhage in patients on chronic anticoagulant drug therapy have been reported.

Dosage: Two Quinidex Extentabs every 8 to 12 hours.

How Supplied: White sugar-coated Extentabs in bottles of 100 and 250 (NDC 0031-6649).

[*Shown in Product Identification Section*]

REGLAN® INJECTABLE ℞

(Metoclopramide Hydrochloride)

Description: Reglan® Injectable is a clear, colorless, sterile solution with a pH of 3.0–5.0; for intravenous administration. Each **2** ml ampul contains:

Metoclopramide base **10 mg**
(as the monohydrochloride monohydrate)

Sodium Metabisulfite, NF 2.96 mg, Sodium Chloride, USP 14 mg, Water for Injection, USP q.s.

Metoclopramide hydrochloride is a white crystalline, odorless substance, freely soluble in water. Chemically, it is 4-amino-5-chloro-N-[2-(diethylamino) ethyl] - 2 - methoxybenzamide monohydrochloride monohydrate. Molecular weight: 354.3.

Actions: Metoclopramide stimulates motility of the upper gastrointestinal tract without stimulating gastric, biliary, or pancreatic secretions. Its mode of action appears to be antagonism of dopaminergic mechanisms, which are physiological inhibitors of gastrointestinal motility. The effect of metoclopramide on motility is not dependent on intact vagal innervation, but it can be abolished by anticholinergic drugs.

Metoclopramide increases the tone and amplitude of gastric (especially antral) contractions, relaxes the pyloric sphincter and the duodenal bulb, and increases peristalsis of the duodenum and jejunum resulting in accelerated gastric emptying and intestinal transit. It increases the resting tone of the lower esophageal sphincter. It has little, if any, effect on the motility of the colon or gallbladder.

Like the phenothiazines and related drugs, which are also dopamine antagonists, metoclopramide produces sedation and may produce extrapyramidal reactions, although these are comparatively rare (See Warnings). Metoclopramide inhibits the central and peripheral effects of apomorphine, induces release of pro-

Continued on next page

Prescribing information on A. H. Robins products listed here is based on official labeling in effect August 1, 1979, with Indications, Contraindications, Warnings, Precautions, Adverse Reactions, and Dosage stated in full.

Robins—Cont.

lactin and increases circulating aldosterone levels.
The onset of action of metoclopramide is 1 to 3 minutes following an intravenous dose and effects persist for 1 to 2 hours. Approximately 85 percent of an oral dose appears in the urine as unchanged drug, sulfate and glucuronide conjugates, a major metabolite 2-[(4-amino-5-chloro-2-methoxy benzoyl)-amino]acetic acid, and other minor unidentified metabolites.
Indications: Single doses of metoclopramide may be used to facilitate small bowel intubation (e.g., for biopsies) in adults and children in whom the tube does not pass the pylorus with conventional maneuvers.
Single doses of metoclopramide may be used to stimulate gastric emptying and intestinal transit of barium in cases where delayed emptying interferes with radiological examination of the stomach and/or small intestine.
Contraindications: Metoclopramide should not be used whenever stimulation of gastrointestinal motility might be dangerous, e.g., in the presence of gastrointestinal hemorrhage, mechanical obstruction, or perforation.
Metoclopramide is contraindicated in patients with pheochromocytoma because the drug may cause a hypertensive crisis, probably due to release of catecholamines from the tumor. Such hypertensive crises may be controlled by phentolamine.
Metoclopramide is contraindicated in patients with known sensitivity or intolerance to the drug.
Metoclopramide should not be used in epileptics or patients receiving other drugs which are likely to cause extrapyramidal reactions, since the frequency and severity of seizures or extrapyramidal reactions may be increased.
Warnings: Extrapyramidal symptoms occur in approximately 1 in 500 patients treated with metoclopramide. These occur more frequently in children and young adults and may occur after a single dose. These most often consist of feelings of restlessness; occasionally they may include involuntary movements of limbs and facial grimacing; rarely, torticollis, oculogyric crisis, rhythmic protusion of tongue, bulbar type of speech or trismus. One dystonic reaction resembling tetanus has been reported.
Precautions: ***General.*** Intravenous injections of metoclopramide should be made slowly over a 1- to 2-minute period, since a transient but intense feeling of anxiety and restlessness, followed by drowsiness, may occur with rapid administration.
Patients should be cautioned about engaging in activities requiring mental alertness for a few hours after the drug has been administered.
Drug Interaction. The effects of metoclopramide on gastrointestinal motility are antagonized by anticholinergic drugs and narcotic analgesics. Additive sedative effects can occur when metoclopramide is given with alcohol, sedatives, hypnotics, narcotics or tranquilizers. Absorption of drugs from the stomach may be diminished (e.g., digoxin) by metoclopramide, whereas absorption of drugs from the small bowel may be accelerated (e.g., acetaminophen, tetracycline, levodopa, ethanol).
Carcinogenesis, Mutagenesis.
Prolactin elevating compounds, such as metoclopramide, have a carcinogenic potential for mammary glands in rodents, which generally can be correlated with the duration and extent of increase in prolactin plasma levels. However, there are major differences between rodents and humans in hormonal and reproductive physiology, and these rodent studies may not be relevant to determining whether such drugs are potential human mammary carcinogens. Therefore, the actual potential of metoclopramide or any other prolactin-inducing agent for mammary carcinogenesis in humans cannot be determined at this time. Human experience with other prolactin-inducing agents suggests that the risk is virtually nonexistent for single dose use of metoclopramide.
Pregnancy. Reproductive studies in rats, mice and rabbits have revealed no evidence of impaired fertility or harm to the fetus due to metoclopramide.
There are no well-controlled studies of the drug in pregnant women. Metoclopramide should be used in pregnant women only when clearly indicated.
Nursing Mothers. It is not known whether this drug is excreted in human milk. As a general rule metoclopramide should not be given to nursing mothers.
Adverse Reactions: The most frequent adverse reactions to metoclopramide are restlessness, drowsiness, fatigue and lassitude, which occur in approximately ten percent of patients. Less frequently, insomnia, headache, dizziness, nausea, or bowel disturbances may occur.
A single instance of supraventricular tachycardia following intramuscular administration has been reported.
Overdosage: Symptoms of overdosage may include drowsiness, disorientation and extrapyramidal reactions. Anticholinergic or antiparkinson drugs or antihistamines with anticholinergic properties may be helpful in controlling the extrapyramidal reactions. Symptoms are self-limiting and usually disappear within 24 hours.
Dosage and Administration: ***To facilitate small bowel intubation:*** If the tube has not passed the pylorus with conventional maneuvers in 10 minutes, a single dose may be administered slowly by the intravenous route over a 1- to 2-minute period.
To aid in radiological examinations: In patients where delayed gastric emptying interferes with radiological examination of the stomach and/or small intestine, a single dose may be administered slowly by the intravenous route over a 1- to 2-minute period.
The recommended dose is: Adults—10 mg metoclopramide base (2 ml).
Children (6–14 years of age)—2.5 to 5 mg metoclopramide base (0.5 to 1 ml); (under 6 years of age)—0.1 mg/kg metoclopramide base.
How Supplied: Each 2 ml ampul of Reglan® Injectable contains 10 mg metoclopramide base (as the monohydrochloride monohydrate). Available in cartons of 5 and 25 ampuls (NDC 0031-6702).

ROBALATE® TABLETS
brand of Dihydroxyaluminum Aminoacetate
0.5 Gm. in each tablet

Action: Robalate is a nonsystemic antacid which does not affect acid-base balance and does not impair renal function. It is non-toxic and does not interfere with normal digestion. Acid Neutralizing Capacity: 7 mEq per tablet.
Indications: To alleviate heartburn, sour stomach, and/or acid indigestion. Also indicated for the symptomatic relief of hyperacidity associated with the diagnosis of peptic ulcer, gastritis, gastric hyperacidity, peptic esophagitis, and hiatal hernia.
Warning: May cause constipation.
Drug Interaction Precaution: Aluminum containing antacids should not be prescribed or recommended for patients taking a prescription antibiotic drug containing any form of tetracycline.
Dosage: The recommended dosage for OTC use for adults is two to four tablets four times daily, between meals and at bedtime. Under the direction and supervision of a physician, the unit dose or frequency of administration may be doubled as needed. Tablets should be chewed before swallowing.
How Supplied: White, compressed tablets engraved AHR in bottles of 100. (NDC 0031-7074).

ROBAMOX® ℞
brand of Amoxicillin
Robicaps®
250 mg and 500 mg
For Oral Suspension
125 mg per 5 ml, 250 mg per 5 ml

Description: Amoxicillin is a semisynthetic penicillin, an analogue of ampicillin, with a broad spectrum of bactericidal activity against gram-positive organisms and many gram-negative pathogens.
Actions: *Pharmacology:* Amoxicillin is stable in the presence of gastric acid and may be given without regard to meals. It is rapidly absorbed after oral administration. It diffuses readily into most body tissues and fluids, with the exception of brain and spinal fluid except when meninges are inflamed. The half-life of amoxicillin is 61.3 minutes. Most of the amoxicillin is excreted unchanged in the urine; its excretion can be delayed by concurrent administration of probenecid. Amoxicillin is not highly protein-bound. In blood serum, amoxicillin is approximately 20 percent protein-bound, as compared with 60 percent for penicillin-G. Following a 1-gm dose and utilizing a special skin window technique to determine levels of the antibiotic, it was noted that therapeutic levels were found in the interstitial fluid.
Orally administered doses of 250 mg and 500 mg amoxicillin capsules result in average peak blood levels one to two hours after administration in the range of 3.5 mcg/ml to 5.0 mcg/ml and 5.5 mcg/ml to 7.5 mcg/ml, respectively.
Orally administered doses of amoxicillin suspension 125 mg/5 ml, and 250 mg/5 ml, result in average peak blood levels one to two hours after administration in the range of 1.5 mcg/ml to 3.0 mcg/ml, and 3.5 mcg/ml to 5.0 mcg/ml, respectively.
Detectable serum levels are observed up to 8 hours after an orally administered dose of amoxicillin. Approximately 60 percent of an orally administered dose of amoxicillin is excreted in the urine within six to eight hours.
Microbiology: Amoxicillin is similar to ampicillin in its bactericidal action against susceptible organisms during the stage of active multiplication. It acts through the inhibition of biosynthesis of cell wall mucopeptides. In vitro studies have demonstrated the susceptibility of most strains of the following gram-positive bacteria: alpha- and beta-hemolytic streptococci, *Streptococcus pneumoniae,* nonpenicillinase-producing staphylococci, and *Streptococcus faecalis.* It is active in vitro against many strains of *Haemophilus influenzae, Neisseria gonorrhoeae, Escherichia coli,* and *Proteus mirabilis.* Because it does not resist destruction by penicillinase, it is not effective against penicillinase-producing bacteria, particularly resistant staphylococci. All strains of Pseudomonas and most strains of Klebsiella and Enterobacter are resistant.
Disc Susceptibility Tests: Quantitative methods that require measurement of zone diameters give the most precise estimates of antibiotic susceptibility. One such procedure* has been recommended for use with discs for testing susceptibility to ampicillin class antibiotics. Interpretations correlate diameter on the disc test with MIC values for amoxicillin. With this procedure, a report from the laboratory of "susceptible" indicates that the infecting organism is likely to respond to therapy. A report of "resistant" indicates that the infecting organism is not likely to respond to therapy. A report of "intermediate susceptibility" suggests that the organism would be susceptible if high dosage is used, or if the infection is confined to tissues and fluids (e.g., urine) in which high antibiotic levels are attained.

* Bauer, A. W., Kirby, W. M. M., Sherris, J.C., and Turck, M.: Antibiotic Testing by a Standardized Single Disc Method, Am. J. Clin. Pathol., 45:493, 1966: Standardized Disc Susceptibility Test, Federal Register 37:20527–29, 1972.

Indications: Amoxicillin is indicated in the treatment of infections due to susceptible strains of the following:
GRAM-NEGATIVE ORGANISMS—*H. influenzae, E. Coli, P. mirabilis, and N. gonorrhoeae.*
GRAM-POSITIVE ORGANISMS—Streptococci (including *Streptococcus faecalis*), *S. pneumoniae,* and nonpenicillinase-producing staphylococci.
Therapy may be instituted prior to obtaining results from bacteriological and susceptibility studies to determine the causative organisms and their susceptibility to amoxicillin.
Indicated surgical procedures should be performed.

Contraindications: A history of a previous hypersensitivity reaction to any of the penicillins is a contraindication.

Warnings: SERIOUS AND OCCASIONALLY FATAL HYPERSENSITIVITY (ANAPHYLACTOID) REACTIONS HAVE BEEN REPORTED IN PATIENTS ON PENICILLIN THERAPY.
ALTHOUGH ANAPHYLAXIS IS MORE FREQUENT FOLLOWING PARENTERAL THERAPY, IT HAS OCCURRED IN PATIENTS ON ORAL PENICILLINS. THESE REACTIONS ARE MORE APT TO OCCUR IN INDIVIDUALS WITH A HISTORY OF SENSITIVITY TO MULTIPLE ALLERGENS.
THERE HAVE BEEN WELL-DOCUMENTED REPORTS OF INDIVIDUALS WITH A HISTORY OF PENICILLIN HYPERSENSITIVITY REACTIONS WHO HAVE EXPERIENCED SEVERE HYPERSENSITIVITY REACTIONS WHEN TREATED WITH A CEPHALOSPORIN. BEFORE THERAPY WITH A PENICILLIN, CAREFUL INQUIRY SHOULD BE MADE CONCERNING PREVIOUS HYPERSENSITIVITY REACTIONS TO PENICILLINS, CEPHALOSPORINS, AND OTHER ALLERGENS.
SERIOUS ANAPHYLACTOID REACTIONS REQUIRE IMMEDIATE EMERGENCY TREATMENT WITH EPINEPHRINE. OXYGEN, INTRAVENOUS STEROIDS AND AIRWAY MANAGEMENT, INCLUDING INTUBATION, SHOULD ALSO BE ADMINISTERED AS INDICATED.

Usage in Pregnancy: Safety for use in pregnancy has not been established.

Precautions: The possibility of superinfections with mycotic organisms or bacterial pathogens should be kept in mind during therapy. In such cases, discontinue the drug and substitute appropriate treatment.
As with any potent drug, periodic assessment of organ system function, including renal, hepatic, and hematopoietic, should be made during prolonged therapy.

Adverse Reactions: As with other penicillins, it may be expected that untoward reactions will be essentially limited to sensitivity phenomena. They are more likely to occur in individuals who have previously demonstrated hypersensitivity to penicillins and in those with history of allergy, asthma, hay fever, or urticaria.
The following adverse reactions have been reported as associated with the use of penicillins.
Gastrointestinal: Glossitis, stomatitis, black, "hairy" tongue, nausea, vomiting, and diarrhea. (These reactions are usually associated with oral dosage forms.)
Hypersensitivity Reactions: Skin rashes and urticaria have been reported frequently. A few cases of exfoliative dermatitis and erythema multiforme have been reported. Anaphylaxis is the most serious reaction experienced and has usually been associated with the parenteral dosage form.
NOTE: Urticaria, other skin rashes, and serum sickness-like reactions may be controlled with antihistamines and, if necessary, systemic corticosteroids. Whenever such reactions occur, amoxicillin should be discontinued unless, in the opinion of the physician, the condition being treated is life threatening and amenable only to amoxicillin therapy. Serious anaphylactic reactions require the immediate use of epinephrine, oxygen, and intravenous steroids.
Liver: Moderate rise in serum glutamic oxaloacetic transaminase (SGOT) has been noted, particularly in infants, but the significance of this finding is unknown.
Hemic and Lymphatic Systems: Anemia, thrombocytopenia, thrombocytopenic purpura, eosinophilia, leukopenia, and agranulocytosis have been reported during therapy with the penicillins. These reactions are usually reversible on discontinuation of therapy and are believed to be hypersensitivity phenomena.

Dosage and Administration: Infections of the ear, nose and throat due to streptococci, pneumococci, nonpenicillinase-producing staphylococi, and *H. influenzae.*
Infections of the genitourinary tract due to *E. coli, Proteus mirabilis,* and *Streptococcus faecalis:*
Infections of the skin and soft tissues due to streptococci, susceptible staphylococci, and *E. coli.*
Usual Dosage: Adults—250 mg every 8 hours. Children: 20 mg/kg/day in divided doses every 8 hours. Children weighing 20 kg or more should be dosed according to the adult recommendations.
In severe infections or those caused by less susceptible organisms: 500 mg every 8 hours for adults, and 40 mg/kg/day in divided doses every 8 hours for children may be needed.
Infections of the lower respiratory tract, due to streptococci, pneumococci, nonpenicillinase-producing staphylococci, and *H. influenzae:*
Usual Dosage: Adults—500 mg every 8 hours. Children: 40 mg/kg/day in divided doses every 8 hours. Children weighing 20 kg or more should be dosed according to the adult recommendations.
Gonorrhea: acute, uncomplicated ano-genital and urethral infections due to *N. Gonorrhoeae:* (males and females)—3 grams as a single oral dose.
Cases of gonorrhoeae with a suspected lesion of syphilis should have dark-field examinations before receiving amoxicillin, and monthly serological tests for a minimum of four months.
Larger doses may be required for stubborn or severe infections. The children's dosage is intended for individuals whose weight will not cause a dosage to be calculated greater than that recommended for adults.
It should be recognized that in the treatment of chronic urinary tract infections, frequent bacteriological and clinical appraisals are necessary. Smaller doses than those recommended above should not be used. Even higher doses may be needed at times. In stubborn infections, therapy may be required for several weeks. It may be necessary to continue clinical and/or bacteriological follow-up for several months after cessation of therapy. Except for gonorrhoeae, treatment should be continued for a mininum of 48 to 72 hours beyond the time that the patient becomes asymptomatic or evidence of bacterial eradication has been obtained. It is recommended that there be at least 10 days treatment for any infection caused by hemolytic streptococci to prevent the occurrence of acute rheumatic fever or glomerulonephritis.

How Supplied: Robamox Robicaps® (amoxicillin capsules) containing 250 mg amoxicillin as the trihydrate, bottles of 100 and 500 (NDC 0031-7117); containing 500 mg amoxicillin as the trihydrate, bottles of 50 (NDC 0031-7127).
[*Shown in Product Identification Section*]
Amoxicillin Powder for Oral Suspension.
Each 5 ml of reconstituted suspension contains amoxicillin trihydrate equivalent to 125 mg or 250 mg amoxicillin.
125 mg/5 ml in 80 ml, 100 ml and 150 ml bottles (NDC 0031-7105).
250 mg/5 ml in 80 ml, 100 ml and 150 ml bottles (NDC 0031-7107).

ROBAXIN® INJECTABLE ℞
brand of Methocarbamol Injection, NF

Composition: Robaxin Injectable is a parenteral dosage form of methocarbamol containing 100 mg of methocarbamol per 1 ml of 50% aqueous polyethylene glycol 300.

Actions: The mechanism of action of methocarbamol in humans has not been established, but may be due to general central nervous system depression. It has no direct action on the contractile mechanism of striated muscle, the motor end plate or the nerve fiber.

Indications: The injectable form of methocarbamol is indicated as an adjunct to rest, physical therapy, and other measures for the relief of discomfort associated with acute, painful musculoskeletal conditions. The mode of action of this drug has not been clearly identified, but may be related to its sedative properties. Methocarbamol does not directly relax tense skeletal muscles in man.

Contraindications: Robaxin Injectable should not be administered to patients with known or suspected renal pathology. This caution is necessary because of the presence of polyethylene glycol 300 in the vehicle.
A much larger amount of polyethylene glycol 300 than is present in recommended doses of Robaxin Injectable is known to have increased pre-existing acidosis and urea retention in patients with renal impairment. Although the amount present in this preparation is well within the limits of safety, caution dictates this contraindication.
Robaxin Injectable is contraindicated in patients hypersensitive to any of the ingredients.

Warnings: Safe use of Robaxin Injectable has not been established with regard to possible adverse effects upon fetal development. Therefore, Robaxin Injectable should not be used in women who are or may become pregnant and particularly during early pregnancy unless in the judgment of the physician the potential benefits outweigh the possible hazards.

Precautions: As with other agents administered either intravenously or intramuscularly, careful supervision of dose and rate of injection should be observed. Rate of injection should not exceed 3 ml per minute—i.e., one 10 ml vial in approximately three minutes. Since Robaxin Injectable is hypertonic, vascular extravasation must be avoided. A recumbent position will reduce the likelihood of side reactions.
Blood aspirated into the syringe does not mix with the hypertonic solution. This phenomenon occurs with many other intravenous preparations. The blood may be safely injected with the methocarbamol, or the injection may be stopped when the plunger reaches the blood, whichever the physician prefers.
The total dosage should not exceed 30 ml (three vials) a day for more than three consecutive days except in the treatment of tetanus.

Continued on next page

Prescribing information on A. H. Robins products listed here is based on official labeling in effect August 1, 1979, with Indications, Contraindications, Warnings, Precautions, Adverse Reactions, and Dosage stated in full.

Robins—Cont.

Caution should be observed in using the injectable form in suspected or known epileptic patients.
Safety and effectiveness in children below the age of 12 years have not been established except in tetanus. See special directions for use in tetanus.
It is not known whether this drug is secreted in human milk. As a general rule, nursing should not be undertaken while a patient is on a drug since many drugs are excreted in human milk.
Methocarbamol may cause a color interference in certain screening tests for 5-hydroxyindoleacetic acid (5-HIAA) and vanilmandelic acid (VMA).
Adverse Reactions: Dizziness, light-headedness, drowsiness, vertigo, fainting, syncope, hypotension, gastrointestinal upset, metallic taste, thrombophlebitis, sloughing at the site of injection, pain at the site of injection, anaphylactic reaction, urticaria, pruritus, rash, conjunctivitis with nasal congestion, flushing, nystagmus, diplopia, mild muscular incoordination, bradycardia, blurred vision, headache, fever. In most cases of syncope there was spontaneous recovery. In others, epinephrine, injectable steroids and/or injectable antihistamines were employed to hasten recovery. Certain of these complaints may have been due to an overly rapid rate of intravenous injection. The onset of convulsive seizures during intravenous administration has been reported, including instances in known epileptics. The psychic trauma of the procedure may have been a contributing factor. Although several observers have reported success in terminating epileptiform seizures with Robaxin Injectable, its administration to patients with epilepsy is not recommended.
Dosage and Administration:
For Intravenous and Intramuscular Use Only.
Total adult dosage should not exceed 30 ml (3 vials) a day for more than 3 consecutive days except in the treatment of tetanus. A like course may be repeated after a lapse of 48 hours if the condition persists. Dosage and frequency of injection should be based on the severity of the condition being treated and therapeutic response noted.
For the relief of symptoms of moderate degree, 10 ml (one vial) may be adequate. Ordinarily this injection need not be repeated, as the administration of the oral form will usually sustain the relief initiated by the injection. For the severest cases or in postoperative conditions in which oral administration is not feasible, 20 to 30 ml (two to three vials) may be required.
Directions For Intravenous Use:
Robaxin Injectable may be administered undiluted directly into the vein at a *maximum rate of three ml per minute.* It may also be added to an intravenous drip of Sodium Chloride Injection (Sterile Isotonic Sodium Chloride Solution for Parenteral Use) or five per cent Dextrose Injection (Sterile 5 per cent Dextrose Solution); one vial given as a single dose should not be diluted to more than 250 ml for I.V. infusion. Care should be exercised to avoid vascular extravasation of this hypertonic solution which may result in thrombophlebitis. It is preferable that the patient be in a recumbent position during and for at least 10 to 15 minutes following the injection.
Directions For Intramuscular Use:
When the intramuscular route is indicated, not more than five ml (one-half vial) should be injected into each gluteal region. The injections may be repeated at eight hour intervals, if necessary. When satisfactory relief of symptoms is achieved, it can usually be maintained with tablets.
NOT RECOMMENDED FOR SUBCUTANEOUS ADMINISTRATION.

Special Directions For Use in Tetanus:
There is clinical evidence which suggests that methocarbamol may have a beneficial effect in the control of the neuromuscular manifestations of tetanus. It does not, however, replace the usual procedure of debridement, tetanus antitoxin, penicillin, tracheotomy, attention to fluid balance, and supportive care. Robaxin Injectable should be added to the regimen as soon as possible.
For adults: Inject one or two vials directly into the tubing of the previously inserted indwelling needle. An additional 10 ml or 20 ml may be added to the infusion bottle so that a total of up to 30 ml (three vials) is given as the initial dose (note Precautions). This procedure should be repeated every six hours until conditions allow for the insertion of a nasogastric tube. Crushed Robaxin (methocarbamol) tablets suspended in water or saline may then be given through this tube. Total daily oral doses up to 24 grams may be required as judged by patient response.
For children: A minimum initial dose of 15 mg/kg is recommended. This dosage may be repeated every six hours as indicated. The maintenance dosage may be given by injection into the tubing or by I.V. infusion with an appropriate quantity of fluid. See directions for I.V. use.
How Supplied: Robaxin Injectable—10 ml single dose vials in packages of 5 and 25 vials (NDC No. 0031-7409).

ROBAXIN® TABLETS ℞

brand of Methocarbamol Tablets, NF
500 mg per tablet

ROBAXIN®-750 TABLETS

brand of Methocarbamol Tablets, NF ℞
750 mg per tablet

Actions: The mechanism of action of methocarbamol in humans has not been established, but may be due to general central nervous system depression. It has no direct action on the contractile mechanism of striated muscle, the motor end plate or the nerve fiber.
Indications: Robaxin (methocarbamol) is indicated as an adjunct to rest, physical therapy, and other measures for the relief of discomforts associated with acute, painful musculoskeletal conditions. The mode of action of this drug has not been clearly identified, but may be related to its sedative properties. Methocarbamol does not directly relax tense skeletal muscles in man.
Contraindications: Robaxin is contraindicated in patients hypersensitive to any of the ingredients.
Warnings: Safe use of Robaxin (methocarbamol) has not been established with regard to possible adverse effects upon fetal development. Therefore, Robaxin should not be used in women who are or may become pregnant and particularly during early pregnancy unless in the judgment of the physician the potential benefits outweigh the possible hazards.
Precautions: Safety and effectiveness in children below the age of 12 years have not been established.
It is not known whether this drug is secreted in human milk. As a general rule, nursing should not be undertaken while a patient is on a drug since many drugs are excreted in human milk.
Methocarbamol may cause a color interference in certain screening tests for 5-hydroxyindoleacetic acid (5-HIAA) and vanilmandelic acid (VMA).
Adverse Reactions: Lightheadedness, dizziness, drowsiness, nausea, allergic manifestations such as urticaria, pruritus, rash, conjunctivitis with nasal congestion, blurred vision, headache, fever.
Dosage and Administration: Robaxin (methocarbamol), 500 mg.—Adults: initial dosage, 3 tablets q.i.d.; maintenance dosage, 2 tablets q.i.d.
Robaxin-750 (methocarbamol), 750 mg—Adults: initial dosage, 2 tablets q.i.d.; maintenance dosage, 1 tablet q.4h. or 2 tablets t.i.d.
Six grams a day are recommended for the first 48 to 72 hours of treatment. (For severe conditions 8 grams a day may be administered.) Thereafter, the dosage can usually be reduced to approximately 4 grams a day.
How Supplied: Robaxin tablets—white scored tablets in bottles of 100 and 500 and in Dis-Co® unit dose packs of 500 (NDC No. 0031-7429).
Robaxin-750—white capsule-shaped tablets in bottles of 100 and 500 and in Dis-Co® unit dose packs of 100 (NDC No. 0031-7449).
[Shown in Product Identification Section]

ROBAXISAL® TABLETS ℞

Description: For oral administration, Robaxisal is available as a pink and white laminated tablet containing:
Methocarbamol, NF....................400 mg
Aspirin, USP....................325 mg
Actions: Robaxisal provides a double approach to the management of discomforts associated with musculoskeletal disorders.
Methocarbamol. The mechanism of action of methocarbamol in humans has not been established, but may be due to general central nervous system depression. It has no direct action on the contractile mechanism of striated muscle, the motor end plate or the nerve fiber.
Aspirin. Aspirin is a mild analgesic with anti-inflammatory and antipyretic activity.
Indications: Robaxisal is indicated as an adjunct to rest, physical therapy, and other measures for the relief of discomfort associated with acute, painful musculoskeletal conditions. The mode of action of methocarbamol has not been clearly identified but may be related to its sedative properties. Methocarbamol does not directly relax tense skeletal muscles in man.
Contraindications: Hypersensitivity to methocarbamol or aspirin.
Precautions: Products containing aspirin should be administered with caution to patients with gastritis or peptic ulceration, or those receiving hypoprothrombinemic anticoagulants.
Methocarbomal may cause a color interference in certain screening tests for 5-hydroxyindoleacetic acid (5-HIAA) and vanilmandelic acid (VMA).
Pregnancy. Safe use of Robaxisal has not been established with regard to possible adverse effects upon fetal development. Therefore, Robaxisal should not be used in women who are or may become pregnant and particularly during early pregnancy unless in the judgment of the physician the potential benefits outweigh the possible hazards.
Nursing Mothers. It is not known whether methocarbamol is secreted in human milk; however, aspirin does appear in human milk in moderate amounts. It can produce a bleeding tendency either by interfering with the function of the infant's platelets or by decreasing the amount of prothrombin in the blood. The risk is minimal if the mother takes the aspirin just after nursing and if the infant has an adequate store of vitamin K.
As a general rule, nursing should not be undertaken while a patient is on a drug.
Pediatric Use. Safety and effectiveness in children 12 years of age and below have not been established.
Use in Activities Requiring Mental Alertness. Robaxisal may rarely cause drowsiness. Until the patient's response has been determined, he should be cautioned against the operation of motor vehicles or dangerous machinery.
Adverse Reactions: The most frequent adverse reaction to methocarbamol is dizziness or lightheadedness and nausea. This occurs in about one in 20–25 patients. Less frequent reactions are drowsiness, blurred vision, head-

ache, fever, allergic manifestations such as urticaria, pruritus, and rash.
Adverse reactions that have been associated with the use of aspirin include: nausea and other gastrointestinal discomfort, gastritis, gastric erosion, vomiting, constipation, diarrhea, angio-edema, asthma, rash, pruritus, urticaria.
Gastrointestinal discomfort may be minimized by taking Robaxisal with food.
Dosage and Administration: Adults and children over 12 years of age: Two tablets four times daily. Three tablets four times daily may be used in severe conditions for one to three days in patients who are able to tolerate salicylates. These dosage recommendations provide respectively 3.2 and 4.8 grams of methocarbamol per day.
Overdosage: Toxicity due to overdosage of methocarbomal is unlikely; however, acute overdosage of aspirin may cause symptoms of salicylate intoxication.
Treatment of Overdosage. Supportive therapy for 24 hours, as methocarbamol is excreted within that time. If salicylate intoxication occurs, especially in children, the hyperpnea may be controlled with sodium bicarbonate. Judicious use of 5% CO_2 with 95% O_2 may be of benefit. Abnormal electrolyte patterns should be corrected with appropriate fluid therapy.
How Supplied: Robaxisal® is supplied as pink and white laminated, compressed tablets in bottles of 100 and 500 and Dis-Co® Unit Dose Packs of 100 (NDC 0031-7469).
[*Shown in Product Identification Section*]

ROBICILLIN VK ℞
brand of
Penicillin V Potassium, USP
for oral use

Description: Penicillin V is the phenoxymethyl analog of penicillin G. The chemical formula is $C_{16}H_{18}N_2O_5S$.
Action and Pharmacology: Penicillin V exerts a bactericidal action against penicillin sensitive microorganisms during the stage of active multiplication. It acts through the inhibition of biosynthesis of cell wall mucopeptide. It is not active against the penicillinase producing bacteria, which include many strains of staphylococci. The drug exerts high in vitro activity against staphylococci (except penicillinase-producing strains), streptococci (groups A, C, G, H, L, and M) and pneumococci. Other organisms sensitive in vitro to penicillin V are **Corynebacterium diphtheriae, Bacillus anthracis**, Clostridia, **Actinomyces bovis, Streptobacillus moniliformis, Listeria monocytogenes,** Leptospira and **N. gonorrhoeae. Treponema pallidum** is extremely sensitive.
Penicillin V has the distinct advantage over penicillin G in resistance to inactivation by gastric acid. It may be given with meals; however, blood levels are slightly higher when the drug is given on an empty stomach. Average blood levels are two to five times higher than the levels following the same dose of oral penicillin G and also show much less individual variation.
Once absorbed, penicillin V is about 80% bound to serum protein. Tissue levels are highest in the kidneys, with lesser amounts in the liver, skin and intestines. Small amounts are found in all other body tissues and the cerebrospinal fluid. The drug is excreted as rapidly as it is absorbed in individuals with normal kidney function; however, recovery of the drug from the urine indicates that only about 25% of the dose given is absorbed. In neonates, young infants and individuals with impaired kidney function, excretion is considerably delayed.
Indications: Penicillin V is indicated in the treatment of mild to moderately severe infections due to penicillin-G sensitive microorganisms that are sensitive to the low serum levels common to this particular dosage form. Therapy should be guided by bacteriological studies (including sensitivity tests) and by clinical response.
Note: Severe pneumonia, empyema, bacteremia, pericarditis, meningitis, and arthritis should not be treated with penicillin V during the acute stage.
Indicated surgical procedures should be performed.
The following infections will usually respond to adequate dosage of Penicillin V:
Streptococcal infections (without bacteremia). Mild to moderate infections of the upper respiratory tract, scarlet fever, and mild erysipelas.
Note: Streptococci in groups A, C, G, H, L, and M are very sensitive to penicillin. Other groups, including group D (enterococcus) are resistant.
Pneumococcal infections. Mild to moderately severe infections of the respiratory tract.
Staphylococcal infections—penicillin G sensitive. Mild infections of the skin and soft tissues.
Note: Reports indicate an increasing number of strains of staphylococci resistant to penicillin G, emphasizing the need for culture and sensitivity studies in treating suspected staphylococcal infections.
Fusospirochetosis (Vincent's gingivitis and pharyngitis)—Mild to moderately severe infections of the oropharynx usually respond to therapy with oral penicillin.
Note: Necessary dental care should be accomplished in infections involving the gum tissue.
Medical conditions in which oral penicillin therapy is indicated as prophylaxis:
For the prevention of recurrence following rheumatic fever and/or chorea: Prophylaxis with oral penicillin on a continuing basis has proven effective in preventing recurrence of these conditions.
To prevent bacterial endocarditis in patients with congenital and/or rheumatic heart lesions who are to undergo dental procedures or minor upper respiratory tract surgery or instrumentation. Prophylaxis should be instituted the day of the procedure and for 2 or more days following. Patients who have a past history of rheumatic fever and are receiving continuous prophylaxis may harbor increased numbers of penicillin-resistant organisms; use of another prophylactic anti-infective agent should be considered. If penicillin is to be used in these patients at surgery, the regular rheumatic fever program should be interrupted 1 week prior to the contemplated surgery. At the time of surgery, penicillin may be reinstituted as a prophylactic measure against the hazards of surgically induced bacteremia.
Note: Oral penicillin should not be used as adjunctive prophylaxis for genitourinary instrumentation or surgery, lower intestinal tract surgery, sigmoidoscopy and childbirth.
Contraindications: A previous hypersensitivity reaction to any penicillin is a contraindication.
Warnings: Serious and occasionally fatal hypersensitivity (anaphylactoid) reactions have been reported in patients on penicillin therapy. Although anaphylaxis is more frequent following parenteral therapy it has occurred in patients on oral penicillins. These reactions are more apt to occur in individuals with a history of sensitivity to multiple allergens.
There have been well documented reports of individuals with a history of penicillin hypersensitivity reactions who have experienced severe hypersensitivity reactions when treated with a cephalosporin. Before therapy with a penicillin, careful inquiry should be made concerning previous hypersensitivity reactions to penicillins, cephalosporins, and other allergens. If an allergic reaction occurs, the drug should be discontinued and the patient treated with the usual agents e.g., pressor amines, antihistamines and corticosteroids.
Precautions: Penicillin should be used with caution in individuals with histories of significant allergies and/or asthma.
The oral route of administration should not be relied upon in patients with severe illness, or with nausea, vomiting, gastric dilatation, cardiospasm or intestinal hypermotility.
Occasionally patients will not absorb therapeutic amounts of orally administered penicillin.
In streptococcal infections, therapy must be sufficient to eliminate the organism (10 days minimum); otherwise the sequelae of streptococcal disease may occur. Cultures should be taken following completion of treatment to determine whether streptococci have been eradicated.
Prolonged use of antibiotics may promote the overgrowth of non-susceptible organisms, including fungi. Should superinfection occur, appropriate measures should be taken.
Adverse Reactions: Although the incidence of reactions to oral penicillins has been reported with much less frequency than following parenteral therapy, it should be remembered that all degrees of hypersensitivity including fatal anaphylaxis, have been reported with oral penicillin.
The most common reactions to oral penicillin are nausea, vomiting, epigastric distress, diarrhea, and black hairy tongue. The hypersensitivity reactions reported are skin eruptions (maculo-papular to exfoliative dermatitis), urticaria and other serum sickness reactions, laryngeal edema and anaphylaxis. Fever and eosinophilia may frequently be the only reaction observed. Hemolytic anemia, leucopenia, thrombocytopenia, neuropathy, and nephropathy are infrequent reactions and usually associated with high doses of parenteral penicillin.
Administration and Dosage: The dosage of penicillin V should be determined according to the sensitivity of the causative microorganisms and the severity of infection, and adjusted to the clinical response of the patient.
The usual dosage recommendations for adults and children 12 years and over are as follows:
Streptococcal infections—mild to moderately severe—of the upper respiratory tract and including scarlet fever, and mild erysipelas; 125 mg (200,000 units) every 6–8 hours for 10 days for mild infections; 250–500 mg (400,000–800,000 units) every 8 hours for 10 days for moderately severe infections.
Pneumococcal infections—mild to moderately severe—of the respiratory tract, including otitis media: 250–500 mg (400,000–800,000 units) every 6 hours until the patient has been afebrile for at least 2 days.
Staphylococcal infections—mild infections of skin and soft tissue (culture and sensitivity tests should be performed): 250–500 mg (400,000–800,000 units) every 6-8 hours.
Fusospirochetosis (Vincent's infection) of the oropharynx. Mild to moderately severe infections: 250mg (400,000 units) every 6-8 hours.
For the prevention of recurrence following rheumatic fever and/or chorea: 125 mg (200,000 units) twice daily on a continuing basis.
To prevent bacterial endocarditis in patients with rheumatic or congenital heart lesions who are to undergo dental or upper respiratory tract surgery or instrumentation: 250 mg (400,000 units) orally the day of the procedure; 500,000 units aqueous penicillin G, I.M. 1 hour before the procedure; and 250 mg (400,000 units) orally every 6 hours for 2 or more days.
Note: Therapy for children under 12 years of age is calculated on the basis of body weight.

Continued on next page

Prescribing information on A. H. Robins products listed here is based on official labeling in effect August 1, 1979, with Indications, Contraindications, Warnings, Precautions, Adverse Reactions, and Dosage stated in full.

Robins—Cont.

For infants and small children the suggested dose is 25,000 to 90,000 units per kg per day in three to six divided doses.
How Supplied:
Penicillin V Potassium for Oral Solution, USP 125 mg. (200,000 Units) per 5 ml. (NDC 0031-8205) and
250 mg. (400,000 Units) per 5 ml. (NDC 0031-8207)—in 100 ml. and 200 ml. bottles.
Penicillin V Potassium Tablets, U.S.P.
250 mg. (400,000 Units)—bottles of 100 and 1,000 tablets (NDC 0031-8217)
500 mg. (800,000 Units)—bottles of 100 tablets and 500 tablets (NDC 0031-8227).
[*Shown in Product Identification Section*]

ROBIMYCIN ROBITABS® ℞
brand of
Erythromycin, USP, enteric-coated tablet—250 mg
For Oral Administration

Description: Erythromycin is produced by a strain of *Streptomyces erythraeus* and belongs to the macrolide group of antibiotics. It is basic and readily forms salts with acids. The base, the stearate salt, and the esters are poorly soluble in water and are suitable for oral administration. Robimycin Tablets, erythromycin base, are specially coated to protect the antibiotic from the inactivating effects of gastric acidity and to permit efficient absorption in the small intestine.
Actions: The mode of action of erythromycin is inhibition of protein synthesis without affecting nucleic acid synthesis. Resistance to erythromycin of some strains of *Haemophilus influenzae* and staphylococci has been demonstrated. Culture and susceptibility testing should be done. If the Kirby-Bauer method of disc susceptibility is used, a 15 mcg. erythromycin disc should give a zone diameter of at least 18 mm. when tested against an erythromycin susceptible organism.
Orally administered erythromycin is readily absorbed by most patients, especially on an empty stomach, but patient variation is observed.
After absorption, erythromycin diffuses readily into most body fluids. In the absence of meningeal inflammation, low concentrations are normally achieved in the spinal fluid, but passage of the drug across the blood-brain barrier increases in meningitis. In the presence of normal hepatic function, erythromycin is concentrated in the liver and excreted in the bile; the effect of hepatic dysfunction on excretion of erythromycin by the liver into the bile is not known. After oral administration, less than 5 percent of the activity of the administered dose can be recovered in the urine. Erythromycin crosses the placental barrier, but fetal plasma levels are low.
Indications: Robimycin is indicated in the treatment of infections due to the following microorganisms:
Streptococcus pyogenes (Group A beta hemolytic streptococcus): For upper and lower respiratory tract, skin, and soft tissue infections of mild to moderate severity.
Injectable benzathine penicillin G is considered by the American Heart Association to be the drug of choice in the treatment and prevention of streptococcal pharyngitis and in long-term prophylaxis of rheumatic fever.
When oral medication is preferred for treatment of the above conditions, penicillin G, V, or erythromycin are alternate drugs of choice. When oral medication is given, the importance of strict adherence by the patient to the prescribed dosage regimen must be stressed. A therapeutic dose should be administered for at least 10 days.
Alpha-hemolytic streptococci (viridans group): For short-term prophylaxis of bacterial endocarditis prior to dental or other operative procedures in patients with a history of rheumatic fever or congenital heart disease who are hypersensitive to penicillin. (Erythromycin is not suitable prior to genitourinary surgery where the organisms likely to lead to bacteremia are gram-negative bacilli or the enterococcus group of streptococci.)
Staphylococcus aureus: For acute infections of skin and soft tissue of mild to moderate severity. Resistant organisms may emerge during treatment.
Streptococcus pneumoniae (Diplococcus pneumoniae): For upper respiratory tract infections (e.g., Otitis media, pharyngitis) and lower respiratory tract infections (e.g., pneumonia) of mild to moderate degree.
Mycoplasma pneumoniae (Eaton agent, PPLO): For respiratory infections due to this organism.
Hemophilus influenzae: For upper respiratory tract infections of mild to moderate severity when used concomitantly with adequate doses of sulfonamides. Not all strains of this organism are susceptible at the erythromycin concentrations ordinarily achieved (see appropriate sulfonamide labeling for prescribing information).
Treponema pallidum: Erythromycin (oral forms only) is an alternate choice of treatment for primary syphilis in patients allergic to the penicillins. In treatment of primary syphilis, spinal fluid examinations should be done before treatment and as part of followup after therapy.
Corynebacterium diphtheriae and C. ***minutissimum:*** As an adjunct to antitoxin, to prevent establishment of carriers, and to eradicate the organism in carriers.
In the treatment of erythrasma.
Entamoeba histolytica: In the treatment of intestinal amebiasis only. Extraenteric amebiasis requires treatment with other agents.
Listeria monocytogenes: Infections due to this organism.
Neisseria gonorrhoeae: Erythromycin lactobionate for injection in conjunction with erythromycin stearate or base orally, as an alternative drug in treatment of acute pelvic inflammatory disease caused by ***N. gonorrhoeae*** in female patients with a history of sensitivity to penicillin. Before treatment of gonorrhea, patients who are suspected of also having syphilis should have a microscopic examination for ***T. pallidum*** (by immunofluorescence or darkfield) before receiving erythromycin, and monthly serologic tests for a minimum of 4 months.
Legionnaires' Disease: Although no controlled clinical efficacy studies have been conducted, *in vitro* and limited preliminary clinical data suggest that erythromycin may be effective in treating Legionnaires' Disease.
Contraindications: Erythromycin is contraindicated in patients with known hypersensitivity to this antibiotic.
Warnings: Usage in pregnancy: Safety for use in pregnancy has not been established.
Precautions: Erythromycin is principally excreted by the liver.
Caution should be exercised in administering the antibiotic to patients with impaired hepatic function.
There have been reports of hepatic dysfunction, with or without jaundice, occurring in patients receiving oral erythromycin products. Although the majority of these cases have been associated with erythromycin estolate, there have been some reports of hepatic dysfunctions in conjunction with the erythromycin base, stearate and ethylsuccinate.
Recent data from studies of erythromycin reveal that its use in patients who are receiving high doses of theophylline may be associated with an increase of serum theophylline levels and potential theophylline toxicity. In case of theophylline toxicity and/or elevated serum theophylline levels, the dose of theophylline should be reduced while the patient is receiving concomitant erythromycin therapy.
Surgical procedures should be performed when indicated.
Adverse Reactions: The most frequent side effects of erythromycin preparations are gastrointestinal, such as abdominal cramping and discomfort, and are dose-related. Nausea, vomiting, and diarrhea occur infrequently with usual oral doses.
During prolonged or repeated therapy, there is a possibility of overgrowth of nonsusceptible bacteria or fungi. If such infections occur, the drug should be discontinued and appropriate therapy instituted.
Mild allergic reactions such as urticaria and other skin rashes have occurred. Serious allergic reactions, including anaphylaxis have been reported.
Dosage and Administration: Optimum blood levels are obtained when doses are given on an empty stomach.
Adults: 250 mg every 6 hours is the usual dose. Dosage may be increased up to 4 or more grams per day according to the severity of the infection.
Children: Age, weight, and severity of the infection are important factors in determining the proper dosage. 30–50 mg/kg/day, in divided doses, is the usual dose. For more severe infections this dose may be doubled.
If dosage is desired on a twice-a-day schedule in either adults or children, one-half of the total daily dose may be given every 12 hours, 1 hour before meals.
In the treatment of streptococcal infections, a therapeutic dosage of erythromycin should be administered for at least 10 days. In continuous ***prophylaxis*** of streptococcal infections in persons with a history of rheumatic heart disease, the dose is 250 mg twice a day.
When used prior to surgery to prevent endocarditis (see Alpha-hemolytic streptococci), a recommended schedule for adults is: 500 mg before the procedure and 250 mg every 6 hours for 4 doses after the procedure. For small children: 30 mg/kg/day divided into three or four evenly spaced doses.
For treatment of primary syphilis: 30–40 grams given in divided doses over a period of 10–15 days.
For treatment of acute pelvic inflammatory disease caused by N. gonorrhoeae: After initial treatment with erythromycin lactobionate for injection (500 mg every 6 hours for 3 days), the oral dosage recommendation is 250 mg every 6 hours for 7 days.
For dysenteric amebiasis: 250 mg four times daily for 10 to 14 days, for adults; 30–50 mg/kg/day in divided doses for 10 to 14 days for children.
For treatment of Legionnaires' Disease: Although optimal doses have not been established, doses utilized in reported clinical data were those recommended above (1 to 4 grams erythromycin base daily in divided doses).
How Supplied: Robimycin Robitabs®† 250 mg (pale green, round) are available in bottles of 100 and 500 (NDC 0031-8317).

†Robitabs® is A. H. Robins' registered trademark for tablets.
[*Shown in Product Identification Section*]

ROBINUL® TABLETS ℞
ROBINUL® FORTE TABLETS ℞
brand of Glycopyrrolate Tablets, NF

Description: Robinul tablets are scored, compressed pink tablets engraved AHR. Each tablet contains:
Glycopyrrolate, NF ....1 mg
Robinul Forte tablets are scored, compressed pink tablets engraved $^{AHR}_{2}$. Each tablet contains:
Glycopyrrolate, NF ....2 mg
Actions: Glycopyrrolate, like other anticholinergic (antimuscarinic) agents, inhibits the

action of acetylcholine on structures innervated by postganglionic cholinergic nerves and on smooth muscles that respond to acetylcholine but lack cholinergic innervation. These peripheral cholinergic receptors are present in the autonomic effector cells of smooth muscle, cardiac muscle, the sinoatrial node, the atrioventricular node, exocrine glands, and, to a limited degree, in the autonomic ganglia. Thus, it diminishes the volume and free acidity of gastric secretions and controls excessive pharyngeal, tracheal, and bronchial secretions.

Glycopyrrolate antagonizes muscarinic symptoms (e.g., bronchorrhea, bronchospasm, bradycardia, and intestinal hypermotility) induced by cholinergic drugs such as the anticholinesterases.

The highly polar quaternary ammonium group of glycopyrrolate limits its passage across lipid membranes, such as the blood-brain barrier, in contrast to atropine sulfate and scopolamine hydrobromide, which are non-polar tertiary amines which penetrate lipid barriers easily.

Indications: For use as adjunctive therapy in the treatment of peptic ulcer.

Contraindications: Glaucoma; obstructive uropathy (for example, bladder neck obstruction due to prostatic hypertrophy); obstructive disease of the gastrointestinal tract (as in achalasia, pyloroduodenal stenosis, etc.); paralytic ileus; intestinal atony of the elderly or debilitated patient; unstable cardiovascular status in acute hemorrhage; severe ulcerative colitis; toxic megacolon complicating ulcerative colitis; myasthenia gravis. Robinul (glycopyrrolate) tablets are contraindicated in those patients with a hypersensitivity to glycopyrrolate.

Warnings: In the presence of a high environmental temperature, heat prostration (fever and heat stroke due to decreased sweating) can occur with use of Robinul.

Diarrhea may be an early symptom of incomplete intestinal obstruction, especially in patients with ileostomy or colostomy. In this instance treatment with this drug would be inappropriate and possibly harmful.

Robinul (glycopyrrolate) may produce drowsiness or blurred vision. In this event, the patient should be warned not to engage in activities requiring mental alertness such as operating a motor vehicle or other machinery, or performing hazardous work while taking this drug.

Theoretically, with overdosage a curare-like action may occur, i.e., neuromuscular blockade leading to muscular weakness and possible paralysis.

Pregnancy. The safety of this drug during pregnancy has not been established. The use of any drug during pregnancy requires that the potential benefits of the drug be weighed against possible hazards to mother and child. Reproduction studies in rats revealed no teratogenic effects from glycopyrrolate; however, the potent anticholinergic action of this agent resulted in diminished rates of conception and of survival at weaning, in a dose-related manner. Other studies in dogs suggest that this may be due to diminished seminal secretion which is evident at high doses of glycopyrrolate. Information on possible adverse effects in the pregnant female is limited to uncontrolled data derived from marketing experience. Such experience has revealed no reports of teratogenic or other fetus-damaging potential. No controlled studies to establish the safety of the drug in pregnancy have been performed.

Nursing Mothers. It is not known whether this drug is secreted in human milk. As a general rule, nursing should not be undertaken while a patient is on a drug since many drugs are excreted in human milk.

Pediatric Use. Since there is no adequate experience in children who have received this drug, safety and efficacy in children have not been established.

Precautions: Use Robinul with caution in the elderly and in all patients with:

- Autonomic neuropathy.
- Hepatic or renal disease.
- Ulcerative colitis—large doses may suppress intestinal motility to the point of producing a paralytic ileus and for this reason may precipitate or aggravate "toxic megacolon," a serious complication of the disease.
- Hyperthyroidism, coronary heart disease, congestive heart failure, cardiac tachyarrhythmias, tachycardia, hypertension and prostatic hypertrophy.
- Hiatal hernia associated with reflux esophagitis, since anticholinergic drugs may aggravate this condition.

Adverse Reactions: Anticholinergics produce certain effects, most of which are extensions of their fundamental pharmacological actions. Adverse reactions to anticholinergics in general may include xerostomia; decreased sweating; urinary hesitancy and retention; blurred vision; tachycardia, palpitations; dilatation of the pupil; cycloplegia; increased ocular tension; loss of taste; headaches; nervousness; mental confusion; drowsiness; weakness; dizziness; insomnia; nausea; vomiting; constipation; bloated feeling; impotence; suppression of lactation; severe allergic reaction or drug idiosyncrasies including anaphylaxis; urticaria and other dermal manifestations.

Robinul (glycopyrrolate) is chemically a quaternary ammonium compound; hence, its passage across lipid membranes, such as the blood-brain barrier, is limited in contrast to atropine sulfate and scopolamine hydrobromide. For this reason the occurrence of CNS related side effects is lower, in comparison to their incidence following administration of anticholinergics which are chemically tertiary amines that can cross this barrier readily.

Overdosage: The symptoms of overdosage of glycopyrrolate are peripheral in nature rather than central.

1. To guard against further absorption of the drug—use gastric lavage, cathartics and/or enemas.
2. To combat peripheral anticholinergic effects (residual mydriasis, dry mouth, etc.) —utilize a quaternary ammonium anticholinesterase, such as neostigmine methylsulfate.
3. To combat hypotension—use pressor amines (norepinephrine, metaraminol) i.v.; and supportive care.
4. To combat respiratory depression—administer oxygen; utilize a respiratory stimulant such as Dopram® i.v.; artificial respiration.

Dosage and Administration: ***The dosage of Robinul or Robinul Forte should be adjusted to the needs of the individual patient to assure symptomatic control with a minimum of adverse reactions. The presently recommended maximum daily dosage of glycopyrrolate is 8 mg.***

Robinul (glycopyrrolate, 1 mg) tablets. The recommended initial dosage of Robinul for adults is one tablet three times daily (in the morning, early afternoon, and at bedtime). Some patients may require two tablets at bedtime to assure overnight control of symptoms. For maintenance, a dosage of one tablet twice a day is frequently adequate.

Robinul Forte (glycopyrrolate, 2 mg) tablets. The recommended dosage of Robinul Forte for adults is one tablet two or three times daily at equally spaced intervals.

Robinul tablets are not recommended for use in children under the age of 12 years.

Drug Interactions: There are no known drug interactions.

How Supplied: Robinul (glycopyrrolate, 1 mg) tablets [NDC 0031-7824]—bottles of 100 and 500.

Robinul Forte (glycopyrrolate, 2 mg) tablets [NDC 0031-7840]—bottles of 100 and 500.

[Shown in Product Identification Section]

ROBINUL® INJECTABLE ℞

brand of Glycopyrrolate Injection, NF

Description: Robinul (glycopyrrolate) is a synthetic anticholinergic agent. Each 1 ml Robinul Injectable contains:

Glycopyrrolate, NF	0.2 mg
Water for Injection, USP	q.s.
Chlorobutanol, USP (preservative)	0.5%

For intramuscular, intravenous or subcutaneous administration as an anticholinergic in the treatment of gastrointestinal disorders.

For intramuscular or intravenous administration in conjunction with anesthesia.

Unlike atropine, glycopyrrolate is completely ionized at physiological pH values.

Robinul Injectable is a clear, colorless liquid; pH 2.0–3.0.

Actions: Glycopyrrolate, like other anticholinergic (antimuscarinic) agents, inhibits the action of acetylcholine on structures innervated by postganglionic cholinergic nerves and on smooth muscles that respond to acetylcholine but lack cholinergic innervation. These peripheral cholinergic receptors are present in the autonomic effector cells of smooth muscle, cardiac muscle, the sinoatrial node, the atrioventricular node, exocrine glands, and, to a limited degree, in the autonomic ganglia. Thus, it diminishes the volume and free acidity of gastric secretions and controls excessive pharyngeal, tracheal, and bronchial secretions.

Glycopyrrolate antagonizes muscarinic symptoms (e.g., bronchorrhea, bronchospasm, bradycardia, and intestinal hypermotility) induced by cholinergic drugs such as the anticholinesterases.

The highly polar quaternary ammonium group of glycopyrrolate limits its passage across lipid membranes, such as the blood-brain barrier, in contrast to atropine sulfate and scopolamine hydrobromide, which are non-polar tertiary amines which penetrate lipid barriers easily.

Peak effects occur approximately 30 to 45 minutes after subcutaneous or intramuscular administration. The vagal blocking effects persist for 2 to 3 hours and the antisialogogue effects persist up to 7 hours, periods longer than for atropine. With intravenous injection, the onset of action is generally evident within one minute.

FOR INTRAMUSCULAR OR INTRAVENOUS ADMINISTRATION IN CONJUNCTION WITH ANESTHESIA

Indications in Anesthesia: Robinul (glycopyrrolate) Injectable is indicated for use as a preoperative antimuscarinic to reduce salivary, tracheobronchial, and pharyngeal secretions; to reduce the volume and free acidity of gastric secretions; and, to block cardiac vagal inhibitory reflexes during induction of anesthesia and intubation. Glycopyrrolate protects against the peripheral muscarinic effects (e.g., bradycardia and excessive secretions) of cholinergic agents such as neostigmine and pyridostigmine given to reverse the neuromuscular blockade due to nondepolarizing muscle relaxants.

Contraindications: There are no absolute contraindications to the use of Robinul Injectable in conjunction with anesthesia except known hypersensitivity to glycopyrrolate.

Warnings: This drug should be used with great caution, if at all, in patients with glaucoma or asthma.

Precautions: ***Usage in Pregnancy.*** The use of any drug in pregnancy, lactation, or in the

Continued on next page

Prescribing information on A. H. Robins products listed here is based on official labeling in effect August 1, 1979, with Indications, Contraindications, Warnings, Precautions, Adverse Reactions, and Dosage stated in full.

Robins—Cont.

childbearing age requires that the potential benefits of the drug be weighed against the possible hazards to mother and child. Reproduction studies in rats and rabbits revealed no teratogenic effects from glycopyrrolate. However, diminished rates of conception and of survival at weaning were observed in rats, in a dose-related manner. Studies in dogs suggest that this may be due to diminished seminal secretion which is evident at high doses of glycopyrrolate.

Use with caution in patients with: myasthenia gravis; coronary artery disease; congestive heart failure; cardiac arrhythmias; hypertension.

The intravenous administration of any anticholinergic in the presence of cyclopropane anesthesia can result in ventricular arrhythmias; therefore, caution should be observed if Robinul (glycopyrrolate) Injectable must be used during cyclopropane anesthesia. If the drug is given in small incremental doses of 0.1 mg or less, the likelihood of producing ventricular arrhythmias is reduced.

Investigate any tachycardia before giving glycopyrrolate since an increase in the heart rate may occur.

Adverse Reactions: Anticholinergics produce certain effects most of which are extensions of their fundamental pharmacological actions. Adverse reactions to anticholinergics in general may include dry mouth; urinary hesitancy and retention; blurred vision due to mydriasis; increased ocular tension; tachycardia; palpitation; decreased sweating; loss of taste; headache; nervousness; drowsiness; weakness; dizziness; insomnia; nausea; vomiting; impotence; suppression of lactation; constipation; bloated feeling; severe allergic reaction or drug idiosyncrasies including anaphylaxis; urticaria and other dermal manifestation; some degree of mental confusion and/or excitement, especially in elderly persons.

Dosage and Administration: Robinul (glycopyrrolate) Injectable may be administered intramuscularly, or intravenously, without dilution, in the following indications:

Adults: ***Preanesthetic Medication.*** The recommended dose of Robinul (glycopyrrolate) Injectable is 0.002 mg (0.01 ml) per pound of body weight by intramuscular injection, given 30 to 60 minutes prior to the anticipated time of induction of anesthesia or at the time the preanesthetic narcotic and/or sedative are administered.

Intraoperative Medication. Robinul (glycopyrrolate) Injectable may be used during surgery to counteract drug-induced or vagal traction reflexes with the associated arrhythmias (e.g., bradycardia). It should be administered intravenously as single doses of 0.1 mg (0.5 ml) and repeated, as needed, at intervals of 2–3 minutes. The usual attempts should be made to determine the etiology of the arrhythmia, and the surgical or anesthetic manipulations necessary to correct parasympathetic imbalance should be performed.

Reversal of Neuromuscular Blockade. The recommended dose of Robinul (glycopyrrolate) Injectable is 0.2 mg (1.0 ml) for each 1.0 mg (1.0 ml) of neostigmine or the equivalent dose of pyridostigmine. In order to minimize the appearance of cardiac side effects, the drugs may be administered simultaneously by intravenous injection and may be mixed in the same syringe.

Children: ***Preanesthetic Medication.*** The recommended dose of Robinul (glycopyrrolate) Injectable in children up to 12 years of age is 0.002 mg to 0.004 mg (0.01 ml to 0.02 ml) per pound of body weight intramuscularly, given 30 to 60 minutes prior to the anticipated time of induction of anesthesia or at the time the preanesthetic narcotic and/or sedative are administered.

Intraoperative Medication. Because of the long duration of action of Robinul (glycopyrrolate) if used as preanesthetic medication, additional Robinul (glycopyrrolate) Injectable for anticholinergic effect intraoperatively is rarely needed; in the event it is required the recommended pediatric dose is 0.002 mg (0.01 ml) per pound of body weight intravenously, not to exceed 0.1 mg (0.5 ml) in a single dose which may be repeated, as needed, at intervals of 2–3 minutes. The usual attempts should be made to determine the etiology of the arrhythmia, and the surgical or anesthetic manipulations necessary to correct parasympathetic imbalance should be performed.

Reversal of Neuromuscular Blockade. The recommended pediatric dose of Robinul (glycopyrrolate) Injectable is 0.2 mg (1.0 ml) for each 1.0 mg (1.0 ml) of neostigmine or the equivalent dose of pyridostigmine. In order to minimize the appearance of cardiac side effects, the drugs may be administered simultaneously by intravenous injection and may be mixed in the same syringe.

NOTE: See below for dosage of Robinul Injectable as an anticholinergic in the treatment of gastrointestinal disorders.

Compatibility With Other Agents: ***Known compatibilities.*** Robinul (glycopyrrolate) Injectable is compatible for mixing and injection with the following: 5% and 10% glucose in water or saline; Demerol® (meperidine) Injectable; morphine sulfate; Innovar® (fentanyl plus droperidol) Injectable; Vistaril® (hydroxyzine) Injectable; Prostigmin® (neostigmine) Injectable; Mestinon® (pyridostigmine) Injectable. Robinul Injectable may be administered via the tubing of a running infusion of physiological saline or lactated Ringer's solution.

Known incompatibilities include the following injectables: sodium bicarbonate; Valium® (diazepam); sodium pentobarbital; various phenothiazines; Dramamine® (dimenhydrinate), and chloramphenicol.

Drug Interaction During Anesthesia. Glycopyrrolate has been used clinically with at least the following medications: a barbiturate (sodium thiopental); narcotic analgesics (morphine, alphaprodine hydrochloride, fentanyl); sedative/tranquilizers (droperidol, diazepam); gaseous anesthetics (nitrous oxide); volatile liquid anesthetics (diethyl ether, halothane, methoxyflurane, enflurane); parenteral anesthetics (ketamine); peripherally-acting skeletal muscle relaxants (succinylcholine, gallamine, d-tubocurarine, pancuronium); cholinergic agents (neostigmine, pyridostigmine); and other anticholinergics (atropine).

There are no known unique or unanticipated drug-drug interactions with other agents except that Robinul (glycopyrrolate) Injectable should be used with caution if at all during cyclopropane anesthesia (see Precautions).

Management of Overdosage: Symptoms of overdosage are peripheral rather than central in nature. To combat peripheral anticholinergic effects, a quaternary ammonium anticholinesterase such as neostigmine methylsulfate may be given in a dose of 1.0 mg for each 1.0 mg of Robinul (glycopyrrolate) Injectable known to have been administered.

****

FOR INTRAMUSCULAR, INTRAVENOUS OR SUBCUTANEOUS ADMINISTRATION AS AN ANTICHOLINERGIC IN THE TREATMENT OF GASTROINTESTINAL DISORDERS

Indications in Gastroenterology: For use as adjunctive therapy for the treatment of peptic ulcer when rapid anticholinergic effect is desired or when oral medication is not tolerated.

Contraindications: Glaucoma, obstructive uropathy (for example, bladder neck obstruction due to prostatic hypertrophy), obstructive disease of the gastrointestinal tract (for example, pyloroduodenal stenosis), paralytic ileus, intestinal atony of the elderly or debilitated patient, unstable cardiovascular status in acute hemorrhage, severe ulcerative colitis, toxic megacolon complicating ulcerative colitis, myasthenia gravis.

Warnings: Robinul (glycopyrrolate) Injectable may be administered without dilution subcutaneously, intramuscularly, or intravenously. However, intravenous administration should be reserved for those clinical situations in which immediate drug effects are essential.

In the presence of a high environmental temperature, heat prostration (fever and heat stroke due to decreased sweating) can occur with use of Robinul (glycopyrrolate).

Diarrhea may be an early symptom of incomplete intestinal obstruction, especially in patients with ileostomy or colostomy. In this instance treatment with Robinul (glycopyrrolate) would be inappropriate and possibly harmful.

Robinul (glycopyrrolate) may produce drowsiness or blurred vision. The patient should be cautioned regarding activities requiring mental alertness such as operating a motor vehicle or other machinery or performing hazardous work while taking this drug.

Theoretically, with overdosage a curarelike action may occur, i.e., neuromuscular blockade leading to muscular weakness and possible paralysis.

Pregnancy. The use of any drug in pregnancy, lactation, or in the childbearing age requires that the potential benefits of the drug be weighed against the possible hazards to mother and child. Reproduction studies in rats and rabbits revealed no teratogenic effects from glycopyrrolate. However, diminished rates of conception and of survival at weaning were observed in rats, in a dose-related manner. Studies in dogs suggest that this may be due to diminished seminal secretion which is evident at high doses of glycopyrrolate.

Nursing Mothers. It is not known whether this drug is secreted in human milk. As a general rule, nursing should not be undertaken while a patient is on a drug since many drugs are excreted in human milk.

Pediatric Use. Since there is no experience in children who have received this drug for gastrointestinal indications, its safety and efficacy in children have not been established.

Precautions: Use Robinul (glycopyrrolate) with caution in the elderly and in all patients with:

- Autonomic neuropathy
- Hepatic or renal disease
- Ulcerative colitis — large doses may suppress intestinal motility to the point of producing a paralytic ileus and for this reason may precipitate or aggravate "toxic megacolon," a serious complication of the disease.
- Hyperthyroidism, coronary heart disease, congestive heart failure, cardiac tachyarrhythmias, tachycardia, hypertension and prostatic hypertrophy.
- Hiatal hernia associated with reflux esophagitis, since anticholinergic drugs may aggravate this condition.

Adverse Reactions: Anticholinergics produce certain effects most of which are extensions of their pharmacologic actions. Adverse reactions to anticholinergics in general may include dry mouth; urinary hesitancy and retention; blurred vision due to mydriasis; increased ocular tension; tachycardia; palpitation; decreased sweating; loss of taste; headache; nervousness; drowsiness; weakness; dizziness; insomnia; nausea; vomiting; impotence; suppression of lactation; constipation; bloated feeling; severe allergic reaction or drug idiosyncrasies including anaphylaxis; urticaria and other dermal manifestations; some degree of mental confusion and/or excitement, especially in elderly persons.

Robinul is chemically a quaternary ammonium compound; hence, its passage across lipid membranes, such as the blood-brain barrier is limited in contrast to atropine sulfate and scopolamine hydrobromide. For this reason the occurrence of CNS related side effects is lower, in comparison to their incidence following administration of anticholinergics which are chemically tertiary amines that can cross this barrier readily.

Management of Overdosage: Symptoms of overdosage are peripheral rather than central in nature. To combat peripheral anticholinergic effects, a quaternary ammonium anticholinesterase such as neostigmine methylsulfate may be given in a dose of 1.0 mg for each 1.0 mg of Robinul (glycopyrrolate) Injectable known to have been administered.

Dosage and Administration: Robinul (glycopyrrolate) Injectable may be administered subcutaneously, intramuscularly, or intravenously without dilution. The usual recommended dose of Robinul (glycopyrrolate) Injectable is 0.1 mg (0.5 ml) administered at 4-hour intervals, 3 or 4 times daily. Where more profound effect is required, 0.2 mg (1.0 ml) may be given. Frequency of administration depends upon individual patient response, but a 4-hour interval between injections is recommended. Some patients may need only a single dose, others may require administration two, three, or four times a day.

NOTE: See above for dosage of Robinul as a preoperative antimuscarinic, for intraoperative use and for reversal of neuromuscular blockade.

Drug Interactions: ***Known Compatibilities.***

Robinul (glycopyrrolate) Injectable is compatible for mixing and injection with the following: 5% and 10% glucose in water or saline; Demerol® (meperidine) Injectable; morphine sulfate; Innovar® (fentanyl plus droperidol) Injectable; Vistaril® (hydroxyzine) Injectable; Mestinon® (pyridostigmine) Injectable. Robinul Injectable may be administered via the tubing of a running infusion of physiological saline or lactated Ringer's solution.

Known incompatibilities include the following injectables: sodium bicarbonate; Valium® (diazepam); sodium pentobarbital; various phenothiazines; Dramamine® (dimenhydrinate), and chloramphenicol.

****

How Supplied: Robinul (glycopyrrolate) Injectable is available in 1 ml single dose vial in cartons of 5 and 25; and 5 ml and 20 ml multiple dose vials (NDC 0031-7890).

ROBINUL®-PH TABLETS ℞
ROBINUL®-PH FORTE TABLETS ℞

Description:

Robinul-PH tablets are scored, compressed blue tablets engraved AHR. Each tablet contains:

Glycopyrrolate, NF .... 1 mg
Phenobarbital, USP .... 16.2 mg
(Warning: May be habit forming)

Robinul-PH Forte tablets are scored, compressed blue tablets engraved $\frac{AHR}{2}$. Each tablet contains:

Glycopyrrolate, NF .... 2 mg
Phenobarbital, USP .... 16.2 mg
(Warning: May be habit forming)

Actions: Glycopyrrolate, like other anticholinergic (antimuscarinic) agents, inhibits the action of acetylcholine on structures innervated by postganglionic cholinergic nerves and on smooth muscles that respond to acetylcholine but lack cholinergic innervation. These peripheral cholinergic receptors are present in the autonomic effector cells of smooth muscle, cardiac muscle, the sinoatrial node, the atrioventricular node, exocrine glands, and, to a limited degree, in the autonomic ganglia. Thus, it diminishes the volume and free acidity of gastric secretions and controls excessive pharyngeal, tracheal, and bronchial secretions.

Glycopyrrolate antagonizes muscarinic symptoms (e.g., bronchorrhea, bronchospasm, bradycardia, and intestinal hypermotility) induced by cholinergic drugs such as the anticholinesterases.

The highly polar quaternary ammonium group of glycopyrrolate limits its passage across lipid membranes, such as the bloodbrain barrier, in contrast to atropine sulfate and scopolamine hydrobromide, which are non-polar tertiary amines which penetrate lipid barriers easily. Phenobarbital produces mild sedation.

Indications

Based on a review of this drug by the National Academy of Sciences—National Research Council and/or other information, FDA has classified the following indications as "possibly" effective:

For use as adjunctive therapy in the treatment of peptic ulcer. ROBINUL-PH HAS NOT BEEN SHOWN TO BE EFFECTIVE IN CONTRIBUTING TO THE HEALING OF PEPTIC ULCER, DECREASING THE RATE OF RECURRENCE OR PREVENTING COMPLICATIONS.

For use as adjunctive therapy in the treatment of irritable bowel syndrome (irritable colon, spastic colon, mucous colitis, acute enterocolitis, and functional gastrointestinal disorders), WHEN NOT RELIEVED BY SUCH MEASURES AS DIET, SEDATION, REASSURANCE, PHYSICIAN INTEREST AND AMELIORATION OF ENVIRONMENTAL FACTORS. Also as adjunctive therapy in the treatment of neurogenic bowel disturbances (including the splenic flexure syndrome and neurogenic colon).

Final classification of these less-than-effective indications requires further investigation.

Contraindications: Glaucoma; obstructive uropathy (for example, bladder neck obstruction due to prostatic hypertrophy); obstructive disease of the gastrointestinal tract (as in achalasia, pyloroduodenal stenosis, etc.); paralytic ileus; intestinal atony of the elderly or debilitated patient; unstable cardiovascular status in acute hemorrhage; severe ulcerative colitis; toxic megacolon complicating ulcerative colitis; myasthenia gravis. Phenobarbital is contraindicated in acute intermittent porphyria. Robinul-PH (glycopyrrolate with phenobarbital) tablets are contraindicated in those patients with a hypersensitivity to glycopyrrolate or phenobarbital and in those patients in whom phenobarbital produces restlessness and/or excitement.

Warnings: Phenobarbital in patients taking anticoagulants may decrease the effect of the anticoagulant and thus require larger doses of the anticoagulant for optimal effect. When the phenobarbital is discontinued, the dose of the anticoagulant may have to be decreased. Barbiturates may thus decrease the action of anticoagulant drugs. (See Drug Interactions section.)

Phenobarbital may be habit-forming and should not be administered to individuals known to be addiction prone or to those with a history of physical and/or psychological dependence upon habit-forming drugs.

Since barbiturates are metabolized in the liver, Robinul-PH should be used with caution and initial small doses in patients with hepatic dysfunction.

In the presence of a high environmental temperature, heat prostration (fever and heat stroke due to decreased sweating) can occur with use of Robinul-PH.

Diarrhea may be an early symptom of incomplete intestinal obstruction, especially in patients with ileostomy or colostomy. In this instance treatment with this drug would be inappropriate and possibly harmful.

Robinul-PH (glycopyrrolate with phenobarbital) may produce drowsiness or blurred vision. In this event, the patient should be warned not to engage in activities requiring mental alertness such as operating a motor vehicle or other machinery, or performing hazardous work while taking this drug.

Theoretically, with overdosage a curarelike action may occur, i.e., neuromuscular blockade leading to muscular weakness and possible paralysis.

Pregnancy. The safety of this drug during pregnancy has not been established. The use of any drug during pregnancy requires that the potential benefits of the drug be weighed against possible hazards to mother and child. Reproduction studies have not been performed on this particular combination in animals. Information on possible adverse effects to the fetus is limited to uncontrolled data derived from marketing experience. Such experience has revealed no reports of teratogenic or other fetus-damaging potential. There are no controlled studies using this combination in animals or humans to determine whether this drug affects fertility in human males or females, has teratogenic potential, or has other adverse effects on the fetus.

Reproduction studies in rats revealed no teratogenic effects from glycopyrrolate; however, the potent anticholinergic action of this agent resulted in diminished rates of conception and of survival at weaning, in a dose-related manner. Other studies in dogs suggest that this may be due to diminished seminal secretion which is evident at high doses of glycopyrrolate.

Nursing Mothers. It is not known whether this drug is secreted in human milk. As a general rule, nursing should not be undertaken while a patient is on a drug since many drugs are excreted in human milk.

Pediatric Use. Since there is no adequate experience in children who have received this drug, safety and efficacy in children have not been established.

Precautions: Use Robinul-PH with caution in the elderly and in all patients with:

- Autonomic neuropathy.
- Hepatic or renal disease.
- Ulcerative colitis—large doses may suppress intestinal motility to the point of producing a paralytic ileus and for this reason may precipitate or aggravate "toxic megacolon," a serious complication of the disease.
- Hyperthyroidism, coronary heart disease, congestive heart failure, cardiac tachyarrhythmias, tachycardia, hypertension and prostatic hypertrophy.
- Hiatal hernia associated with reflux esophagitis, since anticholinergic drugs may aggravate this condition.

Adverse Reactions: Anticholinergics produce certain effects most of which are extensions of their fundamental pharmacologic actions. Adverse reactions to anticholinergics in general may include xerostomia; decreased sweating; urinary hesitancy and retention; blurred vision; tachycardia; palpitations; dilatation of the pupil; cycloplegia; increased ocular tension; loss of taste; headaches; nervousness; mental confusion; drowsiness; weakness; dizziness; insomnia; nausea; vomiting; constipation; bloated feeling; impotence; suppression of lactation; severe allergic reaction or drug

Continued on next page

Prescribing information on A. H. Robins products listed here is based on official labeling in effect August 1, 1979, with Indications, Contraindications, Warnings, Precautions, Adverse Reactions, and Dosage stated in full.

Robins—Cont.

idiosyncrasies including anaphylaxis; urticaria and other dermal manifestations.
Robinul (glycopyrrolate) is chemically a quaternary ammonium compound; hence its passage across lipid membranes, such as the blood-brain barrier, is limited, in contrast to atropine sulfate and scopolamine hydrobromide. For this reason the occurrence of CNS related side effects is lower, in comparison to their incidence following administration of anticholinergics which are chemically tertiary amines that can cross this barrier readily.
Phenobarbital may produce excitement in some patients rather than a sedative effect. An occasional patient may experience musculoskeletal pain. Some patients may acquire a sensitivity to barbiturates and experience allergic phenomena and/or dermatologic responses.
In patients habituated to barbiturates, abrupt withdrawal may produce delirium or convulsions.
Overdosage: The symptoms of overdosage of glycopyrrolate are peripheral in nature rather than central.
1. To guard against further absorption of the drug—use gastric lavage, cathartics and/or enemas.
2. To combat peripheral anticholinergic effects (residual mydriasis, dry mouth, etc.) —utilize a quaternary ammonium anticholinesterase, such as neostigmine methylsulfate.
3. To combat hypotension—use pressor amines (norepinephrine, metaraminol) i.v.; and supportive care.
4. To combat respiratory depression—administer oxygen; utilize a respiratory stimulant such as Dopram® i.v.; artificial respiration.
Overdosage of phenobarbital may lead to sleepiness, mental confusion, and unsteadiness. Treatment should include removal of remaining drug from the stomach by thorough gastric lavage or emesis followed by catharsis, and supportive and symptomatic therapy as indicated.
Dosage and Administration: ***The dosage of Robinul-PH or Robinul-PH Forte should be adjusted to the needs of the individual patient to assure symptomatic control with a minimum of adverse reactions. The presently recommended maximum daily dosage of glycopyrrolate is 8 mg.***
Robinul-PH (glycopyrrolate, 1 mg; phenobarbital, 16.2 mg) tablets. The recommended initial dosage of Robinul-PH for adults is one tablet three times daily (in the morning, early afternoon, and at bedtime). Some patients may require two tablets at bedtime to assure overnight control of symptoms. For maintenance, a dosage of one tablet twice a day is frequently adequate.
Robinul-PH Forte (glycopyrrolate, 2 mg; phenobarbital, 16.2 mg) tablets. The recommended dosage of Robinul-PH Forte for adults is one tablet two or three times daily at equally spaced intervals.
Robinul-PH tablets are not recommended for use in children under the age of 12 years.
Drug Interactions: Phenobarbital and other barbiturates may inhibit the action of anticoagulant drugs. Frequent measurement of the prothrombin time and appropriate adjustment of the anticoagulant dosage are essential when barbiturate intake is initiated, altered or discontinued. Anticoagulant requirements may be increased during barbiturate administration. When the barbiturate is discontinued, the anticoagulant dose may need to be reduced to minimize the risk of hemorrhage.
How Supplied: Robinul-PH (glycopyrrolate, 1 mg; phenobarbital, 16.2 mg) tablets [NDC 0031-7874]—bottles of 100 and 500.
Robinul-PH Forte (glycopyrrolate, 2 mg; phenobarbital, 16.2 mg) tablets [NDC 0031-7880]—bottles of 100 and 500.
[*Shown in Product Identification Section*]

ROBITET® '250' ℞
hydrochloride Robicaps†
(Tetracycline Hydrochloride Capsules, USP)
ROBITET® '500' ℞
hydrochloride Robicaps
(Tetracycline Hydrochloride Capsules, USP)
ROBITET® SYRUP ℞
(Tetracycline, USP)
125 mg per 5 ml

Description: Tetracycline is a broad-spectrum antibiotic prepared from the cultures of certain streptomyces species. Robitet '250' Robicaps are pink and brown hard gelatin capsules each containing 250 mg tetracycline hydrochloride.
Robitet '500' Robicaps are cream and brown hard gelatin capsules each containing 500 mg tetracycline hydrochloride.
Robitet syrup is a cherry flavored suspension containing tetracycline equivalent to 125 mg of tetracycline hydrochloride per teaspoonful (5 ml).
Actions: The tetracyclines are primarily bacteriostatic and are thought to exert their antimicrobial effect by the inhibition of protein synthesis. Tetracyclines are active against a wide range of gram-negative and gram-positive organisms.
The drugs in the tetracycline class have closely similar antimicrobial spectra, and cross-resistance among them is common. Micro-organisms may be considered susceptible if the MIC (minimum inhibitory concentration) is not more than 4.0 mcg./ml. and intermediate if the MIC is 4.0 to 12.5 mcg./ml.
Susceptibility plate testing: A tetracycline disc may be used to determine microbial susceptibility to drugs in the tetracycline class. If the Kirby-Bauer method of disc susceptibility testing is used, a 30 mcg. tetracycline disc should give a zone of at least 19 mm. when tested against a tetracycline-susceptible bacterial strain.
Tetracyclines are readily absorbed and are bound to plasma proteins in varying degree. They are concentrated by the liver in the bile and excreted in the urine and feces at high concentrations and in a biologically active form.
Indications: Tetracycline is indicated in infections caused by the following microorganisms: Rickettsiae (Rocky Mountain spotted fever, typhus fever and the typhus group, Q fever, rickettsialpox and tick fevers), *Mycoplasma pneumoniae* (PPLO, Eaton Agent), Agents of psittacosis and ornithosis, Agents of lymphogranuloma venereum and granuloma inguinale, The spirochetal agent of relapsing fever *(Borrelia recurrentis).*
The following gram-negative micro-organisms: *Haemophilus ducreyi* (chancroid), *Pasteurella pestis* and *Pasteurella tularensis, Bartonella bacilliformis, Bacteroides* species, *Vibrio comma* and *Vibrio fetus, Brucella* species (in conjunction with streptomycin).
Because many strains of the following groups of micro-organisms have been shown to be resistant to tetracyclines, culture and susceptibility testing are recommended.
Tetracycline is indicated for treatment of infections caused by the following gram-negative micro-organisms, when bacteriologic testing indicates appropriate susceptibility to the drug: *Escherichia coli, Enterobacter aerogenes* (formerly *Aerobacter aerogenes), Shigella* species, *Mima* species and *Herellea* species, *Haemophilus influenzae* (respiratory infections), *Klebsiella* species (respiratory and urinary infections).
Tetracycline is indicated for treatment of infections caused by the following gram-positive micro-organisms when bacteriologic testing indicates appropriate susceptibility to the drug:
Streptococcus species: Up to 44 percent of strains of *Streptococcus pyogenes* and 74 percent of *Streptococcus faecalis* have been found to be resistant to tetracycline drugs. Therefore, tetracyclines should not be used for streptococcal disease unless the organism has been demonstrated to be sensitive. For upper respiratory infections due to group A beta-hemolytic streptococci, penicillin is the usual drug of choice, including prophylaxis of rheumatic fever.
Diplococcus pneumoniae, Staphylococcus aureus, skin and soft tissue infections. Tetracyclines are not the drugs of choice in the treatment of any type of staphylococcal infections.
When penicillin is contraindicated, tetracyclines are alternative drugs in the treatment of infections due to: *Neisseria gonorrhoeae, Treponema pallidum* and *Treponema pertenue* (syphilis and yaws), *Listeria monocytogenes, Clostridium* species, *Bacillus anthracis, Fusobacterium fusiforme* (Vincent's infection), *Actinomyces* species.
In acute intestinal amebiasis, the tetracyclines may be a useful adjunct to amebicides.
In severe acne, the tetracyclines may be useful adjunctive therapy.
Tetracyclines are indicated in the treatment of trachoma, although the infectious agent is not always eliminated, as judged by immunofluorescence.
Inclusion conjunctivitis may be treated with oral tetracyclines or with a combination of oral and topical agents.
Contraindication: This drug is contraindicated in persons who have shown hypersensitivity to any of the tetracyclines.
Warnings: THE USE OF DRUGS OF THE TETRACYCLINE CLASS DURING TOOTH DEVELOPMENT (LAST HALF OF PREGNANCY, INFANCY AND CHILDHOOD TO THE AGE OF 8 YEARS) MAY CAUSE PERMANENT DISCOLORATION OF THE TEETH (YELLOW-GRAY-BROWN). This adverse reaction is more common during long-term use of the drugs but has been observed following repeated short-term courses. Enamel hypoplasia has also been reported. TETRACYCLINE DRUGS, THEREFORE, SHOULD NOT BE USED IN THIS AGE GROUP UNLESS OTHER DRUGS ARE NOT LIKELY TO BE EFFECTIVE OR ARE CONTRAINDICATED.
If renal impairment exists, even usual oral or parenteral doses may lead to excessive systemic accumulation of the drug and possible liver toxicity. Under such conditions, lower than usual total doses are indicated and, if therapy is prolonged, serum level determinations of the drug may be advisable.
Photosensitivity manifested by an exaggerated sunburn reaction has been observed in some individuals taking tetracyclines. Patients apt to be exposed to direct sunlight or ultraviolet light should be advised that this reaction can occur with tetracycline drugs, and treatment should be discontinued at the first evidence of skin erythema.
The anti-anabolic action of the tetracyclines may cause an increase in BUN. While this is not a problem in those with normal renal function, in patients with significantly impaired function, higher serum levels of tetracycline may lead to azotemia, hyperphosphatemia, and acidosis.
Usage in pregnancy. (See above "Warnings" about use during tooth development.)
Results of animal studies indicate that tetracyclines cross the placenta, are found in fetal tissues and can have toxic effects on the developing fetus (often related to retardation of skeletal development). Evidence of embryotoxicity has also been noted in animals treated early in pregnancy.
Usage in newborns, infants, and children. (See above "Warnings" about use during tooth development.)

All tetracyclines form a stable calcium complex in any bone forming tissue. A decrease in the fibula growth rate has been observed in prematures given oral tetracycline in doses of 25 mg./kg. every 6 hours. This reaction was shown to be reversible when the drug was discontinued.
Tetracyclines are present in the milk of lactating women who are taking a drug in this class.
Precautions: As with other antibiotic preparations, use of this drug may result in overgrowth of nonsusceptible organisms, including fungi. If superinfection occurs, the antibiotic should be discontinued and appropriate therapy instituted.
In venereal diseases when coexistent syphilis is suspected, darkfield examination should be done before treatment is started and the blood serology repeated monthly for at least 4 months.
Because tetracyclines have been shown to depress plasma prothrombin activity, patients who are on anticoagulant therapy may require downward adjustment of their anticoagulant dosage.
In long-term therapy, periodic laboratory evaluation of organ systems, including hematopoietic, renal and hepatic studies should be performed.
All infections due to Group A beta-hemolytic streptococci should be treated for at least 10 days.
Since bacteriostatic drugs may interfere with the bactericidal action of penicillin, it is advisable to avoid giving tetracycline in conjunction with penicillin.
Adverse Reactions: Gastrointestinal: Anorexia, nausea, vomiting, diarrhea, glossitis, dysphagia, enterocolitis, and inflammatory lesions (with monilial overgrowth) in the anogenital region. These reactions have been caused by both the oral and parenteral administration of tetracyclines.
Skin: maculopapular and erythematous rashes. Exfoliative dermatitis has been reported but is uncommon. Photosensitivity is discussed above. (See "Warnings.")
Renal toxicity: Rise in BUN has been reported and is apparently dose related. (See "Warnings.")
Hypersensitivity reactions: urticaria, angioneurotic edema, anaphylaxis, anaphylactoid purpura, pericarditis and exacerbation of systemic lupus erythematosis.
Bulging fontanels have been reported in young infants following full therapeutic dosage. This sign disappeared rapidly when the drug was discontinued.
Blood: Hemolytic anemia, thrombocytopenia, neutropenia and eosinophilia have been reported.
When given over prolonged periods, tetracyclines have been reported to produce brown-black microscopic discoloration of thyroid glands. No abnormalities of thyroid function studies are known to occur.
Dosage and Administration: Therapy should be continued for at least 24-48 hours after symptoms and fever have subsided.
Concomitant therapy: Antacids containing aluminum, calcium, or magnesium impair absorption and should not be given to patients taking oral tetracycline.
Food and some dairy products also interfere with absorption. Oral forms of tetracycline should be given 1 hour before or 2 hours after meals. Pediatric oral dosage forms should not be given with milk formulas and should be given at least 1 hour prior to feeding.
In patients with renal impairment: (See "Warnings.") Total dosage should be decreased by reduction of recommended individual doses and/or by extending time intervals between doses.
In the treatment of streptococcal infections, a therapeutic dose of tetracycline should be administered for at least 10 days.
ADULTS: Usual daily dose, 1-2 Gm. divided in two or four equal doses, depending on the severity of the infection.
FOR CHILDREN ABOVE EIGHT YEARS OF AGE: Usual daily dose, 10-20 mg. per pound (25-50 mg./kg.) of body weight divided in four equal doses.
For treatment of brucellosis, 500 mg. tetracycline four times daily for 3 weeks should be accompanied by streptomycin. 1 gram intramuscularly twice daily the first week, and once daily the second week.
For treatment of syphilis, a total of 30-40 grams in equally divided doses over a period of 10-15 days should be given. Close followup, including laboratory tests, is recommended.
Treatment of uncomplicated gonorrhea: When penicillin is contraindicated, tetracycline may be used for the treatment of both males and females in the following divided dosage schedule: 1.5 grams initially followed by 0.5 grams q.i.d. for a total of 9.0 grams.
How Supplied: Robitet Robicaps® (Tetracycline Hydrochloride Capsules, USP), 250 mg in bottles of 100 and 1000 (NDC 0031-8417); 500 mg in bottles of 100 and 500 (NDC 0031-8427). Robitet® Syrup, 125 mg per 5 ml, in pint bottles (NDC 0031-8407).

†Robicaps® is A. H. Robins' registered trademark for capsules.

[*Shown in Product Identification Section*]

ROBITUSSIN®
ROBITUSSIN–CF®
ROBITUSSIN–DM®
ROBITUSSIN–PE®

Composition: *Robitussin* contains Guaifenesin, NF 100 mg in 5 ml (1 teaspoonful) of palatable aromatic syrup; alcohol 3.5%. *Robitussin-CF* contains in each 5 ml (1 teaspoonful): Guaifenesin, NF 100 mg, Phenylpropanolamine Hydrochloride, NF 12.5 mg, Dextromethorphan Hydrobromide, NF 10 mg; alcohol 4.75%. *Robitussin-DM* contains in each 5 ml (1 teaspoonful): Guaifenesin, NF 100 mg and Dextromethorphan Hydrobromide, NF 15 mg; alcohol 1.4%. *Robitussin-PE* contains in each 5 ml (1 teaspoonful): Guaifenesin, NF 100 mg and Pseudoephedrine Hydrochloride, NF 30 mg; alcohol 1.4%.
Action and Uses: All four preparations employ the expectorant action of guaifenesin which enhances the output of respiratory tract fluid (RTF). The enhanced flow of less viscid secretions promotes ciliary action, and facilitates the removal of inspissated mucus. As a result, unproductive coughs become more productive and less frequent. *Robitussin* is therefore, useful in combatting coughs associated with the common cold, bronchitis, laryngitis, tracheitis, pharyngitis, pertussis, influenza and measles, and for coughs provoked by chronic paranasal sinusitis. In *Robitussin-CF* the guaifenesin is supplemented with phenylpropanolamine which provides mild vasoconstrictor action resulting in a nasal decongestant effect and dextromethorphan, a synthetic, non-narcotic, centrally-acting cough suppressant. In *Robitussin-DM,* the guaifenesin is supplemented by dextromethorphan. In *Robitussin-PE,* the expectorant action of guaifenesin is supplemented by a sympathomimetic amine, pseudoephedrine, which helps reduce mucosal congestion and edema in the nasal passages.
Contraindications: Hypersensitivity to any of the components. *Robitussin-DM* is also contraindicated in patients who are receiving MAO inhibitors. *Robitussin-CF* and *Robitussin-PE* are also contraindicated in marked hypertension, hyperthyroidism or in patients who are receiving MAO inhibitors or antihypertensive medication.
Precautions: *Robitussin-CF* and *Robitussin-PE* should be administered with caution to patients with hypertension, cardiac disorders, diabetes or peripheral vascular disease. As with all products containing sympathomimetic amines, these products should be used with caution in patients with prostatic hypertrophy or glaucoma.
Note: Guaifenesin has been shown to produce a color interference with certain clinical laboratory determinations of 5-hydroxyindoleacetic acid (5-HIAA) and vanillylmandelic acid (VMA).
Adverse Reactions: No serious side effects have been reported from guaifenesin or dextromethorphan. Possible adverse reactions of *Robitussin-CF* and *Robitussin-PE* include nausea, vomiting, dry mouth, nervousness, insomnia, restlessness or headache.
Dosage: The following dosages are recommended for *Robitussin, Robitussin-CF* and *Robitussin-PE:* Adults and children 12 years of age and over: 2 teaspoonfuls every four hours, not to exceed 12 teaspoonfuls in a 24-hour period; children 6 to under 12 years: 1 teaspoonful every four hours, not to exceed 6 teaspoonfuls in a 24-hour period; children 2 to under 6 years: ½ teaspoonful every four hours, not to exceed 3 teaspoonfuls in a 24-hour period; children under 2 years: use only as directed by physician. *Robitussin-DM:* Adults and children 12 years of age and over: 2 teaspoonfuls every six to eight hours, not to exceed 8 teaspoonfuls in a 24-hour period; children 6 to under 12 years: 1 teaspoonful every six to eight hours, not to exceed 4 teaspoonfuls in a 24-hour period; children 2 to under 6 years: ½ teaspoonful every six to eight hours, not to exceed 2 teaspoonfuls in a 24-hour period; children under 2 years: use only as directed by physician.
How Supplied: *Robitussin* (wine-colored, NDC 0031-8624) and *Robitussin-DM* (cherry-colored, NDC 0031-8684) in bottles of 4 fl. oz., 8 fl. oz., 1 pint and 1 gallon. *Robitussin-CF* (red-colored, NDC 0031-8677) and *Robitussin-PE* (orange-red, NDC 0031-8695) in bottles of 4 fl. oz., 8 fl. oz. and 1 pint. *Robitussin* also available in 1 fl. oz. bottle (4 × 25's) and 5 ml., 10 ml., and 15 ml Dis-Co® Unit Dose Packs (4 × 25's). *Robitussin-DM* also available in 5 ml and 10 ml Dis-Co® Unit Dose Packs (4 × 25's).

ROBITUSSIN A–C® Ⓒ

Robitussin and codeine.
Each 5 ml (1 teaspoonful) contains:
Guaifenesin, NF ....100 mg
Codeine Phosphate, USP ....10 mg
(Warning: May be habit forming)
In a palatable, aromatic syrup
Alcohol 3.5 per cent
Actions: Robitussin A-C combines the expectorant, guaifenesin, with the cough suppressant, codeine. Guaifenesin enhances the output of lower respiratory tract fluid (RTF). The enhanced flow of less viscid secretions promotes ciliary action, and facilitates the removal of inspissated mucus. As a result, dry, unproductive coughs become more productive and less frequent.
Codeine phosphate is favored for its efficacy in low dosage. Robitussin A-C is especially useful when concurrent expectorant and cough suppressant actions are desired.
Indications: Robitussin A-C is useful in combating coughs associated with the common cold, bronchitis, laryngitis, tracheitis, pharyngitis, pertussis, influenza, and measles.
Contraindications: Hypersensitivity to any of the ingredients.
Adverse Reactions: Rarely, nausea, gastrointestinal upset, constipation, and drowsiness

Continued on next page

Prescribing information on A. H. Robins products listed here is based on official labeling in effect August 1, 1979, with Indications, Contraindications, Warnings, Precautions, Adverse Reactions, and Dosage stated in full.

Robins—Cont.

may occur. No serious side effects from guaifenesin have been reported.
Note: Guaifenesin has been shown to produce a color interference with certain clinical laboratory determinations of 5-hydroxyindoleacetic acid (5-HIAA) and vanillylmandelic acid (VMA).
Dosage: Adults and children 12 years of age and over: 2 teaspoonfuls every four hours, not to exceed 12 teaspoonfuls in a 24 hour period; children 6 to under 12 years: 1 teaspoonful every four hours, not to exceed 6 teaspoonfuls in a 24 hour period; children 2 to under 6 years: ½ teaspoonful every four hours, not to exceed 3 teaspoonfuls in a 24 hour period; children under 2 years: use as directed by physician.
How Supplied: Bottles of 2 fl. oz., 4 fl. oz., one pint, and one gallon (NDC 0031-8674).

ROBITUSSIN® -DAC ©

Each 5 ml (1 teaspoonful) contains:

Guaifenesin, NF	100 mg
Pseudoephedrine Hydrochloride, NF	30 mg
Codeine Phosphate, USP	10 mg
(Warning: May be habit forming)	

In a palatable, aromatic syrup
Alcohol 1.4 per cent
Indications: For the temporary relief of cough and nasal congestion as may occur with the common cold or with inhaled irritants.
Contains the expectorant, guaifenesin, which relieves irritated membranes in the respiratory passageways by preventing dryness through increased mucus flow. The nasal decongestant, pseudoephedrine, reduces the swelling of nasal passages. The antitussive, codeine, calms the cough control center and relieves coughing.
Contraindications: Hypersensitivity to any of the ingredients, marked hypertension, hyperthyroidism, or in patients who are receiving MAO inhibitors or antihypertensive medication.
Warnings: Use this product with caution in children under 2 years or in children taking another drug. Prescribe cautiously for patients with persistent or chronic cough such as comes with smoking, asthma, emphysema, or where cough is accompanied by excessive secretions. Caution should be taken in administering this drug to patients with high blood pressure, heart disease or diabetes. In patients with chronic pulmonary disease or shortness of breath, this product should be administered with caution. As with all products containing sympathomimetic amines, use with caution in patients with prostatic hypertrophy or glaucoma. Do not exceed recommended dosage because at higher doses nervousness, dizziness or sleeplessness may occur. May cause or aggravate constipation.
Note: Guaifenesin has been shown to produce a color interference with certain clinical laboratory determinations of 5-hydroxyindoleacetic acid (5-HIAA) and vanillylmandelic acid (VMA).
Adverse Reactions: Agitation, dizziness, insomnia, palpitations or nausea may occur. In such instances, reduction in frequency and/or quantity of dose is indicated.
Recommended Dosage: Adults—1 or 2 teaspoonfuls every four hours, not to exceed 12 teaspoonfuls in a 24 hour period; children 6 to under 12 years: 1 teaspoonful every four hours, not to exceed 6 teaspoonfuls in a 24-hour period; children 2 to under 6 years: ½ teaspoonful every four hours, not to exceed 3 teaspoonfuls in a 24-hour period; children under 2 years: use as directed by a physician.
How Supplied: Robitussin-DAC is available in pints (NDC 0031-8680).

SKELAXIN® TABLETS ℞
brand of metaxalone

Description: Each pale rose, scored tablet contains: metaxalone, 400 mg.
Actions: The mechanism of action of metaxalone in humans has not been established, but may be due to general central nervous system depression. It has no direct action on the contractile mechanism of striated muscle, the motor end plate or the nerve fiber.
Indications: Skelaxin (metaxalone) is indicated as an adjunct to rest, physical therapy, and other measures for the relief of discomforts associated with acute, painful musculoskeletal conditions. The mode of action of this drug has not been clearly identified, but may be related to its sedative properties. Metaxalone does not directly relax tense skeletal muscles in man.
Contraindications: Metaxalone is contraindicated in individuals who have shown hypersensitivity to the drug. Metaxalone should not be administered to patients with a known tendency to drug-induced, hemolytic, or other anemias. It is contraindicated in patients with significantly impaired renal or hepatic function.
Precautions: Elevations in cephalin flocculation tests without concurrent changes in other liver function parameters have been noted. Hence, it is recommended that metaxalone be administered with great care to patients with pre-existing liver damage and that serial liver function studies be performed as required.
False-positive Benedict's tests, due to an unknown reducing substance, have been noted. A glucose-specific test will differentiate findings.
Pregnancy: Reproduction studies have been performed in rats and have revealed no evidence of impaired fertility or harm to the fetus due to mataxalone. Reactions reports from marketing experience have not revealed evidence of fetal injury, but such experience cannot exclude the possibility of infrequent or subtle damage to the human fetus. As with all drugs, metaxalone should be used in women who are or may become pregnant only when clearly needed.
Nursing Mothers: It is not known whether this drug is secreted in human milk. As a general rule, nursing should not be undertaken while a patient is on a drug since many drugs are excreted in human milk.
Pediatric Use: Safety and effectiveness in children 12 years of age and below have not been established.
Adverse Reactions: The most frequent reactions to metaxalone include nausea, vomiting, gastrointestinal upset, drowsiness, dizziness, headache, and nervousness or "irritability." Other adverse reactions are: hypersensitivity reaction, characterized by a light rash with or without pruritus; leukopenia; hemolytic anemia; jaundice.
Dosage: The recommended dose for adults and children over 12 years of age is two tablets (800 mg) three to four times a day.
Management of Overdosage: Gastric lavage and supportive therapy as indicated. (When determining the LD_{50} in rats and mice, progressive sedation, hypnosis and finally respiratory failure were noted as the dosage increased. In dogs, no LD_{50} could be determined as the higher doses produced an emetic action in 15 to 30 minutes), No documented case of major toxicity has been reported.
How Supplied: Skelaxin (metaxalone) is available as a 400 mg, pale rose tablet (scored), bottled in 100's and 500's (NDC 0031-9024).

SULLA® TABLETS ℞
brand of sulfameter
500 mg. tablets

WARNING:
FATALITIES HAVE OCCURRED DUE TO THE DEVELOPMENT OF STEVENS-JOHNSON SYNDROME (ERYTHEMA MULTIFORME EXUDATIVUM) FOLLOWING THE USE OF SULLA (SULFAMETER). THEREFORE, THE PATIENT MUST BE CLOSELY OBSERVED, AND SHOULD A RASH DEVELOP DURING THERAPY WITH SULLA, THE DRUG SHOULD BE DISCONTINUED IMMEDIATELY.
SULLA IS A SULFONAMIDE WHICH MAINTAINS A LONG-LASTING BLOOD LEVEL DUE TO SLOW EXCRETION. BECAUSE OF THE LONG-LASTING BLOOD LEVELS, A SMALLER DOSAGE THAN IS NORMALLY EMPLOYED WITH SHORTER-ACTING SULFONAMIDES SHOULD BE ADMINISTERED. SINCE THE SHORT-ACTING SULFONAMIDES ARE EFFECTIVE FOR THE SAME CONDITIONS, THEIR USE SHOULD BE RULED OUT BEFORE THE LONG-ACTING SULFONAMIDES ARE EMPLOYED.

Sulla (sulfameter) is a unique antibacterial sulfonamide that combines excellent bacteriostatic activity with the advantages of a modern, long-acting drug in low dosage. It is characterized by rapid and uniform absorption with easily maintained, effective bacteriostatic blood, tissue and urine levels on a convenient dosage schedule. Studies have demonstrated its favorable metabolism, including relatively low protein binding and low acetylation, excellent toleration, and high chemotherapeutic action—factors difficult to combine in one agent.
Indications: Sulla (sulfameter) exhibits marked bacteriostatic properties against a wide range of gram-negative and gram-positive organisms which are considered pathogenic in many acute and chronic urinary tract infections. It is more effective when the causative organism is *Escherichia coli, Klebsiella-aerobacter, Paracolon species, Streptococcus species,* or *Staphylococcus species* than it is in conditions due to *Pseudomonas* and *Proteus species.*
Sulla is indicated in the treatment of a wide variety of acute and chronic urinary tract infections. In general, if a favorable clinical and bacteriological response is not obtained within 14 days of treatment, it is unlikely that continued therapy will result in substantial clinical benefits. However, in chronic or recurrent infections, consideration may be given to long-term maintenance therapy (6 weeks to 6 months at full or reduced dosage) if a favorable therapeutic response was attained during the initial course of treatment.
Contraindications: Hypersensitivity to sulfonamide derivatives, including antibacterials, oral hypoglycemics, and thiazides; marked renal or hepatic impairment. Sulla (sulfameter) is not recommended for generalized bacterial infections, including meningitis. This drug should not be given to pregnant women near term or to nursing mothers.
Warnings: (See additional warning at beginning of product listing.)
The usual precautions in sulfonamide therapy should be observed. It is advisable to obtain a complete blood count and urinalysis at serial intervals if the patient is to receive sulfonamide therapy for longer than two weeks. It is important to assure an adequate fluid intake (at least 2,000 to 2,500 ml. daily for an adult) and urinary volume. Attention to fluid intake is particularly pertinent in the presence of fever or dehydration. Since photosensitization may occur, patients should be cautioned against exposure to ultraviolet light or pro-

longed exposure to sunlight. The drug should be discontinued if a reduction in urinary output, alterations in the hematopoietic system or impairment in renal or hepatic function should occur during treatment.
Because of the danger of severe hypoglycemic reactions, Sulla (sulfameter) should be administered with caution to patients receiving oral hypoglycemic agents of the sulfonylurea type.
Usage In Pregnancy:
The use of any drug during pregnancy or lactation requires that the potential benefits of the drug be weighed against possible hazards to the mother and child. Reproduction studies in rats have shown no teratogenic effects with sulfameter although such have been reported with other sulfonamides. In common with other sulfonamides, the treated group produced smaller litter sizes (from 9.4 to 7.4) and a decrease in the number weaned per litter (from 6.3 to 3.5).
Studies designed to determine the safety of administering Sulla during human pregnancy and lactation have not been performed, and clinical experience in such patients is too limited to permit its use in patients who are or are likely to become pregnant unless the potential benefits clearly outweigh the possible risks. Moreover, Sulla (sulfameter) should not be administered to pregnant patients near term nor to nursing mothers because of the increased risk of kernicterus in the offspring.
Precautions: Bacterial organisms differ with respect to their sensitivity to all antibacterial agents, and treatment failures with sulfameter should be expected in the presence of non-sensitive organisms. Therefore, sensitivity tests should be performed when clinically indicated. It must be emphasized, however, that favorable clinical response cannot always be expected even when *in vitro* tests indicate that the organism is sensitive. Sulla (sulfameter) is not effective in viral or rickettsial infections. The drug should be administered with great care and in smaller amounts to patients with impaired renal or hepatic function. Patients with glucose-6-phosphate dehydrogenase deficiency may develop hemolytic anemia if treated with sulfonamides.
Adverse Reactions: Reported and potential adverse reactions to sulfameter are similar in type to those encountered with other sulfonamide drugs and may involve several body systems:

(1) Hematopoietic: granulocytopenia, agranulocytosis, aplastic or hemolytic anemia, thrombocytopenia, methemoglobinemia, hypoprothrombinemia.
(2) Renal: crystalluria, toxic nephrosis.
(3) Hypersensitivity Reactions:
  (a) Vascular: periarteritis.
  (b) Mucocutaneous: purpuric, maculopapular and bullous eruptions, including Stevens-Johnson Syndrome (erythema multiforme exudativum), erythema nodosum, exfoliative dermatitis, lupus erythematosus, urticaria, serum sickness, pruritus, and photosensitization.
  (c) Others: drug fever.
(4) Hepatotoxicity and jaundice.
(5) Neuropsychiatric: peripheral neuritis, mental depression and psychoses.
(6) Miscellaneous: lassitude, anorexia, nausea, vomiting, abdominal pain, arthralgia, headache, fatigue, insomnia, dizziness, vertigo, ataxia and tinnitus.

The incidence of toxic effects should be expected to increase at serum levels above 20-25 mg.% and with repeated courses of treatment with sulfonamide drugs. At recommended dosage in patients with normal or only minimally impaired renal function, serum levels exceeding 20 mg.% are highly unlikely.
Dosage: The following dosage schedule is recommended to rapidly obtain and maintain a peak serum level of approximately 10±3 mg.% (medication given preferably after breakfast):

Recommended Dosage of Sulla

RECOMMENDED DOSAGE	LOADING DOSE First day only (single dose)	DAILY MAINTENANCE Single dose at 24 hour intervals
for patients over 100 pounds or 12 years of age	1500 mg (3 tablets)	500 mg (1 tablet)

ADHERENCE TO THE ABOVE DOSAGE RECOMMENDATIONS IS ESSENTIAL FOR OPTIMAL RESULTS.
Pending additional clinical experience, Sulla should be primarily directed toward those urinary tract infections requiring short-term or intermittent therapy; in any event, continuous administration should not, at the present time, exceed 180 days. Since there has been limited clinical experience in younger age groups, Sulla is not currently recommended for children under the age of 12 years.
How Supplied: Sulla (sulfameter) is available as 500 mg. scored tablets, pale green, in bottles of 100 (NDC 0031-9649).
[Shown in Product Identification Section]

Z-BEC®

One tablet daily provides:

Vitamin Composition	Percentage of U.S. Recommended Daily Allowance (U.S. RDA)	
Vitamin E	150	45.0 I.U.
Vitamin C	1000	600.0 mg
Thiamine (Vitamin B_1)	1000	15.0 mg
Riboflavin (Vitamin B_2)	600	10.2 mg
Niacin	500	100.0 mg
Vitamin B_6	500	10.0 mg
Vitamin B_{12}	100	6.0 mcg
Pantothenic Acid	250	25.0 mg
Mineral Composition		
Zinc	150	22.5 mg*

*22.5 mg zinc (equivalent to zinc content in 100 mg Zinc Sulfate, USP)
Ingredients: Sodium Ascorbate; Niacinamide; Zinc Sulfate; Vitamin E; Lactose; Calcium Pantothenate; Gelatin; Hydroxypropyl Methylcellulose; Povidone; Stearic Acid; Modified Starch; Thiamine Mononitrate; Artificial Color; Pyridoxine Hydrochloride; Riboflavin; Silica; Propylene Glycol; Vanillin; Cyanocobalamin.
Actions and Uses: Z-BEC is a high potency formulation. Its components have important roles in general nutrition, healing of wounds, and prevention of hemorrhage. It is recommended for deficiencies of these components in conditions such as febrile diseases, chronic or acute infections, burns, fractures, surgery, leg ulcers, toxic conditions, physiologic stress, alcoholism, prolonged exposure to high temperature, geriatrics, gastritis, peptic ulcer, and colitis; and in conditions involving special diets and weight-reduction diets.
In dentistry, Z-BEC is recommended for deficiencies of its components in conditions such as herpetic stomatitis, aphthous stomatitis, cheilosis, herpangina and gingivitis.
Precaution: Not intended for the treatment of pernicious anemia.
Dosage: The recommended OTC dosage for adults and children twelve or more years of age, other than pregnant or lactating women, is one tablet daily with food or after meals. Under the direction and supervision of a physician, the dose and frequency of administration may be increased in accordance with the patient's requirements.
How Supplied: Green film-coated, capsule-shaped tablets in bottles of 60 and 500 (NDC 0031-0689).
[Shown in Product Identification Section]

Roche Laboratories
Division of Hoffmann-La Roche Inc.
NUTLEY, NEW JERSEY 07110

Roche Products Inc.
MANATI, PUERTO RICO 00701

ALURATE® ELIXIR ©
(aprobarbital/Roche)

The following text is complete prescribing information based on official labeling in effect August 1, 1979.
Composition: Alurate is an intermediate-acting barbiturate with a duration of action particularly suitable for daytime sedation and nighttime insomnia. It is available as a red elixir providing 40 mg of aprobarbital/Roche per teaspoonful (5 ml) in a pleasant-tasting vehicle containing 20 per cent alcohol.
Indications: For sedation and induction of sleep in all conditions requiring a sedative-hypnotic.
Usual Adult Dosage: As a sedative, 1 teaspoonful three times daily. For mild insomnia, 1 to 2 teaspoonfuls before retiring. For pronounced insomnia, 2 to 4 teaspoonfuls before retiring.
Warning: May be habit forming.
How Supplied: Elixir (red)—bottles of 16 oz.

ANCOBON® ℞
(flucytosine/Roche)

The following text is complete prescribing information based on official labeling in effect August 1, 1979.

> WARNING
> Use with extreme caution in patients with impaired renal function. Close monitoring of hematologic, renal and hepatic status of all patients is essential. These instructions should be thoroughly reviewed before administration of Ancobon.

Description: Flucytosine, an antifungal agent, is a fluorinated pyrimidine chemically related to fluorouracil and floxuridine. Chemically, it is 5-fluorocytosine, a white to off-white crystalline powder, with a molecular weight of 129.1.
Actions: Flucytosine has *in vitro* and *in vivo* activity against Candida and Cryptococcus. The exact mode of action against these fungi is not known. Ancobon is not metabolized significantly when given orally to man.
SUSCEPTIBILITY:
Cryptococcus: Most strains initially isolated from clinical material have shown flucytosine minimal inhibitory concentrations (MIC's) ranging from .46 to 7.8 mcg/ml. Any isolate with an MIC greater than 12.5 mcg/ml is considered resistant. *In vitro* resistance has developed in originally susceptible strains during therapy. It is recommended that clinical cultures for susceptibility testing be taken initially and at weekly intervals during therapy. The initial culture should be reserved as a reference in susceptibility testing of subsequent isolates.
Candida: As high as 40 to 50 percent of the pretreatment clinical isolates of Candida have been reported to be resistant to flucytosine. It is recommended that susceptibility studies be performed as early as possible and be repeated

Continued on next page

Roche—Cont.

during therapy. An MIC value greater than 100 mcg/ml is considered resistant.
Interference with *in vitro* activity of flucytosine occurs in complex or semisynthetic media. In order to rely upon the recommended *in vitro* interpretations of susceptibility, it is essential that the broth medium and the testing procedure used be that described by Shadomy.[1]
Indications: Ancobon is indicated only in the treatment of serious infections caused by susceptible strains of Candida and/or Cryptococcus. Candida: septicemia, endocarditis and urinary system infections have been effectively treated with flucytosine. Limited trials in pulmonary infections justify the use of flucytosine. Cryptococcus: meningitis and pulmonary infections have been treated effectively. Studies in septicemias and urinary tract infections are limited, but good responses have been reported.
Contraindications: Patients with a known hypersensitivity to the drug.
Warnings: Ancobon must be given with extreme caution to patients with impaired renal function. Since Ancobon is excreted primarily by the kidneys, renal impairment may lead to accumulation of the drug. Assays for blood levels of Ancobon should be done in order to determine the adequacy of renal excretion in such patients.[1]
Ancobon must be given with extreme caution to patients with bone marrow depression. Patients may be more prone to depression of bone marrow function if they: 1) have a hematologic disease, 2) are being treated with radiation or drugs which depress bone marrow, or 3) have a history of treatment with such drugs or radiation. Frequent monitoring of hepatic function and of the hematopoietic system is indicated during therapy.
Usage in Pregnancy: Safe use of Ancobon in pregnancy has not been established. NOTE: Teratogenic effects have been seen in rats which metabolize flucytosine to fluorouracil. Use of Ancobon in pregnancy, lactation and in women of childbearing age requires that the potential benefits of therapy be weighed against its possible hazards.
Precautions: Before therapy with Ancobon is instituted, the hematologic and renal status of the patient should be determined (see WARNINGS), and close monitoring of the patient is essential. Liver enzyme levels (alkaline phosphatase, SGOT, SGPT) should be determined at frequent intervals during therapy, as indicated.
Adverse Reactions: Nausea, vomiting, diarrhea, rash, anemia, leukopenia, thrombopenia, and elevation of hepatic enzymes, BUN and creatinine have been reported. Less frequently reported were confusion, hallucinations, headache, sedation and vertigo.
Dosage and Administration: The usual dosage is 50 to 150 mg/kg/day at 6-hour intervals. Nausea or vomiting may be reduced or avoided if the capsules are given a few at a time over a 15-minute period. If the BUN or the serum creatinine is elevated, or if there are other signs of renal impairment, the initial dose should be at the lower level (see WARNINGS).
How Supplied: Capsules, containing 250 mg flucytosine/Roche, green and gray; containing 500 mg flucytosine/Roche, white and gray; bottles of 100.
Reference:

1. Shadomy, S.: *Appl. Microbiol., 17*:871, 1969.

[*Shown in Product Identification Section*]

ARFONAD® ℞
(trimethaphan camsylate/Roche)
Ampuls

The following text is complete prescribing information based on official labeling in effect August 1, 1979.

Description: A thiophanium derivative, Arfonad is a vasodepressor agent used for inducing controlled hypotension. Chemically, trimethaphan camsylate is (+)-1,3-dibenzyldecahydro -2- oxoimidazo [4, 5-c] thieno [1,2-a]-thiolium 2-oxo-10-bornanesulfonate. It has a molecular weight of 596.80.
Arfonad is stable under refrigeration; it should not be frozen, to avoid ampul breakage which may result from ice formation. Each 10-ml ampul contains 500 mg trimethaphan camsylate/Roche compounded with 0.013% sodium acetate and pH adjusted to approximately 5.2 with hydrochloric acid.
Actions: Arfonad is primarily a ganglionic blocking agent. It blocks transmission in autonomic ganglia without producing any preceding or concomitant change in the membrane potentials of the ganglion cells. It does not modify the conduction of impulses in the preganglionic or postganglionic neurones and does not prevent the release of acetylcholine by preganglionic impulses. Arfonad produces ganglionic blockade by occupying receptor sites on the ganglion cells and by stabilizing the postsynaptic membranes against the action of acetylcholine liberated from the presynaptic nerve endings.
In addition to ganglionic blocking, Arfonad may also exert a direct peripheral vasodilator effect. By inducing vasodilation, it causes pooling of blood in the dependent periphery and the splanchnic system. The vasodilation results in a lowering of the blood pressure. Arfonad liberates histamine.
Indications: Arfonad is indicated for the production of controlled hypotension during surgery; for the short term (acute) control of blood pressure in hypertensive emergencies; in the emergency treatment of pulmonary edema in patients with pulmonary hypertension associated with systemic hypertension.
Contraindications: Arfonad is contraindicated in those conditions where hypotension may subject the patient to undue risk, e.g., uncorrected anemia, hypovolemia, shock (both incipient and frank), asphyxia, or uncorrected respiratory insufficiency. Inadequate availability of fluids and inability to replace blood for technical reasons may also constitute contraindications.
Warnings: Arfonad is a powerful hypotensive drug and should always be diluted before use.
It is recommended that the use of Arfonad to produce hypotension in surgical or medical indications be limited to physicians with proper training in this technique. Adequate facilities, equipment and personnel should be available for vigilant monitoring of the circulation since Arfonad is an extremely potent hypotensive agent. Adequate oxygenation must be assured throughout the treatment period, especially in regard to coronary and cerebral circulation.
Arfonad should be used with extreme caution in patients with arteriosclerosis, cardiac disease, hepatic or renal disease, degenerative disease of the central nervous system, Addison's disease, diabetes and patients who are under treatment with steroids.
Usage in Pregnancy: Induced hypotension may have serious consequences upon the fetus.
Precautions: Arfonad should be used with care in patients who have been receiving antihypertensive drugs, since an additive hypotensive effect may occur. It should be used with caution with anesthetic agents, especially spinal anesthetics, which themselves may produce hypotension. Also, use with great caution in the elderly or debilitated, or in children. Because Arfonad liberates histamine, it should be used with caution in allergic individuals. Concomitant therapy with other drugs can modify materially the dose of Arfonad necessary to achieve the desired response.
Diuretic agents may enhance markedly the responses evoked by ganglionic-blocking drugs.
NOTE: Pupillary dilation does not necessarily indicate anoxia or the depth of anesthesia, since Arfonad appears to have a specific effect on the pupil.
Some animal studies indicate that aggressive dosage administration may result in respiratory arrest. Rare cases of respiratory arrest in humans have been reported, although a causal relationship has not been established. It is recommended that the patient's respiratory status be monitored closely, particularly if large doses of Arfonad are used.
Dosage and Administration: Arfonad must always be diluted and administered by intravenous infusion. Solutions should be freshly prepared and any unused portions discarded. For this purpose a 0.1 per cent (1 mg/ml) concentration of Arfonad in 5% Dextrose Injection USP should be employed. Use of other diluents is not recommended, since experience with them has not been reported. The infusion fluid used for administration of Arfonad should not be employed as a vehicle for the simultaneous administration of any other drugs. One (1) ampul of Arfonad—10 ml, 50 mg/ml—should be diluted to 500 ml. Since individual response varies, the rate of administration must be adjusted to the requirements of each patient.
The patient should be positioned so as to avoid cerebral anoxia and, when used in surgery, adequate anesthesia established. Intravenous drip with Arfonad is started at an average rate of 3 to 4 ml (3 to 4 mg) per minute (see chart below). The rate of administration is then adjusted to maintain the desired level of hypotension. Since there is a marked variation of individual response, **frequent blood pressure determinations are essential to maintain proper control.** Rates from as low as 0.3 ml (0.3 mg) per minute to rates exceeding 6 ml (6 mg) per minute have been found necessary in the experience of clinical investigators of Arfonad.

0.1% (1 mg/ml) CONCENTRATION OF ARFONAD

Delivery System Drops/ml	Drops/Min to Obtain 3–4 ml (3–4 mg) Arfonad
10	30–40
15	45–60
60	180–240

For surgical use, administration of Arfonad should be stopped prior to wound closure in order to permit blood pressure to return to normal. A systolic pressure of 100 mm will usually be attained within 10 minutes after stopping Arfonad.
Overdosage: Vasopressor agents may be used to correct undesirable low pressures during surgery or to effect a more rapid return to normotensive levels. Phenylephrine HCl or mephentermine sulfate should be tried initially and nonepinephrine should be reserved for refractory cases.
How Supplied: Ampuls, 10 ml, boxes of 10.

AZO GANTANOL® ℞

The following text is complete prescribing information based on official labeling in effect August 1, 1979.
Composition: Each tablet contains 0.5 Gm sulfamethoxazole/Roche and 100 mg phenazopyridine hydrochloride.
Description: Azo Gantanol combines the antibacterial effectiveness of sulfamethoxazole/Roche (Gantanol®) with the local urinary analgesic activity of phenazopyridine hydrochloride.
Gantanol (sulfamethoxazole/Roche) is an intermediate-dosage sulfonamide. Sulfamethoxazole is an almost white, odorless, tasteless

compound. Chemically, it is N^1-(5-methyl-3-isoxazolyl) sulfanilamide.
Phenazopyridine hydrochloride is a urinary analgesic. Chemically, it is 3-phenylazo-2,6-diaminopyridine hydrochloride.
Sulfonamides exist in the blood as free, conjugated (acetylated and possibly other forms) and protein-bound forms. The "free" form is considered to be the therapeutically active form. It has been shown that approximately 70 per cent of Gantanol is protein bound in the blood;[1] of the unbound portion 80 to 90 per cent is in the nonacetylated form.[2,3] Excretion of sulfonamides is chiefly by the kidneys with glomerular filtration as the primary mechanism.
Actions: The systemic sulfonamides are bacteriostatic agents. The spectrum of activity is similar for all. Sulfonamides competitively inhibit bacterial synthesis of folic acid (pteroylglutamic acid) from para-aminobenzoic acid. Resistant strains are capable of utilizing folic acid precursors or preformed folic acid.
Phenazopyridine hydrochloride has a specific analgesic effect in the urinary tract, promptly relieving pain and burning.
Indications: In adults, urinary tract infections complicated by pain (primarily pyelonephritis, pyelitis and cystitis) due to susceptible organisms (usually *E. coli, Klebsiella-Aerobacter, Staphylococcus aureus, Proteus mirabilis,* and, less frequently, *Proteus vulgaris)* in the absence of obstructive uropathy or foreign bodies.
Important note. In vitro sulfonamide sensitivity tests are not always reliable. The test must be carefully coordinated with bacteriologic and clinical response. When the patient is already taking sulfonamides, follow-up cultures should have aminobenzoic acid added to the culture media.
Currently, the increasing frequency of resistant organisms is a limitation of the usefulness of antibacterial agents including the sulfonamides.
Wide variation in blood levels may result with identical doses. Blood levels should be measured in patients receiving sulfonamides for serious infections. Free sulfonamide blood levels of 5 to 15 mg per 100 ml may be considered therapeutically effective for most infections, with blood levels of 12 to 15 mg per 100 ml optimal for serious infections; 20 mg per 100 ml should be the maximum total sulfonamide level, as adverse reactions occur more frequently above this level.
Contraindications: Children below age 12. Hypersensitivity to sulfonamides. Pregnancy at term and during the nursing period, because sulfonamides pass the placenta and are excreted in the milk and may cause kernicterus. Because Azo Gantanol contains phenazopyridine hydrochloride it is contraindicated in glomerulonephritis, severe hepatitis, uremia, and pyelonephritis of pregnancy with gastrointestinal disturbances.
Warnings: *Usage in Pregnancy:* The safe use of sulfonamides in pregnancy has not been established. The teratogenicity potential of most sulfonamides has not been thoroughly investigated in either animals or humans. However, a significant increase in the incidence of cleft palate and other bony abnormalities of offspring has been observed when certain sulfonamides of the short, intermediate and long-acting types were given to pregnant rats and mice at high oral doses (7 to 25 times the human therapeutic dose).
Deaths associated with the administration of sulfonamides have been reported from hypersensitivity reactions, agranulocytosis, aplastic anemia and other blood dyscrasias.
The presence of clinical signs such as sore throat, fever, pallor, purpura or jaundice may be early indications of serious blood disorders. Complete blood counts should be done frequently in patients receiving sulfonamides.
The frequency of renal complications is considerably lower in patients receiving the more soluble sulfonamides. Urinalysis with careful microscopic examination should be obtained frequently in patients receiving sulfonamides.
Precautions: Sulfonamides should be given with caution to patients with impaired renal or hepatic function and to those with severe allergy or bronchial asthma. In glucose-6-phosphate dehydrogenase-deficient individuals, hemolysis may occur. This reaction is frequently dose-related. Adequate fluid intake must be maintained in order to prevent crystalluria and stone formation.
Adverse Reactions: *Blood dyscrasias:* Agranulocytosis, aplastic anemia, thrombocytopenia, leukopenia, hemolytic anemia, purpura, hypoprothrombinemia and methemoglobinemia.
Allergic reactions: Erythema multiforme (Stevens-Johnson syndrome), generalized skin eruptions, epidermal necrolysis, urticaria, serum sickness, pruritus, exfoliative dermatitis, anaphylactoid reactions, periorbital edema, conjunctival and scleral injection, photosensitization, arthralgia and allergic myocarditis.
Gastrointestinal reactions: Nausea, emesis, abdominal pains, hepatitis, diarrhea, anorexia, pancreatitis and stomatitis.
C.N.S. reactions: Headache, peripheral neuritis, mental depression, convulsions, ataxia, hallucinations, tinnitus, vertigo and insomnia.
Miscellaneous reactions: Drug fever, chills, and toxic nephrosis with oliguria and anuria. Polyarteritis nodosa and L.E. phenomenon have occurred.
The sulfonamides bear certain chemical similarities to some goitrogens, diuretics (acetazolamide and the thiazides) and oral hypoglycemic agents. Goiter production, diuresis and hypoglycemia have occurred rarely in patients receiving sulfonamides. Cross-sensitivity may exist with these agents.
Dosage and Administration: Azo Gantanol is intended for the acute, painful phase of urinary tract infections. The usual dosage in adults is 4 tablets initially followed by 2 tablets morning and evening for up to 3 days. If pain persists, causes other than infection should be sought. After relief of pain has been obtained, continued treatment of the infection with Gantanol (sulfamethoxazole/Roche) may be considered.
NOTE: Patients should be told that the orange-red dye (phenazopyridine HCl) will color the urine soon after ingestion of the medication.
How Supplied: Tablets, red, film-coated, each containing 0.5 Gm sulfamethoxazole/Roche and 100 mg phenazopyridine HCl—bottles of 100 and 500.
References:

1. Struller, T.: *Antibiot. Chemother., 14:* 179, 1968.
2. Boger, W. P., and Gavin, J. J.: *Antibiotics and Chemother., 10*:572, 1960.
3. Brandman, O., and Engelberg, R.: *Curr. Therap. Res., 2*:364, 1960.

[*Shown in Product Identification Section*]

AZO GANTRISIN® ℞

The following text is complete prescribing information based on official labeling in effect August 1, 1979.
Composition: Each tablet contains 0.5 Gm sulfisoxazole/Roche and 50 mg phenazopyridine hydrochloride.
Description: Azo Gantrisin combines the antibacterial effectiveness of sulfisoxazole/Roche (Gantrisin®) with the local urinary analgesic activity of phenazopyridine hydrochloride.
Gantrisin (sulfisoxazole/Roche) is a rapid-acting sulfonamide. Sulfisoxazole is a white to slightly yellowish, odorless, slightly bitter, crystalline powder. It is soluble in alcohol and very slightly soluble in water. Chemically, it is N^1-(3,4-dimethyl-5-isoxazolyl) sulfanilamide.
Phenazopyridine hydrochloride is a urinary analgesic. Chemically, it is 3-phenylazo-2,6-diaminopyridine hydrochloride.
Sulfonamides exist in the blood as free, conjugated (acetylated and possibly other forms) and protein-bound forms. The "free" form is considered to be the therapeutically active form. Approximately 85 per cent of Gantrisin is protein bound in the blood;[1] of the unbound portion 65 to 72 per cent is in the nonacetylated form.[2] Excretion of sulfonamides is chiefly by the kidneys with glomerular filtration as the primary mechanism.
Actions: The systemic sulfonamides are bacteriostatic agents. The spectrum of activity is similar for all. Sulfonamides competitively inhibit bacterial synthesis of folic acid (pteroylglutamic acid) from para-aminobenzoic acid. Resistant strains are capable of utilizing folic acid precursors or preformed folic acid.
Phenazopyridine hydrochloride has a specific analgesic effect in the urinary tract, promptly relieving pain and burning.
Indications: In adults, urinary tract infections complicated by pain (primarily pyelonephritis, pyelitis and cystitis) due to susceptible organisms (usually *E. coli, Klebsiella-Aerobacter, Staphylococcus aureus, Proteus mirabilis,* and, less frequently, *Proteus vulgaris)* in the absence of obstructive uropathy or foreign bodies.
Important note: In vitro sulfonamide sensitivity tests are not always reliable. The test must be carefully coordinated with bacteriologic and clinical response. When the patient is already taking sulfonamides, follow-up cultures should have aminobenzoic acid added to the culture media.
Currently, the increasing frequency of resistant organisms is a limitation of the usefulness of antibacterial agents including the sulfonamides.
Wide variation in blood levels may result with identical doses. Blood levels should be measured in patients receiving sulfonamides for serious infections. Free sulfonamide blood levels of 5 to 15 mg per 100 ml may be considered therapeutically effective for most infections, with blood levels of 12 to 15 mg per 100 ml optimal for serious infections; 20 mg per 100 ml should be the maximum total sulfonamide level, as adverse reactions occur more frequently above this level.
Contraindications: Children below age 12. Hypersensitivity to sulfonamides. Pregnancy at term and during the nursing period, because sulfonamides pass the placenta and are excreted in the milk and may cause kernicterus. Because Azo Gantrisin contains phenazopyridine hydrochloride it is contraindicated in glomerulonephritis, severe hepatitis, uremia, and pyelonephritis of pregnancy with gastrointestinal disturbances.
Warnings: *Usage in Pregnancy:* The safe use of sulfonamides in pregnancy has not been established. The teratogenicity potential of most sulfonamides has not been thoroughly investigated in either animals or humans. However, a significant increase in the incidence of cleft palate and other bony abnormalities of offspring has been observed when certain sulfonamides of the short, intermediate and long-acting types were given to pregnant rats and mice at high oral doses (7 to 25 times the human therapeutic dose).
Deaths associated with the administration of sulfonamides have been reported from hypersensitivity reactions, agranulocytosis, aplastic anemia and other blood dyscrasias.
The presence of clinical signs such as sore throat, fever, pallor, purpura or jaundice may be early indications of serious blood disorders. Complete blood counts should be done frequently in patients receiving sulfonamides.
The frequency of renal complications is considerably lower in patients receiving the more soluble sulfonamides. Urinalysis with careful

Continued on next page

Roche—Cont.

microscopic examination should be obtained frequently in patients receiving sulfonamides.

Precautions: Sulfonamides should be given with caution to patients with impaired renal or hepatic function and to those with severe allergy or bronchial asthma. In glucose-6-phosphate dehydrogenase-deficient individuals, hemolysis may occur. This reaction is frequently dose-related. Adequate fluid intake must be maintained in order to prevent crystalluria and stone formation.

Adverse Reactions: *Blood dyscrasias:* Agranulocytosis, aplastic anemia, thrombocytopenia, leukopenia, hemolytic anemia, purpura, hypoprothrombinemia and methemoglobinemia.

Allergic reactions: Erythema multiforme (Stevens-Johnson syndrome), generalized skin eruptions, epidermal necrolysis, urticaria, serum sickness, pruritus, exfoliative dermatitis, anaphylactoid reactions, periorbital edema, conjunctival and scleral injection, photosensitization, arthralgia and allergic myocarditis.

Gastrointestinal reactions: Nausea, emesis, abdominal pains, hepatitis, diarrhea, anorexia, pancreatitis and stomatitis.

C.N.S. reactions: Headache, peripheral neuritis, mental depression, convulsions, ataxia, hallucinations, tinnitus, vertigo and insomnia.

Miscellaneous reactions: Drug fever, chills, and toxic nephrosis with oliguria and anuria. Polyarteritis nodosa and L.E. phenomenon have occurred.

The sulfonamides bear certain chemical similarities to some goitrogens, diuretics (acetazolamide and the thiazides) and oral hypoglycemic agents. Goiter production, diuresis and hypoglycemia have occurred rarely in patients receiving sulfonamides. Cross-sensitivity may exist with these agents.

Dosage and Administration: Azo Gantrisin is intended for the acute, painful phase of urinary tract infections. The recommended dosage in adults is 4 to 6 tablets initially followed by 2 tablets four times daily for up to 3 days. If pain persists, causes other than infection should be sought. After relief of pain has been obtained, continued treatment of the infection with Gantrisin (sulfisoxazole/Roche) may be considered.

NOTE: Patients should be told that the orange-red dye (phenazopyridine HCl) will color the urine soon after ingestion of the medication.

How Supplied: Tablets, red, film-coated, each containing 0.5 Gm sulfisoxazole/Roche and 50 mg phenazopyridine HCl—bottles of 100 and 500.

References:

1. Struller, T.: *Antibiot. Chemother., 14*:179, 1968.
2. Svec, F. A.; Rhoads, P.S., and Rohr, J.H.: *Arch. Intern. Med., 85*:83, 1950.

[Shown in Product Identification Section]

BACTRIM™ ℞

(trimethoprim and sulfamethoxazole)
Tablets, Suspension,
Pediatric Suspension,
DS (double strength) Tablets

The following text is complete prescribing information based on official labeling in effect October 1, 1979.

Description: Bactrim is a synthetic antibacterial combination product, available in double-strength, notched, capsule-shaped, white tablets, each containing 160 mg trimethoprim and 800 mg sulfamethoxazole; in scored light-green tablets, each containing 80 mg trimethoprim and 400 mg sulfamethoxazole; as a pink, cherry-flavored pediatric suspension and as a pink, fruit-licorice flavored suspension, both forms containing in each teaspoonful (5 ml) the equivalent of 40 mg trimethoprim and 200 mg sulfamethoxazole, compounded with 0.3% alcohol.

Trimethoprim is 2,4-diamino-5-(3,4,5-trimethoxybenzyl) pyrimidine. It is a white to light yellow, odorless, bitter compound with a molecular weight of 290.3.

Sulfamethoxazole is N^1-(5-methyl-3-isoxazolyl)sulfanilamide. It is an almost white in color, odorless, tasteless compound with a molecular weight of 253.28.

Actions: *Microbiology:* Sulfamethoxazole inhibits bacterial synthesis of dihydrofolic acid by competing with *para*-aminobenzoic acid. Trimethoprim blocks the production of tetrahydrofolic acid from dihydrofolic acid by binding to and reversibly inhibiting the required enzyme, dihydrofolate reductase. Thus, Bactrim blocks two consecutive steps in the biosynthesis of nucleic acids and proteins essential to many bacteria.

In vitro studies have shown that bacterial resistance develops more slowly with Bactrim than with trimethoprim or sulfamethoxazole alone.

In vitro serial dilution tests have shown that the spectrum of antibacterial activity of Bactrim includes the common urinary tract pathogens with the exception of *Pseudomonas aeruginosa.* The following organisms are usually susceptible: *Escherichia coli, Klebsiella-Enterobacter, Proteus mirabilis* and indole-positive proteus species.

In addition, the usual spectrum of antimicrobial activity of Bactrim includes the following

REPRESENTATIVE MINIMUM INHIBITORY CONCENTRATION VALUES FOR BACTRIM-SUSCEPTIBLE ORGANISMS
(MIC—mcg/ml)

Bacteria	Trimethoprim Alone	Sulfamethoxazole Alone	TMP/SMX (1:20) TMP	SMX
Escherichia coli	0.05 – 1.5	1.0 – 245	0.05 – 0.5	0.95 – 9.5
Proteus spp. indole positive	0.5 – 5.0	7.35 – 300	0.05 – 1.5	0.95 – 28.5
Proteus mirabilis	0.5 – 1.5	7.35 – 30	0.05 – 0.15	0.95 – 2.85
Klebsiella-Enterobacter	0.15 – 5.0	2.45 – 245	0.05 – 1.5	0.95 – 28.5
Haemophilus influenzae	0.15 – 1.5	2.85 – 95	0.015 – 0.15	0.285 – 2.85
Streptococcus pneumoniae	0.15 – 1.5	7.35 – 24.5	0.05 – 0.15	0.95 – 2.85
Shigella flexneri	<0.01 – 0.04	<0.16 –>320	<0.002 – 0.03	0.04 – 0.625
Shigella sonnei	0.02 – 0.03	0.625 –>320	0.004 – 0.06	0.08 – 1.25

bacterial pathogens isolated from middle ear exudate and from bronchial secretions: *Haemophilus influenzae,* including ampicillin-resistant strains, and *Streptococcus pneumoniae. Shigella flexneri* and *Shigella sonnei* are also usually susceptible.

[See table below].

The recommended quantitative disc susceptibility method (*Federal Register, 37:*20527–20529, 1972; Bauer AW, Kirby WMM, Sherris JC, Turck M: Antibiotic Susceptibility Testing by a Standardized Single Disc Method, *Am J Clin Pathol, 45:*493–496, 1966) may be used for estimating the susceptibility of bacteria to Bactrim. With this procedure, a report from the laboratory of "Susceptible to trimethoprim-sulfamethoxazole" indicates that the infection is likely to respond to therapy with Bactrim. If the infection is confined to the urine, a report of "Intermediate susceptibility to trimethoprim-sulfamethoxazole" also indicates that the infection is likely to respond. A report of "Resistant to trimethoprim-sulfamethoxazole" indicates that the infection is unlikely to respond to therapy with Bactrim.

Human Pharmacology: Bactrim is rapidly absorbed following oral administration. The blood levels of trimethoprim and sulfamethoxazole are similar to those achieved when each component is given alone. Peak blood levels for the individual components occur one to four hours after oral administration. The half-lives of sulfamethoxazole and trimethoprim, 10 and 16 hours respectively, are relatively the same regardless of whether these compounds are administered as individual components or as Bactrim. Detectable amounts of trimethoprim and sulfamethoxazole are present in the blood 24 hours after drug administration. Free sulfamethoxazole and trimethoprim blood levels are proportionately dose dependent. On repeated administration, the steady-state ratio of trimethoprim to sulfamethoxazole levels in the blood is about 1:20.

Sulfamethoxazole exists in the blood as free, conjugated and protein-bound forms; trimethoprim is present as free, protein-bound and metabolized forms. The free forms are considered to be the therapeutically active forms. Approximately 44 percent of trimethoprim and 70 percent of sulfamethoxazole are protein-bound in the blood. The presence of 10 mg percent sulfamethoxazole in plasma decreases the protein binding of trimethoprim to an insignificant degree; trimethoprim does not influence the protein binding of sulfamethoxazole.

Excretion of Bactrim is chiefly by the kidneys through both glomerular filtration and tubular secretion. Urine concentrations of both sulfamethoxazole and trimethoprim are considerably higher than are the concentrations in the blood. When administered together as in Bactrim, neither sulfamethoxazole nor trimethoprim affects the urinary excretion pattern of the other.

Indications and Usage:

URINARY TRACT INFECTIONS: For the treatment of urinary tract infections due to susceptible strains of the following organisms: *Escherichia coli, Klebsiella-Enterobacter, Proteus mirabilis, Proteus vulgaris* and *Proteus morganii.* It is recommended that initial episodes of uncomplicated urinary tract infections be treated with a single effective antibacterial agent rather than the combination.

Note: Currently, the increasing frequency of resistant organisms is a limitation of the usefulness of all antibacterial agents, especially in the treatment of these urinary tract infections.

ACUTE OTITIS MEDIA: For the treatment of acute otitis media in children due to susceptible strains of *Haemophilus influenzae* or *Streptococcus pneumoniae* when in the judgment of the physician Bactrim offers some advantage over the use of other antimicrobial agents. Limited clinical information is presently available on the effectiveness of treat-

ment of otitis media with Bactrim when the infection is due to *Haemophilus influenzae* resistant to ampicillin. To date, there are limited data on the safety of repeated use of Bactrim in children under two years of age. Bactrim is not indicated for prophylactic or prolonged administration in otitis media at any age.

ACUTE EXACERBATIONS OF CHRONIC BRONCHITIS IN ADULTS: For the treatment of acute excerbations of chronic bronchitis due to susceptible strains of *Haemophilus influenzae* or *Streptococcus pneumoniae* when in the judgment of the physician Bactrim offers some advantage over the use of a single antimicrobial agent.

SHIGELLOSIS: For the treatment of enteritis caused by susceptible strains of *Shigella flexneri* and *Shigella sonnei* when antibacterial therapy is indicated.

***PNEUMOCYSTIS CARINII* PNEUMONITIS: Bactrim is also indicated in the treatment of documented *Pneumocystis carinii* pneumonitis. To date, this drug has been tested only in patients 9 months to 16 years of age who were immunosuppressed by cancer therapy.**

Contraindications: Hypersensitivity to trimethoprim or sulfonamides. Pregnancy and during the nursing period (see Reproduction Studies). Infants less than two months of age.

Warnings: BACTRIM SHOULD NOT BE USED IN THE TREATMENT OF STREPTOCOCCAL PHARYNGITIS. Clinical studies have documented that patients with group A β-hemolytic streptococcal tonsillopharyngitis have a greater incidence of bacteriologic failure when treated with Bactrim than do those patients treated with penicillin, as evidenced by failure to eradicate this organism from the tonsillopharyngeal area.

Deaths associated with the administration of sulfonamides have been reported from hypersensitivity reactions, agranulocytosis, aplastic anemia and other blood dyscrasias. Experience with trimethoprim alone is much more limited, but it has been reported to interfere with hematopoiesis in occasional patients. In elderly patients concurrently receiving certain diuretics, primarily thiazides, an increased incidence of thrombopenia with purpura has been reported.

The presence of clinical signs such as sore throat, fever, pallor, purpura or jaundice may be early indications of serious blood disorders. Complete blood counts should be done frequently in patients receiving Bactrim. If a significant reduction in the count of any formed blood element is noted, Bactrim should be discontinued.

Precautions: Bactrim should be given with caution to patients with impaired renal or hepatic function, to those with possible folate deficiency and to those with severe allergy or bronchial asthma. In glucose-6-phosphate dehydrogenase-deficient individuals, hemolysis may occur. This reaction is frequently dose-related. Adequate fluid intake must be maintained in order to prevent crystalluria and stone formation. Urinalyses with careful microscopic examination and renal function tests should be performed during therapy, particularly for those patients with impaired renal function.

It has been reported that Bactrim may prolong the prothrombin time of patients who are receiving the anticoagulant warfarin. This interaction should be kept in mind when Bactrim is given to patients already on anticoagulant therapy, and the coagulation time should be reassessed.

Adverse Reactions: For completeness, all major reactions to sulfonamides and to trimethoprim are included below, even though they may not have been reported with Bactrim.

Blood dyscrasias: Agranulocytosis, aplastic anemia, megaloblastic anemia, thrombopenia, leukopenia, hemolytic anemia, purpura, hypoprothrombinemia and methemoglobinemia.

Allergic reactions: Erythema multiforme, Stevens-Johnson syndrome, generalized skin eruptions, epidermal necrolysis, urticaria, serum sickness, pruritus, exfoliative dermatitis, anaphylactoid reactions, periorbital edema, conjunctival and scleral injection, photosensitization, arthralgia and allergic myocarditis.

Gastrointestinal reactions: Glossitis, stomatitis, nausea, emesis, abdominal pains, hepatitis, diarrhea and pancreatitis.

C.N.S. reactions: Headache, peripheral neuritis, mental depression, convulsions, ataxia, hallucinations, tinnitus, vertigo, insomnia, apathy, fatigue, muscle weakness and nervousness.

Miscellaneous reactions: Drug fever, chills, and toxic nephrosis with oliguria and anuria. Periarteritis nodosa and L. E. phenomenon have occurred.

The sulfonamides bear certain chemical similarities to some goitrogens, diuretics (acetazolamide and the thiazides) and oral hypoglycemic agents. Goiter production, diuresis and hypoglycemia have occurred rarely in patients receiving sulfonamides. Cross-sensitivity may exist with these agents. Rats appear to be especially susceptible to the goitrogenic effects of sulfonamides, and long-term administration has produced thyroid malignancies in the species.

Dosage and Administration: Not recommended for use in infants less than two months of age.

URINARY TRACT INFECTIONS AND SHIGELLOSIS IN ADULTS AND CHILDREN, AND ACUTE OTITIS MEDIA IN CHILDREN:

Adults: The usual adult dosage in the treatment of urinary tract infections is one Bactrium DS (double strength) tablet, two Bactrim tablets or four teaspoonfuls (20 ml) every 12 hours for 10 to 14 days. An identical daily dosge is used for 5 days in the treatment of shigellosis.

Children: The recommended dose for children with urinary tract infections or acute otitis media is 8 mg/kg trimethoprim and 40 mg/kg sulfamethoxazole per 24 hours, given in two divided doses every 12 hours for 10 days. An identical daily dosage is used for 5 days in the treatment of shigellosis. The following table is a guideline for the attainment of this dosage.

Children two months of age or older:

Weight lb	Weight kg	Dose—every 12 hours Teaspoonfuls	Tablets
22	10	1 teasp. (5 ml)	½ tablet
44	20	2 teasp. (10 ml)	1 tablet
66	30	3 teasp. (15 ml)	1½ tablets
88	40	4 teasp. (20 ml)	2 tablets or 1 DS tablet

For patients with renal impairment:

Creatinine Clearance (ml/min)	Recommended Dosage Regimen
Above 30	Usual standard regimen
15–30	½ the usual regimen
Below 15	Use not recommended

ACUTE EXACERBATIONS OF CHRONIC BRONCHITIS IN ADULTS:

The usual adult dosage in the treatment of acute exacerbations of chronic bronchitis is one Bactrim DS (double strength) tablet, two Bactrim tablets or four teaspoonfuls (20 ml) every 12 hours for 14 days.

PNEUMOCYSTIS CARINII PNEUMONITIS:

The recommended dosage for patients with *Pneumocystis carinii* pneumonitis is 20 mg/kg trimethoprim and 100 mg/kg sulfamethoxazole per 24 hours given in equally divided doses every 6 hours for 14 days. In children weighing 80 lbs (36 kgs), the dosage is 1 Bactrim DS (double strength) tablet every 6 hours for 14 days. The following table is a guideline for the attainment of this dosage in children.

Weight lb	Weight kg	Dose—every six hours Teaspoonfuls	Tablets
18	8	1 teasp. (5 ml)	½ tablet
35	16	2 teasp. (10 ml)	1 tablet
53	24	3 teasp. (15 ml)	1½ tablets
70	32	4 teasp. (20 ml)	2 tablets or 1 DS tablet

How Supplied: *Double Strength Tablets,* containing 160 mg trimethoprim and 800 mg sulfamethoxazole—bottles of 100; Tel-E-Dose® packages of 100; Prescription Paks of 20 and 28. Imprint on tablets: BACTRIM-DS ROCHE.

Tablets, containing 80 mg trimethoprim and 400 mg sulfamethoxazole—bottles of 100 and 500; Tel-E-Dose® packages of 100; Prescription Paks of 40.

Pediatric Suspension, containing in each teaspoonful (5 ml) the equivalent of 40 mg trimethoprim and 200 mg sulfamethoxazole; cherry flavored—bottles of 16 oz (1 pint).

Suspension, containing in each teaspoonful (5 ml) the equivalent of 40 mg trimethoprim and 200 mg sulfamethoxazole; fruit-licorice flavored—bottles of 16 oz (1 pint).

Reproduction Studies: In rats, doses of 533 mg/kg sulfamethoxazole or 200 mg/kg trimethoprim produced teratological effects manifested mainly as cleft palates. The highest dose which did not cause cleft palates in rats was 512 mg/kg sulfamethoxazole or 192 mg/kg trimethoprim when administered separately. In two studies in rats, no teratology was observed when 512 mg/kg of sulfamethoxazole was used in combination with 128 mg/kg of trimethoprim. However, in one study, cleft palates were observed in one litter out of 9 when 355 mg/kg of sulfamethoxazole was used in combination with 88 mg/kg of trimethoprim.

In rabbits, trimethoprim administered by intubation from days 8 to 16 of pregnancy at dosages up to 500 mg/kg resulted in higher incidences of dead and resorbed fetuses, particularly at 500 mg/kg. However, there were no significant drug-related teratological effects.

[*Shown in Product Identification Section*]

BEROCCA® TABLETS ℞

The following text is complete prescribing information based on official labeling in effect August 1, 1979.

Composition: Each Berocca Tablet contains:

Thiamine mononitrate (vitamin B_1)	15 mg
Riboflavin (vitamin B_2)	15 mg
Pyridoxine hydrochloride (vitamin B_6)	5 mg
Niacinamide	100 mg
Calcium pantothenate	20 mg
Cyanocobalamin (vitamin B_{12})	5 mcg
Folic acid	0.5 mg
Ascorbic acid (vitamin C)	500 mg

Description: For prophylactic or therapeutic nutritional supplementation, Berocca provides generous amounts of the major B complex vitamins essential in the anabolism of carbohydrate and protein and in hematopoiesis. Berocca also contains therapeutic quantities of ascorbic acid, a substance involved in intracellular reactions such as tissue repair and collagen formation.

Indications: Berocca tablets are indicated for supportive nutritional supplementation in conditions in which water-soluble vitamins are required prophylactically or therapeutically: when requirements are increased, as in febrile

Continued on next page

Roche—Cont.

diseases, before and after surgery, severe burns, hyperthyroidism and pregnancy; gastrointestinal disorders interfering with intake or absorption of water-soluble vitamins; prolonged or wasting diseases; alcoholism and diabetes.

Warning: Not intended for treatment of pernicious anemia or other primary or secondary anemias. Neurologic involvement may develop or progress, despite temporary remission of anemia, in patients with pernicious anemia who receive more than 0.1 mg of folic acid per day and who are inadequately treated with vitamin B_{12}.

Dosage and Administration: One or two tablets daily, as indicated by clinical need.

How Supplied: Bottles of 100 and 500.

[*Shown in Product Identification Section*]

BEROCCA®-C
BEROCCA®-C 500 ℞

The following text is complete prescribing information based on official labeling in effect August 1, 1979.

Description: Berocca-C provides generous amounts of six important B-complex vitamins plus an ample dose of vitamin C (ascorbic acid) in readily absorbable form.

Each 2 ml of Berocca-C contains:

Thiamine HCl (B_1)	10 mg
Riboflavin (B_2) (as riboflavin 5'-phosphate sodium)	10 mg
Niacinamide	80 mg
Pyridoxine HCl (B_6)	20 mg
Dexpanthenol (equivalent to 23.2 mg calcium pantothenate)	20 mg
d-biotin	0.2 mg
Ascorbic acid (C)	100 mg

compounded with 1% benzyl alcohol as preservative and pH adjusted with sodium hydroxide (to approximately 4.2 with the vial, 5.1 with the ampul).

Berocca-C 500 is a duplex package containing one 2-ml ampul of Berocca-C and a separate 2-ml ampul of 400 mg of Vitamin C Sodium Injectable compounded with 0.2% parabens (methyl and propyl) as preservatives, and pH adjusted to 5.5—7.0 with sodium bicarbonate. When the contents of both ampuls are aspirated into the same syringe, the resulting solution (4 ml) will contain equal amounts of the vitamins listed above, with the exception of vitamin C which increases to 500 mg.

Note: the formula of Berocca-C contains a soluble form of riboflavin which permits use of a larger dose and minimizes pain upon injection. While this form of riboflavin causes darkening of the solution which may intensify on prolonged storage, this in no way affects the safety and therapeutic efficacy of the preparation. Berocca-C is ready for immediate use, is stable for at least 18 months and need not be refrigerated.

Indications: Disorders requiring parenteral administration of water-soluble vitamins. Pre- and postoperative treatment; when requirements are increased, as in fever, severe burns, increased metabolism, hyperthyroidism, pregnancy; gastrointestinal disorders interfering with intake or absorption of water-soluble vitamins; prolonged or wasting diseases; alcoholism. In addition to these states indicated above, Berocca-C 500 is particularly useful in severe burns, shock, trauma or other instances when the need for vitamin C is increased out of proportion to that for other vitamins.

Precautions: Occasional sensitivity to thiamine hydrochloride has been reported. When not diluted with infusion fluids, Berocca-C should be injected SLOWLY. Intramuscular administration may cause transient pain.

Side Effects: Occasional hypersensitivity reactions to thiamine hydrochloride have been encountered, principally after repeated intravenous injections of concentrated solutions. Consequently, if the patient has previously received thiamine, subsequent injections should be given with care, and administration discontinued if untoward reactions develop. Pain on intramuscular injection has rarely been reported.

Dosage and Administration: Berocca-C is preferably administered by addition to parenteral infusion fluids—amino acids, glucose solutions, physiologic saline or electrolyte replacement fluids. From 2 ml to 20 ml of Berocca-C per liter of infusion fluid may be added to such solutions.

The contents of a duplex package of Berocca-C 500 (1 ampul of Berocca-C and 1 ampul of Vitamin C Sodium Injectable) should be aspirated into the same syringe—preferably shortly before administration. This preparation may then be added to parenteral infusion fluids—amino acids, glucose solutions, physiologic saline or electrolyte replacement fluids. Four ml of Berocca-C 500 per liter of infusion fluid are usually adequate. If desired, further amounts of vitamin C may be added to such solutions.

A dose of no more than 2 ml of Berocca-C or 4 ml of Berocca-C 500 may also be given undiluted by SLOW intravenous or intramuscular injection. Intravenous injection is usually preferable, since intramuscular administration may cause temporary pain.

Berocca-C may be administered until it is possible to replace it with oral vitamin supplementation.

How Supplied: Berocca-C ampuls: 2 ml, boxes of 10. Vials: 20 ml, boxes of 1. Berocca-C 500 Duplex Package: Contains one 2-ml ampul of Berocca-C and one 2-ml ampul containing 400 mg ascorbic acid—boxes of 10.

CLONOPIN® Ⓒ
(clonazepam/Roche)

The following text is complete prescribing information based on official labeling in effect August 1, 1979.

Description: Chemically, clonazepam is 5-(2-chlorophenyl) -1, 3-dihydro-7-nitro-2H-1,4-benzodiazepin-2-one. It is a light yellow crystalline powder. It has a molecular weight of 315.7.

Actions: In laboratory animals, Clonopin exhibits several pharmacologic properties which are characteristic of the benzodiazepine class of drugs. Convulsions produced in rodents by pentylenetetrazol or electrical stimulation are antagonized, as are convulsions produced by photic stimulation in susceptible baboons. A taming effect in aggressive primates, muscle weakness and hypnosis are likewise produced by Clonopin. In humans it is capable of suppressing the spike and wave discharge in absence seizures (petit mal) and decreasing the frequency, amplitude, duration and spread of discharge in minor motor seizures.

Single oral dose administration of Clonopin to humans gave maximum blood levels of drug, in most cases, within one to two hours. The half-life of the parent compound varied from approximately 18 to 50 hours, and the major route of excretion was in the urine. In humans, five metabolites have been identified. In general, the biotransformation of clonazepam followed two pathways: oxidative hydroxylation at the C-3 position and reduction of the 7-nitro function to form 7-amino and/or 7-acetylamino derivatives.

Indications: Clonopin is useful alone or as an adjunct in the treatment of the Lennox-Gastaut syndrome (petit mal variant), akinetic and myoclonic seizures. In patients with absence seizures (petit mal) who have failed to respond to succinimides, Clonopin may be useful.

In some studies, up to 30% of patients have shown a loss of anticonvulsant activity, often within three months of administration. In some cases, dosage adjustment may reestablish efficacy.

Contraindications: Clonopin should not be used in patients with a history of sensitivity to benzodiazepines, nor in patients with clinical or biochemical evidence of significant liver disease. It may be used in patients with open angle glaucoma who are receiving appropriate therapy, but is contraindicated in acute narrow angle glaucoma.

Warnings: Since Clonopin produces CNS depression, patients receiving this drug should be cautioned against engaging in hazardous occupations requiring mental alertness, such as operating machinery or driving a motor vehicle. They should also be warned about the concomitant use of alcohol or other CNS-depressant drugs during Clonopin therapy (see Drug Interactions).

Usage in Pregnancy: The effects of Clonopin in human pregnancy and nursing infants are unknown.

Recent reports suggest an association between the use of anticonvulsant drugs by women with epilepsy and an elevated incidence of birth defects in children born to these women. Data are more extensive with respect to diphenylhydantoin and phenobarbital, but these are also the most commonly prescribed anticonvulsants; less systematic or anecdotal reports suggest a possible similar association with the use of all known anticonvulsant drugs.

The reports suggesting an elevated incidence of birth defects in children of drug-treated epileptic women cannot be regarded as adequate to prove a definite cause and effect relationship. There are intrinsic methodologic problems in obtaining adequate data on drug teratogenicity in humans; the possibility also exists that other factors, *e.g.*, genetic factors or the epileptic condition itself, may be more important than drug therapy in leading to birth defects. The great majority of mothers on anticonvulsant medication deliver normal infants. It is important to note that anticonvulsant drugs should not be discontinued in patients in whom the drug is administered to prevent seizures because of the strong possibility of precipitating status epilepticus with attendant hypoxia and threat to life. In individual cases where the severity and frequency of the seizure disorder are such that the removal of medication does not pose a serious threat to the patient, discontinuation of the drug may be considered prior to and during pregnancy, although it cannot be said with any confidence that even mild seizures do not pose some hazards to the developing embryo or fetus.

These considerations should be weighed in treating or counseling epileptic women of childbearing potential.

Use of Clonopin in women of childbearing potential should be considered only when the clinical situation warrants the risk. Mothers receiving Clonopin should not breast feed their infants.

In a two-generation reproduction study with Clonopin given orally to rats at 10 or 100 mg/kg/day, there was a decrease in the number of pregnancies and a decrease in the number of offspring surviving until weaning. When Clonopin was administered orally to pregnant rabbits at 0.2, 1.0, 5.0 or 10.0 mg/kg/day, a nondose-related incidence of cleft palates, open eyelids, fused sternebrae and limb defects was observed at the 0.2 and 5.0 mg/kg/day levels. Nearly all of the malformations were seen from one dam in each of the affected dosages.

Usage in Children: Because of the possibility that adverse effects on physical or mental development could become apparent only after many years, a benefit-risk consideration of the long-term use of Clonopin is important in pediatric patients.

Physical and Psychological Dependence: Withdrawal symptoms similar in character to those noted with barbiturates and alcohol have occurred following abrupt discontinuance of benzodiazepine drugs. These symptoms include convulsions, tremor, abdominal and muscle cramps, vomiting and sweating. Addiction-prone individuals, such as drug addicts or alcoholics, should be under careful surveillance when receiving benzodiazepines because of the predisposition of such patients to habituation and dependence.

Precautions: When used in patients in whom several different types of seizure disorders coexist, Clonopin may increase the incidence or precipitate the onset of generalized tonic-clonic seizures (grand mal). This may require the addition of appropriate anticonvulsants or an increase in their dosages. The concomitant use of valproic acid and clonazepam may produce absence status.

Periodic blood counts and liver function tests are advisable during long-term therapy with Clonopin.

The abrupt withdrawal of Clonopin, particularly in those patients on long-term, high-dose therapy, may precipitate status epilepticus. Therefore, when discontinuing Clonopin, gradual withdrawal is essential. While Clonopin is being gradually withdrawn, the simultaneous substitution of another anticonvulsant may be indicated. Metabolites of Clonopin are excreted by the kidneys; to avoid their excess accumulation, caution should be exercised in the administration of the drug to patients with impaired renal function.

Clonopin may produce an increase in salivation. This should be considered before giving the drug to patients who have difficulty handling secretions. Because of this and the possibility of respiratory depression, Clonopin should be used with caution in patients with chronic respiratory diseases.

Adverse Reactions: The most frequently occurring side effects of Clonopin are referable to CNS depression. Experience to date has shown that drowsiness has occurred in approximately 50% of patients and ataxia in approximately 30%. In some cases, these may diminish with time; behavior problems have been noted in approximately 25% of patients. Others, listed by system, are:

Neurologic: Abnormal eye movements, aphonia, choreiform movements, coma, diplopia, dysarthria, dysdiadochokinesis, "glassy-eyed" appearance, headache, hemiparesis, hypotonia, nystagmus, respiratory depression, slurred speech, tremor, vertigo.

Psychiatric: Confusion, depression, forgetfulness, hallucinations, hysteria, increased libido, insomnia, psychosis, suicidal attempt (the behavior effects are more likely to occur in patients with a history of psychiatric disturbances).

Respiratory: Chest congestion, rhinorrhea, shortness of breath, hypersecretion in upper respiratory passages.

Cardiovascular: Palpitations.

Dermatologic: Hair loss, hirsutism, skin rash, ankle and facial edema.

Gastrointestinal: Anorexia, coated tongue, constipation, diarrhea, dry mouth, encopresis, gastritis, hepatomegaly, increased appetite, nausea, sore gums.

Genitourinary: Dysuria, enuresis, nocturia, urinary retention.

Musculoskeletal: Muscle weakness, pains.

Miscellaneous: Dehydration, general deterioration, fever, lymphadenopathy, weight loss or gain.

Hematopoietic: Anemia, leukopenia, thrombocytopenia, eosinophilia.

Hepatic: Transient elevations of serum transaminases and alkaline phosphatase.

Drug Interactions: The CNS-depressant action of the benzodiazepine class of drugs may be potentiated by alcohol, narcotics, barbiturates, nonbarbiturate hypnotics, antianxiety agents, the phenothiazines, thioxanthene and butyrophenone classes of antipsychotic agents, monoamine oxidase inhibitors and the tricyclic antidepressants, and by other anticonvulsant drugs.

Overdosage: Symptoms of Clonopin overdosage, like those produced by other CNS depressants, include somnolence, confusion, coma and diminished reflexes. Treatment includes monitoring of respiration, pulse and blood pressure, general supportive measures and immediate gastric lavage. Intravenous fluids should be administered and an adequate airway maintained. Hypotension may be combated by the use of levarterenol or metaraminol. Methylphenidate or caffeine and sodium benzoate may be given to combat CNS depression. Dialysis is of no known value.

Dosage and Administration: *Infants and Children:* Clonopin is administered orally. In order to minimize drowsiness, the initial dose for infants and children (up to 10 years of age or 30 kg of body weight) should be between 0.01 to 0.03 mg/kg/day but not to exceed 0.05 mg/kg/day given in two or three divided doses. Dosage should be increased by no more than 0.25 to 0.5 mg every third day until a daily maintenance dose of 0.1 to 0.2 mg/kg of body weight has been reached unless seizures are controlled or side effects preclude further increase. Whenever possible, the daily dose should be divided into three equal doses. If doses are not equally divided, the largest dose should be given before retiring.

Adults: The initial dose for adults should not exceed 1.5 mg/day divided into three doses. Dosage may be increased in increments of 0.5 to 1 mg every three days until seizures are adequately controlled or until side effects preclude any further increase. Maintenance dosage must be individualized for each patient depending upon response. Maximum recommended daily dose is 20 mg.

The use of multiple anticonvulsants may result in an increase of depressant adverse effects. This should be considered before adding Clonopin to an existing anticonvulsant regimen.

How Supplied: Scored tablets—0.5 mg, orange; 1 mg, blue; 2 mg, white—Prescription Paks of 100.

[*Shown in Product Identification Section*]

DALMANE® Ⓒ
(flurazepam hydrochloride/Roche)
Capsules

Dalmane is a product of Roche Products Inc., Manati, P.R. 00701.

The following text is complete prescribing information based on official labeling in effect August 1, 1979.

Description: Flurazepam hydrochloride is chemically 7-chloro-1-[2-(diethylamino)ethyl]-5-(*o*-fluorophenyl)-1, 3-dihydro-2*H*-1, 4-benzodiazepin-2-one dihydrochloride. It is a pale yellow, crystalline compound, freely soluble in U.S.P. alcohol and very soluble in water. It has a molecular weight of 460.826.

Actions: In animal studies flurazepam hydrochloride reduced the pressor response to electrical stimulation of the hypothalamus, and increased the arousal threshold to stimulation of the amygdala and hypothalamus; however, the exact site and mode of action are unknown.

Clinical Pharmacology: Flurazepam HCl is rapidly absorbed from the G.I. tract. Flurazepam is rapidly metabolized and is excreted primarily in the urine. The blood level profile of flurazepam and its major metabolites was determined in man following the oral administration of 30 mg daily for 2 weeks. The levels of the intact drug were below the sensitivity limit of the assay. The N_1-hydroxyethyl-flurazepam was measurable only during the early hours after a 30 mg dose and was not detectable after 24 hours. The major metabolite in blood was N_1-desalkyl-flurazepam, which reached steady-state (plateau) levels after 7 days. The half-life of elimination of N_1-desalkyl-flurazepam ranged from 47 to 100 hours. The major urinary metabolite is conjugated N_1-hydroxyethyl-flurazepam which accounts for 22 to 55 percent of the dose. Less than 1% of the dose is excreted in the urine as N_1-desalkyl-flurazepam.

This pharmacokinetic profile may be responsible for the clinical observation that flurazepam is increasingly effective on the second or third night of consecutive use and that for one or two nights after the drug is discontinued both sleep latency and total wake time may still be decreased.

Indications: Dalmane is a hypnotic agent useful in all types of insomnia characterized by difficulty in falling asleep, frequent nocturnal awakenings and/or early morning awakening. Dalmane can be used effectively in patients with recurring insomnia or poor sleeping habits, and in acute or chronic medical situations requiring restful sleep. Sleep laboratory studies have objectively determined that Dalmane is effective for at least 28 consecutive nights of drug administration. Since insomnia is often transient and intermittent, the prolonged use of hypnotics is usually not indicated and should only be undertaken concomitantly with appropriate evaluation of the patient.

Contraindications: Dalmane is contraindicated in patients with known hypersensitivity to the drug.

Warnings: Patients receiving Dalmane should be cautioned about possible combined effects with alcohol and other CNS depressants. Patients should be cautioned against hazardous occupations requiring complete mental alertness such as operating machinery or driving a motor vehicle shortly after ingesting the drug.

***Usage in Pregnancy:* An increased risk of congenital malformations associated with the use of minor tranquilizers (chlordiazepoxide, diazepam and meprobamate) during the first trimester of pregnancy has been suggested in several studies. Dalmane, a benzodiazepine derivative, has not been studied adequately to determine whether it, too, may be associated with an increased risk of fetal abnormality. Because use of these drugs is rarely a matter of urgency, their use during this period should almost always be avoided. The possibility that a woman of childbearing potential may be pregnant at the time of institution of therapy should be considered. Patients should be advised that if they become pregnant during therapy or intend to become pregnant they should communicate with their physician about the desirability of discontinuing the drug.**

Usage in Children: Clinical investigations of Dalmane have not been carried out in children. Therefore, the drug is not currently recommended for use in persons under 15 years of age.

Physical and Psychological Dependence: Physical and psychological dependence have not been reported or observed in persons taking recommended doses of Dalmane. However, as with any hypnotic, caution must be exercised in administering Dalmane to individuals known to be addiction-prone or those whose history suggests they may increase the dosage on their own initiative. It is desirable to limit repeated prescriptions without adequate medical supervision.

Precautions: Since the risk of the development of oversedation, dizziness, confusion and/or ataxia increases substantially with larger doses in elderly and debilitated patients, it is recommended that in such patients the dosage be limited to 15 mg. If Dalmane is to be combined with other drugs having known hypnotic properties or CNS-depressant effects, due consideration should be given to potential additive effects.

Continued on next page

Roche—Cont.

The usual precautions are indicated for severely depressed patients or those in whom there is any evidence of latent depression; particularly the recognition that suicidal tendencies may be present and protective measures may be necessary.
Should Dalmane be used repeatedly, periodic blood counts and liver and kidney function tests should be performed. The usual precautions should be observed in patients with impaired renal or hepatic function.
Adverse Reactions: Dizziness, drowsiness, lightheadedness, staggering, ataxia and falling have occurred, particularly in elderly or debilitated persons. Severe sedation, lethargy, disorientation and coma, probably indicative of drug intolerance or overdosage, have been reported.
Also reported were: headache, heartburn, upset stomach, nausea, vomiting, diarrhea, constipation, gastrointestinal pain, nervousness, talkativeness, apprehension, irritability, weakness, palpitations, chest pains, body and joint pains and genitourinary complaints. There have also been rare occurrences of leukopenia, granulocytopenia, sweating, flushes, difficulty in focusing, blurred vision, burning eyes, faintness, hypotension, shortness of breath, pruritus, skin rash, dry mouth, bitter taste, excessive salivation, anorexia, euphoria, depression, slurred speech, confusion, restlessness, hallucinations, and elevated SGOT, SGPT, total and direct bilirubins, and alkaline phosphatase. Paradoxical reactions, *e.g.,* excitement, stimulation and hyperactivity, have also been reported in rare instances.
Dosage and Administration: Dosage should be individualized for maximal beneficial effects. The usual adult dosage is 30 mg before retiring. In some patients, 15 mg may suffice. In elderly and/or debilitated patients it is recommended that therapy be initiated with 15 mg until individual responses are determined.
Overdosage: Manifestations of Dalmane overdosage include somnolence, confusion and coma. Respiration, pulse and blood pressure should be monitored as in all cases of drug overdosage. General supportive measures should be employed, along with immediate gastric lavage. Intravenous fluids should be administered and an adequate airway maintained. Hypotension and CNS depression may be combated by judicious use of appropriate therapeutic agents. The value of dialysis has not been determined. If excitation occurs in patients following Dalmane overdosage, barbiturates should not be used. As with the management of intentional overdosage with any drug, it should be borne in mind that multiple agents may have been ingested.
How Supplied: Dalmane (flurazepam hydrochloride/Roche) capsules—15 mg, orange and ivory; 30 mg, red and ivory—bottles of 100 and 500; Tel-E-Dose® packages of 100 (4 reverse-numbered boxes of 25 or boxes containing 10 strips of 10), and packages of 120 (4 reverse-numbered boxes of 30); Prescription Paks of 30, available singly and in trays of 10.
Animal Pharmacology and Toxicology: Flurazepam hydrochloride is rapidly absorbed from the gastrointestinal tract and is rapidly metabolized. Studies in rats with ^{14}C-labeled flurazepam hydrochloride indicated that the drug is widely distributed throughout body tissues with no excessive accumulation of drug or metabolite in any one tissue.
The oral LD_{50} was 870 mg/kg in mice, 1232 mg/kg in rats and 568 mg/kg in rabbits. Chronic toxicity studies for one year indicated that the tolerated dose is 80 mg/kg/ day in the rat and 10 mg/kg/day in the dog.
Reproduction Studies: A two-cycle reproduction study in rats was carried out at doses of 5 and 50 mg/kg/day of flurazepam hydrochloride. There were no teratogenic or other adverse effects related to the drug. In a second series of rat reproduction studies doses of 3 and 20 mg/kg/day of flurazepam hydrochloride did not induce changes in fertility and general reproductive performance. There were no teratogenic effects related to the drug or adverse effects in the perinatal and postnatal study. In another reproduction study in rats at doses of 10, 20, 40 and 80 mg/kg/day, no adverse effects on reproduction and no teratological changes were noted.
In rabbits, two sets of teratogenic studies were done. In the first, flurazepam hydrochloride was administered in doses of 5 and 20 mg/kg/day. Twenty-three live litters were obtained in this study. One animal which received 20 mg/kg/day had a litter of nine viable but deformed fetuses. In the second study, the dose of flurazepam hydrochloride was increased to 40 mg/kg/day without the occurrence of abnormalities in all eleven litters. In both studies, there were no significant differences between the control and treated groups in maternal weight, body weight of viable fetuses, fetal body weight and litter size.
Clinical Studies: Dalmane significantly reduced sleep induction time and increased sleep duration in 53 controlled clinical studies on 2010 patients using a double-blind crossover design.
In eight controlled sleep research laboratory studies of 32 insomniac subjects utilizing all-night electroencephalographic (EEG), electromyographic (EMG), and electro-oculographic (EOG) recordings, Dalmane, on average, induced sleep within 17 minutes and provided seven to eight hours of sleep. Of the drugs studied, Dalmane was the only one which consistently decreased sleep latency and number of awakenings while increasing total sleep time. No rebound of dream time as measured by REM (Rapid Eye Movements) was seen after withdrawal of Dalmane in 12 controlled sleep research laboratory studies of 32 insomniac and 23 normal subjects. A minimal decrease of REM time was observed, and a reduction of Stage 4 time was noted after administration of Dalmane.
Eight insomniacs participated in a double-blind crossover sleep research laboratory study in which the effects of Dalmane 30 mg and placebo were compared for 10 consecutive nights. Dalmane reduced sleep latency, number of wakeful periods and time awake, while increasing total sleep time.

[*Shown in Product Identification Section*]

EFUDEX® ℞
(fluorouracil/Roche)

The following text is complete prescribing information based on official labeling in effect August 1, 1979.
Description: Efudex solutions and cream are topical preparations containing the fluorinated pyrimidine 5-fluorouracil, an antineoplastic antimetabolite.
Efudex Solution consists of 2% or 5% fluorouracil/Roche on a weight/weight basis, compounded with propylene glycol, tris(hydroxymethyl)aminomethane, hydroxypropyl cellulose, parabens (methyl and propyl) and disodium edetate.
Efudex Cream contains 5% fluorouracil/Roche in a vanishing cream base consisting of white petrolatum, stearyl alcohol, propylene glycol, polysorbate 60 and parabens (methyl and propyl).
Actions: There is evidence that the metabolism of fluorouracil in the anabolic pathway blocks the methylation reaction of deoxyuridylic acid to thymidylic acid. In this fashion fluorouracil interferes with the synthesis of deoxyribonucleic acid (DNA) and to a lesser extent inhibits the formation of ribonucleic acid (RNA). Since DNA and RNA are essential for cell division and growth, the effect of fluorouracil may be to create a thymine deficiency which provokes unbalanced growth and death of the cell. The effects of DNA and RNA deprivation are most marked on those cells which grow more rapidly and which take up fluorouracil at a more rapid pace. The catabolic metabolism of fluorouracil results in degradative products (e.g., CO_2, urea, α-fluoro-β-alanine) which are inactive.
Studies in man with topical application of ^{14}C-labeled Efudex demonstrated insignificant absorption as measured by ^{14}C content of plasma, urine and respiratory CO_2.
Indications: Efudex is recommended for the topical treatment of multiple actinic or solar keratoses. In the 5% strength it is also useful in the treatment of superficial basal cell carcinomas, when conventional methods are impractical, such as with multiple lesions or difficult treatment sites. The diagnosis should be established prior to treatment, since this new method has not been proven effective in other types of basal cell carcinomas. With isolated, easily accessible lesions, conventional techniques are preferred since success with such lesions is almost 100% with these methods. The success rate with Efudex cream and solution is approximately 93%. This 93% success rate is based on 113 lesions in 54 patients. Twenty-five lesions treated with the solution produced one failure and 88 lesions treated with the cream produced 7 failures.
Contraindications: Efudex is contraindicated in patients with known hypersensitivity to any of its components.
Warnings: If an occlusive dressing is used, there may be an increase in the incidence of inflammatory reactions in the adjacent normal skin. A porous gauze dressing may be applied for cosmetic reasons without increase in reaction.
Prolonged exposure to ultraviolet rays should be avoided while under treatment with Efudex because the intensity of the reaction may be increased.
Usage in Pregnancy: Safety for use in pregnancy has not been established.
Precautions: If Efudex is applied with the fingers, the hands should be washed immediately afterward. Efudex should be applied with care near the eyes, nose and mouth. Solar keratoses which do not respond should be biopsied to confirm the diagnosis. Patients should be forewarned that the reaction in the treated areas may be unsightly during therapy, and, in some cases, for several weeks following cessation of therapy.
Follow-up biopsies should be performed as indicated in the management of superficial basal cell carcinoma.
Adverse Reactions: The most frequently encountered local reactions are pain, pruritus, hyperpigmentation and burning at the site of application. Other local reactions include dermatitis, scarring, soreness, tenderness, suppuration, scaling and swelling.
Also reported are insomnia, stomatitis, irritability, medicinal taste, photosensitivity, lacrimation and telangiectasia, although a causal relationship is remote.
Laboratory abnormalities reported are leukocytosis, thrombocytopenia, toxic granulation and eosinophilia.
Dosage and Administration: When Efudex is applied to a lesion, a response occurs with the following sequence: erythema, usually followed by vesiculation, erosion, ulceration, necrosis and epithelization.
Actinic or solar keratosis: Apply cream or solution twice daily in an amount sufficient to cover the lesions. Medication should be continued until the inflammatory response reaches the erosion, necrosis and ulceration stage, at which time use of the drug should be terminated. The usual duration of therapy is from two to four weeks. Complete healing of the le-

sions may not be evident for one to two months following cessation of Efudex therapy.

Superficial basal cell carcinomas: **Only the 5% strength is recommended.** Apply cream or solution twice daily in an amount sufficient to cover the lesions. Treatment should be continued for at least three to six weeks. Therapy may be required for as long as 10 to 12 weeks before the lesions are obliterated. As in any neoplastic condition, the patient should be followed for a reasonable period of time to determine if a cure has been obtained.

How Supplied: Efudex Solution, 10-ml drop dispensers—containing 2% or 5% fluorouracil/Roche on a weight/weight basis, compounded with propylene glycol, tris(hydroxymethyl)aminomethane, hydroxypropyl cellulose, parabens (methyl and propyl) and disodium edetate.

Efudex Cream, 25-Gm tubes—containing 5% fluorouracil/Roche in a vanishing cream base consisting of white petrolatum, stearyl alcohol, propylene glycol, polysorbate 60 and parabens (methyl and propyl).

ENDEP® ℞
(amitriptyline HCl/Roche)
TABLETS

The following text is complete prescribing information based on official labeling in effect August 1, 1979.

Description: Amitriptyline HCl, a dibenzocycloheptadiene derivative, is a white crystalline compound that is readily soluble in water.

Endep is supplied as round, film-coated, scored tablets, each containing amitriptyline hydrochloride 10 mg, 25 mg, or 50 mg (orange); 75 mg (yellow); 100 mg (peach); or 150 mg (salmon).

Actions: Endep is an antidepressant with an anxiety-reducing, sedative component to its action. Its mechanism of action in man is not known. It is not a monoamine oxidase inhibitor, and it does not act primarily by stimulation of the central nervous system.

Amitriptyline inhibits the membrane pump mechanism responsible for reuptake of norepinephrine into adrenergic neurons. Pharmacologically this action may potentiate or prolong sympathetic activity, since reuptake of norepinephrine is important physiologically in terminating its transmitting actions. This interference with reuptake of norepinephrine is believed by some to underlie the antidepressant activity of amitriptyline.

Indications: For the relief of symptoms of depression. Endogenous depression is more likely to be alleviated than are other depressive states.

Depression accompanied by anxiety.

Contraindications: Endep is contraindicated in patients who have shown prior hypersensitivity to it. It should not be given concomitantly with a monoamine oxidase inhibiting compound. Hyperpyretic crises, severe convulsions and deaths have occurred in patients receiving tricyclic antidepressant and monoamine oxidase inhibiting drugs simultaneously. When it is desired to replace a monoamine oxidase inhibitor with Endep, a minimum of 14 days should be allowed to elapse after the former is discontinued. Endep should then be initiated cautiously with gradual increase in dosage until optimum response is achieved.

This drug is not recommended for use during the acute recovery phase following myocardial infarction.

Warnings: Endep may block the antihypertensive action of guanethidine or similarly acting compounds.

It should be used with caution in patients with a history of seizures and, because of its atropine-like action, in patients with a history of urinary retention, angle-closure glaucoma or increased intraocular pressure. In patients with glaucoma, even average doses may precipitate an attack.

Patients with cardiovascular disorders should be watched closely. Tricyclic antidepressant drugs, including Endep, particularly when given in high doses, have been reported to produce arrhythmias, sinus tachycardia and prolongation of the conduction time. Myocardial infarction and stroke have been reported with drugs of this class.

Close supervision is required when Endep is given to hyperthyroid patients or those receiving thyroid medication.

This drug may impair mental and/or physical abilities required for performance of hazardous tasks, such as operating machinery or driving a motor vehicle.

Usage in Pregnancy: Safe use of Endep during pregnancy and lactation has not been established; therefore, in administering the drug to pregnant patients, nursing mothers or women who may become pregnant, the possible benefits must be weighed against the possible hazards to mother and child.

Animal reproduction studies have been inconclusive, and clinical experience has been limited.

Usage in Children: In view of the lack of experience with the use of this drug in children, it is not recommended at the present time for patients under 12 years of age.

Precautions: Schizophrenic patients may develop increased symptoms of psychosis; patients with paranoid symptomatology may have an exaggeration of such symptoms; manic depressive patients may experience a shift to the manic phase.

In these circumstances the dose of Endep may be reduced or a major tranquilizer may be administered concurrently.

When Endep is given with anticholinergic agents or sympathomimetic drugs, including epinephrine combined with local anesthetics, close supervision and careful adjustment of dosages are required.

Caution is advised if patients receive large doses of ethchlorvynol concurrently. Transient delirium has been reported in patients who were treated with one gram of ethchlorvynol and 75 to 150 mg of amitriptyline HCl.

Endep may enhance the response to alcohol and the effects of barbiturates and other CNS depressants.

The possibility of suicide in depressed patients remains during treatment and until significant remission occurs. This type of patient should not have easy access to large quantities of the drug.

Concurrent administration of Endep and electroshock therapy may increase the hazards associated with such therapy. Such treatment should be limited to patients for whom it is essential.

When possible, the drug should be discontinued several days before elective surgery.

Both elevation and lowering of blood sugar levels have been reported.

Adverse Reactions: ***Note:*** Included in the listing which follows are a few adverse reactions which have not been reported with this specific drug. However, pharmacological similarities among the tricyclic antidepressant drugs require that each of the reactions be considered when Endep is administered.

Cardiovascular: Hypotension, hypertension, tachycardia, palpitation, myocardial infarction, arrhythmias, heart block, stroke.

CNS and Neuromuscular: Confusional states; disturbed concentration; disorientation; delusions; hallucinations; excitement; anxiety; restlessness; insomnia; nightmares; numbness, tingling and paresthesias of the extremities; peripheral neuropathy; incoordination; ataxia; tremors; seizures; alteration in EEG patterns; extrapyramidal symptoms; tinnitus.

Anticholinergic: Dry mouth, blurred vision, disturbance of accommodation, constipation, paralytic ileus, urinary retention, dilatation of urinary tract.

Allergic: Skin rash, urticaria, photosensitization, edema of face and tongue.

Hematologic: Bone marrow depression including agranulocytosis, eosinophilia, purpura, thrombocytopenia.

Gastrointestinal: Nausea, epigastric distress, vomiting, anorexia, stomatitis, peculiar taste, diarrhea, parotid swelling, black tongue.

Endocrine: Testicular swelling and gynecomastia in the male, breast enlargement and galactorrhea in the female, increased or decreased libido, elevation and lowering of blood sugar levels.

Other: Dizziness, weakness, fatigue, headache, weight gain or loss, increased perspiration, urinary frequency, mydriasis, drowsiness, jaundice, alopecia.

Withdrawal Symptoms: Abrupt cessation of treatment after prolonged administration may produce nausea, headache and malaise. These are not indicative of addiction.

Dosage and Administration: Dosage should be initiated at a low level and increased gradually, noting carefully the clinical response and any evidence of intolerance.

Initial Dosage for Adults: Twenty-five mg 3 times a day usually is satisfactory for outpatients. If necessary, this may be increased to a total of 150 mg a day. Increases are made preferably in the late afternoon and/or bedtime doses. A sedative effect may be apparent before the antidepressant effect is noted, but an adequate therapeutic effect may take as long as 30 days to develop.

An alternate method of initiating therapy in outpatients is to begin with 50 to 100 mg at bedtime. This may be increased by 25 to 50 mg as necessary in the bedtime dose to a total of 150 mg per day.

Hospitalized patients may require 100 mg a day initially. This can be increased gradually to 200 mg a day if necessary. A small number of hospitalized patients may need as much as 300 mg a day.

Adolescent and Elderly Patients: In general, lower dosages are recommended for these patients. Ten mg 3 times a day with 20 mg at bedtime may be satisfactory in adolescent and elderly patients who do not tolerate higher dosages.

Maintenance: The usual maintenance dose is 25 mg 2 to 4 times a day. In some patients, 10 mg 4 times a day is sufficient. When satisfactory improvement has been reached, dosage should be reduced to the lowest amount that will maintain relief of symptoms. It is appropriate to continue maintenance therapy 3 months or longer to lessen the possibility of relapse.

Overdosage: All patients suspected of having an overdosage should be admitted to a hospital as soon as possible.

Manifestations: High doses may cause temporary confusion, disturbed concentration or transient visual hallucinations. Overdosage may cause drowsiness; hypothermia; tachycardia and other arrhythmic abnormalities, such as bundle branch block; ECG evidence of impaired conduction; congestive heart failure; dilated pupils; convulsions; severe hypotension; stupor and coma. Other symptoms may be agitation, hyperactive reflexes, muscle rigidity, vomiting, hyperpyrexia or any of those listed under ADVERSE REACTIONS.

In patients with glaucoma, even average doses may precipitate an attack.

Treatment is symptomatic and supportive. Empty the stomach as quickly as possible by emesis or lavage. If the patient is stuporous, but responds to some stimuli, only close watching and nursing care may be required. An ECG should be taken and close monitoring of cardiac function instituted if there is any sign of

Continued on next page

Roche—Cont.

pathology. Maintain an open airway and adequate fluid intake; regulate body temperature. The intravenous administration of 1 to 3 mg of physostigmine salicylate has been reported to reverse the symptoms of amitriptyline poisoning. Anticonvulsants may be given to control convulsions (amitriptyline increases the CNS depressant action but not the anticonvulsant action of barbiturates; therefore, an inhalation anesthetic is recommended for convulsions). Central nervous system depression may be treated with nonconvulsant doses of CNS stimulants. Standard measures should be used to manage cardiac arrhythmias, circulatory shock and metabolic acidosis. Should cardiac failure occur, the use of digitalis should be considered. Close monitoring of cardiac function for at least five days is advised under these circumstances. Cardiac arrhythmias may be treated with neostigmine, pyridostigmine or propranolol.

Dialysis is of no value because of low plasma concentrations of the drug.

Continue treatment for at least 48 hours in patients who do not respond earlier.

Since overdosage is often deliberate, patients may attempt suicide by other means during the recovery phase.

Deaths by deliberate or accidental overdosage have occurred with this class of drugs.

How Supplied: Scored tablets, each containing 10 mg, 25 mg, 50 mg, 75 mg, 100 mg or 150 mg of amitriptyline hydrochloride/Roche—bottles of 100 and 500; Tel-E-Dose® packages of 100; Prescription Paks of 60 (10 mg, 25 mg and 50 mg) or 30 (75 mg, 100 mg and 150 mg).

[*Shown in Product Identification Section*]

FLUOROURACIL ℞
(5-fluorouracil/Roche)
INJECTABLE

The following text is complete prescribing information based on official labeling in effect August 1, 1979.

WARNING
It is recommended that FLUOROURACIL be given only by or under the supervision of a qualified physician who is experienced in cancer chemotherapy and who is well versed in the use of potent antimetabolites. Because of the possibility of severe toxic reactions, it is recommended that patients be hospitalized at least during the initial course of therapy.
These instructions should be thoroughly reviewed before administration of Fluorouracil.

Description: FLUOROURACIL Roche (5-fluorouracil) is a fluorinated pyrimidine belonging to the category of antimetabolites. Fluorouracil resembles the natural uracil molecule in structure, except that a hydrogen atom has been replaced by a fluorine atom in the 5 position.

Actions: There is evidence that the metabolism of fluorouracil in the anabolic pathway blocks the methylation reaction of deoxyuridylic acid to thymidylic acid. In this fashion 5-fluorouracil interferes with the synthesis of deoxyribonucleic acid (DNA) and to a lesser extent inhibits the formation of ribonucleic acid (RNA). Since DNA and RNA are essential for cell division and growth, the effect of fluorouracil may be to create a thymine deficiency which provokes unbalanced growth and death of the cell. The effects of DNA and RNA deprivation are most marked on those cells which grow more rapidly and which take up fluorouracil at a more rapid pace. The catabolic metabolism of fluorouracil results in degradative products (e.g., CO_2, urea, α-fluoro-β-alanine) which are inactive. Following an intravenous injection, no intact drug can be detected in the plasma after three hours. Approximately 15 percent is excreted intact in the urine in six hours, of which over 90 percent is excreted in the first hour. Of the injected intravenous dose 60 to 80 percent is excreted as respiratory CO_2 in 8 to 12 hours.

Indications: Fluorouracil is effective in the palliative management of carcinoma of the colon, rectum, breast, stomach and pancreas in patients who are considered incurable by surgery or other means.

Contraindications: Fluorouracil therapy is contraindicated for patients in a poor nutritional state, those with depressed bone marrow function or those with potentially serious infections.

Warnings: THE DAILY DOSE OF FLUOROURACIL IS NOT TO EXCEED 800 MG. IT IS RECOMMENDED THAT PATIENTS BE HOSPITALIZED DURING THEIR FIRST COURSE OF TREATMENT.

Fluorouracil should be used with extreme caution in poor risk patients with a history of high-dose pelvic irradiation, previous use of alkylating agents or who have a widespread involvement of bone marrow by metastatic tumors or impaired hepatic or renal function. The drug is not intended as an adjuvant to surgery. Although severe toxicity is more likely in poor risk patients, fatalities may be encountered occasionally even in patients in relatively good condition.

Usage in Pregnancy: Safe use of Fluorouracil has not been established with respect to adverse effects on fetal development. Therefore, this drug should not be used during pregnancy, particularly in the first trimester, unless in the judgment of the physician the potential benefits to the patient outweigh the hazards.

Because the risk of mutagenesis has not been evaluated, such possible effects on males and females must be considered.

Combination Therapy: Any form of therapy which adds to the stress of the patient, interferes with nutrition or depresses bone marrow function will increase the toxicity of Fluorouracil.

Precautions: Fluorouracil is a highly toxic drug with a narrow margin of safety. Therefore, patients should be carefully supervised, since therapeutic response is unlikely to occur without some evidence of toxicity. Patients should be informed of expected toxic effects, particularly oral manifestations. White blood counts with differential are recommended before each dose. Severe hematological toxicity, gastrointestinal hemorrhage and even death may result from the use of Fluorouracil despite meticulous selection of patients and careful adjustment of dosage.

Therapy is to be discontinued promptly whenever one of the following signs of toxicity appears:

Stomatitis or *esophagopharyngitis,* At the first visible sign.

Leukopenia (WBC under 3500), or a *rapidly falling white blood count.*

Vomiting, Intractable.

Diarrhea, Frequent bowel movements or watery stools.

Gastrointestinal ulceration and bleeding.

Thrombocytopenia, Platelets under 100,000.

Hemorrhage from any site.

Adverse Reactions: Stomatitis and esophagopharyngitis (which may lead to sloughing and ulceration), diarrhea, anorexia, nausea and emesis are commonly seen during therapy.

Leukopenia usually follows every course of adequate therapy with Fluorouracil. The lowest white blood cell counts are commonly observed between the 9th and 14th days after the first course of treatment, although uncommonly the maximal depression may be delayed for as long as 20 days. By the 30th day the count has usually returned to the normal range.

Alopecia and dermatitis may be seen in a substantial number of cases. Patients should be alerted to the possibility of alopecia as a result of therapy and should be informed that it is a transient effect. The dermatitis most often seen is a pruritic maculopapular rash usually appearing on the extremities and less frequently on the trunk. It is generally reversible and usually responsive to symptomatic treatment. Dry skin and fissuring have also been noted. Photosensitivity, as manifested by erythema or increased pigmentation of the skin, has been observed on occasion. Also noted were photophobia, lacrimation, epistaxis, euphoria, acute cerebellar syndrome (which may persist following discontinuation of treatment) and nail changes, including loss of nails. Myocardial ischemia has also been reported.

Dosage and Administration: *General Instructions:* Administration of Fluorouracil Injectable should be done only intravenously, using care to avoid extravasation. No dilution is required.

All dosages are based on the patient's actual weight. However, the estimated lean body mass (dry weight) is used if the patient is obese or if there has been a spurious weight gain due to edema, ascites or other forms of abnormal fluid retention.

It is recommended that prior to treatment each patient be carefully evaluated in order to estimate as accurately as possible the optimum initial dosage of Fluorouracil.

Dosage: Twelve mg/kg are given intravenously once daily for four successive days. The daily dose should not be more than 800 mg. *If no toxicity is observed,* 6 mg/kg are given on the 6th, 8th, 10th and 12th days unless toxicity occurs. No therapy is given on the 5th, 7th, 9th or 11th days. *Therapy is to be discontinued at the end of the 12th day, even if no toxicity has become apparent.* (See CONTRAINDICATIONS and WARNINGS.)

Poor risk patients or those who are not in adequate nutritional state (see CONTRAINDICATIONS and WARNINGS) should receive 6 mg/kg/day for three days. *If no toxicity is observed,* 3 mg/kg may be given on the 5th, 7th and 9th days *unless toxicity occurs.* No therapy is given on the 4th, 6th or 8th days. The daily dose should not exceed 400 mg.

A sequence of injections on either schedule constitutes a "course of therapy."

Maintenance Therapy: In instances where toxicity has not been a problem, it is recommended that therapy be continued using either of the following schedules:

1. Repeat dosage of first course every 30 days after the last day of the previous course of treatment.
2. When toxic signs resulting from the initial course of therapy have subsided, administer a maintenance dosage of 10 to 15 mg/kg/week as a single dose. Do not exceed 1 Gm per week.

The amount of the drug to be used should take into account the patient's reaction to the previous course and should be adjusted accordingly. Some patients have received from 9 to 45 courses of treatment during periods which ranged from 12 to 60 months.

How Supplied: *Injectable:* 10-ml ampuls (for intravenous use) containing 500 mg 5-fluorouracil in a colorless to faint yellow aqueous solution, with pH adjusted to approximately 9.0 with sodium hydroxide. Boxes of 10.

Note: Although Fluorouracil ampul solution may discolor slightly during storage, the potency and safety are not adversely affected.

Store at room temperature (59° to 86°F). Protect from light. If a precipitate occurs due to exposure to low temperatures, resolubilize by heating to 140°F with vigorous shaking; allow to cool to body temperature before using.

FUDR ℞

(floxuridine/Roche)

The following text is complete prescribing information based on official labeling in effect August 1, 1979.

FOR INTRA-ARTERIAL INFUSION ONLY

WARNING

It is recommended that FUDR be given only by or under the supervision of a qualified physician who is experienced in cancer chemotherapy and intra-arterial drug therapy.

Because of the possibility of severe toxic reactions, all patients should be hospitalized for initiation of treatment.

Description: Floxuridine is a fluorinated pyrimidine belonging to the category of antimetabolites. It is a white to off-white odorless solid, soluble in alcohol and freely soluble in water. The 2% aqueous solution has a pH of 4.0 to 5.5. Chemically, floxuridine is 2′-deoxy-5-fluorouridine with a molecular weight of 246.19.

Actions: When FUDR is given by intra-arterial injection it is apparently rapidly catabolized to 5-fluorouracil. Thus, rapid injection of FUDR produces the same toxic and antimetabolic effects as does 5-fluorouracil. The primary effect is to interfere with the synthesis of deoxyribonucleic acid (DNA) and to a lesser extent inhibit the formation of ribonucleic acid (RNA). However, when FUDR is given by continuous intra-arterial infusion its direct anabolism to FUDR-monophosphate is enhanced, thus increasing the inhibition of DNA.

Indications: FUDR is effective in the palliative management of gastrointestinal adenocarcinoma metastatic to the liver, when given by continuous regional intra-arterial infusion in carefully selected patients who are considered incurable by surgery or other means. Patients with known disease extending beyond an area capable of infusion via a single artery should, except in unusual circumstances, be considered for systemic therapy with other chemotherapeutic agents.

Contraindications: FUDR therapy is contraindicated for patients in a poor nutritional state, those with depressed bone marrow function, or those with potentially serious infections.

Warnings: IT IS IMPERATIVE THAT ALL PATIENTS BE HOSPITALIZED FOR INITIATION OF TREATMENT.

FUDR should be used with extreme caution in poor risk patients with impaired hepatic or renal function or a history of high-dose pelvic irradiation or previous use of alkylating agents. The drug is not intended as an adjuvant to surgery.

Usage in Pregnancy: Safe use of FUDR has not been established with respect to adverse effects on fetal development. Therefore, this drug should not be used during pregnancy, particularly in the first trimester, unless in the judgment of the physician the potential benefits to the patient outweigh the hazards.

Because teratogenicity and mutagenicity have been demonstrated in animals, such possible effects on men and women must be considered.

Combination Therapy: Any form of therapy which adds to the stress of the patient, interferes with nutrition, or depresses bone marrow function will increase the toxicity of FUDR (floxuridine).

Therapy is to be discontinued promptly whenever one of the following signs of toxicity appears:

Stomatitis or esophagopharyngitis, At the first visible sign.

Leukopenia (WBC under 3500), or a rapidly falling white blood count.

Vomiting, Intractable.

Diarrhea, Frequent bowel movements or watery stools.

Gastrointestinal ulceration and bleeding.

Thrombocytopenia, Platelets under 100,000.

Hemorrhage from any site.

Precautions: FUDR is potentially a highly toxic drug with a narrow margin of safety. Therefore, patients should be carefully supervised since therapeutic response is unlikely to occur without some evidence of toxicity. Patients should be informed of expected toxic effects, particularly oral manifestations. Careful monitoring of the white blood count and platelet count is recommended. Severe hematological toxicity, gastrointestinal hemorrhage and even death may result from the use of FUDR despite meticulous selection of patients and careful adjustment of dosage. Although severe toxicity is more likely in poor risk patients, fatalities may be encountered occasionally even in patients in relatively good condition.

Adverse Reactions: The adverse reactions to the arterial infusion of FUDR are generally related to the drug-infused area and can be grouped under the following categories: functional gastrointestinal, mucosal gastrointestinal, hematologic, dermatologic, miscellaneous clinical reactions, laboratory abnormalities and procedural complications of regional arterial infusion.

The more common adverse reactions are nausea, vomiting, diarrhea, enteritis, stomatitis and localized erythema. The more common laboratory abnormalities are anemia, leukopenia, and elevations of alkaline phosphatase, serum transaminase, serum bilirubin and lactic dehydrogenase.

Other adverse reactions are:

Functional gastrointestinal: anorexia, cramps and pain.

Mucosal gastrointestinal: duodenal ulcer, duodenitis, gastritis, gastroenteritis, glossitis and pharyngitis.

Dermatological: alopecia, dermatitis, nonspecific skin toxicity and rash.

Other clinical reactions: fever, lethargy, malaise, and weakness.

Laboratory abnormalities: BSP, prothrombin, total proteins, sedimentation rate and thrombopenia.

Procedural complications of regional arterial infusion: arterial aneurysm, arterial ischemia, arterial thrombosis, bleeding at catheter site, catheter blocked, displaced or leaking, embolism, fibromyositis, infection at catheter site, abscesses and thrombophlebitis.

Dosage and Administration: The recommended therapeutic dose schedule of FUDR by continuous arterial infusion is 0.1 to 0.6 mg/kg/day. The higher dose ranges (0.4 to 0.6 mg) are usually employed for hepatic artery infusion because the liver metabolizes the drug, thus reducing the potential for systemic toxicity. Therapy can be given until adverse reactions appear. When these side effects have subsided, therapy may be resumed. The patient should be maintained on therapy as long as response to FUDR continues. The administration of FUDR is best achieved with the use of an appropriate pump to overcome pressure in large arteries and to ensure a uniform rate of infusion.

How Supplied: 500 mg FUDR (floxuridine/Roche) sterile powder, in a 5-ml vial. This is reconstituted with 5 ml sterile water. Reconstituted vials should be stored under refrigeration (36° to 46°F.) for not more than two weeks.

Clinical Studies: In 349 evaluable patients treated with continuous arterial infusion of FUDR, 144 obtained significant objective response associated with clinical benefit for at least one month, and an additional 14 patients had objective and subjective benefits for at least one year.

GANTANOL® ℞

(sulfamethoxazole/Roche)

TABLETS • SUSPENSION •

DS (double strength) TABLETS

The following text is complete prescribing information based on official labeling in effect August 1, 1979.

Description: Gantanol is an intermediate-dosage sulfonamide. Sulfamethoxazole is an almost white, odorless, tasteless compound. Chemically, it is N^1-(5-methyl-3-isoxazolyl)-sulfanilamide.

In a single dose study using two grams of drug, levels of free sulfamethoxazole achieved in the plasma with the tablet and suspension dosage forms were compared in a group of 19 normal subjects. There was no significant difference between the plasma levels obtained with the two dosage forms. The mean concentration of free sulfamethoxazole in plasma after administration of tablets was:

1½ hours	8.38 mg%
3 hours	12.08 mg%
6 hours	9.82 mg%
9 hours	7.9 mg%
12 hours	6.45 mg%

Administration of Gantanol at the adult recommended dosage of 2 Gm initially followed by 1 Gm every 12 hours for 4 days produced average blood concentrations of 5.8 mg% total sulfonamide and 5.1 mg% free sulfonamide 6 hours following the last dose.

Sulfonamides exist in the blood as free, conjugated (acetylated and possibly other forms) and protein-bound forms. The "free" form is considered to be the therapeutically active form. It has been shown that approximately 70 per cent of Gantanol is protein bound in the blood; of the unbound portion 80 to 90 per cent is in the nonacetylated form. Excretion of sulfonamides is chiefly by the kidneys with glomerular filtration as the primary mechanism.

Actions: The systemic sulfonamides are bacteriostatic agents. The spectrum of activity is similar for all. Sulfonamides competitively inhibit bacterial synthesis of folic acid (pteroylglutamic acid) from para-aminobenzoic acid. Resistant strains are capable of utilizing folic acid precursors or preformed folic acid.

Indications: Acute, recurrent or chronic urinary tract infections (primarily pyelonephritis, pyelitis and cystitis) due to susceptible organisms (usually *E. coli, Klebsiella-Aerobacter,* staphylococcus, *Proteus mirabilis,* and, less frequently, *Proteus vulgaris)* in the absence of obstructive uropathy or foreign bodies.

Meningococcal meningitis prophylaxis when sulfonamide-sensitive group A strains are known to prevail in family groups or larger closed populations. (The prophylactic usefulness of sulfonamides when group B or C infections are prevalent is not proven and in closed population groups may be harmful.)

In acute otitis media due to *Haemophilus influenzae* when used concomitantly with adequate doses of penicillin.

Trachoma. Inclusion conjunctivitis. Nocardiosis. Chancroid. Toxoplasmosis as adjunctive therapy with pyrimethamine. Malaria due to chloroquine-resistant strains of *Plasmodium falciparum,* when used as adjunctive therapy.

Important note. *In vitro* sulfonamide sensitivity tests are not always reliable. The test must be carefully coordinated with bacteriologic and clinical response. When the patient is already taking sulfonamides, follow-up cultures should have aminobenzoic acid added to the culture media.

Currently, the increasing frequency of resistant organisms is a limitation of the usefulness of antibacterial agents including the sulfonamides, especially in the treatment of chronic and recurrent urinary tract infections.

Wide variation in blood levels may result with identical doses. Blood levels should be mea-

Continued on next page

Roche—Cont.

sured in patients receiving sulfonamides for serious infections. Free sulfonamide blood levels of 5 to 15 mg per 100 ml may be considered therapeutically effective for most infections, with blood levels of 12 to 15 mg per 100 ml optimal for serious infections; 20 mg per 100 ml should be the maximum total sulfonamide level, as adverse reactions occur more frequently above this level.

Contraindications: Hypersensitivity to sulfonamides. Infants less than 2 months of age (except in the treatment of congenital toxoplasmosis as adjunctive therapy with pyrimethamine). Pregnancy at term and during the nursing period, because sulfonamides pass the placenta and are excreted in the milk and may cause kernicterus.

Warnings: *Usage in Pregnancy:* The safe use of sulfonamides in pregnancy has not been established. The teratogenicity potential of most sulfonamides has not been thoroughly investigated in either animals or humans. However, a significant increase in the incidence of cleft palate and other bony abnormalities of offspring has been observed when certain sulfonamides of the short, intermediate and long-acting types were given to pregnant rats and mice at high oral doses (7 to 25 times the human therapeutic dose).

The sulfonamides should not be used for the treatment of Group A beta-hemolytic streptococcal infections. In an established infection, they will not eradicate the streptococcus, and therefore will not prevent sequelae such as rheumatic fever and glomerulonephritis.

Deaths associated with the administration of sulfonamides have been reported from hypersensitivity reactions, agranulocytosis, aplastic anemia and other blood dyscrasias.

The presence of clinical signs such as sore throat, fever, pallor, purpura or jaundice may be early indications of serious blood disorders. Complete blood counts should be done frequently in patients receiving sulfonamides.

The frequency of renal complications is considerably lower in patients receiving the more soluble sulfonamides. Urinalysis with careful microscopic examination should be obtained frequently in patients receiving sulfonamides.

At the present time there are insufficient clinical data on prolonged or recurrent therapy in chronic renal diseases of children under 6 years.

Precautions: Sulfonamides should be given with caution to patients with impaired renal or hepatic function and to those with severe allergy or bronchial asthma. In glucose-6-phosphate dehydrogenase-deficient individuals, hemolysis may occur. This reaction is frequently dose-related. Adequate fluid intake must be maintained in order to prevent crystalluria and stone formation.

Adverse Reactions: *Blood dyscrasias:* Agranulocytosis, aplastic anemia, thrombocytopenia, leukopenia, hemolytic anemia, purpura, hypoprothrombinemia and methemoglobinemia.

Allergic reactions: Erythema multiforme (Stevens-Johnson syndrome), generalized skin eruptions, epidermal necrolysis, urticaria, serum sickness, pruritus, exfoliative dermatitis, anaphylactoid reactions, periorbital edema, conjunctival and scleral injection, photosensitization, arthralgia and allergic myocarditis.

Gastrointestinal reactions: Nausea, emesis, abdominal pains, hepatitis, diarrhea, anorexia, pancreatitis and stomatitis.

C.N.S. reactions: Headache, peripheral neuritis, mental depression, convulsions, ataxia, hallucinations, tinnitus, vertigo and insomnia.

Miscellaneous reactions: Drug fever, chills, and toxic nephrosis with oliguria and anuria. Periarteritis nodosa and L.E. phenomenon have occurred.

The sulfonamides bear certain chemical similarities to some goitrogens, diuretics (acetazolamide and the thiazides) and oral hypoglycemic agents. Goiter production, diuresis and hypoglycemia have occurred rarely in patients receiving sulfonamides. Cross-sensitivity may exist with these agents.

Rats appear to be especially susceptible to the goitrogenic effects of sulfonamides, and long-term administration has produced thyroid malignancies in the species.

Dosage and Administration: Systemic sulfonamides are contraindicated in infants under 2 months of age, except in the treatment of congenital toxoplasmosis as adjunctive therapy with pyrimethamine.

The usual dosage schedule is as follows:

Children

Infants (2 Months or Older) and Children	Initial Dose (50-60 mg/kg)	Dose Morning and Evening Daily Thereafter (25-30 mg/kg)
20 lbs	1 tablet or 1 teasp. (0.5 Gm)	½ tablet or ½ teasp. (0.25 Gm)
40 lbs	2 tablets or 2 teasp. (1 Gm)	1 tablet or 1 teasp. (0.5 Gm)
60 lbs	3 tablets or 3 teasp. (1.5 Gm)	1½ tablets or 1½ teasp. (0.75 Gm)
80 lbs	2 DS (double strength) tablets or 4 tablets or 4 teasp. (2 Gm)	1 DS (double strength) tablet or 2 tablets or 2 teasp. (1 Gm)

The maximum dose for children should not exceed 75 mg/kg/24 hours.

Adults		
Mild to Moderate Infections	2 DS (double strength) tablets or 4 tablets or 4 teasp. (2 Gm)	1 DS (double strength) tablet or 2 tablets or 2 teasp. (1 Gm)

Note: One teaspoonful equals 5 ml.

Severe Infections: 2 DS (double strength) tablets, or 4 tablets, or 4 teasp. (2 Gm) initially, followed by 1 DS (double strength) tablet, or 2 tablets, or 2 teasp. (1 Gm) three times daily thereafter.

How Supplied: DS (double strength) tablets, light orange, scored, each containing 1 Gm sulfamethoxazole/Roche—bottles of 100; Tel-E-Dose® packages of 100.

Tablets, green, scored, each containing 0.5 Gm sulfamethoxazole/Roche—bottles of 100 and 500; Tel-E-Dose® packages of 100; Prescription Paks of 50.

Suspension, 10%, 0.5 Gm sulfamethoxazole/Roche per teaspoonful (5 ml), cherry-flavored—bottles of 16 oz (1 pint).

[*Shown in Product Identification Section*]

GANTRISIN® ℞
(sulfisoxazole diolamine/Roche)
OPHTHALMIC SOLUTION
OPHTHALMIC OINTMENT

The following text is complete prescribing information based on official labeling in effect August 1, 1979.

Description: GANTRISIN Ophthalmic Ointment and Solution are sulfonamide preparations specifically for topical ophthalmic use. The solution is a sterile, isotonic preparation containing 4% (40 mg/ml) sulfisoxazole/Roche in the form of the diolamine salt and phenylmercuric nitrate 1:100,000 added as a preservative. It has a physiologic pH, and does not cause significant stinging or burning on application. The ointment is a sterile preparation containing 4% sulfisoxazole in the form of the diolamine salt compounded with white petrolatum, mineral oil and phenylmercuric nitrate 1:50,000 added as a preservative. Both dosage forms are stable at room temperature and do not require refrigeration.

Actions: Sulfonamides exert a bacteriostatic effect against a wide range of gram-positive and gram-negative microorganisms by restricting, through competition with para-aminobenzoic acid, the synthesis of folic acid which bacteria require for growth.

Indications: For the treatment of conjunctivitis, corneal ulcer, and other superficial ocular infections due to susceptible microorganisms, and as an adjunct in systemic sulfonamide therapy of trachoma.

Contraindications: Hypersensitivity to sulfonamide preparations.

Precautions: Gantrisin Ophthalmic Solution and Ointment are incompatible with silver preparations. Ophthalmic ointments may retard corneal healing. Nonsusceptible organisms, including fungi, may proliferate with the use of these preparations. Sulfonamides are inactivated by the para-aminobenzoic acid present in purulent exudates. Should undesirable reactions occur, discontinue administration immediately.

Dosage and Administration: Solution: Instill two to three drops in the eye three or more times daily. Care should be taken not to touch dropper tip to any surface, as contamination of solution may result. Ointment: Instill small amount in the lower conjunctival sac one to three times daily and at bedtime.

How Supplied: Solution: ½-oz bottles with dropper. Ointment: ⅛-oz tubes.

GANTRISIN® ℞
(sulfisoxazole/Roche) Tablets
GANTRISIN® ℞
(acetyl sulfisoxazole/Roche)
Pediatric Suspension and Syrup
LIPO GANTRISIN® ℞
(acetyl sulfisoxazole/Roche)
GANTRISIN® ℞
(sulfisoxazole diolamine/Roche)
Injectable

The following text is complete prescribing information based on official labeling in effect August 1, 1979.

Description: Sulfisoxazole is a white to slightly yellowish, odorless, slightly bitter, crystalline powder. It is soluble in alcohol and very slightly soluble in water. Chemically, it is N^1-(3,4-dimethyl-5-isoxazolyl)sulfanilamide.

Acetyl sulfisoxazole, the tasteless form of sulfisoxazole, is N^1-acetyl sulfisoxazole and must be differentiated from the N^4-acetyl sulfisoxazole which is a metabolite of sulfisoxazole. The injectable form is the 2,2′-iminodiethanol salt of N^1-(3,4-dimethyl-5-isoxazolyl)sulfanilamide.

N^1-acetyl sulfisoxazole is believed to be metabolized to sulfisoxazole by digestive enzymes in the gastrointestinal tract and this enzymatic splitting is presumed responsible for the delayed absorption and attainment of blood levels.[1] With continued administration of N^1-acetyl sulfisoxazole, blood levels approximate those of sulfisoxazole.[1]

Sulfonamides exist in the blood as free, conjugated (acetylated and possibly other forms) and protein-bound forms. The "free" form is considered to be the therapeutically active form.

The concentrations of free and total sulfonamide in the blood with oral doses of 1 Gm sulfisoxazole every 4 hours have been reported as 5.85 mg% and 9.17 mg% respectively, at 24 hours.[2] In adults, doses of 3 Gm of the N^1-acetyl sulfisoxazole every 4 hours produced average blood levels of 8.7 mg%.[3]

With Lipo Gantrisin (acetyl sulfisoxazole/Roche in lipid emulsion), administration of 100 mg/kg every 12 hours produced mean blood levels of free sulfonamide ranging between 8.8 and 16.6 mg% over a 24-hour period; continued administration yielded mean levels of between 11.7 and 16.8 mg% free sulfonamide.[4]

With a dosage schedule of 2 Gm intravenously every 8 hours, average blood levels of 11.7 mg/100 ml free and 16.7 mg/100 ml total were obtained.[2] With subcutaneous injection of 200 mg/kg sulfisoxazole, the average blood level at 12 hours was 10.4 mg% and at 24 hours, 7.1 mg%.[5] With single intramuscular dosage of 2 Gm, the plasma levels peaked from 1 to 4 hours, with average levels of 13.8 mg% of free sulfisoxazole[6] and 16.0 mg% total sulfisoxazole[7] obtained at 2 hours.

Approximately 85% of sulfisoxazole is protein bound in the blood;[8] of the unbound portion 65 to 72% is in the nonacetylated form.[1]

In normal subjects cerebrospinal fluid levels of sulfisoxazole have been reported to range from 8 to 57% of blood levels.[3,9] Higher cerebrospinal fluid levels are found in patients with inflamed meninges.[9]

Excretion of sulfonamides is chiefly by the kidneys with glomerular filtration as the primary mechanism.

Actions: The systemic sulfonamides are bacteriostatic agents. The spectrum of activity is similar for all. Sulfonamides competitively inhibit bacterial synthesis of folic acid (pteroylglutamic acid) from para-aminobenzoic acid. Resistant strains are capable of utilizing folic acid precursors or preformed folic acid.

Indications: Injectable sulfonamides should be used only when oral administration is impractical. Gantrisin is indicated for acute, recurrent or chronic urinary tract infections (primarily cystitis, pyelitis and pyelonephritis) due to susceptible organisms (usually *E. coli, Klebsiella-Aerobacter,* staphylococcus, *Proteus mirabilis,* and, less frequently, *Proteus vulgaris)* in the absence of obstructive uropathy or foreign bodies.

Meningococcal meningitis where the organism has been demonstrated to be susceptible. *Haemophilus influenzae* meningitis as adjunctive therapy with parenteral streptomycin.

Meningococcal meningitis prophylaxis when sulfonamide-sensitive group A strains are known to prevail in family groups or larger closed populations. (The prophylactic usefulness of sulfonamides when group B or C infections are prevalent is not proven and in closed population groups may be harmful.)

In acute otitis media due to *Haemophilus influenzae* when used concomitantly with adequate doses of penicillin.

Trachoma. Inclusion conjunctivitis. Nocardiosis. Chancroid. Toxoplasmosis as adjunctive therapy with pyrimethamine. Malaria due to chloroquine-resistant strains of *Plasmodium falciparum,* when used as adjunctive therapy.

Important note. In vitro sulfonamide sensitivity tests are not always reliable. The test must be carefully coordinated with bacteriologic and clinical response. When the patient is already taking sulfonamides, follow-up cultures should have aminobenzoic acid added to the culture media.

Currently, the increasing frequency of resistant organisms is a limitation of the usefulness of antibacterial agents including the sulfonamides, especially in the treatment of chronic and recurrent urinary tract infections.

Wide variation in blood levels may result with identical doses. Blood levels should be measured in patients receiving sulfonamides for serious infections. Free sulfonamide blood levels of 5 to 15 mg per 100 ml may be considered therapeutically effective for most infections, with blood levels of 12 to 15 mg per 100 ml optimal for serious infections; 20 mg per 100 ml should be the maximum total sulfonamide level, as adverse reactions occur more frequently above this level.

Contraindications: Hypersensitivity to sulfonamides. Infants less than 2 months of age (except in the treatment of congenital toxoplasmosis as adjunctive therapy with pyrimethamine). Pregnancy at term and during the nursing period, because sulfonamides pass the placenta and are excreted in the milk and may cause kernicterus.

Warnings: *Usage in Pregnancy:* The safe use of sulfonamides in pregnancy has not been established. The teratogenicity potential of most sulfonamides has not been thoroughly investigated in either animals or humans. However, a significant increase in the incidence of cleft palate and other bony abnormalities of offspring has been observed when certain sulfonamides of the short, intermediate and long-acting types were given to pregnant rats and mice at high oral doses (7 to 25 times the human therapeutic dose).

The sulfonamides should not be used for the treatment of Group A beta-hemolytic streptococcal infections. In an established infection, they will not eradicate the streptococcus, and therefore will not prevent sequelae such as rheumatic fever and glomerulonephritis.

Deaths associated with the administration of sulfonamides have been reported from hypersensitivity reactions, agranulocytosis, aplastic anemia and other blood dyscrasias.

The presence of clinical signs such as sore throat, fever, pallor, purpura or jaundice may be early indications of serious blood disorders. Complete blood counts should be done frequently in patients receiving sulfonamides.

The frequency of renal complications is considerably lower in patients receiving the more soluble sulfonamides. Urinalysis with careful microscopic examination should be obtained frequently in patients receiving sulfonamides. Occasional severe systemic reactions may follow rapid intravenous administration.

Precautions: Sulfonamides should be given with caution to patients with impaired renal or hepatic function and to those with severe allergy or bronchial asthma. In glucose-6-phosphate dehydrogenase-deficient individuals, hemolysis may occur. This reaction is frequently dose-related. Adequate fluid intake must be maintained in order to prevent crystalluria and stone formation.

Adverse Reactions: *Blood dyscrasias:* Agranulocytosis, aplastic anemia, thrombocytopenia, leukopenia, hemolytic anemia, purpura, hypoprothrombinemia and methemoglobinemia.

Allergic reactions: Erythema multiforme (Stevens-Johnson syndrome), generalized skin eruptions, epidermal necrolysis, urticaria, serum sickness, pruritus, exfoliative dermatitis, anaphylactoid reactions, periorbital edema, conjunctival and scleral injection, photosensitization, arthralgia and allergic myocarditis.

Gastrointestinal reactions: Nausea, emesis, abdominal pains, hepatitis, diarrhea, anorexia, pancreatitis and stomatitis.

C.N.S. reactions: Headache, peripheral neuritis, mental depression, convulsions, ataxia, hallucinations, tinnitus, vertigo and insomnia.

Miscellaneous reactions: Drug fever, chills and toxic nephrosis with oliguria and anuria. Periarteritis nodosa and L.E. phenomenon have occurred. Local reaction may occur with intramuscular injection.

The sulfonamides bear certain chemical similarities to some goitrogens, diuretics (acetazolamide and the thiazides) and oral hypoglycemic agents. Goiter production, diuresis and hypoglycemia have occurred rarely in patients receiving sulfonamides. Cross-sensitivity may exist with these agents.

Rats appear to be especially susceptible to the goitrogenic effects of sulfonamides, and long-term administration has produced thyroid malignancies in the species.

Dosage and Administration: Systemic sulfonamides are contraindicated in infants under 2 months of age, except in the treatment of congenital toxoplasmosis as adjunctive therapy with pyrimethamine. Injectable sulfonamides should be used only when oral administration is impractical.

TABLETS, PEDIATRIC SUSPENSION AND SYRUP (0.5 Gm sulfisoxazole per tablet or the equivalent in each 5-ml teaspoonful of the suspension or syrup)—

Usual dose for infants over 2 months of age and children:

Initial dose: One-half of the 24-hour dose.

Maintenance dose: 150 mg/kg/24 hours or 4 Gm/M²/24 hours—dose to be divided into 4 to 6 doses/24 hours with maximum of 6 Gm/24 hours.

Usual adult dose:

Initial dose: 2 to 4 Gm.

Maintenance dose: 4 to 8 Gm/24 hours, divided into 4 to 6 doses/24 hours.

LIPO GANTRISIN (containing the equivalent of 1 Gm sulfisoxazole in each 5-ml teaspoonful)—

Usual dose for infants over 2 months of age and children:

Initial dose: 60 to 75 mg/kg.

Maintenance dose: 60 to 75 mg/kg twice daily. The maximum dose should not exceed 6 Gm/24 hours.

Usual adult dose:

4 to 5 Gm every twelve hours.

INJECTABLE: For subcutaneous and intravenous administration the 40% solution must be diluted to a concentration of 5% (combine a 5-ml ampul with 35 ml of sterile distilled water). Administration of the drug in combination with parenteral fluids is not recommended. The use of diluents other than sterile distilled water may cause precipitation.

Injectable Gantrisin may be given intramuscularly without dilution.

Usual dose for infants over 2 months of age, children and adults:

Initial dose: One-half of the 24-hour dose.

Maintenance dose: 100 mg/kg/24 hours or 2.25 Gm/M²/24 hours, administered in a 5% solution—

a. Subcutaneous administration, divided into 3 doses/24 hours.

b. Intravenous administration, divided into 4 doses/24 hours. (Administer by slow injection or intravenous drip.)

For example—give 1 ml/kg of 5% solution as an initial dose. This should be followed by 0.50 ml/kg of 5% solution four times daily for intravenous administration or 0.66 ml/kg t.i.d. for subcutaneous administration.

c. Intramuscular administration, divided into 2 or 3 doses/24 hours. Up to 10 ml can be given, but not more than 5 ml in any one site. For children, the volume given intramuscularly in any one site should be correspondingly less than in adults.

How Supplied: *Tablets,* containing 0.5 Gm sulfisoxazole, white, scored—bottles of 100, 500 and 1000; drums of 5000; Tel-E-Dose® packages of 100; Prescription Paks of 100.

Pediatric Suspension, containing, in each teaspoonful (5 ml), the equivalent of approximately 0.5 Gm sulfisoxazole in the form of acetyl sulfisoxazole; raspberry flavored—bottles of 4 oz and 16 oz (1 pint).

Syrup, containing, in each teaspoonful (5 ml), the equivalent of approximately 0.5 Gm sulfisoxazole in the form of acetyl sulfisoxazole; chocolate flavored—bottles of 16 oz (1 pint).

Lipo Gantrisin (acetyl sulfisoxazole/Roche)—the long-acting form—containing, in each teaspoonful (5 ml), the equivalent of 1 Gm sulfisoxazole in the form of acetyl sulfisoxazole in a homogenized mixture containing a readily digestible vegetable oil; vanilla-mint flavored—bottles of 16 oz (1 pint).

Injectable, 5-ml ampuls, containing 2 Gm sulfisoxazole/Roche in the form of the diolamine salt. Each ml of solution contains 400 mg sulfisoxazole/Roche in the form of the diolamine salt compounded with 2 mg sodium metabisulfite. Packages of 10.

References:

1. Randall, L.O., *et al: Antibiot Chemother* *4:*877-885, Aug. 1954.

Continued on next page

Roche—Cont.

2. Svec, F.A., Rhodes, P.S., Rohr, J.H.: *Arch Intern Med 85:*83-90, Jan. 1950.
3. Flake, R.E., *et al: J Lab Clin Med 44:*582-588, Oct. 1954.
4. Krugman, S.: *Ann NY Acad Sci 69:*399-403, Aug. 1957.
5. Price, P.C., Hansen, A.E.: *Texas Rep Biol Med 9:*764-769, Winter 1951.
6. Kaplan, S.A., *et al: J Pharm Sci 61:*773-778, May 1972.
7. Data on file, Hoffmann-La Roche Inc., Nutley, N.J.
8. Struller, T.: *Antibiot Chemother 14:*179-215, 1968.
9. Sarnoff, S.J.: *Proc Soc Exp Biol Med 68:*23-26, May 1948.

[*Shown in Product Identification Section*]

KONAKION® ℞
(phytonadione/Roche)
INJECTABLE
FOR INTRAMUSCULAR USE ONLY

The following text is complete prescribing information based on official labeling in effect August 1, 1979.

Description: Konakion is an essentially clear, aqueous dispersion of vitamin K_1, available for injection by the intramuscular route only. Slight opalescence may occur in the 10 mg ampuls. However, this does not affect the potency, safety or usefulness of the preparation.

The ingredients are as follows: *0.5-ml ampuls:* Each 0.5 ml contains 1 mg phytonadione (vitamin K_1) compounded with 10 mg polysorbate 80, 0.45% phenol as preservative, 10.4 mg propylene glycol, 0.17 mg sodium acetate and 0.00002 ml glacial acetic acid.

1-ml ampuls: Each ml contains 10 mg phytonadione (vitamin K_1) compounded with 40 mg polysorbate 80, 20.7 mg propylene glycol, 0.8 mg sodium acetate and 0.00006 ml glacial acetic acid.

Actions: Konakion possesses the same type and degree of activity as does naturally occurring vitamin K, which is necessary for the synthesis in the liver of prothrombin (factor II), proconvertin (factor VII), plasma thromboplastin component (factor IX), and Stuart factor (factor X).

The prothrombin test is sensitive to the levels of factors II, VII and X. The mechanism by which vitamin K promotes formation of these clotting factors in the liver is not known.

The action of the aqueous dispersion when administered parenterally is generally detectable within an hour or two, and hemorrhage is usually controlled within 3 to 6 hours. A normal prothrombin level may often be obtained in 12 to 14 hours.

In the prophylaxis and treatment of hemorrhagic disease of the newborn, Konakion has demonstrated a greater margin of safety than that of the water-soluble vitamin K analogs.

Indications:
- anticoagulant-induced prothrombin deficiency;
- prophylaxis and therapy of hemorrhagic disease of the newborn;
- hypoprothrombinemia due to oral antibacterial therapy;
- hypoprothrombinemia secondary to factors limiting absorption or synthesis of vitamin K, *e.g.,* obstructive jaundice, biliary fistula, sprue, ulcerative colitis, celiac disease, intestinal resection, cystic fibrosis of the pancreas and regional enteritis;
- other drug-induced hypoprothrombinemia (such as that due to salicylates) where it is definitely shown that the result is due to interference with vitamin K metabolism.

Contraindications: Parenteral use in persons who are hypersensitive to the drug.

Warnings: Konakion promotes the synthesis of prothrombin by the liver and does not directly counteract the effects of the oral anticoagulants; it takes up to two hours for vitamin K to promote prothrombin synthesis. Fresh plasma or blood transfusions may be required for severe blood loss or lack of response to vitamin K. Phytonadione will not counteract the anticoagulant action of heparin.

When vitamin K_1 is used to correct excessive anticoagulant-induced hypoprothrombinemia, anticoagulant therapy still being indicated, the patient is again faced with the clotting hazards existing prior to starting the anticoagulant therapy. Phytonadione is not a clotting agent, but over-zealous therapy with vitamin K may restore conditions which originally permitted thromboembolic phenomena. Dosage, therefore, should be kept as low as possible, and prothrombin time should be checked regularly as clinical conditions indicate.

Repeated large doses of vitamin K are not warranted in liver disease if the response to initial use of the vitamin is unsatisfactory (Koller test). Failure to respond to vitamin K may indicate the presence of a coagulation defect or that the condition being treated is unresponsive to vitamin K.

Effects on reproduction have not been studied in animals. There is no adequate information on whether this drug may affect fertility in human males or females or have a teratogenic potential or other adverse effects on the fetus.

Precautions: Store in a dark place and protect from light at all times.

Temporary resistance to prothrombin-depressing anticoagulants may result, especially when larger doses of phytonadione are used. If relatively large doses have been employed, it may be necessary when reinstituting anticoagulant therapy to use somewhat larger doses of the prothrombin-depressing anticoagulant or to use one which acts on a different principle, such as heparin.

Adverse Reactions: Pain, swelling and tenderness at the injection site have occurred rarely. The possibility of allergic sensitivity, including an anaphylactoid reaction, should be kept in mind.

Although Konakion has a greater margin of safety than the water-soluble vitamin K analogs, hyperbilirubinemia has been reported in the newborn, particularly in prematures when used at 5 to 10 times the recommended dosage. This effect, with its possibility of attendant kernicterus, should be borne in mind if such dosages are deemed necessary.

Dosage and Administration: The human minimum daily requirements for vitamin K have not been established officially. Minimal daily requirements have been estimated at 1 to 5 micrograms per kilogram of body weight for infants and 0.03 micrograms per kilogram for adults. The dietary abundance of vitamin K satisfies the requirements normally except for the neonatal period of 5 to 8 days.

INFANTS

Neonatal hemorrhage due to hypoprothrombinemia:
- *Prophylactic*—1 to 2 mg intramuscularly, immediately after birth.
- *Control*—1 to 2 mg intramuscularly, daily.

ADULTS

Hypoprothrombinemia due to:
- *Anticoagulant therapy* (except of heparin type)—5 to 10 mg I.M. initially; up to 20 mg, if necessary.
- *Antibacterial therapy*—5 to 20 mg I.M.
- *Factors limiting absorption or synthesis*—2 to 20 mg I.M.
- *Other drugs* (*e.g.,* salicylates)—2 to 20 mg I.M.

In older children and adults, injection of Konakion should be in the upper outer quadrant of the buttocks. In infants and young children, the anterolateral aspect of the thighs or the deltoid region is preferred so that danger of sciatic nerve injury is avoided.

Storage: Konakion is stable in the air, but is photosensitive, decomposing with loss of potency on exposure to light. Therefore, it should be stored in a dark place and protected from light at all times. Konakion need not be refrigerated. Store at 59° to 86°F.

How Supplied: Ampuls, 0.5 ml (boxes of 10). Ampuls, 1 ml (boxes of 10).

LAROBEC® TABLETS ℞

The following text is complete prescribing information based on official labeling in effect August 1, 1979.

Each Larobec tablet contains:

Thiamine mononitrate (vitamin B_1 mononitrate)	15 mg
Riboflavin (vitamin B_2)	15 mg
Niacinamide	100 mg
Calcium pantothenate	20 mg
Cyanocobalamin (vitamin B_{12})	5 mcg
Folic acid	0.5 mg
Ascorbic acid (vitamin C)	500 mg

Description: For prophylactic or therapeutic nutritional supplementation concomitant with levodopa therapy in patients with Parkinson's disease and syndrome, Larobec provides high potency dosages of the major B-complex vitamins, without pyridoxine (vitamin B_6) which has been reported[1,2] to reduce the clinical benefits of levodopa therapy. B-complex vitamins are essential in the anabolism of carbohydrate and protein and in hematopoiesis. Larobec also contains therapeutic quantities of ascorbic acid, a substance involved in intracellular reactions such as tissue repair and collagen formation.

Indications: Larobec is indicated for supportive nutritional supplementation when a water-soluble vitamin formula (without pyridoxine) is required prophylactically or therapeutically in patients under treatment with levodopa.

Warning: Administration of vitamin B_6 may be required if signs of pyridoxine deficiency develop. Larobec is not intended for treatment of pernicious anemia or other primary or secondary anemias. Neurologic involvement may develop or progress, despite temporary remission of anemia, in patients with pernicious anemia who receive more than 0.1 mg of folic acid per day and who are inadequately treated with vitamin B_{12}.

Dosage and Administration: One or two tablets daily, as indicated by clinical need.

How Supplied: Orange colored, capsule-shaped tablets—bottles of 100.

References:

1. Duvoisin, R. C., *et al.: Trans. Amer. Neurol. Ass., 94:*81, 1969.
2. Cotzias, G. C.: *J.A.M.A., 210:* 1255, 1969.

[*Shown in Product Identification Section*]

LARODOPA® ℞
(levodopa/Roche)

The following text is complete prescribing information based on official labeling in effect August 1, 1979.

In order to reduce the high incidence of adverse reactions, it is necessary to individualize the therapy and to gradually increase the dosage to the desired therapeutic level.

Description: Chemically, levodopa is (−)-3-(3,4-dihydroxyphenyl)-*L*-alanine. It is a colorless, crystalline compound, slightly soluble in water and insoluble in alcohol, with a molecular weight of 197.2.

Actions: Evidence indicates that the symptoms of Parkinson's disease are related to depletion of striatal dopamine. Since dopamine apparently does not cross the blood-brain barrier, its administration is ineffective in the treatment of Parkinson's disease. However, levodopa, the levo-rotatory isomer of dihydroxyphenylalanine (dopa) which is the metabolic precursor of dopamine, does cross the blood-brain barrier. Presumably it is converted into dopamine in the basal ganglia. This is generally thought to be the mechanism whereby oral levodopa acts in relieving the symptoms of Parkinson's disease.

The major urinary metabolites of levodopa in man appear to be dopamine and homovanillic acid (HVA). In 24-hour urine samples, HVA accounts for 13 to 42 percent of the ingested dose of levodopa.

Indications: Larodopa is indicated in the treatment of idiopathic Parkinson's disease (Paralysis Agitans), postencephalitic parkinsonism, symptomatic parkinsonism which may follow injury to the nervous system by carbon monoxide intoxication, and manganese intoxication. It is indicated in those elderly patients believed to develop parkinsonism in association with cerebral arteriosclerosis.

Contraindications: Monoamine oxidase (MAO) inhibitors and Larodopa should not be given concomitantly and these inhibitors must be discontinued two weeks prior to initiating therapy with Larodopa. Larodopa is contraindicated in patients with known hypersensitivity to the drug and in narrow angle glaucoma. Because levodopa may activate a malignant melanoma, it should not be used in patients with suspicious, undiagnosed skin lesions or a history of melanoma.

Warnings: Larodopa should be administered cautiously to patients with severe cardiovascular or pulmonary disease, bronchial asthma, renal, hepatic or endocrine disease.

Care should be exercised in administering Larodopa to patients with a history of myocardial infarction who have residual atrial, nodal or ventricular arrhythmias. If Larodopa is necessary in this type of patient, it should be used in a facility with a coronary care unit or an intensive care unit.

One must be on the alert for the possibility of upper gastrointestinal hemorrhage in those patients with a past history of active peptic ulcer disease.

All patients should be carefully observed for the development of depression with concomitant suicidal tendencies. Psychotic patients should be treated with caution.

Pyridoxine hydrochloride (vitamin B_6) in oral doses of 10 to 25 mg rapidly reverses the toxic and therapeutic effects of Larodopa. This should be considered before recommending vitamin preparations containing pyridoxine hydrochloride (vitamin B_6).

Usage in Pregnancy: The safety of Larodopa in women who are or who may become pregnant has not been established; hence it should be given only when the potential benefits have been weighed against possible hazards to mother and child. Studies in rodents have shown that levodopa at dosages in excess of 200 mg/kg/day has an adverse effect on fetal and postnatal growth and viability.

Larodopa should not be used in nursing mothers.

Usage in Children: The safety of Larodopa under the age of 12 has not been established.

Precautions: Periodic evaluations of hepatic, hematopoietic, cardiovascular and renal function are recommended during extended therapy in all patients.

Patients with chronic wide angle glaucoma may be treated cautiously with Larodopa, provided the intraocular pressure is well controlled and the patient monitored carefully for changes in intraocular pressure during therapy.

Postural hypotensive episodes have been reported as adverse reactions. Therefore, Larodopa should be administered to patients on antihypertensive drug cautiously (for patients receiving pargyline, see note on MAO inhibitors contraindications), and it may be necessary to adjust the dosage of the antihypertensive drugs.

Adverse Reactions: The most serious adverse reactions associated with the administration of Larodopa having frequent occurrences are: adventitious movements such as choreiform and/or dystonic movements. Other serious adverse reactions with a lower incidence are: cardiac irregularities and/or palpitations, orthostatic hypotensive episodes, bradykinetic episodes (the "on-off" phenomena), mental changes including paranoid ideation and psychotic episodes, depression with or without the development of suicidal tendencies, dementia, and urinary retention.

Rarely, gastrointestinal bleeding, development of duodenal ulcer, hypertension, phlebitis, hemolytic anemia, agranulocytosis, and convulsions have been observed. (The causal relationship between convulsions and Larodopa has not been established.)

Adverse reactions of a less serious nature having a relatively frequent occurrence are the following: anorexia, nausea and vomiting with or without abdominal pain and distress, dry mouth, dysphagia, sialorrhea, ataxia, increased hand tremor, headache, dizziness, numbness, weakness and faintness, bruxism, confusion, insomnia, nightmares, hallucinations and delusions, agitation and anxiety, malaise, fatigue and euphoria. Occurring with a lesser order of frequency are the following: muscle twitching and blepharospasm (which may be taken as an early sign of overdosage; consideration of dosage reduction may be made at this time), trismus, burning sensation of the tongue, bitter taste, diarrhea, constipation, flatulence, flushing, skin rash, increased sweating, bizarre breathing patterns, urinary incontinence, diplopia, blurred vision, dilated pupils, hot flashes, weight gain or loss, dark sweat and/or urine.

Rarely, oculogyric crises, sense of stimulation, hiccups, development of edema, loss of hair, hoarseness, priapism and activation of latent Horner's syndrome have been observed.

Elevations of blood urea nitrogen, SGOT, SGPT, LDH, bilirubin, alkaline phosphatase or protein-bound iodine have been reported; and the significance of this is not known. Occasional reductions in WBC, hemoglobin, and hematocrit have been noted.

Leukopenia has occurred and requires cessation, at least temporarily, of Larodopa administration. The Coombs test has occasionally become positive during extended therapy. Elevations of uric acid have been noted when colorimetric method was used but not when uricase method was used.

Overdosage: For acute overdosage general supportive measures should be employed, along with immediate gastric lavage. Intravenous fluids should be administered judiciously and an adequate airway maintained.

Electrocardiographic monitoring should be instituted and the patient carefully observed for the possible development of arrhythmias; if required, appropriate antiarrhythmic therapy should be given. Consideration should be given to the possibility of multiple drug ingestion by the patient. To date, no experience has been reported with dialysis; hence its value in Larodopa overdosage is not known. Although pyridoxine hydrochloride (vitamin B_6) has been reported to reverse the antiparkinson effects of Larodopa, its usefulness in the management of acute overdosage has not been established.

Dosage and Administration: The optimal daily dose of Larodopa, *i.e.,* the dose producing maximal improvement with tolerated side effects, must be determined and *carefully titrated for each individual patient.* The usual initial dosage is 0.5 to 1 Gm daily, divided in two or more doses with food.

The total daily dosage is then increased gradually in increments not more than 0.75 Gm every three to seven days as tolerated. The usual optimal therapeutic *dosage should not exceed 8 Gm.* The exceptional patient may carefully be given more than 8 Gms as required. In some patients, a significant therapeutic response may not be obtained until six months of treatment.

In the event general anesthesia is required, Larodopa therapy may be continued as long as the patient is able to take fluids and medication by mouth. If therapy is temporarily interrupted, the usual daily dosage may be administered as soon as the patient is able to take oral medication. Whenever therapy has been interrupted for longer periods, dosage should again be adjusted gradually; however, in many cases the patient can be rapidly titrated to his previous therapeutic dosage.

How Supplied: Tablets, pink, scored, each containing levodopa/Roche 0.1 Gm, bottles of 100; 0.25 Gm or 0.5 Gm—bottles of 100 and 500. Capsules, each containing levodopa/Roche 0.1 Gm (pink and scarlet)—bottles of 100; 0.25 Gm (pink and beige) or 0.5 Gm (pink)—bottles of 100 and 500.

[*Shown in Product Identification Section*]

LAROTID® ℞

(amoxicillin/Roche)
CAPSULES and
FOR ORAL SUSPENSION

The following text is complete prescribing information based on official labeling in effect August 1, 1979.

Description: Larotid (amoxicillin/Roche) is a semi-synthetic antibiotic, an analog of ampicillin, with a broad spectrum of bactericidal activity against many gram-positive and gram-negative microorganisms. Chemically, amoxicillin is D-(–)-α-amino-p-hydroxybenzyl penicillin trihydrate.

Actions:

Pharmacology: Amoxicillin is stable in the presence of gastric acid and may be given without regard to meals. It is rapidly absorbed after oral administration. It diffuses readily into most body tissues and fluids, with the exception of brain and spinal fluid, except when meninges are inflamed. The half-life of amoxicillin is 61.3 minutes. Most of the amoxicillin is excreted unchanged in the urine; its excretion can be delayed by concurrent administration of probenecid. Amoxicillin is not highly protein-bound. In blood serum, amoxicillin is approximately 20 percent protein-bound, as compared with 60 percent for penicillin-G.

Orally administered doses of 250 mg and 500 mg amoxicillin capsules result in average peak blood levels one to two hours after administration in the range of 3.5 mcg/ml to 5 mcg/ml and 5.5 mcg/ml to 7.5 mcg/ml, respectively.

Orally administered doses of amoxicillin suspension 125 mg/5 ml and 250 mg/5 ml result in average peak blood levels one to two hours after administration in the range of 1.5 mcg/ml to 3 mcg/ml and 3.5 mcg/ml to 5 mcg/ml, respectively.

Detectable serum levels are observed up to eight hours after an orally administered dose of amoxicillin. Approximately 60 percent of an orally administered dose of amoxicillin is excreted in the urine within six to eight hours. Following a 1-Gm dose and utilizing a special skin window technique to determine levels of the antibiotic, it was noted that therapeutic levels were found in the interstitial fluid.

Microbiology: Larotid is similar to ampicillin in its bactericidal action against susceptible organisms during the stage of active multiplication. It acts through the inhibition of biosynthesis of cell wall mucopeptide. *In vitro* studies have demonstrated the susceptibility of most strains of the following gram-positive bacteria:

Continued on next page

Roche—Cont.

alpha- and beta-hemolytic streptococci, *Diplococcus pneumoniae,* nonpenicillinase-producing staphylococci, and *Streptococcus faecalis.* It is active *in vitro* against many strains of *Hemophilus influenzae, Neisseria gonorrhoeae, Escherichia coli* and *Proteus mirabilis.* Because it does not resist destruction by penicillinase, it is not effective against penicillinase-producing bacteria, particularly resistant staphylococci. All strains of Pseudomonas and most strains of Klebsiella and Enterobacter are resistant.

Disc Susceptibility Tests: Quantitative methods that require measurement of zone diameters give the most precise estimates of antibiotic susceptibility. One such procedure[1] has been recommended for use with discs for testing susceptibility to ampicillin class antibiotics. Interpretations correlate diameters of the disc test with MIC values for amoxicillin. With this procedure, a report from the laboratory of "susceptible" indicates that the infecting organism is likely to respond to therapy. A report of "resistant" indicates that the infecting organism is not likely to respond to therapy. A report of "intermediate susceptibility" suggests that the organism would be susceptible if high dosage is used, or if the infection is confined to tissues and fluids (*e.g.,* urine), in which high antibiotic levels are attained.

Indications: Larotid is indicated in the treatment of infections due to susceptible strains of the following:

Gram-negative organisms: *H. influenzae, E. coli, P. mirabilis* and *N. gonorrhoeae.*

Gram-positive organisms: Streptococci (including *Streptococcus faecalis*), *D. pneumoniae* and nonpenicillinase-producing staphylococci.

Therapy may be instituted prior to obtaining results from bacteriological and susceptibility studies to determine the causative organisms and their susceptibility to amoxicillin.

Indicated surgical procedures should be performed.

Contraindications: The use of this drug is contraindicated in individuals with a history of an allergic reaction to the penicillins.

WARNINGS: SERIOUS AND OCCASIONALLY FATAL HYPERSENSITIVITY (ANAPHYLACTOID) REACTIONS HAVE BEEN REPORTED IN PATIENTS ON PENICILLIN THERAPY. ALTHOUGH ANAPHYLAXIS IS MORE FREQUENT FOLLOWING PARENTERAL THERAPY, IT HAS OCCURRED IN PATIENTS ON ORAL PENICILLINS. THESE REACTIONS ARE MORE LIKELY TO OCCUR IN INDIVIDUALS WITH A HISTORY OF SENSITIVITY TO MULTIPLE ALLERGENS. THERE HAVE BEEN REPORTS OF INDIVIDUALS WITH A HISTORY OF PENICILLIN HYPERSENSITIVITY WHO HAVE EXPERIENCED SEVERE REACTIONS WHEN TREATED WITH CEPHALOSPORINS. BEFORE THERAPY WITH ANY PENICILLIN, CAREFUL INQUIRY SHOULD BE MADE CONCERNING PREVIOUS HYPERSENSITIVITY REACTIONS TO PENICILLINS, CEPHALOSPORINS OR OTHER ALLERGENS. IF AN ALLERGIC REACTION OCCURS, APPROPRIATE THERAPY SHOULD BE INSTITUTED AND DISCONTINUANCE OF AMOXICILLIN THERAPY CONSIDERED. **SERIOUS ANAPHYLACTOID REACTIONS REQUIRE IMMEDIATE EMERGENCY TREATMENT WITH EPINEPHRINE. OXYGEN, INTRAVENOUS STEROIDS AND AIRWAY MANAGEMENT, INCLUDING INTUBATION, SHOULD ALSO BE ADMINISTERED AS INDICATED.**

Usage in Pregnancy: Safety for use in pregnancy has not been established.

Precautions: As with any potent drug, periodic assessment of renal, hepatic and hematopoietic function should be made during prolonged therapy.

The possibility of superinfections with mycotic or bacterial pathogens should be kept in mind during therapy. If superinfections occur (usually involving Enterobacter, Pseudomonas or Candida), the drug should be discontinued and/or appropriate therapy instituted.

Adverse Reactions: As with other penicillins, it may be expected that untoward reactions will be essentially limited to sensitivity phenomena. They are more likely to occur in individuals who have previously demonstrated hypersensitivity to penicillins and in those with a history of allergy, asthma, hay fever or urticaria. The following adverse reactions have been reported as associated with the use of the penicillins:

Gastrointestinal: Nausea, vomiting and diarrhea.

Hypersensitivity Reactions: Erythematous maculopapular rashes and urticaria have been reported.

NOTE: Urticaria, other skin rashes and serum sickness-like reactions may be controlled with antihistamines and, if necessary, systemic corticosteroids. Whenever such reactions occur, amoxicillin should be discontinued, unless, in the opinion of the physician, the condition being treated is life-threatening and amenable only to amoxicillin therapy.

Liver: A moderate rise in serum glutamic oxaloacetic transaminase (SGOT) has been noted, but the significance of this finding is unknown.

Hemic and Lymphatic Systems: Anemia, thrombocytopenia, thrombocytopenic purpura, eosinophilia, leukopenia and agranulocytosis have been reported during therapy with the penicillins. These reactions are usually reversible on discontinuation of therapy and are believed to be hypersensitivity phenomena.

Dosage and Administration: The dosages listed below are those usually recommended. The children's dosage is intended for individuals whose weight will not cause a dosage to be calculated greater than that recommended for adults.

Infections of the ear, nose and throat due to streptococci, pneumococci, nonpenicillinase-producing staphylococci and *H. influenzae;* infections of the genitourinary tract due to *E. coli, Proteus mirabilis* and *Streptococcus faecalis;* infections of the skin and soft tissues due to streptococci, susceptible staphylococci and *E. coli:*

USUAL DOSAGE:

Adults: 250 mg every 8 hours.

Children: 20 mg/kg/day in divided doses every 8 hours.

Children weighing 20 kg or more should be dosed according to the adult recommendations.

In severe infections or those caused by less susceptible organisms:

500 mg every 8 hours for adults and 40 mg/kg/day in divided doses every 8 hours for children may be needed.

Infections of the lower respiratory tract due to streptococci, pneumococci, nonpenicillinase-producing staphylococci and *H. influenzae:*

USUAL DOSAGE:

Adults: 500 mg every 8 hours.

Children: 40 mg/kg/day in divided doses every 8 hours.

Children weighing 20 kg or more should be dosed according to the adult recommendations.

Gonorrhea, acute uncomplicated anogenital and urethral infections due to *N. gonorrhoeae* (males and females):

USUAL DOSAGE:

Adults: 3 grams as a single oral dose.

Prepubertal children: 50 mg/kg amoxicillin combined with 25 mg/kg probenecid as a single dose.

Note: Since probenecid is contraindicated in children under 2 years, this regimen should not be used in these cases.

Cases of gonorrhea with a suspected lesion of syphilis should have dark-field examinations before receiving amoxicillin and monthly serological tests for a minimum of four months.

It should be recognized that in the treatment of chronic urinary tract infections, frequent bacteriological and clinical appraisals are necessary. Smaller doses than those recommended above should not be used. Even higher doses may be needed at times. In stubborn infections, therapy may be required for several weeks. It may be necessary to continue clinical and/or bacteriological follow-up for several months after cessation of therapy. Except for gonorrhea, treatment should be continued for a minimum of 48 to 72 hours beyond the time that the patient becomes asymptomatic or evidence of bacterial eradication has been obtained. It is recommended that there be at least 10 days' treatment for any infection caused by hemolytic streptococci to prevent the occurrence of acute rheumatic fever or glomerulonephritis.

Dosage and Administration of Pediatric Drops: Usual dosage for all indications except infections of the lower respiratory tract:

Under 6 kg (13 lbs): 0.5 ml every 8 hours.

6–8 kg (13–18 lbs): 1 ml every 8 hours.

Infections of the lower respiratory tract:

Under 6 kg (13 lbs): 1 ml every 8 hours.

6–8 kg (13–18 lbs): 2 ml every 8 hours.

Children weighing more than 8 kg (18 lbs) should receive the appropriate dose of the oral suspension 125 mg or 250 mg/5 ml.

After reconstitution, the required amount of suspension should be placed directly on the child's tongue for swallowing. Alternate means of administration are to add the required amount of suspension to formula, milk, fruit juice, water, ginger ale or cold drinks. These preparations should then be taken immediately. To be certain the child is receiving full dosage, such preparations should be consumed in entirety.

Directions for Mixing Oral Suspension: Prepare suspension at time of dispensing as follows: Add the required amount of water (see table below) to the bottle. For ease of preparation, add water in two portions. Shake well after each addition of water. Each teaspoonful (5 ml) will contain 125 mg or 250 mg amoxicillin.

Bottle Size	Amount of Water Required for Reconstitution
80 ml	53 ml
100 ml	66 ml
150 ml	100 ml

Directions for Mixing Pediatric Drops: Add 11 ml of water to the bottle and shake vigorously. Each ml of suspension will contain 50 mg amoxicillin.

NOTE: SHAKE WELL BEFORE USING.

Keep bottle tightly closed. Any unused portion of the reconstituted suspension must be discarded after 14 days. Refrigeration is preferable, but not required.

How Supplied: *Capsules,* containing 250 mg amoxicillin as the trihydrate, beige and brown—bottles of 100 and 500; containing 500 mg amoxicillin as the trihydrate, beige—bottles of 50 and 500; both strengths also supplied in Tel-E-Dose® packages of 100; and in Prescription Paks of 18, available singly and in trays of 10.

Oral suspension: Each 5 ml of reconstituted suspension contains 125 mg or 250 mg amoxicillin as the trihydrate—bottles of 80 ml, 100 ml and 150 ml. Tel-E-Dose® packages of 10; when reconstituted with 5 ml of water, each dose will contain 125 mg or 250 mg amoxicillin as the trihydrate.

Pediatric drops for oral suspension: Each ml of reconstituted suspension contains 50 mg amoxicillin as the trihydrate—bottles of 15 ml.

Reference:

1. Bauer, A. W., *et al.*: Antibiotic Susceptibility Testing by a Standardized Single Disc Method, *Am. J. Clin. Pathol., 45:* 493-496, 1966. Standardized Disc Susceptibility Test, *Fed. Reg., 37:* 20527-20529, 1972.

[*Shown in Product Identification Section*]

LEVO-DROMORAN® Ⓒ

(levorphanol tartrate/Roche)
Ampuls • Vials • Tablets

The following text is complete prescribing information based on official labeling in effect August 1, 1979.

Action: Levo-Dromoran (levorphanol tartrate/Roche) is a highly potent synthetic analgesic with properties and actions similar to those of morphine. It produces a degree of analgesia at least equal to that of morphine and greater than that of meperidine at far smaller doses than either. It is longer acting than either; from 6 to 8 hours of pain relief can be expected with Levo-Dromoran whether given orally or by injection. It is almost as effective orally as it is parenterally. Its safety margin is about equal to that of morphine, but it is less likely to produce nausea, vomiting and constipation.

Indications: Levo-Dromoran is recommended whenever a narcotic-analgesic is required. It is recommended for the relief of pain whether moderate or severe. For example, it may be used in alleviating pain due to biliary and renal colic, myocardial infarction, and severe trauma; intractable pain due to cancer and other tumors; and for postoperative pain relief. Used preoperatively, it allays apprehension, provides prolonged analgesia, reduces thiopental requirements and shortens recovery-room time. Levo-Dromoran is compatible with a wide range of anesthetic agents. It is a useful supplement to nitrous oxide-oxygen anesthesia. It has been given by slow intravenous injection for special indications.

Contraindications: As with the use of morphine, Levo-Dromoran is contraindicated in acute alcoholism, bronchial asthma, increased intracranial pressure, respiratory depression and anoxia.

Warning: May be habit forming. Levo-Dromoran is a narcotic with an addiction liability similar to that of morphine, and for this reason the same precautions should be taken in administering the drug as with morphine. As with all narcotics, Levo-Dromoran should be used in early pregnancy only when expected benefits outweigh risks.

Precautions: To prevent or to counteract narcotic-induced respiratory depression (particularly in parturients and neonates, or during nitrous oxide-oxygen anesthesia with narcotic supplementation), Levo-Dromoran combined with Lorfan® (levallorphan tartrate/Roche) —a narcotic antagonist —is recommended. In appropriate combination [1 part Lorfan to 10 parts Levo-Dromoran] respiratory depression is usually prevented without significantly reducing the pain relief provided by Levo-Dromoran. Lorfan usually acts within 1 minute and its action lasts for 2 to 5 hours.

Adverse Reactions: As is true with the use of any narcotic-analgesic, nausea, emesis and dizziness are not uncommon in the ambulatory patient. Respiratory depression, hypotension, urinary retention and various cardiac arrhythmias have been infrequently reported following the use of Levo-Dromoran, primarily in surgical patients. Occasional allergic reactions in the form of skin rash or urticaria have been reported. Pruritus or sweating are rarely observed.

Dosage and Administration: Good medical practice dictates that the dose of any narcotic-analgesic be appropriate to the degree of pain to be relieved. This is especially important during the postoperative period because (a) residual CNS-depressant effects of anesthetic agents may still be present, and (b) later, gradual lessening of pain may not warrant full narcotizing doses. The average adult dose is 2 mg orally or subcutaneously. The dosage may be increased to 3 mg, if necessary. When Levo-Dromoran is used in combination with the narcotic antagonist Lorfan, the following dosage ratio is recommended: Levo-Dromoran/Lorfan (subcutaneous or I.V.)—10:1 [*e.g.,* 2 mg Levo-Dromoran and 0.2 mg Lorfan].

Antidote for Overdosage: In the event of overdosage of the narcotic, Lorfan is a quick and effective antidote. When the narcotic dosage is of unknown magnitude, Lorfan 1 mg intravenously is usually adequate. If required, one or two additional 0.5 mg doses may be given at 3-minute intervals.

How Supplied: *Ampuls,* 1 ml (boxes of 10). Each ml of solution contains 2 mg levorphanol tartrate/Roche (WARNING: May be habit forming) compounded with 0.2% parabens (methyl and propyl) as preservatives, and sodium hydroxide to adjust pH to approximately 4.3.

Multiple Dose Vials, 10 ml, 2 mg/ml (boxes of 1). Each ml of solution contains 2 mg levorphanol tartrate/Roche (WARNING: May be habit forming) compounded with 0.45% phenol as preservative, and sodium hydroxide to adjust pH to approximately 4.3.

Oral Tablets, 2 mg, scored (bottles of 100). Each tablet contains 2 mg levorphanol tartrate/Roche (WARNING: May be habit forming). Narcotic order required.

[*Shown in Product Identification Section*]

LIBRAX® ℞

Librax is a product of Roche Products Inc., Manati, P.R. 00701

The following text is complete prescribing information based on official labeling in effect August 1, 1979.

Composition: Each capsule contains 5 mg chlordiazepoxide hydrochloride (Librium®) and 2.5 mg clidinium bromide (Quarzan®).

Description: Librax combines in a single capsule formulation the antianxiety action of Librium (chlordiazepoxide hydrochloride/Roche) and the anticholinergic/spasmolytic effects of Quarzan (clidinium bromide/Roche), both exclusive developments of Roche research.

Librium (chlordiazepoxide hydrochloride/Roche) is a versatile therapeutic agent of proven value for the relief of anxiety and tension. It is indicated when anxiety, tension or apprehension are significant components of the clinical profile. It is among the safer of the effective psychopharmacologic compounds.

Chlordiazepoxide hydrochloride is 7-chloro-2-methylamino-5-phenyl-3 H -1, 4-benzodiazepine 4-oxide hydrochloride. A colorless, crystalline substance, it is soluble in water. It is unstable in solution and the powder must be protected from light. The molecular weight is 336.22.

Quarzan (clidinium bromide/Roche) is a synthetic anticholinergic agent which has been shown in experimental and clinical studies to have a pronounced antispasmodic and antisecretory effect on the gastrointestinal tract.

Animal Pharmacology: Chlordiazepoxide hydrochloride has been studied extensively in many species of animals and these studies are suggestive of action on the limbic system of the brain,[1,2,3] which recent evidence indicates is involved in emotional responses.[4,5]

Hostile monkeys were made tame by oral drug doses which did not cause sedation. Chlordiazepoxide hydrochloride revealed a "taming" action with the elimination of fear and aggression.[6] The taming effect of chlordiazepoxide hydrochloride was further demonstrated in rats made vicious by lesions in the septal area of the brain. The drug dosage which effectively blocked the vicious reaction was well below the dose which caused sedation in these animals.[6]

The oral LD_{50} of single doses of chlordiazepoxide hydrochloride, calculated according to the method of Miller and Tainter,[7] is 720 ± 51 mg/kg as determined in mice observed over a period of five days following dosage.

Clidinium bromide is an effective anticholinergic agent with activity approximating that of atropine sulfate against acetylcholine-induced spasms in isolated intestinal strips. On oral administration in mice it proved an effective antisialogogue in preventing pilocarpine-induced salivation. Spontaneous intestinal motility in both rats and dogs is reduced following oral dosing with 0.1 to 0.25 mg/kg. Potent cholinergic ganglionic blocking effects (vagal) are produced with intravenous usage in anesthetized dogs.

Oral doses of 2.5 mg/kg to dogs produced signs of nasal dryness and slight pupillary dilation. In two other species, monkeys and rabbits, doses of 5 mg/kg, p.o., given three times daily for 5 days did not produce apparent secretory or visual changes.

The oral LD_{50} of single doses of clidinium bromide is 860 ± 57 mg/kg as determined in mice observed over a period of 5 days following dosage; the calculations were made according to the method of Miller and Tainter.[7]

Effects on Reproduction: Reproduction studies in rats fed chlordiazepoxide hydrochloride, 10, 20 and 80 mg/kg daily, and bred through one or two matings showed no congenital anomalies, nor were there adverse effects on lactation of the dams or growth of the newborn. However, in another study at 100 mg/kg daily there was noted a significant decrease in the fertilization rate and a marked decrease in the viability and body weight of offspring which may be attributable to sedative activity, thus resulting in lack of interest in mating and lessened maternal nursing and care of the young.[8,9] One neonate in each of the first and second matings in the rat reproduction study at the 100 mg/kg dose exhibited major skeletal defects. Further studies are in progress to determine the significance of these findings.

Two series of reproduction experiments with clidinium bromide were carried out in rats, employing dosages of 2.5 and 10 mg/kg daily in each experiment. In the first experiment clidinium bromide was administered for a 9-week interval prior to mating; no untoward effect on fertilization or gestation was noted. The offspring were taken by caesarean section and did not show a significant incidence of congenital anomalies when compared to control animals. In the second experiment adult animals were given clidinium bromide for ten days prior to and through two mating cycles. No significant effects were observed on fertility, gestation, viability of offspring or lactation, as compared to control animals, nor was there a significant incidence of congenital anomalies in the offspring derived from these experiments.

A reproduction study of Librax was carried out in rats through two successive matings. Oral daily doses were administered in two concentrations: 2.5 mg/kg chlordiazepoxide hydrochloride with 1.25 mg/kg clidinium bromide, or 25 mg/kg chlordiazepoxide hydrochloride with 12.5 mg/kg clidinium bromide. In the first mating no significant differences were noted between the control or the treated groups, with the exception of a slight decrease in the number of animals surviving during lactation among those receiving the highest dosage. As with all anticholinergic drugs, an inhibiting effect on lactation may occur. In the second mating similar results were obtained except for a slight decrease in the number of pregnant females and in the percentage of offspring sur-

Continued on next page

Roche—Cont.

viving until weaning. No congenital anomalies were observed in both matings in either the control or treated groups. Additional animal reproduction studies are in progress.

Indications: Based on a review of this drug by the National Academy of Sciences—National Research Council and/or other information, FDA has classified the indications as follows:
"Possibly" effective: as adjunctive therapy in the treatment of peptic ulcer and in the treatment of the irritable bowel syndrome (irritable colon, spastic colon, mucous colitis) and acute enterocolitis.
Final classification of the less-than-effective indications requires further investigation.

Contraindications: Librax is contraindicated in the presence of glaucoma (since the anticholinergic component may produce some degree of mydriasis) and in patients with prostatic hypertrophy and benign bladder neck obstruction. It is contraindicated in patients with known hypersensitivity to chlordiazepoxide hydrochloride and/or clidinium bromide.

Warnings: As in the case of other preparations containing CNS-acting drugs, patients receiving Librax should be cautioned about possible combined effects with alcohol and other CNS depressants. For the same reason, they should be cautioned against hazardous occupations requiring complete mental alertness such as operating machinery or driving a motor vehicle.

Physical and Psychological Dependence: Physical and psychological dependence have rarely been reported in persons taking recommended doses of Librium (chlordiazepoxide hydrochloride/Roche). However, caution must be exercised in administering Librium to individuals known to be addiction-prone or those whose history suggests they may increase the dosage on their own initiative. Withdrawal symptoms following discontinuation of chlordiazepoxide hydrochloride have been reported.[10] These symptoms (including convulsions) are similar to those seen with barbiturates.

Usage in Pregnancy: **An increased risk of congenital malformations associated with the use of minor tranquilizers (chlordiazepoxide, diazepam and meprobamate) during the first trimester of pregnancy has been suggested in several studies. Because use of these drugs is rarely a matter of urgency, their use during this period should almost always be avoided. The possibility that a woman of childbearing potential may be pregnant at the time of institution of therapy should be considered. Patients should be advised that if they become pregnant during therapy or intend to become pregnant they should communicate with their physicians about the desirability of discontinuing the drug.**

As with all anticholinergic drugs, an inhibiting effect on lactation may occur. (See Animal Pharmacology.)

Management of Overdosage: Manifestations of Librium (chlordiazepoxide hydrochloride/Roche) overdosage include somnolence, confusion, coma and diminished reflexes. Respiration, pulse and blood pressure should be monitored, as in all cases of drug overdosage, although, in general, these effects have been minimal following Librium overdosage.

While the signs and symptoms of Librax overdosage may be produced by either of its components, usually such symptoms will be overshadowed by the anticholinergic actions of Quarzan (clidinium bromide/Roche). The symptoms of overdosage of Quarzan are excessive dryness of mouth, blurring of vision, urinary hesitancy and constipation.

General supportive measures should be employed, along with immediate gastric lavage. Administer physostigmine (Antilirium) 0.5 to 2 mg at a rate of no more than 1 mg per minute. This may be repeated in 1 to 4 mg doses if arrhythmias, convulsions or deep coma recur. Intravenous fluids should be administered and an adequate airway maintained. Hypotension may be combated by the use of Levophed® (levarterenol) or Aramine (metaraminol). Ritalin (methylphenidate) or caffeine and sodium benzoate may be given to combat CNS-depressive effects. Dialysis is of limited value. Should excitation occur, barbiturates should not be used. As with the management of intentional overdosage with any drug, it should be borne in mind that multiple agents may have been ingested.

Precautions: In elderly and debilitated patients, it is recommended that the dosage be limited to the smallest effective amount to preclude the development of ataxia, oversedation, or confusion (not more than two Librax capsules per day initially, to be increased gradually as needed and tolerated). In general, the concomitant administration of Librax and other psychotropic agents is not recommended. If such combination therapy seems indicated, careful consideration should be given to the pharmacology of the agents to be employed—particularly when the known potentiating compounds such as the MAO inhibitors and phenothiazines are to be used. The usual precautions in treating patients with impaired renal or hepatic function should be observed.

Paradoxical reactions to chlordiazepoxide hydrochloride, *e.g.,* excitement, stimulation and acute rage, have been reported in psychiatric patients and should be watched for during Librax therapy. The usual precautions are indicated when chlordiazepoxide hydrochloride is used in the treatment of anxiety states where there is any evidence of impending depression; it should be borne in mind that suicidal tendencies may be present and protective measures may be necessary. Although clinical studies have not established a cause and effect relationship, physicians should be aware that variable effects on blood coagulation have been reported very rarely in patients receiving oral anticoagulants and Librium.

Adverse Reactions:[11] No side effects or manifestations not seen with either compound alone have been reported with the administration of Librax. However, since Librax contains chlordiazepoxide hydrochloride and clidinium bromide, the possibility of untoward effects which may be seen with either of these two compounds cannot be excluded.

When chlordiazepoxide hydrochloride has been used alone the necessity of discontinuing therapy because of undesirable effects has been rare.[12] Drowsiness,[13] ataxia[14] and confusion[9] have been reported in some patients—particularly the elderly and debilitated.[9] While these effects can be avoided in almost all instances by proper dosage adjustment, they have occasionally been observed at the lower dosage ranges. In a few instances syncope has been reported.[15]

Other adverse reactions reported during therapy with Librium include isolated instances of skin eruptions,[13] edema,[16] minor menstrual irregularities,[13] nausea and constipation,[17] extrapyramidal symptoms,[9] as well as increased and decreased libido. Such side effects have been infrequent and are generally controlled with reduction of dosage. Changes in EEG patterns (low-voltage fast activity) have been observed in patients during and after Librium treatment.[18]

Blood dyscrasias,[11] including agranulocytosis,[19] jaundice and hepatic dysfunction[20] have occasionally been reported during therapy with Librium. When Librium treatment is protracted, periodic blood counts and liver function tests are advisable.

Adverse effects reported with use of *Librax* are those typical of anticholinergic agents, *i.e.,* dryness of the mouth, blurring of vision, urinary hesitancy and constipation. Constipation has occurred most often when Librax therapy has been combined with other spasmolytic agents and/or a low residue diet.

Dosage: Because of the varied individual responses to tranquilizers and anticholinergics, the optimum dosage of Librax varies with the diagnosis and response of the individual patient. The dosage, therefore, should be individualized for maximum beneficial effects. The usual maintenance dose is 1 or 2 capsules, 3 or 4 times a day administered before meals and at bedtime.

How Supplied: Librax is available in green capsules, each containing 5 mg chlordiazepoxide hydrochloride (Librium®) and 2.5 mg clidinium bromide (Quarzan®)—bottles of 100 and 500; Tel-E-Dose® packages of 100; Prescription Paks of 50.

References:

1. Schallek, W., *et al:* Arch. Int. Pharmacodyn. *149*:467-483, 1964.
2. Himwich, H. E., *et al:* J. Neuropsych. *3* (Suppl. 1):S15-S26, August 1962.
3. Morillo, A., *et al:* Psychopharmacologia *3* (No. 5):386-394, 1962.
4. MacLean, P. D.: Psychosomatic Med. *17*:355-366, September 1955.
5. Morgan, C. T.: Physiological Psychology, 3rd Ed.; New York, McGraw-Hill, 1965.
6. Randall, L. O. *et al:* J. Pharm. Exper. Therap. *129*:163-171, June 1960.
7. Miller, L. C. and Tainter, M. C.: Proc. Soc. Exp. Biol. Med. 57:261, 1944.
8. Zbinden, G., *et al:* Toxicology and Applied Pharmacology *3*:619-637, November 1961.
9. Data on file, Hoffmann-La Roche Inc., Nutley, New Jersey.
10. Hollister, L. E., *et al:* Psychopharmacologia *2*:63-68, 1961.
11. Bibliography and References available on request from Roche Laboratories.
12. Rickels, K. *et al:* Med. Times *93*:238-245, March 1965.
13. Tobin, J. M. *et al:* J. Amer. Med. Assoc. *174*:1242-1249, November 1960.
14. Jenner, F. A., *et al:* J. Ment. Sci. *107*:575-582, May 1961.
15. Robinson, R. C. V.: Dis. Nerv. System *21*:43-45, March 1960.
16. Rose, J. T.: Amer. J. Psychiat. *120*:899-900, March 1964.
17. Hines, L. R.: Curr. Therap. Res. *2*:227-236, June 1960.
18. Gibbs, F. A. and Gibbs, E. L.: J. Neuropsych., 3 (Suppl. 1):S73-S78, August 1962.
19. Kaelbling, R., *et al:* J. Amer. Med. Assoc. *174*:1863-1865, December 1960.
20. Cacioppo, J., *et al:* Amer. J. Psychiat. *117*:1040-1041, May 1961.

[*Shown in Product Identification Section*]

LIBRIUM® Capsules Ⓒ
(chlordiazepoxide hydrochloride/Roche)
LIBRITABS® Tablets Ⓒ
(chloridiazepoxide/Roche)

Librium Capsules and Libritabs are products of Roche Products Inc., Manati, P. R. 00701.

The following text is complete prescribing information based on official labeling in effect August 1, 1979.

Description: Librium (the original chlordiazepoxide HCl) and Libritabs (the original chlordiazepoxide), prototypes for the benzodiazepine compounds, were synthesized and developed at Hoffmann-La Roche Inc. They are versatile therapeutic agents of proven value for the relief of anxiety and tension, and are among the safer of the effective psychophar-

macologic compounds available as demonstrated by extensive clinical evidence.
Chlordiazepoxide hydrochloride is 7-chloro-2-(methylamino)-5-phenyl-3H-1,4-benzodiazepine 4-oxide hydrochloride. A white to practically white crystalline substance, it is soluble in water. It is unstable in solution and the powder must be protected from light. The molecular weight is 336.22.
Chlordiazepoxide is 7-chloro-2-(methylamino)-5-phenyl-3H-1,4-benzodiazepine 4-oxide. A yellow crystalline substance, it is insoluble in water. The powder must be protected from light. The molecular weight is 299.76.
Actions: Librium (chlordiazepoxide HCl/Roche) and Libritabs (chlordiazepoxide/Roche) have antianxiety, sedative, appetite-stimulating and weak analgesic actions. The precise mechanism of action is not known. The drugs block EEG arousal from stimulation of the brain stem reticular formation. It takes several hours for peak blood levels to be reached and the half-life of the drugs is between 24 and 48 hours. After Librium or Libritabs is discontinued plasma levels decline slowly over a period of several days. Chlordiazepoxide is excreted in the urine, with 1 to 2% unchanged and 3 to 6% as a conjugate.
Indications: Librium and Libritabs are indicated for the relief of anxiety and tension, withdrawal symptoms of acute alcoholism, preoperative apprehension and anxiety, and as an adjunct in the treatment of various disease states in which anxiety and tension are manifested.
The effectiveness of Librium or Libritabs in long-term use, that is, more than 4 months, has not been assessed by systematic clinical studies. The physician should periodically reassess the usefulness of the drug for the individual patient.
Contraindications: Librium and Libritabs are contraindicated in patients with known hypersensitivity to the drug.
Warnings: Chlordiazepoxide hydrochloride and chlordiazepoxide may impair the mental and/or physicial abilities required for the performance of potentially hazardous tasks such as driving a vehicle or operating machinery. Similarly, they may impair mental alertness in children. The concomitant use of alcohol or other central nervous system depressants may have an additive effect. PATIENTS SHOULD BE WARNED ACCORDINGLY.
Physical and Psychological Dependence: Physical and psychological dependence have rarely been reported in persons taking recommended doses of chlordiazepoxide hydrochloride or chlordiazepoxide. However, caution must be exercised in administering chlordiazepoxide hydrochloride or chlordiazepoxide to individuals known to be addiction-prone or those whose histories suggest they may increase the dosage on their own initiative. Withdrawal symptoms following discontinuation of chlordiazepoxide hydrochloride or chlordiazepoxide have been reported. These symptoms (including convulsions) are similar to those seen with barbiturates.

Usage in Pregnancy: An increased risk of congenital malformations associated with the use of minor tranquilizers (chlordiazepoxide, diazepam and meprobamate) during the first trimester of pregnancy has been suggested in several studies. Because use of these drugs is rarely a matter of urgency, their use during this period should almost always be avoided. The possibility that a woman of childbearing potential may be pregnant at the time of institution of therapy should be considered. Patients should be advised that if they become pregnant during therapy or intend to become pregnant they should communicate with their physicians about the desirability of discontinuing the drug.

Precautions: In elderly and debilitated patients, it is recommended that the dosage be limited to the smallest effective amount to preclude the development of ataxia or oversedation (10 mg or less per day initially, to be increased gradually as needed and tolerated). In general, the concomitant administration of Librium or Libritabs and other psychotropic agents is not recommended. If such combination therapy seems indicated, careful consideration should be given to the pharmacology of the agents to be employed—particularly when the known potentiating compounds such as the MAO inhibitors and phenothiazines are to be used. The usual precautions in treating patients with impaired renal or hepatic function should be observed.
Paradoxical reactions, e.g., excitement, stimulation and acute rage, have been reported in psychiatric patients and in hyperactive aggressive children, and should be watched for during Librium or Libritabs therapy. The usual precautions are indicated when Librium or Libritabs is used in the treatment of anxiety states where there is any evidence of impending depression; it should be borne in mind that suicidal tendencies may be present and protective measures may be necessary. Although clinical studies have not established a cause and effect relationship, physicians should be aware that variable effects on blood coagulation have been reported very rarely in patients receiving oral anticoagulants and Librium or Libritabs.
Adverse Reactions: The necessity of discontinuing therapy because of undesirable effects has been rare. Drowsiness, ataxia and confusion have been reported in some patients—particularly the elderly and debilitated. While these effects can be avoided in almost all instances by proper dosage adjustment, they have occasionally been observed at the lower dosage ranges. In a few instances syncope has been reported.
Other adverse reactions reported during therapy include isolated instances of skin eruptions, edema, minor menstrual irregularities, nausea and constipation, extrapyramidal symptoms, as well as increased and decreased libido. Such side effects have been infrequent and are generally controlled with reduction of dosage. Changes in EEG patterns (low-voltage fast activity) have been observed in patients during and after Librium or Libritabs treatment.
Blood dyscrasias (including agranulocytosis), jaundice and hepatic dysfunction have occasionally been reported during therapy. When Librium or Libritabs treatment is protracted, periodic blood counts and liver function tests are advisable.
Dosage and Administration: Because of the wide range of clinical indications for Librium and Libritabs, the optimum dosage varies with the diagnosis and response of the individual patient. The dosage, therefore, should be individualized for maximum beneficial effects.

ADULTS	Usual Daily Dose
Relief of mild and moderate anxiety and tension	5 mg or 10 mg, 3 or 4 times daily
Relief of severe anxiety and tension	20 mg or 25 mg, 3 or 4 times daily
Geriatric patients, or in the presence of debilitating disease	5 mg, 2 to 4 times daily

Preoperative apprehension and anxiety:
On days preceding surgery, 5 to 10 mg orally, 3 or 4 times daily. If used as preoperative medication, 50 to 100 mg I.M.* one hour prior to surgery.

CHILDREN	Usual Daily Dose
Because of the varied response of children to CNS-acting drugs, therapy should be initiated with the lowest dose and increased as required. Since clinical experience in children under 6 years of age is limited, the use of the drug in this age group is not recommended.	5 mg, 2 to 4 times daily (may be increased in some children to 10 mg, 2 or 3 times daily)

For the relief of withdrawal symptoms of acute alcoholism, the parenteral form* is usually used initially. If the drug is administered orally, the suggested initial dose is 50 to 100 mg, to be followed by repeated doses as needed until agitation is controlled—up to 300 mg per day. Dosage should then be reduced to maintenance levels.
*See package insert for Injectable Librium (chlordiazepoxide hydrochloride/Roche).
Management of Overdosage: Manifestations of Librium or Libritabs overdosage include somnolence, confusion, coma and diminished reflexes. Respiration, pulse and blood pressure should be monitored, as in all cases of drug overdosage, although, in general, these effects have been minimal following Librium or Libritabs overdosage. General supportive measures should be employed, along with immediate gastric lavage. Intravenous fluids should be administered and an adequate airway maintained. Hypotension may be combated by the use of Levophed® (levarterenol) or Aramine (metaraminol). Ritalin (methylphenidate) or caffeine and sodium benzoate may be given to combat CNS-depressive effects. Dialysis is of limited value. There have been occasional reports of excitation in patients following chlordiazepoxide hydrochloride or chlordiazepoxide overdosage; if this occurs barbiturates should not be used. As with the management of intentional overdosage with any drug, it should be borne in mind that multiple agents may have been ingested.
How Supplied: Librium (chlordiazepoxide hydrochloride/Roche) capsules—5 mg, green and yellow; 10 mg, green and black; 25 mg, green and white—bottles of 100 and 500; Tel-E-Dose® packages of 100, available in trays of 4 reverse-numbered boxes of 25, and in boxes containing 10 strips of 10; Prescription Paks of 50.
Libritabs (chlordiazepoxide/Roche) tablets—5 mg, 10 mg or 25 mg, green—bottles of 100 and 500.

[*Shown in Product Identification Section*]

LIBRIUM® INJECTABLE Ⓒ
(chlordiazepoxide hydrochloride/Roche)

Librium Injectable is manufactured by Hoffmann-La Roche Inc., Nutley, N. J. 07110 and distributed by Roche Products Inc., Manati, P. R. 00701.

The following text is complete prescribing information based on official labeling in effect August 1, 1979.

Description: Librium (chlordiazepoxide hydrochloride/Roche) is a versatile therapeutic agent of proven value for the relief of anxiety and tension.
Librium is the first of a new class, unrelated chemically and pharmacologically to other types of tranquilizers. Librium promptly relieves anxiety and tension over a wide range of emotional disorders, and is among the safer of the effective psychopharmacologic compounds available.
Chlordiazepoxide hydrochloride is 7-chloro-2-methylamino-5-phenyl-3H-1,4-benzodiazepine 4-oxide hydrochloride. A colorless, crystalline substance, it is soluble in water. It is unstable in solution and the powder must be protected from light. The molecular weight is 336.22.
Animal Pharmacology: The drug has been studied extensively in many species of animals and these studies are suggestive of action on

Continued on next page

Roche—Cont.

the limbic system of the brain,[1,2,3] which recent evidence indicates is involved in emotional responses.[4,5]
Hostile monkeys were made tame by oral drug doses which did not cause sedation. Librium revealed a "taming" action with the elimination of fear and aggression.[6] The taming effect of Librium was further demonstrated in rats made vicious by lesions in the septal area of the brain. The drug dosage which effectively blocked the vicious reaction was well below the dose which caused sedation in these animals.[6]
The LD_{50} of parenterally administered chlordiazepoxide hydrochloride was determined in mice (72 hours) and rats (5 days), and calculated according to the method of Miller and Tainter,[7] with the following results: mice, I.V., 123 ± 12 mg/kg; mice, I.M., 366 ± 7 mg/kg; rats, I.V., 120 ± 7 mg/kg; rats, I.M., >160 mg/kg.
Effects on Reproduction: Reproduction studies in rats fed 10, 20 and 80 mg/kg daily and bred through one or two matings showed no congenital anomalies, nor were there adverse effects on lactation of the dams or growth of the newborn. However, in another study at 100 mg/kg daiy there was noted a significant decrease in the fertilization rate and a marked decrease in the viability and body weight of offspring which may be attributable to sedative activity, thus resulting in lack of interest in mating and lessened maternal nursing and care of the young.[8,9] One neonate in each of the first and second matings in the rat reproduction study at the 100 mg/kg dose exhibited major skeletal defects. Further studies are in progress to determine the significance of these findings.
Indications: Librium is indicated for the relief of anxiety and tension, withdrawal symptoms of acute alcoholism, preoperative apprehension and anxiety, and as an adjunct in the treatment of various disease states in which anxiety and tension are manifested.
Contraindications: Librium is contraindicated in patients with known hypersensitivity to the drug.
Warnings: As in the case of other CNS-acting drugs, patients receiving Librium should be cautioned about possible combined effects with alcohol and other CNS depressants.
As is true of all preparations containing CNS-acting drugs, patients receiving Librium should be cautioned against hazardous occupations requiring complete mental alertness such as operating machinery or driving a motor vehicle.
Physical and Psychological Dependence: Physical and psychological dependence have rarely been reported in persons taking recommended doses of Librium. However, caution must be exercised in administering Librium to individuals known to be addiction-prone or those whose history suggests they may increase the dosage on their own initiative. Withdrawal symptoms following discontinuation of chlordiazepoxide hydrochloride have been reported.[10] These symptoms (including convulsions) are similar to those seen with barbiturates.

Usage in Pregnancy: **An increased risk of congenital malformations associated with the use of minor tranquilizers (chlordiazepoxide, diazepam and meprobamate) during the first trimester of pregnancy has been suggested in several studies. Because use of these drugs is rarely a matter of urgency, their use during this period should almost always be avoided. The possibility that a woman of childbearing potential may be pregnant at the time of institution of therapy should be considered. Patients should be advised that if they become pregnant during therapy or intend to become pregnant they should communicate with their physicians about the desirability of discontinuing the drug.**

Management of Overdosage: Manifestations of Librium overdosage include somnolence, confusion, coma and diminished reflexes. Respiration, pulse and blood pressure should be monitored, as in all cases of drug overdosage, although, in general, these effects have been minimal following Librium overdosage. General supportive measures should be employed, along with immediate gastric lavage. Intravenous fluids should be administered and an adequate airway maintained. Hypotension may be combated by the use of Levophed® (levarterenol) or Aramine (metaraminol). Ritalin (methylphenidate) or caffeine and sodium benzoate may be given to combat CNS-depressive effects. Dialysis is of limited value. There have been occasional reports of excitation in patients following chlordiazepoxide hydrochloride overdosage; if this occurs barbiturates should not be used. As with the management of intentional overdosage with any drug, it should be borne in mind that multiple agents may have been ingested.
Precautions: Librium Injectable (intramuscular or intravenous) is indicated primarily in acute states, and patients receiving this form of therapy should be kept under observation, preferably in bed, for a period of up to three hours. Ambulatory patients should not be permitted to operate a vehicle following an injection. Injectable Librium should not be given to patients in shock or comatose states. Reduced dosage (usually 25 to 50 mg) should be used for elderly or debilitated patients, and for children age twelve or older. In general, the concomitant administration of Librium and other psychotropic agents is not recommended. If such combination therapy seems indicated, careful consideration should be given to the pharmacology of the agents to be employed—particularly when the known potentiating compounds such as the MAO inhibitors and phenothiazines are to be used. The usual precautions in treating patients with impaired renal or hepatic function should be observed.
Paradoxical reactions, *e.g.*, excitement, stimulation and acute rage, have been reported in psychiatric patients and in hyperactive aggressive children, and should be watched for during Librium therapy. The usual precautions are indicated when Librium is used in the treatment of anxiety states where there is any evidence of impending depression; it should be borne in mind that suicidal tendencies may be present and protective measures may be necessary. Although clinical studies have not established a cause and effect relationship, physicians should be aware that variable effects on blood coagulation have been reported very rarely in patients receiving oral anticoagulants and Librium.
Adverse Reactions:[11] The necessity of discontinuing therapy because of undesirable effects has been rare. Drowsiness, ataxia and confusion are more commonly seen in the elderly and debilitated.
Other adverse reactions reported during therapy include isolated instances of syncope, hypotension, tachycardia, skin eruptions, edema, minor menstrual irregularities, nausea and constipation, extrapyramidal symptoms, blurred vision, as well as increased and decreased libido. Such side effects have been infrequent and are generally controlled with reduction of dosage. Similarly, hypotension associated with spinal anesthesia has occurred. Pain following intramuscular injection has been reported. Changes in EEG patterns (low-voltage fast activity) have been observed in patients during and after Librium treatment. Blood dyscrasias, including agranulocytosis, jaundice and hepatic dysfunction, have occasionally been reported during therapy. When Librium treatment is protracted, periodic blood counts and liver function tests are advisable.
Preparation and Administration of Solutions: Solutions of Librium for intramuscular or intravenous use should be prepared aseptically. Sterilization by heating should not be attempted.
Intramuscular: Add 2 ml of *Special Intramuscular Diluent* to contents of 5-ml dry-filled amber ampul of Librium Sterile Powder (100 mg). Avoid excessive pressure in injecting this special diluent into the ampul containing the powder since bubbles will form on the surface of the solution. Agitate gently until completely dissolved. Solution should be prepared immediately before administration. Any unused solution should be discarded. Deep intramuscular injection should be given *slowly* into the upper outer quadrant of the gluteus muscle.
Caution: Although the Librium preparation made with the Intramuscular Diluent has been given intravenously without untoward effects, such administration is not recommended because of the air bubbles which form when the Intramuscular Diluent is added to the Librium Powder. Do not use diluent solution if it is opalescent or hazy.
Intravenous: In most cases, intramuscular injection is the preferred route of administration of Librium Injectable since beneficial effects are usually seen within 15 to 30 minutes. When, in the judgment of the physician, even more rapid action is mandatory, Librium Injectable may be administered intravenously. A suitable solution for intravenous administration may be prepared as follows: Add 5 ml of *sterile physiological saline* or *sterile Water For Injection* to contents of 5-ml dry-filled amber ampul of Librium Sterile Powder (100 mg). Agitate gently until thoroughly dissolved. Solution should be prepared immediately before administration. Any unused portion should be discarded. *Intravenous injection should be given slowly over a one-minute period.*
Caution: Librium solution made with physiological saline or sterile Water For Injection should not be given intramuscularly because of pain on injection.
Dosage: Dosage should be individualized according to the diagnosis and the response of the patient. While 300 mg may be given during a 6-hour period, this dose should not be exceeded in any 24-hour period.

INDICATION	ADULT DOSAGE*
Withdrawal Symptoms of Acute Alcoholism	50 to 100 mg I.M. or I.V. initially; repeat in 2 to 4 hours, if necessary
Acute or Severe Anxiety and Tension	50 to 100 mg I.M. or I.V. initially; then 25 to 50 mg 3 or 4 times daily, if necessary
Preoperative Apprehension and Anxiety	50 to 100 mg I.M. one hour prior to surgery

*Lower doses (usually 25 to 50 mg) should be used for elderly or debilitated patients, and for older children. Since clinical experience in children under 12 years of age is limited, the use of the drug in this age group is not recommended.
In most cases, acute symptoms may be rapidly controlled by parenteral administration so that subsequent treatment, if necessary, may be given orally [See package insert for Oral Librium (chlordiazepoxide hydrochloride/Roche)].
How Supplied: For Parenteral Administration: Ampuls—Duplex package consisting of a 5-ml dry-filled ampul containing 100 mg chlordiazepoxide hydrochloride/Roche in dry crystalline form, and a 2-ml ampul of Special Intramuscular Diluent (for intramuscular administration) compounded with 1.5% benzyl alcohol, 4% polysorbate 80, 20% propylene glycol, 1.6% maleic acid and sodium hydroxide to adjust pH to approximately 3.0. Boxes of 10.
Caution: Before preparing solution for intramuscular or intravenous administration,

please read instructions for PREPARATION AND ADMINISTRATION OF SOLUTIONS.

References:

1. Schallek, W., *et al:* Arch. int. Pharmacodyn. *149*:467–483, 1964.
2. Himwich, H. E., *et al:* J. Neuropsych. *3*(Suppl. 1): S15–S26, 1962.
3. Morillo, A., *et al:* Psychopharmacologia *3*:386–394, 1962.
4. Maclean, P. D.: Psychosomatic Med. *17*:355–366, 1955.
5. Morgan, C. T.: Physiological Psychology, 3rd Ed.; New York, McGraw-Hill, 1965.
6. Randall, L. O., *et al:* J. Pharm. & Exper. Therap. *129*:163–171, 1960.
7. Miller, L. C. and Tainter, M. C.: Proc. Soc. Exp. Biol. & Med. *57*:261, 1944.
8. Zbinden, G., *et al:* Toxicology and Applied Pharmacology *3*:619–637, 1961.
9. Data on file, Hoffmann-La Roche Inc., Nutley, New Jersey.
10. Hollister, L. E., *et al:* Psychopharmacologia 2:63–68, 1961.
11. Bibliography and references are available on request from Roche Laboratories.

LIMBITROL® TABLETS Ⓒ

LIMBITROL 10–25
Each tablet contains 10 mg chlordiazepoxide and 25 mg amitriptyline in the form of the hydrochloride salt.
LIMBITROL 5–12.5
Each tablet contains 5 mg chlordiazepoxide and 12.5 mg amitriptyline in the form of the hydrochloride salt.
Limbitrol is a product of Roche Products Inc., Manati, P.R. 00701.

The following text is complete prescribing information based on official labeling in effect August 1, 1979.

Description: Limbitrol combines in a tablet for oral administration, chlordiazepoxide, an agent for the relief of anxiety and tension, and amitriptyline, an antidepressant.

Chlordiazepoxide is a benzodiazepine with the formula 7-chloro-2-(methylamino)-5-phenyl-3*H*-1,4-benzodiazepine 4-oxide. It is a slightly yellow crystalline material and is insoluble in water. The molecular weight is 299.76.

Amitriptyline is a dibenzocycloheptadiene derivative. The formula is 10,11-dihydro-*N,N*-dimethyl-5H-dibenzo [a, d] cycloheptene-$\Delta^{5,\gamma}$-propylamine hydrochloride. It is a white or practically white crystalline compound that is freely soluble in water. The molecular weight is 313.87.

Actions: Both components of Limbitrol exert their action in the central nervous system. Extensive studies with chlordiazepoxide in many animal species suggest action in the limbic system. Recent evidence indicates that the limbic system is involved in emotional response. Taming action was observed in some species. The mechanism of action of amitriptyline in man is not known, but the drug appears to interfere with the reuptake of norepinephrine into adrenergic nerve endings. This action may prolong the sympathetic activity of biogenic amines.

Indications: Limbitrol is indicated for the treatment of patients with moderate to severe depression associated with moderate to severe anxiety.

The therapeutic response to Limbitrol occurs earlier and with fewer treatment failures than when either amitriptyline or chlordiazepoxide is used alone.

Symptoms likely to respond in the first week of treatment include: insomnia, feelings of guilt or worthlessness, agitation, psychic and somatic anxiety, suicidal ideation and anorexia.

Contraindications: Limbitrol is contraindicated in patients with hypersensitivity to either benzodiazepines or tricyclic antidepressants. It should not be given concomitantly with a monoamine oxidase inhibitor. Hyperpyretic crises, severe convulsions and deaths have occurred in patients receiving a tricyclic antidepressant and a monoamine oxidase inhibitor simultaneously. When it is desired to replace a monoamine oxidase inhibitor with Limbitrol, a minimum of 14 days should be allowed to elapse after the former is discontinued. Limbitrol should then be initiated cautiously with gradual increase in dosage until optimum response is achieved.

This drug is contraindicated during the acute recovery phase following myocardial infarction.

Warnings: Because of the atropine-like action of the amitriptyline component, great care should be used in treating patients with a history of urinary retention or angle-closure glaucoma. In patients with glaucoma, even average doses may precipitate an attack. Severe constipation may occur in patients taking tricyclic antidepressants in combination with anticholinergic-type drugs.

Patients with cardiovascular disorders should be watched closely. Tricyclic antidepressant drugs, particularly when given in high doses, have been reported to produce arrhythmias, sinus tachycardia and prolongation of conduction time. Myocardial infarction and stroke have been reported in patients receiving drugs of this class.

Usage in Pregnancy: Safe use of Limbitrol during pregnancy and lactation has not been established. Because of the chlordiazepoxide component, please note the following:

An increased risk of congenital malformations associated with the use of minor tranquilizers (chlordiazepoxide, diazepam and meprobamate) during the first trimester of pregnancy has been suggested in several studies. Because use of these drugs is rarely a matter of urgency, their use during this period should almost always be avoided. The possibility that a woman of childbearing potential may be pregnant at the time of institution of therapy should be considered. Patients should be advised that if they become pregnant during therapy or intend to become pregnant they should communicate with their physicians about the desirability of discontinuing the drug.

Physical and Psychological Dependence: Experience with Limbitrol is as yet too limited to reasonably assess the combination's potential for physical and psychological dependence. However, since physical and psychological dependence to chlordiazepoxide have been reported rarely, caution must be exercised in administering Limbitrol to individuals known to be addiction-prone or to those whose history suggests they may increase the dosage on their own initiative.

In the so far limited experience with Limbitrol withdrawal symtoms have not been reported. However, withdrawal symptoms following abrupt cessation of prolonged therapy with either component alone have been reported. With amitriptyline, these have been noted to consist of nausea, headache and malaise; for chlordiazepoxide, the symptoms (including convulsions) are similar to those seen with barbiturates.

Precautions: *General:* Use with caution in patients with a history of seizures.

Close supervision is required when Limbitrol is given to hyperthyroid patients or those on thyroid medication.

The usual precautions should be observed when treating patients with impaired renal or hepatic function.

Patients with suicidal ideation should not have easy access to large quantities of the drug. The possibility of suicide in depressed patients remains until significant remission occurs.

Information for the Patient: Because of the sedative effects of Limbitrol, patients should be cautioned about combined effects with alcohol or other CNS depressants. The additive effects may produce a harmful level of sedation and CNS depression.

Patients receiving Limbitrol should be cautioned against engaging in hazardous occupations requiring complete mental alertness, such as operating machinery or driving a motor vehicle.

Essential Laboratory Tests: Patients on prolonged treatment should have periodic liver function tests and blood counts.

Drug and Treatment Interactions: Because of its amitriptyline component, Limbitrol may block the antihypertensive action of guanethidine or compounds with a similar mechanism of action.

The effects of concomitant administration of Limbitrol and other psychotropic drugs have not been evaluated. Sedative effects may be additive.

The drug should be discontinued several days before elective surgery.

Concurrent administration of ECT and Limbitrol should be limited to those patients for whom it is essential.

Pregnancy: See WARNINGS section.

Nursing Mothers: It is not known whether this drug is excreted in human milk. As a general rule, nursing should not be undertaken while a patient is on a drug, since many drugs are excreted in human milk.

Pediatric Use: Safety and effectiveness in children below the age of 12 years have not been established.

Elderly Patients: In elderly and debilitated patients it is recommended that dosage be limited to the smallest effective amount to preclude the development of ataxia, oversedation, confusion or anticholinergic effects.

Adverse Reactions: Adverse reactions to Limbitrol are those associated with the use of either component alone. Most frequently reported were drowsiness, dry mouth, constipation, blurred vision, dizziness and bloating. Other side effects occurring less commonly included vivid dreams, impotence, tremor, confusion and nasal congestion. Many symptoms common to the depressive state, such as anorexia, fatigue, weakness, restlessness and lethargy, have been reported as side effects of treatment with both Limbitrol and amitriptyline.

Granulocytopenia, jaundice and hepatic dysfunction of uncertain etiology have also been observed rarely with Limbitrol. When treatment with Limbitrol is prolonged, periodic blood counts and liver function tests are advisable.

Note: Included in the listing which follows are adverse reactions which have not been reported with Limbitrol. However, they are included because they have been reported during therapy with one or both of the components or closely related drugs.

Cardiovascular: Hypotension, hypertension, tachycardia, palpitations, myocardial infarction, arrhythmias, heart block, stroke.

Psychiatric: Euphoria, apprehension, poor concentration, delusions, hallucinations, hypomania and increased or decreased libido.

Neurologic: Incoordination, ataxia, numbness, tingling and paresthesias of the extremities, extrapyramidal symptoms, syncope, changes in EEG patterns.

Anticholinergic: Disturbance of accommodation, paralytic ileus, urinary retention, dilatation of urinary tract.

Allergic: Skin rash, urticaria, photosensitization, edema of face and tongue, pruritus.

Hematologic: Bone marrow depression including agranulocytosis, eosinophilia, purpura, thrombocytopenia.

Gastrointestinal: Nausea, epigastric distress, vomiting, anorexia, stomatitis, peculiar taste, diarrhea, black tongue.

Continued on next page

Roche—Cont.

Endocrine: Testicular swelling and gynecomastia in the male, breast enlargement, galactorrhea and minor menstrual irregularities in the female and elevation and lowering of blood sugar levels.
Other: Headache, weight gain or loss, increased perspiration, urinary frequency, mydriasis, jaundice, alopecia, parotid swelling.
Overdosage: There has been limited experience with Limbitrol overdosage *per se;* the manifestations of overdosage and recommendations for treatment are based on clinical experience with its components. Primary concern should be with the dangers associated with amitriptyline overdosage. Deaths by deliberate or accidental overdosage have occurred with this class of drugs.
All patients suspected of having an overdosage of Limbitrol should be admitted to a hospital as soon as possible.
Manifestations: High doses may cause drowsiness, temporary confusion, disturbed concentration or transient visual hallucinations. Overdosage may cause hypothermia, tachycardia and other arrhythmias, ECG evidence of impaired conduction (such as bundle branch block), congestive heart failure, dilated pupils, convulsions, severe hypotension, stupor and coma. Other symptoms may be agitation, hyperactive reflexes, muscle rigidity, vomiting, hyperpyrexia or any of those listed under Adverse Reactions.
Treatment: Empty the stomach as quickly as possible by emesis or lavage. In the comatose patient a cuff endotracheal tube should be placed in position prior to either of these measures. The instillation of activated charcoal into the stomach also should be considered. If the patient is stuporous but responds to stimuli, only close observation and nursing care may be required. It is essential to maintain an adequate airway and fluid intake. Body temperature should be watched closely and appropriate measures taken should deviations occur.
The intramuscular or slow intravenous administration of 1 to 3 mg in adults (or 0.5 mg in children) of physostigmine salicylate (Antilirium)[1–3] has been reported to reverse the manifestations of amitriptyline overdosage. Because of its relatively short half-life, additional doses may be needed at intervals of 30 minutes to 2 hours.
Convulsions may be treated by the use of an inhalation anesthetic rather than the use of barbiturates. Cardiac monitoring is advisable, and the cautious use of digitalis or other antiarrhythmic agents should be considered if serious cardiovascular abnormalities occur. Serum potassium levels should be monitored and kept within normal limits by the use of appropriate I.V. fluids. Standard measures including oxygen, I.V. fluids, plasma expanders and corticosteroids may be used to control circulatory shock.
Dialysis is unlikely to be of value, as it has not proven useful in overdosages of either amitriptyline or chlordiazepoxide. Since many suicidal attempts involve multiple drugs including barbiturates, the possibility of dialysis being beneficial for removal of other drugs should not be overlooked.
Treatment should be continued for at least 48 hours, along with cardiac monitoring in patients who do not respond to therapy promptly. Since relapses are frequent, patients should be hospitalized until their conditions remain stable without physostigmine for at least 24 hours.
Since overdosage is often deliberate, patients may attempt suicide by other means during the recovery phase.

References:

1. Granacher RP, Baldessarini RJ: Physostigmine: Its use in acute anticholinergic syndrome with antidepressant and antiparkinson drugs. *Arch Gen Psychiatry 32*:375–380, March 1975.
2. Burks JS, Walker JE, Rumack BH, Ott JE: Tricyclic antidepressant poisoning: Reversal of coma, choreoathetosis, and myoclonus by physostigmine. *JAMA 230*:1405–1407, Dec. 9, 1974.
3. Snyder BD, Blonde L, McWhirter WR: Reversal of amitriptyline intoxication by physostigmine. *JAMA 230*:1433–1434, Dec. 9, 1974.

Dosage and Administration: Optimum dosage varies with the severity of the symptoms and the response of the individual patient. When a satisfactory response is obtained, dosage should be reduced to the smallest amount needed to maintain the remission. The larger portion of the total daily dose may be taken at bedtime. In some patients, a single dose at bedtime may be sufficient. In general, lower dosages are recommended for elderly patients.
Limbitrol 10–25 is recommended in an initial dosage of three or four tablets daily in divided doses; this may be increased to six tablets daily as required. Some patients respond to smaller doses and can be maintained on two tablets daily.
Limbitrol 5–12.5 in an initial dosage of three or four tablets daily in divided doses may be satisfactory in patients who do not tolerate higher doses.
How Supplied: White, film-coated tablets, each containing 10 mg chlordiazepoxide and 25 mg amitriptyline (as the hydrochloride salt) and blue, film-coated tablets, each containing 5 mg chlordiazepoxide and 12.5 mg amitriptyline (as the hydrochloride salt)—bottles of 100 and 500; Tel-E-Dose® packages of 100, available in trays of 4 reverse-numbered boxes of 25, and in boxes containing 10 strips of 10; Prescription Paks of 50.
[*Shown in Product Identification Section*]

LORFAN® ℞
(levallorphan tartrate/Roche)
ampuls • vials

The following text is complete prescribing information based on official labeling in effect August 1, 1979.
Description: Chemically, levallorphan tartrate is (−)-*N*-allyl-3-hydroxymorphinan tartrate. It is chemically related to levorphanol tartrate from which it differs in the replacement of the methyl group on the nitrogen atom by an allyl group. Levallorphan tartrate is a white or practically white, odorless, crystalline powder; it is soluble in water and sparingly soluble in alcohol.
Each ml contains 1 mg levallorphan tartrate/Roche. The pH is adjusted to approximately 4.3 with sodium hydroxide. The solution in ampuls is compounded with 0.2% methyl and propyl parabens and that in vials is compounded with 0.45% phenol as preservatives.
Actions: Lorfan acts as a narcotic antagonist in the presence of a strong narcotic effect. If used in the absence of such a narcotic effect, Lorfan may cause respiratory depression and other undesirable effects.
Indications: For use in the treatment of significant narcotic-induced respiratory depression.
Contraindications: Mild respiratory depression. Narcotic addicts in whom it may produce withdrawal symptoms.
Warnings: Lorfan is ineffective against respiratory depression due to barbiturates, anesthetics, other nonnarcotic agents or pathologic causes, and may increase it.
Precautions: If used in the absence of a narcotic, Lorfan may cause respiratory depression. Artificial respiration with oxygen and other supportive measures should be employed in conjunction with Lorfan in the treatment of significant narcotic-induced respiratory depression. Lorfan does not counteract mild respiratory depression and may increase it. Repeated doses of Lorfan result in decreasing effectiveness and may eventually produce respiratory depression equal to or greater than that produced by narcotics.
Adverse Reactions: Dysphoria, miosis, pseudoptosis, lethargy, dizziness, drowsiness, gastric upset and sweating. Pallor, nausea and a sense of heaviness in the limbs may occur.
In high dosage Lorfan may produce psychotomimetic manifestations such as weird dreams, visual hallucinations, disorientation and feelings of unreality.
In *asphyxia neonatorum,* irritability and a tendency to increased crying may occur.
Dosage and Administration: Administration of Lorfan should be accompanied by the use of other resuscitative measures, such as oxygen or artificial respiration.
Adults: To reverse respiratory depression from narcotic overdosage—1 mg Lorfan intravenously; may be followed, if required, by one or two additional doses of 0.5 mg at 10 to 15 minute intervals. The initial dose should not exceed 1 mg if there is doubt as to whether a narcotic produced the respiratory depression. The total dose should not exceed 3 mg. This regimen may also be employed to overcome narcotic-induced respiratory depression in the parturient woman.
Neonates: To decrease respiratory depression secondary to narcotic administration to the mother, inject 0.05 to 0.1 mg Lorfan (approximately one-tenth the adult dose) into the umbilical cord vein immediately after delivery. If this vein cannot be used, injection may be made intramuscularly or subcutaneously.
Overdosage: Assisted respiration, including a patent airway, the administration of oxygen, and other supportive measures, should be used.
How Supplied: Ampuls, 1 ml, boxes of 10; vials, 10 ml. Each ml contains 1 mg levallorphan tartrate/Roche.

MARPLAN® TABLETS ℞
(isocarboxazid/Roche)

The following text is complete prescribing information based on official labeling in effect August 1, 1979.
Description: Marplan (isocarboxazid/Roche) is an amine-oxidase inhibitor. Chemically, isocarboxazid is 5-methyl-3-isoxazolecarboxylic acid 2-benzylhydrazide.
Isocarboxazid is a colorless, crystalline substance with very little taste.
Actions: Isocarboxazid, a potent inhibitor of amine-oxidase, exhibits antidepressant activity. *In vivo* and *in vitro* studies demonstrated inhibition of amine-oxidase in the brain, heart and liver.
The oral LD_{50} in mice was 171 mg/kg and in rats, 270 mg/kg. In rats administered 120 mg/kg daily for 6 weeks, isocarboxazid produced a reduction of growth rate and appetite. In chronic tolerance studies of 24 weeks duration, hyperexcitability and depression of growth rate occurred in male rats given oral doses of 5 mg/kg/day and in both sexes of this species given 10 mg/kg/day orally. The relevance of these findings to the clinical use of Marplan is not known. No hematologic changes were observed.
Dogs given 15 mg/kg/day for 2 weeks showed emetic effects and a slight lowering of hemoglobin and hematocrit. No adverse effects were noted, however, at doses of 10 mg/kg/day for 6 weeks. Given as successively increasing daily oral doses to a dog, isocarboxazid was tolerated up to 40 mg/kg.
Monkeys given 20 mg/kg/day orally for 2 weeks tolerated the drug with no apparent adverse effects.
Reproduction studies were carried out in rats given 0.5 and 5 mg/kg/day of isocarboxazid as a dietary mixture for 10 weeks prior to mating and continuing through two mating cycles to

the weaning of the second litter. The parent animals remained in good condition throughout the test period. Litters of the treated groups compared favorably with those of the controls. No evidence of teratogenic effects was seen in any of the young.

> INDICATIONS: Based on a review of this drug by the National Academy of Sciences—National Research Council and/or other information, FDA has classified the indications as follows:
> "Probably" effective for the treatment of depressed patients who are refractory to tricyclic antidepressants or electroconvulsive therapy and depressed patients in whom tricyclic antidepressants are contraindicated.
> Final classification of the less-than-effective indications requires further investigation.

Careful selection of candidates for Marplan—with due regard to the symptomatology of the patient and to the properties of the compound—will result in more effective therapy. Complete review of the package insert is advised before initiating treatment.

Contraindications: Marplan is contraindicated in patients with known hypersensitivity to the drug, severe impairment of liver or renal function, congestive heart failure or pheochromocytoma.

The potentiation of sympathomimetic substances by MAO inhibitors may result in *hypertensive crisis;* therefore, patients taking Marplan should not be given *sympathomimetic drugs* (including amphetamines, methyldopa, levodopa, dopamine, and tryptophan as well as epinephrine and norepinephrine) nor *foods with a high concentration of tryptophan* (broad beans) or *tyramine* (cheese, beers, wines, pickled herring, chicken livers, yeast extract). Excessive amounts of caffeine can also cause hypertensive reactions.

These hypertensive crises can be fatal, due to circulatory collapse or intracranial bleeding. Hypertensive crises are characterized by some or all of the following symptoms: occipital headache which may radiate frontally, neck stiffness or soreness, nausea, vomiting, photophobia, dilated pupils, sweating (sometimes with fever and sometimes with cold, clammy skin) and palpitations. Either tachycardia or bradycardia may be present, and can be associated with constricting chest pain. These crises usually occur within several hours after the ingestion of a contraindicated substance. Marplan should be discontinued immediately upon the occurrence of palpitations or frequent headaches.

Recommended treatment in hypertensive crisis: Marplan should be discontinued and therapy to lower blood pressure should be started immediately. A successful method of treatment is with an alpha-adrenergic blocking agent such as phentolamine, 5 mg, I.V., or pentolinium, 3 mg, subcutaneously. These drugs should be administered slowly to avoid excessive hypotension. Fever should be managed by external cooling.

Marplan should not be administered together with or immediately following other MAO inhibitors or dibenzazepines. Such combinations can produce hypertensive crisis, fever, marked sweating, excitation, delirium, tremor, twitching, convulsions, coma, and circulatory collapse. At least 10 days should elapse between the discontinuation of Marplan and the institution of another antidepressant, or the discontinuation of another MAO inhibitor and the institution of Marplan.

Some other amine-oxidase inhibitors commonly used in this country include: pargyline HCl (Eutonyl), phenelzine sulfate (Nardil) and tranylcypromine (Parnate).

Some antidepressants (dibenzazepine derivatives) commonly used in this country include: amitriptyline HCl (Elavil), desipramine HCl (Norpramin, Pertofrane), imipramine HCl (Tofranil), nortriptyline HCl (Aventyl) and protriptyline HCl (Vivactyl).

Patients taking Marplan should not undergo elective surgery requiring general anesthesia. Should spinal anesthesia be essential, consideration should be given to possible combined hypotensive effects of Marplan and the blocking agent. Also, they should not be given cocaine or local anesthetic solutions containing sympathomimetic vasoconstrictors. Marplan should be discontinued at least 10 days prior to elective surgery.

Marplan should not be used in combination with CNS depressants such as narcotics and ethanol (see PRECAUTIONS for barbiturates). Circulatory collapse and death have been reported from the combination of amine-oxidase inhibitors and a single dose of Demerol (meperidine).

Warnings: Because the most serious reactions to Marplan relate to effects on blood pressure, it is not advisable to use this drug in elderly or debilitated patients or in the presence of hypertension, cardiovascular or cerebrovascular disease. Patients with severe or frequent headaches should not be considered as candidates for therapy with Marplan because headaches during therapy may be the first symptom of a hypertensive reaction to the drug.

Marplan should be used with caution in combination with antihypertensive drugs including thiazide diuretics since hypotension may result.

In patients who may be suicidal risks, no single form of treatment, such as Marplan, electroshock or other therapy, should be relied on as a sole therapeutic measure. The strictest supervision, and preferably hospitalization, are advised.

Warning to patient: All patients taking Marplan should be warned against self-medication with proprietary cold, hay fever or reducing preparations, since most of these contain sympathomimetic agents. They should be warned against eating the foods previously mentioned that contain high concentrations of tyramine or tryptophan. Beverages containing caffeine should be used in moderation. Patients should be instructed to report promptly the occurrence of headache or other unusual symptoms.

Use in Children: Marplan is not recommended for use in patients under 16 years of age since there are no controlled studies of safety or efficacy in this group.

Use in Pregnancy: Safe use of Marplan during pregnancy or lactation has not yet been established. Before prescribing Marplan in pregnancy, lactation, or in women of childbearing age, the potential benefit of the drug should be weighed against its possible hazard to mother and child. (See ACTIONS.)

Precautions: Concomitant use of Marplan and other psychotropic agents is not recommended because of possible potentiating effects and decreased margin of safety. This is especially true in patients who may subject themselves to an overdosage of drugs. If combination therapy is indicated, careful consideration should be given to the pharmacology of all agents to be employed. The effects of Marplan may persist for a substantial period after discontinuation of the drug, and this should be borne in mind when another drug is prescribed following Marplan. To avoid potentiation, the physician wishing to terminate treatment with Marplan and begin therapy with another agent should allow for an interval of 10 days.

Marplan should be used cautiously in hyperactive or agitated patients, as well as schizophrenic patients, because it may cause excessive stimulation. Characteristically, in manic-depressive states there may be a tendency for patients to swing from a depressive to a manic phase. If such a swing should occur during Marplan therapy, brief discontinuation of the drug, followed by resumption of therapy at a reduced dosage, is advised.

Clinical evidence indicates only a low incidence of altered liver function or jaundice in patients treated with Marplan. It is difficult to differentiate most cases of drug-induced hepatocellular jaundice from viral hepatitis since they are histopathologically and biochemically indistinguishable. Moreover, many of the clinical signs and symptoms are identical. While some of the few cases of jaundice reported during Marplan therapy may have been drug-induced, the reaction is rare. Nevertheless, Marplan is an amine-oxidase inhibitor and, as with the use of all these agents, it is advisable to watch for hepatic complications. It is suggested that periodic liver function tests, such as bilirubins, alkaline phosphatase or transaminases, be performed during Marplan therapy; use of the drug should be discontinued at the first sign of hepatic dysfunction or jaundice. In patients with impaired renal function, Marplan should be used cautiously to prevent accumulation.

Marplan appears to have varying effects in epileptic patients; while some have a decrease in frequency of seizures, others have more seizures. Appropriate consideration must be given to the latter possibility if Marplan is prescribed for such patients.

All patients taking Marplan should be watched for symptoms of postural hypotension. If such hypotension occurs, the dose should be reduced or the drug discontinued.

Since the MAO inhibitors, including Marplan potentiate hexobarbital hypnosis in animals, the dose of barbiturates if given concomitantly should be reduced.

Since the MAO inhibitors inhibit the destruction of serotonin, which is believed to be released from tissue stores by rauwolfia alkaloids, caution should be exercised when these drugs are used together.

There is conflicting evidence as to whether MAO inhibitors affect glucose metabolism or potentiate hypoglycemic agents. This should be considered if Marplan is used in diabetics.

Adverse Reactions: Marplan is a potent therapeutic agent with a relatively low incidence of adverse reactions. Since Marplan affects many enzyme systems of the body, a variety of side effects may be anticipated. The most frequently noted have been orthostatic hypotension, associated in some patients with falling, disturbances in cardiac rate and rhythm, complaints of dizziness and vertigo, constipation, headache, overactivity, hyperreflexia, tremors and muscle twitching, mania, hypomania, jitteriness, confusion and memory impairment, insomnia, peripheral edema, weakness, fatigue, dryness of the mouth, blurred vision, hyperhidrosis, anorexia and body weight changes, gastrointestinal disturbances, and minor sensitivity reactions such as skin rashes. Isolated cases of akathisia, ataxia, black tongue, coma, dysuria, euphoria, hematologic changes, incontinence, neuritis, photosensitivity, sexual disturbances, spider telangiectases and urinary retention have been reported. These side effects sometimes necessitate discontinuation of therapy. In rare instances, hallucinations have been reported with high dosages, but they have disappeared upon reduction of dosage or discontinuation of therapy. Toxic amblyopia was reported in one psychiatric patient who had received isocarboxazid for about a year; no causal relationship to isocarboxazid was established.

Dosage and Administration: As with other potent drugs, for maximum therapeutic effect the dosage of Marplan must be individually adjusted on the basis of careful observation of the patient. The usual starting dose is 30 mg daily, to be given in single or divided doses.

Continued on next page

Roche—Cont.

Marplan has a cumulative effect; therefore, as soon as clinical improvement is observed, the dosage should be reduced to a maintenance level of 10 to 20 mg daily (or less). Since daily doses larger than 30 mg may cause an increase in the incidence or severity of side effects, it is recommended that this dosage generally not be exceeded. Many patients may show a favorable response to Marplan therapy within a week or less; however, since Marplan acts by directly affecting enzyme metabolism, a beneficial effect may not be seen in some patients for three or four weeks. If no response is obtained by then, continued administration is unlikely to help.

Management of Overdosage: The lethal dose of Marplan in man is not known. There has been one report of a fatality in a patient who ingested 400 mg of Marplan together with an unspecified amount of another drug. Major overdosage may be evidenced by symptoms such as tachycardia, hypotension, coma, convulsions, respiratory depression, sluggish reflexes, pyrexia and diaphoresis; these signs may persist for 8 to 14 days. General supportive measures should be employed, along with immediate gastric lavage or emetics. If the latter are given, the danger of aspiration must be borne in mind. An adequate airway should be maintained, with supplemental oxygen if necessary. The mechanism by which amine-oxidase inhibitors produce hypotension is not fully understood, but there is evidence that these agents block the vascular bed response. Thus it is suggested that plasma may be of value in the management of this hypotension. Administration of pressor amines such as Levophed® (levarterenol bitartrate) may be of limited value (note that their effects may be potentiated by Marplan). Continue treatment for several days until homeostasis is restored. Liver function studies are recommended during the 4 to 6 weeks after recovery, as well as at the time of overdosage. As with the management of intentional overdosage with any drug, it should be borne in mind that multiple agents may have been ingested.

How Supplied: Tablets, 10 mg isocarboxazid each, peach-colored, scored—bottles of 100 and 1000.

[*Shown in Product Identification Section*]

MATULANE® ℞
(procarbazine hydrochloride/Roche)

The following text is complete prescribing information based on official labeling in effect August 1, 1979.

WARNING

It is recommended that MATULANE be given only by or under the supervision of a physician experienced in the use of potent antineoplastic drugs. Adequate clinical and laboratory facilities should be available to patients for proper monitoring of treatment.

The enclosed instructions should be thoroughly reviewed before administration of MATULANE.

Description: Matulane (procarbazine hydrochloride/Roche) has demonstrated an antineoplastic effect against Hodgkin's disease. The mode of cytotoxic action of Matulane has not yet been clearly defined; however, there is evidence that the drug may act by inhibition of protein, RNA and DNA synthesis. No cross-resistance with other chemotherapeutic agents, radiotherapy or steroids has been demonstrated.

Clinical studies, in which the duration of response is at least a month, show an over-all response rate of approximately 50 per cent. This includes both objective regression of disease and associated clinical benefit. These observations have been made in patients who have had prior treatment with radiotherapy and other antineoplastic agents.

The number of patients with malignant diseases other than Hodgkin's disease who have received Matulane therapy is inadequate at this time for any definitive statement regarding efficacy. Therefore, the use of this drug should be limited to Hodgkin's disease.

Chemistry: Procarbazine hydrochloride is *N*-isopropyl-*α*- (2-methylhydrazino) -*p*-toluamide monohydrochloride. It is a white to pale yellow crystalline substance, soluble but unstable in water or aqueous solutions. The molecular weight is 257.76.

Actions: In laboratory studies, procarbazine hydrochloride produced a variety of biologic effects. Among these have been immunosuppression, teratogenesis, carcinogenesis, cytotoxicity with mitotic suppression and chromatin derangement, and an antineoplastic effect against a spectrum of transplanted tumors in mice and rats. The major drug toxicities in acute and chronic animal studies were hematologic with granulocyte depression, thrombocyte depression and anemia. Reticuloendothelial system lymphocytic depletion, marrow cell depression, testicular atrophy and mucous membrane ulceration were further evidence of *in vivo* cytotoxicity.

Distribution of the drug in body fluids, studied in dog and man, showed rapid equilibration between plasma and cerebrospinal fluid after oral administration. Pharmacological studies indicated excellent gastrointestinal absorption. The major portion of drug was excreted in the urine as N-isopropylterephthalamic acid with approximately 25 to 42 per cent appearing during the first 24 hours after administration.

Leukemia and pulmonary tumors in mice, and mammary adenocarcinomas in rats, have been observed subsequent to procarbazine hydrochloride administration in high doses. The oral LD_{50} of procarbazine hydrochloride in mice and rats was determined to be 1320 $\pm$ 66 mg/kg and 785 $\pm$ 34 mg/kg respectively. In rabbits the oral LD_{50} was 147 $\pm$ 11.5 mg/kg.

Indication: Matulane is recommended for the palliative management of generalized Hodgkin's disease and in those patients who have become resistant to other forms of therapy. Although prolongation of survival time may not be evident, amelioration of the disease symptoms and regression of tumors have been demonstrated frequently. The drug should be used as an adjunct to standard modalities of therapy.

Contraindications: Matulane is contraindicated in patients with 1) known hypersensitivity to the drug, or 2) inadequate marrow reserve as demonstrated by bone marrow aspiration. Due consideration of this possible state should be given to each patient who has leukopenia, thrombocytopenia or anemia.

Warnings: To minimize CNS depression and possible synergism, barbiturates, antihistamines, narcotics, hypotensive agents or phenothiazines should be used with caution. Ethyl alcohol should not be used since there may be an Antabuse (disulfiram)-like reaction. Because Matulane exhibits some amine oxidase inhibitory activity, sympathomimetic drugs, tricyclic antidepressant drugs (*e.g.,* amitriptyline HCl, imipramine HCl), and other drugs and foods with known high tyramine content, such as ripe cheese and bananas, should be avoided. A further phenomenon of toxicity common to many hydrazine derivatives is hemolysis and the appearance of Heinz-Ehrlich inclusion bodies in erythrocytes.

Use In Pregnancy: Teratogenicity has been reported in animals. Use of any drug in pregnancy, lactation or in women of childbearing age requires that the potential benefit of the drug be weighed against its possible hazard to mother and child.

Precautions: Undue toxicity may occur if Matulane is used in patients with known impairment of renal and/or hepatic function. When appropriate, hospitalization for the initial course of treatment should be considered. If radiation or a chemotherapeutic agent known to have marrow-depressant activity has been used, an interval of one month or longer without such therapy is recommended before starting treatment with Matulane. The length of this interval may also be determined by evidence of bone marrow recovery based on successive bone marrow studies.

Adverse Reactions: Leukopenia, anemia and thrombopenia occur frequently. Nausea and vomiting are the most commonly reported side effects. Other less frequent gastrointestinal complaints include anorexia, stomatitis, dry mouth, dysphagia, diarrhea and constipation. Pain, including myalgia and arthralgia, chills and fever, sweating, weakness, fatigue, lethargy and drowsiness are often noted. Intercurrent infections, effusion, edema, cough, and pneumonitis have been reported. Bleeding tendencies such as petechiae, purpura, epistaxis, hemoptysis, hematemesis and melena have not been rare. Dermatitis, pruritus, herpes, hyperpigmentation, flushing, alopecia and jaundice have also been noted. Paresthesias and neuropathies, headache, dizziness, depression, apprehension, nervousness, insomnia, nightmares, hallucinations, falling, unsteadiness, ataxia, footdrop, decreased reflexes, tremors, coma, confusion and convulsions have been less common. Hoarseness, tachycardia, retinal hemorrhage, nystagmus, photophobia, photosensitivity, genitourinary symptoms, hypotension and fainting have been rare. Isolated instances of diplopia, inability to focus, papilledema, altered hearing and slurred speech have occurred. Coincidental onset of leukemia during Matulane therapy has been reported in rare instances.

Dosage and Administration:

General Instructions: Baseline laboratory data should be obtained prior to initiation of therapy. The hematologic status as indicated by hemoglobin, hematocrit, white blood count (WBC), differential, reticulocytes and platelets should be monitored closely—at least every 3 or 4 days. Bone marrow depression often occurs 2 to 8 weeks after the start of treatment. If leukopenia occurs, hospitalization of the patient may be needed for appropriate treatment to prevent systemic infection.

Hepatic and renal evaluation are indicated prior to beginning therapy. Urinalysis, transaminase, alkaline phosphatase and blood urea nitrogen should be repeated at least weekly.

Prompt cessation of therapy is recommended if any one of the following occurs:

Central nervous system signs or symptoms such as paresthesias, neuropathies or confusion.

Leukopenia (white blood count under 4000).

Thrombocytopenia (platelets under 100,000).

Hypersensitivity reaction.

Stomatitis—The first small ulceration or persistent spot soreness around the oral cavity is a signal for cessation of therapy.

Diarrhea—Frequent bowel movements or watery stools.

Hemorrhage or bleeding tendencies.

Therapy may be resumed, at the discretion of the physician, after toxic side effects have cleared on clinical evaluation and appropriate laboratory studies. Adjustment to a lower dosage schedule is recommended.

Dosage:

General Instructions: All dosages are based on the patient's actual weight. However, the estimated lean body mass (dry weight) is used if the patient is obese or if there has been a spurious weight gain due to edema, ascites or other forms of abnormal fluid retention.

Adults—To minimize nausea and vomiting experienced by a high percentage of patients beginning Matulane therapy, single or divided doses of 2 to 4 mg/kg/day (to the nearest 50 mg) for the first week are recommended. Daily dosage should then be maintained at 4 to 6 mg/kg/day until the white blood count falls below 4000 per cmm or the platelets fall below 100,000 per cmm or until maximum response is obtained. Upon evidence of hematologic toxicity the drug should be discontinued until there has been satisfactory recovery. Treatment may then be resumed at 1 to 2 mg/kg/day. When maximum response is obtained, the dose may be maintained at 1 to 2 mg/kg/day.

Children—Use of Matulane in children has been quite limited. Very close clinical monitoring is mandatory. Undue toxicity, evidenced by tremors, coma and convulsions, has occurred in a few cases. Dosage, therefore, must be highly individualized. The following dosage schedule is provided as a guideline only.

50 mg daily is recommended for the first week. Daily dosage should then be maintained at 100 mg per square meter of body surface (to the nearest 50 mg) until leukopenia or thrombocytopenia occurs or maximum response is obtained. Upon evidence of hematologic toxicity the drug should be discontinued until there has been satisfactory recovery. Treatment may then be resumed at 50 mg per day. When maximum response is attained, the dose may be maintained at 50 mg daily.

How Supplied: *Capsules:* containing the equivalent of 50 mg procarbazine as the hydrochloride, ivory; bottles of 100.

[*Shown in Product Identification Section*]

MENRIUM® 5-2 ℞

Each tablet contains 5 mg chlordiazepoxide and 0.2 mg water-soluble esterified estrogens.

MENRIUM® 5-4

Each tablet contains 5 mg chlordiazepoxide and 0.4 mg water-soluble esterified estrogens.

MENRIUM® 10-4

Each tablet contains 10 mg chlordiazepoxide and 0.4 mg water-soluble esterified estrogens.

The following text is complete prescribing information based on official labeling in effect August 1, 1979.

Since estrogens are a component of Menrium, please note:

1. ESTROGENS HAVE BEEN REPORTED TO INCREASE THE RISK OF ENDOMETRIAL CARCINOMA.

Three independent case control studies have shown an increased risk of endometrial cancer in postmenopausal women exposed to exogenous estrogens for prolonged periods.[1–3] This risk was independent of the other known risk factors for endometrial cancer. These studies are further supported by the finding that incidence rates of endometrial cancer have increased sharply since 1969 in eight different areas of the United States with population-based cancer reporting systems, an increase which may be related to the rapidly expanding use of estrogens during the last decade.[4] The three case control studies reported that the risk of endometrial cancer in estrogen users was about 4.5 to 13.9 times greater than in nonusers. The risk appears to depend on both duration of treatment[1] and on estrogen dose.[3] In view of these findings, when estrogens are used for the treatment of menopausal symptoms, the lowest dose that will control symptoms should be utilized and medication should be discontinued as soon as possible. When prolonged treatment is medically indicated, the patient should be reassessed on at least a semiannual basis to determine the need for continued therapy. Although the evidence must be considered preliminary, one study suggests that cyclic administration of low doses of estrogen may carry less risk than continuous administration;[3] it therefore appears prudent to utilize such a regimen.

Close clinical surveillance of all women taking estrogens is important. In all cases of undiagnosed persistent or recurring abnormal vaginal bleeding, adequate diagnostic measures should be undertaken to rule out malignancy.

There is no evidence at present that "natural" estrogens are more or less hazardous than "synthetic" estrogens at equiestrogenic doses.

2. ESTROGENS SHOULD NOT BE USED DURING PREGNANCY

The use of female sex hormones, both estrogens and progestogens, during early pregnancy may seriously damage the offspring. It has been shown that females exposed in utero to diethylstilbestrol, a non-steroidal estrogen, have an increased risk of developing, in later life, a form of vaginal or cervical cancer that is ordinarily extremely rare.[5,6] This risk has been estimated as not greater than 4 per 1000 exposures.[7] Furthermore, a high percentage of such exposed women (from 30 to 90 percent) have been found to have vaginal adenosis,[8–12] epithelial changes of the vagina and cervix. Although these changes are histologically benign, it is not known whether they are precursors of malignancy. Although similar data are not available with the use of other estrogens, it cannot be presumed they would not induce similar changes.

Several reports suggest an association between intrauterine exposure to female sex hormones and congenital anomalies, including congenital heart defects and limb reduction defects.[13–16] One case control study[16] estimated a 4.7 fold increased risk of limb reduction defects in infants exposed in utero to sex hormones (oral contraceptives, hormone withdrawal tests for pregnancy, or attempted treatment for threatened abortion). Some of these exposures were very short and involved only a few days of treatment. The data suggest that the risk of limb reduction defects in exposed fetuses is somewhat less than 1 per 1,000. In the past, female sex hormones have been used during pregnancy in an attempt to treat threatened or habitual abortion. There is considerable evidence that estrogens are ineffective for these indications, and there is no evidence from well-controlled studies that progestogens are effective for these uses.

If Menrium is used during pregnancy, or if the patient becomes pregnant while taking this drug, she should be apprised of the potential risks to the fetus, and the advisability of pregnancy continuation.

Description: Menrium affords in a single formulation the psychotropic action of Librium® (chlordiazepoxide/Roche) and hormonal replacement in the form of water-soluble esterified estrogens (expressed in terms of sodium estrone sulfate) to provide comprehensive management of the menopausal syndrome or the climacteric.

Librium (chlordiazepoxide/Roche) is a versatile therapeutic agent of proven value for the relief of anxiety and tension. It is indicated when anxiety, tension or apprehension are significant components of the clinical profile. It is among the safer of the effective psychopharmacologic compounds.

Chlordiazepoxide is 7-chloro-2-methylamino-5-phenyl-3H-1, 4-benzodiazepine 4-oxide. It is a slightly yellow, crystalline material and is insoluble in water. The molecular weight is 299.75.

Water-soluble esterified estrogens provide hormonal replacement in the menopausal patient, the need for which is widely recognized and accepted. Esterified estrogens is a mixture of the sodium salts of the sulfate esters of the estrogenic substances, principally estrone, that are of the type excreted by pregnant mares. It is a white-to buff-colored, amorphous powder, odorless or having a slight, characteristic odor.

Clinical Pharmacology: The estrogenic component of Menrium is water-soluble esterified estrogens—steroidal compounds—which occur naturally. The action of this substance is substantially equal to the action of both conjugated estrogens, also naturally occurring, and synthetic estrogenic substances.

Menopausal changes, such as atrophic changes of the genital tract and breasts due to a slow decline in estrogen secretion, may be reversed by substitution therapy with estrogenic substances.

Estrogens are, in general, completely absorbed following oral administration. Estrogens are detoxified by the liver, and excretion occurs by way of the urine and the feces.

Librium (chlordiazepoxide HCl/Roche) has anti-anxiety and sedative actions. The drug has been studied extensively in many species of animals and these studies are suggestive of action on the limbic system of the brain, which recent evidence indicates is involved in emotional responses. However, the precise mechanism of action in man is not known. The drug blocks EEG arousal from stimulation of the brain stem reticular formation. The mean $\pm$S.E. plasma peak time is 1.4 ($\pm$0.3) hours, and the half-life ranges between 7.1 to 19.8 hours with a mean $\pm$S.E. half-life of 12.0 ($\pm$0.7) hours. After the drug is discontinued, plasma levels are usually at the lowest quantitatively detectable amounts by 48–72 hours. Chlordiazepoxide HCl is excreted in urine with 1% or less unchanged and 12 to 34% recoverable as conjugates.

Indications: Menrium is indicated in the management of the manifestations generally associated with the menopausal syndrome—anxiety and tension, vasomotor complaints and hormonal deficiency states.

MENRIUM HAS NOT BEEN SHOWN TO BE EFFECTIVE FOR ANY PURPOSE DURING PREGNANCY AND ITS USE MAY CAUSE SEVERE HARM TO THE FETUS (SEE BOXED WARNING).

Contraindications: Menrium is contraindicated in patients with known hypersensitivity to chlordiazepoxide and/or esterified estrogens.

Estrogens should not be used in women (or men) with any of the following conditions:

1. Known or suspected cancer of the breast except in appropriately selected patients being treated for metastatic disease.
2. Known or suspected estrogen-dependent neoplasia.
3. Known or suspected pregnancy. (See Boxed Warning.)
4. Undiagnosed abnormal genital bleeding.
5. Active thrombophlebitis or thromboembolic disorders.
6. A past history of thrombophlebitis, thrombosis, or thromboembolic disorders associated with previous estrogen use.

Warnings:

1. *Induction of malignant neoplasms.* Long term continuous administration of natural and synthetic estrogens in certain animal species increases the frequency of carcinomas of the breast, cervix, vagina, and liver. There is now evidence that estrogens increase the risk of carcinoma of the endometrium in humans. (See Boxed Warning.)

Continued on next page

Roche—Cont.

At the present time there is no satisfactory evidence that estrogens given to postmenopausal women increase the risk of cancer of the breast,[17] although a recent long-term followup of a single physician's practice has raised this possibility.[18] Because of the animal data, there is a need for caution in prescribing estrogens for women with a strong family history of breast cancer or who have breast nodules, fibrocystic disease, or abnormal mammograms.

2. *Gall bladder disease.* A recent study has reported a 2- to 3-fold increase in the risk of surgically confirmed gall bladder disease in women receiving postmenopausal estrogens,[17] similar to the 2-fold increase previously noted in users of oral contraceptives.[19,24] In the case of oral contraceptives the increased risk appeared after two years of use.[24]

3. *Effects similar to those caused by estrogen-progestogen oral contraceptives.* There are several serious adverse effects of oral contraceptives, most of which have not, up to now, been documented as consequences of postmenopausal estrogen therapy. This may reflect the comparatively low doses of estrogen used in postmenopausal women. It would be expected that the larger doses of estrogen used to treat prostatic or breast cancer or postpartum breast engorgement are more likely to result in these adverse effects, and, in fact, it has been shown that there is an increased risk of thrombosis in men receiving estrogens for prostatic cancer and women for postpartum breast engorgement.[20–23]

a. *Thromboembolic disease.* It is now well established that users of oral contraceptives have an increased risk of various thromboembolic and thrombotic vascular diseases, such as thrombophlebitis, pulmonary embolism, stroke, and myocardial infarction.[24–31] Cases of retinal thrombosis, mesenteric thrombosis, and optic neuritis have been reported in oral contraceptive users. There is evidence that the risk of several of these adverse reactions is related to the dose of the drug.[32,33] An increased risk of postsurgery thromboembolic complications has also been reported in users of oral contraceptives.[34,35] If feasible, estrogen should be discontinued at least 4 weeks before surgery of the type associated with an increased risk of thromboembolism, or during periods of prolonged immobilization.

While an increased rate of thromboembolic and thrombotic disease in postmenopausal users of estrogens has not been found,[17,36] this does not rule out the possibility that such an increase may be present or that subgroups of women who have underlying risk factors or who are receiving relatively large doses of estrogens may have increased risk. Therefore, estrogens should not be used in persons with active thrombophlebitis or thromboembolic disorders, and they should not be used in persons with a history of such disorders in association with estrogen use. They should be used with caution in patients with cerebral vascular or coronary artery disease and only for those in whom estrogens are clearly needed.

Large doses of estrogen (5 mg conjugated estrogens per day), comparable to those used to treat cancer of the prostate and breast, have been shown in a large prospective clinical trial in men[37] to increase the risk of nonfatal myocardial infarction, pulmonary embolism and thrombophlebitis. When estrogen doses of this size are used, any of the thromboembolic and thrombotic adverse effects associated with oral contraceptive use should be considered a clear risk.

b. *Hepatic adenoma.* Benign hepatic adenomas appear to be associated with the use of oral contraceptives.[38–40] Although benign, and rare, these may rupture and may cause death through intra-abdominal hemorrhage. Such lesions have not yet been reported in association with other estrogen or progestogen preparations but should be considered in estrogen users having abdominal pain and tenderness, abdominal mass, or hypovolemic shock. Hepatocellular carcinoma has also been reported in women taking estrogen-containing oral contraceptives.[39] The relationship of this malignancy to these drugs is not known at this time.

c. *Elevated blood pressure.* Increased blood pressure is not uncommon in women using oral contraceptives. There is now a report that this may occur with the use of estrogens in the menopause[41] and blood pressure should be monitored with estrogen use, especially if high doses are used.

d. *Glucose tolerance.* A worsening of glucose tolerance has been observed in a significant percentage of patients on estrogen-containing oral contraceptives. For this reason, diabetic patients should be carefully observed while receiving estrogen.

4. *Hypercalcemia.* Administration of estrogens may lead to severe hypercalcemia in patients with breast cancer and bone metastases. If this occurs, the drug should be stopped and appropriate measures taken to reduce the serum calcium level.

As in the case of other preparations containing CNS-acting drugs, patients receiving Menrium should be cautioned about possible combined effects with alcohol and other CNS depressants. Other causes of manifestations of the menopausal syndrome, such as pregnancy, should be excluded. As is true of all preparations containing CNS-acting drugs, patients receiving Menrium should be cautioned against hazardous occupations requiring complete mental alertness such as operating machinery or driving a motor vehicle.

Physical and Psychological Dependence: Withdrawal symptoms have not been observed in more than 1300 subjects during clinical trials with Menrium. Physical and psychological dependence have rarely been reported in persons taking recommended doses of Librium. However, caution must be exercised in administering Librium to individuals known to be addiction-prone or those whose history suggests they may increase the dosage on their own initiative. Withdrawal symptoms following discontinuation of chlordiazepoxide hydrochloride have been reported. These symptoms (including convulsions) are similar to those seen with barbiturates.

Precautions:

A. General Precautions.

1. A complete medical and family history should be taken prior to the initiation of any estrogen therapy. The pretreatment and periodic physical examinations should include special reference to blood pressure, breasts, abdomen, and pelvic organs, and should include a Papanicolaou smear. As a general rule, estrogen should not be prescribed for longer than one year without another physical examination being performed.
2. Fluid retention—Because estrogens may cause some degree of fluid retention, conditions which might be influenced by this factor such as epilepsy, migraine, and cardiac or renal dysfunction, require careful observation.
3. Certain patients may develop undesirable manifestations of excessive estrogenic stimulation, such as abnormal or excessive uterine bleeding, mastodynia, etc.
4. Oral contraceptives appear to be associated with an increased incidence of mental depression.[24] Although it is not clear whether this is due to the estrogenic or progestogenic component of the contraceptive, patients with a history of depression should be carefully observed.
5. Preexisting uterine leiomyomata may increase in size during estrogen use.
6. The pathologist should be advised of estrogen therapy when relevant specimens are submitted.
7. Patients with a past history of jaundice during pregnancy have an increased risk of recurrence of jaundice while receiving estrogen-containing oral contraceptive therapy. If jaundice develops in any patient receiving estrogen, the medication should be discontinued while the cause is investigated.
8. Estrogens may be poorly metabolized in patients with impaired liver function and they should be administered with caution in such patients.
9. Because estrogens influence the metabolism of calcium and phosphorus, they should be used with caution in patients with metabolic bone diseases that are associated with hypercalcemia or in patients with renal insufficiency.
10. Because of the effects of estrogens on epiphyseal closure, they should be used judiciously in young patients in whom bone growth is not complete.
11. Certain endocrine and liver function tests may be affected by estrogen-containing oral contraceptives. The following similar changes may be expected with larger doses of estrogen:

a. Increased sulfobromophthalein retention.
b. Increased prothrombin and factors VII, VIII, IX, and X; decreased antithrombin 3; increased norepinephrine-induced platelet aggregability.
c. Increased thyroid binding globulin (TBG) leading to increased circulating total thyroid hormone, as measured by PBI, T4 by column, or T4 by radioimmunoassay. Free T3 resin uptake is decreased, reflecting the elevated TBG; free T4 concentration is unaltered.
d. Impaired glucose tolerance.
e. Decreased pregnanediol excretion.
f. Reduced response to metyrapone test.
g. Reduced serum folate concentration.
h. Increased serum triglyceride and phospholipid concentration.

B. Information for the Patient.

See Text of Patient Package Insert which follows below.

WHAT YOU SHOULD KNOW ABOUT ESTROGENS

Estrogens are female hormones produced by the ovaries. The ovaries make several different kinds of estrogens. In addition, scientists have been able to make a variety of synthetic estrogens. As far as we know, all these estrogens have similar properties and therefore much the same usefulness, side effects, and risks. This leaflet is intended to help you understand what estrogens are used for, the risks involved in their use, and how to use them as safely as possible.

This leaflet includes the most important information about estrogens, but not all the information. If you want to know more, you can ask your doctor or pharmacist to let you read the package insert prepared for the doctor.

Uses of Estrogen: Estrogens are prescribed by doctors for a number of purposes, including:

1. To provide estrogen during a period of adjustment when a woman's ovaries no longer produce it, in order to prevent certain uncomfortable symptoms of estrogen deficiency. (All women normally stop producing estrogens, generally between the ages of 45 and 55; this is called the menopause.)
2. To prevent symptoms of estrogen deficiency when a woman's ovaries have been removed surgically before the natural menopause.
3. To prevent pregnancy. (Estrogens are given along with a progestogen, another female hormone; these combinations are called oral contraceptives or birth control pills. Patient labeling is available to women taking oral contraceptives and they will not be discussed in this leaflet.)
4. To treat certain cancers in women and men.

5. To prevent painful swelling of the breasts after pregnancy in women who choose not to nurse their babies.

THERE IS NO PROPER USE OF ESTROGENS IN A PREGNANT WOMAN.

Estrogens in The Menopause: In the natural course of their lives, all women eventually experience a decrease in estrogen production. This usually occurs between ages 45 and 55 but may occur earlier or later. Sometimes the ovaries may need to be removed before natural menopause by an operation, producing a "surgical menopause."

When the amount of estrogen in the blood begins to decrease, many women may develop typical symptoms: Feelings of warmth in the face, neck, and chest or sudden intense episodes of heat and sweating throughout the body (called "hot flashes" or "hot flushes"). These symptoms are sometimes very uncomfortable. A few women eventually develop changes in the vagina (called "atrophic vaginitis") which cause discomfort, especially during and after intercourse.

Estrogens can be prescribed to treat these symptoms of the menopause. It is estimated that considerably more than half of all women undergoing the menopause have only mild symptoms or no symptoms at all and therefore do not need estrogens. Other woman may need estrogens for a few months, while their bodies adjust to lower estrogen levels. Sometimes the need will be for periods longer than six months. In an attempt to avoid overstimulation of the uterus (womb), estrogens are usually given cyclically during each month of use, that is three weeks of pills followed by one week without pills.

Sometimes women experience nervous symptoms or depression during menopause. There is no evidence that estrogens are effective for such symptoms and they should not be used to treat them, although other treatment may be needed.

You may have heard that taking estrogens for long periods (years) after the menopause will keep your skin soft and supple and keep you feeling young. There is no evidence that this is so, however, and such long-term treatment carries important risks.

Estrogens To Prevent Swelling of The Breasts After Pregnancy: If you do not breast feed your baby after delivery, your breasts may fill up with milk and become painful and engorged. This usually begins about 3 to 4 days after delivery and may last for a few days to up to a week or more. Sometimes the discomfort is severe, but usually it is not and can be controlled by pain relieving drugs such as aspirin and by binding the breasts up tightly. Estrogens can be used to try to prevent the breasts from filling up. While this treatment is sometimes successful, in many cases the breasts fill up to some degree in spite of treatment. The dose of estrogens needed to prevent pain and swelling of the breasts is much larger than the dose needed to treat symptoms of the menopause and this may increase your chances of developing blood clots in the legs or lungs (see below). Therefore, it is important that you discuss the benefits and the risks of estrogen use with your doctor if you have decided not to breast feed your baby.

The Dangers of Estrogens:

1. *Cancer of the uterus.* If estrogens are used in the postmenopausal period for more than a year, there is an increased risk of *endometrial cancer* (cancer of the uterus). Women taking estrogens have roughly 5 to 10 times as great a chance of getting this cancer as women who take no estrogens. To put this another way, while a postmenopausal woman not taking estrogens has 1 chance in 1,000 each year of getting cancer of the uterus, a woman taking estrogens has 5 to 10 chances in 1,000 each year. For this reason *it is important to take estrogens only when you really need them.* The risk of this cancer is greater the longer estrogens are used and also seems to be greater when larger doses are taken. For this reason *it is important to take the lowest dose of estrogen that will control symptoms and to take it only as long as it is needed.* If estrogens are needed for longer periods of time, your doctor will want to reevaluate your need for estrogens at least every six months.

Women using estrogens should report any irregular vaginal bleeding to their doctors; such bleeding may be of no importance, but it can be an early warning of cancer of the uterus. If you have undiagnosed vaginal bleeding, you should not use estrogens until a diagnosis is made and you are certain there is no cancer of the uterus. If you have had your uterus completely removed (total hysterectomy), there is no danger of developing cancer of the uterus.

2. *Other possible cancers.* Estrogens can cause development of other tumors in animals, such as tumors of the breast, cervix, vagina, or liver, when given for a long time. At present there is no good evidence that women using estrogen in the menopause have an increased risk of such tumors, but there is no way yet to be sure they do not; and one study raises the possibility that use of estrogens in the menopause may increase the risk of breast cancer many years later. This is a further reason to use estrogens only when clearly needed. While you are taking estrogens, it is important that you go to your doctor at least once a year for a physical examination. Also, if members of your family have had breast cancer or if you have breast nodules or abnormal mammograms (breast x-rays), your doctor may wish to carry out more frequent examinations of your breasts.

3. *Gall bladder disease.* Women who use estrogens after menopause are more likely to develop gall bladder disease needing surgery as women who do not use estrogens. Birth control pills have a similar effect.

4. *Abnormal blood clotting.* Oral contraceptives increase the risk of blood clotting in various parts of the body. This can result in a stroke (if the clot is in the brain), a heart attack (clot in a blood vessel of the heart), or a pulmonary embolus (a clot which forms in the legs or pelvis, then breaks off and travels to the lungs). Any of these can be fatal.

At this time use of estrogens in the menopause is not known to cause such blood clotting, but this has not been fully studied and there could still prove to be such a risk. It is recommended that if you have had clotting in the legs or lungs or a heart attack or stroke while you were using estrogens or birth control pills, you should not use estrogens (unless they are being used to treat cancer of the breast or prostate). If you have had a stroke or heart attack or if you have angina pectoris, estrogens should be used with great caution and only if clearly needed (for example, if you have severe symptoms of the menopause).

The larger doses of estrogen used to prevent swelling of the breasts after pregnancy have been reported to cause clotting in the legs and lungs.

Special Warning About Pregnancy: You should not receive estrogen if you are pregnant. If this should occur, there is a greater than usual chance that the developing child will be born with a birth defect, although the possibility remains fairly small. A female child may have an increased risk of developing cancer of the vagina or cervix later in life (in the teens or twenties). Every possible effort should be made to avoid exposure to estrogens during pregnancy. If exposure occurs, see your doctor.

Other Effects of Estrogens: In addition to the serious known risks of estrogens described above, estrogens have the following side effects and potential risks:

1. *Nausea and vomiting.* The most common side effect of estrogen therapy is nausea. Vomiting is less common.

2. *Effects on breasts.* Estrogens may cause breast tenderness or enlargement and may cause the breasts to secrete a liquid. These effects are not dangerous.

3. *Effects on the uterus.* Estrogens may cause benign fibroid tumors of the uterus to get larger.

Some women will have menstrual bleeding when estrogens are stopped. But if the bleeding occurs on days you are still taking estrogens you should report this to your doctor.

4. *Effects on liver.* Women taking oral contraceptives develop on rare occasions a tumor of the liver which can rupture and bleed into the abdomen. So far, these tumors have not been reported in women using estrogens in the menopause, but you should report any swelling or unusual pain or tenderness in the abdomen to your doctor immediately.

Women with a past history of jaundice (yellowing of the skin and white parts of the eyes) may get jaundice again during estrogen use. If this occurs, stop taking estrogens and see your doctor.

5. *Other effects.* Estrogens may cause excess fluid to be retained in the body. This may make some conditions worse, such as epilepsy, migraine, heart disease, or kidney disease.

Summary: Estrogens have important uses, but they have serious risks as well. You must decide, with your doctor, whether the risks are acceptable to you in view of the benefits of treatment. Except where your doctor has prescribed estrogens for use in special cases of cancer of the breast or prostate, you should not use estrogens if you have cancer of the breast or uterus, are pregnant, have undiagnosed abnormal vaginal bleeding, clotting in the legs or lungs, or have had a stroke, heart attack or angina, or clotting in the legs or lungs in the past while you were taking estrogens.

You can use estrogens as safely as possible by understanding that your doctor will require regular physical examinations while you are taking them and will try to discontinue the drug as soon as possible and use the smallest dose possible. Be alert for signs of trouble including:

1. Abnormal bleeding from the vagina.
2. Pains in the calves or chest or sudden shortness of breath, or coughing blood (indicating possible clots in the legs, heart, or lungs).
3. Severe headache, dizziness, faintness, or changes in vision (indicating possible developing clots in the brain or eye).
4. Breast lumps (you should ask your doctor how to examine your own breasts).
5. Jaundice (yellowing of the skin).
6. Mental depression.

Based on his or her assessment of your medical needs, your doctor has prescribed this drug for you. Do not give the drug to anyone else.

C. Pregnancy: See Contraindications and Box Warning.

D. Nursing Mothers: As a general principle, the administration of any drug to nursing mothers should be done only when clearly necessary since many drugs are excreted in human milk.

In elderly and debilitated patients, it is recommended that the dosage be limited to the smallest effective amount to preclude the development of ataxia or oversedation (10 mg chlordiazepoxide or less per day initially, to be increased gradually as needed and tolerated). In general, the concomitant administration of Menrium and other psychotropic agents is not recommended. If such combination therapy seems indicated, careful consideration should be given to the pharmacology of the agents to be employed—particularly when the known potentiating compounds such as the MAO inhibitors and phenothiazines are to be used. The usual precautions in treating patients with

Continued on next page

Roche—Cont.

impaired renal or hepatic function should be observed.
Paradoxical reactions to chlordiazepoxide, e.g., excitement, stimulation and acute rage, have been reported in psychiatric patients and should be watched for during Menrium therapy. The usual precautions are indicated when chlordiazepoxide is used in the treatment of anxiety states where there is any evidence of impending depression; it should be borne in mind that suicidal tendencies may be present and protective measures may be necessary. Although clinical studies have not established a cause and effect relationship, physicians should be aware that variable effects on blood coagulation have been reported very rarely in patients receiving oral anticoagulants and Librium.
Adverse Reactions: No side effects or manifestations not seen with either compound alone have been reported with the administration of Menrium. However, since Menrium contains chlordiazepoxide and water-soluble esterified estrogens, the possibility of untoward effects which may be seen with either of these two compounds cannot be excluded.
(See Warnings regarding induction of neoplasia, adverse effects on the fetus, increased incidence of gall bladder disease, and adverse effects similar to those of oral contraceptives, including thromboembolism.) The following additional adverse reactions have been reported with estrogenic therapy, including oral contraceptives:
1. *Genitourinary system.*
Breakthrough bleeding, spotting, change in menstrual flow.
Dysmenorrhea.
Premenstrual-like syndrome.
Amenorrhea during and after treatment.
Increase in size of uterine fibromyomata.
Vaginal candidiasis.
Change in cervical eversion and in degree of cervical secretion.
Cystitis-like syndrome.
2. *Breasts.*
Tenderness, enlargement, secretion.
3. *Gastrointestinal.*
Nausea, vomiting.
Abdominal cramps, bloating.
Cholestatic jaundice.
4. *Skin.*
Chloasma or melasma which may persist when drug is discontinued.
Erythema multiforme.
Erythema nodosum.
Hemorrhagic eruption.
Loss of scalp hair.
Hirsutism.
5. *Eyes.*
Steepening of corneal curvature.
Intolerance to contact lenses.
6. *CNS.*
Headache, migraine, dizziness.
Mental depression.
Chorea.
7. *Miscellaneous.*
Increase or decrease in weight.
Reduced carbohydrate tolerance.
Aggravation of porphyria.
Edema.
Changes in libido.
When chlordiazepoxide has been used alone the necessity of discontinuing therapy because of undesirable effects has been rare. Drowsiness, ataxia and confusion have been reported in some patients—particularly the elderly and debilitated. While these effects can be avoided in almost all instances by proper dosage adjustment, they have occasionally been observed at the lower dosage ranges. In a few instances syncope has been reported.
Other adverse reactions reported during therapy include isolated instances of skin eruptions, edema, minor menstrual irregularities, nausea and constipation, extrapyramidal symptoms, as well as increased and decreased libido. Such side effects have been infrequent and are generally controlled with reduction of dosage. Changes in EEG patterns (low-voltage fast activity) have been observed in patients during and after Librium treatment.
Blood dyscrasias, including agranulocytosis, jaundice and hepatic dysfunction have occasionally been reported during therapy. When Librium treatment is protracted, periodic blood counts and liver function tests are advisable.
Management of Overdosage: Numerous reports of ingestion of large doses of estrogen-containing oral contraceptives by young children indicate that serious ill effects do not occur. Overdosage of estrogen may cause nausea, and withdrawal bleeding may occur in females. Manifestations of Librium overdosage include somnolence, confusion, coma and diminished reflexes. Respiration, pulse and blood pressure should be monitored, as in all cases of drug overdosage, although, in general, these effects have been minimal following Librium overdosage. General supportive measures should be employed, along with immediate gastric lavage. Intravenous fluids should be administered and an adequate airway maintained. Hypotension may be combated by the use of Levophed® (levarterenol) or Aramine (metaraminol). Ritalin (methylphenidate) or caffeine and sodium benzoate may be given to combat CNS-depressive effects. Dialysis is of limited value. There have been occasional reports of excitation in patients following chlordiazepoxide overdosage; if this occurs barbiturates should not be used. As with the management of intentional overdosage with any drug, it should be borne in mind that multiple agents may have been ingested.
Dosage: The lowest dose that will control symptoms should be chosen and medication should be discontinued as promptly as possible.
MENRIUM 5-2—for the majority of patients with the menopausal syndrome or the climacteric having anxiety and tension and hormonal deficiency states requiring estrogen replacement—One tablet, t.i.d.
MENRIUM 5-4—for patients with the menopausal syndrome or the climacteric with anxiety and tension and more severe vasomotor manifestations—One tablet, t.i.d.
MENRIUM 10-4—for patients with the menopausal syndrome or the climacteric with pronounced anxiety and tension and marked vasomotor complaints—One tablet, t.i.d.
Therapy should be continued for 21-day courses, followed by one-week rest periods. While these dosage schedules will prove generally satisfactory, individual adjustment of dosage is desirable, since some patients may obtain satisfactory relief with as little as one tablet daily of Menrium 5-2.
Treated patients with an intact uterus should be monitored closely for signs of endometrial cancer and appropriate diagnostic measures should be taken to rule out malignancy in the event of persistent or recurring abnormal vaginal bleeding.
How Supplied: Menrium 5-2, light green tablets—each tablet contains 5 mg chlordiazepoxide and 0.2 mg water-soluble esterified estrogens—bottles of 100; Menrium 5-4, dark green tablets—each tablet contains 5 mg chlordiazepoxide and 0.4 mg water-soluble esterified estrogens—bottles of 100; Menrium 10-4, purple tablets—each tablet contains 10 mg chlordiazepoxide and 0.4 mg water-soluble esterified estrogens—bottles of 100.

Physician References:

1. Ziel HK, Finkel WD: *N Engl J Med 293*:1167–1170, 1975
2. Smith DC, *et al: N Engl J Med 293*:1164–1167, 1975
3. Mack TM, *et al: N Engl J Med 294*:1262–1267, 1976
4. Weiss NS, Szekely DR, Austin DF: *N Engl J Med 294*:1259–1262, 1976
5. Herbst AL, Ulfelder H, Poskanzer DC: *N Engl J Med 284*:878–881, 1971
6. Greenwald P, *et al: N Engl J Med 285*:390–392, 1971
7. Lanier A, *et al: Mayo Clin Proc 48*:793–799, 1973
8. Herbst A, Kurman R, Scully R: *Obstet Gynecol 40*:287–298, 1972
9. Herbst A, *et al: Am J Obstet Gynecol 118*:607–615, 1974
10. Herbst, A, *et al: N Engl J Med 292*:334–339, 1975
11. Stafl A, *et al: Obstet Gyncecol 43*:118–128, 1974
12. Sherman AI, *et al: Obstet Gynecol 44*:531–545, 1974
13. Gal I, Kirman B, Stern J: *Nature 216*:83, 1967
14. Levy EP, Cohen A, Fraser FC: *Lancet 1*:611, 1973
15. Nora J, Nora A: *Lancet 1*:941–942, 1973
16. Janerich DT, Piper JM, Glebatis DM: *N Engl J Med 291*:697–700, 1974
17. Boston Collaborative Drug Surveillance Program: *N Engl J Med 290*:15–19, 1974
18. Hoover R, *et al: N Engl J Med 295*:401–405, 1976
19. Boston Collaborative Drug Surveillance Program: *Lancet 1*:1399–1404, 1973
20. Daniel DG, Campbell H, Turnbull AC: *Lancet 2*:287–289, 1967
21. The Veterans Administration Cooperative Urological Research Group: *J Urol 98*:516–522, 1967
22. Bailar JC: *Lancet 2*:560, 1967
23. Blackard C, *et al: Cancer 26*:249–256, 1970
24. Royal College of General Practitioners: *J Coll Gen Pract 13*:267–279, 1967
25. Inman WHW, Vessey MP: *Br Med J 2*:193–199, 1968
26. Vessey MP, Doll R: *Br Med J 2*:651–657, 1969
27. Sartwell PE, *et al: Am J Epidemiol 90*:365–380, 1969
28. Collaborative Group for the Study of Stroke in Young Women: *N Engl J Med 288*:871–878, 1973
29. Collaborative Group for the Study of Stroke in Young Women: *JAMA 231*:718–722, 1975
30. Mann JI, Inman WHW: *Br Med J 2*:245–248, 1975
31. Mann JI, *et al: Br Med J 2*:241–245, 1975
32. Inman WHW, *et al: Br Med J 2*:203–209, 1970
33. Stolley PD, *et al: Am J Epidemiol 102*:197–208, 1975
34. Vessey MP, *et al: Br Med J 3*:123–126, 1970
35. Greene GR, Sartwell PE: *Am J Public Health 62*:680–685, 1972
36. Rosenberg L, Armstrong MB, Jick H: *N Engl J Med 294*:1256–1259, 1976
37. Coronary Drug Project Research Group: *JAMA 214*:1303–1313, 1970
38. Baum J, *et al: Lancet 2*:926–928, 1973
39. Mays ET, *et al: JAMA 235*:730–732, 1976
40. Edmondson HA, Henderson B, Benton B: *N Engl J Med 294*:470–472, 1976
41. Pfeffer RI, Van Den Noort S: *Am J Epidemiol 103*:445–456, 1976

[*Shown in Product Identification Section*]

MESTINON® INJECTABLE ℞
(pyridostigmine bromide/Roche)

The following text is complete prescribing information based on official labeling in effect August 1, 1979.
Description: Mestinon Injectable is an active cholinesterase inhibitor. Chemically, pyridostigmine bromide is 3-hydroxy-1-methylpyridinium bromide dimethylcarbamate.
Each ml contains 5 mg pyridostigmine bromide/Roche compounded with 0.2% parabens (methyl and propyl) as preservatives, 0.02% sodium citrate and pH adjusted to approxi-

mately 5.0 with citric acid and, if necessary, sodium hydroxide.

Actions: Mestinon facilitates the transmission of impulses across the myoneural junction by inhibiting the destruction of acetylcholine by cholinesterase. Pyridostigmine is an analog of neostigmine (Prostigmin®) but differs from it clinically by having fewer side effects. Currently available data indicate that pyridostigmine may have a significantly lower degree and incidence of bradycardia, salivation and gastrointestinal stimulation. Animal studies using the injectable form of pyridostigmine and human studies using the oral preparation have indicated that pyridostigmine has a longer duration of action than does neostigmine measured under similar circumstances.

Indications: Mestinon Injectable is useful in the treatment of myasthenia gravis and as a reversal agent or antagonist to nondepolarizing muscle relaxants such as curariform drugs and gallamine triethiodide.

Contraindications: Known hypersensitivity to anticholinesterase agents; intestinal and urinary obstructions of mechanical type.

Warnings: Mestinon Injectable should be used with particular caution in patients with bronchial asthma or cardiac dysrhythmias. Transient bradycardia may occur and be relieved by atropine sulfate. Atropine should also be used with caution in patients with cardiac dysrhythmias. When large doses of Mestinon are administered, as during reversal of muscle relaxants, the prior or simultaneous injection of atropine sulfate is advisable. Because of the possibility of hypersensitivity in an occasional patient, atropine and antishock medication should always be readily available.

As is true of all cholinergic drugs, overdosage of Mestinon may result in cholinergic crisis, a state characterized by increasing muscle weakness which, through involvement of the muscles of respiration, may lead to death. Myasthenic crisis due to an increase in the severity of the disease is also accompanied by extreme muscle weakness and thus may be difficult to distinguish from cholinergic crisis on a symptomatic basis. Such differentiation is extremely important, since increases in doses of Mestinon or other drugs in this class in the presence of cholinergic crisis or of a refractory or "insensitive" state could have grave consequences. Osserman and Genkins[1] indicate that the two types of crisis may be differentiated by the use of Tensilon® (edrophonium chloride) as well as by clinical judgment. The treatment of the two conditions obviously differs radically. Whereas the presence of *myasthenic crisis* requires more intensive anticholinesterase therapy, *cholinergic crisis,* according to Osserman and Genkins,[1] calls for the prompt withdrawal of all drugs of this type. The immediate use of atropine in cholinergic crisis is also recommended. A syringe containing 1 mg of atropine sulfate should be immediately available to be given in aliquots intravenously to counteract severe cholinergic reactions.

Atropine may also be used to abolish or obtund gastrointestinal side effects or other muscarinic reactions; but such use, by masking signs of overdosage, can lead to inadvertent induction of cholinergic crisis.

For detailed information on the management of patients with myasthenia gravis, the physician is referred to one of the excellent reviews such as those by Osserman and Genkins,[2] Grob[3] or Schwab.[4,5]

When used as an antagonist to nondepolarizing muscle relaxants, adequate recovery of voluntary respiration and neuromuscular transmission must be obtained prior to discontinuation of respiratory assistance and there should be continuous patient observation. Satisfactory recovery may be defined by a combination of clinical judgment, respiratory measurements and observation of the effects of peripheral nerve stimulation. If there is any doubt concerning the adequacy of recovery from the effects of the nondepolarizing muscle relaxant, artificial ventilation should be continued until all doubt has been removed.

Usage in Pregnancy: The safety of Mestinon during pregnancy or lactation in humans has not been established. Therefore, use of Mestinon in women who may become pregnant requires weighing the drug's potential benefits against its possible hazards to mother and child.

Adverse Reactions: The side effects of Mestinon are most commonly related to overdosage and generally are of two varieties, muscarinic and nicotinic. Among those in the former group are nausea, vomiting, diarrhea, abdominal cramps, increased peristalsis, increased salivation, increased bronchial secretions, miosis and diaphoresis. Nicotinic side effects are comprised chiefly of muscle cramps, fasciculation and weakness. Muscarinic side effects can usually be counteracted by atropine, but for reasons shown in the preceding section the expedient is not without danger. As with any compound containing the bromide radical, a skin rash may be seen in an occasional patient. Such reactions usually subside promptly upon discontinuance of the medication. Thrombophlebitis has been reported subsequent to intravenous administration.

Dosage and Administration:

For Myasthenia Gravis—To supplement oral dosage, pre- and postoperatively, during labor and postpartum, during myasthenic crisis, or whenever oral therapy is impractical, approximately 1/30th of the oral dose of Mestinon may be given parenterally, either by intramuscular or *very slow* intravenous injection. *The patient must be closely observed for cholinergic reactions, particularly if the intravenous route is used.*

For details regarding the management of myasthenic patients who are to undergo major surgical procedures, see the article by Foldes.[6]

Neonates of myasthenic mothers may have transient difficulty in swallowing, sucking and breathing. Injectable Mestinon may be indicated—by symptomatology and use of the Tensilon® (edrophonium chloride) test—until Mestinon Syrup can be taken. To date the world literature consists of less than 100 neonate patients.[7] Of these only 5 were treated with injectable pyridostigmine, with the vast majority of the remaining neonates receiving neostigmine. Dosage requirements of Mestinon Injectable are minute, ranging from 0.05 mg to 0.15 mg/kg of body weight given intramuscularly. It is important to differentiate between cholinergic and myasthenic crises in neonates. (See WARNINGS.)

Mestinon given parenterally one hour before completion of second stage labor enables patients to have adequate strength during labor and provides protection to infants in the immediate postnatal state. For further information on the use of Mestinon Injectable in neonates of myasthenic mothers, see the article by Namba.[7]

NOTE: For information on a diagnostic test for myasthenia gravis, and on the evaluation and stabilization of therapy, please see product information on Tensilon® (edrophonium chloride/Roche).

For Reversal of Nondepolarizing Muscle Relaxants: When Mestinon Injectable is given intravenously to reverse the action of muscle relaxant drugs, it is recommended that atropine sulfate (0.6 to 1.2 mg) also be given intravenously immediately prior to the Mestinon. Side effects, notably excessive secretions and bradycardia, are thereby minimized. Usually 10 or 20 mg of Mestinon will be sufficient for antagonism of the effects of the nondepolarizing muscle relaxants. Although full recovery may occur within 15 minutes in most patients, others may require a half hour or more. Satisfactory reversal can be evident by adequate voluntary respiration, respiratory measurements and use of a peripheral nerve stimulator device. It is recommended that the patient be well ventilated and a patent airway maintained until complete recovery of normal respiration is assured. Once satisfactory reversal has been attained, recurarization has not been reported. For additional information on the use of Mestinon for antagonism of nondepolarizing muscle relaxants see the article by Katz[8] and McNall.[9]

Failure of Mestinon Injectable to provide prompt (within 30 minutes) reversal may occur, *e.g.,* in the presence of extreme debilitation, carcinomatosis, or with concomitant use of certain broad spectrum antibiotics or anesthetic agents, notably ether. Under these circumstances ventilation must be supported by artificial means until the patient has resumed control of his respiration.

How Supplied: Mestinon is available in 2-ml ampuls (boxes of 10).

References:

1. K. E. Osserman and G. Genkins, *J.A.M.A. 183:*97, 1963.
2. K. E. Osserman and G. Genkins, *New York State J. Med., 61:*2076, 1961.
3. D. Grob, *Arch. Intern. Med., 108:*615, 1961.
4. R. S. Schwab, *New Eng. J. Med., 268:*596, 1963.
5. R. S. Schwab, *New Eng. J. Med., 268:*717, 1963.
6. F. F. Foldes and P. McNall, *Anesthesiology, 23:*837, 1962.
7. T. Namba *et al., Pediatrics, 45:*488, 1970.
8. R. L. Katz, *Anesthesiology, 28:*528, 1967.
9. P. McNall *et al., Anesthesia and Analgesia, 48:*1026, 1969.

MESTINON® ℞

(pyridostigmine bromide/Roche)
TABLETS and SYRUP
TIMESPAN® TABLETS

The following text is complete prescribing information based on official labeling in effect August 1, 1979.

Description: Mestinon is an orally active cholinesterase inhibitor. Chemically, pyridostigmine bromide is 3-hydroxy-1-methylpyridinium bromide dimethylcarbamate.

Actions: Mestinon inhibits the destruction of acetylcholine by cholinesterase and thereby permits freer transmission of nerve impulses across the neuromuscular junction. Pyridostigmine is an analog of neostigmine (Prostigmin®), but differs from it in certain clinically significant respects; for example, pyridostigmine is characterized by a longer duration of action and fewer gastrointestinal side effects.

Indication: Mestinon is useful in the treatment of myasthenia gravis.

Contraindications: Mestinon is contraindicated in mechanical intestinal or urinary obstruction, and particular caution should be used in its administration to patients with bronchial asthma. Care should be observed in the use of atropine for counteracting side effects, as discussed below.

Warnings: Although failure of patients to show clinical improvement may reflect underdosage, it can also be indicative of overdosage. As is true of all cholinergic drugs, overdosage of Mestinon may result in cholinergic crisis, a state characterized by increasing muscle weakness which, through involvement of the muscles of respiration, may lead to death. Myasthenic crisis due to an increase in the severity of the disease is also accompanied by extreme muscle weakness, and thus may be difficult to distinguish from cholinergic crisis on a symptomatic basis. Such differentiation is extremely important, since increases in doses of Mestinon or other drugs of this class in the presence of cholinergic crisis or of a refractory or "insensitive" state could have grave consequences. Osserman and Genkins[1] indicate that the differential diagnosis of the two types of

Continued on next page

Roche—Cont.

crisis may require the use of Tensilon® (edrophonium chloride/Roche) as well as clinical judgment. The treatment of the two conditions obviously differs radically. Whereas the presence of myasthenic crisis suggests the need for more intensive anticholinesterase therapy, the diagnosis of cholinergic crisis, according to Osserman and Genkins,[1] calls for the prompt *withdrawal* of all drugs of this type. The immediate use of atropine in cholinergic crisis is also recommended.

Atropine may also be used to abolish or obtund gastrointestinal side effects or other muscarinic reactions; but such use, by masking signs of overdosage, can lead to inadvertent induction of cholinergic crisis.

For detailed information on the management of patients with myasthenia gravis, the physician is referred to one of the excellent reviews such as those by Osserman and Genkins,[2] Grob[3] or Schwab.[4,5]

Usage in Pregnancy: The safety of Mestinon during pregnancy or lactation in humans has not been established. Therefore, use of Mestinon in women who may become pregnant requires weighing the drug's potential benefits against its possible hazards to mother and child.

Adverse Reactions: The side effects of Mestinon are most commonly related to overdosage and generally are of two varieties, muscarinic and nicotinic. Among those in the former group are nausea, vomiting, diarrhea, abdominal cramps, increased peristalsis, increased salivation, increased bronchial secretions, miosis and diaphoresis. Nicotinic side effects are comprised chiefly of muscle cramps, fasciculation and weakness. Muscarinic side effects can usually be counteracted by atropine, but for reasons shown in the preceding section the expedient is not without danger. As with any compound containing the bromide radical, a skin rash may be seen in an occasional patient. Such reactions usually subside promptly upon discontinuance of the medication.

Dosage and Administration: Mestinon is available in three dosage forms:

Syrup—raspberry-flavored, containing 60 mg pyridostigmine bromide per teaspoonful (5 ml). This form permits accurate dosage adjustment for children and "brittle" myasthenic patients who require fractions of 60-mg doses. It is more easily swallowed, especially in the morning, by patients with bulbar involvement.

Conventional tablets—each containing 60 mg pyridostigmine bromide.

Timespan tablets—each containing 180 mg pyridostigmine bromide. This form provides uniformly slow release, hence prolonged duration of drug action; it facilitates control of myasthenic symptoms with fewer individual doses daily. The immediate effect of a 180-mg Timespan tablet is about equal to that of a 60-mg conventional tablet; however, its duration of effectiveness, although varying in individual patients, averages 2½ times that of a 60-mg dose.

Dosage: The size and frequency of the dosage must be adjusted to the needs of the individual patient.

Syrup and conventional tablets—The average dose is ten 60-mg tablets or ten 5-ml teaspoonfuls daily, spaced to provide maximum relief when maximum strength is needed. In severe cases as many as 25 tablets or teaspoonfuls a day may be required, while in mild cases one to six tablets or teaspoonfuls a day may suffice.

Timespan tablets—One to three 180-mg tablets, once or twice daily, will usually be sufficient to control symptoms; however, the needs of certain individuals may vary markedly from this average. The interval between doses should be at least six hours. For optimum control, it may be necessary to use the more rapidly acting regular tablets or syrup in conjunction with Timespan therapy.

Note: For information on a diagnostic test for myasthenia gravis, and for the evaluation and stabilization of therapy, please see product literature on Tensilon® (edrophonium chloride/Roche).

How Supplied: *Syrup,* 60 mg pyridostigmine bromide per teaspoonful (5 ml) and 5% alcohol—bottles of 16 fluid ounces (1 pint).

Tablets, scored, 60 mg pyridostigmine bromide each—bottles of 100 and 500.

Timespan tablets, scored, 180 mg pyridostigmine bromide each—bottles of 100.

Note: Because of the hygroscopic nature of the Timespan tablets, mottling may occur. This does not affect their efficacy.

References:

1. K. E. Osserman and G. Genkins, *J.A.M.A., 183:*97, 1963.
2. K. E. Osserman and G. Genkins, *New York State J. Med., 61:*2076, 1961.
3. D. Grob, *Arch. Int. Med., 108:*615, 1961.
4. R. S. Schwab, *New England J. Med., 268:*596, 1963.
5. R. S. Schwab, *New England J. Med., 268:*717, 1963.

[*Shown in Product Identification Section*]

NIPRIDE® ℞

(sodium nitroprusside/Roche)

The following text is complete prescribing information based on official labeling in effect August 1, 1979.

Nipride is only to be used as an infusion with sterile 5% dextrose in water. Not for direct injection.
Nipride should be used only when the necessary facilities and equipment for continuous monitoring of blood pressure are available.
If at infusion rates of up to 10 µg/kg/minute, an adequate reduction of blood pressure is not obtained within ten minutes, administration of Nipride should be terminated.
The instructions included herein should be reviewed thoroughly before administration of Nipride.

Description: Nipride (sodium nitroprusside/Roche) in injectable form contains the equivalent of 50 mg of sodium nitroprusside dihydrate (sodium nitrosylpentacyanoferrate [III]) in a 5-ml amber-colored, rubber-stoppered vial. Chemically, sodium nitroprusside is $Na_2Fe(CN)_5NO \cdot 2H_2O$. It is a reddish-brown powder which is soluble in water. In aqueous solution, it is photosensitive and should be protected from light.

Actions: Nipride is a potent, immediate acting, intravenous hypotensive agent. This action is probably due to the nitroso (NO) group. Its effect is almost immediate and ends when the IV infusion is stopped. The brief duration of the drug's action is due to its rapid conversion to thiocyanate. The hypotensive effect is augmented by ganglionic blocking agents, volatile liquid anesthetics (such as halothane and enflurane) and by most other circulatory depressants.

The hypotensive effects of Nipride are caused by peripheral vasodilatation as a result of a direct action on the blood vessels, independent of autonomic innervation. No relaxation is seen in the smooth muscle of the uterus or duodenum *in situ* in animals.

Indications: Nipride is indicated for the immediate reduction of blood pressure of patients in hypertensive crises. Concomitant oral antihypertensive medication should be started while the hypertensive emergency is being brought under control with Nipride. There is no contraindication in using Nipride simultaneously with oral antihypertensive medications.

Nipride is also indicated for producing controlled hypotension during anesthesia in order to reduce bleeding in surgical procedures where surgeon and anesthesiologist deem it appropriate.

Contraindications: Nipride should not be used in the treatment of compensatory hypertension, *e.g.,* arteriovenous shunt or coarctation of the aorta.

The use of Nipride to produce controlled hypotension during surgery is contraindicated in patients with known inadequate cerebral circulation. Nipride is not intended for use during emergency surgery in moribund patients (A.S.A. Risk 5).

Warnings: The following Warnings apply to use of Nipride for controlled hypotension during anesthesia:

1. Tolerance to blood loss, anemia and hypovolemia may be diminished. If possible, preexisting anemia and hypovolemia should be corrected prior to employing controlled hypotension.
2. Hypotensive anesthetic techniques may alter pulmonary ventilation perfusion ratio. Patients intolerant of additional dead air space at ordinary oxygen partial pressure may benefit from higher oxygen partial pressure.
3. Extreme caution should be exercised in patients who are especially poor surgical risks (A.S.A. Class 4 and 4E).

Nipride is only to be used as an infusion with sterile 5% dextrose in water. Not for direct injection.

Infusion rates greater than 10 µg/kg/minute are rarely required. If, at this rate, an adequate reduction in blood pressure is not obtained within 10 minutes, administration of Nipride should be stopped.

Nipride is metabolized to cyanide and then to thiocyanate. If excessive amounts of Nipride are used, thiocyanate toxicity (*e.g.,* tinnitus, blurred vision, delirium) may occur. With gross overdosage, cyanide intoxication is possible (see OVERDOSAGE).

Since cyanide is converted into thiocyanate through the mediation of a hepatic enzyme, rhodanese, Nipride should be used with caution in patients with hepatic insufficiency.

Since thiocyanate inhibits both the uptake and binding of iodine, caution should be exercised in using Nipride in patients with hypothyroidism or severe renal impairment.

Blood levels of thiocyanate should be determined if treatment is to be extended in patients with severe renal dysfunction. Although intravenous infusions of Nipride are not intended for long-term use, as long as blood thiocyanate levels are measured daily and do not exceed 10 mg/100 ml, it is probably safe to continue with the infusion until the patient can be safely treated with oral antihypertensive medications.

Hypertensive patients are more sensitive to the intravenous effect of sodium nitroprusside than are normotensive subjects. Patients who are receiving concomitant antihypertensive medications are more sensitive to the hypotensive effect of sodium nitroprusside and the dosage of Nipride should be adjusted accordingly.

Usage in Pregnancy: The safety of Nipride in women who are or who may become pregnant has not been established; hence, it should be given only when the potential benefits have been weighed against possible hazard to mother and child.

Precautions: Adequate facilities, equipment and personnel should be available for frequent and vigilant monitoring of blood pressure, since the hypotensive effect of Nipride occurs rapidly. When the infusion is slowed or stopped, blood pressure usually begins to rise immediately and returns to pretreatment levels within one to ten minutes. It should be used with caution and initially in low doses in elderly patients, since they may be more sensitive to the hypotensive effects of the drug. Young, vigorous males may require somewhat larger than ordinary doses of sodium nitroprusside for hypotensive anesthesia; however, the infusion rate of 10 μg/kg/minute should not be exceeded. Deepening of anesthesia, if indicated, might permit satisfactory conditions to exist within the recommended dosage range. Because of the rapid onset of action and potency of Nipride, it should preferably be administered with the use of an infusion pump, micro-drip regulator, or any similar device that would allow precise measurement of the flow rate.

Once dissolved in solution, Nipride tends to deteriorate in the presence of light. Therefore, it should be protected from light by wrapping the container of the prepared solution with aluminum foil or other opaque materials. Solutions of Nipride should not be kept or used longer than four hours.

Nipride in aqueous solution yields the nitroprusside ion which reacts with even minute quantities of a wide variety of inorganic and organic substances to form usually highly colored reaction products (blue, green or dark red). If this occurs the infusion should be replaced.

Adverse Reactions: Nausea, retching, diaphoresis, apprehension, headache, restlessness, muscle twitching, retrosternal discomfort, palpitations, dizziness and abdominal pain have been noted with too rapid reduction in blood pressure, but these symptoms rapidly disappeared with slowing of the rate of the infusion or temporary discontinuation of infusion and did not reappear with continued slower rate of administration. Irritation at the infusion site may occur.

One case of hypothyroidism following prolonged therapy with intravenous sodium nitroprusside has been reported. A patient with severe hypertension with uremia received 3900 mg of sodium nitroprusside intravenously over a period of 21 days. This is one of the longest reported intravenous uses of this agent. There was no tachyphylaxis, but the patient developed evidence of hypothyroidism, together with retention of thiocyanate (9.5 mg/100 ml). With peritoneal dialysis the thiocyanate level diminished and the signs of hypothyroidism subsided.

Dosage and Administration: The contents of a 50-mg Nipride vial should be dissolved in 2 to 3 ml of dextrose in water. No other diluent should be used. Depending on the desired concentration, all of the prepared stock solution should be diluted in 250 to 1000 ml of 5 percent dextrose in water and promptly wrapped in aluminum foil or other opaque materials to protect from light. Both the stock solution and the infusion solution should be freshly prepared and any unused portion discarded. The freshly prepared solution for infusion has a very faint brownish tint. If it is highly colored, it should be discarded (see PRECAUTIONS). *Once prepared, the solution should not be kept or used longer than four hours. The infusion fluid used for the administration of Nipride should not be employed as a vehicle for simultaneous administration of any other drug.*

In patients who are not receiving antihypertensive drugs, the average dose of Nipride for both adults and children is 3 μg/kg/minute (range of 0.5 to 10 μg/kg/minute). Usually, at 3 μg/kg/minute, blood pressure can be lowered by about 30 to 40 percent below the pretreatment diastolic levels and maintained. In hypertensive patients receiving concomitant antihypertensive medications, smaller doses are required. In order to avoid excessive levels of thiocyanate and lessen the possibility of a precipitous drop in blood pressure, infusion rates greater than 10 μg/kg/minute should rarely be used. If, at this rate, an adequate reduction of blood pressure is not obtained within 10 minutes, administration of Nipride should be stopped.

1 Vial (50 mg) Nipride in 1000 ml 5% DW (50 μg/ml)
1 Vial (50 mg) Nipride in 500 ml 5% DW (100 μg/ml)
1 Vial (50 mg) Nipride in 250 ml 5% DW (200 μg/ml)

Dose	μg/kg/min
Average	3
Range	0.5 to 10

The intravenous infusion of Nipride should be administered by an infusion pump, micro-drip regulator or any similar device that will allow precise measurement of the flow rate. Care should be taken to avoid extravasation. The rate of administration should be adjusted to maintain the desired antihypertensive or hypotensive effect, as determined by frequent blood pressure determinations. It is recommended that the blood pressure should not be allowed to drop at a too rapid rate and the systolic pressure not be lowered below 60 mmHg. In hypertensive emergencies Nipride infusion may be continued until the patient can safely be treated with oral antihypertensive medications alone.

How Supplied: Nipride injectable is supplied in 5-ml amber-colored vials containing the equivalent of 50 mg sodium nitroprusside dihydrate for reconstitution with dextrose in water—boxes of 1.

Human Pharmacology: Sodium nitroprusside administered intravenously to hypertensive and normotensive patients produced a marked lowering of the arterial blood pressure, slight increase in heart rate, a mild decrease in cardiac output and a moderate diminution in calculated total peripheral vascular resistance.

The decrease in calculated total peripheral vascular resistance suggests arteriolar vasodilatation. The decreases in cardiac and stroke index noted may be due to the peripheral vascular pooling of blood.

In hypertensive patients, moderate depressor doses induce renal vasodilatation roughly equivalent to the decrease in pressure without an appreciable increase in renal blood flow or a decrease in glomerular filtration.

In normotensive subjects, acute reduction of mean arterial pressure to 60 to 75 mmHg by infusion of sodium nitroprusside caused a significant increase in renin activity of renal venous plasma in correlation with the degree of reduction in pressure. Renal response to reduction in pressure was more striking in renovascular hypertensive patients, with significant increase in renin release occurring from the involved kidney at mean arterial pressures ranging from 90 to 137 mmHg. Furthermore, the magnitude of renin release from the involved kidney was significantly greater when compared with that in normotensive subjects, while in the contralateral, uninvolved kidney, no significant release of renin was detected during the reduction of pressure.

Overdosage: The first signs of sodium nitroprusside overdosage are those of profound hypotension. Metabolic acidosis may be an early indication of this overdosage. This may be associated with or followed by dyspnea, headache, vomiting, dizziness, ataxia and loss of consciousness. Sodium nitroprusside should then be immediately discontinued. Massive overdosage may also produce signs similar to those of cyanide poisoning with coma, imperceptible pulse, absent reflexes, widely dilated pupils, pink color, distant heart sounds, hypotension and very shallow breathing. Oxygen alone will not provide relief. Nitrites should be administered to induce methemoglobin formation. Methemoglobin, in turn, combines with cyanide bound to cytochrome oxidase to liberate cytochrome oxidase and form a non-toxic complex, cyanmethemoglobin. Cyanide then gradually dissociates from the latter and is converted by administration of thiosulfate to sodium thiocyanate in the presence of rhodanese.

Treatment: In cases of massive overdosage when signs of cyanide toxicity are present use the following regimen:

1. Discontinue administration of Nipride.
2. Administer amyl nitrite inhalations for 15 to 30 seconds each minute until 3% sodium nitrite solution can be prepared for I.V. administration.
3. Sodium nitrite 3% solution should be injected intravenously at a rate not exceeding 2.5 to 5.0 ml/minute up to a total dose of 10 to 15 ml with careful monitoring of the blood pressure.
4. Following the above steps, inject sodium thiosulfate intravenously, 12.5 Gm in 50 ml of 5% dextrose in water over a ten-minute period.
5. Since signs of overdosage may reappear, the patient must be observed for several hours.
6. If signs of overdosage reappear, sodium nitrite and sodium thiosulfate injections are repeated in one-half of the above doses.
7. During the administration of nitrites and later when thiocyanate formation is taking place, blood pressure may drop but can be corrected with vasopressor agents.

NISENTIL® Ⓒ
(alphaprodine hydrochloride/Roche)
ampuls • vials

The following text is complete prescribing information based on official labeling in effect August 1, 1979.

Description: Nisentil (alphaprodine hydrochloride/Roche) is a rapid-acting, synthetic narcotic analgesic with a short duration of action.

Chemistry: Alphaprodine hydrochloride, a piperidine derivative, is chemically, *dl*-1,3-dimethyl-4-phenyl-4-piperidinol propionate hydrochloride.

Animal Pharmacology: Except for its shorter duration of action, the pharmacologic properties of Nisentil in animals are generally the same as those of morphine. The LD_{50} of alphaprodine hydrochloride in mice is 54 ± 3.9 mg/kg intravenously and 122 ± 5.7 mg/kg subcutaneously; in rats the LD_{50} is 25 ± 1.9 mg/kg intravenously and 71 ± 9 mg/kg subcutaneously.

Indications: Nisentil is useful for obstetric analgesia; for urologic examinations and procedures —particularly cystoscopy; preoperatively in major surgery; in minor surgery where rapid analgesia of brief duration is desirable—especially in orthopedics, ophthalmology, rhinology and laryngology; and for renal or biliary colic, or cardiovascular pain.

Contraindications: Nisentil is contraindicated in patients with known hypersensitivity to the drug.

Warnings: Nisentil is addicting. Narcotic order is required.

The depressant effects of Nisentil are potentiated in the presence of drugs such as barbiturates, general anesthetic agents and some phenothiazines; accordingly, the dosage of Nisentil should be reduced when used concomitantly with such agents. See section *Management of Overdosage* for the treatment of severe respiratory depression.

As with other opiates, Nisentil should be used with extreme caution in conditions such as increased intracranial pressure, hepatic insufficiency, severe CNS depression, myxedema, acute alcoholism, delirium tremens, convulsive disorders and Addison's disease. Narcotic analgesics should be used with extreme caution in patients receiving MAO inhibitors because of the possibility of hypotension.

Nisentil should not be used for relief of chronic pain because its short duration of action would require more frequent administration and might increase the possibility of addiction.

Usage in Pregnancy: While the safety and efficacy of Nisentil have been established as an

Continued on next page

Roche—Cont.

analgesic agent in obstetrics, there is limited experience regarding its use earlier in pregnancy. As is true in all narcotic agents, particularly during the first trimester, use of this drug requires that its potential benefits be weighed against its possible hazards.

Precautions: The intramuscular administration of Nisentil is not recommended because of limited clinical experience with this route of administration. When the drug is given intravenously, special attention should be given to the possibility of respiratory depression. Such depression is especially likely in patients with pulmonary disease and in the elderly or debilitated.

Adverse Reactions: Respiratory depression has been noted occasionally following the administration of Nisentil preoperatively and during labor. This may be severe enough to warrant active measures, particularly in neonatal situations. It is recommended that Lorfan® (levallorphan tartrate/Roche)[1-4] be administered in such cases to combat the respiratory changes. Dizziness, drowsiness, sweating, and urticaria have been reported. Nausea, vomiting, restlessness and confusion are rarely encountered.

Dosage and Administration: The dosages suggested are the usual amounts employed in adults; however, as with any narcotic analgesic, good medical practice dictates the use of the minimal effective dose. *The usual dosage is in the range of 0.4 to 0.6 mg/kg intravenously or 0.4 to 1.2 mg/kg subcutaneously.* Initially, the lower dosage range is recommended, in order to evaluate the patient's response. Thus, *the initial intravenous dose should not exceed 30 mg, nor should the initial subcutaneous dose exceed 60 mg.* The total dose administered by any route should not be more than 240 mg in 24 hours. Whenever this drug is given intravenously, a narcotic antagonist and facilities for resuscitation should be available.

Subcutaneous administration provides analgesic effects within 5 to 10 minutes, lasting about two hours. If required, an additional ¼ dose may be given 30 minutes after the initial dose. The *intravenous* route is recommended when more rapid onset (1 to 2 minutes) and shorter duration (½ to 1 hour) of action are desired. An additional amount of ¼ the initial dosage may be injected after 15 minutes, if required.

Obstetrics: Initially 40 to 60 mg subcutaneously after cervical dilation has begun, repeated as required at two-hour intervals. Nisentil may be combined with scopolamine or atropine, and may be used in conjunction with nerve block or inhalation anesthesia as required.

Urologic procedures, e.g., cystoscopy: Initially 20 to 30 mg intravenously.

Preoperatively in major surgery: Initially 20 to 40 mg subcutaneously, or 10 to 20 mg intravenously.

Minor Surgery: Initially 40 mg subcutaneously, or 20 mg intravenously.

Renal or biliary colic, or cardiovascular pain: Initially 20 to 60 mg subcutaneously, or 20 to 30 mg intravenously.

Children's Dosage: A dosage schedule for use in children under 12 years of age has not been established.

Administration with a Narcotic Antagonist: According to some investigators[5-13] Lorfan (levallorphan tartrate/Roche) is a potent narcotic antagonist which, in proper dosage, selectively antagonizes the respiratory depression due to narcotics. It can be used to help prevent such depression without abolishing analgesia, and it is an effective antidote in the event of overdosage. Lorfan is of particular value in the obstetric patient, the newborn and ambulatory patients. When administered together with Nisentil, it should be given in a ratio of 1 part Lorfan to 50 parts Nisentil. In the obstetric patient, it should be given concomitantly with each dose of Nisentil. If not administered in this fashion, 1 to 2 mg of Lorfan may be injected intravenously 5 to 10 minutes prior to delivery. To prevent narcotic-induced respiratory depression in the newborn, 0.05 to 0.1 mg of Lorfan (approximately one-tenth the adult dose) is injected into the umbilical cord vein immediately after delivery (see section *Management of Overdosage*). In other indications—such as cystoscopy or other endoscopies in ambulatory patients—Lorfan may be employed together with Nisentil in a ratio of 1 part Lorfan to 50 parts Nisentil. For other dosage schedules, see Lorfan package insert. Lorfan is not a narcotic, and a narcotic order is not required.

Management of Overdosage:[1,2] Toxic effects of Nisentil include coma, shallow respiration, cyanosis, hypotension, pinpoint pupils, and early unconsciousness. If these occur, either Lorfan or Nalline (nalorphine hydrochloride) should be given intravenously. When Lorfan is used, inject 1 mg intravenously and repeat in 3 to 5 minutes if necessary. The dose for Nalline (nalorphine hydrochloride) is 5 to 10 mg intravenously, repeated every 15 minutes as necessary to restore adequate respiration. In the presence of apnea, artificial respiration and oxygen therapy should be employed and a patent airway assured. The patient should be carefully observed during the first 24 hours. Body warmth and adequate fluid intake should be maintained. *NOTE:* The use of a narcotic antagonist in a patient addicted to narcotics may precipitate an acute withdrawal syndrome.

How Supplied: Nisentil 1-ml Ampuls, 40 mg/ml (boxes of 10)—Each ml of solution contains 40 mg alphaprodine hydrochloride/Roche (WARNING: May be habit forming) compounded with 0.0875% citric acid and pH adjusted to approximately 4.6 with sodium citrate.

Nisentil 1-ml Ampuls, 60 mg/ml (boxes of 10)—Each ml of solution contains 60 mg alphaprodine hydrochloride/Roche (WARNING: May be habit forming) compounded with 0.0875% citric acid and pH adjusted to approximately 4.6 with sodium citrate.

Nisentil 10-ml Vials, 60 mg/ml—Each ml of solution contains 60 mg alphaprodine hydrochloride/Roche (WARNING: May be habit forming) compounded with 0.45% phenol as preservative, 0.0875% citric acid and pH adjusted to approximately 4.6 with sodium citrate.

References:

1. Auerbach, J. and Coakley, C. S.: *Anesth. & Analg. 35*:460, 1956.
2. Foldes, F. F., *et al.*: *J.A.M.A. 160*:168, 1956.
3. Foldes, F. F., *et al.*: *J.A.M.A. 166*:325, 1958.
4. Foldes, F. F. *et al.*: *Am. J. M. Sc. 233*:153, 1957.
5. Burnett, R. G. and White, C. A.: *Obst. & Gynec. 27*:472, 1966.
6. Hartman, M. M. and Schwab, J. M.: *Surg. Clin. North Am. 43*:1229, 1963.
7. Burbank, P. M.: *Anesth. & Analg. 42*:275, 1963.
8. Backner, D. D., *et al.*: *Am. J. Obst. & Gynec. 74*:271, 1957.
9. Lipson, H. I. and Bradford, H. R.: *J.A.M.A. 163*:1244, 1957.
10. Garnes, H. A.: *J. Urol. 76*:204, 1956.
11. Kepes, E. R. and Margolius, B. R.: *Am. J. Surg. 91*:761, 1956.
12. Belinkoff, S.: *Anesth. & Analg. 35*:246, 1956.
13. Stoelting, V. K. and Hicks, M. L.: *Canad. Anaesth. Soc. J. 3*:107, 1956.

Narcotic order required.

NOLUDAR® 300 CAPSULES ℞
(methyprylon/Roche)

NOLUDAR® TABLETS ℞
(methyprylon/Roche)

The following text is complete prescribing information based on official labeling in effect August 1, 1979.

Description: Methyprylon, a piperidine derivative, is chemically, 3,3-diethyl-5-methyl-2,4-piperidinedione. It is a white crystalline powder, freely soluble in water, having a molecular weight of 183.25.

Noludar is available in three dosage forms: Capsules containing 300 mg of methyprylon/Roche, tablets containing 200 mg of methyprylon/Roche and tablets containing 50 mg of methyprylon/Roche.

Actions: In animal studies, methyprylon has been shown to increase the threshold of the arousal centers in the brainstem. In humans, when taken at bedtime, Noludar usually induces sleep within 45 minutes and provides sleep for 5 to 8 hours.

Mean plasma levels in three subjects following a single 650-mg dose peaked at one to two hours post administration at approximately 7.8 to 10 μg/ml. The levels declined to 3.3 to 7.8 μg/ml at four hours. Trace amounts (0.02 to 0.08 μg/ml) of the dihydro-metabolite were detected in the one to four hour plasma specimens. This dihydro-metabolite is bound approximately 38% to human plasma proteins. Approximately 3% of the dose was recovered in the urine as the intact drug and another 3% as the dihydro-metabolite in the first 24-hour period. Other identified metabolites include the 6-oxo, the 5-hydroxymethyl and the 5-carboxyl derivatives. A spectrophotometric assay for the determination of methyprylon and a flurometric assay for the determination of its dihydro-metabolite in biological media have been reported. A sufficiently sensitive method for the quantitation of all of the metabolites has not yet been reported.

Indications: For use as a hypnotic. In the sleep laboratory it has been objectively determined that Noludar is effective for at least 7 consecutive nights of drug administration. Since insomnia is often transient and intermittent the prolonged use of hypnotics is usually not indicated and should only be undertaken concomitantly with appropriate evaluation of the patient.

Contraindications: Noludar is contraindicated in patients with known hypersensitivity to the drug.

Warnings: Patients receiving Noludar should be cautioned about possible combined effects with alcohol and other CNS depressants. Since Noludar is an effective hypnotic agent, patients should also be cautioned against hazardous occupations requiring complete mental alertness such as operating machinery or driving a motor vehicle shortly after ingesting the drug.

Physical and Psychological Dependence: Physical and psychological dependence have been reported infrequently in patients receiving Noludar therapy. Withdrawal symptoms, when they occur, tend to resemble those associated with the withdrawal of barbiturates and should be treated in a similar fashion. Caution must be exercised in administering Noludar to individuals known to be addiction-prone or those whose history suggests they may increase the dosage on their own initiative. As with all hypnotic agents, good medical practice suggests the desirability of limiting repeated prescriptions without adequate medical supervision.

Usage In Pregnancy: Use of any drug in pregnancy, lactation, or in women of childbearing age requires that the potential benefit of the drug be weighed against its possible hazards to the mother and child.

Usage in Children: Noludar is not recommended in children under 12 years of age.

Precautions: Total daily intake should not exceed 400 mg, as greater amounts do not significantly increase hypnotic benefits. The usual precautions should be observed in the presence of hepatic or renal disorders. If used repeatedly or over prolonged periods of time, periodic blood counts should be made.
Adverse Reactions: At recommended dosages, there have been rare occurrences of morning drowsiness, dizziness, mild to moderate gastric upset (including diarrhea, esophagitis, nausea and vomiting), headache, paradoxical excitation and skin rash. There have been a very few, isolated reports of neutropenia and thrombocytopenia; however, the evidence does not establish that these reactions are related to Noludar.
Dosage: Dosage should be individualized for maximum beneficial effects. The usual adult dosage is 1 capsule (300 mg) or 1 or 2 tablets of 200 mg (200 or 400 mg) before retiring. In children the effective dosage of Noludar varies greatly and, therefore, should also be individualized. Treatment may be initiated with 50 mg and increased up to 200 mg, if required, given at bedtime. The drug is not recommended for use in children under 12 years of age.
Management of Overdosage: Manifestations of Noludar overdosage include somnolence, confusion, coma, constricted pupils, respiratory depression and hypotension. Respiration, pulse and blood pressure should be monitored, as in all cases of drug overdosage. General supportive measures should be employed, along with immediate gastric lavage with precautions to prevent pulmonary aspiration. Appropriate intravenous fluids should be administered and an adequate airway maintained. Hypotension may be combated by the use of levarterenol (Levophed®), metaraminol (Aramine) or other accepted antihypotensive measures. Analeptic agents are believed by some authorities to be of little or no value in the treatment of sedative-hypnotic induced respiratory depression, and their side effects (vomiting, cardiac arrhythmias, convulsions) may be hazardous. If the use of such agents is desired, caffeine and sodium benzoate or pentylenetetrazol (Metrazol) injection may be used, observing due precautions. There are several reports indicating that hemodialysis is of value. Therefore, its use should be considered, especially in those cases where supportive measures are failing and adequate urinary output cannot be maintained. There have been occasional reports of excitation and convulsions in patients following methyprylon overdosage, almost invariably during the recovery phase. Should these occur, barbiturates may be used, but only with great caution. As with the management of intentional overdosage with any drug, it should be borne in mind that multiple agents may have been ingested.
How Supplied: *Capsules,* 300 mg, amethyst and white—bottles of 100 and 500. *Tablets,* 200 mg, scored—bottles of 100. *Tablets,* 50 mg—bottles of 100.
[*Shown in Product Identification Section*]

PANTOPON® Ⓒ
(hydrochlorides of opium alkaloids/Roche)

The following text is complete prescribing information based on official labeling in effect August 1, 1979.
Description: Pantopon contains all the alkaloids of opium in highly purified form free from inert matter—waxes, gums, resins—and in approximately the same proportions in which they occur in nature. Its action is essentially that of opium. It exhibits, therefore, in addition to the action of morphine, the action of codeine, papaverine and other alkaloids present in opium.
Properties: In Pantopon the other alkaloids enhance the sedative and analgesic effects of morphine and tend to minimize its undesirable side reactions. Thus, 1/3 grain (20 mg) of hydrochlorides of opium alkaloids, with a morphine content of only 1/6 grain (10 mg), is therapeutically equivalent to 1/4 grain (15 mg) of morphine. One part of hydrochlorides of opium alkaloids is equivalent to 5 parts of opium.
Indications: Pantopon is indicated in all disorders in which the analgesic, sedative-hypnotic or narcotic effect of an opiate is needed. It is recommended for the relief of severe pain in place of morphine.
Advantages: Pantopon provides all the alkaloids of opium in injectable form. It has a smooth analgesic and hypnotic effect and is not likely to provoke side reactions.
Contraindications: Bronchial asthma, narcotic idiosyncrasies, respiratory depression. Toxicity is manifested by coma, pinpoint pupils, and depressed respiration.
Caution: Pantopon is an addicting drug with an addiction liability equal to morphine, and for this reason the same precautions should be taken in administering the drug as with morphine. Caution should be used in administration to infants, old and debilitated patients and to patients with increased intracranial pressure, toxic psychosis, prostatic obstruction and myxedema.
Warning: May be habit forming. Narcotic order required.
Antidote for Overdosage: The narcotic antagonist Lorfan® (levallorphan tartrate/Roche) is an effective antidote in the event of overdosage.
Dosage and Administration: 20 mg (1/3 grain) hydrochlorides of opium alkaloids—containing 10 mg (1/6 grain) morphine—is usually administered where 15 mg (1/4 grain) morphine is indicated.
Usual Adult Dose: 5 to 20 mg (1/12 to 1/3 grain). Administer only by intramuscular or subcutaneous injection.
How Supplied: Ampuls, 1 ml, containing 20 mg (1/3 grain), boxes of 10. Each ml of solution contains 20 mg hydrochlorides of opium alkaloids/Roche (WARNING: May be habit forming) compounded with 6% alcohol by volume, 136 mg glycerine, 0.2% parabens (methyl and propyl) as preservatives, with either acetic acid or sodium hydroxide, or both, used as necessary to adjust pH to approximately 3.3. Narcotic order required.

PROSTIGMIN® INJECTABLE ℞
(neostigmine methylsulfate/Roche)
Ampuls • Vials

The following text is complete prescribing information based on official labeling in effect August 1, 1979.
Description: Prostigmin (neostigmine methylsulfate/Roche), a cholinergic stimulant, enhances cholinergic action by facilitating the transmission of impulses across the myoneural junction. It inhibits the destruction of acetylcholine by acetylcholinesterase. Its effect is similar to that of physostigmine (eserine) but, in therapeutic doses, it is less likely to cause disturbing side effects. It also has a direct effect on voluntary muscle fibers[1] and possibly on autonomic ganglion cells and neurons of the central nervous system.[2]
Chemically, neostigmine methylsulfate is the dimethylcarbamate of (*m*-hydroxyphenyl) trimethylammonium methylsulfate. It has a molecular weight of 334.4.
Animal Pharmacology: The drug has been studied in many species of animals but most extensively in the cat. These studies indicate that it inhibits or inactivates acetylcholine esterases and thus allows the accumulation of acetylcholine at cholinergic sites. Neostigmine labeled with ^{14}C in one of the methyl groups of the quaternary nitrogen has been used to investigate the excretion and metabolism of neostigmine after administration to cats by stomach tube. About 10% of the dose is excreted in the urine in 5 hours and 20% after 24 hours. Approximately 50% was detected in the intestinal contents and feces 24 hours after administration. The peak concentration in the liver occurs about 2 hours after injection and is equivalent to 2% of the dose.[3]
The LD_{50} of neostigmine methylsulfate in mice is 0.3 ± 0.02 mg/kg intravenously, 0.54 ± 0.03 mg/kg subcutaneously, and 0.395 ± 0.025 mg/kg intramuscularly; in rats the LD_{50} is 0.315 ± 0.019 mg/kg intravenously, 0.445 ± 0.032 mg/kg subcutaneously, and 0.423 ± 0.032 mg/kg intramuscularly.
Indications: Prostigmin is indicated in the prevention and treatment of postoperative distention and urinary retention. It may be utilized as a screening test for early pregnancy. It is of use in the treatment of delayed menstruation. Prostigmin is of particular use in the symptomatic control of myasthenia gravis. It can be used as a diagnostic test for myasthenia gravis; however, Tensilon® (edrophonium chloride/Roche) is usually recommended as a diagnostic test for myasthenia gravis because of its more rapid onset and brief duration of action. Prostigmin can also be used as an antidote for tubocurarine.
Contraindications: Prostigmin is contraindicated in mechanical intestinal or urinary obstruction. It is contraindicated in patients with known sensitivity to the drug.
Precautions: Prostigmin should be used with caution in asthmatic patients. When large doses of Prostigmin are administered, the prior or simultaneous injection of atropine sulfate may be advisable. Separate syringes should be used for the Prostigmin and atropine. Because of the possibility of hypersensitivity in an occasional patient, atropine and antishock medication should always be readily available.
As is true of all cholinergic drugs, overdosage of Prostigmin may result in cholinergic crisis, a state characterized by increasing muscle weakness which, through involvement of the muscles of respiration, may lead to death. Myasthenic crisis due to an increase in the severity of the disease is also accompanied by extreme muscle weakness and thus may be difficult to distinguish from cholinergic crisis on a symptomatic basis. Such differentiation is extremely important, since increases in doses of Prostigmin or other drugs in this class in the presence of cholinergic crisis or of a refractory or "insensitive" state could have grave consequences. Osserman and Genkins[4] indicate that the two types of crises may be differentiated by the use of Tensilon® (edrophonium chloride/Roche) as well as by clinical judgment. The treatment of the two conditions obviously differs radically. Whereas the presence of *myasthenic crisis* requires more intensive anticholinesterase therapy, *cholinergic crisis,* according to Osserman and Genkins,[4] calls for the prompt withdrawal of all drugs of this type. The immediate use of atropine in cholinergic crisis is also recommended.
Atropine may also be used to abolish or obtund gastrointestinal side effects or other muscarinic reactions; but such use, by masking signs of overdosage, can lead to inadvertent induction of cholinergic crisis.
For detailed information on the management of patients with myasthenia gravis, the physician is referred to one of the excellent reviews such as those by Osserman and Genkins[5] or Grob.[6]
Adverse Reactions: The side effects of Prostigmin are most commonly related to overdosage and generally are of two varieties, muscarinic and nicotinic. Among the former group are nausea, vomiting, diarrhea, abdominal cramps, increased salivation, increased bronchial secretions, miosis, and diaphoresis. Nicotinic side effects are comprised chiefly of muscle cramps, fasciculation, and weakness. Muscarinic side effects can usually be counteracted by atropine.

Continued on next page

Roche—Cont.

Dosage: *Prevention of postoperative distention and urinary retention:* One ml of the 1:4000 solution (0.25 mg) subcutaneously or intramuscularly as soon as possible after operation; repeat every 4 to 6 hours for two or three days.
Treatment of postoperative distention: One ml of the 1:2000 solution (0.5 mg) subcutaneously or intramuscularly, as required.
Treatment of urinary retention: One ml of the 1:2000 solution (0.5 mg) subcutaneously or intramuscularly. If urination does not occur within an hour, the patient should be catheterized. After the patient has voided, or the bladder has been emptied, continue the 0.5 mg injections every three hours for at least 5 injections.
Screening test for early pregnancy and treatment of delayed menstruation: One ml of the 1:1000 solution (1 mg) injected intramuscularly daily for three successive days. The patient may be assumed to be pregnant if bleeding does not occur within 72 hours after the third injection, providing pelvic lesions, systemic disease, the menopause and endocrine disorders have been ruled out.
Symptomatic control of myasthenia gravis: One ml of the 1:2000 solution (0.5 mg) subcutaneously or intramuscularly. Subsequent doses should be based on the individual patient's response. In most patients, however, oral treatment with Prostigmin (neostigmine bromide/Roche) tablets, 15 mg each, is adequate for control of symptoms.
As an antidote for tubocurarine: When Prostigmin is administered intravenously, it is recommended that atropine sulfate (0.6 to 1.2 mg) also be given intravenously using separate syringes. Some authorities have recommended that the atropine be injected several minutes before the Prostigmin rather than concomitantly. The usual dose is 0.5 to 2 mg Prostigmin given by *slow* intravenous injection, repeated as required; however, only in exceptional cases should the total dose of Prostigmin exceed 5 mg. It is recommended that the patient be well ventilated and a patent airway maintained until complete recovery of normal respiration is assured. The optimum time to administer the drug is when the patient is being hyperventilated and the carbon dioxide level of the blood is low. It should never be administered in the presence of high concentrations of halothane or cyclopropane. In small children, cardiac cases, and severely ill patients it is advisable to titrate the exact dose of Prostigmin required, using a peripheral nerve stimulator device. In the presence of a bradycardia, the pulse rate should be increased to about 80/minute with atropine before administering neostigmine.
How Supplied: *Prostigmin 1:2000, 1-ml ampuls (boxes of 10)*—Each ml contains 0.5 mg neostigmine methylsulfate/Roche compounded with 0.2% parabens (methyl and propyl) as preservatives and pH adjusted to approximately 5.9 with sodium hydroxide.
Prostigmin 1:4000, 1-ml ampuls (boxes of 10)—Each ml contains 0.25 mg neostigmine methylsulfate/Roche compounded with 0.2% parabens (methyl and propyl) as preservatives and pH adjusted to approximately 5.9 with sodium hydroxide.
Prostigmin 1:1000, 10-ml multiple dose vials—Each ml contains 1 mg neostigmine methylsulfate/Roche compounded with 0.45% phenol as preservative, 0.2 mg sodium acetate, and pH adjusted to approximately 5.9 with acetic acid and sodium hydroxide.
Prostigmin 1:2000, 10-ml multiple dose vials—Each ml contains 0.5 mg neostigmine methylsulfate/Roche compounded with 0.45% phenol as preservative, 0.2 mg sodium acetate, and pH adjusted to approximately 5.9 with acetic acid and sodium hydroxide.

References:

1. Riker, W. F., and Wescoe, W. C.: *J. Pharmacol. & Exper. Therap. 88*:58, 1946.
2. Goodman, L. S., and Gilman, A.: *The Pharmacological Basis of Therapeutics,* 3rd ed., New York, Macmillan, 1965, p. 459.
3. Roberts, J. B., *et al.: Biochem. Pharm. 15*:71, 1966.
4. Osserman, K. E. and Genkins, G.: *J.A.M.A. 183*:97, 1963.
5. Osserman, K. E., and Genkins, G.: *New York J. Med. 61:*2076, 1961.
6. Grob, D.: *Arch. Int. Med. 108*:615, 1961.

PROSTIGMIN® TABLETS ℞
(neostigmine bromide/Roche)

The following text is complete prescribing information based on official labeling in effect August 1, 1979.
Description: Prostigmin (neostigmine bromide/Roche) is a cholinergic drug of proven value in the treatment of myasthenia gravis. Neostigmine bromide is a white crystalline, bitter powder, soluble 1:1 in water, with a molecular weight of 303.22. Chemically it is the dimethylcarbamate of (*m*-hydroxyphenyl) trimethylammonium bromide.
Prostigmin inhibits the destruction of acetylcholine by acetylcholinesterase, thus facilitating transmission of impulses across the myoneural junction. It also has a direct effect on voluntary muscle fibers[1] and possibly on autonomic ganglion cells and neurons of the central nervous system.[2]
Animal Pharmacology: The drug has been studied in many species of animals but most extensively in the cat. These studies indicate that it inhibits or inactivates acetylcholine esterases and thus allows the accumulation of acetylcholine at cholinergic sites. Neostigmine labeled with ^{14}C in one of the methyl groups of the quaternary nitrogen has been used to investigate the excretion and metabolism of neostigmine after administration to cats by stomach tube. About 10% of the dose is excreted in the urine in 5 hours and 20% after 24 hours. Approximately 50% was detected in the intestinal contents and feces 24 hours after administration. The peak concentration in the liver occurs about 2 hours after injection and is equivalent to 2% of the dose. It was concluded that the absorption of ^{14}C-labeled neostigmine after oral administration is slow and prolonged, and that most of the drug that is absorbed is metabolized by the liver.[3]
Indications: Prostigmin is indicated in the symptomatic control of myasthenia gravis. Its greatest usefulness is in prolonged therapy where no difficulty in swallowing is present. In acute myasthenic crisis where difficulty in breathing and swallowing is present, the parenteral form (neostigmine methylsulfate/Roche) should be used, the patient being transferred to the oral form as soon as it can be tolerated.
Contraindications: Prostigmin is contraindicated in patients with known hypersensitivity to the drug. Because of the presence of the bromide ion, it should not be used in patients with a previous history of reaction to bromides. It is contraindicated in patients with mechanical bowel obstruction and in patients with urinary tract infections.
Warnings: As a rule, 15 mg of neostigmine bromide orally is equivalent to 0.5 mg of neostigmine methylsulfate parenterally. This difference is due to the fact that neostigmine bromide is poorly absorbed from the intestinal tract. Large doses should be avoided in situations where there might be an increased absorption rate from the intestinal tract. It should be given with caution when anticholinergic drugs which may slow the intestinal motility are given. It should be used with caution in asthmatic patients.
Management of Overdosage: Although failure of patients to show clinical improvement may reflect underdosage, it can also be indicative of overdosage. As is true of all cholinergic drugs, overdosage of Prostigmin may result in cholinergic crisis, a state characterized by increasing muscle weakness which, through involvement of muscles of respiration, may lead to death. Myasthenic crisis due to an increased severity of the disease is also accompanied by extreme muscle weakness, and thus may be difficult to distinguish from cholinergic crisis on a symptomatic basis. Such differentiation is important, since increases in dosage of Prostigmin in the presence of cholinergic crisis or of a refractory or "insensitive" state could have grave consequences. Osserman and Genkins[4] indicate that the differential diagnosis of the two types of crisis may require the use of Tensilon® (edrophonium chloride/Roche) as well as clinical judgment. The treatment of the two conditions obviously differs radically. Whereas the presence of myasthenic crisis suggests need for more intensive anticholinesterase treatment, the diagnosis of cholinergic crisis calls for the prompt withdrawal of all drugs of this type and the immediate use of atropine.
Atropine may also be used to abolish or reduce gastrointestinal side effects or other muscarinic reactions. It must be remembered, however, that atropine can mask signs of overdosage and thereby lead to induction of cholinergic crisis.
Precautions: Certain antibiotics, especially neomycin,[5] streptomycin, and kanamycin,[6] have a mild but definite nondepolarizing blocking action which may accentuate neuromuscular block. These antibiotics should only be used in the myasthenic patient where definitely indicated, and then careful adjustment should be made of adjunctive anticholinesterase dosage.
Adverse Reactions: Side effects are generally due to an exaggeration of the pharmacological effects. Salivation and fasciculation are the most common. Bowel cramps and diarrhea may occur.
Dosage and Administration: The onset of effect of Prostigmin given orally is slower than that given parenterally, but the duration of action is longer and the intensity of action more uniform. The usual total oral requirement for optimal benefits varies from as little as 15 mg to as much as 375 mg per day. In some instances it may be necessary to exceed these dosages, but the possibility of cholinergic crisis must be borne in mind. The average dose is 10 tablets (150 mg) spread over 24 hours. The interval between doses is of paramount importance; the best dosage schedule must be ascertained by trial and error for each patient and changes made as the need arises. Frequently, therapy is required day and night. Larger portions of the total daily dose may be given at times of greater fatigue (afternoon, mealtimes, etc.). The patient should be encouraged to keep a daily record of his condition to assist the physician in arranging an optimal therapeutic regimen.
How Supplied: Scored white tablets containing 15 mg neostigmine bromide/Roche—bottles of 100 and 1000.

References:

1. Riker, W. F., and Wescoe, W. C.: The Direct Action of Prostigmine on Skeletal Muscle; Its Relationship to the Choline Esters, J. Pharm. Exp. Therap. *88*:58-66, 1946.
2. Goodman, L. S., and Gilman, A.: The Pharmacological Basis of Therapeutics, Third Edition, New York, Macmillan, 1965, p. 459.
3. Roberts, J. B., Thomas, B. H. and Wilson, A.: Excretion and Metabolism of Oral ^{14}C-Neostigmine in the Rat, Biochemical Pharmacology *15*:71-75, 1966.
4. Osserman, K. E., and Genkins, G.: J.A.M.A. *183*:97-101, 1963.
5. Davidson, E. W., *et al.:* Respiratory Depression Following Use of Antibiotics in Pleural

and Pseudocyst Cavities, J.A.M.A. *196*:170-171, 1966.
6. Pindell, M. H.: The Pharmacology of Kanamycin—A Review and New Developments, Ann. N.Y. Acad. Sci. *132*:805-810, 1966.
[*Shown in Product Identification Section*]

QUARZAN® ℞
(clidinium bromide/Roche)
CAPSULES

The following text is complete prescribing information based on official labeling in effect August 1, 1979.

Description: Clidinium bromide is 3-hydroxy-1-methylquinuclidinium bromide benzilate. A white or nearly white crystalline compound, it is soluble in water and has a calculated molecular weight of 432.36.

Clidinium bromide is a quaternary ammonium compound with anticholinergic and antispasmodic activity. Quarzan is available as green and red opaque capsules each containing 2.5 mg clidinium bromide, and green and grey opaque capsules each containing 5 mg clidinium bromide.

Actions: Quarzan inhibits gastrointestinal motility and diminishes gastric acid secretion. Its anticholinergic activity approximates that of atropine sulfate and propantheline bromide.

Indications: Quarzan is effective as adjunctive therapy in peptic ulcer disease. **Quarzan has not been shown to be effective in contributing to the healing of peptic ulcer, decreasing the rate of recurrence or preventing complications.**

Contraindications: Known hypersensitivity to clidinium bromide or to other anticholinergic drugs, glaucoma, obstructive uropathy (for example, bladder neck obstruction due to prostatic hypertrophy), obstructive disease of the gastrointestinal tract (for example, pyloroduodenal stenosis), paralytic ileus, intestinal atony of the elderly or debilitated patient, unstable cardiovascular status in acute hemorrhage, severe ulcerative colitis, toxic megacolon complicating ulcerative colitis, myasthenia gravis.

Warnings: Quarzan may produce drowsiness or blurred vision. The patient should be cautioned regarding activities requiring mental alertness such as operating a motor vehicle or other machinery or performing hazardous work while taking this drug. In the presence of high environmental temperature, heat prostration (fever and heat stroke) may occur with the use of anticholinergics due to decreased sweating. Diarrhea may be an early symptom of incomplete intestinal obstruction, especially in patients with ileostomy or colostomy. Use of anticholinergics in patients with suspected intestinal obstruction would be inappropriate and possibly harmful. With overdosage, a curare-like action may occur, *i.e.*, neuromuscular blockade leading to muscular weakness and possible paralysis.

Usage in Pregnancy: No controlled studies in humans have been performed to establish the safety of the drug in pregnancy. Uncontrolled data derived from clinical usage have failed to show abnormalities attributable to its use. Reproduction studies in rats have failed to show any impaired fertility or abnormality in the fetuses that might be associated with the use of Quarzan. Use of any drug in pregnancy or in women of childbearing potential requires that the pontential benefit of the drug be weighed against the possible hazards to mother and fetus.

Nursing Mothers: As with all anticholinergic drugs, Quarzan may be secreted in human milk and may inhibit lactation. As a general rule, nursing should not be undertaken while a patient is on Quarzan, or the drug should not be used by nursing mothers.

Pediatric Use: Since there is no adequate experience in children who have received this drug, safety and efficacy in children have not been established.

Precautions: Use Quarzan with caution in the elderly and in all patients with autonomic neuropathy, hepatic or renal disease, ulcerative colitis—large doses may suppress intestinal motility to the point of producing a paralytic ileus and for this reason precipitate or aggravate "toxic megacolon," a serious complication of the disease; hyperthyroidism; coronary heart disease; congestive heart failure; cardiac tachy-arrhythmias; tachycardia; hypertension; prostatic hypertrophy; hiatal hernia associated with reflux esophagitis, since anticholinergic drugs may aggravate this condition.

Adverse Reactions: As with other anticholinergic drugs, the most frequently reported adverse effects are dryness of mouth, blurring of vision, urinary hesitancy and constipation. Other adverse effects reported with the use of anticholinergic drugs include decreased sweating, urinary retention, tachycardia, palpitations, dilatation of the pupils, cycloplegia, increased ocular tension, loss of taste, headaches, nervousness, mental confusion, drowsiness, weakness, dizziness, insomnia, nausea, vomiting, bloated feeling, impotence, suppression of lactation and severe allergic reactions or drug idiosyncrasies including anaphylaxis, urticaria and other dermal manifestations.

Overdosage: The symptoms of overdosage with Quarzan progress from an intensification of the usual side effects to CNS disturbances (from restlessness and excitement to psychotic behavior), circulatory changes (flushing, tachycardia, fall in blood pressure, circulatory failure), respiratory failure, paralysis and coma.

Treatment should consist of: *General measures*—(1) gastric lavage, (2) maintenance of adequate airway, using artificial respiration if needed, (3) administration of i.v. fluids, and (4) for fever: alcohol sponging or ice packs.

Specific measures—(1) Antidotes: physostigmine (Antilirium) 0.5 to 2 mg, i.v., repeated as needed up to a total of 5 mg; or pilocarpine, 5 mg, s.c. at intervals until mouth is moist; neostigmine may also be useful. (2) Against excitement: sodium pentothal 2% may be given i.v. or chloral hydrate (100 to 200 ml, 2% solution) *rectally.* (3) Against hypotension and circulatory collapse: levarterenol (Levophed®) or metaraminol (Aramine) infusions. (4) Against CNS depression: caffeine and sodium benzoate. The usefulness of dialysis is not known.

Dosage and Administration: For maximum efficacy, dosage should be individualized according to severity of symptoms and occurrence of side effects. The usual dosage is 2.5 to 5 mg three or four times daily before meals and at bedtime. Dosage in excess of 20 mg daily is usually not required to obtain maximum effectiveness. For the aged or debilitated, one 2.5-mg capsule three times daily before meals is recommended. The desired pharmacological effect of the drug is unlikely to be attained without occasional side effects.

Drug Interactions: No specific drug interactions are known.

How Supplied: Opaque capsules, 2.5 mg, green and red; 5 mg, green and grey—bottles of 100 and 500; Prescription Paks of 50.

[*Shown in Product Identification Section*]

ROCALTROL® ℞
(calcitriol/Roche)
CAPSULES

The following text is complete prescribing information based on official labeling in effect August 1, 1979.

Description: Calcitriol is a colorless, crystalline compound which occurs naturally in humans. It has a calculated molecular weight of 416.65 and is soluble in organic solvents but relatively insoluble in water. Chemically, calcitriol is 9,10-seco(5Z,7E)-5,7,10(19)-cholestatriene-1α,3β, 25-triol.

The other names frequently used for calcitriol are 1,25-dihydroxycholecalciferol, 1,25-hydroxyvitamin D_3, 1,25-DHCC, 1,25$(OH)_2D_3$ and 1,25-diOHC.

Rocaltrol is synthetically manufactured calcitriol and is available as soft gelatin capsules for oral administration in the following strengths: 0.25 mcg (light orange, oval) and 0.5 mcg (dark orange, oblong).

Clinical Pharmacology: The natural supply of vitamin D in man mainly depends on the ultraviolet rays of the sun for conversion of 7-dehydrocholesterol to vitamin D_3 (cholecalciferol). It is now known that vitamin D_3 must be metabolically activated in the liver and the kidney before it is fully active on its target tissues. The initial transformation is catalyzed by a vitamin D_3-25-hydroxylase enzyme (25-OHase) present in the liver, and the product of this reaction is 25-hydroxy-vitamin D_3 [25-$(OH)D_3$]. The latter undergoes hydroxylation in the mitochondria of kidney tissue, and this reaction is activated by the renal 25-hydroxyvitamin D_3-1 alpha-hydroxylase (alpha-OHase) to produce 1,25-$(OH)_2D_3$ (calcitriol), the active form of vitamin D_3.

The two known sites of action of calcitriol are intestine and bone, but additional evidence suggests that it also acts on the kidney and the parathyroid gland. It is the most active known form of vitamin D_3 in stimulating intestinal calcium transport. In acutely uremic rats calcitriol has been shown to stimulate intestinal calcium absorption. It has been suggested that a vitamin D-resistant state exists in uremic patients because of the failure of the kidney to adequately convert precursors to the active compound, calcitriol.

Calcitriol when administered is rapidly absorbed from the intestine. After an oral dose of tritiated calcitriol, the peak concentration of radioactivity in the serum was reported after 4 hours. Vitamin D metabolites are known to be transported in blood, bound to specific plasma proteins. The pharmacologic activity of an administered dose of calcitriol is about 3 to 5 days. Two metabolic pathways for calcitriol seem to have been identified; conversion to 1,24,25-$(OH)_3D_3$ and to an unknown substance with a loss of a side chain at C26 or C27 position.

Indications and Usage: Rocaltrol is indicated in the management of hypocalcemia in patients undergoing chronic renal dialysis. In studies to date, it has been shown to reduce elevated parathyroid hormone levels in some of these patients.

Contraindications: Rocaltrol should not be given to patients with hypercalcemia or evidence of vitamin D toxicity.

Warnings: Since Rocaltrol is the most potent metabolite of vitamin D available, vitamin D and its derivatives should be withheld during treatment.

Aluminum carbonate or hydroxide gel should be used to control serum phosphate levels in patients undergoing dialysis.

Magnesium-containing antacid and Rocaltrol should not be used concomitantly, because such use may lead to the development of hypermagnesemia.

Overdosage of any form of vitamin D is dangerous (see also OVERDOSAGE). Progressive hypercalcemia due to overdosage of vitamin D and its metabolites may be so severe as to require emergency attention. Chronic hypercalcemia can lead to generalized vascular calcification, nephrocalcinosis and other soft-tissue calcification. **The serum calcium times phosphate (Ca × P) product should not be allowed to exceed 70.** Radiographic evaluation of suspect anatomical regions may be useful in the early detection of this condition.

Continued on next page

Roche—Cont.

Precautions:

i) *General:* Excessive dosage of Rocaltrol induces hypercalcemia and in some instances hypercalciuria; therefore, early in treatment during dosage adjustment, serum calcium should be determined twice weekly. A fall in serum alkaline phosphatase levels usually antedates the appearance of hypercalcemia and may be an indication of impending hypercalcemia. Should hypercalcemia develop, the drug should be discontinued immediately. Rocaltrol should be given cautiously to patients on digitalis, because hypercalcemia in such patients may precipitate cardiac arrhythmias.

ii) *Information for the patient:* The patient and his or her parents or spouse should be informed about compliance with dosage instructions, adherence to instructions about diet and calcium supplementation and avoidance of the use of unapproved non-prescription drugs. Patients should also be carefully informed about the symptoms of hypercalcemia (see ADVERSE REACTIONS).

iii) *Essential laboratory tests:* Serum calcium, phosphorus, magnesium and alkaline phosphatase and 24-hour urinary calcium and phosphorous should be determined periodically. During the initial phase of the medication, serum calcium should be determined more frequently (twice weekly).

iv) *Drug interactions:* Cholestyramine has been reported to reduce intestinal absorption of fat soluble vitamins; as such it may impair intestinal absorption of Rocaltrol.

v) *Carcinogenesis, mutagenesis, impairment of fertility:* Long-term studies in animals have not been completed to evaluate the carcinogenic potential of Rocaltrol. There was no evidence of mutagenicity as studied by the Ames Method. No significant effects of Rocaltrol on fertility and/or general reproductive performances were reported.

vi) *Use in pregnancy:* Rocaltrol has been found to be teratogenic in rabbits when given in doses 4 and 15 times the dose recommended for human use. All 15 fetuses in 3 litters at these doses showed external and skeletal abnormalities. However, none of the other 23 litters (156 fetuses) showed significant abnormalities compared with controls. Teratology studies in rats showed no evidence of teratogenic potential. There are no studies in pregnant women.

vii) *Nursing mothers:* It is not known whether this drug is excreted in human milk. As a general rule, nursing should not be undertaken while a patient is on a drug, since many drugs are excreted in human milk.

viii) *Pediatric use:* Safety and efficacy of Rocaltrol in children have not been established.

Adverse Reactions: Since Rocaltrol is believed to be the active hormone which exerts vitamin D activity in the body, adverse effects are, in general, similar to those encountered with excessive vitamin D intake. The early and late signs and symptoms of vitamin D intoxication associated with hypercalcemia include:

a. *Early:* Weakness, headache, somnolence, nausea, vomiting, dry mouth, constipation, muscle pain, bone pain and metallic taste.

b. *Late:* Polyuria, polydipsia, anorexia, weight loss, nocturia, conjunctivitis (calcific), pancreatitis, photophobia, rhinorrhea, pruritus, hyperthermia, decreased libido, elevated BUN, albuminuria, hypercholesterolemia, elevated SGOT and SGPT, ectopic calcification, hypertension, cardiac arrhythmias and, rarely, overt psychosis.

Overdosage: Administration of Rocaltrol to patients in excess of their daily requirements can cause hypercalcemia, hypercalciuria and hyperphosphatemia. High intake of calcium and phosphate concomitant with Rocaltrol may lead to similar abnormalities.

Treatment of Hypercalcemia and Overdosage in Patients on Hemodialysis: General treatment of hypercalcemia (greater than 1 mg/dl above the upper limit of the normal range) consists of immediate discontinuation of Rocaltrol therapy, institution of a low calcium diet and withdrawal of calcium supplements. Serum calcium levels should be determined daily until normocalcemia ensues. Hypercalcemia frequently resolves in two to seven days. When serum calcium levels have returned to within normal limits, Rocaltrol therapy may be reinstituted at a dose of 0.25 mcg/day less than prior therapy. Serum calcium levels should be obtained at least twice weekly after all dosage changes and subsequent dosage titration. Persistent or markedly elevated serum calcium levels may be corrected by dialysis against a calcium-free dialysate.

Treatment of Accidental Overdosage of Rocaltrol: The treatment of acute accidental overdosage of Rocaltrol should consist of general supportive measures. If drug ingestion is discovered within a relatively short time, induction of emesis or gastric lavage may be of benefit in preventing further absorption. If the drug has passed through the stomach, the administration of mineral oil may promote its fecal elimination. Serial serum electrolyte determinations (especially calcium ion), rate of urinary calcium excretion and assessment of electrocardiographic abnormalities due to hypercalcemia should be obtained. Such monitoring is critical in patients receiving digitalis. Discontinuation of supplemental calcium and a low calcium diet are also indicated in accidental overdosage. Due to the relatively short duration of the pharmacological action of calcitriol, further measures are probably unnecessary. Should, however, persistent and markedly elevated serum calcium levels occur, there are a variety of therapeutic alternatives which may be considered, depending on the patient's underlying condition. These include the use of drugs such as phosphates and corticosteroids as well as measures to induce an appropriate forced diuresis. The use of peritoneal dialysis against a calcium-free dialysate has also been reported.

Dosage and Administration: The optimal daily dose of Rocaltrol must be carefully determined for each patient.

The effectiveness of Rocaltrol therapy is predicated on the assumption that each patient is receiving an adequate daily intake of calcium. The RDA for calcium in adults is 1000 mg. To ensure that each patient receives an adequate daily intake of calcium, the physician should either prescribe a calcium supplement or instruct the patient in proper dietary measures.

The recommended initial dose of Rocaltrol is 0.25 mcg/day. If a satisfactory response in the biochemical parameters and clinical manifestations of the disease state are not observed, dosage may be increased by 0.25 mcg/day at two to four-week intervals. During this titration period, serum calcium levels should be obtained at least twice weekly, and if hypercalcemia is noted, the drug should be immediately discontinued until normocalcemia ensues.

Patients with normal or only slightly reduced serum calcium levels may respond to Rocaltrol doses of 0.25 mcg every other day. Most patients undergoing hemodialysis respond to doses between 0.5 and 1 mcg/day.

How Supplied: 0.25 mcg calcitriol in soft gelatin, light orange, oval capsules, imprinted (front) HLR, (back) 143; bottles of 30 and 100. 0.5 mcg calcitriol in soft gelatin, dark orange, oblong capsules, imprinted (front) ROCHE, (back) 144, bottles of 100.

Rocaltrol should be protected from heat and light.

[*Shown in Product Identification Section*]

RONIACOL® ℞
(nicotinyl alcohol/Roche)
TIMESPAN® TABLETS
TABLETS
ELIXIR

The following text is complete prescribing information based on official labeling in effect August 1, 1979.

Description: Roniacol (nicotinyl alcohol/Roche) is a well-tolerated vasodilator which is available in three dosage forms: Timespan Tablets, each providing 150 mg nicotinyl alcohol in the form of the tartrate salt in a sustained-release form; scored Tablets, each containing 50 mg nicotinyl alcohol in the form of the tartrate salt; and port-wine flavored Elixir, containing 50 mg nicotinyl alcohol per teaspoonful (5 ml).

Properties: Roniacol acts selectively by relaxing the musculature of peripheral blood vessels. In the management of conditions associated with deficient circulation, its action is smooth and gradual in onset. When administered in the sustained-release Timespan Tablet, increased blood flow is provided for up to 12 hours with a single dose. Patients usually do not develop tolerance on prolonged medication. The Timespan Tablet releases some of the drug immediately and the remainder continuously over a period of approximately twelve hours, thus increasing the blood flow in ischemic extremities for 10 to 12 hours by specific dilation of peripheral vessels.

INDICATIONS:
Based on a review of this drug by the National Academy of Sciences—National Research Council and/or other information, FDA has classified the indications as follows:
"Possibly" effective: In conditions associated with deficient circulation; *e.g.,* peripheral vascular disease, vascular spasm, varicose ulcers, decubital ulcers, chilblains, Meniere's syndrome and vertigo.
Final classification of the less-than-effective indications requires further investigation.

Caution: Roche Laboratories endorses the principle of caution in the administration of any therapeutic agent to pregnant patients.

Side Effects: Transient flushing, gastric disturbances, minor skin rashes and allergies may occur in some patients, seldom requiring discontinuation of the drug.

Dosage: *Timespan Tablets*—one or two tablets morning and night. *Tablets*—one or two tablets 3 times daily. *Elixir*—one or two teaspoonfuls 3 times daily.

How Supplied: *Timespan Tablets,* containing 150 mg nicotinyl alcohol in the form of the tartrate salt—bottles of 100 and 500. *Tablets,* containing 50 mg nicotinyl alcohol in the form of the tartrate salt—scored, bottles of 100 and 500. *Elixir,* containing 50 mg nicotinyl alcohol per teaspoonful (5 ml) —bottles of 16 oz.

[*Shown in Product Identification Section*]

SOLATENE® ℞
(beta-carotene/Roche)

The following text is complete prescribing information based on official labeling in effect August 1, 1979.

Description: Beta-carotene is a carotenoid pigment occurring naturally in green and yellow vegetables. Chemically, beta-carotene has the empirical formula $C_{40}H_{56}$ and a calculated molecular weight of 536.85. Trans-beta-carotene is a red crystalline compound which is insoluble in water.

Actions: The exact mode of action of beta-carotene in protecting against the deleterious effects of photosensitization in human erythropoietic protoporphyria has not been established. In spite of markedly elevated blood carotene levels, vitamin A levels do not rise above normal. Treated patients become carotenemic and may have slightly yellow skin pigmentation due to accumulation of beta-carotene. The sclera does not become yellow, in contrast to patients with icterus.

Indications: Solatene is a useful agent to ameliorate photosensitivity in patients with erythropoietic protoporphyria.

Contraindications: Beta-carotene is contraindicated in patients with known hypersensitivity to the drug.

Warnings: Beta-carotene has not been shown to be effective as a sunscreen in normal individuals. It should not be used for this effect.

Usage in Pregnancy: The safety of beta-carotene in this dosage range in women who are or who may become pregnant has not been established; hence, it should be given only when the potential benefits have been weighed against possible hazard to mother and child.

Precautions: Beta-carotene should be given with caution to patients with impaired renal or hepatic function, because safety in these conditions has not been established. Patients should be forewarned that their skin may appear slightly yellow while receiving beta-carotene therapy. Since beta-carotene will fulfill normal vitamin A requirements, additional vitamin A should not be prescribed.

Adverse Reactions: Some patients may have occasional looser stools while taking beta-carotene. This reaction is sporadic in appearance and may not require discontinuance of medication.

Dosage and Administration: Solatene may be administered either as a single daily dose or in divided doses, preferably with meals.

Usage in Children: The usual dose for children under 14 is 30 to 150 mg (1 to 5 capsules) per day. Capsules may be opened and contents mixed in orange or tomato juice to aid administration in children.

Usage in Adults: The usual adult dosage is 30 to 300 mg (1 to 10 capsules) per day.

Dosage should be adjusted depending on the severity of the symptoms and the response of the patient. Several weeks of therapy are necessary to accumulate enough beta-carotene in the skin to exert its protective effect. Patients should be instructed not to increase exposure to sunlight until they appear carotenemic (first seen as yellowness of palms and soles). This usually occurs after two to six weeks of therapy. Exposure to the sun should then be increased gradually. The protective effect is not total, and each patient must establish his or her own limits of exposure.

How Supplied: For oral administration, blue and green capsules containing 30 mg of beta-carotene/Roche—bottles of 100. Imprint on capsules: ROCHE 115.

[*Shown in Product Identification Section*]

SYNKAYVITE® ℞

(menadiol sodium diphosphate/Roche)
Injectable

The following text is complete prescribing information based on official labeling in effect August 1, 1979.

Description: Menadiol sodium diphosphate is a synthetic, water-soluble vitamin-K analog. Chemically, it is 2-methyl-1,4-naphthalenediol bis (dihydrogen phosphate) tetrasodium salt.

The composition is as follows: *1 ml ampuls, 5 mg/ml:* Each ml contains 5 mg menadiol sodium diphosphate/Roche compounded with 2.5 mg sodium metabisulfite, 0.45% phenol as preservative, 0.4% sodium chloride for isotonicity and pH adjusted to approximately 8.0 with sodium hydroxide.

1 ml ampuls, 10 mg/ml: Each ml contains 10 mg menadiol sodium diphosphate/Roche compounded with 2.5 mg sodium metabisulfite, 0.45% phenol as preservative, 0.4% sodium chloride for isotonicity and pH adjusted to approximately 8.0 with sodium hydroxide.

2 ml ampuls, 75 mg/2 ml: Each 2 ml contains 75 mg menadiol sodium diphosphate/Roche compounded with 5 mg sodium metabisulfite, 0.45% phenol as preservative, 0.4% sodium chloride for isotonicity and pH adjusted to approximately 8.0 with sodium hydroxide.

Actions: Synkayvite is a synthetic water-soluble derivative of menadione (vitamin K_3) to which it is converted *in vivo*. Its potency is approximately one-half that of menadione. Vitamin K is necessary for the synthesis in the liver of prothrombin (factor II), proconvertin (factor VII), thromboplastin (factor IX) and Stuart factor (factor X). The prothrombin test is sensitive to the levels of factors II, VII and X. The mechanism by which vitamin K promotes formation of these clotting factors in the liver is not known. The action of Synkayvite is generally detectable within an hour or two.

Indications: Synkayvite is indicated in the treatment of hypoprothrombinemia secondary to factors limiting absorption or synthesis of vitamin K, *e.g.*, obstructive jaundice, biliary fistula, sprue, ulcerative colitis, celiac disease, intestinal resection, cystic fibrosis of the pancreas, regional enteritis and antibacterial therapy.

It is also indicated in hypoprothrombinemia secondary to administration of salicylates.

May also be used as a liver function test, although newer methods are available.

Contraindications: Vitamin K, or any of its synthetic analogs, should not be administered to the mother during the last few weeks of pregnancy as a prophylactic measure against physiologic hypoprothrombinemia or hemorrhagic disease of the newborn.

Warnings: In the prophylaxis and treatment of hemorrhagic disease of the newborn, the water-soluble vitamin K analogs are not as safe as Konakion® (phytonadione/Roche).

Synkayvite will not counteract the anticoagulant action of heparin.

Usage in Pregnancy: Effects on reproduction have not been studied in animals. There is no adequate information on whether this drug may affect fertility in human males or females or have a teratogenic potential or other adverse effect on the fetus.

Precautions: Temporary resistance to prothrombin-depressing anticoagulants may result, especially when larger doses of Synkayvite are used. If relatively large doses have been employed, it may be necessary when reinstituting anticoagulant therapy to use larger doses of the prothrombin-depressing anticoagulant, or to use one which acts on a different principle, such as heparin.

Since the liver is the site of metabolic synthesis of prothrombin, hypoprothrombinemia resulting from hepatocellular damage is not corrected by administration of vitamin K. Repeated large doses of vitamin K are not warranted in liver disease if the response to initial use of the vitamin is unsatisfactory (Koller Test). Failure to respond to vitamin K may indicate the presence of a coagulation defect or that the condition being treated is unresponsive to vitamin K.

Adverse Reactions: In adults, bromsulfalein retention and prolongation of prothrombin time have been reported after maximum doses of vitamin K analogs. In infants (particularly premature babies), excessive doses of vitamin K analogs may cause increased bilirubinemia in the first few days of life. This, in turn, may result in kernicterus, which may lead to brain damage or even death. Immaturity is apparently an important factor in the appearance of toxic reactions to vitamin K analogs as full term and larger premature infants demonstrate greater tolerance than smaller premature infants.

Menadione can induce erythrocyte hemolysis in persons having a genetic deficiency of glucose-6-phosphate dehydrogenase in their red blood cells.

In patients with severe hepatic disease, large doses of menadione may further depress liver function.

Occasional allergic reactions, such as skin rash and urticaria, have been reported.

Dosage and Administration: The minimum daily requirements for vitamin K in humans have not been established officially. Minimal daily requirements have been estimated at 1 to 5 micrograms per kilogram for infants and 0.03 micrograms per kilogram for adults. The dietary abundance of vitamin K normally satisfies the requirements except for the neonatal period of 5 to 8 days.

Synkayvite may be injected subcutaneously, intramuscularly or intravenously. The response after intravenous administration may be more prompt, but more sustained action follows intramuscular or subcutaneous use.

The usual recommended dosages are given in the accompanying chart.

[See table above].

USUAL RECOMMENDED DOSAGES FOR SYNKAYVITE INJECTABLE

	ADULTS	CHILDREN
For treatment of hypoprothrombinemia	5 to 15 mg once or twice daily	5 to 10 mg once or twice daily
For liver function test	75 mg intravenously	

Storage: Synkayvite need not be refrigerated. Store at room temperature (59° to 86°F).

How Supplied: 1-ml ampuls (5 mg/ml); 1-ml ampuls (10 mg/ml); and 2-ml ampuls (75 mg/2 ml)—boxes of 10.

SYNKAYVITE® ℞

(menadiol sodium diphosphate/Roche)
Tablets

The following text is complete prescribing information based on official labeling in effect August 1, 1979.

Description: Menadiol sodium diphosphate is a synthetic, water-soluble vitamin-K analog. Chemically, it is 2-methyl-1,4-naphthalenediol bis (dihydrogen phosphate) tetrasodium salt.

Actions: Synkayvite is a synthetic, water-soluble derivative of menadione (vitamin K_3) to which it is converted *in vivo*. Its potency is approximately one-half that of menadione. Vitamin K is necessary for the synthesis in the liver of prothrombin (factor II), proconvertin (factor VII), thromboplastin (factor IX) and Stuart factor (factor X). The prothrombin test is sensitive to the levels of factors II, VII and X. The mechanism by which vitamin K promotes formation of these clotting factors in the liver is not known.

Indications: Vitamin K deficiency secondary to the administration of antibacterial therapy.

Hypoprothrombinemia secondary to obstructive jaundice and biliary fistulas.

Hypoprothrombinemia secondary to administration of salicylates.

Contraindications: Vitamin K, or any of its synthetic analogs, should not be administered to the mother during the last few weeks of pregnancy as a prophylactic measure against

Continued on next page

Roche—Cont.

physiologic hypoprothrombinemia or hemorrhagic disease of the newborn.
Warnings: Synkayvite will not counteract the anticoagulant action of heparin.
Usage in Pregnancy: Effects on reproduction have not been studied in animals. There is no adequate information on whether this drug may affect fertility in human males or females or have a teratogenic potential or other adverse effect on the fetus.
Precautions: Temporary resistance to prothrombin-depressing anticoagulants may result, especially when larger doses of Synkayvite are used. If relatively large doses have been employed, it may be necessary when reinstituting anticoagulant therapy to use somewhat larger doses of the prothrombin-depressing anticoagulant or to use one which acts on a different principle, such as heparin.
Since the liver is the site of metabolic synthesis of prothrombin, hypoprothrombinemia resulting from hepatocellular damage is not corrected by administration of vitamin K. Repeated large doses of vitamin K are not warranted in liver disease if the response to initial use of the vitamin is unsatisfactory (Koller Test). Failure to respond to vitamin K may indicate the presence of a coagulation defect or that the condition being treated is unresponsive to vitamin K.
Adverse Reactions: Bromsulfalein retention and prolongation of prothrombin time have been reported after maximum doses of vitamin K analogs.
Menadione can induce erythrocyte hemolysis in persons having a genetic deficiency of glucose-6-phosphate dehydrogenase in their red blood cells.
In patients with severe hepatic disease, large doses of menadione may further depress liver function.
Occasional allergic reactions, such as skin rash and urticaria, have been reported. There have also been minor instances of gastric upset.
Dosage and Administration: The minimum daily requirements for vitamin K in humans have not been established officially. Minimal daily requirements have been estimated as 0.03 micrograms per kilogram for adults. The dietary abundance of vitamin K normally satisfies the requirements except for the neonatal period of 5 to 8 days.

For hypoprothrombinemia secondary to obstructive jaundice and biliary fistulas... 5 mg daily

For hypoprothrombinemia secondary to the administration of antibacterials or salicylates... 5 to 10 mg daily

How Supplied: Tablets, 5 mg menadiol sodium diphosphate/Roche each—bottles of 100.
[*Shown in Product Identification Section*]

TARACTAN® TABLETS ℞
(chlorprothixene/Roche)
TARACTAN® CONCENTRATE ℞
(chlorprothixene lactate and HCl/Roche)
TARACTAN® AMPULS ℞
(chlorprothixene HCl/Roche)

The following text is complete prescribing information based on official labeling in effect August 1, 1979.
Description: Tablets—each containing 10 mg, 25 mg, 50 mg or 100 mg chlorprothixene. Concentrate—100 mg/5 ml as the lactate and hydrochloride, fruit flavored. Ampuls—25 mg/2 ml as the hydrochloride, with 0.2% parabens (methyl and propyl) added as preservatives and pH adjusted to approximately 3.4 with HCl.
Taractan is a thioxanthene derivative. Chemically, it is the alpha isomer of 2-chloro-*N,N*-dimethylthioxanthene-Δ^9, γ-propylamine. In chemical structure chlorprothixene resembles the phenothiazines; however, in place of the nitrogen (N) in the phenothiazine ring, chlorprothixene carries a carbon atom with a double bond to a side chain.
Actions: EEG changes following the injection of Taractan into cats suggest that it acts on the brain stem. Effects demonstrated were the synchronization of the EEG tracings during rest, a shortening of cortical activation obtained by stimulation of the reticular formation, and modifications of elicited potentials.
Indications: Taractan is indicated for the management of manifestations of psychotic disorders. Taractan has not been shown effective in the management of behavioral complications in patients with mental retardation.
Contraindications: Circulatory collapse, comatose states due to central depressant drugs (alcohol, hypnotics, opiates, etc.) and known sensitivity to the drug are contraindications.
Warnings: *Usage in Pregnancy:* The safety of Taractan during pregnancy or lactation in humans has not been established. Therefore, use of Taractan in women who may become pregnant requires weighing the drug's potential benefits against its possible hazards to mother and child. For the results of reproductive and teratogenic studies in rats and rabbits see ANIMAL PHARMACOLOGY AND TOXICOLOGY.
This drug may impair the mental and/or physical abilities required for the performance of hazardous tasks such as operating machinery or driving a motor vehicle; therefore, the patient should be cautioned accordingly.
As in the case of other CNS-acting drugs, patients receiving Taractan should be cautioned about possible combined effects with alcohol.
The safety and efficacy of Taractan have not been established for oral administration in children under age 6 or for parenteral use in those under age 12.
Precautions: Because of its structural similarity to the phenothiazines, all of the precautions associated with phenothiazine therapy should be considered when patients receive Taractan. Therefore, Taractan should be used with caution in patients who:
—are receiving barbiturates or narcotics, because of additive effects of central nervous system depressants. The dosage of the narcotic or barbiturate should be reduced when given concomitantly with Taractan.
—are receiving atropine or related drugs, because of additive anticholinergic effects.
—have a history of epilepsy. When necessary, Taractan may be used concomitantly with anticonvulsant drugs. However, use of Taractan may lower the convulsive threshold; therefore, an adequate dosage of the anticonvulsant should be maintained.
—are exposed to extreme heat or phosphorous insecticides.
—have cardiovascular disease.
—have respiratory impairment due to acute pulmonary infections or chronic respiratory disorders such as severe asthma or emphysema.

The concurrent use of Taractan and electroshock treatment should be reserved for those patients for whom it is essential, but the hazards may be increased.
Taractan may augment or interfere with the absorption, metabolism or therapeutic activity of other psychotropic drugs and vice versa.
The appearance of signs of blood dyscrasias requires immediate discontinuance of the drug and the institution of appropriate therapy.
The possibility of liver damage, variations in thyroid function, pigmentary retinopathy, lenticular or corneal deposits and development of irreversible dyskinesias should be kept in mind when patients are on prolonged therapy.
When used in the treatment of agitated states accompanying depression, the usual precautions indicated with such patients are necessary, particularly the recognition that a suicidal tendency may be present and protective measures necessary.
Abrupt Withdrawal: Taractan is not known to produce physical dependence. However, gastritis, nausea and vomiting, dizziness and tremulousness have been reported following abrupt cessation of high-dose therapy.
There is sufficient experimental evidence to conclude that chronic administration of antipsychotic drugs which increase prolactin secretion has the potential to induce mammary neoplasms in rodents under the appropriate conditions. There are recognized differences in the physiological role of prolactin between rodents and humans. Since there are, at present, no adequate epidemiological studies, the relevance to human mammary cancer risk from prolonged exposure to Taractan or other antipsychotic drugs is not known.
Adverse Reactions: Not all of the following adverse reactions have been reported with Taractan; however, pharmacological similarities to the various phenothiazine derivatives require that each be considered.
Note: *Sudden death* has occasionally been reported in patients who have received phenothiazines. In some cases death was apparently due to cardiac arrest, in others the cause appeared to be asphyxia due to failure of the cough reflex. In some patients the cause could not be determined nor could it be established that death was due to the phenothiazine.
Drowsiness: May occur particularly during the first or second week, after which it generally disappears. If troublesome, dosage may be lowered.
Jaundice: Incidence is low. It usually occurs between the second and fourth weeks and is regarded as a sensitivity reaction. The clinical picture resembles infectious hepatitis with laboratory features of obstructive jaundice. It is usually reversible; however, chronic jaundice has been reported.
Hematological Disorders: Agranulocytosis, eosinophilia, leukopenia, hemolytic anemia, thrombocytopenic purpura and pancytopenia.
Agranulocytosis: Most cases have occurred between the fourth and tenth weeks of therapy. Patients should be watched closely during that period for the sudden appearance of sore throat or other signs of infection. If white blood count and differential show significant cellular depression, discontinue the drug and start appropriate therapy. However, a slightly lowered white count is not in itself an indication to discontinue the drug.
Cardiovascular: Postural hypotension, tachycardia (especially with sudden marked increase in dosage), bradycardia, cardiac arrest, faintness and dizziness. Occasionally the hypotensive effect may produce a shock-like condition. In the event a vasoconstrictor is required, levarterenol and phenylephrine are the most suitable. Other pressor agents, including epinephrine, should not be used, as a paradoxical further lowering of the blood pressure may ensue.
ECG changes, nonspecific, usually reversible, have been observed in some patients receiving phenothiazine tranquilizers. Their relationship to myocardial damage has not been confirmed.
CNS Effects: Neuromuscular (Extrapyramidal) Reactions: These are usually dosage-related and take three forms: (1) pseudoparkinsonism, (2) akathisia (motor restlessness) and (3) dystonias. Dystonias include spasms of the neck muscles, extensor rigidity of back muscles, carpopedal spasm, eyes rolled back, convulsions, trismus and swallowing difficulties. These resemble serious neurological disorders but usually subside within 48 hours. Management of the extrapyramidal symptoms, depending upon the type and severity, includes sedation, injectable diphenhydramine and the use of antiparkinsonism agents. In rare instances, persistent dyskinesias usually involving the face, tongue and jaw have been reported to last

months, even years, particularly in elderly patients with previous brain damage.
Hyperreflexia has been reported in the newborn when a phenothiazine was used during pregnancy.
Adverse Behavioral Effects: Paradoxical exacerbation of psychotic symptoms.
Other CNS Effects: Cerebral edema. Abnormality of cerebrospinal fluid proteins. Convulsive seizures, particularly in patients with EEG abnormalities or a history of such disorders. Hyperpyrexia.
Allergic Reactions: Urticaria, itching, erythema, photosensitivity (avoid undue exposure to the sun), eczema. Severe reactions including exfoliative dermatitis (rare); contact dermatitis in nursing personnel administering the drug; asthma, laryngeal edema, angioneurotic edema, anaphylactoid reactions.
Endocrine Disorders: Lactation and moderate breast engorgement in females and gynecomastia in males on large doses, changes in libido, false-positive pregnancy tests, amenorrhea, hyperglycemia, hypoglycemia, glycosuria.
Autonomic Reactions: Dry mouth, nasal congestion, constipation, adynamic ileus, myosis, mydriasis, urinary retention.
Special Considerations in Long-Term Therapy: After prolonged administration of high doses, pigmentation of the skin has occurred chiefly in the exposed areas, especially in females on large doses. Ocular changes consisting of deposition of fine particulate matter in the cornea and lens, progressing in more severe cases to star-shaped lenticular opacities; epithelial keratopathies; pigmentary retinopathy.
Persistent Tardive Dyskinesia: As with all antipsychotic agents, tardive dyskinesia may appear in some patients on long-term therapy or may occur after drug therapy has been discontinued. The risk seems to be greater in elderly patients on high-dose therapy, especially females. The symptoms are persistent and in some patients appear to be irreversible. The syndrome is characterized by rhythmical involuntary movements of the tongue, face, mouth, or jaw (*e.g.*, protrusion of tongue, puffing of cheeks, puckering of mouth, chewing movements). Sometimes these may be accompanied by involuntary movements of extremities.
There is no known effective treatment for tardive dyskinesia; antiparkinsonism agents usually do not alleviate the symptoms of this syndrome. It is suggested that all antipsychotic agents be discontinued if these symptoms appear. Should it be necessary to reinstitute treatment, or increase the dosage of the agent, or switch to a different antipsychotic agent, the syndrome may be masked.
It has been reported that fine vermicular movements of the tongue may be an early sign of the syndrome and if the medication is stopped at that time the syndrome may not develop.
Other Adverse Reactions: Enlargement of the parotid gland; increases in appetite and weight; peripheral edema.
The occurrence of a systemic lupus erythematosus-like syndrome has been related to phenothiazine therapy.
Dosage and Administration: Dosage should be individually adjusted according to diagnosis and severity of the condition. In general, small doses should be used initially, and increased to the optimal effective level as rapidly as possible based on therapeutic response. When higher dosage is required, greater sedation may be encountered; therefore, patients should be closely supervised. Lethargy and drowsiness are readily controlled by dosage reduction. Initially, lower doses (10 to 25 mg three or four times daily) should be used for elderly or debilitated patients.
For convenience in prescribing and dispensing, all recommended dosages are expressed as strengths of the active moiety, chlorprothixene.
Taractan may be administered orally as tablets or concentrate. The concentrate, containing 100 mg of the drug per 5 ml teaspoonful, is pleasantly flavored and may be administered alone or in milk, water, fruit juices, coffee and carbonated beverages.

Oral	**Average Daily Dose**
Adults:	Initially, 25 to 50 mg three or four times daily; to be increased as needed. Dosages exceeding 600 mg daily are rarely required.
Children (over 6 years of age):	10 to 25 mg three or four times daily.
Parenteral	
Not to be used in children under the age of 12.	25 to 50 mg I.M. up to three or four times daily.

Pain or induration at the site of injection is minimal. Since postural hypotension may occur in some patients, injection should be given with the patient seated or recumbent. If hypotension does occur, recovery is usually spontaneous; however, the patient should be observed until symptoms of weakness or dizziness pass.
As soon as the acutely agitated patient is brought under control, oral medication should be instituted. The changeover should be made gradually, with oral and parenteral doses being given alternately on the same day, then oral doses only, adjusted to the required maintenance level.
Overdosage: Taractan can be fatal in overdosage in the range of 2.5 to 4 Gm or above. Manifestations of overdosage are drowsiness, coma, respiratory depression, hypotension (which may appear after a delay of several hours and may persist for two to three days), tachycardia, pyrexia and constricted pupils. Convulsions, hyperactivity and hematuria may be seen in the recovery period.
Treatment is essentially symptomatic. Early gastric lavage is recommended, along with supportive measures such as I.V. fluids and the maintenance of an adequate airway. Severe hypotension usually responds to the use of levarterenol or metaraminol. Should coma be prolonged, caffeine and sodium benzoate, or ethamivan may be used, but the possibility must be borne in mind that these may lead to a convulsive episode. Should convulsions occur, the judicious use of sodium amytal is recommended. **Epinephrine must not be used in these patients.**
How Supplied: Tablets—10 mg, 25 mg, 50 mg or 100 mg chlorprothixene—bottles of 100 and 500.
Concentrate—containing, in each teaspoonful, chlorprothixene 100 mg base (as the lactate and hydrochloride)—bottles of 16 fluid ounces (1 pint).
Ampuls—containing chlorprothixene 25 mg/2 ml as the hydrochloride—boxes of 10.
Animal Pharmacology and Toxicology: In mice, the oral LD_{50} of the two oral dosage forms of chlorprothixene were 350 ± 27 mg/kg (as the 2 per cent concentrate) and 220 ± 24 mg/kg (as the tablet form ground and suspended in 5 per cent gum acacia). For the injectable form the intramuscular LD_{50} in mice was greater than 125 mg/kg.
Reproduction Studies: Reproductive and teratological studies in rats and rabbits were performed at levels of 12 and 24 mg/kg. In the rats, a decreased conception rate and an increased incidence of stillborns was noted at both levels. An increased number of resorptions was noted only at the high dose level. There was a decrease in the number of implantation sites at both doses. The number of live fetuses per litter and the mean fetal body weights were reduced slightly at 12 mg/kg and more so at 24 mg/kg. No teratological effects were observed. No deleterious effects on reproduction were seen in rabbits nor were any teratological findings noted.
[*Shown in Product Identification Section*]

TEL-E-DOSE®

Tel-E-Dose is a unit package designed by Roche for convenience in dispensing medications in the hospital and nursing home. Each unit, sealed against contamination and moisture, is clearly identified by product name and strength and carries the control number and expiration date.
Currently available in this package form are the following Roche products: Bactrim™ (80 mg trimethoprim and 400 mg sulfamethoxazole) tablets; Bactrim DS (160 mg trimethoprim and 800 mg sulfamethoxazole) tablets; Dalmane® (flurazepam HCl) capsules, 15 mg, 30 mg; Endep® (amitriptyline HCl) tablets, 10 mg, 25 mg, 50 mg, 75 mg, 100 mg, 150 mg; Gantanol® (sulfamethoxazole) tablets, 0.5 Gm; Gantanol® DS (sulfamethoxazole) tablets, 1 Gm; Gantrisin® (sulfisoxazole) tablets, 0.5 Gm; Larotid® (amoxicillin) capsules, 250 mg, 500 mg; Larotid® (amoxicillin) oral suspension, 125 mg and 250 mg; Librax® (5 mg chlordiazepoxide HCl and 2.5 mg clidinium Br); Librium® (chlordiazepoxide HCl) capsules, 5 mg, 10 mg, 25 mg; Limbitrol (chlordiazepoxide and amitriptyline HCl) tablets, 10-25, 5-12.5; and Valium® (diazepam) tablets, 2 mg, 5 mg, 10 mg.

TENSILON® ℞

(edrophonium chloride/Roche)
Injectable Solution
ampuls • vials

The following text is complete prescribing information based on official labeling in effect August 1, 1979.
Description: Tensilon is a short and rapid-acting cholinergic drug. Chemically, edrophonium chloride is ethyl(*m*-hydroxyphenyl)-dimethylammonium chloride.
10-ml vials: Each ml contains, in a sterile solution, 10 mg edrophonium chloride/Roche compounded with 0.45% phenol and 0.2% sodium sulfite as preservatives, buffered with sodium citrate and citric acid, and pH adjusted to approximately 5.4.
1-ml ampuls: Each ml contains, in a sterile solution, 10 mg edrophonium chloride/Roche compounded with 0.2% sodium sulfite, buffered with sodium citrate and citric acid, and pH adjusted to approximately 5.4.
Actions: Tensilon is an anticholinesterase drug. Its pharmacological action is due primarily to the inhibition or inactivation of acetylcholinesterase at sites of cholinergic transmission. Its effect is manifest within 30 to 60 seconds after injection and lasts an average of 10 minutes.
Indications: Tensilon is recommended for the differential diagnosis of myasthenia gravis and as an adjunct in the evaluation of treatment requirements in this disease. It may also be used for evaluating emergency treatment in myasthenic crises. Because of its brief duration of action, it is not recommended for maintenance therapy in myasthenia gravis.
Tensilon is also useful whenever a curare antagonist is needed to reverse the neuromuscular block produced by curare, tubocurarine, gallamine triethiodide or dimethyl-tubocurarine. It is *not* effective against decamethonium bromide and succinylcholine chloride. It may be used adjunctively in the treatment of respiratory depression caused by curare overdosage.
Contraindications: Known hypersensitivity to anticholinesterase agents; intestinal and urinary obstructions of mechanical type.
Warnings: Whenever anticholinesterase drugs are used for testing, a syringe containing

Continued on next page

Roche—Cont.

1 mg of atropine sulfate should be immediately available to be given in aliquots intravenously to counteract severe cholinergic reactions which may occur in the hypersensitive individual, whether he is normal or myasthenic. Tensilon should be used with caution in patients with bronchial asthma or cardiac dysrhythmias. The transient bradycardia which sometimes occurs can be relieved by atropine sulfate. Isolated instances of cardiac and respiratory arrest following administration of Tensilon have been reported. It is postulated that these are vagotonic effects.

Usage in Pregnancy: The safety of Tensilon during pregnancy or lactation in humans has not been established. Therefore, use of Tensilon in women who may become pregnant requires weighing the drug's potential benefits against its possible hazards to mother and child.

Precautions: Patients may develop "anticholinesterase insensitivity" for brief or prolonged periods. During these periods the patients should be carefully monitored and may need respiratory assistance. Dosages of anticholinesterase drugs should be reduced or withheld until patients again become sensitive to them.

Adverse Reactions: Careful observation should be made for severe cholinergic reactions in the hyperreactive individual. The myasthenic patient in crisis who is being tested with Tensilon should be observed for bradycardia or cardiac standstill and cholinergic reactions if an overdose is given. The following reactions common to anticholinesterase agents may occur, although not all of these reactions have been reported with the administration of Tensilon, probably because of its short duration of action and limited indications: **Eye:** Increased lacrimation, pupillary constriction, spasm of accommodation, diplopia, conjunctival hyperemia. **CNS:** Convulsions, dysarthria, dysphonia, dysphagia. **Respiratory:** Increased tracheobronchial secretions, laryngospasm, bronchiolar constriction, paralysis of muscles of respiration, central respiratory paralysis. **Cardiac:** Arrhythmias (especially bradycardia), fall in cardiac output leading to hypotension. **G.I.:** Increased salivary, gastric and intestinal secretion, nausea, vomiting, increased peristalsis, diarrhea, abdominal cramps. **Skeletal Muscle:** Weakness, fasciculations. **Miscellaneous:** Increased urinary frequency and incontinence, diaphoresis.

Dosage and Administration: *Tensilon Test in the Differential Diagnosis of Myasthenia Gravis:*[1-8]

Intravenous Dosage (Adults): A tuberculin syringe containing 1 ml (10 mg) of Tensilon is prepared with an intravenous needle, and 0.2 ml (2 mg) is injected intravenously within 15 to 30 seconds. The needle is left *in situ. Only* if no reaction occurs after 45 seconds is the remaining 0.8 ml (8 mg) injected. If a cholinergic reaction (muscarinic side effects, skeletal muscle fasciculations and increased muscle weakness) occurs after injection of 0.2 ml (2 mg), the test is discontinued and atropine sulfate 0.4 mg to 0.5 mg is administered intravenously. After one-half hour the test may be repeated.

Intramuscular Dosage (Adults): In adults with inaccessible veins, dosage for intramuscular injection is 1 ml (10 mg) of Tensilon. Subjects who demonstrate hyperreactivity to this injection (cholinergic reaction), should be retested after one-half hour with 0.2 ml (2 mg) of Tensilon intramuscularly to rule out false-negative reactions.

Dosage (Children): The intravenous testing dose of Tensilon in children weighing up to 75 lbs is 0.1 ml (1 mg); above this weight, the dose is 0.2 ml (2 mg). If there is no response after 45 seconds, it may be titrated up to 0.5 ml (5 mg) in children under 75 lbs, given in increments of 0.1 ml (1 mg) every 30 to 45 seconds and up to 1 ml (10 mg) in heavier children. In infants, the recommended dose is 0.05 ml (0.5 mg). Because of technical difficulty with intravenous injection in children, the intramuscular route may be used. In children weighing up to 75 lbs, 0.2 ml (2 mg) is injected intramuscularly. In children weighing more than 75 lbs, 0.5 ml (5 mg) is injected intramuscularly. All signs which would appear with the intravenous test appear with the intramuscular test except that there is a delay of two to ten minutes before a reaction is noted.

Tensilon Test for Evaluation of Treatment Requirements in Myasthenia Gravis: The recommended dose is 0.1 ml to 0.2 ml (1 mg to 2 mg) of Tensilon, administered intravenously one hour after oral intake of the drug being used in treatment.[1-5] Response will be myasthenic in the undertreated patient, adequate in the controlled patient, and cholinergic in the overtreated patient. Responses to Tensilon in myasthenic and nonmyasthenic individuals are summarized in the accompanying chart.[2]
[See table below].

Tensilon Test in Crisis: The term *crisis* is applied to the myasthenic whenever severe respiratory distress with objective ventilatory inadequacy occurs and the response to medication is not predictable. This state may be secondary to a sudden increase in severity of myasthenia gravis (myasthenic crisis), or to overtreatment with anticholinesterase drugs (cholinergic crisis).

When a patient is apneic, controlled ventilation must be secured immediately in order to avoid cardiac arrest and irreversible central nervous system damage. No attempt is made to test with Tensilon until respiratory exchange is adequate. *Dosage used at this time is most important:* If the patient is cholinergic, Tensilon will cause increased oropharyngeal secretions and further weakness in the muscles of respiration. If the crisis is myasthenic, the test clearly improves respiration and the patient can be treated with longer-acting intravenous anticholinesterase medication. When the test is performed, there should not be more than 0.2 ml (2 mg) Tensilon in the syringe. An intravenous dose of 0.1 ml (1 mg) is given initially. The patient's heart action is carefully observed. If, after an interval of one minute, this dose does not further impair the patient, the remaining 0.1 ml (1 mg) can be injected. If no clear improvement of respiration occurs after 0.2 ml (2 mg) dose, it is usually wisest to discontinue all anticholinesterase drug therapy and secure controlled ventilation by tracheostomy with assisted respiration.[5]

For Use as a Curare Antagonist: Tensilon should be administered by intravenous injection in 1 ml (10 mg) doses given slowly over a period of 30 to 45 seconds so that the onset of cholinergic reaction can be detected. This dosage may be repeated whenever necessary. The maximal dose for any one patient should be 4 ml (40 mg). Because of its brief effect, Tensilon should not be given prior to the administration of curare, tubocurarine, gallamine triethiodide or dimethyl-tubocurarine; it should be used at the time when its effect is needed. When given to counteract curare overdosage, the effect of each dose on the respiration should be carefully observed before it is repeated, and assisted ventilation should always be employed.

Drug Interactions: Care should be given when administering this drug to patients with symptoms of myasthenic weakness who are also on anticholinesterase drugs. Since symptoms of anticholinesterase overdose (cholinergic crisis) may mimic underdosage (myasthenic weakness), their condition may be worsened by the use of this drug. (See OVERDOSAGE section for treatment.)

Overdosage: With drugs of this type, muscarine-like symptoms (nausea, vomiting, diarrhea, sweating, increased bronchial and salivary secretions and bradycardia) often appear with overdosage (cholinergic crisis). An important complication that can arise is obstruction of the airway by bronchial secretions. These may be managed with suction (especially if tracheostomy has been performed) and by the use of atropine. Many experts have advocated a wide range of dosages of atropine *(for Tensilon, see atropine dosage below)*, but if there are copious secretions, up to 1.2 mg intravenously may be given initially and repeated every 20 minutes until secretions are controlled. Signs of atropine overdosage such as dry mouth, flush and tachycardia should be avoided as tenacious secretions and bronchial plugs may form. A total dose of atropine of 5 to 10 mg or even more may be required. The following steps should be taken in the management of overdosage of Tensilon:

1. Adequate respiratory exchange should be maintained by assuring an open airway, and the use of assisted respiration augmented by oxygen.
2. Cardiac function should be monitored until complete stabilization has been achieved.
3. Atropine sulfate in doses of 0.4 to 0.5 mg should be administered intravenously. This may be repeated every 3 to 10 minutes. Because of the short duration of action of Tensilon the total dose required will seldom exceed 2 mg.
4. Pralidoxime chloride (a cholinesterase reactivator) may be given intravenously at the rate of 50 to 100 mg per minute; usually the total dose does not exceed 1000 mg. Extreme caution should be exercised in the use of pralidoxime chloride when the cholinergic symptoms are induced by double-bond phosphorous anticholinesterase drugs.[9]
5. If convulsions or shock is present, appropriate measures should be instituted.

How Supplied: *Multiple Dose Vials,* 10 ml. *Ampuls,* 1 ml, boxes of 10.

References:

1. Osserman, K.E. and Kaplan, L.I., *J.A.M.A., 150:*265, 1952.

	Myasthenic*	Adequate**	Cholinergic***
Muscle Strength . . . (ptosis, diplopia, dysphonia, dysphagia, dysarthria, respiration, limb strength)	Increased	No change	Decreased
Fasciculations . . . (orbicularis oculi, facial muscles, limb muscles)	Absent	Present or absent	Present or absent
Side reactions . . . (lacrimation, diaphoresis, salivation, abdominal cramps, nausea, vomiting, diarrhea)	Absent	Minimal	Severe

*Myasthenic Response—occurs in untreated myasthenics and may serve to establish diagnosis; in patients under treatment, indicates that therapy is inadequate.

**Adequate Response—observed in treated patients when therapy is stabilized; a typical response in normal individuals. In addition to this response in nonmyasthenics, the phenomenon of forced lid closure is often observed in psychoneurotics.[1]

***Cholinergic Response—seen in myasthenics who have been overtreated with anticholinesterase drugs.

2. Osserman, K.E., Kaplan, L.I. and Besson, G., *J. Mt. Sinai Hosp., 20:*165, 1953.
3. Osserman, K.E. and Kaplan, L.I., *Arch. Neurol. & Psychiat., 70:*385, 1953.
4. Osserman, K.E. and Teng, P., *J.A.M.A., 160:*153, 1956.
5. Osserman, K.E. and Genkins, G., *Ann. N.Y. Acad. Sci., 135:*312, 1966.
6. Tether, J.E., Second International Symposium Proceedings, Myasthenia Gravis, 1961, p. 444.
7. Tether, J.E., in H.F. Conn: *Current Therapy 1960,* Philadelphia, W. B. Saunders Company, p. 551.
8. Tether, J.E., in H.F. Conn: *Current Therapy 1965,* Philadelphia, W. B. Saunders Company, p. 556.
9. Grob, D. and Johns, R.J., *J.A.M.A., 166:*1855, 1958.

VALIUM® Injectable ℭ
(diazepam/Roche)

The following text is complete prescribing information based on official labeling in effect November 7, 1979.

Description: Each ml contains 5 mg diazepam/Roche compounded with 40% propylene glycol, 10% ethyl alcohol, 5% sodium benzoate and benzoic acid as buffers, and 1.5% benzyl alcohol as preservative.

Diazepam is a benzodiazepine derivative developed through original Roche research. Chemically, diazepam is 7-chloro-1,3-dihydro-1-methyl-5-phenyl-2H-1, 4-benzodiazepin-2-one. It is a colorless crystalline compound, insoluble in water and has a molecular weight of 284.74.

Actions: In animals, diazepam appears to act on parts of the limbic system, the thalamus and hypothalamus, and induces calming effects. Diazepam, unlike chlorpromazine and reserpine, has no demonstrable peripheral autonomic blocking action, nor does it produce extrapyramidal side effects; however, animals treated with diazepam do have a transient ataxia at higher doses. Diazepam was found to have transient cardiovascular depressor effects in dogs. Long-term experiments in rats revealed no disturbances of endocrine function. Injections into animals have produced localized irritation of tissue surrounding injection sites and some thickening of veins after intravenous use.

Indications: Valium is indicated for the symptomatic relief of anxiety and tension associated with anxiety disorders, transient situational disturbances and functional or organic disorders. It is useful in psychoneurotic states manifested by tension, anxiety, apprehension, fatigue, depressive symptoms or agitation.

In acute alcohol withdrawal, Valium may be useful in the symptomatic relief of acute agitation, tremor, impending or acute delirium tremens and hallucinosis.

As an adjunct prior to endoscopic procedures if apprehension, anxiety or acute stress reactions are present, and to diminish the patient's recall of the procedures. (See WARNINGS.)

Valium is a useful adjunct for the relief of skeletal muscle spasm due to reflex spasm to local pathology (such as inflammation of the muscles or joints, or secondary to trauma); spasticity caused by upper motor neuron disorders (such as cerebral palsy and paraplegia); athetosis; stiff-man syndrome; and tetanus.

Injectable Valium is a useful adjunct in status epilepticus and severe recurrent convulsive seizures.

Valium is a useful premedication (the I.M. route is preferred) for relief of anxiety and tension in patients who are to undergo surgical procedures. Intravenously, prior to cardioversion for the relief of anxiety and tension and to diminish the patient's recall of the procedure.

Contraindications: Injectable Valium is contraindicated in patients with a known hypersensitivity to this drug; acute narrow angle glaucoma; and open angle glaucoma unless patients are receiving appropriate therapy.

Warnings: *When used intravenously, the following procedures should be undertaken to reduce the possibility of venous thrombosis, phlebitis, local irritation, swelling, and, rarely, vascular impairment: the solution should be injected slowly, taking at least one minute for each 5 mg (1 ml) given; do not use small veins, such as those on the dorsum of the hand or wrist; extreme care should be taken to avoid intra-arterial administration or extravasation.*

Do not mix or dilute Valium with other solutions or drugs in syringe or infusion flask. If it is not feasible to administer Valium directly I.V., it may be injected slowly through the infusion tubing as close as possible to the vein insertion.

Extreme care must be used in administering Injectable Valium, particularly by the I.V. route, to the elderly, to very ill patients and to those with limited pulmonary reserve because of the possibility that apnea and/ or cardiac arrest may occur. Concomitant use of barbiturates, alcohol or other central nervous system depressants increases depression with increased risk of apnea. Resuscitative equipment including that necessary to support respiration should be readily available.

When Valium is used with a narcotic analgesic, the dosage of the narcotic should be reduced by at least one-third and administered in small increments. In some cases the use of a narcotic may not be necessary.

Injectable Valium should not be administered to patients in shock, coma, or in acute alcoholic intoxication with depression of vital signs. As is true of most CNS-acting drugs, patients receiving Valium should be cautioned against engaging in hazardous occupations requiring complete mental alertness, such as operating machinery or driving a motor vehicle.

Tonic status epilepticus has been precipitated in patients treated with I.V. Valium for petit mal status or petit mal variant status.

Physical and Psychological Dependence: Withdrawal symptoms (similar in character to those noted with barbiturates and alcohol) have occurred following abrupt discontinuance of diazepam (convulsions, tremor, abdominal and muscle cramps, vomiting and sweating). These were usually limited to those patients who had received excessive doses over an extended period of time. Although infrequently seen, milder withdrawal symptoms have also been reported following abrupt discontinuance of benzodiazepines taken continuously, generally at higher therapeutic levels, for at least several months. Consequently, after extended therapy, abrupt discontinuation should generally be avoided and a gradual tapering in dosage followed. Particularly addiction-prone individuals (such as drug addicts or alcoholics) should be under careful surveillance when receiving diazepam or other psychotropic agents because of the predisposition of such patients to habituation and dependence.

Usage in Pregnancy: **An increased risk of congenital malformations associated with the use of minor tranquilizers (diazepam, meprobamate and chlordiazepoxide) during the first trimester of pregnancy has been suggested in several studies. Because use of these drugs is rarely a matter of urgency, their use during this period should almost always be avoided. The possibility that a woman of childbearing potential may be pregnant at the time of institution of therapy should be considered. Patients should be advised that if they become pregnant during therapy or intend to become pregnant they should communicate with their physicians about the desirability of discontinuing the drug.**

In humans, measurable amounts of diazepam were found in maternal and cord blood, indicating placental transfer of the drug. Until additional information is available, Valium Injectable is not recommended for obstetrical use.

Use in Children: Efficacy and safety of parenteral Valium has not been established in the neonate (30 days or less of age).

Prolonged central nervous system depression has been observed in neonates, apparently due to inability to biotransform Valium into inactive metabolites.

In pediatric use, in order to obtain maximal clinical effect with the minimum amount of drug and thus to reduce the risk of hazardous side effects, such as apnea or prolonged periods of somnolence, it is recommended that the drug be given slowly over a three-minute period in a dosage not to exceed 0.25 mg/kg. After an interval of 15 to 30 minutes the initial dosage can be safely repeated. If, however, relief of symptoms is not obtained after a third administration, adjunctive therapy appropriate to the condition being treated is recommended.

Precautions: Although seizures may be brought under control promptly, a significant proportion of patients experience a return to seizure activity, presumably due to the short-lived effect of Valium after I.V. administration. The physician should be prepared to readminister the drug. However, Valium is not recommended for maintenance, and once seizures are brought under control, consideration should be given to the administration of agents useful in longer term control of seizures.

If Valium is to be combined with other psychotropic agents or anticonvulsant drugs, careful consideration should be given to the pharmacology of the agents to be employed—particularly with known compounds which may potentiate the action of Valium, such as phenothiazines, narcotics, barbiturates, MAO inhibitors and other antidepressants. In highly anxious patients with evidence of accompanying depression, particularly those who may have suicidal tendencies, protective measures may be necessary. The usual precautions in treating patients with impaired hepatic function should be observed. Metabolites of Valium are excreted by the kidney; to avoid their excess accumulation, caution should be exercised in the administration to patients with compromised kidney function.

Since an increase in cough reflex and laryngospasm may occur with peroral endoscopic procedures, the use of a topical anesthetic agent and the availability of necessary countermeasures are recommended.

Until additional information is available, injectable diazepam is not recommended for obstetrical use.

Injectable Valium has produced hypotension or muscular weakness in some patients particularly when used with narcotics, barbiturates or alcohol.

Lower doses (usually 2 mg to 5 mg) should be used for elderly and debilitated patients.

Adverse Reactions: Side effects most commonly reported were drowsiness, fatigue and ataxia; venous thrombosis and phlebitis at the site of injection. Other adverse reactions less frequently reported include: *CNS:* confusion, depression, dysarthria, headache, hypoactivity, slurred speech, syncope, tremor, vertigo. *G.I.:* constipation, nausea. *G.U.:* incontinence, changes in libido, urinary retention. *Cardiovascular:* bradycardia, cardiovascular collapse, hypotension. *EENT:* blurred vision, diplopia, nystagmus. *Skin:* urticaria, skin rash. *Other:* hiccups, changes in salivation, neutropenia, jaundice. Paradoxical reactions such as acute hyperexcited states, anxiety, hallucinations, increased muscle spasticity, insomnia, rage, sleep disturbances and stimulation have been reported; should these occur, use of the drug should be discontinued. Minor changes in EEG patterns, usually low-voltage fast activity, have been observed in patients during and af-

Continued on next page

Roche—Cont.

ter Valium therapy and are of no known significance.

	USUAL ADULT DOSAGE	DOSAGE RANGE IN CHILDREN **(I.V. administration should be made slowly)**
Moderate Psychoneurotic Reactions: Manifested by tension-anxiety alone or with depressive symptomatology, agitation, restlessness and psychophysiological disturbances.	2 mg to 5 mg, I.M. or I.V. Repeat in 3 to 4 hours, if necessary.	
Severe Psychoneurotic Reactions: Where severe anxiety, apprehension or agitation exist alone or associated with depressive symptoms.	5 mg to 10 mg, I.M. or I.V. Repeat in 3 to 4 hours, if necessary.	
Acute Alcohol Withdrawal: As an aid in symptomatic relief of acute agitation, tremor, impending or acute delirium tremens and hallucinosis.	10 mg, I.M. or I.V. initially, then 5 mg to 10 mg in 3 to 4 hours, if necessary.	
Endoscopic Procedures: Adjunctively, if apprehension, anxiety or acute stress reactions are present prior to endoscopic procedures. Dosage of narcotics should be reduced by at least a third and in some cases may be omitted. See *Precautions* for peroral procedures.	Titrate I.V. dosage to desired sedative response, such as slurring of speech, with slow administration immediately prior to the procedure. Generally 10 mg or less is adequate, but up to 20 mg I.V. may be given, particularly when concomitant narcotics are omitted. If I.V. cannot be used, 5 mg to 10 mg I.M. approximately 30 minutes prior to the procedure.	
Muscle Spasm: Associated with local pathology, cerebral palsy, athetosis, stiff-man syndrome or tetanus.	5 mg to 10 mg, I.M. or I.V. initially, then 5 mg to 10 mg in 3 to 4 hours, if necessary. For tetanus, larger doses may be required.	For tetanus in infants over 30 days of age, 1 mg to 2 mg I.M. or I.V., slowly, repeated every 3 to 4 hours as necessary. In children 5 years or older, 5 mg to 10 mg repeated every 3 to 4 hours may be required to control tetanus spasms. Respiratory assistance should be available.
Status Epilepticus and Severe Recurrent Convulsive Seizures: In the convulsing patient, the I.V. route is by far preferred. This injection should be administered slowly. However, if I.V. administration is impossible, the I.M. route may be used.	5 mg to 10 mg initially (I.V. preferred). This injection may be repeated if necessary at 10 to 15 minute intervals up to a maximum dose of 30 mg. If necessary, therapy with Valium (diazepam) may be repeated in 2 to 4 hours; however, residual active metabolites may persist, and readministration should be made with this consideration. Extreme caution must be exercised with individuals with chronic lung disease or unstable cardiovascular status.	Infants over 30 days of age and children under 5 years, 0.2 mg to 0.5 mg slowly every 2 to 5 minutes up to a maximum of 5 mg (I.V. preferred). Children 5 years or older, 1 mg every 2 to 5 minutes up to a maximum of 10 mg (slow I.V. administration preferred). Repeat in 2 to 4 hours if necessary. EEG monitoring of the seizure may be helpful.
Preoperative Medication: To relieve anxiety and tension. (If atropine, scopolamine or other premedications are desired, they must be administered in separate syringes.)	10 mg, I.M. (preferred route), before surgery.	
Cardioversion: To relieve anxiety and tension and to reduce recall of procedure.	5 mg to 15 mg, IV., within 5 to 10 minutes prior to the procedure.	

In peroral endoscopic procedures, coughing, depressed respiration, dyspnea, hyperventilation, laryngospasm and pain in throat or chest have been reported.

Because of isolated reports of neutropenia and jaundice, periodic blood counts and liver function tests are advisable during long-term therapy.

Dosage and Administration: Dosage should be individualized for maximum beneficial effect. The usual recommended dose in older children and adults ranges from 2 mg to 20 mg I.M. or I.V., depending on the indication and its severity. In some conditions, e.g., tetanus, larger doses may be required. (See dosage for specific indications.) In acute conditions the injection may be repeated within one hour although an interval of 3 to 4 hours is usually satisfactory. Lower doses (usually 2 mg to 5 mg) and slow increase in dosage should be used for elderly or debilitated patients and when other sedative drugs are administered. (See WARNINGS and ADVERSE REACTIONS.)

For dosage in infants above the age of 30 days and children, see the specific indications below. When intravenous use is indicated, facilities for respiratory assistance should be readily available.

Intramuscular: Injectable Valium should be injected deeply into the muscle.

Intravenous use: (See WARNINGS, particularly for use in children.) The solution should be injected slowly, taking at least one minute for each 5 mg (1 ml) given. Do not use small veins, such as those on the dorsum of the hand or wrist. Extreme care should be taken to avoid intra-arterial administration or extravasation. Do not mix or dilute Valium with other solutions or drugs in syringe or infusion flask. If it is not feasible to administer Valium directly I.V., it may be injected slowly through the infusion tubing as close as possible to the vein insertion.

[See table at left].

Once the acute symptomatology has been properly controlled with Injectable Valium, the patient may be placed on oral therapy with Valium if further treatment is required.

Management of Overdosage:

Manifestations of Valium overdosage include somnolence, confusion, coma, and diminished reflexes. Respiration, pulse and blood pressure should be monitored, as in all cases of drug overdosage, although, in general, these effects have been minimal. General supportive measures should be employed, along with intravenous fluids, and an adequate airway maintained. Hypotension may be combated by the use of Levophed® (levarterenol) or Aramine (metaraminol). Dialysis is of limited value.

How Supplied: Ampuls, 2 ml, boxes of 10; Vials, 10 ml, boxes of 1; Tel-E-Ject® (disposable syringes), 2 ml, boxes of 10.

Animal Pharmacology: Oral LD_{50} of diazepam is 720 mg/kg in mice and 1240 mg/kg in rats. Intraperitoneal administration of 400 mg/kg to a monkey resulted in death on the sixth day.

Reproduction Studies: A series of rat reproduction studies was performed with diazepam in oral doses of 1, 10, 80 and 100 mg/kg given for periods ranging from 60–228 days prior to mating. At 100 mg/kg there was a decrease in the number of pregnancies and surviving offspring in these rats. These effects may be attributable to prolonged sedative activity, resulting in lack of interest in mating and lessened maternal nursing and care of the young. Neonatal survival of rats at doses lower than 100 mg/kg was within normal limits. Several neonates, both controls and experimentals, in these rat reproduction studies showed skeletal or other defects. Further studies in rats at doses up to and including 80 mg/kg/day did not reveal significant teratological effects on the offspring. Rabbits were maintained on doses of 1, 2, 5 and 8 mg/kg from day 6 through day 18 of gestation. No adverse effects on reproduction and no teratological changes were noted.

[*Shown in Product Identification Section*]

VALIUM® TABLETS ℞
(diazepam/Roche)

The following text is complete prescribing information based on official labeling in effect November 7, 1979.

Description: Valium (diazepam/Roche) is a benzodiazepine derivative developed through original Roche research. Chemically, diazepam is 7- chloro - 1,3 - dihydro - 1 - methyl - 5 - phenyl - 2H-1,4-benzodiazepin-2-one. It is a colorless crystalline compound, insoluble in water and has a molecular weight of 284.74.

Pharmacology: In animals Valium appears to act on parts of the limbic system, the thalamus and hypothalamus, and induces calming effects. Valium, unlike chlorpromazine and reserpine, has no demonstrable peripheral autonomic blocking action, nor does it produce extrapyramidal side effects; however, animals treated with Valium do have a transient ataxia at higher doses. Valium was found to have transient cardiovascular depressor effects in dogs. Long-term experiments in rats revealed no disturbances of endocrine function.

Oral LD_{50} of diazepam is 720 mg/kg in mice and 1240 mg/kg in rats. Intraperitoneal administration of 400 mg/kg to a monkey resulted in death on the sixth day.

Reproduction Studies: A series of rat reproduction studies was performed with diazepam in oral doses of 1, 10, 80 and 100 mg/kg. At 100 mg/kg there was a decrease in the number of pregnancies and surviving offspring in these rats. Neonatal survival of rats at doses lower than 100 mg/kg was within normal limits. Several neonates in these rat reproduction studies showed skeletal or other defects. Further studies in rats at doses up to and including 80 mg/kg/day did not reveal teratological effects on the offspring.

In humans, measurable blood levels of Valium were obtained in maternal and cord blood, indicating placental transfer of the drug.

Indications: Valium is indicated for the symptomatic relief of anxiety and tension associated with anxiety disorders, transient situational disturbances and functional or organic disorders. It is useful in psychoneurotic states manifested by tension, anxiety, apprehension, fatigue, depressive symptoms or agitation.

In acute alcohol withdrawal, Valium may be useful in the symptomatic relief of acute agitation, tremor, impending or acute delirium tremens and hallucinosis.

Valium is a useful adjunct for the relief of skeletal muscle spasm due to reflex spasm to local pathology (such as inflammation of the muscles or joints, or secondary to trauma); spasticity caused by upper motor neuron disorders (such as cerebral palsy and paraplegia); athetosis; and stiff-man syndrome.

Oral Valium may be used adjunctively in convulsive disorders, although it has not proved useful as the sole therapy.

The effectiveness of Valium in long-term use, that is, more than 4 months, has not been assessed by systematic clinical studies. The physician should periodically reassess the usefulness of the drug for the individual patient.

Contraindications: Valium is contraindicated in patients with a known hypersensitivity to this drug and, because of lack of sufficient clinical experience, in children under 6 months of age. It may be used in patients with open angle glaucoma who are receiving appropriate therapy, but is contraindicated in acute narrow angle glaucoma.

Warnings: Valium is not of value in the treatment of psychotic patients and should not be employed in lieu of appropriate treatment. As is true of most preparations containing CNS-acting drugs, patients receiving Valium should be cautioned against engaging in hazardous occupations requiring complete mental alertness such as operating machinery or driving a motor vehicle.

As with other agents which have anticonvulsant activity, when Valium is used as an adjunct in treating convulsive disorders, the possibility of an increase in the frequency and/or severity of grand mal seizures may require an increase in the dosage of standard anticonvulsant medication. Abrupt withdrawal of Valium in such cases may also be associated with a temporary increase in the frequency and/or severity of seizures.

Since Valium has a central nervous system depressant effect, patients should be advised against the simultaneous ingestion of alcohol and other CNS-depressant drugs during Valium therapy.

Physical and Psychological Dependence: Withdrawal symptoms (similar in character to those noted with barbiturates and alcohol) have occurred following abrupt discontinuance of diazepam (convulsions, tremor, abdominal and muscle cramps, vomiting and sweating). These were usually limited to those patients who had received excessive doses over an extended period of time. Although infrequently seen, milder withdrawal symptoms have also been reported following abrupt discontinuance of benzodiazepines taken continuously, generally at higher therapeutic levels, for at least several months. Consequently, after extended therapy, abrupt discontinuation should generally be avoided and a gradual tapering in dosage followed. Particularly addiction-prone individuals (such as drug addicts or alcoholics) should be under careful surveillance when receiving diazepam or other psychotropic agents because of the predisposition of such patients to habituation and dependence.

***Usage in Pregnancy:* An increased risk of congenital malformations associated with the use of minor tranquilizers (diazepam, meprobamate and chlordiazepoxide) during the first trimester of pregnancy has been suggested in several studies. Because use of these drugs is rarely a matter of urgency, their use during this period should almost always be avoided. The possibility that a woman of childbearing potential may be pregnant at the time of institution of therapy should be considered. Patients should be advised that if they become pregnant during therapy or intend to become pregnant they should communicate with their physicians about the desirability of discontinuing the drug.**

Management of Overdosage: Manifestations of Valium overdosage include somnolence, confusion, coma and diminished reflexes. Respiration, pulse and blood pressure should be monitored, as in all cases of drug overdosage, although, in general, these effects have been minimal following overdosage. General supportive measures should be employed, along with immediate gastric lavage. Intravenous fluids should be administered and an adequate airway maintained. Hypotension may be combated by the use of Levophed® (levarterenol) or Aramine (metaraminol). Dialysis is of limited value. As with the management of intentional overdosage with any drug, it should be borne in mind that multiple agents may have been ingested.

Precautions: If Valium is to be combined with other psychotropic agents or anticonvulsant drugs, careful consideration should be given to the pharmacology of the agents to be employed—particularly with known compounds which may potentiate the action of Valium, such as phenothiazines, narcotics, barbiturates, MAO inhibitors and other antidepressants. The usual precautions are indicated for severely depressed patients or those in whom there is any evidence of latent depression; particularly the recognition that suicidal tendencies may be present and protective measures may be necessary. The usual precautions in treating patients with impaired renal or hepatic function should be observed.

In elderly and debilitated patients, it is recommended that the dosage be limited to the smallest effective amount to preclude the development of ataxia or oversedation (2 mg to 2½ mg once or twice daily, initially, to be increased gradually as needed and tolerated).

Adverse Reactions: Side effects most commonly reported were drowsiness, fatigue and ataxia. Infrequently encountered were confusion, constipation, depression, diplopia, dysarthria, headache, hypotension, incontinence, jaundice, changes in libido, nausea, changes in salivation, skin rash, slurred speech, tremor, urinary retention, vertigo and blurred vision. Paradoxical reactions such as acute hyperexcited states, anxiety, hallucinations, increased muscle spasticity, insomnia, rage, sleep disturbances and stimulation have been reported; should these occur, use of the drug should be discontinued.

Because of isolated reports of neutropenia and jaundice, periodic blood counts and liver function tests are advisable during long-term therapy. Minor changes in EEG patterns, usually low-voltage fast activity, have been observed in patients during and after Valium therapy and are of no known significance.

Dosage and Administration: Dosage should be individualized for maximum beneficial effect. While the usual daily dosages given below will meet the needs of most patients, there will be some who may require higher doses. In such cases dosage should be increased cautiously to avoid adverse effects.

	USUAL DAILY DOSE
Adults:	
Symptomatic Relief of Tension and Anxiety States and Psychoneurotic States.	Depending upon severity of symptoms —2 mg to 10 mg, 2 to 4 times daily
Symptomatic Relief in Acute Alcohol Withdrawal.	10 mg, 3 or 4 times during the first 24 hours, reducing to 5 mg, 3 or 4 times daily as needed
Adjunctively for Relief of Skeletal Muscle Spasm.	2 mg to 10 mg, 3 or 4 times daily
Adjunctively in Convulsive Disorders.	2 mg to 10 mg, 2 to 4 times daily
Geriatric Patients, or in the presence of debilitating disease.	2 mg to 2½ mg, 1 or 2 times daily initially; increase gradually as needed and tolerated
Children:	
Because of varied responses to CNS-acting drugs, initiate therapy with lowest dose and increase as required. Not for use in children under 6 months.	1 mg to 2½ mg, 3 or 4 times daily initially; increase gradually as needed and tolerated

How Supplied: For oral administration, Valium (diazepam/Roche) scored tablets—2 mg, white; 5 mg, yellow; 10 mg, blue—bottles of 100 and 500; Tel-E-Dose® packages of 100, available in trays of 4 reverse-numbered boxes of 25, and in boxes containing 10 strips of 10; Prescription Paks of 50, available in trays of 10.

[*Shown in Product Identification Section*]

Continued on next page

Roche—Cont.

VI-PENTA® F CHEWABLES ℞
VI-PENTA® F MULTIVITAMIN DROPS
VI-PENTA® F INFANT DROPS
Vitamins with fluoride/Roche

The following text is complete prescribing information based on official labeling in effect August 1, 1979.

Description: VI-PENTA F CHEWABLES provides 11 vitamins with sodium fluoride.

Each chewable tablet contains:

Vitamin A Acetate	5000 I.U.
Ergocalciferol	400 I.U.
Vitamin C (ascorbic acid and sodium ascorbate)	60 mg
Thiamine Mononitrate	1.2 mg
Riboflavin	1.5 mg
Pyridoxine Hydrochloride	1.2 mg
Cyanocobalamin	3 mcg
Biotin	40 mcg
Niacinamide	10 mg
dl-α-Tocopheryl Acetate	2 I.U.
Calcium Pantothenate	10 mg
Fluoride (as Sodium Fluoride)	1 mg

VI-PENTA F MULTIVITAMIN DROPS provides a formulation of 10 vitamins with sodium fluoride in an aqueous, nonalcoholic vehicle.

Each 0.6 ml provides:

Vitamin A Palmitate	5000 I.U.
Ergocalciferol	10 mcg
Ascorbic Acid	50 mg
Thiamine Hydrochloride	1 mg
Riboflavin (as riboflavin-5′-phosphate sodium)	1 mg
Pyridoxine Hydrochloride	1 mg
dl-α-Tocopheryl Acetate	2 I.U.
d-Biotin	30 mcg
Niacinamide	10 mg
D-Panthenol	10 mg
Fluoride (as Sodium Fluoride)	0.5 mg

VI-PENTA F INFANT DROPS provides 4 vitamins with sodium fluoride in an aqueous, nonalcoholic vehicle.

Each 0.6 ml provides:

Vitamin A Palmitate	5000 I.U.
Ergocalciferol	10 mcg
Ascorbic Acid	50 mg
dl-α-Tocopheryl Acetate	2 I.U.
Fluoride (as Sodium Fluoride)	0.5 mg

Indications: VI-PENTA F CHEWABLES offers a comprehensive vitamin supplement together with dietary fluoride to provide daily nutritional support and aid in the prevention of tooth decay in children three years of age and older.

VI-PENTA F MULTIVITAMIN DROPS offers a comprehensive vitamin supplement together with dietary fluoride to provide daily nutritional support and aid in the prevention of tooth decay in infants and children.

VI-PENTA F INFANT DROPS offers a selective vitamin supplement together with dietary fluoride to provide daily nutritional support and aid in the prevention of tooth decay in infants from birth.

Usual Dosage: Where fluoride content of drinking water is known and is less than 0.7 parts per million, *children over 3 years* may be given one VI-PENTA F CHEWABLES tablet daily, chewed or crushed; infants and young children may be given 0.6 ml VI-PENTA F INFANT or MULTIVITAMIN DROPS daily. VI-PENTA F DROPS may be administered by dropping directly on the tongue or mixing with liquids or food.

Precautions: The recommended dosage of VI-PENTA F preparations should not be exceeded, since dental fluorosis may result from continued ingestion of excessive amounts of fluoride.

These preparations should not be used in areas where the fluoride content of drinking water is known to be 0.7 parts per million, or greater. VI-PENTA F preparations should be kept out of reach of children.

Note: VI-PENTA F INFANT and MULTIVITAMIN DROPS should be stored under refrigeration at 2° to 8° C. (36° to 46° F.).

How Supplied: VI-PENTA F CHEWABLES, five fruit flavors and colors, bottles of 100 chewable tablets. VI-PENTA F MULTIVITAMIN DROPS and VI-PENTA F INFANT DROPS, fruit-flavored, bottles of 30 ml, packaged with a calibrated dropper; these products should be dispensed in the original special plastic containers, since contact with glass leads to instability and precipitation.

[*Shown in Product Identification Section*]

VI-PENTA® INFANT DROPS
VI-PENTA® MULTIVITAMIN DROPS

The following text is complete prescribing information based on official labeling in effect August 1, 1979.

Composition: Vi-Penta Infant Drops and Vi-Penta Multivitamin Drops are designed to fill the vitamin needs of specific age groups. (See Composition Table below.)

Vi-Penta Composition Table

Each 0.6 cc of Vi-Penta Infant Drops Provides:		% minimum daily requirements (MDR) Infants (under 1 year)	Young Children (1–6 years)
Vitamin A (as the palmitate)	5000 U.S.P. Units	333%	166%
Vitamin D_2	400 U.S.P. Units	100%	100%
Vitamin C	50 mg	500%	250%
Vitamin E (as *dl-α*-tocopheryl acetate)	2 Int. Units	*	*

Each 0.6 cc of Vi-Penta Multivitamin Drops provides:		% minimum daily requirements (MDR) Infants (under 1 year)	Children (1–6 years)	(6–12 years)
Vitamin A (as the palmitate)	5000 U.S.P. Units	333%	166%	166%
Vitamin D_2	400 U.S.P. Units	100%	100%	100%
Vitamin C	50 mg	500%	250%	250%
Vitamin B_1 (as hydrochloride)	1 mg	400%	200%	133%
Vitamin B_2 (as riboflavin-5′-phosphate sodium)	1 mg	166%	111%	111%
Vitamin B_6	1 mg	*	*	*
Vitamin E (as *dl-α*-tocopheryl acetate)	2 Int. Units	*	*	*
d-Biotin	30 mcg	†	†	†
Niacinamide	10 mg	*	200%	133%
D-Panthenol (equiv. to 11.6 mg Calcium pantothenate)	10 mg	†	†	†

*MDR for these vitamins has not been determined.
†The need for these vitamins in human nutrition has not been established.

Action and Uses: Vi-Penta Drops are water miscible and can be mixed with food or infant formula, or placed directly on the tongue.

Vi-Penta Infant Drops—a selective formula for prevention of vitamin deficiencies in infants and young children. *Vi-Penta Multivitamin Drops*—a comprehensive formula for daily nutritional support in adults as well as children of all ages. It is an especially convenient dosage form when a small volume liquid vitamin supplement is desired, such as to supplement the diets of those patients with conditions which permanently or temporarily impair their ability to swallow, chew or consume normal amounts and/or kinds of food.

Dosage: The average daily dose is 0.6 cc; therapeutic doses should be given according to the needs of the patient.

How Supplied: Vi-Penta Infant Drops and Vi-Penta Multivitamin Drops—fruit flavored, 50-cc bottles packaged with calibrated dropper.

Roerig

A division of Pfizer Pharmaceuticals
235 EAST 42nd STREET
NEW YORK, NY 10017

Product Identification Codes

To provide quick and positive identification of Roerig Division products, we have imprinted the product identification number of the National Drug Code on most tablets and capsules. In order that you may quickly identify a product by its code number, we have compiled below a numerical list of code numbers with their corresponding product names. We are also listing the code numbers by alphabetical order of products.

Numerical Listing

Product Ident. Number	Product
092	Urobiotic®-250 (oxytetracycline HCl 250 mg. with sulfamethizole 250 mg. and phenazopyridine 50 mg.) Capsules
143	Geocillin® (carbenicillin indanyl sodium) Tablets, equivalent to 382 mg. carbenicillin
159	TAO® (troleandomycin) Capsules, 250 mg.
210	Antivert® (meclizine HCl) Tablets, 12.5 mg.
211	Antivert® /25 (meclizine HCl) Tablets, 25 mg.
212	Antivert® /25 (meclizine HCl) Chewable Tablets
220	Sustaire® (theophylline [anhydrous]) Tablets, 100 mg.
221	Sustaire® (theophylline [anhydrous]) Tablets, 300 mg.
254	Marax® (ephedrine sulfate, 25 mg; theophylline, 130 mg; and Atarax® [hydroxyzine HCl], 10 mg) Tablets
294	Cartrax® 10 (hydroxyzine HCl & pentaerythritol tetranitrate) Tablets
295	Cartrax® 20 (hydroxyzine HCl & pentaerythritol tetranitrate) Tablets
504	Heptuna® plus (iron plus vitamins and minerals), Capsules.
560	Atarax® (hydroxyzine HCl) Tablets, 10 mg.
561	Atarax® (hydroxyzine HCl) Tablets, 25 mg.
562	Atarax® (hydroxyzine HCl) Tablets, 50 mg.
563	Atarax® (hydroxyzine HCl) Tablets, 100 mg.

571 Navane® (thiothixene) Capsules, 1 mg.
572 Navane® (thiothixene) Capsules, 2 mg.
573 Navane® (thiothixene) Capsules, 5 mg.
574 Navane® (thiothixene) Capsules, 10 mg.
577 Navane® (thiothixene) Capsules, 20 mg.

Alphabetical Listing

Prod. Ident. Number	Product
210	Antivert® (meclizine HCl) Tablets, 12.5 mg.
211	Antivert® /25 (meclizine HCl) Tablets, 25 mg.
212	Antivert® /25 (meclizine HCl) Chewable Tablets
560	Atarax® (hydroxyzine HCl) Tablets, 10 mg.
561	Atarax® (hydroxyzine HCl) Tablets, 25 mg.
562	Atarax® (hydroxyzine HCl) Tablets, 50 mg.
563	Atarax® (hydroxyzine HCl) Tablets, 100 mg.
294	Cartrax® 10 (hydroxyzine HCl & pentaerythritol tetranitrate) Tablets
295	Cartrax® 20 (hydroxyzine HCl & pentaerythritol tetranitrate) Tablets
143	Geocillin® (carbenicillin indanyl sodium) Tablets equivalent to 382 mg. carbenicillin
504	Heptuna® plus (iron plus vitamins and minerals), Capsules.
254	Marax® (ephedrine sulfate, 25 mg; theophylline, 130 mg; and Atarax® [hydroxyzine HCl], 10 mg) Tablets
571	Navane® (thiothixene) Capsules, 1 mg.
572	Navane® (thiothixene) Capsules, 2 mg.
573	Navane® (thiothixene) Capsules, 5 mg.
574	Navane® (thiothixene) Capsules, 10 mg.
577	Navane® (thiothixene) Capsules, 20 mg.
220	Sustaire® (theophylline [anhydrous]) Tablets, 100 mg.
221	Sustaire® (theophylline [anhydrous]) Tablets, 300 mg.
159	TAO® (troleandomycin) Capsules, 250 mg.
092	Urobiotic®-250 (oxytetracycline HCl 250 mg. with sulfamethizole 250 mg. and phenazopyridine 50 mg.) Capsules

ANTIMINTH® ℞
(pyrantel pamoate)
ORAL SUSPENSION

Actions: Antiminth has demonstrated anthelmintic activity against *Enterobius vermicularis* (pinworm) and *Ascaris lumbricoides* (common roundworm). The anthelmintic action is probably due to the neuromuscular blocking property of the drug.

Antiminth is partially absorbed after an oral dose. Plasma levels of unchanged drug are low. Peak levels (0.05-0.13 μg./ml.) are reached in 1-3 hours. Quantities greater than 50% of administered drug are excreted in feces as the unchanged form, whereas only 7% or less of the dose is found in urine as the unchanged form of the drug and its metabolites.

Indications: For the treatment of ascariasis (common roundworm infection) and enterobiasis (pinworm infection).

Warnings:
Usage in Pregnancy
Reproduction studies have been performed in animals and there was no evidence of propensity for harm to the fetus. The relevance to the human is not known.
There is no experience in pregnant women who have received this drug.
This drug has not been extensively studied in children under two years; therefore, in the treatment of children under the age of two years, the relative benefit/risk should be considered.

Precautions: Minor transient elevations of SGOT have occurred in a small percentage of patients. Therefore, this drug should be used with caution in patients with pre-existing liver dysfunction.

Adverse Reactions: The most frequently encountered adverse reactions are related to the gastrointestinal system.
Gastrointestinal and hepatic reactions: anorexia, nausea, vomiting, gastralgia, abdominal cramps, diarrhea and tenesmus, transient elevation of SGOT.
CNS reactions: headache, dizziness, drowsiness, and insomnia.
Skin reactions: rashes.

Dosage and Administration:
Children and Adults
Antiminth Oral Suspension (50 mg. of pyrantel base/ml.) should be administered in a single dose of 11 mg. of pyrantel base per kg. of body weight (or 5 mg./lb.); maximum total dose 1 gram. This corresponds to a simplified dosage regimen of 1 ml. of Antiminth per 10 lb. of body weight. (One teaspoonful = 5 ml.)
Antiminth (pyrantel pamoate) Oral Suspension may be administered without regard to ingestion of food or time of day, and purging is not necessary prior to, during, or after therapy. It may be taken with milk or fruit juices.

How Supplied: Antiminth Oral Suspension is available as a pleasant tasting caramel flavored suspension which contains the equivalent of 50 mg. pyrantel base per ml., supplied in 60 ml. bottles.

ANTIVERT® TABLETS ℞
(12.5 mg. meclizine HCl)
ANTIVERT®/25 TABLETS ℞
(25 mg. meclizine HCl)
ANTIVERT®/25 CHEWABLE TABLETS ℞
(25 mg. meclizine HCl)

Actions: Antivert is an antihistamine which shows marked protective activity against nebulized histamine and lethal doses of intravenously injected histamine in guinea pigs. It has a marked effect in blocking the vasodepressor response to histamine, but only a slight blocking action against acetylcholine. Its activity is relatively weak in inhibiting the spasmogenic action of histamine on isolated guinea pig ileum.

INDICATIONS

Based on a review of this drug by the National Academy of Sciences-National Research Council and/or other information, FDA has classified the indications as follows:
Effective: Management of nausea and vomiting, and dizziness associated with motion sickness.
Possibly Effective: Management of vertigo associated with diseases affecting the vestibular system.
Final classification of the less than effective indications requires further investigation.

Contraindications: Administration of Antivert during pregnancy or to women who may become pregnant is contraindicated in view of the teratogenic effect of the drug in rats.
The administration of meclizine to pregnant rats during the 12th-15th day of gestation has produced cleft palate in the offspring. Limited studies using doses of over 100 mg./kg./day in rabbits and 10 mg./kg./day in pigs and monkeys did not show cleft palate. Congeners of meclizine have caused cleft palate in species other than the rat.
Meclizine HCl is contraindicated in individuals who have shown a previous hypersensitivity to it.

Warnings: Since drowsiness may, on occasion, occur with use of this drug, patients should be warned of this possibility and cautioned against driving a car or operating dangerous machinery.
USAGE IN CHILDREN:
Clinical studies establishing safety and effectiveness in children have not been done; therefore, usage is not recommended in the pediatric age group.
USAGE IN PREGNANCY:
See "Contraindications."

Adverse Reactions: Drowsiness, dry mouth and, on rare occasions, blurred vision have been reported.

Dosage and Administration:
Motion Sickness:
The initial dose of 25 to 50 mg. of Antivert should be taken one hour prior to embarkation for protection against motion sickness. Thereafter, the dose may be repeated every 24 hours for the duration of the journey.
Vertigo:
For the control of vertigo associated with diseases affecting the vestibular system, the recommended dose is 25 to 100 mg. daily, in divided dosage, depending upon clinical response.

How Supplied:
Antivert—12.5 mg. tablets: Bottles of 100, 1000 and unit dose 100's.
Antivert/25—25 mg. tablets: Bottles of 100, 1000 and unit dose 100's.
Antivert/25 Chewable Tablets—25 mg. scored, pink tablets:
Bottles of 100 and 500.
[*Shown in Product Identification Section*]

ATARAX® ℞
(hydroxyzine hydrochloride)
TABLETS AND SYRUP

Clinical Pharmacology: Atarax is unrelated chemically to the phenothiazines, reserpine, meprobamate, or the benzodiazepines. Atarax is not a cortical depressant, but its action may be due to a suppression of activity in certain key regions of the subcortical area of the central nervous system. Primary skeletal muscle relaxation has been demonstrated experimentally. Bronchodilator activity, and antihistaminic and analgesic effects have been demonstrated experimentally and confirmed clinically. An antiemetic effect, both by the apomorphine test and the veriloid test, has been demonstrated. Pharmacological and clinical studies indicate that hydroxyzine in therapeutic dosage does not increase gastric secretion or acidity and in most cases has mild antisecretory activity. Hydroxyzine is rapidly absorbed from the gastrointestinal tract and Atarax's clinical effects are usually noted within 15 to 30 minutes after oral administration.

Indications: For symptomatic relief of anxiety and tension associated with psychoneurosis and as an adjunct in organic disease states in which anxiety is manifested.
Useful in the management of pruritus due to allergic conditions such as chronic urticaria and atopic and contact dermatoses, and in histamine-mediated pruritus.
As a sedative when used as premedication and following general anesthesia. **Hydroxyzine may potentiate meperidine (Demerol®) and**

Continued on next page

Roerig—Cont.

barbiturates, so their use in pre-anesthetic adjunctive therapy should be modified on an individual basis. Atropine and other belladonna alkaloids are not affected by the drug. Hydroxyzine is not known to interfere with the action of digitalis in any way and it may be used concurrently with this agent.
The effectiveness of hydroxyzine as an antianxiety agent for long term use, that is more than 4 months, has not been assessed by systematic clinical studies. The physician should reassess periodically the usefulness of the drug for the individual patient.
Contraindications: Hydroxyzine, when administered to the pregnant mouse, rat, and rabbit, induced fetal abnormalities in the rat and mouse at doses substantially above the human therapeutic range. Clinical data in human beings are inadequate to establish safety in early pregnancy. Until such data are available, hydroxyzine is contraindicated in early pregnancy.
Hydroxyzine is contraindicated for patients who have shown a previous hypersensitivity to it.
Warnings:
Nursing Mothers: It is not known whether this drug is excreted in human milk. Since many drugs are so excreted, hydroxyzine should not be given to nursing mothers.
Precautions: THE POTENTIATING ACTION OF HYDROXYZINE MUST BE CONSIDERED WHEN THE DRUG IS USED IN CONJUNCTION WITH CENTRAL NERVOUS SYSTEM DEPRESSANTS SUCH AS NARCOTICS, NON-NARCOTIC ANALGESICS AND BARBITURATES. Therefore when central nervous system depressants are administered concomitantly with hydroxyzine their dosage should be reduced.
Since drowsiness may occur with use of this drug, patients should be warned of this possibility and cautioned against driving a car or operating dangerous machinery while taking Atarax. Patients should be advised against the simultaneous use of other CNS depressant drugs, and cautioned that the effect of alcohol may be increased.
Adverse Reactions: Side effects reported with the administration of Atarax (hydroxyzine hydrochloride) are usually mild and transitory in nature.
Anticholinergic: Dry mouth.
Central Nervous System: Drowsiness is usally transitory and may disappear in a few days of continued therapy or upon reduction of the dose. Involuntary motor activity including rare instances of tremor and convulsions have been reported, usually with doses considerably higher than those recommended. Clinically significant respiratory depression has not been reported at recommended doses.
Overdosage: The most common manifestation of Atarax overdosage is hypersedation. As in the management of overdosage with any drug, it should be borne in mind that multiple agents may have been taken.
If vomiting has not occurred spontaneously, it should be induced. Immediate gastric lavage is also recommended. General supportive care, including frequent monitoring of the vital signs and close observation of the patient, is indicated. Hypotension, though unlikely, may be controlled with intravenous fluids and Levophed® (levarterenol), or Aramine® (metaraminol). Do not use epinephrine as Atarax counteracts its pressor action. Caffeine and Sodium Benzoate Injection, U.S.P., may be used to counteract central nervous system depressant effects.
There is no specific antidote. It is doubtful that hemodialysis would be of any value in the treatment of overdosage with hydroxyzine. However, if other agents such as barbiturates have been ingested concomitantly, hemodialysis may be indicated. There is no practical method to quantitate hydroxyzine in body fluids or tissue after its ingestion or administration.
Dosage: For symptomatic relief of anxiety and tension associated with psychoneurosis and as an adjunct in organic disease states in which anxiety is manifested: in adults, 50–100 mg q.i.d.: children under 6 years, 50 mg daily in divided doses and over 6 years, 50–100 mg daily in divided doses.
For use in the management of pruritus due to allergic conditions such as chronic urticaria and atopic and contact dermatoses, and in histamine-mediated pruritus: in adults, 25 mg t.i.d. or q.i.d.; children under 6 years, 50 mg daily in divided doses and over 6 years, 50–100 mg daily in divided doses.
As a sedative when used as a premedication and following general anesthesia: 50–100 mg in adults, and 0.6 mg/kg in children.
When treatment is initiated by the intramuscular route of administration, subsequent doses may be administered orally.
As with all medications, the dosage should be adjusted according to the patient's response to therapy.
Supply:
Atarax Tablets
10 mg: 100's and 500's—orange tablets
25 mg: 100's and 500's—green tablets
50 mg: 100's and 500's—yellow tablets
Atarax 100 Tablets
100 mg: 100's—red tablets
Atarax Syrup
10 mg per teaspoon (5 ml): 1 pint bottles
Alcohol Content—Ethyl Alcohol—0.5% v/v
Bibliography: Available on request.
[Shown in Product Identification Section]

CARTRAX® ℞
(pentaerythritol tetranitrate and hydroxyzine hydrochloride)
TABLETS
For Oral Administration

Actions: Pentaerythritol tetranitrate is a slow acting organic nitrate with a vasodilator action.
Hydroxyzine HCl has been shown clinically to be an effective antianxiety agent. It is not a cortical depressant, but its action may be due to a suppression of activity in certain key regions of the subcortical area of the central nervous system.

Indications
Based on a review of this drug by the National Academy of Sciences-National Research Council and/or other information, the FDA has classified the indications as follows:
Possibly Effective: For the management or treatment of:
1. Angina Pectoris,
2. Angina Decubitus,
3. Precordial Pain,
4. Status Anginosus.

Final classification of these less than effective indications requires further investigation.

Contraindications: This drug is contraindicated in individuals who are hypersensitive to it or any of its components.
Hydroxyzine, when administered to the pregnant mouse, rat, and rabbit induced fetal abnormalities in the rat at doses substantially above the human therapeutic range. Clinical data in human beings are inadequate to establish safety in early pregnancy. Until such data are available, hydroxyzine is contraindicated in early pregnancy.
Precautions: Due to the Atarax (hydroxyzine HCl) component, mild transient drowsiness may occur. Patients should be warned of the possibility and cautioned against driving an automobile or operating dangerous machinery while taking this drug
Like all nitrates PETN may increase intraocular pressure; therefore caution is required in administering this drug to patients with glaucoma. Tolerance to this drug, and cross tolerance to other nitrates and nitrites may occur.
THE POTENTIATING ACTION OF HYDROXYZINE HYDROCHLORIDE, ALTHOUGH MILD, MUST BE TAKEN INTO CONSIDERATION WHEN THE DRUG IS USED IN CONJUNCTION WITH CENTRAL NERVOUS SYSTEM DEPRESSANTS; AND WHEN OTHER CENTRAL NERVOUS SYSTEM DEPRESSANTS ARE ADMINISTERED CONCOMITANTLY WITH HYDROXYZINE THEIR DOSAGE SHOULD BE REDUCED.
Caution should be observed in patients with anemia; however, anemia to date is not considered to be a contraindication to its use.
Adverse Reactions: Cutaneous vasodilatation with flushing may occur and transient episodes of dizziness and weakness as well as other signs of cerebral ischemia and postural hypotension may occur. Side effects of PETN are the same as those of other nitrates, except that these appear to be relatively infrequent and methemoglobinemia has not been demonstrated following prolonged use. Headache is common and may be severe and persistent. Nausea, occasionally observed, tends to disappear after four or five days' medication. This drug can act as a physiologic antagonist to norepinephrine, acetylcholine, histamine, and many other agents. An occasional individual exhibits marked sensitivity to the hypotensive effects of nitrite and severe responses (nausea, vomiting, weakness, restlessness, pallor and collapse) can occur even with usual therapeutic dose. Alcohol may enhance this effect.
Drug rash and/or exfoliative dermatitis may occur.
The amount of Atarax (hydroxyzine hydrochloride) present in CARTRAX has not resulted in disturbing side effects. When used alone specifically as a tranquilizer in the normal dosage range (25 to 50 mg. three or four times a day), side effects are infrequent; even at these higher doses, no serious side effects have been reported and confirmed to date. Those which do occasionally occur are drowsiness, xerostomia and, at extremely high doses, involuntary motor activity including rare instances of tremor and convulsions, all of which may be controlled by reduction of the dosage or discontinuation of the medication. With the relatively low dose of Atarax in CARTRAX, these effects are not likely to occur.
Dosage: CARTRAX is initially administered orally in usual beginning doses of 1 or 2 tablets three to four times daily of the CARTRAX-10 (yellow) tablet.
For dosage flexibility CARTRAX-20 (pink) tablets may be utilized at a level of 1 tablet three to four times a day.
The tablets should be administered before meals for optimal effects.
Dosage schedules should be arranged on an individual basis, with particular attention given to the aged or debilitated patient, with the physician observing the patient for a decrease in the incidence and severity of anginal attacks, improved exercise tolerance, improved electrocardiographic status, and decreased need for nitroglycerin.
How Supplied:
CARTRAX-10: hydroxyzine hydrochloride 10 mg. combined with PETN 10 mg. (yellow tablet).
CARTRAX-20: hydroxyzine hydrochloride 10 mg. combined with PETN 20 mg. (pink tablet).
Both forms are packaged in bottles of 100 tablets.

EMETE-CON® ℞
(benzquinamide hydrochloride)
For Intramuscular and Intravenous Use

Emete-con for injection contains benzquinamide hydrochloride equivalent to 50 mg/vial of benzquinamide. When reconstituted with 2.2 ml of proper diluent, each vial yields 2 ml of a solution containing benzquinamide hydrochloride equivalent to 25 mg/ml of benzquinamide. When reconstituted this product maintains its potency for 14 days at room temperature.

Actions: Benzquinamide HCl exhibited antiemetic, antihistaminic, mild anticholinergic and sedative action in animals. Studies conducted in dogs and human volunteers have demonstrated suppression of apomorphine-induced vomiting; however, relevance to clinical efficacy has not been established. The mechanism of action in humans is unknown. The onset of antiemetic activity in humans usually occurs within 15 minutes.

Benzquinamide metabolism has been studied in animals and in man. In both species, 5-10% of an administered dose is excreted unchanged in the urine. The remaining drug undergoes metabolic transformation in the liver by at least three pathways to a spectrum of metabolites which are excreted in the urine and in the bile, from which the more polar metabolites are not reabsorbed but are excreted in the feces. The half-life in plasma of Emete-con is about 40 minutes. More than 95% of an administered dose was excreted within 72 hours in animal studies using C14-labeled benzquinamide. In blood, benzquinamide is about 58% bound to plasma protein.

Indications: Emete-con is indicated for the prevention and treatment of nausea and vomiting associated with anesthesia and surgery. Since the incidence of postoperative and post-anesthetic vomiting has decreased with the adoption of modern techniques and agents, the prophylactic use of Emete-con should be restricted to those patients in whom emesis would endanger the results of surgery or result in harm to the patient.

Contraindications: Emete-con is contraindicated in individuals who have demonstrated hypersensitivity to the drug.

Warnings:

Use in Pregnancy

No teratogenic effects of benzquinamide were demonstrated in reproduction studies in chick embryos, mice, rats and rabbits. The relevance of these data to the human is not known. However, safe use of this drug in pregnancy has not been established and its use in pregnancy is not recommended.

Use in Children

As the data available at present are insufficient to establish proper dosage in children, the use of Emete-con in children is not recommended.

Intravenous use

Sudden increase in blood pressure and transient arrhythmias (premature ventricular and auricular contractions) have been reported following intravenous administration of benzquinamide. Until a more predictable pattern of the effect of intravenous benzquinamide has been established, the intramuscular route of administration is considered preferable. The intravenous route of administration should be restricted to patients without cardiovascular disease and receiving no pre-anesthetic and/or concomitant cardiovascular drugs.

If patients receiving pressor agents or epinephrine-like drugs are also given benzquinamide, the latter should be given in fractions of the normal dose. Blood pressure should be monitored. Safeguards against hypertensive reactions are particularly important in hypertensive patients.

Precautions: Benzquinamide, like other antiemetics, may mask signs of overdosage of toxic drugs or may obscure diagnosis of such conditions as intestinal obstruction and brain tumor.

Adverse Reactions: The following adverse reactions have been reported in subjects who have received benzquinamide. However, drowsiness appears to be the most common reaction. One case of pronounced allergic reaction has been encountered, characterized by pyrexia and urticaria.

System Affected

Autonomic Nervous System: Dry mouth, shivering, sweating, hiccoughs, flushing, salivation, blurred vision.

Cardiovascular System: Hypertension, hypotension, dizziness, atrial fibrillation, premature auricular and ventricular contractions. Hypertensive episodes have occurred after IM and IV administration.

Central Nervous System: Drowsiness, insomnia, restlessness, headache, excitement, nervousness.

Gastrointestinal System: Anorexia, nausea.

Musculoskeletal System: Twitching, shaking/tremors, weakness.

Skin: Hives/rash.

Other Systems: Fatigue, shaking, chills, increased temperature.

Dosage and Administration:

Intramuscular: 50 mg (0.5 mg/kg–1.0 mg/kg) First dose may be repeated in one hour with subsequent doses every 3-4 hours, as necessary. The precautions applicable to all intramuscular injections should be observed. Emete-con should be injected well within the mass of a larger muscle. The deltoid area should be used only if well developed. Injections should not be made into the lower and mid-thirds of the upper arm. Aspiration of the syringe should be carried out to avoid inadvertent intravascular injection.

Therapeutic blood levels and demonstrable antiemetic activity appear within fifteen minutes of intramuscular administration. When the objective of therapy is the prevention of nausea and vomiting, intramuscular administration is recommended at least fifteen minutes prior to emergence from anesthesia.

Intravenous: 25 mg (0.2 mg/kg–0.4 mg/kg as a single dose) administered slowly (1 ml per 0.5 to 1 minute). Subsequent doses should be given intramuscularly.

The intravenous route of administration should be restricted to patients without cardiovascular disease (See WARNINGS). If it is necessary to use Emete-con intravenously in elderly or debilitated patients, benzquinamide should be administered cautiously and the lower dose range is recommended.

This preparation must be initially reconstituted with 2.2 ml of Sterile Water for Injection, Bacteriostatic Water for Injection with benzyl alcohol or with methylparaben and propylparaben. This procedure yields 2 ml of a solution equivalent to 25 mg benzquinamide/ml, which maintains its potency for 14 days at room temperature.

Overdosage:

Manifestations: On the basis of acute animal toxicology studies, gross Emete-con overdosage in humans might be expected to manifest itself as a combination of Central Nervous System stimulant and depressant effects. This speculation is derived from experimental studies in which intravenous doses of benzquinamide, at least 150 times the human therapeutic dose, were administered to dogs.

Treatment: There is no specific antidote for Emete-con overdosage. General supportive measures should be instituted, as indicated. Atropine may be helpful. Although there has been no direct experience with dialysis, it is not likely to be of value, since benzquinamide is extensively bound to plasma protein.

How Supplied: Emete-con for IM/IV use is available in a vial containing benzquinamide HCl equivalent to 50 mg of benzquinamide in packages of 10 vials.

Caution: Federal law prohibits dispensing without prescription.

GEOCILLIN® ℞
(carbenicillin indanyl sodium)
TABLETS
For Oral Use

Description: Geocillin (carbenicillin indanyl sodium), a semisynthetic penicillin, is the sodium salt of the indanyl ester of Geopen® (carbenicillin disodium). Geocillin is acid stable and well absorbed following oral administration.

Actions:

Microbiology

The antibacterial activity of Geocillin is due to its rapid conversion to carbenicillin by hydrolysis. Though Geocillin provides substantial *in vitro* activity against a variety of both gram-positive and gram-negative microorganisms, the most important aspect of its profile is in its antipseudomonal and antiproteus activity. Because of the high urine levels obtained following administration, Geocillin has demonstrated clinical efficacy in urinary infections due to susceptible strains of:

Escherichia coli
Proteus mirabilis
Proteus morgani
Proteus rettgeri
Proteus vulgaris
Pseudomonas
Enterobacter
Enterococci

In addition, *in vitro* data, not substantiated by clinical studies, indicate the following pathogens to be usually susceptible to Geocillin:

Staphylococcus (non-penicillinase producing)
Streptococcus

Most *Klebsiella* species are often resistant to the action of Geocillin. Some strains of *Pseudomonas* have developed resistance to carbenicillin.

Susceptibility Testing

Geopen (carbenicillin disodium) Susceptibility Powder or 100 mcg. Geopen Susceptibility Discs may be used to determine microbial susceptibility to Geocillin.

Interpretations:

[See table top right on next page].

Interpretations of susceptible, intermediate, and resistant correlate zone size diameters with MIC values. A laboratory report of "susceptible" indicates that the suspected causative microorganism most likely will respond to therapy with carbenicillin. A laboratory report of "resistant" indicates that the infecting microorganism most likely will not respond to therapy. A laboratory report of "intermediate" indicates that the microorganism is most likely susceptible if a high dosage of carbenicillin is used, or if the infection is such that high levels of carbenicillin may be attained as in urine.

Pharmacology

Geocillin is acid stable and well absorbed following oral administration. After absorption, Geocillin is rapidly hydrolyzed to carbenicillin, which is primarily excreted in the urine. In a study utilizing volunteers with normal renal function, the following mean urine levels of carbenicillin were achieved:

[See table bottom left on next page].

Indications: Geocillin (carbenicillin indanyl sodium) is indicated in the treatment of acute and chronic infections of the upper and lower urinary tract and in asymptomatic bacteriuria due to susceptible strains of the following organisms:

Escherichia coli
Proteus mirabilis
Proteus morgani
Proteus rettgeri
Proteus vulgaris
Pseudomonas

Continued on next page

Roerig—Cont.

Enterobacter
Enterococci

Geocillin is also indicated in the treatment of prostatitis due to susceptible strains of the following organisms:

Escherichia coli
Enterococcus (*S. faecalis*)
Proteus mirabilis
Enterobacter sp.

WHEN HIGH RAPID BLOOD AND URINE LEVELS OF ANTIBIOTIC ARE INDICATED, THERAPY WITH GEOPEN (CARBENICILLIN DISODIUM) SHOULD BE INITIATED BY PARENTERAL ADMINISTRATION FOLLOWED, AT THE PHYSICIAN'S DISCRETION, BY ORAL THERAPY.

NOTE: Susceptibility testing should be performed prior to and during the course of therapy to detect the possible emergence of resistant organisms which may develop.

Contraindications: Geocillin is ordinarily contraindicated in patients who have a known penicillin allergy.

Warnings: Serious and occasionally fatal hypersensitivity (anaphylactic) reactions have been reported in patients on oral penicillin therapy. These reactions are more apt to occur in individuals with a history of sensitivity to multiple allergens.

There have been reports of individuals with a history of penicillin hypersensitivity who have experienced severe hypersensitivity reactions when treated with a cephalosporin, and vice versa. Therefore, before therapy with a penicillin, careful inquiry should be made concerning previous hypersensitivity reactions to penicillins, cephalosporins, and other allergens.

SERIOUS ANAPHYLACTOID REACTIONS REQUIRE IMMEDIATE EMERGENCY TREATMENT WITH EPINEPHRINE. OXYGEN, INTRAVENOUS STEROIDS AND AIRWAY MANAGEMENT, INCLUDING INTUBATION, SHOULD ALSO BE ADMINISTERED AS INDICATED.

Usage in Children: Since only limited clinical data is available to date in children, the safety of Geocillin administration in this age group has not yet been established.

Usage in Pregnancy: Safety for use in pregnancy has not been established.

Precautions: Periodic assessment of organ system function including renal, hepatic and hematopoietic systems is recommended during prolonged therapy.

Long term use of Geocillin may result in the overgrowth of nonsensitive organisms. If superinfection occurs during therapy, appropriate measures should be taken.

	Susceptible	Intermediate	Resistant
Pseudomonas aeruginosa and Enterococci			
Inhibition Zone	17 mm or greater*	16 mm–14 mm	13 mm or less
MIC	125 mcg/ml or less	greater than 125 mcg/ml less than 250 mcg/ml	250 mcg/ml or greater
Escherichia coli, Proteus species, and Enterobacter.			
Inhibition Zone	23 mm or greater	22 mm–18 mm	17 mm or less
MIC	15 mcg/ml or less	greater than 20 mcg/ml less than 40 mcg/ml	greater than 40 mcg/ml

*Zone diameter interpretations apply only to results obtained by the Bauer, Kirby, Sherris and Turck method of Susceptibility Testing Am. J. Clin. Path. 45:493, 1966.

Since carbenicillin is excreted by the kidney, patients with severe renal impairment (creatinine clearance of less than 10 ml/min.) will not achieve therapeutic urine levels of carbenicillin.

Adverse Reactions: The following adverse reactions may occur during therapy with Geocillin:

Gastrointestinal Disturbances: Nausea, vomiting, and diarrhea.

Hypersensitivity Reactions: Skin rashes, urticaria, or pruritus have been reported infrequently.

Blood, Hepatic and Renal Studies: As with other penicillins, anemia, thrombocytopenia, leukopenia, neutropenia, and eosinophilia may occur.

Mild SGOT elevations have been observed following Geocillin administration.

Other reactions that have been reported are flatulence, dry mouth, furry tongue, vaginitis, and abdominal cramps.

Dosage and Administration:

Geocillin is available as a coated tablet, to be administered orally.

Usual Adult Dose

URINARY TRACT INFECTIONS	
Escherichia coli, Proteus species, and *Enterobacter*	1-2 tablets 4 times daily
Pseudomonas and Enterococci	2 tablets 4 times daily
PROSTATITIS	
Escherichia coli, Proteus mirabilis, Enterobacter and Enterococcus	2 tablets 4 times daily

		Mean Urine Concentration of Carbenicillin mcg/ml Hours After Initial Dose		
DRUG	DOSE	0–3	3–6	6–24
Geocillin	1 tablet q.6 hr.	1130	352	292
Geocillin	2 tablets q.6 hr.	1428	789	809

Mean serum concentrations of carbenicillin in this study for these dosages are:

		Mean Serum Concentration mcg/ml Hours After Initial Dose								
DRUG	DOSE	½	1	2	4	6	24	25	26	28
Geocillin	1 tablet q.6 hr.	5.1	6.5	3.2	1.9	0.0	0.4	8.8	5.4	0.4
Geocillin	2 tablets q.6 hr.	6.1	9.6	7.9	2.6	0.4	0.8	13.2	12.8	3.8

How Supplied: Geocillin is available as film-coated tablets in bottles of 100's, and unit-dose packages of 100 (10 × 10s). Each tablet contains carbenicillin indanyl sodium equivalent to 382 mg of carbenicillin.

[*Shown in Product Identification Section*]

GEOPEN® ℞

sterile carbenicillin disodium
For Intramuscular and Intravenous Use

Description: Geopen (carbenicillin disodium) is a new semisynthetic injectable penicillin. Geopen is a benzylpenicillin derivative with substitution by an ionizable functional group in the alpha position.

Actions:

Microbiology

Though Geopen has substantial *in vitro* activity against a variety of both gram-positive and gram-negative microorganisms the most important aspect of its profile is in its antipseudomonal and antiproteus effect.

Organisms found to be susceptible to Geopen *in vitro* include the following:

Staphylococcus aureus
(Non-penicillinase producing)
Staphylococcus albus
Diplococcus pneumoniae
Beta-hemolytic Streptococci
Streptococcus faecalis
Hemophilus influenzae
Neisseria species
Enterobacter species
Proteus mirabilis
Proteus morgani
Proteus rettgeri
Proteus vulgaris
Escherichia coli
Salmonella species
Pseudomonas aeruginosa
Anaerobic bacteria, including:
Bacteroides species
Peptostreptococcus species
Peptococcus species
Clostridium species
Fusobacterium species

In vitro synergism between Geopen and gentamicin sulfate in certain strains of *Pseudomonas aeruginosa* has been demonstrated.

Geopen is not stable in the presence of penicillinase.

Most *Klebsiella* species are resistant to the action of Geopen.

Some of the newly emerging pathogenic strains of such microorganisms as *Herellea, Mima, Citrobacter* and *Serratia* have shown susceptibility to Geopen.

Some strains of *Pseudomonas* have developed resistance to Geopen fairly rapidly.

Pharmacology
Geopen is not absorbed orally, hence, it must be administered by the intramuscular or intravenous routes.
Following intramuscular injection, peak blood levels are obtained within 1–2 hours. The administration of probenecid results in somewhat higher and more prolonged serum levels as noted in the table (below).
[See table at right].

CARBENICILLIN BLOOD LEVELS AND URINARY EXCRETION

		SERUM LEVELS mcg/ml								Urinary excretion of administered dose
Dosage	ROUTE	¼ hr.	½ hr.	1 hr.	2 hr.	3 hr.	4 hr.	6 hr.	8 hr.	0–9 hours
500 mg.	IM	8	10	13	9.8	6.5	3.2	0	—	85%
1000 mg.	IM	—	13	18	15	12	7.5	1.7	0.7	74.6%*
2000 mg.	IM	26	38	47	37	25	15	5.9	1.2	79%
1000 mg.	IV	71	45	31	14	8.2	3	0	—	73%
1000 mg. +	IV									
1 Gm. probenecid	Oral	72	55	40	26	17	12	6.5	2.0	74%

*0–24 hr. collection

The **MIC** for many strains of *Pseudomonas* and *Bacteroides fragilis* is relatively high; serum levels of 100 mcg./ml. or greater are required. However, the low degree of toxicity of carbenicillin permits the use of doses large enough to achieve adequate levels for these strains.
Other susceptible organisms usually require serum levels in the range of 10-25 mcg/ml.
Geopen is not highly bound to serum proteins and is excreted unchanged in high concentrations in the urine. After a 0.5 to 2 grams I.M. dose, a urine concentration of 1,000 to 5,000 mcg/ml may be achieved.
Indications: Geopen is primarily indicated in the treatment of infections due to susceptible *Pseudomonas aeruginosa, Proteus* species (particularly indole positive strains) and certain strains of *Escherichia coli.*
By virtue of the very high urinary levels achieved, Geopen is particularly effective in urinary tract infections due to one or more of the above mentioned organisms.
Clinical studies have demonstrated the effectiveness of Geopen in the following infections when due to these organisms:

1. Severe systemic infections and septicemia including meningitis due to *Hemophilus influenzae* and *Streptococcus pneumoniae.* Although Geopen possesses *in vitro* activity against many ampicillin-resistant *H. influenzae,* clinical data are insufficient to recommend its use for treatment of meningitis due to ampicillin-resistant strains.
2. Genitourinary tract infections including those due to *Neisseria gonorrhoeae, Enterobacter* and *Streptococcus faecalis* (enterococcus).
3. Acute and chronic respiratory infections. Though clinical improvement has been shown, bacteriologic cures cannot be expected in patients with chronic respiratory disease and cystic fibrosis.
4. Soft tissue infections.

Geopen is also indicated in the treatment of the following infections due to susceptible anaerobic bacteria:

1. Septicemia.
2. Lower respiratory tract infections such as empyema, anaerobic pneumonitis and lung abscess.
3. Intra-abdominal infections such as peritonitis and intra-abdominal abscess. (Typically resulting from anaerobic organisms resident in the normal gastrointestinal tract.)
4. Infections of the female pelvis and genital tract such as endometritis, pelvic inflammatory disease, pelvic abscess and salpingitis.
5. Skin and soft tissue infections.

Although Geopen (carbenicillin disodium) is indicated primarily in gram-negative infections, its activity against gram-positive organisms should be kept in mind when both gram-positive and gram-negative organisms are isolated (see Actions).
In the treatment of infections due to certain susceptible strains of *Pseudomonas aeruginosa,* clinical efficacy may be enhanced by the use of combined therapy with Geopen (carbenicillin disodium) and gentamicin sulfate in full therapeutic dosages. For additional prescribing information, see the gentamicin sulfate package insert.
NOTE: During therapy, sensitivity testing should be repeated frequently to detect the possible emergence of resistant organisms which may develop, particularly if a suboptimal dose regimen is used.
Contraindications: Geopen is ordinarily contraindicated in patients who have a known penicillin allergy.
Warnings: Serious and occasional fatal hypersensitivity (anaphylactic) reactions have been reported in patients on penicillin therapy. These reactions are more apt to occur in individuals with a history of sensitivity to multiple allergens.
Patients with renal impairment should be observed for bleeding manifestations. Such patients should be dosed strictly according to recommendations (see Dosage and Administration section). If bleeding manifestations appear, the antibiotic should be discontinued and appropriate therapy be instituted.
There have been reports of individuals with a history of penicillin hypersensitivity reactions who have experienced severe hypersensitivity reactions when treated with a cephalosporin. Before therapy with a penicillin, careful inquiry should be made concerning previous hypersensitivity reactions to penicillins, cephalosporins, and other allergens. If an allergic reaction occurs, appropriate therapy should be instituted and discontinuance of carbenicillin therapy considered, unless, in the opinion of the physician the condition being treated is life threatening and amenable only to carbenicillin therapy. The usual agents (antihistamines, pressor amines and corticosteroids) should be readily available.
SERIOUS ANAPHYLACTOID REACTIONS REQUIRE IMMEDIATE EMERGENCY TREATMENT WITH EPINEPHRINE. OXYGEN AND INTRAVENOUS CORTICOSTEROIDS SHOULD ALSO BE ADMINISTERED AS INDICATED.
Usage in Pregnancy
Safety for use in pregnancy has not been established.
Precautions: While Geopen exhibits the characteristic low toxicity of the penicillin group of antibiotics, as with any other potent agent, it is advisable to check periodically for organ system dysfunction, including renal, hepatic and hematopoietic systems, during prolonged therapy.
Emergence of resistant organisms, such as *Klebsiella spp.,* and *Serratia spp.,* which may cause superinfection, should be kept in mind.
Geopen is a disodium salt of carboxybenzylpenicillin and hence each gram of Geopen contains 4.7 mEq. of sodium. In patients where sodium restriction is necessary, such as cardiac patients, periodic electrolyte determinations and monitoring of cardiac status should be made.
In a few patients receiving high doses of Geopen, hypokalemia has been reported. Periodic serum potassium determinations should be made and corrective measures should be implemented when necessary.
As with any penicillin preparation, an allergic response, including anaphylaxis, may occur particularly in a hypersensitive individual.
Cases of gonorrhea with a suspected primary lesion of syphilis should have dark field examinations before treatment. In all other cases where concomitant syphilis is suspected, monthly serological tests should be made for a minimum of 4 months.
Adverse Reactions: The following adverse reactions may occur:
Hypersensitivity reactions: Skin rashes, pruritus, urticaria, drug fever, and anaphylactic reactions.
Gastrointestinal disturbances: Nausea
Hemic and Lymphatic Systems: As with other penicillins, anemia, thrombocytopenia, leukopenia, neutropenia, and eosinophilia may occur.
Blood, Hepatic and Renal Studies: As with other semisynthetic penicillins, SGOT and SGPT elevations have been observed after Geopen administration (particularly in children). In all studies to date, no clinical manifestations of hepatic or renal disorders have been demonstrated.
CNS: As with other penicillins, convulsions or neuromuscular irritability could occur with excessively high serum levels.
Other: Pain at the site of injection after intramuscular and intravenous administration has been reported but is rarely accompanied by induration.
Several uremic patients receiving high doses (24 grams/day) have developed hemorrhagic manifestations associated with abnormalities of coagulation tests such as clotting time and prothrombin time. On withdrawal of the antibiotic, the bleeding ceased. The exact relationship of these findings to carbenicillin therapy is not clear.
Vein Irritation and Phlebitis have been reported occasionally, particularly when undiluted solution was directly injected into the vein.
Dosage and Administration:
[See table on next page].
NEONATES: In the neonate, for severe systemic infections (sepsis) due to susceptible strains of *Pseudomonas, Proteus,* and *E. coli, H. influenzae* and *S. pneumoniae,* the following Geopen (carbenicillin disodium) dosages may be given I.M. or by fifteen (15) minute I.V. infusion:

Infants under 2000 g body weight.
  Initial dose: 100 mg/kg.
  Subsequent doses during first week: 75 mg/kg./8 hrs (225 mg/kg./day)
  After 7 days of age: 100 mg/kg./6 hrs (400 mg/kg./day)
Infants over 2000 g body weight.
  Initial dose: 100 mg/kg.
  Subsequent doses during first 3 days: 75 mg/kg./6 hrs (300 mg/kg./day)
  After 3 days of age: 100 mg/kg./6 hrs (400 mg/kg./day)

NOTE: This dosage schedule should give maximum serum levels of approximately 150-175

Continued on next page

mcg/ml and minimum levels of approximately 50-75 mcg/ml of Geopen.

Dosage and Administration: Indication: Clinical experience indicates that in serious urinary tract and systemic infections intravenous therapy in the higher doses should be used. The recommended maximum dose is 40 g per day. Intramuscular injections should not exceed 2 g per injection.

ADULTS:	*Pseudomonas*	*Proteus and E. coli*	*Enterobacter and S. faecalis*	*Anaerobes*	*H. influenzae and S. pneumoniae*
Urinary Tract Infections					
Serious	200 mg/kg/ day by I.V. drip	200 mg/kg/ day by I.V. drip	200 mg/kg/ day by I.V. drip		
Uncomplicated	1–2 g I.M. or I.V. every 6 hours	1–2 g I.M. or I.V. every 6 hours	1–2 g I.M. or I.V. every 6 hours		
Severe Systemic Infections Septicemia Respiratory Infections Soft Tissue Infections	400–500 mg/ kg/day (30–40 grams) I.V. in divided doses or continuously	300–400 mg/ kg/day (20–30 grams) I.V. in divided doses or continuously		400–500 mg/ kg/day (30–40 grams) I.V. in divided doses or continuously	
Infections complicated by renal insufficiency (Creatinine clearance less than 5 ml/min)		2 g. I.V.(1) every 8–12 hours			

ADULTS:	*Pseudomonas*	*Proteus and E. coli*	*Enterobacter and S. faecalis*	*Anaerobes*	*H. influenzae and S. pneumoniae*
Meningitis					400-500 mg/kg day (30-40 grams) I.V. in divided doses or continuously
During peritoneal dialysis		2 g I.V. every 6 hours			
During hemodialysis		2 g I.V. every 4 hours			

(1) The serum half-life of Geopen in patients with severe renal failure is 12.5 hours. As a consequence 2 grams of Geopen administered intravenously to these patients every 8–12 hours will give Geopen serum levels of approximately 100 mcg/ml, a level notably free of any untoward effects while adequate for treatment of a majority of the infections amenable to Geopen therapy.

Treatment of gonorrhea(2); acute uncomplicated ano-genital and urethral infections due to *N. gonorrhoeae.*

SINGLE 4 g I.M. injection, divided between 2 sites.

(2) Probenecid in a dosage of 1 gram may be administered orally about 30 minutes prior to the I.M. treatment of acute gonorrhoeal infections. For complete information and dosage of probenecid, refer to manufacturer's product information.

CHILDREN:	*Pseudomonas*	*Proteus and E. coli*	*Enterobacter and S. faecalis*	*Anaerobes*	*H. influenzae and S. pneumoniae*
Urinary Tract Infections	50–200 mg/ kg/day in divided doses every 4–6 hours I.M. or I.V.	50–100 mg/ kg/day in divided doses every 4–6 hours I.M. or I.V.	50–200 mg/ kg/day in divided doses every 4–6 hours I.M. or I.V.		
Severe Systemic Infections Septicemia Respiratory Infections Soft Tissue Infections	400–500 mg/ kg/day I.V. in divided doses or by continuous drip	300–400 mg/ kg/day I.M. or I.V. in divided doses		400–500 mg/ kg/day I.V. in divided doses or by continuous drip	
Infections complicated by renal insufficiency (Creatinine clearance less than 5 ml/min)		Clinical data is insufficient to recommend an optimum dose			
Meningitis					400-500 mg/kg day in divided doses or by continuous drip

Gentamicin may be used concurrently with carbenicillin for initial therapy until results of culture and susceptibility studies are known. Seriously ill patients should receive the higher doses. GEOPEN has proved to be useful in infections in which protective mechanisms are impaired, such as in acute leukemia and during therapy with immunosuppressive or oncolytic drugs.

Intramuscular Use

As with all intramuscular preparations, Geopen (carbenicillin disodium) should be injected well within the body of a relatively large muscle.

Adults: The preferred site is the upper outer quadrant of the buttock (i.e., gluteus maximus), or the mid-lateral thigh.

Children: It is recommended that intramuscular injections be given preferably in the midlateral muscles of the thigh. In infants and small children the periphery of the upper outer quadrant of the gluteal region should be used only when necessary, such as in burn patients, in order to minimize the possibility of damage to the sciatic nerve.

The deltoid area should be used only if well developed such as in certain adults and older children, and then only with caution to avoid radial nerve injury. Intramuscular injections should not be made into the lower and midthird of the upper arm. As with all intramuscular injections, aspiration is necessary to help avoid inadvertent injection into a blood vessel.

Intravenous Use

As with all intravenous administrations, particular attention should be directed to insure that the drug is injected only into a vein (including aspiration and proper anatomical site selection) to avoid either intra-arterial injection or extravasation.

Preparation of Solution:

For Intramuscular Use—The 1 g vial should be reconstituted with 2.0 ml. of Sterile Water for Injection. In order to facilitate reconstitution, up to 3.6 ml. of Sterile Water for Injection can be used.

Amount of Diluent to be added to the 1 g Vial	Volume to be Withdrawn for a 1 g Dose
2.0 ml	2.5 ml
2.5 ml	3.0 ml
3.6 ml	4.0 ml

The 2 g vial should be reconstituted with 4.0 ml. of Sterile Water for Injection. In order to facilitate reconstitution, up to 7.2 ml. of Sterile Water for Injection can be used.

Amount of Diluent to be added to the 2 g Vial	Volume to be Withdrawn for a 1 g Dose
4.0 ml	2.5 ml
5.0 ml	3.0 ml
7.2 ml	4.0 ml

The 5 g vial should be reconstituted with 7 ml. of Sterile Water for Injection. In order to facilitate reconstitution, up to 17 ml. of Sterile Water for Injection can be used.

Amount of Diluent to be added to the 5 g Vial	Volume to be Withdrawn for a 1 g Dose
7.0 ml	2.0 ml
9.5 ml	2.5 ml
12.0 ml	3.0 ml
17.0 ml	4.0 ml

After reconstitution, no significant loss of potency occurs for 24 hours at room temperature, and for 72 hours if refrigerated. Any of these unused solutions should be discarded.

For Direct Intravenous Injection—Following reconstitution, each gram should be further diluted by no less than 5 ml of Sterile Water for Injection. In order to avoid vein irritation, the solution should be administered as slowly as possible.

For Intravenous Infusion—Following reconstitution according to directions, Geopen (carbenicillin disodium) may be added to the desired volume of usual intravenous infusion solutions.

WHEN USING THE 2 g, 5 g, AND 10 g PIGGY-BACK UNITS OR BULK PHARMACY PACK FOR. . .

Intravenous Use
As with all intravenous administrations, particular attention should be directed to insure that the drug is injected only into a vein (including aspiration and proper anatomical site selection) to avoid either intra-arterial injection or extravasation.

For Direct Intravenous Injection
The 2 gram vial should be reconstituted with a minimum of 20 ml. Sterile Water for Injection.

Amount of Diluent	Concentration of Solution
100 ml	1 g/50 ml
50 ml	1 g/25 ml
20 ml	1 g/10 ml

The 5 gram vial should be reconstituted with a minimum of 50 ml. of Sterile Water for Injection.

Amount of Diluent	Concentration of Solution
100 ml	1 g/20 ml
50 ml	1 g/10 ml

The 10 gram vial should be reconstituted with a minimum of 95 ml of Sterile Water for Injection.

Amount of Diluent	Concentration of Solution
95 ml	1 g/10 ml

In order to avoid vein irritation, the solution should be administered as slowly as possible. A dilution of 1 g/20 ml or more will further reduce the incidence of vein irritation.
After reconstitution, no significant loss of potency occurs for 24 hours at room temperature and for 72 hours if refrigerated. Any of these unused solutions should be discarded.

Bulk Pharmacy Package
The 30 gram vial should be reconstituted by adding 80 ml of water in two separate 40 ml aliquots. Add 40 ml, shake 25 seconds and add the last 40 ml aliquot and shake for final solution. The resulting solution will contain 300 mg/ml of carbenicillin. Transfer recommended dosage to appropriate intravenous infusion solution.

Reconstituted bulk solution should not be used for direct infusion.

After reconstitution, no significant loss of potency occurs for 24 hours at room temperature and for 72 hours if refrigerated. Any of these unused solutions should be discarded.

For Continuous Intravenous Infusion
After reconstitution as directed, Geopen (carbenicillin disodium) may be added to the desired volume of usual intravenous infusion solutions.
Geopen is stable for 24 hours at room temperature and for 72 hours if stored in a refrigerator when diluted to as low as 10 mg/ml with the following intravenous Infusion Diluents:

Sodium Chloride Injection, USP
Dextrose 5% with 0.225% Sodium Chloride
Dextrose Injection, USP (5%)
Ringer's Injection, USP
Lactated Ringer's Injection, USP
5% Dextrose with Electrolyte No. 48
5% Levugen (Fructose) with Electrolyte No. 75
Invert Sugar 10% in Water
Dextrose 5% and 0.45% Sodium Chloride, USP
5% Alcohol, 5% Dextrose in Water
5% Alcohol, 5% Dextrose in 0.9% Sodium Chloride
5% Dextrose in Alcohol
Maintenance Electrolyte Solution (Electrolyte No. 75)
Pediatric Maintenance Electrolyte Solution (Electrolyte No. 48)

Discard any unused solutions if stored for 24 hours at room temperature, or for 72 hours if refrigerated.
It is recommended that Geopen and gentamicin sulfate not be mixed together in the same IV solution due to the gradual inactivation of gentamicin sulfate under these circumstances. The therapeutic effect of the two drugs remains unimpaired when administered separately.

For Intramuscular Use Only:
Geopen for intramuscular injection ONLY may be diluted with one of the following:

1. 0.5% Lidocaine Hydrochloride (without epinephrine).
2. Bacteriostatic Water containing 0.9% Benzyl Alcohol.

For reconstitution of Geopen with these diluents for intramuscular use ONLY, follow the directions for the amount of diluent in the **PREPARATION OF SOLUTION, For Intramuscular Use section.**
Geopen may be diluted with these solutions and stored for 24 hours at room temperature or for 72 hours when refrigerated. Discard unused solutions stored longer than these time periods.
For full product information, refer to the package insert for Lidocaine Hydrochloride (without epinephrine).
How Supplied: Geopen is available in 1 g, 2 g, and 5 g vials for intramuscular/intravenous use.
Geopen is available in 2 g, 5 g, 10 g Piggyback Units, and 30 g Bulk Pharmacy Pack for intravenous use.

HEPTUNA® PLUS CAPSULES ℞
(Hard Gelatin)
Fortified Oral Hematopoietic Formulation

Each capsule contains:

HEMATOPOIETIC FACTORS
Ferrous Sulfate, dried, U.S.P.
(provides 100 mg. of elemental iron) 311 mg.
Desiccated Liver (Undefatted) ....50 mg.
Vitamin B_{12}, cobalamin concentrate
NF (as Stablets®) ....5 mcg.
With instrinsic factor concentrate
(non-inhibitory) ....25 mg.

VITAMINS
B_1 (thiamine mononitrate, U.S.P.) ....3.1 mg.
B_2 (riboflavin, U.S.P.) ....2 mg.
B_6 (pyridoxine hydrochloride, U.S.P.) .1.6 mg.
Vitamin C (from sodium ascorbate) ...150 mg.
Niacinamide, U.S.P. ....15 mg.
Calcium pantothenate, U.S.P. ....0.9 mg.

MINERALS
Copper (from copper sulfate) ....1 mg.
Molybdenum (from sodium
molybdate) ....0.2 mg.
Calcium (from dibasic calcium
phosphate) ....37.4 mg.
Iodine (from potassium iodide) ....0.05 mg.
Manganese (from manganese
sulfate) ....0.033 mg.
Magnesium (from magnesium sulfate) 2 mg.
Phosphorus (from dibasic calcium
phosphate) ....29 mg.
Potassium (from potassium sulfate) .....1.7 mg.
Stablets U.S. Pat. No. 2,830,933

Heptuna Plus capsules contain the necessary factors for the treatment of anemias amenable to oral therapy plus supplemental amounts of B-complex vitamins and minerals.
Ferrous sulfate compared to other sources of iron provides the highest amounts of iron for utilization in patients with hypochromic anemias.
Sodium ascorbate (source of vitamin C activity) helps to reduce food ferric iron to the ferrous state which increases the utilization of the iron present in the diet.
Pharmacology studies in animals indicate that pyridoxine HCl (vitamin B_6) deficiency may result in a hypochromic microcytic anemia.
Copper is known to be involved in hematopoiesis; the exact role in this area of physiology is still under investigation.
Patients who have an anemia caused by insufficient iron intake may also have a decreased intake of B-complex vitamins and minerals. Supplementary amounts of B-complex vitamins and minerals in Heptuna Plus will help to alleviate possible deficiency in these areas.
Dosage: For many patients one capsule daily will provide sufficient amounts of hematopoietic factors for therapeutic results. If the severity and etiology of the anemia indicate, one capsule three times a day may be prescribed.
Side Effect: In a small per cent of patients, iron therapy causes gastrointestinal irritation. In these patients administering Heptuna Plus with meals or reducing the dosage usually will alleviate the symptoms.
Precautions: Although this product contains Vitamin B_{12} (as Stablets) with intrinsic factor concentrate (non-inhibitory), and desiccated liver, it is not a reliable substitute for parenterally administered cyanocobalamin (Vitamin B_{12}) in the management of pernicious anemia.
Some patients with pernicious anemia may not respond to orally ingested cobalamin concentrate (vitamin B_{12}) and there is no known way to predict which patients will respond or which patients may cease to respond.
Periodic examinations and laboratory studies of pernicious anemia patients are essential and recommended, and should, if necessary, receive Vitamin B_{12} parenterally.
Anemia is a manifestation of an underlying disease, i.e., blood loss, lack of intrinsic factor production, etc. In the treatment of anemia, it is necessary to make an etiological diagnosis.
Supplied: In bottles of 100.
[Shown in Product Identification Section]

MARAX® ℞
(ephedrine sulfate, theophylline, hydroxyzine HCl)
TABLETS AND DF SYRUP

Contents:

	Each Tablet Contains:	Each Teaspoon (5 ml.) Syrup Contains:
Ephedrine Sulfate	25 mg.	6.25 mg.
Theophylline	130 mg.	32.50 mg.
Atarax® (hydroxyzine HCl)	10 mg.	2.5 mg.
Alcohol (Ethyl Alcohol)		5% v/v.

Actions: The action of ephedrine as a vasoconstrictor is well known. It is therefore of significant benefit in symptomatic relief of the congestion occurring in bronchial asthma. As a bronchodilator, it has a slower onset but longer duration of action than does epinephrine, which, in contrast to ephedrine, is not effective upon oral administration.
The diverse actions of theophylline—bronchospasmolytic, cardiovascular, and diuretic—are well established, and make it a particularly useful drug in the treatment of bronchial asthma, both in the acute attack and in the prophylactic therapy of the disease.
Atarax (hydroxyzine HCl) modifies the central stimulatory action of ephedrine preventing excessive excitation in patients on Marax therapy.
In animal studies Atarax (hydroxyzine HCl) has demonstrated antiserotonin activity and antispasmodic potency of a nonspecific nature. Marax-DF Syrup produces an expectorant action wherein the tenacity of the sputum is decreased and the ease of expectoration is increased.

Indications
Based on a review of this drug by the National Academy of Sciences-National Research Council and/or other information, FDA has classified the indications as follows:

Continued on next page

Roerig—Cont.

"Possibly" Effective: For controlling bronchospastic disorders.
Final classification of the less than effective indication requires further investigation.

Contraindications: Because of the ephedrine, Marax is contraindicated in cardiovascular disease, hyperthyroidism, and hypertension. This drug is contraindicated in individuals who have shown hypersensitivity to the drug or its components.
Hydroxyzine, when administered to the pregnant mouse, rat, and rabbit induced fetal abnormalities in the rat at doses substantially above the human therapeutic range. Clinical data in human beings are inadequate to establish safety in early pregnancy. Until such data are available, hydroxyzine is contraindicated in early pregnancy.
Precautions: Because of the ephedrine component this drug should be used with caution in elderly males or those with known prostatic hypertrophy.
The potentiating action of hydroxyzine, although mild, must be taken into consideration when the drug is used in conjunction with central nervous system depressants; and when other central nervous system depressants are administered concomitantly with hydroxyzine their dosage should be reduced.
Patients should be warned—because of the hydroxyzine component—of the possibility of drowsiness occurring and cautioned against driving a car or operating dangerous machinery while taking this drug.
Adverse Reactions: With large doses of ephedrine, excitation, tremulousness, insomnia, nervousness, palpitation, tachycardia, precordial pain, cardiac arrhythmias, vertigo, dryness of the nose and throat, headache, sweating, and warmth may occur. Because ephedrine is a sympathomimetic agent some patients may develop vesical sphincter spasm and resultant urinary hesitation, and occasionally acute urinary retention. This should be borne in mind when administering preparations containing ephedrine to elderly males or those with known prostatic hypertrophy. At the recommended dose for Marax, a side effect occasionally reported is palpitation, and this can be controlled with dosage adjustment, additional amounts of concurrently administered Atarax (hydroxyzine HCl), or discontinuation of the medication. When ephedrine is given three or more times daily patients may develop tolerance after several weeks of therapy.
Theophylline when given on an empty stomach frequently causes gastric irritation accompanied by upper abdominal discomfort, nausea, and vomiting. Administration of the medication after meals will serve to minimize this side effect. Theophylline may cause diuresis and cardiac stimulation. The amount of Atarax (hydroxyzine HCl) present in Marax has not resulted in disturbing side effects. When used alone specifically as a tranquilizer in the normal dosage range (25 to 50 mg. three or four times a day), side effects are infrequent; even at these higher doses, no serious side effects have been reported and confirmed to date. Those which do occasionally occur when Atarax (hydroxyzine HCl) is used alone are drowsiness, xerostomia and, at extremely high doses, involuntary motor activity, unsteadiness of gait, neuromuscular weakness, all of which may be controlled by reduction of the dosage or discontinuation of the medication.
With the relatively low dose of Atarax (hydroxyzine HCl) in Marax, these effects are not likely to occur. In addition, the ataractic action of Atarax (hydroxyzine HCl) may modify the cardiac stimulatory action of ephedrine, and concurrently, increasing the amount of Atarax (hydroxyzine HCl) may control or abolish this undesirable effect of ephedrine.
Dosage and Administration: The dosage of Marax should be adjusted according to the severity of complaints, and the patient's individual toleration.
Tablets: In general, an adult dose of 1 tablet, 2 to 4 times daily, should be sufficient. Some patients are controlled adequately with ½ to 1 tablet at bedtime. The time interval between doses should not be shorter than four hours. The dosage for children over 5 years of age and for adults who are sensitive to ephedrine, is one-half the usual adult dose. Clinical experience to date has been confined to ages above 5 years.
Syrup: The dose for children over 5 years of age is 1 teaspoon (5 ml.), 3 to 4 times daily. Dosage for children 2 to 5 years of age is ½ to 1 teaspoon (2.5-5 ml.), 3 to 4 times daily. Not recommended for children under 2 years of age.
How Supplied: Marax Tablets are available as scored dye free tablets in bottles of 100 and 500.
Marax-DF Syrup is available in pints and gallons as a colorless syrup free of all coal tar dyes, and should be dispensed in amber colored bottles.

[*Shown in Product Identification Section*]

NAVANE® ℞
(thiothixene) CAPSULES
NAVANE®
(thiothixene hydrochloride) CONCENTRATE

Actions: Navane is a psychotropic agent of the thioxanthene series. Navane possesses certain chemical and pharmacological similarities to the piperazine phenothiazines and differences from the aliphatic group of phenothiazines.
Indications: Navane is effective in the management of manifestations of psychotic disorders. Navane has not been evaluated in the management of behavioral complications in patients with mental retardation.
Contraindications: Navane is contraindicated in patients with circulatory collapse, comatose states, central nervous system depression due to any cause, and blood dyscrasias. Navane is contraindicated in individuals who have shown hypersensitivity to the drug. It is not known whether there is a cross sensitivity between the thioxanthenes and the phenothiazine derivatives, but this possibility should be considered.
Warnings:
Usage in Pregnancy—Safe use of Navane during pregnancy has not been established. Therefore, this drug should be given to pregnant patients only when, in the judgment of the physician, the expected benefits from the treatment exceed the possible risks to mother and fetus. Animal reproduction studies and clinical experience to date have not demonstrated any teratogenic effects.
In the animal reproduction studies with Navane, there was some decrease in conception rate and litter size, and an increase in resorption rate in rats and rabbits. Similar findings have been reported with other psychotropic agents. After repeated oral administration of Navane to rats (5 to 15 mg./kg./day), rabbits (3 to 50 mg./kg./day), and monkeys (1 to 3 mg./kg./day) before and during gestation, no teratogenic effects were seen.
Usage in Children—The use of Navane in children under 12 years of age is not recommended because safe conditions for its use have not been established.
As is true with many CNS drugs, Navane may impair the mental and/or physical abilities required for the performance of potentially hazardous tasks such as driving a car or operating machinery, especially during the first few days of therapy. Therefore, the patient should be cautioned accordingly.
As in the case of other CNS-acting drugs, patients receiving Navane (thiothixene) should be cautioned about the possible additive effects (which may include hypotension) with CNS depressants and with alcohol.
Precautions: An antiemetic effect was observed in animal studies with Navane; since this effect may also occur in man, it is possible that Navane may mask signs of overdosage of toxic drugs and may obscure conditions such as intestinal obstruction and brain tumor.
In consideration of the known capability of Navane and certain other psychotropic drugs to precipitate convulsions, extreme caution should be used in patients with a history of convulsive disorders or those in a state of alcohol withdrawal, since it may lower the convulsive threshold. Although Navane potentiates the actions of the barbiturates, the dosage of the anticonvulsant therapy should not be reduced when Navane is administered concurrently.
Though exhibiting rather weak anticholinergic properties, Navane should be used with caution in patients who might be exposed to extreme heat or who are receiving atropine or related drugs.
Use with caution in patients with cardiovascular disease.
Caution as well as careful adjustment of the dosages is indicated when Navane is used in conjunction with other CNS depressants.
Also, careful observation should be made for pigmentary retinopathy, and lenticular pigmentation (fine lenticular pigmentation has been noted in a small number of patients treated with Navane for prolonged periods).
Blood dyscrasias (agranulocytosis, pancytopenia, thrombocytopenic purpura), and liver damage (jaundice, biliary stasis), have been reported with related drugs.
Adverse Reactions:
NOTE: Not all of the following adverse reactions have been reported with Navane. However, since Navane has certain chemical and pharmacologic similarities to the phenothiazines, all of the known side effects and toxicity associated with phenothiazine therapy should be borne in mind when Navane is used.
Cardiovascular effects: Tachycardia, hypotension, lightheadedness, and syncope. In the event hypotension occurs, epinephrine should not be used as a pressor agent since a paradoxical further lowering of blood pressure may result. Nonspecific EKG changes have been observed in some patients receiving Navane. These changes are usually reversible and frequently disappear on continued Navane therapy. The incidence of these changes is lower than that observed with some phenothiazines. The clinical significance of these changes is not known.
CNS effects: Drowsiness, usually mild, may occur although it usually subsides with continuation of Navane therapy. The incidence of sedation appears similar to that of the piperazine group of phenothiazines but less than that of certain aliphatic phenothiazines. Restlessness, agitation and insomnia have been noted with Navane. Seizures and paradoxical exacerbation of psychotic symptoms have occurred with Navane infrequently.
Hyperreflexia has been reported in infants delivered from mothers having received structurally related drugs.
In addition, phenothiazine derivatives have been associated with cerebral edema and cerebrospinal fluid abnormalities.
Extrapyramidal symptoms, such as pseudoparkinsonism, akathisia and dystonia have been reported. Management of these extrapyramidal symptoms depends upon the type and severity. Rapid relief of acute symptoms may require the use of an injectable antiparkinson agent. More slowly emerging symptoms may be managed by reducing the dosage of Navane and/or administering an oral antiparkinson agent.
Persistent Tardive Dyskinesia: As with all antipsychotic agents tardive dyskinesia may ap-

pear in some patients on long term therapy or may occur after drug therapy has been discontinued. The risk seems to be greater in elderly patients on high-dose therapy, especially females. The symptoms are persistent and in some patients appear to be irreversible. The syndrome is characterized by rhythmical involuntary movements of the tongue, face, mouth or jaw (e.g., protrusion of tongue, puffing of cheeks, puckering of mouth, chewing movements). Sometimes these may be accompanied by involuntary movements of extremities.

There is no known effective treatment for tardive dyskinesia; antiparkinsonism agents usually do not alleviate the symptoms of this syndrome. It is suggested that all antipsychotic agents be discontinued if these symptoms appear.

Should it be necessary to reinstitute treatment, or increase the dosage of the agent, or switch to a different antipsychotic agent, the syndrome may be masked.

It has been reported that fine vermicular movements of the tongue may be an early sign of the syndrome and if the medication is stopped at that time, the syndrome may not develop.

Hepatic effects: Elevations of serum transaminase and alkaline phosphatase, usually transient, have been infrequently observed in some patients. No clinically confirmed cases of jaundice attributable to Navane have been reported.

Hematologic effects: As is true with certain other psychotropic drugs, leukopenia and leucocytosis, which are usually transient, can occur occasionally with Navane. Other antipsychotic drugs have been associated with agranulocytosis, eosinophilia, hemolytic anemia, thrombocytopenia and pancytopenia.

Allergic reactions: Rash, pruritus, urticaria, photosensitivity and rare cases of anaphylaxis have been reported with Navane. Undue exposure to sunlight should be avoided. Although not experienced with Navane, exfoliative dermatitis and contact dermatitis (in nursing personnel), have been reported with certain phenothiazines.

Endocrine disorders: Lactation, moderate breast enlargement and amenorrhea have occurred in a small percentage of females receiving Navane (thiothixene). If persistent, this may necessitate a reduction in dosage or the discontinuation of therapy. Phenothiazines have been associated with false positive pregnancy tests, gynecomastia, hypoglycemia, hyperglycemia and glycosuria.

Autonomic effects: Dry mouth, blurred vision, nasal congestion, constipation, increased sweating, increased salivation and impotence have occurred infrequently with Navane therapy. Phenothiazines have been associated with miosis, mydriasis, and adynamic ileus.

Other adverse reactions: Hyperpyrexia, anorexia, nausea, vomiting, diarrhea, increase in appetite and weight, weakness or fatigue, polydipsia, and peripheral edema.

Although not reported with Navane, evidence indicates there is a relationship between phenothiazine therapy and the occurrence of a systemic lupus erythematosus-like syndrome.

NOTE: Sudden deaths have occasionally been reported in patients who have received certain phenothiazine derivatives. In some cases the cause of death was apparently cardiac arrest or asphyxia due to failure of the cough reflex. In others, the cause could not be determined nor could it be established that death was due to phenothiazine administration.

Dosage and Administration: Dosage of Navane should be individually adjusted depending on the chronicity and severity of the condition. In general, small doses should be used initially and gradually increased to the optimal effective level, based on patient response. Some patients have been successfully maintained on once-a-day Navane therapy.

The use of Navane in children under 12 years of age is not recommended because safe conditions for its use have not been established.

In milder conditions, an initial dose of 2 mg. three times daily. If indicated, a subsequent increase to 15 mg./day total daily dose is often effective.

In more severe conditions, an initial dose of 5 mg. twice daily.

The usual optimal dose is 20 to 30 mg. daily. If indicated, an increase to 60 mg./day total daily dose is often effective. Exceeding a total daily dose of 60 mg. rarely increases the beneficial response.

Overdosage: Manifestations include muscular twitching, drowsiness and dizziness. Symptoms of gross overdosage may include CNS depression, rigidity, weakness, torticollis, tremor, salivation, dysphagia, hypotension, disturbances of gait, or coma.

Treatment: Essentially symptomatic and supportive. Early gastric lavage is helpful. Keep patient under careful observation and maintain an open airway, since involvement of the extrapyramidal system may produce dysphagia and respiratory difficulty in severe overdosage. If hypotension occurs, the standard measures for managing circulatory shock should be used (I.V. fluids and/or vasoconstrictors).

If a vasoconstrictor is needed, levarterenol and phenylephrine are the most suitable drugs. Other pressor agents, including epinephrine, are not recommended, since phenothiazine derivatives may reverse the usual pressor action of these agents and cause further lowering of blood pressure.

If CNS depression is present, recommended stimulants include amphetamine, dextroamphetamine, or caffeine and sodium benzoate. Stimulants that may cause convulsions (e. g. picrotoxin or pentylenetetrazol) should be avoided. Extrapyramidal symptoms may be treated with antiparkinson drugs.

There are no data on the use of peritoneal or hemodialysis, but they are known to be of little value in phenothiazine intoxication.

How Supplied: Navane (thiothixene) is available as capsules containing 1 mg., 2 mg., 5 mg., and 10 mg. of thiothixene in bottles of 100, 1,000 and unit-dose pack of 100 (10 × 10's). Navane (thiothixene) is also available as capsules containing 20 mg. of thiothixene in bottles of 100, 500 and unit-dose pack of 100 (10 × 10's).

Navane (thiothixene hydrochloride) Concentrate is available in 120 ml. (4 oz.) bottles with an accompanying dropper calibrated at 2 mg., 4 mg., 5 mg., 6 mg., 8 mg., and 10 mg. and in 30 ml (1 oz.) bottles with an accompanying dropper calibrated at 2 mg, 4 mg, and 5 mg. Each ml. contains thiothixene hydrochloride equivalent to 5 mg. of thiothixene. Contains alcohol, U.S.P. 7.0% v/v. (small loss unavoidable).

[*Shown in Product Identification Section*]

NAVANE® ℞
(thiothixene hydrochloride)
Intramuscular
2 mg./ml. †

Description: Navane (thiothixene hydrochloride) is a thioxanthene derivative. Specifically, it is the *cis* isomer of N,N-dimethyl-9-[3-(4-methyl-1-piperazinyl)-propylidene] thioxanthene-2-sulfonamide.

The thioxanthenes differ from the phenothiazines by the replacement of nitrogen in the central ring with a carbon-linked side chain fixed in space in a rigid structural configuration. An N,N-dimethyl sulfonamide functional group is bonded to the thioxanthene nucleus.

†Navane Intramuscular contains in each ml. thiothixene HCl equivalent to 2 mg. of thiothixene, dextrose 5% w/v, benzyl alcohol 0.9% w/v, and propyl gallate 0.02% w/v.

Actions: Navane is a psychotropic agent of the thioxanthene series. Navane possesses certain chemical and pharmacological similarities to the piperazine phenothiazines and differences from the aliphatic group of phenothiazines. Navane's mode of action has not been clearly established.

Indications: Navane is effective in the management of manifestations of psychotic disorders. Navane has not been evaluated in the management of behavioral complications in patients with mental retardation.

Contraindications: Navane is contraindicated in patients with circulatory collapse, comatose states, central nervous system depression due to any cause, and blood dyscrasias. Navane is contraindicated in individuals who have shown hypersensitivity to the drug. It is not known whether there is a cross sensitivity between the thioxanthenes and the phenothiazine derivatives, but this possibility should be considered.

Warnings: Usage in Pregnancy—Safe use of Navane during pregnancy has not been established. Therefore, this drug should be given to pregnant patients only when, in the judgment of the physician, the expected benefits from treatment exceed the possible risks to mother and fetus. Animal reproductive studies and clinical experience to date have not demonstrated any teratogenic effects.

In the animal reproduction studies with Navane, there was some decrease in conception rate and litter size, and an increase in resorption rate in rats and rabbits, changes which have been similarly reported with other psychotropic agents. After repeated oral administration of Navane to rats (5 to 15 mg./kg./day), rabbits (3 to 50 mg./kg./day), and monkeys (1 to 3 mg./kg./day) before and during gestation, no teratogenic effects were seen. (See Precautions).

Usage in Children—The use of Navane in children under 12 years of age is not recommended because safety and efficacy in the pediatric age group have not been established.

As is true with many CNS drugs, Navane may impair the mental and/or physical abilities required for the performance of potentially hazardous tasks such as driving a car or operating machinery, especially during the first few days of therapy. Therefore, the patient should be cautioned accordingly.

As in the case of other CNS-acting drugs, patients receiving Navane should be cautioned about the possible additive effects (which may include hypotension) with CNS depressants and with alcohol.

Precautions: An antiemetic effect was observed in animal studies with Navane (thiothixene hydrochloride); since this effect may also occur in man, it is possible that Navane may mask signs of overdosage of toxic drugs and may obscure conditions such as intestinal obstruction and brain tumor.

In consideration of the known capability of Navane and certain other psychotropic drugs to precipitate convulsions, extreme caution should be used in patients with a history of convulsive disorders, or those in a state of alcohol withdrawal since it may lower the convulsive threshold. Although Navane potentiates the actions of the barbiturates, the dosage of the anticonvulsant therapy should not be reduced when Navane is administered concurrently.

Caution as well as careful adjustment of the dosage is indicated when Navane is used in conjunction with other CNS depressants other than anticonvulsant drugs.

Though exhibiting rather weak anticholinergic properties, Navane should be used with caution in patients who are known or suspected to have glaucoma, or who might be exposed to extreme heat, or who are receiving atropine or related drugs.

Continued on next page

Roerig—Cont.

Use with caution in patients with cardiovascular disease.
Also, careful observation should be made for pigmentary retinopathy, and lenticular pigmentation (fine lenticular pigmentation has been noted in a small number of patients treated with Navane for prolonged periods).
Blood dyscrasias (agranulocytosis, pancytopenia, thrombocytopenic purpura), and liver damage (jaundice, biliary stasis), have been reported with related drugs.
Undue exposure to sunlight should be avoided. Photosensitive reactions have been reported in patients on Navane.
As with all intramuscular preparations, Navane Intramuscular should be injected well within the body of a relatively large muscle. The preferred sites are the upper outer quadrant of the buttock (i.e., gluteus maximus) and the mid-lateral thigh.
The deltoid area should be used only if well developed such as in certain adults and older children, and then only with caution to avoid radial nerve injury. Intramuscular injections should not be made into the lower and mid-thirds of the upper arm. As with all intramuscular injections, aspiration is necessary to help avoid inadvertent injection into a blood vessel.

Adverse Reactions:

NOTE: Not all of the following adverse reactions have been reported with Navane. However, since Navane has certain chemical and pharmacologic similarities to the phenothiazines, all of the known side effects and toxicity associated with phenothiazine therapy should be borne in mind when Navane is used.
Cardiovascular effects: Tachycardia, hypotension, lightheadedness, and syncope. In the event hypotension occurs, epinephrine should not be used as a pressor agent since a paradoxical further lowering of blood pressure may result. Nonspecific EKG changes have been observed in some patients receiving Navane. These changes are usually reversible and frequently disappear on continued Navane therapy. The clinical significance of these changes is not known.
CNS effects: Drowsiness, usually mild, may occur although it usually subsides with continuation of Navane therapy. The incidence of sedation appears similar to that of the piperazine group of phenothiazines, but less than that of certain aliphatic phenothiazines. Restlessness, agitation and insomnia have been noted with Navane. Seizures and paradoxical exacerbation of psychotic symptoms have occurred with Navane infrequently.
Hyperreflexia has been reported in infants delivered from mothers having received structurally related drugs.
In addition, phenothiazine derivatives have been associated with cerebral edema and cerebrospinal fluid abnormalities.
Extrapyramidal symptoms, such as pseudoparkinsonism, akathisia, and dystonia have been reported. Management of these extrapyramidal symptoms depends upon the type and severity. Rapid relief of acute symptoms may require the use of an injectable antiparkinson agent. More slowly emerging symptoms may be managed by reducing the dosage of Navane and/or administering an oral antiparkinson agent.
Persistent Tardive Dyskinesia: As with all antipsychotic agents tardive dyskinesia may appear in some patients on long term therapy or may occur after drug therapy has been discontinued. The risk seems to be greater in elderly patients on high-dose therapy, especially females. The symptoms are persistent and in some patients appear to be irreversible. The syndrome is characterized by rhythmical involuntary movements of the tongue, face, mouth or jaw (e.g., protrusion of tongue, puffing of cheeks, puckering of mouth, chewing movements). Sometimes these may be accompanied by involuntary movements of extremities.
There is no known effective treatment for tardive dyskinesia; antiparkinsonism agents usually do not alleviate the symptoms of this syndrome. It is suggested that all antipsychotic agents be discontinued if these symptoms appear.
Should it be necessary to reinstitute treatment, or increase the dosage of the agent, or switch to a different antipsychotic agent, the syndrome may be masked.
It has been reported that fine vermicular movements of the tongue may be an early sign of the syndrome and if the medication is stopped at that time, the syndrome may not develop.
Hepatic effects: Elevations of serum transaminase and alkaline phosphatase, usually transient, have been infrequently observed in some patients. No clinically confirmed cases of jaundice attributable to Navane (thiothixene hydrochloride) have been reported.
Hematologic effects: As is true with certain other psychotropic drugs, leukopenia and leucocytosis, which are usually transient, can occur occasionally with Navane. Other antipsychotic drugs have been associated with agranulocytosis, eosinophilia, hemolytic anemia, thrombocytopenia and pancytopenia.
Allergic reactions: Rash, pruritus, urticaria, and rare cases of anaphylaxis have been reported with Navane. Undue exposure to sunlight should be avoided. Although not experienced with Navane, exfoliative dermatitis, contact dermatitis (in nursing personnel), have been reported with certain phenothiazines.
Endocrine disorders: Lactation, moderate breast enlargement and amenorrhea have occurred in a small percentage of females receiving Navane. If persistent, this may necessitate a reduction in dosage or the discontinuation of therapy. Phenothiazines have been associated with false positive pregnancy tests, gynecomastia, hypoglycemia, hyperglycemia, and glycosuria.
Autonomic effects: Dry mouth, blurred vision, nasal congestion, constipation, increased sweating, increased salivation, and impotence have occurred infrequently with Navane therapy. Phenothiazines have been associated with miosis, mydriasis, and adynamic ileus.
Other adverse reactions: Hyperpyrexia, anorexia, nausea, vomiting, diarrhea, increase in appetite and weight, weakness or fatigue, polydipsia and peripheral edema.
Although not reported with Navane, evidence indicates there is a relationship between phenothiazine therapy and the occurrence of a systemic lupus erythematosus-like syndrome.
NOTE: Sudden deaths have occasionally been reported in patients who have received certain phenothiazine derivatives. In some cases the cause of death was apparently cardiac arrest or asphyxia due to failure of the cough reflex. In others, the cause could not be determined nor could it be established that death was due to phenothiazine administration.

Dosage and Administration:

For Intramuscular Use Only

Dosage of Navane should be individually adjusted depending on the chronicity and severity of the condition. In general, small doses should be used initially and gradually increased to the optimal effective level, based on patient response.
Usage in children under 12 years of age is not recommended.
Where more rapid control and treatment of acute behavior is desirable, the intramuscular form of Navane may be indicated. It is also of benefit where the very nature of the patient's symptomatology, whether acute or chronic, renders oral administration impractical or even impossible.
For treatment of acute symptomatology or in patients unable or unwilling to take oral medication, the usual dose is 4 mg. of Navane Intramuscular administered 2 to 4 times daily. Dosage may be increased or decreased depending on response. Most patients are controlled on a total daily dosage of 16 to 20 mg. The maximum recommended dosage is 30 mg./day. An oral form should supplant the injectable form as soon as possible. It may be necessary to adjust the dosage when changing from the intramuscular to oral dosage forms. Dosage recommendations for Navane Capsules and Concentrate can be found in the Navane oral package insert.

Overdosage: Manifestations include muscular twitching, drowsiness, and dizziness. Symptoms of gross overdosage may include CNS depression, rigidity, weakness, torticollis, tremor, salivation, dysphagia, hypotension, disturbances of gait, or coma.
Treatment: Essentially symptomatic and supportive. Keep patient under careful observation and maintain an open airway, since involvement of the extrapyramidal system may produce dysphagia and respiratory difficulty in severe overdosage. If hypotension occurs, the standard measures for managing circulatory shock should be used (I.V. fluids and/or vasoconstrictors).
If a vasoconstrictor is needed, levarterenol and phenylephrine are the most suitable drugs. Other pressor agents, including epinephrine, are not recommended, since phenothiazine derivatives may reverse the usual pressor elevating action of these agents and cause further lowering of blood pressure.
If CNS depression is present, recommended stimulants include amphetamine, dextroamphetamine, or caffeine and sodium benzoate. Picrotoxin or pentylenetetrazol should be avoided. Extrapyramidal symptoms may be treated with antiparkinson drugs.
There are no data on the use of peritoneal or hemodialysis, but they are known to be of little value in phenothiazine intoxication.

How Supplied: Navane (thiothixene hydrochloride) Intramuscular solution is available in a 2 ml. amber glass vial in packages of 10. Each ml. contains thiothixene hydrochloride equivalent to 2 mg. of thiothixene, dextrose 5% w/v, benzyl alcohol 0.9% w/v, and propyl gallate 0.02% w/v.

SUSTAIRE® ℞

theophylline (anhydrous)
SUSTAINED RELEASE TABLETS

Actions: The pharmacologic actions of theophylline are as a bronchodilator, pulmonary vasodilator, and smooth muscle relaxant since the drug directly relaxes the smooth muscle of the bronchial airways and pulmonary blood vessels. Theophylline also possesses other actions typical of the xanthine derivatives: coronary vasodilator, diuretic, cardiac stimulant, and skeletal muscle stimulant. The actions of theophylline may be mediated through inhibition of phosphodiesterase and a resultant increase in intracellular cyclic AMP which could mediate smooth muscle relaxation.
No development of tolerance appears to occur with chronic use of theophylline. The half-life is shortened with cigarette smoking and prolonged in alcoholism, reduced hepatic or renal function, congestive heart failure, and in patients receiving certain antibiotics (see DRUG INTERACTIONS). High fever for prolonged periods may decrease theophylline elimination. Children over six months of age have rapid clearances with average half-lives of approximately 3–5 hours. Newborn infants have extremely slow clearances and half-lives exceeding 24 hours. Older adults with chronic obstructive pulmonary disease, any patients with cor pulmonale or other causes of heart failure, and patients with liver pathology may have much lower clearances with half-lives

that exceed 24 hours. The half-life in nonsmokers averages 7–9 hours.

In single dose studies, SUSTAIRE, administered at 8 mg/kg body weight, produced mean peak theophylline blood levels of 7.5 ± 1.9 mcg/ml at 9.2 ± 1.9 hours following administration. In the multiple dose, steady-state, 3 and 5 day studies, SUSTAIRE achieved remarkably constant intra-subject theophylline levels with an average peak-trough difference of only 4 mcg/ml. This is indicative of smooth and stable maintenance therapeutic theophylline levels throughout a q12h dosing interval.

Indications: Symptomatic relief and/or prevention of asthma and reversible bronchospasm associated with chronic bronchitis and emphysema.

Contraindications: SUSTAIRE is contraindicated in individuals who have shown hypersensitivity to any of its components or xanthine derivatives.

Warnings: Excessive theophylline doses may be associated with toxicity; serum theophylline levels should be monitored to assure maximum benefit with minimum risk. Incidence of toxicity increases at serum levels greater than 20 mcg/ml. High blood levels of theophylline resulting from conventional doses are correlated with clinical manifestations of toxicity in patients with lowered body plasma clearances, patients with liver dysfunction or chronic obstructive lung disease, and patients who are older than 55 years of age—particularly males. There are often no early signs of less serious theophylline toxicity such as nausea and restlessness, which may be the first signs of toxicity. Many patients who have higher theophylline serum levels exhibit a tachycardia. Theophylline products may worsen pre-existing arrhythmias.

Usage in Pregnancy: Safe use in pregnancy has not been established relative to possible adverse effects on fetal development, but neither have adverse effects on fetal development been established. This is, unfortunately, true for most anti-asthmatic medications. Therefore, use of theophylline in pregnant women should be balanced against the risk of uncontrolled asthma.

Precautions: SUSTAIRE TABLETS SHOULD NOT BE CHEWED OR CRUSHED.

Theophylline should not be administered concurrently with other xanthine medications. It should be used with caution in patients with severe cardiac disease, severe hypoxemia, hypertension, hyperthyroidism, acute myocardial injury, cor pulmonale, congestive heart failure, liver disease, in the elderly (particularly males), and in neonates. Great caution should be used in giving theophylline to patients in congestive heart failure since these patients show markedly prolonged theophylline blood level curves. Use theophylline cautiously in patients with history of peptic ulcer. Theophylline may occasionally act as a local irritant to the G.I. tract although gastrointestinal symptoms are more commonly central and associated with high serum concentrations above 20 mcg/ml.

Adverse Reactions: The most consistent adverse reactions are usually due to overdose and are:

Gastrointestinal: nausea, vomiting, epigastric pain, hematemesis, diarrhea.

Central Nervous System: headaches, irritability, restlessness, insomnia, reflex hyperexcitability, muscle twitching, clonic and tonic generalized convulsions.

Cardiovascular: palpitation, tachycardia, extrasystoles, flushing, hypotension, circulatory failure, life threatening ventricular arrhythmias.

Respiratory: tachypnea

Renal: albuminuria, increased excretion of renal tubular cells and red blood cells; potentiation of diuresis.

Others: hyperglycemia and inappropriate ADH syndrome.

Drug Interactions:

Drug	Effect
Theophylline with Furosemide	Increased diuresis
Theophylline with Hexamethonium	Decreased chronotropic effect
Theophylline with Reserpine	Tachycardia
Theophylline with Cyclamycin, TAO® (troleandomycin) Erythromycin or Lincomycin	Increased theophylline blood levels

Overdosage:

Management

A. If potential oral overdose is established and seizure has not occurred:
1) Induce vomiting.
2) Administer a cathartic. (This is particularly important if sustained release preparations have been taken.)
3) Administer activated charcoal.

B. Patient is having a seizure:
1) Establish an airway.
2) Administer O_2
3) Treat the seizure with intravenous diazepam: 0.1 to 0.3 mg/kg up to 10 mg.
4) Monitor vital signs. Maintain blood pressure and provide adequate hydration.

C. Post Seizure Coma:
1) Maintain airway and oxygenation.
2) If a result of oral medication, follow above recommendations to prevent absorption of drug; but intubation and lavage will have to be performed instead of inducing emesis, and the cathartic and charcoal will need to be introduced via a large bore gastric lavage tube.
3) Continue to provide full supportive care and adequate hydration while waiting for drug to be metabolized. In general, the drug is metabolized sufficiently rapidly so as to not warrant consideration of dialysis.

Dosage and Administration: Therapeutic serum levels associated with optimal likelihood for benefit and minimal risk of toxicity are considered to be between 10 and 20 mcg/ml. There is a great variation from patient to patient in dosage needed in order to achieve a therapeutic blood level due to variable rates of elimination. Because of this wide variation from patient to patient, and the relatively narrow therapeutic range, dosage must be individualized.

THE AVERAGE INITIAL CHILDREN'S (UNDER 9 YEARS OF AGE) DOSE IS ONE SUSTAIRE 100 mg TABLET q12h.

THE AVERAGE INITIAL CHILDREN'S (AGES 9–12) DOSE IS ONE HALF (150 mg) OF A SUSTAIRE 300 mg TABLET q12h.

THE AVERAGE INITIAL ADOLESCENT (AGES 12–16) DOSE IS TWO SUSTAIRE 100 mg TABLETS q12h.

THE AVERAGE INITIAL ADULT DOSE IS ONE SUSTAIRE 300 mg TABLET q12h.

If the desired response is not achieved with the above AVERAGE INITIAL DOSAGE recommendations and there are no adverse reactions, the dose may be safely increased by 2–3 mg/kg body weight per day at 3 day intervals until the following MAXIMUM DOSE WITHOUT MEASUREMENT OF SERUM CONCENTRATION or a maximum of 900 mg in any 24 hour period, whichever is less, is attained:

[See table above].

Maximum Dose Without Measurement Of Serum Concentration

	mg per kg body weight*	dose per interval
Children (under 9)	24 mg per day	12 mg q12h**
Children (9–12)	20 mg per day	10 mg q12h
Adolescents (12–16)	18 mg per day	9 mg q12h
Adults	13 mg per day	6.5 mg q12h

*Use ideal body weight for obese patients.
**Some children under 9 may require 8 mg q8h.

If doses higher than those contained in the above MAXIMUM DOSE WITHOUT MEASUREMENT OF SERUM CONCENTRATION are necessary, it is recommended that serum theophylline levels be monitored. Check serum theophylline levels between 3 and 8 hours after a dose. It is important that the patient will have missed *no* doses during the previous 72 hours and that dosing intervals will have been reasonably typical with *no* added doses during that period of time. DOSAGE ADJUSTMENT BASED ON SERUM THEOPHYLLINE MEASUREMENTS WHEN THESE INSTRUCTIONS HAVE NOT BEEN FOLLOWED, MAY RESULT IN RECOMMENDATIONS THAT PRESENT RISK OF TOXICITY TO THE PATIENT.

How Supplied: SUSTAIRE 100 mg and 300 mg Sustained Release Tablets are available in bottles of 100.

Storage Conditions: Keep tightly closed. Store at controlled room temperature 15–30° C (59–86° F).

[*Shown in Product Identification Section*]

TAO® ℞

(troleandomycin)

Capsules and Oral Suspension

Description: TAO (troleandomycin) is a synthetically derived acetylated ester of oleandomycin, an antibiotic elaborated by a species of *Streptomyces antibioticus*. It is a white crystalline compound, insoluble in water, but readily soluble and stable in the presence of gastric juice. The compound has a molecular weight of 814 and corresponds to the empirical formula $C_{41}H_{67}NO_{15}$.

Actions: TAO is an antibiotic shown to be active *in vitro* against the following gram-positive organisms:

Streptococcus pyogenes

Diplococcus pneumoniae

Susceptibility plate testing: If the Kirby-Bauer method of disc sensitivity is used, a 15 mcg. oleandomycin disc should give a zone of over 18 mm. when tested against a troleandomycin sensitive bacterial strain.

Indications:

Diplococcus pneumoniae

Pneumococcal pneumonia due to susceptible strains.

Streptococcus pyogenes

Group A beta-hemolytic streptococcal infections of the upper respiratory tract.

Injectable benzathine penicillin G is considered by the American Heart Association to be the drug of choice in the treatment and prevention of streptococcal pharyngitis and in long term prophylaxis of rheumatic fever.

Troleandomycin is generally effective in the eradication of streptococci from the nasopharynx. However, substantial data establishing the efficacy of TAO in the subsequent prevention of rheumatic fever are not available at present.

Contraindications: Troleandomycin is contraindicated in patients with known hypersensitivity to this antibiotic.

Continued on next page

Roerig—Cont.

Warnings: Usage in Pregnancy: Safety for use in pregnancy has not been established.
The administration of troleandomycin has been associated with an allergic type of cholestatic hepatitis. Some patients receiving troleandomycin for more than two weeks or in repeated courses have shown jaundice accompanied by right upper quadrant pain, fever, nausea, vomiting, eosinophilia, and leukocytosis. The changes have been reversible on discontinuance of the drug. Liver function tests should be monitored in patients on such dosage, and the drug discontinued if abnormalities develop. Reports in the literature have suggested that the concurrent use of ergotamine-containing drugs and troleandomycin may induce ischemic reactions. Therefore, the concurrent use of ergotamine-containing drugs and troleandomycin should be avoided.
Studies in chronic asthmatic patients have suggested that the concurrent use of theophylline and troleandomycin may result in elevated serum concentrations of theophylline. Therefore, it is recommended that patients receiving such concurrent therapy be observed for signs of theophylline toxicity, and that therapy be appropriately modified if such signs develop.
Precautions: Troleandomycin is principally excreted by the liver.
Caution should be exercised in administering the antibiotic to patients with impaired hepatic function.
Adverse Reactions: The most frequent side effects of troleandomycin preparations are gastrointestinal, such as abdominal cramping and discomfort, and are dose related. Nausea, vomiting, and diarrhea occur infrequently with usual oral doses.
During prolonged or repeated therapy, there is a possibility of overgrowth of nonsusceptible bacteria or fungi. If such infections occur, the drug should be discontinued and appropriate therapy instituted.
Mild allergic reactions such as urticaria and other skin rashes have occurred. Serious allergic reactions, including anaphylaxis, have been reported.
Dosage and Administration: Clinical judgment based on the type of infection and its severity should determine dosage within the below listed ranges.
Adults: 250 to 500 mg. 4 times a day
Children: 125 to 250 mg. (3-5 mg./lb. or 6.6 to 11 mg./kg.) every 6 hours
When used in streptococcal infection, therapy should be continued for ten days.
How Supplied:
TAO is supplied as:
Capsules 250 mg.: Each capsule contains troleandomycin equivalent to 250 mg. of oleandomycin; bottle of 100 capsules.
Ready-Mixed Oral Suspension: Each teaspoonful (5 ml.) contains troleandomycin equivalent to 125 mg. of oleandomycin; 60 ml. bottle and pint bottle.
[*Shown in Product Identification Section*]

UROBIOTIC®-250 ℞

Each capsule contains
Oxytetracycline hydrochloride equivalent to 250 mg. oxytetracycline
Sulfamethizole ....250 mg.
Phenazopyridine hydrochloride ....50 mg.

CAPSULES

Actions: Urobiotic-250 is a product designed for use specifically in urinary tract infections. Terramycin (oxytetracycline HCl) is a widely used antibiotic with clinically proved activity against gram-positive and gram-negative bacteria, rickettsiae, spirochetes, large viruses, and certain protozoa. Terramycin is well tolerated and well absorbed after oral administration. It diffuses readily through the placenta and is present in the fetal circulation. It diffuses into the pleural fluid, and under some circumstances, into the cerebrospinal fluid. Oxytetracycline HCl appears to be concentrated in the hepatic system and is excreted in the bile. It is excreted in the urine and in the feces, in high concentrations, in a biologically active form.
Sulfamethizole is a chemotherapeutic agent active against a number of important gram-positive and gram-negative bacteria. This sulfonamide is well absorbed, has a low degree of acetylation, and is extremely soluble. Because of these features and its rapid renal excretion, sulfamethizole has a low order of toxicity and provides prompt and high concentrations of the active drug in the urinary tract.
Phenazopyridine is an orally absorbed agent which produces prompt and effective local analgesia and relief of urinary symptoms by virtue of its rapid excretion in the urinary tract. These effects are confined to the genitourinary system and are not accompanied by generalized sedation or narcosis.

Indications

Based on a review of this drug by the National Academy of Sciences-National Research Council and/or other information, FDA has classified the indications as follows:
"Lacking substantial evidence of effectiveness as a fixed combination":
Urobiotic-250 is indicated in the therapy of a number of genitourinary infections caused by susceptible organisms. These infections include the following: pyelonephritis, pyelitis, ureteritis, cystitis, prostatitis, and urethritis.
Since both Terramycin and sulfamethizole provide effective levels in blood, tissue, and urine, Urobiotic-250 provides a multiple antimicrobial approach at the site of infection. Both antibacterial components are active against the most common urinary pathogens, including *Escherichia coli, Pseudomonas aeruginosa, Aerobacter aerogenes, Streptococcus faecalis, Streptococcus hemolyticus, and Micrococcus pyogenes.* Urobiotic-250 is particularly useful in the treatment of infections caused by bacteria more sensitive to the combination than to either component alone. The combination is also of value in those cases with mixed infections, and in those instances where the causative organism is unknown pending laboratory isolation.
Final classification of the less than effective indications require further investigation. Clinical studies to substantiate the efficacy of Urobiotic-250 are ongoing. Completion of these ongoing studies will provide data for final classification of these indications.

Contraindications: This drug is contraindicated in individuals who have shown hypersensitivity to any of its components.
This drug, because of the sulfonamide component, should not be used in patients with a history of sulfonamide sensitivities, and in pregnant females at term.
Warnings: If renal impairment exists, even usual oral or parenteral doses may lead to excessive systemic accumulation of the drug and possible liver toxicity. Under such conditions, lower than usual doses are indicated and if therapy is prolonged, tetracycline serum level determinations may be advisable.
Oxytetracycline HCl, which is one of the ingredients of Urobiotic-250, may form a stable calcium complex in any bone-forming tissue with no serious harmful effects reported thus far in humans. However, use of oxytetracycline during tooth development (last trimester of pregnancy, neonatal period and early childhood) may cause discoloration of the teeth (yellow-grey-brownish). This effect occurs mostly during long term use of the drug but it also has been observed in usual short treatment courses.
Because of its sulfonamide content, this drug should be used only after critical appraisal in patients with liver damage, renal damage, urinary obstruction, or blood dyscrasias. Deaths have been reported from hypersensitivity reactions, agranulocytosis, aplastic anemia, and other blood dyscrasias associated with sulfonamide administration. When used intermittently, or for a prolonged period, blood counts and liver and kidney function tests should be performed.
Certain hypersensitive individuals may develop a photodynamic reaction precipitated by exposure to direct sunlight during the use of this drug. This reaction is usually of the photoallergic type which may also be produced by other tetracycline derivatives. Individuals with a history of photosensitivity reactions should be instructed to avoid exposure to direct sunlight while under treatment with this or other tetracycline drugs, and treatment should be discontinued at first evidence of skin discomfort.
NOTE: Reactions of a photoallergic nature are exceedingly rare with Terramycin (oxytetracycline HCl). Phototoxic reactions are not believed to occur with Terramycin.
Precautions: As with all antibiotic preparations, use of this drug may result in overgrowth of nonsusceptible organisms, including fungi. If superinfection occurs, the antibiotic should be discontinued and appropriate specific therapy should be instituted. This drug should be used with caution in persons having histories of significant allergies and/or asthma.
Adverse Reactions: Glossitis, stomatitis, proctitis, nausea, diarrhea, vaginitis, and dermatitis, as well as reactions of an allergic nature, may occur during oxytetracycline HCl therapy, but are rare. If adverse reactions, individual idiosyncrasy, or allergy occur, discontinue medication.
With oxytetracycline therapy bulging fontanels in infants and benign intracranial hypertension in adults have been reported in individuals receiving full therapeutic dosages. These conditions disappeared rapidly when the drug was discontinued.
As in all sulfonamide therapy, the following reactions may occur: nausea, vomiting, diarrhea, hepatitis, pancreatitis, blood dyscrasias, neuropathy, drug fever, skin rash, injection of the conjunctiva and sclera, petechiae, purpura, hematuria and crystalluria. The dosage should be decreased or the drug withdrawn, depending upon the severity of the reaction.
Dosage: Urobiotic-250 is recommended in adults only. A dose of 1 capsule four times daily is suggested. In refractory cases 2 capsules four times a day may be used.
Therapy should be continued for a minimum of seven days or until bacteriologic cure in acute urinary tract infections.
To aid absorption of the drug, it should be given at least one hour before or two hours after eating. Aluminum hydroxide gel given with antibiotics has been shown to decrease their absorption and is contraindicated.
Supply: Urobiotic-250 capsules: bottles of 50.
(23-1636-00-3)

Literature Available: Yes.
[*Shown in Product Identification Section*]

Products are cross-indexed by generic and chemical names in the

YELLOW SECTION

Roger Pharmacal, Inc.
P. O. BOX 011022
1654 N. W. 35th STREET
MIAMI, FLORIDA 33142

ETA-LENT ℞
T.D. Capsules
(ethaverine HCl.)
100 mg.

Description: Each capsule* contains:
Ethaverine HCl. ....100 mg.
* In a base to provide prolonged activity.
Action: ETA-LENT is Ethaverine Hydrochloride and acts directly on the smooth muscle cells, without involving the autonomic nervous system or its receptors. It produces smooth muscle relaxation, particularly where spasm exists, affecting the larger blood vessels, especially systemic, peripheral and pulmonary vessels, smooth muscle of the intestines, biliary tree and ureters.
Indications: In peripheral and cerebral vascular insufficiency associated with arterial spasm; also useful as a smooth muscle spasmolytic in spastic conditions of the gastrointestinal and genitourinary tracts.
Contraindications: The use of Ethaverine Hydrochloride is contraindicated in the presence of complete atrioventricular dissociation.
Precautions: As with all vasodilators, ETA-LENT, Ethaverine Hydrochloride should be administered with caution to patients with glaucoma. The safety of ethaverine hydrochloride during pregnancy or lactation has not been established; therefore it should not be used in pregnant women or in women of childbearing age unless, in the judgment of the physician, its use is deemed essential to the welfare of the patient.
Side Effects: Even though the incidence of side effects as reported in the literature is very low, it is possible for a patient to evidence nausea, anorexia, abdominal distress, dryness of the throat, hypotension, malaise, lassitude, drowsiness, flushing, sweating, vertigo, respiratory depression, cardiac depression, cardiac arrhythmia and headache. If these side effects occur, reduce dosage or discontinue medication.
Dosage and Administration: In mild or moderate disease, the usual dose for adults is one capsule three times a day: morning, midafternoon, evening. In more difficult cases, dosage may be increased to two capsules three times a day. It is most effective given early in the course of the vascular disorder. Because of the chronic nature of the disease, long-term therapy is required.
Caution: Federal law prohibits dispensing without prescription.
Supplied: ETA-LENT, Ethaverine Hydrochloride Capsules. Bottles of 50 and bottles of 500.
NDC 12026-119-50.

Important Notice

Before prescribing or administering

any product described in

PHYSICIANS' DESK REFERENCE

always consult the PDR Supplement for

possible new or revised information.

Rorer, Inc., William H.
500 VIRGINIA DRIVE
FORT WASHINGTON, PA 19034

ANANASE® ℞
(bromelains)
Anti-inflammatory enzyme

Description: Ananase (bromelains) is a concentrate of proteolytic enzymes derived from the pineapple plant. Each yellow, enteric coated tablet (Ananase-50) contains 50,000 Rorer Units*. Each orange, enteric coated tablet (Ananase-100) contains 100,000 Rorer Units*.
Actions: Ananase as adjunctive therapy is designed to supplement and augment standard therapeutic procedures for reduction of inflammation and edema, to ease pain, speed healing and accelerate tissue repair. This is the basic purpose of proteolytic enzyme therapy in general.
While the mode of action of proteolytic enzymes has not been finally established, it seems most probable that depolymerization of fibrin and permeability modifications of venules and lymphatics underlie the action.

Indications: Based on a review of this drug by the National Academy of Sciences—National Research Council and/or other information, FDA has classified the indications as follows:
"Possibly effective" for relieving symptomatology related to episiotomy.
"Lacking substantial evidence of effectiveness" for reduction of inflammation and edema in postoperative tissue reactions and in accidental trauma.
Final classification of the less-than-effective indications requires further investigation.

Contraindications: Contraindicated in patients known to be hypersensitive to the drug or to pineapple or its products.
Warnings: USE IN PREGNANCY—Safe use of this drug in pregnancy has not been established.
Due to limited clinical experience, the use of this drug in children 12 years of age and under is not recommended.
Precautions: Ananase should be used with caution in patients with abnormalities of the blood clotting mechanism, such as hemophilia, or with severe hepatic or renal disease. Patients on anticoagulant therapy should be observed carefully because of possible potentiation of the anticoagulant effect by Ananase.
Adverse Reactions: While seldom observed, sensitivity manifested by urticaria or skin rash has occurred. There has been no report of anaphylactoid reaction. One case of hypofibrinogenemia and several cases of menorrhagia and metrorrhagia possibly related to the drug have been reported. Nausea, vomiting or diarrhea have rarely been reported. Adverse reactions are usually reversible upon discontinuation of the drug.
Dosage and Administration:
Usual adult dose: Initially, 100,000 units four times daily. For maintenance, 100,000 units twice daily, or 50,000 units four times daily.
How Supplied: Ananase®-50 (bromelains) is available as yellow tablets of 50,000 Rorer units in bottles of 100 and 500 tablets.
Ananase®-100 (bromelains) is available as orange tablets of 100,000 Rorer units in bottles of 100 and 500 tablets.

* One Rorer Unit of protease activity is defined as that amount of enzyme which will so hydrolyze a standardized casein substrate at pH 7.0 and 25°C as to cause an increase in absorbance at 280 mu of 1 x 10^{-5} per minute of reaction time.
[*Shown in Product Identification Section*]

ASCRIPTIN®
aspirin-Maalox® for relief of pain and inflammation

Formula: Each tablet contains Aspirin (5 grains) 325 mg.; Maalox® (magnesium-aluminum hydroxide) 150 mg.
Description: Ascriptin is an excellent analgesic, antipyretic and anti-inflammatory agent for general use, particularly where there is concern over aspirin-induced gastric distress. When large doses are used, as in arthritis and rheumatic disorders, gastric discomfort is rare.
Indications: As an analgesic for the relief of pain in such conditions as headache, neuralgia, minor injuries and dysmenorrhea. As an analgesic and antipyretic in colds and influenza. As an analgesic and anti-inflammatory agent in arthritis and other rheumatic diseases.
Usual Adult Dose: Two or three tablets, four times daily. For children under 12—at the discretion of the physician.
Supplied: Bottles of 50 and 100 tablets with child-resistant caps. Bottles of 500 tablets. Military Stock #NSN 6505-00-135-2783. V.A. Stock #6505-00-890-1979A [bottles of 500].
[*Shown in Product Identification Section*]

ASCRIPTIN® A/D
Arthritic Doses
Analgesic and antiarthritic
with added Maalox® for increased buffering in Arthritic Doses

Formula: Each capsule shaped tablet contains:
Aspirin ....(5 grains) 325 mg.
Maalox® (magnesium-aluminum hydroxide) ....300 mg.
Description: Ascription® A/D is a highly buffered analgesic, anti-inflammatory and antipyretic agent for use in the treatment of rheumatoid arthritis, osteoarthritis and other arthritic conditions. It is formulated with added Maalox® to provide increased neutralization of gastric acid thus improving the likelihood of GI tolerance when large anti-arthritic doses of aspirin are used.
Indications: As an analgesic, anti-inflammatory and antipyretic agent in rheumatoid arthritis, osteoarthritis and other arthritic conditions.
Usual Adult Dose: Two or three tablets, four times daily, or as directed by the physician for arthritis therapy. For children under twelve, at the discretion of the physician.
Drug Interaction Precaution: Do not use if patient is taking a tetracycline antibiotic.
Supplied: Available in bottles of 100 tablets with child-resistant caps and in special bottles of 500 tablets (without child-resistant closures) for arthritic patients.
[*Shown in Product Identification Section*]

ASCRIPTIN® WITH CODEINE Ⓒ ℞
For severe pain

Formula:
No. 2 Tablet: Each white tablet is marked on one side with the name Rorer and the identification number 132. The other side displays the number 2 which indicates the following contents:
Codeine Phosphate *(warning: may be habit forming)*....................................(¼ grain) 16.2 mg.
Aspirin ....(5 grains) 325 mg.
Maalox® (magnesium-aluminum hydroxide)....................................150 mg.
No. 3 Tablet: Each white tablet is marked on one side with the name Rorer and the identification number 133. The other side displays the

Continued on next page

Rorer—Cont.

number 3 which indicates the following contents:
Codeine Phosphate *(warning: may be habit forming)*................................(½ grain) 32.4 mg.
Aspirin ....(5 grains) 325 mg.
Maalox® (magnesium-aluminum hydroxide)..150 mg.
Description: Ascriptin®, an excellent analgesic, antipyretic and anti-inflammatory, combined with codeine to give effective relief from severe pain with minimal aspirin-induced gastric distress.
Indication: As an analgesic for the relief of pain of all degrees of severity up to that which requires morphine.
Side Effects: Side effects are rare. Nausea, constipation and drowsiness may occur.
Usual Adult Dose: Ascriptin® with Codeine No. 2 (¼ grain): Two tablets every three or four hours when necessary. Ascriptin® with Codeine No. 3 (½ grain): One or two tablets every three or four hours when necessary.
How Supplied: Bottles of 100 tablets. Prescription only. DEA number required.
[*Ascriptin® with Codeine No. 2 Tablets and Ascriptin® with Codeine No. 3 Tablets shown in Product Identification Section.*]

CAMALOX®
High-potency antacid

Description: Camalox® Suspension is a carefully balanced formulation of 200 mg. magnesium hydroxide, 225 mg. aluminum hydroxide and 250 mg. calcium carbonate per teaspoonful (5 ml). This combination of ingredients produces an antacid capability that exceeds that of other leading ethical products in terms of quantity of acid neutralized as well as the speed and duration of antacid activity as measured by laboratory tests. The formulation also minimizes the possibilities of both constipation and diarrhea. Camalox is prepared by a unique process*. This process enhances its texture and vanilla-mint flavor, making it especially palatable even for patients who must take antacids for extended periods.
Camalox® Tablets contain 200 mg. magnesium hydroxide, 225 mg. aluminum hydroxide and 250 mg. calcium carbonate per tablet and have a delicate vanilla-mint flavor. They compare favorably with Camalox Suspension in terms of potency, as well as speed and duration of antacid activity, thus, Camalox Tablets overcome the usual deficiencies of antacid tablets. As measured by the *in vitro* test for acid neutralizing capacity, Camalox Tablets exceed the antacid capabilities of the leading ethical antacid suspensions as well as tablets. In addition, the special manufacturing process* developed by Rorer contributes importantly to the flavor and to the texture of the tablets. Patients can take Camalox Tablets in full dosage day after day without tiring of the taste.
Acid Neutralizing Capacity
Camalox Suspension—36.0 mEq/2 teaspoonfuls
Camalox Tablets—36.0 mEq/2 tablets
Sodium Content
Camalox Suspension—2.5 mg/5 ml
Camalox Tablets—1.5 mg/tablet
Indications: A high potency antacid for the symptomatic relief of hyperacidity associated with the diagnosis of peptic ulcer, gastritis, peptic esophagitis, gastric hyperacidity, heartburn or hiatal hernia.
Directions for Use: Camalox Suspension—two to four teaspoonfuls, four times a day, taken one-half hour after meals and at bedtime, or as directed by a physician.
Camalox Tablets—each Camalox Tablet is equivalent to one teaspoonful of Camalox Suspension. Two to four tablets, well-chewed, one-half to one hour after meals and at bedtime, or as directed by a physician.
Patient Warnings: Do not take more than 16 teaspoonfuls or tablets in a 24-hour period or use the maximum dosage for more than two weeks or use if you have kidney disease except under the advice and supervision of a physician. Keep this and all drugs out of the reach of children.
DRUG INTERACTION PRECAUTION: Do not use with patients taking a prescription antibiotic drug containing any form of tetracycline.
How Supplied: Camalox Suspension—white liquid in convenient 12 fluid ounce (355 ml.) plastic bottles and economical 16 fluid ounce (473 ml.) bottles.
Camalox Tablets—Bottles of 50 tablets and boxes of 100 tablets (in foil strips).
Rationale: Recent studies reveal that clinical symptoms of gastroesophageal reflux correlate with lower esophageal sphincter (LES) incompetency. Although the mechanism of action is unknown, gastric alkalinization has been shown to increase LES pressure.
Camalox is an ideal antacid for the treatment of reflux esophagitis. The balanced formulation of Camalox exerts its neutralizing effect faster and longer than the leading ethical antacids providing prompt symptomatic relief.
Camalox has been shown to produce significant increases in LES pressure providing a physiological barrier against reflux.**
Because Camalox is a high potency antacid with excellent acid neutralizing capacity, fewer and smaller doses are possible.
The refreshing vanilla-mint flavor and smooth texture of Camalox have earned a high level of patient acceptance and wearability. Available in equally effective dosage forms . . . physician-preferred suspension and convenient tablets.

*Patent No. 3,843,778
**Higgs, R.H., Smyth, R.D., and Castell, D.O., Gastric Alkalinization—Effect on Lower-Esophageal-Sphincter Pressure and Serum Gastrin, N. Engl. J. Med. *291*:486-490, 1974.
[*Camalox Tablets shown in Product Identification Section*]

CHARDONNA®-2 Ⓒ ℞
brand of belladonna extract with phenobarbital

REFORMULATED WITHOUT CHARCOAL

Description: Each Chardonna-2 tablet contains: phenobarbital 15 mg. (WARNING: may be habit forming) and belladonna extract 15 mg.
Actions: Chardonna-2 tablets produce antispasmodic, antisecretory and sedative effects. Belladonna acts to inhibit gastric secretion and gastrointestinal motility. The sedative action of phenobarbital allays anxiety accompanying functional gastrointestinal disorders.

Indications: Based on a review of similar drugs by the National Academy of Sciences-National Research Council and/or other information, FDA has classified the indications as follows:
"Possibly effective" as adjunctive therapy in the treatment of peptic ulcer and "possibly effective" in the treatment of irritable bowel syndrome (irritable colon, spastic colon, mucous colitis) and acute enterocolitis.
Final classification of less-than-effective indications requires further investigation.

Contraindications: Chardonna-2 is contraindicated in persons with a known intolerance to any of the ingredients, a history of porphyria or marked impairment of hepatic or renal function, respiratory disease in the presence of dyspnea or obstruction, glaucoma or obstructive uropathy.
Precautions: Use with caution in patients with increased intraocular pressure, prostatic hypertrophy or moderate hepatic or renal disease. Barbiturates are known to stimulate hepatic microsomal enzymes and alter metabolism of certain drugs. Therefore, Chardonna-2 should be used with caution in patients on anticoagulant or corticosteroid therapy. Elderly or debilitated persons may react to barbiturates with marked excitement or depression. Patients should also be warned about the combined effects of central nervous system depressant drugs and alcohol.
Adverse Reactions: Blurred vision, dry mouth, vertigo, tachycardia, urinary retention, flushing or dryness of the skin, drowsiness, lethargy, headache, skin eruptions, nausea and vomiting.
Adult Dosage: Usually given one-half hour before meals and at bedtime. One or two tablets, q.i.d.
How Supplied: Tablets (monogrammed "WHR") — bottles of 100. Prescription only. DEA number required.
[*Shown in Product Identification Section*]

EMETROL®
For nausea and vomiting

Description: Emetrol is an oral solution containing balanced amounts of levulose (fructose) and dextrose (glucose) and orthophosphoric acid with controlled hydrogen ion concentration. Pleasantly mint flavored.
Action: Emetrol quickly relieves nausea and vomiting by local action on the wall of the hyperactive G.I. tract. It reduces smooth-muscle contraction in direct proportion to the amount used. Unlike systemic antiemetics, Emetrol works almost immediately to control both nausea and active vomiting—and it is free from toxicity or side effects.
Indications: For nausea and vomiting.
Advantages:
1. ***Fast action***—works almost immediately by local action on contact with the hyperactive G. I. tract.
2. ***Effectiveness***—reported completely effective in epidemic vomiting—reduces smooth-muscle contractions in direct proportion to the amount used—stops both nausea and active vomiting.
3. ***Safety***—no toxicity or side effects—won't mask symptoms of organic pathology.
4. ***Convenience***—can be recommended over the phone for any member of the family, even the children—no Rx required.
5. ***Patient acceptance***—a low cost that patients appreciate—a pleasant mint flavor that both children and adults like.

Usual dose: *Epidemic and other functional vomiting (intestinal "flu", G.I. grippe, etc.); or nausea and vomiting due to psychogenic factors:* Infants and children, one or two teaspoonfuls at 15 minute intervals until vomiting ceases; adults, one or two tablespoonfuls in same manner. If first dose is rejected, resume dosage schedule in five minutes. *Regurgitation in infants:* One or two teaspoonfuls ten or fifteen minutes before each feeding; in refractory cases, two or three teaspoonfuls one-half hour before feedings. *"Morning sickness":* One or two tablespoonfuls on arising, repeated every three hours or whenever nausea threatens.
Emetrol may also be used in motion sickness and in nausea and vomiting due to drug therapy or inhalation anesthesia; in teaspoonful dosage for young children, tablespoonful dosage for older children and adults.
Important: *DO NOT DILUTE or permit oral fluids immediately before or for at least 15 minutes after dose.*
Supplied: Bottles of 3 fluid ounces (89 ml.) and 1 pint (473 ml.).

FERMALOX®

Hematinic

Formula: Each *uncoated* tablet contains: Ferrous Sulfate 200 mg.; Maalox® (magnesium-aluminum hydroxide) 200 mg.

Advantages: "A less irritating, more easily tolerated medicinal iron compound (Fermalox) fills an important need in the treatment of iron-deficiency states. The demonstration of effective absorption by means of the radioactive iron tracer, plus thousands of clinical cases showing satisfactory rise of hemoglobin level, fully establishes the efficacy of this medicament. In addition, the almost complete absence of the common adverse reactions to ordinary iron medicaments enables the physician to continue use of the drug until a satisfactory therapeutic result is obtained."[1]

Indications: For use as a hematinic in iron-deficiency conditions as may occur with: rapid growth, pregnancy, blood loss, menorrhagia, post-surgical convalescence, pathologic bleeding.

Usual Adult Dose: Two tablets daily; in mild cases dosage may be reduced to one tablet daily.

Supplied: Bottles of 100 tablets with child-resistant caps.

1. *Price, A.H., Erf, L., and Bierly, J.:* **J.A.M.A. 167***:1612 (July 26), 1958.*

[*Shown in Product Identification Section*]

MAALOX®

Antacid

A Balanced Formulation of Magnesium and Aluminum Hydroxides

Description: Maalox Suspension is a balanced combination of magnesium and aluminum hydroxides... first in order of preference for all routine purposes of antacid medication. The high neutralizing power of magnesium hydroxide and the established acid binding capacity of aluminum hydroxide support the reputation of Maalox for reliable antacid action.

MAALOX® No. 1 TABLETS—CHEW OR SWALLOW—200 mg. magnesium hydroxide, 200 mg. aluminum hydroxide.

MAALOX® No. 2 TABLETS—CHEW TABLETS—400 mg. magnesium hydroxide, 400 mg. aluminum hydroxide.

Acid Neutralizing Capacity

Maalox® Suspension—27 mEq/2 teaspoonfuls

Maalox No. 1 Tablets—17 mEq/2 tablets

Maalox No. 2 Tablets—18 mEq/tablet

Sodium Content

Maalox® Suspension—2.5 mg./tsp. (5 ml.) or 0.11 mEq (5 ml.)

Maalox No. 1 Tablets—0.84 mg./tablet or 0.036 mEq/tablet

Maalox No. 2 Tablets—1.80 mg./tablet or 0.078 mEq/tablet

Indications: As an antacid for symptomatic relief of hyperacidity associated with the diagnosis of peptic ulcer, gastritis, peptic esophagitis, gastric hyperacidity, heartburn or hiatal hernia.

Advantages: Many patients prefer Maalox whether they are taking it for occasional heartburn or routinely on an ulcer therapy regimen. Once started on Maalox, patients tend to stay on Maalox because it tastes good, it's effective and it will not cause constipation... three important reasons for Maalox when prolonged therapy is necessary.

Directions for use:

MAALOX® SUSPENSION: Two to four teaspoonfuls, four times a day, taken twenty minutes to one hour after meals and at bedtime, or as directed by a physician.

MAALOX NO. 1 TABLETS: Two to four tablets, well chewed or swallowed with water or milk, twenty minutes to one hour after meals and at bedtime, or as directed by a physician.

MAALOX NO. 2 TABLETS: One or two tablets, well chewed, twenty minutes to one hour after meals and at bedtime, or as directed by a physician. May be followed with milk or water.

Patient Warnings:

Do not take more than 16 teaspoonfuls of Maalox Suspension, 16 Maalox No. 1 Tablets or 8 Maalox No. 2 Tablets in a 24-hour period or use the maximum dosage for more than 2 weeks or use if you have kidney disease, except under the supervision of a physician.

Drug Interaction Precaution: Do not use with patients taking a prescription antibiotic drug containing any form of tetracycline.

Keep this and all drugs out of the reach of children.

Supplied:

MAALOX SUSPENSION is available in bottles of 12 fluid ounces (355 ml.), plastic bottles of 5 fluid ounces (148 ml.) and 26 fluid ounces (769 ml.).

Military Stock #NSN 6505-00-680-0133; V.A. Stock #6505-00-074-0993A [bottles of 6 fluid ounces (177 ml.)].

MAALOX NO. 1 TABLETS (400 mg.) are available in bottles of 100 tablets.

MAALOX NO. 2 TABLETS (800 mg.) available in bottles of 50 and 250 tablets. Also available in boxes of 24 and 100 tablets in easy-to-carry strips.

V.A. Stock #6505-00-993-3507A [boxes of 100 tablets (in cellophane strips)].

[*Maalox No. 1 Tablets and Maalox No. 2 Tablets shown in Product Identification Section*]

MAALOX® PLUS

Antacid-Antiflatulent

☐ **Lemon swiss creme flavor... the taste preferred by physician and patient.**

☐ **Physician-proven Maalox® formula for antacid effectiveness.**

☐ **Simethicone, at a recognized clinical dose, for antiflatulent action.**

Description: Maalox® Plus, a balanced combination of magnesium and aluminum hydroxides plus simethicone, is a non-constipating, lemon-flavored, antacid-antiflatulent.

Composition: To provide symptomatic relief of hyperacidity plus alleviation of gas symptoms, each teaspoonful/tablet contains:

Active Ingredients	Maalox Plus Per Tsp. (5 ml.)	Maalox Plus Per Tablet
Magnesium Hydroxide	200 mg.	200 mg.
Aluminum Hydroxide	225 mg.	200 mg.
Simethicone	25 mg.	25 mg.

To aid in establishing proper dosage schedules, the additional information is provided:

	Minimum Recommended Dosage: Per 2 Tsp. (10 ml.)	Minimum Recommended Dosage: Per 2 Tablets
Acid neutralizing capacity	27 mEq	17 mEq
Sodium content	5.0 mg.	2.8 mg.
Sugar content	None	1.1 gm.
Lactose content	None	None

Indications: As an antacid for symptomatic relief of hyperacidity associated with the diagnosis of peptic ulcer, gastritis, peptic esophagitis, gastric hyperacidity, heartburn or hiatal hernia. As an antiflatulent to alleviate the symptoms of gas, including postoperative gas pain.

Advantages: Among antacids, Maalox Plus is uniquely palatable—an important feature which encourages patients to follow your dosage directions. Maalox Plus has the time proven, nonconstipating, low sodium Maalox formula—useful for those patients suffering from the problems associated with hyperacidity. Additionally, Maalox Plus contains simethicone to alleviate discomfort associated with entrapped gas.

Directions for Use:

MAALOX® PLUS SUSPENSION: Two to four teaspoonfuls, four times a day, taken twenty minutes to one hour after meals and at bedtime, or as directed by a physician.

MAALOX® PLUS TABLETS: Two to four tablets, well chewed, four times a day, taken twenty minutes to one hour after meals and at bedtime, or as directed by a physician.

Patient Warnings: Do not take more than 16 teaspoonfuls or 16 tablets in a 24-hour period or use the maximum dosage for more than two weeks or use if you have kidney disease except under the advice and supervision of a physician.

Drug Interaction Precaution: Do not use with patients taking a prescription antibiotic containing any form of tetracycline. As with all aluminum-containing antacids, Maalox Plus may prevent the proper absorption of the tetracycline.

Keep this and all drugs out of the reach of children.

Supplied:

MAALOX PLUS SUSPENSION is available in a 12 fluid ounce (355 ml.) bottle.

MAALOX PLUS TABLETS are available in bottles of 50 tablets and boxes of 100 tablets in handy portable strips and convenience packs of 12 tablets.

[*Maalox® Plus Tablets shown in Product Identification Section*]

MAALOX® THERAPEUTIC CONCENTRATE

Descriptions and Actions: Maalox® Therapeutic Concentrate is a potent, concentrated, balanced formulation of 300 mg. magnesium hydroxide and 600 mg. aluminum hydroxide per teaspoonful (5 ml.). This formulation produces a therapeutic concentrated antacid that exceeds standard antacids in acid neutralizing capacity and acid consuming capacity.

Maalox® Therapeutic Concentrate is formulated to reduce the need to alter therapy due to treatment induced changes in bowel habits. Palatability is enhanced by a pleasant-tasting peppermint flavor.

Acid Neutralizing Capacity	28.3 mEq/5 ml
Acid Consuming Capacity	49.2/ml*
Sodium Content:	
mg Na/ml	.25
mg Na/mEq ANC	.044

*(ml N/10 HCl/gm)

Indications: Maalox® Therapeutic Concentrate antacid is indicated for the symptomatic relief of hyperacidity associated with the diagnosis of peptic ulcer and other gastrointestinal conditions where a high degree of acid neutralization is desired.

Directions for Use: One or two teaspoonfuls as needed between meals and at bedtime or as directed by a physician. Higher dosage regimens may be employed under the direct super-

Continued on next page

Rorer—Cont.

vision of a physician in the treatment of active peptic ulcer disease.

Patient Warnings

Warning: Do not take more than 8 teaspoonfuls in a 24-hour period, or use the maximum dosage of this product for more than two weeks or use if you have kidney disease except under the advice and supervision of a physician.

Drug Interaction Precaution: Do not take this product if you are presently taking a prescription antibiotic drug containing any form of tetracycline.

In case of accidental overdose, seek professional assistance or contact a poison control center immediately.

How Supplied: Maalox® Therapeutic Concentrate is available in bottles of 12 fluid ounces (355 ml.).

PAREPECTOLIN® Ⓒ
Antidiarrheal

Contains opium ($\frac{1}{4}$ grain) 15 mg. per fluid ounce. *(Warning: may be habit forming.)*

Formula: Each fluid ounce of creamy white suspension contains:

Paregoric (equivalent)........(1 fl. dram) 3.7 ml.
Pectin..................................($2\frac{1}{2}$ grains) 162 mg.
Kaolin ....(85 grains) 5.5 Gm.
(Alcohol 0.69%).

Indications: For symptomatic relief of diarrhea.

Action: The kaolin adsorbs irritants and forms a protective coating on intestinal mucosa. Pectin acts to consolidate the stool. Paregoric is very useful in diarrhea because it has a soothing action and allays griping pains.

Advantages: Because Parepectolin contains paregoric (equivalent), it effectively controls both diarrhea and colicky cramps. It is a stable suspension that tastes good.

Usual Adult Dose: One or two tablespoonfuls after each loose bowel movement for no more than four doses in twelve hours.

Usual Children's Dose: One or two teaspoonfuls after each loose bowel movement for no more than four doses in twelve hours.

Pediatric Dosage:

One year	$\frac{1}{2}$ teaspoonful
Three years	$1\frac{1}{2}$ teaspoonfuls
Six years	2 teaspoonfuls

after each loose bowel movement for no more than four doses in twelve hours.

Supplied: Bottles of 4 (118 ml.) and 8 (237 ml.) fluid ounces.

Ross Laboratories
COLUMBUS, OHIO 43216

ADVANCE®
Nutritional Beverage

Usage: Offers more appropriate nutrition than cow milk for the healthy, growing older baby.

Availability:

Concentrated Liquid; 13-fl-oz cans; 12 per case; No. 03313.

Ready To Feed; 32-fl-oz cans; 6 per case; No. 03301.

Preparation: Standard 16 Cal/fl oz dilution is one part Concentrated Liquid to one part water. Ready To Feed requires no dilution. For hospital use, prebottled ADVANCE is available in the Ross Hospital Formula System.

Composition: Concentrated Liquid

Ingredients: Ⓤ Water, corn syrup, nonfat milk, soy oil, soy protein isolate, corn oil, calcium phosphate tribasic, mono- and diglycerides, soy lecithin, potassium citrate, ascorbic acid, magnesium chloride, carrageenan, ferrous sulfate, zinc sulfate, vitamin A palmitate, vitamin D_3 concentrate, niacinamide, calcium pantothenate, cupric sulfate, alpha-tocopheryl acetate, thiamine chloride hydrochloride, pyridoxine hydrochloride, riboflavin, folic acid and cyanocobalamin.

Approximate Analysis (wt/liter):	Concentrated	Standard Dilution*
Protein	40.0 g	20.0 g
Fat	54.0 g	27.0 g
Carbohydrate	110.0 g	55.0 g
Minerals (Ash)	7.6 g	3.8 g
Calcium	1.02 g	0.51 g
Phosphorus	0.78 g	0.39 g
Sodium (maximum)	0.60 g	0.30 g
Magnesium	128 mg	64 mg
Iron	24 mg	12 mg
Zinc	12 mg	6.0 mg
Copper	1.8 mg	0.9 mg
Iodine	0.12 mg	60 mcg
Water	843 g	920 g
Crude Fiber	0 g	
Calories per fl oz	32	16
Calories per 100 ml	108	54

Vitamins Per Liter (Standard Dilution*)

Vitamin A	2400	I.U.
Vitamin D	400	I.U.
Vitamin E	12	I.U.
Vitamin C	50	mg
Thiamine (Vitamin B_1)	0.75	mg
Riboflavin (Vitamin B_2)	0.90	mg
Niacin (mg equiv.)	10	
Vitamin B_6	0.60	mg
Pantothenic Acid	4.0	mg
Folic Acid	0.10	mg
Vitamin B_{12}	2.5	mcg

*Standard dilution is equal parts ADVANCE Concentrated Liquid and water.

The addition of iron to this beverage conforms to the recommendation of the Committee on Nutrition of the American Academy of Pediatrics.

Composition: Ready To Feed

Ingredients: Ⓤ Water, corn syrup, nonfat milk, soy oil, soy protein isolate, corn oil, calcium phosphate tribasic, mono- and diglycerides, soy lecithin, potassium citrate, ascorbic acid, magnesium chloride, carrageenan, ferrous sulfate, zinc sulfate, vitamin A palmitate, vitamin D_3 concentrate, niacinamide, calcium pantothenate, cupric sulfate, alpha-tocopheryl acetate, thiamine chloride hydrochloride, pyridoxine hydrochloride, riboflavin, folic acid and cyanocobalamin.

Approximate Analysis (wt/liter):

Protein	20.0	g
Fat	27.0	g
Carbohydrate	55.0	g
Minerals (ash)	3.8	g
Calcium	0.51	g
Phosphorus	0.39	g
Sodium (maximum)	0.30	g
Magnesium	64	mg
Iron	12	mg
Zinc	6.0	mg
Copper	0.9	mg
Iodine	60	mcg
Water	920	g
Crude Fiber	0	g
Calories per fl oz	16	
Calories per 100 ml	54	

Vitamins Per Liter:

Vitamin A	2400	I.U.
Vitamin D	400	I.U.
Vitamin E	12	I.U.
Vitamin C	50	mg
Thiamine (Vitamin B_1)	0.75	mg
Riboflavin (Vitamin B_2)	0.90	mg
Niacin (mg equiv.)	10	
Vitamin B_6	0.60	mg
Pantothenic Acid	4.0	mg
Folic Acid	0.10	mg
Vitamin B_{12}	2.5	mcg

The addition of iron to this beverage conforms to the recommendation of the Committee on Nutrition of the American Academy of Pediatrics.

ENSURE®
Liquid Nutrition

Usage: Ensure is a liquid food providing complete, balanced nutrition. Ensure can be used as a full liquid diet, liquid supplement or tube feeding. Ensure is useful whenever the patient's medical, surgical or psychological state precludes normal food intake and/or leads to inadequate nutrition.

Features:

Ensure is complete nutrition. Caloric density: 1.06 Calories per ml, 250 Calories per 8 fl oz, 1000 Calories per quart from a balanced distribution of protein, fat and carbohydrate (caloric distribution: protein, 14%; fat, 31.5%; carbohydrate, 54.5%). Two quarts (2000 Calories) of Ensure meet or surpass 100% of the daily U.S. RDAs for adults or children 4 or more years of age.

Ensure provides protein of high biologic value, a fat source (corn oil) easily digested and low in cholesterol, and a lactose free formulation. Ensure is appropriate for use as a low residue feeding, and has a low osmolality of 450 mOsm/kg water.

Dosage and Administration: Ensure does not require the addition of water for a standard 1 Cal/ml feeding. When used as a sole source of nutrition, the recommended average daily adult consumption is 2 quarts. Additional water, depending on needs of the individual, should be given with or after feedings. Under no circumstances should Ensure be given parenterally.

- Gavage (tube) feeding: Initially, administration of small amounts of a one to one mixture of Ensure and water is recommended until progressively larger amounts and less dilute concentrations can be tolerated. Following adaptation period, Ensure should be given undiluted to meet prescribed caloric intake.
- Oral feeding: Ensure may be used to provide total nutrition or with and between meals for added nutritional support.

Availability:

Ready To Use:

8-fl-oz bottles; 4 six-packs per case; Vanilla, No. 708.

8-fl-oz cans; 4 six-packs per case; Vanilla, No. 711; Chocolate, No.701; Black Walnut, No.703.

32-fl-oz cans; 6 per case; Vanilla, No. 733.

Ross Gavage Feeding Set:

For use with 8-fl-oz bottles; 24 sets per case; No. 61.

Composition:

INGREDIENTS: Ⓤ Water, corn syrup solids, sucrose, sodium and calcium caseinates, corn oil, soy protein isolate, potassium citrate, magnesium chloride, soy lecithin, calcium carbonate, potassium chloride, sodium hexametaphosphate, choline chloride, ascorbic acid, carrageenan, zinc sulfate, ferrous sulfate, alpha-tocopheryl acetate, niacinamide, manganous chloride, cupric sulfate, vitamin D_3 concentrate, vitamin A palmitate, calcium pantothenate, pyridoxine hydrochloride, riboflavin, thiamine chloride hydrochloride, phylloquinone, biotin, potassium iodide, folic acid and cyanocobalamin. Artificial flavoring added.

APPROXIMATE ANALYSIS (g/quart): Protein, 35.2; Fat, 35.2; Carbohydrate, 137.2; Ash, 5.6; Moisture, 798.0. Calories per ml, 1.06; Calories per quart, 1000.

[See table top next page].

ENSURE®
Vari-Flavors® Flavor Pacs

Usage: To help overcome the monotony frequently experienced by patients receiving full liquid diets and liquid supplements.

Vitamins/Minerals	Per Quart	Per 2000 Calories (2 quarts)	Percent U.S. RDA* (2 quarts)
Vitamin A	2500 I.U.	5000 I.U.	100
Vitamin D	200 I.U.	400 I.U.	100
Vitamin E	30 I.U.	60 I.U.	200
Vitamin K_1	0.95 mg	1.9 mg	**
Vitamin C	0.15 g	0.30 g	500
Folic Acid	0.20 mg	0.40 mg	100
Thiamine (Vitamin B_1)	1.5 mg	3.0 mg	200
Riboflavin (Vitamin B_2)	1.7 mg	3.4 mg	200
Vitamin B_6	2.0 mg	4.0 mg	200
Vitamin B_{12}	6.0 mcg	12 mcg	200
Niacin	20 mg	40 mg	200
Choline	0.50 g	1.0 g	**
Biotin	0.15 mg	0.30 mg	100
Pantothenic Acid	5.0 mg	10 mg	100
Sodium	0.70 g	1.4 g	**
Potassium	1.2 g	2.4 g	**
Chloride	1.0 g	2.0 g	**
Calcium	0.50 g	1.0 g	100
Phosphorus	0.50 g	1.0 g	100
Magnesium	0.20 g	0.40 g	100
Iodine	0.075mg	0.15 mg	100
Manganese	2.0 mg	4.0 mg	**
Copper	1.0 mg	2.0 mg	100
Zinc	15 mg	30 mg	200
Iron	9.0 mg	18 mg	100

* For adults and children 4 or more years of age.
**U.S. RDA not established.

Features:

- Five flavors (Pecan, Cherry, Lemon, Orange, Strawberry) offer patients variety and encourage acceptance of liquid diets and liquid supplements.
- Vari-Flavors Flavor Pacs may be added to and will mix readily with Ross Medical Nutritionals—Ensure®, Ensure® Plus, Ensure® Osmolite®, and Vital®.
- Flavor Pacs may be stored for use in the dietary department, at nursing stations, or by patient's bedside.

Availability:
One-gram packets; 24 per dispenser carton.

Pecan	#720
Cherry	#722
Lemon	#724
Orange	#726
Strawberry	#728

Instructions for Use: Tap Pac lightly to shake contents to bottom. Tear off top of packet. Pour contents into suitable dry serving container. Add 8 ounces Vanilla Ensure. Allow flavor to dissolve for a few seconds. Stir until flavor is mixed and serve.

Composition: Dextrose, artificial flavoring and coloring (Strawberry, Cherry, Orange). Dextrose and artificial coloring (Pecan). Dextrose, artificial flavoring, and FD & C Yellow #5 as coloring (Lemon).

When used as directed, Ensure Vari-Flavors contribute only trace amounts of nutrients. The addition of a single Vari-Flavors Pac (1 gram) to an 8-oz serving of Ensure Liquid Nutrition increases caloric density of the serving approximately 4 Calories.

The osmolality of Vanilla Ensure is 450 mOsm/kg of water. When a single Vari-Flavors Flavor Pac is mixed with an 8-oz serving of Ensure, the osmolality will be between 465–480 mOsm/kg of water, depending on the flavor being used.

ENSURE® PLUS
High Calorie Liquid Nutrition

Usage: Ensure Plus is a high calorie liquid food providing complete, balanced nutrition. Caloric density is 1500 Calories per liter, 50% greater than most other liquid feedings. Ensure Plus is intended for use when extra calories and correspondingly higher concentrations of protein and most other nutrients are needed to achieve a required calorie intake in a limited volume. When utilized to provide total nutrition, Ensure Plus can deliver the high-calorie intakes required by severely ill or traumatized patients who are nutritionally depleted, and who may not be able to tolerate large-volume intakes. As a dietary supplement, Ensure Plus can supply extra calories and protein for those patients unable or unwilling to consume adequate nutrition.

Features:
Ensure Plus is complete nutrition. Caloric density: 1.5 Calories per ml, 355 Calories per 8 fl oz, 1420 Calories per quart from a balanced distribution of protein, fat and carbohydrate (caloric distribution: protein, 14.7%; fat, 32.0%; carbohydrate, 53.3%). Vitamin/mineral levels in two quarts (2840 Calories) of Ensure Plus meet or surpass 100% of the U.S. RDAs for adults.

Ensure Plus provides sufficient protein (55 grams/liter) to meet the demands of severe illness. The fat source (corn oil) is easily digested and low in cholesterol, and Ensure Plus is a lactose free feeding. Osmolality (600 mOsm/kg water) is moderate, even though caloric density is 50% greater than standard liquid feedings.

Dosage and Administration: Ensure Plus is ready to use and does not require dilution with water. Additional water, depending on needs of the individual, should be given with or after feedings. Under no circumstances should Ensure Plus be given parenterally.

- **Gavage (tube) feeding:** When initiating Ensure Plus, administration of small amounts of a 1:1 mixture of Ensure Plus and water is recommended until progressively larger amounts and less dilute concentrations can be tolerated. After adaptation period, Ensure Plus should be given undiluted to meet prescribed caloric intake.
- **Oral feeding:** Ensure Plus may be used for total nutrition, or with and between meals for added nutritional support.

Availability: 8-fl-oz bottles; two 12 bottle trays per case; Vanilla, No. 741.
8-fl-oz cans; 4-six packs per case; Vanilla, No. 707; Chocolate, No. 702.

Composition:
INGREDIENTS: Ⓤ Water, corn syrup solids, sodium and calcium caseinates, corn oil, sucrose, soy protein isolate, potassium citrate, magnesium chloride, calcium carbonate, soy lecithin, sodium hexametaphosphate, potassium chloride, choline chloride, ascorbic acid, zinc sulfate, carrageenan, ferrous sulfate, alpha-tocopheryl acetate, niacinamide, manganous chloride, vitamin A palmitate, calcium pantothenate, cupric sulfate, pyridoxine hydrochloride, riboflavin, vitamin D_3 concentrate, thiamine chloride hydrochloride, phylloquinone, biotin, potassium iodide, folic acid and cyanocobalamin. Artificial flavoring added.

APPROXIMATE ANALYSIS (grams/8 fl oz): Protein, 13.0; fat, 12.6; carbohydrate, 47.3; ash, 2.5; moisture, 182.0. Calories per ml, 1.5; Calories per fl oz, 44.4.
[See table at left].

Vitamins/Minerals	Per 8 fl oz	Per Quart	Percent U.S. RDA* (1 Quart)
Vitamin A	625 I.U.	2500 I.U.	50
Vitamin D	50 I.U.	200 I.U.	50
Vitamin E	11.25 I.U.	45 I.U.	150
Vitamin K_1	0.38 mg	1.5 mg	**
Vitamin C	37.5 mg	150 mg	250
Folic Acid	50 mcg	200 mcg	50
Thiamine (Vitamin B_1)	0.63 mg	2.5 mg	165
Riboflavin (Vitamin B_2)	0.65 mg	2.6 mg	150
Vitamin B_6	0.75 mg	3.0 mg	150
Vitamin B_{12}	2.25 mcg	9.0 mcg	150
Niacin	7.5 mg	30 mg	150
Biotin	75 mcg	300 mcg	100
Choline	125 mg	500 mg	**
Pantothenic Acid	2.0 mg	8.0 mg	80
Sodium	0.25 g	1.0 g	**
Potassium	0.45 g	1.8 g	**
Chloride	0.38 g	1.5 g	**
Calcium	0.15 g	0.60 g	60
Phosphorus	0.15 g	0.60 g	60
Magnesium	75 mg	300 mg	75
Manganese	0.50 mg	2.0 mg	**
Iodine	25 mcg	100 mcg	65
Copper	0.38 mg	1.5 mg	75
Iron	3.38 mg	13.5 mg	75
Zinc	5.63 mg	22.5 mg	150

*For adults and children 4 or more years of age.
**U.S. RDA not established.

ISOMIL®
Soy Protein Formula

Usage: As a formula for infants and a beverage for children and adults with allergy or sensitivity to cow milk, and for use as a feeding in disorders where lactose should be avoided: lactose deficiency, lactose intolerance and galactosemia.

Continued on next page

Ross—Cont.

Availability:
Concentrated Liquid; 13-fl-oz cans; 24 per case; No. 02110.
Ready To Feed; (prediluted 20 Cal/fl oz): 32-fl-oz cans; 6 per case; No. 00230.
8-fl-oz cans; 4 six-packs per case; No. 00173.
For hospital use, prebottled ISOMIL is available in the Ross Hospital Formula System.
Preparation:
Concentrated Liquid—Standard 20 Cal/fl oz dilution is one part Concentrated Liquid to one part water.
Composition: Concentrated Liquid
Ingredients: Ⓤ 74% water, 7.3% corn syrup, 5.7% sucrose, 4.2% soy protein isolate, 4.0% coconut oil, 2.7% soy oil, 1.0% modified corn starch, 0.4% calcium phosphate tribasic, 0.19% potassium citrate, 0.14% potassium chloride, mono- and diglycerides, soy lecithin, L-methionine, ascorbic acid, magnesium chloride, carrageenan, sodium chloride, choline chloride, ferrous sulfate, alpha-tocopheryl acetate, zinc sulfate, niacinamide, calcium pantothenate, vitamin A palmitate, cupric sulfate, thiamine chloride hydrochloride, riboflavin, pyridoxine hydrochloride, potassium iodide, phylloquinone, biotin, folic acid, vitamin D_3 concentrate and cyanocobalamin.

Approximate Analysis (wt/liter):	Concentrated	Standard Dilution*
Protein	40.0 g	20.0 g
Fat	72.0 g	36.0 g
Carbohydrate	136.0 g	68.0 g
Minerals (Ash)	7.5 g	3.8 g
Calcium	1.4 g	0.70 g
Phosphorus	1.0 g	0.50 g
Sodium	0.60 g	0.30 g
Potassium	1.42 g	0.71 g
Chloride	1.06 g	0.53 g
Magnesium	0.10 g	50 mg
Iron	24 mg	12 mg
Zinc	10 mg	5.0 mg
Copper	1.0 mg	0.50 mg
Iodine	0.30 mg	0.15 mg
Manganese	0.40 mg	0.2 mg
Water	805.7 g	901.6 g
Crude Fiber	0 g	
Calories per fl oz	40	20
Calories per 100 ml	136	68

Vitamins Per Liter (Standard dilution*):	
Vitamin A	2500 I.U.
Vitamin D	400 I.U.
Vitamin E	15 I.U.
Vitamin C	55 mg
Thiamine (Vitamin B_1)	0.40 mg
Riboflavin (Vitamin B_2)	0.60 mg
Vitamin B_6	0.40 mg
Niacin (mg equiv.)	9.0
Folic acid	0.10 mg
Vitamin B_{12}	3.0 mcg
Pantothenic acid	5.0 mg
Biotin	0.15 mg
Vitamin K_1	0.15 mg

*Standard dilution is one part Isomil Concentrated Liquid to one part water.

Composition: Ready To Feed
Ingredients: Ⓤ 86.4% water, 4.1% corn syrup, 3.2% sucrose, 2.2% soy protein isolate, 2.1% coconut oil, 1.4% soy oil, 0.1% calcium phosphate dibasic, 0.1% potassium citrate, calcium carbonate, potassium chloride, calcium phosphate monobasic, soy lecithin, mono- and diglycerides, carrageenan, ascorbic acid, magnesium chloride, L-methionine, sodium chloride, choline chloride, ferrous sulfate, alpha-tocopheryl acetate, zinc sulfate, niacinamide, calcium pantothenate, vitamin A palmitate, cupric sulfate, riboflavin, thiamine chloride hydrochloride, pyridoxine hydrochloride, potassium iodide, phylloquinone, biotin, folic acid, vitamin D_3 concentrate and cyanocobalamin.

Approximate Analysis (wt/liter):	
Protein	20.0 g
Fat	36.0 g
Carbohydrate	68.0 g
Minerals (Ash)	3.8 g
Calcium	0.70 g
Phosphorus	0.50 g
Sodium	0.30 g
Potassium	0.71 g
Chloride	0.53 g
Magnesium	50 mg
Iron	12 mg
Zinc	5.0 mg
Copper	0.50 mg
Manganese	0.2 mg
Iodine	0.15 mg
Water	901.6 g
Crude Fiber	0 g
Calories per fl oz	20
Calories per 100 ml	68

Vitamins Per Liter:	
Vitamin A	2500 I.U.
Vitamin D	400 I.U.
Vitamin E	15 I.U.
Vitamin C	55 mg
Thiamine (Vitamin B_1)	0.40 mg
Riboflavin (Vitamin B_2)	0.60 mg
Vitamin B_6	0.40 mg
Niacin (mg equiv.)	9.0
Folic acid	0.10 mg
Vitamin B_{12}	3.0 mcg
Pantothenic acid	5.0 mg
Biotin	0.15 mg
Vitamin K_1	0.15 mg

The addition of iron to this formula conforms to the recommendation of the Committee on Nutrition of the American Academy of Pediatrics.

Ensure®
OSMOLITE®
Isotonic Liquid Nutrition

Usage: Osmolite is an isotonic liquid food providing complete, balanced nutrition. Osmolite has been designed for patients particularly sensitive to hyperosmotic feedings who may benefit from an isotonic liquid diet. Osmolite may be used both as an oral and gavage feeding. The mild, unflavored taste of Osmolite also makes this feeding especially appropriate for use with patients experiencing altered or heightened taste perceptions.

Features:

- Complete, balanced nutrition—1.06 Calories per ml, 250 Calories per 8-fl-oz feeding, 1000 Calories per quart from a balanced distribution of protein, fat, and carbohydrate (caloric distribution: protein, 14.0%; fat, 31.4%; carbohydrate, 54.6%). Two quarts (2000 Calories) of Osmolite meet or exceed 100% of the daily U.S. RDAs for adults or children 4 or more years of age.
- Isotonicity—The osmolality is 300 mOsm/kg water, equaling the osmotic pressure of blood plasma. Osmolite will not contribute to osmotically-induced diarrhea and is indicated when feeding problems suggest a sensitivity to hyperosmotic feedings. Isotonicity is achieved without compromising a balanced caloric contribution from energy supplying nutrients.
- Lactose free—Osmolite will not contribute to lactose-associated diarrhea. Polycose® Glucose Polymers is the carbohydrate source, which is a readily available and easily digested source of calories.
- Adequate protein—Protein of high biologic value provides a full complement of amino acids to meet the profile for high quality protein. The total calorie/nitrogen ratio of 178 indicates the effective protein-sparing ability and the effective utilization of available protein.
- Readily absorbed fats—Osmolite contains a high level of essential fatty acids, as well as medium-chain triglycerides as 15% of total calories (50% of fat calories) to facilitate rapid, effective absorption of fat calories. The level of fat is appropriate for dietary management of many long term, chronic care patients. Fat source is low in cholesterol.
- Low fecal residue—Fecal residue is comparable to fecal residue produced by elemental diets.
- Low electrolyte levels—23 mEq of sodium, 23 mEq of potassium, and 23 mEq of chloride per liter permit the use of Osmolite with electrolyte-controlled diets, yet are adequate levels for most hospitalized patients.
- Unflavored taste—The mild, acceptable taste makes Osmolite particularly appropriate for use with patients experiencing altered or heightened taste perceptions (eg, individuals undergoing radiation or chemotherapy treatment). Osmolite is particularly effective orally with patients rejecting conventional, sweet-tasting feedings. The addition of Vari-Flavors® Flavor Pacs helps to combat flavor fatigue experienced by patients receiving full liquid diets and liquid supplements.
- Convenient—Osmolite is ready to use. No mixing is required. Potential for contamination during preparation is reduced. Osmolite may be stored (unopened) and fed at room temperature. Once opened, Osmolite should be covered and refrigerated. Any unused portion should be discarded if not used within 48 hours.

Dosage and Administration: Dilution is not required with Osmolite. When used as a sole source of nutrition, the recommended average daily adult consumption is 2 quarts. Additional fluid requirements should be met by giving water orally with or after feedings, or when flushing the gavage tube.

UNDER NO CIRCUMSTANCES SHOULD OSMOLITE BE GIVEN PARENTERALLY.

- Gavage (tube) feeding: Initially, administration of small amounts of a 1:1 mixture of Osmolite and water is recommended until progressively larger amounts and less dilute concentrations can be tolerated. After the adaptation period, Osmolite should be given undiluted to meet prescribed caloric needs.
- Oral Feeding: Osmolite may be used as a sole source of nutrition or as a supplement with and between meals for added nutritional support. The unflavored taste of Osmolite may encourage the acceptance of liquid nutrition by patients experiencing altered or heightened taste perceptions.

Availability:
Ready To Use:
8-fl-oz bottles; two 12-bottle trays per case; No. 715.
8-fl-oz cans; 4 six-packs per case; No. 709.
32-fl-oz cans; 6 p-r case; No. 738.
For hospital use, prebottled Osmolite is available in 8-fl-oz bottles.
Ross Gavage Feeding Set:
For use with 8-fl-oz bottles; 24 sets per case; No. 61.
Composition:
INGREDIENTS: Water, corn syrup solids, sodium and calcium caseinates, medium-chain triglycerides (fractionated coconut oil), corn oil, soy protein isolate, soy oil, potassium citrate, soy lecithin, tricalcium phosphate, magnesium sulfate, magnesium chloride, choline

chloride, ascorbic acid, carrageenan, zinc sulfate, ferrous sulfate, alpha-tocopheryl acetate, niacinamide, manganous chloride, calcium pantothenate, cupric sulfate, vitamin D_3 concentrate, thiamine chloride hydrochloride, vitamin A palmitate, pyridoxine hydrochloride, riboflavin, phylloquinone, biotin, folic acid, potassium iodide and cyanocobalamin.
APPROXIMATE ANALYSIS (g/quart): - Protein, 35.2; fat, 36.4; carbohydrate, 137.2; ash, 5.1; moisture, 796.3. Calories per ml, 1.06; Calories per fl oz, 31.8.
(See table at right)

Vitamin/Mineral Content of Osmolite

Vitamins/Minerals	Per Quart		Per 2000 Calories (2 Quarts)		Percent U.S.RDA* (2 Quarts)
Vitamin A	2500	I.U.	5000	I.U.	100
Vitamin D	200	I.U.	400	I.U.	100
Vitamin E	30	I.U.	60	I.U.	200
Vitamin K_1	0.95	mg	1.9	mg	**
Vitamin C	0.15	g	0.30	g	500
Folic Acid	0.20	mg	0.40	mg	100
Thiamine (Vitamin B_1)	1.5	mg	3.0	mg	200
Riboflavin (Vitamin B_2)	1.7	mg	3.4	mg	200
Vitamin B_6	2.0	mg	4.0	mg	200
Vitamin B_{12}	6.0	mcg	12	mcg	200
Niacin	20	mg	40	mg	200
Choline	0.50	g	1.0	g	**
Biotin	0.15	mg	0.30	mg	100
Pantothenic Acid	5.0	mg	10	mg	100
Sodium	0.51	g	1.0	g	**
Potassium	0.85	g	1.7	g	**
Chloride	0.76	g	1.5	g	**
Calcium	0.50	g	1.0	g	100
Phosphorus	0.50	g	1.0	g	100
Magnesium	0.20	g	0.40	g	100
Iodine	75	mcg	0.15	mg	100
Manganese	2.0	mg	4.0	mg	**
Copper	1.0	mg	2.0	mg	100
Zinc	15	mg	30	mg	200
Iron	9.0	mg	18	mg	100

* For adults and children 4 or more years of age.
** U.S. RDA not established.

PEDIAFLOR® DROPS ℞
Sodium Fluoride, USP

Composition:
One dropperful (1.0 ml) provides:
Fluoride (as sodium fluoride).................0.5 mg
Indications: For prophylaxis against dental caries.
Contraindications: Should be used only where the fluoride content of the drinking water supply is known to be 0.7 parts per million or less.
Precautions: The recommended dosage should not be exceeded since chronic overdosage of fluoride may result in mottling of tooth enamel and osseous changes. Acute overdosage of fluoride in children may cause excessive salivation and gastrointestinal disturbances.
Dosage: One dropperful or less daily, as directed by physician or dentist.
Availability: 50-ml bottles, calibrated dropper enclosed; Rx; NDC 0074-0101-50.

PEDIALYTE®
Oral Electrolyte Solution

Usage: Maintenance of water and electrolytes during mild to moderate diarrhea in infants and children; for maintenance and replacement of water and electrolytes following corrective parenteral therapy for severe diarrhea.

- Specifically formulated for home management of mild to moderate diarrhea.
- Supplies calories in the form of glucose to help avoid ketosis.
- Ready to use eliminating additional mixing or dilution.
- Identical forms for either home or hospital use.

Availability: 32-fl-oz cans; six per case; NDC 0074-5759-06. For hospital use, prebottled Pedialyte is available in the Ross Hospital Formula System.
Dosage: For maintenance and replacement of losses in mild to moderate diarrhea of infants and young children.[1]
[See table below]
Administration of Pedialyte should begin with discontinuance of usual foods and liquids. Intake of Pedialyte should be adjusted to meet individual needs. Daily intake should be divided into frequent feedings.
Ingredients: Water, dextrose, potassium citrate, sodium chloride, sodium citrate, citric acid, magnesium chloride, and calcium chloride.

WEIGHT (lbs)	7	10	13	17	20	22	24	28	30	32	34	36	38	40
WEIGHT (kg)	3.18	4.54	5.90	7.71	9.07	9.98	10.89	12.70	13.61	14.51	15.42	16.33	17.24	18.14
Approximate Surface Area (square meters)	.21	.26	.30	.35	.40	.44	.47	.53	.58	.61	.64	.67	.71	.74
Pedialyte-Fl oz/day for maintenance	10-14	13-17	15-20	17-23	20-26	22-29	23-31	26-35	29-38	30-40	32-42	33-44	35-47	37-49
Pedialyte-Fl oz/day for maintenance and replacement	15-19	19-24	24-29	29-35	33-40	37-44	40-47	45-54	49-59	52-62	55-66	58-69	61-73	65-77

Above administration guide does not apply to infants less than 1 week of age.
For children 5 years and older: 2 quarts or more daily.

Provides:

	Per 8 fl oz	Per Liter
Sodium (mEq)	7.1	30
Potassium (mEq)	4.7	20
Calcium (mEq)	0.9	4
Magnesium (mEq)	0.9	4
Chloride (mEq)	7.1	30
Citrate (mEq)	6.6	28
Dextrose (grams)	11.8	50
Calories	48	200

Reference:
1. Kaplan, S.A.: Fluid Therapy in Pediatrics, in Current Pediatric Therapy-5, Gellis, S.S.; Kagan, B.M., Philadelphia, W.B. Saunders Company, 1971, pp. 718-719.

PEDIAMYCIN® ℞
Erythromycin Ethylsuccinate, USP

Description: Erythromycin is produced by a strain of *Streptomyces erythraeus* and belongs to the macrolide group of antibiotics. It is basic and readily forms salts with acids. The base, the stearate salt and the esters are poorly soluble in water. Erythromycin ethylsuccinate is an ester of erythromycin suitable for oral administration. The premixed suspension, granules, drops and chewable tablets for oral administration are intended primarily for pediatric use but can also be used in adults.
Pediamycin 400 (erythromycin ethylsuccinate oral suspension), 400 mg erythromycin activity per teaspoonful (5 ml), is a premixed suspension with an appealing cherry flavor, supplied in pint (16-fl-oz) bottles and 100-ml bottles. Its form and flavor make it especially suitable for older children unwilling or unable to swallow capsules or tablets.
Pediamycin Liquid (erythromycin ethylsuccinate oral suspension), 200 mg erythromycin activity per teaspoonful (5 ml), is a premixed suspension with an appealing cherry flavor, supplied in pint (16-fl-oz) bottles and 100-ml bottles. Its form and flavor make it especially suitable for infants and children, and for older children unwilling or unable to swallow capsules or tablets.
Pediamycin Suspension and *Pediamycin Drops* (erythromycin ethylsuccinate for oral suspension), 200 mg erythromycin activity per teaspoonful (5 ml), 100 mg erythromycin activity per dropperful (2.5 ml), are pleasant-tasting cherry-flavored oral suspensions, dispensed as granules of erythromycin ethylsuccinate reconstituted with water. Pediamycin granules are packaged in 60-ml, 100-ml and 150-ml (Suspension), and 50-ml (Drops) bottles. A calibrated dropper is supplied with the 50-ml bottles.
Pediamycin Chewable (erythromycin ethylsuccinate tablets), 200 mg erythromycin activity per tablet, is a pleasant-tasting tablet. The cherry flavor and chewable form encourage cooperation from pediatric patients who are unable to swallow regular tablets or who refuse liquid preparations.
Actions: The mode of action of erythromycin is by inhibition of protein synthesis without affecting nucleic acid synthesis. Resistance to erythromycin of some strains of *Hemophilus influenzae* and staphylococci has been demonstrated. Culture and susceptibility testing should be done. If the Kirby-Bauer method of disc susceptibility is used, a 15 mcg erythromycin disc should give a zone diameter of at least 18 mm when tested against an erythromycin-susceptible organism.
Orally administered erythromycin ethylsuccinate suspensions are readily and reliably absorbed. Pediamycin Chewable is readily and reliably absorbed when chewed. Comparable serum levels of erythromycin are achieved in the fasting and the nonfasting states.
After absorption, erythromycin diffuses readily into most body fluids. In the absence of meningeal inflammation low concentrations

Continued on next page

Ross—Cont.

are normally achieved in the spinal fluid, but passage of the drug across the blood-brain barrier increases in meningitis. In the presence of normal hepatic function, erythromycin is concentrated in the liver and excreted in the bile; the effect of hepatic dysfunction on excretion of erythromycin by the liver into the bile is not known. After oral administration, less than 5 percent of the activity of the administered dose can be recovered in the urine.
Erythromycin crosses the placental barrier but fetal plasma levels are generally low.
Indications: *Streptococcus pyogenes* (Group A beta-hemolytic streptococcus): Upper and lower respiratory tract, skin, and soft tissue infections of mild to moderate severity.
Injectable benzathine penicillin G is considered by the American Heart Association to be the drug of choice in the treatment and prevention of streptococcal pharyngitis and in long-term prophylaxis of rheumatic fever.
When oral medication is preferred for treatment of the above conditions, penicillin G or V, or erythromycin is the alternate drug of choice. When oral medication is given, the importance of strict adherence by the patient to the prescribed dosage regimen must be stressed. A therapeutic dose should be administered for at least 10 days.
Alpha-hemolytic streptococci (viridans group): Short-term prophylaxis of bacterial endocarditis prior to dental or other operative procedures in patients with a history of rheumatic fever or congenital heart disease who are hypersensitive to penicillin. (Erythromycin is not suitable prior to genitourinary surgery where the organisms likely to lead to bacteremia are gram-negative bacilli or the enterococcus group of streptococci.)
Staphylococcus aureus: Acute infections of skin and soft tissue of mild to moderate severity. Resistant organisms may emerge during treatment.
Streptococcus (Diplococcus) pneumoniae: Upper respiratory tract infections (e.g., otitis media, pharyngitis) and lower respiratory tract infections (e.g., pneumonia) of mild to moderate degree.
Mycoplasma pneumoniae (Eaton agent, PPLO): For respiratory infections due to this organism.
Hemophilus influenzae: For upper respiratory tract infections of mild to moderate severity when used concomitantly with adequate doses of sulfonamides. Not all strains of this organism are susceptible at the erythromycin concentrations ordinarily achieved (see appropriate sulfonamide labeling for prescribing information).
Treponema pallidum: Erythromycin is an alternate choice of treatment for primary syphilis in patients allergic to the penicillins. In treatment of primary syphilis, spinal fluid examinations should be done before treatment and as part of follow-up after therapy.
Corynebacterium diphtheriae and *C. minutissimum:* As an adjunct to antitoxin, to prevent establishment of carriers, and to eradicate the organism in carriers.
In the treament of erythrasma.
Entamoeba histolytica: In the treatment of intestinal amebiasis only. Extra-enteric amebiasis requires treatment with other agents.
Listeria monocytogenes: Infections due to this organism.
Legionnaires' Disease: Although no controlled clinical efficacy studies have been conducted, *in vitro* and limited preliminary clinical data suggest that erythromycin may be effective in treating Legionnaires' Disease.
Contraindications: Erythromycin is contraindicated in patients with known hypersensitivity to this antibiotic.

Warnings: Usage during pregnancy and lactation: The safety of erythromycin for use during pregnancy has not been established.
Erythromycin crosses the placental barrier. Erythromycin also appears in breast milk.
Precautions: Erythromycin is principally excreted by the liver. Caution should be exercised in administering the antibiotic to patients with impaired hepatic function. There have been reports of hepatic dysfunction, with or without jaundice occurring in patients receiving oral erythromycin products.
Recent data from studies of erythromycin reveal that its use in patients who are receiving high doses of theophylline may be associated with an increase of serum theophylline levels and potential theophylline toxicity. In case of theophylline toxicity and or elevated serum theophylline levels, the dose of theophylline should be reduced while the patient is receiving concomitant erythromycin therapy.
Surgical procedures should be performed when indicated.

Adverse Reactions: The most frequent side effects of oral erythromycin preparations are gastrointestinal, such as abdominal cramping and discomfort, and are dose related. Nausea, vomiting and diarrhea occur infrequently with usual oral doses.
During prolonged or repeated therapy, there is a possibility of overgrowth of nonsusceptible bacteria or fungi. If such infections occur, the drug should be discontinued and appropriate therapy instituted.
Mild allergic reactions such as urticaria and other skin rashes have occurred. Serious allergic reactions, including anaphylaxis, have been reported.

Dosage and Administration: Erythromycin ethylsuccinate suspensions and chewable tablets may be administered without regard to meals.
For full therapeutic effect, Pediamycin Chewable tablets must be chewed. They should not be swallowed whole.
Children: Age, weight and severity of the infection are important factors in determining the proper dosage. In mild to moderate infections the usual dosage of erythromycin ethylsuccinate for children is 30 to 50 mg/kg/day in equally divided doses. For more severe infections this dosage may be doubled.
Adults: 400 mg erythromycin ethylsuccinate every 6 hours is the usual dose. Dosage may be increased up to 4 g per day according to the severity of the infections.
If twice-a-day dosage is desired in either adults or children, one half of the total daily dose may be given every 12 hours. Doses may also be given three times daily if desired by administering one-third of the total daily dose every 8 hours.
The following approximate dosage schedule is suggested for using *Pediamycin Liquid* (erythromycin ethylsuccinate oral suspension), *Pediamycin Suspension* and *Pediamycin Drops* (erythromycin ethylsuccinate for oral suspension) in the treatment of mild to moderate infections by susceptible organisms.

Body Weight	Dose	Frequency	Approximate Daily Dosage
Under 10 lbs (4.5 kg)	40 mg/kg/day (20 mg/lb/day) in divided doses		
10–15 lbs (4.5 to 6.8 kg)	½ dropperful (50 mg)	4 times/day	
	or		200 mg
	1 dropperful (100 mg)	2 times/day	
15–25 lbs (6.8 11.3 kg)	1 dropperful (100 mg)	4 times/day	
	½ teaspoonful (100 mg)		
	or		400 mg
	2 dropperfuls (200 mg)	2 times/day	
	1 teaspoonful (200 mg)		
25–50 lbs (11.3 to 22.7 kg)	1 teaspoonful (200 mg)	4 times/day	
	or		800 mg
	2 teaspoonfuls (400 mg)	2 times/day	
50–100 lbs (22.7 to 45.4 kg)	1½ teaspoonfuls (300 mg)	4 times/day	
	or		1200 mg
	3 teaspoonfuls (600 mg)	2 times/day	
over 100 lbs (45.4 kg)	2 teaspoonfuls (400 mg)	4 times/day	
	or		1600 mg
	4 teaspoonfuls (800 mg)	2 times/day	

The following approximate dosage schedule is suggested for using *Pediamycin 400* (erythromycin ethylsuccinate oral suspension) in the treatment of mild to moderate infections by susceptible organisms.

Body Weight	Dose	Frequency	Approximate Daily Dosage
25–50 lbs (11.3 to 22.7 kg)	1 teaspoonful (400 mg)	2 times/day	800 mg
50–100 lbs (22.7 to 45.4 kg)	1½ teaspoonfuls (600 mg)	2 times/day	1200 mg
over 100 lbs (45.4 kg)	2 teaspoonfuls (800 mg)	2 times/day	1600 mg

The following approximate dosage schedule is suggested for using Pediamycin Chewable (erythromycin ethylsuccinate tablets) in the treatment of mild to moderate infections by susceptible organisms.

Body Weight	Dose	Frequency	Approximate Daily Dosage
25–50 lbs (11.3 to 22.7 kg)	2 chewables (400 mg)	2 times/day	
	or		800 mg
	1 chewable (200 mg)	4 times/day	
50–100 lbs (22.7 to 45.4 kg)	3 chewables (600 mg)	2 times/day	
	or		1200 mg
	1½ chewables (300 mg)	4 times/day	
over 100 lbs (45.4 kg)	4 chewables (800 mg)	2 times/day	
	or		1600 mg
	2 chewables (400 mg)	4 times/day	

The total daily dosage must be administered in equally divided doses.
In the treatment of streptococcal infections, a therapeutic dosage of erythromycin ethylsuccinate should be administered for at least 10 days. In continuous prophylaxis against recurrences of streptococcal infections in persons

with a history of rheumatic heart disease, the usual dosage is 400 mg twice a day.
When used prior to surgery to prevent endocarditis (see *Alpha-hemolytic streptococci),* a recommended schedule for adults is 800 mg erythromycin ethylsuccinate before the procedure and 400 mg every 6 hours for 4 doses after the procedure. For small children, 30 to 50 mg/kg/day divided into 3 or 4 evenly spaced doses.
For treatment of primary syphilis: Adults: 48 to 64 g given in divided doses over a period of 10 to 15 days.
For intestinal amebiasis: Adults: 400 mg four times daily for 10 to 14 days. Children: 30 to 50 mg/kg/day in divided doses for 10 to 14 days.
For treatment of Legionnaires' Disease: Although optimal doses have not been established, doses utilized in reported clinical data were those recommended above (1.6 to 4 g daily in divided doses).
How Supplied:
Pediamycin 400 (erythromycin ethylsuccinate oral suspension) is supplied in one-pint bottles (NDC 0074-0211-16) and in 100-ml bottles (NDC 0074-0211-13). It provides erythromycin ethylsuccinate equivalent to 400 mg erythromycin per teaspoonful (5 ml).
Pediamycin Liquid (erythromycin ethylsuccinate oral suspension) is supplied in one pint bottles (NDC 0074-0202-16) and in 100-ml bottles (NDC 0074-0202-13). It provides erythromycin ethylsuccinate equivalent to 200 mg of erythromycin per teaspoonful (5 ml).
Pediamycin Suspension (erythromycin ethylsuccinate for oral suspension, U.S.P.) is available for teaspoon dosage in 60-ml (NDC 0074-0206-04), 100-ml (NDC 0074-0206-13) and 150-ml (NDC 0074-0206-09) bottles, in the form of granules to be reconstituted with 46 ml, 77 ml and 115 ml of water, respectively. It provides erythromycin ethylsuccinate equivalent to 200 mg erythromycin per teaspoonful (5 ml).
Pediamycin Drops (erythromycin ethylsuccinate for oral suspension, U.S.P.) is available for dropper dosage in 50-ml bottles (NDC 0074-0207-50), in the form of granules to be reconstituted with 38 ml of water, providing 100 mg of erythromycin activity per dropperful (2.5 ml). Dropper marked for 100 mg (dropperful), 75 mg and 50 mg (half dropperful) doses is enclosed in the carton.
Pediamycin Chewable (erythromycin ethylsuccinate tablets, U.S.P.) is available in packages of 50 scored tablets, cherry-flavored, each containing erythromycin ethylsuccinate equivalent to 200 mg erythromycin (NDC 0074-0205-50). For professional identification each tablet carries the Ross "R", "205", and "CHEW".
[*Shown in Product Identification Section*]
Pediamycin Liquid and *Pediamycin 400* require refrigeration to preserve taste. Refrigeration by patient is not required if used within 14 days.

PEDIAMYCIN® CHEWABLE ℞
Erythromycin Ethylsuccinate Tablet, USP

[*Shown in Product Identification Section*]

PEDIAZOLE® ℞
erythromycin ethylsuccinate and sulfisoxazole acetyl for oral suspension

Description: Pediazole is a combination of erythromycin ethylsuccinate, USP and sulfisoxazole acetyl, USP. When reconstituted with water as directed on the label, the granules form a white, strawberry-banana flavor suspension which provides 200 mg erythromycin activity and the equivalent of 600 mg of sulfisoxazole per teaspoonful (5 ml).
Erythromycin is produced by a strain of *Streptomyces erythraeus* and belongs to the macrolide group of antibiotics. It is basic and readily forms salts and esters. Erythromycin ethylsuccinate is an ester of erythromycin.
Sulfisoxazole acetyl or N^1-acetyl sulfisoxazole is an ester of sulfisoxazole. Chemically, sulfisoxazole is N^1-(3,4-dimethyl-5-isoxazolyl) sulfanilamide.
Actions:
Clinical Pharmacology
Orally administered erythromycin ethylsuccinate suspension is reliably and readily absorbed and serum levels are comparable when administered to patients in either the fasting or non-fasting state. After absorption, erythromycin diffuses readily into most body fluids. In the presence of normal hepatic function, erythromycin is concentrated in the liver and excreted in the bile; the effect of hepatic dysfunction on excretion of erythromycin by the liver into the bile is not known. After oral administration, less than 5 percent of the activity of the administered dose can be recovered in the urine.
Erythromycin crosses the placental barrier but fetal plasma levels are generally low.
Sulfisoxazole acetyl is deacetylated by enzymatic hydrolysis in the gastrointestinal tract from which it is readily absorbed as sulfisoxazole. Sulfisoxazole exists in the blood primarily bound to serum proteins as well as conjugated and in the active or free form. Metabolic pathways include N^4-acetylation and oxidation with approximately 80 percent of an administered dose being excreted by the kidney within 24 hours.
Serum half-life total erythromycin and free sulfisoxazole are about 1.5 and 6 hours, respectively.
Microbiology
Microbiology: Pediazole has been formulated to contain sulfisoxazole for concomitant use with erythromycin. The mode of action of erythromycin is by inhibition of protein synthesis without affecting nucleic acid synthesis. Sulfonamides, including sulfisoxazole, possess bacteriostatic activity. This bacteriostatic agent acts by means of competitively inhibiting bacterial synthesis of folic acid (pteroylglutamic acid) from para-aminobenzoic acid. Resistance to erythromycin blood levels ordinarily achieved has been demonstrated by some strains of *Hemophilus influenzae.* Pediazole is usually active against *Hemophilus influenzae in vitro,* including ampicillin-resistant strains.
Quantitative methods that require measurements of zone diameters give the most precise estimates of antibiotic susceptibility. One such standardized procedure, the ASM-2 method published by the National Committee for Clinical Laboratory Standards (NCCLS), has been recommended for use with discs to test susceptibility to erythromycin and sulfisoxazole. Interpretation involves correlation of the diameters obtained in the disc test with Minimal Inhibitory Concentrations (MIC) values for erythromycin and sulfisoxazole.
If the standardized ASM-2 procedure of disc susceptibility is used, a 15 mcg erythromycin disc should give a zone diameter of at least 18 mm when tested against an erythromycin-sensitive bacterial strain and a 250–300 mcg sulfisoxazole disc should give a zone diameter of at least 17 mm when tested against a sulfisoxazole-sensitive bacterial strain.
In vitro sulfonamide sensitivity tests are not always reliable because media containing excessive amounts of thymidine are capable of reversing the inhibitory effect of sulfonamides which may result in false resistant reports. The tests must be carefully coordinated with bacteriological and clinical responses. When the patient is already taking sulfonamides follow-up cultures should have aminobenzoic acid added to the isolation media but not to subsequent susceptibility test medias.
Indication: For treatment of ACUTE OTITIS MEDIA in children caused by susceptible strains of *Hemophilus influenzae.*
Contraindications: Known hypersensitivity to either erythromycin or sulfonamides.
Infants less than 2 months of age.
Pregnancy at term and during the nursing period, because sulfonamides pass into the placental circulation and are excreted in human breast milk and may cause kernicterus in the infant.
Warnings:
Usage in Pregnancy: (SEE ALSO: CONTRAINDICATIONS) The safe use of erythromycin or sulfonamides in pregnancy has not been established. The teratogenic potential of most sulfonamides has not been thoroughly investigated in either animals or humans. However, a significant increase in the incidence of cleft palate and other bony abnormalities of offspring has been observed when certain sulfonamides of the short, intermediate and long-acting types were given to pregnant rats and mice at high oral doses (7 to 25 times the human therapeutic dose).
Reports of deaths have been associated with sulfonamide administration from hypersensitivity reactions, agranulocytosis, aplastic anemia and other blood dyscrasias. The presence of clinical signs such as sore throat, fever, pallor, purpura or jaundice may be early indications of serious blood disorders. Complete blood counts should be done frequently in patients receiving sulfonamides.
The frequency of renal complications is considerably lower in patients receiving the most soluble sulfonamides such as sulfisoxazole. Urinalysis with careful microscopic examination should be obtained frequently in patients receiving sulfonamides.
Precautions: Erythromycin is principally excreted by the liver. Caution should be exercised in administering the antibiotic to patients with impaired hepatic function. There have been reports of hepatic dysfunction, with or without jaundice occurring in patients receiving oral erythromycin products.
Recent data from studies of erythromycin reveal that its use in patients who are receiving high doses of theophylline may be associated with an increase of serum theophylline levels and potential theophylline toxicity. In case of theophylline toxicity and/or elevated serum theophylline levels, the dose of theophylline should be reduced while the patient is receiving concomitant erythromycin therapy.
Surgical procedures should be performed when indicated.
Sulfonamide therapy should be given with caution to patients with impaired renal or hepatic function and in those patients with a history of severe allergy or bronchial asthma. In the presence of a deficiency in the enzyme glucose-6-phosphate dehydrogenase, hemolysis may occur. This reaction is frequently dose-related. Adequate fluid intake must be maintained in order to prevent crystalluria and renal stone formation.
Adverse Reactions: The most frequent side effects of oral erythromycin preparations are gastrointestinal, such as abdominal cramping and discomfort, and are dose-related. Nausea, vomiting and diarrhea occur infrequently with usual oral doses. During prolonged or repeated therapy, there is a possibility of overgrowth of nonsusceptible bacteria or fungi. If such infections occur, the drug should be discontinued and appropriate therapy instituted. The overall incidence of these latter side effects reported for the combined administration of erythromycin and a sulfonamide is comparable to those observed in patients given erythromycin alone. Mild allergic reactions such as urticaria and other skin rashes have occurred. Serious allergic reactions, including anaphylaxis, have been reported with erythromycin.
The following untoward effects have been associated with the use of sulfonamides:
Blood dyscrasias: Agranulocytosis, aplastic anemia, thrombocytopenia, leukopenia, hemo-

Continued on next page

Ross—Cont.

lytic anemia, purpura, hypoprothrombinemia and methemoglobinemia.
Allergic reactions: Erythema multiforme (Stevens-Johnson syndrome), generalized skin eruptions, epidermal necrolysis, urticaria, serum sickness, pruritus, exfoliative dermatitis, anaphylactoid reactions, periorbital edema, conjunctival and scleral injection, photosensitization, arthralgia and allergic myocarditis.
Gastrointestinal reactions: Nausea, emesis, abdominal pains, hepatitis, diarrhea, anorexia, pancreatitis and stomatitis.
C.N.S. reactions: Headache, peripheral neuritis, mental depression, convulsions, ataxia, hallucinations, tinnitus, vertigo and insomnia.
Miscellaneous reactions: Drug fever, chills and toxic nephrosis with oliguria or anuria. Periarteritis nodosa and L.E. phenomenon have occurred.
The sulfonamides bear certain chemical similarities to some goitrogens, diuretics (acetazolamide and the thiazides) and oral hypoglycemic agents. Goiter production, diuresis and hypoglycemia have occurred rarely in patients receiving sulfonamides. Cross-sensitivity may exist with these agents.
Rats appear to be especially susceptible to the goitrogenic effects of sulfonamides, and long-term administration has produced thyroid malignancies in the species.
Dosage and Administration: PEDIAZOLE SHOULD NOT BE ADMINISTERED TO INFANTS UNDER 2 MONTHS OF AGE BECAUSE OF CONTRAINDICATIONS OF SYSTEMIC SULFONAMIDES IN THIS AGE GROUP.
For Acute Otitis Media in Children:
The recommended dose is 50 mg/kg/day of erythromycin and 150 mg/kg/day, to a maximum of 6 g/day, of sulfisoxazole. Pediazole is to be given in equally divided doses four times a day for 10 days. It may be administered without regard to meals.
The following approximate dosage schedule is recommended for using Pediazole:
Children: Two months of age or older

Weight	Dose—every 6 hours
Less than 8 kg (less than 18 lbs)	Adjust dosage by body weight
8 kg (18 lbs)	½ teaspoonful (2.5 ml)
16 kg (35 lbs)	1 teaspoonful (5 ml)
24 kg (53 lbs)	1 ½ teaspoonfuls (7.5 ml)
over 45 kg (over 100 lbs)	2 teaspoonfuls (10 ml)

How Supplied: Pediazole Suspension is available for teaspoon dosage in 100-ml (**NDC** 0074-8030-13) and 200-ml (**NDC** 0074-8030-53) bottles, in the form of granules to be reconstituted with water. The suspension provides erythromycin ethylsuccinate equivalent to 200 mg erythromycin activity and sulfisoxazole acetyl equivalent to 600 mg sulfisoxazole per teaspoonful (5 ml).

POLYCOSE®
Glucose Polymers

Usage: Polycose, a source of calories solely from carbohydrate, is used to supply calories in persons with increased caloric requirements or persons unable to meet their caloric needs with usual food intake. Polycose may also be utilized to supply carbohydrate calories in protein, electrolyte and fat restricted diets. It may be used to increase the caloric density of traditional foods, liquids, and tube fed diets.
Features:
* Water soluble, therefore, mixes readily with most foods and beverages to increase caloric density.
* Minimally sweet, as compared to glucose and other dietary carbohydrates, which helps improve patient acceptance.
* Rapidly absorbed as glucose with negligible gut residue.
* Osmolality is approximately one-fifth that of pure glucose solutions of comparable caloric density. This helps reduce potential for osmotic diarrhea.
* Low in electrolytes, Polycose may be used in the dietary management of those patients whose intake of electrolytes is restricted.

Dosage and Administration: Polycose may be added to most foods and beverages, or mixed in water, with or without flavoring, in amounts determined by taste, caloric requirement and tolerance. Small, frequent feedings are more desirable than large amounts given infrequently. Polycose may be used for extended periods with diets containing all other essential nutrients, or as an oral adjunct to intravenous administration of nutrients. Polycose is not a balanced diet and should not be used as a sole source of nutrition. If indicated, solutions of Polycose may be administered via gavage tube. Refrigerate any unused dissolved Polycose Powder and opened Polycose Liquid and discard if not used after 24 hours. Concentrated solutions become more viscous when cold; thus serving at room temperature is advised. Not for parenteral use.
Availability:
Powder: 14-ounce (400 g) cans; 6 per case; No. 746.
Liquid: (43% w/w aqueous solution): 4-fl-oz bottles; 48 per case; No. 743.
Composition: Ⓤ
Powder: Glucose polymers derived from controlled hydrolysis of corn starch.
Approximate Analysis (per 100 grams):

Carbohydrate		94 g
Moisture		6 g
Ash	Does not exceed	0.5 g
Calcium	Does not exceed	60 mg (3 mEq)
Sodium	Does not exceed	115 mg (5 mEq)
Potassium	Does not exceed	39 mg (1 mEq)
Chloride	Does not exceed	213 mg (6 mEq)
Phosphorus	Does not exceed	13 mg (2 mEq)

Approximate Caloric Equivalents:
1 Tablespoon (8 g) = 30 Calories; 100 g = 376 Calories
Composition: Ⓤ
Liquid: (43% w/w aqueous solution): Water and glucose polymers derived from controlled hydrolysis of corn starch.
Approximate Analysis (per 100 ml):

Carbohydrate		50g
Moisture		70g
Ash	Does not exceed	0.25g
Calcium	Does not exceed	30mg (1.5 mEq)
Sodium	Does not exceed	58mg (2.5 mEq)
Potassium	Does not exceed	20mg (0.5 mEq)
Chloride	Does not exceed	107mg (3 mEq)
Phosphorus	Does not exceed	6 mg (1 mEq)

Approximate Caloric Equivalents:
1 ml = 2 Calories; 1 fl oz = 60 Calories; 100 ml = 200 Calories.

PRAMET® FA ℞
Vitamin/Mineral Prescription for the Expectant and New Mother

Ingredients: Each Pramet FA Filmtab® Film-Sealed tablet provides:
Vitamins:

Vitamin A (as acetate) 1.2 mg	4000	I.U.
Vitamin D (ergocalciferol, 10 mcg)	400	I.U.
Vitamin C (ascorbic acid)	100	mg
Folic Acid	1	mg
Vitamin B_1 (thiamine mononitrate)	3	mg
Vitamin B_2 (riboflavin)	2	mg
Niacinamide	10	mg
Vitamin B_6 (pyridoxine hydrochloride)	5	mg
Vitamin B_{12} (cyanocobalamin)	3	mcg
Pantothenic Acid (as calcium pantothenate)	0.92	mg

Minerals:

Calcium (as calcium carbonate)	250	mg
Iodine (as calcium iodate)	100	mcg
Elemental Iron+ (300 mg ferrous sulfate USP)	60	mg
Copper (as cupric chloride)	0.15	mg

+ In controlled-release form—Gradumet® U.S. Pat. No. Re. 27,107
Indications: To help prevent vitamin and mineral deficiencies during and after pregnancy and for treatment of megaloblastic anemias. One mg of folic acid has been found to be effective therapy for megaloblastic anemias of pregnancy and lactation.
Warning: Folic acid alone is improper therapy in the treatment of pernicious anemia and other megaloblastic anemias where Vitamin B_{12} is deficient.
Precaution: Folic acid may mask the presence of pernicious anemia in that hematologic remission may occur while neurologic manifestations remain progressive.
Adverse Reaction: Allergic sensitization has been reported following both oral and parenteral administration of folic acid.
Availability: 100-tablet bottles; Rx; NDC 0074-0147-01.
Dosage: One tablet daily, or as directed by physician.
[*Shown in Product Identification Section*]

PRAMILET® FA ℞
Prenatal Vitamin/Mineral Preparation with Folic Acid

Ingredients: Each Pramilet FA Filmtab® Film-Sealed tablet provides:
Vitamins:

Vitamin A (as acetate and palmitate) 1.2 mg	4000	I.U.
Vitamin D (ergocalciferol, 10 mcg)	400	I.U.
Vitamin C (as sodium ascorbate)	60	mg
Folic Acid	1	mg
Vitamin B_1 (thiamine mononitrate)	3	mg
Vitamin B_2 (riboflavin)	2	mg
Niacinamide	10	mg
Vitamin B_6 (pyridoxine hydrochloride)	3	mg
Vitamin B_{12} (cyanocobalamin)	3	mcg
Calcium Pantothenate	1	mg

Minerals:

Calcium (as calcium carbonate)	250	mg
Iodine (as calcium iodate)	100	mcg
Elemental Iron (as ferrous fumarate)	40	mg
Magnesium (as magnesium oxide)	10	mg
Copper (as cupric chloride)	0.15	mg
Zinc (as zinc oxide)	0.085	mg

Indications: To help prevent vitamin and mineral deficiencies during pregnancy and lactation and for treatment of megaloblastic anemias of pregnancy. One mg of folic acid has been found to be effective therapy for megaloblastic anemia of pregnancy.
Availability: 100-tablet bottles; Rx; NDC 0074-0121-01
Dosage: One tablet daily, or as directed by physician.
Warning: Folic acid alone is improper therapy in the treatment of pernicious anemia and other megaloblastic anemias where Vitamin B_{12} is deficient.
Precaution: Folic acid may mask the presence of pernicious anemia in that hematologic remission may occur while neurologic manifestations remain progressive.
Adverse Reaction: Allergic sensitization has been reported following both oral and parenteral administration of folic acid.
[*Shown in Product Identification Section*]

RONDEC-DM™ ℞

Ingredients:	Drops dropperful (1 ml)	Syrup teaspoonful (5 ml)
carbinoxamine maleate	2 mg	4 mg
pseudoephedrine hydrochloride	25 mg	60 mg
dextromethorphan hydrobromide	4 mg	15 mg

alcohol in Drops and Syrup less than 0.6%
Product reformulated January, 1978

	age	dose	frequency
Rondec-DM Drops oral use only	1–3 months	¼ dropperful (¼ ml)	q.i.d.*
	4–6 months	½ dropperful (½ ml)	q.i.d.*
	7–9 months	¾ dropperful (¾ ml)	q.i.d.*
	10–18 months	1 dropperful (1 ml)	q.i.d.*
Rondec-DM Syrup	18 months-5 years	½ teaspoonful (2.5 ml)	q.i.d.*
	adults and children 6 years and older	1 teaspoonful (5 ml)	q.i.d.*

*In mild coughs, less frequent doses may be adequate.

Actions: Antihistamine: carbinoxamine maleate, for histamine blocking that will dry up runny noses and relieve sneezing and itchy, watery eyes.
Decongestant: pseudoephedrine hydrochloride, to decongest swollen mucous membranes of the respiratory tract by vasoconstrictor action, which is similar to that of ephedrine. Pseudoephedrine has been shown in clinical and laboratory tests to have less pressor effect than ephedrine.
Antitussive: dextromethorphan hydrobromide, to control the unproductive cough by elevating the cough threshold with no known liability of addiction.
Indications: RONDEC-DM is indicated for the following disorders:
- nasopharyngitis with postnasal drip
- common cold
- bronchitis and bronchial cough
- recurrent cough due to recurrent respiratory infection

Contraindications: There are no known contraindications for the use of **RONDEC-DM.**
Precautions: Although pseudoephedrine has less pressor effect than ephedrine, use with caution in patients with hypertension.
Because of the antihistamine component, carbinoxamine maleate, patients should be cautioned to exercise care in driving or operating machinery until the possibility of drowsiness is determined.
If a sensitivity reaction or idiosyncrasy should occur, withdraw the drug.
Safety in pregnancy has not been determined. **RONDEC-DM** should be used in pregnant women only when the benefits outweigh the risks.
Adverse Reactions: Those patients particularly sensitive to pseudoephedrine, a sympathomimetic amine, may note mild central nervous system stimulation.
Like all antihistamines, sedation has been observed with the use of carbinoxamine maleate. However, it is generally mild, and tolerance appears to develop rapidly in most cases. Patients particularly sensitive to antihistamines may experience moderate to severe drowsiness.
Mild gastrointestinal disturbance and drowsiness have been observed among patients receiving dextromethorphan hydrobromide. These instances are rare, and no serious side effects have been reported.
Dosage and Administration: Because response to ingredients will vary according to the severity of the illness and the type of patient under treatment, the dosage should be adjusted by age and the clinically determined needs of the individual patient.
Usual Dosage:
[See table above right].
How Supplied: Rondec-DM Drops, grape-flavored, is available in 30-ml bottles for drop-per dosage. Calibrated, shatterproof dropper enclosed in each carton. Container meets safety closure requirements. NDC 0074-5639-30.
RONDEC-DM Syrup, grape-flavored, is available in 16-fl-oz (1-pint) bottles, NDC 0074-5640-16; and 4-fl-oz bottles, NDC 0074-5640-04.
Animal Pharmacology and Toxicology:
Carbinoxamine maleate is an antihistaminic drug with therapeutic index (ratio of median lethal dose to median effective dose in guinea pigs) that is 2 to 50 times that of chlorpheniramine maleate, pheniramine, diphenhydramine and tripelennamine.
Pseudoephedrine hydrochloride is a decongestant with vasoconstrictor action similar to that of ephedrine but has been shown in laboratory animals to have a significantly less effect on blood pressure.
Dextromethorphan hydrobromide is a nonnarcotic antitussive which in cats increased the central threshold for the cough reflex but did not inhibit ciliary activity at dose levels below 5 mg/kg.

RONDEC D™rops ℞
RONDEC S™yrup
RONDEC T™ablet
Antihistamine/Decongestant

Ingredients:
[See table below].

	Tablet each tablet	Syrup—each teaspoonful (5 ml)	Oral Drops—each dropperful (1 ml)
Carbinoxamine maleate	4 mg	4 mg	2 mg
Pseudoephedrine hydrochloride	60 mg	60 mg	25 mg

*Pseudoephedrine equivalent to the hydrochloride.

Actions: Antihistamine: carbinoxamine maleate, for histamine blocking that will dry up runny noses and relieve sneezing and itchy, watery eyes.
Decongestant: pseudoephedrine hydrochloride, to decongest swollen mucous membranes of the respiratory tract by vasoconstrictor action, which is similar to that of ephedrine. Pseudoephedrine has been shown in clinical and laboratory tests to have less pressor effect than ephedrine.
Animal Pharmacology and Toxicology:
Carbinoxamine maleate is an antihistaminic drug with a therapeutic index (ratio of median lethal dose to median effective dose in guinea pigs) that is 2 to 50 times that of chlorpheniramine maleate, pheniramine, diphenhydramine and tripelennamine.
Pseudoephedrine hydrochloride is a decongestant with vasoconstrictor action similar to that of ephedrine but has been shown in laboratory animals to have a significantly less effect on blood pressure.
Indications: RONDEC Drops, **RONDEC** Syrup, and **RONDEC** Tablet are indicated for use in seasonal and perennial allergic rhinitis and vasomotor rhinitis.
Contraindications: There are no known contraindications for use of **RONDEC Drops, RONDEC Syrup,** and **RONDEC Tablet.**
Precautions: Although pseudoephedrine has less pressor effect than ephedrine, use with caution in patients with hypertension.
Because of the antihistamine component, carbinoxamine maleate, patients should be cautioned to exercise care in driving or operating machinery until the possibility of drowsiness is determined.
If sensitivity reaction or idiosyncrasy should occur, withdraw the drug.
Safety for use in pregnancy has not been established. **RONDEC Drops, RONDEC Syrup,** and **RONDEC** Tablet should be used in pregnant women only when the benefits outweigh the risks.
Adverse Reactions: Those patients particularly sensitive to pseudoephedrine, a sympathomimetic amine, may note mild central nervous system stimulation.
Like all antihistamines, sedation has been observed with the use of carbinoxamine maleate. However, it is generally mild, and tolerance appears to develop rapidly in most cases. Patients particularly sensitive to antihistamines may experience moderate to severe drowsiness.
Dosage and Administration: Because response to the ingredients will vary according to the severity of the illness and the type of patient under treatment, the dosage should be adjusted by age and the clinically determined needs of the individual patient.
RONDEC Syrup, and **RONDEC Tablet:**

age	dose	frequency
18 months-5 years	½ teaspoonful (2.5 ml)	4 times a day
adults and children 6 years and older	1 teaspoonful (5 ml) or 1 tablet	4 times a day

RONDEC Drops
oral use only

age	dose	frequency
1–3 months	¼ dropperful (¼ ml)	4 times a day
4–6 months	½ dropperful (½ ml)	4 times a day
7–9 months	¾ dropperful (¾ ml)	4 times a day
10–17 months	1 dropperful (1 ml)	4 times a day

How Supplied: RONDEC Tablet, with Filmtab®, is available in bottles of 100, NDC 0074-5726-13; and bottles of 500, NDC 0074-5726-53. Each tablet marked with Ross R and the number 5726 for professional identification.
RONDEC Syrup, berry-flavored, is available in 16-fl-oz (1-pint) bottles, NDC 0074-5782-16; and 4-fl-oz bottles, NDC 0074-5782-04.
RONDEC Drops, berry-flavored, is available in 30-ml bottles for dropper dosage, NDC 0074-5783-30. Calibrated shatterproof dropper enclosed in each carton. Container meets safety closure requirements.

[*Tablet shown in Product Identification Section*]

Continued on next page

Ross—Cont.

ROSS HOSPITAL FORMULA SYSTEM
Similac® infant formula products for hospital nursery use

SIMILAC 13, Ready To Feed, 13 Cal/fl oz
Availability:
4-fl-oz nursing bottles; 48 per case; No. 408.

SIMILAC 20, Ready To Feed, 20 Cal/fl oz
Availability:
4-fl-oz nursing bottles; 48 per case; No. 415.
8-fl-oz nursing bottles; 24 per case; No. 841.

SIMILAC 24, Ready To Feed, 24 Cal/fl oz
Availability:
4-fl-oz nursing bottles; 48 per case; No. 404.

SIMILAC 24 LBW, Ready To Feed, 24 Cal/fl oz
Availability:
4-fl-oz nursing bottles; 48 per case; No. 422.

SIMILAC 27, Ready To Feed, 27 Cal/fl oz
Availability:
4-fl-oz nursing bottles; 48 per case; No. 427.

SIMILAC WITH IRON 13, Ready To Feed, 13 Cal/fl oz
Availability:
4-fl-oz nursing bottles; 48 per case; No. 413.

SIMILAC WITH IRON 20, Ready To Feed, 20 Cal/fl oz
Availability:
4-fl-oz nursing bottles; 48 per case; No. 426.
8-fl-oz nursing bottles; 24 per case; No. 858.

SIMILAC WITH IRON 24, Ready To Feed, 24 Cal/fl oz
Availability:
4-fl-oz nursing bottles; 48 per case; No. 403.

SIMILAC PM 60/40, Ready To Feed, 20 Cal/fl oz
Availability:
4-fl-oz nursing bottles; 48 per case; No. 424.

ISOMIL 20, Ready To Feed, 20 Cal/fl oz
Availability:
4-fl-oz nursing bottles; 48 per case; No. 406.
8-fl-oz nursing bottles; 24 per case; No. 871.

PEDIALYTE, Ready To Use, NDC 0074-5759-57
Availability:
8-fl-oz nursing bottles; 24 per case; No. 806.

ADVANCE, Ready To Feed
Availability:
8-fl-oz nursing bottles; 24 per case; No. 804.

5% GLUCOSE WATER, Ready To Feed
Availability:
4-fl-oz nursing bottles; 48 per case; No. 405.

10% GLUCOSE WATER, Ready To Feed
Availability:
4-fl-oz nursing bottles; 48 per case; No. 410.

STERILIZED WATER, Ready To Feed
Availability:
4-fl-oz nursing bottles; 48 per case; No. 432.
8-fl-oz nursing bottles; 24 per case; No. 879.

VOLU-FEED®, Ross Volumetric Feeding System
Availability:
Volu-Feed Nursers; 200 per case; No. 40.
Volu-Feed Dispensing Caps; 500 per case; No. 41.

Redi-Nurser® System: Self-contained feeding system with a sterilized nipple attached to a 4-fl-oz nursing bottle is available in nine different varieties of infant feeding.

SIMILAC®
Infant Formula

Usage: When a formula is desired for infants being bottle fed, or as a supplement to breast feeding.
Availability:
Powder: 1-lb cans, measuring scoop enclosed; 12 per case; No. 00139.
Concentrated Liquid: 13-fl-oz cans; 24 per case; No. 00264.
Ready To Feed: (prediluted, 20 Cal/fl oz): 32-fl-oz (quart) cans; 6 per case; No. 00232.
8-fl-oz cans; 4 six-packs per case; No. 00177.
4-fl-oz nursing bottles; 6 per carry-home carton, 8 cartons per case; No. 00480.
8-fl-oz nursing bottles; 6 per carry-home carton, 4 cartons per case; No. 00880.
For hospital use, prebottled SIMILAC is available in the Ross Hospital Formula System.
Preparation:
Powder: Standard 20 Cal/fl oz dilution is 1 level unpacked scoop SIMILAC Powder (8.74 grams) for each 2 fl oz of water.
Concentrated Liquid: Standard 20 Cal/fl oz dilution is 1 part Concentrated Liquid to 1 part water.
Composition: Powder
Ingredients: Ⓤ A powdered, homogenized, modified milk product especially prepared for infant feeding, made from nonfat milk, lactose, coconut and corn oils, sodium citrate, potassium citrate, ascorbic acid, niacinamide, alpha-tocopheryl acetate, zinc sulfate, calcium pantothenate, cupric sulfate, vitamin A palmitate, thiamine chloride hydrochloride, riboflavin, pyridoxine hydrochloride, folic acid, phylloquinone, vitamin D_3 concentrate, manganous chloride and cyanocobalamin.

Approximate Analysis:	Powdered (wt/100 g)	Standard Dilution* (wt/liter)
Fat	27.4 g	36.1 g
Carbohydrate	55.7 g	73.4 g
Protein	11.8 g	15.5 g
Minerals (Ash)	3.1 g	4.1 g
Calcium	0.39 g	0.51 g
Phosphorus	0.30 g	0.39 g
Magnesium	31 mg	41 g
Zinc	3.8 mg	5.0 mg
Copper	0.46 mg	0.60 mg
Iodine	76 mcg	0.10 mg
Manganese	26 mcg	34 mcg
Iron	trace	trace
(This product, like milk, is deficient in iron; an additional 6.8 mg iron per liter should be supplied from other sources.)		
Moisture	2.0 g	900.4 g
Crude Fiber	0 g	
Calories	145 per av oz	20 per fl oz

Vitamins Per Liter (Standard dilution*):	
Vitamin A	2500 I.U.
Vitamin D	400 I.U.
Vitamin E	15 I.U.
Vitamin C	55 mg
Thiamine (Vitamin B_1)	0.65 mg
Riboflavin (Vitamin B_2)	1 mg
Niacin (mg equiv.)	7
Vitamin B_6	0.40 mg
Pantothenic acid	3 mg
Folic acid	0.10 mg
Vitamin K_1	27 mcg
Vitamin B_{12}	1.5 mcg

*Standard dilution is 1 level scoop of Similac Powder to 2 fl oz water.

Composition: Concentrated Liquid
Ingredients: Ⓤ A homogenized, modified milk product especially prepared for infant feeding, made from water, nonfat milk, lactose, coconut and soy oils, mono- and diglycerides, soy lecithin, ascorbic acid, carrageenan, zinc sulfate, niacinamide, alpha-tocopheryl acetate, cupric sulfate, calcium pantothenate, vitamin A palmitate, thiamine chloride hydrochloride, pyridoxine hydrochloride, riboflavin, folic acid, manganous chloride, vitamin D_3 concentrate and cyanocobalamin.

Approximate Analysis (wt/liter):	Concentrated	Standard Dilution*
Fat	72.2 g	36.1 g
Carbohydrate	144.6 g	72.3 g
Protein	31.0 g	15.5 g
Minerals (Ash)	7.2 g	3.6 g
Calcium	1.0 g	0.51 g
Phosphorus	0.77 g	0.39 g
Magnesium	82 mg	41 mg
Zinc	10 mg	5.0 mg
Copper	1.2 mg	0.60 mg
Iodine	0.20 mg	0.10 mg
Manganese	68 mcg	34 mcg
Iron	trace	trace
(This product, like milk, is deficient in iron; an additional 6.8 mg iron per liter should be supplied from other sources.)		
Water	805.9 g	902.0 g
Crude Fiber	0 g	
Calories per fl oz	40	20
Calories per 100 ml	135	68

Vitamins Per Liter (Standard dilution*):	
Vitamin A	2500 I.U.
Vitamin D	400 I.U.
Vitamin E	15 I.U.
Vitamin C	55 mg
Thiamine (Vitamin B_1)	0.65 mg
Riboflavin (Vitamin B_2)	1 mg
Niacin (mg equiv.)	7
Vitamin B_6	0.40 mg
Folic Acid	0.10 mg
Pantothenic acid	3 mg
Vitamin B_{12}	1.5 mcg

*Standard dilution is equal parts Similac Concentrated Liquid and water.

Composition: Ready To Feed
Ingredients: Ⓤ A homogenized, modified milk product especially prepared for infant feeding, made from water, nonfat milk, lactose, coconut and soy oils, mono- and diglycerides, soy lecithin, carrageenan, ascorbic acid, zinc sulfate, niacinamide, alpha-tocopheryl acetate, cupric sulfate, calcium pantothenate, vitamin A palmitate, thiamine chloride hydrochloride, pyridoxine hydrochloride, riboflavin, folic acid, manganous chloride, vitamin D_3 concentrate and cyanocobalamin.

Approximate Analysis:	(wt/liter)
Fat	36.1 g
Carbohydrate	72.3 g
Protein	15.5 g
Minerals (Ash)	3.6 g
Calcium	0.51 g
Phosphorus	0.39 g
Magnesium	41 mg
Zinc	5.0 mg
Copper	0.60 mg
Iodine	0.10 mg
Manganese	34 mcg
Iron	trace
(This product, like milk, is deficient in iron; an additional 6.8 mg iron per liter should be supplied from other sources.)	
Water	902.0 g
Crude Fiber	0 g
Calories per fl oz	20
Calories per 100 ml	68

Vitamins Per Liter:	
Vitamin A	2500 I.U.
Vitamin D	400 I.U.
Vitamin E	15 I.U.
Vitamin C	55 mg
Thiamine (Vitamin B_1)	0.65 mg
Riboflavin (Vitamin B_2)	1 mg
Niacin (mg equiv.)	7
Vitamin B_6	0.40 mg
Folic Acid	0.10 mg
Pantothenic Acid	3 mg
Vitamin B_{12}	1.5 mcg

SIMILAC® PM 60/40
Infant Formula

Usage: Similac PM 60/40 is suitable for those infants who are in the lower range of homeostatic capacity; for those who are problem feeders; those who are predisposed to hypocalcemia, and those whose renal, digestive and/or cardiovascular functions would benefit from lowered mineral and protein levels, as found in human milk.
Availability: Powder only; 1-lb cans, measuring scoop enclosed; six per case; No. 00850.
Preparation: Standard 20 Cal/fl oz dilution is one level, unpacked scoop (enclosed) powder for each 2 fl oz of water.
Higher caloric feedings are prepared by adding 8.56 grams (one level, unpacked scoopful) of Similac PM 60/40 to the following amounts of water:

For:	Water:	Yields:
24 Cal/oz	48 cc	55 cc (1.8 fl oz)
27 Cal/oz	42 cc	49 cc (1.6 fl oz)
30 Cal/oz	37 cc	44 cc (1.5 fl oz)

Ingredients: Ⓤ Demineralized whey solids, coconut oil, lactose, corn oil, calcium sodium caseinate, calcium citrate, potassium chloride, mono- and diglycerides, soy lecithin, potassium phosphate, sodium chloride, magnesium chloride, ascorbic acid, zinc sulfate, niacinamide, vitamin A palmitate, vitamin D_3 concentrate, ferrous sulfate, alpha-tocopheryl acetate, potassium citrate, cupric sulfate, calcium pantothenate, thiamine chloride hydrochloride, riboflavin, pyridoxine hydrochloride, phylloquinone, potassium iodide, folic acid, manganous chloride and cyanocobalamin.

Approximate Analysis:	Powdered (wt/100 g)	Standard Dilution* (wt/liter)
Fat	26.85 g	35.4 g
Protein	11.95 g	15.7 g
Lactalbumin and lactoglobulin	60 %	
Casein	40 %	
Carbohydrate	57.50 g	75.7 g
Minerals (Ash)	1.70 g	2.2 g
Calcium	0.3 g	0.40 g
Phosphorus	0.15 g	0.20 g
Sodium	0.12 g	0.16 g
Potassium	0.44 g	0.58 g
Chloride	0.34 g	0.45 g
Magnesium	32 mg	42 mg
Zinc	3 mg	4.0 mg
Iron	2 mg	2.6 mg
(This product, like milk, is deficient in iron; an additional 4.2 mg iron per liter should be supplied from other sources.)		
Copper	0.30 mg	0.40 mg
Iodine	30 mcg	40 mcg
Manganese	26 mcg	34 mcg
Moisture	2.00	900.5 g
Crude Fiber	0 g	
Calories	145 per av oz	20 per fl oz
Calories per 100 ml		68

Vitamins Per Liter (Standard Dilution*):

Vitamin A	2500 I.U.
Vitamin D	400 I.U.
Vitamin E	15 I.U.
Vitamin C	55 mg
Thiamine (Vitamin B_1)	0.65 mg
Riboflavin (Vitamin B_2)	1 mg
Niacin (mg equiv.)	7.3
Vitamin B_6	0.3 mg
Folic acid	50 mcg
Pantothenic acid	3.0 mg
Vitamin B_{12}	1.5 mcg
Vitamin K_1	27 mcg

*Standard dilution is 1 measure (enclosed) Similac PM 60/40 Powder to 2 fl oz water or 131.7 g of Powder diluted to 1 liter.
Precautions: In conditions where the infant is losing abnormal quantities of one or more electrolytes, it may be necessary to supply electrolytes from sources other than the formula. With premature infants weighing less than 1500 g at birth, it may be necessary to supply an additional source of sodium, calcium and phosphorus during the period of very rapid growth.

SIMILAC® WITH IRON
Infant Formula

Usage: When a formula containing iron is desired for infants being bottle fed or as a supplement to breast feeding.
Availability: Powder: 1-lb cans, measuring scoop enclosed; 12 per case; No. 00360.
Concentrated Liquid; 13-fl-oz cans; 24 cans per case; No. 00414.
Ready To Feed (prediluted, 20 Cal/fl oz):
32-fl-oz (quart) cans; 6 per case; No. 00241.
8-fl-oz cans; 4 six-packs per case; No. 00179.
4-fl-oz nursing bottles; 6 per carry-home carton, 8 cartons per case; No. 06201.
8-fl-oz nursing bottles; 6 per carry-home carton, 4 cartons per case; No. 06202.
For hospital use, prebottled SIMILAC WITH IRON is available in the Ross Hospital Formula System.
Preparation:
Powder: Standard 20 Cal/fl oz dilution is 1 level, unpacked scoop Powder (8.74 grams) for each 2 fl oz of water.
Concentrated Liquid: Standard 20 Cal/fl oz of dilution is 1 part Concentrated Liquid to 1 part water.
Composition: Powder
Ingredients: Ⓤ A powdered, homogenized, modified milk product especially prepared for infant feeding, made from nonfat milk, lactose, coconut and corn oils, sodium citrate, potassium citrate, ascorbic acid, ferrous sulfate, niacinamide, alpha-tocopheryl acetate, zinc sulfate, calcium pantothenate, cupric sulfate, vitamin A palmitate, thiamine chloride hydrochloride, riboflavin, pyridoxine hydrochloride, folic acid, phylloquinone, vitamin D_3 concentrate, manganous chloride and cyanocobalamin.

Approximate Analysis:	Powdered (wt/100 g)	Standard Dilution* (wt/liter)
Fat	27.4 g	36.1 g
Carbohydrate	55.7 g	73.4 g
Protein	11.8 g	15.5 g
Minerals (Ash)	3.1 g	4.1 g
Calcium	0.39 g	0.51 g
Phosphorus	0.30 g	0.39 g
Magnesium	31 mg	41 mg
Iron	9.1 mg	12 mg
Zinc	3.8 mg	5.0 mg
Copper	0.46 mg	0.60 mg
Iodine	76 mcg	0.10 mg
Manganese	26 mcg	34 mcg
Moisture	2.0 g	900.4 g
Crude Fiber	0 g	
Calories	145 per av oz	20 per fl oz

Vitamins Per Liter (Standard dilution*):

Vitamin A	2500 I.U.
Vitamin D	400 I.U.
Vitamin E	15 I.U.
Vitamin C	55 mg
Thiamine (Vitamin B_1)	0.65 mg
Riboflavin (Vitamin B_2)	1 mg
Niacin (mg equiv.)	7
Vitamin B_6	0.40 mg
Pantothenic acid	3 mg
Folic acid	0.10 mg
Vitamin K_1	27 mcg
Vitamin B_{12}	1.5 mcg

*Standard dilution is 1 level scoop of Similac Powder to 2 fl oz water.

Composition: Concentrated Liquid
Ingredients: Ⓤ A homogenized, modified milk product especially prepared for infant feeding, made from water, nonfat milk, lactose, coconut and soy oils, mono- and diglycerides, soy lecithin, ascorbic acid, carrageenan, ferrous sulfate, zinc sulfate, niacinamide, alpha-tocopheryl acetate, potassium citrate, cupric sulfate, calcium pantothenate, vitamin A palmitate, thiamine chloride hydrochloride, pyridoxine hydrochloride, riboflavin, folic acid, manganous chloride, vitamin D_3 concentrate and cyanocobalamin.

Approximate Analysis: (wt/liter)	Concentrated	Standard Dilution*
Fat	72.2 g	36.1 g
Carbohydrate	144.6 g	72.3 g
Protein	31.0 g	15.5 g
Minerals (Ash)	7.4 g	3.7 g
Calcium	1.0 g	0.51 g
Phosphorus	0.77 g	0.39 g
Magnesium	82 mg	41 mg
Iron	24 mg	12 mg
Zinc	10 mg	5.0 mg
Copper	1.2 mg	0.60 mg
Iodine	0.20 mg	0.10 mg
Manganese	68 mcg	34 mcg
Water	805.7 g	901.9 g
Crude Fiber	0 g	
Calories per fl oz	40	20
Calories per 100 ml	135	68

Vitamins Per Liter (Standard dilution*):

Vitamin A	2500 I.U.
Vitamin D	400 I.U.
Vitamin E	15 I.U.
Vitamin C	55 mg
Thiamine (Vitamin B_1)	0.65 mg
Riboflavin (Vitamin B_2)	1 mg
Niacin (mg equiv.)	7
Vitamin B_6	0.40 mg
Folic acid	0.10 mg
Pantothenic acid	3 mg
Vitamin B_{12}	1.5 mcg

*Standard dilution is equal parts Similac With Iron Concentrated Liquid and water.
Composition: Ready To Feed
Ingredients: Ⓤ A homogenized, modified milk product especially prepared for infant feeding, made from water, nonfat milk, lactose, coconut and soy oils, mono- and diglycerides, soy lecithin, carrageenan, ascorbic acid, ferrous sulfate, zinc sulfate, niacinamide, alpha-tocopheryl acetate, potassium citrate, cupric sulfate, calcium pantothenate, vitamin A palmitate, thiamine chloride hydrochloride, pyridoxine hydrochloride, riboflavin, folic acid, manganous chloride, vitamin D_3 concentrate and cyanocobalamin.

Approximate Analysis:	(wt/liter)
Fat	36.1 g
Carbohydrate	72.3 g
Protein	15.5 g
Minerals (Ash)	3.7 g
Calcium	0.51 g
Phosphorus	0.39 g
Magnesium	41 mg
Iron	12 mg
Zinc	5.0 mg
Copper	0.41 mg
Iodine	0.10 mg
Manganese	34 mcg
Water	901.9 g
Crude Fiber	0 g
Calories per fl oz	20
Calories per 100 ml	68

Continued on next page

Ross—Cont.

Vitamins Per Liter:	
Vitamin A	2500 I.U.
Vitamin D	400 I.U.
Vitamin E	15 I.U.
Vitamin C	55 mg
Thiamine (Vitamin B_1)	0.65 mg
Riboflavin (Vitamin B_2)	1 mg
Niacin (mg equiv.)	7
Vitamin B_6	0.40 mg
Folic acid	0.10 mg
Pantothenic acid	3 mg
Vitamin B_{12}	1.5 mcg

The addition of iron to this formula conforms to the recommendation of the Committee on Nutrition of the American Academy of Pediatrics.

VI-DAYLIN® ADC DROPS

Dietary Supplement of Vitamins A, D and C

Usage: Dietary supplement of vitamins A, D and C for infants and children under 4 years of age.

Availability:
50-ml bottles, calibrated dropper enclosed; OTC; NDC 0074-0105-04.

Dosage: One dropperful or less daily, or as directed by the physician.

Composition: One dropperful (1 ml) provides:

Vitamins		% US RDA*	% US RDA**
Vitamin A	1500 I.U.	100	60
Vitamin D	400 I.U.	100	100
Vitamin C	35 mg	100	87

Ingredients: Polysorbate 80, ascorbic acid, sodium ascorbate, vitamin A palmitate, benzoic acid (preservative), methylparaben (preservative), and ergocalciferol in a glycerin-water vehicle with added artificial color and citrus flavoring. Contains only a trace (less than ½%) of alcohol.

* % U.S. Recommended Daily Allowance for infants.

** % U.S. Recommended Daily Allowance for children under 4 years of age.

Product reformulated, November 1977

VI-DAYLIN® DROPS

Multivitamin Supplement

Usage: Multivitamin supplementation for infants and children under 4 years of age.

Availability:
50-ml bottles, calibrated dropper enclosed; OTC; NDC 0074-0103-04.

Dosage: One dropperful, or as directed by the physician.

Composition: One dropperful (1 ml) provides:

Vitamins		% US RDA*	% US RDA**
Vitamin A	1500 I.U.	100	60
Vitamin D	400 I.U.	100	100
Vitamin E	5 I.U.	100	50
Vitamin C	35 mg	100	87
Thiamine (Vitamin B_1)	0.5 mg	100	71
Riboflavin (Vitamin B_2)	0.6 mg	100	75
Niacin	8 mg	100	88
Vitamin B_6	0.4 mg	100	57
Vitamin B_{12}	1.5 mcg	75	50

This product does not contain the essential vitamin folic acid.

Ingredients: Polysorbate 80, ascorbic acid, niacinamide, dl-alpha tocopheryl acetate, benzoic acid (preservative), ferric ammonium citrate (stabilizer), vitamin A palmitate, riboflavin-5′-phosphate sodium, methylparaben (preservative), thiamine hydrochloride, disodium edetate (stabilizer), pyridoxine hydrochloride, ergocalciferol and cyanocobalamin in a glycerin-water vehicle with added artificial flavoring. Contains only a trace (less than ½%) of alcohol.

*% U.S. Recommended Daily Allowance for infants.

**% U.S. Recommended Daily Allowance for children under 4 years of age.

VI-DAYLIN®/F ADC DROPS ℞

ADC Vitamins/Fluoride

Composition: One dropperful (1 ml) provides:
Fluoride 0.25 mg

Vitamins		% US RDA*	% US RDA**
Vitamin A	1500 I.U.	100	60
Vitamin D	400 I.U.	100	100
Vitamin C	35 mg	100	87

Ingredients: Sodium ascorbate, vitamin A palmitate, ascorbic acid, ergocalciferol, sodium fluoride. Alcohol, approximately 0.4%.

* % U.S. Recommended Daily Allowance for infants.

** % U.S. Recommended Daily Allowance for children under 4 years of age.

Indications: As an aid in the prevention of dental caries in infants and children, and in the prophylaxis of Vitamins A, D and C deficiencies.

Contraindications: Should not be used where the fluoride content of the drinking water supply is known to be greater than 0.7 parts per million.

Precautions: The recommended dosage should not be exceeded since chronic overdosage of fluoride may result in mottling of tooth enamel and osseous changes. Acute overdosage of fluoride in children may cause excessive salivation and gastrointestinal disturbances.

Dosage: One dropperful daily or as directed by the physician or dentist.

Availability:
50-ml bottles, calibrated dropper enclosed; Rx; NDC 0074-1106-04.

VI-DAYLIN®/F ADC + IRON DROPS ℞

ADC Vitamins/Fluoride/Iron Supplement

Composition: One dropperful (1.0 ml) provides:
Fluoride 0.25 mg

Vitamins		% US RDA*	% US RDA**
Vitamin A	1500 I. U.	100	60
Vitamin D	400 I. U.	100	100
Vitamin C	35 mg	100	87
Minerals			
Iron	10 mg	66	100

Ingredients: Ascorbic acid, ferrous sulfate, vitamin A palmitate, sodium fluoride and ergocalciferol.

* % U.S. Recommended Daily Allowance for infants.

** % U.S. Recommended Daily Allowance for children under 4 years of age.

Indications: As an aid in the prevention of dental caries in infants and children, and in the prophylaxis of Vitamin A, D and C deficiencies while providing iron supplementation.

Contraindications: Should be used only where the fluoride content of the drinking water supply is known to be 0.7 parts per million or less.

Precautions: The recommended dosage should not be exceeded since chronic overdosage of fluoride may result in mottling of tooth enamel and osseous changes. Acute overdosage of fluoride in children may cause excessive salivation and gastrointestinal disturbances.

Dosage: One dropperful daily or as directed by physician or dentist.

Availability: 50-ml bottles, calibrated dropper enclosed; ℞; NDC 0074-8929-50.

VI-DAYLIN® /F DROPS ℞

Multivitamins/Fluoride

Composition: One dropperful (1.0 ml) provides:
Fluoride 0.25 mg

Vitamins			% US RDA*	% US RDA**
Vitamin A	1500	I.U.	100	60
Vitamin D	400	I.U.	100	100
Vitamin E	5	I.U.	100	50
Vitamin C	35	mg	100	87
Thiamine (Vitamin B_1)	0.5	mg	100	71
Riboflavin (Vitamin B_2)	0.6	mg	100	75
Niacin	8	mg	100	88
Vitamin B_6	0.4	mg	100	57

Ingredients: Ascorbic acid, niacinamide, dl-alpha-tocopheryl acetate, riboflavin-5′-phosphate sodium, sodium fluoride, vitamin A palmitate, thiamine hydrochloride, pyridoxine hydrochloride and ergocalciferol. No artificial sweeteners. Alcohol content less than 0.1%.

* % U.S. Recommended Daily Allowance for infants.

** % U.S. Recommended Daily Allowance for children under 4 years of age.

Indications: As an aid in the prevention of dental caries in infants and children, and in the prophylaxis of appropriate vitamin deficiencies.

Contraindications: Should not be used where the fluoride content of the drinking water supply is known to be greater than 0.7 parts per million.

Precautions: The recommended dosage should not be exceeded since chronic overdosage of fluoride may result in mottling of tooth enamel and osseous changes. Acute overdosage of fluoride in children may cause excessive salivation and gastrointestinal disturbances.

Dosage: One dropperful daily or as directed by the physician or dentist.

Availability: 50-ml bottles, calibrated dropper enclosed; Rx; NDC 0074-1104-04

VI-DAYLIN®/F + IRON DROPS ℞

Multivitamins/Fluoride/Iron Supplement

Composition: One dropperful (1.0 ml) provides:
Fluoride 0.25 mg

Vitamins		% US RDA*	% US RDA**
Vitamin A	1500 I.U.	100	60
Vitamin D	400 I.U.	100	100
Vitamin E	5 I.U.	100	50
Vitamin C	35 mg	100	87
Thiamine (Vitamin B_1)	0.5 mg	100	71
Riboflavin (Vitamin B_2)	0.6 mg	100	75
Niacin	8 mg	100	88
Vitamin B_6	0.4 mg	100	57
Minerals			
Iron	10 mg	66	100

Ingredients: Ascorbic acid, ferrous sulfate, niacinamide, dl-alpha tocopheryl acetate, vitamin A palmitate, riboflavin-5′-phosphate sodium, thiamine hydrochloride, sodium fluoride, pyridoxine hydrochloride and ergocalciferol.

* % U.S. Recommended Daily Allowance for infants.

** % U.S. Recommended Daily Allowance for children under 4 years of age.

Indications: As an aid in the prevention of dental caries in infants and children and in the prophylaxis of appropriate vitamin deficiencies while providing iron supplementation.

Contraindications: Should be used only where the fluoride content of the drinking water supply is known to be 0.7 parts per million or less.
Precautions: The recommended dosage should not be exceeded since chronic overdosage of fluoride may result in mottling of tooth enamel and osseous changes. Acute overdosage of fluoride in children may cause excessive salivation and gastrointestinal disturbances.
Dosage: One dropperful daily or as directed by physician or dentist.
Availability: 50-ml bottles, calibrated dropper enclosed; ℞; NDC 0074-8928-50.

VI-DAYLIN® PLUS IRON DROPS
Multivitamins/Iron Supplement

Usage: Multivitamin supplement with iron for infants and children under 4 years of age.
Availability: 50-ml bottles, calibrated dropper enclosed; OTC; NDC 0074-0116-01.
Dosage: One dropperful daily, or as directed by the physician.
Composition: One dropperful (1 ml) provides:

Vitamins			% US RDA*	% US RDA**
Vitamin A	1500	I.U.	100	60
Vitamin D	400	I.U.	100	100
Vitamin E	5	I.U.	100	50
Vitamin C	35	mg	100	87
Thiamine (Vitamin B_1)	0.5	mg	100	71
Riboflavin (Vitamin B_2)	0.6	mg	100	75
Niacin	8	mg	100	88
Vitamin B_6	0.4	mg	100	57
Vitamin B_{12}	1.5	mcg	75	50
Minerals				
Iron	10	mg	66	100

This product does not contain the essential vitamin folic acid.
Ingredients: Polysorbate 80, ascorbic acid, ferrous sulfate, niacinamide, dl-alpha tocopheryl acetate, sodium ascorbate, vitamin A palmitate, benzoic acid (preservative), riboflavin-5′-phosphate sodium, thiamine hydrochloride, methylparaben (preservative), pyridoxine hydrochloride, ergocalciferol, and cyanocobalamin in a glycerin-water vehicle with added artificial coloring and flavoring.
*% U.S. Recommended Daily Allowance for infants.
** % U.S. Recommended Daily allowance for children under 4 years of age.

VI-DAYLIN® PLUS IRON ADC DROPS
Dietary Supplement of Vitamins A, D and C with Iron

Usage: Dietary supplement of vitamins A, D and C with iron for infants and children under 4 years of age.
Availability: 50-ml bottles; calibrated dropper enclosed; OTC; NDC 0074-0117-01.
Dosage: One dropperful daily, or as directed by the physician.
Composition: One dropperful (1 ml) provides:

Vitamins			% US RDA*	% US RDA**
Vitamin A	1500	I.U.	100	60
Vitamin D	400	I.U.	100	100
Vitamin C	35	mg	100	87
Minerals				
Iron	10	mg	66	100

Ingredients: Polysorbate 80, ferrous sulfate, ascorbic acid, sodium ascorbate, vitamin A palmitate, benzoic acid (preservative), ergocalciferol, and methylparaben (preservative) in a glycerin-water vehicle with added artificial flavoring and coloring.
* % U.S. Recommended Daily Allowance for infants.
** % U.S. Recommended Daily Allowance for children under 4 years of age.
Product reformulated November, 1977

VI-DAYLIN® CHEWABLE
Multivitamin Supplement

Usage: Multivitamin supplement for children under 4 years of age, and adults and children 4 or more years of age.
Availability: 100-tablet bottles; OTC; NDC 0074-4519-13.
Dosage: One tablet daily or as directed by the physician.
Composition: Each chewable tablet contains:

Vitamins			% US RDA*	% US RDA**
Vitamin A	2500	I.U.	100	50
Vitamin D	400	I.U.	100	100
Vitamin E	15	I.U.	150	50
Vitamin C	60	mg	150	100
Folic Acid	0.3	mg	150	75
Thiamine (Vitamin B_1)	1.05	mg	150	70
Riboflavin (Vitamin B_2)	1.2	mg	150	70
Niacin	13.5	mg	150	67
Vitamin B_6	1.05	mg	150	52
Vitamin B_{12}	4.5	mcg	150	75

Ingredients: Sucrose and dextrins, sodium ascorbate, niacinamide, dl-alpha tocopheryl acetate, ascorbic acid, vitamin A palmitate, riboflavin, pyridoxine hydrochloride, thiamine mononitrate, ergocalciferol, folic acid, cyanocobalamin. Made with natural sweeteners, artificial flavoring and artificially colored with natural ingredients.
*% U.S. Recommended Daily Allowance for children under 4 years of age.
**% U.S. Recommended Daily Allowance for adults and children 4 or more years of age.
[Shown in Product Identification Section]

VI-DAYLIN® w/FLUORIDE CHEWABLE ℞
Multivitamins/Fluoride

Composition: Each Chewable tablet contains:
Fluoride (as sodium fluoride) 1 mg

Vitamins			%US RDA*	%US RDA**
Vitamin A (as palmitate, 0.75 mg)	2500	I.U.	100	50
Vitamin D (ergocalciferol, 10 mcg)	400	I.U.	100	100
Vitamin E (dl-alpha tocopheryl acetate)	15	I.U.	150	50
Vitamin C (as sodium ascorbate, 40 mg; ascorbic acid, 20 mg)	60	mg	150	100
Folic Acid	0.2	mg	100	50
Thiamine (thiamine mononitrate)	1.02	mg	150	70
Riboflavin	1.2	mg	150	70
Niacinamide	13.4	mg	150	67
Vitamin B_6 (as pyridoxine hydrochloride)	1.28	mg	150	52
Vitamin B_{12} (cyanocobalamin)	4.5	mcg	150	75

*% US Recommended Daily Allowance for children under 4 years of age.
**% US Recommended Daily Allowance for adults and children 4 or more years of age.
Indications: As an aid in the prevention of dental caries in children and in the prophylaxis of appropriate vitamin deficiencies.
Contraindications: Should not be used where the fluoride content of the drinking water supply is known to be greater than 0.7 parts per million.
Precautions: The recommended use and dosage of Vi-Daylin w/Fluoride Chewable should not be exceeded, since chronic overdosage of fluoride may result in mottling of tooth enamel and osseous changes. Acute overdosage of fluoride in children equivalent to from 10 to 20 Vi-Daylin w/Fluoride tablets may cause excessive salivation and gastrointestinal disturbances.
Dosage: One tablet daily, or as directed by the physician or dentist.
Availability: Bottles of 100 tablets; ℞; NDC 0074-7623-13
[Shown in Product Identification Section]

VI-DAYLIN® + IRON CHEWABLE
Multivitamins/Iron Supplement

Usage: Multivitamin supplement with iron for children under 4 years of age and adults and children 4 or more years of age.
Availability:
100-tablet bottles; OTC; NDC 0074-4520-13.
Dosage: One tablet daily or as directed by the physician.
Composition: Each chewable tablet contains:

Vitamins			% U.S.* RDA	% U.S.** RDA
Vitamin A	2500	I.U.	100	50
Vitamin D	400	I.U.	100	100
Vitamin E	15	I.U.	150	50
Vitamin C	60	mg	150	100
Folic Acid	0.3	mg	150	75
Thiamine (Vitamin B_1)	1.05	mg	150	70
Riboflavin (Vitamin B_2)	1.2	mg	150	70
Niacin	13.5	mg	150	67
Vitamin B_6	1.05	mg	150	52
Vitamin B_{12}	4.5	mcg	150	75
Minerals				
Iron	12	mg	120	66

Ingredients: Sucrose and dextrins, mannitol, sodium ascorbate, niacinamide, ferrous fumarate, dl-alpha tocopheryl acetate, ascorbic acid, vitamin A palmitate, riboflavin, pyridoxine hydrochloride, thiamine mononitrate, ergocalciferol, folic acid, cyanocobalamin. Made with natural sweeteners, artificial flavoring and coloring.
*% U.S. Recommended Daily Allowance for children under 4 years of age.
**%U.S. Recommended Daily Allowance for adults and children 4 or more years of age.
[Shown in Product Identification Section]

VI-DAYLIN® LIQUID
Multivitamin Supplement

Usage: Multivitamin supplement for children under 4 years of age and adults and children 4 or more years of age.
Availability:
16-fl-oz (pint) bottles; OTC; NDC 0074-3606-03.
8-fl-oz bottles; OTC; NDC 0074-3606-02.
Dosage: 1 teaspoonful daily, or as directed by the physician.
Composition: One teaspoonful (5 ml) contains:

Vitamins			% US RDA*	% US RDA**
Vitamin A	2500	I.U.	100	50
Vitamin D	400	I.U.	100	100
Vitamin E	15	I.U.	150	50
Vitamin C	60	mg	150	100
Thiamine (Vitamin B_1)	1.05	mg	150	70
Riboflavin (Vitamin B_2)	1.2	mg	150	70
Niacin	13.5	mg	150	68
Vitamin B_6	1.05	mg	150	50
Vitamin B_{12}	4.5	mcg	150	75

This product does not contain the essential vitamin folic acid.
* % U.S. Recommended Daily Allowance for children under 4 years of age.
** % U.S. Recommended Daily Allowance for adults and children 4 or more years of age.

Continued on next page

Ross—Cont.

Ingredients: Glucose, sucrose, ascorbic acid, polysorbate 80, dl-alpha tocopheryl acetate, niacinamide, acacia, cysteine hydrochloride as stabilizer, benzoic acid (preservative), vitamin A palmitate, methylparaben (preservative), pyridoxine hydrochloride, riboflavin, thiamine hydrochloride, ergocalciferol, and cyanocobalamin in a aqueous vehicle with added natural citrus flavoring and added color. Contains only a trace of alcohol (not more than ½%).

VI-DAYLIN® PLUS IRON LIQUID

Multivitamins Iron Supplement

Usage: Multivitamin supplement with iron for children under 4 years of age and adults and children 4 or more years of age.

Availability:
16-fl-oz (pint) bottles; OTC; NDC 0074-6992-03.
8-fl-oz bottles; OTC; NDC 0074-6992-02.

Dosage: 1 teaspoonful daily or as directed by the physician.

Composition: One teaspoonful (5 ml) contains:

			% US RDA*	% US RDA**
Vitamins				
Vitamin A	2500	I.U.	100	50
Vitamin D	400	I.U.	100	100
Vitamin E	15	I.U.	150	50
Vitamin C	60	mg	150	100
Thiamine (Vitamin B_1)	1:05	mg	150	70
Riboflavin (Vitamin B_2)	1.2	mg	150	70
Niacin	13.5	mg	150	68
Vitamin B_6	1.05	mg	150	50
Vitamin B_{12}	4.5	mcg	150	75
Minerals				
Iron	10	mg	100	55

This product does not contain the essential vitamin folic acid.

* % U.S. Recommended Daily Allowance for children under 4 years of age.

** % U.S. Recommended Daily Allowance for adults and children 4 or more years of age.

Ingredients: Glucose, sucrose, ascorbic acid, ferrous gluconate, polysorbate 80, dl-alpha tocopheryl acetate, niacinamide, acacia, cysteine hydrochloride as stabilizer, benzoic acid (preservative), methylparaben (preservative), vitamin A palmitate, riboflavin-5′-phosphate sodium, pyridoxine hydrochloride, thiamine hydrochloride, propylparaben (preservative), ergocalciferol, and cyanocobalamin in an aqueous vehicle with added natural citrus flavoring and added coloring. Contains only a trace of alcohol (not more than ½%).

VITAL™

Nutritionally Complete Hydrolyzed Diet

Usage: Vital is a hydrolyzed, low-residue feeding intended for use as a source of total or supplemental nutrition for patients with impaired gastrointestinal function (limited digestion/absorption). Vital has been designed to meet the nutritional needs of stressed patients with the following condition:

- Inflammatory bowel disease, including Crohn's disease and ulcerative colitis
- Preoperative bowel preparation and postoperative management
- Diagnostic procedures, such as colon radiography and colonoscopy
- Alimentary tract fistulae
- Cancer, including periods of management by radiation and chemotherapy
- Hypermetabolic conditions, such as those associated with trauma, major burns, multiple fractures, and major sepsis
- Pancreatic insufficiency states
- Short bowel syndrome
- Non specific maldigestive and malabsorptive states

Vital may be utilized not only as a full liquid diet administered by oral or gavage feeding, but also as a liquid supplement.

Features:

- Complete Nutrition—In standard dilution, Vital provides 1 Calorie per ml and 300 Calories per serving (1 packet). Caloric distribution: protein 16.7%; fat, 9.3%; carbohydrate, 74.0%. Five servings (1500 Calories) provide 100% of the U.S. RDAs for essential vitamins and minerals for adults or children 4 or more years of age.
- High levels of nitrogen—Vital provides 62.5 g of protein (10 g nitrogen) in 1500 Calories insuring high levels of available nitrogen for the stressed patient. Vital also supplies a protein system of peptides fortified with free essential amino acids designed for maximum nitrogen absorption. The total Calorie/nitrogen ratio of 150 allows for effective protein sparing and utilization and meets the Calorie/nitrogen ratio recommended for nutritional support of the catabolic patient.
- Good taste—Vital is significantly more palatable and acceptable than diets composed solely of crystalline amino acids. The mild, appealing banana flavor insures better patient acceptance of an elemental feeding with no disturbing aftertaste. The addition of Vari-Flavors® Flavor Pacs helps to combat flavor fatigue experienced by patients receiving full liquid diets and liquid supplements.
- Low osmolality—(450 mOsm/kg water) The lower osmolality of Vital may help to avoid gastrointestinal distress and dumping syndrome commonly associated with elemental feedings.
- Low fecal residue—The fecal residue produced by Vital is comparable to that produced by traditional elemental diets.
- Low Renal Solute Load—(Sodium 17 mEq/-liter, .38 g/liter; Potassium 30 mEq/liter, 1.17 g/liter; Chloride 19 mEq/liter, .67 g/liter). The electrolyte levels are appropriate for electrolyte-restricted diets, yet adequate for most hospitalized patients. Renal solute load is approximately 306 mOsm/liter at standard dilution.

Dosage and Administration:

Mixing Instructions: One packet of Vital (78 g) powder is to be mixed with 255 ml of water for standard dilution of 1 Calorie per ml. Pour 8½ ounces of hot water in a blender. Empty contents of one packet into the blender and blend at low speed until powder dissolves. Prepare no more than the amount intended for a single day's serving. Refrigerate after preparation. Shake before use. Store unopened powder in a cool, dry place. UNDER NO CIRCUMSTANCES SHOULD VITAL BE GIVEN PARENTERALLY.

Additional fluid requirements should be met by giving water orally with or after feedings, or by flushing the gavage tube.

- Gavage (tube) feeding: Initially, administration of small amounts of a 1:1 mixture of Vital and water is recommended until progressively larger amounts and less dilute concentration can be tolerated. After the adaptation period, Vital should be given in standard dilution to meet prescribed caloric needs.
- Oral feeding: Serving banana Vital chilled may enhance its banana flavor and increase palatability. Servings may provide total nutrition or supplemental nutrition with and between meals.

Availability: 2.75-oz (78 g) packets of water-soluble powder (banana flavor); 72 packets per case; No. 765.

Composition:

Ingredients: Glucose oligo- and polysaccharides, enzymatically hydrolyzed proteins (soy, whey and meat), sucrose, corn starch, sunflower oil, dipotassium phosphate, calcium glycerophosphate, L-tyrosine, natural and artificial banana and vanilla flavoring, calcium chloride, L-valine, L-leucine, L-phenylalanine, L-isoleucine, magnesium oxide, L-histidine, choline bitartrate, ascorbic acid, L-threonine, ferrous gluconate, L-tryptophan, alpha-tocopheryl acetate, L-lysine monohydrochloride, vitamin A acetate, niacinamide, calcium pantothenate, zinc oxide, vitamin D_3, manganese acetate, phylloquinone, cupric acetate, sodium riboflavin phosphate (vitamin B_2), pyridoxine hydrochloride, thiamine mononitrate (vitamin B_1), folic acid, biotin and cyanocobalamin.

Approximate Analysis: (grams)	**Per 300 Calories*** (1 packet)	**Per 1500 Calories*** (5 packets)
Protein	12.5	62.5
Fat	3.1	15.5
Carbohydrate	55.5	277.5
Minerals (ash)	1.6	8.0
Moisture	3.9	19.5

* In standard dilution (78 g of Vital [banana] powder mixed in 225 ml of water).

Vitamins/ Minerals	**Per 300 Calories**	**Per 1500 Calories**	**Percent U.S. RDA** 1500 Calories**
Vitamin A, (I.U.)	1000	5000	100
Vitamin D, (I.U.)	80	400	100
Vitamin E, (I.U.)	6	30	100
Vitamin C, mg	18	90	150
Folic acid, mg	0.08	0.4	100
Thiamine (Vitamin B_1), mg	0.3	1.5	100
Riboflavin (Vitamin B_2), mg	0.34	1.7	100
Vitamin B_6, mg	0.4	2	100
Vitamin B_{12}, mcg	1.2	6	100
Niacin, mg	4	20	100
Biotin, mg	0.06	0.3	100
Pantothenic acid, mg	2	10	100
Vitamin K_1, mg	0.4	2	***
Choline, mg	40	200	***
Calcium, mg	200	1000	100
Phosphorus, mg	200	1000	100
Sodium, mg	115	575	***
Potassium, mg	350	1750	***
Chloride, mg	200	1000	***
Magnesium, mg	80	400	100
Iodine, mcg	30	150	100
Manganese, mg	0.4	2	***
Copper, mg	0.4	2	100
Zinc, mg	3	15	100
Iron, mg	3.6	18	100

**% For adults and children 4 or more years of age.

*** % U.S. RDA not established.

IDENTIFICATION PROBLEM?

Consult PDR's

Product Identification Section

where you'll find over 900

products pictured actual size

and in full color.

Rotex Pharmaceuticals, Inc.

3102 CORRINE DRIVE
ORLANDO, FLORIDA 32803

ARTHROGESIC™ TABLETS ℞

Each tablet contains: Magnesium Salicylate 600 mg., Phenyltoloxamine Citrate 30 mg. (NDC 31190-006-01).

NASALSPAN® ℞

Each capsule contains: Chlorpheniramine Maleate 8 mg., d-Pseudoephedrine Hydrochloride 120 mg. (NDC 31190-002-01).

NASALSPAN® EXPECTORANT ℞

Each teaspoonful (5 cc) contains: Pseudoephedrine HCl 30 mg., Dextromethorphan 10 mg., Guaifenesin 50 mg., Sodium Citrate 75 mg., Citric Acid 20 mg. (NDC 31190-007-01).

PODILIQUID® ℞

Each teaspoonful (5 ml) contains: Niacin 50 mg., Glycine 500 mg. in a Palatable Sherry Wine Base. Contains 15% alcohol by volume (NDC 31190-044-01).

ROPRES™ ℞

Each tablet contains: Trichlormethiazide 4 mg., Reserpine 0.1 mg. (NDC 31190-003-01).

ROTHAV®-150 ℞

Each tablet contains: Ethaverine Hydrochloride 150 mg. (NDC 31190-001-01).

ROVITE™

Each tablet contains: Ascorbic Acid 500 mg., Thiamine HCl (Vitamin B-1) 50 mg., Riboflavin (Vitamin B-2) 25 mg., Pyridoxine HCl (Vitamin B-6) 50 mg., Pantothenic Acid as Calcium Panthothenate 50 mg., Niacinamide 50 mg., Vitamin B-12 10 mcg., Zinc Sulfate 40 mg., Magnesium Sulfate 35 mg. (NDC 31190-005-01).

Rowell Laboratories, Inc.

210 MAIN STREET W.
BAUDETTE, MN 56623

COLREX COMPOUND CAPSULES™ Ⓒ
COLREX COMPOUND ELIXIR™ Ⓒ

Composition: COLREX COMPOUND CAPSULES—Codeine Phosphate*, 16 mg.; Acetaminophen, 325 mg.; Phenylephrine HCl, 10 mg.; Chlorpheniramine Maleate, 2 mg.
COLREX COMPOUND ELIXIR—Codeine Phosphate*, 8 mg.; Acetaminophen, 120 mg.; Chlorpheniramine Maleate, 1 mg.; Phenylephrine HCl, 5 mg.; Alcohol 9.5% v/v. SUGAR FREE.
*WARNING: May be habit forming.
Action and Uses: COLREX COMPOUND combines antitussive, antihistaminic, decongestant, analgesic and antipyretic actions.
Indications: Adjunct for temporary relief of cough, congestion, headache and muscle soreness of common colds and upper respiratory infections. Infections should be identified and, if bacterial, given appropriate antimicrobial therapy.
Precautions: Codeine may cause constipation, and an occasional patient may display idiosyncratic response to it. Chlorpheniramine, especially with codeine, may cause drowsiness; use with caution in patients who operate machinery. Phenylephrine may cause gastric upset and, because of its sympathomimetic effect, should be used with caution in cardiovascular disease, thyrotoxicosis and diabetes.
Dosages: COLREX COMPOUND CAPSULES—Adults, 1 or 2 capsules three or four times daily. Children 6 to 12, 1 capsule three or four times daily. Not recommended for children under 6.
COLREX COMPOUND ELIXIR—Children 2 to 6, 1 teaspoonful three or four times daily. Children 6 to 12, 2 teaspoonsful three or four times daily. Adults, 2 to 4 teaspoonsful three or four times daily.
How Supplied: CAPSULES—Yellow, imprinted "ROWELL 0840".
In bottles of 100 and 1000; ELIXIR—In bottles of 60 ml., 480 ml., 1 gallon.

CORTENEMA® ℞
(Hydrocortisone Retention Enema)
Disposable Unit for Rectal Use Only

Each disposable unit (60 ml.) contains: Hydrocortisone, 100 mg. in an aqueous solution containing carboxypolymethylene, polysorbate 80, and methylparaben, 0.18% as a preservative.
Description: CORTENEMA is a convenient disposable single-dose hydrocortisone enema designed for ease of self-administration. Hydrocortisone is a naturally occurring glucocorticoid (adrenal corticosteroid), which similarly as its acetate and sodium hemisuccinate derivatives, is partially absorbed following rectal administration. Absorption studies in ulcerative colitis patients have shown up to 50% absorption of hydrocortisone administered as CORTENEMA and up to 30% of hydrocortisone acetate administered in an identical vehicle.
Actions: CORTENEMA provides the potent anti-inflammatory effect of hydrocortisone. Because this drug is absorbed from the colon, it acts both topically and systemically. Although rectal hydrocortisone, used as recommended for CORTENEMA, has a low incidence of reported adverse reactions, prolonged use presumably may cause systemic reactions associated with oral dosage forms.
Indications: CORTENEMA is indicated as adjunctive therapy in the treatment of ulcerative colitis, especially distal forms, including ulcerative proctitis, ulcerative proctosigmoiditis, and left-sided ulcerative colitis. It has proved useful also in some cases involving the transverse and descending colons.
Contraindications: Systemic fungal infections; and ileocolostomy during the immediate or early postoperative period.
Warnings: In severe ulcerative colitis, it is hazardous to delay needed surgery while awaiting response to medical treatment.
Damage to the rectal wall can result from careless or improper insertion of an enema tip.
In patients on corticosteroid therapy subjected to unusual stress, increased dosage of rapidly acting corticosteroids before, during, and after the stressful situation is indicated.
Corticosteroids may mask some signs of infection, and new infections may appear during their use. There may be decreased resistance and inability to localize infection when corticosteroids are used.
Prolonged use of corticosteroids may produce posterior subcapsular cataracts, glaucoma with possible damage to the optic nerves, and may enhance the establishment of secondary ocular infections due to fungi or viruses.
Usage in pregnancy: Since adequate human reproduction studies have not been done with corticosteroids, the use of these drugs in pregnancy, nursing mothers or women of childbearing potential requires that the possible benefits of the drug be weighed against the potential hazards to the mother and embryo or fetus. Infants born of mothers who have received substantial doses of corticosteroids during pregnancy, should be carefully observed for signs of hypoadrenalism.
Average and large doses of hydrocortisone or cortisone can cause elevation of blood pressure, salt and water retention, and increased excretion of potassium. These effects are less likely to occur with the synthetic derivatives except when used in large doses. Dietary salt restriction and potassium supplementation may be necessary. All corticosteroids increase calcium excretion.
<u>While on corticosteroid therapy patients should not be vaccinated against smallpox. Other immunization procedures should not be undertaken in patients who are on corticosteroids, especially on high dose, because of possible hazards of neurological complications and a lack of antibody response.</u>
If corticosteroids are indicated in patients with latent tuberculosis or tuberculin reactivity, close observation is necessary as reactivation of the disease may occur. During prolonged corticosteroid therapy, these patients should receive chemoprophylaxis.
Precautions: CORTENEMA Hydrocortisone Retention Enema should be used with caution where there is a probability of impending perforation, abscess or other pyogenic infection; fresh intestinal anastomoses; obstruction; or extensive fistulas and sinus tracts. Use with caution in presence of active or latent peptic ulcer; diverticulitis; renal insufficiency; hypertension; osteoporosis; and myasthenia gravis.
Steroid therapy might impair prognosis in surgery by increasing the hazard of infection. If infection is suspected, appropriate antibiotic therapy must be administered, usually in larger than ordinary doses.
Drug-induced secondary adrenocortical insufficiency may occur with prolonged CORTENEMA therapy. This is minimized by gradual reduction of dosage. This type of relative insufficiency may persist for months after discontinuation of therapy; therefore, in any situation of stress occurring during that period, hormone therapy should be reinstituted. Since mineralocorticoid secretion may be impaired, salt and/or a mineralocorticoid should be administered concurrently.
There is an enhanced effect of corticosteroids on patients with hypothyroidism and in those with cirrhosis.
Corticosteroids should be used cautiously in patients with ocular herpes simplex because of possible corneal perforation.
The lowest possible dose of corticosteroid should be used to control the condition under treatment, and when reduction in dosage is possible, the reduction should be gradual.
Psychic derangement may appear when corticosteroids are used, ranging from euphoria, insomnia, mood swings, personality changes, and severe depression, to frank psychotic manifestations. Also, existing emotional instability or psychotic tendencies may be aggravated by corticosteroids.
Aspirin should be used cautiously in conjunction with corticosteroids in hypoprothrombinemia.
Growth and development of infants and children on prolonged corticosteroid therapy should be carefully observed.
Adverse Reactions: Local pain or burning, and rectal bleeding attributed to CORTENEMA have been reported rarely. Apparent exacerbtions or sensitivity reactions also occur rarely. The following adverse reactions should be kept in mind whenever corticosteroids are given by rectal administration.
<u>Fluid and Electrolyte Disturbances:</u> Sodium retention; fluid retention; congestive heart failure in susceptible patients; potassium loss; hypokalemic alkalosis; hypertension. <u>Musculoskeletal:</u> Muscle Weakness; steroid myopathy; loss of muscle mass; osteoporosis; vertebral compression fractures; aseptic necrosis of femoral and humeral heads; pathologic fracture of long bones. <u>Gastrointestinal:</u> Peptic ulcer with possible perforation and hemorrhage; pancrea-

Continued on next page

Rowell—Cont.

titis; abdominal distention; ulcerative esophagitis. Dermatologic: Impaired wound healing; thin fragile skin; petechiae and ecchymoses; facial erythema; increased sweating; may suppress reactions to skin tests. Neurological: Convulsions; increased intracranial pressure with papilledema (pseudo-tumor cerebri) usually after treatment; vertigo; headache. Endocrine: Menstrual irregularities; development of Cushingoid state; suppression of growth in children; secondary adrenocortical and pituitary unresponsiveness, particularly in times of stress, as in trauma, surgery or illness; decreased carbohydrate tolerance; manifestations of latent diabetes mellitus; increased requirements for insulin or oral hypoglycemic agents in diabetics. Ophthalmic: Posterior subcapsular cataracts; increased intraocular pressure; glaucoma; exophthalmos. Metabolic: Negative nitrogen balance due to protein catabolism.

Dosage and Administration: The use of CORTENEMA Hydrocortisone Retention Enema is predicated upon the concomitant use of modern supportive measures such as rational dietary control, sedatives, anti-diarrheal agents, antibacterial therapy, blood replacement if necessary, etc.

The usual course of therapy is one CORTENEMA nightly for 21 days, or until the patient comes into remission both clinically and proctologically. Clinical symptoms usually subside promptly within 3 to 5 days. Improvement in the appearance of the mucosa, as seen by sigmoidoscopic examination, may lag somewhat behind clinical improvement. Difficult cases may require as long as 2 or 3 months of CORTENEMA treatment. Where the course of therapy extends beyond 21 days, CORTENEMA should be discontinued gradually by reducing administration to every other night for 2 or 3 weeks.

If clinical or proctologic improvement fail to occur within 2 or 3 weeks after starting CORTENEMA, discontinue its use.

Symptomatic improvement, evidenced by decreased diarrhea and bleeding; weight gain; improved appetite; lessened fever; and decrease in leukocytosis, may be misleading and should not be used as the sole criterion in judging efficacy. Sigmoidoscopic examination and X-ray visualization are essential for adequate monitoring of ulcerative colitis. Biopsy is useful for differential diagnosis.

Patient instructions for administering CORTENEMA are enclosed in each box of seven units. We recommend that the patient lie on his left side during administration and for 30 minutes thereafter, so that the fluid will distribute throughout the left colon. Every effort should be made to retain the enema for at least an hour and, preferably, all night. This may be facilitated by prior sedation and/or antidiarrheal medication, especially early in therapy, when the urge to evacuate is great.

How Supplied: CORTENEMA Hydrocortisone 100 mg. Retention Enema is supplied as disposable single-dose bottles with lubricated rectal applicator tips, in boxes of seven × 60 ml. (NDC 0032-1904-82) and boxes of one × 60 ml. (NDC 0032-1904-73).

DERMACORT® CREAM ℞
(Buffered 1% Hydrocortisone Cream)
DERMACORT® LOTION 0.5%
(Buffered 0.5% Hydrocortisone Lotion)

Composition: 0.5% hydrocortisone (lotion) 1% hydrocortisone (cream), stearyl alcohol, cetyl alcohol, isopropyl palmitate, citric acid, polyoxyethylene 40 stearate, sodium phosphate, propylene glycol, water, and sorbic acid as a preservative.

Actions: Topical steroids are primarily effective because of their anti-inflammatory, antipruritic and vasoconstrictive actions.

Indications: For relief of the inflammatory manifestations of corticosteroid-responsive dermatoses.

Contraindications: Topical steroids are contraindicated in those patients with a history of hypersensitivity to any of the components of DERMACORT CREAM.

Precautions: If irritation develops, the product should be discontinued and appropriate therapy instituted.

In the presence of an infection, the use of an appropriate antifungal or antibacterial agent should be instituted. If a favorable response does not occur promptly, the corticosteroid should be discontinued until the infection has been adequately controlled.

If extensive areas are treated or if the occlusive technique is used, there will be increased systemic absorption of the corticosteroid and suitable precautions should be taken, particularly in children and infants.

Although topical steroids have not been reported to have an adverse effect on human pregnancy, the safety of their use in pregnant women has not absolutely been established. In laboratory animals, increases in incidence of fetal abnormalities have been associated with exposure of gestating females to topical corticosteroids, in some cases at rather low dosage levels. Therefore, drugs of this class should not be used extensively on pregnant patients, in large amounts, or for prolonged periods of time.

The product is not for ophthalmic use.

Adverse Reactions: The following local adverse reactions have been reported with topical corticosteroids, especially under occlusive dressings: Burning, Itching, Irritation, Dryness, Folliculitis, Hypertrichosis, Acneiform eruptions, Hypopigmentation, Perioral dermatitis, Allergic contact dermatitis, Maceration of the skin, Secondary infection, Skin atrophy, Striae and Miliaria.

Dosage and Administration: Apply to affected areas 3 or 4 times daily. When a favorable response is obtained, reduce dosage gradually and eventually discontinue.

How Supplied: Dermacort Lotion (0.5% Hydrocortisone) in 4 oz plastic squeeze bottle, Dermacort Cream (1% Hydrocortisone) in one pound jar.

DEXONE™ ℞
(Dexamethasone Tablets)

How Supplied:
DEXONE 0.5™ (Dexamethasone 0.5mg) (yellow) embossed "ROWELL 3205"
DEXONE 0.75™ (Dexamethasone 0.75mg) (blue) embossed "ROWELL 3210"
DEXONE 1.5™ (Dexamethasone 1.5mg) (pink) embossed "ROWELL 3215"
DEXONE 4™ (Dexamethasone 4.0 mg) (white) embossed "ROWELL 3220"
Each supplied in bottles of 100's and in unit-dose boxes of 100.

HYDROCIL® PLAIN

A powder containing 50% blond psyllium coating dispersed in pure dextrose.

Hydrocil® is a bulk former useful in the treatment of mild to moderate constipation, nonspecific diarrhea and obesity.

Directions: The usual adult dose of Hydrocil® is one rounded to heaping teaspoonful, briskly stirred in water, milk, fruit juice or other suitable liquid, morning and evening. Follow each dose with another glass of liquid and drink ample amounts of liquid (6–8 glasses) throughout the day. Since Hydrocil® is not a laxative in the usual sense, several days usage may be required for fully satisfactory results.

Keep Hydrocil® and all drugs out of the reach of children. In case of accidental overdose, seek professional assistance or contact a Poison Control Center immediately.

How Supplied: 16 oz. jars.

HYDROCIL® FORTIFIED

A powder containing 50% blond psyllium coating dispersed in pure dextrose, fortified with 30 mg. casanthranol per 6 gm. as a mild laxative. Hydrocil® Fortified provides a mild laxative effect combined with moist, lubricating bulk. It is useful in the treatment of constipation and other conditions as directed by the physician.

Directions: The usual adult dose of Hydrocil® Fortified is one rounded to heaping teaspoonful, briskly stirred in water, milk, fruit juice or other suitable liquid, morning and evening. Follow each dose with another glass of liquid and drink ample amounts of liquid (6–8 glasses) throughout the day.

Warning: Not to be used when abdominal pain, nausea or vomiting are present. Frequent or continued use of this preparation may result in dependence on laxatives.

Keep Hydrocil® Fortified and all drugs out of the reach of children. In case of accidental overdose, seek professional assistance or contact a Poison Control Center immediately.

How Supplied: 16 oz. jars.

LITHONATE® Capsules ℞
LITHOTABS™ Tablets ℞
LITHOBID™ Slow Release Tablets ℞
(not USP)
Brands of Lithium Carbonate
LITHONATE-S™ Syrup ℞
Brand of Lithium Citrate

For Control of Manic Episodes in Manic-Depressive Psychosis.

Caution: Federal law prohibits dispensing without prescription.

> **WARNING**
> Lithium toxicity is closely related to serum lithium levels, and can occur at doses close to therapeutic levels. Facilities for prompt and accurate serum lithium determinations should be available before initiating therapy.

Description:
LITHONATE: Each peach-colored capsule contains 300 mg of lithium carbonate.
LITHOTABS: Each scored white tablet contains 300 mg of lithium carbonate.
LITHOBID: Each film-coated slow-release tablet contains 300 mg of lithium carbonate, 40 mg of sodium chloride, equivalent to 15.7 mg of sodium. This slowly dissolving film-coated tablet is designed to give post-administration serum lithium peaks lower than obtained with conventional oral lithium dosage forms.
LITHONATE-S: Each 5 ml of this lithium citrate syrup contains 8 mEq of lithium ion (Li^+), equivalent to the amount of lithium in 300 mg of lithium carbonate.

Lithium carbonate is a white, light, alkaline powder with molecular formula Li_2CO_3 and molecular weight 73.89. Lithium is an element of the alkali-metal group with atomic number 3, atomic weight 6.94 and an emission line at 671 nm on the flame photometer.

Lithium citrate is prepared in solution from lithium hydroxide and citric acid in a ratio approximating di-lithium citrate.

Indications: Lithium is indicated in the treatment of manic episodes of manic depressive illness. Maintenance therapy prevents or diminishes the intensity of subsequent episodes in those manic-depressive patients with a history of mania.

Typical symptoms of mania include pressure of speech, motor hyperactivity, reduced need for sleep, flight of ideas, grandiosity, elation, poor judgment, aggressiveness, and possibly hostility. When given to a patient experiencing a manic episode, lithium may produce a normalization of symptomatology within 1 to 3 weeks.

Warnings: Lithium should generally not be given to patients with significant renal or cardiovascular disease, severe debilitation or dehydration, or sodium depletion, and to patients receiving diuretics, since the risk of lithium toxicity is very high in such patients. If the psychiatric indication is life-threatening, and if such a patient fails to respond to other measures, lithium treatment may be undertaken with extreme caution, including daily serum lithium determinations and adjustment to the usually low doses ordinarily tolerated by these individuals. In such instances, hospitalization is a necessity.

Lithium toxicity is closely related to serum lithium levels, and can occur at doses close to therapeutic levels (see DOSAGE AND ADMINISTRATION).

Lithium therapy has been reported in some cases to be associated with morphologic changes in the kidneys. The relationship between such changes and renal function has not been established.

Outpatients and their families should be warned that the patient must discontinue lithium therapy and contact his physician if such clinical signs of lithium toxicity as diarrhea, vomiting, tremor, mild ataxia, drowsiness, or muscular weakness occur.

Combined use of haloperidol and lithium: An encephalopathic syndrome (characterized by weakness, lethargy, fever, tremulousness and confusion, extrapyramidal symptoms, leucocytosis, elevated serum enzymes, BUN and FBS) followed by irreversible brain damage has occurred in a few patients treated with lithium plus haloperidol. A causal relationship between these events and the concomitant administration of lithium and haloperidol has not been established; however, patients receiving such combined therapy should be monitored closely for early evidence of neurological toxicity and treatment discontinued promptly if such signs appear.

Usage in Pregnancy: Adverse effects on nidation in rats, embryo viability in mice, and metabolism in-vitro of rat testis and human spermatozoa have been attributed to lithium, as have teratogenicity in submammalian species and cleft palates in mice. Studies in rats, rabbits and monkeys have shown no evidence of lithium-induced teratology.

There are lithium birth registries in the United States and elsewhere; however there are at the present time insufficient data to determine the effects of lithium on human fetuses. Therefore, at this point, lithium should not be used in pregnancy, especially the first trimester, unless in the opinion of the physician, the potential benefits outweigh the possible hazards.

Usage in Children: Since information regarding the safety and effectiveness of lithium in children under 12 years of age is not available, its use in such patients is not recommended at this time.

Precautions: The ability to tolerate lithium is greater during the acute manic phase and decreases when manic symptoms subside (see DOSAGE AND ADMINISTRATION)

The distribution space of lithium approximates that of total body water. Lithium is primarily excreted in urine with insignificant excretion in feces. Renal excretion of lithium is proportional to its plasma concentration. The half-elimination time of lithium is approximately 24 hours. Lithium decreases sodium reabsorption by the renal tubules which could lead to sodium depletion. Therefore, it is essential for the patient to maintain a normal diet, including salt, and an adequate fluid intake (2500–3000 ml.) at least during the initial stabilization period. Decreased tolerance to lithium has been reported to ensue from protracted sweating or diarrhea and, if such occur, supplemental fluid and salt should be administered.

In addition to sweating and diarrhea, concomitant infection with elevated temperatures may also necessitate a temporary reduction or cessation of medication.

Adverse Reactions: Adverse reactions are seldom encountered at serum lithium levels below 1.5 mEq./l., except in the occasional patient sensitive to lithium. Mild to moderate toxic reactions may occur at levels from 1.5 – 2.5 mEq./l., and moderate to severe reactions may be seen at levels from 2.0 – 2.5 mEq./l., depending upon individual response to the drug.

Fine hand tremor, polyuria and mild thirst may occur during initial therapy for the acute manic phase, and may persist throughout treatment. Transient and mild nausea and general discomfort may also appear during the first few days of lithium administration.

These side effects are an inconvenience rather than a disabling condition, and usually subside with continued treatment or a temporary reduction or cessation of dosage. If persistent, a cessation of dosage is indicated.

Diarrhea, vomiting, drowsiness, muscular weakness and lack of coordination may be early signs of lithium intoxication, and can occur at lithium levels below 2.0 mEq./l. At higher levels, giddiness, ataxia, blurred vision, tinnitus and a large output of dilute urine may be seen. Serum lithium levels above 3.0 mEq./l. may produce a complex clinical picture involving multiple organs and organ systems. Serum lithium levels should not be permitted to exceed 2.0 mEq./l. during the acute treatment phase.

The following toxic reactions have been reported and appear to be related to serum lithium levels.

Neuromuscular: tremor, muscle hyperirritability (fasciculations, twitching, clonic movements of whole limbs), ataxia, choreoathetotic movements, hyperactive deep tendon reflexes.

Central Nervous System: blackout spells, epileptiform seizures, slurred speech, dizziness, vertigo, incontinence of urine or feces, somnolence, psychomotor retardation, restlessness, confusion, stupor, coma.

Cardiovascular: cardiac arrhythmia, hypotension, peripheral circulatory collapse.

Gastrointestinal: anorexia, nausea, vomiting, diarrhea.

Genitourinary: albuminuria, oliguria, polyuria, glycosuria.

Dermatologic: drying and thinning of hair, anesthesia of skin, chronic folliculitis, xerosis cutis.

Autonomic Nervous System: blurred vision, dry mouth.

Miscellaneous: fatigue, lethargy, tendency to sleep, dehydration, weight loss, transient scotomata.

Thyroid Abnormalities: Euthyroid goiter and/or hypothyroidism (including myxedema) accompanied by lower T_3 and T_4. I_{131}iodine uptake may be elevated. Underlying thyroid disorders do not constitute a contraindication to lithium treatment; careful monitoring of thyroid function during lithium stabilization and maintenance allows for correction of changing thyroid parameters, if any. They can be treated by prescribing thyroid in these cases.

EEG Changes: diffuse slowing, widening of frequency spectrum, potentiation and disorganization of background rhythm.

EKG Changes: reversible flattening, isoelectricity or inversion of T-waves.

Miscellaneous reactions unrelated to dosage are: transient electroencephalographic and electrocardiographic changes, leucocytosis, headache, diffuse nontoxic goiter with or without hypothyroidism, transient hyperglycemia, generalized pruritis with or without rash, cutaneous ulcers, albuminuria, worsening of organic brain syndromes, excessive weight gain, edematous swelling of ankles or wrists, and thirst or polyuria, sometimes resembling diabetes insipidus.

A single report has been received of the development of painful discoloration of fingers and toes and coldness of the extremities within one day of the starting of treatment of lithium. The mechanism through which these symptoms (resembling Raynaud's Syndrome) developed is not known. Recovery followed discontinuance.

Dosage and Administration:

Acute Mania: Optimal patient response can usually be established and maintained with the following dosages:

LITHONATE	600 mg t.i.d.
LITHOTABS	600 mg t.i.d.
LITHOBID	900 mg b.i.d. or 600 mg t.i.d. (1800 mg per day)
LITHONATE-S	10 ml(2 teaspoons) (16 mEq of lithium) t.i.d.

Such doses will normally produce an effective serum lithium level ranging between 1.0 and 1.5 mEq./l. Dosage must be individualized according to serum levels and clinical response. Regular monitoring of the patient's clinical state and of serum lithium levels is necessary. Serum levels should be determined twice per week during the acute phase, and until the serum level and clinical condition of the patient have been stabilized.

Long-term Control: The desirable serum lithium levels are 0.6 to 1.2 mEq./l. Dosage will vary from one individual to another, but usually the following will maintain this level:

LITHONATE	300 mg t.i.d. or q.i.d.
LITHOTABS	300 mg t.i.d. or q.i.d.
LITHOBID	900 mg to 1200 mg per day given in two or three divided doses.
LITHONATE-S	5 ml (1 teaspoon) (8 mEq of lithium) t.i.d. or q.i.d.

Serum lithium levels in uncomplicated cases receiving maintenance therapy during remission should be monitored at least every two months.

Patients abnormally sensitive to lithium may exhibit toxic signs at serum levels of 1.0 to 1.5 mEq./l. Elderly patients often respond to reduced dosage, and may exhibit signs of toxicity at serum levels ordinarily tolerated by other patients.

N. B.: Blood samples for serum lithium determinations are drawn 8 – 12 hours after the previous dose when lithium concentrations are relatively stable. Total reliance must not be placed on serum levels alone. Accurate patient evaluation requires both clinical and laboratory analysis.

Overdosage: The toxic levels for lithium are close to the therapeutic levels. It is therefore important that patients and their families be cautioned to watch for early toxic symptoms and to discontinue the drug and inform the physician should they occur. Toxic symptoms are listed in detail under ADVERSE REACTIONS.

Treatment: No specific antidote for lithium poisoning is known. Early symptoms of lithium toxicity can usually be treated by reduction or cessation of dosage of the drug and resumption of the treatment at a lower dose after 24 to 48 hours. In severe cases of lithium poisoning, the first and foremost goal of treatment consists of elimination of this ion from the organism.

Treatment is essentially the same as that used in barbiturate poisoning: 1) lavage. 2) correction of fluid and electrolyte imbalance and 3) regulation of kidney functioning. Urea, mannitol, and aminophylline all produce significant increases in lithium excretion. Infection pro-

Continued on next page

Rowell—Cont.

phylaxis, regular chest X-rays, and preservation of adequate respiration are essential.

How Supplied:
LITHONATE (Lithium Carbonate 300 mg) peach colored, No. 2 capsules, imprinted "ROWELL 7512" in red are supplied in bottles of 100's (unit-of-use) and 1000's, and in unit-dose boxes of 100's.
LITHOTABS (Lithium Carbonate 300 mg) scored, white tablets embossed "ROWELL 7516" are supplied in bottles of 100's and 1000's
LITHOBID (Lithium Carbonate 300 mg.) peach-colored, slow-release tablets, imprinted "ROWELL 7514" in red, are supplied in bottles of 100's & 1000's.
LITHONATE-S Lithium Citrate Syrup, 8 mEq of lithium ion per 5 ml (1 teaspoon) is supplied as a sugar-free, raspberry-flavored syrup in bottles of 480 ml.

ORASONE™ ℞
(Prednisone Tablets)

How Supplied:
ORASONE 1™ (Prednisone 1 mg) (pink)
ORASONE 5™ (Prednisone 5 mg) (white)
ORASONE 10™ (Prednisone 10 mg) (blue)
ORASONE 20™ (Prednisone 20 mg) (yellow)
ORASONE 50™ (Prednisone 50 mg) (white)
Each Supplied in bottles of 100's and 1000's and in unit-dose boxes of 100. Tablets are color coded and monogrammed with "ROWELL" and mg strength.

PERIFOAM®

Description: **PERIFOAM** — *Anesthetic, antipruritic, fungistatic, bacteriostatic* — is an efficient aid to male and female personal hygiene in both home and hospital care. Its pure white aerosol foam is transformed quickly to a non-staining, non-oily, self-drying liquid that cleans, deodorizes and soothes sensitive rectal and outer vaginal surfaces. Proven topical anesthetic action, "non-'caine" and non-steroid, also adds temporary relief of surface pain and itching.

Indications For Use: To increase comfort and cleanliness and to prevent itching and scratching which might lead to injury, inflammation or infection of anorectal or vulvovaginal surfaces. Specifically: *After hemorrhoidectomy* and in the care of *external hemorrhoids* and *pruritus ani* or *pruritus scroti. After episiotomy* and in the care of *pruritus vulvae.* Also for temporary relief of anogenital tenderness from diarrhea, constipation or faulty perineal hygiene.

Formulation: Benzalkonium Cl 0.1%, Pramoxine HCl 1.0%, Allantoin 0.3%, Methylparaben 0.15%, Propylparaben 0.05%, Solubilized Lanolin, Witch Hazel 35% (Alcohol approximately 5%) and purified water q.s. to 100%. Also environmentally safe propellant (0.23 oz.) which evaporates on release.

Topical Application: Release a small quantity of **PERIFOAM** — about the size of a quarter — on toilet paper, cleansing tissue, cotton or fingertip. Apply to sensitive anorectal, scrotal or outer vaginal surface. **PERIFOAM** dries by itself and requires no wiping. It may be used as often as needed—both in self-care at home and in office or hospital care of proctologic, postoperative, postpartum and gynecologic patients.

Precautions: For topical anogenital use only—avoid contact with eyes or in nose. Not for prolonged use—if itching or discomfort persists, or if rash or irritation develops, use of **PERIFOAM** should be stopped and the patient should consult his or her physician. Keep all aerosol containers away from heat and keep all medications out of children's reach.

Supplied: **PERIFOAM** is available without ℞ at pharmacies in 1½ oz. aerosol containers.

PROCTOCORT™ ℞
(Buffered 1% Hydrocortisone Cream)

Description: PROCTOCORT Cream is a soothing, non-staining, water-miscible preparation that is buffered to pH 5.0. It contains 1% hydrocortisone in a base containing stearyl alcohol, polyoxyethylene 40 stearate, sodium phosphate, cetyl alcohol, isopropyl palmitate, citric acid, propylene glycol, water, and sorbic acid as a preservative.

Actions: Topical steroids are primarily effective because of their anti-inflammatory, antipruritic, and vasoconstrictive actions.

Indications: For relief of the inflammatory manifestations of corticosteroid-responsive dermatoses.

Contraindications: Topical steroids are contraindicated in those patients with a history of hypersensitivity to any of the components of PROCTOCORT Cream.

Precautions: If irritation develops, the product should be discontinued and appropriate therapy instituted.
In the presence of an infection, the use of an appropriate antifungal or antibacterial agent should be instituted. If a favorable response does not occur promptly, the corticosteroid should be discontinued until the infection has been adequately controlled.
If extensive areas are treated or if the occlusive technique is used, there will be increased systemic absorption of the corticosteroid and suitable precautions should be taken, particularly in children and infants.
Although topical steroids have not been reported to have an adverse effect on human pregnancy, the safety of their use in pregnant women has not absolutely been established. In laboratory animals, increases in incidence of fetal abnormalities have been associated with exposure of gestating females to topical corticosteroids, in some cases at rather low dosage levels. Therefore, drugs of this class should not be used extensively on pregnant patients, in large amounts, or for prolonged periods of time.
The product is not for ophthalmic use.

Adverse Reactions: The following local adverse reactions have been reported with topical corticosteroids, especially under occlusive dressings: Burning, Itching, Irritation, Dryness, Folliculitis, Hypertrichosis, Acneiform eruptions, Hypopigmentation, Perioral dermatitis, Allergic contact dermatitis, Maceration of the skin, Secondary Infection, Skin atrophy, Striae and Miliaria.

Dosage and Administration: Apply to affected areas 3 or 4 times daily. When a favorable response is obtained, reduce dosage gradually and eventually discontinue.

How Supplied: 30 Gram tubes with patient instructions, 12 finger cots and a rectal applicator.

PROCTODON™
(Buffered 1% Diperodon Cream)

Composition: Diperodon HCl 1% and vitamins A and D in a soft, water-miscible cream base.

Action and Uses: PROCTODON provides the local anesthetic action of diperodon HCl, the healing effects of vitamins A and D and the lubricant effect of the soft, cream base buffered to pH 5.5. The buffer re-establishes the normal acidity of the skin and counteracts the alkalinity frequently encountered in the conditions treated. As a lubricant and anesthetic, PROCTODON facilitates rectal digital examinations and alleviates the pain of postoperative bowel movements. Applied to the wound edges, PROCTODON eliminates much of the pain following repair of fistula in ano and pilonidal cyst. It is useful pre- and postoperatively in hemorrhoidectomy and after incision of thrombosed or sclerosed anorectal veins. External or internal application is useful for relief of pain or itching associated with proctitis, papillitis, cryptitis, uncomplicated hemorrhoids and pruritis ani.

Precautions: Where rectal applicator is used, exert great care to avoid injury to rectal wall. If signs of allergic reaction occur, discontinue medication. Burning or stinging may occur in an occasional patient. Irritation or allergic reactions are rarely encountered.

Administration and Dosage: Apply liberally to the affected area, two to four times daily, or in the case of postoperative wound treatment, whenever the dressing is changed. For internal use, PROCTODON may be administered with a lubricated rectal applicator (see precautions) or with a "finger cot".

How Supplied: 30 gram tubes with patient instructions, 12 finger cots and a rectal applicator.

VIO-BEC®
(Therapeutic B Complex with C)

Composition:

Thiamine Mononitrate (B_1)	25 mg.
Riboflavin (B_2)	25 mg.
Pyridoxine HCl (B_6)	25 mg.
Calcium Pantothenate	40 mg.
Niacinamide	100 mg.
Ascorbic Acid	500 mg.

VIO-BEC is a high-potency therapeutic source of B complex vitamins and Vitamin C. It contains only synthetic vitamins (no liver or yeast), therefore, is well tolerated and does not produce unpleasant aftertaste. It does not contain Vitamin B-12 or Folic Acid for they are known to interfere with accurate diagnosis of hematologic status. VIO-BEC is promoted to the medical profession only, for use in conditions requiring high-potency nutritional supplementation.

Action and Uses: VIO-BEC is indicated for treatment of deficiencies in vitamin B complex and vitamin C. It is recommended as a part of the therapeutic regimen in alcoholism, chronic illness, malnutrition, surgery (particularly of the G. I. tract), and other stress conditions leading to increased nutritional demands. Subclinical nutritional deficiencies characterized by anorexia, irritability, fatigability, nervousness and weakness may respond to VIO-BEC.

Dosage: One VIO-BEC capsule daily.

How Supplied: Capsules (brown, imprinted "ROWELL 1216") in bottles of 30, 100, and 1000 and unit dose boxes of 100.

VIO-BEC FORTE™ ℞
Therapeutic B-Complex with Folic Acid, C, E, Zinc and Copper

Composition: Each film-coated tablet contains: Thiamine Mononitrate (B-1) 25 mg., Riboflavin (B-2) 25 mg., Pyridoxine Hydrochloride (B-6) 25 mg., Ascorbic Acid (C) 500 mg., Calcium Pantothenate 40 mg., Nicotinamide 100 mg., dl-alpha Tocopheryl Acetate N.F. (E) 30 I.U., Cyanocobalamin (B-12) 5 mcg., Folic Acid 0.5 mg., Zinc 25 mg. (from Zinc Sulfate), Copper 3 mg. (from Copper Sulfate).

Warnings: Folic acid alone is inappropriate in therapy of pernicious anemia and other megaloblastic anemias where vitamin B-12 is deficient and oral vitamin B-12 is therapeutically ineffective.

Precautions: Folic acid, especially in doses above 1.0 mg./day, may obscure pernicious anemia by temporary hematologic remission while neurologic involvement remains progressive.

Adverse Reactions: Allergic sensitization has been reported after administration of folic acid.

Dosage: As indicated by clinical need, usually 1 tablet daily.

How Supplied: Capsule shaped tablet (film-coated brown and imprinted "ROWELL 1218") in bottles of 100 and unit-dose boxes of 100.

Rystan Company, Inc.

470 MAMARONECK AVE.
WHITE PLAINS, NY 10605

DERIFIL® Tablets and Powder
Water-soluble chlorophyll derivatives

Composition: 100 mg. water-soluble chlorophyll derivatives (Rystan brand, 100% concentration) per tablet or per teaspoonful of prepared solution.
Action and Uses: Oral tablet or solution for control of fecal and urinary odors in colostomy, ileostomy or incontinence; also to deodorize certain necrotic, ulcerative lesions such as decubitus ulcers; also urinary and fecal fistulas and certain breath and body odors not related to faulty hygiene.
Administration and Dosage: In incontinence, one tablet by mouth (or one teaspoonful of solution prepared by dissolving 1 oz. of powder in 1 pint of water) daily at mealtime or any other convenient time. For other conditions, the effective dosage varies with the severity of the odor problem (ordinarily within the range of one to three tablets daily) and is best determined by trial and error. NOTE: Deodorizing effect is cumulative, may require up to seven days to reach maximum. If preferred, tablets may be placed directly in the ostomy appliance.
Side Effects: No toxic effects have been reported from use of DERIFIL, even at high dosage levels for extended periods. A temporary, mild laxative effect may be noted, and the stool is commonly stained dark green. Isolated instances of stomach discomfort or cramps have been reported on high dosages of DERIFIL.
How Supplied: Bottles of 30, 100 and 1000 tablets; 1 oz. and 10 oz. bottles of powder.

PANAFIL® Ointment ℞
PANAFIL®—White Ointment ℞

Composition: PANAFIL contains standardized papain 10%; urea, U.S.P. 10%; and water-soluble chlorophyll derivatives, 0.5% in a hydrophilic base. PANAFIL—White is identical except that the chlorophyll derivatives are omitted.
Action and Uses: For enzymatic debridement and promotion of normal healing (and deodorization, with regular PANAFIL) of surface lesions, particularly where healing is retarded by local infection, necrotic tissue, fibrinous or purulent debris, or eschar.
Administration and Dosage: Apply directly to lesion once or twice daily and cover with gauze. At each redressing, irrigate lesion with mild cleansing solution (*not* hydrogen peroxide solution which may inactivate papain) to remove any accumulation of liquefied necrotic material.
Side Effects: An occasional itching or stinging sensation is sometimes associated with the first application of proteolytic enzymes.
Precautions: Not to be used in eyes.
How Supplied: PANAFIL—1 oz. tubes, 1 lb. jars.
PANAFIL—White—1 oz. tubes.

Products are cross-indexed

by product classifications

in the

BLUE SECTION

SDA Pharmaceuticals, Inc.

919 THIRD AVENUE
NEW YORK, NEW YORK 10022

ANOREXIN™ OTC
Capsules
Anorectic for simple exogenous obesity
contains:
phenylpropanolamine HCl 25 mg
caffeine 100 mg

One-Span™ OTC
Sustained Release Capsules
contains:
phenylpropanolamine HCl 50 mg
caffeine 200 mg

Description: Each capsule contains phenylpropanolamine HCl, an anorexiant, and caffeine, a mild stimulant.
Indication: ANOREXIN is indicated as adjunctive therapy in a regimen of weight reduction based on caloric restriction in the management and control of simple exogenous obesity.
Caution: Do not exceed recommended dosage. Discontinue use if rapid pulse, dizziness or palpitations occur. Do not use if high blood pressure, heart, kidney, diabetes, thyroid or other disease is present, or if pregnant or lactating, nor to be used by anyone under the age of 18, except on physician's advice. Keep this and all drugs out of the reach of children. In case of accidental overdose seek professional assistance or contact a Poison Control Center immediately.
Precaution: Avoid use if taking prescription, anti-hypertensive or anti-depressive drugs containing monoamine oxidase inhibitors or other medication containing sympathomimetic amines. Avoid continuous use longer than 3 months.
Adverse Reactions: Side effects are rare when taken as directed. Nausea or nasal dryness may occasionally occur.
Dosage and Administration:
ANOREXIN™ Capsules: One capsule 30–60 minutes before each meal three times a day with one or two full glasses of water.
ANOREXIN™ One-Span™ Sustained Release Capsules: One capsule with a full glass of water once a day mid-morning (10:00 A.M.)
How Supplied:
ANOREXIN™ Capsules: Bottles of 50, packaged with 1200 calorie ANOREXIN Diet Plan.
ANOREXIN™ One-Span™ Sustained Release Capsules: Bottles of 21; packaged with 1200 calorie ANOREXIN Diet Plan.

> A U.S. Government advisory panel of medical and scientific experts has determined the combination of active ingredients in this product as safe and effective when taken as directed for appetite control to aid in weight reduction by caloric restriction.

Reference: Griboff, Solomon, I., M.D., F.A.C.P. et al., A Double-Blind Clinical Evaluation of a Phenylpropanolamine-Caffeine Combination and a Placebo in the Treatment of Exogenous Obesity, Current Therapeutic Research 17, 6:535, 1975 (June).

Over 7,000 products are

listed alphabetically

in the

PINK SECTION.

Sandoz Pharmaceuticals

(Division of Sandoz, Inc.)
ROUTE 10
EAST HANOVER, NJ 07936

BELLADENAL® ℞
Tablets
BELLADENAL-S®
Tablets

The following prescribing information is based on official labeling in effect on November 1, 1979.
Composition: Each Belladenal *Tablet* and Belladenal-S Tablet contains 0.25 mg Bellafoline® (levorotatory alkaloids of belladonna, as malates), and 50 mg phenobarbital, USP. (Warning: May be habit forming.)
Properties and Therapeutics: Superior antispasmodic/anticholinergic. The natural levorotatory alkaloids of belladonna (Bellafoline) in Belladenal give the antispasmodic-anticholinergic action of belladonna with only minimal central side effects. One Belladenal or Belladenal-S Tablet has the antispasmodic-anticholinergic action of 27 minims of tincture belladonna. Both Belladenal Tablets and Belladenal-S Tablets are scored to permit dosage adjustments necessary for optimal control of symptoms.

> **Indications**
> Based on a review of this drug by the National Academy of Sciences—National Research Council and/or other information, FDA has classified the indications as follows:
> "Possibly" effective: As adjunctive therapy in the treatment of peptic ulcer and in the treatment of the irritable bowel syndrome (irritable colon, spastic colon, mucous colitis) and acute enterocolitis.
> Final classification of the less-than-effective indications requires further investigation.

Contraindications: Glaucoma, elevated intraocular pressure, advanced hepatic or renal disease. Hypersensitivity to any of the components.
Precautions: Due to presence of a barbiturate, may be habit forming. Caution is advised in the elderly.
Side Effects: Urinary retention, blurred vision, dry mouth, flushing or drowsiness may occur.
Dosage and Administration: Belladenal Tablets—Adults: 2 to 4 tablets per day, in divided doses of $\frac{1}{4}$ to $\frac{1}{2}$ tablet. Children: $\frac{1}{4}$ to $\frac{1}{2}$ tablet one to four times daily, according to age. Tablets are scored so that they can be divided easily.
Belladenal-S Tablets—Adults: One tablet in the morning and one at night.
Supplied: Belladenal Tablets (compressed, white, scored) in bottles of 100. Belladenal-S Tablets (compressed, scored tablets of tri-colored pattern: salmon pink, emerald green and white) in bottles of 100.
Company's Product Identification Mark(s): Belladenal Tablets embossed 78-28 on 1 side and scored on reverse side. Belladenal-S Tablets embossed 78-27 on 1 side and scored on reverse side.
[BED-Z11 Issued August 1, 1979]
[*Shown in Product Identification Section*]

Continued on next page

Sandoz—Cont.

CAFERGOT® ℞

(ergotamine tartrate and caffeine) tablets, NF
(ergotamine tartrate and caffeine) suppositories, NF

CAFERGOT® P-B

The following prescribing information is based on official labeling in effect on November 1, 1979.

Description: Each *Cafergot Tablet* contains: 1 mg Gynergen® (ergotamine tartrate, USP) and 100 mg caffeine, USP. Each *Cafergot Suppository* contains: 2 mg Gynergen® (ergotamine tartrate, USP); 100 mg caffeine, USP; tartaric acid, NF; cocoa butter, USP.
Each *Cafergot P-B Tablet* contains: 1 mg Gynergen® (ergotamine tartrate, USP); 100 mg caffeine, USP; 0.125 mg Bellafoline® (levorotatory alkaloids of belladonna, as malates); 30 mg sodium pentobarbital, USP, *(Warning:* May be habit forming). Each *Cafergot P-B Suppository* contains: 2 mg Gynergen® (ergotamine tartrate, USP); 100 mg caffeine, USP; 0.25 mg Bellafoline® (levorotatory alkaloids of belladonna, as malates); 60 mg pentobarbital, NF. (*Warning:* May be habit forming); tartaric acid, NF; malic acid, lactose, USP; theobroma oil, USP.
Cafergot Suppositories and Cafergot P-B Suppositories are *sealed* in foil to afford protection from cocoa butter leakage. If an unavoidable period of exposure to heat softens the suppository, it should be chilled in ice-cold water to solidify it before removing the foil.

Actions: Ergotamine is an alpha adrenergic blocking agent with a direct stimulating effect on the smooth muscle of peripheral and cranial blood vessels and produces depression of central vasomotor centers. The compound also has the properties of serotonin antagonism. In comparison to hydrogenated ergotamine, the adrenergic blocking actions are less pronounced and vasoconstrictive actions are greater.
Caffeine, also a cranial vasoconstrictor, is added to further enhance the vasoconstrictive effect without the necessity of increasing ergotamine dosage.
For individuals experiencing excessive nausea and vomiting during migraine attacks the further addition of the anticholinergic and antiemetic alkaloids of belladonna and pentobarbital for reduction of nervous tension has been provided.
Many migraine patients experience excessive nausea and vomiting during attacks, making it impossible for them to retain any oral medication. In such cases, therefore, the only practical means of medication is through the rectal route where medication may reach the cranial vessels directly, evading the splanchnic vasculature and the liver.

Indications:

Cafergot
Indicated as therapy to abort or prevent vascular headache, e.g., migraine, migraine variants, or so-called "histaminic cephalalgia".

Cafergot P-B
Indicated as therapy to abort or prevent vascular headache complicated by tension and gastrointestinal disturbances.

Contraindications: Peripheral vascular disease, coronary heart disease, hypertension, impaired hepatic or renal function, sepsis and pregnancy. Hypersensitivity to any of the components.

Precautions: Although signs and symptoms of ergotism rarely develop even after long term intermittent use of the orally or rectally administered drugs, care should be exercised to remain within the limits of recommended dosage.

Adverse Reactions: Numbness and tingling of the fingers and toes, muscle pains in the extremities, weakness in the legs, precordial distress and pain, transient tachycardia or bradycardia, nausea, vomiting, localized edema and itching. Drowsiness may occur with Cafergot P-B.

Dosage and Administration: Procedure: For the best results, dosage should start at the first sign of an attack. Adults: *Orally*—2 tablets at start of attack; 1 additional tablet every ½ hour, if needed for full relief (maximum 6 tablets per attack, 10 per week). *Rectally*—1 suppository at start of attack; second suppository after 1 hour, if needed for full relief (maximum 2 suppositories per attack, 5 per week).

Maximum Adult Dosage:
Orally: Total dose for any one attack should not exceed 6 tablets.
Rectally: Two suppositories is the maximum dose for an individual attack.
Total weekly dosage should not exceed 10 tablets or 5 suppositories.
In carefully selected patients, with due consideration of maximum dosage recommendations, administration of the drug at bedtime may be an appropriate short-term preventive measure.

Overdosage: The toxic effects of an acute overdosage of Cafergot are due primarily to the ergotamine component. The amount of caffeine is such that its toxic effects will be overshadowed by those of ergotamine. Symptoms include vomiting; numbness, tingling, pain and cyanosis of the extremities associated with diminished or absent peripheral pulses; hypertension or hypotension; drowsiness, stupor, coma, convulsions and shock. A case has been reported of reversible bilateral papillitis with ring scotomata in a patient who received five times the recommended daily adult dose over a period of 14 days.
Treatment consists of removal of the offending drug by induction of emesis, gastric lavage, and catharsis. Maintenance of adequate pulmonary ventilation, correction of hypotension, and control of convulsions are important considerations. Treatment of peripheral vasospasm should consist of warmth, but not heat, and protection of the ischemic limbs. Vasodilators may be used with benefit but caution must be exercised to avoid aggravating an already existent hypotension.

How Supplied: Cafergot Tablets flesh pink colored, sugar coated. Bottles of 250 and cartons of three SigPak® (dispensing unit) packages, each containing 30 tablets in individual blisters. Cafergot Suppositories (sealed in fuchsia-colored aluminum foil) in boxes of 12. Cafergot P-B Tablets bright green, sugar coated. Bottles of 250 and cartons of three SigPak® (dispensing unit) packages, each containing 30 tablets in individual blisters. Cafergot P-B Suppositories (sealed in blue aluminum foil) in boxes of 12.

Company's Product Identification Mark(s):
Cafergot Tablets imprinted 78-34 on 1 side, CAFERGOT other side.
Cafergot P-B Tablets imprinted 78-36 on 1 side, SANDOZ other side.
Suppositories sealed in aluminum foil bearing Sandoz Trademark with NDC Numbers.

[CAF-Z15 Issued March 1, 1979]
[*Shown in Product Identification Section*]

CEDILANID® ℞

(lanatoside C) tablets

The following prescribing information is based on official labeling in effect on November 1, 1979.
Cedilanid (lanatoside C) is derived from *Digitalis lanata* which is particularly rich in cardioactive glycosides. From this plant the Sandoz Research Laboratories succeeded in isolating three *chemically pure crystalline* glycosides in their initial form. The Committee on Nomenclature for the Council on Pharmacy and Chemistry approved the following scientific terms for these glycosides: lanatoside A, lanatoside B and lanatoside C.
Cedilanid (lanatoside C in pure, crystalline form) is a glycoside not found in the purpurea species.

Indications: Where digitalis is required: cardiac failure with regular rhythm or with fibrillation, flutter or rheumatic heart disease; failure associated with arteriosclerosis and hypertension, valvular diseases or myocardial degenerative disease; auricular fibrillation and paroxysmal tachycardia without heart failure.

Contraindications: Ventricular tachycardia. Hypersensitivity.

WARNINGS

> Digitalis alone or with other drugs has been used in the treatment of obesity. This use of digoxin or other digitalis glycosides is unwarranted. Moreover, since they may cause potentially fatal arrhythmias or other adverse effects, the use of these drugs in the treatment of obesity is dangerous.

Precautions: Digitalized patients should not be given parenteral calcium. Administer Cedilanid (lanatoside C) cautiously to patients recently or presently receiving digitalis. Potassium depletion sensitizes the heart to digitalis intoxication.

Side Effects: Every form of arrhythmia and conduction disturbance can occur as a result of digitalis toxicity. Common symptoms of digitalis overdosage are anorexia, nausea and vomiting, blurred vision, flickering objects of yellow and green color, and disorientation.

Usual Dosage: *Cedilanid* (lanatoside C) is a pure crystalline substance and its therapeutic effect can be readily assessed by the physician. Dosage should be adjusted to the requirement of the individual patient. The following dosage is given as a guide.
Oral Digitalization: The average, total digitalizing dose is 20 tablets (10 mg). A good method of procedure is: first day, 7 tablets; second day, 5 tablets; third day, 4 tablets; thereafter, 3 tablets per day until full digitalization is obtained.
Maintenance Dose: 1 to 3 tablets daily.

Supplied: Tablets, 0.5 mg lanatoside C per tablet. Bottles of 100.

Company's Product Identification Mark:
Tablets imprinted 78–38 on 1 side, SANDOZ on other side.

[CED-ZZ8 Issued September 15, 1978]
[*Shown in Product Identification Section*]

CEDILANID®-D ℞

(deslanoside) injection, NF

The following prescribing information is based on official labeling in effect on November 1, 1979.

Description: The cardiac (or digitalis) glycosides are a closely related group of drugs having in common specific and powerful effects on the myocardium. These drugs are found in a number of plants. The term "digitalis" is used to designate the whole group. Typically, the glycosides are composed of three portions, a steroid nucleus, a lactone ring, and a sugar (hence "glycosides").
Cedilanid-D (deslanoside) is provided as ampul solution containing the cardioactive glycoside, desacetyl lanatoside C. This agent is prepared by controlled alkaline hydrolysis of lanatoside C, a glycoside obtained from digitalis lanata.
Supplied in ampuls of 2 ml. Each 2 ml contains:

deslanoside, NF	0.4 mg
citric acid, USP, q.s. to	pH 6.2±0.3
sodium phosphate, NF	10.6 mg
alcohol, USP	9.8% by vol.
glycerin, USP	15% by wt.

water for injection, USP, q.s. to 2 ml

Action: The digitalis glycosides have qualitatively the same therapeutic effect on the heart. They (1) increase the force of myocardial contraction, (2) increase the refractory period of the atrioventricular (A-V) node, and (3) to a

lesser degree, affect the sinoatrial (S-A) node and conduction system via the parasympathetic and sympathetic nervous systems.
Cedilanid-D (deslanoside) has its onset of action in about 5 minutes after intravenous administration and reaches peak effect in 2-4 hours. Therapeutic action persists for 2 to 5 days.

Indications:

1. "Congestive heart failure," all degrees, is the primary indication. The increased cardiac output results in diuresis and general amelioration of the disturbances characteristic of right (venous congestion, edema) and left (dyspnea, orthopnea, cardiac asthma) heart failure.
   Digitalis, generally, is most effective in "low output" failure and less effective in "high output" (bronchopulmonary insufficiency, infection, hyperthyroidism) heart failure.
   Digitalis should be continued after failure is abolished unless some known precipitating factor is corrected.
2. "Atrial fibrillation"— especially when the ventricular rate is elevated. Digitalis rapidly reduces ventricular rates and eliminates the pulse deficit. Palpitation, precordial distress or weakness are relieved and any concomitant congestive failure ameliorated.
   Digitalis is continued in doses necessary to maintain the desired ventricular rate and other clinical effects.
3. "Atrial flutter" digitalis slows the heart and regular sinus rhythm may appear. Frequently the flutter is converted to atrial fibrillation with a slow ventricular rate. Stopping digitalis at this point may be followed by restoration of sinus rhythm, especially if the flutter was of the paroxysmal type. It is preferable, however, to continue digitalis if failure ensues or if atrial flutter is a frequent occurrence.
4. "Paroxysmal atrial tachycardia" digitalis may be used, especially if it is resistant to lesser measures. Depending on the urgency, a more rapid acting parenteral preparation may be preferable to initiate digitalization, although if failure has ensued or paroxysms recur frequently, digitalis is maintained by oral administration.
   Digitalis is not indicated in sinus tachycardia or premature systoles in the absence of heart failure.

"Cardiogenic shock"—the value of digitalis is not established, but the drug is often employed, especially when the condition is accompanied by pulmonary edema. Digitalis seems to adversely affect shock due to infections.

Contraindications: The presence of toxic effects (See "Overdosage") induced by any digitalis preparation is an absolute contraindication to all of the glycosides.
"Allergy," though rare, does occur. It may not extend to all preparations and another may be tried.
"Ventricular Fibrillation"
"Ventricular tachycardia," unless congestive failure supervenes after a protracted episode not itself due to digitalis.

Warnings: Many of the arrhythmias for which digitalis is advised are identical with those reflecting digitalis intoxication. If the possibility of digitalis intoxication cannot be excluded, cardiac glycosides should be temporarily withheld if permitted by the clinical situation.
The patient with congestive heart failure may complain of nausea and vomiting. These symptoms may also be indications of digitalis intoxication. A clinical determination of the cause of these symptoms must be attempted before further drug administration.

Precautions: "Potassium depletion" sensitizes the myocardium to digitalis and toxicity is apt to develop even with usual dosage. Hypokalemia also tends to reduce the positive inotropic effect of digitalis. Potassium wastage may result from diuretic, corticosteroid, hemodialysis and other therapy. It is apt to accompany malnutrition, old age and long-standing congestive heart failure.
"Acute myocardial infarction," severe pulmonary disease, or far advanced heart failure are apt to be more sensitive to digitalis and more prone to disturbances of rhythm.
"Calcium" affects contractility and excitability of the heart in a manner similar to that of digitalis. Calcium may produce serious arrhythmias in digitalized patients.
"Myxedema"—Digitalis requirements are less because excretion rate is decreased and blood levels are significantly higher.
"Incomplete AV block," especially patients subject to Stokes Adams attacks, may develop advanced or complete heart block. Heart failure in these patients can usually be controlled by other measures and by increasing the heart rate.
"Chronic constrictive pericarditis," is apt to respond unfavorably.
"Idiopathic hypertrophic subaortic stenosis" must be managed extremely carefully. Unless cardiac failure is severe it is doubtful whether digitalis should be employed.
"Renal insufficiency" delays the excretion of digitalis and dosage must be adjusted accordingly in patients with renal disease.
NOTE: This applies also to potassium administration should it become necessary.
Electrical conversion of arrhythmias may require adjustment of digitalis dosage.

Adverse Reactions: Gynecomastia, uncommon.

Overdosage, Toxic Effects: "Gastrointestinal"—anorexia, nausea, vomiting, diarrhea—are the most common early symptoms of overdosages in the adult.
Uncontrolled heart failure may also produce such symptoms.
"Central Nervous System"—headache, weakness, apathy, visual disturbances.
"Cardiac Disturbances"———
Arrhythmias —"ventricular premature beats" is the most common.
Paroxysmal and nonparoxysmal nodal rhythms, atrioventricular (inference) dissociation and paroxysmal atrial tachycardia (PAT) with block are also common arrhythmias due to digitalis overdosage.
Conduction Disturbances—excessive slowing of the pulse is a clinical sign of digitalis overdosage. Atrioventricular block of increasing degree, may proceed to complete heart block.
NOTE: The electrocardiogram is fundamental in determining the presence and nature of these toxic disturbances. Digitalis may also induce other changes (as of the ST segment), but these provide no measure of the degree of digitalization.
TREATMENT OF TOXIC ARRHYTHMIAS: Digitalis is discontinued until after all signs of toxicity are abolished. This may be all that is necessary if toxic manifestations are not severe and appear after the time for peak effect of the drug.
Potassium salts are commonly used. Potassium chloride in divided doses totaling 4 to 6 gm. for adults provided renal function is adequate.
When correction of the arrhythmia is urgent, potassium is administered intravenously in a solution of 5 percent dextrose in water, a total of 40-100 mEq. (40 mEq. per 500 ml.) at the rate of 40 mEq. per hour unless limited by pain due to local irritation.
Additional amounts may be given if the arrhythmia is uncontrolled and the potassium well tolerated.
Electrocardiographic monitoring is indicated to avoid potassium toxicity, e.g. peaking of T waves.
CAUTION: Potassium should not be used and may be dangerous for severe or complete heart block due to digitalis and not related to any tachycardia.
Chelating agents to bind calcium may also be used to counteract the arrhythmia effect of digitalis toxicity, hypokalemia and of elevated serum calcium which may also precipitate digitalis toxicity.
Four grams (0.8 percent solution) of the disodium salt of EDTA is dissolved in 500 ml of 5 percent dextrose in water (50 mg per ml) and administered over a period of 2 hours unless the arrhythmia is controlled before the infusion is completed.
A continuous electrocardiogram should be observed so that the infusion may be promptly stopped when the desired effect is achieved.
Other counteracting agents are: Quinidine, procainamide, and beta adrenergic blocking agents.

Dosage and Administration: "Parenteral" administration should be used only when the drug cannot be taken orally, or rapid digitalization is very urgent.
Parenteral digitalization can be obtained within 12 hours by giving 8 ml (1.6 mg) *either intramuscularly* or *intravenously.* By the I.V. route the dose may be given as one injection or in portions of 4 ml each. By I.M. route, 4 ml portions are injected at each of 2 sites.
After parenteral digitalization with Cedilanid-D (deslanoside) maintenance therapy may be accomplished by starting administration of an oral preparation, within 12 hours.

How Supplied:
Ampuls, 2 ml size (2 ml contains 0.4 mg deslanoside, NF) Boxes of 20 ampuls.
Being chemically pure and of constant potency, deslanoside, NF is standardized by weight; the ampul solution of Cedilanid-D (deslanoside) contains in each 2 ml:

deslanoside, NF	0.4 mg
citric acid, USP q.s. to	pH 6.2±0.3
sodium phosphate, NF	10.6 mg
alcohol, USP	9.8% by vol.
glycerin, USP	15% by wt.
water for injection, USP, q.s. to 2 ml	

[CED-Z15 Issued March 1, 1979]

D.H.E. 45® Injection ℞
(dihydroergotamine mesylate) injection, NF

The following prescribing information is based on official labeling in effect on November 1, 1979.

Description: DHE-45 is hydrogenated ergotamine as the mesylate. It is a clear, colorless, stable ampul solution containing per ml:

dihydroergotamine mesylate, NF	1 mg
methanesulfonic acid/sodium hydroxide	q.s. to pH 3.75±0.5
alcohol, USP	6.1% by vol.
glycerin, USP	15% by wt.
water for injection, USP, q.s. to	1 ml

Actions: Dihydroergotamine is an alpha adrenergic blocking agent with a direct stimulating effect on the smooth muscle of peripheral and cranial blood vessels, and produces depression of central vasomotor centers. The compound also has the properties of serotonin antagonism. In comparison to ergotamine, the adrenergic blocking actions are more pronounced, the vasoconstrictive actions somewhat less pronounced, and there is reduced incidence and degree of nausea and vomiting. Onset of action occurs in 15 to 30 minutes following intramuscular administration and persists for 3-4 hours.
Repeated dosage at 1 hour intervals up to 3 hours may be required to obtain maximal effect.

Indications: As therapy to abort or prevent vascular headache, e.g., migraine, migraine variants, or so-called "histaminic cephalalgia" when rapid control is desired or when other routes of administration are not feasible.

Contraindications: Peripheral vascular disease, coronary heart disease, hypertension,

Continued on next page

Sandoz—Cont.

impaired hepatic or renal function, sepsis and pregnancy. Hypersensitivity.

Adverse Reactions: Numbness and tingling of fingers and toes, muscle pains in the extremities, weakness in the legs, precordial distress and pain, transient tachycardia or bradycardia, nausea, vomiting, localized edema and itching.

Dosage and Administration: *For vascular headache,* 1 ml intramuscularly at first warning sign of headache, repeated at 1 hour intervals to a total of 3 ml. Optimal results are obtained by titrating the dose for several headaches to find the minimal effective dose for each patient and this dose should then be employed at onset of subsequent attacks. Where more rapid effect is desired, the intravenous route may be employed to a maximum of 2 ml. Total weekly dosage should not exceed 6 ml.

Overdosage: Failure to observe the upper limits of repeated parenteral dosage may result in eventual onset of the peripheral toxic signs and symptoms of ergotism. Treatment includes discontinuance of the drug, warmth, vasodilators, and good nursing care to prevent tissue damage.

How Supplied: As a clear, colorless and stable solution in ampuls containing:

dihydroergotamine mesylate, NF	1 mg
methanesulfonic acid/sodium hydroxide	q.s. to pH 3.75±0.5
alcohol, USP	6.1% by vol.
glycerin, USP	15% by wt.
water for injection, USP, q.s. to	1 ml

Ampuls, 1 ml size—boxes of 20.

To assure constant potency, protect the ampuls from light and heat. In the event the ampul solution becomes discolored, it should not be used.

[D.H.E.-Z14 Issued November 1, 1979]

DIAPID® Nasal Spray ℞
(lypressin)

The following prescribing information is based on official labeling in effect on November 1, 1979.

Description: Diapid (lypressin) Nasal Spray contains synthetic lysine-8-vasopressin with an activity of 50 USP Posterior Pituitary (Pressor) Units per ml (0.185 mg/ml). Lysine-8-vasopressin is a polypeptide and is one of the two known naturally occurring molecular forms of mammalian posterior pituitary antidiuretic hormone. This synthetic polypeptide is present as a protein-free substance in Diapid Nasal Spray. Unlike preparations of posterior pituitary antidiuretic hormone of animal origin, Diapid is completely free of oxytocin and foreign proteins. The molecular formula of lysine-8-vasopressin is $C_{46}H_{65}N_{13}O_{12}S_2$.

Action: The principal pharmacologic action of lysine-8-vasopressin, the active ingredient of Diapid (lypressin) Nasal Spray, is similar to that of arginine-8-vasopressin, the posterior pituitary antidiuretic hormone occurring in man. Diapid Nasal Spray increases the rate of reabsorption of solute free water from the distal renal tubules, without significantly modifying the rate of glomerular filtration, producing a fall in free water clearance and an increase in urinary osmolality. The rates of solute and creatinine excretion noted with therapeutic doses of Diapid Nasal Spray suggest that sodium clearance and glomerular filtration rates are essentially unaltered by this hormone. Diapid Nasal Spray is relatively free of oxytocic activity when used within the recommended therapeutic dose levels.

It possesses little pressor activity, the ratio of pressor to antidiuretic activity being in the range of 1:1000.

The antidiuretic effect produced by Diapid Nasal Spray begins rapidly and usually reaches a peak within 30 to 120 minutes. Its usual duration of action is 3 to 8 hours.

Indications: Diapid Nasal Spray is indicated for the control or prevention of the symptoms and complications of diabetes insipidus due to deficiency of endogenous posterior pituitary antidiuretic hormone. These symptoms and complications include polydipsia, polyuria, and dehydration. It is particularly useful in patients with diabetes insipidus who have become unresponsive to other forms of therapy or who experience various types of local and/or systemic reactions, allergic reactions, or other undesirable effects (e.g., excessive fluid retention) from preparations of posterior pituitary antidiuretic hormone of animal origin.

Contraindications: There are no known contraindications to the use of Diapid (lypressin) Nasal Spray.

Warnings: The safety of this drug in pregnancy has not been established. The possibility of risk to the mother and unborn child should be weighed against potential benefits before the drug is administered to women of childbearing age.

Precautions: Cardiovascular pressor effects with Diapid Nasal Spray are minimal or absent when it is administered as a nasal spray in therapeutic doses. Nevertheless, it should be used with caution in patients for whom such effects would not be desirable because mild blood pressure elevation has been noted in unanesthetized subjects who received lypressin intravenously. Large doses intranasally may cause coronary artery constriction and caution should be observed in treating patients with coronary artery disease.

The effectiveness of Diapid (lypressin) Nasal Spray may be lessened in patients with nasal congestion, allergic rhinitis, and upper respiratory infections because these conditions may interfere with absorption of the drug by the nasal mucosa. In this event, larger doses of Diapid Nasal Spray, or adjunctive therapy, may be needed.

Patients with a known sensitivity to anti-diuretic hormone should be tested for sensitivity to Diapid.

Adverse Reactions: With clinical use of Diapid (lypressin) Nasal Spray, adverse reactions have been infrequent and mild. To date, such reactions have included rhinorrhea, nasal congestion, irritation and pruritus of the nasal passages, nasal ulceration, headache, conjunctivitis, heartburn secondary to excessive nasal administration with drippage into the pharynx, and abdominal cramps and increased bowel movements. Inadvertent inhalation of Diapid Nasal Spray has resulted in substernal tightness, coughing, and transient dyspnea. In one patient, an overdose of Diapid Nasal Spray caused marked, but transient, fluid retention. Tolerance or tachyphylaxis to Diapid Nasal Spray has not been reported to date.

Hypersensitivity manifested by a positive skin test.

Dosage and Administration: Patients should be instructed to administer 1 or 2 sprays of Diapid (lypressin) Nasal Spray to one or both nostrils whenever frequency of urination becomes increased or significant thirst develops. (One spray provides approximately 2.0 USP Posterior Pituitary [Pressor] Units.) The usual dosage for adults and children is 1 or 2 sprays in each nostril 4 times daily. An additional dose at bedtime is often helpful to eliminate nocturia, if it is not controlled with the regular daily dosage. For patients requiring more than 2 sprays per nostril every 4 to 6 hours, it is recommended that the time interval between doses be reduced rather than increasing the number of sprays at each dose. (More than 2 or 3 sprays in each nostril usually results in wastage because the unabsorbed excess will drain posteriorly, by way of the nasopharynx, into the digestive tract where it will be inactivated.)

Diapid Nasal Spray permits individualization of dosage necessary to control the symptoms of diabetes insipidus. Patients quickly learn to regulate their dosage in accordance with their degree of polyuria and thirst, and once determined, daily requirements remain fairly stable for months or years. Although most patients require 1 or 2 sprays of Diapid (lypressin) Nasal Spray in each nostril 4 times daily, dosage has ranged from 1 spray per day at bedtime to 10 sprays in each nostril every 3-4 hours. Requirements of the larger doses may represent greater severity of disease or other phenomena, such as poor nasal absorption. A seeming requirement for large doses of lypressin may be due to the presence of mixed hypothalamic-hypophyseal and nephrogenic diabetes insipidus, the latter condition being unresponsive to administration of antidiuretic hormone.

Diapid Nasal Spray is conveniently administered, from a compact and portable, plastic squeeze bottle, by inserting the nozzle of the bottle into the nostril and squeezing once firmly to deliver each short spray.

NOTE: To assure that a uniform, well-diffused spray is delivered, the bottle of Diapid Nasal Spray should be held upright and the patient should be in a vertical position with head upright.

Supplied: Diapid Nasal Spray is supplied in a plastic bottle that contains 8 ml of solution. Each ml of solution contains lypressin (0.185 mg) equivalent to 50 USP Posterior Pituitary (Pressor) Units and the following: propylparaben, USP, methylparaben, USP, sodium phosphate, NF, citric acid, USP, sodium chloride, USP, sorbitol solution, USP, glycerin, USP, sodium acetate, NF, acetic acid, USP, chlorobutanol, USP, (0.1%-0.002%), purified water, USP.

This product has an expiration date of 36 months.

[DIA-Z10 Issued January 27, 1978]

FIOGESIC® Tablets

The following prescribing information is based on official labeling in effect on November 1, 1979.

Composition: Each Tablet contains Calurin® (calcium carbaspirin) 382 mg, equivalent to 300 mg aspirin; phenylpropanolamine hydrochloride, NF 25 mg; pheniramine maleate 12.5 mg; pyrilamine maleate, NF 12.5 mg.

Actions and Uses: For prompt, temporary relief of headache, sinus and nasal congestion, pain and fever due to sinusitis, common cold, or influenza. FIOGESIC promotes sinus and nasal decongestion and drainage with phenylpropanolamine, an orally used alpha adrenergic sympathomimetic approximately equal in potency to ephedrine but with less CNS stimulation, plus two antihistamines, pheniramine maleate and pyrilamine maleate. Calurin®, a freely soluble aspirin complex, alleviates pain and fever.

Contraindications: Sensitivity to any of the ingredients.

Caution: Not for children under 6. Individuals with high blood pressure, heart disease, diabetes, or thyroid disease should use only as directed by a physician. This preparation may cause drowsiness. Do not drive or operate machinery while taking this medication.

Side Effects: Drowsiness, blurred vision, cardiac palpitations, flushing, dizziness, nervousness, or gastrointestinal upsets may occur occasionally.

Dosage: Adults—Two tablets followed by one or two tablets every four hours, up to six per day. Children (6 to 12 years)—one-half to one tablet every four hours up to four tablets per day.

Supplied: Fiogesic Oblong Inlay-Tablets (white with yellow inlay) in bottles of 100.

Company's Product Identification Mark(s): Tablets embossed 78-65 on 1 side, SANDOZ other side.

[*Shown in Product Identification Section*]

FIORINAL® ©

Tablets and Capsules

The following prescribing information is based on official labeling in effect on November 1, 1979.

Description: Each Fiorinal tablet or capsule for oral administration contains: Sandoptal® (butalbital), 50 mg (Warning: May be habit forming); aspirin, USP, 200 mg; phenacetin, USP, 130 mg; caffeine, USP, 40 mg

Butalbital, 5-allyl-5-isobutyl-barbituric acid, a white odorless crystalline powder; is a short- to intermediate-acting barbiturate.

Actions: Pharmacologically, Fiorinal combines the analgesic properties of aspirin-phenacetin-caffeine with the anxiolytic and muscle relaxant properties of Sandoptal.

The clinical effectiveness of Fiorinal in tension headache has been established in double-blind, placebo-controlled, multi-clinic trials. A factorial design study compared Fiorinal with each of its major components, Sandoptal and aspirin-phenacetin-caffeine. This study demonstrated that each component contributes to the efficacy of Fiorinal in the treatment of the target symptoms of tension headache (headache pain, psychic tension, and muscle contraction in the head, neck and shoulder region). For each symptom and the symptom complex as a whole, Fiorinal was shown to have significantly superior clinical effects to either component alone.

Indications: Fiorinal is indicated for the relief of the symptom complex of tension (or muscle contraction) headache.

Contraindications: Hypersensitivity to aspirin, phenacetin, caffeine, or barbiturates. Patients with porphyria.

Warnings:

Drug Dependency: Prolonged use of barbiturates can produce drug dependence, characterized by psychic dependence, and less frequently, physical dependence and tolerance. The abuse liability of Fiorinal is similar to that of other barbiturate-containing drug combinations. Caution should be exercised when prescribing medication for patients with a known propensity for taking excessive quantities of drugs, which is not uncommon in patients with chronic tension headache.

Use in Ambulatory Patients: Fiorinal may impair the mental and/or physical abilities required for the performance of potentially hazardous tasks, such as driving a car or operating machinery. The patient should be cautioned accordingly. Central Nervous System depressant effects of butalbital may be additive with those of other CNS depressants. Concurrent use with other sedative-hypnotics or alcohol should be avoided. When such combined therapy is necessary, the dose of one or more agents may need to be reduced.

Use in Pregnancy: Adequate studies have not been performed in animals to determine whether this drug affects fertility in males or females, has teratogenic potential, or has other adverse effects on the fetus. While there are no well-controlled studies in pregnant women, over twenty years of marketing and clinical experience does not include any positive evidence of adverse effects on the fetus. Although there is no clearly defined risk, such experience cannot exclude the possibility of infrequent or subtle damage to the human fetus. Fiorinal should be used in pregnant women only when clearly needed.

Nursing Mothers: The effects of Fiorinal on infants of nursing mothers are not known. Salicylates and barbiturates are excreted in the breast milk of nursing mothers. The serum levels in infants are believed to be insignificant with therapeutic doses.

Precautions: Salicylates should be used with extreme caution in the presence of peptic ulcer or coagulation abnormalities.

Phenacetin has been reported damaging to the kidneys when taken in large amounts for a long time and should be used with caution in patients with renal disease.

Pediatric Use: Safety and effectiveness in children below the age of 12 have not been established.

Adverse Reactions: The most frequent adverse reactions are drowsiness and dizziness. Less frequent adverse reactions are lightheadedness and gastrointestinal disturbances including nausea, vomiting, and flatulence.

Overdosage: The toxic effects of acute overdosage of Fiorinal are attributable mainly to its barbiturate component, and, to a lesser extent, aspirin. The toxic effects of phenacetin, which may be masked by the barbiturate, may also occur and should not be overlooked. Because toxic effects of caffeine occur in very high dosages only, the possibility of significant caffeine toxicity from Fiorinal overdosage is unlikely. Symptoms attributable to *acute barbiturate poisoning* include drowsiness, confusion, and coma; respiratory depression; hypotension; shock. Symptoms attributable to *acute aspirin poisoning* include hyperpnea; acid-base disturbances with development of metabolic acidosis; vomiting and abdominal pain; tinnitus; hyperthermia; hypoprothrombinemia; restlessness; delirium; convulsions. Symptoms of *acute phenacetin poisoning* include vomiting; chills, hypotension, cyanosis due to methemoglobinemia; convulsions. *Acute caffeine poisoning* may cause insomnia, restlessness, tremor, and delirium; tachycardia and extrasystoles. *Treatment* consists primarily of management of barbiturate intoxication and the correction of the acid-base imbalance due to salicylism. Vomiting should be induced mechanically or with emetics in the conscious patient. Gastric lavage may be used if the pharyngeal and laryngeal reflexes are present and if less than four hours have elapsed since ingestion. A cuffed endotracheal tube should be inserted before gastric lavage of the unconscious patient and when necessary to provide assisted respiration. Diuresis, alkalinization of the urine, and correction of electrolyte disturbances should be accomplished through administration of intravenous fluids such as 1% sodium bicarbonate in 5% dextrose in water. Meticulous attention should be given to maintaining adequate pulmonary ventilation. Correction of hypotension may require the administration of levarterenol bitartrate or phenylephrine hydrochloride by intravenous infusion. In severe cases of intoxication, peritoneal dialysis, hemodialysis, or exchange transfusion may be lifesaving. Hypoprothrombinemia should be treated with Vitamin K, intravenously. Methemoglobinemia over 30% should be treated with methylene blue administered slowly intravenously.

Dosage and Administration: One or two tablets or capsules every four hours. Total daily dose should not exceed six tablets or capsules.

Supplied: Fiorinal Capsules: Color is bright Kelly green and lime green, in packages of 100 and 500. Fiorinal Tablets: White compressed tablets 11 mm. diameter, 5.5 mm. thickness, in packages of 100 and 1000.

Company's Product Identification Mark(s): Tablets imprinted "FIORINAL 78–44" and Capsules imprinted "SANDOZ 78–43".

[FIO-ZZ15 Issued September 9, 1977]

[*Shown in Product Identification Section*]

FIORINAL® with CODEINE ©

Capsules

No. 1, 2 and 3

The following prescribing information is based on official labeling in effect on November 1, 1979.

Composition: Each Fiorinal with Codeine *Capsule* contains: 50 mg Sandoptal® (butalbital), (Warning: May be habit forming.) 40 mg caffeine, USP; 200 mg aspirin, USP; and 130 mg phenacetin, USP.

In addition, Fiorinal with Codeine #1, #2, #3 also contain, respectively, codeine phosphate, USP 7.5 mg (1/8 gr.), 15 mg (1/4 gr.) and 30 mg (1/2 gr.). (Warning: May be habit forming.)

Indications: "Fiorinal with Codeine" raises the threshold of pain and discomfort and can be used in a great variety of painful conditions short of those which require morphine.

Action and Uses: Analgesic, antitussive, and antipyretic. The analgesic-sedative action of Fiorinal complements and increases the time-tested action of codeine. This enhanced analgesic-sedative effect is particularly well-suited for acute, short-range periods of pain and discomfort frequently seen in office practice. The formulation of "Fiorinal with Codeine" provides additional benefits for patients who have developed a cycle of pain, anxiety, tension which reinforces the pain experienced by the patients.

"Fiorinal with Codeine" is indicated for all types of pain associated with medical and surgical aftercare, postpartum pain, dysmenorrhea, neuritis, pleurisy, sciatica, neuralgia, sinusitis, pharyngitis, tonsillitis, otitis, febrile diseases, dental pain following extractions, headache, bursitis, arthritis, rheumatism, low back pain, dislocations, strains, sprains, fractures, etc. The analgesic, antitussive-antipyretic action of this product makes it particularly well-suited for the patient with upper respiratory infections such as acute colds, bronchitis, influenza, and pneumonia.

Contraindication: Hypersensitivity to any of the components.

Precaution: May be habit forming due to presence of codeine and barbiturate.

Side Effects: Nausea, vomiting, constipation, dizziness, skin rash, drowsiness, and miosis are possible side effects. Overdosage is primarily manifested by drowsiness.

Adult Dosage: 1 or 2 capsules, repeated if necessary up to 6 per day, or as directed by physician.

Supplied: Fiorinal with Codeine: 7.5 mg (1/8 gr.), imprinted SANDOZ 78-21, (red and yellow), in bottles of 100; 15 mg (1/4 gr.), imprinted SANDOZ 78-22, (gray and yellow), in bottles of 100; 30 mg (1/2 gr.), imprinted SANDOZ 78-23, (blue and yellow), in bottles of 100.

Fiorinal with Codeine No. 3 (1/2 gr) also in ControlPak® package, 25 capsules (continuous reverse numbered roll of sealed blisters).

Company's Product Identification Mark(s): All capsules imprinted SANDOZ with NDC numbers.

[FIO-Z12 Issued September 4, 1979]

[*Shown in Product Identification Section*]

GYNERGEN® ℞

(ergotamine tartrate) injection, USP

(ergotamine tartrate) tablets, USP

The following prescribing information is based on official labeling in effect on November 1, 1979.

Composition: Each Gynergen *Tablet* contains 1 mg ergotamine tartrate, USP. Gynergen *Injection* contains per ml: 0.5 mg ergotamine tartrate mixture; tartaric acid, NF, q.s. to pH 3.85$\pm$0.15, alcohol, USP, 6.1% by vol.; glycerin, USP, 14.63% by wt.; and water for injection, USP, q.s. to 1 ml.

Continued on next page

Sandoz—Cont.

Action and Uses: Long-term usage has established the fact that Gynergen (ergotamine tartrate) is effective in controlling 90% of acute migraine attacks, so that it is now considered specific for the treatment of this headache syndrome. Being non-narcotic, it has the added virtue of avoiding the dangers inherent in the repeated use of narcotics in the treatment of frequently-recurring headache, such as migraine.
Indications: Vascular headache, e.g. migraine, histaminic cephalalgia (cluster headache).
Contraindications: Peripheral vascular disease, coronary heart disease, hypertension, impaired hepatic or renal function, sepsis, and pregnancy. Hypersensitivity.
Side Effects: Numbness and tingling of fingers and toes, muscle pains in the extremities, weakness in the legs, precordial distress and pain, transient tachycardia or bradycardia, nausea, vomiting, localized edema and itching.
Usual Dose: *By injection:* 0.5-1 ml intramuscularly or subcutaneously for relief of the acute attack. The minimal effective dose should be established for each patient by titrating the amount required to control headaches in that patient. This is best done by starting with an injection of ½ ml at onset of attack and repeating in 40 minutes if required. The total amount required to control the headache should then be employed at the first warning sign of subsequent attacks as the optimal dose for that patient. Maximum dose per week is 2 ml; amount and duration of treatment should be established by attending physician.
Injection Test: Relief of throbbing, recurrent headache following intramuscular injection of 1 ml ergotamine tartrate ampul solution is almost conclusive evidence that the headache is of vascular origin and may serve to confirm the diagnosis.
For oral use: Tablets are provided, each containing 1 mg Gynergen (ergotamine tartrate). Average dose is 2 to 6 tablets per attack. Total weekly dosage should not exceed 10 tablets.
How Supplied: Tablets (ivory gray, sugar-coated) in bottles of 100. Injection in 1 ml (0.5 mg) ampuls in boxes of 20 and 100.
Company's Product Identification Mark(s): Tablets imprinted 78–48 on one side, SANDOZ other side.
Remarks: Protect ergotamine tartrate preparations from light and heat.
[GYN-Z13 Issued August 1, 1979]

HYDERGINE® ℞
Tablets and Sublingual Tablets

The following prescribing information is based on official labeling in effect on November 1, 1979.
Description: Each 1 mg Hydergine tablet contains dihydroergocornine mesylate 0.333 mg, dihydroergocristine mesylate 0.333 mg, and dihydroergocryptine (dihydro-alpha-ergocryptine and dihydro-beta-ergocryptine in the proportion of 2:1) mesylate 0.333 mg, representing a total of 1 mg.
Each 1 mg Hydergine sublingual tablet contains dihydroergocornine mesylate 0.333 mg, dihydroergocristine mesylate 0.333 mg, and dihydroergocryptine (dihydro-alpha-ergocryptine and dihydro-beta-ergocryptine in the proportion of 2:1) mesylate 0.333 mg, representing a total of 1 mg.
Each 0.5 mg Hydergine sublingual tablet contains dihydroergocornine mesylate 0.167 mg, dihydroergocristine mesylate 0.167 mg, and dihydroergocryptine (dihydro-alpha-ergocryptine and dihydro-beta-ergocryptine in the proportion of 2:1) mesylate 0.167 mg, representing a total of 0.5 mg.
Pharmacokinetic Properties: Bioequivalence studies were performed in which Hydergine tablets were administered orally and Hydergine sublingual tablets were administered sublingually to human subjects. Hydergine tablets are rapidly but incompletely absorbed from the gastrointestinal tract. Following administration, the oral tablets resulted in slightly higher peak levels when compared to the sublingual dosage form. Hydergine substance undergoes a rapid first pass liver metabolism and less than 50% of the therapeutic moiety reaches the systemic circulation. The peak plasma levels of single, orally administered doses are achieved within one hour and by 24 hours the plasma levels are not detectable. The mean biologic half life of Hydergine substance is about 3.5 hours.
Actions: There is no specific evidence which clearly establishes the mechanism by which Hydergine tablets and sublingual tablets produce mental effects, nor is there conclusive evidence that the drug particularly affects cerebral arteriosclerosis or cerebrovascular insufficiency.
Indications: Hydergine tablets and sublingual tablets are indicated for the treatment of selected symptoms in elderly patients. Short term clinical studies have demonstrated modest improvement in levels of performance of self care and such symptoms as mood-depression, confusion, unsociability, and dizziness. These symptoms are of unknown etiology and are not specific to any age group or disease. However, to date, only short term studies conducted with elderly patients have been reported.
Contraindications: Hydergine tablets and sublingual tablets are contraindicated in individuals who have previously shown hypersensitivity to the drug.
Precautions: *Practitioners are advised that because the target symptoms are of unknown etiology careful diagnosis should be attempted before prescribing Hydergine tablets and sublingual tablets.*
Adverse Reactions: Hydergine tablets and sublingual tablets have not been found to produce serious side effects. Some sublingual irritation, transient nausea, and gastric disturbances have been reported. Hydergine tablets and sublingual tablets do not possess the vasoconstrictor properties of the natural ergot alkaloids.
Dosage and Administration: 1 mg three times daily.
Alleviation of symptoms is usually gradual and results may not be observed for 3–4 weeks.
How Supplied:
Hydergine tablets (for oral use):
1 mg, round, white, packages of 100 and 500.
Hydergine sublingual tablets:
1 mg, oval, white, packages of 100, & 1000.
0.5 mg, round, white, packages of 100 and 1000.
Company's Product Identification Mark(s):
Hydergine oral tablets 1 mg embossed "HYDERGINE 1" on one side, "78–70" other side.
Hydergine sublingual tablets 1 mg embossed "HYDERGINE" on one side, "78–77" other side.
Hydergine sublingual tablets 0.5 mg embossed "HYDERGINE 0.5" on one side, "78–51" other side.
[HYG–ZZ16 Issued December 1, 1978]
[*Shown in Product Identification Section*]

MELLARIL® ℞
(thioridazine) HCl tablets, USP
(thioridazine) HCl solution, USP
MELLARIL-S™
(thioridazine) base suspension

The following prescribing information is based on official labeling in effect on November 15, 1979.
Description: Mellaril® (thioridazine) is 2-methylmercapto-10-[2- (N-methyl-2-piperidyl) ethyl] phenothiazine
The presence of a thiomethyl radical ($S\text{-}CH_3$) in position 2, conventionally occupied by a halogen, is unique and could account for the greater toleration obtained with recommended doses of thioridazine as well as a greater specificity of psychotherapeutic action.
Clinical Pharmacology: Mellaril is effective in reducing excitement, hypermotility, abnormal initiative, affective tension and agitation through its inhibitory effect on psychomotor functions. Successful modification of such symptoms is the prerequisite for, and often the beginning of, the process of recovery in patients exhibiting mental and emotional disturbances.
Thioridazine's basic pharmacological activity is similar to that of other phenothiazines, but certain specific qualities have come to light which support the observation that the clinical spectrum of this drug shows significant differences from those of the other agents of this class. Minimal antiemetic activity and minimal extrapyramidal stimulation, notably pseudoparkinsonism, are distinctive features of this drug.
Indications: For the management of manifestations of psychotic disorders.
For the short-term treatment of moderate to marked depression with variable degrees of anxiety in adult patients and for the treatment of multiple symptoms such as agitation, anxiety, depressed mood, tension, sleep disturbances, and fears in geriatric patients.
For the treatment of severe behavioral problems in children marked by combativeness and/or explosive hyperexcitable behavior (out of proportion to immediate provocations), and in the short-term treatment of hyperactive children who show excessive motor activity with accompanying conduct disorders consisting of some or all of the following symptoms: impulsivity, difficulty sustaining attention, aggressivity, mood lability, and poor frustration tolerance.
Contraindications: In common with other phenothiazines, Mellaril is contraindicated in severe central nervous system depression or comatose states from any cause. It should also be noted that hypertensive or hypotensive heart disease of extreme degree is a contraindication of phenothiazine administration.
Warnings: It has been suggested in regard to phenothiazines in general, that people who have demonstrated a hypersensitivity reaction (e.g. blood dyscrasias, jaundice) to one may be more prone to demonstrate a reaction to others. Attention should be paid to the fact that phenothiazines are capable of potentiating central nervous system depressants (e.g. anesthetics, opiates, alcohol, etc.) as well as atropine and phosphorus insecticides. Physicians should carefully consider benefit versus risk when treating less severe disorders.
Reproductive studies in animals and clinical experience to date have failed to show a teratogenic effect with Mellaril (thioridazine). However, in view of the desirability of keeping the administration of all drugs to a minimum during pregnancy, Mellaril should be given only when the benefits derived from treatment exceed the possible risks to mother and fetus.
Precautions: Leukopenia and/or agranulocytosis and convulsive seizures have been reported but are infrequent. Mellaril has been shown to be helpful in the treatment of behavioral disorders in epileptic patients, but anticonvulsant medication should also be maintained. Pigmentary retinopathy, which has been observed primarily in patients taking larger than recommended doses, is characterized by diminution of visual acuity, brownish coloring of vision, and impairment of night vision; examination of the fundus discloses deposits of pigment. The possibility of this complication may be reduced by remaining within the recommended limits of dosage.
Where patients are participating in activities requiring complete mental alertness (e.g., driving) it is advisable to administer the phenothiazines cautiously and to increase the dosage

gradually. Female patients appear to have a greater tendency to orthostatic hypotension than male patients. The administration of epinephrine should be avoided in the treatment of drug-induced hypotension in view of the fact that phenothiazines may induce a reversed epinephrine effect on occasion. Should a vasoconstrictor be required, the most suitable are levarterenol and phenylephrine.

It is recommended that a daily dose in excess of 300 mg. be reserved for use only in severe neuropsychiatric conditions.

Adverse Reactions: In the recommended dosage ranges with Mellaril (thioridazine), most side effects are mild and transient.

Central Nervous System: Drowsiness may be encountered on occasion, especially where large doses are given early in treatment. Generally, this effect tends to subside with continued therapy or a reduction in dosage. Pseudoparkinsonism and other extrapyramidal symptoms may occur but are infrequent. Nocturnal confusion, hyperactivity, lethargy, psychotic reactions, restlessness and headache have been reported but are extremely rare.

Autonomic Nervous System: Dryness of mouth, blurred vision, constipation, nausea, vomiting, diarrhea, nasal stuffiness, and pallor have been seen.

Endocrine System: Galactorrhea, breast engorgement, amenorrhea, inhibition of ejaculation, and peripheral edema have been described.

Skin: Dermatitis and skin eruptions of the urticarial type have been observed infrequently. Photosensitivity is extremely rare.

Cardiovascular System: ECG changes have been reported (see Phenothiazine Derivatives: Cardiovascular Effects).

Other: Rare cases described as parotid swelling have been reported following administration of Mellaril (thioridazine).

PHENOTHIAZINE DERIVATIVES: It should be noted that efficacy, indications and untoward effects have varied with the different phenothiazines. It has been reported that old age lowers the tolerance for phenothiazines. The most common neurological side effects in these patients are parkinsonism and akathisia. There appears to be an increased risk of agranulocytosis and leukopenia in the geriatric population. The physician should be aware that the following have occurred with one or more phenothiazines and should be considered whenever one of these drugs is used:

Autonomic Reactions: Miosis, obstipation, anorexia, paralytic ileus.

Cutaneous Reactions: Erythema, exfoliative dermatitis, contact dermatitis.

Blood Dyscrasias: Agranulocytosis, leukopenia, eosinophilia, thrombocytopenia, anemia, aplastic anemia, pancytopenia.

Allergic Reactions: Fever, laryngeal edema, angioneurotic edema, asthma.

Hepatotoxicity: Jaundice, biliary stasis.

Cardiovascular Effects: Changes in the terminal portion of the electrocardiogram, including prolongation of the Q-T interval, lowering and inversion of the T-wave and appearance of a wave tentatively identified as a bifid T or a U wave have been observed in some patients receiving the phenothiazine tranquilizers, including Mellaril (thioridazine). To date, these appear to be due to altered repolarization and not related to myocardial damage. They appear to be reversible. While there is no evidence at present that these changes are in any way precursors of any significant disturbance of cardiac rhythm, it should be noted that several sudden and unexpected deaths apparently due to cardiac arrest have occurred in patients previously showing characteristic electrocardiographic changes while taking the drug. The use of periodic electrocardiograms has been proposed but would appear to be of questionable value as a predictive device. Hypotension, rarely resulting in cardiac arrest.

Extrapyramidal Symptoms: Akathisia, agitation, motor restlessness, dystonic reactions, trismus, torticollis, opisthotonus, oculogyric crises, tremor, muscular rigidity, akinesia.

Persistent Tardive Dyskinesia: As with all antipsychotic agents, tardive dyskinesia may appear in some patients on long-term therapy or may occur after drug therapy has been discontinued. This risk seems to be greater in elderly patients on high-dose therapy, especially females. The symptoms are presistent and in some patients appear to be irreversible. The syndrome is characterized by rhythmical involuntry movements of the tongue, face, mouth or jaw (e.g., protrusion of tongue, puffing of cheeks, puckering of mouth, chewing movements). Sometimes these may be accompanied by involuntary movements of extremities.

There is no known effective treatment for tardive dyskinesia; anti-parkinsonism agents usually do not alleviate the symptoms of this syndrome. It is suggested that all antipsychotic agents be discontinued if these symptoms appear.

Should it be necessary to reinstitute treatment, or increase the dosage of the agent, or switch to a different antipsychotic agent, the syndrome may be masked.

It has been reported that fine vermicular movements of the tongue may be an early sign of the syndrome and if the medication is stopped at that time, the syndrome may not develop.

Endocrine Disturbances: Menstrual irregularities, altered libido, gynecomastia, lactation, weight gain, edema. False positive pregnancy tests have been reported.

Urinary Disturbances: Retention, incontinence.

Others: Hyperpyrexia. Behavioral effects suggestive of a paradoxical reaction have been reported. These include excitement, bizarre dreams, aggravation of psychoses, and toxic confusional states. More recently, a peculiar skin-eye syndrome has been recognized as a side effect following long-term treatment with phenothiazines. This reaction is marked by progressive pigmentation of areas of the skin or conjunctiva and/or accompanied by discoloration of the exposed sclera and cornea. Opacities of the anterior lens and cornea described as irregular or stellate in shape have also been reported. Systemic lupus erythematosus-like syndrome.

Dosage: Dosage must be individualized according to the degree of mental and emotional disburbance. In all cases, the smallest effective dosage should be determined for each patient.

ADULTS: *Psychotic manifestations:* The usual starting dose is 50 to 100 mg. three times a day, with a gradual increment to a maximum of 800 mg. daily if necessary. Once effective control of symptoms has been achieved, the dosage may be reduced gradually to determine the minimum maintenance dose. The total daily dosage ranges from 200 to 800 mg., divided into two to four doses.

For the short-term treatment of moderate to marked depression with variable degrees of anxiety in adult patients and for the treatment of multiple symptoms such as agitation, anxiety, depressed mood, tension, sleep disturbances, and fears in geriatric patients: The usual starting dose is 25 mg. three times a day. Dosage ranges from 10 mg. two to four times a day in milder cases to 50 mg. three or four times a day for more severely disturbed patients. The total daily dosage range is from 20 mg. to a maximum of 200 mg.

CHILDREN: Mellaril (thioridazine) is not intended for children under 2 years of age. For children aged 2 to 12 the dosage of thioridazine hydrochloride ranges from 0.5 to a maximun of 3.0 mg./Kg. per day. For children with moderate disorders 10 mg. two or three times a day is the usual starting dose. For hospitalized, severely disturbed, or psychotic children, 25 mg. two to three times daily is the usual starting dose. Dosage may be increased gradually until optimum therapeutic effect is obtained or the maximum has been reached.

Supplied:

MELLARIL (thioridazine) HCl

Tablets: 10 mg., 15 mg., 25 mg., 50 mg., 100 mg., 150 mg. and 200 mg. thioridazine hydrochloride, USP. Packages of 100 and 1000 tablets. Also, for wholly tax-supported institutions only, packages of 5000 tablets.

Concentrate—30 mg./ml: Each ml. contains 30 mg. thioridazine hydrochloride, USP, alcohol, USP, 3.0% by volume. Immediate containers: Amber glass bottles of 4 fl. oz (118 ml.) and 1 pint packaged as follows:

4 fl. oz bottles, in cartons of 12 bottles, with an accompanying dropper graduated to deliver 10 mg., 25 mg. and 50 mg. of thioridazine hydrochloride, USP. Also, for wholly tax-supported institutions only, gallon cartons of 32 x 4 oz. bottles, each with the same dropper.

1 pint bottles, in gallon cartons of 8 bottles (for Hospital Use Only) with dropper or MELLAMETER® (trademark for dispenser) which delivers 25mg thioridazine hydrochloride, USP, per actuation.

Concentrate—100 mg./ml: Each ml. contains 100 mg. thioridazine hydrochloride, USP, alcohol, 4.2% by volume, *4 fl. oz bottles,* in cartons of 12 bottles, with an accompanying dropper graduated to deliver 100 mg., 150 mg. and 200 mg. of thioridazine hydrochloride.

Remarks: Store and dispense: Below 86°F; tight, amber glass bottle.

The Concentrate may be diluted with distilled water, acidified tap water, or suitable juices. Each dose should be so diluted just prior to administration—preparation and storage of bulk dilutions is not recommended.

MELLARIL-S (thioridazine) base

Suspension—25 mg/5 ml: Each 5 ml contains thioridazine base, equivalent to 25 mg thioridazine hydrochloride, USP. Buttermint-flavored in pint bottles.

Suspension—100 mg/5 ml: Each 5 ml contains thioridazine base, equivalent to 100 mg thioridazine hydrochloride, USP. Buttermint-flavored in pint bottles.

Company's Product Identification Mark(s): All tabs branded MEL with mg strength one side, triangle(s) other side.

[MEL-Z28 Issued November 15, 1979]

[*Shown in Product Identification Section*]

MESANTOIN® Tablets ℞
(mephenytoin) tablets, NF

The following prescribing information is based on official labeling in effect on November 1, 1979.

Description: Mesantoin (mephenytoin) is 3-methyl 5,5-phenyl-ethyl-hydantoin. It may be considered to be the hydantoin homolog of the barbiturate mephobarbital.

Actions: Mephenytoin exhibits pharmacologic effects similar to both diphenylhydantoin and the barbiturates in antagonizing experimental seizures in laboratory animals. Mephenytoin produces behavioral and electroencephalographic effects in man which are similar to those produced by barbiturates.

Indications: For the control of grand mal, focal, Jacksonian, and psychomotor seizures in those patients who have been refractory to less toxic anticonvulsants.

Contraindications: Hypersensitivity to hydantoin products.

Warnings: Mephenytoin should be used only after safer anticonvulsants have been given an adequate trial and have failed.

As with all anticonvulsants, dose reduction must be gradual so as to minimize the risk of precipitating seizures.

Usage in Pregnancy: The effects of mephenytoin in human pregnancy and nursing infants are unknown.

Continued on next page

Sandoz—Cont.

Recent reports suggest an association between the use of anticonvulsant drugs by women with epilepsy and an elevated incidence of birth defects in children born to these women. Data are more extensive with respect to diphenylhydantoin and phenobarbital, but these are also the most commonly prescribed anticonvulsants; less systematic or anecdotal reports suggest a possible similar association with the use of all known anticonvulsant drugs.

The reports suggesting an elevated incidence of birth defects in children of drug-treated epileptic women cannot be regarded as adequate to prove a definite cause and effect relationship. There are intrinsic methodologic problems in obtaining adequate data on drug teratogenicity in humans; the possibility also exists that other factors, e.g., genetic factors or the epileptic condition itself, may be more important than drug therapy in leading to birth defects. The great majority of mothers on anticonvulsant medication deliver normal infants. It is important to note than anticonvulsant drugs should not be discontinued in patients in whom the drug is administered to prevent major seizures because of the strong possibility of precipitating status epilepticus with attendant hypoxia and threat to life. In individual cases where the severity and frequency of the seizure disorder are such that the removal of medication does not pose a serious threat to the patient, discontinuation of the drug may be considered prior to and during pregnancy, although it cannot be said with any confidence that even minor seizures do not pose some hazards to the developing embryo or fetus.

The prescribing physician will wish to weigh these considerations in treating or counseling epileptic women of child-bearing potential.

Precautions: The patient taking Mesantoin (mephenytoin) must be kept under close medical supervision at all times since serious adverse reactions may emerge.

Because the primary site of degradation is the liver, it is recommended that screening tests of liver function precede introduction of the drug. Some patients may show side reactions as the result of individual sensitivity. These reactions can be broken down into three types respectively according to severity: 1) blood dyscrasias; 2) skin and mucous membrane manifestations; and 3) central effects. The blood, skin and mucous membrane manifestations are the more important since they can be more serious in nature. Since mephenytoin has been reported to produce blood dyscrasia in certain instances, the patient must be instructed that in the event any unusual symptoms develop (e.g. sore throat, fever, mucous membrane bleeding, glandular swelling, cutaneous reaction), he must discontinue the drug and report for examination immediately. It is recommended that blood examinations be made (total white cell count and differential count) during the initial phase of administration. Such tests are best made: a) before starting medication; b) after 2 weeks on a low dosage; c) again after 2 weeks when full dosage is reached; d) thereafter, monthly for a year; e) from then on, every 3 months. If the neutrophils drop to between 2500 and 1600/cu.mm., counts are made every 2 weeks. Stop medication if the count drops to 1600.

Adverse Reactions: A number of side effects and toxic reactions have been reported with Mesantoin (mephenytoin) as well as with other hydantoin compounds. Many of these appear to be dose related while others seem to be a manifestation of a hypersensitivity reaction to these drugs.

Blood Dyscrasias

Leukopenia, neutropenia, agranulocytosis, thrombocytopenia and pancytopenia have occurred. Eosinophilia, monocytosis, and leukocytosis have been described. Simple anemia, hemolytic anemia, megaloblastic anemia and aplastic anemia have occurred but are uncommon.

Skin and Mucous Membrane Manifestations

Maculopapular, morbilliform, scarlatiniform, urticarial, purpuric (associted with thrombocytopenia) and non-specific skin rashes have been reported. Exfoliative dermatitis, erythema multiforme (Stevens-Johnson Syndrome), toxic epidermal necrolysis and fatal dermatitides have been described on rare occasions. Skin pigmentation and rashes associated with a lupus erythematosus syndrome have also been reported.

Central Effects

Drowsiness is dose-related and may be reduced by a reduction in dose. Ataxia, diplopia, nystagmus, dysarthria, fatigue, irritability, choreiform movements, depression and tremor have been encountered.

Nervousness, nausea, vomiting, sleeplessness and dizziness may occur during the initial stages of therapy. Generally, these symptoms are transient, often disappearing with continued treatment.

Mental confusion and psychotic disturbances and increased seizures have been reported, but a definite causal relationship with the drug is uncertain.

Miscellaneous

Hepatitis, jaundice and nephrosis have been reported but a definite cause and effect relationship between the drug and these effects has not been established.

Alopecia, weight gain, edema, photophobia, conjunctivitis and gum hyperplasia have been encountered.

Polyarthropathy, pulmonary fibrosis, lupus erythematosus syndrome, and lymphadenopathy which simulates Hodgkin's Disease have also been observed.

Dosage and Administration: Dosage of antiepileptic therapy should be adjusted to the needs of the individual patient. Maintenance dosage is that smallest amount of antiepileptic necessary to suppress seizures completely or reduce their frequency. Optimum dosage is attained by starting with ½ or 1 tablet of Mesantoin (mephenytoin) per day during the first week and thereafter increasing the daily dose by ½ or 1 tablet at weekly intervals. No dose should be increased until it has been taken for at least one week.

The average dose of Mesantoin for adults ranges from 2 to 6 tablets (0.2 to 0.6 Gm.) daily. In some instances it may be necessary to administer as much as 8 tablets or more daily in order to obtain full seizure control. Children usually require from 1 to 4 tablets (0.1 Gm. to 0.4 Gm.) according to nature of seizures and age.

When the physician wishes to replace the anticonvulsant now being employed with Mesantoin (mephenytoin), he should give ½ or 1 tablet of Mesantoin daily during the first week and gradually increase the daily dose at weekly intervals while gradually reducing that of the drug being discontinued. The transition can be made smoothly over a period of three to six weeks. If seizures are not completely controlled with the dose so attained, the daily dose should then be increased by a one-tablet increment at weekly intervals to the point of maximum effect. If the patient had also been receiving phenobarbital, it is well to continue it until the transition is completed, at which time gradual withdrawal of the phenobarbital may be tried.

How Supplied: Each tablet contains 100 mg (1½ gr.) mephenytoin and is scored to permit half-tablet dosage. Packages of 100 and 1,000 tablets. (Pale pink, compressed, scored).

Company's Product Identification Mark(s): Tablets embossed 78-52 and scored on one side, SANDOZ triangle S on other side.

[MES—Z10 Issued November 10, 1975]

[*Shown in Product Identification Section*]

METHERGINE® ℞

(methylergonovine maleate) injection, NF
(methylergonovine maleate) tablets, NF

The following prescribing information is based on official labeling in effect on November 1, 1979.

Description: Each Methergine *Tablet* contains 0.2 mg (1/320 gr.) methylergonovine maleate, NF Methergine *Injection* contains per ml: 0.2 mg (1/320 gr.) methylergonovine maleate, NF; 0.25 mg tartaric acid, NF; 3 mg sodium chloride, USP; and water for injection, USP, q.s. to 1 ml.

Actions: Methergine induces a rapid and sustained tetanic uterotonic effect which shortens the third stage of labor and reduces blood loss. The onset of action after i.v. administration is immediate; after i.m. administration, 2 to 5 minutes, and after oral administration, 5 to 10 minutes.

Indications: For routine management after delivery of the placenta; postpartum atony and hemorrhage; subinvolution. Under full obstetric supervision, it may be given in the second stage of labor following delivery of the anterior shoulder.

Contraindications: Hypertension; toxemia; pregnancy; and hypersensitivity.

Warning: This drug should not be administered i.v. routinely because of the possibility of inducing sudden hypertensive and cerebrovascular accidents. If i.v. administration is considered essential as a lifesaving measure, Methergine should be given slowly over a period of no less than 60 seconds with careful monitoring of blood pressure.

Precautions: Caution should be exercised in the presence of sepsis, obliterative vascular disease, hepatic or renal involvement.

Adverse Reactions: Nausea; vomiting; transient hypertension; dizziness; headache; tinnitus; diaphoresis and palpitation; temporary chest pain; and dyspnea.

Dosage and Administration: Intramuscularly: One ml, 0.2 mg (1/320 grain) after delivery of the anterior shoulder, after delivery of the placenta, or during the puerperium. May be repeated as required, at intervals of 2-4 hours. *Intravenously:* SEE WARNING SECTION. Dosage same as intramuscular. *Orally:* One tablet, 0.2 milligram (1/320 grain) 3 or 4 times daily in the puerperium for a maximum of 1 week.

How Supplied: Tablets in packages of 100 and 1000; Injection in 1 ml ampuls, boxes of 20 and 100.

Remarks: Methergine injection is a clear and colorless solution. In the event the ampul solution becomes discolored, it should not be used.

Company's Product Identification Mark(s): Tablets imprinted 78-54 on 1 side, SANDOZ other side.

[Met-Z13 Issued October 1, 1979]

[*Shown in Product Identification Section*]

PAMELOR® ℞

(nortriptyline HCl), capsules, NF
(nortriptyline HCl) solution, NF

The following prescribing information is based on official labeling in effect on November 1, 1979.

Description: Pamelor (nortriptyline HCl) is 5-(3-methylaminopropylidene)-10, 11-dihydro-5H-dibenzo [a,d] cycloheptene hydrochloride. Its molecular weight is 299.8, and its empirical formula is $C_{19}H_{21}N \cdot HCl$.

Actions: The mechanism of mood elevation by tricyclic antidepressants is at present unknown. Pamelor is not a monoamine oxidase inhibitor. It inhibits the activity of such diverse agents as histamine, 5-hydroxytryptamine, and acetylcholine. It increases the pressor effect of norepinephrine but blocks the pressor response of phenethylamine. Studies suggest that Pamelor interferes with the transport, release, and storage of catecholamines. Operant conditioning techniques

in rats and pigeons suggest that Pamelor has a combination of stimulant and depressant properties.
Indications: Pamelor is indicated for the relief of symptoms of depression. Endogenous depressions are more likely to be alleviated than are other depressive states.
Contraindications: The use of Pamelor or other tricyclic antidepressants concurrently with a monoamine oxidase (MAO) inhibitor is contraindicated. Hyperpyretic crises, severe convulsions, and fatalities have occurred when similar tricyclic antidepressants were used in such combinations. It is advisable to have discontinued the MAO inhibitor for at least two weeks before treatment with Pamelor is started. Patients hypersensitive to Pamelor should not be given the drug.
Cross-sensitivity between Pamelor and other dibenzazepines is a possibility.
Pamelor is contraindicated during the acute recovery period after myocardial infarction.
Warnings: Patients with cardiovascular disease should be given Pamelor only under close supervision because of the tendency of the drug to produce sinus tachycardia and to prolong the conduction time. Myocardial infarction, arrhythmia, and strokes have occurred. The antihypertensive action of guanethidine and similar agents may be blocked. Because of its anticholinergic activity, Pamelor should be used with great caution in patients who have glaucoma or a history of urinary retention. Patients with a history of seizures should be followed closely when Pamelor is administered, inasmuch as this drug is known to lower the convulsive threshold. Great care is required if Pamelor is given to hyperthyroid patients or to those receiving thyroid medication, since cardiac arrhythmias may develop.
Pamelor may impair the mental and/or physical abilities required for the performance of hazardous tasks, such as operating machinery or driving a car; therefore, the patient should be warned accordingly.
Excessive consumption of alcohol in combination with nortriptyline therapy may have a potentiating effect, which may lead to the danger of increased suicidal attempts or overdosage, especially in patients with histories of emotional disturbances or suicidal ideation.
Use in Pregnancy—Safe use of Pamelor during pregnancy and lactation has not been established; therefore, when the drug is administered to pregnant patients, nursing mothers, or women of childbearing potential, the potential benefits must be weighed against the possible hazards. Animal reproduction studies have yielded inconclusive results.
Use in Children—This drug is not recommended for use in children, since safety and effectiveness in the pediatric age group have not been established.
Precautions: The use of Pamelor in schizophrenic patients may result in an exacerbation of the psychosis or may activate latent schizophrenic symptoms. If the drug is given to overactive or agitated patients, increased anxiety and agitation may occur. In manic-depressive patients, Pamelor may cause symptoms of the manic phase to emerge.
Administration of reserpine during therapy with a tricyclic antidepressant has been shown to produce a "stimulating" effect in some depressed patients.
Troublesome patient hostility may be aroused by the use of Pamelor. Epileptiform seizures may accompany its administration, as is true of other drugs of its class.
Close supervision and careful adjustment of the dosage are required when Pamelor is used with other anticholinergic drugs and sympathomimetic drugs.
The patient should be informed that the response to alcohol may be exaggerated.
When it is essential, the drug may be administered with electroconvulsive therapy, although the hazards may be increased. Discontinue the drug for several days, if possible, prior to elective surgery.
The possibility of a suicidal attempt by a depressed patient remains after the initiation of treatment; in this regard, it is important that the least possible quantity of drug be dispensed at any given time.
Both elevation and lowering of blood sugar levels have been reported.
Adverse Reactions: Note: Included in the following list are a few adverse reactions that have not been reported with this specific drug. However, the pharmacologic similarities among the tricyclic antidepressant drugs require that each of the reactions be considered when nortriptyline is administered.
Cardiovascular—Hypotension, hypertension, tachycardia, palpitation, myocardial infarction, arrhythmias, heart block, stroke.
Psychiatric—Confusional states (especially in the elderly) with hallucinations, disorientation, delusions; anxiety, restlessness, agitation; insomnia, panic, nightmares; hypomania; exacerbation of psychosis.
Neurologic—Numbness, tingling, paresthesias of extremities; incoordination, ataxia, tremors; peripheral neuropathy; extrapyramidal symptoms; seizures, alteration in EEG patterns; tinnitus.
Anticholinergic—Dry mouth and, rarely, associated sublingual adenitis; blurred vision, disturbance of accommodation, mydriasis; constipation, paralytic ileus; urinary retention, delayed micturition, dilation of the urinary tract.
Allergic—Skin rash, petechiae, urticaria, itching, photosensitization (avoid excessive exposure to sunlight); edema (general or of face and tongue), drug fever, cross-sensitivity with other tricyclic drugs.
Hematologic—Bone-marrow depression, including agranulocytosis; eosinophilia; purpura; thrombocytopenia.
Gastrointestinal—Nausea and vomiting, anorexia, epigastric distress, diarrhea, peculiar taste, stomatitis, abdominal cramps, black-tongue.
Endocrine—Gynecomastia in the male, breast enlargement and galactorrhea in the female; increased or decreased libido, impotence; testicular swelling; elevation or depression of blood sugar levels.
Other—Jaundice (simulating obstructive); altered liver function; weight gain or loss; perspiration; flushing; urinary frequency, nocturia; drowsiness, dizziness, weakness, fatigue; headache; parotid swelling; alopecia.
Withdrawal Symptoms—Though these are not indicative of addiction, abrupt cessation of treatment after prolonged therapy may produce nausea, headache, and malaise.
Dosage and Administration: Pamelor is not recommended for children.
Pamelor is administered orally in the form of capsules or liquid. Lower than usual dosages are recommended for elderly patients and adolescents. Lower dosages are also recommended for outpatients than for hospitalized patients who will be under close supervision. The physician should initiate dosage at a low level and increase it gradually, noting carefully the clinical response and any evidence of intolerance. Following remission, maintenance medication may be required for a longer period of time at the lowest dose that will maintain remission.
If a patient develops minor side-effects, the dosage should be reduced. The drug should be discontinued promptly if adverse effects of a serious nature or allergic manifestations occur.
Usual Adult Dose—25 mg three or four times daily; dosage should begin at a low level and be increased as required. Doses above 100 mg per day are not recommended. As an alternate regimen, the total daily dosage may be given once-a-day.
Elderly and Adolescent Patients—30 to 50 mg per day, in divided doses, or the total daily dosage may be given once-a-day.
Overdosage: Toxic overdosage may result in confusion, restlessness, agitation, vomiting, hyperpyrexia, muscle rigidity, hyperactive reflexes, tachycardia, ECG evidence of impaired conduction, shock, congestive heart failure, stupor, coma, and C.N.S. stimulation with convulsions followed by respiratory depression. Deaths have occurred following overdosage with drugs of this class.
No specific antidote is known. General supportive measures are indicated, with gastric lavage. Respiratory assistance is apparently the most effective measure when indicated. The use of C.N.S. depressants may worsen the prognosis.
The administration of barbiturates for control of convulsions alleviates an increase in the cardiac work load but should be undertaken with caution to avoid potentiation of respiratory depression.
Intramuscular paraldehyde or diazepam provides anticonvulsant activity with less respiratory depression than do the barbiturates; diazepam seems to be preferred.
The use of digitalis and/or physostigmine may be considered in case of serious cardiovascular abnormalities or cardiac failure.
The value of dialysis has not been established.
How Supplied:
Solution: Pamelor (nortriptyline HCl) NF, equivalent to 10 mg base per 5 ml is supplied in 16-fluid-ounce bottles.
Capsules: Pamelor (nortriptyline HCl) NF, equivalent to 10 mg, 25 mg and 75 mg base, are supplied in bottles of 100. The 10 mg and 25 mg capsules are available in boxes of 100 individually labeled blisters, each containing 1 capsule. The 25 mg capsules are also available in bottles of 500.

[PAM-Z6 Issued November 1, 1979]

[*Shown in Product Identification Section*]

PARLODEL® ℞
(bromocriptine mesylate)

The following prescribing information is based on official labeling in effect on November 1, 1979.
Description: Parlodel® (bromocriptine mesylate) is a potent dopamine receptor agonist that inhibits prolactin secretion. This activity represents a new therapeutic use for specific peptide ergot alkaloid derivatives. Each Parlodel tablet for oral administration contains 2.5 mg bromocriptine (as the mesylate). Parlodel is chemically designated as (1) Ergotaman-3′, 6′, 18-trione, 2-bromo-12′-hydroxy-2′-(1-methylethyl)-5′-(2-methylpropyl)-,(5′*a*) monomethanesulfonate (salt); (2) 2-bromoergocryptine monomethanesulfonate (salt).
Actions: Parlodel® (bromocriptine mesylate) has been shown to be a dopamine receptor agonist in that it activates post-synaptic dopamine receptors. The tubero-infundibular dopaminergic neurons modulate the secretion of prolactin from the anterior pituitary by stimulating the release of prolactin inhibitory factor. Clinically, Parlodel has been shown to significantly reduce plasma levels of prolactin in patients with hyperprolactinemia. Pharmacologic experiments have demonstrated the selectivity and efficacy of bromocriptine in inhibiting prolactin secretion in several mammalian species under various experimental conditions. Studies have shown that bromocriptine suppresses physiological lactation in several species as well as prolactin-dependent tumors at dose levels that do not affect other tropic hormones from the anterior pituitary.
Parlodel (bromocriptine mesylate) is a nonhormonal, nonestrogenic agent which inhibits the secretion of prolactin in humans, with little or no effect on other pituitary hormones, except

Continued on next page

Sandoz—Cont.

in patients with acromegaly, where it lowers elevated blood levels of growth hormone.
In about 75% of cases of galactorrhea associated with amenorrhea, in the absence of demonstrable pituitary tumor, Parlodel therapy suppresses the galactorrhea completely, or almost completely, and reinitiates normal ovulatory menstrual cycles.
Menses are usually reinitiated prior to complete suppression of galactorrhea; the time for this on average is 6-8 weeks. However, some patients respond within a few days.
Galactorrhea may take longer to control depending on the degree of stimulation of the mammary tissue prior to therapy. At least 75% reduction in secretion is usually observed after 8-12 weeks. Some patients may fail to respond even after 24 weeks of therapy.

Human Pharmacology
The pharmacokinetics and metabolism of bromocriptine in human subjects was studied with the help of radioactively labeled drug. It was found that 28% of an oral dose was absorbed from the gastrointestinal tract. The blood levels following a 2.5 mg dose were in the range of 2-3 ng equivalents/ml. The plasma levels were in the range of 4-6 ng equivalents/ml indicating that the red blood cells did not contain appreciable amounts of drug and/or metabolites. *In vitro* experiments showed that the drug was 90-96% bound to serum albumin.
Bromocriptine was completely metabolized prior to excretion. The major route of excretion of absorbed drug was via the bile. Only 2.5-5.5% of the dose was excreted in the urine. Almost all (84.6%) of the administered dose was excreted in the feces in 120 hours.
Indications: Parodel® (bromocriptine mesylate) a dopamine receptor agonist, is indicated for the short-term treatment of amenorrhea/galactorrhea associated with hyperprolactinemia due to varied etiologies, excluding demonstrable pituitary tumors. It is not indicated in patients with normal prolactin levels. Safe use of this drug has not been demonstrated in pregnancy. Parlodel tablets are thus not indicated in the management of infertility.
Contraindications: Sensitivity to any ergot alkaloids.
Warnings: Since hyperprolactinemia with amenorrhea/galactorrhea has been found in patients with pituitary tumors (Forbes-Albright syndrome), a complete evaluation of the sella turcica is advisable before treatment with Parlodel. Although Parlodel therapy will effectively lower plasma levels of prolactin in patients with pituitary tumors, this does not obviate the necessity of radiotherapy or surgical procedures where appropriate.
If pregnancy occurs during Parlodel administration, treatment should be discontinued immediately.
Since it will interfere with lactation, Parlodel should not be administered to nursing mothers.
Safety and efficacy of Parlodel (bromocriptine mesylate) have not been established in children under age 15.
In human studies with Parlodel® (bromocriptine mesylate) there have been approximately 343 infants born to women outside the United States and 26 infants born to women in the United States who took Parlodel during early pregnancy. Among the 343 infants born outside the United States, 11 cases of congenital anomalies have been reported: one case of renal agenesis in a twin, one of pulmonary artery stenosis, one of cleft palate, one of club foot, and one of congenital inguinal hernia, 2 congenital dislocation of the hip, 2 syndactyly, 1 single umbilical artery, 1 with high blood urea (a twin) but no developmental anomalies. All of the 26 infants born in the United States were normal. In addition to these pregnancies, 70 abortions have been reported. Of these 49 were spontaneous and 21 were induced. There were 3 extrauterine pregnancies, 3 intrauterine deaths (20, 24 and 30 weeks), 1 premature birth at 20 weeks, 1 twin birth at 24 weeks and 1 hydatidiform mole.
The reported incidence of congenital malformations and spontaneous abortions within this group of pregnancies does not exceed that generally reported for such occurrences in the population at large. However, it must be noted that the total number of pregnancies reported is an insufficient sample in which to detect any given birth defect, and extrapolation of these data to a greater patient population would be statistically invalid.
Bromocriptine has been investigated in five rabbit studies using two strains to assess potential teratogenic activity; these studies encompassed 740 offspring of mothers treated with the drug. In two of these studies, in which bromocriptine was given before implantation, no significant toxic or teratogenic effect could be found. When the drug was given postimplantation in two other studies using the Yellow-Silver strain, induction of cleft palate was observed in 5/208 offspring of mothers given 100 mg/kg and 300 mg/kg (667 and 2000 times the human doses, respectively). At a dose of 10 mg/kg (67 times the human dose) no teratogenic effects were noted. One cleft palate was observed in 168 concurrent control offspring in the last two studies. In a fifth study there were no teratogenic effects produced in the New Zealand strain of rabbits treated with 100 and 300 mg/kg postimplantation. Random findings in the control and drug groups in all five studies, for which no causal relationship could be found, included renal agenesis and aplasia, missing vertebrae, double rib, aplasia of the gall bladder, and gastrochisis.
Teratogenic studies also were conducted in two strains of rats using doses of bromocriptine as high as 30 mg/kg (200 times the human dose) postimplantation. One instance of aplasia of spinal vertebrae and ribs occurred out of a total of 281 fetuses (0.4%) from dams given 30 mg/kg/day. No malformations were induced with the lower doses. Fertility was not reduced by treatment before mating for 14 days at doses of 1 mg/kg/day and 3 mg/kg/day. No abnormalities were found in stumptail monkeys at a dose of 2 mg/kg/day (13 times the human dose).
Precautions: Treatment of women suffering from amenorrhea/galactorrhea with Parlodel® (bromocriptine mesylate) may result in restoration of fertility. Therefore, patients should be required to use contraceptive measures, other than the oral contraceptives, during treatment with Parlodel. However, since patients often ignore this recommendation and since pregnancy may occur prior to reinitiation of menses, as an additional precaution, a pregnancy test is recommended at least every four weeks during the amenorrheic period, and, once menses are reinitiated, every time a patient misses a menstrual period.
Parlodel therapy has been demonstrated to be effective in the short-term managemment of amenorrhea/galactorrhea only. Data are not available on the safety or effectiveness of its use in long-term continuous dosage, or in patients given repeated courses of treatment following recurrence of amenorrhea/galactorrhea after initial treatment. Recurrence rates are reportedly very high, ranging from 70 to 80% in domestic and foreign studies.
Adverse Reactions: The incidence of adverse effects is quite high (68%) but these are generally mild to moderate in degree. Therapy was discontinued in approximately 6% of patients because of adverse effects. These in decreasing order of frequency are nausea 51%, headache 18%, dizziness 16%, fatigue 8%, abdominal cramps 7%, lightheadedness 6%, vomiting 5%, nasal congestion 5%, constipation 3% and diarrhea 3%.
A slight hypotensive effect may accompany Parlodel® (bromocriptine mesylate) treatment. The occurrence of adverse reactions may be lessened by temporarily reducing dosage to one-half tablet two to three times daily.
Dosage and Administration: The therapeutic dosage of Parlodel is one 2.5 mg tablet, two or three times daily, with meals. The duration of treatment should not exceed six months. It is recommended that treatment commence with one tablet daily, increasing to a therapeutic dosage within the first week, to reduce the possibility of adverse reactions.
How Supplied: Round, white tablets, each containing 2½ mg bromocryptine (as the mesylate) in packages of 30. Embossed PARLODEL 2½ on one side and scored on other side.
Company's Product Identification Mark(s): Tablets embossed "78-17" on one side, "SANDOZ" on the other side.

[PAR-Z3 Issued October 2, 1979]
[*Shown in Product Identification Section*]

PLEXONAL® Tablets ©

The following prescribing information is based on official labeling in effect on November 1, 1979.
Composition: Each Plexonal *Tablet* contains: 45 mg barbital sodium, 25 mg butalbital sodium (Sandoptal® sodium), Warning: May be habit forming. 15 mg phenobarbital sodium, USP, 0.16 mg dihydroergotamine mesylate, NF, 0.08 mg scopolamine hydrobromide, USP.
Properties and Therapeutics: Plexonal provides a sedative-relaxant effect for patients with symptoms such as anxiety, tension, irritability, restlessness and insomnia. A balanced action is achieved through the use of three barbiturates with differing rates of action and dissipation, potentiated by scopolamine and dihydroergotamine.
Indications: Anxiety, tension, nervousness, irritability, apprehension, restlessness, hyperexcitability, insomnia.
Contraindications: Severely depressed or comatose states. Hypersensitivity to any of the components.
Precautions: Use with caution in the presence of hepatic disease, fever, hyperthyroidism, diabetes mellitus, severe anemia. Due to presence of barbiturates, may be habit forming.
Side Effects: Drowsiness, skin rashes, gastrointestinal disturbances may occur.
Dosage: For daytime sedation—1 tablet, 2 to 4 times daily; range, 2 to 6 tablets per day. To promote sleep—2 to 4 tablets, ½ hour before bedtime.
Supplied: Triangular tablets (white, sugar-coated) in bottles of 100.
Company Product Identification Mark(s): Tablets imprinted 78—on 1 side, and—57 other side.

[PLX-Z8 Issued October 26, 1977]
[*Shown in Product Identification Section*]

SANOREX® ©
(mazindol)

The following prescribing information is based on official labeling in effect on November 1, 1979.
Description: Sanorex (mazindol) is an imidazoisoindole anorectic agent. It is chemically designated as 5-p-chloro-phenyl-5-hydroxy-2, 3-dihydro-5H-imidazo (2,1-a) isoindole, a tautomeric form of 2-[2'-(p-chlorobenzoyl) phenyl]-2-imidazoline.
Actions: Sanorex, although an isoindole, has pharmacologic activity similar in many ways to the prototype drugs used in obesity, the amphetamines. Actions include central nervous system stimulation in humans and animals, as well as such amphetamine-like effects in animals as the production of stereotyped behavior. Animal experiments also suggest certain

differences from phenethylamine anorectic drugs, e.g., amphetamine, with respect to site and mechanism of action; for example, mazindol appears to exert its primary effects on the limbic system. The significance of these differences for humans is uncertain. It does not cause brain norepinephrine depletion in animals; on the other hand, it does appear to inhibit storage site uptake of norepinephrine as is suggested by its marked potentiation of the effect of exogenous norepinephrine on blood pressure in dogs (see WARNINGS) and on smooth muscle contraction *in vitro*.

Tolerance has been demonstrated with all drugs of this class in which this phenomenon has been studied.

Drugs used in obesity are commonly known as "anorectics" or "anorexigenics." It has not been established, however, that the action of such drugs in treating obesity is exclusively one of appetite suppression. Other central nervous system actions, or metabolic effects may be involved as well.

Adult obese subjects instructed in dietary management and treated with anorectic drugs, lose more weight on the average than those treated with placebo and diet, as determined in relatively short-term clinical trials.

The average magnitude of increased weight loss of drug-treated patients over placebo-treated patients in studies of anorectics in general is ordinarily only a fraction of a pound a week. The rate of weight loss is greatest in the first weeks of therapy for both drug and placebo subjects and tends to decrease in succeeding weeks.

The amount of weight loss associated with the use of Sanorex (mazindol), as with other anorectic drugs, varies from trial to trial, and the increased weight loss appears to be related in part to variables other than the drugs prescribed, such as the interaction between physician-investigator and the patient, the population treated, and the diet prescribed. The importance of non-drug factors in such weight loss has not been elucidated.

The natural history of obesity is measured in years, whereas, most studies cited are restricted to a few weeks' duration; thus, the total impact of drug-induced weight loss over that of diet alone must be considered clinically limited.

Indication: Sanorex is indicated in the management of exogenous obesity as a short-term (a few weeks) adjunct in a regimen of weight reduction based on caloric restriction. The limited usefulness of agents of this class (see ACTIONS) should be measured against possible risk factors inherent in their use, such as those described below.

Contraindications: Glaucoma; hypersensitivity or idiosyncrasy to Sanorex.

Agitated states.

Patients with a history of drug abuse.

During or within 14 days following the administration of monoamine oxidase inhibitors, (hypertensive crises may result).

Warnings: Tolerance to the effect of many anorectic drugs may develop within a few weeks; if this occurs, the recommended dose should not be exceeded in an attempt to increase the effect; rather, the drug should be discontinued.

Sanorex (mazindol) may impair the ability of the patient to engage in potentially hazardous activities such as operating machinery or driving a motor vehicle; the patient should therefore be cautioned accordingly.

Drug Interactions: Sanorex (mazindol) may decrease the hypotensive effect of guanethidine; patients should be monitored accordingly.

Sanorex may markedly potentiate the pressor effect of exogenous catecholamines. If it should be necessary to give a pressor amine agent (e.g., levarterenol or isoproterenol) to a patient in shock (e.g., from a myocardial infarction) who has recently been taking Sanorex, extreme care should be taken in monitoring blood pressure at frequent intervals and initiating pressor therapy with a low initial dose and careful titration.

Drug Dependence: Sanorex shares important pharmacologic properties with amphetamines. Amphetamines and related stimulant drugs have been extensively abused and can produce tolerance and severe psychologic dependence. In this regard, the manifestations of chronic overdosage or withdrawal of Sanorex have not been determined in humans. Abstinence effects have been observed in dogs after abrupt cessation for prolonged periods. There was some self-administration of the drug in monkeys. EEG studies and "liking" scores in human subjects yielded equivocal results. While the abuse potential of Sanorex (mazindol) has not been further defined, the possibility of dependence should be kept in mind when evaluating the desirability of including Sanorex as part of a weight reduction program.

Usage in Pregnancy: Sanorex was studied in reproduction experiments in rats and rabbits and an increase in neonatal mortality and a possible increased incidence of rib anomalies in rats were observed at relatively high doses. Although these studies have not indicated important adverse effects, use of mazindol by women who are or may become pregnant requires that the potential benefit be weighed against the possible hazard to mother and infant.

Usage in Children: Sanorex is not recommended for use in children under 12 years of age.

Precautions: Insulin requirements in diabetes mellitus may be altered in association with the use of mazindol and the concomitant dietary regimen.

The least amount feasible should be prescribed or dispensed at one time in order to minimize the possibility of overdosage.

Use only with caution in hypertension with monitoring of blood pressure, since evidence is insufficient to rule out a possible adverse effect on blood pressure in some hypertensive patients. The drug is not recommended in severely hypertensive patients. The drug is not recommended for patients with symptomatic cardiovascular disease including arrhythmias.

Adverse Reactions: The most common adverse effects of Sanorex (mazindol) are dry mouth, tachycardia, constipation, nervousness and insomnia.

Cardiovascular: Palpitation, tachycardia.

Central Nervous System: Overstimulation, restlessness, dizziness, insomnia, dysphoria, tremor, headache, depression, drowsiness, weakness.

Gastrointestinal: Dryness of the mouth, unpleasant taste, diarrhea, constipation, nausea, other gastrointestinal disturbances.

Skin: Rash, excessive sweating, clamminess.

Endocrine: Impotence, changes in libido have rarely been observed with Sanorex.

Eye: Treatment of dogs with high doses of Sanorex for long periods resulted in some corneal opacities, reversible on cessation of medication. No such effect has been observed in humans.

Dosage and Administration: Usual dosage is 1 mg three times daily, one hour before meals, or 2 mg once daily, one hour before lunch. The lowest effective dose should be used. To determine the lowest effective dose, therapy with Sanorex may be initiated at 1 mg once a day, and adjusted to the need and response of the patient. Should G.I. discomfort occur, Sanorex may be taken with meals.

Overdosage: There are no data as yet on acute overdosage with Sanorex (mazindol) in humans.

Manifestations of acute overdosage with amphetamines and related substances include restlessness, tremor, rapid respiration, dizziness. Fatigue and depression may follow the stimulatory phase of overdosage. Cardiovascular effects include tachycardia, hypertension and circulatory collapse. Gastrointestinal symptoms include nausea, vomiting and abdominal cramps. While similar manifestations of overdosage may be seen with Sanorex (mazindol), their exact nature has yet to be determined. The management of acute intoxication is largely symptomatic. Data are not available on the treatment of acute intoxication with Sanorex by hemodialysis or peritoneal dialysis, but the substance is poorly soluble except at very acid pH.

How Supplied: Sanorex® (mazindol) is available in 1 mg elliptical, white tablets and in 2 mg round, white scored tablets, in packages of 100.

Company's Product Indentification Mark(s): 1 mg tablets embossed 78- on 1 side, 71 other side. 2 mg tablets scored 78-66 on 1 side, SANDOZ other side.

[SNX-Z8 Issued September 4, 1979]

[*Shown in Product Identification Section*]

SANSERT® ℞

(methysergide maleate) tablets, USP

The following prescribing information is based on official labeling in effect on November 1, 1979.

WARNING

Retroperitoneal Fibrosis, Pleuropulmonary Fibrosis and Fibrotic Thickening of Cardiac Valves May Occur in Patients Receiving Long-term Methysergide Maleate Therapy. Therefore, This Preparation Must be Reserved for Prophylaxis in Patients Whose Vascular Headaches Are Frequent and/or Severe and Uncontrollable and Who Are Under Close Medical Supervision.

(*See Also "Warnings" Section.*)

Composition: Each Sansert tablet contains 2 mg methysergide maleate, USP.

Actions: Sansert (methysergide maleate) has been shown, *in vitro* and *in vivo*, to inhibit or block the effects of serotonin, a substance which may be involved in the mechanism of vascular headaches. Serotonin has been variously described as a central neurohumoral agent or chemical mediator, as a "headache substance" acting directly or indirectly to lower pain threshold (others in this category include tyramine; polypeptides, such as bradykinin; histamine; and acetylcholine), as an intrinsic "motor hormone" of the gastrointestinal tract, and as a "hormone" involved in connective tissue reparative processes. Suggestions have been made by investigators as to the mechanism whereby methysergide produces its clinical effects, but this has not been finally established.

Indications: For the prevention or reduction of intensity and frequency of vascular headaches in the following kinds of patients:

1. Patients suffering from one or more severe vascular headaches per week.
2. Patients suffering from vascular headaches that are uncontrollable or so severe that preventive therapy is indicated regardless of the frequency of the attack.

Contraindications: Pregnancy, peripheral vascular disease, severe arteriosclerosis, severe hypertension, coronary artery disease, phlebitis or cellulitis of the lower limbs, pulmonary disease, collagen diseases or fibrotic processes, impaired liver or renal function, valvular heart disease, debilitated states and serious infections.

Warnings: With long-term, uninterrupted administration, retroperitoneal fibrosis or related conditions—pleuropulmonary fibrosis and cardiovascular disorders with murmurs or vascular bruits have been reported. Patients

Continued on next page

Sandoz—Cont.

must be warned to report immediately the following symptoms: cold, numb, and painful hands and feet; leg cramps on walking; any type of girdle, flank, or chest pain, or any associated symptomatology. Should any of these symptoms develop, methysergide should be discontinued. Continuous administration should not exceed 6 months. There must be a drug-free interval of 3-4 weeks after each 6-month course of treatment. The dosage should be reduced gradually during the last 2-3 weeks of each treatment course to avoid "headache rebound."

The drug is not recommended for use in children.

Precautions: All patients receiving Sansert (methysergide maleate) should remain under constant supervision of the physician and be examined regularly for the development of fibrotic or vascular complications. (See Adverse Reactions).

The manifestations of retroperitoneal fibrosis, pleuropulmonary fibrosis, and vascular shutdown have shown a high incidence of regression once Sansert is withdrawn. These facts should be borne in mind to avoid unnecessary surgical intervention. Cardiac murmurs, which may indicate endocardial fibrosis, have shown varying degrees of regression, with complete disappearance in some and persistence in others.

Sansert has been specifically designed for the prophylaxis of vascular headache and has no place in the management of the acute attack.

Adverse Reactions: Within the recommended dose levels, the following side effects have been reported:

1) Fibrotic Complications

Fibrotic changes have been observed in the retroperitoneal, pleuropulmonary, cardiac, and other tissues, either singly or, very rarely, in combination.

Retroperitoneal Fibrosis: This non-specific fibrotic process is usually confined to the retroperitoneal connective tissue above the pelvic brim and may present clinically with one or more symptoms such as general malaise, fatigue, weight loss, backache, low grade fever (elevated sedimentation rate), urinary obstruction (girdle or flank pain, dysuria, polyuria, oliguria, elevated BUN), vascular insufficiency of the lower limbs (leg pain, Leriche syndrome, edema of legs, thrombophlebitis). The single most useful diagnostic procedure in suspected cases of retroperitoneal fibrosis is intravenous pyelography. Typical deviation and obstruction of one or both ureters may be observed.

Pleuropulmonary Complications: A similar nonspecific fibrotic process, limited to the pleural and immediately subjacent pulmonary tissues, usually presents clinically with dyspnea, tightness and pain in the chest, pleural friction rubs, and pleural effusion. These findings may be confirmed by chest X-ray.

Cardiac Complications: Nonrheumatic fibrotic thickenings of the aortic root and of the aortic and mitral valves usually present clinically with cardiac murmurs and dyspnea.

Other Fibrotic Complications: Several cases of fibrotic plaques simulating Peyronie's disease have been described.

2) Cardiovascular Complications

Encroachment of retroperitoneal fibrosis on the aorta, inferior vena cava and their common iliac branches may result in vascular insufficiency of the lower limbs, the presenting features of which are mentioned under retroperitoneal fibrosis.

Intrinsic vasoconstriction of large and small arteries, involving one or more vessels or merely a segment of a vessel, may occur at any stage of therapy. Depending on the vessel involved, this complication may present with chest pain, abdominal pain, or cold, numb, painful extremities with or without paresthesias and diminished or absent pulses. Progression to ischemic tissue damage has rarely been reported. Prompt withdrawal of the drug at the first signs of impaired circulation is recommended (See Warnings) to obviate such effects. Postural hypotension and tachycardia have also been observed.

3) Gastrointestinal Symptoms

Nausea, vomiting, diarrhea, heartburn, abdominal pain. These effects tend to appear early and can frequently be obviated by gradual introduction of the medication and by administration of the drug with meals.

Constipation and elevation of gastric HCl have also been reported.

4) CNS Symptoms

Insomnia, drowsiness, mild euphoria, dizziness, ataxia, lightheadedness, hyperesthesia, unworldly feelings (described variously as "dissociation," "hallucinatory experiences," etc.). Some of these symptoms may be associated with vascular headaches, per se, and may, therefore, be unrelated to the drug.

5) Dermatological Manifestations

Facial flush, telangiectasia, and nonspecific rashes have rarely been reported. Increased hair loss may occur, but in many instances the tendency has abated despite continued therapy.

6) Edema

Peripheral edema, and more rarely, localized brawny edema may occur.

Dependent edema has responded to lowered doses, salt restriction, or diuretics.

7) Weight Gain

Weight gain may be a reason to caution patients regarding their caloric intake.

8) Hematological Manifestations

Neutropenia, eosinophilia.

9) Miscellaneous

Weakness, arthralgia, myalgia.

Dosage and Administration: Usual adult dose 4 to 8 mg daily. Tablets to be given with meals.

Note: There must be a medication-free interval of 3-4 weeks after every 6-month course of treatment (see WARNINGS).

No pediatric dosage has been established.

If, after a 3-week trial period, efficacy has not been demonstrated, longer administration of Sansert (methysergide maleate) is unlikely to be of benefit.

How Supplied: Bottles of 100 tablets, each tablet containing 2 mg of methysergide maleate, USP.

Company's Product Identification Mark(s): Imprinted 78-58 on 1 side, SANDOZ other side.

[SAN-Z16 Issued May 25, 1979]

[*Shown in Product Identification Section*]

SYNTOCINON® INJECTION ℞

(oxytocin) injection, USP

The following prescribing information is based on official labeling in effect on November 1, 1979.

Description: Syntocinon (oxytocin) injection is a synthetic polypeptide consisting of 8 amino acids. Each ml contains: 10 USP Units (International Units) of 1 mg sodium acetate, USP; 0.5% chlorobutanol, USP; 0.61% by vol. alcohol, USP; acetic acid, USP, q.s. to pH 4 ± 0.3; and water for injection, USP, q.s. to 1 ml.

Action: The pharmacologic and clinical properties of Syntocinon (oxytocin) injection are identical with the naturally occurring oxytocic principle of the posterior lobe of the pituitary. Syntocinon (oxytocin) injection does not contain the amino acids characteristic of vasopressin, and therefore lacks cardiovascular effects. Syntocinon (oxytocin) injection exerts a selective action on the smooth musculature of the uterus, particularly toward the end of pregnancy, during labor and immediately following delivery. Oxytocin stimulates rhythmic contractions of the uterus, increases the frequency of existing contractions, and raises the tone of the uterine musculature.

Indications

> **IMPORTANT NOTICE**
> Syntocinon® (oxytocin) injection is indicated for the medical rather than the elective induction of labor. Available data and information are inadequate to define the benefits to risks considerations in the use of the drug product for elective induction. Elective induction of labor is defined as the initiation of labor for convenience in an individual with a term pregnancy who is free of medical indications.

Antepartum: Syntocinon (oxytocin) injection is indicated for the initiation or improvement of uterine contractions, where this is desirable and considered suitable, in order to achieve early vaginal delivery for fetal or maternal reasons. It is indicated for (1) induction of labor in patients with a medical indication for the initiation of labor, such as Rh problems, maternal diabetes, preeclampsia at or near term, when delivery is in the best interest of mother and fetus or when membranes are prematurely ruptured and delivery is indicated; (2) stimulation or reinforcement of labor, as in selected cases of uterine inertia; (3) management of inevitable, incomplete, or missed abortion.

Postpartum: Syntocinon (oxytocin) injection is indicated to produce uterine contractions during the third stage of labor and to control postpartum bleeding or hemorrhage.

Contraindications: Syntocinon® (oxytocin) injection is contraindicated in any of the following conditions: Significant cephalopelvic disproportion; unfavorable fetal positions or presentations which are undeliverable without conversion prior to delivery, i.e., (transverse lies); in obstetrical emergencies where the benefit-to-risk ratio for either the fetus or the mother favors surgical intervention; in cases of fetal distress where delivery is not imminent; prolonged use in uterine inertia or severe toxemia; hypertonic uterine patterns; patients with hypersensitivity to the drug; induction or augmentation of labor in those cases where vaginal delivery is contraindicated, such as cord presentation or prolapse, total placenta previa, and vasa previa.

Warnings: Syntocinon (oxytocin) injection when given for induction or stimulation of labor, must be administered only by the intravenous route and with adequate medical supervision in a hospital.

Precautions:

1. All patients receiving intravenous oxytocin must be under continuous observation by trained personnel with a thorough knowledge of the drug and qualified to identify complications. A physician qualified to manage any complications should be immediately available.

2. When properly administered, oxytocin should stimulate uterine contractions similar to those seen in normal labor. Overstimulation of the uterus by improper administration can be hazardous to both mother and fetus. Even with proper administration and adequate supervision, hypertonic contractions can occur in patients whose uteri are hypersensitive to oxytocin.

3. Except in unusual circumstances, oxytocin should not be administered in the following conditions: prematurity, borderline cephalopelvic disproportion, previous major surgery on the cervix or uterus including cesarean section, over-distention of the uterus, grand multiparity, or invasive cervical carcinoma. Because of the variability of the combinations of factors which may be present in the conditions listed above, the definition of "unusual circumstances" must be left to the judgment of the physician. The decision can only be made by carefully weighing the potential benefits which oxytocin can provide in a given case against rare but definite potential for the drug to produce hypertonicity or tetanic spasm.

4. Maternal deaths due to hypertensive episodes, subarachnoid hemorrhage, rupture of the uterus, and fetal deaths due to various causes have been reported associated with the use of parenteral oxytocic drugs for induction of labor or for augmentation in the first and second stages of labor.

5. Oxytocin has been shown to have an intrinsic antidiuretic effect, acting to increase water reabsorption from the glomerular filtrate. Consideration should, therefore, be given to the possibility of water intoxication, particularly when oxytocin is administered continuously by infusion and the patient is receiving fluids by mouth.

Adverse Reactions: The following adverse reactions have been reported: Fetal bradycardia, neonatal jaundice, anaphylactic reaction, postpartum hemorrhage, cardiac arrhythmia, fatal afibrionogenemia, nausea, vomiting, premature ventricular contractions and pelvic hematoma.

Excessive dosage or hypersensitivity to the drug may result in uterine hypertonicity, spasm, tetanic contraction, or rupture of the uterus.

The possibility of increased blood loss and afibrinogenemia should be kept in mind when administering the drug.

Severe water intoxication with convulsions and coma has occurred, associated with a slow oxytocin infusion over a 24-hour period. Maternal death due to oxytocin-induced water intoxication has been reported.

Dosage and Administration: Dosage of oxytocin is determined by uterine response. The following dosage information is based upon the various regimens and indications in general use.

A. Induction or Stimulation of Labor

Intravenous infusion (drip method) is the only acceptable method of administration for the induction or stimulation of labor.

Accurate control of the rate of infusion flow is essential. An infusion pump or other such device and frequent monitoring of strength of contractions and fetal heart rate are necessary for the safe administration of oxytocin for the induction or stimulation of labor. If uterine contractions become too powerful, the infusion can be abruptly stopped, and oxytocic stimulation of the uterine musculature will soon wane.

1. An intravenous infusion of non-oxytocin containing solution should be started. Physiologic electrolyte solution should be used except under unusual circumstances.

2. To prepare the usual solution for infusion, the contents of one 1-ml ampule is combined aseptically with 1,000 ml of nonhydrating diluent. The combined solution, rotated in the infusion bottle to insure thorough mixing contains 10 mU/ml. Add the container with dilute oxytocic solution to the system through use of a constant infusion pump or other such device, to control accurately the rate of infusion.

3. The initial dose should be no more than 1-2 mU/min. The dose may be gradually increased in increments of no more than 1 to 2 mU/min. until a contraction pattern has been established, which is similar to normal labor.

4. The fetal heart rate, resting uterine tone, and the frequency, duration, and force of contractions should be monitored.

5. The oxytocin infusion should be discontinued immediately in the event of uterine hyperactivity or fetal distress. Oxygen should be administered to the mother. The mother and the fetus must be evaluated by the responsible physician.

B. Control of Postpartum Uterine Bleeding

1. *Intravenous Infusion (Drip Method):* To control postpartum bleeding, 10 to 40 units of oxytocin may be added to 1,000 ml of a nonhydrating diluent and run at a rate necessary to control uterine atony.

2. *Intramuscular Administration:* 1 ml (10 units) of oxytocin can be given after delivery of the placenta.

How Supplied: Syntocinon Injection in 1 ml (10 USP Units) ampuls; in boxes of 20 and 100.

[SYT-Z15 Issued May 1, 1979]

SYNTOCINON® NASAL SPRAY ℞
(oxytocin)

The following prescribing information is based on official labeling in effect on November 1, 1979.

Description: Each ml. contains 40 USP Units (International Units) Syntocinon (oxytocin) and the following: exsiccated sodium phosphate, NF, citric acid, USP, sodium chloride, USP, glycerin, USP, sorbitol solution, USP, methylparaben, USP, propylparaben, USP, chlorobutanol, USP max. 0.05%, purified water, USP.

Oxytocin is one of the polypeptide hormones of the posterior lobe of the pituitary gland. The pharmacologic and clinical properties of Syntocinon (oxytocin) are identical with *the oxytocic and the galactokinetic* principle of the natural hormone. Syntocinon was synthesized on a commercial scale by Sandoz, and was introduced for clinical use in 1957.

Since oxytocin, a polypeptide, is subject to inactivation by the proteolytic enzymes of the alimentary tract, it is *not absorbed from the gastrointestinal tract.* Intranasal application of the spray preparation, however, is a practical and effective method of administration.

Action: Syntocinon Nasal Spray acts specifically on the myoepithelial elements surrounding the alveoli of the breast, causing them to contract and thus force milk into the larger ducts where it is more readily available to the baby.

Indication: Initial milk let-down.

Contraindications: Pregnancy; hypersensitivity.

Dosage and Administration: One spray into one or both nostrils 2 to 3 minutes before nursing or pumping of breasts.

Note: The squeeze bottle should be held in upright position when administering drug to the nose and patient should be in a sitting position rather than lying down. If preferred, the solution can be instilled in drop form by inverting the squeeze bottle and exerting very gentle pressure on its walls.

Supplied: Syntocinon (oxytocin) Nasal Spray in squeeze bottles containing 2 ml synthetic oxytocin solution or 5 ml synthetic oxytocin solution.

[SYT-ZZ7 Issued October 22, 1976]

Saron Pharmacal Corp.
1640 CENTRAL AVENUE
ST. PETERSBURG, FL 33712

AL-R ℞
6 mg and 12 mg T.D. capsules
(chlorpheniramine maleate)
Antihistamine

How Supplied: Bottles of 100.

ARTHRIN ℞

Description: Each yellow tablet contains 600 mg chelated magnesium salicylate.
Indications: Arthritis.
How Supplied: Bottles of 100.

BUTABELL HMB ℞
Antispasmodic-Anticholinergic-Sedative

Each pink-coated tablet contains:
Butabarbital .... 15 mg
(Warning —may be habit forming)
Hyoscyamine sulfate 0.1037
Atropine sulfate 0.0194
Hyoscine hydrobromide .... 0.0065 mg
How Supplied: Bottles of 100.

CARDABID ℞

Description: Each light purple and clear T.D. capsule contains 2.5 mg nitroglycerin.
Indications: Management, prophylaxis or treatment of angina.
How Supplied: Bottles of 100.

CEREBID ℞

Description: Each red/clear CEREBID TD capsule contains papaverine hydrochloride, 150 mg. Each grey/clear CEREBID-200 TD capsule contains papaverine hydrochloride, 200 mg. Each yellow/clear CEREBID-300 TD capsule contains papaverine hydrochloride, 300 mg.
Indications: For the relief of cerebral and peripheral ischemia.
How Supplied: Bottles of 100.

EMFASEEM ℞

Description: Each blue and white capsule contains:
Dyphylline (Dihydroxy-propyltheophylline) .... 200 mg.
Guaifenesin .... 100 mg.
Indications: Emphysema.
How Supplied: Bottles of 100.

HCV CREME ℞

Contains:
Hydrocortisone Alcohol 1%
Iodochlorhydroxyquin 3%
Indications: Antifungal, Antibacterial, anti-inflammatory topical cream.
How Supplied: 15 gram and 45 gram econopak tubes.

OTALL Ear Drops ℞

Contains:
Pramoxine HCl 1.0%
Hydrocortisone 1.0%
Parachlorometaxylenol 0.1%
Benzalkonium Cl 0.02%
Acetic Acid 2.0%
in a non-aqueous propylene glycol vehicle
Indications: Swimmer's ear.
How Supplied: 10cc measured drop safety-tip plastic bottles.

SAROFLEX ℞
(muscle relaxant)

Each tan capsule contains:
Chlorzoxazone .... 250 mg
Acetaminophen .... 300 mg
How Supplied: Bottles of 100.

SAROLAX ℞
(laxative)

Each brown and yellow capsule contains:
Dioctyl Sodium Sulfosuccinate .... 200 mg
Phenolphthalein Yellow .... 15 mg
Dehydrocholic Acid .... 20 mg
How Supplied: Bottles of 100.

S-PAINACET ©

Each orange capsule-shaped tablet contains:
Propoxyphene HCl .... 65 mg.
Acetaminophen .... 650 mg.
Indications: Pain.
How Supplied: Bottles of 100.

VERSTAT ℞

Each blue capsule contains:
Pentylenetetrazol .... 25 mg
Pheniramine Maleate .... 12.5 mg
Nicotinic Acid .... 50 mg
Indications: Vertigo.
How Supplied: Bottles of 100.

Savage Laboratories
a division of Byk-Gulden, Inc.
1000 MAIN ST.
POST OFFICE BOX 1000
MISSOURI CITY, TEXAS 77459

CHROMAGEN® CAPSULES ℞

Composition: Each maroon soft gelatin capsule contains ferrous fumarate USP 200 mg, ascorbic acid USP 250 mg, cyanocobalamin USP 10 mcg, desiccated stomach substance 100 mg.

Indications: For the treatment of all anemias responsive to oral iron therapy, such as hypochromic anemia associated with pregnancy, chronic or acute blood loss, dietary restriction, metabolic disease and post-surgical convalescence.

Administration and Dosage: Usual adult dose is 1 capsule daily.

Contraindications: Hemochromatosis and hemosiderosis are contraindications to iron therapy.

Side Effects: Average capsule doses in sensitive individuals or excessive dosage may cause nausea, skin rash, vomiting, diarrhea, precordial pain, or flushing of the face and extremities.

Supply:
NDC 0281-4285-53, bottle of 100.
NDC 0281-4285-56, bottle of 500.

CHROMAGEN®-D ℞
(iron dextran injection USP)

Composition: Each ml of Chromagen®-D (iron dextran injection USP), a dark brown, slightly viscous liquid complex of ferric hydroxide and dextran in a 0.9% sodium chloride USP solution contains: the equivalent of 50 mg of elemental iron (as an iron dextran complex) with 0.5% phenol USP as preservative.

Supply: NDC 0281-4290-16, 10 ml multidose vial.

DILOR® Tablets ℞
(dyphylline)

Composition: Each blue, scored tablet contains dyphylline 200 mg; each white scored tablet contains dyphylline 400 mg.

Description: Dyphylline [7-(2,3-Dihydroxypropyl) theophylline] [$C_{10}H_{14}N4\ O_4$] is a white, extremely bitter, amorphous solid, freely soluble in water and soluble to the extent of 2 gm. in 100 ml. alcohol. Dyphylline contains the equivalent of about 70 percent of anhydrous theophylline.

Actions: As a xanthine derivative, dyphylline possesses the peripheral vasodilator and bronchodilator actions characteristic of theophylline. It has diuretic and myocardial stimulant effects, and is effective orally. Dyphylline may show fewer side effects than aminophylline, but its blood levels and possibly its activity are also lower.

Indications: For relief of acute bronchial asthma and for reversible bronchospasm associated with chronic bronchitis and emphysema.

Contraindications: In individuals who have shown hypersensitivity to any of its components. Dyphylline should not be administered concurrently with other xanthine preparations.

Warnings: Status asthmaticus is a medical emergency. Excessive doses may be expected to be toxic.

Usage in Pregnancy: Safe use in pregnancy has not been established relative to possible adverse effects on fetal development. Therefore, dyphylline should not be used in pregnant women unless, in the judgment of the physician, the potential benefits outweigh the possible hazards.

Precautions: Use with caution in patients with severe cardiac disease, hypertension, hyperthyroidism, or acute myocardial injury. Particular caution in dose administration must be exercised in patients with peptic ulcers, since the condition may be exacerbated. Chronic oral administration in high doses (500 to 1,000 mg.) is usually associated with gastrointestinal irritation. Great caution should be used in giving dyphylline to patients in congestive heart failure. Such patients have shown markedly prolonged blood level curves which have persisted for long periods following discontinuation of the drug.

Adverse Reactions: Note: Included in this listing which follows are a few adverse reactions which may not have been reported with this specific drug. However, pharmacological similarities among the xanthine drugs require that each of the reactions be considered when dyphylline is administered. The most consistent adverse reactions are: Gastrointestinal irritation: nausea, vomiting, and epigastric pain, generally preceded by headache, hematemesis, diarrhea. Central nervous system stimulation: irritability, restlessness, insomnia, reflex hyperexcitability, muscle twitching, clonic and tonic generalized convulsions, agitation. Cardiovascular: palpitation, tachycardia, extra systoles, flushing, marked hypotension, and circulatory failure. Respiratory: tachypnea, respiratory arrest. Renal: albuminuria, increased excretion of renal tubule and red blood cells. Others: fever, dehydration.

Dosage and Administration: When administered orally it produces less nausea than aminophylline and other alkaline theophylline compounds. Absorption orally appears to be faster on an empty stomach; preferably the drug is to be given at six hour intervals. Adults: Usual Adult Dose: 15 mg/kg every 6 hours up to 4 times a day. The dosage should be individualized by titration to the condition and response of the patient.

Therapeutic blood levels are considered to be between 10 micrograms/ml. and 20 mcg./ml. Levels above 20 mcg./ml. may produce toxic effects. There is great variation from patient to patient in dosage needed in order to achieve a therapeutic blood level. Also, the duration of action of oral theophylline preparations varies widely from one patient to another. Because of this wide variation from patient to patient and the relatively narrow therapeutic blood level range, dosage must be individualized with monitoring of theophylline blood levels, particularly when prolonged or repeated use is planned. Pulmonary functional measurements before and after a period of treatment allow an objective assessment of whether or not therapy should be continued in patients with chronic bronchitis and emphysema.

Supply: Tablets,
200 mg– NDC 0281-1115-53, bottle of 100.
NDC 0281-1115-57, bottle of 1000.
NDC 0281-1115-63, unit dose, 1 × 100
400 mg– NDC 0281-1116-53, bottle of 100.
NDC 0281-1116-57, bottle of 1000.
NDC 0281-1116-63, unit dose, 1 × 100

Also Available: Dilor Elixir, Dyphylline 160 mg/15 ml; and Dilor Injectable, dyphylline 250 mg/ml.

DILOR-G® ℞

Composition: Each pink, scored tablet contains dyphylline 200 mg, guaifenesin NF 200 mg; oral liquid: each teaspoonful (5 ml) contains dyphylline 100 mg, guaifenesin NF 100 mg.

Supply: Tablets, NDC 0281-1124-53, bottle of 100.
NDC 0281-1124-57, bottle of 1000.
NDC 0281-1124-63, unit dose, 1 × 100.
Liquid, NDC 0281-1127-74, pint.
NDC 0281-1127-76, gallon.

HOMO-TET® ℞
(tetanus immune globulin [human] USP)

Composition: A solution of gamma globulin 16.5%±1.5% prepared from venous blood of human subjects hyperimmunized with tetanus toxoid.

Supply: NDC 0281-7740-11, 250 unit single-dose vial.
NDC 0281-7740-12, 250 unit prefilled disposable syringe.

IMMUGLOBIN® ℞
(Immune Serum Globulin-Human)

Composition: Each ml. contains Gamma Globulin 16.5%±1.5%. Standardized for measles and polio antibody content.

Supply: NDC 0281-7770-16, 10 ml vial.

MEPRED™-40 ℞
MEPRED™-80
(sterile methylprednisolone acetate suspension NF)

Composition: Mepred-40: Each ml contains methylprednisolone acetate USP 40 mg.
Mepred-80: Each ml contains methylprednisolone acetate USP 80 mg.

Supply: Mepred-40, NDC 0281-5201-15, 5 ml vial;
Mepred-80, NDC 0281-5203-15, 5 ml vial.

PHYSPAN™ ℞
(theophylline USP anhydrous, sustained release)

Composition: Each Physpan, blue and clear, sustained release capsule contains 260 mg of theophylline USP anhydrous in a sustained release bead formulation.

Each Physpan, orange and clear, sustaned release capsule contains 130 mg of theophylline USP anhydrous in a sustained release bead formulation.

Indications: For relief and/or prevention of symptoms from asthma and reversible bronchospasm associated with chronic bronchitis and emphysema.

Contraindications: In individuals who have shown hypersensitivity to any of its components.

Warnings: Status asthmaticus is a medical emergency. Optimal therapy frequently requires additional medication including corticosteroids when the patient is not rapidly responsive to bronchodilators.

Excessive theophylline doses may be associated with toxicity; thus serum theophylline levels are recommended to assure maximal benefit without excessive risk. Incidence of toxicity increases at levels greater than 20 mcg/ml. Morphine, curare, and stilbamidine should be used with caution in patients with airflow obstruction since they stimulate histamine release and can induce asthmatic attacks. They may also suppress respiration leading to respiratory failure. Alternative drugs should be chosen whenever possible.

There is an excellent correlation between high blood levels of theophylline resulting from conventional doses and associated clinical manifestations of toxicity in (1) patients with lowered body plasma clearances (due to transient cardiac decompensation), (2) patients with liver dysfunction or chronic obstructive lung disease, (3) patients who are older than 55 years of age, particularly males.

There are often no early signs of less serious theophylline toxicity such as nausea and restlessness, which may appear in up to 50 percent of patients prior to onset of convulsions. Ventricular arrhythmias or seizures may be the first signs of toxicity.

Many patients who have higher theophylline serum levels exhibit a tachycardia.

Theophylline products may worsen pre-existing arrhythmias.

Usage in Pregnancy: Safe use in pregnancy has not been established relative to possible adverse effects on fetal development, but neither have adverse effects on fetal development been established. This is, unfortunately, true for most antiasthmatic medications. Therefore, use of theophylline in pregnant women should be balanced against the risk of uncontrolled asthma.

Precautions: Mean half-life in smokers is shorter than non-smokers; therefore, smokers may require larger doses of theophylline. Theophylline should not be administered concurrently with other xanthine medications. Use with caution in patients with severe cardiac disease, severe hypoxemia, hypertension, hyperthyroidism, acute myocardial injury, cor pulmonale, congestive heart failure, liver disease, and in the elderly (especially males) and in neonates. Great caution should especially be used in giving theophylline to patients in congestive heart failure. Such patients have shown markedly prolonged theophylline blood level curves with theophylline persisting in serum for long periods following discontinuation of the drug.

Use theophylline cautiously in patients with history of peptic ulcer. Theophylline may occasionally act as a local irritant to G.I. tract although gastrointestinal symptoms are more commonly central and associated with serum concentrations over 20 mcg/ml.

Adverse Reactions: The most consistent adverse reactions are usually due to overdose and are:

1. Gastrointestinal: nausea, vomiting, epigastric pain, hematemesis, diarrhea.
2. Central nervous system: headaches, irritability, restlessness, insomnia, reflex hyperexcitability, muscle twitching, clonic and tonic generalized convulsions.
3. Cardiovascular: palpitation, tachycardia, extra systoles, flushing, hypotension, circulatory failure, life threatening ventricular arrhythmias.
4. Respiratory: tachypnea.
5. Renal: albuminuria, increased excretion of renal tubular potentiation or diuresis, and red blood cells.
6. Others: hyperglycemia and inappropriate ADH syndrome.

Dosage and Administration:
CHRONIC ASTHMA:
Theophyllinization is a treatment of first choice for the management of chronic asthma (to prevent symptoms and maintain patent airways). Slow clinical titration is generally preferred to assure acceptance and safety of the medication.

Initial dose: 16 mg/kg/day or 520 mg/day (whichever is lower) in 1-2 divided doses at 12 hour intervals.

Increased dose: The above dosage may be increased in approximately 25% increments at 2-3 day intervals so long as no intolerance is observed until the maximum indicated below is reached.

Maximum dose without measurement of serum concentrations: Not to exceed the following: (WARNING: DO NOT ATTEMPT TO MAINTAIN ANY DOSE THAT IS NOT TOLERATED)

Age <9 years - 24 mg/kg/day
Age 9 - 12 years - 20 mg/kg/day
Age 12-16 years - 18 mg/kg/day
Age >16 years - 13 mg/kg/day or 900 mg/day (WHICHEVER IS LESS)

Therapeutic theophylline serum levels are considered to be between 10 mcg/ml and 20 mcg/ml. Levels above 20 mcg/ml may produce toxic effects. There is a great variation from patient to patient in dosage needed in order to achieve a therapeutic blood level because of variable rates of eliminiation. Because of this wide variation from patient to patient and the relatively narrow therapeutic blood level range, dosage must be individualized, and monitoring of theophylline serum levels is highly recommended. Dosage should be calculated on the basis of lean (ideal) body weight where mg/kg dosage is stated.

How Supplied: Capsules: 130 mg-NDC 0281-1239-53, bottle of 100; 260 mg-NDC 0281-1242-53, bottle of 100.

See package insert for full information.

TRACILON™ ℞
(sterile triamcinolone diacetate suspension NF)

Composition: Each ml of Tracilon contains triamcinolone diacetate NF 40 mg.
Supply: NDC 0281-5240-15, 5 ml vial.

ZIPAN-25® and ZIPAN-50® ℞
(promethazine hydrochloride USP)

Composition: ZiPAN-25: Each ml contains promethazine hydrochloride USP 25 mg; ZiPAN-50: Each ml contains promethazine hydrochloride USP 50 mg.

Supply:
ZIPAN-25, NDC 0281-1410-16, 10 ml vial.
NDC 0281-1410-24, 25 × 1 ml ampules.
ZIPAN-50, NDC 0281-1411-16, 10 ml vial.
NDC 0281-1411-24, 25 × 1 ml ampules.

Schattner Company, The R.
Pharmaceutical Division
4000 MASSACHUSETTS AVE., N.W.
WASHINGTON, DC 20016

ORADERM® LIP BALM
(Effective surface anesthetic and antiseptic)

Composition: A hypo-allergenic, "ALL-WEATHER™", lip balm incorporating sodium phenolate, sodium tetraborate and phenol in a specially prepared protective base containing an anionic emulsifier.

Action: ORADERM is both an anesthetic and antiseptic hypo-allergenic lip balm containing no "caines" or antibiotics. It is specifically designed to maintain lip hygiene by reducing the oral bacterial flow and to relieve local dryness, soreness and irritations. It protects against infection while bringing symptomatic relief. Lasting surface anesthesia is obtained, usually in seconds. ORADERM is an effective antimicrobial against a wide range of gram negative and gram positive bacteria and fungi for infection control. ORADERM is a soothing protectant which cools and promotes healing of the lip tissues.

Indications: ORADERM may be used in adjunctive therapy, as a topical *anesthetic* and *antiseptic* in labial manifestations of systemic disease. It is indicated for prompt temporary symptomatic relief of pain and discomfort associated with: *sunburn, windburn, cold sores* (lesions and cracking), *dryness* (from fever, mouth breathing and lip licking), *herpetic lesions* (fever blisters), *dermatitis venenata* (from lipstick), cheilitis (chronic and simplex), *perleche* (angular stomatitis), *abrasions* (lip biting, etc.)

Hypo-allergenic: In controlled university studies, ORADERM was found to be non-toxic, non-sensitizing and hypo-allergenic.

Administration: Apply liberally to the labial tissues, as often as necessary.

How Supplied: Pocket-size 1/8 oz.
NO PRESCRIPTION NECESSARY.

MEMORANDUM

Schering Corporation
GALLOPING HILL ROAD
KENILWORTH, NJ 07033

A and D Ointment
REG. T.M.

How Supplied: A and D Ointment is available in 1½-ounce (42.5 g) and 4-ounce (113 g) tubes and 1-pound (454 g) jars.
For complete prescribing information, contact the Schering Professional Services Department.

AFRIN®
brand of oxymetazoline hydrochloride, USP
Nasal Spray 0.05%
Menthol Nasal Spray 0.05%
Nose Drops 0.05%
Pediatric Nose Drops 0.025%

How Supplied: AFRIN **Nasal Spray** 0.05% (1:2000), 15 ml. and 30 ml. plastic squeeze bottles.
AFRIN **Menthol Nasal Spray** 0.05% (1:2000), 15 ml. plastic squeeze bottle.
AFRIN **Nose Drops,** 0.05% (1:2000), 20 ml. dropper bottle.
AFRIN **Pediatric Nose Drops,** 0.025% (1:4000), 20 ml. dropper bottle.
For complete prescribing information, contact the Schering Professional Services Department.

AFRINOL™ ℞
brand of pseudoephedrine sulfate
Long-Acting Decongestant REPETABS® Tablets

Description: Each AFRINOL Long-Acting Decongestant REPETABS (brand of repeat-action tablets) Tablet contains 120 mg. pseudoephedrine sulfate equally distributed between the tablet coating and a barrier-coated core. Following ingestion, the active ingredient in the coating is quickly liberated; release of the active ingredient in the core is delayed for several hours after ingestion of the tablet.
Pseudoephedrine is one of the naturally occurring alkaloids obtained from various species of the plant *Ephedra*. The chemical name for pseudoephedrine sulfate is: benzenemethanol, α-[1-(methylamino)ethyl]-, [*S*(*R**,*R**)]-, sulfate.
Actions: Pseudoephedrine sulfate, a sympathomimetic amine, is an orally effective nasal decongestant. The mucous membrane of the respiratory tract is decongested through action on the sympathetic nerves. Drowsiness does not result, and in the normotensive adult, little or no pressor effect occurs with the recommended oral dosage.
Indications: AFRINOL Long-Acting Decongestant REPETABS Tablets are indicated for the relief of nasal congestion and eustachian tube congestion. Analgesics, antihistamines, and antibiotics may be administered concurrently, when indicated.
Contraindications: In patients with severe hypertension, severe coronary artery disease, hyperthyroidism and in those receiving monoamine oxidase (MAO) inhibitor therapy, sympathomimetic amines are contraindicated. AFRINOL Long-Acting Decongestant REPETABS Tablets are also contraindicated in patients who have shown hypersensitivity or idiosyncrasy to adrenergic agents, which may be manifested by insomnia, dizziness, weakness, tremor or arrhythmias.
This product should *not* be used in children less than 12 years of age.
Because of the higher than usual risk for infants from sympathomimetics, this drug is contraindicated in nursing mothers.
Warnings: Sympathomimetic amines should be administered with caution to patients with hypertension, diabetes mellitus, ischemic heart disease, increased intraocular pressure or prostatic hypertrophy. Central nervous system stimulation and convulsions or cardiovascular collapse with accompanying hypotension may be produced by sympathomimetics.
Use in the Elderly (approximately 60 years and older): The elderly are more likely to have adverse reactions to sympathomimetics, such as hallucinations, convulsions, CNS depression, and death. For this reason, before considering the use of a repeat-action formulation, the safe use of a short-acting sympathomimetic should be demonstrated for the particular elderly patient.
Do not exceed recommended dosage.
Use in Pregnancy: Safety for use of this product during pregnancy has not been established.
Precautions: Pseudoephedrine should be used with caution in patients with cardiovascular disease.
Adverse Reactions: The following adverse reactions have been associated with sympathomimetic drugs: fear, anxiety, tenseness, restlessness, tremor, weakness, pallor, respiratory difficulty, dysuria, insomnia, hallucinations, convulsions, CNS depression, arrhythmias, and cardiovascular collapse with hypotension. Ephedrine-like reactions in hyperreactive individuals include: palpitations, tachycardia, hypertension, headache, dizziness or nausea.
Dosage and Administration: For adults and children 12 years of age and over: One tablet twice daily (every 12 hours).
Drug Interactions: Sympathomimetics increase the effect of monoamine oxidase inhibitors with resultant toxic effects. The antihypertensive effects of methyldopa, mecamylamine, reserpine and veratrum alkaloids may be reduced by sympathomimetics. Beta-adrenergic blocking agents may also interact with sympathomimetics.
How Supplied: AFRINOL Long-Acting Decongestant REPETABS Tablets, blue, sugar-coated tablets branded in white with the Schering trademark and product identification numbers, 258; bottle of 100.

[*Shown in Product Identification Section.*]

AKRINOL® ℞
brand of acrisorcin, NF
Cream

How Supplied: AKRINOL Cream, 2 mg/g, 50 g tube.
For complete prescribing information, contact the Schering Professional Services Department.

BECAUSE® CONTRACEPTOR®
Vaginal Contraceptive Foam

How Supplied: Disposable 10 gm CONTRACEPTOR containing six applications of BECAUSE contraceptive foam.
For complete prescribing information, contact the Schering Professional Services Department.
[*Shown in Product Identification Section*]

CELESTONE® ℞
brand of betamethasone, NF
Cream

How Supplied: CELESTONE Cream 0.2%, 15-gram tube, box of one.
For complete prescribing information, contact the Schering Professional Services Department.

CELESTONE® ℞
brand of betamethasone, NF
Tablets

Description: Glucocorticoids are adrenocortical steroids, both naturally occurring and synthetic, that are readily absorbed from the gastrointestinal tract. A derivative of prednisolone, CELESTONE has a 16β-methyl group that enhances the anti-inflammatory action of the molecule and reduces the sodium- and water-retaining properties of the fluorine atom bound at carbon 9.
The formula for betamethasone is $C_{22}H_{29}FO_5$ and has a molecular weight of 392.47. Chemically, it is 9-fluoro-11β, 17,21-trihydroxy-16β-methylpregna-1,4-diene-3,20-dione.
Betamethasone is a white to practically white, odorless, crystalline powder. It melts at about 240°C with some decomposition. Betamethasone is sparingly soluble in acetone, alcohol, dioxane, and methanol; very slightly soluble in chloroform and ether; and is insoluble in water.
Each CELESTONE **Tablet** contains 0.6 mg. betamethasone.
Actions: Naturally occurring glucocorticoids (hydrocortisone and cortisone), which also have salt-retaining properties, are used as replacement therapy in adrenocortical deficiency states. Their synthetic analogs, such as betamethasone, are primarily used for their potent anti-inflammatory effects in disorders of many organ systems.
Glucocorticoids, such as betamethasone, cause profound and varied metabolic effects. In addition, they modify the body's immune response to diverse stimuli.
Indications:
Endocrine disorders: primary or secondary adrenocortical insufficiency (hydrocortisone or cortisone is the first choice; synthetic analogs may be used in conjunction with mineralocorticoids where applicable; in infancy mineralocorticoid supplementation is of particular importance).
congenital adrenal hyperplasia
nonsuppurative thyroiditis
hypercalcemia associated with cancer
Rheumatic disorders: as adjunctive therapy for short-term administration (to tide the patient over an acute episode or exacerbation) in:
psoriatic arthritis
rheumatoid arthritis, including juvenile rheumatoid arthritis (selected cases may require low-dose maintenance therapy)
ankylosing spondylitis
acute and subacute bursitis
acute nonspecific tenosynovitis
acute gouty arthritis
post-traumatic osteoarthritis
synovitis of osteoarthritis
epicondylitis
Collagen diseases: during an exacerbation or as maintenance therapy in selected cases of:
systemic lupus erythematosus
acute rheumatic carditis
Dermatologic diseases:
pemphigus
bullous dermatitis herpetiformis
severe erythema multiforme (Stevens-Johnson syndrome)
exfoliative dermatitis
mycosis fungoides
severe psoriasis
severe seborrheic dermatitis
Allergic states: control of severe or incapacitating allergic conditions intractable to adequate trials of conventional treatment:
seasonal or perennial allergic rhinitis
serum sickness
bronchial asthma
contact dermatitis
atopic dermatitis
drug hypersensitivity reactions
Ophthalmic diseases: severe acute and chronic allergic and inflammatory processes involving the eye and its adnexa, such as:
allergic conjunctivitis
keratitis
allergic corneal marginal ulcers
herpes zoster ophthalmicus
iritis and iridocyclitis
chorioretinitis
anterior segment inflammation
diffuse posterior uveitis and choroiditis
optic neuritis
sympathetic ophthalmia

Respiratory diseases:
symptomatic sarcoidosis
Loffler's syndrome not manageable by other means
berylliosis
fulminating or disseminated pulmonary tuberculosis when used concurrently with appropriate antituberculous chemotherapy
aspiration pneumonitis
Hematologic disorders:
idiopathic thrombocytopenic purpura in adults
secondary thrombocytopenia in adults
acquired (autoimmune) hemolytic anemia
erythroblastopenia (RBC anemia)
congenital (erythroid) hypoplastic anemia
Neoplastic dieases: for palliative management of:
leukemias and lymphomas in adults
acute leukemia of childhood
Edematous states: to induce a diuresis or remission of proteinuria in the nephrotic syndrome, without uremia, of the idiopathic type or that due to lupus erythematosus.
Gastrointestinal diseases: to tide the patient over a critical period of the disease in:
ulcerative colitis
regional enteritis
Miscellaneous: tuberculous meningitis with subarachnoid block or impending block when used concurrently with appropriate antituberculous chemotherapy; trichinosis with neurologic or myocardial involvement.

Contraindications: CELESTONE **Tablets** are contraindicated in systemic fungal infections.

Warnings: In patients on corticosteroid therapy subjected to unusual stress, increased dosage of rapidly acting corticosteroids before, during, and after the stressful situation is indicated.

Corticosteroids may mask some signs of infection, and new infections may appear during their use. There may be decreased resistance and inability to localize infection when corticosteroids are used.

Prolonged use of corticosteroids may produce posterior subcapsular cataracts, glaucoma with possible damage to the optic nerves, and may enhance the establishment of secondary ocular infections due to fungi or viruses.

Average and large doses of hydrocortisone or cortisone can cause elevation of blood pressure, salt and water retention, and increased excretion of potassium. These effects are less likely to occur with the synthetic derivatives except when used in large doses. Dietary salt restrictions and potassium supplementation may be necessary. All corticosteroids increase calcium excretion.

While on corticosteroid therapy patients should not be vaccinated against smallpox. Other immunization procedures should not be undertaken in patients who are on corticosteroids, especially on high doses, because of possible hazards of neurological complications and a lack of antibody response.

The use of CELESTONE **Syrup** and **Tablets** in active tuberculosis should be restricted to those cases of fulminating or disseminated tuberculosis in which the corticosteroid is used for the management of the disease in conjunction with an appropriate antituberculous regimen.

If corticosteroids are indicated in patients with latent tuberculosis or tuberculin reactivity, close observation is necessary as reactivation of the disease may occur. During prolonged corticosteroid therapy, these patients should receive chemoprophylaxis.

Usage in pregnancy: Since adequate human reproduction studies have not been done with corticosteroids, the use of these drugs in pregnancy, nursing mothers or women of childbearing potential requires that the possible benefits of the drug be weighed against the potential hazards to the mother and embryo or fetus. Infants born of mothers who have received substantial doses of corticosteroids during pregnancy should be carefully observed for signs of hypoadrenalism.

Precautions: Drug-induced secondary adrenocortical insufficiency may be minimized by gradual reduction of dosage. This type of relative insufficiency may persist for months after discontinuation of therapy; therefore, in any situation of stress occurring during that period, hormone therapy should be reinstituted. Since mineralocorticoid secretion may be impaired, salt and/or a mineralocorticoid should be administered concurrently.

There is an enhanced effect of corticosteroids on patients with hypothyroidism and in those with cirrhosis.

Corticosteroids should be used cautiously in patients with ocular herpes simplex because of possible corneal perforation.

The lowest possible dose of corticosteroid should be used to control the condition under treatment, and when reduction in dosage is possible, the reduction should be gradual.

Psychic derangements may appear when corticosteroids are used, ranging from euphoria, insomnia, mood swings, personality changes, and severe depression to frank psychotic manifestations. Also, existing emotional instability or psychotic tendencies may be aggravated by corticosteroids.

Aspirin should be used cautiously in conjunction with corticosteroids in hypoprothrombinemia.

Steroids should be used with caution in nonspecific ulcerative colitis, if there is a probability of impending perforation, abscess or other pyogenic infection; diverticulitis; fresh intestinal anastomoses; active or latent peptic ulcer; renal insufficiency; hypertension; osteoporosis; and myasthenia gravis.

Growth and development of infants and children on prolonged corticosteroid therapy should be carefully observed.

Adverse Reactions:
Fluid and electrolyte disturbances: sodium retention, fluid retention, congestive heart failure in susceptible patients, potassium loss, hypokalemic alkalosis, hypertension.
Musculoskeletal: muscle weakness, steroid myopathy, loss of muscle mass, osteoporosis, vertebral compression fractures, aseptic necrosis of femoral and humeral heads, pathologic fractures of long bones.
Gastrointestinal: peptic ulcer with possible perforation and hemorrhage, pancreatitis, abdominal distention, ulcerative esophagitis.
Dermatologic: impaired wound healing, thin fragile skin, petechiae and ecchymoses, facial erythema, increased sweating, may suppress reactions to skin tests.
Neurological: convulsions, increased intracranial pressure with papilledema (pseudotumor cerebri) usually after treatment, vertigo, headache.
Endocrine: menstrual irregularities; development of Cushingoid state; suppression of growth in children; secondary adrenocortical and pituitary unresponsiveness, particularly in times of stress, as in trauma, surgery or illness; decreased carbohydrate tolerance; manifestations of latent diabetes mellitus; increased requirements of insulin or oral hypoglycemic agents in diabetics.
Ophthalmic: posterior subcapsular cataracts, increased intraocular pressure, glaucoma, exophthalmos.
Metabolic: negative nitrogen balance due to protein catabolism.

Dosage and Administration: The initial dosage of CELESTONE may vary from 0.6 mg. to 7.2 mg. per day depending on the specific disease entity being treated. In situations of less severity lower doses will generally suffice, while in selected patients higher initial doses may be required. The initial dosage should be maintained or adjusted until a satisfactory response is noted. If after a reasonable period of time there is a lack of satisfactory clinical response, betamethasone should be discontinued and the patient transferred to other appropriate therapy. IT SHOULD BE EMPHASIZED THAT DOSAGE REQUIREMENTS ARE VARIABLE AND MUST BE INDIVIDUALIZED ON THE BASIS OF THE DISEASE UNDER TREATMENT AND THE RESPONSE OF THE PATIENT. After a favorable response is noted, the proper maintenance dosage should be determined by decreasing the initial drug dosage in small decrements at appropriate time intervals until the lowest dosage which will maintain an adequate clinical response is reached. It should be kept in mind that constant monitoring is needed in regard to drug dosage. Included in the situations which may make dosage adjustments necessary are changes in clinical status secondary to remissions or exacerbations in the disease process, the patient's individual drug responsiveness, and the effect of patient exposure to stressful situations not directly related to the disease entity under treatment; in this latter situation it may be necessary to increase the dosage of betamethasone for a period of time consistent with the patient's condition. If after long-term therapy the drug is to be stopped, it is recommended that it be withdrawn gradually rather than abruptly.

How Supplied: CELESTONE **Tablets,** 0.6 mg., pink, compressed, scored tablets impressed with the Schering trademark and product identification letters, BDA, or numbers, 011; bottles of 100 and 500. Also available, CELESTONE Tablet Pack (For Six Day Therapy), 0.6 mg., 21 tablets and CELESTONE **Syrup,** 0.6 mg. per 5 ml., orange-red colored liquid; 4 oz. bottle.
Protect **Syrup** from light.

[*Shown in Product Identification Section*]

CELESTONE® Phosphate ℞
brand of betamethasone sodium phosphate, NF
Injection

Description: CELESTONE Phosphate Injection is an aqueous solution containing in each ml.: 4.0 mg. betamethasone sodium phosphate equivalent to 3.0 mg. betamethasone alcohol; 10 mg. dibasic sodium phosphate; 0.1 mg. edetate disodium; 3.2 mg. sodium bisulfite; and 5.0 mg. phenol as preservative. The pH is adjusted to approximately 8.5 with sodium hydroxide.

Actions: Naturally occurring glucocorticoids (hydrocortisone), which also have salt-retaining properties, are used as replacement therapy in adrenocortical deficiency states. Their synthetic analogs are primarily used for their potent anti-inflammatory effects in disorders of many organ systems.

Glucocorticoids cause profound and varied metabolic effects. In addition, they modify the body's immune responses to diverse stimuli.

Indications: When oral therapy is not feasible, CELESTONE Phosphate Injection for **intravenous or intramuscular use** is indicated as follows:

Endocrine disorders: Primary or secondary adrenocortical insufficiency (hydrocortisone or cortisone is the drug of choice; synthetic analogs may be used in conjunction with mineralocorticoids where applicable; in infancy, mineralocorticoid supplementation is of particular importance). Acute adrenocortical insufficiency (hydrocortisone or cortisone is the drug of choice; mineralocorticoid supplementation may be necessary, particularly when synthetic analogs are used). Preoperatively and in the event of serious trauma or illness, in patients

Continued on next page

Information on Schering products appearing on these pages is effective as of September 30, 1979.

Schering—Cont.

with known adrenal insufficiency or when adrenocortical reserve is doubtful. Shock unresponsive to conventional therapy if adrenocortical insufficiency exists or is suspected. Congenital adrenal hyperplasia. Nonsuppurative thyroiditis.

Rheumatic disorders: As adjunctive therapy for short-term administration (to tide the patient over an acute episode or exacerbation) in: post-traumatic osteoarthritis; synovitis of osteoarthritis; rheumatoid arthritis; acute and subacute bursitis; epicondylitis; acute nonspecific tenosynovitis; acute gouty arthritis; psoriatic arthritis; ankylosing spondylitis; juvenile rheumatoid arthritis.

Collagen diseases: During an exacerbation or as maintenance therapy in selected cases of: systemic lupus erythematosus; acute rheumatic carditis.

Dermatologic diseases: Pemphigus; severe erythema multiforme (Stevens-Johnson syndrome); exfoliative dermatitis; bullous dermatitis herpetiformis; severe seborrheic dermatitis; severe psoriasis.

Allergic states: Control of severe or incapacitating allergic conditions intractable to adequate trials of conventional treatment in: bronchial asthma; contact dermatitis; atopic dermatitis; serum sickness; seasonal or perennial allergic rhinitis; drug hypersensitivity reactions; urticarial transfusion reactions; acute noninfectious laryngeal edema (epinephrine is the drug of first choice).

Ophthalmic diseases: Severe, acute and chronic allergic and inflammatory processes involving the eye, such as: herpes zoster ophthalmicus; iritis, iridocyclitis; chorioretinitis; diffuse posterior uveitis and choroiditis; optic neuritis; sympathetic ophthalmia; anterior segment inflammation.

Gastrointestinal diseases: To tide the patient over a critical period of disease in: ulcerative colitis—(systemic therapy); regional enteritis—(systemic therapy).

Respiratory diseases: Symptomatic sarcoidosis; berylliosis; fulminating or disseminated pulmonary tuberculosis, when concurrently accompanied by appropriate antituberculous chemotherapy; aspiration pneumonitis.

Hematologic disorders: Acquired (autoimmune) hemolytic anemia; idiopathic thrombocytopenic purpura in adults (I.V. only; I.M. administration is contraindicated).

Neoplastic diseases: For palliative management of: leukemias and lymphomas in adults; acute leukemia of childhood.

Edematous state: To induce diuresis or remission of proteinuria in the nephrotic syndrome, without uremia, of the idiopathic type or that due to lupus erythematosus.

Miscellaneous: Tuberculous meningitis with subarachnoid block or impending block when concurrently accompanied by appropriate antituberculous chemotherapy.

When the strength and dosage form of the drug lend the preparation to the treatment of the condition, the **intra-articular or soft tissue administration** of CELESTONE Phosphate Injection is indicated as adjunctive therapy for short-term administration (to tide the patient over an acute episode or exacerbation) in: synovitis of osteoarthritis; rheumatoid arthritis; acute and subacute bursitis; acute gouty arthritis; epicondylitis; acute nonspecific tenosynovitis; post-traumatic osteoarthritis.

When the strength and dosage form of the drug lend the preparation to the treatment of the condition, the **intralesional administration** of CELESTONE Phosphate Injection is indicated for: keloids; localized hypertrophic, infiltrated, inflammatory lesions of lichen planus, psoriatic plaques, granuloma annulare, and lichen simplex chronicus (neurodermatitis); discoid lupus erythematosus; necrobiosis lipoidica diabeticorum; alopecia areata.

Contraindications: CELESTONE Phosphate Injection is contraindicated in systemic fungal infections.

Warnings: In patients on corticosteroid therapy subjected to any unusual stress, increased dosage of rapidly acting corticosteroids before, during, and after the stressful situation is indicated.

Corticosteroids may mask some signs of infection, and new infections may appear during their use. There may be decreased resistance and inability to localize infection when corticosteroids are used.

Prolonged use of corticosteroids may produce posterior subcapsular cataracts, glaucoma with possible damage to the optic nerves, and may enhance the establishment of secondary ocular infections due to fungi or viruses.

Average and large doses of cortisone or hydrocortisone can cause elevation of blood pressure, salt and water retention, and increased excretion of potassium. These effects are less likely to occur with the synthetic derivatives except when used in large doses. Dietary salt restriction and potassium supplementation may be necessary. All corticosteroids increase calcium excretion.

While on Corticosteroid Therapy Patients Should Not Be Vaccinated Against Smallpox. Other Immunization Procedures Should Not Be Undertaken in Patients Who are on Corticosteroids, Especially in High Doses, Because of Possible Hazards of Neurological Complications and Lack of Antibody Response.

The use of CELESTONE Phosphate Injection in active tuberculosis should be restricted to those cases of fulminating or disseminated tuberculosis in which the corticosteroid is used for the management of the disease in conjunction with appropriate antituberculous regimen.

If corticosteroids are indicated in patients with latent tuberculosis or tuberculin reactivity, close observation is necessary as reactivation of the disease may occur. During prolonged corticosteroid therapy, these patients should receive chemoprophylaxis.

Because rare instances of anaphylactoid reactions have occurred in patients receiving parenteral corticosteroid therapy, appropriate precautionary measures should be taken prior to administration, especially when the patient has a history of allergy to any drug.

Usage in pregnancy: Since adequate human reproduction studies have not been done with corticosteroids, the use of these drugs in pregnancy, nursing mothers, or women of childbearing potential requires that the possible benefits of the drug be weighed against the potential hazards to the mother and embryo or fetus. Infants born to mothers who have received substantial doses of corticosteroids during pregnancy should be carefully observed for signs of hypoadrenalism.

Precautions: Drug-induced secondary adrenocortical insufficiency may be minimized by gradual reduction of dosage. This type of relative insufficiency may persist for months after discontinuation of therapy; therefore, in any situation of stress occurring during that period, hormone therapy should be reinstituted. Since mineralocorticoid secretion may be impaired, salt and/or a mineralocorticoid should be administered concurrently.

There is an enhanced effect of corticosteroids in patients with hypothyroidism and in those with cirrhosis.

Corticosteroids should be used cautiously in patients with ocular herpes simplex for fear of corneal perforation.

The lowest possible dose of corticosteroid should be used to control the condition under treatment, and when reduction in dosage is possible, the reduction must be gradual.

Psychic derangements may appear when corticosteroids are used, ranging from euphoria, insomnia, mood swings, personality changes, and severe depression to frank psychotic manifestations. Also, existing emotional instability or psychotic tendencies may be aggravated by corticosteroids.

Aspirin should be used cautiously in conjunction with corticosteroids in hypoprothrombinemia.

Steroids should be used with caution in nonspecified ulcerative colitis, if there is a probability of impending perforation, abscess or other pyogenic infection, also in diverticulitis, fresh intestinal anastomoses, active or latent peptic ulcer, renal insufficiency, hypertension, osteoporosis, and myasthenia gravis. Growth and development of infants and children on prolonged corticosteroid therapy should be carefully followed.

The following additional precautions also apply for parenteral corticosteroids. Intra-articular injection of a corticosteroid may produce systemic as well as local effects.

Appropriate examination of any joint fluid present is necessary to exclude a septic process. A marked increase in pain accompanied by local swelling, further restriction of joint motion, fever, and malaise are suggestive of septic arthritis. If this complication occurs and the diagnosis of sepsis is confirmed, appropriate antimicrobial therapy should be instituted.

Local injection of a steroid into a previously infected joint is to be avoided.

Corticosteroids should not be injected into unstable joints.

The slower rate of absorption by intramuscular administration should be recognized.

Adverse Reactions:

Fluid and electrolyte disturbances: sodium retention; fluid retention; congestive heart failure in susceptible patients; potassium loss; hypokalemic alkalosis; hypertension.

Musculoskeletal: muscle weakness; steroid myopathy; loss of muscle mass; osteoporosis; vertebral compression fractures; aseptic necrosis of femoral and humeral heads; pathologic fracture of long bones.

Gastrointestinal: peptic ulcer with possible subsequent perforation and hemorrhage; pancreatitis; abdominal distention; ulcerative esophagitis.

Dermatologic: impaired wound healing; thin fragile skin; petechiae and ecchymoses; facial erythema; increased sweating; may suppress reactions to skin tests.

Neurological: convulsions; increased intracranial pressure with papilledema (pseudotumor cerebri) usually after treatment; vertigo; headache.

Endocrine: menstrual irregularities; development of Cushingoid state; suppression of growth in children; secondary adrenocortical and pituitary unresponsiveness, particularly in times of stress, as in trauma, surgery or illness; decreased carbohydrate tolerance; manifestations of latent diabetes mellitus; increased requirements for insulin or oral hypoglycemic agents in diabetics.

Ophthalmic: posterior subcapsular cataracts; increased intraocular pressure; glaucoma; exophthalmos.

Metabolic: negative nitrogen balance due to protein catabolism.

The following *additional* adverse reactions are also related to parenteral corticosteroid therapy: rare instances of blindness associated with intralesional therapy around the face and head; hyperpigmentation or hypopigmentation; subcutaneous and cutaneous atrophy; sterile abscess; postinjection flare (following intra-articular use); charcot-like arthropathy.

Dosage and Administration: The initial dosage of parenterally administered betamethasone may vary up to 9.0 mg. per day depending on the specific disease entity being treated. In situations of less severity, lower doses will generally suffice while in selected patients higher initial doses may be required. Usually the parenteral dosage ranges are one-third to

one-half the 12-hourly oral dose. However, in certain overwhelming, acute, life-threatening situations, administration in dosages exceeding the usual dosages may be justified and may be in multiples of the oral dosages.
The initial dosage should be maintained or adjusted until a satisfactory response is noted. If after a reasonable period of time there is a lack of satisfactory clinical response, CELESTONE Phosphate Injection should be discontinued and the patient transferred to other appropriate therapy. *It Should Be Emphasized that Dosage Requirements are Variable and Must Be Individualized on the Basis of the Disease Under Treatment and the Response of the Patient.* After a favorable response is noted, the proper maintenance dosage should be determined by decreasing the initial drug dosage in small decrements at appropriate time intervals until the lowest dosage which will maintain an adequate clinical response is reached. It should be kept in mind that constant monitoring is needed in regard to drug dosage. Included in the situations which may make dosage adjustments necessary are changes in clinical status secondary to remissions or exacerbations in the disease process, the patient's individual drug responsiveness, and the effect of patient exposure to stressful situations not directly related to the disease entity under treatment; in this latter situation it may be necessary to increase dosage of CELESTONE Phosphate Injection for a period of time consistent with the patient's condition. If after long-term therapy the drug is to be stopped, it is recommended that it be withdrawn gradually rather than abruptly.
How Supplied: CELESTONE Phosphate Injection, 4.0 mg. per ml. (equivalent to 3.0 mg. per ml. betamethasone alcohol), supplied in 1 ml. ampules and 5 ml. multiple-dose vials.
Protect from freezing.

CELESTONE® SOLUSPAN® * ℞

brand of sterile betamethasone sodium phosphate
and betamethasone acetate suspension, NF
6 mg. per ml.

FOR INTRAMUSCULAR, INTRABURSAL, INTRA-ARTICULAR, PERIARTICULAR, INTRADERMAL, AND INTRALESIONAL INJECTION.
Description: Each ml. of sterile aqueous suspension of CELESTONE SOLUSPAN* Suspension contains: 3.0 mg. betamethasone as betamethasone sodium phosphate; 3.0 mg. betamethasone acetate; 7.1 mg. dibasic sodium phosphate; 3.4 mg. monobasic sodium phosphate; 0.1 mg. edetate disodium; and 0.2 mg. benzalkonium chloride.
Actions: Naturally occurring glucocorticoids (hydrocortisone), which also have salt-retaining properties, are used as replacement therapy in adrenocortical deficiency states. Their synthetic analogs are primarily used for their potent anti-inflammatory effects in disorders of many organ systems.
Betamethasone sodium phosphate, a soluble ester, provides prompt activity, while betamethasone acetate is only slightly soluble and affords sustained activity.
Glucocorticoids cause profound and varied metabolic effects. In addition, they modify the body's immune responses to diverse stimuli.
Indications: When oral therapy is not feasible and the strength, dosage form, and route of administration of the drug reasonably lend the preparation to the treatment of the condition, CELESTONE SOLUSPAN Suspension for **intramuscular use** is indicated as follows:
Endocrine disorders: Primary or secondary adrenocortical insufficiency (hydrocortisone or cortisone is the drug of choice; synthetic analogs may be used in conjunction with mineralocorticoids where applicable; in infancy, mineralocorticoid supplementation is of particular importance).
Acute adrenocortical insufficiency (hydrocortisone or cortisone is the drug of choice; mineralocorticoid supplementation may be necessary, particularly when synthetic analogs are used).
Preoperatively and in the event of serious trauma or illness, in patients with known adrenal insufficiency or when adrenocortical reserve is doubtful. Shock unresponsive to conventional therapy if adrenocortical insufficiency exists or is suspected. Congenital adrenal hyperplasia. Nonsuppurative thyroiditis.
Rheumatic disorders: As adjunctive therapy for short-term administration (to tide the patient over an acute episode or exacerbation) in: post-traumatic osteoarthritis; synovitis of osteoarthritis; rheumatoid arthritis; acute and subacute bursitis; epicondylitis; acute nonspecific tenosynovitis; acute gouty arthritis; psoriatic arthritis; ankylosing spondylitis; juvenile rheumatoid arthritis.
Collagen disease: During an exacerbation or as maintenance therapy in selected cases of: systemic lupus erythematosus; acute rheumatic carditis.
Dermatologic diseases: Pemphigus: severe erythema multiforme (Stevens-Johnson syndrome); exfoliative dermatitis; bullous dermatitis herpetiformis; severe seborrheic dermatitis; severe psoriasis.
Allergic states: Control of severe or incapacitating allergic conditions intractable to adequate trials of conventional treatment in: bronchial asthma; contact dermatitis; atopic dermatitis; serum sickness; seasonal or perennial allergic rhinitis; drug hypersensitivity reactions; urticarial transfusion reactions; acute noninfectious laryngeal edema (epinephrine is the drug of first choice).
Ophthalmic diseases: Severe, acute and chronic allergic and inflammatory processes involving the eye, such as: herpes zoster ophthalmicus; iritis, iridocyclitis; chorioretinitis; diffuse posterior uveitis and choroiditis; optic neuritis; sympathetic ophthalmia; anterior segment inflammation.
Gastrointestinal diseases: To tide the patient over a critical period of disease in: ulcerative colitis—(systemic therapy); regional enteritis—(systemic therapy).
Respiratory diseases: Symptomatic sarcoidosis; berylliosis; fulminating or disseminated pulmonary tuberculosis, when concurrently accompanied by appropriate antituberculous chemotherapy; aspiration pneumonitis.
Hematologic disorders: Acquired (autoimmune) hemolytic anemia.
Neoplastic diseases: For palliative management of: leukemias and lymphomas in adults; acute leukemia of childhood.
Edematous state: To induce diuresis or remission of proteinuria in the nephrotic syndrome, without uremia, of the idiopathic type or that due to lupus erythematosus.
Miscellaneous: Tuberculous meningitis with subarachnoid block or impending block when concurrently accompanied by appropriate antituberculous chemotherapy.
When the strength and dosage form of the drug lend the preparation to the treatment of the condition, the **intra-articular or soft tissue administration** of CELESTONE SOLUSPAN Suspension is indicated as adjunctive therapy for short-term administration (to tide the patient over an acute episode or exacerbation) in: synovitis of osteoarthritis; rheumatoid arthritis; acute and subacute bursitis; acute gouty arthritis; epicondylitis; acute nonspecific tenosynovitis; post-traumatic osteoarthritis.
When the strength and dosage form of the drug lend the preparation to the treatment of the condition, the **intralesional administration** of CELESTONE SOLUSPAN Suspension is indicated for: keloids; localized hypertrophic, infiltrated, inflammatory lesions of lichen planus, psoriatic plaques, granuloma annulare, and lichen simplex chronicus (neurodermatitis); discoid lupus erythematosus; necrobiosis lipoidica diabeticorum; alopecia areata.

Contraindications:
CELESTONE SOLUSPAN Suspension is contraindicated in systemic fungal infections.

Warnings: CELESTONE SOLUSPAN should not be administered intravenously.
In patients on corticosteroid therapy subjected to any unusual stress, increased dosage of rapidly acting corticosteroids before, during, and after the stressful situation is indicated.
Corticosteroids may mask some signs of infection, and new infections may appear during their use. There may be decreased resistance and inability to localize infection when corticosteroids are used.
Prolonged use of corticosteroids may produce posterior subcapsular cataracts, glaucoma with possible damage to the optic nerves, and may enhance the establishment of secondary ocular infections due to fungi or viruses.
Average and large doses of cortisone or hydrocortisone can cause elevation of blood pressure, salt and water retention, and increased excretion of potassium. These effects are less likely to occur with the synthetic derivatives except when used in large doses. Dietary salt restriction and potassium supplementation may be necessary. All corticosteroids increase calcium excretion.
While on Corticosteroid Therapy Patients Should Not Be Vaccinated Against Smallpox. Other Immunization Procedures Should Not Be Undertaken in Patients Who Are on Corticosteroids, Especially in High Doses, Because of Possible Hazards of Neurological Complications and Lack of Antibody Response.
The use of CELESTONE SOLUSPAN Suspension in active tuberculosis should be restricted to those cases of fulminating or disseminated tuberculosis in which the corticosteroid is used for the management of the disease in conjunction with appropriate antituberculous regimen.
If corticosteroids are indicated in patients with latent tuberculosis or tuberculin reactivity, close observation is necessary as reactivation of the disease may occur. During prolonged corticosteroid therapy, these patients should receive chemoprophylaxis.
Because rare instances of anaphylactoid reactions have occurred in patients receiving parenteral corticosteroid therapy, appropriate precautionary measures should be taken prior to administration, especially when the patient has a history of allergy to any drug.
Usage in pregnancy: Since adequate human reproduction studies have not been done with corticosteroids, the use of these drugs in pregnancy, nursing mothers, or women of childbearing potential requires that the possible benefits of the drug be weighed against the potential hazards to the mother and embryo or fetus. Infants born of mothers who have received substantial doses of corticosteroids during pregnancy should be carefully observed for signs of hypoadrenalism.

Precautions: Drug-induced secondary adrenocortical insufficiency may be minimized by gradual reduction of dosage. This type of relative insufficiency may persist for months after discontinuation of therapy; therefore, in any situation of stress occurring during that period, hormone therapy should be reinstituted. Since mineralocorticoid secretion may be impaired, salt and/or a mineralocorticoid should be administered concurrently.

Continued on next page

Information on Schering products appearing on these pages is effective as of September 30, 1979.

* Brand of rapid repository injectable.

Schering—Cont.

There is an enhanced effect of corticosteroids in patients with hypothyroidism and in those with cirrhosis.
Corticosteroids should be used cautiously in patients with ocular herpes simplex for fear of corneal perforation.
The lowest possible dose of corticosteroid should be used to control the condition under treatment, and when reduction in dosage is possible, the reduction must be gradual.
Psychic derangements may appear when corticosteroids are used, ranging from euphoria, insomnia, mood swings, personality changes, and severe depression to frank psychotic manifestations. Also, existing emotional instability or psychotic tendencies may be aggravated by corticosteroids.
Aspirin should be used cautiously in conjunction with corticosteroids in hypoprothrombinemia.
Steroids should be used with caution in nonspecific ulcerative colitis, if there is a probability of impending perforation, abscess or other pyogenic infection, also in diverticulitis, fresh intestinal anastomoses, active or latent peptic ulcer, renal insufficiency, hypertension, osteoporosis, and myasthenia gravis.
Growth and development of infants and children on prolonged corticosteroid therapy should be carefully followed.
The following additional precautions also apply for parenteral corticosteroids. Intra-articular injection of a corticosteroid may produce systemic as well as local effects.
Appropriate examination of any joint fluid present is necessary to exclude a septic process.
A marked increase in pain accompanied by local swelling, further restriction of joint motion, fever, and malaise are suggestive of septic arthritis. If this complication occurs and the diagnosis of sepsis is confirmed, appropriate antimicrobial therapy should be instituted.
Local injection of a steroid into a previously infected joint is to be avoided.
Corticosteroids should not be injected into unstable joints.
The slower rate of absorption by intramuscular administration should be recognized.
Adverse Reactions:
Fluid and electrolyte disturbances: sodium retention; fluid retention; congestive heart failure in susceptible patients; potassium loss; hypokalemic alkalosis; hypertension.
Musculoskeletal: muscle weakness; steroid myopathy; loss of muscle mass; osteoporosis; vertebral compression fractures; aseptic necrosis of femoral and humeral heads; pathologic fracture of long bones.
Gastrointestinal: peptic ulcer with possible subsequent perforation and hemorrhage; pancreatitis; abdominal distention; ulcerative esophagitis.
Dermatologic: impaired wound healing; thin fragile skin; petechiae and ecchymoses; facial erythema; increased sweating; may suppress reactions to skin tests.
Neurological: convulsions; increased intracranial pressure with papilledema (pseudotumor cerebri) usually after treatment; vertigo; headache.
Endocrine: menstrual irregularities; development of Cushingoid state; suppression of growth in children; secondary adrenocortical and pituitary unresponsiveness, particularly in times of stress, as in trauma, surgery, or illness; decreased carbohydrate tolerance; manifestations of latent diabetes mellitus; increased requirements for insulin or oral hypoglycemic agents in diabetics.
Ophthalmic: posterior subcapsular cataracts; increased intraocular pressure; glaucoma; exophthalmos.
Metabolic: negative nitrogen balance due to protein catabolism.
The following *additional* adverse reactions are related to parenteral corticosteroid therapy: rare instances of blindness associated with intralesional therapy around the face and head; hyperpigmentation or hypopigmentation; subcutaneous and cutaneous atrophy; sterile abscess; post-injection flare (following intra-articular use); charcot-like arthropathy.
Dosage and Administration: The initial dosage of CELESTONE SOLUSPAN Suspension may vary from 0.5 to 9.0 mg. per day depending on the specific disease entity being treated. In situations of less severity, lower doses will generally suffice while in selected patients higher initial doses may be required. Usually the parenteral dosage ranges are one-third to one-half the oral dose given every 12 hours. However, in certain overwhelming, acute, life-threatening situations, administration in dosages exceeding the usual dosages may be justified and may be in multiples of the oral dosages.
The initial dosage should be maintained or adjusted until a satisfactory response is noted. If after a reasonable period of time there is a lack of satisfactory clinical response, CELESTONE SOLUSPAN Suspension should be discontinued and the patient transferred to other appropriate therapy. *It Should Be Emphasized That Dosage Requirements Are Variable and Must Be Individualized on the Basis of the Disease Under Treatment and the Response of the Patient.* After a favorable response is noted, the proper maintenance dosage should be determined by decreasing the initial drug dosage in small decrements at appropriate time intervals until the lowest dosage which will maintain an adequate clinical response is reached. It should be kept in mind that constant monitoring is needed in regard to drug dosage. Included in the situations which may make dosage adjustments necessary are changes in clinical status secondary to remissions or exacerbations in the disease process, the patient's individual drug responsiveness, and the effect of patient exposure to stressful situations not directly related to the disease entity under treatment; in this latter situation it may be necessary to increase the dosage of CELESTONE SOLUSPAN Suspension for a period of time consistent with the patient's condition. If after long-term therapy the drug is to be stopped, it is recommended that it be withdrawn gradually rather than abruptly.
If coadministration of a local anesthetic is desired, CELESTONE SOLUSPAN Suspension may be mixed with 1% or 2% lidocaine hydrochloride, using the formulations which do not contain parabens. Similar local anesthetics may also be used. Diluents containing methylparaben, propylparaben, phenol, etc., should be avoided since these compounds may cause flocculation of the steroid. The required dose of CELESTONE SOLUSPAN Suspension is first withdrawn from the vial into the syringe. The local anesthetic is then drawn in, and the syringe shaken briefly. **Do not inject local anesthetics into the vial of CELESTONE SOLUSPAN Suspension.**
Bursitis, tenosynovitis, peritendinitis. In acute subdeltoid, subacromial, olecranon, and prepatellar bursitis, one intrabursal injection of 1.0 ml. CELESTONE SOLUSPAN Suspension can relieve pain and restore full range of movement. Several intrabursal injections of corticosteroids are usually required in recurrent acute bursitis and in acute exacerbations of chronic bursitis. Partial relief of pain and some increase in mobility can be expected in both conditions after one or two injections. Chronic bursitis may be treated with reduced dosage once the acute condition is controlled. In tenosynovitis and tendinitis, three or four local injections at intervals of one to two weeks between injections are given in most cases. Injections should be made into the affected tendon sheaths rather than into the tendons themselves. In ganglions of joint capsules and tendon sheaths, injection of 0.5 ml. directly into the ganglion cysts has produced marked reduction in the size of the lesions. *Rheumatoid arthritis and osteoarthritis.* Following intra-articular administration of 0.5 to 2.0 ml. of CELESTONE SOLUSPAN Suspension, relief of pain, soreness, and stiffness may be experienced. Duration of relief varies widely in both diseases. Intra-articular Injection—CELESTONE SOLUSPAN Suspension is well tolerated in joints and periarticular tissues. There is virtually no pain on injection, and the "secondary flare" that sometimes occurs a few hours after intra-articular injection of corticosteroids has not been reported with CELESTONE SOLUSPAN Suspension. Using sterile technique, a 20- to 24-gauge needle on an empty syringe is inserted into the synovial cavity, and a few drops of synovial fluid are withdrawn to confirm that the needle is in the joint. The aspirating syringe is replaced by a syringe containing CELESTONE SOLUSPAN Suspension and injection is then made into the joint.

Recommended Doses for Intra-articular Injection

Size of joint	Location	Dose (ml.)
Very Large	Hip	1.0-2.0
Large	Knee, Ankle, Shoulder	1.0
Medium	Elbow, Wrist	0.5-1.0
Small (Metacarpophalangeal, interphalangeal) (Sternoclavicular)	Hand Chest	0.25-0.5

A portion of the administered dose of CELESTONE SOLUSPAN Suspension is absorbed systemically following intra-articular injection. In patients being treated concomitantly with oral or parenteral corticosteroids, especially those receiving large doses, the systemic absorption of the drug should be considered in determining intra-articular dosage.
Dermatologic conditions. In intralesional treatment, 0.2 ml./sq. cm. of CELESTONE SOLUSPAN Suspension is injected intradermally (not subcutaneously) using a tuberculin syringe with a 25-gauge, ½-inch needle. Care should be taken to deposit a uniform depot of medication intradermally. A total of no more than 1.0 ml. at weekly intervals is recommended. *Disorders of the foot.* A tuberculin syringe with a 25-gauge, ¾-inch needle is suitable for most injections into the foot. The following doses are recommended at intervals of three days to a week.

Diagnosis	CELESTONE SOLUSPAN Suspension Dose (ml.)
Bursitis	
under heloma durum or heloma molle	0.25-0.5
under calcaneal spur	0.5
over hallux rigidus or digiti quinti varus	0.5
Tenosynovitis, periostitis of cuboid	0.5
Acute gouty arthritis	0.5-1.0

How Supplied: CELESTONE SOLUSPAN Suspension, 5 ml. multiple-dose vial, box of one. Shake well before using. Store between 2° and 25°C (36° and 77°F).

CHLOR-TRIMETON®
brand of chlorpheniramine maleate, USP
REPETABS® Tablets 8 mg
Tablets
Syrup

How Supplied: CHLOR-TRIMETON REPETABS Tablets, 8 mg, sugar-coated, yellow tablets branded in red with the Schering trademark and product identification letters CC or numbers, 374; box of 24, bottles of 100 and 1000, canister of 5000.
CHLOR-TRIMETON **Tablets,** 4 mg., yellow, compressed, scored tablets impressed with the Schering trademark and product identification letters, TW, or numbers, 080; box of 24, bottles of 100 and 1000; canisters of 5000.
CHLOR-TRIMETON **Syrup,** 2 mg. per 5 ml., blue-green-colored liquid; 4-fluid ounce (473 ml.) and 128-fluid ounce (3.8 liters) bottles.
For complete prescribing information, contact the Schering Professional Services Department.
[*Shown in Product Identification Section*]

CHLOR-TRIMETON® ℞
brand of chlorpheniramine maleate, USP
REPETABS® Tablets 12 mg
Injection

Description: CHLOR-TRIMETON is chlorpheniramine maleate, USP, an antihistamine having the chemical name, 2-[*p*-Chloro-α-[2-(dimethylamino)ethyl] benzyl] pyridine maleate (1:1).
CHLOR-TRIMETON REPETABS (brand of repeat-action tablets) **Tablets** contain 12 mg. chlorpheniramine maleate, USP; the dosage is equally divided between an outer layer for rapid absorption and an inner core protected by a special timed barrier for release three to six hours after ingestion.
CHLOR-TRIMETON **Injection,** 10 mg/ml, is intended for intravenous, intramuscular or subcutaneous injection; each ml. contains 10 mg. chlorpheniramine maleate, USP and water for injection q.s. CHLOR-TRIMETON **Injection,** 100 mg/ml, is intended for intramuscular or subcutaneous administration (not for intravenous use); each ml. contains 100 mg. chlorpheniramine maleate, USP and water for injection q.s.
Actions: CHLOR-TRIMETON is an antihistamine with anticholinergic (drying) and sedative side effects. Antihistamines appear to compete with histamine for cell receptor sites on effector cells.
Indications:
CHLOR-TRIMETON **Injection** is indicated for use in the following conditions when use of the oral form of the drug is impractical: amelioration of allergic reactions to blood or plasma; in anaphylaxis as an adjunct to epinephrine and other standard measures after the acute symptoms have been controlled; for other uncomplicated allergic conditions of the immediate type when oral therapy is impossible or contraindicated.
CHLOR-TRIMETON REPETABS **Tablets** are indicated for the treatment of perennial and seasonal allergic rhinitis; vasomotor rhinitis; allergic conjunctivitis due to inhalant allergens and foods; mild, uncomplicated allergic skin manifestations of urticaria and angioedema; amelioration of allergic reactions to blood or plasma; dermographism. They are also indicated as therapy for anaphylactic reactions adjunctive to epinephrine and other standard measures after the acute manifestations have been controlled.
Contraindications: Use in Newborn or Premature Infants: This drug should not be used in newborn or premature infants.
Use in Nursing Mothers: Because of the higher risk of antihistamines for infants generally and for newborns and prematures in particular, antihistamine therapy is contraindicated in nursing mothers.
Use in Lower Respiratory Disease: Antihistamines should not be used to treat lower respiratory tract symptoms, including asthma.
Antihistamines are also contraindicated in the following conditions: hypersensitivity to chlorpheniramine maleate and other antihistamines of similar chemical structure; monoamine oxidase inhibitor therapy (See Drug Interactions Section).
Warnings: Antihistamines should be used with considerable caution in patients with: narrow angle glaucoma; stenosing peptic ulcer; pyloroduodenal obstruction; symptomatic prostatic hypertrophy; bladder neck obstruction.
Use in Children: In infants and children especially, antihistamines in overdosage may cause hallucinations, convulsions or death.
As in adults, antihistamines may diminish mental alertness in children. In the young child particularly, they may produce excitation.
Use in Pregnancy: Experience with this drug in pregnant women is inadequate to determine whether there exists a potential for harm to the developing fetus.
Use with CNS Depressants: Chlorpheniramine maleate has additive effects with alcohol and other CNS depressants (hypnotics, sedatives, tranquilizers, etc.).
Use in Activities Requiring Mental Alertness: Patients should be warned about engaging in activities requiring mental alertness, such as driving a car or operating appliances, machinery, etc.
Use in The Elderly (approximately 60 years or older): Antihistamines are more likely to cause dizziness, sedation, and hypotension in elderly patients.
Precautions: Chlorpheniramine maleate has an atropine-like action and therefore should be used with caution in patients with: a history of bronchial asthma; increased intraocular pressure; hyperthyroidism; cardiovascular disease; hypertension.
Adverse Reactions: Slight to moderate drowsiness occurs relatively infrequently with chlorpheniramine maleate. Other possible side effects common to antihistamines in general include:
General: urticaria, drug rash, anaphylactic shock, photosensitivity, excessive perspiration, chills, dryness of mouth, nose, and throat.
Cardiovascular System: hypotension, headache, palpitations, tachycardia, extrasystoles.
Hematologic System: hemolytic anemia, thrombocytopenia, agranulocytosis.
Nervous System: sedation, dizziness, disturbed coordination, fatigue, confusion, restlessness, excitation, nervousness, tremor, irritability, insomnia, euphoria, paresthesias, blurred vision, diplopia, vertigo, tinnitus, acute labyrinthitis, hysteria, neuritis, convulsions.
Gastrointestinal System: epigastric distress, anorexia, nausea, vomiting, diarrhea, constipation.
Genitourinary System: urinary frequency, difficult urination, urinary retention, early menses.
Respiratory System: thickening of bronchial secretions, tightness of chest and wheezing, nasal stuffiness.
Dosage and Administration: DOSAGE SHOULD BE INDIVIDUALIZED ACCORDING TO THE NEEDS AND RESPONSE OF THE PATIENT.
CHLOR-TRIMETON REPETABS **Tablets** — Adults: one 12 mg. tablet at bedtime or every 8 to 10 hours during the day.
CHLOR-TRIMETON **Injection**—For amelioration of allergic reactions to blood or plasma: 10 to 20 mg. administered as a single dose; the maximum recommended dose for 24 hours is 40 mg.
In anaphylaxis as an adjunct to epinephrine and other standard measures after the acute symptoms have been controlled: 10 to 20 mg. administered intravenously as a single dose.
For other uncomplicated allergic conditions of the immediate type when oral therapy is impossible or contraindicated: 5 to 20 mg. administered as a single dose.
Note: CHLOR-TRIMETON **Injection,** 100 mg/ml, is intended for intramuscular or subcutaneous use only and is not to be used when intravenous administration is indicated. Intradermal administration is not recommended.
CHLOR-TRIMETON **Injection,** 10 mg/ml, is intended for intravenous, intramuscular, or subcutaneous administration.
Overdosage: In the event of overdosage, emergency treatment should be started immediately. *Manifestations* of antihistamine overdosage may vary from central nervous system depression (sedation, apnea, cardiovascular collapse) to stimulation (insomnia, hallucinations, tremors or convulsions). Other signs and symptoms may be dizziness, tinnitus, ataxia, blurred vision and hypotension. Stimulation is particularly likely in children, as are atropine-like signs and symptoms (dry mouth; fixed, dilated pupils; flushing; hyperthermia and gastrointestinal symptoms).
Treatment—The patient should be induced to vomit, even if emesis has occurred spontaneously. Pharmacologic vomiting by the administration of ipecac syrup is a preferred method. However, vomiting should not be induced in patients with impaired consciousness. The action of ipecac is facilitated by physical activity and by the administration of eight to twelve fluid ounces of water. If emesis does not occur within fifteen minutes, the dose of ipecac should be repeated. Precautions against aspiration must be taken, especially in infants and children. Following emesis, any drug remaining in the stomach may be adsorbed by activated charcoal administered as a slurry with water. If vomiting is unsuccessful, or contraindicated, gastric lavage should be performed. Isotonic and one-half isotonic saline are the lavage solutions of choice. Saline cathartics, such as milk of magnesia, draw water into the bowel by osmosis and, therefore, may be valuable for their action in rapid dilution of bowel content. After emergency treatment the patient should continue to be medically monitored.
Treatment of the signs and symptoms of overdosage is symptomatic and supportive. Stimulants (analeptic agents) should not be used. Vasopressors may be used to treat hypotension. Short acting barbiturates, diazepam or paraldehyde may be administered to control seizures. Hyperpyrexia, especially in children, may require treatment with tepid water sponge baths or a hypothermic blanket. Apnea is treated with ventilatory support.
Drug Interactions: MAO inhibitors prolong and intensify the anticholinergic (drying) effects of antihistamines.
How Supplied: CHLOR-TRIMETON REPETABS **Tablets,** 12 mg., sugar-coated, orange tablets branded in black with the Schering trademark and product identification letters, AAE or numbers, 009; bottles of 100 and 1000, canister of 5000.
CHLOR-TRIMETON **Injection,** 10 mg/ml, 1 ml. ampules; box of 100.
CHLOR-TRIMETON **Injection,** 100 mg/ml, 2 ml. multiple-dose vials; box of one.
CHLOR-TRIMETON **Injection** should be protected from light to prevent discoloration.

[*Shown in Product Identification Section*]

Continued on next page

Information on Schering products appearing on these pages is effective as of September 30, 1979.

Schering—Cont.

CHLOR-TRIMETON® Decongestant Tablets

How Supplied: CHLOR-TRIMETON Decongestant Tablets—boxes of 24's and 48's.
For complete prescribing information, contact the Schering Professional Services Department.
[Shown in Product Identification Section]

CHLOR-TRIMETON® Expectorant

How Supplied: CHLOR-TRIMETON Expectorant, 16 fl. oz. (473 ml) bottles.
For complete prescribing information, contact the Schering Professional Services Department.

COD LIVER OIL CONCENTRATE
Tablets
Capsules
Tablets with Vitamin C

How Supplied: Cod Liver Oil Concentrate Tablets: bottles of 100 and 240. Cod Liver Oil Concentrate Capsules: bottles of 40 and 100. Cod Liver Oil Concentrate Tablets with Vitamin C: bottles of 100 tablets.
For complete prescribing information, contact the Schering Professional Services Department.
[Shown in Product Identification Section]

CORICIDIN® Tablets
CORICIDIN 'D'® Decongestant Tablets
CORICIDIN® Cough Syrup
CORICIDIN® Decongestant Nasal Mist

How Supplied: CORICIDIN Tablets—bottles of 12, 24, 60, 100 and 1000. Dispensing Package, box of 100 packets, 4 tablets in each packet.
CORICIDIN 'D' Decongestant Tablets—bottles of 12, 24, 50, and 100. Dispensing Package, box of 100 packets, 4 tablets in each packet.
CORICIDIN Cough Syrup—bottles of 4 oz. (118 ml).
CORICIDIN Decongestant Nasal Mist—Plastic squeeze bottles of ⅔ fl. oz. (20 ml).
For complete prescribing information, contact the Schering Professional Services Department.
[Shown in Product Identification Section]

CORICIDIN® MEDILETS®
Tablets for Children
CORICIDIN® DEMILETS®
Tablets for Children
CORICIDIN® Children's Cough Syrup

How Supplied: CORICIDIN MEDILETS Tablets—boxes of 24 and 36, individually wrapped in a child's protective pack.
CORICIDIN DEMILETS Tablets—boxes of 24 and 36, individually wrapped in a child's protective pack.
CORICIDIN Children's Cough Syrup—bottles of 4 fl. oz. (118 ml).
For complete prescribing information, contact the Schering Professional Services Department.
[Shown in Product Identification Section]

CORICIDIN® Extra Strength Sinus Headache Tablets

How Supplied: Box of 24.
For complete prescribing information, contact the Schering Professional Services Department.
[Shown in Product Identification Section]

CORILIN® Infant Liquid ℞

How Supplied: CORILIN Infant Liquid, bottle of one fluid ounce (30 ml.) with calibrated dropper; red-colored liquid.
For complete prescribing information, contact the Schering Professional Services Department.

DEMAZIN®
REPETABS® Tablets
Syrup

How Supplied: DEMAZIN REPETABS **Tablets**, blue, sugar-coated tablets branded in red with the Schering trademark and either product identification letters, ADD or numbers, 133; box of 24 tablets and bottles of 100 and 1000.
DEMAZIN **Syrup**, blue-colored liquid, bottles of 4 fluid ounces (118 ml.) and 128 fluid ounces (1 gallon).
For complete prescribing information, contact the Schering Professional Services Department.
[Shown in Product Identification Section]

DIPROSONE® ℞
brand of betamethasone dipropionate, USP
Aerosol 0.1% w/w
(Potency expressed as betamethasone)
For Dermatologic Use Only—
Not For Ophthalmic Use

Description: DIPROSONE is betamethasone dipropionate, USP (9-fluoro-11β,17,21-trihydroxy-16β -methyl pregna-1, 4-diene-3,20-dione 17,21-dipropionate).
DIPROSONE Aerosol contains 6.4 mg. betamethasone dipropionate, USP, equivalent to 5.0 mg. betamethasone in a vehicle of mineral oil and caprylic/capric triglyceride. It also contains 10% isopropyl alcohol and sufficient inert propellent of hydrocarbon (propane and isobutane) to make 85 grams. The spray deposits betamethasone dipropionate, equivalent to approximately 0.1% betamethasone in a nonvolatile, almost invisible film. A three-second spray delivers betamethasone dipropionate equivalent to approximately 0.06 mg. betamethasone.
Actions: DIPROSONE Aerosol is primarily effective because of its anti-inflammatory, antipruritic, and vasoconstrictive actions.
Indications: DIPROSONE Aerosol is indicated solely for the adjunctive topical management for the relief of inflammatory manifestations of acute contact dermatitis. DIPROSONE Aerosol has not been shown to be effective in any steroid-responsive dermatosis other than contact dermatitis.
As with all topical steroid aerosols, the use of occlusive dressings is not recommended.
Contraindications: DIPROSONE Aerosol is contraindicated in those patients with a history of hypersensitivity to any of the components of the preparation.
Warnings: Keep away from eyes or other mucous membranes.
Use only as directed; intentional misuse by deliberately concentrating and inhaling the contents can be harmful or fatal.
Avoid freezing of the tissue by not spraying for more than three seconds, at a distance of not less than six inches.
Contents under pressure. Do not puncture. Flammable mixture, do not use or store near heat or open flame. Exposure to temperatures above 120° Fahrenheit may cause bursting. Never throw container into fire or incinerator. Keep out of the reach of children.
Precautions: If irritation develops with the use of DIPROSONE Aerosol, treatment should be discontinued and appropriate therapy instituted.
In the presence of an infection, the use of an appropriate antifungal or antibacterial agent should be instituted. If a favorable response does not occur promptly, the corticosteroid should be discontinued until the infection has been adequately controlled.
It should be recognized that any of the side effects reported following systemic use of corticosteroids, including adrenal suppression, may also occur following their topical use, especially in infants and children. Systemic absorption of topically applied steroids will be increased if extensive body surface areas are treated. Therefore, under these circumstances, suitable precautions should be taken when long-term use is anticipated, particularly in infants and children.
Although topical steroids have not been reported to have an adverse effect on human pregnancy, the safety of their use in pregnant women has not been absolutely established. In laboratory animals, increases in incidence of fetal abnormalities have been associated with exposure of gestating females to topical corticosteroids. In some cases at rather low dosage levels. Therefore, drugs of this class should not be used on pregnant patients in large amounts or for prolonged periods of time.
DIPROSONE Aerosol is not for ophthalmic use.
Adverse Reactions: The following local adverse reactions have been reported with topical corticosteroid preparations: burning; itching; irritation; dryness; folliculitis; hypertrichosis; acneiform eruptions; hypopigmentation; perioral dermatitis; allergic contact dermatitis; maceration of the skin; secondary infection; skin atrophy; striae; miliaria.
Dosage and Administration: The container may be held upright or inverted during use. The spray should be directed onto the affected area from a distance of not less than six inches and applied for only three seconds. For most effective and economical use, a three-second spray is sufficient to cover an area about the size of the hand.
Apply sparingly to the affected skin area three times a day.
How Supplied: DIPROSONE Aerosol, 0.1%, 85-gram spray can.
Store between 35° and 86°F (2° and 30° C).

DIPROSONE® ℞
brand of betamethasone dipropionate, USP
Cream 0.05%
(Potency expressed as betamethasone)
For Dermatologic Use Only—
Not For Ophthalmic Use

Description: DIPROSONE is betamethasone dipropionate, USP (9-Fluoro-11β,17,21-trihydroxy-16β-methylpregna-1, 4-diene-3, 20-dione 17,21-dipropionate).
Each gram of DIPROSONE Cream 0.05% contains 0.64 mg. betamethasone dipropionate, USP (equivalent to 0.5 mg. betamethasone) in a hydrophilic, emollient cream consisting of purified water, mineral oil, white petrolatum, polyethylene glycol 1000 monocetyl ether, cetostearyl alcohol, phosphoric acid, and monobasic sodium phosphate with 4-chloro-*m*-cresol as preservative.
Actions: DIPROSONE Cream is primarily effective because of its anti-inflammatory, antipruritic, and vasoconstrictive actions.
Indications: DIPROSONE Cream is indicated for the relief of the inflammatory manifestations of corticosteroid-responsive dermatoses.
Contraindications: DIPROSONE Cream is contraindicated in those patients with a history of hypersensitivity to any of the components of such preparations.
Precautions: If irritation develops with the use of DIPROSONE Cream, treatment should be discontinued and appropriate therapy instituted.
In the presence of an infection, the use of an appropriate antifungal or antibacterial agent should be instituted. If a favorable response does not occur promptly, the corticosteroid should be discontinued until the infection has been adequately controlled.
It should be recognized that any of the side effects reported following systemic use of corticosteroids, including adrenal suppression, may also occur following their topical use, especially in infants and children. Systemic absorption of topically applied steroids will be in-

creased if extensive body surface areas are treated or if the occlusive technique is used. Therefore, under these circumstances, suitable precautions should be taken when long-term use is anticipated, particularly in infants and children.
Although topical steroids have not been reported to have an adverse effect on human pregnancy, the safety of their use in pregnant women has not been absolutely established. In laboratory animals, increases in incidence of fetal abnormalities have been associated with exposure of gestating females to topical corticosteroids, in some cases at rather low dosage levels. Therefore, drugs of this class should not be used on pregnant patients in large amounts or for prolonged periods of time.
DIPROSONE Cream is not for ophthalmic use.
Adverse Reactions: The following local adverse reactions have been reported with topical corticosteroids, especially under occlusive dressings: burning; itching; irritation; dryness; folliculitis; hypertrichosis; acneiform eruptions; hypopigmentation; perioral dermatitis; allergic contact dermatitis; maceration of the skin; secondary infection; skin atrophy; striae; miliaria.
Dosage and Administration: Apply a thin film of DIPROSONE Cream to the affected skin areas twice daily, in the morning and at night. Clinical studies of DIPROSONE have indicated that applications twice a day are generally adequate.
How Supplied: DIPROSONE Cream 0.05% is supplied in 15- and 45-gram tubes, boxes of one.
Store between 35° and 86° F.

DIPROSONE® ℞
brand of betamethasone dipropionate, USP
Lotion 0.05% w/w
Ointment 0.05%
(Potency expressed as betamethasone)
For Dermatologic Use Only–Not for Opthalmic Use

Description: DIPROSONE is betamethasone dipropionate, USP (9-Fluoro-11β,17,21-trihydroxy-16β-methylpregna-1, 4-diene-3, 20-dione 17,21-dipropionate).
Each gram of DIPROSONE **Lotion** 0.05% w/w contains 0.64 mg betamethasone dipropionate (equivalent to 0.5 mg. betamethasone) in a vehicle consisting of isopropyl alcohol (46.8%) and purified water slightly thickened with carbomer 934P; the pH is adjusted to approximately 4.7 with sodium hydroxide.
Each gram of DIPROSONE **Ointment** 0.05% contains 0.64 mg. betamethasone dipropionate (equivalent to 0.5 mg. betamethasone) in an ointment base of mineral oil and white petrolatum.
Actions: DIPROSONE **Lotion** and **Ointment** are primarily effective because of their anti-inflammatory, antipruritic, and vasoconstrictive actions.
Indications: DIPROSONE **Lotion** and **Ointment** are indicated for the relief of the inflammatory manifestations of corticosteroid-responsive dermatoses.
Contraindications: DIPROSONE **Lotion** and **Ointment** are contraindicated in those patients with a history of hypersensitivity to any of the components of the preparations.
Precautions: If irritation develops with the use of DIPROSONE **Lotion** or **Ointment**, treatment should be discontinued and appropriate therapy instituted.
In the presence of an infection, the use of an appropriate antifungal or antibacterial agent should be instituted. If a favorable response does not occur promptly, the corticosteroid should be discontinued until the infection has been adequately controlled.
It should be recognized that any of the side effects reported following systemic use of corticosteroids, including adrenal suppression, may also occur following their topical use, especially in infants and children. Systemic absorption of topically applied steroids will be increased if extensive body surface areas are treated or if the occlusive technique is used. Therefore, under these circumstances, suitable precautions should be taken when long-term use is anticipated, particularly in infants and children.
Although topical steroids have not been reported to have an adverse effect on human pregnancy, the safety of their use in pregnant women has not been absolutely established. In laboratory animals, increases in incidence of fetal abnormalities have been associated with exposure of gestating females to topical corticosteroids, in some cases at rather low dosage levels. Therefore, drugs of this class should not be used on pregnant patients in large amounts or for prolonged periods of time.
DIPROSONE **Lotion** and **Ointment** are not for ophthalmic use.
Adverse Reactions: The following local adverse reactions have been reported with topical corticosteroids, especially under occlusive dressings: burning; itching; irritation; dryness; folliculitis, hypertrichosis; acneiform eruptions; hypopigmentation; perioral dermatitis; allergic contact dermatitis; maceration of the skin; secondary infection; skin atrophy; striae; miliaria.
Dosage and Administration:
DIPROSONE **Lotion**
Apply a few drops of DIPROSONE **Lotion** to the affected skin areas and massage gently until it disappears. Apply twice daily, in the morning and at night.
For the most effective and economical use, apply nozzle to affected area and gently squeeze bottle.
DIPROSONE **Ointment**
Apply a small quantity of DIPROSONE **Ointment** to the affected skin areas twice daily, in the morning and at night.
How Supplied: DIPROSONE **Lotion** 0.05% w/w is supplied in 20 ml. (18.7g) and 60 ml. (56.2g) plastic squeeze bottles; boxes of one.
Protect from light. Store between 35° and 86°F.
DIPROSONE **Ointment** 0.05% is supplied in 15- and 45-gram tubes; boxes of one.
Store between 35° and 86°F.

DISOPHROL® ℞
brand of dexbrompheniramine maleate, NF and pseudoephedrine sulfate
Chronotab® Tablets

Description: Each DISOPHROL CHRONOTAB (brand of sustained-action tablet) Tablet contains 6 mg. dexbrompheniramine maleate, NF and 120 mg. pseudoephedrine sulfate. These two active components are equally distributed between the tablet coating and a sustained-release core. Following ingestion, the active components in the coating are rapidly released; subsequently, the active components in the core are slowly released.
Dexbrompheniramine maleate is an antihistamine having the chemical name, (+)-2-[*p*-bromo-α-[2- (dimethylamino) ethyl] benzyl] pyridine maleate (1:1). Pseudoephedrine, also known as d-isoephedrine, is one of the naturally occurring alkaloids obtained from various species of the plant, *Ephedra.*
Actions: DISOPHROL combines the antihistaminic actions of dexbrompheniramine maleate with the vasoconstrictive properties of pseudoephedrine sulfate.
Dexbrompheniramine maleate is the dextroisomer of brompheniramine maleate, a racemic compound that is among the most potent of available antihistamines. That the dextro-isomer is responsible for nearly all the antihistaminic activity of racemic brompheniramine has been shown by comparative bio-assays of the racemic drug and its two isomeric forms. Studies of oral activity in guinea pigs have demonstrated that the d-isomer is approximately twice as potent as racemic brompheniramine, and about thirty times more potent than the l-isomer. Further, comparative studies of acute oral toxicity in guinea pigs have revealed that the d-form is no more toxic than the racemic mixture and less toxic than the l-form of the drug. The high potency and therapeutic index of dexbrompheniramine maleate, observed in animal studies, are reflected in the results of clinical investigation.
Pseudoephedrine Sulfate Like ephedrine, isoephedrine occurs in racemic and stereoisomeric forms. Pharmacologically, the most active forms are levo-ephedrine and dextro-isoephedrine, the racemic forms being essentially only as potent as the content of these two isomers.
The pharmacodynamic effects of ephedrine and isoephedrine are qualitatively similar but differ quantitatively in certain important respects. Given by the oral route for relief of nasal congestion, isoephedrine and ephedrine have approximately the same activity. In effective oral dosage, however, isoephedrine is less likely to give rise to unwanted cardiovascular and central effects.
The usefulness of an orally administered vasoconstrictor for shrinkage of congested nasal mucosa has been emphasized by a number of authors. In this regard, it has been pointed out that peroral administration of the drug has several advantages: (a) it produces a gradual but sustained decongestant effect, causing little, if any, "rebound" congestion; (b) it facilitates shrinkage of swollen mucosa in upper respiratory areas that are relatively inaccessible to topically applied sprays or drops; (c) it relieves nasal obstruction without the additional irritation which may result from local medication.
Indications: DISOPHROL CHRONOTAB Tablets are indicated for the relief of symptoms of upper respiratory mucosal congestion in seasonal and perennial nasal allergies, eustachian tube congestion, acute rhinitis, and rhinosinusitis.
Contraindications: DISOPHROL CHRONOTAB Tablets should not be given to children under 12 years of age.
DISOPHROL should not be administered to pregnant women or nursing mothers until the safety of this preparation for use during gestation and lactation is established.
DISOPHROL is also contraindicated in patients with severe hypertension and coronary artery disease.
Warnings: As in the case of other preparations containing central nervous system-acting drugs, patients receiving DISOPHROL should be cautioned about possible additive effects with alcohol and other central nervous system depressants (hypnotics, sedatives, tranquilizers). For the same reason, they should be cautioned against hazardous occupations requiring complete mental alertness, such as operating machinery or driving a motor vehicle.
Precautions: Pseudoephedrine-containing preparations should be used with caution in the presence of: hypertension; coronary artery disease; any other cardiovascular disease; glaucoma; prostatic hypertrophy; hyperthyroidism; diabetes.
Adverse Reactions: The physician should be alert to the possibility of any of the adverse reactions which have been observed with sym-

Continued on next page

Information on Schering products appearing on these pages is effective as of September 30, 1979.

Schering—Cont.

pathomimetic and antihistaminic drugs. These include: drowsiness; confusion; restlessness; nausea; vomiting; drug rash; vertigo; palpitation; anorexia; dizziness; dysuria due to vesicle sphincter spasm; headache; insomnia; anxiety; tension; weakness; tachycardia; angina; sweating; blood pressure elevation; mydriasis; gastric distress; abdominal cramps; central nervous system stimulation; circulatory collapse.

Dosage and Administration: Adults and Children 12 or More Years of Age: One DISOPHROL CHRONOTAB Tablet in the morning and one at bedtime. In exceptional cases, administration of one tablet every eight hours may be required.

How Supplied: DISOPHROL CHRONOTAB Tablets, sugar-coated, cherry-red tablets branded in black with either the product identification code, 85-WMH, or one of the Schering trademarks and the numbers, 231; bottle of 100.

[*Shown in Product Identification Section*]

DRIXORAL® ℞

brand of dexbrompheniramine maleate, NF and pseudoephedrine sulfate
Sustained-Action Tablets

Description: Each DRIXORAL Sustained-Action Tablet contains 6 mg. dexbrompheniramine maleate, NF and 120 mg. pseudoephedrine sulfate. These two active ingredients are equally distributed between the tablet coating and a sustained-release core. Following ingestion, the active components in the coating are quickly liberated; subsequently, the active components in the core are slowly released.

Dexbrompheniramine maleate is an antihistamine having the chemical name, (+)-2-[*p*-bromo-α-[2-(dimethylamino)ethyl]benzyl] pyridine maleate (1:1). Pseudoephedrine is one of the naturally occurring alkaloids obtained from various species of the plant *Ephedra.*

Actions: DRIXORAL Sustained-Action Tablets combine the antihistaminic actions of dexbrompheniramine maleate with the vasoconstrictive properties of pseudoephedrine sulfate.

Indications: DRIXORAL Sustained-Action Tablets are indicated for the relief of symptoms of upper respiratory mucosal congestion in seasonal and perennial nasal allergies, acute rhinitis, rhinosinusitis and eustachian tube blockage.

Contraindications: DRIXORAL should not be given to children under 12 years of age. DRIXORAL should not be administered to pregnant women or nursing mothers, until the safety of this preparation for use during gestation and lactation is established.

DRIXORAL is contraindicated in patients with severe hypertension and coronary artery disease.

Warnings: As in the case of other preparations containing central nervous system-acting drugs, patients receiving DRIXORAL should be cautioned about possible additive effects with alcohol and other central nervous system depressants, such as hypnotics, sedatives and tranquilizers.

Patients receiving DRIXORAL should also be cautioned against hazardous occupations requiring complete mental alertness, such as operating machinery or driving a motor vehicle.

Precautions: Preparations containing pseudoephedrine should be used cautiously in patients with the following conditions: hypertension; coronary artery disease or any other cardiovascular disease; glaucoma; prostatic hypertrophy; hyperthyroidism; diabetes.

Adverse Reactions: The physician should be alert to the possibility of any of the adverse reactions which have been observed with sympathomimetic and antihistaminic drugs. These include: drowsiness; confusion; restlessness; nausea; vomiting; drug rash; vertigo; palpitation; anorexia; dizziness; dysuria due to vesicle sphincter spasm; headache; insomnia; anxiety; tension; weakness; tachycardia; angina; sweating; blood pressure elevation; mydriasis; gastric distress; abdominal cramps; central nervous system stimulation; circulatory collapse.

Dosage and Administration: For adults and children over 12 years: one tablet in the morning and one at bedtime. In exceptional cases, one tablet every eight hours may be required.

How Supplied: DRIXORAL Sustained-Action Tablets, green, sugar-coated tablets branded in black with one of the Schering trademarks and product identification numbers 445 or letters AMN or the product name; bottle of 100.

[*Shown in Product Identification Section*]

EMKO® PRE-FIL®

Vaginal Contraceptive Foam

How Supplied: EMKO PRE-FIL Contraceptive Foam, 30 gm can with applicator and purse. Refill can without applicator and purse in 60 gm size. Both sizes feature a unique weighing cap that indicates when a new supply of foam is needed.

For complete prescribing information, contact the Schering Professional Services Department.

[*Shown in Product Identification Section*]

EMKO® Vaginal Contraceptive Foam

How Supplied: EMKO Contraceptive Foam, 40 gm can with applicator and storage purse. Refill cans without applicator and purse available in 40 gm and 90 gm sizes. All sizes feature a unique weighing cap that indicates when a new foam supply is needed.

For complete prescribing information, contact the Schering Professional Services Department.

[*Shown in Product Identification Section*]

ESTINYL® ℞

brand of ethinyl estradiol, USP
Tablets

BOXED WARNINGS

1. ESTROGENS HAVE BEEN REPORTED TO INCREASE THE RISK RATIO OF ENDOMETRIAL CARCINOMA.

Three independent case control studies have reported an increased risk ratio of endometrial cancer in postmenopausal women exposed to exogenous estrogens for prolonged periods.[1–3] This risk ratio was independent of the other risk factors for endometrial cancer. These studies are further supported by the report that incidence rates of endometrial cancer have increased sharply since 1969 in eight different areas of the United States with population-based cancer reporting systems, an increase which may be related to the rapidly expanding use of estrogens during the last decade.[4]

The three case control studies reported that the risk ratio of endometrial cancer in estrogen users was about 4.5 to 13.9 times greater than in nonusers. The risk ratio appears to depend on both duration of treatment[1] and on estrogen dose.[3] In view of these reports, when estrogens are used for the treatment of menopausal symptoms, the lowest dose that will control symptoms should be utilized and medication should be discontinued as soon as possible. When prolonged treatment is medically indicated, the patient should be reassessed on at least a semiannual basis to determine the need for continued therapy.

Although the evidence must be considered preliminary, one study suggests that cyclic administration of low doses of estrogen may carry less risk than continuous administration[3]; it therefore appears prudent to utilize such a regimen.

Close clinical surveillance of all women taking estrogens is important. In all cases of undiagnosed persistent or recurring abnormal vaginal bleeding, adequate diagnostic measures should be undertaken to rule out malignancy.

There is no evidence at present that "natural" estrogens are more or less hazardous than "synthetic" estrogens at equiestrogenic doses.

2. ESTROGENS SHOULD NOT BE USED DURING PREGNANCY.

The use of estrogens during early pregnancy may seriously damage the offspring. It has been reported that females exposed in utero to diethylstilbestrol, a non-steroidal estrogen, may have an increased risk of developing in later life a form of vaginal or cervical cancer that is ordinarily extremely rare.[5,6] This risk has been estimated statistically as not greater than 4 per 1000 exposures.[7] In certain studies, a high percentage of such exposed women (from 30 to 90 percent) have been found to have vaginal adenosis,[8–11] epithelial changes of the vagina and cervix. Although these changes are histologically benign, it is not known whether they are precursors of malignancy. Although similar data are not available with the use of other estrogens, it cannot be presumed they would not induce similar changes.

Several reports suggest an association between intrauterine fetal exposure to female sex hormones and congenital anomalies, including congenital heart defects and limb reduction defects.[12–15] One case control study[15] estimated a 4.7 fold increased risk of limb reduction defects in infants exposed in utero to sex hormones (oral contraceptives, hormone withdrawal tests for pregnancy, or attempted treatment for threatened abortion). Some of these exposures were very short and involved only a few days of treatment. The data suggest that the risk of limb reduction defects in exposed fetuses is somewhat less than 1 per 1000.

In the past, estrogens have been used during pregnancy to treat threatened or habitual abortion. There is considerable evidence that estrogens are ineffective for these indications.

If ESTINYL is used during pregnancy, or if the patient becomes pregnant while taking this drug, she should be apprised of the potential risks to the fetus, and the advisability of pregnancy continuation.

Description: ESTINYL Tablets contain ethinyl estradiol, a potent synthetic estrogen having the chemical name, 19-Nor-17α-pregna-1,3,5(10)-trien-20-yne-3,17-diol.

ESTINYL for oral administration is available in tablets containing 0.02, 0.05, or 0.5 mg. ethinyl estradiol, USP.

Clinical Pharmacology: Ethinyl estradiol promotes growth of the endometrium and thickening, stratification and cornification of the vagina. It causes growth of the ducts of the mammary gland, but inhibits lactation. It also inhibits the anterior pituitary and causes capillary dilatation, fluid retention and protein anabolism.

Indications: ESTINYL Tablets are indicated in the treatment of: 1) Moderate to severe *vasomotor* symptoms associated with the menopause. (There is no evidence that estrogens are effective for nervous symptoms or depression which might occur during menopause, and they should not be used to treat these conditions.) 2) Female hypogonadism. 3) Prostatic carcinoma—palliative therapy of advanced disease. 4) Breast cancer (for palliation only) in appropriately selected women, such as those who are more than 5 years postmenopausal with progressing inoperable or radiation-resistant disease.

ESTINYL HAS NOT BEEN SHOWN TO BE EFFECTIVE FOR ANY PURPOSE DURING PREGNANCY AND ITS USE MAY CAUSE SEVERE HARM TO THE FETUS (SEE BOXED WARNING ABOVE).

Contraindications: Estrogens should not be used in women (or men) with any of the following conditions:

1. Known or suspected cancer of the breast except in appropriately selected patients being treated for metastatic disease.
2. Known or suspected estrogen-dependent neoplasia.
3. Known or suspected pregnancy (See Boxed Warning).
4. Undiagnosed abnormal genital bleeding.
5. Active thrombophlebitis or thromboembolic disorders.
6. A past history of thrombophlebitis, thrombosis or thromboembolic disorders associated with previous estrogen use (except when used in treatment of breast or prostatic malignancy).

Warnings: 1. *Induction of malignant neoplasms.* Long-term continuous administration of natural and synthetic estrogens in certain animal species increases the frequency of carcinomas of the breast, cervix, vagina, and liver. There is now evidence that estrogens increase the risk of carcinoma of the endometrium in humans. (See Boxed Warning.)

At the present time there is no satisfactory evidence that estrogens given to postmenopausal women increase the risk of cancer of the breast,[16] although a recent long-term follow-up of a single physician's practice has raised this possibility.[17] Because of the animal data, there is a need for caution in prescribing estrogens for women with a strong family history of breast cancer or who have breast nodules, fibrocystic disease, or abnormal mammograms. Estrogens have been reported to be associated with carcinoma of the male breast and suspicious lesions in males receiving estrogen therapy should be investigated accordingly.

2. *Gallbladder disease.* A recent study has reported a 2- to 3-fold increase in the risk of surgically confirmed gallbladder disease in women receiving postmenopausal estrogens,[16] similar to the 2-fold increase previously noted in users of oral contraceptives.[18,22] In the case of oral contraceptives, the increased risk appeared after two years of use.[22]

3. *Effects similar to those caused by estrogen-progestagen oral contraceptives.* There are several serious adverse effects of oral contraceptives, most of which have not, up to now, been documented as consequences of postmenopausal estrogen therapy. This may reflect the comparatively low doses of estrogen used in postmenopausal women. It would be expected that the larger doses of estrogen used to treat prostatic or breast cancer are more likely to result in these adverse effects, and, in fact, it has been shown that there is an increased risk of thrombosis in men receiving estrogens for prostatic cancer.[19–22]

a. *Thromboembolic disease* It is now well established that users of oral contraceptives have an increased risk of various thromboembolic and thrombotic vascular diseases, such as thrombophlebitis, pulmonary embolism, stroke and myocardial infarction.[22–29] Cases of retinal thrombosis, mesenteric thrombosis, and optic neuritis have been reported in oral contraceptive users. There is evidence that the risk of several of these adverse reactions is related to the dose of the drug.[30,31] An increased risk of postsurgery thromboembolic complications has also been reported in users of oral contraceptives.[32,33] If feasible, estrogen should be discontinued at least 4 weeks before surgery of the type associated with an increased risk of thromboembolism, or during periods of immobilization.

While an increased rate of thromboembolic and thrombotic disease in postmenopausal users of estrogen has not been found,[16,34] this does not rule out the possibility that such an increase may be present or that subgroups of women who have underlying risk factors or who are receiving relatively large doses of estrogens may have increased risk. Therefore, estrogens should not be used in persons with active thrombophlebitis or thromboembolic disorders, and they should not be used (except in treatment of malignancy) in persons with a history of such disorders in association with estrogen use. They should be used with caution in patients with cerebral vascular or coronary artery disease and only for those in whom estrogens are clearly needed.

Large doses of estrogen (5 mg. conjugated estrogens per day), comparable to those used to treat cancer of the prostate and breast, have been shown in a large prospective clinical trial in men[35] to increase the risk of nonfatal myocardial infarction, pulmonary embolism and thrombophlebitis. When estrogen doses of this size are used, any of the thromboembolic and thrombotic adverse effects associated with oral contraceptive use should be considered a clear risk.

b. *Hepatic adenoma* Benign hepatic adenomas appear to be associated with the use of oral contraceptives.[36–38] Although benign, and rare, these may rupture and may cause death through intra-abdominal hemorrhage. Such lesions have not yet been reported in association with other estrogen or progestagen preparations but should be considered in estrogen users having abdominal pain and tenderness, abdominal mass, or hypovolemic shock. Hepatocellular carcinoma has also been reported in women taking estrogen-containing oral contraceptives.[37] The relationship of this malignancy to these drugs is not known at this time.

c. *Elevated blood pressure* Increased blood pressure is not uncommon in women using oral contraceptives. There is now a report that this may occur with use of estrogens in the menopause[39] and blood pressure should be monitored with estrogen use, especially if high doses are used.

d. *Glucose tolerance* A worsening of glucose tolerance has been observed in a significant percentage of patients on estrogen-containing oral contraceptives. For this reason, diabetic patients should be carefully observed while receiving estrogen.

4. *Hypercalcemia* Administration of estrogens may lead to severe hypercalcemia in patients with breast cancer and bone metastases. If this occurs, the drug should be stopped and appropriate measures taken to reduce the serum calcium level.

Precautions:

General Precautions

1. A complete medical and family history should be taken prior to the initiation of any estrogen therapy. The pretreatment and periodic physical examinations should include special reference to blood pressure, breasts, abdomen, and pelvic organs, and should include a Papanicolaou smear. As a general rule, estrogen should not be prescribed for longer than one year without another physical examination being performed.
2. Fluid retention—Because estrogens may cause some degree of fluid retention, conditions which might be influenced by this factor, such as epilepsy, migraine, and cardiac or renal dysfunction, require careful observation.
3. Certain patients may develop undesirable manifestations of excessive estrogenic stimulation, such as abnormal or excessive uterine bleeding, mastodynia, etc.
4. Oral contraceptives appear to be associated with an increased incidence of mental depression.[22] Although it is not clear whether this is due to the estrogenic or progestagenic component of the contraceptive, patients with a history of depression should be carefully observed.
5. Preexisting uterine leiomyomata may increase in size during estrogen use.
6. The pathologist should be advised of estrogen therapy when relevant specimens are submitted.
7. Patients with a past history of jaundice during pregnancy have an increased risk of recurrence of jaundice while receiving estrogen-containing oral contraceptive therapy. If jaundice develops in any patient receiving estrogen, the medication should be discontinued while the cause is investigated.
8. Estrogens may be poorly metabolized in patients with impaired liver function and they should be administered with caution in such patients.
9. Because estrogens influence the metabolism of calcium and phosphorus, they should be used with caution in patients with metabolic bone diseases that are associated with hypercalcemia or in patients with renal insufficiency.
10. Because of the effects of estrogens on epiphyseal closure, they should be used judiciously in young patients in whom bone growth is not complete.
11. Certain endocrine and liver function tests may be affected by estrogen-containing oral contraceptives. The following similar changes may be expected with larger doses of estrogen: Increased sulfobromophthalein retention; increased prothrombin and factors VII, VIII, IX, and X; decreased antithrombin 3; increased norepinephrine-induced platelet aggregation; increased thyroid binding globulin (TBG) leading to increased circulating total thyroid hormone, as measured by PBI, T4 by column, or T4 by radioimmunoassay. Free T3 resin uptake is decreased, reflecting the elevated TBG; free T4 concentration is unaltered; impaired glucose tolerance; decreased pregnanediol excretion; reduced response to metyrapone test; reduced serum folate concentration; increased serum triglyceride and phospholipid concentration.

Information for the Patient: See text of Patient Package Insert.

Pregnancy Category X. See Contraindications and Boxed Warning above.

Nursing Mothers: As a general principle, the administration of any drug to nursing mothers should be done only when clearly necessary, since many drugs are excreted in human milk.

Adverse Reactions: (See Warnings regarding induction of neoplasia, adverse effects on the fetus, increased incidence of gallbladder disease, and adverse effects similar to those of oral contraceptives, including thromboembolism.) The following additional adverse reactions have been reported with estrogenic therapy, including oral contraceptives:

Genitourinary system: Breakthrough bleeding, spotting, change in menstrual flow; dysmenorrhea; premenstrual-like syndrome; amenorrhea during and after treatment; increase in size of uterine fibromyomata; vaginal candidiasis; change in cervical eversion and in degree of cervical secretion; cystitis-like syndrome.

Breasts: Tenderness, enlargement, secretion.

Gastrointestinal: Nausea, vomiting; abdominal cramps, bloating; cholestatic jaundice.

Skin: Chloasma or melasma which may persist when drug is discontinued; erythema mul-

Continued on next page

Information on Schering products appearing on these pages is effective as of September 30, 1979.

Schering—Cont.

tiforme; erythema nodosum; hemorrhagic eruption; loss of scalp hair; hirsutism.
Eyes: Steepening of corneal curvature; intolerance to contact lenses.
CNS: Headache, migraine, dizziness; mental depression; chorea.
Miscellaneous: Increase or decrease in weight; reduced carbohydrate tolerance; aggravation of porphyria; edema; changes in libido.

Acute Overdosage: Numerous reports of ingestion of large doses of estrogen-containing oral contraceptives by young children indicate that serious ill effects do not occur. Overdosage of estrogen may cause nausea, and withdrawal bleeding may occur in females.

Dosage and Administration: 1. *Given cyclically for short-term use only.*
For treatment of moderate to severe *vasomotor* symptoms associated with the menopause: The lowest dose that will control symptoms should be chosen and medication should be discontinued as promptly as possible. Administration should be cyclic (eg, 3 weeks on and 1 week off). Attempts to discontinue or taper medication should be made at 3- to 6-month intervals. The usual dosage range is one 0.02 mg. or 0.05 mg. tablet daily. In some instances, the effective dose may be as low as one 0.02 mg. tablet every other day. A useful dosage schedule for early menopause, while spontaneous menstruation continues, is 0.05 mg. once a day for twenty-one days and then a rest period for seven days. This can be continued cyclically indefinitely adding a progestational agent during the latter part of the cycle. For the initial treatment of the late menopause, the same regimen is indicated with the 0.02 mg. ESTINYL Tablet for the first few cycles, after which the 0.05 mg. dosage may be substituted. In more severe cases, such as those due to surgical and roentgenologic castration, one 0.05 mg. tablet may be administered three times daily at the start of treatment. With adequate clinical improvement, usually obtainable in a few weeks, the dosage may be reduced to one 0.05 mg. tablet daily and the patient continued thereafter on a maintenance dosage as in the average case. At the discretion of the physician, a progestational agent may be added during the latter part of a planned cycle.
2. *Given cyclically.*
Female hypogonadism: One 0.05 mg. tablet is given one to three times daily during the first two weeks of a theoretical menstrual cycle. This is followed by progesterone during the last half of the arbitrary cycle. This regimen is continued for three to six months. The patient is then allowed to go untreated for two months to determine whether or not she can maintain the cycle without hormonal therapy. If not, additional courses of therapy may be prescribed.
3. *Given chronically.*
Inoperable progressing prostatic cancer: From three 0.05 mg. to four 0.5 mg. tablets may be administered daily for palliation.
Inoperable progressing breast cancer in appropriately selected postmenopausal women (See Indications): Two 0.5 mg. tablets three times daily for palliation.
Treated patients with an intact uterus should be monitored closely for signs of endometrial cancer and appropriate diagnostic measures should be taken to rule out malignancy in the event of persistent or recurring abnormal vaginal bleeding.

How Supplied: ESTINYL Tablets 0.02 mg., beige, sugar-coated tablets branded in black with the Schering trademark and either product indentification numbers, 298, or letters, ER; bottles of 100 and 250.
ESTINYL Tablets 0.05 mg., pink, sugar-coated tablets branded in black with the Schering trademark and either product identification numbers, 070, or letters, EM; bottles of 100 and 250.
ESTINYL Tablets 0.5 mg., peach-colored, compressed, scored tablets impressed with the Schering trademark and either product identification numbers, 150, or letters, EP; bottle of 100.
Patient package inserts are being dispensed with this product. They are available to physicians upon request. Physician references available on request.

[*Shown in Product Identification Section*]

ETRAFON® ℞

brand of perphenazine, NF—amitriptyline hydrochloride, USP
ETRAFON 2-10 TABLETS (2-10)
ETRAFON-A TABLETS (4-10)
ETRAFON TABLETS (2-25)
ETRAFON-FORTE TABLETS (4-25)

Description: ETRAFON Tablets contain perphenazine, NF and amitriptyline hydrochloride, USP. Perphenazine is a piperazinyl phenothiazine having the chemical formula, $C_{21}H_{26}ClN_3OS$. Amitriptyline hydrochloride is a dibenzocycloheptadiene derivative having the chemical formula, $C_{20}H_{23}N.HCl$.

Actions: ETRAFON combines the tranquilizing action of perphenazine with the antidepressant properties of amitriptyline hydrochloride. Perphenazine acts on the central nervous system and has a greater behavioral potency than other phenothiazine derivatives whose side chains do not contain a piperazine moiety. Amitriptyline hydrochloride is a tricyclic antidepressant. It is not a monoamine oxidase inhibitor, but its mechanism of action in man is not known.

Indications: ETRAFON Tablets are indicated for the treatment of patients with moderate to severe anxiety and/or agitation and depressed mood; patients with depression in whom anxiety and/or agitation are moderate or severe; patients with anxiety and depression associated with chronic physical disease; patients in whom depression and anxiety cannot be clearly differentiated.
Schizophrenic patients who have associated symptoms of depression should be considered for therapy with ETRAFON.

Contraindications: ETRAFON is contraindicated in drug-associated, central-nervous-system depression (from barbiturates, alcohol, narcotics, analgesics, or antihistamines); in the presence of existing blood dyscrasias; bone marrow depression; pre-existing liver damage; and in patients who are hypersensitive to any of its components.
ETRAFON should not be given concomitantly with a monoamine oxidase inhibiting compound. Hyperpyretic crises, severe convulsions and deaths have occurred in patients receiving tricyclic antidepressant and monoamine oxidase inhibiting drugs simultaneously. In patients who have been receiving a monoamine oxidase inhibitor, it is recommended that two weeks or longer elapse before the start of treatment with ETRAFON Tablets to permit recovery from the effects of the MAO inhibitor and to avoid possible potentiation. Treatment with ETRAFON Tablets should be initiated cautiously in such patients, with gradual increase in dosage until a satisfactory response is obtained.
Amitriptyline hydrochloride is not recommended for use during the acute recovery phase following myocardial infarction.

Warnings: ETRAFON should not be given concomitantly with guanethidine or similarly acting compounds, since amitriptyline, like other tricyclic antidepressants, may block the antihypertensive effect of these compounds.
Because of the anticholinergic activity of amitriptyline hydrochloride, ETRAFON should be used with caution in patients with glaucoma, increased ocular pressure, and those in whom urinary retention is present or anticipated. In patients with angle-closure glaucoma even average doses may precipitate an attack.
Perphenazine can lower the convulsive threshold in susceptible individuals; it should be used with caution in patients with convulsive disorders. If the patient is being treated with an anticonvulsant agent, increased dosage of that agent may be required when ETRAFON Tablets are used concomitantly.
Patients with cardiovascular disorders should be watched closely. Tricyclic antidepressant drugs, including amitriptyline hydrochloride, particularly when given in high doses, have been reported to produce arrhythmias, sinus tachycardia, and prolongation of the conduction time. Myocardial infarction and stroke have been reported with drugs of this class.
Close supervision is required when amitriptyline hydrochloride is given to hyperthyroid patients or those receiving thyroid medication.
ETRAFON Tablets may impair the mental and/or physical abilities required for the performance of potentially hazardous tasks, such as driving a car or operating machinery.

Usage in Pregnancy: Safe use of ETRAFON during pregnancy and lactation has not been established; therefore, in administering the drug to pregnant patients, nursing mothers, or women who may become pregnant, the possible benefits must be weighed against the possible hazards to mother and child.

Usage in Children: Since a dosage for children has not been established, ETRAFON is not recommended for use in children.

Precautions: The possibility of suicide in depressed patients remains during treatment and until significant remission occurs. This type of patient should not have easy access to large quantities of this drug.

Perphenazine

As with all phenothiazine compounds, perphenazine should not be used indiscriminately. Caution should be observed in giving it to patients who have previously exhibited severe adverse reactions to other phenothiazines or to imipramine.
Some of the untoward actions of perphenazine tend to appear more frequently when high doses are used. However, as with other phenothiazine compounds, patients receiving perphenazine in any dosage should be kept under close supervision.
The antiemetic effect of perphenazine may obscure signs of toxicity due to overdosage of other drugs, or render more difficult the diagnosis of disorders such as brain tumors or intestinal obstruction.
A significant, not otherwise explained, rise in body temperature may suggest individual intolerance to perphenazine, in which case ETRAFON should be discontinued.
If hypotension develops, epinephrine should not be administered, since its action is blocked and partially reversed by perphenazine. Severe, acute hypotension has occurred with the use of phenothiazines and is of particular concern in patients with mitral insufficiency or pheochromocytoma.
Since phenothiazines can potentiate the action of central nervous system depressants (opiates, analgesics, antihistamines, barbiturates, alcohol), less than the usual dosage of these agents is required when they are administered concomitantly with ETRAFON. Patients should be cautioned that their response to alcohol may be increased while they are being treated with ETRAFON. The risk of suicide and the danger of overdose may be increased in patients who use alcohol excessively due to its potentiation of the drug's effect.
Phenothiazines also potentiate the effects of atropine, heat, and phosphorous insecticides and should be used with caution in patients exposed to any of these agents.

Amitriptyline Hydrochloride

In manic-depressive psychosis, depressed patients may experience a shift toward the manic phase if they are treated with an antidepressant drug. Patients with paranoid symptomatology may have an exaggeration of such symptoms. The tranquilizing effect of ETRAFON has seemed to reduce the likelihood of this effect.

When amitriptyline hydrochloride is given with anticholinergic agents or sympathomimetic drugs, including epinephrine combined with local anesthetics, close supervision and careful adjustment of dosages are required.

Paralytic ileus may occur in patients taking tricyclic antidepressants in combination with anticholinergic-type drugs.

Concurrent use of large doses of ethchlorvynol should be used with caution, since transient delirium has been reported in patients receiving this drug in combination with amitriptyline hydrochloride.

This drug may enhance the response to alcohol and the effects of barbiturates and other CNS depressants.

Concurrent administration of amitriptyline hydrochloride and electroshock therapy may increase the hazards of therapy. Such treatment should be limited to patients for whom it is essential.

Discontinue the drug several days before elective surgery, if possible.

Both elevation and lowering of blood sugar levels have been reported.

Adverse Reactions: Adverse reactions to ETRAFON Tablets are the same as those to its components, perphenazine and amitriptyline hydrochloride. There have been no reports of effects peculiar to the combination of these components in ETRAFON Tablets.

Perphenazine

Extrapyramidal reactions: opisthotonus, trismus, torticollis, retrocollis, aching and numbness of the limbs, motor restlessness, oculogyric crisis, hyperreflexia, dystonia, including protrusion, discoloration, aching and rounding of the tongue, tonic spasm of the masticatory muscles, tight feeling in the throat, slurred speech, dysphagia, akathisia, dyskinesia, parkinsonism, and ataxia. Their incidence and severity usually increase with an increase in dosage, but there is considerable individual variation in the tendency to develop such symptoms. Extrapyramidal symptoms can usually be controlled by the concomitant use of effective antiparkinsonian drugs, such as benztropine mesylate, and/or by reduction in dosage. In some instances, however, these reactions may persist after discontinuation of treatment with perphenazine.

Persistent tardive dyskinesia: As with all antipsychotic agents, tardive dyskinesia may appear in some patients on long-term therapy or may appear after drug therapy has been discontinued. The risk appears to be greater in elderly patients on high-dose therapy, especially females. The symptoms are persistent and in some patients appear to be irreversible. The syndrome is characterized by rhythmical, involuntary movements of the tongue, face, mouth or jaw (eg, protrusion of tongue, puffing of cheeks, puckering of mouth, chewing movements). Sometimes these may be accompanied by involuntary movements of the extremities. There is no known effective treatment for tardive dyskinesia; antiparkinsonism agents usually do not alleviate the symptoms of this syndrome. It is suggested that all antipsychotic agents be discontinued if these symptoms appear. Should it be necessary to reinstitute treatment, or increase the dosage of the agent, or switch to a different antipsychotic agent, the syndrome may be masked. It has been reported that fine, vermicular movements of the tongue may be an early sign of the syndrome, and if the medication is stopped at that time the syndrome may not develop.

Allergic reactions: photosensitivity, pruritus, erythema, urticaria, eczema, exfoliative dermatitis, asthma, anaphylactoid reactions, laryngeal edema and angioneurotic edema. In extremely rare instances, individual idiosyncrasy or hypersensitivity to phenothiazines has resulted in cerebral edema, circulatory collapse and death.

Autonomic reactions: dry mouth or salivation, nausea, vomiting; anorexia, constipation, obstipation, urinary frequency or incontinence, blurred vision, nasal congestion, hypertension, hypotension, tachycardia, and a change in the pulse rate occasionally may occur. Significant autonomic effects have been infrequent in patients receiving less than 24 mg. perphenazine daily.

Other reactions: peripheral edema, reversed epinephrine effect, hyperglycemia, endocrine disturbances (lactation, galactorrhea, gynecomastia, disturbances in the menstrual cycle), altered cerebrospinal fluid proteins, increase in PBI not attributable to an increase in thyroxine, paradoxical excitement, headache, ECG abnormalities (quinidine-like effect), and systemic lupus erythematosus-like syndrome, reactivation of psychotic processes, paranoid-like reactions, catatonia and the production of catatonic-like states have been described.

The following adverse reactions, though rare, have also been reported to be associated with perphenazine treatment: agranulocytosis, jaundice, hyperpigmentation of the skin, grand mal convulsions, failure of ejaculation.

The possibility exists that the following reactions, which have been seen with phenothiazine therapy, may occur with ETRAFON Tablets: certain blood dyscrasias (pancytopenia, thrombocytopenic purpura, leukopenia, eosinophilia); liver damage (billary stasis); polyphagia; photophobia.

Pigmentary retinopathy has been reported to occur after administration of some phenothiazines with a piperidylethyl side chain, but not with perphenazine which has a piperazine side chain.

Pigmentation of the cornea and lens has been reported to occur after long-term administration of some phenothiazines. Although it has not been reported in patients receiving ETRAFON, the possibility that it might occur should be considered.

Hypnotic effects appear to be minimal, particularly in patients who are permitted to remain active.

A few patients have reported lassitude, muscle weakness, and mild insomnia.

Amitriptyline Hydrochloride

Although activation of latent schizophrenia has been reported with antidepressant drugs, including amitriptyline hydrochloride, it may be prevented with ETRAFON Tablets in some cases because of the antipsychotic effect of perphenazine. A few instances of epileptiform seizures have been reported in chronic schizophrenic patients during treatment with amitriptyline hydrochloride.

Note: Included in the listing which follows are a few adverse reactions which have not been reported with this specific drug. However, pharmacological similarities among the tricyclic antidepressant drugs require that each of the reactions be considered when amitriptyline hydrochloride is administered.

Allergic: Rash, pruritus, urticaria, photosensitization, edema of face and tongue.

Anticholinergic: Dry mouth, blurred vision, disturbance of accommodation, constipation, paralytic ileus, urinary retention, dilatation of urinary tract.

Cardiovascular: Hypotension, hypertension, tachycardia, palpitations, myocardial infarction, arrhythmias, heart block, stroke.

CNS and Neuromuscular: Confusional states, disturbed concentration, disorientation, delusions, hallucinations, excitement, jitteriness, anxiety, restlessness, insomnia, nightmares, numbness, tingling, and paresthesias of the extremities, peripheral neuropathy, incoordination, ataxia, tremors, seizures, alteration in EEG patterns, extrapyramidal symptoms, tinnitus.

Endocrine: Testicular swelling and gynecomastia in the male, breast enlargement and galactorrhea in the female, increased or decreased libido, elevation and lowering of blood sugar levels, syndrome of inappropriate ADH (antidiuretic hormone secretion).

Gastrointestinal: Nausea, epigastric distress, heartburn, vomiting, anorexia, stomatitis, peculiar taste, diarrhea, parotid swelling, black tongue. Rarely hepatitis has occurred (including altered liver function and jaundice).

Hematologic: Bone marrow depression including agranulocytosis, leukopenia, eosinophilia, purpura, thrombocytopenia.

Other: Dizziness, weakness, fatigue, headache, weight gain or loss, increased perspiration, urinary frequency, mydriasis, drowsiness, jaundice, alopecia.

Withdrawal Symptoms: Abrupt cessation of treatment after prolonged administration may produce nausea, headache, and malaise. These are not indicative of addiction.

Dosage and Administration:

Initial Dosage

In psychoneurotic patients whose anxiety and depression warrant combined therapy, one ETRAFON Tablet (2–25) or one ETRAFON-FORTE Tablet (4–25) three or four times a day is recommended.

In elderly patients, adolescents and other patients as indicated, one ETRAFON-A Tablet (4–10) may be administered three or four times a day as initial dosage. This dosage may be adjusted as required to produce an adequate response.

In more severely ill patients with schizophrenia, two ETRAFON-FORTE Tablets (4–25) three times a day are recommended as the initial dosage. If necessary, a fourth dose may be given at bedtime. The total daily dosage should not exceed nine tablets.

Maintenance Dosage

Depending on the condition being treated, the onset of therapeutic response may vary from a few days to a few weeks or even longer. After a satisfactory response is noted, dosage should be reduced to the smallest amount necessary to obtain relief from the symptoms for which ETRAFON Tablets are being administered. A useful maintenance dosage is one ETRAFON Tablet (2–25) or one ETRAFON-FORTE Tablet (4–25) two to four times a day. In some patients, maintenance dosage is required for many months.

ETRAFON 2–10 Tablets (2–10) and ETRAFON-A Tablets (4–10) can be used to increase flexibility in adjusting maintenance dosage to the lowest amount consistent with relief of symptoms.

Overdosage:

Manifestations—High doses may cause temporary confusion, disturbed concentration, or transient visual hallucinations. Overdosage may cause drowsiness; hypothermia; tachycardia and other arrhythmic abnormalities—for example, bundle branch block; ECG evidence of impaired conduction; congestive heart failure; dilated pupils; convulsions; severe hypotension; stupor; and coma. Other symptoms may be agitation, hyperactive reflexes, muscle rigidity, vomiting, hyperpyrexia, or any of the adverse reactions listed for perphenazine or amitriptyline hydrochloride.

Overdosage with tricyclic antidepressants (TCAs), such as imipramine, doxepin, or amitriptyline may result in plasma TCA levels of

Continued on next page

Information on Schering products appearing on these pages is effective as of September 30, 1979.

Schering—Cont.

1,000 ng/ml or higher. Such levels more accurately define patients who are at risk for major medical complications of overdosage than does the amount of drug ingested based on patient history. In one study, all patients with TCA levels of this magnitude had a QRS duration of 100 msec or more on a routine ECG within the first 24 hours following overdose.

In the absence of TCA blood level determinations, a QRS of 100 msec or more suggests a greater likelihood of serious complications.

Treatment—To treat hypotension, levarterenol (norepinephrine) may be used, but not epinephrine.

Treatment is symptomatic and supportive. There is no specific antidote. The stomach should be emptied as quickly as possible by emesis. All patients suspected of having taken an overdose should be hospitalized as soon as possible. Gastric lavage should be performed at the hospital following emesis. Because of perphenazine's antiemetic effect, saline emetics are not recommended, since retention of the saline load could result in hypernatremia. After gastric lavage, 20 to 30 g. of activated charcoal may be given every four to six hours during the first 24 to 48 hours after ingestion of the overdose. An electrocardiogram should be taken and close monitoring of cardiac function instituted if there is any sign of abnormality. An open airway and adequate fluid intake should be maintained. Body temperature should be regulated.

The intravenous administration of 1 to 3 mg. physostigmine salicylate has been reported to reverse the symptoms of tricyclic antidepressant poisoning and therefore, should be considered in the symptomatic treatment of the central anticholinergic effects due to overdosage with ETRAFON Tablets. Because physostigmine is rapidly metabolized, it should be readministered as required, especially if life-threatening signs, such as arrhythmias, convulsions or deep coma recur or persist.

Standard measures (oxygen, intravenous fluids, corticosteroids) should be used to manage circulatory shock or metabolic acidosis. Cardiac arrhythmias may be treated with neostigmine, pyridostigmine or propranolol. Digitalis should be considered for cardiac failure. Close monitoring of cardiac function is advisable for not less than five days.

Anticonvulsants (an inhalation anesthetic, diazepam or paraldehyde) are recommended for control of convulsions, since amitriptyline and perphenazine increase the central nervous system depressant action, but not the anticonvulsant action of barbiturates.

If acute symptoms of parkinsonism result from perphenazine intoxication, benztropine mesylate or diphenhydramine may be administered.

Central nervous system depression may be treated with nonconvulsant doses of CNS stimulants.

Dialysis is of no value because of low plasma concentrations of the drug.

Continue treatment for at least 48 hours in patients who do not respond earlier.

Since overdosage is often deliberate, patients may attempt suicide by other means during the recovery phase.

Deaths by deliberate or accidental overdosage have occurred with this class of drugs.

How Supplied: ETRAFON 2–10 Tablets (perphenazine 2 mg. and amitriptyline hydrochloride 10 mg.): deep yellow, sugar-coated tablets branded in blue-black with the Schering trademark and either product identification letters, ANA or numbers, 287; bottles of 100 and 500 and box of 100 for unit-dose dispensing (10 strips of 10 tablets each).

ETRAFON Tablets (perphenazine 2 mg. and amitriptyline hydrochloride 25 mg.): pink, sugar-coated tablets branded in red with the Schering trademark and either product identification letters, ANC or numbers, 598; bottles of 100 and 500 and box of 100 for unit-dose dispensing (10 strips of 10 tablets each).

ETRAFON-A Tablets (perphenazine 4 mg. and amitriptyline hydrochloride 10 mg.): orange, sugar-coated tablets branded in blue-black with the Schering trademark and either product identification letters, ANB or numbers, 119; bottles of 100 and 500 and box of 100 for unit-dose dispensing (10 strips of 10 tablets each).

ETRAFON-FORTE Tablets (perphenazine 4 mg. and amitriptyline hydrochloride 25 mg.): red, sugar-coated tablets branded in blue with the Schering trademark and either product identification letters, ANE or numbers, 720; bottles of 100 and 500 and box of 100 for unit dose dispensing (10 strips of 10 tablets each).

[*Shown in Product Identification Section*]

FULVICIN® P/G ℞

brand of griseofulvin ultramicrosize Tablets

Description: FULVICIN P/G Tablets contain ultramicrosize crystals of griseofulvin, an antibiotic derived from a species of *Penicillium*. Griseofulvin crystals are partly dissolved in polyethylene glycol 6000 and partly dispersed throughout the tablet matrix.

Each FULVICIN P/G Tablet contains 125 mg. or 250 mg. griseofulvin ultramicrosize.

Actions: Microbiology Griseofulvin is fungistatic with *in vitro* activity against various species of *Microsporum, Epidermophyton,* and *Trichophyton*. It has no effect on bacteria or on other genera of fungi.

Human Pharmacology Following oral administration, griseofulvin is deposited in the keratin precursor cells and has a greater affinity for diseased tissue. The drug is tightly bound to the new keratin which becomes highly resistant to fungal invasions.

Controlled bioavailability studies of FULVICIN P/G have demonstrated comparable values to blood levels regarded as adequate. The efficiency of gastrointestinal absorption of ultramicrocrystalline griseofulvin is approximately twice that of the conventional microsized griseofulvin. This factor permits the oral intake of half as much griseofulvin per tablet but there is no evidence, at this time, that this confers any significant clinical differences in regard to safety and efficacy.

Indications: FULVICIN P/G Tablets are indicated for the treatment of ringworm infections of the skin, hair, and nails, namely: tinea corporis, tinea pedis, tinea cruris, tinea barbae, tinea capitis, tinea unguium (onychomycosis) when caused by one or more of the following genera of fungi: *Trichophyton rubrum, Trichophyton tonsurans, Trichophyton mentagrophytes, Trichophyton interdigitale, Trichophyton verrucosum, Trichophyton megninii, Trichophyton gallinae, Trichophyton crateriforme, Trichophyton sulphureum, Trichophyton schoenleinii, Microsporum audounii, Microsporum canis, Microsporum gypseum,* and *Epidermophyton floccosum.*

Note: Prior to therapy, the type of fungi responsible for the infection should be identified. The use of this drug is not justified in minor or trivial infections which will respond to topical agents alone.

Griseofulvin is not effective in the following: bacterial infections, candidiasis (moniliasis), histoplasmosis, actinomycosis, sporotrichosis, chromoblastomycosis, coccidioidomycosis, North American blastomycosis, cryptococcosis (torulosis), tinea versicolor, and nocardiosis.

Contraindications: This drug is contraindicated in patients with porphyria, hepatocellular failure, and in individuals with a history of sensitivity to griseofulvin.

Warnings: *Prophylactic Usage:* Safety and efficacy of griseofulvin for prophylaxis of fungal infections have not been established.

Animal Toxicology: Chronic feeding of griseofulvin, at levels ranging from 0.5–2.5% of the diet, resulted in the development of liver tumors in several strains of mice, particularly in males. Smaller particle sizes result in an enhanced effect. Lower oral dosage levels have not been tested. Subcutaneous administration of relatively small doses of griseofulvin once a week during the first three weeks of life has also been reported to induce hepatomata in mice. Although studies in other animal species have not yielded evidence of tumorogenicity, these studies were not of adequate design to form a basis for conclusions in this regard.

In subacute toxicity studies, orally administered griseofulvin produced hepatocellular necrosis in mice, but this has not been seen in other species. Disturbances in porphyrin metabolism have been reported in griseofulvin-treated laboratory animals. Griseofulvin has been reported to have a colchicine-like effect on mitosis and cocarcinogenicity with methylcholanthrene in cutaneous tumor induction in laboratory animals.

Usage in Pregnancy: The safety of this drug during pregnancy has not been established.

Animal Reproduction Studies: It has been reported in the literature that griseofulvin was found to be embryotoxic and teratogenic on oral administration to pregnant rats. Pups with abnormalities have been reported in the litters of a few bitches treated with griseofulvin. Additional animal reproduction studies are in progress.

Suppression of spermatogenesis has been reported to occur in rats, but investigation in man failed to confirm this.

Precautions: Patients on prolonged therapy with any potent medication should be under close observation. Periodic monitoring of organ system function, including renal, hepatic, and hematopoietic, should be done.

Since griseofulvin is derived from species of *Penicillium*, the possibility of cross sensitivity with penicillin exists; however, known penicillin-sensitive patients have been treated without difficulty.

Since a photosensitivity reaction is occasionally associated with griseofulvin therapy, patients should be warned to avoid exposure to intense natural or artificial sunlight. Should a photosensitivity reaction occur, lupus erythematosus may be aggravated.

Griseofulvin decreases the activity of warfarin-type anticoagulants so that patients receiving these drugs concomitantly may require dosage adjustment of the anticoagulant during and after griseofulvin therapy.

Barbiturates usually depress griseofulvin activity, and concomitant administration may require a dosage adjustment of the antifungal agent.

Adverse Reactions: When adverse reactions occur, they are most commonly of the hypersensitivity type, such as skin rashes, urticaria, and rarely, angioneurotic edema, and may necessitate withdrawal of therapy and appropriate countermeasures. Paresthesias of the hands and feet have been reported rarely after extended therapy. Other side effects reported occasionally are oral thrush, nausea, vomiting, epigastric distress, diarrhea, headache, fatigue, dizziness, insomnia, mental confusion, and impairment of performance of routine activities.

Proteinuria and leukopenia have been reported rarely. Administration of the drug should be discontinued if granulocytopenia occurs.

When rare, serious reactions occur with griseofulvin, they are usually associated with high dosages, long periods of therapy, or both.

Dosage and Administration: Accurate diagnosis of the infecting organism is essential. Identification should be made either by direct

microscopic examination of a mounting of infected tissue in a solution of potassium hydroxide or by culture on an appropriate medium.
Medication must be continued until the infecting organism is completely eradicated as indicated by appropriate clinical or laboratory examination. Representative treatment periods are tinea capitis, 4 to 6 weeks; tinea corporis, 2 to 4 weeks; tinea pedis, 4 to 8 weeks; tinea unguium—depending on rate of growth—fingernails, at least 4 months; toenails, at least 6 months.
General measures in regard to hygiene should be observed to control sources of infection or reinfection. Concomitant use of appropriate topical agents is usually required particularly in treatment of tinea pedis. In some forms of athlete's foot, yeasts and bacteria may be involved as well as fungi. Griseofulvin will not eradicate the bacterial or monilial infection.
Adults: Daily administration of 250 mg. (as a single dose or in divided amounts) will give a satisfactory response in most patients with tinea corporis, tinea cruris, and tinea capitis. For those fungus infections more difficult to eradicate, such as tinea pedis and tinea unguium, a divided daily dosage of 500 mg. is recommended.
Children: Approximately 2.5 mg. per pound of body weight per day is an effective dose for most children. On this basis, the following dosage schedule is suggested: Children weighing 30 to 50 pounds—62.5 mg. to 125 mg. daily. Children weighing over 50 pounds—125 mg. to 250 mg. daily.
Children 2 years of age and younger—dosage has not been established.
Clinical experience with griseofulvin in children with tinea capitis indicates that a single daily dose is effective. Clinical relapse will occur if the medication is not continued until the infecting organism is eradicated.
How Supplied: FULVICIN P/G Tablets, 125 mg., white, compressed, scored tablets impressed with the Schering trademark and product identification numbers, 228; bottle of 100.
FULVICIN P/G Tablets, 250 mg., white, compressed, scored tablets impressed with the Schering trademark and product identification numbers, 507; bottle of 100.
Store at controlled room temperature 59°F to 86°F (15°C to 30°C).

[*Shown in Product Identification Section*]

FULVICIN-U/F® ℞
brand of griseofulvin (microsize), USP
Tablets

Description: Griseofulvin is an antibiotic derived from a species of *Penicillium.* A special process furnishes griseofulvin of microsize crystals offering a greater and more effective surface area for increased gastrointestinal absorption.
Actions: Microbiology: Griseofulvin is fungistatic with *in vitro* activity against various species of *Microsporum, Epidermophyton,* and *Trichophyton.* It has no effect on bacteria or on other genera of fungi.
Human Pharmacology: Griseofulvin absorption from the gastrointestinal tract varies considerably among individuals mainly because of insolubility of the drug in aqueous media of the upper G.I. tract. The peak serum level found in fasting adults given 0.5 g. occurs at about four hours and ranges between 0.5 to 2.0 mcg./ml. The serum level may be increased by giving the drug with a meal with a high fat content.
Griseofulvin is deposited in the keratin precursor cells and has a greater affinity for diseased tissue. The drug is tightly bound to the new keratin which becomes highly resistant to fungal invasions.
Indications: FULVICIN-U/F Tablets are indicated for the treatment of ringworm infections of the skin, hair, and nails, namely: tinea corporis, tinea pedis, tinea cruris, tinea barbae, tinea capitis, tinea unguium (onychomycosis) when caused by one or more of the following genera of fungi: *Trichophyton rubrum, Trichophyton tonsurans, Trichophyton mentagrophytes, Trichophyton interdigitale, Trichophyton verrucosum, Trichophyton megninii, Trichophyton gallinae, Trichophyton crateriforme, Trichophyton sulphureum, Trichophyton schoenleinii, Microsporum audouinii, Microsporum canis, Microsporum gypseum,* and *Epidermophyton floccosum.*
Note: Prior to therapy, the type of fungi responsible for the infection should be identified. The use of this drug is not justified in minor or trivial infections which will respond to topical agents alone.
Griseofulvin is not effective in the following: bacterial infections, candidiasis (moniliasis), histoplasmosis, actinomycosis, sporotrichosis, chromoblastomycosis, coccidioidomycosis, North American blastomycosis, cryptococcosis (torulosis), tinea versicolor, and nocardiosis.
Contraindications: This drug is contraindicated in patients with porphyria, hepatocellular failure, and in individuals with a history of sensitivity to griseofulvin.
Warnings: Prophylactic usage: Safety and efficacy of griseofulvin for prophylaxis of fungal infections have not been established.
Animal toxicology: Chronic feeding of griseofulvin, at levels ranging from 0.5-2.5% of the diet, resulted in the development of liver tumors in several strains of mice, particularly in males. Smaller particle sizes result in an enhanced effect. Lower oral dosage levels have not been tested. Subcutaneous administration of relatively small doses of griseofulvin, once a week, during the first three weeks of life has also been reported to induce hepatomata in mice. Although studies in other animal species have not yielded evidence of tumorogenicity, these studies were not of adequate design to form a basis for conclusions in this regard.
In subacute toxicity studies, orally administered griseofulvin produced hepatocellular necrosis in mice, but this has not been seen in other species. Disturbances in porphyrin metabolism have been reported in griseofulvin-treated laboratory animals. Griseofulvin has been reported to have a colchicine-like effect on mitosis and cocarcinogenicity with methylcholanthrene in cutaneous tumor induction in laboratory animals.
Usage in pregnancy: The safety of this drug during pregnancy has not been established.
Animal reproduction studies: It has been reported in the literature that griseofulvin was found to be embryotoxic and teratogenic on oral administration to pregnant rats. Pups with abnormalities have been reported in the litters of a few bitches treated with griseofulvin. Additional animal reproduction studies are in progress.
Suppression of spermatogenesis has been reported to occur in rats, but investigation in man failed to confirm this.
Precautions: Patients on prolonged therapy with any potent medication should be under close observation. Periodic monitoring of organ system functions, including renal, hepatic, and hematopoietic, should be done.
Since griseofulvin is derived from species of *Penicillium,* the possibility of cross sensitivity with penicillin exists; however, known penicillin-sensitive patients have been treated without difficulty.
Since a photosensitivity reaction is occasionally associated with griseofulvin therapy, patients should be warned to avoid exposure to intense natural or artificial sunlight. Should a photosensitivity reaction occur, lupus erythematosus may be aggravated.
Griseofulvin decreases the activity of warfarin-type anticoagulants so that patients receiving these drugs concomitantly may require dosage adjustment of the anticoagulant during and after griseofulvin therapy.
Barbiturates usually depress griseofulvin activity and concomitant administration may require a dosage adjustment of the antifungal agent.
Adverse Reactions: When adverse reactions occur, they are most commonly of the hypersensitivity type, such as skin rashes, urticaria, and rarely, angioneurotic edema, and may necessitate withdrawal of therapy and appropriate countermeasures. Paresthesias of the hands and feet have been reported rarely after extended therapy. Other side effects reported occasionally are oral thrush, nausea, vomiting, epigastric distress, diarrhea, headache, fatigue, dizziness, insomnia, mental confusion, and impairment of performance of routine activities.
Proteinuria and leukopenia have been reported rarely. Administration of the drug should be discontinued if granulocytopenia occurs.
When rare, serious reactions occur with griseofulvin, they are usually associated with high dosages, long periods of therapy, or both.
Dosage and Administration: Accurate diagnosis of the infecting organism is essential. Identification should be made either by direct microscopic examination of a mounting of infected tissue in a solution of potassium hydroxide or by culture on an appropriate medium.
Medication must be continued until the infecting organism is completely eradicated as indicated by appropriate clinical or laboratory examination. Representative treatment periods are for tinea capitis, four to six weeks; tinea corporis, two to four weeks; tinea pedis, four to eight weeks; tinea unguium, depending on the rate of growth, fingernails, at least four months; toenails, at least six months.
General measures in regard to hygiene should be observed to control sources of infection or reinfection. Concomitant use of appropriate topical agents is usually required, particularly in treatment of *tinea pedis.* In some forms of athlete's foot, yeasts and bacteria may be involved as well as fungi. Griseofulvin will not eradicate the bacterial or monilial infection.
Adults: Daily administration of 500 mg. (as a single dose or in divided amounts), will give a satisfactory response in most patients with tinea corporis, tinea cruris, and tinea capitis. For those fungus infections more difficult to eradicate, such as tinea pedis and tinea unguium, daily dosage of 1.0 g. is recommended.
Children: Approximately 5 mg. per pound of body weight per day is an effective dose for most children. On this basis the following dosage schedule for children is suggested:
Children weighing 30 to 50 pounds—125 mg. to 250 mg. daily.
Children weighing over 50 pounds—250 mg. to 500 mg. daily.
How Supplied: FULVCIN-U/F Tablets, 250 mg.: white, compressed, scored tablets impressed with the Schering trademark and product identification letters, AUF, or numbers, 948; bottles of 60 and 250.
FULVICIN-U/F Tablets, 500 mg.: white, compressed, scored tablets impressed with the Schering trademark and product identification letters, AUG, or numbers, 496; bottles of 60 and 250.

[*Shown in Product Identification Section*]

Continued on next page

Information on Schering products appearing on these pages is effective as of September 30, 1979.

Schering—Cont.

GARAMYCIN® ℞

brand of gentamicin sulfate, USP
Cream 0.1%
and
Ointment 0.1%
For Dermatologic Use

Description: Each gram of GARAMYCIN **Cream** 0.1% contains 1.7 mg. gentamicin sulfate, USP equivalent to 1.0 mg. gentamicin base, with 1.0 mg. methylparaben and 4.0 mg. butylparaben as preservatives, in a bland emulsion-type vehicle composed of stearic acid, propylene glycol monostearate, isopropyl myristate, propylene glycol, polysorbate 40, sorbitol solution and purified water.

Each gram of GARAMYCIN **Ointment** 0.1% contains 1.7 mg. gentamicin sulfate, USP equivalent to 1.0 mg. gentamicin base, with 0.5 mg. methylparaben and 0.1 mg. propylparaben as preservatives in a bland, unctuous petrolatum base.

Actions: GARAMYCIN, a wide-spectrum antibiotic, provides highly effective topical treatment in primary and secondary bacterial infections of the skin. GARAMYCIN may clear infections that have not responded to other topical antibiotic agents. In impetigo contagiosa and other primary skin infections, treatment three or four times daily with GARAMYCIN usually clears the lesions promptly. In secondary skin infections, GARAMYCIN facilitates the treatment of the underlying dermatosis by controlling the infection. Bacteria susceptible to the action of GARAMYCIN include sensitive strains of streptococci (group A beta-hemolytic, alpha-hemolytic), *Staphylococcus aureus* (coagulase positive, coagulase negative, and some penicillinase-producing strains), and the gram-negative bacteria, *Pseudomonas aeruginosa, Aerobacter aerogenes, Escherichia coli, Proteus vulgaris,* and *Klebsiella pneumoniae.*

Indications: *Primary skin infections:* Impetigo contagiosa, superficial folliculitis, ecthyma, furunculosis, sycosis barbae, and pyoderma gangrenosum. *Secondary skin infections:* Infectious eczematoid dermatitis, pustular acne, pustular psoriasis, infected seborrheic dermatitis, infected contact dermatitis (including poison ivy), infected excoriations, and bacterial superinfections of fungal or viral infections.

Note: GARAMYCIN is a bactericidal agent that is not effective against viruses or fungi in skin infections. GARAMYCIN is useful in the treatment of infected skin cysts and certain other skin abscesses when preceded by incision and drainage to permit adequate contact between the antibiotic and the infecting bacteria. Good results have been obtained in the treatment of infected stasis and other skin ulcers, infected superficial burns, paronychia, infected insect bites and stings, infected lacerations and abrasions, and wounds from minor surgery. Patients sensitive to neomycin can be treated with gentamicin, although regular observation of patients sensitive to topical antibiotics is advisable when such patients are treated with any topical antibiotic. GARAMYCIN **Ointment** helps retain moisture and has been useful in infection on dry eczematous or psoriatic skin. GARAMYCIN **Cream** is recommended for wet, oozing primary infections, and greasy, secondary infections, such as pustular acne or infected seborrheic dermatitis. If a water-washable preparation is desired, GARAMYCIN **Cream** is preferable. GARAMYCIN **Ointment** and **Cream** have been used successfully in infants over one year of age as well as in adults and children.

Contraindications: This drug is contraindicated in individuals with a history of sensitivity reactions to any of its components.

Precautions: Use of topical antibiotics occasionally allows overgrowth of nonsusceptible organisms, including fungi. If this occurs, or if irritation, sensitization, or superinfection develops, treatment with gentamicin should be discontinued and appropriate therapy instituted.

Adverse Reactions: In patients with dermatoses treated with gentamicin, irritation (erythema and pruritus) that did not usually require discontinuance of treatment has been reported in a small percentage of cases. There was no evidence of irritation or sensitization, however, in any of these patients patch-tested subsequently with gentamicin on normal skin. Possible photosensitization has been reported in several patients but could not be elicited in these patients by reapplication of gentamicin followed by exposure to ultraviolet radiation.

Dosage and Administration: A small amount of GARAMYCIN **Cream** or **Ointment** should be applied gently to the lesions three or four times daily. The area treated may be covered with a gauze dressing if desired. In impetigo contagiosa, the crusts should be removed before application of GARAMYCIN to permit maximum contact between the antibiotic and the infection. Care should be exercised to avoid further contamination of the infected skin. Infected stasis ulcers have responded well to GARAMYCIN under gelatin packing.

How Supplied: GARAMYCIN **Cream** 0.1%, and GARAMYCIN **Ointment** 0.1%, 15 g. tubes.
Store away from heat.

GARAMYCIN® ℞

brand of gentamicin sulfate, U.S.P.
Ophthalmic Solution—Sterile
Ophthalmic Ointment—Sterile
Each ml. or gram contains gentamicin sulfate equivalent to 3.0 mg. gentamicin

Description: Gentamicin sulfate is a water-soluble antibiotic of the aminoglycoside group active against a wide variety of pathogenic gram-negative and gram-positive bacteria.

GARAMYCIN **Ophthalmic Solution** is a sterile, aqueous solution buffered to approximately pH 7 for use in the eye. Each ml. contains gentamicin sulfate (equivalent to 3.0 mg. gentamicin), disodium phosphate, monosodium phosphate, sodium chloride, and benzalkonium chloride as a preservative.

GARAMYCIN **Ophthalmic Ointment** is a sterile ointment, each gram containing gentamicin sulfate (equivalent to 3.0 mg. gentamicin) in a bland base of white petrolatum, with methylparaben and propylparaben as preservatives.

Actions: The gram-positive bacteria against which gentamicin sulfate is active include coagulase-positive and coagulase-negative staphylococci, including certain strains that are resistant to penicillin; Group A beta-hemolytic and nonhemolytic streptococci; and *Diplococcus pneumoniae.* The gram-negative bacteria against which gentamicin sulfate is active include certain strains of *Pseudomonas aeruginosa,* indole-positive and indole-negative *Proteus* species, *Escherichia coli, Klebsiella pneumoniae* (Friedlander's bacillus), *Haemophilus influenza* and *Haemophilus aegyptius* (Koch-Weeks bacillus), *Aerobacter aerogenes, Moraxella lacunata* (diplobacillus of Morax-Axenfeld), and *Neisseria* species, including *Neisseria gonorrhoeae.* Although significant resistant organisms have not been isolated from patients treated with gentamicin at the present time, this may occur in the future as resistance has been produced with difficulty *in vitro* by repeated exposures.

Indications: GARAMYCIN **Ophthalmic Solution** and **Ointment** are indicated in the topical treatment of infections of the external eye and its adnexa caused by susceptible bacteria. Such infections embrace conjunctivitis, keratitis and keratoconjunctivitis, corneal ulcers, blepharitis and blepharoconjunctivitis, acute meibomianitis, and dacryocystitis.

Contraindications: GARAMYCIN **Ophthalmic Solution** and **Ointment** are contraindicated in patients with known hypersensitivity to any of the components.

Warnings: GARAMYCIN **Ophthalmic Solution** is not for injection. It should never be injected subconjunctivally, nor should it be directly introduced into the anterior chamber of the eye.

Precautions: Prolonged use of topical antibiotics may give rise to overgrowth of nonsusceptible organisms, such as fungi. Should this occur, or if irritation or hypersensitivity to any component of the drug develops, discontinue use of the preparation and institute appropriate therapy.

Ophthalmic ointments may retard corneal healing.

Adverse Reactions: Transient irritation has been reported with the use of GARAMYCIN **Ophthalmic Solution.**

Occasional burning or stinging may occur with the use of GARAMYCIN **Ophthalmic Ointment.**

Dosage and Administration: GARAMYCIN **Ophthalmic Solution:** instill one or two drops into the affected eye every four hours. In severe infections, dosage may be increased to as much as two drops once every hour.

GARAMYCIN **Ophthalmic Ointment:** apply a small amount to the affected eye two to three times a day.

How Supplied: GARAMYCIN **Ophthalmic Solution—Sterile,** 5 ml. plastic dropper bottle, sterile, boxes of one and six. Store away from heat.

GARAMYCIN **Ophthalmic Ointment—Sterile,** ⅛ ounce tube, boxes of one and six. Store away from heat.

GARAMYCIN® Injectable ℞

brand of gentamicin sulfate injection, USP
40 mg. per ml.
Each ml. contains gentamicin sulfate, USP equivalent to 40 mg. gentamicin.
For Parenteral Administration

WARNINGS

Patients treated with aminoglycosides should be under close clinical observation because of the potential toxicity associated with their use.

As with other aminoglycosides, GARAMYCIN Injectable is potentially nephrotoxic. The risk of nephrotoxicity is greater in patients with impaired renal function and in those who receive high dosage or prolonged therapy.

Neurotoxicity manifested by ototoxicity, both vestibular and auditory, can occur in patients treated with GARAMYCIN Injectable primarily in those with pre-existing renal damage and in patients with normal renal function treated with higher doses and/or for longer periods than recommended. Other manifestations of neurotoxicity may include numbness, skin tingling, muscle twitching and convulsions.

Renal and eighth cranial nerve function should be closely monitored, especially in patients with known or suspected reduced renal function at onset of therapy and also in those whose renal function is initially normal but who develop signs of renal dysfunction during therapy. Urine should be examined for decreased specific gravity, increased excretion of protein, and the presence of cells or casts. Blood urea nitrogen, serum creatinine, or creatinine clearance should be determined periodically. When feasible, it is recommended that serial audiograms be obtained in patients old enough to be tested, particularly high-risk patients. Evidence of ototoxicity (dizziness, vertigo, tinnitus, roaring in the ears or hearing loss) or nephrotoxicity requires dosage adjustment or discontinuance of the drug. As with the other aminoglycosides, on rare occasions changes in renal and eighth cranial nerve function may not become manifest until soon after completion of therapy.

Serum concentrations of aminoglycosides should be monitored when feasible to assure adequate levels and to avoid potentially toxic levels. When monitoring gentamicin peak concentrations, dosage should be adjusted so that prolonged levels above 12 mcg/ml are avoided. When monitoring gentamicin trough concentrations, dosage should be adjusted so that levels above 2 mcg/ml are avoided. Excessive peak and/or trough serum concentrations of aminoglycosides may increase the risk of renal and eighth cranial nerve toxicity. In the event of overdose or toxic reactions, hemodialysis or peritoneal dialysis will aid in removal of gentamicin from the blood.

Concurrent and/or sequential systemic or topical use of other potentially neurotoxic and/or nephrotoxic drugs, such as cisplatin, cephaloridine, kanamycin, amikacin, neomycin, polymyxin B, colistin, paromomycin, streptomycin, tobramycin, vancomycin, and viomycin, should be avoided. Other factors which may increase patient risk of toxicity are advanced age and dehydration.

The concurrent use of gentamicin with potent diuretics, such as ethacrynic acid or furosemide, should be avoided, since certain diuretics by themselves may cause ototoxicity. In addition, when administered intravenously, diuretics may enhance aminoglycoside toxicity by altering the antibiotic concentration in serum and tissue.

Description: Gentamicin sulfate, USP, a water-soluble antibiotic of the aminoglycoside group, is derived from *Micromonospora purpurea*, an actinomycete. GARAMYCIN Injectable is a sterile, aqueous solution for parenteral administration. Each ml. contains gentamicin sulfate. USP equivalent to 40 mg. gentamicin base, 1.8 mg. methylparaben and 0.2 mg. propylparaben as preservatives, 3.2 mg. sodium bisulfite, and 0.1 mg. edetate disodium.

Clinical Pharmacology: After intramuscular administration of GARAMYCIN Injectable, peak serum concentrations usually occur between 30 and 60 minutes and serum levels are measurable for six to eight hours. When gentamicin is administered by intravenous infusion over a two-hour period, the serum concentrations are similar to those obtained by intramuscular administration.

In patients with normal renal function, peak serum concentrations of gentamicin (mcg/ml) are usually up to four times the single intramuscular dose (mg/kg); for example, a 1.0 mg/kg injection in adults may be expected to result in a peak serum concentration up to 4 mcg/ml; a 1.5 mg/kg dose may produce levels up to 6 mcg/ml. While some variation is to be expected due to a number of variables such as age, body temperature surface area and physiologic differences, the individual patient given the same dose tends to have similar levels in repeated determinations. Gentamicin administered at 1.0 mg/kg every eight hours for the usual 7- to 10-day treatment period to patients with normal renal function does not accumulate in the serum.

Gentamicin, like all aminoglycosides, may accumulate in the serum and tissues of patients treated with higher doses and for prolonged periods, particularly in the presence of impaired renal function. In adult patients, treatment with gentamicin dosages of 4 mg/kg/day or higher for seven to ten days may result in a slight, progressive rise in both peak and trough concentrations. In patients with impaired renal function, gentamicin is cleared from the body more slowly than in patients with normal renal function. The more severe the impairment, the slower the clearance. (Dosage must be adjusted.)

Since gentamicin is distributed in extracellular fluid, peak serum concentrations may be lower than usual in adult patients who have a large volume of this fluid. Serum concentrations of gentamicin in febrile patients may be lower than those in afebrile patients given the same dose. When body temperature returns to normal serum concentrations of the drug may rise. Febrile and anemic states may be associated with a shorter than usual serum half-life. (Dosage adjustment is usually not necessary.)

In severely burned patients, the half-life may be significantly decreased and resulting serum concentrations may be lower than anticipated from the mg/kg dose.

Protein binding studies have indicated that the degree of gentamicin binding is low; depending upon the methods used for testing, this may be between 0 and 30%.

After initial administration to patients with normal renal function, generally 70% or more of the gentamicin dose is recoverable in the urine in 24 hours, concentrations in urine above 100 mcg/ml may be achieved. Little, if any, metabolic transformation occurs; the drug is excreted principally by glomerular filtration. After several days of treatment, the amount of gentamicin excreted in the urine approaches the daily dose administered. As with other aminoglycosides, a small amount of the gentamicin dose may be retained in the tissues, especially in the kidneys. Minute quantities of aminoglycosides have been detected in the urine weeks after drug administration was discontinued. Renal clearance of gentamicin is similar to that of endogenous creatinine.

In patients with marked impairment of renal function, there is a decrease in the concentration of aminoglycosides in urine and in their penetration into defective renal parenchyma. This decreased drug excretion, together with the potential nephrotoxicity of aminoglycosides, should be considered when treating such patients who have urinary tract infections.

Probenecid does not affect renal tubular transport of gentamicin.

The endogenous creatinine clearance rate and the serum creatinine level have a high correlation with the half-life of gentamicin in serum. Results of these tests may serve as guides for adjusting dosage in patients with renal impairment (see DOSAGE AND ADMINISTRATION).

Following parenteral administration, gentamicin can be detected in serum, lymph, tissues, sputum, and in pleural, synovial, and peritoneal fluids. Concentrations in renal cortex sometimes may be eight times higher than the usual serum levels. Concentrations in bile, in general, have been low and have suggested minimal biliary excretion. Gentamicin crosses the peritoneal as well as the placental membranes. Since aminoglycosides diffuse poorly into the subarachnoid space after parenteral administration, concentrations of gentamicin in cerebrospinal fluid are often low and dependent upon dose, rate of penetration, and degree of meningeal inflammation. There is minimal penetration of gentamicin into ocular tissues following intramuscular or intravenous administration.

Microbiology: *In vitro* tests have demonstrated that gentamicin is a bactericidal antibiotic which acts by inhibiting normal protein synthesis in susceptible microorganisms. It is active against a wide variety of pathogenic bacteria including *Escherichia coli, Proteus* species, (indole-positive and indole-negative), *Pseudomonas aeruginosa*, species of the *Klebsiella-Enterobacter-Serratia* group. *Citrobacter* species and *Staphylococcus* species (including penicillin- and methicillin-resistant strains). Gentamicin is also active *in vitro* against species of *Salmonella* and *Shigella*. The following bacteria are usually resistant to aminoglycosides; *Streptococcus pneumoniae*, most species of streptococci, particularly group D and anaerobic organisms, such as *Bacteroides* species or *Clostridium* species.

In vitro studies have shown that an aminoglycoside combined with an antibiotic that interferes with cell wall synthesis may act synergistically against some group D streptococcal strains. The combination of gentamicin and penicillin G has a synergistic bactericidal effect against virtually all strains of *Streptococcus faecalis* and its varieties *(S. faecalis* var. *liquifaciens, S. faecalis* var. *zymogenes), S. faecium* and *S. durans*. An enhanced killing effect against many of these strains has also been shown *in vitro* with combinations of gentamicin and ampicillin, carbenicillin, nafcillin, or oxacillin.

The combined effect of gentamicin and carbenicillin is synergistic for many strains of *Pseudomonas aeruginosa*. *In vitro* synergism against other gram-negative organisms has been shown with combinations of gentamicin and cephalosporins.

Gentamicin may be active against clinical isolates of bacteria resistant to other aminoglycosides. Bacteria resistant to one aminoglycoside may be resistant to one or more other aminoglycosides. Bacterial resistance to gentamicin is generally developed slowly.

Susceptibility Testing: If the disc method of susceptibility testing used is that described by Bauer *et al. (Am J Clin Path* 45:493, 1966; *Federal Register* 37:20527-20529, 1972), a disc containing 10 mcg. of gentamicin should give a zone of inhibition of 13mm. or more to indicate susceptibility of the infecting organism. A zone of 12mm. or less indicates that the infecting organism is likely to be resistant. In certain conditions it may be desirable to do additional susceptibility testing by the tube or agar dilution method; gentamicin substance is available for this purpose.

Indications and Usage: GARAMYCIN Injectable is indicated in the treatment of serious infections caused by susceptible strains of the following microorganisms: *Pseudomonas aeruginosa, Proteus* species (indole-positive and indole-negative). *Escherichia coli, Klebsiella-Enterobacter-Serratia* species, *Citrobacter* species and *Staphylococcus* species (coagulase-positive and coagulase-negative).

Clinical studies have shown GARAMYCIN Injectable to be effective in bacterial neonatal sepsis; bacterial septicemia; and serious bacterial infections of the central nervous system (meningitis), urinary tract, respiratory tract, gastrointestinal tract (including peritonitis), skin, bone and soft tissue (including burns).

Aminoglycosides, including gentamicin, are not indicated in uncomplicated initial episodes of urinary tract infections unless the causative organisms are susceptible to these antibiotics and are not susceptible to antibiotics having less potential for toxicity.

Specimens for bacterial culture should be obtained to isolate and identify causative organisms and to determine their susceptibility to gentamicin.

GARAMYCIN may be considered as initial therapy in suspected or confirmed gram-negative infections, and therapy may be instituted before obtaining results of susceptibility testing. The decision to continue therapy with this drug should be based on the results of suscepti-

Continued on next page

Information on Schering products appearing on these pages is effective as of September 30, 1979.

Schering—Cont.

bility tests, the severity of the infection, and the important additional concepts contained in the "WARNINGS Box" above. If the causative organisms are resistant to gentamicin, other appropriate therapy should be instituted.
In serious infections when the causative organisms are unknown GARAMYCIN may be administered as initial therapy in conjunction with a penicillin-type or cephalosporin-type drug before obtaining results of susceptibility testing. If anaerobic organisms are suspected as etiologic agents, consideration should be given to using other suitable antimicrobial therapy in conjunction with gentamicin. Following identification of the organism and its susceptibility, appropriate antibiotic therapy should then be continued.
GARAMYCIN has been used effectively in combination with carbenicillin for the treatment of life-threatening infections caused by *Pseudomonas aeruginosa*. It has also been found effective when used in conjunction with a penicillin-type drug for the treatment of endocarditis caused by group D streptococci.
GARAMYCIN Injectable has also been shown to be effective in the treatment of serious staphylococcal infections. While not the antibiotic of first choice, GARAMYCIN Injectable may be considered when penicillins or other less potentially toxic drugs are contraindicated and bacterial susceptibility tests and clinical judgment indicate its use. It may also be considered in mixed infections caused by susceptible strains of staphylococci and gram-negative organisms.
In the neonate with suspected bacterial sepsis or staphylococcal pneumonia, a penicillin-type drug is also usually indicated as concomitant therapy with gentamicin.
Contraindications: Hypersensitivity to gentamicin is a contraindication to its use. A history of hypersensitivity or serious toxic reactions to other aminoglycosides may contraindicate use of gentamicin because of the known cross-sensitivity of patients to drugs in this class.
Warnings: (See "WARNINGS Box" above.)
Precautions: Neurotoxic and nephrotoxic antibiotics may be absorbed in significant quantities from body surfaces after local irrigation or application. The potential toxic effect of antibiotics administered in this fashion should be considered.
Increased nephrotoxicity has been reported following concomitant administration of aminoglycoside antibiotics and cephalosporins.
Neuromuscular blockade and respiratory paralysis have been reported in the cat receiving high doses (40 mg/kg) of gentamicin. The possibility of these phenomena occurring in man should be considered if aminoglycosides are administered by any route to patients receiving anesthetics, or to patients receiving neuromuscular blocking agents, such as succinylcholine, tubocurarine, or decamethonium, or in patients receiving massive transfusions of citrate-anticoagulated blood. If neuromuscular blockade occurs, calcium salts may reverse it.
Aminoglycosides should be used with caution in patients with neuromuscular disorders, such as myasthenia gravis or parkinsonism, since these drugs may aggravate muscle weakness because of their potential curare-like effects on the neuromuscular junction.
Elderly patients may have reduced renal function which may not be evident in the results of routine screening tests, such as BUN or serum creatinine. A creatinine clearance determination may be more useful. Monitoring of renal function during treatment with gentamicin, as with other aminoglycosides, is particularly important in such patients.
Cross-allergenicity among aminoglycosides has been demonstrated.
Patients should be well hydrated during treatment.
Although the *in vitro* mixing of gentamicin and carbenicillin results in a rapid and significant inactivation of gentamicin, this interaction has not been demonstrated in patients with normal renal function who received both drugs by different routes of administration. A reduction in gentamicin serum half-life has been reported in patients with severe renal impairment receiving carbenicillin concomitantly with gentamicin.
Treatment with gentamicin may result in overgrowth of nonsusceptible organisms. If this occurs, appropriate therapy is indicated.
See "WARNINGS Box" regarding concurrent use of potent diuretics and regarding concurrent and/or sequential use of other neurotoxic and/or nephrotoxic antibiotics and for other essential information.
Usage in Pregnancy—Safety for use in pregnancy has not been established.
Adverse Reactions: *Nephrotoxicity:* Adverse renal effects, as demonstrated by the presence of casts, cells, or protein in the urine or by rising BUN, NPN, serum creatinine or oliguria, have been reported. They occur more frequently in patients with a history of renal impairment and in patients treated for longer periods or with larger dosage than recommended.
Neurotoxicity: Serious adverse effects on both vestibular and auditory branches of the eighth nerve have been reported, primarily in patients with renal impairment and in patients on high doses and/or prolonged therapy. Symptoms include dizziness, vertigo, tinnitus, roaring in the ears and also hearing loss, which, as with the other aminoglycosides, may be irreversible. Hearing loss is usually manifested initially by diminution of high-tone acuity. Other factors which may increase the risk of toxicity include excessive dosage, dehydration and previous exposure to other ototoxic drugs.
Numbness, skin tingling, muscle twitching and convulsions have also been reported.
Note: The risk of toxic reactions is low in patients with normal renal function who do not receive GARAMYCIN Injectable at higher doses or for longer periods of time than recommended.
Other reported adverse reactions possibly related to gentamicin include: respiratory depression, lethargy, confusion, depression, visual disturbances, decreased appetite, weight loss, and hypotension and hypertension; rash, itching, urticaria, generalized burning, laryngeal edema, anaphylactoid reactions, fever, and headache, nausea, vomiting, increased salivation, and stomatitis; purpura, pseudotumor cerebri, acute organic brain syndrome, pulmonary fibrosis, alopecia, joint pain, transient hepatomegaly, and splenomegaly.
Laboratory abnormalities possibly related to gentamicin include: increased levels of serum transaminase (SGOT, SGPT), serum LDH and bilirubin; decreased serum calcium, magnesium, sodium and potassium; anemia, leukopenia, granulocytopenia, transient agranulocytosis, eosinophilia, increased and decreased reticulocyte counts, and thrombocytopenia.
While local tolerance of GARAMYCIN Injectable is generally excellent, there has been an occasional report of pain at the injection site. Subcutaneous atrophy or fat necrosis suggesting local irritation has been reported rarely.
Overdosage: In the event of overdose or toxic reactions, hemodialysis or peritoneal dialysis will aid in the removal of gentamicin from the blood.
Dosage and Administration: GARAMYCIN Injectable may be given intramuscularly or intravenously. The patient's pretreatment body weight should be obtained for calculation of correct dosage. The dosage of aminoglycosides in obese patients should be based on an estimate of the lean body mass. It is desirable to limit the duration of treatment with aminoglycosides to short term.

PATIENTS WITH NORMAL RENAL FUNCTION

Adults: The recommended dosage of GARAMYCIN Injectable for patients with serious infections and normal renal function is 3 mg/kg/day, administered in three equal doses every eight hours (Table I).
For patients with life-threatening infections, dosages up to 5 mg/kg/day may be administered in three or four equal doses. This dosage should be reduced to 3 mg/kg/day as soon as clinically indicated (Table I).
It is desirable to measure both peak and trough serum concentrations of gentamicin to determine the adequacy and safety of the dosage. When such measurements are feasible, they should be carried out periodically during therapy to assure adequate but not excessive drug levels. For example, the peak concentration (at 30 to 60 minutes after intramuscular injection) is expected to be in the range of 4 to 6 mcg/ml. When monitoring peak concentrations after intramuscular or intravenous administration, dosage should be adjusted so that prolonged levels above 12 mcg/ml are avoided. When monitoring trough concentrations (just prior to the next dose), dosage should be adjusted so that levels above 2 mcg/ml are avoided. Determination of the adequacy of a serum level for a particular patient must take into consideration the susceptibility of the causative organism, the severity of the infection, and the status of the patient's host-defense mechanisms.
In patients with extensive burns, altered pharmacokinetics may result in reduced serum concentrations of aminoglycosides. In such patients treated with gentamicin, measurement of serum concentrations is recommended as a basis for dosage adjustment.

TABLE I
DOSAGE SCHEDULE GUIDE FOR ADULTS WITH NORMAL RENAL FUNCTION
(Dosage at Eight-Hour Intervals)
40 mg. per ml.

Patient's Weight* kg (lb)	Usual Dose For Serious Infections 1 mg/kg q8h (3 mg/kg/day)		Dose for Life-Threatening Infections (Reduce as Soon as Clinically Indicated) 1.7 mg/kg q8h** (5 mg/kg/day)	
	mg/dose q8h	ml/dose	mg/dose q8h	ml/dose
40 (88)	40	1.0	66	1.6
45 (99)	45	1.1	75	1.9
50 (110)	50	1.25	83	2.1
55 (121)	55	1.4	91	2.25
60 (132)	60	1.5	100	2.5
65 (143)	65	1.6	108	2.7
70 (154)	70	1.75	116	2.9
75 (165)	75	1.9	125	3.1
80 (176)	80	2.0	133	3.3
85 (187)	85	2.1	141	3.5
90 (198)	90	2.25	150	3.75
95 (209)	95	2.4	158	4.0
100 (220)	100	2.5	166	4.2

* The dosage of aminoglycosides in obese patients should be based on an estimate of the lean body mass.
** For q6h schedules, dosage should be recalculated.

Children: 6 to 7.5 mg/kg/day. (2.0 to 2.5 mg/kg administered every 8 hours.)
Infants and Neonates: 7.5 mg/kg/day. (2.5 mg/kg administered every 8 hours.)
Premature or Full-Term Neonates One Week of Age or Less: 5 mg/kg/day. (2.5 mg/kg administered every 12 hours).
For further information concerning the use of gentamicin in infants and children, see

GARAMYCIN Pediatric Injectable Product Information.

The usual duration of treatment for all patients is seven to ten days. In difficult and complicated infections, a longer course of therapy may be necessary. In such cases monitoring of renal, auditory, and vestibular functions is recommended, since toxicity is more apt to occur with treatment extended for more than ten days. Dosage should be reduced if clinically indicated.

For Intravenous Administration

The intravenous administration of gentamicin may be particularly useful for treating patients with bacterial septicemia or those in shock. It may also be the preferred route of administration for some patients with congestive heart failure, hematologic disorders, severe burns, or those with reduced muscle mass. For intermittent intravenous administration in adults, a single dose of GARAMYCIN Injectable may be diluted in 50 to 200 ml. of sterile isotonic saline solution or in a sterile solution of dextrose 5% in water, in infants and children, the volume of diluent should be less. The solution may be infused over a period of one-half to two hours.

The recommended dosage for intravenous and intramuscular administration is identical. GARAMYCIN Injectable should not be physically premixed with other drugs, but should be administered separately in accordance with the recommended route of administration and dosage schedule.

PATIENT WITH IMPAIRED RENAL FUNCTION

Dosage must be adjusted in patients with impaired renal function. Whenever possible serum concentrations of gentamicin should be monitored. One method of dosage adjustment is to increase the interval between administration of the usual doses. Since the serum creatinine concentration has a high correlation with the serum half-life of gentamicin, this laboratory test may provide guidance for adjustment of the interval between doses. The interval between doses (in hours) may be approximated by multiplying the serum creatinine level (mg/100 ml) by 8. For example, a patient weighing 60 kg. with a serum creatinine level of 2.0 mg/100 ml could be given 60 mg. (1 mg/kg) every 16 hours (2 × 8).

In patients with serious systemic infections and renal impairment, it may be desirable to administer the antibiotic more frequently but in reduced dosage. In such patients, serum concentrations of gentamicin should be measured so that adequate but not excessive levels result. A peak and trough concentration measured intermittently during therapy will provide optimal guidance for adjusting dosage. After the usual initial dose, a rough guide for determining reduced dosage at eight-hour intervals is to divide the normally recommended dose by the serum creatinine level (Table II). For example, after an initial dose of 60 mg. (1 mg/kg), a patient weighing 60 kg. with a serum creatinine level of 2.0 mg/100 ml could be given 30 mg. every eight hours (60÷2). It should be noted that the status of renal function may be changing over the course of the infectious process.

It is important to recognize that deteriorating renal function may require a greater reduction in dosage than that specified in the above guidelines for patients with stable renal impairment.

TABLE II
DOSAGE ADJUSTMENT GUIDE FOR PATIENTS WITH RENAL IMPAIRMENT
(Dosage at Eight-Hour Intervals After the Usual Initial Dose)

Serum Creatinine (mg %)	Approximate Creatinine Clearance Rate ($ml/min/1.73M^2$)	Percent of Usual Doses Shown in Table I
≤ 1.0	> 100	100
1.1–1.3	70–100	80
1.4–1.6	55–70	65
1.7–1.9	45–55	55
2.0–2.2	40–45	50
2.3–2.5	35–40	40
2.6–3.0	30–35	35
3.1–3.5	25–30	30
3.6–4.0	20–25	25
4.1–5.1	15–20	20
5.2–6.6	10–15	15
6.7–8.0	< 10	10

In adults with renal failure undergoing hemodialysis, the amount of gentamicin removed from the blood may vary depending upon several factors including the dialysis method used. An eight-hour hemodialysis may reduce serum concentrations of gentamicin by approximately 50%. The recommended dosage at the end of each dialysis period is 1 to 1.7 mg/kg depending upon the severity of infection. In children, a dose of 2 mg/kg may be administered.

The above dosage schedules are not intended as rigid recommendations but are provided as guides to dosage when the measurement of gentamicin serum levels is not feasible.

A variety of methods are available to measure gentamicin concentrations in body fluids; these include microbiologic, enzymatic and radioimmunoassay techniques.

How Supplied: GARAMYCIN Injectable, 40 mg. per ml., for parenteral administration, is supplied in 2 ml. (80 mg.) vials, boxes of 1 and 25; 20 ml. (800 mg) vials, box of 5; and in 1.5 ml. (60 mg.) and 2 ml. (80 mg.) disposable syringes, each in boxes of 1 and 10.

Also available, GARAMYCIN Pediatric Injectable, 10 mg. per ml., for parenteral administration, supplied in 2 ml. (20 mg) vials; box of one. GARAMYCIN Injectable is a clear, stable solution that requires no refrigeration.

JANUARY 1979

Schering Pharmaceutical Corporation (P.R.)
An Affiliate of Schering Corporation
Kenilworth, N.J. 07033

[*Shown in Product Identification Section*]

GARAMYCIN® PEDIATRIC Injectable ℞

brand of gentamicin sulfate injection, USP 10 mg. per ml.

Each ml. contains gentamicin sulfate, USP equivalent to 10 mg. gentamicin.

For Parenteral Administration

WARNINGS

Patients treated with aminoglycosides should be under close clinical observation because of the potential toxicity associated with their use.

As with other aminoglycosides, GARAMYCIN Pediatric Injectable is potentially nephrotoxic. The risk of nephrotoxicity is greater in patients with impaired renal function and in those who receive high dosage or prolonged therapy.

Neurotoxicity manifested by ototoxicity, both vestibular and auditory, can occur in patients treated with GARAMYCIN Pediatric Injectable, primarily in those with pre-existing renal damage and in patients with normal renal function treated with higher doses and/or for longer periods than recommended. Other manifestations of neurotoxicity may include numbness, skin tingling, muscle twitching, and convulsions.

Renal and eighth cranial nerve function should be closely monitored, especially in patients with known or suspected reduced renal function at onset of therapy and also in those whose renal function is initially normal but who develop signs of renal dysfunction during therapy. Urine should be examined for decreased specific gravity, increased excretion of protein, and the presence of cells or casts.. Blood urea nitrogen, serum creatinine, or creatinine clearance should be determined periodically. When feasible, it is recommended that serial audiograms be obtained in patients old enough to be tested, particularly high-risk patients. Evidence of ototoxicity (dizziness, vertigo, tinnitus, roaring in the ears or hearing loss) or nephrotoxicity requires dosage adjustment or discontinuance of the drug. As with the other aminoglycosides, on rare occasions changes in renal and eighth cranial nerve function may not become manifest until soon after completion of therapy.

Serum concentrations of aminoglycosides should be monitored when feasible to assure adequate levels and to avoid potentially toxic levels. When monitoring gentamicin peak concentrations, dosage should be adjusted so that prolonged levels above 12 mcg/ml are avoided. Excessive peak and/or trough serum concentrations of aminoglycosides may increase the risk of renal and eighth cranial nerve toxicity. In the event of overdose or toxic reactions, hemodialysis or peritoneal dialysis will aid in the removal of gentamicin from the blood. In the newborn infant, exchange transfusions may also be considered.

Concurrent and/or sequential systemic or topical use of other potentially neurotoxic and/or nephrotoxic drugs, such as cisplatin, cephaloridine, kanamycin, amikacin, neomycin, polymyxin B, colistin, paromomycin, streptomycin, tobramycin, vancomycin, and viomycin, should be avoided. Another factor which may increase patient risk of toxicity is dehydration.

The concurrent use of gentamicin with potent diuretics, such as ethacrynic acid or furosemide, should be avoided, since certain diuretics by themselves may cause ototoxicity. In addition, when administered intravenously, diuretics may enhance aminoglycoside toxicity by altering the antibiotic concentration in serum and tissue.

Description: Gentamicin sulfate, USP, a water-soluble antibiotic of the aminoglycoside group, is derived from *Micromonospora purpurea,* an actinomycete. GARAMYCIN Pediatric Injectable is a sterile, aqueous solution for parenteral administration. Each ml. contains gentamicin sulfate, USP equivalent to 10 mg. gentamicin base, 1.3 mg. methylparaben and 0.2 mg. propylparaben as preservatives, 3.2 mg. sodium bisulfate; and 0.1 mg. edetate disodium.

Clinical Pharmacology: After intramuscular administration of GARAMYCIN Pediatric Injectable, peak serum concentrations usually occur between 30 and 60 minutes and serum levels are measurable for 6 to 12 hours. In infants, a single dose of 2.5 mg/kg usually provides a peak serum level in the range of 3 to 5 mcg/ml. When gentamicin is administered by intravenous infusion over a two-hour period, the serum concentrations are similar to those

Information on Schering products appearing on these pages is effective as of September 30, 1979.

Continued on next page

Schering—Cont.

obtained by intramuscular administration. Age markedly affects the peak concentrations: in one report, a 1 mg/kg dose produced mean peak concentrations of 1.58, 2.03, and 2.81 mcg/ml in patients 6 months to 5 years old, 5 to 10 years old, and over 10 years old, respectively.
In infants one week to six months of age, the half-life is 3 to 3½ hours. In full-term and large premature infants less than one week old, the appropriate serum half-life of gentamicin is 5½ hours. In small premature infants, the half-life is inversely related to birth weight. In premature infants weighing less than 1500 grams, the half-life is 11½ hours; in those weighing 1500 to 2000 grams, the half-life is 8 hours; in those weighing over 2000 grams, the half-life is approximately 5 hours. While some variation is to be expected due to a number of variables such as age, body temperature, surface area and physiologic differences, the individual patient given the same dose tends to have similar levels in repeated determinations.
Gentamicin, like all aminoglycosides, may accumulate in the serum and tissues of patients treated with higher doses and for prolonged periods, particularly in the presence of impaired or immature renal function. In patients with immature or impaired renal function, gentamicin is cleared from the body more slowly than in patients with normal renal function. The more severe the impairment, the slower the clearance. (Dosage must be adjusted.)
Since gentamicin is distributed in extracellular fluid, peak serum concentrations may be lower than usual in patients who have a large volume of this fluid. Serum concentrations of gentamicin in febrile patients may be lower than those in afebrile patients given the same dose. When body temperature returns to normal, serum concentrations of the drug may rise. Febrile and anemic states may be associated with a shorter than usual serum half-life. (Dosage adjustment is usually not necessary.) In severely burned patients, the half-life may be significantly decreased and resulting serum concentrations may be lower than anticipated from the mg/kg/dose.
Protein binding studies have indicated that the degree of gentamicin binding is low, depending upon the methods used for testing, this may be between 0 and 30%.
In neonates less than 3 days old, approximately 10% of the administered dose is excreted in 12 hours; in infants 5 to 40 days old, approximately 40% is excreted over the same period. Excretion of gentamicin correlates with postnatal age and creatinine clearance. Thus, with increasing postnatal age and concomitant increase in renal maturity, gentamicin is excreted more rapidly. Little, if any, metabolic transformation occurs; the drug is excreted principally by glomerular filtration. After several days of treatment, the amount of gentamicin excreted in the urine approaches, but does not equal, the daily dose administered. As with other aminoglycosides, a small amount of the gentamicin dose may be retained in the tissues, especially in the kidneys. Minute quantities of aminoglycosides have been detected in the urine of some patients weeks after drug administration was discontinued. Renal clearance of gentamicin is similar to that of endogenous creatinine.
In patients with marked impairment of renal function, there is a decrease in the concentration of aminoglycosides in urine and in their penetration into defective renal parenchyma. This decreased drug excretion, together with the potential nephrotoxicity of aminoglycosides, should be considered when treating such patients who have urinary tract infections.
Probenecid does not affect renal tubular transport of gentamicin.
The endogenous creatinine clearance rate and the serum creatinine level have a high correlation with the half-life of gentamicin in serum. Results of these tests may serve as guides for adjusting dosage in patients with renal impairment (see DOSAGE AND ADMINISTRATION).
Following parenteral administration, gentamicin can be detected in serum, lymph, tissues, sputum, and in pleural, synovial, and peritoneal fluids. Concentrations in renal cortex sometimes may be eight times higher than the usual serum levels. Concentrations in bile, in general, have been low and have suggested minimal biliary excretion. Gentamicin crosses the peritoneal as well as the placental membranes. Since aminoglycosides diffuse poorly into the subarachnoid space after parenteral administration, concentrations of gentamicin in cerebrospinal fluid are often low and dependent upon dose, rate of penetration, and degree of meningeal inflammation. There is minimal penetration of gentamicin into ocular tissues following intramuscular or intravenous administration.
Microbiology: *In vitro* tests have demonstrated that gentamicin is a bactericidal antibiotic which acts by inhibiting normal protein synthesis in susceptible microorganisms. It is active against a wide variety of pathogenic bacteria including *Escherichia coli, Proteus* species (indole-positive and indole-negative). *Pseudomonas aeruginosa,* species of *Klebsiella-Enterobacter-Serratia* group, *Citrobacter* species, and *Staphylococcus* species (including penicillin- and methicillin-resistant strains). Gentamicin is also active *in vitro* against species of *Salmonella* and *Shigella.* The following bacteria are usually resistant to aminoglycosides. *Streptococcus pneumoniae,* most species of streptococci, particularly group D and anaerobic organisms, such as *Bacteroides* species or *Clostridium* species.
In vitro studies have shown that an aminoglycoside combined with an antibiotic that interferes with cell wall synthesis may act synergistically against some group D streptococcal strains. The combination of gentamicin and penicillin G has a synergistic bacterial effect against virtually all strains of *Streptococcus faecalis* and its varieties *(S. faecalis* var. *liquifaciens, S. faecalis* var. *zymogenes), S. faecium* and *S. durans.* An enhanced killing effect against many of these strains has also been shown *in vitro* with combinations of gentamicin and ampicillin, carbenicillin, nafcillin, or oxacillin.
The combined effect of gentamicin and carbenicillin is synergistic for many strains of *Pseudomonas aeruginosa. In vitro* synergism against other gram-negative organisms has been shown with combinations of gentamicin and cephalosporins.
Gentamicin may be active against clinical isolates of bacteria resistant to other aminoglycosides. Bacteria resistant to one aminoglycoside may be resistant to one or more other aminoglycosides. Bacterial resistance to gentamicin is generally developed slowly.
Susceptibility Testing: If the disc method of susceptibility testing used is that described by Bauer *et al (Am J Clin Path* 45:493, 1966; *Federal Register* 37:20527–20529, 1972), a disc containing 10 mcg. of gentamicin should give a zone of inhibition of 13 mm. or more to indicate susceptibility of the infecting organism. A zone of 12 mm. or less indicates that the infecting organism is likely to be resistant. In certain conditions it may be desirable to do additional susceptibility testing by the tube or agar dilution method; gentamicin substance is available for this purpose.
Indications and Usage: GARAMYCIN Pediatric Injectable is indicated in the treatment of serious infections caused by susceptible strains of the following microorganisms: *Pseudomonas aeruginosa, Proteus* species (indole-positive and indole-negative), *Escherichia coli, Klebsiella-Enterobacter-Serratia* species, *Citrobacter* species, and *Staphylococcus* species (coagulase-positive and coagulase-negative).
Clinical studies have shown GARAMYCIN Pediatric Injectable to be effective in bacterial neonatal sepsis; bacterial septicemia; and serious bacterial infections of the central nervous system (meningitis), urinary tract, respiratory tract, gastrointestinal tract (including peritonitis), skin, bone and soft tissue (including burns).
Aminoglycosides, including gentamicin, are not indicated in uncomplicated initial episodes of urinary tract infections unless the causative organisms are susceptible to these antibiotics and are not susceptible to antibiotics having less potential for toxicity.
Specimens for bacterial culture should be obtained to isolate and identify causative organisms and to determine their susceptibility to gentamicin.
GARAMYCIN may be considered as initial therapy in suspected or confirmed gram-negative infections, and therapy may be instituted before obtaining results of susceptibility testing. The decision to continue therapy with this drug should be based on the results of susceptibility tests, the severity of the infection, and the important additional concepts contained in the "WARNINGS Box" above. If the causative organisms are resistant to gentamicin, other appropriate therapy should be instituted.
In serious infections when the causative organisms are unknown, GARAMYCIN may be administered as initial therapy in conjunction with a penicillin-type or cephalosporin-type drug before obtaining results of susceptibility testing. If anaerobic organisms are suspected as etiologic agents, consideration should be given to using other suitable antimicrobial therapy in conjunction with gentamicin. Following identification of the organism and its susceptibility, appropriate antibiotic therapy should then be continued.
GARAMYCIN has been used effectively in combination with carbenicillin for the treatment of life-threatening infections caused by *Pseudomonas aeruginosa.* It has also been found effective when used in conjunction with a penicillin-type drug for the treatment of endocarditis caused by group D streptococci.
GARAMYCIN Pediatric Injectable has also been shown to be effective in the treatment of serious staphylococcal infections. While not the antibiotic of first choice, GARAMYCIN Pediatric Injectable may be considered when penicillins or other less potentially toxic drugs are contraindicated and bacterial susceptibility tests and clinical judgment indicate its use. It may also be considered in mixed infections caused by susceptible strains of staphylococci and gram-negative organisms.
In the neonate with suspected bacterial sepsis or staphylococcal pneumonia, a penicillin-type drug is also usually indicated as concomitant therapy with gentamicin.
Contraindications: Hypersensitivity to gentamicin is a contraindication to its use. A history of hypersensitivity or serious toxic reactions to other aminoglycosides may contraindicate use of gentamicin because of the known cross-sensitivity of patients to drugs in this class.
Warnings: (See "WARNINGS Box" above.)
Precautions: Neurotoxic and nephrotoxic antibiotics may be absorbed in significant quantities from body surfaces after local irrigation or application. The potential toxic effect of antibiotics administered in this fashion should be considered.
Increased nephrotoxicity has been reported following concomitant adminstration of aminoglycoside antibiotics and cephalosporins. Neuromuscular blockade and respiratory paralysis have been reported in the cat receiving high doses (40 mg/kg) of gentamicin. The possi-

bility of these phenomena occurring in man should be considered if aminoglycosides are administered by any route to patients receiving anesthetics, or to patients receiving neuromuscular blocking agents, such as succinylcholine, tubocurarine, or decamethonium, or in patients receiving massive transfusions of citrate anticoagulated blood. If neuromuscular blockade occurs, calcium salts may reverse it.
Aminoglycosides should be used with caution in patients with neuromuscular disorders, such as myasthenia gravis or parkinsonism, since these drugs may aggravate muscle weakness because of their potential curare-like effects on the neuromuscular junction.
Cross-allergenicity among aminoglycosides has been demonstrated.
Patients should be well hydrated during treatment.
Although the *in vitro* mixing of gentamicin and carbenicillin results in a rapid and significant inactivation of gentamicin, this interaction has not been demonstrated in patients with normal renal function who received both drugs by different routes of administration. A reduction in gentamicin serum half-life has been reported in patients with severe renal impairment receiving carbenicillin concomitantly with gentamicin.
Treatment with gentamicin may result in overgrowth of nonsusceptible organisms. If this occurs, appropriate therapy is indicated.
See "WARNINGS Box" regarding concurrent and/or sequential use of other neurotoxic and/or nephrotoxic antibiotics and for other essential information.
Usage in Pregnancy—Safety for use in pregnancy has not been established.
Adverse Reactions: *Nephrotoxicity* Adverse renal effects, as demonstrated by the presence of casts, cells or protein in the urine or by rising BUN, NPN, serum creatinine or oliguria, have been reported. They occur more frequently in patients treated for longer periods or with larger dosages than recommended.
Neurotoxicity Serious adverse effects on both vestibular and auditory branches of the eighth nerve have been reported, primarily in patients with renal impairment and in patients on high doses and/or prolonged therapy. Symptoms include dizziness, vertigo, tinnitus, roaring in the ears and also hearing loss, which, as with the other aminoglycosides, may be irreversible. Hearing loss is usually manifested initially by diminution of high-tone acuity. Other factors which may increase the risk of toxicity include excessive dosage, dehydration and previous exposure to other ototoxic drugs.
Numbness, skin tingling, muscle twitching and convulsions have also been reported.
Note: The risk of toxic reactions is low in neonates, infants and children with normal renal function who do not receive GARAMYCIN Pediatric Injectable at higher doses or for longer periods of time than recommended.
Other reported adverse reactions possibly related to gentamicin include: respiratory depression, lethargy, confusion, depression, visual disturbances, decreased appetite, weight loss and hypotension and hypertension; rash, itching, urticaria, generalized burning, laryngeal edema, anaphylactoid reactions, fever, and headache; nausea, vomiting, increased salivation, and stomatitis; purpura, pseudotumor cerebri, acute organic brain syndrome, pulmonary fibrosis, alopecia, joint pain, transient hepatomegaly, and splenomegaly.
Laboratory abnormalities possibly related to gentamicin include: increased levels of serum transaminase (SGOT, SGPT), serum LDH and bilirubin; decreased serum calcium, magnesium, sodium, and potassium; anemia, leukopenia, granulocytopenia, transient agranulocytosis, eosinophilia, increased and decreased reticulocyte counts, and thrombocytopenia.
When local tolerance of GARAMYCIN Pediatric Injectable is generally excellent, there has been an occasional report of pain at the injection site. Subcutaneous atrophy or fat necrosis suggesting local irritation has been reported rarely.
Overdosage: In the event of overdose or toxic reactions, hemodialysis or peritoneal dialysis will aid in the removal of gentamicin from the blood. In the newborn infant, exchange transfusions may also be considered.
Dosage and Administration: GARAMYCIN Pediatric Injectable may be given intramuscularly or intravenously.The patient's pretreatment body weight should be obtained for calculation of correct dosage. The dosage of aminoglycosides in obese patients should be based on an estimate of the lean body mass. It is desirable to limit the duration of treatment with aminoglycosides to short term.

PATIENTS WITH NORMAL RENAL FUNCTION

Children: 6 to 7.5 mg/kg/day. (2.0 to 2.5 mg/kg administered every 8 hours.)
Infants and Neonates: 7.5 mg/kg/day. (2.5 mg/kg administered every 8 hours.)
Premature or Full-Term Neonates One Week of Age or Less: 5 mg/kg/day. (2.5 mg/kg administered every 12 hours.)
It is desirable to measure both peak and trough serum concentrations of gentamicin to determine the adequacy and safety of the dosage. When such measurements are feasible, they should be carried out periodically during therapy to assure adequate but not excessive drug levels. For example, the peak concentration (at 30 to 60 minutes after intramuscular injection) is expected to be in the range of 3 to 5 mcg/ml. When monitoring peak concentrations after intramuscular or intravenous administration dosage should be adjusted so that prolonged levels above 12 mcg/ml are avoided. When monitoring trough concentrations (just prior to the next dose), dosage should be adjusted so that levels above 2 mcg/ml are avoided. Determination of the adequacy of a serum level for a particular patient must take into consideration the susceptibility of the causative organism, the severity of the infection, and the status of the patient's host-defense mechanisms.
In patients with extensive burns, altered pharmacokinetics may result in reduced serum concentrations of aminoglycosides. In such patients treated with gentamicin, measurement of serum concentrations is recommended as a basis for dosage adjustment.
The usual duration of treatment is seven to ten days. In difficult and complicated infections, a longer course of therapy may be necessary. In such cases monitoring of renal, auditory, and vestibular functions is recommended, since toxicity is more apt to occur with treatment extended for more than ten days. Dosage should be reduced if clinically indicated.

For Intravenous Administration

The intravenous administration of gentamicin may be particularly useful for treating patients with bacterial septicemia or those in shock. It may also be the preferred route of administration for some patients with congestive heart failure, hematologic disorders, severe burns, or those with reduced muscle mass. For intermittent intravenous administration, a single dose of GARAMYCIN Pediatric Injectable may be diluted in sterile isotonic saline solution or in a sterile solution of dextrose 5% in water. The solution may be infused over a period of one-half to two hours.
The recommended dosage of intravenous and intramuscular administration is identical.
GARAMYCIN Pediatric Injectable should not be physically premixed with other drugs, but should be administered separately in accordance with the recommended route of administration and dosage schedule.

PATIENTS WITH IMPAIRED RENAL FUNCTION

Dosage must be adjusted in patients with impaired renal function. Whenever possible, serum concentrations of gentamicin should be monitored. One method of dosage adjustment is to increase the interval between administration of the usual doses. Since the serum creatinine concentration has a high correlation with the serum half-life of gentamicin, this laboratory test may provide guidance for adjustment of the interval between doses. In adults, the interval between doses (in hours) may be approximated by multiplying the serum creatinine level (mg/100 ml) by 8. For example, a patient weighing 60 kg. with a serum creatinine level of 2.0 mg/100 ml could be given 60 mg. (1 mg/kg) every 16 hours (2×8). These guidelines may be considered when treating infants and children with serious renal impairment.
In patients with serious systemic infections and renal impairment, it may be desirable to administer the antibiotic more frequently but in reduced dosage. In such patients, serum concentrations of gentamicin should be measured so that adequate but not excessive levels result. A peak and trough concentration measured intermittently during therapy will provide optimal guidance for adjusting dosage. After the usual initial dose, a rough guide for determining reduced dosage at eight-hour intervals is to divide the normally recommended dose by the serum creatinine level (Table 1). For example, after an initial dose of 20 mg. (2.0 mg/kg), a child weighing 10 kg with a serum creatinine level of 2.0 mg/100 ml could be given 10 mg. every eight hours ($20 \div 2$). It should be noted that the status of renal function may be changing over the course of the infectious process. It is important to recognize that deteriorating renal function may require a greater reduction in dosage than that specified in the above guidelines for patients with stable renal impairment.

TABLE 1
DOSAGE ADJUSTMENT GUIDE FOR PATIENTS WITH RENAL IMPAIRMENT
(Dosage at Eight-Hour Intervals After the Usual Initial Dose)

Serum Creatinine (mg %)	Approximate Creatinine Clearance Rate (ml/min/1.73M^2)	Percent of Usual Doses Shown Above
≤ 1.0	> 100	100
1.1–1.3	70–100	80
1.4–1.6	55–70	65
1.7–1.9	45–55	55
2.0–2.2	40–45	50
2.3–2.5	35–40	40
2.6–3.0	30–35	35
3.1–3.5	25–30	30
3.6–4.0	20–25	25
4.1–5.1	15–20	20
5.2–6.6	10–15	15
6.7–8.0	< 10	10

In patients with renal failure undergoing hemodialysis, the amount of gentamicin removed from the blood may vary depending upon several factors including the dialysis method used. An eight-hour hemodialysis may reduce serum concentrations of gentamicin by approximately 50%. In children, the recommended dose at the end of each dialysis period is 2.0 to 2.5 mg/kg depending upon the severity of infection.

Continued on next page

Information on Schering products appearing on these pages is effective as of September 30, 1979.

Schering—Cont.

The above dosage schedules are not intended as rigid recommendations but are provided as guides to dosage when the measurement of gentamicin serum levels is not feasible.
A variety of methods are available to measure gentamicin concentrations in body fluids; these include microbiologic, enzymatic and radioimmunoassay techniques.
How Supplied: GARAMYCIN Pediatric Injectable, 10 mg. per ml., for parenteral administration, supplied in 2 ml. (20 mg.) vials; box of one.
Also available, GARAMYCIN Injectable, 40 mg. per ml., for parenteral administration, supplied in 2 ml. (80 mg.) vials, boxes of 1 and 25; 20 ml (800 mg) vials, box of 5; and in 1.5 ml. (60 mg.) and 2 ml. (80 mg.) disposable syringes, each in boxes of 1 and 10.
GARAMYCIN Pediatric Injectable is a clear, stable solution that requires no refrigeration.
JANUARY 1979
Schering Pharmaceutical Corporation (P.R.)
An Affiliate of Schering Corporation
Kenilworth, N.J. 07033

[*Shown in Product Identification Section*]

GARAMYCIN® Intrathecal ℞
brand of gentamicin sulfate, USP
Injection 2.0 mg/ml
FOR DIRECT ADMINISTRATION INTO THE CEREBROSPINAL FLUID SPACES OF THE CENTRAL NERVOUS SYSTEM

WARNINGS
GARAMYCIN Intrathecal Injection is intended as adjunctive therapy in patients with central nervous system infections. Since patients considered for treatment with GARAMYCIN Intrathecal Injection will usually be receiving concomitant treatment with intramuscular or intravenous gentamicin sulfate, all warnings and precautions for this or other concomitantly administered agents must be observed. Moreover, when the drug is administered by more than one route, additive effects must be considered. (See GARAMYCIN Injectable or GARAMYCIN Pediatric Injectable Product Information.) Laboratory studies in animals have shown that gentamicin sulfate, when administered directly into the central nervous system, has caused neurologic disturbances, including adverse effects on the eighth cranial nerve. The risk of direct administration of a potentially neurotoxic drug into the cerebrospinal fluid spaces of the central nervous system must be weighed against the potential benefit to be derived from this route of administration.

Description: Gentamicin sulfate, USP, a water-soluble antibiotic of the aminoglycoside group, is derived from *Micromonospora purpurea*, an antinomycete. GARAMYCIN Intrathecal Injection is a sterile, aqueous solution for direct administration into the cerebrospinal fluid spaces of the central nervous system. Each ml. contains: gentamicin sulfate, USP equivalent to 2.0 mg. gentamicin base; and 8.5 mg. sodium chloride.
Clinical Pharmacology: Since gentamicin sulfate and other aminoglycosides diffuse poorly into the subarachnoid space after systemic administration, concentrations of these antibiotics in the lumbar or ventricular cerebrospinal fluid (CSF) are often low. Following intramuscular or intravenous administration of the usual doses, gentamicin concentrations in CSF in the absence of infection are usually less than 1 mcg/ml. In acute meningitis, slightly higher concentrations are obtained but these vary and are usually well below the peak serum concentration. CSF concentrations which are attained following intravenous or intramuscular administration of gentamicin sulfate tend to become lower as meningeal inflammation subsides. GARAMYCIN Intrathecal Injections are intended to increase the concentration of gentamicin in the CSF when used as part of the management of patients with central nervous system infections.
When GARAMYCIN Intrathecal Injection is given concomitantly with systemically administered gentamicin sulfate, the CSF levels are substantially increased depending upon the location of the injection. Peak CSF concentrations which follow intralumbar administration generally occur at 1 to 6 hours after injection. Factors which affect the concentration of gentamicin in the CSF following injection into cerebrospinal fluid spaces are the dose administered, the site of the injection (intralumbar, intraventricular), the volume in which the dose is diluted, and the presence or absence of obstruction to the CSF flow. There appears to be considerable inter-patient variation.
The half-life of gentamicin in the CSF of adults who received intralumbar injections is approximately 5.5 hours; this is somewhat longer than that in serum.
In one pharmacokinetic study in adults, a 3 to 4 mg. intralumbar injection resulted in a mean CSF concentration of 6.2 mcg/ml 24 hours after injection. The mean CSF concentration was noted to decrease with time; during days 1 through 6 of treatment with GARAMYCIN Intrathecal Injection by the intralumbar route, the mean 24-hour concentration was 9.9 mcg/ml, while during days 7 through 13, the mean concentration was 3.7 mcg/ml.
In another study in adults, CSF levels were measured at varying intervals after intralumbar administration of gentamicin sulfate. During days 1 through 6 of treatment, a 4 mg. dose produced a mean CSF level of 2.4 mcg/ml 24 hours after injection, while during days 7 through 13, the same dose produced a mean 24-hour level of 0.5 mcg/ml.
Following intralumbar administration there may be limited upward diffusion of the drug, presumably because of the direction of the CSF flow. Intraventricular administration produces high concentrations in the ventricles and throughout the central nervous system. Adequate levels will usually result from dosing every 24 hours, but it is desirable to manage each patient's infection with serial monitoring of gentamicin serum and CSF concentrations.
Microbiology: *In vitro* tests have demonstrated that gentamicin is a bactericidal antibiotic which acts by inhibiting normal protein synthesis in susceptible microorganisms. It is active against a wide variety of pathogenic bacteria including *Escherichia coli, Proteus* species (indole-positive and indole-negative), *Pseudomonas aeruginosa*, species of the *Klebsiella-Enterobacter-Serratia* group, *Citrobacter* species, and *Staphlococcus* species (including penicillin- and methicillin-resistant strains). Gentamicin is also active *in vitro* against species of *Salmonella* and *Shigella.* The following bacteria are usually resistant to aminoglycosides: *Streptococcus pneumoniae,* most species of streptococci, particularly group D and anaerobic organisms, such as *Bacteroides* species or *Clostridium* species.
In vitro studies have shown that an aminoglycoside combined with an antibiotic that interferes with cell wall synthesis may act synergistically against some group D streptococcal strains. The combination of gentamicin sulfate and penicillin G has a synergistic bactericidal effect against virtually all strains of *Streptococcus faecalis* and its varieties (*S. faecalis* var. *liquifaciens, S. faecalis* var. *zymogenes), S. faecium* and *S. durans.* An enhanced killing effect against many of these strains has also been shown *in vitro* with combinations of gentamicin and ampicillin, carbenicillin, nafcillin, or oxacillin.
The combined effect of gentamicin and carbenicillin is synergistic for many strains of *Pseudomonas aeruginosa.*
Gentamicin may be active against clinical isolates of bacteria resistant to other aminoglycosides. However, bacteria resistant to one aminoglycoside may be resistant to one or more other aminoglycosides.
Susceptibility Testing: If the disc method of susceptibility testing used is that described by Bauer *et al* (*Am J Clin Path* **45**:493, 1966; *Federal Register* **37**:20527–20529, 1972), a disc containing 10 mcg. of gentamicin, when tested against a bacterial strain susceptible to gentamicin, should give a zone of inhibition of $\geq$ 13 mm. A zone of $\leq$ 12 mm. indicates resistance. In certain conditions it may be desirable to do additional susceptibility testing by the broth or agar dilution method; gentamicin substance is available for this purpose.
Indications and Usage: GARAMYCIN Intrathecal Injection is indicated as adjunctive therapy to systemically administered gentamicin sulfate in the treatment of serious central nervous system infections (meningitis, ventriculitis) caused by susceptible *Pseudomonas* species.
Bacteriologic tests should be performed to determine that the causative organisms are *Pseudomonas* species susceptible to gentamicin.
Contraindications: Hypersensitivity to gentamicin sulfate is a contraindication to its use. A history of hypersensitivity or serious toxic reactions to aminoglycosides may also contraindicate use of gentamicin sulfate because of the known cross-sensitivity of patients to drugs in this class.
Warnings: (See "WARNINGS Box" above and the WARNINGS listed in the Product Information for GARAMYCIN Injectable and GARAMYCIN Pediatric Injectable.)
Precautions: (See PRECAUTIONS listed in the Product Information for GARAMYCIN Injectable and GARAMYCIN Pediatric Injectable.)
In a patient with a seven-year history of multiple sclerosis who was treated with gentamicin sulfate by intralumbar injection, disseminated microscopic lesions of the brain stem were reported at autopsy. Lesions observed were: tissue rarefaction with loss and marked swelling of axis cylinders with occasional calcification, loss of oligodendroglia and astroglia, and a poor inflammatory response.
Safety and efficacy in children below the age of three months have not been established.
Adverse Reactions: Local tolerance to GARAMYCIN Intrathecal Injection has been good. Local reactions of arachnoiditis or burning at the injection site have been reported rarely.
Because the recommended dosage of GARAMYCIN Intrathecal Injection is low, the potential for systemic adverse effects is minimal. However, GARAMYCIN Intrathecal Injection is recommended as adjunctive therapy with other antibiotics, such as parenteral gentamicin sulfate, which should be administered in full therapeutic dosages. Evidence of eighth nerve dysfunction, changes in renal function, leg cramps, rash, fever, convulsions, and an increase in cerebrospinal fluid protein have been reported in patients who were treated concomitantly with GARAMYCIN Intrathecal Injection and the parenteral preparation of gentamicin.
Administration of excessive (40 to 160 mg.) doses of the parenteral formulation of gentamicin sulfate (which contains a preservative system) by the various intrathecal routes has been reported to produce neuromuscular disturbances, e.g., ataxia, paresis, and incontinence.
Dosage and Administration: GARAMYCIN Intrathecal Injection is intended for adminis-

tration directly into the cerebrospinal fluid spaces of the central nervous system.

The dosage will vary depending upon factors, such as age and weight of the patient, site of injection, degree of obstruction to cerebrospinal fluid flow and the amount of cerebrospinal fluid estimated to be present. In general, the recommended dose for infants 3 months of age and older (see PRECAUTIONS) and children is 1 to 2 mg. once a day. For adults, 4 to 8 mg. may be administered once a day.

Administration of GARAMYCIN Intrathecal Injection should be continued as long as sensitive organisms are demonstrated in the cerebrospinal fluid. Since the intralumbar or intraventricular dose is administered immediately after specimens are taken for laboratory study, treatment should usually be continued for at least one day after negative results have been obtained from CSF cultures and/or stained smears.

The suggested method for administering GARAMYCIN Intrathecal Injection into the lumbar area is as follows: the desired quantity of GARAMYCIN Intrathecal Injection is drawn up carefully from the ampule into a 5- or 10-ml. sterile syringe. After the lumbar puncture is performed and a specimen of the spinal fluid is removed for laboratory tests, the syringe containing GARAMYCIN Intrathecal Injection is inserted into the hub of the spinal needle. A quantity of cerebrospinal fluid (approximately 10% of the estimated total CSF volume) is allowed to flow into the syringe and mix with the GARAMYCIN Intrathecal Injection. The resultant solution is then injected over a period of 3 to 5 minutes with the bevel of the needle directed upward.

If the cerebrospinal fluid is grossly purulent, or if it is unobtainable, GARAMYCIN Intrathecal Injection may be diluted with sterile normal saline before injection.

GARAMYCIN Intrathecal Injection may also be administered directly into the subdural space or directly into the ventricles, including administration by use of an implanted reservoir.

How Supplied: GARAMYCIN Intrathecal Injection, 2.0 mg. per ml., is supplied in 2 ml. ampules; box of 25.

NOTE: This preparation does not contain any preservative. Once opened, contents should be used immediately and unused portions should be discarded.

Animal Pharmacology and Toxicology: In dogs, an 8-hour perfusion of the ventriculosubarachnoid system with a solution containing 40 mcg/ml (~5 mg. or ~0.3 mg/kg) gentamicin produced no seizure activity or change in vital signs during administration. No morphological changes were observed when the dogs were sacrificed at 10 and 90 days following infusion.

The effects of repeated intrathecal injections of gentamicin at 0.1 and 0.3 mg/kg were evaluated in tranquilized beagle puppies. Transient flaccid paralysis was observed on the first day when the drug was administered rapidly (i.e., in less than 5 seconds), but no adverse effects were observed thereafter when the drug was administered less rapidly (i.e., over a period of approximately 30 seconds). No drug-related changes were found on histological examination of the cerebellum, brain stem or cephalic cord. In cats, gentamicin administered intracisternally at one-hour intervals in doses of up to 50 mg/kg did not produce any abnormalities in the electroencephalogram. In another study in cats, gentamicin sulfate given daily by the intracisternal route for up to 7 days caused neurologic disturbances, including adverse effects on the eighth cranial nerve.

In rabbits intracisternal injection of gentamicin at doses 50 and 100 times the therapeutic dose produced peak CSF concentrations of 160 and 180 mcg/ml, respectively. These doses were associated with changes in the myelin sheath predominantly of the lateral columns of the upper cervical cord, and some changes in glial cells and lesions in the medulla oblongata. In addition to a high incidence of mortality, the animals demonstrated weakness, ataxia and paralysis. At doses of one and ten times the therapeutic dose (providing peak levels of 16.5 and 40 mcg/ml CSF), no morphologic changes occurred and there were no drug-related symptoms identified.

GITALIGIN® ℞

brand of gitalin
Tablets

How Supplied: GITALIGIN Tablets, 0.5 mg., light green, scored, compressed tablets impressed with the Schering trademark and product identification letters, WAR, or numbers 617; bottles of 100.

For complete prescribing information, contact the Schering Professional Services Department.

[*Shown in Product Identification Section*]

GYNE-LOTRIMIN® ℞

brand of clotrimazole
Vaginal Cream 1%

Description: GYNE-LOTRIMIN is clotrimazole [1-(*o*-Chloro-α, α-diphenylbenzyl) imidazole], a synthetic antifungal agent having the chemical formula, $C_{22}H_{17}ClN_2$.

Each applicatorful of GYNE-LOTRIMIN Vaginal Cream contains approximately 50 mg. clotrimazole dispersed in sorbitan monostearate, polysorbate 60, cetyl esters wax, cetostearyl alcohol, 2-octyldodecanol, purified water, and as preservative, benzyl alcohol (1%).

Actions: Clotrimazole is a broad-spectrum antifungal agent that inhibits the growth of pathogenic yeasts. Clotrimazole exhibits fungicidal activity *in vitro* against *Candida albicans* and other species of the genus *Candida*.

No single-step or multiple-step resistance to clotrimazole has developed during successive passages of *Candida albicans*.

Indications: GYNE-LOTRIMIN Vaginal Cream is indicated for the local treatment of patients with vulvovaginal candidiasis (moniliasis). As GYNE-LOTRIMIN Vaginal Cream has been shown to be effective only for candidal vulvovaginitis, the diagnosis should be confirmed by KOH smears and/or cultures. Other pathogens commonly associated with vulvovaginitis (*Trichomonas* and *Hemophilus vaginalis*) should be ruled out by appropriate laboratory methods.

Studies have shown that women taking oral contraceptives had a cure rate similar to those not taking oral contraceptives

Contraindications: GYNE-LOTRIMIN Vaginal Cream is contraindicated in women who have shown hypersensitivity to any of the components of the preparation.

Precautions: *Laboratory Test:* If there is a lack of response to GYNE-LOTRIMIN Vaginal Cream, appropriate microbiological studies should be repeated to confirm the diagnosis and rule out other pathogens before instituting another course of antimycotic therapy.

Application of ^{14}C-labeled clotrimazole has shown negligible absorption (peak serum level of 0.01 mcg/ml 24 hours after insertion of vaginal cream containing 50 mg. of active drug) from both normal and inflamed human vaginal mucosa.

Usage in Pregnancy: While GYNE-LOTRIMIN Vaginal Cream has not been studied in the first trimester of pregnancy, use in the second and third trimesters has not been associated with ill effects.

Adverse Reactions: Three (0.5%) of the 653 patients treated with GYNE-LOTRIMIN Vaginal Cream reported complaints during therapy that were possibly drug related. Vaginal burning occurred in one patient; erythema, irritation and burning in another; intercurrent cystitis was reported in the third.

Dosage and Administration: GYNE-LOTRIMIN Vaginal Cream has been found to be effective when used from seven to fourteen days; studies have shown that patients treated for fourteen days had a significantly higher cure rate. The recommended dose is one applicatorful a day for seven to fourteen consecutive days; using the applicator supplied, insert one applicatorful of cream (approximately 5 grams) intravaginally preferably at bedtime.

How Supplied: GYNE-LOTRIMIN Vaginal Cream 1% is supplied in 45-gram tubes with a measured-dose applicator; box of one for seven-day treatment; box of two for fourteen-day treatment.

Store between 35° and 86°F (2° and 30°C).

[*Shown in Product Identification Section*]

GYNE-LOTRIMIN® ℞

brand of clotrimazole
Vaginal Tablets

Description: GYNE-LOTRIMIN is clotrimazole [1-(*o*-Chloro-α,α-diphenylbenzyl) imidazole], a synthetic antifungal agent having the chemical formula, $C_{22}H_{17}ClN_2$.

Each GYNE-LOTRIMIN Vaginal Tablet contains 100 mg. clotrimazole dispersed in lactose, providone, corn starch and magnesium stearate.

Actions: Clotrimazole is a broad-spectrum antifungal agent that inhibits the growth of pathogenic yeasts. Clotrimazole exhibits fungicidal activity *in vitro* against *Candida albicans* and other species of the genus *Candida*.

No single-step or multiple-step resistance to clotrimazole has developed during successive passages of *Candida albicans*.

Indications: GYNE-LOTRIMIN Vaginal Tablets are indicated for the local treatment of vulvovaginal candidiasis. The diagnosis should be confirmed by KOH smears and/or cultures. In randomized double-blind trials where GYNE-LOTRIMIN Vaginal Tablets were compared to Nystatin Vaginal Tablets, cure rates were similar.

Contraindications: GYNE-LOTRIMIN Vaginal Tablets are contraindicated in women who have shown hypersensitivity to this drug.

Precautions: Laboratory Tests: If there is a lack of response to GYNE-LOTRIMIN, appropriate microbiological studies should be repeated to confirm the diagnosis and rule out other pathogens.

Application of ^{14}C-labeled clotrimazole has shown negligible absorption (peak of 0.03 mcg/ml of serum 24 hours after insertion of a 100 mg. Tablet) from both normal and inflamed human vaginal mucosa.

Usage in Pregnancy: While GYNE-LOTRIMIN Vaginal Tablets have not been studied in the first trimester of pregnancy, use in the second and third trimesters has not been associated with ill effects. Follow-up reports now available on 41 neonates of 107 pregnant patients reveal no adverse effects or complications attributable to GYNE-LOTRIMIN therapy.

Adverse Reactions: Eleven (1.6%) of the 689 patients treated with GYNE-LOTRIMIN reported complaints during therapy that were possibly drug-related. Mild burning occurred in four patients while other complaints, such as skin rash, lower abdominal cramps, slight urinary frequency, and burning or irritation in the sexual partner, occurred rarely. In no case

Continued on next page

Information on Schering products appearing on these pages is effective as of September 30, 1979.

Schering—Cont.

was it necessary to discontinue treatment with GYNE-LOTRIMIN.

Dosage and Administration: The recommended dose is one tablet a day for seven consecutive days; using the applicator supplied, insert one tablet intravaginally preferably at bedtime. In the event of treatment failure, other pathogens commonly responsible for vaginitis should be ruled out before instituting another course of antimycotic therapy. There are no studies to show whether a second course of clotrimazole would be effective in patients who fail to respond to the initial course.

How Supplied: GYNE- LOTRIMIN Vaginal Tablets, 100 mg., white, tear-drop-shaped, uncoated tablets impressed with the Schering trademark and product identification numbers, 734; supplied in strip of seven tablets with plastic applicator and patient instructions, box of one.

Do not store above 35°C (95°F).

[*Shown in Product Identification Section*]

GYNETONE® ℞

brand of estrogen-androgen

Tablets

BOXED WARNINGS

1. ESTROGENS HAVE BEEN REPORTED TO INCREASE THE RISK RATIO OF ENDOMETRIAL CARCINOMA.

Three independent case control studies have reported an increased risk ratio of endometrial cancer in postmenopausal women exposed to exogenous estrogens for prolonged periods.[1–3] This risk ratio was independent of the other risk factors for endometrial cancer. These studies are further supported by the report that incidence rates of endometrial cancer have increased sharply since 1969 in eight different areas of the United States with population-based cancer reporting systems, an increase which may be related to the rapidly expanding use of estrogens during the last decade.[4]

The three case control studies reported that the risk ratio of endometrial cancer in estrogen users was about 4.5 to 13.9 times greater than in nonusers. The risk ratio appears to depend on both duration of treatment[1] and on estrogen dose.[3] In view of these reports, when estrogens are used for the treatment of menopausal symptoms, the lowest dose that will control symptoms should be utilized and medication should be discontinued as soon as possible. When prolonged treatment is medically indicated, the patient should be reassessed on at least a semiannual basis to determine the need for continued therapy. Although the evidence must be considered preliminary, one study suggests that cyclic administration of low doses of estrogen may carry less risk than continuous administration[3]; it therefore appears prudent to utilize such a regimen.

Close clinical surveillance of all women taking estrogens is important. In all cases of undiagnosed persistent or recurring abnormal vaginal bleeding, adequate diagnostic measures should be undertaken to rule out malignancy.

There is no evidence at present that "natural" estrogens are more or less hazardous than "synthetic" estrogens at equiestrogenic doses.

2. ESTROGENS SHOULD NOT BE USED DURING PREGNANCY.

The use of estrogens during early pregnancy may seriously damage the offspring. It has been reported that females exposed in utero to diethylstilbestrol, a non-steroidal estrogen, may have an increased risk of developing in later life a form of vaginal or cervical cancer that is ordinarily extremely rare.[5,6] This risk has been estimated statistically as not greater than 4 per 1000 exposures.[7] In certain studies, a high percentage of such exposed women (from 30 to 90 percent) have been found to have vaginal adenosis,[8–11] epithelial changes of the vagina and cervix. Although these changes are histologically benign, it is not known whether they are precursors of malignancy. Although similar data are not available with the use of other estrogens, it cannot be presumed they would not induce similar changes.

Several reports suggest an association between intrauterine fetal exposure to female sex hormones and congenital anomalies, including congenital heart defects and limb reduction defects.[12–15] One case control study[15] estimated a 4.7 fold increased risk of limb reduction defects in infants exposed in utero to sex hormones (oral contraceptives, hormone withdrawal tests for pregnancy, or attempted treatment for threatened abortion). Some of these exposures were very short and involved only a few days of treatment. The data suggest that the risk of limb reduction defects in exposed fetuses is somewhat less than 1 per 1000.

In the past, estrogens have been used during pregnancy to treat threatened or habitual abortion. There is considerable literature which reports that estrogens may be ineffective for these indications.

If GYNETONE is used during pregnancy, or if the patient becomes pregnant while taking this drug, she should be apprised of the potential risks to the fetus, and the advisability of pregnancy continuation.

Description: GYNETONE Tablets for oral administration contain ethinyl estradiol, USP and methyltestosterone, USP. Ethinyl estradiol is an estrogen having the chemical name, 19-Nor-17α-pregna-1,3,5(10)-trien-20-yne-3,17-diol. Methyltestosterone is an androgen having the chemical name, 17β-Hydroxy-17-methylandrost-4-en-3-one.

Each GYNETONE ".02" Tablet contains .02 mg. ethinyl estradiol and 5 mg. methyltestosterone. Each GYNETONE ".04" Tablet contains .04 mg. ethinyl estradiol and 10 mg. methyltestosterone.

Clinical Pharmacology: Combined estrogen and androgen therapy is used to avoid breakthrough and withdrawal bleeding from estrogen therapy alone in menopausal women.

Indications: GYNETONE Tablets are indicated for the treatment of moderate to severe *vasomotor* symptoms associated with the menopause in those patients not improved by estrogen alone. (There is no evidence that estrogens are effective for nervous symptoms or depression which might occur during menopause, and they should not be used to treat these conditions.)

GYNETONE HAS NOT BEEN SHOWN TO BE EFFECTIVE FOR ANY PURPOSE DURING PREGNANCY AND ITS USE MAY CAUSE SEVERE HARM TO THE FETUS (SEE BOXED WARNING ABOVE).

Contraindications: Estrogens should not be used in women with any of the following conditions:

1. Known or suspected cancer of the breast except in appropriately selected patients being treated for metastatic disease.
2. Known or suspected estrogen-dependent neoplasia.
3. Known or suspected pregnancy (See Boxed Warning).
4. Undiagnosed abnormal genital bleeding.
5. Active thrombophlebitis or thromboembolic disorders.
6. A past history of thrombophlebitis, thrombosis, or thromboembolic disorders associated with previous estrogen use (except when used in the treatment of breast malignancy).

Androgens are contraindicated in patients with cardiac, hepatic or renal decompensation and in those with hypercalcemia or liver function impairment. Androgens are also contraindicated in patients easily stimulated.

Warnings: 1. *Induction of malignant neoplasms.* Long-term continuous administration of natural and synthetic estrogens in certain animal species increases the frequency of carcinomas of the breast, cervix, vagina, and liver. There is now evidence that estrogens increase the risk of carcinoma of the endometrium in humans. (See Boxed Warning.)

At the present time there is no satisfactory evidence that estrogens given to postmenopausal women increase the risk of cancer of the breast,[16] although a recent long-term follow-up of a single physician's practice has raised this possibility.[17] Because of the animal data, there is a need for caution in prescribing estrogens for women with a strong family history of breast cancer or who have breast nodules, fibrocystic disease, or abnormal mammograms.

2. *Gallbladder disease.* A recent study has reported a 2- to 3-fold increase in the risk of surgically confirmed gallbladder disease in women receiving postmenopausal estrogens,[16] similar to the 2-fold increase previously noted in users of oral contraceptives.[18,23] In the case of oral contraceptives, the increased risk appeared after two years of use.[23]

3. *Effects similar to those caused by estrogen-progestagen oral contraceptives.* There are several serious adverse effects of oral contraceptives, most of which have not, up to now, been documented as consequences of postmenopausal estrogen therapy. This may reflect the comparatively low doses of estrogen used in postmenopausal women. It would be expected that the larger doses of estrogen used to treat prostatic or breast cancer or postpartum breast engorgement are more likely to result in these adverse effects, and, in fact, it has been shown that there is an increased risk of thrombosis in men receiving estrogens for prostatic cancer and women for postpartum breast engorgement.[19–22]

a. *Thromboembolic disease.* It is now well established that users of oral contraceptives have an increased risk of various thromboembolic and thrombotic vascular diseases, such as thrombophlebitis, pulmonary embolism, stroke, and myocardial infarction.[23–30] Cases of retinal thrombosis, mesenteric thrombosis and optic neuritis have been reported in oral contraceptive users. There is evidence that the risk of several of these adverse reactions is related to the dose of the drug.[31,32] An increased risk of postsurgery thromboembolic complications has also been reported in users of oral contraceptives.[33,34] If feasible, estrogen should be discontinued at least 4 weeks before surgery of the type associated with an increased risk of thromboembolism, or during periods of prolonged immobilization.

While an increased rate of thromboembolic and thrombotic disease in postmenopausal users of estrogens has not been found,[16,35] this does not rule out the possibility that such an increase may be present or that subgroups of women who have underlying risk factors or who are receiving relatively large doses of estrogens may have increased risk. Therefore, estrogens should not be used in persons with active thrombophlebitis or thromboembolic disorders and they should not be used (except in treatment of malignancy) in persons with a history of such disorders in association with estrogen use. They should be used with caution in patients with cerebral vascular or coronary artery disease and only for those in whom estrogens are clearly needed.

Large doses of estrogen (5 mg. conjugated estrogens per day), comparable to those used to treat cancer of the prostate and breast, have been shown in a large prospective clinical trial in men[36] to increase the risk of nonfatal myocardial infarction, pulmonary embolism and thrombophlebitis. When estrogen doses of this size are used, any of the thromboembolic and thrombotic adverse effects associated with oral contraceptive use should be considered a clear risk.

b. *Hepatic adenoma.* Benign hepatic adenomas appear to be associated with the use of oral contraceptives.[37-39] Although benign, and rare, these may rupture and may cause death through intra-abdominal hemorrhage. Such lesions have not yet been reported in association with other estrogen or progestagen preparations but should be considered in estrogen users having abdominal pain and tenderness, abdominal mass, or hypovolemic shock. Hepatocellular carcinoma has also been reported in women taking estrogen-containing oral contraceptives.[38] The relationship of this malignancy to these drugs is not known at this time.

c. *Elevated blood pressure.* Increased blood pressure is not uncommon in women using oral contraceptives. There is now a report that this may occur with use of estrogens in the menopause[40] and blood pressure should be monitored with estrogen use, especially if high doses are used.

d. *Glucose tolerance.* A worsening of glucose tolerance has been observed in a significant percentage of patients on estrogen-containing oral contraceptives. For this reason, diabetic patients should be carefully observed while receiving estrogen.

4. *Hypercalcemia.* Administration of estrogens and androgens may lead to severe hypercalcemia in patients with breast cancer and bone metastases. If this occurs, the drug should be stopped and appropriate measures taken to reduce the serum calcium level. Hypercalcemia may also occur in immobilized patients treated with androgens.

5. *Virilization.* Watch female patients closely for signs of virilization. Some effects, such as voice changes, may not be reversible even when the drug is stopped.

6. *Cholestatic hepatitis with jaundice.* Discontinue the drug if cholestatic hepatitis with jaundice appears or if liver function tests become abnormal.

Precautions:

General Precautions

1. A complete medical and family history should be taken prior to the initiation of any estrogen therapy. The pretreatment and periodic physical examinations should include special reference to blood pressure, breasts, abdomen, and pelvic organs, and should include a Papanicolaou smear. As a general rule, estrogen should not be prescribed for longer than one year without another physical examination being performed.

2. Fluid retention—Because estrogens and androgens may cause some degree of sodium and water retention, conditions which might be influenced by this factor, such as epilepsy, migraine, and cardiac, renal or hepatic dysfunction, require careful observation.

3. Certain patients may develop undesirable manifestations of excessive estrogenic stimulation, such as abnormal or excessive uterine bleeding, mastodynia, etc.

4. Oral contraceptives appear to be associated with an increased incidence of mental depression.[23] Although it is not clear whether this is due to the estrogenic or progestagenic component of the contraceptive, patients with a history of depression should be carefully observed.

5. Preexisting uterine leiomyomata may increase in size during use.

6. The pathologist should be advised of estrogen therapy when relevant specimens are submitted.

7. Patients with a past history of jaundice during pregnancy have an increased risk of recurrence of jaundice while receiving estrogen-containing oral contraceptive therapy. If jaundice develops in any patient receiving estrogen, the medication should be discontinued while the cause is investigated.

8. Estrogens may be poorly metabolized in patients with impaired liver function and they should be administered with caution in such patients.

9. Because estrogens influence the metabolism of calcium and phosphorus, they should be used with caution in patients with metabolic bone diseases that are associated with hypercalcemia or in patients with renal insufficiency.

10. Because of the effects of estrogens on epiphyseal closure, they should be used judiciously in young patients in whom bone growth is not complete.

11. Certain endocrine and liver function tests may be affected by estrogen-containing oral contraceptives. The following similar changes may be expected with larger doses of estrogen: Increased sulfobromophthalein retention; increased prothrombin and factors VII, VIII, IX, and X; decreased antithrombin 3; increased norepinephrine-induced platelet aggregation; increased thyroid binding globulin (TBG) leading to increased circulating total thyroid hormone, as measured by PBI, T4 by column, or T4 by radioimmunoassay. Free T3 resin uptake is decreased, reflecting the elevated TBG; free T4 concentration is unaltered; impaired glucose tolerance; decreased pregnanediol excretion; reduced response to metyrapone test; reduced serum folate concentration; increased serum triglyceride and phospholipid concentration.

The PBI may decrease during androgen therapy without clinical significance.

Pregnancy Category X: See Contraindications and Boxed Warning above.

Nursing Mothers: As a general principle, the administration of any drug to nursing mothers should be done only when clearly necessary, since many drugs are excreted in human milk.

Adverse Reactions: (See Warnings regarding induction of neoplasia, adverse effects on the fetus, increased incidence of gallbladder disease, and adverse effects similar to those of oral contraceptives, including thromboembolism.) The following additional adverse reactions have been reported with estrogens and androgens:

Genitourinary system: Breakthrough bleeding, spotting, change in menstrual flow; dysmenorrhea; premenstrual-like syndrome; amenorrhea during and after treatment; increase in size of uterine fibromyomata; vaginal candidiasis; change in cervical eversion and in degree of cervical secretion; cystitis-like syndrome.

Breasts: Tenderness, enlargement, secretion.

Gastrointestinal: Nausea, vomiting; abdominal cramps, bloating; cholestatic jaundice.

Skin: Chloasma or melasma which may persist when drug is discontinued; erythema multiforme; erythema nodosum; hemorrhagic eruption; loss of scalp hair; hirsutism; acne.

Eyes: Steepening of corneal curvature; intolerance to contact lenses.

CNS: Headache, migraine, dizziness; mental depression; chorea.

Miscellaneous: Increase or decrease in weight; reduced carbohydrate tolerance; hypercalcemia; aggravation of porphyria; edema; virilization in females; changes in libido; hypersensitivity, including skin manifestations and anaphylactoid reactions.

Acute Overdosage: Numerous reports of ingestion of large doses of estrogen-containing oral contraceptives by young children indicate that serious ill effects do not occur. Overdosage of estrogen may cause nausea, and withdrawal bleeding may occur in females. Excessive quantities of androgen may cause masculinizing effects, such as acne vulgaris, coarsening of body hair, growth of beard, baldness, hoarseness, deepening of the voice and enlargement of the clitoris.

Dosage and Administration: *Given cyclically for short-term use only.*

For treatment of moderate to severe *vasomotor* symptoms associated with the menopause: The lowest dose that will control symptoms should be chosen and medication should be discontinued as promptly as possible. Administration should be cyclic (eg, 3 weeks on and 1 week off). Attempts to discontinue or taper medication should be made at 3- to 6-month intervals. The usual dosage range is one or two GYNETONE ".04" Tablets or one to four GYNETONE ".02" Tablets daily. As soon as menopausal symptoms are controlled, a maintenance dosage of one GYNETONE ".02" Tablet daily or every other day will be adequate in most cases.

Treated patients with an intact uterus should be monitored closely for signs of endometrial cancer and appropriate diagnostic measures should be taken to rule out malignancy in the event of persistent or recurring abnormal vaginal bleeding.

How Supplied: GYNETONE ".02" Tablets, sugar-coated, salmon-pink tablets branded in red with the Schering trademark and either product identification letters, AMT, or numbers, 800; bottle of 100.

GYNETONE ".04" Tablets, sugar-coated, green tablets branded in black with the Schering trademark and either product identification letters, AMU, or numbers, 490; bottle of 100.

Patient package inserts are being dispensed with this product. They are available to physicians upon request. Physicians references available on request.

[*Shown in Product Identification Section*]

HYPERSTAT® I.V. ℞

brand of diazoxide, USP

Injection

FOR INTRAVENOUS USE IN HOSPITALIZED PATIENTS ONLY

Description: HYPERSTAT I.V. Injection is a rapidly acting antihypertensive agent. Each ampule (20 ml.) contains 300 mg. diazoxide USP, a nondiuretic benzothiadiazine derivative, in a clear, colorless, aqueous solution; the pH is adjusted to approximately 11.6 with sodium hydroxide. Diazoxide is 7-chloro-3-methyl-2*H*-1, 2, 4-benzothiadiazine 1, 1-dioxide.

Actions: HYPERSTAT I.V. Injection produces a prompt reduction in blood pressure by relaxing smooth muscle in the peripheral arterioles. Cardiac output is increased as blood pressure is reduced by diazoxide; coronary and cerebral blood flow are maintained. Renal blood flow is increased after an initial decrease. Diazoxide has no known direct action on the central nervous system.

Patients refractory to other antihypertensive agents usually remain responsive to diazoxide. Diazoxide is extensively bound to serum protein (>90%). The plasma half-life is 28 ± 8.3 hours; however, the duration of its antihypertensive effect is variable, generally lasting less than 12 hours. Although an antihypertensive response has been obtained with slow intravenous injection, in general, a greater antihypertensive effect is obtained with rapid intravenous administration.

Continued on next page

Information on Schering products appearing on these pages is effective as of September 30, 1979.

Schering—Cont.

Indications: HYPERSTAT I.V. Injection is indicated for the emergency reduction of blood pressure in malignant hypertension in hospitalized patients, when prompt and urgent decrease of diastolic pressure is required. Treatment with orally effective antihypertensive agents should be instituted as soon as the hypertensive emergency is controlled.
HYPERSTAT I.V. Injection is ineffective against hypertension due to pheochromocytoma.
Contraindications: HYPERSTAT I.V. Injection should not be used in the treatment of compensatory hypertension, such as that associated with aortic coarctation or arteriovenous shunt.
The drug should not be used in patients hypersensitive to diazoxide or other thiazides, unless the potential benefits outweigh the possible risks.
Warnings: Hypotension may occasionally result from the administration of HYPERSTAT I.V. If hypotension severe enough to require therapy occurs, it will usually respond to the administration of sympathomimetic agents, such as norepinephrine.
Hyperglycemia occurs in the majority of patients, but usually requires treatment only in patients with diabetes mellitus; it will respond to the usual management, including insulin. Therefore, blood glucose levels should be monitored, especially in patients with diabetes or in those requiring multiple injections of diazoxide. Hyperglycemia and hyperosmolar coma associated with transient cataracts developed in one infant receiving repeated daily doses of oral diazoxide. The disturbed carbohydrate metabolism was successfully treated with insulin. Cataracts have been observed in a few animals receiving repeated daily doses of intravenous or oral diazoxide.
Since diazoxide causes sodium retention, repeated injections may precipitate edema and congestive heart failure. This retention responds characteristically to diuretic agents if adequate renal function exists. It should be noted that concurrently administered thiazides may potentiate the antihypertensive, hyperglycemic, and hyperuricemic actions of diazoxide (See DRUG INTERACTIONS).
Since increased volume of extracellular fluid may be a cause of treatment failure in nonresponsive patients, it may be advisable to reduce this increased volume by means of a diuretic agent.
Although no evidence of excessive anticoagulant effects has been reported, patients, especially those who are hypoalbuminemic and receive HYPERSTAT I.V. Injection and coumarin or its derivatives, may require reduction in dosage of the anticoagulant (See DRUG INTERACTIONS).
HYPERSTAT I.V. Injection should be administered with caution to patients being treated concurrently with methyldopa or reserpine, or with drugs which act by direct peripheral vasodilatation, especially hydralazine, the nitrites and papaverine-like compounds.
Usage in Pregnancy: The safety of HYPERSTAT I.V. Injection in pregnancy has not yet been established.
Information is not available concerning the passage of HYPERSTAT in breast milk. However, it is known that diazoxide crosses the placental barrier and appears in cord blood. Like other thiazides, the drug may produce fetal or neonatal hyperbilirubinemia, thrombocytopenia, altered carbohydrate metabolism, and possibly other adverse reactions that have occurred in adults.
Usage in Children: The safety of HYPERSTAT I.V. Injection in children has not yet been established.
Precautions: HYPERSTAT (diazoxide) I.V. Injection is a potent antihypertensive agent requiring close monitoring of the patient's blood pressure at frequent intervals. Its administration may occasionally cause hypotension requiring treatment with sympathomimetic drugs. Therefore, adequate facilities to treat such untoward reactions should be available when HYPERSTAT I.V. Injection is used.
HYPERSTAT I.V. Injection should be administered only into a peripheral vein. Because the alkalinity of the solution is irritating to tissue, extravascular injection or leakage should be avoided; subcutaneous administration has produced inflammation and pain without subsequent necrosis. If leakage into subcutaneous tissue occurs, the area should be treated conservatively.
Maximal antihypertensive effects occur after rapid administration (within 30 seconds) into the vein; a slower injection may fail to reduce blood pressure or produce a very brief response.
As with any potent antihypertensive agent, HYPERSTAT I.V. Injection should be used with care in patients who have impaired cerebral or cardiac circulation, that is, patients in whom abrupt and brief reductions in blood pressure might be detrimental or those in whom concurrent tachycardia may be deleterious.
Special attention is required for patients with diabetes mellitus and those in whom retention of salt and water may present serious problems (See Warnings). Nondiabetic patients may have a transient, reversible, and clinically insignificant increase in blood glucose following HYPERSTAT I.V. Injection.
Since peritoneal dialysis or hemodialysis can reduce levels of diazoxide in the blood, patients undergoing dialysis may require more than one injection.
Adverse Reactions:
Frequent and serious adverse reactions: Sodium and water retention after repeated injections, especially important in patients with impaired cardiac reserve; hyperglycemia frequently requiring treatment in diabetic patients, especially after repeated injections.
Infrequent but serious adverse reactions: Hypotension to shock levels; myocardial ischemia, usually transient but possibly leading to thrombosis and manifested by angina, atrial and ventricular arrhythmias, and marked electrocardiographic changes; cerebral ischemia, usually transient but possibly leading to thrombosis and manifested by unconsciousness, convulsions, paralysis, confusion or focal neurological deficit, such as numbness of the hands; persistent retention of nitrogenous wastes after repeated injections; sensitivity reactions, such as rash, leukopenia, and fever. Rarely, acute pancreatitis has been reported. Papilledema, induced by plasma volume expansion secondary to the administration of diazoxide, was reported in one patient who had received eleven injections over a twenty-two day period.
Other adverse reactions: Vasodilative phenomena, such as orthostatic hypotension, sweating, flushing, and generalized or localized sensations of warmth; supraventricular tachycardia and palpitation; bradycardia; various transient neurological findings secondary to alterations in regional blood flow to the brain, such as headache (sometimes throbbing), dizziness, lightheadedness, sleepiness (also reported as lethargy, somnolence or drowsiness), euphoria or "funny feeling", ringing in the ears and momentary hearing loss, and weakness of short duration; chest discomfort or nonanginal "tightness in the chest"; transient hyperglycemia in nondiabetic patients; transient retention of nitrogenous wastes; and various respiratory and gastrointestinal findings secondary to the relaxation of smooth muscle, such as dyspnea, cough and choking sensation; nausea and vomiting and/or abdominal discomfort, anorexia, alteration in taste, parotid swelling, salivation, dry mouth, lacrimation, ileus, constipation and diarrhea. Also, warmth or pain along the injected vein; cellulitus without sloughing and/or phlebitis at the site of extravasation; back pain; and increased nocturia. Apprehension or anxiety, malaise and blurred vision occurred on single occasions.
Drug Interactions: Since diazoxide is highly bound to serum protein, it may displace other substances which are also bound to protein, such as bilirubin or coumarin and its derivatives, resulting in higher blood levels of these substances. A drug interaction has also been reported for oral diazoxide and diphenylhydantoin, such that their concomitant administration may result in a loss of seizure control. These potential interactions must be considered when administering HYPERSTAT I.V. Injection. The concomitant administration of diazoxide with thiazides or other commonly used potent diuretics may potentiate the hyperglycemic, hyperuricemic, and antihypertensive effects of diazoxide. HYPERSTAT I.V. Injection should be administered with caution to patients being treated concurrently with methyldopa or reserpine, or with drugs which act by direct peripheral vasodilatation, especially hydralazine, the nitrites and papaverine-like compounds.
Overdosage: Overdosage of HYPERSTAT I.V. Injection may cause an undesirable hypotension. Usually, this can be controlled with sympathomimetic agents, such as norepinephrine; failure of the blood pressure to rise in response to such an agent suggests that the hypotension may have been caused by something other than diazoxide. Excessive hyperglycemia resulting from overdosage will respond to conventional therapy of hyperglycemia.
Diazoxide may be removed from the blood by peritoneal dialysis or hemodialysis.
Animal Pharmacology and Toxicology: In studies involving a number of species, including the rat, cat, dog, and monkey, diazoxide has been shown to exert significant antihypertensive actions through its direct effect on peripheral arterioles, which neither impairs cardiac function nor seriously diminishes perfusion of kidneys. In addition, in each species tested, including the rat, dog, and monkey, diazoxide elicits hyperglycemia, increased serum-free fatty acids and decreased plasma insulin levels by a mechanism thought to involve both suppression of insulin release and enhanced catecholamine action.
Although the data are not conclusive, reproduction and teratology studies in several species of animals indicate that diazoxide, when administered during the critical period of embryo formation, may interfere with normal fetal development, possibly through altered glucose metabolism. Parturition was occasionally prolonged in animals treated at term.
Dosage and Administration: HYPERSTAT I.V. Injection is administered undiluted and rapidly by intravenous injection. It should only be given into a peripheral vein. Do not administer it intramuscularly, subcutaneously, or into body cavities. Avoid extravasation of the drug into subcutaneous tissues.
The response to HYPERSTAT I.V. Injection varies from patient to patient. Generally, blood pressure decreases within five minutes, often within one to two minutes, to the lowest level achieved. The blood pressure increases relatively rapidly in the next 10 to 30 minutes, and then more slowly over the following two to 12 hours, nearly reaching but rarely exceeding the pretreatment level. The response to successive injections is frequently better than that to the initial injection.
Treatment of hypertensive emergencies with HYPERSTAT I.V. Injection should be limited to a few days and a regimen of oral antihypertensive medications should be instituted as soon as possible.

With the patient recumbent, the contents of one 20 ml. ampule containing 300 mg. of HYPERSTAT I.V. Injection are administered intravenously in 30 seconds or less. Slow intravenous injection may fail to reduce the blood pressure or may produce an exceedingly short response.
Specific dosage is required in children or in unusually large or small patients. This dosage may be calculated on the basis of 5 mg/kg body weight (0.3 ml/kg) (See WARNINGS).
A second administration of HYPERSTAT I.V. Injection may be required for a satisfactory reduction in blood pressure if the first injection fails to give an adequate response within 30 minutes.
Repeated administration of HYPERSTAT I.V. Injection at intervals of four to 24 hours usually will maintain the blood pressure below pretreatment levels until a regimen of oral antihypertensive medication becomes effective. The interval between injections may be adjusted by the duration of the response to each injection. It is usually unnecessary to continue treatment with HYPERSTAT I.V. Injection for more than four to five days.
Following the use of HYPERSTAT I.V. Injection, the blood pressure should be monitored closely until it has stabilized. Thereafter, measurements taken hourly during the balance of the effect will indicate any unusual response. A further decrease in blood pressure at 30 minutes or more after injection should be investigated for causes other than the action of HYPERSTAT I.V. Injection. It is preferable that the patient remain recumbent for half an hour after injection. In ambulatory patients, the blood pressure should be measured with the patient standing before surveillance is ended.
Since repeated administration of HYPERSTAT I.V. Injection can lead to sodium and water retention, administration of a diuretic may be necessary both for maximal blood pressure reduction and to avoid congestive failure.
How Supplied: HYPERSTAT I.V. Injection is supplied in a 20 ml. ampule containing diazoxide 300 mg. in a clear, colorless aqueous solution; box of one ampule.
Protect from light and freezing.
Store between 36° and 86°F (2° and 30°C).

[*Shown in Product Identification Section*]

LOTRIMIN® ℞
brand of clotrimazole
Cream 1%
For Dermatologic Use

Description: LOTRIMIN is clotrimazole [1-(*o*-chloro-*α*,*α*-diphenylbenzyl) imidazole], a synthetic antifungal agent having the chemical formula, $C_{22}H_{17}ClN_2$.
Each gram of LOTRIMIN Cream contains 10 mg. clotrimazole in a vanishing cream base of sorbitan monostearate, polysorbate 60, cetyl esters wax, cetostearyl alcohol, 2-octyldodecanol, purified water and, as preservative, benzyl alcohol (1%).
Actions: Clotrimazole is a broad-spectrum, antifungal agent that inhibits the growth of pathogenic dermatophytes, yeasts, and *Malassezia furfur*. Clotrimazole exhibits fungicidal activity *in vitro* against isolates of *Trichophyton rubrum, Trichophyton mentagrophytes, Epidermophyton floccosum, Microsporum canis,* and *Candida albicans.*
No single-step or multiple-step resistance to clotrimazole has developed during successive passages of *Candida albicans* and *Trichophyton mentagrophytes.*
Indications: LOTRIMIN Cream is indicated for the topical treatment of the following dermal infections: tinea pedis, tinea cruris, and tinea corporis due to *Trichophyton rubrum, Trichophyton mentagrophytes, Epidermophyton floccosum,* and *Microsporum canis;* candidiasis due to *Candida albicans;* and tinea versicolor due to *Malassezia furfur.*
Contraindications: LOTRIMIN Cream is contraindicated in individuals who have shown hypersensitivity to any of its components.
Warnings: LOTRIMIN Cream is not for opthalmic use.
Precautions: In the first trimester of pregnancy, LOTRIMIN Cream should be used only when considered essential to the welfare of the patient.
If irritation or sensitivity develops with the use of LOTRIMIN, treatment should be discontinued and appropriate therapy instituted.
Adverse Reactions: The following adverse reactions have been reported in connection with the use of this product: erythema, stinging, blistering, peeling, edema, pruritus, urticaria, and general irritation of the skin.
Dosage and Administration: Gently massage sufficient LOTRIMIN Cream into the affected and surrounding skin areas twice a day, in the morning and evening.
Clinical improvement, with relief of pruritus, usually occurs within the first week of treatment. If a patient shows no clinical improvement after four weeks of treatment with LOTRIMIN, the diagnosis should be reviewed.
How Supplied: LOTRIMIN Cream 1% is supplied in 15- and 30-gram tubes; boxes of one.
Store between 35° and 86°F.

[*Shown in Product Identification Section*]

LOTRIMIN® ℞
brand of clotrimazole
Solution 1%
For Dermatologic Use

Description: LOTRIMIN is clotrimazole [1-(*o*-chloro-*α*,*α*-diphenylbenzyl) imidazole], a synthetic antifungal agent having the chemical formula, $C_{22}H_{17}ClN_2$.
Each ml. of LOTRIMIN Solution contains 10 mg. clotrimazole in a nonaqueous vehicle of polyethylene glycol 400.
Actions: Clotrimazole is a broad-sprectrum, antifungal agent that inhibits the growth of pathogenic dermatophytes, yeasts, and *Malassezia furfur.* Clotrimazole exhibits fungicidal activity *in vitro* against isolates of *Trichiphyton rubrum, Trichophyton mentagrophytes, Epidermophyton floccosum, Microsporum canis,* and *Candida albicans.*
No single-step or multiple-step resistance to clotrimazle has developed during successive passages of *Candida albicans* and *Trichophyton mentagrophytes.*
Indications: LOTRIMIN Solution is indicated for the topical treatment of the following dermal infections: tinea pedis, tinea cruris, and tinea corporis due to *Trichophyton rubrum, Trichophyton mentagrophytes, Epidermophyton floccosum,* and *Microsporum canis;* candidiasis due to *Candida albicans;* and tinea versicolor due to *Malassezia furfur.*
Contraindications: LOTRIMIN Solution is contraindicated in individuals who have shown hypersensitivity to any of its components.
Warnings: LOTRIMIN Solution is not for ophthalmic use.
Precautions: In the first trimester of pregnancy, LOTRIMIN Solution should be used only when considered essential to the welfare of the patient.
If irritation or sensitivity develops with the use of LOTRIMIN, treatment should be discontinued and appropriate therapy instituted.
Adverse Reactions: The following adverse reactions have been reported in connection with the use of this product: erythema, stinging, blistering, peeling, edema, pruritus, urticaria, and general irritation of the skin.
Dosage and Administration: Gently massage sufficient LOTRIMIN Solution into the affected and surrounding skin areas twice a day, in the morning and evening.
Clinical improvement, with relief of pruritus, usually occurs within the first week of treatment. If a patient shows no clinical improvement after four weeks of treatment with LOTRIMIN, the diagnosis should be reviewed.
How Supplied: LOTRIMIN Solution 1% is supplied in 10 ml. and 30 ml. plastic bottles; boxes of one.
Store between 35° and 86° F.

[*Shown in Product Identification Section*]

METICORTELONE® Acetate ℞
brand of prednisolone acetate, USP
Aqueous Suspension–Sterile

How Supplied: METICORTELONE Acetate Aqueous Suspension, 25 mg. per ml., 5 ml. multiple-dose vial, boxes of one and six.
For complete prescribing information, contact the Schering Professional Services Department.

METICORTEN® ℞
brand of prednisone, U.S.P.
Tablets

How Supplied: METICORTEN **Tablets** (1 mg.): white, unscored, compressed tablets impressed with the Schering trademark and product identification letters, KEM or numbers, 843; bottle of 100.
METICORTEN **Tablets** (5 mg.): white, scored, compressed tablets impressed with the Schering trademark and product identification letters, ABB or numbers, 172; bottles of 100.
For complete prescribing information, contact the Schering Professional Services Department.
[*Shown in Product Identification Section*]

METI-DERM® ℞
brand of prednisolone, USP
Aerosol

How Supplied: METI-DERM Aerosol, 115-gram spray can.
For complete prescribing information, contact the Schering Professional Services Department.

METI-DERM® ℞
brand of prednisolone, USP
Cream 0.5%

How Supplied: METI-DERM Cream 0.5%, 10- and 25-gram tubes; boxes of one.
For complete prescribing information, contact the Schering Professional Services Department.

METIMYD® ℞
brand of prednisolone acetate USP and sulfacetamide sodium, USP
Ophthalmic Suspension—Sterile
Ophthalmic Ointment—Sterile

Description: METIMYD Ophthalmic **Suspension** is a sterile preparation containing in each ml.: 5 mg. prednisolone acetate, USP; 100 mg. sulfacetamide sodium, USP; 5 mg. phenylethyl alcohol and 0.25 mg. benzalkonium chloride as preservatives; disodium hydrogen phosphate, sodium dihydrogen phosphate, tyloxapol, sodium thiosulfate, edetate disodium, and purified water.
METIMYD Ophthalmic **Ointment** is a sterile preparation, each gram containing 5 mg. prednisolone acetate and 100 mg. sulfacetamide sodium, with 0.5 mg. methylparaben and 0.1 mg. propylparaben as preservatives, in a bland

Continued on next page

Information on Schering products appearing on these pages is effective as of September 30, 1979.

Schering—Cont.

unctuous base of mineral oil and white petrolatum.
Actions: METIMYD combines the anti-inflammatory action of prednisolone acetate with the antibacterial properties of sulfacetamide sodium, which is active against most microorganisms which cause external ocular infection. The high solubility of sulfacetamide sodium in water, its low alkalinity, and the almost total lack of irritant action on local application to delicate tissues make it particularly suitable for ophthalmologic use.

Indications

Based on a review of this drug by the National Academy of Sciences—National Research Council and/or other information, FDA has classified the indications as follows:
"Possibly" effective: for the treatment of the following inflammatory and allergic conditions affecting the eyelids and anterior segment of the eye. EYELIDS: allergic blepharitis, blepharitis associated with seborrheic dermatitis and other nonpurulent types of blepharitis. CONJUNCTIVA: allergic conjunctivitis, i.e., vernal, phlyctenular, and other nonpurulent forms of conjunctivitis including those associated with hay fever, and conjunctivitis due to physical agents such as foreign bodies, chemicals (acids, alkalies) and other irritants. CORNEA, SCLERA, IRIS, AND UVEA: interstitial, postoperative, and sclerosing keratitis; chemical and thermal burns of the cornea; corneal ulcer; herpes zoster ophthalmicus; phlyctenular keratoconjunctivitis; corneal neovascularization; scleritis; episcleritis; acute, chronic, and traumatic iridocyclitis.
Final classification of the less-than-effective indications requires further investigation.

In deep-seated infections, such as endophthalmitis, panophthalmitis, and orbital cellulitis, or when systemic infection threatens, specific oral (antibiotic, sulfonamide) therapy should be employed. Local treatment may be used as adjunctive therapy.
Contraindications: The contraindications for METIMYD are the same as those for other corticosteroid-sulfonamide preparations. Topical ophthalmic corticosteroid preparations and combinations are contraindicated in: early acute herpes simplex and the early acute stages of most other viral diseases of the cornea and conjunctiva; active tuberculosis of the anterior segment of the eye; fungal disease of the cornea, conjunctiva and lids; acute purulent untreated infections of the eye which, like other diseases caused by microorganisms, may be masked or enhanced by the presence of the steroid.
METIMYD Ophthalmic **Suspension** and **Ointment** are contraindicated in individuals with known or suspected sensitivity to sulfonamides or to any of the ingredients of the preparation.
Precautions: Whenever it is suspected that the infection is caused by organisms non-sensitive to sulfonamides, supplemental therapy with appropriate antibiotic agents should be included. If the infection fails to respond promptly, the medication should be discontinued and other appropriate measures started.
Extended use of topical steroid therapy may cause increased intraocular pressure in certain individuals. In prolonged therapy, it is advisable that intraocular pressure be checked frequently. In those diseases causing thinning of the cornea, perforation has been known to have occurred with the use of topical steroids. The protracted use of topical corticosteroids in the eye reportedly has been rarely associated with the development of posterior subcapsular cataracts. As with any antibacterial preparation, prolonged use may result in overgrowth of non-susceptible organisms, including fungi. If superinfection occurs, appropriate measures should be instituted.
Sulfonamides are inactivated by the para-aminobenzoic acid present in purulent exudates. METIMYD Ophthalmic **Suspension** and **Ointment** are incompatible with silver preparations. Ophthalmic ointments may retard corneal healing.
Sensitization may recur when a sulfonamide is readministered irrespective of the route of administration, and cross sensitivity between different sulfonamides may occur. If signs of sensitivity or other untoward reactions occur, discontinue use of the preparation.
Adverse Reactions: Sulfacetamide sodium may cause transient stinging or burning, or local irritation.
Although sensitivity reactions to sulfacetamide sodium are rare, an isolated incident of Stevens-Johnson syndrome was reported in a patient who had experienced a previous bullous drug reaction to an orally administered sulfonamide, and a single instance of local hypersensitivity was reported which progressed to a fatal syndrome resembling systemic lupus erythematosus.
Dosage and Administration: Dosage should be adjusted according to the specific needs of the patient.
METIMYD Ophthalmic **Suspension:** Two or three drops should be instilled into the conjunctival sac every hour or two during the day, and less often at night until a favorable response is obtained. Thereafter, the dosage may be reduced, but care should be taken not to discontinue therapy prematurely.
METIMYD Ophthalmic **Ointment:** A thin film should be applied three or four times daily and once or twice at night. In chronic conditions, withdrawal of treatment should be carried out by gradually decreasing the frequency of application.
How Supplied: METIMYD Ophthalmic **Suspension,** 5 ml. dropper bottle, box of one. **Store away from heat, as clumping may occur on long standing at high temperatures. Shake well before using. Protect from light.**
METIMYD Ophthalmic **Ointment,** 3.5 g applicator tube, box of one. **Store away from heat.**

METRETON® ℞
brand of prednisolone sodium phosphate
(0.5% prednisolone phosphate equivalent)
Ophthalmic Solution—Sterile

Description: METRETON Ophthalmic Solution is a clear, sterile, aqueous solution. Each ml. contains 5.5 mg. prednisolone sodium phosphate (equivalent to 5.0 mg. prednisolone phosphate), disodium edetate, monobasic sodium phosphate, dibasic sodium phosphate, tyloxapol, purified water, U.S.P.; sodium hydroxide to adjust pH to approximately 7.8; benzalkonium chloride and phenylethyl alcohol are added as preservatives.
Actions: METRETON Ophthalmic Solution inhibits the inflammatory response to inciting agents of a mechanical, chemical or immunological nature. No generally accepted explanation of this steroid property has been advanced.
Indications: METRETON Ophthalmic Solution is indicated for the treatment of the following conditions. *Ophthalmic:* steroid-responsive inflammatory conditions of the palpebral and bulbar conjunctiva, cornea and anterior segment of the globe, such as allergic conjunctivitis, acne rosacea, superficial punctate keratitis, herpes zoster keratitis, iritis, cyclitis, selected infective conjunctivitis when the inherent hazard of steroid use is accepted to obtain an advisable diminution in edema and inflammation; corneal injury from chemical or thermal burns or penetration of foreign bodies.
Otic: steroid-responsive inflammatory conditions of the external auditory meatus, such as allergic otitis externa, selected purulent and nonpurulent infective otitis externa when the hazard of steroid use is accepted to obtain an advisable diminution in edema and inflammation.
Contraindications: METRETON Ophthalmic Solution should not be used in acute superficial herpes simplex keratitis or in other viral infections of the cornea and conjunctiva, such as vaccinia and varicella.
This drug is contraindicated in patients with perforation of a drum membrane.
METRETON Ophthalmic Solution is contraindicated in patients with tuberculosis of the eye and in those with fungal diseases of ocular or auricular structures.
Hypersensitivity to a component of this medication contraindicates its use.
Warnings: METRETON Ophthalmic Solution is not effective in mustard gas keratitis and in Sjogren's keratoconjunctivitis.
Steroids should be used with great caution in the treatment of stromal herpes simplex; frequent slit-lamp microscopy is mandatory.
Prolonged use of this medication may result in glaucoma, damage to the optic nerve, defects in visual acuity and fields of vision, posterior subcapsular cataract formation, or may aid in the establishment of secondary ocular infections from pathogens liberated from ocular tissues.
In those diseases causing thinning of the cornea or sclera, perforation has been known to occur with the use of topical steriods.
Acute, purulent, untreated infection of the eye or ear may be masked or activity enhanced by the presence of steroid medication.
Usage in Pregnancy The safety of intensive or protracted use of topical steroids during pregnancy has not been substantiated.
Precautions: Since fungal infections of the cornea are particularly prone to develop coincidentally with long-term local steroid applications, fungus invasion must be considered in any persistent corneal ulceration where a steroid is in use or has been used.
Intraocular pressure should be checked frequently.
Adverse Reactions: Glaucoma with optic nerve damage, visual acuity and field defects, posterior subcapsular cataract formation, secondary ocular infections from pathogens, including herpes simplex liberated from ocular tissues, perforation of the globe.
Viral and fungal infections of the cornea may be exacerbated by the application of steroids.
Rarely, stinging or burning may occur.
Dosage and Administration: The duration of treatment will vary with the type of lesion and may extend from a few days to several weeks, depending on therapeutic response. Relapses, more common in chronic, active lesions than in self-limited conditions, usually respond to retreatment.
Eye Instill one or two drops of METRETON Ophthalmic Solution into the conjunctival sac every hour during the day and every two hours during the night as initial therapy. When a favorable response is observed, reduce dosage to one drop every four hours. Later, further reduction in dosage to one drop three or four times daily may suffice to control symptoms.
Ear Clean the aural canal thoroughly and sponge dry. Instill the solution directly into the aural canal. A suggested initial dosage is three or four drops two or three times a day. When a favorable response is obtained, reduce dosage gradually and eventually discontinue.
If preferred, the aural canal may be packed with a gauze wick saturated with solution. Keep the wick moist with the preparation and remove from the ear after 12 to 24 hours.

Treatment may be repeated as often as necessary at the discretion of the physician.

How Supplied: METRETON Ophthalmic Solution, 5-ml. plastic dropper bottle, box of one.

Store away from heat. Protect from light.

MOL-IRON®

Tablets
Liquid
CHRONOSULE Capsules
Tablets with Vitamin C
CHRONOSULE Capsules with Vitamin C

How Supplied: MOL-IRON Tablets—maroon colored tablets, bottles of 100 and 1000; MOL-IRON Liquid—bottles of 16 fl. oz.; MOL-IRON CHRONOSULE Capsules—bottles of 30 and 250; MOL-IRON Tablets with Vitamin C—bottles of 100; MOL-IRON CHRONOSULE Capsules with Vitamin C—bottles of 50.

For complete prescribing information, contact the Schering Professional Services Department.

[*Shown in Product Identification Section*]

NAQUA® ℞

brand of trichlormethiazide, NF
Tablets

Description: NAQUA Tablets contain trichlormethiazide, an antihypertensive agent and diuretic of the benzothiadiazine series having the chemical formula, $C_8H_8Cl_3N_3O_4S_2$. Each NAQUA Tablet contains 2 or 4 mg. trichlormethiazide.

Actions: The mechanism of action results in an interference with the renal tubular mechanism of electrolyte reabsorption. At maximal therapeutic dosage all thiazides are approximately equal in their diuretic potency. The mechanism whereby thiazides function in the control of hypertension is unknown.

Indications: NAQUA Tablets are indicated as adjunctive therapy in edema associated with congestive heart failure, hepatic cirrhosis, and corticosteroid and estrogen therapy.

NAQUA Tablets have also been found useful in edema due to various forms of renal dysfunction, such as: nephrotic syndrome; acute glomerulonephritis; and chronic renal failure.

NAQUA Tablets are indicated in the management of hypertension either as the sole therapeutic agent or to enhance the effectiveness of other antihypertensive drugs in the more severe forms of hypertension.

Usage in Pregnancy The routine use of diuretics in an otherwise healthy woman is inappropriate and exposes the mother and fetus to unnecessary hazard. Diuretics do not prevent development of toxemia in pregnancy, and there is no satisfactory evidence that they are useful in the treatment of developed toxemia. Edema during pregnancy may arise from pathological causes or from the physiologic and mechanical consequences of pregnancy. Thiazides are indicated in pregnancy when edema is due to pathologic causes, just as they are in the absence of pregnancy (however, see WARNINGS, below). Dependent edema in pregnancy, resulting from restriction of venous return by the expanded uterus, is properly treated through elevation of the lower extremities and use of support hose; use of diuretics to lower intravascular volume in this case is illogical and unnecessary. There is hypervolemia during normal pregnancy which is harmful to neither the fetus nor the mother (in the absence of cardiovascular disease), but which is associated with edema, including generalized edema, in the majority of pregnant women. If this edema produces discomfort, increased recumbency will often provide relief. In rare instances, this edema may cause extreme discomfort which is not relieved by rest. In these cases, a short course of diuretics may provide relief and may be appropriate.

Contraindications: NAQUA Tablets are contraindicated in patients with anuria.

Hypersensitivity to this or other sulfonamide-derived drugs is a contraindication to the use of this product.

Warnings: Thiazides should be used with caution in severe renal disease. In patients with renal disease, thiazides may precipitate azotemia. Cumulative effects of the drug may develop in patients with impaired renal function. Thiazides should be used with caution in patients with impaired hepatic function or progressive liver disease, since minor alterations of fluid and electrolyte balance may precipitate hepatic coma.

Thiazides may add to or potentiate the action of other antihypertensive drugs. Potentiation occurs with ganglionic or peripheral adrenergic blocking drugs.

Sensitivity reactions may occur in patients with a history of allergy or bronchial asthma. The possibility of exacerbation or activation of systemic lupus erythematosus has been reported.

Usage in Pregnancy Thiazides cross the placental barrier and appear in cord blood. The use of thiazides in pregnant women requires that the anticipated benefit be weighed against possible hazards to the fetus. These hazards include fetal or neonatal jaundice, thrombocytopenia, and possibly other adverse reactions which have occurred in the adult.

Nursing Mothers Thiazides appear in breast milk. If use of the drug is deemed essential, the patient should stop nursing.

Precautions: Periodic determination of serum electrolytes to detect possible electrolyte imbalance should be performed at appropriate intervals.

All patients receiving thiazide therapy should be observed for clinical signs of fluid or electrolyte imbalance, namely, hyponatremia, hypochloremic alkalosis, and hypokalemia. Serum and urine electrolyte determinations are particularly important when the patient is vomiting excessively or receiving parenteral fluids. Medication such as digitalis may also influence serum electrolytes. Warning signs, irrespective of cause, are: dryness of mouth, thirst, weakness, lethargy, drowsiness, restlessness, muscle pains or cramps, muscular fatigue, hypotension, oliguria, tachycardia, and gastrointestinal disturbances such as nausea and vomiting.

Hypokalemia may develop with thiazides as with any other potent diuretic, especially with brisk diuresis, when severe cirrhosis is present, or during concomitant use of corticosteroids or ACTH.

Interference with adequate oral electrolyte intake will also contribute to hypokalemia. Digitalis therapy may exaggerate metabolic effects of hypokalemia especially with reference to myocardial activity.

Any chloride deficit is generally mild and usually does not require specific treatment except under extraordinary circumstances (as in liver disease or renal disease). Dilutional hyponatremia may occur in edematous patients in hot weather; appropriate therapy is water restriction, rather than administration of salt, except in rare instances when the hyponatremia is life threatening. In actual salt depletion, appropriate replacement is the therapy of choice.

Hyperuricemia may occur or frank gout may be precipitated in certain patients receiving thiazide therapy.

Insulin requirements in diabetic patients may be increased, decreased, or unchanged. Latent diabetes mellitus may become manifest during thiazide administration.

Thiazide drugs may increase the responsiveness to tubocurarine.

The antihypertensive effects of the drug may be enhanced in the post-sympathectomy patient.

Thiazides may decrease arterial responsiveness to norepinephrine. This diminution is not sufficient to preclude effectiveness of the pressor agent for therapeutic use.

If progressive renal impairment becomes evident, as indicated by a rising nonprotein nitrogen or blood urea nitrogen, a careful reappraisal of therapy is necessary with consideration given to withholding or discontinuing diuretic therapy.

Thiazides may decrease serum PBI levels without signs of thyroid disturbance.

Adverse Reactions: *Gastrointestinal System Reactions:* anorexia; gastric irritation; nausea; vomiting; cramping; diarrhea; constipation; jaundice (intrahepatic cholestatic jaundice); pancreatitis.

Central Nervous System Reactions: dizziness; vertigo; paresthesias; headache; xanthopsia.

Hematologic Reactions: leukopenia; agranulocytosis; thrombocytopenia; aplastic anemia.

Dermatologic—Hypersensitivity Reactions: purpura; photosensitivity; rash; urticaria; necrotizing angiitis (vasculitis, cutaneous vasculitis).

Cardiovascular Reaction: Orthostatic hypotension may occur and may be aggravated by alcohol, barbiturates or narcotics.

Other: hyperglycemia; glycosuria; hyperuricemia; muscle spasm; weakness; restlessness.

Whenever adverse reactions are moderate or severe, thiazide dosage should be reduced or therapy withdrawn.

Dosage and Administration: Therapy should be individualized according to patient response. This therapy should be titrated to gain maximal therapeutic response as well as the minimal dose possible to maintain that therapeutic response.

Edematous Conditions The usual dosage of NAQUA Tablets for diuretic effect is 1 to 4 mg. daily.

Hypertension The usual dosage of NAQUA Tablets for antihypertensive effect is 2 to 4 mg. daily.

How Supplied: NAQUA Tablets, 2 mg., pink, clover-shaped, compressed tablets impressed with the letter S and product identification letters, AHG, or numbers 822; bottles of 100 and 1000.

NAQUA Tablets, 4 mg., aqua, clover-shaped, compressed tablets impressed with the letter S and product identification letters, AHH, or numbers 547; bottles of 100 and 1000.

[*Shown in Product Identification Section*]

NAQUIVAL® ℞

brand of trichlormethiazide, NF—reserpine, USP
Tablets

> **Warning**
> This fixed combination drug is not indicated for initial therapy of hypertension. Hypertension requires therapy titrated to the individual patient. If the fixed combination represents the dosage so determined, its use may be more convenient in patient management. The treatment of hypertension is not static, but must be reevaluated as conditions in each patient warrant.

Description: Each NAQUIVAL Tablet contains 4 mg. NAQUA® (brand of trichlormethiazide, NF) and 0.1 mg. reserpine, USP. Trichlormethiazide is an antihypertensive agent and diuretic of the benzothiadiazine series having the chemical formula, $C_8H_8Cl_3N_3O_4S_2$. The

Continued on next page

Information on Schering products appearing on these pages is effective as of September 30, 1979.

Schering—Cont.

antihypertensive agent, reserpine, is a rauwolfia alkaloid having the chemical formula, $C_{33}H_{40}N_2O_9$.
Actions: NAQUIVAL Tablets combine the antihypertensive and diuretic properties of trichlormethiazide with the antihypertensive actions of reserpine; maximum antihypertensive effects are achieved with minimal doses of each ingredient.
Indications: NAQUIVAL Tablets are indicated for the treatment of hypertension (see box warning).
Contraindications: NAQUIVAL Tablets are contraindicated in patients with anuria.
Hypersensitivity to this or other sulfonamide-derived drugs is a contraindication to the use of this product.
The routine use of diuretics in an otherwise healthy pregnant woman with or without mild edema is contraindicated and possibly hazardous.
The presence of an active peptic ulcer, ulcerative colitis, or severe depression contraindicates the use of reserpine.
Warnings: NAQUIVAL Tablets should be withdrawn at least three weeks prior to elective surgery or electroconvulsive therapy because of the reserpine activity.
If parenteral antihypertensive therapy is indicated for a patient receiving NAQUIVAL Tablets, the physician should be alert to the possible synergism of reserpine and trichlormethiazide with such drugs, especially those administered by rapid infusion, e.g., diazoxide.
Sympathomimetics should be used with caution in patients who are receiving reserpine, since its antihypertensive effects may be reduced.
NAQUIVAL Tablets should be used with caution in severe renal disease. In patients with renal disease, thiazides may precipitate azotemia. Cumulative effects of the drug may develop in patients with impaired renal function.
Thiazides should be used with caution in patients with impaired hepatic function or progressive liver disease, since minor alterations of fluid and electrolyte balance may precipitate hepatic coma.
Thiazides may be additive or potentiative of the action of other antihypertensive drugs. Potentiation occurs with ganglionic or peripheral adrenergic blocking drugs or vasodilators.
Sensitivity reactions may occur in patients with a history of allergy or bronchial asthma.
The possibility of exacerbation or activation of systemic lupus erythematosus has been reported.
Usage in Pregnancy Usage of thiazides in women of childbearing age requires that the potential benefits of the drug be weighed against its possible hazards to the fetus. These hazards include fetal or neonatal jaundice, thrombocytopenia, and possibly other adverse reactions which have occurred in the adult.
The safety of reserpine for use during pregnancy or lactation has not been established; therefore, it should be used in pregnant patients or in women of childbearing age only when, in the judgment of the physician, its use is deemed essential to the welfare of the patient.
Nursing Mothers Thiazides cross the placental barrier and appear in cord blood and breast milk.
Precautions: Periodic determination of serum electrolytes to detect possible electrolyte imbalance should be performed at appropriate intervals.
All patients receiving thiazide therapy should be observed for clinical signs of fluid or electrolyte imbalance, namely, hyponatremia, hypochloremic alkalosis, and hypokalemia. Serum and urine electrolyte determinations are particularly important when the patient is vomiting excessively or receiving parenteral fluids. Medication such as digitalis may also influence serum electrolytes. Warning signs, irrespective of cause, are: dryness of mouth, thirst, weakness, lethargy, drowsiness, restlessness, muscle pains or cramps, muscular fatigue, hypotension, oliguria, tachycardia, and gastrointestinal disturbances such as nausea and vomiting.
Hypokalemia may develop with thiazides as with any other potent diuretic, especially with brisk diuresis, when severe cirrhosis is present, or during concomitant use of corticosteroids or ACTH.
Interference with adequate oral electrolyte intake will also contribute to hypokalemia. Digitalis therapy may exaggerate metabolic effects of hypokalemia especially with reference to myocardial activity.
Any chloride deficit is generally mild and usually does not require specific treatment except under extraordinary circumstances (as in liver disease or renal disease). Dilutional hyponatremia may occur in edematous patients in hot weather; appropriate therapy is water restriction, rather than administration of salt, except in rare instances when the hyponatremia is life threatening. In actual salt depletion, appropriate replacement is the therapy of choice.
Hyperuricemia may occur or frank gout may be precipitated in certain patients receiving thiazide therapy.
Insulin requirements in diabetic patients may be increased, decreased, or unchanged. Latent diabetes mellitus may become manifest during thiazide administration.
Thiazide drugs may increase the responsiveness to tubocurarine.
The antihypertensive effects of the drug may be enhanced in the post-sympathectomy patient.
Thiazides may decrease arterial responsiveness to norepinephrine. This diminution is not sufficient to preclude effectiveness of the pressor agent for therapeutic use.
If progressive renal impairment becomes evident, as indicated by a rising nonprotein nitrogen or blood urea nitrogen, a careful reappraisal of therapy is necessary with consideration given to withholding or discontinuing diuretic therapy.
Thiazides may decrease serum PBI levels without signs of thyroid disturbance.
Reserpine may augment secretory and motor activity of the gastrointestinal tract, and gastric hyperacidity, peptic ulceration and mucous colitis may develop. Patients undergoing emergency surgery should be watched for precipitous falls in blood pressure; vasopressor agents such as levarterenol should be available.
Reserpine may precipitate biliary colic in patients with gallstones.
Because of the decreased sympathetic tone caused by reserpine catecholamine depletion, special care should be exercised in treating patients with a history of bronchial asthma.
Adverse Reactions: *Autonomic Reactions:* nasal stuffiness; dryness of the mouth; blurred vision; flushing of the face.
Gastrointestinal System Reactions: anorexia; gastric irritation; nausea; vomiting; cramping; diarrhea; constipation; jaundice (intrahepatic cholestatic jaundice); pancreatitis.
Central Nervous System Reactions: dizziness; vertigo; parasthesias; headache; xanthopsia; depression; central nervous system sensitization manifested as dull sensorium, deafness, glaucoma, uveitis, and optic atrophy.
Hematologic Reactions: leukopenia; agranulocytosis; thrombocytopenia; aplastic anemia.
Dermatologic—Hypersensitivity Reactions: purpura; photosensitivity; rash; urticaria; necrotizing angiitis (vasculitis, cutaneous vasculitis).
Cardiovascular Reactions: Ectopic cardiac rhythms, particularly when used concurrently with digitalis; orthostatic hypotension may occur and may be aggravated by alcohol, barbiturates or narcotics.
Other: hyperglycemia; glycosuria; hyperuricemia; muscle spasm; weakness; restlessness; drowsiness; weight gain; dyspnea; dyskinesia; impotence and decreased libido; conjunctival injection.
Whenever adverse reactions are moderate or severe, NAQUIVAL dosage should be reduced or therapy withdrawn.
Dosage and Administration: The dosage of NAQUIVAL should be determined by individual titration (see box warning).
Initial dosage with NAQUIVAL is frequently one tablet twice a day, with reduction to maintenance levels as therapeutic benefits become manifest. When NAQUIVAL is used with ganglionic blocking agents, careful downward adjustment of these drugs should be made to avoid precipitous blood pressure falls.
How Supplied: NAQUIVAL Tablets: peach-colored, scored, compressed tablets impressed with the Schering Trademark and product identification letters, AHT or numbers, 394; bottles of 100 and 500.

[*Shown in Product Identification Section*]

OPTIMINE® ℞

brand of azatadine maleate
Tablets

Description: OPTIMINE is azatadine maleate, an antihistamine having the chemical formula, $C_{20}H_{22}N_2 \cdot 2C_4H_4O_4$. Each OPTIMINE Tablet contains 1 mg. azatadine maleate.
Actions: Azatadine maleate is an antihistamine with antiserotonin, anticholinergic (drying), and sedative effects. Antihistamines appear to compete with histamine for cell receptor sites on effector cells. Azatadine maleate is related chemically to cyproheptadine.
Indications: OPTIMINE Tablets are indicated for the treatment of perennial and seasonal allergic rhinitis; and chronic urticaria.
Contraindications:
Use in Newborn or Premature Infants
This drug should not be used in newborn or premature infants.
Use in Nursing Mothers
Because of the higher risk of antihistamines for infants generally and for newborns and prematures in particular, antihistamine therapy is contraindicated in nursing mothers.
Use in Lower Respiratory Disease
Antihistamines should NOT be used to treat lower respiratory tract symptoms including asthma.
Antihistamines are also contraindicated in the following conditions: hypersensitivity to azatadine maleate and other antihistamines of similar chemical structure; monamine oxidase inhibitor therapy (See DRUG INTERACTIONS Section).
Warnings: Antihistamines should be used with considerable caution in patients with:
Narrow angle glaucoma
Stenosing peptic ulcer
Pyloroduodenal obstruction
Symptomatic prostatic hypertrophy
Bladder neck obstruction
Use in Children
In infants and children especially, antihistamines in overdosage may cause hallucinations, convulsions, or death.
As in adults, antihistamines may diminish mental alertness in children. In the young child, particularly, they may produce excitation.
Use in Pregnancy
Experience with this drug in pregnant women is inadequate to determine whether there exists a potential for harm to the developing fetus.

Use with CNS Depressants
Azatadine maleate has additive effects with alcohol and other CNS depressants (hypnotics, sedatives, tranquilizers, etc.).
Use in Activities Requiring Mental Alertness
Patients should be warned about engaging in activities requiring mental alertness, such as driving a car or operating appliances, machinery, etc.
Use in Patients approximately 60 years or older
Antihistamines are more likely to cause dizziness, sedation, and hypotension in elderly patients.

Precautions: Azatadine maleate has an atropine-like action and, therefore, should be used with caution in patients with:
- A history of bronchial asthma
- Increased intraocular pressure
- Hyperthyroidism
- Cardiovascular disease
- Hypertension

Adverse Reactions: The most frequent adverse reactions are underlined:
General: Urticaria, drug rash, anaphylactic shock, photosensitivity, excessive perspiration, chills, dryness of mouth, nose and throat.
Cardiovascular System: Hypotension, headache, palpitations, tachycardia, extrasystoles.
Hematologic System: Hemolytic anemia, thrombocytopenia, agranulocytosis.
Nervous System: Sedation, sleepiness, dizziness, disturbed coordination, fatigue, confusion, restlessness, excitation, nervousness, tremor, irritability, insomnia, euphoria, paresthesias, blurred vision, diplopia, vertigo, tinnitus, acute labyrinthitis, hysteria, neuritis, convulsions.
Gastrointestinal System: Epigastric distress, anorexia, nausea, vomiting, diarrhea, constipation.
Genitourinary System: Urinary frequency, difficult urination, urinary retention, early menses.
Respiratory System: Thickening of bronchial secretions, tightness of chest and wheezing, nasal stuffiness.

Drug Interactions: MAO inhibitors prolong and intensify the anticholinergic (drying) effects of antihistamines.

Overdosage: In the event of overdosage, emergency treatment should be started immediately.
Manifestations of antihistamine overdosage may vary from central nervous system depression (sedation, apnea, diminished mental alertness, cardiovascular collapse) to stimulation (insomnia, hallucinations, tremors or convulsions) to death. Other signs and symptoms may be dizziness, tinnitus, ataxia, blurred vision and hypotension. Stimulation is particularly likely in children, as are atropine-like signs and symptoms (dry mouth; fixed, dilated pupils; flushing; hyperthermia and gastrointestinal symptoms).
Treatment—The patient should be induced to vomit, even if emesis has occurred spontaneously. Pharmacologic vomiting by the administration of ipecac syrup is a preferred method. However, vomiting should not be induced in patients with impaired consciousness. The action of ipecac is facilitated by physical activity and by the administration of eight to twelve fluid ounces of water. If emesis does not occur within fifteen minutes, the dose of ipecac should be repeated. Precautions against aspiration must be taken especially in infants and children. Following emesis, any drug remaining in the stomach may be adsorbed by activated charcoal administered as a slurry with water. If vomiting is unsuccessful, or contraindicated, gastric lavage should be performed. Isotonic and one-half isotonic saline are the lavage solutions of choice. Saline cathartics, such as milk of magnesia, draw water into the bowel by osmosis and, therefore, may be valuable for their action in rapid dilution of bowel content. After emergency treatment the patient should continue to be medically monitored.
Treatment of the signs and symptoms of overdosage is symptomatic and supportive. Stimulants (analeptic agents) should not be used. Vasopressors may be used to treat hypotension. Short acting barbiturates, diazepam or paraldehyde may be administered to control seizures. Hyperpyrexia, especially in children, may require treatment with tepid water sponge baths or a hypothermic blanket. Apnea is treated with ventilatory support.

Dosage and Administration: DOSAGE SHOULD BE INDIVIDUALIZED ACCORDING TO THE NEEDS AND THE RESPONSE OF THE PATIENT.
The usual adult dosage is 1 or 2 mg. twice a day.
OPTIMINE TABLETS ARE NOT INTENDED FOR USE IN CHILDREN UNDER 12 YEARS OF AGE.

How Supplied: OPTIMINE Tablets, 1 mg., white, compressed, scored tablets impressed with the Schering trademark and product identification numbers, 282; bottle of 100.

[*Shown in Product Identification Section*]

OPTIMYD® ℞

brand of prednisolone sodium phosphate, USP and sulfacetamide sodium, USP (0.5% Prednisolone Phosphate Equivalent and 10% Sulfacetamide Sodium)
Ophthalmic Solution—Sterile

Description: OPTIMYD Ophthalmic Solution contains in each ml. 5.5 mg. prednisolone sodium phosphate, USP (equivalent to 5.0 mg. of prednisolone phosphate) and 100 mg. of sulfacetamide sodium; sodium thiosulfate, tyloxapol, edetate disodium, monobasic sodium phosphate, dibasic sodium phosphate; sodium hydroxide to adjust pH; purified water, benzalkonium chloride 0.025% and phenylethyl alcohol 0.5% are added as preservatives. It is a clear, sterile aqueous solution.

Actions: OPTIMYD Ophthalmic Solution combines in an aqueous vehicle the anti-inflammatory effect of prednisolone sodium phosphate and the antibacterial action of sulfacetamide sodium. Prednisolone sodium phosphate effectively suppresses the acute exudative phase of many inflammatory conditions involving the anterior segment of the eye, while sulfacetamide sodium exerts a bacteriostatic action against a wide spectrum of sensitive ocular pathogens. Because of their aqueous solubilities and their virtual lack of irritant action, both active ingredients are particularly well adapted to topical ophthalmic therapy.

Indications: OPTIMYD is indicated in the following inflammatory and allergic conditions affecting the eyelids and anterior segment of the eye.
EYELIDS: allergic blepharitis, blepharitis associated with seborrheic dermatitis, and other nonpurulent types of blepharitis.
CONJUNCTIVA: allergic conjunctivitis, i.e., vernal, phlyctenular and other nonpurulent forms of conjunctivitis including that associated with hay fever, and conjunctivitis due to physical agents such as foreign bodies, chemicals (acids, alkalies) and other irritants.
CORNEA, SCLERA, IRIS, UVEA: interstitial, postoperative and sclerosing keratitis; chemical and thermal burns of the cornea; corneal ulcer; herpes zoster ophthalmicus; phlyctenular keratoconjunctivitis; corneal neovascularization; scleritis; episcleritis; acute, chronic and traumatic iridocyclitis.
In deep-seated infections, such as endophthalmitis, panophthalmitis or when systemic infection threatens, specific oral (antibiotic, sulfonamide) therapy should be employed. Local treatment may be used as adjunctive therapy.

Contraindications: Like other topical ophthalmic preparations containing corticosteroids, OPTIMYD Ophthalmic Solution should not be used in acute herpes simplex or in the acute stages of other viral infections of the cornea and conjunctiva.
OPTIMYD Ophthalmic Solution is also contraindicated in the presence of active tuberculosis of the anterior segment of the eye, in fungal infections, and in untreated acute purulent infections of the eye which, like other microorganisms, may be masked or enchanced by the presence of the steroid.
OPTIMYD Ophthalmic Solution is contraindicated in individuals with known or suspected sensitivity to sulfonamides or to any of the ingredients of the preparation.

Precautions: Whenever it is suspected that the infection is caused by organisms non-sensitive to sulfonamides, supplemental therapy with appropriate antibiotic agents should be included. If the infection fails to respond promptly, the medication should be discontinued and other indicated measures started. Prolonged use of topical steroid therapy may cause increased intraocular pressure in certain individuals, and hence, it is advisable that intraocular pressure be checked at regular intervals. In those diseases causing thinning of the cornea, perforation has been known to have occurred with the use of topical steroids.
The protracted use of topical corticosteroids in the eye reportedly has been rarely associated with the development of posterior subcapsular cataracts. Non-susceptible organisms, including fungi, may proliferate with the use of the preparation: if superinfection occurs, appropriate measures should be instituted. Sulfonamides are inactivated by the para-aminobenzoic acid present in purulent exudates. OPTIMYD Ophthalmic Solution is incompatible with silver preparations.
Sensitization may recur when a sulfonamide is readministered irrespective of the route of administration, and cross sensitivity between different sulfonamides may occur. If signs of sensitivity or other untoward reactions occur, discontinue use of the preparation.

Adverse Reactions: Sulfacetamide sodium may cause transient stinging or burning, or local irritation.
Although sensitivity reactions to sulfacetamide sodium are rare, an isolated incident of Stevens-Johnson syndrome was reported in a patient who had experienced a previous bullous drug reaction to an orally administered sulfonamide, and a single instance of local hypersensitivity was reported which progressed to a fatal syndrome resembling systemic lupus erythematosus.

Dosage and Administration: Instill one or two drops of OPTIMYD Ophthalmic Solution into the conjunctival sac every hour during the acute stage; thereafter gradually reduce the frequency of application to a maintenance dose of one or two drops every three to four hours. The duration of treatment will vary with the type and severity of the lesion and should be adjusted according to the patient's progress.

How Supplied: OPTIMYD Ophthalmic Solution, 5 ml. plastic dropper bottle; box of one.
Store away from heat and protect from light.

Continued on next page

Information on Schering products appearing on these pages is effective as of September 30, 1979.

Schering—Cont.

ORETON® ℞
brand of testosterone, NF
Pellets for Subcutaneous Implantation

How Supplied: ORETON Pellets for Subcutaneous Implantation, 75 mg., one Pellet per vial, box of three vials.
For complete prescribing information, contact the Schering Professional Services Department.

ORETON® Methyl ℞
brand of methyltestosterone, USP
Tablets
Buccal Tablets

Description: ORETON Methyl is methyltestosterone, a synthetic androgen having the chemical name, 17β-hydroxy-17-methylandrost-4-en-3-one. It occurs as white or creamy white crystals or crystalline powder and is practically insoluble in water but dissolves readily in organic solvents. It is stable in air, slightly hygroscopic, and affected by light.
ORETON Methyl **Tablets** contain methyltestosterone, USP in strengths of 10 mg. and 25 mg.
Each ORETON Methyl **Buccal Tablet** contains 10 mg. methyltestosterone, USP.
Actions: The androgenic action of methyltestosterone is responsible for maintenance of secondary sexual characteristics, as well as for development of accessory sexual organs in the male. In the eunuch and eunuchoid male androgens stimulate as well as maintain the secondary sexual characteristics.
Androgens influence the closure of epiphyseal lines.
In males and some females, administration of androgens reduces urinary excretion of nitrogen, sodium, potassium, chloride, phosphorus and water.
When administered orally methyltestosterone, unlike testosterone, is sufficiently stable to escape extensive inactivation in the liver.
Testosterone is probably not the active form of the hormone. It is converted by a reductase in target tissues to the more active dihydrotestosterone, which binds to a cytoplasmic protein receptor and is transferred to the nucleus. Increased RNA polymerase activity and increased synthesis of specific RNA and protein result.
The precise mode of action on the target tissues is unknown.
Indications:
In the male: ORETON Methyl is indicated for the treatment of: eunuchoidism and eunuchism; male climacteric when these symptoms are secondary to androgen deficiency; impotence due to androgen deficiency; postpuberal cryptorchidism with evidence of hypogonadism.
In the female: ORETON Methyl is indicated for: prevention of postpartum breast pain and engorgement. There is no satisfactory evidence that this drug prevents or suppresses lactation.
ORETON Methyl is also indicated for palliation of androgen-responsive, advancing, inoperable mammary cancer in women who are more than one year, but less than five years post-menopausal or who have been proven to have a hormone-dependent tumor, as shown by previous beneficial response to castration.
Contraindications: Methyltestosterone is contraindicated in carcinoma of the male breast; known or suspected carcinoma of the prostate; cardiac, hepatic, or renal decompensation; hypercalcemia; impaired liver function; patients easily sexually stimulated; pregnancy; and breast feeding.
A history of hypersensitivity or toxic reactions to methyltestosterone contraindicates its use.
Warnings: Hypercalcemia may occur in immobilized patients and in breast cancer patients. In patients with cancer, hypercalcemia may indicate progression of bony metastases, in which case the drug should be discontinued. Watch female patients closely for signs of virilization. Some effects, such as voice changes, may not be reversible even when the drug is stopped.
Precautions: Patients with cardiac, renal or hepatic derangement may retain sodium and water with resulting edema formation.
Males, especially the elderly, may become overly stimulated.
Priapism or excessive sexual stimulation may develop. Males, especially the elderly, may become overly stimulated. In treating males for symptoms of climacteric, avoid stimulation to the point of increasing the nervous, mental and physical activities beyond the patient's cardiovascular capacity.
Oligospermia and reduced ejaculatory volume may occur after prolonged administration or excessive dosage.
Hypersensitivity and gynecomastia may occur. When any of these effects appear, the androgen should be stopped; if restarted, a lower dosage should be utilized. Use cautiously in young boys to avoid possible premature epiphyseal closure.
The PBI may decrease during androgen therapy without clinical significance.
Adverse Reactions: The side effects of androgen are dependent in large part on dosage. The following adverse reactions have been reported to occur with methyltestosterone: hypersensitivity, including skin manifestations and anaphylactoid reactions; decreased ejaculatory volume; oligospermia; gynecomastia; priapism; hypercalcemia, especially in immobile patients and those with metastatic breast carcinoma; virilization in females, including acne vulgaris, coarsening of body hair, growth of beard, baldness, hoarseness, deepening of the voice, enlargement of clitoris; creatinura.
Buccal tablets may cause stomatitis.
Significant alterations in libido have been reported.
Electrolyte and water retention may occur with attendant possible complications such as edema, dyspnea, confusion and perspiring extremities.
Other than possible nausea, no signs or symptoms would be expected from a single excessive dose of androgens.
BSP elevations, rises in transaminase levels, and cholestatic jaundice may be produced by steroid therapy. If tests show these abnormalities, it is recommended that they be repeated after the drug has been withdrawn for two months. If the androgen is restarted, a lower dosage should be used.
There have been rare reports of hepatocellular neoplasms and peliosis hepatis in association with long-term androgenic-anabolic steroid therapy.
Dosage and Administration: Dosage must be strictly individualized. Daily requirements are best administered in divided doses. The following chart is suggested as an average daily dose guide. Duration of therapy will depend upon the response of the condition being treated and the appearance of adverse reactions.
Note: Buccal tablets have approximately twice the potency of the orally ingested hormone.
[See table below].
Administration of Buccal Tablets: ORETON Methyl **Buccal Tablets** should not be swallowed, since the hormone is meant to be absorbed through the mucous membranes. Place buccal tablet in the upper or lower buccal pouch between the gum and cheek. Avoid eating, drinking, chewing, or smoking while the buccal tablet is in place. Proper oral hygienic measures are particularly important after the use of buccal tablets.
How Supplied: ORETON Methyl **Buccal Tablets,** 10 mg., compressed, lavender-colored, oval tablets impressed with the Schering trademark and product identification letters, BE, or numbers, 970; bottle of 100. Note: Color of tablets may fade; potency and effectiveness are not impaired.
ORETON Methyl **Tablets,** 10 mg., compressed, white, round tablets impressed with the Schering trademark and product identification letters, JD, or numbers, 311; bottle of 100.
ORETON Methyl **Tablets,** 25 mg., compressed, peach-colored, round tablets impressed with the Schering trademark and product identification letters, JE, or numbers, 499; bottle of 100.

[*Shown in Product Identification Section*]

TOTAL AVERAGE DAILY DOSE

Indications	ORETON Methyl Buccal Tablets	ORETON Methyl Tablets
In the male:		
eunuchism and eunuchoidism	5 to 20 mg.	10 to 40 mg.
male climacteric and impotency	5 to 20 mg.	10 to 40 mg.
postpuberal cryptorchidism	15 mg.	30 mg.
In the female:		
postpartum breast pain and engorgement (3 to 5 days)	40 mg.	80 mg.
breast cancer	100 mg.	200 mg.

ORETON® Propionate ℞
brand of testosterone propionate, U.S.P.
Buccal Tablets

How Supplied: ORETON Propionate Buccal Tablets (10 mg.): compressed, oval, pink tablets impressed with the Schering trademark and product identification letters, BJ, or numbers 675; bottle of 100
For complete prescribing information, contact the Schering Professional Services Department.
[*Shown in Product Identification Section*]

OTOBIONE® Otic Suspension ℞

How Supplied: OTOBIONE Otic Suspension, 5 ml. amber glass bottle with sterile dropper packaged separately, units of six.
For complete prescribing information, contact the Schering Professional Services Department.

PERMITIL® ℞
brand of fluphenazine hydrochloride, USP
Tablets, Oral Concentrate, CHRONOTAB® Tablets

Description: PERMITIL **Tablets, Oral Concentrate,** and CHRONOTAB (brand of repeat-action tablet) **Tablets** are formulations of fluphenazine hydrochloride, a phenothia- zine of the piperazine group. PERMITIL CHRONOTAB **Tablets** contain fluphenazine hydrochloride equally distributed between the tablet coating and the core.
Actions: Fluphenazine hydrochloride has actions at all levels of the central nervous system, as well as on other organ systems. However, the mechanism of action is not known.
Indications: PERMITIL **Tablets, Oral Concentrate,** and CHRONOTAB **Tablets** are indicated for the management of manifestations of psychotic disorders.

PERMITIL has not been shown effective in the management of behavioral complications in patients with mental retardation.

Contraindications: PERMITIL is contraindicated in comatose or greatly depressed states due to central nervous system depressants.

Phenothiazines are contraindicated in patients with suspected or established subcortical brain damage, with or without hypothalamic damage, since a hyperthermic reaction with temperatures in excess of 104°F may occur in such patients, sometimes not until 14 to 16 hours after drug administration. Total body ice-packing is recommended for such a reaction; antipyretics may also be useful.

Phenothiazine compounds should not be used in patients receiving large doses of hypnotics.

Patients with special medical disorders, such as mitral insufficiency or pheochromocytoma and patients who have exhibited idiosyncrasy to other centrally acting drugs may experience severe reactions to phenothiazines.

The presence of bone marrow depression, blood dyscrasias, liver damage, or renal insufficiency precludes the use of fluphenazine hydrochloride.

Warnings: Fluphenazine hydrochloride may impair the mental and/or physical abilities required for the performance of hazardous tasks, such as driving a car or operating machinery; therefore, the patient should be warned accordingly.

The use of alcohol should be avoided since additive effects and hypotention may occur.

Since there is no adequate experience in children who have received this drug, safety and efficacy in children have not been established.

Usage in pregnancy: Safe use of fluphenazine hydrochloride during pregnancy and lactation has not been established; therefore, in administering the drug to pregnant patients, nursing mothers, or women who may become pregnant, the possible benefits must be weighed against the possible hazards to mother and child.

Precautions: Fluphenazine hydrochloride should be used cautiously in patients who have developed cholestatic jaundice, dermatoses, or other allergic reactions to phenothiazine derivatives.

Psychotic patients on large doses of a phenothiazine drug who are undergoing surgery should be watched carefully for possible hypotensive phenomena. Moreover, reduced amounts of anesthetics or central nervous system depressants may be necessary.

Hepatic function, blood, and renal function should be checked periodically. The appearance of signs of blood dyscrasias requires the discontinuance of the drug and institution of appropriate therapy. Renal function in patients on long-term therapy should be monitored; if blood urea nitrogen (BUN) becomes abnormal, treatment with fluphenazine hydrochloride should be discontinued.

Use with caution in patients who are receiving barbiturates, narcotics, or other central nervous system depressants. Because phenothiazines may prolong and intensify the central nervous system depressant action, a low initial dose is recommended.

Use with caution in patients who are receiving atropine or related drugs because of additive anticholinergic effects and also in patients who will be exposed to extreme heat or phosphorus insecticides.

In patients who are seizure prone, phenothiazines may lower the convulsive threshold. Adequate anticonvulsant medication must be maintained concomitantly.

Use with caution in patients suffering from respiratory impairment due to acute pulmonary infections, or in chronic respiratory disorders, such as severe asthma or emphysema.

The antiemetic effect may obscure the diagnosis of such conditions as brain tumor, intestinal obstruction, and toxicity of other drugs.

In general, phenothiazines, including fluphenazine hydrochloride, do not produce psychic dependence. Gastritis, nausea and vomiting, dizziness, and tremulousness have been reported following abrupt cessation of high-dose therapy. Reports suggest that these symptoms can be reduced by continuing concomitant antiparkinson agents for several weeks after the phenothiazine is withdrawn.

The possibility of liver damage, corneal and lenticular deposits, and irreversible dyskinesias should be kept in mind when patients are on long-term therapy.

Adverse Reactions: Not all of the following adverse reactions have been reported with this specific drug; however, pharmacological similarities among various phenothiazine derivatives require that each be considered. In the case of the piperazine group (of which fluphenazine hydrochloride is an example), the extrapyramidal symptoms are more common, and others (eg, sedative effects, jaundice, and blood dyscrasias) are less frequently seen.

Sudden death has occasionally been reported in patients who have received phenothiazines. In some cases, the death was apparently due to cardiac arrest; in others, the cause appeared to be asphyxia due to failure of the cough reflex. In some patients, the cause could not be determined, nor could it be established that the death was due to the phenothiazine.

Drowsiness may occur particularly during the first or second week, after which it generally disappears. If troublesome, lower the dosage.

Jaundice usually occurs between the second and fourth weeks and is regarded as a sensitivity reaction. Incidence is low. The clinical picture resembles infectious hepatitis with laboratory features of obstructive jaundice. It is usually reversible; however, chronic jaundice has been reported. An increase in cephalin flocculation, sometimes accompanied by alterations in other liver function tests, has been reported in patients receiving fluphenazine hydrochloride who have had no clinical evidence of liver damage.

Hematological disorders occurring include agranulocytosis, eosinophilia, leukopenia, hemolytic anemia, thrombocytopenic purpura, and pancytopenia. Most cases of agranulocytosis have occurred between the fourth and tenth weeks of therapy. Patients should be watched closely during that period for the sudden appearance of sore throat or other signs of infection. If white blood and differential counts show significant cellular depression, discontinue the drug and start appropriate therapy. However, a slightly lowered white count is not in itself an indication to discontinue the drug.

Cardiovascular disorders include postural hypotension, tachycardia (especially with sudden marked increase in dosage), bradycardia, cardiac arrest, faintness, and dizziness. Occasionally, the hypotensive effect may produce a shock-like condition. In the event a vasoconstrictor is required, levarterenol and phenylephrine are the most suitable. Other pressor agents, including epinephrine, should not be used because the blood pressure may be lowered further.

ECG changes, nonspecific, usually reversible, have been observed in some patients receiving phenothiazine tranquilizers.

CNS effects including neuromuscular (extrapyramidal) reactions are usually dosage related and take three forms (1) pseudoparkinsonism, (2) akathisia (motor restlessness), and (3) dystonias. Dystonias include spasms of the neck muscles, extensor rigidity of back muscles, carpopedal spasm, eyes rolled back, convulsions, trismus, and swallowing difficulties. These resemble serious neurological disorders but usually subside within 48 hours. Management of the extrapyramidal symptoms, depending upon the type and severity, includes sedation, injectable diphenhydramine, and the use of antiparkinsonism agents.

Persistent tardive dyskinesia: As with all antipsychotic agents, tardive dyskinesia may appear in some patients on long-term therapy or may appear after drug therapy has been discontinued. The risk appears to be greater in elderly patients on high-dose therapy, especially females. The symptoms are persistent and in some patients appear to be irreversible. The syndrome is characterized by rhythmical involuntary movements of the tongue, face, mouth or jaw (eg, protrusion of tongue, puffing of cheeks, puckering of mouth, chewing movements). Sometimes these may be accompanied by involuntary movements of extremities. There is no known effective treatment for tardive dyskinesia; anti-parkinsonism agents usually do not alleviate the symptoms of this syndrome. It is suggested that all antipsychotic agents be discontinued if these symptoms appear. Should it be necessary to reinstitute treatment, or increase the dosage of the agent, or switch to a different antipsychotic agent, the syndrome may be masked. It has been reported that fine vermicular movements of the tongue may be an early sign of the syndrome, and if the medication is stopped at that time, the syndrome may not develop.

Hyperreflexia has been reported in the newborn when a phenothiazine was used during pregnancy.

Other CNS effects include cerebral edema; abnormality of cerebrospinal fluid proteins; convulsive seizures, particularly in patients with EEG abnormalities or a history of such disorders; and headaches.

Adverse behavioral effects include paradoxical exacerbation of psychotic symptoms, catatonic-like states, paranoid reactions, lethargy, restlessness, hyperactivity, nocturnal confusion, and bizarre dreams.

Allergic reactions include urticaria, itching, erythema, and photosensitivity (avoid undue exposure to the sun), and eczema. Severe reactions include exfoliative dermatitis (rare), contact dermatitis in nursing personnel administering the drug, asthma, laryngeal edema, angioneurotic edema, anaphylactoid reactions, and fever.

Endocrine disorders include lactation and moderate breast enlargement in females and gynecomastia in males on large doses, changes in libido, inhibition of ejaculation, false positive pregnancy tests, amenorrhea, hyperglycemia, hypoglycemia, and glycosuria.

Autonomic reactions include dry mouth, nasal congestion, pallor, constipation, adynamic ileus, myosis, mydriasis, urinary retention, fecal impaction, incontinence, nausea, vomiting, diarrhea, salivation, polyuria, perspiration, blurred vision, glaucoma, and bladder paralysis.

Special considerations in long-term therapy include pigmentation of the skin, occurring chiefly in the exposed areas; ocular changes consisting of deposition of fine particulate matter in the cornea and lens, progression in more severe cases to star-shaped lenticular opacities; epithelial keratopathies; and pigmentary retinopathy.

Other adverse reactions include alterations in appetite and weight, peripheral edema, parotid swelling (rare), hyperpyrexia, and systemic lupus erythematosus-like syndrome.

Dosage and Administration: In all cases the smallest effective dose should be used. Doses should be initiated at a low level and increased gradually to determine clinical response. Patients who are acutely ill may respond to lower doses than those who are chronically ill. Acutely ill patients may require a rapid increase of dosage. Elderly and debilitated patients and adolescents may respond to low dosages. Outpatients should receive smaller dos-

Continued on next page

Information on Schering products appearing on these pages is effective as of September 30, 1979.

Schering—Cont.

ages than are given to hospitalized patients who are under close supervision.
Adults: The total daily dose ranges from 0.5 mg. to 10 mg. and is usually administered in divided doses. In general, a daily dose in excess of 3 mg. is rarely necessary. A dose in excess of 20 mg. should be used with caution.
Administration of an adequate dose should be continued for sufficiently long periods in order to obtain maximum benefits. After maximum therapeutic response is obtained, dosage may be decreased gradually to a maintenance level.
Geriatric patients: Reduced dosage is usually recommended.
PERMITIL **Oral Concentrate** is a palatable liquid preparation, suitable for administration with the following diluents: water, saline, Seven-Up, homogenized milk, carbonated orange beverage, and pineapple, apricot, prune, orange, V-8, grape, tomato, and grapefruit juices.
PERMITIL CHRONOTAB **Tablets** are suggested for those conditions in which a prolonged effect from a single tablet is desired.
Overdosage: Manifestations One of three clinical pictures may be seen: (1) extreme somnolence; patient can usually be roused, but if permitted, will fall asleep; general condition is usually satisfactory; the skin, though pale, is warm and dry; slight blood pressure, respiratory, and pulse changes may occur but are not a problem; (2) mild to moderate drop in blood pressure (patient may be conscious or unconscious); skin is markedly gray but warm and dry; nail beds are pink; respiration is slow and regular; pulse is strong but the rate slightly increased; (3) severe hypotension, possibly accompanied by weakness, cyanosis, perspiration, rapid thready pulse and respiratory depression.
Treatment Essentially symptomatic and supportive. Early gastric lavage and intestinal purges may help. Centrally acting emetics will not help because of the antiemetic effect of fluphenazine hydrochloride. Give hot tea or coffee.
Severe hypotension usually responds to measures described under hypotensive effects (ADVERSE REACTIONS: Cardiovascular). Additional measures include pressure bandages to lower limbs, oxygen, and intravenous fluids.
Avoid stimulants that may cause convulsions (eg, picrotoxin and pentylenetetrazol).
Limited experience with dialysis indicates that it is not helpful.
How Supplied: PERMITIL **Tablets,** 0.25 mg., sugar-coated, bright green tablets branded in black with the Schering trademark and product identification letters, WBK, or numbers, 122; bottle of 100.
PERMITIL **Tablets,** 2.5 mg., compressed, scored, light orange, oval tablets impressed with the Schering trademark and product identification letters, WDR, or numbers, 442; bottle of 100.
PERMITIL **Tablets,** 5 mg., compressed, scored, purple-pink, oval tablets impressed with the Schering trademark and product identification letters, WFF, or numbers, 550; bottle of 100.
PERMITIL **Tablets,** 10 mg., compressed, scored, light red, oval tablets impressed with the Schering trademark and product identification letters, WFG, or numbers, 316; bottle of 1000.
PERMITIL **Oral Concentrate,** 5 mg. per ml., a straw-colored, unflavored syrup; bottle of 4 fluid ounces (118 ml), with dropper calibrated both in mg. of fluphenazine hydrochloride and in ml. of concentrate. **Protect from light and dispense only in amber bottles.**
PERMITIL CHRONOTAB **Tablets,** 1 mg., sugar-coated, yellow tablets branded in black with the Schering trademark and product identification letters, WKJ, or numbers, 840; bottles of 60 and 250.

[*Shown in Product Identification Section*]

POLARAMINE® ℞
brand of dexchlorpheniramine maleate, NF
REPETABS® Tablets
Syrup
Expectorant
Tablets

Description: POLARAMINE products contain dexchlorpheniramine maleate, NF, an antihistamine having the chemical name, (+)-2-[*p*-chloro-α-[2-(dimethylamino) ethyl]benzyl] pyridine maleate (1:1). It is available as REPETABS (brand of repeat-action tablets) **Tablets,** 2 or 3 mg. in an outer layer for prompt effect and 2 or 3 mg. in an inner core for release three to six hours after ingestion; **Syrup,** 2 mg. per 5 ml., in a pleasant-tasting vehicle containing approximately six percent alcohol; **Expectorant,** 2 mg. dexchlorpheniramine maleate, 20 mg. pseudoephedrine sulfate, 100 mg. guaifenesin, NF and 7.2% alcohol per 5 ml.; and 2 mg. **Tablets.**
Actions: Dexchlorpheniramine maleate effectively antagonizes many of the characteristic effects of histamine and is therefore of value clinically in the prevention and relief of many allergic manifestations.
POLARAMINE **Expectorant** combines the antihistaminic actions of dexchlorpheniramine maleate with the vasoconstrictive properties of pseudoephedrine sulfate; guaifenesin increases respiratory tract fluid output and eases expectoration.
Indications: POLARAMINE REPETABS **Tablets, Syrup,** and **Tablets** are indicated for the symptomatic relief of some of the allergic conditions, such as hay fever, urticaria, angioedema, vasomotor rhinitis, allergic eczema, atopic dermatitis, contact dermatitis (including poisoning by ivy or oak), drug and serum reactions, insect bites, pruritus ani and vulvae, and pruritus of nonspecific origin. Allergic migraine and allergic asthma exhibit a variable but often beneficial response. Some cases of asthma, spasmodic bronchial cough and migraine respond favorably to POLARAMINE **Tablets** or **Syrup.** POLARAMINE **Tablets** and **Syrup** can be used for the prevention and treatment of allergic reactions to injections of allergic substances.
POLARAMINE **Expectorant** is indicated for relief of coughs and complications associated with allergic disorders and allergic manifestations of respiratory illnesses, such as hay fever, vasomotor rhinitis and selected cases of asthma.
Precautions: Since drowsiness may occur, caution patients against engaging in mechanical operations requiring alertness, such as driving an automobile, until their response has been determined.
Although pseudoephedrine in the **Expectorant** causes virtually no pressor effect in normotensive patients, it should be used with caution in patients with hypertension.
Adverse Reactions: One of the principle advantages of POLARAMINE is its relative freedom from side effects, such as are frequently encountered with some antihistamine drugs. Certain patients may, however, respond to antihistamine drugs by becoming drowsy, dizzy or nauseated. Other possible side effects include restlessness, dry mouth, weakness, anorexia, headache, nervousness, polyuria, heartburn, diplopia, sweating, dysuria, and very rarely, dermatitis.
Dosage and Administration: REPETABS **Tablets,** 4 mg.: Adults—Usual dosage is one in the morning and one before retiring. For the treatment of certain resistant cases, it may be desirable to administer two REPETABS **Tablets** in the morning and two at night.
REPETABS **Tablets,** 6 mg.: Adults—Usual dose is one REPETABS **Tablet** in the morning and one before retiring. For the treatment of certain resistant cases, it may be desirable to administer one every 8 hours.
Syrup: Adults—one teaspoonful 3 or 4 times daily; Children under 12—one-half teaspoonful 3 or 4 times daily; Infants—one-quarter teaspoonful 3 or 4 times daily.
Expectorant: Adults—one or two teaspoonfuls 3 or 4 times daily; Children 6 to 12 years—one-half to one teaspoonful 3 or 4 times daily; Children 2 to 6 years—one-quarter to one-half teaspoonful 3 or 4 times daily.
Tablets: Adults—one tablet 3 or 4 times daily; in some patients, one-half tablet is adequate. Children under 12 years—one-half tablet 3 or 4 times daily; infants—one-quarter tablet is sufficient.
How Supplied: POLARAMINE REPETABS **Tablets,** 4 mg., light red, sugar-coated, oval tablets branded in blue-black with the Schering trademark and product identification letters, AGA or numbers 095; bottle of 100.
POLARAMINE REPETABS **Tablets,** 6 mg., bright red, sugar-coated, oval tablets branded in white with the Schering trademark and product identification letters, AGB or numbers 148; bottles of 100 and 1000.
POLARAMINE **Syrup,** 2 mg. per 5 ml., red-orange-colored liquid; 16 fluid ounce (473 ml) bottle.
POLARAMINE **Expectorant,** 2 mg. per 5 ml., orange-colored liquid; 16 fluid ounce (473 ml) bottle.
POLARAMINE **Tablets,** 2 mg., red, compressed, oval tablets impressed with the Schering trademark and product identification letters, AGT or numbers 820; bottle of 100.

[*Shown in Product Identification Section*]

PRANTAL® ℞
brand of diphemanil methylsulfate, NF
Tablets

How Supplied: PRANTAL Tablets, 100 mg., bottle of 100.
For complete prescribing information, contact the Schering Professional Services Department.
[*Shown in Product Identification Section*]

PROGLYCEM® ℞
brand of diazoxide, USP
Capsules
Suspension
FOR ORAL ADMINISTRATION

Description: PROGLYCEM (diazoxide; 7-chloro-3-methyl-2*H*-1, 2, 4-benzothiadiazine 1, 1-dioxide) is a benzothiadiazine derivative. PROGLYCEM **Capsules** contain either 50 or 100 mg. diazoxide, USP. The **Suspension** contains 50 mg. of diazoxide, USP in each milliliter and has a chocolate-mint flavor; alcohol content is approximately 7.25%.
Actions: Diazoxide administered orally produces a prompt dose-related increase in blood glucose level, due primarily to an inhibition of insulin release from the pancreas, and also to an extrapancreatic effect.
The hyperglycemic effect begins within an hour and generally lasts no more than eight hours in the presence of normal renal function.
PROGLYCEM decreases the excretion of sodium and water, resulting in fluid retention which may be clinically significant.
The effects on blood pressure are usually not marked with the oral preparation. This contrasts with the intravenous preparation of diazoxide (see Adverse Reactions).
Other pharmacologic actions of PROGLYCEM include increased pulse rate; increased serum uric acid levels due to decreased excretion; increased serum levels of free fatty acids; decreased chloride excretion; decreased para-aminohippuric acid (PAH) clearance with no

appreciable effect on glomerular filtration rate.
The concomitant administration of a benzothiazide diuretic may intensify the hyperglycemic and hyperuricemic effects of PROGLYCEM. In the presence of hypokalemia, hyperglycemic effects are also potentiated.
PROGLYCEM-induced hyperglycemia is reversed by the administration of insulin or tolbutamide.
The inhibition of insulin release by PROGLYCEM is antagonized by alpha-adrenergic blocking agents.
PROGLYCEM is extensively bound (more than 90%) to serum proteins, and is excreted by the kidneys. The plasma half-life following i.v. administration is 28±8.3 hours. Limited data on oral administration revealed a half-life of 24 and 36 hours in two adults. In four children aged four months to six years, the plasma half-life varied from 9.5 to 24 hours on long-term oral administration. The half-life may be prolonged following overdosage, and in patients with impaired renal function.

Indications: PROGLYCEM (oral diazoxide) is useful in the management of hypoglycemia due to hyperinsulinism associated with the following conditions:
Adults: Inoperable islet cell adenoma or carcinoma, or extrapancreatic malignancy.
Infants and Children: Leucine sensitivity, islet cell hyperplasia, nesidioblastosis, extrapancreatic malignancy, islet cell adenoma, or adenomatosis. PROGLYCEM may be used preoperatively as a temporary measure, and postoperatively, if hypoglycemia persists.
PROGLYCEM should be used only after a diagnosis of hypoglycemia due to one of the above conditions has been definitely established. When other specific medical therapy or surgical management either has been unsuccessful or is not feasible, treatment with PROGLYCEM should be considered.

Contraindications: The use of PROGLYCEM for functional hypoglycemia is contraindicated. The drug should not be used in patients hypersensitive to diazoxide or to other thiazides unless the potential benefits outweigh the possible risks.

Warnings: The antidiuretic property of diazoxide may lead to significant fluid retention, which in patients with compromised cardiac reserve, may precipitate congestive heart failure. The fluid retention will respond to conventional therapy with diuretics.
It should be noted that concomitantly administered thiazides may potentiate the hyperglycemic and hyperuricemic actions of diazoxide (see Drug Interactions and Animal Pharmacology and Toxicology).
Ketoacidosis and nonketotic hyperosmolar coma have been reported in patients treated with recommended doses of PROGLYCEM usually during intercurrent illness. Prompt recognition and treatment are essential (see Overdosage), and prolonged surveillance following the acute episode is necessary because of the long drug half-life of approximately 30 hours. The occurrence of these serious events may be reduced by careful education of patients regarding the need for monitoring the urine for sugar and ketones and for prompt reporting of abnormal findings and unusual symptoms to the physician.
Transient cataracts occurred in association with hyperosmolar coma in an infant, and subsided on correction of the hyperosmolarity. Cataracts have been observed in several animals receiving daily doses of intravenous or oral diazoxide.
Usage in Pregnancy: Reproduction studies using the oral preparation in rats have revealed increased fetal resorptions and delayed parturition, as well as fetal skeletal anomalies; evidence of skeletal and cardiac teratogenic effects in rabbits has been noted with intravenous administration. The drug has also been demonstrated to cross the placental barrier in animals and cause degeneration of the fetal pancreatic beta cells (see Animal Pharmacology and Toxicology). Since there are no adequate data on fetal effects of this drug when given to pregnant women, safety in pregnancy has not been established. When the use of PROGLYCEM in pregnant women is considered, the indications should be limited to those specified above for adults (see Indications), and the potential benefits to the mother must be weighed against possible harmful effects to the fetus.

Precautions: Treatment with PROGLYCEM should be initiated under close clinical supervision, with careful monitoring of blood glucose and clinical response until the patient's condition has stabilized. This usually requires several days. If not effective in two to three weeks, the drug should be discontinued.
Prolonged treatment requires regular monitoring of the urine for sugar and ketones, especially under stress conditions, with prompt reporting of any abnormalities to the physician. Additionally, blood sugar levels should be monitored periodically by the physician to determine the need for dose adjustment.
The effects of diazoxide on the hematopoietic system and the level of serum uric acid should be kept in mind; the latter should be considered particularly in patients with hyperuricemia or a history of gout.
In some patients, higher blood levels have been observed with the liquid than with the capsule formulation of PROGLYCEM. Dosage should be adjusted as necessary in individual patients if changed from one formulation to the other.
Since the plasma half-life of diazoxide is prolonged in patients with impaired renal function, a reduced dosage should be considered. Serum electrolyte levels should also be evaluated for such patients.
The antihypertensive effect of other drugs may be enhanced by PROGLYCEM, and this should be kept in mind when administering it concomitantly with antihypertensive agents.
Because of protein binding, administration of PROGLYCEM with coumarin or its derivatives may require reduction in the dosage of the anticoagulant, although there has been no reported evidence of excessive anticoagulant effect. In addition, PROGLYCEM may possibly displace bilirubin from albumin; this should be kept in mind particularly when treating newborns with increased bilirubinemia.

Adverse Reactions:
Frequent and Serious: *Sodium and fluid retention* is most common in young infants and in adults and may precipitate congestive heart failure in patients with compromised cardiac reserve. It usually responds to diuretic therapy (see Drug Interactions).
Infrequent but Serious: Diabetic ketoacidosis and hyperosmolar nonketotic coma may develop very rapidly. Conventional therapy with insulin and restoration of fluid and electrolyte balance are usually effective if instituted promptly. Prolonged surveillance is essential in view of the long half-life of PROGLYCEM (see Overdosage).
Other frequent adverse reactions are: *Hirsutism* of the lanugo type, mainly on the forehead, back and limbs, occurs most commonly in children and women and may be cosmetically unacceptable. It subsides on discontinuation of the drug.
***Hyperglycemia* or *glycosuria* may require re**duction in dosage in order to avoid progression to ketoacidosis or hyperosmolar coma.
***Gastrointestinal intolerance* may include anorexia, nausea, vomiting, abdominal pain, ileus, diarrhea, transient loss of taste. *Tachycardia, palpitations, increased levels of serum uric acid* are common.**
***Thrombocytopenia* with or without *purpura* may require discontinuation of the drug. *Neutropenia* is transient, is not associated with increased susceptibility to infection, and ordinarily does not require discontinuation of the drug. *Skin rash, headache, weakness,* and *malaise* may also occur.**
Other adverse reactions which have been observed are:
Cardiovascular: Hypotension occurs occasionally, which may be augmented by thiazide diuretics given concurrently. A few cases of transient hypertension, for which no explanation is apparent, have been noted. Chest pain has been reported rarely.
Hematologic: eosinophilia; decreased hemoglobin/hematocrit; excessive bleeding; decreased IgG. *Hepato-renal:* increased SGOT, alkaline phosphatase; azotemia, decreased creatinine clearance, reversible nephrotic syndrome, decreased urinary output, hematuria, albuminuria. *Neurologic:* anxiety, dizziness, insomnia, polyneuritis, paresthesia, pruritus, extrapyramidal signs. *Ophthalmologic:* transient cataracts, subconjunctival hemorrhage, ring scotoma, blurred vision, diplopia, lacrimation. *Skeletal, integumentary;* monilial dermatitis, herpes, advance in bone age; loss of scalp hair. *Systemic:* fever, lymphadenopathy. *Other:* gout, acute pancreatitis/pancreatic necrosis, galactorrhea, enlargement of lump in breast.

Drug Interactions: Since diazoxide is highly bound to serum protein, it may displace other substances which are also bound to protein, such as bilirubin or coumarin and its derivatives, resulting in higher blood levels of these substances. A drug interaction has also been reported for oral diazoxide and diphenylhydantoin, such that their concomitant administration may result in a loss of seizure control. These potential interactions must be considered when administering PROGLYCEM Capsules or Suspension. The concomitant administration of thiazides or other commonly used potent diuretics may potentiate the hyperglycemic and hyperuricemic effects of diazoxide.

Dosage and Administration: Patients should be under close clinical observation when treatment with PROGLYCEM is initiated. The clinical response and blood glucose level should be carefully monitored until the patient's condition has stabilized satisfactorily; in most instances, this may be accomplished in several days. If administration of PROGLYCEM is not effective after two or three weeks, the drug should be discontinued.
The dosage of PROGLYCEM must be individualized based on the severity of the hypoglycemic condition and the blood glucose level and clinical response of the patient. The dosage should be adjusted until the desired clinical and laboratory effects are produced with the least amount of the drug. Special care should be taken to assure accuracy of dosage in infants and young children.
Adults and children: The usual daily dosage is 3 to 8 mg/kg, divided into two or three equal doses every 8 or 12 hours. In certain instances, patients with refractory hypoglycemia may require higher dosages. Ordinarily, an appropriate starting dosage is 3 mg/kg/day, divided into three equal doses every eight hours. Thus, an average adult would receive a starting dosage of approximately 200 mg. daily.
Infants and newborns: The usual daily dosage is 8 to 15 mg/kg, divided into two or three equal doses every 8 or 12 hours. An appropriate starting dosage is 10 mg/kg/day, divided into three equal doses every eight hours.

Overdosage: An overdosage of PROGLYCEM causes marked hyperglycemia which may be associated with ketoacidosis. It will respond to prompt insulin administration and restoration of fluid and electrolyte balance. Because of the

Continued on next page

Information on Schering products appearing on these pages is effective as of September 30, 1979.

Schering—Cont.

drug's long half-life (approximately 30 hours), the symptoms of overdosage require prolonged surveillance for periods up to seven days, until the blood sugar level stabilizes within the normal range. One investigator reported successful lowering of diazoxide blood levels by peritoneal dialysis in one patient and by hemodialysis in another.

How Supplied: PROGLYCEM **Capsules,** 50 mg., half opaque, orange and half clear capsules, branded in black with the Schering trademark and product identification letters, PBA, or numbers, 205; bottle of 100.

PROGLYCEM **Capsules,** 100 mg., opaque orange capsules, branded in black with the Schering trademark and product identification letters, PBB, or numbers, 830; bottle of 100.

PROGLYCEM **Suspension,** 50 mg/ml, a chocolate-mint flavored suspension; bottle of 30 ml. with dropper calibrated to deliver 10, 20, 30, 40 and 50 mg. diazoxide. Shake well before each use. Protect from light.

Animal Pharmacology and Toxicology: Oral diazoxide in the mouse, rat, rabbit, dog, pig, and monkey produces a rapid and transient rise in blood glucose levels. In dogs, increased blood glucose is accompanied by increased free fatty acids, lactate, and pyruvate in the serum. In mice, a marked decrease in liver glycogen and an increase in the blood urea nitrogen level occur.

In acute toxicity studies, the LD_{50} for oral diazoxide suspension is >5000 mg/kg in the rat, >522 mg/kg in the neonatal rat, between 1900 and 2572 mg/kg in the mouse, and 210 mg/kg in the guinea pig. Although the oral LD_{50} was not determined in the dog, a dosage of up to 500 mg/kg was well tolerated.

In subacute oral toxicity studies, diazoxide at 400 mg/kg in the rat produced growth retardation, edema, increases in liver and kidney weights, and adrenal hypertrophy. Daily dosages up to 1080 mg/kg for three months produced hyperglycemia, an increase in liver weight and an increase in mortality. In dogs given oral diazoxide at approximately 40 mg/kg/day for one month, no biologically significant gross or microscopic abnormalities were observed. Cataracts, attributed to markedly disturbed carbohydrate metabolism, have been observed in a few dogs given repeated daily doses of oral or intravenous diazoxide. The lenticular changes resembled those which occur experimentally in animals with increased blood sugar levels. In chronic toxicity studies, rats given a daily dose of 200 mg/kg diazoxide for 52 weeks had a decrease in weight gain and an increase in heart, liver, adrenal, and thyroid weights. Mortality in drug-treated and control groups was not different. Dogs treated with diazoxide at dosages of 50, 100, and 200 mg/kg/day for 82 weeks had higher blood glucose levels than controls. Mild bone marrow stimulation and increased pancreas weights were evident in the drug-treated dogs; several developed inguinal hernias, one had a testicular seminoma, and another had a mass near the penis. Two females had inguinal mammary swellings. The etiology of these changes was not established. There was no difference in mortality between drug-treated and control groups. In a second chronic oral toxicity study, dogs given milled diazoxide at 50, 100, and 200 mg/kg/day had anorexia and severe weight loss, causing death in a few. Hematologic, biochemical, and histologic examinations did not indicate any cause of death other than inanition. After one year of treatment, there is no evidence of herniation or tissue swelling in any of the dogs.

When diazoxide was administered at high dosages concomitantly with either chlorothiazide to rats or trichlormethiazide to dogs, increased toxicity was observed. In rats, the combination was nephrotoxic; epithelial hyperplasia was observed in the collecting tubules. In dogs, a diabetic syndrome was produced which resulted in ketosis and death. Neither of the drugs given alone produced these effects.

Although the data are inconclusive, reproduction and teratology studies in several species of animals indicate that diazoxide, when administered during the critical period of embryo formation, may interfere with normal fetal development, possibly through altered glucose metabolism. Parturition was occasionally prolonged in animals treated at term. Intravenous administration of diazoxide to pregnant sheep, goats, and swine produced in the fetus an appreciable increase in blood glucose level and degeneration of the beta cells of the islets of Langerhans. The reversibility of these effects was not studied.

[Shown in Product Identification Section]

PROGYNON® ℞

brand of estradiol, NF
Pellets for Subcutaneous Implantation

How Supplied: PROGYNON Pellets for Subcutaneous Implantation, 25 mg., white or creamy white, cylindrical, sterile pellets packaged in individual vials; box of three vials.

Patient package inserts are being dispensed with this product. They are available to physicians upon request. For complete prescribing information, contact the Schering Professional Services Department. Physicians references available on request.

RELA® ℞

brand of carisoprodol
Tablets

How Supplied: RELA Tablets (350 mg.): pink, sugar-coated, round tablets branded in brown with the Schering trademark and either product identification letters, AHR or numbers, 160; bottle of 100.

For complete prescribing information, contact the Schering Professional Services Department.

[Shown in Product Identification Section]

SEBIZON® ℞

brand of sulfacetamide sodium, USP
Lotion

How Supplied: SEBIZON Lotion 85 g. plastic squeeze tube, box of one.

For complete prescribing information, contact the Schering Professional Services Department.

Sodium SULAMYD® ℞

brand of sulfacetamide sodium, USP
Ophthalmic Solution 30%—Sterile
Ophthalmic Solution 10%—Sterile
Ophthalmic Ointment 10%—Sterile

Description: Sodium SULAMYD is available in three ophthalmic forms:

Ophthalmic Solution 30% contains in each ml. of sterile aqueous solution 300 mg. sulfacetamide sodium, USP, 1.5 mg. sodium thiosulfate, with 0.5 mg. methylparaben and 0.1 mg. propylparaben added as preservatives, and sodium dihydrogen phosphate as buffer.

Ophthalmic Solution 10% contains in each ml. of sterile aqueous solution 100 mg. sulfacetamide sodium, USP, 3.1 mg. sodium thiosulfate, and 5 mg. methylcellulose, with 0.5 mg. methylparaben and 0.1 mg. propylparaben added as preservatives and sodium dihydrogen phosphate as buffer.

Ophthalmic Ointment 10% is a sterile ointment, each gram containing 100 mg. sulfacetamide sodium, USP, with 0.5 mg. methylparaben, 0.1 mg. propylparaben and 0.25 mg. benzalkonium chloride added as preservatives, and sorbitan monolaurate and water in a bland, unctuous, petrolatum base.

Actions: Sodium SULAMYD exerts a bacteriostatic effect against a wide range of gram-positive and gram-negative microorganisms by restricting, through competition with para-aminobenzoic acid, the synthesis of folic acid which bacteria require for growth.

Indications: Sodium SULAMYD is indicated for the treatment of conjunctivitis, corneal ulcer, and other superficial ocular infections due to susceptible microorganisms, and as adjunctive treatment in systemic sulfonamide therapy of trachoma.

Contraindications: Sodium SULAMYD is contraindicated in individuals with known or suspected sensitivity to sulfonamides or to any of the ingredients of the preparations.

Precautions: Sodium SULAMYD products are incompatible with silver preparations. Ophthalmic ointments may retard corneal healing. Non-susceptible organisms, including fungi, may proliferate with the use of these preparations. Sulfonamides are inactivated by the para-aminobenzoic acid present in purulent exudates.

Sensitization may recur when a sulfonamide is re-administered irrespective of the route of administration, and cross sensitivity between different sulfonamides may occur. If signs of sensitivity or other untoward reactions occur, discontinue use of the preparation.

Adverse Reactions: Sulfacetamide sodium may cause local irritation. Transient stinging or burning has been reported with the 30% solution of sulfacetamide sodium.

Although sensitivity reactions to sulfacetamide sodium are rare, an isolated incident of Stevens-Johnson syndrome was reported in a patient who had experienced a previous bullous drug reaction to an orally administered sulfonamide and a single instance of local hypersensitivity was reported which progressed to a fatal syndrome resembling systemic lupus erythematosus.

Dosage and Administration: Sodium SULAMYD Ophthalmic Solution 30%. *For conjunctivitis or corneal ulcer:* instill one drop into lower conjunctival sac every two hours or less frequently according to severity of infection. *For trachoma:* Two drops every two hours; concomitant systemic sulfonamide therapy is indicated.

Sodium SULAMYD Ophthalmic Solution 10%. One or two drops into the lower conjunctival sac every two or three hours during the day and less often at night.

Sodium SULAMYD Ophthalmic Ointment 10%. Apply a small amount four times daily and at bedtime. The ointment may be used adjunctively with either of the solution forms.

How Supplied: Sodium SULAMYD Ophthalmic Ointment 10%, 3.5 gram tube, box of one. **Store away from heat.**

Sodium SULAMYD Ophthalmic Solution 30%, 15 ml. dropper bottle, box of one. **Store in a cool place (8° to 15°C–46° to 59°F).**

Sodium SULAMYD Ophthalmic Solution 10%, 5 ml. dropper bottle, box of 25; 15 ml. dropper bottle, box of one. **Store in a cool place (8° to 15°C–46° to 59°F).**

On long standing, sulfonamide solutions will darken in color and should be discarded.

SOLGANAL® ℞

brand of sterile aurothioglucose
Suspension, USP
For Intramuscular Injection Only

Description: SOLGANAL is a sterile, intramuscular suspension of aurothioglucose, USP in sesame oil with 2 percent aluminum monostearate and 1 mg. per ml. propylparaben added as preservative. Aurothioglucose contains approximately 50 percent gold.

Actions: Although the mechanism of action is unknown, aurothioglucose's predominant action appears to be suppression of the synovitis of active rheumatoid disease. Aurothioglucose is gradually absorbed following intramuscular injection, producing a prolonged effect which is therapeutically desirable.

Indications: SOLGANAL Suspension is indicated for the adjunctive treatment of rheumatoid arthritis, both of the adult and juvenile types. Laboratory and clinical tests indicate that, as compared with many gold preparations, SOLGANAL is well tolerated by most patients.

Contraindications: Gold therapy is contraindicated in severe uncontrolled diabetes, severe debilitation, renal disease, hepatic dysfunction or a history of infectious hepatitis, marked hypertension, heart failure, systemic lupus erythematosus, Sjögren's syndrome in rheumatoid arthritis, and in patients with a history of agranulocytosis or hemorrhagic diathesis. Patients with blood dyscrasias, those who have recently had radiation, and those who have developed severe toxicity from previous exposure to gold or other heavy metals should not receive SOLGANAL Suspension.

Pregnancy is a contraindication to the use of this product because certain gold compounds have been shown to be teratogenic in rats and rabbits.

Urticaria, eczema and colitis are also contraindications to the use of the metal.

Concomitant use of antimalarials, immunosuppressants, phenylbutazone or oxyphenbutazone is contraindicated because of their potential to cause blood dyscrasias.

Warnings: The possibility of severe toxic reactions should always be kept in mind when using chrysotherapy. Physicians planning to use gold therapy should become thoroughly familiar with the behavior of this drug by observation of its use in a clinic or treatment center. The patient should be informed of the possibility of toxic reactions and of the need to report promptly any symptoms suggesting toxicity.

Before treatment is started a complete blood count, platelet count and urinalysis should be done to serve as reference points. Pregnancy should be positively ruled out. Throughout the treatment period, urinalysis should be repeated prior to each injection, and complete blood and platelet counts should be performed every two weeks. A platelet count is indicated any time that purpura or ecchymoses occurs. Before each injection the physician should see the patient to check for adverse reactions. Weekly inquiry should be made regarding pruritus, sore mouth and indigestion. The following signs should be considered danger signals of gold toxicity, and no additional injections should be given unless further studies reveal some other cause for their presence: rapid reduction of hemoglobin, leukopenia (WBC count) below 4000/cu mm, eosinophilia above 5%, platelet count decrease below 100,000/cu mm, albuminuria, hematuria, pruritus, dermatitis, stomatitis and jaundice.

Gold is poorly tolerated by aged patients.

SOLGANAL Suspension should be used with extreme caution in patients with: hypersensitivity to medications, skin rash, a history of renal or liver disease.

In long-term toxicity studies, renal adenomas developed in rats receiving a gold product similar to SOLGANAL Suspension at high dose levels (2 mg/kg weekly for 45 weeks, followed by 6 mg/kg daily for 47 weeks). The adenomas were histologically similar to those produced by chronic administration of experimental gold compounds and other heavy metals, such as lead. No reports of renal adenomas in man have been received in association with the use of SOLGANAL Suspension.

Adverse Reactions: At any time during treatment or many months thereafter, adverse reactions may occur.

Cutaneous reactions: Dermatitis is the most common reaction. Pruritus should be considered a warning signal of an impending cutaneous reaction. Erythema and occasionally the more severe reactions, such as papular, vesicular and exfoliative dermatitis leading to alopecia and shedding of the nails, may occur. Chrysiasis has been reported, especially on photoexposed areas. Gold dermatitis may be aggravated by exposure to sunlight, or an actinic rash may develop.

Mucous membrane reactions: Stomatitis is the second most common adverse reaction. Shallow ulcers on the buccal membranes, on the borders of the tongue and on the palate, diffuse glossitis or gingivitis may be preceded by the sensation of metallic taste. Careful oral hygiene is important. Inflammation of the upper respiratory tract, pharyngitis, gastritis, colitis, tracheitis and vaginitis have also been reported. Conjunctivitis is rare.

Renal reactions: Nephrotic syndrome or glomerulitis with hematuria, which is usually relatively mild, subsides completely if recognized early and treatment is discontinued. These may become severe and chronic if treatment is continued after onset of the reactions. Therefore, it is important to perform a urinalysis before each injection and to discontinue treatment promptly if proteinuria or hematuria develops.

Hematologic reactions: Although rare, blood dyscrasias, including granulocytopenia, agranulocytosis, thrombocytopenia with or without purpura, leukopenia, eosinophilia, panmyelopathy, hemorrhagic diathesis, hypoplastic and aplastic anemia, have been reported.

Nitritoid and allergic reactions: These reactions, which may resemble anaphylactoid effects, include flushing, fainting, dizziness, sweating, malaise and weakness.

Less common but more severe effects include: anaphylactic shock, syncope, bradycardia, thickening of the tongue, difficulty in swallowing and breathing, and angioneurotic edema. These may occur up to ten minutes following an injection and at any time during the course of therapy. If they are observed, treatment with aurothioglucose should be discontinued.

Miscellaneous reactions: On rare occasions, gastrointestinal symptoms, ie, nausea, vomiting, colic, anorexia, abdominal cramps, diarrhea, ulcerative enterocolitis and headache, which may be attributed to gold therapy, have been reported.

There have been rare reports of iritis, corneal ulcers, and gold deposits in ocular tissues.

Other reported reactions include encephalitis, immunological destruction of the synovia, EEG abnormalities, hepatitis with jaundice, toxic hepatitis, acute yellow atrophy, peripheral neuritis, gold bronchitis, pulmonary injury manifested by interstitial pneumonitis, fibrosis and partial or complete hair loss.

Arthralgia may occur for one or two days after an injection.

Dosage and Administration: *Adults* The usual dosage schedule for the intramuscular administration of SOLGANAL is as follows: first dose, 10 mg.; second and third doses, 25 mg.; fourth and subsequent doses, 50 mg. The interval between doses is one week. The 50 mg. dose is continued at weekly intervals until 0.8 to 1.0 g. SOLGANAL has been given. If the patient has improved and has exhibited no signs of toxicity, the 50 mg. dose may be continued many months longer, at three- to four-week intervals. A weekly dose above 50 mg. is usually unnecessary and contraindicated; the tendency in gold therapy is toward lower dosage. With this in mind, it may eventually be established that a 25 mg. dose is the one of choice.

Children six to twelve years—one-fourth of the adult dose, governed chiefly by body weight.

SOLGANAL should be injected *intramuscularly,* never intravenously. The vial should be thoroughly shaken in order to suspend all of the active material. Heating the vial to body temperature (by immersion in warm water) will facilitate drawing the suspension into the syringe. An 18-gauge, 1½-inch needle is recommended for depositing the preparation deep into the muscular tissue. For obese patients, an 18-gauge, 2-inch needle may be used. The site usually selected for injection is the upper outer quadrant of the gluteal region.

NOTE: Shake the vial in horizontal position before the dose is withdrawn. Needle and syringe must be dry.

Management of Adverse Reactions: In the event of toxic reactions, gold therapy should be discontinued immediately.

In the presence of mild reactions, it is usually sufficient to discontinue the administration of SOLGANAL for a short period and then to resume treatment with smaller doses.

Dermatitis and pruritus may respond to soothing lotions, other appropriate antipruritic treatment, or topical glucocorticoids, if indicated. Chrysiasis may be treated with strong iodine solution.

If dermatitis or stomatitis becomes severe or spreads, systemic glucocorticoid treatment may be indicated. For renal, hematologic and most other adverse reactions, glucocorticoids may be required in larger doses and for a longer time than for dermatologic reactions. Often this treatment may be required for many months because of gold's slow elimination from the body.

If severe adverse reactions do not improve with steroid treatment in patients who received large doses of gold, a chelating agent, such as dimercaprol, may be used. In one case it was reported that D-penicillamine was beneficial in the treatment of gold-induced thrombocytopenia.

In the presence of severe or idiosyncratic reactions, treatment with SOLGANAL Suspension should not be reinstituted.

How Supplied: SOLGANAL Suspension is available in 10 ml. multiple-dose vials containing 5% (50 mg/ml) aurothioglucose in oil suspension; box of one.

Protect from light. Store between 0°–30°C (32°–86°F). Shake well before using.

SUNRIL® PREMENSTRUAL CAPSULES

How Supplied: SUNRIL® Premenstrual Capsules are pink and lavender capsules; bottle of 100.

For complete prescribing information, contact the Schering Professional Services Department.

THEOVENT™ ℞

brand of theophylline anhydrous, USP Long-Acting Capsules

Description: THEOVENT Long-Acting Capsules are a specially formulated preparation of theophylline anhydrous which is gradually released for prolonged therapeutic effect after oral administration. The product is formulated so that the entire dose is not released in the stomach, thereby minimizing exposure of the gastric mucosa to the potentially irritating effects of theophylline. Each capsule contains 125 mg. or 250 mg. of anhydrous theophylline, USP.

Theophylline is 1*H*-Purine-2,6-dione, 3,7-dihydro-1,3-dimethyl-, monohydrate or anhydrous, a xanthine compound having the chemical formula, $C_7H_8N_4O_2 \cdot H_20$ (monohydrate). It is a white, odorless, crystalline powder which is stable in air and has a bitter taste. It contains not less than 98.5% and not more than 101.0% of the labeled amount of $C_7H_8N_4O_2$, calculated on the dried basis.

Continued on next page

Information on Schering products appearing on these pages is effective as of September 30, 1979.

Schering—Cont.

Clinical Pharmacology: Theophylline directly relaxes the smooth muscle of the bronchial airways and pulmonary blood vessels, thus acting mainly as a bronchodilator, pulmonary vasodilator and smooth muscle relaxant. It produces an increase in vital capacity and counteracts the entrapment of residual air. Its bronchodilating action helps relieve wheezing, coughing, and other respiratory symptoms associated with reversible bronchospasm.

Theophylline also possesses other actions typical of the xanthine derivatives: coronary vasodilator; diuretic; and skeletal muscle, cardiac, and cerebral stimulation. Its actions may be mediated through inhibition of phosphodiesterase and a resultant increase in intracellular cyclic AMP which could mediate smooth muscle relaxation. Theophylline also inhibits the release of histamine by mast cells at concentrations higher than those attained clinically.

In vitro theophylline has been shown to react synergistically with beta agonists (e.g., isoproterenol), that increase intracellular cyclic AMP through the stimulation of adenyl cyclase, but synergism has not been demonstrated in clinical studies. More data are needed to determine if theophylline and beta agonists have clinically important additive effects.

Apparently, tolerance has not developed with chronic use of theophylline.

In usual patient populations the elimination characteristics of theophylline are as follows:

Patient Population	Theophylline Plasma Clearance Rates (means ± S.D.)	Average Half-life (means ± S.D.)
Children (over 6 months of age)	1.45 ± .58 ml/kg/min	3.7 ± 1.1 hrs.
Adult non-smokers with uncomplicated asthma	.65 ± .19 ml/kg/min	8.7 ± 2.2 hrs.

The half-life is shortened by cigarette smoking and also by low carbohydrate, high protein diet. Conversely, the half-life is prolonged by high carbohydrate, low protein diet and also in patients with alcoholism, reduced hepatic or renal function, congestive heart failure, and in patients receiving certain antibiotics, such as TAO (troleandomycin), erthromycin, lincomycin or clindamycin. High fever for prolonged periods may decrease theophylline elimination.

Although THEOVENT Long-Acting Capsules are not indicated for young children or infants, it should be noted that newborn infants have extremely slow clearances and half-lives exceeding 24 hours. In infants 3 to 6 months old, these elimination characteristics are similar to those in older children.

Older adults with chronic obstructive pulmonary disease, any patients with cor pulmonale or other causes of heart failure, and patients with liver pathology may have much lower clearances with half-lives that may exceed 24 hours.

The half-life of theophylline in smokers (of 1 to 2 packs of cigarettes per day) averaged 4 to 5 hours among various studies, much shorter than the half-life in non-smokers, which averaged about 7 to 9 hours. The increase in theophylline clearance caused by smoking is probably the result of induction of drug-metabolizing enzymes. After cessation of smoking, normalization of theophylline pharmacokinetics may not occur for 3 months to 2 years.

In a well-controlled study in normal adult males, a single dose of 500 mg. THEOVENT, administered as two capsules each containing 250 mg., resulted in a mean peak plasma concentration of 7.5 mcg/ml at 4.6 hours after administration. The relative bioavailability was essentially complete when compared to that of a standard theophylline syrup. In chronic therapy of patients requiring higher than average doses, the gradual absorption of THEOVENT Long-Acting Capsules, as compared with that of non-sustained release theophylline products, may minimize the fluctuation (peaks and troughs) in serum concentrations and permit longer intervals between dosing.

Indications: THEOVENT Long-Acting Capsules are indicated for relief and/or prevention of reversible bronchospasm associated with asthma, chronic bronchitis or emphysema. Theophyllinization is a treatment of first choice for the management of chronic asthma to prevent symptoms and maintain patent airways.

Contraindications: This product is contraindicated in individuals who have shown hypersensitivity to any of its components, to aminophylline, or to other xanthines (theobromine or caffeine).

Warnings: Status asthmaticus is a medical emergency. When the patient is not rapidly responsive to bronchodilators, optimal therapy frequently requires additional medication, including corticosteroids. Severe episodes of bronchospasm may require inhalant and/or parenteral therapy or a rapidly acting theophylline preparation.

Because excessive theophylline doses may be associated with toxicity, periodic measurement of theophylline serum levels is recommended to assure maximal benefit without excessive risk. The incidence of toxicity increases at serum levels greater than 20 mcg/ml.

High serum levels of theophylline may result from conventional doses in association with clinical manifestations of toxicity in certain clinical situations such as: patients with lowered body plasma clearances (due to transient cardiac decompensation); patients with liver dysfunction or chronic obstructive lung disease; patients who are more than 55 years of age, particularly males.

Although early signs of theophylline toxicity, such as nausea and restlessness, are often seen, in some cases more serious signs such as ventricular arrhythmias or convulsions may be the first signs of toxicity.

It is important that doses not tolerated be discontinued. In such situations if therapy is to be resumed, it should be at a lower dosage after all signs of toxicity have disappeared.

Tachycardia may occur in many patients who have higher theophylline serum levels. Theophylline products may worsen preexisting arrhythmias.

Usage in Pregnancy: As with most anti-asthmatic medications, safe use in pregnancy has not been established relative to possible adverse effects on fetal development, but neither have adverse effects on fetal development been established. Theophylline levels have been found in cord serum. The potential risks of uncontrolled asthma in pregnant women should be balanced against the possible risks to the fetus.

Usage in Nursing Mothers: It has been reported that theophylline distributes readily into breast milk; therefore, the drug should not be used in nursing women.

Precautions: Theophylline should not be administered concurrently with other xanthine medications. Use theophylline with caution in patients with severe cardiac disease, arrhythmias, acute myocardial injury, congestive heart failure, cor pulmonale, hypertension, severe hypoxemia, hyperthyroidism, liver or renal disease, dehydration, and in the elderly (especially males over 55 years of age). In patients with a history of peptic ulcer, the condition may be exacerbated. Theophylline may occasionally act as a local gastrointestinal irritant, especially in high doses and chronic use, but gastrointestinal symptoms are more commonly central and associated with serum concentrations exceeding 20 mcg/ml.

Factors known to influence body clearance of theophylline are: cigarette smoking (increased clearance), age (decreasing clearance with increasing age), congestive heart failure (decreased clearance), liver disease (decreased clearance), pulmonary edema (decreased clearance), concurrent infection (decreased clearance), concomitant use of erythromycin, troleandomycin, clindamycin or lincomycin (decreased clearance). In the presence of any of the above factors, it is advisable to monitor theophylline serum levels periodically. Other circumstances in which it is advisable to monitor serum levels include: unexplained poor control of asthmatic signs and symptoms; occurrence of toxic symptoms; addition or removal of other drugs from the therapeutic regimen which affect the metabolism of theophylline; use of unusually high doses.

Adverse Reactions: Most adverse reactions are usually due to overdose and include:

Gastrointestinal: nausea, vomiting, epigastric pain, hematemesis, diarrhea.

Central nervous system: headaches, irritability, restlessness, insomnia, reflex hyperexcitability, muscle twitching, clonic and tonic generalized convulsions.

Cardiovascular: palpitations, tachycardia, extrasystoles, flushing, hypotension, circulatory failure, life-threatening ventricular arrhythmias.

Respiratory: tachypnea.

Renal: albuminuria, increased excretion of renal tubular and red blood cells; potentiation of diuresis.

Others: hyperglycemia and inappropriate anti-diuretic hormone syndrome.

Drug Interactions: Toxic synergism with ephedrine has been documented and may occur with some other sympathomimetic bronchodilators. Recent controlled studies suggest that the addition of ephedrine to dosage regimens of theophylline results in an increase in toxic effects, but not in efficacy when compared to theophylline alone.

Following is a list of drugs and the effects seen from their interactions with theophylline:

DRUG	EFFECT
lithium carbonate	increased excretion of lithium carbonate
propranolol	antagonism of propranolol
furosemide	increased diuresis
reserpine	tachycardia
troleandomycin, erythromycin, lincomycin, clindamycin	increased theophylline blood levels

DOSAGE AND ADMINISTRATION: THE USUAL INITIAL DOSAGE FOR ADULTS AND CHILDREN 12 YEARS AND OLDER IS ONE OR TWO 250 MG. CAPSULES EVERY 12 HOURS.

THE USUAL INITIAL DOSAGE FOR CHILDREN 6 THROUGH 11 YEARS OF AGE IS ONE OR TWO 125 MG. CAPSULES EVERY 12 HOURS.

DOSAGE MUST BE ADJUSTED ACCORDING TO THE NEEDS AND RESPONSE OF THE PATIENT. Therapeutic serum levels of theophylline are considered to be between 10 and 20 mcg/ml; higher levels may produce toxic effects. There is wide interpatient variation in the dosage needed to achieve and maintain therapeutic serum levels. Because of these wide variations and the relatively narrow range between therapeutic and toxic serum levels, dosage must be individualized, and serum level monitoring is recommended particularly when prolonged use is planned. (See also CLINICAL PHARMACOLOGY, WARNINGS, and PRECAUTIONS sections.)

Dosage should be calculated on the basis of lean (ideal) body weight. Theophylline does not distribute into fatty tissue.

Giving theophylline with food may prevent the rare case of stomach irritation; although absorption may be slower, it is still complete.

Adults and children 12 years and older: generally an initial dose of 12 mg/kg/day in divided doses will produce theophylline serum levels which do not exceed 20 mcg/ml. The dose may be increased by 2 mg/kg/day every 2 days until the desired therapeutic response is achieved if no systemic side effects are encountered.

At doses above 20 mg/kg/day, serum levels of theophylline should be monitored. The usual initial dosage for this age group is one or two 250 mg. capsules every 12 hours. This dosage may be increased by 125 mg. per dose every 2 days up to a dosage of 750 mg. every 12 hours. Daily doses exceeding 1500 mg. should be used cautiously with monitoring of theophylline serum levels. If required, the total daily dose may also be administered in 3 divided doses.

Children 6 through 11 years: generally an initial dose of 20 mg/kg/day in divided doses will not produce toxic serum levels. The dose may be increased by 2 mg/kg/day every two days until the desired therapeutic response is achieved if no systemic side effects are encountered. At doses above 34 mg/kg/day, theophylline serum levels should be monitored. The usual initial dosage in this age group is one or two 125 mg. capsules every 12 hours. This dosage may be increased every 2 days up to a dosage of 375 mg. every 12 hours. Daily doses exceeding 750 mg. should be used cautiously with monitoring of theophylline serum levels. If required, the total daily dose may also be administered in 3 divided doses.

Patients currently maintained on non-sustained release theophylline or aminophylline products: The total daily dose of a non-sustained release product may be replaced by the equivalent amount of anhydrous theophylline given as THEOVENT Long-Acting Capsules, administered in 2 or 3 divided doses.

Measurement of serum theophylline concentrations: In order to achieve optimal therapeutic dosage, monitoring of serum theophylline concentrations is recommended. For purposes of these measurements, serum should be obtained at the time of peak drug absorption (4–6 hours after ingestion). In the preceding 48 hours, dosage should have been reasonably typical of the prescribed regimen and no doses should have been missed or added. DOSAGE ADJUSTMENT BASED ON SERUM THEOPHYLLINE MEASUREMENTS WHEN THESE INSTRUCTIONS HAVE NOT BEEN FOLLOWED MAY RESULT IN RECOMMENDATIONS THAT PRESENT RISK OF TOXICITY TO THE PATIENT.

Overdosage: Management: Emergency treatment should be started immediately.

A. If overdose is established and seizure has not occurred:
   1. Induce vomiting, even if emesis has occurred spontaneously. Pharmacologic vomiting by the administration of ipecac syrup is a preferred method. However, emesis should not be induced in patients with impaired consciousness. The action of ipecac is facilitated by physical activity and the administration of eight to twelve ounces of water. If emesis does not occur within 15 minutes, the dose of ipecac should be repeated. Precautions against aspiration must be taken, especially in infants and children. If vomiting is unsuccessful or contraindicated, gastric lavage should be performed.
   2. Administer a cathartic (this is particularly important if a sustained-release preparation has been taken).
   3. Administer activated charcoal
B. If the patient is having a seizure:
   1. Establish an airway
   2. Administer oxygen
   3. Treat the seizure with intravenous diazepam 0.1 to 0.3 mg/kg up to 10 mg.
   4. Monitor vital signs, maintain blood pressure and provide adequate hydration.
C. Post-Seizure Coma
   1. Maintain airway and oxygenation
   2. Follow above recommendations to prevent absorption of drug, but perform intubation and lavage instead of inducing emesis. Introduce the cathartic and charcoal via a large bore gastric lavage tube.
   3. Continue to provide full supportive care and adequate hydration while waiting for the drug to be metabolized. This generally occurs rapidly enough so that consideration of dialysis is not warranted.
D. General

Treatment is symptomatic and supportive. Stimulants (analeptic agents) should not be used. If atrial arrhythmia occurs during treatment with theophylline, lidocaine should be administered with caution, since both drugs may produce accelerated atrioventricular conduction.

Intravenous fluids may be required to overcome dehydration, acid-base imbalance, and hypotension; the latter may also be treated with vasopressors. Apnea will require ventilatory support. Hyperpyrexia, especially in children, may be treated with tepid water sponge baths or a hypothermic blanket. Theophylline serum levels should be monitored until they fall below 20 mcg/ml. After emergency treatment medical monitoring should be continued. In one case of massive overdose, charcoal hemoperfusion over a six-hour period rapidly removed theophylline from the serum, with notable clinical improvement. Charcoal hemoperfusion should be considered in patients with severe theophylline intoxication as a possible means of preventing irreversible central nervous system damage.

E. Animal studies suggest that phenobarbital may decrease theophylline toxicity, but at present there are insufficient data to recommend it as a treatment for theophylline overdosage.

How Supplied: THEOVENT Long-Acting Capsules, 125 mg., dark green and yellow capsules, branded in blue with the Schering trademark and product identification numbers, 402; bottles of 100 and 500.

THEOVENT Long-Acting Capsules, 250 mg., dark green and clear capsules, branded in blue with the Schering trademark and product identification numbers, 753; bottles of 100 and 500.

Store between 2° and 30°C (36° and 86°F).

TINACTIN®
brand of tolnaftate, USP
Cream 1% • Solution 1% • Powder 1% • Powder (1%) Aerosol

How Supplied: TINACTIN **Cream** 1%, 15 g., collapsible tube with dispensing tip. TINACTIN **Solution** 1%, 10 ml. plastic squeeze bottle. TINACTIN **Powder** 1%, 45 g. plastic container. TINACTIN **Powder** (1%) **Aerosol**, 100 g. spray can.

For complete prescribing information, contact the Schering Professional Services Department.

TINDAL® ℞
brand of acetophenazine maleate, NF
Tablets

Description: TINDAL Tablets contain acetophenazine maleate, a phenothiazine of the piperazine group. Each TINDAL Tablet contains 20 mg. acetophenazine maleate, NF.

How Supplied: TINDAL Tablets, 20 mg., sugar-coated, salmon-colored tablets branded in brown with the Schering trademark and product identification letters, BBA or numbers 968; bottles of 100.

For complete prescribing information, contact the Schering Professional Services Department.

[*Shown in Product Identification Section*]

TREMIN® ℞
brand of trihexyphenidyl hydrochloride, USP
Tablets

How Supplied: TREMIN Tablets 2 mg.: white, compressed, scored tablets impressed with the Schering trademark and product identification letters, AKH or numbers, 892; bottle of 100.

TREMIN Tablets, 5 mg.: white (formerly gray), compressed, scored tablets impressed with the Schering trademark and product identification letters, AKJ or numbers, 596; bottle of 100.

For complete prescribing information, contact the Schering Professional Services Department.

[*Shown in Product Identification Section*]

TRILAFON® ℞
brand of perphenazine, NF
Tablets
REPETABS® Tablets
Concentrate
Injection

Description: TRILAFON products contain perphenazine, NF (4-[3-(2-Chlorophenothiazin-10-yl)propyl]-1-piperazineethanol), a piperazinyl phenothiazine having the chemical formula, $C_{21}H_{26}ClN_3OS$. It is available as **Tablets,** 2, 4, 8 and 16 mg.; REPETABS (brand of repeat-action tablets) **Tablets,** 4 mg. in an outer layer for immediate effect and 4 mg. in an inner core for release three to six hours later; **Concentrate,** 16 mg. perphenazine per 5 ml. and alcohol less than 0.1%; and **Injection,** perphenazine 5 mg., disodium citrate 24.6 mg., sodium bisulfite 2 mg., and Water for Injection, USP, per 1 ml.

Actions: Perphenazine has actions at all levels of the central nervous system, particularly the hypothalamus. However, the site and mechanism of action are not known.

Indications: Perphenazine is indicated for use in the management of the manifestations of psychotic disorders; and for the control of severe nausea and vomiting in adults.

TRILAFON has not been shown effective in the management of behavioral complications in patients with mental retardation.

Contraindications: TRILAFON is contraindicated in drug-associated, central nervous system depression (barbiturates, alcohol, narcotics, analgesics, antihistamines). Perphenazine is contraindicated in the presence of existing blood dyscrasias, bone marrow depression and pre-existing liver damage, and in patients who are hypersensitive to perphenazine.

TRILAFON **Injection** should not be given to patients in coma or severely depressed states.

Warnings: Perphenazine can lower the convulsive threshold in susceptible individuals; it should be used with caution in patients with convulsive disorders. If the patient is being treated with an anticonvulsant agent, increased dosage of that agent may be required when perphenazine is used concomitantly.

Perphenazine may impair the mental and/or physical abilities required for the performance of potentially hazardous tasks, such as driving a car or operating machinery.

Perphenazine is not recommended for children under 12 years of age.

Perphenazine should be used with caution in patients with psychic depression.

Continued on next page

Information on Schering products appearing on these pages is effective as of September 30, 1979.

Schering—Cont.

Usage in Pregnancy: Safe use of TRILAFON during pregnancy and lactation has not been established; therefore, in administering the drug to pregnant patients, nursing mothers, or women who may become pregnant, the possible benefits must be weighed against the possible hazards to mother and child.

Precautions: The possibility of suicide in depressed patients remains during treatment and until significant remission occurs. This type of patient should not have easy access to large quantities of this drug.

As with all phenothiazine compounds, perphenazine should not be used indiscriminately. Patients who have had any severe reaction to phenothiazines or to imipramine should be treated cautiously under close medical supervision.

Some of the untoward actions of perphenazine tend to appear more frequently when high doses are used. However, as with other phenothiazine compounds, patients receiving perphenazine in any dosage should be kept under close supervision.

The antiemetic effect of perphenazine can obscure signs of toxicity due to overdosage of other drugs, or mask the symptoms of disease (eg, brain tumor or intestinal obstruction).

A significant rise in body temperature may indicate an idiosyncratic reaction to perphenazine; treatment with perphenazine should be stopped if this occurs.

If hypotension develops, epinephrine should not be used because its action is blocked and partly reversed by perphenazine. Severe, acute hypotension has occurred with the use of phenothiazines and is of particular concern in patients with mitral insufficiency or pheochromocytoma.

Contact dermatitis has been reported with a perphenazine solution; therefore, contact of hands or clothing by those handling perphenazine solutions should be avoided.

Potentiation: Since phenothiazines can potentiate the central nervous system depressant actions of opiates, analgesics, antihistamines, barbiturates, and alcohol, less than the usual dosage of these agents is required when they are administered concomitantly with TRILAFON. Patients should be cautioned that their response to alcohol may be increased while they are being treated with TRILAFON. The risk of suicide and the danger of overdose may be increased in patients who use alcohol excessively because of its potentiation of the drug's effect.

Phenothiazines also potentiate the effects of atropine, heat, and phosphorus insecticides, and should be used with caution in persons exposed to these agents.

Adverse Reactions: *Extrapyramidal reactions:* opisthotonus, trismus, torticollis, retrocollis, aching and numbness of the limbs, motor restlessness, oculogyric crisis, hyperreflexia, dystonia, including protrusion, discoloration, aching and rounding of the tongue, tonic spasm of the masticatory muscles, tight feeling in the throat, slurred speech, dysphagia, akathisia, dyskinesia, parkinsonism, and ataxia. Their incidence and severity usually increase with an increase in dosage, but there is considerable individual variation in the tendency to develop such symptoms. Extrapyramidal symptoms can usually be controlled by the concomitant use of effective antiparkinsonian drugs, such as benztropine mesylate, and/or by reduction in dosage. In some instances, however, these reactions may persist after discontinuation of treatment with perphenazine.

Persistent tardive dyskinesia: As with all antipsychotic agents, tardive dyskinesia may appear in some patients on long-term therapy or may appear after drug therapy has been discontinued. The risk appears to be greater in elderly patients on high-dose therapy, especially females. The symptoms are persistent and in some patients appear to be irreversible. The syndrome is characterized by rhythmical, involuntary movements of the tongue, face, mouth or jaw (eg, protrusion of tongue, puffing of cheeks, puckering of mouth, chewing movements). Sometimes these may be accompanied by involuntary movements of the extremities. There is no known effective treatment for tardive dyskinesia; antiparkinsonism agents usually do not alleviate the symptoms of this syndrome. It is suggested that all antipsychotic agents be discontinued if these symptoms appear. Should it be necessary to reinstitute treatment, or increase the dosage of the agent, or switch to a different antipsychotic agent, the syndrome may be masked. It has been reported that fine, vermicular movements of the tongue may be an early sign of the syndrome, and if the medication is stopped at that time the syndrome may not develop.

Allergic reactions: photosensitivity, pruritus, erythema, urticaria, eczema, exfoliative dermatitis, asthma, anaphylactoid reactions, local and generalized edema. In extremely rare instances, individual idiosyncrasy or hypersensitivity to phenothiazines has resulted in cerebral edema, circulatory collapse and death.

Autonomic reactions: dry mouth or salivation, nausea, vomiting, anorexia, constipation, obstipation, urinary frequency or incontinence, blurred vision, nasal congestion, hypertension, hypotension, tachycardia, and a change in the pulse rate occasionally may occur. Significant autonomic effects have been infrequent in patients receiving less than 24 mg. perphenazine daily.

Other reactions: reversed epinephrine effect, hyperglycemia, endocrine disturbances (lactation, galactorrhea, gynecomastia, disturbances in the menstrual cycle), altered cerebrospinal fluid proteins, increase in PBI not attributable to an increase in thyroxine, paradoxical excitement, headache, ECG abnormalities (quinidine-like effect), and systemic lupus erythematosus-like syndrome, reactivation of psychotic processes, paranoid-like reactions, and the production of catatonic-like states have been described.

The following adverse reactions, though rare, have also been reported to be associated with perphenazine treatment: agranulocytosis, jaundice, hyperpigmentation of the skin, grand mal convulsions, failure of ejaculation.

The possibility exists that the following reactions, which have been seen with phenothiazine therapy, may occur with TRILAFON Tablets: certain blood dyscrasias (pancytopenia, thrombocytopenic purpura, leukopenia, eosinophilia); liver damage (biliary stasis); polyphagia; photophobia.

Pigmentary retinopathy has been reported to occur after administration of some phenothiazines with a piperidylethyl side chain, but not with perphenazine which has a piperazine side chain.

Pigmentation of the cornea and lens has been reported to occur after long-term administration of some phenothiazines. Although it has not been reported in patients receiving TRILAFON, the possibility that it might occur should be considered.

Hypnotic effects appear to be minimal, particularly in patients who are permitted to remain active.

A few patients have reported lassitude, muscle weakness, and mild insomnia.

Side effects with intramuscular TRILAFON **Injection** have been infrequent and transient. Dizziness or significant hypotension after treatment with TRILAFON **Injection** is a rare occurrence.

Dosage and Administration: Dosage must be individualized and adjusted according to the severity of the condition and the response obtained. As with all potent drugs, the best dose is the lowest dose that will produce the desired clinical effect. Since extrapyramidal symptoms increase in frequency and severity with increased dosage, it is important to employ the lowest effective dose. These symptoms have disappeared upon reduction of dosage, withdrawal of the drug or administration of an anti-parkinsonian agent.

Prolonged administration of doses exceeding 24 mg. daily should be reserved for hospitalized patients or patients under continued observation for early detection and management of adverse reactions. An antiparkinsonian agent, such as trihexyphenidyl hydrochloride or benztropine mesylate, is valuable in controlling drug-induced, extrapyramidal symptoms.

TRILAFON **Tablets** and REPETABS **Tablets**

Suggested dosages for **Tablets** and REPETABS **Tablets** for various conditions follow:

Moderately disturbed non-hospitalized psychotic patients:

Tablets 4 to 8 mg. t.i.d., or one or two REPETABS **Tablets** b.i.d., initially; reduce as soon as possible to minimum effective dosage.

Hospitalized psychotic patients: **Tablets** 8 to 16 mg. b.i.d. to q.i.d. or one to four REPETABS **Tablets** b.i.d.; avoid dosages in excess of 64 mg. daily.

Severe nausea and vomiting in adults: **Tablets** 8 to 16 mg. daily in divided doses or one REPETABS **Tablet** b.i.d.; 24 mg. occasionally may be necessary; early dosage reduction is desirable. Two REPETABS **Tablets** may be administered in acute cases.

TRILAFON **Injection**—Intramuscular Administration

The injection is used when rapid effect and prompt control of acute or intractable conditions is required or when oral administration is not feasible. TRILAFON **Injection**, administered by deep intramuscular injection, is well tolerated. The injection should be given with the patient seated or recumbent, and the patient should be observed for a short period after administration.

Therapeutic effect is usually evidenced in 10 minutes and is maximal in 1 to 2 hours. The average duration of effective action is 6 hours, occasionally 12 to 24 hours.

Pediatric dosage has not yet been established. Children over 12 years may receive the lowest limit of adult dosage.

The usual initial dose is 5 mg. (1 ml.). This may be repeated every 6 hours. Ordinarily, the total daily dosage should not exceed 15 mg. in ambulatory patients or 30 mg. in hospitalized patients. When required for satisfactory control of symptoms in severe conditions, an initial 10 mg. intramuscular dose may be given. Patients should be placed on oral therapy as soon as practicable. Generally, this may be achieved within 24 hours. In some instances, however, patients have been maintained on injectable therapy for several months. It has been established that TRILAFON **Injection** is more potent than TRILAFON **Tablets**. Therefore, equal or higher dosage should be used when the patient is transferred to oral therapy after receiving the injection.

Psychotic conditions: While 5 mg. of the **Injection** has a definite tranquilizing effect, it may be necessary to use 10 mg. doses to initiate therapy in severely agitated states. Most patients will be controlled and amenable to oral therapy within a maximum of 24 to 48 hours. Acute conditions (hysteria, panic reaction) often respond well to a single dose, whereas in chronic conditions, several injections may be required. When transferring patients to oral therapy, it is suggested that increased dosage be employed to maintain adequate clinical control. This should be followed by gradual reduction to the minimal effective maintenance dose.

Severe nausea and vomiting in adults: To obtain rapid control of vomiting, administer 5 mg. (1 ml.); in rare instances it may be necessary to increase the dosage to 10 mg.; in gen-

eral, higher dosage should be given only to hospitalized patients.
TRIFALON **Injection**—Intravenous Administration
The intravenous administration of TRILAFON **Injection** is seldom required. This route of administration should be used with particular caution and care and only when absolutely necessary to control severe vomiting, intractable hiccoughs, or acute conditions, such as violent retching during surgery. Its use should be limited to recumbent, hospitalized adults in doses not exceeding 5 mg. When employed in this manner, intravenous injection ordinarily should be given as a diluted solution by either fractional injection or a slow drip infusion. In the surgical patient, slow infusion of not more than 5 mg. is preferred. When administered in divided doses, TRILAFON **Injection** should be diluted to 0.5 mg/ml (1 ml. mixed with 9 ml. of physiologic saline solution), and not more than 1 mg. per injection given at not less than one- to two-minute intervals. Intravenous injection should be discontinued as soon as symptoms are controlled and should not exceed 5 mg. The possibility of hypotensive and extrapyramidal side effects should be considered and appropriate means for management kept available. Blood pressure and pulse should be monitored continuously during intravenous administration. Pharmacologic and clinical studies indicate that intravenous administration of norepinephrine should be useful in alleviating the hypotensive effect.
TRILAFON **Concentrate**
In hospitalized psychotic patients, the usual dosage range is 8 to 16 mg. b.i.d. to q.i.d., depending on the severity of symptoms and individual response. Although a number of investigators have employed higher dosage, a total daily dose of more than 64 mg. ordinarily is not required. The **Concentrate** should be diluted with fruit juice, milk, coffee, carbonated beverage or other suitable liquid vehicle prior to administration. Mixtures with tea are not recommended. Suggested dilution is approximately two fluid ounces of diluent for each 5 ml. (16 mg.) teaspoonful of TRILAFON **Concentrate.** For convenience in measuring smaller doses, a graduated dropper marked to measure 8 mg. or 4 mg. is supplied with each bottle.
Overdosage: *Manifestations*—Overdosage of perphenazine primarily involves the extrapyramidal mechanism and produces the same side effects described above under Adverse Reactions, but to a more marked degree. It is usually evidenced by stupor or coma; children may have convulsive seizures.
Treatment—To treat hypotension, levarterenol (norepinephrine) may be used, but not epinephine.
Treatment is symptomatic and supportive. There is no specific antidote. The stomach should be emptied as quickly as possible by emesis. All patients suspected of having taken an overdose should be hospitalized as soon as possible. Gastric lavage should be performed at the hospital following emesis. Because of perphenazine's antiemetic effect, saline emetics are not recommended, since retention of the saline load could result in hypernatremia. After gastric lavage, 20 to 30 g. of activated charcoal may be given every four to six hours during the first 24 to 48 hours after ingestion of the overdose. An electrocardiogram should be taken and close monitoring of cardiac function instituted if there is any sign of abnormality. An open airway and adequate fluid intake should be maintained. Body temperature should be regulated.
Standard measures (oxygen, intravenous fluids, corticosteroids) should be used to manage circulatory shock or metabolic acidosis. Cardiac arrhythmias may be treated with neostigmine, pyridostigmine or propranolol. Digitalis should be considered for cardiac failure. Close monitoring of cardiac function is advisable for not less than five days.
Anticonvulsants (an inhalation anesthetic, diazepam or paraldehyde) are recommended for control of convulsions, since perphenazine increases the central nervous system depressant action, but not the anticonvulsant action of barbiturates.
If acute symptoms of parkinsonism result from perphenazine intoxication, benztropine mesylate or diphenhydramine may be administered.
Central nervous system depression may be treated with nonconvulsant doses of CNS stimulants.
Dialysis is of no value because of low plasma concentrations of the drug.
Continue treatment for at least 48 hours in patients who do not respond earlier.
Since overdosage is often deliberate, patients may attempt suicide by other means during the recovery phase.
Deaths by deliberate or accidental overdosage have occurred with this class of drugs.
How Supplied: TRILAFON **Tablets** (2 mg.): gray, sugar-coated tablets branded in blue-black with the Schering trademark and either product identification letters, ADH, or numbers, 705; bottles of 100 and 500.
TRILAFON **Tablets** (4 mg.): gray, sugar-coated tablets branded in green with the Schering trademark and either product identification letters, ADK, or numbers, 940; bottles of 100 and 500.
TRILAFON **Tablets** (8 mg.): gray, sugar-coated tablets branded in blue with the Schering trademark and either product identification letters, ADJ, or numbers 313; bottles of 100 and 500.
TRILAFON **Tablets** (16 mg.): gray, sugar-coated tablets branded in red with the Schering trademark and either product identification letters, ADM, or numbers, 077; bottles of 100 and 500.
TRILAFON REPETABS **Tablets** (8 mg.): white, sugar-coated tablets branded in gray with the Schering trademark and either product identification letters, ADX, or numbers, 141; bottle of 100.
TRILAFON **Concentrate**, 16 mg. per 5 ml., 4 fluid ounce (118 ml.) bottle with graduated dropper. The **Concentrate** is light-sensitive and should be dispensed in amber bottles. **Protect from light.**
TRILAFON **Injection**, 5 mg. per ml., 1-ml. ampul for intramuscular or intravenous use, box of 100. Keep package closed to protect from light. Exposure may cause discoloration. Slight yellowish discoloration will not alter potency or therapeutic efficacy; if markedly discolored, ampul should be discarded.

[*Shown in Product Identification Section*]

VALISONE® ℞

brand of betamethasone valerate, NF
Aerosol 0.15% w/w (as betamethasone)
For Dermatologic Use Only—
Not For Ophthalmic Use

Description: VALISONE contains betamethasone valerate, NF (9-Fluoro-11β,17,21-trihydroxy-16 β-methylpregna-1, 4-diene-3, 20-dione 17-valerate).
VALISONE Aerosol contains 9.1 mg. betamethasone valerate, NF equivalent to 7.5 mg. betamethasone, in a vehicle of mineral oil and caprylic/capric triglyceride. It also contains 10% isopropyl alcohol and sufficient inert propellant of hydrocarbon (propane and isobutane) to make 85 grams. The spray deposits betamethasone valerate equivalent to approximately 0.15% betamethasone in a nonvolatile, almost invisible film. A three-second spray delivers betamethasone valerate equivalent to approximately 0.09 mg. betamethasone.
Actions: VALISONE Aerosol is primarily effective because of its anti-inflammatory, antipruritic, and vasoconstrictive actions.
Indications: VALISONE Aerosol is indicated solely for the adjunctive topical management for the relief of inflammatory manifestations of acute contact dermatitis. As with all topical steroid aerosols, the use of occlusive dressings is not recommended.
Contraindications: VALISONE Aerosol is contraindicated in those patients with a history of hypersensitivity to any of the components of the preparation.
Warnings: Keep away from eyes or other mucous membranes.
Use only as directed; intentional missuse by deliberately concentrating and inhaling the contents can be harmful or fatal.
Avoid freezing of the tissue by not spraying for more than three seconds, at a distance of not less than six inches.
Contents under pressure. Do not puncture. Flammable mixture, do not use or store near heat or open flame. Exposure to temperatures above 120° Fahrenheit may cause bursting. Never throw container into fire or incinerator. Keep out of the reach of children.
Precautions: If irritation develops with use of VALISONE Aerosol, treatment should be discontinued and appropriate therapy instituted.
In the presence of an infection, the use of an appropriate antifungal or antibacterial agent should be instituted. If a favorable response does not occur promptly, the corticosteroid should be discontinued until the infection has been adequately controlled.
It should be recognized that any of the side effects reported following systemic use of corticosteroids, including adrenal suppression, may also occur following their topical use, especially in infants and children. Systemic absorption of topically applied steroids will be increased if extensive body surface areas are treated. Therefore, under these circumstances, suitable precautions should be taken when long-term use is anticipated, particularly in infants and children.
Although topical steroids have not been reported to have an adverse effect on human pregnancy, the safety of their use in pregnant women has not been absolutely established. In laboratory animals, increases in incidence of fetal abnormalities have been associated with exposure of gestating females to topical corticosteroids, in some cases at rather low dosage levels. Therefore, drugs of this class should not be used on pregnant patients in large amounts or for prolonged periods of time.
VALISONE Aerosol is not for ophthalmic use.
Adverse Reactions: The following local adverse reactions have been reported with topical corticosteroid preparations: burning; itching; irritation; dryness; folliculitis; hypertrichosis; acneiform eruptions; hypopigmentation; perioral dermatitis; allergic contact dermatitis; maceration of the skin; secondary infection; skin atrophy; striae; miliaria.
Dosage and Administration: The container may be held upright or inverted during use. The spray should be directed onto the affected area from a distance of not less than 6 inches and applied for only 3 seconds.
For most effective and economical use, a three-second spray is sufficient to cover an area about the size of the hand.
Apply the medication three to four times a day.
How Supplied: VALISONE Aerosol, 0.15% w/w, 85-gram spray can.
Store between 35° and 86° F (2° and 30°C).

Continued on next page

Information on Schering products appearing on these pages is effective as of September 30, 1979.

Schering—Cont.

VALISONE® ℞
brand of betamethasone valerate, NF
Cream 0.1%
For Dermatologic Use Only–Not For Ophthalmic Use

Description: VALISONE contains betamethasone valerate, NF (9-Fluoro-11β,17,21-trihydroxy-16β-methylpregna-1, 4-diene-3, 20-dione 17-valerate).
Each gram of VALISONE Cream 0.1% contains 1.2 mg. betamethasone valerate, NF (equivalent to 1.0 mg. betamethasone) in a soft, white, hydrophilic cream of water, mineral oil, petrolatum, polyethylene glycol 1000 monocetyl ether, cetostearyl alcohol, monobasic sodium phosphate, and phosphoric acid; 4-chloro-*m*-cresol is present as a preservative.
VALISONE Cream contains no parabens.
Actions: VALISONE Cream is primarily effective because of its anti-inflammatory, antipruritic, and vasoconstrictive actions.
Indications: VALISONE Cream is indicated for the relief of the inflammatory manifestations of corticosteroid-responsive dermatoses.
Contraindications: VALISONE Cream is contraindicated in those patients with a history of hypersensitivity to any of the components of the preparation.
Precautions: If irritation develops with the use of VALISONE Cream, treatment should be discontinued and appropriate therapy instituted.
In the presence of an infection, the use of an appropriate antifungal or antibacterial agent should be instituted. If a favorable response does not occur promptly, the corticosteroid should be discontinued until the infection has been adequately controlled.
It should be recognized that any of the side effects reported following systemic use of corticosteroids, including adrenal suppression, may also occur following their topical use, especially in infants and children. Systemic absorption of topically applied steroids will be increased if extensive body surface areas are treated or if the occlusive technique is used. Therefore, under these circumstances, suitable precautions should be taken when long-term use is anticipated, particularly in infants and children.
Although topical steroids have not been reported to have an adverse effect on human pregnancy, the safety of their use in pregnant women has not been absolutely established. In laboratory animals, increases in incidence of fetal abnormalities have been associated with exposure of gestating females to topical corticosteroids, in some cases at rather low dosage levels. Therefore, drugs of this class should not be used on pregnant patients in large amounts or for prolonged periods of time.
Valisone Cream is not for ophthalmic use.
Adverse Reactions: The following local adverse reactions have been reported with topical corticosteroids, especially under occlusive dressings; burning; itching; irritation; dryness; folliculitis; hypertrichosis; acneiform eruptions; hypopigmentation; perioral dermatitis; allergic contact dermatitis; maceration of the skin; secondary infection; skin atrophy; striae; miliaria.
Dosage and Administration: Apply a thin film of VALISONE Cream to the affected skin areas one to three times a day. Clinical Studies of VALISONE have indicated that dosage only once or twice a day is often feasible and effective.
How Supplied: VALISONE Cream 0.1% is supplied in 5-, 15-, and 45-gram tubes; boxes of one.
Store away from heat.

VALISONE® ℞
brand of betamethasone valerate, NF
Lotion 0.1%
Ointment 0.1%
For Dermatologic Use Only–Not for Ophthalmic Use

Description: VALISONE contains betamethasone valerate, NF (9-Fluoro-11β,17,21-trihydroxy-16β-methylpregna-1, 4-diene-3, 20-dione 17-valerate).
VALISONE **Lotion** 0.1% contains in each gram betamethasone valerate, equivalent to 1.0 mg. betamethasone in a vehicle consisting of isopropyl alcohol (47.5%) and water slightly thickened with carboxy vinyl polymer; the pH is adjusted to approximately 4.7 with sodium hydroxide.
Each gram of VALISONE **Ointment** 0.1% contains 1.2 mg. betamethasone valerate (equivalent to 1.0 mg. betamethasone) in an ointment base of liquid and white petrolatum, and hydrogenated lanolin.
VALISONE **Ointment** contains no parabens.
Actions: VALISONE **Lotion** and **Ointment** are primarily effective because of their anti-inflammatory, antipruritic, and vasoconstrictive actions.
Indications: VALISONE **Lotion** and **Ointment** are indicated for the relief of the inflammatory manifestations of corticosteroid-responsive dermatoses.
Contraindications: VALISONE **Lotion** and **Ointment** are contraindicated in those patients with a history of hypersensitivity to any of the components of the preparations.
Precautions: If irritation develops with the use of VALISONE **Lotion** or **Ointment**, treatment should be discontinued and appropriate therapy instituted.
In the presence of an infection, the use of an appropriate antifungal or antibacterial agent should be instituted. If a favorable response does not occur promptly, the corticosteroid should be discontinued until the infection has been adequately controlled.
It should be recognized that any of the side effects reported following systemic use of corticosteroids, including adrenal suppression, may also occur following their topical use, especially in infants and children. Systemic absorption of topically applied steroids will be increased if extensive body surface areas are treated or if the occlusive technique is used. Therefore, under these circumstances, suitable precautions should be taken when long-term use is anticipated, particularly in infants and children.
Although topical steroids have not been reported to have an adverse effect on human pregnancy, the safety of their use in pregnant women has not been absolutely established. In laboratory animals, increases in incidence of fetal abnormalities have been associated with exposure of gestating females to topical corticosteroids, in some cases at rather low dosage levels. Therefore, drugs of this class should not be used on pregnant patients in large amounts or for prolonged periods of time.
VALISONE **Lotion** and **Ointment** are not for ophthalmic use.
Adverse Reactions: The following local adverse reactions have been reported with topical corticosteroids, especially under occlusive dressings: burning; itching; irritation; dryness; folliculitis; hypertrichosis; acneiform eruptions; hypopigmentation; perioral dermatitis; allergic contact dermatitis; maceration of the skin; secondary infection; skin atrophy; striae; miliaria.
Dosage and Administration:
VALISONE **Lotion**
Apply a few drops of VALISONE **Lotion** to the affected area and massage lightly until it disappears. Apply twice daily, in the morning and at night. Dosage may be increased in stubborn cases. Following improvement, apply once daily.
For the most effective and economical use, apply nozzle to affected area and gently squeeze bottle.
VALISONE **Ointment**
Apply a thin film of VALISONE **Ointment** to the affected skin areas one to three times a day.
Clinical studies of VALISONE have indicated that dosage only once or twice a day is often feasible and effective.
How Supplied: VALISONE **Lotion** 0.1% (containing 1.0 mg. betamethasone as the valerate per gram of lotion) is available in 20 ml. and 60 ml. plastic squeeze bottles; boxes of one.
Protect from light. Store between 59° and 86° F.
VALISONE **Ointment** 0.1% is supplied in 5-, 15-, and 45-gram tubes; boxes of one.
Store away from heat.

VALISONE® ℞
brand of betamethasone valerate, NF
Reduced Strength Cream 0.01%

How Supplied: VALISONE Reduced Strength Cream, 0.01%, is supplied in 15- and 60-gram tubes; boxes of one.
For complete prescribing information, contact the Schering Professional Services Department.

VANCERIL® Inhaler ℞
brand of beclomethasone dipropionate
FOR ORAL INHALATION ONLY

Description: Beclomethasone dipropionate, the active component of VANCERIL Inhaler, is an anti-inflammatory steroid having the chemical name 9-Chloro-11β,17-21-trihydroxy-16 β-methylpregna-1,4-diene-3, 20-dione 17,21-dipropionate.
VANCERIL Inhaler is a metered-dose aerosol unit containing a microcrystalline suspension of beclomethasone dipropionate-trichloromonofluoromethane clathrate in a mixture of propellants (trichloromonofluoromethane and dichlorodifluoromethane) with oleic acid. Each canister contains beclomethasone dipropionate-trichloromonofluoromethane clathrate having a molecular proportion of beclomethasone dipropionate to trichloromonofluoromethane between 3:1 and 3:2. Each actuation delivers from the mouthpiece a quantity of clathrate equivalent to 42 mcg. of beclomethasone dipropionate. The contents of one canister provide at least 200 oral inhalations.
Clinical Pharmacology: Beclomethasone 17,21-dipropionate is a diester of beclomethasone, a synthetic corticosteriod which is chemically related to prednisolone. Beclomethasone differs from prednisolone only in having a chlorine at the 9-alpha and a methyl group at the 16-beta position in place of hydrogen. Animal studies showed that beclomethasone dipropionate has potent anti-inflammatory activity. When administered systemically to mice, the anti-inflammatory activity was accompanied by other typical features of glucocorticoid action including thymic involution, liver glycogen deposition, and pituitary-adrenal suppression. However, after systemic administration to rats, the anti-inflammatory action was associated with little or no effect on other tests of glucocorticoid activity.
Beclomethasone dipropionate is sparingly soluble and is poorly mobilized from subcutaneous or intramuscular injection sites. However, systemic absorption occurs after all routes of administration. When given to animals in the form of an aerosolized suspension of the trichloromonofluoromethane clathrate, the drug is deposited in the mouth and nasal passages, the trachea and principal bronchi, and in the lung; a considerable portion of the drug is also swallowed. Absorption occurs rapidly from all respiratory and gastrointestinal tissues, as indicated by the rapid clearance of radioac-

tively labeled drug from local tissues and appearance of tracer in the circulation. There is no evidence of tissue storage of beclomethasone dipropionate or its metabolites. Lung slices can metabolize beclomethasone dipropionate rapidly to beclomethasone 17-monopropionate and more slowly to free beclomethasone (which has very weak anti-inflammatory activity). However, irrespective of the route of administration (injection, oral, or aerosol), the principal route of excretion of the drug and its metabolites is the feces. Less than 10% of the drug and its metabolites is excreted in the urine. In humans, 12% to 15% of an orally administered dose of beclomethasone dipropionate was excreted in the urine as both conjugated and free metabolites of the drug.

The mechanisms responsible for the anti-inflammatory action of beclomethasone dipropionate are unknown. The precise mechanism of the aerosolized drug's action in the lung is also unknown.

Indications: VANCERIL Inhaler is indicated only for patients who require chronic treatment with corticosteroids for control of the symptoms of bronchial asthma. Such patients would include those already receiving systemic corticosteroids, and selected patients who are inadequately controlled on a non-steroid regimen and in whom steroid therapy has been withheld because of concern over potential adverse effects.

VANCERIL Inhaler is NOT indicated:

1. For relief of asthma which can be controlled by bronchodilators and other non-steroid medications.
2. In patients who require systemic corticosteroid treatment infrequently.
3. In the treatment of non-asthmatic bronchitis.

Contraindications: VANCERIL Inhaler is contraindicated in the primary treatment of status asthmaticus or other acute episodes of asthma where intensive measures are required.

Hypersensitivity to any of the ingredients of this preparation contraindicates its use.

Warnings:

Particular care is needed in patients who are transferred from systemically active corticosteroids to VANCERIL Inhaler because deaths due to adrenal insufficiency have occurred in asthmatic patients during and after transfer from systemic corticosteroids to aerosal beclomethasone dipropionate. After withdrawal from systemic corticosteroids, a number of months are required for recovery of hypothalamic-pituitary-adrenal (HPA) function. During this period of HPA suppression, patients may exhibit signs and symptoms of adrenal insufficiency when exposed to trauma, surgery or infections, particularly gastroenteritis. Although VANCERIL Inhaler may provide control of asthmatic symptoms during these episodes, it does NOT provide the systemic steroid which is necessary for coping with these emergencies. During periods of stress or a severe asthmatic attack, patients who have been withdrawn from systemic corticosteroids should be instructed to resume systemic steroids (in large doses) immediately and to contact their physician for further instruction. These patients should also be instructed to carry a warning card indicating that they may need supplementary systemic steroids during periods of stress or a severe asthma attack. To assess the risk of adrenal insufffficiency in emergency situations, routine tests of adrenal cortical function, including measurement of early morning resting cortisol levels, should be performed periodically in all patients. An early morning resting cortisol level may be accepted as normal only if it falls at or near the normal mean level.

Localized infections with *Candida albicans* or *Aspergillus niger* have occurred frequently in the mouth and pharynx and occasionally in the larynx. Positive cultures for oral *Candida* may be present in up to 75% of patients. Although the frequency of clinically apparent infection is considerably lower, these infections may require treatment with appropriate antifungal therapy or discontinuance of treatment with VANCERIL Inhaler.

VANCERIL Inhaler is not to be regarded as a bronchodilator and is not indicated for rapid relief of bronchospasm.

Patients should be instructed to contact their physician immediately when episodes of asthma which are not responsive to bronchodilators occur during the course of treatment with VANCERIL. During such episodes, patients may require therapy with systemic corticosteroids.

There is no evidence that control of asthma can be achieved by the administration of VANCERIL in amounts greater than the recommended doses.

Transfer of patients from systemic steroid therapy to VANCERIL Inhaler may unmask allergic conditions previously suppressed by the systemic steroid therapy, e.g., rhinitis, conjunctivitis, and eczema.

Precautions: During withdrawal from oral steroids, some patients may experience symptoms of systemically active steroid withdrawal, e.g., joint and/or muscular pain, lassitude and depression, despite maintenance or even improvement of respiratory function (See DOSAGE AND ADMINISTRATION for details).

In responsive patients, beclomethasone dipropionate may permit control of asthmatic symptoms without suppression of HPA function, as discussed below (See CLINICAL STUDIES). Since beclomethasone dipropionate is absorbed into the circulation and can be systemically active, the beneficial effects of VANCERIL Inhaler in minimizing or preventing HPA dysfunction may be expected only when recommended dosages are not exceeded.

The long-term effects of beclomethasone dipropionate in human subjects are still unknown. In particular, the local effects of the agent on developmental or immunologic processes in the mouth, pharynx, trachea, and lung are unknown. There is also no information about the possible long-term systemic effects of the agent.

In a one-year oral inhalation study in beagle dogs, narrowed or irregular tracheal caliber was observed on postmortem examination of the treated dogs, but not in the control dogs. Further, the possibility of a drug-related interference with sexual maturation or function of female dogs was suggested by this study (See ANIMAL PHARMACOLOGY AND TOXICOLOGY). The relevance to patients of both of these findings following prolonged administration of the drug is not known.

The potential effects of VANCERIL on acute, recurrent, or chronic pulmonary infections, including active or quiescent tuberculosis, are not known. Similarly, the potential effects of long-term administration of the drug on lung or other tissues are unknown.

Pulmonary infiltrates with eosinophilia may occur in patients on VANCERIL Inhaler therapy. Although it is possible that in some patients this state may become manifest because of systemic steroid withdrawal when inhalational steroids are administered, a causative role for beclomethasone dipropionate and/or its vehicle cannot be ruled out.

Use in Pregnancy: Glucocorticoids are known teratogens in rodent species and beclomethasone dipropionate is no exception.

Teratology studies were done in rats, mice, and rabbits treated with subcutaneous beclomethasone dipropionate. Beclomethasone dipropionate was found to produce fetal resorptions, cleft palate, agnathia, microstomia, absence of tongue, delayed ossification and partial agenesis of the thymus. Well-controlled trials relating to fetal risk in humans are not available. Glucocorticoids are secreted in human milk. It is not known whether beclomethasone dipropionate would be secreted in human milk but it is safe to assume that it is likely. The use of beclomethasone dipropionate in pregnancy, nursing mothers, or women of childbearing potential requires that the possible benefits of the drug be weighed against the potential hazards to the mother, embryo, or fetus. Infants born of mothers who have received substantial doses of corticosteroids during pregnancy should be carefully observed for hypoadrenalism.

Adverse Reactions: Deaths due to adrenal insufficiency have occurred in asthmatic patients during and after transfer from systemic corticosteroids to aerosol beclomethasone dipropionate (See WARNINGS).

Suppression of HPA function (reduction of early morning plasma cortisol levels) have been reported in adult patients who received 1600 mcg. daily doses of VANCERIL for one month. A few patients on VANCERIL have complained of hoarseness or dry mouth. Bronchospasm and rash have been reported rarely.

Dosage and Administration: Adults: The usual dosage is two inhalations (84 mcg.) given three or four times a day. In patients with severe asthma, it is advisable to start with 12 to 16 inhalations a day and adjust the dosage downward according to the response of the patient. The maximal daily intake should not exceed 20 inhalations, 840 mcg. (0.84 mg.), in adults.

Children 6 to 12 years of age: The usual dosage is one or two inhalations (42 to 84 mcg.) given three or four times a day according to the response of the patient. The maximal daily intake should not exceed ten inhalations, 420 mcg. (0.42 mg.), in children 6 to 12 years of age. Insufficient clinical data exist with respect to the administration of VANCERIL Inhaler in children below the age of 6. Rinsing the mouth after inhalation is advised.

Patients receiving bronchodilators by inhalation should be advised to use the bronchodilator before VANCERIL Inhaler in order to enhance penetration of beclomethasone dipropionate into the bronchial tree. After use of an aerosol bronchodilator, several minutes should elapse before use of the VANCERIL Inhaler to reduce the potential toxicity from the inhaled fluorocarbon propellants in the two aerosols.

Different considerations must be given to the following groups of patients in order to obtain the full therapeutic benefit of VANCERIL Inhaler.

Patients not receiving systemic steroids: The use of VANCERIL Inhaler is straightforward in patients who are inadequately controlled with non-steroid medications but in whom systemic steroid therapy has been withheld because of concern over potential adverse reactions. In patients who respond to VANCERIL, an improvement in pulmonary function is usually apparent within one to four weeks after the start of VANCERIL Inhaler.

Patients receiving systemic steroids: In those patients dependent on systemic steroids, transfer to VANCERIL and subsequent management may be more difficult because recovery from impaired adrenal function is usually slow. Such suppression has been known to last for up to 12 months. Clinical studies, however,

Continued on next page

Information on Schering products appearing on these pages is effective as of September 30, 1979.

Schering—Cont.

have demonstrated that VANCERIL may be effective in the management of these asthmatic patients and may permit replacement or significant reduction in the dosage of systemic corticosteroids.
The patient's asthma should be reasonably stable before treatment with VANCERIL Inhaler is started. Initially, the aerosol should be used concurrently with the patient's usual maintenance dose of systemic steroid. After approximately one week, gradual withdrawal of the systemic steroid is started by reducing the daily or alternate daily dose. The next reduction is made after an interval of one or two weeks, depending on the response of the patient. Generally, these decrements should not exceed 2.5 mg. of prednisone or its equivalent. A slow rate of withdrawal cannot be overemphasized. During withdrawal, some patients may experience symptoms of systemically active steroid withdrawal, e.g., joint and/or muscular pain, lassitude and depression, despite maintenance or even improvement of respiratory function. Such patients should be encouraged to continue with the Inhaler but should be watched carefully for objective signs of adrenal insufficiency, such as hypotension and weight loss. If evidence of adrenal insufficiency occurs, the systemic steroid dose should be boosted temporarily and thereafter further withdrawal should continue more slowly.
During periods of stress or a severe asthma attack, transfer patients will require supplementary treatment with systemic steroids. Exacerbations of asthma which occur during the course of treatment with VANCERIL Inhaler should be treated with a short course of systemic steroid which is gradually tapered as these symptoms subside. There is no evidence that control of asthma can be achieved by administration of VANCERIL in amounts greater than the recommended doses.
Directions for Use: Illustrated patient instructions for proper use accompany each package of VANCERIL Inhaler.
CONTENTS UNDER PRESSURE. Do not puncture. Do not use or store near heat or open flame. Exposure to temperatures above 120°F. may cause bursting. Never throw container into fire or incinerator. Keep out of reach of children.
How Supplied: VANCERIL Inhaler 16.89 canister; box of one. It is supplied with an oral adapter and patient's instructions; (NDC-0085-0736-04).
Animal Pharmacology and Toxicology: Studies in a number of animal species including rats, rabbits, and dogs have shown no unusual toxicity during acute experiments. However, the effects of beclomethasone dipropionate in producing signs of glucocorticoid excess during chronic administration by various routes were dose related.
Particular note is made of a one-year study in dogs (beagles) which were given beclomethasone dipropionate in the form of the aerosolized suspension of the trichloromonofluoromethane clathrate; some of the animals also received supplementary treatment with oral beclomethasone. The animals which were given the larger treatment doses of beclomethasone dipropionate trichloromonofluoromethane clathrate, with or without oral beclomethasone dipropionate, developed severe Cushing's syndrome, associated with suppression of pituitary-adrenal function, delayed growth and sexual maturation, obesity, fatty infiltration of the liver, etc. Even in the absence of severe Cushing's syndrome, the following adverse reactions were noted in the young beagles (age 17 weeks at beginning of study): (1) There was a high incidence of convulsions and uncoordinated movements which were attributed to excessive fluorocarbon propellant and/or the possible anoxia caused by the mode of administration of the aerosol. (2) On post-mortem examination narrowed or irregular tracheal caliber was noted in the treated, but not in the control groups. (3) In female animals, the possibility of a drug-related interference with sexual maturation or function was suggested by the ovarian and uterine weights which were disproportionately low in relation to body size. It is unknown whether these observations in beagles have any relationship to possible adverse effects of prolonged administration of the drug in man, and additional studies will be carried out to clarify this matter.
Clinical Studies: The effects of beclomethasone dipropionate on hypothalamic-pituitary-adrenal (HPA) function have been evaluated in adult volunteers. There was no suppression of early morning plasma cortisol concentrations when beclomethasone dipropionate was administered in a dose of 1000 mcg./day for one month as an aerosol or for three days by intramuscular injection. However, partial suppression of plasma cortisol concentration was observed when beclomethasone dipropionate was administered in doses of 2000 mcg./day either intramuscularly or by aerosol. Immediate suppression of plasma cortisol concentrations was observed after single doses of 4000 mcg. of beclomethasone dipropionate.
In one study, the effects of beclomethasone dipropionate on HPA function were examined in patients with asthma. There was no change in basal early morning plasma cortisol concentrations or in the cortisol responses to tetracosactrin (ACTH 1:24) stimulation after daily administration of 400, 800 or 1200 mcg. of beclomethasone dipropionate for 28 days. After daily administration of 1600 mcg. each day for 28 days, there was a slight reduction in basal cortisol concentrations and a statistically significant ($p < .01$) reduction in plasma cortisol responses to tetracosactrin stimulation. The effects of a more prolonged period of beclomethasone dipropionate administration on HPA function have not been evaluated. However, a number of investigators have noted that when systemic corticosteroid therapy in asthmatic subjects can be replaced with recommended doses of beclomethasone dipropionate, there is gradual recovery of endogenous cortisol concentrations to the normal range. There is still no documented evidence of recovery from other adverse systemic corticosteroid-induced reactions during prolonged therapy of patients with beclomethasone dipropionate.
Clinical experience has shown that some patients with bronchial asthma who require corticosteroid therapy for control of symptoms can be partially or completely withdrawn from systemic corticosteroid if therapy with beclomethasone dipropionate aerosol is substituted. Beclomethasone dipropionate aerosol is not effective for all patients with bronchial asthma or at all stages of the disease in a given patient.
The early clinical experience has revealed several new problems which may be associated with the use of beclomethasone dipropionate by inhalation for treatment of patients with bronchial asthma:
1. There is a risk of adrenal insufficiency when patients are transferred from systemic corticosteroids to aerosol beclomethasone dipropionate. Although the aerosol may provide adequate control of asthma during the transfer period, it does not provide the systemic steroid which is needed during acute stress situations. Deaths due to adrenal insufficiency have occurred in asthmatic patients during and after transfer from systemic corticosteroids to aerosol beclomethasone dipropionate. (See WARNINGS.)
2. Transfer of patients from systemic steroid therapy to beclomethasone dipropionate aerosol may unmask allergic conditions which were previously controlled by the systemic steroid therapy, e.g., rhinitis, conjunctivitis, and eczema.
3. Localized infections with *Candida albicans* or *Aspergillus niger* have occurred frequently in the mouth and pharynx and occasionally in the larynx. It has been reported that up to 75% of the patients who receive prolonged treatment with beclomethasone dipropionate have positive oral cultures for *Candida albicans.* The incidence of clinically apparent infection is considerably lower but may require therapy with appropriate antifungal agents or discontinuation of treatment with beclomethasone dipropionate aerosol.
The long-term effects of beclomethasone dipropionate in human subjects are still unknown. In particular, the local effects of the agent on developmental or immunologic processes in the mouth, pharynx, trachea and lung are unknown. There is also no information about the possible long-term systemic effects of the agent. The possible relevance of the data in animal studies to results in human subjects cannot be evaluated.

[*Shown in Product Identification Section*]

Information on Schering products appearing on these pages is effective as of September 30, 1979.

Schmid Products Company

Division of Schmid Laboratories, Inc.
ROUTE 46 WEST
LITTLE FALLS, NEW JERSEY 07424

RAMSES® BENDEX® ℞
FLEXIBLE CUSHIONED DIAPHRAGM
(Arc-ing Spring)

Composition: Noted for its unusual rim design—a rust-resistant arc-ing spring encased in a cushion of soft rubber tubing. The BENDEX Diaphragm retains all the features of the regular RAMSES Diaphragm, *plus the hinge mechanism.* Lateral flexibility supplies the proper degree of spring tension without discomfort, permitting complete freedom of movement while maintaining anterior-posterior rigidity and a spermtight fit against the vaginal walls.
Action and Uses: Provides complete comfort and safety to the patient with structural abnormalities such as cystocele or rectocele. Use does not impair future planned pregnancy and does not alter female physiology. Recommended for use with RAMSES Contraceptive Vaginal Jelly in combined technique of conception control.
Note: See under RAMSES Contraceptive Vaginal Jelly for full disclosure.
Administration and Dosage: Easily inserted, slips readily into place without the use of an introducer, and easily removed. Insert diaphragm up to one hour before coitus, according to instructions in "Information for Patients" in package circular. Diaphragm should be left in place at least 8 hours after coitus.
Side Effects: None.
Precautions: None.
Contraindications: None.
How Supplied: RAMSES BENDEX Diaphragm: Package #603, Bendex and 1¼ oz. tube of Ramses Vaginal Jelly; package #703, Bendex zipper kit. Diaphragms prescribed in sizes 65–90 mm.

RAMSES® ℞
FLEXIBLE CUSHIONED DIAPHRAGM

Composition: A coral-colored rim with a dome of pure gum rubber. Rim construction: spring coil encased in soft rubber to buffer spring

pressure; flexible in all planes, thus permitting ready adjustment to muscular action of vagina.
Action and Uses: Provides dependable barrier to sperm, with complete comfort to patient. Use does not impair future planned pregnancy and does not impair female physiology. Recommended for use with RAMSES Contraceptive Vaginal Jelly in combined technique of conception control.
Note: See under RAMSES Contraceptive Vaginal Jelly for full disclosure.
Administration and Dosage: Easily inserted, placed and removed. Insert diaphragm up to one hour before coitus, according to instructions for "Information for Patients" in package circular. Diaphragm should be left in place at least 8 hours after last coitus.
Side Effects: None.
Precautions: None.
Contraindications: None.
How Supplied: RAMSES DIAPHRAGM: Package #602; diaphragm and 1¼ oz. tube RAMSES Vaginal Jelly, package #701 diaphragm, introducer, and 3 oz. tube RAMSES Vaginal Jelly in zipper kit. Diaphragms prescribed in sizes 50–95 mm.

RAMSES® CONTRACEPTIVE VAGINAL JELLY

Composition: Active agents, nonoxynol-9 5%, boric acid 1%, ethyl alcohol 5%, in a jelly base.
Action and Uses: For conception control by jelly-alone technique or with a diaphragm. Immobilizes sperm and maintains an occlusive barrier. Will not liquefy at body temperature, water-miscible and nonstaining, unobtrusively fragrant, acceptable to *both* partners. Use does not impair future planned pregnancy.
Administration and Dosage: Easily administered with nonbreakable, plastic applicator, easily cleaned. Full instructions provided in package circular.
Jelly-Alone Technique:
1. Place threaded applicator tip over mouth of jelly tube. Turn it gently until applicator is firmly attached.
2. Pull plunger back about ½ inch. Squeeze tube from bottom until applicator fills to ridge marked. Unscrew applicator from tube and insert into the vagina.
3. Holding applicator between thumb and third finger, press plunger with index finger as far as it will go. This deposits correct amount of protective jelly in front of cervix.

Jelly-Diaphragm Technique: Applicator not necessary.
Deposit about 1 teaspoonful of RAMSES Jelly directly from tube into dome of diaphragm. Lubricate entire rim with jelly to facilitate insertion and provide additional protection.
Side Effects: No significant side effects reported to date.
Precautions: RAMSES Vaginal Jelly should not be removed from vagina for at least 8 hours after intercourse. While douching is not necessary, a douche of 2 quarts of warm water may be used for the removal of jelly. A new application of RAMSES Vaginal Jelly is required before each act of coitus.
Contraindications: None.
How Supplied: No. 3 Set: 3-oz. tube and measured-dose applicator. Refills available in 3-oz. (No. 2) and 5-oz. (No. 5) economy size tubes.

SAF-T-COIL® ℞
Intra-Uterine Contraceptive Device

U.S. Patents 3,374,788; 3,234,938; 3,590,816; and 3,630,190.

Description: Saf-T-Coil is a double coil intrauterine contraceptive device made of a plastic material, Ethylene-vinyl acetate copolymer, with barium sulfate added for radiopacity and release agents. The Saf-T-Coil is provided sterile in three sizes. Saf-T-Coil 33-S, the standard size, is 37 mm in width by 32 mm in length. Saf-T-Coil 32-S, the intermediate size, is 29 mm in width and 30 mm in length. Saf-T-Coil 25-S Nullip, the small size is 25 mm in width by 20 mm in length. The components in the package include the Saf-T-Coil with monofilament nylon sutures. In addition, disposable plastic insertion tube with adjustable blue stop, plastic plunger, and uterine sound are included (packages containing 33-SX, 32-SX, and 25-SX Nullip do not include the uterine sound).
Mode of Action: The exact mechanism by which the inert Saf-T-Coil attains effective conception control has not been conclusively demonstrated. IUD's seem to interfere in some manner with nidation in the endometrium, probably through foreign body reaction in the uterus.
Indications: Saf-T-Coil is indicated for contraception.
Contraindications: IUD's should not be inserted when the following conditions exist:
1. Pregnancy or suspicion of pregnancy.
2. Abnormalities of the uterus resulting in distortion of the uterine cavity.
3. Acute pelvic inflammatory disease or a history of repeated pelvic inflammatory disease.
4. Post partum endometritis or infected abortion in the past 3 months.
5. Known or suspected uterine or cervical malignancy including unresolved, abnormal "Pap" smear.
6. Genital bleeding of unknown etiology.
7. Untreated acute cervicitis until infection is controlled.

Warnings:
1. Pregnancy—a. Long-term effects. Long-term effects on the off-spring when pregnancy occurs with Saf-T-Coil in place are unknown.
b. Septic abortion. Reports have indicated an increased incidence of septic abortion associated in some instances with septicemia, septic shock, and death in patients becoming pregnant with an IUD in place. Most of these reports have been associated with the midtrimester of pregnancy. In some cases, the initial symptoms have been insidious and not easily recognized. If pregnancy should occur with an IUD in place, the IUD should be removed if the string is visible or, if removal proves to be or would be difficult, termination of the pregnancy should be considered and offered the patient as an option bearing in mind that the risks associated with an elective abortion increase with gestational age.
c. Continuation of pregnancy: If the patient chooses to continue the pregnancy, she must be warned of the increased risk of spontaneous abortion and of the increased risk of sepsis, including death if the pregnancy continues with the IUD in place. The patient must be closely observed and she must be advised to report all abnormal symptoms, such as flu-like syndrome, fever, abdominal cramping, and pain, bleeding, or vaginal discharge, immediately because generalized symptoms of septicemia may be insidious.
2. Ectopic pregnancy. a. A pregnancy that occurs with an IUD in place is more likely to be ectopic than a pregnancy occurring without an IUD in place. Accordingly, patients who become pregnant while using the IUD should be carefully evaluated for the possibility of an ectopic pregnancy.
b. Special attention should be directed to patients with delayed menses, slight metrorrhagia and/or unilateral pelvic pain and to those patients who wish to terminate a pregnancy because of IUD failure to determine whether ectopic pregnancy has occurrred.
3. Pelvic infection. Pelvic infection may occur with the IUD in place and at times results in the development of tubo-ovarian abscesses or general peritonitis. Appropriate aerobic and anaerobic bacteriological studies should be done and antibiotic therapy initiated. If the infection does not show a marked clinical improvement within 24 to 48 hours, the IUD should be removed and the continuing treatment reassessed based upon the results of culture and sensitivity tests.
4. Embedment. Partial penetration or lodging of the IUD in the endometrium can result in difficult removals.
5. Perforation. Partial or total perforation of the uterine wall or cervix may occur with the use of IUD's. The possibility of perforation must be kept in mind during insertion and at the time of any subsequent examination. If perforation occurs, the IUD should be removed. Adhesions, foreign body reactions, and intestinal obstruction may result if an IUD is left in the peritoneal cavity.

Precautions:
1. Patient counseling. Prior to insertion the physician, nurse, or other trained health professional must provide the patient with the Patient Brochure. The patient should be given the opportunity to read the brochure and discuss fully any questions she may have concerning the IUD as well as other methods of contraception.
2. Patient evaluation and clinical considerations. a. A complete medical history should be obtaned to determine conditions that might influence the selection of an IUD. Physical examination should include a pelvic examination, "Pap" smear, gonorrhea culture and, if indicated, appropriate tests for other forms of venereal disease.
b. The uterus should be carefully sounded prior to insertion to determine the degree of patency of the endocervical canal and the internal os, and the direction and depth of the uterine cavity. In occasional cases, severe cervical stenosis may be encountered. Do not use excessive force to overcome this resistance.
c. The uterus should sound to a depth of 6 to 8 centimeters (cm). Insertion of an IUD into a uterine cavity measuring less than 6.5 cm by sounding may increase the incidence of expulsion, bleeding and pain.
d. The possibility of insertion in the presence of an existing undetermined pregnancy is reduced if insertion is performed during or shortly following a menstrual period. The IUD should not be inserted post partum or postabortion until involution of the uterus is completed. The incidence of perforation and expulsion is greater if involution is not completed.
e. IUD's should be used with caution in those patients who have anemia or a history of menorrhagia or hypermenorrhea. Patients experiencing menorrhagia and/or metrorrhagia following IUD insertion may be at risk for the development of hypochromic microcytic anemia. Also, IUD's should be used with caution in patients receiving anticoagulants or having a coagulopathy.
f. Syncope, bradycardia, or other neurovascular episodes may occur during insertion or removal of IUD's especially in patients with a previous disposition to these conditions.
g. Patients with valvular or congenital heart disease are more prone to develop subacute bacterial endocarditis than patients who do not have valvular or congenital heart disease. Use of an IUD in these patients may represent a potential source of septic emboli.
h. Use of an IUD in those patients with acute cervicitis should be postponed until proper treatment has cleared up the infection.
i. Since an IUD may be expelled or displaced, patients should be reexamined and evaluated shortly after the first postinsertion menses, but definitely within 3 months after insertion. Thereafter, annual examina-

Continued on next page

Schmid—Cont.

tion with appropriate medical and laboratory examination should be carried out.

j. The patient should be told that some bleeding and cramps may occur during the first few weeks after insertion, but if these symptoms continue or are severe she should report them to her physician. She should be instructed on how to check after each menstrual period to make certain that the thread still protrudes from the cervix, and she should be cautioned that there is no contraceptive protection if the IUD is expelled. She should be cautioned not to pull on the thread and displace the IUD. If partial expulsion occurs, removal is indicated and a new IUD may be inserted.

k. The use of medical diathermy (shortwave and microwave) in patients with metal-containing IUD's may cause heat injury to the surrounding tissue. Therefore, medical diathermy to the abdominal and sacral areas should not be used.*

Adverse Reactions: These adverse reactions are not listed in any order of frequency or severity.

Reported adverse reactions include: endometritis, spontaneous abortion, septic abortion, septicemia, perforation of the uterus and cervix, embedment, fragmentation of the IUD, pelvic infection, vaginitis, leukorrhea, cervical erosion, pregnancy, ectopic pregnancy, difficult removal, complete or partial expulsion of the IUD, intermenstrual spotting, prolongation of menstrual flow, anemia, pain and cramping, dysmenorrhea, backaches, dyspareunia, neurovascular episodes including bradycardia and syncope secondary to insertion. Perforation into the abdomen has been followed by abdominal adhesions, intestinal penetration, intestinal obstruction, and cystic masses in the pelvis.

Directions for Use:

Insertion Technique

Preparation for Insertion: For insertion of Saf-T-Coil 33-S, 32-S and 25-S Nullip use Saf-T-Sound where indicated (physician use own appropriate uterine sound for 33-SX, 32-SX and 25-SX Nullip). To facilitate insertion, have at hand sponges, an antiseptic solution and sterile speculum, tenaculum, uterine sound and scissors.

1) Cleanse vagina and cervix with an antiseptic solution.
2) Peel the transparent cover of the sterile package about ⅓ length and remove Saf-T-Sound.
3) Gently probe the cervical canal with the uterine sound to determine the depth, position and direction of the uterus and to check for any abnormality.
4) Leave the sound in position for a few moments to slightly dilate the cervix, to align the cervical canal, and to ease the way for passage of the insertion tube.
5) Remove the sound and note the depth of the uterine cavity.

Loading the Insertion Tube

1) With the Saf-T-Coil on the package insert card, position the adjustable blue stop on the insertion tube 1.5 cm less than the depth of the uterine cavity as measured by the uterine sound. Rotate the blue stop, if necessary, to be sure its tabs are in the same plane as coils of Saf-T-Coil. Bend insertion tube (containing Saf-T-Coil) to approximate the natural curvature of the canal as determined with the uterine sound. Grasping the protruding end of the plunger, slowly pull Saf-T-Coil into insertion tube until nodule on the end of the coil contacts the distal end of the insertion tube and remains in place.

NOTE: Do not hold Saf-T-Coil in the insertion tube more than 5 minutes to prevent loss of its 'memory'.

Push plunger back into insertion tube as far as possible without advancing Saf-T-Coil.

Introducing Device into Uterus

While holding the tenaculum in one hand, gently introduce the distal end of the loaded insertion tube into the cervical os. Carefully advance it into the uterus until the blue stop is flush with the cervix, keeping the tabs of the blue stop parallel to the frontal plane of the body.

Meticulous care should be exercised at this point to avoid excessive pressure against the fundus.

Depositing the Saf-T-Coil

Hold plunger in place and retract insertion tube over the plunger. This releases Saf-T-Coil, without pressure, into proper position within the uterine cavity. (If there is any question as to its having attained its proper position, withdraw at once into the insertion tube and reinsert as described above).

Completing the Insertion

Wait a full minute, to allow Saf-T-Coil to assume its original configuration. Withdraw the insertion tube until the sutures become visible. With scissors, clip sutures leaving about 2 inches of sutures exposed. (Sutures may be shortened at a later date, if desired).

Do not leave patient unattended. Observe patient several minutes after insertion for signs of syncope, severe cramping, abnormal bleeding, or extrusion of the coil.

Clinical Studies: Different event rates have been recorded with the use of different IUD's. Inasmuch as these rates are usually derived from separate studies conducted by different investigators in several population groups, they cannot be compared with precision. Furthermore, event rates tend to be lower as clinical experience is expanded, possibly due to retention in the clinical study of those patients who accept the treatment regimen and do not discontinue due to adverse reactions or pregnancy. In clinical trials conducted by Tietze (1967), Solish and Majzlin (1968), Tietze and Lewit (1970), Hayes (1973) and Laufe, *et al* (1974) with the Saf-T-Coil, use effectiveness was determined as follows for parous and nulliparous women, as tabulated by the life table method. (Rates are expressed as events per 100 women through 12 and 24 months of use). This experience is based on 46,721 women/months of use including 4,231 women who completed 12 months of use and 1,842 women who completed 24 months of use.

[See table below].

	12 Months		24 Months	
	Parous	Nulliparous	Parous	Nulliparous
Pregnancy	2.4 (0.42-2.8)	—	3.1 (0.42-3.8)	—
Expulsion	18.3 (7.8-29.0)	—	18.8 (9.0-21.5)	—
Medical removal	15.6 (4.8-18.7)	—	23.2 (9.0-27.0)	—
Continuation rate	70.4 (55.2-88.0)	—	59.8 (57.0-81.5)	—

References:

Hayes, O.J.: *A Clinical Evaluation of the Intrauterine Device for Control of Contraception.* South. Med. J. 66:254 (1973).

Laufe, L.E., Brickner, P.B., Ryser, P.E., and Ammer, J.L.: *An Evaluation of the Use-Effectiveness of the Saf-T-Coil in Private Practice.* Contraception 9:23 (1974).

Solish, G.I. and Majzlin, G.: *The Majzlin Spring IUCD.* Presented at the Sixth Annual Meeting of the Am. Assoc. of Planned Parenthood Physicians, Apr. 16-17, 1968.

Tietze, C. and Lewit, S.: *Evaluation of Intrauterine Devices: Ninth Progress Report of the Operative Statistical Program.* Studies in Family Planning. A publication of The Population Council. No. 55, (1970).

Tietze, C.: *Report of a New IUD: The Double Coil.* Advances in Planned Parenthood, III:85 (1967).

Long Term Experience: An additional extensive study extending for five years relating actual field experience of the Florida Public Health Clinics has been reported. That study included 27,712 patients with 541,248 women months of use of the Saf-T-Coil. Event rates reported include 0.8% for pregnancy, 11.9% for expulsion, 8.0% for medical removal and continuation rate increased from 75% in 1967 to 80% in 1971. That study indicates that physicians and other medical personnel of diverse background and training are able to achieve outstanding use-effectiveness with the Saf-T-Coil when the device is properly inserted.

Reference:

Caraway, A.F., and Vaughn, B.J.: *Florida's Five Year Experience with the Double Coil IUD.* J. Reprod. Med. 10:170 (1973).

How Supplied: SAF-T-COIL is available in three sizes: 33-S (standard) for the multiparous patient; 32-S (intermediate) for the primiparous patient and the person who cannot accommodate the 33-S; and 25-S Nullip (small) for the nulliparous patient. Each package of SAF-T-COIL (33-S, 32-S, and 25-S Nullip) is enclosed with a SAF-T-SOUND in a sterile, peel package. SAF-T-SOUND is a sterile, disposable intrauterine probe that assists in more accurate placement of the SAF-T-COIL. SAF-T-COIL 33-SX, 32-SX and 25-SX Nullip are also available without the SAF-T-SOUND included in the package. Physician instructions and patient instructions are provided with each package. There are six SAF-T-COIL units per carton. SAF-T-COIL/SAF-T-SOUND units are available from Surgical Supply Dealers.

Federal law restricts this device to sale by or on the order of a physician.

*Not associated with Saf-T-Coil.

VAGISEC® Liquid
VAGISEC® PLUS Suppositories ℞

Composition: VAGISEC Liquid—active ingredients: Polyoxyethylene nonyl phenol, sodium edetate, sodium dioctyl sulfosuccinate. 3 gram VAGISEC PLUS Suppositories contain 9-aminoacridine hydrochloride 6 mg., polyoxyethylene nonyl phenol 5.25 mg., sodium edetate .66 mg., and sodium dioctyl sulfosuccinate 0.07 mg. in a polyethylene glycol base containing glycerin and citric acid.

Action: The polyoxyethylene nonyl phenol, sodium edetate and sodium dioctyl sulfosuccinate in combination, is a complex (Vagisec Liquid) long proven as an effective trichomonacide. The 9-aminoacridine is a broad spectrum antibacterial of extensive medical acceptance for the topical treatment of bacterial infections.

Indications: For the specific treatment of vaginitis caused by *Trichomonas vaginalis*, as well as mixed vaginal infections complicated by a bacterial moiety. For continued vaginal cleanliness, Vagisec Liquid makes a pleasant douche. It deodorizes, and leaves a clean, refreshed feeling.

Precautions: Therapeutic Treatment: Recurrence of vaginitis often indicates extravaginal foci or infection in cervical, vestibular and urethral glands, or reinfection by the sexual partner. During treatment, it is recommended that the patient refrain from intercourse or the partner should wear a prophylactic. To prevent flare-up after completion of therapy, the patient is advised to continue with VAGISEC Liquid as a regular douche.

Douche: use Vagisec Liquid for continued vaginal cleanliness, but no more than twice weekly unless otherwise directed by physician.

Contraindication: Douching is not recommended for pregnant patients. Vagisec Liquid and Vagisec Plus Suppositories are spermicidal and should not be used on days when the patient is trying to conceive.
Side Effects: No significant side effects reported to date. Any minor irritation is alleviated by discontinuance of douche for a single day.
Administration and Dosage: *Office Treatment (Adult):* For the treatment of vaginal trichomoniasis and mixed vaginal infections, best results are obtained by scrubbing the vagina with VAGISEC Liquid, diluted 1:100, by the physician in the office: 3 scrubs the first week, 2 the second. A suppository is inserted after each office scrub in the Liquid/Suppository regimen. Patient should be instructed to continue treatment at home. *Home Treatment:* Liquid/Suppository regimen: In all instances, the combination douche and suppositories are recommended for home use. The usual home treatment is VAGISEC Liquid Douche in the morning, followed by a VAGISEC PLUS Suppository inserted deep in the vagina and a second suppository inserted in like manner at bedtime daily, for a period of 14 days. For those physicians who feel it important to treat the patient through the complete menstrual cycle the Liquid/Suppository regimen may be continued throughout the month. It is advisable to continue treatment through two menstrual periods. Treatment should be omitted the night and morning preceding an office visit. Patients should be reexamined 3 days after home treatment has been discontinued. The full course of therapy must be completed to eliminate the infecting microorganisms from the vagina. In chronic or stubborn cases, therapy may be repeated with no interval between courses. During treatment, patient should refrain from intercourse, or the partner should wear a prophylactic. No patient should be considered cured until vaginal smears or cultures, taken at monthly intervals for 3 months following treatment, show absence of trichomonads and a return to the normal vaginal flora.
Douche for complete feminine hygiene: Premix one teaspoonful of VAGISEC Liquid Concentrate thoroughly in small amount of water in separate container. Then pour into douche bag and add sufficient warm water to make one quart mixture. Stir well. Use according to the proper douching technique described in the package insert.
How Supplied: VAGISEC Liquid — 4 oz. plastic bottle. VAGISEC PLUS suppositories-box of 28-3 gram suppositories, foil-wrapped, with inserter. Federal law prohibits dispensing VAGISEC PLUS suppositories without prescription.

Sclavo Inc.
5 MANSARD COURT
WAYNE, NEW JERSEY 07470

THE FOLLOWING IS A PRELIMINARY LISTING ONLY:
COMPLETE INFORMATION FOR THE BELOW LISTED PRODUCTS IS FURNISHED IN THE PACKAGING.

ANTIRABIES SERUM ℞
(equine), Purified, U.S.P.

How Supplied: 1,000 U. vial.

CHOLERA VACCINE ℞
U.S.P.

1.5ml vial; 20 ml vial

DIPHTHERIA ANTITOXIN ℞
(equine), Refined, U.S.P.

How Supplied: 10,000 U/5cc vial; 20,000 U/10cc vial.

DIPHTHERIA TOXOID, ADSORBED, U.S.P. ℞

How Supplied: 5cc vial.

DIPHTHERIA AND TETANUS TOXOIDS ADSORBED, USP ℞
(For Pediatric Use)

How Supplied: 5 ml vial, 0.5 ml vial.

SclavoTest®-PPD ℞
Tuberculin Purified Protein Derivative (PPD)
Multiple Puncture Device

For product information, consult Diagnostic Product Information Section.

TETANUS ANTITOXIN ℞
(equine), Refined, U.S.P.

How Supplied: 1,500 U. vial; 20,000 U. vial.

TETANUS TOXOID, ADSORBED, U.S.P. ℞

How Supplied: 5cc vial, 0.5cc vial.

TETANUS AND DIPHTHERIA TOXOIDS ADSORBED, USP ℞
(For Adult Use)

How Supplied: 5 ml vial, 0.5 ml vial.

Scot-Tussin Pharmacal Co., Inc.
50 CLEMENCE STREET
POST OFFICE BOX 8217
CRANSTON, RI 02920

Scot-Tussin National Drug Code

NDC 0372	Product
0001-04	SCOT-TUSSIN® Syrup
0001-16	
0001-28	
0002-04	SCOT-TUSSIN® Sugar-Free
0002-16	
0002-28	
0008-16	S-T DECONGEST™ Sugar-Free, Dye Free
0006-04	S-T EXPECTORANT™ Sugar-Free, Dye Free
0006-16	
0006-28	
0017-16	TUSSIREX™ w/CODEINE Syrup
0017-28	
0018-16	TUSSIREX™ w/CODEINE Sugar-Free
0018-28	

S-T FORTE™ Syrup
S-T FORTE™ SUGAR-FREE ©
(Formerly: SCOT-TUSSIN FORTE)

This is the text of the latest official Package Circular dated Nov. '69.
Alcohol 5% by volume.
Caution: Federal Law prohibits dispensing without a prescription.
Composition: Each oz. (30 ml) contains:
Hydrocodone Bitartrate, N.F. ....15 mg.
(Warning: May be habit forming.)
Phenylephrine HCl U.S.P. ....30 mg.
Phenylpropanolamine HCl, N.F. ....30 mg.
Pheniramine Maleate, N.F. ....80 mg.
Guaifenesin, N.F. ....480 mg.
Administration and Dosage:
Average Adult Dosage: One teaspoonful 3 or 4 times a day as indicated, not to exceed 4 teasp. in any 24 hours.
Children: 6 to 12 years, half teasp. 3 or 4 times a day as indicated, not to exceed 2 teasp. in any 24 hours.
Children: 3 to 6 years, ½ teasp.; 1 to 3 years 20 drops; 6 mos. to 1 year 10 drops.
Side Effects: S-T Forte is usually well tolerated, but if drowsiness or nausea or other side effects occur, discontinue its use immediately. Keep this and all medications out of the reach of children.
Action and Uses: S-T Forte, "The 5-action cough medicine", gives 5-action symptomatic relief of stubborn coughs and nasal congestion due to colds or hay fever. It contains: HYDROCODONE BITARTRATE, N.F., an excellent narcotic antitussive. PHENYLEPHRINE HCl U.S.P., an orally effective vasoconstrictor for relief of nasal congestion and bronchial spasm. PHENYLPROPANOLAMINE HCl, N.F., a well known decongestant used to shrink engorged mucous membranes caused by hay fever and allergic rhinitis. PHENIRAMINE MALEATE, N.F., one of the most potent antihistamines on a weight basis. GUAIFENESIN, N.F., an effective expectorant in the treatment of coughs.
Precautions and Contraindications: S-T Forte contains Hydrocodone Bitartrate and may be habit forming; therefore should be used with caution and only when indicated, not for a prolonged period of time. It should be used with caution in patients sensitive to antihistamines and to sympathomimetic products, or patients suffering with arteriosclerosis, hypertension or hyperthyroidism Patients taking S-T Forte should not drive vehicles or operate machinery.
How Supplied:
Syrup: Pints NDC 0372-0004-16; Gallons NDC 0372-0004-28.
Sugar-Free: Pints NDC 0372-0005-16; Gallons NDC 0372-0005-28.
S-T Forte is a schedule 3 controlled substance.

VITA-PLUS H™
(Hematinic)
SUGAR-FREE Liquid

Preliminary listing only.
Complete information furnished in the packaging.
Each teaspoonful (5 ml.) contains:
1-Lysine Mono HCl .... 100 mg.
Vitamin B_1 .... 10 mg.
Vitamin B_{12} (Cobalamin Conc.) .... 25 mcgm.
Vitamin B_6 .... 5 mg.
Iron Pyrophosphate soluble .... 100 mg.
(Equivalent to 22 mg. elemental iron)
In a palatable Sorbitol Base.
How Supplied: 4 oz. NDC 0372-0021-04
8 oz. NDC 0372-0021-08

IDENTIFICATION PROBLEM?

Consult PDR's

Product Identification Section

where you'll find over 900

products pictured actual size

and in full color.

Searle Laboratories
Division of Searle Pharmaceuticals Inc.
Box 5110
CHICAGO, ILLINOIS 60680

Searle & Co.*
SAN JUAN, PUERTO RICO 00936

Alphabetic Product Listing

List#	Prod. ID# (NDC†), Form, Strength
46	*Aldactazide, 1011, Tablet, 25 mg./25 mg.
39	*Aldactone, 1001, Tablet, 25 mg.
97	Aminophyllin, 1203, Ampul I.M., 500 mg./2 ml.
96	Aminophyllin, 1213, Ampul I.V., 250 mg./10 ml.
95	Aminophyllin, 1223, Ampul I.V., 500 mg./20 ml.
18	Aminophyllin, 1231, Tablet, 100 mg.
44	Aminophyllin, 1251, Tablet, 200 mg.
47	Amodrine, 1291, Tablet
43	Anavar, 1401, Tablet, 2.5 mg.
40	*Banthīne, 1501, Tablet, 50 mg.
152	Cu-7, 708, Unit
159	Comfolax, 1552, Capsule, 100 mg.
196	Comfolax-*plus*, 1572, Capsule, 100 mg./30 mg.
163	*Demulen Compack, 71, Tablet
172	*Demulen Refill, 71, Tablet
181	*Demulen Triopak, 71, Tablet
156	*Demulen-28 Compack, 71 (0081) Tablet
164	*Demulen-28 Refill, 71 (0081), Tablet
251	Diulo, 501, Tablet, 2½ mg.
273	Diulo, 511, Tablet, 5 mg.
285	Diulo, 521, Tablet, 10 mg.
74	Dramamine, 1724, Vial, 250 mg./5 ml.
34	Dramamine, 1703, Ampul, 50 mg./1 ml.
73	Dramamine, 1736, Liquid, 12.5 mg./4 ml.
72	Dramamine, 1701, Tablets, 50 mg.
71	Dramamine, 1715, Suppos., 100 mg.
112	Dramamine Unit-Dose, 1701, Tablet, 50 mg.
56	*Enovid, 51, Tablet, 5 mg.
22	*Enovid Calendar-Pack, 51, Tablet, 5 mg.
67	*Enovid, 101, Tablet, 10 mg.
27	*Enovid-E Compack, 131 (0121), Tablet
98	*Enovid-E Refill, 131 (0121), Tablet
153	*Enovid-E 21 Compack, 131, Tablet
191	*Enovid-E 21 Refill, 131, Tablet
111	*Flagyl, 1831, Tablet, 250 mg.
1093	Icy Hot 3½ oz. (2008), Balm
1097	Icy Hot 7 oz. (2008), Balm
10914	Icy Hot 14 oz. (2008), Balm
33	Ketochol, 2101, Tablet, 250 mg.
81	*Lomotil, 61, Tablet, 2.5 mg.
107	*Lomotil Audit Pack, 61, Tablet, 2.5 mg.
94	*Lomotil Liquid, 66, 2.5 mg./5 ml.
154	Mark-7 Sound, 709, Unit
5407	Metamucil 7 oz., 2209, Powder
5414	Metamucil 14 oz., 2209, Powder
5421	Metamucil 21 oz., 2209, Powder
1716	Metamucil Instant-Mix 16s, (2219), Packet
1730	Metamucil Instant-Mix 30s, (2219), Packet
123	Norpace, 2752, Capsule, 100 mg.
906	Norpace, 2762, Capsule, 150 mg.
24	*Ovulen Compack, 401 (0411), Tablet
59	*Ovulen Refill, 401 (0411), Tablet
129	*Ovulen-21 Compack, 401, Tablet
137	*Ovulen-21 Refill, 401, Tablet
133	*Ovulen-21 Triopak, 401, Tablet
130	*Ovulen-28 Compack, 401 (0421), Tablet,
141	*Ovulen-28 Refill, 401 (0421), Tablet
150	*Ovulen-28 Triopak,401(0421), Tablet
30	*Pro-Banthīne, 624, Vial, 30 mg.
28	*Pro-Banthīne, 601, Tablet, 15 mg.
121	*Pro-Banthīne Unit Dose, 601, Tablet, 15 mg.
9	*Pro-Banthīne 611, Tablet, 7½ mg.
29	*Pro-Banthīne with Phenobarbital, 631, Tablet, 15 mg./15 mg.
132	*Pro-Banthīne/Pheno Unit Dose, 631, Tablet, 15 mg./15 mg.
31	*Pro-Banthīne with Dartal, 641, Tablet, 15 mg./5 mg.

*Product of Searle & Co.
†When the Product ID# is not the same as the NDC#, the NDC# appears in parentheses.

Searle Laboratories
Division of Searle Pharmaceuticals Inc.
BOX 5110
CHICAGO, ILLINOIS 60680

AMINOPHYLLIN Injection ℞
(aminophylline)

Description: Each ampul of Aminophyllin contains an aqueous solution of aminophylline, a complex containing approximately 85% anhydrous theophylline and 15% ethylenediamine. Ampuls for intravenous injection contain 10 ml. (250 mg.) or 20 ml. (500 mg.). Ampuls for intramuscular injection contain 2 ml. (500 mg.) with 2% of benzyl alcohol and 58 mg. excess ethylenediamine per gram of aminophylline.

Clinical Pharmacology: Aminophylline directly relaxes the smooth muscle of the bronchial airways and pulmonary blood vessels, thus acting mainly as a bronchodilator, pulmonary vasodilator and smooth muscle relaxant. The drug also possesses other actions typical of the xanthine derivatives: coronary vasodilator, diuretic, cardiac stimulant, cerebral stimulant and skeletal muscle stimulant. Aminophylline is well known for its ability to increase the depth and rate of respiration.

In the body aminophylline is converted to its component parts: theophylline, the active ingredient, and ethylenediamine. Theophylline is converted by the liver to three major metabolites: 1, 3-dimethyluric acid, 1-methyluric acid, and 3-methylxanthine. These metabolites are excreted by the kidneys.

There is wide interpatient variability in the rate of clearance of theophylline. This is manifested by wide ranges of theophylline half-life seen in various patients ranging from four to ten hours after administration of aminophylline to adults. The mean half-life has been reported to be 5.2 hours. Children metabolize theophylline more rapidly, in general, with theophylline half-lives ranging from 1.4 to 7.8 hours and a mean half-life of 3.6 hours in children ages 4 to 15.

The half-life of theophylline is shortened with cigarette smoking which increases the clearance rate of theophylline. In patients with significant impairment of hepatic or renal function, and in patients with congestive heart failure, the half-life of theophylline is prolonged.

Indications: Aminophyllin is indicated for bronchial asthma, status asthmaticus, congestive heart failure, Cheyne-Stokes respiration, the reduction of exertional dyspnea in emphysema patients, and for cardiac paroxysmal dyspnea. It is also useful as a diuretic agent.

Contraindications: Patients with a history of hypersensitivity to aminophylline or theophylline should not be treated with Aminophyllin.

The drug should not be administered with other xanthine preparations. (See *PRECAUTIONS* regarding intake of coffee, tea, cola beverages and chocolate.)

Aminophyllin (aminophylline) should not be administered to patients with active peptic ulcer disease, since it may increase the volume and acidity of gastric secretions. Occasionally in such patients, the need for intravenous Aminophyllin may be so urgent that the physician will choose to give a course of Aminophyllin with concomitant therapy, as appropriate, for the peptic ulcer disease.

Warnings: Intravenous doses given too rapidly or excessive doses by any route of administration may be expected to be toxic, causing gastrointestinal, central nervous system, cardiovascular and/or respiratory symptoms (see *OVERDOSAGE*). Some children may be unusually sensitive to aminophylline. Toxic synergism with ephedrine and other sympathomimetic drugs may occur.

Caution should be used when aminophylline is given to patients in congestive heart failure. Serum levels in such patients may persist longer than expected. The same applies to patients with impaired liver function.

Use in Pregnancy: Safe use in pregnancy has not been established relative to possible adverse effects on fetal development. Therefore, Aminophyllin (aminophylline) should not be used in pregnant women unless, in the judgment of the physician, the potential benefits outweigh the possible hazards.

Precautions: Use with caution in patients with severe cardiac or hepatic disease, hypertension, hyperthyroidism, or acute myocardial injury. In patients with a history of peptic ulcer, this disease may be exacerbated.

The concurrent administration of aminophylline and ephedrine or other sympathomimetic drugs increases the toxicity potential and may result in symptoms of overdosage due to the additive pharmacological effects of these compounds.

The intramuscular administration of Aminophyllin (aminophylline) is painful.

When blood levels of theophylline are measured by spectrophotometric methods, coffee, tea, cola beverages, chocolate and acetaminophen contribute to falsely high values.

Adverse Reactions: The most frequently encountered adverse reactions observed with *therapeutic* amounts of aminophylline are:

1. Gastrointestinal: Nausea, vomiting, anorexia, and/or gastrointestinal distress.
2. Central nervous system: Nervousness, agitation, headache, dizziness, vertigo, lightheadedness.
3. Cardiovascular: Palpitation, tachycardia and/or other arrhythmias, flushing, and hypotension.
4. Respiratory: Increase in respiratory rate.
5. Dermatologic: Urticaria, skin rash.

Overdosage: The most consistent reactions observed with *toxic* overdoses of aminophylline are:

1. Gastrointestinal: Anorexia, nausea, vomiting, hematemesis.
2. Central nervous system: Nervousness, agitation, headache, vertigo, hyperreflexia, fasciculations, stupor, coma, and convulsions. (Convulsions are especially prone to occur in cases of overdosage in infants and small children.)
3. Cardiovascular: Tachycardia or other arrhythmias, diaphoresis, hypotension and, rarely, vasomotor collapse.
4. Respiratory: Tachypnea and hyperventilation. Respiratory arrest may occur.
5. Renal: Albuminuria and microhematuria may occur.
6. General systemic effects: Syncope, collapse, fever and dehydration, hyperthermia.

Management of Toxic Symptoms:
1. Discontinue drug immediately.
2. There is no known specific antidote.
3. Treatment is supportive and symptomatic.
4. Avoid administration of sympathomimetic drugs.

5. Intravenous fluids, oxygen and other supportive measures to prevent hypotension; correct dehydration and acid-base imbalance.
6. For hyperthermia, use a cooling blanket or give sponge baths as necessary.
7. Maintain patent airway and use artificial respiration in case of respiratory depression.
8. Control convulsions with appropriate parenteral medication(s) such as short-acting barbiturates, diazepam, or phenytoin.
9. Monitor serum theophylline levels until below 20 mcg./ml.

Dosage and Administration: *NOTE:* Before deciding upon the initial dose of intravenous or intramuscular Aminophyllin (aminophylline), the amount of aminophylline/theophylline received by the patient during the previous 12 to 24 hours should be ascertained. The dosages suggested below apply to patients who have normal cardiac and hepatic function and have had no aminophylline/theophylline therapy for at least 24 hours.

INTRAVENOUS ADMINISTRATION: In adults, 250 to 500 mg. Aminophyllin (5 to 6 mg./kg. of body weight) should initially be given slowly over a 20-minute period. The intravenous ampuls come in 10 ml. (250 mg.) or 20 ml. (500 mg.) sizes. This solution can either be injected very slowly by syringe or, more conveniently, may be infused in a small quantity (usually 100 to 200 ml.) of 5% dextrose in water or saline. This solution is sometimes given "piggy back" through an I.V. system already in place. The therapeutic effects can be expected to last for six to eight hours if adequate supportive management such as hydration, correction of electrolyte and pH imbalance and ventilatory assistance is provided. However, the initial 20-minute intravenous infusion can be immediately followed by continuous infusion of approximately 0.9 mg./kg./hr. This infusion can then be adjusted up or down according to the needs of the patient.

If congestive heart failure is present, the initial dose and subsequent doses of Aminophyllin should be decreased by 20 to 25 percent. Similarly, if hepatic impairment exists, the dose may need to be reduced.

Serum theophylline levels are valuable, especially where the response has been unsatisfactory. Serum concentrations of 10 to 20 mcg./ml. are considered to be in the therapeutic range.

Individuals differ in the amount of Aminophyllin required mainly because of differences in their rates of drug clearance.

In *children,* who generally metabolize aminophylline and theophylline more rapidly than adults, approximately 6 mg./kg. of body weight should initially be given intravenously over a 20-minute period. By noting the clinical response (and serum theophylline levels if available) the dosage for further intermittent or continuous infusions can be determined. Usual maintenance doses are 3.5 to 4.0 mg./kg. of body weight every six to eight hours with the Aminophyllin diluted in an intravenous solution.

Oral therapy should be substituted for intravenous Aminophyllin (aminophylline) as soon as adequate improvement is achieved.

INTRAMUSCULAR ADMINISTRATION: For *adults,* the usual dose is 5 to 6 mg./kg. of body weight every six to eight hours as required. Smaller doses may be adequate in some patients. For *children,* the doses required may be somewhat higher on an mg./kg. basis.

Drug Interactions: Studies in patients receiving the antibiotics troleandomycin or erythromycin concurrently with theophylline preparations have demonstrated that elevated serum levels of theophylline may result. Therefore, such patients should be watched carefully for signs of toxicity to theophylline and the dose of Aminophyllin decreased if necessary. If ephedrine or other sympathomimetic drugs are given concomitantly with Aminophyllin (aminophylline), toxic synergism may occur. Cigarette-smoking will increase the rate of metabolism of theophylline which may increase the dosage requirements of Aminophyllin (aminophylline).

INTRAVENOUS ADMIXTURE INCOMPATIBILITY: Although there have been reports of aminophylline precipitating in acidic media, these reports do not apply to the dilute solutions found in intravenous infusions. Aminophyllin should not be mixed in a syringe with other drugs but should be added separately to the intravenous solution.

Because of the alkalinity of aminophylline-containing solutions, drugs known to be alkali-labile should be avoided in admixtures. These would include isoproterenol HCl, epinephrine HCl, levarterenol bitartrate and penicillin G potassium.

When an intravenous solution containing Aminophyllin is given "piggy back," the intravenous system already in place should be turned off while the Aminophyllin (aminophylline) is infused if there is a potential problem with admixture incompatibility.

How Supplied: *For Intravenous Injection:* 10 ml. (250 mg.) or 20 ml. (500 mg.) ampuls, aqueous solution, U.S.P.; cartons of 5 and 25, and boxes of 100.

For Intramuscular Injection: 2 ml. (500 mg.) ampuls, aqueous solution with 2 percent of benzyl alcohol; cartons of 5, 25, and 100.

AMINOPHYLLIN Tablets ℞
(aminophylline)

Description: Each tablet contains 100 or 200 mg. of aminophylline U.S.P., a soluble complex containing approximately 85% anhydrous theophylline and 15% ethylenediamine. Aminophylline is white or slightly yellowish granules or powder, having a slight ammoniacal odor and a bitter taste.

Actions: Aminophylline directly relaxes the smooth muscle of the bronchial airways and pulmonary blood vessels, thus acting mainly as a bronchodilator, pulmonary vasodilator and smooth muscle relaxant. The drug also possesses other actions typical of the xanthine derivatives: coronary vasodilator, diuretic, cardiac stimulant, cerebral stimulant and skeletal muscle stimulant.

Indications: Aminophyllin Tablets are indicated for the relief of acute bronchial asthma and for reversible bronchospasm associated with chronic bronchitis and emphysema.

Contraindications: Aminophylline should not be administered to patients with active peptic ulcer disease, since it may increase the volume and acidity of gastric secretions.

Patients with a history of hypersensitivity to aminophylline or theophylline should not be treated with the drug.

Aminophylline should not be administered with other xanthine preparations.

Warnings: Excessive doses may be expected to be toxic. Some children may be unusually sensitive to aminophylline. Toxic synergism with ephedrine and other sympathomimetic bronchodilator drugs may occur.

Usage in Pregnancy. Safe use in pregnancy has not been established relative to possible adverse effects on fetal development. Therefore, aminophylline should not be used in pregnant women unless, in the judgment of the physician, the potential benefits outweigh the possible hazards.

Precautions: Use with caution in patients with severe cardiac disease, hypertension, hyperthyroidism, or acute myocardial injury. Particular caution in dose administration must be exercised in patients with a history of peptic ulcer since the condition may be exacerbated. Chronic oral administration in high doses may be associated with gastrointestinal irritation.

Caution should be used in giving aminophylline to patients in congestive heart failure. Serum levels in such patients have persisted for long periods following discontinuation of the drug.

The addition of ephedrine or other sympathomimetic drugs to regimens of aminophylline increases the toxicity potential and may result in symptoms of overdosage, due to the additive pharmacological effects of these compounds.

Adverse Reactions: The most consistent adverse reactions observed with *therapeutic* amounts of aminophylline are:

1. Gastrointestinal: Nausea, vomiting, anorexia, bitter aftertaste, dyspepsia, heavy feeling in the stomach and gastrointestinal distress.
2. Central nervous system: Dizziness, vertigo, light-headedness, headache, nervousness, insomnia and agitation.
3. Cardiovascular: Palpitation, tachycardia, flushing and extrasystoles.
4. Respiratory: Increase in respiratory rate.
5. Dermatologic: Urticaria.

Overdosage: The most consistent reactions observed with *toxic* overdoses of aminophylline are:

1. Gastrointestinal: Nausea, vomiting, epigastric pain, hematemesis and diarrhea.
2. Central nervous system: In addition to those cited above, the patient may exhibit hyperreflexia, fasciculations, and clonic and tonic convulsions. These are especially prone to occur in cases of overdosage in infants and small children.
3. Cardiovascular: In addition to those outlined above, marked hypotension and circulatory failure may be manifest.
4. Respiratory: Tachypnea and respiratory arrest may occur.
5. Renal: Albuminuria and microhematuria may occur. Increased excretion of renal tubular cells has been observed.
6. General systemic effects: Syncope, collapse, fever and dehydration.

Treatment of Toxic Symptoms:

1. Discontinue drug immediately.
2. There is no known specific antidote.
3. Gastric lavage.
4. Emetic medication may be of value.
5. Avoid administration of sympathomimetic drugs.
6. Intravenous fluids, oxygen and other supportive measures to prevent hypotension and overcome dehydration.
7. Central nervous system stimulation and seizures may respond to short-acting barbiturates.
8. Monitor serum levels until below 20 mcg./ml.

Dosage and Administration: The oral dose for adults should be adjusted according to the need and response of the patient. Usually a daily dose in the range of 600 to 1600 mg., administered in 3 or 4 divided doses, will provide the desired therapeutic effect. Similarly, the dose for children should be adjusted according to the response. An oral dose of 12 mg./kg./24 hours, administered in four divided doses, will usually provide the desired therapeutic effect in children.

Therapeutic serum levels are considered to be between 10 mcg./ml. and 20 mcg./ml. Levels above 20 mcg./ml. may produce toxic effects. There is great variation from patient to patient in dosage needed to achieve a therapeutic serum level and in the duration of action of oral aminophylline. Because of these wide variations and the relatively narrow therapeutic serum-level range, dosage must be individualized with monitoring of theophylline serum levels, particularly when prolonged use is planned.

How Supplied: Aminophyllin Tablets are supplied as:

Continued on next page

Searle Labs.—Cont.

Round, white, scored tablets with SEARLE debossed on one side and 1231 on the other side, each tablet containing 100 mg. of aminophylline; bottles of 100 and 1,000.
Oval, white, scored tablets with SEARLE debossed on one side and 1251 on the other side, each tablet containing 200 mg. of aminophylline; bottles of 100 and 1,000.
[*Shown in Product Identification Section*]

COMFOLAX®
(dioctyl sodium sulfosuccinate U.S.P.)

Description: Each translucent, soft gelatin capsule of Comfolax contains 100 mg. of dioctyl sodium sulfosuccinate U.S.P., a wetting agent and fecal softener for the gentle promotion of bowel regularity.
Actions: Through its surface-active properties it encourages easy, strain-free elimination in patients with hemorrhoids or other painful anorectal disorders. This non-habit-forming agent is highly acceptable for bowel management of patients with chronic, spastic, atonic and pregnancy constipation; it is especially useful in convalescing or senile patients since its gentle non-stimulant action does not increase the peristaltic activity of the bowel unnecessarily.
Dosage and Administration: One or two capsules daily for adults and for children over 12 years of age. In stubborn constipation adult dosage may be increased to two capsules twice daily. The softening effect of Comfolax is usually apparent in one to three days after the first capsule is taken.
When limitations in the diet or lack of bowel tonicity make the addition of bulk advisable, Metamucil®, alone or with Comfolax, should be considered.
Because of its dosage size, Comfolax is not recommended for use by children less than 12 years of age.
How Supplied: In bottles of 60 capsules.
Product Identification Mark(s): Capsules are bright green and oval shaped, imprinted with SEARLE 1552.
Is This Product O.T.C.: Yes.
[*Shown in Product Identification Section*]

COMFOLAX-*plus*®
(dioctyl sodium sulfosuccinate with casanthranol)

Description: Each soft gelatin capsule of Comfolax-*plus* contains 100 mg. of dioctyl sodium sulfosuccinate U.S.P., a wetting agent, and 30 mg. of casanthranol, a gentle bowel stimulant. This combination provides highly effective laxative action for the prompt, gentle relief of bowel sluggishness and irregularity.
Actions: Dioctyl sodium sulfosuccinate dissolves readily in the intestinal tract, lowering surface tension of fluids and softening bowel content to maintain a soft fecal mass. Casanthranol has a selective action on the bowel, gently stimulating propulsion and elimination. Comfolax-*plus* usually works overnight, giving prompt relief of constipation. After initial relief has been obtained with Comfolax-*plus*, most recurrent constipation problems will respond sufficiently to Comfolax® alone.
When used in preparation for surgical procedures Comfolax-*plus* will provide predictable and relatively rapid evacuation of the bowel; it may be used safely during the convalescent period to counteract the bowel sluggishness encountered during inactivity and debilitation.
Warnings: Do not use when abdominal pain, nausea or vomiting is present. Frequent or prolonged use of this preparation may result in dependence on laxatives.
Dosage and Administration: For adults, one or two capsules at bedtime for one or two days. Thereafter, one capsule daily as needed.
Because of its dosage size, Comfolax-*plus* is not recommended for use by children less than 12 years of age.
How Supplied: In bottles of 60 capsules.
Product Identification Mark(s): Two-tone green, oval-shaped capsules, imprinted with SEARLE 1572.
Is This Product O.T.C.: Yes.
[*Shown in Product Identification Section*]

DIULO™ ℞
(metolazone)

Each DIULO tablet contains 2½, 5, or 10 mg. of metolazone.
Description: DIULO (metolazone) has the molecular formula $C_{16}H_{16}ClN_3O_3S$ and a molecular weight of 365.84. The chemical name is 7-chloro-1,2,3,4-tetrahydro-2-methyl-4-oxo-3-o-tolyl-6-quinazolinesulfonamide. Metolazone is only sparingly soluble in water, but more soluble in plasma, blood, alkali, and organic solvents.
Actions: DIULO (metolazone) is a diuretic/saluretic/antihypertensive drug. The action of DIULO results in an interference with the renal tubular mechanism of electrolyte reabsorption. The mechanism of this action is unknown. DIULO acts primarily to inhibit sodium reabsorption at the cortical diluting site and in the proximal convoluted tubule. Sodium and chloride ions are excreted in approximately equivalent amounts. The increased delivery of sodium to the distal-tubular exchange site may result in increased potassium excretion.
DRUG INTERACTION STUDIES: In animals pretreated with metolazone, the drug did not alter the characteristic effect of heparin on clotting time nor protamine antagonism; dicumarol on prothrombin time nor Vitamin K antagonism; the response of guanethidine, reserpine and hydralazine to cardiovascular parameters nor the pressor response of the subsequent dose of norepinephrine.
Metolazone and furosemide, administered concurrently have produced marked diuresis in some patients whose edema or ascites was refractory to treatment with maximum recommended doses of these or other diuretics administered alone. The mechanism of this interaction is not known.
In clinical usage, metolazone does not inhibit carbonic anhydrase. Its proximal action has been evidenced in humans by increased excretion of phosphate and magnesium ions, by markedly increased fractional excretion of sodium in patients with severely compromised glomerular filtration, and in animals by the results of micropuncture studies. Decrease in calcium ion excretion has not been noted.
At maximum therapeutic dosage DIULO is approximately equal to thiazide diuretics in its diuretic potency. However, DIULO may produce diuresis in patients with glomerular filtration rates below 20 ml./min.
When DIULO is given, diuresis and saluresis usually begin within one hour and persist for 12 to 24 hours depending on dosage. Maximum effect occurs about two hours after administration. At the higher recommended dosages, effect may be prolonged beyond 24 hours. *A single daily dose is recommended.* For most patients the duration of effect can be varied by adjusting the daily dose.
The prolonged duration of action of DIULO is attributed to protein binding and enterohepatic recycling. A small amount of DIULO is metabolized and the fraction so changed is nontoxic. The primary route of excretion is renal.
The mechanism whereby diuretics function in the control of hypertension is unknown; both renal and extra-renal actions may be involved.
An antihypertensive effect may be seen as early as three to four days after DIULO has been started. Administration for three to four weeks, however, is usually required for optimum antihypertensive effect.
Indications: DIULO (metolazone) is indicated in the management of hypertension either as the sole therapeutic agent or to enhance the effectiveness of other antihypertensive drugs in the more severe forms of hypertension.
DIULO (metolazone) is indicated for the treatment of salt and water retention including
— edema accompanying congestive heart failure
— edema accompanying renal diseases, including the nephrotic syndrome, and states of diminished renal function.

Usage in Pregnancy: The routine use of diuretics in an otherwise healthy woman is inappropriate and exposes mother and fetus to unnecessary hazard. Diuretics do not prevent development of toxemia of pregnancy, and there is no satisfactory evidence that they are useful in the treatment of developed toxemia.
Edema during pregnancy may arise from pathological causes or from the physiologic and mechanical consequences of pregnancy. DIULO is indicated in pregnancy when edema is due to pathologic causes, just as it is in the absence of pregnancy (however, see *Warnings*, below). Dependent edema in pregnancy, resulting from restriction of venous return by the expanded uterus, is properly treated through elevation of the lower extremities and use of support hose; use of diuretics to lower intravascular volume in this case is illogical and unnecessary. There is hypervolemia during normal pregnancy which is harmful to neither the fetus nor the mother (in the absence of cardiovascular disease), but which is associated with edema, including generalized edema, in the majority of pregnant women. If this edema produces discomfort, increased recumbency will often provide relief. In rare instances, this edema may cause extreme discomfort which is not relieved by rest. In these cases, a short course of diuretics may provide relief and may be appropriate.
Contraindications: Anuria.
Hepatic coma or pre-coma; known allergy or hypersensitivity to metolazone.
Warnings: While not reported to date, cross-allergy theoretically may occur when DIULO (metolazone) is given to patients known to be allergic to sulfonamide-derived drugs, thiazides, or quinethazone.
Hypokalemia may occur, with consequent weakness, cramps, and cardiac dysrhythmias. Hypokalemia is a particular hazard in digitalized patients; dangerous or fatal arrhythmias may be precipitated.
Azotemia and hyperuricemia may be noted or precipitated during the administration of DIULO. Infrequently, gouty attacks have been reported in persons with history of gout.
If azotemia and oliguria worsen during treatment of patients with severe renal disease, DIULO should be discontinued.
Until additional data have been obtained, DIULO is not recommended for patients in the pediatric age group.
Unusually large or prolonged effects on volume and electrolytes may result when DIULO and furosemide are administered concurrently. It is recommended that concurrent administration of these diuretics for treatment of resistant edema be started under hospital conditions in order to provide for adequate monitoring.
When DIULO is used with other antihypertensive drugs, particular care must be taken, especially during initial therapy. Dosage of other antihypertensive agents, especially the ganglionic blockers, should be reduced.
DIULO may be given with a potassium-sparing diuretic when indicated. In this circumstance, diuresis may be potentiated and dosages should be reduced. Potassium retention and hyperkalemia may result; the serum potassium should be determined frequently. Potas-

sium supplementation is contraindicated when a potassium-sparing diuretic is given.

Usage in Pregnancy: DIULO crosses the placental barrier and appears in cord blood. The use of DIULO in pregnant women requires that the anticipated benefit be weighed against possible hazards to the fetus. These hazards include fetal or neonatal jaundice, thrombocytopenia, and possibly other adverse reactions which have occurred in the adult.

Nursing Mothers: Metolazone appears in breast milk. If use of the drug is deemed essential, the patient should stop nursing.

Precautions: Periodic determination of serum electrolytes to detect possible electrolyte imbalance should be performed at appropriate intervals. Blood urea nitrogen, uric acid, and glucose levels should be assessed at intervals during diuretic therapy.

All patients receiving DIULO (metolazone) therapy should be observed for clinical signs of fluid and/or electrolyte imbalance; namely, hyponatremia, hypochloremic alkalosis, and hypokalemia. Serum and urine electrolyte determinations are particularly important when the patient is vomiting excessively or receiving parenteral fluids. Medication such as digitalis may also influence serum electrolytes. Warning signs, irrespective of cause, are: dryness of mouth, thirst, weakness, lethargy, drowsiness, restlessness, muscle pains or cramps, muscular fatigue, hypotension, oliguria, tachycardia, and gastrointestinal disturbances such as nausea and vomiting.

The serum potassium should be determined at regular intervals, and potassium supplementation instituted whenever indicated. Hypokalemia will be more common in association with intensive or prolonged diuretic therapy, with concomitant steroid or ACTH therapy, and with inadequate electrolyte intake.

While not reported to date for metolazone, related diuretics have increased responsiveness to tubocurarine and decreased arterial responsiveness to norepinephrine. Accordingly, it may be advisable to discontinue DIULO three days before elective surgery.

Caution should be observed when administering DIULO to hyperuricemic or gouty patients. DIULO exerts minimal effects on glucose metabolism; insulin requirements may be affected in diabetics, and hyperglycemia and glycosuria may occur in patients with latent diabetes.

Chloride deficit and hypochloremic alkalosis may occur. In patients with severe edema accompanying cardiac failure or renal disease, a low-salt syndrome may be produced; hot weather and a low-salt diet will contribute.

Caution should be observed when administering DIULO to patients with severely impaired renal function. As most of the drug is excreted by the renal route, cumulative effects may be seen in this circumstance.

Orthostatic hypotension may occur; this may be potentiated by alcohol, barbiturates, narcotics, or concurrent therapy with other antihypertensive drugs.

While not reported for metolazone, use of other diuretics has been associated on rare occasions with pathological changes in the parathyroid glands, with hypercalcemia and hypophosphatemia. This possibility should be kept in mind with clinical use of DIULO.

Adverse Reactions: Adverse reactions encountered during therapy with potent medications should be considered in two groups: those that represent extension of the expected pharmacologic actions of the drug, and those which are pharmacologically unexpected, idiosyncratic, specially toxic, due to allergy or hypersensitivity, or due to unexplained causes.

For DIULO (metolazone), adverse reactions constituting extensions of the expected pharmacologic actions of this potent diuretic/saluretic/antihypertensive drug may include:

Gastrointestinal reactions: constipation.

Central nervous system reactions: syncope, dizziness, drowsiness.

Cardiovascular reactions: orthostatic hypotension, excessive volume depletion, hemoconcentration, venous thrombosis.

Other reactions: dryness of the mouth, symptomatic and asymptomatic hypokalemia, hyponatremia, hypochloremia; hypochloremic alkalosis, hyperuricemia, hyperglycemia, glycosuria, increase in BUN or creatinine, fatigue, muscle cramps or spasm, weakness, restlessness.

In the second classification, adverse reactions to DIULO may include:

Gastrointestinal reactions: nausea, vomiting, anorexia, diarrhea, abdominal bloating, epigastric distress, intrahepatic cholestatic jaundice, hepatitis.

Central nervous system reactions: vertigo, headache.

Hematologic reactions: leukopenia.

Dermatologic-hypersensitivity reactions: urticaria and other skin rashes.

Cardiovascular reactions: palpitation, chest pain.

Other reactions: chills, acute gouty attacks.

Adverse reactions which have occurred with other diuretics, but which have not been reported to date with metolazone, include: pancreatitis, paresthesias, xanthopsia, agranulocytosis, thrombocytopenia, aplastic anemia, purpura, photosensitivity, and necrotizing angiitis (cutaneous vasculitis). These reactions should be considered as possible occurrences with clinical usage of DIULO.

Whenever adverse reactions are moderate or severe, DIULO dosage should be reduced or therapy withdrawn.

Dosage and Administration: Therapy should be individualized according to patient response. Programs of therapy with DIULO (metolazone) should be titrated to gain a maximal initial therapeutic response, and to determine the minimal dose possible to maintain that therapeutic response.

DIULO is a potent drug with a prolonged, 12- to 24-hour duration of action. When an initially-desired therapeutic effect has been obtained, it is ordinarily advisable to reduce the dosage of DIULO to a lower maintenance level. The time interval required for the initial higher-dosage regimen may vary from days in edematous states to three or four weeks in the treatment of elevated blood pressure.

The daily dosage depends on the severity of each patient's condition, sodium intake, and responsiveness. Therefore, dosage adjustment is usually necessary during the course of therapy. A decision to reduce the daily dosage of DIULO from a higher induction level to a lower maintenance level should be based on the results of thorough clinical and laboratory evaluations. If antihypertensive drugs or diuretics are given concurrently with DIULO, careful dosage adjustment may be necessary.

Usual Dosage

Suitable initial dosages will usually fall in the ranges given:

Edema of cardiac failure: DIULO 5-10 mg., once daily

Edema of renal disease: DIULO 5-20 mg., once daily

Mild to moderate essential hypertension:
DIULO 2½-5 mg., once daily

For patients with congestive cardiac failure who tend to experience paroxysmal nocturnal dyspnea, it is usually advisable to employ a dosage near the upper end of the range, to ensure prolongation of diuresis and saluresis for a full 24-hour period.

How Supplied: DIULO (metolazone) is provided as: pink 2½-mg. tablets, blue 5-mg. tablets, and yellow 10-mg. tablets in bottles of 100.

[*Shown in Product Identification Section*]

DRAMAMINE® Ampuls ℞
DRAMAMINE® Liquid
DRAMAMINE® Supposicones® ℞
DRAMAMINE® Tablets
DRAMAMINE® Vials ℞
(dimenhydrinate)

Description: Dimenhydrinate is the chlorotheophylline salt of the antihistaminic agent diphenhydramine. Dimenhydrinate contains not less than 53% and not more than 56% of diphenhydramine, and not less than 44% and not more than 47% of 8-chlorotheophylline, calculated on the dried basis.

Actions: While the precise mode of action of dimenhydrinate is not known, it has a depressant action on hyperstimulated labyrinthine function.

Indications: Dramamine is indicated for the prevention and treatment of the nausea, vomiting or vertigo of motion sickness.

Warning: Caution should be used when Dramamine is given in conjunction with certain antibiotics which may cause ototoxicity, since Dramamine is capable of masking ototoxic symptoms and an irreversible state may be reached.

Precautions and Adverse Reactions: Drowsiness may be experienced by some patients, especially on high dosage, although this action frequently is not undesirable in some conditions for which the drug is used. However, because of possible drowsiness patients taking Dramamine should be cautioned against operating automobiles or dangerous machinery.

Dosage and Administration: *Adults*—Nausea or vomiting may be expected to be controlled for approximately four hours with 50 mg. of Dramamine, and prevented by a similar dose every four hours. Its administration may be attended by some degree of drowsiness in some patients, and 100 mg. every four hours may be given in conditions in which drowsiness is not objectionable or is even desirable.

For *intramuscular administration* each milliliter (50 mg.) of solution is injected as needed, but for *intravenous therapy* each milliliter (50 mg.) of solution is diluted in 10 ml. of Sodium Chloride Injection U.S.P. and injected over a period of two minutes.

Dramamine for injection is supplied in 1-ml. constricted ampuls and in 5-ml. serum-type vials, each containing 50 mg. per ml. of Dramamine dissolved in a solution containing 5% benzyl alcohol, 50% propylene glycol and water q.s.

Dramamine Supposicones are administered rectally to adults by inserting one 100-mg. Supposicone above the anal sphincter once or twice daily.

Children—The following oral dosage schedule should provide therapeutic relief or prophylactic protection:

8 to 12 years: 25 to 50 mg. three times daily. Younger children should use Dramamine liquid, but only on the advice of a physician.

The liquid dosage form will be particularly useful for children in whom fractional doses are required; also such doses may be obtained by dividing the scored tablet.

The intramuscular dosage of Dramamine Injection for children should be 1.25 mg./kg. of body weight or 37.5 mg./m^2 of body surface, four times a day, up to 300 mg. daily.

How Supplied: Dramamine (dimenhydrinate) is supplied in the following dosage forms and package sizes:

For oral use—scored yellow tablets of 50 mg., U.S.P., with SEARLE debossed on one side and 1701 on the other side, bottles of 36, 100, 1,000 and 2,500, packets of 12 tablets, and cartons of 100 unit-dose individually blister-sealed tablets; liquid, 12.5 mg. per 4 ml., ethyl alcohol 5%, bottles of 16 ounces, and Junior®, 3 ounces.

Continued on next page

Searle Labs.—Cont.

For parenteral use—ampuls, 1 ml. (50 mg.); cartons of 5, 25 and 100; *vials,* serum type, 5 ml. (250 mg.); cartons of 5, 25 and 100.
For rectal use—Supposicones®, 100 mg.; boxes of 12 and twelve boxes of 12.

[*Tablets are shown in Product Identification Section*]

METAMUCIL®
(psyllium hydrophilic mucilloid)

Description: Metamucil is a bulk laxative which furnishes a smoothage effect and provides a bland, nonirritating bulk which promotes natural elimination. It contains refined hydrophilic mucilloid, a highly efficient dietary fiber, derived from the husk of the psyllium seed (*Plantago ovata*). An equal amount of dextrose, a carbohydrate, is added as a dispersing agent. Each dose furnishes less than 0.01 gm. of sodium and about 14 calories.
Actions: Metamucil is uniform, instantly miscible, palatable and nonirritative in the gastrointestinal tract. It is indicated for its smoothage effect in the management of chronic constipation, in irritable bowel syndrome, as adjunctive therapy in constipation of duodenal ulcer and diverticular disease, in the bowel management of patients with hemorrhoids, and for constipation during pregnancy, convalescence and senility.
Dosage and Administration: The usual adult dosage is one rounded teaspoonful (7 gm.) stirred into a glass of cool water or other suitable liquid, taken orally one to three times a day depending on the need and response. It may require continuing use for 2 or 3 days to provide optimal benefit. Best results are observed if each dose is followed by an additional glass of liquid.
Contraindications: Intestinal obstruction, fecal impaction.
How Supplied: Powder, containers of 7 oz., 14 oz., and 21 oz.
Is This Product O.T.C.: Yes.

INSTANT MIX METAMUCIL®
(psyllium hydrophilic mucilloid)

Description: Premeasured single-dose packets for oral use. Each packet contains $3\frac{1}{2}$ grams of refined hydrophilic mucilloid, a highly efficient dietary fiber, derived from the husk of the psyllium seed (*Plantago ovata*), together with citric acid, sodium bicarbonate, sucrose, and natural and artificial flavoring. Each dose contains 0.25 gm. of sodium and about 3 calories.
Actions: Instant Mix Metamucil, effervescent and requiring no stirring, is uniform, instantly miscible, palatable, and nonirritative in the gastrointestinal tract. It is indicated for its smoothage effect in the management of chronic constipation, in irritable bowel syndrome, as adjunctive therapy in constipation of duodenal ulcer and diverticular disease, in the bowel management of patients with hemorrhoids, and for constipation during pregnancy, convalescence and senility.
Dosage and Administration: The usual adult dosage is the contents of one packet, taken one to three times daily as follows: 1. Entire contents of a packet are poured into a standard 8-ounce water glass. 2. The glass is slowly filled with cool water. 3. Entire contents are drunk immediately. (An additional glass of water may be taken for best results.)
Contraindications: Intestinal obstruction, fecal impaction.
Precaution: Its sodium content of 0.25 gm. per dose should be considered when prescribed to patients on a restricted sodium diet.
How Supplied: Cartons of 16 and of 30 single-dose packets.
Is This Product O.T.C.: Yes.

NORPACE® CAPSULES ℞
(disopyramide phosphate)

Description: Norpace (disopyramide phosphate) is an antiarrhythmic drug available for oral administration in capsules containing 100 mg. or 150 mg. of disopyramide base, present as the phosphate. The base content of the phosphate salt is 77.6%. The chemical name of Norpace is α-[2-(diisopropylamino) ethyl]-α-phenyl-2-pyridineacetamide phosphate.
Norpace is freely soluble in water, and the free base (pKa 8.36) has an aqueous solubility of 1 mg./ml. The chloroform:water partition coefficient of the base is 3.1 at pH 7.2.
Norpace is a racemic mixture of *d*- and *l*- isomers. This drug is not chemically related to other antiarrhythmic drugs.
Clinical Pharmacology:
Mechanisms of action. Norpace (disopyramide phosphate) is a Type 1 antiarrhythmic drug (i.e., similar to procainamide and quinidine): transmembrane action potential studies in animals have shown that it decreases the rate of diastolic depolarization (phase 4) in cells with augmented automaticity, decreases the upstroke velocity (phase 0) and increases the action potential duration of normal cardiac cells. Norpace has also been shown to decrease the disparity in refractoriness between infarcted and adjacent normally perfused myocardium in experimental studies in the dog. The drug has no effect on alpha- or beta-adrenergic receptors in animal studies.
Electrophysiology. His-Purkinje studies in man involving the intravenous administration of Norpace have demonstrated that at therapeutic blood levels Norpace shortens the sinus node recovery time, lengthens the effective refractory period of the atrium and has a minimal effect on the effective refractory period of the AV node. Little effect has been shown on AV nodal conduction time, His-Purkinje conduction time, or QRS duration in human studies, although prolonged AV nodal and intraventricular conduction time have been observed in the dog. Electrophysiology studies in man have demonstrated prolongation of conduction in accessory pathways.
Hemodynamics. At recommended oral doses, Norpace rarely produces significant alterations of blood pressure (but see *Warnings*). Hemodynamic studies of intravenously administered Norpace in patients with coronary artery disease have revealed minimal cardiac depression, with approximately a 10% reduction of cardiac output. Intravenous injection (2 mg./kg. over 3 minutes) produced a transient and moderate increase in heart rate and in total peripheral resistance.
Anticholinergic activity. Norpace possesses anticholinergic properties and has been shown in tests to be about 0.06% as potent as atropine *in vitro.* Oral Norpace has little or no effect on resting sinus rate. Its anticholinergic activity may affect the gastrointestinal and/or urogenital systems (see *Warnings* and *Adverse Reactions*). These effects may be transitory or may disappear upon reduction of dose.
Pharmacokinetics. Following oral administration Norpace (disopyramide phosphate) is rapidly and almost completely absorbed. Peak plasma levels are usually attained within two hours after a dose. The usual therapeutic plasma levels are 2–4 mcg./ml. At these concentrations disopyramide in the blood is approximately equally distributed between plasma and erythrocytes. In the rat, the uptake and elimination characteristics of disopyramide in the myocardium are similar to those in the plasma. Plasma protein binding of disopyramide in humans varies with the drug concentration. At therapeutic concentrations the protein binding is approximately 50%.
The mean plasma half-life of disopyramide in healthy humans is 6.7 hours with a range of 4 to 10 hours; it lies between 5 and 8 hours in approximately three fourths of these subjects. In four patients with impaired renal function (creatinine clearance less than 40 ml./min.), disopyramide half-life values have been 8 to 18 hours.
In healthy men the urinary and fecal excretions of disopyramide and its metabolites account for approximately 80% and 10% of the dose, respectively. About 50% of a given dose of disopyramide is excreted in the urine as the unchanged drug, about 20% as the mono-N-dealkylated metabolite and 10% as other metabolites. The plasma concentration of the major metabolite is approximately one tenth that of disopyramide. Altering the urinary pH in man does not affect the plasma half-life or the amount of disopyramide excreted in the urine.
Toxicology. Plasma levels that are consistently toxic have not been defined in man, but are thought to exceed 9 mcg./ml. in patients with compensated left ventricular function. In patients with poorly compensated left ventricular function, hypotension or worsened congestive heart failure may occur. This may be associated with the negative inotropic properties of the drug and/or its potential to modify conduction within compromised specialized conduction tissue (see *Overdosage*).
Indications: Norpace should be prescribed only after appropriate electrocardiographic assessment.
Norpace (disopyramide phosphate) is indicated for suppression and prevention of recurrence of the following cardiac arrhythmias when they occur singly or in combination:

1. Unifocal premature (ectopic) ventricular contractions
2. Premature (ectopic) ventricular contractions of multifocal origin
3. Paired premature ventricular contractions (couplets)
4. Episodes of ventricular tachycardia (persistent ventricular tachycardia is ordinarily treated with D.C. cardioversion)

Norpace is equally effective in treating the above arrhythmias in both digitalized and nondigitalized patients. Norpace is also equally effective in the treatment of primary cardiac arrhythmias and those which occur in association with organic heart disease including coronary artery disease. Oral Norpace (disopyramide phosphate) has not been adequately studied in patients with acute myocardial infarction or in patients with persistent ventricular tachycardia or atrial arrhythmias. Type 1 antiarrhythmic drugs are usually not effective in treating arrhythmias secondary to digitalis intoxication and, therefore, Norpace is not indicated for such cases.
The value of antiarrhythmic drugs in preventing sudden death in patients with serious ventricular ectopic activity has not been established.
Clinical Trials
1. In a clinical trial involving 120 patients with ventricular and atrial ectopic activity, a four-week lead-in placebo period was followed by eight weeks of Norpace treatment (400–800 mg./day) and a four-week lead-out placebo period. Dose adjustment was not allowed. Ectopic activity was monitored by four 9-hour daytime Holter recordings for each patient, one in each placebo period and two during Norpace treatment.
Of the 76 patients with at least 60 ectopic beats per hour, 31 had a decrease of at least 75% in mean ectopic activity and 16 had a 50–75% decrease, compared with the mean placebo rate. Six patients had ventricular tachycardia during both placebo periods but not during either Norpace period. There was no instance in which this arrhythmia was seen in both Norpace periods but not in either placebo period. Twelve patients had bigeminy during both placebo periods but not in either Norpace period; seven patients had trigeminy (3 of these also had bigeminy) during both placebo periods but not in either Norpace period. In contrast, only two patients had one or both of these ar-

rhythmias during both of the Norpace periods but not during either placebo period.

2. One hundred twenty-four patients were studied in an eight-week randomized double-blind comparison of Norpace (600 mg./day) and quinidine sulfate (1300 mg./day). Changes in ectopic activity were monitored by means of five 9-hour daytime Holter recordings for each patient. The effect of the two drugs was approximately equal in suppression of ventricular arrhythmias. Suppression of ectopic activity by 75% or more, compared with the baseline, occurred in approximately 50% of the patients in each treatment group. Norpace-treated patients experienced less severe side effects, especially gastrointestinal effects, resulting in significantly fewer dropouts (10% Norpace, 30% quinidine). Complete abolition of ectopic activity occurred in less than 10% of both groups of patients. Occasional increases of ectopic activity by more than 75% were seen. Among the 56 Norpace patients who completed the trial, seven (12%) had such increases, five on one recording and one each on two and on three recordings. Of the 40 quinidine patients who completed the study, two patients (5%) had such increases, one on a single recording and one on three recordings.

3. The acute effects of oral Norpace were studied in 69 patients who received a 300-mg. loading dose followed by maintenance therapy at 150–200 mg. q. 6 h. for the next three days. Of the 46 patients with at least one PVC per minute and/or more than one episode of coupled PVCs, ventricular tachycardia, R on T or supraventricular tachycardia, 23 patients showed at least a 75% decrease in PVCs, and 6 additional patients had a more than 50% decrease within 2.5 hours. Of the 44 patients evaluable during the next 72 hours, 25 (57%) manifested at least a 75% decrease in PVCs while 6 patients had a 50–75% decrease. Of the 19 patients with episodes of ventricular tachycardia during the placebo period, 15 (79%) experienced complete or greater than 75% suppression during treatment. One patient without ventricular tachycardia during placebo treatment developed it while on Norpace. In 13 patients with inadequately suppressed arrhythmias on 150 mg. every 6 hours, dosage of Norpace was increased to 800 to 1200 mg./day. In 9 of these 13 patients there was a detectable increase in plasma drug level and a clear enhancement of antiarrhythmic effect.

Contraindications: Norpace (disopyramide phosphate) is contraindicated in the presence of cardiogenic shock, preexisting second- or third-degree AV block (if no pacemaker is present), or known hypersensitivity to the drug.

Warnings:

Hypotension. Severe hypotension following Norpace administration has been observed, primarily in patients with primary cardiomyopathy or inadequately compensated congestive heart failure. If hypotension develops Norpace should be discontinued promptly (unless the hypotension is due to cardiac arrhythmia) and subsequently may be restarted at a lower dosage level without an initial loading dose. Under such circumstances, patients should be closely monitored.

Heart failure. Norpace should not be used in the presence of poorly compensated or uncompensated congestive heart failure unless the heart failure is exacerbated by or caused by an arrhythmia and proper treatment including optimal digitalization has been accomplished. Norpace (disopyramide phosphate) may then be useful in suppressing the ectopy. Careful monitoring is essential under these circumstances.

In patients with marginally compensated heart failure or with a history of heart failure, the administration of Norpace may worsen cardiac decompensation. In these patients, progressing congestive heart failure should generally be treated with cardiac glycosides and diuretics and the course of treatment closely followed. The dose of Norpace should be reduced or Norpace should be discontinued if adequate control of congestive failure is not attained.

Concomitant antiarrhythmic therapy—The concomitant use of Norpace with other Type 1 antiarrhythmic agents (such as quinidine or procainamide) and/or propranolol should be reserved for patients with life-threatening arrhythmias who are demonstrably unresponsive to single agent antiarrhythmic therapy. Such use may produce serious negative inotropic effects, or may excessively prolong conduction. This should be considered particularly in patients with any degree of cardiac decompensation or those with a prior history thereof. Patients receiving more than one antiarrhythmic drug must be carefully monitored.

Heart block. If first-degree heart block develops in a patient receiving Norpace, the dosage should be reduced. If the block persists despite reduction of dosage, continuation of the drug must depend upon weighing the benefit being obtained against the risk of higher degrees of heart block. Development of second- or third-degree AV block or unifascicular, bifascicular or trifascicular block requires discontinuation of Norpace therapy, unless the ventricular rate is adequately controlled by a temporary or implanted ventricular pacemaker.

Anticholinergic activity. Because of its anticholinergic properties, Norpace should not be used in patients with glaucoma or in patients with urinary retention unless adequate overriding measures are taken; these consist of the topical application of potent miotics (e.g., pilocarpine) for patients with glaucoma, and catheter drainage or operative relief for patients with urinary retention. Urinary retention may occur in patients of either sex as a consequence of Norpace administration, but males with benign prostatic hypertrophy are at particular risk. In patients with a family history of glaucoma, intraocular pressure should be measured before initiating Norpace therapy. Norpace should be used with special care in patients with myasthenia gravis since its anticholinergic properties could precipitate a myasthenic crisis in such patients.

Precautions:

QRS widening. Although it is unusual, significant widening (greater than 25%) of the QRS complex may occur during Norpace administration; in such cases Norpace (disopyramide phosphate) should be discontinued.

Q-T prolongation. As with other Type 1 antiarrhythmic drugs, prolongation of the Q-T interval (corrected) and worsening of the arrhythmia may occur, particularly in response to higher doses. Patients who have evidenced prolongation of the Q-T interval in response to quinidine may be at particular risk. If a Q-T prolongation of greater than 25% is observed and if ectopy continues, the patient should be monitored closely, and consideration be given to discontinuing Norpace.

Atrial tachyarrhythmias. Patients with atrial flutter or fibrillation should be digitalized prior to Norpace administration to ensure that drug-induced enhancement of AV conduction does not result in an increase of ventricular rate beyond physiologically acceptable limits.

Conduction abnormalities. Care should be taken when prescribing Norpace for patients with sick sinus syndrome (bradycardia-tachycardia syndrome), Wolff-Parkinson-White syndrome (WPW), or bundle branch block. The effect of Norpace (disopyramide phosphate) in these conditions is uncertain at present.

Cardiomyopathy. Patients with myocarditis or other cardiomyopathy may develop significant hypotension in response to the usual dosage of Norpace, probably due to cardiodepressant mechanisms. Therefore, a loading dose of Norpace should not be given to such patients and initial dosage and subsequent dosage adjustments should be made under close supervision (see *Dosage and Administration*).

Drug interactions. Other antiarrhythmic drugs (e.g., quinidine, procainamide, lidocaine, propranolol) have occasionally been used concurrently with Norpace but no specific drug interaction studies have been conducted (see *Warnings*). Excessive widening of the QRS complex and/or prolongation of the Q-T interval may occur in these situations.

Renal impairment. More than 50% of disopyramide is excreted in the urine unchanged. Therefore Norpace dosage should be reduced in patients with impaired renal function (see *Dosage and Administration*). The electrocardiogram should be carefully monitored for prolongation of PR interval, evidence of QRS widening or other signs of overdosage (see *Overdosage*).

Hepatic impairment. Hepatic impairment also causes an increase in the plasma half-life of disopyramide. Dosage should be reduced for patients with such impairment. The electrocardiogram should be carefully monitored for signs of overdosage (see *Overdosage*).

Hypokalemia. Antiarrhythmic drugs may be ineffective in patients with hypokalemia. Therefore, any potassium deficit should be corrected before instituting Norpace therapy.

Pregnancy. Reproduction studies in rats and teratology studies performed both in rats and in rabbits have revealed minimal evidence of impaired fertility. No fetal anomalies were attributable to Norpace. However, well-controlled studies of Norpace have not been performed in pregnant women and experience with Norpace during pregnancy is limited; therefore the possibility of damage to the fetus cannot be excluded. Norpace has been reported to stimulate contractions of the pregnant uterus. Norpace (disopyramide phosphate) should be used in pregnant women only when it is clearly indicated and the benefit/risk ratio has been carefully evaluated.

Labor and delivery. It is not known whether the use of Norpace during labor or delivery has immediate or delayed adverse effects on the fetus, or whether it prolongs the duration of labor or increases the need for forceps delivery or other obstetric intervention.

Nursing mothers. Whether disopyramide is excreted in human milk is unknown. However, studies in rats have shown that the concentration of disopyramide and its metabolites is between one and three times greater in milk than it is in plasma. Therefore, if use of the drug is deemed essential, an alternative method of infant feeding should be instituted.

Pediatrics. The safety and effectiveness of Norpace in children have not been established.

Adverse Reactions: The adverse reactions which were reported in clinical trials encompass observations in 713 patients, including 100 patients studied for at least two years. The most common adverse reactions are associated with the anticholinergic properties of the drug. Urinary retention, although relatively uncommon (2%), is the most serious anticholinergic effect.

The following reactions were reported in 10–40% of patients:

Anticholinergic: dry mouth (40%), urinary hesitancy (10–20%)

The following reactions were reported in 3–9% of patients:

Anticholinergic: constipation, blurred vision, dry nose/eyes/throat

Genitourinary: urinary frequency and urgency

Gastrointestinal: nausea, pain/bloating/gas

The following reactions were reported in 1–3% of patients:

Anticholinergic: urinary retention

General: dizziness, general fatigue/muscle weakness, headache, malaise

Continued on next page

Searle Labs.—Cont.

Cardiovascular: hypotension (see *Warnings*), congestive heart failure (see *Warnings*), cardiac conduction disturbances (see *Warnings*), edema/weight gain, shortness of breath, syncope, chest pain
Gastrointestinal: anorexia, diarrhea, vomiting
Dermatologic: generalized rash/dermatoses
Central nervous system: nervousness
The following reactions, reported in less than 1%, occurred under circumstances where a causal relationship is uncertain and are therefore mentioned to alert the physician to a possible relationship: impotence, depression, insomnia, and dysuria.
There have been reports of hypoglycemia in association with Norpace administration, usually in patients with impaired liver function. Rarely, acute psychosis has been reported following Norpace therapy, with prompt return to normal mental status when therapy was stopped. Infrequent occurrences of reversible cholestatic jaundice have been reported in association with disopyramide therapy as have rare instances of reversible agranulocytosis. The physician should be aware of these possible reactions and should discontinue Norpace therapy promptly if they occur.
Dosage and Administration: The dosage of Norpace (disopyramide phosphate) must be individualized for each patient on the basis of response and tolerance. The usual adult dosage of Norpace is 400 to 800 mg. per day given in divided doses four times daily. The recommended dosage schedule for most adults is 150 mg. every six hours. For patients whose body weight is less than 110 pounds (50 kg.), the recommended dosage is 100 mg. every six hours.

For patients with cardiomyopathy or possible cardiac decompensation, a loading dose, as discussed below, should not be given and initial dosage should be limited to 100 mg. of Norpace every six hours. Subsequent dosage adjustments should be made gradually, with close monitoring for the possible development of hypotension and/or congestive heart failure (see *Warnings*).

For patients with moderate renal insufficiency (creatinine clearance greater than 40 ml./min.) or hepatic insufficiency, Norpace dosage of 100 mg. every six hours is recommended, with or without an initial loading dose of 200 mg.

For patients with severe renal insufficiency (C_{cr} less than 40 ml./min.) the recommended dosage regimen is 100 mg. (with or without an initial loading dose of 200 mg.) given approximately every half-life ($T\frac{1}{2}$). See the table below for the relationship between creatinine clearance and the approximate maintenance-dosing interval:

NORPACE DOSAGE INTERVAL FOR PATIENTS WITH RENAL INSUFFICIENCY

Creatinine clearance (ml./min.)	40–15	15–5	5–1
Approximate maintenance-dosing interval	q. 10 hr.	q. 20 hr.	q. 30 hr.

For patients in whom rapid control of ventricular arrhythmia is essential, an initial loading dose of 300 mg. of Norpace (200 mg. for patients whose body weight is less than 110 pounds) is recommended, followed by the appropriate maintenance dosage. Therapeutic effects are usually attained 30 minutes to three hours after administration of a 300-mg. loading dose. If there is no response nor evidence of toxicity within six hours of the loading dose, 200 mg. every six hours may be prescribed instead of the usual 150 mg. If there is no response to this dosage within 48 hours, either Norpace should then be discontinued or the physician should consider hospitalizing the patient for careful monitoring while subsequent doses of 250 or 300 mg. every six hours are given. A limited number of patients with severe refractory ventricular tachycardia have tolerated daily doses of Norpace up to 1600 mg. per day (400 mg. every 6 hours) resulting in disopyramide plasma levels up to 9 mcg./ml. If such treatment is warranted, it is essential that patients be hospitalized for close evaluation and continuous monitoring.
Transferring to Norpace. The following dosage schedule based on theoretical considerations rather than experimental data is suggested for transferring patients with normal renal function from either quinidine sulfate or procainamide therapy (Type 1 antiarrhythmic agents) to Norpace therapy.

Norpace may be started using the regular maintenance schedule **without a loading dose** 6–12 hours after the last dose of quinidine sulfate or 3–6 hours after the last dose of procainamide.

In patients where withdrawal of quinidine sulfate or procainamide is likely to produce life-threatening arrhythmias, the physician should consider hospitalization of the patient.
Overdosage: No specific antidote for Norpace has been identified. Treatment of overdosage should be supportive and may include the administration of isoproterenol and/or dopamine, hemodialysis, intra-aortic balloon counterpulsation and mechanically assisted respiration.
In vitro studies with human blood have demonstrated good dialyzability for disopyramide. Its clearance was 33 ml./min. at a blood flow of 250 ml./min. when an initial plasma concentration of 22 mcg./ml. was dialyzed using an artificial kidney (Cordis-DOW-4).
On the basis of animal studies toxic plasma levels of disopyramide might be expected to produce excessive widening of the QRS complex and Q-T interval, worsening of congestive heart failure, hypotension, varying kinds and degrees of conduction disturbance, bradycardia and finally asystole. Obvious anticholinergic effects might also be observed. The electrocardiogram should be monitored and supportive therapy with vasopressors, sympathomimetics, cardiac glycosides and diuretics should be given as required.
How Supplied: Norpace (disopyramide phosphate) is supplied in hard gelatin capsules containing either 100 mg. or 150 mg. of disopyramide base.
Norpace 100-mg. capsules are white and orange, with markings SEARLE and 2752.
Norpace 150-mg. capsules are brown and orange, with markings SEARLE and 2762.
Available in bottles of 100 and 500 capsules.
[*Shown in Product Identification Section*]

The preceding prescribing information for Searle Laboratories products was current on November 1, 1979.

Products are cross-indexed by

generic and chemical names

in the

YELLOW SECTION

Searle & Co.
SAN JUAN, PUERTO RICO 00936

ALDACTAZIDE® ℞
(spironolactone with hydrochlorothiazide)

> **Warning**
> Spironolactone, an ingredient of Aldactazide, has been shown to be a tumorigen in chronic toxicity studies in rats (see *Warnings*). Aldactazide should be used only in those conditions described under *Indications*. Unnecessary use of this drug should be avoided.
> Fixed-dose combination drugs are not indicated for initial therapy of edema or hypertension. Edema or hypertension requires therapy titrated to the individual patient. If the fixed combination represents the dosage so determined, its use may be more convenient in patient management. The treatment of hypertension and edema is not static, but must be reevaluated as conditions in each patient warrant.

Description: Each tablet of Aldactazide contains 25 mg. of spironolactone (Aldactone®) and 25 mg. of hydrochlorothiazide.
Spironolactone is 17-hydroxy-7α-mercapto-3-oxo-17α-pregn-4-ene-21-carboxylic acid γ-lactone acetate. Hydrochlorothiazide is 6-chloro-3,4-dihydro-2H-1,2,4-benzothiadiazine-7-sulfonamide 1,1-dioxide.
Actions: Aldactazide is a combination of two diuretic agents with different but complementary mechanisms and sites of action, thereby providing additive diuretic and antihypertensive effects. Additionally, the spironolactone component helps to minimize the potassium loss characteristically induced by the thiazide component.
The diuretic effect of spironolactone is mediated through its action as a specific pharmacologic antagonist of aldosterone, primarily by competitive binding of receptors at the aldosterone-dependent sodium-potassium exchange site in the distal convoluted renal tubule. Hydrochlorothiazide promotes the excretion of sodium and water primarily by inhibiting their reabsorption in the cortical diluting segment of the renal tubule.
Aldactazide is effective in significantly lowering the systolic and diastolic blood pressure in many patients with essential hypertension, even when aldosterone secretion is within normal limits.
Both spironolactone and hydrochlorothiazide reduce exchangeable sodium, plasma volume, body weight and blood pressure. The diuretic and antihypertensive effects of the individual components are potentiated when spironolactone and hydrochlorothiazide are given concurrently.
Clinical Pharmacology: In the human, the bioavailability of both spironolactone and hydrochlorothiazide from orally administered Aldactazide tablets is approximately 90 percent when compared with equivalent doses of the individual components administered in an optimally-absorbed solution (spironolactone in polyethylene glycol 400).
Spironolactone is rapidly and extensively metabolized. The primary metabolite is canrenone which attains peak serum levels at two to four hours following single oral administration. Canrenone plasma concentrations decline in two distinct phases, being rapid in the first 12 hours and slower from 12 to 96 hours. The log-linear phase half-life of canrenone, following multiple doses of Aldactone (spironolactone), is between 13 and 24 hours. Both spironolactone and canrenone are more than 90-percent bound to plasma proteins. The me-

tabolites of spironolactone are excreted primarily in urine, but also in bile.
Hydrochlorothiazide is rapidly absorbed following oral administration. Onset of action is observed within one hour and persists for 6 to 12 hours. Plasma concentrations attain peak levels at one to two hours and decline with a half-life of four to five hours. Hydrochlorothiazide undergoes only slight metabolic alteration and is excreted in urine. It is distributed throughout the extracellular space, with essentially no tissue accumulation except in the kidney.

Indications: Spironolactone, an ingredient of Aldactazide, has been shown to be a tumorigen in chronic toxicity studies in rats (see *Warnings* section). Aldactazide should be used only in those conditions described below. Unnecessary use of this drug should be avoided.
Aldactazide is indicated for:

Edematous conditions for patients with:

Congestive heart failure: For the management of edema and sodium retention when the patient is only partially responsive to, or is intolerant of, other therapeutic measures. The treatment of diuretic-induced hypokalemia in patients with congestive heart failure when other measures are considered inappropriate. The treatment of patients with congestive heart failure taking digitalis when other therapies are considered inadequate or inappropriate.

Cirrhosis of the liver accompanied by edema and/or ascites: Aldosterone levels may be exceptionally high in this condition. Aldactazide is indicated for maintenance therapy together with bed rest and the restriction of fluid and sodium.

The nephrotic syndrome: For nephrotic patients when treatment of the underlying disease, restriction of fluid and sodium intake, and the use of other diuretics do not provide an adequate response.

Essential hypertension

For patients with essential hypertension in whom other measures are considered inadequate or inappropriate. In hypertensive patients for the treatment of a diuretic-induced hypokalemia when other measures are considered inappropriate.

Usage in Pregnancy. The routine use of diuretics in an otherwise healthy woman is inappropriate and exposes mother and fetus to unnecessary hazard. Diuretics do not prevent development of toxemia of pregnancy, and there is no satisfactory evidence that they are useful in the treatment of developing toxemia.
Edema during pregnancy may arise from pathologic causes or from the physiologic and mechanical consequences of pregnancy. Aldactazide is indicated in pregnancy when edema is due to pathologic causes just as it is in the absence of pregnancy (however, see *Warnings* section). Dependent edema in pregnancy, resulting from restriction of venous return by the expanded uterus, is properly treated through elevation of the lower extremities and use of support hose; use of diuretics to lower intravascular volume in this case is unsupported and unnecessary. There is hypervolemia during normal pregnancy which is harmful to neither the fetus nor the mother (in the absence of cardiovascular disease), but which is associated with edema, including generalized edema, in the majority of pregnant women. If this edema produces discomfort, increased recumbency will often provide relief. In rare instances, this edema may cause extreme discomfort which is not relieved by rest. In these cases, a short course of diuretics may provide relief and may be appropriate.

Contraindications: Aldactazide is contraindicated in patients with anuria, acute renal insufficiency, significant impairment of renal function or hyperkalemia and in patients who are allergic to thiazide diuretics or to other sulfonamide-derived drugs. Aldactazide may also be contraindicated in acute or severe hepatic failure.

Warnings: Potassium supplementation, either in the form of medication or as a diet rich in potassium, should not ordinarily be given in association with Aldactazide therapy. Excessive potassium intake may cause hyperkalemia in patients receiving Aldactazide (see *Precautions* section). Aldactazide should not be administered concurrently with other potassium-sparing diuretics.
Sulfonamide derivatives, including thiazides, have been reported to exacerbate or activate systemic lupus erythematosus.
Spironolactone has been shown to be a tumorigen in chronic toxicity studies performed in rats, with its proliferative effects manifested on endocrine organs and the liver. In one study using 25, 75 and 250 times the usual daily human dose (2 mg./kg.) there was a statistically significant dose-related increase in benign adenomas of the thyroid and testes. In female rats there was a statistically significant increase in malignant mammary tumors at the mid-dose only. In male rats there was a dose-related increase in proliferative changes in the liver. At the highest dosage level (500 mg./kg.) the range of effects included hepatocytomegaly, hyperplastic nodules and hepatocellular carcinoma; the last was not statistically significant at a value of $p = 0.05$.

Precautions: Patients receiving Aldactazide therapy should be carefully evaluated for possible disturbances of fluid and electrolyte balance. Hyperkalemia may occur in patients with impaired renal function or excessive potassium intake and can cause cardiac irregularities which may be fatal. Consequently, no potassium supplement should ordinarily be given with Aldactazide. Hyperkalemia can be treated promptly by the rapid intravenous administration of glucose (20 to 50 percent) and regular insulin, using 0.25 to 0.5 units of insulin per gram of glucose. This is a temporary measure to be repeated as required. Aldactazide should be discontinued and potassium intake (including dietary potassium) restricted.
Hypokalemia may develop as a result of profound diuresis, particularly when Aldactazide is used concomitantly with loop diuretics, glucocorticoids or ACTH. Hypokalemia may exaggerate the effects of digitalis therapy. Potassium depletion may induce signs of digitalis intoxication at previously tolerated dosage levels.
Warning signs of possible fluid and electrolyte imbalance include dryness of the mouth, thirst, weakness, lethargy, drowsiness, restlessness, muscle pains or cramps, muscular fatigue, hypotension, oliguria, tachycardia and gastrointestinal symptoms.
Aldactazide therapy may cause a transient elevation of BUN. This appears to represent a concentration phenomenon rather than renal toxicity, since the BUN returns to normal after Aldactazide is discontinued. Progressive elevation of BUN is suggestive of the presence of preexisting renal impairment.
Dilutional hyponatremia, manifested by dryness of the mouth, thirst, lethargy and drowsiness, and confirmed by a low serum sodium level, may be induced, especially when Aldactazide is administered in combination with other diuretics. A true low-salt syndrome may rarely develop with Aldactazide therapy and may be manifested by increasing mental confusion similar to that observed with hepatic coma. This syndrome is differentiated from dilutional hyponatremia in that it does not occur with obvious fluid retention. Its treatment requires that diuretic therapy be discontinued and sodium administered.
Gynecomastia may develop in association with the use of spironolactone, and physicians should be alert to its possible onset. The development of gynecomastia appears to be related to both dosage level and duration of therapy and is normally reversible when Aldactazide is discontinued. In rare instances some breast enlargement may persist.
Thiazides have been demonstrated to alter the metabolism of uric acid and carbohydrates, with possible development of hyperuricemia, gout and decreased glucose tolerance. Thiazides may temporarily exaggerate abnormalities of glucose metabolism in diabetic patients or cause abnormalities to appear in patients with latent diabetes.
Both spironolactone and hydrochlorothiazide reduce the vascular responsiveness to norepinephrine. Therefore, caution should be exercised in the management of patients subjected to regional or general anesthesia while they are being treated with Aldactazide. Thiazides may also increase the responsiveness to tubocurarine. The antihypertensive effects of hydrochlorothiazide may be enhanced in patients who have undergone sympathectomy.
Pathologic changes in the parathyroid gland with hypercalcemia and hypophosphatemia have been observed in patients on prolonged thiazide therapy. Thiazides may also decrease serum PBI levels without evidence of alteration of thyroid function.
Usage in Pregnancy. Spironolactone or its metabolites may, and hydrochlorothiazide does, cross the placental barrier. Therefore, the use of Aldactazide in pregnant women requires that the anticipated benefit be weighed against possible hazards to the fetus. These hazards include fetal or neonatal jaundice, thrombocytopenia, and possible other adverse reactions which have been reported in the adult.
Nursing Mothers. Canrenone, a metabolite of spironolactone, and hydrochlorothiazide appear in breast milk. If use of these drugs is deemed essential, an alternative method of infant feeding should be instituted.

Adverse Reactions: Gynecomastia is observed not infrequently. Other adverse reactions that have been reported in association with the use of spironolactone are: gastrointestinal symptoms including cramping and diarrhea, drowsiness, lethargy, headache, maculopapular or erythematous cutaneous eruptions, urticaria, mental confusion, drug fever, ataxia, inability to achieve or maintain erection, irregular menses or amenorrhea, postmenopausal bleeding, hirsutism and deepening of the voice. Carcinoma of the breast has been reported in patients taking spironolactone, but a cause and effect relationship has not been established.
Adverse reactions reported in association with the use of thiazides include: gastrointestinal symptoms (anorexia, nausea, vomiting, diarrhea, abdominal cramps), purpura, thrombocytopenia, leukopenia, agranulocytosis, dermatologic symptoms (cutaneous eruptions, pruritus, erythema multiforme), paresthesia, acute pancreatitis, jaundice, dizziness, vertigo, headache, xanthopsia, photosensitivity, necrotizing angiitis, aplastic anemia, orthostatic hypotension, muscle spasm, weakness and restlessness.
Adverse reactions are usually reversible upon discontinuation of Aldactazide.

Dosage and Administration: Optimal dosage should be established by individual titration of the components (see Box Warning).

Edema in adults (*congestive heart failure, hepatic cirrhosis or nephrotic syndrome*). The usual maintenance dose of Aldactazide is one tablet four times daily but may range from one to eight tablets daily depending on the response to the initial titration. In some instances it may be desirable to administer separate tablets of either Aldactone (spironolactone) or hydrochlorothiazide in addition to Aldactazide in order to provide optimal individual therapy.
The onset of diuresis with Aldactazide occurs promptly and, due to prolonged effect of the

Continued on next page

Searle & Co.—Cont.

spironolactone component, persists for two to three days after Aldactazide is discontinued.
Edema in children. The usual daily maintenance dose of Aldactazide should be that which provides 0.75 to 1.5 mg. of spironolactone per pound of body weight (1.65 to 3.3 mg./kg.).
Essential hypertension. Although the dosage will vary depending on the results of titration of the individual ingredients, many patients will be found to have an optimal response to the amount of hydrochlorothiazide and spironolactone contained in two to four tablets of Aldactazide per day.
Concurrent potassium supplementation is not recommended when Aldactazide is used in the long-term management of hypertension or in the treatment of most edematous conditions, since the spironolactone content of Aldactazide is usually sufficient to minimize loss induced by the hydrochlorothiazide component.
How Supplied: Aldactazide is supplied as scored, ivory-colored tablets with SEARLE and 1011 debossed on the scored side and ALDACTAZIDE on the other side, each tablet containing 25 mg. of Aldactone (spironolactone) and 25 mg. of hydrochlorothiazide; bottles of 100, 500, 1,000 and 2,500, and cartons of 100 unit-dose individually blister-sealed tablets.
[*Shown in Product Identification Section*]

ALDACTONE® ℞
(spironolactone, U.S.P.)

> **Warning**
> Spironolactone has been shown to be a tumorigen in chronic toxicity studies in rats (see *Warnings*). Aldactone should be used only in those conditions described under *Indications*. Unnecessary use of this drug should be avoided.

Description: Each Aldactone tablet contains 25 mg. of spironolactone. Spironolactone is 17-hydroxy-7α-mercapto-3-oxo-17α-pregn-4-ene-21-carboxylic acid γ-lactone acetate.
Actions: Aldactone (spironolactone) is a specific pharmacologic antagonist of aldosterone, acting primarily through competitive binding of receptors at the aldosterone-dependent sodium-potassium exchange site in the distal convoluted renal tubule. Aldactone causes increased amounts of sodium and water to be excreted, while potassium is retained. Aldactone acts both as a diuretic and as an antihypertensive drug by this mechanism. It may be given alone or with other diuretic agents which act more proximally in the renal tubule.
Increased levels of the mineralocorticoid, aldosterone, are present in primary and secondary hyperaldosteronism. Edematous states in which secondary aldosteronism is usually involved include congestive heart failure, hepatic cirrhosis, and the nephrotic syndrome. By competing with aldosterone for receptor sites, Aldactone provides effective therapy for the edema and ascites in those conditions. Aldactone counteracts secondary aldosteronism induced by the volume depletion and associated sodium loss caused by active diuretic therapy.
Aldactone is effective in lowering the systolic and diastolic blood pressure in patients with primary hyperaldosteronism. It is also effective in most cases of essential hypertension, despite the fact that aldosterone secretion may be within normal limits in benign essential hypertension.
Through its action in antagonizing the effect of aldosterone, Aldactone inhibits the exchange of sodium for potassium in the distal renal tubule and helps to prevent potassium loss.
Aldactone has not been demonstrated to elevate serum uric acid, to precipitate gout or to alter carbohydrate metabolism.
Clinical Pharmacology: In the human, the bioavailability of spironolactone from orally administered Aldactone tablets exceeds 90 percent when compared with an optimally-absorbed solution (spironolactone in polyethylene glycol 400). Spironolactone is rapidly and extensively metabolized. The primary metabolite is canrenone which attains peak serum levels at two to four hours following single oral administration. Canrenone plasma concentrations decline in two distinct phases, being rapid in the first 12 hours and slower from 12 to 96 hours. The log-linear phase half-life of canrenone, following multiple doses of Aldactone, is between 13 and 24 hours. Both spironolactone and canrenone are more than 90-percent bound to plasma proteins. The metabolites of spironolactone are excreted primarily in urine, but also in bile.
Indications: Aldactone (spironolactone) is indicated in the management of:
Primary hyperaldosteronism for:
Establishing the diagnosis of primary hyperaldosteronism by therapeutic trial.
Short-term preoperative treatment of patients with primary hyperaldosteronism.
Long-term maintenance therapy for patients with discrete aldosterone-producing adrenal adenomas who are judged to be poor operative risks, or who decline surgery.
Long-term maintenance therapy for patients with bilateral micro- or macronodular adrenal hyperplasia (idiopathic hyperaldosteronism).
Edematous conditions for patients with:
Congestive heart failure: For the management of edema and sodium retention when the patient is only partially responsive to, or is intolerant of, other therapeutic measures. Aldactone is also indicated for patients with congestive heart failure taking digitalis when other therapies are considered inappropriate.
Cirrhosis of the liver accompanied by edema and/or ascites: Aldosterone levels may be exceptionally high in this condition. Aldactone is indicated for maintenance therapy together with bed rest and the restriction of fluid and sodium.
The nephrotic syndrome: For nephrotic patients when treatment of the underlying disease, restriction of fluid and sodium intake, and the use of other diuretics do not provide an adequate response.
Essential hypertension
Usually in combination with other drugs, Aldactone is indicated for patients who cannot be treated adequately with other agents or for whom other agents are considered inappropriate.
Hypokalemia
For the treatment of patients with hypokalemia when other measures are considered inappropriate or inadequate. Aldactone is also indicated for the prophylaxis of hypokalemia in patients taking digitalis when other measures are considered inadequate or inappropriate.
Usage in Pregnancy. The routine use of diuretics in an otherwise healthy woman is inappropriate and exposes mother and fetus to unnecessary hazard. Diuretics do not prevent development of toxemia of pregnancy, and there is no satisfactory evidence that they are useful in the treatment of developing toxemia.
Edema during pregnancy may rise from pathologic causes or from the physiologic and mechanical consequences of pregnancy.
Aldactone is indicated in pregnancy when edema is due to pathologic causes just as it is in the absence of pregnancy (however, see *Warnings* section). Dependent edema in pregnancy, resulting from restriction of venous return by the expanded uterus, is properly treated through elevation of the lower extremities and use of support hose; use of diuretics to lower intravascular volume in this case is unsupported and unnecessary. There is hypervolemia during normal pregnancy which is harmful to neither the fetus nor the mother (in the absence of cardiovascular disease), but which is associated with edema, including generalized edema, in the majority of pregnant women. If this edema produces discomfort, increased recumbency will often provide relief. In rare instances, this edema may cause extreme discomfort which is not relieved by rest. In these cases, a short course of diuretics may provide relief and may be appropriate.
Contraindications: Aldactone is contraindicated for patients with anuria, acute renal insufficiency, significant impairment of renal function, or hyperkalemia.
Warnings: Potassium supplementation, either in the form of medication or as a diet rich in potassium, should not ordinarily be given in association with Aldactone therapy. Excessive potassium intake may cause hyperkalemia in patients receiving Aldactone (see *Precautions* section). Aldactone should not be administered concurrently with other potassium-sparing diuretics.
Spironolactone has been shown to be a tumorigen in chronic toxicity studies performed in rats, with its proliferative effects manifested on endocrine organs and the liver. In one study using 25, 75 and 250 times the usual daily human dose (2 mg./kg.) there was a statistically significant dose-related increase in benign adenomas of the thyroid and testes. In female rats there was a statistically significant increase in malignant mammary tumors at the mid-dose only. In male rats there was a dose-related increase in proliferative changes in the liver. At the highest dosage level (500 mg./kg.) the range of effects include hepatocytomegaly, hyperplastic nodules and hepatocellular carcinoma; the last was not statistically significant at a value of $p = 0.05$.
Precautions: Because of the diuretic action of Aldactone (spironolactone), patients should be carefully evaluated for possible disturbances of fluid and electrolyte balance. Hyperkalemia may occur in patients with impaired renal function or excessive potassium intake and can cause cardiac irregularities which may be fatal. Consequently, no potassium supplement should ordinarily be given with Aldactone. Hyperkalemia can be treated promptly by the rapid intravenous administration of glucose (20 to 50 percent) and regular insulin, using 0.25 to 0.5 units of insulin per gram of glucose. This is a temporary measure to be repeated as required. Aldactone should be discontinued and potassium intake (including dietary potassium) restricted.
Hyponatremia, manifested by dryness of the mouth, thirst, lethargy and drowsiness, and confirmed by a low serum sodium level, may be caused or aggravated, especially when Aldactone is administered in combination with other diuretics.
Gynecomastia may develop in association with the use of spironolactone, and physicians should be alert to its possible onset. The development of gynecomastia appears to be related to both dosage level and duration of therapy and is normally reversible when Aldactone is discontinued. In rare instances some breast enlargement may persist.
Aldactone therapy may cause a transient elevation of BUN, especially in patients with preexisting renal impairment. Aldactone may cause mild acidosis.
When used in combination with other diuretics or antihypertensive agents Aldactone potentiates their effects. Therefore, the dosage of such drugs, particularly the ganglionic blocking agents, should be reduced by at least 50 percent when Aldactone is added to the regimen.
Spironolactone reduces the vascular responsiveness to norepinephrine. Therefore, caution should be exercised in the management of pa-

tients subjected to regional or general anesthesia while they are being treated with Aldactone.

Usage in Pregnancy. Spironolactone or its metabolites may cross the placental barrier. Therefore, the use of Aldactone in pregnant women requires that the anticipated benefit be weighed against possible hazard to the fetus.

Nursing Mothers. Canrenone, a metabolite of spironolactone, appears in breast milk. If use of the drug is deemed essential, an alternative method of infant feeding should be instituted.

Adverse Reactions: Gynecomastia is observed not infrequently. Other adverse reactions that have been reported in association with Aldactone are: gastrointestinal symptoms including cramping and diarrhea, drowsiness, lethargy, headache, maculopapular or erythematous cutaneous eruptions, urticaria, mental confusion, drug fever, ataxia, inability to achieve or maintain erection, irregular menses or amenorrhea, postmenopausal bleeding, hirsutism and deepening of the voice. Carcinoma of the breast has been reported in patients taking spironolactone, but a cause and effect relationship has not been established.

Adverse reactions are usually reversible upon discontinuation of the drug.

Dosage and Administration: **Primary hyperaldosteronism.** Aldactone may be employed as an initial diagnostic measure to provide presumptive evidence of primary hyperaldosteronism while patients are on normal diets.

Long test: Aldactone (spironolactone) is administered at a daily dosage of 400 mg. for three to four weeks. Correction of hypokalemia and of hypertension provides presumptive evidence for the diagnosis of primary hyperaldosteronism.

Short test: Aldactone is administered at a daily dosage of 400 mg. for four days. If serum potassium increases during Aldactone administration but drops when Aldactone is discontinued, a presumptive diagnosis of primary hyperaldosteronism should be considered.

After the diagnosis of hyperaldosteronism has been established by more definitive testing procedures, Aldactone may be administered in doses of 100 to 400 mg. daily in preparation for surgery. For patients who are considered unsuitable for surgery, Aldactone may be employed for long-term maintenance therapy at the lowest effective dosage determined for the individual patient.

Edema in adults (*congestive heart failure, hepatic cirrhosis or nephrotic syndrome*). An initial daily dosage of 100 mg. of Aldactone administered in divided doses is recommended, but may range from one to eight tablets (25 to 200 mg.) daily. When given as the sole agent for diuresis, Aldactone should be continued for at least five days at the initial dosage level, after which it may be adjusted to the optimal therapeutic or maintenance level. If, after five days, an adequate diuretic response to Aldactone has not occurred, a second diuretic which acts more proximally in the renal tubule may be added to the regimen. Because of the additive effect of Aldactone when administered concurrently with such diuretics, an enhanced diuresis usually begins on the first day of combined treatment; combined therapy is indicated when more rapid diuresis is desired. The dosage of Aldactone should remain unchanged when other diuretic therapy is added.

Edema in children. The initial daily dosage should provide approximately 1.5 mg. of Aldactone per pound of body weight (3.3 mg./kg.) administered in divided doses. For small children, Aldactone tablets may be pulverized and administered as a suspension in cherry syrup, N.F. When refrigerated, such a suspension is stable for one month.

Essential hypertension. For adults, an initial daily dosage of 50 to 100 mg. of Aldactone administered in divided doses is recommended. Aldactone may also be given with diuretics which act more proximally in the renal tubule or with other antihypertensive agents. Treatment with Aldactone should be continued for at least two weeks, since the maximum response may not occur before this time. Subsequently, dosage should be adjusted according to the response of the patient.

Hypokalemia. Aldactone in a dosage ranging from 25 mg. to 100 mg. daily is useful in treating a diuretic-induced hypokalemia, when oral potassium supplements or other potassium-sparing regimens are considered inappropriate.

How Supplied: Aldactone is supplied as scored, light tan tablets of 25 mg. each with SEARLE and 1001 debossed on the scored side and ALDACTONE on the other side; bottles of 100, 500, 1,000, and 2,500, and cartons of 100 unit-dose individually blister-sealed tablets.

[*Shown in Product Identification Section*]

DEMULEN® ℞
DEMULEN-28® ℞
(ethynodiol diacetate with ethinyl estradiol)

OVULEN® ℞
OVULEN-21® ℞
OVULEN-28® ℞
(ethynodiol diacetate with mestranol)

ENOVID-E® ℞
ENOVID-E® 21 ℞
(norethynodrel with mestranol)

ENOVID® 5 mg. ℞
(norethynodrel with mestranol)

Description:

Demulen and Demulen-28. Each white tablet contains 1 mg. of ethynodiol diacetate and 50 mcg. of ethinyl estradiol. Each pink tablet in the Demulen-28 package is a placebo, containing no active ingredients.

Ovulen, Ovulen-21 and Ovulen-28. Each white tablet contains 1 mg. of ethynodiol diacetate and 0.1 mg of mestranol. Each pink tablet in the Ovulen-28 package is a placebo, containing no active ingredients.

Enovid-E and Enovid-E 21. Each tablet contains 2.5 mg. of norethynodrel and 0.1 mg. of mestranol.

Enovid 5 mg. Each tablet contains 5 mg. of norethynodrel and 75 mcg. of mestranol.

The chemical name for norethynodrel is 17α-ethynyl-17-hydroxy-5(10)-estren-3-one, for mestranol it is 3-methoxy-19-nor-17α-pregna-1,3,5(10)-trien-20-yn-17-ol, for ethynodiol diacetate it is 19-nor-17α-pregn-4-en-20-yne-3β,17-diol diacetate and for ethinyl estradiol it is 19-nor-17α-pregna-1, 3, 5(10)-trien-20-yne-3,17-diol.

Therapeutic Class: Oral contraceptive
Estrogen-progestogen combination (Enovid 5 mg. only)

Clinical Pharmacology: Combination oral contraceptives act primarily through the mechanism of gonadotropin suppression due to the estrogenic and progestational activity of their components. Although the primary mechanism of action is inhibition of ovulation, alterations in the genital tract, including changes in the cervical mucus (which reduce sperm penetration) and the endometrium (which reduce the likelihood of implantation) may also contribute to contraceptive effectiveness.

Enovid 5 mg., when used for the treatment of endometriosis, may be administered to induce changes in areas of endometriosis similar to those that occur during pregnancy. In many instances when Enovid 5 mg. is taken continuously the areas of endometriosis develop a decidua-like response followed by necrosis, which may result in destruction of the abnormally located tissue and resolution of the lesions.

Indications and Usage: Demulen, Ovulen, Enovid-E and Enovid 5 mg. are indicated for the prevention of pregnancy in women who elect to use oral contraceptives as a method of contraception.

Enovid 5 mg. is also indicated for the treatment of endometriosis; for the treatment of hypermenorrhea and for the production of cyclic withdrawal bleeding.

NOTE: The contraindication, warning, precaution, and adverse reaction information in this leaflet also applies when Enovid 5 mg. is prescribed for indications other than contraception.

Oral contraceptives are highly effective. The pregnancy rate in women using conventional combination oral contraceptives (containing 35 mcg. or more of ethinyl estradiol or 50 mcg. or more of mestranol) is generally reported to be less than one pregnancy per 100 woman-years of use. Slightly higher rates (somewhat more than one pregnancy per 100 woman-years of use) are reported for some combination products containing 35 mcg. or less of ethinyl estradiol, and rates on the order of three pregnancies per 100 woman-years are reported for the progestogen-only oral contraceptives.

These rates are derived from separate studies conducted by different investigators in several population groups and, therefore, a precise comparison cannot be made. Furthermore, pregnancy rates tend to be lower as clinical studies are continued, possibly due to selective retention in the longer studies of those patients who accept the treatment regimen and do not discontinue as a result of adverse reactions, pregnancy or other reasons. In Table 1 ranges of pregnancy rates as reported in the literature[1] are shown for other means of contraception. The efficacy of these means of contraception, except for the IUD, depends upon the degree of adherence to the method.

Table 1
Pregnancies per 100 Woman-Years

Method	*Range*
IUD	<1 to 6
Diaphragm with spermicidal cream or gel	2 to 20
Condom	3 to 36
Spermicidal aerosol foams	2 to 29
Spermicidal gels and creams	4 to 36
Periodic abstinence (rhythm), all types	<1 to 47
1. Calendar method	14 to 47
2. Temperature method	1 to 20
3. Temperature method (intercourse only in post-ovulatory phase)	<1 to 7
4. Mucus method	1 to 25
No contraception	60 to 80

Dose-related Risk of Thromboembolism from Oral Contraceptives: One study showed a positive association between the dose of estrogens in oral contraceptives and the risk of thromboembolism[2] (see *Warning* No. 1). For this reason, it is prudent and in keeping with good principles of therapeutics to minimize exposure to estrogen. The oral contraceptive product prescribed for any given patient should be that product which contains the least amount of estrogen that is compatible with an acceptable pregnancy rate and patient acceptance. It is recommended that new users of oral contraceptives be started on preparations containing 50 mcg. or less of estrogen.

Contraindications: Oral contraceptives should not be used in women with any of the following conditions:

1. Thrombophlebitis, thromboembolic disorders, cerebral vascular disease, myocardial infarction or coronary artery disease, or a past history of these conditions.
2. Known or suspected carcinoma of the breast.
3. Known or suspected estrogen-dependent neoplasia.
4. Undiagnosed abnormal vaginal bleeding.
5. Known or suspected pregnancy (see *Warning* No. 5).

Continued on next page

Searle & Co.—Cont.

6. Markedly impaired liver function.
7. Past or present, benign or malignant liver tumors (see *Warning* No. 4).

WARNINGS

Cigarette-smoking increases the risk of serious cardiovascular side effects from oral contraceptive use. This risk increases with age and with heavy smoking (15 or more cigarettes per day) and is quite marked in women over 35 years of age. Women who use oral contraceptives should be strongly advised not to smoke.

The use of oral contraceptives is associated with increased risk of several serious conditions including venous and arterial thromboembolism, thrombotic and hemorrhagic stroke, myocardial infarction, visual disorders, hepatic tumors, gallbladder disease, hypertension, and fetal abnormalities. Practitioners prescribing oral contraceptives should be familiar with the following information relating to these and other risks.

1. *Thromboembolic Disorders and Other Vascular Problems.* An increased risk of thromboembolic and thrombotic disease associated with the use of oral contraceptives is well established. One study in Great Britain[3] demonstrated an increased relative risk for fatal venous thromboembolism; 2 British[4,5] and 3 U.S. studies[6–8] demonstrated an increased relative risk for nonfatal venous thromboembolism. Two U.S. studies[6,9,10] demonstrated an increased relative risk for stroke, which had not been shown in prior British studies.[3–5] In these studies it was estimated that users of oral contraceptives were 1.9 to 11 times more likely than nonusers to manifest these diseases without evident cause (Table 2). In a British study of idiopathic deep vein thrombosis and pulmonary embolism, the projected annual hospitalization rates for women aged 16–40 were 47 per 100,000 users and 5 for nonusers.[77] In one British mortality study,[3] overall excess mortality due to pulmonary embolism or stroke was on the order of 1.3 to 3.4 deaths annually per 100,000 users and increased with age.

Cerebrovascular Disorders: In a collaborative U.S. study[9,10] of cerebrovascular disorders in women with and without predisposing causes, it was estimated that the risk of hemorrhagic stroke was 2.0 times greater in users than in nonusers, and the risk of thrombotic stroke was 4.0[10] to 9.5[9] times greater in users than in nonusers (Table 2). Analysis of mortality trends in 21 countries indicates that, since oral contraceptives first became available, changes in mortality from nonrheumatic heart disease and hypertension, cerebrovascular disease, and all nonrheumatic cardiovascular disease among women aged 15 to 44 years have been associated with changes in the prevalence of oral contraceptive use in each country.[11]

Table 2. *Summary of Relative Risks of Thromboembolic Disorders and Other Vascular Problems in Oral Contraceptive Users Compared with Nonusers.*

Disorders	*Relative Risk*
Idiopathic thromboembolic disease	2 to 11 times greater
Postsurgery thromboembolic complications	4 to 7 times greater
Thrombotic stroke	4 to 9.5 times greater
Hemorrhagic stroke	2.0 to 2.3 times greater
Myocardial infarction	2 to 12 times greater

In May 1974 the Royal College of General Practitioners[12] issued an interim report of its continuing large-scale prospective study comparing a user with a nonuser group. It stated: "A statistically significant higher rate of reporting of cerebrovascular accidents in Takers is evident, but the numbers are too small to justify an estimation of the degree of risk." This study also reported a higher incidence of superficial and deep vein thrombosis in users, the former being correlated with the progestogen dose.[92] The RCGP data suggest[92] that the presence of varicose veins substantially increases the risk of superficial venous thrombosis of the leg, the risk depending upon the severity of the varicosities. The same may be true for deep vein thrombosis, but low numbers preclude a thorough analysis. A 1977 analysis of data from this study was reported[13] to show a 5-fold increased mortality from circulatory diseases, mainly from myocardial infarction and hemorrhagic stroke, in users. The excess mortality was associated with age, smoking and duration of use.

In October 1976 an interim report was issued on the long-term follow-up study of the British Family Planning Association.[14] There was a highly significant association between oral contraceptive use and stroke, although total numbers were small in this study also. The increase in risk of venous thrombosis and pulmonary embolism among users was about 4-fold and was statistically highly significant. In a later report[15] it was noted that mortality from circulatory diseases was significantly greater in users.

Myocardial Infarction: An increased risk of myocardial infarction associated with the use of oral contraceptives has been reported in Great Britain,[16–19] confirming a previously suspected association.[3] The morbidity study[16,17] found that the greater the number of underlying risk factors for coronary artery disease (cigarette-smoking, hypertension, hypercholesterolemia, obesity, diabetes, history of pre-eclamptic toxemia) the higher the risk of developing myocardial infarction, regardless of whether the patient was an oral contraceptive user or not. Oral contraceptives were considered an additional risk factor.

The annual excess rate of fatal myocardial infarction in British oral contraceptive users was estimated to be approximately 3.5 cases per 100,000 women users in the 30- to 39-year age group and 20 per 100,000 women users in the 40- to 44-year age group.[19] (These estimates are based on British vital statistics, which show acute myocardial infarction death rates 2 to 3 times less than in the U.S. for women in these age groups. In an attempt to extrapolate these figures to U.S. women it was estimated that the annual excess rates in users are 25.7 cases per 100,000 for women aged 30–39 with predisposing conditions, versus 1.5 cases without; corresponding estimates for women aged 40–44 were 86.2 versus 5.1.[78]) The annual excess rate of hospitalization for nonfatal myocardial infarction in married British oral contraceptive users was estimated to be approximately 3.5 per 100,000 women users in the 30- to 39-year age group and 47 per 100,000 women users in the 40- to 44-year age group.[16]

Smoking is considered a major predisposing condition to myocardial infarction. In terms of relative risk, it has been estimated[20] that oral contraceptive users who do not smoke are about twice as likely to have a fatal myocardial infarction as nonusers who do not smoke. Oral contraceptive users who are also smokers have about a 5-fold increased risk of fatal infarction compared to users who do not smoke, but about a 10- to 12-fold increased risk compared to nonusers who do not smoke. Furthermore, the amount of smoking is also an important factor. In determining the importance of these relative risks, however, the baseline rates for various age groups, as shown in Table 3, must be given serious consideration. The importance of other predisposing conditions mentioned above in determining relative and absolute risks has not been quantified; it is likely that the same synergistic action exists, but perhaps to a lesser extent.

Similar findings relating nonfatal myocardial infarction, oral contraceptives, smoking, and age were subsequently published in the U.S.[91]

Table 3. *Estimated Annual Mortality Rate per 100,000 Women from Myocardial Infarction by Use of Oral Contraceptives, Smoking Habits, and Age in Years[20]*

	Myocardial infarction			
	Women aged 30–39		Women aged 40–44	
Smoking habits	Users	Nonusers	Users	Nonusers
All smokers ..	10.2	2.6	62.0	15.9
Heavy*	13.0	5.1	78.7	31.3
Light	4.7	0.9	28.6	5.7
Nonsmokers .	1.8	1.2	10.7	7.4
Smokers and nonsmokers	5.4	1.9	32.8	11.7

*15 or more cigarettes per day

Risk of Dose: Reports of thromboembolism following the use of oral contraceptives containing 50 mcg. or more of estrogen received by drug safety committees in Great Britain, Sweden and Denmark were compared with the distribution expected from market research estimates of sales.[2] A positive correlation was found between the dose of estrogen and the reporting of thromboembolism, including coronary thrombosis, in excess of that predicted by sales estimates. Preparations containing 100 mcg. or more of estrogen were associated with a higher risk of thromboembolism than those containing 50–80 mcg. of estrogen. The authors' analysis did suggest, however, that the quantity of estrogen may not be the sole factor involved. Any influence on the part of the progestogens was not considered, which may have been responsible for certain discrepancies in the data. No significant differences were detected between preparations containing the same dose of estrogen nor between the two estrogens ethinyl estradiol and mestranol. Careful epidemiologic studies to determine the degree of thromboembolic risk associated with progestogen-only oral contraceptives have not been performed. Cases of thromboembolic disease have been reported in women using these products, and they should not be presumed to be free of excess risk.

The relative risk of oral contraceptive use one month prior to hospitalization for various types of thromboembolism was calculated in a

U.S. retrospective case-control study.[8] If no account is taken of the relative estrogenic potency of different estrogens and if any possible influence of the different progestogenic components is ignored, the products employed may be divided into those containing less than 100 mcg. and those containing 100 mcg. or more of estrogen. For all cases combined, the larger dose category was associated with only a slightly higher relative risk; for the idiopathic subgroup, the relative risk was approximately doubled with the larger estrogen content, but the confidence limits overlapped considerably and the differences, therefore, were not statistically significant. Apparently there was no significant increased relative risk for the subgroup with predispositions to thromboembolism.

The risk of thromboembolic and thrombotic disorders, in both users and nonusers of oral contraceptives, increases with age. Oral contraceptives have been considered an independent risk factor for these events.

Estimate of Excess Mortality from Circulatory Diseases: A large prospective study[13] carried out in the U.K. provided estimates of the mortality rate per 100,000 women per year from diseases of the circulatory system for users and nonusers of oral contraceptives according to age, smoking habits, and duration of use. The overall excess death rate annually from circulatory diseases for oral contraceptive users was estimated to be 20 per 100,000 (ages 15–34—12/100,000; ages 35–44—33/100,000; ages 45–49—140/100,000), the risk being concentrated in older women, in those with a long duration of use, and in cigarette-smokers. It was not possible, however, to examine the interrelationships of age, smoking, and duration of use, nor to compare the effects of continuous versus intermittent use. Although a 10-fold increase in death rate due to circulatory diseases in users for 5 or more years was estimated, all of these deaths occurred in women 35 or older. Until larger numbers of women under 35 with continuous use for 5 or more years are available, it is not possible to assess the magnitude of the relative risk for this younger age group. This study suggested that risk of circulatory disease may persist after the pill is discontinued.

The available data from a variety of sources have been analyzed[21] to estimate the risk of death associated with various methods of contraception. The estimates of risk of death for each method included the combined risk of the contraceptive method (e.g., thromboembolic and thrombotic disease in the case of oral contraceptives) plus the risk attributable to pregnancy or abortion in the event of method failure. This latter risk varies with the effectiveness of the contraceptive method. The findings of this analysis are shown in Figure 1.[21] The study concluded that the mortality associated with all methods of birth control is low and below that associated with childbirth, except for that associated with oral contraceptives in women over 40 who smoke. (The rates given for pill only/smokers for each age group are for smokers as a class. For "heavy" smokers (more than 15 cigarettes a day), the rates given would be about double; for "light" smokers (less than 15 cigarettes a day),[20] about 50 percent.) The mortality associated with oral contraceptive use in nonsmokers over 40 is higher than with any other method of contraception in that age group. The lowest mortality is associated with the condom or diaphragm backed up by early legal abortion.

Figure 1. Estimated annual number of deaths associated with control of fertility and no control per 100,000 nonsterile women, by regimen of control and age of woman

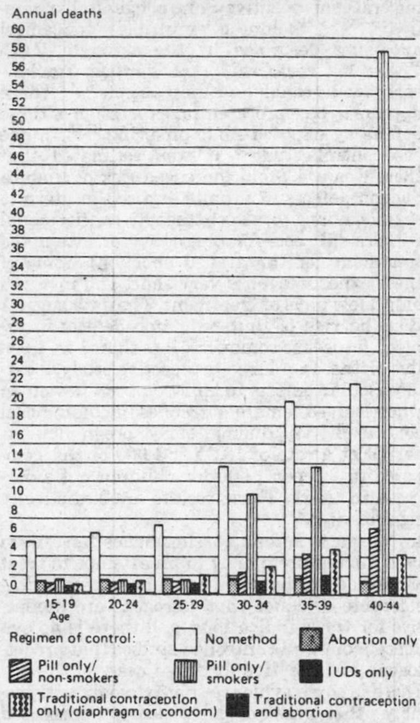

The risk of thromboembolic and thrombotic disease associated with oral contraceptives increases with age after approximately age 30 and, for myocardial infarction, is further increased by hypertension, hypercholesterolemia, obesity, diabetes, or history of preeclamptic toxemia and especially by cigarette-smoking.[20,78,79]

Based on the data currently available, the following table gives a gross estimate of the risk of death from circulatory disorders associated with the use of oral contraceptives:

Table 4. *Smoking Habits and Other Predisposing Conditions—Risk Associated with Use of Oral Contraceptives*

Age	Below 30	30–39	40+
Heavy smokers	C	B	A
Light smokers	D	C	B
Nonsmokers (no predisposing conditions)	D	C,D	C
Nonsmokers (other predisposing conditions)	C	C,B	B,A

A—Use associated with very high risk.
B—Use associated with high risk.
C—Use associated with moderate risk.
D—Use associated with low risk.

The physician and patient should be alert to the earliest manifestations of thromboembolic and thrombotic disorders (e.g., thrombophlebitis, pulmonary embolism, cerebrovascular insufficiency, coronary artery disease or myocardial infarction, retinal thrombosis, and mesenteric thrombosis). Should any of these occur or be suspected, the drug should be discontinued immediately.

A 4- to 7-fold increased risk of postsurgery thromboembolic complications has also been reported in oral contraceptive users.[22,23] If feasible, oral contraceptives should be discontinued at least 4 weeks before elective surgery or during periods of prolonged immobilization. Oral contraceptives should not be resumed until at least 4 weeks after surgery.

Among patients with thromboembolic disease, the results of retrospective studies suggest the possibility of an increased risk for users who are of blood types A, B, or AB as compared with those of type O.

2. *Ocular Lesions.* There have been reports of neuro-ocular lesions such as optic neuritis or retinal thrombosis associated with the use of oral contraceptives. Discontinue medication if there is unexplained, gradual or sudden, partial or complete loss of vision; proptosis or diplopia; papilledema; or any evidence of retinal vascular lesions. Appropriate diagnostic and therapeutic measures should be instituted.

3. *Carcinoma.* Long-term continuous administration of either natural or synthetic estrogens in certain animal species increases the frequency of certain carcinomas and/or nonmalignant neoplasms, such as those of the breast, uterus, cervix, vagina, ovary, liver, and pituitary. Certain synthetic progestogens, none currently contained in oral contraceptives, have been noted to increase the incidence of mammary nodules, benign and malignant, in dogs. There is now evidence that estrogens increase the risk of carcinoma of the endometrium in humans.

In several independent, retrospective case-control studies,[24–28,80,93] an increased relative risk (2.2 to 13.9 times) was reported, associating endometrial carcinoma with the prolonged use of estrogens in postmenopausal women who took estrogen replacement medication to relieve menopausal symptoms. This risk was independent of the other known risk factors for endometrial cancer and appeared to depend on both duration of treatment[24,27,28] and estrogen dose.[26–28] These findings are supported by the observation that incidence rates of endometrial cancer have increased sharply since 1969 in 8 different areas of the U.S. with population-based cancer-reporting systems, an increase which may be related to the rapidly expanding use of estrogens during the past decade.[29]

There is no evidence at present that "natural" estrogens are more or less hazardous than "synthetic" estrogens at equi-estrogenic doses. One publication[30] reported on the first 30 cases submitted by physicians to a registry of cases of adenocarcinoma of the endometrium in women under 40 on oral contraceptives. Of the adenocarcinomas found in women without predisposing risk factors for adenocarcinoma of the endometrium (e.g., irregular bleeding at the time oral contraceptives were first given, polycystic ovaries) nearly all occurred in women who had used a sequential oral contraceptive. These products are no longer marketed. No statistical association has been reported suggesting an increased risk of endometrial cancer in users of conventional combination or progestogen-only oral contraceptives, although individual cases have been reported.

Several studies[7,31–35] have shown no increased risk of breast cancer to women taking oral contraceptives or estrogens. In one study,[36,37] however, while no overall increased risk of breast cancer was noted in women treated with oral contraceptives, a greater risk was suggested for the subgroups of oral contraceptive users with documented benign breast disease and for long-term (2–4 years) users. One other study[38] indicated an increasing risk of breast cancer in women taking menopausal estrogens, which increased with duration of follow-up. A reduced occurrence of benign breast tumors in users of oral contraceptives has been well documented.[7,12,14,31,36,39,40]

Some epidemiologic studies[41,81–84] have suggested an increased risk of cervical dysplasia, erosion, and carcinoma in long-term pill users; however, cause and effect has not been estab-

Continued on next page

Searle & Co.—Cont.

lished. There have been other reports of microglandular dysplasia of the cervix in users.
In summary, there is at present no confirmed evidence from human studies of an increased risk of cancer associated with oral contraceptives.[42] Close clinical surveillance of all women taking oral contraceptives is, nevertheless, essential. In all cases of undiagnosed persistent or recurrent abnormal vaginal bleeding, nonfunctional causes should be borne in mind and appropriate diagnostic measures should be taken to rule out malignancy. Women who have a strong family history of breast cancer or who have breast nodules, fibrocystic disease, recurrent cystic mastitis, abnormal mammograms, or cervical dysplasia should be monitored with particular care if they elect to use oral contraceptives.
4. *Hepatic Lesions (adenomas, hepatomas, hamartomas, regenerating nodules, focal nodular hyperplasia, hemangiomas, hepatocellular carcinoma, etc.).* Benign hepatic adenomas and other hepatic lesions have been associated with the use of oral contraceptives.[43-46,85] One study[46] reported that oral contraceptive formulations with high "hormonal potency" were associated with a higher risk than lower-potency formulations. Although benign, these hepatic lesions may rupture and may cause death through intra-abdominal hemorrhage. This has been reported in short-term as well as long-term users of oral contraceptives. Two studies related risk with duration of use of the contraceptive, the risk being much greater after 4 or more years of oral contraceptive use.[45,46] While such hepatic lesions are rare, they should be considered in women presenting with abdominal pain and tenderness, abdominal mass or shock. Patients with liver tumors have demonstrated variable clinical features, which may make preoperative diagnosis difficult. About one quarter of the cases presented because of abdominal masses; up to one half had signs and symptoms of acute intraperitoneal hemorrhage. Routine radiological and laboratory studies may not be helpful. Liver scans may clearly show a focal defect. Hepatic arteriography or computed tomography may be useful procedures in diagnosing primary liver neoplasms.
A few cases of hepatocellular carcinoma have been reported in women taking oral contraceptives.[44] The relationship of these drugs to this type of malignancy is not known at this time. Oral contraceptives are contraindicated if there are past or present, benign or malignant liver tumors.
5. *Use in or Immediately Preceding Pregnancy, Birth Defects in Offspring, and Malignancy in Offspring.* The use of female sex hormones, both estrogens and progestogens, during early pregnancy may seriously damage the offspring. It has been reported that females exposed in utero to diethylstilbestrol and other nonsteroidal estrogens have an increased risk of developing in later life a form of vaginal or cervical cancer that is ordinarily extremely rare.[47,48] This risk has been estimated to be on the order of 1 in 1,000 exposures or less.[49,50] Although there is no evidence at the present time that oral contraceptives further enhance the risk of developing this type of malignancy, such patients should be monitored with particular care if they elect to use oral contraceptives instead of other methods of contraception. Furthermore, a high percentage of such exposed women (from 30–90%) have been found to have adenosis (epithelial changes) of the vagina and cervix.[51–55] Although these changes are histologically benign, it is not known whether this condition is a precursor of malignancy. Male children so exposed may develop abnormalities of the urogenital tract.[56–58] Although similar data are not available for the use of other estrogens, it cannot be presumed that they would not induce similar changes.
Several reports suggest an association between fetal exposure to female sex hormones, including oral contraceptives, and congenital anomalies,[59–64,94] including multiple congenital anomalies described by the acronym VACTERL, for vertebral, anal, cardiac, tracheoesophageal, renal, and limb defects.[61,62] There appears to be a preferential expression of these defects by exposed male offspring.[63,65] In one case-control study[63] it was estimated that there was a 4.7-fold increased risk of limb-reduction defects in infants exposed in utero to sex hormones (oral contraceptives, hormonal withdrawal tests for pregnancy or attempted treatment for threatened abortion). Some of these exposures were very short and involved only a few days of treatment. The data suggest that the risk of limb-reduction defects in exposed fetuses is somewhat less than 1 in 1,000 live births. In a large prospective study,[64] cardiovascular defects in children born to women who received female hormones, including oral contraceptives, during early pregnancy occurred at a rate of 18.2 per 1,000 births, compared to 7.8 per 1,000 for children not so exposed in utero. These results are statistically significant.
In the past, female sex hormones have been used during pregnancy in an attempt to treat threatened or habitual abortion. There is considerable evidence that estrogens are ineffective for these indications, and there is no evidence from well-controlled studies that progestogens are effective for these uses.
There is some evidence that triploidy and possibly other types of polyploidy are increased among abortuses from women who become pregnant soon after stopping oral contraceptives.[66] Embryos with these anomalies are virtually always aborted spontaneously. Whether there is an overall increase in spontaneous abortion of pregnancies conceived soon after stopping the oral contraceptives is unknown.
The safety of this product in pregnancy has not been demonstrated. Pregnancy should be ruled out before initiating or continuing the contraceptive regimen. Pregnancy should always be considered if withdrawal bleeding does not occur. It is recommended that for any patient who has missed 2 consecutive periods, pregnancy should be ruled out before continuing the contraceptive regimen. If the patient has not adhered to the prescribed schedule, the possibility of pregnancy should be considered at the time of the first missed period, and further use of oral contraceptives should be withheld until pregnancy has been ruled out. If pregnancy is confirmed, the patient should be apprised of the potential risks to the fetus, and the advisability of continuation of the pregnancy should be discussed in the light of these risks.
It is recommended that women who discontinue oral contraceptives with the intent of becoming pregnant use an alternative form of contraception for a period of time before attempting to conceive. Many clinicians recommend 3 months, although no precise information is available on which to base this recommendation.
The administration of progestogen-only or progestogen-estrogen combinations to induce withdrawal bleeding should not be used as a test of pregnancy.
6. *Gallbladder Disease.* Reports of studies[7,8,12,14,33] indicate an increased risk for surgically confirmed gallbladder disease in users of oral contraceptives or estrogens. In one study,[12] an increased risk appeared after 2 years of use and doubled after 4 or 5 years of use. In one of the other studies[7] an increased risk was apparent between 6 and 12 months of use.
7. *Carbohydrate and Lipid Metabolism.* A decrease in glucose tolerance has been observed in a significant percentage of patients on oral contraceptives. For this reason, prediabetic and diabetic patients should be carefully observed while receiving oral contraceptives. An increase in triglycerides and total phospholipids has been observed in patients receiving oral contraceptives.[67] The clinical significance of this finding remains to be defined.
8. *Elevated Blood Pressure.* An increase in blood pressure has been reported in patients receiving oral contraceptives.[12,69] There is evidence that the degree of hypertension may correlate directly with increasing dosage of progestogen.[86] In some women, hypertension may occur within a few months of beginning oral contraceptive use. The prevalence of hypertension in users is low in the first year of use, and may be no higher than that in a comparable group of nonusers. The prevalence in users increases, however, with longer exposure and, in the fifth year of use, is 2½ to 3 times the reported prevalence in the first year. Age is also strongly correlated with the development of hypertension in oral contraceptive users.
Women with a history of elevated blood pressure (hypertension), pre-existing renal disease, a history of toxemia or elevated blood pressure during pregnancy, a familial tendency to hypertension or its consequences, or a history of excessive weight gain or fluid retention during the menstrual cycle may be more likely to develop elevation of blood pressure when given oral contraceptives and, therefore, should be monitored closely.[68] Even though elevated blood pressure may remain within the "normal" range, the clinical implications of elevations should not be ignored and close surveillance is indicated, particularly for women with other risk factors for cardiovascular disease or stroke.[69] High blood pressure may or may not persist after discontinuation of the oral contraceptive.
9. *Headache.* The onset or exacerbation of migraine or development of headache of a new pattern which is recurrent, persistent, or severe, requires discontinuation of oral contraceptives and evaluation of the cause.
10. *Bleeding Irregularities.* Breakthrough bleeding, spotting, and amenorrhea are frequent reasons for discontinuance of oral contraceptives. In breakthrough bleeding, as in all cases of irregular vaginal bleeding, nonfunctional causes should be borne in mind. In patients with undiagnosed persistent or recurrent abnormal vaginal bleeding, adequate diagnostic measures are indicated to rule out pregnancy or malignancy. If a pathologic basis has been excluded, passage of time or a change to another formulation may correct the bleeding problem. A change to an oral contraceptive with a higher estrogen content, while potentially useful in minimizing menstrual irregularity, should be made only when considered necessary since this may increase the risk of thromboembolic disease.
Women with a past history of oligomenorrhea or secondary amenorrhea or young women who have not established regular cycles may have a tendency to remain anovulatory or to become amenorrheic after discontinuation of oral contraceptives. Women with these preexisting problems should be informed of these possibilities and encouraged to use other contraceptive methods. Post-use anovulation, possibly prolonged, may also occur in women without previous irregularities. A higher incidence of galactorrhea and of pituitary tumors (e.g., adenomas) has been associated with amenorrhea in former users compared with nonusers.[87] One study[70] reported a 16-fold increased prevalence of pituitary prolactin-secreting tumors among patients with postpill amenorrhea when galactorrhea was present.
11. *Ectopic Pregnancy.* Contraceptive failure may result in either ectopic or intrauterine pregnancy. In failures with combination-type oral contraceptives, the ratio of ectopic to intrauterine pregnancies is no higher than in women who are not receiving oral contracep-

tives. It has been suggested, however, that there may be an increased risk of ectopic pregnancy after discontinuance of an oral contraceptive.

12. *Breast Feeding.* Oral contraceptives given in the postpartum period may interfere with lactation. There may be a decrease in the quantity and quality of the breast milk. Furthermore, a small fraction of the hormonal agents in oral contraceptives has been identified in the milk of mothers receiving these drugs.[71,88,89] The effects, if any, on the breastfed child have not been determined. If feasible, the use of oral contraceptives should be deferred until the infant has been weaned.

13. *Infertility.* There is evidence of fertility impairment in women discontinuing oral contraceptives in comparison with those discontinuing other methods.[14,90] The impairment appears to be independent of the duration of use. While the impairment diminishes with time, there is still an appreciable difference in the results in nulliparous women 30 months after discontinuation of birth control; the difference is negligible after 42 months. For parous women the difference is no longer apparent 30 months after cessation of contraception.

Precautions:

General. 1. A complete medical and family history should be taken and a thorough physical examination should be performed prior to the initiation of oral contraceptives. The pretreatment and periodic physical examinations should include special reference to blood pressure, breasts, abdomen and pelvic organs, including a Papanicolaou smear and relevant laboratory tests. As a general rule, oral contraceptives should not be prescribed for longer than one year without the performance of another physical examination (see *Warnings*).

2. Pre-existing uterine leiomyomata may increase in size during oral contraceptive use.

3. Oral contraceptives appear to be associated with an increased incidence of mental depression. Therefore, patients with a history of depression should be carefully observed and the drug discontinued if depression recurs to a serious degree. Patients becoming significantly depressed while taking oral contraceptives should stop the medication and use an alternate method of contraception in an attempt to determine whether the symptom is drug related.

4. Oral contraceptives may cause some degree of fluid retention. They should be prescribed with caution, and only with careful monitoring, in patients with conditions which might be aggravated by fluid retention, such as convulsive disorders, migraine syndrome, asthma, or cardiac, hepatic or renal dysfunction.

5. Patients with a past history of jaundice during pregnancy have an increased risk of recurrence of jaundice and should be carefully observed while receiving oral contraceptives. If jaundice develops in any patient receiving such drugs, the medication should be discontinued while the cause is investigated.

6. Steroid hormones may be poorly metabolized in patients with impaired liver function and should be administered with caution in such patients. Oral contraceptives are contraindicated in patients with markedly impaired liver function.

7. Oral contraceptive users may have disturbances in normal tryptophan metabolism, which may result in a relative pyridoxine deficiency. The clinical significance of this is unknown, although megaloblastic anemia has been reported.

8. Serum folate levels may be depressed by oral contraceptive therapy. Since the pregnant woman is predisposed to folate deficiency and the incidence of folate deficiency increases with lengthening gestation, it is possible that if a woman becomes pregnant shortly after stopping oral contraceptives, she may have a greater chance of developing folate deficiency and complications attributed to this deficiency.

9. The pathologist should be advised of oral contraceptive therapy when relevant specimens are submitted.

10. Certain endocrine and liver function tests may be affected by estrogen-containing oral contraceptives. Therefore, it is recommended that any abnormal tests be repeated after the drug has been withdrawn for two months. The following alterations in laboratory results have been observed with the use of oral contraceptives:

a. Hepatic function: Increased sulfobromophthalein retention and other abnormalities in tests of liver function.
b. Coagulation tests: Increased prothrombin and coagulation factors VII, VIII, IX and X; decreased antithrombin III; increased platelet aggregability.
c. Thyroid function: Increased thyroid-binding globulin (TBG) leading to increased circulating total thyroid hormone, as measured by protein-bound iodine (PBI) or T^4 by column or radioimmunoassay. Free T^3 resin uptake is decreased, reflecting the elevated TBG; free T^4 concentration is unaltered.
d. Decreased pregnanediol excretion.
e. Reduced response to metyrapone test.
f. Increased blood transcortin and corticosteroid levels.
g. Increased blood triglyceride and phospholipid concentrations.
h. Reduced serum folate concentration.
i. Impaired glucose tolerance.
j. Altered plasma levels of trace minerals, e.g., increased ceruloplasmin.

11. The influence of prolonged oral contraceptive therapy on pituitary, ovarian, adrenal, hepatic, or uterine function, or on the immune response, has not been established.

12. Treatment with oral contraceptives may mask the onset of the climacteric. (See *Warnings* section regarding risks in this age group.)

Information for the Patient. See patient labeling printed at end.

Drug Interactions. Oral contraceptives may be rendered less effective and increased incidence of breakthrough bleeding may occur by virtue of drug interaction with rifampicin, isoniazid, ampicillin, neomycin, penicillin V, chloramphenicol, sulfonamides, nitrofurantoin, barbiturates, phenytoin, primidone, phenylbutazone, analgesics, tranquilizers and antimigraine preparations.[72–74] Oral contraceptives may alter the effectiveness of other types of drugs, such as oral anticoagulants, anticonvulsants, tricyclic antidepressants, antihypertensive agents (e.g., guanethidine), vitamins and hypoglycemic agents.[72]

Carcinogenesis. See *Warnings* No. 3 and 4 for information on the carcinogenic potential of oral contraceptives.

Pregnancy. Pregnancy category X. See *Contraindication* No. 5 and *Warning* No. 5.

Nursing Mothers. See *Warning* No. 12.

Adverse Reactions: An increased risk of the following serious adverse reactions has been associated with the use of oral contraceptives (see *Warnings*).

- Thrombophlebitis and thrombosis
- Pulmonary embolism
- Myocardial infarction and coronary thrombosis
- Cerebral thrombosis
- Cerebral hemorrhage
- Hypertension
- Gallbladder disease
- Benign adenomas and other hepatic lesions, with or without intra-abdominal bleeding
- Congenital anomalies

There is evidence of an association between the following conditions and the use of oral contraceptives, although confirmatory studies have not been done:

- Mesenteric thrombosis
- Budd-Chiari syndrome
- Neuro-ocular lesions, e.g., retinal thrombosis and optic neuritis

The following adverse reactions have been reported in patients receiving oral contraceptives and are believed to be drug related:

- Nausea and vomiting
  (Usually the most common adverse reactions, occurring in approximately 10% or less of patients during the first cycle. Other reactions, as a general rulc, are seen much less frequently or only occasionally.)
- Gastrointestinal symptoms (e.g., abdominal cramps and bloating)
- Breakthrough bleeding
- Spotting
- Change in menstrual flow
- Dysmenorrhea
- Amenorrhea during and after use
- Infertility after discontinuation
- Edema
- Chloasma or melasma, which may persist when the drug is discontinued
- Breast changes: tenderness, enlargement and secretion
- Change in weight (increase or decrease)
- Change in cervical erosion and secretion
- Endocervical hyperplasia
- Possible diminution in lactation when given immediately post partum
- Cholestatic jaundice
- Migraine
- Increase in size of uterine leiomyomata
- Rash (allergic)
- Mental depression
- Reduced tolerance to carbohydrates
- Vaginal candidiasis
- Change in corneal curvature (steepening)
- Intolerance to contact lenses

The following adverse reactions or conditions have been reported in users of oral contraceptives, and the association has been neither confirmed nor refuted:

- Premenstrual-like syndrome
- Cataracts
- Changes in libido
- Chorea
- Changes in appetite
- Cystitis-like syndrome
- Headache
- Paresthesia
- Nervousness
- Dizziness
- Auditory disturbances
- Rhinitis
- Fatigue
- Backache
- Hirsutism
- Loss of scalp hair
- Erythema multiforme
- Erythema nodosum
- Hemorrhagic eruption
- Itching
- Vaginitis
- Porphyria
- Impaired renal function
- Anemia
- Pancreatitis
- Hepatitis
- Colitis
- Gingivitis
- Lupus erythematosus
- Rheumatoid arthritis
- Pituitary tumors (e.g., adenoma), with amenorrhea and/or galactorrhea after use
- Endometrial, cervical, and breast carcinoma (see *Warning* No. 3)

Acute Overdosage: Serious ill effects have not been reported following the acute ingestion of large doses of oral contraceptives by young children.[75,76] Overdosage may cause nausea, and withdrawal bleeding might occur in females.

Dosage and Administration: Contraception: Demulen, Demulen-28, Ovulen, Ovulen-21, Ovulen-28, Enovid-E, Enovid-E 21, and Enovid 5 mg.

Continued on next page

Searle & Co.—Cont.

To achieve maximum contraceptive effectiveness, oral contraceptives must be taken exactly as directed and at intervals of 24 hours.
IMPORTANT: The patient should be instructed to use an additional method of protection until after the first week of administration *in the initial cycle.* The possibility of ovulation and conception prior to initiation of use should be considered.
Ovulen, Enovid-E or Enovid 5 mg. 20-Tablet Dosage Schedule: The patient should take one tablet daily for twenty consecutive days beginning each 20-tablet course on day 5 of her menstrual cycle or eight days after taking the last pill from the previous cycle, whichever occurs first. The first day of menstruation is counted as day 1.
Demulen, Demulen-28, Ovulen-21, Ovulen-28 and Enovid-E 21 Dosage Schedules: The Demulen, Ovulen-21 and Enovid-E 21 Compack® tablet dispensers contain 21 tablets arranged in three numbered rows of 7 tablets each.
The Ovulen-28 and Demulen-28 tablet dispensers contain 21 white active tablets arranged in three numbered rows of 7 tablets each, followed by a fourth row of 7 pink placebo tablets. Days of the week are printed above the tablets, starting with Sunday on the left.
Two dosage schedules are described, one of which may be more convenient or suitable than the other for an individual patient.
Schedule #1: Sunday Start: The patient begins taking Demulen, Demulen-28, Ovulen-21, Ovulen-28 or Enovid-E 21 from the first row of her package, one tablet daily, starting on the first Sunday after the onset of menstruation. If the patient's period begins on a Sunday she takes her first tablet that very same day. The twenty-first tablet or the twenth-eighth tablet, depending on whether the patient is taking the 21- or 28-tablet course, will then be taken on a Saturday.
Subsequent Cycles:
21-tablet course—The patient begins a new 21-tablet course on the eighth day, Sunday, after taking her last tablet. All subsequent cycles will also begin on Sunday, one tablet being taken each day for three weeks followed by a week of no pill-taking.
28-tablet course—The patient begins a new 28-tablet course on the next day, Sunday, and all subsequent cycles will also begin on Sunday, one tablet being taken each and every day.
With a Sunday start schedule, a woman whose period begins on the day of or one to four days before taking the first tablet should expect a diminution of flow and fewer menstrual days. The initial cycle will likely be shortened by from one to five days. Thereafter, cycles should be about 28 days in length.
Schedule #2: Day 5 Start: The patient begins taking Demulen, Ovulen-21 or Enovid-E 21 from the first row of her package, one tablet daily, starting with the pill day which corresponds to day 5 of her menstrual cycle; the first day of menstruation is counted as day 1. After the last (Saturday) tablet in row #3 has been taken, if any remain in the first row, the patient completes her 21-tablet schedule starting with Sunday in row #1.
Subsequent Cycles: The patient begins a new 21-tablet course on the eighth day after taking her last tablet, again starting the same day of the week on which she began her first course. All subsequent cycles will also begin on that same day, one tablet being taken each day for three weeks followed by a week of no pill-taking.
Postpartum Administration. Ovulen, Ovulen-21, and Ovulen-28 oral contraceptives may be prescribed at the first postpartum examination regardless of whether or not the patient has experienced spontaneous menstruation. In non-nursing mothers administration may be initiated immediately after delivery if desired or on the first Sunday after delivery. If preferred the tablets may be started on the day the patient leaves the hospital. (For nursing mothers see *Warning* No. 12.)
Hypermenorrhea: Production of Cyclic Withdrawal Bleeding: Enovid 5 mg. only. Most patients with hypermenorrhea may be expected to respond to Enovid 5 mg. therapy within 24 to 48 hours. Regular withdrawal bleeding may then be induced by cyclic administration. Vaginal bleeding at times other than the regular menstrual period requires that a diagnosis be established prior to beginning therapy.
For emergency control of severe bleeding in patients with hypermenorrhea give 20–30 mg. of Enovid 5 mg. daily until the bleeding is controlled, then reduce the daily dose to 10 mg. and continue through day 24 of the cycle. Then discontinue Enovid 5 mg. and withdrawal flow usually will begin approximately two to three days later.
Cyclic withdrawal bleeding may be produced after treatment in this initial cycle by giving the patient 5–10 mg. of Enovid 5 mg. daily from day 5 through day 24 of the next two or three cycles. A new course of Enovid 5 mg. should be started on day 5 of her menstrual cycle or eight days after the last pill from the previous cycle, whichever occurs first. The first day of menstruation is counted as day 1.
Endometriosis: Enovid 5 mg. only. A daily dose of Enovid 5 mg. should be given for six to nine months or longer on the following schedule: 5 or 10 mg. should be given for two weeks beginning on day 5 of a menstrual cycle. This daily dose should be given continuously (without cyclic interruption) and increased 5 or 10 mg. at two-week intervals until the patient is receiving 20 mg. daily. This dose of 20 mg. should be continued for six to nine months and further increased (up to 40 mg. daily) if breakthrough bleeding occurs.
Therapy may be discontinued after six months if the disease is mild and the lesions are no longer palpable. If the disorder is more severe continue treatment for nine months or longer. When surgery is contemplated prior administration of Enovid 5 mg. may facilitate the surgical procedure. (See *Warning* No. 1 concerning discontinuation prior to elective surgery.)
Special Notes: *Spotting or Breakthrough Bleeding.* If spotting (bleeding insufficient to require a pad) or breakthrough bleeding (heavier bleeding similar to a menstrual flow) occurs when used for contraception the patient should continue taking her tablets as directed. The incidence of spotting or breakthrough bleeding when used for contraception is minimal, most frequently occurring in the first cycle. Ordinarily spotting or breakthrough bleeding will stop within a week. Usually the patient will begin to cycle regularly within two or three courses of tablet-taking. If breakthrough bleeding occurs while the patient is taking Enovid 5 mg. for hypermenorrhea she should immediately increase the daily dosage by 5 or 10 mg. until bleeding has been controlled for three days, after which the original dosage usually may be resumed. In the event of spotting or breakthrough bleeding organic causes should be borne in mind. (See *Warning* No. 10.)
Missed Menstrual Periods. Withdrawal flow will normally occur two or three days after the last active tablet is taken. Failure of withdrawal bleeding ordinarily does not mean that the patient is pregnant, providing the dosage schedule has been correctly followed. (See *Warning* No. 5.)
If the patient has *not* adhered to the prescribed dosage regimen, the possibility of pregnancy should be considered after the first missed period and oral contraceptives should be withheld until pregnancy has been ruled out.
If the patient has adhered to the prescribed regimen and misses two consecutive periods, pregnancy should be ruled out before continuing the contraceptive regimen.
The first intermenstrual interval after discontinuing the tablets is usually prolonged; consequently, a patient for whom a 28-day cycle is usual might not begin to menstruate for 35 days or longer. Ovulation in such prolonged cycles will occur correspondingly later in the cycle. Post-treatment cycles after the first one, however, are usually typical for the individual woman prior to taking tablets. (See *Warnings* No. 10 and 11.)
Missed Tablets (Contraception). If a woman misses taking one active tablet the missed tablet should be taken as soon as it is remembered. In addition, the next tablet should be taken at the usual time. If two consecutive tablets are missed the dosage should be doubled for the next two days. The regular schedule should then be resumed, but an additional method of protection is recommended for the remainder of the cycle.
While there is little likelihood of ovulation if only one active tablet is missed, the possibility of spotting or breakthrough bleeding is increased and should be expected if two or more successive active tablets are missed. However, the possibility of ovulation increases with each successive day that scheduled active tablets are missed.
If one or more pink placebo tablets of Demulen-28 or Ovulen-28 are missed the Demulen-28 or Ovulen-28 schedule should be resumed on the following Sunday (the eighth day after the last white tablet was taken). Omission of placebo tablets in the 28-tablet courses does not increase the possibility of conception provided that this schedule is followed.
How Supplied:
Demulen: Each white Demulen tablet is round in shape, with a debossed SEARLE on one side and 71 on the other side, and contains 1 mg. of ethynodiol diacetate and 50 mcg. of ethinyl estradiol.
Demulen is packaged in cartons of 6 Compack tablet dispensers of twenty-one tablets each, in cartons of 12 and 48 Compack refills of twenty-one tablets each, and in cartons of 10 Triopak™ tablet containers, each Triopak containing 1 Compack tablet dispenser and 2 refills of twenty-one tablets each.
Demulen-28 is packaged in cartons of 6 Compack tablet dispensers and in cartons of 12 Compack refills. Each Compack and refill contain twenty-one white Demulen tablets and seven pink placebo tablets. (Placebo tablets have a debossed SEARLE on one side and a "P" on the other side.)
Ovulen: Each white Ovulen tablet is pentagonal in shape, with a debossed SEARLE on one side and 401 on the other side, and contains 1 mg. of ethynodiol diacetate and 0.1 mg. of mestranol.
Ovulen is packaged in cartons of 6 Compack tablet dispensers of twenty tablets each, and in cartons of 12 Compack refills of twenty tablets each.
Ovulen-21. Ovulen-21 is packaged in cartons of 6 Compack tablet dispensers of twenty-one tablets each; in cartons of 12 and 48 Compack refills of twenty-one tablets each, and in cartons of 10 and boxes of 100 Triopak™ tablet containers, each Triopak containing 1 Compack tablet dispenser and 2 refills of twenty-one tablets each.
Ovulen-28. Ovulen-28 is packaged in cartons of 6 Compack tablet dispensers and in cartons of 12 Compack refills. Each Compack and refill contain twenty-one white Ovulen tablets and seven pink placebo tablets. (Placebo tablets have a debossed SEARLE on one side and a "P" on the other side.)
Enovid-E: Each *Enovid-E* tablet is pale pink, round in shape, with a debossed SEARLE E on one side and 131 on the other side, and contains 2.5 mg. of norethynodrel and 0.1 mg. of mestra-

nol. Enovid-E is packaged in cartons of 6 Compack tablet dispensers of twenty tablets each, and in cartons of 12 Compack refills of twenty tablets each for Compack tablet dispensers.
Enovid-E 21 is packaged in cartons of 6 Compack tablet dispensers of 21 tablets each, and in cartons of 12 Compack refills of 21 tablets each.
Enovid 5 mg.: Each Enovid 5 mg. tablet is pink, round in shape, with a debossed SEARLE 5 on one side and 51 on the other side, and contains 5 mg. of norethynodrel and 75 mcg. of mestranol. Enovid 5 mg. is packaged in cartons of 6 Calendar-Pack™ tablet dispensers of twenty tablets each and in bottles of 100 tablets each.

References:

1. Population Reports, Series H, No. 2 (May) 1974; Series I, No. 1 (June) 1974; Series B, No. 2 (Jan.) 1975; Series H, No. 3 (Jan.) 1975; Series H, No. 4 (Jan.) 1976; Population Information Program, Geo. Washington U. Medical Center, Washington, D.C. **2.** Inman, W. H. W., et al.: Br. Med. J. *2*:203 (April 25) 1970. **3.** Inman, W. H. W., et al.: Br. Med. J. *2*:193 (April 27) 1968. **4.** Royal College of General Practitioners: J. Coll. Gen. Pract. *13*:267 (May) 1967. **5.** Vessey, M. P., et al.: Br. Med. J. *2*:651 (June 14) 1969. **6.** Sartwell, P. E., et al.: Am. J. Epidemiol. *90*:365 (Nov.) 1969. **7.** Boston Collaborative Drug Surveillance Programme: Lancet *1*:1399 (June 23) 1973. **8.** Stolley, P.D., et al.: Am. J. Epidemiol. *102*:197 (Sept.) 1975. **9.** Collaborative Group for the Study of Stroke in Young Women: N. Engl. J. Med. *288*:871 (April 26) 1973.
10. Collaborative Group for the Study of Stroke in Young Women: J.A.M.A. *231*:718 (Feb. 17) 1975. **11.** Beral, V.: Lancet *2*:1047 (Nov. 13) 1976. **12.** Royal College of General Practitioners: Oral Contraceptives and Health, New York, Pitman Publ. Corp., May 1974. **13.** Beral V.: Lancet *2*:727 (Oct. 8) 1977. **14.** Vessey, M., et al.: J. Biosoc. Sci. *8*:373 (Oct.) 1976. **15.** Vessey, M., et al.: Lancet *2*:731 (Oct. 8) 1977. **16.** Mann, J. I., et al.: Br. Med. J. *2*:241 (May 3) 1975. **17.** Mann, J. I., et al.: Br. Med. J. *3*:631 (Sept. 13) 1975. **18.** Mann, J. I., et al.: Br. Med. J. *2*:245 (May 3) 1975. **19.** Mann, J. I., et al.: Br. Med. J. *2*:445 (Aug. 21) 1976.
20. Jain, A. K.: Stud. Fam. Plann. *8*:50 (March) 1977. **21.** Tietze, C.: Fam. Plann. Perspect. *9*:74 (March-April) 1977. **22.** Vessey, M. P., et al.: Br. Med. J. *3*:123 (July 18) 1970. **23.** Greene, G. R., et al.: Am. J. Public Health *62*:680 (May) 1972. **24.** Ziel, H. K., et al.: N. Engl. J. Med. *293*:1167 (Dec. 4) 1975. **25.** Smith, D. C., et al.: N. Engl. J. Med. *293*:1164 (Dec. 4) 1975. **26.** Mack, T. M., et al.: N. Engl. J. Med. *294*:1262 (June 3) 1976. **27.** Gray, L. A., et al.: Obstet. Gynecol. *49*:385 (April) 1977. **28.** McDonald, T. W., et al.: Am. J. Obstet. Gynecol. *127*:572 (March 15) 1977. **29.** Weiss, N. S., et al.: N. Engl. J. Med. *294*:1259 (June 3) 1976.
30. Silverberg, S. G., et al.: Cancer *39*:592 (Feb.) 1977. **31.** Vessey, M. P., et al.: Br. Med. J. *3*:719 (Sept. 23) 1972. **32.** Vessey, M. P., et al.: Lancet *1*:941 (April 26) 1975. **33.** Boston Collaborative Drug Surveillance Program: N. Engl. J. Med. *290*:15 (Jan. 3) 1974. **34.** Arthes, F. G., et al.: Cancer *28*:1391 (Dec.) 1971. **35.** Casagrande, J., et al.: J. Natl. Cancer Inst. *56*:839 (April) 1976. **36.** Fasal, E., et al.: J. Natl. Cancer Inst. *55*:767 (Oct.) 1975. **37.** Paffenbarger, R. S., et al.: Cancer *49*:1887 (April Suppl.) 1977. **38.** Hoover, R., et al.: N. Engl. J. Med. *295*:401 (Aug. 19) 1976. **39.** Kelsey, J. L., et al.: Am. J. Epidemiol. *107*:236 (March) 1978.
40. Ory, H., et al.: N. Engl. J. Med. *294*:419 (Feb. 19) 1976. **41.** Stern, E., et al.: Science *196*:1460 (June 24) 1977. **42.** Population Reports, Series A, No. 4 (May) 1977: Population Information Program, Geo. Washington U. Medical Center, Washington, D.C. **43.** Baum, J. K., et al.: Lancet *2*:926 (Oct. 27) 1973. **44.** Mays, E. T., et al.: J.A.M.A. *235*:730 (Feb. 16) 1976. **45.** Edmondson, H. A., et al.: N. Engl. J. Med. *294*:470 (Feb. 26) 1976. **46.** Rooks, J. B., et al.: Internat. J. Gynaecol. Obstet. *15*:143, 1977. **47.** Herbst, A. L., et al.: N. Engl. J. Med. *284*:878 (April 22) 1971. **48.** Greenwald, P., et al.: N. Engl. J. Med. *285*:390 (Aug. 12) 1971. **49.** Lanier, A. P., et al.: Mayo Clin. Proc. *48*:793 (Nov.) 1973.
50. Herbst, A. L., et al.: Am. J. Obstet. Gynecol. *128*:43 (May 1) 1977. **51.** Herbst, A. L., et al.: Obstet. Gynecol. *40*:287 (Sept.) 1972. **52.** Herbst, A. L., et al.: Am. J. Obstet. Gynecol. *118*:607 (March 1) 1974. **53.** Herbst, A. L., et al.: N. Engl. J. Med. *292*:334 (Feb. 13) 1975. **54.** Stafl, A., et al.: Obstet. Gynecol. *43*:118 (Jan.) 1974. **55.** Sherman, A. I., et al.: Obstet. Gynecol. *44*:531 (Oct.) 1974. **56.** Bibbo, M., et al.: J. Reprod. Med. *15*:29 (July) 1975. **57.** Gill, W., et al.: J. Reprod. Med. *16*:147 (April) 1976. **58.** Henderson, B., et al.: Pediatrics *58*:505 (Oct.) 1976. **59.** Gal, I., et al.: Nature *216*:83 (Oct. 7) 1967.
60. Levy, E. P., et al.: Lancet *1*:611 (March 17) 1973. **61.** Nora, J. J., et al.: Lancet *1*:941 (April 28) 1973. **62.** Nora, A. H., et al.: Arch. Environ. Health *30*:17 (Jan.) 1975; Adv. Plann. Parent. *12*:156, 1978. **63.** Janerich, D. T., et al.: N. Engl. J. Med. *291*:697 (Oct. 3) 1974. **64.** Heinonen, O. P., et al.: N. Engl. J. Med. *296*:67 (Jan. 13) 1977. **65.** Nora, J. J., et al.: N. Engl. J. Med. *291*:731 (Oct. 3) 1974. **66.** Carr, D. H.: Can. Med. Assoc. J. *103*:343 (Aug. 15 & 29) 1970. **67.** Wynn, V., et al.: Lancet *2*:720 (Oct. 1) 1966. **68.** Laragh, J. H.: Am. J. Obstet. Gynecol. *126*:141 (Sept.) 1976. **69.** Fisch, I. R., et al.: J.A.M.A. *237*:2499 (June 6) 1977.
70. Van Campenhout, J., et al.: Fertil. Steril. *28*:728 (July) 1977. **71.** Laumas, K. R., et al.: Am. J. Obstet. Gynecol. *98*:411 (June 1) 1967. **72.** Stockley, I.: Pharmaceut. J. *216*:140 (Feb. 14) 1976. **73.** Hempel, E., et al.: Drugs *12*:442 (Dec.) 1976. **74.** Bessot, J.-C., et al.: Nouv. Presse Med. *6*:1568 (April 30) 1977. **75.** Francis, W. G., et al.: Can. Med. Assoc. J. *92*:191 (Jan. 23) 1965. **76.** Verhulst, H. L., et al.: J. Clin. Pharmacol. 7:9 (Jan.-Feb.) 1967. **77.** Vessey, M. P., et al.: Br. Med. J. *2*:199 (April 27) 1968. **78.** Ory, H. W.: J.A.M.A. *237*:2619 (June 13) 1977. **79.** Jain, A. K.: Am. J. Obstet. Gynecol. *126*:301 (Oct. 1) 1976.
80. Ziel, H. K., et al.: Am. J. Obstet. Gynecol. *124*:735 (April 1) 1976. **81.** Peritz, E., et al.: Am. J. Epidemiol. *106*:462 (Dec.) 1977. **82.** Ory, H. W., et al.: in Garattini, S., and Berendes, H. (eds.), Pharmacology of Steroid Contraceptive Drugs, Raven Press, N.Y., 1977. **83.** Goldacre, M. J., et al.: Br. Med. J. *1*:748 (March 25) 1978. **84.** Meisels, A., et al.: Cancer *40*:3076 (Dec.) 1977. **85.** Klatskin, G.: Gastroenterology *73*:386 (Aug.) 1977. **86.** Kay, C. R.: Lancet *1*:624 (March 19) 1977. **87.** March, C. M., et al.: Fertil. Steril. *28*:346 (March) 1977. **88.** Saxena, B. N., et al.: Contraception *16*:605 (Dec.) 1977. **89.** Nilsson, S., et al.: Contraception *17*:131 (Feb.) 1978.
90. Vessey, M. P., et al.: Br. Med. J. *1*:265 (Feb. 4) 1978. **91.** Jick, H., et al.: J.A.M.A. *239*:1403, 1407 (April 3) 1978. **92.** Kay, C. R.: J. Royal Coll. Gen. Pract. *28*:393 (July) 1978. **93.** Hoogerland, D. L., et al.: Gynecol. Oncol. *6*:451 (Oct.) 1978. **94.** Lorber, C. A., et al.: Fertil. Steril. *31*:21 (Jan.) 1979.

Brief Summary of Patient Labeling

Cigarette-smoking increases the risk of serious adverse effects on the heart and blood vessels from oral contraceptive use. This risk increases with age and with heavy smoking (15 or more cigarettes per day) and is quite marked in women over 35 years of age. Women who use oral contraceptives should not smoke.

In the detailed leaflet, "What You Should Know About Oral Contraceptives," which you have received, the risks and benefits of oral contraceptives are discussed in much more detail. This leaflet also provides information on other forms of contraception. Please take time to read it carefully for it may have been recently revised.
If you have any questions or problems regarding this information, contact your doctor.

Oral contraceptives taken as directed are about 99% effective in preventing pregnancy. (The mini-pill, however, is somewhat less effective.) Forgetting to take your pills increases the chance of pregnancy.

Women who have or have had clotting disorders, cancer of the breast or sex organs, unexplained vaginal bleeding, stroke, heart attack, chest pains on exertion (angina pectoris), liver tumors, markedly impaired liver function, or who suspect they may be pregnant should not use oral contraceptives.

Most side effects of the pill are not serious. The most common side effects are nausea, vomiting, bleeding between menstrual periods, weight gain, and breast tenderness. However, proper use of oral contraceptives requires that they be taken under your doctor's continuing supervision, because they can be associated with serious side effects which may be fatal. Fortunately, these are very uncommon. The serious side effects are:

1. Blood clots in the legs, arms, lungs, brain, heart, eyes, abdomen or elsewhere in the body.
2. Bleeding in the brain (hemorrhage) as a result of bursting of a blood vessel.
3. Disorders of vision.
4. Liver tumors, which may rupture and cause severe bleeding.
5. Birth defects if the pill is taken during pregnancy.
6. High blood pressure.
7. Gallbladder disease.

The symptoms associated with these serious side effects are discussed in the detailed leaflet given you with your supply of pills. Notify your doctor if you notice any unusual physical disturbance while taking the pill.

Breast cancer and other cancers have developed in certain animals when given the estrogens in oral contraceptives for long periods. These findings suggest that oral contraceptives may also cause cancer in humans. However, studies to date in women taking currently marketed oral contraceptives have not confirmed that oral contraceptives cause cancer in humans.

Caution: Oral contraceptives are of no value in the prevention or treatment of venereal disease.

Detailed Patient Labeling: What You Should Know About Oral Contraceptives

Oral contraceptives ("the pill") are the most effective way (except for sterilization) to prevent pregnancy if you follow the directions for their use and are careful not to skip doses or take them irregularly. They are also convenient and, for most women, free of serious or unpleasant side effects. Oral contraceptives must always be taken under the continuing supervision of a doctor.

It is important that any woman who considers using an oral contraceptive understands the risks involved. Although the oral contraceptives have important advantages over other methods of contraception, they have certain risks that no other method has. Only you can decide whether the advantages are worth these risks. This leaflet will tell you about the most important risks. It will explain how you can help your doctor prescribe the pill as safely as possible by telling him/her about yourself and being alert for the earliest signs of trouble. And it will tell you how to use the pill properly, so that it will be as effective as possible. THERE IS MORE DETAILED INFORMATION AVAILABLE IN THE LEAFLET PREPARED FOR DOCTORS. Your pharmacist can show

Continued on next page

Searle & Co.—Cont.

you a copy; you may need your doctor's help in understanding parts of it.

Enovid 5 mg. can be prescribed not only for contraception, but also as a treatment for endometriosis and as a treatment for hypermenorrhea and regulating periods. If you are taking Enovid 5 mg. for one of these other conditions besides contraception the warning information in the detailed leaflet also applies, so please read this leaflet.

Caution: Oral contraceptives are of no value in the prevention or treatment of venereal disease.

Cigarette-smoking increases the risk of serious adverse effects on the heart and blood vessels from oral contraceptive use. This risk increases with age and with heavy smoking (15 or more cigarettes per day) and is quite marked in women over 35 years of age. Women who use oral contraceptives should not smoke.

Who Should Not Use Oral Contraceptives: You should not use oral contraceptives:

A. If you have *ever* had any of the following:
   1. Blood clots in the legs, lungs or elsewhere in the body.
   2. Stroke (clots or bleeding in the brain).
   3. Heart attack or chest pains on exertion (angina pectoris).
   4. Liver tumor.

B. If you *now* have any of the following:
   1. Known or suspected cancer of the breast or sex organs, such as the womb (uterus), vagina, or cervix.
   2. Unusual vaginal bleeding that has not been diagnosed by your doctor.
   3. Known or suspected pregnancy (one or more menstrual periods missed).
   4. Markedly impaired liver function.

C. If you have scanty or irregular periods or are a young woman without a regular cycle, you should use another method of contraception because, if you use the pill, you may have difficulty becoming pregnant or may fail to have menstrual periods after discontinuing the pill.

Deciding to Use Oral Contraceptives. If you do not have any of the conditions listed above and are thinking about using oral contraceptives, to help you decide, you need information about the advantages and risks of oral contraceptives and of other contraceptive methods as well. This leaflet describes the advantages and risks of oral contraceptives. Except for sterilization, the intrauterine device (IUD) and abortion, which have their own specific risks, the only risks of other methods of contraception are those due to pregnancy should the method fail. Your doctor can answer questions you may have with respect to other methods of contraception, and further questions you may have on oral contraceptives after reading this leaflet.

1. *What Oral Contraceptives Are and How They Work.*

Oral contraceptives are of two types. The most common, often simply called "the pill," is a *combination* of an estrogen and a progestogen, the two kinds of female hormones. The amount of estrogen and progestogen can vary, but the amount of estrogen is more important because both the effectiveness and some of the dangers of oral contraceptives have been related to the amount of estrogen. This "combination" oral contraceptive works principally by preventing release of an egg from the ovary during the cycle in which the pills are taken. When the amount of estrogen is 50 micrograms or more, and the pill is taken as directed, oral contraceptives are more than 99% effective (that is, there would be less than one pregnancy in 100 women using the pill for one year). Pills that contain 20 to 35 micrograms of estrogen vary slightly in effectiveness, ranging from 98% to more than 99% effective.

The second type of oral contraceptive, often called the "mini-pill," contains only a progestogen. It works in part by preventing release of an egg from the ovary, but also by keeping sperm from reaching the egg and by making the womb (uterus) less receptive to any fertilized egg that reaches it. The mini-pill is less effective than the combination oral contraceptive, about 97% effective. In addition, the mini-pill has a tendency to cause irregular bleeding, which may be quite inconvenient, or cessation of bleeding entirely. The mini-pill is used despite its lower effectiveness in the hope that it will prove not to have some of the serious side effects of the estrogen-containing pill, but it is not yet certain that the mini-pill does in fact have fewer serious side effects. The following discussion, while based mainly on information about the combination pills, should be considered to apply as well to the mini-pill.

2. *Other Nonsurgical Ways to Prevent Pregnancy.*

As this leaflet will explain, oral contraceptives have several serious risks. Other methods of contraception have lesser risks or none at all. They are also less effective than oral contraceptives, but, used properly, may be effective enough for many women. The following table gives reported pregnancy rates (the number of women out of 100 who would become pregnant in one year) for these methods:

Pregnancies per 100 Women per Year

Method	*Range*
Intrauterine device (IUD)	less than 1 to 6
Diaphragm with spermicidal cream or jelly	2 to 20
Condom (rubber)	3 to 36
Spermicidal aerosol foams	2 to 29
Spermicidal jellies or creams	4 to 36
Periodic abstinence (rhythm), all types	less than 1 to 47
1. Calendar method	14 to 47
2. Temperature method	1 to 20
3. Temperature method (intercourse only in postovulatory phase)	less than 1 to 7
4. Mucus method	1 to 25
No contraception	60 to 80

These figures (except for the IUD) vary widely because people differ in how well they use each method. Very faithful users of the various methods obtain the best results, except for users of the periodic abstinence (rhythm) calendar method. Effective use of these methods, except for the IUD, requires somewhat more effort than simply taking a single pill every day, but it is an effort that many couples undertake successfully. Your doctor can tell you a great deal more about these methods of contraception and their effectiveness.

3. *The Dangers of Oral Contraceptives.*

a. *Circulatory Disorders (Blood Clots, Strokes and Heart Attacks).* Blood clots occasionally form in the blood vessels of the body and, though rare, are the most common of the serious side effects of oral contraceptives. Clotting can result in a stroke (a clot in the brain), a heart attack (a clot in a blood vessel of the heart), or a pulmonary embolus (a clot that forms in the legs or abdominal region, then breaks off and travels to the lungs), or loss of a limb (a clot in a blood vessel in, or leading to, an arm or leg). Clots can also form in the blood vessels of the intestines or liver. Any of these events can be fatal (lead to death). Clots also occur rarely in the blood vessels of the eye, resulting in blindness or impairment of vision in that eye. There is some evidence that the risk of clotting may increase with higher estrogen doses. It is therefore important for your doctor to keep the dose of estrogen as low as possible, so long as the oral contraceptive used has an acceptable pregnancy rate and doesn't cause unacceptable changes in the menstrual pattern. Furthermore, cigarette-smoking by oral contraceptive users increases the risk of serious adverse effects on the heart and blood vessels. This risk increases with age and with heavy smoking (15 or more cigarettes per day) and begins to become quite marked in women over 35 years of age. For this reason, women who use oral contraceptives should not smoke.

The risk of abnormal clotting increases with age in both users and nonusers of oral contraceptives, but the increased risk with the oral contraceptives appears to be present at all ages.

For oral contraceptive users in general, it has been estimated that in women between the ages of 15 and 34 the risk of death due to a circulatory disorder is about 1 in 12,000 per year, whereas for nonusers the rate is about 1 in 50,000 per year. In the age group 35 to 44, the risk is estimated to be about 1 in 2,500 per year for oral contraceptive users and about 1 in 10,000 per year for nonusers. The risk increases with advancing age, with long duration of use, and in cigarette-smokers. The effects on the circulatory system may persist after the pill is discontinued.

For women aged 16 to 40 it is estimated that about 1 in 2,000 using oral contraceptives will be hospitalized each year because of abnormal clotting in the veins or lungs. Among nonusers of the same age, about 1 in 20,000 would be hospitalized each year for these disorders.

The risk of abnormal blood clotting may be greater if your blood type is A, B, or AB rather than type O.

Strokes are caused by a bursting blood vessel in the brain (hemorrhage) or a loss of blood circulation to the brain due to blood clots. When they occur, paralysis of all or part of the body may result; death can result. The risk of strokes due to clots or hemorrhages in the brain has been reported to be increased in pill users when compared with nonusers.

It has been estimated that pill users are twice as likely as nonusers to have a stroke due to a bursting blood vessel in the brain. It has further been estimated that pill users are 4 to 10 times as likely as nonusers to have a stroke due to clotting in a blood vessel in or leading to the brain.

It has been reported that women using the pill may have a greater risk of heart attack than nonusers. Even without the pill the risk of having a heart attack increases with age and is also increased by additional risk factors such as high blood pressure, high blood cholesterol, obesity, diabetes, cigarette-smoking, or the occurrence during pregnancy of high blood pressure, swelling of the legs, or protein in the urine. Without any risk factors present, the use of oral contraceptives alone may double the risk of heart attack. However, the combination of cigarette-smoking, especially heavy smoking, and oral contraceptive use greatly increases the risk of heart attack. Oral contraceptive users who smoke are about five times more likely to have a heart attack than users who do not smoke and about ten times more likely to have a heart attack than nonusers who do not smoke. It has been estimated that users between the ages of 30 and 39 who smoke have about a 1 in 10,000 chance each year of having a fatal heart attack compared to about a 1 in 50,000 chance in users who do not smoke, and about a 1 in 100,000 chance in nonusers who do not smoke. In the age group 40 to 44, the risk is about 1 in 1,700 per year for users who smoke compared to about 1 in 10,000 for users who do not smoke and to about 1 in 14,000 per year for nonusers who do not smoke. Heavy smoking (about 15 cigarettes or more a day) further increases the risk. If you do not smoke and have none of the other heart attack risk factors described above, you will have a smaller risk than listed. If you have several heart attack risk factors, the risk may be considerably greater than listed.

The above are average figures for Great Britain; comparable estimates for the U.S. have been higher.

Oral contraceptives should never be used at any age by women who have had a stroke, a heart attack, or chest pains on exertion (angina pectoris), or who have had blood clots in the legs, lungs or elsewhere.

Anyone using the pill who has severe leg or chest pains, coughs up blood, has difficulty in breathing, severe headache or vomiting, dizziness or fainting, disturbances of vision or speech, weakness, numbness, or pain in an arm or leg should call her doctor immediately and stop taking the pill, and use another method of contraception.

b. *Formation of tumors.* When certain animals are given the female sex hormone estrogen (which is an ingredient in oral contraceptives) continuously for long periods, cancers may develop in organs such as the breast, cervix, vagina, liver, womb, ovary, and pituitary. These findings suggest that oral contraceptives may cause cancer in humans. However, studies to date in women taking currently marketed oral contraceptives have not confirmed that oral contraceptives cause cancer in humans, but it remains possible they will be discovered in the future to do so. Several studies have found no increase in breast cancer in users, although it has been suggested that oral contraceptives might cause an increase in breast cancer in women who already have benign (noncancerous) breast disease (for example, cysts) or in long-term (2–4 years) users.

Women with a family history of breast cancer or who have breast nodules (lumps), fibrocystic disease (breast cysts), or abnormal mammograms (x-ray pictures of the breasts) or who were exposed to the estrogen diethylstilbestrol (DES) during their mother's pregnancy, or who have abnormal Pap smears should be followed very closely by their doctors if they choose to use oral contraceptives instead of another method of contraception. Many studies have shown that women taking oral contraceptives have less risk of getting benign (noncancerous) breast disease than those who have not used oral contraceptives. There is strong evidence that estrogens (one component of combination-type oral contraceptives), when given for periods of more than one year to women after the menopause (change-of-life), increase the risk of cancer of the womb (uterus). There is also some evidence that the sequential oral contraceptive, a kind of oral contraceptive that is no longer sold, may increase the risk of cancer of the womb. There is no evidence, however, that the oral contraceptives now available increase the risk of this type of cancer, although some individual cases have been reported. Cancer of the cervix may develop more readily in long-term users of the pill, particularly if they have had pre-existing abnormal Pap smears. Cervical erosion and cell abnormalities have been reported to be more frequent in pill users.

Very rarely, oral contraceptive users may have a noncancerous tumor of the liver. These tumors do not spread, but they may rupture and cause internal bleeding, which may be fatal. This has been reported in short-term as well as long-term users. One study reported that oral contraceptive products with a high "hormonal potency" were associated with a higher risk than lower-potency products. A few cases of cancer of the liver have been reported in women using oral contraceptives, but it is not yet known whether the drug caused them.

c. *Dangers to the developing baby if oral contraceptives are used in or immediately preceding pregnancy.* Oral contraceptives should not be taken by pregnant women because they may damage the developing baby. There is an increased risk to the baby of abnormalities of such parts of the body as the backbone, anus, heart, windpipe, esophagus, kidneys, arms and legs. In addition, the developing female child whose mother has received DES, a synthetic estrogen, during pregnancy has a risk of getting cancer of the vagina or cervix in her teens or young adulthood. This risk is estimated to be about 1 in 1,000 exposures or less. Abnormalities of the urinary and sex organs have been reported in DES-exposed male babies as well. It is possible that other estrogens, such as the estrogens in oral contraceptives, could have the same effect in the baby if the mother takes them during pregnancy.

Occasionally women who are taking the pill miss periods. It has been reported to occur as frequently as several times each year in some women, depending on various factors such as age and prior history. (Your doctor is the best source of information about this.) The pill should not be used when you are pregnant or suspect you may be pregnant. Very rarely, women who are using the pill as directed become pregnant. The likelihood of becoming pregnant is higher if you occasionally miss one or two pills. Therefore, if you miss a period you should consult your physician before continuing to take the pill. If you miss a period, especially if you have not taken the pill regularly, you should use an alternative method of contraception until pregnancy has been ruled out; if you have missed more than one pill at any time, you should immediately start using an additional method of contraception and complete your pill cycle.

You should not attempt to become pregnant for at least three months after discontinuing oral contraceptives. Use another method of contraception during this period of time. The reason for this is that during this period there may be an increased risk of "miscarriage" and deformity to the baby. Whether there is an overall increase in "miscarriage" in women who become pregnant soon after stopping the pill as compared with women who did not use the pill is not known, but it is possible that there may be.

If, however, you do become pregnant soon after stopping oral contraceptives, and do not have a miscarriage, there is no evidence that the baby has an increased risk of being abnormal.

d. *Gallbladder disease.* Women who use oral contraceptives have a greater risk than nonusers of having gallbladder disease requiring surgery. The increased risk may first appear within one year of use and may double after 4 or 5 years of use.

e. *Other side effects of oral contraceptives.* Some women using oral contraceptives experience unpleasant side effects from the pill which are not dangerous and are not likely to damage their health. Some of these side effects are similar to symptoms women experience in early pregnancy and may be temporary. Your breasts may feel tender, be enlarged or have a discharge; nausea and vomiting or other stomach or intestinal problems may occur; you may gain or lose weight, and your ankles may swell. A spotty darkening of the skin, particularly of the face, is possible and may persist after the drug is discontinued. An allergic or other type of rash or vaginal yeast infection might occur. You may notice unexpected vaginal bleeding, change in discharge or changes in your menstrual period. Irregular bleeding is frequently seen when using the mini-pill or the combination oral contraceptives containing less than 50 micrograms of estrogen. These should all be reported to your doctor.

Other side effects include worsening of migraine, asthma, convulsive disorders (such as epilepsy) and kidney, liver or heart disease because of a tendency for water to be retained in the body when oral contraceptives are used. Other side effects are painful periods; growth of pre-existing fibroid tumors of the womb; mental depression; and liver problems with jaundice (yellowing of the whites of the eyes or of the skin). Your doctor may find that levels of sugar and fatty substances in your blood are elevated; the long-term effects of these changes are not known. Some women develop high blood pressure while taking oral contraceptives, which ordinarily, but not always, returns to the original levels when the oral contraceptive is stopped. The degree of blood pressure rise may be related to the amount of progestogen in the pill. Women with a history of increased blood pressure, kidney disease, or toxemia during pregnancy (increased blood pressure, swelling of the legs, protein in the urine, or convulsions), or a family tendency to high blood pressure or its consequences (stroke, heart disease, kidney disease, blood vessel problems) or a history of excessive weight gain or swelling of the legs during their menstrual cycle, may be more likely to develop increased blood pressure when given oral contraceptives and, therefore, should have their blood pressure taken frequently. High blood pressure predisposes one to stroke, heart attacks, kidney disease, and other diseases of the blood vessels. The effect of prolonged use of oral contraceptives on several of your organs (pituitary, liver, ovaries, womb, and adrenals) or immune system is not known at this time.

Other conditions, although not proved to be caused by oral contraceptives, are occasionally reported. These include more frequent urination and some discomfort when urinating, kidney disease, nervousness, dizziness, hearing problems, inflammation of the nasal passages, loss of scalp hair, an increase in body hair, an increase or decrease in sex drive, appetite changes, gum disease, cataracts, a need for a change in contact lens prescription or inability to use contact lenses, tiredness, backache, vaginal infections, itching, anemia, headache, symptoms similar to those you get before a period, breast, womb, and cervical cancer, inflammation of the pancreas, liver or colon, chorea (spasmodic movements), burning or prickly sensation, and rheumatoid arthritis.

After you stop using oral contraceptives, there may be a delay before you are able to become pregnant or before you resume having menstrual periods. This is especially true of women who had irregular menstrual cycles prior to the use of oral contraceptives.

One study showed that this delay in becoming pregnant can persist to 30 months after stopping the pill, especially if you have never had children, and does not depend on how long you have used the pill. Very rarely there may be secretions from the breast associated with the absence of periods, which might be due to a noncancerous tumor of the pituitary gland requiring surgery. This may occur more frequently in former users of the pill than in nonusers. As discussed previously, you should wait at least three months after stopping the pill before you try to become pregnant. There is a possibility that more tubal pregnancies (which require surgery) will occur immediately after stopping oral contraceptives. During the first three months after stopping oral contraceptives, use another form of contraception. You should consult your doctor before resuming use of oral contraceptives after childbirth, especially if you plan to nurse your baby. Drugs in oral contraceptives are known to appear in the milk, and the long-range effect on babies is not known at this time. Furthermore, oral contraceptives may cause a decrease in your milk supply as well as in the quality of the milk.

4. *Comparison of the Risks of Oral Contraceptives and Other Contraceptive Methods.*

The many studies on the risks and effectiveness of oral contraceptives and other methods of contraception have been analyzed to estimate the risk of death associated with various methods of contraception. This risk has two parts: (a) the risk of the method itself (for example, the risk that oral contraceptives might

Continued on next page

Searle & Co.—Cont.

cause death due to abnormal blood clotting), and (b) the risk of death due to pregnancy or abortion in the event the method fails. The results of this analysis are shown in the following bar graph. The height of the bars indicates the number of deaths per 100,000 women each year. There are six sets of bars, each set referring to a specific age group of women. Within each set of bars, there is a single bar for each of the different contraceptive methods.

For oral contraceptives, there are two bars —one for smokers and the other for nonsmokers. The analysis is based on present knowledge and new information could, of course, alter it. The analysis shows that the risk of death from all methods of birth control is low and below that associated with the risks of childbirth, *except for oral contraceptives in women over 40 who smoke.* The risk of death associated with pill use in nonsmokers over 40 is higher than with any other method of contraception in that age group. It shows that the lowest risk of death is associated with the condom or diaphragm (traditional contraception) backed up by early legal abortion in case of failure of the condom or diaphragm to prevent pregnancy. Also, at any age, the risk of death (due to unexpected pregnancy) from use of traditional contraception, even without a backup of abortion, is generally the same as, or less than, that from use of oral contraceptives.

Figure 1. Estimated annual number of deaths associated with control of fertility and no control per 100,000 nonsterile women, by regimen of control and age of woman

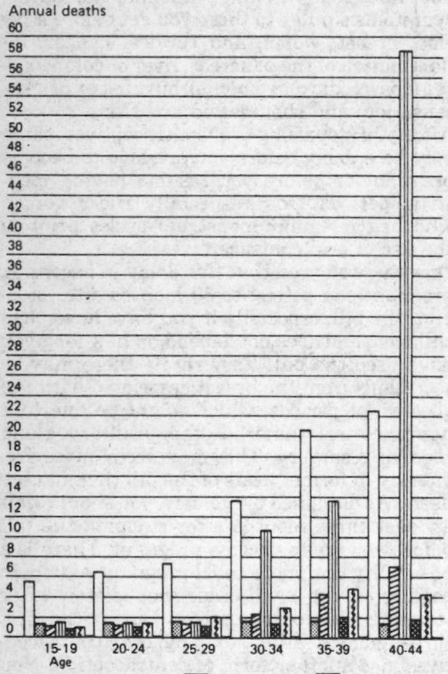

How to Use Oral Contraceptives as Safely and Effectively as Possible, Once You Have Decided to Use Them:

1. *What to Tell Your Doctor.* You can make use of the pill as safe as possible, by telling your doctor if you have any of the following:

a. Conditions that mean you should not use oral contraceptives:

If you have *ever* had any of the following:

(1) Blood clots in the legs, lungs or elsewhere in the body.
(2) Stroke (clots or bleeding in the brain).
(3) Heart attack or chest pains on exertion (angina pectoris).
(4) Liver tumor.

If you *now* have any of the following:

(1) Known or suspected cancer of the breast or sex organs such as of the womb, vagina, or cervix.
(2) Unusual vaginal bleeding that has not been diagnosed.
(3) Known or suspected pregnancy (one or more menstrual periods missed).
(4) Markedly impaired liver function.

b. Inform your doctor of the following conditions since s/he will want to watch them closely or they might cause him/her to suggest another method of contraception:

A family history of breast cancer
Breast nodules (lumps), fibrocystic disease (breast cysts), abnormal mammograms (x-ray pictures of the breasts), or abnormal Pap smears
Diabetes
High blood pressure
High blood cholesterol
Cigarette-smoking
Migraine
Heart or kidney disease
Asthma
Problems during a prior pregnancy
Epilepsy
Mental depression
Fibroid tumors of the womb
History of jaundice (yellowing of the whites of the eyes or of the skin)
Gallbladder disease
Varicose veins
Tuberculosis
Plans for elective surgery
Previous problems with your periods (irregularities)
Use of any of the following kinds of drugs, which might interact with the pill: antibiotics, sulfa drugs, drugs for epilepsy or migraine, painkillers, tranquilizers, sedatives or sleeping pills, blood-thinning drugs, vitamins, drugs being used for the treatment of depression, high blood pressure, or high blood sugar (diabetes)

c. Once you are using oral contraceptives, you should be alert for signs of a serious adverse effect and call your doctor immediately if any of these occur:

Sharp pain in the chest, coughing up blood, or sudden shortness of breath (indicating possible clots in the lungs).
Pain in the calf (possible clot in the leg).
Crushing chest pain or heaviness (indicating possible heart attack).
Sudden severe headache or vomiting, dizziness or fainting, disturbance of vision or speech, or weakness or numbness in an arm or leg (indicating a possible stroke).
Sudden partial or complete loss of vision (indicating a possible clot in the blood vessels of the eye).
Abnormal vaginal bleeding.
Breast lumps (you should ask your doctor to show you how to examine your own breasts).
Severe and/or persistent pain or a mass in the abdomen (indicating a possible tumor of the liver, which might have ruptured).
Severe depression.
Yellowing of the whites of the eyes or of the skin (jaundice).
Unusual swelling.
Other unusual conditions.

2. *How to Take the Pill So That It is Most Effective. Dosage Schedules.* See later sections in this leaflet concerning spotting, breakthrough bleeding, forgotten pills and missed menstruation.

When you first begin to use the pill, you should use an additional method of protection until you have taken your first seven pills.

To remove a pill, press down on it. The pill will drop through a hole in the bottom of the Compack®.

The "20-pill" Schedule. Ovulen®, Enovid-E®, and Enovid® 5 mg. may be prescribed on the 20-pill schedule.

The Enovid 5 mg. package is a Calendar-Pack™. Sometimes Enovid 5 mg. is dispensed in a bottle.

Your Compack is round if your physician has prescribed Ovulen or Enovid-E for you on the 20-pill schedule. It contains 20 tablets arranged in three circles.

Take a pill each day for 20 consecutive days, beginning each pill cycle on day 5 after your period starts, just as you did during the first pill cycle, or on the eighth day after having taken the last pill, whichever occurs first. Count the day you start to menstruate as day 1. Continue this 20-pill schedule, cycle after cycle, regardless of whether your flow has or has not ceased when you start or whether you happen to spot or experience unexpected (breakthrough) bleeding during a cycle.

You will probably have your periods about every 27 days.

The Two "three weeks on—one week off" Schedules. Your Compack is rectangular in shape if your doctor has prescribed Demulen®, Ovulen-21, or Enovid-E 21. It contains 21 tablets arranged in three numbered rows with the days of the week printed above them.

Day-5 Schedule. If you are to begin on day 5, count the day you start to menstruate as day 1 and determine which day to start. Start in row #1 with the pill under the day which corresponds to day 5 after your flow began. Continue to take one pill each day on consecutive days of the week.

After the last (Saturday) pill in row #3 has been taken, if any remain in the first row, complete your 21-pill schedule by taking one pill daily starting with Sunday in row #1. Then stop for one week before starting to take the pills again. Begin your next pill cycle on the same day of the week that you began the first cycle.

Sunday Schedule. Start taking the pills on the first Sunday after your period begins unless your period begins on Sunday. If your period begins on Sunday start taking the pill that very same day.

Begin in row #1 and take your pills, one each day on consecutive days, for three weeks (21 days), then stop taking them for one week (7 days) before starting to take the pills again on Sunday.

Whether you begin on "day 5" or on Sunday, continue taking your pills as directed, month after month, regardless of whether your flow has or has not ceased or whether you may have experienced spotting or unexpected (breakthrough) bleeding during your pill cycle. You will probably have your period about every 28 days.

The "Pill-a-day" Schedule. Your Compack is rectangular in shape if your doctor has prescribed Demulen-28 or Ovulen-28. It contains 28 pills arranged in four numbered rows of seven pills each with the days of the week printed above them.

You must take your pills in order, one pill each day. Begin with the Sunday pill in row #1.

1—Start taking the pills on the first Sunday after your period begins unless your period begins on Sunday. *If your period begins on Sunday start taking the pills that very same day.*

2—Continue to take one pill each day on consecutive days of the week.

3—After the Saturday pill in row #1 has been taken begin taking pills in row #2 and so on until the Saturday pill in row #4 has been taken.

4—Replace the Refill in your Compack at once and begin a new pill cycle the next day, starting with the Sunday pill in row #1.

You will probably have your period about every 28 days, while you are taking the pink pills. Continue your pill-a-day schedule, month after month, regardless of whether your flow ceases while you are taking the pink pills, or whether

you experienced spotting or unexpected (breakthrough) bleeding during a cycle.
Take your pill faithfully every "pill day"!
It is important that you take a pill without fail every "pill day" at intervals of 24 hours for two reasons. First, your ovaries may release an egg and therefore you may become pregnant if you do not take your pills regularly. Second, you may spot or start to flow between your periods. This may be inconvenient.
Take your pill at the same time every day!
You are probably wondering why the same time of day is important. By taking your pill at the same time every day it becomes a good habit and you are much less likely to forget. You may wish to keep your pills in the medicine cabinet near your toothbrush as a reminder to take them when you brush your teeth at night. The best time to take your daily pill may be either with your evening meal or at bedtime. You may find it helpful to associate your pill-taking with something else you do every day at a particular time.
Another very important reason for you to take your pills as "regular as clockwork" is that you are protected best when you take one every 24 hours; they are made to work that way. Just remember that once every day is not the same as once every 24 hours. Here is why. Suppose you were to take your Monday pill in the morning when you get up, and then not take your Tuesday pill till the evening before you go to bed. True, you will have taken a pill each day, on Monday and on Tuesday—but the time between pill-taking will probably have been more than 36 hours, or more than 1½ days! You might spot. Chances are you would still be protected and would not get pregnant, but why risk it when it is so easy to guarantee yourself maximal protection by taking your pill faithfully every pill day and at the same time every pill day?
In summary, you should take the pills exactly as directed and at intervals of 24 hours in order to achieve maximum contraceptive effectiveness.
Spotting. This is a slight staining between your menstrual periods which may not even require a pad. Some women spot even though they take their pills exactly as directed. Many women spot although they have never taken the pills. Spotting does not mean that your ovaries are releasing an egg. Spotting may be the result of irregular pill-taking. Getting back on schedule will usually stop it.
If you should spot while taking the pills you should not be alarmed because spotting usually stops by itself within a few days. It seldom occurs after the first pill cycle. Consult your doctor if spotting persists for more than a few days or if it occurs after the second cycle.
Unexpected (Breakthrough) Bleeding. Unexpected (breakthrough) bleeding does not mean your ovaries have released an egg. It seldom occurs, but when it does happen it is most common in the first pill cycle. It is a flow much like a regular period, requiring the use of a pad or tampon.
If you experience breakthrough bleeding use a pad or tampon and continue with your schedule. Usually your periods will become regular within a few cycles. Breakthrough bleeding will seldom bother you again.
Consult your doctor if breakthrough bleeding does not stop within a week or if it occurs after the second cycle.
Forgotten Pills. There is little likelihood of your getting pregnant if only one active pill is missed; however, the possibility increases with each successive day that the scheduled active pills are missed. If you forget to take a pill one day, take two the next day—the one you forgot as soon as you remember and your regular pill at your usual time.
If you forget your pills (except the inactive colored pills in Demulen-28 or Ovulen-28) on two consecutive days, do not be surprised if you spot or start to flow. You should take two pills each day for the next two days and use an additional method of protection for the remainder of the cycle.
If you are using Demulen-28 or Ovulen-28 and forget to take one or more colored pills, begin a new cycle on the next Sunday; use a new package and start taking the white pills. Missing the colored pills does not increase your chances of getting pregnant providing the white pill schedule has been followed.
Missed Menstruation. At times there may be no menstrual period after a cycle of pills. Therefore, if you miss one menstrual period but have taken the pills *exactly as you were supposed to,* continue as usual into the next cycle. You may wish to call your doctor. If you have not taken the pills correctly and miss a menstrual period, *you may be pregnant* and should stop taking oral contraceptives until your doctor determines whether or not you are pregnant. Until you can get to your doctor, use another form of contraception. If two consecutive menstrual periods are missed, you should stop taking the pills until it is determined whether you are pregnant. If you do become pregnant while using oral contraceptives, you should discuss the risks to the developing baby with your doctor.
3. *Periodic Examinations.* Your doctor will take a complete medical and family history before prescribing oral contraceptives. At that time and about once a year thereafter, s/he will generally examine your blood pressure, breasts, abdomen, and internal female organs (including a "Pap" smear test for cancer of the cervix) and perform certain laboratory tests. Certain health problems or conditions in your medical or family history may require that your doctor see you more frequently while you are taking the pill.
4. *Using Enovid for Purposes Other Than Contraception.* Since dosage schedules for these uses must be individualized for each patient, please follow the directions of your doctor.
Summary: Oral contraceptives are the most effective method, except sterilization, for preventing pregnancy. Other methods, when used conscientiously, are also very effective and have fewer risks. The serious side effects of oral contraceptives are uncommon and the pill is a very convenient method for preventing pregnancy.
Women who use oral contraceptives should not smoke.
If you have certain conditions or have had these conditions in the past, you should not use oral contraceptives because of increased risk. These conditions are listed in this leaflet. If you do not have these conditions, and decide to use the pill, please read this leaflet carefully so that you can use the pill safely and effectively. Be certain to read new revisions of this leaflet. Based on your doctor's assessment of your medical needs, this drug has been prescribed for you. Do not give it to anyone else.
See your doctor regularly, ask any questions you may have about the use of the pill, and report any special problems that may arise.
[*These products are shown in Product Identification Section.*]

ENOVID–E® ℞
ENOVID–E® 21 ℞
(norethynodrel with mestranol)

See Demulen under Searle & Co. for Enovid-E and Enovid-E 21 prescribing information.
[*Shown in Product Identification Section.*]

ENOVID® 5 mg. ℞
(norethynodrel with mestranol)

See Demulen under Searle & Co. for Enovid 5 mg. prescribing information.
[*Shown in Product Identification Section.*]

FLAGYL® ℞
(metronidazole)

Warning
Metronidazole has been shown to be carcinogenic in mice and possibly carcinogenic in rats. (See *Warnings.*) Unnecessary use of the drug should be avoided. Its use should be reserved for the conditions described in the *Indications* section below.

Description: Flagyl is 1-(β-hydroxyethyl)-2-methyl-5-nitroimidazole.
Actions: Metronidazole possesses direct trichomonacidal and amebacidal activity against *Trichomonas vaginalis* and *Entamoeba histolytica. In vitro* the MIC for most strains of *T. vaginalis* is less than 1 mcg./ml. Metronidazole is usually well absorbed after oral administration with the peak serum concentrations usually occurring between one and two hours. Serum concentrations are proportional to the administered dose. After a single 2-gram oral dose, serum metronidazole concentrations (chemical assay) were approximately 40 mcg./ml. Studies reveal no significant bioavailability differences in males and females. Due to weight differences, the resulting serum concentrations in males are generally lower but still well above the therapeutic range.
The half-life of elimination of metronidazole from the serum is approximately seven hours. In the urine, which is the major route of drug elimination, both unchanged metronidazole and several metabolites are present. The metabolites result primarily from oxidation of side chains and glucuronide conjugation. Metronidazole concentrations approximately equivalent to those in the serum appear in the saliva and breast milk during treatment.
Indications: *Symptomatic Trichomoniasis.* Flagyl is indicated for the treatment of symptomatic trichomoniasis in females and in males when the presence of the trichomonad has been confirmed by appropriate laboratory procedures (wet smears and/or cultures).
Asymptomatic Trichomoniasis. Flagyl (metronidazole) is indicated in the treatment of asymptomatic females when the organism is associated with endocervicitis, cervicitis, or cervical erosion. Since there is evidence that presence of the trichomonad can interfere with accurate assessment of abnormal cytological smears, additional smears should be performed after eradication of the parasite.
Treatment of Asymptomatic Consorts. T. vaginalis infection is a venereal disease. Therefore, asymptomatic sexual partners of treated patients should be treated simultaneously if the organism has been found to be present, in order to prevent reinfection of the partner. The decision as to whether to treat an asymptomatic male partner who has a negative culture or one for whom no culture has been attempted is an individual one. In making this decision, it should be noted that there is evidence that women may become reinfected if the consort is not treated. Also, since there can be considerable difficulty in isolating the organism from the asymptomatic male carrier, negative smears and cultures cannot be relied upon in this regard. In any event, the consort should be treated with Flagyl in cases of reinfection.
Amebiasis. Flagyl is indicated in the treatment of acute intestinal amebiasis (amebic dysentery) and amebic liver abscess.
Contraindications: Flagyl is contraindicated in patients with evidence of or history of blood dyscrasia because upon occasion a mild leukopenia has been observed during its administration. However, no persistent hematologic abnormalities have been observed in animal or clinical studies.

Continued on next page

Searle & Co.—Cont.

Flagyl (metronidazole) is also contraindicated in patients with active organic disease of the central nervous system. (See *Adverse Reactions.*)
Flagyl is contraindicated during the first trimester of pregnancy. (See *Warnings.*)
Flagyl is also contraindicated in patients with a prior history of hypersensitivity to metronidazole.
Warnings: *Usage During Pregnancy and Lactation.* Flagyl crosses the placental barrier and enters the fetal circulation rapidly; when administered to nursing mothers it is secreted in the breast milk. Although Flagyl has not been shown to be teratogenic in either animal or human studies, data are not adequate to rule out a possible teratogenic effect; therefore, Flagyl should not be used in the first trimester of pregnancy. In addition, since Flagyl has been shown to be tumorigenic in rodents, it is recommended that the use of Flagyl (metronidazole) for trichomoniasis in the second and third trimesters and during lactation should be restricted to those in whom local palliative treatment has been inadequate to control symptoms. If used during lactation, an alternate method of infant feeding may be elected.
Tumorigenicity Studies in Rodents. Metronidazole has shown evidence of tumorigenic activity in a number of studies involving chronic, oral administration in mice and rats.
Most prominent among the effects in the mouse was the promotion of pulmonary tumorigenesis. This has been observed in all five reported studies in that species, including one study in which the animals were dosed on an intermittent schedule (administration during every fourth week only). The published results of one of the mouse studies indicate an increase in the incidence of malignant lymphomas as well as pulmonary neoplasms associated with lifetime feeding of the drug. All these effects are statistically significant.
Two long-term toxicity studies in the rat have been completed. There was a statistically significant increase in the incidence of various neoplasms, particularly mammary tumors, among female rats administered metronidazole over that noted in the concurrent female control groups.
Two lifetime tumorigenicity studies in hamsters have been performed and reported to be negative.
Metronidazole has been reported to potentiate the anticoagulant effect of coumarin and warfarin resulting in a prolongation of prothrombin time. This possible drug interaction should be considered when Flagyl is prescribed for patients on this type of anticoagulant therapy.
Precautions: Metronidazole is a nitroimidazole and mild leukopenia has been reported during its administration. Therefore, total and differential leukocyte counts are recommended before and after treatment with the drug, especially if a second course is necessary.
Flagyl may interfere with certain chemical analyses for serum glutamic oxalacetic transaminase.
Alcoholic beverages should not be consumed during Flagyl (metronidazole) therapy because abdominal cramps, nausea, vomiting, headaches and flushing may occur.
The appearance of abnormal neurologic signs demands the prompt discontinuation of Flagyl therapy.
Known or previously unrecognized candidiasis may present more prominent symptoms during therapy with Flagyl and requires treatment with a candicidal agent. Vaginitis due to organisms other than *Trichomonas vaginalis* does not respond to Flagyl (metronidazole). In amebic liver abscess, metronidazole therapy does not obviate the need for aspiration of pus.
Adverse Reactions: By far the most common adverse reactions have been referable to the gastrointestinal tract, particularly nausea, sometimes accompanied by headache, anorexia and occasionally vomiting, diarrhea, epigastric distress and abdominal cramping; constipation has also been reported. A metallic, sharp, unpleasant taste is not unusual. Furry tongue, glossitis and stomatitis have occurred; these may be associated with a sudden overgrowth of *Candida* which may occur during effective therapy. Proliferation of *Candida* also may occur in the vagina.
A moderate leukopenia may be observed occasionally. If this occurs, the total leukocyte count may be expected to return to normal after the course of medication is completed.
If patients receiving Flagyl drink alcoholic beverages, they may experience abdominal distress, nausea, vomiting, flushing or headache. A modification of the taste of alcoholic beverages has also been reported.
Dizziness, vertigo, incoordination, ataxia and convulsive seizures have been reported. Confusion, irritability, depression, weakness, insomnia, and a mild erythematous eruption have been experienced as have fleeting joint pains sometimes resembling "serum sickness," and peripheral neuropathy, characterized mainly by numbness or paresthesia of an extremity. Since persistent peripheral neuropathy has been reported in some patients receiving prolonged administration of Flagyl, such subjects should be specifically warned about these reports and should be told to stop the drug and report immediately if any neurological symptoms occur.
Urticaria, flushing, nasal congestion, dryness of the mouth (or vagina or vulva), pruritus, dysuria, cystitis and a sense of pelvic pressure have been reported. Very rarely dyspareunia, fever, polyuria, incontinence, decrease of libido, proctitis and pyuria have occurred in patients receiving the drug.
Instances of a darkened urine have been reported and this manifestation has been the subject of a special investigation. Although the pigment which is probably responsible for this phenomenon has not been positively identified, it is almost certainly a metabolite of Flagyl. It seems certain that it is of no clinical significance and may be encountered only when Flagyl (metronidazole) is administered in higher-than-recommended doses.
Flattening of the T-wave may be seen in electrocardiographic tracings.
Dosage and Administration:
Trichomoniasis: *In the Female:*
Studies have demonstrated the efficacy of one-day therapy with 2 grams of Flagyl given either as a single dose or in divided doses of four 250-mg. tablets given twice in one day. There is some indication from controlled comparative studies that cure rates, as determined by vaginal smears, signs and symptoms, may be higher after a seven-day course of treatment, i.e., 250 mg. three times daily for seven days, than after the one-day treatment regimen.
The dosage regimen should be individualized. Single dose treatment can assure compliance, especially if administered under supervision, in those patients who cannot be relied on to continue the seven-day regimen. A seven-day course of treatment may minimize reinfection of the female long enough to treat sexual contacts. Further, some patients may tolerate one course of therapy better than the other. For example, the short treatment requires the patient to take 8 tablets in one day, while with the seven-day course of treatment only 3 tablets a day are necessary.
Pregnant patients should not be treated during the first trimester with either regimen. If treated during the second or third trimester, the one-day course of therapy should not be used as it results in higher serum levels which reach the fetal circulation. (See Pregnancy *Warnings.*)
When repeat courses of the drug are required, it is recommended that an interval of four to six weeks elapse between courses and that the presence of the trichomonad be reconfirmed by appropriate laboratory measures. Total and differential leukocyte counts should be made before and after re-treatment.
In the Male: Treatment should be individualized as above.
Amebiasis: *Adults:*
For acute intestinal amebiasis (acute amebic dysentery): 750 mg. orally three times daily for 5 to 10 days.
For amebic liver abscess:
500 mg. or 750 mg. orally three times daily for 5 to 10 days.
Children:
35 to 50 mg./kg. of body weight/24 hours, divided into three doses, orally for 10 days.
How Supplied: *For oral use*—White tablets of 250 mg. with SEARLE debossed on one side of tablets and 1831 on the other side; bottles of 100, 250 and 1,000.
[*Shown in Product Identification Section*]

•LOMOTIL® Liquid Ⓒ
•LOMOTIL® Tablets Ⓒ
(diphenoxylate hydrochloride with atropine sulfate)

Description: Each Lomotil tablet and each 5 ml. of Lomotil liquid contain:
diphenoxylate hydrochloride........... 2.5 mg.
(Warning: May be habit forming)
atropine sulfate............................. 0.025 mg.
Important Information: Lomotil is classified as a Schedule V substance by federal law; however, diphenoxylate hydrochloride is chemically related to the narcotic meperidine. In case of overdosage or individual hypersensitivity, reactions similar to those after meperidine or morphine overdosage may occur. Therefore, treatment of these patients is similar to that for meperidine or morphine intoxication, in which prolonged and careful monitoring is essential, since respiratory depression may be evidenced as late as 30 hours after ingestion and may recur in spite of an initial response to Narcan® (naloxone hydrochloride). LOMOTIL IS *NOT* AN INNOCUOUS DRUG AND DOSAGE RECOMMENDATIONS SHOULD BE STRICTLY ADHERED TO, ESPECIALLY IN CHILDREN. THIS MEDICATION SHOULD BE KEPT OUT OF REACH OF CHILDREN.
Actions: Lomotil acts by slowing intestinal motility.
Indications: Lomotil is effective as adjunctive therapy in the management of diarrhea.
Contraindications: Lomotil is contraindicated in children less than 2 years of age due to the decreased margin of safety in younger age groups. Lomotil is also contraindicated in patients with a known hypersensitivity to diphenoxylate hydrochloride or atropine and in patients who are jaundiced. Lomotil is contraindicated in the treatment of diarrhea associated with pseudomembranous enterocolitis, which may occur during, or up to several weeks following, treatment with antibiotics such as clindamycin (Cleocin®) or lincomycin (Lincocin®).
Warnings: Lomotil should be used with special caution in young children because of the greater variability of response in this age group. The use of Lomotil does not preclude the administration of appropriate fluid and electrolyte therapy. Dehydration, particularly in younger children, may further influence the variability of response to Lomotil and may predispose to delayed diphenoxylate intoxication. Drug-induced inhibition of peristalsis may result in fluid retention in the colon which may further aggravate dehydration and electrolyte imbalance. If severe dehydration or electrolyte imbalance is manifested, Lomotil should be withheld until appropriate corrective therapy has been initiated.

Since the chemical structure of diphenoxylate hydrochloride is similar to that of meperidine hydrochloride, the concurrent use of Lomotil with monoamine oxidase inhibitors may, in theory, precipitate hypertensive crisis.
Lomotil should be used with extreme caution in patients with cirrhosis and other advanced hepatic disease and in all patients with abnormal liver function tests, since hepatic coma may be precipitated.
Diphenoxylate hydrochloride may potentiate the action of barbiturates, tranquilizers and alcohol. Therefore, the patient should be closely observed when these medications are used concomitantly.
Usage in pregnancy: The use of any drug during pregnancy, lactation or in women of childbearing age requires that the potential benefits of the drug be weighed against any possible hazard to the mother and child. Effects of diphenoxylate hydrochloride or atropine sulfate may be evident in the infants of nursing mothers taking Lomotil since these compounds are excreted in breast milk.
Precautions: Addiction to (dependency on) diphenoxylate hydrochloride is theoretically possible at high dosage. Therefore the recommended dosage should not be exceeded.
Because of the structural and pharmacologic similarity of diphenoxylate hydrochloride to drugs with a definite addiction potential, Lomotil should be administered with considerable caution to patients who are receiving addicting drugs, to individuals known to be addiction prone, or to those whose histories suggest they may increase the dosage on their own initiative.
In some patients with acute ulcerative colitis, agents which inhibit intestinal motility or prolong intestinal transit time have been reported to induce toxic megacolon. Consequently, patients with acute ulcerative colitis should be carefully observed and Lomotil therapy should be discontinued promptly if abdominal distention occurs or if other untoward symptoms develop.
Because a subtherapeutic dose of atropine has been added to the diphenoxylate hydrochloride to discourage deliberate overdosage, there should be strict observance of the contraindications, warnings, and precautions for the use of atropine.
In children, Lomotil should be used with caution since signs of atropinism may occur even with recommended doses, particularly in patients with Down's syndrome.
Adverse Reactions: Atropine effects, such as dryness of the skin and mucous membranes, flushing, hyperthermia, tachycardia and urinary retention may occur, especially in children. Other adverse reactions reported with Lomotil use are:

Nausea	Malaise
Sedation	Drowsiness (sedation effect)
Vomiting	Coma
Swelling of the gums	Lethargy
Abdominal discomfort	Anorexia
	Restlessness
Respiratory depression	Euphoria
	Pruritus
Numbness of the extremities	Angioneurotic edema
Headache	Giant urticaria
Dizziness	Paralytic ileus
Depression	Toxic megacolon

Dosage and Administration: *Adults:* The recommended initial dosage is two Lomotil tablets four times daily or 10 ml. (two regular teaspoonfuls) of Lomotil liquid four times daily (20 mg. per day). Most patients will require this dosage until initial control has been achieved, after which the dosage may be reduced to meet individual requirements. Control may often be maintained with as little as 5 mg. (two tablets or 10 ml. of liquid) daily.
Children: Lomotil is contraindicated in children under 2 years of age. Lomotil should be used with special caution in young children due to the variable response in this age group.
In children 2 to 12 years of age use Lomotil liquid. Do not use Lomotil tablets for this age group.
For children 2 to 12 years of age, the recommended initial dosage of Lomotil liquid is 0.3 to 0.4 mg./kg. daily administered in divided doses. The following schedule will usually fulfill dosage requirements:

Age:	*Dosage:*
2 to 5 years (13 to 20 kg.)	4 ml. (2 mg.) t.i.d.
5 to 8 years (20 to 27 kg.)	4 ml. (2 mg.) q.i.d.
8 to 12 years (27 to 36 kg.)	4 ml. (2 mg.) 5 times daily

Reduction of dosage may be made as soon as initial control of symptoms has been achieved. Maintenance dosage may be as low as one fourth of the initial daily dosage.
Do not exceed recommended dosage.
OVERDOSAGE: *Diagnosis and Treatment.* Caution patients to adhere strictly to recommended dosage schedules. The medication should be kept out of reach of children, since accidental overdosage may result in severe, even fatal, respiratory depression. In the event of overdosage (initial signs may include dryness of the skin and mucous membranes, flushing, hyperthermia and tachycardia followed by lethargy or coma, hypotonic reflexes, nystagmus, pinpoint pupils and respiratory depression), gastric lavage, establishment of a patent airway and possibly mechanically assisted respiration are advised.
The narcotic antagonist Narcan® (naloxone hydrochloride) may be used in the treatment of respiratory depression caused by narcotic analgesics or pharmacologically related compounds such as Lomotil. When Narcan is administered intravenously the onset of action is generally apparent within two minutes. Narcan may also be administered subcutaneously or intramuscularly, providing a slightly less-rapid onset of action but a more prolonged effect.
To counteract respiratory depression caused by Lomotil overdosage, the following dosage schedule for Narcan should be followed:
Adult dosage: The usual initial adult dose of Narcan is 0.4 mg. (1 ml.) administered intravenously. If respiratory function does not adequately improve after the initial dose the same I.V. dose may be repeated at 2- to 3-minute intervals.
Children: The usual initial dose of Narcan for children is 0.01 mg./kg. of body weight administered intravenously and repeated at 2- to 3-minute intervals if necessary.
Following the initial improvement of respiratory function, repeat doses of Narcan may be required in response to recurrent respiratory depression. Supplemental intramuscular doses of Narcan may be utilized to produce a longer-lasting effect.
Since the duration of action of diphenoxylate hydrochloride is longer than that of naloxone hydrochloride, improvement of respiration following administration may be followed by recurrent respiratory depression. Consequently, continuous observation is necessary until the effect of diphenoxylate hydrochloride on respiration (which effect may persist for many hours) has passed. The period of observation should extend over at least 48 hours, preferably under continuous hospital care.
It should be noted that, although signs of overdosage and respiratory depression may not be evident soon after ingestion of diphenoxylate hydrochloride, respiratory depression may occur from 12 to 30 hours later.
How Supplied:
Tablets—white, with SEARLE debossed on one side and 61 on the other side and containing 2.5 mg. of diphenoxylate hydrochloride and 0.025 mg. (1/2,400 grain) of atropine sulfate; bottles of 100, 500, 1,000 and 2,500, cartons of ten 30-Pack dispensers, cartons of 100 unit-dose individually blister-sealed tablets, and Audit Packs of 100 (2 cartons of 50) individually blister-sealed tablets.
Liquid—containing 2.5 mg. of diphenoxylate hydrochloride and 0.025 mg. (1/2,400 grain) of atropine sulfate per 5 ml.; bottles of 2 oz.
A plastic dropper calibrated in increments of one-half ml. (¼mg.) with a capacity of 2 ml. (1 mg.) accompanies each 2-oz. bottle of Lomotil liquid. Only this plastic dropper should be used when measuring Lomotil liquid for administration.
Note: 1. Lomotil is classified as a Schedule V substance by federal law.
2. The subtherapeutic amount of atropine sulfate is included in Lomotil to discourage deliberate overdosage.

[*Shown in Product Identification Section*]

OVULEN® ℞
OVULEN-21® ℞
OVULEN-28® ℞
(ethynodiol diacetate with mestranol)

See Demulen under Searle & Co. for Ovulen prescribing information.

[*Shown in Product Identification Section*]

PRO-BANTHĪNE® Tablets ℞
(propantheline bromide)

Description: Pro-Banthīne tablets contain 15 mg. or 7½ mg. of propantheline bromide, (2-hydroxyethyl)diisopropylmethylammonium bromide xanthene-9-carboxylate.
Clinical Pharmacology: Pro-Banthīne inhibits gastrointestinal motility and diminishes gastric acid secretion. The drug also inhibits the action of acetylcholine at the postganglionic nerve endings of the parasympathetic nervous system.
After oral administration to man, propantheline bromide is extensively metabolized primarily by hydrolysis to the inactive materials xanthene-9-carboxylic acid and (2-hydroxyethyl)diisopropylmethylammonium bromide, approximately half of which occurs in the gastrointestinal tract prior to its absorption. After a single 15-mg. oral dose of carbon-14 labeled drug given to a healthy man, 390 ng./ml. peak plasma concentration of total-^{14}C material is attained at 6 hours. Unmetabolized drug represents only a small proportion of the total-^{14}C materials. The plasma half-life of the total-^{14}C material is about 9 hours and approximately 70 percent of the dose is excreted in the urine, mostly as metabolites. The urinary excretion of the intact propantheline is about 5 percent after oral administration, and about 20 percent after intravenous administration.
Indications: Pro-Banthīne is effective as adjunctive therapy in the treatment of peptic ulcer.
Contraindications: Pro-Banthīne (propantheline bromide) is contraindicated in patients with:
1. Glaucoma, since mydriasis is to be avoided.
2. Obstructive disease of the gastrointestinal tract (pyloroduodenal stenosis, achalasia, paralytic ileus, etc).
3. Obstructive uropathy (prostatism).
4. Intestinal atony of elderly or debilitated patients.
5. Severe ulcerative colitis or toxic megacolon complicating ulcerative colitis.
6. Hiatal hernia associated with reflux esophagitis.
7. Unstable cardiovascular adjustment in acute hemorrhage.
8. Myasthenia gravis.

Warnings: In the presence of a high environmental temperature, heat prostration (fever and heat stroke due to decreased sweating) can occur with the use of Pro-Banthīne.

Continued on next page

Searle & Co.—Cont.

Diarrhea may be an early symptom of incomplete intestinal obstruction, especially in patients with ileostomy or colostomy. In this instance treatment with Pro-Banthīne would be inappropriate and possibly harmful.
Pro-Banthīne may produce drowsiness or blurred vision. The patient should be cautioned regarding activities requiring mental alertness, such as operating a motor vehicle or other machinery or performing hazardous work, while taking this drug.
With overdosage, a curare-like action may occur, i.e., neuromuscular blockade leading to muscular weakness and possible paralysis.
Patients with severe cardiac disease should be given this medication with caution if an increase in heart rate is undesirable.
Use in Pregnancy: Reproduction studies have not been performed in animals. Information on possible adverse effects to the fetus is limited to uncontrolled data derived from marketing experience. Such experience has revealed no evidence of toxicity to mother or fetus. There are no controlled studies in animals or humans to determine whether this drug affects fertility in human males or females, has teratogenic potential, or has other adverse effects on the fetus. It should be used during pregnancy only when, in the opinion of the physician, the benefits outweigh any possible risk.
Use in Nursing Mothers: Information regarding the secretion of Pro-Banthīne (propantheline bromide) in breast milk is limited to uncontrolled data derived from marketing experience. Such experience does not suggest that significant quantities of Pro-Banthīne are secreted in breast milk.
Pediatric Use: Since there is inadequate experience with the use of Pro-Banthīne in children, safety and efficacy in children have not been established.
Precautions: Varying degrees of urinary hesitancy may be evidenced by patients with prostatic hypertrophy. In such patients urinary retention may be avoided if they are advised to micturate at the time of taking the medication.
Pro-Banthīne (propantheline bromide) should be used with caution in the elderly and in all patients with autonomic neuropathy, hepatic or renal disease, hyperthyroidism, coronary heart disease, congestive heart failure, cardiac tachyarrhythmias, or hypertension.
In patients with ulcerative colitis, large doses of Pro-Banthīne may suppress intestinal motility to the point of producing paralytic ileus and, for this reason, may precipitate or aggravate toxic megacolon, a serious complication of the disease.
Adverse Reactions: Varying degrees of drying of salivary secretions may occur as well as decreased sweating. Ophthalmic side effects include blurred vision, mydriasis, cycloplegia, and increased ocular tension. Other reported adverse reactions include urinary hesitancy and retention, tachycardia, palpitations, loss of the sense of taste, headache, nervousness, mental confusion, drowsiness, weakness, dizziness, insomnia, nausea, vomiting, constipation, bloated feeling, impotence, suppression of lactation, and allergic reactions or drug idiosyncracies including anaphylaxis, urticaria and other dermal manifestations.
Overdosage: The symptoms of overdosage with Pro-Banthīne progress from an intensification of the usual side effects to CNS disturbances (from restlessness and excitement to psychotic behavior), circulatory changes (flushing, fall in blood pressure, circulatory failure), respiratory failure, paralysis and coma.
Measures to be taken are (1) immediate lavage of the stomach and (2) injection of physostigmine 0.5 to 2 mg. intravenously, and repeated as necessary up to a total of 5 mg. Fever may be treated symptomatically (alcohol sponging, ice packs).
Excitement of a degree which demands attention may be managed with sodium thiopental 2% solution given slowly intravenously or chloral hydrate (100–200 ml. of a 2% solution) by rectal infusion. In the event of progression of the curare-like effect to paralysis of the respiratory muscles, artificial respiration should be instituted and maintained until effective respiratory action returns.
Dosage and Administration: The usual initial adult dose of Pro-Banthīne tablets is 15 mg. taken 30 minutes before each meal and 30 mg. at bedtime (a total of 75 mg. daily). Subsequent dosage adjustment should be made according to the patient's individual response and tolerance. The administration of one 7½-mg. tablet three times a day is convenient for patients with mild manifestations and for geriatric patients and for those of small stature.
Drug Interactions: Concurrent use of Pro-Banthīne (propantheline bromide) with slow-dissolving tablets of digoxin may cause increased serum digoxin levels. This interaction can be avoided by using only those digoxin tablets that rapidly dissolve by U.S.P. standards. Anticholinergics may delay absorption of other medication given concomitantly. Excessive cholinergic blockade may occur if Pro-Banthīne is given concomitantly with belladonna alkaloids or synthetic and semisynthetic anticholinergic agents (e.g., antispasmodics, antiparkinsonism agents), phenothiazine, tricyclic antidepressants, quinidine, antihistamines, or procainamide.
How Supplied: *For oral use:* Tablets: Pro-Banthīne 15-mg. tablets are sugar coated, peach colored, with SEARLE imprinted on one side and 601 on the other side; bottles of 100, 500, 1,000 and 2,500, and cartons containing 100 unit-dose, individually blister-sealed tablets.
Pro-Banthīne 7½-mg. tablets are sugar coated, white, with SEARLE imprinted on one side and 611 on the other side; bottles of 100 and 500.
[*Shown in Product Identification Section*]

PRO-BANTHĪNE® 7½-mg. Tablets ℞
(propantheline bromide)

See Pro-Banthīne Tablets for prescribing information including 7½-mg. tablets.
[*Shown in Product Identification Section*]

PRO-BANTHĪNE® for Injection ℞
(propantheline bromide)

Description: Each serum-type vial of Pro-Banthīne contains 30 mg. of propantheline bromide, (2-hydroxyethyl)diisopropylmethylammonium bromide xanthene-9-carboxylate.
For *Clinical Pharmacology* see Pro-Banthīne Tablets.
Indications: Pro-Banthīne is effective as adjunctive therapy in the treatment of peptic ulcer.
Parenterally administered Pro-Banthīne is also effective in reducing duodenal motility to facilitate the diagnostic radiologic procedure, hypotonic duodenography.
For *Contraindications, Warnings, Precautions, Adverse Reactions* and *Overdosage* see Pro-Banthīne Tablets.
Dosage and Administration:
Peptic Ulcer
For patients unable to retain oral medication or having a severe condition requiring vigorous therapy, Pro-Banthīne for Injection (propantheline bromide) is available in 30-mg. vials. Initial parenteral medication for an adult is usually 30 mg. every six hours intramuscularly or intravenously. Subsequent dosage adjustment to the patient's requirements and tolerance should be made. For maintenance therapy, approximately one half of the initial dose (15 mg. every six hours) will fulfill the needs of most patients.
Hypotonic Duodenography
Intramuscular: 30 to 60 mg. of Pro-Banthīne administered by the intramuscular route 5 to 10 minutes prior to the diagnostic procedure is recommended for reducing duodenal motility to facilitate hypotonic duodenography.
Intravenous: 30 to 60 mg. of Pro-Banthīne (propantheline bromide) given by slow intravenous administration immediately prior to the initiation of the diagnostic procedure of hypotonic duodenography may be utilized as an alternate method. The rate of administration should not exceed 2 ml. (6 mg.) per minute.
Preparation of Solution
For intramuscular use the solution is prepared by sterilizing the rubber cap with alcohol and injecting 1 ml. of Sterile Water for Injection U.S.P. into the vial. For intravenous use 10 ml. of Sodium Chloride Injection U.S.P. is recommended as a diluent. A solution stored under refrigeration and properly protected from contamination will remain usable for up to two weeks.
For *Drug Interactions* see Pro-Banthīne Tablets.
How Supplied:
For parenteral use: Each 2-ml. serum-type vial is made of clear glass; white powder fill; 30-mg. vials; cartons of 5, 25, and 100.

PRO-BANTHĪNE® with DARTAL® ℞

Description: Each aqua-colored tablet contains 15 mg. of propantheline bromide, (2-hydroxyethyl) diisopropylmethylammonium bromide xanthene-9-carboxylate, and 5 mg. of thiopropazate hydrochloride, 4-[3-(2-chlorophenothiazin-10-yl) propyl]-1-piperazineethanol acetate dihydrochloride.
Actions: Pro-Banthīne inhibits gastrointestinal propulsive motility and decreases gastric acid secretion. The drug also inhibits the action of acetylcholine at the postganglionic nerve endings of the parasympathetic nervous system. Dartal (thiopropazate hydrochloride) produces depression of the central nervous system, thus reducing agitation and psychomotor hyperactivity.

Indications:

Based on a review of this drug by the National Academy of Sciences—National Research Council and/or other information, FDA has classified the indication as follows:
"Possibly" effective: as adjunctive therapy in the treatment of peptic ulcer.
Final classification of the less-than-effective indication requires further investigation.

Contraindications: Pro-Banthīne with Dartal is contraindicated in patients with glaucoma since mydriasis is to be avoided.
Warnings: *Pro-Banthīne:* Patients with severe cardiac disease should be given this medication with caution if even a slight increase in heart rate is undesirable.
Dartal: Do not give this drug to patients under the influence of barbiturates, alcohol or narcotics. Administer Dartal cautiously to epileptic patients or those in depressed states. Discontinue Dartal immediately if convulsions occur or the state of depression deepens.
Precautions: *Pro-Banthīne:* Varying degrees of urinary hesitancy may be evidenced by elderly patients with prostatic hypertrophy. In such patients urinary retention may be avoided if they are advised to micturate at the time of taking the medication.
Dartal: Patients with liver disease will tolerate small doses of Dartal, but caution is necessary as hepatic coma has occurred with similar drugs.

Hypersensitivity to Dartal may occur rarely in patients who are known to be hypersensitive to drugs of a similar nature.
Since Dartal has not been studied extensively in pregnant women, it must be used with caution during pregnancy.
Pro-Banthīne with Dartal contains thiopropazate hydrochloride, a tranquilizing drug. There is sufficient experimental evidence to conclude that chronic administration of antipsychotic drugs which increase prolactin secretion has the potential to induce mammary neoplasms in rodents under the appropriate conditions. There are recognized differences in the physiological role of prolactin between rodents and humans. Since there are, at present, no adequate epidemiological studies, the relevance to human mammary cancer risk from prolonged exposure to thiopropazate hydrochloride and other antipsychotic drugs is not known.
This product contains FD&C Yellow No. 5 (tartrazine) which may cause allergic-type reactions (including bronchial asthma) in certain susceptible individuals. Although the overall incidence of FD&C Yellow No. 5 (tartrazine) sensitivity in the general population is low, it is frequently seen in patients who also have aspirin hypersensitivity.
Adverse Reactions: *Pro-Banthīne:* Patients commonly complain of dryness of the mouth or blurring of vision, especially at high dosages. These complaints when reported are usually minor, disappear on continued treatment and necessitate no adjustment of dosage. Occasionally, however, they may be severe enough to require reduction in dosage, and then morning and/or noon doses may be reduced, while evening and night doses are maintained in order to provide maximal protection against high night secretions.
On a theoretical basis a curare-like action, although not reported, may occur with considerable overdosage. Under such circumstances loss of control of voluntary muscles will occur, the most important manifestation being the loss of control of the respiratory muscles. Such patients must receive prompt and continuing artificial respiration until the drug effect has been exhausted.
Dartal: The following adverse reactions have been associated with its use: pseudoparkinsonism (associated with high dosage, including muscular rigidity, fixed facies, tremor, ataxia, festinant gait and drooling), blurring of vision, xerostomia, hypotension, nasal congestion, leukopenia (rare), generalized erythema, constipation and allergic purpura.
Theoretically, since Dartal is a phenothiazine, side effects characteristic of this group of compounds may occur. Among these side effects, none of which have been known to occur with this drug, are the following: grand mal convulsions, altered cerebrospinal proteins, cerebral edema, atropine potentiation, potentiation of the effects of heat or of phosphorus insecticides, autonomic reactions, endocrine disturbances, reversed epinephrine effect, hyperpyrexia and pigmentary retinopathy.
Dosage and Administration: The average dose schedule of Pro-Banthīne with Dartal for adults is one tablet three times daily. One or two additional tablets daily may be indicated in the individual patient.
How Supplied: Each compression-coated aqua-colored tablet has SEARLE debossed on one side and 641 on the other side, and contains 15 mg. of propantheline bromide and 5 mg. of thiopropazate hydrochloride; bottles of 100 and 500.

PRO-BANTHĪNE® with PHENOBARBITAL Tablets ℞
(Warning: may be habit forming)

Each Pro-Banthīne with Phenobarbital tablet contains:

propantheline bromide .... 15 mg.
phenobarbital .... 15 mg.
(Warning: May be habit forming)

Propantheline bromide is (2-hydroxyethyl) diisopropylmethylammonium bromide xanthene-9-carboxylate.
For *Clinical Pharmacology* see Pro-Banthīne Tablets.

Indications:

Based on a review of this drug by the National Academy of Sciences—National Research Council and/or other information, FDA has classified the indications as follows:
"Possibly" effective: as adjunctive therapy in the treatment of peptic ulcer and in the treatment of the irritable bowel syndrome (irritable colon, spastic colon, mucous colitis, acute enterocolitis, and functional gastrointestinal disorders).
Final classification of the less-than-effective indications requires further investigation.

For *Contraindications, Warnings, Precautions, Adverse Reactions,* and *Overdosage* see Pro-Banthīne Tablets.
Dosage and Administration: The usual *adult dosage* of Pro-Banthīne with Phenobarbital is one or two tablets three or four times daily.
For *Drug Interactions* see Pro-Banthīne Tablets.
How Supplied: *For Oral Use:* Tablets: Pro-Banthīne with Phenobarbital tablets containing 15 mg. of propantheline bromide and 15 mg. of phenobarbital are sugar coated, ivory colored, with SEARLE imprinted on one side and 631 on the other side; bottles of 100, 500, 1,000, and 2,500, and cartons containing 100 unit-dose, individually blister-sealed tablets.
[*Shown in Product Identification Section*]

The preceding prescribing information for Searle & Co. was current as of November 1, 1979.

Serono Laboratories, Inc.
11 BROOKS DRIVE
BRAINTREE, MA 02184

ASELLACRIN® ℞
(somatropin)
For Intramuscular Injection

Description: Asellacrin (somatropin) is a sterile, lyophilized, purified somatropic hormone extracted from the human pituitary gland.
The potency of Asellacrin (somatropin) is determined by bioassay in hypophysectomized rats and is designated in International Units (IU). Each 10 ml vial contains 10 IU somatropin and 40 mg of mannitol, and the pH is adjusted between 6 and 8 with hydrochloric acid and or sodium hydroxide.
Clinical Pharmacology: Asellacrin (somatropin) stimulates linear growth in patients with pituitary growth hormone deficiency.
Asellacrin (somatropin) is an anabolic agent that stimulates intracellular transport of amino acids and net retention of nitrogen, phosphorus and potassium. The intestinal absorption and urinary excretion of calcium are both increased. The serum concentration of phosphorus and alkaline phosphatase are increased. The synthesis of chondroitin sulfate and collagen, as well as the urinary excretion of hydroxyproline are also stimulated by Asellacrin (somatropin). Asellacrin (somatropin) stimulates intracellular lipolysis, increases the plasma concentration of free fatty acids and stimulates the oxidation of fatty acids. Intracellular glucose metabolism is inhibited, and there is decreased sensitivity to the action of insulin in response to the chronic administration of Asellacrin (somatropin).
Indications and Usage: Growth failure due to a deficiency of pituitary growth hormone is the only indication of Ascellacrin (somatropin) administration. Patients must have growth failure as evidenced by a growth rate that is subnormal for age in the absence of any cause other than growth hormone deficiency. Growth hormone deficiency must be documented by demonstrating failure of the serum growth hormone concentration to increase above 5–7 mg/ml in response to two standard stimuli. Standard stimuli which may be used are hypoglycemia, intravenous arginine, oral levodopa, intramuscular glucagon, or suitable modifications of these procedures.
Contraindications: Asellacrin (somatropin) is ineffective, and should not be used, in patients with closed epiphyses.
Asellacrin (somatropin) is contraindicated in the face of any progression of an underlying intracranial lesion.
Precautions: Asellacrin (somatropin) should be used only by physicians experienced in the diagnosis and management of patients with pituitary growth hormone deficiency.
Because of its diabetogenic actions, which include the induction of hyperglycemia and ketosis, Asellacrin (somatropin) should be used with caution in patients with diabetes mellitus or with a family history of diabetes mellitus. Regular urine testing for evidence of glycosuria should be carried out in all patients.
Subcutaneous administration of Asellacrin (somatropin) may lead to local lipoatrophy or lipodystrophy and may enhance the development of neutralizing antibodies. The injections must be intramuscular and the injection site should be rotated.
Bone age must be monitored annually during Asellacrin (somatropin) administration, especially in patients who are pubertal and/or receiving concomitant thyroid replacement therapy. Under these circumstances, epiphyseal maturation may progress rapidly to closure.
Concomitant glucocorticoid therapy may inhibit the response to Asellacrin (somatropin) and should not exceed 10–15 mg hydrocortisone equivalent/M^2 body surface area during the administration of Asellacrin (somatropin).
Patients with growth hormone deficiency secondary to an intracranial lesion should be examined frequently for progression or recurrence of the underlying disease process.
Adverse Reactions: Antibodies to somatropin are formed in 30–40% of the patients who have received somatropin prepared by similar methods. In general, these antibodies are not neutralizing and do not interfere with the response to Asellacrin (somatropin) administration. Approximately 5% of treated patients developed neutralizing antibodies and failed to respond to somatropin. Therefore, testing for anti-somatropin antibodies should be carried out in any patient with well-documented growth hormone deficiency who fails to respond to therapy.
Dosage and Administration: Reconstitute each vial with 5 ml of Bacteriostatic Water for Injection (U.S.P.) only. Each vial of reconstituted Asellacrin (somatropin) provides 2 IU somatropin per ml, 10 IU per vial.
It is recommended that Asellacrin (somatropin) be given initially as 1 ml (2 IU) intramuscularly, three times a week, with a minimum of 48 hours between injections.
If at any time during continuous Asellacrin (somatropin) administraion the growth rate does not exceed 2.5 cm (1 in) in a 6-month period, the dose may be doubled for the next six months. This may be done with or without the

Continued on next page

Serono—Cont.

presence of antibodies to Asellacrin (somatropin). If there is still no satisfactory response, Asellacrin (somatropin) should be discontinued and the patient reinvestigated.

Treatment should be discontinued when the patient has reached a satisfactory adult height, when the epiphyses have fused, or when the patient ceases to respond to Asellacrin (somatropin) administration.

Storage: Unreconstituted vials of Asellacrin (somatropin) may be stored at room temperature (15°–30°C/59°–86°F).

Reconstituted vials must be refrigerated (2°–8°C/36°–46°F) and used within one month.

How Supplied: Each vial contains 10 IU somatropin in sterile, lyophillized form. There are four vials per carton.

Asellacrin (somatropin) will be supplied directly to physicians for patients who show clinical and laboratory evidence of growth hormone deficiency. Forms for providing supporting clinical and laboratory information to qualify patients for treatment may be obtained from MEDICAL AFFAIRS, Medical Research Dept., SERONO LABORATORIES, INC., Braintree, MA 02184.

Manufactured Expressly for:
SERONO LABORATORIES, INC.
Braintree, MA 02184 U.S.A.
by:
Ben Venue Laboratories, Inc., Bedford, OH 44146

PERGONAL® ℞
(menotropins)

Description: Pergonal® (menotropins) is a purified preparation of gonadotropins extracted from the urine of postmenopausal women. Each ampule of Pergonal® (menotropins) contains 75 I.U. of follicle-stimulating hormone (FSH) activity and 75 I.U. of luteinizing hormone (LH) activity.

Pergonal® (menotropins) is biologically standardized for FSH and LH (ICSH) gonadotropin activities in terms of the Second International Reference Preparation for Human Menopausal Gonadotropins established in September, 1964, by the Expert Committee on Biological Standards of the World Health Organization.

Actions: Pergonal® (menotropins) administered for nine to twelve days produces ovarian follicular growth in women who do not have primary ovarian failure. Treatment with Pergonal® (menotropins) in most instances results only in follicular growth and maturation. In order to effect ovulation, HCG (human chorionic gonadotropin) must be given following the administration of Pergonal® (menotropins) when clinical assessment of the patient indicates that sufficient follicular maturation has occurred.

Indications: Pergonal® (menotropins) and HCG given in a sequential manner are indicated for the induction of ovulation and pregnancy in the anovulatory infertile patient in whom the cause of anovulation is secondary and is not due to primary ovarian failure.

Pergonal® (menotropins) has proven effective in treating infertility in women with the following diagnoses: primary amenorrhea, secondary amenorrhea, secondary amenorrhea with galactorrhea, polycystic ovary syndrome, anovulatory cycles, irregular menses.

Selection of Patients:

1. Before treatment with Pergonal® (menotropins) is instituted, a thorough gynecologic and endocrinologic evaluation must be performed. This should include a hysterosalpingogram (to rule out uterine and tubal pathology) and documentation of anovulation by means of basal body temperature, serial vaginal smears, examination of cervical mucus, determination of urinary pregnanediol and endometrial biopsy.
2. Primary ovarian failure should be excluded by the determination of urinary gonadotropin.
3. Careful examination should be made to rule out the presence of an early pregnancy.
4. In patients with irregular bleeding, cancer of the endometrium and other possible organic causes of such bleeding should be ruled out before starting Pergonal® (menotropins) therapy.
5. Evaluation of the husband should be included in the workup.

Contraindications:

1. A high level of urinary gonadotropin indicating primary ovarian failure.
2. The presence of overt thyroid and adrenal dysfunction.
3. An organic intracranial lesion such as a pituitary tumor.
4. The presence of any cause of infertility other than anovulation, as stated in the indications.
5. In patients with abnormal bleeding of undetermined origin.
6. In patients with ovarian cysts or enlargement not due to polycystic ovary syndrome.
7. Pregnancy.

Warning: Pergonal® (menotropins) is a drug that should only be used by physicians who are thoroughly familiar with infertility problems. It is a potent gonadotropic substance capable of causing mild to severe adverse reactions. It must be used with a great deal of care.

Precautions:

1. Diagnosis Prior to Therapy.
   Careful attention should be given to diagnosis in candidates for Pergonal® (menotropins) therapy. (See sections headed "Indications" and "Selection of Patients").
2. Overstimulation of the Ovary During Pergonal® (menotropins) Therapy.
   In order to minimize the hazard associated with the occasional abnormal ovarian enlargement associated with Pergonal® (menotropins)-HCG therapy, the lowest dose consistent with expectation of good results should be used.
   Mild to moderate uncomplicated ovarian enlargement which may be accompanied by abdominal distension and/or abdominal pain occurs in approximately 20% of those treated with Pergonal® (menotropins) and HCG, and generally regresses without treatment within two or three weeks.
   The hyperstimulation syndrome characterized by sudden ovarian enlargement accompanied by ascites with or without pain and/or pleural effusion occurs in approximately 0.4% of patients when the recommended dose is administered. In studies performed, the overall incidence of the hyperstimulation syndrome was 1.3%.
   If hyperstimulation occurs, treatment should be stopped and the patient hospitalized. The hyperstimulation syndrome develops rapidly over a period of three to four days and generally occurs during the two week period immediately following treatment. The phenomenon of hemoconcentration associated with fluid loss in the abdominal cavity has been seen to occur and should be thoroughly assessed in the following manner: 1) fluid intake and output, 2) weight, 3) hematocrit, 4) serum and urinary electrolytes, and 5) urine specific gravity.
   These determinations are to be performed daily or more often if the need arises. Treatment is primarily symptomatic and would consist primarily of bed rest, fluid and electrolyte replacement and analgesics if needed. The ascitic fluid should never be removed because of the potential danger of injury to the ovary.
   Hemoperitoneum may occur from ruptured ovarian cysts. This is usually the result of pelvic examination. If this does occur, and if bleeding becomes such that surgery is required, the conservative approach with partial resection of the enlarged ovary or ovaries is generally adequate.
   Intercourse should be prohibited in those patients in whom significant ovarian enlargement occurs after ovulation because of the danger of hemoperitoneum resulting from ruptured ovarian cysts.
3. Arterial Thromboembolism
   Arterial thromboembolism following Pergonal® (menotropins) and HCG therapy has been reported in two patients, one of whom died (1).
4. Multiple Births
   Of the pregnancies following therapy with Pergonal® (menotropins) and HCG, 80% have resulted in single births and 20% in multiple births, most of which have been twins. Fifteen percent of the total pregnancies resulted in twins, of which 93% were viable (78 surviving infants from 43 sets of twins). Five percent of the total pregnancies have resulted in three or more conceptuses, of which only 20% were viable (nine surviving infants from three sets of triplets, four surviving infants from four sets of quadruplets, and no surviving infants from four sets of quintuplets). The patient and her husband should be advised of the frequency and potential hazards of multiple pregnancy before starting treatment.

Adverse Reactions:

1. Ovarian Enlargement
2. Hyperstimulation Syndrome
3. Hemoperitoneum
4. Arterial Thromboembolism
   (For details on these four adverse reactions, please refer to 'Precautions' above.)
5. Sensitivity to Pergonal® (menotropins)
   Three patients experienced febrile reactions after the administration of Pergonal® (menotropins). It is not clear whether or not these were pyrogenic responses or possibly allergic reactions.
6. Defects at Birth
   From 287 completed pregnancies following Pergonal® (menotropins)-HCG therapy, five incidents of birth defects have been reported. One infant had multiple congenital anomalies consisting of imperforate anus, aplasia of the sigmoid colon, third degree hypospadias, cecovesicle fistula, bifid scrotum, meningocele, bilateral internal tibial torsion, and right metatarsus adductus. Another infant was born with an imperforate anus and possible congenital heart lesions; another had a supernumerary digit; another was born with hypospadias and exstrophy of the bladder; and the fifth child had Down's syndrome. None of the investigators felt that these defects were drug-related.

Dosage and Administration:

FOR INTRAMUSCULAR ADMINISTRATION

1. Treatment for induction of ovulation
   Treatment with Pergonal® (menotropins) in most instances results only in follicular growth and maturation. In order to effect ovulation, HCG must be given following the administration of Pergonal® (menotropins) when clinical assessment of the patient indicates that sufficient follicular maturation has occurred. This is indirectly estimated by the estrogenic effect upon the target organs. These indices of estrogenic activity include:
   a) changes in the vaginal smear
   b) appearance and volume of the cervical mucus
   c) Spinnbarkeit, and
   d) ferning of the cervical mucus.
   If available, the urinary excretion of estrogens is a more reliable index of follicular maturation.
   The clinical confirmation of ovulation, with the exception of pregnancy, is obtained by indirect indices of progesterone production.

The indices most generally used are as follows:
a) a rise in basal body temperature
b) change of the cervical mucus from a "fern" pattern to a "cellular" pattern.
c) vaginal cytology characteristic of the luteal phase of the menstrual cycle
d) increase in urinary pregnanediol, and
e) menstruation following the shift in basal body temperature
Because of the subjectivity of the various tests for the determination of follicular maturation and ovulation, it cannot be over-emphasized that the physician should choose tests with which he is thoroughly familiar.

2. Dosage of Pergonal® (menotropins)
The dose of Pergonal® (menotropins) to produce maturation of the follicle must be individualized for each patient. It is recommended that the initial dose to any patient should be 75 I.U. of FSH and 75 I.U. of LH (one ampule) per day, **ADMINISTERED INTRAMUSCULARLY** for nine to twelve days followed by HCG, 10,000 I.U., one day after the last dose of Pergonal® (menotropins). The hyperstimulation syndrome has never occurred with administration of 75 I.U. of FSH and 75 I.U. of LH (one ampule) per day for up to twelve days. Administration of Pergonal® (menotropins) should not exceed 12 days. The patient should be treated until indices of estrogenic activity, as indicated under Item 1 above, are equivalent to or greater than those of the normal individual. If urinary estrogen determinations are available, they may be useful as a guide to therapy. If the total estrogen excretion is less than 100 mcg/24 hours or the estriol excretion is less than 50 mcg/24 hours prior to HCG administration, the hyperstimulation syndrome is less likely to occur. If the estrogen values are greater than this, it is not advisable to administer HCG because the hyperstimulation syndrome is more likely to occur.
If the ovaries are abnormally enlarged on the last day of Pergonal® (menotropins) therapy, HCG should not be administered in this course of therapy; this will reduce the chances of development of the hyperstimulation syndrome. If there is evidence of ovulation but no pregnancy, repeat this dosage regime for at least two more courses before increasing the dose of of Pergonal® (menotropins) to 150 I.U. of FSH and 150 I.U. of LH (two ampules) per day for nine to twelve days. As before, this dose should be followed by 10,000 I.U. of HCG one day after the last dose of Pergonal® (menotropins). 150 I.U. of FSH and 150 I.U. of LH (two ampules) of Pergonal® (menotropins) per day have proven to be the most effective dose. If evidence of ovulation is present, but pregnancy does not ensue, repeat the same dose for two more courses. Doses larger than this are not recommended.
During treatment with both Pergonal® (menotropins) and HCG and during a two-week post-treatment period, patients should be examined at least every other day for signs of excessive ovarian stimulation. It is recommended that Pergonal® (menotroins) administration be stopped if the ovaries became abnormally enlarged or abdominal pain occurs. Most of the ovarian hyperstimulation occurs after treatment has been discontinued and reaches its maximum at about seven to ten days post-ovulation. Patients should be followed for at leat two weeks after HCG administration.
The couple should be encouraged to have intercourse daily, beginning on the day prior to the administration of HCG until ovulation becomes apparent from the indices employed for the determination of progestational activity. Care should be taken to insure insemination.

	% Pts. Ovul.	% Pts. Preg.	% Abort	Multi Preg.	% Twins	% 3 or More Conceptuses	% Hyperstim. Syndr.
Primary Amenorrhea	62	22	14	25	25	0	0
Secondary Amen.	61	28	24	28	18	10	1.9
Secondary Amen. with Galactorrhea	77	42	21	41	31	10	1.2
Polycystic Ovaries	76	26	39	17	17	0	1.1
Anovulatory Cycles	77	24	15	14	9	5	2.0
Miscellaneous	83	20	36	2	2	0	0.1

In the light of the foregoing indices and parameters mentioned, it should become obvious that, unless a physician is willing to devote considerable time to these patients and be familiar with and conduct the necessary laboratory studies, he should not use Pergonal® (menotropins).

3. How to Administer Pergonal® (menotropins).
Dissolve the contents of one ampule of Pergonal® (menotropins) in one to two ml of sterile saline and **ADMINISTER INTRAMUSCULARLY** immediately. Any unused reconstituted material should be discarded.

How Supplied: Each ampule of Pergonal® (menotropins) contains 75 I.U. of FSH and 75 I.U. of LH (ICSH) plus 10 mg lactose in a lyophilized form. By biological assay, one I.U. of LH for the Second International Reference Preparation (IRP) for HMG is biologically equivalent to approximately ½ I.U. of human chorionic gonadotropin (HCG).

Clinical Studies: The results of the clinical experience and effectiveness of the administration of Pergonal® (menotropins) to 1,286 patients in 3,002 courses of therapy are summarized below. The values include patients who were treated with other than the recommended dosage regime. The values for the presently recommended dosage regime are essentially the same, except for the fact that the hyperstimulation syndrome has not occurred with administration of 75 I.U. of Pergonal® (menotropins) per day for 9 to 12 days and the incidence of the hyperstimulation syndrome with administration of 150 I.U. of Pergonal® (menotropins) per day for 9 to 12 days has not exceeded 0.4%.

	%
Patients ovulating	75
Patients pregnant	25
Patients aborting	25*
Multiple pregnancies	20†
Twins	15†
Three or more conceptuses	5†
Fetal abnormalities	1.7†
Hyperstimulation syndrome	1.3

*Based on total pregnancies
†Based on total deliveries (births & abortions)

Results by diagnosis group are summarized below. (These values include patients who were treated with other than the present recommended dosage regime).
[See table above].

References:

1. Mozes M., Bogokowsky H., Antebi E., et al: Thromboembolic phenomena after ovarian stimulation with human gonadotropins. **Lancet 2:** 1213-1215, 1965.

PROFASI® HP ℞
(Chorionic gonadotropin for Injection)

Description: Human chorionic gonadotropin (HCG), a polypeptide hormone produced by the human placenta, is composed of an alpha and a beta sub-unit. The alpha sub-unit is essentially identical to the alpha sub-units of the human pituitary gonadotropins, luteinizing-hormone (LH) and follicle-stimulating hormone (FSH), as well as to the alpha sub-unit of human thyroid-stimulating hormone (TSH). The beta sub-units of these hormones differ in amino acid sequence. Chorionic Gonadotropin is derived from the urine of pregnant women. It is standardized by a biological assay procedure.

Actions: The action of HCG is virtually identical to that of pituitary-LH, although HCG appears to have a small degree of FSH activity as well. It stimulates production of gonadal steroid hormones by stimulating the interstitial cells (Leydig cells) of the testis to produce androgens and the corpus luteum of the ovary to produce progesterone. Androgen stimulation in the male leads to the development of secondary sex characteristics and may stimulate testicular descent when no anatomical impediment to descent is present. This descent is usually reversible when HCG is discontinued. During the normal menstrual cycle, LH participates with FSH in the development and maturation of the normal ovarian follicle, and the mid-cycle LH surge triggers ovulation. HCG can substitute for LH in this function.
During a normal pregnancy, HCG secreted by the placenta maintains the corpus luteum after LH secretion decreases, supporting continued secretion of estrogen and progesterone and preventing menstruation.
HCG HAS NO KNOWN EFFECT ON FAT MOBILIZATION, APPETITE OR SENSE OF HUNGER, OR BODY FAT DISTRIBUTION.

Indications: HCG HAS NOT BEEN DEMONSTRATED TO BE EFFECTIVE ADJUNCTIVE THERAPY IN THE TREATMENT OF OBESITY. THERE IS NO SUBSTANTIAL EVIDENCE THAT IT INCREASES WEIGHT LOSS BEYOND THAT RESULTING FROM CALORIC RESTRICTION, THAT IT CAUSES A MORE ATTRACTIVE OR "NORMAL" DISTRIBUTION OF FAT, OR THAT IT DECREASES THE HUNGER AND DISCOMFORT ASSOCIATED WITH CALORIE-RESTRICTED DIETS.

1. Prepubertal cryptorchidism not due to anatomical obstruction. In general, HCG is thought to induce testicular descent in situations when descent would have occurred at puberty. HCG thus may help predict whether or not orchiopexy will be needed in the future. Although, in some cases, descent following HCG administration is permanent, in most cases, the response is temporary. Therapy is usually instituted between the ages of 4 and 9.
2. Selected cases of hypogonadotropic hypogonadism (hypogonadism secondary to a pituitary deficiency) in males.
3. Induction of ovulation and pregnancy in the anovulatory, infertile woman in whom the cause of anovulation is secondary and not due to primary ovarian failure, and who has been appropriately pre-treated with human menopausal gonadotropins.

Contraindications: Precocious puberty, prostatic carcinoma or other androgen-dependent neoplasm, prior allergic reaction to HCG.

Warnings: HCG should be used in conjunction with human menopausal gonadotropins only by physicians experienced with infertility problems who are familiar with the criteria for patient selection, contraindications, warnings, precautions, and adverse reactions described in the package insert for menotropins. The principal serious adverse reactions during this use are: (1) Ovarian hyperstimulation, a syn-

Continued on next page

Serono—Cont.

drome of sudden ovarian enlargement, ascites with or without pain, and/or pleural effusion, (2) Rupture of ovarian cysts with resultant hemoperitoneum, (3) Multiple births, and (4) Arterial thromboembolism.

Precautions: Induction of androgen secretion by HCG may induce precocious puberty in patients treated for cryptorchidism. Therapy should be discontinued if signs of precocious puberty occur.

Since androgens may cause fluid retention, HCG should be used with caution in patients with cardiac or renal disease, epilepsy, migraine, or asthma.

Adverse Reactions: Headache, irritability, restlessness, depression, fatigue, edema, precocious puberty, gynecomastia, pain at the site of injection.

Dosage and Administration (Intramuscular Use Only): The dosage regimen employed in any particular case will depend upon the indication for use, the age and weight of the patient, and the physician's preference. The following regimens have been advocated by various authorities.

Prepubertal cryptorchidism not due to anatomical obstruction

1. 4,000 U.S.P. Units three times weekly for three weeks.
2. 5,000 U.S.P. Units every second day for four injections.
3. 15 injections of 500 to 1,000 U.S.P. Units over a period of six weeks.
4. 500 U.S.P. Units three times weekly for four to six weeks. If this course of treatment is not successful, another is begun one month later, giving 1,000 U.S.P. Units per injection.

Selected cases of hypogonadotropic hypogonadism in males

1. 500 to 1,000 U.S.P. Units three times a week for three weeks, followed by the same dose twice a week for three weeks.
2. 4,000 U.S.P. Units three times weekly for six to nine months, following which the dosage may be reduced to 2,000 U.S.P. Units three times weekly for an additional three months.

Induction of ovulation and pregnancy in the anovulatory, infertile woman in whom the cause of anovulation is secondary and not due to primary ovarian failure and who has been appropriately pre-treated with human menotropins (See prescribing information for menotropins for dosage and administration for that drug product).

5,000 to 10,000 U.S.P. Units one day following the last dose of menotropins. (A dosage of 10,000 U.S.P. Units is recommended in the labeling for menotropins).

IMPORTANT: USE COMPLETELY WITHIN 60 DAYS AFTER RECONSTITUTION. REFRIGERATE AFTER RECONSTITUTION.

How Supplied: The freeze-dried, stabilized active principle is supplied in a two vial package including Bacteriostatic Water for Injection as diluent.

When reconstituted, each vial contains in U.S.P. Units:

[See table below].

The product is assayed in accord with the U.S.P. method and potencies refer to U.S.P. Units (International Units) defined in terms of the U.S.P. Chorionic Gonadotropin Reference Standard.

Caution: Federal law prohibits dispensing without prescription.

Directions for Reconstitution: Withdraw sterile air from lyophilized vial and inject into diluent vial. Remove 10 ml. from diluent and add to lyophilized vial; agitate gently until solution is complete.

VIAL SIZE:*	10 ml.	**10 ml.**	30 ml.	10 ml.
Chorionic Gonadotropin	5,000 U.	**10,000 U.**	15,000 U.	20,000 U.
Mannitol, U.S.P.	50 mg.	**100 mg.**	150 mg.	200 mg.
Benzyl Alcohol, N.F.	0.9%	**0.9%**	0.9%	0.9%

with Sodium Phosphate Dibasic and Sodium Phosphate Monobasic to adjust pH.

** Only available in 10,000 U.*

Smith Kline & French Laboratories

Division of SmithKline Corporation
1500 SPRING GARDEN ST.
P.O. BOX 7929
PHILADELPHIA, PA 19101

SK&F Co.

Carolina, P.R. 00630
Subsidiary of SmithKline Corporation

SK&F Lab Co.

Carolina, P.R. 00630
Subsidiary of SmithKline Corporation

Menley & James Laboratories

a SmithKline company
P.O. BOX 8082
PHILADELPHIA, PA 19101

SK&F PRODUCT CODE INDEX

Code	Product, Form and Strength
A70	'Anspor' Capsules 250 mg.
A71	'Anspor' Capsules 500 mg.
A90	'Benzedrine' *Spansule* capsules 15 mg.
A91	'Benzedrine' Tablets 5 mg.
A92	'Benzedrine' Tablets 10 mg.
C26	'Combid' *Spansule* capsules
C44	'Compazine' *Spansule* capsules 10 mg.
C46	'Compazine' *Spansule* capsules 15 mg.
C47	'Compazine' *Spansule* capsules 30 mg.
C49	'Compazine' *Spansule* capsules 75 mg.
C60	'Compazine' Suppositories 2 ½ mg.
C61	'Compazine' Suppositories 5 mg.
C62	'Compazine' Suppositories 25 mg.
C66	'Compazine' Tablets 5 mg.
C67	'Compazine' Tablets 10 mg.
C69	'Compazine' Tablets 25 mg.
D14	'Cytomel' Tablets 5 mcg.
D16	'Cytomel' Tablets 25 mcg.
D17	'Cytomel' Tablets 50 mcg.
D62	'Darbid' Tablets 5 mg.
D91	'Dexamyl' *Spansule* capsules No. 1
D92	'Dexamyl' *Spansule* capsules No. 2
D93	'Dexamyl' Tablets
E12	'Dexedrine' *Spansule* capsules 5 mg.
E13	'Dexedrine' *Spansule* capsules 10 mg.
E14	'Dexedrine' *Spansule* capsules 15 mg.
E19	'Dexedrine' Tablets 5 mg.
E33	'Dibenzyline' Capsules 10 mg.
E90	*'Dyazide' Capsules
H06	*'Dyrenium' Capsules 50 mg.
H07	*'Dyrenium' Capsules 100 mg.
H24	††'Ecotrin' Tablets 5 gr.
J07	'Eskalith' Capsules 300 mg.
J09	'Eskalith' Tablets 300 mg.
J66	'Eskatrol' *Spansule* capsules
K31	††'Feosol' *Spansule* capsules
K32	††'Feosol' Tablets
K33	'Feosol Plus' Capsules
K60	††'Fortespan' Capsules
K77	'Hispril' *Spansule* capsules 5 mg.
N10	††'Ornacol' Capsules
N23	'Ornade' *Spansule* capsules
N17	††'Ornex' Capsules
N71	'Parnate' Tablets 10 mg.
S90	'Selacryn' Tablets 250 mg.
120	'SK-Amitriptyline' Tablets 10 mg.
121	'SK-Amitriptyline' Tablets 25 mg.
123	'SK-Amitriptyline' Tablets 50 mg.
124	'SK-Amitriptyline' Tablets 75 mg.
131	'SK-Amitriptyline' Tablets 100 mg.
132	'SK-Amitriptyline' Tablets 150 mg.
101	'SK-Ampicillin' Capsules 250 mg.
102	'SK-Ampicillin' Capsules 500 mg.
107	'SK-Ampicillin' Tablets 125 mg.
174	'SK-APAP' Tablets 325 mg.
173	'SK-APAP' Tablets 650 mg.
494	'SK-APAP' with Codeine Tablets 300 mg./15 mg.
496	'SK-APAP' with Codeine Tablets 300 mg./30 mg.
497	'SK-APAP' with Codeine Tablets 300 mg./60 mg.
133	'SK-Bamate' Tablets 200 mg.
134	'SK-Bamate' Tablets 400 mg.
193	'SK-Bisacodyl' Tablets 5 mg.
176	'SK-Chloral Hydrate' Capsules 500 mg.
419	'SK-Chlorothiazide' Tablets 250 mg.
420	'SK-Chlorothiazide' Tablets 500 mg.
374	'SK-Dexamethasone' Tablets 0.5 mg.
376	'SK-Dexamethasone' Tablets 0.75 mg.
377	'SK-Dexamethasone' Tablets 1.5 mg.
122	'SK-Digoxin' Tablets 0.25 mg.
303	'SK-Diphenhydramine' Capsules 25 mg.
304	'SK-Diphenhydramine' Capsules 50 mg.
423	'SK-Diphenoxylate' Tablets
367	'SK-Erythromycin' Tablets 250 mg.
369	'SK-Erythromycin' Tablets 500 mg.
363	'SK-Hydrochlorothiazide' Tablets 25 mg.
364	'SK-Hydrochlorothiazide' Tablets 50 mg.
441	'SK-Lygen' Capsules 5 mg.
442	'SK-Lygen' Capsules 10 mg.
443	'SK-Lygen' Capsules 25 mg.
129	'SK-Niacin' Tablets 50 mg.
130	'SK-Niacin' Tablets 100 mg.
111	'SK-Penicillin G' Tablets 400,000 units
112	'SK-Penicillin G' Tablets 800,000 units
116	'SK-Penicillin VK' Tablets 250 mg.
117	'SK-Penicillin VK' Tablets 500 mg.
136	'SK-Phenobarbital' Tablets 15 mg.
137	'SK-Phenobarbital' Tablets 30 mg.
321	'SK-Pramine' Tablets 10 mg.
322	'SK-Pramine' Tablets 25 mg.
323	'SK-Pramine' Tablets 50 mg.
339	'SK-Prednisone' Tablets 5 mg.
171	'SK-Quinidine Sulfate' Tablets 200 mg.
169	'SK-Reserpine' Tablets 0.25 mg.
463	'SK-65' Capsules 65 mg.
467	'SK-65 Compound' Capsules
474	'SK-65 APAP' Tablets
163	'SK-Soxazole' Tablets 500 mg.
126	'SK-Tetracycline' Capsules 250 mg.
127	'SK-Tetracycline' Capsules 500 mg.
403	'SK-Triamcinolone' Tablets 2 mg.
404	'SK-Triamcinolone' Tablets 4 mg.
406	'SK-Triamcinolone' Tablets 8 mg.
S03	*'Stelazine' Tablets 1 mg.
S04	*'Stelazine' Tablets 2 mg.
S06	*'Stelazine' Tablets 5 mg.
S07	*'Stelazine' Tablets 10 mg.
T13	†'Tagamet' Tablets 300 mg.
S72	††'Teldrin' Timed-Release capsules 8 mg.
S73	††'Teldrin' Timed-Release capsules 12 mg.
T01	'Temaril' *Spansule* capsules 5 mg.
T03	'Temaril' Tablets 2.5 mg.
T63	'Thorazine' *Spansule* capsules 30 mg.
T64	'Thorazine' *Spansule* capsules 75 mg.
T66	'Thorazine' *Spansule* capsules 150 mg.
T67	'Thorazine' *Spansule* capsules 200 mg.
T69	'Thorazine' *Spansule* capsules 300 mg.
T70	'Thorazine' Suppositories 25 mg.
T71	'Thorazine' Suppositories 100 mg.
T73	'Thorazine' Tablets 10 mg.
T74	'Thorazine' Tablets 25 mg.
T76	'Thorazine' Tablets 50 mg.

T77 'Thorazine' Tablets 100 mg.
T79 'Thorazine' Tablets 200 mg.
V24 ††'Troph-Iron' Tablets
V43 ††'Trophite' Tablets
V71 'Tuss-Ornade' *Spansule* capsules
V90 'Urispas' Tablets 100 mg.
X42 'Vontrol' Tablets 25 mg.

---

*A product of SK&F Co., Carolina, P.R. 00630, Subsidiary of SmithKline Corporation, Philadelphia, Pa.
†A product of SK&F Lab Co., Carolina, P.R. 00630, Subsidiary of SmithKline Corporation, Philadelphia, Pa.
††A product of Menley & James Laboratories, Professional Products Division, a SmithKline company, Philadelphia, Pa.

ACNOMEL® CREAM AND CAKE††
acne therapy

Description: *Cream*—sulfur, 8%; resorcinol, 2%; alcohol, 11% (w/w); in a stable, grease-free, flesh-tinted vehicle. Standard strength for home application, morning or night. *Cake* (half strength)—sulfur, 4%; resorcinol, 1%; a washable, flesh-tinted cake base; in a handy compact for convenient use away from home.
Action and Uses: Acnomel provides effective acne therapy. Easily applied, flesh-tinted, it conceals as it heals. Because Acnomel is virtually invisible when applied, it is well accepted by even the most self-conscious person.
Directions: Wash and dry affected areas thoroughly. Apply a thin coating with fingertips or a moist sponge two or three times daily. Do not rub in.
Warning: If undue skin irritation develops or increases, discontinue use and consult physician. Do not apply to acutely inflamed area. Keep out of eyes and off eyelids. Keep this and all medicines out of reach of children. In case of accidental ingestion, contact a physician or poison control center immediately.
How Supplied: *Cream*—in specially lined 1 oz. tubes. *Cake*—handy 1 oz. plastic containers.
Remarks: Do not dilute or compound. When prescribing write for original container.

---

††Acnomel® Cream and Cake are products of Menley & James Laboratories, Professional Products Division, a SmithKline company.

ANCEF® ℞
(brand of sterile cefazolin sodium)
(lyophilized)

Description: Ancef® (sterile cefazolin sodium, SK&F) is a semisynthetic cephalosporin for parenteral administration. It is the sodium salt of 3-{[(5-methyl-1,3,4-thiadiazol-2-yl)-thio] methyl} -8-oxo-7- [2- (1H-tetrazol-1-yl) acetamido] -5-thia-1-azabicyclo [4.2.0] oct-2-ene-2- carboxylic acid. The sodium content is 46 mg. per gram of cefazolin.
Actions: Microbiology: *In vitro* tests demonstrate that the bactericidal action of cephalosporins results from inhibition of cell wall synthesis. Ancef (sterile cefazolin sodium, SK&F) is active against the following organisms *in vitro:*
Staphylococcus aureus (penicillin-sensitive and penicillin-resistant)
Group A beta-hemolytic streptococci and other strains of streptococci (many strains of enterococci are resistant)
Streptococcus pneumoniae (formerly *D. pneumoniae*)
Escherichia coli
Proteus mirabilis
Klebsiella species
Enterobacter aerogenes
Hemophilus influenzae
Most strains of *Enterobacter cloacae* and indole positive Proteus (*P. vulgaris, P. morgani, P. rettgeri*) are resistant. Methicillin-resistant staphylococci, serratia, pseudomonas, mima, herellea species are almost uniformly resistant to cefazolin.
Human Pharmacology: The following tables demonstrate the blood levels and duration of cefazolin following the administration of 'Ancef'.

TABLE 1
Duration of Blood Levels of Cefazolin

250 mg. I.M. Dose (Figures are μg./ml.)

	Time After Injection in Hours				
	½	1	2	4	6
CEFAZOLIN	15.5	17.0	13.0	5.1	2.5

TABLE 2
500 mg. I.M. Dose (Figures are μg./ml.)

	Time After Injection in Hours					
	½	1	2	4	6	8
CEFAZOLIN	36.2	36.8	37.9	15.5	6.3	3.0

TABLE 3
1 gram I.M. Dose (Figures are μg./ml.)

	Time After Injection in Hours						
	½	1	2	4	6	8	10
CEFAZOLIN*	60.1	63.8	54.3	29.3	13.2	7.1	<4.1

*Average of the two studies
Clinical pharmacology studies in patients hospitalized with infections indicate that Ancef (sterile cefazolin sodium, SK&F) produces mean peak serum levels approximately equivalent to those seen in normal volunteers.
In a study (using normal volunteers) of constant intravenous infusion with dosages of 3.5 mg./kg. for 1 hour (approximately 250 mg.) and 1.5 mg./kg. the next two hours (approximately 100 mg.), 'Ancef' produced a steady serum level at the third hour of approximately 28 μg./ml.
The following table shows the average serum concentration and average half life of cefazolin after I.V. injection of a single 1 gram dose of 'Ancef'.

TABLE 4
1 gram I.V. Dose (Figures are μg./ml.)

	Time After Injection, Min.			
	5	15	30	60
CEFAZOLIN	188.4	135.8	106.8	73.7

1 gram I.V. Dose (Figures are μg./ml.)

	Time After Injection, Min.			
	120	240	Peak	Half-life in Hours
CEFAZOLIN	45.6	16.5	190.0	1.4

Controlled studies on adult normal volunteers, receiving 1 gram 4 times a day for 10 days, monitoring CBC, SGOT, SGPT, bilirubin, alkaline phosphatase, BUN, creatinine, and urinalysis, indicated no clinically significant changes attributed to 'Ancef'.
'Ancef' is excreted unchanged in the urine. In the first six hours approximately 60% of the drug is excreted in the urine and this increases to 70%-80% within 24 hours. 'Ancef' achieves peak urine concentrations of approximately 2400 μg./ml. and 4000 μg./ml. respectively following 500 mg. and 1 gram intramuscular doses.
Bile levels in patients without obstructive biliary disease can reach or exceed serum levels by up to five times; however, in patients with obstructive biliary disease, bile levels of 'Ancef' are considerably lower than serum levels (<1.0 μg./ml.). In synovial fluid, the 'Ancef' level becomes comparable to that reached in serum at about four hours after drug administration. Studies of cord blood show prompt transfer of 'Ancef' across the placenta. 'Ancef' is present in very low concentrations in the milk of nursing mothers.
Disc Susceptibility Tests
Quantitative methods that require measurement of zone diameters give the most precise estimates of antibiotic susceptibility. One such procedure* has been recommended for use with discs for testing susceptibility to cephalosporin class antibiotics. Interpretations correlate diameters of the disc test with MIC values for 'Ancef'. With this procedure, a report from the laboratory of "susceptible" indicates that the infecting organism is likely to respond to therapy. A report of "resistant" indicates that the infecting organism is not likely to respond to therapy. A report of "intermediate susceptibility" suggests that the organism would be susceptible if high dosage is used, or if the infection is confined to tissues and fluids (e.g., urine) in which high antibiotic levels are attained.
Indications: Ancef (sterile cefazolin sodium, SK&F) is indicated in the treatment of the following serious infections due to susceptible organisms:
RESPIRATORY TRACT INFECTIONS due to *Streptococcus pneumoniae* (formerly *D. pneumoniae*), *Klebsiella* species, *Hemophilus influenzae, Staphylococcus aureus* (penicillin-sensitive and penicillin-resistant), and group A beta-hemolytic streptococci.
Injectable benzathine penicillin is considered to be the drug of choice in treatment and prevention of streptococcal infections, including the prophylaxis of rheumatic fever.
'Ancef' is effective in the eradication of streptococci from the nasopharynx; however, data establishing the efficacy of 'Ancef' in the subsequent prevention of rheumatic fever are not available at present.
URINARY TRACT INFECTIONS due to *Escherichia coli, Proteus mirabilis, Klebsiella* species, and some strains of enterobacter and enterococci.
SKIN STRUCTURE INFECTIONS due to *Staphylococcus aureus* (penicillin-sensitive and penicillin-resistant), group A beta-hemolytic streptococci and other strains of streptococci.
BILIARY TRACT INFECTIONS due to *Escherichia coli*, various strains of streptococci, *Proteus mirabilis, Klebsiella* species and *Staphylococcus aureus.*
BONE AND JOINT INFECTIONS due to *Staphylococcus aureus.*
GENITAL INFECTIONS (i.e., prostatitis, epididymitis) due to *Escherichia coli, Proteus mirabilis, Klebsiella* species, and some strains of enterococci.
SEPTICEMIA due to *Streptococcus pneumoniae* (formerly *D. pneumoniae*), *Staphylococcus aureus* (penicillin-sensitive and penicillin-resistant), *Proteus mirabilis, Escherichia coli,* and *Klebsiella* species.

Continued on next page

Smith Kline & French—Cont.

ENDOCARDITIS due to *Staphylococcus aureus* (penicillin-sensitive and penicillin-resistant) and group A beta-hemolytic streptococci.

Appropriate culture and susceptibility studies should be performed to determine susceptibility of the causative organism to 'Ancef'.

Contraindications: ANCEF (STERILE CEFAZOLIN SODIUM, SK&F) IS CONTRAINDICATED IN PATIENTS WITH KNOWN ALLERGY TO THE CEPHALOSPORIN GROUP OF ANTIBIOTICS.

Warnings: BEFORE CEFAZOLIN THERAPY IS INSTITUTED, CAREFUL INQUIRY SHOULD BE MADE CONCERNING PREVIOUS HYPERSENSITIVITY REACTIONS TO CEPHALOSPORINS AND PENICILLIN. CEPHALOSPORIN C DERIVATIVES SHOULD BE GIVEN CAUTIOUSLY IN PENICILLIN-SENSITIVE PATIENTS.

SERIOUS ACUTE HYPERSENSITIVITY REACTIONS MAY REQUIRE EPINEPHRINE AND OTHER EMERGENCY MEASURES.

There is some clinical and laboratory evidence of partial cross-allergenicity of the penicillins and the cephalosporins. Patients have been reported to have had severe reactions (including anaphylaxis) to both drugs.

Any patient who has demonstrated some form of allergy, particularly to drugs, should receive antibiotics cautiously. No exception should be made with regard to 'Ancef'.

Usage in Pregnancy: Safety of this product for use during pregnancy has not been established.

Usage in Infants: Safety for use in prematures and infants under 1 month of age has not been established.

Precautions: Prolonged use of Ancef (sterile cefazolin sodium, SK&F) may result in the overgrowth of nonsusceptible organisms. Careful clinical observation of the patient is essential.

When 'Ancef' is administered to patients with low urinary output because of impaired renal function, lower daily dosage is required (see dosage instructions). A false positive reaction for glucose in the urine of patients on 'Ancef' has occurred with Clinitest® tablets solution.

Adverse Reactions: The following reactions have been reported:

Hypersensitivity: Drug fever, skin rash, vulvar pruritus, and eosinophilia have occurred.

Blood: Neutropenia, leukopenia, thrombocythemia, and positive direct and indirect Coombs tests have occurred.

Hepatic and Renal: Transient rise in SGOT, SGPT, BUN and alkaline phosphatase levels has been observed without clinical evidence of renal or hepatic impairment.

Gastrointestinal: Nausea, anorexia, vomiting, diarrhea, oral candidiasis (oral thrush) have been reported.

Other: Pain at site of injection after intramuscular administration has occurred, some with induration. Phlebitis at site of injection has been noted. Other reactions include genital and anal pruritus, genital moniliasis, and vaginitis.

Dosage and Administration: Ancef (sterile cefazolin sodium, SK&F) may be administered intramuscularly or intravenously after reconstitution.

DILUTION TABLE*

Vial Size	Diluent to be Added	Approximate Available Volume	Approximate Average Concentration
250 mg.	2.0 ml.	2.0 ml.	125 mg./ml.
500 mg.	2.0 ml.	2.2 ml.	225 mg./ml.
1 gram	2.5 ml.	3.0 ml.	330 mg./ml.

* See labeling on "Piggyback" Vials (500 mg. and 1 gram) and Pharmacy Bulk Vials (5 and 10 grams) for their reconstitution directions.

Intramuscular Administration—Reconstitute with Sterile Water for Injection, Bacteriostatic Water for Injection or Sodium Chloride Injection, according to the dilution table above. Shake well until dissolved. 'Ancef' should be injected into a large muscle mass. Pain on injection is infrequent with 'Ancef'. Reconstituted 'Ancef' is stable for 24 hours at room temperature and for 96 hours if stored under refrigeration.

Intravenous Administration—Ancef (sterile cefazolin sodium, SK&F) may be administered by intravenous injection or by continuous or intermittent infusion. Total daily dosages are the same as with intramuscular injection.

Intermittent intravenous infusion: 'Ancef' can be administered along with primary intravenous fluid management programs in a volume control set or in a separate, secondary I.V. bottle. Reconstituted 500 mg. or 1 gram of 'Ancef' may be diluted in 50 to 100 ml. of one of the following intravenous solutions:

- Sodium Chloride Injection
- 5% or 10% Dextrose Injection
- 5% Dextrose in Lactated Ringer's Injection
- 5% Dextrose and 0.9% Sodium Chloride Injection (also may be used with 5% Dextrose and 0.45% or 0.2% Sodium Chloride Injection)
- Lactated Ringer's Injection
- Invert Sugar 5% or 10% in Sterile Water for Injection
- Ringer's Injection
- 5% Sodium Bicarbonate in Sterile Water for Injection

'Ancef' is stable in these intravenous fluids for 24 hours at room temperature and 96 hours if stored under refrigeration (5°C).

Direct intravenous injection: Dilute the reconstituted 500 mg. or 1 gram of 'Ancef' in 10 ml. of Sterile Water for Injection. Inject solution slowly over 3 to 5 minutes. May be administered directly into vein or through tubing for patient receiving the above parenteral fluids.

Usual Adult Dosage

Type of Infection	Dose	Frequency
Moderate to severe infections	500 mg. to 1 gram	every 6 to 8 hrs.
Mild infections caused by susceptible gram + cocci	250 mg. to 500 mg.	every 8 hours
Acute, uncomplicated urinary tract infections	1 gram	every 12 hours
Pneumococcal pneumonia	500 mg.	every 12 hours
Severe, life-threatening infections (e.g., endocarditis, septicemia)*	1 gram to 1.5 grams	every 6 hours

*In rare instances, doses of up to 12 grams of 'Ancef' per day have been used.

'Ancef' may be used in patients with reduced renal function with the following dosage adjustments: Patients with a creatinine clearance of 55 ml./min. or greater or a serum creatinine of 1.5 mg.% or less can be given full doses. Patients with creatinine clearance rates of 35 to 54 ml./min. or serum creatinine of 1.6 to 3.0 mg.% can also be given full doses but dosage should be restricted to at least 8 hour intervals. Patients with creatinine clearance rates of 11 to 34 ml./min. or serum creatinine of 3.1 to 4.5 mg.% should be given ½ the usual dose every 12 hours. Patients with creatinine clearance rates of 10 ml./min. or less or serum creatinine of 4.6 mg.% or greater should be given ½ the usual dose every 18 to 24 hours. All reduced dosage recommendations apply after an initial loading dose appropriate to the severity of the infection.

Pediatric Dosage

In children, a total daily dosage of 25 to 50 mg. per kg. (approximately 10 to 20 mg. per pound) of body weight, divided into three or four equal doses, is effective for most mild to moderately severe infections. Total daily dosage may be increased to 100 mg. per kg. (45 mg. per pound) of body weight for severe infections. Since safety for use in premature infants and in infants under one month has not been established, the use of 'Ancef' in these patients is not recommended.

Pediatric Dosage Guide

Weight		25 mg./kg./Day Divided into 3 Doses		25 mg./kg./Day Divided into 4 Doses	
Lbs.	Kg.	Approximate Single Dose mg./q8h	Vol. (ml.) needed with dilution of 125 mg./ml.	Approximate Single Dose mg./q6h	Vol. (ml.) needed with dilution of 125 mg./ml.
10	4.5	40 mg.	0.35 ml.	30 mg.	0.25 ml.
20	9.0	75 mg.	0.60 ml.	55 mg.	0.45 ml.
30	13.6	115 mg.	0.90 ml.	85 mg.	0.70 ml.
40	18.1	150 mg.	1.20 ml.	115 mg.	0.90 ml.
50	22.7	190 mg.	1.50 ml.	140 mg.	1.10 ml.

Weight		50 mg./kg./Day Divided into 3 Doses		50 mg./kg./Day Divided into 4 Doses	
Lbs.	Kg.	Approximate Single Dose mg./q8h	Vol. (ml.) needed with dilution of 225 mg./ml.	Approximate Single Dose mg./q6h	Vol. (ml.) needed with dilution of 225 mg./ml.
10	4.5	75 mg.	0.35 ml.	55 mg.	0.25 ml.
20	9.0	150 mg.	0.70 ml.	110 mg.	0.50 ml.
30	13.6	225 mg.	1.00 ml.	170 mg.	0.75 ml.
40	18.1	300 mg.	1.35 ml.	225 mg.	1.00 ml.
50	22.7	375 mg.	1.70 ml.	285 mg.	1.25 ml.

In children with mild to moderate renal impairment (creatinine clearance of 70 to 40 ml./min.), 60 percent of the normal daily dose given in equally divided doses every 12 hours should be sufficient. In patients with moderate impairment (creatinine clearance of 40 to 20 ml./min.), 25 percent of the normal daily dose given in equally divided doses every 12 hours should be adequate. Children with severe renal impairment (creatinine clearance of 20 to 5 ml./min.) may be given 10 percent of the normal daily dose every 24 hours. All dosage recommendations apply after an initial loading dose.

How Supplied: Ancef (sterile cefazolin sodium, SK&F)—supplied in vials equivalent to 250 mg., 500 mg. or 1 gram of cefazolin; in "Piggyback" Vials for intravenous admixture equivalent to 500 mg. or 1 gram of cefazolin; and in Pharmacy Bulk Vials equivalent to 5 grams or 10 grams of cefazolin.

Military—Vial, 1 gram, 6505-01-010-0832; vial, 500 mg., 6505-01-010-0833.

*Bauer, A.W.; Kirby, W.M.M.; Sherris, J.C., and Turck, M.: Antibiotic Testing by a Standardized Single Disc Method, Am. J. Clin. Path. 45:493, 1966. Standardized Disc Susceptibility Test, Federal Register 39:19182-19184, 1974.

ANSPOR® ℞
(brand of cephradine)
Capsules, 250 mg. and 500 mg.
and
For Oral Suspension, 125 mg./5 ml. and 250 mg./5 ml.

Description: Anspor (cephradine, SK&F) is a semisynthetic cephalosporin antibiotic chemically designated as 7-[D-2-amino-2-(1,4-cyclohexadien-1-yl) acetamido]-3-methyl-8-oxo-5-thia-1-azabicyclo [4.2.0] -oct-2-ene-2-carboxylic acid.

Actions: Human Pharmacology: Anspor (cephradine, SK&F) is acid stable. It is rapidly absorbed after oral administration in the fasting state. Following doses of 250 mg. and 500 mg. in normal adult volunteers, average peak serum levels within one hour were approximately 9 and 16.5 mcg. per ml. respectively. The presence of food in the gastrointestinal tract delays the absorption but does not affect the total amount of cephradine absorbed. Over 90 percent of the drug is excreted unchanged in the urine within 6 hours. Peak urine concentrations are approximately 1600 mcg. per ml. following a 250 mg. dose and 3200 mcg. per ml. following a 500 mg. dose.

Microbiology: *In vitro* tests demonstrate that the cephalosporins are bactericidal because of their inhibition of cell-wall synthesis. Cephradine is active against the following organisms *in vitro:*

- Beta-hemolytic streptococci
- Staphylococci, including coagulase-positive, coagulase-negative, and penicillinase-producing strains
- *Streptococcus pneumoniae* (formerly *D. pneumoniae*)
- *Escherichia coli*
- *Proteus mirabilis*
- *Klebsiella* sp.
- *Hemophilus influenzae*

Note—Some strains of enterococci (*Streptococcus faecalis*) are resistant to cephradine. It is not active against most strains of *Enterobacter* sp., *Pr. morganii*, and *Pr. vulgaris*. It has no activity against *Pseudomonas* or *Herellea* species. When tested by *in vitro* methods, staphylococci exhibit cross-resistance between cephradine and methicillin-type antibiotics.

Disc Susceptibility Tests: Quantitative methods that require measurement of zone diameters give the most precise estimates of antibiotic susceptibility. One recommended procedure (21 CFR § 460.1) uses cephalosporin class discs for testing susceptibility; interpretations correlate zone diameters of this disc test with MIC values for cephradine. With this procedure, a report from the laboratory of "resistant" indicates that the infecting organism is not likely to respond to therapy. A report of "intermediate susceptibility" suggests that the organism would be susceptible if the infection is confined to the urinary tract, as high antibiotic levels can be obtained in the urine, or if high dosage is used in other types of infection.

Indications: Anspor (cephradine, SK&F) Capsules and 'Anspor' for Oral Suspension are indicated in the treatment of the following infections when caused by susceptible strains of designated microorganisms:

Infections of the respiratory tract (e.g., tonsillitis, pharyngitis, and lobar pneumonia) caused by group A beta-hemolytic streptococci and *Streptococcus pneumoniae* (formerly *D. pneumoniae*).

(Penicillin is the usual drug of choice in the treatment and prevention of streptococcal infections, including the prophylaxis of rheumatic fever. 'Anspor' is generally effective in the eradication of streptococci from the nasopharynx; substantial data establishing the efficacy of 'Anspor' in the subsequent prevention of rheumatic fever are not available at present.)

Otitis media caused by group A beta-hemolytic streptococci, *Streptococcus pneumoniae* (formerly *D. pneumoniae*), *Hemophilus influenzae* and staphylococci.

Infections of the skin and soft tissues caused by staphylococci.

Infections of the urinary tract, including prostatitis, caused by *Escherichia coli, Pr. mirabilis,* and *Klebsiella* sp.

Note—Culture and susceptibility tests should be initiated prior to and during therapy. Renal function studies should be performed when indicated.

Contraindications: Cephradine is contraindicated in patients with known hypersensitivity to the cephalosporin group of antibiotics.

Warnings: BEFORE CEPHRADINE THERAPY IS INSTITUTED, CAREFUL INQUIRY SHOULD BE MADE CONCERNING PREVIOUS HYPERSENSITIVITY REACTIONS TO CEPHALOSPORINS AND PENICILLIN. CEPHALOSPORIN C DERIVATIVES SHOULD BE GIVEN CAUTIOUSLY IN PENICILLIN-SENSITIVE PATIENTS.

SERIOUS ACUTE HYPERSENSITIVITY REACTIONS MAY REQUIRE EPINEPHRINE AND OTHER EMERGENCY MEASURES.

There is some clinical and laboratory evidence of partial cross-allergenicity of the penicillins and the cephalosporins. Patients have been reported to have had severe reactions (including anaphylaxis) to both drugs.

Any patient who has demonstrated some form of allergy, particularly to drugs, should receive antibiotics cautiously. No exception should be made with regard to 'Anspor'.

Usage in Pregnancy and Lactation: Although no teratogenic or antifertility effects were seen in reproduction studies in mice and rats receiving up to four times the maximum human dose, the safety of this drug for use in human pregnancy has not been established. The benefits of the drug in pregnant women should be weighed against a possible risk to the fetus. Cephradine is secreted in breast milk during lactation.

Precautions: Patients should be followed carefully so that any side effects or unusual manifestations of drug idiosyncrasy may be detected. If a hypersensitivity reaction occurs, the drug should be discontinued and the patient treated with the usual agents, e.g., pressor amines, antihistamines, or corticosteroids.

Administer cephradine with caution in the presence of markedly impaired renal function. In patients with known or suspected renal impairment, careful clinical observation and appropriate laboratory studies should be made prior to and during therapy as cephradine accumulates in the serum and tissues. See DOSAGE AND ADMINISTRATION section for information on treatment of patients with impaired renal function.

Prolonged use of antibiotics may promote the overgrowth of nonsusceptible organisms. Should superinfection occur during therapy, appropriate measures should be taken.

After treatment with cephradine, a false positive reaction for glucose in the urine may occur with Benedict's solution, Fehling's solution, or with Clinitest® tablets, but not with enzyme-based tests such as Clinistix® and Tes-Tape®.

A false positive direct Coombs test has been reported after treatment with other cephalosporins; therefore, it should be recognized that a positive Coombs test may be due to the drug.

Indicated surgical procedures should be performed in conjunction with antibiotic therapy.

Adverse Reactions: As with other cephalosporins, untoward reactions are limited essentially to gastrointestinal disturbances and to hypersensitivity phenomena. The latter are more likely to occur in individuals who have previously demonstrated hypersensitivity and those with a history of allergy, asthma, hay fever, or urticaria.

The following adverse reactions have been reported following the use of cephradine:

Gastrointestinal: Glossitis, nausea, vomiting, diarrhea or loose stools, abdominal pain and heartburn were reported by some patients.

Skin and Hypersensitivity Reactions: Mild urticaria or skin rash, pruritus, and joint pains were reported by very few patients.

Blood: Mild, transient eosinophilia, leukopenia and neutropenia have been reported.

Liver: Transient mild rise of SGOT, SGPT, and total bilirubin has been observed with no evidence of hepatocellular damage.

Renal: Transitory rises in BUN have been observed in some patients treated with cephalosporins; their frequency increases in patients over 50 years old. In adults for whom serum creatinine determinations were performed, the rise in BUN was not accompanied by a rise in serum creatinine.

Other adverse reactions have included dizziness and tightness in the chest and candidal vaginitis.

Dosage and Administration: Anspor (cephradine, SK&F) may be given without regard to meals. **Adults:** For skin and soft-tissue and respiratory tract infections (other than lobar pneumonia), the usual dose is 250 mg. every 6 hours or 500 mg. every 12 hours. For acute infections of the urinary tract, including prostatitis, and pneumococcal lobar pneumonia, the usual dose is 500 mg. every 6 hours or 1 gram every 12 hours. Severe or chronic infections may require larger doses.

Children: No adequate information is available on the efficacy of b.i.d. regimens in children under nine months of age. The usual dose in children over nine months of age is 25 to 50 mg./kg./day administered in equally divided doses every 6 or 12 hours. For otitis media due to *H. influenzae*, doses are from 75 to 100 mg./kg./day administered in equally divided doses every 6 or 12 hours. The maximum dose should not exceed 4 grams per day.

All patients, regardless of age and weight: Larger doses (up to 1 gram, q.i.d.) may be given for severe or chronic infections.

As with antibiotic therapy generally, therapy should be continued for a minimum of 48 to 72 hours after the patient becomes asymptomatic or evidence of bacterial eradication has been obtained. In infections caused by group A beta-hemolytic streptococci, a minimum of 10 days of treatment is recommended to guard against the risk of rheumatic fever or glomerulonephritis. In the treatment of chronic urinary tract infection, frequent bacteriologic and clinical appraisal is necessary during therapy and may be necessary for several months afterwards. Persistent infections may require treatment for several weeks. Prolonged intensive therapy is recommended for prostatitis. Doses smaller than those indicated are not recommended. Doses for children should not exceed doses recommended for adults.

Patients with Impaired Renal Function

Not on Dialysis: The following initial dosage schedule is suggested as a guideline based on creatinine clearance. Further modification in the dosage schedule may be required because of individual variations in absorption.

Creatinine Clearance	Dose	Time Interval
>20 ml./min.	500 mg.	6 hours
5–20 ml./min.	250 mg.	6 hours
<5 ml./min.	250 mg.	12 hours

On Chronic, Intermittent Hemodialysis:
250 mg. Start
250 mg. at 12 hours
250 mg. 36–48 hours (after start)

Children may require dosage modification proportional to their weight and severity of infection.

How Supplied: Anspor (cephradine, SK&F) is available as 'Anspor' Capsules which provide 250 mg. or 500 mg. of cephradine. 'Anspor' is

Continued on next page

Smith Kline & French—Cont.

also available as 'Anspor' for Oral Suspension which, after reconstitution, provides 125 mg. or 250 mg. of cephradine per 5 ml. teaspoonful in a pleasant, fruit-flavored suspension.
Military—Capsules, 250 mg., 100's, 6505-01-009-9531.

[*Shown in Product Identification Section*]

BENZEDREX® INHALER ††
nasal decongestant

Composition: Each Benzedrex Inhaler is packed with propylhexedrine, 250 mg.; menthol, 12.5 mg.; and aromatics.
Action and Uses: It relieves—*in a matter of seconds*—the congestion of head colds and hay fever. Also useful for the relief of ear block and pressure pain in air travelers.
Benzedrex rarely causes undesirable stimulation or interferes with sleep.
Directions: Insert in nostril. Close other nostril. Inhale twice. Treat other nostril the same way. Avoid excessive use.
Inhaler loses potency after 2 or 3 months' use but some aroma may linger.
Warning: Keep this and all medicines out of reach of children. In the case of accidental overdose or ingestion of contents, seek professional assistance or contact a poison control center immediately.
How Supplied: In single plastic tubes.

††Benzedrex is a product of Menley & James Laboratories, Professional Products Division, a SmithKline company.

BENZEDRINE® Ⓒ
(brand of amphetamine sulfate)
SPANSULE® CAPSULES and TABLETS

Warning:

AMPHETAMINES HAVE A HIGH POTENTIAL FOR ABUSE. THEY SHOULD THUS BE TRIED ONLY IN WEIGHT REDUCTION PROGRAMS FOR PATIENTS IN WHOM ALTERNATIVE THERAPY HAS BEEN INEFFECTIVE. ADMINISTRATION OF AMPHETAMINES FOR PROLONGED PERIODS OF TIME IN OBESITY MAY LEAD TO DRUG DEPENDENCE AND MUST BE AVOIDED. PARTICULAR ATTENTION SHOULD BE PAID TO THE POSSIBILITY OF SUBJECTS OBTAINING AMPHETAMINES FOR NON-THERAPEUTIC USE OR DISTRIBUTION TO OTHERS, AND THE DRUGS SHOULD BE PRESCRIBED OR DISPENSED SPARINGLY.

Description: Benzedrine (amphetamine sulfate, SK&F) is a racemic mixture of the dextro and levo isomers of amphetamine sulfate, a sympathomimetic amine of the amphetamine group. Chemically, amphetamine is *dl*-alphamethylphenethylamine, and is present in all forms of 'Benzedrine' as the neutral sulfate.
Spansule® sustained release capsules—Each 'Spansule' sustained release capsule contains amphetamine sulfate, 15 mg., so prepared that an initial dose is released promptly and the remaining medication is released gradually over a prolonged period.
Tablets—Each tablet contains amphetamine sulfate, 5 mg. or 10 mg.
Actions: Amphetamines are sympathomimetic amines with CNS stimulant activity. Peripheral actions include elevation of systolic and diastolic blood pressures and weak bronchodilator and respiratory stimulant action.
There is neither specific evidence which clearly establishes the mechanism whereby amphetamines produce mental and behavioral effects in children, nor conclusive evidence regarding how these effects relate to the condition of the central nervous system.
Drugs of this class used in obesity are commonly known as "anorectics" or "anorexigenics." It has not been established, however, that the action of such drugs in treating obesity is primarily one of appetite suppression. Other central nervous system actions, or metabolic effects, may be involved, for example.
Adult obese subjects instructed in dietary management and treated with "anorectic" drugs lose more weight on the average than those treated with placebo and diet, as determined in relatively short-term clinical trials.
The magnitude of increased weight loss of drug-treated patients over placebo-treated patients is only a fraction of a pound a week. The rate of weight loss is greatest in the first weeks of therapy for both drug and placebo subjects and tends to decrease in succeeding weeks. The origins of the increased weight loss due to the various possible drug effects are not established. The amount of weight loss associated with the use of an "anorectic" drug varies from trial to trial, and the increased weight loss appears to be related in part to variables other than the drug prescribed, such as the physician-investigator, the population treated, and the diet prescribed. Studies do not permit conclusions as to the relative importance of the drug and nondrug factors on weight loss.
The natural history of obesity is measured in years, whereas the studies cited are restricted to a few weeks' duration; thus, the total impact of drug-induced weight loss over that of diet alone must be considered clinically limited.
'Benzedrine' *Spansule* capsules are formulated to release the active drug substance *in vivo* in a more gradual fashion than the standard formulation, as demonstrated by blood levels. The formulation has not been shown superior in effectiveness over the same dosage of the standard, noncontrolled-release formulations given in divided doses.
Indications: Benzedrine (amphetamine sulfate, SK&F) is indicated:
1. **In Narcolepsy.**
2. As an integral part of a total treatment program which typically includes other remedial measures (psychological, educational, social) for a stabilizing effect in children with a behavioral syndrome characterized by the following group of developmentally inappropriate symptoms: moderate to severe distractibility, short attention span, hyperactivity, emotional lability and impulsivity. The diagnosis of this syndrome should not be made with finality when these symptoms are only of comparatively recent origin. Nonlocalizing (soft) neurological signs, learning disability, and abnormal EEG may or may not be present, and a diagnosis of central nervous system dysfunction may or may not be warranted.
3. **In Exogenous Obesity,** as a short-term (a few weeks) adjunct in a regimen of weight reduction based on caloric restriction, for patients refractory to alternative therapy, e.g., repeated diets, group programs, and other drugs. The limited usefulness of amphetamines (see ACTIONS) should be weighed against possible risks inherent in use of the drug, such as those described below.

Contraindications: Advanced arteriosclerosis, symptomatic cardiovascular disease, moderate to severe hypertension, hyperthyroidism, known hypersensitivity or idiosyncrasy to the sympathomimetic amines, glaucoma.
Agitated states.
Patients with a history of drug abuse.
During or within 14 days following the administration of monoamine oxidase inhibitors (hypertensive crises may result).
Warnings: When tolerance to the "anorectic" effect develops, the recommended dose should not be exceeded in an attempt to increase the effect; rather, the drug should be discontinued.
Amphetamines may impair the ability of the patient to engage in potentially hazardous activities such as operating machinery or vehicles; the patient should therefore be cautioned accordingly.
Drug Dependence: Amphetamines have been extensively abused. Tolerance, extreme psychological dependence, and severe social disability have occurred. There are reports of patients who have increased the dosage to many times that recommended. Abrupt cessation following prolonged high dosage administration results in extreme fatigue and mental depression; changes are also noted on the sleep EEG.
Manifestations of chronic intoxication with amphetamines include severe dermatoses, marked insomnia, irritability, hyperactivity, and personality changes. The most severe manifestation of chronic intoxication is psychosis, often clinically indistinguishable from schizophrenia.
Usage in Pregnancy: Safe use in pregnancy has not been established. Reproduction studies in mammals at high multiples of the human dose have suggested both an embryotoxic and teratogenic potential. Use of amphetamines by women who are or who may become pregnant, and especially those in the first trimester of pregnancy, requires that the potential benefit be weighed against the possible hazard to mother and infant.
Usage in Children: Amphetamines are not recommended for use as anorectic agents in children under 12 years of age, or in children under 3 years of age with the behavioral syndrome described under INDICATIONS.
Clinical experience suggests that in psychotic children, administration of amphetamines may exacerbate symptoms of behavior disturbance and thought disorder.
Data are inadequate to determine whether chronic administration of amphetamines may be associated with growth inhibition; therefore, growth should be monitored during treatment.
Precautions: Caution is to be exercised in prescribing amphetamines for patients with even mild hypertension.
Insulin requirements in diabetes mellitus may be altered in association with the use of amphetamines and the concomitant dietary regimen.
Amphetamines may decrease the hypotensive effect of guanethidine.
The least amount feasible should be prescribed or dispensed at one time in order to minimize the possibility of overdosage.
Drug treatment is not indicated in all cases of the behavioral syndrome and should be considered only in light of the complete history and evaluation of the child. The decision to prescribe amphetamines should depend on the physician's assessment of the chronicity and severity of the child's symptoms and their appropriateness for his/her age. Prescription should not depend solely on the presence of one or more of the behavioral characteristics.
When these symptoms are associated with acute stress reactions, treatment with amphetamines is usually not indicated.
Long-term effects of amphetamines in children have not been well established.
Adverse Reactions: *Cardiovascular:* Palpitation, tachycardia, elevation of blood pressure. *Central nervous system:* Overstimulation, restlessness, dizziness, insomnia, euphoria, dysphoria, tremor, headache; rarely, psychotic episodes at recommended doses. *Gastrointestinal:* Dryness of the mouth, unpleasant taste, diarrhea, constipation, other gastrointestinal disturbances. Anorexia and weight loss may occur as undesirable effects when amphetamines are used for other than the anorectic effect. *Allergic:* Urticaria. *Endocrine:* Impotence, changes in libido.

Dosage and Administration: Regardless of indication, amphetamines should be administered at the lowest effective dosage and dosage should be individually adjusted. Late evening doses—particularly with the 'Spansule' capsule form—should be avoided because of the resulting insomnia.

Narcolepsy: Usual dose 5 to 60 milligrams per day in divided doses, depending on the individual patient response.

Narcolepsy seldom occurs in children under 12 years of age; however, when it does, Benzedrine (amphetamine sulfate, SK&F) may be used. The suggested initial dose for patients aged 6–12 is 5 mg. daily; daily dose may be raised in increments of 5 mg. at weekly intervals until optimal response is obtained. In patients 12 years of age and older, start with 10 mg. daily; daily dosage may be raised in increments of 10 mg. at weekly intervals until optimal response is obtained. If bothersome adverse reactions appear (e.g., insomnia or anorexia), dosage should be reduced. 'Spansule' capsules may be used for once-a-day dosage wherever appropriate. With tablets, give first dose on awakening; additional doses (1 or 2) at intervals of 4 to 6 hours.

Behavioral Syndrome in Children: Not recommended for children under 3 years of age.

In children from 3 to 5 years of age, start with 2.5 mg. daily; daily dosage may be raised in increments of 2.5 mg. at weekly intervals until optimal response is obtained.

In children 6 years of age and older, start with 5 mg. once or twice daily; daily dosage may be raised in increments of 5 mg. at weekly intervals until optimal response is obtained. Only in rare cases will it be necessary to exceed a total of 40 milligrams per day.

'Spansule' capsules may be used for once-a-day dosage wherever appropriate.

With tablets, give first dose on awakening; additional doses (1 or 2) at intervals of 4 to 6 hours.

Where possible, drug administration should be interrupted occasionally to determine if there is a recurrence of behavioral symptoms sufficient to require continued therapy.

Exogenous Obesity: Usual dosage is one 15 mg. 'Spansule' capsule—or 2 if required—daily, taken in the morning, or up to 30 mg. daily by tablets, taken in divided doses of 5 to 10 mg. 30 to 60 minutes before meals. Not recommended for this use in children under 12 years of age.

Overdosage: SYMPTOMS—Manifestations of acute overdosage with amphetamines include restlessness, tremor, hyperreflexia, rapid respiration, confusion, assaultiveness, hallucinations, panic states.

Fatigue and depression usually follow the central stimulation.

Cardiovascular effects include arrhythmias, hypertension or hypotension and circulatory collapse. Gastrointestinal symptoms include nausea, vomiting, diarrhea, and abdominal cramps. Fatal poisoning is usually preceded by convulsions and coma.

TREATMENT—Management of acute amphetamine intoxication is largely symptomatic and includes gastric lavage and sedation with a barbiturate. Experience with hemodialysis or peritoneal dialysis is inadequate to permit recommendation in this regard. Acidification of the urine increases amphetamine excretion. If acute, severe hypertension complicates amphetamine overdosage, administration of intravenous phentolamine (Regitine®, CIBA) has been suggested. However, a gradual drop in blood pressure will usually result when sufficient sedation has been achieved.

Since much of the 'Spansule' capsule medication is coated for gradual release, therapy directed at reversing the effects of the ingested drug and at supporting the patient should be continued for as long as overdosage symptoms remain. Saline cathartics are useful for hastening the evacuation of pellets that have not already released medication.

How Supplied: 'Spansule' capsules—15 mg., in bottles of 50. **Tablets**—5 mg. and 10 mg., in bottles of 100.

[*Shown in Product Identification Section*]

COMBID® SPANSULE® CAPSULES ℞

Description: Each 'Combid' *Spansule* capsule contains 10 mg. of prochlorperazine, as the maleate, and isopropamide iodide equivalent to 5 mg. of isopropamide.

The prochlorperazine component is so prepared that an initial dose is released promptly and the remaining medication is released gradually over a prolonged period. The isopropamide iodide component is not in sustained release form because it can provide 10 to 12 hours of antisecretory-antispasmodic action.

Actions: A single 'Combid' *Spansule* capsule b.i.d. (every 12 hours) can provide the following actions: (1) reduction of gastric secretion, (2) inhibition of spasm and motility, (3) relief of anxiety and tension, and (4) control of nausea and vomiting.

Indications

Based on a review of this drug by the National Academy of Sciences—National Research Council and/or other information, FDA has classified the indications as follows:

Possibly effective: As adjunctive therapy in peptic ulcer and in the irritable bowel syndrome (irritable colon, spastic colon, mucous colitis, functional gastrointestinal disorders); functional diarrhea.

Final classification of the less-than-effective indications requires further investigation.

Contraindications: Known hypersensitivity to prochlorperazine maleate and/or isopropamide iodide, existing drug-induced C.N.S. depression, glaucoma, pyloric obstruction, prostatic hypertrophy, bladder neck obstruction, obstructive intestinal lesions and/or ileus, bone marrow depression, jaundice, hepatic disease, blood dyscrasias.

Children under 12 years of age.

Because of the antiemetic action of the prochlorperazine component, 'Combid' *Spansule* capsules should not be used where nausea and vomiting are believed to be a manifestation of intestinal obstruction or brain tumor.

Warnings: Use cautiously in patients with a past history of jaundice, hepatic abnormality or blood dyscrasias. Because of possible additive effects, caution patients about concomitant use of alcohol and other C.N.S. depressants. Also, caution patients about activities requiring alertness (e.g., operating vehicles or machinery).

Usage in Pregnancy: Use of any drug in pregnancy, lactation, or in women who may bear children requires that the potential benefit of the drug be weighed against its possible hazards to the mother and child. As with all anticholinergic drugs, an inhibiting effect on lactation may occur.

Precautions: Patients who have shown a sensitivity reaction to other drugs may be more liable to have such a reaction to prochlorperazine. Use 'Combid' cautiously in elderly patients. Since the iodine in isopropamide iodide may alter PBI test results and will suppress I^{131} uptake, it is suggested that 'Combid' *Spansule* capsules be discontinued one week prior to these tests. Also, iodine skin rash may occur rarely.

Adverse Reactions:

Isopropamide Iodide: Xerostomia (dry mouth); urinary hesitancy and retention; tachycardia; palpitation; mydriasis (dilatation of the pupils); cycloplegia; blurred vision; constipation; bloated feeling; nausea; dysphagia; fever; nasal congestion.

Prochlorperazine or Other Phenothiazine Derivatives: Adverse reactions with different phenothiazines vary in type, frequency, and mechanism of occurrence, i.e., some are dose-related, while others involve individual patient sensitivity. Some adverse reactions may be more likely to occur, or occur with greater intensity, in patients with special medical problems, e.g., patients with mitral insufficiency or pheochromocytoma have experienced severe hypotension following recommended doses of certain phenothiazines.

Not all of the following adverse reactions have been observed with every phenothiazine derivative, but they have been reported with one or more and should be borne in mind when drugs of this class are administered.

Extrapyramidal symptoms (opisthotonos, oculogyric crisis, hyperreflexia, dystonia, akathisia, dyskinesia, pseudo-parkinsonism) have been reported. (These symptoms usually subside several hours after 'Combid' is discontinued; if troublesome to the patient, mild sedation or injectable 'Benadryl'* may be useful.)

As with all antipsychotic agents, persistent or tardive dyskinesia may appear after long-term therapy—especially in elderly female patients on high doses. Symptoms are persistent and in some patients irreversible. The syndrome is characterized by rhythmical involuntary movements of the tongue, face, mouth or jaw, sometimes accompanied by involuntary movements of extremities. Fine vermicular movements of the tongue may be an early sign; if these appear, discontinuation of medication is suggested.

Other adverse reactions include drowsiness; dizziness; grand mal convulsions; altered cerebrospinal fluid proteins; cerebral edema; intensification and prolongation of the action of central nervous system depressants (opiates, analgesics, antihistamines, barbiturates, alcohol), atropine, heat, organophosphorus insecticides; autonomic reactions (dryness of mouth, nasal congestion, headache, nausea, constipation, obstipation, adynamic ileus, inhibition of ejaculation); reactivation of psychotic processes, catatonic-like states; hypotension (sometimes fatal); cardiac arrest; blood dyscrasias (pancytopenia, thrombocytopenic purpura, leukopenia, agranulocytosis, eosinophilia); liver damage (jaundice, biliary stasis); endocrine disturbances (lactation, galactorrhea, gynecomastia, menstrual irregularities, false positive pregnancy tests); skin disorders (photosensitivity, itching, erythema, urticaria, eczema up to exfoliative dermatitis); other allergic reactions (asthma, laryngeal edema, angioneurotic edema, anaphylactoid reactions); peripheral edema; reversed epinephrine effect; hyperpyrexia; a systemic lupus erythematosus-like syndrome; pigmentary retinopathy; with prolonged administration of substantial doses, skin pigmentation, epithelial keratopathy, and lenticular and corneal deposits.

EKG changes—particularly nonspecific, usually reversible Q and T wave distortions—have been observed in some patients receiving phenothiazine tranquilizers. Their relationship to myocardial damage has not been confirmed.

Although phenothiazines cause neither psychic nor physical dependence, sudden discontinuance in long-term psychiatric patients may cause temporary symptoms, e.g., nausea and vomiting, dizziness, tremulousness.

Note: There have been occasional reports of sudden death in patients receiving phenothiazines. In some cases, the cause appeared to be asphyxia due to failure of the cough reflex. In others, the cause could not be determined. There is not sufficient evidence to establish a relationship between such deaths and the administration of phenothiazines.

Continued on next page

Smith Kline & French—Cont.

Dosage and Administration: *Adults and children over 12*—One 'Combid' *Spansule* capsule b.i.d. (every 12 hours). Some patients may require only one capsule every 24 hours (on arising). Only the exceptional patient will require two capsules in the morning and two at night.

Overdosage: (See also Adverse Reactions)
Symptoms of 'Combid' overdosage may be those of either isopropamide iodide or prochlorperazine overdosage.

Isopropamide Iodide: *Symptoms*—May include dryness of mouth, dysphagia, thirst, blurred vision, dilated pupils, photophobia, fever, rapid pulse and respiration, disorientation. Depression and circulatory collapse may result from severe overdosage.

Treatment—Gastric lavage, repeated several times.

Respiratory depression should be promptly treated by the use of oxygen and stimulants. If marked excitement is present, one of the short-acting barbiturates, chloral hydrate, or gas anesthesia may be used. Otherwise do not administer sedation. Hyperpyrexia may be treated with physical cooling measures. Force fluids by mouth or, if necessary, by intravenous administration.

While pilocarpine or similar drugs are sometimes recommended for the relief of dry mouth, many authorities feel that these drugs are not indicated, since they relieve the minor peripheral effect but do not influence the more serious central effects and, thus, may merely mask signs of drug activity. If photophobia occurs, the patient should be kept in a darkened room. It is not known whether isopropamide is dialyzable.

Prochlorperazine: *Symptoms*—Primarily involvement of the extrapyramidal mechanism producing some of the dystonic reactions described above.

Symptoms of central nervous system depression to the point of somnolence or coma. Agitation and restlessness may also occur. Other possible manifestations include convulsions, fever, and autonomic reactions such as hypotension, dry mouth and ileus.

Treatment—Essentially symptomatic and supportive. Early gastric lavage is helpful. Keep patient under observation and maintain an open airway, since involvement of extrapyramidal mechanism may produce dysphagia and respiratory difficulty in severe overdosage. **Do not attempt to induce emesis because a dystonic reaction of the head or neck may develop that could result in aspiration of vomitus.** Extrapyramidal symptoms may be treated with anti-parkinsonism drugs, barbiturates, or 'Benadryl'.

If administration of a stimulant is desirable, amphetamine, dextroamphetamine, or caffeine with sodium benzoate is recommended. Stimulants that may cause convulsions (e.g., picrotoxin or pentylenetetrazol) should be avoided.

If hypotension occurs, the standard measures for managing circulatory shock should be initiated. If it is desirable to administer a vasoconstrictor, 'Levophed' and 'Neo-Synephrine'† are most suitable. Other pressor agents, including epinephrine, are not recommended because phenothiazine derivatives may reverse the usual elevating action of these agents and cause a further lowering of blood pressure.

Limited experience indicates that phenothiazines are *not* dialyzable.

Special note on 'Spansule' capsules—Since much of the 'Spansule' capsule medication is coated for gradual release, therapy directed at reversing the effects of the ingested drugs and at supporting the patient should be continued for as long as overdosage symptoms remain. Saline cathartics are useful for hastening evacuation of pellets that have not already released medication.

How Supplied: In bottles of 50 and 500; in Single Unit Packages of 100 (intended for institutional use only).

Military—Capsules, 500's, 6505-00-935-9817

---

*Trademark Reg. U.S. Pat. Off.: 'Benadryl' for diphenhydramine hydrochloride, Parke-Davis.
†'Levophed' and 'Neo-Synephrine' are the trademarks (Reg. U.S. Pat. Off.) of Winthrop Laboratories for its brands of levarterenol and phenylephrine respectively.

[*Shown in Product Identification Section*]

COMPAZINE® ℞
(brand of prochlorperazine)

Description: Tablets—Each tablet contains 5 mg., 10 mg., or, for severe neuropsychiatric conditions, 25 mg. of prochlorperazine as the maleate.

Spansule® sustained release capsules—Each 'Spansule' capsule contains 10 mg., 15 mg., 30 mg., or, for severe neuropsychiatric conditions, 75 mg. of prochlorperazine as the maleate, so prepared that an initial dose is released promptly and the remaining medication is released gradually over a prolonged period. (In general, dosage recommendations for other oral forms of the drug may be applied to 'Spansule' capsules on the basis of the total daily dose in milligrams.)

Ampuls, 2 ml. (5 mg./ml.)—Each ml. contains, in aqueous solution, 5 mg. prochlorperazine as the edisylate, 1 mg. sodium sulfite, 1 mg. sodium bisulfite, 8 mg. sodium phosphate and 12 mg. sodium biphosphate.

Multiple-dose Vials, 10 ml. (5 mg./ml.)—Each ml. contains, in aqueous solution, 5 mg. prochlorperazine as the edisylate, 5 mg. sodium biphosphate, 12 mg. sodium tartrate, 0.9 mg. of sodium saccharin and 0.75% benzyl alcohol as preservative.

Disposable Syringes, 2 ml. (5 mg./ml.)—Each ml. contains, in aqueous solution, 5 mg. prochlorperazine as the edisylate, 5 mg. sodium biphosphate, 12 mg. sodium tartrate, 0.9 mg. sodium saccharin, and 0.75% benzyl alcohol as preservative.

Suppositories—Each suppository contains 2½ mg., 5 mg., or 25 mg. of prochlorperazine; with glycerin, glyceryl monopalmitate, glyceryl monostearate, hydrogenated cocoanut oil fatty acids and hydrogenated palm kernel oil fatty acids.

Syrup—Each 5 ml. (one teaspoonful) contains 5 mg. of prochlorperazine as the edisylate.

Concentrate (intended for institutional use only)—Each ml. contains 10 mg. of prochlorperazine as the edisylate.

N.B. The Concentrate dosage form is primarily for use in severe neuropsychiatric conditions when oral medication is preferred and other oral forms are considered impractical. The Concentrate is not intended for use in children.

Indications: Management of the manifestations of psychotic disorders; management of psychoneurotic patients displaying primarily symptoms of moderate to severe anxiety and tension; and for control of severe nausea and vomiting.

'Compazine' has not been shown effective in the management of behavioral complications in patients with mental retardation.

Contraindications: In comatose or greatly depressed states due to central nervous system depressants; and in the presence of bone marrow depression. Do not use in pediatric surgery.

Warnings: The extrapyramidal symptoms which can occur secondary to 'Compazine' may be confused with the central nervous system signs of an undiagnosed primary disease responsible for the vomiting, e.g., Reye's syndrome or other encephalopathy. The use of 'Compazine' and other potential hepatotoxins should be avoided in children and adolescents whose signs and symptoms suggest Reye's syndrome.

Patients who have demonstrated a hypersensitivity reaction (e.g., blood dyscrasias, jaundice) with a phenothiazine should not be re-exposed to any phenothiazine, including Compazine (prochlorperazine, SK&F), unless in the judgment of the physician the potential benefits of treatment outweigh the possible hazard.

'Compazine' may impair mental and/or physical abilities, especially during the first few days of therapy. Therefore, caution patients about activities requiring alertness (e.g., operating vehicles or machinery).

Phenothiazines may intensify or prolong the action of central nervous system depressants (e.g., alcohol, anesthetics, narcotics).

Usage in Pregnancy: Safety for the use of 'Compazine' during pregnancy has not been established. Therefore, it is recommended that the drug be given to pregnant patients only when, in the judgment of the physician, the potential benefits outweigh the possible hazards.

Precautions: The antiemetic action of 'Compazine' may mask the signs and symptoms of overdosage of other drugs and may obscure the diagnosis and treatment of other conditions such as intestinal obstruction, brain tumor, and Reye's syndrome (See WARNINGS).

Aspiration of vomitus has occurred in a few post-surgical patients who have received 'Compazine' as an antiemetic. Although no causal relationship has been established, this possibility should be borne in mind during surgical aftercare.

Deep sleep, from which patients can be aroused, and coma have been reported, usually with overdosage.

To lessen the likelihood of adverse reactions related to drug accumulation, patients on long-term therapy, particularly on high doses, should be evaluated periodically to decide whether the maintenance dosage could be lowered, or drug therapy could be discontinued.

Children with acute illnesses (e.g., chickenpox, C.N.S. infections, measles, gastroenteritis) or dehydration seem to be much more susceptible to neuromuscular reactions, particularly dystonias, than are adults. In such patients, the drug should be used only under close supervision.

Adverse Reactions: Drowsiness, dizziness, amenorrhea, blurred vision, skin reactions and hypotension may occur. Cholestatic jaundice, leukopenia and agranulocytosis have occurred. There have been a few observations of fatty changes in the livers of patients who have died while receiving the drug. No causal relationship has been established.

Neuromuscular (Extrapyramidal) Reactions
These symptoms are seen in a significant number of hospitalized mental patients. They may be characterized by motor restlessness, be of the dystonic type, or they may resemble parkinsonism.

Depending on the severity of symptoms, dosage should be reduced or discontinued. If therapy is reinstituted, it should be at a lower dosage. Should these symptoms occur in children or pregnant patients, the drug should be stopped and not reinstituted. In most cases barbiturates by suitable route of administration will suffice. (Or, injectable 'Benadryl'* may be useful.) In more severe cases, the administration of an anti-parkinsonism agent, except levodopa, usually produces rapid reversal of symptoms. Suitable supportive measures such as maintaining a clear airway and adequate hydration should be employed.

Motor Restlessness: Symptoms may include agitation or jitteriness and sometimes insomnia. These symptoms often disappear spontaneously. At times these symptoms may be similar to the original neurotic or psychotic symptoms. Dosage should not be increased until these side effects have subsided.

If this phase becomes too troublesome, the symptoms can usually be controlled by a reduction of dosage or concomitant administration of a barbiturate.

Dystonias: Symptoms may include: spasm of the neck muscles, sometimes progressing to torticollis; extensor rigidity of back muscles, sometimes progressing to opisthotonos; carpopedal spasm, trismus, swallowing difficulty, oculogyric crisis and protrusion of the tongue. These usually subside within a few hours, and almost always within 24 to 48 hours, after the drug has been discontinued.

In mild cases, reassurance or a barbiturate is often sufficient. *In moderate cases,* barbiturates will usually bring rapid relief. *In more severe adult cases,* the administration of an anti-parkinsonism agent, except levodopa, usually produces rapid reversal of symptoms. *In children,* reassurance and barbiturates will usually control symptoms. (Or, injectable 'Benadryl' may be useful.)

Pseudo-parkinsonism: Symptoms may include: mask-like facies; drooling; tremors; pillrolling motion; cogwheel rigidity; and shuffling gait. Reassurance and sedation are important. In most cases these symptoms are readily controlled when an anti-parkinsonism agent is administered concomitantly. Anti-parkinsonism agents should be used only when required. Generally, therapy of a few weeks to two or three months will suffice. After this time patients should be evaluated to determine their need for continued treatment. (Note: Levodopa has not been found effective in pseudo-parkinsonism.) Occasionally it is necessary to lower the dosage of 'Compazine' or to discontinue the drug.

Persistent Tardive Dyskinesia: As with all antipsychotic agents, tardive dyskinesia may appear in some patients on long-term therapy or may appear after drug therapy has been discontinued. The risk appears to be greater in elderly patients on high-dose therapy, especially females. The symptoms are persistent and in some patients appear to be irreversible. The syndrome is characterized by rhythmical involuntary movements of the tongue, face, mouth or jaw (e.g., protrusion of tongue, puffing of cheeks, puckering of mouth, chewing movements). Sometimes these may be accompanied by involuntary movements of extremities.

There is no known effective treatment for tardive dyskinesia; anti-parkinsonism agents do not alleviate the symptoms of this syndrome. It is suggested that all antipsychotic agents be discontinued if these symptoms appear. Should it be necessary to reinstitute treatment, or increase the dosage of the agent, or switch to a different antipsychotic agent, the syndrome may be masked.

It has been reported that fine vermicular movements of the tongue may be an early sign of the syndrome and if the medication is stopped at that time the syndrome may not develop.

Contact Dermatitis: Avoid getting the Concentrate and Injection solutions on hands or clothing because of the possibility of contact dermatitis.

Adverse Reactions Reported with Compazine (prochlorperazine, SK&F) or Other Phenothiazine Derivatives: Adverse reactions with different phenothiazines vary in type, frequency, and mechanism of occurrence, i.e., some are dose-related, while others involve individual patient sensitivity. Some adverse reactions may be more likely to occur, or occur with greater intensity, in patients with special medical problems, e.g., patients with mitral insufficiency or pheochromocytoma have experienced severe hypotension following recommended doses of certain phenothiazines.

Not all of the following adverse reactions have been observed with every phenothiazine derivative, but they have been reported with one or more and should be borne in mind when drugs of this class are administered: extrapyramidal symptoms (opisthotonos, oculogyric crisis, hyperreflexia, dystonia, akathisia, dyskinesia, parkinsonism) some of which have lasted months and even years—particularly in elderly patients with previous brain damage; grand mal convulsions; altered cerebrospinal fluid proteins; cerebral edema; intensification and prolongation of the action of central nervous system depressants (opiates, analgesics, antihistamines, barbiturates, alcohol), atropine, heat, organophosphorus insecticides; autonomic reactions (dryness of mouth, nasal congestion, headache, nausea, constipation, obstipation, adynamic ileus, inhibition of ejaculation); reactivation of psychotic processes, catatonic-like states; hypotension (sometimes fatal); cardiac arrest; blood dyscrasias (pancytopenia, thrombocytopenic purpura, leukopenia, agranulocytosis, eosinophilia); liver damage (jaundice, biliary stasis); endocrine disturbances (lactation, galactorrhea, gynecomastia, menstrual irregularities, false positive pregnancy tests); skin disorders (photosensitivity, itching, erythema, urticaria, eczema up to exfoliative dermatitis); other allergic reactions (asthma, laryngeal edema, angioneurotic edema, anaphylactoid reactions); peripheral edema; reversed epinephrine effect; hyperpyrexia; a systemic lupus erythematosus-like syndrome; pigmentary retinopathy; with prolonged administration of substantial doses, skin pigmentation, epithelial keratopathy, and lenticular and corneal deposits.

EKG changes—particularly nonspecific, usually reversible Q and T wave distortions—have been observed in some patients receiving phenothiazine tranquilizers. Their relationship to myocardial damage has not been confirmed.

Although phenothiazines cause neither psychic nor physical dependence, sudden discontinuance in long-term psychiatric patients may cause temporary symptoms, e.g., nausea and vomiting, dizziness, tremulousness.

Note: There have been occasional reports of sudden death in patients receiving phenothiazines. In some cases, the cause appeared to be asphyxia due to failure of the cough reflex. In others, the cause could not be determined. There is not sufficient evidence to establish a relationship between such deaths and the administration of phenothiazines.

Dosage and Administration: Note on Injection: It is recommended that Compazine (prochlorperazine, SK&F) Injection not be mixed with other agents in the syringe. This solution should be protected from light. Slight yellowish discoloration will not alter potency. If markedly discolored, solution should be discarded.

Note on Concentrate: When the Concentrate is to be used, add the desired dosage of Concentrate to 60 ml. (2 fl. oz.) or more of diluent *just prior to administration.* This will insure palatability and stability. Vehicles suggested for dilution are: tomato or fruit juice, milk, simple syrup, orange syrup, carbonated beverages, coffee, tea, or water. Semisolid foods (soups, puddings, etc.) may also be used. The Concentrate is light sensitive; it should be protected from light and dispensed in amber bottles. *Refrigeration is not required.*

Dosage and Administration—Adults:
(For children's dosage and administration, see below.) Dosage should be increased more gradually in debilitated or emaciated patients.

Elderly Patients: In general, dosages in the lower range are sufficient for most elderly patients. Since they appear to be more susceptible to hypotension and neuromuscular reactions, such patients should be observed closely. Dosage should be tailored to the individual, response carefully monitored, and dosage adjusted accordingly. Dosage should be increased more gradually in elderly patients.

1. To Control Severe Nausea and Vomiting or to Control Excessive Anxiety: Adjust dosage to the response of the individual. Begin with the lowest recommended dosage.

Oral Dosage: Usually 5 or 10 mg. 3 or 4 times daily; by 'Spansule' capsule, usually one 15 mg. capsule on arising or one 10 mg. capsule q12h.

Rectal Dosage: 25 mg. twice daily.

I.M. Dosage: Initially 5 to 10 mg. (1-2 ml.) injected *deeply* into the upper outer quadrant of the buttock. If necessary, repeat every 3 or 4 hours. Total I.M. dosage should not exceed 40 mg. per day.

Subcutaneous administration is not advisable because of local irritation.

2. Adult Surgery (for severe nausea and vomiting): Total parenteral dosage should not exceed 40 mg. per day. Hypotension is a possibility if the drug is given by I.V. injection or infusion.

I.M. Dosage: 5 to 10 mg. (1-2 ml.) 1 to 2 hours before induction of anesthesia (repeat once in 30 minutes, if necessary), or to control acute symptoms during and after surgery (repeat once if necessary).

I.V. Injection: 5 to 10 mg. (1-2 ml.) 15 to 30 minutes before induction of anesthesia, or to control acute symptoms during or after surgery. Repeat once if necessary.

I.V. Infusion: 20 mg. (4 ml.) per liter of isotonic solution. Add to I.V. infusion 15 to 30 minutes before induction.

3. In Adult Psychiatry: Adjust dosage to the response of the individual and according to the severity of the condition. Begin with the lowest recommended dose. Although response ordinarily is seen within a day or two, longer treatment is usually required before maximal improvement is seen.

Oral Dosage: *In relatively mild conditions,* as seen in private psychiatric practice or in outpatient clinics, dosage is 5 or 10 mg. 3 or 4 times daily.

In moderate to severe conditions, for hospitalized or adequately supervised patients, usual starting dosage is 10 mg. 3 or 4 times daily. Increase dosage gradually until symptoms are controlled or side effects become bothersome. When dosage is increased by small increments every 2 or 3 days, side effects either do not occur or are easily controlled. Some patients respond satisfactorily on 50 to 75 mg. daily.

In more severe disturbances, optimum dosage is usually 100 to 150 mg. daily.

I.M. Dosage: For immediate control of severely disturbed adults, inject an initial dose of 10 to 20 mg. (2-4 ml.) *deeply* into the upper outer quadrant of the buttock. Many patients respond shortly after the first injection. If necessary, however, repeat the initial dose every 2 to 4 hours (or, in resistant cases, every hour) to gain control of the patient. More than 3 or 4 doses are seldom necessary. After control is achieved, switch patient to an oral form of the drug at the same dosage level or higher. If, in rare cases, parenteral therapy is needed for a prolonged period, give 10 to 20 mg. (2-4 ml.) every 4 to 6 hours. Pain and irritation at the site of injection have seldom occurred.

Subcutaneous administration is not advisable because of local irritation.

Dosage and Administration—Children:
Do not use in pediatric surgery.

Children seem more prone to develop extrapyramidal reactions, even on moderate doses. Therefore, use lowest effective dosage. Tell parents not to exceed prescribed dosage, since the possibility of adverse reactions increases as dosage rises.

Occasionally the patient may react to the drug with signs of restlessness and excitement; if this occurs, do not administer additional doses. Take particular precaution in administering the drug to children with acute illnesses or dehydration (see under Dystonias).

When writing a prescription for the $2\frac{1}{2}$ mg. size suppository, write "$2\frac{1}{2}$," not "2.5"; this

Continued on next page

Smith Kline & French—Cont.

will help avoid confusion with the 25 mg. adult size.

1. Severe Nausea and Vomiting in Children: 'Compazine' should generally not be used in children under 20 pounds in weight or two years of age. It should not be used in conditions for which children's dosages have not been established. Dosage and frequency of administration should be adjusted according to the severity of the symptoms and the response of the patient. The duration of activity following intramuscular administration may last up to 12 hours. Subsequent doses may be given by the same route if necessary.

Oral or Rectal Dosage: More than one day's therapy is seldom necessary.

Weight	Usual Dosage	Not to Exceed
under 20 lbs.	not recommended	
20-29 lbs.	2½ mg. 1 or 2 times a day	7.5 mg. per day
30-39 lbs.	2½ mg. 2 or 3 times a day	10 mg. per day
40-85 lbs.	2½ mg. 3 times a day or 5 mg. 2 times a day	15 mg. per day

I.M. Dosage: Calculate each dose on the basis of 0.06 mg. of the drug per lb. of body weight; give by deep I.M. injection. Control is usually obtained with one dose.

2. In Child Psychiatry:

Oral or Rectal Dosage: For children 2 to 12 years, starting dosage is 2½ mg. 2 or 3 times daily. Do not give more than 10 mg. the first day. Then increase dosage according to patient's response.

FOR AGES 2-5, total daily dosage usually does not exceed 20 mg.

FOR AGES 6-12, total daily dosage usually does not exceed 25 mg.

I.M. Dosage: For ages under 12, calculate each dose on the basis of 0.06 mg. of Compazine (prochlorperazine, SK&F) per lb. of body weight; give by deep I.M. injection. Control is usually obtained with one dose. After control is achieved, switch the patient to an oral form of the drug at the same dosage level or higher.

Overdosage: (See also Adverse Reactions.)

Symptoms—Primarily involvement of the extrapyramidal mechanism producing some of the dystonic reactions described above.

Symptoms of central nervous system depression to the point of somnolence or coma. Agitation and restlessness may also occur. Other possible manifestations include convulsions, fever, and autonomic reactions such as hypotension, dry mouth and ileus.

Treatment—Essentially symptomatic and supportive. Early gastric lavage is helpful. Keep patient under observation and maintain an open airway, since involvement of the extrapyramidal mechanism may produce dysphagia and respiratory difficulty in severe overdosage. **Do not attempt to induce emesis because a dystonic reaction of the head or neck may develop that could result in aspiration of vomitus.** Extrapyramidal symptoms may be treated with anti-parkinsonism drugs, barbiturates, or 'Benadryl'.

If administration of a stimulant is desirable, amphetamine, dextroamphetamine, or caffeine with sodium benzoate is recommended. Stimulants that may cause convulsions (e.g., picrotoxin or pentylenetetrazol) should be avoided.

If hypotension occurs, the standard measures for managing circulatory shock should be initiated. If it is desirable to administer a vasoconstrictor, 'Levophed' and 'Neo-Synephrine'† are most suitable. Other pressor agents, including epinephrine, are not recommended because phenothiazine derivatives may reverse the usual elevating action of these agents and cause a further lowering of blood pressure. Limited experience indicates that phenothiazines are *not* dialyzable.

Special note on 'Spansule' capsules—Since much of the 'Spansule' capsule medication is coated for gradual release, therapy directed at reversing the effects of the ingested drug and at supporting the patient should be continued for as long as overdosage symptoms remain. Saline cathartics are useful for hastening evacuation of pellets that have not already released medication.

How Supplied: Tablets—5 and 10 mg., in bottles of 100 and 1000; in Single Unit Packages of 100 (intended for institutional use only). For use in severe neuropsychiatric conditions, 25 mg., in bottles of 100 and 1000.

'Spansule' capsules—10, 15 and 30 mg., in bottles of 50 and 500; in Single Unit Packages of 100 (intended for institutional use only). For use in severe neuropsychiatric conditions, 75 mg., in bottles of 50. **Ampuls**—2 ml. (5 mg./ml.), in boxes of 10, 100 and 500. **Multiple-dose Vials**—10 ml. (5 mg./ml.), in boxes of 1, 20 and 100.

Disposable Syringes—2 ml. (5 mg./ml.), individually packaged in boxes of 10 and 100.

Suppositories—2½ mg. (for young children), 5 mg. (for older children) and 25 mg. (for adults), in boxes of 12. **Syrup**—5 mg./teaspoonful (5 ml.), in 4 fl. oz. bottles. **Concentrate** (intended for institutional use only)—10 mg./ml., in 4 fl. oz. bottles, and in cartons of 36 bottles.

Military—Injection 2 ml., 100's, 6505-00-656-1610; Suppositories 2½ mg., 12's, 6505-00-133-5213; 25 mg., 12's, 6505-00-133-5214; Tablets 5 mg., 1000's, 6505-00-022-1328, and S.U.P. 100's 6505-00-118-2563; 10 mg., 1000's, 6505-00-022-1329.

*Trademark Reg. U.S. Pat. Off.: 'Benadryl' for diphenhydramine hydrochloride, Parke-Davis.

†'Levophed' and 'Neo-Synephrine' are the trademarks (Reg. U.S. Pat. Off.) of Winthrop Laboratories for its brands of levarterenol and phenylephrine respectively.

[*Shown in Product Identification Section*]

CYTOMEL® TABLETS ℞
(brand of liothyronine sodium)
[L-triiodothyronine]

Description: 'Cytomel' contains liothyronine (L-triiodothyronine or LT_3) as the sodium salt. 25 mcg. of liothyronine is equivalent to approximately 1 grain of desiccated thyroid or thyroglobulin and 0.1 mg. of L-thyroxine.

Actions: 'Cytomel' contains liothyronine sodium, a synthetic form of a natural thyroid hormone, with all pharmacologic activities of the natural substance. Thyroid hormone acts to promote the synthesis of protein. It increases the metabolic rate of the body, presumably by, among other things, increasing oxygen consumption, altering enzymes (particularly those that affect growth), and altering the permeability of the mitochondrial membranes of cells.

Since liothyronine sodium is not firmly bound to serum protein, 'Cytomel' is readily available to body tissues. Following oral administration, about 85% of the dose is absorbed from the gastrointestinal tract. The onset of activity of liothyronine sodium is rapid, occurring within a few hours. Maximum pharmacologic response occurs within two or three days, providing early clinical response. The biological half-life is about 2½ days. The drug has a rapid cutoff of activity which permits quick dosage adjustment and facilitates control of the effects of overdosage, should they occur.

'Cytomel' can be used in patients allergic to desiccated thyroid or thyroid extract derived from pork or beef.

Indications:

1. Cytomel (liothyronine sodium, SK&F) is indicated for thyroid replacement in patients with inadequate endogenous thyroid hormone production. These include mild hypofunction, cretinism, and myxedema. Replacement therapy will be effective only in manifestations of hypothyroidism.
2. Simple (non-toxic) goiter: 'Cytomel' may be used therapeutically in an attempt to reduce the size of such a goiter.
3. For use in the T_3 suppression test to differentiate suspected *hyper*thyroidism from euthyroidism. (See special instructions under Dosage and Administration.)

Contraindication: Uncorrected adrenal insufficiency.

Warnings:

> Drugs with thyroid hormone activity, alone or together with other therapeutic agents, have been used for the treatment of obesity. In euthyroid patients, doses within the range of daily hormonal requirements are ineffective for weight reduction. Larger doses may produce serious or even life-threatening manifestations of toxicity, particularly when given in association with sympathomimetic amines such as those used for their anorectic effects.

Cytomel (liothyronine sodium, SK&F) should not be used in the presence of cardiovascular disease unless thyroid-replacement therapy is clearly indicated. In such cases, it should be used with caution and initiated at a low dosage, with due consideration for its relatively rapid onset of action. Starting dosage is 5 mcg. daily, and should be increased by no more than 5 mcg. increments at two-week intervals.

Morphologic hypogonadism and nephrosis should be ruled out before the drug is administered. If hypopituitarism is present, the adrenal deficiency must be corrected prior to starting the drug.

Myxedematous patients are very sensitive to thyroid; dosage should be started at a very low level and increased gradually.

Severe and prolonged hypothyroidism can lead to a decreased level of adrenocortical activity commensurate with the lowered metabolic state. When thyroid-replacement therapy is administered, the metabolism increases at a greater rate than adrenocortical activity. This can precipitate adrenocortical insufficiency. Therefore, in severe and prolonged hypothyroidism, supplemental adrenocortical steroids may be necessary.

In rare instances the administration of thyroid hormone may precipitate a hyperthyroid state or may aggravate existing hyperthyroidism.

Precautions: Since liothyronine sodium is not as firmly bound to serum protein as thyroxine, the PBI usually remains at levels below normal during full replacement therapy using Cytomel (liothyronine sodium, SK&F).

As with all thyroid preparations, thyroid gland function reflected by ^{131}I thyroid uptake may be depressed by 'Cytomel', particularly when dosage exceeds 75 mcg. daily. This effect disappears rapidly, and useful ^{131}I thyroid uptake values may be obtained usually within two weeks following discontinuance of the drug.

Adverse Reactions: Overdosage will produce signs and symptoms of hyperthyroidism, such as nervousness, cardiac arrhythmias, angina pectoris, and menstrual irregularities. (See Overdosage section.) Medication should be interrupted until symptoms disappear, then resumed in smaller doses. Therapy can usually be resumed after one or two days.

In rare instances, allergic skin reactions have been reported.

Dosage and Administration: Optimum dosage is usually determined by the patient's clinical response. Confirmatory tests include: Radioactive Iodine T_3 Resin Uptake, BMR, Thyro Binding Index (TBI), and the Achilles Tendon Reflex test.

Once-a-day dosage is recommended; although Cytomel (liothyronine sodium, SK&F) has a rapid cutoff, its metabolic effects persist for a few days following discontinuance.

Mild Hypothyroidism: Recommended starting dosage is 25 mcg. daily. Daily dosage then may be increased by 12.5 or 25 mcg. every one or two weeks. Usual maintenance dose is 25–75 mcg. daily. Smaller doses may be fully effective in some patients, while dosage of 100 mcg. daily may be required in others.

Myxedema: Recommended starting dosage is 5 mcg. daily. This may be increased by 5 to 10 mcg. daily every one or two weeks. When 25 mcg. daily is reached, dosage may often be increased by 12.5 or 25 mcg. every one or two weeks. Usual maintenance dose is 50 to 100 mcg. daily.

Cretinism: Since the mother provides little or no thyroid hormone to the fetus, infants with thyroid dysfunction will require replacement therapy from birth. Treatment should be initiated as early as possible to avoid permanent physical and mental changes.

Recommended starting dosage is 5 mcg. daily, with a 5 mcg. increment every three to four days until the desired response is achieved. Infants a few months old may require only 20 mcg. daily for maintenance. At 1 year, 50 mcg. daily may be required. Above 3 years, full adult dosage may be necessary.

Simple (non-toxic) goiter: Recommended starting dosage is 5 mcg. daily. This dosage may be increased by 5 to 10 mcg. daily every one or two weeks. When 25 mcg. daily is reached, dosage may be increased every week or two by 12.5 or 25 mcg. Usual maintenance dosage is 75 mcg. daily.

In the elderly or in children, therapy should be started with 5 mcg. daily and increased only by 5 mcg. increments at the recommended intervals.

When switching a patient to 'Cytomel' from thyroid, L-thyroxine or thyroglobulin, discontinue the other medication, initiate 'Cytomel' at a low dosage, and increase gradually according to the patient's response. When selecting a starting dosage, bear in mind that this drug has a rapid onset of action, and that residual effects of the other thyroid preparation may persist for the first several weeks of therapy.

Special Instructions for T_3 Suppression Test: When ^{131}I Thyroid Uptake is in the borderline-high range, administer 75-100 mcg. of Cytomel (liothyronine sodium, SK&F) daily for 7 days, then repeat ^{131}I Thyroid Uptake test. In the hyperthyroid patient, 24-hour ^{131}I Thyroid Uptake will not be affected significantly. In the euthyroid patient, 24-hour ^{131}I Thyroid Uptake will drop to less than 20%.

Overdosage: *Symptoms*—Headache, irritability, nervousness, sweating, tachycardia, increased bowel motility, and menstrual irregularities. Angina pectoris or congestive heart failure may be induced or aggravated. Shock may also develop. Massive overdosage may result in symptoms resembling thyroid storm. Chronic excessive dosage will produce the signs and symptoms of hyperthyroidism. *Treatment*—In shock, supportive measures and treatment of unrecognized adrenal insufficiency should be considered.

How Supplied: In three dosage strengths: 5 mcg. tablets in bottles of 100; 25 mcg. tablets (scored) in bottles of 100 and 1000; and 50 mcg. tablets (scored) in bottles of 100.

Military—Tablets 5 mcg., 100's, 6505-00-660-1609; 25 mcg., 1000's, 6505-00-066-4875.

[*Shown in Product Identification Section*]

DARBID® TABLETS, 5 mg. ℞
(brand of isopropamide iodide)

Description: Each tablet contains isopropamide iodide equivalent to 5 mg. of isopropamide.

Chemically, Darbid (isopropamide iodide, SK&F) is 3-carbamoyl-3, 3-diphenylpropyl) diisopropylmethyl ammonium iodide.

Actions: Darbid (isopropamide iodide, SK&F) is a synthetic anticholinergic that produces 10- to 12-hour gastric acid antisecretory effect and gastrointestinal antispasmodic response in man.

Indications

Based on a review of this drug by the National Academy of Sciences—National Research Council and/or other information, FDA has classified the indications as follows:

Effective: As adjunctive therapy in peptic ulcer.

Probably effective: In the irritable bowel syndrome (irritable colon, spastic colon, mucous colitis, acute enterocolitis, and functional gastrointestinal disorders).

Final classification of the less-than-effective indications requires further investigation.

IT SHOULD BE NOTED AT THIS POINT IN TIME THAT THERE IS A LACK OF CONCURRENCE AS TO THE VALUE OF ANTICHOLINERGICS IN THE TREATMENT OF GASTRIC ULCER. IT HAS NOT BEEN SHOWN CONCLUSIVELY WHETHER ANTICHOLINERGIC DRUGS AID IN THE HEALING OF A PEPTIC ULCER, DECREASE THE RATE OF RECURRENCES, OR PREVENT COMPLICATION.

FUNCTIONAL DISORDERS ARE OFTEN RELIEVED BY VARYING COMBINATIONS OF SEDATIVES, REASSURANCE, PHYSICIAN INTEREST, AMELIORATION OF ENVIRONMENTAL FACTORS, ETC.

To be effective, dosage must be titrated to the individual patient's needs.

Contraindications: Glaucoma; obstructive uropathy (e.g., bladder neck obstruction due to prostatic hypertrophy); obstructive disease of the gastrointestinal tract (as in achalasia, pyloroduodenal stenosis, etc.); obstructive or paralytic ileus, intestinal atony of the elderly or debilitated patient; unstable cardiovascular status in acute hemorrhage; severe ulcerative colitis; toxic megacolon complicating ulcerative colitis; myasthenia gravis.

Warnings: In the presence of a high environmental temperature, heat prostration (fever and heat stroke due to decreased sweating) can occur.

In patients with diarrhea due to incomplete intestinal obstruction (especially those with ileostomy or colostomy), treatment with Darbid (isopropamide iodide, SK&F) would be inappropriate and possibly harmful.

'Darbid' may produce drowsiness or blurred vision. In this event, the patient should be warned not to engage in activities requiring mental alertness such as operating a motor vehicle or other machinery or perform hazardous work while taking this drug.

Usage in Pregnancy: In pregnancy, lactation, and in women who may bear children, the potential benefits of the drug must be weighed against possible hazards.

Precautions: Use cautiously in elderly patients.

Since the iodine in isopropamide iodide may alter PBI test results and will suppress I^{131} uptake, it is suggested that therapy be discontinued one week prior to these tests. Also, iodine skin rash may occur rarely.

Use with caution in patients with:

Autonomic neuropathy.

Hepatic or renal disease.

Ulcerative colitis (large doses may suppress intestinal motility to the point of producing paralytic ileus, and the use of this drug may precipitate or aggravate the serious complication of toxic megacolon).

Hyperthyroidism, coronary heart disease, congestive heart failure, cardiac arrhythmia, hypertension and nonobstructing prostatic hypertrophy.

Hiatal hernia associated with reflux esophagitis (anticholinergic drugs may aggravate this condition).

It should be noted that the use of anticholinergic drugs in the treatment of gastric ulcer may produce a delay in gastric emptying time (antral stasis) and, thus, complicate therapy.

Do not rely on the use of the drug in the presence of complication of biliary tract disease.

Investigate any tachycardia before giving anticholinergic (atropine-like) drugs, since they may increase the heart rate.

With overdosage, a curare-like action may occur.

Adverse Reactions: Anticholinergics produce certain pharmacological effects which may be desirable or undesirable, depending upon the individual patient's response. The physician must delineate these.

Adverse reactions which have occurred with Darbid (isopropamide iodide, SK&F) include: xerostomia (dry mouth); urinary hesitancy and retention; blurred vision; tachycardia; palpitations; mydriasis (dilatation of the pupils); cycloplegia; constipation; bloated feeling; nausea; dysphagia; fever; and nasal congestion.

Other adverse reactions possible with anticholinergics include: increased ocular tension; loss of taste; headaches; nervousness; drowsiness; weakness; dizziness; insomnia; vomiting; impotence; suppression of lactation; severe allergic reaction or drug idiosyncrasies including anaphylaxis; urticaria and other dermal manifestations; some degree of mental confusion and/or excitement, especially in elderly persons.

Decreased sweating may occur. It should be noted that adrenergic innervation of the eccrine sweat glands on the palms and soles makes complete control of sweating impossible. An end point of complete anhidrosis cannot occur because large doses of drug would be required, and this would produce severe side effects from parasympathetic paralysis.

Dosage and Administration: Not for use in children under 12. Adults and children over 12—Usual starting dose is one 5 mg. tablet b.i.d. (every 12 hours). Patients with severe symptoms may require two 5 mg. tablets b.i.d., or more. Dosage should be individualized and titrated to the patient's need for greatest therapeutic effect.

Overdosage: Involves the cardiovascular, respiratory, gastrointestinal, central and peripheral nervous systems.

SYMPTOMS—May include dryness of mouth, dysphagia, thirst, blurred vision, dilated pupils, photophobia, fever, rapid pulse and respiration, disorientation. Depression and circulatory collapse may result from severe overdosage. TREATMENT—Gastric lavage, repeated several times.

Respiratory depression should be promptly treated by the use of oxygen and stimulants. If marked excitement is present, one of the short-acting barbiturates, chloral hydrate, or gas anesthesia may be used. Otherwise do not administer sedation. Hyperpyrexia may be treated with physical cooling measures. Force fluids by mouth or, if necessary, by intravenous administration.

While pilocarpine or similar drugs are sometimes recommended for the relief of dry mouth, many authorities feel that these drugs are not

Continued on next page

Smith Kline & French—Cont.

indicated, since they relieve the minor peripheral effect but do not influence the more serious central effects and, thus, may merely mask signs of drug activity. If photophobia occurs, the patient should be kept in a darkened room.
How Supplied: In bottles of 50.
[*Shown in Product Identification Section*]

DEXAMYL® SPANSULE® CAPSULES and TABLETS ©

Amphetamines have a significant potential for abuse. In view of their short-term anorectic effect and rapid development of tolerance, they should be used with extreme caution and only for limited periods of time in weight-reduction programs.

Description: 'Dexamyl' contains dextroamphetamine sulfate and amobarbital. Dextroamphetamine sulfate is the dextro isomer of the compound *d, l*-amphetamine sulfate, a sympathomimetic amine of the amphetamine group. Chemically, dextroamphetamine is *d*-alpha-methylphenethylamine, and is present as the neutral sulfate. Amobarbital is 5-ethyl-5-isopentylbarbituric acid [Warning, may be habit forming].

Spansule® sustained release capsules—Each 'Spansule' capsule No. 2 (standard strength) contains 15 mg. of dextroamphetamine sulfate and 1½ gr. (97 mg.) of amobarbital, derivative of barbituric acid [Warning, may be habit forming]. Each 'Spansule' capsule No. 1 (lower strength) contains 10 mg. of dextroamphetamine sulfate and 1 gr. (65 mg.) of amobarbital [Warning, may be habit forming]. Both strengths are so prepared that an initial dose is released promptly and the remaining medication is released gradually over a prolonged period.

Tablets—Each tablet contains 5 mg. of dextroamphetamine sulfate and ½ gr. (32 mg.) of amobarbital [Warning, may be habit forming].

Actions: Dextroamphetamine sulfate is a sympathomimetic amine with CNS stimulant activity. Peripheral actions include elevation of systolic and diastolic blood pressures and weak bronchodilator and respiratory stimulant action. The anorectic effect diminishes after a few weeks. Amobarbital, a derivative of barbituric acid, reduces the possibility of wakefulness and excitation which may occur in some patients on dextroamphetamine sulfate alone. The 'Spansule' capsule dosage form provides the convenience of once-a-day dosage.

Indications: Exogenous obesity, as a short-term (a few weeks) adjunct in a regimen of weight reduction based on caloric restriction.[1,2,3]

Contraindications: Advanced arteriosclerosis, symptomatic cardiovascular disease, moderate to severe hypertension, hyperthyroidism, known hypersensitivity or idiosyncrasy to the sympathomimetic amines.
Agitated states.
Porphyria.
Patients with a history of drug abuse.
During or within 14 days following the administration of monoamine oxidase inhibitors; hypertensive crises may result.

Warnings: Tolerance to the anorectic effect usually develops within a few weeks. When this occurs, the recommended dose should not be exceeded in an attempt to increase the effect; rather, the drug should be discontinued. Amphetamines may mask extreme fatigue. Caution patients about activities requiring alertness (e.g., operating vehicles or machinery).

Drug Dependence: Amphetamines have a significant potential for abuse. Tolerance and extreme psychological dependence have occurred. There are reports of patients who have increased dosage to many times that recommended. For these reasons, care should be used in the selection of candidates for 'Dexamyl' therapy. Should dependence occur, gradual withdrawal of the medication is recommended. Abrupt cessation following prolonged high dosage administration results in extreme fatigue and mental depression and barbiturate withdrawal symptoms; changes have also been noted on the sleep EEG. Manifestations of chronic intoxication with amphetamines include severe dermatoses, marked insomnia, irritability, hyperactivity, and personality changes. The most severe manifestation of chronic intoxication is psychosis, often clinically indistinguishable from schizophrenia.

Usage in Pregnancy: Safe use in pregnancy has not been established. Reproductive studies in mammals at high multiples of the human dose of amphetamines have suggested an embryotoxic and a teratogenic potential. Use of amphetamines by women who are or who may become pregnant, and especially those in the first trimester of pregnancy, requires that the potential benefit be weighed against the possible hazard to mother and infant.

Usage in Children: 'Dexamyl' is not recommended for use in children under 12 years of age.

Precautions: Use with caution in mild hypertension.
Medications containing barbiturates should be administered with caution to patients with decreased liver function, since a prolongation of effect may occur. The possibility of an additive effect with alcohol should be kept in mind. Insulin requirements in diabetes mellitus may be altered in association with the use of amphetamines and the concomitant dietary regimen.
Amphetamines may decrease the hypotensive effect of guanethidine.
The smallest quantity feasible should be prescribed or dispensed at one time in order to minimize the possibility of overdosage.

Adverse Reactions: Dextroamphetamine sulfate—*Cardiovascular:* Palpitation, tachycardia, elevation of blood pressure. *Central Nervous System:* Overstimulation, restlessness, dizziness, insomnia, euphoria, dyskinesia, dysphoria, tremor, headache; rarely, psychotic episodes at recommended doses. *Gastrointestinal:* Dryness of the mouth, unpleasant taste, diarrhea, other gastrointestinal disturbances. Anorexia and weight loss may occur as undesirable effects when amphetamines are used for other than the anorectic effect. *Allergic:* Urticaria. *Endocrine:* Impotence, changes in libido.
Amobarbital—Idiosyncrasy, in the form of excitement, hangover, or pain; hypersensitivity reactions, especially in patients with asthma, urticaria or angioneurotic edema.

Dosage and Administration: 'Dexamyl' should be administered at the lowest effective dosage, and dosage should be individually adjusted. Time of administration should receive special attention—particularly with the 'Spansule' capsule form—because of possible insomnia. Late evening medication should be avoided.
'Spansule' capsules—Usual dosage is one capsule taken in the morning. Not recommended for use in children under 12 years of age.
Tablets—Usual dosage is one tablet 2 or 3 times daily, 30 to 60 minutes before meals. Not recommended for use in children under 12 years of age.
NOTE: Appetite depressants are usually most effective for therapy periods of 4 to 8 weeks.[4,5] Should patients become tolerant to the anorectic effect, it is advisable to discontinue the medication for 2 to 4 weeks before reinstituting therapy if a longer period of anorectic treatment is indicated at this point.

Overdosage: *Symptoms*—Excessive stimulation or excessive sedation, which may reach the point of shock in some cases. **Excessive stimulation**—Central effects may include restlessness, dizziness, increased reflexes, tremor, insomnia, tenseness and irritability; also, confusion, assaultiveness, hallucinations and panic states. Fatigue and depression usually follow central stimulation. Cardiovascular effects may include chilliness, pallor or flushing, sweating, palpitation, hypertension or hypotension, headache, extrasystoles and other arrhythmias, anginal pain, circulatory collapse and syncope. Gastrointestinal effects include nausea, vomiting, diarrhea and abdominal cramps. Severe poisoning may result in convulsion and coma.
Excessive sedation—Symptoms may include respiratory depression, depression of superficial and deep reflexes, constriction of pupils to a slight degree (although in severe poisoning they may dilate), decreased urine formation, and coma.
Treatment—In both excessive stimulation and excessive sedation, treatment should consist primarily of symptomatic therapy, including gastric lavage, and supportive therapy in the case of shock. The urine pH is a significant factor in determining the rate of excretion of the components of 'Dexamyl'. **Excessive stimulation**—In addition to gastric lavage and other usual measures (emesis and catharsis), sedatives should be given when indicated. For this purpose a *non-barbiturate* tranquilizer should be used. To provide a basal level of sedation, one or more doses of such medication may be given by mouth or, if necessary, by intramuscular injection. This may be repeated as often as necessary and in quantities sufficient to control the symptoms. In general, the hypertension which may result from massive overdosage of the dextroamphetamine sulfate component does not require treatment. A gradual drop in blood pressure will usually result when sufficient sedation has been administered. In the presence of severe hypotension the usual procedures employed for shock should be instituted. Experience with hemodialysis or peritoneal dialysis in amphetamine overdosage is not adequate to permit recommendations in this regard. **Excessive sedation**—In addition to gastric lavage, administration of i.v. fluids and maintenance of blood pressure, body temperature and adequate respiratory exchange are recommended. An artificial kidney will increase the rate of removal of barbiturates from body fluids. Caution should be exercised, as the abrupt withdrawal of high doses of amobarbital may result in convulsions.
Since much of the 'Spansule' capsule medication is coated for gradual release, therapy directed at reversing the effects of the ingested drugs and at supporting the patient should be continued for as long as overdosage symptoms remain. Saline cathartics are useful for hastening evacuation of pellets that have not already released medication.

How Supplied: 'Dexamyl' Spansule capsules No. 1 and No. 2, in bottles of 50; **Tablets**, in bottles of 100.

References:

1. Rosenberg, P.: The Use of Mood Ameliorating Agents in the Treatment of Psychogenic Obesity, *Am. Pract. & Digest Treat. 4:*818 (Dec.) 1953.
2. Thorpe, G.: Treating Overweight Patients, *J.A.M.A. 165:*1361 (Nov. 16) 1957.
3. Shapiro, R., and Michaile, K.: The Use of Sustained-Release *d*-Amphetamine-Amobarbital Preparation in the Treatment of Obesity, *Internat. Rec. Med. 169:*638 (Oct.) 1956.
4. Mayer, J.: Some Aspects of the Problem of Regulation of Food Intake and Obesity, *New England J. Med. 274:*722 (Mar. 31) 1966.
5. Musgrave, P.W.: Rapid Weight Reduction for Aircrews, *Aerospace Med. 33:*1332 (Nov.) 1962.

[*Shown in Product Identification Section*]

DEXEDRINE® ℂ
(brand of dextroamphetamine sulfate)
SPANSULE® CAPSULES,
TABLETS and ELIXIR

Warning:

AMPHETAMINES HAVE A HIGH POTENTIAL FOR ABUSE. THEY SHOULD THUS BE TRIED ONLY IN WEIGHT REDUCTION PROGRAMS FOR PATIENTS IN WHOM ALTERNATIVE THERAPY HAS BEEN INEFFECTIVE. ADMINISTRATION OF AMPHETAMINES FOR PROLONGED PERIODS OF TIME IN OBESITY MAY LEAD TO DRUG DEPENDENCE AND MUST BE AVOIDED. PARTICULAR ATTENTION SHOULD BE PAID TO THE POSSIBILITY OF SUBJECTS OBTAINING AMPHETAMINES FOR NON-THERAPEUTIC USE OR DISTRIBUTION TO OTHERS, AND THE DRUGS SHOULD BE PRESCRIBED OR DISPENSED SPARINGLY.

Description: Dexedrine (dextroamphetamine sulfate, SK&F) is the dextro isomer of the compound *d,l*-amphetamine sulfate, a sympathomimetic amine of the amphetamine group. Chemically, dextroamphetamine is *d*-alpha-methylphenethylamine, and is present in all forms of 'Dexedrine' as the neutral sulfate.

Spansule® sustained release capsules—Each 'Spansule' sustained release capsule contains dextroamphetamine sulfate, 5 mg., 10 mg., or 15 mg., so prepared that an initial dose is released promptly and the remaining medication is released gradually over a prolonged period.

Tablets—Each tablet contains dextroamphetamine sulfate, 5 mg.

Elixir—Each 5 ml. (one teaspoonful) contains dextroamphetamine sulfate, 5 mg., and alcohol, 10%.

Actions: Amphetamines are sympathomimetic amines with CNS stimulant activity. Peripheral actions include elevation of systolic and diastolic in blood pressures and weak bronchodilator and respiratory stimulant action.

There is neither specific evidence which clearly establishes the mechanism whereby amphetamines produce mental and behavioral effects in children, nor conclusive evidence regarding how these effects relate to the condition of the central nervous system.

Drugs of this class used in obesity are commonly known as "anorectics" or "anorexigenics." It has not been established, however, that the action of such drugs in treating obesity is primarily one of appetite suppression. Other central nervous system actions, or metabolic effects, may be involved, for example.

Adult obese subjects instructed in dietary management and treated with "anorectic" drugs lose more weight on the average than those treated with placebo and diet, as determined in relatively short-term clinical trials.

The magnitude of increased weight loss of drug-treated patients over placebo-treated patients is only a fraction of a pound a week. The rate of weight loss is greatest in the first weeks of therapy for both drug and placebo subjects and tends to decrease in succeeding weeks. The origins of the increased weight loss due to the various possible drug effects are not established. The amount of weight loss associated with the use of an "anorectic" drug varies from trial to trial, and the increased weight loss appears to be related in part to variables other than the drug prescribed, such as the physician-investigator, the population treated, and the diet prescribed. Studies do not permit conclusions as to the relative importance of the drug and nondrug factors on weight loss.

The natural history of obesity is measured in years, whereas the studies cited are restricted to a few weeks' duration; thus, the total impact of drug-induced weight loss over that of diet alone must be considered clinically limited.

'Dexedrine' *Spansule* capsules are formulated to release the active drug substance *in vivo* in a more gradual fashion than the standard formulation, as demonstrated by blood levels. The formulation has not been shown superior in effectiveness over the same dosage of the standard, noncontrolled-release formulations given in divided doses.

Indications: Dexedrine (dextroamphetamine sulfate, SK&F) is indicated:

1. **In Narcolepsy.**
2. As an integral part of a total treatment program which typically includes other remedial measures (psychological, educational, social) for a stabilizing effect in children with a behavioral syndrome characterized by the following group of developmentally inappropriate symptoms: moderate to severe distractibility, short attention span, hyperactivity, emotional lability, and impulsivity. The diagnosis of this syndrome should not be made with finality when these symptoms are only of comparatively recent origin. Nonlocalizing (soft) neurological signs, learning disability, and abnormal EEG may or may not be present, and a diagnosis of central nervous system dysfunction may or may not be warranted.
3. **In Exogenous Obesity,** as a short-term (a few weeks) adjunct in a regimen of weight reduction based on caloric restriction, for patients refractory to alternative therapy, e.g., repeated diets, group programs, and other drugs. The limited usefulness of amphetamines (see ACTIONS) should be weighed against possible risks inherent in use of the drug, such as those described below.

Contraindications: Advanced arteriosclerosis, symptomatic cardiovascular disease, moderate to severe hypertension, hyperthyroidism, known hypersensitivity or idiosyncrasy to the sympathomimetic amines, glaucoma.

Agitated states.

Patients with a history of drug abuse.

During or within 14 days following the administration of monoamine oxidase inhibitors (hypertensive crises may result).

Warnings: When tolerance to the "anorectic" effect develops, the recommended dose should not be exceeded in an attempt to increase the effect; rather, the drug should be discontinued.

Amphetamines may impair the ability of the patient to engage in potentially hazardous activities such as operating machinery or vehicles; the patient should therefore be cautioned accordingly.

Drug Dependence: Amphetamines have been extensively abused. Tolerance, extreme psychological dependence, and severe social disability have occurred. There are reports of patients who have increased the dosage to many times that recommended. Abrupt cessation following prolonged high dosage administration results in extreme fatigue and mental depression; changes are also noted on the sleep EEG.

Manifestations of chronic intoxication with amphetamines include severe dermatoses, marked insomnia, irritability, hyperactivity, and personality changes. The most severe manifestation of chronic intoxication is psychosis, often clinically indistinguishable from schizophrenia.

Usage in Pregnancy: Safe use in pregnancy has not been established. Reproduction studies in mammals at high multiples of the human dose have suggested both an embryotoxic and a teratogenic potential. Use of amphetamines by women who are or who may become pregnant, and especially those in the first trimester of pregnancy, requires that the potential benefit be weighed against the possible hazard to mother and infant.

Usage in Children: Amphetamines are not recommended for use as anorectic agents in children under 12 years of age, or in children under 3 years of age with the behavioral syndrome described under INDICATIONS.

Clinical experience suggests that in psychotic children, administration of amphetamines may exacerbate symptoms of behavior disturbance and thought disorder.

Data are inadequate to determine whether chronic administration of amphetamines may be associated with growth inhibition; therefore, growth should be monitored during treatment.

Precautions: Caution is to be exercised in prescribing amphetamines for patients with even mild hypertension.

Insulin requirements in diabetes mellitus may be altered in association with the use of amphetamines and the concomitant dietary regimen.

Amphetamines may decrease the hypotensive effect of guanethidine.

The least amount feasible should be prescribed or dispensed at one time in order to minimize the possibility of overdosage.

Drug treatment is not indicated in all cases of the behavioral syndrome and should be considered only in light of the complete history and evaluation of the child. The decision to prescribe amphetamines should depend on the physician's assessment of the chronicity and severity of the child's symptoms and their appropriateness for his/her age. Prescription should not depend solely on the presence of one or more of the behavioral characteristics.

When these symptoms are associated with acute stress reactions, treatment with amphetamines is usually not indicated.

Long-term effects of amphetamines in children have not been well established.

Adverse Reactions: *Cardiovascular:* Palpitation, tachycardia, elevation of blood pressure. *Central nervous system:* Overstimulation, restlessness, dizziness, insomnia, euphoria, dyskinesia, dysphoria, tremor, headache; rarely, psychotic episodes at recommended doses. *Gastrointestinal:* Dryness of the mouth, unpleasant taste, diarrhea, constipation, other gastrointestinal disturbances. Anorexia and weight loss may occur as undesirable effects when amphetamines are used for other than the anorectic effect. *Allergic:* Urticaria. *Endocrine:* Impotence, changes in libido.

Dosage and Administration: Regardless of indication, amphetamines should be administered at the lowest effective dosage and dosage should be individually adjusted. Late evening doses—particularly with the 'Spansule' capsule form—should be avoided because of the resulting insomnia.

Narcolepsy: Usual dose 5 to 60 milligrams per day in divided doses, depending on the individual patient response.

Narcolepsy seldom occurs in children under 12 years of age; however, when it does, Dexedrine (dextroamphetamine sulfate, SK&F) may be used. The suggested initial dose for patients aged 6-12 is 5 mg. daily; daily dose may be raised in increments of 5 mg. at weekly intervals until optimal response is obtained. In patients 12 years of age and older, start with 10 mg. daily; daily dosage may be raised in increments of 10 mg. at weekly intervals until optimal response is obtained. If bothersome adverse reactions appear (e.g., insomnia or anorexia), dosage should be reduced. 'Spansule' capsules may be used for once-a-day dosage wherever appropriate. With tablets or elixir, give first dose on awakening; additional doses (1 or 2) at intervals of 4 to 6 hours.

Behavioral Syndrome in Children: Not recommended for children under 3 years of age.

In children from 3 to 5 years of age, start with 2.5 mg. daily, by tablet or elixir; daily dosage

Continued on next page

Smith Kline & French—Cont.

may be raised in increments of 2.5 mg. at weekly intervals until optimal response is obtained.
In children 6 years of age and older, start with 5 mg. once or twice daily; daily dosage may be raised in increments of 5 mg. at weekly intervals until optimal response is obtained. Only in rare cases will it be necessary to exceed a total of 40 milligrams per day.
'Spansule' capsules may be used for once-a-day dosage wherever appropriate.
With tablets or elixir, give first dose on awakening; additional doses (1 or 2) at intervals of 4 to 6 hours.
Where possible, drug administration should be interrupted occasionally to determine if there is a recurrence of behavioral symptoms sufficient to require continued therapy.
Exogenous Obesity: Usual dosage is one 10 or 15 mg. 'Spansule' capsule daily, taken in the morning, or up to 30 mg. daily by tablets or elixir, taken in divided doses of 5 to 10 mg. 30 to 60 minutes before meals. Not recommended for this use in children under 12 years of age.
Overdosage: SYMPTOMS—Manifestations of acute overdosage with amphetamines include restlessness, tremor, hyperreflexia, rapid respiration, confusion, assaultiveness, hallucinations, panic states.
Fatigue and depression usually follow the central stimulation.
Cardiovascular effects include arrhythmias, hypertension or hypotension and circulatory collapse. Gastrointestinal symptoms include nausea, vomiting, diarrhea, and abdominal cramps. Fatal poisoning is usually preceded by convulsions and coma.
TREATMENT—Management of acute amphetamine intoxication is largely symptomatic and includes gastric lavage and sedation with a barbiturate. Experience with hemodialysis or peritoneal dialysis is inadequate to permit recommendation in this regard. Acidification of the urine increases amphetamine excretion. If acute, severe hypertension complicates amphetamine overdosage, administration of intravenous phentolamine (Regitine®, CIBA) has been suggested. However, a gradual drop in blood pressure will usually result when sufficient sedation has been achieved.
Since much of the 'Spansule' capsule medication is coated for gradual release, therapy directed at reversing the effects of the ingested drug and at supporting the patient should be continued for as long as overdosage symptoms remain. Saline cathartics are useful for hastening the evacuation of pellets that have not already released medication.
How Supplied: 'Spansule' capsules—5 mg., in bottles of 50; 10 mg. and 15 mg., in bottles of 50 and 500. **Tablets**—bottles of 100 and 1000. **Elixir**—16 fl. oz. (473 ml.) bottles.
Military—Tablets 5 mg., 100's, 6505-00-106-8715.
[*Shown in Product Identification Section*]

DIBENZYLINE® Capsules ℞
(brand of phenoxybenzamine hydrochloride)

Description: Each capsule contains phenoxybenzamine hydrochloride, 10 mg.
Actions: Dibenzyline (phenoxybenzamine hydrochloride, SK&F) is a long-acting, adrenergic, α-receptor blocking agent which can produce and maintain "chemical sympathectomy" by oral administration. It increases blood flow to the skin, mucosa and abdominal viscera, and lowers both supine and erect blood pressures. It has no effect on the parasympathetic system.

Indications
Based on a review of this drug by The National Academy of Sciences—National Research Council and/or other information, FDA has classified the indications as follows:
Effective: Pheochromocytoma, to control episodes of hypertension and sweating. If tachycardia is excessive, it may be necessary to use a beta-blocking agent concomitantly.
Possibly effective: Vasospastic peripheral vascular disease associated with increased α-adrenergic activity such as Raynaud's syndrome, acrocyanosis and frostbite sequelae.
Final classification of the less-than-effective indications requires further investigation.

Contraindications: Conditions where a fall in blood pressure may be undesirable.
Warning: 'Dibenzyline'-induced *alpha*-adrenergic blockade leaves *beta*-adrenergic receptors unopposed. Compounds that stimulate both types of receptors may therefore produce an exaggerated hypotensive response and tachycardia.
Precautions: Administer with caution in patients with marked cerebral or coronary arteriosclerosis or renal damage. Adrenergic blocking effect may aggravate symptoms of respiratory infections.
Dibenzyline (phenoxybenzamine hydrochloride, SK&F) should not be used in diseases involving the larger blood vessels where direct-acting vasodilators are preferred therapy.
Adverse Reactions: Nasal congestion, miosis, postural hypotension, tachycardia and inhibition of ejaculation may occur. These so-called "side effects" are actually evidence of adrenergic blockade and vary according to the degree of blockade. Furthermore, they tend to decrease as therapy is continued. Gastrointestinal irritation has also been reported.
Dosage and Administration: The dosage should be adjusted to fit the needs of each patient. Small initial doses should be *slowly* increased until the desired effect is obtained or the side effects from blockade become troublesome. *After each increase, the patient should be observed on that level for at least 4 days before instituting another increase.* The dosage should be carried to a point where symptomatic relief and/or objective improvement are obtained, but not so high that the side effects from blockade become troublesome.
Initially, 10 mg. daily. After at least 4 days, the daily dosage may be increased by 10 mg., and similarly increased thereafter until optimum dosage is reached. Dosage range is usually 20–60 mg. daily. NOTE: At least 2 weeks are usually required to reach the optimal dosage level in most patients. At this time improvement in these patients will usually be observed. But it may be several more weeks before the *full* benefits of the drug become apparent.
Overdosage: *Symptoms*—These are largely the result of block of the sympathetic nervous system and of the circulating epinephrine. They may include postural hypotension resulting in dizziness or fainting; tachycardia, particularly postural; vomiting; lethargy; shock.
Treatment—When symptoms and signs of overdosage exist, discontinue the drug. Treatment of circulatory failure, if present, is a prime consideration. In cases of mild overdosage, recumbent position with legs elevated usually restores cerebral circulation. In the more severe cases, the usual measures to combat shock should be instituted. Usual pressor agents are *not* effective. Epinephrine is contraindicated because it stimulates both α and β receptors; since α receptors are blocked, the net effect of epinephrine administration is vasodilation and a further drop in blood pressure (epinephrine reversal).
The patient may have to be kept flat for 24 hours or more in the case of overdose, as the effect of the drug is prolonged. Leg bandages and an abdominal binder may shorten the period of disability.
I.V. infusion of levarterenol bitartrate* may be used to combat severe hypotensive reactions, because it stimulates α receptors primarily. Although Dibenzyline (phenoxybenzamine hydrochloride, SK&F) is an α adrenergic blocking agent, a sufficient dose of levarterenol bitartrate will overcome this effect.
How Supplied: Bottles of 100.

*Available as Levophed® Bitartrate (brand of levarterenol bitartrate) from Winthrop Laboratories.
[*Shown in Product Identification Section*]

DYAZIDE® Capsules ℞

('Dyazide' is a product of SK&F Co., Carolina, P.R. 00630, Subsidiary of SmithKline Corporation, Philadelphia, Pa.)

Warning:
This fixed combination drug is not indicated for initial therapy of edema or hypertension. Edema or hypertension requires therapy titrated to the individual patient. If the fixed combination represents the dosage so determined, its use may be more convenient in patient management. The treatment of hypertension and edema is not static, but must be reevaluated as conditions in each patient warrant.

Description: Each maroon and white 'Dyazide' capsule contains 50 mg. of Dyrenium® (brand of triamterene) and 25 mg. of hydrochlorothiazide.
Dyrenium (triamterene, SK&F CO.) is 2, 4, 7-triamino-6-phenylpteridine. Hydrochlorothiazide is 6-chloro-3, 4-dihydro-2H-1, 2, 4-benzothiadiazine-7-sulfonamide 1, 1-dioxide.
Action: 'Dyazide' is a diuretic/antihypertensive drug product that combines two natriuretics, each of which complements the action of the other. The hydrochlorothiazide component blocks the reabsorption of sodium and chloride ions, and thereby increases the quantity of sodium traversing the distal tubule and the volume of water excreted. A portion of the additional sodium presented to the distal tubule is exchanged there for potassium and hydrogen ions. With continued use of hydrochlorothiazide and depletion of sodium, compensatory mechanisms tend to increase this exchange and may produce excessive loss of potassium, hydrogen and chloride ions. Hydrochlorothiazide also decreases the excretion of calcium and uric acid, may increase the excretion of iodide and may reduce glomerular filtration rate. The exact mechanism of the antihypertensive effect of hydrochlorothiazide is not known.
The triamterene component of 'Dyazide' exerts its diuretic effect on the distal renal tubule to inhibit the reabsorption of sodium in exchange for potassium and hydrogen ions. Its natriuretic activity is limited by the amount of sodium reaching its site of action. Although it blocks the increase in this exchange that is stimulated by mineralocorticoids (chiefly aldosterone) it is not a competitive antagonist of aldosterone and its activity can be demonstrated in adrenalectomized rats and patients with Addison's disease. As a result the dose of triamterene required is not proportionally related to the level of mineralocorticoid activity, but is dictated by the response of the individual patient, and the kaliuretic effect of concomitantly administered drugs. By inhibiting the distal tubular exchange mechanism, triamterene maintains or increases the sodium excretion and reduces the excess loss of potassium, hydrogen, and chloride ions induced by hydrochlorothiazide. As with hydrochlorothiazide, triamterene may reduce glomerular fil-

tration and renal plasma flow. Via this mechanism it may reduce uric acid excretion although it has no tubular effect on uric acid reabsorption or secretion. Triamterene does not affect calcium excretion. No predictable antihypertensive effect has been demonstrated for triamterene.

Duration of diuretic activity and effective dosage range of the hydrochlorothiazide and triamterene components of 'Dyazide' are similar. Onset of diuresis with 'Dyazide' takes place within one hour, peaks at two-three hours and tapers off during the subsequent seven to nine hours.

Indications: This combination drug finds its usefulness primarily in the treatment of edema. Any usefulness of triamterene when used with a thiazide in hypertension will derive from its potassium sparing effect. Either its main diuretic effect or potassium sparing effect when used with a thiazide drug should be determined by individual titration. (See box warning.)

When the fixed combination represents the dosage determined by titration, 'Dyazide' is indicated as adjunctive therapy in edema associated with congestive heart failure, hepatic cirrhosis and the nephrotic syndrome. It is also indicated in corticosteroid and estrogen induced edema and idiopathic edema.

When the potassium sparing action of its 'Dyrenium' component is warranted and the fixed combination represents the dosage determined by titration, 'Dyazide' is indicated in the management of hypertension as determined by individual dosage titration of all agents employed. (See box warning.)

Usage in Pregnancy. The routine use of diuretics in an otherwise healthy woman is inappropriate and exposes mother and fetus to unnecessary hazard. Diuretics do not prevent development of toxemia of pregnancy, and there is no satisfactory evidence that they are useful in the treatment of developed toxemia. Edema during pregnancy may arise from pathological causes or from the physiologic and mechanical consequences of pregnancy. Diuretics are indicated in pregnancy when edema is due to pathologic causes, just as they are in the absence of pregnancy (however, see Warnings, below). Dependent edema in pregnancy, resulting from restriction of venous return by the expanded uterus, is properly treated through elevation of the lower extremities and use of support hose; use of diuretics to lower intravascular volume in this case is illogical and unnecessary. There is hypervolemia during normal pregnancy which is harmful to neither the fetus nor the mother (in the absence of cardiovascular disease), but which is associated with edema, including generalized edema, in the majority of pregnant women. If this edema produces discomfort, increased recumbency will often provide relief. In rare instances, this edema may cause extreme discomfort which is not relieved by rest. In these cases, a short course of diuretics may provide relief and may be appropriate.

Contraindications: 'Dyazide' is contraindicated for further use in patients who exhibit anuria or progressive renal dysfunction, including increasing oliguria and increasing azotemia or in patients who develop hyperkalemia while on the drug.

'Dyazide' should not be used in patients with pre-existing elevated serum potassium, as is sometimes seen in patients with impaired renal function. Increasing hepatic dysfunction in patients on 'Dyazide' contraindicates further use of the preparation. Hypersensitivity to either drug in the preparation or to other sulfonamide-derived drugs is a contraindication.

Warnings: Patients should not be placed on dietary potassium supplements or potassium salts in conjunction with 'Dyazide' unless they develop hypokalemia or their dietary intake of potassium is markedly impaired. Because of the potassium conserving effect of Dyrenium (triamterene, SK&F CO.), hypokalemia is an uncommon occurrence with the use of 'Dyazide'. If the need for supplementary potassium is demonstrated by repeated low serum potassium determinations a form other than potassium tablets should be used since these have been implicated in the development of nonspecific small bowel lesions consisting of stenosis with or without ulceration.

Abnormal elevation of serum potassium, though uncommon, is potentially the most severe electrolyte disturbance with 'Dyazide' therapy. Hyperkalemia has been reported and in some cases has been associated with cardiac irregularities. Hyperkalemia is more likely to occur in patients who are severely ill, with relatively small urine volumes (less than one liter per day), or in elderly or diabetic patients with confirmed or suspected renal insufficiency. Acute transient hyperkalemia has been observed during intravenous glucose tolerance testing of diabetics dosed with the Dyrenium (triamterene, SK&F CO.) component of 'Dyazide'. Fatalities due to hyperkalemia have been reported, accordingly no potassium supplements should ordinarily be given with 'Dyazide' therapy, and periodic determinations of serum potassium should be made. If hyperkalemia develops, withdraw 'Dyazide', substitute a thiazide alone, and restrict potassium intake.

If hyperkalemia is present or suspected, an electrocardiogram should be obtained. If the ECG shows no widening of the QRS or arrhythmia in the presence of hyperkalemia, it is usually sufficient to discontinue 'Dyazide' and any potassium supplementation and substitute a thiazide alone. Sodium polystyrene sulfonate (Kayexalate®, Winthrop) may be administered to enhance the excretion of excess potassium. **The presence of a widened QRS complex or arrhythmia in association with hyperkalemia requires prompt additional therapy.** For tachyarrhythmia, infuse 44 mEq. of sodium bicarbonate or 10 ml. of 10% calcium gluconate or calcium chloride over several minutes. For asystole, bradycardia or A-V block transvenous pacing is also recommended.

The effect of calcium and sodium bicarbonate is transient and repeated administration may be required. When indicated by the clinical situation, excess K^+ may be removed by dialysis or oral or rectal administration of Kayexalate®. Infusion of glucose and insulin has also been used to treat hyperkalemia.

Usage in Pregnancy. Thiazides cross the placental barrier and appear in cord blood. The use of thiazides in pregnant women requires that the anticipated benefit be weighed against possible hazards to the fetus. These hazards include fetal or neonatal jaundice, thrombocytopenia, and possibly other adverse reactions which have occurred in the adult.

Nursing Mothers. Thiazides appear and triamterene may appear in breast milk. If use of the drug product is deemed essential, the patient should stop nursing.

Usage in Children

Adequate information on the use of 'Dyazide' in children is not available.

Precautions: Electrolyte imbalance, often encountered in such conditions as heart failure, renal disease, or cirrhosis of the liver, may also be aggravated by diuretics, and should be considered during 'Dyazide' therapy when using high doses for prolonged periods or in patients on a salt-restricted diet. Serum determinations of electrolytes should be performed, and are particularly important if the patient is vomiting excessively or receiving fluids parenterally. Possible fluid and electrolyte imbalance may be indicated by such warning signs as: dry mouth, thirst, weakness, lethargy, drowsiness, restlessness, muscle pain or cramps, muscular fatigue, hypotension, oliguria, tachycardia, and gastrointestinal symptoms.

Because of the potassium sparing characteristic of Dyrenium (triamterene, SK&F CO.), hypokalemia is uncommon with 'Dyazide' but may occur in some cases when the 'Dyrenium' component is unable to completely compensate for the potassium wasting effect of the hydrochlorothiazide component or the disease. The myocardial effects of digitalis may be exaggerated in patients with hypokalemia. In these patients signs of digitalis intoxication may be produced by previously tolerated doses of digitalis.

'Dyazide' may produce an elevated blood urea nitrogen level, creatinine level, or both. This apparently is secondary to a reversible reduction of glomerular filtration rate or a depletion of intravascular fluid volume (prerenal azotemia) rather than renal toxicity; levels return to normal when 'Dyazide' is discontinued. Elevated levels are seldom seen with every-other-day therapy. If azotemia increases, discontinue 'Dyazide'. Periodic BUN or serum creatinine determinations should be made, especially in elderly patients and in patients with suspected or confirmed renal insufficiency.

Thiazides can precipitate hepatic coma in patients with severe liver disease. Potassium depletion induced by the thiazide may be important in this connection. Administer 'Dyazide' cautiously and be alert for such early signs of impending coma as confusion, drowsiness and tremor; if mental confusion increases discontinue 'Dyazide' for a few days. Attention must be given to other factors that may precipitate hepatic coma, such as blood in the gastrointestinal tract or pre-existing potassium depletion.

'Dyazide' is usually not used concomitantly with spironolactone. If it is, determine serum potassium levels frequently, since both the 'Dyrenium' component in 'Dyazide' and spironolactone can cause potassium retention and elevated serum potassium levels. Two deaths have been reported in patients receiving concomitant spironolactone and 'Dyrenium' or 'Dyazide'. In one case dosage recommendations were exceeded, in the other serum electrolytes were not properly monitored.

Patients should be observed regularly for the possible occurrence of blood dyscrasias, liver damage, or other idiosyncratic reactions. There have been reports of blood dyscrasias in patients receiving 'Dyrenium'. Leukopenia, thrombocytopenia, agranulocytosis, and aplastic anemia have been reported with the thiazides. Cirrhotics with splenomegaly may have marked variations in their blood pictures—including thrombocyte and leukocyte levels—which are not related to drug therapy. Since the 'Dyrenium' component of 'Dyazide' is a weak folic acid antagonist, it may contribute to the appearance of megaloblastosis in cases where folic acid stores are depleted. Periodic blood studies in these patients are recommended.

The antihypertensive effects of 'Dyazide' may be enhanced in the post-sympathectomy patient.

Thiazides may cause hyperglycemia and glycosuria, and alter insulin requirements in diabetes. 'Dyazide' may have similar effects. Hyperuricemia may be observed, with possible occurrence of gout. Dyrenium (triamterene, SK&F CO.) may cause a decreasing alkali reserve with the possibility of metabolic acidosis.

Thiazides have been shown to decrease arterial responsiveness to norepinephrine (an effect attributed to loss of sodium) and to increase the paralyzing effect of non-depolarizing muscle relaxants such as tubocurarine (an effect attributed to potassium loss); consequently caution should be observed in patients undergoing surgery.

'Dyrenium' and quinidine have similar fluorescence spectra; thus, 'Dyazide' will interfere with the fluorescent measurement of quinidine.

Continued on next page

Smith Kline & French—Cont.

Lithium generally should not be given with diuretics because they reduce its renal clearance and increase the risk of lithium toxicity. Read circulars for lithium preparations before use of such concomitant therapy with 'Dyazide'.

Adverse Reactions: Side effects observed in association with the use of 'Dyazide' include: muscle cramps, weakness, dizziness, headache and dry mouth; anaphylaxis, rash, urticaria, photosensitivity, purpura and other dermatological conditions; nausea and vomiting, diarrhea, constipation, and other gastrointestinal disturbances. (Such nausea can usually be prevented by giving the drug after meals.)

It should be noted that symptoms of nausea and vomiting can also be indicative of electrolyte imbalance (see Precautions).

Thiazides alone have been known to cause necrotizing vasculitis, paresthesias, icterus, pancreatitis, xanthopsia, and, rarely, allergic pneumonitis.

Newborn, whose mothers had received thiazides during pregnancy, in rare instances have developed thrombocytopenia or pancreatitis.

Dosage and Administration: As determined by individual titration. (See box warning.)

Adults:

The usual dose is one or two capsules twice daily after meals. Some patients may be maintained on one capsule daily or every other day. Maximum daily dose should not exceed four capsules, and at this dosage, the incidence of side effects may increase.

Since 'Dyazide' has an antihypertensive effect, hypotensive drugs used concomitantly should be added at reduced dosage—at least one half the usual dosage—particularly if it is a ganglionic blocking agent. Adjust dosage as indicated.

Children:

Adequate information on the use of 'Dyazide' in children is not available.

Note: Potassium supplementation used concurrently with other diuretics should be discontinued when titrating with Dyrenium (triamterene, SK&F CO.). They should not be reinstituted when the patient is placed on 'Dyazide' unless the triamterene component does not completely compensate for the potassium loss.

Overdosage: Electrolyte imbalance is the major concern (See Warnings section). Symptoms reported include: polyuria, nausea, vomiting, weakness, lassitude, fever, flushed face, and hyperactive deep tendon reflexes. If hypotension occurs, it may be treated with pressor agents such as levarterenol to maintain blood pressure. Carefully evaluate the electrolyte pattern and fluid balance. Induce immediate evacuation of the stomach through emesis or gastric lavage. There is no specific antidote.

How Supplied: In bottles of 100 and 1000 capsules; in Single Unit Packages of 100 (intended for institutional use only).

[*Shown in Product Identification Section*]

DYRENIUM® ℞
(brand of triamterene)

('Dyrenium' is a product of SK&F Co., Carolina, P.R. 00630, Subsidiary of SmithKline Corporation, Philadelphia, Pa.)

Description: Each capsule contains triamterene, 50 mg. or 100 mg.

Dyrenium (triamterene, SK&F CO.) is 2,4,7-triamino-6-phenylpteridine.

Action: Dyrenium (triamterene, SK&F CO.) has a unique mode of action; it inhibits the reabsorption of sodium ions in exchange for potassium and hydrogen ions at that segment of the distal tubule under the control of adrenal mineralocorticoids (especially aldosterone). This activity takes place through a direct effect on the renal tubule and not by competitive aldosterone antagonism; it is not directly related to the level of aldosterone secretion.

The fraction of filtered sodium reaching this distal tubular exchange site is relatively small, and the amount which is exchanged depends on the level of mineralocorticoid activity. Thus, the degree of natriuresis and diuresis produced by inhibition of the exchange mechanism is necessarily limited. Increasing the amount of available sodium and the level of mineralocorticoid activity by the use of more proximally-acting diuretics will increase the degree of diuresis and potassium conservation.

'Dyrenium' occasionally causes increases in serum potassium which, in some instances, can result in hyperkalemia. It does not produce alkalosis because it does not cause excessive excretion of titratable acid and ammonium.

Indications: Dyrenium (triamterene, SK&F CO.) is indicated in the treatment of edema associated with congestive heart failure, cirrhosis of the liver, and the nephrotic syndrome; also in steroid-induced edema, idiopathic edema, and edema due to secondary hyperaldosteronism.

'Dyrenium' may be used alone or with other diuretics either for its added diuretic effect or its potassium-conserving potential. It also promotes increased diuresis when patients prove resistant or only partially responsive to thiazides or other diuretics because of secondary hyperaldosteronism.

Usage in Pregnancy. The routine use of diuretics in an otherwise healthy woman is inappropriate and exposes mother and fetus to unnecessary hazard. Diuretics do not prevent development of toxemia of pregnancy, and there is no satisfactory evidence that they are useful in the treatment of developed toxemia.

Edema during pregnancy may arise from pathological causes or from the physiologic and mechanical consequences of pregnancy. Diuretics are indicated in pregnancy when edema is due to pathologic causes, just as they are in the absence of pregnancy (however, see Warnings, below). Dependent edema in pregnancy, resulting from restriction of venous return by the expanded uterus, is properly treated through elevation of the lower extremities and use of support hose; use of diuretics to lower intravascular volume in this case is illogical and unnecessary. There is hypervolemia during normal pregnancy which is harmful to neither the fetus nor the mother (in the absence of cardiovascular disease), but which is associated with edema, including generalized edema, in the majority of pregnant women. If this edema produces discomfort, increased recumbency will often provide relief. In rare instances, this edema may cause extreme discomfort which is not relieved by rest. In these cases, a short course of diuretics may provide relief and may be appropriate.

Contraindications: Anuria. Severe or progressive kidney disease or dysfunction with the possible exception of nephrosis. Severe hepatic disease. Hypersensitivity to the drug.

Dyrenium (triamterene, SK&F CO.) should not be used in patients with pre-existing elevated serum potassium, as is sometimes seen in patients with impaired renal function or azotemia, or in patients who develop hyperkalemia while on the drug. Potassium supplements, either as medication or as a potassium-rich diet, should not be used with 'Dyrenium'.

Warnings: Patients should be observed regularly for the possible occurrence of blood dyscrasias, liver damage, or other idiosyncratic reactions. There have been reports of blood dyscrasias in patients receiving Dyrenium (triamterene, SK&F CO.)

Periodic BUN and serum potassium determinations should be made to check kidney function, especially in patients with suspected or confirmed renal insufficiency. It is particularly important to make serum potassium determinations in elderly or diabetic patients receiving the drug; these patients should be observed carefully for possible adverse serum potassium increases.

'Dyrenium' is usually not used concomitantly with spironolactone. If it is, however, the physician should frequently determine serum potassium levels, since both of these agents can cause potassium retention and, in some instances, hyperkalemia.

Usage in Pregnancy. Triamterene has been shown to cross the placental barrier and appear in the cord blood of ewes; this may occur in humans. The use of 'Dyrenium' in pregnant women requires that the anticipated benefit be weighed against possible hazards to the fetus. These possible hazards include adverse reactions which have occurred in the adult.

Nursing Mothers. Triamterene appears in cow's milk; this may occur in humans. If use of the drug is deemed essential, the patient should stop nursing.

Precautions: Dyrenium (triamterene, SK&F CO.) tends to conserve potassium rather than to promote its excretion as do many diuretics and, occasionally, can cause increases in serum potassium which, in some instances, can result in hyperkalemia. In rare instances, hyperkalemia has been associated with cardiac irregularities.

Hyperkalemia will rarely occur in patients with adequate urinary output, but it is a possibility if large doses are used for considerable periods of time.* If hyperkalemia is observed, 'Dyrenium' should be withdrawn. Because 'Dyrenium' conserves potassium, it has been theorized that in patients who have received intensive therapy or been given the drug for prolonged periods, a rebound kaliuresis could occur upon abrupt withdrawal. In such patients withdrawal of 'Dyrenium' should be gradual.

Electrolyte imbalance often encountered in such diseases as congestive heart failure, renal disease, or cirrhosis may be aggravated or caused independently by any effective diuretic agent including 'Dyrenium'. The use of full doses of a diuretic when salt intake is restricted can result in a low-salt syndrome.

'Dyrenium' can cause mild nitrogen retention which is reversible upon withdrawal of the drug and is seldom observed with intermittent (every-other-day) therapy.

By the very nature of their illness, cirrhotics with splenomegaly sometimes have marked variations in their blood pictures. Since 'Dyrenium' is a weak folic acid antagonist, it may contribute to the appearance of megaloblastosis in cases where folic acid stores have been depleted. Therefore, periodic blood studies in these patients are recommended.

Although 'Dyrenium' has not proved to be a consistent antihypertensive agent, the physician should be aware of a possible lowering of blood pressure. Concomitant use with antihypertensive drugs may result in an additive effect.

'Dyrenium' may cause a decreasing alkali reserve with the possibility of metabolic acidosis.

'Dyrenium' and quinidine have similar fluorescence spectra; thus, 'Dyrenium' will interfere with the fluorescent measurement of quinidine.

Lithium generally should not be given with diuretics because they reduce its renal clearance and increase the risk of lithium toxicity. Read circulars for lithium preparations before use of such concomitant therapy with 'Dyrenium'.

Adverse Reactions: There have been occasional reports of diarrhea, nausea and vomiting, and other gastrointestinal disturbances. Such nausea can usually be prevented by giving the drug after meals. Weakness, headache, dry mouth, anaphylaxis, photosensitivity, and rash have also been reported. Only rarely has

it been necessary to discontinue therapy because of these side effects.
It should be noted that symptoms of nausea and vomiting can also be indicative of electrolyte imbalance (see Precautions).
Note on Gout and Diabetes: In special studies, investigators found that Dyrenium (triamterene, SK&F CO.) has little or no effect on serum uric acid levels or carbohydrate metabolism. However, it has elevated uric acid, especially in persons predisposed to gouty arthritis.
Dosage and Administration: **Adult Dosage**
Dosage should be titrated to the needs of the individual patient. When used alone, the usual starting dose is 100 mg. twice daily after meals. When combined with another diuretic, the total daily dosage of each agent should usually be lowered initially, and then adjusted to the patient's needs. The total daily dosage should not exceed 300 mg.
Onset of action is 2–4 hours after ingestion. Most patients will respond to Dyrenium (triamterene, SK&F CO.) during the first day of treatment. Maximum therapeutic effect, however, may not be seen for several days. Duration of diuresis depends on several factors, especially renal function, but it generally tapers off 7–9 hours after administration.
When 'Dyrenium' is added to other diuretic therapy or when patients are switched to 'Dyrenium' from other diuretics, all potassium supplementation should be discontinued.
Overdosage: In the event of overdosage it can be theorized that electrolyte imbalance would be the major concern, with particular attention to possible hyperkalemia. Other symptoms that might be seen would be nausea and vomiting, other g.i. disturbances, and weakness. It is conceivable that some hypotension could occur. As with an overdose of any drug, immediate evacuation of the stomach should be induced through emesis and gastric lavage. Careful evaluation of the electrolyte pattern and fluid balance should be made. There is no specific antidote.
How Supplied: 50 mg. capsules, in bottles of 100, in Single Unit Packages of 100 (intended for institutional use only). 100 mg. capsules in bottles of 100 and 1000, in Single Unit Packages of 100 (intended for institutional use only).
Military—Capsules 100 mg., 100's, 6505-00-982-9143.

---

*In making laboratory checks, blood samples require careful handling to prevent hemolysis on standing with resulting false serum potassium readings.

[*Shown in Product Identification Section*]

ECOTRIN® ††
Enteric-coated Aspirin

Composition: Each Ecotrin tablet contains 325 mg. (5 gr.) aspirin, specially processed with Duentric® coating to prevent disintegration in the stomach and minimize the possibility of consequent gastric irritation.
Indications: When your physician recommends regular use of aspirin, Ecotrin may be taken—particularly for temporary relief of minor aches and pains of arthritis and rheumatism. The Ecotrin tablet has a Duentric® coating which protects against gastric upset caused by plain, uncoated aspirin. Because Ecotrin passes through the stomach before dissolving in the intestine, initial relief may take longer.
Usual Dosage: 1 or 2 tablets every 4 hours, as necessary. Do not exceed 12 tablets in 24 hours unless directed by a physician.
High aspirin dosage is recommended in arthritis and rheumatic conditions (40–80 gr. daily) and in acute rheumatic fever (up to 120 gr. daily), in divided doses. In arthritic and rheumatic conditions, concomitant use of Ecotrin often permits a reduction in steroid dosage.
Warning: If under medical care, do not use without physician's approval. If pain persists more than 10 days or redness is present, or in arthritic or rheumatic conditions affecting children under 12, consult a physician immediately. Discontinue use if dizziness, ringing in ears, or impaired hearing occurs.
Keep this and all medicines out of reach of children. In case of accidental overdose, contact a physician or poison control center immediately.
EASY-OPENING CAP available on 250 tablet bottle—intended for households without children.
How Supplied: 5 grain tablets, in bottles of 100, 250 and 1000.

---

††Ecotrin is a product of Menley & James Laboratories, Professional Products Division, a SmithKline company.

[*Shown in Product Identification Section*]

ESKALITH® ℞
(brand of lithium carbonate)

> **WARNING**
> Lithium toxicity is closely related to serum lithium levels, and can occur at doses close to therapeutic levels. Facilities for prompt and accurate serum lithium determinations should be available before initiating therapy.

Description: 'Eskalith' contains lithium carbonate, a white, light alkaline powder with molecular formula Li_2CO_3 and molecular weight 73.89. Lithium is an element of the alkali-metal group with atomic number 3, atomic weight 6.94 and an emission line at 671 nm on the flame photometer.
Actions: Preclinical studies have shown that lithium alters sodium transport in nerve and muscle cells and effects a shift toward intraneuronal metabolism of catecholamines, but the specific biochemical mechanism of lithium action in mania is unknown.
Indications: Eskalith (lithium carbonate, SK&F) is indicated in the treatment of manic episodes of manic-depressive illness. Maintenance therapy prevents or diminishes the intensity of subsequent episodes in those manic-depressive patients with a history of mania.
Typical symptoms of mania include pressure of speech, motor hyperactivity, reduced need for sleep, flight of ideas, grandiosity, elation, poor judgment, aggressiveness, and possibly hostility. When given to a patient experiencing a manic episode, 'Eskalith' may produce a normalization of symptomatology within 1 to 3 weeks.
Warnings: Lithium should generally not be given to patients with significant renal or cardiovascular disease, severe debilitation or dehydration, or sodium depletion, and to patients receiving diuretics, since the risk of lithium toxicity is very high in such patients. If the psychiatric indication is life-threatening, and if such a patient fails to respond to other measures, lithium treatment may be undertaken with extreme caution, including daily serum lithium determinations and adjustment to the usually low doses ordinarily tolerated by these individuals. In such instances, hospitalization is a necessity.
Lithium therapy has been reported in some cases to be associated with morphologic changes in the kidneys. The relationship between such changes and renal function has not been established.
An encephalopathic syndrome (characterized by weakness, lethargy, fever, tremulousness and confusion, extrapyramidal symptoms, leukocytosis, elevated serum enzymes, BUN and FBS) followed by irreversible brain damage has occurred in a few patients treated with lithium plus haloperidol. A causal relationship between these events and the concomitant administration of lithium and haloperidol has not been established; however, patients receiving such combined therapy should be monitored closely for early evidence of neurologic toxicity and treatment discontinued promptly if such signs appear. The possibility of similar adverse interactions with other antipsychotic medication exists.
Lithium toxicity is closely related to serum lithium levels, and can occur at doses close to therapeutic levels (see DOSAGE AND ADMINISTRATION).
Outpatients and their families should be warned that the patient must discontinue lithium carbonate therapy and contact his physician if such clinical signs of lithium toxicity as diarrhea, vomiting, tremor, mild ataxia, drowsiness, or muscular weakness occur.
Lithium carbonate may impair mental and/or physical abilities. Caution patients about activities requiring alertness (e.g., operating vehicles or machinery).
Lithium may prolong the effects of neuromuscular blocking agents. Therefore, neuromuscular blocking agents should be given with caution to patients receiving lithium.
Usage in Pregnancy: Adverse effects on nidation in rats, embryo viability in mice, and metabolism *in vitro* of rat testes and human spermatozoa have been attributed to lithium, as have teratogenicity in submammalian species and cleft palates in mice. Studies in rats, rabbits and monkeys have shown no evidence of lithium-induced teratology.
There are lithium birth registries in the United States and elsewhere; however there are at the present time insufficient data to determine the effects of lithium carbonate on human fetuses. Therefore, at this point, lithium should not be used in pregnancy, especially during the first trimester, unless in the opinion of the physician, the potential benefits outweigh possible hazards.
Usage in Nursing Mothers: Lithium is excreted in human milk. Nursing should not be undertaken during lithium therapy except in rare and unusual circumstances where, in the view of the physician, the potential benefits to the mother outweigh possible hazards to the child.
Usage in Children: Since information regarding the safety and effectiveness of lithium carbonate in children under 12 years of age is not available, its use in such patients is not recommended at this time.
Precautions: The ability to tolerate lithium is greater during the acute manic phase and decreases when manic symptoms subside (see DOSAGE AND ADMINISTRATION).
The distribution space of lithium approximates that of total body water. Lithium is primarily excreted in urine with insignificant excretion in feces. Renal excretion of lithium is proportional to its plasma concentration. The half-life of elimination of lithium is approximately 24 hours. Lithium decreases sodium reabsorption by the renal tubules which could lead to sodium depletion. Therefore, it is essential for the patient to maintain a normal diet, including salt, and an adequate fluid intake (2500–3000 ml.) at least during the initial stabilization period. Decreased tolerance to lithium has been reported to ensue from protracted sweating or diarrhea and, if such occur, supplemental fluid and salt should be administered.
In addition to sweating and diarrhea, concomitant infection with elevated temperatures may also necessitate a temporary reduction or cessation of medication.
Previously existing underlying thyroid disorders do not necessarily constitute a contraindication to lithium treatment; where hypothy-

Continued on next page

Smith Kline & French—Cont.

roidism exists, careful monitoring of thyroid function during lithium stabilization and maintenance allows for correction of changing thyroid parameters, if any; where hypothyroidism occurs during lithium stabilization and maintenance, supplemental thyroid treatment may be used.

Adverse Reactions: Adverse reactions are seldom encountered at serum lithium levels below 1.5 mEq./l., except in the occasional patient unusually sensitive to lithium. Mild to moderate toxic reactions may occur at levels from 1.5 to 2.5 mEq./l., and moderate to severe reactions may be seen at levels from 2.0 to 2.5 mEq./l., depending upon the individual response to the drug.

Fine hand tremor, polyuria, and mild thirst may occur during initial therapy for the acute manic phase, and may persist throughout treatment. Transient and mild nausea and general discomfort may also appear during the first few days of lithium administration.

These side effects are an inconvenience rather than a disabling condition, and usually subside with continued treatment or a temporary reduction or cessation of dosage. If persistent, a cessation of dosage is indicated.

Diarrhea, vomiting, drowsiness, muscular weakness, and lack of coordination may be early signs of lithium intoxication, and can occur at lithium levels below 2.0 mEq./l. At higher levels, ataxia, giddiness, tinnitus, blurred vision, and a large output of dilute urine may be seen. Serum lithium levels above 3.0 mEq./l. may produce a complex clinical picture, involving multiple organs and organ systems. Serum lithium levels should not be permitted to exceed 2.0 mEq./l. during the acute treatment phase.

The following reactions have been reported and appear to be related to serum lithium levels, including levels within the therapeutic range: **Neuromuscular**—tremor, muscle hyperirritability (fasciculations, twitching, clonic movements of whole limbs), ataxia, choreoathetotic movements, hyperactive deep tendon reflex; **Central Nervous System**—blackout spells, epileptiform seizures, slurred speech, dizziness, vertigo, incontinence of urine or feces, somnolence, psychomotor retardation, restlessness, confusion, stupor, coma; **Cardiovascular**—cardiac arrhythmia, hypotension, peripheral circulatory collapse; **Gastrointestinal**—anorexia, nausea, vomiting, diarrhea; **Genitourinary**—albuminuria, oliguria, polyuria, glycosuria; **Dermatologic**—drying and thinning of hair, alopecia, anesthesia of skin, chronic folliculitis, exacerbation of psoriasis, xerosis cutis; **Autonomic**—blurred vision, dry mouth; **Thyroid Abnormalities**—euthyroid goiter and/or hypothyroidism (including myxedema) accompanied by lower T_3 and T_4. I^{131} uptake may be elevated. (See Precautions.) Paradoxically, rare cases of hyperthyroidism have been reported. **EEG Changes**—diffuse slowing, widening of the frequency spectrum, potentiation and disorganization of background rhythm; **EKG Changes**—reversible flattening, isoelectricity or inversion of T-waves; **Miscellaneous**—fatigue, lethargy, transient scotomata, dehydration, weight loss, tendency to sleep.

Miscellaneous reactions unrelated to dosage include: transient electroencephalographic and electrocardiographic changes, leukocytosis, headache, diffuse nontoxic goiter with or without hypothyroidism, transient hyperglycemia, generalized pruritus with or without rash, cutaneous ulcers, albuminuria, worsening of organic brain syndromes, excessive weight gain, edematous swelling of ankles or wrists, thirst or polyuria, sometimes resembling diabetes insipidus, and metallic taste.

A single report has been received of the development of painful discoloration of fingers and toes and coldness of the extremities within one day of the starting of treatment with lithium. The mechanism through which these symptoms (resembling Raynaud's syndrome) developed is not known. Recovery followed discontinuance.

Dosage and Administration:

Acute Mania—Optimal patient response to Eskalith (lithium carbonate, SK&F) can usually be established and maintained with 600 mg. t.i.d. Such doses will normally produce the desired serum lithium level ranging between 1.0 and 1.5 mEq./l.

Dosage must be individualized according to serum levels and clinical response. Regular monitoring of the patient's clinical state and serum lithium levels is necessary. Serum levels should be determined twice per week during the acute phase, and until the serum level and clinical condition of the patient have been stabilized.

Long-Term Control—The desirable serum lithium levels are 0.6 to 1.2 mEq./l. Dosage will vary from one individual to another, but usually 300 mg. t.i.d. or q.i.d. will maintain this level. Serum lithium levels in uncomplicated cases receiving maintenance therapy during remission should be monitored at least every two months.

Patients abnormally sensitive to lithium may exhibit toxic signs at serum levels of 1.0 to 1.5 mEq./l. Elderly patients often respond to reduced dosage, and may exhibit signs of toxicity at serum levels ordinarily tolerated by other patients.

N.B.: Blood samples for serum lithium determinations should be drawn immediately prior to the next dose when lithium concentrations are relatively stable (i.e., 8–12 hours after the previous dose). Total reliance must not be placed on serum levels alone. Accurate patient evaluation requires both clinical and laboratory analysis.

Overdosage: The toxic levels for lithium are close to the therapeutic levels. It is therefore important that patients and their families be cautioned to watch for early toxic symptoms and to discontinue the drug and inform the physician should they occur. Toxic symptoms are listed in detail under ADVERSE REACTIONS.

Treatment: No specific antidote for lithium poisoning is known. Early symptoms of lithium toxicity can usually be treated by reduction or cessation of dosage of the drug and resumption of the treatment at a lower dose after 24 to 48 hours. In severe cases of lithium poisoning, the first and foremost goal of treatment consists of elimination of this ion from the patient. Treatment is essentially the same as that used in barbiturate poisoning: 1) gastric lavage, 2) correction of fluid and electrolyte imbalance, and 3) regulation of kidney function. Urea, mannitol, and aminophylline all produce significant increases in lithium excretion. Hemodialysis is an effective and rapid means of removing the ion from the severely toxic patient. Infection prophylaxis, regular chest X-rays and preservation of adequate respiration are essential.

How Supplied: 300 mg. capsules in bottles of 100 and 500; 300 mg. scored tablets in bottles of 100.

[*Shown in Product Identification Section*]

ESKATROL® SPANSULE® CAPSULES Ⓒ

Amphetamines have a significant potential for abuse. In view of their short-term anorectic effect and rapid development of tolerance, they should be used with extreme caution and only for limited periods of time in weight-reduction programs.

Description: 'Eskatrol' contains dextroamphetamine sulfate and prochlorperazine. Dextroamphetamine sulfate is the dextro isomer of the compound *d, l*-amphetamine sulfate, a sympathomimetic amine of the amphetamine group. Chemically, dextroamphetamine is *d*-alpha-methylphenethylamine, and is present in 'Eskatrol' as the neutral sulfate. Prochlorperazine is 2-chloro-10 [3-(4-methyl -1- piperazinyl)-propyl]-phenothiazine, and is present in 'Eskatrol' as the maleate.

Each 'Eskatrol' *Spansule* capsule contains dextroamphetamine sulfate, 15 mg., and prochlorperazine, 7.5 mg., as the maleate, so prepared that an initial dose is released promptly and the remaining medication is released gradually over a prolonged period.

Actions: Dextroamphetamine sulfate is a sympathomimetic amine with CNS stimulant activity. Peripheral actions include elevation of systolic and diastolic blood pressures and weak bronchodilator and respiratory stimulant action. The anorectic effect diminishes after a few weeks. Prochlorperazine, a nonsedative tranquilizer, minimizes the stimulation which may occur in some patients on dextroamphetamine sulfate alone. The 'Spansule' capsule dosage form provides the convenience of once-a-day dosage.

Indications

Based on a review of this drug by the National Academy of Sciences—National Research Council and/or other information, FDA has classified the indications as follows:

Possibly effective: In exogenous obesity, as a short-term (a few weeks) adjunct in a regimen of weight reduction based on caloric restriction.

Final classification of the less-than-effective indications requires further investigation.

Contraindications: Advanced arteriosclerosis, symptomatic cardiovascular disease, moderate to severe hypertension, hyperthyroidism, known hypersensitivity or idiosyncrasy to the sympathomimetic amines.

Agitated states.

Patients with a history of drug abuse, phenothiazine-induced jaundice or blood dyscrasias, or in the presence of bone marrow depression.

During or within 14 days following the administration of monoamine oxidase inhibitors; hypertensive crises may result.

Lactating (nursing) mothers.

Because of the antiemetic action of the prochlorperazine component, 'Eskatrol' *Spansule* capsules should not be used where nausea and vomiting are believed to be a manifestation of intestinal obstruction or brain tumor.

Warnings: Tolerance to the anorectic effect usually develops within a few weeks. When this occurs, the recommended dose should not be exceeded in an attempt to increase the effect; rather, the drug should be discontinued.

Amphetamines may mask extreme fatigue which can impair the ability to perform potentially hazardous activities such as operating machinery or driving motor vehicles; patients should be cautioned accordingly.

Drug Dependence: Amphetamines have a significant potential for abuse. Tolerance and extreme psychological dependence have occurred. There are reports of patients who have increased dosage to many times that recommended. For these reasons, care should be used in the selection of candidates for 'Eskatrol' therapy. Should psychological dependence occur, discontinue medication. Abrupt cessation following prolonged high dosage of amphetamines results in extreme fatigue and mental depression; changes have also been noted on the sleep EEG.

Manifestations of chronic intoxication with amphetamines include severe dermatoses, marked insomnia, irritability, hyperactivity, and personality changes. The most severe manifestation of chronic intoxication is psychosis, often clinically indistinguishable from schizophrenia.

Usage in Pregnancy: Safe use in pregnancy has not been established. Reproductive studies in mammals at high multiples of the human dose of amphetamines have suggested an embryotoxic and a teratogenic potential. Use of amphetamines by women who are or who may become pregnant, and especially those in the first trimester of pregnancy, requires that the potential benefit be weighed against the possible hazard to mother and infant.

Usage in Children: Amphetamines are not recommended for use as anorectic agents in children under 12 years of age.

Precautions: Use with caution in mild hypertension.

Insulin requirements in diabetes mellitus may be altered in association with the use of amphetamines and the concomitant dietary regimen.

Amphetamines may decrease the hypotensive effect of guanethidine.

The smallest quantity feasible should be prescribed or dispensed at one time in order to minimize the possibility of overdosage.

Although prochlorperazine has little or no clinically significant potentiating activity, phenothiazines may intensify and prolong the action of central nervous system depressants including alcohol. If hypotension should occur, epinephrine should not be used, since there may be a reversal of its usual hypertensive effect.

Adverse Reactions: Dextroamphetamine sulfate: *Cardiovascular:* Palpitation, tachycardia, elevation of blood pressure. *Central Nervous System:* Overstimulation, restlessness, dizziness, insomnia, euphoria, dyskinesia, dysphoria, tremor, headache; rarely, psychotic episodes at recommended doses. *Gastrointestinal:* Dryness of the mouth, unpleasant taste, diarrhea, other gastrointestinal disturbances. *Allergic:* Urticaria. *Endocrine:* Impotence, changes in libido.

Prochlorperazine: Sedation, dizziness, hypotension, tachycardia, dry mouth, skin rash, tinnitus, vertigo, nasal congestion, miosis, lethargy, cholestatic jaundice, leukopenia, agranulocytosis, extrapyramidal or parkinsonism-like symptoms (spasticity, painful constriction of skeletal muscles, or myotonia dystonica, chiefly those of the head, neck, and shoulders, sometimes resulting in dislocations and fractures, opisthotonos, oculogyric crises, carpopedal spasms, dystonias and persistent tardive dyskinesia), convulsions, catatonic-like reactions, and reversal of epinephrine effects.

Adverse Reactions Reported with Prochlorperazine or Other Phenothiazine Derivatives: Adverse reactions with different phenothiazines vary in type, frequency, and mechanism of occurrence, i.e., some are dose-related, while others involve individual patient sensitivity. Some adverse effects may be more likely to occur, or occur with greater intensity, in patients with special medical problems, e.g., patients with mitral insufficiency or pheochromocytoma have experienced severe hypotension following recommended doses of certain phenothiazines. Not all of the following adverse reactions have been observed with every phenothiazine derivative, but they have been reported with one or more and should be borne in mind when drugs of this class are administered: extrapyramidal symptoms (opisthotonos, oculogyric crisis, hyperreflexia, dystonia, akathisia, dyskinesia, parkinsonism) some of which, in rare instances, have lasted months and even years—particularly in elderly patients with previous brain damage; grand mal convulsions; altered cerebrospinal fluid proteins; cerebral edema; intensification and prolongation of the action of central nervous system depressants (opiates, analgesics, antihistamines, barbiturates, alcohol), atropine, heat, organophosphorus insecticides; autonomic reactions (dryness of mouth, nasal congestion, headache, nausea, constipation, obstipation, adynamic ileus, inhibition of ejaculation); reactivation of psychotic processes, catatonic-like states; hypotension (sometimes fatal); cardiac arrest; blood dyscrasias (pancytopenia, thrombocytopenic purpura, leukopenia, agranulocytosis, eosinophilia); liver damage (jaundice, biliary stasis); endocrine disturbances (lactation, galactorrhea, gynecomastia, menstrual irregularities, false positive pregnancy tests); skin disorders (photosensitivity, itching, erythema, urticaria, eczema up to exfoliative dermatitis); other allergic reactions (asthma, laryngeal edema, angioneurotic edema, anaphylactoid reactions); peripheral edema, reversed epinephrine effect; hyperpyrexia; a systemic lupus erythematosus-like syndrome; pigmentary retinopathy; with prolonged administration of substantial doses, skin pigmentation, epithelial keratopathy, and lenticular and corneal deposits.

EKG changes—particularly nonspecific, usually reversible Q and T wave distortions—have been observed in some patients receiving phenothiazine tranquilizers. Their relationship to myocardial damage has not been confirmed.

Although phenothiazines cause neither psychic nor physical dependence, sudden discontinuance in long-term psychiatric patients may cause temporary symptoms, e.g., nausea and vomiting, dizziness, tremulousness.

Note: There have been occasional reports of sudden death in patients receiving phenothiazines. In some cases, the cause appeared to be asphyxia due to failure of the cough reflex. In others, the cause could not be determined. There is not sufficient evidence to establish a relationship between such deaths and the administration of phenothiazines.

Dosage and Administration: One capsule daily, taken in the morning. If appetite control is desired through evening hours, shift dose to midmorning. Late afternoon or evening medication should be avoided because of the resulting insomnia. Not recommended in children under 12 years of age.

NOTE: Appetite depressants are usually most effective for therapy periods of 4 to 8 weeks. Should patients become tolerant to the anorectic effect, it is advisable to discontinue the medication for 2 to 4 weeks before reinstituting therapy if a longer period of anorectic treatment is indicated at this point.

Overdosage: (See also Adverse Reactions) Symptoms of 'Eskatrol' overdosage may be those of either dextroamphetamine sulfate or prochlorperazine overdosage.

Dextroamphetamine sulfate: *Symptoms*—These are usually extensions of the therapeutic actions of the drug. Central effects may include restlessness, dizziness, increased reflexes, tremor, insomnia, tenseness and irritability; also, confusion, assaultiveness, hallucinations and panic states. Fatigue and depression usually follow central stimulation. Cardiovascular reactions may include chilliness, pallor or flushing, sweating, palpitation, hypertension or hypotension, headache, extrasystoles and other arrhythmias, anginal pain, circulatory collapse and syncope. Gastrointestinal effects include nausea, vomiting, diarrhea and abdominal cramps. Severe poisoning may result in convulsions and coma. *Treatment*—The treatment of overdosage with dextroamphetamine sulfate is essentially symptomatic. In addition to gastric lavage and catharsis, sedatives should be given when indicated. For this purpose the barbiturates, either orally or parenterally, are generally used. To provide a basal level of sedation, one or more doses of sodium amobarbital may be given by mouth or, if necessary, by intramuscular injection. This may be repeated as often as necessary and in quantities sufficient to control the symptoms. In general, the hypertension which may result from massive overdosage of dextroamphetamine sulfate does not require treatment. A gradual drop in blood pressure will usually result when sufficient sedation has been administered. In the presence of severe hypotension the usual procedures employed for shock should be instituted (see below, treatment of hypotension due to prochlorperazine overdosage). If the urine is alkaline, excretion of the dextroamphetamine sulfate component may be diminished. Experience with hemodialysis or peritoneal dialysis in amphetamine overdosage is inadequate to permit recommendations in this regard.

Prochlorperazine: *Symptoms*—Primarily involvement of the extrapyramidal mechanism producing some of the dystonic reactions described above.

Symptoms of central nervous system depression to the point of somnolence or coma. Agitation and restlessness may also occur. Other possible manifestations include convulsions, fever, and autonomic reactions such as hypotension, dry mouth and ileus.

Treatment—Essentially symptomatic and supportive. Early gastric lavage is helpful. Keep patient under observation and maintain an open airway, since involvement of the extrapyramidal mechanism may produce dysphagia and respiratory difficulty in severe overdosage. **Do not attempt to induce emesis because a dystonic reaction of the head or neck may develop that could result in aspiration of vomitus.** Extrapyramidal symptoms may be treated with anti-parkinsonism drugs, barbiturates, or 'Benadryl'.*

If administration of a stimulant is desirable, amphetamine, dextroamphetamine, or caffeine with sodium benzoate is recommended. Stimulants that may cause convulsions (e.g., picrotoxin or pentylenetetrazol) should be avoided.

If hypotension occurs, the standard measures for managing circulatory shock should be initiated. If it is desirable to administer a vasoconstrictor, 'Levophed' and 'Neo-Synephrine'† are most suitable. Other pressor agents, including epinephrine, are not recommended because phenothiazine derivatives may reverse the usual elevating action of these agents and cause a further lowering of blood pressure.

Limited experience indicates that phenothiazines are *not* dialyzable.

Special note on 'Spansule' capsules—Since much of the 'Spansule' capsule medication is coated for gradual release, therapy directed at reversing the effects of the ingested drugs and at supporting the patient should be continued for as long as overdosage symptoms remain. Saline cathartics are useful for hastening evacuation of pellets that have not already released medication.

How Supplied: Bottles of 50 capsules.

*Trademark Reg. U.S. Pat. Off.: 'Benadryl' for diphenhydramine hydrochloride, Parke-Davis.
†'Levophed' and 'Neo-Synephrine' are the trademarks (Reg. U.S. Pat. Off.) of Winthrop Laboratories for its brands of levarterenol and phenylephrine respectively.

[*Shown in Product Identification Section*]

FEOSOL® ELIXIR††
Hematinic

Description: Feosol Elixir, an unusually palatable iron elixir, provides the body with ferrous sulfate—iron in its most efficient form. The standard elixir for simple iron deficiency and iron-deficiency anemia when the need for such therapy has been determined by a physician.

Each 5 ml. (1 teaspoonful) contains ferrous sulfate USP, 220 mg. (44 mg. of elemental iron); alcohol, 5%

Usual Dosage: *Adults*—1 to 2 teaspoonfuls three times daily. *Children*—½ to 1 teaspoonful three times daily preferably between

Continued on next page

Smith Kline & French—Cont.

meals. *Infants*—as directed by physician. Mix with water or fruit juice to avoid temporary staining of teeth; do not mix with milk or wine-based vehicles.
Warning: The treatment of any anemic condition should be under the advice and supervision of a physician. Since oral iron products interfere with absorption of oral tetracycline antibiotics, these products should not be taken within two hours of each other. Occasional gastrointestinal discomfort (such as nausea) may be minimized by taking with meals and by beginning with one teaspoonful the first day, two the second, etc. until the recommended doage is reached. Iron-containing medication may occasionally cause constipation or diarrhea, and liquids may cause temporary staining of the teeth (this is less likely when diluted). Keep this and all medicines out of reach of children. In case of accidental overdose, contact a physician or poison control center immediately.
How Supplied: A clear orange liquid in 12 fl. oz. bottles.
Also Available: Feosol® Tablets, Feosol® Spansule capsules.

††Feosol Elixir is a product of Menley & James Laboratories, Professional Products Division, a SmithKline company.

FEOSOL® SPANSULE® CAPSULES††
Hematinic

Description: Feosol *Spansule* capsules provide the body with ferrous sulfate—iron in its most efficient form—for simple iron deficiency and iron-deficiency anemia, when the need for such therapy has been determined by a physician.
The special *Spansule* capsule formulation—ferrous sulfate in pellets—reduces stomach upset, a common problem with iron.
Formula: Each capsule contains 167 mg. of dried ferrous sulfate USP (50 mg. of elemental iron), equivalent to 250 mg. of ferrous sulfate USP.
Usual Dosage: *Adults and Children*—One to two Feosol *Spansule* capsules daily, depending on severity of iron deficiency. Children too young to swallow the capsule can be given the contents in a spoonful of soft, cool food (aplesauce, custard, etc.) *Children under 6*—Use Feosol® Elixir.
Warning: The treatment of any anemic condition should be under the advice and supervision of a physician. Since oral iron products interfere with absorption of oral tetracycline antibiotics, these products should not be taken within two hours of each other. Keep this and all medicines out of reach of children. In case of accidental overdose, contact a physician or poison control center immediately. Iron containing medicine may occasionally cause constipation or diarrhea.
How Supplied: Bottles of 30 and 500 capsules; in Single Unit Packages of 100 capsules (intended for institutional use only).
Also available in Tablets and Elixir.

††Feosol *Spansule* capsules are a product of Menley & James Laboratories, Professional Products Division, a SmithKline company.
[*Shown in Product Identification Section*]

FEOSOL® TABLETS††
Hematinic

Description: Feosol Tablets provide the body with ferrous sulfate, iron in its most efficient form, for iron deficiency and iron-deficiency anemia when the need for such therapy has been determined by a physician. The distinctive triangular-shaped tablet has a special coating to prevent oxidation and improve palatability.
Formula: Each tablet contains 200 mg. of dried ferrous sulfate USP (65 mg. of elemental iron), equivalent to 325 mg. (5 grains) of ferrous sulfate USP.
Usual Dosage: *Adults*—one tablet 3 to 4 times daily, after meals and upon retiring. *Children 6 to 12 years*—one tablet three times a day after meals. *Children under 6 years and infants*—use Feosol® Elixir.
Warning: The treatment of any anemic condition should be under the advice and supervision of a physician. Since oral iron products interfere with absorption of oral tetracycline antibiotics, these products should not be taken within two hours of each other.
Occasional gastrointestinal discomfort (such as nausea) may be minimized by taking with meals and by beginning with one tablet the first day, two the second, etc. until the recommended dosage is reached. Iron-containing medication may occasionally cause constipation or diarrhea.
Keep this and all medicines out of reach of children. In case of accidental overdose, contact a physician or poison control center immediately.
How Supplied: Bottles of 100 and 1000 tablets; in Single Unit Packages of 100 tablets (intended for institutional use only).
Also available in Spansule® capsules and Elixir.

††Feosol Tablets are a product of Menley & James Laboratories, Professional Products Division, a SmithKline company.
[*Shown in Product Identification Section*]

FEOSOL PLUS® ℞
(Modified Formula)

Description: Each 'Feosol Plus' capsule contains:

Ferrous sulfate, dried (equivalent to 325 mg. ferrous sulfate USP; 65 mg. of elemental iron)	200 mg.
Folic acid	0.4 mg.
Ascorbic acid (C)	50 mg.
Thiamine hydrochloride (B_1)	2 mg.
Riboflavin (B_2)	2 mg.
Pyridoxine hydrochloride (B_6)	2 mg.
Vitamin B_{12} (Activity Equiv.)	5 mcg.
Nicotinic acid (Niacin)	20 mg.

Indications: For use in iron deficiency and iron-deficiency anemia where additional vitamins are indicated.
Warning: The use of folic acid in patients who have or may develop pernicious anemia involves a serious hazard of permitting progressive degeneration of the spinal cord while treating the anemia characteristic of the disease. Parenterally administered cyanocobalamin (Vitamin B_{12}) is the therapy of choice in pernicious anemia and should be employed in patients receiving folic acid unless pernicious anemia has been ruled out.
Precaution: Since oral iron products interfere with absorption of oral tetracycline antibiotics, these products should not be taken within two hours of each other.
Adverse Reactions: Adverse reactions with 'Feosol Plus' are primarily those due to the iron content, e.g., occasional gastrointestinal discomfort (such as nausea), dose-related bowel effects (such as constipation or diarrhea). Gastrointestinal effects may be minimized by administration with meals.
Dosage and Administration: Two capsules daily after meals, depending on the degree of iron deficiency. *Children 4 years of age and over*—one or two capsules daily.
Overdosage: Symptoms and treatment same as for 'Feosol' Tablets.
How Supplied: Bottles of 100 capsules.
[*Shown in Product Identification Section*]

FORTESPAN®††
Therapeutic Multivitamins

Description: For the treatment of multiple vitamin deficiencies.
Formula: Each Fortespan capsule contains:

Ascorbic acid (Vitamin C)	150 mg.
Thiamine mononitrate (Vitamin B_1)	6 mg.
Riboflavin (Vitamin B_2 as the phosphate)	6 mg.
Nicotinamide	60 mg.
Pyridoxine HCl (Vitamin B_6)	6 mg.
Vitamin A	10,000 International Units
Vitamin D	400 International Units
Vitamin B_{12} (cyanocobalamin)	15 mcg.
Pantothenic acid (as *dl*-panthenol)	6 mg.

Usual Dosage: One Fortespan capsule at breakfast or as directed by physician.
Warning: Keep this and all medicines out of reach of children. In case of accidental overdose, contact a physician or poison control center immediately.
How Supplied: Bottles of 30 and 100 capsules.

††Fortespan is a product of Menley & James Laboratories, Professional Products Division, a SmithKline company.
[*Shown in Product Identification Section*]

HISPRIL® ℞
(brand of diphenylpyraline hydrochloride)
SPANSULE® CAPSULES 5 mg.

Description: Hispril®, brand of diphenylpyraline HCl, is an antihistamine.
Each 'Spansule' capsule contains diphenylpyraline hydrochloride, 5 mg., so prepared that an initial dose is released promptly and the remaining medication is released gradually over a prolonged period.
Actions: Diphenylpyraline hydrochloride is an antihistamine with anticholinergic (drying) and sedative side effects. Antihistamines appear to compete with histamine for cell receptor sites on effector cells.
Indications: For the symptomatic treatment of perennial and seasonal allergic rhinitis; vasomotor rhinitis; allergic conjunctivitis due to inhalant allergens and foods; mild, uncomplicated allergic skin manifestations of urticaria and angioedema; amelioration of allergic reactions to blood or plasma; dermographism; and as therapy for anaphylactic reactions adjunctive to epinephrine and other standard measures after the acute manifestations have been controlled.
Contraindications:
Use in Newborn or Premature Infants—This drug should *not* be used in newborn or premature infants.
Use in Nursing Mothers—Because of the higher risk of antihistamines for infants generally and for newborns and prematures in particular, antihistamine therapy is contraindicated in nursing mothers.
Use in Lower Respiratory Disease—Antihistamines *should NOT* be used to treat lower respiratory tract symptoms including asthma.
Antihistamines are also contraindicated in the following conditions:
- Hypersensitivity to diphenylpyraline hydrochloride and other antihistamines of similar chemical structure
- Monoamine oxidase inhibitor therapy (See Drug Interactions section)

Warnings: Antihistamines should be used with considerable caution in patients with:
- Narrow angle glaucoma
- Stenosing peptic ulcer
- Pyloroduodenal obstruction
- Symptomatic prostatic hypertrophy
- Bladder neck obstruction

Use in Children—In infants and children, especially, antihistamines in *overdosage* may cause hallucinations, convulsions, or death.
As in adults, antihistamines may diminish mental alertness in children. In the young

child, particularly, they may produce excitation.

Use in Pregnancy—Experience with this drug in pregnant women is inadequate to determine whether there exists a potential for harm to the developing fetus.

Use with CNS Depressants—Diphenylpyraline hydrochloride has additive effects with alcohol and other CNS depressants (hypnotics, sedatives, tranquilizers, etc.).

Use in Activities Requiring Mental Alertness—Patients should be warned about engaging in activities requiring mental alertness as driving a car or operating appliances, machinery, etc.

Use in the Elderly (approximately 60 years or older)—Antihistamines are more likely to cause dizziness, sedation, and hypotension in the elderly than in younger patients.

Precautions: Diphenylpyraline hydrochloride has an atropine-like action and, therefore, should be used with caution in patients with:

History of bronchial asthma
Increased intraocular pressure
Hyperthyroidism
Cardiovascular disease
Hypertension

Drug Interactions—MAO inhibitors prolong and intensify the anticholinergic (drying) effects of antihistamines.

Adverse Reactions: The most frequent adverse reactions are underlined:

1. **General:** Urticaria, drug rash, anaphylactic shock, photosensitivity, excessive perspiration, chills, dryness of mouth, nose, and throat.
2. **Cardiovascular System:** Hypotension, headache, palpitations, tachycardia, extrasystoles.
3. **Hematologic System:** Hemolytic anemia, thrombocytopenia, agranulocytosis.
4. **Nervous System:** Sedation, sleepiness, dizziness, disturbed coordination, fatigue, confusion, restlessness, excitation, nervousness, tremor, irritability, insomnia, euphoria, paresthesias, blurred vision, diplopia, vertigo, tinnitus, acute labyrinthitis, hysteria, neuritis, convulsions.
5. **G.I. System:** Epigastric distress, anorexia, nausea, vomiting, diarrhea, constipation.
6. **G.U. System:** Urinary frequency, difficult urination, urinary retention, early menses.
7. **Respiratory System:** Thickening of bronchial secretions, tightness of chest and wheezing, nasal stuffiness.

Overdosage: Antihistamine overdosage reactions may vary from central nervous system depression to stimulation. Stimulation is particularly likely in children. Atropine-like signs and symptoms—dry mouth; fixed, dilated pupils; flushing; and gastrointestinal symptoms may also occur. Marked cerebral irritation, resulting in jerking of muscles and possible convulsions, may be followed by deep stupor.

If vomiting has not occurred spontaneously the patient should be induced to vomit. This is best done by having him drink a glass of water or milk after which he should be made to gag. Precautions against aspiration must be taken, especially in infants and children.

If vomiting is unsuccessful gastric lavage is indicated within 3 hours after ingestion and even later if large amounts of milk or cream were given beforehand. Isotonic or ½ isotonic saline is the lavage solution of choice.

Saline cathartics, as milk of magnesia, by osmosis draw water into the bowel and, therefore, are valuable for their action in rapid dilution of bowel content.

Do not treat CNS depression with analeptics which might precipitate convulsions. Use only short-acting depressants to treat convulsions. **Stimulants** should *not* be used.

If a vasoconstrictor is required for hypotension, levarterenol bitartrate, USP, may be used. Other pressor agents, including epinephrine, should not be used as they may cause a paradoxical further lowering of blood pressure.

Special note on 'Spansule' capsules—Since much of the 'Spansule' capsule medication is coated for gradual release, therapy directed at reversing the effects of the ingested drug and at supporting the patient should be continued for as long as overdosage symptoms remain. Saline cathartics are useful for hastening evacuation of pellets that have not already released medication.

Dosage and Administration: DOSAGE SHOULD BE INDIVIDUALIZED ACCORDING TO THE NEEDS AND THE RESPONSE OF THE PATIENT.

Adults—One capsule (5 mg.), q12h.

Older Children (6–12 years)—One 5 mg. capsule daily is usually sufficient. The physician should bear in mind that in children a higher incidence and a greater degree of antihistaminic side effects may be encountered. Do not use in children under 6 years.

How Supplied: Bottles of 50 capsules.

[*Shown in Product Identification Section*]

ORNACOL®††

Relieves coughing and nasal congestion.

Description: Ornacol is specifically formulated for temporary relief from coughing and nasal congestion due to the common cold and sinusitis.

Ornacol contains no sedatives or antihistamines and, therefore, does not produce drowsiness in most people. This makes it especially suited for working people and others who must remain alert.

Composition: Each red and gray Ornacol Cough & Cold Capsule contains: 30 mg. dextromethorphan hydrobromide; 25 mg. phenylpropanolamine hydrochloride.

Each teaspoonful (5 ml.) of Ornacol Cough & Cold Liquid contains: 15 mg. phenylpropanolamine hydrochloride; alcohol 8%.

Dosage: Ornacol Capsules: *Adults and children over 12*—one capsule four times a day. *Children*—use Ornacol Liquid.

Ornacol Liquid: *Adults and children over 12*—two teaspoonfuls four times a day. *Children (4–12)*—one teaspoonful four times a day. *Children (2–4)*—one half teaspoonful four times a day.

Warning: Persistent cough may indicate the presence of a serious condition. Persons with a high fever or persistent cough should not use this preparation unless directed by a physician.

Individual with high blood pressure, heart disease, diabetes or thyroid disease should use only as directed by a physician. If relief does not occur within three days, discontinue use and consult a physician.

Keep this and all medicines out of reach of children. In case of accidental overdose, contact a physician or a poison control center immediately.

Supplied: Ornacol Cough & Cold Capsules in packages of 20 and bottles of 100. Ornacol Cough & Cold Liquid in 4 fl. oz. bottles.

††Ornacol is a product of Menley & James Laboratories, Professional Products Division, a SmithKline company.

[*Shown in Product Identification Section*]

ORNADE® SPANSULE® CAPSULES ℞

Description: Each 'Spansule' capsule contains 8 mg. of chlorpheniramine maleate and 50 mg. of phenylpropanolamine hydrochloride, so prepared that an initial dose is released promptly and the remaining medication is released gradually over a prolonged period; and isopropamide iodide equivalent to 2.5 mg. of isopropamide. Because isopropamide iodide, a synthetic anticholinergic, can provide 10 to 12 hours of antisecretory action, this component is not in sustained release form.

Actions: 'Ornade' provides relief of sneezing, running nose, weeping and other symptoms of nasal congestion. Its formula contains a drying agent, isopropamide iodide, in addition to a nasal decongestant and an antihistamine.

Indications

Based on a review of this drug by the National Academy of Sciences—National Research Council and/or other information, FDA has classified the indications as follows:

Possibly effective: For relief of upper respiratory tract congestion and hypersecretion associated with vasomotor rhinitis and allergic rhinitis, and for prolonged relief.

Lacking in substantial evidence of effectiveness: For relief of nasal congestion and hypersecretion associated with the common cold and sinusitis. Final classification of the less-than-effective indications requires further investigation.

Contraindications: Hypersensitivity to any of the components; concurrent MAO inhibitor therapy; severe hypertension; bronchial asthma; coronary artery disease; stenosing peptic ulcer; pyloroduodenal or bladder neck obstruction. Do not use in children under 6 years.

Warnings: Caution patients about activities requiring alertness (e.g., operating vehicles or machinery). Patients should also be warned about the possible additive effects of alcohol and other CNS depressants.

Usage in Pregnancy: Safe use in pregnancy has not been established. This drug should be used in pregnancy, nursing mothers or by women who might bear children only when the potential benefits have been weighed against the possible hazards to the mother and child. However, 'Ornade' has had extensive clinical use in pregnant patients without known deleterious effect. Rat reproduction studies with low drug doses have shown no teratogenic effect. As with all anticholinergics, an inhibitory effect on lactation may occur.

Effect on PBI Determination and I^{131} Uptake: The iodine in isopropamide iodide may alter the PBI determination and will suppress I^{131} uptake. Therefore, thyroid function tests unaffected by exogenous iodides should be substituted.

Precautions: Use with caution in persons with cardiovascular disease, glaucoma, prostatic hypertrophy, hyperthyroidism.

Adverse Reactions: Drowsiness; excessive dryness of nose, throat or mouth; nervousness; or insomnia may occur on rare occasions with 'Ornade', but are usually mild and transitory. Other reported adverse reactions are: nausea, vomiting, epigastric distress, diarrhea, rash, dizziness, weakness, tightness of chest, angina pain, abdominal pain, irritability, palpitation, headache, incoordination, tremor, difficulty in urination, dysuria, thrombocytopenia, leukopenia, convulsions, hypertension, hypotension, anorexia, constipation, visual disturbances. Isopropamide iodide may cause signs of iodine toxicity, such as acne and parotitis.

Dosage and Administration: (Not for use in children under 6 years of age.) Adults and children over 6—One 'Ornade' *Spansule* capsule q12h.

Overdosage: *Symptoms*—May include dryness of mouth, dysphagia, thirst, blurred vision, dilated pupils, photophobia, fever, rapid pulse and respiration, disorientation, and either excitation or depression of the central nervous system.

Treatment—Gastric lavage, repeated several times. Since much of the 'Spansule' capsule medication is coated for gradual release, saline cathartics should be administered to hasten

Continued on next page

Smith Kline & French—Cont.

evacuation of pellets that have not already released medication.
Respiratory depression should be treated promptly by the use of oxygen and stimulants. If marked excitement is present, one of the short-acting barbiturates or chloral hydrate may be used.
How Supplied: In bottles of 50 and 500; in Single Unit Packages of 100 (intended for institutional use only).
Military—Capsules, 500's, 6505-00-014-1028.
[*Shown in Product Identification Section*]

ORNADE 2® Liquid for Children

Description: Each 5 ml. teaspoonful of 'Ornade 2' Liquid for Children contains 12.5 mg. of phenylpropanolamine hydrochloride, 2 mg. of chlorpheniramine maleate, and alcohol 5%.
Actions: Phenylpropanolamine hydrochloride provides vasoconstriction similar to that of ephedrine but with less CNS stimulation. Chlorpheniramine maleate is an antihistamine (H_1-receptor antagonist) with anticholinergic (drying) and sedative side effects. Antihistamines appear to compete with histamine for H_1-receptor sites on effector cells.
Indications: For relief of runny nose, sneezing, itchy nose or throat, itchy and watery eyes or nasal congestion as may occur in the common cold or in allergic rhinitis such as hay fever.
Contraindications: Hypersensitivity to either ingredient, severe hypertension or severe coronary artery disease. 'Ornade 2' Liquid for Children should NOT be used to treat lower respiratory tract conditions such as asthma. As in any product containing a sympathomimetic, 'Ornade 2' Liquid for Children should NOT be used in patients taking MAO inhibitors.
Adverse Reactions: Drowsiness; excessive dryness of nose, throat or mouth; nervousness or insomnia may occur on rare occasions with 'Ornade 2' Liquid for Children but is usually mild and transitory. Other reported adverse reactions with the components of this formulation include: nausea, vomiting, epigastric distress, diarrhea, rash, dizziness, weakness, tightness of chest, angina pain, abdominal pain, irritability, palpitation, headache, incoordination, tremor, difficulty in urination, dysuria, thrombocytopenia, leukopenia, convulsions, hypertension, hypotension, anorexia, constipation, visual disturbances.
Dosage: Adults and children 12 and over—2 teaspoonfuls every four hours. Children 6 to 12—1 teaspoonful every four hours. For children 2 to 6 years, oral dosage is ½ teaspoon every 4 to 6 hours. Do not exceed 6 doses in 24 hours.
Note: Because 'Ornade 2' Liquid for Children may be purchased without a prescription, the following warnings and information appear on package labelling:
"**Warnings:** May cause drowsiness. Use caution in activities requiring alertness (e.g., operating vehicles or heavy machinery).
"Do not take this product if you are presently taking a prescription antihypertensive or antidepressant drug containing a monoamine oxidase inhibitor except on the advice of a physician. Individuals with asthma, glaucoma, high blood pressure, heart disease, enlarged prostate, diabetes or thyroid disease should use only under the advice and supervision of a physician.
"Avoid alcoholic beverages while taking this product. Do not exceed recommended dosage because at higher doses nervousness, dizziness, or sleeplessness may occur. May cause excitability, especially in children.
"If symptoms do not improve within 7 days or are accompanied by high fever, consult your physician before continuing use.
"Keep this and all drugs out of the reach of children. In case of accidental overdose, seek professional assistance or contact a poison control center immediately."
Overdosage: Symptoms may vary from central nervous system depression to stimulation. Also, atropine-like signs and symptoms (dry mouth; fixed, dilated pupils; flushing, etc.) as well as gastrointestinal symptoms may occur. Marked cerebral irritation resulting in jerking of muscles and possible convulsions may be followed by deep stupor and respiratory failure. Acute hypertension or cardiovascular collapse with accompanying hypotension may occur.
Treatment of Overdosage: Immediate evacuation of the stomach should be induced by emesis and gastric lavage. Respiratory depression should be treated promptly with oxygen. Do not treat respiratory or CNS depression with analeptics which might precipitate convulsions; if convulsions or marked CNS excitement occur, only short-acting barbiturates or chloral hydrate should be used.
Supplied: In 4 fl. oz. bottles with safety closure and 16 fl. oz. bottles.

ORNEX®††
decongestant/analgesic

Composition: Each blue and white Ornex capsule contains: 18 mg. phenylpropanolamine hydrochloride; 325 mg. acetaminophen.
Action: For temporary relief of nasal congestion, headache, aches, pains and fever due to colds, sinusitis and flu. No antihistamine drowsiness.
Dosage: Adults—TWO CAPSULES every 4 hours. Do not exceed 8 capsules in 24 hours. Children (6 to 12 years)—ONE CAPSULE every 4 hours. Do not exceed 4 capsules in 24 hours.
Warning: Do not give to children under 6 years or use for more than 10 days, unless directed by physician. Individuals with high blood pressure, heart disease, diabetes or thyroid disease should use only as directed by physician. Keep this and all medicines out of reach of children. In case of accidental overdose, contact a physician or poison control center immediately.
Supplied: In consumer packages of 24 and 48 capsules, in bottles of 100 capsules. Also, Dispensary Packages of 800 capsules for industrial dispensaries and student health clinics only.

††Ornex is a product of Menley & James Laboratories Professional Products Division, a SmithKline company.
[*Shown in Product Identification Section*]

PAREDRINE® 1% ℞
(brand of hydroxyamphetamine hydrobromide)
with BORIC ACID, OPHTHALMIC SOLUTION

Description: Hydroxyamphetamine hydrobromide, 1%, in distilled water. Made tear-isotonic with 2% boric acid, and preserved with thimerosal, 1:50,000.
Action: Dilates the pupil; probably by stimulating the dilator muscles of the iris.
Indication: To dilate the pupil; produces a pupillary dilatation which lasts for a few hours.
Contraindication: Narrow-angle glaucoma.
Precautions: Use with caution in patients with hypertension, hyperthyroidism and diabetes.
Adverse Reactions: With widely dilated pupils there will likely be increased intraocular pressure, photophobia and blurring of vision.
Dosage and Administration: Instil 1 or 2 drops into the conjunctival sac.
Overdosage: *Symptoms*—Dilatation of pupils. *Treatment*—Dilute pilocarpine (1%) may be administered if desired. Instil one drop at intervals. Repeat as necessary. **Accidental ingestion**—*Symptoms*—These may include marked rise in blood pressure, palpitation, cardiac arrhythmias, substernal discomfort, headache, sweating, nausea, vomiting and gastrointestinal irritation. *Treatment*—Sedation is indicated. Further treatment is symptomatic. Shock, if present, should be treated promptly. If hypertension is prominent, measures should be taken to lower blood pressure.
How Supplied: ½ fl. oz. bottles.

PARNATE® ℞
(brand of tranylcypromine sulfate)

Before prescribing, the physician should be familiar with the entire contents of this prescribing information.
Description: Each tablet contains tranylcypromine sulfate equivalent to 10 mg. of tranylcypromine.
Chemically, tranylcypromine sulfate is (±)-*trans*-2-phenylcyclopropylamine sulfate (2:1).
Action: Tranylcypromine is a non-hydrazine monoamine oxidase inhibitor with a rapid onset of activity. It increases the concentration of epinephrine, norepinephrine, and serotonin in storage sites throughout the nervous system, and in theory, this increased concentration of monoamines in the brainstem is the basis for its antidepressant activity. When tranylcypromine is withdrawn, monoamine oxidase activity is recovered in 3 to 5 days, although the drug is excreted in 24 hours.

Indications
Based on a review of this drug by the National Academy of Sciences—National Research Council and/or other information, FDA has classified the indications as follows:
Probably effective: For symptomatic relief of severe reactive or endogenous depression in hospitalized or closely supervised patients who have not responded to other antidepressant therapy.
Final classification of the less-than-effective indications requires further investigation.

Summary of Contraindications: Parnate (tranylcypromine sulfate, SK&F) should not be administered in combination with any of the following: MAO inhibitors or dibenzazepine derivatives; sympathomimetics (including amphetamines); some central nervous system depressants (including narcotics and alcohol); antihypertensive, diuretic, antihistaminic, sedative or anesthetic drugs; cheese or other foods with a high tyramine content; or excessive quantities of caffeine.
Parnate (tranylcypromine sulfate, SK&F) should not be administered to any patient beyond 60 years of age or with a confirmed or suspected cerebrovascular defect or to any patient with cardiovascular disease, hypertension or history of headache.
(For complete discussion of contraindications and warnings, see below.)
Contraindications: Parnate (tranylcypromine sulfate, SK&F) is contraindicated:
1. In patients with cerebrovascular defects or cardiovascular disorders
Parnate (tranylcypromine sulfate, SK&F) should not be administered to any patient with a confirmed or suspected cerebrovascular defect or to any patient with cardiovascular disease or hypertension. The drug should also be withheld from individuals beyond the age of 60 because of the possibility of existing cerebral sclerosis with damaged vessels.
2. In the presence of pheochromocytoma
Parnate (tranylcypromine sulfate, SK&F) should not be used in the presence of pheochromocytoma since such tumors secrete pressor substances.

3. In combination with MAO inhibitors or with dibenzazepine derivatives
Parnate (tranylcypromine, SK&F) should not be administered together or in rapid succession with other MAO inhibitors or with dibenzazepine derivatives. Hypertensive crises or severe convulsive seizures may occur in patients receiving such combinations.
In patients being transferred to 'Parnate' from another MAO inhibitor or from a dibenzazepine derivative, allow a medication-free interval of at least a week, then initiate 'Parnate' using half the normal starting dosage for at least the first week of therapy. Similarly, at least a week should elapse between the discontinuance of 'Parnate' and the administration of another MAO inhibitor or a dibenzazepine derivative.
Other MAO inhibitors presently known to be marketed in this country:

Generic Name	Trademark
Isocarboxazid	'Marplan' (Roche Laboratories)
Pargyline HCl	'Eutonyl' (Abbott Laboratories)
Pargyline HCl and methyclothiazide	'Eutron' (Abbott Laboratories)
Phenelzine sulfate	'Nardil' (Warner-Chilcott Laboratories)

Dibenzazepine derivatives and other tricyclic drugs presently known to be marketed in this country:

Generic Name	Trademark
Amitriptyline	'Elavil' (Merck Sharp & Dohme) 'SK-Amitriptyline' (Smith Kline &French)
Perphenazine and amitriptyline	'Etrafon' (Schering) 'Triavil' (Merck Sharp & Dohme)
Desipramine	'Norpramin' (Merrell-National) 'Pertofrane' (USV)
Imipramine	'Imavate' (Robins) 'Presamine' (USV) 'SK-Pramine' (Smith Kline &French) 'Tofranil' (Geigy Pharmaceuticals)
Nortriptyline	'Aventyl' (Eli Lilly & Co.)
Protriptyline	'Vivactil' (Merck Sharp & Dohme)
Doxepin	'Adapin' (Pennwalt) 'Sinequan' (Pfizer)
Carbamazepine	'Tegretol' (Geigy Pharmaceuticals)
Cyclobenzaprine HCl	'Flexeril' (Merck Sharp & Dohme)

4. In combination with sympathomimetics
Parnate (tranylcypromine sulfate, SK&F) should not be administered in combination with sympathomimetics, including amphetamines, and over-the-counter drugs such as cold, hay fever or weight-reducing preparations that contain vasoconstrictors.
During 'Parnate' therapy, it appears that certain patients are particularly vulnerable to the effects of sympathomimetics when the activity of certain enzymes is inhibited. Use of sympathomimetics and compounds such as methyldopa, dopamine, levodopa and tryptophane with 'Parnate' may precipitate hypertension, headache, and related symptoms.
5. In combination with cheese or other foods with a high tyramine content
Hypertensive crises have sometimes occurred during Parnate (tranylcypromine sulfate, SK&F) therapy after ingestion of foods with a high tyramine content. In general, the patient should avoid protein foods in which aging or protein breakdown is used to increase flavor. In particular, patients should be instructed not to take foods such as cheese (particularly strong or aged varieties), sour cream, Chianti wine, sherry, beer, pickled herring, liver, canned figs, raisins, bananas or avocados (particularly if overripe), chocolate, soy sauce, the pods of broad beans (fava beans), yeast extracts, or meat prepared with tenderizers.
Additional Contraindications: In general, the physician should bear in mind the possibility of a lowered margin of safety when Parnate (tranylcypromine sulfate, SK&F) is administered in combination with potent drugs.
1. 'Parnate' should not be used in combination with some central nervous system depressants such as narcotics and alcohol, or with hypotensive agents. A marked potentiating effect on these classes of drugs has been reported.
2. Anti-parkinsonism drugs should be used with caution in patients receiving 'Parnate' since severe reactions have been reported.
3. 'Parnate' should not be used in patients with a history of liver disease or in those with abnormal liver function tests.
4. Excessive use of caffeine in any form should be avoided in patients receiving 'Parnate'.
Warning to Physicians: Parnate (tranylcypromine sulfate, SK&F) is a potent agent with the capability of producing serious side effects. 'Parnate' is not recommended in those severe endogenous depressions in which electroconvulsive therapy is the treatment of choice or in those depressive reactions where other antidepressant drugs may be effective. **It should be reserved for patients who are either hospitalized or under close supervision and who have not responded satisfactorily to other antidepressant therapy.**
Before prescribing, the physician should be completely familiar with the full material on dosage, side effects, and contraindications on these pages, with the principles of MAO inhibitor therapy and the side effects of this class of drugs. Also, the physician should be familiar with the symptomatology of mental depressions and alternate methods of treatment to aid in the careful selection of patients for 'Parnate' therapy. In depressed patients, the possibility of suicide should always be considered and adequate precautions taken.
Pregnancy Warning: Use of any drug in pregnancy, during lactation, or in women of childbearing age requires that the potential benefits of the drug be weighed against its possible hazards to mother and child. Animal reproductive studies show that Parnate (tranylcypromine sulfate, SK&F) passes through the placental barrier into the fetus of the rat. Also, it passes into milk of the lactating dog. The absence of a harmful action of 'Parnate' on fertility or on postnatal development by either prenatal treatment or from the milk of treated animals has not been demonstrated.
Warning to the Patient: Patients should be instructed to report promptly the occurrence of headache or other unusual symptoms.
Patients should be warned against eating the foods listed in Section 5 under Contraindications while on Parnate (tranylcypromine sulfate, SK&F) therapy. Also, they should be told not to drink alcoholic beverages.
Patients should be warned against self-medication with proprietary (over-the-counter) drugs such as cold, hay fever or weight-reducing preparations that contain pressor agents. They should be advised not to consume excessive amounts of caffeine in any form.
Warnings: Hypertensive Crises: The most important reaction associated with Parnate (tranylcypromine, SK&F) is the occurrence of hypertensive crises which have sometimes been fatal.
These crises are characterized by some or all of the following symptoms: occipital headache which may radiate frontally, palpitation, neck stiffness or soreness, nausea or vomiting, sweating (sometimes with fever and sometimes with cold, clammy skin) and photophobia. Either tachycardia or bradycardia may be present, and associated constricting chest pain and dilated pupils may occur. **Intracranial bleeding, sometimes fatal in outcome, has been reported in association with the paradoxical increase in blood pressure.**
In all patients taking 'Parnate' blood pressure should be followed closely to detect evidence of any pressor response. It is emphasized that full reliance should not be placed on blood pressure readings, but that the patient should also be observed frequently.
Therapy should be discontinued immediately upon the occurrence of palpitation or frequent headaches during 'Parnate' therapy. These signs may be prodromal of a hypertensive crisis.

Important: Recommended treatment in hypertensive crises

If a hypertensive crisis occurs, Parnate (tranylcypromine sulfate, SK&F) should be discontinued and therapy to lower blood pressure should be instituted immediately. Headache tends to abate as blood pressure is lowered. On the basis of present evidence, phentolamine (available as 'Regitine'*) is recommended. (The dosage reported for phentolamine is 5 mg. i.v.) Care should be taken to administer this drug slowly in order to avoid producing an excessive hypotensive effect. Fever should be managed by means of external cooling. Other symptomatic and supportive measures may be desirable in particular cases. Do not use parenteral reserpine.
Precautions: Hypotension—Hypotension has been observed during Parnate (tranylcypromine sulfate, SK&F) therapy. Symptoms of postural hypotension are seen most commonly but not exclusively in patients with pre-existent hypertension; blood pressure usually returns rapidly to pretreatment levels upon discontinuation of the drug. At doses above 30 mg. daily, postural hypotension is a major side effect and may result in syncope. Dosage increases should be made more gradually in patients showing a tendency toward hypotension at the beginning of therapy. Postural hypotension may be relieved by having the patient lie down until blood pressure returns to normal. Also, when 'Parnate' is combined with those phenothiazine derivatives or other compounds known to cause hypotension, the possibility of additive hypotensive effects should be considered.
Other Precautions: In depressed patients, the possibility of suicide should always be considered and adequate precautions taken. Exclusive reliance on drug therapy to prevent suicidal attempts is unwarranted, as there may be a delay in the onset of therapeutic effect or an increase in anxiety and agitation. Also, of course, some patients fail to respond to drug therapy or may respond only temporarily.
MAO inhibitors may have the capacity to suppress anginal pain that would otherwise serve as a warning of myocardial ischemia. The usual precautions should be observed in patients with impaired renal function since there is a possibility of accumulative effects in such patients.
Although excretion is rapid, inhibition of MAO may persist for a few days. It is, therefore, suggested that the drug be discontinued seven days before elective surgery to allow time for recovery of enzymatic activity before anesthetic agents are given.
Because the influence of Parnate (tranylcypromine sulfate, SK&F) on the convulsive threshold is variable in animal experiments, suitable precautions should be taken if epileptic patients are treated.
Some MAO inhibitors have contributed to hypoglycemic episodes in diabetic patients receiving insulin or oral hypoglycemic agents. There-

Continued on next page

Smith Kline & French—Cont.

fore, 'Parnate' should be used with caution in diabetics using these drugs.
'Parnate' may aggravate coexisting symptoms in depression, such as anxiety and agitation.
Use 'Parnate' with caution in hyperthyroid patients because of their increased sensitivity to pressor amines.
'Parnate' should be administered with caution to patients receiving disulfiram (Antabuse®†). In a single study, rats given high intraperitoneal doses of *d* or *l* isomers of tranylcypromine sulfate plus disulfiram experienced severe toxicity including convulsions and death. Additional studies in rats given high oral doses of racemic tranylcypromine sulfate ('Parnate') and disulfiram produced no adverse interaction.

Adverse Reactions: Overstimulation which may include increased anxiety, agitation and manic symptoms is usually evidence of excessive therapeutic action. Dosage should be reduced, or a phenothiazine tranquilizer should be administered concomitantly.
Patients may experience restlessness or insomnia; may notice some weakness, drowsiness, episodes of dizziness, or dry mouth; or may report nausea, diarrhea, abdominal pain, or constipation. Most of these effects can be relieved by lowering the dosage or by giving suitable concomitant medication.
Tachycardia, significant anorexia, edema, palpitation, blurred vision, chills, and impotence have each been reported.
Headaches without blood pressure elevation have occurred.
Rare instances of hepatitis and skin rash have been reported.
Tinnitus, muscle spasm and tremors, paresthesia and urinary retention have been reported so rarely that the role of Parnate (tranylcypromine sulfate, SK&F) cannot be established.
Blood toxicity has not been reported.

Dosage and Administration: Dosage should be adjusted to the requirements of the individual patient. Improvement should be seen within 48 hours to three weeks after starting therapy.

1. Recommended starting dosage is 20 mg. per day—10 mg. in the morning and 10 mg. in the afternoon.
2. This dosage may be continued for two weeks.
3. If no signs of a response appear, dosage may be increased to 30 mg. daily—20 mg. in the morning and 10 mg. in the afternoon.
4. This dosage may be continued for a week. If no improvement occurs, continued administration is unlikely to be beneficial.
5. When a satisfactory response is obtained, dosage may usually be reduced to a maintenance level.
6. Some patients will be maintained on 20 mg. per day; many will need only 10 mg. daily.
7. Although dosages above 30 mg. daily have been used, the physician should bear in mind that the likelihood of side effects increases as dosage is raised.
8. When ECT is being administered concurrently, 10 mg. b.i.d. can usually be given during the series, then reduced to 10 mg. daily for maintenance therapy.

Dosage increases should be made in increments of 10 mg. per day and ordinarily at intervals of one to three weeks. It is important that the lowest effective dose be used.
Reduction from peak to maintenance dosage is desirable before withdrawal. If withdrawn prematurely, original symptoms will recur. Although no tendency to produce rebound depressions of greater intensity has been seen, this is a theoretical possibility.

Overdosage: *Symptoms:* The characteristic symptoms that may be caused by overdosage are usually those described on the preceding pages.
However, an intensification of these symptoms and sometimes severe additional manifestations may be seen, depending on the degree of overdosage and on individual susceptibility. Some patients exhibit insomnia, restlessness and anxiety, progressing in severe cases to agitation, mental confusion and incoherence. Hypotension, dizziness, weakness and drowsiness may occur, progressing in severe cases to extreme dizziness and shock. A few patients have displayed hypertension with severe headache and other symptoms. Rare instances have been reported in which hypertension was accompanied by twitching or myoclonic fibrillation of skeletal muscles with hyperpyrexia, sometimes progressing to generalized rigidity and coma.
Treatment: Gastric lavage is helpful if performed early. Treatment should normally consist of general supportive measures, close observation of vital signs and steps to counteract specific symptoms as they occur, since MAO inhibition may persist. The management of hypertensive crises is described under Hypertensive Crises.
External cooling is recommended if hyperpyrexia occurs. Barbiturates have been reported to help relieve myoclonic reactions, but frequency of administration should be controlled carefully because Parnate (tranylcypromine sulfate, SK&F) may prolong barbiturate activity. When hypotension requires treatment, the standard measures for managing circulatory shock should be initiated. If pressor agents are used, the rate of infusion should be regulated by careful observation of the patient because an exaggerated pressor response sometimes occurs in the presence of MAO inhibition. Remember that the toxic effect of 'Parnate' may be delayed or prolonged following the last dose of the drug. Therefore, the patient should be closely observed for at least a week.

How Supplied: Tablets, containing tranylcypromine sulfate equivalent to 10 mg. of tranylcypromine, in bottles of 100 and 1000.

Clinical Studies: There have been only a small number of controlled studies (e.g., 1,2,3,4) of the effectiveness of Parnate (tranylcypromine sulfate, SK&F) in comparison to placebo or other antidepressant drugs, embracing comparatively few subjects. These and other studies disclose a remarkably high incidence, about 50 per cent, of favorable placebo effect and a statistically significant but small superiority of 'Parnate' and other antidepressant drugs over placebo. No statistically significant superiority of 'Parnate' over other antidepressant drugs, including other MAO inhibitors, has been regularly demonstrated. However, clinical experience also indicates that some patients who fail to respond satisfactorily to one therapy may respond to another.

References:

1. Bartholomew, A.A.: An evaluation of tranylcypromine ('Parnate') in the treatment of depression, *M. J. Australia 1:*655 (May 5) 1962.
2. Khanna, J.L., et al.: A study of certain effects of tranylcypromine, a new antidepressant, *J. New Drugs 3:*227, 1963.
3. Spear, F.G., et al.: A comparison of subjective responses to imipramine and tranylcypromine, *Brit. J. Psychiat. 110:*53, 1964.
4. Janacek, J., et al.: Pargyline and tranylcypromine in the treatment of hospitalized depressed patients, *J. New Drugs 3:*309, 1963.

*Trade Mark Reg. U.S. Pat. Off.: 'Regitine' for phentolamine mesylate, U.S.P., CIBA.
†Trademark of Ayerst Laboratories

[*Shown in Product Identification Section*]

PRAGMATAR® OINTMENT††

Description: Cetyl alcohol-coal tar distillate, 4%; precipitated sulfur, 3%; salicylic acid, 3%—in an oil-in-water emulsion base.

Action and Uses: Pragmatar is highly effective in a wide range of common skin disorders both in adults and in children: seborrheic affections, especially of the scalp, including dandruff and "cradle cap"; subacute and chronic dermatitis; eczematous eruptions; fungous infections, including "athlete's foot"; etc. *Note:* For use in infants and when otherwise desired, Pragmatar may be diluted by mixing a few drops of water with a small quantity of the ointment in the palm of the hand.

Precautions: Keep out of eyes and off eyelids. Use with care near the groin or on acutely inflamed areas. Do not use on blistered surfaces. If rash or irritation develops, discontinue use.

Administration and Dosage: *On the scalp:* Part hair and massage into small areas before retiring. Apply sparingly but thoroughly to entire scalp. Remove with a light shampoo the following morning. Use no more often than once daily. *On other areas:* Use small quantities, confining application to affected surfaces. Apply no more often than once daily.

Warning: Keep this and all medicines out of reach of children. In case of accidental ingestion, contact a physician or poison control center immediately.

How Supplied: 1 oz. tubes.

††Pragmatar Ointment is a product of Menley & James Laboratories, Professional Products Division, a SmithKline company.

QUOTANE® OINTMENT††

Description: Quotane Ointment contains dimethisoquin hydrochloride, 0.5%; preserved with thimerosal 1:50,000; in a white, water-miscible emulsion base.

Action and Uses: Quotane relieves pain, itching and burning of minor skin conditions such as pruritus ani and vulvae, contact dermatitis (poison ivy, etc.), skin manifestations of systemic disease (chickenpox, measles, etc.), allergic dermatitis, sunburn, insect bites, stasis dermatitis, fungous infections, lichen planus, eczema, neurodermatitis, prickly heat, urticaria, intertrigo, scabies (after specific antiparasitic treatment), mild burns, neurotic excoriations, diaper rash.
It is not related chemically to the various "-caine" type preparations and has a low index of sensitization.
Quotane Ointment is generally useful in dry dermatologic conditions, especially those that have become cracked and fissured; and in irritation due to hemorrhoids, or rectal itching.

Precautions: Do not use in the eyes or on the eyelids. Do not apply to bleeding hemorrhoids or to extensive areas. Not for prolonged use; if the condition for which preparation is used persists, or if a rash or irritation develops, discontinue use.

Administration: Apply a light coating when necessary, not more than 4 times daily, or as directed by physician. Use special applicator for itching hemorrhoids (do not apply to bleeding hemorrhoids).
If the condition for which the preparation is used persists, or if a rash or irritation develops, discontinue use and consult physician.
Keep tube tightly closed to prevent drying.

Warning: Quotane Ointment should not be used in the eyes or on eyelids. Do not apply to bleeding hemorrhoids or to extensive areas. Not for prolonged use. Keep this and all drugs out of reach of children. In case of accidental ingestion, contact a physician or poison control center immediately.

How Supplied: In 1 oz. tubes (with rectal applicator).

Remarks: Not compatible with tannic acid.

††Quotane Ointment is a product of Menley & James Laboratories, Professional Products Division, a SmithKline company.

SELACRYN® ℞
(brand of ticrynafen)

Description: 'Selacryn' (brand of ticrynafen) is [2,3-dichloro-4-(2-thienylcarbonyl)-phenoxy] acetic acid.

Clinical Pharmacology:

Actions: Three principal actions have been established: antihypertensive, diuretic and uricosuric.

Antihypertensive: 'Selacryn' (brand of ticrynafen) provides a significant and consistent antihypertensive effect at doses of 250 to 500 mg. per day. Little additional antihypertensive effect is obtained at higher doses. Initially, this effect is provided primarily through reduction of plasma volume due to the diuretic properties of the compound. The long-term, consistent antihypertensive effect of 'Selacryn' may involve both renal and extrarenal mechanisms; the exact antihypertensive mechanisms of diuretics are not known. 'Selacryn' does not significantly lower blood pressure in normotensive subjects.

Diuretic: The major site of diuretic action of 'Selacryn', like the thiazides, is in the cortical diluting segment of the distal convoluted tubule of the nephron.

The diuretic and natriuretic effects of 'Selacryn' are dose related through the therapeutic range of 250 mg. once daily to 500 mg. twice daily. Little additional diuretic effect is obtained with higher doses. The diuretic and natriuretic effects begin in one hour after oral administration, reach a maximum in two to four hours, and continue for 12 to 24 hours depending upon the dosage and the individual response of the subject. The urinary excretion of sodium, chloride and potassium produced by 250 mg. of 'Selacryn' is equivalent to that produced by 50 mg. of hydrochlorothiazide.

Uricosuric: 'Selacryn' causes a prompt, consistent reduction in both normal and elevated serum uric acid levels. As with the diuretic activity, the reduction in serum uric acid with 'Selacryn' is dose related through the range of 125 mg. to 250 mg. per day. Little additional uricosuric effect is obtained with higher doses. A 125 mg. dose of 'Selacryn' lowers serum uric acid levels to about the same extent as 500 mg. of probenecid.

Pyrazinamide suppression studies demonstrate that reduction of serum uric acid is produced through inhibition of urate reabsorptive mechanisms at both pre- and post-secretory sites in the proximal tubule, resulting in enhanced urinary excretion of both filtered and secreted uric acid. In crystal equilibration studies in normal volunteers, 'Selacryn', by virtue of its inherent diuretic effect, did not significantly increase the degree of urinary saturation of either uric acid or monosodium urate.

In vitro, 'Selacryn' has no significant inhibitory activity upon xanthine oxidase. There is no enhanced excretion of the oxypurines, xanthines, or hypoxanthines, indicating that 'Selacryn' does not interfere with purine metabolism.

The administration of 'Selacryn' (250 mg.) with other diuretics (hydrochlorothiazide 50 mg., furosemide 40 mg., acetazolamide 500 mg.) can produce additive diuretic and natriuretic effects, while the reduction of serum uric acid and uricosuric effects of 'Selacryn' are maintained.

Pharmacokinetics: 'Selacryn' (brand of ticrynafen) is rapidly absorbed and is cleared from the body by metabolism and by excretion in the urine. Following administration of 250 mg., significant plasma levels of 'Selacryn' are apparent within one hour, with maximum plasma concentration reached at two to three hours. 'Selacryn' is rapidly cleared from plasma, with a half-life of approximately two hours. 'Selacryn' appears essentially unchanged in plasma although traces of oxidized and reduced metabolites are also present. Approximately 80% of 'Selacryn' is excreted in the urine, 34% as the parent drug.

Short-Term (Six Weeks) Therapy

	No. Patients	Supine Diastolic Blood Pressure (mmHg.)			Serum Uric Acid (mg. %)		
		Predrug	6 Wks.	Reduction	Predrug	6 Wks.	Change
'Selacryn' (250 mg. once or twice daily)	66	105	92	13	6.1	3.3	−2.8
Hydrochlorothiazide (50 mg. once or twice daily)	59	105	93	12	6.4	8.0	+1.6
Placebo	25	103	100	3	6.7	6.6	−0.1

Long-Term (Six Months) Therapy

	No. Patients	Supine Diastolic Blood Pressure (mmHg.)			Serum Uric Acid (mg. %)		
		Predrug	6 Mos.	Reduction	Predrug	6 Mos.	Change
'Selacryn' (250 mg. once or twice daily)	71	101	87	14	6.2	4.0	−2.2
Hydrochlorothiazide (50 mg. once or twice daily)	72	100	87	13	6.1	7.3	+1.2

Clinical Studies:

Hypertension: Double-blind multi-investigator studies were carried out in hypertensive patients with supine diastolic blood pressure of 95–115 mmHg. In short- and long-term studies, 'Selacryn' (brand of ticrynafen) effectively and consistently lowered blood pressure to the same degree as hydrochlorothiazide. The results of representative studies are given below. [See table above].

Patients from the double-blind studies were continued on 'Selacryn' (250 mg. or 500 mg. daily); supine diastolic pressure was controlled at levels of 90 mmHg. or less in about 75% of the patients. Approximately 50% of the patients received concomitant therapy with non-diuretic antihypertensive agents such as propranolol or methyldopa.

Congestive Cardiac Failure: Double-blind studies of six to 12 weeks' duration comparing the effects of 'Selacryn' (250 or 500 mg. daily) and hydrochlorothiazide (50 or 100 mg. daily) in patients with congestive cardiac failure of various etiologies showed that 'Selacryn' and hydrochlorothiazide were equally effective in controlling signs and symptoms of congestive cardiac failure. Patients treated with 'Selacryn' had a significant decrease in serum uric acid levels, whereas those treated with hydrochlorothiazide had an increase or no significant change in serum uric acid levels.

Indications: 'Selacryn' (brand of ticrynafen) is indicated in the management of hypertension, with or without hyperuricemia, either as the sole therapeutic agent or to enhance the effectiveness of other antihypertensive drugs in the more severe forms of hypertension. Because of its uricosuric activity, 'Selacryn' will not increase serum uric acid levels, as other diuretic agents usually do.

'Selacryn' is indicated in the management of salt and water retention states associated with congestive cardiac failure.

Use in Pregnancy. Routine use of diuretics during normal pregnancy is inappropriate and exposes mother and fetus to unnecessary hazard. Diuretics do not prevent development of toxemia of pregnancy and there is no satisfactory evidence that they are useful in the treatment of toxemia.

Edema during pregnancy may arise from pathologic causes or from the physiologic and mechanical consequences of pregnancy. Diuretics are indicated in pregnancy when edema is due to pathologic causes, just as they are in the absence of pregnancy (however, see WARNINGS below). Dependent edema in pregnancy, resulting from restriction of venous return by the gravid uterus, is properly treated through elevation of the lower extremities and use of support stockings. Use of diuretics to lower intravascular volume in this instance is inappropriate. During normal pregnancy there is hypervolemia which is not harmful to the fetus or the mother in the absence of cardiovascular disease. However, it may be associated with edema, rarely generalized edema. If such edema causes discomfort, increased recumbency will often provide relief. Rarely this edema may cause extreme discomfort which is not relieved by rest. In these instances, a short course of diuretic therapy may provide relief and be appropriate.

Contraindications: Anuria, severe or progressive renal disease, hypersensitivity to the drug, and known renal uric acid calculi.

Warnings:

Interaction with Anticoagulants: *'Selacryn' (brand of ticrynafen) potentiates the action of oral anticoagulants.* Therefore, caution should be exercised when these drugs are used together. *In vitro* studies indicate that 'Selacryn' can compete with warfarin-type anticoagulants for the same protein-binding sites to cause an increase in free warfarin. When used with 'Selacryn', anticoagulant dosage should be reduced to one-quarter or one-half of the maintenance dose, and during titration of dosage the prothrombin time should be carefully monitored until stabilized.

Potassium-Sparing Diuretics: Marked elevation of BUN and creatinine has been seen in some patients who received 'Selacryn' and triamterene. Therefore, such a combination is not recommended.

Patients with Impaired Liver Function: 'Selacryn', like the thiazides, is not considered appropriate therapy in hepatic ascites and its use is not recommended in such patients. In severely ill hepatic ascites patients treated with 'Selacryn', elevations of BUN (up to 44 mg.%) and serum creatinine (up to 4.5 mg.%) have been observed. Such elevations were not seen

Continued on next page

Smith Kline & French—Cont.

in ambulatory cirrhotic patients with mild ascites.

Patients with Impaired Renal Function: In patients with progressive or advanced renal disease, 'Selacryn' may precipitate azotemia. Cumulative effects of diuretics may develop in patients with impaired renal function. Frequent electrolyte, creatinine and BUN determinations should be performed early in therapy and periodically thereafter during treatment. If renal impairment progresses, 'Selacryn' should be discontinued.

Usage in Pregnancy: There has been no experience to date with the use of 'Selacryn' in pregnant patients. However, animal studies have demonstrated that 'Selacryn' crosses the placental barrier. Teratology studies have shown no effects attributable to 'Selacryn'. Routine use of diuretics during normal pregnancy is inappropriate and exposes mother and fetus to unnecessary hazard. 'Selacryn' should not be used in pregnant patients unless in the judgment of the physician the anticipated benefits outweigh the potential risks.

Nursing Mothers: It is not known whether 'Selacryn' is excreted in human milk. As a general rule, nursing should not be undertaken while a patient is on a drug since many drugs are excreted in human milk. 'Selacryn' is excreted in the milk of animals.

Precautions:

FLUID INTAKE: Substantial uricosuria occurs within hours after the first dose of 'Selacryn' (brand of ticrynafen) is given; for this reason, hypertensive patients changing from other diuretics should be instructed to discontinue the diuretic and increase fluid intake for three days before beginning 'Selacryn' therapy. Where feasible, diuretics should be discontinued for one to two days in patients with congestive cardiac failure. Fluid intake should be increased for up to three days before and three days after initiation of therapy (to a total of approximately 1500 cc. per day) in patients who may be dehydrated (e.g., patients with excessive alcohol intake, severe vomiting or diarrhea), particularly if the patients are hyperuricemic or when 'Selacryn' is instituted as a replacement for other diuretics.

In well-hydrated patients, initial doses of 'Selacryn' usually produce sufficient diuresis so that supplemental fluids and alkalinization of urine are not necessary.

Patients with Gout: Any drug with uricosuric or diuretic activity, including 'Selacryn', may precipitate acute attacks of gout. Therapeutic doses of colchicine are recommended to control the acute attack, during which treatment with 'Selacryn' may be continued.

Glucose Metabolism: 'Selacryn' exerts effects on glucose metabolism similar to those observed with thiazide diuretics. Insulin requirements may be affected in diabetics, and hyperglycemia and glycosuria may occur in patients with latent diabetes.

BUN/Serum Creatinine: Elevation of BUN and/or serum creatinine can occur during diuretic therapy. These effects usually revert to baseline values during continued therapy or upon withdrawal of the drug.

Electrolyte Imbalance: All patients receiving diuretic therapy should be observed for clinical signs of fluid or electrolyte imbalance, i.e., hypokalemia, hyponatremia and hypochloremic alkalosis. Periodic determination of electrolytes to detect possible electrolyte imbalance should be performed at appropriate intervals. Serum and urine electrolyte determinations are particularly important when the patient is vomiting excessively or receiving parenteral fluids. Medication such as digitalis may also influence serum electrolytes. Warning signs, irrespective of cause, are dryness of mouth, thirst, weakness, lethargy, drowsiness, restlessness, muscle pains or cramps, muscular fatigue, hypotension, oliguria, tachycardia and gastrointestinal disturbances such as nausea or vomiting. Hypokalemia can sensitize or exaggerate the response of the heart to the toxic effects of digitalis (i.e., increased ventricular irritability). Any chloride deficit is generally mild and usually does not require specific treatment except under extraordinary circumstances (as in liver disease or renal disease).

Cytotoxic Agents: Drugs with uricosuric activity should be used with caution in patients receiving cytotoxic agents. Since cytotoxic agents result in increased uric acid formation, and some are nephrotoxic, use of cytotoxic drugs with uricosuric drugs requires individualization of dosage and management.

Pediatric Usage: Safety and effectiveness of 'Selacryn' in children have not been established.

Drug Interactions:

Protein-Bound Drugs: 'Selacryn' (brand of ticrynafen) potentiates the action of oral anticoagulants; when these agents are used concomitantly, anticoagulant dosage should be reduced to one-quarter or one-half of the maintenance dose and prothrombin time carefully monitored until stabilized **(See Warnings)**.

Because *in vitro* studies with tolbutamide, phenytoin (diphenylhydantoin), and warfarin have shown competition for protein-binding sites, caution should be exercised when 'Selacryn' is administered with other drugs that are highly protein bound.

Potassium-Sparing Diuretics: Marked elevation of BUN and creatinine has been seen in some patients who received 'Selacryn' and triamterene. Therefore, such a combination is not recommended.

Organic Acids: Like other uricosurics, 'Selacryn' may compete with some compounds for excretion sites in the nephron. This results in decreased excretion and increased plasma levels of these agents. Some of the compounds which may compete with 'Selacryn' for excretion are aminohippuric acid (PAH), penicillin, phenolsulfonphthalein (PSP), and salicylates. 'Selacryn' causes a decrease in the excretion of penicillin and PSP.

Salicylates have a slight inhibitory effect on the uricosuric action of 'Selacryn'.

Lithium: Lithium generally should not be given with diuretics because they reduce its renal clearance and increase the risk of lithium toxicity. Read circulars for lithium preparations before use of such concomitant therapy with 'Selacryn'.

Adverse Reactions: Adverse reactions seen with 'Selacryn' (brand of ticrynafen) in controlled studies were approximately the same as those seen with hydrochlorothiazide. Except where noted, the following adverse effects seen with 'Selacryn' have been reported in a small number of patients, e.g., approximately 1 in 100. **Gastrointestinal:** anorexia, nausea, vomiting, dyspepsia, cramping, diarrhea, constipation; **Central nervous system:** dizziness/lightheadedness (totaled approximately 9 in 100), headache (approximately 4 in 100), paresthesia, syncope, vertigo, somnolence, insomnia; **Cardiovascular:** orthostatic hypotension, palpitation; **Hypersensitivity:** rash, urticaria, pruritus, rare cases of fever and interstitial nephritis, which cleared on withdrawal of the drug, have been reported; however, no causal relationship has been established. **Other:** fatigue/tiredness (approximately 4 in 100), hyperglycemia, glycosuria, muscle cramps, weakness, bitter taste and dryness in mouth, exacerbation of gout, renal colic or costovertebral pain. Abnormal liver function tests and jaundice have been reported in a few patients treated with 'Selacryn' (brand of ticrynafen); however, no causal relationship has been established.

Occasionally in patients switched to 'Selacryn' from another diuretic, there have been reports of nausea, vomiting, flank pain, azotemia, oliguria and, rarely, anuria. These effects were reversible after 'Selacryn' was discontinued. These cases occurred when patients were switched to 'Selacryn' without a washout period or without adequate hydration **(See Precautions)**.

The following adverse reactions have not been reported to date with 'Selacryn' but have occurred with thiazides or other diuretics: pancreatitis, sialadenitis, xanthopsia, purpura, photosensitivity, necrotizing angiitis, Stevens-Johnson syndrome, respiratory distress, anaphylactic reaction, leukopenia, agranulocytosis, thrombocytopenia, aplastic anemia, restlessness and transient blurred vision.

Dosage and Administration: Adequate fluid intake should be maintained in all patients. Fluid intake should be increased for up to three days before and three days after initiation of therapy in dehydrated patients or in patients in whom 'Selacryn' (brand of ticrynafen) is instituted as a replacement for other diuretics **(See Precautions)**.

Hypertension: Diuretic therapy should be interrupted for three days before starting 'Selacryn'. The usual adult starting dose is one 250 mg. tablet daily. Depending upon the response of the patient, after two to four weeks dosage may be increased to 500 mg. as a single daily dose or one 250 mg. tablet twice a day. Although reduction of blood pressure may be seen within two to three days, three to four weeks may be required to achieve optimal therapeutic effect.

When used with other antihypertensive agents, the dose of such other drugs should be reduced by one-half. Titrate to achieve optimal response.

Salt and water retention states ***associated with congestive cardiac failure.*** Diuretic therapy should be interrupted for one to two days before starting 'Selacryn'. The usual adult starting dose is one 250 mg. tablet daily. Depending upon the response of the patient, dosage may be increased to 500 mg. as a single daily dose or one 250 mg. tablet twice a day. Daily dosage should not exceed 1000 mg.

Accidental Overdose: Diuretic overdosage may cause excessive diuresis with hypovolemia, postural hypotension and severe electrolyte imbalance. Excessive uric acid excretion with massive doses of 'Selacryn' (brand of ticrynafen) may have the potential of producing urate nephropathy and renal failure. Appropriate therapy for overdosage should include restoration of fluid and electrolyte balance. Alkalinization of urine with sodium bicarbonate should be considered if the acid-base status of the patient permits. When alkali is administered, the acid-base balance of the patient should be frequently monitored by laboratory tests.

How Supplied: 'Selacryn' (brand of ticrynafen) tablets are supplied as light blue, round, scored, monogrammed tablets of 250 mg. in bottles of 100, and in Single Unit Packages of 100 (intended for institutional use only).

SK-LINE®

SK-AMITRIPTYLINE™ ℞
(amitriptyline HCl, SK&F)

Tablets: 10 mg. (No. 120), 25 mg. (No. 121), 50 mg. (No. 123), 75 mg. (No. 124), 100 mg. (No. 131), 150 mg. (No. 132).

SK-AMPICILLIN® ℞
(ampicillin, SK&F)

Capsules: 250 mg. (No. 101), 500 mg. (No. 102).
Tablets: 125 mg. (No. 107).
For Oral Suspension: 125 mg./5 ml. (No. 103), 250 mg./5 ml. (No. 104), 100 mg./ml. (No. 109).

SK-AMPICILLIN-N® ℞
(sterile ampicillin sodium, SK&F)

Injection: 500 mg. (No. 106).

SK-APAP™ OTC
(acetaminophen, SK&F)

Tablets: 325 mg. (No. 174), 650 mg. (No. 173).
Elixir: 120 mg./5 ml. (contains alcohol) (No. 175).

SK-APAP™ with CODEINE Ⓒ
(acetaminophen, codeine)

Tablets: 300 mg./15 mg. (No. 494), 300 mg./30 mg. (No. 496), 300 mg./60 mg. (No. 497).

SK-BAMATE™ Ⓒ
(meprobamate, SK&F)

Tablets: 200 mg. (No. 133), 400 mg. (No. 134).

SK-BISACODYL™ OTC
(bisacodyl, SK&F)

Tablets: 5 mg. (No. 193).

SK-CHLORAL HYDRATE™ Ⓒ
(chloral hydrate, SK&F)

Capsules: 500 mg. (No. 176).

SK-CHLOROTHIAZIDE™ ℞
(chlorothiazide, SK&F)

Tablets: 250 mg. (No. 419), 500 mg. (No. 420).

SK-DEXAMETHASONE™ ℞
(dexamethasone, SK&F)

Tablets: 0.5 mg. (No. 374), 0.75 mg. (No. 376), 1.5 mg. (No. 377).

SK-DIGOXIN™ ℞
(digoxin, SK&F)

Tablets: 0.25 mg. (No. 122).

SK-DIPHENHYDRAMINE™ ℞
(diphenhydramine hydrochloride, SK&F)

Capsules: 25 mg. (No. 303), 50 mg. (No. 304).
Elixir: 12.5 mg./5 ml. (No. 305).

SK-DIPHENOXYLATE™ Ⓒ
(diphenoxylate HCl, atropine sulfate)

Tablets: 2.5 mg./.025 mg. (No. 423).

SK-ERYTHROMYCIN™ ℞
(erythromycin stearate, SK&F)

Tablets: 250 mg. (No. 367), 500 mg. (No. 369).

SK-HYDROCHLOROTHIAZIDE™ ℞
(hydrochlorothiazide, in SK&F)

Tablets: 25 mg. (No. 363), 50 mg. (No. 364).

SK-LYGEN® Ⓒ
(chlordiazepoxide hydrochloride, SK&F)

Capsules: 5 mg. (No. 441), 10 mg. (No. 442), 25 mg. (No. 443).

SK-NIACIN™ OTC
(niacin, SK&F)

Tablets: 50 mg. (No. 129), 100 mg. (No. 130).

SK-PENICILLIN G™ ℞
(penicillin G potassium, SK&F)

Tablets: 400,000 units (No. 111), 800,000 units (No. 112).
For Oral Solution: 200,000 units/5 ml. (No. 113), 400,000 units/5 ml. (No. 114).

SK-PENICILLIN VK™ ℞
(penicillin V potassium, SK&F)

Tablets: 250 mg. (No. 116), 500 mg. (No. 117).
For Oral Solution: 125 mg./5 ml. (No. 118), 250 mg./5 ml. (No. 119).

SK-PHENOBARBITAL™ Ⓒ
(phenobarbital, SK&F)

Tablets: 15 mg. (No. 136), 30 mg. (No. 137).

SK-PRAMINE™ ℞
(imipramine hydrochloride, SK&F)

Tablets: 10 mg. (No. 321), 25 mg. (No. 322), 50 mg. (No. 323).

SK-PREDNISONE™ ℞
(prednisone, SK&F)

Tablets: 5 mg. (No. 339).

SK-QUINIDINE SULFATE™ ℞
(quinidine sulfate, SK&F)

Tablets: 200 mg. (No. 171).

SK-RESERPINE™ ℞
(reserpine, SK&F)

Tablets: 0.25 mg. (No. 169).

SK-65® Ⓒ
(propoxyphene hydrochloride, SK&F)

Capsules: 65 mg. (No. 463).

SK-65 APAP® Ⓒ

Each tablet: 65 mg. propoxyphene HCl, 650 mg. acetaminophen (No. 474).

SK-65® COMPOUND Ⓒ

Each capsule: 65 mg. propoxyphene HCl, 227 mg. aspirin, 162 mg. phenacetin, 32.4 mg. caffeine (No. 467).

SK-SOXAZOLE™ ℞
(sulfisoxazole, SK&F)

Tablets: 500 mg. (No. 163).

SK-TETRACYCLINE™ CAPSULES ℞
(tetracycline hydrochloride, SK&F)

250 mg. (No. 126), 500 mg. (No. 127).

SK-TETRACYCLINE™ SYRUP ℞
(tetracycline oral suspension, SK&F)

125 mg./5 ml. (No. 125).

SK-TRIAMCINOLONE™ ℞
(triamcinolone, SK&F)

Tablets: 2 mg. (No. 403), 4 mg. (No. 404), 8 mg. (No. 406).

STELAZINE® ℞
(brand of trifluoperazine hydrochloride)

('Stelazine' is a product of SK&F Co., Carolina, P.R. 00630, Subsidiary of SmithKline Corp., under trademark license from SmithKline Corp., Philadelphia, Pa.)

Description: Tablets—Each tablet contains trifluoperazine, 1 mg., 2 mg., 5 mg., or 10 mg., as the hydrochloride.

Multiple-dose Vials, 10 ml. (2 mg./ml.)—Each ml. contains, in aqueous solution, trifluoperazine, 2 mg., as the hydrochloride; sodium tartrate, 4.75 mg.; sodium biphosphate, 11.6 mg.; sodium saccharin, 0.3 mg.; benzyl alcohol, 0.75%, as preservative.

Concentrate (intended for institutional use only)—Each ml. contains trifluoperazine, 10 mg., as the hydrochloride.

N.B.: The Concentrate is for use in severe neuropsychiatric conditions when oral medication is preferred and other oral forms are considered impractical.

Indications
Based on a review of this drug by the National Academy of Sciences—National Research Council and/or other information, FDA has classified the indications as follows:
Effective: For the management of the manifestations of psychotic disorders.
Possibly effective: To control excessive anxiety, tension and agitation as seen in neuroses or associated with somatic conditions.
'Stelazine' has not been shown effective in the management of behavioral complications in patients with mental retardation.
Final classification of the less-than-effective indications requires further investigation.

Contraindications: Comatose or greatly depressed states due to central nervous system depressants, and in cases of existing blood dyscrasias, bone marrow depression and pre-existing liver damage.

Warnings: Patients who have demonstrated a hypersensitivity reaction (e.g., blood dyscrasias, jaundice) with a phenothiazine should not be re-exposed to any phenothiazine, including Stelazine (trifluoperazine HCl, SK&F), unless in the judgment of the physician the potential benefits of treatment outweigh the possible hazard.

'Stelazine' may impair mental and/or physical abilities, especially during the first few days of therapy. Therefore, caution patients about activities requiring alertness (e.g., operating vehicles or machinery).

Usage in Pregnancy: Animal reproductive studies and clinical experience to date have not demonstrated any teratogenic effect from Stelazine (trifluoperazine HCl, SK&F). However, as with any medication, it should be used in pregnant patients only when, in the judgment of the physician, it is necessary for the welfare of the patient.

Precautions: Agranulocytosis, thrombocytopenia, pancytopenia and anemia have been reported in patients receiving the drug. Jaundice of the cholestatic type of hepatitis or liver damage has been reported.

One result of therapy may be an increase in mental and physical activity. For example, a few patients with angina pectoris have complained of increased pain while taking the drug. Therefore, angina patients should be observed carefully and, if an unfavorable response is noted, the drug should be withdrawn.

Because hypotension has occurred, large doses and parenteral administration should be avoided in patients with impaired cardiovascular systems.

Since certain phenothiazines have been reported to produce retinopathy, the drug should be discontinued if ophthalmoscopic examination or visual field studies should demonstrate retinal changes.

The antiemetic effect of 'Stelazine' may mask signs of overdosage of toxic drugs or obscure the diagnosis of conditions such as intestinal obstruction and brain tumor.

If agents such as sedatives, narcotics, anesthetics, tranquilizers, or alcohol are used either simultaneously or successively with the drug, the possibility of an undesirable additive depressant effect should be considered.

With prolonged administration at high dosages, the possibility of cumulative effects, with sudden onset of severe central nervous system or vasomotor symptoms, should be kept in mind.

To lessen the likelihood of adverse reactions related to drug accumulation, patients on long-

Continued on next page

Smith Kline & French—Cont.

term therapy, particularly on high doses, should be evaluated periodically to decide whether the maintenance dosage could be lowered, or drug therapy could be discontinued.

Adverse Reactions: Drowsiness, dizziness, skin reactions, rash, dry mouth, insomnia, amenorrhea, fatigue, muscular weakness, anorexia, lactation, blurred vision and neuromuscular (extrapyramidal) reactions.

Neuromuscular (Extrapyramidal) Reactions

These symptoms are seen in a significant number of hospitalized mental patients. They may be characterized by motor restlessness, be of the dystonic type, or they may resemble parkinsonism.

Depending on the severity of symptoms, dosage should be reduced or discontinued. If therapy is reinstituted, it should be at a lower dosage. Should these symptoms occur in children or pregnant patients, the drug should be stopped and not reinstituted. In most cases barbiturates by suitable route of administration will suffice. (Or, injectable 'Benadryl'* may be useful.) In more severe cases, the administration of an anti-parkinsonism agent, except levodopa, usually produces rapid reversal of symptoms. Suitable supportive measures such as maintaining a clear airway and adequate hydration should be employed.

Motor Restlessness: Symptoms may include agitation or jitteriness and sometimes insomnia. These symptoms often disappear spontaneously. At times these symptoms may be similar to the original neurotic or psychotic symptoms. Dosage should not be increased until these side effects have subsided.

If this phase becomes too troublesome, the symptoms can usually be controlled by a reduction of dosage or concomitant administration of a barbiturate.

Dystonias: Symptoms may include: spasm of the neck muscles, sometimes progressing to torticollis; extensor rigidity of back muscles, sometimes progressing to opisthotonos; carpopedal spasm, trismus, swallowing difficulty, oculogyric crisis and protrusion of the tongue. These usually subside within a few hours, and almost always within 24 to 48 hours, after the drug has been discontinued.

In mild cases, reassurance or a barbiturate is often sufficient. *In moderate cases,* barbiturates will usually bring rapid relief. *In more severe adult cases,* the administration of an anti-parkinsonism agent, except levodopa, usually produces rapid reversal of symptoms. Also, intravenous caffeine with sodium benzoate seems to be effective. *In children,* reassurance and barbiturates will usually control symptoms. (Or, injectable 'Benadryl' may be useful.)

Pseudo-parkinsonism: Symptoms may include: mask-like facies; drooling; tremors; pillrolling motion; cogwheel rigidity; and shuffling gait. Reassurance and sedation are important. In most cases these symptoms are readily controlled when an anti-parkinsonism agent is administered concomitantly. Anti-parkinsonism agents should be used only when required. Generally, therapy of a few weeks to two or three months will suffice. After this time patients should be evaluated to determine their need for continued treatment. (Note: Levodopa has not been found effective in pseudo-parkinsonism.) Occasionally it is necessary to lower the dosage of 'Stelazine' or to discontinue the drug.

Persistent Tardive Dyskinesia: As with all antipsychotic agents, tardive dyskinesia may appear in some patients on long-term therapy or may appear after drug therapy has been discontinued. The risk appears to be greater in elderly patients on high-dose therapy, especially females. The symptoms are persistent and in some patients appear to be irreversible. The syndrome is characterized by rhythmical involuntary movements of the tongue, face, mouth or jaw (e.g., protrusion of tongue, puffing of cheeks, puckering of mouth, chewing movements). Sometimes these may be accompanied by involuntary movements of extremities.

There is no known effective treatment for tardive dyskinesia; anti-parkinsonism agents do not alleviate the symptoms of this syndrome. It is suggested that all antipsychotic agents be discontinued if these symptoms appear. Should it be necessary to reinstitute treatment, or increase the dosage of the agent, or switch to a different antipsychotic agent, the syndrome may be masked.

It has been reported that fine vermicular movements of the tongue may be an early sign of the syndrome and if the medication is stopped at that time the syndrome may not develop.

Adverse Reactions Reported with Stelazine (trifluoperazine HCl, SK&F) or Other Phenothiazine Derivatives: Adverse effects with different phenothiazines vary in type, frequency, and mechanism of occurrence, i.e., some are dose-related, while others involve individual patient sensitivity. Some adverse effects may be more likely to occur, or occur with greater intensity, in patients with special medical problems, e.g., patients with mitral insufficiency or pheochromocytoma have experienced severe hypotension following recommended doses of certain phenothiazines.

Not all of the following adverse reactions have been observed with every phenothiazine derivative, but they have been reported with one or more and should be borne in mind when drugs of this class are administered: extrapyramidal symptoms (opisthotonos, oculogyric crisis, hyperreflexia, dystonia, akathisia, dyskinesia, parkinsonism) some of which have lasted months and even years—particularly in elderly patients with previous brain damage; grand mal convulsions; altered cerebrospinal fluid proteins; cerebral edema; intensification and prolongation of the action of central nervous system depressants (opiates, analgesics, antihistamines, barbiturates, alcohol), atropine, heat, organophosphorus insecticides; autonomic reactions (dryness of mouth, nasal congestion, headache, nausea, constipation, obstipation, adynamic ileus, inhibition of ejaculation); reactivation of psychotic processes, catatonic-like states; hypotension (sometimes fatal); cardiac arrest; blood dyscrasias (pancytopenia, thrombocytopenic purpura, leukopenia, agranulocytosis, eosinophilia); liver damage (jaundice, biliary stasis); endocrine disturbances (lactation, galactorrhea, gynecomastia, menstrual irregularities, false positive pregnancy tests); skin disorders (photosensitivity, itching, erythema, urticaria, eczema up to exfoliative dermatitis); other allergic reactions (asthma, laryngeal edema, angioneurotic edema, anaphylactoid reactions); peripheral edema; reversed epinephrine effect; hyperpyrexia; a systemic lupus erythematosus-like syndrome; pigmentary retinopathy; with prolonged administration of substantial doses, skin pigmentation, epithelial keratopathy, and lenticular and corneal deposits.

EKG changes—particularly nonspecific, usually reversible Q and T wave distortions—have been observed in some patients receiving phenothiazine tranquilizers. Their relationship to myocardial damage has not been confirmed.

Although phenothiazines cause neither psychic nor physical dependence, sudden discontinuance in long-term psychiatric patients may cause temporary symptoms, e.g., nausea and vomiting, dizziness, tremulousness.

Note: There have been occasional reports of sudden death in patients receiving phenothiazines. In some cases, the cause appeared to be asphyxia due to failure of the cough reflex. In others, the cause could not be determined. There is not sufficient evidence to establish a relationship between such deaths and the administration of phenothiazines.

Dosage and Administration: Dosage should be adjusted to the needs of the individual. The lowest effective dosage should always be used. Dosage should be increased more gradually in debilitated or emaciated patients. When maximum response is achieved, dosage may be reduced gradually to a maintenance level. Because of the inherent long action of the drug, patients may be controlled on convenient b.i.d. administration; some patients may be maintained on once-a-day administration.

When Stelazine (trifluoperazine HCl, SK&F) is administered by intramuscular injection, equivalent oral dosage may be substituted once symptoms have been controlled.

Elderly Patients: In general, dosages in the lower range are sufficient for most elderly patients. Since they appear to be more susceptible to hypotension and neuromuscular reactions, such patients should be observed closely. Dosage should be tailored to the individual, response carefully monitored, and dosage adjusted accordingly. Dosage should be increased more gradually in elderly patients.

1. Adult Dosage

Oral (for office patients and outpatients): 1 or 2 mg. twice daily. It is seldom necessary to exceed 4 mg. a day except in patients with more severe conditions and in discharged mental patients.

Oral (for hospitalized patients or those under close supervision): Usual starting dosage is 2 mg. to 5 mg. b.i.d. (Small or emaciated patients should always be started on the lower dosage.) Most patients will show optimum response on 15 mg. or 20 mg. daily, although a few may require 40 mg. a day or more. Optimum therapeutic dosage levels should be reached within two or three weeks.

When the Concentrate dosage form is to be used, it should be added to 60 ml. (2 fl. oz.) or more of diluent *just prior to administration* to insure palatability and stability. Vehicles suggested for dilution are: tomato or fruit juice, milk, simple syrup, orange syrup, carbonated beverages, coffee, tea, or water. Semisolid foods (soup, puddings, etc.) may also be used.

Intramuscular (for prompt control of severe symptoms): Usual dosage is 1 mg. to 2 mg. (½-1 ml.) by deep intramuscular injection q4-6h, p.r.n. More than 6 mg. within 24 hours is rarely necessary.

Only in very exceptional cases should intramuscular dosage exceed 10 mg. within 24 hours. Injections should not be given at intervals of less than 4 hours because of a possible cumulative effect.

Note: Stelazine (trifluoperazine HCl, SK&F) Injection has been usually well tolerated and there is little, if any, pain and irritation at the site of injection.

The Injection should be protected from light. Exposure may cause discoloration. Slight yellowish discoloration will not alter potency or efficacy. If markedly discolored, the solution should be discarded.

2. Dosage for Psychotic Children

Dosage should be adjusted to the weight of the child and severity of the symptoms. These dosages are for children, ages 6 to 12, who are hospitalized or under close supervision.

Oral: The starting dosage is 1 mg. administered once a day or b.i.d. Dosage may be increased gradually until symptoms are controlled or until side effects become troublesome.

While it is usually not necessary to exceed dosages of 15 mg. daily, some older children with severe symptoms may require higher dosages.

Intramuscular: There has been little experience with the use of Stelazine (trifluoperazine HCl, SK&F) Injection in children. However, if it is necessary to achieve rapid control of severe symptoms, 1 mg. (½ ml.) of the drug may be administered intramuscularly once or twice a day.

Overdosage: (See also under Adverse Reactions.)
Symptoms—Primarily involvement of the extrapyramidal mechanism producing some of the dystonic reactions described above.
Symptoms of central nervous system depression to the point of somnolence or coma. Agitation and restlessness may also occur. Other possible manifestations include convulsions, fever, and autonomic reactions such as hypotension, dry mouth and ileus.
Treatment—Essentially symptomatic and supportive. Early gastric lavage is helpful. Keep patient under observation and maintain an open airway, since involvement of the extrapyramidal mechanism may produce dysphagia and respiratory difficulty in severe overdosage. **Do not attempt to induce emesis because a dystonic reaction of the head or neck may develop that could result in aspiration of vomitus.** Extrapyramidal symptoms may be treated with anti-parkinsonism drugs, barbiturates, or 'Benadryl'. If administration of a stimulant is desirable, amphetamine, dextroamphetamine, or caffeine with sodium benzoate is recommended. Stimulants that may cause convulsions (e.g., picrotoxin or pentylenetetrazol) should be avoided.
If hypotension occurs, the standard measures for managing circulatory shock should be initiated. If it is desirable to administer a vasoconstrictor, 'Levophed' and 'Neo-Synephrine'† are most suitable. Other pressor agents, including epinephrine, are not recommended because phenothiazine derivatives may reverse the usual elevating action of these agents and cause a further lowering of blood pressure.
Limited experience indicates that phenothiazines are *not* dialyzable.

How Supplied:
Tablets, 1 mg. and 2 mg., in bottles of 100 and 1000; in Single Unit Packages of 100 (intended for institutional use only).
For psychiatric patients who are hospitalized or under close supervision:
Tablets, 5 mg. and 10 mg., in bottles of 100 and 1000; in Single Unit Packages of 100 (intended for institutional use only).
Multiple-dose Vials, 10 ml. (2 mg./ml.), in boxes of 1 and 20.
Concentrate (intended for institutional use only)—10 mg./ml., in 2 fl. oz. bottles and in cartons of 12 bottles.
Each bottle is packaged with a graduated dropper.
The Concentrate form is light-sensitive. For this reason, it should be protected from light and dispensed in amber bottles. *Refrigeration is not required.*
Note: Although there is little likelihood of contact dermatitis due to the drug, persons with known sensitivity to phenothiazine drugs should avoid direct contact.
Military—Tablets 1 mg., 1000's, 6505-00-022-1336, and S.U.P. 100's, 6505-00-132-0132; 2 mg., 1000's, 6505-00-022-1337; 5 mg., 1000's, 6505-00-022-1338; 10 mg., 1000's 6505-00-180-5973, and S.U.P. 100's, 6505-00-132-0188.

*Trademark Reg. U.S. Pat. Off.: 'Benadryl' for diphenhydramine hydrochloride, Parke-Davis.
†'Levophed' and 'Neo-Synephrine' are the trademarks (Reg. U.S. Pat. Off.) of Winthrop Laboratories for its brands of levarterenol and phenylephrine respectively.

[*Shown in Product Identification Section*]

STOXIL® ℞
(brand of idoxuridine)

Description: 'Stoxil' Ophthalmic Solution contains idoxuridine (5-iodo-2'-deoxyuridine) 0.1% (1 mg./ml.) in distilled water; sterile when packaged. Preserved with thimerosal, 1:50,000. 'Stoxil' Ophthalmic Ointment contains idoxuridine 0.5% (5 mg./ gram) in a petrolatum base. (White petrolatum and liquid petrolatum are inactive ingredients.)
Actions: Inhibits replication of herpes simplex virus by irreversibly inhibiting the incorporation of thymidine into the viral DNA.
Indications: Stoxil (idoxuridine, SK&F) is indicated only in the treatment of herpes simplex keratitis.
Epithelial infections, especially initial attacks, characterized by the presence of a dendritic figure, have responded better than *stromal infections.*[1,2] Recurrences are common. 'Stoxil' will often control the infection, but will have no effect on the accumulated scarring, vascularization or on the resultant progressive loss of vision.
Contraindications: 'Stoxil' Solution or Ointment is contraindicated in patients with known or suspected hypersensitivity to any of its components.
Precautions: General: Some strains of herpes simplex appear to be resistant to the action of Stoxil (idoxuridine, SK&F). If there is no response in *epithelial infections* after seven or eight days of treatment, other forms of therapy should be considered.
The recommended frequency and duration of administration should not be exceeded.
'Stoxil' is not effective in corneal inflammations following herpes simplex keratitis in which the virus is not present.
Corticosteroids can accelerate the spread of a viral infection and are usually contraindicated in herpes simplex keratitis.
Boric acid should not be administered during the course of therapy since it may cause irritation in the presence of 'Stoxil'.
To insure that the stability of the preparation is maintained, 'Stoxil' Ophthalmic Solution should not be mixed with other medications.
Usage in Pregnancy: Idoxuridine should be administered with caution in pregnancy or in women of childbearing potential. Idoxuridine has been reported to cross the placental barrier and to produce fetal malformations in Japanese albino rabbits when administered topically to the eyes of pregnant females in doses similar to those used clinically, but did not produce malformations in New Zealand white rabbits when administered ocularly, dermally, or intraperitoneally in doses much higher than the doses used in the preceding study. Idoxuridine has also been reported to produce fetal malformations in the rat after intraperitoneal and oral administration of high doses and in the mouse but not in the rat after subcutaneous administration.
Nursing Mothers: It is not known whether idoxuridine is secreted in human milk. As a general rule, nursing should not be undertaken while a patient is on drug therapy since many drugs and their metabolites are excreted in human milk.
Mutagenic Potential: Idoxuridine has been reported to cause chromosome aberrations in mice and to cause mutations in mammalian cells in culture (e.g., diploid human lymphoblasts and mouse lymphoma cells), *Drosophila melanogaster,* and in a host-mediated assay system utilizing mammalian cells. In other tests, idoxuridine has not been found to exhibit mutagenic activity in the dominant lethal assay in the mouse, in the Salmonella assay, or in the micronucleus assay.
Oncogenic Potential: The studies performed to date on idoxuridine are inadequate for assessment of carcinogenicity. This cytotoxic drug should be regarded as being potentially carcinogenic. It can inhibit DNA synthesis or function and is incorporated into the DNA of mammalian cells as well as into the genome of DNA viruses.
Adverse Reactions: Occasionally, some irritation, pain, pruritus, inflammation, or edema will be experienced in the eye or lids. Allergic reactions, although rare, have been reported. Photophobia has occurred. The occasional appearance of corneal clouding, stippling and small punctate defects in the corneal epithelium have been observed. However, the punctate defects may be a manifestation of the infection since healing usually takes place without interruption of therapy and these defects have been observed in untreated herpes simplex keratitis.
Administration and Dosage:
Ophthalmic Solution—Initially, place one drop in each infected eye every hour during the day and every two hours at night. Continue the initial dosage until definite improvement has taken place, as evidenced by loss of staining with fluorescein. Dosage may then be reduced to one drop every two hours during the day and every four hours at night. In order to minimize recurrences, Stoxil (idoxuridine, SK&F) therapy should be continued at this reduced dosage for three to five days after healing appears to be complete.
Ophthalmic Ointment—Recommended dosage is five instillations daily, given approximately q4h with the last dose h.s. The Ointment is placed inside the conjunctival sac of the infected eye. It is advisable to continue therapy for three to five days after healing appears to be complete.
Patients should be observed at frequent intervals. In *epithelial infections,* improvement is usually seen within seven to eight days. If the patient continues to improve, therapy should be continued, usually not longer than 21 days.
In the management of herpes simplex with stromal lesions, corneal edema, or iritis, topical corticosteroids may be used with 'Stoxil' depending on the judgment of the physician. Such combined therapy may be used for as long as the condition warrants. It is important that 'Stoxil' therapy be continued a few days after the steroid has been withdrawn.
Antibiotics may be used with 'Stoxil' to control secondary infections, and atropine preparations may be employed adjunctively as indicated.
Overdosage: *Topical*—Quantitative overdosage in the eye is highly unlikely, since the eye quickly expels fluid or ointment in excess of the limited capacity of the conjunctival sac. However, overdosage by means of too frequent administration (see recommended dosage) is possible. In this event, small defects might appear on the epithelium of the cornea. If overly frequent administration does produce such effects, therapy should be discontinued, either temporarily or permanently, as indicated after close observation of the progress of the infection.
Accidental Ingestion—All available data indicate that the minimum systemic dose that will produce toxic effects is many times greater than the quantity in a commercial bottle (15 mg.) or tube (20 mg.). Also, metabolic breakdown and excretion take place very rapidly. Thus, no untoward consequences should be expected from the accidental ingestion of even an entire bottle of the Ophthalmic Solution or tube of Ophthalmic Ointment and no treatment is indicated.
How Supplied: 0.1% Ophthalmic Solution (1 mg./ml.), in 15 ml. bottles with dropper; 0.5% Ophthalmic Ointment (5 mg./gram) in 4 gram tubes.
Military—Solution 15 ml., 6505-00-763-6821; Ointment 4 grams, 6505-00-932-0682.
Notes on Stability: Stoxil (idoxuridine, SK&F) Ophthalmic Solution should be stored in refrigerator until dispensed. 'Stoxil' Ophthalmic Ointment does not require refrigeration.
References:

1. Laibson, P.R., and Leopold, I.H.: An Evaluation of Double-Blind IDU Therapy in 100 Cases of Herpetic Keratitis, Tr. Am. Acad. Ophth. *68*:22, 1964.
2. Gold, J.A., et al.: The Epidemiology and Chemotherapy of Herpes Simplex Keratitis and Herpes Simplex Skin Infections, Ann. New York Acad. Sc. *130*:209 (July 30) 1965.

Continued on next page

Smith Kline & French—Cont.

TAGAMET® ℞
(brand of cimetidine tablets and cimetidine hydrochloride injection)

Description: 'Tagamet' (brand of cimetidine) is a histamine H_2 receptor antagonist. Chemically it is *N*″-cyano-N-methyl-*N*′-[2-[[(5-methyl-1H-imidazol-4-yl)methyl] thio]-ethyl]-guanidine.
(The injection dosage form contains cimetidine as the hydrochloride.)
Cimetidine has a bitter taste and characteristic odor.
Tablets: Each tablet contains 300 mg. of cimetidine.
Vials: Each 2 ml. vial contains, in aqueous solution, cimetidine hydrochloride equivalent to cimetidine, 300 mg.; phenol, 10 mg.
Multiple-dose Vials: 8 ml. (300 mg./2 ml.)—Each 2 ml. contains, in aqueous solution, cimetidine hydrochloride equivalent to cimetidine, 300 mg.; phenol, 10 mg.
Clinical Pharmacology: 'Tagamet' (brand of cimetidine) competitively inhibits the action of histamine at the histamine H_2 receptors of the parietal cells and thus represents a new class of pharmacological agents, the histamine H_2-receptor antagonists.
'Tagamet' is not an anticholinergic agent. Studies have shown that 'Tagamet' inhibits both daytime and nocturnal basal gastric acid secretion. 'Tagamet' also inhibits gastric acid secretion stimulated by food, histamine, pentagastrin, caffeine and insulin.

Antisecretory Activity

1) **Acid Secretion:** *Basal:* Oral 'Tagamet' 300 mg. inhibited basal gastric acid secretion by 100% for at least two hours and by at least 90% throughout the 4 hour study in fasting duodenal ulcer patients.
The gastric pH in all subjects was increased to 5.0 or greater for at least 2¼ hours.
Nocturnal: Nighttime basal secretion in fasting duodenal ulcer patients was inhibited by a 300 mg. dose of 'Tagamet' by 100% for at least one hour and by a mean of 89% over a seven hour period. Gastric pH was increased to 5.0 or greater in most of the patients for three to four hours.
'Tagamet' 300 mg. reduced non-stimulated acid concentration by 70–100% and the nonstimulated volume of gastric secretion by 20–50%.
Food Stimulated: During the first hour after a standard experimental meal, oral 'Tagamet' 300 mg. inhibited gastric acid secretion in duodenal ulcer patients by at least 50%. During the subsequent two hours 'Tagamet' inhibited gastric acid secretion by at least 75%.
The effect of a 300 mg. breakfast dose of 'Tagamet' continued for at least four hours and there was partial suppression of the rise in gastric acid secretion following the luncheon meal in duodenal ulcer patients. This suppression of gastric acid output was enhanced and could be maintained by another 300 mg. dose of 'Tagamet' given with lunch.
In another study, 'Tagamet' 300 mg. given with the meal increased gastric pH as compared with placebo.

	Mean Gastric pH	
	'Tagamet'	Placebo
1 hour	3.5	2.6
2 hours	3.1	1.6
3 hours	3.8	1.9
4 hours	6.1	2.2

The effects of oral 'Tagamet' 300 mg. and propantheline bromide on food-stimulated gastric acid secretion were compared in 7 duodenal ulcer patients. Propantheline bromide was titrated to maximally tolerated dosages—the average dose was 45 mg. 'Tagamet' 300 mg. reduced gastric acid output by 67% vs. 27% ($p<0.05$) for propantheline bromide.
Chemically Stimulated: Oral 'Tagamet' significantly inhibited gastric acid secretion stimulated by betazole (an isomer of histamine), pentagastrin, caffeine and insulin as follows:

Stimulant	Stimulant Dose	'Tagamet'	% Inhibition
Betazole	1.5mg/kg (sc)	300mg (po)	85% at 2½ hours
Pentagastrin	6mcg/kg/hr (iv)	100mg/hr (iv)	60% at 1 hour
Caffeine	5mg/kg/hr (iv)	300mg (po)	100% at 1 hour
Insulin	0.03 units/kg/hr (iv)	100mg/hr (iv)	82% at 1 hour

When food and betazole were used to stimulate secretion, inhibition of hydrogen ion concentration usually ranged from 45–75% and the inhibition of volume ranged from 30–65%.
2) **Pepsin:** Oral 'Tagamet' 300 mg. reduced total pepsin output as a result of the decrease in volume of gastric juice.
3) **Intrinsic Factor:** Intrinsic factor secretion was studied with betazole as a stimulant. Oral 'Tagamet' 300 mg. inhibited the rise in intrinsic factor concentration produced by betazole, but some intrinsic factor was secreted at all times.
4) **Serum Gastrin:** A single oral dose of 'Tagamet' 300 mg. augments the normal serum gastrin increase in response to a meal. This effect is probably attributable to the action of the drug in inhibiting food-stimulated gastric acid secretion. 'Tagamet' does not increase nocturnal serum gastrin levels in fasting patients. Studies of serum gastrin levels in short-term therapy have shown a slight or no increase. Studies are continuing for evaluation of the long-term effects, if any, of 'Tagamet' on serum gastrin.

Other

Lower Esophageal Sphincter Pressure and Gastric Emptying
'Tagamet' has no effect on lower esophageal sphincter (LES) pressure or the rate of gastric emptying.

Pharmacokinetics
'Tagamet' is rapidly absorbed after oral administration and peak levels occur in 45-90 minutes. The half-life of 'Tagamet' is approximately 2 hours. Both oral and parenteral (IV or IM) administration provide comparable periods of therapeutically effective blood levels; blood concentrations remain above that required to provide 80% inhibition of basal gastric acid secretion for 4-5 hours following a dose of 300 mg.
The principal route of excretion of 'Tagamet' is the urine. Following parenteral administration, most of the drug is excreted as the parent compound; following oral administration, the drug is more extensively metabolized, the sulfoxide being the major metabolite. Following a single oral dose, 48% of the drug is recovered from the urine after 24 hours as the parent compound. Following IV or IM administration, approximately 75% of the drug is recovered from the urine after 24 hours as the parent compound.

Clinical Trials:

Duodenal Ulcer
In worldwide double-blind clinical studies, endoscopically evaluated duodenal ulcer healing rates with 'Tagamet' (brand of cimetidine) were consistently higher than those of the placebo controls. In many of the studies, these differences were statistically significant.
In a multicenter, double-blind controlled U.S. study on endoscopically diagnosed duodenal ulcers earlier healing was seen in the 'Tagamet' patients as shown below:

	'Tagamet'†	Placebo†
Inpatients		
week 1	15/43 (35%)	12/51 (24%)
week 2	24/43 (56%*)	18/49 (37%)
Outpatients		
week 1	20/87 (23%)	14/91 (15%)
week 2	12/26 (46%*)	7/27 (26%)
week 4	16/28 (57%)	13/27 (48%)
week 6	22/29 (76%)	17/27 (63%)

†All patients were permitted p.r.n. antacids for relief of pain.
*$p<0.05$

In this study, 'Tagamet'-treated patients reported a general reduction in both daytime and nocturnal pain, and they also consumed less antacid.
Duodenal ulcer is a chronic, recurrent disease. While short-term treatment with 'Tagamet' can result in complete healing of the ulcer, the standard 4–6 week treatment period should not be expected to alter the subsequent course of ulcer recurrence. A follow-up of double-blind studies has shown that there was no difference in frequency or time to onset of recurrences between the treated and control groups.

Pathological Hypersecretory Conditions (such as Zollinger-Ellison Syndrome)
'Tagamet' significantly inhibited gastric acid secretion and reduced occurrence of diarrhea, anorexia and pain in patients with pathological hypersecretion associated with Zollinger-Ellison Syndrome, systemic mastocytosis and multiple endocrine adenomas. Use of 'Tagamet' was also followed by healing of intractable ulcers.

Indications: 'Tagamet' (brand of cimetidine) is indicated in:
(1) Short-term treatment of duodenal ulcer (up to 8 weeks).
(2) The treatment of pathological hypersecretory conditions (i.e., Zollinger-Ellison Syndrome, systemic mastocytosis, multiple endocrine adenomas).
Concomitant antacids should be given as needed for relief of pain.
Studies available to date do not provide evidence of safety of cimetidine in uncomplicated duodenal ulcer for periods of more than 8 weeks.

Contraindications: There are no known contraindications to the use of 'Tagamet' (brand of cimetidine). However, the physician should refer to the Precautions section regarding usage in pregnant, nursing, or pediatric patients.

Precautions: In a 24-month toxicity study conducted in rats, at dose levels of 150, 378 and 950 mg./kg./day (approximately 9 to 56 times the recommended human dose), a statistically significant, higher incidence of benign Leydig cell tumors was seen in the drug-treated groups compared to controls. These tumors were common in control groups as well as treated groups and the difference became apparent only in aged rats.
In reproduction studies performed in rats, mice and rabbits, there was no evidence of impaired mating performance, fertility or harm to the fetus due to 'Tagamet' (brand of cimetidine).
Symptomatic response to 'Tagamet' therapy does not preclude the presence of a gastric malignancy.
Drug Interaction: Potentiation of warfarin-type anticoagulants has been observed with concomitant 'Tagamet' administration. For this reason, close monitoring of prothrombin time is recommended, and adjustment of the anticoagulant dose may be necessary when these drugs are administered concomitantly.

Usage in Pregnancy: There has been no experience to date with the use of 'Tagamet' in pregnant patients. However, animal studies have demonstrated that 'Tagamet' crosses the placental barrier. Teratology studies (100–950 mg./kg./day) have shown no effects attributable to 'Tagamet' on litter parameters or early development of the young.

'Tagamet' should not be used in pregnant patients or women of childbearing potential unless, in the judgment of the physician, the anticipated benefits outweigh the potential risks.

Nursing Mothers: It is not known whether 'Tagamet' is excreted in human milk. As a general rule, nursing should not be undertaken while a patient is on a drug since many drugs are excreted in human milk. 'Tagamet' is secreted in the milk of animals.

Pediatric Use: Clinical experience in children is limited. Therefore, 'Tagamet' therapy cannot be recommended for children under 16, unless, in the judgment of the physician, anticipated benefits outweigh the potential risks. In very limited experience, doses of 20–40 mg./kg. per day have been used.

Adverse Reactions: Mild and transient diarrhea, muscular pain, dizziness and rash have been reported in a small number of patients, e.g., approximately 1 in 100, during treatment with 'Tagamet' (brand of cimetidine).

Mild gynecomastia has been reported in a few patients treated for one month or longer. In patients being treated for pathological hypersecretory states, this occurred in about 4 percent of cases while in all others the incidence was about 3 patients in 1000. No evidence of induced endocrine dysfunction was found, and the condition remained unchanged or returned toward normal with continuing 'Tagamet' treatment.

A few cases of reversible confusional states have been reported, usually in elderly and/or severely ill patients, such as those with renal insufficiency or organic brain syndrome; overdosage may have played a role in some cases. These confusional states generally cleared within 24 hours of drug withdrawal.

A few cases of neutropenia have been reported in patients receiving 'Tagamet'. Because these patients had serious concomitant illnesses and were receiving drugs and/or treatment known to produce neutropenia, a cause and effect relationship cannot be established.

Regularly observed small increases in plasma creatinine have been reported. These did not progress with continued therapy and disappeared at the end of therapy.

Some increases in serum transaminase and rare cases of fever and interstitial nephritis, which cleared on withdrawal of the drug, have been reported.

Dosage and Administration:

Duodenal Ulcer

The recommended adult oral dosage for duodenal ulcer is 300 mg. four times a day, with meals and at bedtime.

Concomitant antacids should be given as needed for relief of pain.

While healing with 'Tagamet' often occurs during the first week or two, treatment should be continued for 4–6 weeks unless healing has been demonstrated by endoscopic examination.

Pathological Hypersecretory Conditions (such as Zollinger-Ellison Syndrome)

Recommended adult oral dosage: 300 mg. four times a day with meals and at bedtime. In some patients it may be necessary to administer 'Tagamet' 300 mg. doses more frequently. Doses should be adjusted to individual patient needs, but should not usually exceed 2400 mg. per day and should continue as long as clinically indicated.

Parenteral Administration

In some hospitalized patients with pathological hypersecretory conditions or intractable ulcers, or in patients who are unable to take oral medication, 'Tagamet' may be administered parenterally according to the following recommendations:

Intramuscular injection: 300 mg. q 6 hours (no dilution necessary). Transient pain at the site of injection has been reported.

Intravenous injection: 300 mg. q 6 hours. Dilute 'Tagamet' Injection, 300 mg., in Sodium Chloride Injection (0.9%) or other compatible i.v. solution (see STABILITY OF 'TAGAMET' INJECTION) to a total volume of 20 ml. and inject over 1-2 minutes.

Intermittent intravenous infusion: 300 mg. q 6 hours. Dilute 'Tagamet' Injection, 300 mg., in 100 ml. of Dextrose Injection (5%) or other compatible i.v. solution (see STABILITY OF 'TAGAMET' INJECTION) and infuse over 15–20 minutes. In some patients it may be necessary to increase dosage. When this is necessary the increases should be made by more frequent administration of a 300 mg. dose, but should not exceed 2400 mg. per day.

Dosage Adjustment for Patients with Impaired Renal Function

Patients with severely impaired renal function have been treated with 'Tagamet'. However, such usage has been very limited. On the basis of this experience the recommended dosage is 300 mg. q 12 hours orally or by intravenous injection. Should the patient's condition require, the frequency of dosing may be increased to q 8 hours or even further with caution. In severe renal failure accumulation may occur and the lowest frequency of dosing compatible with an adequate patient response should be used. Hemodialysis reduces the level of circulating 'Tagamet'. Ideally, the dosage schedule should be adjusted so that the timing of a scheduled dose coincides with the end of hemodialysis.

Stability of 'Tagamet' Injection

'Tagamet' (brand of cimetidine) Injection is stable for 48 hours at normal room temperature when added to or diluted with most commonly used intravenous solutions, e.g., Sodium Chloride Injection (0.9%), Dextrose Injection (5% or 10%), Lactated Ringer's Solution, 5% Sodium Bicarbonate Injection.

Overdosage: The usual measures to remove unabsorbed material from the gastrointestinal tract, clinical monitoring and supportive therapy should be employed. Studies in animals indicate that toxic doses are associated with respiratory failure and tachycardia which may be controlled by assisted respiration and the administration of a beta-blocker.

Human experience with gross overdosage is limited. However, in the few cases which have been reported, doses up to 10 grams have not been associated with any untoward effects.

How Supplied:

Pale Green Tablets: 300 mg. tablets in bottles of 100 and Single Unit Packages of 100 (intended for institutional use only).

[*Shown in Product Identification Section*]

Injection: 300 mg./2 ml. in single-dose vials and in 8 ml. multiple-dose vials, in packages of 10.

TELDRIN®††

Chlorpheniramine maleate

TIMED-RELEASE ALLERGY CAPSULES, 8 mg. and 12 mg.

Description: Each Teldrin Timed-Release capsule contains chlorpheniramine maleate, 8 mg. or 12 mg., so formulated that a portion of the antihistamine dose is released initially, and the remaining medication is released gradually over a prolonged period.

Indications: Teldrin provides up to 12 hours of relief from hay fever/upper respiratory allergy symptoms: sneezing; runny nose; itchy, watery eyes.

Dosage: DOSAGE SHOULD BE INDIVIDUALIZED ACCORDING TO THE NEEDS AND THE RESPONSE OF THE USER.

Adults and children over 12 years of age: One 12 mg. capsule in the morning; or one 12 mg. capsule q12h. Children 6 to 12 years of age: One 8 mg. capsule daily. Not recommended for children less than 6 years of age, less than 46 kg. in weight, or having a surface area of less than one square meter. In children less than 6 years of age, a liquid antihistamine preparation is usually indicated.

Warning: Do not take this product if patient has asthma, glaucoma or difficulty in urination due to enlargement of the prostate gland, except under the advice and supervision of a physician.

Do not drive or operate heavy machinery as this preparation may cause drowsiness. Avoid alcoholic beverages while taking this product. May cause excitability especially in children. Keep this and all medicines out of the reach of children. In case of accidental overdose, contact a physician or poison control center immediately.

How Supplied: 8 mg. and 12 mg. Timed-Release capsules in packages of 12 capsules, in bottles of 50 and 500; in Single Unit Packages of 100 (intended for institutional use only).

††Teldrin is a product of Menley & James Laboratories, Professional Products Division, a SmithKline company.

[*Shown in Product Identification Section*]

TEMARIL® ℞

(brand of trimeprazine tartrate)

Tablets, Syrup and Spansule® capsules

Description: 'Temaril', available as trimeprazine tartrate, a phenothiazine derivative, is 10-[3-(dimethylamino)-2-methylpropyl]-phenothiazine tartrate.

Trimeprazine tartrate is a white to off-white odorless, crystalline powder readily soluble in water.

Tablets—Each tablet contains trimeprazine tartrate equivalent to 2.5 mg. of trimeprazine.

Syrup—Each 5 ml. (one teaspoonful) contains trimeprazine tartrate equivalent to 2.5 mg. of trimeprazine, and alcohol, 5.7%.

Spansule® sustained release capsules—Each 'Spansule' capsule contains trimeprazine tartrate equivalent to 5 mg. of trimeprazine, so prepared that an initial dose is released promptly and the remaining medication is released gradually over a prolonged period.

Actions: Temaril (trimeprazine tartrate, SK&F), a phenothiazine, possesses antipruritic and antihistaminic properties with anticholinergic (drying) and sedative side effects.

Indications

Based on a review of this drug by the National Academy of Sciences—National Research Council and/or other information, FDA has classified the indications as follows:

Effective: For symptomatic relief of pruritic symptoms in urticaria.

Possibly effective: For relief of pruritic symptoms in neurodermatitis, allergic dermatitis, contact dermatitis, atopic dermatitis, chickenpox, pruritus ani and vulvae.

Final classification of the less-than-effective indications requires further investigation.

Contraindications: Temaril (trimeprazine tartrate, SK&F) is contraindicated: in comatose patients; in patients who have received large amounts of central nervous system depressants (alcohol, barbiturates, narcotics, etc.); in patients with bone marrow depression; in patients who have demonstrated an idiosyncrasy

Continued on next page

Smith Kline & French—Cont.

or hypersensitivity to 'Temaril' or other phenothiazines; in newborn or premature children; and in nursing mothers. It should not be used in children who are acutely ill and/or dehydrated, as there is an increased susceptibility to dystonias in such patients.

Warnings: Temaril (trimeprazine tartrate, SK&F) may impair the mental and/or physical ability required for the performance of potentially hazardous tasks, such as driving a vehicle or operating machinery. Similarly, it may impair mental alertness in children. The concomitant use of alcohol or other central nervous system depressants may have an additive effect. Patients should be warned accordingly.

'Temaril' should be used with extreme caution in patients with:

- Asthmatic attack
- Narrow-angle glaucoma
- Prostatic hypertrophy
- Stenosing peptic ulcer
- Pyloroduodenal obstruction
- Bladder neck obstruction
- Patients receiving monoamine oxidase inhibitors

Usage in Pregnancy: The safe use of 'Temaril' has not been established with respect to the possible adverse effects upon fetal development. Therefore, it should not be used in women of childbearing potential. Jaundice and prolonged extrapyramidal symptoms have been reported in infants whose mothers received phenothiazines during pregnancy.

Usage in Children: 'Temaril' should be used with caution, as administration in the young child may result in excitation. Overdosage may produce hallucinations, convulsions and sudden death.

Usage in Elderly Patients (60 years or older): Elderly patients are more prone to develop the following side effects from phenothiazines:

- Hypotension
- Syncope
- Toxic confusional states
- Extrapyramidal symptoms, especially parkinsonism
- Excessive sedation

Precautions: Temaril (trimeprazine tartrate, SK&F) may significantly affect the actions of other drugs. It may increase, prolong or intensify the sedative action of central nervous system depressants such as anesthetics, barbiturates or alcohol. When 'Temaril' is administered concomitantly the dose of a narcotic or barbiturate should be reduced to ¼ or ½ the usual amount. In the patient with pain, receiving treatment with narcotics, excessive amounts of 'Temaril' may lead to restlessness and motor hyperactivity. 'Temaril' can block and even reverse the usual pressor effect of epinephrine.

'Temaril' should be used cautiously in persons with acute or chronic respiratory impairment, particularly children, as it may suppress the cough reflex.

This drug should be used cautiously in persons with cardiovascular disease, impairment of liver function, or those with a history of ulcer disease.

Since 'Temaril' has a slight antiemetic action, it may obscure signs of intestinal obstruction, brain tumor, or overdosage of toxic drugs.

Adverse Reactions: Temaril (trimeprazine tartrate, SK&F) may produce adverse reactions attributable to both phenothiazines and antihistamines.

Note: Not all of the following adverse reactions have been reported with 'Temaril'; however, pharmacological similarities among the phenothiazine derivatives require that each be considered when 'Temaril' is administered. There have been occasional reports of sudden death in patients receiving phenothiazine derivatives chronically.

C.N.S. Effects: Drowsiness is the most common C.N.S. effect of this drug. Extrapyramidal reactions (opisthotonos, dystonia, akathisia, dyskinesia, parkinsonism) occur, particularly with high doses. (See Overdosage section for management of extrapyramidal symptoms). Hyperreflexia has been reported in the newborn when a phenothiazine was used during pregnancy. Other reported reactions include dizziness, headache, lassitude, tinnitus, incoordination, fatigue, blurred vision, euphoria, diplopia, nervousness, insomnia, tremors and grand mal seizures, excitation, catatonic-like states, neuritis and hysteria, oculogyric crises, disturbing dreams/nightmares, pseudoschizophrenia, and intensification and prolongation of the action of C.N.S. depressants (opiates, analgesics, antihistamines, barbiturates, alcohol), atropine, heat, organophosphorus insecticides.

Cardiovascular Effects: Postural hypotension is the most common cardiovascular effect of phenothiazines. Reflex tachycardia may be seen. Bradycardia, faintness, dizziness and cardiac arrest have been reported. ECG changes, including blunting of T waves and prolongation of the Q-T interval, may be seen.

Gastrointestinal: Anorexia, nausea, vomiting, epigastric distress, diarrhea, constipation, and dry mouth may occur. Increased appetite and weight gain have also been reported.

Genitourinary: Urinary frequency and dysuria, urinary retention, early menses, induced lactation, gynecomastia, decreased libido, inhibition of ejaculation and false positive pregnancy tests have been reported.

Respiratory: Thickening of bronchial secretions, tightness of the chest, wheezing and nasal stuffiness may occur.

Allergic Reactions: These include urticaria, dermatitis, asthma, laryngeal edema, angioneurotic edema, photosensitivity, lupus erythematosus-like syndrome and anaphylactoid reactions.

Other Reported Reactions: Leukopenia, agranulocytosis, pancytopenia, hemolytic anemia, elevation of plasma cholesterol levels and thrombocytopenic purpura have been reported. Jaundice of the obstructive type has also been reported; it is usually reversible but chronic jaundice has been reported. Erythema, peripheral edema, and stomatitis have been reported. High or prolonged glucose tolerance curves, glycosuria, elevated spinal fluid proteins and reversed epinephrine effects may also occur.

Long-Term Therapy Considerations: After prolonged phenothiazine administration at high dosage, pigmentation of the skin has occurred, chiefly in the exposed areas. Ocular changes consist of the appearance of lenticular and corneal opacities, epithelial keratopathies and pigmentary retinopathy. Vision may be impaired.

Dosage and Administration:

Tablets and Syrup:

Adults Usual dosage is 2.5 mg. q.i.d.

Children over three years: Usual dosage is 2.5 mg. h.s., or t.i.d. if needed.

Children 6 months to 3 years: Usual dosage is 1.25 mg. (½ teaspoonful of syrup) h.s., or t.i.d. if needed.

'Spansule' capsules:

Adults: Usual daily dosage is 1 capsule q12h.

Children over 6 years of age: 1 capsule daily. This product form is not recommended for children under 6 years of age. Use tablets or syrup for their dosage flexibility.

Because some side effects appear to be dose-related, it is important to use the lowest effective dosage.

Drug Interactions: MAO inhibitors and thiazide diuretics prolong and intensify the anticholinergic effects of 'Temaril'. Combined use of MAO inhibitors and phenothiazines may result in hypertension and extrapyramidal reactions.

Narcotics: The C.N.S. depressant and analgesic effects of narcotics are potentiated by phenothiazines.

The following drugs may result in potentiation of phenothiazine effects:

- Oral contraceptives
- Progesterone
- Reserpine
- Nylidrin hydrochloride

Management of Overdosage: Signs and symptoms of 'Temaril' overdosage range from mild depression of the central nervous system and cardiovascular system to profound hypotension, respiratory depression and unconsciousness. Stimulation may be evident, especially in children and geriatric patients. Atropine-like signs and symptoms—dry mouth, fixed, dilated pupils, flushing, etc.—as well as gastrointestinal symptoms may occur. The treatment of overdosage is essentially symptomatic and supportive. Early gastric lavage may be beneficial. **Do not administer emetics or attempt to induce vomiting because a dystonic reaction of the head or neck might result in aspiration of vomitus.** Extrapyramidal symptoms may be treated with antiparkinsonism drugs, barbiturates, or 'Benadryl'.*

Avoid analeptics, which may cause convulsions. Severe hypotension usually responds to the administration of levarterenol or phenylephrine. EPINEPHRINE SHOULD NOT BE USED, since its use in a patient with partial adrenergic blockade may further lower the blood pressure. Additional measures include oxygen and intravenous fluids. Limited experience with dialysis indicates that it is not helpful.

Special note on 'Spansule' capsules—Since much of the 'Spansule' capsule medication is coated for gradual release, therapy directed at reversing the effects of the ingested drug and at supporting the patient should be continued for as long as overdosage symptoms remain. Saline cathartics are useful for hastening evacuation of pellets that have not already released medication.

How Supplied:

'Temaril' Tablets—2.5 mg. trimeprazine/tablet in bottles of 100 and 1000; Single Unit Packages of 100 (intended for institutional use only).

'Temaril' Syrup—2.5 mg. trimeprazine/5 ml. (teaspoonful) and alcohol 5.7%, in 4 fl. oz. bottles.

'Temaril' Spansule capsules—5 mg. trimeprazine/capsule in bottles of 50; Single Unit Packages of 100 (intended for institutional use only).

Military—Tablets 2.5 mg., 1000's, 6505-00-935-9826.

*Trademark Reg. U.S. Pat. Off.: 'Benadryl' for diphenhydramine hydrochloride, Parke-Davis.

[*Shown in Product Identification Section*]

THORAZINE® ℞
(brand of chlorpromazine)

Description: Thorazine (chlorpromazine, SK&F) is 10-(3-dimethylaminopropyl)-2-chlorphenothiazine, a dimethylamine derivative of phenothiazine. It is present in oral and injectable forms as the hydrochloride salt, and in the suppositories as the base.

Actions: The precise mechanism whereby the therapeutic effects of chlorpromazine are produced is not known. The principal pharmacological actions are psychotropic. It also exerts sedative and antiemetic activity. Chlorpromazine has actions at all levels of the central nervous system—primarily at subcortical levels—as well as on multiple organ systems. Chlorpromazine has strong antiadrenergic and weaker peripheral anticholinergic activity;

ganglionic blocking action is relatively slight. It also possesses slight antihistaminic and antiserotonin activity.

Indications

Based on a review of this drug by the National Academy of Sciences—National Research Council and/or other information, FDA has classified the indications as follows:

Effective: For the management of the manifestations of psychotic disorders.

To control nausea and vomiting.

For control of the manifestations of manic-depressive illness (manic phase).

For relief of intractable hiccups.

Prior to surgery, to control restlessness and apprehension.

For control of acute intermittent porphyria.

As an adjunct in the treatment of tetanus.

Probably effective: In mild alcohol withdrawal, to reduce agitation, tension, nausea and vomiting in patients under close supervision.

For the control of moderate to severe agitation, hyperactivity or aggressiveness in disturbed children.

Possibly effective: In cancer and severe pain: to reduce apprehension and suffering; to reduce narcotic requirements.

For control of excessive anxiety, tension and agitation as seen in neuroses.

Final classification of the less-than-effective indications requires further investigation.

Contraindications: Comatose states, presence of large amounts of C.N.S. depressants (alcohol, barbiturates, narcotics, etc.), and in the presence of bone marrow depression.

Warnings: The extrapyramidal symptoms which can occur secondary to 'Thorazine' may be confused with the central nervous system signs of an undiagnosed primary disease responsible for the vomiting, e.g., Reye's syndrome or other encephalopathy. The use of 'Thorazine' and other potential hepatotoxins should be avoided in children and adolescents whose signs and symptoms suggest Reye's syndrome.

Patients who have demonstrated a hypersensitivity reaction (e.g., blood dyscrasias, jaundice with a phenothiazine) should not be re-exposed to any phenothiazine, including Thorazine (chlorpromazine, SK&F), unless in the judgment of the physician the potential benefits of treatment outweigh the possible hazard.

'Thorazine' may impair mental and/or physical abilities, especially during the first few days of therapy. Therefore, caution patients about activities requiring alertness (e.g., operating vehicles or machinery).

The use of alcohol with this drug should be avoided due to possible additive effects and hypotension.

'Thorazine' may counteract the antihypertensive effect of guanethidine and related compounds.

Usage in Pregnancy: Safety for the use of 'Thorazine' during pregnancy has not been established; therefore, it is recommended that the drug be given to pregnant patients only when, in the judgment of the physician, it is essential. The potential benefits should clearly outweigh possible hazards. There are reported instances of jaundice or prolonged extrapyramidal signs in newborn infants whose mothers had received 'Thorazine'.

Reproductive studies in rodents have demonstrated a potential for embryotoxicity, increased neonatal mortality and nursing transfer of the drug. Tests in the offspring of the drug-treated rodents demonstrate decreased performance. The possibility of permanent neurological damage cannot be excluded.

Nursing Mothers: There is evidence that chlorpromazine is excreted in the breast milk of nursing mothers.

Precautions: Thorazine (chlorpromazine, SK&F) should be administered cautiously to persons with cardiovascular or liver disease.

Because of its C.N.S. depressant effect, 'Thorazine' should be used with caution in patients with chronic respiratory disorders such as severe asthma, emphysema and acute respiratory infections, particularly in children.

Because 'Thorazine' can suppress the cough reflex, aspiration of vomitus is possible.

Thorazine (chlorpromazine, SK&F) prolongs and intensifies the action of C.N.S. depressants such as anesthetics, barbiturates and narcotics. When 'Thorazine' is administered concomitantly, about $\frac{1}{4}$ to $\frac{1}{2}$ the usual dosage of such agents is required. When 'Thorazine' is not being administered to reduce requirements of C.N.S. depressants, it is best to stop such depressants before starting 'Thorazine' treatment. These agents may subsequently be reinstated at low doses and increased as needed.

Note: 'Thorazine' does *not* intensify the anticonvulsant action of barbiturates. Therefore, dosage of anticonvulsants, including barbiturates, should *not* be reduced if 'Thorazine' is started. Instead, start 'Thorazine' at low doses and increase as needed.

Use with caution in persons who will be exposed to extreme heat, organophosphorus insecticides, and in persons receiving atropine or related drugs.

To lessen the likelihood of adverse reactions related to drug accumulation, patients on long-term therapy, particularly on high doses, should be evaluated periodically to decide whether the maintenance dosage could be lowered, or drug therapy could be discontinued.

Antiemetic Effect: The antiemetic action of 'Thorazine' may mask the signs and symptoms of overdosage of other drugs and may obscure the diagnosis and treatment of other conditions such as intestinal obstruction, brain tumor, and Reye's syndrome (See WARNINGS).

Abrupt Withdrawal: Like other phenothiazines, Thorazine (chlorpromazine, SK&F) is not known to cause psychic dependence and does not produce tolerance or addiction. There may be, however, following abrupt withdrawal of high-dose therapy, some symptoms resembling those of physical dependence such as gastritis, nausea and vomiting, dizziness and tremulousness. These symptoms can usually be avoided or reduced by gradual reduction of the dosage or by continuing concomitant anti-parkinsonism agents for several weeks after 'Thorazine' is withdrawn.

Adverse Reactions: Drowsiness, usually mild to moderate, may occur, particularly during the first or second week, after which it generally disappears. If troublesome, dosage may be lowered.

Jaundice: Over-all incidence has been low, regardless of indication or dosage. Most investigators conclude it is a sensitivity reaction. Most cases occur between the second and fourth weeks of therapy. The clinical picture resembles infectious hepatitis, with laboratory features of obstructive jaundice, rather than those of parenchymal damage. It is usually promptly reversible on withdrawal of the medication; however, chronic jaundice has been reported.

There is no conclusive evidence that pre-existing liver disease makes patients more susceptible to jaundice. Alcoholics with cirrhosis have been successfully treated with Thorazine (chlorpromazine, SK&F) without complications. Nevertheless, the medication should be used cautiously in patients with liver disease. Patients who have experienced jaundice with a phenothiazine should not, if possible, be re-exposed to 'Thorazine' or other phenothiazines.

If fever with grippe-like symptoms occurs, test for increased bilirubin or for bile in urine. If tests are positive, stop treatment.

Liver function tests in jaundice induced by the drug may mimic extrahepatic obstruction; withhold exploratory laparotomy until extrahepatic obstruction is confirmed.

Hematological Disorders, including agranulocytosis, eosinophilia, leukopenia, hemolytic anemia, thrombocytopenic purpura, and pancytopenia, though rare, have been reported.

Agranulocytosis—Observe patients regularly for sudden appearance of sore throat or other signs of infection. If white blood counts and differential smears indicate cellular depression, stop treatment and start antibiotic and other suitable therapy.

Most cases have occurred between the 4th and 10th weeks of therapy; patients should be watched closely during that period.

Moderate suppression of white blood cells is not an indication for stopping treatment unless accompanied by the symptoms described above.

Cardiovascular:

Hypotensive Effects—Postural hypotension, simple tachycardia, momentary fainting and dizziness may occur after the first injection; occasionally after subsequent injections; rarely, after the first oral dose. Usually recovery is spontaneous and symptoms disappear within $\frac{1}{2}$ to 2 hours. Occasionally, these effects may be more severe and prolonged, producing a shock-like condition.

To minimize hypotension after initial injection, keep patient lying down and observe for at least $\frac{1}{2}$ hour. To control hypotension, place patient in head-low position with legs raised. If a vasoconstrictor is required, 'Levophed' and 'Neo-Synephrine'* are the most suitable. Other pressor agents, including epinephrine, should not be used as they may cause a paradoxical further lowering of blood pressure.

EKG Changes—particularly nonspecific, usually reversible Q and T wave distortions—have been observed in some patients receiving phenothiazine tranquilizers, including Thorazine (chlorpromazine, SK&F). Their relationship to myocardial damage has not been confirmed.

Note: Sudden death, apparently due to cardiac arrest, has been reported, but there is not sufficient evidence to establish a relationship between such deaths and the administration of the drug.

C.N.S. Effects:

Neuromuscular (Extrapyramidal) Reactions, closely resembling parkinsonism, and motor restlessness have occurred most frequently in psychiatric patients receiving high dosages. Dystonic reactions have been reported occasionally. Such symptoms usually disappear soon after dosage is lowered, the drug temporarily withdrawn, and/or concomitant administration of an anti-parkinsonism agent. (Note: Levodopa has not been found effective in relief of these neuromuscular reactions.) In severe cases suitable supportive measures such as maintaining a clear airway and adequate hydration should be used. When 'Thorazine' is reinstituted, it should be at a lower dosage.

Hyperreflexia has been reported in the newborn.

Persistent Tardive Dyskinesia—As with all antipsychotic agents, tardive dyskinesia may appear in some patients on long-term therapy or may appear after drug therapy has been discontinued. The risk appears to be greater in elderly patients on high-dose therapy, especially females. The symptoms are persistent and in some patients appear to be irreversible. The syndrome is characterized by rhythmical involuntary movements of the tongue, face, mouth or jaw (e.g., protrusion of tongue, puffing of cheeks, puckering of mouth, chewing movements). Sometimes these may be accom-

Continued on next page

Smith Kline & French—Cont.

panied by involuntary movements of extremities.

There is no known effective treatment for tardive dyskinesia; anti-parkinsonism agents usually do not alleviate the symptoms of this syndrome. It is suggested that all antipsychotic agents be discontinued if these symptoms appear. Should it be necessary to reinstitute treatment, or increase the dosage of the agent, or switch to a different antipsychotic agent, the syndrome may be masked.

It has been reported that fine vermicular movements of the tongue may be an early sign of the syndrome and if the medication is stopped at that time the syndrome may not develop.

Adverse Behavioral Effects—Psychotic symptoms and catatonic-like states have been reported rarely.

Other C.N.S. Effects—Cerebral edema has been reported.

Convulsive seizures (*petit mal* and *grand mal*) have been reported, particularly in patients with EEG abnormalities or history of such disorders.

Abnormality of the cerebrospinal fluid proteins has also been reported.

Allergic Reactions of a mild urticarial type or photosensitivity are seen. Avoid undue exposure to sun. More severe reactions, including exfoliative dermatitis, have been reported occasionally.

Contact dermatitis has been reported in nursing personnel; accordingly, the use of rubber gloves when administering 'Thorazine' liquid or injectable is recommended.

Endocrine Disorders: Lactation and moderate breast engorgement may occur in females on large doses. If persistent, lower dosage or withdraw drug. False-positive pregnancy tests have been reported, but are less likely to occur when a serum test is used. Amenorrhea and gynecomastia have also been reported. Hyperglycemia, hypoglycemia and glycosuria have been reported.

Autonomic Reactios: Occasional dry mouth; nasal congestion; constipation; adynamic ileus; urinary retention, miosis and mydriasis.

Special Considerations in Long-Term Therapy: Skin pigmentation and ocular changes have occurred in some patients taking substantial doses of Thorazine (chlorpromazine, SK&F) for prolonged periods.

Skin Pigmentation—Rare instances of skin pigmentation have been observed in hospitalized mental patients, primarily females who have received the drug usually for three years or more in dosages ranging from 500 mg. to 1500 mg. daily. The pigmentary changes, restricted to exposed areas of the body, range from an almost imperceptible darkening of the skin to a slate gray color, sometimes with a violet hue. Histological examination reveals a pigment, chiefly in the dermis, which is probably a melanin-like complex. The pigmentation may fade following discontinuance of the drug.

Ocular Changes—Ocular changes have occurred more frequently than skin pigmentation and have been observed both in pigmented and nonpigmented patients receiving Thorazine (chlorpromazine, SK&F) usually for two years or more in dosages of 300 mg. daily and higher. Eye changes are characterized by deposition of fine particulate matter in the lens and cornea. In more advanced cases, star-shaped opacities have also been observed in the anterior portion of the lens. The nature of the eye deposits has not yet been determined. A small number of patients with more severe ocular changes have had some visual impairment. In addition to these corneal and lenticular changes, epithelial keratopathy and pigmentary retinopathy have been reported. Reports suggest that the eye lesions may regress after withdrawal of the drug.

Since the occurrence of eye changes seems to be related to dosage levels and/or duration of therapy, it is suggested that long-term patients on moderate to high dosage levels have periodic ocular examinations.

Etiology—The etiology of both of these reactions is not clear, but exposure to light, along with dosage/duration of therapy, appears to be the most significant factor. If either of these reactions is observed, the physician should weigh the benefits of continued therapy against the possible risks and, on the merits of the individual case, determine whether or not to continue present therapy, lower the dosage, or withdraw the drug.

Other Adverse Reactions: Mild fever may occur after large I.M. doses. Hyperpyrexia has been reported. Increases in appetite and weight sometimes occur. Peripheral edema and a systemic lupus erythematosus-like syndrome have been reported.

Note: There have been occasional reports of sudden death in patients receiving phenothiazines. In some cases, the cause appeared to be asphyxia due to failure of the cough reflex. In others, the cause could not be determined. There is not sufficient evidence to establish a relationship between such deaths and the administration of phenothiazines.

Dosage and Administration: Adjust dosage to individual and the severity of his condition, recognizing that the milligram for milligram potency relationship among all dosage forms has not been precisely established clinically. It is important to increase dosage until symptoms are controlled. Dosage should be increased more gradually in debilitated or emaciated patients. In continued therapy, gradually reduce dosage to the lowest effective maintenance level, after symptoms have been controlled for a reasonable period.

In general, dosage recommendations for other oral forms of the drug may be applied to Spansule® brand sustained release capsules on the basis of total daily dosage in milligrams.

Increase parenteral dosage only if hypotension has not occurred. Before using I.M., see Important Notes on Injection.

Elderly Patients: In general, dosages in the lower range are sufficient for most elderly patients. Since they appear to be more susceptible to hypotension and neuromuscular reactions, such patients should be observed closely. Dosage should be tailored to the individual, response carefully monitored, and dosage adjusted accordingly. Dosage should be increased more gradually in elderly patients.

General Medicine:

Adults: EXCESSIVE ANXIETY, TENSION AND AGITATION—*Oral:* 10 mg. t.i.d. or q.i.d., or 25 mg. b.i.d. or t.i.d. MORE SEVERE CASES—*Oral:* 25 mg. t.i.d. After 1 or 2 days, daily dosage may be increased by 20 to 50 mg. semiweekly, until patient becomes calm and cooperative. (Maximum improvement may not be seen for weeks or even months.) Continue optimum dosage for 2 weeks; then gradually reduce to maintenance level. Daily dosage of 200 mg. is not unusual. Some patients require higher dosages (e.g., 800 mg. daily is not uncommon in discharged mental patients).

PROMPT CONTROL OF SEVERE SYMPTOMS—*I.M.:* 25 mg. (1 ml.). If necessary, repeat in 1 hour. Subsequent doses should be oral, 25 to 50 mg. t.i.d.

NAUSEA AND VOMITING—*Oral:* 10 to 25 mg. q4-6h, p.r.n., increased, if necessary. *I.M.:* 25 mg. (1 ml.). If no hypotension occurs, give 25 to 50 mg. q3-4h, p.r.n., until vomiting stops. Then switch to oral dosage. *Rectal:* One 100 mg. suppository q6-8h, p.r.n. In some patients, half this dose will do.

INTRACTABLE HICCUPS—*Oral:* 25 to 50 mg. t.i.d. or q.i.d. If symptoms persist for 2-3 days, give 25 to 50 mg. (1-2 ml.) I.M. Should symptoms persist, use *slow* I.V. infusion with patient flat in bed: 25 to 50 mg. (1-2 ml.) in 500 to 1,000 ml. of saline. Follow blood pressure closely.

MILD ALCOHOL WITHDRAWAL—Depending on the condition of the patient—(1) *I.M.:* 25 to 50 mg. (1-2 ml.). Repeat, if necessary. Start subsequent oral dosages at 25 to 50 mg. t.i.d. (2) *Oral:* 50 mg. followed by 25 to 50 mg. t.i.d. or, (3) *Oral:* 10 mg. t.i.d. or q.i.d., or 25 mg. b.i.d. or t.i.d. Note: Stuporous patients should sleep off alcohol effects before treatment is begun.

CANCER AND SEVERE PAIN—*I.M.:* 25 mg. (1 ml.) b.i.d. or t.i.d. *Oral:* 10 mg. t.i.d. or q.i.d., or 25 mg. b.i.d. or t.i.d. Note: Reduce dosage of concomitant narcotics and sedatives to ¼ or ½.

ACUTE INTERMITTENT PORPHYRIA—*Oral:* 25 to 50 mg. t.i.d. or q.i.d. Can usually be discontinued after several weeks, but maintenance therapy may be necessary for some patients. *I.M.:* 25 mg. (1 ml.) t.i.d. or q.i.d. until patient can take oral therapy.

TETANUS—*I.M.:* 25 to 50 mg. (1-2 ml.) given 3 or 4 times daily, usually in conjunction with barbiturates. Total doses and frequency of administration must be determined by the patient's response, starting with low doses and increasing gradually. *I.V.:* 25 to 50 mg. (1-2 ml.). Dilute to at least 1 mg. per ml. and administer at a rate of 1 mg. per minute.

Children: NAUSEA AND VOMITING—Thorazine (chlorpromazine, SK&F) should generally not be used in children under 6 months of age. It should not be used in conditions for which children's dosages have not been established. Dosage and frequency of administration should be adjusted according to the severity of the symptoms and response of the patient. The duration of activity following intramuscular administration may last up to 12 hours. Subsequent doses may be given by the same route if necessary. *Oral:* ¼ mg./lb. body weight q4-6h (e.g., 40 lb. child—10 mg. q4-6h). *Rectal:* ½ mg./lb. body weight q6-8h, p.r.n. (e.g., 20-30 lb. child —half of a 25 mg. suppository q6-8h). *I.M.:* ¼ mg./lb. body weight q6-8h, p.r.n. *Maximum I.M. Dosage:* Children up to 5 yrs. (or 50 lbs.), not over 40 mg./day; 5-12 yrs. (or 50-100 lbs.), not over 75 mg./day except in severe cases. (For mental and emotional disorders, see Psychiatry, below.)

TETANUS—*I.M.* or *I.V.:* ¼ mg./lb. body weight q6-8h. When given I.V., dilute to at least 1 mg./ml. and administer at rate of 1 mg. per 2 minutes. In children up to 50 lbs., do not exceed 40 mg. daily; 50 to 100 lbs., do not exceed 75 mg., except in severe cases.

Surgery:

Adults: PREOPERATIVE—*Oral:* 25 to 50 mg., 2 to 3 hours before the operation. *I.M.:* 12.5 to 25 mg. (0.5-1 ml.), 1 to 2 hours before operation. DURING SURGERY—Administer only to control acute nausea and vomiting. *I.M.:* 12.5 mg. (0.5 ml.). Repeat in ½ hour if necessary and if no hypotension occurs. *I.V.:* 2 mg. per fractional injection, at 2-minute intervals. Do not exceed 25 mg. Dilute to 1 mg./ml., i.e., 1 ml. (25 mg.) mixed with 24 ml. of saline. POSTOPERATIVE—*Oral:* 10 to 25 mg. q4-6h, p.r.n. *I.M.:* 12.5 to 25 mg. (0.5-1 ml.). Repeat in 1 hour if necessary and if no hypotension occurs.

Children: Thorazine (chlorpromazine, SK&F) should generally not be used in children under 6 months of age except where potentially lifesaving. It should not be used in conditions for which specific children's dosages have not been established. PREOPERATIVE—¼ mg./lb. body weight, either *orally* 2 to 3 hours before operation, or *I.M.* 1 to 2 hours before. DURING SURGERY—*I.M.:* ⅛ mg./lb. body weight. Repeat in ½ hour if necessary and if no hypotension occurs. *I.V.:* 1 mg. per fractional injection at 2-minute intervals and not exceeding recommended I.M. dosage. Always dilute to 1 mg./ml., i.e., 1 ml. (25 mg.) mixed with 24 ml. of saline. POSTOPERATIVE—¼ mg./lb. body weight, either *orally* q4-6h, p.r.n., or *I.M.* Repeat in 1 hour if necessary and if no hypotension occurs.

Psychiatry:
Increase dosage gradually until symptoms are controlled. Maximum improvement may not be seen for weeks or even months. Continue optimum dosage for 2 weeks; then gradually reduce dosage to the lowest effective maintenance level.

Adults: OFFICE PATIENTS OR OUTPATIENTS—*Oral:* 10 mg. t.i.d. or q.i.d., or 25 mg. b.i.d. or t.i.d. MORE SEVERE CASES — *Oral:* 25 mg. t.i.d. After 1 or 2 days, daily dosage may be increased by 20-50 mg. at semiweekly intervals until patient becomes calm and cooperative. PROMPT CONTROL OF SEVERE SYMPTOMS—*I.M.:* 25 mg. (1 ml.). If necessary, repeat in 1 hour. Subsequent doses should be oral, 25-50 mg. t.i.d.
HOSPITALIZED PATIENTS: ACUTELY AGITATED, MANIC, OR DISTURBED—*I.M.:* 25 mg. (1 ml.). If necessary, give additional 25 to 50 mg. injection in 1 hour. Increase subsequent I.M. doses gradually over several days—up to 400 mg. q4-6h in exceptionally severe cases —until patient is controlled. Usually patient becomes quiet and cooperative within 24 to 48 hours and oral doses may be substituted and increased until the patient is calm. 500 mg. a day is generally sufficient. While gradual increases to 2,000 mg. a day or more may be necessary, there is usually little therapeutic gain to be achieved by exceeding 1,000 mg. a day for extended periods. In general, dosage levels should be lower in the elderly, the emaciated and the debilitated. LESS ACUTELY AGITATED PATIENTS—*Oral:* 25 mg. t.i.d. Increase gradually until effective dose is reached—usually 400 mg. daily.

Children: OFFICE PATIENTS OR OUTPATIENTS—Select route of administration according to severity of patient's condition and increase dosage gradually as required. *Oral:* ¼ mg./lb. body weight q4-6h, p.r.n. (e.g., for 40 lb. child—10 mg. q4-6h). *Rectal:* ½ mg./lb. body weight q6-8h, p.r.n. (e.g., for 20-30 lb. child —half a 25 mg. suppository q6-8h). *I.M.:* ¼ mg./lb. body weight q6-8h, p.r.n.
HOSPITALIZED PATIENTS—As with outpatients, start with low doses and increase dosage gradually. In severe behavior disorders or psychotic conditions, higher dosages (50-100 mg. daily, and in older children, 200 mg. daily or more) may be necessary. *Maximum I.M. Dosage:* Children up to 5 years (or 50 lbs.), not over 40 mg./day; 5-12 years (or 50-100 lbs.), not over 75 mg./day except in unmanageable cases.

Important Notes on Injection: Inject slowly, deep into upper outer quadrant of buttock.
Because of possible hypotensive effects, reserve parenteral administration for bedfast patients or for acute ambulatory cases, and keep patient lying down for at least ½ hour after injection. If irritation is a problem, dilute Injection with saline or 2% procaine; mixing with other agents in the syringe is not recommended. Subcutaneous injection is not advised. Avoid injecting undiluted Thorazine (chlorpromazine, SK&F) into vein. I.V. route is only for severe hiccups and surgery.
Because of the possibility of contact dermatitis, avoid getting solution on hands or clothing. Protect from light, or discoloration may occur. Slight yellowing will not alter potency. Discard if markedly discolored.

Note on Concentrate: When the Concentrate is to be used, add the desired dosage of Concentrate to 60 ml. (2 fl. oz.) or more of diluent *just prior to administration.* This will insure palatability and stability. Vehicles suggested for dilution are: tomato or fruit juice, milk, simple syrup, orange syrup, carbonated beverages, coffee, tea, or water. Semisolid foods (soups, puddings, etc.) may also be used. The Concentrate is light sensitive; it should be protected from light and dispensed in amber glass bottles. *Refrigeration is not required.*

Overdosage: (See also Adverse Reactions.)
Symptoms—Primarily symptoms of central nervous system depression to the point of somnolence or coma. Hypotension and extrapyramidal symptoms.
Other possible manifestations include agitation and restlessness, convulsions, fever, autonomic reactions such as dry mouth and ileus, EKG changes and cardiac arrhythmias.
Treatment—Essentially symptomatic and supportive. Early gastric lavage is helpful. Keep patient under observation and maintain an open airway, since involvement of the extrapyramidal mechanism may produce dysphagia and respiratory difficulty in severe overdosage. **Do not attempt to induce emesis because a dystonic reaction of the head or neck may develop that could result in aspiration of vomitus.** Extrapyramidal symptoms may be treated with anti-parkinsonism drugs, barbiturates, or 'Benadryl'†.
If administration of a stimulant is desirable, amphetamine, dextroamphetamine, or caffeine with sodium benzoate is recommended. Stimulants that may cause convulsions (e.g., picrotoxin or pentylenetetrazol) should be avoided.
If hypotension occurs, the standard measures for managing circulatory shock should be initiated. If it is desirable to administer a vasoconstrictor, 'Levophed' and 'Neo-Synephrine' are most suitable. Other pressor agents, including epinephrine, are not recommended because phenothiazine derivatives may reverse the usual elevating action of these agents and cause a further lowering of blood pressure.
Limited experience indicates that phenothiazines are *not* dialyzable.
Special note on 'Spansule' capsules—Since much of the 'Spansule' capsule medication is coated for gradual release, therapy directed at reversing the effects of the ingested drug and at supporting the patient should be continued for as long as overdosage symptoms remain. Saline cathartics are useful for hastening evacuation of pellets that have not already released medication.

How Supplied: Tablets—Each tablet contains chlorpromazine hydrochloride, 10 mg., 25 mg. or 50 mg., in bottles of 100 and 1000; in Single Unit Packages of 100 (intended for institutional use only). For use in severe neuropsychiatric conditions, 100 mg. and 200 mg., in bottles of 100 and 1000; in Single Unit Packages of 100 (intended for institutional use only).
Spansule® brand of sustained release capsules—Each 'Spansule' capsule contains chlorpromazine hydrochloride, so prepared that an initial dose is released promptly and the remaining medication is released gradually over a prolonged period. Available as 30 mg., 75 mg., 150 mg. or 200 mg., in bottles of 50 and 500; in Single Unit Packages of 100 (intended for institutional use only). For use in severe neuropsychiatric conditions, 300 mg., in bottles of 50; in Single Unit Packages of 100 (intended for institutional use only).
Ampuls—1 ml. and 2 ml. (25 mg./ml.), in boxes of 10, 100 and 500. Each ml. contains, in aqueous solution, chlorpromazine hydrochloride, 25 mg.; ascorbic acid, 2 mg.; sodium bisulfite, 1 mg.; sodium sulfite, 1 mg.; sodium chloride, 6 mg.
Multiple-dose Vials—10 ml. (25 mg./ml.), in boxes of 1, 20 and 100. Each ml. contains, in aqueous solution, chlorpromazine hydrochloride, 25 mg.; ascorbic acid, 2 mg.; sodium bisulfite, 1 mg.; sodium sulfite, 1 mg.; sodium chloride, 1 mg. Contains benzyl alcohol, 2%, as a preservative.
Syrup—Each 5 ml. (one teaspoonful) contains chlorpromazine hydrochloride, 10 mg., in 4 fl. oz. bottles.
Suppositories—Each suppository contains chlorpromazine, 25 mg. or 100 mg., glycerin, glyceryl monopalmitate, glyceryl monostearate, hydrogenated cocoanut oil fatty acids, hydrogenated palm kernel oil fatty acids, in boxes of 12.
Concentrate (intended for institutional use only)—*30 mg./ml.:* Each ml. contains chlorpromazine hydrochloride, 30 mg., in 4 fl. oz. bottles, in cartons of 36 bottles, and in 1 gallon bottles. *100 mg./ml.:* Each ml. contains chlorpromazine hydrochloride, 100 mg., in 8 fl. oz. bottles, in cartons of 12.
Military—Concentrate 30 mg./ml., 4 fl.oz., 6505-00-660-1664; Injection 2 ml., 6's, 6505-00-597-5843; Tablets 25 mg., S.U.P. 100's, 6505-00-118-2529, and 1000's, 6505-00-022-1326; Tablets 50 mg., S.U.P. 100's, 6505-00-132-0371, and 1000's, 6505-00-022-1327; Tablets 100 mg., S.U.P. 100's, 6505-00-132-0372, and 1000's, 6505-00-935-9820.

---

*'Levophed' and 'Neo-Synephrine' are the trademarks (Reg. U.S. Pat. Off.) of Winthrop Laboratories for its brands of levarterenol and phenylephrine respectively.
†Trademark Reg. U.S. Pat. Off.: 'Benadryl' for diphenhydramine hydrochloride, Parke-Davis.
[*Shown in Product Identification Section*]

TROPH-IRON®††
Vitamins B_1, B_{12} and Iron

Description: Each 5 ml. (1 teaspoonful) and each tablet contains thiamine hydrochloride (vitamin B_1), 10 mg.; vitamin B_{12}, 25 mcg.; elemental iron, 30 mg., present as soluble ferric pyrophosphate.
Indications: For deficiencies of vitamins B_1, B_{12} and iron.
Dosage and Administration: Adults and children 4 years of age and over: One 5 ml. teaspoonful or one tablet daily—or as directed by physician. Children under 4 years: ½ teaspoonful daily.
The treatment of any anemic condition should be under the advice and supervision of a physician. Since oral iron products interfere with absorption of oral tetracycline antibiotics, these products should not be taken within two hours of each other.
Iron-containing medications may occasionally cause gastrointestinal discomfort, such as nausea, constipation or diarrhea.
Warning: Keep this and all medicines out of reach of children. In case of accidental overdose, contact a physician or poison control center immediately.
How Supplied: Liquid—a clear red liquid in 4 fl. oz. (118 ml.) bottles; Tablets—bottles of 50. (While its effectiveness is in no way affected, Troph-Iron liquid may darken as it ages.)

---

††Troph-Iron liquid and tablets are products of Menley & James Laboratories, Professional Products Division, a SmithKline company.
[*Shown in Product Identification Section*]

TROPHITE®††
Vitamins B_1 and B_{12}

Description: Each 5 ml. (1 teaspoonful) and each tablet contains thiamine hydrochloride (vitamin B_1), 10 mg.; and vitamin B_{12}, 25 mcg.
Indications: For deficiencies of vitamins B_1 and B_{12}.
Dosage and Administration: Adults and children 4 years of age and over: One 5 ml. teaspoonful or one tablet daily—or as directed by physician. Children under 4 years: ½ teaspoonful daily.
Trophite Liquid may be mixed with water, milk, or fruit or vegetable juices immediately before taking.
Warning: Keep this and all medicines out of reach of children. In case of accidental over-

Continued on next page

Smith Kline & French—Cont.

dose, contact a physician or poison control center immediately.
How Supplied: Liquid—4 fl. oz. (118 ml.) bottles. Tablets—bottles of 50.

††Trophite Liquid and Tablets are products of Menley & James Laboratories, Professional Products Division, a SmithKline company.
[*Shown in Product Identification Section*]

TUSS-ORNADE® ℞
SPANSULE® CAPSULES and LIQUID

Description: Each 'Tuss-Ornade' *Spansule* capsule contains 20 mg. of caramiphen edisylate; 8 mg. of chlorpheniramine maleate; and 50 mg. of phenylpropanolamine hydrochloride, so prepared that an initial dose is released promptly and the remaining medication is released gradually over a prolonged period; and isopropamide iodide equivalent to 2.5 mg. of isopropamide. Because isopropamide iodide, a synthetic anticholinergic, can provide 10 to 12 hours of antisecretory action, this component is not in sustained release form.
Each 5 ml. teaspoonful of 'Tuss-Ornade' Liquid contains 5 mg. of caramiphen edisylate; 2 mg. of chlorpheniramine maleate; 15 mg. of phenylpropanolamine hydrochloride; isopropamide iodide equivalent to 0.75 mg. of isopropamide; and alcohol, 7.5%.
Actions: 'Tuss-Ornade' provides relief of coughing, sneezing, running nose, weeping and other symptoms of nasal congestion. Its formula contains an antitussive, nasal decongestant, antihistamine and a drying agent.

Indications

Based on a review of this drug by the National Academy of Sciences—National Research Council and/or other information, FDA has classified the indications as follows:
Lacking in substantial evidence of effectiveness as a fixed combination: For relief from coughing, upper respiratory congestion and hypersecretion associated with the common cold, sinusitis, vasomotor rhinitis and allergic rhinitis.
Final classification of the less-than-effective indications requires further investigation.

Contraindications: Hypersensitivity to any of the components; concurrent MAO inhibitor therapy; severe hypertension; bronchial asthma; coronary artery disease; stenosing peptic ulcer; pyloroduodenal or bladder neck obstruction. Do not use 'Tuss-Ornade' Liquid in children under 15 lbs. or in children less than six months of age. Do not use 'Tuss-Ornade' *Spansule* capsules in children under 12 years of age.
Warnings: Caution patients about activities requiring alertness (e.g., operating vehicles or machinery). Patients should also be warned about the possible additive effects of alcohol and other CNS depressants.
Usage in Pregnancy: Safe use in pregnancy has not been established. This drug should be used in pregnancy, nursing mothers or by women who might bear children only when the potential benefits have been weighed against the possible hazards to the mother and child. However, 'Tuss-Ornade' has had extensive clinical use in pregnant patients without known deleterious effect. Rat reproduction studies with low drug doses have shown no teratogenic effect. As with all anticholinergics, an inhibitory effect on lactation may occur.
Effect on PBI Determination and I^{131} Uptake: The iodine in isopropamide iodide may alter the PBI determination and will suppress I^{131} uptake. Therefore, thyroid function tests unaffected by exogenous iodides should be substituted.
Precautions: Use with caution in persons with cardiovascular disease, glaucoma, prostatic hypertrophy, hyperthyroidism.
Adverse Reactions: Drowsiness; excessive dryness of nose, throat or mouth; nervousness; or insomnia may occur on rare occasions with 'Tuss-Ornade', but are usually mild and transitory. Other reported adverse reactions are: nausea, vomiting, epigastric distress, diarrhea, rash, dizziness, weakness, tightness of chest, angina pain, abdominal pain, irritability, palpitation, headache, incoordination, tremor, difficulty in urination, dysuria, thrombocytopenia, leukopenia, convulsions, hypertension, hypotension, anorexia, constipation, visual disturbances. Isopropamide iodide may cause signs of iodine toxicity, such as acne and parotitis.
Dosage and Administration: 'Tuss-Ornade' *Spansule* capsules (Not for use in children under 12 years of age): Adults and children over 12 years of age—one 'Tuss-Ornade' *Spansule* capsule q12h.
'Tuss-Ornade' Liquid: Do not use in children under 15 lbs. or children less than six months of age. Adults, 1 to 2 teaspoonfuls 3 or 4 times a day; children (over 25 lbs.), 1 teaspoonful 3 or 4 times a day; children (15-25 lbs.), ½ teaspoonful 3 or 4 times a day.
Overdosage: *Symptoms*—May include dryness of mouth, dysphagia, thirst, blurred vision, dilated pupils, photophobia, fever, rapid pulse and respiration, disorientation, dizziness, nausea, fainting, tachycardia, and either excitation or depression of the central nervous system.
Treatment—Gastric lavage, repeated several times. Since much of the 'Spansule' capsule medication is coated for gradual release, saline cathartics should be administered to hasten evacuation of pellets that have not already released medication.
Respiratory depression should be treated promptly by the use of oxygen and stimulants. If marked excitement is present, one of the short-acting barbiturates or chloral hydrate may be used.
Supplied: 'Tuss-Ornade' *Spansule* capsules: In bottles of 50 and 500 capsules.
'Tuss-Ornade' Liquid: an orange-pineapple flavored liquid in 16 fl. oz. bottles.
[*Shown in Product Identification Section*]

URISPAS® ℞
(brand of flavoxate HCl)
100 mg. tablets
Urinary tract spasmolytic

Description: Urispas (brand of flavoxate HCl) is a synthetic antispasmodic offered specifically for the relief of symptoms associated with various urologic disorders. 'Urispas' exerts its effect directly on the muscle.
Chemically, flavoxate hydrochloride is 2-piperidinoethyl 3-methyl-4-oxo-2-phenyl-4*H*-1-benzopyran-8-carboxylate hydrochloride. The empirical formula of flavoxate hydrochloride is $C_{24}H_{25}NO_4 \bullet HCl$.
Action: Flavoxate hydrochloride counteracts smooth muscle spasm of the urinary tract.
Indications: Urispas (brand of flavoxate HCl) is indicated for symptomatic relief of dysuria, urgency, nocturia, suprapubic pain, frequency and incontinence as may occur in cystitis, prostatitis, urethritis, urethrocystitis/urethrotrigonitis. 'Urispas' is not indicated for definitive treatment, but is compatible with drugs used for the treatment of urinary tract infections.
Contraindications: Urispas (brand of flavoxate HCl) is contraindicated in patients who have any of the following obstructive conditions: pyloric or duodenal obstruction, obstructive intestinal lesions or ileus, achalasia, gastrointestinal hemorrhage, and obstructive uropathies of the lower urinary tract.
Warnings: Urispas (brand of flavoxate HCl) should be given cautiously in patients with suspected glaucoma.
Usage in Pregnancy—Safety in women who are or may become pregnant has not been established. Therefore, Urispas (brand of flavoxate HCl) should not be given except when the expected benefits outweigh the possible hazards.
Usage in Children—This drug cannot be recommended for infants and children under 12 years of age because safety and efficacy have not been demonstrated in this age group.
Precautions: In the event of drowsiness and blurred vision, the patient should not operate a motor vehicle or machinery or participate in activities where alertness is required.
Adverse Reactions: Adverse reactions reported include nausea and vomiting, dry mouth, nervousness, vertigo, headache, drowsiness, blurred vision, increased ocular tension, disturbance in eye accommodation, urticaria and other dermatoses, mental confusion especially in the elderly patient, dysuria, tachycardia and palpitation, hyperpyrexia, eosinophilia and leukopenia (1 case which was reversible upon discontinuation of the drug).
Dosage and Administration: Adults and children over twelve years of age: one or two 100 mg. tablets three or four times a day. With improvement of symptoms, the dose may be reduced. This drug cannot be recommended for infants and children under 12 years of age because safety and efficacy have not been demonstrated in this age group.
How Supplied: 100 mg. tablets, in bottles of 100; in Single Unit Packages of 100 (intended for institutional use only).
Military—Tablets, 100 mg., 100's, 6505-00-172-3420.
[*Shown in Product Identification Section*]

VONTROL® ℞
(brand of diphenidol)

'Vontrol' may cause hallucinations, disorientation, or confusion. For this reason, its use is limited to patients who are hospitalized or under comparable, continuous, close, professional supervision. Even then, the physician should carefully weigh the benefits against the possible risks and give due consideration to alternate therapeutic measures.

Description: 'Vontrol', α, α-diphenyl-1-piperidinebutanol, is a compound not related to the antihistamines, phenothiazines, barbiturates, or other agents with antivertigo or antiemetic action.
Actions: 'Vontrol' (diphenidol, SK&F) apparently exerts a specific antivertigo effect on the vestibular apparatus to control vertigo and inhibits the chemoreceptor trigger zone to control nausea and vomiting.
Indications (See Warnings):
1) VERTIGO—'Vontrol' is indicated in peripheral (labyrinthine) vertigo and associated nausea and vomiting, as seen in such conditions as: Meniere's disease, middle- and inner-ear surgery (labyrinthitis).
2) NAUSEA AND VOMITING—'Vontrol' is indicated in the control of nausea and vomiting, as seen in such conditions as: postoperative states, malignant neoplasms and labyrinthine disturbances.

Contraindications: Known hypersensitivity to the drug is a contraindication. Anuria is a contraindication. (Since approximately 90% of the drug is excreted in the urine, renal shutdown could cause systemic accumulation.)
Warnings: 'Vontrol' (diphenidol, SK&F) may cause hallucinations, disorientation or confusion. For this reason, its use is limited to patients who are hospitalized or under comparable, continuous, close, professional supervision. Even then, the physician should carefully weigh the benefits against the possible risks

and give due consideration to alternate therapeutic measures.

The incidence of auditory and visual hallucinations, disorientation and confusion appears to be less than ½% or approximately one in 350 patients. The reaction has usually occurred within three days of starting the drug in recommended dosage and has subsided spontaneously usually within three days after discontinuation of the drug. Patients on 'Vontrol' should be observed closely and in the event of such a reaction the drug should be stopped.

Usage in Pregnancy: Use of any drug in pregnancy, lactation or in women of childbearing age requires that the potential benefits of the drug be weighed against its possible hazards to the mother and child.

In animal teratogenesis and reproduction studies of 'Vontrol' (diphenidol, SK&F), there were no significant differences between drug-treated groups and untreated control groups, except as noted under animal Reproduction Studies (see "Pharmacology [animal]").

In 936 patients who received 'Vontrol' during pregnancy, the incidences of normal and abnormal birth were comparable to those reported in the literature for the average population of pregnant patients. And in no instance was there any evidence that 'Vontrol' played a part in birth abnormality (see "In Pregnancy").

'Vontrol' is not indicated for use in nausea and vomiting of pregnancy, since the therapeutic value and safety in this indication have not yet been determined.

Precautions: The antiemetic action of 'Vontrol' (diphenidol, SK&F) may mask signs of overdose of drugs (e.g., digitalis) or may obscure diagnosis of conditions such as intestinal obstruction and brain tumor.

Although there have been no reports of blood dyscrasias with 'Vontrol', patients should be observed regularly for any idiosyncratic reactions.

'Vontrol' has a weak peripheral anticholinergic effect and should be used with care in patients with glaucoma, obstructive lesions of the gastrointestinal and genitourinary tracts, such as stenosing peptic ulcer, prostatic hypertrophy, pyloric and duodenal obstruction, and organic cardiospasm.

Intravenous administration to persons with a history of sinus tachycardia may be undesirable because this procedure may initiate an attack in such patients.

Several patients were reported to have had a transient decrease in systolic and diastolic blood pressure, up to 20 mm. Hg., following parenteral use of 'Vontrol'.

Adverse Reactions: Auditory and visual hallucinations, disorientation and confusion have been reported. Drowsiness, overstimulation, depression, sleep disturbance, dry mouth, g.i. irritation (nausea and indigestion), or blurred vision may occur.

Rarely, slight dizziness, skin rash, malaise, headache, or heartburn may occur. Mild jaundice of questionable relationship to the use of 'Vontrol' (diphenidol, SK&F) has been reported. Slight, transient lowering of blood pressure has been reported in a few patients.

(See laboratory studies under "Pharmacology [human]").

Dosage and Administration (See Warnings): Adults—for Vertigo or Nausea and Vomiting:

Tablets: The usual dose is one tablet (25 mg.) every four hours as needed. Some patients may require two tablets (50 mg.).

Injection—Intramuscular: For rapid control of acute symptoms, 1 to 2 ml. (20-40 mg.) of injection solution by deep intramuscular injection. Another 1 ml. may be injected after one hour if symptoms persist. Thereafter, 1 to 2 ml. every four hours as needed.

Injection—Intravenous (hospitalized patients): For rapid control of acute symptoms, 1 ml. (20 mg.) of injection solution may be injected directly or through venoclysis already in operation. Another 1 ml. may be injected after one hour if symptoms persist. Thereafter, switch to an I.M. or oral dosage route.

It should seldom be necessary to exceed a total daily dose of 300 mg.

NOTE: Subcutaneous administration is not recommended. Care should be taken to avoid subcutaneous or perivenous infiltration.

Children—for Nausea and Vomiting: These recommendations are for nausea and vomiting only. There has been no experience with 'Vontrol' in vertigo in children.

Unit doses in children are best calculated by body weight: usually 0.4 mg./lb. orally; 0.2 mg./lb. intramuscularly (see table).

Children's doses usually should not be given more often than every four hours. However, if symptoms persist after the first dose, an oral or intramuscular dose may be repeated after one hour. Thereafter, doses may be given every four hours as needed.

The total dose in 24 hours should not exceed 2.5 mg./lb. orally, or 1.5 mg./lb. intramuscularly.

NOTE: The drug is not recommended for use in infants under six months or 25 pounds. Intravenous or subcutaneous administration is not recommended in children of any age.

PEDIATRIC DOSAGE TABLE

Weight	Intramuscular	Oral
25 to 50 lbs.	¼ to ½ ml. (5–10 mg.) by deep injection	—
50 to 75 lbs.	½ to ¾ ml. (10–15 mg.) by deep injection	One tablet (25 mg.)
75 to 100 lbs.	¾ to 1 ml. (15–20 mg.) by deep injection	

Overdosage: In the event of overdosage, the patient should be managed according to his symptoms. Treatment is essentially supportive, with maintenance of blood pressure and respiration, plus careful observation. With oral overdosage early gastric lavage may be indicated depending on the amount of overdose and nature of symptoms.

How Supplied:

Ampuls, 2 ml. (20 mg./ml.), boxes of 10—Each ml. contains, in aqueous solution, 20 mg. diphenidol as the hydrochloride, 7.8 mg. sodium tartrate, 5 mg. tartaric acid, and 0.5% phenol as preservative.

Tablets, in bottles of 100—Each tablet contains 25 mg. diphenidol as the hydrochloride.

Pharmacology (animal): 'Vontrol' (diphenidol, SK&F) exerts its antiemetic effect primarily by inhibiting the chemoreceptor trigger zone, as evidenced by its activity in blocking emesis induced by apomorphine in dogs. In this regard 'Vontrol', as the hydrochloride salt, has a potency equal to the potent phenothiazine antiemetic, chlorpromazine hydrochloride. In animals 'Vontrol' has only weak parasympatholytic activity and no significant sedative, tranquilizing or antihistaminic action or effects on blood pressure, heart rate, respiration or the electrocardiogram.

Subacute and chronic toxicity studies in rats and dogs, in which large doses of 'Vontrol', as the hydrochloride salt, were administered orally and intramuscularly for periods up to one year, revealed no significant effects on hematology, liver function, kidney function or blood glucose determinations. Histological examination of the animals' tissues did not reveal any significant lesions attributable to administration of 'Vontrol'.

Reproduction Studies: Teratogenesis and reproduction studies were carried out in rats and rabbits. In rats, 'Vontrol' (diphenidol, SK&F), as the hydrochloride salt, was fed daily to male and female animals in doses of 20 mg./kg. and 40 mg./kg. (approximately three and six times the maximum recommended daily dose in adult humans) for 60 days before mating, and during mating, gestation and lactation for each of two litters. There were no significant differences between drug-treated and untreated control groups with regard to conception rate, litter size, live birth or viability in either of the two litters. There was no congenital anomaly among the offspring. In rabbits, 'Vontrol', as the hydrochloride salt, was fed in the diets in doses of 5 mg./kg. or 75 mg./kg. (approximately equal to, and 12 times as much as, the maximum recommended daily dose in adult humans) from the first day of gestation through the 26th or 27th day of gestation, when the young were delivered by Cesarean section. There were no significant differences between drug-treated and control groups with regard to number and weight of fetuses, numbers of resorption sites or viable fetuses. There was also no statistically significant difference between drug-treated and control groups with regard to the total percentage of underdeveloped fetuses. However, when data were calculated on the basis of a ratio between underdeveloped fetuses and number of pregnant does, an adverse dose-related effect was observed in the high-dose test group.

Pharmacology (human): Three double-blind controlled studies comparing 'Vontrol' (diphenidol, SK&F) to placebo were carried out: one in 32 male volunteers over a four-week period; one in 45 volunteers of whom 15 were studied for 12 weeks and 17 for 24 weeks; and one in 48 volunteers of whom 36 were studied for 12 weeks.

In the first study 'Vontrol', as the hydrochloride salt, was given orally in daily doses that were started at 75 mg. during the first week and graduated up to 200 mg. by the fourth week. In the second study, one group received 'Vontrol' orally, as the hydrochloride salt, titrated up to 500 mg. daily, then down to 200 mg. daily; another group received a maximum of 200 mg. daily. In the third study, patients received oral doses of 200 mg. to 300 mg. of 'Vontrol' daily, as the hydrochloride or pamoate salts.

The studies included these laboratory determinations: complete blood counts (including hemoglobin and hematocrit determinations), urinalyses (including microscopic examination), serum alkaline phosphatase, serum bilirubin, and bromsulphalein retention. The studies also included records of weight and blood pressure and, in one, electrocardiograms. In two of these studies, clinical laboratory changes were seen among volunteers in both treated and control groups. The changes included: extrasystoles, white cells in the urine, increase in prothrombin time, rise in hematocrit, rise in leucocytes, rise in eosinophils, and rise or reduction in neutrophils. At no time in any study did changes in the treated group differ significantly from those in the control group.

'Vontrol', as the hydrochloride salt, was given orally to 17 children (aged five to 15). Total daily doses ranged from 90 to 240 mg. Complete blood counts and, in some patients, urinalyses were done before treatment and after approximately four days of treatment. There was no significant difference between pre- and post-treatment laboratory determinations in any child. No side effects were seen.

Excretion: Following oral administration of 'Vontrol' (diphenidol, SK&F) to dogs, as the hydrochloride or pamoate salts, and to humans, as the hydrochloride salt, peak blood concentration of the drug generally occurs in one and a half to three hours. In dogs and rats, virtually all of an oral dose of C^{14}-labeled 'Vontrol' is excreted in the urine and feces within three to

Continued on next page

Smith Kline & French—Cont.

four days, as determined by radioactivity counts. Approximately the same percentage of an administered dose appeared in the urine of dogs following either oral administration of the hydrochloride salt or rectal administration of the free base.

In Pregnancy: Investigators kept follow-up records on 936 patients who had received 'Vontrol' (diphenidol, SK&F) at some time during pregnancy, primarily during the first trimester.

Of the 936 women, 864 (92%) had normal births of normal infants.

Seventy-two (8%) of the women experienced some birth abnormality. Of the 72, six patients had premature but otherwise normal infants, 40 patients aborted, 10 had stillbirths, and 16 had infants with miscellaneous defects. These included hernias, congenital heart defects, hydrocephalus, internal strabismus, anencephalus, enlarged thyroid, and hypospadia. These incidences of abnormal birth are lower than those generally reported in the literature for the average population of pregnant patients. And in no instance was there any evidence that the administration of 'Vontrol' played a part in birth abnormality.

[*Shown in Product Identification Section*]

Smith, Miller & Patch

Division of Cooper Vision P.R., Inc.
P.O. BOX 367
SAN GERMAN, PUERTO RICO 00753

OPHTHALMIC PRODUCTS

For information on SMP prescription and OTC ophthalmic products, consult the Physicians' Desk Reference For Ophthalmology. For literature, service items or sample material, contact your SMP representative. See a complete listing of products in the Manufacturers' Index section of this book.

South Laboratories, Inc.

P.O. BOX 341658
CORAL GABLES, FLORIDA 33134

BETONAL CAP ℞

Description: Each capsule contains, Vitamin A 10,000 I.U. Vitamin D 400 I.U. Vitamin B-1 10 mg., Vitamin B2 10 mg. Vitamin B-6 5 mg., Vitamin C 200 mg., Niacinamine 100 mg. D-Calcium Pantothenate 25 mg. Vitamin B12 5 mcg. Folic Acid 1 mg.

Actions: BETONAL CAP is recommended for deficiencies of Vitamin C and the B-Complex Vitamins, Folic Acid and Cyanocobalamin (Vitamin B12) which are essential for the growth and reproduction of cells and for hematopoiesis.

Contraindications: Folic Acid is contraindicated in patients with untreated and uncomplicated pernicious anemia and in those with anaphylactic sensitivity. Cyanocobalamin is contraindicated in patients with sensitivity to cobalt or Cyanocobalamin (Vitamin B12).

Adverse Reaction: Allergic sentization has been reported following administration of Folic Acid.

Dosage: One or two capsules daily.

Caution: Federal law prohibits dispensing without prescription.

How Supplied:
Betonal Cap: Bottles of 60 gelatin capsules
Betonal Plus: Bottles of 4 fluid oz.
Betonal 12: Bottles of 6 fluid oz.
Betonal Injectable: 10 ml. multiple dose vial

Squibb & Sons, Inc., E. R.

GENERAL OFFICES
P.O. BOX 4000
PRINCETON, NJ 08540

UNILOG®
(Tablet and Capsule Identification Code)
NUMERICAL INDEX

Unilog Number **Product**

111 Vitamin A Capsules USP 10,000 I.U.
113 Velosef '250' Capsules (Cephradine Capsules) 250 mg.
114 Velosef '500' Capsules (Cephradine Capsules) 500 mg.
147 Velosef Tablets (Cephradine Tablets) 1 g.
160 Ethril '250' (Erythromycin Stearate Tablets USP) 250 mg.
161 Ethril '500' (Erythromycin Stearate Tablets USP) 500 mg.
164 Pentids Tablets (Penicillin G Potassium Tablets USP) 200,000 u.
165 Pentids '400' Tablets (Penicillin G Potassium Tablets USP) 400,000 u.
168 Pentids '800' Tablets (Penicillin G Potassium Tablets USP) 800,000 u.
194 Vitamin C Tablets 100 mg.
196 Vitamin C Tablets 250 mg.
197 Vitamin C Tablets 500 mg.
201 Aspirin Tablets USP, 324 mg. (5 gr.)
204 B Complex Vitamin Tablets
230 Trimox '250' Capsules (Amoxicillin Capsules) 250 mg.
231 Trimox '500' Capsules (Amoxicillin Capsules) 500 mg.
355 Valadol Tablets (Acetaminophen Tablets USP) 325 mg. (5 gr.)
429 Florinef Acetate (Fludrocortisone Acetate Tablets USP) 0.1 mg.
431 Pronestyl Tablets (Procainamide Hydrochloride Tablets) 250 mg.
434 Pronestyl Tablets (Procainamide Hydrochloride Tablets) 375 mg.
438 Pronestyl Tablets (Procainamide Hydrochloride Tablets) 500 mg.
455 Oragrafin Sodium Capsules (Ipodate Sodium Capsules USP) 500 mg.
457 Mycostatin Vaginal Tablets (Nystatin Vaginal Tablets USP) 100,000 u.
478 Engran-HP Tablets (Multi-Vitamin and Multi-Mineral Supplement)
504 Kenacort (Triamcinolone Tablets NF) 2 mg.
512 Kenacort (Triamcinolone Tablets NF) 4 mg.
518 Kenacort (Triamcinolone Tablets NF) 8 mg.
520 B Complex with Vitamin C Tablets
535 Theragran Hematinic (Therapeutic Formula Vitamin Tablets with Hematinics)
537 Niacin Tablets NF, 500 mg.
549 Iron with Vitamin C Tablets
573 Ora-Testryl (Fluoxymesterone Tablets USP) 5 mg.
580 Mycostatin Oral Tablets (Nystatin Tablets USP) 500,000 u.
598 Neomycin Sulfate Tablets USP, 500 mg.
603 Sumycin '500' Tablets (Tetracycline Hydrochloride Tablets NF) 500 mg.
605 Naturetin-2.5 (Bendroflumethiazide Tablets NF) 2.5 mg.
606 Naturetin-5 (Bendroflumethiazide Tablets NF) 5 mg.
610 Niacin Tablets NF, 25 mg.
611 Niacin Tablets NF, 50 mg.
612 Niacin Tablets NF, 100 mg.
615 Propoxyphene Hydrochloride Capsules USP, 65 mg.
618 Naturetin-10 (Bendroflumethiazide Tablets NF) 10 mg.
619 Propoxyphene Hydrochloride and APC Capsules USP
623 Noctec Capsules (Chloral Hydrate Capsules USP) 250 mg. (3¾ grains)
626 Noctec Capsules (Chloral Hydrate Capsules USP) 500 mg. (7½ grains)
637 Nydrazid Tablets (Isoniazid Tablets USP) 100 mg.
648 Veetids '500' Tablets (Penicillin V Potassium Tablets USP) 500 mg. (800,000 u.)
649 Trigot (Sublingual Tablets) 0.5 mg.
654 Trigot (Sublingual Tablets) 1 mg.
655 Sumycin '250' Capsules (Tetracycline Hydrochloride Capsules USP) 250 mg.
663 Sumycin '250' Tablets (Tetracycline Hydrochloride Tablets NF) 250 mg.
684 Veetids '250' Tablets (Penicillin V Potassium Tablets USP) 250 mg. (400,000 u.)
689 Teslac Tablets (Testolactone Tablets NF) 250 mg.
690 Teslac Tablets (Testolactone Tablets NF) 50 mg.
693 Hydrochlorothiazide Tablets USP, 25 mg.
694 Hydrochlorothiazide Tablets USP, 50 mg.
713 Raudixin (Rauwolfia Serpentina Tablets NF) 50 mg.
718 Chlordiazepoxide Hydrochloride Capsules USP, 5 mg.
727 Chlordiazepoxide Hydrochloride Capsules USP, 10 mg.
736 Chlordiazepoxide Hydrochloride Capsules USP, 25 mg.
756 Pronestyl Capsules (Procainamide Hydrochloride Capsules USP) 375 mg.
757 Pronestyl Capsules (Procainamide Hydrochloride Capsules USP) 500 mg.
758 Pronestyl Capsules (Procainamide Hydrochloride Capsules USP) 250 mg.
763 Sumycin '500' Capsules (Tetracycline Hydrochloride Capsules USP) 500 mg.
767 Mysteclin-F '125' Capsules (Tetracycline - Amphotericin B Capsules) 125 mg. c̄ 25 mg.
769 Rauzide Tablets (50 mg. powdered Rauwolfia serpentina with 4 mg. bendroflumethiazide)
776 Raudixin (Rauwolfia Serpentina Tablets NF) 100 mg.
779 Mysteclin-F Capsules (Tetracycline - Amphotericin B Capsules) 250 mg. c̄ 50 mg.
780 Rau-Sed (Reserpine Tablets USP) 0.25 mg.
788 Vitamin B_{12} Capsules 25 mcg.

823 **Theragran Tablets**
825 **Theragran-M Tablets**
829 **Chlorothiazide Tablets USP,** 500 mg.
830 **Hydrea Capsules**
(Hydroxyurea Capsules USP) 500 mg.
863 **Prolixin Tablets**
(Fluphenazine Hydrochloride Tablets USP) 1 mg.
864 **Prolixin Tablets**
(Fluphenazine Hydrochloride Tablets USP) 2.5 mg.
876 **Trigesic Tablets**
(Analgesic Compound)
877 **Prolixin Tablets**
(Fluphenazine Hydrochloride Tablets USP) 5 mg.
887 **Terfonyl Tablets**
(Trisulfapyrimidines Tablets USP) 500 mg.
889 **Vitamin E Capsules** 100 I.U.
915 **Vitamin B_1 Tablets** 50 mg.
916 **Vitamin B_1 Tablets** 100 mg.
917 **Amitid Tablets**
(Amitriptyline Hydrochloride Tablets USP) 10 mg.
918 **Amitid Tablets**
(Amitriptyline Hydrochloride Tablets USP) 25 mg.
921 **Vesprin Tablets**
(Triflupromazine Hydrochloride Tablets NF) 10 mg.
922 **Vesprin Tablets**
(Triflupromazine Hydrochloride Tablets NF) 25 mg.
923 **Vesprin Tablets**
(Triflupromazine Hydrochloride Tablets NF) 50 mg.
942 **Amitid Tablets**
(Amitriptyline Hydrochloride Tablets USP) 50 mg.
943 **Amitid Tablets**
(Amitriptyline Hydrochloride Tablets USP) 75 mg.
955 **Amitid Tablets**
(Amitriptyline Hydrochloride Tablets USP) 100 mg.
956 **Prolixin Tablets**
(Fluphenazine Hydrochloride Tablets USP) 10 mg.
971 **Principen '250' Capsules**
(Ampicillin Capsules USP) 250 mg.
974 **Principen '500' Capsules**
(Ampicillin Capsules USP) 500 mg.

AMITID™ ℞
(Amitriptyline Hydrochloride Tablets USP)

Description: Amitriptyline hydrochloride, a dibenzocycloheptadiene derivative, is a white or practically white, crystalline compound that is freely soluble in water. Chemically, amitriptyline hydrochloride is a 10,11-dihydro-*N,N*-dimethyl-5*H*-dibenzo [*a,d*]cycloheptene-Δ^{5}, γ-propylamine hydrochloride. The molecular weight is 313.87. The empirical formula is $C_{20}H_{23}N.HCl$.
Amitid (Amitriptyline Hydrochloride Tablets USP) is available for oral administration as FILMLOK® tablets providing 10, 25, 50, 75, and 100 mg. amitriptyline hydrochloride. (Filmlok is a Squibb trademark for veneer-coated tablets.)

Clinical Pharmacology: Amitriptyline is an antidepressant agent with an anxiety-reducing, sedative component to its action. Its mechanism of action in man is not known. It is not a monoamine oxidase inhibitor and it does not act primarily by stimulation of the central nervous system.
Amitriptyline inhibits the membrane pump mechanism responsible for reuptake of norepinephrine into adrenergic neurons. Pharmacologically this action may potentiate or prolong sympathetic activity, since reuptake of norepinephrine is important physiologically in terminating its transmitting actions. This interference with reuptake of norepinephrine is believed by some to underlie the antidepressant activity of amitriptyline.

Indications and Usage: For the relief of symptoms of depression. Endogenous depression is more likely to be alleviated than are other depressive states.

Contraindications: Amitriptyline is contraindicated in patients who have shown prior hypersensitivity to it. It should not be given concomitantly with a monoamine oxidase inhibiting compound. Hyperpyretic crises, severe convulsions, and deaths have occurred in patients receiving tricyclic antidepressant and monoamine oxidase inhibiting drugs simultaneously. When it is desired to replace a monoamine oxidase inhibitor with amitriptyline, a minimum of 14 days should be allowed to elapse after the former is discontinued. Amitriptyline hydrochloride should then be initiated cautiously with gradual increase in dosage until optimum response is achieved.
This drug is not recommended for use during the acute recovery phase following myocardial infarction.

Warnings: Amitriptyline may block the antihypertensive action of guanethidine or similarly-acting compounds.
It should be used with caution in patients with a history of seizures and, because of its atropine-like action, in patients with a history of urinary retention, narrow-angle glaucoma or increased intraocular pressure. In patients with narrow-angle glaucoma, even average doses may precipitate an attack.
Patients with cardiovascular disorders should be watched closely. Tricyclic antidepressant drugs, including amitriptyline, particularly when given in high doses, have been reported to produce arrhythmias, sinus tachycardia, and prolongation of the conduction time. Myocardial infarction and stroke have been reported with drugs of this class.
Close supervision is required when amitriptyline is given to hyperthyroid patients or those receiving thyroid medication.
This drug may impair mental and/or physical abilities required for performance of hazardous tasks, such as operating machinery or driving a motor vehicle.
In patients who may use alcohol excessively, it should be borne in mind that the potentiation may increase the danger inherent in any suicide attempt or overdosage.

Usage in Pregnancy: Safe use of amitriptyline during pregnancy and lactation has not been established; therefore, in administering the drug to pregnant patients, nursing mothers, or women who may become pregnant, the possible benefits must be weighed against the possible hazards to mother and child.
Animal reproduction studies have been inconclusive and clinical experience has been limited.

Usage in Children: In view of the lack of experience with the use of this drug in children, it is not recommended at the present time for patients under 12 years of age.

Precautions: Schizophrenic patients may develop increased symptoms of psychosis; patients with paranoid symptomatology may have an exaggeration of such symptoms; manic depressive patients may experience a shift to the manic phase. In these circumstances the dose of amitriptyline may be reduced or a major tranquilizer may be administered concurrently.
When this drug is given with anticholinergic agents or sympathomimetic drugs, including epinephrine combined with local anesthetics, close supervision and careful adjustment of dosages are required. Paralytic ileus may occur in patients taking tricyclic antidepressants in combination with anticholinergic-type drugs.
Caution is advised if patients receive large doses of ethchlorvynol concurrently. Transient delirium has been reported in patients who were treated with one gram of ethchlorvynol and 75 to 150 mg. of amitriptyline hydrochloride.
Amitriptyline may enhance the response to alcohol and the effects of barbiturates and other CNS depressants.
The possibility of suicide in depressed patients remains during treatment and until significant remission occurs. Potentially suicidal patients should not have easy access to large quantities of the drug. Prescriptions should be written for the smallest amount feasible.
Concurrent administration of amitriptyline and electroshock therapy may increase the hazards associated with such therapy. Such treatment should be limited to patients for whom it is essential.
When possible, the drug should be discontinued several days before elective surgery.
Both elevation and lowering of blood sugar levels have been reported.
Amitriptyline should be used with caution in patients with impaired liver function.

Adverse Reactions: NOTE—Included in the listing which follows are a few adverse reactions which have not been reported with this specific drug. However, pharmacological similarities among the tricyclic antidepressant drugs require that each of the reactions be considered when amitriptyline is administered.
Cardiovascular: Hypotension, hypertension, tachycardia, palpitation, myocardial infarction, arrhythmias, heart block, and stroke.
CNS and Neuromuscular: Confusional states; disturbed concentration; disorientation; delusions; hallucinations; excitement; anxiety; restlessness; insomnia; nightmares; numbness, tingling, and paresthesias of the extremities; peripheral neuropathy; incoordination; ataxia; tremors; seizures; alteration in EEG patterns; extrapyramidal symptoms; tinnitus; and syndrome of inappropriate ADH (antidiuretic hormone) secretion.
Anticholinergic: Dry mouth, blurred vision, disturbance of accommodation, increased intraocular pressure, constipation, paralytic ileus, urinary retention, and dilatation of the urinary tract.
Allergic: Skin rash, urticaria, photosensitization, and edema of face and tongue.
Hematologic: Bone marrow depression including agranulocytosis, leukopenia, eosinophilia, purpura, and thrombocytopenia.
Gastrointestinal: Nausea, epigastric distress, vomiting, anorexia, stomatitis, peculiar taste, diarrhea, parotid swelling, and black tongue. Rarely hepatitis (including altered liver function and jaundice).
Endocrine: Testicular swelling and gynecomastia in the male, breast enlargement and galactorrhea in the female, increased or decreased libido, and elevation and lowering of blood sugar levels.
Other: Dizziness, weakness, fatigue, headache, weight gain or loss, increased perspiration, urinary frequency, mydriasis, drowsiness, and alopecia.
Withdrawal Symptoms: Abrupt cessation of treatment after prolonged administration may produce nausea, headache, and malaise. These are not indicative of addiction.

Dosage and Administration: Dosage should be initiated at a low level and increased gradually, noting carefully the clinical response and any evidence of intolerance.

Initial Oral Dosage for Adults: Twenty-five mg. three times a day is usually satisfactory for outpatients. If necessary this may be increased to a total of 150 mg. a day. Increases are made preferably in the late afternoon and/or bedtime doses. The sedative effect may be apparent before the antidepressant effect is noted, but an adequate therapeutic effect may take as long as 30 days to develop.
An alternate method of initiating therapy in outpatients is to begin with 50 to 100 mg. ami-

Squibb—Cont.

triptyline hydrochloride at bedtime. This may be increased by 25 to 50 mg. as necessary in the bedtime dose to a total of 150 mg. per day. Hospitalized patients may require 100 mg. a day initially. This can be increased gradually to 200 mg. a day if necessary. A small number of hospitalized patients may need as much as 300 mg. a day.

Adolescent and Elderly Patients: In general, lower dosages are recommended for these patients. Ten mg. three times a day with 20 mg. at bedtime may be satisfactory in adolescent and elderly patients who do not tolerate higher dosages.

Maintenance: The usual maintenance dosage is 25 mg. two to four times a day. In some patients 10 mg. four times a day is sufficient. For maintenance therapy, the total daily dosage may be given in a single dose preferably at bedtime. When satisfactory improvement has been reached, dosage should be reduced to the lowest amount that will maintain relief of symptoms. It is appropriate to continue maintenance therapy three months or longer to lessen the possibility of relapse.

Usage in Children: In view of the lack of experience with the use of this drug in children, it is not recommended at the present time for patients under 12 years of age.

Overdosage: Manifestations—High doses may cause temporary confusion, disturbed concentration, or transient visual hallucinations. Overdosage may cause drowsiness; hypothermia; tachycardia and other arrhythmic abnormalities, such as bundle branch block; ECG evidence of impaired conduction; congestive heart failure; dilated pupils; convulsions; severe hypotension; stupor; and coma. Other symptoms may be agitation, hyperactive reflexes, muscle rigidity, vomiting, hyperpyrexia, or any of those listed under ADVERSE REACTIONS.

All patients suspected of having taken an overdosage should be admitted to a hospital as soon as possible.

Treatment—Treatment is symptomatic and supportive. Empty the stomach as quickly as possible by emesis followed by gastric lavage upon arrival at the hospital. Following gastric lavage, activated charcoal may be administered. Twenty to 30 g. of activated charcoal may be given every four to six hours during the first 24 to 48 hours after ingestion. An ECG should be taken and close monitoring of cardiac function instituted if there is any sign of abnormality. Maintain an open airway and adequate fluid intake; regulate body temperature.

The intravenous administration of 1 to 3 mg. of physostigmine salicylate has been reported to reverse the symptoms of tricyclic antidepressant poisoning. Because physostigmine is rapidly metabolized, the dosage of physostigmine should be repeated as required particularly if life threatening signs such as arrhythmias, convulsions, and deep coma recur or persist after the initial dosage of physostigmine.

Standard measures should be used to manage circulatory shock and metabolic acidosis. Cardiac arrhythmias may be treated with neostigmine, pyridostigmine, or propranolol. Should cardiac failure occur, the use of digitalis should be considered. Close monitoring of cardiac function for not less than five days is advisable. Anticonvulsants may be given to control convulsions. Amitriptyline increases the CNS depressant action, but not the anticonvulsant action of barbiturates; therefore, an inhalation anesthetic, diazepam, or paraldehyde is recommended for control of convulsions.

Dialysis is of no value because of low plasma concentrations of the drug.

Since overdosage is often deliberate, patients may attempt suicide by other means during the recovery phase.

Deaths by deliberate or accidental overdosage have occurred with this class of drugs.

How Supplied: Amitid (Amitriptyline Hydrochloride Tablets USP) is available for oral administration as FILMLOK tablets providing 10, 25, 50, 75, and 100 mg. amitriptyline hydrochloride. The 10 mg., 25 mg., and 50 mg. tablets are available in bottles of 100 and 1000; the 75 mg. and 100 mg. tablets are available in bottles of 100.

Storage: Store at room temperature; protect from light; avoid excessive heat.

CARDIOGRAFIN® ℞
(Diatrizoate Meglumine Injection USP 85%)

(See Diagnostic Section)

CHOLOGRAFIN® MEGLUMINE ℞
(Iodipamide Meglumine Injection USP 52%)

(See Diagnostic Section)

CRYSTICILLIN® 300 A.S. ℞
CRYSTICILLIN® 600 A.S. ℞
(Sterile Penicillin G Procaine Suspension USP)

Description: Crysticillin 300 A.S. and Crysticillin 600 A.S. are aqueous suspensions providing 300,000 u. per ml. and 600,000 u. per 1.2 ml. (500,000 u./ml.) penicillin G procaine, respectively. The vials providing 300,000 u. per ml. also contain 0.13% methylparaben, 0.02% propylparaben, and 0.25% phenol as preservatives; 0.5% lecithin; 0.5% povidone; 1% sodium citrate; not more than 0.01% sodium formaldehyde sulfoxylate; and 0.075% sodium carboxymethylcellulose. The vials providing 600,000 u. per 1.2 ml. also contain 0.13% methylparaben, 0.02% propylparaben, and 0.18% phenol as preservatives; 0.3% povidone; 1% sodium citrate; 0.05% sodium carboxymethylcellulose; not more than 0.03% sodium formaldehyde sulfoxylate; and 2.3% lecithin.

Clinical Pharmacology: Penicillin G is bactericidal against penicillin-sensitive microorganisms during the stage of active multiplication. It acts by inhibiting biosynthesis of cell-wall mucopeptide. It is not active against the penicillinase-producing bacteria, which include many strains of staphylococci. Penicillin G is highly active *in vitro* against staphylococci (except penicillinase-producing strains), streptococci (groups A, C, G, H, L, and M), and pneumococci. Other organisms sensitive *in vitro* to penicillin G are *N. gonorrhoeae, Corynebacterium diphtheriae, Bacillus anthracis,* Clostridia, *Actinomyces bovis, Streptobacillus moniliformis, Listeria monocytogenes,* and Leptospira; *Treponema pallidum* is extremely sensitive.

Sensitivity plate testing: If the Kirby-Bauer method of disc sensitivity is used, a 10 u. penicillin disc should give a zone greater than 28 mm. when tested against a penicillin-sensitive bacterial strain.

Penicillin G procaine is an equimolar compound of procaine and penicillin G administered intramuscularly as a suspension. It dissolves slowly at the site of injection, giving a plateau type of blood level at about four hours which falls slowly during the next 15 to 20 hours.

Approximately 60 percent of penicillin G is bound to serum protein. The drug is distributed throughout the body tissues in widely varying amounts. Highest levels are found in the kidneys with lesser amounts in the liver, skin, and intestines. Penicillin G penetrates into all other tissues to a lesser degree with a very small level found in the cerebrospinal fluid. The drug is excreted rapidly by tubular excretion in patients with normal kidney function. In neonates and young infants, and in individuals with impaired kidney function, excretion is considerably delayed. Approximately 60 to 90 percent of a dose of parenteral penicillin G is excreted in the urine within 24 to 36 hours.

Indications and Usage: Crysticillin 300 A.S. and Crysticillin 600 A.S. (Sterile Penicillin G Procaine Suspension USP) are indicated in the treatment of moderately severe infections due to penicillin G-sensitive microorganisms. Therapy should be guided by bacteriological studies, including sensitivity tests, and by clinical response. Note: severe pneumonia, empyema, bacteremia, pericarditis, meningitis, peritonitis, and septic arthritis are better treated with aqueous penicillin G during the acute stage; when high, sustained serum levels are required, aqueous penicillin G, either I.M. or I.V. should be used.

The following infections will usually respond to adequate dosage:

Streptococcal infections Group A without bacteremia—Moderately severe to severe infections of the upper respiratory tract, skin and soft tissue infections, scarlet fever, and erysipelas. Note: streptococci in groups A, C, H, G, L, and M are very sensitive to penicillin G. Other groups, including group D (enterococcus) are resistant. Aqueous penicillin is recommended for streptococcal infections with bacteremia.

Pneumococcal infections—Moderately severe infections of the respiratory tract.

Staphylococcal infections — penicillin G-sensitive — Moderately severe infections of the skin and soft tissues. Note: reports indicate an increasing number of strains of staphylococci resistant to penicillin G, emphasizing the need for culture and sensitivity studies in treating suspected staphylococcal infections. Indicated surgical procedures should be performed.

Vincent's gingivitis and pharyngitis (fusospirochetosis)—Moderately severe infections of the oropharynx. Note: necessary dental care should be accomplished in infections involving the gum tissue.

Syphilis (*T. pallidum*)—All stages; **Gonorrheal infections** (acute and chronic—without bacteremia)—With adequate recommended doses; **Treponema**—Yaws, Bejel, Pinta; **Diphtheria**—as an adjunct to antitoxin for the prevention of the carrier state; **Anthrax; Rat-bite fever** (*S. moniliformis* and *S. minus*); **Erysipeloid.**

Subacute bacterial endocarditis (group A streptococcus)—Only in extremely sensitive infections. **Prophylaxis against bacterial endocarditis**—May be given to patients with congenital and/or rheumatic heart lesions who are to undergo dental or upper respiratory tract surgery or instrumentation. Prophylaxis should be instituted the day of the procedure and continued for two or more days afterwards. Note: since patients who have a past history of rheumatic fever and are receiving continuous prophylaxis may harbor increased numbers of penicillin-resistant organisms, use of another prophylactic antiinfective agent should be considered. If penicillin is to be used in these patients at surgery, the regular rheumatic fever program should be interrupted one week prior to the contemplated surgery. At the time of surgery, penicillin may be reinstituted as a prophylactic measure against the hazards of surgically-induced bacteremia.

Contraindications: Contraindicated in patients with a history of hypersensitivity to procaine or any penicillin.

Warnings: Serious and occasional fatal hypersensitivity (anaphylactoid) reactions have been reported in patients on penicillin therapy. Although anaphylaxis is more frequent following parenteral administration, it has occurred in patients on oral penicillins. These reactions are more apt to occur in individuals with a history of sensitivity to multiple allergens.

There have been well-documented reports of individuals with a history of penicillin hypersensitivity who have experienced severe hy-

persensitivity reactions when treated with cephalosporins. Before therapy with a penicillin, careful inquiry should be made concerning previous hypersensitivity reactions to penicillins, cephalosporins, and other allergens. If an allergic reaction occurs, the drug should be discontinued and the patient treated with the usual agents, e.g., pressor amines, antihistamines, and corticosteroids. Serious anaphylactoid reactions are not controlled by antihistamines alone, and require such emergency measures as the immediate use of epinephrine, aminophylline, oxygen, and intravenous corticosteroids.

Immediate toxic reactions to procaine may occur in some individuals, particularly when a large single dose is administered in the treatment of gonorrhea (4.8 million u.). These reactions may be manifested by mental disturbances including anxiety, confusion, agitation, depression, weakness, seizures, hallucinations, combativeness, and expressed "fear of impending death." The reactions noted in carefully controlled studies occurred in approximately one in 500 patients treated for gonorrhea. Reactions are transient, lasting from 15 to 30 minutes.

Precautions: Penicillin should be used with caution in individuals with histories of significant allergies and/or asthma.

A small percentage of patients are sensitive to procaine. If there is a history of sensitivity, make the usual test: inject intradermally 0.1 ml. of a 1 to 2% procaine hydrochloride solution. Development of an erythema, wheal, flare or eruption indicates procaine sensitivity. Sensitivity should be treated by the usual methods, and procaine penicillin preparations should not be used. Antihistamines appear beneficial in the treatment of procaine reactions.

The use of antibiotics may result in overgrowth of nonsusceptible organisms. Constant observation of the patient is essential. If new infections due to bacteria or fungi appear during therapy, the drug should be discontinued and appropriate measures taken. Whenever allergic reactions occur, penicillin should be withdrawn unless, in the opinion of the physician, the condition being treated is life-threatening and amenable only to penicillin therapy.

Care should be taken to avoid accidental intravenous administration.

In prolonged therapy with penicillin, and particularly with high dosage schedules, periodic evaluation of the renal and hematopoietic systems is recommended.

In streptococcal infections, therapy must be sufficient to eliminate the organism (10 days minimum); otherwise the sequelae of streptococcal disease may occur. Cultures should be taken following the completion of treatment to determine whether streptococci have been eradicated.

In suspected staphylococcal infections, proper laboratory studies, including sensitivity tests, should be performed.

When treating gonococcal infections in which primary or secondary syphilis may be suspected, proper diagnostic procedures, including darkfield examinations, should be done. In all cases in which concomitant syphilis is suspected, monthly serological tests should be made for at least four months. All cases of penicillin-treated syphilis should receive clinical and serological examinations every six months for at least two or three years.

Adverse Reactions: Penicillin is a substance of low toxicity, but does possess a significant index of sensitization. The hypersensitivity reactions reported are skin rashes ranging from maculopapular eruptions to exfoliative dermatitis; urticaria; and serum sickness-like reactions including chills, fever, edema, arthralgia, and prostration. Hemolytic anemia, leukopenia, thrombocytopenia, neuropathy, and nephropathy are infrequent reactions and are usually associated with high doses of parenteral penicillin. Severe and often fatal anaphylaxis has been reported; these reactions require emergency measures (see WARNINGS). As with other treatments for syphilis, the Jarisch-Herxheimer reaction has been reported.

Procaine toxicity manifestations have been reported (see WARNINGS). Procaine hypersensitivity reactions have not been reported with this drug.

Dosage and Administration:

For intramuscular use only

The product is ready for immediate injection after vigorous shaking of the vial to insure a uniform suspension.

Injection is made rapidly by the intramuscular route. The preferred site is the upper outer quadrant of the gluteal area. Injections are easier to make and there is less likelihood of needle blockage if a small bore syringe is used; use a 20-gauge needle. Avoid using a syringe with a loosely-fitting plunger as crystals may creep between the walls and cause it to "freeze". Remove the needle and plunger from the syringe soon after injection to prevent "freezing" of the remaining crystals.

The usual dosage recommendation is as follows:

Streptococcal infections (Group A)—moderately severe to severe tonsillitis, erysipelas, scarlet fever, infections of the upper respiratory tract, and skin and soft tissue infections: 600,000 to 1,200,000 u. daily for a minimum of 10 days.

Pneumococcal infections (uncomplicated)—moderately severe: 600,000 to 1,200,000 u. daily.

Staphylococcal infections—moderately severe to severe: 600,000 to 1,200,000 u. daily.

Vincent's gingivitis and pharyngitis (fusospirochetosis): 600,000 to 1,200,000 u. daily.

Syphilis—*Primary, secondary and latent* with a negative spinal fluid in adults and children over 12 years of age: 600,000 u. daily for eight days—total 4,800,000 u.; *Late* (tertiary, neurosyphilis and latent syphilis with positive or no spinal fluid examination): 600,000 u. daily for 10 to 15 days—total 6 to 9 million u.; *Congenital* (under 32 kg. [70 lb.] body weight): 10,000 u./kg./day for 10 days.

Gonorrheal infections (uncomplicated): 4.8 million u. divided into at least two doses at one visit for males and females; one gram of oral probenecid is given 30 minutes before the injections. Follow-up cultures should be obtained from the original site(s) of infection 7 to 14 days after therapy. In women, it is also desirable to obtain culture test-of-cure from both the endocervical and anal canals. Note: gonorrheal endocarditis should be treated intensively with aqueous penicillin G.

Yaws, Bejel, and Pinta—treat same as syphilis in corresponding stage of disease.

Diphtheria—*adjunctive therapy with antitoxin:* 300,000 to 600,000 u. daily; **Anthrax**—cutaneous: 600,000 to 1,200,000 u. daily; **Rat-bite fever** (*S. moniliformis* and *S. minus*) and **Erysipeloid:** 600,000 to 1,200,000 u. daily.

Bacterial endocarditis (group A streptococcus)—only in extremely sensitive infections: 600,000 to 1,200,000 u. daily.

Prophylaxis against bacterial endocarditis—to prevent bacterial endocarditis in patients with rheumatic or congenital heart lesions who are to undergo dental or upper respiratory tract surgery or instrumentation: 1,000,000 u. of aqueous penicillin G combined with 600,000 u. of penicillin G procaine (aqueous) given I.M. one-half to one hour prior to the procedure, then 500 mg. of penicillin V (oral) every six hours for eight doses.

How Supplied: Crysticillin 300 A.S. (Sterile Penicillin G Procaine Suspension USP) is available in 10 ml. vials; Crysticillin 600 A.S. is available in 12 ml. vials.

Storage: Store below 15° C. (59° F.); avoid freezing.

CYSTOGRAFIN® ℞
(Diatrizoate Meglumine Injection USP 30%)

(See Diagnostic Section)

DELATESTRYL® ℞
(Testosterone Enanthate Injection USP)

Description: Delatestryl is a sterile solution of testosterone enanthate for intramuscular use.

Clinical Pharmacology: Delatestryl is intended for androgen therapy, particularly when prolonged action is desirable. Following a single intramuscular injection, the androgenic effect is sustained over a period of about four weeks. This continuous flow of hormone is thought to resemble closely the endogenous production of testosterone.

Testosterone enanthate is primarily used for its protein anabolic effect and its catabolic inhibiting effect on tissue. Nitrogen balance is improved with anabolic agents but only when there is sufficient intake of calories and protein. Whether this positive nitrogen balance is of primary benefit in the utilization of protein-building dietary substances has not been established.

Enhancement of protein anabolism is manifest by conservation of sodium, nitrogen, phosphorus, potassium, sulfur, and water in the proportions of physiologic protein tissues, and of calcium with additional phosphorus in the proportions of physiologic osseous tissues.

Certain clinical effects and adverse reactions demonstrate the androgenic properties of this class of drugs. Complete dissociation of anabolic and androgenic effects has not been achieved. The actions of anabolic steroids are therefore similar to those of male sex hormones with the possibility of causing serious disturbances of growth and sexual development if given to young children. They suppress the gonadotropic functions of the pituitary and may exert a direct effect upon the testes.

Indications and Usage: In males, Delatestryl (Testosterone Enanthate Injection USP) is indicated in the treatment of eunuchism, eunuchoidism, deficiency after castration, male climacteric-like symptoms when these are secondary to androgen deficiency, and oligospermia.

Contraindications: Androgens are contraindicated in male patients with prostatic or breast cancer, in those elderly patients in whom overstimulation is to be avoided, and in those cases of benign prostatic hypertrophy with obstructive symptoms. Androgens are also contraindicated in patients with nephrosis or the nephrotic phase of nephritis.

Precautions: If symptomatic hypercalcemia occurs, discontinue androgen therapy and institute appropriate measures.

Caution is required in administering androgens to patients with cardiac, renal, or hepatic disease. Edema may occur occasionally. Concomitant administration with adrenal steroids or ACTH may add to the edema.

Anabolic steroids may increase sensitivity to anticoagulants. Dosage of the anticoagulant may have to be decreased in order to maintain the prothrombin time at the desired therapeutic level.

Anabolic steroids have been shown to alter glucose tolerance tests. Diabetics should be followed carefully and the insulin or oral hypoglycemic dosage adjusted accordingly.

Serum cholesterol may increase or decrease during therapy. Because of its hypercholesterolemic effects, caution is required when administering this drug to patients with a history of myocardial infarction or coronary artery disease. Serial determinations of serum cholesterol should be made and therapy adjusted accordingly. A cause and effect relationship between myocardial infarction and hypercholesterolemia has not been established.

Squibb—Cont.

Inhibition of testicular function and decrease in ejaculatory volume may occur when the drug is administered in doses greater than those used for replacement therapy in hypogonadal males.

Adverse Reactions: In males, the following postpubertal adverse reactions have occurred: inhibition of testicular function, testicular atrophy and oligospermia, impotence, chronic priapism, gynecomastia, epididymitis, and bladder irritability. In addition, the following reactions are known to occur with anabolic steroids: increased or decreased libido, flushing of the skin, acne, habituation, excitation and sleeplessness, chills, leukopenia, and bleeding in patients on concomitant anticoagulant therapy. There have been rare reports of hepatocellular neoplasms and peliosis hepatis in association with long-term androgenic-anabolic steroid therapy.

Intramuscular preparations of anabolic steroids have been associated with urticaria at the injection site, postinjection induration, and furunculosis.

Alterations may occur in the following clinical laboratory tests: metyrapone test, fasting blood sugar (FBS), and glucose tolerance test; thyroid function tests [decrease in protein-bound iodine (PBI), thyroxine-binding capacity, and radioactive iodine uptake, and an increase in T_3 uptake by the red blood cells or resin; free thyroxine levels remain normal and the altered tests usually persist for two to three weeks after stopping anabolic therapy]; electrolytes (retention of sodium, chloride, water, potassium, calcium, and inorganic phosphates); blood coagulation tests (increase in clotting factors II, V, VII, and X); and miscellaneous laboratory tests (decreased creatinine and creatine excretion lasting up to two weeks after discontinuing therapy and increased 17-ketosteroid excretion).

Dosage and Administration: When properly given, injections of Delatestryl are well tolerated. Care should be taken to inject the preparation deeply into the gluteal muscle following the usual precautions for intramuscular administration. In general, total doses above 400 mg. per month are not required because of the prolonged action of the preparation. Injections more frequently than every two weeks are rarely indicated. NOTE: Use of a wet needle or wet syringe may cause the solution to become cloudy; however, this does not affect the potency of the material.

In male hypogonadism (i.e., eunuchism, eunuchoidism, severe deficiency after castration, male climacteric-like symptoms when secondary to androgen deficiency), the suggested dosage is 200 to 400 mg. every four weeks. Androgen therapy is regarded as replacement therapy, being effective only as long as continued.

In the treatment of oligospermia, the suggested dosage is 100 to 200 mg. every four to six weeks for the development and maintenance of testicular tubular function; for suppression and rebound stimulation, the recommended dosage is 200 mg. every week for 6 to 12 weeks.

How Supplied: Delatestryl (Testosterone Enanthate Injection USP) is available in multiple dose vials of 5 ml. and Unimatic® single-dose preassembled syringes of 1 ml. Each ml. of sterile solution provides 200 mg. testosterone enanthate in sesame oil with 0.5% chlorobutanol (chloral derivative) as a preservative. (The Unimatic single dose preassembled syringe has a 20-gauge needle and is 1½" long.)

Storage: Vials should be stored at room temperature. Warming and shaking the vial will redissolve any crystals that may have formed during storage at low temperatures. Unimatic single-dose preassembled syringes should be stored at room temperature.

ENGRAN®-HP
(Multi-Vitamin and Multi-Mineral Supplement)

Engran-HP is a multi-vitamin and multi-mineral supplement for pregnant or lactating women.

Usage: Two tablets daily.

Two tablets provide		Percent U.S. RDA*
Vitamins		
Vitamin A (2.4 mg.)	8000 I.U.	100
Vitamin D (10 mcg.)	400 I.U.	100
Vitamin E (30 mg.)	30 I.U.	100
Vitamin C	60 mg.	100
Folic Acid	0.8 mg.	100
Thiamine (Vitamin B_1)	1.7 mg.	100
Riboflavin (Vitamin B_2)	2 mg.	100
Niacin	20 mg.	100
Vitamin B_6	2.5 mg.	100
Vitamin B_{12}	8 mcg.	100
Minerals		
Calcium	650 mg.	50
Iodine	150 mcg.	100
Iron	18 mg.	100
Magnesium	100 mg.	22

*U.S. Recommended Daily Allowances

How Supplied: In bottles of 100 tablets.

Storage: Store at room temperature; avoid excessive heat.

EPI*CLEAR®
(Squibb Acne Products)

Description: EPI*CLEAR Squibb Acne Products comprise a comprehensive line of acne hygiene products.

Indications: Intended as an aid in the treatment of acne vulgaris.

How Supplied: EPI*CLEAR Squibb Acne Kit —Each kit contains 1 bar (4 oz.) of EPI*CLEAR Squibb Acne Soap for Oily Skin containing 6.3% sulfated surfactants and hydrocarbon hydrotropes, 1 bottle (1 fl. oz.) of EPI*CLEAR Squibb Acne Lotion containing 10% sulfur and 10% alcohol, and 1 tube (2.7 oz.) of EPI*CLEAR Squibb Scrub Cleanser for Acne (fine) containing 38% aluminum oxide particles in a surfactant cleansing base.

Also available as individual items are the following:

EPI*CLEAR Squibb Scrub Cleanser for Acne containing aluminum oxide particles in a surfactant cleansing base—38% (fine) 5.5 oz. jars, 52% (medium) 6 oz. jars, and 65% (coarse) 6.5 oz. jars.

EPI*CLEAR Squibb Acne Lotion containing 10% sulfur and 10% alcohol—1 fl. oz. bottle.

EPI*CLEAR Squibb Acne Soap for Oily Skin containing 6.3% sulfated surfactants and hydrocarbon hydrotropes—4 oz. bars.

EPI*CLEAR Squibb Antiseptic Lotion for Acne containing 5% or 10% benzoyl peroxide in a greaseless water-washable base—1 fl. oz. bottles.

ETHRIL® '250' ℞
ETHRIL® '500' ℞
(Erythromycin Stearate Tablets USP)

Description: Erythromycin is produced by a strain of *Streptomyces erythreus* and belongs to the macrolide group of antibiotics. It is basic and readily forms salts with acids. The base, the stearate salt, and the esters are poorly soluble in water and are suitable for oral administration.

Ethril '250' and Ethril '500' (Erythromycin Stearate Tablets USP) are available for oral administration as FILMLOK® tablets providing erythromycin stearate equivalent to 250 mg. and 500 mg. erythromycin respectively. Ethril '500' tablets contain FD&C Yellow No. 5 (tartrazine). (FILMLOK is a Squibb trademark for veneer-coated tablets.)

Actions: Erythromycin is a protein-synthesis inhibitor—without, itself, affecting nucleic acid synthesis. Resistance to erythromycin by some strains of *Hemophilus influenzae* and staphylococci has been demonstrated. Culture and susceptibility testing should be done. If the Kirby-Bauer method of disc susceptibility is used, a 15 mcg. erythromycin disc should give a zone diameter of at least 18 mm. when tested against an erythromycin-susceptible organism.

Orally administered erythromycin is readily absorbed by most patients, especially on an empty stomach, but patient variation has been observed.

After absorption, erythromycin diffuses readily into most body fluids. In the absence of meningeal inflammation, low concentrations are normally achieved in the spinal fluid, but passage of the drug across the blood-brain barrier increases in meningitis. In the presence of normal hepatic function, erythromycin is concentrated in the liver and excreted in the bile; the effect of hepatic dysfunction on excretion of erythromycin by the liver into the bile is not known. After oral administration, less than 5 percent of the activity of the administered dose can be recovered in the urine.

Erythromycin crosses the placental barrier, but fetal plasma levels are low.

Indications: *Streptococcus pyogenes* (Group A beta-hemolytic streptococci)—Upper and lower respiratory tract, skin, and skin structures infections of mild to moderate severity. Sterile Penicillin G Benzathine Suspension USP is considered by the American Heart Association to be the drug of choice in the treatment and prevention of streptococcal pharyngitis and in long-term prophylaxis of rheumatic fever. When oral medication is preferred for the treatment of streptococcal pharyngitis, penicillin G, V, or erythromycin are alternate drugs of choice. When oral medication is given, the importance of strict adherence to the prescribed dosage regimen by the patient must be stressed. A therapeutic dose should be administered for at least 10 days.

Alpha-hemolytic streptococci (viridans group)—Short-term prophylaxis against bacterial endocarditis prior to dental or other operative procedures in patients with a history of rheumatic fever or congenital heart disease who are hypersensitive to penicillin. (Erythromycin is not suitable prior to genitourinary surgery where the organisms likely to lead to bacteremia are gram-negative bacilli or the enterococcus group of streptococci.)

Staphylococcus aureus—Acute infections of skin and skin structures of mild to moderate severity. Resistance may develop during treatment.

Streptococcus pneumoniae (formerly *Diplococcus pneumoniae*)—Upper respiratory tract infections (e.g., otitis media, pharyngitis) and lower respiratory tract infections (e.g., pneumonia) of mild to moderate degree.

Mycoplasma pneumoniae (Eaton agent, PPLO) —In the treatment of primary atypical pneumonia, when due to this organism.

Hemophilus influenzae: Upper respiratory tract infections of mild to moderate severity when used concomitantly with adequate doses of sulfonamides. Not all strains of this organism are susceptible at the erythromycin concentrations ordinarily achieved (see appropriate sulfonamide labeling for prescribing information).

Treponema pallidum—Erythromycin is an alternate choice of treatment for primary syphilis in patients allergic to the penicillins. Patients who are suspected of having syphilis should have a microscopic examination for *T. pallidum* (by immunofluorescence or darkfield) before receiving erythromycin and monthly tests for a minimum of four months. In the treatment of primary syphilis, spinal fluid examinations should be done before treatment and as part of follow-up after therapy.

Corynebacterium diphtheriae and *C. minutissimum*—As an adjunct to antitoxin, to prevent establishment of carriers and to eradicate

the organism in carriers. In the treatment of erythrasma.
Entamoeba histolytica—In the treatment of intestinal amebiasis only. Extraenteric amebiasis requires treatment with other agents.
Listeria monocytogenes—Infections due to this organism.
Neisseria gonorrhoeae—Erythromycin lactobionate for injection in conjunction with erythromycin stearate orally, as an alternative drug in the treatment of acute pelvic inflammatory disease caused by *N. gonorrhoeae* in female patients with a history of sensitivity to penicillin. Before treatment of gonorrhea, patients who are suspected of having syphilis should have a microscopic examination for *T. pallidum* (by immunofluorescence or darkfield) before receiving erythromycin and monthly tests for a minimum of four months.
Legionnaires' disease—Although no controlled clinical efficacy studies have been conducted, *in vitro* and limited preliminary clinical data suggest that erythromycin may be effective in treating Legionnaires' disease.
Contraindications: Erythromycin is contraindicated in patients with known hypersensitivity to this antibiotic.
Warning: Usage in Pregnancy—Safety for use in pregnancy has not been established.
Precautions: Erythromycin is excreted principally by the liver. Caution should be exercised in administering the antibiotic to patients with impaired hepatic function. There have been reports of hepatic dysfunction, with or without jaundice, occurring in patients receiving oral erythromycin products.
Recent data from studies of erythromycin reveal that its use in patients who are receiving high doses of theophylline may be associated with an increase of serum theophylline levels and potential theophylline toxicity. In case of theophylline toxicity and/or elevated serum theophylline levels, the dose of theophylline should be reduced while the patient is receiving concomitant erythromycin therapy.
Surgical procedures should be performed when indicated.
Ethril '500' (Erythromycin Stearate Tablets USP) contains FD&C Yellow No. 5 (tartrazine) which may cause allergic-type reactions (including bronchial asthma) in certain susceptible individuals. Although the overall incidence of FD&C Yellow No. 5 (tartrazine) sensitivity in the general population is low, it is frequently seen in patients who also have aspirin hypersensitivity.
Adverse Reactions: The most frequent side effects of erythromycin preparations are gastrointestinal, such as abdominal cramping and discomfort; these are dose-related. Nausea, vomiting, and diarrhea occur infrequently with usual oral doses.
During prolonged or repeated therapy, there is a possibility of overgrowth of nonsusceptible bacteria or fungi. If such infections occur, the drug should be discontinued and appropriate therapy instituted.
Mild allergic reactions such as urticaria and other skin rashes have occurred. Serious allergic reactions, including anaphylaxis, have been reported.
Dosage and Administration: Optimum blood levels are obtained when doses are given on an empty stomach.
Adults: The usual dose is 250 mg. every six hours. Dosage may be increased up to 4 or more grams per day according to the severity of the infection.
Children: Age, weight, and severity of the infection are important factors in determining the proper dosage. The usual dosage, in divided doses, is 30 to 50 mg./kg./day. For more severe infections this dose may be doubled.
If dosage is desired on a twice-a-day schedule in either adults or children, one half of the total daily dose may be given every 12 hours, one hour before meals.
In the treatment of streptococcal infections, a therapeutic dosage of erythromycin should be administered for at least 10 days. In continuous *prophylaxis* of streptococcal infections in persons with a history of rheumatic heart disease, the dose is 250 mg. twice a day.
When used prior to surgery to prevent endocarditis (see alpha-hemolytic streptococci), a recommended schedule for adults is 500 mg. one and one-half to two hours before the procedure; and 250 mg. every six hours for the remainder of that day and for the two days following the procedure (or longer in the case of delayed healing). For small children, the dose is 20 mg./kg. orally one and one-half to two hours before the procedure; and 10 mg./kg. every six hours for the remainder of that day and for the two days following the procedure (or longer in the case of delayed healing).
For treatment of primary syphilis, the dose is 30 to 40 g. given in divided doses over a period of 10 to 15 days.
For treatment of acute pelvic inflammatory disease caused by *N. gonorrhoeae,* 500 mg. erythromycin lactobionate for injection every six hours for three days, followed by one Ethril '250' (Erythromycin Stearate Tablets USP) every six hours for seven days.
For dysenteric amebiasis, the dose for adults is 250 mg. four times daily for 10 to 14 days; for children, the dose is 30 to 50 mg./kg./day in divided doses for 10 to 14 days.
For treatment of Legionnaires' disease—Although optimal doses have not been established, doses utilized in reported clinical data were 1 to 4 grams erythromycin stearate or base daily in divided doses.
How Supplied: 250 mg. in bottles of 100 and 500; 500 mg. in bottles of 50.
Storage: Store at room temperature; avoid excessive heat. Keep from light to prevent discoloration.
[*Shown in Product Identification Section*]

FLORINEF® ACETATE ℞
(Fludrocortisone Acetate Tablets USP)

Description: Fludrocortisone acetate is a synthetic adrenocortical steroid possessing very potent mineralocorticoid properties and high glucocorticoid activity, available for oral administration as scored tablets providing 0.1 mg. fludrocortisone acetate per tablet.
Clinical Pharmacology: The physiologic action of fludrocortisone acetate is similar to that of hydrocortisone. However, the effects of fludrocortisone acetate, particularly on electrolyte balance, but also on carbohydrate metabolism, are considerably heightened and prolonged. In small oral doses, fludrocortisone acetate produces marked sodium retention and increased urinary potassium excretion. It also causes a rise in blood pressure, apparently because of these effects on electrolyte levels.
In larger doses, fludrocortisone acetate inhibits endogenous adrenal cortical secretion, thymic activity, and pituitary corticotropin excretion; promotes the deposition of liver glycogen; and, unless protein intake is adequate, induces negative nitrogen balance.
Indications and Usage: Florinef Acetate is indicated as partial replacement therapy for primary and secondary adrenocortical insufficiency in Addison's disease and for the treatment of salt-losing adrenogenital syndrome.
Contraindications: Corticosteroids are contraindicated in patients with systemic fungal infections.
Warnings: BECAUSE OF ITS MARKED EFFECT ON SODIUM RETENTION, THE USE OF FLUDROCORTISONE ACETATE IN THE TREATMENT OF CONDITIONS OTHER THAN THOSE INDICATED HEREIN IS NOT ADVISED.
Corticosteroids may mask some signs of infection, and new infections may appear during their use. There may be decreased resistance and inability to localize infection when corticosteroids are used. If an infection occurs during fludrocortisone acetate therapy, it should be promptly controlled by suitable antimicrobial therapy.
Prolonged use of corticosteroids may produce posterior subcapsular cataracts, glaucoma with possible damage to the optic nerves, and may enhance the establishment of secondary ocular infections due to fungi or viruses.
Average and large doses of hydrocortisone or cortisone can cause elevation of blood pressure, salt and water retention, and increased excretion of potassium. These effects are less likely to occur with the synthetic derivatives except when used in large doses. However, since fludrocortisone acetate is a potent mineralocorticoid, both the dosage and salt intake should be carefully monitored in order to avoid the development of hypertension, edema, or weight gain. **Periodic checking of serum electrolyte levels is advisable during prolonged therapy; dietary salt restriction and potassium supplementation may be necessary.** All corticosteroids increase calcium excretion.
Patients should not be vaccinated against smallpox while on corticosteroid therapy. Other immunization procedures should not be undertaken in patients who are on corticosteroids, especially on high dose, because of possible hazards of neurological complications and a lack of antibody response.
The use of Florinef Acetate (Fludrocortisone Acetate Tablets USP) in patients with active tuberculosis should be restricted to those cases of fulminating or disseminated tuberculosis in which the corticosteroid is used for the management of the disease in conjunction with an appropriate antituberculous regimen. If corticosteroids are indicated in patients with latent tuberculosis or tuberculin reactivity, close observation is necessary since reactivation of the disease may occur. During prolonged corticosteroid therapy these patients should receive chemoprophylaxis.
Precautions: Adverse reactions to corticosteroids may be produced by too rapid withdrawal or by continued use of large doses.
To avoid drug-induced adrenal insufficiency, supportive dosage may be required in times of stress (such as trauma, surgery, or severe illness) both during treatment with fludrocortisone acetate and for a year afterwards.
There is an enhanced corticosteroid effect in patients with hypothyroidism and in those with cirrhosis.
Corticosteroids should be used cautiously in patients with ocular herpes simplex because of possible corneal perforation.
The lowest possible dose of corticosteroid should be used to control the condition being treated. A gradual reduction in dosage should be made when possible.
Psychic derangements may appear when corticosteroids are used. These may range from euphoria, insomnia, mood swings, personality changes, and severe depression to frank psychotic manifestations. Existing emotional instability or psychotic tendencies may also be aggravated by corticosteroids.
Aspirin should be used cautiously in conjunction with corticosteroids in patients with hypoprothrombinemia.
Corticosteroids should be used with caution in patients with nonspecific ulcerative colitis if there is a probability of impending perforation, abscess, or other pyogenic infection. Corticosteroids should also be used cautiously in patients with diverticulitis, fresh intestinal anastomoses, active or latent peptic ulcer, renal insufficiency, hypertension, osteoporosis, acute glomerulonephritis, vaccinia, varicella, exanthema, Cushing's syndrome, antibiotic-resistant infections, diabetes mellitus, congestive heart failure, chronic nephritis, thromboembolitic tendencies, thrombophlebitis, con-

Continued on next page

Squibb—Cont.

vulsive disorders, metastatic carcinoma, and myasthenia gravis.
Growth and development of infants and children on prolonged corticosteroid therapy should be carefully observed.
Usage in Pregnancy: Adequate reproduction studies have not been performed in animals to determine whether this drug affects fertility in males or females, has teratogenic potential, or has other adverse effects on the fetus. There are no well-controlled studies in pregnant women, but marketing experience does not include any positive evidence of adverse effects on the fetus. Although there is no clearly defined risk, such experience cannot exclude the possibility of infrequent or subtle damage to the human fetus. Fludrocortisone acetate should be used in pregnant women only when clearly needed.
The use of this drug in nursing mothers or women of childbearing potential requires that the possible benefits of the drug be weighed against the potential hazards.
Infants born of mothers who have received substantial doses of fludrocortisone acetate during pregnancy should be carefully observed for signs of hypoadrenalism.
Adverse Reactions: In the recommended small dosages, the side effects seen with cortisone and its derivatives are not usually a problem with fludrocortisone. However, the following untoward effects should be kept in mind, particularly when this agent is used over a prolonged period of time or in conjunction with cortisone or a similar glucocorticoid:
Fluid and electrolyte disturbances—sodium retention, fluid retention, congestive heart failure in susceptible patients, potassium loss, hypokalemic alkalosis, and hypertension.
Musculoskeletal—muscle weakness, steroid myopathy, loss of muscle mass, osteoporosis, vertebral compression fractures, aseptic necrosis of femoral and humeral heads, pathologic fracture of long bones, and spontaneous fractures.
Gastrointestinal—peptic ulcer with possible perforation and hemorrhage, pancreatitis, abdominal distention, and ulcerative esophagitis.
Dermatologic—impaired wound healing, thin fragile skin, bruising, petechiae and ecchymoses, facial erythema, increased sweating, subcutaneous fat atrophy, purpura, striae, hyperpigmentation of the skin and nails, hirsutism, and acneform eruptions; reactions to skin tests may be suppressed.
Neurological—convulsions, increased intracranial pressure with papilledema (pseudotumor cerebri) usually after treatment, vertigo, headache, and severe mental disturbances.
Endocrine—menstrual irregularities; development of the cushingoid state; suppression of growth in children; secondary adrenocortical and pituitary unresponsiveness, particularly in times of stress (e.g., trauma, surgery, or illness); decreased carbohydrate tolerance; manifestations of latent diabetes mellitus; and increased requirements for insulin or oral hypoglycemic agents in diabetics.
Ophthalmic—posterior subcapsular cataracts, increased intraocular pressure, glaucoma, and exophthalmos.
Metabolic—hyperglycemia, glycosuria, and negative nitrogen balance due to protein catabolism.
Other adverse reactions that may occur following the administration of a corticosteroid are necrotizing angiitis, thrombophlebitis, aggravation or masking of infections, insomnia, syncopal episodes, and anaphylactoid reactions.
Dosage and Administration:
Addison's Disease
In Addison's disease, the combination of Florinef Acetate (Fludrocortisone Acetate Tablets USP) with a glucocorticoid such as hydrocortisone or cortisone provides substitution therapy approximating normal adrenal activity with minimal risks of unwanted effects.
The usual dose is 0.1 mg. of Florinef Acetate daily, although dosage ranging from 0.1 mg. three times a week to 0.2 mg. daily has been employed. In the event transient hypertension develops as a consequence of therapy, the dose should be reduced to 0.05 mg. daily. Florinef Acetate is preferably administered in conjunction with cortisone (10 mg. to 37.5 mg. daily in divided doses) or hydrocortisone (10 mg. to 30 mg. daily in divided doses).
Salt-Losing Adrenogenital Syndrome
The recommended dosage for treating the salt-losing adrenogenital syndrome is 0.1 mg. to 0.2 mg. of Florinef Acetate daily.
How Supplied: Florinef Acetate (Fludrocortisone Acetate Tablets USP) for oral administration is supplied in bottles of 100 scored tablets providing 0.1 mg. fludrocortisone acetate per tablet.
Storage: Store at room temperature; avoid excessive heat.

FOLLUTEIN ℞
(Chorionic Gonadotropin for Injection USP)

Description: Human chorionic gonadotropin (HCG), a polypeptide hormone produced by the human placenta, is composed of an alpha and a beta sub-unit. The alpha sub-unit is essentially identical to the alpha sub-units of the human pituitary gonadotropins, luteinizing hormone (LH) and follicle-stimulating hormone (FSH), as well as to the alpha sub-unit of human thyroid-stimulating hormone (TSH). The beta sub-units of these hormones differ in amino acid sequence.
Follutein is a sterile, lyophilized, highly purified powder of the anterior pituitary-like hormone, HCG, isolated from gravid human urine. Each vial provides 10,000 USP Units of chorionic gonadotropin, with 83 mg. sodium chloride, and sodium hydroxide to adjust the pH of the reconstituted solution. When reconstituted with the accompanying 10 ml. sterile, aqueous diluent, each ml. provides 1,000 USP Units chorionic gonadotropin with 0.5% phenol as a preservative, and sodium hydroxide or hydrochloric acid to adjust the pH to 6.0 to 8.0. At the time of manufacture, the air in the diluent container is replaced by nitrogen.
To reconstitute the preparation, simply add the sterile diluent to the vial containing the powder. If necessary, less than the total amount of diluent may be added to the vial to provide solutions of higher concentration.
Actions: The action of HCG is virtually identical to that of pituitary LH, although HCG appears to have a small degree of FSH activity as well. It stimulates production of gonadal steroid hormones by stimulating the interstitial cells (Leydig cells) of the testis to produce androgens and the corpus luteum of the ovary to produce progesterone. Androgen stimulation in the male leads to the development of secondary sex characteristics and may stimulate testicular descent when no anatomical impediment to descent is present. This descent is usually reversible when HCG is discontinued. During the normal menstrual cycle, LH participates with FSH in the development and maturation of the normal ovarian follicle, and the mid-cycle LH surge triggers ovulation. HCG can substitute for LH in this function.
During a normal pregnancy, HCG secreted by the placenta maintains the corpus luteum after LH secretion decreases, supporting continued secretion of estrogen and progesterone and preventing menstruation. HCG HAS NO KNOWN EFFECT ON FAT MOBILIZATION, APPETITE OR SENSE OF HUNGER, OR BODY FAT DISTRIBUTION.
Indications: HCG HAS NOT BEEN DEMONSTRATED TO BE EFFECTIVE ADJUNCTIVE THERAPY IN THE TREATMENT OF OBESITY. THERE IS NO SUBSTANTIAL EVIDENCE THAT IT INCREASES WEIGHT LOSS BEYOND THAT RESULTING FROM CALORIC RESTRICTION, THAT IT CAUSES A MORE ATTRACTIVE OR "NORMAL" DISTRIBUTION OF FAT, OR THAT IT DECREASES THE HUNGER AND DISCOMFORT ASSOCIATED WITH CALORIE-RESTRICTED DIETS.
Follutein (Chorionic Gonadotropin for Injection USP) is indicated for:
A. Prepubertal cryptorchidism not due to anatomical obstruction. In general, HCG is thought to induce testicular descent in situations when descent would have occurred at puberty. HCG thus may help predict whether or not orchiopexy will be needed in the future. Although, in some cases, descent following HCG administration is permanent, in most cases, the response is temporary. Therapy is usually instituted between the ages of four and nine.
B. Selected cases of hypogonadotropic hypogonadism (hypogonadism secondary to a pituitary deficiency) in males.
C. Induction of ovulation and pregnancy in the anovulatory, infertile woman in whom the cause of anovulation is secondary and not due to primary ovarian failure, and who has been appropriately pre-treated with human menotropins.
Contraindications: HCG is contraindicated in individuals experiencing precocious puberty, in patients with prostatic carcinoma or other androgen dependent neoplasia, or individuals who have exhibited prior allergic reaction to HCG.
Warnings: HCG should be used in conjunction with human menopausal gonadotropins only by physicians experienced with infertility problems who are familiar with the criteria for patient selection, contraindications, warnings, precautions, and adverse reactions described in the package insert for menotropins. The principal serious adverse reactions during this use are: (1) Ovarian hyperstimulation, a syndrome of sudden ovarian enlargement, ascites with or without pain, and/or pleural effusion, (2) Rupture of ovarian cysts with resultant hemoperitoneum, (3) Multiple births, and (4) Arterial thromboembolism.
Precautions: Induction of androgen secretion by HCG may induce precocious puberty in patients treated for cryptorchidism. Therapy should be discontinued if signs of precocious puberty occur.
Since androgens may cause fluid retention, HCG should be used with caution in patients with cardiac or renal disease, epilepsy, migraine, or asthma.
If hypogonadism due to pituitary dysfunction has existed over a period of several years, irreparable testicular damage may have occurred, and response to therapy with chorionic gonadotropin may not be satisfactory. Stimulation therapy is not recommended in the treatment of hypogonadism due to disturbances which have their primary origin in the testes.
Adverse Reactions: Adverse reactions associated with the administration of HCG are: headache, irritability, restlessness, depression, fatigue, edema, precocious puberty, gynecomastia, and pain at the site of injection.
Dosage and Administration: Follutein (Chorionic Gonadotropin for Injection USP) should be administered by intramuscular injection only.
The dosage regimen employed in any particular case will depend upon the indication for use, the age and weight of the patient, and the physician's preference. The following regimens have been advocated by various authorities.
A. *Prepubertal cryptorchidism not due to anatomical obstruction*
(1) 4,000 USP Units three times weekly for three weeks.

(2) 5,000 USP Units every second day for four injections.
(3) 15 injections of 500 to 1,000 USP Units over a period of six weeks.
(4) 500 USP Units three times weekly for four to six weeks. If this course of treatment is not successful, another is begun one month later, giving 1,000 USP Units per injection.

B. *Selected cases of hypogonadotropic hypogonadism in males*
(1) 500 to 1,000 USP Units three times a week for three weeks, followed by the same dose twice a week for three weeks.
(2) 4,000 USP Units three times weekly for six to nine months, following which the dosage may be reduced to 2,000 USP Units three times weekly for an additional three months.

C. *Therapy in conjunction with human menotropins*
Induction of ovulation and pregnancy in the anovulatory, infertile woman in whom the cause of anovulation is secondary and not due to primary ovarian failure and who has been appropriately pre-treated with human menotropins (see prescribing information for menotropins for dosage and administration for that drug product).
5,000 to 10,000 USP Units one day following the last dose of menotropins (a dosage of 10,000 USP Units is recommended in the labeling for menotropins).

How Supplied: Follutein (Chorionic Gonadotropin for Injection USP) is supplied in combination packages: each package contains one vial providing 10,000 USP Units sterile chorionic gonadotropin powder and one ampul providing 10 ml. sterile diluent.

Storage: After reconstitution the preparation should be stored in a refrigerator. When refrigerated, the solution retains its potency for two months; thereafter potency slowly diminishes.

FUNGIZONE® ℞
(Amphotericin B) CREAM/LOTION/OINTMENT

Description: Fungizone Cream (Amphotericin B Cream) contains the antifungal antibiotic Amphotericin B USP at a concentration of 3% (30 mg./gram) in a pleasantly tinted aqueous vehicle, which also contains titanium dioxide, thimerosal, propylene glycol, cetearyl alcohol (and) ceteareth-20, white petrolatum, methylparaben, propylparaben, sorbitol solution, glyceryl monostearate, polyethylene glycol monostearate, simethicone, and sorbic acid.
Fungizone Lotion (Amphotericin B Lotion) contains the antifungal antibiotic Amphotericin B USP at a concentration of 3% (30 mg./ml.) in a tinted aqueous lotion vehicle, which is pleasantly scented, and also contains thimerosal, titanium dioxide, guar gum, propylene glycol, cetyl alcohol, stearyl alcohol, sorbitan monopalmitate, polysorbate 20, glyceryl monostearate, polyethylene glycol monostearate, simethicone, sorbic acid, methylparaben, and propylparaben.
Fungizone Ointment (Amphotericin B Ointment) contains the antifungal antibiotic Amphotericin B USP at a concentration of 3% (30 mg./gram) in a tinted form of Plastibase® (Plasticized Hydrocarbon Gel), a polyethylene and mineral oil gel base with titanium dioxide.

Clinical Pharmacology: Amphotericin B is an antibiotic with antifungal activity which is produced by a strain of *Streptomyces nodosus.* It has been shown to exhibit greater *in vitro* activity than nystatin against *Candida* (Monilia) *albicans.* In clinical studies involving cutaneous and mucocutaneous candidal infections, results with topical preparations of amphotericin B were comparable to those obtained with nystatin in similar formulations.
Although amphotericin B exhibits some *in vitro* activity against the superficial dermatophytes (ringworm organisms), it has not demonstrated an effectiveness *in vivo* on topical application. Amphotericin B has no significant effect either *in vitro* or clinically against gram-positive or gram-negative bacteria, or viruses.

Indications: Fungizone (Amphotericin B) topical preparations are indicated in the treatment of cutaneous and mucocutaneous mycotic infections caused by Candida (Monilia) species.

Contraindications: The preparations are contraindicated in patients with a history of hypersensitivity to any of their components.

Precautions: Should a reaction of hypersensitivity occur the drug should be immediately withdrawn and appropriate measures taken.

Adverse Reactions: Fungizone Cream (Amphotericin B Cream) —No evidence of any systemic toxicity or side effects has been observed during or following the use of the Cream. The preparation is usually well tolerated by all age groups. It is not a primary irritant and apparently has only a slight sensitizing potential. It may have a "drying" effect on some skin, and local irritation characterized by erythema, pruritus, or a burning sensation sometimes occurs, particularly in intertriginous areas.
Fungizone Lotion (Amphotericin B Lotion) —No evidence of any systemic toxicity or side effects has been observed during or following even prolonged, intensive and extensive application of the Lotion. The preparation is extremely well tolerated by all age groups, including infants, even when therapy must be continued for many months. It is not a primary irritant and apparently has only a slight sensitizing potential. Local intolerance, which seldom occurs, has included increased pruritus with or without other subjective or objective evidence of local irritation, or exacerbation of preexisting candidal lesions. Allergic contact dermatitis is rare.
Fungizone Ointment (Amphotericin B Ointment)—No evidence of any systemic toxicity or side effects has been observed during or following even prolonged, intensive and extensive application of the Ointment. The preparation is usually well tolerated by all age groups. It is not a primary irritant and apparently has only a slight sensitizing potential. However, it is well to remember that any oleaginous ointment vehicle may occasionally irritate when applied to moist, intertriginous areas.

Dosage and Administration: Fungizone (Amphotericin B) Cream, Lotion, or Ointment should be applied liberally to the candidal lesions two to four times daily. Duration of therapy depends on individual patient response. Intertriginous lesions usually respond within a few days, and treatment may be completed in one to three weeks. Similarly, candidiasis of the diaper area, perleche, and glabrous skin lesions usually clear in one to two weeks. Interdigital (erosio) lesions may require two to four weeks of intensive therapy; paronychias also require relatively prolonged therapy, and those onychomycoses which respond may require several months or more of treatment. (Relapses are frequently encountered in the last three clinical conditions.)
NOTE: When rubbed into the lesion, the Cream discolors the skin minimally. The Lotion and Ointment do not stain the skin when thoroughly rubbed into the lesion although nail lesions may be stained. The patient should be informed that any discoloration of fabrics from the Cream may be removed by handwashing the fabric with soap and warm water, that any discoloration of fabrics from the Lotion is readily removed with soap and warm water, or that any discoloration of fabrics from the Ointment may be removed by applying a standard cleaning fluid.

How Supplied: Fungizone Cream (Amphotericin B Cream) is supplied in tubes of 20 grams.
Fungizone Lotion (Amphotericin B Lotion) is supplied in 30 ml. plastic squeeze bottles (Military Depot Item, NSN 6505-00-890-1486).
Fungizone Ointment (Amphotericin B Ointment) is supplied in tubes of 20 grams.

Storage: Store the Cream and Lotion at room temperature; avoid freezing. Store the Ointment at room temperature.

FUNGIZONE® INTRAVENOUS ℞
(Amphotericin B for Injection USP)

> **WARNING**
> This drug should be used *primarily* for treatment of patients with progressive and potentially fatal fungal infections; it should not be used to treat the common clinically inapparent forms of fungal disease which show only positive skin or serologic tests.

Description: Fungizone Intravenous (Amphotericin B for Injection USP) is an antifungal antibiotic derived from a strain of *Streptomyces nodosus.* Crystalline amphotericin B is insoluble in water; therefore, the antibiotic is "solubilized" by the addition of sodium desoxycholate to form a mixture which provides a colloidal dispersion for parenteral administration.

Actions:
Microbiology
Amphotericin B shows a high order of *in vitro* activity against many species of fungi. *Histoplasma capsulatum, Coccidiodes immitis, Candida* species, *Blastomyces dermatitidis, Rhodotorula, Cryptococcus neoformans, Sporotrichum schenckii, Mucor mucedo,* and *Aspergillus fumigatus* are all inhibited by concentrations of amphotericin B ranging from 0.03 to 1.0 mcg./ml. *in vitro.* The antibiotic is without effect on bacteria, rickettsiae, and viruses.
Clinical Pharmacology
Amphotericin B is fungistatic or fungicidal depending on the concentration obtained in body fluids and the susceptibility of the fungus. The drug probably acts by binding to sterols in the fungus cell membrane with a resultant change in membrane permeability which allows leakage of a variety of small molecules. Mammalian cell membranes also contain sterols and it has been suggested that the damage to human cells and fungal cells may share common mechanisms.
An initial intravenous infusion of 1 to 5 mg. of amphotericin B per day, gradually increased to 0.65 mg./kg. daily, produces peak plasma concentrations of approximately 2 to 4 mcg./ml. which can persist between doses since the plasma half-life of amphotericin B is about 24 hours. (For recommended dosages, see the DOSAGE AND ADMINISTRATION section.) It has been reported that amphotericin B is highly bound (>90%) to plasma proteins and is poorly dialyzable.
Amphotericin B is excreted very slowly by the kidneys with two to five percent of a given dose being excreted in biologically active form. After treatment is discontinued, the drug can be detected in the urine for at least seven weeks. The cumulative urinary output over a seven-day period amounts to approximately 40 percent of the amount of drug infused.
Details of tissue distribution and possible metabolic pathways are not known.

Indications: Fungizone Intravenous should be administered primarily to patients with progressive, potentially fatal infections. This potent drug should not be used to treat the common inapparent forms of fungal disease which show only positive skin or serologic tests.
Fungizone Intravenous (Amphotericin B for Injection USP) is specifically intended to treat cryptococcosis (torulosis); North American blastomycosis; the disseminated forms of moniliasis, coccidioidomycosis, and histoplasmosis; mucormycosis (phycomycosis) caused by species of the genera *Mucor, Rhizopus, Absidia, Entomophthora,* and *Basidiobolus;* sporotrichosis (*Sporothrix schenckii* [formerly *Sporotri-*

Continued on next page

Squibb—Cont.

chum schenckii]); aspergillosis (*Aspergillus fumigatus*).

Amphotericin B may be helpful in the treatment of American mucocutaneous leishmaniasis, but is not the drug of choice in primary therapy.

Contraindications: This product is contraindicated in those patients who have shown hypersensitivity to it unless, in the opinion of the physician, the condition requiring treatment is life-threatening and amenable only to amphotericin B therapy.

Warnings: Amphotericin B is frequently the only effective treatment available for potentially fatal fungal disease. In each case, its possible life-saving benefit must be balanced against its untoward and dangerous side effects.

Usage in Pregnancy: Safety for use in pregnancy has not been established; therefore, it should be used during pregnancy only if the possible benefits to be derived outweigh the potential risks involved.

Precautions: Prolonged therapy with amphotericin B is usually necessary. Unpleasant reactions are quite common when the drug is given parenterally at therapeutic dosage levels. **Some of these reactions are potentially dangerous.** Hence, amphotericin B should be used parenterally only in hospitalized patients or those under close clinical observation by medically trained personnel and should be reserved for those patients in whom a diagnosis of the progressive, potentially fatal forms of susceptible mycotic infections has been firmly established, preferably by positive culture or histologic study.

Corticosteroids should not be administered concomitantly unless they are necessary to control drug reactions. Other nephrotoxic antibiotics and antineoplastic agents such as nitrogen mustard should not be given concomitantly except with great caution.

Laboratory facilities must be available to perform blood urea nitrogen and serum creatinine or endogenous creatinine clearance tests. These determinations should be made at least weekly during therapy. If the BUN exceeds 40 mg. per 100 ml. or the serum creatinine exceeds 3.0 mg. per 100 ml. the drug should be discontinued or the dosage markedly reduced until renal function is improved. Weekly hemograms and serum potassium determinations are also advisable. Low serum magnesium levels have also been noted during treatment with amphotericin B. Therapy should be discontinued if liver function test results (elevated bromsulphalein, alkaline phosphatase and bilirubin) are abnormal.

Whenever medication is interrupted for a period longer than seven days, therapy should be resumed by starting with the lowest dosage level, e.g., 0.25 mg./kg. of body weight, and increased gradually as outlined under DOSAGE AND ADMINISTRATION.

Adverse Reactions: While some few patients may tolerate full intravenous doses of amphotericin B without difficulty, most will exhibit some intolerance, often at less than the full therapeutic dosage. They may be made less severe by giving aspirin, antihistamines, and antiemetics. Administration of the drug on alternate days may decrease anorexia and phlebitis. Intravenous administration of small doses of adrenal corticosteroids just prior to or during the amphotericin B infusion may decrease febrile reactions. The dosage and duration of such corticosteroid therapy should be kept to a minimum. Adding a small amount of heparin to the infusion may lessen the incidence of thrombophlebitis. Extravasation may cause chemical irritation.

The adverse reactions that are most commonly observed are: fever (sometimes with shaking chills); headache; anorexia; weight loss; nausea and vomiting; malaise; dyspepsia; diarrhea; generalized pain including muscle and joint pains, cramping epigastric pain, and local venous pain at the injection site with phlebitis and thrombophlebitis; and normochromic, normocytic anemia. Abnormal renal function including hypokalemia, azotemia, hyposthenuria, renal tubular acidosis and nephrocalcinosis is also commonly observed, and usually improves upon interruption of therapy; however, some permanent impairment often occurs, especially in those patients receiving large amounts (over 5 g.) of amphotericin B. Supplemental alkali medication may decrease renal tubular acidosis complications.

The following adverse reactions occur less frequently or rarely: anuria; oliguria; cardiovascular toxicity including arrhythmias, ventricular fibrillation, cardiac arrest, hypertension, and hypotension; coagulation defects; thrombocytopenia; leukopenia; agranulocytosis; eosinophilia; leukocytosis; melena or hemorrhagic gastroenteritis; maculopapular rash; hearing loss; tinnitus; transient vertigo; blurred vision or diplopia; peripheral neuropathy; convulsions and other neurologic symptoms; pruritus (without rash); anaphylactoid reactions; acute liver failure; and flushing.

Dosage and Administration: Fungizone Intravenous (Amphotericin B for Injection USP) should be administered by *slow* intravenous infusion. Intravenous infusion should be given over a period of approximately six hours observing the usual precautions for intravenous therapy. The recommended concentration for intravenous infusion is 0.1 mg./ml. (1 mg./10 ml.).

Dosage must be adjusted to the specific requirements of each patient since tolerance to amphotericin B varies individually. Therapy is usually instituted with a daily dose of 0.25 mg./kg. of body weight and **gradually** increased as tolerance permits. There are insufficient data presently available to define total dosage requirements and duration of treatment necessary for eradication of mycoses such as phycomycosis. The optimal dose is unknown. Total daily dosage may range up to 1.0 mg./kg. of body weight or alternate day dosages ranging up to 1.5 mg./kg. Several months of therapy are usually necessary; a shorter period of therapy may produce an inadequate response and lead to relapse.

CAUTION: Under no circumstances should a total daily dosage of 1.5 mg./kg. be exceeded.

Therapy with intravenous amphotericin B for sporotrichosis has ranged up to nine months. The usual dose per injection is 20 mg.

Aspergillosis has been treated with amphotericin B intravenously for a period up to 11 months with a total dose up to 3.6 g.

Rhinocerebral phycomycosis, a fulminating disease, generally occurs in association with diabetic ketoacidosis. It is, therefore, imperative that rapid restoration of diabetic control be instituted before successful treatment with Fungizone Intravenous (Amphotericin B for Injection USP) can be accomplished. In contradistinction, pulmonary phycomycosis, which is more common in association with hematologic malignancies, is often an incidental finding at autopsy. A cumulative dose of at least 3 g. of amphotericin B is recommended. Although a total dose of 3 to 4 g. will infrequently cause lasting renal impairment, this would seem a reasonable minimum where there is clinical evidence of invasion of the deep tissues; since rhinocerebral phycomycosis usually follows a rapidly fatal course, the therapeutic approach must necessarily be more aggressive than that used in more indolent mycoses.

Preparation of Solutions: Reconstitute as follows: An initial concentrate of 5 mg. amphotericin B per ml. is first prepared by rapidly expressing 10 ml. Sterile Water for Injection USP *without a bacteriostatic agent* directly into the lyophilized cake, using a sterile needle (minimum diameter: 20 gauge) and syringe. Shake the vial immediately until the colloidal solution is clear. The infusion solution, providing 0.1 mg. amphotericin B per ml., is then obtained by further dilution (1:50) with 5% Dextrose Injection USP *of pH above 4.2*. The pH of each container of Dextrose Injection should be ascertained before use. Commercial Dextrose Injection usually has a pH above 4.2; however, if it is below 4.2, then 1 or 2 ml. of buffer should be added to the Dextrose Injection before it is used to dilute the concentrated solution of amphotericin B. The recommended buffer has the following composition:

Dibasic sodium phosphate (anhydrous)	1.59 g.
Monobasic sodium phosphate (anhydrous)	0.96 g.
Water for Injection USP	qs. 100.0 ml.

The buffer should be sterilized before it is added to the Dextrose Injection, either by filtration through a bacterial retentive stone, mat, or membrane, or by autoclaving for 30 minutes at 15 lb. pressure (121° C.).

CAUTION: Aseptic technique must be strictly observed in all handling, since no preservative or bacteriostatic agent is present in the antibiotic or in the materials used to prepare it for administration. **All entries into the vial or into the diluents must be made with a sterile needle. Do not reconstitute with saline solutions. The use of any diluent other than the ones recommended or the presence of a bacteriostatic agent** (e.g., benzyl alcohol) **in the diluent may cause precipitation of the antibiotic. Do not use the initial concentrate or the infusion solution if there is any evidence of precipitation or foreign matter in either one.**

An in-line membrane filter may be used for intravenous infusion of amphotericin B; **however, the mean pore diameter of the filter should not be less than 1.0 micron in order to assure passage of the antibiotic dispersion.**

How Supplied: Fungizone Intravenous is supplied in vials as a sterile lyophilized cake (which may partially reduce to powder following manufacture) providing 50 mg. amphotericin B and 41 mg. sodium desoxycholate with 20.2 mg. sodium phosphates as a buffer. At the time of manufacture, the air in the container is replaced by nitrogen.

Storage: Prior to reconstitution, Fungizone Intravenous (Amphotericin B for injection USP) should be stored in the refrigerator, protected against exposure to light. The concentrate (5 mg. amphotericin B per ml. after reconstitution with 10 ml. Sterile Water for Injection USP) may be stored in the dark, at room temperature for 24 hours, or at refrigerator temperatures for one week with minimal loss of potency and clarity. Any unused material should then be discarded. Solutions prepared for intravenous infusion (0.1 mg. or less amphotericin B per ml.) should be used promptly after preparation and should be protected from light during administration.

GASTROGRAFIN® ℞

(Diatrizoate Meglumine and Diatrizoate Sodium Solution USP)

(See Diagnostic Section)

HALOG® ℞

(Halcinonide)

CREAM/OINTMENT/SOLUTION

Description: Halog preparations contain the active synthetic corticosteroid halcinonide. The chemical name is (11β,16α)-21-Chloro-9-fluoro-11-hydroxy-16, 17-[(1-methylethylidene) bis-(oxy)] pregn-4-ene-3,20-dione.

Halog Cream 0.025% (Halcinonide Cream 0.025%) contains 0.25 mg. halcinonide per gram in a specially formulated cream base consisting of glyceryl monostearate NF XII, cetyl alcohol, cetyl esters wax, polysorbate 60, propylene glycol, dimethicone 350, and purified water. Halog Cream 0.1% (Halcinonide Cream 0.1%) contains 1 mg. halcinonide per gram in a specially formulated cream base consisting of glyceryl monostearate NF XII, cetyl alcohol, isopropyl palmitate, dimethicone 350, polysorbate 60, titanium dioxide, propylene glycol, and purified water.

Halog Ointment 0.025% (Halcinonide Ointment 0.025%) contains 0.25 mg. halcinonide per gram in Plastibase® (Plasticized Hydrocarbon Gel), a polyethylene and mineral oil gel base with polyethylene glycol 400, polyethylene glycol 6000 distearate, polyethylene glycol 300, polyethylene glycol 1540, and butylated hydroxytoluene as a preservative. Halog Ointment 0.1% (Halcinonide Ointment 0.1%) contains 1 mg. halcinonide per gram in Plastibase® (Plasticized Hydrocarbon Gel), a polyethylene and mineral oil gel base with polyethylene glycol 400, polyethylene glycol 6000 distearate, polyethylene glycol 300, polyethylene glycol 1540, and butylated hydroxytoluene as a preservative.

Halog Solution 0.1% (Halcinonide Solution 0.1%) contains 1 mg. halcinonide per ml. with edetate disodium, polyethylene glycol 300, purified water, and butylated hydroxytoluene as a preservative.

Actions: Halcinonide preparations are primarily effective because of their anti-inflammatory, antipruritic and vasoconstrictive actions.

Indications: Halog (Halcinonide) preparations are indicated for relief of the inflammatory manifestations of corticosteroid-responsive dermatoses.

Contraindications: Topical steroids are contraindicated in those patients with a history of hypersensitivity to any of the components of the preparations.

Precautions:

General: If irritation develops, the product should be discontinued and appropriate therapy instituted.

In the presence of an infection, the use of an appropriate antifungal or antibacterial agent should be instituted. If a favorable response does not occur promptly, the corticosteroid should be discontinued until the infection has been adequately controlled.

If extensive areas are treated or if the occlusive technique is used, there will be increased systemic absorption of the corticosteroid and suitable precautions should be taken, particularly in children and infants.

These preparations are not for ophthalmic use.

Usage in Pregnancy: Although topical steroids have not been reported to have an adverse effect on human pregnancy, the safety of their use in pregnant women has not been absolutely established. In laboratory animals, increases in incidence of fetal abnormalities have been associated with exposure of gestating females to topical corticosteroids—in some cases at rather low dosage levels. Therefore, drugs of this class should not be used extensively on pregnant patients, in large amounts, or for prolonged periods of time.

Occlusive Dressing Technique: The use of occlusive dressing increases the percutaneous absorption of corticosteroids. For patients with extensive lesions it may be preferable to use a sequential approach, occluding one portion of the body at a time. The patient should be kept under close observation if treated with the occlusive technique over large areas and over a considerable period of time. Occasionally, a patient who has been on prolonged therapy, especially occlusive therapy, may develop symptoms of steroid withdrawal when the medication is stopped. Thermal homeostasis may be impaired if large areas of the body are covered. Use of the occlusive dressing should be discontinued if elevation of the body temperature occurs. Occasionally, a patient may develop a sensitivity reaction to a particular occlusive dressing material or adhesive and a substitute material may be necessary.

If infection develops, discontinue the use of the occlusive dressing and institute appropriate antimicrobial therapy.

Adverse Reactions: The following local adverse reactions have been reported with topical corticosteroids, especially under occlusive dressings: burning sensations, itching, irritation, dryness, folliculitis, hypertrichosis, acneform eruptions, hypopigmentation, perioral dermatitis, allergic contact dermatitis, maceration of the skin, secondary infection, skin atrophy, striae, and miliaria.

Dosage and Administration: Halog Cream 0.025% (Halcinonide Cream 0.025%) or Halog Cream 0.1% (Halcinonide Cream 0.1%): Apply to the affected area two to three times daily. Rub in gently.

Halog Ointment 0.025% (Halcinonide Ointment 0.025%) or Halog Ointment 0.1% (Halcinonide Ointment 0.1%): Apply a thin film to the affected area two to three times daily.

Halog Solution 0.1% (Halcinonide Solution 0.1%): Apply to the affected area two to three times daily.

Occlusive Dressing Technique: Particularly resistant lesions of chronic dermatoses such as psoriasis and neurodermatitis may require the use of a halcinonide preparation under occlusive dressings.

Halog Cream (Halcinonide Cream) 0.025% and 0.1%: Gently rub a small amount of the cream into the lesion until it disappears. Reapply the preparation leaving a thin coating on the lesion and cover with a pliable nonporous film. The frequency of changing dressings is best determined on an individual basis. Good results have been obtained by applying the cream under an occlusive dressing in the evening and removing the dressing in the morning (i.e., 12-hour occlusion). When utilizing the 12-hour occlusion regimen, additional cream should be applied, without occlusion, during the day. Reapplication is essential at each dressing change.

Halog Ointment 0.025% (Halcinonide Ointment 0.025%) or Halog Ointment 0.1% (Halcinonide Ointment 0.1%): Apply a thin film of the ointment to the lesion and cover with a pliable nonporous film. The frequency of changing dressings is best determined on an individual basis. It may be convenient to apply the ointment under an occlusive dressing in the evening and to remove the dressing in the morning (i.e., 12-hour occlusion). When utilizing the 12-hour occlusion regimen, additional ointment should be applied, without occlusion, during the day. Reapplication is essential at each dressing change.

Halog Solution 0.1% (Halcinonide Solution 0.1%): Apply the solution to the lesion and cover with a pliable nonporous film. The frequency of changing dressings is best determined on an individual basis. It may be convenient to apply the solution under an occlusive dressing in the evening and to remove the dressing in the morning (i.e., 12-hour occlusion). When utilizing the 12-hour occlusion regimen, additional solution should be applied, without occlusion, during the day. Reapplication is essential at each dressing change.

How Supplied:

0.025% Cream: Tubes of 15 g. and 60 g.; jars of 240 g. (8 oz.).

0.1% Cream: Tubes of 15 g., 30 g., and 60 g.; jars of 240 g. (8 oz.) [Tubes of 60 g. V.A. Depot Item, NSN6505-01-007-9895A].

0.025% Ointment: Tubes of 15 g. and 60 g.; jars of 240 g. (8 oz.).

0.1% Ointment: Tubes of 15 g. 30 g., and 60 g.; jars of 240 g. (8 oz.).

0.1% Solution: Plastic squeeze bottles of 20 ml. and 60 ml.

Storage: Store the 0.025% and 0.1% Creams at room temperature; avoid excessive heat (104° F). Store the 0.025% and 0.1% Ointments at room temperature; avoid excessive heat (104° F). Store the Solution at room temperature; avoid freezing and temperatures above 104° F.

HYDREA® ℞
(Hydroxyurea Capsules USP)

Description: Hydrea (Hydroxyurea Capsules USP) is an antineoplastic agent, available for oral use as capsules providing 500 mg. hydroxyurea. Capsules contain FD&C Yellow No. 5 (tartrazine). Hydroxyurea occurs as an essentially tasteless, white crystalline powder.

Actions: Mechanism of Action

The precise mechanism by which hydroxyurea produces its cytotoxic effects cannot, at present, be described. However, the reports of various studies in tissue culture in rats and man lend support to the hypothesis that hydroxyurea causes an immediate inhibition of DNA synthesis without interfering with the synthesis of ribonucleic acid or of protein. This hypothesis explains why, under certain conditions, hydroxyurea may induce teratogenic effects.

Three mechanisms of action have been postulated for the increased effectiveness of concomitant use of hydroxyurea therapy with irradiation on squamous cell (epidermoid) carcinomas of the head and neck. *In vitro* studies utilizing Chinese hamster cells suggest that hydroxyurea (1) is lethal to normally radioresistant S-stage cells, and (2) holds other cells of the cell cycle in the G1 or pre-DNA synthesis stage where they are most susceptible to the effects of irradiation. The third mechanism of action has been theorized on the basis of *in vitro* studies of HeLa cells: it appears that hydroxyurea, by inhibition of DNA synthesis, hinders the normal repair process of cells damaged but not killed by irradiation, thereby decreasing their survival rate; RNA and protein syntheses have shown no alteration.

Absorption, Metabolism, Fate and Excretion

After oral administration in man, hydroxyurea is readily absorbed from the gastrointestinal tract. The drug reaches peak serum concentrations within 2 hours; by 24 hours the concentration in the serum is essentially zero. Approximately 80% of an oral or intravenous dose of 7 to 30 mg./kg. may be recovered in the urine within 12 hours.

Animal Pharmacology and Toxicology

The oral LD_{50} of hydroxyurea is 7330 mg./kg. in mice and 5780 mg./kg. in rats, given as a single dose.

In subacute and chronic toxicity studies in the rat, the most consistent pathological findings were an apparent dose-related mild to moderate bone marrow hypoplasia as well as pulmonary congestion and mottling of the lungs. At the highest dosage levels (1260 mg./kg./day for 37 days then 2520 mg./kg./day for 40 days), testicular atrophy with absence of spermatogenesis occurred; in several animals, hepatic cell damage with fatty metamorphosis was noted. In the dog, mild to marked bone marrow depression was a consistent finding except at the lower dosage levels. Additionally, at the higher dose levels (140 to 420 mg. or 140 to 1260 mg./kg./week given 3 or 7 days weekly for 12 weeks), growth retardation, slightly increased blood glucose values and hemosiderosis of the liver or spleen were found; reversible spermatogenic arrest was noted. In the monkey, bone marrow depression, lymphoid atrophy of the spleen and degenerative changes in the epithelium of the small and large intestines were found. At the higher, often lethal, doses (400 to 800 mg./kg./day for 7 to 15 days), hemorrhage and congestion were found in the lungs, brain and urinary tract. Cardiovascular effects (changes in heart rate, blood pressure, orthostatic hypotension, EKG changes) and

Continued on next page

Squibb—Cont.

hematological changes (slight hemolysis, slight methemoglobinemia) were observed in some species of laboratory animals at doses exceeding clinical levels.

Indications: Significant tumor response to Hydrea (Hydroxyurea Capsules USP) has been demonstrated in melanoma, resistant chronic myelocytic leukemia, and recurrent, metastatic, or inoperable carcinoma of the ovary.

Hydrea used concomitantly with irradiation therapy is intended for use in the local control of primary squamous cell (epidermoid) carcinomas of the head and neck, excluding the lip.

Contraindications: Hydroxyurea is contraindicated in patients with marked bone marrow depression, i.e., leukopenia (less than 2500 WBC) or thrombocytopenia (less than 100,000), or severe anemia.

Warnings: Treatment with hydroxyurea should not be initiated if bone marrow function is markedly depressed (—see CONTRAINDICATIONS). Bone marrow suppression may occur, and leukopenia is generally its first and most common manifestation. Thrombocytopenia and anemia occur less often, and are seldom seen without a preceding leukopenia. However, the recovery from myelosuppression is rapid when therapy is interrupted. It should be borne in mind that bone marrow depression is more likely in patients who have previously received radiotherapy or cytotoxic cancer chemotherapeutic agents; hydroxyurea should be used cautiously in such patients.

Patients who have received irradiation therapy in the past may have an exacerbation of post-irradiation erythema.

Severe anemia must be corrected with whole blood replacement before initiating therapy with hydroxyurea.

Erythrocytic abnormalities: megaloblastic erythropoiesis, which is self-limiting, is often seen early in the course of hydroxyurea therapy. The morphologic change resembles pernicious anemia, but is not related to vitamin B_{12} or folic acid deficiency. Hydroxyurea may also delay plasma iron clearance and reduce the rate of iron utilization by erythrocytes, but it does not appear to alter the red blood cell survival time.

Hydroxyurea should be used with caution in patients with marked renal dysfunction.

Elderly patients may be more sensitive to the effects of hydroxyurea, and may require a lower dose regimen.

Usage in Pregnancy—Drugs which affect DNA synthesis, such as hydroxyurea, may be potential mutagenic agents. The physician should carefully consider this possibility before administering this drug to male or female patients who may contemplate conception.

Hydrea (Hydroxyurea Capsules USP) is a known teratogenic agent in animals. Therefore, hydroxyurea should not be used in women who are or may become pregnant unless in the judgment of the physician the potential benefits outweigh the possible hazards.

Precautions: Therapy with Hydrea requires close supervision. The complete status of the blood, including bone marrow examination, if indicated, as well as kidney function and liver function should be determined prior to, and repeatedly during, treatment. The determination of the hemoglobin level, total leukocyte counts, and platelet counts should be performed at least once a week throughout the course of Hydrea (Hydroxyurea Capsules USP) therapy. If the white blood cell count decreases to less than 2500/mm^3, or the platelet count to less than 100,000/mm^3, therapy should be interrupted until the values rise significantly toward normal levels. Anemia, if it occurs, should be managed with whole blood replacement, without interrupting hydroxyurea therapy.

Hydroxyurea capsules contain FD&C Yellow No. 5 (tartrazine) which may cause allergic-type reactions (including bronchial asthma) in certain susceptible individuals. Although the overall incidence of FD&C Yellow No. 5 (tartrazine) sensitivity in the general population is low, it is frequently seen in patients who also have aspirin hypersensitivity.

Adverse Reactions: Adverse reactions have been primarily bone marrow depression (leukopenia, anemia, and occasionally thrombocytopenia), and less frequently gastrointestinal symptoms (stomatitis, anorexia, nausea, vomiting, diarrhea, and constipation), and dermatological reactions such as maculopapular rash, and facial erythema. Dysuria and alopecia occur very rarely. Large doses may produce moderate drowsiness. Neurological disturbances have occurred extremely rarely and were limited to headache, dizziness, disorientation, hallucinations, and convulsions. Hydroxyurea occasionally may cause temporary impairment of renal tubular function accompanied by elevations in serum uric acid, BUN, and creatinine levels. Abnormal BSP retention has been reported.

Adverse reactions observed with combined hydroxyurea and irradiation therapy are similar to those reported with the use of hydroxyurea alone. These effects primarily include bone marrow depression (anemia and leukopenia), and gastric irritation. Almost all patients receiving an adequate course of combined hydroxyurea and irradiation therapy will demonstrate concurrent leukopenia. Platelet depression (less than 100,000 cells/mm^3) has occurred rarely and only in the presence of marked leukopenia. Gastric distress has also been reported with irradiation alone and in combination with hydroxyurea therapy.

It should be borne in mind that therapeutic doses of irradiation alone produce the same adverse reactions as hydroxyurea; combined therapy may cause an increase in the incidence and severity of these side effects.

Although inflammation of the mucous membranes at the irradiated site (mucositis) is attributed to irradiation alone, some investigators believe that the more severe cases are due to combination therapy.

Dosage and Administration: Because of the rarity of melanoma, resistant chronic myelocytic leukemia, carcinoma of the ovary, and carcinomas of the head and neck in children, dosage regimens have not been established.

All dosage should be based on the patient's actual or ideal weight, whichever is less.

NOTE: If the patient prefers, or is unable to swallow capsules, the contents of the capsules may be emptied into a glass of water and taken immediately. Some inert material used as a vehicle in the capsule may not dissolve, and may float on the surface.

Solid Tumors

Intermittent Therapy: 80 mg./kg. administered orally as a *single* dose every *third* day

Continuous Therapy: 20 to 30 mg./kg. administered orally as a *single* dose *daily*

The intermittent dosage schedule offers the advantage of reduced toxicity since patients on this dosage regimen have rarely required complete discontinuance of therapy because of toxicity.

Concomitant Therapy with Irradiation (*Carcinoma of the head and neck*)—80 mg./kg. administered orally as a *single* dose every *third* day.

Administration of Hydrea (Hydroxyurea Capsules USP) should be begun at least seven days before initiation of irradiation and continued during radiotherapy as well as indefinitely afterwards provided that the patient may be kept under adequate observation and evidences no unusual or severe reactions.

Irradiation should be given at the maximum dose considered appropriate for the particular therapeutic situation; adjustment of irradiation dosage is not usually necessary when Hydrea is used concomitantly.

Resistant Chronic Myelocytic Leukemia

Until the intermittent therapy regimen has been evaluated, CONTINUOUS therapy (20 to 30 mg./kg. administered orally as a *single* dose *daily*) is recommended.

An adequate trial period for determining the antineoplastic effectiveness of Hydrea is 6 weeks of therapy. When there is regression in tumor size or arrest in tumor growth, therapy should be continued indefinitely. Therapy should be interrupted if the white blood cell count drops below 2500/mm^3, or the platelet count below 100,000/mm^3. In these cases, the counts should be re-checked after 3 days, and therapy resumed when the counts rise significantly toward normal values. Since the hematopoietic rebound is prompt, it is usually necessary to omit only a few doses. If prompt rebound has not occurred during combined hydroxyurea and irradiation therapy, irradiation may also be interrupted. However, the need for postponement of irradiation has been rare; radiotherapy has usually been continued using the recommended dosage and technique. Anemia, if it occurs, should be corrected with whole blood replacement, without interrupting hydroxyurea therapy. Because hematopoiesis may be compromised by extensive irradiation or by other antineoplastic agents, it is recommended that Hydrea be administered cautiously to patients who have recently received extensive radiation therapy or chemotherapy with other cytotoxic drugs.

Pain or discomfort from inflammation of the mucous membranes at the irradiated site (mucositis) is usually controlled by measures such as topical anesthetics and orally administered analgesics. If the reaction is severe, hydroxyurea therapy may be temporarily interrupted; if it is extremely severe, irradiation dosage may, in addition, be temporarily postponed. However, it has rarely been necessary to terminate these therapies.

Severe gastric distress, such as nausea, vomiting, and anorexia resulting from combined therapy may usually be controlled by temporary interruption of Hydrea (Hydroxyurea Capsules USP) administration; rarely has the additional interruption of irradiation been necessary.

How Supplied: Bottles of 100.

Storage: Store at room temperature; avoid excessive heat.

[*Shown in Product Identification Section*]

INSULIN, SQUIBB

Squibb carries a long line of U-40, U-80, and U-100 insulins. Squibb Insulins are manufactured under exacting quality controls and meet all official standards for purity, stability, consistency, and sterility. All U-40 insulins have red caps with labels printed in red. All U-80 insulins have green caps with labels printed in green. All U-100 insulins have orange caps with labels printed in black and with an identifying symbol: R = U-100 Insulin Injection, G = U-100 Globin Zinc Insulin Injection, N = U-100 Isophane Insulin Suspension, L = U-100 Lente® Insulin, P = U-100 Protamine Zinc Insulin Suspension, S = U-100 Semilente® Insulin, and U = U-100 Ultralente® Insulin. The following is a list along with a brief description of each of the insulin preparations available from Squibb.

INSULIN INJECTION USP

Insulin Injection USP (also called regular, unmodified, ordinary, or plain insulin) is a clear, colorless liquid. This is a fast-acting form of insulin with a short duration of action. Its ef-

fect is evident in approximately one-half to 1 hour, reaches its peak in approximately 2 to 3 hours, and persists for approximately 6 hours.
How Supplied: U-40 (40 units per ml.), U-80 (80 units per ml.), and U-100 (100 units per ml.) in 10 ml. vials.

GLOBIN ZINC INSULIN INJECTION USP

Globin Zinc Insulin Injection USP, also referred to as Globin Insulin with Zinc, is a clear, yellowish liquid. This is an intermediate acting form of insulin; its effect is evident in approximately 2 hours, reaches its peak in approximately 8 to 16 hours, and persists for approximately 24 hours.
How Supplied: U-40 (40 units per ml.), U-80 (80 units per ml.), and U-100 (100 units per ml.) in 10 ml. vials.

ISOPHANE INSULIN SUSPENSION USP
(NPH Insulin)

Isophane Insulin Suspension USP, also referred to as NPH Insulin, is a cloudy suspension. This is an intermediate acting form of insulin; its effect is evident in approximately one to one and one-half hours, reaches its peak in approximately 8 to 12 hours, and persists for approximately 24 hours.
How Supplied: U-40 (40 units per ml.), U-80 (80 units per ml.), and U-100 (100 units per ml.) in vials of 10 ml.

LENTE® Insulin
(Insulin Zinc Suspension USP)

Lente Insulin is a cloudy suspension. This is an intermediate acting form of insulin; its effect is evident in approximately one to one and one-half hours, reaches its peak in approximately 8 to 12 hours, and persists for approximately 24 hours.
How Supplied: U-40 (40 units per ml.), U-80 (80 units per ml.), and U-100 (100 units per ml.) in 10 ml. vials. [Lente® is licensed T.M. of Novo Terapeutisk Laboratorium A/S.]

PROTAMINE ZINC INSULIN SUSPENSION USP

Protamine Zinc Insulin Suspension USP, also referred to as PZI Insulin, is a cloudy suspension. This is a long acting form of insulin; its effect is evident in approximately 4 to 8 hours, reaches its peak in approximately 14 to 20 hours, and persists for approximately 36 hours.
How Supplied: U-40 (40 units per ml.), U-80 (80 units per ml.), and U-100 (100 units per ml.) in 10 ml. vials

SEMILENTE® Insulin
(Prompt Insulin Zinc Suspension USP)

Semilente Insulin is a cloudy suspension. This is a fast acting form of insulin with a short duration of action. Its effect is evident in approximately one-half to one hour, reaches its peak in approximately 5 to 7 hours, and persists for approximately 12 to 16 hours.
How Supplied: U-40 (40 units per ml.), U-80 (80 units per ml.), and U-100 (100 units per ml.) in 10 ml. vials.
[Semilente® is licensed T.M. of Novo Terapeutisk Laboratorium A/S.]

ULTRALENTE® Insulin
(Extended Insulin Zinc Suspension USP)

Ultralente Insulin is a cloudy suspension. This is a long acting form of insulin; its effect is evident in approximately 4 to 8 hours, reaches its peak in approximately 16 to 18 hours, and persists for more than 36 hours.
How Supplied: U-40 (40 units per ml.), U-80 (80 units per ml.), and U-100 (100 units per ml.) in 10 ml. vials.
[Ultralente® is licensed T.M. of Novo Terapeutisk Laboratorium A/S.]

KENACORT® TABLETS ℞
(Triamcinolone Tablets NF)
KENACORT® DIACETATE SYRUP ℞
(Triamcinolone Diacetate Syrup NF)

How Supplied: Kenacort Tablets are available in potencies of 2, 4, or 8 mg. triamcinolone per tablet; each tablet is scored to facilitate flexibility of dosage. The syrup provides 4.85 mg. triamcinolone diacetate anhydrous (equivalent to 4 mg. triamcinolone) per 5 ml. teaspoonful.
Kenacort Tablets (Triamcinolone Tablets NF) (scored), 2 mg., and 8 mg., bottles of 50; 4 mg., bottles of 30 and 100. Kenacort Diacetate Syrup (Triamcinolone Diacetate Syrup NF), bottles of 120 ml.

KENALOG® ℞
(Triamcinolone Acetonide)
CREAM/LOTION/OINTMENT/SPRAY

Description: Kenalog Creams, Lotions, Ointments, and Spray contain the active synthetic corticosteroid triamcinolone acetonide. Chemically, triamcinolone acetonide is pregna-1,4-diene-3,20-dione, 9-fluoro-11,21-dihydroxy-16, 17-[(1-methylethylidene) bis (oxy)]-, (11β,16α)-.
Each gram of Kenalog Cream 0.025% (Triamcinolone Acetonide Cream USP 0.025%), Kenalog Cream 0.1% (Triamcinolone Acetonide Cream USP 0.1%), and Kenalog Cream 0.5% (Triamcinolone Acetonide Cream USP 0.5%) provides 0.25 mg., 1 mg., or 5 mg. triamcinolone acetonide, respectively, in a vanishing cream base containing propylene glycol, cetearyl alcohol (and) ceteareth-20, white petrolatum, sorbitol solution, glyceryl monostearate, polyethylene glycol monostearate, simethicone, sorbic acid, and purified water.
Each ml. of Kenalog Lotion 0.025% (Triamcinolone Acetonide Lotion 0.025%) and Kenalog Lotion 0.1% (Triamcinolone Acetonide Lotion 0.1%) provides 0.25 mg. and 1 mg. triamcinolone acetonide, respectively, in a lotion base containing propylene glycol, cetyl alcohol, stearyl alcohol, sorbitan monopalmitate, polysorbate 20, simethicone, and purified water.
Each gram of Kenalog Ointment 0.025% (Triamcinolone Acetonide Ointment USP 0.025%), Kenalog Ointment 0.1% (Triamcinolone Acetonide Ointment USP 0.1%), and Kenalog Ointment 0.5% (Triamcinolone Acetonide Ointment USP 0.5%) provides 0.25 mg., 1 mg., or 5 mg. triamcinolone acetonide, respectively, in Plastibase® (Plasticized Hydrocarbon Gel), a polyethylene and mineral oil gel base.
Kenalog Spray (Triamcinolone Acetonide Aerosol NF) is **for dermatologic use only.** A two-second application, which covers an area approximately the size of the hand, delivers an amount of triaminolone acetonide not exceeding 0.2 mg. After spraying, the nonvolatile vehicle remaining on the skin contains approximately 0.2% triamcinolone acetonide. Each gram of spray provides 0.147 mg. triamcinolone acetonide in a vehicle of isopropyl palmitate, dehydrated alcohol (10.3%), and isobutane propellant.
Actions: Triamcinolone Acetonide Creams, Lotions, Ointments, and Spray are primarily effective because of their anti-inflammatory, antipruritic, and vasoconstrictive actions.
Indications: Triamcinolone Acetonide Cream 0.025%, 0.1%, and 0.5%, Triamcinolone Acetonide Lotion 0.025% and 0.1%, Triamcinolone Acetonide Ointment 0.025%, 0.1%, and 0.5%, and Triamcinolone Acetonide Aerosol Spray are indicated for relief of the inflammatory manifestations of corticosteroid-responsive dermatoses.
Contraindication: Topical steroids are contraindicated in those patients with a history of hypersensitivity to any of the components of the preparations.
Precautions: General—If irritation develops, the product should be discontinued and appropriate therapy instituted.
In the presence of an infection, the use of an appropriate antifungal or antibacterial agent should be instituted. If a favorable response does not occur promptly, the corticosteroid should be discontinued until the infection has been adequately controlled.
If extensive areas are treated or if the occlusive technique is used, there will be increased systemic absorption of the corticosteroid and suitable precautions should be taken, particularly in children and infants.
These preparations are not for ophthalmic use. When Kenalog Spray (Triamcinolone Acetonide Aerosol NF) is used about the face, the eyes should be covered and inhalation of the spray should be avoided.
Usage in Pregnancy—Although topical steroids have not been reported to have an adverse effect on human pregnancy, the safety of their use in pregnant women has not been absolutely established. In laboratory animals, increases in incidence of fetal abnormalities have been associated with exposure of gestating females to topical corticosteroids — in some cases at rather low dosage levels. Therefore, drugs of this class should not be used extensively on pregnant patients, in large amounts, or for prolonged periods of time.
Occlusive Dressing Technique—The use of occlusive dressings increases the percutaneous absorption of corticosteroids. For patients with extensive lesions it may be preferable to use a sequential approach, occluding one portion of the body at a time. The patient should be kept under close observation if treated with the occlusive technique over large areas and over a considerable period of time. Occasionally, a patient who has been on prolonged therapy, especially occlusive therapy, may develop symptoms of steroid withdrawal when the medication is stopped. Thermal homeostasis may be impaired if large areas of the body are covered. Use of the occlusive dressing should be discontinued if elevation of the body temperature occurs. Occasionally, a patient may develop a sensitivity reaction to a particular occlusive dressing material or adhesive and a substitute material may be necessary.
If infection develops, discontinue the use of the occlusive dressing and institute appropriate antimicrobial therapy.
Adverse Reactions: The following local adverse reactions have been reported with topical corticosteroids, especially under occlusive dressings: burning sensations, itching, irritation, dryness, folliculitis, hypertrichosis, acneform eruptions, hypopigmentation, perioral dermatitis, allergic contact dermatitis, maceration of the skin, secondary infection, skin atrophy, striae, and miliaria.
Dosage and Administration: Kenalog Cream 0.025% (Triamcinolone Acetonide Cream USP 0.025%): Apply to the affected area two to four times daily. Rub in gently.
Kenalog Cream 0.1% (Triamcinolone Acetonide Cream USP 0.1%) and Kenalog Cream 0.5% (Triamcinolone Acetonide Cream USP 0.5%): Apply, as appropriate, to the affected area two to three times daily. Rub in gently.
Kenalog Lotion 0.025% (Triamcinolone Acetonide Lotion 0.025%): Apply to the affected area two to four times daily. Rub in gently.
Kenalog Lotion 0.1% (Triamcinolone Acetonide Lotion 0.1%): Apply to the affected area two to three times daily. Rub in gently.
Kenalog Ointment 0.025% (Triamcinolone Acetonide Ointment USP 0.025%): Apply a thin film to the affected area two to four times daily.

Continued on next page

Squibb—Cont.

Kenalog Ointment 0.1% (Triamcinolone Acetonide Ointment USP 0.1%) and Kenalog Ointment 0.5% (Triamcinolone Acetonide Ointment USP 0.5%): Apply a thin film, as appropriate, to the affected area two to three times daily.

Kenalog Spray (Triamcinolone Acetonide Aerosol NF): Directions for the use of the spray can are provided on the label. The preparation may be applied to any area of the body, but when it is sprayed about the face, care should be taken to see that the eyes are covered, and that inhalation of the spray is avoided. Three or four applications daily are generally adequate.

Occlusive Dressing Technique: Kenalog Cream 0.025%, 0.1%, and 0.5% (Triamcinolone Acetonide Cream USP): Gently rub a small amount of the cream into the lesion until it disappears. Reapply the preparation leaving a thin coating on the lesion and cover with a pliable nonporous film. If needed, additional moisture may be provided by covering the lesion with a dampened clean cotton cloth before the plastic film is applied or by briefly soaking the affected area in water. The frequency of changing dressings is best determined on an individual basis. Reapplication is essential at each dressing change.

Kenalog Lotion 0.025% and 0.1% (Triamcinolone Acetonide Lotion): Gently rub a small amount of the lotion into the lesion until it disappears. Reapply the preparation leaving a thin coating on the lesion and cover with a pliable nonporous film. If needed, additional moisture may be provided by covering the lesion with a dampened clean cotton cloth before the plastic film is applied or by briefly soaking the affected area in water. The frequency of changing dressings is best determined on an individual basis. Reapplication is essential at each dressing change.

Kenalog Ointment, 0.025%, 0.1% and 0.5% (Triamcinolone Acetonide Ointment USP): Apply a thin coat of the ointment to the affected area and cover with a pliable nonporous film. If desired, the lesion may be moistened with a dampened clean cotton cloth before the ointment and plastic film are applied. The frequency of changing dressings is best determined on an individual basis. Reapplication is essential at each dressing change.

Kenalog Spray (Triamcinolone Acetonide Aerosol NF): Spray a small amount of the preparation into the lesion and cover with a pliable nonporous film. If needed, additional moisture may be provided by covering the lesion with a dampened clean cotton cloth before the plastic film is applied or by briefly soaking the affected area in water. The frequency of changing dressings is best determined on an individual basis. Reapplication is essential at each dressing change.

How Supplied:

0.025% Cream: Tubes of 15 g. and 80 g.; jars of 240 g. (8 oz.) and 2.38 kg. (5.25 lb.).

0.1% Cream: Tubes of 15 g., 60 g., and 80 g.; jars of 240 g. (8 oz.) and 2.38 kg. (5.25 lb.).

0.5% Cream: Tubes of 20 g. and jars of 240 g. (8 oz.).

0.025% Lotion: 60 ml. plastic squeeze bottles.

0.1% Lotion: 15 ml. and 60 ml. plastic squeeze bottles [60 ml. bottle, V.A. Depot Item NSN6505-00-282-5118A].

0.025% Ointment: Tubes of 15 g. and 80 g.; jars of 240 g. (8 oz.).

0.1% Ointment: Tubes of 15 g., 60 g., and 80 g.; jars of 240 g. (8 oz.) [240 g. jars, V.A. Depot Item, NSN6505-00-764-0598A].

0.5% Ointment: Tubes of 20 g. and jars of 240 g. (8 oz.).

Spray: Aerosol cans (each can supplied with a spray tube applicator) of 23 g. and 63 g. [63 g. cans, Military Depot Item, NSN6505-01-066-1325].

Storage: Store the creams and lotions at room temperature; avoid freezing. Store the ointments at room temperature. Store the spray at room temperature; avoid excessive heat.

KENALOG-H™ CREAM 0.1% ℞

(Triamcinolone Acetonide Cream USP 0.1%)

Description: Kenalog-H Cream 0.1% (Triamcinolone Acetonide Cream USP 0.1%) contains the active synthetic corticosteroid triamcinolone acetonide. Chemically, triamcinolone acetonide is pregna-1,4-diene-3,20-dione,9-fluoro-11,21-dihydroxy-16, 17-[(1-methylethylidene)bis(oxy)]-,(11β,16α)-.

Each gram of the cream provides 1 mg. triamcinolone acetonide in a specially formulated hydrophilic vanishing cream base containing propylene glycol, dimethicone 350, castor oil, cetearyl alcohol (and) ceteareth-20, propylene glycol stearate, white petrolatum, and purified water. This formulation is water-washable, greaseless, and nonstaining, with moisturizing and emollient properties.

Actions: Kenalog-H Cream 0.1% is primarily effective because of its anti-inflammatory, antipruritic, and vasoconstrictive actions.

Indications: Kenalog-H Cream 0.1% (Triamcinolone Acetonide Cream USP 0.1%) is indicated for relief of the inflammatory manifestations of corticosteroid-responsive dermatoses.

Contraindications: Topical steroids are contraindicated in those patients with a history of hypersensitivity to any of the components of the cream.

Precautions: General—If irritation develops, the product should be discontinued and appropriate therapy instituted.

In the presence of an infection, the use of an appropriate antifungal or antibacterial agent should be instituted. If a favorable response does not occur promptly, the corticosteroid should be discontinued until the infection has been adequately controlled.

If extensive areas are treated or if the occlusive technique is used, there will be increased systemic absorption of the corticosteroid and suitable precautions should be taken, particularly in children and infants.

The product is not for ophthalmic use.

Usage in Pregnancy—Although topical steroids have not been reported to have an adverse effect on human pregnancy, the safety of their use in pregnant women has not been absolutely established. In laboratory animals, increases in incidence of fetal abnormalities have been associated with exposure of gestating females to topical corticosteroids—in some cases, at rather low dosage levels. Therefore, drugs of this class should not be used extensively on pregnant patients, in large amounts, or for prolonged periods of time.

Occlusive Dressing Technique—The use of occlusive dressings increases the percutaneous absorption of corticosteroids. For patients with extensive lesions it may be preferable to use a sequential approach, occluding one portion of the body at a time. The patient should be kept under close observation if treated with the occlusive technique over large areas and over a considerable period of time. Occasionally, a patient who has been on prolonged therapy, especially occlusive therapy, may develop symptoms of steroid withdrawal when the medication is stopped. Thermal homeostasis may be impaired if large areas of the body are covered. Use of the occlusive dressing should be discontinued if elevation of the body temperature occurs. Occasionally, a patient may develop a sensitivity reaction to a particular occlusive dressing material or adhesive and a substitute material may be necessary.

If infection develops, discontinue the use of the occlusive dressing and institute appropriate antimicrobial therapy.

Adverse Reactions: The following local adverse reactions have been reported with topical corticosteroids, especially under occlusive dressings: burning sensations, itching, irritation, dryness, folliculitis, hypertrichosis, acneform eruptions, hypopigmentation, perioral dermatitis, allergic contact dermatitis, maceration of the skin, secondary infection, skin atrophy, striae, and miliaria.

Dosage and Administration: Apply Kenalog-H Cream 0.1% (Triamcinolone Acetonide Cream USP 0.1%) to the affected area two to three times daily. Rub in gently.

Occlusive Dressing Technique—Gently rub a small amount of the cream into the lesion until it disappears. Reapply the preparation leaving a thin coating on the lesion and cover with a pliable nonporous film. If needed, additional moisture may be provided by covering the lesion with a dampened clean cotton cloth before the plastic film is applied or by briefly soaking the affected area in water.

The frequency of changing dressings is best determined on an individual basis. Reapplication is essential at each dressing change.

How Supplied: Kenalog-H Cream 0.1% (Triamcinolone Acetonide Cream USP 0.1%) is supplied in 15 g. and 60 g. tubes.

Storage: Store at room temperature; avoid freezing.

KENALOG®-40 INJECTION ℞

(Sterile Triamcinolone Acetonide Suspension USP)

NOT FOR INTRAVENOUS OR INTRADERMAL USE

Description: Kenalog-40 Injection provides a synthetic corticosteroid with marked anti-inflammatory action. Each ml. of the sterile, aqueous suspension provides 40 mg. of triamcinolone acetonide, with sodium chloride for isotonicity, 0.9% (w/v) benzyl alcohol as a preservative, 0.75% sodium carboxymethylcellulose, and 0.04% polysorbate 80. Sodium hydroxide or hydrochloric acid may be present to adjust pH to 5.0 to 7.5. At the time of manufacture, the air in the container is replaced by nitrogen.

Actions: Naturally occurring glucocorticoids (hydrocortisone), which also have salt-retaining properties, are used as replacement therapy in adrenocortical deficiency states. Their synthetic analogs are primarily used for their potent anti-inflammatory effects in disorders of many organ systems.

Glucocorticoids cause profound and varied metabolic effects. In addition, they modify the body's immune responses to diverse stimuli.

Kenalog-40 Injection has an extended duration of effect which may be permanent, or sustained over a period of several weeks. Studies indicate that following a single intramuscular dose of 60 to 100 mg. of triamcinolone acetonide, adrenal suppression occurs within 24 to 48 hours and then gradually returns to normal, usually in 30 to 40 days. This finding correlates closely with the extended duration of therapeutic action achieved with the drug.

Indications:

Intramuscular

Where oral therapy is not feasible or is temporarily undesirable in the judgment of the physician, Kenalog-40 Injection (Sterile Triamcinolone Acetonide Suspension USP) is indicated for intramuscular use as follows:

1. *Endocrine disorders*—Primary or secondary adrenocortical insufficiency (hydrocortisone or cortisone is the drug of choice; synthetic analogs may be used in conjunction with mineralocorticoids where applicable; in infancy, mineralocorticoid supplementation is of particular importance).

Acute adrenocortical insufficiency (hydrocortisone or cortisone is the drug of choice; mineralocorticoid supplementation may be necessary, particularly when synthetic analogs are used).

Preoperatively and in the event of serious trauma or illness, in patients with known adrenal insufficiency or when adrenocortical reserve is doubtful.
Shock unresponsive to conventional therapy if adrenocortical insufficiency exists or is suspected.
Congenital adrenal hyperplasia. Nonsuppurative thyroiditis.
2. *Rheumatic disorders*—As adjunctive therapy for short-term administration (to tide the patient over an acute episode or exacerbation) in: posttraumatic osteoarthritis; synovitis of osteoarthritis; rheumatoid arthritis; acute and subacute bursitis; epicondylitis; acute nonspecific tenosynovitis; acute gouty arthritis; psoriatic arthritis; ankylosing spondylitis; juvenile rheumatoid arthritis.
3. *Collagen diseases*—During an exacerbation or as maintenance therapy in selected cases of: systemic lupus erythematosus; acute rheumatic carditis.
4. *Dermatologic diseases*—Pemphigus; severe erythema multiforme (Stevens-Johnson syndrome); exfoliative dermatitis; bullous dermatitis herpetiformis; severe seborrheic dermatitis; severe psoriasis.
5. *Allergic states*—Control of severe or incapacitating allergic conditions intractable to adequate trials of conventional treatment in: bronchial asthma; contact dermatitis; atopic dermatitis; serum sickness; seasonal or perennial allergic rhinitis; drug hypersensitivity reactions; urticarial transfusion reactions; acute noninfectious laryngeal edema (epinephrine is the drug of first choice).
6. *Ophthalmic diseases*—Severe acute and chronic allergic and inflammatory processes involving the eye, such as: herpes zoster ophthalmicus; iritis; irridocyclitis; chorioretinitis; diffuse posterior uveitis and choroiditis; optic neuritis; sympathetic ophthalmia; anterior segment inflammation.
7. *Gastrointestinal diseases*—To tide the patient over a critical period of disease in: ulcerative colitis (systemic therapy); regional enteritis (systemic therapy).
8. *Respiratory diseases*—Symptomatic sarcoidosis; berylliosis; fulminating or disseminated pulmonary tuberculosis when concurrently accompanied by appropriate antituberculous chemotherapy; aspiration pneumonitis.
9. *Hematologic disorders*—Acquired (autoimmune) hemolytic anemia.
10. *Neoplastic diseases*—For palliative management of: leukemias and lymphomas in adults; acute leukemia of childhood.
11. *Edematous state*—To induce diuresis or remission of proteinuria in the nephrotic syndrome, without uremia, of the idiopathic type or that due to lupus erythematosus.
12. *Miscellaneous*—Tuberculous meningitis with subarachnoid block or impending block when concurrently accompanied by appropriate antituberculous chemotherapy.

Intra-Articular

Kenalog-40 Injection (Sterile Triamcinolone Acetonide Suspension USP) is indicated for intra-articular or intrabursal administration, and for injections into tendon sheaths, as adjunctive therapy for short-term administration (to tide the patient over an acute episode or exacerbation) in: synovitis of osteoarthritis; rheumatoid arthritis; acute and subacute bursitis; acute gouty arthritis; epicondylitis; acute nonspecific tenosynovitis; posttraumatic osteoarthritis.

Contraindications: Corticosteroids are contraindicated in patients with systemic fungal infections. Intramuscular corticosteroid preparations are contraindicated for idiopathic thrombocytopenic purpura.

Warnings: Because it is a suspension, the preparation should **not** be administered intravenously. Strict aseptic technique is mandatory. This preparation is not recommended for children under six years of age.
When patients who are receiving corticosteroid therapy are subjected to unusual stress, increased dosage of rapidly acting corticosteroids is indicated before, during, and after the stressful situation.
Corticosteroids may mask some signs of infection, and new infections may appear during their use. There may be decreased resistance and inability to localize infection when corticosteroids are used. If an infection occurs during corticosteroid therapy, it should be promptly controlled by suitable antimicrobial therapy (see PRECAUTIONS).
Prolonged use of corticosteroids may produce posterior subcapsular cataracts, glaucoma with possible damage to the optic nerves, and may enhance the establishment of secondary ocular infections due to fungi or viruses.
Average and large doses of hydrocortisone or cortisone can cause elevation of blood pressure, salt and water retention, and increased excretion of potassium. These effects are less likely to occur with the synthetic derivatives except when they are used in large doses; dietary salt restriction and potassium supplementation may be necessary (see PRECAUTIONS). All corticosteroids increase calcium excretion.
Patients should not be vaccinated against smallpox while on corticosteroid therapy. Other immunization procedures should not be undertaken in patients who are on corticosteroids, especially on high dose, because of possible hazards of neurological complications and a lack of antibody response.
The use of triamcinolone acetonide in patients with active tuberculosis should be restricted to those cases of fulminating or disseminated tuberculosis in which the corticosteroid is used for the management of the disease in conjunction with an appropriate antituberculous regimen. If corticosteroids are indicated in patients with latent tuberculosis or tuberculin reactivity, close observation is necessary since reactivation of the disease may occur. During prolonged corticosteroid therapy, these patients should receive chemoprophylaxis.
Because rare instances of anaphylactoid reactions have occurred in patients receiving parenteral corticosteroid therapy, appropriate precautionary measures should be taken prior to administration, especially when the patient has a history of allergy to any drug.
Unless a **deep** intramuscular injection is given, local atrophy is likely to occur. (For recommendations on injection techniques, see DOSAGE AND ADMINISTRATION.) Due to the significantly higher incidence of local atrophy when the material is injected into the deltoid area, this injection site should be avoided in favor of the gluteal area. Only very unusual circumstances would warrant injection into the deltoid area.

Usage in Pregnancy: Since adequate human reproduction studies have not been done with corticosteroids, the use of these drugs in pregnancy, nursing mothers, or women of childbearing potential requires that the possible benefits of the drug be weighed against the potential hazards to the mother and the embryo, fetus, or nursing infant. Infants born of mothers who have received substantial doses of corticosteroids during pregnancy should be carefully observed for signs of hypoadrenalism.

Precautions: Drug-induced secondary adrenocortical insufficiency may be minimized by a gradual reduction of dosage. This type of relative insufficiency may persist for months after discontinuation of therapy; therefore, in any situation of stress (such as trauma, surgery, or severe illness) occurring during that period, hormone therapy should be reinstituted. Since mineralocorticoid secretion may be impaired, salt and/or a mineralocorticoid should be administered concurrently.
There is an enhanced corticosteroid effect in patients with hypothyroidism and in those with cirrhosis.
Corticosteroids should be used cautiously in patients with ocular herpes simplex because of possible corneal perforation.
The lowest possible dose of corticosteroid should be used to control the condition being treated. A gradual reduction in dosage should be made when possible.
Psychic derangements may appear when corticosteroids are used. These may range from euphoria, insomnia, mood swings, personality changes and severe depression to frank psychotic manifestations. Existing emotional instability or psychotic tendencies may also be aggravated by corticosteroids.
Aspirin should be used cautiously in conjunction with corticosteroids in patients with hypoprothrombinemia.
Corticosteroids should be used with caution in patients with nonspecific ulcerative colitis if there is a probability of impending perforation, abscess, or other pyogenic infection. Corticosteroids should also be used cautiously in patients with diverticulitis, fresh intestinal anastomoses, active or latent peptic ulcer, renal insufficiency, hypertension, osteoporosis, acute glomerulonephritis, vaccinia, varicella, exanthema, Cushing's syndrome, antibiotic resistant infections, diabetes mellitus, congestive heart failure, chronic nephritis, thromboembolitic tendencies, thrombophlebitis, convulsive disorders, metastatic carcinoma, and myasthenia gravis.
Growth and development of infants and children on prolonged corticosteroid therapy should be carefully observed.
Although therapy with Kenalog-40 Injection (Sterile Triamcinolone Acetonide Suspension USP) will ameliorate symptoms, it is in no sense a cure and the hormone has no effect on the cause of the inflammation. Therefore, this method of treatment does not obviate the need for the conventional measures usually employed.
Intra-articular injection of a corticosteroid may produce systemic as well as local effects.
The inadvertent injection of the suspension into the soft tissues surrounding a joint is not harmful, but may lead to the occurrence of systemic effects, and is the most common cause of failure to achieve the desired local results.
Following intra-articular steroid therapy, patients should be specifically warned to avoid overuse of joints in which symptomatic benefit has been obtained. Negligence in this matter may permit an increase in joint deterioration that will more than offset the beneficial effects of the steroid. To detect deterioration, follow-up x-ray examination is suggested in selected cases.
Overdistention of the joint capsule and deposition of steroid along the needle track should be avoided in intra-articular injection since this may lead to subcutaneous atrophy.
Corticosteroids should not be injected into unstable joints. Repeated intra-articular injection may in some cases result in instability of the joint. In selected cases, particularly when repeated injections are given, x-ray follow-up is suggested.
An increase in joint discomfort has seldom occurred. A marked increase in pain accompanied by local swelling, further restriction of joint motion, fever, and malaise are suggestive of a septic arthritis. If these complications should appear, and the diagnosis of septic arthritis is confirmed, administration of triamcinolone acetonide should be stopped, and antimicrobial therapy should be instituted immediately and continued for 7 to 10 days after all evidence of infection has disappeared. Appropriate examination of any joint fluid present is necessary to exclude a septic process.
Local injection of a steroid into a previously infected joint is to be avoided.

Continued on next page

Squibb—Cont.

Kenalog-40 Injection (Sterile Triamcinolone Acetonide Suspension USP) should be administered only with full knowledge of characteristic activity of, and varied responses to, adrenocortical hormones. Like other potent corticosteroids, triamcinolone acetonide should be used under close clinical supervision. Triamcinolone acetonide can cause elevation of blood pressure, salt and water retention, and increased potassium and calcium excretion necessitating dietary salt restriction and potassium supplementation. Edema may occur in the presence of renal disease with a fixed or decreased glomerular filtration rate.
During prolonged therapy, **a liberal protein intake is essential** for counteracting the tendency to gradual weight loss sometimes associated with negative nitrogen balance, wasting and weakness of skeletal muscles.
When local or systemic microbial infections are present, therapy with triamcinolone acetonide is not recommended, but may be employed with caution and only in conjunction with appropriate antibiotic or chemotherapeutic medication. Triamcinolone acetonide may mask signs of infection and enhance dissemination of the infecting organism. Hence, all patients receiving triamcinolone acetonide should be watched for evidence of intercurrent infection. Should infection occur, vigorous, appropriate anti-infective therapy should be initiated. If possible, abrupt cessation of steroids should be avoided because of the danger of superimposing adrenocortical insufficiency on the infectious process.
Menstrual irregularities may occur, and this possibility should be mentioned to female patients past menarche.
In peptic ulcer, recurrence may be asymptomatic until perforation or hemorrhage occurs. Long-term adrenocorticoid therapy may evoke hyperacidity or peptic ulcer; therefore, as a prophylactic measure, an ulcer regimen and the administration of an antacid are highly recommended. X-rays should be taken in peptic ulcer patients complaining of gastric distress, or when therapy is prolonged. Whether or not changes are observed, an ulcer regimen is recommended.
As with other corticosteroids, the possibility of other severe reactions should be considered. If such reactions should occur, appropriate corrective measures should be instituted and use of the drug discontinued.
Continued supervision of the patient after termination of triamcinolone acetonide therapy is essential, since there may be a sudden reappearance of severe manifestations of the disease for which the patient was treated.
Adverse Reactions: Following Administration by Any Route — Patients should be watched closely for the following adverse reactions which may be associated with any corticosteroid therapy:
Fluid and electrolyte disturbances — sodium retention, fluid retention, congestive heart failure in susceptible patients, potassium loss, cardiac arrhythmias or ECG changes due to potassium deficiency, hypokalemic alkalosis, and hypertension.
Musculoskeletal — muscle weakness, fatigue, steroid myopathy, loss of muscle mass, osteoporosis, vertebral compression fractures, delayed healing of fractures, aseptic necrosis of femoral and humeral heads, pathologic fractures of long bones, and spontaneous fractures.
Gastrointestinal — peptic ulcer with possible subsequent perforation and hemorrhage, pancreatitis, abdominal distention, and ulcerative esophagitis.
Dermatologic — impaired wound healing, thin fragile skin, petechiae and ecchymoses, facial erythema, increased sweating, purpura, striae, hirsutism, acneform eruptions, lupus erythematosus-like lesions and suppressed reactions to skin tests.
Neurological — convulsions, increased intracranial pressure with papilledema (pseudotumor cerebri) usually after treatment, vertigo, headache, neuritis or paresthesias, and aggravation of pre-existing psychiatric conditions.
Endocrine — menstrual irregularities; development of the cushingoid state; suppression of growth in children; secondary adrenocortical and pituitary unresponsiveness, particularly in times of stress (e.g., trauma, surgery, or illness); decreased carbohydrate tolerance; manifestations of latent diabetes mellitus and increased requirements for insulin or oral hypoglycemic agents in diabetics.
Ophthalmic — posterior subcapsular cataracts, increased intraocular pressure, glaucoma, and exophthalmos.
Metabolic — hyperglycemia, glycosuria, and negative nitrogen balance due to protein catabolism.
Others — necrotizing angiitis, thrombophlebitis, thromboembolism, aggravation or masking of infections, insomnia, syncopal episodes, and anaphylactoid reactions.
Following Intramuscular Administration — Severe pain has been reported in a few cases. Sterile abscess formation, subcutaneous and cutaneous atrophy, hyperpigmentation and hypopigmentation and charcot-like arthropathy have also occurred.
Following Intra-articular Administration — Undesirable reactions have included postinjection flare, transient pain, occasional irritation at the injection site, sterile abscess formation, hyperpigmentation and hypopigmentation, charcot-like arthropathy and occasional brief increase in joint discomfort.

Dosage and Administration:

General

The initial dose of Kenalog-40 Injection (Sterile Triamcinolone Acetonide Suspension USP) may vary from 2.5 to 60 mg. per day depending on the specific disease entity being treated (see **Dosage** section below). In situations of less severity, lower doses will generally suffice while in selected patients higher initial doses may be required. Usually the parenteral dosage ranges are one-third to one-half the oral dose given every 12 hours. However, in certain overwhelming, acute, life-threatening situations, administration of dosages exceeding the usual dosages may be justified and may be in multiples of the oral dosages.
The initial dosage should be maintained or adjusted until a satisfactory response is noted. If after a reasonable period of time there is a lack of satisfactory clinical response, Kenalog-40 Injection should be discontinued and the patient transferred to other appropriate therapy. **IT SHOULD BE EMPHASIZED THAT DOSAGE REQUIREMENTS ARE VARIABLE AND MUST BE INDIVIDUALIZED ON THE BASIS OF THE DISEASE UNDER TREATMENT AND THE RESPONSE OF THE PATIENT.** After a favorable response is noted, the proper maintenance dosage should be determined by decreasing the initial drug dosage in small increments at appropriate time intervals until the lowest dosage which will maintain an adequate clinical response is reached. It should be kept in mind that constant monitoring is needed in regard to drug dosage. Included in the situations which may make dosage adjustments necessary are changes in clinical status secondary to remissions or exacerbations in the disease process, the patient's individual drug responsiveness, and the effect of patient exposure to stressful situations not directly related to the disease entity under treatment; in this latter situation it may be necessary to increase the dosage of Kenalog-40 Injection for a period of time consistent with the patient's condition. If after long-term therapy the drug is to be stopped, it is recommended that it be withdrawn gradually rather than abruptly.

Dosage

Systemic: Although Kenalog-40 Injection (Sterile Triamcinolone Acetonide Suspension USP) may be administered intramuscularly for initial therapy, most physicians prefer to adjust the dose orally until adequate control is attained. Intramuscular administration provides a sustained or depot action which can be used to supplement or replace initial oral therapy. With intramuscular therapy, greater supervision of the amount of steroid used is made possible in the patient who is inconsistent in following an oral dosage schedule. In maintenance therapy, the patient-to-patient response is not uniform and, therefore, the dose must be individualized for optimal control.
For **adults and children over 12 years of age,** the suggested initial dose is 60 mg., **injected deeply into the gluteal muscle.** Subcutaneous fat atrophy may occur if care is not taken to inject the preparation intramuscularly. Dosage is usually adjusted within the range of 40 to 80 mg., depending upon patient response and duration of relief. However, some patients may be well controlled on dosages as low as 20 mg. or less. Patients with hay fever or pollen asthma who are not responding to pollen administration and other conventional therapy may obtain a remission of symptoms lasting throughout the pollen season after one injection of 40 to 100 mg.
For **children from 6 to 12 years of age,** the suggested initial dose is 40 mg., although dosage depends more on the severity of symptoms than on age or weight. There is insufficient clinical experience with Kenalog-40 Injection to recommend its use in children under six years of age.
Local: For intra-articular or intrabursal administration and for injection into tendon sheaths, the initial dose of Kenalog-40 Injection (Sterile Triamcinolone Acetonide Suspension USP) may vary from 2.5 to 5 mg. for smaller joints and from 5 to 15 mg. for larger joints depending on the specific disease entity being treated. (A more dilute form of Sterile Triamcinolone Acetonide Suspension USP is available—see ALSO AVAILABLE.) For adults, doses up to 10 mg. for smaller areas and up to 40 mg. for larger areas have usually been sufficient to alleviate symptoms. Single injections into several joints for multiple locus involvement, up to a total of 80 mg., have been given without undue reactions. A single local injection of triamcinolone acetonide is frequently sufficient, but several injections may be needed for adequate relief of symptoms. The lower dosages in the initial dosage range of triamcinolone acetonide may produce the desired effect when the corticosteroid is administered to provide a localized concentration. The site of the injection and the volume of the injection should be carefully considered when triamcinolone acetonide is administered for this purpose.

Administration

General: Shake the vial before use to insure a uniform suspension. After withdrawal, inject without delay to prevent settling in the syringe. Careful technique should be employed to avoid the possibility of entering a blood vessel or introducing infection.
Routine laboratory studies, such as urinalysis, two-hour postprandial blood sugar, determination of blood pressure and body weight and a chest x-ray should be made at regular intervals during prolonged therapy. Upper GI x-rays are desirable in patients with an ulcer history or significant dyspepsia.
Systemic: For systemic therapy, injection should be made **deeply into the gluteal muscle** to insure intramuscular delivery (see WARNINGS). For adults, a minimum needle length of 1 ½ inches is recommended. In obese patients, a longer needle may be required. Use alternate sites for subsequent injections.
Local: For treatment of joints, the usual intra-articular injection technique, as described

in standard textbooks, should be followed. If an excessive amount of synovial fluid is present in the joint, some, but not all, should be aspirated to aid in the relief of pain and to prevent undue dilution of the corticosteroid.

With intra-articular or intrabursal administration, and with injection of the drug into tendon sheaths, the use of a local anesthetic may often be desirable. When a local anesthetic is used, its package insert should be read with care and all the precautions connected with its use should be observed. It should be injected into the surrounding soft tissues prior to the injection of the corticosteroid. A small amount of the anesthetic solution may be instilled into the joint.

In treating acute nonspecific tenosynovitis, care should be taken to insure that the injection of the corticosteroid is made into the tendon sheath rather than the tendon substance.

Epicondylitis (tennis elbow) may be treated by infiltrating the preparation into the area of greatest tenderness.

How Supplied: In vials of 1, 5, and 10 ml. [5 ml. vial—Military Depot Item, NSN 6505-00-885-6216 and V.A. Depot Item, NSN6505-00-885-6216A].

Also Available: Kenalog-10 Injection (Sterile Triamcinolone Acetonide Suspension USP) providing 10 mg. triamcinolone acetonide per ml., with sodium chloride for isotonicity, 0.9% (w/v) benzyl alcohol as a preservative, 0.75% sodium carboxymethylcellulose, and 0.04% polysorbate 80. See package insert for full information.

Storage: Store at room temperature; avoid freezing.

KENALOG®-10 INJECTION ℞
(Sterile Triamcinolone Acetonide Suspension USP)
NOT FOR INTRAVENOUS USE

Description: Kenalog-10 Injection provides a synthetic corticosteroid with marked anti-inflammatory action. Each ml. of the sterile aqueous suspension provides 10 mg. triamcinolone acetonide, with sodium chloride for isotonicity, 0.9% (w/v) benzyl alcohol as a preservative, 0.75% sodium carboxymethylcellulose, and 0.04% polysorbate 80; sodium hydroxide or hydrochloric acid may be present to adjust pH. At the time of manufacture, the air in the container is replaced by nitrogen.

Actions: Naturally occurring glucocorticoids (hydrocortisone), which also have salt-retaining properties, are used as replacement therapy in adrenocortical deficiency states. Their synthetic analogs are primarily used for their potent anti-inflammatory effects in disorders of many organ systems.

Glucocorticoids cause profound and varied metabolic effects. In addition, they modify the body's immune responses to diverse stimuli.

Indications: Intra-Articular—Kenalog-10 Injection is indicated for intra-articular or intrabursal administration, and for injections into tendon sheaths, as adjunctive therapy for short-term administration (to tide the patient over an acute episode or exacerbation) in: synovitis of osteoarthritis, rheumatoid arthritis, acute and subacute bursitis, acute gouty arthritis, epicondylitis, acute nonspecific tenosynovitis, and post-traumatic osteoarthritis.

Intradermal—Intralesional administration of Kenalog-10 Injection is indicated for the treatment of keloids, discoid lupus erythematosus, necrobiosis lipoidica diabeticorum, alopecia areata, and localized hypertrophic, infiltrated, inflammatory lesions of: lichen planus, psoriatic plaques, granuloma annulare, and lichen simplex chronicus (neurodermatitis).

Contraindications: Corticosteroids are contraindicated in patients with systemic fungal infections.

Warnings: Because it is a suspension, the preparation should *not* be administered intravenously. Strict aseptic technique is mandatory.

When patients who are receiving corticosteroid therapy are subjected to unusual stress, increased dosage of rapidly acting corticosteroids is indicated before, during, and after the stressful situation.

Corticosteroids may mask some signs of infection, and new infections may appear during their use. There may be decreased resistance and inability to localize infection when corticosteroids are used. If an infection occurs during corticosteroid therapy, it should be promptly controlled by suitable antimicrobial therapy (see PRECAUTIONS).

Prolonged use of corticosteroids may produce posterior subcapsular cataracts, glaucoma with possible damage to the optic nerves, and may enhance the establishment of secondary ocular infections due to fungi or viruses.

Average and large doses of hydrocortisone or cortisone can cause elevation of blood pressure, salt and water retention, and increased excretion of potassium. These effects are less likely to occur with the synthetic derivatives except when they are used in large doses; dietary salt restriction and potassium supplementation may be necessary (see PRECAUTIONS). All corticosteroids increase calcium excretion.

Patients should not be vaccinated against smallpox while on corticosteroid therapy. Other immunization procedures should not be undertaken in patients who are on corticosteroids, especially on high dose, because of possible hazards of neurological complications and a lack of antibody response.

The use of triamcinolone acetonide in patients with active tuberculosis should be restricted to those cases of fulminating or disseminated tuberculosis in which the corticosteroid is used for the management of the disease in conjunction with an appropriate antituberculous regimen. If corticosteroids are indicated in patients with latent tuberculosis or tuberculin reactivity, close observation is necessary since reactivation of the disease may occur. During prolonged corticosteroid therapy these patients should receive chemoprophylaxis.

Because rare instances of anaphylactoid reactions have occurred in patients receiving parenteral corticosteroid therapy, appropriate precautionary measures should be taken prior to administration, especially when the patient has a history of allergy to any drug.

Usage in Pregnancy—Since adequate human reproduction studies have not been done with corticosteroids, the use of these drugs in pregnancy, nursing mothers, or women of childbearing potential requires that the possible benefits of the drug be weighed against the potential hazards to the mother and the embryo, fetus, or nursing infant. Infants born of mothers who have received substantial doses of corticosteroids during pregnancy should be carefully observed for signs of hypoadrenalism.

Precautions: Drug-induced secondary adrenocortical insufficiency may be minimized by a gradual reduction of dosage. This type of relative insufficiency may persist for months after discontinuation of therapy; therefore, in any situation of stress (such as trauma, surgery, or severe illness) occurring during that period, hormone therapy should be reinstituted. Since mineralocorticoid secretion may be impaired, salt and/or a mineralocorticoid should be administered concurrently.

There is an enhanced corticosteroid effect in patients with hypothyroidism and in those with cirrhosis.

Corticosteroids should be used cautiously in patients with ocular herpes simplex because of possible corneal perforation.

The lowest possible dose of corticosteroid should be used to control the condition being treated. A gradual reduction in dosage should be made when possible.

Psychic derangements may appear when corticosteroids are used. These may range from euphoria, insomnia, mood swings, personality changes, and severe depression, to frank psychotic manifestations. Existing emotional instability or psychotic tendencies may also be aggravated by corticosteroids.

Aspirin should be used cautiously in conjunction with corticosteroids in patients with hypoprothrombinemia.

Corticosteroids should be used with caution in patients with nonspecific ulcerative colitis if there is a probability of impending perforation, abscess, or other pyogenic infection. Corticosteroids should also be used cautiously in patients with diverticulitis, fresh intestinal anastomoses, active or latent peptic ulcer, renal insufficiency, hypertension, osteoporosis, acute glomerulonephritis, vaccinia, varicella, exanthema, Cushing's syndrome, antibiotic resistant infections, diabetes mellitus, congestive heart failure, chronic nephritis, thromboembolitic tendencies, thrombophlebitis, convulsive disorders, metastatic carcinoma, and myasthenia gravis.

Growth and development of infants and children on prolonged corticosteroid therapy should be carefully observed.

Although therapy with Kenalog-10 Injection (Sterile Triamcinolone Acetonide Suspension USP) will ameliorate symptoms, it is in no sense a cure and the hormone has no effect on the cause of the inflammation. Therefore, this method of treatment does not obviate the need for the conventional measures usually employed.

Intra-articular injection of a corticosteroid may produce systemic as well as local effects. The inadvertent injection of the suspension into the soft tissues surrounding a joint is not harmful, but may lead to the occurrence of systemic effects, and is the most common cause of failure to achieve the desired local results.

Following intra-articular steroid therapy, patients should be specifically warned to avoid overuse of joints in which symptomatic benefit has been obtained. Negligence in this matter may permit an increase in joint deterioration that will more than offset the beneficial effects of the steroid. To detect deterioration, follow-up x-ray examination is suggested in selected cases.

Overdistention of the joint capsule and deposition of steroid along the needle track should be avoided in intra-articular injection since this may lead to subcutaneous atrophy.

Corticosteroids should not be injected into unstable joints. Repeated intra-articular injection may in some cases result in instability of the joint. In selected cases, particularly when repeated injections are given, x-ray follow-up is suggested.

An increase in joint discomfort has seldom occurred. A marked increase in pain accompanied by local swelling, further restriction of joint motion, fever, and malaise are suggestive of a septic arthritis. If these complications should appear, and the diagnosis of septic arthritis is confirmed, administration of triamcinolone acetonide should be stopped, and antimicrobial therapy should be instituted immediately and continued for 7 to 10 days after all evidence of infection has disappeared. Appropriate examination of any joint fluid present is necessary to exclude a septic process.

Local injection of a steroid into a previously infected joint is to be avoided.

Kenalog-10 Injection (Sterile Triamcinolone Acetonide Suspension USP) should be administered only with full knowledge of characteristic activity of, and varied responses to, adrenocortical hormones. Like other potent corticosteroids, triamcinolone acetonide should be used under close clinical supervision. Triamcinolone acetonide can cause elevation of blood

Continued on next page

Squibb—Cont.

pressure, salt and water retention, and increased potassium and calcium excretion necessitating dietary salt restriction and potassium supplementation. Edema may occur in the presence of renal disease with a fixed or decreased glomerular filtration rate.
During prolonged therapy, *a liberal protein intake is essential* for counteracting the tendency to gradual weight loss sometimes associated with negative nitrogen balance, wasting and weakness of skeletal muscles.
When local or systemic microbial infections are present, therapy with triamcinolone acetonide is not recommended, but may be employed with caution and only in conjunction with appropriate antibiotic or chemotherapeutic medication. Triamcinolone acetonide may mask signs of infection and enhance dissemination of the infecting organism. Hence, all patients receiving triamcinolone acetonide should be watched for evidence of intercurrent infection. Should infection occur, vigorous, appropriate anti-infective therapy should be initiated. If possible, abrupt cessation of steroids should be avoided because of the danger of superimposing adrenocortical insufficiency on the infectious process.
Menstrual irregularities may occur, and this possibility should be mentioned to female patients past menarche.
In peptic ulcer, recurrence may be asymptomatic until perforation or hemorrhage occurs. Long-term adrenocorticoid therapy may evoke hyperacidity or peptic ulcer; therefore, as a prophylactic measure, an ulcer regimen and the administration of an antacid are highly recommended. X-rays should be taken in peptic ulcer patients complaining of gastric distress, or when therapy is prolonged. Whether or not changes are observed, an ulcer regimen is recommended.
As with other corticosteroids, the possibility of other severe reactions should be considered. If such reactions should occur, appropriate corrective measures should be instituted and use of the drug discontinued.
Continued supervision of the patient after termination of triamcinolone acetonide therapy is essential since there may be a sudden reappearance of severe manifestations of the disease for which the patient was treated.
Adverse Reactions: Undesirable reactions following intra-articular administration of the preparation have included post-injection flare, transient pain, occasional local irritation at the injection site, sterile abscesses, hyper- and hypopigmentation, charcot-like arthropathy, and occasional brief increase in joint discomfort; following intradermal administration, rare instances of blindness associated with intralesional therapy around the face and head, transient local discomfort, sterile abscesses, hyper- and hypopigmentation, and subcutaneous and cutaneous atrophy (which usually disappears, unless the basic disease process is itself atrophic) have occurred.
Since systemic absorption may occasionally occur with intra-articular or other local administration, patients should be watched closely for the following adverse reactions which may be associated with any corticosteroid therapy:
Fluid and electrolyte disturbances—sodium retention, fluid retention, congestive heart failure in susceptible patients, potassium loss, cardiac arrhythmias or ECG changes due to potassium deficiency, hypokalemic alkalosis, and hypertension.
Musculoskeletal—muscle weakness, fatigue, steroid myopathy, loss of muscle mass, osteoporosis, vertebral compression fractures, delayed healing of fractures, aseptic necrosis of femoral and humeral heads, pathologic fractures of long bones, and spontaneous fractures.
Gastrointestinal—peptic ulcer with possible subsequent perforation and hemorrhage, pancreatitis, abdominal distention, and ulcerative esophagitis.
Dermatologic—impaired wound healing, thin fragile skin, petechiae and ecchymoses, facial erythema, increased sweating, purpura, striae, hirsutism, acneform eruptions, lupus erythematosus-like lesions and suppressed reactions to skin tests.
Neurological—convulsions, increased intracranial pressure with papilledema (pseudo-tumor cerebri) usually after treatment, vertigo, headache, neuritis or paresthesias, and aggravation of pre-existing psychiatric conditions.
Endocrine—menstrual irregularities; development of the cushingoid state; suppression of growth in children; secondary adrenocortical and pituitary unresponsiveness, particularly in times of stress (e.g., trauma, surgery, or illness); decreased carbohydrate tolerance; manifestations of latent diabetes mellitus and increased requirements for insulin or oral hypoglycemic agents in diabetics.
Ophthalmic—posterior subcapsular cataracts, increased intraocular pressure, glaucoma, and exophthalmos.
Metabolic—hyperglycemia, glycosuria, and negative nitrogen balance due to protein catabolism.
Others—necrotizing angiitis, thrombophlebitis, thromboembolism, aggravation or masking of infections, insomnia, syncopal episodes, and anaphylactoid reactions.
Dosage and Administration:
Dosage: The initial dose of Kenalog-10 Injection (Sterile Triamcinolone Acetonide Suspension USP) for intra-articular or intrabursal administration and for injection into tendon sheaths may vary from 2.5 mg. to 5 mg. for smaller joints and from 5 to 15 mg. for larger joints depending on the specific disease entity being treated. Single injections into several joints for multiple locus involvement, up to a total of 20 mg. or more, have been given without incident. For intradermal administration, the initial dose of triamcinolone acetonide will vary depending upon the specific disease entity being treated but should be limited to 1.0 mg. (0.1 ml.) per injection site, since larger volumes are more likely to produce cutaneous atrophy. Multiple sites (separated by one centimeter or more) may be so injected, keeping in mind that the greater the *total* volume employed the more corticosteroid becomes available for possible systemic absorption and subsequent corticosteroid effects. Such injections may be repeated, if necessary, at weekly or less frequent intervals.
The lower dosages in the initial dosage range of triamcinolone acetonide may produce the desired effect when the corticosteroid is administered to provide a localized concentration. The site of the injection and the volume of the injection should be carefully considered when triamcinolone acetonide is administered for this purpose. The initial dosage should be maintained or adjusted until a satisfactory response is noted. If after a reasonable period of time there is a lack of satisfactory clinical response, Kenalog-10 Injection should be discontinued and the patient transferred to other appropriate therapy. IT SHOULD BE EMPHASIZED THAT DOSAGE REQUIREMENTS ARE VARIABLE AND MUST BE INDIVIDUALIZED ON THE BASIS OF THE DISEASE UNDER TREATMENT AND THE RESPONSE OF THE PATIENT. After a favorable response is noted, the proper maintenance dosage should be determined by decreasing the initial drug dosage in small increments at appropriate time intervals until the lowest dosage which will maintain an adequate clinical response is reached. It should be kept in mind that constant monitoring is needed in regard to drug dosage. Included in the situations which may make dosage adjustments necessary are changes in clinical status secondary to remissions or exacerbations in the disease process, the patient's individual drug responsiveness, and the effect of patient exposure to stressful situations not directly related to the disease entity under treatment; in this latter situation it may be necessary to increase the dosage of Kenalog-10 Injection (Sterile Triamcinolone Acetonide Suspension USP) for a period of time consistent with the patient's condition. If the drug is to be stopped after long-term therapy, it is recommended that it be withdrawn gradually rather than abruptly.
Administration: Shake the vial before use to insure a uniform suspension. After withdrawal, inject without delay to prevent settling in the syringe. Careful technique should be employed to avoid the possibility of entering a blood vessel or introducing infection.
Routine laboratory studies, such as urinalysis, two-hour postprandial blood sugar, determination of blood pressure and body weight, and a chest x-ray should be made at regular intervals during prolonged therapy. Upper GI x-rays are desirable in patients with an ulcer history or significant dyspepsia.
For treatment of joints, the usual intra-articular injection technique, as described in standard textbooks, should be followed. If an excessive amount of synovial fluid is present in the joint, some, but not all, should be aspirated to aid in the relief of pain and to prevent undue dilution of the steroid.
With intra-articular or intrabursal administration, and with injection of Kenalog-10 Injection into tendon sheaths, the use of a local anesthetic may often be desirable. When a local anesthetic is used, its package insert should be read with care and all the precautions connected with its use should be observed. It should be injected into the surrounding soft tissues prior to the injection of the corticosteroid. A small amount of the anesthetic solution may be instilled into the joint.
In treating acute nonspecific tenosynovitis, care should be taken to insure that the injection of Kenalog-10 Injection is made into the tendon sheath rather than the tendon substance. Epicondylitis (tennis elbow) may be treated by infiltrating the preparation into the area of greatest tenderness.
For treatment of dermal lesions, Kenalog-10 Injection is injected directly into the lesion, i.e., intradermally or sometimes subcutaneously. For accuracy of dosage measurement and ease of administration, it is preferable to employ a tuberculin syringe and a small-bore needle (23- to 25-gauge). Ethyl chloride spray may be used to alleviate the discomfort of the injection.
How Supplied: Kenalog-10 Injection (Sterile Triamcinolone Acetonide Suspension USP) is supplied in multiple-dose vials of 5 ml. providing 10 mg. triamcinolone acetonide per ml.
Storage: Store at room temperature; avoid freezing.

KENALOG® IN ORABASE® ℞
(Triamcinolone Acetonide Dental Paste USP)

Description: Each gram of Kenalog in Orabase provides 1 mg. (0.1%) triamcinolone acetonide in emollient dental paste containing gelatin, pectin, and carboxymethylcellulose sodium in Plastibase® (Plasticized Hydrocarbon Gel), a polyethylene and mineral oil gel base.
Actions: Triamcinolone acetonide is a synthetic corticosteroid which possesses anti-inflammatory, antipruritic, and antiallergic action. The emollient dental paste acts as an adhesive vehicle for applying the active medication to the oral tissues. The vehicle provides a protective covering which may serve to temporarily reduce the pain associated with oral irritation.
Indications: Kenalog in Orabase (Triamcinolone Acetonide Dental Paste USP) is indicated for adjunctive treatment and for the tempo-

rary relief of symptoms associated with oral inflammatory lesions and ulcerative lesions resulting from trauma.

Contraindications: This preparation is contraindicated in patients with a history of hypersensitivity to any of its components.

Because it contains a corticosteroid, the preparation is contraindicated in the presence of fungal, viral, or bacterial infections of the mouth or throat.

Warning: Usage in Pregnancy—Safe use of this preparation during pregnancy has not been established with respect to possible adverse reactions upon fetal development; therefore, it should not be used in women of childbearing potential and particularly during early pregnancy unless, in the judgment of the physician or dentist, the potential benefits outweigh the possible hazards.

Precautions: Patients with tuberculosis, peptic ulcer or diabetes mellitus should not be treated with any corticosteroid preparation without the advice of the patient's physician.

It should be borne in mind that the normal defensive responses of the oral tissues are depressed in patients receiving topical corticosteroid therapy. Virulent strains of oral microorganisms may multiply without producing the usual warning symptoms of oral infections.

The small amount of steroid released when the preparation is used as recommended makes systemic effects very unlikely; however, they are a possibility when topical corticosteroid preparations are used over a long period of time.

If local irritation or sensitization should develop, the preparation should be discontinued and appropriate therapy instituted.

If significant regeneration or repair of oral tissues has not occurred in seven days, additional investigation into the etiology of the oral lesion is advised.

Adverse Reactions: Prolonged administration may elicit the adverse reactions known to occur with systemic steroid preparations; for example, adrenal suppression, alteration of glucose metabolism, protein catabolism, peptic ulcer activations, and others. These are usually reversible and disappear when the hormone is discontinued.

Dosage and Administration: Press a small dab (about one-quarter of an inch) to the lesion until a thin film develops. A larger quantity may be required for coverage of some lesions. For optimal results use only enough to coat the lesion with a thin film. Do not rub in. Attempting to spread this preparation may result in a granular, gritty sensation and cause it to crumble. After application, however, a smooth, slippery film develops.

The preparation should be applied at bedtime to permit steroid contact with the lesion throughout the night. Depending on the severity of symptoms, it may be necessary to apply the preparation two or three times a day, preferably after meals. If significant repair or regeneration has not occurred in seven days, further investigation is advisable.

How Supplied: 5 gram tubes (Military Depot Item, NSN 6505-00-926-8913).

Storage: Store at room temperature.

KINEVAC® ℞
(Sincalide for Injection)

(See Diagnostic Section)

MEDOTOPES® ℞
(Radiopharmaceuticals)

(See Diagnostic Section)

MYCOLOG® ℞
(Nystatin—Neomycin Sulfate—Gramicidin—Triamcinolone Acetonide)
CREAM AND OINTMENT

Description: Mycolog (Nystatin—Neomycin Sulfate—Gramicidin—Triamcinolone Acetonide) is available as a cream in an aqueous vanishing cream base and as an ointment in Plastibase® (Plasticized Hydrocarbon Gel), a polyethylene and mineral oil gel base. Each gram of the cream or ointment provides 100,000 units nystatin, neomycin sulfate equivalent to 2.5 mg. neomycin base, 0.25 mg. gramicidin and 1 mg. triamcinolone acetonide. The cream also contains polysorbate 60, alcohol, aluminum hydroxide concentrated wet gel, titanium dioxide, glyceryl monostearate, polyethylene glycol monostearate, simethicone, sorbic acid, propylene glycol, ethylenediamine hydrochloride, white petrolatum, cetearyl alcohol (and) ceteareth-20, methylparaben, propylparaben, and sorbitol solution.

Actions: Triamcinolone acetonide is primarily effective because of its anti-inflammatory, antipruritic, and vasoconstrictive actions. Nystatin provides specific anticandidal activity and the two topical antibiotics, neomycin and gramicidin, provide antibacterial activity.

Indications

Based on a review of these drugs by the National Academy of Sciences—National Research Council and/or other information, FDA has classified the indications as follows:

Possibly effective: In
- cutaneous candidiasis
- superficial bacterial infections
- the following conditions when complicated by candidal and/or bacterial infection: atopic, eczematoid, stasis, nummular, contact, or seborrheic dermatitis; neurodermatitis and dermatitis venenata
- infantile eczema
- lichen simplex chronicus
- the Cream is also possibly effective in pruritus ani and pruritus vulvae

Final classification of the less-than-effective indications requires further investigation.

Contraindications: Topical steroids are contraindicated in viral diseases of the skin, such as vaccinia and varicella. The preparations are also contraindicated in fungal lesions of the skin except candidiasis, and in those patients with a history of hypersensitivity to any of their components.

The preparations are not for ophthalmic use nor should they be applied in the external auditory canal of patients with perforated eardrums.

Topical steroids should not be used when circulation is markedly impaired.

Warnings: Because of the potential hazard of nephrotoxicity and ototoxicity, prolonged use or use of large amounts of these products should be avoided in the treatment of skin infections following extensive burns, trophic ulceration, and other conditions where absorption of neomycin is possible.

Usage in Pregnancy: Although topical steroids have not been reported to have an adverse effect on the fetus, the safety of topical steroid preparations during pregnancy has not been absolutely established; therefore, they should not be used extensively on pregnant patients, in large amounts, or for prolonged periods of time.

Precautions: As with any antibiotic preparation, prolonged use may result in overgrowth of nonsusceptible organisms, including fungi other than *Candida.* Constant observation of the patient is essential. Should superinfection due to nonsusceptible organisms occur, suitable concomitant antimicrobial therapy must be administered. If a favorable response does not occur promptly, application of Mycolog (Nystatin—Neomycin Sulfate—Gramicidin—Triamcinolone Acetonide) Cream or Ointment should be discontinued until the infection is adequately controlled by other anti-infective measures.

If extensive areas are treated or if the occlusive technique is used, the possibility exists of increased systemic absorption of the corticosteroid and suitable precautions should be taken.

If irritation develops, the product should be discontinued and appropriate therapy instituted.

Adverse Reactions: Hypersensitivity to nystatin is extremely uncommon. Sensitivity reactions following the topical use of gramicidin are rarely encountered. Hypersensitivity to neomycin has been reported and articles in the current medical literature indicate an increase in its prevalence.

The following local adverse reactions have been reported with topical corticosteroids either with or without occlusive dressings: burning sensations, itching, irritation, dryness, folliculitis, secondary infection, skin atrophy, striae, miliaria, hypertrichosis, acneform eruptions, maceration of the skin and hypopigmentation. Contact sensitivity to a particular dressing material or adhesive may occur occasionally.

Ototoxicity and nephrotoxicity have been reported.

Dosage and Administration: *Mycolog Cream* (Nystatin—Neomycin Sulfate—Gramicidin—Triamcinolone Acetonide Cream) —Rub into affected areas two to three times daily.

Mycolog Ointment (Nystatin—Neomycin Sulfate—Gramicidin—Triamcinolone Acetonide Ointment)—Apply a thin film to the affected areas two to three times daily.

Occlusive Dressing Technique—Cream: Gently rub a small amount of the Cream into the lesion until it disappears. Reapply the Cream leaving a thin coating on the lesion and cover with a pliable nonporous film. If needed, additional moisture may be provided by covering the lesion with a dampened clean cotton cloth before the plastic film is applied or by briefly soaking the affected area in water.

The frequency of changing dressings is best determined on an individual basis. Reapplication is essential at each dressing change.

Ointment: Apply the Ointment leaving a thin coating on the lesion and cover with a pliable nonporous film. If needed, additional moisture may be provided by covering the lesion with a dampened clean cotton cloth before the plastic film is applied or by briefly soaking the affected area in water.

The frequency of changing dressings is best determined on an individual basis. Reapplication is essential at each dressing change.

How Supplied: Both preparations are available in tubes of 15, 30, and 60 g. They are also available in jars of 120 g. (4 oz.) for hospital or institutional use only. [Cream in 15 g. tubes—Military Depot Item, NSN6505-00-961-5504 and V.A. Depot Item, NSN6505-00-961-5504A; Cream in 120 g. (4 oz.) jars—V.A. Depot Item, NSN6505-00-772-0245A; Ointment in 15 g. tubes—V.A. Depot Item, NSN6505-00-772-0244A.]

Storage: Store the cream at room temperature; avoid freezing. Store the ointment at room temperature.

Continued on next page

Squibb—Cont.

MYCOSTATIN® CREAM ℞
(Nystatin Cream)
MYCOSTATIN OINTMENT ℞
(Nystatin Ointment USP)
MYCOSTATIN TOPICAL POWDER ℞
(Nystatin Topical Powder)

Description: Mycostatin Cream (Nystatin Cream) contains the antifungal antibiotic Nystatin USP at a concentration of 100,000 units per gram in an aqueous, perfumed vanishing cream base containing aluminum hydroxide concentrated wet gel, titanium dioxide, propylene glycol, cetearyl alcohol (and) ceteareth-20, white petrolatum, sorbitol solution, glyceryl monostearate, polyethylene glycol monostearate, sorbic acid and simethicone.
Mycostatin Ointment (Nystatin Ointment USP) provides 100,000 units Nystatin USP per gram in *Plastibase*® (Plasticized Hydrocarbon Gel), a polyethylene and mineral oil gel base.
Mycostatin Topical Powder (Nystatin Topical Powder) provides, in each gram, 100,000 units Nystatin USP dispersed in Talc USP.
Clinical Pharmacology: Nystatin is an antifungal antibiotic which is both fungistatic and fungicidal *in vitro* against a wide variety of yeasts and yeast-like fungi. It probably acts by binding to sterols in the cell membrane of the fungus with a resultant change in membrane permeability allowing leakage of intracellular components. Nystatin is a polyene antibiotic of undetermined structural formula that is obtained from *Streptomyces noursei*, and is the first well tolerated antifungal antibiotic of dependable efficacy for the treatment of cutaneous, oral and intestinal infections caused by *Candida* (Monilia) *albicans* and other Candida species. It exhibits no appreciable activity against bacteria.
Nystatin provides specific therapy for all localized forms of candidiasis. Symptomatic relief is rapid, often occurring within 24 to 72 hours after the initiation of treatment. Cure is effected both clinically and mycologically in most cases of localized candidiasis.
Indications and Usage: Mycostatin topical preparations are indicated in the treatment of cutaneous or mucocutaneous mycotic infections caused by *Candida* (Monilia) *albicans* and other Candida species.
Contraindications: Mycostatin topical preparations are contraindicated in patients with a history of hypersensitivity to any of their components.
Precautions: Should a reaction of hypersensitivity occur the drug should be immediately withdrawn and appropriate measures taken.
Adverse Reactions: Nystatin is virtually nontoxic and nonsensitizing and is well tolerated by all age groups including debilitated infants, even on prolonged administration. If irritation on topical application should occur, discontinue medication.
Dosage and Administration: The cream and the ointment should be applied liberally to affected areas twice daily or as indicated until healing is complete. The powder should be applied to candidal lesions two or three times daily until lesions have healed. For fungal infection of the feet caused by Candida species, the powder should be dusted freely on the feet as well as in shoes and socks. The cream is usually preferred to the ointment in candidiasis involving intertriginous areas; very moist lesions, however, are best treated with the topical dusting powder.
The preparations do not stain skin or mucous membranes and they provide a simple, convenient means of treatment.
How Supplied: Mycostatin Cream (Nystatin Cream) is supplied in tubes of 15 g. and 30 g. Mycostatin Ointment (Nystatin Ointment USP) is supplied in tubes of 15 g. and 30 g.
Mycostatin Topical Powder (Nystatin Topical Powder) is supplied in plastic squeeze bottles of 15 g. (½ oz.) [Military Depot Item, NSN 6505-00-890-1218].
Storage: Store the cream at room temperature; avoid freezing. Store the ointment at room temperature. Store the topical powder at room temperature; avoid excessive heat.

MYCOSTATIN® ORAL SUSPENSION ℞
(Nystatin Oral Suspension USP)

Description: Nystatin is an antifungal antibiotic which is both fungistatic and fungicidal *in vitro* against a wide variety of yeasts and yeast-like fungi. It is a polyene antibiotic of undetermined structural formula that is obtained from *Streptomyces noursei.* Mycostatin Oral Suspension is provided for oral administration containing 100,000 units nystatin per ml. in a vehicle containing 50% sucrose; not more than 1% alcohol by volume.
Clinical Pharmacology: Nystatin probably acts by binding to sterols in the cell membrane of the fungus with a resultant change in membrane permeability allowing leakage of intracellular components. It exhibits no appreciable activity against bacteria or trichomonads.
Following oral administration, nystatin is sparingly absorbed with no detectable blood levels when given in the recommended doses. Most of the orally administered nystatin is passed unchanged in the stool.
Indications and Usage: Mycostatin Oral Suspension is indicated for the treatment of candidiasis in the oral cavity.
Contraindication: The preparation is contraindicated in patients with a history of hypersensitivity to any of its components.
Precautions:
Usage in Pregnancy—No adverse effects or complications have been attributed to nystatin in infants born to women treated with nystatin.
Adverse Reactions: Nystatin is virtually nontoxic and nonsensitizing and is well tolerated by all age groups including debilitated infants, even on prolonged administration. Large oral doses have occasionally produced diarrhea, gastrointestinal distress, nausea, and vomiting.
Dosage and Administration: INFANTS—2 ml. (200,000 units nystatin) four times daily (1 ml. in each side of mouth).
NOTE: Limited clinical studies in premature and low birth weight infants indicate that 1 ml. four times daily is effective.
CHILDREN AND ADULTS—4-6 ml. (400,000 to 600,000 units nystatin) four times daily (one-half of dose in each side of mouth). The preparation should be retained in the mouth as long as possible before swallowing.
Continue treatment for at least 48 hours after perioral symptoms have disappeared and cultures returned to normal.
How Supplied: Mycostatin Oral Suspension (Nystatin Oral Suspension USP) is available in 60 ml. bottles as a pleasant-tasting, ready-to-use suspension containing 100,000 units nystatin per ml. A calibrated dropper is supplied with each bottle of suspension.
Storage: Store at room temperature; avoid freezing.

MYCOSTATIN® ORAL TABLETS ℞
(Nystatin Tablets USP)

Description: Nystatin is an antifungal antibiotic which is both fungistatic and fungicidal *in vitro* against a wide variety of yeasts and yeast-like fungi. It is a polyene antibiotic of undetermined structural formula that is obtained from *Streptomyces noursei.* Mycostatin Oral Tablets are provided for oral administration as coated tablets containing 500,000 units nystatin. The tablets contain FD&C Yellow No. 5 (tartrazine).
Clinical Pharmacology: Nystatin probably acts by binding to sterols in the cell membrane of the fungus with a resultant change in membrane permeability allowing leakage of intracellular components. It exhibits no appreciable activity against bacteria or trichomonads.
Following oral administration, nystatin is sparingly absorbed with no detectable blood levels when given in the recommended doses. Most of the orally administered nystatin is passed unchanged in the stool.
Indications and Usage: Mycostatin Oral Tablets (Nystatin Tablets USP) are intended for the treatment of intestinal candidiasis.
Contraindications: Mycostatin Oral Tablets are contraindicated in patients with a history of hypersensitivity to any of their components.
Precautions: **Usage in Pregnancy**—No adverse effects or complications have been attributed to nystatin in infants born to women treated with nystatin.
Mycostatin Oral Tablets contain FD&C Yellow No. 5 (tartrazine) which may cause allergic-type reactions (including bronchial asthma) in certain susceptible individuals. Although the overall incidence of FD&C Yellow No. 5 (tartrazine) sensitivity in the general population is low, it is frequently seen in patients who also have aspirin hypersensitivity.
Adverse Reactions: Nystatin is virtually nontoxic and nonsensitizing and is well tolerated by all age groups including debilitated infants, even on prolonged administration. Large oral doses have occasionally produced diarrhea, gastrointestinal distress, nausea and vomiting.
Dosage and Administration: The usual therapeutic dosage is one to two tablets (500,000 to 1,000,000 units nystatin) three times daily. Treatment should generally be continued for at least 48 hours after clinical cure to prevent relapse.
How Supplied: Mycostatin Oral Tablets (Nystatin Tablets USP) are available for oral administration as FILMLOK® tablets providing 500,000 units nystatin per tablet in bottles of 100 and UNIMATIC® cartons of 100. (Filmlok is a Squibb trademark for veneer-coated tablets.) [Military Depot Item, NSN6505-00-118-1949.]
Storage: Store at room temperature; avoid excessive heat.
[*Shown in Product Identification Section*]

MYCOSTATIN® VAGINAL TABLETS ℞
(Nystatin Vaginal Tablets USP)

Description: Mycostatin Vaginal Tablets are provided as diamond-shaped, individually foil wrapped, compressed tablets containing 100,000 units of nystatin dispersed in lactose with ethyl cellulose, stearic acid, and starch.
Clinical Pharmacology: Nystatin is an antifungal antibiotic which is both fungistatic and fungicidal *in vitro* against a wide variety of yeasts and yeast-like fungi. It probably acts by binding to sterols in the cell membrane of the fungus with a resultant change in membrane permeability allowing leakage of intracellular components. Nystatin is a polyene antibiotic of undetermined structural formula that is obtained from *Streptomyces noursei.* It exhibits no appreciable activity against bacteria or trichomonads.
Indications and Usage: Mycostatin Vaginal Tablets are effective for the local treatment of vulvovaginal candidiasis (moniliasis). The diagnosis should be confirmed, prior to therapy, by KOH smears and/or cultures. Other pathogens commonly associated with vulvovaginitis (Trichomonas and *Hemophilus vaginalis*) do not respond to nystatin and should be ruled out by appropriate laboratory methods.
Contraindications: This preparation is contraindicated in patients with a history of hypersensitivity to any of its components.

Precautions: **General**—Discontinue treatment if sensitization or irritation is reported during use.

Laboratory Tests—If there is a lack of response to Mycostatin Vaginal Tablets (Nystatin Vaginal Tablets USP), appropriate microbiological studies should be repeated to confirm the diagnosis and rule out other pathogens before instituting another course of antimycotic therapy.

Usage in Pregnancy: No adverse effects or complications have been attributed to nystatin in infants born to women treated with nystatin vaginal tablets.

Adverse Reactions: Nystatin is virtually nontoxic and nonsensitizing and is well tolerated by all age groups, even on prolonged administration. Rarely, irritation or sensitization may occur (see PRECAUTIONS).

Dosage and Administration: The usual dosage is one tablet (100,000 units nystatin) daily for two weeks. The tablets should be deposited high in the vagina by means of the applicator. "Instructions for the Patient" are enclosed in each package.

Even though symptomatic relief may occur within a few days, treatment should be continued for the full course.

It is important that therapy be continued during menstruation. Adjunctive measures such as therapeutic douches are unnecessary and sometimes inadvisable. Cleansing douches may be used by nonpregnant women, if desired, for esthetic purposes.

How Supplied: Mycostatin Vaginal Tablets (Nystatin Vaginal Tablets USP) are available in packages of 15 and 30 individually foil wrapped tablets (100,000 units nystatin each) with applicator, and in UNIMATIC® cartons of 50 single-dose packs per carton—each cello-protected single-dose pack consists of one individually foil wrapped tablet (100,000 units nystatin), one applicator and one "Instructions for the Patient" leaflet.

Storage: Store in refrigerator below 15° C (59° F).

[*Shown in Product Identification Section*]

MYSTECLIN-F® CAPSULES ℞
(Tetracycline—Amphotericin B Capsules)
MYSTECLIN-F® SYRUP ℞
(Tetracycline—Amphotericin B Syrup)

> Recently, a panel of the National Academy of Sciences—National Research Council has stated that in its informed judgment Mysteclin-F is ineffective as a fixed combination. Further, it stated, "The Panel is not aware of evidence of proved efficacy of this combination in the prevention of disease due to monilial organisms, although suppression of growth of monilia may be accomplished. It should be noted that the apparent reduction of organisms in the feces may be an artifact due to residual antibiotic activity and thus may not reflect the true state in the patient. It is preferable, in the Panel's opinion, to prescribe antifungal drugs when clinically indicated, rather than to use them indiscriminately as 'prophylaxis' against an uncommon clinical entity seen during therapy with tetracyclines and other antibiotics."

Mysteclin-F Capsules (Tetracycline—Amphotericin B Capsules) are available in two potencies: the equivalent of 250 mg. tetracycline hydrochloride with 50 mg. amphotericin B, and the equivalent of 125 mg. tetracycline hydrochloride with 25 mg. amphotericin B, both buffered with potassium metaphosphate. Mysteclin-F Syrup (Tetracycline—Amphotericin B Syrup) is a fruit-flavored syrup containing, in each 5 ml. teaspoonful, tetracycline equivalent to 125 mg. tetracycline hydrochloride, buffered with potassium metaphosphate, and 25 mg. amphotericin B.

Clinical Pharmacology: Mysteclin-F (Tetracycline—Amphotericin B) Capsules and Syrup have been designed to provide simultaneous antimicrobial therapy and anticandidal prophylaxis, a concept first developed by Squibb.

The preparations, which contain the broad spectrum antibiotic tetracycline, well known for its pronounced antimicrobial effect against a wide range of pathogenic organisms, produce exceptionally high initial tetracycline blood levels as well as excellent diffusion to tissues and body fluids.

Furthermore, these preparations also contain **prophylactic** amounts of the antifungal antibiotic, amphotericin B. This antibiotic, first isolated and described by the Squibb Institute for Medical Research, is substantially more active *in vitro* against *Candida* strains than nystatin, and has been widely used by the intravenous route in the treatment of many deep-seated mycotic infections.

Given orally, amphotericin B is extremely well tolerated and is virtually nontoxic in prophylactic doses. Although poorly absorbed from the gut, amphotericin B has a high degree of activity against *Candida* species in the intestinal tract and prevents the overgrowth of these organisms commonly associated with broad spectrum antibiotic therapy (amphotericin B has no antibacterial activity). By suppressing overgrowth of *Candida* in the gastrointestinal tract, thereby minimizing a possible reservoir of this organism, Mysteclin-F (Tetracycline—Amphotericin B) provides added protection for the patient against troublesome, or even serious, candidal superinfections, e.g., intestinal (diarrheal), anogenital, vulvovaginal, mucocutaneous candidiasis.

Note: Microorganisms that have become insensitive to one tetracycline invariably exhibit cross-resistance to other tetracyclines. In addition, gram-negative bacilli made tetracycline resistant may also show cross-resistance to chloramphenicol.

Indications and Usage: Candidal overgrowth occurs in a large number of patients taking broad spectrum antibiotics. Although it is impossible to predict exactly which patient will develop candidal complications and which will not, certain types of patients are known to be particularly susceptible to candidiasis. Among these are elderly or debilitated patients; patients on high or prolonged antibiotic dosage; diabetics; infants; patients on corticoid therapy; patients who have developed candidiasis on previous broad spectrum therapy; women, particularly during pregnancy. Because the danger of candidal complications is greatest in these patients, they are potential candidates for therapy with Mysteclin-F.

Mysteclin-F (Tetracycline—Amphotericin B) Capsules and Syrup are indicated for the many common infections, including those of the respiratory, gastrointestinal and genitourinary systems, which are amenable to tetracycline therapy. Infections caused by gram-positive and gram-negative bacteria, spirochetes, viruses of the lymphogranuloma-psittacosis-trachoma group, rickettsiae and *Endamoeba histolytica* can be expected to respond. Because of the wide range of antimicrobial activity, the preparations are particularly useful in the treatment of mixed infections due to susceptible organisms.

Mysteclin-F (Tetracycline—Amphotericin B) Capsules and Syrup are also a useful part of the armamentarium in the management of chronic cases of acne vulgaris which, in the judgment of the clinician, require long-term treatment. The cystic and pustular forms of this condition respond most satisfactorily to tetracycline therapy; the papular form may also show improvement in some individuals. Because long-term maintenance therapy with tetracycline is involved, the presence of amphotericin B in the product is a particular advantage, helping to guard against the risk of candidal overgrowth.

Note: A number of strains of staphylococci and streptococci have shown resistance to tetracyclines. A few strains of pneumococci, *E. coli* and shigellae also have been reported as resistant. Indicated laboratory studies, including sensitivity tests, should be performed.

Contraindications: These products should not be used in persons with a history of hypersensitivity to any of their components.

Warnings: THE USE OF DRUGS OF THE TETRACYCLINE CLASS DURING TOOTH DEVELOPMENT (LAST HALF OF PREGNANCY, INFANCY, AND CHILDHOOD TO AGE OF EIGHT YEARS) MAY CAUSE PERMANENT DISCOLORATION OF THE TEETH (YELLOW-GRAY-BROWN). This reaction is more common during long-term use of the drugs but has been observed following repeated short-term courses. Enamel hypoplasia has also been reported. TETRACYCLINE DRUGS, THEREFORE, SHOULD NOT BE USED IN THIS AGE GROUP UNLESS OTHER DRUGS ARE NOT LIKELY TO BE EFFECTIVE OR ARE CONTRAINDICATED.

If renal impairment exists, even usual oral or parenteral doses may lead to excessive systemic accumulation of the drug and possible liver toxicity. Under such conditions, lower-than-usual doses are indicated and if therapy is prolonged, tetracycline serum level determinations may be advisable.

Certain hypersensitive individuals may develop a photodynamic reaction precipitated by exposure to direct sunlight during the use of this drug. This reaction is usually of the photoallergic type which may also be produced by other tetracycline derivatives. Individuals with a history of photosensitivity reactions should be instructed to avoid exposure to direct sunlight while under treatment with this or other tetracycline drugs and treatment should be discontinued at first evidence of skin discomfort.

NOTE: Photosensitization reactions have occurred most frequently with demethylchlortetracycline, less with chlortetracycline and very rarely with oxytetracycline and tetracycline.

Precautions: As with any antibiotic preparation, prolonged use may result in overgrowth of nonsusceptible organisms. Constant observation of the patient is essential. Should superinfection occur, the preparation should be discontinued and/or appropriate therapy instituted. *Note:* Superinfection of the bowel by staphylococci may be life threatening.

Tetracycline may form a stable calcium complex in any bone forming tissue with no serious harmful effects reported thus far in humans. However, use of tetracycline during tooth development (i.e., latter half of gestation, neonatal period and early childhood) may cause discoloration of the teeth (i.e., yellow-gray-brownish). This effect occurs mostly during long-term use of the drug but it has also been observed in usual short treatment courses.

During long-term therapy, periodic assessment of organ system function, including renal, hepatic, and hematopoietic systems, should be made.

Increased intracranial pressure with bulging fontanels has been observed in infants taking therapeutic doses of tetracycline. Occurrence has been rare and all signs and symptoms have disappeared rapidly upon cessation of treatment.

Since sensitivity reactions are more likely to occur in persons with a history of allergy, asthma, hay fever, or urticaria, the preparation should be used with caution in such individuals. Cross-sensitization among the various tetracyclines is extremely common.

Continued on next page

Squibb—Cont.

In the treatment of gonorrhea, patients with a suspected lesion of syphilis should have dark-field examinations before receiving tetracycline and monthly serologic tests for a minimum of three months.
The use of tetracycline in staphylococcal infections does not preclude the need for indicated surgical procedures.
Adverse Reactions: Oral administration of amphotericin B is usually well tolerated.
The following adverse reactions have been reported with tetracycline preparations:
Gastrointestinal irritation (anorexia, epigastric distress, nausea, vomiting) as well as bulky loose stools, and diarrhea may occur. Glossitis, stomatitis, enterocolitis, proctitis, and pruritus ani may occur in some patients. Black hairy tongue, sore throat, dysphagia, and hoarseness have also been reported. However, tetracycline is generally well tolerated, undesirable gastrointestinal side effects occurring significantly less frequently than with the two analogues, oxytetracycline and chlortetracycline.
Tetracyclines may also cause maculopapular and erythematous skin rashes. A rare case of exfoliative dermatitis has been reported. Photosensitivity, manifested by an exaggerated sunburn reaction has been observed in some individuals (see *Warnings*). Onycholysis and discoloration of the nails have been reported rarely.
Rise in BUN has been reported and is apparently dose related. Urinary loss of nitrogen has been observed in some patients receiving tetracyclines and may result in negative nitrogen balance. Increased excretion of sodium has also been reported. The development of peptic ulcers and bleeding has been observed in uremic patients receiving tetracyclines.
Hypersensitivity reactions may include urticaria, serum sickness-like reactions (fever, rash, arthralgia), angioneurotic edema, and anaphylactoid shock. If allergic reactions occur, or if an individual idiosyncrasy appears, tetracycline therapy should be discontinued.
Increased intracranial pressure with bulging fontanels has been reported in infants following full therapeutic doses of tetracycline. This symptom disappears rapidly when administration of tetracycline is discontinued (see *Precautions*).
The use of tetracycline during the mineralization phase of tooth development (latter half of gestation, neonatal period, and early childhood) may cause discoloration of the teeth (yellow-gray-brownish) which may sometimes be accompanied by enamel hypoplasia (see *Warnings*).
Anemia, thrombocytopenic purpura, neutropenia, and eosinophilia have been reported. Tetracyclines may delay blood coagulation.
Hepatic cholestasis has been reported rarely, and is usually associated with high dosage levels of tetracycline.
Dosage and Administration: Dosage should be based on the tetracycline content.
Adults: For the many common infections amenable to tetracycline therapy, adults should receive a minimum of 250 mg. four times daily. Higher dosages, such as 500 mg. four times daily, may be required for severe infections or for those infections which do not respond to the smaller dose. **For children above eight years of age:** In general, the pediatric dosage should supply 10 to 20 mg. tetracycline per pound of body weight each day, in divided doses, depending on the type and severity of the infection.
Representative pediatric dosages of Mysteclin-F Syrup (Tetracycline—Amphotericin B Syrup) are as follows: 20 lbs.: ½ teaspoonful q.i.d.; 40 lbs.: 1 teaspoonful q.i.d.; 60 lbs: 1½ teaspoonfuls q.i.d.; 80 lbs.: 2 teaspoonfuls q.i.d.
Oral forms of tetracycline should be given one hour before or two hours following meals. Pediatric dosage forms (oral) should not be given with milk formulas or other calcium containing food, and should be given at least one hour prior to feeding.
Treatment of most common infections should continue for 24 to 48 hours after symptoms and fever subside. However, if the capsules or syrup are used in the treatment of streptococcal infections due to susceptible organisms, therapy should be continued for a full 10 days to guard against the risk of rheumatic fever or glomerulonephritis. Higher dosage and even more prolonged therapy is necessary for subacute bacterial endocarditis and may be required in certain staphylococcal infections.
In chronic cases of acne vulgaris which, in the judgment of the clinician, require long-term treatment, the recommended initial dosage of the capsules or syrup is 1 gram daily in divided doses. When improvement is noted, usually within one week, dosage should be gradually reduced to maintenance levels ranging from 125 to 500 mg. daily. In some patients it may be possible to maintain adequate remission of lesions with alternate-day or intermittent therapy. Tetracycline therapy of acne vulgaris should augment the other standard measures known to be of value.
How Supplied: *Mysteclin-F Capsules (Tetracycline—Amphotericin B Capsules) are available in bottles of 16 and 100 and Unimatic® single-dose cartons of 100.
*Mysteclin-F '125' Capsules (Tetracycline —Amphotericin B Capsules) are available in bottles of 100.
Mysteclin-F Syrup (Tetracycline—Amphotericin B Syrup) is available in bottles of 60 ml. and 240 ml. (8 oz.)
Storage: Store the capsules at room temperature; avoid excessive heat; keep tightly closed. Store the syrup below 30°C. (86°F.); protect from light; keep tightly closed.
*[*Shown in Product Identification Section*]

NATURETIN®-2.5 ℞
NATURETIN®-5 ℞
NATURETIN®-10 ℞
(Bendroflumethiazide Tablets NF)

Description: Naturetin is a benzothiadiazine derivative containing a benzyl and a trifluoromethyl group. It is a potent oral diuretic and antihypertensive agent available as compressed tablets providing 2.5, 5, or 10 mg. bendroflumethiazide. The tablets contain FD&C Yellow No. 5 (tartrazine).
Actions: The mechanism of action results in an interference with the renal tubular mechanism of electrolyte reabsorption. At maximal therapeutic dosage all thiazides are approximately equal in their diuretic potency. The mechanism whereby thiazides function in the control of hypertension is unknown.
Indications: Naturetin is indicated as adjunctive therapy in edema associated with congestive heart failure, hepatic cirrhosis, and corticosteroid and estrogen therapy.
Naturetin has also been found useful in edema due to various forms of renal dysfunction, such as: nephrotic syndrome, acute glomerulonephritis, and chronic renal failure.
Naturetin (Bendroflumethiazide Tablets NF) is indicated in the management of hypertension either as the sole therapeutic agent or to enhance the effectiveness of other antihypertensive drugs in the more severe forms of hypertension.
Usage in Pregnancy—The routine use of diuretics in an otherwise healthy woman is inappropriate and exposes mother and fetus to unnecessary hazard. Diuretics do not prevent development of toxemia of pregnancy, and there is no satisfactory evidence that they are useful in the treatment of developed toxemia. Edema during pregnancy may arise from pathological causes or from the physiologic and mechanical consequences of pregnancy. Thiazides are indicated in pregnancy when edema is due to pathologic causes, just as they are in the absence of pregnancy (see WARNINGS). Dependent edema in pregnancy, resulting from restriction of venous return by the expanded uterus, is properly treated through elevation of the lower extremities and use of support hose; use of diuretics to lower intravascular volume in this case is illogical and unnecessary. There is hypervolemia during normal pregnancy which is harmful to neither the fetus nor the mother (in the absence of cardiovascular disease), but which is associated with edema, including generalized edema, in the majority of pregnant women. If this edema produces discomfort, increased recumbency will often provide relief. In rare instances, this edema may cause extreme discomfort which is not relieved by rest. In these cases, a short course of diuretics may provide relief and may be appropriate.
Contraindications: Bendroflumethiazide is contraindicated in anuria.
It is also contraindicated in patients who have previously demonstrated hypersensitivity to it or other sulfonamide-derived drugs.
Warnings: Bendroflumethiazide should be used with caution in severe renal disease. In patients with renal disease, thiazides may precipitate azotemia. Cumulative effects of the drug may develop in patients with impaired renal function.
Thiazides should be used with caution in patients with impaired hepatic function or progressive liver disease, since minor alterations of fluid and electrolyte balance may precipitate hepatic coma.
Thiazides may be additive or may potentiate the action of other antihypertensive drugs. Potentiation occurs with ganglionic or peripheral adrenergic blocking drugs.
Sensitivity reactions may occur in patients with a history of allergy or bronchial asthma. The possibility of exacerbation or activation of systemic lupus erythematosus has been reported.
Usage in Pregnancy—Thiazides cross the placental barrier and appear in cord blood. The use of thiazides in pregnant women requires that the anticipated benefit be weighed against possible hazards to the fetus. These hazards include fetal or neonatal jaundice, thrombocytopenia, and possibly other adverse reactions which have occurred in the adult.
Nursing Mothers—Thiazides appear in breast milk. If use of the drug is deemed essential, the patient should stop nursing.
Precautions: Periodic determination of serum electrolytes to detect possible electrolyte imbalance should be performed at appropriate intervals.
All patients receiving thiazide therapy should be observed for clinical signs of fluid or electrolyte imbalance; namely, hyponatremia, hypochloremic alkalosis, and hypokalemia. Serum and urine electrolyte determinations are particularly important when the patient is vomiting excessively or receiving parenteral fluids. Medication such as digitalis may also influence serum electrolytes. Warning signs, irrespective of cause, are: dryness of the mouth, thirst, weakness, lethargy, drowsiness, restlessness, muscle pains or cramps, muscular fatigue, hypotension, oliguria, tachycardia, and gastrointestinal disturbances such as nausea and vomiting.
Hypokalemia may develop with thiazides as with any other pótent diuretic, especially with brisk diuresis, when severe cirrhosis is present, or during concomitant use of corticosteroids or ACTH.
Interference with adequate oral electrolyte intake will also contribute to hypokalemia. Digitalis therapy may exaggerate metabolic effects of hypokalemia especially with reference to myocardial activity.
Any chloride deficit is generally mild and usually does not require specific treatment except under extraordinary circumstances (as in liver

disease or renal disease). Dilutional hyponatremia may occur in edematous patients in hot weather; appropriate therapy is water restriction, rather than administration of salt except in rare instances when the hyponatremia is life threatening. In actual salt depletion, appropriate replacement is the therapy of choice. Hyperuricemia may occur or frank gout may be precipitated in certain patients receiving thiazide therapy.
Insulin requirements in diabetic patients may be increased, decreased, or unchanged. Latent diabetes mellitus may become manifest during thiazide administration.
Thiazide drugs may increase the responsiveness to tubocurarine.
The antihypertensive effects of the drug may be enhanced in the postsympathectomy patient.
Thiazides may decrease arterial responsiveness to norepinephrine. This diminution is not sufficient to preclude effectiveness of the pressor agent for therapeutic use. If emergency surgery is indicated, preanesthetic and anesthetic agents should be administered in reduced dosage.
If progressive renal impairment becomes evident, as indicated by a rising nonprotein nitrogen or blood urea nitrogen, a careful reappraisal of therapy is necessary with consideration given to withholding or discontinuing diuretic therapy.
Thiazides may decrease serum PBI levels without signs of thyroid disturbance.
This product contains FD&C Yellow No. 5 (tartrazine) which may cause allergic-type reactions (including bronchial asthma) in certain susceptible individuals. Although the overall incidence of FD&C Yellow No. 5 (tartrazine) sensitivity in the general population is low, it is frequently seen in patients who also have aspirin hypersensitivity.
Adverse Reactions: *Gastrointestinal System:* anorexia, gastric irritation, nausea, vomiting, cramping, diarrhea, constipation, jaundice (intrahepatic cholestatic jaundice), and pancreatitis. *Central Nervous System:* dizziness, vertigo, paresthesia, headache, and xanthopsia. *Hematologic:* leukopenia, agranulocytosis, thrombocytopenia, and aplastic anemia. *Dermatologic-Hypersensitivity:* purpura, photosensitivity, rash, urticaria, and necrotizing angiitis (vasculitis, cutaneous vasculitis). *Cardiovascular:* orthostatic hypotension may occur and may be aggravated by alcohol, barbiturates or narcotics. *Other*: hyperglycemia, glycosuria, occasional metabolic acidosis in diabetic patients, hyperuricemia, allergic glomerulonephritis, muscle spasm, weakness, and restlessness.
Whenever adverse reactions are moderate or severe, thiazide dosage should be reduced or therapy withdrawn.
Dosage and Administration: Therapy should be individualized according to patient response. This therapy should be titrated to gain maximal therapeutic response as well as the minimal dose possible to maintain that therapeutic response.
Diuretic: The usual dose is 5 mg. once daily, preferably given in the morning. To initiate therapy, doses up to 20 mg. may be given once daily or divided into two doses. A single daily dose of 2.5 to 5 mg. should suffice for maintenance.
Alternatively, intermittent therapy may be advantageous in many patients. By administering the preparation every other day or on a three to five day per week schedule, electrolyte imbalance is less likely to occur; however, the possibility still exists.
In general, the lowest dosage that achieves the therapeutic response should be employed.
Antihypertensive: The suggested initial dosage is 5 to 20 mg. daily. Maintenance dosage may range from 2.5 to 15 mg. per day, depending on the individual response of the patient. When the diuretic is used with other antihypertensive agents, lower maintenance doses for each drug are usually sufficient.
How Supplied: 2.5 mg. in bottles of 100; 5 mg. (scored) in bottles of 100 and 1000; 10 mg. (scored) in bottles of 100.
Storage: Store at room temperature; avoid excessive heat.
[*Shown in Product Identification Section*]

NOCTEC® CAPSULES ℞ Ⓒ
(Chloral Hydrate Capsules USP)
NOCTEC SYRUP ℞ Ⓒ
(Chloral Hydrate Syrup USP)

Description: Noctec is an effective sedative and hypnotic agent.
Actions: Chloral hydrate is the oldest member of the hypnotic group of drugs and is still considered to be one of the best sedative agents. Somnifacient doses promptly produce drowsiness and sedation, followed by quiet, sound sleep within an hour. The action of the drug is confined to the cerebral hemispheres. Blood pressure and respiration are depressed only slightly more than in normal sleep and reflexes are not greatly depressed, so that the patient can be awakened and completely aroused. In contrast to barbiturates or other sedatives, "hangover" and depressant aftereffects are only rarely encountered. With the commonly employed therapeutic dosage, preliminary excitement is rare and tolerance and cumulation are unlikely. Although the drug is detoxified in the liver and subsequently eliminated by the kidney, moderately impaired function of either organ is not a contraindication for the usual therapeutic doses.
Indications: Noctec is indicated for nocturnal sedation in all types of patients and especially for the ill, the young, and the elderly patient. In candidates for surgery, it is a satisfactory preoperative sedative that allays anxiety and induces sleep without depressing respiration or cough reflex. When combined with barbiturates, Noctec (Chloral Hydrate) is a useful hypnotic and sedative during the first stage of labor. In postoperative care and control of pain, it is a valuable adjunct to opiates and analgesics.
Contraindications: Chloral hydrate is contraindicated in patients with marked hepatic or renal impairment; it is also contraindicated in patients who have previously exhibited an idiosyncrasy or hypersensitivity to the drug.
Warnings: Chloral hydrate may be habit forming.
Chloral hydrate must be used with caution in patients receiving any of the coumarin or coumarin related anticoagulants. When chloral hydrate is added to or subtracted from the therapeutic regimen, or when changes in dosage of chloral hydrate are contemplated, the effect of the sedative on prothrombin time deserves special attention.
Precautions: The physician should be aware that the concomitant administration of alcohol and chloral hydrate, both of which are central nervous system depressants, may significantly potentiate the sedative action of chloral hydrate.
Continued use of therapeutic doses of chloral hydrate has been shown to be without deleterious effect on the heart. Large doses of chloral hydrate, however, should not be used in patients with *severe* cardiac disease.
Accidental overdosage should be treated with gastric lavage.
Adverse Reactions: With the exception of gastric irritation which may occur in some patients, there are few unfavorable effects. Excitement and delirium are rarely encountered and tolerance and addiction are quite uncommon.
Dosage and Administration: The capsules should be taken with a full glass of liquid. The syrup may be administered in a half glass of water, fruit juice or ginger ale.
ADULTS: The usual *hypnotic* dose is 500 mg. to 1 gram, taken 15 to 30 minutes before bedtime or one-half hour before surgery. The usual *sedative* dose is 250 mg. three times daily after meals. Generally, single doses or daily dosage should not exceed 2 grams.
CHILDREN: The usual daily *hypnotic* dosage is 50 mg./kg. of body weight, with a maximum of 1 gram per single dose. Daily dosage may be given in divided doses, if indicated. The *sedative* dosage is half of the hypnotic dosage.
How Supplied: Noctec is available for oral use as capsules providing 250 mg. (3¾ grains) and 500 mg. (7½ grains) and as an aromatic, flavored syrup supplying 500 mg. (7½ grains) per 5 ml. teaspoonful. *Noctec Capsules (Chloral Hydrate Capsules USP) (red), 250 mg. (3¾ gr.) in bottles of 100; and 500 mg. (7½ gr.) in bottles of 100 and Unimatic® Single-Dose Packs of 25 and 100. [500 mg. capsules in Unimatic® packages of 100—V.A. Depot Item, NSN 6505-00-481-1934A.] Noctec Syrup (Chloral Hydrate Syrup USP) (orange-flavored), bottles of 473 ml. (1 pt.) and 3.8 liters (1 gal.) and Unimatic Single-Dose bottles in cartons of 4 X 25 bottles (5 ml. each bottle).
Storage: Store the capsules and the syrup at room temperature; avoid excessive heat.
*[*Shown in Product Identification Section*]

NYDRAZID® TABLETS ℞
(Isoniazid Tablets USP)
NYDRAZID® INJECTION ℞
(Isoniazid Injection USP)

WARNING
Severe and sometimes fatal hepatitis associated with isoniazid therapy may occur and may develop even after many months of treatment. The risk of developing hepatitis is age related. Approximate case rates by age are: 0 per 1,000 for persons under 20 years of age, 3 per 1,000 for persons in the 20 to 34 year age group, 12 per 1,000 for persons in the 35 to 49 year age group, 23 per 1,000 for persons in the 50 to 64 year age group, and 8 per 1,000 for persons over 65 years of age. The risk of hepatitis is increased with daily consumption of alcohol. Precise data to provide a fatality rate for isoniazid-related hepatitis is not available; however, in a US Public Health Service Surveillance Study of 13,838 persons taking isoniazid, there were 8 deaths among 174 cases of hepatitis.
Therefore, patients given isoniazid should be carefully monitored and interviewed at monthly intervals. Serum transaminase concentration becomes elevated in about 10 to 20 percent of patients, usually during the first few months of therapy but it can occur at any time. Usually enzyme levels return to normal despite continuance of drug but in some cases progressive liver dysfunction occurs. Patients should be instructed to report immediately any of the prodromal symptoms of hepatitis, such as fatigue, weakness, malaise, anorexia, nausea, or vomiting. If these symptoms appear or if signs suggestive of hepatic damage are detected, isoniazid should be discontinued promptly since continued use of the drug in these cases has been reported to cause a more severe form of liver damage.
Patients with tuberculosis should be given appropriate treatment with alternative drugs. If isoniazid must be reinstituted, it should be reinstituted only after symptoms and laboratory abnormalities have cleared. The drug should be restarted in very small and gradually increasing doses and should be withdrawn immediately if

Continued on next page

Squibb—Cont.

there is any indication of recurrent liver involvement.
Preventive treatment should be deferred in persons with acute hepatic diseases.

Description: Isoniazid is the hydrazide of isonicotinic acid and is available as Nydrazid Tablets (Isoniazid Tablets USP) providing 100 mg. isoniazid per tablet and as Nydrazid Injection (Isoniazid Injection USP) in vials providing 100 mg. isoniazid per ml. and containing 0.25% chlorobutanol (chloral derivative) as a preservative; the pH has been adjusted to 6.0 to 7.0 with sodium hydroxide or hydrochloric acid. At the time of manufacture, the air in the container is replaced by nitrogen.

Actions: Isoniazid acts against actively growing tubercle bacilli.

Within one to two hours after oral administration, isoniazid produces peak blood levels which decline to 50 percent or less within six hours. It diffuses readily into all body fluids (cerebrospinal, pleural, and ascitic), tissues, organs, and excreta (saliva, sputum, and feces). The drug also passes through the placental barrier and into milk in concentrations comparable to those in the plasma. From 50 to 70 percent of a dose of isoniazid is excreted in the urine in 24 hours.

Isoniazid is metabolized primarily by acetylation and dehydrazination. The rate of acetylation is genetically determined. Approximately 50 percent of Blacks and Caucasians are "slow inactivators" and the rest are "rapid inactivators"; the majority of Eskimos and Orientals are "rapid inactivators."

The rate of acetylation does not significantly alter the effectiveness of isoniazid. However, slow acetylation may lead to higher blood levels of the drug and thus an increase in toxic reactions.

Pyridoxine (B_6) deficiency is sometimes observed in adults with high doses of isoniazid and is considered probably due to its competition with pyridoxal phosphate for the enzyme apotryptophanase.

Indications: Nydrazid Tablets (Isoniazid Tablets USP) and Nydrazid Injection (Isoniazid Injection USP) are recommended for all forms of tuberculosis in which organisms are susceptible.

Intramuscular administration is intended for use whenever administration by the oral route is not possible.

Isoniazid is recommended for preventive therapy for the following groups, in order of priority:

1. Household members and other close associates of persons with recently diagnosed tuberculous disease.
2. Positive tuberculin skin test reactors with findings on the chest roentgenogram consistent with nonprogressive tuberculous disease, in whom there are neither positive bacteriologic findings nor a history of adequate chemotherapy.
3. Newly infected persons.
4. Positive tuberculin skin test reactors in the special clinical situations as follows: prolonged therapy with adrenocorticosteroids; immunosuppressive therapy; some hematologic and reticuloendothelial diseases, such as leukemia or Hodgkin's disease; diabetes mellitus; silicosis; after gastrectomy.
5. Other positive tuberculin reactors under 35 years of age.
   The risk of hepatitis must be weighed against the risk of tuberculosis in positive tuberculin reactors over the age of 35. However, the use of isoniazid is recommended for those with the additional risk factors listed above (1 to 4) and on an individual basis in situations where there is likelihood of serious consequences to contacts who may become infected.

Contraindications: Previous isoniazid-associated hepatic injury; severe adverse reactions to isoniazid, such as drug fever, chills, and arthritis; acute liver disease of any etiology.

Warnings: See the boxed warning.

Precautions: All drugs should be stopped and an evaluation made at the first sign of a hypersensitivity reaction. If isoniazid therapy must be reinstituted, the drug should be given only after symptoms have cleared. The drug should be restarted in very small and gradually increasing doses and should be withdrawn immediately if there is any indication of recurrent hypersensitivity reaction.

Use of isoniazid should be carefully monitored in the following:

1. Patients who are receiving phenytoin concurrently. Isoniazid may decrease the excretion of phenytoin or may enhance its effects. To avoid phenytoin intoxication, appropriate dosage adjustment of the anticonvulsant should be made.
2. Daily users of alcohol. Daily ingestion of alcohol may be associated with a higher incidence of isoniazid hepatitis.
3. Those patients with current chronic liver disease or severe renal dysfunction.

Periodic ophthalmologic examinations during isoniazid therapy are recommended when visual symptoms occur.

Usage in Pregnancy and Lactation: It has been reported that in both rats and rabbits, isoniazid may exert an embryocidal effect when administered orally during pregnancy, although no isoniazid-related congenital anomalies have been found in reproduction studies in mammalian species (mice, rats, and rabbits). Isoniazid should be prescribed during pregnancy only when therapeutically necessary. The benefit of preventive therapy should be weighed against a possible risk to the fetus. Preventive treatment generally should be started after delivery because of the increased risk of tuberculosis for new mothers.

Since isoniazid is known to cross the placental barrier and to pass into maternal breast milk, neonates and breast-fed infants of isoniazid-treated mothers should be carefully observed for any evidence of adverse effects.

Carcinogenesis: Isoniazid has been reported to induce pulmonary tumors in a number of strains of mice.

Adverse Reactions: The most frequent reactions are those affecting the nervous system and the liver.

Nervous system: Peripheral neuropathy is the most common toxic effect. It is dose related, occurs most often in the malnourished and in those predisposed to neuritis (e.g., alcoholics and diabetics), and is usually preceded by paresthesias of the feet and hands. The incidence is higher in "slow inactivators."

Other neurotoxic effects which are uncommon with conventional doses are convulsions, toxic encephalopathy, optic neuritis and atrophy, memory impairment, and toxic psychosis.

Gastrointestinal: Nausea, vomiting, and epigastric distress.

Hepatic: Elevated serum transaminases (SGOT, SGPT), bilirubinemia, bilirubinuria, jaundice, and occasionally severe and sometimes fatal hepatitis. The common prodromal symptoms are anorexia, nausea, vomiting, fatigue, malaise, and weakness. Mild and transient elevation of serum transaminase levels occurs in 10 to 20 percent of persons taking isoniazid. The abnormality usually occurs in the first four to six months of treatment but can occur at any time during therapy. In most instances, enzyme levels return to normal without need to discontinue medication. In occasional instances, progressive liver damage occurs with accompanying symptoms. In these cases, the drug should be discontinued immediately. The frequency of progressive liver damage increases with age. It is rare in individuals under 20, but occurs in up to 2.3 percent of those over 50 years of age.

Hematologic: Agranulocytosis; hemolytic, sideroblastic, or aplastic anemia; throbocytopenia; and eosinophilia.

Hypersensitivity: Fever, skin eruptions (morbilliform, maculopapular, purpuric, or exfoliative), lymphadenopathy, and vasculitis.

Metabolic and endocrine: Pyridoxine deficiency, pellagra, hyperglycemia, metabolic acidosis, and gynecomastia.

Miscellaneous: Rheumatic syndrome and systemic lupus erythematosus-like syndrome. Local irritation has been observed at the site of intramuscular injection.

Overdosage: Signs and Symptoms — Isoniazid overdosage produces signs and symptoms within 30 minutes to three hours after ingestion. Nausea, vomiting, dizziness, slurring of speech, blurring of vision, and visual hallucinations (including bright colors and strange designs) are among the early manifestations. With marked overdosage, respiratory distress and CNS depression, progressing rapidly from stupor to profound coma, are to be expected along with severe, intractable seizures. Severe metabolic acidosis, acetonuria, and hyperglycemia are typical laboratory findings.

Treatment—Untreated or inadequately treated cases of gross isoniazid overdosage can terminate fatally, but good response has been reported in most patients brought under adequate treatment within the first few hours after drug ingestion.

Secure the airway and establish adequate respiratory exchange. Gastric lavage within the first two to three hours is advised, but should not be attempted until convulsions are under control. To control convulsions, administer I.V. short-acting barbiturates and I.V. pyridoxine (usually 1 mg./mg. isoniazid ingested).

Obtain blood samples for immediate determination of gases, electrolytes, BUN, glucose, etc.; type and crossmatch blood in preparation for possible hemodialysis.

Rapid control of metabolic acidosis is fundamental to management. Give I.V. sodium bicarbonate at once and repeat as needed, adjusting subsequent dosage on the basis of laboratory findings (i.e., serum sodium, pH, etc.).

Forced osmotic diuresis must be started early and should be continued for some hours after clinical improvement to hasten renal clearance of the drug and help prevent relapse. Fluid intake and output should be monitored.

Hemodialysis is advised for severe cases; if this is not available, peritoneal dialysis can be used along with forced diuresis.

Along with measures based on initial and repeated determination of blood gases and other laboratory tests as needed, meticulous respiratory and other intensive care should be utilized to protect against hypoxia, hypotension, aspiration pneumonitis, etc.

Note: For preventive therapy of tuberculous infection it is recommended that physicians be familiar with the joint recommendations of the American Thoracic Society, American Lung Association, and the Center for Disease Control, as published in the American Review of Respiratory Disease, Vol. 110, No. 3, September, 1974, or CDC's Morbidity and Mortality Weekly Report, Vol. 24, No. 8, February 22, 1975.

Dosage and Administration: Nydrazid Tablets (Isoniazid Tablets USP) and Nydrazid Injection (Isoniazid Injection USP) are used in conjunction with other effective antituberculous agents. If the bacilli become resistant, therapy must be changed to agents to which the bacilli are susceptible.

Usual Oral or Parenteral Dosage—

For Treatment of Tuberculosis—Adults: 5 mg./kg. up to 300 mg. daily in a single dose.

Infants and Children: 10 to 20 mg./kg. depending on severity of infection (up to 300 to 500 mg. daily) in a single dose.

For Preventive Therapy—Adults: 300 mg. per day in a single dose.
Infants and Children: 10 mg./kg. (up to 300 mg. daily) in a single dose.
Continuous administration of isoniazid for a sufficient period of time is an essential part of the regimen because relapse rates are higher if chemotherapy is stopped prematurely. In the treatment of tuberculosis, resistant organisms may multiply and their emergence during the treatment may necessitate a change in the regimen.
Concomitant administration of pyridoxine (B_6) is recommended in the malnourished and in those predisposed to neuropathy (e.g., alcoholics and diabetics).
How Supplied: Nydrazid Tablets (Isoniazid Tablets USP) are available for oral use providing 100 mg. isoniazid per tablet. Bottles of 100 and 1000.
Nydrazid Injection (Isoniazid Injection USP) is available for intramuscular use in vials providing 100 mg. isoniazid per ml. Vials of 10 ml.
Storage: Store Nydrazid (Isoniazid) preparations at room temperature.
The parenteral form of the drug may crystallize at low temperatures. If this occurs, warm the vial to room temperature before use to redissolve the crystals.
Bottles of isoniazid tablets should be kept tightly closed; avoid excessive heat.

OPHTHAINE® SOLUTION ℞
(Proparacaine Hydrochloride Ophthalmic Solution 0.5%)

Description: Ophthaine Solution is a sterile, aqueous solution containing 0.5% proparacaine hydrochloride with glycerin as a stabilizer, sodium hydroxide or hydrochloric acid to adjust the pH, and 0.2% chlorobutanol (chloral derivative) and benzalkonium chloride as antimicrobial preservatives. At the time of manufacture, the air in the container is replaced by nitrogen.
Action: Ophthaine Solution is a rapid acting local anesthetic suitable for ophthalmic use. With a single drop, the onset of anesthesia occurs in approximately 13 seconds and persists for 15 minutes or longer.
The main site of anesthetic action is the nerve cell membrane where proparacaine interferes with the large transient increase in the membrane permeability to sodium ions that is normally produced by a slight depolarization of the membrane. As the anesthetic action progressively develops in a nerve, the threshold for electrical stimulation gradually increases and the safety factor for conduction decreases; when this action is sufficiently well developed, block of conduction is produced.
The exact mechanism whereby proparacaine and other local anesthetics influence the permeability of the cell membrane is unknown; however, several studies indicate that local anesthetics may limit sodium ion permeability by closing the pores through which the ions migrate in the lipid layer of the nerve cell membrane. This limitation prevents the fundamental change necessary for the generation of the action potential.
Indications: Ophthaine Solution (Proparacaine Hydrochloride Ophthalmic Solution) is indicated for topical anesthesia in ophthalmic practice. Representative ophthalmic procedures in which the preparation provides good local anesthesia include measurement of intraocular pressure (tonometry), removal of foreign bodies and sutures from the cornea, conjunctival scraping in diagnosis and gonioscopic examination; it is also indicated for use as a topical anesthetic prior to surgical operations such as cataract extraction.
Contraindications: This preparation is contraindicated in patients with known hypersensitivity to proparacaine.
Warning: Prolonged use of a topical ocular anesthetic may produce permanent corneal opacification with accompanying loss of vision.
Precautions: Proparacaine should be used cautiously and sparingly in patients with known allergies, cardiac disease, or hyperthyroidism. The long-term toxicity of proparacaine is unknown; prolonged use may possibly delay wound healing. Although exceedingly rare with ophthalmic application of local anesthetics, it should be borne in mind that systemic toxicity (manifested by central nervous system stimulation followed by depression) may occur.
Protection of the eye from irritating chemicals, foreign bodies and rubbing during the period of anesthesia is very important. Tonometers soaked in sterilizing or detergent solutions should be thoroughly rinsed with sterile distilled water prior to use. Patients should be advised to avoid touching the eye until the anesthesia has worn off.
Adverse Reactions: Pupillary dilatation or cycloplegic effects have rarely been observed with proparacaine hydrochloride. The drug appears to be safe for use in patients sensitive to other local anesthetics, but local or systemic sensitivity occasionally occurs. Instillation of proparacaine in the eye at recommended concentration and dosage usually produces little or no initial irritation, stinging, burning, conjunctival redness, lacrimation, or increased winking. However, some local irritation and stinging may occur several hours after the instillation.
Rarely, a severe, immediate-type, apparently hyperallergic corneal reaction may occur which includes acute, intense and diffuse epithelial keratitis; a gray, ground-glass appearance; sloughing of large areas of necrotic epithelium; corneal filaments and, sometimes, iritis with descemetitis.
Allergic contact dermatitis with drying and fissuring of the fingertips has been reported.
Softening and erosion of the corneal epithelium and conjunctival congestion and hemorrhage have been reported.
Dosage and Administration: *Deep anesthesia as in cataract extraction*—Instill 1 drop every 5 to 10 minutes for 5 to 7 doses.
Removal of sutures—Instill 1 or 2 drops 2 or 3 minutes before removal of stitches.
Removal of foreign bodies—Instill 1 or 2 drops prior to operating.
Tonometry—Instill 1 or 2 drops immediately before measurement.
How Supplied: 15 ml. plastic squeeze bottles with dropper tips.
Storage: Store bottle in carton to protect from light until bottle is empty. Ophthaine Solution (Proparacaine Hydrochloride Ophthalmic Solution) may be stored at room temperature until first use. Refrigerate opened bottle to retard discoloration of solution. Do not use a discolored solution. Keep bottle tightly closed.

ORAGRAFIN® CALCIUM GRANULES ℞
(Ipodate Calcium for Oral Suspension USP)
ORAGRAFIN® SODIUM CAPSULES ℞
(Ipodate Sodium Capsules USP)

(See Diagnostic Section)

O-V STATIN® ℞
(oral/vaginal therapy pack)

O-V STATIN (oral/vaginal therapy pack) is designed specifically to provide a convenient therapy pack for use in the treatment of coexisting intestinal candidiasis and vulvovaginal candidiasis.
Mycostatin® Oral Tablets
(Nystatin Tablets USP)
Mycostatin® Vaginal Tablets
(Nystatin Vaginal Tablets USP)
Description: Nystatin is an antifungal antibiotic which is both fungistatic and fungicidal *in vitro* against a wide variety of yeasts and yeast-like fungi. It is a polyene antibiotic of undetermined structural formula that is obtained from *Streptomyces noursei.*
MYCOSTATIN ORAL TABLETS (Nystatin Tablets USP) are provided for oral administration as coated tablets containing 500,000 units nystatin. Mycostatin Oral Tablets contain FD&C Yellow No. 5 (tartrazine).
MYCOSTATIN VAGINAL TABLETS (Nystatin Vaginal Tablets USP) are provided as diamond-shaped, individually foil wrapped, compressed tablets containing 100,000 units nystatin dispersed in lactose with ethyl cellulose, stearic acid and starch.
Clinical Pharmacology: Nystatin probably acts by binding to sterols in the cell membrane of the fungus with a resultant change in membrane permeability allowing leakage of intracellular components. It exhibits no appreciable activity against bacteria or trichomonads.
Following oral administration, nystatin is sparingly absorbed with no detectable blood levels when given in the recommended doses. Most of the orally administered nystatin is passed unchanged in the stool.
Indications and Usage: O-V STATIN oral/vaginal therapy pack [Mycostatin Oral Tablets (Nystatin Tablets USP) and Mycostatin Vaginal Tablets (Nystatin Vaginal Tablets USP)] is indicated for use in the treatment of coexisting intestinal candidiasis and vulvovaginal candidiasis.
MYCOSTATIN VAGINAL TABLETS (Nystatin Vaginal Tablets USP) are effective for the local treatment of vulvovaginal candidiasis (moniliasis). The diagnosis should be confirmed, prior to therapy, by KOH smears and/or cultures. Other pathogens commonly associated with vulvovaginitis (Trichomonas and *Hemophilus vaginalis*) do not respond to nystatin and should be ruled out by appropriate laboratory methods.
Contraindications: Both preparations are contraindicated in patients with a history of hypersensitivity to any of their components.
Precautions: General—Discontinue treatment if sensitization or irritation is reported during intravaginal use.
Mycostatin Oral Tablets contain FD&C Yellow No. 5 (tartrazine) which may cause allergic-type reactions (including bronchial asthma) in certain susceptible individuals. Although the overall incidence of FD&C Yellow No. 5 (tartrazine) sensitivity in the general population is low, it is frequently seen in patients who also have aspirin hypersensitivity.
Laboratory Tests—If there is a lack of response to MYCOSTATIN VAGINAL TABLETS (Nystatin Vaginal Tablets USP), appropriate microbiological studies should be repeated to confirm the diagnosis and rule out other pathogens before instituting another course of antimycotic therapy.
Usage in Pregnancy: No adverse effects or complications have been attributed to nystatin in infants born to women treated with nystatin oral or vaginal tablets.
Adverse Reactions: Nystatin is virtually nontoxic and nonsensitizing and is well tolerated by all age groups, even on prolonged administration. Large oral doses have occasionally produced diarrhea, gastrointestinal distress, nausea and vomiting. Rarely, irritation or sensitization on intravaginal use may occur (see PRECAUTIONS).
Dosage and Administration: MYCOSTATIN ORAL TABLETS—The usual therapeutic dosage is one to two tablets (500,000 to 1,000,000 units nystatin) three times daily. Treatment should generally be continued for at least 48 hours after clinical cure to prevent relapse.
MYCOSTATIN VAGINAL TABLETS—The usual dosage is one tablet (100,000 units ny-

Continued on next page

Squibb—Cont.

statin) daily for two weeks. The tablets should be deposited high in the vagina by means of the applicator. "Instructions for the Patient" are enclosed in each package.
Even though symptomatic relief may occur within a few days, treatment should be continued for the full course.
It is important that therapy be continued during menstruation. Adjunctive measures such as therapeutic douches are unnecessary and sometimes inadvisable. Cleansing douches may be used by nonpregnant women, if desired, for esthetic purposes.
How Supplied: O-V STATIN oral/vaginal therapy pack—containing one bottle of 21 MYCOSTATIN ORAL TABLETS (Nystatin Tablets USP, 500,000 units nystatin each) and 14 individually foil wrapped MYCOSTATIN VAGINAL TABLETS (Nystatin Vaginal Tablets USP, 100,000 units nystatin each) with one plastic applicator and one "Instructions for the Patient" leaflet.
Storage: Store in refrigerator below 15° C (59° F).

PENICILLIN G POTASSIUM FOR INJECTION USP ℞

Description: Penicillin G Potassium for Injection USP is crystalline penicillin G potassium as a sterile powder. The preparation contains approximately 27 mg. citrate buffer (composed of sodium citrate and not more than 0.94 mg. of citric acid) with approximately 1.7 mEq. potassium and 0.3 mEq. sodium per million units of penicillin.
Actions: Penicillin G is bactericidal against penicillin-sensitive microorganisms during the stage of active multiplication. It acts by inhibiting biosynthesis of cell-wall mucopeptide. It is not active against the penicillinase-producing bacteria, which include many strains of staphylococci. Penicillin G is highly active *in vitro* against staphylococci (except penicillinase-producing strains), streptococci (groups A, C, G, H, L, and M) and pneumococci. Other organisms sensitive *in vitro* to penicillin G are *N. gonorrhoeae, Corynebacterium diphtheriae, Bacillus anthracis,* Clostridia, *Actinomyces bovis, Streptobacillus moniliformis, Listeria monocytogenes* and Leptospira; *Treponema pallidum* is extremely sensitive. Some species of gram-negative bacilli are sensitive to moderate to high concentrations of penicillin G obtained with intravenous administration. These include most strains of *Escherichia coli,* all strains of *Proteus mirabilis,* Salmonella and Shigella and some strains of *Enterobacter aerogenes* (formerly *Aerobacter aerogenes*) and *Alcaligenes faecalis.*
Sensitivity plate testing: If the Kirby-Bauer method of disc sensitivity is used, a 10 u. penicillin disc should give a zone greater than 28 mm. when tested against a penicillin-sensitive bacterial strain.
Aqueous penicillin G is rapidly absorbed following both intramuscular and subcutaneous injection. Approximately 60 percent of the total dose of 300,000 u. is excreted in the urine within this five-hour period. Therefore, high and frequent doses are required to maintain the elevated serum levels desirable in treating certain severe infections in individuals with normal kidney function. In neonates and young infants, and in individuals with impaired kidney function, excretion is considerably delayed.
Indications: Penicillin G Potassium for Injection USP is indicated in the treatment of severe infections caused by penicillin G-sensitive microorganisms when rapid and high penicillinemia is required. Therapy should be guided by bacteriological studies, including sensitivity tests, and by clinical response.
The following infections will usually respond to adequate dosage:
Streptococcal infections. Note: streptococci in groups A, C, H, G, L, and M are very sensitive to penicillin G. Some group D organisms are sensitive to the high serum levels obtained with aqueous penicillin G. Aqueous penicillin G potassium is the penicillin dosage form of choice for bacteremia, empyema, severe pneumonia, pericarditis, endocarditis, meningitis and other severe infections caused by sensitive strains of the gram-positive species listed above.
Pneumococcal infections; Staphylococcal infections—penicillin G-sensitive; **Anthrax; Actinomycosis; Clostridial infections** (including tetanus); **Diphtheria** (to prevent the carrier state); **Erysipeloid endocarditis** (Erysipelothrix insidiosa); **Vincent's gingivitis and pharyngitis** (fusospirochetosis)—Severe infections of the oropharynx (Note: necessary dental care should be accomplished in infections involving gum tissue.), and **lower respiratory tract and genital area infections** due to *F. fusiformisans* spirochetes; **Gram-negative bacillary infections** (bacteremias)—*(E. coli, E. aerogenes, A. faecalis,* Salmonella, Shigella and *P. mirabilis);* **Listeria infections** *(L. monocytogenes);* **Meningitis and endocarditis; Pasteurella infections** *(P. multocida); Bacteremia* and *meningitis;* **Ratbite fever** *(S. minus* or *S. moniliformis);* **Gonorrheal endocarditis and arthritis** *(N. gonorrhoeae);* **Syphilis** *(T. pallidum) including congenital syphilis;* **Meningococcic meningitis.**
Prophylaxis against bacterial endocarditis in patients with rheumatic or congenital heart disease when undergoing dental or upper respiratory tract surgery or instrumentation, surgery of the lower intestinal tract, childbirth, and instrumentation of the genitourinary tract. Note: because patients who have a past history of rheumatic fever and are receiving continuous prophylaxis may harbor increased numbers of penicillin-resistant organisms, use of another prophylactic anti-infective agent should be considered. If penicillin is to be used in these patients at surgery, the regular rheumatic fever program should be interrupted one week prior to the contemplated surgery. At the time of surgery, penicillin may be reinstituted as a prophylactic measure against the hazards of surgically-induced bacteremia.
Contraindications: Contraindicated in patients with a history of hypersensitivity to any penicillin.
Warnings: Serious and occasional fatal hypersensitivity (anaphylactoid) reactions have been reported in patients on penicillin therapy. Although anaphylaxis is more frequent following parenteral administration, it has occurred in patients on oral penicillins. These reactions are more apt to occur in individuals with a history of sensitivity to multiple allergens.
There have been well-documented reports of individuals with a history of penicillin hypersensitivity who have experienced severe hypersensitivity reactions when treated with cephalosporins. Before therapy with a penicillin, careful inquiry should be made concerning previous hypersensitivity reactions to penicillins, cephalosporins, and other allergens. If an allergic reaction occurs, the drug should be discontinued and the patient treated with the usual agents, e.g., pressor amines, antihistamines, and corticosteroids. Serious anaphylactoid reactions are not controlled by antihistamines alone, and require such emergency measures as the immediate use of epinephrine, aminophylline, oxygen, and intravenous corticosteroids.
Precautions: Penicillin should be used with caution in individuals with histories of significant allergies and/or asthma.
In prolonged therapy with penicillin and particularly with high dosage schedules, periodic evaluation of the renal and hematopoietic systems is recommended.
In streptococcal infections, therapy must be sufficient to eliminate the organism (ten days minimum); otherwise the sequelae of streptococcal disease may occur. Cultures should be taken following the completion of treatment to determine whether streptococci have been eradicated.
In high doses (above 10 million u.), intravenous aqueous penicillin G potassium should be administered slowly because of the adverse effects of electrolyte imbalance from the potassium content of the penicillin. The patient's renal, cardiac and vascular status should be evaluated and if impairment of function is suspected or known to exist, a reduction in the total dosage should be considered. Frequent evaluation of electrolyte balance, and renal and hematopoietic function is recommended during therapy when high doses of intravenous aqueous penicillin G potassium are used.
Prolonged use of antibiotics may promote overgrowth of nonsusceptible organisms, including fungi. Should superinfection occur, appropriate measures should be taken. Indwelling intravenous catheters encourage superinfections and should be avoided whenever possible.
Therapy of susceptible infections should be accompanied by any indicated surgical procedures. In suspected staphylococcal infections, proper laboratory studies, including sensitivity tests, should be performed.
When treating gonococcal infections in which primary or secondary syphilis may be suspected, proper diagnostic procedures, including darkfield examinations, should be done. In all cases in which concomitant syphilis is suspected, monthly serological tests should be made for at least four months. All cases of penicillin-treated syphilis should receive clinical and serological examinations every six months for at least two or three years.
Adverse Reactions: Penicillin is a substance of low toxicity but does possess a significant index of sensitization.
The hypersensitivity reactions reported are skin rashes ranging from maculopapular eruptions to exfoliative dermatitis; urticaria; and serum sickness-like reactions including chills, fever, edema, arthralgia and prostration. Severe and occasionally fatal anaphylaxis has occurred (see WARNINGS).
Hemolytic anemia, leukopenia, thrombocytopenia, neuropathy, and nephropathy are rarely observed adverse reactions and are usually associated with high intravenous dosage.
Urticaria, other skin rashes, and serum sickness-like reactions may be controlled by antihistamines and, if necessary, corticosteroids. Whenever such reactions occur, penicillin should be discontinued unless, in the opinion of the physician, the condition being treated is life-threatening and amenable only to penicillin therapy. Patients given continuous intravenous therapy with penicillin G potassium in high dosage (10 million to 100 million u. daily) may suffer severe or even fatal potassium poisoning, particularly if renal insufficiency is present. Hyperreflexia, convulsions and coma may be indicative of this syndrome.
The Jarisch-Herxheimer reaction has been reported in patients treated for syphilis.
Dosage and Administration: Penicillin G Potassium for Injection USP may be given intramuscularly or by continuous intravenous drip.
The 10,000,000 and 20,000,000 u. preparations of Penicillin G Potassium for Injection USP should be administered by intravenous infusion only.
The usual dosage recommendation is as follows:
Severe infections due to susceptible strains of streptococci, pneumococci, and staphylococci; bacteremia, pneumonia, endocarditis, pericarditis, empyema, meningitis and other severe infections: a minimum of 5 million u. daily.
Anthrax: a minimum of 5 million u./day in divided doses until cure is effected; **Actinomy-**

cosis: 1 to 6 million u./day for cervicofacial cases; 10 to 20 million u./day for thoracic and abdominal disease; **Clostridial infections** (as adjunctive therapy to antitoxin): 20 million u./day; **Diphtheria**—adjunctive therapy to antitoxin for prevention of the carrier state: 300,000 to 400,000 u./day in divided doses for 10 to 12 days; **Erysipeloid:** *Endocarditis:* 2 to 20 million u./day for 4 to 6 weeks: **Fusospirochetal infections** (fusospirochetosis)—severe infections of the oropharynx, lower respiratory tract and genital area: 5 to 10 million u./day; **Gram-negative bacillary infections** *(E. coli, E. aerogenes, A. faecalis,* Salmonella, Shigella and *P. mirabilis): Bacteremia:* 20 to 80 million u./day; **Listeria infections** *(L. monocytogenes): Neonates:* 500,000 to 1 million u./day; *Adults with meningitis:* 15 to 20 million u./day for 2 weeks; *Adults with endocarditis:* 15 to 20 million u./day for 4 weeks; **Pasteurella infections** *(P. multocida): Bacteremia* and *meningitis:* 4 to 6 million u./day for 2 weeks; **Rat-bite fever** *(S. minus* or *S. moniliformis):* 12 to 15 million u./day for 3 to 4 weeks.

Gonorrheal endocarditis and arthritis: a minimum of 5 million u. daily.

Syphilis—aqueous penicillin G potassium may be used in the treatment of acquired and congenital syphilis but, because of the necessity of frequent dosage, hospitalization is recommended. Dosage and duration of therapy is determined by the age of the patient and the stage of the disease.

Meningococcic meningitis: 1 to 2 million u. I.M. every 2 hours or continuous I.V. drip of 20 to 30 million u./day.

Prophylaxis against bacterial endocarditis in patients with rheumatic or congenital heart disease when undergoing dental or other operative procedures: 600,000 u. aqueous penicillin G procaine mixed with 200,000 u. of aqueous penicillin G one hour prior to procedure and once daily for the two days following the procedure.

Preparation of Solutions: Solutions of penicillin should be prepared as follows: Loosen powder. Hold vial horizontally and rotate it while *slowly* directing the stream of diluent against the wall of the vial. Shake vial vigorously after all the diluent has been added. Depending on the route of administration, use Sterile Water for Injection USP, isotonic Sodium Chloride Injection USP, or Dextrose Injection USP. NOTE: Penicillins are rapidly inactivated in the presence of carbohydrate solutions at alkaline pH.

RECONSTITUTION: **1,000,000 u. vial**—add 9.6 ml., 4.6 ml., or 3.6 ml. diluent to provide 100,000 u., 200,000 u., or 250,000 u. per ml., respectively; **5,000,000 u. vial**—add 23 ml., 18 ml., 8 ml., or 3 ml. diluent to provide 200,000 u., 250,000 u., 500,000 u., or 1,000,000 u. per ml., respectively. *For I.V. infusion only:* **10,000,000 u. vial**—add 15.5 ml. or 5.4 ml. diluent to provide 500,000 u. or 1,000,000 u. per ml., respectively; **20,000,000 u. vial**—add 31.6 ml. diluent to provide 500,000 u. per ml.

How Supplied: Penicillin G Potassium for Injection USP is available in vials providing 1, 5, 10, and 20 million units of crystalline penicillin G potassium.

Storage: The dry powder is relatively stable and may be stored at room temperature without significant loss of potency. Sterile solutions may be kept in the refrigerator one week without significant loss of potency. Solutions prepared for intravenous infusion are stable at room temperature for at least 24 hours.

PENICILLIN G SODIUM FOR INJECTION NF ℞

Description: Penicillin G Sodium for Injection NF is crystalline penicillin G sodium as a sterile powder. The preparation contains 28 mg. citrate buffer (composed of sodium citrate, and not more than 0.92 mg. citric acid) and 2.0 mEq. sodium per million units of penicillin.

Actions: Penicillin G is bactericidal against penicillin-sensitive microorganisms during the stage of active multiplication. It acts by inhibiting biosynthesis of cell-wall mucopeptide. It is not active against the penicillinase-producing bacteria, which include many strains of staphylococci. Penicillin G is highly active *in vitro* against staphylococci (except penicillinase-producing strains), streptococci (groups A, C, G, H, L, and M) and pneumococci. Other organisms sensitive *in vitro* to penicillin G are *N. gonorrhoeae, Corynebacterium diphtheriae, Bacillus anthracis,* Clostridia, *Actinomyces bovis, Streptobacillus moniliformis, Listeria monocytogenes* and Leptospira; *Treponema pallidum* is extremely sensitive. Some species of gram-negative bacilli are sensitive to moderate to high concentrations of penicillin G obtained with intravenous administration. These include most strains of *Escherichia coli,* all strains of *Proteus mirabilis,* Salmonella and Shigella and some strains of *Enterobacter aerogenes* (formerly *Aerobacter aerogenes*) and *Alcaligenes faecalis.*

Sensitivity plate testing: If the Kirby-Bauer method of disc sensitivity is used, a 10 u. penicillin disc should give a zone greater than 28 mm. when tested against a penicillin-sensitive bacterial strain.

Aqueous penicillin G is rapidly absorbed following both intramuscular and subcutaneous injection. Approximately 60 percent of the total dose of 300,000 u. is excreted in the urine within this five-hour period. Therefore, high and frequent doses are required to maintain the elevated serum levels desirable in treating certain severe infections in individuals with normal kidney function. In neonates and young infants, and in individuals with impaired kidney function, excretion is considerably delayed.

Indications: Penicillin G Sodium for Injection NF is indicated in the treatment of severe infections caused by penicillin G-sensitive microorganisms when rapid and high penicillinemia is required. Therapy should be guided by bacteriological studies, including sensitivity tests, and by clinical response.

The following infections will usually respond to adequate dosage:

Streptococcal infections. Note: streptococci in groups A, C, H, G, L, and M are very sensitive to penicillin G. Some group D organisms are sensitive to the high serum levels obtained with aqueous penicillin G. Aqueous penicillin G sodium is the penicillin dosage form of choice for bacteremia, empyema, severe pneumonia, pericarditis, endocarditis, meningitis and other severe infections caused by sensitive strains of the gram-positive species listed above.

Pneumococcal infections; Staphylococcal infections—penicillin G-sensitive; **Anthrax; Actinomycosis; Clostridial infections** (including tetanus); **Diphtheria** (to prevent the carrier state); **Erysipeloid endocarditis** (Erysipelothrix insidiosa); **Vincent's gingivitis and pharyngitis** (fusospirochetosis)—Severe infections of the oropharynx (Note: necessary dental care should be accomplished in infections involving gum tissue.), and **lower respiratory tract and genital area infections** due to *F. fusiformisans* spirochetes; **Gram-negative bacillary infections** (bacteremias)—*(E. coli, E. aerogenes, A. faecalis,* Salmonella, Shigella and *P. mirabilis);* **Listeria infections** *(L. monocytogenes);* **Meningitis and endocarditis; Pasteurella infections** *(P. multocida): Bacteremia* and *meningitis;* **Rat-bite fever** *(S. minus* or *S. moniliformis);* **Gonorrheal endocarditis and arthritis** *(N. gonorrhoeae);* **Syphilis** *(T. pallidum) including congenital syphilis;* **Meningococcic meningitis.**

Prophylaxis against bacterial endocarditis in patients with rheumatic or congenital heart disease when undergoing dental or upper respiratory tract surgery or instrumentation, surgery of the lower intestinal tract, childbirth, and instrumentation of the genitourinary tract. Note: because patients who have a past history of rheumatic fever and are receiving continuous prophylaxis may harbor increased numbers of penicillin-resistant organisms, use of another prophylactic anti-infective agent should be considered. If penicillin is to be used in these patients at surgery, the regular rheumatic fever program should be interrupted one week prior to the contemplated surgery. At the time of surgery, penicillin may be reinstituted as a prophylactic measure against the hazards of surgically-induced bacteremia.

Contraindications: Contraindicated in patients with a history of hypersensitivity to any penicillin.

Warnings: Serious and occasional fatal hypersensitivity (anaphylactoid) reactions have been reported in patients on penicillin therapy. Although anaphylaxis is more frequent following parenteral administration, it has occurred in patients on oral penicillins. These reactions are more apt to occur in individuals with a history of sensitivity to multiple allergens.

There have been well-documented reports of individuals with a history of penicillin hypersensitivity who have experienced severe hypersensitivity reactions when treated with cephalosporins. Before therapy with a penicillin, careful inquiry should be made concerning previous hypersensitivity reactions to penicillins, cephalosporins, and other allergens. If an allergic reaction occurs, the drug should be discontinued and the patient treated with the usual agents, e.g., pressor amines, antihistamines, and corticosteroids. Serious anaphylactoid reactions are not controlled by antihistamines alone, and require such emergency measures as the immediate use of epinephrine, aminophylline, oxygen, and intravenous corticosteroids.

Precautions: Penicillin should be used with caution in individuals with histories of significant allergies and/or asthma.

In prolonged therapy with penicillin and particularly with high dosage schedules, periodic evaluation of the renal and hematopoietic systems is recommended.

In streptococcal infections, therapy must be sufficient to eliminate the organism (10 days minimum); otherwise the sequelae of streptococcal disease may occur. Cultures should be taken following the completion of treatment to determine whether streptococci have been eradicated.

In high doses (above 10 million u.), intravenous aqueous penicillin G sodium should be administered slowly because of the adverse effects of electrolyte imbalance from the sodium content of the penicillin. The patient's renal, cardiac and vascular status should be evaluated and if impairment of function is suspected or known to exist, a reduction in the total dosage should be considered. Frequent evaluation of electrolyte balance, and renal and hematopoietic function is recommended during therapy when high doses of intravenous aqueous penicillin G sodium are used.

Prolonged use of antibiotics may promote overgrowth of nonsusceptible organisms, including fungi. Should superinfection occur, appropriate measures should be taken. Indwelling intravenous catheters encourage superinfections and should be avoided whenever possible.

Therapy of susceptible infections should be accompanied by any indicated surgical procedures. In suspected staphylococcal infections, proper laboratory studies, including sensitivity tests, should be performed.

When treating gonococcal infections in which primary or secondary syphilis may be suspected, proper diagnostic procedures, including darkfield examinations, should be done. In all cases in which concomitant syphilis is suspected, monthly serological tests should be made for at least four months. All cases of peni-

Continued on next page

Squibb—Cont.

cillin-treated syphilis should receive clinical and serological examinations every six months for at least two or three years.

Adverse Reactions: Penicillin is a substance of low toxicity but does possess a significant index of sensitization.

The hypersensitivity reactions reported are skin rashes ranging from maculopapular eruptions to exfoliative dermatitis; urticaria; and serum sickness-like reactions including chills, fever, edema, arthralgia and prostration. Severe and occasionally fatal anaphylaxis has occurred (see WARNINGS).

Hemolytic anemia, leukopenia, thrombocytopenia, neuropathy, and nephropathy are rarely observed adverse reactions and are usually associated with high intravenous dosage. Urticaria, other skin rashes, and serum sickness-like reactions may be controlled by antihistamines and, if necessary, corticosteroids. Whenever such reactions occur, penicillin should be discontinued unless, in the opinion of the physician, the condition being treated is life-threatening and amenable only to penicillin therapy. High dosage of penicillin G sodium may result in congestive heart failure due to high sodium intake.

The Jarisch-Herxheimer reaction has been reported in patients treated for syphilis.

Dosage and Administration: Penicillin G Sodium for Injection NF may be given intramuscularly or by continuous intravenous drip. The usual dosage recommendation is as follows:

Severe infections due to susceptible strains of streptococci, pneumococci, and staphylococci; bacteremia, pneumonia, endocarditis, pericarditis, empyema, meningitis and other severe infections: a minimum of 5 million u. daily.

Anthrax: a minimum of 5 million u./day in divided doses until cure is effected; **Actinomycosis:** 1 to 6 million u./day for cervicofacial cases; 10 to 20 million u./day for thoracic and abdominal disease; **Clostridial infections** (as adjunctive therapy to antitoxin): 20 million u./day; **Diphtheria**—adjunctive therapy to antitoxin for prevention of the carrier state: 300,000 to 400,000 u./day in divided doses for 10 to 12 days; **Erysipeloid:** *Endocarditis:* 2 to 20 million u./day for 4 to 6 weeks: **Fusospirochetal infections** (fusospirochetosis)—severe infections of the oropharynx, lower respiratory tract and genital area: 5 to 10 million u./day; **Gram-negative bacillary infections** *(E. coli, E. aerogenes, A. faecalis,* Salmonella, Shigella and *P. mirabilis); Bacteremia:* 20 to 80 million u./day; **Listeria infections** *(L. monocytogenes): Neonates:* 500,000 to 1 million u./day; *Adults with meningitis:* 15 to 20 million u./day for 2 weeks; *Adults with endocarditis:* 15 to 20 million u./day for 4 weeks; **Pasteurella infections** *(P. multocida): Bacteremia* and *meningitis:* 4 to 6 million u./day for 2 weeks; **Rat-bite fever** *(S. minus* or *S. moniliformis):* 12 to 15 million u./day for 3 to 4 weeks.

Gonorrheal endocarditis and arthritis: a minimum of 5 million u. daily.

Syphilis—aqueous penicillin G sodium may be used in the treatment of acquired and congenital syphilis but, because of the necessity of frequent dosage, hospitalization is recommended. Dosage and duration of therapy is determined by the age of the patient and the stage of the disease.

Meningococcic meningitis: 1 to 2 million u. I.M. every 2 hours or continuous I.V. drip of 20 to 30 million u./day.

Prophylaxis against bacterial endocarditis in patients with rheumatic or congenital heart disease when undergoing dental or other operative procedures: 600,000 u. aqueous penicillin G procaine mixed with 200,000 u. of aqueous penicillin G one hour prior to procedure; and once daily for the two days following the procedure.

Preparation of Solutions: Solutions of penicillin should be prepared as follows: Loosen powder. Hold vial horizontally and rotate it while *slowly* directing the stream of diluent against the wall of the vial. Shake vial vigorously after all the diluent has been added. Depending on the route of administration, use Sterile Water for Injection USP, isotonic Sodium Chloride Injection USP, or Dextrose Injection USP. NOTE: Penicillins are rapidly inactivated in the presence of carbohydrate solutions at alkaline pH.

Reconstitute with 23 ml., 18 ml., 8 ml., or 3 ml. diluent to provide concentrations of 200,000 u., 250,000 u., 500,000 u., or 1,000,000 u. per ml., respectively.

How Supplied: In vials providing 5 million units of crystalline penicillin G sodium.

Storage: The dry powder is relatively stable and may be stored at room temperature without significant loss of potency. Sterile solutions may be kept in the refrigerator one week without significant loss of potency. Solutions prepared for intravenous infusion are stable at room temperature for at least 24 hours.

PENTIDS® TABLETS ℞
PENTIDS® '400' TABLETS ℞
PENTIDS® '800' TABLETS ℞
(Penicillin G Potassium Tablets USP)
PENTIDS® FOR SYRUP ℞
PENTIDS® '400' FOR SYRUP ℞
(Penicillin G Potassium for Oral Solution)

Description: Pentids Tablets, Pentids '400' Tablets and Pentids '800' Tablets (Penicillin G Potassium Tablets USP) are scored, compressed uncoated tablets of crystalline penicillin G potassium. Pentids '800' Tablets contain FD&C Yellow No. 5 (tartrazine).

Pentids for Syrup and Pentids '400' for Syrup (Penicillin G Potassium for Oral Solution) provide penicillin G potassium in flavored powder forms for preparation as syrups when liquid oral penicillin therapy is indicated, especially for infants and children. Pentids for Syrup and Pentids '400' for Syrup contain FD&C Yellow No. 5 (tartrazine).

Clinical Pharmacology: Penicillin G is bactericidal against penicillin-susceptible microorganisms during the stage of active multiplication. It acts by inhibiting biosynthesis of cell-wall mucopeptide. It is not active against the penicillinase-producing bacteria, which include many strains of staphylococci.

Penicillin G is highly active *in vitro* against staphylococci (except penicillinase-producing strains), streptococci (groups A, C, G, H, L, and M) and pneumococci. Other organisms susceptible *in vitro* to penicillin G are *Neisseria gonorrhoeae, Corynebacterium diphtheriae, Bacillus anthracis,* Clostridia, *Actinomyces bovis, Streptobacillus moniliformis, Listeria monocytogenes,* and Leptospira; *Treponema pallidum* is extremely susceptible. Some species of gram-negative bacilli are susceptible to moderate to high concentrations of penicillin G obtained with intravenous administration. These include most strains of *Escherichia coli,* all strains of *Proteus mirabilis,* Salmonella and Shigella and some strains of *Enterobacter aerogenes* (formerly *Aerobacter aerogenes*) and *Alcaligenes faecalis.*

Oral preparations of penicillin G are only slightly affected by normal gastric acidity (pH 2 to 3.5); however, a pH below 2.0 may partially or totally inactivate penicillin G. Oral penicillin G is absorbed in the upper small intestine, chiefly the duodenum; however, serum level and urinary excretion data indicate that only approximately 30 percent of the dose is absorbed. For this reason four to five times the dose of oral penicillin G must be given to obtain a blood level comparable to that obtained with parenteral penicillin G. Since gastric acidity, stomach emptying time, and other factors affecting absorption may vary considerably, serum levels may be appreciably reduced to nontherapeutic levels in certain individuals.

Approximately 60 percent of penicillin G is bound to serum protein. The drug is distributed throughout the body tissues in widely varying amounts. Highest levels are found in the kidneys with lesser amounts in the liver, skin, and intestines. Penicillin G penetrates into all other tissues to a lesser degree with very limited amounts found in the cerebrospinal fluid. The drug is excreted rapidly by tubular excretion in patients with normal kidney function. In neonates and young infants, and in individuals with impaired kidney function, excretion is considerably delayed. Normally, approximately 20 percent of a dose of oral penicillin G is excreted in the urine.

Indications and Usage: Pentids (Penicillin G Potassium) are indicated in the treatment of mild to moderately severe infections due to penicillin G-susceptible microorganisms. Therapy should be guided by bacteriological studies, including susceptibility tests, and by clinical response. Note: severe pneumonia, empyema, bacteremia, pericarditis, meningitis, and septic arthritis should not be treated with oral penicillin G during the acute stage.

Indicated surgical procedures should be performed.

The following infections will usually respond to adequate dosage:

Streptococcal infections Group A without bacteremia—Mild to moderate infections of the upper respiratory tract, skin and skin structures infections, scarlet fever, and mild erysipelas. Note: streptococci in groups A, C, G, H, L, and M are very susceptible to penicillin G. Other groups, including group D (enterococcus) are resistant.

Pneumococcal infections—Mild to moderately severe infections of the respiratory tract.

Staphylococcal infections — penicillin G-susceptible—Mild infections of the skin and skin structures. Note: reports indicate an increasing number of strains of staphylococci resistant to penicillin G, emphasizing the need for culture and susceptibility studies in treating suspected staphylococcal infections.

Vincent's gingivitis and pharyngitis (fusospirochetosis)—Mild to moderately severe infections of the oropharynx usually respond to oral penicillin G. Note: necessary dental care should be accomplished in infections involving gum tissue.

Medical conditions in which oral penicillin G therapy is indicated as prophylaxis: (A) *For the prevention of recurrence following rheumatic fever and/or chorea.* Prophylaxis with oral penicillin G on a continuing basis is effective in preventing recurrence of these conditions.

(B) *To prevent bacterial endocarditis* in patients with congenital and/or rheumatic heart lesions who are to undergo dental procedures or minor upper respiratory tract surgery or instrumentation. Prophylaxis should be instituted the day of the procedure and for two or more days afterwards. Patients who have a past history of rheumatic fever and are receiving continuous prophylaxis may harbor increased numbers of penicillin-resistant organisms; use of another prophylactic antiinfective agent should be considered. If penicillin is to be used in these patients at surgery, the regular rheumatic fever program should be interrupted one week prior to the contemplated surgery. At the time of surgery, penicillin may be reinstituted as a prophylactic measure against the hazards of surgically-induced bacteremia. Note: oral penicillin G should not be used as adjunctive prophylaxis for genitourinary instrumentation or surgery, lower intestinal tract surgery, sigmoidoscopy, and child birth.

(C) *Prevention of bacteremia following tooth extraction.*

Contraindications: Contraindicated in patients with a history of hypersensitivity to any penicillin.

Warnings: Serious and occasional fatal hypersensitivity (anaphylactoid) reactions have been reported in patients on penicillin therapy. Although anaphylaxis is more frequent following parenteral administration, it has occurred in patients on oral penicillins. These reactions are more apt to occur in individuals with a history of sensitivity to multiple allergens.

There have been well-documented reports of individuals with a history of penicillin hypersensitivity who have experienced severe hypersensitivity reactions when treated with cephalosporins. Before therapy with a penicillin, careful inquiry should be made concerning previous hypersensitivity reactions to penicillins, cephalosporins, and other allergens. If an allergic reaction occurs, the drug should be discontinued and the patient treated with the usual agents, e.g., pressor amines, antihistamines, and corticosteroids. Serious anaphylactoid reactions are not controlled by antihistamines alone, and require such emergency measures as the immediate use of epinephrine, aminophylline, oxygen, and intravenous corticosteroids.

Precautions: Penicillin should be used with caution in individuals with histories of significant allergies and/or asthma.

The oral route of administration should not be relied upon in patients with severe illness, or with nausea, vomiting, gastric dilatation, cardiospasm or intestinal hypermotility.

Occasional patients will not absorb therapeutic amounts of orally administered penicillin.

In streptococcal infections, therapy must be sufficient to eliminate the organism (10 days minimum); otherwise the sequelae of streptococcal disease may occur. Cultures should be taken following completion of treatment to determine whether streptococci have been eradicated.

Prolonged use of antibiotics may promote the overgrowth of nonsusceptible organisms, including fungi. Should superinfection occur, appropriate measures should be taken.

In prolonged therapy with penicillin, and particularly with high dosage schedules, periodic evaluation of the renal and hematopoietic systems is recommended.

Pentids '800' Tablets (Penicillin G Potassium Tablets USP), Pentids for Syrup (Penicillin G Potassium for Oral Solution), and Pentids '400' for Syrup contain FD&C Yellow No. 5 (tartrazine) which may cause allergic-type reactions (including bronchial asthma) in certain susceptible individuals. Although the overall incidence of FD&C Yellow No. 5 (tartrazine) sensitivity in the general population is low, it is frequently seen in patients who also have aspirin hypersensitivity.

Adverse Reactions: Although the incidence of reactions to oral penicillins has been reported with much less frequency than following parenteral therapy, it should be remembered that all degrees of hypersensitivity, including fatal anaphylaxis, have been reported with oral penicillin.

The most common reactions to oral penicillin are nausea, vomiting, epigastric distress, diarrhea, and black hairy tongue. The hypersensitivity reactions reported are skin rashes ranging from maculopapular to exfoliative dermatitis; urticaria; serum sickness-like reactions including chills, fever, edema, arthralgia, and prostration; laryngeal edema; and anaphylaxis. Fever and eosinophilia may frequently be the only reactions observed. Hemolytic anemia, leukopenia, thrombocytopenia, neuropathy, and nephropathy are infrequent reactions usually associated with high doses of parenteral penicillin. Urticaria, other skin rashes, and serum sickness-like reactions may be controlled by antihistamines and, if necessary, corticosteroids. Whenever such reactions occur, penicillin should be discontinued unless, in the opinion of the physician, the condition being treated is life-threatening and amenable only to penicillin therapy. Serious anaphylactoid reactions require emergency measures (see WARNINGS).

An occasional patient may complain of sore mouth or tongue, as with any oral penicillin preparation.

Dosage and Administration: The dosage of penicillin G should be determined according to the susceptibility of the causative microorganisms and the severity of infection, and adjusted to the clinical response of the patient.

Therapy for children under 12 years of age is calculated on the basis of body weight. For infants and small children the suggested dose is 15 to 56 mg. (25,000 to 90,000 u.) per kg./day in three to six divided doses.

For maximum absorption of penicillin, dosage should be given on an empty stomach. Thus, a dose of 200,000 units should be administered one-half hour before or at least two hours after meals. The blood concentration with a dose of 400,000 units is sufficiently high to inhibit susceptible bacteria when the antibiotic is given without regard to meals but, as can be expected, the resultant concentration will be higher when it is given before meals.

The usual dosage recommendation for adults and children 12 years and over is as follows:

Streptococcal infections—mild to moderately severe—of the upper respiratory tract and including otitis media, scarlet fever and mild erysipelas: 125 mg. (200,000 u.) t.i.d. or q.i.d. for 10 days for mild infections; 250 mg. (400,000 u.) t.i.d. for 10 days for moderately severe infections; alternatively, 500 mg. (800,000 u.) may be given b.i.d.

Pneumococcal infections—mild to moderately severe—of the respiratory tract, including otitis media: 250 mg. (400,000 u.) q.i.d. until the patient has been afebrile for at least two days.

Staphylococcal infections—mild infections of skin and skin structures (culture and susceptibility tests should be performed): 125 to 250 mg. (200,000 to 400,000 u.) t.i.d. or q.i.d. until infection is cured.

Vincent's gingivitis and pharyngitis (fusospirochetosis)—mild to moderately severe infections of the oropharynx: 250 mg. (400,000 u.) t.i.d. or q.i.d.

Medical conditions in which oral penicillin therapy is indicated as prophylaxis: *For the prevention of recurrence following rheumatic fever and/or chorea:* 125 mg. (200,000 u.) twice daily on a continuing basis. *To prevent bacterial endocarditis* in patients with congenital and/or rheumatic heart lesions who are to undergo dental procedures or minor upper respiratory tract surgery or instrumentation: 750 mg. (1,200,000 u.) oral penicillin G potassium one hour before the procedure and then 375 mg. (600,000 u.) every six hours for the remainder of that day and for the two days following the procedure (or longer in the case of delayed healing).

How Supplied: *Pentids, *Pentids '400' and *Pentids '800' Tablets (Penicillin G Potassium Tablets USP) are available for oral administration as scored, uncoated tablets which provide 125 mg. (200,000 units), 250 mg. (400,000 units) and 500 mg. (800,000 units) crystalline penicillin G potassium, respectively, equivalent to 120 mg., 240 mg. and 480 mg. of penicillin G sodium reference standard; the tablets are buffered with calcium carbonate. Pentids Tablets, in bottles of 100; Pentids '400' Tablets in bottles of 16 and 100 and Unimatic® cartons of 100; and Pentids '800' Tablets in bottles of 30 and 100.

Pentids for Syrup and Pentids '400' for Syrup (Penicillin G Potassium for Oral Solution) are available for oral administration as powders that, when prepared as directed, provide fruit-flavored syrups respectively containing 125 mg. (200,000 units) and 250 mg. (400,000 units) of penicillin G potassium (equivalent to 120 mg. and 240 mg. penicillin G sodium reference standard) per 5 ml. teaspoonful; both preparations are buffered with sodium phosphates. Pentids for Syrup and Pentids '400' for Syrup in 100 ml. and 200 ml. bottles.

Storage: Penicillin G Potassium Tablets—Store at room temperature; avoid excessive heat; keep bottle tightly closed.

Penicillin G Potassium for Oral Solution—Store at room temperature prior to preparation of syrup; store syrup in refrigerator; keep bottle tightly closed; discard unused portion after 14 days.

*[*Shown in Product Identification Section*]

PRINCIPEN® '250' CAPSULES ℞
PRINCIPEN® '500' CAPSULES ℞
(Ampicillin Capsules USP)
PRINCIPEN® '125' FOR ORAL SUSPENSION ℞
PRINCIPEN® '250' FOR ORAL SUSPENSION ℞
(Ampicillin for Oral Suspension USP)

Description: Principen (Ampicillin Trihydrate), a semisynthetic penicillin derived from the basic penicillin nucleus, 6- aminopenicillanic acid, is available for oral administration as Principen '250' Capsules and Principen '500' Capsules (Ampicillin Capsules USP) which provide ampicillin trihydrate equivalent to 250 mg. and 500 mg. ampicillin, respectively. It is also available as Principen '125' for Oral Suspension and Principen '250' for Oral Suspension (Ampicillin for Oral Suspension USP) which provide, after mixing, ampicillin trihydrate equivalent to 125 mg. and 250 mg. ampicillin, respectively, per 5 ml. teaspoonful.

Actions: Human Pharmacology: Ampicillin is bactericidal at low concentrations and is clinically effective not only against the gram-positive organisms usually susceptible to penicillin G but also against a variety of gram-negative organisms. It is stable in the presence of gastric acid and is well absorbed from the gastrointestinal tract. It diffuses readily into most body tissues and fluids; however, penetration into the cerebrospinal fluid and brain occurs only with meningeal inflammation. Ampicillin is excreted largely unchanged in the urine; its excretion can be delayed by concurrent administration of probenecid which inhibits the renal tubular secretion of ampicillin. In blood serum, ampicillin is the least bound of all the penicillins; an average of about 20 percent of the drug is bound to the plasma proteins as compared to 60 to 90 percent for the other penicillins. The administration of a 500 mg. dose of ampicillin trihydrate capsules results in an average peak blood serum level of approximately 3.0 mcg./ml.; the average peak serum level for the same dose of ampicillin trihydrate for oral suspension is approximately 3.4 mcg./ml.

Microbiology: The following microorganisms show *in vitro* sensitivity to ampicillin:

GRAM-POSITIVE—strains of alpha- and beta-hemolytic streptococci, *Streptococcus pneumoniae* (formerly *Diplococcus pneumoniae*), those strains of staphylococci which do not produce penicillinase, *Clostridium* sp., *Bacillus anthracis, Corynebacterium xerose,* and most strains of enterococci.

GRAM-NEGATIVE—*Hemophilus influenzae; Neisseria gonorrhoeae* and *N. meningitidis; Proteus mirabilis;* and many strains of Salmonella (including *S. typhosa*), Shigella, and *Escherichia coli.*

NOTE: Ampicillin is inactivated by penicillinase and therefore is ineffective against penicillinase-producing organisms including certain strains of staphylococci, *Pseudomonas aeruginosa, P. vulgaris, Klebsiella pneumoniae, Enterobacter aerogenes* (formerly *Aerobacter aerogenes*), and some strains of *E. coli.* Ampicillin is not active against Rickettsia, Mycoplasma, and "large viruses" (Miyagawanella).

Continued on next page

Squibb—Cont.

TESTING FOR SUSCEPTIBILITY: The invading organism should be cultured and its sensitivity demonstrated as a guide to therapy. If the Kirby-Bauer method of disc sensitivity is used, a 10 mcg. ampicillin disc should be used to determine the relative *in vitro* susceptibility.

Indications: Principen Capsules (Ampicillin Capsules USP) and Principen for Oral Suspension (Ampicillin for Oral Suspension USP) are primarily indicated for the treatment of genitourinary, respiratory, and gastrointestinal tract infections caused by susceptible strains of gram-negative bacteria (including Shigella, *S. typhosa* and other Salmonella, *E. coli, H. influenzae, N. gonorrhoeae* and *N. meningitidis,* and *P. mirabilis).* Ampicillin may also be indicated in certain infections due to susceptible gram-positive bacteria: penicillin G-sensitive staphylococci, streptococci, pneumococci, and enterococci.

Bacteriology studies to determine the causative organisms and their sensitivity to ampicillin should be performed. Therapy may be instituted prior to the results of sensitivity testing.

Contraindications: A history of a previous hypersensitivity reaction to any of the penicillins is a contraindication. Ampicillin is also contraindicated in infections caused by penicillinase-producing organisms.

Warnings: Serious and occasional fatal hypersensitivity (anaphylactoid) reactions have been reported in patients on penicillin therapy. Although anaphylaxis is more frequent following parenteral administration, it has occurred in patients on oral penicillins. These reactions are more apt to occur in individuals with a history of sensitivity to multiple allergens.

There have been well-documented reports of individuals with a history of penicillin hypersensitivity who have experienced severe hypersensitivity reactions when treated with cephalosporins. Before therapy with a penicillin, careful inquiry should be made concerning previous hypersensitivity reactions to penicillins, cephalosporins, and other allergens. If an allergic reaction occurs, the drug should be discontinued and the patient treated with the usual agents, e.g., pressor amines, antihistamines, and corticosteroids. **Serious anaphylactoid reactions require immediate emergency treatment with epinephrine. Oxygen, intravenous steroids and airway management, including intubation, should also be administered as indicated.**

Usage in Pregnancy: The safety of this drug for use in pregnancy has not been established.

Precautions: Prolonged use of antibiotics may promote the overgrowth of nonsusceptible organisms, including fungi. Should superinfection occur, appropriate measures should be taken.

Cases of gonococcal infection with a suspected lesion of syphilis should have darkfield examinations ruling out syphilis before receiving ampicillin. Patients who do not have suspected lesions of syphilis and are treated with ampicillin should have a follow-up serologic test for syphilis each month for four months to detect syphilis that may have been masked by treatment for gonorrhea. Patients with gonorrhea who also have syphilis should be given additional appropriate parenteral penicillin treatment.

Treatment with ampicillin does not preclude the need for surgical procedures, particularly in staphylococcal infections.

In prolonged therapy, and particularly with high dosage schedules, periodic evaluation of the renal, hepatic, and hematopoietic systems is recommended.

Adverse Reactions: As with other penicillins, it may be expected that untoward reactions will be essentially limited to sensitivity phenomena. They are more likely to occur in individuals who have previously demonstrated hypersensitivity to penicillin and in those with a history of allergy, asthma, hay fever, or urticaria.

The following adverse reactions have been reported as associated with the use of ampicillin:

Gastrointestinal: glossitis, stomatitis, nausea, vomiting, enterocolitis, pseudomembranous colitis, and diarrhea. These reactions are usually associated with oral dosage forms of the drug.

Hypersensitivity Reactions: an erythematous, mildly pruritic, maculopapular skin rash has been reported fairly frequently. The rash, which usually does not develop within the first week of therapy, may cover the entire body including the soles, palms, and oral mucosa. The eruption usually disappears in 3 to 7 days. Other hypersensitivity reactions that have been reported are: skin rash, pruritus, urticaria, erythema multiforme, and an occasional case of exfoliative dermatitis. Anaphylaxis is the most serious reaction experienced and has usually been associated with the parenteral dosage form of the drug.

NOTE: Urticaria, other skin rashes, and serum sickness-like reactions may be controlled by antihistamines, and, if necessary, systemic corticosteroids. Whenever such reactions occur, ampicillin should be discontinued unless, in the opinion of the physician, the condition being treated is life-threatening and amenable only to ampicillin therapy. Serious anaphylactoid reactions require emergency measures (see WARNINGS).

Liver: moderate elevation in serum glutamic oxaloacetic transaminase (SGOT) has been noted, but the significance of this finding is unknown.

Hemic and Lymphatic Systems: anemia, thrombocytopenia, thrombocytopenic purpura, eosinophilia, leukopenia, and agranulocytosis have been reported during therapy with penicillins. These reactions are usually reversible on discontinuation of therapy and are believed to be hypersensitivity phenomena.

Other adverse reactions that have been reported with the use of ampicillin are laryngeal stridor and high fever. An occasional patient may complain of sore mouth or tongue as with any oral penicillin preparation.

Dosage and Administration: *Adults, and children weighing over 20 kg.:* **For genitourinary or gastrointestinal tract infections other than gonorrhea in men and women,** the usual dose is 500 mg. q.i.d. in equally spaced doses; severe or chronic infections may require larger doses. For the treatment of gonorrhea in both men and women, a single oral dose of 3.5 grams of ampicillin administered simultaneously with 1.0 gram of probenecid is recommended. Physicians are cautioned to use no less than the above recommended dosage for the treatment of gonorrhea. Follow-up cultures should be obtained from the original site(s) of infection 7 to 14 days after therapy. In women, it is also desirable to obtain culture test-of-cure from both the endocervical and anal canals. Prolonged intensive therapy is needed for complications such as prostatitis and epididymitis. For **respiratory tract infections,** the usual dose is 250 mg. q.i.d. in equally spaced doses.

Children weighing 20 kg. or less: For **genitourinary or gastrointestinal tract infections,** the usual dose is 100 mg./kg./day total, q.i.d. in equally divided and spaced doses. For **respiratory infections,** the usual dose is 50 mg./kg./day total, in equally divided and spaced doses 3 to 4 times daily.

All patients, irrespective of age and weight: Larger doses may be required for severe or chronic infections. Although ampicillin is resistant to degradation by gastric acid, like all antibiotics given orally it should be administered at least two hours after or one-half hour before meals for maximal absorption. Except for the single dose regimen for gonorrhea referred to above, therapy should be continued for a minimum of 48 to 72 hours after the patient becomes asymptomatic or evidence of bacterial eradication has been obtained. In infections caused by hemolytic strains of streptococci, a minimum of 10 days' treatment is recommended to guard against the risk of rheumatic fever or glomerulonephritis. In the treatment of chronic urinary or gastrointestinal infections, frequent bacteriologic and clinical appraisal is necessary during therapy and may be necessary for several months afterwards. Stubborn infections may require treatment for several weeks. Smaller doses than those indicated above should not be used. Doses for children should not exceed doses recommended for adults.

How Supplied: Principen is available for oral administration as *Principen '250' Capsules and *Principen '500' Capsules (Ampicillin Capsules USP) which provide ampicillin trihydrate equivalent to 250 mg. and 500 mg. ampicillin, respectively; the 250 mg. potency in bottles of 100 and 500 and Unimatic® Single Dose Packs of 100 and 500; the 500 mg. potency in bottles of 16, 100, and 500 and Unimatic Single Dose Packs of 100 and 500. It is also available for oral administration as Principen '125' for Oral Suspension and Principen '250' for Oral Suspension (Ampicillin for Oral Suspension USP) which provide, after mixing, pleasantly flavored suspensions containing ampicillin trihydrate equivalent to 125 mg. and 250 mg. ampicillin, respectively, per 5 ml. teaspoonful; both potencies in 80, 100, 150, and 200 ml. bottles, and in Unimatic® cartons of 4 × 25 bottles (5 ml. each bottle).

Storage: Principen Capsules—Store at room temperature; avoid excessive heat; keep bottle tightly closed.

Principen for Oral Suspension—Store at room temperature prior to preparation of suspension; after preparation of suspension, store at room temperature and discard unused portion after 7 days or store in refrigerator and discard unused portion after 14 days; keep bottle tightly closed.

*[*Shown in Product Identification Section*]

PRINCIPEN® with PROBENECID ℞
(Ampicillin—Probenecid Capsules)

Description: Ampicillin trihydrate is a semisynthetic penicillin derived from the basic penicillin nucleus, 6-aminopenicillanic acid. Probenecid is a uricosuric and renal tubular blocking agent. Principen with Probenecid is provided in single-dose bottles containing nine capsules; each capsule contains ampicillin trihydrate equivalent to 389 mg. ampicillin and 111 mg. probenecid (9 capsules contain ampicillin trihydrate equivalent to 3.5 g. ampicillin and 1 g. probenecid).

Actions: Ampicillin is stable in the presence of gastric acid and is well absorbed from the gastrointestinal tract. It diffuses readily into most body tissues and fluids; however, penetration into the cerebrospinal fluid and brain occurs only with meningeal inflammation. Ampicillin is excreted largely unchanged in the urine; its excretion is delayed by concurrent administration of probenecid which inhibits the renal tubular secretion of ampicillin. In blood serum, ampicillin is the least bound of all the penicillins; an average of about 20 percent of the drug is bound to the plasma proteins as compared to 60 to 90 percent for the other penicillins. Probenecid inhibits the tubular reabsorption of urate, thus increasing the urinary excretion of uric acid and decreasing serum uric acid levels. It also inhibits the tubular secretion of penicillin and usually increases penicillin plasma levels by any route the antibiotic is given. A two-fold to four-fold elevation has been demonstrated for various penicillins.

Ampicillin is inactivated by penicillinase and therefore is ineffective against penicillinase-producing organisms.

Indications: Principen with Probenecid (Ampicillin—Probenecid Capsules) is indicated for the treatment of uncomplicated infection (urethral, endocervical, or rectal) caused by *Neisseria gonorrhoeae* in men and women.

Urethritis and the presence of gram-negative diplococci in urethral smears is strong presumptive evidence of gonorrhea. Culture or fluorescent antibody studies will confirm the diagnosis.

Susceptibility studies should be performed with recurrent infections or when resistant strains are encountered. Therapy may be instituted prior to obtaining results of susceptibility testing.

Contraindications: A history of a previous hypersensitivity reaction to any of the penicillins or to probenecid is a contraindication.

Probenecid is not recommended in persons with known blood dyscrasias or uric acid kidney stones or during an acute attack of gout. It is not recommended in conjunction with ampicillin in the presence of known renal impairment.

Warnings: Serious and occasional fatal hypersensitivity (anaphylactoid) reactions have been reported in patients on penicillin therapy. Although anaphylaxis is more frequent following parenteral administration, it has occurred in patients on oral penicillins. These reactions are more apt to occur in individuals with a history of sensitivity to multiple allergens.

There have been well-documented reports of individuals with a history of penicillin hypersensitivity who have experienced severe hypersensitivity reactions when treated with cephalosporins. Before therapy with a penicillin, careful inquiry should be made concerning previous hypersensitivity reactions to penicillins, cephalosporins, and other allergens. If an allergic reaction occurs, the patient should be treated with the usual agents, e.g., pressor amines, antihistamines, and corticosteroids. **Serious anaphylactoid reactions require immediate emergency treatment with epinephrine. Oxygen, intravenous steroids, and airway management, including intubation, should also be administered as indicated.**

Usage in Pregnancy: The safety of these drugs for use in pregnancy has not been established.

Precautions: Cases of gonococcal infection with a suspected lesion of syphilis should have darkfield examinations ruling out syphilis before receiving ampicillin. Patients who do not have suspected lesions of syphilis and are treated with ampicillin should have a follow-up serologic test for syphilis each month for four months to detect syphilis that may have been masked by treatment for gonorrhea. Patients with gonorrhea who also have syphilis should be given additional appropriate parenteral penicillin treatment.

Adverse Reactions: Ampicillin—As with other penicillins, it may be expected that untoward reactions will be essentially limited to sensitivity phenomena. They are more likely to occur in individuals who have previously demonstrated hypersensitivity to penicillin and in those with a history of allergy, asthma, hay fever, or urticaria.

The following adverse reactions have been reported as associated with the use of ampicillin:

Gastrointestinal: glossitis, stomatitis, nausea, vomiting, enterocolitis, pseudomembranous colitis, and diarrhea. These reactions are usually associated with oral dosage forms of the drug.

Hypersensitivity Reactions: An erythematous, mildly pruritic, maculopapular skin rash has been reported fairly frequently. The rash, which usually does not develop within the first week of therapy, may cover the entire body including the soles, palms, and oral mucosa. The eruption usually disappears in three to seven days. Other hypersensitivity reactions that have been reported are: skin rash, pruritus, urticaria, erythema multiforme, and an occasional case of exfoliative dermatitis. Anaphylaxis is the most serious reaction experienced and has usually been associated with the parenteral dosage form of the drug.

NOTE: Urticaria, other skin rashes, and serum sickness-like reactions may be controlled by antihistamines, and, if necessary, systemic corticosteroids. Serious anaphylactoid reactions require emergency measures (see WARNINGS).

Liver: Moderate elevation in serum glutamic oxaloacetic transaminase (SGOT) has been noted, but the significance of this finding is unknown.

Hemic and Lymphatic Systems: Anemia, thrombocytopenia, thrombocytopenic purpura, eosinophilia, leukopenia, and agranulocytosis have been reported during therapy with penicillins. These reactions are usually reversible on discontinuation of therapy and are believed to be hypersensitivity phenomena.

Probenecid—The following are the principal adverse reactions which have been reported as associated with the use of probenecid, generally with more prolonged or repeated administration: hypersensitivity reactions (including anaphylaxis), nephrotic syndrome, hepatic necrosis, aplastic anemia; also other anemias, including hemolytic anemia related to genetic deficiency of glucose-6-phosphate dehydrogenase.

Dosage and Administration: For the treatment of gonorrhea in both men and women—3.5 g. ampicillin and 1 g. probenecid (9 capsules) is administered as a single dose.

Physicians are cautioned to use no less than the above recommended dosage.

Follow-up cultures should be obtained from the original site(s) of infection 7 to 14 days after therapy. In women, it is also desirable to obtain culture test-of-cure from both the endocervical and anal canals.

How Supplied: Principen with Probenecid (Ampicillin—Probenecid Capsules) is provided in single-dose bottles containing nine capsules; each capsule contains ampicillin trihydrate equivalent to 389 mg. ampicillin and 111 mg. probenecid (9 capsules contain ampicillin trihydrate equivalent to 3.5 g. ampicillin and 1 g. probenecid).

Storage: Store at room temperature; avoid excessive heat.

PROLIXIN® INJECTION ℞
(Fluphenazine Hydrochloride Injection USP)
PROLIXIN® TABLETS ℞
(Fluphenazine Hydrochloride Tablets USP)
PROLIXIN® ELIXIR ℞
(Fluphenazine Hydrochloride Elixir USP)

Description: Prolixin is a trifluoromethyl phenothiazine derivative.

Prolixin Injection (Fluphenazine Hydrochloride Injection USP) is available in multiple dose vials providing 2.5 mg. fluphenazine hydrochloride per ml. **FOR INTRAMUSCULAR USE ONLY.** The preparation also includes sodium chloride for isotonicity, sodium hydroxide or hydrochloric acid to adjust the pH to 4.8 to 5.2, and 0.1% methylparaben and 0.01% propylparaben as preservatives. At the time of manufacture, the air in the vials is replaced by nitrogen.

Prolixin Tablets (Fluphenazine Hydrochloride Tablets USP) are available for oral administration as tablets providing 1, 2.5, 5, and 10 mg. fluphenazine hydrochloride. Prolixin 2.5, 5, and 10 mg. tablets contain FD&C Yellow No. 5 (tartrazine).

Prolixin Elixir (Fluphenazine Hydrochloride Elixir USP) is available as an elixir for oral administration which provides 0.5 mg. fluphenazine hydrochloride per ml. (2.5 mg. per 5 ml. teaspoonful) and contains 14% alcohol by volume.

Clinical Pharmacology: Prolixin has activity at all levels of the central nervous system as well as on multiple organ systems. The mechanism whereby its therapeutic action is exerted is unknown.

Indications and Usage: Prolixin (Fluphenazine Hydrochloride) Injection, Tablets, and Elixir are indicated in the management of manifestations of psychotic disorders.

Fluphenazine hydrochloride has not been shown effective in the management of behavorial complications in patients with mental retardation.

Contraindications: Phenothiazines are contraindicated in patients with suspected or established subcortical brain damage, in patients receiving large doses of hypnotics, and in comatose or severely depressed states. The presence of blood dyscrasia or liver damage precludes the use of fluphenazine hydrochloride. Prolixin (Fluphenazine Hydrochloride) is contraindicated in patients who have shown hypersensitivity to fluphenazine; cross-sensitivity to phenothiazine derivatives may occur.

Warnings: The use of this drug may impair the mental and physical abilities required for driving a car or operating heavy machinery.

Potentiation of the effects of alcohol may occur with the use of this drug.

Since there is no adequate experience in children who have received this drug, safety and efficacy in children have not been established.

Usage in Pregnancy: The safety for the use of this drug during pregnancy has not been established; therefore, the possible hazards should be weighed against the potential benefits when administering this drug to pregnant patients.

Precautions: Because of the possibility of cross-sensitivity, fluphenazine hydrochloride should be used cautiously in patients who have developed cholestatic jaundice, dermatoses or other allergic reactions to phenothiazine derivatives.

Prolixin Tablets (Fluphenazine Hydrochloride Tablets USP) 2.5, 5, and 10 mg. contain FD&C Yellow No. 5 (tartrazine) which may cause allergic-type reactions (including bronchial asthma) in certain susceptible individuals. Although the overall incidence of FD&C Yellow No. 5 (tartrazine) sensitivity in the general population is low, it is frequently seen in patients who also have aspirin hypersensitivity.

Psychotic patients on large doses of a phenothiazine drug who are undergoing surgery should be watched carefully for possible hypotensive phenomena. Moreover, it should be remembered that reduced amounts of anesthetics or central nervous system depressants may be necessary.

The effects of atropine may be potentiated in some patients receiving fluphenazine because of added anticholinergic effects.

Fluphenazine hydrochloride should be used cautiously in patients exposed to extreme heat or phosphorus insecticides; in patients with a history of convulsive disorders since grand mal convulsions have been known to occur; and in patients with special medical disorders such as mitral insufficiency or other cardiovascular diseases and pheochromocytoma.

The possibility of liver damage, pigmentary retinopathy, lenticular and corneal deposits, and development of irreversible dyskinesia should be remembered when patients are on prolonged therapy.

There is sufficient experimental evidence to conclude that chronic administration of antipsychotic drugs which increase prolactin secretion has the potential to induce mammary neoplasms in rodents under the appropriate conditions. There are recognized differences in the physiological role of prolactin between rodents and humans. Since there are, at present, no

Continued on next page

Squibb—Cont.

adequate epidemiological studies, the relevance to human mammary cancer risk from prolonged exposure to fluphenazine hydrochloride and other antipsychotic drugs is not known.

Abrupt Withdrawal: In general, phenothiazines do not produce psychic dependence; however, gastritis, nausea and vomiting, dizziness, and tremulousness have been reported following abrupt cessation of high dose therapy. Reports suggest that these symptoms can be reduced if concomitant antiparkinsonian agents are continued for several weeks after the phenothiazine is withdrawn.

Facilities should be available for periodic checking of hepatic function, renal function and the blood picture. Renal function of patients on long-term therapy should be monitored; if BUN (blood urea nitrogen) becomes abnormal, treatment should be discontinued.

As with any phenothiazine, the physician should be alert to the possible development of "silent pneumonias" in patients under treatment with fluphenazine hydrochloride.

Adverse Reactions: *Central Nervous System*—The side effects most frequently reported with phenothiazine compounds are extrapyramidal symptoms including pseudoparkinsonism, dystonia, dyskinesia, akathisia, oculogyric crises, opisthotonos, and hyperreflexia. Most often these extrapyramidal symptoms are reversible; however, they may be persistent (see below). With any given phenothiazine derivative, the incidence and severity of such reactions depend more on individual patient sensitivity than on other factors, but dosage level and patient age are also determinants.

Extrapyramidal reactions may be alarming, and the patient should be forewarned and reassured. These reactions can usually be controlled by administration of antiparkinsonian drugs, such as Benztropine Mesylate or intravenous Caffeine and Sodium Benzoate Injection, and by subsequent reductions in dosage.

Persistent Tardive Dyskinesia: As with all antipsychotic agents, tardive dyskinesia may appear in some patients on long-term therapy or may occur after drug therapy has been discontinued. The risk seems to be greater in elderly patients on high-dose therapy, especially females. The symptoms are persistent and in some patients appear to be irreversible. The syndrome is characterized by rhythmical involuntary movements of the tongue, face, mouth, or jaw (e.g., protrusion of tongue, puffing of cheeks, puckering of mouth, chewing movements). Sometimes these may be accompanied by involuntary movements of the extremities. There is no known effective treatment for tardive dyskinesia; antiparkinsonism agents usually do not alleviate the symptoms of this syndrome. It is suggested that all antipsychotic agents be discontinued if these symptoms appear. Should it be necessary to reinstitute treatment, or increase the dosage of the agent, or switch to a different antipsychotic agent, the syndrome may be masked. It has been reported that fine vermicular movements of the tongue may be an early sign of the syndrome and if the medication is stopped at that time, the syndrome may not develop.

Drowsiness or lethargy, if they occur, may necessitate a reduction in dosage; the induction of a catatonic-like state has been known to occur with dosages of fluphenazine far in excess of the recommended amounts. As with other phenothiazine compounds, reactivation or aggravation of psychotic processes may be encountered.

Phenothiazine derivatives have been known to cause, in some patients, restlessness, excitement, or bizarre dreams.

Autonomic Nervous System—Hypertension and fluctuation in blood pressure have been reported with fluphenazine hydrochloride.

Hypotension has rarely presented a problem with fluphenazine. However, patients with pheochromocytoma, cerebral vascular or renal insufficiency, or a severe cardiac reserve deficiency such as mitral insufficiency appear to be particularly prone to hypotensive reactions with phenothiazine compounds and should therefore be observed closely when the drug is administered. If severe hypotension should occur, supportive measures including the use of intravenous vasopressor drugs should be instituted immediately. Levarterenol Bitartrate Injection is the most suitable drug for this purpose; *epinephrine should not be used* since phenothiazine derivatives have been found to reverse its action, resulting in a further lowering of blood pressure.

Autonomic reactions including nausea and loss of appetite, salivation, polyuria, perspiration, dry mouth, headache, and constipation may occur. Autonomic effects can usually be controlled by reducing or temporarily discontinuing dosage.

In some patients, phenothiazine derivatives have caused blurred vision, glaucoma, bladder paralysis, fecal impaction, paralytic ileus, tachycardia, or nasal congestion.

Metabolic and Endocrine—Weight change, peripheral edema, abnormal lactation, gynecomastia, menstrual irregularities, false results on pregnancy tests, impotency in men and increased libido in women have all been known to occur in some patients on phenothiazine therapy.

Allergic Reactions—Skin disorders such as itching, erythema, urticaria, seborrhea, photosensitivity, eczema and even exfoliative dermatitis have been reported with phenothiazine derivatives. The possibility of anaphylactoid reactions occurring in some patients should be borne in mind.

Hematologic—Routine blood counts are advisable during therapy since blood dyscrasias including leukopenia, agranulocytosis, thrombocytopenic or nonthrombocytopenic purpura, eosinophilia, and pancytopenia have been observed with phenothiazine derivatives. Furthermore, if any soreness of the mouth, gums, or throat, or any symptoms of upper respiratory infection occur and confirmatory leukocyte count indicates cellular depression, therapy should be discontinued and other appropriate measures instituted immediately.

Hepatic—Liver damage as manifested by cholestatic jaundice may be encountered, particularly during the first months of therapy; treatment should be discontinued if this occurs. An increase in cephalin flocculation, sometimes accompanied by alterations in other liver function tests, have been reported in patients receiving fluphenazine hydrochloride who have had no clinical evidence of liver damage.

Others—Sudden, unexpected and unexplained deaths have been reported in hospitalized psychotic patients receiving phenothiazines. Previous brain damage or seizures may be predisposing factors; high doses should be avoided in known seizure patients. Several patients have shown sudden flare-ups of psychotic behavior patterns shortly before death. Autopsy findings have usually revealed acute fulminating pneumonia or pneumonitis, aspiration of gastric contents, or intramyocardial lesions.

Although this is not a general feature of fluphenazine, potentiation of central nervous system depressants (opiates, analgesics, antihistamines, barbiturates, alcohol) may occur.

The following adverse reactions have also occurred with phenothiazine derivatives: systemic lupus erythematosus-like syndrome, hypotension severe enough to cause fatal cardia arrest, altered electrocardiographic and electroencephalographic tracings, altered cerebrospinal fluid proteins, cerebral edema, asthma, laryngeal edema and angioneurotic edema; with long-term use—skin pigmentation, and lenticular and corneal opacities.

Dosage and Administration: *Prolixin Injection (Fluphenazine Hydrochloride Injection USP)*—The average well-tolerated parenteral starting dose for adult psychotic patients is 1.25 mg. (0.5 ml.) intramuscularly. Depending on the severity and duration of symptoms, initial total daily parenteral dosage may range from 2.5 to 10.0 mg. and should be divided and given at 6- to 8-hour intervals.

The smallest amount that will produce the desired results must be carefully determined for each individual since optimal dosage levels of this potent drug vary from patient to patient. In general, the parenteral dose for fluphenazine has been found to be approximately ⅓ to ½ the oral dose. Treatment may be instituted with a *low initial dosage*, which may be increased, if necessary, until the desired clinical effects are achieved. Dosages exceeding 10.0 mg. intramuscularly daily should be used with caution.

When symptoms are controlled, oral maintenance therapy can generally be instituted, often with single daily doses. Continued treatment, by the oral route if possible, is needed to achieve maximum therapeutic benefits; further adjustments in dosage may be necessary during the course of therapy to meet the patient's requirements.

Prolixin (Fluphenazine Hydrochloride) Tablets and Elixir—Depending on severity and duration of symptoms, total daily oral dosage for *adult* psychotic patients may range initially from 2.5 to 10.0 mg. and should be divided and given at 6- to 8-hour intervals.

The smallest amount that will produce the desired results must be carefully determined for each individual since optimal dosage levels of this potent drug vary from patient to patient. In general, the oral dose has been found to be approximately two to three times the parenteral dose of fluphenazine. Treatment is best instituted with a *low initial dosage*, which may be increased, if necessary, until the desired clinical effects are achieved. Oral dosages exceeding 20.0 mg. daily should be used with caution.

When symptoms are controlled, dosage can generally be reduced gradually to daily oral maintenance doses of 1.0 or 5.0 mg., often given as a single daily dose. Continued treatment is needed to achieve maximum therapeutic benefits; further adjustments in dosage may be necessary during the course of therapy to meet the patient's requirements.

For psychotic patients who have been stabilized on a fixed daily dosage of Prolixin (Fluphenazine Hydrochloride) Tablets or Elixir, conversion of therapy from oral fluphenazine hydrochloride dosage forms to the long-acting injectable Prolixin Decanoate® may be indicated [see package insert for Prolixin Decanoate (Fluphenazine Decanoate Injection) for conversion information].

For *geriatric* patients, the suggested starting dose is 1.0 to 2.5 mg. orally daily, adjusted according to the response of the patient.

Prolixin Injection (Fluphenazine Hydrochloride Injection USP) is useful when psychotic patients are unable or unwilling to take oral therapy.

How Supplied: Prolixin Injection (Fluphenazine Hydrochloride Injection USP) is available as a sterile, aqueous solution providing 2.5 mg. fluphenazine hydrochloride per ml. in multiple-dose vials of 10 ml.

*Prolixin Tablets (Fluphenazine Hydrochloride Tablets USP) are available for oral administration as sugar-coated tablets providing 1, 2.5, 5, and 10 mg. fluphenazine hydrochloride. — 1 mg. (pink) and 10 mg. (coral) in bottles of 50 and 500; 2.5 mg. (yellow) and 5 mg. (green) in bottles of 50 and 500 and Unimatic® Single Dose Packs of 100 [2.5 mg in bottles of 500—V.A. Depot Item, NSN6505-00-764-

4322A; 5 mg. in bottles of 500—V.A. Depot Item, NSN6505-00-951-4750A.]

Prolixin Elixir (Fluphenazine Hydrochloride Elixir USP) is available as an elixir for oral administration which provides 0.5 mg. fluphenazine hydrochloride per ml. (2.5 mg. per 5 ml. teaspoonful)—(orange-flavored and colored) in bottles of 473 ml. (1 pint) and in 60 ml. dropper assembly bottles with dropper calibrated at 0.5 ml. (0.25 mg.), 1 ml. (0.5 mg.), 1.5 ml. (0.75 mg.), and 2 ml. (1 mg.). [1 pint bottles—V.A. Depot Item, NSN6505-00-764-5042A.]

Storage: Prolixin Injection should be protected from exposure to light. Parenteral solutions may vary in color from essentially colorless to light amber. If a solution has become any darker than light amber or is discolored in any other way, it should not be used. Store at room temperature; avoid freezing.

Store the tablets and elixir at room temperature; protect from light; keep tightly closed. Tablets: avoid excessive heat. Elixir: avoid freezing.

*[*Shown in Product Identification Section*]

PROLIXIN DECANOATE® ℞
(Fluphenazine Decanoate Injection)

Description: Prolixin Decanoate is the decanoate ester of a trifluoromethyl phenothiazine derivative. It is a highly potent behavior modifier with a markedly extended duration of effect. Prolixin Decanoate is available for intramuscular or subcutaneous administration, providing 25 mg. fluphenazine decanoate per ml. in a sesame oil vehicle with 1.2% (w/v) benzyl alcohol as a preservative. At the time of manufacture, the air in the vials is replaced by nitrogen.

Clinical Pharmacology: The basic effects of fluphenazine decanoate appear to be no different from those of fluphenazine hydrochloride, with the exception of duration of action. The esterification of fluphenazine markedly prolongs the drug's duration of effect without unduly attenuating its beneficial action.

Prolixin Decanoate has activity at all levels of the central nervous system as well as on multiple organ systems. The mechanism whereby its therapeutic action is exerted is unknown.

Fluphenazine differs from other phenothiazine derivatives in several respects: it is more potent on a milligram basis, it has less potentiating effect on central nervous system depressants and anesthetics than do some of the phenothiazines and appears to be less sedating, and it is less likely than some of the older phenothiazines to produce hypotension (nevertheless, appropriate cautions should be observed—see sections on PRECAUTIONS and ADVERSE REACTIONS).

Indications and Usage: Prolixin Decanoate is indicated in the management of manifestations of schizophrenia.

Fluphenazine decanoate has not been shown effective in the management of behavioral complications in patients with mental retardation.

Contraindications: Phenothiazines are contraindicated in patients with suspected or established subcortical brain damage.

Phenothiazine compounds should not be used in patients receiving large doses of hypnotics.

Prolixin Decanoate is contraindicated in comatose or severely depressed states.

The presence of blood dyscrasia or liver damage precludes the use of fluphenazine decanoate.

Fluphenazine decanoate is not intended for use in children under 12 years of age.

Prolixin Decanoate (Fluphenazine Decanoate Injection) is contraindicated in patients who have shown hypersensitivity to fluphenazine; cross-sensitivity to phenothiazine derivatives may occur.

Warnings: The use of this drug may impair the mental and physical abilities required for driving a car or operating heavy machinery.

Physicians should be alert to the possibility that severe adverse reactions may occur which require immediate medical attention.

Potentiation of the effects of alcohol may occur with the use of this drug.

Since there is no adequate experience in children who have received this drug, safety and efficacy in children have not been established.

Usage in Pregnancy—The safety for the use of this drug during pregnancy has not been established; therefore, the possible hazards should be weighed against the potential benefits when administering this drug to pregnant patients.

Precautions: Because of the possibility of cross-sensitivity, fluphenazine decanoate should be used cautiously in patients who have developed cholestatic jaundice, dermatoses, or other allergic reactions to phenothiazine derivatives.

Psychotic patients on large doses of a phenothiazine drug who are undergoing surgery should be watched carefully for possible hypotensive phenomena. Moreover, it should be remembered that reduced amounts of anesthetics or central nervous system depressants may be necessary.

The effects of atropine may be potentiated in some patients receiving fluphenazine because of added anticholinergic effects.

Fluphenazine decanoate should be used cautiously in patients exposed to extreme heat or phosphorus insecticides.

The preparation should be used with caution in patients with a history of convulsive disorders since grand mal convulsions have been known to occur.

Use with caution in patients with special medical disorders such as mitral insufficiency or other cardiovascular diseases and pheochromocytoma.

The possibility of liver damage, pigmentary retinopathy, lenticular and corneal deposits, and development of irreversible dyskinesia should be remembered when patients are on prolonged therapy.

Outside state hospitals or other psychiatric institutions, fluphenazine decanoate should be administered under the direction of a physician experienced in the clinical use of psychotropic drugs, particularly phenothiazine derivatives. Furthermore, facilities should be available for periodic checking of hepatic function, renal function, and the blood picture. Renal function of patients on long-term therapy should be monitored; if BUN (blood urea nitrogen) becomes abnormal, treatment should be discontinued.

As with any phenothiazine, the physician should be alert to the possible development of "silent pneumonias" in patients under treatment with fluphenazine decanoate.

There is sufficient experimental evidence to conclude that chronic administration of antipsychotic drugs which increase prolactin secretion has the potential to induce mammary neoplasms in rodents under the appropriate conditions. There are recognized differences in the physiological role of prolactin between rodents and humans. Since there are, at present, no adequate epidemiological studies, the relevance to human mammary cancer risk from prolonged exposure to fluphenazine decanoate and other antipsychotic drugs is not known.

Adverse Reactions: *Central Nervous System*—The side effects most frequently reported with phenothiazine compounds are extrapyramidal symptoms including pseudoparkinsonism, dystonia, dyskinesia, akathisia, oculogyric crises, opisthotonos, and hyperreflexia. Muscle rigidity sometimes accompanied by hyperthermia has been reported following use of fluphenazine decanoate. Most often these extrapyramidal symptoms are reversible; however, they may be persistent (see below). The frequency of such reactions is related in part to chemical structure; one can expect a higher incidence with fluphenazine decanoate than with less potent piperazine derivatives or with straight-chain phenothiazines such as chlorpromazine. With any given phenothiazine derivative, the incidence and severity of such reactions depend more on individual patient sensitivity than on other factors, but dosage level and patient age are also determinants.

Extrapyramidal reactions may be alarming, and the patient should be forewarned and reassured. These reactions can usually be controlled by administration of antiparkinsonian drugs, such as Benztropine Mesylate or intravenous Caffeine and Sodium Benzoate Injection, and by subsequent reduction in dosage.

Persistent Tardive Dyskinesia: As with all antipsychotic agents, tardive dyskinesia may appear in some patients on long-term therapy or may occur after drug therapy has been discontinued. The risk seems to be greater in elderly patients on high-dose therapy, especially females. The symptoms are persistent and in some patients appear to be irreversible. The syndrome is characterized by rhythmical involuntary movements of the tongue, face, mouth or jaw (e.g., protrusion of tongue, puffing of cheeks, puckering of mouth, chewing movements). Sometimes these may be accompanied by involuntary movements of the extremities. There is no known effective treatment for tardive dyskinesia; antiparkinsonism agents usually do not alleviate the symptoms of this syndrome. It is suggested that all antipsychotic agents be discontinued if these symptoms appear. Should it be necessary to reinstitute treatment, or increase the dosage of the agent, or switch to a different antipsychotic agent, the syndrome may be masked. It has been reported that fine vermicular movements of the tongue may be an early sign of the syndrome and if the medication is stopped at that time, the syndrome may not develop.

Drowsiness or lethargy, if they occur, may necessitate a reduction in dosage; the induction of a catatonic-like state has been known to occur with dosages of fluphenazine far in excess of the recommended amounts. As with other phenothiazine compounds, reactivation or aggravation of psychotic processes may be encountered.

Phenothiazine derivatives have been known to cause, in some patients, restlessness, excitement, or bizarre dreams.

Autonomic Nervous System—Hypertension and fluctuations in blood pressure have been reported with fluphenazine.

Hypotension has rarely presented a problem with fluphenazine. However, patients with pheochromocytoma, cerebral vascular or renal insufficiency, or a severe cardiac reserve deficiency such as mitral insufficiency appear to be particularly prone to hypotensive reactions with phenothiazine compounds, and should therefore be observed closely when the drug is administered. If severe hypotension should occur, supportive measures including the use of intravenous vasopressor drugs should be instituted immediately. Levarterenol Bitartrate Injection is the most suitable drug for this purpose; *epinephrine should not be used* since phenothiazine derivatives have been found to reverse its action, resulting in a further lowering of blood pressure.

Autonomic reactions including nausea and loss of appetite, salivation, polyuria, perspiration, dry mouth, headache, and constipation may occur. Autonomic effects can usually be controlled by reducing or temporarily discontinuing dosage.

In some patients, phenothiazine derivatives have caused blurred vision, glaucoma, bladder paralysis, fecal impaction, paralytic ileus, tachycardia, or nasal congestion.

Continued on next page

Squibb—Cont.

Metabolic and Endocrine—Weight change, peripheral edema, abnormal lactation, gynecomastia, menstrual irregularities, false results on pregnancy tests, impotency in men and increased libido in women have all been known to occur in some patients on phenothiazine therapy.
Allergic Reactions—Skin disorders such as itching, erythema, urticaria, seborrhea, photosensitivity, eczema and even exfoliative dermatitis have been reported with phenothiazine derivatives. The possibility of anaphylactoid reactions occurring in some patients should be borne in mind.
Hematologic—Routine blood counts are advisable during therapy since blood dyscrasias including leukopenia, agranulocytosis, thrombocytopenic or nonthrombocytopenic purpura, eosinophilia, and pancytopenia have been observed with phenothiazine derivatives. Furthermore, if any soreness of the mouth, gums, or throat, or any symptoms of upper respiratory infection occur and confirmatory leukocyte count indicates cellular depression, therapy should be discontinued and other appropriate measures instituted immediately.
Hepatic—Liver damage as manifested by cholestatic jaundice may be encountered, particularly during the first months of therapy; treatment should be discontinued if this occurs. An increase in cephalin flocculation, sometimes accompanied by alterations in other liver function tests, has been reported in patients receiving the enanthate ester of fluphenazine (a closely related compound) who have had no clinical evidence of liver damage.
Others—Sudden, unexpected and unexplained deaths have been reported in hospitalized psychotic patients receiving phenothiazines. Previous brain damage or seizures may be predisposing factors; high doses should be avoided in known seizure patients. Several patients have shown sudden flare-ups of psychotic behavior patterns shortly before death. Autopsy findings have usually revealed acute fulminating pneumonia or pneumonitis, aspiration of gastric contents, or intramyocardial lesions.
Although this is not a general feature of fluphenazine, potentiation of central nervous system depressants (opiates, analgesics, antihistamines, barbiturates, alcohol) may occur. The following adverse reactions have also occurred with phenothiazine derivatives: systemic lupus erythematosus-like syndrome, hypotension severe enough to cause fatal cardiac arrest, altered electrocardiographic and electroencephalographic tracings, altered cerebrospinal fluid proteins, cerebral edema, asthma, laryngeal edema, and angioneurotic edema; with long-term use—skin pigmentation and lenticular and corneal opacities.
Injections of fluphenazine decanoate are extremely well tolerated, local tissue reactions occurring only rarely.
Dosage and Administration: Prolixin Decanoate (Fluphenazine Decanoate Injection) may be given intramuscularly or subcutaneously. A dry syringe and needle of at least 21 gauge should be used. Use of a wet needle or syringe may cause the solution to become cloudy.
To begin therapy with Prolixin Decanoate the following regimens are suggested:
For *most patients*, a dose of 12.5 to 25 mg. (0.5 to 1 ml.) may be given to initiate therapy. The onset of action generally appears between 24 and 72 hours after injection and the effects of the drug on psychotic symptoms becomes significant within 48 to 96 hours. Subsequent injections and the dosage interval are determined in accordance with the patient's response. When administered as maintenance therapy, a single injection may be effective in controlling schizophrenic symptoms up to four weeks or longer. The response to a single dose has been found to last as long as six weeks in a few patients on maintenance therapy.
It may be advisable that patients who have had no history of taking phenothiazines should be treated initially with a shorter-acting form of fluphenazine (see HOW SUPPLIED section for the availability of the shorter-acting fluphenazine hydrochloride dosage forms) before administering the decanoate to determine the patient's response to fluphenazine and to establish appropriate dosage. For psychotic patients who have been stabilized on a fixed daily dosage of Prolixin® Tablets (Fluphenazine Hydrochloride Tablets USP) or Prolixin Elixir (Fluphenazine Hydrochloride Elixir USP), conversion of therapy from these short-acting oral forms to the long-acting injectable Prolixin Decanoate may be indicated.
Appropriate dosage of Prolixin Decanoate should be individualized for each patient and responses carefully monitored. No precise formula can be given to convert to use of Prolixin Decanoate; however, a controlled multicentered study*, in patients receiving oral doses from 5 to 60 mg. fluphenazine hydrochloride daily, showed that 20 mg. fluphenazine hydrochloride daily was equivalent to 25 mg. (1 ml.) Prolixin Decanoate every three weeks. This represents an approximate conversion ratio of 0.5 ml. (12.5 mg.) of decanoate every three weeks for every 10 mg. of fluphenazine hydrochloride daily.
Once conversion to Prolixin Decanoate is made, careful clinical monitoring of the patient and appropriate dosage adjustment should be made at the time of each injection.
Severely agitated patients may be treated with a rapid-acting phenothiazine compound such as Prolixin Injection (Fluphenazine Hydrochloride Injection USP—see package insert accompanying that product for complete information). When acute symptoms have subsided, 25 mg. (1 ml.) of Prolixin Decanoate may be administered; subsequent dosage is adjusted as necessary.
"Poor risk" patients (those with known hypersensitivity to phenothiazines or with disorders that predispose to undue reactions): Therapy may be initiated cautiously with oral or parenteral fluphenazine hydrochloride (see package inserts accompanying these products for complete information). When the pharmacologic effects and an appropriate dosage are apparent, an equivalent dose of Prolixin Decanoate may be administered. Subsequent dosage adjustments are made in accordance with the response of the patient.
The optimal amount of the drug and the frequency of administration must be determined for each patient, since dosage requirements have been found to vary with clinical circumstances as well as with individual response to the drug.
Dosage should not exceed 100 mg. If doses greater than 50 mg. are deemed necessary, the next dose and succeeding doses should be increased cautiously in increments of 12.5 mg.
How Supplied: Prolixin Decanoate (Fluphenazine Decanoate Injection) is available in 1 ml. Unimatic® single dose preassembled syringes, 1 ml. cartridge-needle units, and 5 ml. vials, providing 25 mg. fluphenazine decanoate per ml. [5 ml. vial—V.A. Depot Item, NSN 6505-00-264-7759A; preassembled syringe—V.A. Depot Item, NSN 6505-00-282-3788A.] Prolixin (fluphenazine) is also available for oral administration as Prolixin Tablets (Fluphenazine Hydrochloride Tablets USP) providing 1, 2.5, 5, and 10 mg. fluphenazine hydrochloride per tablet, and Prolixin Elixir (Fluphenazine Hydrochloride Elixir USP) providing 0.5 mg. fluphenazine hydrochloride per ml. (2.5 mg. per 5 ml. teaspoonful).
Storage: Store at room temperature; avoid freezing and excessive heat. Protect from light.

*The Initiation of Long-Term Pharmacotherapy in Schizophrenia: Dosage and Side Effect Comparisons Between Oral and Depot Fluphenazine; N.R. Schooler; Pharmakopsych. 9:159-169, 1976.

PROLIXIN ENANTHATE® ℞
(Fluphenazine Enanthate Injection USP)

Description: Prolixin Enanthate is an esterified trifluoromethyl phenothiazine derivative. It is a highly potent behavior modifier with a markedly extended duration of effect. Prolixin Enanthate is available for intramuscular or subcutaneous administration, providing 25 mg. fluphenazine enanthate per ml. in a sesame oil vehicle with 1.5% (w/v) benzyl alcohol as a preservative. At the time of manufacture, the air in the vials is replaced by nitrogen.
Clinical Pharmacology: The basic effects of fluphenazine enanthate appear to be no different from those of fluphenazine hydrochloride, with the exception of duration of action. The esterification of fluphenazine markedly prolongs the drug's duration of effect without unduly attenuating its beneficial action. The onset of action generally appears between 24 to 72 hours after injection, and the effects of the drug on psychotic symptoms become significant within 48 to 96 hours. Amelioration of symptoms then continues for 1 to 3 weeks or longer, with an average duration of effect of about 2 weeks.
Fluphenazine has activity at all levels of the central nervous system as well as on multiple organ systems. The mechanism whereby its therapeutic action is exerted is unknown.
Fluphenazine differs from other phenothiazine derivatives in several respects: it is more potent on a milligram basis, it has less potentiating effect on central nervous system depressants and anesthetics than do some of the phenothiazines and appears to be less sedating, and it is less likely than some of the older phenothiazines to produce hypotension (nevertheless, appropriate cautions should be observed—see sections on PRECAUTIONS and ADVERSE REACTIONS).
Indications and Usage: Prolixin Enanthate is indicated in the management of manifestations of psychotic disorders.
Prolixin Enanthate has not been shown effective in the management of behavorial complications in patients with mental retardation.
Contraindications: Phenothiazines are contraindicated in patients with suspected or established subcortical brain damage.
Phenothiazine compounds should not be used in patients receiving large doses of hypnotics.
Prolixin Enanthate (Fluphenazine Enanthate Injection USP) is contraindicated in comatose or severely depressed states.
The presence of blood dyscrasia or liver damage precludes the use of fluphenazine enanthate.
Fluphenazine enanthate is not intended for use in children under 12 years of age.
Prolixin Enanthate is contraindicated in patients who have shown hypersensitivity to fluphenazine; cross-sensitivity to phenothiazine derivatives may occur.
Warnings: The use of this drug may impair the mental and physical abilities required for driving a car or operating heavy machinery.
Physicians should be alert to the possibility that severe adverse reactions may occur which require immediate medical attention.
Potentiation of the effects of alcohol may occur with the use of this drug.
Since there is no adequate experience in children who have received this drug, safety and efficacy in children have not been established.
Usage in Pregnancy—The safety for the use of this drug during pregnancy has not been established; therefore, the possible hazards should be weighed against the potential benefits when administering the drug to pregnant patients.

Precautions: Because of the possibility of cross-sensitivity, fluphenazine enanthate should be used cautiously in patients who have developed cholestatic jaundice, dermatoses, or other allergic reactions to phenothiazine derivatives.

Psychotic patients on large doses of a phenothiazine drug who are undergoing surgery should be watched carefully for possible hypotensive phenomena. Moreover, it should be remembered that reduced amounts of anesthetics or central nervous system depressants may be necessary.

The effects of atropine may be potentiated in some patients receiving fluphenazine because of added anticholinergic effects.

Fluphenazine enanthate should be used cautiously in patients exposed to extreme heat or phosphorus insecticides.

The preparation should be used with caution in patients with a history of convulsive disorders since grand mal convulsions have been known to occur.

Use with caution in patients with special medical disorders such as mitral insufficiency or other cardiovascular diseases and pheochromocytoma.

The possibility of liver damage, pigmentary retinopathy, lenticular and corneal deposits, and development of irreversible dyskinesia should be remembered when patients are on prolonged therapy.

Outside state hospitals or other psychiatric institutions, fluphenazine enanthate should be administered under the direction of a physician experienced in the clinical use of psychotropic drugs, particularly phenothiazine derivatives. Furthermore, facilities should be available for periodic checking of hepatic function, renal function, and the blood picture. Renal function of patients on long-term therapy should be monitored; if BUN (blood urea nitrogen) becomes abnormal, treatment should be discontinued.

As with any phenothiazine, the physician should be alert to the possible development of "silent pneumonias" in patients under treatment with fluphenazine enanthate.

There is sufficient experimental evidence to conclude that chronic administration of antipsychotic drugs which increase prolactin secretion has the potential to induce mammary neoplasms in rodents under the appropriate conditions. There are recognized differences in the physiological role of prolactin between rodents and humans. Since there are, at present, no adequate epidemiological studies, the relevance to human mamary cancer risk from prolonged exposure to fluphenazine enanthate and other antipsychotic drugs is not known.

Adverse Reactions: *Central Nervous System:* The side effects most frequently reported with phenothiazine compounds are extrapyramidal symptoms including pseudoparkinsonism, dystonia, dyskinesia, akathisia, oculogyric crises, opisthotonos, and hyperreflexia. Most often these extrapyramidal symptoms are reversible; however, they may be persistent (see below). The frequency of such reactions is related in part to chemical structure; one can expect a higher incidence with fluphenazine enanthate than with less potent piperazine derivatives or with straight-chain phenothiazines such as chlorpromazine. With any given phenothiazine derivative, the incidence and severity of such reactions depend more on individual patient sensitivity than on other factors, but dosage level and patient age are also determinants.

Extrapyramidal reactions may be alarming, and the patient should be forewarned and reassured. These reactions can usually be controlled by administration of antiparkinsonian drugs, such as Benztropine Mesylate or intravenous Caffeine and Sodium Benzoate Injection, and by subsequent reduction in dosage.

Persistent Tardive Dyskinesia: As with all antipsychotic agents, tardive dyskinesia may appear in some patients on long-term therapy or may occur after drug therapy has been discontinued. The risk seems to be greater in elderly patients on high-dose therapy, especially females. The symptoms are persistent and in some patients appear to be irreversible. The syndrome is characterized by rhythmical involuntary movements of the tongue, face, mouth or jaw (e.g., protrusion of tongue, puffing of cheeks, puckering of mouth, chewing movements). Sometimes these may be accompanied by involuntary movements of the extremities. There is no known effective treatment for tardive dyskinesia; antiparkinsonism agents usually do not alleviate the symptoms of this syndrome. It is suggested that all antipsychotic agents be discontinued if these symptoms appear. Should it be necessary to reinstitute treatment, or increase the dosage of the agent, or switch to a different antipsychotic agent, the syndrome may be masked. It has been reported that fine vermicular movements of the tongue may be an early sign of the syndrome and if the medication is stopped at that time, the syndrome may not develop.

Drowsiness or lethargy, if they occur, may necessitate a reduction in dosage; the induction of a catatonic-like state has been known to occur with dosages of fluphenazine far in excess of the recommended amounts. As with other phenothiazine compounds, reactivation or aggravation of psychotic processes may be encountered.

Phenothiazine derivatives have been known to cause, in some patients, restlessness, excitement, or bizarre dreams.

Autonomic Nervous System: Hypertension and fluctuations in blood pressure have been reported with fluphenazine enanthate.

Hypotension has rarely presented a problem with fluphenazine. However, patients with pheochromocytoma, cerebral vascular or renal insufficiency, or a severe cardiac reserve deficiency such as mitral insufficiency appear to be particularly prone to hypotensive reactions with phenothiazine compounds and should therefore be observed closely when the drug is administered. If severe hypotension should occur, supportive measures including the use of intravenous vasopressor drugs should be instituted immediately. Levarterenol Bitartrate Injection is the most suitable drug for this purpose; *epinephrine should not be used* since phenothiazine derivatives have been found to reverse its action, resulting in a further lowering of blood pressure.

Autonomic reactions including nausea and loss of appetite, salivation, polyuria, perspiration, dry mouth, headache, and constipation may occur. Autonomic effects can usually be controlled by reducing or temporarily discontinuing dosage.

In some patients, phenothiazine derivatives have caused blurred vision, glaucoma, bladder paralysis, fecal impaction, paralytic ileus, tachycardia, or nasal congestion.

Metabolic and Endocrine: Weight change, peripheral edema, abnormal lactation, gynecomastia, menstrual irregularities, false results on pregnancy tests, impotency in men and increased libido in women have all been known to occur in some patients on phenothiazine therapy.

Allergic Reactions: Skin disorders such as itching, erythema, urticaria, seborrhea, photosensitivity, eczema and even exfoliative dermatitis have been reported with phenothiazine derivatives. The possibility of anaphylactoid reactions occurring in some patients should be borne in mind.

Hematologic: Routine blood counts are advisable during therapy since blood dyscrasias including leukopenia, agranulocytosis, thrombocytopenic or nonthrombocytopenic purpura, eosinophilia, and pancytopenia have been observed with phenothiazine derivatives. Furthermore, if any soreness of the mouth, gums, or throat, or any symptoms of upper respiratory infection occur and confirmatory leukocyte count indicates cellular depression, therapy should be discontinued and other appropriate measures instituted immediately.

Hepatic: Liver damage as manifested by cholestatic jaundice may be encountered, particularly during the first months of therapy; treatment should be discontinued if this occurs. An increase in cephalin flocculation, sometimes accompanied by alterations in other liver function tests, has been reported in patients receiving fluphenazine enanthate who have had no clinical evidence of liver damage.

Others: Sudden, unexpected and unexplained deaths have been reported in hospitalized psychotic patients receiving phenothiazines. Previous brain damage or seizures may be predisposing factors; high doses should be avoided in known seizure patients. Several patients have shown sudden flare-ups of psychotic behavior patterns shortly before death. Autopsy findings have usually revealed acute fulminating pneumonia or pneumonitis, aspiration of gastric contents, or intramyocardial lesions.

Although this is not a general feature of fluphenazine, potentiation of central nervous system depressants (opiates, analgesics, antihistamines, barbiturates, alcohol) may occur.

The following adverse reactions have also occurred with phenothiazine derivatives: systemic lupus erythematosus-like syndrome, hypotension severe enough to cause fatal cardiac arrest, altered electrocardiographic and electroencephalographic tracings, altered cerebrospinal fluid proteins, cerebral edema, asthma, laryngeal edema and angioneurotic edema; with long-term use—skin pigmentation and lenticular and corneal opacities.

Injections of fluphenazine enanthate are extremely well tolerated, local tissue reactions occurring only rarely.

Dosage and Administration: Prolixin Enanthate (Fluphenazine Enanthate Injection USP) may be given intramuscularly or subcutaneously. A dry syringe and needle of at least 21 gauge should be used. Use of a wet needle or syringe may cause the solution to become cloudy.

To begin therapy with Prolixin Enanthate the following regimens are suggested:

For *most patients* a dose of 25 mg. (1 ml.) every 2 weeks should prove to be adequate, and therapy may be started on that basis. Subsequent adjustments in the amount and the dosage interval may be made, if necessary, in accordance with the patient's response.

It may be advisable that patients who have had no history of taking phenothiazines should be treated initially with a shorter-acting form of fluphenazine before administering the enanthate to determine the patient's response to fluphenazine and to establish appropriate dosage. Since the dosage comparability of the shorter-acting forms of fluphenazine to the longer-acting enanthate is not known, special caution should be exercised when switching from the shorter-acting forms to the enanthate.

Severely agitated patients may be treated initially with a rapid-acting phenothiazine compound such as Prolixin Injection (Fluphenazine Hydrochloride Injection USP—see package insert accompanying that product for complete information). When acute symptoms have subsided, 25 mg. (1 ml.) of Prolixin Enanthate may be administered; subsequent dosage is adjusted as necessary.

"Poor risk" patients (those with known hypersensitivity to phenothiazines, or with disorders that predispose to undue reactions): Therapy may be initiated cautiously with oral or parenteral fluphenazine hydrochloride (see package inserts accompanying these products for complete information). When the pharmacologic effects and an appropriate dosage are apparent, an equivalent dose of Prolixin Enanthate

Continued on next page

Squibb—Cont.

may be administered. Subsequent dosage adjustments are made in accordance with the response of the patient.
The optimal amount of the drug and the frequency of administration must be determined for each patient, since dosage requirements have been found to vary with clinical circumstances as well as with individual response to the drug. Although in a large series of patients the optimal dose was usually 25 mg. every 2 weeks, the amount required ranged from 12.5 to 100 mg. (0.5 to 4 ml.). The interval between doses ranged from 1 week to 3 weeks in most instances. The response to a single dose was found to last as long as 6 weeks in a few patients on maintenance therapy.
Dosage should not exceed 100 mg. If doses greater than 50 mg. are deemed necessary, the next dose and succeeding doses should be increased cautiously in increments of 12.5 mg.
How Supplied: Prolixin Enanthate (Fluphenazine Enanthate Injection USP) is available in 5 ml. vials and in 1 ml. Unimatic® single dose preassembled syringes providing 25 mg. fluphenazine enanthate per ml. [5 ml. vial-V.A. Depot Item, NSN 6505-00-812-2531A; preassembled syringe-V.A. Depot Item, NSN 6505-00-286-7604A].
Storage: Store at room temperature; avoid freezing and excessive heat. Protect from light.

PRONESTYL® CAPSULES ℞
(Procainamide Hydrochloride Capsules USP)
PRONESTYL® TABLETS ℞
(Procainamide Hydrochloride Tablets)

> The prolonged administration of procainamide often leads to the development of a positive anti-nuclear antibody (ANA) test with or without symptoms of lupus erythematosus-like syndrome. If a positive ANA titer develops, the benefit/risk ratio related to continued procainamide therapy should be assessed. This may necessitate consideration of alternative antiarrhythmic therapy.

Description: Pronestyl is the amide analogue of procaine hydrochloride. It is available for oral administration as capsules and FILMLOK® tablets in potencies of 250 mg., 375 mg., and 500 mg. Pronestyl 375 mg. and 500 mg. capsules and Pronestyl tablets contain FD&C Yellow No. 5 (tartrazine). (FILMLOK is a Squibb trademark for veneer-coated tablets.)
Actions: Procainamide depresses the excitability of cardiac muscle to electrical stimulation and slows conduction in the atrium, the bundle of His, and the ventricle. The refractory period of the atrium is considerably more prolonged than that of the ventricle. Contractility of the heart is usually not affected, nor is cardiac output decreased to any extent unless myocardial damage exists. In the absence of any arrhythmia, the heart rate may occasionally be accelerated by conventional doses, suggesting that the drug possesses anticholinergic properties. Larger doses can induce atrioventricular block and ventricular extrasystoles which may proceed to ventricular fibrillation. These effects on the myocardium are reflected in the electrocardiogram; a widening of the QRS complex occurs most consistently; less regularly, the P-R and Q-T intervals are prolonged, and the QRS and T waves show some decrease in voltage.
The action of procainamide begins almost immediately after intramuscular or intravenous administration. Plasma levels after intramuscular injection are at their peak in 15 to 60 minutes. Following oral administration, plasma levels of the drug are comparable to those obtained parenterally, and are maximal within an hour; therapeutic levels are usually attained in half that time.
Therapeutic plasma levels have been reported to be 3 to 10 mcg./ml., with those for the majority of patients in the range of 4 to 8 mcg./ml. Procainamide is less readily hydrolyzed than procaine, and plasma levels decline slowly—about 10% to 20% per hour. The drug is excreted primarily in the urine, about 10% as free and conjugated p-aminobenzoic acid and about 60% in the unchanged form. The fate of the remainder is unknown.
Indications: Pronestyl (Procainamide Hydrochloride) Capsules and Tablets are indicated in the treatment of premature ventricular contractions and ventricular tachycardia, atrial fibrillation, and paroxysmal atrial tachycardia.
Contraindications: It has been suggested that procainamide be contraindicated in patients with myasthenia gravis. Hypersensitivity to the drug is an absolute contraindication; in this connection, cross sensitivity to procaine and related drugs must be borne in mind. Procainamide should not be administered to patients with complete atrioventricular heart block. Procainamide is also contraindicated in cases of second degree and third degree A-V block unless an electrical pacemaker is operative.
Precautions: During administration of the drug, evidence of untoward myocardial responses should be carefully watched for in all patients. In the presence of an abnormal myocardium, procainamide may at times produce untoward responses. In atrial fibrillation or flutter, the ventricular rate may increase suddenly as the atrial rate is slowed. Adequate digitalization reduces but does not abolish this danger. If myocardial damage exists, ventricular tachysystole is particularly hazardous. Correction of atrial fibrillation, with resultant forceful contractions of the atrium, may cause a dislodgment of mural thrombi and produce an embolic episode. However, it has been suggested that in a patient who is already discharging emboli, procainamide is more likely to stop than to aggravate the process.
Attempts to adjust the heart rate in a patient who has developed ventricular tachycardia during an occlusive coronary episode should be carried out with extreme caution. Caution is also required in marked disturbances of atrioventricular conduction such as second degree and third degree A-V block, bundle branch block, or severe digitalis intoxication, where the use of procainamide may result in additional depression of conduction and ventricular asystole or fibrillation.
Since patients with severe organic heart disease and ventricular tachycardia may also have complete heart block which is difficult to diagnose under these circumstances, this complication should always be kept in mind when treating ventricular arrhythmias with procainamide. If the ventricular rate is significantly slowed by procainamide without attainment of regular atrioventricular conduction, the drug should be stopped and the patient reevaluated as asystole may result under these circumstances.
In patients receiving normal dosage, but who have both liver and kidney disease, symptoms of overdosage (principally ventricular tachycardia and severe hypotension) may occur due to drug accumulation.
Instances of a syndrome resembling lupus erythematosus have been reported in connection with oral maintenance procainamide therapy. The mechanism of this syndrome is uncertain. Polyarthralgia, arthritis, and pleuritic pain are common symptoms; to a lesser extent fever, myalgia, skin lesions, pleural effusion and pericarditis may occur. Rare cases of thrombocytopenia or Coombs positive hemolytic anemia have been reported which may be related to this syndrome. Patients receiving procainamide for extended periods of time or in whom symptoms suggestive of a lupus-like reaction appear should have anti-nuclear antibody titers measured at regular intervals. If there is a rising titer (anti-nuclear antibody) or clinical symptoms of LE appear, the benefit/risk ratio related to continued procainamide therapy should be assessed (see boxed Warning). The LE syndrome may be reversible upon discontinuance of the drug. If discontinuation of the drug does not cause remission of the symptoms, steroid therapy may be effective. If the syndrome develops in a patient with recurrent life-threatening arrhythmias not controllable by other antiarrhythmic agents, steroid suppressive therapy may be used concomitantly with procainamide.
Pronestyl Capsules (Procainamide Hydrochloride Capsules USP) 375 mg. and 500 mg. and Pronestyl Tablets (Procainamide Hydrochloride Tablets) contain FD&C Yellow No. 5 (tartrazine) which may cause allergic-type reactions (including bronchial asthma) in certain susceptible individuals. Although the overall incidence of FD&C Yellow No. 5 (tartrazine) sensitivity in the general population is low, it is frequently seen in patients who also have aspirin hypersensitivity.
Adverse Reactions: Hypotension following oral administration is rare. Serious disturbances of cardiac rhythm such as ventricular asystole or fibrillation are more common with intravenous administration.
Large oral doses of procainamide may sometimes produce anorexia, nausea, urticaria, and/or pruritus.
A syndrome resembling lupus erythematosus has been reported in patients on oral maintenance therapy (see PRECAUTIONS). Reactions consisting of fever and chills have also been reported, including a case with fever and chills plus nausea, vomiting, abdominal pain, acute hepatomegaly, and a rise in serum glutamic oxaloacetic transaminase following single doses of the drug. Bitter taste, diarrhea, weakness, mental depression, giddiness, and psychosis with hallucinations have been reported. The possibility of such untoward effects should be borne in mind.
Hypersensitivity reactions such as angioneurotic edema and maculopapular rash have also occurred.
Agranulocytosis has occasionally followed the repeated use of the drug, and deaths have occurred. Therefore, routine blood counts are advisable during maintenance procainamide therapy. The patients should be instructed to report any soreness of the mouth, throat, or gums, unexplained fever or any symptoms of upper respiratory tract infection. If any of these should occur, and leukocyte counts indicate cellular depression, procainamide therapy should be discontinued and appropriate treatment should be instituted immediately.
Dosage and Administration: Oral administration is preferred for treatment of arrhythmias which do not require immediate suppression, or to continue treatment after control of serious arrhythmias with Pronestyl Injection (Procainamide Hydrochloride Injection USP) or other antiarrhythmic therapy.
Intravenous therapy for the treatment of serious arrhythmias including those following myocardial infarctions should be limited to use in hospitals where monitoring facilities are available (see package insert accompanying Pronestyl Injection [Procainamide Hydrochloride Injection USP] for complete information).
If oral procainamide therapy is continued for appreciable periods, electrocardiograms should be made occasionally to determine the need for the drug.
Oral dose: For ventricular tachycardia, an initial dose of 1 gram orally followed thereafter by a *total daily dose* of 50 mg./kg. of body weight given at 3 hour intervals. The suggested oral dosage for premature ventricular contractions is 50 mg./kg. of body weight daily given in divided doses at 3 hour intervals.

To provide 50 mg./kg./day: give patients weighing less than 120 lbs. 250 mg. q. 3 hours; give patients between 120 and 200 lbs. 375 mg. q. 3 hours; and give patients over 200 lbs. 500 mg. q. 3 hours. This dosage schedule is for use as a guide for treating the average patient but all patients must be considered on an individual basis.

In atrial fibrillation and paroxysmal atrial tachycardia, an initial dose of 1.25 g. may be followed in one hour by 0.75 g. if there have been no electrocardiographic changes. A dose of 0.5 to 1 g. may then be given every 2 hours until arrhythmia is interrupted or the limit of tolerance is reached. Suggested maintenance dosage is 0.5 to 1 g. every 4 to 6 hours.

How Supplied: Pronestyl Capsules (Procainamide Hydrochloride Capsules USP) providing 250 mg. and 500 mg. are available in bottles of 100 and 1000, and UNIMATIC® single dose cartons of 100. The capsules which provide 375 mg. are available in bottles of 100 and UNIMATIC single dose cartons of 100 [375 mg. capsules in bottles of 100, Military Depot Item, 6505-01-015-1846]. Pronestyl Tablets (Procainamide Hydrochloride Tablets) providing 250 mg., 375 mg., and 500 mg. are available in bottles of 100 and Unimatic single-dose cartons of 100; the 250 mg. and 500 mg. tablets are also available in bottles of 1000.

Storage: Store the capsules and tablets at room temperature; avoid excessive heat.

[*Shown in Product Identification Section*]

PRONESTYL® INJECTION ℞
(Procainamide Hydrochloride Injection USP)

Description: Procainamide hydrochloride is the amide analogue of procaine hydrochloride. It is available for parenteral use as a sterile, aqueous solution providing 100 mg. or 500 mg. per ml. The 100 mg./ml. potency contains 0.9% (w/v) benzyl alcohol and 0.09% sodium bisulfite as preservatives; pH adjusted to 4.0–6.0 with hydrochloric acid or sodium hydroxide; the 500 mg./ml. potency contains 0.1% methylparaben and not more than 0.2% sodium bisulfite as preservatives; pH adjusted with hydrochloric acid or sodium hydroxide. At the time of manufacture, the air in the containers is replaced by nitrogen.

Actions: Procainamide depresses the excitability of cardiac muscle to electrical stimulation and slows conduction in the atrium, the bundle of His, and the ventricle. The refractory period of the atrium is considerably more prolonged than that of the ventricle. Contractility of the heart is usually not affected, nor is cardiac output decreased to any extent unless myocardial damage exists. In the absence of any arrhythmia, the heart rate may occasionally be accelerated by conventional doses, suggesting that the drug possesses anticholinergic properties. Larger doses can induce atrioventricular block and ventricular extrasystoles which may proceed to ventricular fibrillation. These effects on the myocardium are reflected in the electrocardiogram; a widening of the QRS complex occurs most consistently; less regularly, the P-R and Q-T intervals are prolonged, and the QRS and T waves show some decrease in voltage.

The action of procainamide begins almost immediately after intramuscular or intravenous administration. Plasma levels after intramuscular injection are at their peak in 15 to 60 minutes. Following oral administration, plasma levels of the drug are comparable to those obtained parenterally, and are maximal within an hour; therapeutic levels are usually attained in half that time.

Therapeutic plasma levels have been reported to be 3 to 10 mcg./ml., with those for the majority of patients in the range of 4 to 8 mcg./ml. Procainamide is less readily hydrolyzed than procaine, and plasma levels decline slowly—about 10% to 20% per hour. The drug is excreted primarily in the urine, about 10% as free and conjugated p-aminobenzoic acid and about 60% in the unchanged form. The fate of the remainder is unknown.

Indications: Pronestyl Injection (Procainamide Hydrochloride Injection USP) is indicated in the treatment of ventricular extrasystoles and tachycardia, atrial fibrillation, paroxysmal atrial tachycardia, and cardiac arrhythmias associated with anesthesia and surgery.

Contraindications: It has been suggested that procainamide be contraindicated in patients with myasthenia gravis. Hypersensitivity to the drug is an absolute contraindication; in this connection, cross sensitivity to procaine and related drugs must be borne in mind. Procainamide should not be administered to patients with complete atrioventricular heart block. Procainamide is also contraindicated in cases of high-degree A-V block unless an electrical pacemaker is operative.

Precautions: During administration of the drug, evidence of untoward myocardial responses should be carefully watched for in all patients. In the presence of an abnormal myocardium, procainamide may at times produce untoward responses. In atrial fibrillation or flutter, the ventricular rate may increase suddenly as the atrial rate is slowed. Adequate digitalization reduces, but does not abolish this danger. If myocardial damage exists, ventricular tachysystole is particularly hazardous. Correction of atrial fibrillation, with resultant forceful contractions of the atrium, may cause a dislodgment of mural thrombi and produce an embolic episode. However, it has been suggested that in a patient who is already discharging emboli, procainamide is more likely to stop than to aggravate the process.

Attempts to adjust the heart rate in a patient who has developed ventricular tachycardia during an occlusive coronary episode should be carried out with extreme caution. Caution is also required in marked disturbances of atrioventricular conduction such as A-V block, bundle branch block, or severe digitalis intoxication, where the use of procainamide may result in additional depression of conduction and ventricular asystole or fibrillation.

Parenteral administration should be monitored electrocardiographically whenever practicable. If electrocardiograms give evidence of impending heart block, parenteral administration should be discontinued at once. Since patients with severe organic heart disease and ventricular tachycardia may also have complete heart block which is difficult to diagnose under these circumstances, this complication should always be kept in mind when treating ventricular arrhythmias with procainamide (especially parenterally). If the ventricular rate is significantly slowed by procainamide without attainment of regular atrioventricular conduction, the drug should be stopped and the patient re-evaluated as asystole may result under these circumstances.

In patients receiving normal dosage, but who have both liver and kidney disease, symptoms of overdosage (principally ventricular tachycardia and severe hypotension) may occur due to drug accumulation.

Instances of a syndrome resembling lupus erythematosus have been reported in connection with oral maintenance procainamide therapy. The mechanism of this syndrome is uncertain. Polyarthralgia, arthritis, and pleuritic pain are common symptoms; to a lesser extent fever, myalgia, skin lesions, pleural effusion and pericarditis may occur. Rare cases of thrombocytopenia or Coombs positive hemolytic anemia have been reported which may be related to this syndrome. Patients receiving procainamide for extended periods of time or in whom symptoms suggestive of a lupus-like reaction appear should have anti-nuclear antibody titers measured at regular intervals. The drug should be discontinued if there is a rising titer (anti-nuclear antibody) or clinical symptoms of LE appear. The LE syndrome may be reversible upon discontinuance of the drug. If discontinuation of the drug does not cause remission of the symptoms, steroid therapy may be effective. If the syndrome develops in a patient with recurrent life-threatening arrhythmias not controllable by other antiarrhythmic agents, steroid suppressive therapy may be used concomitantly with procainamide.

Adverse Reactions: Because procainamide is a peripheral vasodilator, intravenous administration may produce transient but at times severe lowering of blood pressure, particularly in conscious patients. Intramuscular injection is less likely to be accompanied by serious falls in blood pressure. Serious disturbances of cardiac rhythm such as ventricular asystole or fibrillation are also more common with intravenous administration. Precautionary measures to be followed during intravenous injection are given in the section on "DOSAGE AND ADMINISTRATION".

A syndrome resembling lupus erythematosus has been reported in patients on oral maintenance therapy (see PRECAUTIONS). Reactions consisting of fever and chills have also been reported, including a case with fever and chills plus nausea, vomiting, abdominal pain, acute hepatomegaly, and a rise in serum glutamic oxaloacetic transaminase following single doses of the drug. Bitter taste, diarrhea, weakness, mental depression, giddiness, and psychosis with hallucinations have been reported. The possibility of such untoward effects should be borne in mind.

Hypersensitivity reactions such as angioneurotic edema and maculopapular rash have also occurred.

Agranulocytosis has occasionally followed the repeated use of the drug, and deaths have occurred. Therefore, routine blood counts are advisable during maintenance procainamide therapy. The patients should be instructed to report any soreness of the mouth, throat, or gums, unexplained fever or any symptoms of upper respiratory tract infection. If any of these should occur, and leukocyte counts indicate cellular depression, procainamide therapy should be discontinued and appropriate treatment should be instituted immediately.

Dosage and Administration: Oral administration is preferred for treatment of arrhythmias which do not require immediate suppression, or to continue treatment after control of serious arrhythmias with Pronestyl Injection (Procainamide Hydrochloride Injection USP) or other antiarrhythmic therapy.

Intravenous therapy for the treatment of serious arrhythmias including those following myocardial infarction should be limited to use in hospitals where monitoring facilities are available.

Both the 100 mg./ml. and 500 mg./ml. concentrations of Pronestyl Injection (Procainamide Hydrochloride Injection USP) should be diluted prior to intravenous use to facilitate control of dosage rate.

Intramuscular dose: Intramuscular administration may be preferable to the oral route in patients with vomiting, in those who are to receive nothing *per os* before surgery, or in those in whom there is reason to believe absorption may be unreliable. A dose of 0.5 to 1 g. may be given intramuscularly, repeated every four to eight hours until oral therapy is possible.

Intravenous dose: CAUTION—Intravenous use of procainamide hydrochloride may be accompanied by a hypotensive response, sometimes marked, if the dose is excessive or administration too rapid. Therefore, to initiate therapy, the intravenous dose should be diluted in 5% Dextrose Injection USP prior to administration to facilitate control of dosage rate; the dose should be administered at a rate not

Continued on next page

Squibb—Cont.

greater than 25 to 50 mg. per minute by either direct intravenous administration or infusion. Slow administration allows for some initial tissue distribution.

Direct Intravenous Administration—To reduce the possibility of a hypotensive response, 100 mg. doses may be administered every five minutes by direct slow intravenous injection, at a rate not exceeding 50 mg. in any one minute, until the arrhythmia is suppressed or the maximum dosage of 1 g. has been administered. Blood pressure must be taken and the electrocardiogram read before each dose. Some effects may be seen after the first 100 or 200 mg., and it is unusual to require more than 500 to 600 mg. to achieve satisfactory antiarrhythmic effects.

To maintain therapeutic levels, an infusion may then be started at a rate of 2 to 6 mg. procainamide per minute (see Table entitled "DILUTIONS AND RATES FOR INTRAVENOUS INFUSIONS") depending on the patient's body weight, circulatory condition and renal function.

Intravenous Infusion—An alternative method of achieving and then maintaining a therapeutic plasma concentration is to infuse 500 to 600 mg. of procainamide at a constant rate over a period of 25 to 30 minutes and then changing to another infusion for maintenance at a rate of 2 to 6 mg./min. (see Table entitled "DILUTIONS AND RATES FOR INTRAVENOUS INFUSIONS").

Intravenous therapy should be terminated as soon as the patient's basic cardiac rhythm appears to be stabilized and, if indicated, the patient should be placed on oral antiarrhythmic maintenance therapy. A period of about three to four hours (one half-life) should elapse after the last intravenous dose of procainamide before administering the first oral dose of procainamide.

Intravenous administration should be monitored electrocardiographically. Excessive widening of the QRS complex or prolongation of the P-R interval suggests the occurrence of myocardial toxicity. Patients should be kept in a supine position and blood pressure should be measured almost continuously during administration. If the fall in blood pressure exceeds 15 mm Hg, administration should be temporarily discontinued. Phenylephrine Hydrochloride Injection USP or Levarterenol Bitartrate Injection USP should be available to counteract severe hypotensive responses.

[See table below].

Surgical Use: For cardiac arrhythmias associated with anesthesia and surgery, the suggested parenteral dose is 0.1 to 0.5 g., preferably given intramuscularly.

How Supplied: Pronestyl Injection (Procainamide Hydrochloride Injection USP) is available as sterile, aqueous solutions in 10 ml. vials providing 100 mg. procainamide hydrochloride per ml. or 2 ml. vials providing 500 mg. procainamide hydrochloride per ml.

The solutions, which are colorless initially, may develop a slightly yellow color in time. This does not indicate a change which would prevent its use, but a solution any darker than light amber or discolored in any other way should not be used.

Pronestyl is also available for oral administration as Pronestyl Tablets (Procainamide Hydrochloride Tablets) and Pronestyl Capsules (Procainamide Hydrochloride Capsules USP) providing 250 mg., 375 mg., and 500 mg. procainamide hydrochloride (see package inserts accompanying the products for complete information).

Storage: Store Pronestyl Injection between 50° and 80° F.

DILUTIONS AND RATES FOR INTRAVENOUS INFUSIONS*

Approximate Final Concentration	Infusion Bottle Size (ml.)	ml. of Pronestyl (100 mg./ml.) to be added	ml. of Pronestyl (500 mg./ml.) to be added	Infusion Rate
0.2% (2 mg./ml.)	500	10	2	1–3 ml./min.
	250	5	1	
0.4% (4 mg./ml.)	500	20	4	0.5–1.5 ml./min.
	250	10	2	

* CAUTION: The flow rate of all intravenous infusion solutions must be closely monitored. These dilutions are calculated to deliver 2 to 6 mg. per minute at the infusion rates listed.

RAUDIXIN® ℞

(Rauwolfia Serpentina Tablets NF)
Whole Root—Biologically Standardized

Description: Raudixin contains Powdered Rauwolfia Serpentina NF, a hypotensive agent prepared from the powdered whole root of *Rauwolfia serpentina* Benth. The powdered rauwolfia serpentina in Raudixin contains not less than 0.15 percent and not more than 0.2 percent of reserpine-rescinnamine group alkaloids, calculated as reserpine. This product contains FD&C Yellow No. 5 (tartrazine).

Actions: Rauwolfia serpentina probably produces its antihypertensive effects through depletion of tissue stores of catecholamines (epinephrine and norepinephrine) from peripheral sites. By contrast, its sedative and tranquilizing properties are thought to be related to depletion of 5-hydroxytryptamine from the brain.

Rauwolfia serpentina is characterized by slow onset of action and sustained effect. Both its cardiovascular and central nervous system effects may persist following withdrawal of the drug.

Indications: Raudixin (Rauwolfia Serpentina Tablets NF) is indicated in the treatment of mild essential hypertension. It is also useful as adjunctive therapy with other antihypertensive agents in the more severe forms of hypertension.

Raudixin is also indicated for the relief of symptoms in agitated psychotic states (e.g., schizophrenia), primarily in those individuals unable to tolerate phenothiazine derivatives or those who also require antihypertensive medication.

Contraindications: The preparation is contraindicated in patients who have previously demonstrated hypersensitivity to rauwolfia. In this regard, it should be remembered that a past history of bronchial asthma or allergy may increase the possibility of drug sensitivity reactions. It is also contraindicated in patients with mental depression (especially with suicidal tendencies), active peptic ulcer, ulcerative colitis, and in patients receiving electroconvulsive therapy.

Warnings: Extreme caution should be exercised in treating patients with a history of mental depression. Discontinue the drug at the first sign of despondency, early morning insomnia, loss of appetite, impotence, or self-deprecation. Drug-induced depression may persist for several months after drug withdrawal and may be severe enough to result in suicide.

Usage in Pregnancy: Usage of rauwolfia preparations in women of childbearing age requires that the potential benefits of the drug be weighed against its possible hazards to the fetus. The hazards of using rauwolfia preparations include increased respiratory secretions, nasal congestion, cyanosis and anorexia in infants born to rauwolfia alkaloid-treated mothers.

Nursing Mothers: Rauwolfia preparations cross the placental barrier and appear in cord blood and breast milk.

Precautions: Because rauwolfia preparations increase gastrointestinal motility and secretion, this drug should be used cautiously in patients with a history of peptic ulcer, ulcerative colitis, or gallstones where biliary colic may be precipitated. Patients on high dosage should be observed carefully at regular intervals to detect possible reactivation of peptic ulcer.

Caution should be exercised when treating hypertensive patients with renal insufficiency since they adjust poorly to lowered blood pressure levels.

Use Rauwolfia serpentina cautiously with digitalis and quinidine since cardiac arrhythmias have occurred with rauwolfia preparations.

Preoperative withdrawal of rauwolfia serpentina does not insure that circulatory instability will not occur. It is important that the anesthesiologist be aware of the patient's drug intake and consider this in the overall management since hypotension has occurred in patients receiving rauwolfia preparations. Anticholinergic and/or adrenergic drugs (metaraminol, norepinephrine) have been employed to treat adverse vagocirculatory effects.

This product contains FD&C Yellow No. 5 (tartrazine) which may cause allergic-type reactions (including bronchial asthma) in certain susceptible individuals. Although the overall incidence of FD&C Yellow No. 5 (tartrazine) sensitivity in the general population is low, it is frequently seen in patients who also have aspirin hypersensitivity.

Adverse Reactions: *Gastrointestinal System*—hypersecretion, nausea, vomiting, anorexia, and diarrhea. *Central Nervous System*—drowsiness, depression, nervousness, paradoxical anxiety, nightmares, rare Parkinsonian syndrome, C.N.S. sensitization manifested by dull sensorium, deafness, glaucoma, uveitis, and optic atrophy. *Cardiovascular*—angina-like symptoms, arrhythmias, particularly when used concurrently with digitalis or quinidine, and bradycardia. *Other*—nasal congestion, pruritus, rash, dryness of mouth, dizziness, headache, dyspnea, purpura, impotence or decreased libido, dysuria, muscular aches, conjunctival injection, weight gain, and extrapyramidal tract symptoms.

These reactions are usually reversible and disappear when the drug is discontinued.

Water retention with edema in patients with hypertensive vascular disease may occur rarely, but the condition generally clears with cessation of therapy, or with the administration of a diuretic agent.

Dosage and Administration: For adults, the average oral dose is 200 to 400 mg. daily, given in divided doses in the morning and evening. Higher doses should be used cautiously because serious mental depression and other side effects may be considerably increased. (Orally, 200 to 300 mg. of powdered whole root is equiv-

alent to 0.5 mg. of reserpine.) Maintenance doses may vary from 50 to 300 mg. per day given as a single dose or as two divided doses. Concomitant use of rauwolfia serpentina and ganglionic blocking agents, guanethidine, veratrum, hydralazine, methyldopa, chlorthalidone, or thiazides necessitates careful titration of dosage with each agent.
Dosage for adolescents, children and the aged should be proportionately less than the usual adult dosage.
How Supplied: Raudixin (Rauwolfia Serpentina Tablets NF) is available for oral use as 50 and 100 mg. coated tablets, in bottles of 100 and 1000.
Storage: Store at room temperature; avoid excessive heat; keep bottle tightly closed.
[*Shown in Product Identification Section*]

RAU-SED® ℞
(Reserpine Tablets USP)

Description: Rau-Sed provides the crystalline alkaloid reserpine derived from the root of various species of *Rauwolfia*.
Actions: Reserpine probably produces its antihypertensive effects through depletion of tissue stores of catecholamines (epinephrine and norepinephrine) from peripheral sites. By contrast, its sedative and tranquilizing properties are thought to be related to depletion of 5-hydroxytryptamine from the brain.
Reserpine is characterized by slow onset of action and sustained effect. Both its cardiovascular and central nervous system effects may persist following withdrawal of the drug.
Indications: Rau-Sed is indicated in the treatment of mild essential hypertension. It is also useful as adjunctive therapy with other antihypertensive agents in the more severe forms of hypertension.
Rau-Sed (Reserpine Tablets USP) is also indicated for use in the relief of symptoms in agitated psychotic states (e.g., schizophrenia), primarily in those individuals unable to tolerate phenothiazine derivatives or those who also require antihypertensive medication.
Contraindications: The preparation is contraindicated in patients who have previously demonstrated hypersensitivity to rauwolfia alkaloids. In this regard, it should be remembered that a past history of bronchial asthma or allergy may increase the possibility of drug sensitivity reactions. Reserpine is also contraindicated in patients with mental depression (especially with suicidal tendencies), active peptic ulcer, ulcerative colitis, and in patients receiving electroconvulsive therapy.
Warnings: Extreme caution should be exercized in treating patients with a history of mental depression. Discontinue the drug at the first sign of despondency, early morning insomnia, loss of appetite, impotence, or self-deprecation. Drug-induced depression may persist for several months after drug withdrawal and may be severe enough to result in suicide.
Usage in Pregnancy: Usage of reserpine in women of childbearing age requires that the potential benefits of the drug be weighed against its possible hazards to the fetus. The hazards of using reserpine include increased respiratory secretions, nasal congestion, cyanosis and anorexia in infants born to reserpine-treated mothers.
Nursing Mothers: Reserpine crosses the placental barrier and appears in cord blood and breast milk.
Precautions: Because rauwolfia preparations increase gastrointestinal motility and secretion, this drug should be used cautiously in patients with a history of peptic ulcer, ulcerative colitis, or gallstones where biliary colic may be precipitated. Patients on high dosage should be observed carefully at regular intervals to detect possible reactivation of peptic ulcer.
Caution should be exercised when treating hypertensive patients with renal insufficiency since they adjust poorly to lowered blood pressure levels.
Use reserpine cautiously with digitalis and quinidine since cardiac arrhythmias have occurred with reserpine preparations.
Preoperative withdrawal of reserpine does not insure that circulatory instability will not occur. It is important that the anesthesiologist be aware of the patient's drug intake and consider this in the overall management since hypotension has occurred in patients receiving rauwolfia preparations. Anticholinergic and/or adrenergic drugs (metaraminol, norepinephrine) have been employed to treat adverse vagocirculatory effects.
Adverse Reactions: *Gastrointestinal System*—hypersecretion, nausea, vomiting, anorexia, and diarrhea. *Central Nervous System*—drowsiness, depression, nervousness, paradoxical anxiety, nightmares, rare Parkinsonian syndrome, C.N.S. sensitization manifested by dull sensorium, deafness, glaucoma, uveitis, and optic atrophy. *Cardiovascular*—angina-like symptoms, arrhythmias, particularly when used concurrently with digitalis or quinidine, and bradycardia. *Other*—nasal congestion, pruritus, rash, dryness of mouth, dizziness, headache, dyspnea, purpura, impotence or decreased libido, dysuria, muscular aches, conjunctival injection, weight gain, and extrapyramidal tract symptoms.
These reactions are usually reversible and disappear when the drug is discontinued.
Water retention with edema in patients with hypertensive vascular disease may occur rarely, but the condition generally clears with cessation of therapy, or with the administration of a diuretic agent.
Dosage and Administration: *Hypertension:* For the average patient not receiving other antihypertensive agents, the usual initial oral dose of Rau-Sed (Reserpine Tablets USP) is 0.5 mg. daily for 1 or 2 weeks. For maintenance, reduce the dose to 0.1 mg. to 0.25 mg. daily. Higher doses should be used with caution because serious mental depression and other side effects may be increased considerably.
Psychiatric disorders: The average initial oral dose is 0.5 mg. daily with a range of 0.1 mg. to 1.0 mg. Adjust dosage upward or downward according to the patient's response.
Note: Dosage for adolescents, children, and elderly or severely debilitated patients should be proportionately lower than the adult dosage.
Concomitant use of reserpine with ganglionic blocking agents, guanethidine, veratrum, hydralazine, methyldopa, chlorthalidone, or thiazides necessitates careful titration of dosage with each agent.
How Supplied: For oral use as tablets providing 0.25 mg. reserpine, bottles of 1000.
Storage: Store at room temperature; avoid excessive heat; keep bottle tightly closed.

RAUZIDE® ℞
(Powdered Rauwolfia Serpentina [50 mg.] with Bendroflumethiazide [4 mg.])

Description: Rauzide is Powdered Rauwolfia Serpentina (RAUDIXIN®) with Bendroflumethiazide (NATURETIN®). The Powdered Rauwolfia Serpentina in Rauzide contains not less than 0.15 percent and not more than 0.2 percent of reserpine-rescinnamine group alkaloids, calculated as reserpine. The preparation has been designed specifically to combine the antihypertensive effects of both rauwolfia and bendroflumethiazide for the treatment of hypertension, and may be useful in those patients not adequately benefited by either component alone. This product contains FD&C Yellow No. 5 (tartrazine).
Actions: The mechanism of action of bendroflumethiazide results in an interference with the renal tubular mechanism of electrolyte reabsorption. At maximal therapeutic dosage all thiazides are approximately equal in their diuretic potency. The mechanism whereby thiazides function in the control of hypertension is unknown.
Rauwolfia serpentina probably produces its antihypertensive effects through depletion of tissue stores of catecholamines (epinephrine and norepinephrine) from peripheral sites. By contrast, its sedative and tranquilizing properties are thought to be related to depletion of 5-hydroxytryptamine from the brain.
Rauwolfia serpentina is characterized by slow onset of action and sustained effect. Both its cardiovascular and central nervous system effects may persist following withdrawal of the drug.
Either of the components of Rauzide, when administered alone, may produce a reduction of blood pressure in hypertension. When the two agents are administered simultaneously, the action of the one appears to supplement that of the other so that a hypotensive effect may be produced which is greater than that produced by either agent alone. Thus, hypertension which does not adequately respond to either drug alone may frequently respond to the combination of both drugs.
Indications: Rauzide is indicated for hypertension (see box under WARNINGS).
Contraindications: The preparation is contraindicated in patients who have previously demonstrated hypersensitivity to thiazides or other sulfonamide-derived drugs, or rauwolfia. In this regard, it should be remembered that a past history of bronchial asthma or allergy may increase the possibility of drug sensitivity reactions.
Bendroflumethiazide is contraindicated in anuria.
The routine use of diuretics in otherwise healthy pregnant women with or without mild edema is contraindicated and possibly hazardous.
Rauwolfia serpentina is contraindicated in patients with mental depression (especially with suicidal tendencies), active peptic ulcer, ulcerative colitis, and in patients receiving electroconvulsive therapy.
Warnings:

> This fixed combination drug is not indicated for initial therapy of hypertension. Hypertension requires therapy titrated to the individual patient. If the fixed combination represents the dosage so determined, its use may be more convenient in patient management. The treatment of hypertension is not static, but must be reevaluated as conditions in each patient warrant.

Bendroflumethiazide should be used with caution in severe renal disease. In patients with renal disease, thiazides may precipitate azotemia. Cumulative effects of the drug may develop in patients with impaired renal function.
Thiazides should be used with caution in patients with impaired hepatic function or progressive liver disease, since minor alterations of fluid and electrolyte balance may precipitate hepatic coma.
Thiazides may be additive or may potentiate the action of other antihypertensive drugs. Potentiation occurs with ganglionic or peripheral adrenergic blocking drugs.
Sensitivity reactions may occur in patients with a history of allergy or bronchial asthma. The possibility of exacerbation or activation of systemic lupus erythematosus has been reported.
When using rauwolfia serpentina, extreme caution should be exercised in treating patients with a history of mental depression. Discontinue the drug at the first sign of despon-

Continued on next page

Squibb—Cont.

dency, early morning insomnia, loss of appetite, impotence, or self-deprecation. Drug-induced depression may persist for several months after drug withdrawal and may be severe enough to result in suicide.

Usage in Pregnancy—Usage of thiazides and rauwolfia preparations in women of childbearing age requires that the potential benefits of the drug be weighed against its possible hazards to the fetus. The hazards of using thiazides include fetal or neonatal jaundice, thrombocytopenia and possibly other adverse reactions which have occurred in the adult. The hazards of using rauwolfia preparations include increased respiratory secretions, nasal congestion, cyanosis and anorexia in infants born to rauwolfia alkaloid-treated mothers.

Nursing mothers—Thiazides and rauwolfia preparations cross the placental barrier and appear in cord blood and breast milk.

Precautions: This product contains FD&C Yellow No. 5 (tartrazine) which may cause allergic-type reactions (including bronchial asthma) in certain susceptible individuals. Although the overall incidence of FD&C Yellow No. 5 (tartrazine) sensitivity in the general population is low, it is frequently seen in patients who also have aspirin hypersensitivity.

Bendroflumethiazide—Periodic determination of serum electrolytes to detect possible electrolyte imbalance should be performed at appropriate intervals.

All patients receiving thiazide therapy should be observed for clinical signs of fluid or electrolyte imbalance; namely, hyponatremia, hypochloremic alkalosis, and hypokalemia. Serum and urine electrolyte determinations are particularly important when the patient is vomiting excessively or receiving parenteral fluids. Medication such as digitalis may also influence serum electrolytes. Warning signs, irrespective of cause, are: dryness of the mouth, thirst, weakness, lethargy, drowsiness, restlessness, muscle pains or cramps, muscular fatigue, hypotension, oliguria, tachycardia, and gastrointestinal disturbances such as nausea and vomiting.

Hypokalemia may develop with thiazides as with any other potent diuretic, especially with brisk diuresis, when severe cirrhosis is present, or during concomitant use of corticosteroids or ACTH.

Interference with adequate oral electrolyte intake will also contribute to hypokalemia. Digitalis therapy may exaggerate metabolic effects of hypokalemia especially with reference to myocardial activity.

Any chloride deficit is generally mild and usually does not require specific treatment except under extraordinary circumstances (as in liver disease or renal disease). Dilutional hyponatremia may occur in edematous patients in hot weather; appropriate therapy is water restriction, rather than administration of salt except in rare instances when the hyponatremia is life threatening. In actual salt depletion appropriate replacement is the therapy of choice.

Hyperuricemia may occur or frank gout may be precipitated in certain patients receiving thiazide therapy.

Insulin requirements in diabetic patients may be increased, decreased, or unchanged. Latent diabetes mellitus may become manifest during thiazide administration.

Thiazide drugs may increase the responsiveness to tubocurarine.

The antihypertensive effects of the drug may be enhanced in the post-sympathectomy patient.

Thiazides may decrease arterial responsiveness to norepinephrine. This diminution is not sufficient to preclude effectiveness of the pressor agent for therapeutic use. If emergency surgery is indicated, preanesthetic and anesthetic agents should be administered in reduced dosage.

If progressive renal impairment becomes evident, as indicated by a rising nonprotein nitrogen or blood urea nitrogen, a careful reappraisal of therapy is necessary with consideration given to withholding or discontinuing diuretic therapy.

Thiazides may decrease serum PBI levels without signs of thyroid disturbance.

Rauwolfia serpentina—Because rauwolfia preparations increase gastrointestinal motility and secretion, this drug should be used cautiously in patients with a history of peptic ulcer, ulcerative colitis, or gallstones where biliary colic may be precipitated. Patients on high dosage should be observed carefully at regular intervals to detect possible reactivation of peptic ulcer.

Caution should be exercised when treating hypertensive patients with renal insufficiency since they adjust poorly to lowered blood pressure levels.

Use Rauwolfia serpentina cautiously with digitalis and quinidine since cardiac arrhythmias have occurred with rauwolfia preparations.

Preoperative withdrawal of rauwolfia serpentina does not insure that circulatory instability will not occur. It is important that the anesthesiologist be aware of the patient's drug intake and consider this in the overall management since hypotension has occurred in patients receiving rauwolfia preparations. Anticholinergic and/or adrenergic drugs (metaraminol, norepinephrine) have been employed to treat adverse vagocirculatory effects.

Adverse Reactions: Bendroflumethiazide: *Gastrointestinal System*—anorexia, gastric irritation, nausea, vomiting, cramping, diarrhea, constipation, jaundice (intrahepatic cholestatic jaundice), and pancreatitis. *Central Nervous System*—dizziness, vertigo, paresthesias, headache, and xanthopsia. *Hematologic*—leukopenia, agranulocytosis, thrombocytopenia, and aplastic anemia. *Dermatologic-Hypersensitivity*—purpura, photosensitivity, rash, urticaria, and necrotizing angiitis (vasculitis, cutaneous vasculitis). *Cardiovascular*—Orthostatic hypotension may occur and may be aggravated by alcohol, barbiturates or narcotics. *Other*—hyperglycemia, glycosuria, occasional metabolic acidosis in diabetic patients, hyperuricemia, allergic glomerulonephritis, muscle spasm, weakness, and restlessness. Whenever adverse reactions are moderate or severe, thiazide dosage should be reduced or therapy withdrawn.

Rauwolfia serpentina: *Gastrointestinal System*—hypersecretion, nausea, vomiting, anorexia, and diarrhea. *Central Nervous System*—drowsiness, depression, nervousness, paradoxical anxiety, nightmares, rare Parkinsonian syndrome, C.N.S. sensitization manifested by dull sensorium, deafness, glaucoma, uveitis, and optic atrophy. *Cardiovascular*—angina-like symptoms, arrhythmias, particularly when used concurrently with digitalis or quinidine, and bradycardia. *Other*—nasal congestion, pruritus, rash, dryness of mouth, dizziness, headache, dyspnea, purpura, impotence or decreased libido, dysuria, muscular aches, conjunctival injection, weight gain, and extrapyramidal tract symptoms.

These reactions are usually reversible and disappear when the drug is discontinued.

Dosage and Administration: As determined by individual titration (see box under WARNINGS). Usual dosage may range from 1 to 4 tablets daily.

How Supplied: Rauzide is available as tablets providing 50 mg. powdered rauwolfia serpentina and 4 mg. bendroflumethiazide. Bottles of 100 and 1000.

Storage: Store at room temperature; avoid excessive heat; keep bottle tightly closed.

[*Shown in Product Identification Section*]

RENOGRAFIN® -60 ℞
(Diatrizoate Meglumine and Diatrizoate Sodium Injection USP)

(See Diagnostic Section)

RENOGRAFIN® -76 ℞
(Diatrizoate Meglumine and Diatrizoate Sodium Injection USP)

(See Diagnostic Section)

RENO-M-30® ℞
(Diatrizoate Meglumine Injection USP 30%)

(See Diagnostic Section)

RENO-M-60® ℞
(Diatrizoate Meglumine Injection USP 60%)

(See Diagnostic Section)

RENO-M-DIP® ℞
(Diatrizoate Meglumine Injection USP 30%) For Intravenous Drip Infusion

(See Diagnostic Section)

RENOVIST® ℞
(Diatrizoate Meglumine and Diatrizoate Sodium Injection USP)

(See Diagnostic Section)

RENOVIST® II ℞
(Diatrizoate Meglumine and Diatrizoate Sodium Injection USP)

(See Diagnostic Section)

RENOVUE®-65 ℞
(Iodamide Meglumine Injection)

(See Diagnostic Section)

RENOVUE®-DIP ℞
(Iodamide Meglumine Injection 24%)

(See Diagnostic Section)

RUBRAMIN PC® ℞
(Cyanocobalamin Injection USP)

Description: Rubramin PC (Vitamin B_{12}) is a clear, sterile, aqueous solution with a characteristic red color. The cobalt content of the 100 mcg./ml. and 1000 mcg./ml. Rubramin PC is 4 mcg./ml. and 40 mcg./ml., respectively. The preparation contains 1% (w/v) benzyl alcohol as a preservative and sodium chloride for isotonicity; the pH has been adjusted with sodium hydroxide or hydrochloric acid.

Actions: Vitamin B_{12} is essential to growth, cell reproduction, hematopoiesis, nucleoprotein and myelin synthesis.

Within 48 hours after injection of 100 to 1000 mcg. of vitamin B_{12}, 50 to 98% of the injected dose may appear in the urine. The major portion is excreted within the first 8 hours.

Indications: Rubramin PC is indicated for vitamin B_{12} deficiency due to malabsorption occurring in Addisonian (pernicious) anemia, gastrointestinal pathology, dysfunction or surgery, fish tapeworm infestation, gluten enteropathy, sprue, and concomitant folic acid deficiency. It is also indicated in pregnancy, thyrotoxicosis, hemolytic anemia, hemorrhage, malignancy, hepatic and renal disease because of increased requirements for vitamin B_{12}. Rubramin PC (Cyanocobalamin Injection USP) is also suitable for use as the flushing dose in the Schilling (vitamin B_{12} absorption) Test for pernicious anemia.

Contraindications: This preparation is contraindicated in patients who are sensitive to cobalt or vitamin B_{12}.

Warnings: The preparation should be protected from sunlight.

If a vitamin B_{12} deficiency is allowed to progress for more than 3 months, permanent degenerative spinal cord lesions may occur; such

lesions have been observed when folic acid is used as the sole hematopoietic agent.
Patients who have early Leber's disease (hereditary optic nerve atrophy) have been found to suffer severe and swift optic atrophy when treated with vitamin B_{12}.
Hypokalemia and sudden death may occur when severe megaloblastic anemia is treated intensively. Lack of therapeutic response may be due to infection, uremia, concomitant treatment with chloramphenicol or misdiagnosis.
The preparation should not be administered intravenously.
Precautions: Before administering vitamin B_{12}, an intradermal test dose is recommended for patients known to be sensitive to cobalamines.
Most antibiotics, methotrexate, and pyrimethamine invalidate folic acid and vitamin B_{12} diagnostic microbiological blood assays.
Colchicine, para-aminosalicylic acid or excessive alcohol intake longer than 2 weeks may produce malabsorption of vitamin B_{12}. Doses of vitamin B_{12} exceeding 10 mcg. daily may produce a hematologic response in patients who have a folate deficiency. Indiscriminate administration of vitamin B_{12} may mask the true diagnosis of pernicious anemia. A dietary deficiency of only vitamin B_{12} is rare. Multiple vitamin deficiency is expected in any dietary deficiency.
Adverse Reactions: Mild transient diarrhea, polycythemia vera, peripheral vascular thrombosis, itching, transitory exanthema, feeling of swelling of entire body, pulmonary edema and congestive heart failure early in treatment, anaphylactic shock and death.
Dosage and Administration:
A. General Rules
In patients with Addisonian (pernicious) anemia, parenteral therapy with vitamin B_{12} is the recommended method of treatment and will be required for the remainder of the patient's life. Oral therapy is not dependable. Serum potassium must be watched closely the first 48 hours; and potassium should be replaced if necessary. Reticulocyte plasma count, vitamin B_{12} and folic acid levels must be obtained prior to treatment and between the fifth and seventh day of therapy.
In patients with other types of vitamin B_{12} deficiency due to malabsorption, the malabsorption should be corrected. In all patients a well balanced dietary intake should be prescribed and poor dietary habits should be corrected.
B. Treatment of Vitamin B_{12} Deficiency:
Thirty micrograms daily for 5 to 10 days followed by 100 mcg. monthly injected intramuscularly or deep subcutaneously. Folic acid should be administered concomitantly early in the treatment unless folic acid levels are adequate.
In patients having normal intestinal absorption where the vitamin B_{12} deficiency is due to increased requirements, an oral therapeutic multivitamin preparation containing 15 mcg. vitamin B_{12} should be given daily for 1 month.
C. Schilling Test:
The flushing dose is 1000 mcg.
How Supplied: Rubramin PC (Cyanocobalamin Injection USP) is available in 10 ml. multiple-dose vials providing 100 mcg. cyanocobalamin per ml. and in 1 ml. and 10 ml. multiple-dose vials providing 1000 mcg. cyanocobalamin per ml. Both potencies are also available in 1 ml. UNIMATIC® single-dose preassembled syringes; the syringes have 22-gauge, 1¼-inch needles.
Storage: Store at room temperature; avoid freezing.

SINOGRAFIN® ℞
(Diatrizoate Meglumine and Iodipamide Meglumine Injection)

(See Diagnostic Section)

STOMAHESIVE®
(Peristomal Covering)

Stomahesive is a covering which can be applied to the skin around the stoma of an ostomate or the skin around a fistula to protect against contact of skin with exudates. It may also be applied to pressure points of the immobile patient to help preserve skin integrity and help prevent ulceration. It is available as wafers containing gelatin, pectin, sodium carboxymethylcellulose, and polyisobutylene.
Stomahesive is for use with colostomies, ileostomies, and ileal bladders. When applied as directed, it helps protect against drainage with an effective skintight adhesion that permits an ostomy appliance to remain intact for up to seven days.
How Supplied: Boxes of 5 4″ x 4″ wafers and boxes of 3 8″ x 8″ wafers. Both packages contain application instructions and cutting guides.

STOMAHESIVE® WAFER WITH SUR-FIT® APPLIANCE SYSTEM

The Stomahesive Wafer with Sur-Fit Appliance System is a two-piece system which consists of a 4″ × 4″ Stomahesive Wafer with Sur-Fit Flange and a Sur-Fit Pouch with matching size Sur-Fit Flange.
The round, plastic Sur-Fit Flange is welded to the surface of a Stomahesive Wafer and to a Sur-Fit Pouch. The flanges of the pouch and wafer snap together and fit precisely to insure a leak-free seal between the pouch and wafer to help prevent skin irritation from drainage around the stoma.
When applied as directed, the Stomahesive Wafer helps protect against drainage with an effective skintight adhesion around the stoma. The Sur-Fit Pouch can be removed whenever necessary without disturbing the Stomahesive Wafer with Flange for up to seven full days.
The Sur-Fit Appliance System provides a secure, comfortable, easy-to-use appliance system for all types of colostomies and ileostomies.
How Supplied: Stomahesive Wafer with Sur-Fit Flange—boxes of five 4″ × 4″ wafers with flange openings of 1½″, 1¾″, 2¼″, and 2¾″.
Sur-Fit Pouches—Small opaque drainable, 10″; Standard opaque drainable, 12″; Standard transparent drainable, 12″; Closed-End opaque. All pouches are available with flange openings of 1½″, 1¾″, 2¼″, and 2¾″ except for the transparent pouch which is not available in the 1½″ flange size.
Also available—Belts suitable for use with the Sur-Fit Appliance System, adjustable up to approximately 50″.

SUCOSTRIN® ℞
(Succinylcholine Chloride Injection USP)

CAUTION
Succinylcholine should be used only when apparatus for assisted or controlled respiration with oxygen is available, and should be administered only by persons well versed in the use of such apparatus.
The intravenous injection of procaine or the parenteral use of all antibiotics, except for the penicillins, may intensify the action of succinylcholine.
Description: Sucostrin (Succinylcholine Chloride Injection USP) is a potent skeletal-muscle relaxant for parenteral use. Each ml. of the aqueous preparation provides the equivalent of either 20, 50, or 100 mg. of anhydrous succinylcholine chloride with 0.1% methylparaben and 0.01% propylparaben as preservatives. At the time of manufacture, the air in the container is replaced by nitrogen. The pH is adjusted to 3.0 to 4.5 with hydrochloric acid or sodium hydroxide. Sodium chloride is added to the 20 mg. potency for isotonicity. The 50 and 100 mg. potencies are intended for addition to infusion solutions to be given by intravenous drip.
Actions: Succinylcholine promptly induces complete, but very brief, relaxation of skeletal muscle by persistent depolarization of the motor-end plates of skeletal muscle. Muscular paralysis is preceded by a transient stimulation of skeletal muscle. This initial stimulation is responsible for the muscle fibrillations which are observed shortly after administration of the drug. The sequence of muscular relaxation proceeds from the head and neck, to the shoulder, limbs, abdomen and intercostal muscles to the diaphragm. Recovery of normal muscle tone follows the reverse order.
Following intravenous injection of a suitable dose, the drug produces complete muscular relaxation within 30 to 60 seconds. Maximal muscular paralysis persists about two minutes and muscle tone generally returns to normal within the next four minutes. On intramuscular injection, onset of maximum relaxation of jaw muscles may vary from 75 seconds to three minutes following drug administration. Muscular relaxation of longer duration can be achieved by repeated injections at appropriate intervals or by continuous intravenous infusion. The degree of muscular relaxation can be altered within 30 to 60 seconds by changing the rate of infusion.
The effects of the drug disappear promptly upon discontinuation of the intravenous infusion. In the usual doses, succinylcholine normally has no effect on the cardiovascular system (see PRECAUTIONS). The drug does not affect autonomic nerve transmission or intestinal motility and is only a weak histamine liberator when given in the commonly employed clinical doses. It should be noted that the drug is not an anesthetic and does not impair sensory perception.
Succinylcholine is rapidly hydrolyzed by the pseudocholinesterase of the blood plasma into two normal metabolites, succinic acid and choline. The low toxicity of the drug and the lack of cumulative effect following repeated administration is due to its prompt enzymatic destruction. Correlation has been found between pseudocholinesterase levels in the plasma and duration of effect of the drug.
Indications: Succinylcholine chloride is indicated as an adjunct to anesthesia to induce skeletal muscle relaxation. It may also be employed to reduce the intensity of muscle contractions of pharmacologically or electrically induced convulsions.
Contraindication: Succinylcholine is contraindicated in patients with known hypersensitivity to the drug.
Warnings: SUCCINYLCHOLINE SHOULD NOT BE ADMINISTERED UNLESS FACILITIES FOR INTUBATION, ARTIFICIAL RESPIRATION, AND ADMINISTRATION OF OXYGEN THERAPY ARE INSTANTANEOUSLY AVAILABLE. THE CLINICIAN MUST BE PREPARED TO ASSIST OR CONTROL RESPIRATION.
When succinylcholine is given over a prolonged period, the characteristic depolarization block of the myoneural junction may change to a nondepolarizing block which results in prolonged respiratory depression or apnea. Under such circumstances, small repeated doses of neostigmine or edrophonium preceded by atropine may act as antagonists. A nerve stimulator may be used to ascertain the type of neuromuscular blockade. If a depolarization block is present both fast (tetanic) and slow (twitch) rates of nerve stimulation are well sustained and post-tetanic facilitation is absent. If a nondepolarizing block is present, there is post-tetanic facilitation and "fade" of successive stimuli on both fast (tetanic) and slow (twitch) rates of nerve stimulation. (The package inserts for neostigmine and edropho-

Continued on next page

Squibb—Cont.

nium should be consulted for complete prescribing information.)

The concurrent use of a depolarizing and a nondepolarizing (competitive) muscle relaxant is not recommended since a prolonged mixed block may occur (see PRECAUTIONS). In this instance, the dominant feature of the block may be determined by the use of a nerve stimulator as described above and treatment administered accordingly.

Because succinylcholine is rapidly hydrolyzed in alkaline solution, it is incompatible with sodium thiopental; separate injections are therefore preferable.

Succinylcholine is rapidly hydrolyzed to the intermediate metabolite succinylmonocholine. This metabolite, due to its slower rate of hydrolysis, can possibly accumulate and cause prolonged paralysis of the patient.

Usage in pregnancy: The safe use of succinylcholine has not been established with respect to the possible adverse effects upon fetal development. Therefore, it should not be used in women of childbearing potential and particularly during early pregnancy unless, in the judgment of the physician, the potential benefits outweigh the potential hazards.

Precautions: Respiratory depression or prolonged apnea may occur if succinylcholine is given in amounts greater than those recommended. Generally, doses of 30 mg. or less given to adult patients as a single injection, or 2.5 mg./minute by infusion, do not cause complete or prolonged respiratory paralysis although transient apnea usually occurs at the time of maximal effect. Spontaneous respiration generally returns in a few seconds, or at most, in three or four minutes. *Unless spontaneous respiration begins promptly, it is essential to initiate and continue controlled respiration with oxygen. Hyperventilation should be avoided, however, since this will prolong apnea* (see WARNINGS). Complete or prolonged respiratory paralysis frequently follows the administration of doses twice this size (i.e., over 1 mg./kg. of body weight) and requires similar treatment.

Sensitivity to the effects of succinylcholine occurs in patients whose pseudocholinesterase levels are low. This condition has occurred rarely as an inherited deficiency. Succinylcholine should be used cautiously in these patients as well as in patients with myasthenia gravis, renal failure, or disturbed electrolyte balance, and also in those exposed to cholinesterase inhibitors such as diisopropylfluorophosphate (DFP) or diethyl-p-nitrophenylthiophosphate. In such cases, fresh whole blood or plasma may be indicated to replenish cholinesterase levels.

Succinylcholine has been reported to cause an increase in intraocular tension which may prove harmful in operations for cataract. Succinylcholine should therefore be used with caution in ophthalmic surgery. In glaucoma patients, the increase in intraocular tension does not appear sufficient to cause ill effects.

If a curare-type muscle relaxant is used in conjunction with succinylcholine, its effect should be permitted to wear off before succinylcholine is administered.

Because of the possibility of muscle fasciculation following the administration of succinylcholine, the drug should be used cautiously in patients with fractures to avoid additional trauma.

Succinylcholine should be administered with great caution to patients with severe burns, those who are digitalized, or those recovering from severe trauma, since serious cardiac arrhythmias or cardiac arrest may result. Caution should also be observed in patients who are paraplegic, who have suffered spinal cord injury, or have degenerative or dystrophic neuromuscular disease, as such patients tend to become severely hyperkalemic when succinylcholine is given.

Adverse Reactions: Adverse reactions consist primarily of an extension of the drug's pharmacological actions. Profound and prolonged muscle relaxation may occur resulting in respiratory depression to the point of apnea. Hyperthermia, muscle pain, bradycardia, hypotension, cardiac arrhythmia, and increased salivation may occur following the use of succinylcholine.

Dosage and Administration: SINGLE INTRAVENOUS INJECTION: The average dose required to produce muscular relaxation of short duration is 20 mg. given over a period of 10 to 30 seconds. Some patients respond satisfactorily to doses as small as 10 mg., while others require 30 mg. or more. With higher doses, respiratory depression can usually be anticipated (see PRECAUTIONS).

Premedication with atropine or scopolamine is advised to prevent excessive salivation. Sucostrin (Succinylcholine Chloride Injection USP) is administered *after* narcosis has been induced with an inhalation agent or intravenous barbiturate. An initial test dose of 10 mg. may be used to determine the sensitivity of the patient and his recovery time. If moderate relaxation follows the test dose, 20 mg. will probably be needed for adequate relaxation; if only minimal relaxation follows the test dose, 30 mg. may be needed for adequate relaxation. Since the effect of a given dose generally wears off completely in a few minutes, subsequent doses must be calculated as though no previous dose had been given.

Relaxation prior to endotracheal intubation generally occurs in 30 to 40 seconds after the injection of succinylcholine. The jaws will be relaxed and the cords can be seen with a laryngoscope. If the cord reflexes have been abolished, the tube can be passed at once. An anesthetic lubricating jelly may be smeared on the tip of the endotracheal tube to aid in the insertion. More succinylcholine should be given if relaxation is not complete.

For *electroshock therapy,* the premedication and the muscle relaxant should be given in an amount and at such times, with respect to the time of shock, that the convulsion will be slight and will be followed almost at once by spontaneous respiration. Generally only about one minute should elapse between the injection of succinylcholine and the shock. The following schedule has been found satisfactory by many therapists:

1. Atropine (0.6 mg. [1/100 gr.]) or (0.32 mg. [1/200 gr.]) each of atropine and scopolamine is given 30 to 40 minutes before the shock.
2. Sodium thiopental (400 to 600 mg.) is given intravenously two to three minutes before the shock.
3. Succinylcholine chloride (10 to 30 mg.) is injected intravenously approximately one minute before the shock, usually through the same needle as that used for thiopental, but from a different syringe.
4. Pure oxygen is then administered for 45 seconds and a gauze roll placed between the teeth.
5. The shock is then given. If apnea is observed after the shock, oxygen is again administered.

INFUSION: For prolonged surgical procedures good muscular relaxation without respiratory arrest is necessary. The intravenous infusion of succinylcholine makes possible the maintenance of any desired level of paralysis over several hours. The drug, usually in a strength of 0.2%, is infused in 5% Dextrose Injection USP or Sodium Chloride Injection USP, the flow usually being adjusted between 1 to 2 ml. (2 to 4 mg.)/minute. The degree of relaxation may be adjusted in 30 to 60 seconds by changing the rate of infusion.

Premedication should include atropine or atropine and scopolamine. An appropriate anesthetic is given and the infusion begun. When it is desired to employ inhalation anesthesia through an endotracheal tube, the infusion of succinylcholine is continued until the jaw is relaxed and the laryngeal reflex obtunded. The patient may be apneic at this time and ventilation should be commenced as soon as the airway has been connected to the anesthesia machine. The infusion of succinylcholine should be stopped or slowed until the respiratory pattern returns. Generally, respiration will resume within one-half to three minutes following cessation of the infusion; meanwhile, controlled respiration with an anesthetic-oxygen mixture should be maintained.

The aim of succinylcholine administration should be to provide adequate relaxation while still maintaining the patient's respiratory pattern. Ideally, therefore, respiration should be assisted rather than controlled.

By altering the rate of infusion, different degrees of muscular relaxation can be provided as required. A more rapid flow may be needed, for example, for opening the peritoneum, during the initial explorations, or at the time of wound closure, than when the definite procedure is underway and packs and retractors are in place.

INTRAMUSCULAR INJECTION IN INFANTS AND CHILDREN: The suggested dosage for infants and children is 1.5 mg./lb. of body weight; a maximum total dose of 150 mg. should not be exceeded. The drug should be given by deep intramuscular injection, high into the deltoid muscle.

Premedication with atropine is advised. With a dosage regimen of 1.5 mg. succinylcholine chloride per lb. of body weight, cyclopropane is generally the most efficient anesthetic for intubation, while larger intramuscular doses are usually required with less potent anesthetics. It should be noted that respiratory depression may be expected to increase with increasing doses of succinylcholine. If the muscle relaxant is injected immediately after consciousness is lost, intubation can proceed during plane 1, third stage of cyclopropane anesthesia. A period of hyperventilation with oxygen is recommended prior to the removal of the mask and exposure of the larynx to maintain the patient during the unavoidable interruption in ventilation caused by intubation.

How Supplied: Sucostrin (Succinylcholine Chloride Injection USP) is available as an aqueous solution in vials or ampuls as follows: Sucostrin Injection, providing the equivalent of 20 mg. anhydrous succinylcholine chloride per ml., in 10 ml. vials; Sucostrin for Infusion, providing the equivalent of 50 mg. anhydrous succinylcholine chloride per ml., in 10 ml. ampuls; Sucostrin High Potency, providing the equivalent of 100 mg. anhydrous succinylcholine chloride per ml., in 10 ml. vials.

Storage: Vials and ampuls should be stored in the refrigerator. Freshly prepared infusion solutions should be refrigerated until used; at room temperature, they are stable for 24 hours without significant loss of potency.

SUMYCIN® '250' TABLETS ℞
SUMYCIN® '500' TABLETS ℞
(Tetracycline Hydrochloride Tablets NF)
SUMYCIN® '250' CAPSULES ℞
SUMYCIN® '500' CAPSULES ℞
(Tetracycline Hydrochloride Capsules USP)
SUMYCIN® SYRUP ℞
(Tetracycline Oral Suspension USP)

Description: Sumycin '250' and Sumycin '500' Tablets (Tetracycline Hydrochloride Tablets NF) are available for oral administration as FILMLOK® tablets providing 250 mg. and 500 mg. tetracycline hydrochloride, respectively. (FILMLOK is a Squibb trademark for veneer-coated tablets.)

Sumycin '250' and Sumycin '500' Capsules (Tetracycline Hydrochloride Capsules USP)

contain 250 mg. and 500 mg. crystalline tetracycline hydrochloride, respectively.
Sumycin Syrup (Tetracycline Oral Suspension USP) is a suspension containing, in each 5 ml. teaspoonful, tetracycline equivalent to 125 mg. tetracycline hydrochloride.

Clinical Pharmacology: The tetracyclines are primarily bacteriostatic antibiotics and are thought to exert their antimicrobial effect by the inhibition of protein synthesis. Tetracyclines are active against a wide range of gram-negative and gram-positive organisms.
The drugs in the tetracycline class have closely similar antimicrobial spectra. Microorganisms that have become insensitive to one tetracycline invariably exhibit cross-resistance to other tetracyclines. In addition, gram-negative bacilli made tetracycline-resistant may also show cross-resistance to chloramphenicol. Microorganisms may be considered susceptible if the MIC (minimum inhibitory concentration) is not more than 4 mcg./ml. and intermediate if the MIC is 4 to 12.5 mcg./ml.
Susceptibility plate testing: A tetracycline disc may be used to determine microbial susceptibility to drugs in the tetracycline class. If the Kirby-Bauer method of disc sensitivity is used, a 30 mcg. tetracycline disc should give a zone of at least 19 mm. when tested against a tetracycline-susceptible bacterial strain.
Tetracyclines are readily absorbed and are bound to plasma proteins in varying degree. They are concentrated by the liver in the bile and excreted in the urine and feces at high concentrations and in a biologically active form.

Indications and Usage: Tetracycline is indicated in infections caused by the following microorganisms.
Rickettsiae: Rocky mountain spotted fever, typhus fever and the typhus group, Q fever, rickettsialpox, tick fevers, *Mycoplasma pneumoniae* (PPLO, Eaton agent), agents of psittacosis and ornithosis, agents of *Lymphogranuloma venereum* and *Granuloma inguinale*, and the spirochetal agent of relapsing fever *(B. recurrentis).*
The following gram-negative organisms: *H. ducreyi* (chancroid), *Pasteurella pestis* and *Past. tularensis, Bartonella bacilliformis,* Bacteroides, *Vibrio comma* and *V. fetus,* and Brucella organisms (in conjunction with streptomycin).
Because many strains of the following groups of microorganisms have been shown to be resistant to tetracyclines, culture and susceptibility testing are recommended.
The following gram-negative organisms, when bacteriologic testing indicates appropriate susceptibility to the drug: *E. coli, Enterobacter aerogenes* (formerly *A. aerogenes*), Shigella, *Mima, Herellea, H. influenzae* (respiratory infections), and Klebsiella infections (respiratory and urinary).
The following gram-positive organisms when bacteriologic testing indicates appropriate susceptibility to the drug:
1) Streptococcus species: Up to 44 percent of strains of *Streptococcus pyogenes* and 74 percent of *Streptococcus faecalis* have been found to be resistant to tetracycline drugs. Therefore, tetracyclines should not be used for streptococcal disease unless the organism has been demonstrated to be sensitive.
(For upper respiratory infections due to group A beta-hemolytic streptococci, penicillin is the usual drug of choice including prophylaxis of rheumatic fever.)
2) *D. pneumoniae.*
3) *Staphylococcus aureus* (skin and soft tissue infections). Tetracyclines are not the drugs of choice in the treatment of any type of staphylococcal infections.
When penicillin is contraindicated, tetracyclines are alternative drugs in the treatment of infections due to: *N. gonorrhoeae, T. pallidum* and *T. pertenue* (syphilis and yaws), *Listeria monocytogenes,* Clostridia, *B. anthracis, Fusobacterium fusiforme* (Vincent's infection), and *Actinomyces.*
In acute intestinal amebiasis, the tetracyclines may be a useful adjunct to amebicides.
In severe acne the tetracyclines may be useful adjunctive therapy.
Tetracyclines are indicated in the treatment of trachoma, although the infectious agent is not always eliminated, as judged by immunofluorescence.
Inclusion conjunctivitis may be treated with oral tetracyclines or with a combination of oral and topical agents.

Contraindications: This drug is contraindicated in persons who have shown hypersensitivity to any of the tetracyclines.

Warnings: THE USE OF DRUGS OF THE TETRACYCLINE CLASS DURING TOOTH DEVELOPMENT (LAST HALF OF PREGNANCY, INFANCY AND CHILDHOOD TO THE AGE OF EIGHT YEARS) MAY CAUSE PERMANENT DISCOLORATION OF THE TEETH (YELLOW-GRAY-BROWN). This reaction is more common during long-term use of the drugs but has been observed following repeated short-term courses. Enamel hypoplasia has also been reported. TETRACYCLINE DRUGS, THEREFORE, SHOULD NOT BE USED IN THIS AGE GROUP UNLESS OTHER DRUGS ARE NOT LIKELY TO BE EFFECTIVE OR ARE CONTRAINDICATED.
If renal impairment exists, even usual oral or parenteral doses may lead to excessive systemic accumulation of the drug and possible liver toxicity. Under such conditions, lower than usual doses are indicated and, if therapy is prolonged, serum level determinations of the drug may be advisable. The antianabolic action of tetracycline may cause an increase in BUN. While this is not a problem in those with normal renal function, in patients with significantly impaired function, higher serum levels of tetracycline may lead to azotemia, hyperphosphatemia, and acidosis.
Photosensitivity, manifested by an exaggerated sunburn reaction, has been observed in some individuals taking tetracyclines. Patients apt to be exposed to direct sunlight or ultraviolet light should be advised that this reaction can occur with tetracycline drugs, and treatment should be discontinued at the first evidence of skin erythema. NOTE: Photosensitization reactions have occurred most frequently with demeclocycline, less with chlortetracycline, and very rarely with oxytetracycline and tetracycline.

Usage in Pregnancy: (See WARNINGS about use during tooth development.)
Results of animal studies indicate that tetracyclines cross the placenta, are found in fetal tissues and can have toxic effects on the developing fetus (often related to retardation of skeletal development). Evidence of embryotoxicity has also been noted in animals treated early in pregnancy.

Usage in Newborns, Infants, and Children: (See WARNINGS about use during tooth development.)
Tetracyclines form a stable calcium complex in any bone-forming tissue. A decrease in the fibula growth rate has been observed in prematures given oral tetracycline in doses of 25 mg./kg. every six hours. This reaction was shown to be reversible when the drug was discontinued.
Tetracyclines are present in the milk of lactating women who are taking a drug in this class.

Precautions: As with other antibiotics, use of this drug may result in overgrowth of nonsusceptible organisms, including fungi. If superinfection occurs, the antibiotic should be discontinued and appropriate therapy instituted. Note: Superinfection of the bowel by staphylococci may be life-threatening.
In venereal diseases when coexistent syphilis is suspected, patients should have darkfield examinations before treatment is started and the blood serology should be repeated monthly for at least four months.
Because the tetracyclines have been shown to depress plasma prothrombin activity, patients who are on anticoagulant therapy may require downward adjustment of their anticoagulant dosage.
During long-term therapy, periodic laboratory evaluation of organ systems, including hematopoietic, renal and hepatic studies should be performed.
All infections due to group A beta-hemolytic streptococci should be treated for at least 10 days.
Since bacteriostatic drugs may interfere with the bactericidal action of penicillin, it is advisable to avoid giving tetracycline in conjunction with penicillin.
Since sensitivity reactions are more likely to occur in persons with a history of allergy, asthma, hay fever, or urticaria, the preparation should be used with caution in such individuals.

Adverse Reactions: Gastrointestinal: anorexia, epigastric distress, nausea, vomiting, diarrhea, bulky loose stools, stomatitis, sore throat, glossitis, black hairy tongue, dysphagia, hoarseness, enterocolitis, and inflammatory lesions (with candidal overgrowth) in the anogenital region, including proctitis and pruritus ani. These reactions have been caused by both the oral and parenteral administration of tetracyclines but are less frequent after parenteral use.
Skin: maculopapular and erythematous rashes. Exfoliative dermatitis has been reported but is uncommon. Onycholysis and discoloration of the nails have been reported rarely. Photosensitivity has occurred (see WARNINGS).
Renal toxicity: rise in BUN has been reported and is apparently dose-related (see WARNINGS).
Hepatic cholestasis has been reported rarely, and is usually associated with high dosage levels of tetracycline.
Hypersensitivity reactions: urticaria, angioneurotic edema, anaphylaxis, anaphylactoid purpura, pericarditis, exacerbation of systemic lupus erythematosus, and serum sickness-like reactions, as fever, rash, and arthralgia.
When given over prolonged periods, tetracyclines have been reported to produce brown-black microscopic discoloration of thyroid glands. No abnormalities of thyroid function studies are known to occur.
Bulging fontanels have been reported in young infants following full therapeutic dosage. This sign disappeared rapidly when the drug was discontinued.
Blood: anemia, hemolytic anemia, thrombocytopenia, thrombocytopenic purpura, neutropenia and eosinophilia have been reported.
Dizziness and headache have been reported.

Dosage and Administration: Adults: Usual daily dose is 1 to 2 g.; for mild to moderate infections: 500 mg. b.i.d. or 250 mg. q.i.d.; higher dosages such as 500 mg. q.i.d. may be required for severe infections.
For children above eight years of age: Usual daily dose is 10 to 20 mg./lb. (25 to 50 mg./kg.) body weight divided in four equal doses.
Representative pediatric dosages for the syrup on a q.i.d. basis are as follows: 20 lbs.—½ teaspoonful; 40 lbs.—1 teaspoonful; 60 lbs.—1½ teaspoonfuls; and 80 lbs.—2 teaspoonfuls.
Therapy should be continued for at least 24 to 48 hours after symptoms and fever have subsided.
The treatment of brucellosis, 500 mg. tetracycline four times daily for three weeks should be accompanied by streptomycin, 1 g. intramuscularly twice daily the first week and once daily the second week.
For treatment of gonorrhea, the recommended dose is 1.5 g. initially, then 0.5 g. every six hours until a total of 9 g. have been given.

Continued on next page

Squibb—Cont.

For treatment of syphilis, a total of 30 to 40 g. in equally divided doses over a period of 10 to 15 days should be given. Close followup, including laboratory tests, is recommended.
In cases of severe acne which, in the judgment of the clinician, require long-term treatment, the recommended initial dosage is 1 g. daily in divided doses. When improvement is noted, usually within one week, dosage should be gradually reduced to maintenance levels ranging from 125 mg. to 500 mg. daily. In some patients it may be possible to maintain adequate remission of lesions with alternate-day or intermittent therapy. Tetracycline therapy of acne should augment the other standard measures known to be of value.
In patients with renal impairment (see WARNINGS) total dosage should be decreased by reduction of recommended individual doses and/or by extending time intervals between doses.
In the treatment of streptococcal infections, a therapeutic dose of tetracycline should be administered for at least 10 days.
Concomitant therapy: Antacids containing aluminum, calcium, or magnesium impair absorption and should not be given to patients taking oral tetracycline.
Foods and some dairy products also interfere with absorption. Oral forms of tetracycline should be given one hour before or two hours after meals. Pediatric oral dosage forms should not be given with milk formulas and should be given at least one hour prior to feeding.
How Supplied: *Sumycin '250' Tablets (Tetracycline Hydrochloride Tablets NF) are available for oral administration as tablets containing 250 mg. tetracycline hydrochloride in bottles of 100 and 1000. *Sumycin '500' Tablets are available for oral administration as tablets containing 500 mg. tetracycline hydrochloride in bottles of 100 and 500. *Sumycin '250' Capsules (Tetracycline Hydrochloride Capsules USP) are available for oral administration as capsules containing 250 mg. tetracycline hydrochloride in bottles of 100 and 1000 and in Unimatic® Single-Dose Packs of 100. *Sumycin '500' Capsules are available for oral administration as capsules containing 500 mg. tetracycline hydrochloride in bottles of 100 and 500 and in Unimatic Single-Dose Packs of 100.
Sumycin Syrup (Tetracycline Oral Suspension USP) is available as a fruit-flavored suspension containing, in each 5 ml. teaspoonful, tetracycline equivalent to 125 mg. tetracycline hydrochloride buffered with potassium metaphosphate in bottles of 60 ml. and 473 ml. (1 pint).
Storage: Store the tablets and capsules at room temperature; avoid excessive heat. Store the syrup below 30° C (86° F); avoid freezing; protect from light; keep bottle tightly closed.
*[*Shown in Product Identification Section*]

TESLAC® SUSPENSION ℞
(Sterile Testolactone Suspension NF)
FOR INTRAMUSCULAR USE

TESLAC® TABLETS ℞
(Testolactone Tablets NF)

Description: Teslac (Testolactone) contains testolactone which is chemically designated as D-Homo-17a-oxaandrosta-1, 4-diene-3, 17-dione (1-dehydrotestololactone, or Δ^1-testololactone). Testolactone is a white, odorless, crystalline solid, soluble in ethanol and slightly soluble in water.
Each ml. of Teslac Suspension provides 100 mg. testolactone, with sodium chloride for isotonicity, 0.9% (w/v) benzyl alcohol as a preservative, 0.75% sodium carboxymethylcellulose, and 0.04% polysorbate 80. Sodium hydroxide or hydrochloric acid is used to adjust the pH to 5.0 to 7.5.
Teslac Tablets are available for oral administration as tablets containing 50 mg. and 250 mg. testolactone.
Actions: The precise mechanism by which testolactone produces its clinical antineoplastic effects is unknown at present.
Although the chemical configuration of testolactone is similar to that of certain androgenic hormones, it is devoid of androgenic activity in the doses commonly employed.
Teslac was found to be effective in approximately 15% of patients with advanced or disseminated mammary cancer evaluated according to the following criteria: 1) those with a measurable decrease in size of all demonstrable tumor masses; 2) those in whom more than 50% of non-osseous lesions decreased in size although all bone lesions remained static; and 3) those in whom more than 50% of total lesions improved while the remainder were static.
Indications: Teslac Suspension (Sterile Testolactone Suspension NF) and Teslac Tablets (Testolactone Tablets NF) are recommended as adjunctive therapy in the palliative treatment of advanced or disseminated breast cancer in postmenopausal women when hormonal therapy is indicated. It may also be used in women who were diagnosed as having had disseminated breast carcinoma when premenopausal, in whom ovarian function has been subsequently terminated.
Contraindications: Testolactone is contraindicated in the treatment of breast cancer in men.
Warnings: Usage in Pregnancy: Since safe use of testolactone has not been established with respect to adverse effects upon fetal development, and since this preparation is intended for use only in postmenopausal women, testolactone should not be used during pregnancy.
Precautions: Plasma calcium levels should be routinely determined in any patient receiving therapy for mammary cancer, particularly during periods of active remission of bony metastases. If hypercalcemia occurs, appropriate measures should be instituted.
Adverse Reactions: Parenteral administration of the drug occasionally may result in slight pain at the injection site, local inflammation, and/or irritation.
Other signs and symptoms have been reported in association with the use of this drug but, in these instances, it is often impossible to determine the relationship of the underlying disease and drug administration to the reported reaction. Such reactions include maculopapular erythema, increase in blood pressure, paresthesia, aches and edema of the extremities, glossitis, anorexia, and nausea and vomiting. Alopecia alone and with associated nail growth disturbance have been reported rarely; these side effects subsided without interruption of treatment.
Dosage and Administration: The intramuscular dose is 100 mg. 3 times per week. The recommended oral dose is 250 mg. q.i.d.
In order to evaluate the response, therapy with testolactone should be continued for a minimum of three months unless there is active progression of the disease.
Shake the vial of Teslac Suspension (Sterile Testolactone Suspension NF) vigorously before use to insure a uniform suspension. Inject immediately to prevent settling in the syringe.
The parenteral preparation should be administered by deep intramuscular injection. The preferred site is the upper outer quadrant of the gluteal area. Aspiration and proper anatomical selection of injection site should be observed in order to avoid inadvertent injection into a blood vessel or major nerve. Deposition in the subcutaneous tissues should be avoided; accidental injection into these tissues may cause pain and induration which can be alleviated by applying an ice pack. For adults, a minimum needle length of one and one-half inches is recommended. In obese patients, a longer needle may be required. Use alternate sites for subsequent injections.
How Supplied: Teslac Suspension is available for intramuscular administration as a sterile aqueous suspension providing 100 mg. testolactone per ml. in multiple-dose vials of 5 ml.
Teslac Tablets are available for oral administration as tablets containing 50 mg. or 250 mg. testolactone in bottles of 100.
Storage: Store Teslac Suspension (Sterile Testolactone Suspension NF) at room temperature; avoid freezing. Store Teslac Tablets (Testolactone Tablets NF) at room temperature; avoid excessive heat.

THERAGRAN HEMATINIC® ℞
(Therapeutic Formula Vitamin Tablets with Hematinics)

Description: Theragran Hematinic Tablets are designed for oral therapy of iron-deficiency anemias and other nutritional deficiency states. This product contains FD&C Yellow No. 5 (tartrazine).
Each tablet contains:

Vitamin A Acetate	(8,333 IU) 2.5 mg.
Vitamin D (Ergocalciferol)	(133 IU) 3.3 mcg.
Thiamine Mononitrate	3.3 mg.
Riboflavin	3.3 mg.
Pyridoxine Hydrochloride	3.3 mg.
Niacinamide	33.3 mg.
Calcium Pantothenate	11.7 mg.
Vitamin E (dl-α-Tocopheryl Acetate)	(5 IU) 5 mg.
Copper (as Sulfate)	0.67 mg.
Magnesium (as Carbonate)	41.7 mg.
Iron, elemental (as Ferrous Fumarate)	66.7 mg.
Vitamin B_{12} (as Cyanocobalamin)	50 mcg.
Folic Acid	0.33 mg.
Vitamin C (as Sodium Ascorbate)	100 mg.

Actions: The vitamins and the dietary minerals are fundamentally involved in vital metabolic processes, where they usually serve as oxidizing and reducing agents and as factors in various enzyme systems. These essential nutrients are so closely interrelated that the lack of any one may affect the body requirements of others. Thus, when a single dietary deficiency becomes clinically manifest, other nutritional insufficiencies are almost inevitable: for example, in iron-deficiency anemias due to inadequacy in the diet, the likelihood exists that the diet is also low in other basic requirements. Such multiple insufficiencies are especially apt to occur in times of increased growth or stress, as in pregnancy and lactation, when nutritional requirements are high. Dietary deficiencies are also more likely to occur in persons whose diets are unsatisfactory because of restrictions or personal idiosyncrasies; in the elderly, who often neglect good eating habits, especially when living alone; and in persons suffering from conditions known to affect the requirements, absorption, utilization, or rate of destruction and excretion of vitamins or minerals.
Theragran Hematinic Tablets provide elemental iron in the form of ferrous fumarate. The ferrous form of iron is regarded to be less likely to produce gastric disturbances than the ferric salts, is best absorbed, and is the most completely utilized form of oral iron.
Indications: Theragran Hematinic Tablets are indicated in the treatment of many of the common anemias, including hypochromic microcytic anemia, nutritional macrocytic anemia, macrocytic or microcytic anemia of pregnancy, and tropical and nontropical sprue.
Theragran Hematinic Tablets are particularly useful in the treatment of anemias primarily due to iron deficiency, especially when complicated by deficiencies of other nutrients or when nutritional requirements are high. The preparation is thus particularly beneficial in the anemias associated with dietary inadequacy which are commonly characterized by malaise and chronic fatigue, the anemias at-

tending convalescence, the anemias frequently encountered in late childhood, early adolescence and old age, the anemia associated with menorrhagia, and the anemias of women from menarche to menopause.

Theragran Hematinic Tablets may also be beneficial in other conditions involving dietary insufficiencies that can be corrected with the ingredients supplied by the tablets, and in conditions characterized by alteration in the absorption, utilization, or elimination of these ingredients.

Contraindications: Hemochromatosis and hemosiderosis are contraindications to iron therapy.

Warning: Folic acid alone is improper therapy in the treatment of pernicious anemia and other megaloblastic anemias where vitamin B_{12} is deficient.

Precautions: Since iron-deficiency anemia may be a manifestation of a basic systemic disturbance such as recurrent blood loss, the underlying cause of the anemia should be determined and corrected if possible.

The ingredients in Theragran Hematinic are not sufficient nor are they intended for the treatment of pernicious anemia. The possibility of pernicious anemia should be excluded before treatment. While folic acid may correct the blood picture of pernicious anemia, it may not ameliorate the attendant neurologic involvement. Parenteral use of vitamin B_{12} is recommended to assure essential medical supervision of the patient.

This product contains FD&C Yellow No. 5 (tartrazine) which may cause allergic-type reactions (including bronchial asthma) in certain susceptible individuals. Although the overall incidence of FD&C Yellow No. 5 (tartrazine) sensitivity in the general population is low, it is frequently seen in patients who also have aspirin hypersensitivity.

Adverse Reactions: Allergic sensitization has been reported following both oral and parenteral administration of folic acid.

Dosage and Administration: In adults, therapy may be initiated with 1 Theragran Hematinic Tablet three times daily. Dosage may be adjusted according to the response of the patient. Since ferrous fumarate is not likely to cause gastric upsets, dosage need not be given at mealtime.

How Supplied: Theragran Hematinic Tablets are available in bottles of 90.

Storage: Store at room temperature; avoid excessive heat.

[*Shown in Product Identification Section*]

THERAGRAN® LIQUID
(High Potency Vitamin Supplement)

Each 5 ml. teaspoonful contains:

			Percent US RDA*
Vitamin A	(3 mg)	10,000 IU	200
Vitamin D	(10 mcg)	400 IU	100
Vitamin C		200 mg	333
Thiamine		10 mg	667
Riboflavin		10 mg	588
Niacin		100 mg	500
Vitamin B_6		4.1 mg	205
Vitamin B_{12}		5 mcg	83
Pantothenic Acid		21.4 mg	214

*US Recommended Daily Allowance

Usage: For 12 year olds and older—1 teaspoonful daily.

The following statement appears on the label: **"USE OF THIS PRODUCT MAY BE HAZARDOUS TO YOUR HEALTH. THIS PRODUCT CONTAINS SACCHARIN WHICH HAS BEEN DETERMINED TO CAUSE CANCER IN LABORATORY ANIMALS".**

How Supplied: In bottles of 4 fl. oz.

Storage: Store at room temperature; avoid excessive heat.

THERAGRAN® TABLETS
(High Potency Vitamin Supplement)

Each tablet contains:

			Percent US RDA*
Vitamin A	(3 mg)	10,000 IU	200
Vitamin D	(10 mcg)	400 IU	100
Vitamin E	(15 mg)	15 IU	50
Vitamin C		200 mg	333
Thiamine		10.3 mg	687
Riboflavin		10 mg	588
Niacin		100 mg	500
Vitamin B_6		4.1 mg	205
Vitamin B_{12}		5 mcg	83
Pantothenic Acid		18.4 mg	184

*US Recommended Daily Allowance

Usage: For 12 year olds and older—1 tablet daily.

How Supplied: Bottles of 1000; Handy Packs of 30, 60, 100, and 180; and Unimatic® cartons of 100.

Storage: Store at room temperature; avoid excessive heat.

[*Shown in Product identification Section*]

THERAGRAN–M® TABLETS
(High Potency Vitamin Supplement with Minerals)

Each tablet contains:

			Percent US RDA*
Vitamins			
Vitamin A	(3 mg)	10,000 IU	200
Vitamin D	(10 mcg)	400 IU	100
Vitamin E	(15 mg)	15 IU	50
Vitamin C		200 mg	333
Thiamine		10.3 mg	687
Riboflavin		10 mg	588
Niacin		100 mg	500
Vitamin B_6		4.1 mg	205
Vitamin B_{12}		5 mcg	83
Pantothenic Acid		18.4 mg	184
Minerals			
Iodine		150 mcg	100
Iron		12 mg	67
Magnesium		65 mg	16
Copper		2 mg	100
Zinc		1.5 mg	10
Manganese		1 mg	**

*US Recommended Daily Allowance
**US RDA not established

Usage: For 12 year olds and older —1 tablet daily.

How Supplied: Bottles of 1000; Handy Packs of 30, 60, 100, and 180; and Unimatic® cartons of 100.

Storage: Store at room temperture; avoid excessive heat.

[*Shown in Product Identification Section*]

THERAGRAN–Z™ TABLETS
(High Potency Vitamin-Mineral Supplement with Zinc)

Each tablet contains:

			Percent US RDA*
Vitamins			
Vitamin A	(3 mg)	10,000 IU	200
Vitamin D	(10 mcg)	400 IU	100
Vitamin E	(15 mg)	15 IU	50
Vitamin C		200 mg	333
Thiamine		10.3 mg	687
Riboflavin		10 mg	588
Niacin		100 mg	500
Vitamin B_6		4.1 mg	205
Vitamin B_{12}		5 mcg	83
Pantothenic Acid		18.4 mg	184
Minerals			
Iodine		150 mcg	100
Iron		12 mg	67
Copper		2 mg	100
Zinc		22.5 mg	150
Manganese		1 mg	**

*US Recommended Daily Allowance
**US RDA not established

Usage: For 12 year olds and older — 1 tablet daily.

How Supplied: Bottles of 30, 60, and 100.

Storage: Store at room temperature; avoid excessive heat.

TRIMOX® '250' CAPSULES ℞
TRIMOX® '500' CAPSULES ℞
(Amoxicillin Capsules)
TRIMOX® '125' FOR ORAL SUSPENSION ℞
TRIMOX® '250' FOR ORAL SUSPENSION ℞
(Amoxicillin for Oral Suspension)

Description: Trimox (Amoxicillin) is a semisynthetic antibiotic, an analog of ampicillin, with a broad spectrum of bactericidal activity against many Gram-positive and Gram-negative microorganisms. Chemically it is D-(-)-alpha-amino-p-hydroxybenzyl penicillin trihydrate.

Clinical Pharmacology: Amoxicillin is stable in the presence of gastric acid and may be given without regard to meals. It is rapidly absorbed after oral administration. It diffuses readily into most body tissues and fluids, with the exception of brain and spinal fluid, except when meninges are inflamed. The half-life of amoxicillin is 61.3 minutes. Most of the amoxicillin is excreted unchanged in the urine; its excretion can be delayed by concurrent administration of probenecid. Amoxicillin is not highly protein-bound. In blood serum, amoxicillin is approximately 20 percent protein-bound as compared to 60 percent for penicillin G.

Orally administered doses of 250 mg. and 500 mg. amoxicillin capsules result in average peak blood levels one to two hours after administration in the range of 3.5 mcg./ml. to 5.0 mcg./ml. and 5.5 mcg./ml. to 7.5 mcg./ml. respectively.

Orally administered doses of amoxicillin suspension 125 mg./5 ml. and 250 mg./5 ml. result in average peak blood levels one to two hours after administration in the range of 1.5 mcg./ml. to 3.0 mcg./ml. and 3.5 mcg./ml. to 5.0 mcg./ml. respectively.

Detectable serum levels are observed up to 8 hours after an orally administered dose of amoxicillin. Following a 1 g. dose and utilizing a special skin window technique to determine levels of the antibiotic, it was noted that therapeutic levels were found in the interstitial fluid. Approximately 60 percent of an orally administered dose of amoxicillin is excreted in the urine within six to eight hours.

Microbiology: Trimox (Amoxicillin) is similar to ampicillin in its bactericidal action against susceptible organisms during the stage of active multiplication. It acts through the inhibition of biosynthesis of cell wall mucopeptides. *In vitro* studies have demonstrated the susceptibility of most strains of the following Gram-positive bacteria: alpha- and beta-hemolytic streptococci, *Streptococcus pneumoniae* (formerly *Diplococcus pneumoniae*), nonpenicillinase-producing staphylococci, and *Streptococcus faecalis.* It is active *in vitro* against many strains of *Hemophilus influenzae, Neisseria gonorrhoeae, Escherichia coli* and *Proteus mirabilis.* Because it does not resist destruction by penicillinase, it is *not* effective against penicillinase-producing bacteria, particularly resistant staphylococci. All strains of Pseudomonas and most strains of Klebsiella and Enterobacter are resistant.

Disc Susceptibility Tests: Quantitative methods that require measurement of the diameters of zones of inhibition of microbial growth give the most precise estimates of antibiotic susceptibility. One recommended procedure (21 CFR Sec. 460.1) uses discs for testing susceptibility

Continued on next page

Squibb—Cont.

to ampicillin-class antibiotics. Interpretations correlate diameters of the disc test with MIC values for amoxicillin. With this procedure, a report from the laboratory of "susceptible" indicates that the infecting organism is likely to respond to therapy. A report of "resistant" indicates that the infecting organism is not likely to respond to therapy. A report of "intermediate susceptibility" suggests that the organism would be susceptible if high dosage is used, or if the infection is confined to tissues and fluids (e.g., urine) in which high antibiotic levels are attained.

Indications: Trimox (Amoxicillin) is indicated in the treatment of infections due to susceptible strains of the following:

Gram-negative organisms — *H. influenzae, E. coli, P. mirabilis* and *N. gonorrhoeae.*

Gram-positive organisms — Streptococci (including *Streptococcus faecalis*), *S. pneumoniae* and nonpenicillinase-producing staphylococci.

Therapy may be instituted prior to obtaining results from bacteriological and susceptibility studies to determine the causative organisms and their susceptibility to amoxicillin.

Indicated surgical procedures should be performed.

Contraindications: The use of this drug is contraindicated in individuals with a history of an allergic reaction to any of the penicillins.

Warnings: Serious and occasionally fatal hypersensitivity (anaphylactoid) reactions have been reported in patients on penicillin therapy. Although anaphylaxis is more frequent following parenteral therapy, it has occurred in patients on oral penicillins. These reactions are more likely to occur in individuals with a history of sensitivity to multiple allergens. There have been reports of individuals with a history of penicillin hypersensitivity who have experienced severe reactions when treated with a cephalosporin. Before therapy with any penicillin, careful inquiry should be made concerning previous hypersensitivity reactions to penicillins, cephalosporins, or other allergens. If an allergic reaction occurs, appropriate therapy should be instituted and discontinuance of amoxicillin therapy considered. **Serious anaphylactoid reactions require immediate emergency treatment with epinephrine. Oxygen, intravenous steroids, and airway management, including intubation, should also be administered as indicated.**

Precautions: As with any potent drug, periodic assessment of renal, hepatic and hematopoietic function should be made during prolonged therapy.

The possibility of superinfections with mycotic or bacterial pathogens should be kept in mind during therapy. If superinfections occur (usually involving Enterobacter, Pseudomonas or Candida), amoxicillin should be discontinued and/or appropriate therapy instituted.

Usage in Pregnancy: Safety for use in pregnancy has not been established.

Adverse Reactions: As with other penicillins, it may be expected that untoward reactions will be essentially limited to sensitivity phenomena. They are more likely to occur in individuals who have previously demonstrated hypersensitivity to penicillins and in those with a history of allergy, asthma, hay fever or urticaria. The following adverse reactions have been reported as associated with the use of the penicillins:

Gastrointestinal: Glossitis, stomatitis, black "hairy" tongue, nausea, vomiting and diarrhea.

Hypersensitivity Reactions: Erythematous maculopapular rashes, urticaria, and a few cases of exfoliative dermatitis and erythema multiforme have been reported. Anaphylaxis is the most serious reaction experienced and has usually been associated with parenteral dosage forms (See WARNINGS).

NOTE: Urticaria, other skin rashes and serum sickness-like reactions may be controlled with antihistamines and, if necessary, systemic corticosteroids. Whenever such reactions occur, amoxicillin should be discontinued unless, in the opinion of the physician, the condition being treated is life-threatening and amenable only to amoxicillin therapy.

Liver: A moderate rise in serum glutamic oxaloacetic transaminase (SGOT) has been noted, but the significance of this finding is unknown.

Hemic and Lymphatic Systems: Anemia, thrombocytopenia, thrombocytopenic purpura, eosinophilia, leukopenia and agranulocytosis have been reported during therapy with the penicillins. These reactions are usually reversible on discontinuation of therapy and are believed to be hypersensitivity phenomena.

Dosage and Administration: **Infections of the ear, nose and throat** due to streptococci, pneumococci, nonpenicillinase-producing staphylococci and *H. influenzae;* **Infections of the genitourinary tract** due to *E. coli, P. mirabilis* and *S. faecalis;* **Infections of the skin and soft tissues** due to streptococci, susceptible staphylococci and *E. coli:*

USUAL DOSAGE:

Adults: 250 mg. every 8 hours

Children: 20 mg./kg./day in divided doses every 8 hours

Children weighing 20 kg. or more should be dosed according to the adult recommendations.

In severe infections or those caused by less susceptible organisms:

500 mg. every 8 hours for adults and 40 mg./kg./day in divided doses every 8 hours for children may be needed.

Infections of the lower respiratory tract due to streptococci, pneumococci, nonpenicillinase-producing staphylococci and *H. influenzae:*

USUAL DOSAGE:

Adults: 500 mg. every 8 hours

Children: 40 mg./kg./day in divided doses every 8 hours

Children weighing 20 kg. or more should be dosed according to the adult recommendations.

Gonorrhea, acute uncomplicated ano-genital and urethral infections due to *N. gonorrhoeae* (males and females):

3 grams as a single oral dose

Cases of gonorrhea with a suspected lesion of syphilis should have darkfield examinations before receiving amoxicillin, and monthly serological tests for a minimum of four months.

General: Larger doses may be required for stubborn or severe infections.

The children's dosage is intended for individuals whose weight will not cause a dosage to be calculated greater than that recommended for adults.

It should be recognized that in the treatment of chronic urinary tract infections frequent bacteriological and clinical appraisals are necessary. Smaller doses than those recommended above should not be used. Even higher doses may be needed at times. In stubborn infections, therapy may be required for several weeks. It may be necessary to continue clinical and/or bacteriological follow-up for several months after cessation of therapy. Except for gonorrhea, treatment should be continued for a minimum of 48 to 72 hours beyond the time that the patient becomes asymptomatic or evidence of bacterial eradication has been obtained. It is recommended that there be at least 10 days' treatment for any infection caused by hemolytic streptococci to prevent the occurrence of acute rheumatic fever or glomerulonephritis.

Preparation and Storage of Oral Suspensions: Prepare the suspension at the time of dispensing. Add the total amount of water as directed on the labeling of the package being dispensed. **Shake well before using.** Discard any unused suspension after 7 days if stored at room temperature, or after 14 days if stored under refrigeration.

How Supplied: Trimox (Amoxicillin) is available for oral administration as *Trimox '250' Capsules and *Trimox '500' Capsules (Amoxicillin Capsules) which provide amoxicillin trihydrate equivalent to 250 mg. and 500 mg. amoxicillin, respectively. The 250 mg. capsules are available in bottles of 100 and 500 and in Unimatic® cartons of 100. The 500 mg. capsules are available in bottles of 50 and 500 and in Unimatic cartons of 100. Trimox is also available as Trimox '125' for Oral Suspension and Trimox '250' for Oral Suspension (Amoxicillin for Oral Suspension) which provide, after preparation, pleasantly flavored suspensions containing amoxicillin trihydrate equivalent to 125 mg. and 250 mg. amoxicillin, respectively, per 5 ml. teaspoonful. Available in bottles of 80, 100, and 150 ml. and Unimatic® cartons of 4 × 25 single-dose bottles, 5 ml. per bottle.

Storage: Store Trimox Capsules (Amoxicillin Capsules) and Trimox for Oral Suspension (Amoxicillin for Oral Suspension) (dry form) at room temperature.

*[*Shown in Product Identification Section*]

VALADOL®

(Acetaminophen)

Tablets and Liquid

Valadol is a non-salicylate antipyretic and analgesic which is available in tablet and liquid forms. Valadol contains no aspirin; therefore, it can be used by many persons who are unable to take aspirin because of aspirin-induced stomach upset.

Valadol tablets are intended for the temporary relief of minor muscular aches and pains, menstrual pains, and simple headaches. Valadol tablets reduce fever and the minor discomfort due to colds and flu. Valadol tablets are also recommended for temporary relief of minor aches and pains of arthritis and rheumatism. Valadol liquid is a pleasant-tasting liquid intended for use in children. Valadol liquid is intended for the temporary relief of minor muscular aches and pains, and minor discomfort due to teething, immunization, tonsillectomy, colds and flu. Valadol liquid is also intended for reduction of fever due to colds and flu.

Dosage:

Valadol tablets: Adults—1 to 2 tablets 3 or 4 times a day. Children 6 to 12 years of age—½ to 1 tablet 3 or 4 times a day. (Dosage for children under 6 years of age should be as directed by physician.)

Valadol liquid: Children 6 to 12 years of age—2 teaspoonfuls 3 or 4 times a day. Children 3 to 6 years of age—1 teaspoonful 3 or 4 times a day. (Dosage for children under 3 years of age should be as directed by physician.)

Note—The following appears on Valadol Tablets label: "Consult a physician for use by children under 6 or for use longer than 10 days. Caution: If pain persists for more than 10 days, or redness is present, or in conditions affecting children under 12 years of age, consult a physician immediately."

The following appears on Valadol Liquid labels: "Consult a physician for use by children under 3 or for use longer than 10 days."

The following appears on all Valadol products labels. "Warning: Keep this and all medicines out of the reach of children. In case of accidental overdosage, contact a physician immediately."

How Supplied: *Valadol Tablets, 325 mg. (5 gr.) acetaminophen per tablet, bottles of 100 and 500. Valadol Liquid, 120 mg. (2 gr.) acetaminophen per 5 ml. teaspoonful (alcohol 9%), bottles of 4 fl. oz.

Storage: Store Valadol tablets at room temperature; avoid excessive heat. Store Valadol liquid at room temperature; avoid freezing.

*[*Shown in Product Identification Section*]

VEETIDS® '250' TABLETS ℞
VEETIDS® '500' TABLETS ℞
(Penicillin V Potassium Tablets USP)
VEETIDS® '125' FOR ORAL SOLUTION ℞
VEETIDS® '250' FOR ORAL SOLUTION ℞
(Penicillin V Potassium for Oral Solution USP)

Description: Veetids (Penicillin V Potassium) is the potassium salt of semisynthetically-produced penicillin V. Veetids '250' Tablets and Veetids '125' for Oral Solution contain FD&C Yellow No. 5 (tartrazine).

Clinical Pharmacology: Penicillin V is bactericidal against penicillin-susceptible microorganisms during the stage of active multiplication. It acts by inhibiting biosynthesis of cell-wall mucopeptide. It is not active against the penicillinase-producing bacteria, which include many strains of staphylococci. Penicillin V is highly active *in vitro* against staphylococci (except penicillinase-producing strains), streptococci (groups A, C, G, H, L, and M) and pneumococci. Other organisms susceptible *in vitro* to penicillin V are *Corynebacterium diphtheriae, Bacillus anthracis,* Clostridia, *Actinomyces bovis, Streptobacillus moniliformis, Listeria monocytogenes,* Leptospira and *Neisseria gonorrhoeae; Treponema pallidum* is extremely susceptible.

Penicillin V is more resistant to inactivation by gastric acid than penicillin G; however, it has the same bacterial spectrum as penicillin G. It may be given with meals; however, blood levels are slightly higher when the drug is given on an empty stomach. Average blood levels are two to five times higher than the levels following the same dose of oral penicillin G and also show much less individual variation.

Once absorbed, penicillin V is about 75 percent bound to serum protein. Highest levels are found in the kidneys, with lesser amounts in the liver, skin, and intestines. Penicillin V penetrates into all other tissues to a lesser degree with a very small level found in the cerebrospinal fluid. The drug is excreted rapidly by tubular excretion in patients with normal kidney function. In neonates and young infants, and in individuals with impaired kidney function, excretion is considerably delayed.

Indications and Usage: Veetids (Penicillin V Potassium) are indicated in the treatment of mild to moderately severe infections due to penicillin-susceptible microorganisms. Therapy should be guided by bacteriological studies, including susceptibility tests, and by clinical response. Note: severe pneumonia, empyema, bacteremia, pericarditis, meningitis, and septic arthritis should not be treated with penicillin V during the acute stage.

Indicated surgical procedures should be performed.

The following infections will usually respond to adequate oral dosage:

Streptococcal infections Group A without bacteremia—Mild to moderate infections of the upper respiratory tract (including otitis media), scarlet fever, and mild erysipelas. Note: streptococci in groups A, C, G, H, L, and M are very susceptible to penicillin. Other groups including group D (enterococcus) are resistant.

Pneumococcal infections—Mild to moderately severe infections of the respiratory tract, including otitis media.

Staphylococcal infections — penicillin-susceptible—Mild infections of the skin and skin structures. Note: reports indicate an increasing number of strains of staphylococci resistant to penicillin, emphasizing the need for culture and susceptibility studies in treating suspected staphylococcal infections.

Vincent's gingivitis and pharyngitis (fusospirochetosis)—Mild to moderately severe infections of the oropharynx usually respond to oral penicillin. Note: necessary dental care should be accomplished in infections involving gum tissue.

Medical conditions in which oral penicillin therapy is indicated as prophylaxis: *For the prevention of recurrence following rheumatic fever and/or chorea.* Prophylaxis with oral penicillin on a continuing basis is effective in preventing recurrence of these conditions. *To prevent bacterial endocarditis* in patients with congenital and/or rheumatic heart lesions who are to undergo dental procedures or minor upper respiratory tract surgery or instrumentation. Prophylaxis should be instituted the day of the procedure and for two or more days afterwards. Patients who have a past history of rheumatic fever and are receiving continuous prophylaxis may harbor increased numbers of penicillin-resistant organisms; use of another prophylactic anti-infective agent should be considered. If penicillin is to be used in these patients at surgery, the regular rheumatic fever program should be interrupted one week prior to the contemplated surgery. At the time of surgery, penicillin may be reinstituted as a prophylactic measure against the hazards of surgically-induced bacteremia. Note: oral penicillin should not be used as adjunctive prophylaxis for genitourinary instrumentation or surgery, lower intestinal tract surgery, sigmoidoscopy and childbirth.

Contraindications: Contraindicated in patients with a history of hypersensitivity to any penicillin.

Warnings: Serious and occasional fatal hypersensitivity (anaphylactoid) reactions have been reported in patients on penicillin therapy. Although anaphylaxis is more frequent following parenteral administration, it has occurred in patients on oral penicillins. These reactions are more apt to occur in individuals with a history of sensitivity to multiple allergens.

There have been well-documented reports of individuals with a history of penicillin hypersensitivity who have experienced severe hypersensitivity reactions when treated with cephalosporins. Before therapy with a penicillin, careful inquiry should be made concerning previous hypersensitivity reactions to penicillins, cephalosporins, and other allergens. If an allergic reaction occurs, the drug should be discontinued and the patient treated with the usual agents, e.g., pressor amines, antihistamines, and corticosteroids. Serious anaphylactoid reactions are not controlled by antihistamines alone, and require such emergency measures as the immediate use of epinephrine, aminophylline, oxygen, and intravenous corticosteroids.

Concomitant use of oral neomycin therapy should be avoided since malabsorption of penicillin V potassium has been reported.

Precautions: Penicillin should be used with caution in individuals with histories of significant allergies and/or asthma.

The oral route of administration should not be relied upon in patients with severe illness, or with nausea, vomiting, gastric dilatation, cardiospasm or intestinal hypermotility.

Occasional patients will not absorb therapeutic amounts of orally administered penicillin.

In streptococcal infections, therapy must be sufficient to eliminate the organism (10 days minimum); otherwise the sequelae of streptococcal disease may occur. Cultures should be taken following completion of treatment to determine whether streptococci have been eradicated.

Prolonged use of antibiotics may promote the overgrowth of nonsusceptible organisms, including fungi. Should superinfection occur, appropriate measures should be taken.

In prolonged therapy with penicillin, and particularly with high dosage schedules, periodic evaluation of the renal and hematopoietic systems is recommended.

Veetids '250' Tablets and Veetids '125' for Oral Solution contain FD&C Yellow No. 5 (tartrazine) which may cause allergic-type reactions (including bronchial asthma) in certain susceptible individuals. Although the overall incidence of FD&C Yellow No. 5 (tartrazine) sensitivity in the general population is low, it is frequently seen in patients who also have aspirin hypersensitivity.

Adverse Reactions: Although the incidence of reactions to oral penicillins has been reported with much less frequency than following parenteral therapy, it should be remembered that all degrees of hypersensitivity, including fatal anaphylaxis, have been reported with oral penicillin.

The most common reactions to oral penicillin are nausea, vomiting, epigastric distress, diarrhea, and black hairy tongue. The hypersensitivity reactions reported are skin rashes ranging from maculopapular to exfoliative dermatitis; urticaria; serum sickness-like reactions including chills, fever, edema, arthralgia, and prostration; laryngeal edema; and anaphylaxis. Fever and eosinophilia may frequently be the only reactions observed. Hemolytic anemia, leukopenia, thrombocytopenia, neuropathy, and nephropathy are infrequent reactions usually associated with high doses of parenteral penicillin. Urticaria, other skin rashes, and serum sickness-like reactions may be controlled by antihistamines and, if necessary, corticosteroids. Whenever such reactions occur, penicillin should be discontinued unless, in the opinion of the physician, the condition being treated is life-threatening and amenable only to penicillin therapy. Serious anaphylactoid reactions require emergency measures (see WARNINGS).

An occasional patient may complain of sore mouth or tongue, as with any oral penicillin preparation.

Dosage and Administration: The dosage of Veetids (Penicillin V Potassium) should be determined according to the susceptibility of the causative microorganism and the severity of the infection, and adjusted to the clinical response of the patient.

For Therapeutic Use

Dosage for *children under 12 years* of age is calculated on the basis of body weight. For *infants and small children* the suggested dose is 15 to 56 mg. (25,000 to 90,000 u.) per kg./day in three to six divided doses.

The usual dosage recommendations for *adults and children 12 years and over* are as follows:

Streptococcal infections—mild to moderately severe—of the upper respiratory tract and including otitis media, scarlet fever and mild erysipelas: 125 mg. (200,000 u.) t.i.d. or q.i.d. for 10 days for mild infections; 250 mg. (400,000 u.) t.i.d. for 10 days for moderately severe infections; for mild to moderately severe streptococcal pharyngitis: 500 mg. (800,000 u.) b.i.d. may be used as an alternative regimen.

Pneumococcal infections—mild to moderately severe—of the respiratory tract, including otitis media: 250 to 500 mg. (400,000 to 800,000 u.) q.i.d. until the patient has been afebrile for at least two days.

Staphylococcal infections—mild infections of skin and skin structures (culture and susceptibility tests should be performed): 250 mg. (400,000 u.) t.i.d. or q.i.d., or 500 mg. (800,000 u.) t.i.d.

Vincent's gingivitis and pharyngitis (fusospirochetosis)—mild to moderately severe infections of the oropharynx: 250 mg. (400,000 u.) t.i.d. or q.i.d., or 500 mg. t.i.d.

Continued on next page

Squibb—Cont.

For Prophylactic Use

For the prevention of recurrence following rheumatic fever and/or chorea: *Adults*—125 mg. (200,000 u.) b.i.d. on a continuing basis. Dosage for *children under 12 years* of age is calculated on the basis of body weight. For *infants and small children* the suggested dose is 15 to 56 mg. (25,000 to 90,000 u.) per kg./day in three to six divided doses.

To prevent bacterial endocarditis in patients with rheumatic or congenital heart lesions who are to undergo dental or upper respiratory tract surgery or instrumentation: *Adults and children more than 60 lbs.*—2 g. (3,200,000 u.) 30 minutes to one hour before the procedure and then 500 mg. (800,000 u.) every six hours for eight doses. *Children less than 60 lbs.*—1 g. (1,600,000 u.) 30 minutes to one hour before the procedure and then 250 mg. (400,000 u.) every six hours for eight doses.

How Supplied: *Veetids '250' Tablets and *Veetids '500' Tablets (Penicillin V Potassium Tablets USP) are available for oral administration as FILMLOK® tablets providing penicillin V potassium equivalent to 250 mg. (400,000 units) and 500 mg. (800,000 units), respectively, of penicillin V. (Filmlok is a Squibb trademark for veneer-coated tablets.) Bottles of 100 and Unimatic® cartons of 100.

Veetids '125' for Oral Solution and Veetids '250' for Oral Solution (Penicillin V Potassium for Oral Solution USP) are available as powders that, when constituted as directed, provide pleasantly flavored solutions containing penicillin V potassium equivalent to 125 mg. (200,000 units) and 250 mg. (400,000 units), respectively, of penicillin V per 5 ml. teaspoonful. Bottles of 100 ml. and 200 ml.

Storage: Store Veetids Tablets at room temperature; avoid excessive heat. Store Veetids for Oral Solution in dry form at room temperature; after preparation of the solution, store in refrigerator and discard unused portion after 14 days.

*[*Shown in Product Identification Section*]

VELOSEF® '250' CAPSULES ℞
VELOSEF® '500' CAPSULES ℞
(Cephradine Capsules)
VELOSEF® TABLETS 1 GRAM ℞
(Cephradine Tablets)
VELOSEF® '125' FOR ORAL SUSPENSION ℞
VELOSEF® '250' FOR ORAL SUSPENSION ℞
(Cephradine for Oral Suspension)

Description: Velosef is a semisynthetic cephalosporin antibiotic chemically designated as 7-[D-2-amino-2-(1,4-cyclohexadien-1-yl) acetamido] -3-methyl-8-oxo-5-thia-l-azabicyclo [4.2.0] oct-2-ene-2-carboxylic acid.

Actions: *Clinical Pharmacology*—Velosef (Cephradine, Squibb) is acid stable. It is rapidly absorbed after oral administration in the fasting state. Following single doses of 250 mg., 500 mg., and 1 g. in normal adult volunteers, average peak serum concentrations within one hour were approximately 9 mcg./ml., 16.5 mcg./ml., and 24.2 mcg./ml., respectively. The presence of food in the gastrointestinal tract delays absorption but does not affect the total amount of cephradine absorbed. Over 90 percent of the drug is excreted unchanged in the urine within six hours. Peak urine concentrations are approximately 1600 mcg./ml., 3200 mcg./ml., and 4000 mcg./ml. following single doses of 250 mg., 500 mg., and 1 g., respectively.

Microbiology—*In vitro* tests demonstrate that the cephalosporins are bactericidal because of their inhibition of cell-wall synthesis. Cephradine is active against the following organisms *in vitro:*

Group A beta-hemolytic streptococci
Staphylococci, including coagulase-positive, coagulase-negative, and penicillinase-producing strains
Streptococcus pneumoniae (formerly *Diplococcus pneumoniae*)
Escherichia coli
Proteus mirabilis
Klebsiella species
Hemophilus influenzae

Cephradine is not active against most strains of *Enterobacter* species, *P. morganii*, and *P. vulgaris*. It has no activity against *Pseudomonas* or *Herellea* species. When tested by *in vitro* methods, staphylococci exhibit cross-resistance between cephradine and methicillin-type antibiotics.

Note—Most strains of enterococci (*Streptococcus faecalis*) are resistant to cephradine.

Disc Susceptibility Tests—Quantitative methods that require measurement of zone diameters give the most precise estimates of antibiotic susceptibility. One recommended procedure (21 CFR Sec. 460.1) uses cephalosporin class discs for testing susceptibility; interpretations correlate zone diameters of this disc test with MIC values for cephradine. With this procedure, a report from the laboratory of "resistant" indicates that the infecting organism is not likely to respond to therapy. A report of "intermediate susceptibility" suggests that the organism would be susceptible if the infection is confined to the urinary tract, as high antibiotic levels can be obtained in the urine, or if high dosage is used in other types of infection.

Indications: Velosef Capsules (Cephradine Capsules), Velosef Tablets (Cephradine Tablets), and Velosef for Oral Suspension (Cephradine for Oral Suspension) are indicated in the treatment of the following infections when caused by susceptible strains of the designated microorganisms:

RESPIRATORY TRACT INFECTIONS (e.g., tonsillitis, pharyngitis, and lobar pneumonia) caused by group A beta-hemolytic streptococci and *S. pneumoniae* (formerly *D. pneumoniae*).

[Penicillin is the usual drug of choice in the treatment and prevention of streptococcal infections, including the prophylaxis of rheumatic fever. Velosef is generally effective in the eradication of streptococci from the nasopharynx; substantial data establishing the efficacy of Velosef (Cephradine, Squibb) in the subsequent prevention of rheumatic fever are not available at present.]

OTITIS MEDIA caused by group A beta-hemolytic streptococci, *S. pneumoniae* (formerly *D. pneumoniae*), *H. influenzae*, and staphylococci.

SKIN AND SKIN STRUCTURES INFECTIONS caused by staphylococci (penicillin-susceptible and penicillin-resistant) and beta-hemolytic streptococci.

URINARY TRACT INFECTIONS, including prostatitis, caused by *E. coli*, *P. mirabilis*, *Klebsiella* species, and enterococci (*S. faecalis*). The high concentrations of cephradine achievable in the urinary tract will be effective against many strains of enterococci for which disc susceptibility studies indicate relative resistance. It is to be noted that among beta-lactam antibiotics, ampicillin is the drug of choice for enterococcal urinary tract (*Streptococcus faecalis*) infection.

Note—Culture and susceptibility tests should be initiated prior to and during therapy. Renal function studies should be performed when indicated.

Contraindications: Cephradine is contraindicated in patients with known hypersensitivity to the cephalosporin group of antibiotics.

Warnings: *In penicillin-sensitive patients, cephalosporin derivatives should be used with great caution. There is clinical and laboratory evidence of partial cross-allergenicity of the penicillins and the cephalosporins, and there are instances of patients who have had reactions to both drug classes (including anaphylaxis after parenteral use).*

Any patient who has demonstrated some form of allergy, particularly to drugs, should receive antibiotics, including Velosef (Cephradine, Squibb), cautiously and then only when absolutely necessary.

Usage in Pregnancy and Lactation: Although no teratogenic or anti-fertility effects were seen in reproduction studies in mice and rats receiving up to four times the maximum human dose, the safety of this drug for use in human pregnancy has not been established. The benefits of the drug in pregnant women should be weighed against a possible risk to the fetus. Cephradine is secreted in breast milk during lactation.

Precautions: Patients should be followed carefully so that any side effects or unusual manifestations of drug idiosyncrasy may be detected. If a hypersensitivity reaction occurs, the drug should be discontinued and the patient treated with the usual agents, e.g., pressor amines, antihistamines, or corticosteroids.

Administer cephradine with caution in the presence of markedly impaired renal function. In patients with known or suspected renal impairment, careful clinical observation and appropriate laboratory studies should be made prior to and during therapy as cephradine accumulates in the serum and tissues. See DOSAGE AND ADMINISTRATION section for information on treatment of patients with impaired renal function.

Prolonged use of antibiotics may promote the overgrowth of nonsusceptible organisms. Should superinfection occur during therapy, appropriate measures should be taken.

After treatment with cephradine, a false positive reaction for glucose in the urine may occur with Benedict's solution, Fehling's solution, or with Clinitest® tablets, but not with enzyme-based tests such as Clinistix® and Tes-Tape®.

A false positive direct Coombs test has been reported after treatment with other cephalosporins; therefore, it should be recognized that a positive Coombs test may be due to the drug.

Indicated surgical procedures should be performed in conjunction with antibiotic therapy.

Adverse Reactions: As with other cephalosporins, untoward reactions are limited essentially to gastrointestinal disturbances and, on occasion, to hypersensitivity phenomena. The latter are more likely to occur in individuals who have previously demonstrated hypersensitivity and those with a history of allergy, asthma, hay fever, or urticaria.

The following adverse reactions have been reported following the use of cephradine:

Gastrointestinal: Glossitis, nausea, vomiting, diarrhea or loose stools, abdominal pain and heartburn were reported by some patients.

Skin and Hypersensitivity Reactions: Mild urticaria or skin rash, pruritus, and joint pains were reported by very few patients.

Blood: Mild, transient eosinophilia, leukopenia, and neutropenia have been reported.

Liver: Transient mild rise of SGOT, SGPT, and total bilirubin have been observed with no evidence of hepatocellular damage.

Renal: Transitory rises in BUN have been observed in some patients treated with cephalosporins; their frequency increases in patients over 50 years old. In adults for whom serum creatinine determinations were performed, the rise in BUN was not accompanied by a rise in serum creatinine.

Other adverse reactions have included dizziness and tightness in the chest and candidal vaginitis.

Dosage and Administration: Velosef (Cephradine, Squibb) may be given without regard to meals.

Adults: For respiratory tract infections (other than lobar pneumonia) and skin and skin structures infections, the usual dose is 250 mg. every 6 hours or 500 mg. every 12 hours.

For lobar pneumonia and urinary tract infections, including prostatitis, the usual dose is 500 mg. every 6 hours or 1 g. every 12 hours. Severe or chronic infections may require larger doses.

Children: No adequate information is available on the efficacy of b.i.d. regimens in children under nine months of age. The usual dose in children over nine months of age is 25 to 50 mg./kg./day administered in equally divided doses every 6 or 12 hours. For otitis media due to *H. influenzae*, doses are from 75 to 100 mg./kg./day administered in equally divided doses every 6 or 12 hours, but should not exceed 4 g. per day. Dosage for children should not exceed dosage recommended for adults.

All patients, regardless of age and weight: Larger doses (up to 1 gram q.i.d.) may be given for severe or chronic infections.

As with antibiotic therapy in general, treatment should be continued for a minimum of 48 to 72 hours after the patient becomes asymptomatic or evidence of bacterial eradication has been obtained. In infections caused by group A beta-hemolytic streptococci, a minimum of 10 days of treatment is recommended to guard against the risk of rheumatic fever or glomerulonephritis. In the treatment of chronic urinary tract infection, frequent bacteriologic and clinical appraisal is necessary during therapy and may be necessary for several months afterwards. Persistent infections may require treatment for several weeks. Prolonged intensive therapy is recommended for prostatitis. Doses smaller than those indicated are not recommended.

Patients With Impaired Renal Function

A modified dosage schedule in patients with decreased renal function is necessary. Each patient should be considered individually; the following reduced dosage schedule is recommended as a guideline, based on the creatinine clearance (ml./min./1.73 m^2). In adults, the initial loading dose is 750 mg. of Velosef (Cephradine, Squibb) and the maintenance dose is 500 mg. at the time intervals listed below:

Creatinine Clearance	Time Interval
> 20 ml./min.	6–12 hours
15–19 ml./min.	12–24 hours
10–14 ml./min.	24–40 hours
5–9 ml./min.	40–50 hours
< 5 ml./min.	50–70 hours

Further modification of the dosage schedule may be necessary in children.

How Supplied: Velosef is available as *Velosef '250' Capsules and *Velosef '500' Capsules (Cephradine Capsules) providing 250 mg. and 500 mg. cephradine per capsule, respectively, and as *Velosef Tablets (Cephradine Tablets) providing 1 g. cephradine per tablet. The Capsules are available in bottles of 24 and 100 and Unimatic® cartons of 100. The Tablets are available in bottles of 24.

Velosef is also available as Velosef '125' for Oral Suspension and Velosef '250' for Oral Suspension (Cephradine for Oral Suspension) which, after constitution, provide 125 mg. and 250 mg. cephradine, respectively, per 5 ml. teaspoonful in a pleasant fruit-flavored suspension. Bottles of 100 ml. and 200 ml.

Storage: Velosef Capsules—Do not store above 86°F.; keep bottle tightly closed. Velosef Tablets—Do not store above 86°F.; keep bottle tightly closed. Velosef for Oral Suspension—Prior to constitution, store at room temperature; avoid excessive heat. After constitution, the suspension may be stored at room temperature or in refrigerator; when the suspension is stored at room temperature, discard unused portion after 7 days; when the suspension is stored in the refrigerator, discard unused portion after 14 days.

*[*Shown in Product Identification Section*]

VELOSEF® for INFUSION ℞
(Sterile Cephradine)
Sodium-Free

Description: Velosef (Cephradine, Squibb) is a semisynthetic cephalosporin antibiotic. Chemically, Velosef is designated as 7-[D-2-amino-2- (1, 4-cyclohexadien-1-yl) acetamido]-3-methyl-8-oxo-5-thia-1-azabicyclo [4.2.0] oct-2-ene-2-carboxylic acid.

Velosef for Infusion is sterile cephradine, a white powder for constitution and intravenous administration by drip infusion; it is available in infusion bottles containing 2 g. cephradine. At the time of manufacture, the air in the container is replaced by nitrogen.

Actions: *Clinical Pharmacology:* Pharmacokinetic studies with Velosef for Injection (Sterile Cephradine for Injection) (containing sodium carbonate) and Velosef for Infusion (Sterile Cephradine) (sodium-free) performed by drip infusion demonstrate bioequivalence for these formulations. The mean steady-state concentration of cephradine maintained in the sera of nine normal adult volunteers during infusion of either solution was approximately 3 mcg. per ml. for each mg. of cephradine infused per hour per kg. of body weight. Serum half-life, serum clearance, and apparent volume of distribution were equivalent following intravenous infusion of either preparation.

Figure 1 depicts mean serum concentrations after administration of Velosef for Infusion (Sterile Cephradine) to nine normal adult volunteers at the average rate of 380 mg. cephradine per hour (5.3 mg./kg./hr.) over a four-hour period; the mean cephradine level rises rapidly and approaches a mean steady-state concentration of 17 mcg./ml. in approximately 1.5 hours. After the infusion is discontinued, the cephradine concentration decreases exponentially, declining to 1.5 mcg./ml. at 6.5 hours.

Figure 1

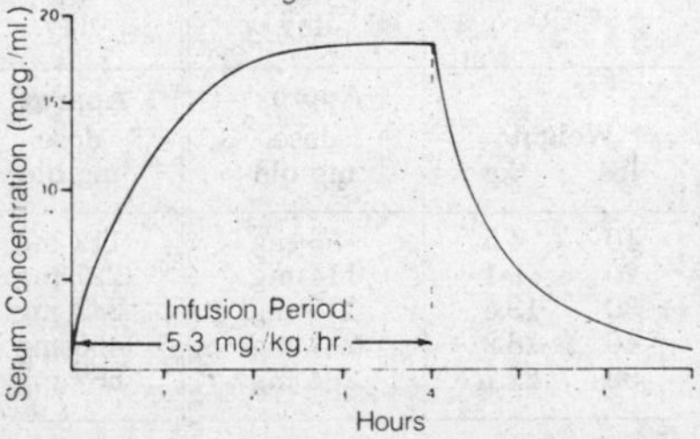

Cephradine is excreted unchanged in the urine. Between 1.5 and 4 hours after the start of the infusion depicted in Figure 1, cephradine is excreted in urine at a mean rate of 312 mg./hr.; a high concentration of cephradine in the urine exists during this period with a mean concentration of 885 mcg./ml. Studies with Velosef for Injection (Sterile Cephradine for Injection) demonstrate that probenecid slows tubular excretion of cephradine and increases serum concentration.

Assays of bone obtained at surgery have shown that cephradine penetrates bone tissue.

Microbiology: In Vitro tests demonstrate that the cephalosporins are bactericidal because of their inhibition of cell-wall synthesis. Cephradine is active against the following organisms *in vitro:* group A beta-hemolytic streptococci; staphylococci, including coagulase-positive, coagulase-negative, and penicillinase-producing strains; *Escherichia coli; Streptococcus pneumoniae* (formerly *Diplococcus pneumoniae*); *Proteus mirabilis; Klebsiella* species; and *Hemophilus influenzae.*

It is not active against most strains of *Enterobacter* species, *Proteus morganii,* and *Proteus vulgaris.* It has no activity against *Pseudomonas* or *Herellea* species. When tested by *in vitro* methods, staphylococci exhibit cross-resistance between cephradine and methicillin-type antibiotics.

NOTE—Most strains of enterococci (*Streptococcus faecalis*) are resistant to cephradine.

Disc Susceptibility Tests: Quantitative methods that require measurement of zone diameters give the most precise estimates of antibiotic susceptibility. One recommended procedure (21 CFR Sec. 460.1) uses cephalosporin class discs for testing susceptibility; interpretations correlate zone diameters of this disc test with MIC values for cephradine. With this procedure, a report from the laboratory of "resistant" indicates that the infecting organism is not likely to respond to therapy. A report of "intermediate susceptibility" suggests that the organism would be susceptible if the infection is confined to the urinary tract, as high antibiotic levels can be obtained in the urine, or if high dosage is used in other types of infection.

Indications: Velosef for Infusion (Sterile Cephradine) is indicated in the treatment of the following serious infections when caused by susceptible strains of the designated microorganisms:

RESPIRATORY TRACT INFECTIONS due to *Streptococcus pneumoniae* (formerly *Diplococcus pneumoniae*), *Klebsiella* species, *H. influenzae, Staphylococcus aureus* (penicillin-susceptible and penicillin-resistant), and group A beta-hemolytic streptococci.

[Penicillin is the usual drug of choice in the treatment and prevention of streptococcal infections, including the prophylaxis of rheumatic fever. Velosef (Cephradine, Squibb) is generally effective in the eradication of streptococci from the nasopharynx; substantial data establishing the efficacy of Velosef (Cephradine, Squibb) in the subsequent prevention of rheumatic fever are not available at present.]

URINARY TRACT INFECTIONS due to *E. coli, Pr. mirabilis,* and *Klebsiella* species.

SKIN AND SKIN STRUCTURES INFECTIONS due to *S. aureus* (penicillin-susceptible and penicillin-resistant) and group A beta-hemolytic streptococci.

BONE INFECTIONS due to *S. aureus* (penicillin-susceptible and penicillin-resistant).

SEPTICEMIA due to *Streptococcus pneumoniae* (formerly *Diplococcus pneumoniae*), *S. aureus* (penicillin-susceptible and penicillin-resistant), *Pr. mirabilis,* and *E. coli.*

NOTE—Culture and susceptibility tests should be initiated prior to and during therapy. Renal function studies should be performed when indicated.

Contraindications: Cephradine is contraindicated in patients with known hypersensitivity to the cephalosporin group of antibiotics.

Warnings: *In penicillin-sensitive patients, cephalosporin C derivatives should be used with great caution. There is clinical and laboratory evidence of partial cross-allergenicity of the penicillins and the cephalosporins, and there are instances of patients who have had reactions to both drug classes (including fatal anaphylaxis after parenteral use).*

Any patient who has demonstrated some form of allergy, particularly to drugs, should receive antibiotics, including cephradine, cautiously and then only when absolutely necessary. Serious anaphylactoid reactions require immediate emergency treatment with epinephrine. Oxygen, intravenous steroids, and airway management, including intubation, should also be administered as indicated.

Usage in Pregnancy and Lactation: Although no teratogenic or antifertility effects were seen in reproduction studies in mice and rats receiving up to four times the maximum human dose, the safety of this drug for use in human pregnancy has not been established. The benefits of the drug in pregnant women should be weighed against a possible risk to the fetus. Cephradine is secreted in breast milk during lactation.

Continued on next page

Squibb—Cont.

Usage in Infants: Cephradine has been effectively used in this age group, but all laboratory parameters have not been extensively studied in infants one month to one year of age; therefore, in the treatment of children in this age group, the benefits of the drug to the risk involved must be considered.
Since safety for use in premature infants and in infants under one month of age has not been established, the use of cephradine by infusion should be based on careful consideration of the benefits of the drug against the risk involved.
Precautions: Prolonged use of antibiotics may promote the overgrowth of nonsusceptible organisms. Should superinfection occur during therapy, appropriate measures should be taken.
When cephradine is administered to patients with markedly impaired renal function, lower daily dosage is required. (See DOSAGE AND ADMINISTRATION.) In patients with known or suspected renal impairment, careful clinical observation and appropriate laboratory studies should be conducted because cephradine in the usual recommended dosage will accumulate in the serum and tissues.
Increased nephrotoxicity has been reported following concomitant administration of cephalosporins and aminoglycoside antibiotics.
Patients should be followed carefully so that any side effects or unusual manifestations of drug idiosyncrasy may be detected. If a hypersensitivity reaction occurs, the drug should be discontinued and the patient treated with the usual agents, e.g., pressor amines, antihistamines, or corticosteroids.
After treatment with cephradine, a false-positive reaction for glucose in the urine may occur with Benedict's Solution, Fehling's Solution, or with Clinitest® tablets, but not with enzyme-based tests such as Clinistix®, and Tes-Tape®.
As with other cephalosporins, positive direct Coombs tests have been infrequently reported.
To reduce the risk of phlebitis from intravenous infusion, the injection site should be changed at appropriate intervals during long-term therapy.
Adverse Reactions: As with other cephalosporins, untoward reactions are limited essentially to gastrointestinal disturbances and, on occasion, to hypersensitivity phenomena. The latter are more likely to occur in individuals who have previously demonstrated hypersensitivity and those with a history of allergy, asthma, hay fever, or urticaria.
The following adverse reactions have been reported following the use of cephradine:
Gastrointestinal: Glossitis, nausea, vomiting, diarrhea or loose stools, tenesmus, and abdominal pain.
Skin and Hypersensitivity Reactions: Mild urticaria or skin rash, edema, erythema, pruritus, joint pains, and drug fever.
Blood: Mild, transient eosinophilia, leukopenia, and neutropenia.
Liver: Instances of elevated SGOT and SGPT of approximately 10 percent and 2 percent of patients, respectively, have been observed; also, a few cases of elevated total bilirubin, alkaline phosphatase and LDH have been observed. In most patients, values tended to return to normal after the end of therapy.
Renal: Mild elevations in BUN have been observed in some patients treated with cephalosporins; their frequency increases in patients over 50 years old and in children under three. In adults for whom serum creatinine determinations were performed, the rise in BUN was not accompanied by a rise in serum creatinine.
Other adverse reactions are headache, dizziness, dyspnea, paresthesia, candidal overgrowth, candidal vaginitis, isolated instances of hepatomegaly, and thrombophlebitis at the site of injection.

Dosage and Administration: Velosef for Infusion (Sterile Cephradine) may be administered by continuous or intermittent intravenous infusion. The infusion bottle is designed to be suspended from an I.V. stand and may also be used in any administration procedure where sequential administration of infusion solutions is intended.
Adults: The usual daily dosage of Velosef for Infusion is 2 to 4 g. of cephradine given in equally divided doses four times a day (e.g., 500 mg. to 1 g. q.i.d.). In bone infections the usual dosage is 1 g. q.i.d. A daily dose of 2 g. is adequate in uncomplicated pneumonia, skin and skin structures infections, and most urinary tract infections. In severe infections, the dosage may be increased.
The maximum daily dose should not exceed 8 g. per day.
Infants and Children: The usual dosage range of Velosef for Infusion is 50 to 100 mg./kg./day (approximately 23 to 45 mg./lb./day) in equally divided doses four times a day and should be determined by age, weight of the patient, and severity of the infection being treated.
All laboratory parameters have not been extensively studied in infants under one year of age; therefore, in the treatment of children in this age group, the benefits of the drug to the risk involved must be considered. In newborn infants, accumulation of other cephalosporin-class antibiotics (with resultant prolongation of drug half-life) has been reported.
The maximum daily pediatric dose should not exceed doses recommended for adults.

PEDIATRIC DOSAGE GUIDE

Weight lbs	Weight kg	50 mg/kg/day Approx. dose mg qid	100 mg/kg/day Approx. dose mg qid
10	4.5	56 mg	112 mg
20	9.1	114 mg	227 mg
30	13.6	170 mg	340 mg
40	18.2	227 mg	455 mg
50	22.7	284 mg	567 mg

As with antibiotic therapy generally: therapy should be continued for a minimum of 48 to 72 hours after the patient becomes asymptomatic or evidence of bacterial eradication has been obtained; in infections caused by group A beta-hemolytic streptococci, a minimum of 10 days of treatment is recommended to guard against the risk of rheumatic fever or glomerulonephritis; in the treatment of chronic urinary tract infection, frequent bacteriologic and clinical appraisal is necessary during therapy and may be necessary for several months afterwards; persistent infections may require treatment for several weeks; doses smaller than those indicated above should not be used.
Parenteral therapy may be followed by oral Velosef (Cephradine, Squibb) either as capsules or as an oral suspension.
Velosef for Infusion (Sterile Cephradine) should be administered only by intravenous infusion.
Renal Impairment Dosage: A modified dosage schedule in patients with decreased renal function is necessary. Each patient should be considered individually; the following reduced dosage schedule is recommended as a guideline, based on the creatinine clearance (ml./min./1.73m^2).
In adults, the initial loading dose is 750 mg. of Velosef and the maintenance dose is 500 mg. at the time intervals listed below:

Creatinine Clearance	Time Interval
> 20 ml./min.	6 - 12 hours
15 - 19 ml./min.	12 - 24 hours
10 - 14 ml./min.	24 - 40 hours
5 - 9 ml./min.	40 - 50 hours
< 5 ml./min.	50 - 70 hours

Further modification of the dosage schedule may be necessary in children.
Constitution and Storage: The choice of I.V. solution and the volume to be employed are dictated by fluid and electrolyte management. Suitable I.V. solutions are: 5% Dextrose Injection USP, Lactated Ringer's Injection USP, 10% Dextrose Injection USP, Dextrose and Sodium Chloride Injection USP (5% : 0.9% or 5% : 0.45%), 10% Invert Sugar in Water for Injection, Normosol®-R, Ionosol® B with Dextrose 5%, Sodium Chloride Injection USP, or Sodium Lactate Injection USP (M/6 sodium lactate). **Do not use Sterile Water for Injection.** Aseptically add 150 ml. or 200 ml. of the I.V. solution to the infusion bottle for approximate concentrations of 13.3 mg./ml. or 10 mg./ml., respectively. *Note: Complete solution of the preparation requires a minimum of 150 ml. of diluent. Shake well until dissolved.*
Infusion solutions prepared as directed above retain potency for 48 hours at room temperature, or one week under refrigeration (5° C.). Unused solutions must be discarded after these time periods. Constituted solutions may vary in color from nearly colorless to light yellow. Store Velosef for Infusion (Sterile Cephradine) at room temperature in dry form; avoid excessive heat. Protect the dry form and constituted solutions from concentrated light or direct sunlight.
Extemporaneous mixtures with other antibiotics or drugs are not recommended.
How Supplied: Velosef for Infusion (Sterile Cephradine) is available in intravenous infusion bottles (200 ml. size) containing 2 g. cephradine.

VELOSEF® for INJECTION ℞

(Sterile Cephradine for Injection)

Description: Velosef is a semisynthetic cephalosporin antibiotic. Chemically, Velosef is designated as 7-[D-2-amino-2-(1,4-cyclohexadien-1-yl) acetamido]-3-methyl-8-oxo-5- thia-1-azabicyclo- [4.2.0] oct-2-ene-2-carboxylic acid. Velosef for Injection is a sterile powder for reconstitution available in vials containing 250 mg., 500 mg., or 1 g. cephradine; and bottles containing 2 g. or 4 g. cephradine; the preparations also contain 79 mg., 157 mg., 315 mg., 630 mg., or 1.26 g. anhydrous sodium carbonate, respectively. The sodium content is approximately 136 mg. (6 mEq.) per gram of cephradine. At the time of manufacture, the air in the container is replaced by nitrogen.
Actions: *Clinical Pharmacology*—Table I indicates the blood levels following intramuscular administration of a 500 mg. or 1 g. dose to normal adults.
[See table on next page].
Figure I depicts representative mean serum concentrations after administration of a 500 mg. and 1 g. I.M. dose, and a 500 mg. oral dose of cephradine. Areas beneath the curves for the 500 mg. oral and I.M. dose are equivalent.

Figure I
VELOSEF FOR INJECTION
(Sterile Cephradine for Injection)

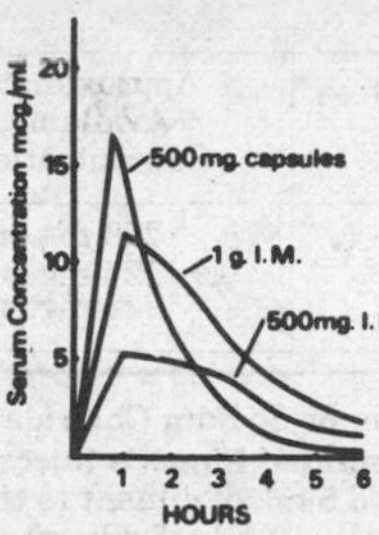

A single intravenous dose of 1 g. cephradine resulted in serum levels of approximately 86 mcg./ml. at 5 minutes, 50 mcg./ml. at 15 minutes, 26 mcg./ml. at 30 minutes, and 12 mcg./ml. at 60 minutes; these levels declined to 1 mcg./ml. at four hours.

Velosef (Cephradine, Squibb) is excreted unchanged in the urine. The kidneys excrete 57–80 percent of an intramuscular dose in the first six hours; this results in a high urine concentration, e.g., a mean urine concentration of 313 mcg./ml. within a six hour period following a 500 mg. I.M. dose. Probenecid slows tubular excretion and increases serum concentration.

Assays of bone obtained at surgery have shown that cephradine penetrates bone tissue.

Microbiology—*In vitro* tests demonstrate that the cephalosporins are bactericidal because of their inhibition of cell-wall synthesis. Cephradine is active against the following organisms *in vitro:* group A beta-hemolytic streptococci; staphylococci, including coagulase-positive, coagulase-negative, and penicillinase-producing strains; *Escherichia coli; Streptococcus pneumoniae* (formerly *Diplococcus pneumoniae); Proteus mirabilis; Klebsiella* species; and *Hemophilus influenzae.*

It is not active against most strains of *Enterobacter* species, *Proteus morganii,* and *Proteus vulgaris.* It has no activity against *Pseudomonas* or *Herellea* species. When tested by *in vitro* methods, staphylococci exhibit cross-resistance between cephradine and methicillin-type antibiotics.

NOTE—Most strains of enterococci (*Streptococcus faecalis*) are resistant to cephradine.

Disc Susceptibility Tests—Quantitative methods that require measurement of zone diameters give the most precise estimates of antibiotic susceptibility. One recommended procedure (21 CFR § 460.1) uses cephalosporin class discs for testing susceptibility; interpretations correlate zone diameters of this disc test with MIC values for cephradine. With this procedure, a report from the laboratory of "resistant" indicates that the infecting organism is not likely to respond to therapy. A report of "intermediate susceptibility" suggests that the organism would be susceptible if the infection is confined to the urinary tract, as high antibiotic levels can be obtained in the urine, or if high dosage is used in other types of infection.

Indications: Velosef (Sterile Cephradine for Injection) is indicated in the treatment of the following serious infections when caused by susceptible strains of the designated microorganisms:

RESPIRATORY TRACT INFECTIONS due to *Streptococcus pneumoniae* (formerly *Diplococcus pneumoniae*), *Klebsiella* species, *H. influenzae, Staphylococcus aureus* (penicillin-susceptible and penicillin-resistant), and group A beta-hemolytic streptococci.

[Penicillin is the usual drug of choice in the treatment and prevention of streptococcal infections, including the prophylaxis of rheumatic fever. Velosef is generally effective in the eradication of streptococci from the nasopharynx; substantial data establishing the efficacy of Velosef in the subsequent prevention of rheumatic fever are not available at present.]

URINARY TRACT INFECTIONS due to *E. coli, Pr. mirabilis,* and *Klebsiella* species.

SKIN AND SKIN STRUCTURES INFECTIONS due to *S. aureus* (penicillin-susceptible and penicillin-resistant) and group A beta-hemolytic streptococci.

BONE INFECTIONS due to *S. aureus* (penicillin-susceptible and penicillin-resistant).

SEPTICEMIA due to *Streptococcus pneumoniae* (formerly *Diplococcus pneumoniae), S. aureus* (penicillin-susceptible and penicillin-resistant), *Pr. mirabilis,* and *E. coli.*

NOTE—Culture and susceptibility tests should be initiated prior to and during therapy. Renal function studies should be performed when indicated.

Contraindications: Cephradine is contraindicated in patients with known hypersensitivity to the cephalosporin group of antibiotics.

Warnings: *In penicillin sensitive patients, cephalosporin C derivatives should be used with great caution. There is clinical and laboratory evidence of partial cross-allergenicity of the penicillins and the cephalosporins, and there are instances of patients who have had reactions to both drug classes (including fatal anaphylaxis after parenteral use).*

Any patient who has demonstrated some form of allergy, particularly to drugs, should receive antibiotics, including Velosef (Cephradine, Squibb), cautiously and then only when absolutely necessary. Serious anaphylactoid reactions require immediate emergency treatment with epinephrine. Oxygen, intravenous steroids, and airway management, including intubation, should also be administered as indicated.

Usage in Pregnancy and Lactation—Although no teratogenic or anti-fertility effects were seen in reproduction studies in mice and rats receiving up to four times the maximum human dose, the safety of this drug for use in human pregnancy has not been established. The benefits of the drug in pregnant women should be weighed against a possible risk to the fetus. Cephradine is secreted in breast milk during lactation.

Usage in Infants—Velosef (Sterile Cephradine for Injection) has been effectively used in this age group, but all laboratory parameters have not been extensively studied in infants one month to one year of age; therefore, in the treatment of children in this age group, the benefits of the drug to the risk involved must be considered.

Since safety for use in premature infants and in infants under one month of age has not been established, the use of cephradine by injection or infusion should be based on careful consideration of the benefits of the drug against the risk involved.

Precautions: Prolonged use of antibiotics may promote the overgrowth of nonsusceptible organisms. Should superinfection occur during therapy, appropriate measures should be taken.

When Velosef is administered to patients with markedly impaired renal function lower daily dosage is required. (See DOSAGE AND ADMINISTRATION.) In patients with known or suspected renal impairment, careful clinical observation and appropriate laboratory studies should be conducted because cephradine in the usual recommended dosage will accumulate in the serum and tissues.

Increased nephrotoxicity has been reported following concomitant administration of cephalosporins and aminoglycoside antibiotics.

Patients should be followed carefully so that any side effects or unusual manifestations of drug idiosyncrasy may be detected. If a hypersensitivity reaction occurs, the drug should be discontinued and the patient treated with the usual agents, e.g., pressor amines, antihistamines, or corticosteroids.

After treatment with cephradine, a false-positive reaction for glucose in the urine may occur with Benedict's solution, Fehling's solution, or with Clinitest® tablets, but not with enzyme-based tests such as Clinistix®, and Tes-Tape®.

As with other cephalosporins, positive direct Coombs tests have been infrequently reported.

Velosef for Injection is physically compatible with most commonly used intravenous fluids and electrolyte solutions (such as 5% Dextrose Injection or Sodium Chloride Injection or M/6 sodium lactate); however, it is *not* compatible with Lactated Ringer's Injection because of the incompatibility between calcium ions and the sodium carbonate present in Velosef for Injection (Sterile Cephradine for Injection).

Adverse Reactions: As with other cephalosporins, untoward reactions are limited essentially to gastrointestinal disturbances and, on occasion, to hypersensitivity phenomena. The latter are more likely to occur in individuals who have previously demonstrated hypersensitivity and those with a history of allergy, asthma, hay fever, or urticaria.

The following adverse reactions have been reported following the use of cephradine:

Gastrointestinal: Glossitis, nausea, vomiting, diarrhea or loose stools, tenesmus and abdominal pain.

Skin and Hypersensitivity Reactions: Mild urticaria or skin rash, edema, erythema, pruritus, joint pains and drug fever.

Blood: Mild, transient eosinophilia, leukopenia and neutropenia.

Liver: Instances of elevated SGOT and SGPT of approximately 10 percent and 2 percent of patients, respectively, have been observed; also, a few cases of elevated total bilirubin, alkaline phosphatase and LDH have been observed. In most patients, values tended to return to normal after the end of therapy.

Renal: Mild elevations in BUN have been observed in some patients treated with cephalo-

Continued on next page

TABLE I
VELOSEF FOR INJECTION
(Sterile Cephradine for Injection)

	MEAN TIME TO PEAK SERUM LEVELS Minutes		MEAN PEAK SERUM CONCENTRATION mcg./ml.		MEAN SERUM CONCENTRATION AT 1 HR. - mcg./ml.	
	500 mg. I.M.	1 g. I.M.	500 mg. I.M.	1 g. I.M.	500 mg. I.M.	1 g. I.M.
MALES	49 (41–59)*	52 (45–61)	6.3 (5.5–7.2)	13.6 (12.2–15.1)	6.2 (5.5–6.9)	12.4 (11.0–14.0)
FEMALES	98 (87–111)	128 (103–157)	5.8 (5.1–6.6)	9.9 (8.7–11.2)	4.3 (3.5–5.2)	6.0 (4.4–8.1)

*Figures in parentheses are 95% confidence limits.

Squibb—Cont.

sporins; their frequency increases in patients over 50 years old and in children under three. In adults for whom serum creatinine determinations were performed, the rise in BUN was not accompanied by a rise in serum creatinine. Other adverse reactions are headache, dizziness, dyspnea, paresthesia, candidal overgrowth, candidal vaginitis, isolated instances of hepatomegaly, and thrombophlebitis at the site of injection.

Pain on intramuscular injection has been experienced by some patients. Since sterile abscesses have been reported following accidental subcutaneous injection, the preparation should be administered by deep intramuscular injection.

Dosage and Administration: *Adults*—The usual daily dosage of Velosef for Injection (Sterile Cephradine for Injection) is 2 to 4 g. of cephradine given in equally divided doses four times a day intramuscularly or intravenously (e.g., 500 mg. to 1 g. q.i.d.). In bone infections the usual dosage is 1 g. q.i.d. administered intravenously. A dosage of 500 mg. q.i.d. is adequate in uncomplicated pneumonia, skin and skin structures and most urinary tract infections. In severe infections, the dose may be increased by giving injections every four hours or by increasing the dose.

The maximum daily dose should not exceed 8 g. per day.

Infants and Children—The usual dosage range of Velosef is 50 to 100 mg./ kg./day (approximately 23–45 mg./lb./day) in equally divided doses four times a day and should be regulated by age, weight of the patient and severity of the infection being treated.

All laboratory parameters have not been extensively studied in infants under one year of age; therefore, in the treatment of children in this age group, the benefits of the drug to the risk involved must be considered. In newborn infants, accumulation of other cephalosporin-class antibiotics (with resultant prolongation of drug half-life) has been reported.

The maximum daily pediatric dose should not exceed doses recommended for adults.

[See table entitled "Pediatric Dosage Guide".]

As with antibiotic therapy generally: therapy should be continued for a minimum of 48 to 72 hours after the patient becomes asymptomatic or evidence of bacterial eradication has been obtained; in infections caused by group A beta-hemolytic streptococci, a minimum of 10 days of treatment is recommended to guard against the risk of rheumatic fever or glomerulonephritis; in the treatment of chronic urinary tract infection, frequent bacteriologic and clinical appraisal is necessary during therapy and may be necessary for several months afterwards; persistent infections may require treatment for several weeks; doses smaller than those indicated above should not be used.

VELOSEF FOR INJECTION
(Sterile Cephradine for Injection)

PEDIATRIC DOSAGE GUIDE

Weight lbs.	kg.	50 mg./kg./day: Approx. single dose mg. q. 6 h.	50 mg./kg./day: Volume needed @ 208 mg./ml. dilution	100 mg./kg./day: Approx. single dose mg. q. 6 h.	100 mg./kg./day: Volume needed @ 227 mg./ml.
10	4.5	56 mg.	0.27 ml.	112 mg.	0.5 ml.
20	9.1	114 mg.	0.55 ml.	227 mg.	1 ml.
30	13.6	170 mg.	0.82 ml.	340 mg.	1.5 ml.
40	18.2	227 mg.	1.1 ml.	455 mg.	2 ml.
50	22.7	284 mg.	1.4 ml.	567 mg.	2.5 ml.

VELOSEF FOR INJECTION
(Sterile Cephradine for Injection)

I.M. DILUTION TABLE

Vial Size	Volume of Diluent	Approximate Available Volume	Approximate Available Concentration
250 mg.	1.2 ml.	1.2 ml.	208 mg./ml.
500 mg.	2.0 ml.	2.2 ml.	227 mg./ml.
1 g.	4.0 ml.	4.5 ml.	222 mg./ml.

Parenteral therapy may be followed by oral Velosef either as capsules or as an oral suspension.

Velosef (Sterile Cephradine for Injection) may be given intravenously or by deep intramuscular injection. To minimize pain and induration, intramuscular injections should be made into a large muscle mass, such as the gluteus or lateral aspect of the thigh.

Renal Impairment Dosage—A modified dosage schedule in patients with decreased renal function is necessary. Each patient should be considered individually; the following reduced dosage schedule is recommended as a guideline, based on the creatinine clearance (ml./min./1.73m^2).

In adults, the initial loading dose is 750 mg. of Velosef (Sterile Cephradine for Injection) and the maintenance dose is 500 mg. at the time intervals listed below.

Creatinine Clearance	Time Interval
> 20 ml./min.	6–12 hours
15–19 ml./min.	12–24 hours
10–14 ml./min.	24–40 hours
5–9 ml./min.	40–50 hours
< 5 ml./min.	50–70 hours

Further modification of the dosage schedule may be necessary in children.

Reconstitution and Storage:

For I.M. Use.—Aseptically add Sterile Water for Injection or Bacteriostatic Water for Injection (containing 0.9% [w/v] benzyl alcohol, or 0.12% methylparaben and 0.014% propylparaben) according to the following table [i.e., the table entitled "I.M. Dilution Table"].

Intramuscular solutions should be used within two hours at room temperature; if stored in the refrigerator at 5° C., solutions retain full potency for 24 hours. Reconstituted solutions may vary in color from light straw to yellow; however, this does not affect the potency.

For I.V. Use—Velosef (Sterile Cephradine for Injection) may also be administered by direct intravenous injection or by continuous or intermittent infusion. A 3 mcg./ml. serum concentration can be maintained for each mg. of cephradine per kg. body weight per hour of infusion.

For Direct I.V. Administration: Suitable diluents are Sterile Water for Injection, 5% Dextrose Injection, or Sodium Chloride Injection. **Do not use Lactated Ringer's Injection.**

Aseptically add 5 ml. of diluent to the 250 mg. or 500 mg. vials, 10 ml. of diluent to the 1 g. vial, or 20 ml. of diluent to the 2 g. bottle; withdraw entire contents. The solution may be slowly injected directly into a vein over a three to five minute period or may be given as a supplementary injection through the injection site on the administration set when the infusion solution is compatible with cephradine. These Velosef (Cephradine, Squibb) solutions should be used within two hours when held at room temperature; if stored at 5° C., the solutions retain full potency for 24 hours.

For Continuous or Intermittent I.V. Infusion: Suitable intravenous infusion solutions for Velosef are 5% or 10% Dextrose Injection; Sodium Chloride Injection; Sodium Lactate Injection (M/6 sodium lactate); Dextrose and Sodium Chloride Injection (5% : 0.9%) or (5% : 0.45%); 10% Invert Sugar in Water for Injection; Normosol®-R, and Ionosol® B with Dextrose 5%. Sterile Water for Injection may be used as an I.V. infusion solution for Velosef at a concentration of 30 to 50 mg./ml. (30 mg./ml. is approximately isotonic). **Do not use Lactated Ringer's Injection.**

a) To prepare a Velosef solution for transfer into an I.V. infusion bottle, aseptically add 10 ml., 20 ml., or 40 ml. of Sterile Water for Injection or a suitable infusion solution, respectively, to the 1 g. vial, or 2 g. or 4 g. bottles. Promptly withdraw the entire contents of the resulting solution and aseptically transfer to an I.V. infusion bottle. Intravenous infusion solutions containing Velosef at a concentration of five percent (50 mg./ml.) or less retain potency as noted under (b) below. The choice of I.V. infusion solution and the volume to be employed are dictated by fluid and electrolyte management.

b) Velosef (Sterile Cephradine for Injection) may be infused directly from the 2 g. or 4 g. I.V. bottle. Reconstitute the 2 g. bottle with 40 ml. and the 4 g. bottle with 80 ml. of a suitable intravenous infusion solution; attach an I.V. administration set directly to the Sterile Cephradine for Injection I.V. infusion bottle. The 2 g. and 4 g. I.V. bottles are designed to be suspended from an I.V. stand.

Intravenous infusion solutions containing Velosef retain full potency for 10 hours at room temperature or 48 hours at 5° C.; infusion solutions of Velosef in Sterile Water for Injection that are frozen immediately after reconstitution in the original container are stable for as long as six weeks when stored at −20° C.

For prolonged infusions, replace the infusion every 10 hours with a freshly prepared solution.

Extemperaneous mixtures of Velosef for Injection with other antibiotics are not recommmended.

Protect solutions of Velosef from concentrated light or direct sunlight. Velosef for Injection may be stored at room temperature prior to reconstitution; avoid excessive heat; protect from light.

How Supplied: Velosef for Injection (Sterile Cephradine for Injection) is available for intramuscular or intravenous use in vials containing 250 mg., 500 mg., or 1 g. cephradine; and for intravenous use in 100 ml. infusion bottles containing 2 g. or 4 g. cephradine.

VESPRIN® INJECTION ℞
(Triflupromazine Hydrochloride Injection NF)
VESPRIN® TABLETS ℞
(Triflupromazine Hydrochloride Tablets NF)
VESPRIN® HIGH-POTENCY SUSPENSION ℞
(Triflupromazine Oral Suspension NF)

Description: Vesprin is a phenothiazine derivative. It is available for parenteral use in multiple dose vials providing 10 or 20 mg. triflupromazine hydrochloride per ml. and in 1 ml. Unimatic® single dose preassembled syringes providing 10 mg. triflupromazine hydrochloride per ml., with 1.5% (w/v) benzyl alcohol as a preservative and sodium chloride for isotonicity. The pH has been adjusted to 4.5-5.2 with sodium hydroxide or hydrochloric acid. At the time of manufacture, the air in the vials is replaced by nitrogen.
Vesprin is also available for oral use as tablets providing 10, 25, and 50 mg. triflupromazine hydrochloride and as a suspension providing triflupromazine equivalent to 50 mg. triflupromazine hydrochloride per 5 ml. teaspoonful (10 mg. per ml.). Vesprin Tablets, 25 mg. and 50 mg., contain FD&C Yellow No. 5 (tartrazine).
Clinical Pharmacology: Experimental and clinical studies suggest that the phenothiazine derivatives act on the hypothalamus. These drugs are believed to depress various components of the mesodiencephalic activating system, which is involved in the control of basal metabolism and body temperature, wakefulness, vasomotor tone, emesis, and hormonal balance. In addition, the drugs exert a peripheral autonomic effect in varying degrees. However, the site and mode of action of phenothiazine derivatives including triflupromazine have not been completely elucidated.
Indications and Usage: Oral: Vesprin (Triflupromazine) is effective for oral use in the management of the manifestations of psychotic disorders (excluding psychotic depressive reactions) and for the control of severe nausea and vomiting.
Parenteral: Vesprin Injection (Triflupromazine Hydrochloride Injection NF) is effective in the management of the manifestations of psychotic disorders (excluding psychotic depressive reactions) and for the control of severe nausea and vomiting.
Triflupromazine has not been shown effective in the management of behavioral complications in patients with mental retardation.
Contraindications: Phenothiazines are contraindicated in patients with suspected or established subcortical brain damage, with or without hypothalamic damage, since a hyperthermic reaction with temperatures in excess of 104° F. may occur in such patients, sometimes not until 14 to 16 hours after drug administration. Total body ice-packing is recommended for such a reaction; antipyretics may also be useful.
Phenothiazine compounds should not be used in patients receiving large doses of hypnotics. As with other phenothiazine compounds, triflupromazine is contraindicated in comatose or severely depressed states.
The presence of blood dyscrasia or liver damage precludes the use of triflupromazine.
Warnings: The extrapyramidal symptoms which can occur secondary to administration of triflupromazine may be confused with the central nervous system signs of an undiagnosed primary disease responsible for the vomiting, e.g., Reye Syndrome or other encephalopathy. The use of triflupromazine and other potential hepatotoxins should be avoided in children and adolescents whose signs and symptoms suggest Reye Syndrome.
The use of this drug may impair the mental and physical abilities required for driving a car or operating heavy machinery.
Potentiation of the effects of alcohol may occur with the use of this drug.
Usage in Pregnancy—The safety for the use of this drug during pregnancy has not been established; therefore, the possible hazards should be weighed against the potential benefits when administering this drug to pregnant patients.
Precautions: Antiemetic Effect: The antiemetic action of triflupromazine may mask the signs and symptoms of overdosage of other drugs and may obscure the diagnosis and treatment of other conditions such as intestinal obstruction, brain tumor, and Reye Syndrome (see WARNINGS).
Because of the possibility of cross-sensitivity, this drug should be used cautiously in patients who have developed cholestatic jaundice, dermatoses, or other allergic reactions to phenothiazine derivatives.
Psychotic patients on large doses of a phenothiazine drug who are undergoing surgery should be watched carefully for possible hypotensive phenomena. Moreover, it should be remembered that reduced amounts of anesthetics or central nervous system depressants may be necessary. It is generally not recommended that triflupromazine be used prior to spinal anesthesia.
Although this is not a general feature of triflupromazine, potentiation of central nervous system depressants (opiates, analgesics, antihistamines, barbiturates, alcohol) may occur. The effects of atropine may be potentiated in some patients receiving triflupromazine.
Phenothiazines should be used with caution in patients with a history of convulsive disorders, since grand mal convulsions have been known to occur.
Patients with special medical disorders such as mitral insufficiency or pheochromocytoma and patients who have exhibited idiosyncrasy to other centrally-acting drugs may experience severe reactions to phenothiazine compounds.
The parenteral administration of triflupromazine may sometimes cause postural hypotension; to preclude its occurrence, patients should be kept under close clinical supervision, in a recumbent position if necessary.
Facilities should be available for periodic checking of hepatic function, renal function and the blood picture. Renal function of patients on long-term therapy should be monitored; if BUN (blood urea nitrogen) becomes abnormal, treatment should be discontinued.
As with any phenothiazine, the physician should be alert to the possible development of "silent pneumonias" in patients under treatment with triflupromazine.
There is sufficient experimental evidence to conclude that chronic administration of antipsychotic drugs which increase prolactin secretion has the potential to induce mammary neoplasms in rodents under the appropriate conditions. There are recognized differences in the physiological role of prolactin between rodents and humans. Since there are, at pesent, no adequate epidemiological studies, the relevance to human mammary cancer risk from prolonged exposure to triflupromazine and other antipsychotic drugs is not known.
Vesprin Tablets (Triflupromazine Hydrochloride Tablets NF), 25 mg. and 50 mg., contain FD&C Yellow No. 5 (tartrazine) which may cause allergic-type reactions (including bronchial asthma) in certain susceptible individuals. Although the overall incidence of FD&C Yellow No. 5 (tartrazine) sensitivity in the general population is low, it is frequently seen in patients who also have aspirin hypersensitivity.
Adverse Reactions: *Central Nervous System*—The side effects most frequently reported with phenothiazine compounds are extrapyramidal symptoms including pseudoparkinsonism, dystonia, dyskinesia, akathisia, oculogyric crises, opisthotonos, and hyperreflexia. Most often these extrapyramidal symptoms are reversible; however, they may be persistent (see below). With any given phenothiazine derivative, the incidence and severity of such reactions depend more on individual patient sensitivity than on other factors, but dosage level and patient age are also determinants.
Extrapyramidal reactions may be alarming, and the patient should be forewarned and reassured. These reactions can usually be controlled by administration of antiparkinsonian drugs such as Benztropine Mesylate and by subsequent reduction in dosage.
Persistent Tardive Dyskinesia—As with all antipsychotic agents, tardive dyskinesia may appear in some patients on long-term therapy or may occur after drug therapy has been discontinued. The risk seems to be greater in elderly patients on high-dose therapy, especially females. The symptoms are persistent and in some patients appear to be irreversible. The syndrome is characterized by rhythmical involuntary movements of the tongue, face, mouth, or jaw (e.g., protrusion of tongue, puffing of cheeks, puckering of mouth, chewing movements). Sometimes these may be accompanied by involuntary movements of the extremities. There is no known effective treatment for tardive dyskinesia; antiparkinsonism agents usually do not alleviate the symptoms of this syndrome. It is suggested that all antipsychotic agents be discontinued if these symptoms appear. Should it be necessary to reinstitute treatment, or increase the dosage of the agent, or switch to a different antipsychotic agent, the syndrome may be masked. It has been reported that fine vermicular movements of the tongue may be an early sign of the syndrome and if the medication is stopped at that time, the syndrome may not develop.
Drowsiness or lethargy, if they occur, may necessitate a reduction in dosage; the induction of a catatonic-like state has been known to occur with dosages far in excess of the recommended amounts. As with other phenothiazine compounds, reactivation or aggravation of psychotic processes may be encountered.
Phenothiazine derivatives have been known to cause, in some patients, restlessness, excitement, or bizarre dreams.
Autonomic Nervous System—Hypertension and fluctuation in blood pressure have been reported with triflupromazine.
Patients with pheochromocytoma, cerebral vascular or renal insufficiency appear to be particularly prone to hypotensive reactions with phenothiazine compounds and should therefore be observed closely when the drug is administered. If severe hypotension should occur, supportive measures including the use of intravenous vasopressor drugs should be instituted immediately. Levarterenol Bitartrate Injection and Phenylephrine Hydrochloride Injection are suitable drugs for this purpose. *Epinephrine should not be used* since phenothiazine derivatives have been found to reverse its action, resulting in a further lowering of blood pressure.
Autonomic reactions including nausea and loss of appetite, salivation, polyuria, perspiration, dry mouth, headache, and constipation may occur. Autonomic effects can usually be controlled by reducing or temporarily discontinuing dosage.
In some patients, phenothiazine derivatives have caused blurred vision, glaucoma, bladder paralysis, fecal impaction, paralytic ileus, tachycardia, or nasal congestion.
Metabolic and Endocrine—Weight change, peripheral edema, abnormal lactation, gynecomastia, menstrual irregularities, false results on pregnancy tests, impotency in men, and increased libido in women have all been known to occur in some patients on phenothiazine therapy.
Allergic Reactions—Skin disorders such as itching, erythema, urticaria, seborrhea, photo-

Continued on next page

Squibb—Cont.

sensitivity, eczema, and even exfoliative dermatitis have been reported with phenothiazine derivatives. The possibility of anaphylactoid reactions occuring in some patients should be borne in mind.

Hematologic—Routine blood counts are advisable during therapy since blood dyscrasias including leukopenia, agranulocytosis, thrombocytopenic or nonthrombocytopenic purpura, eosinophilia, and pancytopenia have been observed with phenothiazine derivatives. Furthermore, if any soreness of the mouth, gums, or throat, or any symptoms of upper respiratory infection occur and confirmatory leukocyte count indicates cellular depression, therapy should be discontinued and other appropriate measures instituted immediately.

Hepatic—Liver damage as manifested by cholestatic jaundice or biliary stasis have been observed with phenothiazine derivatives, particularly during the first months of therapy; treatment should be discontinued if this occurs. An increase in cephalin flocculation, sometimes accompanied by alterations in other liver function tests has been reported in patients receiving phenothiazines who have had no clinical evidence of liver damage.

Others—Sudden, unexpected, and unexplained deaths have been reported in hospitalized psychotic patients receiving phenothiazines. Previous brain damage or seizures may be predisposing factors; high doses should be avoided in known seizure patients. Several patients have shown sudden flare-ups of psychotic behavior patterns shortly before death. Autopsy findings have usually revealed acute fulminating pneumonia or pneumonitis, aspiration of gastric contents, or intramyocardial lesions.

The following adverse reactions have also occurred with phenothiazine derivatives: systemic lupus erythematosus-like syndrome, hypotension severe enough to cause fatal cardiac arrest, altered electrocardiographic and electroencephalographic tracings, altered cerebrospinal fluid proteins, cerebral edema, potentiation of heat and of phosphorus insecticides, asthma, laryngeal edema, angioneurotic edema, and pigmentary retinopathy; with long-term use—skin pigmentation, and lenticular and corneal opacities.

Dosage and Administration: Psychotic Disorders—*Institutionalized Adult Patients:* Optimum dosage levels must be determined individually in each patient. The recommended initial dose for oral therapy is 100 mg. up to a maximum total daily dose of 150 mg. After treatment is instituted, the daily dosage should be adjusted until the desired clinical effect is obtained. Continued treatment is necessary to achieve maximum therapeutic benefits. In some patients, optimum clinical improvement may occur only after prolonged treatment. When symptoms are controlled, dosage can generally be reduced gradually to maintenance levels.

The recommended intramuscular dose is 60 mg. up to a maximum total daily dose of 150 mg.

Noninstitutionalized Adult Patients: Use the same regimen as outlined for institutionalized patients.

For patients on *maintenance therapy* following institutional care, the recommended oral dose is 30 mg. up to a maximum total daily dose of 150 mg.

Children: As in adult therapy, optimum dosage levels must be determined individually for each patient. The recommended oral dosage schedule is 2 mg./kg. (1 mg./lb.) up to a maximum total daily dose of 150 mg. in divided doses. For maintenance therapy, dosage should be increased or decreased to meet individual requirements.

When intramuscular use is indicated in children, the recommended range is 0.2 to 0.25 mg./kg. ($^1/_{10}$ to $^1/_8$ mg./lb.) up to a maximum total daily dose of 10 mg. The drug should not be administered to children under 2½ years of age.

Nausea and Vomiting—For adults, the recommended dosage range for prophylaxis as well as for treatment is 1 mg. up to a maximum total daily dose of 3 mg. intravenously or 5 to 15 mg. as a single dose which may be repeated every four hours up to a maximum total daily dose of 60 mg. intramuscularly. The recommended dosage range for oral prophylaxis is 20 mg. up to a maximum total daily dose of 30 mg. For elderly or debilitated patients, the recommended intramuscular dosage is 2.5 mg. up to a maximum total daily dose of 15 mg.

Triflupromazine should generally not be used in children under 2½ years of age. It should not be used in conditions for which children's dosages have not been established. Dosage and frequency of administration should be adjusted according to the severity of the symptoms and response of the patient. The duration of activity following intramuscular administration may last up to 12 hours. Subsequent doses may be given by the same route if necessary.

For children, the recommended dosage is 0.2 mg./kg. ($^1/_{10}$ mg./lb.) up to a maximum total daily dose of 10 mg. divided into three doses orally or a range of 0.2 to 0.25 mg./kg. ($^1/_{10}$ to $^1/_8$ mg./lb.) up to a maximum total daily dose of 10 mg. intramuscularly. Intravenous administration is not recommended for children.

How Supplied: Vesprin Injection (Triflupromazine Hydrochloride Injection NF) is available in multiple dose vials of 1 ml. providing 20 mg. per ml., multiple dose vials of 10 ml. providing 10 mg. per ml., and in 1 ml. Unimatic® single dose preassembled syringes providing 10 mg. per ml.

Vesprin Tablets (Triflupromazine Hydrochloride Tablets NF) are available in potencies of 10 mg., 25 mg. and 50 mg. in bottles of 50 and 500.

Vesprin High-Potency Suspension (Triflupromazine Oral Suspension NF) is available as a flavored suspension providing triflupromazine equivalent to 50 mg. triflupromazine hydrochloride per 5 ml. teaspoonful (10 mg. per ml.) in bottles of 120 ml.

Storage: Store the injection, tablets and oral suspension at room temperature; protect from light. Injection: avoid freezing. Parenteral solutions may vary in color from essentially colorless to light amber. If a solution has become any darker than light amber or is discolored in any other way it should not be used. Tablets: keep tightly closed; avoid excessive heat. Oral suspension: keep tightly closed; avoid excessive heat and freezing.

VIGRAN® TABLETS
(Multi-Vitamin Supplement)

Vigran is a multi-vitamin supplement for adults and children 4 or more years of age.

One tablet daily provides:		Percent US RDA*
Vitamin A (1.5 mg.)	5000 IU	100
Vitamin D (10 mcg.)	400 IU	100
Vitamin E (30 mg.)	30 IU	100
Vitamin C	60 mg.	100
Folic Acid	0.4 mg.	100
Thiamine	1.5 mg.	100
Riboflavin	1.7 mg.	100
Niacin	20 mg.	100
Vitamin B_6	2 mg.	100
Vitamin B_{12}	6 mcg.	100

*U.S. Recommended Daily Allowances

Usage: One FILMLOK® tablet daily for adults and children 4 or more years of age. (FILMLOK® is a Squibb trademark for veneer-coated tablets.)

How Supplied: Bottles of 100 and 1000 and packages of 2 bottles of 100.

Storage: Store at room temperature; avoid excessive heat.

VIGRAN® plus IRON
(Multi-Vitamin Supplement with Iron)

Vigran plus Iron is a multi-vitamin supplement with iron for adults and children 4 or more years of age.

One tablet daily provides:		Percent US RDA*
Vitamin A (1.5 mg.)	5000 IU	100
Vitamin D (10 mcg.)	400 IU	100
Vitamin E (30 mg.)	30 IU	100
Vitamin C	60 mg.	100
Folic Acid	0.4 mg.	100
Thiamine	1.5 mg.	100
Riboflavin	1.7 mg.	100
Niacin	20 mg.	100
Vitamin B_6	2 mg.	100
Vitamin B_{12}	6 mcg.	100
Iron	27 mg.	150

*U.S. Recommended Daily Allowances

Usage: One tablet daily for adults and children 4 or more years of age.

How Supplied: Bottles of 90 and packages of 2 bottles of 90.

Storage: Store at room temperature; avoid excessive heat.

For information on Squibb products, write to: Squibb Professional Services Department, Lawrenceville-Princeton Road, Princeton, N.J. 08540

Standard Process Laboratories, Inc.
2023 WEST WISCONSIN AVENUE
MILWAUKEE, WISCONSIN 53201

CHLOROPHYLL COMPLEX PERLES

Composition: Crude, natural chlorophyll extracted from Alfalfa and Tillandsia is a steroid rich source of fat soluble natural Vitamin K (6 Perles supply 3.3 mg. of Vitamin K). Vitamin K is indicated to be essential to the normal function of the liver and the formation of prothrombin, one of the normal constituents of the blood.

Action and Uses: Prothrombin is one of the several clotting agents in the blood. (Ref. #1) On the other hand, *water soluble* extracts of chlorophyll, being chemically altered from their natural form, contain no vitamins. Doses of synthetic Vitamin K have produced hemolytic anemia in rats and the toxicity of *synthetic* Vitamin K is attributed to increased breakdown of the red blood cells, (Ref. #2) whereas it is interesting to note, that administering *natural, fat soluble* Vitamin K, causes a prompt response by the body with the formation of prothrombin. The blood returns to its normal composition. (Ref. #3)

Administration: Three to six perles per day or as directed.

How Supplied: CHLOROPHYLL COMPLEX PERLES in bottles of 60 and 350.

Also Available: CHLOROPHYLL, FAT SOLUBLE OINTMENT in 1½-oz. tube.

References: (1) and (3) *Yearbook of Agriculture,* 1959, (U.S. Government Publication) pages 137-138. (2) *Recommended Dietary Allowances,* (Seventh Edition-1968), National Research Council Publication No. 1694, page 30.

ZYPAN TABLETS
An Enzymatic Digestive Supplement for Common Indigestion

Description: Each ZYPAN TABLET contains 1.0 gr. Pancreatin, plus 0.5 gr. of other Pancreas extracts, 1.5 gr. Pepsin (1:3000), 2.75 gr.

Betaine Hydrochloride and 0.15 gr. Ammonium Chloride.
ZYPAN is a source of digestive enzymes as derived from fresh, frozen beef pancreas (as pancreatin), with betaine hydrochloride as a source of hydrochloric acid, and ammonium chloride as an acidifying agent. Pancreatin is a source of multiple digestive enzymes, notably as follows: (1) Trypsin, which breaks down *protein* into amino acids, (2) Diastase, which converts *starch* to an absorbable form, and (3) Lipase, which assists in the digestion of *fats*.
Indications: When intestinal fermentative processes result in such conditions as flatulence, bloating, and fullness after meals; a lack of digestive enzymes may be present. A long-term inability to absorb foods, because of incomplete digestion, may affect the general health. Deficient protein digestion should be a primary concern, and mere increase of protein in the diet may not correct a deficiency as efficiently as when aided by the proteolytic enzymes.
Administration: One to two tablets with each meal, or as directed.
How Supplied: Bottles of 100 tablets.

Star Pharmaceuticals, Inc.
P. O. BOX 600431
16499 N.E. 19TH AVE.
N. MIAMI BEACH, FL 33160

MICROSUL® 0.5 Gm. ℞
NDC 0076-0104-03 & 04

Each tablet contains: Sulfamethizole 0.5 Gm.

MICROSUL® 1.0 Gm. ℞
NDC 0076-0202-03 & 04

Each tablet contains: Sulfamethizole 1.0 Gm.

MICROSUL-A® ℞
NDC 0076-0105-03 & 04

Each tablet contains: Sulfamethizole 0.5 Gm. with Phenazopyridine HCl 50 mg.

NITREX® 50 mg. ℞
NDC 0076-0401-03 & 04

Each tablet contains: Nitrofurantoin USP 50 mg.

NITREX® 100 mg. ℞
NDC 0076-0402-03 & 04

Each tablet contains: Nitrofurantoin USP 100 mg.

PROSED® ℞
NDC 0076-0107-03 & 04

Each tablet contains: Methenamine 40.8 mg., Methylene blue 5.4 mg., Phenyl Salicylate 18.1 mg., Atropine sulfate 0.03 mg., Hyocyamine 0.03 mg., Benzoic acid 4.5 mg.

STAR-OTIC® OTC
Antibacterial-Antifungal Otic Solution
NDC 0076-0300-03

Each 15 cc. contains: Aluminum Acetate (Modified Burow's Solution), Acetic Acid 1.0%, Boric Acid 1.0% in Propylene Glycol Vehicle.

URO-KP-NEUTRAL® ℞
NDC 0076-0109-03 & 04

Each 6 light-orange capsule shaped tablets contain:

Sodium	1361 mg.
Potassium	298.6 mg.
Phosphorous	1037 mg.

derived from Sodium Phosphate Dibasic Anhydrous and Potassium Phosphate Dibasic Anhydrous.

UROLENE BLUE® ℞
NDC 0076-0501-03 & 04

Each tablet contains: Methylene blue USP 65 mg.

VESICHOLINE® ℞
NDC 0076-0701-03 & 04

Each tablet contains: Bethanechol chloride NF 25 mg. FOR ORAL USE.

VIRILON® ℞
NDC 0076-0301-03 & 04

Each capsule contains: Methyltestosterone USP 10 mg. in controlled release pellets.

Steri-Med Inc.
POST OFFICE BOX 459
LINDENHURST, NY 11757

LEVODOPA ℞

> Toward reducing the high incidence of adverse reactions, it is necessary to individualize the therapy and to gradually increase the dosage to the desired therapeutic level.

Description: Chemically, levodopa is (—)—3—(3, 4-dihydroxyphenyl)-L-alanine. It is a colorless, crystalline compound, slightly soluble in water and insoluble in alcohol, with a molecular weight of 197.2.
Actions: Evidence indicates that the symptoms of Parkinson's disease are related to depletion of striatal dopamine. Since dopamine apparently does not cross the blood-brain barrier, its administration is ineffective in the treatment of Parkinson's disease. However, levodopa, the levorotatory isomer of dihydroxyphenylalanine (dopa) which is the metabolic precursor of dopamine, does cross the blood-brain barrier. Presumably it is converted into dopamine in the basal ganglia. This is generally thought to be the mechanism whereby oral levodopa acts in relieving the symptoms of Parkinson's disease.
The major urinary metabolites of levodopa in man appear to be dopamine and homovanillic acid (HVA). In 24 hour urine samples, HVA accounts for 13 to 42 percent of the ingested dose of levodopa.
Indications: Levodopa is indicated in the treatment of idiopathic Parkinson's disease (Paralysis Agitans), post encephalitic parkinsonism, symptomatic parkinsonism which may follow injury to the nervous system by carbon monoxide intoxication, and manganese intoxication. It is indicated in those elderly patients believed to develop parkinsonism in association with cerebral arteriosclerosis.
Contraindications: Monoamine oxidase (MAO) inhibitors and levodopa should not be given concomitantly and these inhibitors must be discontinued two weeks prior to initiating therapy with levodopa. Levodopa is contraindicated in patients with known hypersensitity to the drug and in narrow angle glaucoma.
Warnings: Levodopa should be administered cautiously to patients with severe cardiovascular or pulmonary disease, bronchial asthma, renal, hepatic or endocrine disease.
Care should be exercised in administering levodopa to patients with a history of myocardial infarction who have residual atrial, nodal or ventricular arrhythmias. If levodopa is necessary in this type of patient, it should be done in a facility with a coronary care unit or an intensive care unit.
One must be on the alert for the possibility of upper gastrointestinal hemorrhage in those patients with a past history of active peptic ulcer disease.
All patients should be carefully observed for the development of depression with concomitant suicidal tendencies. Psychotic patients should be treated with caution.
Pyridoxine hydrochloride (vitamin B6) in oral doses of 10 to 25 mg rapidly reverses the toxic and therapeutic effects of levodopa. This should be considered before recommending vitamin preparations containing pyridoxine hydrochloride (vitamin B6).
Usage in Pregnancy: The safety of levodopa in women who are or who may become pregnant has not been established; hence, it should be given only when the potential benefits have been weighed against possible hazards to mother and child. Studies in rodents have shown that levodopa at dosages in excess of 200 mg/kg/day has an adverse effect on fetal and post natal growth and viability.
Levodopa should not be used in nursing mothers.
Usage in children: The safety of levodopa under the age of 12 has not been established.
Precautions: Periodic evaluations of hepatic, hematopoietic, cardiovascular and renal function are recommended during extended therapy in all patients.
Patients with chronic wide angle glaucoma may be treated cautiously with levodopa provided the intra-ocular pressure is well controlled and the patient monitored carefully for changes in intra-ocular pressure during therapy.
Postural hypotensive episodes have been reported as adverse reactions. Therefore, levodopa should be administered to patients on antihypertensive drugs cautiously (for patients receiving pargyline, see note on MAO inhibitors under CONTRA-INDICATIONS), and it may be necessary to adjust the dosage of antihypertensive drugs.
Adverse Reactions: The most serious adverse reactions associated with the administration of levodopa having frequent occurrences are: adventitious movements such as choreiform and/or dystonic movements. Other serious adverse reactions with a lower incidence are: cardiac irregularities and/or palpitations, orthostatic hypotensive epidsodes, bradykinetic episodes (the "on-off" phenomena), mental changes including paranoid ideation and psychotic episodes, depression with or without the development of suicidal tendencies, dementia, and urinary retention.
Rarely gastrointestinal bleeding, development of duodenal ulcer, hypertension, phlebitis, hemolytic anemia, agranulocytosis, and convulsions have been observed. (The causal relationship between convulsions and levodopa has not been established.)
Adverse reactions of a less serious nature having a relatively frequent occurrence are the following: anorexia, nausea, and vomiting with or without abdominal pain and distress, dry mouth, dysphagia, sialorrhea, ataxia, increased head tremor, headache, dizziness, numbness, weakness and faintness, bruxism, confusion, insomnia, nightmares, hallucinations and delusions, agitation and anxiety, malaise, fatigue and euphoria. Occurring with a lesser order of frequency are the following: muscle twitching and blepharospasm (which may be taken as an early sign of overdosage; consideration of dosage reduction may be made at this time), trismus, burning sensation of the tongue, bitter taste, diarrhea, constipation, flatulence, flushing, skin rash, increased sweating, bizarre breathing patterns, urinary incontinence, diplopia, blurred vision, dilated pupils, hot flashes, weight gain or loss, dark sweat and/or urine.
Rarely, oculogyric crises, sense of stimulation, hiccups, development of edema, loss of hair, hoarseness, priapism and activation of latent Horner's syndrome have been observed.

Continued on next page

Steri-Med—Cont.

Elevation of blood urea nitrogen, SGOT, SGPT, LDH, bilirubin, alkaline phosphatase or protein bound iodine have been reported; and the significance of this is not known. Occasional reductions in WBC, hemoglobin, and hematocrit have been noted.
Leukopenia has occurred and requires cessation at least temporarily, of levodopa administration. The Coomb's test has occasionally become positive during extended therapy. Elevations of uric acid have been noted when colormetric method was used but not when uricase method was used.
Dosage and Administration: The optimal daily dose of levodopa i.e. the dose producing maximal improvement with tolerated side effects, must be determined and **carefully titrated for each individual patient.** The usual initial dosage is 0.5 to 1 Gm daily, divided in two or more doses with food.
The total daily dosage is then increased gradually in increments not more than 0.75 Gm every three to seven days as tolerated. The usual optimal therapeutic **dosage should not exceed 8 Gm.** The exceptional patient may carefully be given more than 8 Gm as required. In some patients, a significant therapeutic response may not be obtained until six months of treatment.
In the event general anesthesia is required, levodopa therapy may be continued as long as the patient is able to take fluids and medication by mouth. If therapy is temporarily interrupted, the usual daily dosage may be administered as soon as the patient is able to take oral medication. Whenever therapy has been interrupted for long periods, dosage should again be adjusted gradually, however, in many cases the patient can be rapidly titrated to his previous therapeutic dosage.
Overdosage: For acute overdosage general supportive measures should be employed, along with immediate gastric lavage. Intravenous fluids should be administered judiciously and an adequate airway maintained.
Electrocardiographic monitoring should be instituted and the patient carefully observed for the possible development of arrhythmias: if required, appropriate antiarrhythmic therapy should be given. Consideration should be given to the possibility of multiple drug ingestion by the patient. To date, no experience has been reported with dialysis; hence its value in levodopa overdosage is not known. Although pyridoxine hydrochloride (vitamin B6) has been reported to reverse the antiparkinson effects of levodopa, its usefulness in the management of acute overdosage has not been established.
How Supplied: Levodopa is supplied in capsules containing 125 mg (opaque orange), 250 mg (opaque pink & brown) and 500 mg (opaque pink).

NITROFURANTOIN TABLETS U.S.P. ℞

Description: Nitrofurantoin is 1-[(5-nitrofurfurylidene) amino] hydantoin, a synthetic, crystalline, yellow, stable compound.
Actions: Nitrofurantoin is an antibacterial agent for specific urinary tract infections. It is bacteriostatic in low concentrations (1:100,000 to 1:200,000) and in vitro is considered to be bactericidal in higher concentrations. Its presumed mode of action is based upon its interference with several bacterial enzyme systems. Nitrofurantoin is rapidly excreted in the urine. It is highly soluble in urine to which it may impart a brown color.
Indications: Nitrofurantoin is indicated for the treatment of pyelonephritis, pyelitis, and cystitis when due to susceptible E. coli, enterococci, S. Aureus (not indicated for the treatment of associated renal cortical or perinephric abscesses), and certain strains of Klebsiella, Aerobacter Proteus, and Pseudomonas.
Contraindications: Anuria, oliguria, or significant impairment of renal function are contraindications to therapy with this drug. Treatment of this type of patient carries an increased risk of toxicity because of impaired excretion of the drug. For this same reason, this drug is much less effective under these circumstances.
The drug is contraindicated in pregnant patients at term as well as infants under 3 months of age because of the possibility of hemolytic anemia due to immature enzyme systems (gluthathione instability).
The drug is contraindicated in those patients with known hypersensitivity to nitrofurantoin.
Warnings: Cases of hemolytic anemia of the primaquine sensitivity type have been induced by nitrofurantoin. The hemolysis appears to be linked to a glucose-6-phosphate dehydrogenase deficiency in the red blood cells of the affected patients. This deficiency is found in 10 percent of Negroes and a small percentage of ethnic groups of Mediterranean and Near-Eastern origin. Any sign of hemolysis is an indication to discontinue the drug.
Pseudomonas is the organism most commonly implicated in superinfections in patients treated with nitrofurantoin.
Usage in Pregnancy: The safety of nitrofurantoin during pregnancy and lactation has not been established. It should not be used in women of childbearing potential unless the expected benefits outweigh the possible hazards.
Precautions: Peripheral neuropathy may occur with nitrofurantoin therapy; this may become severe or irreversible. Fatalities have been reported. Predisposing conditions such as renal impairment, anemia, diabetes, electrolyte imbalance, vitamin B deficiency, and debilitating disease may enhance such occurrence.
Acute, subacute or chronic pulmonary reaction has been observed in patients treated with nitrofurantoin. If these reactions occur, the drug should be withdrawn and appropriate measures should be taken.
Insidious onset of pulmonary reactions (diffuse interstitial pneumonitis, or pulmonary fibrosis, or both) in patients on long-term therapy warrants close monitoring of these patients.
Adverse Reactions: Gastrointestinal reactions: Anorexia, nausea, emesis are the most frequent reactions; less frequently, abdominal pain and diarrhea; rarely hepatitis. This dose-related toxicity reaction can be minimized by reduction of dosage, especially in the female patient.
Hypersensitivity reactions: Pulmonary sensitivity reactions, which can be acute, subacute, or chronic.
Acute reaction is commonly manifested by fever, chills, cough, chest pain, dyspnea, pulmonary infiltration with consolidation or pleural effusion on X-ray, and eosinophilia. The acute reactions usually occur within the first week of treatment and resolve with cessation of the drug therapy.
Subacute or chronic pulmonary reaction is associated with prolonged therapy. Insidious onset of malaise, dyspnea on exertion, cough, altered pulmonary function and roentgenographic and histologic findings of diffuse interstitial pneumonitis or fibrosis or both are common manifestations. Impaired pulmonary function may result even after cessation of the drug therapy.
Dermatologic reactions: Maculopapular, erythematous, or eczematous eruption, pruritis, urticaria, and angioedema.
Other sensitivity reactions: Anaphylaxis, asthmatic attack in patients with history of asthma, cholestatic jaundice, drug fever, and arthralgia.
Hematologic reactions: Hemolytic anemia, granulocytopenia, eosinophilia, and megaloblastic anemia.
Neurological reactions: Peripheral neuropathy, headache, dizziness, nystagmus, and drowsiness.
Miscellaneous reactions: Transient Alopecia; superinfections in the genito-urinary tract by resistant organisms.
Dosage and Administration:
Adult: 50—100 mg. four times a day
Children: should be calculated on the basis of 5–7 mg./kg. of body weight per 24 hours to be given in divided doses four times a day (contraindicated under 3 months).
Administration: Nitrofurantoin may be given with food or milk to minimize gastric upset.
The drug should be continued for at least 3 days after sterility of the urine is obtained. Continued infection indicates the need for reevaluation.
If the drug is to be used for long-term suppressive therapy, reduction of dosage should be considered.
How Supplied: Nitrofurantoin, U.S.P., is supplied in the form of 50 mg. and 100 mg. scored, compressed tablets.

Stiefel Laboratories, Inc.
2801 PONCE DE LEON BLVD.
CORAL GABLES, FL 33134

DUOFILM® ℞

Composition: Salicylic Acid USP, 16.7% and Lactic Acid USP, 16.7% in Flexible Collodion, USP.
Indications: DUOFILM is indicated as a keratolytic agent for the removal of benign epithelial tumors such as common warts.
Dosage and Administration: Prior to the application of DUOFILM, soak the affected area in hot water for at least five minutes. Dry thoroughly with a clean towel.
Apply two to four drops of DUOFILM directly to the wart using the plastic applicator. Each drop should be permitted to dry before re-application of the liquid. Care should be taken to see that DUOFILM is not applied to the surrounding skin. A Band-Aid® or similar bandage should then be applied lightly.
Treatment should take place once daily and continue as directed by physician.
(NOTE: Special patient instruction sheets are available on request.)
Contraindications: Diabetics or patients with impaired blood circulation should not use DUOFILM. Do not use on moles, birthmarks or unusual warts with hair growing from them.
Precautions: For external use only.
DUOFILM is highly flammable and should be kept away from fire or flame. Keep bottle tightly capped when not in use. Store at controlled room temperature.
If spilled on mucous membranes or in eyes, flush with water, remove precipitated collodion and flush with water for an additional 15 minutes.
How Supplied: DUOFILM is available in ½ oz. bottles with plastic applicators.

LASAN® UNGUENT ℞
(formerly Lasan Pomade)

Composition: Lasan Unguent contains 0.4% Anthralin, U.S.P., in a base containing cetyl alcohol, mineral oil and sodium lauryl sulfate with salicylic acid as a preservative.
Actions: Use of Lasan Unguent provides the inhibiting action of Anthralin in an ointment base suitable for skin and scalp usage. Anthralin has been shown to inhibit enzyme metabolism and reduce mitotic turnover.
Indications: Used as an aid in the treatment of psoriasis.

Dosage and Administration: When used on the skin: At bedtime, apply Lasan Unguent carefully to plaque sites, making certain that it does not get on unaffected areas. A protective film of petrolatum applied to the areas surrounding the plaques may be helpful. In the morning, remove any remaining Unguent with warm liquid petrolatum followed by a bath.
When used on the scalp: Massage Lasan Unguent carefully into the affected areas of the scalp. Before applying, a protective film of petrolatum should be applied to the uninvolved scalp margin and ears. Care should be taken to avoid scalp margins and the accumulation of excessive material behind the ears. The scalp should be cleansed the following morning with a shampoo. Tar shampoos, such as Polytar®, may prove to be a useful adjunct.
Treatment should not be discontinued until scales are removed, lesions flattened and no palpable differences exist between the site of the lesions and normal surrounding skin.
Contraindications: Do not use in presence of renal disease or on areas of the skin where inflammation is present. Use only on quiescent or chronic patches and not in acute eruptions.
Precautions: For external use only. Do not permit the product to come in contact with the eyes since conjunctivitis may result. Exercise due care when applying to the face or intertriginous skin areas. If irritation develops or redness is observed on adjacent normal skin, discontinue use and notify physician. Wash hands thoroughly and carefully after using. Anthralin may stain fabrics or skin and may temporarily discolor gray or white hair. Discoloration of hair fades slowly when applications are reduced but the stained keratin at the scalp margins usually desquamates in four to seven days. The use of plastic gloves when applying the Unguent will prevent fingernail staining. The use of a plastic cap at bedtime will prevent staining of the pillow.
How Supplied: 4 ounce jars
Literature Available: Patient Instruction Sheets

PANOXYL® 5, PANOXYL® 10 GELS ℞

Composition: PanOxyl 5 contains 5% Benzoyl Peroxide. PanOxyl 10 contains 10% Benzoyl Peroxide. PanOxyl 5 and PanOxyl 10 also contain 20% ethyl alcohol and polyoxyethylene lauryl ether in a gel base formulated with colloidal magnesium aluminum silicate, hydroxypropylmethylcellulose, citric acid and purified water.
Action and Uses: The topical use of PanOxyl 5 and PanOxyl 10 provides therapeutic control of acne through drying and desquamative action, as well as providing antibacterial activity.
Indications: Use as an aid in the treatment of acne.
Dosage and Administration: Apply 1 or more times daily to affected areas. Washing the face with soap and water prior to application greatly enhances the efficacy of the medication.
Contraindications: Patients with a known sensitivity to benzoyl peroxide should not employ these medications.
Precautions: For external use only. Avoid contact with the eyes or mucosal membranes. Very fair individuals should always be started on a single application at bedtime, allowing the medication to remain on the skin overnight. PanOxyl may bleach colored fabrics.
How Supplied: 2 oz. and 4 oz. plastic tubes.

PANOXYL® AQ 2½ ACNE GEL ℞
PANOXYL® AQ 5 ACNE GEL ℞
PANOXYL® AQ 10 ACNE GEL ℞

Composition: PanOxyl AQ 2½ contains 2½% benzoyl peroxide in a gel base formulated with purified water, polyoxyethylene lauryl ether, propylene glycol, sodium lauryl sulfate, carbomer 934P and di-isopropanolamine.
PanOxyl AQ 5 contains 5% benzoyl peroxide in a gel base formulated with purified water, polyoxyethylene lauryl ether, propylene glycol, sodium lauryl sulfate, carbomer 934P and di-isopropanolamine.
PanOxyl AQ 10 contains 10% benzoyl peroxide in a gel base formulated with purified water, polyoxyethylene lauryl ether, propylene glycol, sodium lauryl sulfate, carbomer 934P and di-isopropanolamine.
Caution: Federal Law prohibits dispensing without a prescription.
Action and Uses: The topical use of PanOxyl AQ 2½, PanOxyl AQ 5, and PanOxyl AQ 10 provides therapeutic control of acne through drying and desquamative action, as well as providing antiseptic activity.
Indications: Use as an aid in the treatment of acne.
Dosage and Administration: After washing as instructed, apply 1 or 2 times daily to affected areas.
Contraindications: Patients with a known sensitivity to benzoyl peroxide should not employ these medications.
Precautions: For external use only. Do not permit products to come in contact with the eyes or mucosal membranes. Keep this and all drugs out of reach of children. Very fair individuals should always be started on a single application at bedtime, allowing the medication to remain on the skin overnight. PanOxyl AQ may bleach hair and colored fabrics. Keep from heat.
Package Information: PanOxyl AQ 2½, PanOxyl AQ 5, and PanOxyl AQ 10 are supplied in 2.0 ounce and 4.0 ounce plastic tubes.

SULFOXYL® LOTION REGULAR ℞
SULFOXYL® LOTION STRONG

Composition: Sulfoxyl Lotion regular contains 5% benzoyl peroxide and 2% sulfur; Sulfoxyl Lotion Strong contains 10% benzoyl peroxide and 5% sulfur, each in a lotion base formulated with polyethylene glycol monostearate, stearic acid, glyceryl monostearate, isopropyl palmitate, propylene glycol, zinc soap and purified water.
Indications: Use as a topical aid in the treatment of acne.
Dosage and Administration: After cleansing the skin, smooth Sulfoxyl Lotion gently into the affected areas, once daily for three days. If no discomfort is felt, frequency of application can then be increased to twice daily. The amount of drying and desquamation can be modified by adjusting the dosage schedule.
Contraindications: Patients with a known sensitivity to benzoyl peroxide, sulfur or any of the other formulation ingredients should not use these medications.
Precautions: For external use only. Avoid contact with eyes, mucous membranes and sensitive areas of the neck. Notify physician if excessive dryness or irritation occurs or increases.
Keep from heat.
Caution: Patients should be warned that these formulations may bleach colored linens, towels and apparel.
How Supplied: 1.0 ounce plastic bottles.

Over 7,000 products are

listed alphabetically

in the

PINK SECTION.

Stuart Pharmaceuticals
Div. of ICI Americas Inc.
WILMINGTON, DELAWARE 19897

ALternaGEL™
Liquid
High-Potency Aluminum Hydroxide Antacid

Composition: ALternaGEL is available as a white, pleasant-tasting, high-potency aluminum hydroxide liquid antacid.
Each 5 ml teaspoonful contains 600 mg aluminum hydroxide (equivalent to dried gel, USP) providing 12 milliequivalents (mEq) of acid-neutralizing capacity (ANC), and less than 2 mg (.087 mEq) of sodium per teaspoonful.
Action and Uses: ALternaGEL is indicated for the symptomatic relief of hyperacidity associated with peptic ulcer, gastritis, peptic esophagitis, gastric hyperacidity, hiatal hernia, and heartburn.
ALternaGEL will be of special value to those patients for whom magnesium-containing antacids are undesirable, such as patients with renal insufficiency, patients requiring control of attendant G.I. complications resulting from steroid or other drug therapy, and patients experiencing the laxation which may result from magnesium or combination antacid regimens.
Dosage and Administration: One or two teaspoonfuls, as needed, between meals and at bedtime, or as directed by a physician. May be followed by a sip of water if desired.
Warnings: As with all medications, ALternaGEL should be kept out of the reach of children.
Except under the advice and supervision of a physician, more than 18 teaspoonfuls should not be taken in a 24-hour period, or the maximum recommended dosage taken for more than two weeks.
ALternaGEL may cause constipation.
Drug Interaction Precaution: ALternaGEL should not be taken concurrently with an antibiotic containing any form of tetracycline.
How Supplied: ALternaGEL is available in bottles of 12 fluid ounces and 5 fluid ounces. NDC 0038-0860.

BUCLADIN®-S SOFTAB™ Tablets ℞
(buclizine hydrochloride)

Description: Buclizine hydrochloride is 1-(p-tert-Butylbenzyl) -4- (p-chloro- α -phenylbenzyl) piperazine dihydrochloride. Each tablet contains 50 mg. buclizine hydrochloride.
Actions: BUCLADIN-S (buclizine hydrochloride) acts centrally to suppress nausea and vomiting.

Indications: Based on a review of this drug by the National Academy of Sciences—National Research Council and/or other information, FDA has classified the indications as follows:
Effective: Management of nausea, vomiting, and dizziness associated with motion sickness.
Possibly Effective: Management of nausea, vomiting, and vertigo which may occur in a variety of conditions including labyrinthitis and Meniere's syndrome.
Final classification of the less than effective indications requires further investigation.

Contraindications: Buclizine hydrochloride, when administered to the pregnant rat, induced fetal abnormalities at doses above the human therapeutic range. Clinical data are not adequate to establish nonteratogenicity in early pregnancy. Until such data are available, buclizine hydrochloride is contraindicated for use in early pregnancy. Buclizine hydrochlo-

Continued on next page

Stuart—Cont.

ride is contraindicated in individuals who have shown a previous hypersensitivity to it.
Warnings: Since drowsiness may occur with use of this drug, patients should be warned of this possibility and cautioned against engaging in activities requiring mental alertness, such as driving a car, or operating heavy machinery or appliances. Safe and effective dosage in children has not been established.
Precaution: This product contains FD&C Yellow #5 (tartrazine) which may cause allergic-type reactions (including bronchial asthma) in certain susceptible individuals. Although the overall incidence of FD&C Yellow #5 (tartrazine) sensitivity in the general population is low, it is frequently seen in patients who also have aspirin hypersensitivity.
Adverse Reactions: Occasionally drowsiness, dryness of mouth, headache, and jitteriness are encountered.
Dosage and Administration: BUCLADIN-S (buclizine hydrochloride) SOFTAB Tablets can be taken without swallowing water. Place the SOFTAB tablet in the mouth and allow it to dissolve, or the tablet may be chewed or swallowed whole.
Adults: One tablet usually serves to alleviate nausea. In severe cases, three tablets a day may be taken. The usual maintenance dosage is one tablet twice daily. In the prevention of motion sickness, one tablet taken at least ½ hour before beginning travel usually suffices. For extended travel, a second tablet may be taken after 4 to 6 hours.
How Supplied: Bottles of 100 scored, yellow, SOFTAB Tablets, embossed front "STUART", reverse "864". NDC 0038-0864.
[*Shown in Product Identification Section*]

CARI-TAB® SOFTAB® Tablets ℞
(fluoride with multivitamins)

Composition: Each tablet contains: Fluoride (as 1.1 mg. sodium fluoride), 0.5 mg.; Vitamin A (as palmitate), 2,000 USP units; Vitamin D (ergocalciferol), 200 USP units; Vitamin C (as ascorbic acid, and sodium ascorbate), 75 mg.
Indications: As an aid in promoting the development of caries-resistant teeth and in preventing deficiencies of vitamins A, D, and C. Controlled studies show that fluoride must be provided in adequate amounts to infants and children by daily dietary supplementation, if natural sources are deficient, through at least the first ten years to achieve maximal anticariogenic effect.
CARI-TAB SOFTAB provides a pleasant tasting, raspberry flavored, convenient form for administering an optimal amount of fluoride and those vitamins which are essential to the formation of normal bones and teeth.
Caution: Dental fluorosis (mottling) may result from exceeding the recommended dose. In hypersensitive individuals, fluorides occasionally cause skin eruptions such as atopic dermatitis, eczema, or urticaria. Gastric distress, headache, and weakness have also been reported. These hypersensitive reactions usually disappear promptly after discontinuation of the fluoride.
Dosage and Administration: Infants and Children under three years of age - one tablet daily. For infant use, tablet should be crushed and mixed with food or formula.
Children three years of age and older - two tablets daily after a meal. Tablets may be chewed or allowed to dissolve in the mouth.
Important Note: A daily fluoride intake of 0.5 mg. from birth through age three years, and 1.0 mg. from three to ten years, either from drinking water or a dietary supplement such as CARI-TAB, is recommended. In areas where the water supply is insufficiently fluoridated, supplemental fluoride dosage must be adjusted accordingly. One quart of water with a fluoride content of one part per million (ppm) provides approximately 1.0 mg. of fluoride. CARI-TAB should not be used in geographical areas in which the concentration of fluoride in the drinking water is greater than 0.7 ppm or the combined daily intake from water and other sources exceeds recommended daily intake.
How Supplied: Bottles of 100 pink colored, scored SOFTAB tablets, embossed front "STUART", reverse "680". NDC 0038-0680.

DIALOSE® Capsules
Stool Softener

Composition: Each capsule contains dioctyl potassium sulfosuccinate, 100 mg.
Action and Uses: DIALOSE is indicated for treating constipation due to hardness, or lack of moisture in the intestinal contents. DIALOSE is an effective stool softener, whose gentle action will help to restore normal bowel function gradually, without griping or acute discomfort.
Dosage and Administration:
Adults: Initially, one capsule three times a day.
Children, 6 years and over: One capsule at bedtime, or as directed by physician.
Children, under 6 years: As directed by physician.
It is helpful to increase the daily intake of fluids by taking a glass of water with each dose. When adequate laxation is obtained, the dose may be adjusted to meet individual needs.
How Supplied: Bottles of 36, 100, and 500 pink capsules, printed "STUART 470". Also available in 100 capsule unit dose boxes (10 strips of 10 capsules each).
NDC 0038-0470.
[*Shown in Product Identification Section*]

DIALOSE® PLUS Capsules
Stool Softener
***plus* Peristaltic Activator**

Composition: Each capsule contains: dioctyl potassium sulfosuccinate, 100 mg. and casanthranol, 30 mg.
Action and Uses: DIALOSE PLUS is indicated for the treatment of constipation generally associated with any of the following: hardness, or lack of moisture in the intestinal contents, or decreased intestinal motility.
DIALOSE PLUS combines the advantages of the stool softener, dioctyl potassium sulfosuccinate, with the peristaltic activating effect of casanthranol.
Warning: As with any laxative, DIALOSE PLUS should not be used when abdominal pain, nausea, or vomiting are present. Frequent or prolonged use may result in dependence on laxatives.
Dosage and Administration:
Adults: Initially, one capsule two times a day.
Children: As directed by physician.
When adequate laxation is obtained the dose may be adjusted to meet individual needs.
It is helpful to increase the daily intake of fluids by taking a glass of water with each dose.
How Supplied: Bottles of 36, 100, and 500 yellow capsules, printed "STUART 475". Also available in 100 capsule unit dose boxes (10 strips of 10 capsules each).
NDC 0038-0475.
[*Shown in Product Identification Section*]

EFFERSYLLIUM® Instant Mix
Bulk Laxative

Composition: Each rounded teaspoonful, or individual packet (7 g.) contains psyllium hydrocolloid, 3 g.
Actions and Uses: EFFERSYLLIUM produces a soft, lubricating bulk which promotes natural elimination.
EFFERSYLLIUM is not a one-dose, fast-acting purgative or cathartic. Administration for several days may be needed to establish regularity.
Effersyllium contains less than 7 mg. sodium per rounded teaspoonful.
Dosage and Administration:
Adults: One rounded teaspoonful, or one packet, in a glass of water one to three times a day, or as directed by physician.
Children, 6 years and over: One level teaspoonful, or one-half packet (3.5 g.) in one-half glass of water at bedtime, or as directed by physician. *Children, under 6 years:* As directed by physician.
Note: To avoid caking, always use a dry spoon to remove EFFERSYLLIUM from its container. Dosage should be placed in a dry glass. Add water, stir and drink immediately. REPLACE CAP TIGHTLY. KEEP IN A DRY PLACE.
Warning: As with all medications, keep out of the reach of children.
How Supplied: Bottles of 9 oz. and 16 oz. of tan, granular powder. Convenient pouch package 7 g. per packet in boxes of 12 or 24.
NDC 0038-0440.

FERANCEE®
Chewable Tablets

Composition: Each tablet contains: iron (from 200 mg. ferrous fumarate), 67 mg. and Vitamin C (as ascorbic acid, 49 mg. and sodium ascorbate, 114 mg.), 150 mg.
Action and Uses: A pleasant tasting hematinic for iron-deficiency anemias, FERANCEE is particularly useful when chronic blood loss, onset of menses, or pregnancy create additional demands for iron supplementation. Because ferrous fumarate is unusually well-tolerated, FERANCEE can be administered between meals when iron absorption is maximal. The peach-cherry flavored chewable tablets dissolve quickly in the mouth and may be either chewed or swallowed.
Dosage and Administration:
Adults: Two tablets daily, or as directed by physician.
Children over 6 years of age: One tablet daily, or as directed by physician.
Children under 6 years of age: As directed by physician.
How Supplied: Bottles of 100 brown and yellow, two-layer tablets embossed "STUART 650" on brown layer. A childproof cap is standard on each bottle as a safeguard against accidental ingestion by children.
NDC 0038-0650.
[*Shown in Product Identification Section*]

FERANCEE®-HP Tablets

Composition: Each tablet contains: iron (from 330 mg. ferrous fumarate), 110 mg.; Vitamin C (as ascorbic acid, 350 mg. and sodium ascorbate, 281 mg.), 600 mg.
Action and Uses: FERANCEE-HP is a high potency formulation of iron and vitamin C and is intended for use as either:
(1) intensive therapy for the acute and/or severe iron deficiency anemia where a high intake of elemental iron is required, or
(2) a maintenance hematinic for those patients needing a daily iron supplement to maintain normal hemoglobin levels.

The use of well-tolerated ferrous fumarate provides high levels of elemental iron with a low incidence of gastric distress. The inclusion of 600 mg. of Vitamin C per tablet serves to maintain more of the iron in the absorbable ferrous state.
Precautions: Because FERANCEE-HP contains 110 mg. of elemental iron per tablet, it is recommended that its use be limited to adults, i.e. over age 12 years. As with all medication, FERANCEE-HP should be kept out of the reach of children.

Dosage and Administration:
For acute and/or severe iron deficiency anemia, two or three tablets per day taken one tablet per dose after meals. (Each tablet provides 110 mg. elemental iron).
For maintenance of normal hemoglobin levels in most patients with a history of recurring iron deficiency anemia, one tablet per day taken after a meal should be sufficient.
How Supplied: FERANCEE-HP is supplied in bottles of 60 red, film coated, oval shaped tablets.
NDC 0038-0863.
Note: A childproof safety cap is standard on each bottle of 60 tablets as a safeguard against accidental ingestion by children.
[*Shown in Product Identification Section*]

HIBICLENS® Antimicrobial Skin Cleanser
(chlorhexidine gluconate)

Description: HIBICLENS is an antimicrobial skin cleanser possessing bactericidal activities. HIBICLENS contains 4% chlorhexidine gluconate, a chemically unique hexamethylenebis (biguanide), in a mild, sudsing base adjusted to pH 5.0–6.5 for optimal activity and stability as well as compatability with the normal pH of the skin.
Action: HIBICLENS is bactericidal on contact and has a persistent antimicrobial effect against a wide range of microorganisms, including gram-positive bacteria, and gram-negative bacteria such as *Pseudomonas aeruginosa*. The effectiveness of HIBICLENS is not signficantly reduced by the presence of organic matter, such as pus or blood.[1]
In a study[2] simulating surgical use, the immediate bactericidal effect of HIBICLENS after a single six-minute scrub resulted in a 99.9% reduction in resident bacterial flora, with a reduction of 99.98% after the eleventh scrub. Reductions on surgically gloved hands were maintained over the six-hour test period.
HIBICLENS displays persistent antimicrobial action. In one study[2], 93% of a radiolabeled formulation of HIBICLENS remained present on uncovered skin after five hours.
Indications: HIBICLENS is indicated for use as a surgical scrub, as a health-care personnel handwash, and as a skin wound cleanser.
Safety: The extensive use of chlorhexidine gluconate for over 20 years outside the United States has produced no evidence of absorption of the compound through intact skin. The potential for producing skin reactions is extremely low. HIBICLENS can be used many times a day without causing irritation, dryness, or discomfort. When used for cleaning superficial wounds, HIBICLENS will neither cause additional tissue injury nor delay healing.
Precautions: HIBICLENS is for topical use only. The sudsing formulation may be irritating to the eyes. If HIBICLENS should get into the eyes, rinse out promptly and thoroughly with water.
Keep out of ears. Chlorhexidine gluconate, like various other antimicrobial agents, has been reported to cause deafness when instilled in the middle ear. In the presence of a perforated eardrum particular care should be taken to prevent exposure of inner ear tissues to HIBICLENS.
HIBICLENS should not be used by persons with sensitivity to any of its components. Adverse reactions, including dermatitis and photosensitivity, are rare, but if they do occur, discontinue use. Keep this and all other drugs out of the reach of children. Avoid excessive heat (104°F).
Directions for Use:
As a surgical scrub: Wet hands and forearms to the elbows with warm water. (Avoid using very cold or very hot water.) Dispense about 5 ml. of HIBICLENS into cupped hands. Spread over both hands. Scrub hands and forearms for 3 minutes without adding water... using a brush or sponge. (Avoid using extremely hard-bristled brushes.) While scrubbing, pay particular attention to fingernails, cuticles, and interdigital spaces. (Do not use pressure to produce additional lather.) Rinse thoroughly with warm water. Dispense about 5 ml. of HIBICLENS into cupped hands. Wash for an additional 3 minutes. (No need to use brush or sponge.) Then rinse thoroughly. Dry thoroughly.
As a health-care personnel handwash: Wet hands with warm water. (Avoid using very cold or very hot water.) Dispense about 5 ml. of HIBICLENS into cupped hands. Wash for 15 seconds. (Do not use excessive pressure to produce additional lather.) Rinse thoroughly with warm water. Dry thoroughly.
As a skin wound cleanser: Rinse the wound area with water. Apply a small amount of HIBICLENS to the wound and wash gently to remove dirt and debris. Rinse again thoroughly.
How Supplied: In plastic disposable bottles: for general handwashing locations, 4 oz. and 8 oz. with dispenser caps, and 16 oz. filled globes; for surgical scrub areas, 32 oz. and 1 gal. The 32 oz. bottle is designed for a special foot-operated wall dispenser. A hand-operated wall dispenser is available for the 16 oz. globe. Hand pumps are available for 16 oz., 32 oz., and 1 gal. sizes. NDC 0038-0575
References:

1. Lowbury, EJL, and Lilly, HA: The effect of blood on disinfection of surgeons' hands, Brit. J. Surg. 61:19–21 (Jan.) 1974.
2. Peterson AF, Rosenberg A, Alatary SD: Comparative evaluation of surgical scrub preparations, Surg. Gynecol. Obstet. 146:63–65 (Jan.) 1978.

[*Shown in Product Identification Section*]

HIBITANE® Tincture (Tinted)
HIBITANE® Tincture (Non-tinted)
(chlorhexidine gluconate)
Patient Preoperative Skin Preparation

Description: HIBITANE Tincture is a patient preoperative skin preparation possessing both a rapid and persistent antimicrobial effect against a wide range of microorganisms. It contains 0.5% chlorhexidine gluconate in 70% isopropyl alcohol.
Actions and Uses: HIBITANE Tincture offers wide-range bactericidal activity for the preparation of the skin at the surgical site and prior to skin puncture or vessel puncture. It provides rapid action on contact and maintains persistent antimicrobial effect, not being significantly affected by pus or blood. HIBITANE Tincture (Tinted) contains a skin colorant to provide visible demarcation of the skin. HIBITANE Tincture (Non-tinted) is slightly colored, but will not tint the skin. Both products are nondetergent and ready to use without dilution.
Cautions: Keep out of eyes and ears. If HIBITANE Tincture should get into eyes or ears, rinse immediately and thoroughly with water. Chlorhexidine gluconate has been reported to cause deafness when instilled in the middle ear through perforated ear drums. Irritation or other adverse reactions such as dermatitis or photosensitivity are rare, but if they do occur, discontinue use. HIBITANE Tincture may be irritating if used on mucosal tissue. Keep this and all other drugs out of the reach of children. Avoid excessive heat (104°F).
Directions for Use: Apply HIBITANE Tincture liberally to surgical site and swab for at least 2 minutes. Dry with a sterile towel. Repeat this procedure for and additional 2 minutes, and allow skin to air dry.
How Supplied: In plastic disposable bottles of 4 oz. and 1 gal.
HIBITANE® Tincture (Tinted) NDC 0038-580
HIBITANE® Tincture (Non-tinted) NDC 0038-583
[*Shown in Product Identification Section*]

KASOF® Capsules
High Strength Stool Softener

Composition: Each KASOF capsule contains dioctyl potassium sulfosuccinate, 240 mg.
Action and Uses: KASOF provides a highly efficient wetting action to restore moisture to the bowel, thus softening the stool to prevent straining. KASOF is especially valuable for the severely constipated, as well as patients with anorectal disorders, such as hemorrhoids and anal fissures. KASOF is ideal for patients with any condition that can be complicated by straining at stool, for example, cardiac patients. The action of KASOF does not interfere with normal peristalsis and generally does not cause griping or extreme sensation of urgency. KASOF is sodium-free, containing a unique potassium formulation, without the problems associated with sodium intake. The simple, one-a-day dosage helps assure patient compliance in maintaining normal bowel function.
Dosage and Administration: Adults: 1 KASOF capsule daily for several days, or until bowel movements are normal and gentle. It is helpful to increase the daily intake of fluids by drinking a glass of water with each dose.
How Supplied: KASOF is available in bottles of 30 and 60 brown, gelatin capsules, printed "Stuart 380".
NDC 0038-0380.
[*Shown in Product Identification Section*]

KINESED® Tablets ℞
(belladonna alkaloids and phenobarbital)

Description: KINESED is a balanced formulation providing the effective spasmolytic and anticholinergic action of the belladonna alkaloids and the sustained sedative effect of phenobarbital.
Composition: Each chewable, fruit-flavored, scored, oval tablet contains:
Phenobarbital........16 mg.
(Warning: May be habit forming)
Hyoscyamine Sulfate........0.1 mg.
Atropine Sulfate........0.02 mg.
Scopolamine Hydrobromide........0.007 mg.
Action: The belladonna alkaloids (atropine sulfate, hyoscyamine sulfate, scopolamine hydrobromide) depress the activity of the post-ganglionic fibers of smooth muscle and secretory glands. Within recommended doses, effects on the central nervous system should be absent or minimal.
Phenobarbital is included to provide a mild sedative effect. The smooth, even sedative action of phenobarbital is well suited for the control of anxiety, tension, or other emotional overlay often associated with many functional disorders.

Indications:
Based on a review of this drug by the National Academy of Sciences—National Research Council, and/or other information, FDA has classified the indications as follows:
Possibly effective as adjunctive therapy in the treatment of peptic ulcer and in the treatment of the irritable bowel syndrome (irritable colon, spastic colon, mucous colitis) and acute enterocolitis.

Contraindications: Contraindicated in patients hypersensitive to belladonna alkaloids or barbiturates, and in patients with glaucoma or advanced hepatic or renal disease.
Precautions: As with any parasympathc lytic agent, administer with caution to patien

Continued on next p

Stuart—Cont.

with incipient glaucoma, bladder neck obstruction, or urinary bladder atony. Prolonged use of barbiturates may result in habituation.
Side Effects: Atropine-like side reactions such as blurred vision, oral dryness, and difficult urination, may occur at high doses, but are only rarely noted at recommended dosages.
Dosage and Administration:
Adults: One or two tablets, three or four times daily; chewed, or swallowed with liquids.
Children, 2 to 12 Years: One-half to one tablet, three or four times daily; chewed, or swallowed with liquids.
How Supplied:
Bottles of 100 and 500 scored, oval, fruit-flavored, orange, chewable tablets, embossed front "STUART," reverse "220." NDC 0038-0220.
[*Shown in Product Identification Section*]

MUCOPLEX® Tablets

Composition: Each tablet contains: Heprofax® (Liver Fraction A, 375 mg. and Liver Fraction 2, 375 mg.), 750 mg.; riboflavin, 1.5 mg.; Vitamin B_{12} (cyanocobalamin), 5 mcg.
Action and Uses: MUCOPLEX is a supplement which provides liver, riboflavin and Vitamin B_{12}.
Heprofax is added to this product as an additional source of Vitamin B Complex factors.
Dosage and Administration: One or two tablets three times daily after meals; or as directed by physician or dentist. Three tablets provide 375% of the Minimum Daily Requirement of riboflavin. The MDR of Vitamin B_{12} has not been determined.
How Supplied: Bottles of 100 brown, capsule-shaped tablets.
NDC 0038-0420.

MULVIDREN® SOFTAB® Tablets

Composition: Each tablet contains: Vitamin A (as palmitate), 4,000 USP units; Vitamin D (ergocalciferol), 400 USP units; Vitamin C (as ascorbic acid, 25 mg. and sodium ascorbate, 56 mg.), 75 mg.; thiamine mononitrate, 2 mg.; riboflavin, 2 mg.; Vitamin B_6 (as pyridoxine hydrochloride), 1.2 mg.; Vitamin B_{12} (cyanocobalamin), 3 mcg.; calcium pantothenate, 3 mg.; niacinamide, 10 mg.
Action and Uses: For daily vitamin supplementation. MULVIDREN is a pleasant tasting SOFTAB tablet specially constructed to dissolve quickly in the mouth, or may be swallowed. If liquid is preferred, dissolve tablet in a teaspoonful of water, or fruit juice.
Dosage and Administration: One tablet daily or as directed by physician.
How Supplied: Bottles of 100 pineapple-flavored SOFTAB tablets, embossed front "STUART", reverse "310".
NDC 0038-0310.

MULVIDREN®-F SOFTAB® Tablets ℞
(fluoride with multivitamins)

Composition: Each tablet contains: fluoride (as 2.2 mg. sodium fluoride), 1 mg.; Vitamin A (as palmitate), 4,000 USP units; Vitamin D (ergocalciferol), 400 USP units; Vitamin C (as ascorbic acid, and sodium ascorbate), 75 mg.; thiamine mononitrate, 2 mg.; riboflavin, 2 mg.; Vitamin B_6 (as pyridoxine hydrochloride), 1.2 mg.; Vitamin B_{12} (cyanocobalamin), 3 mcg.; niacinamide, 10 mg.; calcium pantothenate, 3 mg.
Action and Uses: As an aid in promoting the development of caries-resistant teeth, MULVIDREN-F provides a source of daily fluoride supplementation in addition to full nutritional amounts of vitamins. Controlled studies show that a definite decrease in the incidence of dental caries is obtained in children receiving an optimal nutritional supply of fluoride. These studies indicate that in order to achieve maximal anticariogenic effect, fluoride must be provided throughout the stages of tooth formation and calcification. Thus, fluoride should be provided in adequate amounts to the child from birth through at least the first ten years of life. Fluoride should be made available continuously throughout this period by daily dietary supplementation if natural sources are deficient. MULVIDREN-F SOFTAB is a well-accepted and convenient form of administering fluoride for both topical and systemic effects.
Dosage and Administration: It is necessary to know the fluoride content and the daily intake of drinking water in order to adjust the dosage of this product correctly.
Children, three years of age and older: One tablet daily after a meal. Tablets may be chewed or allowed to dissolve in the mouth.
Infants and Children, under three years of age: One-half tablet daily. For infant use, tablet should be crushed and mixed with food or formula.
Important Note: It is recommended that a daily fluoride intake of 0.5 mg. should be received from birth through the age of three and 1.0 mg. from the age of three to ten years, either from drinking water or from a dietary supplement such as MULVIDREN-F. In areas where fluoride is present in the water supply but in insufficient amounts, the dosage of MULVIDREN-F must be adjusted accordingly. One quart of water with a fluoride content of one part per million (ppm) provides approximately 1.0 mg. of fluoride. MULVIDREN-F should not be used in geographical areas in which the concentration of fluoride in the drinking water is greater than 0.7 ppm or the combined daily intake from water and other sources exceeds recommended daily intake.
Precautions: Dental fluorosis (mottling) may result from exceeding the recommended dose. In hypersensitive individuals, fluorides occasionally cause skin eruptions such as atopic dermatitis, eczema or urticaria. Gastric distress, headache and weakness have also been reported. These hypersensitivity reactions usually disappear promptly after discontinuation of the fluoride. In rare cases, a delay in the eruption of teeth has been reported.
How Supplied: Bottles of 100 orange colored SOFTAB tablets, embossed front "STUART", reverse "710".
NDC 0038-0710.
[*Shown in Product Identification Section*]

MYLANTA®
Liquid and Tablets
Antacid/Antiflatulent

Composition: Each chewable tablet or each 5 ml. (one teaspoonful) of liquid contains:

Aluminum hydroxide (Dried Gel, USP in tablet and equiv. to Dried Gel, USP in liquid)	200 mg.
Magnesium hydroxide	200 mg.
Simethicone	20 mg.

Sodium Content: 0.68 mg. (0.03 mEq) sodium per 5 ml. teaspoonful of liquid; 0.77 mg. (0.03 mEq) per tablet.
Acid Neutralizing Capacity: Each teaspoonful of MYLANTA liuqid will neutralize 12.7 mEq of acid. Each MYLANTA tablet will neutralize 11.5 mEq.
Actions and Uses: MYLANTA, a well-balanced combination of two antacids and simethicone, is effective for the relief of symptoms associated with gastric hyperacidity, and mucus-entrapped air or "gas". These indications include:

- Common heartburn (pyrosis)
- Hiatal hernia
- Peptic esophagitis
- Gastritis
- Peptic ulcer

The soft, easy-to-chew tablets and exceptionally pleasant tasting liquid encourage patients' acceptance, thereby minimizing the skipping of prescribed doses. MYLANTA is appropriate whenever there is a need for effective relief of temporary gastric hyperacidity and mucus-entrapped gas.
Dosage and Administration: One or two teaspoonfuls of liquid or one or two tablets, well-chewed, every two to four hours between meals and at bedtime, or as directed by physician.
Warning: Magnesium hydroxide and other magnesium salts, in the presence of renal insufficiency, may cause central nervous system depression and other symptoms of hypermagnesemia.
Drug Interaction Precaution: Do not use this product for any patient receiving a prescription antibiotic containing any form of tetracycline.
How Supplied: MYLANTA is available as a white, pleasant tasting liquid suspension, and as a two-layer yellow and white chewable tablet, embossed on yellow layer "STUART 620". Liquid supplied in bottles of 5 oz. and 12 oz. Tablets supplied in boxes of individually wrapped 40's and 100's, economy size bottles of 180, and consumer convenience packs of 48. Also available as liquid unit-dose cups of ½ oz. and 1 oz.
NDC 0038-0610 (liquid). NDC 0038-0620 (tablets).
[*Shown in Product Identification Section*]

MYLANTA®-II
Liquid and Tablets
High Potency Antacid/Antiflatulent

Composition: Each chewable tablet or each 5 ml. (one teaspoonful) of liquid contains:

Aluminum hydroxide (Dried Gel, USP in tablet and equiv. to Dried Gel, USP in liquid)	400 mg.
Magnesium hydroxide	400 mg.
Simethicone	30 mg.

Sodium Content: 1.14 mg. (0.05 mEq) sodium per 5 ml. teaspoonful of liquid; 1.3 mg. (0.06 mEq) per tablet.
Acid Neutralizing Capacity: Each teaspoonful of MYLANTA-II liquid will neutralize 25.4 mEq. of acid. Each MYLANTA-II tablet will neutralize 23.0 mEq.
Actions and Uses: MYLANTA-II is a high-potency antacid with an antiflatulent. The soft, easy-to-chew tablets and exceptionally pleasant tasting liquid encourage patient acceptance, thereby minimizing the skipping of prescribed doses. MYLANTA-II is effective in relieving the symptoms of gastric hyperacidity, and mucus-entrapped gas associated with peptic ulcer, and other conditions involving a high output of gastric acid. The high potency of MYLANTA-II is achieved through its concentration of noncalcium antacid ingredients. Thus MYLANTA-II can produce both rapid and long lasting neutralization without the acid rebound associated with calcium carbonate. The balanced formula of aluminum and magnesium hydroxides minimizes undesirable bowel effects. Simethicone is effective for the relief of concomitant symptoms due to mucus-entrapped gas and swallowed air.
Dosage and Administration: One or two teaspoonfuls of liquid, or one or two tablets, well-chewed, between meals and at bedtime, or as directed by physician.
Because patients with peptic ulcer vary greatly in both acid output and gastric emptying time, the amount and schedule of dosages should be varied accordingly.
Warning: Magnesium hydroxide and other magnesium salts, in the presence of renal insufficiency, may cause central nervous system depression and other symptoms of hypermagnesemia.
Drug Interaction Precaution: Do not use this product for any patient receiving a prescription antibiotic containing any form of tetracycline.

How Supplied: MYLANTA-II is available as a white, pleasant tasting liquid suspension, and a two-layer green and white chewable tablet, embossed on green layer "STUART 851". Liquid supplied in 12 oz. bottles. Tablets supplied in boxes of 60 individually wrapped chewable tablets. Also available for hospital use in liquid unit dose cups of ½ oz. and 1 oz., and 5 oz. bottles.
NDC 0038-0852 (liquid). NDC 0038-0851 (tablets).
[Shown in Product Identification Section]

MYLICON® Tablets and Drops
Antiflatulent

Composition: Each tablet or 0.6 ml. of drops contains simethicone, 40 mg.
Action and Uses: For relief of the painful symptoms of excess gas in the digestive tract. MYLICON is a valuable adjunct in the treatment of many conditions in which the retention of gas may be a problem, such as: postoperative gaseous distention, air swallowing, functional dyspepsia, peptic ulcer, spastic or irritable colon, diverticulitis.
The defoaming action of MYLICON relieves flatulence by dispersing and preventing the formation of mucus-surrounded gas pockets in the gastrointestinal tract. MYLICON acts in the stomach and intestines to change the surface tension of gas bubbles enabling them to coalesce; thus the gas is freed and is eliminated more easily by belching or passing flatus.
Dosage and Administration:
Tablets—One or two tablets four times daily after meals and at bedtime. May also be taken as needed or as directed by a physician. TABLETS SHOULD BE CHEWED THOROUGHLY.
Drops—0.6 ml. four times daily after meals and at bedtime. May also be taken as needed or as directed by a physician. Shake well before using.
How Supplied: Bottles of 100 and 500 white, scored, chewable tablets, embossed front "STUART", reverse "450," and dropper bottles of 30 ml. pink, pleasant tasting liquid. Also available in 100 tablet unit dose boxes (10 strips of 10 tablets each).
NDC 0038-0450 (tablets).
NDC 0038-0630 (drops).
[Shown in Product Identification Section]

MYLICON®-80 Tablets
High-Capacity Antiflatulent

Composition: Each tablet contains simethicone, 80 mg.
Action and Uses: For relief of the painful symptoms of excess gas in the digestive tract. MYLICON-80 is a high capacity antiflatulent for adjunctive treatment of many conditions in which the retention of gas may be a problem, such as the following: air swallowing, functional dyspepsia, postoperative gaseous distention, peptic ulcer, spastic or irritable colon, diverticulitis.
MYLICON-80 has a defoaming action that relieves flatulence by dispersing and preventing the formation of mucus-surrounded gas pockets in the gastrointestinal tract. MYLICON-80 acts in the stomach and intestines to change the surface tension of gas bubbles enabling them to coalesce; thus, the gas is freed and is eliminated more easily by belching or passing flatus.
Dosage and Administration: One tablet four times daily after meals and at bedtime. May also be taken as needed or as directed by a physician. TABLETS SHOULD BE CHEWED THOROUGHLY.
How Supplied: Bottles of 100 and economical convenience packages of individually wrapped 12 and 48 pink, scored, chewable tablets embossed "STUART 858". Also available in 100 tablet unit dose boxes (10 strips of 10 tablets each).
NDC 0038-0858.
[Shown in Product Identification Section]

NOLVADEX® 10 mg. Tablets ℞
(tamoxifen citrate)

Description: Nolvadex (tamoxifen citrate) tablets for oral administration contain 15.2 mg. of tamoxifen citrate, which is equivalent to 10 mg. of tamoxifen. It is a nonsteroidal antiestrogen.
Chemically, Nolvadex is the trans-isomer of a triphenylethylene derivative. The chemical name is (Z)-2-[4-(1,2-diphenyl-1-butenyl) phenoxy]-N, N-dimethylethanamine 2-hydroxy-1, 2, 3-propanetricarboxylate(1:1).
Nolvadex is intended only for oral administration; the tablets should be protected from heat and light.
Clinical Pharmacology: Nolvadex is a nonsteroidal agent which has demonstrated potent antiestrogenic properties in animal test systems. The antiestrogenic effects may be related to its ability to compete with estrogen for binding sites in target tissues such as breast. Tamoxifen inhibits the induction of rat mammary carcinoma induced by dimethylbenzanthracene (DMBA), and causes the regression of already established DMBA-induced tumors. In this rat model, tamoxifen appears to exert its antitumor effects by binding to estrogen receptors.
In cytosols derived from human breast adenocarcinomas, tamoxifen competes with estradiol for estrogen receptor protein.
Preliminary pharmacokinetics in women using radio-labeled tamoxifen has shown that most of the radioactivity is slowly excreted in the feces, with only small amounts appearing in urine. The drug is excreted mainly as conjugates, with unchanged drug and hydroxylated metabolites accounting for 30% of the total.
Blood levels of total radioactivity following single oral doses of approximately 0.3 mg./kg. reached peak values of 0.06–0.14 μg/ml. at 4–7 hours after dosing, with only 20–30% of the drug present as tamoxifen. There was an initial half-life of 7–14 hours with secondary peaks four or more days later. The prolongation of blood levels and fecal excretion is believed to be due to enterohepatic circulation.
Indications and Usage: Nolvadex has proven useful in the palliative treatment of advanced breast cancer in postmenopausal women. Available evidence indicates that patients who have had a recent negative estrogen receptor assay are unlikely to respond to Nolvadex.
Contraindications: There are no known contraindications to the use of Nolvadex.
Warnings: Nolvadex may have oncogenic activity in animals; the possibility of this potential in humans should be considered. Safe use in pregnancy has not been established. Nolvadex is teratogenic in rats and rabbits with evidence of skeletal abnormalities. Nolvadex also affects reproductive functions in rats at dose levels somewhat higher than the human dose. Safe use in pregnancy has not been established.
Ocular changes have been reported in a few patients treated for periods greater than one year with Nolvadex at doses at least four times the highest recommended daily dose of 40 mg. The ocular changes consist of retinopathy and, in some patients, there are also corneal changes and a decrease in visual acuity. Ophthalmologic examinations of selected patients receiving long-term therapy with Nolvadex at recommended doses have not detected any ocular pathology attributable to the drug.
As with other additive hormonal therapy (estrogens and androgens), hypercalcemia has been reported in some breast cancer patients with bone metastases within a few weeks of starting treatment with Nolvadex. If hypercalcemia does occur, appropriate measures should be taken and, if severe, Nolvadex should be discontinued.
Precautions: Nolvadex should be used cautiously in patients with existing leukopenia or thrombocytopenia. Observations of leukopenia and thrombocytopenia occasionally have been made, but it is uncertain if these effects are due to Nolvadex therapy. Transient decreases in platelet counts, usually to 50,000–100,000/ cu. mm., infrequently lower, have been occasionally reported in patients taking Nolvadex for breast cancer. No hemorrhagic tendency has been recorded and the platelet counts returned to normal levels even though treatment with Nolvadex continued. Periodic complete blood counts, including platelet counts, may be appropriate.
Usage in Pregnancy: Safe use in pregnancy has not been established.
Adverse Reactions: The most frequent adverse reactions to Nolvadex are hot flashes, nausea, and vomiting. These may occur in up to one-fourth of patients, but are rarely severe enough to require discontinuation of treatment.
Less frequently reported adverse reactions are vaginal bleeding, vaginal discharge, menstrual irregularities, and skin rash. Usually these have not been of sufficient severity to require dosage reduction or discontinuation of treatment.
Increased bone and tumor pain, and also local disease flare have occurred, which are sometimes associated with a good tumor response. Patients with increased bone pain may require additional analgesics. Patients with soft tissue disease may have sudden increases in the size of preexisting lesions, sometimes associated with marked erythema within and surrounding the lesions, and/or the development of new lesions. When they occur, the bone pain or disease flare are seen shortly after starting Nolvadex and generally subside rapidly.
Other adverse reactions which are seen infrequently are hypercalcemia, peripheral edema, distaste for food, pruritus vulvae, depression, dizziness, light-headedness, and headache.
If adverse reactions are severe, it is sometimes possible to control them by a simple reduction of dosage without loss of control of the disease.
Overdosage: Overdosage in humans has not been reported. Doses up to 100 mg./m²b.i.d. have been used in clinical trials with no appreciable increase in serious adverse reactions over those reported at recommended dosage. Signs observed at the highest doses following studies to determine LD_{50} in animals were respiratory difficulties and convulsions. No specific treatment for overdosage is known; treatment must be symptomatic.
Dosage and Administration: One or two 10 mg. tablets twice a day (morning and evening).
How Supplied: Nolvadex tablets are white, round, biconvex tablets, embossed "Stuart 600," containing tamoxifen as the citrate in an amount equivalent to 10 mg. of tamoxifen. The tablets are available in bottles of 60 and 250 tablets. The tablets should be protected from heat and light. NDC0038-0600.
[Shown in Product Identification Section]

OREXIN® SOFTAB® Tablets

Composition: Each tablet contains: thiamine mononitrate, 10 mg.; Vitamin B_6 (as pyridoxine hydrochloride), 5 mg.; and Vitamin B_{12} (cyanocobalamin), 25 mcg.
Action and Uses: OREXIN is a high-potency vitamin supplement providing thiamine mononitrate and Vitamins B_6 and B_{12}.
OREXIN SOFTAB tablets are specially formulated to dissolve quickly in the mouth. They may be chewed or swallowed. Dissolve tablet in a teaspoonful of water or fruit juice if liquid is preferred.

Continued on next page

Stuart—Cont.

Dosage and Administration: One tablet daily, or as directed by physician.
How Supplied: Bottles of 100 pale pink SOF-TAB tablets, embossed "STUART".
NDC 0038-0280

PROBEC®-T Tablets

Composition: Each tablet contains: Vitamin C (as ascorbic acid, 67 mg. and sodium ascorbate, 600 mg.), 600 mg.; thiamine mononitrate, 15 mg.; riboflavin, 10 mg.; Vitamin B_6 (as pyridoxine hydrochloride), 5 mg.; Vitamin B_{12} (cyanocobalamin), 5 mcg.; niacinamide, 100 mg.; calcium pantothenate, 20 mg.
Action and Uses: PROBEC-T is a high-potency B complex supplement with 600 mg. of Vitamin C in easy to swallow odorless tablets.
Dosage and Administration: One tablet a day with a meal, or as directed by physician.
How Supplied: Bottles of 60, salmon colored, capsule-shaped tablets.
NDC 0038-0840.
[*Shown in Product Identification Section*]

SORBITRATE® Tablets ℞
(isosorbide dinitrate)

Description: SORBITRATE (isosorbide dinitrate) is an organic nitrate that is designated chemically as 1,4:3,6-dianhydrosorbitol-2,5-dinitrate.
The potency of the following available ascorbic acid, 67 mg. maintained under normal ascorbate, 600 mg.),
CHEWABLE SORBITRATE
5 mg. Chewable Tablets. Each green, round, scored tablet contains 5 mg. of isosorbide dinitrate.
10 mg. Chewable Tablets. Each yellow, round, scored tablet contains 10 mg. of isosorbide dinitrate.
SORBITRATE Sublingual
2.5 mg. Sublingual Tablets. Each white, round tablet contains 2.5 mg. of isosorbide dinitrate.
5 mg. Sublingual Tablets. Each pink, round tablet contains 5 mg. of isosorbide dinitrate.
SORBITRATE Oral
5 mg. Oral Tablets. Each green, oval-shaped, scored tablet contains 5 mg. of isosorbide dinitrate.
10 mg. Oral Tablets. Each yellow, oval-shaped, scored tablet contains 10 mg. of isosorbide dinitrate.
20 mg. Oral Tablets. Each blue, oval-shaped, scored tablet contains 20 mg. of isosorbide dinitrate.
SORBITRATE SA
Sustained Action Tablets. Each yellow, round 40 mg. compression coated tablet contains 10 mg. isosorbide dinitrate in the outer coat and 30 mg. in the inner core (sustained action base).
Mode of Action: The mechanism of action of SORBITRATE (isosorbide dinitrate) in the relief of angina pectoris is unknown at this time, although the basic pharmacologic action is to relax smooth muscle.
Since therapy at the present time is essentially empirical, clinical improvement is generally measured by a decrease in the severity of the symptoms of angina pectoris and the need for medication. Specifically, SORBITRATE reduces in number and severity the incidence of angina pectoris attacks, with concomitant reduction in nitroglycerin intake.
In the evaluation of isosorbide dinitrate in angina pectoris, clinical improvement has been customarily measured subjectively. Individual patterns of angina pectoris differ widely as does the symptomatic response to antianginal agents. In conjunction with the total management of patients with angina pectoris, isosorbide dinitrate has been generally accepted as safe and widely regarded as useful.

Indications:
Based on a review of this drug by The National Academy of Sciences—National Research Council and/or other information, FDA has classified the indications as follows:
Probably effective: Sublingual and chewable dosage forms of SORBITRATE are indicated for the treatment of acute anginal attacks and for prophylaxis in situations likely to provoke such attacks.

Possibly effective: Oral dosage forms of SORBITRATE are indicated for the relief of angina pectoris (pain of coronary artery disease). They are not intended to abort the acute anginal episode, but they are widely regarded as useful in the prophylactic treatment of angina pectoris.
Final classification of the less-than-effective indications requires further investigation.

Contraindications: A history of sensitivity to the drug.
Warnings: Data supporting the use of nitrates during the early days of the acute phase of myocardial infarction (the period during which clinical and laboratory findings are unstable) are insufficient to establish safety.
Precautions: Tolerance to this drug and cross tolerance to other nitrites and nitrates may occur. All SORBITRATE forms (except Sublinguals and 20 mg. Oral) contain FD&C Yellow No. 5 (tartrazine) which may cause allergic-type reactions (including bronchial asthma) in certain susceptible individuals. Although the overall incidence of FD&C Yellow No. 5 (tartrazine) sensitivity in the general population is low, it is frequently seen in patients who also have aspirin hypersensitivity.
Adverse Reactions: Headache is the most common adverse reaction and may be severe and persistent. Lowering the dose and the use of analgesics will help control the headaches which usually diminish or disappear as therapy is continued. Cutaneous vasodilation with flushing may occur. Transient episodes of dizziness and weakness, as well as other signs of cerebral ischemia associated with postural hypotension, may occasionally develop. This drug can act as a physiological antagonist to norepinephrine, acetylcholine, histamine, and many other agents. An occasional individual exhibits marked sensitivity to the hypotensive effects of nitrates and severe responses (nausea, vomiting, weakness, restlessness, pallor, perspiration, and collapse) can occur even with the usual therapeutic dose. Alcohol may enhance this effect. Drug rash and/or exfoliative dermatitis may occasionally occur.
Dosage and Administration:
Route: Chewable, sublingual, sustained action, and oral tablets.
Initiating Therapy: In starting patients on SORBITRATE (isosorbide dinitrate) it is necessary to adjust the dosage until the smallest effective dose is determined. This is of particular importance in employing chewable tablets. Occasionally, severe hypotensive responses may occur with this dosage form, even with doses as low as 5 mg.
Individual Dose: 2.5 to 10 mg. is the range commonly used although doses up to 30 mg. have frequently been employed. The oral and chewable tablets are scored for more accurate dosage adjustment when necessary. The usual dose for sustained action tablets is one 40 mg. tablet.
Dosage Schedule: Smallest effective dose necessary for the prevention and treatment of pain of an anginal attack. CHEWABLE SORBITRATE and SORBITRATE Sublingual may be taken P.R.N. for prompt relief of anginal pain, or at 4 to 6 hour intervals. SORBITRATE Oral may be taken 3 to 4 times daily. SORBITRATE SA sustained action oral tablets may be taken at 12 hour intervals. Although the onset of effect and the duration of effect of coronary nitrates may be quite variable, following are the generally reported ranges of these values for SORBITRATE.
Onset of Effect:
Chewable and Sublingual: 2 to 5 minutes
Oral and Sustained Action: 15 to 30 minutes
Duration of Effect:
Chewable and Sublingual: 1 to 2 hours
Oral: Estimated to be 4 to 6 hours
Sustained Action: Estimated to be up to 12 hours at a continuous controlled rate
It is recommended that the oral dosage be taken on an empty stomach. If vascular headache cannot be effectively controlled by ordinary measures, dosages may be taken with meals to minimize this side effect.
How Supplied: CHEWABLE SORBITRATE (isosorbide dinitrate) **5 mg.** green, round, scored tablets (embossed front "STUART", reverse "810") are supplied in bottles of 100 and 500. Also available in unit dose packages of 100. NDC 0038-0810.
CHEWABLE SORBITRATE (isosorbide dinitrate) **10 mg.** yellow, round, scored tablets (embossed front "STUART," reverse "815") are supplied in bottles of 100. Also available in unit dose packages of 100. NDC 0038-0815.
SORBITRATE (isosorbide dinitrate) **Sublingual 2.5 mg.** white, round tablets are supplied in bottles of 100 and 500. Also available in unit dose packages of 100. NDC 0038-0853.
SORBITRATE (isosorbide dinitrate) **Sublingual 5 mg.** pink, round tablets are supplied in bottles of 100 and 500. Also available in unit dose packages of 100. NDC 0038-0760.
SORBITRATE (isosorbide dinitrate) **Oral 5 mg.** green, oval-shaped, scored tablets (embossed front "STUART", reverse "770") are supplied in bottles of 100 and 500. Also available in unit dose packages of 100. NDC 0038-0770.
SORBITRATE (isosorbide dinitrate) **Oral 10 mg.** yellow, oval-shaped, scored tablets (embossed front "STUART", reverse "780") are supplied in bottles of 100 and 500. Also available in unit dose packages of 100. NDC 0038-0780.
SORBITRATE (isosorbide dinitrate) **Oral 20 mg.** blue, oval-shaped, scored tablets (embossed front "STUART", reverse "820") are supplied in bottles of 100. Also available in unit dose packages of 100. NDC 0038-0820.
SORBITRATE SA (isosorbide dinitrate) **Oral Sustained Action 40 mg.** yellow, round tablets (embossed front "STUART", reverse "880") are supplied in bottles of 100. Also available in unit dose packages of 100. NDC 0038-0880.
[*Shown in Product Identification Section*]

THE STUART FORMULA® Liquid

Composition: Each teaspoonful (5 ml.) contains:
__Vitamins:__ Vitamin A (as palmitate), 3,333 USP units; Vitamin D (ergocalciferol), 333 USP units; thiamine hydrochloride, 1.33 mg.; riboflavin, 1.33 mg.; Vitamin B_6 (as pyridoxine hydrochloride), 0.067 mg.; niacin and niacinamide, 10 mg.; panthenol, 1.43 mg.; Vitamin E (d-alpha tocopheryl as acetate) 0.1 I.U.
__Minerals:__ iron (from 25 mg. ferrous sulfate), 5 mg.; manganese (from manganese sulfate), 0.33 mg.
The above ingredients are supplied in a malt base which provides natural B-complex vitamins.
Actions and Uses: The STUART FORMULA Liquid provides a balanced formula at the maintenance level, including B-complex.
Dosage and Administration: One teaspoonful (5 ml.) daily or as directed by physician. Best taken after meals.
How Supplied: In 16 oz. pint bottles of amber colored liquid. A childproof safety cap is stan-

dard on each 16 oz. bottle as a safeguard against accidental ingestion by children.
NDC 0038-0010.

THE STUART FORMULA® Tablets

Composition: Each tablet contains:
Vitamins: Vitamin A (as palmitate), 5000 I.U.; Vitamin D (ergocalciferol), 400 I.U.; Vitamin E (as dl-alpha tocopheryl acetate), 15 I.U.; Vitamin C (as ascorbic acid), 60 mg.; folic acid, 0.4 mg.; thiamine (as thiamine mononitrate), 1.5 mg.; riboflavin, 1.7 mg.; niacin (as niacinamide), 20 mg.; Vitamin B_6 (as pyridoxine hydrochloride), 2 mg.; Vitamin B_{12} (cyanocobalamin), 6 mcg.
Minerals: calcium 160 mg.; phosphorus, 125 mg.; iodine, 150 mcg.; iron (from 54 mg. ferrous fumarate) 18 mg.; magnesium, 100 mg.
Actions and Uses: The STUART FORMULA tablet provides a well-balanced multivitamin/multimineral formula intended for use as a daily dietary supplement for adults and children over age four.
Dosage and Administration: One tablet daily or as directed by a physician.
How Supplied: Bottles of 100, 250 and 500 white round tablets. Childproof safety caps are standard on the 100 and 250 tablet bottles as a safeguard against accidental ingestion by children.
NDC 0038-0866
[Shown in Product Identification Section]

STUART HEMATINIC® Liquid

Composition: Each teaspoonful (5 ml.) contains: iron (from 190 mg. ferrous gluconate), 22 mg.; Liver Fraction 1, 54 mg.; thiamine hydrochloride, 1.7 mg.; riboflavin, 1.7 mg.; Vitamin B_6 (as pyridoxine hydrochloride), 0.5 mg.; niacinamide, 10 mg.; panthenol, 1.43 mg.
Action and Uses: For the treatment of iron deficiency anemia and deficiencies of B-complex vitamins. Contains ferrous gluconate, a well-tolerated source of iron. Liver Fraction 1 is added to this product as an additional source of vitamin B-complex factors. A pleasant tasting hematinic liquid.
Dosage and Administration:
Adults: Two tablespoonfuls (30 ml.) daily.
Children, over 6 years: Three teaspoonfuls (15 ml.) daily.
Children, 2 to 6 years: Two teaspoonfuls (10 ml.) daily.
Infants to 2 years: As directed by physician.
It is suggested that the daily dosage be divided into two or three equal portions, each portion to be taken with or after a meal and followed by water.
How Supplied: 16 oz. pint bottles of caramel-colored liquid. A childproof safety cap is standard on each 16 oz. bottle as a safeguard against accidental ingestion by children.
NDC 0038-0050.

STUART PRENATAL® Tablets

Composition: Each tablet contains:

Vitamins:	% U.S. RDA*	
A (as acetate)	100%	8,000 I.U.
D (ergocalciferol)	100%	400 I.U.
E (as dl-alpha tocopheryl acetate)	100%	30 I.U.
C (ascorbic acid)	100%	60 mg.
Folic Acid	100%	0.8 mg.
Thiamine (as thiamine mononitrate)	100%	1.7 mg.
Riboflavin	100%	2 mg.
Niacin (as niacinamide)	100%	20 mg.
B_6 (as pyridoxine hydrochloride)	160%	4 mg.
B_{12} (cyanocobalamin)	100%	8 mcg.
Minerals:		
Calcium (from 679 mg. calcium sulfate anhydrous)	15%	200 mg.
Iodine (from potassium iodide)	100%	150 mcg.
Iron (from 182 mg. ferrous fumarate)	333%	60 mg.
Magnesium (from magnesium oxide)	22%	100 mg.

* Recommended Daily Allowance
Action and Uses: STUART PRENATAL is a multivitamin/multimineral supplement for pregnant and lactating women. It provides vitamins equal to 100% or more of the U.S. RDA for pregnant and lactating women, plus essential minerals, including 60 mg. of elemental iron as well-tolerated ferrous fumarate, and 200 mg. of elemental calcium (non-alkalizing and phosphorus-free). Stuart Prenatal also contains .8 mg. folic acid.
Dosage and Administration: During and after pregnancy, one tablet daily after a meal, or as directed by a physician.
How Supplied: Bottles of 100 and 500 pink capsule-shaped tablets. A childproof safety cap is standard on 100 tablet bottles as a safeguard against accidental ingestion by children.
NDC 0038-0270.
(Shown in Product Identification Section)

STUART PRENATAL® with Folic Acid Tablets ℞

Composition: Each tablet contains:
Vitamins: Vitamin A (as acetate), 6,000 USP units; Vitamin D (ergocalciferol), 400 USP Units; Vitamin C (ascorbic acid), 100 mg.; thiamine mononitrate, 3 mg.; riboflavin, 3 mg.; Vitamin B_6 (as pyridoxine hydrochloride), 10 mg.; Vitamin B_{12} (cyanocobalamin), 5 mcg.; niacinamide, 20 mg.; calcium pantothenate, 5.44 mg.; folic acid, 0.3 mg.
Minerals: iron (from 197 mg. ferrous fumarate), 65 mg.; calcium (from 1.2 g. calcium sulfate anhydrous), 350 mg.
Action and Uses: STUART PRENATAL with FOLIC ACID is indicated in pregnancy and during lactation to provide vitamin and mineral nutritional supplementation. Each tablet provides 350 mg. phosphorus-free calcium, and 65 mg. elemental iron. STUART PRENATAL with FOLIC ACID is high in pyridoxine hydrochloride and Vitamin C. Folic acid is added to aid in the prevention of megaloblastic anemia.
Precaution: Folic acid may partially correct the hematological damage due to Vitamin B_{12} deficiency of pernicious anemia, while the associated neurological damage progresses.
Dosage and Administration: One tablet daily, to be taken after a meal, or as directed by physician.
How Supplied: Bottles of 100 light blue colored capsule-shaped tablets. A childproof safety cap is standard on each 100 tablet bottle as a safeguard against accidental ingestion by children.
NDC 0038-0800.
[Shown in Product Identification Section]

STUART THERAPEUTIC® Multivitamin Tablets

Composition: Each tablet contains: Vitamin A (as acetate), 10,000 USP units; Vitamin D (ergocalciferol), 400 USP units; Vitamin C (as ascorbic acid, 22 mg. and sodium ascorbate, 200 mg.), 200 mg.; thiamine mononitrate, 10 mg.; riboflavin, 10 mg.; Vitamin B_6 (as pyridoxine hydrochloride), 5 mg.; Vitamin B_{12} (cyanocobalamin), 5 mcg.; niacinamide, 100 mg.; calcium pantothenate, 20 mg.
Action and Uses:
STUART THERAPEUTIC MULTIVITAMIN is a high-potency, multivitamin supplement in small, easy to swallow, capsule-shaped tablets.
Dosage and Administration: One tablet daily. Do not exceed stated dosage except on the advice of a physician.
How Supplied: Bottles of 100 deep orange, small, capsule-shaped tablets.
NDC 0038-0060.

STUARTINIC® Tablets

Composition: Each tablet contains: iron (from 300 mg. ferrous fumarate), 100 mg.; Vitamin C (as ascorbic acid, 300 mg. and sodium ascorbate, 225 mg.), 500 mg.; Vitamin B_{12} (cyanocobalamin), 25 mcg.; thiamine mononitrate, 6 mg.; riboflavin, 6 mg.; Vitamin B_6 (as pyridoxine hydrochloride), 1 mg.; niacinamide, 20 mg.; calcium pantothenate, 10 mg.
Action and Uses: STUARTINIC is a complete hematinic for patients with history of iron deficiency anemia who also lack adequate amounts of B-complex vitamins due to poor diet.
The use of well-tolerated ferrous fumarate in STUARTINIC provides a high level of elemental iron with a low incidence of gastric distress. The inclusion of 500 mg. of Vitamin C per tablet serves to maintain more of the iron in the absorbable ferrous state. The B-complex vitamins improve nutrition where B-complex deficient diets contribute to the anemia.
Precautions: Because STUARTINIC contains 100 mg. of elemental iron per tablet, use should be confined to adults, i.e. over age 12 years. As with all medications, STUARTINIC should be kept out of the reach of children.
Dosage and Administration: One tablet daily taken after a meal to maintain normal hemoglobin levels in most patients with chronic iron deficiency anemia resulting from inadequate diet. Higher doses of STUARTINIC can be taken as directed by the physician.
How Supplied: STUARTINIC is supplied in bottles of 60 and 500 yellow, film coated, oval shaped tablets. NDC 0038-0862.
Note: A childproof safety cap is standard on each bottle of 60 tablets. The physician should prescribe or recommend the bottle of 60 tablets, where appropriate, to provide that additional safeguard against accidental ingestion by children.
[Shown in Product Identification Section]

STUARTNATAL® 1+1 Tablets ℞

Composition: Each tablet contains:

Vitamins:	% U.S. RDA*	
A (as acetate)	100%	8,000 I.U.
D (ergocalciferol)	100%	400 I.U.
E (as dl-alpha tocopheryl acetate)	100%	30 I.U.
C (ascorbic acid)	150%	90 mg.
Folic Acid	125%	1 mg.
Thiamine (as thiamine mononitrate)	150%	2.55 mg.
Riboflavin	150%	3 mg.
Niacin (as niacinamide)	100%	20 mg.
B_6 (as pyridoxine hydrochloride)	400%	10 mg.
B_{12} (cyanocobalamin)	150%	12 mcg.
Minerals:		
Calcium (from 679 mg. calcium sulfate anhydrous)	15%	200 mg.
Iodine (from potassium iodide)	100%	150 mcg.
Iron (from 197 mg. ferrous fumarate)	361%	65 mg.
Magnesium (from magnesium oxide)	22%	100 mg.

*Recommended Daily Allowance
Action and Uses: STUARTNATAL 1+1 is indicated to provide more potent vitamin and mineral supplementation throughout pregnancy and during the postnatal period—for both the lactating and non-lactating mother. Each tablet provides vitamins equal to 100% or more of U.S. RDA for pregnant and lactating women plus essential minerals, including 1 full grain of elemental iron and 200 mg. of elemen-

Continued on next page

Stuart—Cont.

tal calcium (non-alkalizing and phosphorus-free). STUARTNATAL 1+1 also offers 1 mg. folic acid to aid in the prevention of megaloblastic anemia.
Precaution: Folic acid may partially correct the hematological damage due to Vitamin B_{12} deficiency of pernicious anemia, while the associated neurological damage progresses.
Dosage and Administration: During and after pregnancy, one tablet daily after a meal, or as directed by a physician.
How Supplied: Bottles of 100 and 500 light yellow capsule-shaped tablets. A childproof safety cap is standard on 100 tablet bottles as a safeguard against accidental ingestion by children.
NDC 0038-0850.
(Shown in Product Identification Section)

THERON® Tablets

Composition: Each tablet contains:
Vitamins: Vitamin A (as acetate), 10,000 USP Units; Vitamin D (ergocalciferol), 400 USP units; Vitamin C (as ascorbic acid, 34 mg. and sodium ascorbate, 300 mg.), 300 mg.; thiamine mononitrate, 15 mg.; riboflavin, 10 mg.; Vitamin B_6 (as pyridoxine hydrochloride), 5 mg.; Vitamin B_{12} (cyanocobalamin), 5 mcg.; niacinamide, 100 mg.; calcium pantothenate, 20 mg.
Minerals: calcium (from calcium sulfate), 100 mg.; iron (from 45 mg. ferrous fumarate), 15 mg.; manganese (from manganese sulfate), 1 mg.; zinc (from zinc sulfate), 1.5 mg.
Action and Uses: THERON is a high-potency multivitamin supplement with minerals added in easy to take, capsule-shaped tablet form.
Dosage and Administration: One tablet daily. Do not exceed stated dosage except on the advice of a physician.
How Supplied: Bottles of 100 peach, capsule-shaped tablets.
NDC 0038-0230.

SugarLo Company

3540 ATLANTIC AVENUE
POST OFFICE BOX 1017
ATLANTIC CITY, NJ 08404

LACTAID®
(lactase enzyme)

Description: Each 5 drop dosage contains not less than 1000 NLU (Neutral Lactase Units) of Beta-D-galactosidase derived from Kluyveromyces lactis yeast. The enzyme is in a liquid carrier of glycerol (50%), water (30%), and inert yeast dry matter (20%) 4–5 drops hydrolyzes approximately 70% of the lactose in 1 quart of milk at refrigerator temperature, @ 42°F–6°C in 24 hours, or will do the same in 2 hours @ 85°F–30°C. Additional time and/or enzyme required for 100% lactose conversion. 1 U.S. quart of milk will contain approximately 50 gm lactose prior to lactose hydrolysis and will contain 15 gm or less, after. Hydrolysis converts the lactose into its simple sugar components, glucose and galactose.
Actions: Converts the disaccharide lactose into its monosugar components, glucose and galactose.
Indications: Lactase insufficiency in the patient, suspected from g.i. disturbances after consumption of milk or milk content products: e.g., bloat, distension, flatulence, diarrhea; or identified by a lactose tolerance test.
Precautions: Diabetics should be aware that the milk sugar will now be metabolically available and must be taken into account (25 gm glucose and 25 gm galactose per quart). No reports received of any diabetics' reactions. Galactosemics may not have milk in any form, lactase enzyme modified or not.
Usage: Added to milk. 4–5 drops per quart depending on level of lactose conversion desired.
Toxicity: Animal studies @ 4% of enzyme by body weight (equivalent of 24,000-5 drop dosages in a 50-kilo human) showed no effects. LD_{50} not achievable. LactAid is not a drug but a food which modifies another food to make it more digestible.
Other Uses: Veterinary indications: treatment of milk for animals with gastric surgery; sick young animals; sick or healthy older animals.
How Supplied: Retail sale units of 4, 12 or 30 dosages at 5 drops per dose. Bulk institutional size also available. Sample and full product information to doctors, dietitians and institutions, on request. Also from dairies in some locations in U.S. as ready to drink hydrolyzed LactAid milk, with the enzyme modification having been done at the dairy to a 70% conversion level. Persons who find this 70% level to be inadequate can further modify the milk at home by utilizing the LactAid liquid drops covered in this description. Any person unable to locate LactAid in the store can order direct from SugarLo Company at retail.

Surgikos

A Johnson & Johnson Company
501 GEORGE STREET
NEW BRUNSWICK, NJ 08903

SURGICEL™ Absorbable Hemostat ℞
(oxidized regenerated cellulose)
For surgical use

(For dental applications of this product, reference should be made to the package insert for dental use.)

Description: SURGICEL Absorbable Hemostat is a chemically-sterilized, absorbable knitted fabric prepared by the controlled oxidation of regenerated cellulose. The fabric is white with a pale yellow cast and has a faint, caramel-like aroma. It is strong and can be sutured or cut without fraying. It is stable and can be stored at controlled room temperature. A slight discoloration may occur with age, but this does not affect performance.
Actions: The mechanism of action whereby SURGICEL accelerates clotting is not completely understood, but it appears to be a physical effect rather than any alteration of the normal physiologic clotting mechanism. After SURGICEL Absorbable Hemostat has been saturated with blood, it swells into a brownish or black gelatinous mass which aids in the formation of a clot, thereby serving as a hemostatic adjunct in the control of local hemorrhage. When used properly in minimal amounts, SURGICEL is absorbed from the sites of implantation with practically no tissue reaction. Absorption depends upon several factors including the amount used, degree of saturation with blood, and the tissue bed.
Indications: SURGICEL Absorbable Hemostat (oxidized regenerated cellulose) is used adjunctively in surgical procedures to assist in the control of capillary, venous, and small arterial hemorrhage when ligation or other conventional methods of control are impractical or ineffective.
Contraindications: Although packing or wadding sometimes is medically necessary, SURGICEL Absorbable Hemostat should not be used in this manner unless it is to be removed after hemostasis is achieved.
SURGICEL should not be used for implantation in bone defects, such as fractures, since there is a possibility of interference with callus formation and a theoretical chance of cyst formation.
When SURGICEL is used to help achieve hemostasis around the spinal cord in laminectomies, or around the optic nerve and chiasm, it must always be removed after hemostasis is achieved since it will swell and could exert unwanted pressure.
SURGICEL should not be used to control hemorrhage from large arteries.
SURGICEL should not be used on non-hemorrhagic serous oozing surfaces, since body fluids other than whole blood, such as serum, do not react with SURGICEL to produce satisfactory hemostatic effect.
Warnings: SURGICEL Absorbable Hemostat is supplied sterile and should not be autoclaved because autoclaving causes physical breakdown of the product.
SURGICEL is not intended as a substitute for careful surgery and the proper use of sutures and ligatures.
Closing SURGICEL in a contaminated wound without drainage may lead to complications and should be avoided.
The hemostatic effect of SURGICEL is greater when it is applied dry; therefore it should not be moistened with water or saline.
SURGICEL should not be impregnated with anti-infective agents or with other materials such as buffering or hemostatic substances. Its hemostatic effect is not enhanced by the addition of thrombin, the activity of which is destroyed by the low pH of the product.
Although SURGICEL Absorbable Hemostat may be left *in situ* when necessary, it is advisable to remove it once hemostasis is achieved. It *must* always be removed from the site of application after use in laminectomy procedures and from foramina in bone when hemostasis is obtained. This is because SURGICEL, by swelling, may cause nerve damage by pressure in a bony confine. Paralysis has been reported when used around the spinal cord, particularly in surgery for herniated intervertebral disc.
Precautions: Use only as much SURGICEL Absorbable Hemostat as is necessary for hemostasis, holding it in place until bleeding stops. Remove any excess before surgical closure in order to facilitate absorption and minimize the possibility of foreign body reaction.
SURGICEL should be applied loosely against the bleeding surface. Wadding or packing should be avoided, especially within rigid cavities, where swelling may interfere with normal function or possibly cause necrosis.
In urological procedures, minimal amounts of SURGICEL should be used and care must be exercised to prevent plugging of the urethra, ureter, or a catheter by dislodged portions of the product.
Since absorption of SURGICEL could be prevented in chemically cauterized areas, its use should not be preceded by application of silver nitrate or any other escharotic chemicals.
If SURGICEL is used temporarily to line the cavity of large open wounds, it should be placed so as not to overlap the skin edges. It should also be removed from open wounds by forceps or by irrigation with sterile water or saline solution after bleeding has stopped.
Precautions should be taken in otorhinolaryngologic surgery to assure that none of the material is aspirated by the patient. (Examples: controlling hemorrhage after tonsillectomy and controlling epistaxis.)
Care should be taken not to apply SURGICEL too tightly when it is used as a wrap during vascular surgery (See "ADVERSE REACTIONS" section).
Adverse Reactions: "Encapsulation" of fluid and foreign body reactions have been reported. There have been two reports of stenotic effect when SURGICEL Absorbable Hemostat has been applied as a wrap during vascular surgery. Although it has not been established that the stenosis was directly related to the use of SURGICEL, it is important to be cautious and avoid applying the material tightly as a wrapping.
Possible prolongation of drainage in cholecystectomies and difficulty passing urine per urethra after prostatectomy have been reported.

There has been one report of a blocked ureter after kidney resection, in which postoperative catheterization was required.
Occasional reports of "burning" and "stinging" sensations and sneezing when SURGICEL has been used as packing in epistaxis, are believed due to the low pH of the product.
Burning has been reported when SURGICEL was applied after nasal polyp removal and after hemorrhoidectomy. Headache, burning, stinging, and sneezing in epistaxis and other rhinological procedures, and stinging when SURGICEL was applied on surface wounds (varicose ulcerations, dermabrasions, and donor sites) also have been reported.
Dosage and Administration: Sterile technique should be observed in removing SURGICEL Absorbable Hemostat from its container. The glass container should be wiped with antiseptic. The cap should then be removed and SURGICEL withdrawn from the container with dry sterile forceps. Minimal amounts of SURGICEL of appropriate size are laid on the bleeding site or held firmly against the tissues until hemostasis is obtained.
Opened, unused SURGICEL should be discarded, because it cannot be resterilized.
How Supplied: Sterile SURGICEL Absorbable Hemostat (oxidized regenerated cellulose) is supplied as knitted fabric strips in sealed glass vials in the following sizes:
2″ × 14″
4″ × 8″
2″ × 3″
½″ × 2″

Clinical Studies: SURGICEL Absorbable Hemostat (oxidized regenerated cellulose) has been found useful in helping to control capillary or venous bleeding in a variety of surgical applications, including abdominal, thoracic, neurosurgical, and orthopedic, as well as in otorhinolaryngologic procedures. Examples include gallbladder surgery, partial hepatectomy, hemorrhoidectomy, resections or injuries of the pancreas, spleen, kidney, prostate, bowel, breast or thyroid, and in amputations.[1,3]
SURGICEL has been applied as a surface dressing on donor sites and superficial open wounds, controlling bleeding adequately, and causing no delay in healing or interference with epithelization.[4,6] It also has been applied after dermabrasion, punch biopsy, excision biopsy, curettage, finger and toenail removal, and to traumatic wounds. In the foregoing applications, bleeding was controlled and the SURGICEL was absorbed from the sites where it was applied.[5]
In cardiovascular surgery, investigators have found SURGICEL useful in helping to control bleeding from implanted textile grafts, including those of the abdominal aorta.[2,7] Such grafts may leak or weep considerably, even when preclotted, but this seepage can be controlled by covering the graft with a layer or two of SURGICEL after the graft is in place and before releasing the proximal and distal clamps. When the flow has been reestablished and all bleeding controlled, the fabric either can be removed or left *in situ*, since absorption of SURGICEL has been shown to occur without constriction of the graft or other untoward incident when proper wrapping technique is employed.
Otorhinolaryngologic experience with SURGICEL includes adjunctive use in controlling bleeding resulting from epistaxis, tonsillectomy, adenoidectomy, removal of nasal polyps, repair of deviated septum, tympanoplasty, stapes surgery, surgery for sinusitis, and removal of tumors.[8,9]
SURGICEL has been reported useful as a hemostatic adjunct in such gynecologic procedures as oophorectomy, hysterectomy, conization of the cervix, and repair of cystorectocele.[1,10]

References:

1. Degenshein, G., Hurwitz, A., and S. Ribacoff: Experience with regenerated oxidized cellulose. ***New York State Journal of Medicine 63*** (18):2639-2643, 1963.
2. Hurwitt, E.: A new absorbable hemostatic packing. ***Bulletin de la Societe Internationale de Chirurgie XXI*** (3):237-242, 1962.
3. Venn, R.: Reduction of postsurgical blood-replacement needs with Surgicel hemostatis. ***Medical Times 93*** (10):1113-1116, 1965.
4. Miller, J., Ginsberg, M., McElfatrick, G., and H. Johnson: Clinical experience with oxidized regenerated cellulose. ***Experimental Medicine and Surgery 19*** (2-3):202-206, (June-Sept.) 1961.
5. Blau, S., Kanof, N., and L. Simonson: Absorbable hemostatic gauze SURGICEL in dermabrasions and dermatologic surgery. ***Acta Dermato-Venerelogica 40*** :358-361, 1960.
6. Shea, P., Jr.: Management of the donor site: a new dressing technic. ***Journal of the Medical Association of Georgia 51*** (9):437-440, 1962.
7. Denck, H.: Use of resorbable oxycellulose in surgery. ***Chirurg 33*** (11):486-488, 1962.
8. Tibbels, E., Jr.: Evaluation of a new method of epistaxis management. ***Laryngoscope LXXIII*** (3):306-314, 1963.
9. Huggins, S.: Control of hemorrhage in otorhinolaryngologic surgery with oxidized regenerated cellulose. ***Eye, Ear, Nose and Throat Monthly 48*** (7):(July) 1969.
10. Crisp, W. E. Shalauta, H., and W. A. Bennett: Shallow conization of the cervix. ***Obstetrics and Gynecology 31*** (6):755-758, 1968.

SURGIKOS ARTEGRAFT*

Description: The SURGIKOS Artegraft** is composed of a section of specially selected bovine carotid artery which has been subjected to enzymatic digestion with ficin and tanned with dialdehyde starch.
Actions: The function and action of the artegraft is simply to serve as a substitute conduit for blood where bypass or replacement of occluded or diseased arterial segments is required or to establish a conduit for hemodialysis.
Indications: The artegraft is intended for use distal to the aorta as a segmental arterial replacement, as an arterial bypass, as an arteriovenous shunt where more conventional methods have proven inadequate, or as an arterial patch graft.
The use of the artegraft for femoropopliteal bypass should be reserved for those patients where the autologous saphenous vein is absent or inadequate. It is also not recommended for reconstruction across the knee joint. However, in the absence of other viable alternatives, the surgeon may well find the benefit to risk ratio warrants its use as an attempted limb salvage procedure.
Contraindications:
1. The SURGIKOS Artegraft should not be used in venous or low pressure systems.
2. Once the package seal is broken, the graft should be used immediately; any left-over material should be discarded.
3. The graft should not be used after the expiration date imprinted on the label; this is based on a period of three years from the date of manufacture.

Warnings:
1. After the artegraft has been removed from the container in the manner prescribed to preserve its sterility, it should be gently and thoroughly washed and rinsed to minimize carry-over of preserving fluid. For aseptic removal and wash procedures, please see DOSAGE AND ADMINISTRATION Section.
2. Silk is not recommended for anastomosis. This suture occasionally was found to give rise to thick suture-line pannus in the dog.
3. The prosthesis is not to be used unless the capacity of the run-off vessel is adequate, as shown by pre-operative arteriography. Artegraft selection must be of comparable cross-sectional diameter to the host artery, particularly at the distal end, in order to avoid early thrombosis.
4. A minimum of ten days should be allowed after implantation before puncturing the graft with needles for hemodialysis. If edema appears around or distal to the graft, this should be allowed to resolve before cannulation.
5. Thrombosis of the graft has been reported from inadvertent external compression. Patients and those administering dialysis should be cautioned against compression of the graft for prolonged periods.

Precautions:
1. In the event of early occlusion, re-exploration of the graft and removal of the thrombus with a Fogarty catheter or other means often results in effective restoration of long-term patency. This procedure is somewhat easier to perform in the case of the artegraft than with other prostheses.
2. Some surgeons recommend systemic heparinization of the patient after completion of the preparatory dissection, with or without subsequent neutralization with protamine sulfate. Others rely on the periodic injection of diluted heparin into the arterial tree during the period of vascular clamping and anastomosis. Post-operative heparinization is usually not employed.
3. During implantation, scrupulous technic is essential to avoid twisting and to achieve meticulous approximation at the suture lines.
4. Clinical evidence suggests that subfascial, rather than subcutaneous, implantation in the lower extremity is the more satisfactory procedure.

For precautions regarding true aneurysms, please see ADVERSE REACTIONS Section.
Adverse Reactions: Pseudointima formation and less frequently pseudodiaphragm formation may occur. Disruption of anastomoses, especially in the presence of infection, has been observed. In a few cases, transient low grade fever, the etiology of which has not been obvious, has been experienced. In humans, immunologically-mediated rejection of the artegraft has not been demonstrated.
An occasional true aneurysm has been reported (in a recent survey, the cumulative average incidence of true aneurysms in artegraft was found to be about 5% in 5 years, based upon life table methods). In view of this, patients with implanted artegrafts should be observed so that appropriate action can be taken if an aneurysm should occur. For the same reason, the artegraft is not recommended for use in the young, where there is a long life expectancy.
The complications encountered when the artegraft is used as an A-V shunt for dialysis include thrombosis, infection, aneurysm, and bleeding and/or hematoma. The true incidence of these will vary depending upon the frequency with which the graft is needle-punctured, the length of time the graft has been implanted and, very importantly, the condition of the patient, since the graft is recommended for use when more conventional measures prove inadequate. Less frequent complications include "steal syndrome", and, in patients with heart disease, a significant incidence of high output congestive heart failure secondary to an arteriovenous shunt.
Dosage and Administration: To remove the artegraft aseptically from its glass container, the container should be held in a semi-upright position. After carefully removing the cap without contaminating the rim of the con-

Continued on next page

Surgikos—Cont.

tainer, the mandrel supporting the graft and the graft itself should be lifted from the vial with a long fine-tipped thumb forcep. As soon as the graft itself becomes accessible, it should be grasped and removed from the vial with the mandrel, care being taken not to touch the outside rim of the vial.
The surgeon should immerse the graft in a large basin of sterile 0.9% sodium chloride solution and using a syringe irrigates the graft's lumen at least seven or eight times with sterile 0.9% sodium chloride solution. A final irrigation and immersion should be performed in heparin-saline solution (2,500 units of heparin in 4 oz. of sterile 0.9% sodium chloride solution). The graft is now considered ready for insertion into the patient.
The graft number and its length and diameter should be recorded on the patient's chart, as well as the actual length of graft inserted into the patient.
Since the SURGIKOS Artegraft is intended as a conduit for arterial blood, no specific rules can be laid down as to the number and size of artegrafts to be used in any given case, since individual requirements will vary widely.
However, in meeting specific exigencies, accepted vascular surgical techniques should be employed, including the use of non-crushing clamps to control the host artery and very gentle handling of the ends of the graft itself. Precise anastomosis without tension, bulging or twisting is mandatory.
The use of fine non-cutting rather than cutting-type needles helps avoid trouble-some punctate bleeding at the anastomotic sites, particularly in the smaller diameter grafts.
If troublesome bleeding does occur, it may readily be controlled by simply applying a small bit of artegraft as a patch to the bleeding area in a reverse manner so that adventitia is in direct contact with adventitia.
In order to avoid possible snarling of the suture in the rather shaggy adventitia of the graft, it has been found convenient to start the stitch in the host artery rather than starting it in the graft. In so doing, care should be exercised to avoid the possibility of displacing an atheromatous plaque.
How Supplied: The SURGIKOS Artegraft is packaged in a specially designed glass tube containing a sterilizing solution prepared with one per cent propylene oxide in 40 per cent aqueous U.S.P. ethyl alcohol. Each tube is enclosed in a foam lined set-up box for protection during shipment and storage.
The length and outside diameter of each artegraft are specified on the box and tube labels. The internal diameter of the artegraft is approximately 1mm less than the outside diameter. The availability of graft diameters and lengths are dependent upon the animal source. Diameters of 6mm to 10mm and lengths of 20cm to 45cm are readily available upon request. Artegrafts with 5mm diameters are sometimes available in limited quantities. Grafts longer than 45cm (48cm maximum) are sometimes available.
The approximate desired length and diameter of each graft should be specified when ordering; the nearest available size will be supplied.

*U.S. Adopted Name for arterial graft of bovine origin.
**U.S. Patent No. 3,093,439.

Survival Technology, Inc.
7801 WOODMONT AVENUE
BETHESDA, MD 20014

LIDOPEN® Auto-Injector ℞
Lidocaine Hydrochloride for Intramuscular Injection
for Cardiac Arrhythmias
LIDOPEN®
lidocaine hydrochloride 300 mg. (3 ml. 10% solution)
Differs from U.S.P.: pH 3.7–5.7

Description: Lidocaine hydrochloride: acetamide, 2- (diethylamino)- N- (2, 6-dimethylphenyl)-, monohydrochloride.
Lidocaine Hydrochloride Injection, intramuscular for Cardiac Arrhythmias, is a sterile solution prepared from lidocaine with the aid of hydrochloric acid in water for injection.
Each LidoPen® contains 300 mg. lidocaine hydrochloride, 3 mg. disodium edetate, 3 mg. methylparaben, sodium hydroxide in sufficient quantity to adjust pH to 5.2 in 3.0 ml. water for injection.
Actions: Lidocaine hydrochloride is reported to increase the electrical stimulation threshold of the ventricle during diastole and, thereby, exert an antiarrhythmic effect. In the dosage recommended, lidocaine hydrochloride produces no change in systolic arterial blood pressure, absolute refractory period, or myocardial contractility.
Clinical studies in which cardiac arrhythmias were monitored indicated that the onset and duration of antiarrhythmic activity of intramuscular lidocaine hydrochloride are correlated with the attained blood levels of lidocaine hydrochloride.
The relative blood levels in normal volunteers obtained by a "conventional" intravenous infusion and following the LidoPen® Auto-Injector can be determined by reference to the accompanying chart.
Approximately 90% of an administered dose of lidocaine hydrochloride is metabolized in the liver. Less than 10% of the drug is excreted unchanged via the kidneys.
Indications: Lidocaine hydrochloride is indicated in the management of cardiac arrhythmias, particularly those of ventricular origin, such as occur with acute myocardial infarction.

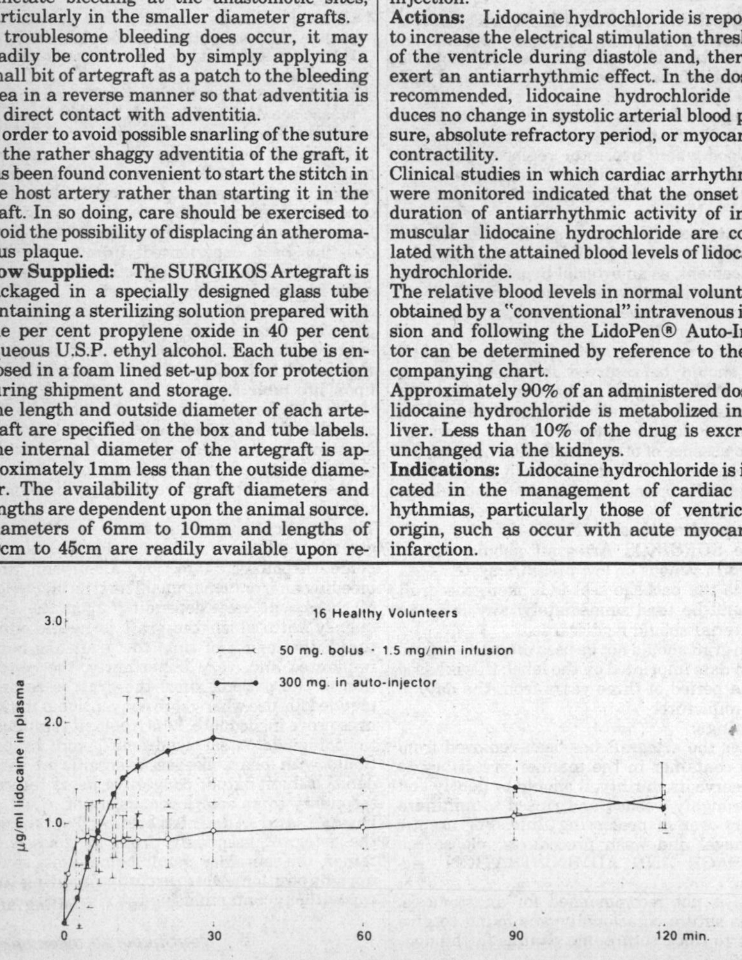

The selection of the intramuscular route of administration (single dose) is justified in the following circumstances:
1. By a physician in whose opinion the potential benefits outweigh the possible risks even when ECG equipment is not available to verify the arrhythmia.
2. By, or under the supervision of, a physician, including mobile coronary care units, when facilities for intravenous administration are not readily available; or under circumstances where maintaining continuous intravenous therapy is difficult or impossible.
3. For use in the prehospital phase of suspected acute myocardial infarction by a patient who has transmitted his electrocardiogram with a CardioBeeper®, whose electrocardiogram demonstrates the presence of a ventricular arrhythmia and who is instructed to self-administer the LidoPen® Auto-Injector by qualified medical personnel.

Contraindications: Lidocaine hydrochloride is contraindicated in patients with known hypersensitivity to local anesthetics of the amide type; in patients with STOKES-ADAMS Syndrome, Wolff-Parkinson-White Syndrome; or severe degrees of sinoatrial, atrioventricular, or intraventricular block.
Warnings: EVERY EFFORT SHOULD BE MADE TO AVOID POSSIBLE INADVERTENT INTRAVASCULAR ADMINISTRATION THROUGH APPROPRIATE SELECTION OF INJECTION SITE SUCH AS THIGH OR DELTOID. DO NOT INJECT INTO BUTTOCK. Monitoring with an electrocardiograph is recommended when lidocaine hydrochloride is administered by the intramuscular route. In emergency situations when a ventricular rhythm disorder is suspected and electrocardiographic equipment is not available, a single dose may be administered when the physician in attendance has determined that the potential benefits outweigh the possible risks. If possible, emergency resuscitative equipment and drugs should be immediately available to manage potential adverse reactions involving the cardiovascular, respiratory, or central nervous system.
Occasional acceleration of ventricular rate may occur when lidocaine hydrochloride is administered to patients with atrial fibrillation.
The intramuscular use of lidocaine hydrochloride may result in an increase in creatine phosphokinase levels. Thus, the use of the enzyme determination without isoenzyme separation, as a diagnostic test for the presence of acute myocardial infarction, may be compromised by the use of intramuscular lidocaine hydrochloride.
Usage in Pregnancy: It is not known whether lidocaine hydrochloride may have adverse effects upon fetal development. The benefits of the drug to the mother should be weighed against possible risk to the fetus.
Usage in Children: Intramuscular lidocaine hydrochloride is not recommended for pediatric use, since evidence concerning proper use in children is not available.
Precautions: Caution should be employed in the repeated use of lidocaine hydrochloride in patients with severe liver or renal disease because accumulation may occur and lead to toxic phenomena since lidocaine hydrochloride is metabolized mainly in the liver and excreted by the kidneys. This drug should also be used with caution in patients with hypovolemia and shock and all forms of heart block. (See Contraindications and Warnings.)
Adverse Reactions: The following types of systemic reactions have been reported with lidocaine hydrochloride administration:
1. Central Nervous System: light-headedness; drowsiness; dizziness; apprehension; euphoria; tinnitus; blurred or double vision; vomiting; sensations of heat, cold or

numbness; twitching; tremors; convulsions; unconsciousness; respiratory depression and arrest.
2. Cardiovascular System: hypotension; bradycardia; cardiovascular collapse and cardiac arrest.
3. Allergic reactions may occur but are infrequent. There have been no reports of cross-sensitivity between lidocaine hydrochloride and procainamide or between lidocaine hydrochloride and quinidine.

Soreness at the injection site following intramuscular injections has occasionally been reported.

Management of Adverse Reactions:
1. In the case of severe reaction, do not continue or repeat administration of the drug.
2. Institute emergency resuscitative procedures including maintenance of patient airway and cardiopulmonary resuscitation if required.
3. For severe convulsions, parenteral administration of a rapidly acting anticonvulsant may be used by persons appropriately trained in the use of these drugs and the management of the cardiovascular and respiratory depression which may result. Resuscitative equipment should be available.

Dosage and Administration: A physician who prescribes this device for the patient must take appropriate steps to insure that his patient understands the indications and use of this device including review with the patient, in detail, the patient package insert and operation of the Auto-Injector.
Inject the contents of 1 LidoPen® Auto-Injector (300 mg. lidocaine hydrochloride, 3 ml, 10% solution) intramuscularly into the anterolateral aspect of the thigh or deltoid region of the arm. See Detailed Instructions below.
As soon as possible, and when indicated, patients should be changed to an intravenous infusion of lidocaine hydrochloride or to an oral antiarrhythmic preparation for maintenance therapy. However, if necessary, an additional intramuscular injection may be made after an interval of 60–90 minutes. IT SHOULD BE MADE CLEAR TO THE PATIENT THAT THIS SECOND INJECTION SHOULD NOT BE MADE WITHOUT FURTHER INSTRUCTION BY QUALIFIED MEDICAL PERSONNEL.
Detailed Instructions: (See Directions for Use in the PATIENT INFORMATION AND INSTRUCTIONS Section.)
PATIENT INFORMATION AND INSTRUCTIONS FOR SELF-ADMINISTRATION OF THE LidoPen® Auto-Injector BY PATIENTS EQUIPPED WITH A CardioBeeper®.
A separate booklet containing this information will be made available to the patient.
Introduction: As part of the early management of a heart attack, your physician has prescribed for you a drug—lidocaine hydrochloride contained in an automatic injector—The LidoPen® Auto-Injector.
This drug has been shown to be valuable in the management of certain abnormal heart rhythms which sometimes accompany heart attacks. As with all other drugs, it is not without risk. UNDER NO CIRCUMSTANCES SHOULD IT BE USED WITHOUT SPECIFIC INSTRUCTIONS TO DO SO BY QUALIFIED MEDICAL PERSONNEL.
Therefore, your physician has taken steps to provide you with a CardioBeeper® with which to transmit your heart rate and rhythm by conventional telephone.
Be certain to review the information contained in this booklet and practice with the use of the CardioBeeper®.
The LidoPen® Auto-Injector: The LidoPen® Auto-Injector is a disposable, prefilled automatic injection device containing 300 mg. lidocaine hydrochloride.
- Keep the LidoPen® Auto-Injector with you at all times.
- It should not be kept in excessive heat or cold.
- You should note the expiration date on the LidoPen® Auto-Injector and make sure yours is replaced prior to that date.

When to Use the LidoPen® Auto-Injector: If you experience the signs and symptoms described to you by your physician as suggesting a possible heart attack, immediately telephone your physician, or center designated by your physician, and transmit your electrocardiogram by CardioBeeper®. You will then be instructed whether or not you are to use the LidoPen® Auto-Injector, and what else you should do.
Directions for Use: When, as described above, you have been instructed to use the LidoPen® Auto-Injector, proceed as follows:
1. Remove gray safety.
2. Place black end on thickest part of thigh and press hard till injector functions.
3. Hold firmly in place for ten seconds, then remove. Massage the area of injection for 10 seconds.

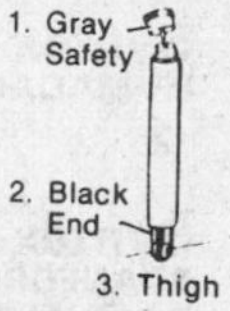

UNLESS ABSOLUTELY NECESSARY, DO NOT ATTEMPT TO OPERATE A MOTOR VEHICLE AFTER USE OF THE Lido-Pen® Auto-Injector.
Proceed as instructed by physician.
How Supplied: Packages containing 4 LidoPen® Auto Injectors and 1 Training Aid Auto Injector or Box of 12 LidoPen® Auto Injectors. NDC 11704-221-02
[Shown in Product Identification Section]

Sween Corporation
P.O. BOX 3404
MANKATO, MN 56001

FORDUSTIN'®
Body Powder

Composition: A non-caking natural corn starch based body powder with methylbenzethonium chloride 1:1200. National Drug Code 11701-005.
Action and Uses: Lubrication of skin subject to excoriation from friction. Helps absorb perspiration to aid in the protection of the skin from perspiration irritation.
Precautions and Adverse Reactions: None. Transmission electron microscopy and electron diffraction examinations of Fordustin' powder found the product free of any form of fibrous material (asbestiform minerals included) or inorganic materials.
Administration and Dosage: Apply liberally to areas subject to friction and perspiration irritations.
How Supplied: 8-oz. and 3-oz. containers.

PERI–CARE®
Water Resistant Ointment for Perineal Protection

Composition: A soft petrolatum ointment with parachlorometaxylenol, casein, natural vitamins A and D, and methylbenzethonium chloride. National Drug Code 11701-010.
Action and Uses: Used in the perineal area, Peri-Care provides a protective barrier against urine, feces, and post operative drainage.
Contraindications: None.
Precautions and Adverse Reactions: For external use only. Peri-Care ointment is not an eye or a skin irritant, nor is it toxic by oral ingestion (LD_{50} found to be greater than 40 ml/kg body weight).
Administration and Dosage: Apply liberally in the perineal area for protection from yeast infections when medications are given, and to protect perineal area against fecal enzymes, and urine.
How Supplied: 2-oz. and 8-oz. jars.

PERI-WASH®
Perineal Area Cleanser

Composition: A skin surfactant and feces and urine emulsifier with methylbenzethonium chloride 1:1200. Normal pH. National Drug Code 11701-014.
Action and Uses: Peri-Wash is used for daily care of the perineal area. It is indicated for cleansing of perineal areas afflicted with dermatitis and ammonia dermatitis associated with diarrhea. Through the process of emulsification, Peri-Wash makes the removal of fecal matter from the skin easier, thereby reducing the irritation and formation of denuded skin around the anus. Peri-Wash reduces or eliminates the ammonia odors from urine or feces. Peri-Wash is used for cleansing peristomal skin, in ostomy appliances and urine collecting appliances for control of offensive odors. Additional uses for odor control: Cleaning bed pans, urinals, wheel chairs, soiled linens and garments, and hands.
Precautions and Adverse Reactions: For external use only. Use should be discontinued if irritation develops. Peri-Wash is not a skin irritant, nor is it toxic by oral ingestion (LD_{50} found to be 16.2 ml/kg body weight. Peri-Wash is an eye irritant (sodium lauryl sulfate) and should be rinsed thoroughly from eyes if accidental contact occurs.
Administration and Dosage: Apply liberally to perineal area. Wash and rinse with clean warm water in the normal manner.
How Supplied: 4 fl. oz. and 8 fl. oz. bottles with spray fitment, in addition to larger bulk sizes.

SURGI–KLEEN™
Skin cleanser and shampoo

Description: Surfactants blended with lanolin derivatives and Methylbenzethonium Chloride with a normal pH. Rinses free easily to insure that no residues remain on the skin or in the hair. National Drug Code 11701-003.
Directions: Surgi-Kleen may be used full strength or diluted one part to three parts of water.
For Regular Bathing: Apply diluted product to moistened wash cloth and gently wash skin, rinse and pat dry.
For Shampooing: Apply diluted or undiluted to moistened hair. Massage hair and scalp until lather develops. Then rinse and lather again. A very small quantity of Surgi-Kleen will develop a thick, rich lather when hair is clean.
Precautions and Adverse Reactions: For external use only. Use should be discontinued if irritation develops. Surgi-Kleen is not a skin irritant, nor is it toxic by oral ingestion (LD_{50} found to be greater than 16 ml/kg body weight). Surgi-Kleen is an eye irritant (sodium lauryl sulfate) and should be rinsed thoroughly from eyes if accidental contact occurs.
How Supplied: 16 fl. oz. bottles with flip-top caps, in addition to larger bulk sizes.

SWEEN CREAM™
Protective Cream

Composition: A vanishing cream with methylbenzethonium chloride, dewaxed fraction of lanolin, and natural vitamins A and D. National Drug Code 11701-002.
Action and Uses: Sween Cream is used for long-term care of incontinent, geriatric, ostomy, and para/quadraplegic skin. Apply as needed to red, sore, irritated skin such as urine scald, diaper rash, diarrheal breakdowns, rectal itch, psoriasis, minor burns, chaffing and

Continued on next page

Sween—Cont.

itching. Also apply to folds of skin subject to perspiration irritation, to dry or cracked skin and to pressure sore areas. For ostomy patients, apply a small amount around stoma area before attaching appliance to protect skin, relieve itching, and improve tape adhesion.
Precautions and Adverse Reactions: For external use only. Use should be discontinued if irritation or other signs develop. Sween Cream is not an eye or skin irritant nor is it toxic by oral ingestion (LD_{50} greater than 40 ml/kg body weight).
Administration and Dosage: Apply liberally as required.
How Supplied: 2-oz. and 9-oz. jars.

SWEEN KARAYA POWDER—ANTIMICROBIAL

Composition: Karaya gum powder with parachlorametaxylenol. National Drug Code 11701-019.
Action and Uses: Sween karaya gum powder is antimicrobial against a broad range of pathogens. For more detailed information, refer to package inserts and literature. Sween Karaya Powder is hygroscopic and provides a protective barrier when used in the treatment of abraded or excoriated skin.
Precautions: For external use only. If irritation develops, discontinue use immediately and consult physician. Keep away from eyes. Keep out of reach of children.
How Supplied: 85-gm. containers with fliptop.

WHIRL-SOL®
Skin Conditioner

Composition: Mineral oil, peg-6 oleate, lanolin oil, D&C green number 6. National Drug Code 11701-001.
Action and Uses: Whirl-Sol is a completely water dispersible oil easily absorbed by the skin to aid in the relief of dry, pruritic conditions. Whirl-Sol helps soothe and restore skin to a more elastic and pliable condition. It is an effective aid in treating skin problems such as soap dermatitis, pruritus senilis and hiemalis, chronic atopic dermatitis, asteatosis, xerosis, ichthyosis, psoriasis, etc. Whirl-Sol promotes a normal healthy skin with natural-like oils.
Administration: Whirl-Sol is always used with water. It is added, one or two capfuls to whirlpool bathing systems, regular bath tubs, or wash basins. Apply to washcloth for use in the shower.
Precautions: Guard against slipping in tub or shower. Whirl-Sol is not an eye or a skin irritant, nor is it toxic by oral ingestion. The acute oral LD_{50} was found to be greater than 40 ml/kg body weight.
How Supplied: 8 fl. oz. and 16 fl. oz. bottles in addition to larger bulk sizes.

XTRACARE® II
Moisturizing Body Lotion

Composition: A thick-bodied, high moisturizing cream consisting of water, cetyl alcohol, propylene glycol, lanolin oil, beeswax, sodium lauryl sulfate, Quaternium-15, fragrance and methylbenzethonium chloride.
National Drug Code 11701-004.
Action and Uses: Xtracare II is an unusually rich moisturizer which serves as an exceptional massage vehicle for the entire body. Its creamy consistency applies easily and uniformly to soothe and moisturize skin. The special emollient and humectant properties provide long lasting retardation of skin moisture evaporation. This leaves the skin feeling smooth, cool and comfortable without greasiness and tackiness or interference of normal skin respiration. Apply as needed for back rubs, dry skin problems and physical therapy. Especially suited for foot and lower leg care. Liberal application recommended before applying plaster casts.
Contraindications: None.
Precautions and Adverse Reactions: For External Use Only. Xtracare II is not a primary skin or eye irritant, nor is it toxic by oral ingestion.
Administration and Dosage: Apply liberally as often as needed for dry skin management. Use as a massage lubricant for back rubs and for therapeutic muscle massage.
How Supplied: 4 fl. oz. and 8 fl. oz. bottles with dispenser caps, in addition to larger bulk sizes.

Syntex (F.P.) Inc.
HUMACAO, PUERTO RICO 00661

Syntex Laboratories, Inc
STANFORD INDUSTRIAL PARK
PALO ALTO, CA 94304

Syntex Puerto Rico, Inc.
HUMACAO, PUERTO RICO 00661

ANADROL®-50 ℞
(oxymetholone)
50 mg. Tablets

A product of Syntex Laboratories, Inc.

Description: Anadrol-50 contains 50 mg. of the steroid, oxymetholone, which has the chemical name 17 β-hydroxy-2-(hydroxymethylene)-17-methyl-5α-androstan-3-one.
Action: Anadrol-50 is a potent anabolic and androgenic drug. It enhances the production and urinary excretion of erythropoietin in patients with anemias due to bone marrow failure and often stimulates erythropoiesis in anemias due to deficient red cell production.
Indications: Anadrol-50 is indicated in the treatment of anemias caused by deficient red cell production. Acquired aplastic anemia, congenital aplastic anemia, myelofibrosis and the hypoplastic anemias due to the administration of myelotoxic drugs often respond. Anadrol-50 should not replace other supportive measures such as transfusion, correction of iron, folic acid, vitamin B_{12} or pyridoxine deficiency, antibacterial therapy and the appropriate use of corticosteroids.
Contraindications: Since anabolic agents are generally contraindicated in the following situations, before instituting therapy, the clinician must weigh the risk involved against the patients' needs.

1. Carcinoma of the prostate or breast in male patients.
2. Pregnancy—primarily because of masculinization of the fetus.
3. Infancy. Since evidence of beneficial effect in prematures and newborns is lacking, and consequences of the use of anabolic steroids in these patients are unknown, their use is not recommended.
4. Nephrosis or the nephrotic phase of nephritis.
5. Hypersensitivity.
6. Hepatic dysfunction.

Warnings: Anabolic steroids do not enhance athletic ability.
Precautions:
1. *Hepatotoxicity*
Hepatotoxic effects, including jaundice, are common with the prescribed dosage. Clinical jaundice may be painless, with or without pruritus. It may also be associated with acute hepatic enlargement and right-upper quadrant pain, which has been mistaken for acute (surgical) obstruction of the bile duct. Drug-induced jaundice is usually reversible when the medication is discontinued. Continued therapy has been associated with hepatic coma and death. Because of the hepatotoxicity associated with Anadrol-50 (oxymetholone) administration, periodic liver function tests are recommended. Hepatocellular carcinoma and peliosis hepatis,[1] a rare condition of ill-defined etiology consisting of blood-filled cysts in the liver, have been observed in patients with congenital and acquired aplastic anemia treated with oxymetholone and other androgens for prolonged periods. In some cases withdrawal of the drug has been associated with regression of the hepatic lesions.
2. *Virilization*
In the female virilization may occur. Amenorrhea usually occurs in the adult female, even in the presence of thrombocytopenia. Concomitant administration of large doses of progestational agents to control menorrhagia is not recommended.
3. *Iron deficiency*
The development of iron deficiency anemia, manifested by a low serum iron and decreased percent saturation of transferrin, has been observed in some patients treated with Anadrol-50 (oxymetholone). Periodic determination of the serum iron and iron binding capacity is recommended. If iron deficiency is detected, it should be appropriately treated with supplementary iron.
4. Leukemia has been observed in patients with aplastic anemia treated with oxymetholone. The role, if any, of oxymetholone is unclear because malignant transformation has been seen in blood dyscrasias and leukemia has been reported in patients with aplastic anemia who have not been treated with oxymetholone.
5. Caution is required in administering these agents to patients with cardiac, renal, or hepatic disease. Edema, with or without congestive heart failure, may occur occasionally. Concomitant administration with adrenal steroids or ACTH may add to the edema. This is generally controllable with appropriate diuretic and/or digitalis therapy.
6. Hypercalcemia may develop both spontaneously and as a result of hormonal therapy in women with disseminated breast carcinoma. If it develops while on this agent, the drug should be stopped.
7. Anabolic steroids may increase sensitivity to anticoagulants. Dosage of the anticoagulant may have to be decreased in order to maintain the prothrombin time at the desired therapeutic level.
8. Anabolic steroids have been shown to alter glucose tolerance tests. Diabetics should be followed carefully and the insulin or oral hypoglycemic dosage adjusted accordingly.
9. Anabolic steroids should be used with caution in patients with benign prostatic hypertrophy.
10. Serum cholesterol may increase or decrease during therapy. Therefore, caution is required in administering these agents to patients with a history of myocardial infarction or coronary artery disease. Serial determinations of serum cholesterol should be made and therapy adjusted accordingly.

Adverse Reactions:
1. *Hepatotoxicity* is the most serious adverse reaction associated with anabolic steroid therapy. Reversible increase in BSP retention occurs early and appears to be directly related to the dose. Increase in serum bilirubin, with or without an increase in the serum alkaline phosphatase and transaminases (SGOT and SGPT) indicate a higher degree of excretory dysfunction. Clinical jaundice, which is reversible when the drug is discontinued, may occur. The histologic picture is one of intrahepatic cholestasis with little or no cellular damage. Continued therapy may be associated with hepatic coma and death.

2. Virilization is the most common undesirable effect associated with anabolic steroid therapy. Acne occurs frequently in all age groups.
Prepuberal male: The first signs of virilization in the prepuberal male are phallic enlargement and an increase in frequency of erection. Hirsutism and increased skin pigmentation may also occur.
Postpuberal male: Inhibition of testicular function with oligospermia: decrease in seminal volume, alteration in libido, and impotence may occur with prolonged or intensive anabolic therapy. Gynecomastia, and testicular atrophy may occur. Chronic priapism, male-pattern of hair loss, epididymitis and bladder irritability have been reported. In females, hirsutism, hoarseness or deepening of the voice, clitoral enlargement, alteration of libido, and menstrual irregularities and male-pattern baldness may occur. The voice change and clitoral enlargement are usually irreversible even after prompt discontinuance of therapy. The use of estrogens in combination with androgens will not prevent virilization in females.
3. Other adverse reactions associated with anabolic/androgenic therapy include: muscle cramps, nausea, excitation and sleeplessness, chills, bleeding in patients on concomitant anticoagulant therapy, premature closure of epiphyses in children, vomiting and diarrhea.
4. Alterations in these clinical laboratory tests:

a. The metyrapone test
b. The FBS and glucose tolerance test
c. The thyroid function tests: a decrease in the PBI, in thyroxine-binding capacity and radioactive iodine uptake and an increase in T^3 uptake by the rbc's or resin may occur. Free thyroxine is normal. Altered tests usually persist for 2-3 weeks after stopping anabolic therapy.
d. The electrolytes: retention of sodium, chlorides, water, potassium, phosphates and calcium.
e. Increased or decreased serum cholesterol.
f. Suppression of clotting factors II, V, VII, and X.
g. Increased creatine and creatinine excretion lasting up to two weeks after discontinuing therapy.
h. Decreased 17-ketosteroid excretion.

Dosage and Administration: The recommended daily dose in children and adults, 1-5 mg./kg. body weight per day. The usual effective dose is 1-2 mg./kg./day but higher doses may be required and the dose should be individualized. Response is not often immediate and a minimum trial of three to six months should be given. Following remission, some patients may be maintained without the drug; others may be maintained on an established lower daily dosage. A continued maintenance dose is usually necessary in patients with congenital aplastic anemia.
Availability: Anadrol-50 (oxymetholone) is available in bottles of 100 white scored tablets imprinted with the code "2902" and "Syntex".

---

[1]Zak, F. G., Peliosis Hepatis. Am. J. Path. 26:1-15, (Jan.) 1950.

[Shown in Product Identification Section]

BREVICON® ℞
(norethindrone with ethinyl estradiol)
Tablets

NORINYL® ℞
(norethindrone with mestranol)
Tablets

NOR-Q.D.® ℞
(norethindrone)
Tablets 0.35 mg.
Oral Contraceptives

Products of Syntex (F.P.) Inc.

Description: **BREVICON 21-DAY** Tablets provide an oral contraceptive regimen consisting of 21 blue tablets containing norethindrone 0.5 mg. with ethinyl estradiol 0.035 mg.
BREVICON 28-DAY Tablets provide a continuous oral contraceptive regimen consisting of 21 blue tablets containing norethindrone 0.5 mg. with ethinyl estradiol 0.035 mg. and 7 orange tablets containing inert ingredients.
NORINYL 1 + 50 21-DAY Tablets provide an oral contraceptive regimen consisting of 21 white tablets containing norethindrone 1 mg. with mestranol 0.05 mg.
NORINYL 1 + 80 21-DAY Tablets provide an oral contraceptive regimen consisting of 21 yellow tablets containing norethindrone 1 mg. with mestranol 0.08 mg.
NORINYL 1 + 50 28-DAY Tablets provide a continuous oral contraceptive regimen consisting of 21 white tablets containing norethindrone 1 mg. with mestranol 0.05 mg. and 7 orange tablets containing inert ingredients.
NORINYL 1 + 80 28-DAY Tablets provide a continuous oral contraceptive regimen consisting of 21 yellow tablets containing norethindrone 1 mg. with mestranol 0.08 mg. and 7 orange tablets containing inert ingredients.
NORINYL 2 mg. Tablets provide an oral contraceptive regimen consisting of 20 white tablets containing norethindrone 2 mg. and mestranol 0.1 mg.
NOR-Q.D. (norethindrone) Tablets provide a continuous oral contraceptive regimen of one yellow norethindrone 0.35 mg. tablet daily.
Norethindrone is a potent progestational agent with the chemical name 17-hydroxy-19-nor-17α-pregn-4-en-20-yn-3-one. Ethinyl estradiol is an estrogen with the chemical name 19-nor-17α-pregna-1, 3, 5(10) -trien-20-yne-3, 17-diol. Mestranol is an estrogen with the chemical name 3-methoxy-19-nor-17α-pregna-1, 3, 5(10) -trien-20-yn-17-ol.

Clinical Pharmacology: Combination oral contraceptives act primarily through the mechanism of gonadotrophin suppression due to the estrogenic and progestational activity of the ingredients. Although the primary mechanism of action is inhibition of ovulation, alterations in the genital tract including changes in the cervical mucus (which increase the difficulty of sperm penetration) and the endometrium (which reduce the likelihood of implantation) may also contribute to contraceptive effectiveness.
The primary mechanism through which NOR-Q.D. prevents conception is not known, but progestogen-only contraceptives are known to alter the cervical mucus, exert a progestational effect on the endometrium, interfering with implantation, and, in some patients, suppress ovulation.

Indications and Usage: Oral contraceptives are indicated for the prevention of pregnancy in women who elect to use oral contraceptives as a method of contraception. NORINYL 2 mg. is also indicated in the treatment of hypermenorrhea.
Oral contraceptives are highly effective. The pregnancy rate in women using conventional combination oral contraceptives (containing 35 mcg. or more of ethinyl estradiol or 50 mcg. or more of mestranol) is generally reported as less than one pregnancy per 100 woman-years of use. Slightly higher rates (somewhat more than 1 pregnancy per 100 woman-years of use) are reported for some combination products containing 35 mcg. or less of ethinyl estradiol, and rates on the order of 3 pregnancies per 100 woman-years are reported for the progestogen-only oral contraceptives.
These rates are derived from separate studies conducted by different investigators in several population groups and cannot be compared precisely. Furthermore, pregnancy rates tend to be lower as clinical studies are continued, possibly due to selective retention in the longer studies of those patients who accept the treatment regimen and do not discontinue as a result of adverse reactions, pregnancy, or other reasons.
In clinical trials with BREVICON, 1,168 patients completed 16,345 cycles and a total of 3 pregnancies was reported. This represents a pregnancy rate of 0.22 per 100 woman-years. The dropout rate for medical reasons, as observed in the clinical trials conducted with BREVICON, appears to be somewhat higher than observed with higher dose combination products. The dropout rate due to menstrual disorders and irregularities was also somewhat higher, dropouts being equally split between menstrual disorders and irregularities and other medical reasons attributable to the drug.
In clinical trials with NORINYL 1 + 50 21-DAY, 3,852 patients completed 45,937 cycles and a total of 10 pregnancies was reported. This represents a pregnancy rate of 0.26 per 100 woman-years. In clinical trials with NORINYL 1 + 50 28-DAY, 1,590 patients completed 7,330 cycles and a total of 3 pregnancies was reported. This represents a pregnancy rate of 0.5 per 100 woman-years. In clinical trials with NORINYL 1 + 80 21- and 28-DAY, 3,464 patients completed 34,068 cycles and a total of 5 pregnancies was reported. This represents a pregnancy rate of 0.18 per 100 woman-years. In clinical trials with NORINYL 2 mg. 6,097 patients completed 121,233 cycles and a total of 13 pregnancies was reported. This represents a pregnancy rate of 0.13 per 100 woman-years. In clinical trials with NOR-Q.D. (norethindrone) 2,963 patients completed 25,901 cycles of therapy and a total of 55 pregnancies was reported. This represents an average pregnancy rate of 2.54 per 100 women-years. A higher pregnancy rate of 3.72 was recorded in "fresh" patients (those who had never taken oral contraceptives prior to starting NOR-Q.D. therapy) to a large extent because of incorrect tablet intake. This compares to the lower pregnancy rate of 1.95 recorded in "changeover" patients (those switched from other oral contraceptives). This difference was found to be statistically significant. Furthermore, an even greater statistically significant difference in pregnancy rates between these two groups was found during the first six months of NOR-Q.D. therapy. Therefore, it is especially important for "fresh" patients to strictly adhere to the regimen.
Table 1 gives ranges of pregnancy rates reported in the literature[1] for other means of contraception. The efficacy of these means of contraception (except the IUD) depends upon the degree of adherence to the method.

TABLE 1. *Pregnancies per 100 Woman-Years*
IUD, less than 1–6;
Diaphragm with spermicidal products (creams or jellies), 2–20;
Condom, 3–36;
Aerosol foams, 2–29;
Jellies and creams, 4–36;
Periodic abstinence (rhythm) all types, less than 1–47;
—Calendar method, 14–47;
—Temperature method, 1–20;
—Temperature method—intercourse only in post-ovulatory phase, less than 1–7;
—Mucus method, 1–25;
No contraception, 60–80.

Dose-Related Risk of Thromboembolism From Oral Contraceptives. Studies have shown a positive association between the dose of estrogens in oral contraceptives and the risk of thromboembolism[2,3]. For this reason, it is prudent and in keeping with good principles of therapeutics to minimize exposure to estrogen. The oral contraceptive product prescribed for any given patient should be that product which contains the least amount of estrogen that is compatible with an acceptable pregnancy rate and patient acceptance. It is recommended that new acceptors of oral contraceptives

Continued on next page

Syntex—Cont.

should be started on preparations containing 0.05 mg or less of estrogen.

Contraindications:

1. Known or suspected pregnancy (see Warning No. 5).
2. Oral contraceptives should not be used in women who have or have had any of the following conditions:
   a. Thrombophlebitis or thromboembolic disorders.
   b. Cerebral vascular or coronary artery disease.
   c. Markedly impaired liver function.
   d. Known or suspected carcinoma of the breast.
   e. Known or suspected estrogen dependent neoplasia.
   f. Undiagnosed abnormal genital bleeding.

Warnings:

Cigarette smoking increases the risk of serious cardiovascular side effects from oral contraceptive use. This risk increases with age and with heavy smoking (15 or more cigarettes per day) and is quite marked in women over 35 years of age. Women who use oral contraceptives should be strongly advised not to smoke.

The use of oral contraceptives is associated with increased risk of several serious conditions including thromboembolism, stroke, myocardial infarction, liver tumor, gall bladder disease, visual disturbances, fetal abnormalities, and hypertension. Practitioners prescribing oral contraceptives should be familiar with the following information relating to these risks.

1. *Thromboembolic Disorders and Other Vascular Problems:* An increased risk of thromboembolic and thrombotic disease associated with the use of oral contraceptives is well established. One British study[4] demonstrated an increased relative risk for fatal venous thromboembolism, two British[5,6] and three American[3,7,8] studies demonstrated an increased relative risk to non-fatal venous thromboembolism. These studies estimate that users of oral contraceptives are 4 to 11 times more likely than nonusers to develop these diseases without evident cause (Table 2).

Cerebrovascular Disorders. Two American studies[7,9,10] demonstrated an increased relative risk for stroke, which had not been shown in prior British studies[4–6]. In a collaborative American study[9,10] of cerebrovascular disorders in women with and without predisposing causes, it was estimated that the relative risk of hemorrhagic stroke was 2.0 times greater in users than nonusers and the relative risk of thrombotic stroke was 4 to 9.5 times greater in users than in nonusers (Table 2). A British long-term, follow-up study[11] reported in 1976 a highly significant association between oral contraceptive use and stroke. Another British long-term, follow-up study[12] had suggested such an association in 1974, but the number of cases was too small to estimate the risk.

Myocardial Infarction. An increased relative risk of myocardial infarction associated with the use of oral contraceptives has been reported[13–15], confirming a previously suspected association[4]. One study[11,12] conducted in the United Kingdom found, as expected, that the greater the number of underlying risk factors for coronary artery disease (cigarette smoking, hypertension, hypercholesterolemia, obesity, diabetes, history of preeclamptic toxemia) the higher the risk of developing myocardial infarction, regardless of whether the patient was an oral contraceptive user or not. Oral contraceptives, however, were found to be an additional risk factor.

In terms of relative risk, it has been estimated[16,17] that oral contraceptive users who do not smoke (smoking is considered a major predisposing condition to myocardial infarction) are about twice as likely to have a fatal myocardial infarction as nonusers who do not smoke. Oral contraceptive users who are also smokers have about a 5-fold increased risk of fatal infarction compared to users who do not smoke, and about a 10- to 12-fold increased risk compared to nonusers who do not smoke. Furthermore, the number of cigarettes smoked is also an important factor. In determining the importance of these relative risks, however, the baseline rates for various age groups, as shown in Table 3, must be given serious consideration. (The estimates in Table 3 are based on British vital statistics which show acute myocardial infarction death rate 2- to 3-times less than in the U.S. for women in these age groups; consequently, actual U.S. death rates could be higher than those in Table 3[17].) The importance of other predisposing conditions mentioned above in determining relative and absolute risks has not been quantified; other synergistic actions may exist.

TABLE 2. *Summary of relative risk of thromboembolic disorders and other vascular problems in oral contraceptive users compared to nonusers*

	Relative risk, times greater
Idiopathic thromboembolic disease	4–11
Post surgery thromboembolic complications	4–6
Thrombotic stroke	4–9.5
Hemorrhagic stroke	2
Myocardial infarction	2–12

TABLE 3. *Estimated[16] annual mortality rate per 100,000 women from myocardial infarction by use of oral contraceptives, smoking habits, and age (in years)*

	Myocardial infarction			
	Women aged 30–39		Women aged 40–44	
Smoking habits	Users	Non-users	Users	Non-users
All smokers	10.2	2.6	62.0	15.9
Heavy*	13.0	5.1	78.7	31.3
Light	4.7	0.9	28.6	5.7
Nonsmokers	1.8	1.2	10.7	7.4
Smokers and nonsmokers	5.4	1.9	32.8	11.7

*Heavy smoker: 15 or more cigarettes per day.

Risk of Dose. In an analysis of data derived from several national adverse reaction reporting systems[2], British investigators concluded that the risk of thromboembolism including coronary thrombosis is directly related to the dose of estrogen used in oral contraceptives. Preparations containing 0.1 mg or more of estrogen were associated with a higher risk of thromboembolism than those containing 0.05–0.08 mg of estrogen. Their analysis did suggest, however, that the quantity of estrogen may not be the sole factor involved. This finding has been supported by a study in the United States[3]. Careful epidemiological studies to determine the degree of thromboembolic risk associated with progestogen-only oral contraceptives have not been performed. Cases of thromboembolic disease have been reported in women using these products, and they should not be presumed to be free of excess risk.

Estimate of Excess Mortality from Circulatory Diseases. A large British prospective study[12,18] estimated[18] the mortality rate per 100,000 women per year from diseases of the circulatory system for users and nonusers of oral contraceptives according to age, smoking habits, and duration of use. The overall excess death rate annually from circulatory diseases for oral contraceptive users was estimated to be 20 per 100,000 (ages 15–34—5/100,000; ages 35–44—33/100,000; ages 45–49—140/100,000). The risk is concentrated in older women, in those with a long duration of use, and in cigarette smokers, and may persist after discontinuation of oral contraceptive use. It was not possible, however, to examine the interrelationships of age, smoking, and duration of use, nor to compare the effects of continuous vs. intermittent use. Although the study showed a 10-fold increase in death due to circulatory diseases in users for 5 or more years, all of these deaths occurred in women 35 or older. Until larger numbers of women under 35 with continuous use for 5 or more years are available, it is not possible to assess the magnitude of the relative risk for this younger age group.

The available data from a variety of sources have been analyzed[19] to estimate the risk of death associated with various methods of contraception. The estimates of risk of death for each method include the combined risk of the contraceptive method (e.g., thromboembolic and thrombotic disease in the case of oral contraceptives) plus the risk attributable to pregnancy or abortion in the event of method failure. This latter risk varies with the effectiveness of the contraceptive method. The findings of this analysis are shown in Figure 1 below[19]. The study concluded that the mortality associated with all methods of birth control is low and below that of childbirth, with the exception of oral contraceptives in women over 40 who smoke. (The rates given for pill only/smokers for each age group are for smokers as a class. For "heavy" smokers (more than 15 cigarettes a day), the rates given would be about double; for "light" smokers (less than 15 cigarettes a day), about 50 percent.) The lowest mortality is associated with the condom or diaphragm backed up by early abortion. The study also concluded that oral contraceptive users who smoke, especially those over the age of 30, have a greater mortality risk than oral contraceptive users who do not smoke.

Figure 1. Annual number of deaths associated with control of fertility and no control per 100,000 nonsterile women, by regimen of control and age of woman

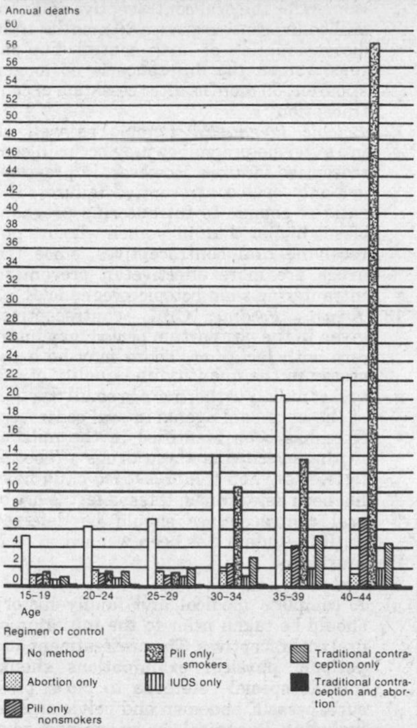

The risk of thromboembolic and thrombotic disease associated with oral contraceptives increases with age after approximately age 30 and, for myocardial infarction, is further increased by hypertension, hyperlipidemias, obesity, diabetes, or history of preeclamptic toxemia and especially by cigarette smoking[16,17].

Based on the data currently available, the following chart gives a gross estimate of the risk of death from circulatory disorders associated with the use of oral contraceptives:

Smoking Habits and Other Predisposing Conditions—Risk Associated with Use of Oral Contraceptives

Age	Below 30	30–39	40+
Heavy smokers	C	B	A
Light smokers	D	C	B
Nonsmokers (no predisposing conditions)	D	C, D	C
Nonsmokers (other predisposing conditions)	C	C, B	B, A

A—Use associated with very high risk.
B—Use associated with high risk.
C—Use associated with moderate risk.
D—Use associated with low risk.

The physician and the patient should be alert to the earliest manifestations of thromboembolic and thrombotic disorders (e.g., thrombophlebitis, pulmonary embolism, cerebrovascular insufficiency, coronary occlusion, retinal thrombosis, and mesenteric thrombosis). Should any of these occur or be suspected, the drug should be discontinued immediately.

A four- to six-fold increased risk of post-surgery thromboembolic complications has been reported in oral contraceptive users[20,21]. If feasible, oral contraceptives should be discontinued at least 4 weeks before surgery of a type associated with an increased risk of thromboembolism or prolonged immobilization.

Among patients with thromboembolic disease, the results of retrospective studies suggest the possibility of an increased risk for users who are of blood types A, B, or AB, as compared with those of type O.

2. *Ocular Lesions:* There have been reports of neuro-ocular lesions such as optic neuritis or retinal thrombosis associated with the use of oral contraceptives. Discontinue oral contraceptive medication if there is unexplained, sudden or gradual, partial or complete loss of vision; onset of proptosis or diplopia; papilledema; or retinal vascular lesions; and institute appropriate diagnostic and therapeutic measures.
3. *Carcinoma:* Long-term continuous administration of either natural or synthetic estrogen in certain animal species increases the frequency of certain adenomas, benign or malignant, such as those of the breast, cervix, vagina, uterus, ovary, pituitary and liver. Certain synthetic progestogens, none currently contained in oral contraceptives, have been noted to increase the incidence of mammary nodules, benign and malignant, in dogs.

Several retrospective case-control studies[22–27] have reported an increased relative risk (3.1 to 13.9 times) associating endometrial carcinoma with the prolonged use of estrogens in postmenopausal women who took estrogen replacement medication to relieve menopausal symptoms. One publication[28] reported on the first 30 cases submitted by physicians to a registry of cases of adenocarcinoma of the endometrium in women under 40 on oral contraceptives. Of the adenocarcinomas found in women without predisposing risk factors for adenocarcinoma of the endometrium (e.g., irregular bleeding at the time oral contraceptives were first given, polycystic ovaries) nearly all occurred in women who had used a sequential oral contraceptive. These products are no longer marketed. No statistical association has been reported suggesting an increased risk of endometrial cancer in users of conventional combination or progestogen-only oral contraceptives, although individual cases have been reported.

Several studies[8,29–33] have shown no increased risk of breast cancer to women taking oral contraceptives or estrogens. In one study[34,35], however, while no overall increased risk of breast cancer was noted in women treated with oral contraceptives, a greater risk was suggested for the subgroups of oral contraceptive users with documented benign breast disease and for long-term (2–4 years) users. One other study[38] indicated an increasing risk of breast cancer in women taking menopausal estrogens, which increased with duration of follow-up. A reduced occurrence of benign breast tumors in users of oral contraceptives has been well documented[8,11,12,29,34,37,38].

In a prospective study[39] of women with cervical dypslasia, there was an increase in severity and of conversion to cancer *in situ* in oral contraceptive users compared with nonusers. This became statistically significant after 3 to 4 years of use. Nonreversal of dysplasia within the first 6 months of pill use was suggested to be predictive of progression after prolonged exposure. There have been other reports of microglandular hyperplasia of the cervix in users of oral contraceptives.

In summary, there is at present no confirmed evidence from human studies of an increased risk of cancer associated with oral contraceptives. Close clinical surveillance of all women taking oral contraceptives is, nevertheless, essential. In all cases of undiagnosed persistent or recurrent abnormal vaginal bleeding, appropriate diagnostic measures should be taken to rule out malignancy. Women with a strong family history of breast cancer or who have breast nodules, fibrocystic disease or abnormal mammograms should be monitored with particular care if they elect to use oral contraceptives instead of other methods of contraception.

4. *Liver Tumors:* Sudden severe abdominal pain or shock may be due to rupture and hemorrhage of a liver tumor. There have been reports associating benign or malignant liver tumors with oral contraceptive use[40–44]. This has been reported in short-term as well as long-term users of oral contraceptives. One study[44] showed that oral contraceptive formulations with high hormonal potency were associated with a higher risk than lower potency formulations. Two studies[41,44] relate risk with duration of use, the risk being much greater after 4 or more years of use. Although it is an uncommon lesion, it should be considered in women presenting with an "acute abdomen". The tumor may cause serious or fatal hemorrhage. Patients with liver tumors have demonstrated variable clinical features which may make preoperative diagnosis difficult. Some cases presented because of right upper quadrant masses, while most had signs and symptoms of acute intraperitoneal hemorrhage. Routine radiological and laboratory studies may not be helpful. Liver scans may clearly show a focal defect. Hepatic arteriography may be a useful procedure in diagnosing primary liver neoplasm.
5. *Use in or Immediately Preceding Pregnancy, Birth Defects in Offspring, and Malignancy in Female Offspring:* The use of female sex hormones—both estrogenic and progestational agents—during early pregnancy may seriously damage the offspring. It has been shown that females exposed *in utero* to diethylstilbestrol, a nonsteroidal estrogen, have an increased risk of developing in later life a form of vaginal or cervical cancer that is ordinarily extremely rare[45,46]. This risk has been estimated to be of the order of 1 in 1,000 exposures or less[47,48]. Although there is no evidence at the present time that oral contraceptives further enhance the risk of developing this type of malignancy, such patients should be monitored with particular care if they elect to use oral contraceptives instead of other methods of contraception.

Furthermore, a high percentage of women exposed to diethylstilbestrol (from 30 to 90%) have been found to have epithelial changes of the vagina and cervix[49–53]. Although these changes are histologically benign, it is not known whether this condition is a precursor of vaginal malignancy. Male children so exposed may develop abnormalities of the urogenital tract[54–56]. Although similar data are not available with the use of other estrogens, it cannot be presumed that they would not induce similar changes.

An increased risk of congenital anomalies, including heart defects and limb defects, has been reported following use of sex hormones, including oral contraceptives, in pregnancy[57–61]. In one case-control study[60] it was estimated that there was a 4.7-fold

Continued on next page

Syntex—Cont.

increased relative risk of limb-reduction defects in infants exposed *in utero* to sex hormones (oral contraceptives, hormonal withdrawal tests for pregnancy or attempted treatment for threatened abortion). Some of these exposures were very short and involved only a few days of treatment. The data suggest that the risk of limb-reduction defects in exposed fetuses is somewhat less than 1 in 1,000 live births. In a large prospective study[61], cardiovascular defects in children born to women who received female hormones, including oral contraceptives, during early pregnancy occurred at a rate of 18.2 per 1,000 births, compared to 7.8 per 1,000 for children not so exposed *in utero*. These results are statistically significant.

In the past, female sex hormones have been used during pregnancy in an attempt to treat threatened or habitual abortion. There is considerable evidence that estrogens are ineffective for these indications, and there is no evidence from well controlled studies that progestogens are effective for these uses.

There is some evidence that triploidy and possibly other types of polyploidy are increased among abortuses from women who become pregnant soon after ceasing oral contraceptives.[62]. Embryos with these anomalies are virtually always aborted spontaneously. Whether there is an overall increase in spontaneous abortion of pregnancies conceived soon after stopping oral contraceptives is unknown.

If the patient has not adhered to the prescribed schedule, the possibility of pregnancy should be considered at the time of the first missed period (or after 45 days from the last menstrual period if progestogen-only contraceptives are used) and further use of oral contraceptives should be withheld until pregnancy has been ruled out. It is recommended that for any patient who has missed two consecutive periods, pregnancy should be ruled out before continuing the contraceptive regimen. If pregnancy is confirmed, the patient should be apprised of the potential risks to the fetus and the advisability of continuation of the pregnancy should be discussed in the light of these risks.

It is also recommended that women who discontinue oral contraceptives with the intent of becoming pregnant use an alternate form of contraception for a period of time before attempting to conceive. Many clinicians recommend 3 months, although no precise information is available on which to base this recommendation.

The administration of progestogen-only or progestogen-estrogen combinations to induce withdrawal bleeding should not be used as a test of pregnancy.

6. *Gall Bladder Disease:* Studies[3,8,11,12,31] report an increased risk of gall bladder disease in users of oral contraceptives or estrogens. In one study[12], an increased risk appeared after 2 years of use and doubled after 4 or 5 years of use. In another study[8], an increased risk was apparent between 6 and 12 months of use.
7. *Carbohydrate and Lipid Metabolic Effects:* A decrease in glucose tolerance has been observed in a significant percentage of patients on oral contraceptives. For this reason, prediabetic and diabetic patients should be carefully observed while receiving oral contraceptives.

   An increase in triglycerides and total phospholipids has been observed in patients receiving oral contraceptives[63]. The clinical significance of this finding is unknown.
8. *Elevated Blood Pressure:* An increase in blood pressure has been reported[12,64] with oral contraceptive use. In some women, hypertension may occur within a few months of beginning oral contraceptive use. In the first year of use, the prevalence of women with hypertension is low in users and may be no higher than that of a comparable group of nonusers. The prevalence in users increases, however, with longer exposure, and in the fifth year of use is two and a half to three times the reported prevalence in the first year. Age is also strongly correlated with the development of hypertension in oral contraceptive users. Women with a history of elevated blood pressure (hypertension), preexisting renal disease, a history of toxemia or elevated blood pressure during pregnancy, a familial tendency to hypertension or its consequences, or a history of excessive weight gain or fluid retention during the menstrual cycle may be more likely to develop elevation of blood pressure when given oral contraceptives and, therefore, should be monitored closely[65]. Even though elevated blood pressure may remain within the "normal" range, the clinical implications of elevations should not be ignored and close surveillance is indicated, particularly for women with other risk factors for cardiovascular disease or stroke[64]. High blood pressure may or may not persist after discontinuation of the oral contraceptive.
9. *Headache:* The onset or exacerbation of migraine or development of headache of a new pattern which is recurrent, persistent, or severe, requires discontinuation of oral contraceptives and evaluation of the cause.
10. *Bleeding Irregularities:* Breakthrough bleeding, spotting, and missed menses are frequent reasons for patients discontinuing oral contraceptives. In breakthrough bleeding, as in all cases of irregular bleeding from the vagina, nonfunctional causes should be borne in mind. In undiagnosed persistent or recurrent abnormal bleeding from the vagina, adequate diagnostic measures are indicated to rule out pregnancy or malignancy. If pathology has been excluded, time or a change to another formulation may solve the problem. Changing to an oral contraceptive with a higher estrogen content, while potentially useful in minimizing menstrual irregularity, should be done only if necessary since this may increase the risk of thromboembolic disease.

    Women with a past history of oligomenorrhea or secondary amenorrhea or young women without regular cycles may have a tendency to remain anovulatory or to become amenorrheic after discontinuation of oral contraceptives. Women with these preexisting problems should be advised of this possibility and encouraged to use other contraceptive methods.

    Post-use anovulation, possibly prolonged, may also occur in women without previous irregularities. A higher incidence of galactorrhea and of pituitary tumors (e.g., adenomas) has been associated with amenorrhea in former users compared with nonusers[66,67]. One study[67] reported a 16-fold increased prevalence of pituitary prolactin-secreting tumors among patients with postpill amenorrhea when galactorrhea was present.
11. *Infertility:* There is evidence of impairment of fertility in women discontinuing oral contraceptives in comparison with those discontinuing other methods of contraception. The impairment appears to be independent of the duration of use of the preparations. While the impairment diminishes with time, there is still an appreciable difference in the results in nulliparous women for the oral contraceptive and nonoral contraceptive groups 30 months after discontinuation of birth control. For parous women the difference is no longer apparent 30 months after cessation of contraception[11].
12. *Ectopic Pregnancy:* Ectopic as well as intrauterine pregnancy may occur in contraceptive failures. However, in progestogen-only oral contraceptive failures, the ratio of ectopic to intrauterine pregnancies is higher than in women who are not receiving oral contraceptives, since the drugs are more effective in preventing intrauterine than ectopic pregnancies.
13. *Breast Feeding:* Oral contraceptives given in the postpartum period may interfere with lactation. There may be a decrease in the quantity and quality of the breast milk. Furthermore, a small fraction of the hormonal agents in oral contraceptives has been identified in the milk of mothers receiving these drugs[67]. The effects, if any, on the breast fed child have not been determined. If feasible, the use of oral contraceptives should be deferred until the infant has been weaned.

Precautions:

General

1. A complete medical and family history should be taken prior to the initiation of oral contraceptives. The pretreatment and periodic physical examinations should include special reference to blood pressure, breasts, abdomen and pelvic organs, including Papanicolaou smear and relevant laboratory tests. As a general rule, oral contraceptives should not be prescribed for longer than 1 year without another physical examination being performed.
2. Under the influence of estrogen-progestogen preparations, preexisting uterine leiomyomata may increase in size.
3. Patients with a history of psychic depression should be carefully observed and the drug discontinued if depression recurs to a serious degree. Patients becoming significantly depressed while taking oral contraceptives should stop the medication and use an alternate method of contraception in an attempt to determine whether the symptom is drug related.
4. Oral contraceptives may cause some degree of fluid retention. They should be prescribed with caution, and only with careful monitoring, in patients with conditions which might be aggravated by fluid retention, such as convulsive disorders, migraine syndrome, asthma or cardiac, hepatic or renal insufficiency.
5. Patients with a past history of jaundice during pregnancy have an increased risk of recurrence of jaundice while receiving oral contraceptive therapy. If jaundice develops in any patient receiving such drugs, the medication should be discontinued.
6. Steroid hormones may be poorly metabolized in patients with impaired liver function and should be administered with caution in such patients.
7. Oral contraceptive users may have disturbances in normal tryptophan metabolism which may result in a relative pyridoxine deficiency. The clinical significance of this is unknown.
8. Serum folate levels may be depressed by oral contraceptive therapy. Since the pregnant woman is predisposed to the development of folate deficiency and the incidence of folate deficiency increases with increasing gestation, it is possible that if a woman becomes pregnant shortly after stopping oral contraceptives, she may have a

greater chance of developing folate deficiency and complications attributed to this deficiency.

9. The pathologist should be advised of oral contraceptive therapy when relevant specimens are submitted.
10. Certain endocrine and liver function tests and blood components may be affected by estrogen-containing oral contraceptives. For example:
    a. Increased sulfobromophthalein retention.
    b. Increased prothrombin and factors VII, VIII, IX, and X; decreased antithrombin 3; increased norepinephrine-induced platelet aggregability.
    c. Increased thyroid binding globulin (TBG) leading to increased circulating total thyroid hormone, as measured by protein-bound iodine (PBI), T4 by column, or T4 by radioimmunoassay. Free T3 resin uptake is decreased, reflecting the elevated TBG, free T4 concentration is unaltered.
    d. Decreased pregnanediol excretion.
    e. Reduced response to metyrapone test.

DRUG INTERACTIONS

Oral contraceptions may be rendered less effective by virtue of drug interaction with rifampin, isoniazid, ampicillin, neomycin, penicillin V, chloramphenicol, sulfonamides, nitrofurantoin, barbiturates, phenytoin, primidone, analgesics, tranquilizers and antimigraine preparations[69–71]. Oral contraceptives may alter the effectiveness of other types of drugs, such as oral anticoagulants, anticonvulsants, tricyclic antidepressants, antihypertensive agents (e.g., guanethidine), vitamins and hypoglycemic agents[69].

INFORMATION FOR THE PATIENT

See accompanying detailed patient leaflet.

CARCINOGENESIS

See Warnings section for information on the carcinogenic potential of oral contraceptives.

PREGNANCY

Pregnancy category X. See Contraindications and Warnings.

NURSING MOTHERS

See Warnings.

Adverse Reactions: An increased risk of the following serious adverse reactions has been associated with the use of oral contraceptives (see Warnings):

- Thrombophlebitis, thrombosis
- Pulmonary embolism
- Coronary thrombosis
- Cerebral thrombosis
- Mesenteric thrombosis
- Liver tumors
- Cerebral hemorrhage
- Hypertension
- Gall bladder disease
- Congenital anomalies
- Neuro-ocular lesions, e.g., retinal thrombosis and optic neuritis

The following adverse reactions have been reported in patients receiving oral contraceptives and are believed to be drug related:

- Bleeding irregularities
  - Breakthrough bleeding
  - Spotting
  - Missed menses during treatment
  - Amenorrhea after treatment
- Gastrointestinal symptoms
  - Nausea
  - Vomiting
  - Bloating
  - Abdominal cramps
- Dysmenorrhea
- Infertility after discontinuance of treatment
- Edema
- Chloasma or melasma which may persist after drug is discontinued
- Breast changes: tenderness, enlargement, and secretion
- Intolerance to contact lenses
- Change in corneal curvature (steepening)
- Change in weight (increase or decrease)
- Change in cervical erosion and cervical secretion
- Possible diminution in lactation when given immediately postpartum
- Cholestatic jaundice
- Migraine
- Increase in size of uterine leiomyomata
- Rash (allergic)
- Mental depression
- Reduced tolerance to carbohydrates
- Vaginal candidiasis
- Prolaction-secreting pituitary tumors

The following adverse reactions have been reported in users of oral contraceptives, and the association has been neither confirmed nor refuted:

- Premenstrual-like syndrome
- Cataracts
- Changes in libido
- Chorea
- Changes in appetite
- Cystitis-like syndrome
- Headache
- Nervousness
- Dizziness
- Hirsutism
- Loss of hair
- Erythema multiforme
- Erythema nodosum
- Hemorrhagic eruption
- Vaginitis
- Porphyria
- Impaired renal function

Acute Overdose: Serious ill effects have not been reported following acute ingestion of large doses of oral contraceptives by young children. Overdosage may cause nausea. Withdrawal bleeding may occur in females.

Dosage and Administration: To achieve maximum contraceptive effectiveness, oral contraceptives must be taken exactly as directed and at intervals not exceeding 24 hours.

21-Day Regimen Dosage Schedule: The dosage for the initial cycle of therapy is one tablet taken each evening at bedtime from DAY 5 through DAY 25 of the menstrual cycle, counting the first day of menstrual flow as DAY 1. No tablets are taken for 7 days, then, whether bleeding has stopped or not, a new course is started of one tablet a day for 21 days. This institutes a three weeks on, one week off dosage regimen.

28-Day Regimen Dosage Schedule: The dosage for the initial cycle of therapy is one tablet taken daily beginning with DAY 5 of the menstrual cycle, counting the first day of menstrual flow as DAY 1. Tablets are taken without interruption as follows: Beginning with Tablet 1, take one tablet each evening at bedtime for 21 days, through Tablet 21. Then take orange Tablets 22 through 28, one each evening at bedtime, for 7 days. After all 28 tablets have been taken, whether bleeding has stopped or not, repeat the same dosage schedule beginning on the following day.

NORINYL 2 mg. Tablets: To prevent conception, one tablet is taken each evening at bedtime for 20 days beginning on DAY 5 of the menstrual cycle, counting the first day of menstrual flow as DAY 1. In the vast majority of women on this schedule menses occur within two to three days following the termination of each 20-day course, but tend to be scantier than normal menses. In those cases where withdrawal bleeding may be delayed until 4, 5 or 6 days after the 20-day course of therapy, the patient should start the next course of medication on the 7th day following completion of the previous 20-day course. For the treatment of hypermenorrhea, one tablet is taken each evening at bedtime from day 5 through day 24 of each menstrual cycle.

Even if spotting or breakthrough bleeding should occur, continue the medication according to the schedule. Should spotting or breakthrough bleeding persist, your physician should be notified.

Use of oral contraceptives in the event of a missed menstrual period:

1. If the patient has not adhered to the prescribed dosage regimen, the possibility of pregnancy should be considered after the first missed period and oral contraceptives should be withheld until pregnancy has been ruled out.
2. If the patient has adhered to the prescribed regimen and misses two consecutive periods, pregnancy should be ruled out before continuing the contraceptive regimen.

NOR-Q.D.® (norethindrone) is administered as a continuous daily dosage regimen starting on the first day of menstruation, i.e., one tablet each day, every day of the year. Tablets should be taken at the same time each day and continued daily, without interruption, whether bleeding occurs or not. This is especially important for patients new to progestogen alone oral contraception. The patient should be advised that if prolonged bleeding occurs, she should consult her physician. In the non-nursing mother, NOR-Q.D. may be prescribed in the post-partum period either immediately or at the first post-partum examination whether or not menstruation has resumed.

The risk of pregnancy increases with each tablet missed. If the patient misses one tablet, she should be instructed to take it as soon as she remembers and also to take her next tablet at the regular time which means she will be taking two tablets on that day. If she misses two tablets in a row, she should take one of the missed tablets as soon as she remembers, discard the other missed tablet, and take her regular tablet for that day at the proper time. Furthermore, she should use an additional method of contraception in addition to taking NOR-Q.D. until menses has appeared or pregnancy has been excluded. If more than two tablets in a row have been missed, NOR-Q.D. should be discontinued immediately and an additional method of contraception should be used until menses has appeared or pregnancy has been excluded. Whether or not the patient has adhered to the prescribed schedule, if she does not have a period within 45 days of her last period, she should stop taking NOR-Q.D. and depend upon a method of nonhormonal contraception until pregnancy has been ruled out.

How Supplied:

BREVICON® 21-DAY Tablets (21 blue norethindrone 0.5 mg. with ethinyl estradiol 0.035 mg. tablets) are available in MEMORETTE® Tablet Dispensers, each containing 21 tablets. Also supplied are 21-tablet refills. BREVICON® 28-DAY Tablets (21 blue norethindrone 0.5 mg. with ethinyl estradiol 0.035 mg. tablets followed by 7 orange tablets) are available in MEMORETTE Tablet Dispensers, each containing 28 tablets. Also supplied are 28-tablet refills.

NORINYL® 1 + 50 21-DAY Tablets (21 white norethindrone 1 mg. with mestranol 0.05 mg. tablets) and NORINYL® 1 + 80 21-DAY Tablets (21 yellow norethindrone 1 mg. with mestranol 0.08 mg. tablets) are available in MEMORETTE® Tablet Dispensers, each containing 21 tablets. Also supplied are 21-tablet refills. NORINYL 1 + 50 28-DAY Tablets (21 white norethindrone 1 mg. with mestranol 0.05 mg. tablets followed by 7 orange inert tablets) and NORINYL 1 + 80 28-DAY Tablets (21 yellow norethindrone 1 mg. with mestranol 0.08 mg. tablets followed by 7 orange inert tablets) are available in MEMORETTE Tablet Dispensers, each containing 28 tablets. Also supplied are 28-tablet refills. NORINYL® 2 mg. Tablets (20 white norethindrone 2 mg. with mestranol 0.1 mg. tablets) are available in MEMORETTE® Tablet Dispensers, each con-

Continued on next page

Syntex—Cont.

taining 20 tablets. Also supplied are 20-tablet refills.
NOR-Q.D.® (norethindrone) (as yellow-colored unscored tablets) is available in 42-tablet dispensers.

References:

[1] Population Reports, Series H, Number 2, May 1974; Series I, Number 1, June 1974: Series B, Number 2, January 1975; Series H, Number 3, January 1975; Series H, Number 4, January 1976 (published by the Population Information Program, The George Washington University Medical Center, 2001 S St. NW, Washington, D. C.).
[2] Inman, W., et al.: *Brit Med J* 2:203–209, 1970.
[3] Stolley, P., et al.: *Am J Epidemiol* 102:197–208, 1975.
[4] Inman, W., et al.: *Brit Med J* 2:193–199, 1968.
[5] Royal College of General Practitioners: *J Coll Gen Pract* 13:267–279, 1967.
[6] Vessey, M., et al.: *Brit Med J* 2:651–657, 1969.
[7] Sartwell, P., et al.: *Am J Epidemiol* 90:365–380, 1969.
[8] Boston Collaborative Drug Surveillance Program: *Lancet* 1:1399–1404, 1973.
[9] Collaborative Group for the Study of Stroke in Young Women: *N Engl J Med* 288:871–878, 1973.
[10] Collaborative Group for the Study of Stroke in Young Women: *JAMA* 231:718–722, 1975.
[11] Vessey, M., et al.: *J Biosoc Sci* 8:373–427, (Oct.) 1976.
[12] Royal College of General Practitioners: Oral Contraceptives and Health, London, Pitman, 1974.
[13] Mann, J., et al.: *Brit Med J* 2:245–248, 1975.
[14] Mann, J., et al.: *Brit Med J* 2:445–447, 1976.
[15] Mann, J., et al.: *Brit Med J* 2:241–245, 1975.
[16] Jain, A.: *Studies in Family Planning* 8:50–54, 1977.
[17] Ory, H.: *JAMA* 237:2619–2622, (June 13) 1977.
[18] Beral, V.: *Lancet* 2:727–731, 1977.
[19] Tietze, C.: *Family Planning Perspectives* 9:74–76, 1977.
[20] Vessey, M., et al.: *Brit Med J* 3:123–126, 1970.
[21] Greene, G., et al.: *Am J Pub Health* 62:680–685, 1972.
[22] Ziel, H., et al.: *N Engl J Med* 293:1167–1170, 1975.
[23] Gordon, J., et al.: *N Engl J Med* 297:570–571, (Sept. 15) 1977.
[24] Smith, D., et al.: *N Engl J Med* 293:1164–1167, 1975.
[25] Mack, T., et al.: *N Engl J Med* 294:1262–1267, 1976.
[26] Gray, L., et al.: *Obstet Gyncecol* 49:385–389, (April) 1977.
[27] McDonald, T., et al.: *Am J Obstet Gynecol* 127:572–580, (Mar. 20) 1977.
[28] Silverberg, S., et al.: *Cancer* 39:592–598, (Feb.) 1977).
[29] Vessey, M., et al.: *Brit Med J* 3:719–724, 1972.
[30] Vessey, M., et al.: *Lancet* 1:941–943, 1975.
[31] Boston Collaborative Drug Surveillance Program: *N Engl J Med* 290:15–19, 1974.
[32] Arthes, F., et al.: *Cancer* 28:1391–1394, 1971.
[33] Casagrande, J., et al.: *J Natl Cancer Inst* 56:839–841, (April) 1976).
[34] Fasal, E., et al.: *J Natl Cancer Inst* 55:767–773, 1975.
[35] Paffenbarger, R., et al.: *Cancer* 49:1887–1891, (April Suppl.) 1977.
[36] Hoover, R., et al.: *N Engl J Med* 295:401–405, (Aug. 19) 1976.
[37] Kelsey, J., et al.: *Internat J Epidemiol* 3:333–340, 1974.
[38] Ory, H., et al.: *N Engl J Med* 294:419–422, 1976.
[39] Stern, E., et al.: *Science* 196:1460–1462, (June 24) 1977.
[40] Mays, E., et al.: *JAMA* 235:730–732, 1976.
[41] Edmondson, H., et al.: *N Engl J Med* 294:470–472, 1976.
[42] Murphy, G.: *Am Col of Surg Bull*, (April) 1977.
[43] Klatskin, G.: *Gastroent* 73:386–394, (Aug.) 1977.
[44] Center for Disease Control: *Morbidity and Mortality Weekly Rpt* 26:293–294, (Sept. 9) 1977.
[45] Herbst, A., et al.: *N Engl J Med* 284:878–881, 1971.
[46] Greenwald, P., et al.: *N Engl J Med* 285:390–392, 1971.
[47] Lanier, A., et al.: *Mayo Clin Pro* 48:793–799, 1973.
[48] Herbst, A., et al.: *Am J Obstet Gynecol* 128:43–50, 1977.
[49] Herbst, A., et al.: *Obstet Gyncecol* 40:287–298, 1972.
[50] Herbst, A., et al.: *Am J Obstet Gyncecol* 118:607–615, 1974.
[51] Herbst, A., et al.: *N Engl J Med* 292:334–339, 1975.
[52] Stafl, A., et al.: *Obstet Gynecol* 43:118–128, 1974.
[53] Sherman, A., et al.: *Obstet Gynecol* 44:531–545, 1974.
[54] Bibbo, M., et al.: *Jour of Repro Med* 15:29–32, 1975.
[55] Gill, W., et al.: *Jour of Repro Med* 16:147–153, 1976.
[56] Henderson, B., et al.: *Pediatrics* 58:505–507, 1976.
[57] Gal, I., et al.: *Nature* 216:83, 1967.
[58] Levy, E., et al.: *Lancet* 1:611, 1973.
[59] Nora, J., et al.: *Lancet* 1:941–942, 1973.
[60] Janerich, D., et al.: *N Engl J Med* 291:697–700, 1974.
[61] Heinonen, O., et al.: *N Engl J Med* 296:67–70, 1977.
[62] Carr, D.: *Canad Med Assoc J* 103:343–348, 1970.
[63] Wynn, V., et al.: *Lancet* 2:720–723, 1966.
[64] Fisch, I., et al.: *JAMA* 273:2499–2503, (June 6) 1977.
[65] Laragh, J.: *Am J Obstet Gynecol* 126:141–147, (Sept.) 1976.
[66] March, C., et al.: *Fertil and Steril* 28:346, (Mar.) 1977.
[67] Van Campenhout, J., et al.: *Fertil and Steril* 28:728–732, (July) 1977.
[68] Laumas, K., et al.: *Am J Obstet Gynecol* 98:411–413, 1967.
[69] Stockley, I.: *Pharm J* 216:140–143, (Feb. 14) 1976.
[70] Hempel, E., et al.: *Drugs* 12:442–448, (Dec.) 1976.
[71] Bessot, J.-C., et al.: *Nouv Press Med* 6:1568, (Apr. 30) 1977.

Detailed Patient Labeling: Oral contraceptives ("the pill") are the most effective way (except for sterilization) to prevent pregnancy. They are also convenient and, for most women, free of serious or unpleasant side effects. Oral contraceptives must always be taken under the continuous supervision of a physician.

It is important that any woman who considers using an oral contraceptive understand the risks involved. Although the oral contraceptives have important advantages over the other methods of contraception, they have certain risks that no other method has. Only you can decide whether the advantages are worth these risks. This leaflet will tell you about the most important risks. It will explain how you can help your doctor prescribe the pill as safely as possible by telling him/her about yourself and being alert for the earliest signs of trouble. And it will tell you how to use the pill properly, so that it will be as effective as possible. There is more detailed information available in the leaflet prepared for doctors. If you need further help, ask your physician or pharmacist.

Who Should Not Use Oral Contraceptives:

A. If you have any of the following conditions you should not use the pill:
1. Unusual vaginal bleeding that has not yet been diagnosed.
2. Known or suspected pregnancy.

B. If you have or have had any of the following conditions you should not use the pill:
1. Heart attack or stroke.
2. Clots in the legs, lungs, brain, heart or elsewhere.
3. Chest pain (angina pectoris).
4. Known or suspected cancer of the breast or sex organs.
5. Severe liver disease.

C. Cigarette smoking increases the risk of serious adverse effects on the heart and blood vessels from oral contraceptive use. This risk increases with age and with heavy smoking (15 or more cigarettes per day) and is quite marked in women over 35 years of age. Women who use oral contraceptives should not smoke.

D. If you have scanty or irregular periods or are a young woman without a regular cycle, you should use another method of contraception because, if you use the pill, you may have difficulty becoming pregnant or may fail to have menstrual periods after discontinuing the pill.

What You Should Know About Oral Contraceptives: This leaflet describes the advantages and risks of oral contraceptives. Except for sterilization, the IUD and abortion, which have their own exclusive risks, the only risks of other methods of contraception are those due to pregnancy should the method fail or not be used conscientiously. Your doctor can answer questions you may have with respect to methods of contraception.

1. What Oral Contraceptives Are and How They Work. Oral contraceptives are of two types. The most common, often simply called "the pill", is a combination of an estrogen and a progestogen, the two kinds of female hormones. The amount of estrogen and progestogen can vary, but the amount of estrogen is most important because both the effectiveness and some of the dangers of oral contraceptives are related to the amount of estrogen. This kind of oral contraceptive works principally by preventing release of an egg from the ovary. When the amount of estrogen is 0.05 milligrams or more, and the pill is taken as directed, oral contraceptives are more than 99% effective (i.e., there would be less than one pregnancy if 100 women used the pill for 1 year). Pills that contain 0.02 to 0.035 milligrams of estrogen vary slightly in effectiveness, ranging from 98% to more than 99% effective.

The second type of oral contraceptive, often called the "mini-pill", contains only a progestogen. It works in part by preventing release of an egg from the ovary but also by keeping sperm from reaching the egg and by making the uterus (womb) less receptive to any fertilized egg that reaches it. The mini-pill is less effective than the combination oral contraceptive, about 97% effective. In addition, the progestogen-only pill has a tendency to cause irregular bleeding which may be quite inconvenient, or cessation of bleeding entirely. The progestogen-only pill is used despite its lower effectiveness in the hope that it will prove not to have some of the serious side effects of the estrogen-containing pill (see below) but it is not yet certain that the mini-pill does in fact have fewer serious side effects. The discussion below, while based mainly on information about the combination pills, should be considered to apply as well to the mini-pill.

2. Other Nonsurgical Ways to Prevent Pregnancy. As this leaflet will explain, oral contraceptives have several serious risks. Some

other methods of contraception have lesser risks. They are usually less effective than oral contraceptives, but, used properly, may be effective enough for many women. The following table gives reported pregnancy rates (the number of women out of 100 who would become pregnant in 1 year) for these methods:

Pregnancies per 100 Women per Year
Intrauterine device (IUD), less than 1–6;
Diaphragm with spermicidal products (creams or jellies), 2–20;
Condom (rubber), 3–36;
Aerosol foams, 2–29;
Jellies and creams, 4–36;
Periodic abstinence (rhythm), all types, less than 1–47;
—Calendar method, 14–47;
—Temperature method, 1–20;
—Temperature method—intercourse only in post-ovulatory phase, less than 1–7;
—Mucus method, 1–25;
No contraception, 60–80.

The figures (except for the IUD) vary widely because people differ in how well they use each method. Very faithful users of the various methods, with the exception of the calendar method of periodic abstinence (rhythm), may achieve lower pregnancy rates than those given above, which are the average results for large groups of women. Except for the IUD, effective use of these methods requires somewhat more effort than simply taking a single pill every evening, but it is an effort that many couples undertake successfully. Your doctor can tell you a great deal more about these methods of contraception.

3. The Dangers of Oral Contraceptives

a. *Circulatory disorders (abnormal blood clots, strokes, and heart attacks).* Blood clots (in various blood vessels of the body) are the most common of the serious side effects of oral contraceptives. A clot can result in a stroke (if the clot is in the brain), a heart attack (if the clot is in a blood vessel of the heart), a pulmonary embolus (a clot which forms in the legs or pelvis, then breaks off and travels to the lungs), or loss of a limb (a clot in a blood vessel in or leading to an arm or leg). Any of these can cause death or disability. Clots also occur rarely in the blood vessels of the eye, resulting in blindness or impairment of vision in that eye. There is evidence that the risk of clotting increases with higher estrogen doses. It is therefore important to keep the dose of estrogen as low as possible, so long as the oral contraceptive used has an acceptable pregnancy rate and doesn't cause unacceptable changes in the menstrual pattern.

The risk of abnormal clotting increases with age in both users and nonusers of oral contraceptives, but the increased risk from the contraceptive appears to be present at all ages. The risk may be greater if your blood type is A, B, or AB rather than O.

In addition to blood-clotting disorders, it has been estimated that women taking oral contraceptives are twice as likely as nonusers to have a stroke due to rupture of a blood vessel in the brain.

Furthermore, cigarette smoking by oral contraceptive users increases the risk of serious adverse effects on the heart and blood vessels. This risk increases with age and with heavy smoking (15 or more cigarettes per day) and becomes quite marked in women over 35 years of age. For this reason, women who use oral contraceptives should not smoke.

For oral contraceptive users in general, it has been estimated that in women between the ages of 15 and 34 the risk of death due to a circulatory disorder is about 1 in 12,000 per year, whereas for nonusers the rate is about 1 in 50,000 per year. In the age group 35 to 44, the risk is estimated to be about 1 in 2,500 per year for oral contraceptive users and about 1 in 10,000 per year for nonusers. The risk is concentrated in older women, in those with a long duration of use, and in cigarette smokers. The effects on the circulatory system may persist after oral contraceptives are discontinued.

Even without the pill the risk of having a heart attack increases with age and is also increased by such heart attack risk factors as high blood pressure, high cholesterol, obesity, diabetes, and cigarette smoking. Without any risk factors present, the use of oral contraceptives alone may double the risk of heart attack. However, the combination of cigarette smoking, especially heavy smoking, and oral contraceptive use greatly increases the risk of heart attack. Oral contraceptive users who smoke are about 5 times more likely to have a heart attack than users who do not smoke and about 10 times more likely to have a heart attack than nonusers who do not smoke. It has been estimated that users between the ages of 30 and 39 who smoke have about a 1 in 10,000 chance each year of having a fatal heart attack compared to about a 1 in 50,000 chance in users who do not smoke, and about a 1 in 100,000 chance in nonusers who do not smoke.

In the age group 40 to 44, the risk is about 1 in 1,700 per year for users who smoke compared to about 1 in 10,000 for users who do not smoke and to about 1 in 14,000 per year for nonusers who do not smoke. These are average figures for Great Britain; comparable estimates for the U.S. may be higher. Heavy smoking (about 15 cigarettes or more a day) further increases the risk. If you do not smoke and have none of the other heart attack risk factors described above, you will have a smaller risk than listed. If you have several heart attack risk factors, the risk may be considerably greater than listed.

b. *Formation of tumors.* Studies have found that when certain animals are given the female sex hormone estrogen, which is an ingredient of oral contraceptives, continuously for long periods, cancers may develop in the breast, cervix, vagina, uterus, ovary, pituitary and liver.

These findings suggest that oral contraceptives may cause cancer in humans. However, studies to date in women taking currently marketed oral contraceptives have not confirmed that oral contraceptives cause cancer in humans. Several studies have found no increase in breast cancer in users, although one study suggested oral contraceptives might cause an increase in breast cancer in women who already have benign breast disease (e.g., cysts).

Women with a strong family history of breast cancer or who have breast nodules, fibrocystic disease, or abnormal mammograms or who were exposed to DES (diethylstilbestrol), an estrogen, during their mother's pregnancy must be followed very closely by their doctors if they choose to use oral contraceptives instead of another method of contraception. Many studies have shown that women taking oral contraceptives have less risk of getting benign breast disease than those who have not used oral contraceptives. Strong evidence has emerged that estrogens (one component of oral contraceptives) when given alone (unaccompanied by progestogen) for periods of more than one year to women after the menopause, increase the risk of cancer of the uterus (womb). There is also some evidence that a kind of oral contraceptive which is no longer marketed, the sequential oral contraceptive, may increase the risk of cancer of the uterus. There remains no evidence, however, that the oral contraceptives now available (containing estrogen and progestogen in combination or progestogen alone) increase the risk of this cancer. Cancer of the cervix may develop more readily in long-term (3–4 years) users of the pill who had preexisting abnormal Pap smears.

Benign or malignant liver tumors have been associated with short-term as well as long-term oral contraceptive use. The benign (non-malignant) tumors do not spread, but they may rupture and produce internal bleeding, which may cause death.

c. *Dangers to a developing child if oral contraceptives are used in or immediately preceding pregnancy.* Oral contraceptives should not be taken by pregnant women because they may damage the developing child. An increased risk of birth defects, including heart defects and limb defects, has been associated with the use of sex hormones, including oral contraceptives, in pregnancy. In addition, the developing female child whose mother has received DES (diethylstilbestrol), an estrogen, during pregnancy has a risk of getting cancer of the vagina or cervix in her teens or young adulthood. This risk is estimated to be about 1 in 1,000 exposures or less. Abnormalities of the urinary and sex organs have been reported in male offspring so exposed. It is possible that other estrogens, such as the estrogens in oral contraceptives, could have the same effect in the child if the mother takes them during pregnancy.

If you stop taking oral contraceptives to become pregnant, your doctor may recommend that you use another method of contraception for a short while. The reason for this is that there is evidence from studies in women who have had "miscarriages" soon after stopping the pill, that the lost fetuses are more likely to be abnormal. Whether there is an overall increase in "miscarriage" in women who become pregnant soon after stopping the pill as compared with women who do not use the pill is not known, but it is possible that there may be. If, however, you do become pregnant soon after stopping oral contraceptives, and do not have a miscarriage, there is no evidence that the baby has an increased risk of being abnormal.

d. *Gallbladder disease.* Women who use oral contraceptives have a greater risk than nonusers of having gallbladder disease requiring surgery. The increased risk may first appear within 1 year of use and may double after 4 to 5 years of use.

e. *Other side effects of oral contraceptives.* Some women using oral contraceptives experience unpleasant side effects that are not dangerous and are not likely to damage their health. Some of these may be temporary. Your breasts may feel tender, nausea and vomiting may occur, you may gain or lose weight, and your ankles may swell. A spotty darkening of the skin, particularly of the face, is possible and may persist. Many of these effects are seen more frequently with combination oral contraceptives containing 0.05 milligrams or more of estrogen. You may notice unexpected vaginal bleeding or changes in your menstrual period. Irregular bleeding is frequently seen when using the mini-pill or combination oral contraceptives containing less than 0.05 milligrams of estrogen.

More serious side effects include worsening of migraine, asthma, epilepsy, and kidney or heart disease because of a tendency for water to be retained in the body when oral contraceptives are used. Other side effects are growth of preexisting fibroid tumors of the uterus; mental depression; and liver problems with jaundice (yellowing of the skin). Your doctor may find that levels of sugar and fatty substances in your blood are elevated; the long-term effects of these changes are not known. Some women develop high blood pressure while taking oral contraceptives, which may persist after discontinuation. High blood pressure may lead to serious disease of the kidney and circulatory system. Your physician may wish to check your blood pressure more frequently if you have a history of toxemia of pregnancy, kidney disease or increased blood pressure.

Other reactions have been reported occasionally. These include more frequent urination and some discomfort when urinating, kidney disease, nervousness, dizziness, an increase in or loss of hair, an increase or decrease in sex

Continued on next page

Syntex—Cont.

drive, appetite changes, cataracts, and a need for a change in contact lens prescription or inability to use contact lenses.

After you stop using oral contraceptives, your ability to menstruate or become pregnant may be impaired. This impairment may be greater if you have never been pregnant.

As discussed previously, you should wait a few months after stopping the pill before you try to become pregnant. During these few months, use another form of contraception. You should consult your physician before resuming use of oral contraceptives after childbirth, especially if you plan to nurse your baby. Drugs in oral contraceptives are known to appear in the milk, and the long-range effect on infants is not known. Furthermore, oral contraceptives may cause a decrease in your milk supply as well as in the quality of the milk.

4. Comparison of the Risks of Oral Contraceptives and Other Contraceptive Methods. The many studies on the risks and effectiveness of oral contraceptives and other methods of contraception have been analyzed to estimate the risk of death associated with various methods of contraception. This risk has two parts: (a) the risk associated with the method itself (e.g., the risk that an oral contraceptive user will die due to abnormal clotting), and (b) the risk associated with failure of the method (death due to pregnancy or abortion). The results of this analysis are shown in the bar graph below. The height of the bars is the estimated number of deaths per 100,000 women each year. There are six sets of bars, each set referring to a specific age group of women. Within each set of bars, there are two bars for oral contraceptive users, one referring to users who smoke and one referring to users who do not smoke, and five bars for other contraceptive methods including one bar representing no method of contraception. ("Traditional contraception" means diaphragm or condom.)

Figure 1. Annual number of deaths associated with control of fertility and no control per 100,000 nonsterile women, by regimen of control and age of woman

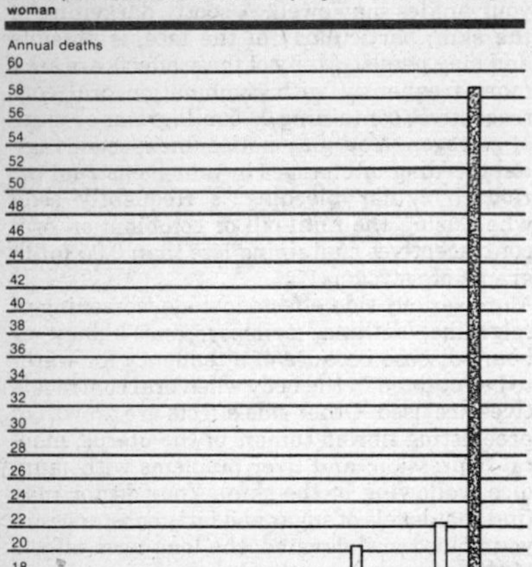

This analysis is based on present knowledge and new information could, of course, alter it. The analysis shows that the risk of death from all methods of birth control is low compared to the risks of childbirth, *except for oral contraceptives in women over 40 who smoke.* It shows that the lowest risk of death is associated with the condom or diaphragm (traditional contraception) backed up by early abortion in case of failure of the condom or diaphragm to prevent pregnancy. Also, at any age the risk of death (due to unexpected pregnancy) from use of traditional contraception even without a backup of abortion is generally the same as, or less than, that from use of oral contraceptives.

Careful Use of Oral Contraceptives:

1. Tell Your Doctor About Any Of The Following:

a. Present or past conditions that mean you should not use oral contraceptives:
Clots in the legs, lungs or elsewhere
A stroke, heart attack, or chest pain (angina pectoris)
Known or suspected cancer of the breast or sex organs
Severe liver disease
Irregular or scanty menstrual periods before starting to take the pill

b. Present conditions that mean you should not use oral contraceptives:
Unusual vaginal bleeding that has not yet been diagnosed.
Known or suspected pregnancy.

c. Conditions that your doctor will want to watch closely or which might cause him to suggest another method of contraception:
A family history of breast cancer
Breast nodules, fibrocystic disease of the breast, or an abnormal mammogram
Diabetes
High blood pressure
High cholesterol
Cigarette smoking
Migraine headaches
Heart or kidney disease
Epilepsy
Mental depression
Fibroid tumors of the uterus
Gallbladder disease
Asthma
Problems during a prior pregnancy
Plans for elective surgery
History of jaundice

d. Use of any of the following kinds of drugs, which might interact with the pill: antibiotics, sulfa drugs, drugs for epilepsy or migraine, pain killers, tranquilizers, sedatives or sleeping pills, blood thinning drugs, vitamins, drugs being used for the treatment of depression, high blood pressure, or high blood sugar (diabetes).

e. Once you are using oral contraceptives, you should be alert for signs of a serious adverse effect and call your doctor if they occur:
Sharp pain in the chest, coughing blood, or sudden shortness of breath (indicating possible clots in the lungs)
Pain in the calf (possible clot in the leg)
Crushing chest pain or heaviness (indicating possible heart attack)
Sudden severe headache or vomiting, dizziness or fainting, disturbance of vision or speech, or weakness or numbness in an arm or leg (indicating a possible stoke)
Sudden partial or complete loss of vision (indicating a possible clot in the eye)
Breast lumps (you should ask your doctor to show you how to examine your own breasts)
Severe pain or mass in the abdomen (indicating a possible tumor of the liver)
Severe depression
Yellowing of the skin (jaundice)
Unusual swelling.

2. How to Take the Pill So That It is Most Effective

Your physician has prescribed one of the following dosage schedules. Please follow the instructions appropriate for your schedule.

20-Day Schedule: Counting the onset of flow as day 1, take the first pill on day 5 of the menstrual cycle whether or not the flow has stopped. Take another pill the same time each day, preferably at bedtime, for 20 days. Then wait for 7 days, during which time a menstrual period usually occurs, and begin taking 1 pill every day on the 8th day after you took your last pill, whether or not the menstrual flow has stopped. This cycle is repeated 20 days on pills and 7 days off pills until time for the physician's examination and pill refill. If you are taking NORINYL® 2 mg Tablets for the control of excessive bleeding (hypermenorrhea), your physician may instruct you to stop taking the pills after 3 cycles to determine the need for further treatment. The information contained in this leaflet regarding who should not use the pill, the dangers of the pill and safe use of the pill applies to the use of the pill for hypermenorrhea, as well as for contraception.

21-Day Schedule: Counting the onset of flow as day 1, take the first pill on day 5 of the menstrual cycle whether or not the flow has stopped. Take another pill the same time each day, preferably at bedtime, for 21 days. Then wait for 7 days, during which time a menstrual period usually occurs, and begin taking 1 pill every day on the 8th day after you took your last pill, whether or not the menstrual flow has stopped. This cycle is repeated 21 days on pills and 7 days off pills until time for the physician's examination and pill refill.

28-Day Schedule: Counting the onset of flow as day 1, take the first pill on day 5 of the menstrual cycle whether or not the flow has stopped. Take another pill the same time each day, preferably at bedtime, for 21 days. Then take pills 22 through 28 (which are a different color) and expect a menstrual period during this week. Pills 22 through 28 contain no active drug and are included simply for your convenience—to eliminate the need for counting days. After all 28 pills have been taken, whether bleeding has stopped or not, take the first pill of the next cycle without any interruption. With the 28-day package, pills are taken every day of the year with no gap between cycles.

Important Additional Instructions for the 20-Day, 21-Day and 28-Day Schedules

The prescribed dosage schedule must be followed exactly. The chance of becoming pregnant increases with each pill missed. If you miss one pill, you should take it as soon as you remember and also take your next pill at the regular time, which means you will be taking two pills on that day. If you miss two pills in a row, you should take one of the missed pills as soon as you remember, discard the other missed pill, and take your regular pill for that day at the proper time. Furthermore, you should use an additional method of contraception in addition to taking your pills for the remainder of the cycle. If more than 2 pills in a row have been missed, discontinue taking your pills immediately and use an additional method of contraception until you have a period or your doctor determines that you are not pregnant. Missing pills numbered 22–28 (orange pills) in the 28-day schedule does not increase your chances of becoming pregnant. At times there may be no menstrual period after a cycle of pills. Therefore, if you miss one menstrual period but have taken the pills *exactly as you were supposed to,* continue as usual into the next cycle. If you have not taken the pills correctly, and have missed a menstrual period, *you may be pregnant* and should stop taking oral contraceptives until your doctor determines whether or not you are pregnant. Until you can get to your doctor, use another form of contraception. If two consecutive menstrual periods are missed, you should stop taking pills until it is determined whether you are pregnant. If you do become pregnant while using oral contraceptives, you should discuss the risks to the developing child with your doctor.

Even if spotting or breakthrough bleeding should occur, continue the medication according to the schedule. Should spotting or breakthrough bleeding persist you should notify your physician.

NOR-Q.D.® (norethindrone) Tablets 0.35 mg. Schedule: Take the first pill on the first day of the menstrual flow, and take another pill each day, every day of the year. The pill should be taken at the same time of day, preferably at bedtime, and *continued daily, without interruption, whether bleeding occurs or not.* If prolonged bleeding occurs, you should consult your physician.

The chance of becoming pregnant increases with each pill missed. If you miss one pill, you should take it as soon as you remember and also take your next pill at the regular time, which means you will be taking two pills on that day. If you miss two pills in a row you should take one of the missed pills as soon as you remember, discard the other missed pill, and take your regular pill for that day at the proper time. Furthermore, you should use an additional method of contraception in addition to taking NOR-Q.D.® until you have a period or your doctor determines you are not pregnant. If more than 2 pills in a row have been missed, NOR-Q.D. should be discontinued immediately and an additional method of contraception should be used until you have a period or your doctor determines that you are not pregnant.

Whether or not you have missed a pill, if you have not had a period within 45 days of your last period, *you may be pregnant.* You should stop taking NOR-Q.D. until your doctor determines whether or not you are pregnant. Until you can get to your doctor, use another form of contraception. If you do become pregnant while using NOR-Q.D., you should discuss the risks to the developing child with your doctor.

3. Periodic Examination

Your doctor will take a complete medical and family history before prescribing oral contraceptives. At that time and about once a year thereafter, he will generally examine your blood pressure, breasts, abdomen, and pelvic organs (including a Papanicolaou smear).

Summary: Oral contraceptives are the most effective method, except sterilization, for preventing pregnancy. Other methods, when used conscientiously, are also very effective and have fewer risks. The serious risks of oral contraceptives are uncommon and the "pill" is a very convenient method of preventing pregnancy.

If you have certain conditions or have had these conditions in the past, you should not use oral contraceptives because the risk is too great. These conditions are listed in this leaflet. If you do not have these conditions, and decide to use the "pill", please read this leaflet carefully so that you can use the "pill" most safely and effectively.

Based on his or her assessment of your medical needs, your doctor has prescribed this drug for you. Do not give the drug to anyone else.

[*Shown in Product Identification Section*]

CARMOL® 10 OTC

10% urea lotion for total body dry skin care.

A product of Syntex Laboratories, Inc.
(See PDR For Nonprescription Drugs)

CARMOL® 20 OTC

20% Urea Cream Extra strength for rough, dry skin

A product of Syntex Laboratories, Inc.
(See PDR For Nonprescription Drugs)

CARMOL® HC ℞

(hydrocortisone acetate) Cream 1%

A product of Syntex Laboratories, Inc.

Description: CARMOL HC contains micronized hydrocortisone acetate, USP, 10 mg./g., in a water-washable vanishing cream containing urea (10%), purified water, stearic acid, isopropyl myristate, PPG-26 oleate, isopropyl palmitate, propylene glycol, triethanolamine, cetyl alcohol, carbomer 940, sodium bisulfite, sodium laureth sulfate, edetate disodium, xanthan gum; scented with hypoallergenic perfume. CARMOL HC is non-lipid, non-occlusive and hypoallergenic; it contains no mineral oil, petrolatum, lanolin or parabens.

Actions: Topical steroids are primarily effective because of their anti-inflammatory, antipruritic and vasoconstrictive actions.

Indications: For relief of the inflammatory manifestations of corticosteroid-responsive dermatoses.

Contraindications: Topical steroids are contraindicated in those patients with a history of hypersensitivity to any of the components of the preparation.

Precautions: If irritation develops, the product should be discontinued and appropriate therapy instituted.

In the presence of an infection, the use of an appropriate antifungal or antibacterial agent should be instituted. If a favorable response does not occur promptly, the corticosteroid should be discontinued until the infection has been adequately controlled.

If extensive areas are treated or if the occlusive technique is used there will be increased systemic absorption of the corticosteroid and suitable precautions should be taken, particularly in children and infants.

Although topical steroids have not been reported to have an adverse effect on human pregnancy, the safety of their use in pregnant women has not absolutely been established. In laboratory animals, increases in incidences of fetal abnormalities have been associated with exposure of gestating females to topical corticosteroids, in some cases at rather low dosage levels. Therefore, drugs of this class should not be used extensively on pregnant patients, in large amounts, or for prolonged periods of time.

CARMOL® HC Cream is not for ophthalmic use.

Adverse Reactions: The following local adverse reactions have been reported with topical corticosteroids, especially under occlusive dressings: burning, itching, irritation, dryness, folliculitis, hypertrichosis, acneform eruptions, hypopigmentation, perioral dermatitis, allergic contact dermatitis, maceration of the skin, secondary infection, skin atrophy, striae, miliaria.

Dosage and Administration: Apply to affected areas 3 or 4 times daily.

How Supplied: CARMOL HC (hydrocortisone acetate) Cream, 1%, is supplied in 1 oz. tubes and 4 oz. jars. Protect from excessive heat.

CHO-FREE® Formula Base OTC

Carbohydrate Free and Milk Free Infant Formula Base.

A product of Syntex Laboratories, Inc.
(See PDR For Nonprescription Drugs)

EVEX® ℞

(Esterified Estrogens) TABLETS

A product of Syntex Laboratories, Inc.

1. ESTROGENS HAVE BEEN REPORTED TO INCREASE THE RISK OF ENDOMETRIAL CARCINOMA.

Three independent case control studies have shown an increased risk of endometrial cancer in post-menopausal women exposed to exogenous estrogens for prolonged periods.[1–3] This risk was independent of the other known risk factors for endometrial cancer. These studies are further supported by the finding that incidence rates of endometrial cancer have increased sharply since 1969 in eight different areas of the United States with population-based cancer reporting systems, an increase which may be related to the rapidly expanding use of estrogens during the last decade.[4]

The three case control studies reported that the risk of endometrial cancer in estrogen users was about 4.5 to 13.9 times greater than in nonusers. The risk appears to depend on both duration of treatment[1] and on estrogen dose.[3] In view of these findings, when estrogens are used for the treatment of menopausal symptoms, the lowest dose that will control symptoms should be utilized and medication should be discontinued as soon as possible. When prolonged treatment is medically indicated, the patient should be reassessed on at least a semiannual basis to determine the need for continued therapy. Although the evidence must be considered preliminary, one study suggests that cyclic administration of low doses of estrogen may carry less risk than continuous administration;[3] it therefore appears prudent to utilize such a regimen.

Close clinical surveillance of all women taking estrogens is important. In all cases of undiagnosed persistent or recurring abnormal vaginal bleeding, adequate diagnostic measures should be undertaken to rule out malignancy.

There is no evidence at present that "natural" estrogens are more or less hazardous than "synthetic" estrogens at equiestrogenic doses.

2. ESTROGENS SHOULD NOT BE USED DURING PREGNANCY.

The use of female sex hormones, both estrogens and progestogens, during early pregnancy may seriously damage the offspring. It has been shown that females exposed *in utero* to diethylstilbestrol, a non-

Continued on next page

Syntex—Cont.

steroidal estrogen, have an increased risk of developing in later life a form of vaginal or cervical cancer that is ordinarily extremely rare.[5,6] This risk has been estimated as not greater than 4 per 1000 exposures.[7] Furthermore, a high percentage of such exposed women (from 30 to 90 percent) have been found to have vaginal adenosis, epithelial changes of the vagina and cervix.[8–12] Although these changes are histologically benign, it is not known whether they are precursors of malignancy. Although similar data are not available with the use of other estrogens, it cannot be presumed they would not induce similar changes.

Several reports suggest an association between intrauterine exposure to female sex hormones and congenital anomalies, including congenital heart defects and limb reduction defects.[13–16] One case control study[16] estimated a 4.7 fold increased risk of limb reduction defects in infants exposed *in utero* to sex hormones (oral contraceptives, hormone withdrawal tests for pregnancy, or attempted treatment for threatened abortion). Some of these exposures were very short and involved only a few days of treatment. The data suggest that the risk of limb reduction defects in exposed fetuses is somewhat less than 1 per 1000.

In the past, female sex hormones have been used during pregnancy in an attempt to treat threatened or habitual abortion. There is considerable evidence that estrogens are ineffective for these indications, and there is no evidence from well controlled studies that progestogens are effective for these uses.

If EVEX is used during pregnancy, or if the patient becomes pregnant while taking this drug, she should be apprised of the potential risks to the fetus, and the advisability of pregnancy continuation.

Description: EVEX (esterified estrogens) tablets for oral administration contain either 0.625 mg. or 1.25 mg. of purified, esterified, orally active, water soluble estrogens expressed as sodium estrone sulfate.

Clinical Pharmacology: Estrogens promote growth of the endometrium; promote thickening, stratification, and cornification of the vagina; cause growth of mammary gland ducts; and inhibit the anterior pituitary gland. The ability of estrogens to promote the development of both primary and secondary sex characteristics is of benefit in female hypogonadism, where estrogens provide a substitute for deficient ovarian function.

Indications: EVEX tablets are indicated in the treatment of:

1. Moderate to severe *vasomotor* symptoms associated with the menopause. (There is no evidence that estrogens are effective for nervous symptoms or depression which might occur during menopause, and they should not be used to treat these conditions.)
2. Atrophic vaginitis.
3. Kraurosis vulvae.
4. Female hypogonadism.
5. Female castration.
6. Primary ovarian failure.
7. Breast cancer (for palliation only) in appropriately selected women and men with metastatic disease.
8. Prostatic carcinoma—palliative therapy of advanced disease.

EVEX HAS NOT BEEN SHOWN TO BE EFFECTIVE FOR ANY PURPOSE DURING PREGNANCY AND ITS USE MAY CAUSE SEVERE HARM TO THE FETUS (SEE BOXED WARNING).

Contraindications: Estrogens should not be used in women (or men) with any of the following conditions:

1. Known or suspected cancer of the breast except in appropriately selected patients being treated for metastatic disease.
2. Known or suspected estrogen-dependent neoplasia.
3. EVEX can cause fetal damage when administered to pregnant women. EVEX is contraindicated in women who are or may become pregnant. If this drug is used during pregnancy, or if the patient becomes pregnant while taking this drug, the patient should be apprised of the potential risks to the fetus, and the possibility of termination of the pregnancy should be discussed in the light of those risks. (See boxed warning).
4. Undiagnosed abnormal genital bleeding.
5. Active thrombophlebitis or thromboembolic disorders.
6. A past history of thrombophlebitis or thromboembolic disorders associated with previous estrogen use (except when used in treatment of breast or prostatic malignancy).

Warnings:

1. *Induction of malignant neoplasms.* Long term continuous administration of natural and synthetic estrogens in certain animal species increases the frequency of carcinomas of the breast, cervix, vagina, and liver. There is now evidence that estrogens increase the risk of carcinoma of the endometrium in humans. (See boxed warning.) At the present time there is no satisfactory evidence that estrogens given to postmenopausal women increase the risk of cancer of the breast,[18] although a recent long-term followup of a single physician's practice has raised this possibility.[18a] Because of the animal data there is a need for caution in prescribing estrogens for women with a strong family history of breast cancer or who have breast nodules, fibrocystic disease, or abnormal mammograms.
2. *Gall bladder disease.* A recent study has reported a 2 to 3-fold increase in the risk of surgically confirmed gall bladder disease in women receiving postmenopausal estrogens,[18] similar to the 2-fold increase previously noted in users of oral contraceptives.[19,24] In the case of oral contraceptives, the increased risk appeared after two years of use.[24]
3. *Effects similar to those caused by estrogen-progestogen oral contraceptives.* There are several serious adverse effects of oral contraceptives, most of which have not, up to now, been documented as consequences of postmenopausal estrogen therapy. This may reflect the comparatively low doses of estrogen used in postmenopausal women. It would be expected that the larger doses of estrogen used to treat prostatic or breast cancer or postpartum breast enlargement are more likely to result in these adverse effects, and, in fact, it has been shown that there is an increased risk of thrombosis in men receiving estrogens for prostatic cancer and women for postpartum breast engorgement.[20–23]

   a. *Thromboembolic disease.* It is now well established that users of oral contraceptives have an increased risk of various thromboembolic and thrombotic vascular diseases, such as thrombophlebitis, pulmonary embolism, stroke, and myocardial infarction.[24–31] Cases of retinal thrombosis, mesenteric thrombosis and optic neuritis have been reported in oral contraceptive users. There is evidence that the risk of several of these adverse reactions is related to the dose of the drug.[32,33] An increased risk of post-surgery thromboembolic complications has also been reported in users of oral contraceptives.[34,35] If feasible, estrogen should be discontinued at least 4 weeks before surgery of the type associated with an increased risk of thromboembolism, or during periods of prolonged immobilization.

   While an increased rate of thromboembolic and thrombotic disease in postmenopausal users of estrogens has not been found[18,36] this does not rule out the possibility that such an increase may be present or that subgroups of women who have underlying risk factors or who are receiving relatively large doses of estrogen may have increased risk. Therefore estrogens should not be used in persons with active thrombophlebitis or thromboembolic disorders, and they should not be used (except in treatment of malignancy) in persons with a history of such disorders in association with estrogen use. They should be used with caution in patients with cerebral vascular or coronary artery disease and only for those women in whom estrogens are clearly needed.

   Large doses of estrogen (5 mg. esterified estrogens per day), comparable to those used to treat cancer of the prostate and breast, have been shown in a large prospective clinical trial in men[37] to increase the risk of nonfatal myocardial infarction, pulmonary embolism and thrombophlebitis. When estrogen doses of this size are used, any of the thromboembolic and thrombotic adverse effects associated with oral contraceptive use should be considered a clear risk.

   b. *Hepatic adenoma.* Benign hepatic adenomas appear to be associated with the use of oral contraceptives.[38–40] Although benign, and rare, these may rupture and may cause death through intraabdominal hemorrhage. Such lesions have not yet been reported in association with other estrogen or progestogen preparations but should be considered in estrogen users having abdominal pain and tenderness, abdominal mass, or hypovolemic shock. Hepatocellular carcinoma has also been reported in women taking estrogen-containing oral contraceptives.[39] The relationship of this malignancy to these drugs is not known at this time.

   c. *Elevated blood pressure.* Increased blood pressure is not uncommon in women using oral contraceptives. There is now a report that this may occur with use of estrogens in the menopause[41] and blood pressure should be monitored with estrogen use, especially if high doses are used.

   d. *Glucose tolerance.* A worsening of glucose tolerance has been observed in a significant percentage of patients on estrogen-containing oral contraceptives. For this reason, diabetic patients should be carefully observed while receiving estrogen.
4. *Hypercalcemia.* Administration of estrogens may lead to severe hypercalcemia in patients with breast cancer and bone metastases. If this occurs, the drug should be stopped and appropriate measures taken to reduce the serum calcium level.

Precautions:

A. General Precautions.

1. A complete medical and family history should be taken prior to the initiation of any estrogen therapy. The pretreatment and periodic physical examinations should include special reference to blood pressure, breasts, abdomen, and pelvic organs, and should include a Papanicolaou smear. As a general rule, estrogen should not be prescribed for longer than one year without another physical examination being performed.

2. Fluid retention—Because estrogens may cause some degree of fluid retention, conditions which might be influenced by this factor such as epilepsy, migraine, and cardiac or renal dysfunction, require careful observation.
3. Certain patients may develop undesirable manifestations of excessive estrogenic stimulation, such as abnormal or excessive uterine bleeding, mastodynia, etc.
4. Oral contraceptives appear to be associated with an increased incidence of mental depression.[24] Although it is not clear whether this is due to the estrogenic or progestogenic component of the contraceptive, patients with a history of depression should be carefully observed.
5. Preexisting uterine leiomyomata may increase in size during estrogen use.
6. The pathologist should be advised of estrogen therapy when relevant specimens are submitted.
7. Patients with a past history of jaundice during pregnancy have an increased risk of recurrence of jaundice while receiving estrogen-containing oral contraceptive therapy. If jaundice develops in any patient receiving estrogen, the medication should be discontinued while the cause is investigated.
8. Estrogens may be poorly metabolized in patients with impaired liver function and they should be administered with caution in such patients.
9. Because estrogens influence the metabolism of calcium and phosphorus, they should be used with caution in patients with metabolic bone diseases that are associated with hypercalcemia or in patients with renal insufficiency.
10. Because of the effects of estrogens on epiphyseal closure, they should be used judiciously in young patients in whom bone growth is not complete.
11. Certain endocrine and liver function tests may be affected by estrogen-containing oral contraceptives. The following similar changes may be expected with larger doses of estrogen:
    a. Increased sulfobromophthalein retention.
    b. Increased prothombin and factors VII, VIII, IX, and X; decreased antithrombin 3; increased norepinephrine-induced platelet aggregability.
    c. Increased thyroid binding globulin (TBG) leading to increased circulating total thyroid hormone, as measured by PBI, T4 by column or T4 by radioimmunoassay. Free T3 resin uptake is decreased, reflecting the elevated TBG; free T4 concentration is unaltered.
    d. Impaired glucose tolerance.
    e. Decreased pregnanediol excretion.
    f. Reduced response to metyrapone test.
    g. Reduced serum folate concentration.
    h. Increased serum triglyceride and phospholipid concentration.

B. Pregnancy Category X
See Contraindications and boxed warning.
C. Nursing Mothers
As a general principle, the administration of any drug to nursing mothers should be done only when clearly necessary since many drugs are excreted in human milk.

Adverse Reactions: (See Warnings regarding induction of neoplasia, adverse effects on the fetus, increased incidence of gall bladder disease, and adverse effects similar to those of oral contraceptives, including thromboembolism.) The following additional adverse reactions have been reported with estrogenic therapy, including oral contraceptives:

1. Genitourinary system
Breakthrough bleeding
Spotting
Change in menstrual flow
Dysmenorrhea
Premenstrual-like syndrome
Amenorrhea during and after treatment
Increase in size of uterine fibromyomata
Vaginal candidiasis
Change in cervical eversion and in degree of cervical secretion
Cystitis-like syndrome

2. Breasts
Tenderness, enlargement, secretion

3. Gastrointestinal
Nausea, vomiting
Abdominal cramps, bloating
Cholestatic jaundice

4. Skin
Chloasma or melasma which may persist when drug is discontinued
Erythema multiforme
Erythema nodosum
Hemorrhagic eruption
Loss of scalp hair
Hirsutism

5. Eyes
Steepening of corneal curvature
Intolerance to contact lenses

6. CNS
Headache, migraine, dizziness
Mental depression
Chorea

7. Miscellaneous
Increase or decrease in weight
Reduced carbohydrate tolerance
Aggravation of porphyria
Edema
Changes in libido

Acute Overdosage: Numerous reports of ingestion of large doses of estrogen-containing oral contraceptives by young children indicate that serious ill effects do not occur. Overdosage of estrogen may cause nausea, and withdrawal bleeding may occur in females.

Dosage and Administration:

1. Given cyclically for short term use only:
For treatment of moderate to severe *vasomotor* symptoms, atrophic vaginitis, or kraurosis vulvae associated with the menopause.
The lowest dose that will control symptoms should be chosen and medication should be discontinued as promptly as possible.
Administration should be cyclic (e.g., 3 weeks on and 1 week off).
Attempts to discontinue or taper medication should be made at 3 to 6 month intervals.
The usual dosage ranges are as follows:

Severe vasomotor symptoms: 0.625 mg. to 1.25 mg. daily, depending on severity of symptoms. Dosage may be increased to 2.5 mg. or 3.75 mg. daily if necessary to control symptoms. Dosage should be individualized and titrated according to response.

Atrophic vaginitis and kraurosis vulvae: 1.25 mg. to 3.75 mg. daily for kraurosis vulvae and 0.3 mg. to 1.25 mg. daily for atrophic vaginitis, depending on tissue response. Careful diagnostic evaluation of vulvar lesions is indicated before therapy is instituted.

2. Given cyclically:
Female hypogonadism, female castration, and primary ovarian failure: EVEX is administered for 21 days in a dosage of 2.5 mg. to 7.5 mg. daily. If bleeding occurs before this regimen is concluded, therapy should be discontinued. This same regimen should be resumed following 7 days of no medication, thereby instituting a 3 weeks on, 1 week off dosage regimen.

3. Given chronically:
Inoperable progressing prostatic cancer: For temporary relief of local discomfort, 1.25 mg. to 2.5 mg. daily. Effectiveness can be judged by symptomatic response to therapy and by phosphatase determinations.

Inoperable progressing breast cancer in appropriately selected men and postmenopausal women (see Indications): A dose of up to 10 mg. three times daily over a period of at least three months has been used. Side effects are common in such large doses. Dose adjustment to therapeutic response is important. Treated patients with an intact uterus should be monitored closely for signs of endometrial cancer and appropriate diagnostic measures should be taken to rule out malignancy in the event of persistent or recurring abnormal vaginal bleeding.

References:

[1] Ziel, H. K. and W. D. Finkel, "Increased Risk of Endometrial Carcinoma Among Users of Conjugated Estrogens," *New England Journal of Medicine,* 293:1167-1170, 1975.
[2] Smith, D. C., R. Prentice, D. J. Thompson, and W. L. Hermann, "Association of Exogenous Estrogen and Endometrial Carcinoma," *New England Journal of Medicine,* 293:1164-1167, 1975.
[3] Mack, T. M., M. C. Pike, B. E. Henderson, R. I. Pfeffer, V. R. Gerkins, M. Arthur, and S. E. Brown, "Estrogens and Endometrial Cancer in a Retirement Community," *New England Journal of Medicine,* 294:1262-1267, 1976.
[4] Weiss, N. S., D. R. Szekely, and D. F. Austin, "Increasing Incidence of Endometrial Cancer in the United States," *New England Journal of Medicine,* 294:1259-1262, 1976.
[5] Herbst, A. L., H. Ulfelder, and D. C. Poskanzer, "Adenocarcinoma of Vagina," *New England Journal of Medicine,* 284:878-881, 1971.
[6] Greenwald, P., J. Barlow, P. Nasca, and W. Burnett, "Vaginal Cancer after Maternal Treatment with Synthetic Estrogens," *New England Journal of Medicine,* 285:390-392, 1971.
[7] Lanier, A., K. Noller, D. Decker, L. Elveback, and L. Kurland, "Cancer and Stilbestrol. A Follow-up of 1719 Persons Exposed to Estrogens *In Utero* and Born 1943-1959," *Mayo Clinic Proceedings,* 48:793-799, 1973.
[8] Herbst, A., R. Kurman, and R. Scully, "Vaginal and Cervical Abnormalities After Exposure to Stilbestrol *In Utero,*" *Obstetrics and Gynecology,* 40:287-298, 1972.
[9] Herbst, A., S. Robboy, G. Macdonald, and R. Scully, "The Effects of Local Progesterone on Stilbestrol-Associated Vaginal Adenosis," *American Journal of Obstetrics and Gynecology,* 118:607-615, 1974.
[10] Herbst, A., D. Poskanzer, S. Robboy, L. Friedlander, and R. Scully, "Prenatal Exposure to Stilbestrol, A Prospective Comparison of Exposed Female Offspring with Unexposed Controls," *New England Journal of Medicine,* 292:334-339, 1975.
[11] Stafi, A., R. Mattingly, D. Foley, and W. Fetherston, "Clinical Diagnosis of Vaginal Adenosis," *Obstetrics and Gynecology,* 43: 118-128, 1974.
[12] Sherman, A. I., M. Goldrath, A. Berlin, V. Vakhariya, F. Banooni, W. Michaels, P. Goodman, S. Brown, "Cervical-Vaginal Adenosis After *In Utero* Exposure to Synthetic Estrogens," *Obstetrics and Gynecology,* 44:531-545, 1974.
[13] Gal, I., B. Kirman, and J. Stern, "Hormone Pregnancy Tests and Congenital Malformation," *Nature* 216:83, 1967.
[14] Levy, E. P., A. Cohen, and F. C. Fraser, "Hormone Treatment During Pregnancy and Congenital Heart Defects," *Lancet,* 1:611, 1973.
[15] Nora, J. and A. Nora, "Birth Defects and Oral Contraceptives," *Lancet,* 1:941-942, 1973.
[16] Janerich, D. T., J. M. Piper, and D. M. Glebatis, "Oral Contraceptives and Congenital Limb-Reduction Defects," *New England Journal of Medicine,* 291:697-700, 1974.
[17] "Estrogens for Oral or Parenteral Use," *Federal Register,* 40:8212, 1975.

Continued on next page

Syntex—Cont.

[18] Boston Collaborative Drug Surveillance Program "Surgically Confirmed Gall Bladder Disease, Venous Thromboembolism and Breast Tumors in Relation to Post-Menopausal Estrogen Therapy." *New England Journal of Medicine,* 290:15-19, 1974.

[18a] Hoover, R., L. A. Gray, Sr., P. Cole, and B. MacMahon, "Menopausal Estrogens and Breast Cancer," *New England Journal of Medicine,* 295:401-405, 1976.

[19] Boston Collaborative Drug Surveillance Program, "Oral Contraceptives and Venous Thromboembolic Disease, Surgically Confirmed Gall Bladder Disease, and Breast Tumors," *Lancet* 1:1399-1404, 1973.

[20] Daniel, D. G., H. Campbell, and A. C. Turnbull, "Puerperal Thromboembolism and Suppression of Lactation," *Lancet,* 2: 287-289, 1967.

[21] The Veterans Administration Cooperative Urological Research Group, "Carcinoma of the Prostate: Treatment Comparisons," *Journal of Urology,* 98:516-522, 1967.

[22] Bailer, J. C., "Thromboembolism and Oestrogen Therapy," *Lancet,* 2:560, 1967.

[23] Blackard, C., R. Doe, G. Mellinger, and D. Byar, "Incidence of Cardiovascular Disease and Death in Patients Receiving Diethylstilbestrol for Carcinoma of the Prostate," *Cancer,* 26:249-256, 1970.

[24] Royal College of General Practitioners, "Oral Contraception and Thromboembolic Disease," *Journal of the Royal College of General Practitioners,* 13:267-279, 1967.

[25] Inman, W. H. W., and M. P. Vessey, "Investigation of Deaths from Pulmonary, Coronary, and Cerebral Thrombosis and Embolism in Women of Child-Bearing Age," *British Medical Journal,* 2:193-199, 1968.

[26] Vessey, M. P. and R. Doll, "Investigation of Relation Between Use of Oral Contraceptives and Thromboembolic Disease. A Further Report," *British Medical Journal,* 2:651-657, 1969.

[27] Sartwell, P. E., A. T. Masi, F. G. Arthes, G. R. Greene, and H. E. Smith, "Thromboembolism and Oral Contraceptives: An Epidemiological Case Control Study," *American Journal of Epidemiology,* 90:365-380, 1969.

[28] Collaborative Group for the Study of Stroke in Young Women, "Oral Contraception and Increased Risk of Cerebral Ischemia or Thrombosis," *New England Journal of Medicine,* 288:871-878, 1973.

[29] Collaborative Group for the Study of Stroke in Young Women, "Oral Contraceptives and Stroke in Young Women: Associated Risk Factors", *Journal of the American Medical Association,* 231:718-723, 1975.

[30] Mann, J. I. and W. H. W. Inman, "Oral Contraceptives and Death fom Myocardial Infarction," *British Medical Journal,* 2:245-248, 1975.

[31] Mann, J. I., M. P. Vessey, M. Thorogood, and R. Doll, "Myocardial Infarction in Young Women with Special Reference to Oral Contraceptive Practice," *British Medical Journal,* 2:241-245, 1975.

[32] Inman, W. H. W., V. P. Vessey, B. Westerholm, and A. Engelund, "Thromboembolic Disease and the Steroidal Content of Oral Contraceptives," *British Medical Journal,* 2:203-209, 1970.

[33] Stolley, P. D., J. A. Tonascia, M. S. Tockman, P. E. Sartwell, A. H. Rutledge, and M. P. Jacobs, "Thrombosis with Low-Estrogen Oral Contraceptives," *American Journal of Epidemiology,* 102:197-208, 1975.

[34] Vessey, M. P., R. Doll, A. S. Fairbairn, and G. Glober, "Post-Operative Thromboembolism and the Use of the Oral Contraceptives," *British Medical Journal,* 3:123-126, 1970.

[35] Greene, G. R. and P. E. Sartwell, "Oral Contraceptive Use in Patients with Thromboembolism Following Surgery, Trauma or Infection," *American Journal of Public Health,* 62:680-685, 1972.

[36] Rosenberg, L., M. B. Armstrong, and H. Jick, "Myocardial Infarction and Estrogen Therapy in Postmenopausal Women," *New England Journal of Medicine,* 294:1256-1259, 1976.

[37] Coronary Drug Project Research Group, "The Coronary Drug Project: Initial Findings Leading to Modifications of Its Research Protocol, *Journal of the American Medical Association,* 214:1303-1313, 1970.

[38] Baum, J., F. Holtz, J. J. Bookstein, and E. W. Klein, "Possible Association between Benign Hepatomas and Oral Contraceptives," *Lancet,* 2:926-928, 1973.

[39] Mays, E. T., W. M. Christopherson, M. M. Mahr, and H. C. Williams, "Hepatic Changes in Young Women Ingesting Contraceptive Steroids, Hepatic Hemorrhage and Primary Hepatic Tumors," *Journal of the American Medical Association,"* 235:730-782, 1976.

[40] Edmondson, H. A., B. Henderson, and B. Benton, "Liver Cell Adenomas Associated with the Use of Oral Contraceptives," *New England Journal of Medicine,* 294:470-472, 1976.

[41] Pfeiffer, R. I. and S. Van Den Noort, "Estrogen Use and Stroke Risk in Postmenopausal Women," *American Journal of Epidemiology,* 103:445-456, 1976.

How Supplied: EVEX (esterified estrogens) is supplied as film-coated tablets in two potencies in bottles of 100 tablets: 0.625 mg. (orange) and 1.25 mg. (pink).

Patient Labeling

What You Should Know About Estrogens: Estrogens are female hormones produced by the ovaries. The ovaries make several different kinds of estrogens. In addition, scientists have been able to make a variety of synthetic estrogens. As far as we know, all these estrogens have similar properties and therefore much the same usefulness, side effects, and risks. This leaflet is intended to help you understand what estrogens are used for, the risks involved in their use, and how to use them as safely as possible.

This leaflet includes the most important information about estrogens, but not all the information. If you want to know more, you can ask your doctor or pharmacist to let you read the package insert prepared for the doctor.

Uses of Estrogen: Estrogens are prescribed by doctors for a number of purposes, including:

1. To provide estrogen during a period of adjustment when a woman's ovaries no longer produce it, in order to prevent certain uncomfortable symptoms of estrogen deficiency. (All women normally stop producing estrogens, generally between the ages of 45 and 55; this is called the menopause.)
2. To prevent symptoms of estrogen deficiency when a woman's ovaries have been removed surgically before the natural menopause.
3. To treat certain cancers in women and men.
4. To prevent painful swelling of the breasts after pregnancy in women who choose not to nurse their babies, although the usefulness of this treatment is limited and EVEX is not indicated for this use.

THERE IS NO PROPER USE OF ESTROGENS IN A PREGNANT WOMAN.

Estrogens in the Menopause: In the natural course of their lives all women eventually experience a decrease in estrogen production. This usually occurs between ages 45 and 55 but may occur earlier or later. Sometimes the ovaries may need to be removed before natural menopause by an operation, producing a "surgical menopause."

When the amount of estrogen in the blood begins to decrease, many women may develop typical symptoms: feelings of warmth in the face, neck, and chest or sudden intense episodes of heat and sweating throughout the body (called "hot flashes" or "hot flushes"). These symptoms are sometimes very uncomfortable. A few women eventually develop changes in the vagina (called "atrophic vaginitis") which cause discomfort, especially during and after intercourse.

Estrogens can be prescribed to treat these symptoms of the menopause. It is estimated that considerably more than half of all women undergoing the menopause have only mild symptoms or no symptoms at all and therefore do not need estrogens. Other women may need estrogens for a few months, while their bodies adjust to lower estrogen levels. Sometimes the need will be for periods longer than six months. In an attempt to avoid over-stimulation of the uterus (womb), estrogens are usually given cyclically during each month of use, that is, three weeks of pills followed by one week without pills.

Sometimes women experience nervous symptoms or depression during menopause. There is no evidence that estrogens are effective for such symptoms and they should not be used to treat them, although other treatment may be needed.

You may have heard that taking estrogens for long periods (years) after the menopause will keep your skin soft and supple and keep you feeling young. There is no evidence that this is so, however, and such long-term treatment carries important risks.

The Dangers of Estrogens:

1. *Cancer of the uterus.* When estrogens are used, there is an increased risk of endometrial cancer (cancer of the uterus), particularly with prolonged use. Women taking estrogens have roughly 5 to 10 times as great a chance of getting this cancer as women who take no estrogens. To put this another way, while a postmenopausal woman not taking estrogens has one chance in a 1,000 each year of getting cancer of the uterus, a woman taking estrogens has 5 to 10 chances in 1,000 each year. For this reason *it is important to take estrogens only when you really need them.*

The risk of this cancer is greater the longer estrogens are used and also seems to be greater when larger doses are taken. For this reason *it is important to take the lowest dose of estrogen that will control symptoms and to take it only as long as it is needed.* If estrogens are needed for longer periods of time, your doctor will want to reevaluate your need for estrogens at least every six months.

Women using estrogens should report any irregular vaginal bleeding to their doctors; such bleeding may be of no importance, but it can be an early warning of cancer of the uterus. If you have undiagnosed vaginal bleeding, you should not use estrogens until a diagnosis is made and you are certain there is no cancer of the uterus. If you have had your uterus completely removed (total hysterectomy), there is no danger of developing cancer of the uterus.

2. *Other possible cancers.* Estrogens can cause development of other tumors in animals, such as tumors of the breast, cervix, vagina, or liver, when given for a long time. At present there is no good evidence that women using estrogen in the menopause have an increased risk of such tumors, but there is no way yet to be sure they do not; and one study raises the possibility that use of estrogens in the menopause may increase the risk of breast cancer many years later. This is a further reason to use estrogens only when clearly needed. While you are taking estrogens, it is important that you go to your doctor at least once a year for a physical examination. Also, if members of your family have had breast cancer or if you have breast nodules or abnormal mammograms (breast x-rays), your doctor may wish to carry out more frequent examinations of your breasts.

3. *Abnormal Blood Clotting.* Oral contraceptives, which contain estrogens, increase the risk of blood clotting in various parts of the body. Use of estrogens alone in the menopause is not known to cause such blood clotting, but this has not been fully studied. Estrogens in large doses in the male have been shown to increase the risk of abnormal blood clotting. Abnormal blood clotting can result in a stroke (if the clot is in the brain), a heart attack (clot in a blood vessel of the heart), or a pulmonary embolus (a clot which forms in the legs or pelvis, then breaks off and travels to the lungs). Any of these can be fatal or can lead to serious disability.
If you have had clotting in the legs or lungs, or have had a stroke or heart attack, or if you have angina pectoris, estrogens should be used with great caution and only if clearly needed. Estrogens should not be used at all if you have had any of these conditions while you were using estrogens or birth control pills previously (unless they are being used to treat cancer of the breast or prostate).
Larger doses of estrogens have been shown to increase the risk of abnormal blood clotting; therefore the dosage should be kept as low as possible.
4. *Gall bladder disease.* Women who use estrogens after the menopause are more likely to develop gall bladder disease needing surgery than women who do not use estrogens. Birth control pills have a similar effect.
Special Warning About Pregnancy: You should not use estrogens if you are pregnant. If this should occur, there is a greater than usual chance that the developing child will be born with a birth defect, although the possibility remains fairly small. A female child may have an increased risk of developing cancer of the vagina or cervix later in life (in the teens or twenties). Every possible effort should be made to avoid exposure to estrogens during pregnancy. If exposure occurs, see your doctor.
Other Effects of Estrogens: In addition to the serious known risks described above, estrogens have the following side effects and potential risks:
1. *Nausea and vomiting.* The most common side effect of estrogen therapy is nausea. Vomiting is less common.
2. *Effects on breasts.* Estrogens may cause breast tenderness or enlargement and may cause the breasts to secrete a liquid. These effects are not dangerous.
3. *Effects on the uterus.* Estrogens may cause benign fibroid tumors of the uterus to get larger.
Some women will have menstrual bleeding when estrogens are stopped. But if the bleeding occurs on days you are still taking estrogens you should report this to your doctor.
4. *Effects on liver.* Women taking oral contraceptives, which contain estrogens, on rare occasions develop a tumor of the liver which can rupture and bleed into the abdomen. You should report any swelling or unusual pain or tenderness in the abdomen to your doctor immediately.
Women with a past history of jaundice (yellowing of the skin and white parts of the eyes) may get jaundice again during estrogen use. If this occurs, stop taking estrogens and see your doctor.
5. *Other effects.* Estrogens may cause excess fluid to be retained in the body. This may make some conditions worse, such as epilepsy, migraine, heart disease, or kidney disease.
Summary: Estrogens have important uses, but they have serious risks as well. You must decide, with your doctor, whether the risks are acceptable to you in view of the benefits of treatment. Except where your doctor has prescribed estrogens for use in special cases of cancer of the breast or prostate, you should not use estrogens if you have cancer of the breast or uterus, are pregnant, have undiagnosed abnormal vaginal bleeding, clotting in the legs or lungs, or have had a stroke, heart attack or angina, or clotting in the legs or lungs in the past while you were taking estrogens.
You can use estrogens as safely as possible by understanding that your doctor will require regular physical examinations while you are taking them and will try to discontinue the drug as soon as possible and use the smallest dose possible. Be alert for signs of trouble including:
1. Abnormal bleeding from the vagina.
2. Pains in the calves or chest or sudden shortness of breath, or coughing blood (indicating possible clots in the legs, heart, or lungs).
3. Severe headache, dizziness, faintness, or changes in vision (indicating possible developing clots in the brain or eye).
4. Breast lumps (you should ask your doctor how to examine your own breasts).
5. Jaundice (yellowing of the skin).
6. Mental depression.
Based on his or her assessment of your medical needs, your doctor has prescribed this drug for you. Do not give this drug to anyone else.

KATO® (potassium chloride for oral solution) 20 mEq. (1.5 g. KCl) ℞

A product of Syntex Puerto Rico, Inc.

Description: Spray-dried tomato powder containing 20 mEq potassium (equivalent to 1.5 g. KCl) per 6 grams powder (one dose) with natural and synthetic flavors, spices and colors. Benzoic acid and potassium benzoate added as preservatives. When reconstituted as directed, makes a pleasantly flavored, low sodium tomato juice drink. Each daily dose (2 packets) contains less than 10 mg. sodium.
Indications: The prevention or correction of potassium deficit, particularly when accompanied by hypochloremic alkalosis in conjunction with thiazide diuretic therapy, in digitalis intoxication, or as the result of long-term corticosteroid therapy, low dietary intake of potassium, or excessive vomiting or diarrhea.
Contraindications: Potassium is contraindicated in severe renal impairment involving oliguria, anuria or azotemia; in untreated Addison's disease, familial periodic paralysis, acute dehydration, heat cramps, hyperkalemia from any cause. Potassium chloride should not be employed in patients receiving potassium-sparing agents such as aldosterone antagonists and triamterene.
Precautions: KATO is a concentrate and should be taken only after reconstituting with water as directed. This preparation, like other potassium supplements, must be properly diluted to avoid the possibility of gastrointestinal irritation. Do not use in patients with low urinary output or renal decompensation. Administer with caution; it is impossible to assess accurately the daily dose required. Excessive dosage may result in potassium intoxication. Frequent checks of the clinical status of the patient, ECG and/or plasma potassium level should be made. High plasma concentrations of potassium ion may cause death through cardiac depression, arrhythmias or arrest. Use with caution in patients with cardiac disease.
Adverse Reactions: Vomiting, diarrhea, nausea, and abdominal discomfort may occur. Gross overdosage may produce signs and symptoms of potassium intoxication: mental confusion, listlessness, paresthesia of the extremities, weakness and heaviness of legs, flaccid paralysis, hyperkalemia. ECG abnormalities, fall in blood pressure, cardiac arrhythmias and heart block. The characteristic changes in the ECG are disappearance of the P wave, widening and slurring of QRS complex, changes of the S-T segment, tall peaked T waves, etc.
Toxicity: Potassium intoxication may result from overdosage of potassium or from therapeutic dosage in conditions stated under "Contraindications." Hyperkalemia, when detected, must be treated immediately because lethal levels can be reached in a few hours.
Treatment of Hyperkalemia: 1. Dextrose solution 10% or 25% containing 10 units of crystalline insulin per 20 g. dextrose, given I.V. in a dose of 300cc to 500cc in an hour. 2. Adsorption and exchange or potassium using sodium or ammonium cycle cation exchange resin, orally or as retention enema. 3. Hemodialysis or peritoneal dialysis. 4. Elimination of potassium-containing foods and medicaments. Warning: Digitalis toxicity can be precipitated by lowering the plasma potassium concentration too rapidly in digitalized patients.
Administration and Dosage: Mix with water to make a pleasant tomato juice drink. Each 6 gram unit dose packet provides 20 mEq of potassium. Usual adult dose—1 packet of KATO mixed with about 2 ounces of water twice daily—supplies 40 mEq potassium per day. Take with meals or follow with ½ glass of water. Larger doses may be required, but should be administered under close supervision because of the possibility of potassium intoxication.
How Supplied: Cartons of 30 and 120 6 gram unit dose packets, 20 mEq each.

LIDEX® (fluocinonide) CREAM 0.05% OINTMENT 0.05% ℞

LIDEX®-E (fluocinonide) CREAM 0.05% ℞

TOPSYN® (fluocinonide) GEL 0.05% ℞

Products of Syntex Laboratories, Inc.

Description: LIDEX preparations contain the active compound fluocinonide; TOPSYN gel also contains the active compound fluocinonide. Fluocinonide, which is the 21-acetate ester of fluocinolone acetonide, has the chemical formula 6α, 9-difluoro-11β, 16α, 17, 21-tetrahydroxypregna-1, 4-diene-3, 20-dione, cyclic 16, 17-acetal with acetone 21-acetate.
LIDEX cream contains fluocinonide 0.5 mg./g. in FAPG® cream, a specially formulated cream base consisting of stearyl alcohol, polyethylene glycol 6000, propylene glycol, 1,2,6-hexanetriol and citric acid. This white cream vehicle is greaseless, non-staining, anhydrous and completely water miscible. The base provides emollient and hydrophilic properties.
LIDEX ointment contains fluocinonide 0.5 mg./g. in a specially formulated ointment base consisting of Amerchol CAB (mixture of sterols and higher alcohols), white petrolatum, propylene carbonate and propylene glycol. It provides the occulsive and emollient effects desirable in an ointment.
In these formulations, the active ingredient is totally in solution.
LIDEX-E cream contains fluocinonide 0.5 mg./g. in a water-washable aqueous emollient base of stearyl alcohol, cetyl alcohol, mineral oil, propylene glycol, sorbitan monostearate, polysorbate 60, citric acid and purified water.
TOPSYN gel contains fluocinonide 0.5 mg./g. in a specially formulated gel base consisting of propylene glycol, propyl gallate, disodium edetate, and Carbopol 940 (carboxypolymethylene) with NaOH and/or HCl added to adjust the pH. This clear, colorless, thixotropic vehicle is greaseless, non-staining and completely water miscible. In this formulation, the active ingredient is totally in solution.
Actions: LIDEX preparations and TOPSYN gel are primarily effective because of their anti-inflammatory, antipruritic and vasoconstrictor actions.

Continued on next page

Syntex—Cont.

Indications: For relief of the inflammatory manifestations of corticosteroid-responsive dermatoses.
Contraindications: Topical steroids are contraindicated in those patients with a history of hypersensitivity to any of the components of the preparation.
Precautions: If irritation develops, the cream should be discontinued and appropriate therapy instituted.
In the presence of an infection, the use of an appropriate antifungal or antibacterial agent should be instituted. If a favorable response does not occur promptly, the corticosteroid cream should be discontinued until the infection has been adequately controlled.
If extensive areas are treated or if occlusive technique is used, there will be increased systemic absorption of the corticosteroid and suitable precautions should be taken, particularly in children and infants.
Although topical steroids have not been reported to have an adverse effect on human pregnancy, the safety of their use in pregnant women has not absolutely been established. In laboratory animals, increases in incidences of fetal abnormalities have been associated with exposure of gestating females to topical corticosteroids, in some cases at rather low dosage levels. Therefore, drugs of this class should not be used extensively on pregnant patients, in large amounts or for prolonged periods of time. LIDEX preparations and TOPSYN gel are not for ophthalmic use.
Adverse Reactions: The following local adverse reactions have been reported with topical corticosteroids: burning, itching, irritation, dryness, folliculitis, hypertrichosis, acneform eruptions, hypopigmentation, perioral dermatitis, allergic contact dermatitis, maceration of the skin, secondary infection, skin atrophy, striae, miliaria.
Dosage and Administration: A small amount should be gently massaged into the affected area three or four times daily, as needed.
How Supplied:
LIDEX (fluocinonide)
Cream 0.05%—15g., 30g. and 60g. tubes.
Ointment 0.05%—15g., 30g. and 60g. tubes.
LIDEX-E
Cream 0.05%—15g., 30g. and 60g. tubes.
TOPSYN
Gel 0.05%—15g., 30g. and 60g. tubes.

METHAKOTE® Diaper Rash Cream OTC

A product of Syntex Laboratories, Inc.
(See PDR For Nonprescription Drugs)

NAPROSYN® ℞
(naproxen)
Tablets

A product of Syntex Puerto Rico, Inc.

Description: NAPROSYN tablets for oral administration contain 250 mg. of naproxen. NAPROSYN, a non-steroidal anti-inflammatory agent, is related to the arylacetic acid class of drugs. The chemical name is (+)6-methoxy-α-methyl-2-naphthaleneacetic acid.
Naproxen is an odorless, white to off-white crystalline substance. It is lipid soluble, practically insoluble in water at low pH and freely soluble in water at high pH.
Clinical Pharmacology: NAPROSYN is a non-steroidal agent which has demonstrated anti-inflammatory, analgesic and antipyretic properties in classical animal test systems. In patients with rheumatoid arthritis the anti-inflammatory action has been shown by a reduction in joint swelling, a reduction in pain, a reduction in duration of morning stiffness, a reduction in disease activity as assessed by both the investigator and patient, and increased mobility as demonstrated by a reduction in walking time.
It exhibits an anti-inflammatory effect even in adrenalectomized animals and, therefore, its action is not mediated through the pituitary-adrenal axis. It is not a corticosteroid. It inhibits prostaglandin synthesis but beyond this its mode of action is unknown.
Reproduction studies in rats have shown naproxen to be associated with prolonged labor and difficult parturition when given during late pregnancy. Evidence suggests that this may be due to decreased uterine contractility resulting from the inhibition of prostaglandin synthesis.
Although NAPROSYN relieves certain symptoms and reduces certain clinical manifestations associated with rheumatoid arthritis, there is no evidence that it alters the progressive course of the underlying disease.
In man, NAPROSYN appears to be completely absorbed from the gastrointestinal tract after oral administration. Peak plasma levels following each dose are attained in 2–4 hours with steady-state conditions normally achieved after 4–5 doses. It has a mean biological half-life of approximately 13 hours. At therapeutic levels NAPROSYN is greater than 99% bound to serum albumin.
Approximately 95% of a naproxen dose is excreted in the urine, primarily as unchanged naproxen, 6-0-desmethyl naproxen or their conjugates. The rate of excretion has been found to coincide closely with the rate of drug disappearance from the plasma.
Indications and Usage: NAPROSYN is indicated for relief of the signs and symptoms of rheumatoid arthritis. It is indicated in the treatment of acute flares and in the long-term management of the disease. The safety and effectiveness of NAPROSYN have not been established in those rheumatoid arthritis patients which are designated by the American Rheumatism Association as Functional Class IV (incapacitated, largely or wholly bedridden or confined to a wheelchair; little or no self care).
Improvement in patients treated with NAPROSYN for rheumatoid arthritis has been demonstrated by a reduction in joint swelling, a reduction in pain, a reduction in duration of morning stiffness, a reduction in disease activity as assessed by both the investigator and patient, and by increased mobility as demonstrated by a reduction in walking time.
In clinical studies in patients with rheumatoid arthritis, NAPROSYN has been shown to be comparable to aspirin in controlling the aforementioned measures of disease activity but the frequency and severity of the milder gastrointestinal adverse effects (nausea, dyspepsia, heartburn) and nervous system adverse effects (tinnitus, dizziness, lightheadedness) were less than in the aspirin-treated patients. It is not known whether NAPROSYN causes less peptic ulceration than aspirin.
NAPROSYN may be used safely in combination with gold salts and/or corticosteroids; however, in controlled clinical trials, NAPROSYN added to the regimen of patients receiving corticosteroids did not appear to cause greater improvement over that seen with corticosteroids alone. Whether NAPROSYN could be used in conjunction with partially effective doses of corticosteroid for a "steroid-sparing" effect has not been adequately studied. NAPROSYN added to the regimen of patients receiving gold salts did result in greater improvement. The use of NAPROSYN in combination with salicylates is not recommended because data are inadequate to demonstrate the NAPROSYN produces greater improvement over that achieved with aspirin alone. Further, there is some evidence that aspirin increases the rate of excretion of NAPROSYN.
Controlled trials to establish the safety and effectiveness of NAPROSYN in children have not been conducted.
Generally, improvement due to NAPROSYN has not been found to be dependent on age, sex, severity or duration of disease.
Contraindications: NAPROSYN is contraindicated in patients who have shown hypersensitivity to it. Because the potential exists for cross-sensitivity reactions, NAPROSYN should not be given to patients in whom aspirin or other non-steroidal anti-inflammatory drugs induce the syndrome of asthma, rhinitis or urticaria.
Warnings: NAPROSYN should be given under close supervision to patients prone to upper gastrointestinal tract disease and only after consulting the ADVERSE REACTIONS Section. Gastrointestinal bleeding, sometimes severe, and occasionally fatal, has been reported in patients receiving NAPROSYN (see ADVERSE REACTIONS). In patients with active peptic ulcer and active rheumatoid arthritis, attempts should be made to treat the arthritis with non-ulcerogenic drugs, such as gold. If NAPROSYN must be given, the patient should be under close supervision for signs of ulcer perforation or severe gastrointestinal bleeding.
Precautions: The safety of this drug in pregnancy and lactation has not been established and its use during these events is therefore not recommended. Reproduction studies have been performed in rats, rabbits and mice. In rats, pregnancy was prolonged when naproxen was given before the onset of labor; when it was given after the delivery process had begun, labor was protracted. Similar results have been found with those non-steroidal anti-inflammatory drugs which inhibit prostaglandin synthetase.
Naproxen readily crosses the placental barrier. It has been found in the milk of lactating women at a concentration of approximately 1% of that found in the plasma.
In vitro studies have shown that NAPROSYN, because of its affinity for protein, may displace from their binding sites other drugs which are also albumin-bound and may consequently lead to drug interactions. Theoretically, NAPROSYN itself could likewise be displaced. In a patient receiving bishydroxycoumarin or warfarin, the addition of NAPROSYN to therapy could prolong the prothrombin time. Patients receiving both drugs should be under careful observation. Similarly, patients receiving NAPROSYN and a hydantoin, sulfonamide or sulfonylurea should be observed for signs of toxicity to these drugs.
In chronic studies in mice and rats, high doses of NAPROSYN caused nephritis. Since NAPROSYN is eliminated to a large extent from the body by urinary excretion via glomerular filtration, the drug should be used with great caution in patients with significantly impaired renal function and the monitoring of serum creatinine and/or creatinine clearance is advised in these patients. Additionally, a reduction in daily dosage should be anticipated to avoid the possibility of excessive drug accumulation. In clinical trials a few patients developed mild elevations in BUN. The significance of this is unknown.
If steroid dosage is reduced or eliminated during NAPROSYN therapy, the steroid dosage should be reduced slowly and the patients must be observed closely for any evidence of adverse effects, including adrenal insufficiency and exacerbation of symptoms of rheumatoid arthritis.
Studies to date have not shown changes in the eye attributable to NAPROSYN administration; however, because of adverse eye findings in animal studies with some other non-steroidal anti-inflammatory drugs, it is recommended that ophthalmologic studies be carried out within a reasonable period of time after

starting chronic NAPROSYN therapy and at periodic intervals therafter.
Caution should be exercised by patients whose activities require alertness if they experience drowsiness, dizziness, vertigo or depression during NAPROSYN therapy.
Peripheral edema has been observed in some patients receiving NAPROSYN. Although sodium retention has not been found in metabolic studies, it is possible that patients with questionable or compromised cardiac function may be at greater risk when taking NAPROSYN.
NAPROSYN decreases platelet aggregation and prolongs bleeding time. This effect should be kept in mind when bleeding times are determined.
Patients with initial hemoglobin values of 10 grams or less who are to receive long-term NAPROSYN therapy should have hemoglobin values determined frequently.
The administration of NAPROSYN may result in increased urinary values for 17-ketogenic steroids because of an interaction between the drug and/or its metabolites with m-dinitrobenzene used in this assay. Although 17-hydroxycorticosteroid measurements (Porter-Sibler test) do not appear to be artifactually altered, it is suggested that NAPROSYN therapy be temporarily discontinued 72 hours before adrenal function tests are performed.
Adverse Reactions: Adverse reactions related to the gastrointestinal tract were reported in approximately 1 in 7 patients. In decreasing order of frequency they were: heartburn, nausea, dyspepsia, abdominal pain, constipation, stomatitis, diarrhea, vomiting, melena and gastrointestinal bleeding.
Among 737 patients treated with NAPROSYN during the course of clinical trials in the United States (256 treated for more than two years), 15 cases of peptic ulceration were reported. About half were on concomitant corticosteroid and/or salicylate therapy and about a third had a prior history of peptic ulcer. Gastrointestinal bleeding, including seven potentially serious cases, was also reported in this population. These were not always preceded by premonitory gastrointestinal symptoms. Although most of the patients with serious bleeding were receiving concomitant therapy and had a history of peptic ulcer disease, it should be kept in mind that NAPROSYN also has the potential for causing gastrointestinal bleeding on its own. In foreign marketing experience, there have been a number of fatalities due to gastrointestinal bleeding in patients who were receiving NAPROSYN. A cause-effect relationship in these patients was not established.
Adverse reactions related to the central nervous system were reported in approximately 1 in 12 patients. In decreasing order of frequency they were: headache, drowsiness, dizziness, lightheadedness, vertigo, inability to concentrate and depression.
Adverse reactions related to the skin were reported in approximately 1 in 20 patients. In decreasing order of frequency they were: itching (pruritus), skin eruptions, sweating, ecchymoses, skin rashes, urticaria and purpura.
Adverse reactions related to special senses were reported in approximately 1 in 20 patients. In decreasing order of frequency they were: tinnitus, visual disturbances and hearing disturbances.
Adverse reactions related to the cardiovascular system were reported in approximately 1 in 50 patients. In decreasing order of frequency they were: edema, palpitations and dyspnea. Thirst was reported in approximately 1 in 100 patients.
Rare reactions include angioneurotic edema, thrombocytopenia, agranulocytosis and jaundice.
Overdosage: Should a patient ingest a large number of NAPROSYN tablets, accidentally or purposefully, the stomach may be emptied and usual supportive measures employed. Animal studies suggest that the prompt administration of 5 grams of activated charcoal would tend to reduce markedly the absorption of the drug.
Four cases of significant accidental overdose have been reported in adults. In each case drug doses ranged from 1,900 mg. to 3,000 mg. daily (four to six times the usual daily dose of 500 mg.) for periods of from three to seven days. With the exception of one patient who exhibited some drowsiness, heartburn and a single episode of vomiting, there was no evidence of toxicity or late sequelae from 5 to 15 months later.
The plasma level curves of naproxen have been evaluated in several studies. While the areas under the plasma drug concentration vs. time curves were found to increase proportionally with doses up to 500 mg. b.i.d., larger doses resulted in a less than proportional increase. As incomplete absorption of the drug was eliminated as a factor, it appears that this effect is due to accelerated renal clearance of disproportionately increased amounts of non-protein bound drug. However, whether this effect increases or decreases the toxicity of NAPROSYN has not been established.
Dosage and Administration: The recommended starting dose of NAPROSYN in rheumatoid arthritis is 250 mg., orally, twice daily (morning and evening). During long-term administration the dose may be adjusted up or down depending on the clinical response of the patient. A lower daily dose may suffice for long-term administration. Daily doses higher than 750 mg. are not recommended. The morning and evening doses do not have to be equal in size and the administration of NAPROSYN more frequently than twice daily is not necessary.
Controlled trials to establish the safety and effectiveness of NAPROSYN in children have not been conducted.
Symptomatic improvement usually begins within two weeks. However, if improvement is not seen within this period, a trial for an additional two weeks should be considered.
How Supplied: NAPROSYN is available in scored tablets of 250 mg. (yellow) in bottles of 100 and 500 tablets each.
U. S. Pat. No. 3,904,682
Other U. S. Patents Pending
[*Shown in Product Identification Section*]

NEO-MULL-SOY® OTC
Concentrated Liquid
Milk-Free Soy Isolate Formula

A product of Syntex Laboratories, Inc.
(See PDR For Nonprescription Drugs)

NEO-SYNALAR® ℞
CREAM
[neomycin sulfate 0.5%
(0.35% neomycin base),
fluocinolone acetonide 0.025%]

A product of Syntex Laboratories, Inc.

Description: NEO-SYNALAR cream contains fluocinolone acetonide, which has the chemical formula 6α, 9α-difluoro-16α-hydroxyprednisolone-16, 17-acetonide. The cream contains neomycin sulfate 5 mg./g. (3.5 mg./g. neomycin base) and fluocinolone acetonide 0.25 mg./g. in a water-washable aqueous base of stearic acid, propylene glycol, sorbitan monostearate and monooleate, polysorbate 60 and purified water with methylparaben and propylparaben as preservatives.
Actions: Topical steroids are primarily effective because of their anti-inflammatory, antipruritic and vasoconstrictive actions.

Indications:
Based on a review of this drug by the National Academy of Sciences—National Research Council and/or other information, FDA has classified the indications as follows:
"Possibly" effective:
For topical use in the adjunctive management of acute or chronic dermatoses where the dermatoses are initially infected or develop infection during treatment, when such infections are caused by organisms susceptible to neomycin.
These include: atopic dermatitis, neurodermatitis, contact dermatitis, seborrheic dermatitis, eczematous dermatitis, pruritus ani, lichen simplex chronicus, postanal surgical infections, nummular eczema, stasis dermatitis, intertrigo, exfoliative dermatitis and intertriginous psoriasis.
Final classification of the less-than-effective indications requires further investigation.

Contraindications: Topical steroids are contraindicated in those patients with a history of hypersensitivity to any of the components of the preparation.
Warnings: If local infection should continue or become severe, or in the presence of systemic infection, appropriate systemic antibacterial therapy, based on susceptibility testing, should be considered.
Because of the potential hazard of nephrotoxicity and ototoxicity, prolonged use or use of large amounts of this product should be avoided in the treatment of skin infections following extensive burns, trophic ulceration, and other conditions where absorption of neomycin is possible.
There are articles in the current medical literature that indicate an increase in the prevalence of persons sensitive to neomycin.
Precautions: If irritation develops, the cream should be discontinued and appropriate therapy instituted.
As with all antibiotics, prolonged use may result in over-growth of nonsusceptible organisms. If superinfection occurs, appropriate measures should be taken.
If extensive areas are treated or if occlusive technique is used, there will be increased systemic absorption of the corticosteroid and suitable precautions should be taken, particularly in children and infants.
Although topical steroids have not been reported to have an adverse effect on human pregnancy, the safety of their use in pregnant women has not absolutely been established. In laboratory animals, increases in incidences of fetal abnormalities have been associated with exposure of gestating females to topical corticosteroids, in some cases at rather low dosage levels. Therefore, drugs of this class should not be used extensively on pregnant patients, in large amounts or for prolonged periods of time.
NEO-SYNALAR cream is not for ophthalmic use.
Adverse Reactions: The following local adverse reactions have been reported with topical corticosteroids: burning, itching, irritation, dryness, folliculitis, hypertrichosis, acneform eruptions, hypopigmentation, perioral dermatitis, allergic contact dermatitis, maceration of the skin, secondary infection, skin atrophy, striae, miliaria.
The following adverse reactions have been reported with the topical use of neomycin: ototoxicity and nephrotoxicity.
Dosage and Administration: A small amount should be applied lightly to the affected skin area two or three times daily, as needed, and rubbed in gently and thoroughly until it disappears. Since NEO-SYNALAR® cream is a water-washable vanishing cream, it is easily applied and leaves no traces.
How Supplied: NEO-SYNALAR cream—15, 30 and 60 g. tubes.

Continued on next page

Syntex—Cont.

NORINYL® ℞
(norethindrone with mestranol)
Tablets

Refer to entry under BREVICON® (norethindrone with ethinyl estradiol) Tablets.

NOR-Q.D.® ℞
(norethindrone)
0.35 mg. Tablets

Refer to entry under BREVICON® (norethindrone with ethinyl estradiol) Tablets.

SYNALAR® ℞
(fluocinolone acetonide)
CREAM 0.025%
CREAM 0.01%
OINTMENT 0.025%
TOPICAL SOLUTION 0.01%

SYNALAR-HP® ℞
(fluocinolone acetonide)
CREAM 0.2%

Products of Syntex Laboratories, Inc.

Description: SYNALAR (fluocinolone acetonide) and SYNALAR-HP (fluocinolone acetonide) have the chemical name 6α, 9α-difluoro-16α-hydroxyprednisolone-16, 17-acetonide.

SYNALAR cream contains fluocinolone acetonide 0.25 mg./g. or 0.1 mg./g. in a water-washable aqueous base of stearic acid, propylene glycol, sorbitan monostearate and monooleate, polysorbate 60, purified water and citric acid with methylparaben and propylparaben as preservatives.

SYNALAR ointment contains fluocinolone acetonide 0.25 mg./g. in a white petrolatum U.S.P. vehicle.

SYNALAR topical solution contains fluocinolone acetonide 0.1 mg./g. in a water-washable base of propylene glycol with citric acid.

SYNALAR-HP cream contains fluocinolone acetonide 2 mg./g. in a water-washable aqueous base of stearyl alcohol, cetyl alcohol, mineral oil, propylene glycol, sorbitan monostearate, polysorbate 60, purified water and citric acid with methylparaben and propylparaben as perservatives.

Action: Topical steroids are primarily effective because of their anti-inflammatory, antipruritic and vasoconstrictive actions.

Indications: For relief of the inflammatory manifestations of corticosteroid-responsive dermatoses.

Contraindications: Topical steroids are contraindicated in those patients with a history of hypersensitivity to any of the components of the preparation.

SYNALAR-HP® (fluocinolone acetonide) cream 0.2% should not be used on infants up to two years of age.

Precautions: If irritation develops, the cream should be discontinued and appropriate therapy instituted.

In the presence of an infection, the use of an appropriate antifungal or antibacterial agent should be instituted. If a favorable response does not occur promptly, the corticosteroid cream should be discontinued until the infection has been adequately controlled.

If extensive areas are treated or if occlusive technique is used, there will be increased systemic absorption of the corticosteroid and suitable precautions should be taken, particularly in children and infants.

Although topical steroids have not been reported to have an adverse effect on human pregnancy, the safety of their use in pregnant women has not absolutely been established. In laboratory animals, increases in incidences of fetal abnormalities have been associated with exposure of gestating females to topical corticosteroids, in some cases at rather low dosage levels. Therefore, drugs of this class should not be used extensively on pregnant patients, in large amounts or for prolonged periods of time.

SYNALAR and SYNALAR-HP products are not for ophthalmic use.

SYNALAR-HP cream should not be used for prolonged periods and the quantity per day should not exceed 2 g. of formulated material.

Adverse Reactions: The following local adverse reactions have been reported with topical corticosteroids: burning, itching, irritation, dryness, folliculitis, hypertrichosis, acneform eruptions, hypopigmentation, perioral dermatitis, allergic contact dermatitis, maceration of the skin, secondary infection, skin atrophy, striae, miliaria.

Dosage and Administration:

Open Therapy

Apply three or four times daily as follows: A sparing amount, sufficient to cover the affected area, should be spread evenly over the surface and rubbed in gently until it disappears. In hairy sites, the hair should be parted to allow direct contact with the lesion.

Occlusive Dressing Technique

Apply directly to the affected area, leaving a visible thin coat on the surface. Cover completely with a pliable non-porous film. Changes of dressing may be done once or twice daily as determined on an individual basis by the physician.

Some plastic films may be flammable and due care should be exercised in their use. Similarly, caution should be employed when such films are used on children or left in their proximity, to avoid the possibility of accidental suffocation.

How Supplied:

SYNALAR (fluocinolone acetonide)

Cream 0.025%—15, 30 and 60 g. tubes and 120 and 425 g. jars.

Cream 0.01%—15, 45 and 60 g. tubes.

Ointment 0.025%—15, 30 and 60 g. tubes and 425 g. jars.

Topical Solution 0.01%—20 cc. and 60 cc. plastic squeeze bottles.

SYNALAR-HP® (fluocinolone acetonide) Cream 0.2%—12 g. tubes.

SYNEMOL® ℞
(fluocinolone acetonide)
CREAM 0.025%

A product of Syntex Laboratories, Inc.

Description: SYNEMOL (fluocinolone acetonide) has the chemical name 6α,9α-difluoro-16α-hydroxyprednisolone-16, 17-acetonide. The cream contains fluocinolone acetonide 0.25 mg./g. in a water-washable aqueous emollient base of stearyl alcohol, cetyl alcohol, mineral oil, propylene glycol, sorbitan monostearate, polysorbate 60, purified water, and citric acid.

Actions: SYNEMOL (fluocinolone acetonide) cream is primarily effective because of its anti-inflammatory, antipruritic and vasoconstrictor action.

Indications: For relief of the inflammatory manifestations of corticosteroid-responsive dermatoses.

Contraindications: Topical steroids are contraindicated in those patients with a history of hypersensitivity to any of the components of the preparation.

Precautions: If irritation develops, the cream should be discontinued and appropriate therapy instituted.

In the presence of an infection, the use of an appropriate antifungal or antibacterial agent should be instituted. If a favorable response does not occur promptly, the corticosteroid cream should be discontinued until the infection has been adequately controlled.

If extensive areas are treated or if occlusive technique is used, there will be increased systemic absorption of the corticosteroid and suitable precautions should be taken, particularly in children and infants.

Although topical steroids have not been reported to have an adverse effect on human pregnancy, the safety of their use in pregnant women has not absolutely been established. In laboratory animals, increases in incidences of fetal abnormalities have been associated with exposure of gestating females to topical corticosteroids, in some cases at rather low dosage levels. Therefore, drugs of this class should not be used extensively on pregnant patients, in large amounts or for prolonged periods of time.

SYNEMOL® (fluocinolone acetonide) cream is not for ophthalmic use.

Adverse Reactions: The following local adverse reactions have been reported with topical corticosteroids: burning, itching, irritation, dryness, folliculitis, hypertrichosis, acneform eruptions, hypopigmentation, perioral dermatitis, allergic contact dermatitis, maceration of the skin, secondary infection, skin atrophy, striae, miliaria.

Dosage and Administration:

Open Therapy

SYNEMOL® (fluocinolone acetonide) cream should be applied three or four times daily as follows: a sparing amount, sufficient to cover the affected area, should be spread evenly over the surface and rubbed in gently until it disappears. In hairy sites, the hair should be parted to allow direct contact with the lesion.

Occlusive Dressing Technique

Apply SYNEMOL cream directly to the affected area, leaving a visible thin coat on the surface. Cover completely with a pliable non-porous film. Changes of dressing may be done once or twice daily as determined on an individual basis by the physician.

Some plastic films may be flammable and due care should be exercised in their use. Similarly, caution should be employed when such films are used on children or left in their proximity, to avoid the possibility of accidental suffocation.

How Supplied: Synemol® (fluocinolone acetonide) Cream 0.025%—15, 30 and 60 g. tubes.

TOPIC® OTC
Benzyl alcohol gel
Relieves itching

A product of Syntex Laboratories, Inc.

(See PDR For Nonprescription Drugs)

VAGITROL® ℞
Cream
Suppositories

Products of Syntex Laboratories, Inc.

Description: Vagitrol cream is a water miscible, absorptive cream with the following formula:

Sulfanilamide	15.0%
Allantoin	2.0%
Aminacrine hydrochloride	0.2%

with lactose, stearic acid, cetyl alcohol, triethanolamine, sodium lauryl sulfate and glycerin with methylparaben and propylparaben as preservatives, buffered with lactic acid to a pH of approximately 4.5

The Vagitrol cream base has a very low surface tension that permits rapid and thorough dispersion into the folds of the vaginal mucous membrane.

Each Vagitrol soft gelatin suppository contains:

Sulfanilamide	1.05 g.
Allantoin	0.14 g.
Aminacrine hydrochloride	0.014 g.

in a water miscible absorptive base consisting of lactose, polyethylene glycol 400, polysorbate 80, polyethylene glycol 4000, glycerin, lactic acid, and coloring with methylparaben and propylparaben as preservatives. Each suppository is equivalent to one applicatorful of Vagitrol cream.

Actions: Local antimicrobial activity of sulfanilamide and aminacrine hydrochloride against *Haemophilus vaginalis* and other susceptible microorganisms.

Vagitrol is formulated to inhibit growth of pathogenic organisms without attacking vaginal tissues. It is buffered to a pH of approximately 4.5 resembling that of the normal vagina; this acidity discourages pathogenic organisms and at the same time provides a favorable environment for eventual recolonization by the acid-producing Döderlein bacilli normally found in the vagina.

Whenever possible, treatment should be based on specific diagnoses established with sound clinical and laboratory methods.

Indications:
Based on a review of this drug by the National Academy of Sciences-National Research Council and/or other information. FDA has classified the indications as follows:

"Probably" effective: For the relief of symptoms of vulvovaginitis where isolation of the specific organism responsible (usually *Trichomonas vaginalis, Candida albicans*, or *Haemophilus vaginalis*) is not possible.

NOTE.—When the offending organism is known, treatment with a specific agent known to be active against that microorganism is preferred.

"Possibly" effective: For the treatment of trichomoniasis, vulvovaginal candidiasis, and vaginitis due to *Haemophilus vaginalis* or other susceptible bacteria.

Final classification of the less-than-effective indications requires further investigation.

Contraindications: Hypersensitivity to sulfonamides or to the ingredients of this product. Kidney disease.

Warnings: *Use in Pregnancy:* The safe use of sulfonamides in pregnancy has not been established. The teratogenic potential of most sulfonamides has not been thoroughly investigated in either animals or humans. However, a significant increase in the incidence of cleft palate and other bony abnormalities of offspring has been observed when certain sulfonamides of the short, intermediate and long acting types were given to pregnant rats and mice at high oral doses (7 to 25 times the human therapeutic dose).

The usefulness of antibacterial agents, including the sulfonamides, is limited due to the increasing frequency of resistant organisms.

Deaths associated with the administration of sulfonamides have been reported from hypersensitivity reactions, agranulocytosis, aplastic anemia, and other blood dyscrasias. The presence of clinical signs such as sore throat, fever, pallor, purpura, or jaundice may be early indications.

If evidence of systemic toxicity occurs, the medication should be discontinued.

Precautions: Sulfonamides should be given with caution to patients with impaired renal or hepatic function and to those with severe allergy or bronchial asthma.

Adequate fluid intake must be maintained in order to prevent crystalluria and stone formation.

In glucose-6-phosphate dehydrogenase deficient individuals, hemolysis may occur. This reaction is frequently dose-related.

Adverse Reactions: Blood dyscrasias: Agranulocytosis, aplastic anemia, thrombocytopenia, leukopenia, hemolytic anemia, purpura, hypoprothrombinemia and methemoglobinemia.

Allergic reactions: Erythema multiforme (Stevens-Johnson Syndrome), generalized skin eruptions, epidermal necrolysis, urticaria, serum sickness, pruritus, exfoliative dermatitis, anaphylactoid reactions, periorbital edema, conjunctival and scleral injection, photosensitization, arthralgia, and allergic myocarditis.

Gastrointestinal reactions: Nausea, emesis, abdominal pains, hepatitis, diarrhea, anorexia, pancreatitis, and stomatitis.

C.N.S. reactions: Headache, peripheral neuritis, mental depression, convulsions, ataxia, hallucinations, tinnitus, vertigo and insomnia.

Miscellaneous reactions: Drug fever, chills, and toxic nephrosis with oliguria and anuria. Periarteritis nodosum and L.E. phenomenon have occurred.

The sulfonamides bear certain chemical similarities to some goitrogens, diuretics (acetazolamide and the thiazides), and oral hypoglycemic agents. Goiter production, diuresis, and hypoglycemia have occurred rarely in patients receiving sulfonamides. Cross-sensitivity may exist with these agents.

Rats appear to be especially susceptible to the goitrogenic effects of sulfonamides, and long-term administration has produced thyroid malignancies in the species.

Dosage and Administration: One applicatorful (about 6 g.) or suppository intravaginally once or twice daily. Improvements in symptoms should occur within a few days, but treatment should be continued through one complete menstrual cycle unless a definite diagnosis is made and specific therapy initiated.

If there is no response within a few days or if symptoms recur, the drug should be discontinued and another attempt made by appropriate laboratory methods to isolate the organism responsible (*Trichomonas vaginalis, Candida albicans, Haemophilus vaginalis*) and institute specific therapy.

Douching with a suitable solution before insertion may be recommended for hygienic purposes. A pad may be used to protect the underclothing if necessary.

How Supplied:
Vagitrol cream
4 oz. tubes with applicator
Vagitrol suppositories
16 vaginal suppositories with applicator

Thex Corporation
202 GREEN STREET
SAN FRANCISCO, CA 94111

CANTHARONE® ℞
Cantharidin Collodion

Composition: 0.7% cantharidin in a film-forming vehicle containing acetone, ethocel and flexible collodion. Ether 35%, alcohol 11%.

Indications: Cantharone is intended for removal of benign epithelial growths: warts (including ordinary, periungual, subungual, plantar and palpebral warts) and molluscum contagiosum. It is designed for topical application by or under the supervision of a physician. Its simplicity and the absence of instruments and manipulation commend Cantharone to the physician treating children.

Advantages: Simple and painless to apply. No advance preparation. No knives, needles or cauteries. Leaves no scar because it is selectively destructive; does not affect tissue layers below the epidermis; contains no randomly destructive acids. Clinically proved effective.

Directions: *Ordinary and periungual warts*—No cutting or prior treatment is required. (Occasionally nails must be trimmed to expose subungual warts to medication.) Apply Cantharone directly to the lesion; cover the growth completely using an applicator stick. Allow a few seconds for a thin membrane to form and cover with a piece of non-porous plastic adhesive tape, e.g., Blenderm. Instruct patient to remove tape in 24 hours and replace with a loose Band-Aid. On next visit remove necrotic tissue and reapply Cantharone to any growth remaining. Defer second treatment if inflammation is intense. A single application usually suffices for normally keratinized skin. *Plantar warts*—Pare away keratin covering the wart; avoid cutting viable tissue. Using an applicator stick, apply Cantharone to the wart, repeating until a generous amount has been applied. Allow to dry until a film forms, then apply a protective cut-out cushion and secure with non-porous plastic adhesive tape (Blenderm). Leave in place for a week, then debride. If any viable wart tissue remains after debridement, reapply a small amount of Cantharone and bandage as above. Three or more such treatments may be required for large lesions. When destruction of wart is complete, the healed site will appear smooth, with normal skin lines.

Palpebral warts—Using a toothpick or fine probe, apply a small amount of Cantharone to the surface of the wart. Avoid touching surrounding normal skin or applying inside the eyelashes. Leave lesion uncovered. Repeat in a week or ten days if any growth remains.

Molluscum contagiousum—Coat each lesion with a thin film of Cantharone. In one week, treat any new lesions the same way and retreat any resistant lesions with Cantharone, this time covering with a small piece of occlusive tape. The tape should be removed in 6 to 8 hours.

Warnings: Cantharidin is a strong vesicant and Cantharone may produce blisters if it comes in contact with normal skin or mucous membrane. If spilled on skin, wipe off at once, using acetone, alcohol or tape remover. Then wash vigorously with warm soapy water and rinse well. If spilled on mucous membranes or in eyes, flush with water, remove precipitated collodion, and flush with water for an additional 15 minutes.

Patients vary in their sensitivity to cantharidin and in rare cases tingling, burning or extreme tenderness may develop. In these cases the patient should remove tape and soak the area in cool water for 10 to 15 minutes, repeating as required for relief. If soreness persists, puncture blister using sterile technique, apply antiseptic and cover with a Band-Aid. It is advisable to treat only one or two lesions on the first visit, until the sensitivity of the patient is known. For external use only.

Adverse Reactions: The development of annular warts following Cantharone therapy has been reported in a small percentage of patients. These lesions are superficial and, although they may alarm some patients, present little problem. Treatment consists of patient reassurance and retreatment using either Cantharone or other procedures.

There has been one report of chemical lymphangitis following use of Cantharone in combination with salicylic acid plaster.

How Supplied: 7.5 ml bottles.

Literature: Reprints available.

THEX® FORTE Capsules
High Potency Vitamin C and B Complex

Composition: Each capsule provides:

Ascorbic Acid	500 mg
Thiamine Mononitrate	25 mg
Riboflavin	15 mg
Pyridoxine Hydrochloride	5 mg
Niacinamide	100 mg
Calcium Pantothenate	10 mg

Contains no folic acid, no vitamin B_{12}.

Action and Uses: Thex Forte Capsules provide massive doses of water-soluble vitamins for those clinical situations in which saturation vitamin therapy is indicated. These conditions may include convalescence following surgery, burns or trauma; nutritional management of patients suffering from febrile disor-

Continued on next page

Thex—Cont.

ders, chronic infections or gastrointestinal disorders; malnutrition in geriatric or alcoholic patients; prolonged antibiotic therapy; or concurrent vitamin B complex and vitamin C deficiencies.
Dosage: Adults: one or two capsules daily.
How Supplied: Bottles of 30 and 100.

Thompson Medical Company, Inc.
919 THIRD AVENUE
NEW YORK, NEW YORK 10022

EXTRA STRENGTH APPEDRINE® OTC
Anorectic for Weight Control

Each tablet contains:	
phenylpropanolamine HCl	35 mg
caffeine	100 mg
Each three tablets contain:	
Vitamin A	5000 IU
Vitamin D	400 IU
Vitamin E	30 IU
Vitamin C (Ascorbic Acid)	60 mg
Folic Acid	0.4 mg
Vitamin B_1 (Thiamine HCl)	1.5 mg
Vitamin B_2 (Riboflavin)	1.7 mg
Niacinamide	20 mg
Vitamin B_6 (Pyridoxine HCl)	2 mg
Vitamin B_{12} (Cyanocobalamin)	6 mcg
d-Calcium Pantothenate	10 mg

Description: Each tablet contains phenylpropanolamine HCl, an anorexiant and caffeine, a mild stimulant and one third of the recommended daily adult requirement of major vitamins.
Indications: Extra Strength APPEDRINE is indicated as adjunctive therapy in the management of simple exogenous obesity in a regimen of weight reduction and control based on caloric restriction.
Caution: Do not exceed recommended dosage. Discontinue use if rapid pulse, dizziness or palpitations occur. Do not use if high blood pressure, heart, diabetes, kidney, thyroid or other disease is present or if pregnant, nursing or by anyone under the age of 18 except on the advice of a physician. Keep this and all drugs out of the reach of children. In case of accidental overdose, seek professional assistance or contact a Poison Control Center immediately.
Precaution: Avoid use if taking prescription, anti-hypertensive and anti-depressive drugs containing monoamine oxidase inhibitors or other medication containing sympathomimetic amines. Avoid continuous use longer than 3 months.
Adverse Reactions: Side effects are rare when taken as directed. Nausea or nasal dryness may occasionally occur.
Dosage and Administration: Adults: One tablet 30–60 minutes before each meal three times a day with one or two full glasses of water.
How Supplied: Extra Strength APPEDRINE® packages of 30 and 60 tablets packaged with 1200 Calorie Extra Strength Appedrine Diet Plan.

ASPERCREME™

Description: 10% Triethanolamine Salicylate in a pleasantly scented lotion and cream.
Actions: External analgesic with rapid penetration and absorption.
Indications: An effective salicylate analgesic for temporary relief from minor pains of arthritis, rheumatism and muscular aches. Moderately effective in relieving the sensation of burning and tingling, frequently occurring in the hands and feet of elderly patients.
Contraindications: Do not use in patients manifesting idiosyncrasy to salicylates.
Warning: Use only as directed. If pain persists for more than ten days or in arthritic or rheumatic conditions affecting children under twelve years of age, consult a physician immediately. Keep out of reach of children.
Precautions: For external use only. Occasionally where this product has been used extensively, moderate peeling of the skin may occur. This is a normal reaction to salicylates on the skin, and should not warrant discontinuance of the use of the product.
Dosage and Administration: Apply to painful areas with gentle massage until absorbed into skin, three or four times daily, especially before retiring. Relief lasts for hours.
How Supplied: Lotion; 6 oz plastic bottle. Cream; 3 oz plastic tube.
References: Golden, Emanuel L., M.D., A Double-Blind Comparison of Orally Ingested Aspirin and a Topically Applied Salicylate Cream in the Relief of Rheumatic Pain, Current Therapeutic Research, 24, 5:524, 1978 (Sept.).

CONTROL™ Capsules OTC
Prolonged action anorectic for weight control containing
phenylpropanolamine HCl 75 mg

Description: Phenylpropanolamine HCl is a sympathomimetic, related to ephedrine but with less CNS stimulation. Useful as an anorexiant.
Indication: CONTROL is indicated as adjunctive therapy in a regimen of weight reduction based on caloric restriction in the management and control of simple exogenous obesity.
Caution: For Adults use only.
Do not exceed recommended dose. If nervousness, dizziness, sleeplessness, rapid pulse, palpitations or other symptoms occur discontinue medication and consult your physician. If you have, or are being treated for high blood pressure, heart, diabetes, thyroid or other disease, or while pregnant, or nursing or under the age of 18 do not take this drug except under the advice of a physician. Keep this and all drugs out of the reach of children. In case of accidental overdose seek professional assistance or contact a Poison Control Center immediately.
Precaution: Avoid use if taking prescription, anti-hypertensive and anti-depressive drugs containing monoamine oxidase inhibitors or other medication containing sympathomimetic amines. Avoid continuous use for longer than 3 months.
Adverse Reactions: Side effects are rare when taken as directed. Nausea or nasal dryness may occasionally occur.
Dosage and Administration: One capsule with a full glass of water once a day at midmorning (10:00 A.M.).
How Supplied: CONTROL™ Capsules—Packages of 14, 28 and 56 capsules, packaged with 1200 Calorie CONTROL Diet Plan.

> A U.S. Government advisory panel of medical and scientific experts has determined that active ingredient in this product is safe and effective when taken as directed for appetite control to aid in weight reduction by caloric restriction.

Reference: Griboff, Solomon, I., M.D., F.A.C.P. et al., A Double-Blind Clinical Evaluation of a Phenylpropanolamine-Caffeine Combination and a Placebo in the Treatment of Exogenous Obesity, Current Therapeutic Research 17, 6:535, 1975 (June).

DEXATRIM™ Capsules OTC
Prolonged action anorectic for weight control contains

phenylpropanolamine HCl	**50 mg**
caffeine	**200 mg**

DEXATRIM™ Extra Strength Capsules OTC

phenylpropanolamine	**75 mg**
caffeine	**200 mg**

Description: Phenylpropanolamine hydrochloride is a sympathomimetic, related to ephedrine but with less CNS stimulation. Useful as an anorexiant. Caffeine is a mild stimulant.
Indication: DEXATRIM and Extra Strength DEXATRIM Capsules are indicated as adjunctive therapy in a regimen of weight reduction based on caloric restriction in the management and control of simple exogenous obesity.
Studies comparing DEXATRIM to prescription anorexiants have shown DEXATRIM to be equally effective in helping to suppress appetite and in resultant weight loss. DEXATRIM, however, unlike prescription products, has been shown to induce little to no untoward CNS effects. When DEXATRIM was compared to mazindol in a six-week, double-blind study employing 67 outpatients[1] similar weight losses were reported for all subjects. DEXATRIM patients reported no significant adverse effects, while 18% of the mazindol patients reported side effects which included nervousness, nausea and insomnia.
In a six week double-blind parallel study comparing phenylpropanolamine HCl to diethylpropion similar weight losses occurred in 62 clinically obese patients. Ninety-six percent of the patients receiving phenylpropanolamine HCl and 87% of the patients receiving diethylpropion lost weight.[2]
Caution: Do not exceed recommended dosage. Discontinue use if rapid pulse, dizziness or palpitations occur. Do not use if high blood pressure, heart, diabetes, kidney, thyroid or other disease is present or if pregnant, nursing or by anyone under the age of 18 except on the advice of a physician. Keep this and all drugs out of the reach of children. In case of accidental overdose seek professional assistance or contact a Poison Control Center immediately.
Precaution: Avoid use if taking prescription, anti-hypertensive and anti-depressive drugs containing monoamine oxidase inhibitors or other medication containing sympathomimetic amines. Avoid continuous use for longer than 3 months.
Adverse Reactions: Side effects are rare when taken as directed. Nausea or nasal dryness may occasionally occur.
Dosage and Administration:
DEXATRIM™ Capsules: One capsule with a full glass of water mid-morning (10:00 AM)
Extra Strength DEXATRIM™ Capsules: One capsule with a full glass of water mid-morning (10:00 AM)
How Supplied:
DEXATRIM™ Capsules: Packages of 28 or 56 with 1200 calorie DEXATRIM Diet Plan
Extra Strength DEXATRIM™ Capsules:- Packages of 20 and 40 with 1200 calorie DEXATRIM Diet Plan.

> A U.S. Government advisory panel of medical and scientific experts has determined the combination of active ingredients in this product as safe and effective when taken as directed for appetite control to aid in weight reduction by caloric restriction.

1. Report on file, Professional Services, Thompson Medical Company, Inc. 919 Third Avenue, New York, New York 10022.
2. Report on file, Professional Services, Thompson Medical Company, Inc. 919

Third Avenue, New York, New York 10022.

Super Strength PROLAMINE™ Capsules OTC
Continous Action Anorectic for Weight Control

Each capsule contains:

phenylpropanolamine HCl	50 mg
caffeine	140 mg

Description: Each capsule contains phenylpropanolamine hydrochloride an anorexiant and caffeine, a mild stimulant.
Indication: Super Strength PROLAMINE is indicated as adjunctive therapy in the regimen of weight reduction based on caloric restriction in the management and control of simple exogenous obesity.
In a six week double-blind study of 70 obese patients comparing phenylpropanolamine HCl to a placebo, 35% of the subjects taking phenylpropanolamine HCl experienced a weight loss of 8 pounds or more. Only 9% of the subjects taking placebo lost that amount of weight. Results were statistically significant at the 0.05 probability level.[1]
Caution: Do not exceed recommended dosage. Discontinue use if rapid pulse, dizziness, or palpitations occur. Do not take if you have high blood pressure, heart disease, diabetes, kidney, thyroid, or other disease or if pregnant or lactating. Keep this and all drugs out of the reach of children. In case of accidental overdose seek professional assistance or contact a Poison Control Center immediately.
Precaution: Avoid use if taking prescription, anti-hypertensive and anti-depressive drugs containing monoamine oxidase inhibitors or other medication containing sympathomimetic amines. Avoid continuous use for longer than 3 months.
Adverse Reactions: Side effects are rare when taken as directed. Nausea or nasal dryness may occasionally occur.
Dosage and Administration: One capsule at 10 A.M. and 1 capsule at 4 P.M.
How Supplied: Super Strength PROLAMINE™ Capsules: Packages of 20 and 50 packaged with 1200 Calorie PROLAMINE Diet Plan.

A U.S. Government advisory panel of medical and scientific experts has determined the combination of active ingredients in this product as safe and effective when taken as directed for appetite control to aid in weight reduction by caloric restriction.

1. Report on file, Professional Services, Thompson Medical Company, Inc. 919 Third Avenue, New York, New York 10022

Travenol Laboratories, Inc.
Parenteral Products Division
ONE BAXTER PARKWAY
DEERFIELD, ILLINOIS 60015

AMIGEN® ℞
(Protein Hydrolysate Injection, USP-Casein) Injections †

Description: AMIGEN (Protein Hydrolysate Injections, USP-Casein) Injections are sterile, nonpyrogenic solutions of alpha-amino acids and low molecular weight peptides derived from casein by hydrolysis using pancreatic proteolytic enzymes.
The pH of AMIGEN (Protein Hydrolysate) Injections is adjusted with sulfurous acid. The pH ranges between 5.0 and 6.0. Sodium Bisulfite, USP, 0.05% and potassium metabisulfite, 0.056% are added as stabilizers.

AMIGEN Injection	Approx kcal/l	Approx mOs/l	Electrolytes* mEq/l Na+	K+	Ca++	Mg++	Cl−	HPO_4−
AMIGEN Injection, 5%	170	430	35	19	5	2	20	30
AMIGEN Injection, 5%; Dextrose, 5%	340	682	35	19	5	2	20	30
AMIGEN Injection, 10%**	340	860	60	31	10	4	44	60

*The excess of cations is balanced by anions of the amino acids and stabilizers.
** To be diluted aseptically with desired carbohydrate solution.

Total nitrogen is approximately 6.5 g/l in 5% AMIGEN Injection and 13.0 g/l in 10% AMIGEN Injection; alpha-amino nitrogen is typically 55 to 60% of total nitrogen.
†Available as TRAVAMIN® (Protein Hydrolysate Injection, USP casein)

Approximate Amino Acid Content of 5% AMIGEN (Protein Hydrolysate) Injection

Essential Amino Acids mg/100 ml		Non-essential Amino Acids mg/100 ml	
Leucine	410	Glutamic Acid	1300
Lysine	310	Proline	450
Valine	310	Aspartic Acid	350
Isoleucine	260	Serine	300
Phenylalanine	200	Arginine	180
Threonine	190	Alanine	150
Methionine	130	Glycine	110
Histidine	130	Tyrosine	60
Tryptophan	35		

Approximate calories, osmolarities and milliequivalents of electrolytes:
[See table above].
Actions: AMIGEN (Protein Hydrolysate) Injections provide a biologically utilizable source material for protein synthesis, when administered with non-protein calories (such as hypertonic dextrose solution or lipid emulsion). Administered peripherally after appropriate dilution or with minimal calorie supplementation, (such as 5% dextrose), it enhances the conservation of body protein.
Indications: AMIGEN (Protein Hydrolysate) Injections are indicated as an adjunct in the prevention of nitrogen loss or in the treatment of negative nitrogen balance in patients where: (1) the alimentary tract, by the oral, gastrostomy or jejunostomy route, cannot or should not be used, (2) gastrointestinal absorption of protein is impaired, or (3) metabolic requirements for protein are subsantially increased, as with extensive burns.
Central Vein Administration: Central vein infusion should be considered when amino acid solutions are to be admixed with hypertonic dextrose to promote protein synthesis for hypercatabolic or depleted patients or those requiring long-term parenteral nutrition.
Peripheral Vein Administration: For patients in whom the central vein route is not indicated, amino acid solutions mixed with low dextrose concentrations may be infused by peripheral vein when supplemented with fat emulsion.
Protein Sparing: Dilute amino acid solutions *for peripheral administration* may be used in patients who exemplify no clinically significant protein malnutrition. The purpose of the solution is to replace protein losses which occur in relation to an intercurrent phenomenon which is known or suspected to be productive of a protein loss condition for a short or moderate period of time. Protein sparing can be achieved by peripheral infusion of amino acid solutions.
Contraindications:
1. Patients with renal failure-anuria
2. Patients with severe liver disease-hepatic coma
3. Hypersensitivity to one or more amino acids

Warnings:
1. Proper administration of AMIGEN (Protein Hydrolysate) Injections requires a knowledge of fluid and electrolyte balance and nutrition as well as clinical expertise in recognition and treatment of the complications which may occur FREQUENT CLINICAL EVALUATION AND LABORATORY DETERMINATIONS ARE NECESSARY FOR PROPER MONITORING DURING ADMINISTRATION. Studies should include blood sugar, serum proteins, kidney and liver function tests, electrolytes, hemogram, carbon dioxide combining power or content, serum and urine osmolarities, and blood ammonia levels.
2. Administration of protein hydrolysate injection to a patient with hepatic insufficiency may result in serum amino acid imbalances, hyperammonemia, stupor and coma.
   Hyperammonemia is of SPECIAL SIGNIFICANCE IN INFANTS as it can result in mental retardation. This reaction appears to be dose-related and more likely to develop during prolonged therapy. This reaction appears to be related to a deficiency of the urea cycle amino acids of genetic or product origin. It is essential that blood ammonia be measured frequently in infants.
   Conservative doses of AMIGEN (Protein Hydrolysate) Injections should be given to patients with known or suspected hepatic dysfunction. Should symptoms of hyperammonemia develop, administration should be discontinued and the patient's clinical status re-evaluated.
3. Administration of protein hydrolysate injection in the presence of impaired renal function presents special dangers associated with retention of electrolytes.
4. The safety of the use of protein hydrolysate injection in pregnant women has not been demonstrated.
5. Do not administer unless solution is clear.

Precautions:
1. It is essential to provide adequate calories concurrently if parenterally administered protein hydrolysate is to be retained by the body and utilized for protein synthesis. Concentrated dextrose solutions are an effective source of such calories.
2. With the administration of AMIGEN (Protein Hydrolysate) Injections in combination with highly concentrated dextrose solutions, hyperglycemia, glycosuria, and hyperosmolar syndrome may result. Blood and urine glucose should be monitored on a routine basis in patients receiving this therapy.
3. Sudden cessation in administration of a concentrated dextrose solution may result in insulin reaction due to continued endogenous insulin production.
   Parenteral nutrition mixtures should be withdrawn slowly.
4. AMIGEN (Protein Hydrolysate) Injections contain electrolytes, however, supplementation may be required. Particular attention should be given to minitoring serum potassium and phosphate levels.
5. Strongly hypertonic nutrient solutions should be administered through an indwelling intravenous catheter with the tip located in the superior vena cava.
6. Care should be taken to avoid circulatory overload, particularly in patients with cardiac insufficiency.
7. Depending on shipping and storage conditions, trace amounts of Tyrosine may crystallize out of 10% AMIGEN (Protein Hy-

Continued on next page

Travenol—Cont.

drolysate) Injection. The Tyrosine may be redissolved by warming the bottle in a water bath for approximately one hour and gradually cooling to 25-35°C. It is necessary that this be done before the addition of the carbohydrate diluent.

Special Precautions: Administration of protein hydrolysate injection and other nutrients via central venous catheter may be associated with complications which can be prevented or minimized by careful attention to all aspects of the procedure. This includes attention to solution preparation, administration, and patient monitoring. IT IS ESSENTIAL THAT A CAREFULLY PREPARED PROTOCOL, BASED ON CURRENT MEDICAL PRACTICES BE FOLLOWED, PREFERABLY BY AN EXPERIENCED TEAM.

Although a detailed discussion of the complications is beyond the scope of this insert, the following summary lists those based on current literature.

1. **Technical:** The placement of a central venous catheter should be regarded as a surgical procedure. The physician should be fully acquainted with various techniques of catheter insertion as well as recognition and treatment of complications. For details of techniques and placement sites consult the medical literature. X-ray is the best means of verifying catheter placement. Complications known to occur from the placement of central venous catheters are pneumothorax, hemothorax, hydrothorax, artery puncture and transection, injury to the brachial plexus, malposition of the catheter, formation of arterio-venous fistula, phlebitus thrombosis, cardiac arrhythmia and catheter embolus.
2. **Septic:** The constant risk of sepsis is present during administration of the solution. Since contaminated solutions and infusion catheters are potential sources of infection, it is imperative that the preparation of the solution and the placement and care of catheters be accomplished under controlled aseptic conditions. If fever develops, the solution, its delivery system and the site of the indwelling catheter should be changed.
   Solutions ideally should be prepared in the hospital pharmacy under a laminar flow hood. The key factor in their preparation is careful aseptic technique to avoid inadvertent touch contamination during mixing of solutions and addition of other nutrients.
   Solutions should be used promptly after mixing. Any storage should be under refrigeration and limited to a brief period of time, preferably less than 24 hours.
3. **Metabolic:** The following metabolic complications have been reported: metabolic acidosis, hypophosphatemia, alkalosis, hyperglycemia and glycosuria, osmotic diuresis and dehydration, rebound hypoglycemia, elevated liver enzymes, hypo and hypervitaminosis, electrolyte imbalances, and hyperammonemia. Frequent clinical evaluation and laboratory determinations are necessary, especially during the first few days of therapy, to prevent or minimize these complications.

Adverse Reactions: See Warnings and Special precautions.

Dosage and Administration: The total daily dose of the solution depends on the patient's metabolic requirement and clinical response. The determination of nitrogen balance and accurate daily body weights, corrected for fluid balance, are probably the best means of assessing individual nitrogen requirements.

Central Vein Administration: Hypertonic mixtures of protein hydrolysate and dextrose may be safely administered by continuous infusion through a central venous catheter with the tip located in the vena cava. Typically 500 ml of 10% AMIGEN (Protein Hydrolysate) Injection mixed with 500 ml of 50% dextrose injection, electrolytes and vitamins are administered over an 8 hour period. (If the rate of administration should fall behind schedule, no attempt to catch up to planned intake should be made.) In addition to meeting nitrogen needs, the administration rate is governed, especially during the first few days of therapy, by the patient's tolerance to dextrose. Daily intake of protein hydrolysate and dextrose should be increased gradually to the maximum required dose as indicated by frequent determinations of urine and blood sugar levels.

Recommended daily dietary allowances* for protein range from 2.2 g/kg of body weight for infants to 56 g of protein per day for adults weighing 70 kg. Associated carbohydrate calories should be administered in a quantity of approximately 40 kcals/kg/day. For the initial treatment of trauma or protein calorie malnutrition, higher doses of protein with corresponding quantities of carbohydrate will be necessary to promote adequate patient response to therapy. The severity of the illness being treated is the primary consideration in determining proper dose level.

Care should be exercised to insure the maintenance of proper levels of serum potassium. It may be necessary to enhance the already present quantity of this electrolyte in the AMIGEN (Protein Hydrolysate) Injections, depending primarily on the amount of carbohydrate administrered to and metabolized by the patient. All serum electrolytes should be monitored frequently, especially phosphate, magnesium, and chloride. Quantities of 60–180 mEq of potassium per day have been used with adequate clinical effect.

In many patients provision of adequate calories in the form of hypertonic dextrose may require the administration of exogenous insulin to prevent hyperglycemia and glycosuria. Parenteral nutrition may be started with infusates containing lower concentrations of dextrose; dextrose content may be gradually increased to estimated caloric needs as the patient's glucose tolerance increases.

Sudden cessation in administration of a concentrated dextrose solution may result in insulin reaction due to continued endogenous insulin production. Such solutions should be withdrawn slowly.

Peripheral Vein Administration: For patients requiring parenteral nutrition in whom the central vein route is not indicated, AMIGEN (Protein Hydrolysate) Injection can be mixed with low concentration dextrose solutions and administered by peripheral vein with fat emulsions.

For example, 5% AMIGEN (Protein Hydrolysate) and 5% Dextrose Injection provides in each liter 30 g of utilizable protein and 170 carbohydrate calories with an osmolarity of approximately 682 mOs/l.

Parenteral fat emulsion provides approximately 1.1 calories per ml and may be administered along with amino acid—dextrose solutions through a Y-type administrtion set to supplement caloric intake. Fat, however, should not be the sole caloric intake since studies have indicated that glucose is more nitrogen sparing in the stressed patient.

Protein Sparing: For well-nourished patients who require short-term parenteral support, 5% AMIGEN (Protein Hydrolysate) and 5% Dextrose Injection can be administered peripherally.

*Food and Nutrition Board National Academy of Sciences—National Research Council (Revised 1974).

Note: It is recommended that all intravenous administration apparatus be replaced at least every 24 hours.

How Supplied:
5% AMIGEN (Protein Hydrolysate) Injection 1000 ml 1A6104
10% AMIGEN (Protein Hydrolysate) Injection 500 ml in 1000 ml bottles 1A6304
5% AMIGEN (Protein Hydrolysate) and 5% Dextrose Injection 1000 ml 1A6114

TRAVASOL® (Amino Acid) Injections with Electrolytes ℞
TRAVASOL® (Amino Acid) Injections without Electrolytes

Description: TRAVASOL (Amino Acid) Injections are sterile, nonpyrogenic hypertonic solutions of essential and non-essential L-amino acids provided with or without electrolytes for intravenous administration.

Each 100 ml of TRAVASOL (Amino Acid) Injections with Electrolytes and without Electrolytes contains:

	5.5%	8.5%
L-Amino Acids	5.5 g	8.5 g
Total Nitrogen	924 mg	1.42 g
Approximate pH	6.0	6.0
Essential Amino Acids	**5.5%**	**8.5%**
L-Leucine	340 mg	526 mg
L-Phenylalanine	340 mg	526 mg
L-Methionine	318 mg	492 mg
L-Lysine (added as the hydrochloride salt)	318 mg	492 mg
L-Isoleucine	263 mg	406 mg
L-Valine	252 mg	390 mg
L-Histidine	241 mg	372 mg
L-Threonine	230 mg	356 mg
L-Tryptophan	99 mg	152 mg
Non-essential Amino Acids	**5.5%**	**8.5%**
L-Alanine	1.14 g	1.76 g
Aminoacetic Acid	1.14 g	1.76 g
L-Arginine	570 mg	880 mg
L-Proline	230 mg	356 mg
L-Tyrosine	22 mg	34 mg

In addition to the above, TRAVASOL (Amino Acid) Injections with Electrolytes contain in each 100 ml:

Electrolytes	**5.5%**	**8.5%**
Soldium Acetate, Hydrous, USP	431 mg	594 mg
Dibasic Potassium Phosphate	522 mg	522 mg
Sodium Chloride, USP	224 mg	154 mg
Magnesium Chloride, USP	102 mg	102 mg

TRAVASOL (Amino Acid) Injections with Electrolytes contain the following milliequivalents:

Electrolyte	**5.5%**	**8.5%**
Sodium	70 mEq/l	70 mEq/l
Potassium	60 mEq/l	60 mEq/l
Magnesium	10 mEq/l	10 mEq/l
Acetate*	100 mEq/l	135 mEq/l
Chloride	70 mEq/l	70 mEq/l
Phosphate (as $HPO_4^{=}$)	60 mEq/l (30 mM)	60 mEq/l (30 mM)

*Acetate is added as sodium acetate and as acetic acid used for pH adjustment.

TRAVASOL (Amino Acid) Injections without Electrolytes contain the following anion profiles in mEq/l:

Anion	**5.5%**	**8.5%**
Acetate (1)	35 mEq/l	52 mEq/l
Chloride (2)	22 mEq/l	34 mEq/l

(1) derived from pH adjustment with acetic acid
(2) contributed by the L-Lysine Hydrochloride

Approximately 3 mEq/l Sodium Bisulfite, USP is added as stabilizer to all TRAVASOL (Amino Acid) Injections.

Actions: TRAVASOL (Amino Acid) Injections administered via central vein provide biologically utilizable source material for protein synthesis when used with concentrated calorie sources (such as hypertonic dextrose or fat emulsion), electrolytes, vitamins and minerals. Administered peripherally after appropriate dilution or with minimal calorie supplementation (such as 5% dextrose), it enhances the conservation of body protein.

Indications: TRAVASOL (Amino Acid) Injections are indicated as an adjunct in the offsetting of nitrogen loss or in the treatment of negative nitrogen balance in patients where: (1) the alimentary tract, by the oral, gastrostomy or jejunostomy route, cannot or should not be used, (2) gastrointestinal absorption of protein is impaired, or (3) metabolic requirements for protein are substantially increased, as with extensive burns.

Central Vein Administration: Central vein infusion should be considered when amino acid solutions are to be admixed with hypertonic dextrose to promote protein synthesis such as for hypercatabolic or depleted patients or those requiring long term parenteral nutrition.

Peripheral Vein Administration: For patients in whom the central vein route is not indicated, amino acid solutions mixed with low dextrose concentrations may be infused by peripheral vein when supplemented with fat emulsion.

Protein Sparing: Dilute amino acid solutions for **peripheral administration** may be used in patients who exemplify no clinically significant protein malnutrition. The purpose of the solution is to replace protein losses which occur in relation to an intercurrent phenomenon which is known or suspected to be productive of a protein loss condition for a short or moderate period of time. Protein sparing can be achieved by peripheral infusion of amino acid solutions with or without dextrose.

Contraindications:

1. Patients with renal failure—anuria [for TRAVASOL (Amino Acid) Injection with Electrolytes only]
2. Patients with severe liver disease—hepatic coma
3. Hypersensitivity to one or more amino acids.

Warnings:

1. Proper administration of TRAVASOL (Amino Acid) Injections requires a knowledge of fluid and electrolyte balance and nutrition as well as clinical expertise in recognition and treatment of the complications which may occur. FREQUENT CLINICAL EVALUATION AND LABORATORY DETERMINATIONS ARE NECESSARY FOR PROPER MONITORING DURING ADMINISTRATION. Studies should include blood sugar, serum proteins, kidney and liver function tests, electrolytes, hemogram, carbon dioxide combining power or content, serum osmolarities, blood cultures and blood ammonia levels.
2. Administration of amino acid solutions to a patient with hepatic insufficiency may result in serum amino acid imbalances, hyperammonemia, stupor and coma.
   Hyperammonemia is of SPECIAL SIGNIFICANCE IN INFANTS. This reaction appears to be related to a deficiency of the urea cycle amino acids of genetic or product origin. It is essential that blood ammonia be measured frequently in infants.
   Conservative doses of TRAVASOL (Amino Acid) Injection should be given to patients with known or suspected hepatic dysfunction. Should symptoms of hyperammonemia develop, administration should be discontinued and the patient's clinical status reevaluated.
3. Administration of amino acid solutions in the presence of impaired renal function presents special issues associated with retention of electrolytes.
4. The safety of the use of amino acid solutions in pregnant women has not been demonstrated.
5. Do not administer unless solution is clear. This solution should not be administered simultaneously with blood through the same infusion set because of the possiblity of pseudoagglutination.

Precautions:

1. It is essential to provide adequate calories concurrently if parenterally administered amino acids are to be retained by the body and utilized for protein synthesis. Concentrated dextrose solutions are an effective source of such calories.
2. With the administration of TRAVASOL (Amino Acid) Injection in combination with highly concentrated dextrose solutions, hyperglycemia, glycosuria, and hyperosmolar syndrome may result. Blood and urine glucose should be monitored on a routine basis in patients receiving this therapy.
3. Sudden cessation in administration of a concentrated dextrose solution may result in insulin reaction due to continued endogenous insulin production. Parenteral nutrition mixtures should be withdrawn slowly.
4. TRAVASOL (Amino Acid) Injection with Electrolytes contains sufficient electrolytes to provide for most parenteral nutritional needs with the possible exception of potassium where supplementation may be required. However, replacement of exceptional electrolyte loss due to nasogastric suction, fistula drainage, or unusual tissue exudation may be necessary. Particular attention should be given to monitoring serum potassium levels.
   Electrolytes may be added to the TRAVASOL (Amino Acid) Injections without Electrolytes as dictated by the patient's electrolyte profile.
5. Commonly reported complications of parenteral nutrition, hyperammonemia and hyperchloremic metabolic acidosis, were not observed during clinical studies with TRAVASOL (Amino Acid) Injection. While the potassium, phosphate, metabolizable acetate anion, and amino acid profiles in TRAVASOL (Amino Acid) Injections with Electrolytes were designed to minimize or prevent occurrences of these imbalances, the physician should be aware of appropriate counter-measures if they become necessary.
6. Strongly hypertonic nutrient solutions should be administered through an indwelling intravenous catheter with the tip located in the superior vena cava.
7. Care should be taken to avoid circulatory overload, particularly in patients with cardiac insufficiency.
8. During protein sparing therapy in the absence of supporting carbohydrate metabolism, an accumulation of ketone bodies in the blood often occurs. Correction of ketonemia usually can be accomplished by administering some carbohydrates.
9. Protein sparing therapy is useful for periods up to 10–12 days. Patients requiring nutritional support thereafter should be placed on oral or parenteral regimens that employ adequate non-protein calorie components.

Special Precautions: Administration of amino acid solutions and other nutrients via central or peripheral venous catheter may be associated with complications which can be prevented or minimized by careful attention to all aspects of the procedure. This includes attention to solution preparation, administration, and patient montioring. IT IS ESSENTIAL THAT A CAREFULLY PREPARED PROTOCOL, BASED ON CURRENT MEDICAL PRACTICES, BE FOLLOWED, PREFERABLY BY AN EXPERIENCED TEAM.

Although a detailed discussion of the complications is beyond the scope of this insert, the following summary lists those based on current literature:

1. **Technical:** The placement of a central venous catheter should be regarded as a surgical procedure. The physician should be fully acquainted with various techniques of catheter insertion as well as recognition and treatment of complications. For details of techniques and placement sites consult the medical literature. X-ray is the best means of verifying catheter placement. Complications known to occur from the placement of central venous catheters are pneuothorax, hemothorax, hydrothorax, artery puncture and transection, injury to the brachial plexus, malposition of the catheter, formation of arterio-venous fistula, phlebitis, thrombosis, cardiac arrhythmia and catheter embolus.
2. **Septic:** The constant risk of sepsis is present during administration of parenteral nutrition solution. Since contaminated solutions and infusion catheters are potential sources of infection, it is imperative that the preparation of the solution and the placement and care of catheters be accomplished under controlled aseptic conditions. If fever develops, the solution, its delivery system and the site of the indwelling catheter should be changed.
   Solutions ideally should be prepared in the hospital pharmacy under a laminar flow hood. The key factor in their preparation is careful aseptic technique to avoid inadvertent touch contamination during mixing of solutions and addition of other nutrients.
   Solutions should be used promptly after mixing. Any storage should be under refrigeration and limited to a brief period of time, preferably less than 24 hours.
3. **Metabolic:** The following metabolic complications have been reported: metabolic acidosis, hypophosphatemia, alkalosis, hyperglycemia and glycosuria, osmotic diuresis and dehydration, rebound hypoglycemia, elevated liver enzymes, hypo and hypervitaminosis, electrolyte imbalances, and hyperammonemia. Frequent clinical evaluation and laboratory determinations are necessary, especially during the first few days of therapy, to prevent or minimize these complications.

Adverse Reactions: See Warnings and Special Precautions.

Dosage and Administration: The total daily dose of these solutions depends on the patient's metabolic requirement and clinical response. The determination of nitrogen balance and accurate daily body weights, corrected for fluid balance, are probably the best means of assessing individual nitrogen requirements.

Recommended Dietary Allowances* of protein range from approximately 0.8 g/kg of body weight for adults to 2.2 g/kg for infants. It must be recognized, however, that protein as well as caloric requirements in traumatized or malnourished patients may be substantially increased. Daily amino acid doses of approximately 1.0 to 1.5 g/kg of body weight for adults and 2 to 3 g/kg of body weight for infants with adequate calories and generally sufficient to satisfy protein needs and promote positive nitrogen balance.

For the initial treatment of trauma or protein calorie malnutrition, higher doses of protein with corresponding quantities of carbohydrate will be necessary to promote adequate patient response to therapy. The severity of the illness being treated is the primary consideration in determining proper dose level. Such higher doses, especially in infants, must be accompanied by more frequent laboratory evaluation.

For protein sparing in well-nourished patients not receiving significant additional calories, amino acid dosages of 1.0 to 1.7 g/kg/day reduce nitrogen losses and spare body protein. If daily increases in BUN in the range of 10–15 mg% for more than three days should occur, then protein sparing therapy should be discontinued and a regimen with full-protein calorie substrates should be adopted.

*Food and Nutrition Board National Academy of Sciences—National Research Council (Revised 1974).

Continued on next page

Travenol—Cont.

Care should be exercised to insure the maintenance of proper levels of serum potassium. Quantities of 60–180 mEq of potassium per day have been used with adequate clinical effect. It may be necessary to enhance the already present quantity of this electrolyte in TRAVASOL (Amino Acid) Injections with Electrolytes, depending primarily on the amount of carbohydrate administered to and metabolized by the patient. All serum electrolytes should be monitored frequently, especially phosphate, magnesium, and chloride.

Patients receiving TRAVASOL (Amino Acid) Injections without Electrolytes should be monitored (carefully) and their electrolyte requirements individualized.

Central Vein Administration: Hypertonic mixtures of amino acids and dextrose may be administered safely by continuous infusion through a central vein catheter with the tip located in the vena cava. Typically 500 ml of TRAVASOL (Amino Acid) Injection mixed with 500 ml of 50% Dextrose Injection, electrolytes (if indicated) and vitamins is administered over an 8 hour period. (If the rate of administration should fall behind schedule, no attempt to "catch up" to planned intake should be made.) In addition to meeting nitrogen needs, the administration rate is governed, especially during the first few days of therapy, by the patient's tolerance to dextrose. Daily intake of amino acids and dextrose should be increased gradually to the maximum required dose as indicated by frequent determinations of urine and blood sugar levels.

In many patients, provision of adequate calories in the form of hypertonic dextrose may require the administration of exogenous insulin to prevent hyperglycemia and glycosuria.

Parenteral nutrition may be started with infusates containing lower concentrations of dextrose; dextrose content may be gradually increased to estimated caloric needs as the patient's glucose tolerance increases.

Sudden cessation in administration of a concentrated dextrose solution may result in insulin reaction due to continued endogenous insulin production. Such solutions should be withdrawn slowly.

Peripheral Vein Administration: For patients requiring parenteral nutrition in whom the central vein route is not indicated, TRAVASOL (Amino Acid) Injection can be mixed with low concentration dextrose solutions and administered by peripheral vein with fat emulsions.

For example, to prepare a solution of 2.75% TRAVASOL (Amino Acid) Injection in 5% dextrose, aseptically transfer 500 ml of 5.5% TRAVASOL (Amino Acid) Injection with Electrolytes and 500 ml of 10% dextrose to a liter intravenous container. Each liter of the resultant solution provides 28.9 g of protein equivalent and 170 carbohydrate calories with an osmolarity of approximately 680 mOs/l.

Parenteral fat emulsion provides approximately 1.1 calories per ml and may be administered along with amino acid-dextrose solutions through a Y-type administration set to supplement caloric intake. Fat, however, should not be the sole caloric intake since studies have indicated that glucose is more nitrogen sparing in the stressed patient.

Protein Sparing: For well-nourished patients who require short-term parenteral support, TRAVASOL (Amino Acid) Injection can be administered peripherally with or without carbohydrate calories. Such infusates can be prepared by dilution of TRAVASOL (Amino Acid) Injection with Sterile Water for Injection or 5% dextrose solutions to prepare isotonic or slightly hypertonic solutions which may be administered by peripheral vein. For example, a 2.75% TRAVASOL (Amino Acid) Injection solution can be prepared by the aseptic transfer of 500 ml of 5.5% TRAVASOL (Amino Acid) Injection with Electrolytes to a half-filled intravenous liter container of Sterile Water for Injection. The resultant solution contains 2.75% amino acids, and provides 28.9 g of protein equivalent with an osmolarity of approximately 425 mOs/l.

Route: Peripheral or central vein.

Storage: It is recommended that all intravenous administration apparatus be replaced at least every 24 hours.

L-Amino Acid Solutions should be protected from light until immediately prior to use.

Protect from excessive heat (above 40°C) and freezing.

How Supplied: TRAVASOL (Amino Acid) Injection with Electrolytes and without Electrolytes are available in 5.5% and 8.5% concentrations and are supplied in 500 ml containers.

3.5% TRAVASOL® M ℞
(Amino Acid) Injection with Electrolyte 45

Description: 3.5% TRAVASOL M (Amino Acid) Injection with Electrolyte 45 is a sterile, nonpyrogenic hypertonic solution of essential and nonessential L-amino acids and electrolytes having an osmolarity of 450 mOs/l. It contains 35 g/l (5.9 g nitrogen) of amino acids and 45 mEq/l of cations. The pH is approximately 6.0.

Each 100 ml of 3.5% TRAVASOL M (Amino Acid) Injection with Electrolyte 45 contains:

L-Amino Acids	3.5 g
Total nitrogen	588 mg
Approximate pH	6.0
Essential Amino Acids	
L-Leucine	217 mg
L-Phenylalanine	217 mg
L-Methionine	203 mg
L-Lysine (added as the hydrochloride salt)	203 mg
L-Isoleucine	168 mg
L-Valine	161 mg
L-Histidine	154 mg
L-Threonine	147 mg
L-Tryptophan	63 mg
Non-essential Amino Acids	
L-Alanine	728 mg
Aminoacetic Acid	728 mg
L-Arginine	364 mg
L-Proline	147 mg
L-Tyrosine	14 mg
Electrolytes	
Sodium Acetate, Hydrous, USP	218 mg
Dibasic Potassium Phosphate	131 mg
Sodium Chloride, USP	35 mg
Magnesium Chloride, USP	51 mg

3.5% TRAVASOL M (Amino Acid) Injection with Electrolyte 45 contains the following milliequivalents of electrolytes.

Electrolytes	
Sodium	25 mEq/l
Potassium	15 mEq/l
Magnesium	5 mEq/l
Acetate*	54 mEq/l
Chloride	25 mEq/l
Phosphate (as $HPO_4=$)	15 mEq/l

*Acetate is added as sodium acetate and as acetic acid used for pH adjustment.

Approximately 3 mEq/l Sodium Bisulfite, USP is added as stabilizer.

Actions: 3.5% TRAVASOL M (Amino Acid) Injection with Electrolyte 45 is intended for protein sparing therapy, the diminution of net protein losses.

Indications: 3.5% TRAVASOL M (Amino Acid) Injection with Electrolyte 45 is designed <u>for peripheral administration</u> for use in patients who before administration of the solution have exemplified no clinically significant protein malnutrition. The purpose of the solution is to replace protein losses which occur in relation to an intercurrent phenomenon which is known or suspected to be productive of a protein loss condition for a short or moderate period of time.

Contraindications:
1. Patients with renal failure—anuria
2. Patients with severe liver disease
3. Hypersensitivity to one or more amino acids

Warnings:
1. Proper administraion of 3.5% TRAVASOL M (Amino Acid) Injection with Electrolyte 45 solution requires a knowledge of fluid and electrolyte balance and an appreciation for the role of protein sparing therapy in relation to other forms of nutritional support.
2. Administration of amino acid solutions to a patient with hepatic insufficiency may result in serum amino acid imbalances, hyperammonemia, stupor, and coma. The use of 3.5% TRAVASOL M (Amino Acid) Injection with Electrolyte 45 in such patients should be considered very carefully by the physicians, and the benefits of protein sparing therapy should outweigh the risk of adverse results.
3. The safety of the use of amino acid solutions has not been demonstrated in pregnant women. In such patients protein sparing therapy would seem unlikely to have an application that would supervene unknown risks.
4. Do not administer unless this solution is clear. This solution should not be given simultaneously with blood through the same infusion set because of the possibility of pseudoagglutination.

Precautions:
1. The electrolyte profile of 3.5% TRAVASOL M (Amino Acid) Injection with Electrolyte 45 favors the intracellular ions and has been planned for protein sparing therapy. Losses greater than normal should be monitored and replaced in the usual fashion.
2. Protein sparing therapy is useful for periods up to 10–12 days. Patients requiring nutritional support thereafter should be placed on oral or parenteral regimens that employ adequate non-protein calorie components.
3. Care should be taken to avoid circulatory overload, particularly in patients with cardiac insufficiency.
4. In the absence of supporting carbohydrate metabolism, an accumulation of ketone bodies in the blood often occurs. Correction of ketonemia usually can be accomplished by administering some carbohydrates.
5. Though not anticipated, if daily increases in BUN in the range of 10–15 mg% for more than 3 days should occur, then protein sparing therapy should be discontinued and a regimen with full non-protein calorie substrate should be adopted.

Adverse Reactions: See Warnings and Precautions.

Dosage and Administration: As a general matter protein sparing therapy is implemented by administering 3.5% TRAVASOL M (Amino Acid) Injection with Electrolyte 45 solution and any desired supporting electrolytes. The tonicity of this solution will allow comfortable administration into a peripheral vein. Approximately 3 liters of the solution per 24 hour period will provide optimal results. When used postoperatively the therapy should begin with 1000 ml on the first post-operative day; thereafter, an increase to the 3000 ml level is typical.

3.5% TRAVASOL M (Amino Acid) Injection with Electrolyte 45 is <u>not recommended for central venous administration.</u>

<u>NOTE:</u> It is recommended that all intravenous administration apparatus be replaced at least every 24 hours.

How Supplied: 3.5% TRAVASOL M (Amino Acid) Injection with Electrolyte 45 is supplied in 500 ml and 1000 ml containers.

Trimen Laboratories, Inc.

Pharmaceutical Division
80 TWENTY-SIXTH STREET
PITTSBURGH, PA 15222

BELLERMINE-O.D™ CAPSULES ℞
Belladonna Ergotamine

Each long-acting capsule contains:
Phenobarbital ....40.0 mg.
(Warning: May be habit forming)
Ergotamine tartrate ....0.6 mg.
Belladonna alkaloids ....0.2 mg.
How Supplied: Bottles of 100's, chocolate and clear with white beads, imprinted "TRIMEN".

FE-O.D.® TABLET
(Hematinic)

Each Tablet contains: 300 mg. Fe Fumarate*, 500 mg. Ascorbic Acid
*In a special time release base.
How Supplied: Bottles of 100's, yellow, oval tablet, embossed with logo.

FLEXAPHEN™ CAPSULES ℞
Skeletal Muscle Relaxant and Analgesic

How Supplied: Bottles of 100s, tan capsule imprinted "TRIMEN".
Each capsule contains:
Chlorzoxazone ....250 mg.
Acetaminophen ....300 mg.

HYDREX® TABLETS ℞
(Benzthiazide 50 mg.)
Diuretic-Antihypertensive

How Supplied: Bottles of 100's, white, scored tablet embossed with logo.

KORIGESIC® TABLETS ℞
Analgesic Decongestant

Each Tablet contains: 4 mg. Chlorpheniramine Maleate, 14 mg. Phenylpropanolamine Hydrochloride, 5 mg. Phenylephrine Hydrochloride, 150 mg. Salicylamide, 120 mg. Phenacetin, 30 mg. Caffeine.
How Supplied: Bottles of 100's, two-layer, scored blue and white tablet, embossed with logo.

LAXATYL™ TABLETS
Stool Softener and Stimulant Laxative

Each tablet contains: 60 mg. dioctyl sodium sulfosuccinate USP and 50 mg. danthron N.F.
How Supplied: Bottles of 100's, sugar-coated tan, round tablet imprinted with logo.

NATACOMP-FA® TABLETS ℞
Multivitamin, Multimineral supplement for pregnant or lactating women

How Supplied: Bottles of 100's and 500's pink, oval, film coated tablet.

SORATE® ℞
Isosorbide Dinitrate

How Supplied:
Sorate®-5 Chewable as 5 mg orange, round, scored, chewable tablet, embossed with logo.
Sorate®-2.5 Sublingual as 2.5 mg lavender tablet.
Sorate®-5 Sublingual as 5 mg light green oval shaped tablet.
Sorate®-10 Tablets as 10 mg light blue, round scored tablet, embossed with logo.
Sorate®-40 Capsules as 40 mg long-acting, opaque purple and clear with white beads imprinted TRIMEN.

VIOPAN-T™ TABLETS
High Potency Vitamin Mineral Formula

How Supplied: Red, film coated tablet, embossed with TRIMEN.

Tutag Pharmaceuticals, Inc.

2599 W. MIDWAY BLVD.
BROOMFIELD, COLORADO 80020

AQUATAG® ℞
(benzthiazide tablets, N.F.)

Description: AQUATAG (benzthiazide) is a potent, orally active, nonmercurial, diuretic agent. It is effective orally in producing diuresis in edema states. AQUATAG (benzthiazide) is mildly antihypertensive in its own right and enhances the action of other antihypertensive drugs when used in combination.
AQUATAG (benzthiazide), a sulfamyl benzothiadiazine derivative, presents an apparently different mechanism of action from that of the carbonic anhydrase inhibitors. AQUATAG (benzthiazide) is designated generically as benzthiazide, and chemically as 3-benzylthiomethyl-6-chloro-7 sulfamyl-1, 2, 4-benzothiadiazine-1, 1-dioxide. Its empirical formula is $C_{15}H_{14}O_4N_3S_3Cl$. It is an odorless, white crystalline compound, readily soluble in alkaline solution. AQUATAG (benzthiazide) is 5 to 20 times as potent, on a weight basis, as chlorothiazide.
Actions: Benzthiazide affects the renal tubular mechanism of electrolyte reabsorption. At maximal therapeutic dosage all thiazides are approximately equal in their diuretic potency. Benzthiazide increases excretion of sodium and chloride in approximately equivalent amounts. Natriuresis causes a secondary loss of potassium and bicarbonate. The mechanism of the antihypertensive effect of thiazides is unknown. Benzthiazide does not affect normal blood pressure.
Onset of action of Benzthiazide occurs in 2 hours and the peak effect at about 4 hours. Its action persists for approximately 6 to 12 hours. Benzthiazide is eliminated rapidly by the kidney.
Indications: AQUATAG (benzthiazide) is indicated as adjunctive therapy in edema associated with congestive heart failure, hepatic cirrhosis and corticosteroid and estrogen therapy. AQUATAG (benzthiazide) has also been found useful in edema due to various forms of renal dysfunction such as:
Nephrotic syndrome;
Acute glomerulonephritis; and
Chronic renal failure.
Benzthiazide is indicated in the management of hypertension either as the sole therapeutic agent or to enhance the effectiveness of other antihypertensive drugs in the more severe forms of hypertension.
Usage in Pregnancy: The routine use of diuretics in an otherwise healthy woman is inappropriate and exposes mother and fetus to unnecessary hazard. Diuretics do not prevent development of toxemia of pregnancy, and there is no satisfactory evidence that they are useful in the treatment of developed toxemia.
Edema during pregnancy may arise from pathological causes or from the physiologic and mechanical consequences of pregnancy. Thiazides are indicated in pregnancy when edema is due to pathologic causes, just as they are in the absence of pregnancy (however, see Warnings, below). Dependent edema in pregnancy, resulting from restriction of venous return by the expanded uterus, is properly treated through elevation of the lower extremities and use of support hose; use of diuretics to lower intravascular volume in this case is illogical and unnecessary. There is hypervolemia during normal pregnancy which is harmful to neither the fetus nor the mother (in the absence of cardiovascular disease), but which is associated with edema, including generalized edema, in the majority of pregnant women. If this edema produces discomfort, increased recumbency will often provide relief. In rare instances, this edema may cause extreme discomfort which is not relieved by rest. In these cases, a short course of diuretics may provide relief and may be appropriate.
Contraindications: Anuria.
Hypersensitivity to this or other sulfonamide-derived drugs.
Warnings: Thiazides should be used with caution in severe renal disease. In patients with renal disease, thiazides may precipitate azotemia, Cumulative effects of the drug may develop in patients with impaired renal function.
Thiazides should be used with caution in patients with impaired hepatic function or progressive liver disease, since minor alterations of fluid and electrolyte balance may precipitate hepatic coma.
Thiazides may add to or potentiate the action of other antihypertensive drugs. Potentiation occurs with ganglionic or peripheral adrenergic blocking drugs.
Sensitivity reactions may occur in patients with a history of allergy or bronchial asthma.
The possibility of exacerbation or activation of systemic lupus erythematosus has been reported.
Usage in Pregnancy: Thiazides cross the placental barrier and appear in cord blood. The use of thiazides in pregnant women requires that the anticipated benefit be weighed against possible hazards to the fetus. These hazards include fetal or neonatal jaundice, thrombocytopenia, and possibly other adverse reactions which have occurred in the adult.
Nursing Mothers: Thiazides appear in breast milk. If use of the drug is deemed essential, the patient should stop nursing.
Precautions: Periodic determination of serum electrolytes to detect possible electrolyte imbalance should be performed at appropriate intervals.
All patients receiving thiazide therapy should be observed for clinical signs of fluid or electrolyte imbalance; namely, hyponatremia, hypochloremic alkalosis, and hypokalemia. Serum and urine electrolyte determinations are particularly important when the patient is vomiting excessively or receiving parenteral fluids. Medication such as digitalis may also influence serum electrolytes. Warning signs, irrespective of cause, are: Dryness of mouth, thirst, weakness, lethargy, drowsiness, restlessness, muscle pains or cramps, muscular fatigue, hypotension, oliguria, tachycardia, and gastrointestinal disturbances such as nausea and vomiting.
Hypokalemia may develop especially with brisk diuresis, when severe cirrhosis is present, or during concomitant use of corticosteroids or ACTH.
Interference with adequate oral electrolyte intake will also contribute to hypokalemia. Hypokalemia can sensitize or exaggerate the response of the heart to the toxic effects of digitalis (e.g., increased ventricular irritability). Hypokalemia may be avoided or treated by use of potassium supplements such as foods with a high potassium content.
Any chloride deficit is generally mild and usually does not require specific treatment except under extraordinary circumstances (as in liver disease or renal disease). Dilutional hyponatremia may occur in edematous patients in hot weather; appropriate therapy is water restriction rather than administration of salt except in rare instances when the hyponatremia is life threatening. In actual salt depletion, appropriate replacement is the therapy of choice.

Continued on next page

Tutag—Cont.

Hyperuricemia may occur or frank gout may be precipitated in certain patients receiving thiazide therapy. Insulin requirements in diabetic patients may be increased, decreased, or unchanged. Diabetes mellitus which has been latent may become manifest during thiazide administration.
Thiazide drugs may increase the responsiveness to tubocurarine.
The antihypertensive effects of the drug may be enhanced in the postsympathectomy patient. Thiazides may decrease arterial responsiveness to norepinephrine. This diminution is not sufficient to preclude effectiveness of the pressor agent for therapeutic use.
If progressive renal impairment becomes evident, consider withholding or discontinuing diuretic therapy.
Thiazides may decrease serum PBI levels without signs of thyroid disturbance. Calcium excretion is decreased by thiazides.
Pathological changes in the parathyroid gland with hypercalcemia and hypophosphatemia have been observed in a few patients on prolonged thiazide therapy. The common complications of hyperparathyroidism such as renal lithiasis, bone resorption, and peptic ulceration have not been seen. Thiazides should be discontinued before carrying out tests for parathyroid function.
Adverse Reactions:
A. Gastrointestinal System
1. anorexia
2. gastric irritation
3. nausea
4. vomiting
5. cramping
6. diarrhea
7. constipation
8. jaundice (intrahepatic cholestatic jaundice)
9. pancreatitis
10. sialadenitis

B. Central Nervous System
1. dizziness
2. vertigo
3. paresthesias
4. headache
5. xanthopsia

C. Hematologic
1. leukopenia
2. agranulocytosis
3. thrombocytopenia
4. aplastic anemia

D. Cardiovascular
1. Orthostatic hypotension (may be aggravated by alcohol, barbiturates, or narcotics).

E. Hypersensitivity
1. purpura
2. photosensitivity
3. rash
4. urticaria
5. necrotizing angiitis (vasculitis) (cutaneous vasculitis)
6. fever
7. respiratory distress including pneumonitis
8. anaphylactic reactions

F. Other
1. hyperglycemia
2. glycosuria
3. hyperuricemia
4. muscle spasm
5. weakness
6. restlessness
7. transient blurred vision

Whenever adverse reactions are moderate or severe, thiazide dosage should be reduced or therapy withdrawn.
Dosage and Administration: Therapy should be individualized according to patient response. This therapy should be titrated to gain maximal therapeutic response as well as the minimal dose possible to maintain that therapeutic response.
Adults: For Diuresis: The usual adult dosage for diuretic effects is 50 to 200mg. daily in divided doses.
For Control of Hypertension: The usual adult dosage for antihypertensive effects is 50 to 200mg. daily in divided doses.
How Supplied: As 25mg. scored tablets in bottles of 100 and 1000. As 50mg. scored tablets in bottles of 28, 100 and 1000.
Caution: Federal law prohibits dispensing without prescription.
[*Shown in Product Identification Section*]

BACARATE® TABLETS Ⓔ ℞
(phendimetrazine tartrate)
35 mg.

Description: Phendimetrazine Tartrate (+) 3, 4 Dimethyl-2 phenylmorpholine tartrate. Phendimetrazine is a white, odorless powder with a bitter taste. It is soluble in water, methanol and ethanol. It has a molecular weight of 341. For clinical use, phendimetrazine tartrate is available as a 35mg. scored tablet.
Actions: Phendimetrazine Tartrate is a sympathomimetic amine with pharmacological activity similar to the prototype drugs of this class used in obesity, the amphetamines. Actions include central nervous system stimulation and elevation of blood pressure. Tachyphylaxis and tolerance have been demonstrated with all drugs of this class in which these phenomena have been looked for. Drugs of this class used in obesity are commonly known as "anorectics" or "anorexigenics". It has not been established, however, that the action of such drugs in treating obesity is primarily one of appetite suppression. Other central nervous system actions, or metabolic effects, may be involved, for example. Adult obese subjects instructed in dietary management and treated with "anorectic" drugs, lose more weight on the average than those treated with placebo and diet, as determined in relatively short-term clinical trials.
The magnitude of increased weight loss of drug-treated patients over placebo-treated patients is only a fraction of a pound a week. The rate of weight loss is greatest in the first weeks of therapy for both drug and placebo subjects and tends to decrease in succeeding weeks. The possible origins of the increased weight loss due to the various drug effects are not established. The amount of weight loss associated with the use of an "anorectic" drug varies from trial to trial, and the increased weight loss appears to be related in part to variables other than the drug prescribed, such as the physician-investigator, the population treated, and the diet prescribed. Studies do not permit conclusions as to the relative importance of the drug and non-drug factors on weight loss.
The natural history of obesity is measured in years, whereas the studies cited are restricted to a few weeks duration; thus, the total impact of drug-induced weight loss over that of diet alone must be considered clinically limited.
Indications: Phendimetrazine tartrate is indicated in the management of exogenous obesity as a short-term adjunct (a few weeks) in a regimen of weight reduction based on caloric restriction. The limited usefulness of agents of this class (see ACTIONS) should be measured against possible risk factors inherent in their use such as those described below.
Contraindications: Advanced arteriosclerosis, symptomatic cardiovascular disease, moderate to severe hypertension, hyperthyroidism, known hypersensitivity, or idiosyncrasy to the sympathomimetic amines, glaucoma.
Agitated states.
Patients with a history of drug abuse.
During or within 14 days following the administration of monoamine oxidase inhibitors, hypertensive crises may result.
Warnings: Tolerance to the anorectic effect usually develops within a few weeks. When this occurs, the recommended dose should not be exceeded in an attempt to increase the effect; rather, the drug should be discontinued. Phendimetrazine Tartrate may impair the ability of the patient to engage in potentially hazardous activities such as operating machinery or driving a motor vehicle; the patient should therefore be cautioned accordingly.
Drug Dependence: Phendimetrazine Tartrate is related chemically and pharmacologically to the amphetamines. Amphetamines and related stimulant drugs have been extensively abused, and the possibility of abuse of Phendimetrazine Tartrate should be kept in mind when evaluating the desirability of including a drug as part of a weight reduction program. Abuse of amphetamines and related drugs may be associated with intense psychological dependence and severe social dysfunction. There are reports of patients who have increased the dosage to many times that recommended. Abrupt cessation following prolonged high dosage administration results in extreme fatigue and mental depression; changes are also noted on the sleep EEG. Manifestations of chronic intoxication with anorectic drugs include severe dermatoses, marked insomnia, irritability, hyperactivity, and personality changes. The most severe manifestation of chronic intoxications is psychosis, often clinically indistinguishable from schizophrenia.
Usage in Pregnancy: The safety of phendimetrazine tartrate in pregnancy and lactation has not been established. Therefore, use cautiously in women of childbearing age. The potential benefit must be weighed against the possible hazard to the mother and infant.
Usage in Children: Phendimetrazine tartrate is not recommended for use in children under 12 years of age.
Precaution: Caution is to be exercised in prescribing Phendimetrazine Tartrate for patients with even mild hypertension.
Insulin requirements in diabetes mellitus may be altered in association with the use of Phendimetrazine Tartrate and the concomitant dietary regimen. Phendimetrazine Tartrate may decrease the hypotensive effect of guanethidine. The least amount feasible should be prescribed or dispensed at one time in order to minimize the possibility of overdosage.
Adverse Reactions: **Cardiovascular:** Palpitation, tachycardia, elevation of blood pressure.
Central Nervous System: Overstimulation, restlessness, dizziness, insomnia, euphoria, dysphoria, tremor, headache; rarely psychotic episodes at recommended doses.
Gastrointestinal: Dryness of the mouth, unpleasant taste, diarrhea, constipation, other gastrointestinal disturbances.
Allergic: Urticaria.
Endocrine: Impotence, changes in libido.
Dosage and Administration: Usual Adult Dose: Dosage should be individualized to obtain an adequate response with the lowest effective dose. In some cases 17½mg. per dose may be adequate.
1 tablet (35mg.) b.i.d. or t.i.d. one hour before meals. Dosage should not exceed 2 tablets t.i.d.
Overdosage: Manifestations of acute overdosage may include restlessness, tremor, hyperreflexia, rapid respiration, confusion, assaultiveness, hallucinations, panic states.
Fatigue and depression usually follow the central stimulation.
Cardiovascular effects include arrhythmias, hypertension or hypotension and circulatory collapse. Gastrointestinal symptoms include nausea, vomiting, diarrhea, and abdominal cramps. Fatal poisoning usually terminates in convulsions and coma. Management of acute intoxication is largely symptomatic and includes lavage and sedation with a barbiturate. Experience with hemodialysis or peritoneal

dialysis is inadequate to permit recommendation in this regard. Acidification of the urine increases Phendimetrazine Tartrate excretion. Intravenous phentolamine (Regitine) has been suggested for possible acute, severe hypertension, if this complicates overdosage.
How Supplied: Each tablet contains 35mg. Phendimetrazine Tartrate, in bottles of 42, 100 and 1000.
Caution: Federal law prohibits dispensing without prescription.
[*Shown in Product Identification Section*]

ESCOT® CAPSULES

Description: Each capsule contains:
Bismuth Aluminate....100 mg.
Aluminum Hydroxide Coprecipitate 130 mg.
Magnesium Carbonate
Magnesium Trisilicate....160 mg.
Indications: As an antacid to alleviate the following symptoms: heartburn, sour stomach, and/or acid indigestion.
Warning: Do not take more than the recommended daily dosage unless directed by a physician. May cause constipation or have laxative effect when taken in maximum dose.
Drug Interaction Precautions: Do not take this capsule if you are presently taking a prescription antibiotic drug containing any form of tetracycline.
Directions For Use: One to two capsules 3 or 4 times daily. The dosage for persons with severe renal disease should be under the direction of a physician.
Literature available on request.
How Supplied: Bottles of 100.
[*Shown in Product Identification Section*]

LO-TUSSIN™ ©

Description: Each 5ml. (one teaspoonful) contains:
Codeine Phosphate, USP....10mg.
(**Warning:** May be habit forming.)
Pseudoephedrine Hydrochloride, NF....30mg.
Guaifenesin, NF....100mg.
Grape/Cherry/Raspberry flavor
Actions: Lo-Tussin combines the effectiveness of codeine as a centrally acting antitussive, with the sympathomimetic nasal decongestant effects of pseudoephedrine, and the expectorant action of guaifenesin which relieves irritated membranes in the respiratory passageways by preventing dryness through increased mucus flow.
Indications: For the temporary relief of the concurrent symptoms of dry, nonproductive cough and nasal congestion.
Directions: **Adults:** 2 teaspoonsful every 4 hours, not to exceed 6 doses in 24 hours.
Children 6–12 years: 1 teaspoonful every 4 hours, not to exceed 6 doses in 24 hours.
Children 2–5 years: ½ teaspoonful every 4 hours, not to exceed 6 doses in 24 hours.
For children under 2 years there is no recommended dosage, except under the advice and supervision of a physician.
Warnings: The codeine component may cause or aggravate constipation. Do not give this product to children under 2 years except under the advise and supervision of a physician. Do not give this product to children taking other medications except under the advice and supervision of a physician. Do not take this product for persistent or chronic cough such as occurs with smoking, asthma, or emphysema, or where cough is accompanied by excessive secretions, except under the advice and supervision of a physician. Do not take this product if you have chronic pulmonary disease or shortness of breath except under the advice and supervision of a physician. Do not exceed recommended dosage because at higher doses nervousness, dizziness, or sleeplessness may occur. If symptoms do not improve within 7 days, or are accompanied by a high fever, consult a physician before continuing use. Do not take this preparation if you have high blood pressure, heart disease, diabetes, or thyroid disease except under the advice and supervision of a physician.
KEEP THIS AND ALL DRUGS OUT OF THE REACH OF CHILDREN. IN CASE OF ACCIDENTAL OVERDOSE, SEEK PROFESSIONAL ASSISTANCE OR CONTACT A POISON CONTROL CENTER IMMEDIATELY.
Caution: A persistent cough may be a sign of a serious condition. If cough persists for more than 1 week, tends to recur, or is accompanied by high fever, rash, or persistent headache, consult a physician.
Drug Interaction Precaution: Do not take this product if you are presently taking a prescription antihypertensive or antidepressant drug containing a monoamine oxidase inhibitor, except under the advice and supervision of a physician.
How Supplied: Bottles of 473ml. (1 pint).

NEOTEP® GRANUCAPS* ℞

Description: Each red and clear banded Granucap* contains:
Chlorpheniramine Maleate....9 mg.
Phenylephrine Hydrochloride....21 mg.
Actions: NEOTEP is a combination of potent antihistamine and decongestant. Chlorpheniramine maleate is one of the most active of antihistaminic drugs. It is used both for therapy and prophylaxis in conditions when antihistamines may be effective. Its characteristic action is antagonism of histamine in the symptomatic treatment of various allergic diseases. The major use of phenylephrine is as a nasal decongestant.
Indications: Pollinosis or hay fever, Rose fever and allergies of the respiratory tract. Symptomatic relief from sneezing, rhinorrhea, and itching of eyes, nose and throat is generally accomplished through the use of NEOTEP Granucaps.
Contraindications: Hypersensitivity to either of the components. All antihistamine therapy should be withdrawn prior to skin testing for allergy.
Warning: Use with caution in patients subject to hyperthyroidism, hypertension, or coronary artery disease.
Precautions: Patients should be cautioned that drowsiness, though rarely a problem, may be encountered with the use of NEOTEP and that this may affect the operation of machinery or automobiles.
Use in Pregnancy: Women of child bearing age and nursing mothers should use NEOTEP only when the potential benefits of the drug have been weighed against the possible hazardous effect to mother and child.
Adverse Reactions: Average or large doses may cause drowsiness, headache, xerostomia, anorexia, nausea, vomiting, dizziness, nervousness, insomnia, palpitations, dysuria.
Dosage and Administration: One NEOTEP Granucap at 12 hour intervals.
Overdosage: Overdosage may produce a mixture of depressive and excitatory effects. Treatment is of a symptomatic nature and includes oxygen, gastric lavage and usual supporting measures.
How Supplied: Bottles of 100 and 1000.
Caution: Federal law prohibits dispensing without prescription.
*Granucap—T.M. Reg.—the medication in each "Granucap" is made available in a base to provide prolonged activity.
[*Shown in Product Identification Section*]

NORMACID® TABLETS
Digestant

Description: Each tablet contains:
Betaine HCl....440 mg.
Pepsin....100 mg.
Each tablet provides the equivalent of 28.6 ml. of 0.1 Normal hydrochloric acid or approximately 15 minims of diluted hydrochloric acid.
Indications: Normacid® assists digestion in gastric hypoacidity by gradual release of hydrochloric acid and pepsin.
Dosage: One tablet during each meal, or as directed by physician
How Supplied: Bottles of 100 (NDC 0124-1095-01).
[*Shown in Product Identification Section*]

QUINITE™ TABLETS ℞

Each tablet contains:
Quinine sulfate....260mg.
Aminophylline....195mg.
Actions: Quinine acts on skeletal muscle by two mechanisms; it increases the refractory period by direct action on the muscle fiber, and it also decreases the excitability of the motor end-plate by a curariform action. The mechanism of action of aminophylline is not fully established; it may be due to increase in blood flow, a depolarization of the muscle membrane, or an increase in metabolic rate of muscle.
Indications: For the prevention and treatment of nocturnal recumbency leg muscle cramps, including those associated with arthritis, diabetes, varicose veins, thrombophlebitis, arteriosclerosis, and static foot deformities.
Contraindications: Because of the quinine content, Quinite is contraindicated in women of child-bearing potential, in pregnancy, in patients with known quinine sensitivity, and in patients with glucose-6-phosphate dehydrogenase deficiency. Hemolysis (with the potential for hemolytic anemia) has been associated with a G-6-PD deficiency in patients taking quinine.
Precautions: Thrombocytopenic purpura may follow the administration of quinine in highly sensitive patients. Recovery will follow withdrawal of the medication. Cinchona alkaloids, including quinine, have the potential to depress the hepatic enzyme system that synthesizes the vitamin K-dependent factors. The resulting hypoprothrombinemic effect may enhance the action of warfarin and other oral anticoagulants.
Adverse Reactions: Aminophylline may produce intestinal cramps in some instances, and quinine may produce symptoms of cinchonism, such as tinnitus, dizziness, and gastrointestinal disturbances. If ringing in the ears, deafness, skin rash, or visual disturbances occur, the drug should be discontinued.
Dosage and Administration: 1 tablet upon retiring. When necessary, 1 additional tablet may be taken following the evening meal.
How Supplied: Bottles of 30, 100 and 500 tablets.
[*Shown in Product Identification Section*]

SULADYNE® TABLETS ℞
(sulfamethizole, sulfadiazine, phenazopyridine HCl)

Composition: Each tablet contains: sulfamethizole, 125mg.; sulfadiazine, 125mg.; Azodyne® (phenazopyridine hydrochloride), 75mg.
Actions and Uses: SULADYNE® is recommended for the treatment of acute urinary tract infections. Sulfamethizole, is extremely soluble, absorbed rapidly and almost completely from the intestinal tract into the blood stream. It is excreted rapidly by way of the kidneys, with the result that a high concentration of active drug is established in the urinary

Continued on next page

Tutag—Cont.

tract 1 to 2 hours after ingestion. The lower degree of acetylation of sulfamethizole assures greater effectiveness with minimum renal toxicity. It may be administered to patients sensitive to other sulfonamides, since there is little cross-sensitization.
Phenazopyridine HCl has a long clinical history of successful use. Phenazopyridine is an orally absorbed agent which produces prompt and effective local analgesia and relief of the pain and burning of urinary symptoms such as dysuria, frequency and urgency by virtue of its rapid excretion in the urinary tract. These effects are confined to the genitourinary system and are not accompanied by generalized sedation or narcosis.
Suladyne® is a bacteriostatic chemotherapeutic agent active against, a number of important gram-positive and gram-negative bacteria. In adults, it is indicated in the treatment of urinary tract infections (primarily pyelonephritis, pyelitis, and cystitis) complicated by pain in the absence of obstructive uropathy or foreign bodies when these infections are caused by susceptible strains of the following organisms: Escherichia coli, Klebsiella-Enterobacter, Staphylococcus aureus, Proteus mirabilis, and Proteus vulgaris, in the absence of obstructive uropathy or foreign bodies.
Important note: In vitro sulfonamide sensitivity tests are not always reliable. The test must be carefully coordinated with bacteriologic and clinical response. When the patient is already taking sulfonamides, follow-up cultures should have aminobenzoic acid added to the culture media.
Currently, the increasing frequency of resistant organisms is a limitation of the usefulness of antibacterial agents, including the sulfonamides, especially in the treatment of recurrent and complicated urinary tract infections.
Wide variation in blood levels may result with identical doses. Blood levels should be measured in patients receiving sulfonamides for serious infections. Free sulfonamide blood levels of 5–15mg. per 100ml. may be considered therapeutically effective for most infections, with blood levels of 12–15mg. per 100ml. Optimal for serious infections; 20mg. per 100ml, should be the maximum total sulfonamide level, as adverse reactions occur more frequently above this level.
Contraindications: Children below age 12. Hypersensitivity to sulfonamides. Pregnancy at term and during the nursing period, because sulfonamides pass the placenta and are excreted in the milk and may cause kernicterus. Because Suladyne® contains phenazopyridine hydrochloride it is contraindicated in glomerulonephritis severe hepatitis, uremia, and pyelonephritis of pregnancy with gastrointestinal disturbances. The drug should not be used in patients with a history of sensitivity to one of the components; or in prematures, neonates, pregnant females at term; or in patients with chronic glomerulonephritis, uremia, severe hepatitis, hepatic or renal failure, or severe pyelitis of pregnancy.
Warnings: Sulfonamides should not be used to treat group A streptococci infections or their sequelae. The occurrence of sore throat, fever, pallor, purpura, or jaundice during sulfonamide administration may be an early indication of serious blood dyscrasias.
Deaths associated with the administration of sulfonamides have been reported from hypersensitivity reactions, agranulocytosis, aplastic anemia, and other blood dyscrasias.
The frequency of renal complications is considerably lower in patients receiving the more soluble sulfonamides. However, frequent, complete blood counts and renal function tests should be carried out during sulfonamide treatment. Microscopic urinalysis should be done once a week when a patient is treated for longer than two weeks. Urine cultures should be made to confirm eradication of bacteriuria.
USAGE IN PREGNANCY: The safe use of sulfonamides in pregnancy has not been established. The teratogenicity potential of most sulfonamides has not been thoroughly investigated in either animals or humans. However, a significant increase in the incidence of cleft palate and other bony abnormalities of offspring has been observed when certain sulfonamides of the short, intermediate, and long-acting types were given to pregnant rats and mice at high oral doses (7 to 25 times the human dose.)
Precautions: To allay any possible apprehension, patients should be told that this medication may color the urine orange or red.
The usual precautions used in sulfonamide therapy should be observed, including the maintenance of an adequate fluid intake. Sulfonamides should be used with caution in patients with severe allergy or bronchial asthma. Severe impairment of hepatic or renal function, and in patients with glucose-6-phosphate dehydrogenase deficiency since sulfas may cause hemolysis in this latter group.
Adverse Reactions: BLOOD DYSCRASIAS. Agranulocytosis, apalstic anemia, thrombocytopenia, leukopenia, hemolytic anemia, purpura, hypoprothrombinemia, and methemoglobinemia.
ALLERIC REACTIONS. Erythema multiforme (Stevens-Johnson Sydrome), generalized skin eruptions, epidermal necrolysis, urticaria, serum sickness, pruritus, exfoliative dermatitis, anaphylactoid reactions, periorbital edema, conjunctival and scleral injection, photosensitization, arthralgia, and allergic myocarditis.
GASTROINTESTINAL REACTIONS. Nausea, emesis, abdominal pains, hepatitis, diarrhea, anorexia, pancreatitis, and stomatitis.
C.N.S. REACTIONS. Headache, peripheral neuritis, mental depression, convulsions, ataxia, hallucinations, tinnitus, vertigo, and insomnia.
MISCELLANEOUS REACTIONS. Drug fever, chills, and toxic nephrosis with oliguria and anuria. Periarteritis nodosum and L.E. phenomenon have occurred.
The sulfonamides bear certain chemical similarities to some goitrogens, diuretics (acetazolamide and the thiazides), and oral hypoglycemic agents. Goiter production, diuresis, and hypolgycemia have occurred rarely in patients receiving sulfonamides. Cross-sensitivity may exist with these agents.
Rats appear to be especially susceptible to the goiterogenic effects of sulfonamides, and long-term administration has produced thyroid malignancies in the species.
Dosage and Administration: Adults—two tablets, four times a day, or as directed by physician.
How Supplied: Small, round, maroon-colored tablets in bottles of 100 tablets.
Caution: Federal law prohibits dispensing without prescription.
[*Shown in Product Identification Section*]

UNPROCO® CAPSULES ℞

Description: Each capsule contains:

Guaifenesin, N.F.	200 mg.
Dextromethorphan HBr	30 mg.

Action and Uses: Unproco Capsules combine the expectorant action of Guaifenesin with the cough suppressing action of Dextromethorphan Hydrobromide. Guaifenesin, an effective long lasting expectorant, significantly increases the respiratory tract fluid. The enhanced flow of secretions exerts a demulcent effect on the tracheobronchial mucosa, promotes ciliary action and facilitates the removal of viscid secretions.
Dextromethorphan Hydrobromide, a non-narcotic cough suppressant, has the antitussive effectiveness of codeine but does not have its addiction liability, nor does it cause codeine-like side effects, such as constipation, anorexia and sedation. UNPROCO enhances the productivity of the cough by stimulating the secretion of fluids of the bronchial tree. As a result, the dry unproductive cough becomes more productive and less frequent.
UNPROCO is useful for the symptomatic relief of those respiratory conditions associated with dry, unproductive cough and in the presence of mucus in the respiratory tract.
UNPROCO is ideally suited for the relief of dry unproductive coughing associated with the common cold, influenza, acute and chronic bronchitis, tracheitis, laryngitis and pharyngitis.
Contraindications: Hypersensitivity to either component.
Dosage and Administration: Adults, one capsule every four hours.
How Supplied: Available in bottles of 20, 100 and 500.
Caution: Federal law prohibits dispensing without prescription.
[*Shown in Product Identification Section*]

USV Laboratories, Division
USV Pharmaceutical Corp.
TUCKAHOE, NY 10707

USV Laboratories Inc.
MANATI, P.R. 00701

USV (P.R.) Development Corp.
MANATI, P.R. 00701

AQUASOL® A DROPS OTC

Composition: Oil-soluble vitamin A water solubilized with polysorbate 20 for faster, better absorption and utilization. Drops provide 5,000 I.U. vitamin A per 0.1 ml.
Actions: There is evidence that aqueous vitamin A produces a more rapid increase in the blood concentration and higher blood levels than the oily form of the vitamin.
Administration and Dosage: As a dietary supplement 0.1 ml. (3 drops) for adults and children 4 or more years of age provides 100% of the U.S. RDA; 2 drops for children under 4, 133%.
How Supplied: *Drops:* 5,000 I.U. per 0.1 ml., bottles of 30 ml., with dropper.

AQUASOL® A CAPSULES ℞
(water-miscible vitamin A)
50,000 I.U. (15 mg.)
25,000 I.U. (7.5 mg.)

Composition: Oil-soluble vitamin A—water solubilized with polysorbate 20 to enable better absorption and utilization particularly in conditions in which absorption or utilization of fats and fat-soluble substances is impaired—50,000 and 25,000 I.U. per capsule.
Actions: Beta-carotene, retinol and retinal have effective and reliable vitamin A activity. Retinal and retinol are in chemical equilibrium in the body and have equivalent antixerophthalmic activity. Retinal combines with the rod pigment, opsin, in the retina to form rhodopsin, necessary for visual dark adaptation. Vitamin A prevents retardation of growth and preserves the epithelial cells integrity. Normal adult liver storage is sufficient to satisfy two years' requirements of vitamin A.
Indication: AQUASOL A Capsules are effective for the treatment of vitamin A deficiency.

Contraindications: Hypervitaminosis A; sensitivity to any of the ingredients of this preparation.
Warnings: Avoid overdosage. Keep out of the reach of children.
Use in pregnancy: Safety of amounts exeeding 6,000 I.U. of vitamin A daily during pregnancy has not been established at this time. From the standpoint of the fetus, therefore, the use of vitamin A in excess of the recommended dietary allowance during normal pregnancy should be avoided. Animal reproduction studies have shown fetal abnormalities in several species, associated with overdosage. Malformations of the central nervous system, the eye, the palate and the urogenital tract are recorded.
Precautions: Protect from light.
Vitamin A administration from fortified foods, dietary supplements, self-administered drugs and prescription drug sources should be evaluated. Prolonged daily dose administration over 25,000 I.U. vitamin A should be under close supervision. Blood level assays are not a direct measure of liver storage. Liver storage should be adequate before discontinuing therapy. Single vitamin A deficiency is rare. Multiple vitamin deficiency is expected in any dietary deficiency.
Women on oral contraceptives have shown a significant increase in plasma vitamin A levels.
Adverse Reactions: See Overdosage.
Dosage and Administration: For adults and children over eight years of age:
a. Severe deficiency: 100,000 I.U. daily for three days followed by 50,000 I.U. daily for two weeks.
b. Follow-up therapy: 10,000 to 20,000 I.U. daily for two months.
Poor dietary habits should be corrected and an abundant and well-balanced dietary intake should be prescribed.
Overdosage: The following amounts have been found to be toxic. Toxicity manifestations depend on the age, dosage units and duration of administration.
Acute toxicity—Single dose (25,000 I.U./Kg. body weight)
Infant: 350,000 I.U.
Adult: Over 2 million I.U.
Chronic toxicity (4,000 I.U./Kg. body weight for 6 to 15 months)
3 to 6 months old: 18,500 I.U. (water dispersed)/day for one to three months
Adult: 1 million I.U. daily for three days
Adult: 50,000 I.U. daily for longer than 18 months
Adult: 500,000 I.U. daily for two months
Hypervitaminosis A Syndrome:
1. *General manifestations:* Fatigue, malaise, lethargy, abdominal discomfort, anorexia and vomiting.
2. *Specific manifestations:*
a. Skeletal: slow growth, hard tender cortical thickening over the radius and tibia, migratory arthralgia and premature closure of the epiphysis.
b. Central Nervous System: irritability, headache, and increased intracranial pressure as manifested by bulging fontanels, papilledema, exophthalmos.
c. Dermatologic: fissures of the lips, drying and cracking of the skin, alopecia, scaling, massive desquamation and increased pigmentation.
d. Systemic: hypomenorrhea, hepatosplenomegaly, jaundice, leukopenia, vitamin A plasma level over 1200 I.U./100 cc.
The treatment of hypervitaminosis A consists of immediate withdrawal of the vitamin along with symptomatic and supportive treatment.
How Supplied: AQUASOL A CAPSULES (water-miscible vitamin A) 50,000 I.U. vitamin A, bottles of 100 and 500; 25,000 I.U. vitamin A, bottles of 100.
[*Shown in Product Identification Section*]

AQUASOL® E — OTC
(Aqueous Vitamin E Supplements, Oral)

Composition: Three potencies, 30 I.U., 100 I.U. and 400 I.U. vitamin E per capsule; water-solubilized for more rapid and more complete absorption than oily vitamin E. Drops, 50 I.U. vitamin E per cc. in aqueous solution.
How Supplied: 30 and 100 I.U. Capsules, bottles of 100; 400 I.U. capsules, bottles of 30. Drops, 15 cc.
[*Shown in Product Identification Section*]

ARLIDIN® — ℞
(nylidrin HCl)
Vasodilator/Vasorelaxant

Arlidin is a product of USV Laboratories Inc., Manati, P.R. 00701.

Description: Tablets of 6 and 12 mg. nylidrin HCl.
Actions: Arlidin acts predominantly by beta-receptor stimulation. Beta stimulation with Arlidin has been demonstrated in a variety of isolated tissues from rabbits, guinea pigs and dogs. It has been shown to dilate arterioles in skeletal muscle and to increase cardiac output in the anesthetized dog and cat and in unanesthetized man.

Indications: Based on a review of this drug by the National Academy of Sciences—National Research Council and/or other information, FDA has classified the indications as follows:
"Possibly" effective whenever an increase in blood supply is desirable in vasospastic disorders such as:
Peripheral vascular disease: arteriosclerosis obliterans, thromboangiitis obliterans, diabetic vascular disease, night leg cramps, Raynaud's phenomenon and disease, ischemic ulcer, frostbite, acrocyanosis, acroparesthesia, thrombophlebitis, cold feet, legs and hands.
Circulatory disturbances of the inner ear: primary cochlear cell ischemia, cochlear stria vascular ischemia, macular or ampullar ischemia and other disturbances due to labyrinthine artery spasm or obstruction.
Final classification of the less-than-effective indications requires further investigation.

Contraindications: Acute myocardial infarction, paroxysmal tachycardia, progressive angina pectoris and thyrotoxicosis.
Warnings: In patients with cardiac disease such as tachyarrhythmias and uncompensated congestive heart failure, the benefit/risk ratio should be weighed prior to therapy and reconsidered at intervals during treatment.
Adverse Reactions: Trembling, nervousness, weakness, dizziness (not associated with labyrinthine artery insufficiency), palpitations, nausea and vomiting may occur. Postural hypotension, while not reported, may also occur.
Dosage: Orally, 3 to 12 mg. three or four times a day.
How Supplied: ARLIDIN (nylidrin HCl)—White, scored tablets, 6 mg. and 12 mg. Bottles of 100 and 1000. Unit-dose blister packs, boxes of 100 (10 x 10 strips).
NSN 6505-00-685-5435A, V.A. Depots (6 mg., 1000s).
Date of last revision: Sept. 1976.
[*Shown in Product Identification Section*]

AZOLID® Tablets — ℞
(phenylbutazone USP) 100 mg.
AZOLID®-A Capsules — ℞

Composition: Each capsule provides 100 mg. phenylbutazone USP, 100 mg. dried aluminum hydroxide gel, and 150 mg. magnesium trisilicate.

Nonhormonal antiarthritic anti-inflammatory agent

Important Note: AZOLID cannot be considered a simple analgesic and should never be administered casually. Each patient should be carefully evaluated before treatment is started and should remain constantly under the close supervision of the physician. The following cautions should be observed:
1. Therapy should not be initiated until a careful detailed history and complete physical and laboratory examination, including a complete hemogram and urinalysis, etc., of the patient have been made. These examinations should be made at regular, frequent intervals throughout the duration of this drug therapy.
2. Patients should be carefully selected, avoiding those in whom it is contraindicated as well as those who will respond to ordinary therapeutic measures, or those who cannot be observed at frequent intervals.
3. Patients taking this drug should be warned not to exceed the recommended dosage, since this may lead to toxic effects, and should discontinue the drug and report to the physician immediately any sign of:
   a. Fever, sore throat, lesions in the mouth (symptoms of blood dyscrasia).
   b. Dyspepsia, epigastric pain, symptoms of anemia, unusual bleeding, unusual bruising, black or tarry stools or other evidence of intestinal ulceration.
   c. Skin rashes.
   d. Significant weight gain or edema.
4. A trial period of one week of therapy is considered adequate to determine the therapeutic effect of the drug. In the absence of a favorable response, therapy should be discontinued.
   In the elderly (sixty years and over) the drug should be restricted to short-term treatment periods only—if possible, one week maximum.
5. BEFORE PRESCRIBING AZOLID FOR AN INDIVIDUAL PATIENT, READ THOROUGHLY THE INFORMATION CONTAINED UNDER EACH HEADING WHICH FOLLOWS:

Description and Actions: AZOLID is closely related chemically and pharmacologically, including toxic effects, to the well-known pyrazolines (pyrazole compounds) amidopyrine and antipyrine.
Chemically, AZOLID is 4-butyl-1,2-diphenyl-3,5-pyrazolidinedione. It is entirely unrelated to the steroid hormones. It has anti-inflammatory and antipyretic action as well as analgesic and mild uricosuric properties resulting in symptomatic relief only. THE DISEASE PROCESS ITSELF IS UNALTERED BY THIS DRUG.
Indications: The leading indications in which AZOLID affords relief are:
Gout
Rheumatoid Arthritis
Rheumatoid Spondylitis
Osteoarthritis
Psoriatic Arthritis
Acute Superficial Thrombophlebitis*
Painful Shoulder (peritendinitis, capsulitis, bursitis, and acute arthritis of that joint)
*Cumulative clinical experience has demonstrated that phenylbutazone is remarkably effective in the treatment of those cases of superficial venous thrombosis, regardless of location, in which acute perivascular inflammation is a major source of symptoms and disability.
The analgesic, antipyretic, anti-inflammatory actions of phenylbutazone are manifested as

Continued on next page

USV—Cont.

prompt relief of pain, lysis of fever and diminution of swelling, tenderness and local heat.
Phenylbutazone is especially useful in allowing early ambulation. It may be used in conjunction with other therapeutic measures, such as anticoagulants, bed rest, elevation of the limb, use of pressure bandages, or surgical evacuation of the clot.

Contraindications:

1. Age
   AZOLID is contraindicated in children fourteen years or less and in senile patients.
2. Gastrointestinal Problems
   Patients with a history or symptoms of gastrointestinal inflammation or ulceration, including severe or recurrent or persistent dyspepsia, should not be treated with the drug.
3. AZOLID is contraindicated in patients with the history of, or presence of: drug allergy; blood dyscrasias; renal, hepatic or cardiac dysfunction; hypertension; thyroid disease; systemic edema; salivary gland enlargement due to the drug; stomatitis due to the drug; polymyalgia rheumatica and temporal arteritis.
4. Concurrent Therapy
   Phenylbutazone is contraindicated when the patient is receiving other potent chemotherapeutic agents.
5. Concomitant Anticoagulant Therapy
   Phenylbutazone should not be given to patients on long-term anticoagulant therapy.

Warnings:

GENERAL TOXICITY

1. The known factors affecting the incidence of toxic reactions are: age, weight, dosage, duration of therapy, existence of concomitant diseases, and concurrent potent chemotherapy.
   Careful instructions to, and observations of, the individual patient are essential to the prevention of serious, life-threatening adverse reactions. This is especially true in the *aging* (40 years and over) who have an increased susceptibility to the toxicity of the drug.
   The lowest effective dose for the specific patient should be the continuous goal of therapy with this drug.
   In each patient, the risk of severe, and even fatal drug reactions must be weighed against the possible drug benefits initially unpredictable for the individual.
2. **IN ELDERLY PATIENTS**
   (60 years of age and over)

AZOLID should be restricted to treatment periods of *one week* duration. The appearance of clinical edema is an indication to discontinue treatment with the drug.

PREGNANCY

Animal reproduction studies thus far, though inconclusive, exhibit evidences of embryotoxicity.
Therefore, it is recommended that the drug be used with caution in the first trimester of pregnancy, weighing the potential risks against the benefits. Pregnant women and nursing mothers should receive phenylbutazone with caution since the drug may appear in cord blood and breast milk.

HEMATOLOGY

Blood Dyscrasias Serious, even fatal blood dyscrasias, including aplastic anemia, due to phenylbutazone, may occur suddenly despite regular repeated hemograms, and may become manifest many days or weeks after cessation of the drug.
Any significant change in the total white count, relative decrease in granulocytes, appearance of immature forms, or fall in hematocrit should be a signal for immediate cessation of therapy and a complete hematologic investigation.
Unexplained Bleeding Unexplained bleeding involving the CNS, adrenal glands, and gastrointestinal tract, has occurred due to therapy with this drug.

ANTIDIABETIC AND SULFONAMIDE-TYPE AGENTS

Phenylbutazone may potentiate the pharmacologic action of insulin, sulfonylurea, and sulfonamide-type agents. Patients receiving such concomitant therapy should be carefully observed for this effect.

THYROID-INHIBITION

Phenylbutazone reduces the iodine uptake by the thyroid. Both nontoxic and toxic goiters and myxedema due to therapy with this drug have been reported.

BLURRED VISION

The development of blurred vision while on this drug can be a significant toxic symptom worthy of a complete ophthalmological examination.

CLINICAL EDEMA

In patients *under sixty years of age* swelling of the ankles or face alone may be prevented by reducing the dosage. Otherwise, the appearance of clinical edema is an indication to discontinue the drug.

Precautions: Because of the unpredictability and severity of the potential side effects of AZOLID therapy IN ALL PATIENTS, the following should be accomplished at *regular* intervals:

1. A careful detailed history for the disease being treated and the detection of the earliest signs of adverse reactions.
2. A complete physical examination including check of the patient's weight.
3. A COMPLETE *WEEKLY* (especially for the aging), or EVERY TWO-WEEK BLOOD CHECK.
4. Any additional laboratory studies pertinent to the individual case.
5. Each patient should be warned to report immediately to his doctor the occurrence of fever, sore throat, oral lesions, salivary gland enlargement, black or tarry stools, weight gain, edema and any other sign or symptom pertinent to the individual case.
6. While on the drug, patients should be cautioned about participation in activity necessitating alertness and coordination, as driving a car, etc.

LEUKEMIA

Although a definite causal relationship to phenylbutazone therapy has not been firmly established, cases of leukemia have been reported in patients with a history of short- and long-term therapy with the drug. The overwhelming majority of these patients were over forty years of age. It should also be recognized that arthritic-type pains can be the presenting symptom of leukemia.
In some patients, phenylbutazone may cause an activation of symptoms of systemic lupus erythematosus. In such cases the drug should be discontinued.

Adverse Reactions: AZOLID is a potent drug; its misuse can lead to serious results. Detailed information on its use should be thoroughly reviewed before undertaking therapy.

GASTROINTESTINAL: Ulcerative esophagitis; acute and reactivated gastric and duodenal ulcer with perforation and hemorrhage; ulceration and perforation of large bowel; occult gastrointestinal bleeding with anemia; gastritis; epigastric pain; hematemesis; dyspepsia; nausea, vomiting and diarrhea; abdominal distention.

HEMATOLOGIC: Agranulocytosis, aplastic anemia, hemolytic anemia, anemia due to blood loss including occult gastrointestinal bleeding, thrombocytopenia, pancytopenia, leukemia, leukopenia, bone marrow depression.

FLUID, ELECTROLYTE DISTURBANCES: Sodium and chloride retention, water retention and edema, plasma dilution, respiratory alkalosis, metabolic acidosis.

HEPATIC: Fatal and nonfatal hepatitis (cholestasis may or may not be prominent).

DERMATOLOGIC: Petechiae, purpura without thrombocytopenia, toxic pruritus, erythema nodosum. See ALLERGIC REACTIONS for further dermatologic involvement.

ALLERGIC REACTIONS: All allergic reactions require *prompt* and *permanent withdrawal* of phenylbutazone.
Erythema multiforme; Stevens-Johnson Syndrome, Lyell's Syndrome, toxic necrotizing epidermolysis; exfoliative dermatitis; serum sickness; hypersensitivity angiitis (polyarteritis); anaphylactic shock; urticaria; arthralgia; fever; rashes.

RENAL: Proteinuria, hematuria, oliguria, anuria, renal failure with azotemia, glomerulonephritis, acute tubular necrosis, nephrotic syndrome, bilateral renal cortical necrosis, renal stones, ureteral obstruction with uric acid crystals due to the uricosuric action of this drug, impaired renal function.

CARDIOVASCULAR: Cardiac decompensation, hypertension, pericarditis, diffuse interstitial myocarditis with muscle necrosis, perivascular granulomata, aggravation of temporal arteritis in patients with polymyalgia rheumatica.

OCULAR: Optic neuritis, blurred vision, retinal hemorrhage, toxic amblyopia, retinal detachment.

OTIC: Hearing loss.

METABOLIC-ENDOCRINE: Hyperglycemia, thyroid hyperplasia, toxic goiter, association of hypothyroidism and hyperthyroidism (causal relationship not established).

CNS: Agitation, confusional states, lethargy.

CNS REACTIONS ASSOCIATED WITH OVERDOSAGE: Convulsions, euphoria, psychosis, depression, headaches, hallucinations, giddiness, vertigo, coma, hyperventilation, insomnia.

MISCELLANEOUS: Ulcerative stomatitis, salivary gland enlargement.

Dosage and Administration:

IN CHILDREN AND IN SENILE PATIENTS

AZOLID is contraindicated in children fourteen years of age or less, and in senile patients.

IN ELDERLY PATIENTS

(sixty years and over)
Every effort must be made to discontinue therapy on, or as soon as possible after the *seventh day,* because of the exceedingly high risk of severe, fatal toxic reactions in this group.

IN ALL PATIENTS

For the individual patient, the efficacy and the safety of phenylbutazone is unpredictable. Therefore:

1. The goal of therapy should be SHORT-TERM relief of SEVERE symptoms to a level tolerable to the SMALLEST possible drug dosage.
2. When improvement of symptoms occurs, prompt efforts to rapidly reduce the dosage should be made repeatedly, until complete drug discontinuation is achieved.
3. The action of the drug is usually manifest by the third to fourth day of treatment. Therefore, do not continue therapy beyond a week in the absence of a favorable result.
4. To minimize gastric upset, it should always be taken immediately before or after meals or with a full glass of milk. AZOLID-A capsules should be substituted if dyspeptic symptoms occur following the administration of AZOLID tablets.
5. See WARNINGS SECTION entitled GENERAL TOXICITY.

Dosage: In selecting the appropriate dosage in any specific case, consideration should be given to the patient's age, weight, general health, and any other factors that may influence his response to the drug.
Dosage Regimen in Rheumatoid Arthritis, Rheumatoid Spondylitis, Osteoarthritis, Psori-

atic Arthritis and Painful Shoulder: Initial Dosage: The initial daily dosage in adults ranges from 300 mg. to 600 mg., divided into three or four equal doses. In most instances, it is unnecessary to exceed 400 mg. daily to ensure maximum therapeutic response.

A trial period of one week of therapy is considered adequate to determine the therapeutic effect of the drug. In the absence of a favorable response, therapy should be discontinued.

Maintenance Dosage: When improvement is obtained, dosage should be promptly decreased to the minimum effective level necessary to maintain relief. This maintenance dosage should not exceed 400 mg. daily because of possible cumulative toxic effects. Satisfactory response is often achieved with as little as 100 to 200 mg. daily.

Dosage Regimen in Acute Gouty Arthritis: The treatment of acute gouty arthritis calls for a somewhat different dosage regimen. In this condition, best results are obtained from an initial dose of 400 mg., followed by 100 mg. every four hours until articular inflammation subsides, usually within four days. This therapy should not be continued beyond a period of one week.

Dosage Regimen in Acute Superficial Thrombophlebitis: Best results have been obtained with a dosage of 600 mg. daily in divided doses for the first two or three days, followed by a reduction to 300 mg. daily. Usual duration of treatment is five to seven days and only rarely must therapy be extended beyond ten days.

Overdosage:

Signs and Symptoms: Include any of the following: nausea, vomiting, epigastric pain, excessive perspiring, tinnitus, difficulty in hearing, edema (sodium retention), hypertension, cyanosis, respiratory depression, agitation, hallucinations, stupor, convulsions, coma, hematuria, and oliguria. Hepatomegaly, jaundice, and ulceration of the buccal or gastrointestinal mucosa have been reported as late manifestations of massive overdosage.

Reported laboratory abnormalities following overdosage include: respiratory or metabolic acidosis, impaired hepatic or renal function, and abnormalities of formed blood elements.

Treatment: In the alert patient, empty the stomach promptly by induced emesis followed by lavage. In the obtunded patient, secure the airway with a cuffed endotracheal tube before beginning lavage (do not induce emesis). Maintain adequate respiratory exchange, do not use respiratory stimulants. Treat shock with appropriate supportive measures. Control seizures with intravenous diazepam or short-acting barbiturates. Dialysis may be helpful if renal function is impaired.

How Supplied: AZOLID (phenylbutazone) 100 mg. tablets (yellow, coated), bottles of 100 and 1000. AZOLID-A capsules (yellow and white), bottles of 100 and 1000.

NSN 6505-00-181-7888 (Azolid 100s), NSN 6505-00-181-7895 (Azolid 1000s), Military Depots

NSN 6505-00-063-8323 (Azolid 1000s), VA Depots

[*Shown in Product Identification Section*]

CERESPAN® ℞
(papaverine HCl)
in sustained-release micro-dialysis cells

Composition: Each capsule provides 150 mg. papaverine hydrochloride in micro-dialysis cells, uniquely processed for sustained release of medication to provide prolonged therapeutic effect.

Actions and Uses: The main actions of papaverine are exerted on cardiac and various smooth muscles. It relaxes the smooth musculature of the larger blood vessels, especially coronary, systemic peripheral, cerebral and pulmonary arteries. This relaxation may be prominent if spasm exists. The muscle cell is not paralyzed by papaverine, and still responds to drugs and other stimuli causing contraction. The antispasmodic effect is a direct one, and unrelated to muscle innervation. Papaverine is practically devoid of effects on the central nervous system.

Perhaps by its direct vasodilating action on cerebral blood vessels, papaverine increases cerebral blood flow and decreases cerebral vascular resistance in normal subjects; oxygen consumption is unaltered. These effects may explain the benefit reported from the drug in cerebral vascular encephalopathy.

Like quinidine, papaverine acts directly on heart muscle to depress conduction and prolong the refractory period. These direct actions provide the basis for its clinical trial in abrogating atrial and ventricular premature systoles and ominous ventricular arrhythmias.

The coronary vasodilator action could be an additional factor of therapeutic value when such rhythms are secondary to insufficiency or occlusion of the coronary arteries.

In patients with acute coronary thrombosis, the occurrence of ventricular rhythms is serious and requires measures designed to decrease myocardial irritability. Papaverine may have advantages over quinidine, used for a similar purpose, in that it may be given in an emergency by the intravenous route, does not depress myocardial contraction or cause cinchonism, and produces coronary vasodilation.

Indications: For the relief of cerebral and peripheral ischemia associated with arterial spasm and myocardial ischemia complicated by arrhythmias.

Precautions: Use with caution in patients with glaucoma. Hepatic hypersensitivity has been reported with gastrointestinal symptoms, jaundice, eosinophilia and altered liver function tests. Discontinue drug if these occur.

Side Effects: Although occurring rarely, the reported side effects of papaverine include nausea, abdominal distress, anorexia, constipation or diarrhea, skin rash, malaise, drowsiness, vertigo, sweating, and headache.

Administration and Dosage: One capsule every 12 hours. In difficult cases administration may be increased to one capsule every 8 hours, or two capsules every 12 hours.

How Supplied: Bottles of 100 and 1000; drums of 5000; unit-dose blister packs, boxes of 100 (10 x 10 strips).

[*Shown in Product Identification Section*]

DEMI-REGROTON™ ℞
Oral antihypertensive

See under Regroton®.

DORIDEN® Ⓒ
(glutethimide NF)

Doriden is a product of USV (P.R.) Development Corp., Manati, P.R. 00701.

Composition: Each tablet provides 0.5 Gm., or 0.25 Gm. glutethimide. Each capsule provides 0.5 Gm. glutethimide.

Description: Doriden is a piperidinedione derivative; occurs as a white, crystalline powder; is practically insoluble in water, soluble in alcohol.

Clinical Pharmacology: Doriden is erratically absorbed from the gastrointestinal tract. Following single oral doses of 500 mg., wide variations in absorption of the drug were observed, and the peak plasma concentration occurred from one to six hours after administration. The average plasma half-life is 10–12 hours. Glutethimide is a racemate; both isomers are hydroxylated, the d-isomer on the piperidinedione ring and the l-isomer on the phenyl substituent. Both hydroxylates are conjugated with glucuronic acid; the glucuronides pass into the enterohepatic circulation, and thence are excreted in the urine. Less than 2% of a usual dose is excreted in the urine unchanged. About 50% of the drug is bound to plasma proteins.

Glutethimide exhibits pronounced anticholinergic activity, which is manifested by mydriasis, inhibition of salivary secretions and intestinal motility.

Indications: Glutethimide has been shown to be effective as a hypnotic for three to seven days. It is not indicated for chronic administration. Should insomnia persist, a drug-free interval of one or more weeks should elapse before retreatment is considered. Attempts should be made to find alternative non-drug therapy in chronic insomnia.

Contraindications: Glutethimide is contraindicated in patients with known hypersensitivity to the drug. It is also contraindicated in patients with porphyria.

Warnings: The patient should be warned about the possible additive effects when glutethimide is taken concomitantly with other central nervous system depressants such as alcohol.

The patient on Doriden must be warned against driving a car or operating dangerous machinery while on the drug, since glutethimide may impair the ability to perform hazardous activities requiring mental alertness or physical coordination.

Glutethimide induces hepatic microsomal enzymes resulting in increased metabolism of coumarin anticoagulants and decreased anticoagulant response.

Physical and Psychological Dependence: Both physical and psychological dependence have occurred: therefore patients should be carefully evaluated before prescribing Doriden. Ordinarily, an amount adequate for one week is sufficient. The patient should be reevaluated before represcribing, after an interval of one or more weeks. Withdrawal symptoms include nausea, abdominal discomfort, tremors, convulsions, and delirium. Newborn infants of mothers dependent on glutethimide may also exhibit withdrawal symptoms. In the presence of dependence, dosage should be reduced gradually.

Usage in Pregnancy: The lack of adverse effects of glutethimide on fetal development has not been established. Therefore its use in pregnancy is not recommended.

Usage in Children: Glutethimide is *not* recommended for use in children, since its safety and effectiveness in the pediatric age group have *not* been established.

Precautions: For elderly or debilitated patients, the initial daily dosage should not exceed 0.5 Gm. at bedtime, in order to avoid oversedation.

Adverse Reactions: With recommended doses, there have been rare reports of nausea, hangover, paradoxical excitation, and blurring of vision. Rarely, acute hypersensitivity reactions, porphyria, and blood dyscrasias such as thrombocytopenic purpura, aplastic anemia, or leukopenia, have been reported. Osteomalacia has been reported after long-term use of Doriden. A generalized skin rash may occur, in which case the drug should be withdrawn. This rash usually clears spontaneously within a few days after drug withdrawal. Occasionally, a purpuric or urticarial rash may occur; exfoliative dermatitis has been reported rarely.

Dosage and Administration: For use as a hypnotic, dosage should be individualized. The usual adult dosage is 0.25 to 0.5 Gm. at bedtime.

Overdosage:

Acute Overdosage: The single acute lethal dose of glutethimide in humans ranges from 10 Gm. to 20 Gm. Although the majority of fatalities have resulted from single doses in this range, patients have died from single doses as low as 5 Gm. and have recovered from single doses as high as 35 Gm. A single oral dose of 5 Gm. usually produces severe intoxication. A plasma level of 3 mg./100 ml. is indicative of

Continued on next page

USV—Cont.

severe poisoning, but the level may be higher if the patient is tolerant to the drug. However, the level may also be lower because of sequestration of the drug in body fat depots and in the gastrointestinal tract. A lower level does not preclude the possibility of severe poisoning; therefore, the extent of intoxication may not be accurately reflected by single glutethimide plasma level determinations. Serial determinations are mandatory for proper patient evaluation.
Ingestion of acutely excessive dosage of glutethimide can give rise to a life-threatening situation. The effects of glutethimide are exaggerated by concomitant ingestion of other hypnotics or sedatives such as alcohol, barbiturates, etc., and suicidal efforts commonly involve multiple drugs of the sedative-hypnotic-tranquilizer types.
Signs and Symptoms: The principal signs and symptoms caused by glutethimide intoxication vary in severity in ratio to the ingested dosage, in general, and are indistinguishable from those caused by barbiturate intoxication. The degree of CNS depression often fluctuates, possibly due to irregular absorption of the drug and/or accumulation of an active toxic metabolite, 4-hydroxy-2-ethyl-2-phenyl-glutarimide (4-HG). They are: CNS depression, including coma *(profound and prolonged in severe intoxication)*; hypothermia, which may be followed by fever even without apparent infection; depressed or lost deep tendon reflexes; depression or absence of corneal and pupillary reflexes; dilatation of pupils; depressed or absent response to painful stimuli; inadequate ventilation (even with relatively normal respiratory rate), sometimes with cyanosis; sudden apnea, especially with manipulation such as gastric lavage or endotracheal intubation; diminished or absent peristalsis. Severe hypotension unresponsive to volume expansion, tonic muscular spasms, twitching and convulsions may occur.
Treatment: As with all forms of acute intoxication, the sooner adequate treatment is instituted, the better the prognosis. Early and vigorous cardiopulmonary supportive measures should be employed and should include:
1) Maintenance of a patent airway with assisted ventilation if necessary.
2) Monitoring of vital signs and level of consciousness.
3) Continuous electrocardiogram to detect arrhythmias.
4) Maintenance of blood pressure with plasma volume expanders and, if absolutely essential, pressor drugs.
Blood for glutethimide levels and other chemical determinations should be obtained as well as arterial blood for blood gas determinations. Vomiting should be induced if the patient is fully conscious. Gastric lavage should be done in all cases regardless of elapsed time since drug ingestion, with due caution to prevent aspiration of gastric contents or respiratory arrest during manipulation, including prior insertion of a cuffed endotracheal tube or employment of tracheostomy. Lavage with a 1:1 mixture of castor oil and water is capable of removing larger amounts of glutethimide from the stomach than with aqueous lavage. Fifty ml. of castor oil should be left in the stomach as a cathartic.
Intestinal lavage is used to remove unabsorbed Doriden from the intestines (100–250 ml. of 20–40% sorbitol or mannitol). If emesis or gastric lavage cannot be effected in the fully conscious patient, delay absorption of Doriden by giving one pint of water, milk or fruit juice; flour or cornstarch suspension, or activated charcoal in water. Follow up as soon as possible with production of emesis or gastric lavage.
Adequate respiratory gas exchange must be maintained and may require tracheostomy and mechanical assistance. If coma is prolonged, urine output must be monitored and maintained, while preventing overhydration which might contribute to pulmonary or cerebral edema.
In *Severe Intoxication*, in addition to intensive supportive measures and symptomatic care, consideration should be given to dialysis or hemoperfusion in the following circumstances: Grade III or Grade IV coma, but the level of coma per se is not a mandatory indication for the procedure. Hemodialysis may also be required when renal shutdown or impaired renal function are manifest and in life-threatening overdose situations complicated by (a) pulmonary edema, (b) heart failure, (c) circulatory collapse, (d) significant liver disease, (e) major metabolic disturbance, (f) uremia. While aqueous hemodialysis is less effective for glutethimide than for readily water-soluble compounds that are not bound by proteins or sequestered in body fat depots, glutethimide blood levels may decline more rapidly with hemodialysis and the duration of coma may be shortened; efficacy of the procedure, however, is largely controversial. As long as significant amounts of glutethimide remain in fat depots or as an unabsorbed bolus in the intestinal tract, the fall in serum level accelerated by hemodialysis may be followed by increased absorption into the bloodstream on termination of dialysis and may require further dialysis.
Recent clinical data indicate that use of pure food-grade soybean oil as the dialysate enhances removal of glutethimide and some other lipidsoluble substances by means of hemodialysis. Peritoneal dialysis, while able to remove some glutethimide, apparently is of minimal value.
Hemoperfusion appears to be a promising technique for eliminating glutethimide from the body. Charcoal hemoperfusion utilizing acrylic hydrogel microencapsulation of activated charcoal has been reported to be simpler and more effective than hemodialysis. Similarly, a microcapsule artificial kidney has been developed utilizing activated charcoal granules encapsulated with cellulose nitrate and albumin. *Resin* hemoperfusion utilizing a column containing Amerberlite XAD-2 has demonstrated exceptionally high clearance capabilities in glutethimide intoxication and has been reported to be clinically superior to hemodialysis in patients with profound life-threatening coma and potentially lethal blood concentrations of intoxicant drugs.
Drug extraction techniques should be continued for at least two hours after the patient regains consciousness. Glutethimide is highly lipid soluble and, therefore, rapidly accumulated in lipoid tissue. As the drug is removed from the bloodstream by any technique, it is gradually released from fat storage depots back into the bloodstream. Even after substantial quantities of the drug have been extracted, this blood-level rebound can cause coma to persist or recur.
As in the case of any prolonged coma, appropriate antibiotic therapy is indicated if pulmonary or other infection intervenes.
Chronic Overdosage: Signs and symptoms of chronic glutethimide intoxication (and for all drugs producing barbiturate-alcohol type of dependence in chronic overdosage) include impairment of memory and ability to concentrate, impaired gait, ataxiá, tremors, hyporeflexia, and slurring of speech. Abrupt discontinuance of glutethimide after prolonged overdosage will in most cases cause withdrawal reactions ranging from nervousness and anxiety to grand mal seizures, and may include abdominal cramping, chills, numbness of extremities, and dysphagia.
Treatment: Chronic glutethimide intoxication may be treated by gradual, stepwise reduction of dosage over a period of days or weeks. Watch patient carefully. If withdrawal reactions occur, they can be controlled by readministration of glutethimide, or substitution of pentobarbital, and subsequent gradual withdrawal.
How Supplied: *Tablets,* 0.5 Gm. (white, scored); bottles of 100, 500, 1000 and Strip Dispensers of 100. *Tablets,* 0.25 Gm. (white, scored); bottles of 100 and 1000. *Capsules,* 0.5 Gm. (blue and white); bottles of 100.
NSN 6505-00-616-9069A, V.A. Depots (0.5 Gm. tablets, 1000s).
[*Shown in Product Identification Section*]

HISTASPAN® ℞
(chlorpheniramine maleate)
in sustained-release micro-dialysis cells

Composition: Each capsule provides 8 mg. or 12 mg. chlorpheniramine maleate in microdialysis cells, uniquely processed for sustained release of medication to provide prolonged therapeutic effect.
Indications: Perennial and seasonal allergic rhinitis; vasomotor rhinitis; allergic conjunctivitis due to inhalant allergens and foods; mild, uncomplicated allergic skin manifestations of urticaria and angioedema; amelioration and prevention of allergic reactions to blood or plasma in patients with a known history of such reactions; dermographism; as therapy for anaphylactic reactions adjunctive to epinephrine and other standard measures after the acute manifestations have been controlled.
Contraindication: Known hypersensitivity to the drug.
Precautions: Since drowsiness or dizziness may occur, patients should be cautioned about driving or operating machinery.
Adverse Reactions: May include drowsiness, dizziness, dry mouth, disturbed coordination, blurred vision, G.I. disturbance, tachycardia, headache, nervousness, weakness, and urinary disturbances.
Dosage: *8 mg. capsules:* children over age 6 and adults, one capsule in the morning and one at night (q. 12 h.). *12 mg. capsules:* adults and children over age 12, one capsule in the morning and one at night (q. 12 h.).
How Supplied: 8 mg. and 12 mg. capsules, bottles of 100 and 1000.
[*Shown in Product Identification Section*]

HISTASPAN-D® ℞
in sustained-release micro-dialysis cells

Composition: Each Histaspan-D capsule provides 8 mg. Histaspan® (chlorpheniramine maleate), 20 mg. phenylephrine hydrochloride, and 2.5 mg. methscopolamine nitrate in sustained-release micro-dialysis cells, uniquely processed for sustained release of medication to provide prolonged therapeutic effect.
Action: Histaspan-D combines the highly effective and widely used antihistamine, chlorpheniramine maleate, with a decongestant, phenylephrine hydrochloride, and a drying agent, methscopolamine nitrate, for relief of rhinorrhea, sneezing, lacrimation, nasal congestion, and other respiratory symptoms accompanying the common cold, sinusitis, hay fever and similar allergic conditions. Prolonged therapeutic effect is obtained by sustained release of medication through the micro-dialysis process.
Indications: One capsule q. 12 h. usually provides relief of rhinorrhea, sneezing, lacrimation, itching of eyes and nose, and nasal congestion accompanying upper respiratory infections such as the common cold and sinusitis; and hay fever and similar allergic conditions.
Contraindications: Hypersensitivity to any component of the drug, glaucoma, paralytic ileus, pyloric obstruction and prostatic hypertrophy.
Precautions: Use with caution in diabetes mellitus, hyperthyroidism, hypertension, cardiovascular disease, debilitated patients with chronic lung disease, in the aged and in chil-

dren under age 12. Since blurred vision, drowsiness and dizziness may occur, patients should be cautioned about driving or operating machinery.
Adverse Reactions: May include drowsiness, dizziness, blurred vision, and excessive dryness of the nose, throat and mouth. Other possible adverse reactions to individual components, infrequently seen, include photophobia, tachycardia, gastrointestinal symptoms, increased irritability or excitement, flushing, incoordination, headache, nervousness, weakness and urinary disturbances.
Administration and Dosage: Adults and children over age 12, one capsule in the morning and one at night (q. 12 h.).
How Supplied: Bottles of 100 and 1000.
[*Shown in Product Identification Section*]

HISTASPAN®-PLUS ℞
in sustained-release micro-dialysis cells

Composition: Each Histaspan-Plus capsule provides 8 mg. Histaspan® (chlorpheniramine maleate) and 20 mg. phenylephrine hydrochloride in sustained-release micro-dialysis cells, uniquely processed for sustained release of medication to provide prolonged therapeutic effect.
Actions and Uses: Antihistaminic and decongestant for relief of nasal congestion and other respiratory symptoms accompanying the common cold, sinusitis, hay fever and similar allergic conditions.
Contraindication: Hypersensitivity to any component of the drug.
Precautions: Use with caution in diabetes mellitus, hyperthyroidism, hypertension and cardiovascular disease. Since blurred vision, drowsiness or dizziness may occur, patients should be cautioned about driving or operating machinery.
Adverse Reactions: May include drowsiness, dizziness, blurred vision, dry mouth, disturbed coordination, G.I. disturbance, tachycardia, headache, nervousness, weakness and urinary disturbances.
Dosage: Adults and children over age 12, one capsule every 12 hours.
How Supplied: Bottles of 100.
[*Shown in Product Identification Section*]

HYGROTON® ℞
(chlorthalidone USP)
Oral antihypertensive-diuretic

Hygroton is a product of USV Laboratories Inc., Manati, P.R. 00701.

Composition: Each tablet provides 25 mg., 50 mg. or 100 mg. chlorthalidone.
Description: Hygroton is a monosulfamyl diuretic which differs chemically from thiazide diuretics in that a double-ring system is incorporated in its structure.
Actions: Hygroton is an oral diuretic with prolonged action (48-72 hours) and low toxicity. The diuretic effect of the drug occurs within two hours of an oral dose and continues for up to 72 hours. It produces copious diuresis with greatly increased excretion of sodium and chloride. At maximal therapeutic dosage, chlorthalidone is approximately equal in its diuretic effect to comparable maximal therapeutic doses of benzothiadiazine diuretics. The site of action appears to be the cortical diluting segment of the ascending limb of Henle's loop of the nephron.
Indications: Diuretics such as Hygroton are indicated in the management of hypertension either as the sole therapeutic agent or to enhance the effect of other antihypertensive drugs in the more severe forms of hypertension.
Hygroton is indicated as adjunctive therapy in edema associated with congestive heart failure, hepatic cirrhosis, and corticosteroid and estrogen therapy.
Hygroton has also been found useful in edema due to various forms of renal dysfunction such as nephrotic syndrome, acute glomerulonephritis, and chronic renal failure.
Usage in Pregnancy: The routine use of diuretics in an otherwise healthy woman is inappropriate and exposes mother and fetus to unnecessary hazard. Diuretics do not prevent development of toxemia of pregnancy, and there is no satisfactory evidence that they are useful in the treatment of developed toxemia. Edema during pregnancy may arise from pathological causes or from the physiologic and mechanical consequences of pregnancy. Chlorthalidone is indicated in pregnancy when edema is due to pathologic causes, just as it is in the absence of pregnancy (however, see Warnings, below). Dependent edema in pregnancy, resulting from restriction of venous return by the expanded uterus, is properly treated through elevation of the lower extremities and use of support hose; use of diuretics to lower intravascular volume in this case is illogical and unnecessary. There is hypervolemia during normal pregnancy which is harmful to neither the fetus nor the mother (in the absence of cardiovascular disease), but which is associated with edema, including generalized edema, in the majority of pregnant women. If this edema produces discomfort, increased recumbency will often provide relief. In rare instances, this edema may cause extreme discomfort which is not relieved by rest. In these cases, a short course of diuretics may provide relief and may be appropriate.
Contraindications: Anuria.
Hypersensitivity to chlorthalidone or other sulfonamide-derived drugs.
Warnings: Should be used with caution in severe renal disease. In patients with renal disease, chlorthalidone or related drugs may precipitate azotemia. Cumulative effects of the drug may develop in patients with impaired renal function.
Chlorthalidone should be used with caution in patients with impaired hepatic function or progressive liver disease, since minor alterations of fluid and electrolyte balance may precipitate hepatic coma.
Chlorthalidone may add to or potentiate the action of other antihypertensive drugs. Potentiation occurs with ganglionic or peripheral adrenergic blocking drugs.
Sensitivity reactions may occur in patients with a history of allergy or bronchial asthma. The possibility of exacerbation or activation of systemic lupus erythematosus has been reported with thiazide diuretics, which are structurally related to chlorthalidone. However, systemic lupus erythematosus has not been reported following chlorthalidone administration.
USAGE IN PREGNANCY: Reproduction studies in various animal species at multiples of the human dose showed no significant level of teratogenicity; no fetal or congenital abnormalities were observed. Animal data should not be extrapolated for clinical application.
Thiazides cross the placental barrier and appear in cord blood. The use of chlorthalidone and related drugs in pregnant women requires that the anticipated benefits of the drug be weighed against possible hazards to the fetus. These hazards include fetal or neonatal jaundice, thrombocytopenia, and possibly other adverse reactions which have occurred in the adult.
NURSING MOTHERS: Thiazides cross the placental barrier and appear in breast milk. If use of the drug is deemed essential, the patient should stop nursing.
Precautions: Periodic determination of serum electrolytes to detect possible electrolyte imbalance should be performed at appropriate intervals.
All patients receiving chlorthalidone should be observed for clinical signs of fluid or electrolyte imbalance; namely, hyponatremia, hypochloremic alkalosis, and hypokalemia. Serum and urine electrolyte determinations are particularly important when the patient is vomiting excessively or receiving parenteral fluids. Medication such as digitalis may also influence serum electrolytes. Warning signs, irrespective of cause, are: Dryness of mouth, thirst, weakness, lethargy, drowsiness, restlessness, muscle pains or cramps, muscular fatigue, hypotension, oliguria, tachycardia, and gastrointestinal disturbances such as nausea and vomiting.
Hypokalemia may develop with chlorthalidone as with any other potent diuretic, especially with brisk diuresis, when severe cirrhosis is present, or during concomitant use of corticosteroids or ACTH.
Interference with adequate oral electrolyte intake will also contribute to hypokalemia. Digitalis therapy may exaggerate metabolic effects of hypokalemia especially with reference to myocardial activity.
Any chloride deficit is generally mild and usually does not require specific treatment except under extraordinary circumstances (as in liver disease or renal disease). Dilutional hyponatremia may occur in edematous patients in hot weather; appropriate therapy is water restriction, rather than administration of salt except in rare instances when the hyponatremia is life threatening. In actual salt depletion, appropriate replacement is the therapy of choice.
Hyperuricemia may occur or frank gout may be precipitated in certain patients receiving chlorthalidone.
Insulin requirements in diabetic patients may be increased, decreased, or unchanged. Latent diabetes mellitus may become manifest during chlorthalidone administration.
Chlorthalidone and related drugs may increase the responsiveness to tubocurarine.
The antihypertensive effects of the drug may be enhanced in the postsympathectomy patient.
Chlorthalidone and related drugs may decrease arterial responsiveness to norepinephrine. This diminution is not sufficient to preclude effectiveness of the pressor agent for therapeutic use.
If progressive renal impairment becomes evident, as indicated by a rising nonprotein nitrogen or blood urea nitrogen, a careful reappraisal of therapy is necessary with consideration given to withholding or discontinuing diuretic therapy.
Chlorthalidone and related drugs may decrease serum PBI levels without signs of thyroid disturbance.
Adverse Reactions: *Gastrointestinal System Reactions:* anorexia, gastric irritation, nausea, vomiting, cramping, diarrhea, constipation, jaundice (intrahepatic cholestatic jaundice), pancreatitis; *Central Nervous System Reactions:* dizziness, vertigo, paresthesias, headache, xanthopsia; *Hematologic Reactions:* leukopenia, agranulocytosis, thrombocytopenia, aplastic anemia; *Dermatologic—Hypersensitivity Reactions:* purpura, photosensitivity, rash, urticaria, necrotizing angiitis (vasculitis) (cutaneous vasculitis), Lyell's syndrome (toxic epidermal necrolysis); *Cardiovascular Reaction:* Orthostatic hypotension may occur and may be aggravated by alcohol, barbiturates or narcotics. *Other Adverse Reactions:* hyperglycemia, glycosuria, hyperuricemia, muscle spasm, weakness, restlessness, impotence.
Whenever adverse reactions are moderate or severe, chlorthalidone dosage should be reduced or therapy withdrawn.
Dosage and Administration: Therapy should be individualized according to patient response. This therapy should be titrated to gain maximal therapeutic response as well as the minimal dose possible to maintain that therapeutic response. A single dose given in the

Continued on next page

USV—Cont.

morning with food is recommended; divided doses are unnecessary.

Hypertension. *Initiation:* Therapy should be initiated with a dose of 25 mg. or 50 mg. as a single daily dose. In some patients a 100 mg. dose may lower the blood pressure further but dosage above this level usually does not increase effectiveness. Increases in serum uric acid and decreases in serum potassium are dose-related over the 25-100 mg./day range.

Maintenance: Maintenance doses may often be lower than initial doses and should be adjusted according to the individual patient. Effectiveness is well sustained during continued use.

Edema. *Initiation:* Adults, initially 50 to 100 mg. daily, or 100 mg. on alternate days. Some patients may require 150 to 200 mg. at these intervals, or up to 200 mg. daily. Dosages above this level, however, do not usually produce a greater response.

Maintenance: Maintenance doses may often be lower than initial doses and should be adjusted according to the individual patient. Effectiveness is well sustained during continued use.

Overdosage: Symptoms of overdosage include nausea, weakness, dizziness and disturbances of electrolyte balance. There is no specific antidote, but gastric lavage is recommended, followed by supportive treatment. Where necessary, this may include intravenous dextrose-saline with potassium, administered with caution.

How Supplied: HYGROTON (chlorthalidone). White, single-scored tablets of 100 mg. and aqua tablets of 50 mg. in bottles of 100, 1000 and 5000; unit-dose blister packs, boxes of 100 (10 × 10 strips). Also, 25 mg. peach-color tablets in bottles of 100 and 1000; unit-dose blister packs, boxes of 100 (10 × 10 strips). NSN 6505-00-074-9914A (100 mg., 100s), NSN 6505-00-065-4246A (100 mg., 1000s), V.A. Depots; NSN 6505-00-074-9914 (100 mg., 100s), Military Depots.

Animal Pharmacology: Biochemical studies in animals have suggested reasons for the prolonged effect of chlorthalidone. Absorption from the gastrointestinal tract is slow, due to its low solubility. After passage to the liver, some of the drug enters the general circulation, while some is excreted in the bile, to be reabsorbed later. In the general circulation, it is distributed widely to the tissues, but is taken up in highest concentrations by the kidneys, where amounts have been found 72 hours after ingestion, long after it has disappeared from other tissues. The drug is excreted unchanged in the urine.

[*Shown in Product Identification Section*]

M.V.I.® ℞
(Multi-Vitamin Infusion)

Composition: Each 10 cc. ampul† or 5 cc. Concentrate vial†† provides:

Ascorbic acid (C)	500 mg.
Vitamin A*	10,000 I.U.
Vitamin D* (ergocalciferol)	1,000 I.U.
Thiamine HCl (B_1)	50 mg.
Riboflavin (B_2)**	10 mg.
Niacinamide	100 mg.
Pyridoxine HCl (B_6)	15 mg.
Dexpanthenol	25 mg.
Vitamin E* (dl-alpha tocopheryl acetate)	5 I.U.

†with sorethytan laurate 1%, sodium hydroxide 1%, butylated hydroxytoluene 0.003%, butylated hydroxyanisole 0.0008%; and gentisic acid ethanolamide 2% as preservative.

††with propylene glycol 30% and gentisic acid ethanolamide 2% as stabilizers and preservatives, sodium hydroxide for pH adjustment, sorethytan laurate 1.6%, butylated hydroxytoluene 0.006%, butylated hydroxyanisole 0.0015%.

*Oil-soluble vitamins A, D and E water solubilized with sorethytan laurate.

**In Concentrate as riboflavin-5-phosphate.

ORIGINAL "AQUEOUS" MULTIVITAMIN FORMULA FOR INTRAVENOUS INFUSION:

M.V.I. (Multi-Vitamin Infusion) makes available a combination of important oil-soluble and water-soluble vitamins in an aqueous solution, formulated specially for incorporation in intravenous infusions. Through special processing techniques developed in the research laboratories of USV Pharmaceutical Corporation, the liposoluble vitamins A, D and E have been solubilized in an aqueous medium, permitting intravenous administration of these vitamins.

Indications: *In Emergency Feedings*
Surgery, extensive burns, fractures and other trauma, severe infectious diseases, comatose states, etc. may provoke a "stress" situation with profound alterations in the body's metabolic demands and consequent tissue depletion of nutrients. As a result, wound healing may be impaired, enzyme activity disturbed, hematopoietic tissues affected; hypoproteinemia and edema may appear; convalescence is thus prolonged.

In such patients M.V.I. (administered in intravenous fluids under proper dilution) contributes optimum vitamin intake toward maintaining the body's normal resistance and repair processes.

Directions for Use: M.V.I. is ready for immediate use when added to intravenous infusion fluids.

For intravenous feeding, one daily dose of 10 cc. of M.V.I. or 5 cc. of M.V.I. Concentrate added directly to not less than 500 cc., preferably 1,000 cc., of intravenous dextrose, saline or similar infusion solutions ... plasma, protein hydrolysates, etc.

Precaution: Allergic reaction has been known to occur following intravenous administration of solutions containing thiamine.

Caution: Not to be given as a direct undiluted intravenous injection as it may give rise to dizziness, faintness, etc.

Therapeutic Note: Intravenous use should be discontinued as early as practical in favor of an oral vitamin preparation, if needed.

How Supplied: M.V.I.—10 cc. ampuls, boxes of 25 and 100. NSN 6505-00-455-9955/NSN 6505-00-424-9808A. M.V.I. CONCENTRATE —5 cc. vials, boxes of 25. NSN 6505-00-212-6156A. Available in 100s only.

[*Shown in Product Identification Section*]

NITROSPAN® ℞
(nitroglycerin)
in sustained-release capsules

Composition: Each capsule provides 2.5 mg. or 6.5 mg. nitroglycerin in a sustained-release vehicle processed to release medication gradually and continuously for prolonged therapeutic effect.

Actions: The mechanism of action of nitroglycerin in the relief of angina pectoris is not as yet known. However, its main pharmacologic action is to relax smooth muscle, principally in the smaller blood vessels, thus dilating arterioles and capillaries, especially in the coronary circulation. In therapeutic doses, nitroglycerin is thought to increase the blood supply to the myocardium which may in turn relieve myocardial ischemia, the possible functional basis for the pain of angina pectoris.

In Nitrospan the micro-dialysis cells permit smooth, continuous release of nitroglycerin, requiring only the presence of fluid in the gastrointestinal tract.

Indications: Based on a review of this drug by the National Academy of Sciences—National Research Council and/or other information, FDA has classified the indication as follows:
"Possibly" effective: For the management, prophylaxis, or treatment of anginal attacks.
Final classification of the less-than-effective indication requires further investigation.

Contraindications: Acute or recent myocardial infarction, severe anemia, closed-angle glaucoma, postural hypotension, increased intracranial pressure and idiosyncrasy to the drug.

Warnings: Nitrospan Capsules must be swallowed. FOR ORAL, NOT SUBLINGUAL USE. This form of the drug is not intended for immediate relief of anginal attacks.

Precautions: Intraocular pressure may be increased; therefore, caution is required in administering to patients with glaucoma. Tolerance to this drug and cross-tolerance to other organic nitrites and nitrates may occur. If blurring of vision, dryness of mouth or lack of benefit occurs, the drug should be discontinued.

Adverse Reactions: Severe and persistent headaches, cutaneous flushing, dizziness and weakness. Occasionally, drug rash or exfoliative dermatitis, and nausea and vomiting may occur; these responses may disappear with a decrease in dosage. Adverse effects are enhanced by ingestion of alcohol, which appears to increase absorption from the gastrointestinal tract.

Dosage and Administration: Administer the smallest effective dose 2 or 3 times daily at 8- to 12-hour intervals, unless clinical response suggests a different regimen. Discontinue if not effective.

How Supplied: Capsules: 2.5 mg. (light green and clear), bottles of 100; 6.5 mg. (dark green and clear), bottles of 60.
NSN 6505-00-998-5871A (2.5 mg.), V.A. Depots.

[*Shown in Product Identification Section*]

OXALID® Tablets ℞
(oxyphenbutazone) 100 mg.

A potent anti-inflammatory agent

Composition: Each tablet provides 100 mg. oxyphenbutazone.

Important Note: OXALID cannot be considered a simple analgesic and should never be administered casually. Each patient should be carefully evaluated before treatment is started and should remain constantly under the close supervision of the physician. The following cautions should be observed:

1. Therapy should not be initiated until a careful detailed history and complete physical and laboratory examination, including a complete hemogram and urinalysis, etc., of the patient have been made. These examinations should be made at regular, frequent intervals throughout the duration of this drug therapy.
2. Patients should be carefully selected, avoiding those in whom it is contraindicated as well as those who will respond to ordinary therapeutic measures, or those who cannot be observed at frequent intervals.
3. Patients taking this drug should be warned not to exceed the recommended dosage, since this may lead to toxic effects, and should discontinue the drug and report to the physician immediately any sign of:
   a. Fever, sore throat, lesions in the mouth (symptoms of blood dyscrasia).
   b. Dyspepsia, epigastric pain, symptoms of anemia, unusual bleeding, unusual bruising, black or tarry stools or other evidence of intestinal ulceration.

c. Skin rashes.
d. Significant weight gain or edema.

4. A trial period of one week of therapy is considered adequate to determine the therapeutic effect of the drug. In the absence of a favorable response, therapy should be discontinued.
In the elderly (sixty years and over) the drug should be restricted to short-term treatment periods only—if possible, *one week* maximum.
5. BEFORE PRESCRIBING OXALID FOR AN INDIVIDUAL PATIENT, READ THOROUGHLY THE INFORMATION CONTAINED UNDER EACH HEADING WHICH FOLLOWS:

Description and Actions: OXALID is closely related chemically and pharmacologically, including toxic effects, to the well-known pyrazolines (pyrazole compounds) amidopyrine and antipyrine.
Chemically, OXALID is 4-butyl-1-(*p*-hydroxyphenyl) 2-phenyl-3,5-pyrazolidinedione monohydrate, the parahydroxy analog of phenylbutazone, USP.
It has anti-inflammatory and antipyretic action as well as analgesic and mild uricosuric properties resulting in symptomatic relief only. THE DISEASE PROCESS ITSELF IS UNALTERED BY THIS DRUG.

Indications: The leading indications in which OXALID affords relief are the following:
Rheumatoid Arthritis
Rheumatoid Spondylitis
Psoriatic Arthritis
Osteoarthritis
Gout
Painful Shoulder (peritendinitis, capsulitis, bursitis, and acute arthritis of that joint)
Acute Superficial Thrombophlebitis
Severe forms of a variety of local inflammatory conditions (see below)

Pharmacologic and Clinical Development: In animals, oxyphenbutazone inhibits or suppresses experimentally produced inflammatory lesions. This action apparently does not involve pituitary-adrenal function and does not impair immunity responses. The compound also shows analgesic and antipyretic activity. In the human, these properties have been demonstrated clinically in many types of painful inflammation.
Inflammation *per se* is frequently of questionable value as a defensive mechanism, and may be clearly detrimental. Edema, deposition of fibrin, leukocytic infiltration, vascular stasis and increased tissue turgor may delay final healing, produce excessive fibrosis, and restrict function. Pain and tenderness are often disabling and contribute to loss of function. OXALID is a practical therapeutic tool for resolving or modifying such inflammation, thus relieving pain and promoting restoration of normal function. Unlike some other pyrazole derivatives, oxyphenbutazone has no significant uricosuric activity.
Oxyphenbutazone continues under clinical investigation in a wide variety of inflammatory conditions. However, it is *not* indicated for the treatment of trivial disturbances, and many of the disorders for which it has been found useful must be considered experimental indications pending further evaluation.
In inflammatory conditions not involving prolonged or fatal disease, oxyphenbutazone should be used only when the severity of the condition balances the potential toxicity. With short periods of therapy, this potential is substantially reduced. Effective control of postoperative, post-traumatic and some types of infectious inflammation with short courses (2 to 7 days) of oxyphenbutazone therapy has been reported. Treatment of such acute inflammatory conditions with OXALID, using all recommended precautions, is advisable under the following circumstances: a) when the inflammatory process involves a closed space or produces pressure on vital organs or seriously embarrasses normal function; b) when severe pain due to inflammation is not readily controlled by the usual analgesics; c) where the success of a surgical procedure is jeopardized by inflammation; d) when severe disability due to inflammatory reaction is not relieved by conventional measures. In all such cases, customary specific measures such as antibiotics, incision and drainage, etc., should be instituted concomitantly when indicated.
It is the clinical impression of most observers that oxyphenbutazone exerts beneficial effects in many cases of superficial thrombophlebitis. Oxyphenbutazone apparently relieves local pain, an action dependent upon its specific anti-inflammatory activity, and distinct from its antipyretic or central analgesic properties. Oxyphenbutazone should not be used as a substitute for anticoagulant therapy to control potential embolization, especially with deep vein thrombosis.
In the chronic arthritides, OXALID can be expected to relieve pain and improve function in a majority of cases. Improvement, once obtained, can usually be maintained on low dosage. In benign conditions, such as simple osteoarthritis, the use of OXALID should be restricted to acute exacerbations and to patients who do not respond to simple analgesics.
Comparative pharmacologic studies in rats have demonstrated that oxyphenbutazone has considerably less ulcerogenic activity than phenylbutazone. Clinical observations of better gastric tolerances consistent with this finding have been reported. Nevertheless, the utmost caution should be exercised when OXALID is administered to patients with a history of peptic ulcer.

Contraindications:
1. Age
OXALID is contraindicated in children fourteen years or less and in senile patients.
2. Gastrointestinal Problems
Patients with a history or symptoms of gastrointestinal inflammation or ulceration, including severe or recurrent or persistent dyspepsia, should not be treated with the drug.
3. OXALID is contraindicated in patients with the history of, or presence of: drug allergy; blood dyscrasias; renal, hepatic or cardiac dysfunction; hypertension; thyroid disease; systemic edema; salivary gland enlargement due to the drug; stomatitis due to the drug; polymyalgia rheumatica and temporal arteritis.
4. Concurrent Therapy
Oxyphenbutazone is contraindicated when the patient is receiving other potent chemotherapeutic agents.
5. Concomitant Anticoagulant Therapy
Oxyphenbutazone should not be given to patients on long-term anticoagulant therapy.

Warnings:

GENERAL TOXICITY
1. The known factors affecting the incidence of toxic reactions are: age, weight, dosage, duration of therapy, existence of concomitant diseases, and concurrent potent chemotherapy.
Careful instructions to, and observations of, the individual patient are essential to the prevention of serious, life-threatening adverse reactions. This is especially true in the *aging* (40 years and over) who have an increased susceptibility to the toxicity of the drug.
The lowest effective dose for the specific patient should be the continuous goal of therapy with this drug.
In each patient, the risk of severe, and even fatal drug reactions must be weighed against the possible drug benefits initially unpredictable for the individual.
2. IN ELDERLY PATIENTS
(60 years of age and over)
OXALID should be restricted to treatment periods of *one week* duration. The appearance of clinical edema is an indication to discontinue treatment with the drug.

PREGNANCY
Animal reproduction studies thus far, though inconclusive, exhibit evidences of embryotoxicity.
Therefore, it is recommended that the drug be used with caution in the first trimester of pregnancy, weighing the potential risks against the benefits. Pregnant women and nursing mothers should receive oxyphenbutazone with caution since the drug may appear in cord blood and breast milk.

HEMATOLOGY
Blood Dyscrasias
Serious, even fatal blood dyscrasias, including aplastic anemia, due to oxyphenbutazone may occur suddenly despite regular repeated hemograms, and may become manifest many days or weeks after cessation of the drug.
Any significant change in the total white count, relative decrease in granulocytes, appearance of immature forms, or fall in hematocrit should be a signal for immediate cessation of therapy and a complete hematologic investigation.
Unexplained Bleeding
Unexplained bleeding involving the CNS, adrenal glands, and gastrointestinal tract, has occurred due to therapy with this drug.

ANTIDIABETIC AND SULFONAMIDE-TYPE AGENTS
Oxyphenbutazone may potentiate the pharmacologic action of insulin, sulfonylurea, and sulfonamide-type agents. Patients receiving such concomitant therapy should be carefully observed for this effect.

THYROID-INHIBITION
Oxyphenbutazone reduces the iodine uptake by the thyroid. Both nontoxic and toxic goiters and myxedema due to therapy with this drug have been reported.

BLURRED VISION
The development of blurred vision while on this drug can be a significant toxic symptom worthy of a complete ophthalmological examination.

CLINICAL EDEMA
In patients *under sixty years of age* swelling of the ankles or face alone may be prevented by reducing the dosage. Otherwise, the appearance of clinical edema is an indication to discontinue the drug.

Precautions: Because of the unpredictability and severity of the potential side effects of OXALID therapy IN ALL PATIENTS, the following should be accomplished at *regular* intervals:
1. A careful detailed history for the disease being treated and the detection of the earliest signs of adverse reactions.
2. A complete physical examination including check of the patient's weight.
3. A COMPLETE *WEEKLY* (especially for the aging), or EVERY TWO-WEEK BLOOD CHECK.
4. Any additional laboratory studies pertinent to the individual case.
5. Each patient should be warned to report immediately to his doctor the occurrence of fever, sore throat, oral lesions, salivary gland enlargement, black or tarry stools, weight gain, edema and any other sign or symptom pertinent to the individual case.
6. While on the drug, patients should be cautioned about participation in activity necessitating alertness and coordination, as driving a car, etc.

LEUKEMIA
Although a definite causal relationship to oxyphenbutazone therapy has not been firmly established, cases of leukemia have been reported in patients with a history of short- and long-term therapy with the drug. The overwhelming majority of these patients were over forty years of age. It should also be recognized

Continued on next page

USV—Cont.

that arthritic-type pains can be the presenting symptom of leukemia.
In some patients, oxyphenbutazone may cause an activation of symptoms of systemic lupus erythematosus. In such cases, the drug should be discontinued.
Adverse Reactions: OXALID is a potent drug; its misuse can lead to serious results. Detailed information on its use should be thoroughly reviewed before undertaking therapy.
GASTROINTESTINAL: Ulcerative esophagitis; acute and reactivated gastric and duodenal ulcer with perforation and hemorrhage; ulceration and perforation of large bowel; occult gastrointestinal bleeding with anemia; gastritis; epigastric pain; hematemesis; dyspepsia; nausea, vomiting and diarrhea; abdominal distention.
HEMATOLOGIC: Agranulocytosis, aplastic anemia, hemolytic anemia, anemia due to blood loss including occult gastrointestinal bleeding, thrombocytopenia, pancytopenia, leukemia, leukopenia, bone marrow depression.
FLUID, ELECTROLYTE DISTURBANCES: Sodium and chloride retention, water retention and edema, plasma dilution, respiratory alkalosis, metabolic acidosis.
HEPATIC: Fatal and nonfatal hepatitis (cholestasis may or may not be prominent).
DERMATOLOGIC: Petechiae, purpura without thrombocytopenia, toxic pruritus, erythema nodosum. See ALLERGIC REACTIONS for further dermatologic involvement.
ALLERGIC REACTIONS: All allergic reactions require *prompt* and *permanent withdrawal* of OXALID.
Erythema multiforme; Stevens-Johnson Syndrome, Lyell's Syndrome, toxic necrotizing epidermolysis; exfoliative dermatitis; serum sickness; hypersensitivity angiitis (polyarteritis); anaphylactic shock; urticaria; arthralgia; fever; rashes.
RENAL: Proteinuria, hematuria, oliguria, anuria, renal failure with azotemia, glomerulonephritis, acute tubular necrosis, nephrotic syndrome, bilateral renal cortical necrosis, renal stones, ureteral obstruction with uric acid crystals due to the uricosuric action of this drug, impaired renal function.
CARDIOVASCULAR: Cardiac decompensation, hypertension, pericarditis, diffuse interstitial myocarditis with muscle necrosis, perivascular granulomata, aggravation of temporal arteritis in patients with polymyalgia rheumatica.
OCULAR: Optic neuritis, blurred vision, retinal hemorrhage, toxic amblyopia, retinal detachment.
OTIC: Hearing loss.
METABOLIC-ENDOCRINE: Hyperglycemia, thyroid hyperplasia, toxic goiter, association of hypothyroidism and hyperthyroidism (causal relationship not established).
CNS: Agitation, confusional states, lethargy.
CNS REACTIONS ASSOCIATED WITH OVERDOSAGE: Convulsions, euphoria, psychosis, depression, headaches, hallucinations, giddiness, vertigo, coma, hyperventilation, insomnia.
MISCELLANEOUS: Ulcerative stomatitis, salivary gland enlargement.
Dosage and Administration:
IN CHILDREN AND IN SENILE PATIENTS
OXALID is contraindicated in children fourteen years of age or less, and in senile patients.
IN ELDERLY PATIENTS
(sixty years and over)
Every effort must be made to discontinue therapy on, or as soon as possible after the *seventh day,* because of the exceedingly high risk of severe, fatal toxic reactions in this group.
IN ALL PATIENTS
For the individual patient, the efficacy and the safety of oxyphenbutazone is unpredictable. Therefore:
1. The goal of therapy should be SHORT-TERM relief of SEVERE symptoms to a level tolerable to the SMALLEST possible drug dosage.
2. When improvement of symptoms occurs, prompt efforts to rapidly reduce the dosage should be made repeatedly, until complete drug discontinuation is achieved.
3. The action of the drug is usually manifest by the third to fourth day of treatment. Therefore, do not continue therapy beyond a week in the absence of a favorable result.
4. To minimize gastric upset, it should always be taken immediately before or after meals or with a full glass of milk.
5. See WARNINGS SECTION entitled GENERAL TOXICITY.
Dosage: In selecting the appropriate dosage in any specific case, consideration should be given to the patient's age, weight, general health, and any other factors that may influence his response to the drug.
Dosage Regimen in Chronic Inflammatory Conditions such as Rheumatoid Arthritis, Rheumatoid Spondylitis, Osteoarthritis, and Psoriatic Arthritis: Initial Dosage: The initial dosage in adults ranges from 300 mg. to 600 mg. daily, divided into 3 or 4 equal doses. In most instances, it is unnecessary to exceed 400 mg. daily to ensure maximum therapeutic response. A trial period of one week of therapy is considered adequate to determine the therapeutic effect of the drug. In the absence of a favorable response, therapy should be discontinued.
Maintenance Dosage: When improvement is obtained, the dosage should be promptly decreased to the minimum effective level to maintain relief. This maintenance dosage should not exceed 400 mg. per day because of possible cumulative toxic effects. Satisfactory effect is often achieved with as little as 100 to 200 mg. daily.
Dosage Regimen in Acute Gouty Arthritis: The treatment of acute gouty arthritis calls for a somewhat different dosage regimen. In this condition, best results are obtained from an initial dose of 400 mg. followed by 100 mg. every 4 hours until articular inflammation subsides, usually within 4 days. The dosage should not be continued beyond a period of one week.
Dosage Regimen in Acute Superficial Thrombophlebitis: Best results have been obtained with a dosage of 600 mg. per day in divided doses for the first 2 or 3 days, followed by a reduction to 300 mg. daily. Usual duration of treatment is 5 to 7 days and only rarely must therapy be extended beyond 10 days.
In severe forms of a variety of acute local inflammatory conditions, satisfactory therapeutic results can usually be achieved with a short 2- to 7-day course of therapy. Relief of pain and resolution of swelling, redness and induration is frequently achieved with these limited periods of treatment. In general, 400 to 600 mg. daily in divided doses for the first 2 or 3 days is recommended. Subsequent doses of 300 mg. daily are usually adequate.
In the treatment of transient conditions, such as painful shoulder, medication should be discontinued a few days following relief of symptoms; in the event of relapse, therapy may be resumed as needed to control symptoms. In the treatment of more chronic disorders, medication may be continued at the minimal effective level required to maintain relief and freedom from acute exacerbations. Medication should be discontinued whenever toxic symptoms appear or whenever blood studies indicate any significant reduction in the formed elements.
Overdosage:
Signs and Symptoms: Include any of the following: nausea, vomiting, epigastric pain, excessive perspiring, tinnitus, difficulty in hearing, edema (sodium retention), hypertension, cyanosis, respiratory depression, agitation, hallucinations, stupor, convulsions, coma, hematuria, and oliguria. Hepatomegaly, jaundice, and ulceration of the buccal or gastrointestinal mucosa have been reported as late manifestations of massive overdosage.
Reported laboratory abnormalities following overdosage include: respiratory or metabolic acidosis, impaired hepatic or renal function, and abnormalities of formed blood elements.
Treatment: In the alert patient, empty the stomach promptly by induced emesis followed by lavage. In the obtunded patient, secure the airway with a cuffed endotracheal tube before beginning lavage (do not induce emesis). Maintain adequate respiratory exchange, do not use respiratory stimulants. Treat shock with appropriate supportive measures. Control seizures with intravenous diazepam or short-acting barbiturates. Dialysis may be helpful if renal function is impaired.
How Supplied: 100 mg. Tablets (white, round, sugar coated), bottles of 100 and 1000.
[*Shown in Product Identification Section*]

PANTHODERM® OTC
Lotion and Cream

Composition: Panthoderm Lotion and Panthoderm Cream contain dexpanthenol 2% in a water-miscible cream base.
Indications: Panthoderm relieves itching and may aid healing of skin lesions by stimulating epithelization and granulation in mild eczemas and dermatoses; itching skin, minor wounds, insect bites, poison ivy and poison oak, minor skin irritations. Also, in infants and children—diaper rash, chafing, mild skin irritations.
Administration: Apply directly to affected areas once or twice daily, or more often as needed.
How Supplied: *Lotion:* Bottles of 4 fl. oz. *Cream:* 1 oz. tube, 2 oz. and 1 lb. jars.

PERTOFRANE® ℞
(desipramine hydrochloride NF)

Pertofrane is a product of USV Laboratories Inc., Manati, P.R. 00701.
Composition: Each capsule provides 25 mg. or 50 mg. desipramine hydrochloride.
Description: PERTOFRANE is a metabolite of imipramine hydrochloride. It is a dibenzazepine derivative, representing the desmethyl analog of imipramine hydrochloride. Chemically, it is 10,11-dihydro-5-[3-(methylamino) propyl]-5H-dibenz [b,f] azepine Monohydrochloride, and differs from the parent substance by having only one methyl group on the side chain nitrogen.
Desipramine hydrochloride is a white, crystalline substance with a molecular weight of 302.8. It is soluble to the extent of about 10% w/v in water, and melts within a range of 5° between 208-218°C.
Actions: PERTOFRANE has been found in some studies to have a more rapid onset of action than imipramine; antidepressant efficacy is similar though potency on a weight basis may be less. The earliest manifestations consist mainly of an increase in psychomotor activity. Full treatment benefit is seldon attained before the end of the second week.
PERTOFRANE is not a monoamine oxidase inhibitor and does not act primarily as a central nervous system stimulant. Like all tricyclic antidepressants, PERTOFRANE blocks the reuptake of norepinephrine by adrenergic nerve terminals. Demethylated analogs such as desipramine are more potent in increasing norepinephrine turnover rate than the methylated compounds. However, the exact mechanism of action of tricyclics in depression is still unknown.
A mechanism of action proposed for antidepressant drugs, the biogenic amine theory,

postulates that some, if not all, depression is associated with a deficiency or depletion of catecholamines and that some antidepressant drugs increase the amount of amine available at the synaptic receptor.

Desipramine is metabolized in the liver and approximately 70% is excreted in the urine.

Indications: PERTOFRANE is indicated for the relief of mental depression (see Note before How Supplied section for additional information on depressive symptomatologies often responsive to this drug).

Contraindications: The use of PERTOFRANE concomitantly or within two weeks of the administration of MAO inhibitors, is contraindicated. Hyperpyretic crises or severe convulsive seizures may occur in patients receiving such combinations. The potentiation of adverse reactions can be serious, or even fatal. When it is desired to substitute PERTOFRANE in patients receiving a monoamine oxidase inhibitor, as long an interval should elapse as the clinical situation allows, with a minimum of 14 days. Initial dosage should be low and increases should be gradual and cautiously prescribed.

The drug is contraindicated following recent myocardial infarction.

Patients with a known hypersensitivity to tricyclic antidepressants should not be given PERTOFRANE.

Warnings: As with other potent antidepressants, an activation of the psychosis may occasionally be observed in schizophrenic patients. Due to the drug's atropine-like effects and sympathomimetic potentiation, PERTOFRANE should be used only with the greatest care in patients with narrow-angle glaucoma and with urethral or ureteral spasm.

Likewise, only when patient need outweighs the risk of serious adverse reactions should the drug be used in the presence of any of the following conditions: severe coronary heart disease with EKG abnormalities, progressive heart failure, angina pectoris, paroxysmal tachycardia and active seizure disorder (this agent has been shown to lower the seizure threshold).

In some instances, desipramine and the parent compound, imipramine, have been shown to block the pharmacologic action of the antihypertensive, guanethidine, and related adrenergic neuron-blocking agents.

Hypertensive episodes have been observed during surgery in patients on desipramine hydrochloride therapy.

The concurrent use of other central nervous system drugs or alcohol may potentiate the adverse effects of desipramine hydrochloride. Since many such drugs may be used during surgery, it is recommended that desipramine hydrochloride be discontinued for as long as the clinical situation will allow prior to elective surgery.

In patients who may use alcohol excessively, it should be borne in mind that the potentiation may increase the danger inherent in any suicide attempt or overdosage.

Patients should be cautioned about the possibility of impaired ability to operate a motor vehicle or other dangerous machinery.

Usage in Pregnancy: Although teratogenic studies in mice, rats and rabbits have revealed no adverse effects, safe use of this drug in women who are or may become pregnant has not been definitely established. Therefore, PERTOFRANE should be withheld from these women unless the clinical situation warrants the potential risk.

In view of the lack of experience in children, the drug is not recommended for use in patients under twelve years of age.

Elderly and adolescent patients can usually be managed on lower dosage than that recommended for other patients and may not tolerate higher doses as well because of an increased incidence of adverse reactions.

Precautions: It should be kept in mind that the possibility of suicide in seriously depressed patients is inherent in the illness and may persist until remission occurs. These patients require careful supervision and protective measures during therapy.

Anxiety and increased agitation have been reported, particularly where depression is not the primary disorder. A shift to hypomanic or manic excitement may occur during therapy. Such reactions may necessitate discontinuation of the drug.

Although the anticholinergic activity of the drug is weak, in susceptible patients and in those receiving anticholinergic drugs (including antiparkinsonism agents), atropine-like effects may be more pronounced (e.g. paralytic ileus).

Caution should be observed in prescribing the drug in hyperthyroid patients and in those receiving thyroid medications. Transient cardiac arrhythmias have occurred in rare instances.

In all patients undergoing extended courses of therapy, periodic blood and liver studies for signs of toxicity should supplement careful clinical observations.

Adverse Reactions: PERTOFRANE is well tolerated by most patients and severe complications or adverse reactions are infrequent. Those most often reported cause little discomfort and seldom require discontinuation of the drug.

Nervous System: Dizziness, drowsiness, insomnia, headache and disturbed visual accommodation have been reported with the drug. In addition, tremor, unsteadiness, tinnitus and paresthesias have been reported. Occasionally, mild extrapyramidal activity, falling and neuromuscular incoordination have been seen. A confusional state (with such symptoms as hallucinations and disorientation) may be produced, particularly in older patients and at higher dosage, and may require discontinuation of the drug. Changes in EEG patterns have been observed. Epileptiform seizures may occur. A reduction in dosage may help control some of these adverse reactions.

Gastrointestinal Tract: Anorexia, dryness of the mouth, nausea, epigastric distress, constipation and diarrhea have been reported in patients receiving PERTOFRANE.

Skin: Skin rashes (including photosensitization), perspiration and flushing sensations have been reported during therapy.

Liver: Transient jaundice, apparently of an obstructive nature, and liver damage have been observed in rare cases. Elevation in transaminase and changes in alkaline phosphatase have occurred and should indicate repeated liver-function profiles. If progressive elevation occurs, the drug should be discontinued.

Blood Elements: Bone-marrow depression, agranulocytosis, thrombocytopenia and purpura have been reported. If these occur, the drug should be discontinued. Transient eosinophilia has been observed in some instances.

Cardiovascular System: Orthostatic hypotension and tachycardia have been observed but seldom require discontinuation of treatment. Patients who require concomitant vasodilating therapy should be carefully supervised, particularly during the initial phases.

Genitourinary System: Urinary frequency or retention and impotence have been reported.

Endocrine System: Occasional hormonal effects, including gynecomastia, galactorrhea and breast enlargement have been reported with PERTOFRANE. In addition, decreased libido and estrogenic effect have been noted. The exact relationship of these adverse effects to the administration of the drug has not been established.

Sensitivity: Urticaria and rare instances of drug fever and cross-sensitivity with imipramine have been observed.

Dosage and Administration: All Patients Except Geriatric and Adolescent: The usual dosage range is from 75 to 150 mg./day in divided doses or as a single daily dose. Titration to a maintenance dose should be based on clinical response and tolerance by starting in the low dose range and increasing dosage when required. When necessary, dosage may be increased, after initiation of therapy, up to 200 mg. daily in divided doses. Continued therapy at the optimal dosage level should be maintained during the active phase of the depression.

It is recommended that a lower maintenance dosage be continued for at least two months after a satisfactory response has been achieved. This, too, may be given on a once-daily schedule for convenience and compliance.

In cases of relapse due to premature withdrawal of the drug, a prompt response may be obtained by immediate resumption of treatment.

Geriatric and Adolescent Patients: Elderly and adolescent patients can usually be managed on lower dosage and may not tolerate higher doses as well as other patients. Therapy in these age groups may be initiated with 25 to 50 mg. daily. Dosage may be increased according to response and tolerance to a maximum of 100 mg. daily. It is recommended that a lower maintenance dosage be continued for at least two months after a satisfactory response has been achieved. Therapy may be given in divided doses or as a single daily dose.

Overdosage:

Signs and Symptoms: These may vary in severity depending on several factors, including the amount absorbed, age, interval between ingestion and start of treatment, etc. In infants and young children, especially, acute overdosage in any amount must be considered serious and potentially fatal.

CNS abnormalities may include drowsiness, stupor, coma, ataxia, restlessness, agitation, hyperactive reflexes, muscle rigidity, athetoid and choreiform movements, and convulsions.

Cardiac abnormalities may include arrhythmia, tachycardia, ECG evidence of impaired conduction, and signs of congestive failure.

Respiratory depression, cyanosis, hypotension, shock, vomiting, hyperpyrexia, mydriasis, and diaphoresis may also be present.

Treatment: Because CNS involvement, respiratory depression and cardiac arrhythmia can occur suddenly, hospitalization and close observation are necessary, even when the amount ingested is thought to be small or the initial degree of intoxication appears slight or moderate. All patients with ECG abnormalities should have continuous cardiac monitoring for at least 72 hours and be closely observed until well after cardiac status has returned to normal; relapses may occur after apparent recovery.

The *slow* intravenous administration of physostigmine salicylate has been reported to reverse most of the cardiovascular and CNS effects of overdosage with tricyclic antidepressants. In adults, 1 to 3 mg. has been reported to be effective. In children, start with 0.5 mg. and repeat at 5 minute intervals to determine the minimum effective dose; do not exceed 2 mg. Because of the short duration of action of physostigmine, repeat the effective dose at 30 to 60 minute intervals, as necessary. Avoid rapid injection to reduce the possibility of physostigmine-induced convulsions.

In the alert patient, empty the stomach promptly by induced emesis followed by lavage. In the obtunded patient, secure the airway with a cuffed endotracheal tube before beginning lavage (do not induce emesis). Continue lavage for 24 hours or longer, depending on the apparent severity of intoxication. Use normal or half-normal saline to avoid water intoxication, especially in children. Instilla-

Continued on next page

USV—Cont.

tion of activated charcoal slurry may help reduce absorption of desipramine.
Minimize external stimulation to reduce the tendency to convulsions. If anticonvulsants are necessary, diazepam, short-acting barbiturates, paraldehyde or methocarbamol may be useful. Do not use barbiturates if MAO inhibitors have been taken recently.
Maintain adequate respiratory exchange. Do not use respiratory stimulants.
Shock should be treated with supportive measures, such as intravenous fluids, oxygen and corticosteroids. Digitalis may increase conduction abnormalities and further irritate an already sensitized myocardium. If congestive heart failure necessitates rapid digitalization, particular care must be exercised.
Hyperpyrexia should be controlled by whatever external means are available, including ice packs and cooling sponge baths, if necessary.
Hemodialysis, peritoneal dialysis, exchange transfusions and forced diuresis have been generally reported as ineffective because of the rapid fixation of desipramine in tissues. Blood desipramine levels may not correlate with the degree of intoxication, and are unreliable indicators in the clinical management of the patient.
Note: Depressions which are most responsive to PERTOFRANE may be described in terms of "target symptoms." These include:
Despondency, sadness and depressed mood
Fatigue
Lack of interest and emotional response
Helplessness, hopelessness, pessimism and despair
Feelings of incapacity and inferiority
Psychomotor retardation and inhibition
Delusions of guilt and unworthiness
Psychosomatic complaints
Insomnia
Anorexia and weight loss
Depression-related anxiety and agitation
Suicidal drive
It should be borne in mind that these "target symptoms" of depression assume their proper significance only after careful history, physical and mental evaluations and other investigative procedures have confirmed a diagnosis of one of the several types of depression.
How Supplied: 25 mg. Capsules (pink), bottles of 100 and 1000 (NSN 6505-00-913-0382A—V.A. Depots); 50 mg. Capsules (maroon and pink), bottles of 100 and 1000.
[*Shown in Product Identification Section*]

PRESAMINE™ ℞
(imipramine hydrochloride USP)

Composition: Each tablet provides 25 mg., or 50 mg. imipramine hydrochloride for oral administration.
Description: PRESAMINE, the original tricyclic antidepressant, is a member of the dibenzazepine group of compounds. It is designated 5-[3-(Dimethylamino) propyl]-10, 11-dihydro-5H-dibenz [b, f] azepine Monohydrochloride. Its molecular weight is 316.9 and its empirical formula is $C_{19}H_{24}N_2$.HCl.
Imipramine hydrochloride is a white, crystalline substance that turns yellowish or reddish on long exposure to light. It is easily soluble in water, fairly soluble in acetone or alcohol, but almost insoluble in ether. It melts at 170-174°C.
Actions: The mechanism of action of imipramine hydrochloride is not definitely known. However, it does not act primarily by stimulation of the central nervous system. The clinical effect is hypothesized as being due to potentiation of adrenergic synapses by blocking uptake of norepinephrine at nerve endings. The mode of action of the drug in controlling childhood enuresis is thought to be apart from its antidepressant effect.
Indications: *Depression:* For the relief of symptoms of depression. Endogenous depression is more likely to be alleviated than other depressive states.
Childhood Enuresis: May be useful as temporary adjunctive therapy in reducing enuresis in children aged 6 years and older, after possible organic causes have been excluded by appropriate tests. In patients having daytime symptoms of frequency and urgency, examination should include voiding cystourethrography and cystoscopy, as necessary. The effectiveness of treatment may decrease with continued drug administration.
Contraindications: The concomitant use of monoamine oxidase inhibiting compounds is contraindicated. Hyperpyretic crises or severe convulsive seizures may occur in patients receiving such combinations. The potentiation of adverse effects can be serious, or even fatal. When it is desired to substitute PRESAMINE in patients receiving a monoamine oxidase inhibitor, as long an interval should elapse as the clinical situation will allow, with a minimum of 14 days. Initial dosage should be low and increases should be gradual and cautiously prescribed.
The drug is contraindicated during the acute recovery period after a myocardial infarction. Patients with a known hypersensitivity to this compound should not be given the drug. The possibility of cross-sensitivity to other dibenzazepine compounds should be kept in mind.
Warnings:
Usage in Pregnancy: Safe use of imipramine during pregnancy and lactation has not been established; therefore, in administering the drug to pregnant patients, nursing mothers, or women of childbearing potential, the potential benefits must be weighed against the possible hazards. Animal reproduction studies have yielded inconclusive results. (See also Animal Pharmacology & Toxicology.) There have been clinical reports of congenital malformation associated with the use of this drug, but a causal relationship has not been confirmed.
Extreme caution should be used when this drug is given to:
Patients with cardiovascular disease because of the possibility of conduction defects, arrhythmias, myocardial infarction, strokes and tachycardia
Patients with increased intraocular pressure, history of narrow-angle glaucoma, or history of urinary retention because of the drug's anticholinergic properties
Hyperthyroid patients or those on thyroid medication because of the possibility of cardiovascular toxicity
Patients with a history of seizure disorder because this drug has been shown to lower the seizure threshold
Patients receiving guanethidine or similar agents since PRESAMINE may block the pharmacologic effects of these drugs.
Usage in Children: Administration of the drug in pediatric conditions other than enuresis or in children younger than 6 years is not recommended. Since drug treatment of enuresis may mask genitourinary disease, the latter should be ruled out by appropriate tests prior to initiating PRESAMINE. (See Indications.) Safety in long-term chronic use in children has not been established. After an adequate trial with a favorable response, consideration should be given to instituting a drug-free period.
Since the drug may impair the mental and/or physical abilities required for the performance of potentially hazardous tasks, such as operating an automobile or machinery, the patient should be cautioned accordingly.
Precautions: It should be kept in mind that the possibility of suicide in seriously depressed patients is inherent in the illness and may persist until significant remission occurs. Such patients should be carefully supervised during the early phase of treatment with PRESAMINE and may require hospitalization. Prescriptions should be written for the smallest amount feasible.
Hypomanic or manic episodes may occur, particularly in patients with cyclic disorders. Such reactions may necessitate discontinuation of the drug. If needed, PRESAMINE may be resumed in lower dosage when these episodes are relieved. Administration of a tranquilizer may be useful in controlling such episodes.
Prior to elective surgery, imipramine hydrochloride should be discontinued for as long as the clinical situation will allow.
An activation of the psychosis may occasionally be observed in schizophrenic patients and may require reduction of dosage and the addition of a phenothiazine.
In occasional susceptible patients or in those receiving anticholinergic drugs (including antiparkinsonism agents) in addition, the atropine-like effects may become more pronounced (e.g., paralytic ileus). Close supervision and careful adjustment of dosage are required when this drug is administered concomitantly with anticholinergic or sympathomimetic drugs.
Avoid the use of preparations, such as decongestants and local anesthetics, which contain any sympathomimetic amine (e.g., adrenalin, noradrenalin), since it has been reported that tricyclic antidepressants can potentiate the effects of catecholamines.
Patients should be warned that the concomitant use of alcoholic beverages may be associated with exaggerated effects.
Both elevation and lowering of blood sugar levels have been reported.
Concurrent administration of imipramine hydrochloride with electroshock therapy may increase the hazards; such treatment should be limited to those patients for whom it is essential, since there is limited clinical experience.
Adverse Reactions:
Note: Although the listing that follows includes a few adverse reactions that have not been reported with this specific drug, the pharmacological similarities among the tricyclic antidepressant drugs require that each of the reactions be considered when imipramine is administered.
Cardiovascular: Hypotension, hypertension, tachycardia, palpitation, myocardial infarction, arrhythmias, heart block, stroke, falls.
Psychiatric: Confusional states (especially in the elderly) with hallucinations, disorientation, delusions; anxiety, restlessness, agitation; insomnia and nightmares; hypomania; exacerbation of psychosis.
Neurological: Numbness, tingling, paresthesias of extremities; incoordination, ataxia, tremors; peripheral neuropathy; extrapyramidal symptoms; seizures, alterations in EEG patterns; tinnitus.
Anticholinergic: Dry mouth, and, rarely, associated sublingual adenitis; blurred vision, disturbances of accommodation, mydriasis; constipation, paralytic ileus; urinary retention, delayed micturition, dilation of the urinary tract.
Allergic: Skin rash, petechiae, urticaria, itching, photosensitization (avoid excessive exposure to sunlight); edema (general or of face and tongue), drug fever, cross-sensitivity with desipramine.
Hematologic: Bone marrow depression including agranulocytosis; eosinophilia; purpura; thrombocytopenia. Leukocyte and differential counts should be performed in any patient who develops fever and sore throat during therapy; the drug should be discontinued if there is evidence of pathological neutrophil depression.
Gastrointestinal: Nausea and vomiting, anorexia, epigastric distress, diarrhea; peculiar taste, stomatitis, abdominal cramps, black tongue.
Endocrine: Gynecomastia in the male; breast enlargement and galactorrhea in the female; increased or decreased libido, impotence; tes-

ticular swelling; elevation or depression of blood sugar levels.

Other: Jaundice (simulating obstructive); altered liver function; weight gain or loss; perspiration; flushing; urinary frequency; drowsiness, dizziness, weakness and fatigue; headache, parotid swelling, alopecia.

Withdrawal Symptoms: Though not indicative of addiction, abrupt cessation of treatment after prolonged therapy may produce nausea, headache and malaise.

Note: In enuretic children treated with PRESAMINE, the most common adverse reactions have been nervousness, sleep disorders, tiredness, and mild gastrointestinal disturbances. These usually disappear during continued drug administration or when dosage is decreased. Other reactions which have been reported include constipation, convulsions, anxiety, emotional instability, syncope, and collapse. All of the adverse effects reported with adult use should be considered.

Dosage and Administration: Lower dosages are recommended for elderly patients and adolescents. Lower dosages are also recommended for outpatients as compared to hospitalized patients who will be under close supervision. Dosage should be initiated at a low level and increased gradually, noting carefully the clinical response and any evidence of intolerance. Following remission, maintenance medication may be required for a longer period of time, at the lowest dose that will maintain remission.

Oral:

Usual Adult Dose: Hospitalized patients—Initially, 100 mg./day in divided doses gradually increased to 200 mg./day as required. If no response after two weeks, increase to 250-300 mg./day.

Outpatients—Initially, 75 mg./day increased to 150 mg./day. Dosages over 200 mg./day are not recommended. Maintenance, 50-150 mg./day.

Adolescent and geriatric patients—Initially, 30-40 mg./day; it is generally not necessary to exceed 100 mg./day.

Childhood Enuresis: Initially, an oral dose of 25 mg./day should be tried in children age 6 and older. Medication should be given one hour before bedtime. If a satisfactory response does not occur within one week, increase the dose to 50 mg. nightly in children under 12 years; children over 12 may receive up to 75 mg. nightly. A daily dose greater than 75 mg. does not enhance efficacy and tends to increase side effects. Evidence suggests that in early night bedwetters, the drug is more effective given earlier and in divided amounts; i.e., 25 mg. in mid-afternoon, repeated at bedtime. Dosage should be gradually tapered off; this may reduce the tendency to relapse. Children who relapse when the drug is discontinued do not always respond to a subsequent course of treatment.

Overdosage:

Signs and Symptoms: These may vary in severity depending on several factors, including the amount absorbed, age, interval between ingestion and start of treatment, etc. In infants and young children, especially, acute overdosage in any amount must be considered serious and potentially fatal.

CNS abnormalities may include drowsiness, stupor, coma, ataxia, restlessness, agitation, hyperactive reflexes, muscle rigidity, athetoid and choreiform movements, and convulsions.

Cardiac abnormalities may include arrhythmia, tachycardia, ECG evidence of impaired conduction, and signs of congestive failure.

Respiratory depression, cyanosis, hypotension, shock, vomiting, hyperpyrexia, mydriasis, and diaphoresis may also be present.

Treatment: Because CNS involvement, respiratory depression and cardiac arrhythmia can occur suddenly, hospitalization and close observation are necessary, even when the amount ingested is thought to be small or the initial degree of intoxication appears slight or moderate. All patients with ECG abnormalities should have continuous cardiac monitoring for at least 72 hours and be closely observed until well after cardiac status has returned to normal; relapses may occur after apparent recovery.

The *slow* intravenous administration of physostigmine salicylate has been reported to reverse most of the cardiovascular and CNS effects of overdosage with tricyclic antidepressants. In adults, 1 to 3 mg. has been reported to be effective. In children, start with 0.5 mg. and repeat at 5 minute intervals to determine the minimum effective dose; do not exceed 2 mg. Because of the short duration of action of physostigmine, repeat the effective dose at 30 to 60 minute intervals, as necessary. Avoid rapid injection to reduce the possibility of physostigmine-induced convulsions.

In the alert patient, empty the stomach promptly by induced emesis followed by lavage. In the obtunded patient, secure the airway with a cuffed endotracheal tube before beginning lavage (do not induce emesis). Continue lavage for 24 hours or longer, depending on the apparent severity of intoxication. Use normal or half-normal saline to avoid water intoxication, especially in children. Instillation of activated charcoal slurry may help reduce absorption of imipramine.

Minimize external stimulation to reduce the tendency to convulsions. If anticonvulsants are necessary, diazepam, short-acting barbiturates, paraldehyde or methocarbamol may be useful. Do not use barbiturates if MAO inhibitors have been taken recently.

Maintain adequate respiratory exchange. Do not use respiratory stimulants.

Shock should be treated with supportive measures, such as intravenous fluids, oxygen and corticosteroids. Digitalis may increase conduction abnormalities and further irritate an already sensitized myocardium. If congestive heart failure necessitates rapid digitalization, particular care must be exercised.

Hyperpyrexia should be controlled by whatever external means are available, including ice packs and cooling sponge baths, if necessary.

Hemodialysis, peritoneal dialysis, exchange transfusions and forced diuresis have been generally reported as ineffective because of the rapid fixation of imipramine in tissues. Blood imipramine levels may not correlate with the degree of intoxication, and are unreliable indicators in the clinical management of the patient.

How Supplied: PRESAMINE (imipramine hydrochloride) tablets: 25 mg. (tan, round, sugar coated), bottles of 100, 1000 and 5000; 50 mg. (dark blue, round, sugar coated), bottles of 100, 1000 and 5000.

Animal Pharmacology and Toxicology:

A. *Acute:* Oral LD_{50} ranges are as follows:

Rat 355 to 682 mg./kg.

Dog 100 to 215 mg./kg.

Depending on the dosage in both species, toxic signs proceeded progressively from depression, irregular respiration and ataxia to convulsions and death.

B. *Reproduction/Teratogenic:* The overall evaluation may be summed up in the following manner:

Oral: Independent studies in three species (rat, mouse and rabbit) revealed that when imipramine hydrochloride is administered orally in doses up to approximately 2½ times the maximum human dose in the first two species and up to 25 times the maximum human dose in the third species, the drug is essentially free from teratogenic potential. In the three species studied, only one instance of fetal abnormality occurred (in the rabbit) and in that study there was likewise an abnormality in the control group. However, evidence does exist from the rat studies that some systemic and embryotoxic potential is demonstrable. This is manifested by reduced litter size, a slight increase in the stillborn rate and a reduction in the mean birth weight.

Parenteral: In contradistinction to the oral data, imipramine hydrochloride does exhibit a slight but definite teratogenic potential when administered by the subcutaneous route. Drug effects on both the mother and fetus in the rabbit are manifested in higher resorption rates and decrease in mean fetal birth weights, while teratogenic findings occurred at a level of 5 times the maximum human dose. In the mouse, teratogenicity occurred at 1½ and 6½ times the maximum human dose, but no teratogenic effects were seen at levels 3 times the maximum human dose. Thus, in the mouse the findings are equivocal.

[*Shown in Product Identification Section*]

REGROTON® ℞
DEMI-REGROTON® ℞
Oral antihypertensives

Regroton and Demi-Regroton are products of USV Laboratories Inc., Manati, P.R. 00701.

Composition: Each REGROTON tablet provides 50 mg. chlorthalidone USP and 0.25 mg. reserpine USP. Each DEMI-REGROTON tablet provides 25 mg. chlorthalidone USP and 0.125 mg. reserpine USP.

Description: REGROTON and DEMI-REGROTON are drug combinations of two well-known antihypertensive agents, chlorthalidone and reserpine.

Chemistry: A monosulfamyl diuretic, chlorthalidone differs from thiazide diuretics in that a double-ring system is incorporated in its structure. Chemically, it is 2-Chloro-5-(1-hydroxy-3-oxo-1-isoindolinyl) benzenesulfonamide.

Reserpine is a pure crystalline alkaloid from the root of Rauwolfia serpentina.

Actions: The pharmacologic effects are those of the constituent drugs. Chlorthalidone produces a saluretic effect in humans, beginning within two hours after an oral dose and continuing for as long as 72 hours. Copious diuresis is produced, with greatly increased excretion of sodium and chloride.

Reserpine, because it reduces arterial blood pressure and exerts a sedative effect, is particularly useful in the therapy of hypertension with related emotional disturbance. Reserpine is characterized by slow onset of action and sustained effect. Both its cardiovascular and central nervous system effects may persist following withdrawal of the drug. (See Precautions.)

Both chlorthalidone and reserpine have prolonged action, and the combination is thus able to exert a smooth and concerted effect over a long period. The two drugs appear to enhance each other, and this gives the combination a high degree of effectiveness. When considered necessary, the combination may be prescribed together with other antihypertensive agents, which may then be given in lower dosage with lessened chance of side reactions.

Indication: Treatment of hypertension. (See box warning.)

Contraindications: Mental depression, demonstrated hypersensitivity, and most cases of severe renal or hepatic diseases are the only contraindications.

Warnings:

These fixed combination drugs are not indicated for initial therapy of hypertension. Hypertension requires therapy titrated to the individual patient. If the fixed combination represents the dosage so determined, its use may be more convenient in patient management. The treatment of hypertension is not static, but

Continued on next page

USV—Cont.

must be reevaluated as conditions in each patient warrant.

These drugs should be used with caution in severe renal disease, since products containing chlorthalidone or similar drugs may precipitate azotemia. Cumulative effects of the drug may develop in patients with impaired renal function.
They should be used with caution in patients with impaired hepatic function or progressive liver disease, since minor alterations of fluid and electrolyte balance may precipitate hepatic coma.
REGROTON or DEMI-REGROTON may add to or potentiate the action of other antihypertensive drugs. Potentiation occurs with ganglionic or peripheral adrenergic blocking drugs.
Sensitivity reactions may occur in patients with a history of allergy or bronchial asthma.
Discontinue the drug in patients in whom mental depression develops while on the drug (the possibility of suicide should be kept in mind). In patients who have had depression, the drug should not be started. Electroshock therapy should not be given to patients taking reserpine, since severe and even fatal reactions have occurred. The drug should be stopped at least seven days before giving electroshock therapy.
In susceptible patients, peptic ulcer may be precipitated or activated, in which case REGROTON should be discontinued.
Usage in Pregnancy: Reproduction studies with chlorthalidone in various animal species at multiples of the human dose showed no significant level of teratogenicity; no fetal or congenital abnormalities were observed. Animal data should not be extrapolated for clinical application.
Thiazides cross the placental barrier and appear in cord blood. The use of chlorthalidone and related drugs in pregnant women requires that the anticipated benefits of the drug be weighed against possible hazards to the fetus. These hazards include fetal or neonatal jaundice, thrombocytopenia, and possibly other adverse reactions which have occurred in the adult.
REGROTON or DEMI-REGROTON should be used with care in nursing mothers since thiazides and reserpine cross the placental barrier and appear in cord blood and breast milk. Increased respiratory secretions, nasal congestion, cyanosis and anorexia may occur in infants born to reserpine-treated mothers. If use of the drug is deemed essential, the patient should stop nursing.
Precautions: Antihypertensive therapy with chlorthalidone/reserpine combinations should always be initiated cautiously in postsympathectomy patients and in those receiving ganglionic blocking agents, other potent antihypertensive drugs, or curare. At least a one-half reduction in the usual dosage of such agents may be advisable. Careful and continuous supervision of patients on such multiple-drug regimens is necessary.
Since some patients receiving Rauwolfia preparations have experienced hypotension when undergoing surgery, it may be advisable to discontinue chlorthalidone/reserpine combination drugs therapy about two weeks prior to elective surgical procedures. Emergency surgery may be carried out by using, if necessary, anticholinergic or adrenergic drugs to prevent vagocirculatory responses; other supportive measures may be used as indicated.
Because of the possibility of progression of renal damage, periodic kidney function tests are indicated. In case of a rising BUN, the drug should be stopped.
The drug should be discontinued in cases of aggravated liver dysfunction (hepatic coma may be precipitated).
Periodic determination of serum electrolytes to detect possible electrolyte imbalance should be performed at appropriate intervals.
All patients receiving chlorthalidone should be observed for clinical signs of fluid or electrolyte imbalance; namely, hyponatremia, hypochloremic alkalosis, and hypokalemia. Serum and urine electrolyte determinations are particularly important when the patient is vomiting excessively or receiving parenteral fluids. Medication such as digitalis may also influence serum electrolytes. Warning signs, irrespective of cause, are: Dryness of mouth, thirst, weakness, lethargy, drowsiness, restlessness, muscle pains or cramps, muscular fatigue, hypotension, oliguria, tachycardia, and gastrointestinal disturbances such as nausea and vomiting.
Hypokalemia may develop with chlorthalidone as with any other potent diuretic, especially with brisk diuresis, when severe cirrhosis is present, or during concomitant use of corticosteroids or ACTH.
Interference with adequate oral electrolyte intake will also contribute to hypokalemia. Digitalis therapy may exaggerate metabolic effects of hypokalemia especially with reference to myocardial activity.
Any chloride deficit is generally mild and usually does not require specific treatment except under extraordinary circumstances (as in liver disease or renal disease). Dilutional hyponatremia may occur in edematous patients in hot weather; appropriate therapy is water restriction, rather than administration of salt except in rare instances when the hyponatremia is life threatening. In actual salt depletion, appropriate replacement is the therapy of choice.
Hyperuricemia may occur or frank gout may be precipitated in certain patients receiving chlorthalidone.
Insulin requirements in diabetic patients may be increased, decreased, or unchanged. Latent diabetes mellitus may become manifest during chlorthalidone administration.
Chlorthalidone and related drugs may decrease arterial responsiveness to norepinephrine. This diminution is not sufficient to preclude effectiveness of the pressor agent for therapeutic use.
Chlorthalidone and related drugs may decrease serum PBI levels without signs of thyroid disturbance.
Because reserpine increases gastrointestinal motility and secretion, REGROTON or DEMI-REGROTON should be used cautiously in patients with ulcerative colitis or gallstones, where biliary colic may be precipitated. In susceptible patients, bronchial asthma may occur.
Adverse Reactions: Clinical trials indicate that the combination of chlorthalidone with reserpine is generally well tolerated. The adverse reactions most frequently seen include anorexia, gastric irritation, nausea, vomiting, diarrhea, constipation, nasal congestion, muscle cramps, dizziness, weakness, headache, drowsiness, and mental depression. Skin rashes, urticaria, and a case of ecchymosis have been reported. (Other dermatologic manifestations may occur—see below.)
A decreased glucose tolerance evidenced by hyperglycemia and glycosuria may develop inconsistently. This condition—usually reversible on discontinuation of therapy—responds to control with antidiabetic treatment. Diabetics and those predisposed should be checked regularly.
Hyperuricemia may be observed on occasion and acute attacks of gout have been precipitated. In cases where prolonged and significant elevation of blood uric acid concentration is considered potentially deleterious, concomitant use of a uricosuric agent is effective in reversing hyperuricemia without loss of diuretic and/or antihypertensive activity.
In addition to the reactions listed above, certain adverse reactions attributable to the drugs' components are shown below. Since REGROTON and DEMI-REGROTON combine chlorthalidone and reserpine in relatively small doses, such reactions may be less than when those drugs are used in full dosage.
Chlorthalidone: Idiosyncratic drug reactions such as aplastic anemia, purpura, thrombocytopenia, leukopenia, agranulocytosis, necrotizing angiitis and Lyell's syndrome (toxic epidermal necrolysis) have occurred, but are rare.
The remote possibility of pancreatitis should be considered when epigastric pain or unexplained gastrointestinal symptoms develop after prolonged administration.
Other reported reactions include restlessness, transient myopia, impotence or dysuria, and orthostatic hypotension, which may be potentiated when chlorthalidone is combined with alcohol, barbiturates or narcotics. Since jaundice, xanthopsia, paresthesia, and photosensitization have been documented in related compounds, the possibility of these reactions should be kept in mind.
Reserpine: The sedative effect of reserpine may lead to drowsiness or lassitude in some patients. Frequently, this effect disappears with continued administration. Nasal stuffiness sometimes occurs. Gastrointestinal reactions include increased gastric secretions, loose stools, or increased bowel frequency.
Symptoms of mental depression may occur in a small percentage of patients, although the recommended dosage of REGROTON contains substantially less reserpine than that usually implicated in such reactions. The same is true of other rare side effects recorded for reserpine, which include bradycardia and ectopic cardiac rhythms (especially when used with digitalis), pruritus, eruptions and/or flushing of skin, angina pectoris, headache, dizziness, paradoxical anxiety, nightmare, dull sensorium, muscular aches, a reversible paralysis agitans-like syndrome, blurred vision, conjunctival injection, uveitis, optic atrophy and glaucoma, increased susceptibility to colds, dyspnea, weight gain, decreased libido or impotence, dryness of the mouth, deafness, and anorexia.
Dosage and Administration:
Selection of drug and dosage should be determined by individual titration. (See box warning.) According to the requirement, the recommended dose of either REGROTON or DEMI-REGROTON is usually *one tablet once a day.* Some patients may require two tablets once a day. Divided doses are unnecessary, and a single dose given in the morning with food is recommended.
Maintenance: Maintenance dosage must be individually adjusted. Mild cases may be adequately controlled with one DEMI-REGROTON tablet daily. Optimal lowering of elevated blood pressure may require two weeks or more in some cases because of the slow onset of action of reserpine.
Combination With Other Drugs: In more severe cases, if the response to a chlorthalidone/reserpine combination alone is inadequate, potent antihypertensives may be added gradually in dosages at least 50% lower than those usually employed. Such patients should be supervised carefully and continuously. As soon as desired blood pressure levels have been attained, the lowest effective maintenance dosage should be followed.
Overdosage: Adverse reactions resulting from accidental acute overdosage may include nausea, weakness, dizziness, syncope, and disturbances of electrolyte balance. There is no specific antidote. However, the following is recommended: gastric lavage followed by supportive treatment, including intravenous dextrose-saline with potassium chloride if necessary, to be given with the usual caution. If marked hypotension results from overdosage, it can be treated with vasopressor drugs.

How Supplied: REGROTON is available as pink, round, single-scored tablets, in bottles of 100 and 1000; DEMI-REGROTON as white, round tablets, bottles of 100.
Animal Pharmacology: In animal biochemical studies, chlorthalidone is absorbed slowly from the gastrointestinal tract, due to low solubility. After passage to the liver, some of the drug enters the general circulation, while some is excreted in the bile, to be reabsorbed later. In the general circulation, the drug is distributed widely to the tissues, but is taken up in the highest concentrations in the kidneys, where amounts have been found 72 hours after ingestion, long after it has disappeared from other tissues. The drug is excreted unchanged in the urine. The high renal concentration of chlorthalidone may be causally associated with the prolonged saluretic effect of the drug. Chlorthalidone appears to inhibit sodium and chloride reabsorption in the cortical diluting segment of ascending limb of Henle's loop. The reduction of plasma volume following diuresis is a probable mechanism in the initial antihypertensive action of the drug.
Reserpine probably produces its sedative and hypotensive effects through a depletion in tissue stores of catecholamines. The antihypertensive action of reserpine is probably due to loss of epinephrine and norepinephrine from peripheral sites. By contrast, its sedative and tranquilizing properties are thought to be related to depletion of 5-hydroxytryptamine from the brain.
[*Shown in Product Identification Section*]

VORANIL® Ⓒ
(clortermine HCl)

Description: Voranil is an oral anorectic agent, *o*-chloro-*αα*-dimethylphenylethylamine hydrochloride.
Actions: Voranil is a sympathomimetic amine with pharmacologic activity similar to the prototype drugs of this class used in obesity, the amphetamines. Actions include central nervous system stimulation and elevation of blood pressure. Tolerance has been demonstrated with all drugs of this class in which this phenomenon has been looked for.
Drugs of this class used in obesity are commonly known as "anorectics" or "anorexigenics." It has not been established, however, that the action of such drugs in treating obesity is primarily one of appetite suppression. Other central nervous system actions, or metabolic effects may be involved.
Adult obese subjects instructed in dietary management and treated with anorectic drugs lose more weight on the average than those treated with placebo and diet, as determined in relatively short-term clinical trials.
The magnitude of increased weight loss of drug-treated patients over placebo-treated patients is only a fraction of a pound a week. The rate of weight loss is greatest in the first weeks of therapy for both drug and placebo subjects and tends to decrease in succeeding weeks. The possible origins of the increased weight loss due to the various drug effects are not established. The amount of weight loss associated with the use of an anorectic drug varies from trial to trial, and the increased weight loss appears to be related in part to variables other than the drugs prescribed, such as the physician-investigator, the population treated, and the diet prescribed. Studies do not permit conclusions as to the relative importance of the drug and non-drug factors on weight loss.
The natural history of obesity is measured in years, whereas the studies cited are restricted to a few weeks duration; thus, the total impact of drug-induced weight loss over that of diet alone must be considered clinically limited.
Indication: Voranil is indicated in the management of exogenous obesity as a short-term (a few weeks) adjunct in a regimen of weight reduction based on caloric restriction. The limited usefulness of agents of this class (see ACTIONS) should be measured against possible risk factors inherent in their use such as those described below.
Contraindications: Hyperthyroidism, known hypersensitivity, or idiosyncrasy to the sympathomimetic amines, glaucoma.
Agitated states.
Patients with a history of drug abuse.
During or within 14 days following the administration of monoamine oxidase inhibitors (hypertensive crises may result).
Warnings: When tolerance to the anorectic effect develops, the recommended dose should not be exceeded in an attempt to increase the effect; rather, the drug should be discontinued.
Voranil may impair the ability of the patient to engage in potentially hazardous activities such as operating machinery or driving a motor vehicle; the patient should therefore be cautioned accordingly.
Drug Dependence: The drug is related chemically and pharmacologically to the amphetamines. Amphetamines and related stimulant drugs have been extensively abused, and the possibility of abuse of clortermine should be kept in mind when evaluating the desirability of including a drug as part of a weight reduction program. Abuse of amphetamines and related drugs may be associated with intense psychological dependence and severe social dysfunction. There are reports of patients who have increased the dosage to many times that recommended. Abrupt cessation following prolonged high dosage administration results in extreme fatigue and mental depression; changes are also noted on the sleep EEG. Manifestations of chronic intoxication with anorectic drugs include severe dermatoses, marked insomnia, irritability, hyperactivity, and personality changes. The most severe manifestation of chronic intoxication is psychosis, often clinically indistinguishable from schizophrenia.
Usage in Pregnancy: Reproduction studies in animals at multiples of the human dose showed no interference with the course of pregnancy; slight delays in skeletal ossification of fetuses occurred in some animals. There was a 20 per cent reduction in conception rate when rats of both sexes were fed approximately 16-19 times the human dose.
Use of Voranil by women who are or may become pregnant requires that the potential benefit be weighed against the possible hazard to mother and infant.
Usage in Children: Voranil is not recommended for use in children under 12 years of age.
Precautions: Use only with caution in hypertension with monitoring of blood pressure since evidence is insufficient to rule out a possible adverse effect on blood pressure in some hypertensive patients. The drug is not recommended in severely hypertensive patients. The drug is not recommended for patients with symptomatic cardiovascular disease, including arrhythmias.
Insulin requirements in diabetes mellitus may be altered in association with the use of Voranil and the concomitant dietary regimen.
Amphetamines may decrease the hypotensive effect of guanethidine. The least amount of Voranil feasible should be prescribed or dispensed at one time in order to minimize the possibility of overdosage.
Adverse Reactions: *Cardiovascular:* Palpitation, tachycardia, elevation of blood pressure.
Central Nervous System: Overstimulation, restlessness, dizziness, insomnia, euphoria, dysphoria, tremor, headache; rarely, psychotic episodes at recommended doses.
Gastrointestinal: Dryness of the mouth, unpleasant taste, diarrhea, constipation, other gastrointestinal disturbances.
Allergic: Urticaria.
Endocrine: Impotence, changes in libido.
Dosage and Administration: Adult: One 50 mg. tablet daily at mid-morning. Not recommended for children under 12 years of age.
Overdosage: Manifestations of acute overdosage with anorectic agents of this type may include the following: restlessness, agitation, tremors, confusion, assaultiveness, hallucinations, hyperreflexia and muscle twitching. Fatigue and depression usually follow the central stimulation. Cardiovascular effects may include arrhythmias, palpitations, hypertension or hypotension and circulatory collapse. Gastrointestinal symptoms include nausea, vomiting, diarrhea, and abdominal cramps. Fatal poisoning usually terminates in convulsions and coma.
Management of acute intoxication is largely symptomatic and includes induction of emesis or gastric lavage, maintenance of adequate circulation and respiratory exchange. Protect the patient against self-injury and disturbing external stimuli. Efficacy of peritoneal dialysis or extracorporeal hemodialysis for anorectic agents of this type has not been established.
Severe hypertensive reactions to clortermine have not been observed. However, if these should occur, the use of intravenous phentolamine (Regitine) has been suggested on pharmacological grounds.
How Supplied: Tablets, 50 mg. (pale yellow); bottles of 100.
[*Shown in Product Identification Section*]

Ulmer Pharmacal Company

(Div. of Physicians and Hospitals Supply Company)
2440 FERNBROOK LANE
MINNEAPOLIS, MN 55441

ANDOIN

Composition: Contains Vitamins A and D with 1% Allantoin in a special hydrous emollient base.
Action and Uses: Promotes healing as it soothes and softens the skin when used on bedridden patients, or for minor burns, diaper rash, superficial sores, dryness and sunburn.
Administration: Apply locally to area one to three times a day as needed. Burns and sores may be bandaged as a protective measure.
Caution: For External Use Only—Do not use around eyes. If infection is present, irritation increases, or if condition does not improve, consult a physician.
Supplied:

One ounce	Catalog No. NDC 0127-1040-04
One pound	Catalog No. NDC 0127-1040-14

BU-LAX®
(Dioctyl Sodium Sulfosuccinate Capsules)
(Stool Softener)

Composition: Two potencies, 100 mg. and 250 mg. Dioctyl Sodium Sulfosuccinate per capsule.
Action and Uses: Stool softener for use in treating and avoiding constipation.
Administration and Dosage: Adults: 1 or 2 capsules daily or as directed by a physician. The effect on the stools may not be apparent until 1-3 days after first oral dose.
How Supplied:

Bu-Lax® capsules, 100 mg.	
NDC 0127-1160-01	Bottles of 100
NDC 0127-1160-11	Bottles of 1000
Bu-Lax® capsules, 250 mg.	
NDC 0127-1165-01	Bottles of 100
NDC 0127-1165-11	Bottles of 1000

Continued on next page

Ulmer—Cont.

BU-LAX® PLUS
(Dioctyl Sodium Sulfosuccinate with Casanthranol Capsules)
(Stool Softener/Laxative)

Composition: Each capsule contains: Dioctyl Sodium Sulfosuccinate, 100 mg.; Casanthranol, 30 mg.
Action and Uses: BU-LAX PLUS is a laxative and stool softener for use in the management of chronic or temporary constipation.
Administration and Dosage: 1 capsule daily or as directed by a physician.
Warning: As with any laxative, BU-LAX PLUS should not be used when abdominal pain, nausea or vomiting are present. Frequent or prolonged use of this preparation may result in dependence on laxatives.
How Supplied:

Bu-Lax® Plus capsules

NDC 0127-1170-01	Bottles of 100
NDC 0127-1170-11	Bottles of 1000

PENTAZYME®
Digestant

Composition:
Each orange enteric coated tablet contains:
Outer Coating:
Pepsin .... 150 mg
Inner Core (Enteric coated):
Wilzyme 400
(pancreatic enzyme concentrate) .... 100 mg
Ox Bile Extract .... 100 mg
Cellulase .... 10 mg
Each tablet contains sufficient digestive activity measured under simulated physiological conditions to digest in one hour: 15 gm. protein, 40 gm. starch, 8 gm. fat and up to 6 gm. cellulose.
Action: As a digestive aid and supplement to insufficiency of natural digestive enzymes. Useful when faulty digestion causes flatulence, fullness and epigastric distress.
Pentazyme releases pepsin in the acid medium of the stomach to aid in the digestion of protein. The core of the enteric-coated tablet dissolves in the small intestine and releases the pancreatic enzyme concentrate, ox bile extract and cellulase. The pancreatic enzyme concentrate aids in the intestinal digestion of starch, fat and protein. Cellulase helps digest fiber in vegetables, i.e.: corn and cabbage. Ox bile extract assists in the activation of lipase, emulsifies fat and aids in the absorption of certain foodstuffs.
Contraindications: Contraindicated in bile tract or gall bladder disease, or hypersensitivity to any of the ingredients. Rash may occur with hypersensitivity to any of the ingredients.
Precautions: Slight stool looseness may occur.
Dosage: One or two tablets taken with each meal, or immediately after meal.
How Supplied:

NDC 000127-1696-01	Bottles of 100
NDC 000127-1696-05	Bottles of 500

TOKOLS®
(Vitamin E Capsules)

Composition: Three potencies, 100 I.U., 200 I.U. and 400 I.U. Vitamin E, d-alpha-Tocopheryl Acetate, from natural vegetable oil.
Dosage: One capsule daily as vitamin supplement or as directed by physician.
How Supplied: Tokols® capsules, 100 I.U.

NDC 0127-2155-01	Bottles of 100
NDC 0127-2155-11	Bottles of 1000
Tokols® capsules, 200 I.U.	
NDC 0127-2160-01	Bottles of 100
Tokols® capsules, 400 I.U.	
NDC 0127-2165-01	Bottles of 100
NDC 0127-2165-05	Bottles of 500

ULCORT LOTION ½% and 1% ℞
(Hydrocortisone Alcohol Lotion ½% and 1%)
ULCORT CREAM 1%
(Hydrocortisone Cream 1%)

Composition:
Lotion
Micronized Hydrocortisone Alcohol 5 mg./g. (0.5%) or 10 mg./g. (1.0%) in a water washable base. The vehicle contains Stearic Acid, Propylene Glycol, Amerchol L-101, Isopropyl Myristate, Cetyl Alcohol, Monodiglycerides, Polysorbate 80, Sorbitan Monooleate, Methylparaben, Propylparaben and a scent in water (1% contains FD&C Blue #1).
Cream
These preparations contain Hydrocortisone in a pH adjusted Hydrophilic Base containing Stearyl Alcohol, Stearic Acid, Sodium Lauryl Sulfate, Triethanolamine, Glycerin, Citric Acid, Purified Water, and preserved with Methylparaben and Propylparaben.
Actions: Topical steroids are primarily effective because of their anti-inflammatory, antipruritic and vasoconstrictive actions.
Indications: For relief of the inflammatory manifestations of corticosteroid-responsive dermatoses.
Contraindications: Topical steroids are contraindicated in those patients with a history of hypersensitivity to any of the components of the preparation.
Precautions: If irritation develops, the product should be discontinued and appropriate therapy instituted.
In the presence of an infection, the use of appropriate antifungal or antibacterial agents should be instituted. If a favorable response does not occur promptly, the corticosteroid should be discontinued until the infection has been adequately controlled.
If extensive areas are treated or if the occlusive technique is used, there will be increased systemic absorption of the corticosteroid and suitable precautions should be taken particularly in children and infants.
Although topical steroids have not been reported to have an adverse effect on human pregnancy, the safety of their use in pregnant women has not absolutely been established. In laboratory animals, increases in incidence of fetal abnormalities have been associated with exposure of gestating females to topical corticosteroids, in some cases at rather low dosage levels. Therefore, drugs of this class should not be used extensively on pregnant patients, or in large amounts, or for prolonged periods of time.
This preparation is not for ophthalmic use.
Adverse Reactions: The following local adverse reactions have been reported with topical corticosteroids, especially under occlusive dressings: burning, itching, irritation, dryness, folliculitis, secondary infection, skin atrophy, striae, hypertrichosis, acneiform eruption, hypopigmentation, maceration of the skin, miliaria, perioral dermatitis and allergic contact dermatitis.
Dosage and Administration: Apply to affected areas 3 or 4 times daily.
Caution: Federal law prohibits dispensing without prescription.
How Supplied:
Lotion
½%, Bottles of 4 ounces, *NDC* 0127-1830-79
1%, Bottles of 2 ounces, *NDC* 0127-1832-77.
Cream
1 ounce tube *NDC* 0127-1826-04
1 pound jar *NDC* 0127-1826-14.

VASOSPAN® ℞
(Papaverine Hydrochloride 150 mg.)
Sustained Release Capsules

Description: Each capsule contains: Papaverine Hydrochloride . . . 150 mg. In special base that provides for prolonged therapeutic effect. Papaverine hydrochloride is a benzylisoquinoline alkaloid prepared synthetically or obtained from opium. Papaverine is chemically and pharmacologically distinct from morphine; it does not contain a phenanthrene group as do morphine and codeine and does not evoke tolerance or addiction.
Actions: The main actions of Papaverine are exerted on cardiac and smooth muscle. Like a quinidine, Papaverine acts directly on the heart muscle to depress conduction and prolong the refractory period. Papaverine relaxes various smooth muscles. This relaxation may be prominent if spasm exists. The muscle cell is not paralyzed by Papaverine, and still responds to drugs and other stimuli causing contraction. The anti-spasmodic effect is a direct one, and unrelated to muscle innervation. Papaverine is practically devoid of effects on the central nervous system.
Papaverine relaxes the smooth musculature of the large blood vessels, especially coronary, systemic peripheral, and pulmonary arteries. Perhaps by its direct vasodilating action on cerebral blood vessels Papaverine increases cerebral blood flow and decreases cerebral vascular resistance in normal subjects; oxygen consumption is unaltered. These effects may explain the benefit reported from the drug in cerebrovascular encephalopathy.
The direct actions of Papaverine on the heart to depress conduction and irritability and to prolong the refractory period of the myocardium, provide the basis for its clinical trial in abrogating atrial and ventricular premature systoles and omious ventricular arrhythmias. The coronary vasodilator action could be an additional factor of therapeutic value when such rhythms are secondary to insufficiency or occulusion of the coronary arteries.
In patients with acute coronary thrombosis, the occurence of ventricular rhythms is serious and requires measures designed to decrease myocardial irritability. Papaverine may have advantages over quinidine, used for a similar purpose in that it may be given in an emergency by the intravenous route, does not depress myocardial contraction or cause cinchonism and produces coronary vasodilation.
Indications: Smooth muscle relaxant, including arterial. For relief of cerebral and peripheral ischemia associated with arterial spasm and myocardial ischemia complicated by arrhythmias.
Warnings: Federal law prohibits dispensing without prescription.
Precautions: Use with caution in patients with glaucoma. Hepatic sensitivity has been reported with gastrointestinal symptoms, jaundice, eosinophilla, and altered liver function tests. Discontinue medication if these symptoms occur. If drowsiness occurs, patients should be warned against operating motor vehicles or engaging in activities requiring alertness.
Adverse Reactions: Although infrequent may produce nausea, abdominal distress, anorexia constipation, sweating, malaise, vertigo, drowsiness, headache, skin rash and diarrhea.
Dosage: Adults, one capsule every 12 hours. In difficult cases dosage may be increased to one capsule every eight hours or two capsules every 12 hours.
How Supplied:
Bottles of 100 Capsules, ***NDC*** 0127-1930-01
Bottles of 500 Capsules, ***NDC*** 0127-1930-05

VLEMINCKX'
(Sulfurated Lime Solution)

Composition: A saturated solution of Calcium Polysulfides, principally Calcium Pentasulfide and Calcium Thiosulfate.
Indications: For management of scabies and certain resistant non-inflammatory dermatoses such as the papular and cystic forms of acne vulgaris or other dermatoses which may respond to sulfur treatment. The use solution has a mild dequamation action.

Directions For Use: For treatment of scabies—dilute solution 1:9 with hot water. Wash the affected part thoroughly with soap and apply dilution as a hot compress one or two times daily. Apply for three days unless directed by physician.
For treatment of acne or other dermatoses—follow directions above using dilutions from 1:32 to 1:9. Frequency of use and use dilution may vary as treatment requires and according to tolerance of patient.
Warning: If any irritation appears, stop treatment immediately and consult your physician. Keep away from eyes. In case of contact, flush eyes thoroughly. Avoid contact with non-stainless metals. FOR EXTERNAL USE ONLY.
How Supplied:
Catalog No. NDC 0127-3350-02
One Pint Bottles

Upjohn Company, The
KALAMAZOO, MI 49001

UPJOHN PRODUCT IDENTIFICATION CODE. All products manufactured by The Upjohn Company have been assigned a National Drug Code (NDC) number. That portion of the number indicating product and strength has been or will be imprinted on each Upjohn tablet or capsule. This number along with the Upjohn imprint which also appears on the tablet or capsule will provide for prompt and positive identification.

Code #	Product	Strength
11	**FEMINONE®** Tablets (Ethinyl Estradiol Tablets, U.S.P.)	0.05 mg
12	**CORTEF®** Tablets (Hydrocortisone Tablets, U.S.P.)	5 mg
13	**FERROUS SULFATE** Tablets, U.S.P.	325 mg
14	**HALOTESTIN®** Tablets (Fluoxymesterone Tablets, U.S.P.) *See Product Identification Section*	2 mg
15	**CORTISONE ACETATE** Tablets, U.S.P.	5 mg
18	**DIDREX™** Tablets Ⓒ (benzphetamine hydrochloride) *See Product Identification Section*	25 mg
19	**HALOTESTIN®** Tablets (Fluoxymesterone Tablets, U.S.P.) *See Product Identification Section*	5 mg
21	**CARDRASE®** Tablets (Ethoxzolamide Tablets, U.S.P.)	125 mg
22	**MEDROL®** Tablets (Methylprednisolone Tablets, N.F.) *See Product Identification Section*	8 mg
23	**CORTISONE ACETATE** Tablets, U.S.P.	10 mg
24	**DIDREX™** Tablets (benzphetamine hydrochloride) *See Product Identification Section*	50 mg
25	**DELTA-CORTEF®** Tablets (Prednisolone Tablets, U.S.P.)	5 mg
31	**CORTEF®** Tablets (Hydrocortisone Tablets, U.S.P.)	10 mg
32	**DELTASONE®** Tablets (Prednisone Tablets, U.S.P.) *See Product Identification Section*	2.5 mg.
34	**CORTISONE ACETATE** Tablets, U.S.P.	25 mg
36	**HALOTESTIN®** Tablets (Fluoxymesterone Tablets, U.S.P.) *See Product Identification Section*	10 mg
38	**HALODRIN®** Tablets (fluoxymesterone and ethinyl estradiol)	
44	**CORTEF®** Tablets (Hydrocortisone Tablets, U.S.P.)	20 mg
45	**DELTASONE®** Tablets (Prednisone Tablets, U.S.P.) *See Product Identification Section*	5 mg
49	**MEDROL®** Tablets (Methylprednisolone Tablets, N.F.) *See Product Identification Section*	2 mg
50	**PROVERA®** Tablets (Medroxyprogesterone Acetate Tablets, U.S.P.) *See Product Identification Section*	10 mg
51	**RESERPOID®** Tablets (Reserpine Tablets, U.S.P.)	0.1 mg
53	**ALPHADROL®** Tablets (Fluprednisolone Tablets)	1.5 mg
56	**MEDROL®** Tablets (Methylprednisolone Tablets, N.F.) *See Product Identification Section*	4 mg
61	**PAMINE®** Tablets (Methscopolamine Bromide, N.F.) *See Product Identification Section*	2.5 mg
64	**PROVERA®** Tablets (Medroxyprogesterone Acetate Tablets, U.S.P.) *See Product Identification Section*	2.5 mg
65	**RESERPOID®** Tablets (Reserpine Tablets, U.S.P.)	0.25 mg
70	**TOLINASE®** Tablets (Tolazamide, U.S.P.) *See Product Identification Section*	100 mg
73	**MEDROL®** Tablets (Methylprednisolone Tablets, N.F.) *See Product Identification Section*	16 mg
77	**ORTHOXINE®** Tablets (methoxyphenamine hydrochloride)	100 mg
78	**RESERPOID®** Tablets (Reserpine Tablets, U.S.P.)	1 mg
81	**ADEFLOR CHEWABLE®** Tablets Fluoride and vitamins *See Product Identification Section*	0.5 mg
82	**PHENOBARBITAL AND BELLADONNA,** No. 1, Tablets	Ⓒ
83	**SPECIAL FORMULA,** No. 2, Tablets	
84	**THYROID** Tablets, U.S.P.	1 gr.
85	**PHENOBARBITAL** Tablets, U.S.P.	Ⓒ ½ gr.
92	**ADEFLOR CHEWABLE®** Tablets Fluoride and vitamins *See Product Identification Section*	1 mg
95	**PHENOBARBITAL AND BELLADONNA,** No. 2, Tablets	
100	**ORINASE®** Tablets (Tolbutamide Tablets, U.S.P.) *See Product Identification Section*	0.5 Gm
101	**ALBAMYCIN®** Capsules (sodium novobiocin capsules)	250 mg
102	**ASPIRIN** Tablets, U.S.P.	5 grs.
103	**E-MYCIN®** Tablets (erythromycin enteric-coated tablets) *See Product Identification Section*	250 mg
106	**DIOSTATE D™** Tablets Vitamin, calcium and phosphorus supplement	
109	**CEBEFORTIS®** Tablets Vitamins B and C	
110	**PYRROXATE®** Capsules	
111	**SIGTAB®** Tablets High potency vitamin supplement	
114	**TOLINASE®** Tablets (Tolazamide Tablets, U.S.P.) *See Product Identification Section*	250 mg
115	**ADEFLOR M™** Tablets Vitamins and minerals with fluoride	
119	**UPJOHN VITAMIN C** Tablets	250 mg
121	**LONITEN®** Tablets (minoxidil) *See Product Identification Section*	2.5 mg
122	**CEBENASE®** Tablets	
132	**CEBETINIC®** Tablets Iron and vitamin supplement	
137	**LONITEN®** Tablets (minoxidil) *See Product Identification Section*	10 mg
149	**UNICAP T®** Tablets Vitamins with minerals	
155	**MEDROL®** Tablets (Methylprednisolone Tablets, N.F.) *See Product Identification Section*	24 mg
165	**DELTASONE®** Tablets (Prednisone Tablets, U.S.P.) *See Product Identification Section*	20 mg
176	**MEDROL®** Tablets (Methylprednisolone Tablets, N.F.) *See Product Identification Section*	32 mg
191	**UNICAP®** Plus Iron Tablets	
193	**DELTASONE®** Tablets (Prednisone Tablets, U.S.P.) *See Product Identification Section*	10 mg
195	**PANMYCIN®** Tablets (Tetracycline Hydrochloride Tablets, N.F.) *See Product Identification Section*	250 mg
198	**UNICAP CHEWABLE®** Tablets Multivitamin	
225	**CLEOCIN HCl™** Capsules (Clindamycin HCl Capsules, U.S.P.) *See Product Identification Section*	150 mg
243	**ALKETS®** Tablets	
251	**CALCIUM GLUCONATE** Flavored Wafers	15 grs.
267	**FERRITRINSIC®** Tablets	
272	**CALCIUM LACTATE** Tablets, N.F.	650 mg
284	**UNICAP M®** Tablets Vitamins with minerals	
310	**PANMYCIN®** Tablets (Tetracycline Hydrochloride Tablets, N.F.) *See Product Identification Section*	500 mg
331	**CLEOCIN HCl™** Capsules (Clindamycin HCl Capsules, U.S.P.) *See Product Identification Section*	75 mg
336	**LINCOCIN®** Pediatric Capsules (Lincomycin Hydrochloride Capsules, U.S.P.)	250 mg
348	**UNICAP SENIOR®** Tablets Vitamins with minerals	
363	**ZYMACAP®** Capsules Multivitamins	
366	**UPJOHN VITAMIN E** Capsules	200 I.U.
388	**DELTASONE®** Tablets (Prednisone Tablets, U.S.P.) *See Product Identification Section*	50 mg
412	**MAOLATE®** Tablets (chlorphenesin carbamate) *See Product Identification Section*	400 mg
477	**TOLINASE®** Tablets (Tolazamide Tablets, U.S.P.) *See Product Identification Section*	500 mg
500	**LINCOCIN®** Capsules (Lincomycin Hydrochloride Capsules, U.S.P.)	500 mg
521	**MYCIFRADIN®** Tablets (Neomycin Sulfate Tablets, U.S.P.)	0.5 Gm
586	**UTICILLIN VK®** Tablets (Penicillin V Potassium Tablets, U.S.P.) *See Product Identification Section*	250 mg
653	**ORTHOXINE®** and Aminophylline Capsules	
655	**P-A-C®** Compound Capsules (Aspirin, Phenacetin and Caffeine capsules)	
664	**P-A-C®** Compound Tablets, Green (Aspirin, Phenacetin and Caffeine Tablets)	
671	**UTICILLIN VK®** Tablets (Penicillin V Potassium Tablets, U.S.P.) *See Product Identification Section*	500 mg
677	**P-A-C®** Compound Tablets, Pink (Aspirin, Phenacetin and Caffeine Tablets)	
686	**P-A-C®** with Codeine Tablets	Ⓒ ¼ gr.
692	**P-A-C®** Compound Tablets, White (Aspirin, Phenacetin and Caffeine	

Continued on next page

Information on these Upjohn products is based on labeling in effect on November 1, 1979. Further information on dosage and administration, side effects, precautions and contraindications for these and other Upjohn products may be obtained from either the package insert or Medical Services, The Upjohn Company, Kalamazoo, Michigan.

Upjohn—Cont.

	Tablets)	
701	**ORINASE®** Tablets (Tolbutamide Tablets, USP) *See Product Identification Section*	250 mg
705	**P-A-C®** with Codeine Ⓒ Capsules	½ gr.
716	**P-A-C®** with Codeine Ⓒ Tablets	½ gr.
730	**PHENOLAX®** Wafers (Phenolphthalein)	
733	**MOTRIN®** Tablets (ibuprofen)	300 mg
742	**MOTRIN®** Tablets (ibuprofen) *See Product Identification Section*	600 mg
750	**MOTRIN®** Tablets (ibuprofen) *See Product Identification Section*	400 mg
782	**PANMYCIN®** Capsules (Tetracycline Hydrochloride Capsules, U.S.P.) *See Product Identification Section*	250 mg
815	**PYRROXATE®** Tablets	
829	**PENSYN™** Capsules (Ampicillin Capsules, U.S.P.) *See Product Identification Section*	250 mg
831	**PYRROXATE®** with Codeine Ⓒ Capsules	¼ gr
873	**SUPER D® Perles** (Oleovitamins A and D Capsules, N.F.)	
949	**URACIL MUSTARD** Capsules	1 mg
977	**PENSYN™** Capsules (Ampicillin Capsules, U.S.P.) *See Product Identification Section*	500 mg
984	**VITAMIN E** Capsules	75 I.U.

ADEFLOR CHEWABLE® TABLETS ℞

Composition: Each 0.5 mg or 1 mg tablet contains:

Fluoride (as sodium fluoride)	0.5 mg or 1 mg
Vitamin A	4000 Int. Units
Vitamin D	400 Int. Units
Ascorbic Acid (as sodium ascorbate)	75 mg
Thiamine Mononitrate	2 mg
Riboflavin	2 mg
Niacinamide	18 mg
Pyridoxine Hydrochloride	1 mg
Calcium Pantothenate	5 mg
Cyanocobalamin	2 mcg

The palatable cherry-flavored *Adeflor Chewable* Tablets 0.5 mg or raspberry-flavored 1 mg tablets may be chewed, dissolved in the mouth or swallowed whole.

How Supplied:

0.5 mg	Bottles of 100	*NDC 0009-0081-01*
	Bottles of 500	*NDC 0009-0081-02*
1 mg	Bottles of 100	*NDC 0009-0092-01*
	Bottles of 500	*NDC 0009-0092-02*

[*Shown in Product Identification Section*]

ADEFLOR® DROPS ℞

Composition: Each 0.6 ml contains:

Fluoride (as sodium fluoride)	0.5 mg
Vitamin A	2000 Int. Units
Vitamin D	400 Int. Units
Ascorbic Acid (C)	50 mg
Pyridoxine Hydrochloride (B_6)	1 mg

How Supplied: Aqueous solution in calibrated dropper bottles.

30 ml *NDC 0009-0211-01*
50 ml *NDC 0009-0211-02*

BACITRACIN USP STERILE POWDER ℞
For Intramuscular Use

Warning

Nephrotoxicity: Bacitracin in parenteral (intramuscular) therapy may cause renal failure due to tubular and glomerular necrosis. Its use should be restricted to infants with staphylococcal pneumonia and empyema when due to organisms shown to be susceptible to bacitracin. It should be used only where adequate laboratory facilities are available and when constant supervision of the patient is possible.
Renal function should be carefully determined prior to and daily during therapy. The recommended daily dose should not be exceeded and fluid intake and urinary output maintained at proper levels to avoid kidney toxicity. If renal toxicity occurs the drug should be discontinued. The concurrent use of other nephrotoxic drugs, particularly streptomycin, kanamycin, polymyxin B, polymyxin E (colistin), neomycin, and viomycin, should be avoided.

Description: Bacitracin is a white to pale buff, hygroscopic powder, odorless or having a slight odor. It is freely soluble in water; insoluble in acetone, chloroform, and ether. While soluble in alcohol, methanol, and glacial acetic acid, there is some insoluble residue. It is precipitated from its solutions and inactivated by many of the heavy metals.

Actions: Bacitracin, an antibiotic substance derived from cultures of *Bacillus subtilis* (Tracey), exerts pronounced antibacterial action *in vitro* against a variety of gram-positive and a few gram-negative organisms. However, among systemic diseases, only staphylococcal infections qualify for consideration of bacitracin therapy. Bacitracin is assayed against a standard and its activity is expressed in units, 1 mg having a potency of not less than 50 units.
Susceptibility plate testing: If the Kirby-Bauer method of disk susceptibility is used, a 10-unit bacitracin disk should give a zone of over 13 mm when tested against a bacitracin-susceptible strain of *Staphylococcus aureus*.
Absorption of bacitracin following intramuscular injection is rapid and complete. A dose of 200 or 300 units/kg every 6 hours gives serum levels of 0.2 to 2 mcg/ml in individuals with normal renal function. The drug is excreted slowly by glomerular filtration. It is widely distributed in all body organs and is demonstrable in ascitic and pleural fluids after intramuscular injection.

Indications: In accord with the statements in the "Warning Box" the use of intramuscular bacitracin is limited to the treatment of infants with pneumonia and empyema caused by staphylococci shown to be susceptible to the drug.

Contraindications: This drug is contraindicated in those individuals with a history of previous hypersensitivity or toxic reaction to it.

Precautions: See "Warning Box" for precautions in regard to kidney toxicity associated with intramuscular use of bacitracin.
Adequate fluid intake should be maintained orally, or if necessary, by parenteral method.
As with other antibiotics, use of this drug may result in overgrowth of nonsusceptible organisms, including fungi. If superinfection occurs, appropriate therapy should be instituted.

Adverse Reactions:

Nephrotoxic reactions. Albuminuria, cylindruria, azotemia. Rising blood levels without any increase in dosage.

Other reactions. Nausea and vomiting. Pain at site of injection. Skin rashes.

Dosage and Administration:

TO BE ADMINISTERED INTRAMUSCULARLY ONLY

Infant dose: For infants under 2500 grams—900 units/kg/24 hours in 2 or 3 divided doses. For infants over 2500 grams— 1,000 units/kg/24 hours, in 2 or 3 divided doses. Intramuscular injections of the solution should be given in the upper outer quadrant of the buttocks, alternating right and left and avoiding multiple injections in the same region because of the transient pain following injection.

Preparation of Solutions—Should be dissolved in Sodium Chloride Injection containing 2 percent procaine hydrochloride. The concentration of the antibiotic in the solution should not be less than 5,000 units per ml nor more than 10,000 units per ml.
Reconstitution of the 50,000 unit vial with 9.8 ml of diluent and the 10,000 unit vial with 2.0 ml of diluent will result in a concentration of 5,000 units per ml.

Storage Conditions: Store the unreconstituted product in a refrigerator 2°–8° C (36°–46° F). Solutions are stable for one week when stored in a refrigerator 2°–8° C (36°–46° F).

How Supplied:

Vials of 10,000 units	*NDC 0009-0224-01*
Vials of 50,000 units	*NDC 0009-0233-01*

Code 810 160 000

CLEOCIN HCl™ CAPSULES ℞
(Clindamycin HCl Capsules, USP)

150 mg (100's):
NSN 6505-00-159-4892 (M & VA)

WARNING

Clindamycin therapy has been associated with severe colitis which may end fatally. Therefore, it should be reserved for serious infections where less toxic antimicrobial agents are inappropriate, as described in the Indications section. It should not be used in patients with nonbacterial infections, such as most upper respiratory tract infections. Studies indicate a toxin(s) produced by *Clostridia* is one primary cause of antibiotic associated colitis. Cholestyramine and colestipol resins have been shown to bind the toxin *in vitro*. See WARNINGS section. The colitis is usually characterized by severe, persistent diarrhea and severe abdominal cramps and may be associated with the passage of blood and mucus. Endoscopic examination may reveal pseudomembranous colitis.
When significant diarrhea occurs, the drug should be discontinued or, if necessary, continued only with close observation of the patient. Large bowel endoscopy has been recommended.
Antiperistaltic agents such as opiates and diphenoxylate with atropine (Lomotil) may prolong nd/or worsen the condition. Diarrhea, colitis, and pseudomembranous colitis have been observed to begin up to several weeks following cessation of therapy with clindamycin.

Description: *Cleocin HCl* Capsules (clindamycin hydrochloride) contain clindamycin hydrochloride, equivalent to 75 mg or 150 mg of clindamycin. *Cleocin HCl* is the hydrated hydrochloride salt of clindamycin. Clindamycin is a semi-synthetic antibiotic produced by a 7(S)-chloro-substitution of the 7(R)-hydroxyl group of the parent compound lincomycin.

Actions:

Microbiology: Clindamycin has been shown to have *in vitro* activity against isolates of the following organisms:

Aerobic gram positive cocci, including:
Staphylococcus aureus
Staphylococcus epidermidis
(penicillinase and nonpenicillinase producing strains). When tested by *in vitro* methods some staphylococcal strains originally resistant to erythromycin rapidly develop resistance to clindamycin.
Streptococci (except *S. faecalis*)
Pneumococci

Anaerobic gram negative bacilli, including:
Bacteroides species (including *Bacteroides fragilis* group and *Bacteroides melaninogenicus* group)

Fusobacterium species

Anaerobic gram positive nonsporeforming bacilli, including;

Propionibacterium

Eubacterium

Actinomyces species

Anaerobic and microaerophilic gram positive cocci, including:

Peptococcus species

Peptostreptococcus species

Microaerophilic streptococci

Clostridia: Clostridia are more resistant than most anaerobes to clindamycin. Most *Clostridium perfringens* are susceptible, but other species, eg, *Clostridium sporogenes* and *Clostridium tertium*, are frequently resistant to clindamycin. Susceptibility testing should be done.

Cross resistance has been demonstrated between clindamycin and lincomycin.

Antagonism has been demonstrated between clindamycin and erythromycin.

Human Pharmacology. Serum level studies with a 150 mg oral dose of *Cleocin HCl* (clindamycin hydrochloride) in 24 normal adult volunteers showed that *Cleocin* (clindamycin) was rapidly absorbed after oral administration. An average peak serum level of 2.50 mcg/ml was reached in 45 minutes; serum levels averaged 1.51 mcg/ml at 3 hours and 0.70 mcg/ml at 6 hours. Absorption of an oral dose is virtually complete (90%), and the concomitant administration of food does not appreciably modify the serum concentrations; serum levels have been uniform and predictable from person to person and dose to dose. Serum level studies following multiple doses of *Cleocin HCl* (clindamycin hydrochloride) for up to 14 days show no evidence of accumulation or altered metabolism of drug.

Serum half-life of *Cleocin* (clindamycin) is increased slightly in patients with markedly reduced renal function. Hemodialysis and peritoneal dialysis are not effective in removing *Cleocin* from the serum.

Concentrations of *Cleocin* in the serum increased linearly with increased dose. Serum levels exceed the MIC (minimum inhibitory concentration) for most indicated organisms for at least six hours following administration of the usually recommended doses. *Cleocin* is widely distributed in body fluids and tissues (including bones). The average biological half-life is 2.4 hours. Approximately 10% of the bioactivity is excreted in the urine and 3.6% in the feces; the remainder is excreted as bio-inactive metabolites.

Doses of up to 2 gm of *Cleocin HCl* per day for 14 days have been well tolerated by healthy volunteers, except that the incidence of gastrointestinal side effects is greater with the higher doses.

No significant levels of clindamycin are attained in the cerebrospinal fluid, even in the presence of inflamed meninges.

Indications: Clindamycin is indicated in the treatment of serious infections caused by susceptible anaerobic bacteria.

Clindamycin is also indicated in the treatment of serious infections due to susceptible strains of streptococci, pneumococci, and staphylococci. Its use should be reserved for penicillin-allergic patients or other patients for whom, in the judgment of the physician, a penicillin is inappropriate. Because of the risk of colitis, as described in the WARNING box, before selecting clindamycin the physician should consider the nature of the infection and the suitability of less toxic alternatives (eg, erythromycin).

Anaerobes: Serious respiratory tract infections such as empyema, anaerobic pneumonitis and lung abscess; serious skin and soft tissue infections; septicemia; intra-abdominal infections such as peritonitis and intra-abdominal abscess (typically resulting from anaerobic organisms resident in the normal gastrointestinal tract); infections of the female pelvis and genital tract such as endometritis, nongonococcal tubo-ovarian abscess, pelvic cellulitis and postsurgical vaginal cuff infection.

Streptococci: Serious respiratory tract infections; serious skin and soft tissue infections.

Staphylococci: Serious respiratory tract infections; serious skin and soft tissue infections.

Pneumococci: Serious respiratory tract infections.

Bacteriologic studies should be performed to determine the causative organisms and their susceptibility to clindamycin.

In Vitro Susceptibility Testing: A standardized disk testing procedure* is recommended for determining susceptibility of aerobic bacteria to clindamycin. A description is contained in the *Cleocin* Susceptibility Disk insert. Using this method, the laboratory can designate isolates as resistant, intermediate, or susceptible. Tube or agar dilution methods may be used for both anaerobic and aerobic bacteria. When the directions in the *Cleocin* Susceptibility Powder insert are followed, an MIC of 1.6 mcg/ml may be considered susceptible; MICs of 1.6 to 4.8 mcg/ml may be considered intermediate and MICs greater than 4.8 mcg/ml may be considered resistant.

Cleocin (clindamycin) Susceptibility Disks 2 mcg. See package insert for use.

Cleocin (clindamycin) Susceptibility Powder 20 mg. See package insert for use.

For anaerobic bacteria the minimal inhibitory concentration (MIC) of clindamycin can be determined by agar dilution and broth dilution (including microdilution) techniques. If MICs are not determined routinely, the disk broth method is recommended for routine use. THE KIRBY-BAUER DISK DIFFUSION METHOD AND ITS INTERPRETIVE STANDARDS ARE NOT RECOMMENDED FOR ANAEROBES.

*Bauer, A.W., Kirby, W.M.M., Sherris, J.C., Turck, M.; Antibiotic susceptibility testing by a standardized single disc method, *Am. J. Clin. Path.* 45:493-496, 1966. Standardized Disc Susceptibility Test, *Federal Register* 37:20527-29, 1972.

Contraindications: *Cleocin HCl* (clindamycin hydrochloride) is contraindicated in individuals with a history of hypersensitivity to preparations containing clindamycin or lincomycin.

Warnings:

See WARNING box. Studies indicate a toxin(s) produced by *Clostridia* is one primary cause of antibiotic associated colitis.[1–5] Cholestyramine and colestipol resins have been shown to bind the toxin *in vitro*. Mild cases of colitis may respond to drug discontinuance alone. Moderate to severe cases should be managed with fluid, electrolyte and protein supplementation as indicated. Systemic corticoids and corticoid retention enemas may help relieve the colitis. Other causes of colitis should also be considered.

A careful inquiry should be made concerning previous sensitivities to drugs and other allergens.

Usage in Pregnancy - Safety for use in pregnancy has not been established.

Usage in Newborns and Infants: When *Cleocin HCl* (clindamycin hydrochloride) is administered to newborns and infants, appropriate monitoring of organ system functions is desirable.

Nursing Mothers—Clindamycin has been reported to appear in breast milk in ranges of 0.7 to 3.8 mcg/ml.

Usage in Meningitis: Since clindamycin does not diffuse adequately into the cerebrospinal fluid, the drug should not be used in the treatment of meningitis.

Antagonism has been demonstrated between *Cleocin* and erythromycin *in vitro*. Because of possible clinical significance, these two drugs should not be administered concurrently.

1. Bartlett JG, et al: Antibiotic associated Pseudomembranous Colitis Due to Toxin-producing *Clostridia*. *N Engl J Med* 298(10):531-534, 1978.
2. George RH, et al: Identification of *Clostridium difficile* as a cause of Pseudomembranous Colitis. *Br Med J* 6114:669-671, 1978.
3. Larson HE, Price AB: Pseudomembranous Colitis Presence of Clostridial Toxin, *Lancet* 8052/3:1312-1314, 1977.
4. Rifkin GD, Fekety FR, Silva J: Antibiotic-induced Colitis Implication of a Toxin Neutralized by *Clostridium sordellii* Antitoxin. *Lancet* 8048:1103-1106, 1977.
5. Bailey WR, Scott EG: Diagnostic Microbiology. The CV Mosby Company, St. Louis, 1978.

Precautions: Review of experience to date suggests that a subgroup of older patients with associated severe illness may tolerate diarrhea less well. When clindamycin is indicated in these patients, they should be carefully monitored for change in bowel frequency.

Cleocin HCl (clindamycin hydrochloride) should be prescribed with caution in individuals with a history of gastrointestinal disease, particularly colitis.

Cleocin HCl should be prescribed with caution in atopic individuals.

During prolonged therapy, periodic liver and kidney function tests and blood counts should be performed.

Indicated surgical procedures should be performed in conjunction with antibiotic therapy.

The use of *Cleocin HCl* occasionally results in overgrowth of nonsusceptible organisms—particularly yeasts. Should superinfections occur, appropriate measures should be taken as indicated by the clinical situation.

Patients with very severe renal disease and/or very severe hepatic disease accompanied by severe metabolic aberrations should be dosed with caution, and serum clindamycin levels monitored during high-dose therapy.

Clindamycin has been shown to have neuromuscular blocking properties that may enhance the action of other neuromuscular blocking agents. Therefore, it should be used with caution in patients receiving such agents.

This product contains FD&C Yellow No. 5 (tartrazine) which may cause allergic-type reactions (including bronchial asthma) in certain susceptible individuals. Although the overall incidence of FD&C Yellow No. 5 (tartrazine) sensitivity in the general population is low, it is frequently seen in patients who also have aspirin hypersensitivity.

Adverse Reactions: The following reactions have been reported with the use of clindamycin.

Gastrointestinal: Abdominal pain, esophagitis, nausea, vomiting and diarrhea. (See **Warning** Box)

Hypersensitivity Reactions: Maculopapular rash and urticaria have been observed during drug therapy. Generalized mild to moderate morbilliform-like skin rashes are the most frequently reported of all adverse reactions. Rare instances of erythema multiforme, some resembling Stevens-Johnson syndrome, have been associated with clindamycin. A few cases of anaphylactoid reactions have been reported. If a hypersensitivity reaction occurs, the drug should be discontinued. The usual agents (epinephrine, corticosteroids, antihistamines) should be available for emergency treatment of serious reactions.

Continued on next page

Information on these Upjohn products is based on labeling in effect on November 1, 1979. Further information on dosage and administration, side effects, precautions and contraindications for these and other Upjohn products may be obtained from either the package insert or Medical Services, The Upjohn Company, Kalamazoo, Michigan.

Upjohn—Cont.

Liver: Jaundice and abnormalities in liver function tests have been observed during clindamycin therapy.
Hematopoietic: Transient neutropenia (leukopenia) and eosinophilia have been reported. Reports of agranulocytosis and thrombocytopenia have been made. No direct etiologic relationship to concurrent clindamycin therapy could be made in any of the foregoing.
Musculoskeletal: Rare instances of polyarthritis have been reported.

Dosage and Administration:
If significant diarrhea occurs during therapy, this antibiotic should be discontinued. (See **Warning** box).
Adults: *Serious infections*—150 to 300 mg every 6 hours. *More severe infections*—300 to 450 mg every 6 hours.
Children: *Serious infections*—8 to 16 mg/kg/day (4 to 8 mg/lb/day) divided into three or four equal doses. *More severe infections*—16 to 20 mg/kg/day (8 to 10 mg/lb/day) divided into three or four equal doses.
To avoid the possibility of esophageal irritation, *Cleocin HCl* (clindamycin hydrochloride) capsules should be taken with a full glass of water.
In the treatment of anaerobic infections, *Cleocin Phosphate*™ Sterile Solution (clindamycin phosphate injection) should be used initially. This may be followed by oral therapy with *Cleocin HCl* capsules or *Cleocin Pediatric®* Flavored Granules (clindamycin palmitate *HCl*) at the discretion of the physician.
In cases of β-hemolytic streptococcal infections, treatment should continue for at least 10 days.
How Supplied: *Cleocin HCl* (clindamycin hydrochloride) is available as:
75 mg Capsules. Each capsule contains clindamycin hydrochloride equivalent to 75 mg clindamycin base.
Bottles of 100 *NDC 0009-0331-02*
150 mg Capsules. Each capsule contains clindamycin hydrochloride equivalent to 150 mg clindamycin base.
Bottles of 16 *NDC 0009-0225-01*
Bottles of 100 *NDC 0009-0225-02*
Unit Dose Package (100) *NDC 0009-0225-03*
Toxicology: Animal toxicity studies showed the following:
LD_{50} I.P. Administration—Mouse ....361 mg/kg
LD_{50} I.V. Administration—Mouse ....245 mg/kg
LD_{50} Oral Administration—Rat ....2,618 mg/kg
One year oral toxicity studies in Spartan Sprague-Dawley rats and Beagle dogs at levels of 30, 100 and 300 mg/kg/day (3 grams/day per dog) have shown *Cleocin HCl* to be well tolerated. No appreciable difference in pathological findings has been obtained in *Cleocin HCl* treated groups of animals from comparable control groups. Rats receiving *Cleocin HCl* Capsules (clindamycin hydrochloride) at 600 mg/kg/day for six months tolerated the drug well; however, dogs dosed at this level vomited, would not eat, and lost weight.
Code 810 570 002
[*Shown in Product Identification Section*]

CLEOCIN PEDIATRIC® FLAVORED GRANULES ℞
(Clindamycin Palmitate HCl for Oral Solution, NF)
Not for Injection

WARNING
Clindamycin therapy has been associated with severe colitis which may end fatally. Therefore, it should be reserved for serious infections where less toxic antimicrobial agents are inappropriate, as described in the Indications Section. It should not be used in patients with nonbacterial infections, such as most upper respiratory tract infections. Studies indicate a toxin(s) produced by *Clostridia* is one primary cause of antibiotic associated colitis. Cholestyramine and colestipol resins have been shown to bind the toxin *in vitro*. See WARNINGS section. The colitis is usually characterized by severe, persistent diarrhea and severe abdominal cramps and may be associated with the passage of blood and mucus. Endoscopic examination may reveal pseudomembranous colitis.
When significant diarrhea occurs, the drug should be discontinued or, if necessary, continued only with close observation of the patient. Large bowel endoscopy has been recommended.
Antiperistaltic agents such as opiates and diphenoxylate with atropine (Lomotil) may prolong and/or worsen the condition. Diarrhea, colitis, and pseudomembranous colitis have been observed to begin up to several weeks following cessation of therapy with clindamycin.

Description: *Cleocin Pediatric* Flavored Granules (clindamycin palmitate HCl) is a preparation of clindamycin palmitate hydrochloride, flavored granules for reconstitution which contains the equivalent of 75 mg clindamycin base in each 5 ml. Clindamycin palmitate hydrochloride is a water soluble hydrochloride salt of the ester of clindamycin and palmitic acid. Clindamycin is a semi-synthetic antibiotic produced by a 7(S)-chloro-substitution of the 7(R)-hydroxyl group of the parent compound lincomycin.
Actions:
Microbiology: Although clindamycin palmitate HCl is inactive *in vitro*, rapid *in vivo* hydrolysis converts this compound to the antibacterially active clindamycin.
Clindamycin has been shown to have *in vitro* activity against isolates of the following organisms:
Aerobic gram positive cocci, including:
- *Staphylococcus aureus*
- *Staphylococcus epidermidis* (penicillinase and non-penicillinase producing strains). When tested by *in vitro* methods some staphylococcal strains originally resistant to erythromycin rapidly develop resistance to clindamycin.
- Streptococci (except *S. faecalis*)
- Pneumococci

Anaerobic gram negative bacilli, including:
- Bacteroides species (including *Bacteroides fragilis* group and *Bacteroides melaninogenicus* group)
- Fusobacterium species

Anaerobic gram positive nonsporeforming bacilli, including:
- Propionibacterium
- Eubacterium
- Actinomyces species

Anaerobic and microaerophilic gram positive cocci, including:
- Peptococcus species
- Peptostreptococcus species
- Microaerophilic streptococci

Clostridia: Clostridia are more resistant than most anaerobes to clindamycin. Most *Clostridium perfringens* are susceptible, but other species, eg, *Clostridium sporogenes* and *Clostridium tertium* are frequently resistant to clindamycin. Susceptibility testing should be done.
Cross resistance has been demonstrated between clindamycin and lincomycin.
Antagonism has been demonstrated between clindamycin and erythromycin.
Human Pharmacology: Blood level studies comparing *Cleocin Pediatric* with *Cleocin HCl*™ Capsules (clindamycin HCl) show that both products reach their peak active serum levels at the same time, indicating a rapid hydrolysis of the palmitate to the clindamycin base.
Cleocin is widely distributed in body fluids and tissues (including bones). Approximately 10% of the biological activity is excreted in the urine. The average biological half-life after doses of *Cleocin Pediatric* is approximately two hours in children.
Serum half-life of *Cleocin* is increased slightly in patients with markedly reduced renal function. Hemodialysis and peritoneal dialysis do not appreciably affect the half-life of *Cleocin* in the serum.
Serum level studies with *Cleocin Pediatric* in normal children weighing 50-100 lbs given 2, 3 or 4 mg/kg every 6 hours (8, 12 or 16 mg/kg/day) demonstrated mean peak clindamycin serum levels of 1.24, 2.25 and 2.44 mcg/ml respectively, one hour after the first dose. By the fifth dose, the 6-hour serum concentration had reached equilibrium. Peak serum concentrations after this time would be about 2.46, 2.98 and 3.79 mcg/ml with doses of 8, 12, 16 mg/kg/day, respectively. Serum levels have been uniform and predictable from person to person and dose to dose. Multiple-dose studies in newborns and infants up to 6 months of age show that the drug does not accumulate in the serum and is excreted rapidly. Serum levels exceed the MICs for most indicated organisms for at least six hours following administration of the usually recommended doses of *Cleocin Pediatric* in adults and children.
No significant levels of clindamycin are attained in the cerebrospinal fluid, even in the presence of inflamed meninges.
Indications: Clindamycin is indicated in the treatment of serious infections caused by susceptible anaerobic bacteria.
Clindamycin is also indicated in the treatment of serious infections due to susceptible strains of streptococci, pneumococci, and staphylococci. Its use should be reserved for penicillin-allergic patients or other patients for whom, in the judgment of the physician, a penicillin is inappropriate. Because of the risk of colitis, as described in the WARNING box, before selecting clindamycin the physician should consider the nature of the infection and the suitability of less toxic alternatives (eg, erythromycin).
Anaerobes: Serious respiratory tract infections such as empyema, anaerobic pneumonitis and lung abscess; serious skin and soft tissue infections; septicemia; intra-abdominal infections such as peritonitis and intra-abdominal abscess (typically resulting from anaerobic organisms resident in the normal gastrointestinal tract); infections of the female pelvis and genital tract such as endometritis, nongonococcal tubo-ovarian abscess, pelvic cellulitis and postsurgical vaginal cuff infection.
Streptococci: Serious respiratory tract infections; serious skin and soft tissue infections.
Staphylococci: Serious respiratory tract infections; serious skin and soft tissue infections.
Pneumococci: Serious respiratory tract infections.
Bacteriologic studies should be performed to determine the causative organisms and their susceptibility to clindamycin.
In Vitro Susceptibility Testing: A standardized disk testing procedure* is recommended for determining susceptibility of aerobic bacteria to clindamycin. A description is contained in the *Cleocin* Susceptibility Disk insert. Using this method, the laboratory can designate isolates as resistant, intermediate, or susceptible. Tube or agar dilution methods may be used for both anaerobic and aerobic bacteria. When the directions in the *Cleocin* Susceptibility Powder insert are followed, an MIC (minimal inhibitory concentration) of 1.6 mcg/ml may be considered susceptible; MICs of 1.6 to 4.8 mcg/ml may be considered intermediate and MICs

greater than 4.8 mcg/ml may be considered resistant.

Cleocin (clindamycin) Susceptibility Disks 2 mcg. See package insert for use.

Cleocin (clindamycin) Susceptibility Powder 20 mg. See package insert for use.

For anaerobic bacteria the minimal inhibitory concentration (MIC) of clindamycin can be determined by agar dilution and broth dilution (including microdilution) techniques. If MICs are not determined routinely, the disk broth method is recommended for routine use. THE KIRBY-BAUER DISK DIFFUSION METHOD AND ITS INTERPRETIVE STANDARDS ARE NOT RECOMMENDED FOR ANAEROBES.

---

*Bauer, A.W., Kirby, W.M.M., Sherris, J.C., Turck, M.: Antibiotic susceptibility testing by a standardized single disc method, *Am. J. Clin. Path.*, **45**:493-496, 1966. Standardized Disc Susceptibility Test, *Federal Register* **37**:20527-29, 1972.

Contraindications: This drug is contraindicated in individuals with a history of hypersensitivity to preparations containing clindamycin or lincomycin.

Warnings:
See WARNING box. Studies indicate a toxin(s) produced by *Clostridia* is one primary cause of antibiotic associated colitis.[1–5] Cholestyramine and colestipol resins have been shown to bind the toxin *in vitro*. Mild cases of colitis may respond to drug discontinuance alone. Moderate to severe cases should be managed promptly with fluid, electrolyte and protein supplementation as indicated. Systemic corticoids and corticoid retention enemas may help relieve the colitis. Other causes of colitis should also be considered.

A careful inquiry should be made concerning previous sensitivities to drugs and other allergens.

Usage in Pregnancy—Safety for use in pregnancy has not been established.

Usage in Newborns and Infants: When *Cleocin Pediatric* (clindamycin palmitate HCl) is administered to newborns and infants, appropriate monitoring of organ system functions is desirable.

Nursing Mothers—Clindamycin has been reported to appear in breast milk in ranges of 0.7 to 3.8 mcg/ml.

Usage in Meningitis: Since clindamycin does not diffuse adequately into the cerebrospinal fluid, the drug should not be used in the treatment of meningitis.

Antagonism has been demonstrated between *Cleocin* (clindamycin) and erythromycin *in vitro*. Because of possible clinical significance, these two drugs should not be administered concurrently.

1. Bartlett JG, et al: Antibiotic associated Pseudomembranous Colitis Due to Toxin-producing *Clostridia*. *N Engl J Med* 298(10):531-534, 1978.
2. George RH, et al: Identification of *Clostridium difficile* as a cause of Pseudomembranous Colitis. *Br Med J* 6114:669-671, 1978.
3. Larson HE, Price AB: Pseudomembranous Colitis Presence of Clostridial Toxin. *Lancet* 8052/3:1312-1314, 1977.
4. Rifkin GD, Fekety FR, Silva J: Antibiotic-induced Colitis Implication of a Toxin Neutralized by *Clostridium sordellii* Antitoxin. *Lancet* 8048:1103-1106, 1977.
5. Bailey WR, Scott EG: Diagnostic Microbiology. The CV Mosby Company, St. Louis, 1978.

Precautions: Review of experience to date suggests that a subgroup of older patients with associated severe illness may tolerate diarrhea less well. When clindamycin is indicated in these patients, they should be carefully monitored for change in bowel frequency.

Cleocin Pediatric (clindamycin palmitate HCl) should be prescribed with caution in individuals with a history of gastrointestinal disease, particularly colitis.

Cleocin Pediatric should be prescribed with caution in atopic individuals.

During prolonged therapy periodic liver and kidney function tests and blood counts should be performed.

Indicated surgical procedures should be performed in conjunction with antibiotic therapy.

The use of *Cleocin Pediatric* may result in overgrowth of nonsusceptible organisms—particularly yeasts. Should superinfections occur, appropriate measures should be taken as indicated by the clinical situation.

Patients with very severe renal disease and/or very severe hepatic disease accompanied by severe metabolic aberrations should be dosed with caution, and serum clindamycin levels monitored during high-dose therapy.

Clindamycin has been shown to have neuromuscular blocking properties that may enhance the action of other neuromuscular blocking agents. Therefore, it should be used with caution in patients receiving such agents.

Adverse Reactions: The following reactions have been reported with the use of clindamycin.

Gastrointestinal: Abdominal pain, nausea, vomiting and diarrhea. (See **Warning** box)

Hypersensitivity Reactions: Maculopapular rash and urticaria have been observed during drug therapy. Generalized mild to moderate morbilliform-like skin rashes are the most frequently reported of all adverse reactions. Rare instances of erythema multiforme, some resembling Stevens-Johnson syndrome, have been associated with clindamycin. A few cases of anaphylactoid reactions have been reported. If a hypersensitivity reaction occurs, the drug should be discontinued. The usual agents (epinephrine, corticosteroids, antihistamines) should be available for emergency treatment of serious reactions.

Liver: Jaundice and abnormalities in liver function tests have been observed during clindamycin therapy.

Hematopoietic: Transient neutropenia (leukopenia) and eosinophilia have been reported. Reports of agranulocytosis and thrombocytopenia have been made. No direct etiologic relationship to concurrent clindamycin therapy could be made in any of the foregoing.

Musculoskeletal: Rare instances of polyarthritis have been reported.

Dosage and Administration: If significant diarrhea occurs during therapy, this antibiotic should be discontinued. (See **Warning** box.)

Concomitant administration of food does not adversely affect the absorption of *Cleocin Pediatric* (clindamycin palmitate HCl).

Serious infections: 8-12 mg/kg/day (4-6 mg/lb/day) divided into 3 or 4 equal doses.

Severe infections: 13-16 mg/kg/day (6.5-8 mg/lb/day) divided into 3 or 4 equal doses.

More severe infections: 17-25 mg/kg/day (8.5-12.5 mg/lb/day) divided into 3 or 4 equal doses.

In children weighing 10 kg or less, ½ teaspoon (37.5 mg) three times a day should be considered the minimum recommended dose.

In the treatment of anaerobic infections, *Cleocin Phosphate* ™ (clindamycin phosphate) should be used initially. This may be followed by oral therapy with *Cleocin Pediatric* or *Cleocin HCl* (clindamycin HCl) at the discretion of the physician.

NOTE: In cases of β-hemolytic streptococcal infections, treatment should be continued for at least 10 days.

Reconstitution instructions:
When reconstituted with water as follows, each 5 ml (teaspoon) of solution contains clindamycin palmitate HCl equivalent to 75 mg clindamycin base.

Reconstitute bottles of 100 ml and 200 ml with **75 ml** and **150 ml** of water respectively. Add a large portion of the water and shake vigorously; add the remainder of the water and shake until the solution is uniform.

Storage conditions:
Store unreconstituted product at controlled room temperature 15°-30°C (59°-86°F).

Do **NOT** refrigerate the reconstituted solution; when chilled, the solution may thicken and be difficult to pour. The solution is stable for 2 weeks at room temperature.

How Supplied: *Cleocin Pediatric* Flavored Granules (clindamycin palmitate HCl for oral solution) is available in the following sizes:

100 ml bottles *NDC 0009-0760-04*
200 ml bottles *NDC 0009-0760-03*

When reconstituted as directed, each bottle yields a solution containing 75 mg of clindamycin base per 5 ml.

Code 810 568 002

CLEOCIN PHOSPHATE™ ℞
STERILE SOLUTION
(Clindamycin Phosphate Injection, NF)
For Intramuscular and Intravenous Use

2 ml ampoule:
NSN 6505-00-138-8474 (M)
NSN 6505-00-279-7560A (VA)
4 ml ampoule:
NSN 6505-00-139-1318 (M)
NSN 6505-00-279-7565A (VA)

WARNING

Clindamycin therapy has been associated with severe colitis which may end fatally. Therefore, it should be reserved for serious infections where less toxic antimicrobial agents are inappropriate, as described in the Indications Section. It should not be used in patients with nonbacterial infections, such as most upper respiratory tract infections. Studies indicate a toxin(s) produced by *Clostridia* is one primary cause of antibiotic associated colitis. Cholestyramine and colestipol resins have been shown to bind the toxin *in vitro*. See WARNINGS section. The colitis is usually characterized by severe, persistent diarrhea and severe abdominal cramps and may be associated with the passage of blood and mucus. Endoscopic examination may reveal pseudomembranous colitis.

When significant diarrhea occurs, the drug should be discontinued or, if necessary, continued only with close observation of the patient. Large bowel endoscopy has been recommended.

Antiperistaltic agents such as opiates and diphenoxylate with atropine (Lomotil) may prolong and/or worsen the condition. Diarrhea, colitis, and pseudomembranous colitis have been observed to begin up to several weeks following cessation of therapy with clindamycin.

Description: *Cleocin Phosphate* Sterile Solution (clindamycin phosphate injection) is a sterile solution of a water soluble ester of clindamycin and phosphoric acid which contains the equivalent of 150 mg clindamycin base, 5 mg benzyl alcohol and 0.5 mg disodium edetate in each ml of water for injection. Clindamycin is a semi-synthetic antibiotic produced by a 7(S)-chloro-substitution of the 7(R)-hydroxyl group of the parent compound lincomycin.

Continued on next page

Information on these Upjohn products is based on labeling in effect on November 1, 1979. Further information on dosage and administration, side effects, precautions and contraindications for these and other Upjohn products may be obtained from either the package insert or Medical Services, The Upjohn Company, Kalamazoo, Michigan.

Upjohn—Cont.

Actions:

Microbiology: Although clindamycin phosphate is inactive *in vitro*, rapid *in vivo* hydrolysis converts this compound to the antibacterially active clindamycin.

Clindamycin has been shown to have *in vitro* activity against isolates of the following organisms:

Aerobic gram positive cocci, including:
Staphylococcus aureus
Staphylococcus epidermidis
(penicillinase and nonpenicillinase producing strains). When tested by *in vitro* methods some staphylococcal strains originally resistant to erythromycin rapidly develop resistance to clindamycin.
Streptococci (except *S. faecalis*)
Pneumococci

Anaerobic gram negative bacilli, including:
Bacteroides species (including *Bacteroides fragilis* group and *Bacteroides melaninogenicus* group)
Fusobacterium species

Anaerobic gram positive nonsporeforming bacilli, including:
Propionibacterium
Eubacterium
Actinomyces species

Anaerobic and microaerophilic gram positive cocci, including:
Peptococcus species
Peptostreptococcus species
Microaerophilic streptococci

Clostridia: Clostridia are more resistant than most anaerobes to clindamycin. Most *Clostridium perfringens* are susceptible, but other species, eg, *Clostridium sporogenes* and *Clostridium Tertium* are frequently resistant to clindamycin. Susceptibility testing should be done.

Cross resistance has been demonstrated between clindamycin and lincomycin.

Antagonism has been demonstrated between clindamycin and erythromycin.

Human Pharmacology:

Biologically inactive clindamycin phosphate is rapidly converted to active clindamycin.

By the end of short-term intravenous infusion, peak serum levels of active clindamycin are reached. Biologically inactive clindamycin phosphate disappears rapidly from the serum; the average disappearance half-life is 6 minutes; however, the serum disappearance half-life of active clindamycin is about 3 hours in adults and 2 ½ hours in children.

After intramuscular injection of clindamycin phosphate, peak levels of active clindamycin are reached within 3 hours in adults and 1 hour in children. Serum level curves may be constructed from IV peak serum levels as given in Table 1 by application of disappearance half-lives listed above.

Serum levels of clindamycin can be maintained above the *in vitro* minimum inhibitory concentrations for most indicated organisms by administration of clindamycin phosphate every 8-12 hours in adults and every 6-8 hours in children, or by continuous intravenous infusion. An equilibrium state is reached by the third dose.

The disappearance half-life of clindamycin is increased slightly in patients with markedly reduced renal or hepatic function; dosage schedules need not be modified in the presence of mild or moderate renal or hepatic disease.

No significant levels of clindamycin are attained in the cerebrospinal fluid, even in the presence of inflamed meninges.

Serum assays for active clindamycin require an inhibitor to prevent *in vitro* hydrolysis of clindamycin phosphate.

[See table below].

Indications: Clindamycin is indicated in the treatment of serious infections caused by susceptible anaerobic bacteria.

Clindamycin is also indicated in the treatment of serious infections due to susceptible strains of streptococci, pneumococci, and staphylococci. Its use should be reserved for penicillin-allergic patients or other patients for whom, in the judgment of the physician, a penicillin is inappropriate. Because of the risk of colitis, as described in the WARNING box, before selecting clindamycin the physician should consider the nature of the infection and the suitability of less toxic alternatives (e.g., erythromycin).

Anaerobes: Serious respiratory tract infections such as empyema, anaerobic pneumonitis and lung abscess; serious skin and soft tissue infections; septicemia; intra-abdominal infections such as peritonitis and intra-abdominal abscess (typically resulting from anaerobic organisms resident in the normal gastrointestinal tract); infections of the female pelvis and genital tract such as endometritis, nongonococcal tubo-ovarian abscess, pelvic cellulitis and postsurgical vaginal cuff infection.

Streptococci: Serious respiratory tract infections; serious skin and soft tissue infections; septicemia.

Staphylococci: Serious respiratory tract infections; serious skin and soft tissue infections; septicemia; acute hematogenous osteomyelitis.

Pneumococci: Serious respiratory tract infections.

Adjunctive Therapy: In the surgical treatment of chronic bone and joint infections due to susceptible organisms.

Indicated surgical procedures should be performed in conjunction with antibiotic therapy. Bacteriologic studies should be performed to determine the causative organisms and their susceptibility to clindamycin.

In Vitro Susceptibility Testing: A standardized disk testing procedure* is recommended for determining susceptibility of aerobic bacteria to clindamycin. A description is contained in the *Cleocin* Susceptibility Disk insert. Using this method, the laboratory can designate isolates as resistant, intermediate, or susceptible. Tube or agar dilution methods may be used for both anaerobic and aerobic bacteria. When the directions in the *Cleocin* Susceptibility Powder insert are followed, an MIC (minimal inhibitory concentration) of 1.6 mcg/ml may be considered susceptible; MICs of 1.6 to 4.8 mcg/ml may be considered intermediate and MICs greater than 4.8 mcg/ml may be considered resistant.

Cleocin (clindamycin) Susceptibility Disks 2 mcg. See package insert for use.

Cleocin (clindamycin) Susceptibility Powder 20 mg. See package insert for use.

For anaerobic bacteria the minimal inhibitory concentration (MIC) of clindamycin can be determined by agar dilution and broth dilution (including microdilution) techniques. If MICs are not determined routinely, the disk broth method is recommended for routine use. The KIRBY-BAUER DISK DIFFUSION METHOD AND ITS INTERPRETIVE STANDARDS ARE NOT RECOMMENDED FOR ANAEROBES.

*Bauer, A.W., Kirby, W.M.M., Sherris, J.C., Turck, M.: Antibiotic susceptibility testing by a standardized single disc method, *Am. J. Clin. Path.*, **45**:493-496, 1966. Standardized Disc Susceptibility Test, *Federal Register* **37**:20527-29, 1972.

Contraindications: This drug is contraindicated in individuals with a history of hypersensitivity to preparations containing clindamycin or lincomycin.

Warnings:

See WARNING box. Studies indicate a toxin(s) produced by *Clostridia* is one primary cause of antibiotic associated colitis.[1–5] Cholestyramine and colestipol resins have been shown to bind the toxin *in vitro*. Mild cases of colitis may respond to drug discontinuance alone. Moderate to severe cases should be managed promptly with fluid, electrolyte and protein supplementation as indicated. Systemic corticoids and corticoid retention enemas may help relieve the colitis. Other causes of colitis should also be considered.

A careful inquiry should be made concerning previous sensitivities to drugs and other allergens.

Usage in Pregnancy—Safety for use in pregnancy has not been established.

Usage in Newborns and infants: When *Cleocin Phosphate* (clindamycin phosphate) is administered to newborns and infants, appropriate monitoring of organ system functions is desirable.

Nursing Mothers—Clindamycin has been reported to appear in breast milk in ranges of 0.7 to 3.8 mcg/ml.

Usage in Meningitis: Since clindamycin does not diffuse adequately into the cerebrospinal fluid, the drug should not be used in the treatment of meningitis.

Antagonism has been demonstrated between *Cleocin* and erythromycin *in vitro*. Because of possible clinical significance, these two drugs should not be administered concurrently.

SERIOUS ANAPHYLACTOID REACTIONS REQUIRE IMMEDIATE EMERGENCY TREATMENT WITH EPINEPHRINE. OXYGEN AND INTRAVENOUS CORTICOSTEROIDS SHOULD ALSO BE ADMINISTERED AS INDICATED.

1. Bartlett JG, et al: Antibiotic associated Pseudomembranous Colitis Due to Toxin-producing *Clostridia. N Engl J Med* 298(10):531-534, 1978.
2. George RH, et al: Identification of *Clostridium difficile* as a cause of Pseudomembranous Colitis. *Br Med J* 6114:669-671, 1978.
3. Larson HE, Price AB: Pseudomembranous Colitis Presence of Clostridial Toxin. *Lancet* 8052/3:1312-1314, 1977.
4. Rifkin GD, Fekety FR, Silva J: Antibiotic-induced Colitis Implication of a Toxin Neu-

Table 1. Average Peak Serum Concentrations After Dosing with Clindamycin Phosphate

Dosage Regimen	Clindamycin mcg/ml	Clindamycin Phosphate mcg/ml
Healthy Adult Males (Post equilibrium)		
300 mg IV in 10 min, q8h	7	15
600 mg IV in 20 min, q8h	10	23
900 mg IV in 30 min, q12h	11	29
1200 mg IV in 45 min, q12h	14	49
300 mg IM q8h	6	3
600 mg IM q12h*	9	3
Children (first dose)*		
5-7 mg/kg IV in 1 hr	10	
3-5 mg/kg IM	4	
5-7 mg/kg IM	8	

*Data in this group from patients being treated for infection

tralized by *Clostridium sordellii* Antitoxin. *Lancet* 8048:1103-1106, 1977.
5. Bailey WR, Scott EG: Diagnostic Microbiology. The CV Mosby Company, St. Louis, 1978.

Precautions: Review of experience to date suggests that a subgroup of older patients with associated severe illness may tolerate diarrhea less well. When clindamycin is indicated in these patients, they should be carefully monitored for change in bowel frequency.

Cleocin Phosphate (clindamycin phosphate) should be prescribed with caution in individuals with a history of gastrointestinal disease, particularly colitis.

Cleocin Phosphate should be prescribed with caution in atopic individuals.

During prolonged therapy periodic liver and kidney function tests and blood counts should be performed.

Indicated surgical procedures should be performed in conjunction with antibiotic therapy.

The use of *Cleocin Phosphate* may result in overgrowth of nonsusceptible organisms—particularly yeasts. Should superinfections occur, appropriate measures should be taken as indicated by the clinical situation.

Cleocin Phosphate should not be injected intravenously undiluted as a bolus, but should be infused over at least 10-60 minutes as directed in the **Dosage and Administration** Section.

Patients with very severe renal disease and/or very severe hepatic disease accompanied by severe metabolic aberrations should be dosed with caution, and serum clindamycin levels monitored during high-dose therapy.

Clindamycin has been shown to have neuromuscular blocking properties that may enhance the action of other neuromuscular blocking agents. Therefore, it should be used with caution in patients receiving such agents.

Adverse Reactions: The following reactions have been reported with the use of clindamycin.

Gastrointestinal: Abdominal pain, nausea, vomiting and diarrhea (See **Warning** box).

Hypersensitivity Reactions: Maculopapular rash and urticaria have been observed during drug therapy. Generalized mild to moderate morbilliform-like skin rashes are the most frequently reported of all adverse reactions. Rare instances of erythema multiforme, some resembling Stevens-Johnson syndrome, have been associated with clindamycin. A few cases of anaphylactoid reactions have been reported. If a hypersensitivity reaction occurs, the drug should be discontinued. The usual agents (epinephrine, corticosteroids, antihistamines) should be available for emergency treatment of serious reactions.

Liver: Jaundice and abnormalities in liver function tests have been observed during clindamycin therapy.

Hematopoietic: Transient neutropenia (leukopenia) and eosinophilia have been reported. Reports of agranulocytosis and thrombocytopenia have been made. No direct etiologic relationship to concurrent clindamycin therapy could be made in any of the foregoing.

Musculoskeletal: Rare instances of polyarthritis have been reported.

Local Reactions: Pain, induration and sterile abscess have been reported after intramuscular injection and thrombophlebitis after intravenous infusion. Reactions can be minimized or avoided by giving deep intramuscular injections and avoiding prolonged use of indwelling intravenous catheters.

Dosage and Administration:

If significant diarrhea occurs during therapy, this antibiotic should be discontinued. (See **Warning** box).

Adults

Parenteral (IM or IV Administration):

Serious infections due to aerobic gram-positive cocci and the more sensitive anaerobes (NOT generally including *Bacteroides fragilis, Peptococcus* species and *Clostridium* species other than *Clostridium perfringens*):

600–1200 mg/day in 2, 3 or 4 equal doses

More severe infections, particularly those due to proven or suspected *Bacteroides fragilis, Peptococcus* species, or *Clostridium* species other than *Clostridium perfringens:*

1200–2700 mg/day in 2, 3 or 4 equal doses

For more serious infections, these doses may have to be increased. In life threatening situations due to aerobes or anaerobes, these doses may be increased. Doses of as much as 4800 mg daily have been given intravenously to adults. See **Dilution and Infusion Rates** section below.

Alternatively, drug may be administered in the form of a single rapid infusion of the first dose followed by continuous IV infusion as follows:

To maintain serum clindamycin levels	Rapid infusion rate	Maintenance infusion rate
Above 4 mcg/ml	10 mg/min for 30 min	0.75 mg/min
Above 5 mcg/ml	15 mg/min for 30 min	1.00 mg/min
Above 6 mcg/ml	20 mg/min for 30 min	1.25 mg/min

[See table above].

Children (over 1 month of age)

Parenteral (IM or IV Administration):

Serious infections:

15–25 mg/kg/day in 3 or 4 equal doses

More severe infections:

25–40 mg/kg/day in 3 or 4 equal doses

As an alternative to dosing on a body weight basis, children may be dosed on the basis of square meters body surface: 350 mg/m^2/day for serious infections and 450 mg/m^2/day for more severe infections.

In severe infections it is recommended that children be given no less than 300 mg/day regardless of body weight.

Parenteral therapy may be changed to oral clindamycin (Pediatric or HCl) when the condition warrants and at the discretion of the physician.

In cases of β-hemolytic streptococcal infections, treatment should be continued for at least 10 days.

Dilution and Infusion Rates

Single IM injections of greater than 600 mg are not recommended. Clindamycin phosphate must be diluted prior to IV administration to a dilution of 300 mg in 50 ml or more of diluent. Infusion rates are as follows:

Dose	*Diluent*	*Time*
300 mg	50 ml	10 min
600 mg	100 ml	20 min
900 mg	150 ml	30 min
1200 mg	200 ml	45 min

Administration of more than 1200 mg in a single 1-hour infusion is not recommended.

Dilution and Compatibility

Physical and biological compatibility studies monitored for 24 hours at room temperature have demonstrated no inactivation or incompatibility with the use of *Cleocin Phosphate* (clindamycin phosphate) in IV solutions containing NaCl, glucose, calcium or potassium and solutions containing vitamin B complex in concentrations usually used clinically. No incompatibility has been demonstrated with the antibiotics cephalothin, kanamycin, gentamicin, penicillin or carbenicillin.

The following drugs are physically incompatible with *Cleocin Phosphate:* ampicillin, diphenylhydantoin, barbiturates, aminophylline, calcium gluconate, and magnesium sulfate.

How Supplied: Each ml *Cleocin Phosphate* Sterile Solution (clindamycin phosphate) contains clindamycin phosphate equivalent to 150 mg clindamycin base; 5 mg benzyl alcohol; 0.5 mg disodium edetate; and water for injection, qs. When necessary, pH is adjusted with sodium hydroxide and/or hydrochloric acid.

The following sizes are available:

2 ml ampoule (300 mg)

5-pack *NDC 0009-0870-01*

100-pack *NDC 0009-0870-03*

4 ml ampoule (600 mg)

5-pack *NDC 0009-0775-01*

100-pack *NDC 0009-0775-03*

Code 810 020 001

[*Shown in Product Identification Section*]

COLESTID® GRANULES ℞
(colestipol hydrochloride)

How Supplied: *Colestid* Granules (colestipol hydrochloride) is available as follows:

Box of 30–5 gram packets *NDC 0009-0260-01*

500 gram bottle *NDC 0009-0260-02*

Each packet or each level scoop supplies 5 grams of Colestid.

CORTEF® ACETATE OINTMENT ℞
(Hydrocortisone Acetate Ointment, U.S.P.)

How Supplied: In two concentrations—10 mg (1%) or 25 mg (2.5%) hydrocortisone acetate per gram.

1%	5 Gm tubes	*NDC 0009-0273-01*
	20 Gm tubes	*NDC 0009-0273-02*
2.5%	5 Gm tubes	*NDC 0009-0289-01*
	20 Gm tubes	*NDC 0009-0289-02*

CORTEF® TABLETS ℞
(Hydrocortisone Tablets, USP)

How Supplied: Scored tablets in 3 strengths.

5 mg	Bottles of 50	*NDC 0009-0012-01*
10 mg	Bottles of 100	*NDC 0009-0031-01*
20 mg	Bottles of 100	*NDC 0009-0044-01*

CORTISONE ACETATE USP
STERILE AQUEOUS SUSPENSION
For Intramuscular Use Only
NOT FOR INTRAVENOUS USE

How Supplied: Cortisone Acetate USP, Sterile Aqueous Suspension 25 mg per ml. Each ml contains: 25 mg cortisone acetate; also 4.9 mg sodium carboxymethylcellulose, low viscosity; 3.93 mg polysorbate 80; 8.8 mg sodium chloride; 8.8 mg benzyl alcohol; water for injection qs.

When necessary, pH was adjusted with sodium hydroxide and/or hydrochloric acid.

20 ml vial *NDC 0009-0314-01*

CORTISONE ACETATE TABLETS, USP ℞

How Supplied: Scored tablets in 3 strengths.

5 mg	Bottles of 50	*NDC 0009-0015-01*
10 mg	Bottles of 100	*NDC 0009-0023-01*
25 mg	Bottles of 100	*NDC 0009-0034-01*
	Bottles of 500	*NDC 0009-0034-02*

Continued on next page

Information on these Upjohn products is based on labeling in effect on November 1, 1979. Further information on dosage and administration, side effects, precautions and contraindications for these and other Upjohn products may be obtained from either the package insert or Medical Services, The Upjohn Company, Kalamazoo, Michigan.

Upjohn—Cont.

CYTOSAR-U® ℞
STERILE POWDER
(sterile cytarabine, USP)

For intravenous and subcutaneous use only

> **WARNING**
> Only physicians experienced in cancer chemotherapy should use *Cytosar-U* Sterile Powder.
> For induction therapy patients should be treated in a facility with laboratory and supportive resources sufficient to monitor drug tolerance and protect and maintain a patient compromised by drug toxicity. The main toxic effect of *Cytosar-U* is bone marrow suppression with leukopenia, thrombocytopenia and anemia. Less serious toxicity includes nausea, vomiting, diarrhea and abdominal pain, oral ulceration, and hepatic dysfunction.
> The physician must judge possible benefit to the patient against known toxic effects of this drug in considering the advisability of therapy with *Cytosar-U*. Before making this judgment or beginning treatment, the physician should be familiar with the following text.

Description: *Cytosar-U* Sterile Powder contains cytarabine (1-β-D-arabinofuranosylcytosine; cytosine arabinoside). Cytarabine is a synthetic nucleoside which differs from the normal nucleosides cytidine and deoxycytidine in that the sugar moiety is arabinose rather than ribose or deoxyribose.

Cytosar-U is an antineoplastic agent for parenteral administration. It is available as a sterile freeze-dried preparation in two sizes:

100 mg vials—when prepared as directed, each ml contains:
20 mg cytarabine (Supplied with 5 ml ampoule of Bacteriostatic Water for Injection with 0.9% Benzyl Alcohol w/v).

500 mg vials—when prepared as directed, each ml contains:
50 mg cytarabine (Supplied with 10 ml ampoule of Bacteriostatic Water for Injection with 0.9% Benzyl Alcohol w/v).

When necessary, the pH of *Cytosar-U* was adjusted with hydrochloric acid and/or sodium hydroxide.

Pharmacology:

Cell Culture Studies

Cytarabine is cytotoxic to a wide variety of proliferating mammalian cells in culture. It exhibits cell phase specificity, primarily killing cells undergoing DNA synthesis (S-phase) and under certain conditions blocking the progression of cells from the G_1 phase to the S-phase. Although the mechanism of action is not completely understood, it appears that cytarabine acts through the inhibition of DNA polymerase. A limited, but significant, incorporation of cytarabine into both DNA and RNA has also been reported. Extensive chromosomal damage, including chromatoid breaks, have been produced by cytarabine and malignant transformation of rodent cells in culture has been reported. Deoxycytidine prevents or delays (but does not reverse) the cytotoxic activity.

Cell culture studies have shown an antiviral effect.[1] However, efficacy against herpes zoster or smallpox could not be demonstrated in controlled clinical trials.[2–4]

Cellular Resistance and Sensitivity

Cytarabine is metabolized by deoxycytidine kinase and other nucleotide kinases to the nucleotide triphosphate, an effective inhibitor of DNA polymerase; it is inactivated by a pyrimidine nucleoside deaminase which converts it to the nontoxic uracil derivative. It appears that the balance of kinase and deaminase levels may be an important factor in determining sensitivity or resistance of the cell to cytarabine.

Animal Studies

In experimental studies with mouse tumors, cytarabine was most effective in those tumors with a high growth fraction. The effect was dependent on the treatment schedule; optimal effects were achieved when the schedule (multiple closely spaced doses or constant infusion) ensured contact of the drug with the tumor cells when the maximum number of cells were in the susceptible S-phase. The best results were obtained when courses of therapy were separated by intervals sufficient to permit adequate host recovery.

Human Pharmacology

Cytosar-U (cytarabine) is rapidly metabolized and is not effective orally; less than 20 percent of the orally administered dose is absorbed from the gastrointestinal tract.

Following rapid intravenous injection of *Cytosar-U* labeled with tritium, the disappearance from plasma is biphasic. There is an initial distributive phase with a half-life of about 10 minutes, followed by a second elimination phase with a half-life of about 1 to 3 hours. After the distributive phase, over 80 percent of plasma radioactivity can be accounted for by the inactive metabolite 1-β-D-arabinofuranosyluracil (ara-U). Within 24 hours about 80 percent of the administered radioactivity can be recovered in the urine, approximately 90 percent of which is excreted as ara-U.

Relatively constant plasma levels can be achieved by continuous intravenous infusion.

After subcutaneous or intramuscular administration of *Cytosar-U* labeled with tritium, peak-plasma levels of radioactivity are achieved about 20 to 60 minutes after injection and are considerably lower than those after intravenous administration.

Cerebrospinal fluid levels of cytarabine are low in comparison to plasma levels after single intravenous injection. However, in one patient in whom cerebrospinal levels were examined after 2 hours of constant intravenous infusion, levels approached 40 percent of the steady state plasma level. With intrathecal administration, levels of cytarabine in the cerebrospinal fluid declined with a first order half-life of about 2 hours. Because cerebrospinal fluid levels of deaminase are low, little conversion to ara-U was observed.

Immunosuppressive Action

Cytosar-U (cytarabine) is capable of obliterating immune responses in man during administration with little or no accompanying toxicity.[5,6] Suppression of antibody responses to E-coli-VI antigen and tetanus toxoid have been demonstrated. This suppression was obtained during both primary and secondary antibody responses.

Cytosar-U also suppressed the development of cell-mediated immune responses such as delayed hypersensitivity skin reaction to dinitrochlorobenzene. However, it had no effect on already established delayed hypersensitivity reactions.

Following 5-day courses of intensive therapy with *Cytosar-U* the immune response was suppressed, as indicated by the following parameters: macrophage ingress into skin windows; circulating antibody response following primary antigenic stimulation; lymphocyte blastogenesis with phytohemagglutinin. A few days after termination of therapy there was a rapid return to normal.[7]

Indications and Usage: *Cytosar-U* (cytarabine) is indicated primarily for induction and maintenance of remission in acute myelocytic leukemia of both adults and children. It has also been found useful in the treatment of other leukemias, such as acute lymphocytic leukemia, chronic myelocytic leukemia (blast phase) and erythroleukemia. *Cytosar-U* may be used alone or in combination with other antineoplastic agents; the best results are often obtained with combination therapy.

Cytosar-U has been used experimentally in a variety of neoplastic diseases. In general, few patients with solid tumors have benefited.

Remissions induced by *Cytosar-U* not followed by maintenance treatment have been brief. Maintenance therapy has extended these and provided useful and comfortable remissions with relatively little toxicity.

Acute Myelocytic Leukemia

The following tables outline the results of treatment with *Cytosar-U* alone and in combination with other chemotherapeutic agents, in the treatment of acute myelocytic leukemia in adults and children.

The treatment regimens outlined in the tables should not be compared for efficacy. These were independent studies with a number of variables involved, such as patient population, duration of disease, and previous treatment.

[See table on next page].

The responsiveness and course of childhood acute myelocytic leukemia (AML) appears to be different from that in adults.[21–23] Numerous studies show response rates to be higher in children than in adults with similar treatment schedules. Experience indicates that at least with induction and initial drug responsiveness, childhood AML appears to be more similar to childhood acute lymphocytic leukemia (ALL) than to its adult variant.

Acute Lymphocytic Leukemia

Cytosar-U has been used in the treatment of acute lymphocytic leukemia in both adults and children. When *Cytosar-U* was used with other antineoplastic agents as part of a total therapy program, results were equal to or better than reported with such programs which did not include *Cytosar-U*.[24,25] Used singly, or in combination with other agents, *Cytosar-U* has also been effective in treating patients who had relapsed on other therapy. Table III summarizes the results obtained in previously treated patients. Since these are independent studies with such variables as patient population, duration of disease and previous treatment, results shown should not be used for comparing the efficacy of the outlined treatment programs.

Intrathecal Use in Meningeal Leukemia

Cytosar-U has been used intrathecally in acute leukemia in doses ranging from 5 mg/m^2 to 75 mg/m^2 of body surface area. The frequency of administration varied from once a day for 4 days to once every 4 days. The most frequently used dose was 30 mg/m^2 every 4 days until cerebrospinal fluid findings were normal, followed by one additional treatment.[34–38] The dosage schedule is usually governed by the type and severity of central nervous system manifestations and the response to previous therapy.

Prophylactic therapy following the successful treatment of the acute meningeal episode may be useful. The physician should familiarize himself with the current literature before instituting such a program.

Cytosar-U given intrathecally may cause systemic toxicity and careful monitoring of the hemopoietic system is indicated. Modification of other anti-leukemia therapy may be necessary. Major toxicity is rare. The most frequently reported reactions after intrathecal administration were nausea, vomiting and fever; these reactions are mild and self-limiting. Paraplegia has been reported in at least three instances.[39] Necrotizing leukoencephalopathy occurred in 5 children; these patients had also been treated with intrathecal methotrexate and hydrocortisone, as well as by central nervous system radiation.[40] Isolated neurotoxicity has been reported.[41] Blindness occurred in two patients in remission whose treatment had consisted of combination systemic chemotherapy, prophylactic central nervous system radiation and intrathecal *Cytosar-U*.[42]

Focal leukemic involvement of the central nervous system may not respond to intrathecal

TABLE I
ACUTE MYELOCYTIC LEUKEMIA
REMISSION INDUCTION
ADULTS

Drug-Dosage Schedule*	No. Patients Evaluated	Complete Remissions	Investigator
(CYTOSAR-U) SINGLE-DRUG THERAPY			
(infusion)			
10 mg/m² 12 hrs/day	12	2 (17%)	Ellison[8] (1968)
30 mg/m² 12 hrs/day	41	10 (24%)	
10 mg/m² 24 hrs/day	9	2 (22%)	
30 mg/m² 24 hrs/day	36	2 (6%)	
(infusion) 200 mg/m² 24 hrs/5 days	36	9 (25%)	Bodey[9] (1969)
10 mg/m² IV injection initially, then infusions of 30 mg/m²/12 hrs or 60 mg/m²/day for 4 days	49	21 (43%)	Goodell[10] (1970)
(infusion therapy)			Southwest
800 mg/m²/2 days	53	12 (23%)	Oncology
1000 mg/m²/5 days	60	24 (40%)	Group[11] (1974)
100 mg/m²/day 1 hr infusion	49	7 (14%)	Carey[12] (1975)
5–12.5 mg/kg/12 hour infusion following IV synchronizing dose**	5	5 (100%)	Lampkin[13] (1976)
COMBINED THERAPY			
Cytosar-U-thioguanine	36	15 (42%)	Gee[14] (1969)
Cytosar-U-thioguanine	64	28 (44%)	Grann[15] (1974)
Cytosar-U-cyclophosphamide-prednisone-vincristine	66	32 (48%)	Bodey[16] (1974)
Cytosar-U-thioguanine	88	49 (56%)	Clarkson[17] (1975)
Cytosar-U-cyclophosphamide-vincristine	50	23 (46%)	Curtis[18] (1975)

*Unless otherwise stated all doses given until drug effect—modifications then based on hematologic response. See references
**Highly experimental-requires ability to study mitotic indices

TABLE II
ACUTE MYELOCYTIC LEUKEMIA
REMISSION INDUCTION
CHILDREN (21 and under)

Drug Therapy	No. Patients Evaluated	Complete Remissions	Investigator
Cytosar-U (5–12.5 mg/kg following IV synchronizing dose**)	16	12 (75%)	Lampkin[13] (1976)
Cytosar-U-cyclophosphamide-vincristine	60	27 (45%)	Sonley[19] (1971)
Cytosar-U-thioguanine-doxorubicin	11	8 (72%)	Hagbin[20] (1975)
Cytosar-U-thioguanine	47	20 (43%)	Pizzo[21] (1976)
Cytosar-U-cyclophosphamide	12	7 (58%)	

**Highly experimental-requires ability to study mitotic indices

Cytosar-U and may better be treated with radiotherapy.

Although severe reactions attributable to the diluent are uncommon, many investigators prefer to use a special diluent for intrathecal use which is physiologically similar to the spinal fluid (Elliott's B Solution).[43]

Contraindications: *Cytosar-U* (cytarabine) is contraindicated in those patients who are hypersensitive to the drug.

Warnings: *Cytosar-U* (cytarabine) is a potent bone marrow suppressant. Therapy should be started cautiously in patients with pre-existing drug-induced bone marrow suppression. Patients receiving this drug must be under close medical supervision and, during induction therapy, should have leukocyte and platelet counts performed daily. Bone marrow examinations should be performed frequently after blasts have disappeared from the peripheral blood. Facilities should be available for management of complications of bone marrow suppression (infection resulting from granulocytopenia and other impaired body defenses, and hemorrhage secondary to thrombocytopenia). One case of anaphylaxis that resulted in acute cardiopulmonary arrest and required resuscitation has been reported. This occurred immediately after the intravenous administration of *Cytosar-U*.

Use in Pregnancy

Cytosar-U is known to be teratogenic in some animal species. Use of this drug in women who are or who may become pregnant should be

Continued on next page

Information on these Upjohn products is based on labeling in effect on November 1, 1979. Further information on dosage and administration, side effects, precautions and contraindications for these and other Upjohn products may be obtained from either the package insert or Medical Services, The Upjohn Company, Kalamazoo, Michigan.

Upjohn—Cont.

undertaken only after due consideration of potential benefit and potential hazard to both mother and child.

In five reported cases on the use of *Cytosar-U* during pregnancy, in combination with other cytotoxic agents, four normal infants were delivered (one weighed only 2,250 grams).[44–47] In the fifth case, the patient had a therapeutic abortion at 24 weeks following four weeks of therapy with cytarabine and thioguanine; a trisomy C chromosal abnormality was found in the chorionic tissue. No congenital abnormalities were observed in the fetus. Therapy had been initiated in these patients between the 20th and 28th week of gestation.

Because of the potential for abnormalies with cytotoxic therapy, particularly during the first trimester, a patient who is or who becomes pregnant while on *Cytosar-U* should be apprised of the potential risk to the fetus and the advisability of pregnancy continuation. There is a definite, but considerably lesser, risk if therapy is initiated during the second or third trimester. Although normal infants have been delivered to patients treated after the first trimester of pregnancy, follow-up of such infants would be advisable.

Precautions: Patients receiving *Cytosar-U* (cytarabine) must be monitored closely. Frequent platelet and leukocyte counts and bone marrow examinations are mandatory. Consider suspending or modifying therapy when drug-induced marrow depression has resulted in a platelet count under 50,000 or a polymorphonuclear granulocyte count under 1000 per cu. mm. Counts of formed elements in the peripheral blood may continue to fall after the drug is stopped and reach lowest values after drug-free intervals of 12 to 24 days. When indicated, restart therapy when definite signs of marrow recovery appear (on successive bone marrow studies). Patients whose drug is withheld until "normal" peripheral blood values are attained may escape from control.

When large intravenous doses are given quickly, patients are frequently nauseated and may vomit for several hours postinjection. This problem tends to be less severe when the drug is infused.

The human liver apparently detoxifies a substantial fraction of an administered dose. Use the drug with caution and at reduced dose in patients whose liver function is poor.

Periodic checks of bone marrow, liver and kidney functions should be performed in patients receiving *Cytosar-U.*

Like other cytotoxic drugs, *Cytosar-U* may induce hyperuricemia secondary to rapid lysis of neoplastic cells. The clinician should monitor the patient's blood uric acid level and be prepared to use such supportive and pharmacologic measures as might be necessary to control this problem.

Adverse Reactions:

Expected Reactions

Because *Cytosar-U* (cytarabine) is a bone marrow suppressant, anemia, leukopenia, thrombocytopenia, megaloblastosis and reduced reticulocytes can be expected as a result of its administration. The severity of these reactions are dose and schedule dependent.[48] Cellular changes in the morphology of bone marrow and peripheral smears can be expected.[49]

Following 5-day constant infusions or acute injections of 50 mg/m^2 to 600 mg/m^2, white cell depression follows a biphasic course. Regardless of initial count, dosage level, or schedule, there is an initial fall starting the first 24 hours with a nadir at days 7–9. This is followed by a brief rise which peaks around the twelfth day. A second and deeper fall reaches nadir at days 15–24. Then there is rapid rise to above baseline in the next 10 days. Platelet depression is noticeable at 5 days with a peak depression occurring between days 12–15. Thereupon, a rapid rise to above baseline occurs in the next 10 days.[50]

Most Frequent Adverse Reactions

- anorexia
- nausea
- vomiting
- diarrhea
- oral and anal inflammation or ulceration
- hepatic dysfunction
- fever
- rash
- thrombophlebitis
- bleeding (all sites)

Nausea and vomiting are most frequent following rapid intravenous injection.

Less Frequent Adverse Reactions

- sepsis
- pneumonia
- cellulitis at injection site
- skin ulceration
- urinary retention
- renal dysfunction
- neuritis or neural toxicity
- sore throat
- esophageal ulceration
- esophagitis
- chest pain
- abdominal pain
- freckling
- jaundice
- conjunctivitis (may occur with rash)
- dizziness
- alopecia
- anaphylaxis (See WARNINGS)

[See table below].

Dosage and Administration: *Cytosar-U* (cytarabine) is not active orally. The schedule and method of administration varies with the program of therapy to be used. *Cytosar-U* may be given by intravenous infusion or injection or subcutaneously. Thrombophlebitis has occurred at the site of drug injection or infusion in some patients, and rarely patients have noted pain and inflammation at subcutaneous injection sites. In most instances, however, the drug has been well tolerated.

Patients can tolerate higher total doses when they receive the drug by rapid intravenous injection as compared with slow infusion. This phenomenon is related to the drug's rapid inactivation and brief exposure of susceptible normal and neoplastic cells to significant levels after rapid injection. Normal and neoplastic cells seem to respond in somewhat parallel fashion to these different modes of administration and no clear-cut clinical advantage has been demonstrated for either.

Clinical experience accumulated to date suggests that success with *Cytosar-U* is dependent more on adeptness in modifying day-to-day dosage to obtain maximum leukemic cell kill with tolerable toxicity than on the basic treatment schedule chosen at the outset of therapy. Toxicity necessitating dosage alteration almost always occurs.

In many chemotherapeutic programs, *Cytosar-U* is used in combination with other cytotoxic drugs. The addition of these cytotoxic drugs has necessitated changes and dose alterations. The dosage schedules for combination therapy outlined below have been reported in the literature (see references).

Dosage Schedules:

Acute myelocytic leukemia—induction remission, adults

Cytosar-U (cytarabine)—200 mg/m^2 daily by continuous infusion for 5 days (120 hours)—total dose 1000 mg/m^2. This course is repeated approximately every 2 weeks. Modifications must be made and based on hematologic response.

Combined Chemotherapy

Before instituting a program of combined chemotherapy, the physician should be familiar with adverse reactions, precautions, contraindications, and warnings applicable to all the drugs involved in the program.

Cytosar-U and thioguanine [14,15,17]

Cytosar U: 3.0 mg/kg every 12 hours by IV injection

Thioguanine: 2.5 mg/kg every 12 hours (orally)

Both drugs are given until bone marrow becomes hypoplastic. This usually takes from 1

TABLE III
ACUTE LYMPHATIC LEUKEMIA
REMISSION INDUCTION
PREVIOUSLY TREATED PATIENTS

ADULTS AND CHILDREN

Drug Therapy	No. of Patients Evaluated	Complete Remissions	Response	Investigator
Cytosar-U 3–5 mg/kg/day (IV injection)	43	2 (5%)	15 (35%)	Howard[26] (1968)
Cytosar-U-asparaginase	9	8 (89%)	8 (89%)	McElwain[27] (1969)
Cytosar-U-cyclophosphamide	11	7 (64%)	9 (82%)	Bodey[28] (1970)
Cytosar-U-prednisone	83		(49%)	Nesbit[29] (1970)
Cytosar-U 150–200 mg/m^2/5 days (infusion)	34	1 (3%)	4 (12%)	Wang[30] (1970)
Cytosar-U 25 mg/kg/twice weekly (infusion)	74	24 (32%)	29 (39%)	Traggis[31] (1971)
Cytosar-U-asparaginase	22	13 (59%)	15 (68%)	Ortega[32] (1972)
Cytosar-U-thioguanine	19	9 (47%)	9 (47%)	Bryan[33] (1974)

week to 10 days. Following a 10 to 20 day rest period the cycle is started again.

Cytosar-U, cyclophosphamide, vincristine, prednisone[16]

Cytosar-U: 100 mg/m^2/day for 5 days (rapid IV injection in divided doses-every 8 hours).

Cyclophosphamide: 100 mg/m^2/day for 5 days (rapid IV injection in divided doses-every 8 hours).

Vincristine: 2 mg by rapid IV injection, day 1 only.

Prednisone: 25 mg four times daily for 5 days.

Courses of therapy are initiated at 2-week intervals, the second course being given without regard to peripheral blood cell counts and appearance of bone marrow. When there is rapid recovery of blast cells in the peripheral blood, further courses can be reinstituted at less than the 2-week intervals. Therapy should be delayed when the bone marrow is hypocellular or if severe infection or hemorrhage develop. The dosage schedule is continued until the patient is in complete remission or until progressive disease is apparent after a minimum of five courses.

Dosage for subsequent courses is determined by the patient's response and the condition of the bone marrow.

Acute myelocytic leukemia-maintenance, adults

Maintenance programs are modifications of induction programs and, in general, use similar schedules of drug therapy as were used during induction. Most programs have a greater time spacing between courses of therapy during remission maintenance.

Acute myelocytic leukemia-induction and maintenance in children

Numerous studies have shown that childhood AML responds better than adult AML given similar regimens. Where the adult dosage is stated in terms of body weight or surface area, the children's dosage may be calculated on the same basis. When specified amounts of a drug are indicated for the adult dosage, these should be adjusted for children on the basis of such factors as age, body weight or body surface area.

Acute lymphocytic leukemia

In general, dosage schedules are similar to those used in acute myelocytic leukemia with some modifications. For dosage recommendations see referenced literature in Table III.

Dosage Modification—The dosage of *Cytosar-U* must be modified or suspended when signs of serious hematologic depression appear. In general, consider discontinuing the drug if the patient has less than 50,000 platelets or 1000 polymorphonuclear granulocytes per cu mm in his peripheral blood. These guidelines may be modified depending on signs of toxicity in other systems and on the rapidity of fall in formed blood elements. Restart the drug when there are signs of marrow recovery and the above platelet and granulocyte levels have been attained. Withholding therapy until the patient's blood values are normal may result in escape of the patient's disease from control by the drug.

How Supplied: Store unreconstituted product at controlled room temperature: 15°–30°C (59°–86°F). *Cytosar-U* Sterile Powder (cytarabine) is available as a freeze-dried preparation in multidose vials of two sizes:

100 mg* vial—Must be reconstituted with 5 ml of Bacteriostatic Water for Injection with Benzyl Alcohol 0.9% w/v, the resulting solution contains 20 mg of cytarabine per ml.

500 mg* vial—Must be reconstituted with 10 ml of Bacteriostatic Water for Injection with Benzyl Alcohol 0.9% w/v, the resulting solution contains 50 mg of cytarabine per ml.

*When necessary, the pH was adjusted with hydrochloric acid and/or sodium hydroxide.

In this form the drug is suitable for intravenous or subcutaneous administration. The pH of the reconstituted solution is about 5. THESE SOLUTIONS MAY BE STORED AT CONTROLLED ROOM TEMPERATURE 15°–30°C (59°–86°F) FOR 48 HOURS. DISCARD ANY SOLUTION IN WHICH A SLIGHT HAZE DEVELOPS.

Chemical Stability in Infusion Solutions

Chemical stability studies were performed by ultraviolet assay on *Cytosar-U* infusion solutions. These studies showed that when the reconstituted *Cytosar-U* Sterile Powder (cytarabine) was added to Water for Injection, 5% Dextrose in Water or Sodium Chloride Injection, 94 to 96 percent of the cytarabine was present after 192 hours storage at room temperature.

References:

1. Zaky DA, Betts RF, Douglas RG, et al: Varicella-Zoster Virus and Subcutaneous Cytarabine: Correlation of In Vitro Sensitivities to Blood Levels, Antimicrob Agents Chemother *7*:229–232, 1975
2. Davis CM, VanDarsarl JV, Coltman CA Jr: Failure of Cytarabine in Varicella-Zoster Infections, JAMA *224*:122–123, 1973
3. Betts RF, Zaky DA, Douglas RG, et al: Ineffectiveness of Subcutaneous Cytosine Arabinoside in Localized Herpes Zoster, Ann Intern Med *82*:778–783, 1975
4. Dennis DT, Doberstyn EB, Awoke S, et al: Failure of Cytosine Arabinoside in Treating Smallpox; A Double-blind Study, Lancet *2*:377–379, 1974
5. Gray GD: ARA-C and Derivatives as Examples of Immunosuppressive Nucleoside Analogs, Ann NY Acad Sci *255*:372–379, 1975
6. Mitchell MS, Wade ME, DeConti RC, et al: Immunosuppressive Effects of Cytosine Arabinoside and Methotrexate in Man, Ann Intern Med *70*:535–547, 1969
7. Frei E, Ho DHW, Bodey GP, et al: Pharmacologic and Cytokinetic Studies of Arabinosyl Cytosine. In *Unifying Concepts of Leukemia*, Bibl. Hematol. No. 39. Karger, Basel 1973, pp 1085–1097
8. Ellison RR, Holland JF, Weil M, et al: Arabinosyl Cytosine: A Useful Agent in the Treatment of Acute Leukemia in Adults, Blood *32*:507–523, 1968
9. Bodey GP, Freireich EJ, Monto RW, et al: Cytosine Arabinoside (NSC-63878) Therapy for Acute Leukemia in Adults, Cancer Chemother Rep *53*:59–66, 1969
10. Goodell B, Leventhal B, Henderson E: Cytosine Arabinoside in Acute Granulocytic Leukemia, Clin Pharmacol Ther *12*:599–606, 1970
11. Southwest Oncology Group: Cytarabine for Acute Leukemia in Adults, Arch Intern Med *133*:251–259, 1974
12. Carey RW, Ribas-Mundo M, Ellison RR, et al: Comparative Study of Cytosine Arabinoside Therapy Alone and Combined with Thioguanine, Mercaptopurine or Daunorubicin in Acute Myelocytic Leukemia, Cancer *36*:1560–1566, 1975
13. Lampkin BC, McWilliam NB, Mauer AM, et al: Manipulation of the Mitotic Cycle in the Treatment of Acute Myelogenous Leukaemia, Brit J Haematol *32*:29–40, 1976
14. Gee TS, Yu KP, Clarkson BD: Treatment of Adult Acute Leukemia with Arabinosylcytosine and Thioguanine, Cancer *23*:1019–1032, 1969
15. Grann V, Erichson R, Flannery J, et al: The Therapy of Acute Granulocytic Leukemia in Patients More Than Fifty Years Old, Ann Int Med *80*:15–20, 1974
16. Bodey GP, Coltman CA, Freireich EJ, et al: Chemotherapy of Acute Leukemia; Comparison of Cytarabine Alone and in Combination with Vincristine, Prednisone, and Cyclophosphamide, Arch Intern Med *133*:260–266, 1974
17. Clarkson BD, Dowling MD, Gee TS, et al: Treatment of Acute Leukemia in Adults, Cancer *36*:775–795, 1975
18. Curtis JE, Cowan DH, Bergsagel DE, et al: Acute Leukemia in Adults: Assessment of Remission Induction with Combination Chemotherapy by Clinical and Cell-Culture Criteria, Canad Med Assoc J *113*:289–294, 1975
19. Sonley MJ, Nesbit M, Thatcher LG, et al: Cytosine Arabinoside, Cyclophosphamide and Vincristine in Children with Acute Myelogenous Leukemia, Proc Am Assoc Cancer Res *12*:87, 1971
20. Haghbin M: Acute Non-lymphoblastic Leukemia; Clinical and Morphological Characterization, Mod Prob Pediatr *16*:39–58, 1975
21. Pizzo PA, Henderson ES, Leventhal BG: Acute Myelogenous Leukemia in Children: A Preliminary Report of Combination Chemotherapy, J Pediatr *88*:125–130, 1976
22. Report of the Medical Research Council's Working Party on Leukaemia in Adults: Treatment of Acute Myeloid Leukaemia with Daunorubicin, Cytosine Arabinoside, Mercaptopurine, L-Asparaginase, Prednisone and Thioguanine: Results of Treatment with Five Multiple-Drug Schedules, Brit J Haematol *27*:373–389, 1974
23. Ansari BM, Thompson EN, Whittaker JA: A Comparative Study of Acute Myeloblastic Leukaemia in Children and Adults, Brit J Haematol *31*:269–277, 1975
24. Gee TS, Haghbin M, Dowling MD Jr, et al: Acute Lymphoblastic Leukemia in Adults and Children; Differences in Response with Similar Therapeutic Regimens, Cancer *37*:1256–1264, 1976
25. Spiers ASD, Roberts PD, Marsh GW, et al: Acute Lymphoblastic Leukaemia: Cyclical Chemotherapy with three Combinations of Four Drugs (COAP-POMP-CART Regimen). Brit Med J *4*:614–617, 1975
26. Howard JP, Albo V, Newton WA Jr: Cytosine Arabinoside: Results of a Cooperative Study in Acute Childhood Leukemia, Cancer *21*:341–345, 1968
27. McElwain TJ, Hardisty RM: Remission Induction with Cytosine Arabinoside and L-Asparaginase in Acute Lymphoblastic Leukaemia, Brit Med J *4*:596–598, 1969
28. Bodey GP, Rodriguez, V, Hart J, et al: Therapy of Acute Leukemia with the Combination of Cytosine Arabinoside (NSC-63878) and Cyclophosphamide (NSC-26271), Cancer Chemother Rep *54*:255–262, 1970
29. Nesbit ME Jr, Hammond D: Cytosine Arabinoside (ARAC) and Prednisone Therapy of Previously Treated Acute Lymphoblastic and Undifferentiated Leukemia (ALL/AUL) of Childhood, Proc Am Assoc Cancer Res *11*:59, 1970
30. Wang JJ, Selawry OS, Vietti TJ, et al: Prolonged Infusion of Arabinosyl Cytosine in Childhood Leukemia, Cancer *25*:1–6, 1970

Continued on next page

Information on these Upjohn products is based on labeling in effect on November 1, 1979. Further information on dosage and administration, side effects, precautions and contraindications for these and other Upjohn products may be obtained from either the package insert or Medical Services, The Upjohn Company, Kalamazoo, Michigan.

Upjohn—Cont.

31. Traggis DG, Dohlwitz A, Das L, et al: Cytosine Arabinoside in Acute Leukemia of Childhood, Cancer *28*:815–818, 1971
32. Ortega JA, Finklestein JZ, Ertell, et al: Effective Combination Treatment of Advanced Acute Lymphocytic Leukemia with Cytosine Arabinoside (NSC-63878) and L-Asparaginase (NSC-109229), Cancer Chemother Rep *56*:363–368, 1972
33. Bryan JH, Henderson ES, Leventhal BG: Cytosine Arabinoside and 6- Thioguanine in Refractory Acute Lymphocytic Leukemia, Cancer *33*:539–544, 1974
34. Proceedings of the Chemotherapy Conference on ARA-C: Development and Application (Cytosine Arabinoside Hydrochloride—NSC 63878), Oct. 10, 1969
35. Lay HN, Colebatch JH, Ekert H: Experiences with Cytosine Arabinoside in Childhood Leukaemia and Lymphoma, Med J Aust *2*:187–192, 1971
36. Halikowski B, Cyklis R, Armata J, et al: Cytosine Arabinoside Administered Intrathecally in Cerebromeningeal Leukemia, Acta Paediat Scand *59*:164–168, 1970
37. Wang JJ, Pratt CB: Intrathecal Arabinosyl Cytosine in Meningeal Leukemia, Cancer *25*:531–534, 1970
38. Band PR, Holland JF, Bernard J, et al: Treatment of Central Nervous System Leukemia with Intrathecal Cytosine Arabinoside, Cancer *32*:744–748, 1973
39. Saiki JH, Thompson S, Smith F, et al: Paraplegia Following Intrathecal Chemotherapy, Cancer *29*:370–374, 1972
40. Rubinstein LJ, Herman MM, Long TF, et al: Disseminated Necrotizing Leukoencephalopathy: A Complication of Treated Central System Leukemia and Lymphoma, Cancer *35*:291–305, 1975
41. Marmont Am, Damasio EE: Neurotoxicity of Intrathecal Chemotherapy for Leukaemia, Brit Med J *4*:47, 1973
42. Margileth DA, Poplack DG, Pizzo PA, et al: Blindness During Remission in Two Patients with Acute Lymphoblastic Leukemia, Cancer *39*:58–61, 1977
43. Duttera MJ, Gallelli JF, Kleinman LM, et al: Intrathecal Methotrexate, Lancet *1*:540, 1972
44. Pawliger DF, McLean FW, Noyes WD: Normal Fetus After Cytosine Arabinoside Therapy, Ann Intern Med *74*:1012, 1971
45. Raich PC, Curet LB: Treatment of Acute Leukemia During Pregnancy, Cancer *36*:861–862, 1975
46. The Upjohn Company, Personal Communications, 1972-1973
47. Maurer LH, Forcier RJ, McIntyre OR: Fetal Group C Trisomy After Cytosine Arabinoside and Thioguanine, Ann Intern Med *75*:809–810, 1971
48. Frei E III, Bickers JN, Hewlett JS, et al: Dose Schedule and Antitumor Studies of Arabinosyl Cytosine (NSC 63878), Cancer Res *29*:1325–1332, 1969
49. Bell WR, Whang JJ, Carbone PP, et al: Cytogenetic and Morphologic Abnormalities in Human Bone Marrow Cells during Cytosine Arabinoside Therapy, J. Hematol *27*:771–781, 1966
50. Burke PJ, Serpick AA, Carbone PP, et al: A Clinical Evaluation of Dose and Schedule of Administration of Cytosine Arabinoside (NSC 63878), Cancer Res *28*:274–279, 1968

Animal Toxicology: Toxicity of cytarabine in experimental animals, as well as activity, is markedly influenced by the schedule of administration. For example, in mice the LD_{10} for single intraperitoneal administration is greater than 6000 mg/m^2. However, when administered in 8 doses, each separated by 3 hours, the LD_{10} is less than 750 mg/m^2 total dose. Similarly, although a total dose of 1920 mg/m^2 administered as 12 injections at 6-hour intervals was lethal to beagle dogs (severe bone marrow hypoplasia with evidence of liver and kidney damage), dogs receiving the same total dose administered as 8 injections (again at 6-hour intervals) over a 48-hour period survived with minimal signs of toxicity. The most consistent observation in surviving dogs was elevated transaminase levels. In all experimental species the primary limiting toxic effect is marrow suppression with leukopenia. In addition, cytarabine causes abnormal cerebellar development in the neonatal hamster and is teratogenic to the rat fetus.
Code 810 126 000

DELTA-CORTEF® TABLETS ℞
(Prednisolone Tablets, U.S.P.)

How Supplied: 5 mg scored tablets.
Bottles of 100 *NDC 0009-0025-01*
Bottles of 500 *NDC 0009-0025-02*

DELTASONE® TABLETS ℞
(Prednisone Tablets, USP)

How Supplied: Scored tablets in the following strength and sizes:

2.5 mg	Bottles of 100	*NDC 0009-0032-01*
5 mg	Bottles of 100	*NDC 0009-0045-01*
	Bottles of 500	*NDC 0009-0045-02*
	Dosepak™ Unit of use (21)	*NDC 0009-0045-04*
	Unit Dose Package (100)	*NDC 0009-0045-05*
10 mg	Bottles of 100	*NDC 0009-0193-01*
	Bottles of 500	*NDC 0009-0193-02*
	Unit Dose Packages (100)	*NDC 0009-0193-03*
20 mg	Bottles of 100	*NDC 0009-0165-01*
	Bottles of 500	*NDC 0009-0165-02*
	Unit dose Packages (100)	*NDC 0009-0165-03*
50 mg	Bottles of 100	*NDC 0009-0388-01*
	Unit dose Packages (100)	*NDC 0009-0388-02*

Code 810 342 000
[*Shown in Product Identification Section*]

DEPO-MEDROL® STERILE AQUEOUS SUSPENSION ℞
(Sterile Methylprednisolone Acetate Suspension, NF)
NOT FOR INTRAVENOUS USE

40 mg/ml (1 ml vial):
NSN 6505-00-952-0267 (M)
40 mg/ml (5 ml vial):
NSN 6505-00-890-1186A (M & VA)

Description: Methylprednisolone acetate is the 6-methyl derivative of prednisolone. It is a white or practically white, odorless, crystalline powder which melts at about 215° with some decomposition. It is soluble in dioxane, sparingly soluble in acetone, in alcohol, in chloroform, and in methanol, and slightly soluble in ether. It is practically insoluble in water.
The chemical name for methylprednisolone acetate is pregna-1, 4-diene-3, 20-dione, 21-(acetyloxy)-11, 17-dihydroxy-6-methyl-,(6α, 11β)- and the molecular weight is 416.51.
Depo-Medrol Sterile Aqueous Suspension (methylprednisolone acetate) is an anti-inflammatory glucocorticoid in a sterile aqueous suspension for intramuscular, intra-articular, soft tissue or intralesional injection. It is available in three strengths: 20 mg/ml; 40 mg/ml; 80 mg/ml.
[See table below].

Each ml of these preparations contains:	**20 mg**	**40 mg**	**80 mg**
Methylprednisolone Acetate	20 mg	40 mg	80 mg
Also			
Polyethylene Glycol 4000	29.6 mg	29 mg	28 mg
Sodium Chloride	8.9 mg	8.7 mg	8.5 mg
Myristyl-gamma-picolinium Chloride	0.19 mg	0.19 mg	0.19 mg
Water for Injection	qs	qs	qs

When necessary, pH was adjusted with Sodium Hydroxide and/or Hydrochloric Acid. The pH of the finished product remains within the NF specified range; ie, 3.5 to 7.0.

Actions: Naturally occurring glucocorticoids (hydrocortisone), which also have salt retaining properties, are used in replacement therapy in adrenocortical deficiency states. Their synthetic analogs are used primarily for their potent anti-inflammatory effects in disorders of many organ systems.
Glucocorticoids cause profound and varied metabolic effects. In addition, they modify the body's immune response to diverse stimuli.

Indications

A. FOR INTRAMUSCULAR ADMINISTRATION

When oral therapy is not feasible and the strength, dosage form, and route of administration of the drug reasonably lend the preparation to the treatment of the condition, the intramuscular use of *Depo-Medrol* (methylprednisolone acetate) is indicated as follows:

1. **Endocrine Disorders**
   - Primary or secondary adrenocortical insufficiency (hydrocortisone or cortisone is the drug of choice; synthetic analogs may be used in conjunction with mineralocorticoids where applicable; in infancy, mineralocorticoid supplementation is of particular importance)
   - Acute adrenocortical insufficiency (hydrocortisone or cortisone is the drug of choice; mineralocorticoid supplementation may be necessary, particularly when synthetic analogs are used)
   - Preoperatively and in the event of serious trauma or illness, in patients with known adrenal insufficiency or when adrenocortical reserve is doubtful
   - Congenital adrenal hyperplasia
   - Hypercalcemia associated with cancer
   - Nonsuppurative thyroiditis
2. **Rheumatic Disorders**
   As adjunctive therapy for short-term administration (to tide the patient over an acute episode or exacerbation) in:
   - Post-traumatic osteoarthritis
   - Synovitis of osteoarthritis
   - Rheumatoid arthritis, including juvenile rheumatoid arthritis (selected cases may require low-dose maintenance therapy)
   - Acute and subacute bursitis
   - Epicondylitis
   - Acute nonspecific tenosynovitis
   - Acute gouty arthritis
   - Psoriatic arthritis
   - Ankylosing spondylitis
3. **Collagen Diseases**
   During an exacerbation or as maintenance therapy in selected cases of:
   - Systemic lupus erythematosus
   - Systemic dermatomyositis (polymyositis)
   - Acute rheumatic carditis
4. **Dermatologic Diseases**
   - Pemphigus
   - Severe erythema multiforme (Stevens-Johnson syndrome)
   - Exfoliative dermatitis
   - Bullous dermatitis herpetiformis
   - Severe seborrheic dermatitis
   - Severe psoriasis

Mycosis fungoides

5. **Allergic States**
Control of severe or incapacitating allergic conditions intractable to adequate trials of conventional treatment in:
Bronchial asthma
Contact dermatitis
Atopic dermatitis
Serum sickness
Seasonal or perennial allergic rhinitis
Drug hypersensitivity reactions
Urticarial transfusion reactions
Acute noninfectious laryngeal edema (epinephrine is the drug of first choice)

6. **Ophthalmic Diseases**
Severe acute and chronic allergic and inflammatory processes involving the eye, such as:
Herpes zoster ophthalmicus
Iritis, iridocyclitis
Chorioretinitis
Diffuse posterior uveitis and choroiditis
Optic neuritis
Sympathetic ophthalmia
Anterior segment inflammation
Allergic conjunctivitis
Allergic corneal marginal ulcers
Keratitis

7. **Gastrointestinal Diseases**
To tide the patient over a critical period of the disease in:
Ulcerative colitis (systemic therapy)
Regional enteritis (systemic therapy)

8. **Respiratory Diseases**
Symptomatic sarcoidosis
Berylliosis
Fulminating or disseminated pulmonary tuberculosis when used concurrently with appropriate antituberculous chemotherapy
Loeffler's syndrome not manageable by other means
Aspiration pneumonitis

9. **Hematologic Disorders**
Acquired (autoimmune) hemolytic anemia
Secondary thrombocytopenia in adults
Erythroblastopenia (RBC anemia)
Congenital (erythroid) hypoplastic anemia

10. **Neoplastic Diseases**
For palliative management of:
Leukemias and lymphomas in adults
Acute leukemia of childhood

11. **Edematous States**
To induce diuresis or remission of proteinuria in the nephrotic syndrome, without uremia, of the idiopathic type or that due to lupus erythematosus

12 **Nervous System**
Acute exacerbations of multiple sclerosis

13. **Miscellaneous**
Tuberculous meningitis with subarachnoid block or impending block when used concurrently with appropriate antituberculous chemotherapy
Trichinosis with neurologic or myocardial involvement

B. FOR INTRA-ARTICULAR OR SOFT TISSUE ADMINISTRATION
Depo-Medrol is indicated as adjunctive therapy for short-term administration (to tide the patient over an acute episode or exacerbation) in:
Synovitis of osteoarthritis
Rheumatoid arthritis
Acute and subacute bursitis
Acute gouty arthritis
Epicondylitis
Acute nonspecific tenosynovitis
Post-traumatic osteoarthritis

C. FOR INTRALESIONAL ADMINISTRATION
Depo-Medrol is indicated for intralesional use in the following conditions:
Keloids
Localized hypertrophic, infiltrated inflammatory lesions of:
lichen planus, psoriatic plaques, granuloma annulare, and lichen simplex chronicus (neurodermatitis)
Discoid lupus erythematosus
Necrobiosis lipodica diabeticorum
Alopecia areata
Depo-Medrol also may be useful in cystic tumors of an aponeurosis or tendon (ganglia).

Contraindications: Systemic fungal infections.

Warnings: While crystals of adrenal steroids in the dermis suppress inflammatory reactions, their presence may cause disintegration of the cellular elements and physiochemical changes in the ground substance of the connective tissue. The resultant infrequently occurring dermal and/or subdermal changes may form depressions in the skin at the injection site. The degree to which this reaction occurs will vary with the amount of adrenal steroid injected. Regeneration is usually complete within a few months or after all crystals of the adrenal steroid have been absorbed.

In order to minimize the incidence of dermal and subdermal atrophy, care must be exercised not to exceed recommended doses in injections. Multiple small injections into the area of the lesion should be made whenever possible. The technique of intra-articular and intramuscular injection should include precautions against injection or leakage into the dermis. Injection into the deltoid muscle should be avoided because of a high incidence of subcutaneous atrophy.

In patients on corticosteroid therapy subjected to any unusual stress, increased dosage of rapidly acting corticosteroids before, during, and after the stressful situation is indicated.

Corticosteroids may mask some signs of infection, and new infections may appear during their use. There may be decreased resistance and inability to localize infection when corticosteroids are used. Do not use intra-articularly, intrabursally or for intratendinous administration for *local* effect in the presence of acute infection.

Prolonged use of corticosteroids may produce posterior subcapsular cataracts, glaucoma with possible damage to the optic nerves, and may enhance the establishment of secondary ocular infections due to fungi or viruses.

Usage in pregnancy. Since adequate human reproduction studies have not been done with corticosteroids, the use of these drugs in pregnancy, nursing mothers, or women of childbearing potential requires that the possible benefits of the drug be weighed against the potential hazards to the mother and embryo or fetus. Infants born of mothers who have received substantial doses of corticosteroids during pregnancy should be carefully observed for signs of hypoadrenalism.

Average and large doses of cortisone or hydrocortisone can cause elevation of blood pressure, salt and water retention, and increased excretion of potassium. These effects are less likely to occur with the synthetic derivatives except when used in large doses. Dietary salt restriction and potassium supplementation may be necessary. All corticosteroids increase calcium excretion.

While on corticosteroid therapy patients should not be vaccinated against smallpox. Other immunization procedures should not be undertaken in patients who are on corticosteroids, especially in high doses, because of possible hazards of neurological complications and lack of antibody response.

The use of *Depo-Medrol* (methylprednisolone acetate) in active tuberculosis should be restricted to those cases of fulminating or disseminated tuberculosis in which the corticosteroid is used for the management of the disease in conjunction with appropriate antituberculous regimen.

If corticosteroids are indicated in patients with latent tuberculosis or tuberculin reactivity, close observation is necessary as reactivation of the disease may occur. During prolonged corticosteroid therapy, these patients should receive chemoprophylaxis.

Because rare instances of anaphylactoid reactions have occurred in patients receiving parenteral corticosteroid therapy, appropriate precautionary measures should be taken prior to administration especially when the patient has a history of allergy to any drug.

Precautions: Drug-induced secondary adrenocortical insufficiency may be minimized by gradual reduction of dosage. This type of relative insufficiency may persist for months after discontinuation of therapy; therefore, in any situation of stress occurring during that period, hormone therapy should be reinstituted. Since mineralocorticoid secretion may be impaired, salt and/or a mineralocorticoid should be administered concurrently.

There is an enhanced effect of corticosteroids in patients with hypothyroidism and in those with cirrhosis.

Corticosteroids should be used cautiously in patients with ocular herpes simplex for fear of corneal perforation.

The lowest possible dose of corticosteroid should be used to control the condition under treatment, and when reduction in dosage is possible, the reduction must be gradual.

Psychic derangements may appear when corticosteroids are used, ranging from euphoria, insomnia, mood swings, personality changes, and severe depression to frank psychotic manifestations. Also, existing emotional instability or psychotic tendencies may be aggravated by corticosteroids.

Aspirin should be used cautiously in conjunction with corticosteroids in hypoprothrombinemia.

Steroids should be used with caution in nonspecific ulcerative colitis, if there is a probability of impending perforation, abscess or other pyogenic infection. Caution must also be used in diverticulitis, fresh intestinal anastomoses, active or latent peptic ulcer, renal insufficiency, hypertension, osteoporosis, and myasthenia gravis, when steroids are used as direct or adjunctive therapy.

Growth and development of infants and children on prolonged corticosteroid therapy should be carefully followed.

The following additional precautions apply for parenteral corticosteroids. Intra-articular injection of a corticosteroid may produce systemic as well as local effects.

Appropriate examination of any joint fluid present is necessary to exclude a septic process. A marked increase in pain accompanied by local swelling, further restriction of joint motion, fever, and malaise are suggestive of septic arthritis. If this complication occurs and the diagnosis of sepsis is confirmed, appropriate antimicrobial therapy should be instituted.

Local injection of a steroid into a previously infected joint is to be avoided.

Corticosteroids should not be injected into unstable joints.

The slower rate of absorption by intramuscular administration should be recognized.

Continued on next page

Information on these Upjohn products is based on labeling in effect on November 1, 1979. Further information on dosage and administration, side effects, precautions and contraindications for these and other Upjohn products may be obtained from either the package insert or Medical Services, The Upjohn Company, Kalamazoo, Michigan.

Upjohn—Cont.

Although controlled clinical trials have shown corticosteroids to be effective in speeding the resolution of acute exacerbations of multiple sclerosis, they do not show that corticosteroids affect the ultimate outcome or natural history of the disease. The studies do show that relatively high doses of corticosteroids are necessary to demonstrate a significant effect. (See **Dosage And Administration**).

Since complications of treatment with glucocorticoids are dependent on the size of the dose and the duration of treatment, a risk/benefit decision must be made in each individual case as to dose and duration of treatment and as to whether daily or intermittent therapy should be used.

Adverse Reactions:

Fluid and electrolyte disturbances:

Sodium retention
Fluid retention
Congestive heart failure in susceptible patients
Potassium loss
Hypokalemic alkalosis
Hypertension

Musculoskeletal:

Muscle weakness
Steroid myopathy
Loss of muscle mass
Osteoporosis
Vertebral compression fractures
Aseptic necrosis of femoral and humeral heads
Pathologic fracture of long bones

Gastrointestinal:

Peptic ulcer with possible subsequent perforation and hemorrhage
Pancreatitis
Abdominal distention
Ulcerative esophagitis

Dermatologic:

Impaired wound healing
Thin fragile skin
Petechiae and ecchymoses
Facial erythema
Increased sweating
May suppress reactions to skin tests

Neurological:

Convulsions
Increased intracranial pressure with papilledema (pseudotumor cerebri) usually after treatment
Vertigo
Headache

Endocrine:

Menstrual irregularities
Development of Cushingoid state
Suppression of growth in children
Secondary adrenocortical and pituitary unresponsiveness, particularly in times of stress, as in trauma, surgery or illness
Decreased carbohydrate tolerance
Manifestations of latent diabetes mellitus
Increased requirements for insulin or oral hypoglycemic agents in diabetes

Ophthalmic:

Posterior subcapsular cataracts
Increased intraocular pressure
Glaucoma
Exophthalmos

Metabolic:

Negative nitrogen balance due to protein catabolism

The following *additional* adverse reactions are related to parenteral corticosteroid therapy:

Rare instances of blindness associated with intralesional therapy around the face and head
Hyperpigmentation or hypopigmentation
Subcutaneous and cutaneous atrophy
Sterile abscess
Postinjection flare, following intra-articular use
Charcot-like arthropathy
Arachnoiditis has been reported following intrathecal administration

Dosage And Administration: Because of possible physical incompatibilities, *Depo-Medrol* (methylprednisolone acetate) should not be diluted or mixed with other solutions.

A. Administration for Local Effect

Therapy with *Depo-Medrol* does not obviate the need for the conventional measures usually employed. Although this method of treatment will ameliorate symptoms, it is in no sense a cure and the hormone has no effect on the cause of the inflammation.

1. Rheumatoid and Osteoarthritis. The dose for intra-articular administration depends upon the size of the joint and varies with the severity of the condition in the individual patient. In chronic cases, injections may be repeated at intervals ranging from one to five or more weeks depending upon the degree of relief obtained from the initial injection. The doses in the following table are given as a general guide:

Size of Joint	*Examples*	*Range of Dosage*
Large	Knees Ankles Shoulders	20 to 80 mg
Medium	Elbows Wrists	10 to 40 mg
Small	Metacarpophalangeal Interphalangeal Sternoclavicular Acromioclavicular	4 to 10 mg

Procedure: It is recommended that the anatomy of the joint involved suspension. reviewed before attempting intra-articular injection. In order to obtain the full anti-inflammatory effect it is important that the injection be made into the synovial space. Employing the same sterile technique as for a lumbar puncture, a sterile 20 to 24 gauge needle (on a dry syringe) is quickly inserted into the synovial cavity. Procaine infiltration is elective. The aspiration of only a few drops of joint fluid proves the joint space has been entered by the needle. *The injection site for each joint is determined by that location where the synovial cavity is most superficial and most free of large vessels and nerves.* With the needle in place, the aspirating syringe is removed and replaced by a second syringe containing the desired amount of *Depo-Medrol.* The plunger is then pulled outward slightly to aspirate synovial fluid and to make sure the needle is still in the synovial space. After injection, the joint is moved gently a few times to aid mixing of the synovial fluid and the suspension. The site is covered with a small sterile dressing.

Suitable sites for intra-articular injection are the knee, ankle, wrist, elbow, shoulder, phalangeal, and hip joints. Since difficulty is not infrequently encountered in entering the hip joint, precautions should be taken to avoid any large blood vessels in the area. Joints not suitable for injection are those that are anatomically inaccessible such as the spinal joints and those like the sacroiliac joints that are devoid of synovial space. Treatment failures are most frequently the result of failure to enter the joint space. Little or no benefit follows injection into surrounding tissue. If failures occur when injections into the synovial spaces are certain, as determined by aspiration of fluid, repeated injections are usually futile. Local therapy does not alter the underlying disease process, and whenever possible comprehensive therapy including physiotherapy and orthopedic correction should be employed.

Following intra-articular steroid therapy, care should be taken to avoid overuse of joints in which symptomatic benefit has been obtained. Negligence in this matter may permit an increase in joint deterioration that will more than offset the beneficial effects of the steroid. Unstable joints should not be injected. Repeated intra-articular injection may in some cases result in instability of the joint. X-ray follow-up is suggested in selected cases to detect deterioration.

If a local anesthetic is used prior to injection of *Depo-Medrol,* the anesthetic package insert should be read carefully and all the precautions observed.

2. Bursitis. The area around the injection site is prepared in a sterile way and a wheal at the site made with 1 percent procaine hydrochloride solution. A 20 to 24 gauge needle attached to a dry syringe is inserted into the bursa and the fluid aspirated. The needle is left in place and the aspirating syringe changed for a small syringe containing the desired dose. After injection, the needle is withdrawn and a small dressing applied.

3. Miscellaneous: Ganglion, Tendinitis, Epicondylitis. In the treatment of conditions such as tendinitis or tenosynovitis, care should be taken, following application of a suitable antiseptic to the overlying skin, to inject the suspension into the tendon sheath rather than into the substance of the tendon. The tendon may be readily palpated when placed on a stretch. When treating conditions such as epicondylitis, the area of greatest tenderness should be outlined carefully and the suspension infiltrated into the area. For ganglia of the tendon sheaths, the suspension is injected directly into the cyst. In many cases, a single injection causes a marked decrease in the size of the cystic tumor and may effect disappearance. The usual sterile precautions should be observed, of course, with each injection.

The dose in the treatment of the various conditions of the tendinous or bursal structures listed above varies with the condition being treated and ranges from 4 to 30 mg. In recurrent or chronic conditions, repeated injections may be necessary.

4. Injections for Local Effect in Dermatologic Conditions. Following cleansing with an appropriate antiseptic such as 70% alcohol, 20 to 60 mg of the suspension is injected into the lesion. It may be necessary to distribute doses ranging from 20 to 40 mg by repeated local injections in the case of large lesions. Care should be taken to avoid injection of sufficient material to cause blanching since this may be followed by a small slough. One to four injections are usually employed, the intervals between injections varying with the type of lesion being treated and the duration of improvement produced by the initial injection.

B. Administration for Systemic Effect

The intramuscular dosage will vary with the condition being treated. When employed as a temporary substitute for oral therapy, a single injection during each 24-hour period of a dose of the suspension equal to the total daily oral dose of *Medrol*® (methylprednisolone) is usually sufficient. When a prolonged effect is desired, the weekly dose may be calculated by multiplying the daily oral dose by 7 and given as a single intramuscular injection.

Dosage must be individualized according to the severity of the disease and response of the patient. For infants and children, the recommended dosage will have to be reduced, but dosage should be governed by the severity of the condition rather than by strict adherence to the ratio indicated by age or body weight.

Hormone therapy is an adjunct to, and not a replacement for, conventional therapy. Dosage must be decreased or discontinued gradually when the drug has been administered for more than a few days. The severity, prognosis and expected duration of the disease and the reaction of the patient to medication are primary factors in determining dosage. If a period of spontaneous remission occurs in a chronic condition, treatment should be discontinued. Routine laboratory studies, such as urinalysis, two-hour postprandial blood sugar, determination of blood pressure and body weight, and a chest X-ray should be made at regular intervals during prolonged therapy. Upper GI X-rays are desirable in patients with an ulcer history or significant dyspepsia.

In patients with the **adrenogenital syndrome**, a single intramuscular injection of 40 mg every two weeks may be adequate. For maintenance of patients with **rheumatoid arthritis**, the weekly intramuscular dose will vary from 40 to 120 mg. The usual dosage for patients with **dermatologic lesions** benefited by systemic corticoid therapy is 40 to 120 mg *Depo-Medrol* Sterile Aqueous Suspension administered intramuscularly at weekly intervals for one to four weeks. In acute severe dermatitis due to poison ivy, relief may result within 8 to 12 hours following intramuscular administration of a single dose of 80 to 120 mg. In chronic contact dermatitis repeated injections at 5 to 10 day intervals may be necessary. In seborrheic dermatitis, a weekly dose of 80 mg may be adequate to control the condition.

Following intramuscular administration of 80 to 120 mg to asthmatic patients, relief may result within 6 to 48 hours and persist for several days to two weeks. Similarly in patients with allergic rhinitis (hay fever) an intramuscular dose of 80 to 120 mg may be followed by relief of coryzal symptoms within six hours persisting for several days to three weeks.

If signs of stress are associated with the condition being treated, the dosage of the suspension should be increased. If a rapid hormonal effect of maximum intensity is required, the intravenous administration of highly soluble methylprednisolone sodium succinate is indicated.

Multiple Sclerosis

In treatment of acute exacerbations of multiple sclerosis daily doses of 200 mg of prednisolone for a week followed by 80 mg every other day for 1 month have been shown to be effective (4 mg of methylprednisolone is equivalent to 5 mg of prednisolone).

How Supplied: *Depo-Medrol* Sterile Aqueous Suspension (methylprednisolone acetate) is available in the following strengths and sizes:

20 mg/ml	5 ml vial	*NDC 0009-0274-01*
40 mg/ml	1 ml vial	*NDC 0009-0280-01*
	5 ml vial	*NDC 0009-0280-02*
	10 ml vial	*NDC 0009-0280-03*
80 mg/ml	1 ml vial	*NDC 0009-0306-01*
	1 ml *U-Ject®* Disposable Syringe	*NDC 0009-0306-04*
	5 ml vial	*NDC 0009-0306-02*

Code 810 341 000

[*Shown in Product Identification Section*]

DEPO-PROVERA® STERILE AQUEOUS SUSPENSION ℞

(Sterile Medroxyprogesterone Acetate Suspension, USP)

100 mg/ml
5 ml vial
NSN 6505-00-207-7965 (M)
400 mg/ml
2.5 ml vial
NSN 6505-01-059-9006 (VA)
10 ml vial
NSN 6505-01-059-9005 (VA)

WARNING

THE USE OF PROGESTATIONAL AGENTS DURING THE FIRST FOUR MONTHS OF PREGNANCY IS NOT RECOMMENDED

Progestational agents have been used beginning with the first trimester of pregnancy in an attempt to prevent habitual abortion or treat threatened abortion. There is no adequate evidence that such use is effective and there is evidence of potential harm to the fetus when such drugs are given during the first four months of pregnancy. Furthermore, in the vast majority of women, the cause of abortion is a defective ovum, which progestational agents could not be expected to influence. In addition, the use of progestational agents, with their uterine-relaxant properties, in patients with fertilized defective ova may cause a delay in spontaneous abortion. Therefore, the use of such drugs during the first four months of pregnancy is not recommended.

Several reports suggest an association between intrauterine exposure to female sex hormones and congenital anomalies, including congenital heart defects and limb reduction defects[1–5]. One study[4] estimated a 4.7-fold increased risk of limb reduction defects in infants exposed in utero to sex hormones (oral contraceptives, hormone withdrawal tests for pregnancy, or attempted treatment for threatened abortion). Some of these exposures were very short and involved only a few days of treatment. The data suggest that the risk of limb reduction defects in exposed fetuses is somewhat less than 1 in 1000.

If the patient is exposed to *Depo-Provera* Sterile Aqueous Suspension (medroxyprogesterone acetate) during the first four months of pregnancy or if she becomes pregnant while taking this drug, she should be apprised of the potential risks to the fetus.

Description: Medroxyprogesterone acetate is a derivative of progesterone and is active by the parenteral and oral routes of administration. It is a white to off-white, odorless crystalline powder, stable in air, melting between 200 and 210° C. It is freely soluble in chloroform, soluble in acetone and dioxane, sparingly soluble in alcohol and methanol, slightly soluble in ether and insoluble in water.

The chemical name for medroxyprogesterone acetate is Pregn-4-ene-3,20-dione, 17-(acetyloxy)-6-methyl-, (6α)-.

Depo-Provera (medroxyprogesterone acetate) is a sterile aqueous suspension for intramuscular injection available in 2 strengths, 100 mg/ml and 400 mg/ml medroxyprogesterone acetate.

Each ml of the **100 mg/ml** suspension contains:

Medroxyprogesterone Acetate	100 mg
Also	
Polyethylene Glycol 4000	27.6 mg
Polysorbate 80	1.84 mg
Sodium Chloride	8.3 mg
Methylparaben	1.65 mg
Propylparaben	0.18 mg
Water for Injection	qs

Each ml of the **400 mg/ml** suspension contains:

Medroxyprogesterone Acetate	400 mg
Polyethylene Glycol 4000	20.3 mg
Sodium Sulfate Anhydrous	11 mg
Myristyl-gamma-picolinium Chloride	1.7 mg
Water for Injection	qs

When necessary, pH was adjusted with sodium hydroxide and/or hydrochloric acid.

Actions: *Depo-Provera* (medroxyprogesterone acetate) administered parenterally in the recommended doses to women with adequate endogenous estrogen transforms proliferative endometrium into secretory endometrium.

Depo-Provera inhibits (in the usual dose range) the secretion of pituitary gonadotropin which, in turn, prevents follicular maturation and ovulation.

Because of its prolonged action and the resulting difficulty in predicting the time of withdrawal bleeding following injection, *Depo-Provera* is not recommended in secondary amenorrhea or dysfunctional uterine bleeding. In these conditions oral therapy is recommended.

Indications: Adjunctive therapy and palliative treatment of inoperable, recurrent, and metastatic endometrial carcinoma or renal carcinoma.

Contraindications:

1. Thrombophlebitis, thromboembolic disorders, cerebral apoplexy or patients with a past history of these conditions.
2. Carcinoma of the breast.
3. Undiagnosed vaginal bleeding.
4. Missed abortion.
5. As a diagnostic test for pregnancy.
6. Known sensitivity to *Depo-Provera* (medroxyprogesterone acetate).

Warnings:

1. The physician should be alert to the earliest manifestations of thrombotic disorders (thrombophlebitis, cerebrovascular disorders, pulmonary embolism, and retinal thrombosis). Should any of these occur or be suspected, the drug should be discontinued immediately.
2. Long term toxicology studies in the monkey, dog and rat disclose:
   1) Beagle dogs receiving 75 mg/kg and 3 mg/kg every 90 days developed mammary nodules, as did some of the control animals. The nodules appearing in the control animals were intermittent in nature, whereas the nodules in the drug treated animals were larger, more numerous, persistent, and there were two high dose animals that developed breast malignancies.
   2) Two of the monkeys receiving 150 mg/kg every 90 days developed undifferentiated carcinoma of the uterus. No uterine malignancies were found in monkeys receiving 30 mg/kg, 3 mg/kg, or placebo every 90 days. Transient mammary nodules were found during the study in the control, 3 mg/kg and 30 mg/kg groups, but not in the 150 mg/kg group. At sacrifice, the only nodules extant were in three of the monkeys in the 30 mg/kg group. Upon histopathologic examination these nodules have been determined to be hyperplastic.
   3) No uterine or breast abnormalities were revealed in the rat.

The relevance of any of these findings with respect to humans has not been established.

3. The use of *Depo-Provera* (medroxyprogesterone acetate) for contraception is investigational since there are unresolved questions relating to its safety for this indication. Therefore, this is not an approved indication.
4. Discontinue medication pending examination if there is sudden partial or complete loss of vision, or if there is a sudden onset of proptosis, diplopia or migraine. If examination reveals papilledema or retinal vascular lesions, medication should be withdrawn.
5. Usage in pregnancy (See WARNING Box).
6. Retrospective studies of morbidity and mortality in Great Britain and studies of morbidity in the United States have shown a statistically significant association between thrombophlebitis, pulmonary embolism, and cerebral thrombosis and embolism and the use of oral contraceptives.[6–9] The estimate of the relative risk of thromboembolism in the study by Vessey and

Continued on next page

Information on these Upjohn products is based on labeling in effect on November 1, 1979. Further information on dosage and administration, side effects, precautions and contraindications for these and other Upjohn products may be obtained from either the package insert or Medical Services, The Upjohn Company, Kalamazoo, Michigan.

Upjohn—Cont.

Doll[8] was about sevenfold, while Sartwell and associates[9] in the United States found a relative risk of 4.4, meaning that the users are several times as likely to undergo thromboembolic disease without evident cause as non-users. The American study also indicated that the risk did not persist after discontinuation of administration, and that it was not enhanced by long continued administration. The American study was not designed to evaluate a difference between products.

7. Following repeated injections, amenorrhea and infertility may persist for periods up to 18 months and occasionally longer.
8. The physician should be alert to the earliest manifestations of impaired liver function.

Precautions:

1. The pretreatment physical examination should include special reference to breast and pelvic organs, as well as Papanicolaou smear.
2. Because progestogens may cause some degree of fluid retention, conditions which might be influenced by this factor, such as epilepsy, migraine, asthma, cardiac or renal dysfunction, require careful observation.
3. In cases of breakthrough bleeding, as in all cases of irregular bleeding per vaginum, nonfunctional causes should be borne in mind. In cases of undiagnosed vaginal bleeding, adequate diagnostic measures are indicated.
4. Patients who have a history of psychic depression should be carefully observed and the drug discontinued if the depression recurs to a serious degree.
5. Any possible influence of prolonged progestin therapy on pituitary, ovarian, adrenal, hepatic or uterine functions awaits further study.
6. A decrease in glucose tolerance has been observed in a small percentage of patients on estrogen-progestin combination drugs. The mechanism of this decrease is obscure. For this reason, diabetic patients should be carefully observed while receiving progestin therapy.
7. The age of the patient constitutes no absolute limiting factor although treatment with progestins may mask the onset of the climacteric.
8. The pathologist should be advised of progestin therapy when relevant specimens are submitted.
9. Because of the occasional occurrence of thrombotic disorders, (thrombophlebitis, pulmonary embolism, retinal thrombosis, and cerebrovascular disorders) in patients taking estrogen-progestin combinations and since the mechanism is obscure, the physician should be alert to the earliest manifestation of these disorders.

Information for the Patient

See Patient Information at the end of the insert.

The patient insert should be given to all premenopausal women, except those in whom childbearing is impossible.

Adverse Reactions: (See WARNING Box for possible adverse effects on the fetus).

In a few instances there have been undesirable sequelae at the site of injection, such as residual lump, change in color of skin or sterile abscess.

The following adverse reactions have been associated with the use of *Depo-Provera* (medroxyprogesterone acetate).

Breast—In a few instances, breast tenderness or galactorrhea have occurred.

Psychic—An occasional patient has experienced nervousness, insomnia, somnolence, fatigue or dizziness.

Thromboembolic Phenomena—Thromboembolic phenomena including thrombophlebitis and pulmonary embolism have been reported.

Skin and Mucous Membranes—Sensitivity reactions ranging from pruritus, urticaria, angioneurotic edema to generalized rash and anaphylaxis have occasionally been reported. Acne, alopecia, or hirsutism have been reported in a few cases.

Gastrointestinal—Rarely, nausea has been reported. Jaundice, including neonatal jaundice, has been noted in a few instances.

Miscellaneous—Rare cases of headache and hyperpyrexia have been reported.

The following adverse reactions have been observed in women taking progestins including *Depo-Provera:*

breakthrough bleeding
spotting
change in menstrual flow
amenorrhea
edema
change in weight
(increase or decrease)
changes in cervical erosion and
cervical secretions
cholestatic jaundice
rash (allergic) with and
without pruritus
melasma or chloasma
mental depression

A statistically significant association has been demonstrated between use of estrogen-progestin combination drugs and the following serious adverse reactions: thrombophlebitis; pulmonary embolism and cerebral thrombosis and embolism. For this reason patients on progestin therapy should be carefully observed.

Although available evidence is suggestive of an association, such a relationship has been neither confirmed nor refuted for the following serious adverse reactions: neuro-ocular lesions, eg, retinal thrombosis and optic neuritis.

The following adverse reactions have been observed in patients receiving estrogen-progestin combination drugs:

rise in blood pressure in susceptible individuals
premenstrual-like syndrome
changes in libido
changes in appetite
cystitis-like syndrome
headache
nervousness
dizziness
fatigue
backache
hirsutism
loss of scalp hair
erythema multiforme
erythema nodosum
hemorrhagic eruption
itching

In view of these observations, patients on progestin therapy should be carefully observed.

The following laboratory results may be altered by the use of estrogen-progestin combination drugs:

Increased sulfobromophthalein retention and other hepatic function tests.
Coagulation tests: increase in prothrombin factors VII, VIII, IX and X.
Metyrapone test.
Pregnanediol determination.
Thyroid function: increase in PBI, and butanol extractable protein bound iodine and decrease in T^3 uptake values.

Dosage and Administration: The suspension is intended for intramuscular administration only.

Endometrial or renal carcinoma—doses of 400 mg to 1000 mg of *Depo-Provera* (medroxyprogesterone acetate) per week are recommended initially. If improvement is noted within a few weeks or months and the disease appears stabilized, it may be possible to maintain improvement with as little as 400 mg per month. Medroxyprogesterone acetate is not recommended as primary therapy, but as adjunctive and palliative treatment in advanced inoperable cases including those with recurrent or metastatic disease.

How Supplied: *Depo-Provera* sterile aqueous suspension (medroxyprogesterone acetate) is available in 2 strengths:

100 mg/ml:	
5 ml vials	NDC 0009-0248-02
400 mg/ml:	
1 ml unit dose	
U-ject® Disposable Syringe	NDC 0009-0626-03
2.5 ml vial	NDC 0009-0626-01
10 ml vial	NDC 0009-0626-02

References:

1. Gal I, Kirman B, Stern J: Hormonal pregnancy tests and congenital malformation. Nature *216*:83, 1967.
2. Levy EP, Cohen A, Fraser FC: Hormone treatment during pregnancy and congenital heart defects. Lancet *1*:611, 1973.
3. Nora JJ, Nora AH: Birth defects and oral contraceptives. Lancet *1*:941–942, 1973.
4. Janerich DT, Piper JM, Glebatis DM: Oral contraceptives and congenital limb-reduction defects. N Engl J Med *291*:697–700, 1974.
5. Heinonen OP, Slone D, Monson RR, et al: Cardiovascular birth defects and antenatal exposure to female sex hormones. N Engl J Med *296*:67–70, 1977.
6. Royal College of General Practitioners: Oral contraception and thromboembolic disease. J Coll Gen Pract *13*:267–279, 1967.
7. Inman WHW, Vessey MP: Investigation of deaths from pulmonary, coronary, and cerebral thrombosis and embolism in women of child-bearing age. Br Med J *2*:193–199, 1968.
8. Vessey MP, Doll R: Investigation of relation between use of oral contraceptives and thromboembolic disease. A further report. Br Med J *2*:651–657, 1969.
9. Sartwell PE, Masi AT, Arthes FG, et al: Thromboembolism and oral contraceptives: An epidemiological case-control study. Am J Epidemiol *90*:365–380, 1969.

The text of the patient insert for progesterone and progesterone-like drugs is set forth below.

Patient Information: *Depo-Provera* Sterile Aqueous Suspension contains a progesterone (medroxyprogesterone acetate). The information below is that which the U.S. Food and Drug Administration requires be provided for all patients taking progesterones. The information below relates only to the risk to the unborn child associated with use of progesterone during pregnancy. For further information on the use, side effects and other risks associated with this product, ask your doctor.

WARNING FOR WOMEN

There is an increased risk of birth defects in children whose mothers take this drug during the first four months of pregnancy.

Medroxyprogesterone acetate is similar to the progesterone hormones naturally produced by the body. Progesterone and progesterone-like drugs are used to treat menstrual disorders, to test if the body is producing certain hormones, and to treat some forms of cancer in women. They have been used as a test for pregnancy but such use is no longer considered safe because of possible damage to a developing baby. Also, more rapid methods for testing for pregnancy are now available.

These drugs have also been used to prevent miscarriage in the first few months of pregnancy. No adequate evidence is available to show that they are effective for this purpose. Furthermore, most cases of early miscarriage are due to causes which could not be helped by these drugs.

There is an increased risk of birth defects, such as heart or limb defects, if progesterone and

progesterone-like drugs are taken during the first four months of pregnancy.
The exact risk of taking this drug early in pregnancy and having a baby with a birth defect is not known. However, one study found that babies born to women who had taken sex hormones (such as progesterone-like drugs) during the first three months of pregnancy were 4 to 5 times more likely to have abnormalities of the arms or legs than if their mothers had not taken such drugs. Some of these women had taken these drugs for only a few days. The chance that an infant whose mother had taken this drug will have this type of defect is about 1 in 1,000.
If you take *Depo-Provera* Sterile Aqueous Suspension and later find you were pregnant when you took it, be sure to discuss this with your doctor as soon as possible.
Code 810 597 000

DEPO®-TESTOSTERONE ℞
STERILE SOLUTION
(Testosterone Cypionate Injection, USP)
For Intramuscular Use Only

How Supplied: *Depo*-Testosterone Sterile Solution is available in the following packages:
50 mg per ml. Each ml contains 50 mg testosterone cypionate, also 5 mg chlorobutanol anhydrous (chloral deriv.), in 874 mg cottonseed oil with 0.1% oxystearin.
10 ml vial *NDC 0009-0303-01*
100 mg per ml. Each ml contains 100 mg testosterone cypionate, also 9 mg benzyl alcohol, in 828 mg cottonseed oil with 0.1% oxystearin.
1 ml vial *NDC 0009-0347-01*
10 ml vial *NDC 0009-0347-02*
200 mg per ml. Each ml contains 200 mg testosterone cypionate, also 0.2 ml benzyl benzoate, 9 mg benzyl alcohol, in 560 mg cottonseed oil with 0.1% oxystearin.
1 ml vial *NDC 0009-0417-01*
10 ml vial *NDC 0009-0417-02*

DIDREX™ TABLETS Ⓒ ℞
(benzphetamine hydrochloride tablets)

Description: Benzphetamine hydrochloride is d-N-benzyl-N, α-dimethylphenethylamine hydrochloride, a white crystalline powder readily soluble in water, 95% ethanol and chloroform.
Actions: *Didrex* Tablets (benzphetamine hydrochloride) are a sympathomimetic amine with pharmacologic activity similar to the prototype drugs of this class used in obesity, the amphetamines. Actions include central nervous system stimulation and elevation of blood pressure. Tachyphylaxis and tolerance have been demonstrated with all drugs of this class in which these phenomena have been looked for.
Drugs of this class used in obesity are commonly known as "anorectics" or "anorexigenics." It has not been established, however, that the action of such drugs in treating obesity is primarily one of appetite suppression. Other central nervous system actions, or metabolic effects, may be involved, for example.
Adult obese subjects instructed in dietary management and treated with "anorectic" drugs, lose more weight on the average than those treated with placebo and diet, as determined in relatively short term clinical trials.
The magnitude of increased weight loss of drug treated patients over placebo treated patients is only a fraction of a pound a week. The rate of weight loss is greatest in the first weeks of therapy for both drug and placebo subjects and tends to decrease in succeeding weeks. The possible origins of the increased weight loss due to the various drug effects are not established. The amount of weight loss associated with the use of an "anorectic" drug varies from trial to trial, and the increased weight loss appears to be related in part to variables other than the drug prescribed, such as the physician-investigator, the population treated, and the diet prescribed. Studies do not permit conclusions as to the relative importance of the drug and nondrug factors on weight loss.
The natural history of obesity is measured in years, whereas the studies cited are restricted to a few weeks duration; thus, the total impact of drug induced weight loss over that of diet alone must be considered clinically limited.
Indications: *Didrex* (benzphetamine hydrochloride) is indicated in the management of exogenous obesity as a short term adjunct (a few weeks) in a regimen of weight reduction based on caloric restriction. The limited usefulness of agents of this class (see **Actions**) should be measured against possible risk factors inherent in their use such as those described above.
Contraindications: *Didrex* (benzphetamine hydrochloride) is contraindicated in patients with advanced arteriosclerosis, symptomatic cardiovascular disease, moderate to severe hypertension, hyperthyroidism, known hypersensitivity or idiosyncrasy to sympathomimetic amines, and agitated states, and in patients with a history of drug abuse.
Hypertensive crises have resulted when sympathomimetic amines have been used concomitantly or within 14 days following use of monamine oxidase inhibitors. *Didrex* should not be used concomitantly with other CNS stimulants.
Warnings:
Drug Dependence: *Didrex* (benzphetamine hydrochloride) is related chemically and pharmacologically to the amphetamines. Amphetamines and related stimulant drugs have been extensively abused, and the possibility of abuse of *Didrex* should be kept in mind when evaluating the desirability of including a drug as part of a weight reduction program. Abuse of amphetamines and related drugs may be associated with intense psychological dependence and severe social dysfunction. There are reports of patients who have increased the dosage to many times that recommended. Abrupt cessation following prolonged high dosage administration results in extreme fatigue and mental depression; changes are also noted on the sleep EEG. Manifestations of chronic intoxication with anorectic drugs include severe dermatoses, marked insomnia, irritability, hyperactivity, and personality changes. The most severe manifestation of chronic intoxication is psychosis, often clinically indistinguishable from schizophrenia.
Usage in Pregnancy—Safe use in pregnancy has not been established. Reproductive studies in mammals at high multiples of the human dose on some anorectic drugs have suggested both an embryotoxic and a teratogenic potential for this type of drug. Therefore, use of *Didrex* by women who are or who may become pregnant, and especially those in the first trimester of pregnancy, requires that the potential benefit be weighed against the possible hazard to mother and infant.
Usage in Children—Use of benzphetamine hydrochloride is not recommended in children under 12 years of age.
Precautions: Insulin requirements in diabetes mellitus may be altered in association with use of anorexigenic drugs and the concomitant dietary restrictions.
Psychological disturbances have been reported in patients who receive an anorectic agent together with a restrictive dietary regimen.
Didrex Tablets, 25 mg, contain FD&C Yellow No. 5 (tartrazine) which may cause allergic-type reactions (including bronchial asthma) in certain susceptible individuals. Although the overall incidence of FD&C Yellow No. 5 (tartrazine) sensitivity in the general population is low, it is frequently seen in patients who also have aspirin hypersensitivity.
Adverse Reactions: The following have been associated with the use of benzphetamine hydrochloride:
Overstimulation, restlessness, dizziness, insomnia, gastrointestinal disturbances, nausea, diarrhea, palpitation, tachycardia, elevation of blood pressure, tremor, sweating, headache, dryness of the mouth or unpleasant taste, urticaria and other allergic reactions involving the skin, changes in libido; rarely, psychotic episodes at recommended dosage; depression following withdrawal of drug.
Dosage and Administration: Dosage should be individualized according to the response of the patient. The suggested dosage ranges from 25 to 50 mg one to three times daily. Treatment should begin with 25 to 50 mg once daily with subsequent increase in individual dose or frequency according to response. A single daily dose is preferably given in mid-morning or mid-afternoon, according to the patient's eating habits. In an occasional patient it may be desirable to avoid late afternoon administration. Use of benzphetamine hydrochloride is not recommended in children under 12 years of age.
Treatment of Overdosage: (See **Warnings**) Information concerning the effects of overdosage with *Didrex* (benzphetamine hydrochloride) is extremely limited. The following is based on experience with other anorexiants.
Management of acute amphetamine intoxication is largely symptomatic and includes sedation with a barbiturate. If hypertension is marked the use of a nitrite or rapidly acting alpha receptor blocking agent should be considered. Experience with hemodialysis or peritoneal dialysis is inadequate to permit recommendations in this regard.
How Supplied: *Didrex* Tablets (benzphetamine hydrochloride) are available as press-coated tablets in 2 strengths:
25 mg (unscored)
Bottles of 100 *NDC 0009-0018-01*
50 mg (scored)
Bottles of 100 *NDC 0009-0024-01*
Bottles of 500 *NDC 0009-0024-02*
Code 810 735 000
[*Shown in Product Identification Section*]

E-MYCIN® TABLETS ℞
(erythromycin enteric-coated tablets)
Each tablet contains 250 mg of erythromycin as the free base

Description: Erythromycin is produced by a strain of *Streptomyces erythraeus* and belongs to the macrolide group of antibiotics. It is basic and readily forms salts with acids. The base is a white to off-white crystals or powder slightly soluble in water, soluble in alcohol, in chloroform, and in ether. *E-Mycin* Tablets (erythromycin enteric-coated tablets) are specially coated to protect the contents from the inactivating effects of gastric acidity and to permit efficient absorption of the antibiotic in the small intestine.
Actions: The mode of action of erythromycin is inhibition of protein synthesis without affecting nucleic acid synthesis. Resistance to erythromycin of some strains of *Haemophilus influenzae* and staphylococci has been demonstrated. Culture and susceptibility testing should be done. If the Kirby-Bauer method of disk susceptibility is used, a 15 mcg erythromycin disk should give a zone diameter of at least 18 mm when tested against an erythromycin susceptible organism.

Continued on next page

Information on these Upjohn products is based on labeling in effect on November 1, 1979. Further information on dosage and administration, side effects, precautions and contraindications for these and other Upjohn products may be obtained from either the package insert or Medical Services, The Upjohn Company, Kalamazoo, Michigan.

Upjohn—Cont.

Bioavailability data are available from The Upjohn Company.
E-Mycin (erythromycin enteric-coated tablets) is well absorbed and may be given without regard to meals.
After absorption, erythromycin diffuses readily into most body fluids. In the absence of meningeal inflammation, low concentrations are normally achieved in the spinal fluid but passage of the drug across the blood-brain barrier increases in meningitis. In the presence of normal hepatic function, erythromycin is concentrated in the liver and excreted in the bile; the effect of hepatic dysfunction on excretion of erythromycin by the liver into the bile is not known. After oral administration, less than 5 percent of the activity of the administered dose can be recovered in the urine.
Erythromycin crosses the placental barrier but fetal plasma levels are low.
Indications:
Streptococcus pyogenes (Group A beta hemolytic streptococcus): For upper and lower respiratory tract, skin, and soft tissue infections of mild to moderate severity.
Injectable benzathine penicillin G is considered by the American Heart Association to be the drug of choice in the treatment and prevention of streptococcal pharyngitis and in long-term prophylaxis of rheumatic fever.
When oral medication is preferred for treatment of the above conditions, penicillin G, V, or erythromycin are alternate drugs of choice.
When oral medication is given, the importance of strict adherence by the patient to the prescribed dosage regimen must be stressed. A therapeutic dose should be administered for at least 10 days.
Alpha-hemolytic streptococci (viridans group): For short-term prophylaxis of bacterial endocarditis prior to dental or other operative procedures in patients with a history of rheumatic fever or congenital heart disease who are hypersensitive to penicillin. (Erythromycin is not suitable prior to genitourinary surgery where the organisms likely to lead to bacteremia are gram-negative bacilli or the enterococcus group of streptococci.)
Staphylococcus aureus: For acute infections of skin and soft tissue of mild to moderate severity. Resistant organisms may emerge during treatment.
Streptococcus pneumoniae (Diplococcus pneumoniae): For upper respiratory tract infections (eg, otitis media, pharyngitis) and lower respiratory tract infections (eg, pneumonia) of mild to moderate degree.
Mycoplasma pneumoniae (Eaton agent, PPLO): For respiratory infections due to this organism.
Hemophilus influenzae: For upper respiratory tract infections of mild to moderate severity when used concomitantly with adequate doses of sulfonamides. Not all strains of this organism are susceptible at the erythromycin concentrations ordinarily achieved (see appropriate sulfonamide labeling for prescribing information).
Treponema pallidum: Erythromycin is an alternate choice of treatment for primary syphilis in patients allergic to the penicillins. In treatment of primary syphilis, spinal fluid examinations should be done before treatment and as part of follow-up after therapy.
Corynebacterium diphtheriae and **C. minutissimum:** As an adjunct to antitoxin, to prevent establishment of carriers, and to eradicate the organism in carriers.
In the treatment of erythrasma.
Entamoeba histolytica: In the treatment of intestinal amebiasis only. Extraenteric amebiasis requires treatment with other agents.
Listeria monocytogenes: Infections due to this organism.
Neisseria gonorrhoeae: Erythromycin lactobionate for injection in conjunction with erythromycin base orally, as an alternative drug in treatment of acute pelvic inflammatory disease caused by *N. gonorrhoeae* in female patients with a history of sensitivity to penicillin. Before treatment of gonorrhea, patients who are suspected of also having syphilis should have a microscopic examination for *T. pallidum* (by immunofluorescence or darkfield) before receiving erythromycin, and monthly serologic tests for a minimum of 4 months.
Legionnaires Disease: Although no controlled clinical efficacy studies have been conducted, *in vitro* and limited preliminary clinical data suggest that erythromycin can be effective in treating Legionnaires Disease.
Contraindications: Erythromycin is contraindicated in patients with known hypersensitivity to this antibiotic.
Warning: Usage in pregnancy: Safety for use in pregnancy has not been established.
Precautions: Erythromycin is principally excreted by the liver. Caution should be exercised in administering the antibiotic to patients with impaired hepatic function.
There have been reports of hepatic dysfunction, with or without jaundice, occurring in patients receiving oral erythromycin products.
Recent data from studies of erythromycin reveal that its use in patients who are receiving high doses of theophylline may be associated with an increase of serum theophylline levels and potential theophylline toxicity. In cases of theophylline toxicity and/or elevated serum theophylline levels, the dose of theophylline should be reduced while the patient is receiving concomitant erythromycin therapy.
Surgical procedures should be performed when indicated.
Adverse Reactions: The most frequent side effects of erythromycin preparations are gastrointestinal, such as abdominal cramping and discomfort, and are dose related. Nausea, vomiting, and diarrhea occur infrequently with usual oral doses.
During prolonged or repeated therapy, there is a possibility of overgrowth of nonsusceptible bacteria or fungi. If such infections occur, the drug should be discontinued and appropriate therapy instituted.
Mild allergic reactions such as urticaria and other skin rashes have occurred. Serious allergic reactions, including anaphylaxis, have been reported.
Dosage and Administration: *E-Mycin* Tablets (erythromycin enteric-coated tablets) are well absorbed when given orally immediately after meals or between meals on an empty stomach.
Adults: The usual dose is 250 mg four times daily.
If twice a day dosage is desired, the recommended dose is 500 mg every 12 hours.
Dosage may be increased up to 4 or more grams per day according to the severity of the infection. Twice-a-day dosing is not recommended when doses larger than 1 gram daily are administered.
Children: Age, weight, and severity of the infection are important factors in determining the proper dosage. 30 to 50 mg/kg/day, in divided doses, is the usual dose. For more severe infections, this dose may be doubled.
In the treatment of streptococcal infections, a therapeutic dosage of erythromycin should be administered for at least 10 days. In continuous **prophylaxis** of streptococcal infections in persons with a history of rheumatic heart disease, the dose is 250 mg twice a day.
When used prior to surgery to prevent endocarditis (see **Alpha-hemolytic streptococci**), the American Heart Association recommended schedule for adults is: 1 gram orally 1½–2 hours prior to the procedure and then 500 mg orally every 6 hours for 8 doses. For children: 20 mg/kg orally 1½–2 hours prior to the procedure and then 10 mg/kg every 6 hours for 8 doses.
For treatment of primary syphilis: 30 to 40 grams given in divided doses over a period of 10 to 15 days.
For treatment of acute pelvic inflammatory disease caused by *N. gonorrhoeae:* After initial treatment with erythromycin lactobionate for injection (500 mg every 6 hours for 3 days), the oral dosage recommendation is 250 mg every 6 hours for 7 days.
For dysenteric amebiasis: 250 mg four times daily for 10 to 14 days, for adults; 30 to 50 mg/kg/day in divided doses for 10 to 14 days, for children.
For treatment of Legionnaires Disease: Although optimal doses have not been established, doses utilized in reported clinical data were those recommended above (1 to 4 grams erythromycin base daily in divided doses).
Treatment of Overdosage: The drug is virtually nontoxic, though some individuals may exhibit gastric intolerance to even therapeutic amounts. Allergic reactions associated with acute overdosage should be handled in the usual manner—that is, by the administration of adrenalin, corticosteroids, and antihistamines as indicated and the prompt elimination of unabsorbed drug, in addition to all needed supportive measures.
How Supplied: Enteric-coated tablets containing 250 mg erythromycin in the following packages:

Bottles of 100	*NDC 0009-0103-02*
Bottles of 500	*NDC 0009-0103-15*
Unit dose packages (100)	*NDC 0009-0103-03*

Code 810 386 000
[*Shown in Product Identification Section*]

E-MYCIN E™ LIQUID ℞
(erythromycin ethylsuccinate oral suspension)

Description: Erythromycin is produced by a strain of *Streptomyces erythraeus* and belongs to the macrolide group of antibiotics. It is basic and readily forms salts with acids. The base, the stearate salt, and the esters are poorly soluble in water. Erythromycin ethylsuccinate is an ester of erythromycin suitable for oral administration.
The pleasant tasting oral suspensions are supplied ready for oral administration. The ready made suspensions are intended primarily for pediatric use but can also be used in adults.
Actions: The mode of action of erythromycin is by inhibition of protein synthesis without affecting nucleic acid synthesis. Resistance to erythromycin of some strains of *Haemophilus influenzae* and staphylococci has been demonstrated. Culture and susceptibility testing should be done. If the Kirby-Bauer method of disk susceptibility is used, a 15 mcg erythromycin disk should give a zone diameter of at least 18 mm when tested against an erythromycin susceptible organism.
Orally administered erythromycin ethylsuccinate suspensions are readily and reliably absorbed. Comparable serum levels of erythromycin are achieved in the fasting and nonfasting states.
After absorption, erythromycin diffuses readily into most body fluids. In the absence of meningeal inflammation low concentrations are normally achieved in the spinal fluid, but passage of the drug across the blood-brain barrier increases in meningitis. In the presence of normal hepatic function, erythromycin is concentrated in the liver and excreted in the bile; the effect of hepatic dysfunction on excretion of erythromycin by the liver into the bile is not known. After oral administration, less than five percent of the activity of the administered dose can be recovered in the urine.
Erythromycin crosses the placental barrier but fetal plasma levels are generally low.
Indications:
Streptococcus pyogenes (Group A beta-hemolytic streptococcus): Upper and lower respira-

tory tract, skin, and soft tissue infections of mild to moderate severity.
Injectable benzathine penicillin G is considered by the American Heart Association to be the drug of choice in the treatment and prevention of streptococcal pharyngitis and in long-term prophylaxis of rheumatic fever.
When oral medication is preferred for treatment of the above conditions, penicillin G, V or erythromycin are alternate drugs of choice.
When oral medication is given, the importance of strict adherence by the patient to the prescribed dosage regimen must be stressed. A therapeutic dose should be administered for at least ten days.
Alpha-hemolytic streptococci (viridans group): Short-term prophylaxis of bacterial endocarditis prior to dental or other operative procedures in patients with a history of rheumatic fever or congenital heart disease who are hypersensitive to penicillin. (Erythromycin is not suitable prior to genitourinary surgery where the organisms likely to lead to bacteremia are gram-negative bacilli or the enterococcus group of streptococci.)
Staphylococcus aureus: Acute infections of skin and soft tissue of mild to moderate severity. Resistant organisms may emerge during treatment.
Steptococcus pneumoniae (Diplococcus pneumoniae): Upper respiratory tract infections (eg, otitis media, pharyngitis) and lower respiratory tract infections (eg, pneumonia) of mild to moderate degree.
Mycoplasma pneumoniae (Eaton agent, PPLO): For respiratory infections due to this organism.
Haemophilus influenzae: For upper respiratory tract infections of mild to moderate severity when used concomitantly with adequate doses of sulfonamides. Not all strains of this organism are susceptible at the erythromycin concentrations ordinarily achieved (see appropriate sulfonamide labeling for prescribing information).
Treponema pallidum: Erythromycin is an alternate choice of treatment for primary syphilis in patients allergic to the penicillins. In treatment of primary syphilis, spinal fluid examinations should be done before treatment and as part of followup after therapy.
Corynebacterium diphtheriae and *C. minutissimum:* As an adjunct to antitoxin, to prevent establishment of carriers, and to eradicate the organism in carriers.
In the treatment of erythrasma.
Entamoeba histolytica: In the treatment of intestinal amebiasis only. Extraenteric amebiasis requires treatment with other agents.
Listeria monocytogenes: Infections due to this organism.
Legionnaires' Disease: Although no controlled clinical efficacy studies have been conducted, *in vitro* and limited preliminary clinical data suggest that erythromycin may be effective in treating Legionnaires' Disease.
Contraindications: Erythromycin is contraindicated in patients with known hypersensitivity to this antibiotic.
Warnings: Usage in pregnancy: Safety for use in pregnancy has not been established.
Precautions: Erythromycin is principally excreted by the liver. Caution should be exercised in administering the antibiotic to patients with impaired hepatic function.
There have been reports of hepatic dysfunction, with or without jaundice, occurring in patients receiving oral erythromycin products. Recent data from studies of erythromycin reveal that its use in patients who are receiving high doses of theophylline may be associated with an increase of serum theophylline levels and potential theophylline toxicity. In cases of theophylline toxicity and/or elevated serum theophylline levels, the dose of theophylline should be reduced while the patient is receiving concomitant erythromycin therapy.

Surgical procedures should be performed when indicated.
Adverse Reactions: The most frequent side effects of erythromycin preparations are gastrointestinal, such as abdominal cramping and discomfort, and are dose related. Nausea, vomiting, and diarrhea occur infrequently with usual oral doses.
Mild allergic reactions such as urticaria and other skin rashes have occurred. Serious allergic reactions, including anaphylaxis, have been reported.
Dosage and Administration: *E-Mycin E* Liquid (erythromycin ethylsuccinate oral suspension) may be administered without regard to meals.
Children: Age, weight, and severity of the infection are important factors in determining the proper dosage. In mild to moderate infections the usual dosage of *E-Mycin E* for children is 30 to 50 mg/kg/day in equally divided doses. For more severe infections this dosage may be doubled.
The following dosage schedule is suggested for mild to moderate infections:

BODY WEIGHT	TOTAL DAILY DOSE
Under 10 lbs	30–50 mg/kg/day 15–25 mg/lb/day
10 to 15 lbs	200 mg
16 to 25 lbs	400 mg
26 to 50 lbs	800 mg
51 to 100 lbs	1200 mg
over 100 lbs	1600 mg

Adults: 400 mg *E-Mycin E* every six hours is the usual dose. Dosage may be increased up to 4 grams per day according to the severity of the infection.
If twice-a-day dosage is desired in either adults or children, one-half of the total daily dose may be given every 12 hours.
In the treatment of streptococcal infections, a therapeutic dosage of erythromycin ethylsuccinate should be administered for at least 10 days. In continuous prophylaxis against recurrences of streptococcal infections in persons with a history of rheumatic heart disease, the usual dosage is 400 mg twice a day.
When used prior to surgery to prevent endocarditis (see *Alpha-hemolytic streptococci),* a recommended schedule for adults is 800 mg *E-Mycin E* before the procedure and 400 mg every 6 hours for 4 doses after the procedure. For small children, 30 to 50 mg/kg/day divided into 3 or 4 evenly spaced doses.
For treatment of primary syphilis: Adults: 48 to 64 grams given in divided doses over a period of 10 to 14 days.
For intestinal amebiasis: Adults: 400 mg four times daily for 10 to 14 days. Children: 30 to 50 mg/kg/day in divided doses for 10 to 14 days.
For treatment of Legionnaires' Disease: Although optimal doses have not been established, doses utilized in reported clinical data were those recommended above (1 to 4 grams daily in divided doses).
How Supplied: *E-Mycin E* Liquid (erythromycin ethylsuccinate oral suspension) is supplied in the following sizes:

200 mg/5 ml	500 ml bottle NDC 0009-0939-01
400 mg/5 ml	500 ml bottle NDC 0009-0940-01

Each 5 ml (one teaspoonful) contains erythromycin ethylsuccinate equivalent to erythromycin 200 mg or 400 mg. Preserved with methylparaben.
Store in a refrigerator to preserve taste until dispensed. Refrigeration by patient is not required if used within 14 days.

Code NOF-1
[*Shown in Product Identification Section*]

FLORONE® CREAM 0.05% ℞
(diflorasone diacetate)

Description: Each gram of *Florone* Cream (diflorasone diacetate) contains 0.5 mg diflorasone diacetate in a cream base.
Chemically, diflorasone diacetate is: 6α, 9α-difluoro-11β, 17, 21-trihydroxy-16β-methylpregna-1,4-diene-3,20-dione 17,21 diacetate.
Florone Cream contains diflorasone diacetate in an emulsified and hydrophilic cream base consisting of propylene glycol, stearic acid, polyoxyethylene 20 sorbitan monostearate, sorbitan monostearate and monooleate, sorbic acid, citric acid and water. The corticosteroid is formulated as a solution in the vehicle using 15 percent propylene glycol to optimize drug delivery.
Actions: *Florone* Cream (diflorasone diacetate) is effective because of its anti-inflammatory, antipruritic and vasoconstrictor action.
Indications: *Florone* Cream (diflorasone diacetate) is intended for topical use as adjunctive therapy for the relief of inflammatory manifestations of acute and chronic corticosteroid-responsive dermatoses.
Contraindications: Topical steroids are contraindicated in vaccinia and varicella. Topical steroids are contraindicated in those patients with a history of hypersensitivity to any of the components of the preparation.
Precautions: If irritation develops, the cream should be discontinued and appropriate therapy instituted.
In the presence of an infection, the use of an appropriate antifungal or antibacterial agent should be instituted. If a favorable response does not occur promptly, the corticosteroid cream should be discontinued until the infection has been adequately controlled.
If extensive areas are treated, the possibility exists of increased systemic absorption and suitable precautions should be taken.
Although topical steroids have not been reported to have an adverse effect on human pregnancy, the safety of their use in pregnant women has not been absolutely established. Studies in rats show increased numbers of fetal abnormalities in groups treated with topical corticosteroids. Therefore, they should not be used extensively in pregnant patients, in large amounts or for prolonged periods of time.
Occlusive Dressing Technique—The use of occlusive dressing increases the percutaneous absorption of corticosteroids; their extensive use increases the possibility of systemic effects. For patients with extensive lesions it may be preferable to use a sequential approach, occluding one portion of the body at a time. The patient should be kept under close observation if treated with the occlusive technique over large areas and over a considerable period of time. Occasionally, a patient who has been on prolonged therapy, especially occlusive therapy, may develop symptoms of steroid withdrawal when the medication is stopped. Thermal homeostatis may be impaired if large areas of the body are covered. Use of the occlusive dressing should be discontinued if elevation of the body temperature occurs. Occasionally, a patient may develop a sensitivity reaction to a particular occlusive dressing material or adhesive and a substitute material may be

Continued on next page

Information on these Upjohn products is based on labeling in effect on November 1, 1979. Further information on dosage and administration, side effects, precautions and contraindications for these and other Upjohn products may be obtained from either the package insert or Medical Services, The Upjohn Company, Kalamazoo, Michigan.

Upjohn—Cont.

necessary. If infection develops, discontinue the use of the occlusive dressing and institute appropriate antimicrobial therapy.
Florone Cream (diflorasone diacetate) is not for ophthalmic use.
Adverse Reactions: The following adverse reactions have been reported with topical corticosteroids: burning, itching, irritation, striae, skin atrophy, secondary infection, dryness, folliculitis, hypertrichosis, acneiform eruptions and hypopigmentation. The following may occur more frequently with occlusive dressings: maceration of the skin, secondary infection, skin atrophy, striae, and miliaria.
Dosage and Administration: A small amount of cream should be gently massaged into the affected area two to four times daily, as needed.
How Supplied: *Florone* Cream 0.05% (diflorasone diacetate), is available in 15, 30 and 60 gram tubes.

15 gram tube	NDC 0009-0199-07
30 gram tube	NDC 0009-0199-03
60 gram tube	NDC 0009-0199-05

Code 810 471 000
[*Shown in Product Identification Section*]

FLORONE® OINTMENT, 0.05% ℞
(diflorasone diacetate)

Description: Each gram of *Florone* Ointment (diflorasone diacetate) contains 0.5 mg diflorasone diacetate in an ointment base:
Chemically, diflorasone diacetate is: 6α,9α-difluoro 11β, 17, 21 trihydroxy-16β methylpregna-1,4-diene-3,20-dione 17,21 diacetate.
Florone ointment contains 0.5 mg/gram of diflorasone diacetate in an emollient, occlusive base consisting of polyoxypropylene 15-stearyl ether, stearic acid, lanolin alcohol and white petrolatum.
Actions: *Florone* Ointment (diflorasone diacetate) is effective because of its anti-inflammatory, antipruritic and vasoconstrictor actions.
Indications: *Florone* Ointment (diflorasone diacetate) is intended for topical use as adjunctive therapy for the relief of inflammatory manifestations of corticosteroid-responsive dermatoses.
Contraindications: Topical steroids are contraindicated in vaccinia and varicella and in those patients with a history of hypersensitivity to any of the components of the preparations. *Florone* Ointment (diflorasone diacetate) is not for ophthalmic use.
Precautions: If irritation develops, the ointment should be discontinued and appropriate therapy instituted.
In the presence of an infection, the use of an appropriate anti-fungal or anti-bacterial agent should be instituted. If a favorable response does not occur promptly, the corticosteroid ointment should be discontinued until the infection has been adequately controlled.
If extensive areas are treated, the possibility exists of increased systemic absorption and suitable precautions should be taken.
Although topical steroids have not been reported to have an adverse effect on pregnancy, the safety of their use in pregnant females has not been absolutely established. Studies in rats show increased numbers of fetal abnormalities in groups treated with topical corticosteroids. Therefore, they should not be used extensively on pregnant patients, in large amounts or for prolonged periods of time.
Adverse Reactions: The following adverse reactions have been reported with topical corticosteroids: burning, itching, irritation, striae, skin atrophy, secondary infection, dryness, folliculitis, hypertrichosis, acneiform eruptions, and hypopigmentation. The following may occur more frequently with occlusive dressings: maceration of the skin, secondary infection, skin atrophy, striae, and miliaria.
Dosage and Administration: Apply a thin film of *Florone* Ointment (diflorasone diacetate) to the affected skin areas one to three times a day.
Occlusive Dressing Technique
The use of occlusive dressings increases the percutaneous absorption of corticosteroids; their extensive use increases the possibility of systemic effects. For patients with extensive lesions it may be preferable to use a sequential approach, occluding one portion of the body at a time. The patient should be kept under close observation if treated with occlusive technique over large areas and over a considerable period of time. Occasionally, a patient who has been on prolonged therapy, especially occlusive therapy, may develop symptoms of steroid withdrawal when the medication is stopped. Thermal homeostasis may be impaired if large areas of the body are covered. Use of the occlusive dressing should be discontinued if elevation of the body temperature occurs. Occasionally, a patient may develop a sensitivity reaction to a particular occlusive dressing material or adhesive and a substitute material may be necessary. If infection develops, discontinue the use of the occlusive dressing and institute appropriate antimicrobial therapy.
How Supplied: *Florone* Ointment (diflorasone diacetate) 0.05% is supplied in 15, 30 and 60 gram tubes.

15 gram tube	NDC 0009-0917-01
30 gram tube	NDC 0009-0917-02
60 gram tube	NDC 0009-0917-03

Code 810 462 000
[*Shown in Product Identification Section*]

GELFOAM® STERILE SPONGE (ABSORBABLE GELATIN SPONGE, USP)

Size 12-7 mm:
NSN 6510-00-080-2053 (M)
Size 100:
NSN 6510-00-080-2054 (M)
Dental Packs, Size 4:
NSN 6510-00-064-4858 (M)

How Supplied: ***Gelfoam* Sterile Sponge (Absorbable Gelatin Sponge, USP)** is available as:
Size 12-3 mm. Each measures 20 x 60 x 3 mm, packaged in boxes containing 4 individually wrapped sponges.
NDC 0009-0301-01
Size 12-7 mm. Each measures 20 x 60 x 7 mm, packaged in boxes of 12 sponges in individual envelopes. Also packaged in a jar of 4 sponges.
Box NDC 0009-0315-03
Jar NDC 0009-0315-02
Size 50, 100 or 200. Sponges measure 80 x 62.5 x 10 mm, 80 x 125 x 10 mm, or 80 x 250 x 10 mm, respectively. Packaged in boxes of 4 (Size 50) or boxes of 6 (Sizes 100 and 200) in individual envelopes.

Size 50	*NDC 0009-0323-01*
Size 100	*NDC 0009-0342-01*
Size 200	*NDC 0009-0349-01*

***Gelfoam* Compressed, Size 100 (USP)** For application in dry state. Sponges measure 80 x 125 mm and are available in boxes of 6 sponges in individual envelopes.
NDC 0009-0353-01
***Gelfoam* Dental Packs (USP), Size 2 or 4.** Each measures 10 x 20 x 7 mm or 20 x 20 x 7 mm, respectively, packaged in jars of 15 packs.
Size 2 NDC 0009-0379-01
Size 4 NDC 0009-0396-01
***Gelfoam* Packs (USP), Size 2 cm or 6 cm.** Packs measure 40 x 2 cm, or 40 x 6 cm, respectively. Packaged in single jars (Size 2) or in boxes of 6 packs in individual envelopes (Size 6).
Size 2 NDC 0009-0364-01
Size 6 NDC 0009-0371-01
***Gelfoam* Prostatectomy Cones, (USP), Size 13 cm or 18 cm** (for use with Foley bag catheter). Each cone diameter measures 13 cm or 18 cm, respectively. Packaged in boxes of 6 cones in individual envelopes.
Size 13 cm NDC 0009-0449-01
Size 18 cm NDC 0009-0457-01

GELFOAM® STERILE POWDER
(Absorbable Gelatin Powder)

How Supplied: *Gelfoam* Sterile Powder (absorbable gelatin powder) is supplied in jars containing 1 gram.
NDC 0009-0433-01

HALOTESTIN® TABLETS ℞
(Fluoxymesterone Tablets, USP)

10 mg-100s
NSN 6505-01-053-8669A (VA)
Description: Fluoxymesterone is a white or practically white odorless, crystalline powder, melting at about 240° C. with some decomposition. It is practically insoluble in water, sparingly soluble in alcohol and slightly soluble in chloroform.
Actions: In the eunuch and eunuchoid male, androgens act to stimulate and maintain the secondary sexual characteristics associated with the adult male. Androgens influence closure of the epiphyseal lines.
In males and some females, administration of androgens reduces urinary excretion of nitrogen, sodium, potassium, chloride, phosphorus and water.
Indications:
In the male
The primary indication in the male is replacement therapy in conditions associated with a deficiency or absence of endogenous testicular hormone. Androgen therapy prevents the development of atrophic changes in the accessory male sex organs following castration; as long as replacement therapy is continued, these organs can be maintained in a relatively normal state.
1. Eunuchoidism and eunuchism.
2. Climacteric symptoms when these are secondary to androgen deficiency.
3. Those symptoms of panhypopituitarism related to hypogonadism. Appropriate adrenocortical and thyroid hormone replacement therapy are still necessary, however, and are actually of primary importance.
4. Impotence due to androgen deficiency.
5. Delayed puberty, provided it has been definitely established as such, and it is not just a familial trait.

In the female
1. Prevention of postpartum breast pain and engorgement. There is no satisfactory evidence that this drug prevents or suppresses lactation.
2. Palliation of androgen responsive, advancing, inoperable mammary cancer, in women who are more than 1 year, but less than 5 years postmenopausal, or who have been proven to have a hormone-dependent tumor as shown by previous beneficial response to castration.

Contraindications:
Carcinoma of the male breast
Carcinoma known or suspected of the prostate
Cardiac, hepatic or renal decompensation
Hypercalcemia
Liver function impairment
Prepubertal males
Pregnancy
Patients easily stimulated
Warnings:
Hypercalcemia may occur in immobilized patients and in patients with breast cancer. In patients with cancer this may indicate progression of bony metastasis. If this occurs the drug should be discontinued.
Watch female patients closely for signs of virilization. Some effects such as voice changes may not be reversible even when the drug is stopped.
Discontinue the drug if cholestatic hepatitis with jaundice appears or liver tests become abnormal.
Precautions: Patients with cardiac, renal or hepatic derangement may retain sodium and

water thus forming edema. Priapism or excessive sexual stimulation may develop. Males, especially the elderly, may become overly stimulated. Oligospermia and reduced ejaculatory volume may occur after prolonged administration or excessive dosage. Hypersensitivity and gynecomastia may occur. When any of these affects appear the androgen should be stopped and if restarted, a lower dosage should be utilized.

Halotestin Tablets (fluoxymesterone) may increase sensitivity to oral anticoagulants. Dosage of the anticoagulant may require reduction in order to maintain a satisfactory therapeutic hypoprothrombinemia.

The PBI may decrease during androgen therapy without clinical significance.

Adverse Reactions:

- Acne
- Decreased ejaculatory volume
- Gynecomastia
- Edema
- Hypersensitivity, including skin manifestations and anaphylactoid reactions
- Priapism
- Hypercalcemia (especially in immobile patients and those with metastatic breast carcinoma)
- Virilization in females
- Cholestatic jaundice

There have been rare reports of hepatocellular neoplasms and peliosis hepatis in association with long-term androgenic-anabolic steroid therapy.

Dosage and Administration: The dosage will vary depending upon the individual, the condition being treated, its severity, and prior androgenic therapy. The total daily oral dose may be administered singly or in divided (three or four) doses.

Male Hypogonadism—For complete replacement in eunuchs and eunuchoid patients, a daily dose of 2 to 10 mg will suffice in the majority of patients. It is usually preferable to begin treatment with full therapeutic doses which are later adjusted to individual requirements. Priapism is indicative of excessive dosage and is an indication for temporary withdrawal of the drug.

Impotence due to Testicular Deficiency; Male Climacteric—In impotency due to testicular insufficiency, this preparation may be administered in doses ranging from 2 to 10 mg daily. A similar dose may be employed in males with the climacteric syndrome.

Inoperable Carcinoma of the Breast in the Female—The recommended total daily dose for palliative therapy in advanced inoperable carcinoma of the breast is 15 to 30 mg. Because of its short action, fluoxymesterone should be administered to patients in divided, rather than single, daily doses to ensure more stable blood levels. In general, it appears necessary to continue therapy for at least one month for a satisfactory subjective response, and for 2 to 3 months for an objective response.

Postpartum Breast Engorgement—To lessen the degree and duration of painful breast engorgement, a dose of 2.5 mg may be administered when active labor has started. Thereafter, a daily dose of 5 to 10 mg, preferably in divided doses, may be given for 4 to 5 days.

How Supplied: Scored tablets containing 2 mg, 5 mg or 10 mg fluoxymesterone in the following sizes:

2 mg	Bottles of 100	*NDC 0009-0014-01*
5 mg	Bottles of 100	*NDC 0009-0019-06*
10 mg	Bottles of 30	*NDC 0009-0036-03*
	Bottles of 100	*NDC 0009-0036-04*

Code NMF-1

[*Shown in Product Identification Section*]

STERILE SOLUTION
HEPARIN SODIUM INJECTION, USP ℞

Composition:

From beef lung each ml of the 1,000 and 5,000 USP units per ml preparations contains: Heparin Sodium 1,000 or 5,000 USP units; 9 mg Sodium Chloride; 9 mg Benzyl Alcohol; water for injection qs. Each ml of the 10,000 units per ml preparations contains: Heparin Sodium 10,000 USP units; 9 mg Benzyl Alcohol; water for injection qs.

How Supplied: Sterile solution containing heparin sodium derived from beef lung in the following strengths and sizes:

From beef lung:

1,000 USP Units per ml

10 ml vial	*NDC 0009-0268-01*
30 ml vial	*NDC 0009-0268-02*

5,000 USP Units per ml

1 ml vial	*NDC 0009-0291-02*
10 ml vial	*NDC 0009-0291-01*

10,000 USP Units per ml

1 ml vial	*NDC 0009-0317-01*
4 ml vial	*NDC 0009-0317-02*

LINCOCIN® CAPSULES, STERILE SOLUTION, SYRUP ℞
(Lincomycin Hydrochloride, USP)

WARNING

Lincomycin can cause severe colitis which may end fatally. Therefore, it should be reserved for serious infections where less toxic antimicrobial agents are inappropriate, as described in the Indications Section. It should not be used in patients with nonbacterial infections, such as most upper respiratory tract infections. Studies indicate a toxin(s) produced by *Clostridia* is one primary cause of antibiotic associated colitis. The colitis is usually characterized by severe, persistent diarrhea and severe abdominal cramps and may be associated with the passage of blood and mucus. Endoscopic examination may reveal pseudomembranous colitis.

When significant diarrhea occurs, the drug should be discontinued or, if necessary, continued only with close observation of the patient. Large bowel endoscopy has been recommended.

Antiperistaltic agents such as opiates and diphenoxylate with atropine (Lomotil) may prolong and/or worsen the condition. Diarrhea, colitis, and pseudomembranous colitis have been observed to begin up to several weeks following cessation of therapy with lincomycin.

Description: Lincomycin hydrochloride is the monohydrated salt of lincomycin, a substance produced by the growth of a member of the *lincolnensis* group of *Streptomyces lincolnensis* (Fam. *Streptomycetaceae*). It is a white, or practically white, crystalline powder and is odorless or has a faint odor. Its solutions are acid and are dextrorotatory. Lincomycin hydrochloride is freely soluble in water; soluble in dimethylformamide and very slightly soluble in acetone.

Actions: Microbiology—*Lincocin* (lincomycin hydrochloride) has been shown to be effective against most of the common gram-positive pathogens. Depending on the sensitivity of the organism and concentration of the antibiotic, it may be either bactericidal or bacteriostatic. Cross resistance has not been demonstrated with penicillin, chloramphenicol, ampicillin, cephalosporins or the tetracyclines. Despite chemical differences, lincomycin exhibits antibacterial activity similar but not identical to the macrolide antibiotics (e.g. erythromycin). Some cross resistance (with erythromycin) including a phenomenon known as dissociated cross resistance or macrolide effect has been reported. Microorganisms have not developed resistance to *Lincocin* rapidly when tested by *in vitro* or *in vivo* methods. Staphylococci develop resistance to *Lincocin* in a slow, step-wise manner based on *in vitro*, serial subculture experiments. This pattern of resistance development is unlike that shown for streptomycin.

Studies indicate that *Lincocin* does not share antigenicity with penicillin compounds.

Biological Studies—*In vitro* studies indicate that the spectrum of activity includes *Staphylococcus aureus, Staphylococcus albus, β-hemolytic Streptococcus, Streptococcus viridans, Diplococcus pneumoniae, Clostridium tetani, Clostridium perfringens, Corynebacterium diphtheriae and Corynebacterium acnes.*

NOTE: The drug is not active against most strains of *Streptococcus faecalis*, nor against *Neisseria gonorrhoeae, Neisseria meningitidis, Hemophilus influenzae*, or other gram-negative organisms or yeasts.

Human Pharmacology—*Lincocin* is absorbed rapidly after a 500 mg oral dose, reaching peak levels in 2 to 4 hours. Levels are maintained above the MIC (minimum inhibitory concentration) for most gram-positive organisms for 6 to 8 hours. Urinary recovery of drug in a 24-hour period ranges from 1.0 to 31 percent (mean: 4.0) after a single oral dose of 500 mg. Tissue level studies indicate that bile is an important route of excretion. Significant levels have been demonstrated in the majority of body tissues. Although the drug is not present in significant amounts in the spinal fluid of normal volunteers, it has been demonstrated in the spinal fluid of one patient with pneumococcal meningitis.

Intramuscular administration of a single dose of 600 mg produces a peak serum level at 30 minutes with detectable levels persisting for 24 hours. Urinary excretion after this dose ranges from 1.8 to 24.8 percent (mean: 17.3).

The intravenous infusion over a 2-hour interval of 600 mg of *Lincocin* (lincomycin hydrochloride) in 500 ml of 5 percent glucose in distilled water yields therapeutic levels for 14 hours. Urinary excretion ranges from 4.9 to 30.3 percent (mean: 13.8).

The biological half-life, after oral, intramuscular or intravenous administration is 5.4 ± 1.0 hours.

Hemodialysis and peritoneal dialysis do not effectively remove lincomycin from the blood.

Indications: Lincomycin is indicated in the treatment of serious infections due to susceptible strains of streptococci, pneumococci, and staphylococci. Its use should be reserved for penicillin-allergic patients or other patients for whom, in the judgment of the physician, a penicillin is inappropriate. Because of the risk of colitis, as described in the WARNING box, before selecting lincomycin the physician should consider the nature of the infection and the suitability of less toxic alternatives (e.g., erythromycin).

Lincocin has been demonstrated to be effective in the treatment of staphylococcal infections resistant to other antibiotics and susceptible to lincomycin. Staphylococcal strains resistant to *Lincocin* have been recovered; culture and susceptibility studies should be done in conjunction with *Lincocin* therapy. In the case of macrolides, partial but not complete cross resistance may occur (see **Microbiology**). The drug

Continued on next page

Information on these Upjohn products is based on labeling in effect on November 1, 1979. Further information on dosage and administration, side effects, precautions and contraindications for these and other Upjohn products may be obtained from either the package insert or Medical Services, The Upjohn Company, Kalamazoo, Michigan.

Upjohn—Cont.

may be administered concomitantly with other antimicrobial agents when indicated.

Contraindications: This drug is contraindicated in patients previously found to be hypersensitive to lincomycin or clindamycin. It is not indicated in the treatment of minor bacterial infections or viral infections.

WARNINGS:
See WARNING box. Studies indicate a toxin(s) produced by *Clostridia* is one primary cause of antibiotic associated colitis.[1–5] Mild cases of colitis may respond to drug discontinuance alone. Moderate to severe cases should be managed promptly with fluid, electrolyte and protein supplementation as indicated. Systemic corticoids and corticoid retention enemas may help relieve the colitis. Other causes of colitis should also be considered.

A careful inquiry should be made concerning previous sensitivities to drugs and other allergens.

Usage in Pregnancy—Safety for use in pregnancy has not been established.

Usage in Newborn—Until further clinical experience is obtained, *Lincocin* (lincomycin hydrochloride) is not indicated in the newborn.

Nursing Mothers—*Lincocin* has been reported to appear in breast milk in ranges of 0.5 to 2.4 mcg/ml.

1. Bailey, WR, Scott, EG, *Diagnostic Microbiology*CV Mosby Company, St. Louis, 1978.
2. Bartlett, JG, et al, "Clindamycin-associated Colitis due to a Toxin-producing Species of *Clostridium* in Hamsters" *J. Inf. Dis.* **136**(5): 701–705, (November) 1977.
3. Larson, HE, Price, AB, "Pseudomembranous Colitis: Presence of Clostridial Toxin," *Lancet*, 1312–1314 (December) 24 and 31, 1977.
4. Lusk, RH, et al, "Clindamycin-Induced Enterocolitis in Hamsters", *J. Inf. Dis.* **137**(4): 464–474 (April) 1978.
5. "Antibiotic-associated Colitis: A Progress Report", *British Med. J.* **1**:669–671 (March 18) 1978.

Precautions: Review of experience to date suggests that a subgroup of older patients with associated severe illness may tolerate diarrhea less well. When *Lincocin* (lincomycin hydrochloride) is indicated in these patients, they should be carefully monitored for change in bowel frequency.

Lincocin should be prescribed with caution in individuals with a history of gastrointestinal disease, particularly colitis.

Lincocin, like any drug, should be used with caution in patients with a history of asthma or significant allergies.

The use of antibiotics occasionally results in overgrowth of nonsusceptible organisms—particularly yeasts. Should superinfections occur, appropriate measures should be taken. When patients with pre-existing monilial infections require *Lincocin* therapy, concomitant antimonilial treatment should be given.

During prolonged *Lincocin* therapy, periodic liver function studies and blood counts should be performed.

Since adequate data are not yet available in patients with pre-existing liver disease, its use in such patients is not recommended at this time unless special clinical circumstances so indicate.

Lincomycin has been shown to have neuromuscular blocking properties that may enhance the action of other neuromuscular blocking agents. Therefore, it should be used with caution in patients receiving such agents.

Indicated surgical procedures should be performed in conjunction with antibiotic therapy.

Adverse Reactions:

Gastrointestinal—Glossitis, stomatitis, nausea, vomiting. Persistent diarrhea, enterocolitis and pruritus ani. (See **Warning** box)

Hematopoietic: Neutropenia, leukopenia, agranulocytosis and thrombocytopenic purpura have been reported. There have been rare reports of aplastic anemia and pancytopenia in which *Lincocin* (lincomycin hydrochloride) could not be ruled out as the causative agent.

Hypersensitivity Reactions—Hypersensitivity reactions such as angioneurotic edema, serum sickness and anaphylaxis have been reported, some of these in patients known to be sensitive to penicillin. Rare instances of erythema multiforme, some resembling Stevens-Johnson syndrome, have been associated with *Lincocin*. If an allergic reaction should occur, the drug should be discontinued and the usual agents (epinephrine, corticosteroids, antihistamines) should be available for emergency treatment.

Skin and Mucous Membranes—Skin rashes, urticaria and vaginitis and rare instances of exfoliative and vesiculobullous dermatitis have been reported.

Liver—Although no direct relationship of *Lincocin* (lincomycin hydrochloride) to liver dysfunction has been established, jaundice and abnormal liver function tests (particularly elevations of serum transaminase) have been observed in a few instances.

Cardiovascular—Instances of hypotension following parenteral administration have been reported, particularly after too rapid intravenous administration. Rare instances of cardiopulmonary arrest have been reported after too rapid intravenous administration. (See **Dosage and Administration**).

Special Senses—Tinnitus and vertigo have been reported occasionally.

Local Reactions—Patients have demonstrated excellent local tolerance to intramuscularly administered *Lincocin* (lincomycin hydrochloride). Reports of pain following injection have been infrequent. Intravenous administration of *Lincocin* in 250 to 500 ml of 5 percent glucose in distilled water or normal saline produced no local irritation or phlebitis.

Physical Compatibilities:

Physically compatible for 24 hours at room temperature unless otherwise indicated.

Infusion Solutions
Dextrose in Water, 5% and 10%
Dextrose in Saline, 5% and 10%
Ringer's Solution
Sodium Lactate 1/6 Molar
Travert 10%—Electrolyte No. 1
Dextran in Saline 6% w/v

Vitamins in Infusion Solutions
B-Complex
B-Complex with Ascorbic Acid

Antibiotics in Infusion Solutions
Penicillin G Sodium (Satisfactory for 4 hours)
Cephalothin
Tetracycline HCl
Cephaloridine
Colistimethate (Satisfactory for 4 hours)
Ampicillin
Methicillin
Chloramphenicol
Polymyxin B Sulfate

Physically Incompatible With:
Novobiocin
Kanamycin

IT SHOULD BE EMPHASIZED THAT THE COMPATIBLE AND INCOMPATIBLE DETERMINATIONS ARE PHYSICAL OBSERVATIONS ONLY, NOT CHEMICAL DETERMINATIONS. ADEQUATE CLINICAL EVALUATION OF THE SAFETY AND EFFICACY OF THESE COMBINATIONS HAS NOT BEEN PERFORMED.

Dosage and Administration:
If significant diarrhea occurs during therapy, this antibiotic should be discontinued. (See **Warning** box).

Oral—**Adults:** *Serious infections*—500 mg 3 times per day (500 mg approximately every 8 hours). *More severe infections*—500 mg or more 4 times per day (500 mg or more approximately every 6 hours). **Children over 1 month of age:** *Serious infections*—30 mg/kg/day (15 mg/lb/day) divided into 3 or 4 equal doses. *More severe infections*—60 mg/kg/day (30 mg/lb/day) divided into 3 or 4 equal doses.

With β-hemolytic streptococcal infections, treatment should continue for at least 10 days to diminish the likelihood of subsequent rheumatic fever or glomerulonephritis.

NOTE: For optimal absorption it is recommended that nothing be given by mouth except water for a period of one to two hours before and after oral administration of *Lincocin* (lincomycin hydrochloride).

Intramuscular—**Adults:** *Serious infections*—600 mg (2 ml) intramuscularly every 24 hours. *More severe infections*—600 mg (2 ml) intramuscularly every 12 hours or more often. **Children over 1 month of age:** *Serious infections*—one intramuscular injection of 10 mg/kg (5 mg/lb) every 24 hours. *More severe infections*—one intramuscular injection of 10 mg/kg (5 mg/lb) every 12 hours or more often.

Intravenous—**Adults:** The intravenous dose will be determined by the severity of the infection. For serious infections doses of 600 mg (2 ml) to 1 gm are given every 8-12 hours. For more severe infections these doses may have to be increased. In life-threatening situations daily intravenous doses of as much as 8 grams have been given. Intravenous doses are given on the basis of 1 gm of *Lincocin* diluted in **not less than** 100 ml of appropriate solution (see **Physical Compatibilities**) and infused over a period of not less than one hour.

Dose	Vol. Diluent	Time
600 mg	100 ml	1 hr
1 gm	100 ml	1 hr
2 gm	200 ml	2 hr
3 gm	300 ml	3 hr
4 gm	400 ml	4 hr

These doses may be repeated as often as required to the limit of the maximum recommended daily dose of 8 gm.

Children over 1 month of age: 10-20 mg/kg/day (5-10 mg/lb/day) depending on the severity of the infection may be infused in divided doses as described above for adults.

NOTE: Severe cardiopulmonary reactions have occurred when this drug has been given at greater than the recommended concentration and rate.

[See table at left].

Subconjunctival Injection—0.25 ml (75 mg) injected subconjunctivally will result in ocular fluid levels of antibiotic (lasting for at least 5 hours) with MIC's sufficient for most susceptible pathogens.

Patients with diminished renal function: *When Lincocin therapy is required in individuals with severe impairment of renal function, an appropriate dose is 25 to 30% of that recommended for patients with normally functioning kidneys.*

How Supplied:
Lincocin is available as:

250 mg Pediatric Capsules: Each capsule contains lincomycin hydrochloride equivalent to lincomycin base 250 mg.

Bottles of 24 *NDC 0009-0336-01*

500 mg Capsules: Each capsule contains lincomycin hydrochloride equivalent to lincomycin base 500 mg.

Bottles of 24 *NDC 0009-0500-01*
Bottles of 100 *NDC 0009-0500-02*

Sterile Solution: Each ml contains lincomycin hydrochloride equivalent to lincomycin base 300 mg; also Benzyl Alcohol, 9 mg; Water for injection, qs—available in single dose 2 ml syringes, in 2 ml and 10 ml vials.

2 ml *U-Ject®* *NDC 0009-0600-01*
Disposable Syringe
2 ml vial *NDC 0009-0555-01*
10 ml vial *NDC 0009-0555-02*

Syrup: Each 5 ml (teaspoonful) contains lincomycin hydrochloride equivalent to lincomycin base 250 mg.

60 ml bottles *NDC 0009-0444-01*

Animal Pharmacology: *In vivo* experimental animal studies demonstrated the effectiveness of *Lincocin* (lincomycin hydrochloride) in protecting animals infected with *Streptococcus viridans, β-hemolytic Streptococcus, Staphylococcus aureus, Diplococcus pneumoniae* and *Leptospira pomona.* It was ineffective in *Klebsiella, Pasteurella, Pseudomonas, Salmonella* and *Shigella* infections.

Clinical Studies: Experience with 345 obstetrical patients receiving this drug revealed no ill effects related to pregnancy.

Code 810 378 000

LONITEN® TABLETS ℞
(minoxidil)

Warnings: *Loniten* Tablets contain the powerful antihypertensive agent, minoxidil, which may produce serious adverse effects. It can cause pericardial effusion, occasionally progressing to tamponade, and angina pectoris may be exacerbated. *Loniten* should be reserved for severely hypertensive patients who do not respond adequately to maximum therapeutic doses of a diuretic and two other antihypertensive agents.

In experimental animals, minoxidil caused several kinds of myocardial lesions as well as other adverse cardiac effects (see Cardiac Lesions in Animals).

Loniten must be administered under close supervision, usually concomitantly with therapeutic doses of a beta-adrenergic blocking agent to prevent tachycardia and increased myocardial workload. It must also usually be given with a diuretic, frequently one acting in the ascending limb of the loop of Henle, to present serious fluid accumulation. Patients with malignant hypertension and those already receiving guanethidine (see Warnings) should be hospitalized when *Loniten* is first administered so that they can be monitored to avoid too rapid, or large orthostatic, decreases in blood pressure.

Description: *Loniten* Tablets contain minoxidil, an antihypertensive peripheral vasodilator. The chemical name for minoxidil is 2, 4-diamino-6-piperidinopyrimidine-3-oxide (mw = 209.25). It occurs as a white or off-white, odorless, crystalline solid that is soluble in water to the extent of approximately 2 mg/ml; is readily soluble in propylene glycol or ethanol; and is almost insoluble in acetone, chloroform or ethyl acetate.

Clinical Pharmacology:

1. General Pharmacologic Properties

Minoxidil is an orally effective direct acting peripheral vasodilator that reduces elevated systolic and diastolic blood pressure by decreasing peripheral vascular resistance. Microcirculatory blood flowin animals is enhanced or maintained in all systemic vascular beds. In man, forearm and renal vascular resistance decline; forearm blood flow increases while renal blood flow and glomerular filtration rate are preserved.

Because it causes peripheral vasodilation, minoxidil elicits a number of predictable reactions. Reduction of peripheral arteriolar resistance and the associated fall in blood pressure trigger sympathetic, vagal inhibitory, and renal homeostatic mechanisms, including an increase in renin secretion, that lead to increased cardiac rate and output and salt and water retention. These adverse effects can usually be minimized by concomitant administration of a diuretic and a beta-adrenergic blocking agent or other sympathetic nervous system suppressant.

Minoxidil does not interfere with vasomotor reflexes and therefore does not produce orthostatic hypotension. The drug does not enter the central nervous system in experimental animals in significant amounts, and it does not affect CNS function in man.

2. Effects on Blood Pressure

The extent and time-course of blood pressure reduction by minoxidil do not correspond closely to its concentration in plasma. After an effective single oral dose, blood pressure usually starts to decline within one-half hour, reaches a minimum between 2 and 3 hours and recovers at an arithmetically linear rate of about 30%/day. The total duration of effect is approximately 75 hours. When minoxidl is administered chronically, once or twice a day, the time required to achieve maximum effect on blood pressure with a given daily dose is inversely related to the size of the dose. Thus, maximum effect is achieved on 10 mg/day within 7 days, on 20 mg/day within 5 days, and on 40 mg/day within 3 days.

The blood pressure response to minoxidil is linearly related to the logarithm of the dose administered. The slope of this log-linear dose-response relationship is proportional to the extent of hypertension and approaches zero at a supine diastolic blood pressure of approximately 85 mmHg.

3. Absorption and Metabolism

Minoxidil is at least 90% absorbed from the GI tract in experimental animals and man. Plasma levels of the parent drug reach maximum within the first hour and decline rapidly thereafter. The average plasma half-life in man is 4.2 hours. Approximtely 90% of the administered drug is metabolized, predominantly by conjugation with glucuronic acid at the N-oxide position in the pyrimidine ring, but also by conversion to more polar products. Known metabolites exert much less pharmacologic effect than minoxidil itself; all are excreted principally in the urine. Minoxidil does not bind to plasma proteins, and its renal clearance corresponds to the glomerular filtration rate. In the absence of functional renal tissue, minoxidil and its metabolites can be removed by hemodialysis.

4. Cardiac Lesions in Animals

Minoxidil produced two types of cardiac lesions in non-primate species:

(a) Dog atrial lesion—

Daily oral doses of 0.5 mg/kg for several days to 1 month or longer produced a grossly visible hemorrhagic lesion of the right atrium of the dog. This lesion has not been seen in other species. Microscopic examination showed replacement of myocardial cells by proliferating fibroblasts and angioblasts; phagocytosis; and hemosiderin accumulation in macrophages.

(b) Papillary muscle lesion—

Short term treatment (about 3 days) in several species (dog, rat, minipig) produced necrosis of the papillary muscles, and, in some cases subendocardial areas of the left ventricle, lesions similar to those produced by other peripheral dilators and by beta-adrenergic receptor agonists such as isoproterenol and epinephrine. These are thought to result from myocardial ischemia resulting from reflex sympathetic or vagal withdrawal-induced tachycardia in combination with hypotension. These lesions were reduced in incidence and severity by betaadrenergic receptor blockade.

(c) *Hemorrhagic lesions* were seen in many parts of the heart, mainly in the epicardium, endocardium, and walls of small coronary arteries and arterioles, after acute minoxidil treatment in dogs, and left atrial hemorrhagic lesions were seen in minipigs.

In addition to these lesions, longer term studies in rats, dogs, and monkeys showed cardiac hypertrophy and (in rats) cardiac dilation. In monkeys, hydrochlorothiazide partly reversed the increased heart weight, suggesting it may be related to fluid overload. In a one-year dog study, serosanguinous pericardial fluid was seen.

Autopsies of 79 patients who died from various causes and who had received minoxidil did not reveal right atrial or other hemorrhagic pathology of the kind seen in dogs. Instances of necrotic areas in the papillary muscles were seen, but these occurred in the presence of known pre-existing ischemic heart disease and did not appear different from, or more common than, lesions seen in patients never exposed to minoxidil. Studies to date cannot rule out the possibility that minoxidil can be associated with cardiac damage in humans.

Indications and Usage: Because of the potential for serious adverse effects, *Loniten* (minoxidil) is indicated only in the treatment of severe hypertension that is symptomatic or associated with target organ damage and is not manageable with maximum therapeutic doses of a diuretic plus two other antihypertensive drugs. At the present time use in milder degrees of hypertension is not recommended because the benefit-risk relationship in such patients has not been defined.

When used according to its indication, *Loniten* reduced supine diastolic blood pressure by 20 mmHg or to 90 mmHg or less in approximately 75% of the patients studied.

Contraindications: *Loniten* (minoxidil) is contraindicated in pheochromocytoma, because it may stimulate secretion of catecholamines from the tumor through its antihypertensive action.

Warnings:

1. Salt and Water Retention; Congestive Heart Failure—concomitant use of an adequate diuretic is required—

Loniten (minoxidil) must usually be administered concomitantly with a diuretic adequate to prevent fluid retention and possible congestive heart failure; a high ceiling (loop) diuretic is *almost always* required. Body weight should be monitored closely. If *Loniten* is used without a diuretic, retention of several hundred milliequivalents of salt and corresponding volumes of water can occur within a few days, leading to increased plasma and interstitial fluid volume and local or generalized edema. Diuretic treatment alone, or in combination with restricted salt intake, will usually minimize fluid retention, although reversible edema did develop in approximately 10% of nondialysis patients so treated. Diuretic effectiveness was limited mostly by disease-related impaired renal function. The condition of patients with preexisting congestive heart failure occasionally deteriorated in association with fluid retention although because of the fall in blood pressure (reduction of afterload), more than twice as many improved than worsened. Rarely, refractory fluid retention may require discontinuation of *Loniten.* Provided that the patient is under close medical supervision, it may be possible to resolve refractory salt retention by discontinuing *Loniten* for 1 or 2 days and then

Continued on next page

Information on these Upjohn products is based on labeling in effect on November 1, 1979. Further information on dosage and administration, side effects, precautions and contraindications for these and other Upjohn products may be obtained from either the package insert or Medical Services, The Upjohn Company, Kalamazoo, Michigan.

Upjohn—Cont.

resuming treatment in conjunction with vigorous diuretic therapy.

2. Concomitant Treatment to Prevent Tachycardia is Usually Required—*Loniten* increases the heart rate. This increase can be partly or entirely prevented by the concomitant administration of a beta-adrenergic blocking drug or other sympathetic nervous system suppressant. The ability of beta-adrenergic blocking agents to minimize papillary muscle lesions in animals is further reason to utilize such an agent concomitantly. Round-the-clock effectiveness of the sympathetic suppressant should be assured. In addition, angina may worsen or appear for the first time during *Loniten* treatment, probably because of the increased oxygen demands associated with increased heart rate and cardiac output. This can usually be prevented by sympathetic blockade.

3. Pericardial Effusion and Tamponade—Pericardial effusion, occasionally with tamponade, has been observed in about 3% of treated patients not on dialysis, especially those with inadequate or compromised renal function. Although in many cases, the pericardial effusion was associated with a connective tissue disease, the uremic syndrome, congestive heart failure, or marked fluid retention, there have been instances in which these potential causes of effusion were not present. Patients should be observed closely for any suggestion of a pericardial disorder, and echocardiographic studies should be carried out if suspicion arises. More vigorous diuretic therapy, dialysis, pericardiocentesis, or surgery may be required. If the effusion persists, withdrawal of *Loniten* should be considered in light of other means of controlling the hypertension and the patient's clinical status.

4. *Interaction with Guanethidine:* Although minoxidil does not itself cause orthostatic hypotension, its administration to patients already receiving guanethidine can result in profound orthostatic effects. If at all possible, guanethidine should be discontinued well before minoxidil is begun. Where this is not possible, minoxidil therapy should be started in the hospital and the patient should remain institutionalized until severe orthostatic effects are no longer present or the patient has learned to avoid activities that provoke them.

5. *Hazard of Rapid Control of Blood Pressure:* In patients with very severe blood pressure elevation, too rapid control of blood pressure, especially with intravenous agents, can precipitate cerebrovascular accidents and myocardial infarction. Although such events have not been unequivocally associated with minoxidil use, total experience is limited at present.

Any patient with malignant hypertension should have initial treatment with minoxidil carried out in a hospital setting, both to assure that blood pressure is falling and to assure that it is not falling more rapidly than intended.

Precautions:

1. General—(a) **Monitor fluid and electrolyte balance and body weight** (see Warning: Salt and Water Retention).

(b) **Observe patients for signs and symptoms of pericardial effusion** (see Warning: Pericardial Effusion and Tamponade).

(c) **Use after myocardial infarction**—*Loniten* has not been used in patients who have had a myocardial infarction within the preceding month. It is possible that a reduction of arterial pressure with *Loniten* might further limit blood flow to the myocardium, although this might be compensated by decreased oxygen demand because of lower blood pressure.

(d) **Hypersensitivity**—Possible hypersensitivity to *Loniten*, manifested as a skin rash, has been seen in less than 1% of patients; whether the drug should be discontinued when this occurs depends on treatment alternatives.

(e) **Renal failure or dialysis patients** may require smaller doses of *Loniten* and should have close medical supervision to prevent exacerbation of renal failure or precipitation of cardial failure.

2. Patient Information—The patient should be made fully aware of the importance of continuing all of his antihypertensive medications and of the nature of symptoms that would suggest fluid overload. A patient brochure has been prepared and is included with each *Loniten* package. The text of this brochure is reprinted below.

3. Carcinogenesis, Mutagenesis and Impairment of Fertility—Twenty-two month carcinogenicity studies in rats at doses 15 times the human dose did not provide evidence of tumorigenicity. The drug was not mutagenic in the Salmonella (Ames) test.

Rats receiving up to five times the human dose of minoxidil had a reduction in conception rate, possibly related to drug treatment. There was no evidence of increased fetal resorptions in rats but they did occur in rabbits.

4. Use in Pregnancy-Teratogenic Effects—Pregnancy Category C. Minoxidil has been shown to reduce the conception rate in rats and to show evidence of increased fetal absorption in rabbits when administered at five times the human dose. There was no evidence of teratogenic effects in rats and rabbits. There are no adequate and well controlled studies in pregnant women. *Loniten* should be used during pregnancy only if the potential benefit justifies the potential risk to the fetus.

5. Nursing Mothers—It is not known whether this drug is secreted in human milk. As a general rule, nursing should not be undertaken while a patient is on *Loniten*.

6. Use in Pediatrics—Total use in children has been limited to date, particularly in infants. The recommendations under Dosage and Administration can be considered only a rough guide at present and careful titration is essential.

Adverse Reactions:

1. Salt and Water Retention (see Warning: Concomitant Use of Adequate Diuretic is Required)—Temporary edema developed in 7% of patients who were not edematous at the start of therapy.

2. Pericardial Effusion and Tamponade (see Warnings).

3. Hypertrichosis—Elongation, thickening, and enhanced pigmentation of fine body hair are seen in about 80% of patients taking *Loniten* (minoxidil). This develops within 3 to 6 weeks after starting therapy. It is usually first noticed on the temples, between the eyebrows, between the hairline and the eyebrows, or in the side-burn area of the upper lateral cheek, later extending to the back, arms, legs, and scalp. Upon discontinuation of *Loniten*, new hair growth stops, but 1 to 6 months may be required for restoration to pretreatment appearance. No endocrine abnormalities have been found to explain the abnormal hair growth; thus, it is hypertrichosis without virilism. Hair growth is especially disturbing to children and women and such patients should be thoroughly informed about this effect before therapy with *Loniten* is begun.

4. Miscellaneous—Breast tenderness developed in less than 1% of patients.

5. Altered Laboratory Findings—(a) ECG changes—changes in direction and magnitude of the ECG T-waves occur in approximately 60% of patients treated with *Loniten*. In rare instances a large negative amplitude of the T-wave may encroach upon the S-T segment, but the S-T segment is not independently altered. These changes usually disappear with continuance of treatment and revert to the pretreatment state if *Loniten* is discontinued. No symptoms have been associated with these changes, nor have there been alterations in blood cell counts or in plasma enzyme concentrations that would suggest myocardial damage. Long-term treatment of patients manifesting such changes has provided no evidence of deteriorating cardiac function. At present the changes appear to be nonspecific and without identifiable clinical significance. (b) Effects of hemodilution—Hematocrit, hemoglobin and erythrocyte count usually fall about 7% initially and then recover to pretreatment levels. (c) Other—Alkaline phosphatase increased varyingly without other evidence of liver or bone abnormality. Serum creatinine increased an average of 6% and BUN slightly more, but later declined to pretreatment levels.

Overdosage: There have been only a few instances of deliberate or accidental overdosage with *Loniten* (minoxidil). One patient recovered after taking 50 mg of *Loniten* together with 500 mg of a barbiturate. When exaggerated hypotension is encountered, it is most likely to occur in association with residual sympathetic nervous system blockade from previous therapy (guanethidine-like effects or alpha-adrenergic blockage), which prevents the usual compensatory maintenance of blood pressure. Intravenous administration of normal saline will help to maintain blood pressure and facilitate urine formation in these patients. Sympathomimetic drugs such as norepinephrine or epinephrine should be avoided because of their excessive cardiac stimulating action. Phenylephrine, angiotensin II, vasopressin, and dopamine all reverse hypotension due to *Loniten*, but should only be used if underperfusion of a vital organ is evident.

Dosage and Administration:

Patients over 12 years of age: The recommended initial dosage of *Loniten* (minoxidil) is 5 mg given as a single daily dose. Daily dosage can be increased to 10, 20 and then to 40 mg in single or divided doses if required for optimum blood pressure control. The effective dosage range is usually 10 to 40 mg per day. The maximum recommended dosage is 100 mg per day.

Patients under 12 years of age: The initial dosage is 0.2 mg/kg *Loniten* as a single daily dose. The dosage may be increased in 50 to 100% increments until optimum blood pressure control is achieved. The effective dosage range is usually 0.25 to 1.0 mg/kg/day. The maximum recommended dosage is 50 mg daily. (see **6. Use in Pediatrics** under **Precautions**).

Dose frequency: The magnitude of within-day fluctuation of arterial pressure during therapy with *Loniten* is directly proportional to the extent of pressure reduction. If supine diastolic pressure has been reduced less than 30 mmHg, the drug need be administered only once a day; if supine diastolic pressure has been reduced more than 30 mmHg, the daily dosage should be divided into two equal parts.

Frequency of dosage adjustment: Dosage must be titrated carefully according to individual response. Intervals between dosage adjustments normally should be at least 3 days since the full response to a given dose is not obtained for at least that amount of time. **Where a more rapid management of hypertension is required, dose adjustments can be made every 6 hours if the patient is carefully monitored.**

Concomitant therapy: Diuretic and beta-blocker or other sympathetic nervous system supressant.

Diuretics: *Loniten* must be used in conjunction with a diuretic in patients relying on renal function for maintaining salt and water balance. Diuretics have been used at the following dosages when starting therapy with *Loniten:* hydrochlorothiazide (50 mg, b.i.d.) or other thiazides at equieffective dosage; Chlorthalidone (50 to 100 mg, once daily); furosemide (40 mg, b.i.d.)

If excessive salt and water retention results in a weight gain of more than 5 pounds, diuretic therapy should be changed to furosemide; if the patient is already taking furosemide, dosage should be increased in accordance with the patient's requirements.

Beta-blocker or other sympathetic nervous system suppressants: When therapy with *Loniten* is begun, the dosage of a beta-adrenergic receptor blocking drug should be the equivalent of 80 to 160 mg of propranolol per day in divided doses.

If beta-blockers are contraindicated, methyldopa (250 to 750 mg, b.i.d.) may be used instead. Methyldopa must be given for at least 24 hours before starting therapy with *Loniten* because of the delay in the onset of methyldopa's action. Limited clinical experience indicates that clonidine may also be used to prevent tachycardia induced by *Loniten;* the usual dosage is 0.1 to 0.2 mg twice daily.

Sympathetic nervous system suppressants may not completely prevent an increase in heart rate due to *Loniten* but usually do prevent tachycardia. Typically, patients receiving a beta-blocker prior to initiation of therapy with *Loniten* have a bradycardia and can be expected to have an increase in heart rate toward normal when *Loniten* is added. When treatment with *Loniten* and beta-blocker or other sympathetic nervous system suppressant are begun simultaneously, their opposing cardiac effects usually nullify each other, leading to little change in heart rate.

How Supplied: *Loniten* (minoxidil) is supplied as round, scored white tablets. Dosage strengths are imprinted on one convex surface. The following strengths and container sizes are available:

Strength	Container and Size	NDC Number
2.5 mg	Bottles of 100	0009-0121-01
10 mg	Bottles of 100	0009-0137-01

Patient Information: *Loniten* Tablets contain minoxidil, a powerful medicine for the treatment of high blood pressure. *Loniten* is used for the treatment of severe hypertension that is difficult to control. It must usually be taken with other medicines.

Be absolutely sure to take all of your medicines for high blood pressure according to your doctor's instructions. Do not stop taking *Loniten* unless your doctor tells you to. Do not give any of your medicine to other people.

It is important that you look for the warning signals of certain undesired effects of *Loniten*. Call your doctor if they occur. Your doctor will need to see you regularly while you are taking *Loniten*. Be sure to keep all your appointments or to arrange for new ones if you must miss one.

Do not hesitate to call your doctor if any discomforts or problems occur.

The information here is intended to help you take *Loniten* properly. It does not tell you all there is to know about *Loniten*. There is a more technical leaflet that you may request from the pharmacist; you may need your doctor's help in understanding parts of that leaflet.

What is *Loniten?*

Loniten Tablets contain minoxidil which is a powerful drug for lowering the blood pressure. It works by relaxing and enlarging certain small blood vessels so that blood flows through them more easily.

Why lower blood pressure?

Your doctor has prescribed *Loniten* to lower your blood pressure and protect vital parts of your body. Uncontrolled blood pressure can cause stroke, heart failure, blindness, kidney failure, and heart attacks.

Most people with high blood pressure need to take medicines to treat it for their whole lives.

Who should take *Loniten?*

There are many people with high blood pressure, but most of them do not need *Loniten*. *Loniten* is used ONLY when your doctor decides that:

1. your high blood pressure is severe;
2. your high blood pressure is causing symptoms or damage to vital organs; and
3. other medicines did not work well enough or had very disturbing side effects.

Loniten should be taken only when a doctor prescribes it. Never give any of your *Loniten* Tablets, or any other high blood pressure medicine, to a friend or relative.

Pregnancy: In some cases doctors may prescribe *Loniten* for women who are pregnant or who are planning to have children. However, its safe use in pregnancy has not been established. Laboratory animals had a reduced ability to become pregnant and a reduced survival of offspring while taking *Loniten*. If you are pregnant or are planning to become pregnant, be sure to tell your doctor.

How to take *Loniten*.

Usually, your doctor will prescribe two other medicines along with *Loniten*. These will help lower blood pressure and will help prevent undesired effects of *Loniten*.

Often, when a medicine like *Loniten* lowers blood pressure, your body tries to return the blood pressure to the original, higher level. It does this by holding on to water and salt (so there will be more fluid to pump) and by making your heart beat faster.

To prevent this, your doctor will usually prescribe a water tablet to remove the extra salt and water from your body (a diuretic dye-u-RET-tic) and another medicine to slow your heart beat.

You must follow your doctor's instructions exactly, taking all the prescribed medicines, in the right amounts, each day. These medicines will decrease the side effects you might otherwise have and will also help keep your blood pressure down.

You may take *Loniten* with water or other liquids, either with or between meals.

Loniten Tablets come in two strengths (2 ½ milligrams and 10 milligrams) that are marked on each tablet. Pay close attention to the tablet markings to be sure you are taking the correct strength. Your doctor may prescribe half a tablet; the tablets are scored (partly cut on one side) so that you can easily break them.

When you first start taking *Loniten*, your doctor may need to see you often in order to adjust your dosage. Take all your medicine according to the schedule prescribed by your doctor. **Do not skip any doses. If you should forget a dose of *Loniten*, wait until it is time for your next dose, then continue with your regular schedule. Remember: do not stop taking *Loniten*, or any of your other high blood pressure medicines, without checking with your doctor.** Make sure that any doctor treating or examining you knows that you are taking high blood pressure medicines, including *Loniten*.

Warning Signals: Even if you take all your medicines correctly, you may have side effects. Some of these are serious and you should be on the lookout for them. **If any of the following warning signals occur, you must call your doctor immediately:**

1. *Increase in heart rate*—You should measure your heart rate by counting your pulse rate **while you are resting.** If you have an increase of 20 beats or more a minute over your normal pulse, contact your doctor immediately. If you do not know how to take your pulse rate, ask your doctor. Also ask your doctor how often to check your pulse.
2. *Rapid weight gain of more than 5 pounds*—You should weigh yourself daily. If you quickly gain five or more pounds, or if there is any swelling or puffiness in the face, hands, ankles, or stomach area, this could be a sign that you are retaining body fluids. Your doctor may have to change your drugs or change the dose of your drugs. You may also need to reduce the amount of salt you eat. A smaller weight gain (2 to 3 pounds) often occurs when treatment is started. You may lose this extra weight with continued treatment.
3. *Increased difficulty in breathing*, especially when lying down. This too may be due to an increase of body fluids. It can also happen because your high blood pressure is getting worse. In either case, you might require treatment with other medicines.
4. *New or worsening of pain in the chest, arm, or shoulder or signs of severe indigestion*—These could be signs of serious heart problems.
5. *Dizziness, lighteadedness or fainting*—These can be signs of high blood pressure or they may be side effects from one of the medicines. Your doctor may need to change or adjust the dosage of the medicines you are taking.

Other Side Effects: *Loniten* can cause side effects that are annoying but not dangerous. Do not stop taking the drug because of these side effects without talking to your doctor.

Hair growth: About 8 out of every 10 patients who have taken *Loniten* noticed that fine **body hair grew darker or longer** on certain parts of the body. This happened about three to six weeks after beginning treatment. The hair may first be noticed on the forehead and temples, between the eyebrows, or on the upper part of the cheeks. Later, hair may grow on the back, arms, legs, or scalp. Although hair growth may not be noticeable to some patients, it often is bothersome in women and children. **Unwanted hair can be controlled with a hair remover or by shaving.** The extra hair is not permanent, it disappears within 1 to 6 months of stopping *Loniten*. Nevertheless, **you should not stop taking *Loniten* without first talking to your doctor.**

A few patients have developed a rash or breast tenderness while taking *Loniten* Tablets (minoxidil), but this is unusual.

Code 810 384 002

[Shown in Product Identification Section]

MAOLATE® TABLETS ℞
(chlorphenesin carbamate)

500's
NSN 6505-00-998-7143A (M & VA)

How Supplied: Scored tablets containing 400 mg chlorphenesin carbamate are available in the following packages.

Bottles of 50	*NDC 0009-0412-01*
Bottles of 500	*NDC 0009-0412-02*
Unit dose package (100)	*NDC 0009-0412-03*

[Shown in Product Identification Section]

MEDROL® ACETATE OINTMENT ℞
(methylprednisolone acetate)
For External Use Only

How Supplied: In two concentrations-2.5 mg (0.25%) or 10 mg (1.0%) methylprednisolone acetate per gram.

0.25%	7.5 Gm tubes	*NDC 0009-0483-01*
	30 Gm tubes	*NDC 0009-0483-02*
	1½ oz tubes	*NDC 0009-0483-03*
1%	7.5 Gm tubes	*NDC 0009-0505-01*
	30 Gm tubes	*NDC 0009-0505-02*
	1½ oz tubes	*NDC 0009-0505-03*

MEDROL ENPAK® KIT ℞
(Methylprednisolone Acetate for Enema, USP)

This product is prepared specifically for administration as a retention enema.
Not for injection

Description: Methylprednisolone Acetate is the 6-methyl derivative of prednisolone. It is a

Continued on next page

Information on these Upjohn products is based on labeling in effect on November 1, 1979. Further information on dosage and administration, side effects, precautions and contraindications for these and other Upjohn products may be obtained from either the package insert or Medical Services, The Upjohn Company, Kalamazoo, Michigan.

Upjohn—Cont.

white or practically white, odorless, crystalline powder which melts at about 215° with some decomposition. It is soluble in dioxane, sparingly soluble in acetone, in alcohol, in chloroform, and in methanol, and slightly soluble in ether. It is practically insoluble in water.
Each bottle contains:
Methylprednisolone Acetate....................40 mg
Also Sodium Chloride and Polysorbate 80
Actions: Naturally occurring glucocorticoids (hydrocortisone), which also have salt-retaining properties, are used as replacement therapy in adrenocortical deficiency states. Their synthetic analogs are primarily used for their potent anti-inflammatory effects in disorders of many organ systems.
Glucocorticoids cause profound and varied metabolic effects. In addition, they modify the body's immune responses to diverse stimuli.

Indications
Based on a review of this drug by the National Academy of Sciences—National Research Council and/or other information, FDA has classified the indications as follows:
Probably Effective
As a retention enema for the adjunctive treatment of ulcerative colitis.
Final classification of the less-than-effective indications requires further investigation.

Contraindications: Systemic fungal infections.
Warnings: In patients on corticosteroid therapy subjected to any unusual stress, increased dosage of rapidly acting corticosteroids before, during, and after the stressful situation is indicated.
Corticosteroids may mask some signs of infection, and new infections may appear during their use. There may be decreased resistance and inability to localize infection when corticosteroids are used.
Prolonged use of corticosteroids may produce posterior subcapsular cataracts, glaucoma with possible damage to the optic nerves, and may enhance the establishment of secondary ocular infections due to fungi or viruses.
Usage in Pregnancy. Since adequate human reproduction studies have not been done with corticosteroids, the use of these drugs in pregnancy, nursing mothers, or women of childbearing potential requires that the possible benefits of the drug be weighed against the potential hazards to the mother and embryo or fetus. Infants born of mothers who have received substantial doses of corticosteroids during pregnancy should be carefully observed for signs of hypoadrenalism.
Average and large doses of cortisone or hydrocortisone can cause elevation of blood pressure, salt and water retention, and increased excretion of potassium. These effects are less likely to occur with the synthetic derivatives except when used in large doses. Dietary salt restriction and potassium supplementation may be necessary. All corticosteroids increase calcium excretion.
While on corticosteroid therapy patients should not be vaccinated against smallpox. Other immunization procedures should not be undertaken in patients who are on corticosteroids, especially in high doses, because of possible hazards of neurological complications and lack of antibody response.
The use of methylprednisolone acetate in active tuberculosis should be restricted to those cases of fulminating or disseminated tuberculosis in which the corticosteroid is used for the management of the disease in conjunction with appropriate antituberculous regimen.
If corticosteroids are indicated in patients with latent tuberculosis or tuberculin reactivity, close observation is necessary as reactivation of the disease may occur. During prolonged corticosteroid therapy, these patients should receive chemoprophylaxis.
Precautions: Drug induced secondary adrenocortical insufficiency may be minimized by gradual reduction of dosage. This type of relative insufficiency may persist for months after discontinuation of therapy; therefore, in any situation of stress occurring during that period, hormone therapy should be reinstituted. Since mineralocorticoid secretion may be impaired, salt and/or a mineralocorticoid should be administered concurrently.
There is an enhanced effect of corticosteroids in patients with hypothyroidism and in those with cirrhosis.
Corticosteroids should be used cautiously in patients with ocular herpes simplex for fear of corneal perforation.
The lowest possible dose of corticosteroid should be used to control the condition under treatment, and when reduction in dosage is possible, the reduction must be gradual.
Psychic derangements may appear when corticosteroids are used, ranging from euphoria, insomnia, mood swings, personality changes, and severe depression to frank psychotic manifestations. Also, existing emotional instability or psychotic tendencies may be aggravated by corticosteroids.
Aspirin should be used cautiously in conjunction with corticosteroids in hypoprothrombinemia.
Steroids should be used with caution in nonspecific ulcerative colitis, if there is a probability of impending perforation, abscess or other pyogenic infection, also in diverticulitis, fresh intestinal anastomoses, active or latent peptic ulcer, renal insufficiency, hypertension, osteoporosis, and myasthenia gravis.
Growth and development of infants and children on prolonged corticosteroid therapy should be carefully followed.
Adverse Reactions:
Fluid and electrolyte disturbances:
- Sodium retention
- Fluid retention
- Congestive heart failure in susceptible patients
- Potassium loss
- Hypokalemic alkalosis
- Hypertension

Musculoskeletal:
- Muscle weakness
- Steroid myopathy
- Loss of muscle mass
- Osteoporosis
- Vertebral compression fractures
- Aseptic necrosis of femoral and humeral heads
- Pathologic fracture of long bones

Gastrointestinal:
- Peptic ulcer with possible subsequent perforation and hemorrhage
- Pancreatitis
- Abdominal distention
- Ulcerative esophagitis

Dermatologic:
- Impaired wound healing
- Thin fragile skin
- Petechiae and ecchymoses
- Facial erythema
- Increased sweating
- May suppress reactions to skin tests

Neurological:
- Convulsions
- Increased intracranial pressure with papilledema (pseudotumor cerebri) usually after treatment
- Vertigo
- Headache

Endocrine:
- Menstrual irregularities
- Development of Cushingoid state
- Suppression of growth in children
- Secondary adrenocortical and pituitary unresponsiveness, particularly in times of stress, as in trauma, surgery, or illness
- Decreased carbohydrate tolerance
- Manifestations of latent diabetes mellitus
- Increased requirements for insulin or oral hypoglycemic agents in diabetics

Ophthalmic:
- Posterior subcapsular cataracts
- Increased intraocular pressure
- Glaucoma
- Exophthalmos

Metabolic:
- Negative nitrogen balance due to protein catabolism

Dosage and Administration: A dose of 40 mg administered as a retention enema or by continuous drip three to seven times weekly for periods of two or more weeks has been shown to be a useful adjunct in the treatment of some patients with ulcerative colitis. Other accepted therapeutic measures should be instituted.
Directions for using *Medrol Enpak* Kit (methylprednisolone acetate).
1. Transfer contents of one glass bottle into plastic bottle, add 30 to 180 ml (1 to 6 fl oz) of warm water and shake until all solid material is suspended.
2. Place clamp in open position. Remove cap from plastic calibrated bottle and insert bottle top into green filler cap of plastic bag. With plastic bag in lower position than clamp, slowly squeeze the bottle and transfer contents into plastic bag. Close green cap tightly.
3. Slide clamp to convenient position. Close clamp on tubing, invert plastic bag and hang it in convenient location.
4. Fill plastic tubing completely with liquid by operating clamp. When tube is full, close clamp.
5. Moisten end of tubing. Insert in rectum and gradually open clamp.
6. By manipulating clamp, adjust flow into drip-chamber at the rate of 1 to 2 drops per second or at such a rate that the urge to defecate is not stimulated.
7. Allow to flow by gravity. Do not squeeze bag. Shake bottle every half-hour during administration.

How Supplied: Each *Medrol Enpak* Kit contains one administration unit and 6 bottles of *Medrol*® Acetate ointment (methylprednisolone acetate), 40 mg
NDC 0009-0435-01
Also available: Refill boxes of 12 bottles.
NDC 0009-0474-01
Code 810 562 000

MEDROL® TABLETS ℞
(Methylprednisolone Tablets, NF)
4 mg (500's):
NSN 6505-00-050-3068A (VA)
16 mg (50's):
NSN 6505-00-764-4358A (VA)

Description: Glucocorticoids are adrenocortical steroids, both naturally occurring and synthetic, which are readily absorbed from the gastrointestinal tract. Methylprednisolone occurs as a white to practically white, odorless, crystalline powder. It is sparingly soluble in alcohol, in dioxane, and in methanol, slightly soluble in acetone, and in chloroform, and very slightly soluble in ether. It is practically insoluble in water.
The chemical name for methylprednisolone is pregna-1, 4-diene-3, 20-dione,11, 17, 21-trihydroxy-6-methyl-,(6α, 11β)- and the molecular weight is 374.48.
Medrol Tablets (methylprednisolone) are available as scored tablets in the following strengths: 2 mg, 4 mg, 8 mg, 16 mg, 24 mg, 32 mg.

Actions: Naturally occurring glucocorticoids (hydrocortisone and cortisone), which also have salt-retaining properties, are used as replacement therapy in adrenocortical deficiency states. Their synthetic analogs are primarily used for their potent anti-inflammatory effects in disorders of many organ systems. Glucocorticoids cause profound and varied metabolic effects. In addition, they modify the body's immune responses to diverse stimuli.

Indications: *Medrol* Tablets (methylprednisolone) are indicated in the following conditions:

1. **Endocrine Disorders**
   Primary or secondary adrenocortical insufficiency (hydrocortisone or cortisone is the first choice; synthetic analogs may be used in conjunction with mineralocorticoids where applicable; in infancy mineralocorticoid supplementation is of particular importance).
   Congenital adrenal hyperplasia
   Nonsuppurative thyroiditis
   Hypercalcemia associated with cancer
2. **Rheumatic Disorders**
   As adjunctive therapy for short-term administration (to tide the patient over an acute episode or exacerbation) in:
   Psoriatic arthritis
   Rheumatoid arthritis, including juvenile rheumatoid arthritis (selected cases may require low-dose maintenance therapy)
   Ankylosing spondylitis
   Acute and subacute bursitis
   Acute nonspecific tenosynovitis
   Acute gouty arthritis
   Post-traumatic osteoarthritis
   Synovitis of osteoarthritis
   Epicondylitis
3. **Collagen Diseases**
   During an exacerbation or as maintenance therapy in selected cases of:
   Systemic lupus erythematosus
   Acute rheumatic carditis
   Systemic dermatomyositis (polymyositis)
4. **Dermatologic Diseases**
   Pemphigus
   Bullous dermatitis herpetiformis
   Severe erythema multiforme (Stevens-Johnson syndrome)
   Exfoliative dermatitis
   Mycosis fungoides
   Severe psoriasis
   Severe seborrheic dermatitis
5. **Allergic States**
   Control of severe or incapacitating allergic conditions intractable to adequate trials of conventional treatment:
   Seasonal or perennial allergic rhinitis
   Serum sickness
   Bronchial asthma
   Drug hypersensitivity reactions
   Contact dermatitis
   Atopic dermatitis
6. **Ophthalmic Diseases**
   Severe acute and chronic allergic and inflammatory processes involving the eye and its adnexa such as:
   Allergic corneal marginal ulcers
   Herpes zoster ophthalmicus
   Anterior segment inflammation
   Diffuse posterior uveitis and choroiditis
   Sympathetic ophthalmia
   Allergic conjunctivitis
   Keratitis
   Chorioretinitis
   Optic neuritis
   Iritis and iridocyclitis
7. **Respiratory Diseases**
   Symptomatic sarcoidosis
   Loeffler's syndrome not manageable by other means
   Berylliosis
   Fulminating or disseminated pulmonary tuberculosis when used concurrently with appropriate antituberculous chemotherapy
   Aspiration pneumonitis
8. **Hematologic Disorders**
   Idiopathic thrombocytopenic purpura in adults
   Secondary thrombocytopenia in adults
   Acquired (autoimmune) hemolytic anemia
   Erythroblastopenia (RBC anemia)
   Congenital (erythroid) hypoplastic anemia
9. **Neoplastic Diseases**
   For palliative management of:
   Leukemias and lymphomas in adults
   Acute leukemia of childhood
10. **Edematous States**
   To induce a diuresis or remission of proteinuria in the nephrotic syndrome, without uremia, of the idiopathic type or that due to lupus erythematosus.
11. **Gastrointestinal diseases**
   To tide the patient over a critical period of the disease in:
   Ulcerative colitis
   Regional enteritis
12. **Nervous System**
   Acute exacerbations of multiple sclerosis
13. **Miscellaneous**
   Tuberculous meningitis with subarachnoid block or impending block when used concurrently with appropriate antituberculous chemotherapy.
   Trichinosis with neurologic or myocardial involvement

Contraindications: Systemic fungal infections.

Warnings: In patients on corticosteroid therapy subjected to unusual stress, increased dosage of rapidly acting corticosteroids before, during, and after the stressful situation is indicated.

Corticosteroids may mask some signs of infection and new infections may appear during their use. There may be decreased resistance and inability to localize infection when corticosteroids are used.

Prolonged use of corticosteroids may produce posterior subcapsular cataracts, glaucoma with possible damage to the optic nerves, and may enhance the establishment of secondary ocular infections due to fungi or viruses.

Usage in pregnancy: Since adequate human reproduction studies have not been done with corticosteroids, the use of these drugs in pregnancy, nursing mothers or women of childbearing potential requires that the possible benefits of the drug be weighed against the potential hazards to the mother and embryo or fetus. Infants born of mothers who have received substantial doses of corticosteroids during pregnancy should be carefully observed for signs of hypoadrenalism.

Average and large doses of hydrocortisone or cortisone can cause elevation of blood pressure, salt and water retention, and increased excretion of potassium. These effects are less likely to occur with the synthetic derivatives except when used in large doses. Dietary salt restriction and potassium supplementation may be necessary. All corticosteroids increase calcium excretion.

While on corticosteroid therapy patients should not be vaccinated against smallpox. Other immunization procedures should not be undertaken in patients who are on corticosteroids, especially on high dose, because of possible hazards of neurological complications and a lack of antibody response.

The use of *Medrol* Tablets (methylprednisolone) in active tuberculosis should be restricted to those cases of fulminating or disseminated tuberculosis in which the corticosteroid is used for the management of the disease in conjunction with an appropriate antituberculous regimen.

If corticosteroids are indicated in patients with latent tuberculosis or tuberculin reactivity, close observation is necessary as reactivation of the disease may occur. During prolonged corticosteroid therapy, these patients should receive chemoprophylaxis.

Precautions: Drug-induced secondary adrenocortical insufficiency may be minimized by gradual reduction of dosage. This type of relative insufficiency may persist for months after discontinuation of therapy; therefore, in any situation of stress occurring during that period, hormone therapy should be reinstituted. Since mineralocorticoid secretion may be impaired, salt and/or a mineralocorticoid should be administered concurrently.

There is an enhanced effect of corticosteroids on patients with hypothyroidism and in those with cirrhosis.

Corticosteroids should be used cautiously in patients with ocular herpes simplex because of possible corneal perforation.

The lowest possible dose of corticosteroid should be used to control the condition under treatment, and when reduction in dosage is possible, the reduction should be gradual.

Psychic derangements may appear when corticosteroids are used, ranging from euphoria, insomnia, mood swings, personality changes and severe depression, to frank psychotic manifestations. Also, existing emotional instability or psychotic tendencies may be aggravated by corticosteroids.

Aspirin should be used cautiously in conjunction with corticosteroids in hypoprothrombinemia.

Steroids should be used with caution in nonspecific ulcerative colitis, if there is a probability of impending perforation, abscess or other pyogenic infection; diverticulitis; fresh intestinal anastomoses; active or latent peptic ulcer; renal insufficiency; hypertension; osteoporosis; and myasthenia gravis.

Growth and development of infants and children on prolonged corticosteroid therapy should be carefully observed.

Although controlled clinical trials have shown corticosteroids to be effective in speeding the resolution of acute exacerbations of multiple sclerosis, they do not show that corticosteroids affect the ultimate outcome or natural history of the disease. The studies do show that relatively high doses of corticosteroids are necessary to demonstrate a significant effect. (See **Dosage and Administration**)

Since complications of treatment with glucocorticoids are dependent on the size of the dose and the duration of treatment, a risk/benefit decision must be made in each individual case as to dose and duration of treatment and as to whether daily or intermittent therapy should be used.

The 24 mg tablet contains FD&C Yellow No. 5 (tartrazine) which may cause allergic-type reactions (including bronchial asthma) in certain susceptible individuals. Although the overall incidence of FD&C Yellow No. 5 (tartrazine) sensitivity in the general population is low, it is frequently seen in patients who also have aspirin hypersensitivity.

Continued on next page

Information on these Upjohn products is based on labeling in effect on November 1, 1979. Further information on dosage and administration, side effects, precautions and contraindications for these and other Upjohn products may be obtained from either the package insert or Medical Services, The Upjohn Company, Kalamazoo, Michigan.

Upjohn—Cont.

Adverse Reactions:

Fluid and Electrolyte Disturbances
- Sodium retention
- Fluid retention
- Congestive heart failure in susceptible patients
- Potassium loss
- Hypokalemic alkalosis
- Hypertension

Musculoskeletal
- Muscle weakness
- Steroid myopathy
- Loss of muscle mass
- Osteoporosis
- Vertebral compression fractures
- Aseptic necrosis of femoral and humeral heads
- Pathologic fracture of long bones

Gastrointestinal
- Peptic ulcer with possible perforation and hemorrhage
- Pancreatitis
- Abdominal distention
- Ulcerative esophagitis

Dermatologic
- Impaired wound healing
- Thin fragile skin
- Petechiae and ecchymoses
- Facial erythema
- Increased sweating
- May suppress reactions to skin tests

Neurological
- Increased intracranial pressure with papilledema (pseudo-tumor cerebri) usually after treatment
- Convulsions
- Vertigo
- Headache

Endocrine
- Development of Cushingoid state
- Suppression of growth in children
- Secondary adrenocortical and pituitary unresponsiveness, particularly in times of stress, as in trauma, surgery or illness.
- Menstrual irregularities
- Decreased carbohydrate tolerance
- Manifestations of latent diabetes mellitus
- Increased requirements for insulin or oral hypoglycemic agents in diabetics

Ophthalmic
- Posterior subcapsular cataracts
- Increased intraocular pressure
- Glaucoma
- Exophthalmos

Metabolic
- Negative nitrogen balance due to protein catabolism

Dosage and Administration:

The initial dosage of *Medrol* Tablets (methylprednisolone) may vary from 4 mg to 48 mg per day depending on the specific disease entity being treated. In situations of less severity lower doses will generally suffice while in selected patients higher initial doses may be required. The initial dosage should be maintained or adjusted until a satisfactory response is noted. If after a reasonable period of time there is a lack of satisfactory clinical response, *Medrol* should be discontinued and the patient transferred to other appropriate therapy. IT SHOULD BE EMPHASIZED THAT DOSAGE REQUIREMENTS ARE VARIABLE AND MUST BE INDIVIDUALIZED ON THE BASIS OF THE DISEASE UNDER TREATMENT AND THE RESPONSE OF THE PATIENT.

After a favorable response is noted, the proper maintenance dosage should be determined by decreasing the initial drug dosage in small decrements at appropriate time intervals until the lowest dosage which will maintain an adequate clinical response is reached. It should be kept in mind that constant monitoring is needed in regard to drug dosage. Included in the situations which may make dosage adjustments necessary are changes in clinical status secondary to remissions or exacerbations in the disease process, the patient's individual drug responsiveness, and the effect of patient exposure to stressful situations not directly related to the disease entity under treatment; in this latter situation it may be necessary to increase the dosage of *Medrol* for a period of time consistent with the patient's condition. If after long-term therapy the drug is to be stopped, it is recommended that it be withdrawn gradually rather than abruptly.

Multiple Sclerosis

In treatment of acute exacerbations of multiple sclerosis daily doses of 200 mg of prednisolone for a week followed by 80 mg every other day for 1 month have been shown to be effective (4 mg of methylprednisolone is equivalent to 5 mg of prednisolone).

ADT™ Alternate Day Therapy

Alternate day therapy is a corticosteroid dosing regimen in which twice the usual daily dose of corticoid is administered every other morning. The purpose of this mode of therapy is to provide the patient requiring long-term pharmacologic dose treatment with the beneficial effects of corticoids while minimizing certain undesirable effects, including pituitary-adrenal suppression, the Cushingoid state, corticoid withdrawal symptoms, and growth suppression in children.

The rationale for this treatment schedule is based on two major premises: (a) the anti-inflammatory or therapeutic effect of corticoids persists longer than their physical presence and metabolic effects and (b) administration of the corticosteroid every other morning allows for re-establishment of more nearly normal hypothalamic-pituitary-adrenal (HPA) activity on the off-steroid day.

A brief review of the HPA physiology may be helpful in understanding this rationale. Acting primarily through the hypothalamus a fall in free cortisol stimulates the pituitary gland to produce increasing amounts of corticotropin (ACTH) while a rise in free cortisol inhibits ACTH secretion. Normally the HPA system is characterized by diurnal (circadian) rhythm. Serum levels of ACTH rise from a low point about 10 pm to a peak level about 6 am. Increasing levels of ACTH stimulate adrenal cortical activity resulting in a rise in plasma cortisol with maximal levels occurring between 2 am and 8 am. This rise in cortisol dampens ACTH production and in turn adrenal cortical activity. There is a gradual fall in plasma corticoids during the day with lowest levels occurring about midnight.

The diurnal rhythm of the HPA axis is lost in Cushing's disease, a syndrome of adrenal cortical hyperfunction characterized by obesity with centripetal fat distribution, thinning of the skin with easy bruisability, muscle wasting with weakness, hypertension, latent diabetes, osteoporosis, electrolyte imbalance, etc. The same clinical findings of hyperadrenocorticism may be noted during long-term pharmacologic dose corticoid therapy administered in conventional daily divided doses. It would appear, then, that a disturbance in the diurnal cycle with maintenance of elevated corticoid values during the night may play a significant role in the development of undesirable corticoid effects. Escape from these constantly elevated plasma levels for even short periods of time may be instrumental in protecting against undesirable pharmacologic effects.

During conventional pharmacologic dose corticosteroid therapy, ACTH production is inhibited with subsequent suppression of cortisol production by the adrenal cortex. Recovery time for normal HPA activity is variable depending upon the dose and duration of treatment. During this time the patient is vulnerable to any stressful situation. Although it has been shown that there is considerably less adrenal suppression following a single morning dose of prednisolone (10 mg) as opposed to a quarter of that dose administered every 6 hours, there is evidence that some suppressive effect on adrenal activity may be carried over into the following day when pharmacologic doses are used. Further, it has been shown that a single dose of certain corticosteroids will produce adrenal cortical suppression for two or more days. Other corticoids, including methylprednisolone, hydrocortisone, prednisone, and prednisolone, are considered to be short acting (producing adrenal cortical suppression for 1¼ to 1½ days following a single dose) and thus are recommended for alternate day therapy.

The following should be kept in mind when considering alternate day therapy:

1) Basic principles and indications for corticosteroid therapy should apply. The benefits of *ADT* should not encourage the indiscriminate use of steroids.

2) *ADT* is a therapeutic technique primarily designed for patients in whom long-term pharmacologic corticoid therapy is anticipated.

3) In less severe disease processes in which corticoid therapy is indicated, it may be possible to initiate treatment with *ADT*. More severe disease states usually will require daily divided high dose therapy for initial control of the disease process. The initial suppressive dose level should be continued until satisfactory clinical response is obtained, usually four to ten days in the case of many allergic and collagen diseases. It is important to keep the period of initial suppressive dose as brief as possible particularly when subsequent use of alternate day therapy is intended.

Once control has been established, two courses are available: (a) change to *ADT* and then gradually reduce the amount of corticoid given every other day *or* (b) following control of the disease process reduce the daily dose of corticoid to the lowest effective level as rapidly as possible and then change over to an alternate day schedule. Theoretically, course (a) may be preferable.

4) Because of the advantages of *ADT*, it may be desirable to try patients on this form of therapy who have been on daily corticoids for long periods of time (eg, patients with rheumatoid arthritis). Since these patients may already have a suppressed HPA axis, establishing them on *ADT* may be difficult and not always successful. However, it is recommended that regular attempts be made to change them over. It may be helpful to triple or even quadruple the daily maintenance dose and administer this every other day rather than just doubling the daily dose if difficulty is encountered. Once the patient is again controlled, an attempt should be made to reduce this dose to a minimum.

5) As indicated above, certain corticosteroids, because of their prolonged suppressive effect on adrenal activity, are not recommended for alternate day therapy (eg, dexamethasone and betamethasone).

6) The maximal activity of the adrenal cortex is between 2 am and 8 am, and it is minimal between 4 pm and midnight. Exogenous corticosteroids suppress adrenocortical activity the least, when given at the time of maximal activity (am).

7) In using *ADT* it is important, as in all therapeutic situations, to individualize and tailor the therapy to each patient. Complete control of symptoms will not be possible in all patients. An explanation of the benefits of *ADT* will help the patient to understand and tolerate the possible flare-up in symptoms which may occur in the latter part of the off-steroid day. Other symptomatic therapy may be added or increased at this time if needed.

8) In the event of an acute flare-up of the disease process, it may be necessary to return to a full suppressive daily divided corticoid dose for control. Once control is again established alternate day therapy may be reinstituted.

9) Although many of the undesirable features of corticosteroid therapy can be minimized by *ADT*, as in any therapeutic situation, the physician must carefully weigh the benefit-risk ratio for each patient in whom corticoid therapy is being considered.

How Supplied:
Medrol Tablets (methylprednisolone) are available in the following strengths and sizes:

2 mg	Bottles of 30	*NDC 0009-0049-01*
	Bottles of 100	*NDC 0009-0049-02*
4 mg	Bottles of 30	*NDC 0009-0056-01*
	Bottles of 100	*NDC 0009-0056-02*
	Bottles of 500	*NDC 0009-0056-03*
	Unit Dose Package (100)	*NDC 0009-0056-05*
	Dosepak™ Unit of use (21 tablets)	*NDC 0009-0056-04*
8 mg	Bottles of 25	*NDC 0009-0022-01*
16 mg	Bottles of 50	*NDC 0009-0073-01*
	ADT Pak® (14 tablets)	*NDC 0009-0073-02*
24 mg	Bottles of 25	*NDC 0009-0155-01*
32 mg	Bottles of 25	*NDC 0009-0176-01*

Code 810 487 000

[*Shown in Product Identification Section*]

MOTRIN® TABLETS ℞
(ibuprofen)

Description: *Motrin* (ibuprofen) is (±)-2-(*p*-isobutylphenyl) propionic acid. It is a white powder with a melting point of 74–77°C and is very slightly soluble in water (< 1 mg/ml) and readily soluble in organic solvents such as ethanol and acetone.
Motrin is a nonsteroidal anti-inflammatory agent. It is available in 300, 400 and 600 mg tablets for oral administration.
Clinical Pharmacology: *Motrin* (ibuprofen) is a nonsteroidal anti-inflammatory agent that possesses analgesic and antipyretic activities. Its mode of action, like that of other nonsteroidal anti-inflammatory agents, is not known; however, its therapeutic action is not due to pituitary-adrenal stimulation. *Motrin* does not alter the course of the underlying disease.
In patients treated with *Motrin* for rheumatoid arthritis and osteoarthritis, the anti-inflammatory action of *Motrin* has been shown by reduction in joint swelling, reduction in pain, reduction in duration of morning stiffness, reduction in disease activity as assessed by both the investigator and patient; and by improved functional capacity as demonstrated by an increase in grip strength, a delay in the time to onset of fatigue, and a decrease in time to walk 50 feet.
Motrin is rapidly absorbed when administered orally. Peak serum ibuprofen levels are generally attained one to two hours after administration. With single doses ranging from 200 mg to 800 mg, a dose-response relationship exists between amount of drug administered and the integrated area under the serum drug concentration vs time curve. There is no evidence of drug accumulation or enzyme induction.
The administration of *Motrin* Tablets either under fasting conditions or immediately before meals yields quite similar serum ibuprofen concentration-time profiles. When *Motrin* is administered immediately after a meal, there is a reduction in the rate of absorption but no appreciable decrease in the extent of absorption. The bioavailability of *Motrin* is minimally altered by the presence of food.
Motrin is rapidly metabolized and eliminated in the urine. The excretion of *Motrin* is virtually complete 24 hours after the last dose. The serum half-life of *Motrin* is 1.8 to 2.0 hours.
Studies have shown that following ingestion of the drug, 45% to 79% of the dose was recovered in the urine within 24 hours as metabolite A (25%), (+)-2-[*p*-(2hydroxymethylpropyl)-phenyl] propionic acid and metabolite B (37%), (+)-2-[*p*(2carboxypropyl)-phenyl] propionic acid; the percentages of free and conjugated ibuprofen were approximately 1% and 14%, respectively.
Indications and Usage: *Motrin* (ibuprofen) is indicated for relief of the signs and symptoms of rheumatoid arthritis and osteoarthritis. It is indicated in the treatment of acute flares and in the long-term management of these diseases. The safety and effectiveness of *Motrin* have not been established in those rheumatoid arthritis patients who are designated by the American Rheumatism Association as Functional Class IV (incapacitated, largely or wholly bedridden, or confined to wheelchair; little or no self-care).
In patients treated with *Motrin* for rheumatoid arthritis and osteoarthritis, the anti-inflammatory action of *Motrin* has been shown by reduction in joint swelling, reduction in pain, reduction in duration of morning stiffness, reduction in disease activity as assessed by both the investigator and patient; and by improved functional capacity as demonstrated by an increase in grip strength, a delay in the time to onset of fatigue, and a decrease in time to walk 50 feet.
In clinical studies in patients with rheumatoid arthritis and osteoarthritis, *Motrin* has been shown to be comparable to aspirin in controlling the aforementioned signs and symptoms of disease activity and to be associated with a statistically significant reduction in the milder gastrointestinal side effects (see ADVERSE REACTIONS). *Motrin* may be well tolerated in some patients who have had gastrointestinal side effects with aspirin, but these patients when treated with *Motrin* should be carefully followed for signs and symptoms of gastrointestinal ulceration and bleeding. Although it is not definitely known whether *Motrin* causes less peptic ulceration than aspirin, in one study involving 885 patients with rheumatoid arthritis treated for up to one year, there were no reports of gastric ulceration with *Motrin* whereas frank ulceration was reported in 13 patients in the aspirin group (statistically significant $p < .001$).
In clinical studies in patients with rheumatoid arthritis, *Motrin* has been shown to be comparable to indomethacin in controlling the aforementioned signs and symptoms of disease activity and to be associated with a statistically significant reduction of the milder gastrointestinal (see ADVERSE REACTIONS) and CNS side effects.
Motrin may be used in combination with gold salts and/or corticosteroids. When *Motrin* and placebo were compared in gold-treated rheumatoid arthritis patients, *Motrin* was consistently more effective in relieving symptoms than was placebo. However, it cannot be inferred that *Motrin* potentiates the effect of gold on the underlying disease. Whether or not *Motrin* can be used in conjunction with partially effective doses of corticosteroid for a "steroid-sparing" effect, and result in greater improvement, has not been adequately studied.
Motrin is also indicated for relief of mild to moderate pain.
Since there have been no controlled clinical trials to demonstrate whether or not there is any beneficial effect or harmful interaction with the use of *Motrin* in conjunction with aspirin, the combination cannot be recommended (see **Drug Interactions**).
Controlled clinical trials to establish the safety and effectiveness of *Motrin* in children have not been conducted.
Contraindications: *Motrin* (ibuprofen) should not be used in patients who have previously exhibited hypersensitivity to it, or in individuals with the syndrome of nasal polyps, angioedema and bronchospastic reactivity to aspirin or other nonsteroidal anti-inflammatory agents (see WARNINGS).
Warnings: Anaphylactoid reactions have occurred in patients with known aspirin hypersensitivity (see CONTRAINDICATIONS).
Peptic ulceration and gastrointestinal bleeding, sometimes severe, have been reported in patients receiving *Motrin* (ibuprofen). Peptic ulceration, perforation, or severe gastrointestinal bleeding can have a fatal outcome, and although a few such reports have been received with *Motrin*, a cause and effect relationship has not been established. *Motrin* should be given under close supervision to patients with a history of upper gastrointestinal tract disease, and only after consulting the ADVERSE REACTIONS section.
In patients with active peptic ulcer and active rheumatoid arthritis, attempts should be made to treat the arthritis with nonulcerogenic drugs, such as gold. If *Motrin* must be given, the patient should be under close supervision for signs of ulcer perforation or gastrointestinal bleeding.
Precautions: Blurred and/or diminished vision, scotomata, and/or changes in color vision have been reported. If a patient develops such complaints while receiving *Motrin* (ibuprofen), the drug should be discontinued and the patient should have an ophthalmologic examination.
Fluid retention and edema have been reported in association with *Motrin;* therefore, the drug should be used with caution in patients with a history of cardiac decompensation.
Motrin, like other nonsteroidal anti-inflammatory agents, can inhibit platelet aggregation but the effect is quantitatively less and of shorter duration than that seen with aspirin. *Motrin* has been shown to prolong bleeding time (but within the normal range) in normal subjects. Because this prolonged bleeding effect may be exaggerated in patients with underlying hemostatic defects, *Motrin* should be used with caution in persons with intrinsic coagulation defects and those on anticoagulant therapy.
Patients on *Motrin* should report to their physicians signs or symptoms of gastrointestinal ulceration or bleeding, blurred vision or other eye symptoms, skin rash, weight gain, or edema.
In order to avoid exacerbation of disease or adrenal insufficiency, patients who have been on prolonged corticosteroid therapy should have their therapy tapered slowly rather than discontinued abruptly when *Motrin* is added to the treatment program.
Drug Interactions
Coumarin-type anticoagulants. Several short-term controlled studies failed to show that *Motrin* significantly affected prothrombin times or a variety of other clotting factors when administered to individuals on coumarin-type anticoagulants. However, because bleeding has been reported when *Motrin* and other nonsteroidal anti-inflammatory agents have been administered to patients on coumarin-type anticoagulants, the physician should be cautious when administering *Motrin* to patients on anticoagulants.
Aspirin. Animal studies show that aspirin given with nonsteroidal anti-inflammatory agents, including *Motrin*, yields a net decrease in anti-inflammatory activity with lowered blood levels of the nonaspirin drug. Single dose bioavailability studies in normal volunteers have failed to show an effect of aspirin on *Motrin* blood levels. Correlative clinical studies have not been done.

Continued on next page

Information on these Upjohn products is based on labeling in effect on November 1, 1979. Further information on dosage and administration, side effects, precautions and contraindications for these and other Upjohn products may be obtained from either the package insert or Medical Services, The Upjohn Company, Kalamazoo, Michigan.

Upjohn—Cont.

Pregnancy
Reproductive studies conducted in rats and rabbits at doses somewhat less than the maximal clinical dose did not demonstrate evidence of developmental abnormalities. These data are inadequate to provide reasonable assurance that the drug will not have an adverse effect on the fetus. *Motrin* (ibuprofen) has been shown to inhibit prostaglandin synthesis and release. The same effect has been demonstrated by other nonsteroidal and anti-inflammatory drugs and has been associated with an increased incidence of dystocia and delayed parturition in pregnant animals when such drugs were administered late in pregnancy. Administration of *Motrin* is not recommended during pregnancy.

Nursing Mothers
In limited studies, an assay capable of detecting 1 mcg/ml did not demonstrate *Motrin* in the milk of lactating mothers. However, because of the limited nature of the studies, *Motrin* is not recommended for use in nursing mothers.

Adverse Reactions:

Incidence greater than 1%

Gastrointestinal: The most frequent type of adverse reaction occurring with *Motrin* (ibuprofen) is gastrointestinal. In controlled clinical trials the percentage of patients reporting one or more gastrointestinal complaints ranged from 4% to 16%. Such complaints included nausea*, epigastric pain*, heartburn*, diarrhea, abdominal distress, nausea and vomiting, indigestion, constipation, abdominal cramps or pain, fullness of the GI tract (bloating and flatulence).

In controlled studies when *Motrin* was compared to aspirin and indomethacin in equally effective doses, the overall incidence of gastrointestinal complaints was about half that seen in either the aspirin- or indomethacin-treated patients.

Other reactions observed during controlled clinical trials which were greater than 1 in 100:

Central Nervous System: dizziness*, headache, nervousness.

Dermatologic: rash* (including maculopapular type), pruritus.

Special Senses: tinnitus

Metabolic: decreased appetite, edema, fluid retention. Fluid retention generally responds promptly to drug discontinuation (see PRECAUTIONS).

*Reactions occurring in 3% to 9% of patients treated with *Motrin*. (Those reactions occurring in less than 3% of the patients are unmarked.)

Incidence less than 1 in 100

The following adverse reactions, occurring less frequently than 1 in 100, were reported in controlled clinical trials and through voluntary reports since marketing. The probability of a causal relationship exists between *Motrin* and these adverse reactions:

Gastrointestinal: gastric or duodenal ulcer with bleeding and/or perforation, gastrointestinal hemorrhage, melena

Dermatologic: vesiculobullous eruptions, urticaria, erythema multiforme

Central Nervous System: depression, insomnia

Special Senses: amblyopia (blurred and/or diminished vision, scotomata and/or changes in color vision). Any patient with eye complaints during *Motrin* therapy should have an ophthalmologic examination which includes central visual fields (see PRECAUTIONS).

Hematologic: leukopenia and decreases in hemoglobin and hematocrit

Cardiovascular: congestive heart failure in patients with marginal cardiac function, elevated blood pressure

Causal relationship unknown

Other reactions have been reported but occurred under circumstances where a causal relationship could not be established. However, in these rarely reported events, the possibility cannot be excluded. Therefore these observations are being listed to serve as alerting information to the physician.

Gastrointestinal: Hepatitis, jaundice, abnormal liver function

Central Nervous System: Paresthesias, hallucinations, dream abnormalities

Dermatologic: Alopecia, Stevens-Johnson syndrome

Special Senses: Conjunctivitis, diplopia, optic neuritis

Hematologic: Hemolytic anemia, thrombocytopenia, granulocytopenia, bleeding episodes (eg., purpura, epistaxis, hematuria, menorrhagia)

Allergic: Fever, serum sickness, lupus erythematosus syndrome

Endocrine: Gynecomastia, hypoglycemic reaction

Cardiovascular: Arrhythmias (sinus tachycardia, sinus bradycardia, palpitations)

Renal: Decreased creatinine clearance, polyuria, azotemia

Overdosage: Approximately 1½ hours after the reported ingestion of from 7 to 10 *Motrin* Tablets (ibuprofen) (400 mg), a 19-month old child weighing 12 kg was seen in the hospital emergency room, apneic and cyanotic, responding only to painful stimuli. This type of stimulus, however, was sufficient to induce respiration. Oxygen and parenteral fluids were given; a greenish-yellow fluid was aspirated from the stomach with no evidence to indicate the presence of *Motrin*. Two hours after ingestion the child's condition seemed stable; she still responded only to painful stimuli and continued to have periods of apnea lasting from 5 to 10 seconds. She was admitted to intensive care and sodium bicarbonate was administered as well as infusions of dextrose and normal saline. By four hours post-ingestion she could be aroused easily, sit by herself and respond to spoken commands. Blood level of ibuprofen was 102.9 μg/ml approximately 8½ hours after accidental ingestion. At 12 hours she appeared to be completely recovered.

In two other reported cases where children (each weighing approximately 10 kg) had taken six tablets for an estimated acute intake of approximately 120 mg/kg, there were no signs of acute intoxication or late sequelae. Blood level in one child 90 minutes after ingestion was 700 μg/ml—about 10 times the peak levels seen in absorption-excretion studies.

A 19-year old male who had taken 8,000 mg of *Motrin* over a period of a few hours complained of dizziness, and nystagmus was noted. After hospitalization, parenteral hydration and three days' bed rest, he recovered with no reported sequelae.

In cases of acute overdosage, the stomach should be emptied by vomiting or lavage, though little drug will likely be recovered if more than an hour has elapsed since ingestion. Because the drug is acidic and is excreted in the urine, it is theoretically beneficial to administer alkali and induce diuresis.

Dosage and Administration:

Rheumatoid arthritis and osteoarthritis, including flare-ups of chronic disease:

Suggested Dosage: 300 mg, 400 mg, or 600 mg t.i.d. or q.i.d. The dose of *Motrin* (ibuprofen) should be tailored to each patient, and may be lowered or raised depending on the severity of symptoms either at time of initiating drug therapy or as the patient responds or fails to respond.

In general, patients with rheumatoid arthritis seem to require higher doses of *Motrin* than do patients with osteoarthritis.

The smallest dose of *Motrin* that yields acceptable control should be employed.

A therapeutic response to *Motrin* therapy is sometimes seen in a few days to a week but most often is observed by two weeks. After a satisfactory response has been achieved, the patient's dose should be reviewed and adjusted as required.

Mild to moderate pain:
400 mg every 4 to 6 hours as necessary for relief of pain.

Do not exceed 2,400 mg total daily dose. If gastrointestinal complaints occur, administer *Motrin* with meals or milk.

How Supplied:

***Motrin* Tablets, 300 mg** (white)	
Bottles of 60	NDC 0009-0733-01
Bottles of 500	NDC 0009-0733-02
***Motrin* Tablets, 400 mg** (orange)	
Bottles of 500	NDC 0009-0750-02
Unit-dose package of 100	NDC 0009-0750-06
Unit of Use bottles of 100	NDC 0009-0750-25
***Motrin* Tablets, 600 mg** (peach)	
Bottles of 60	NDC 0009-0742-01
Bottles of 500	NDC 0009-0742-02

Code 810 015 001

[*Shown in Product Identification Section*]

MYCIFRADIN® TABLETS ℞
(Neomycin Sulfate Tablets, USP)

MYCIFRADIN® ℞
ORAL SOLUTION
(Neomycin Sulfate Oral Solution, USP)

Description: Neomycin is an antibiotic obtained from the metabolic products of the actinomycete *Streptomyces fradiae*.

Actions: Neomycin is poorly absorbed from the normal gastrointestinal tract. The small absorbed fraction is rapidly excreted with normal kidney function. The unabsorbed portion of the drug (approximately 97 percent) is eliminated unchanged in the feces.

Growth of most intestinal bacteria is rapidly suppressed following oral administration of neomycin, with the suppression persisting for 48-72 hours. Nonpathogenic yeasts and occasionally resistant strains of *Enterobacter aerogenes* (formerly *Aerobacter aerogenes*) replace the intestinal bacteria.

Indications: Suppression of intestinal bacteria. Neomycin may be indicated when suppression of the normal bacterial flora of the bowel is desirable for either short or long term adjunctive therapy.

Hepatic Coma. Prolonged administration has been shown to be effective adjunctive therapy in hepatic coma by reduction of the ammonia-forming bacteria in the intestinal tract. The subsequent reduction in blood ammonia has resulted in neurologic improvement.

Diarrhea due to Enteropathogenic Escherichia coli. Diarrhea due to enteropathogenic *Escherichia coli* may be effectively treated with neomycin sulfate. When this diarrhea occurs in epidemic form, all patients and carriers should be treated concurrently.

Contraindications: Neomycin sulfate oral preparations are contraindicated in the presence of intestinal obstruction and in individuals with a history of hypersensitivity to the drug.

WARNING: BECAUSE OF REPORTED CASES OF DEAFNESS FOLLOWING THE ORAL USE OF NEOMYCIN AND THE POTENTIAL NEPHROTOXIC EFFECTS, PATIENTS SHOULD BE UNDER CLOSE CLINICAL OBSERVATION INCLUDING AUDIOMETRIC TESTING BEFORE AND DURING LONG TERM THERAPY.

Patients with renal insufficiency may develop toxic blood levels of the drug unless doses are properly regulated. If renal insufficiency develops during treatment, the dosage should be reduced or the antibiotic discontinued. Urine and blood examinations and audiometric tests should be given prior to and during extended therapy in individuals with hepatic and/or

renal disease to avoid nephrotoxicity and eighth nerve damage from improper dosage.
Usage in Pregnancy: Safety for use in pregnancy has not been established.
Precautions: Caution should be taken in concurrent use of other ototoxic and/or nephrotoxic antimicrobial drugs while neomycin is administered orally. These include streptomycin, kanamycin, polymyxin B, colistin, viomycin, gentamicin and cephaloridine.
The concurrent use of potent diuretics such as ethacrynic acid, furosemide, urea and mannitol (particularly when the diuretics are given intravenously) should be avoided. They may cause cumulative adverse effects of the neomycin on the kidney and auditory nerve.
Prolonged use of oral neomycin may result in overgrowth of nonsusceptible organisms, particularly fungi. If this occurs, appropriate therapy should be instituted.
Adverse Reactions: The most common adverse reactions to oral neomycin are nausea, vomiting and diarrhea. The "Malabsorption Syndrome" characterized by increased fecal fat, decreased serum carotene and fall in xylose absorption has been reported with prolonged therapy. Nephrotoxicity and ototoxicity have been reported following prolonged and high dosage therapy in hepatic coma.
Dosage and Administration: Hepatic Coma—For use as an adjunct in the management of hepatic coma, the following regimen has been found useful.

1. Withdraw protein from diet. Avoid use of diuretic agents.
2. Supportive therapy including transfusions as indicated.
3. *Mycifradin* (neomycin) orally in doses of 4 to 12 grams per day (8 to 24 tablets) in divided doses. Treatment should be continued over a period of five to six days during which time protein should be returned incrementally to the diet.
4. Chronic hepatic insufficiency may require doses of up to 4 grams (8 tablets) per day, over an indefinite period.

Infectious Diarrhea—*Mycifradin* may be administered in doses of 50 mg/kg/day for two to three days in divided doses to treat infectious diarrhea due to enteropathic *Escherichia coli.* In adults, a dose of 3 grams per day is ordinarily sufficient to obtain optimal benefit in responsive cases. For treatment or prevention of diarrhea in infants and younger children, *Mycifradin* Oral Solution is recommended as a preferable dosage form.
Preoperative preparation in abdominal surgery—The following regimen, in the absence of obstruction or other contraindications, has been employed for a 2 to 3 day preparation:

1. Low residue diet.
2. The total daily dose for preoperative bowel preparation in children or adults is calculated on the basis of 40 mg of *Mycifradin* per pound of body weight and is administered in six equally divided doses (one dose every 4 hours). The first dose is given immediately after a saline cathartic.

The following regimen may be used for a 24-hour preparation in an adult:

1. Low residue diet.
2. Cathartic.
3. One gram *Mycifradin* every hour for four doses, followed by 1 gram every 4 hours for the balance of the 24 hours.

Preoperative treatment is usually 24 hours and should not extend beyond 72 hours.
How Supplied:
***Mycifradin* Tablets** 0.5 Gm.
Bottles of 20 *NDC 0009-0521-01*
Bottles of 100 *NDC 0009-0521-02*
Bottles of 500 *NDC 0009-0521-03*
***Mycifradin* Oral Solution**, 125 mg neomycin sulfate per 5 ml.
2 oz bottles *NDC 0009-0513-01*
Pint bottles *NDC 0009-0513-02*
Code MBD-2

NEO-DELTA-CORTEF® OPHTHALMIC SUSPENSION ℞
(neomycin sulfate-prednisolone acetate)

Description: Each ml contains prednisolone acetate 2.5 mg (0.25%), neomycin sulfate 5 mg (equivalent to 3.5 mg neomycin), also myristyl-gamma-picolinium chloride, sodium citrate, polyethylene glycol 4000, povidone, and water for injection. When necessary, the pH was adjusted with sodium hydroxide and/or hydrochloric acid.
Actions: *Delta-Cortef®* (prednisolone) exerts a marked anti-inflammatory effect in the same manner as does hydrocortisone, i.e., through a controlling influence on vascular permeability and on the cellular, fibrous and amorphous components of connective tissue. In anti-inflammatory activity prednisolone is more potent than hydrocortisone and a concentration of 0.25% of prednisolone acetate is highly effective on topical application in inflammatory conditions of the anterior ocular segment. Local application to the eye often gives rapid relief of pain and photophobia, particularly in lesions of the cornea. This effect is believed due to the controlling action of the hormone on the inflammatory process rather than to a specific analgesic effect. By inhibiting fibroblastic proliferation, symblepharon formation in chemical and thermal burns may be prevented, and through decreased scar formation and reduced formation of new blood vessels clearer corneas may result.
Topically applied prednisolone acetate is usually rapidly effective, particularly in acute inflammatory conditions of the conjunctiva, sclera, cornea and anterior uveal tract. Chronic conditions respond more slowly and relapses are more frequent. In the presence of laboratory or clinical evidence of infection of the eye in traumatic conditions, and following intraocular surgery, the inflammatory reaction may be effectively inhibited by prednisolone and the bacterial infection controlled by neomycin. In generalized uveitis and inflammatory diseases of the posterior segment, systemic corticosteroid therapy should be employed.
Neomycin is an antibacterial substance derived from cultures of the soil organism *Streptomyces fradiae.* It exhibits a wider spectrum of antibacterial activity than either bacitracin, streptomycin or penicillin. Its antimicrobial range includes both gram-positive and gram-negative organisms commonly responsible for ocular infections; such as, staphylococci, *Escherichia coli,* Morax-Axenfeld diplobacillus, *Hemophilus influenzae* (Koch-Weeks), and many strains of *Proteus* and *Pseudomonas* organisms. It is not active against fungi. Neomycin rarely causes resistant strains of microorganisms to develop; in addition, it is unusually nontoxic for human epithelial cells in tissue culture and is nonirritating in therapeutic concentrations.

Indications

Based on a review of this drug by the National Academy of Sciences—National Research Council and/or other information, FDA has classified the indications as follows:
Possibly Effective:
Topical application of this preparation is indicated in the following conditions when complicated by infection due to neomycin-sensitive organisms:
Eye
Phlyctenular keratoconjunctivitis
Nonspecific superficial keratitis
Acne rosacea keratitis
Allergic conjunctivitis
Sclerokeratitis
Episcleritis
Traumatic Keratitis
Final classification of the less-than-effective indications requires further investigation.

Contraindications: Topical therapy with this preparation is contraindicated in the presence of tuberculous, fungal and acute purulent infections of the eye and in the presence of certain viral infections of the cornea and conjunctiva such as herpes simplex keratitis (dendritic ulcer), vaccinia and varicella, and in those individuals with a history of sensitivity to any of its components.
Precautions: *Neo-Delta-Cortef* Ophthalmic Suspension (neomycin sulfate-prednisolone acetate) is usually well tolerated; but if signs of irritation or sensitivity should develop, application should be discontinued. According to current medical literature, there has been an increase in the prevalence of neomycin hypersensitivity.
Repeated local application of corticoids to the eye for prolonged periods may result in increased intraocular pressure or posterior subcapsular cataract formation in certain individuals. For the former reason intraocular pressures should be determined regularly in such patients.
Perforation of the cornea, while infrequent, has occurred during treatment of herpes zoster ophthalmicus with corticoids. Also, in rare instances, scleral perforation resembling scleromalacia perforans has occurred during prolonged local therapy with these agents.
The prolonged use of antibiotic containing preparations may result in overgrowth of nonsusceptible organisms—particularly monilia. If new infections appear during treatment, appropriate antibiotic therapy should be instituted, and, if such is not available, as in the case of herpes simplex keratitis, therapy with this agent should be discontinued as well. The safety of the use of topical steroid preparations during pregnancy has not been fully established. Therefore, steroids should not be used unnecessarily during pregnancy or for prolonged periods of time.
The sterility may not persist after the bottle has been opened. Patients should be instructed to take appropriate measure to avoid contamination, especially when applying the preparation to open lesions of the eye.
Administration: For beginning treatment in acute ocular inflammation, one or two drops may be placed in the conjunctival sac every hour during the day and every two hours at night. When improvement occurs, the dosage may be reduced to one drop three or four times daily.
How Supplied: Available in 5 ml dropper bottles.
NDC 0009-0645-01
Code NBK-2

Continued on next page

Information on these Upjohn products is based on labeling in effect on November 1, 1979. Further information on dosage and administration, side effects, precautions and contraindications for these and other Upjohn products may be obtained from either the package insert or Medical Services, The Upjohn Company, Kalamazoo, Michigan.

Upjohn—Cont.

ORINASE® TABLETS ℞
(Tolbutamide Tablets, USP)
30s
NSN 6505-01-061-3651 (VA)
200s:
NSN 6505-00-982-9069 (M)
500s:
NSN 6505-00-079-8722A (VA)

Description: Tolbutamide is 1-butyl-3-*p*-tolylsulfonylurea, which is a pure white crystalline compound practically insoluble in water but forming water soluble salts with alkalies. It has a molecular weight of 270.34; its molecular formula is $C_{12}H_{18}N_2O_3S$.
This is an oral antidiabetes agent which effectively restores blood sugar to normal ranges in selected diabetic patients. *Orinase* Tablets (tolbutamide) diminishes glycosuria and alleviates such symptoms as pruritus, polyuria, polydipsia, polyphagia. While most commonly used as the sole therapeutic agent in the management of mild to moderately severe adult-type diabetes, it has also been found of value as an adjuvant to insulin therapy in the stabilization of certain cases of labile diabetes. Such combination therapy not infrequently results in significant reduction of insulin requirement, greater freedom from threat of hypoglycemic reaction, and marked subjective improvement.
Mode of Action: Numerous studies have provided convincing evidence that the major, if not sole, mode of action of tolbutamide is that of stimulation of synthesis and release of endogenous insulin.
One factor relative to mechanism is conclusively established—that is, *Orinase (tolbutamide) will not lower blood sugar in the human subject who has no pancreatic beta cells.* Whether this agent has any significant effect after total pancreatectomy when insulin is being injected is still a moot question. If *Orinase* does exert an insulin sparing effect (and available data on this point are controversial), the mechanism of the action remains to be elucidated. It has been demonstrated that tolbutamide does not alter the rate at which labeled iodo-insulin disappears from the blood.
The Blood Sugar Lowering Effect: The blood sugar lowering effect is independent of the pituitary, adrenocortical, and neural mechanisms that exert a regulatory effect on carbohydrate metabolism. *Orinase* (tolbutamide) does not inhibit the hyperglycemic response induced by epinephrine or glucagon, and it has no effect on the renal threshold for glucose excretion.
The administration of 3 grams of *Orinase* to either nondiabetics or tolbutamide-responsive diabetics will, in both instances, occasion a gradual lowering of blood sugar. Increasing the dose to 6 grams does not usually cause a response which is significantly different from that produced by a 3 gram dose. Nondiabetics show a very slight fall in blood sugar with the lowest level being reached four to five hours after dose administration. On the other hand, tolbutamide-responsive diabetics show a marked reduction of blood sugar to euglycemic levels. In these patients some decrease in blood sugar is discernible after the first hour and the nadir is seen 5 hours or more following administration. This difference between responsive diabetic and nondiabetic types of response has been emphasized in studies which employed specially prepared solutions of *Orinase* sodium. A summary of the results of these studies follows.
In nondiabetic human subjects—After the oral administration of a 3 gram dose of *Orinase* solution, healthy fasting adults usually exhibit a 30% or greater reduction in blood sugar within one hour, following which the blood sugar gradually returns to the fasting level over a period of 6 to 12 hours. With a 6 gram oral dose, the maximal fall in blood sugar is usually not significantly different from that produced by an oral dose of 3 grams. The hypoglycemic response after an oral dose of 50 mg per Kg of body weight is essentially the same as is induced by the intravenous injection of 0.1 unit of insulin per Kg of body weight.
In diabetic patients—Unlike the nondiabetic subject whose hypoglycemic response is maximal within the first hour after taking *Orinase* solution, the tolbutamide-responsive diabetic patient shows a gradually progressive blood sugar lowering effect, the maximal response being reached between 5 to 8 hours after ingestion of a single 3 gram dose; the blood sugar then rises gradually and by the 24th hour has usually returned to the pretest level. While the time of occurrence of the maximal reduction in blood sugar differs in the nondiabetic subject and the tolbutamide-responsive diabetic patient, the magnitude of the reduction, when expressed in terms of percent of the pretest blood sugar, tends to be similar. For example: in one study comparing the blood sugar lowering effect of *Orinase* (single oral dose of 50 mg per Kg of body weight) in 50 healthy adult subjects and 133 tolbutamide-responsive diabetic patients, the maximal decrease in blood sugar averaged 45.9 $\pm$ 1.8% for the normal group and 46.3 $\pm$ 1.5% for the diabetic group; the respective average mean decreases in blood sugar over the 5 hour observation period were 31.7 $\pm$ 1.4% for the normal subjects and 31.8 $\pm$ 1.2% for the diabetic patients.
Significance of the Molecular Structure: Tolbutamide is a sulfonamide but *not a sulfanilamide* derivative. While closely related to the so-called "sulfa" drugs, it differs in one important aspect. All "sulfa" drugs commonly used for treating infections have an amino group (either free or substituted) attached to the benzene ring at the *para* position. In tolbutamide, however, the amino group is replaced by a methyl group. This fundamental change in the molecular structure results in the following important characteristics of *Orinase* (tolbutamide).

1. It is devoid of chemotherapeutic effect; it *has no antibacterial activity.*
2. It cannot be measured in body fluids by the method of Bratton and Marshall.
3. It cannot be acetylated; the principal metabolite excreted in the urine is 1-butyl-3-*p*-carboxyphenylsulfonylurea.

Absorption, Degradation, and Excretion: When administered orally, *Orinase* (tolbutamide) is readily absorbed from the gastrointestinal tract. As it has no *p*-amino group, it cannot be acetylated, which is one of the common modes of metabolic degradation for the antibacterial sulfonamides. However, the presence of the *p*-methyl group renders *Orinase* susceptible to oxidation and this appears to be the principal manner of its metabolic degradation in man. The *p*-methyl group is oxidized to form a carboxyl group, converting *Orinase* into the totally inactive metabolite 1-butyl-3-*p*-carboxyphenylsulfonylurea, which can be recovered in the urine within 24 hours in amounts accounting for up to 75% of the administered dose.
Characteristics of the Metabolite:
Activity—The *Orinase* (tolbutamide) metabolite has no detectable pharmacologic effects. It has been administered orally in doses up to 6 grams and intravenously in doses up to 3 grams to normal and diabetic subjects and found devoid of hypoglycemic or other action. (When given intravenously, 71% of the 3 gram dose was excreted in the urine.)
Solubility—The tolbutamide metabolite is highly soluble over the critical acid range of urinary pH values, and its solubility increases with increase in pH. The measured solubility at pH 5 is 280 mg per 100 ml, increasing to 2000 mg per 100 ml at pH 5.5; at pH 6, by extrapolation, the solubility becomes 30,000 mg per 100 ml. Because of the marked solubility of the *Orinase* metabolite, crystalluria does not occur.
"Pseudo-albuminuria"—On very rare occasions, urine containing the tolbutamide metabolite may give a false-positive reaction for albumin by the usual test (acidification after boiling) since this procedure causes the metabolite to precipitate as flocculent particles. This problem may be circumvented by the use of bromphenol strips.
Information for modification of the sulfosalicylic acid and Esbach's tests will be supplied on request.
Indications: The principal clinical indication for *Orinase* (tolbutamide) is diabetes mellitus of the stable type without acute complications such as acidosis or ketosis. This form of diabetes has been variously described as relatively mild adult, maturity-onset, or nonketotic type. In certain patients with labile diabetes, its use as a supplement to insulin therapy may effect stabilization of the diabetic condition and reduce insulin requirement.
Tolbutamide has been demonstrated to be exceptionally well tolerated. Certain patients removed from chlorpropamide therapy because of intolerance to usual therapeutic doses have subsequently been managed successfully on *Orinase.*
Selection of Patients: The basic requirement for *Orinase* (tolbutamide) therapy is that the diabetes be adult or maturity-onset in character. The patient most likely to be responsive is one in whom the disease is relatively mild and stable and has developed sometime after the age of 30 years.
At present there is no reliable index whereby one may determine in advance the responsiveness of patients who qualify as candidates. History of an episode of diabetic coma does not necessarily disqualify a patient as a suitable candidate, but history of repeated episodes of acidosis or coma would serve as a contraindication. The only reliable method of determining responsiveness is therapeutic trial with *Orinase* for a period of at least 7 days. If the patient is already on insulin, it should be slowly withdrawn as response to *Orinase* is observed. If, during this trial period, there is absence of ketonuria plus a satisfactory reduction in blood sugar and glycosuria, the patient is responsive. The patient is considered nonresponsive if any of the following appear: ketonuria, increasing glycosuria, unsatisfactory lowering or persistent elevation of the blood sugar, or failure to obtain and hold clinical improvement.
Use in Early, Mild Diabetes: There is now considerable evidence, obtained from studies in animals and in patients with mild tolbutamide-responsive diabetes, that improvement in pancreatic beta cell function with consequent improvement in glucose tolerance occurs with prolonged administration of *Orinase* (tolbutamide). Therapy in the early, asymptomatic diabetic has produced normalization or improvement in glucose tolerance which has persisted up to 52 months. This improvement may occur after a few months of therapy, but in some instances improvement has taken place only after 10 to 14 months of continuous *Orinase* administration. Accordingly, in patients with mild, asymptomatic diabetes in whom glucose tolerance remains abnormal despite dietary therapy, it has been recommended that tolbutamide be administered in usual dosage over prolonged periods of time. Progress should be followed in these patients with glucose tolerance determinations at intervals of three to six months.
Although the long term effect of this therapy in the development of the complications of diabetes is unknown, as with other forms of antidiabetes therapy, it can reasonably be expected that improvement in the glucose tolerance or its restoration to normal may have a salutary effect on the course of the disease.

Contraindications: *Orinase* (tolbutamide) alone is not effective in juvenile or growth-onset diabetes nor in diabetes of the unstable, brittle type. Therefore, treatment of such cases requires the use of insulin, although *Orinase* may be used adjunctively when indicated.

Orinase should not be used in diabetes complicated by acidosis, ketosis, or coma; and in the presence of other acute complications such as fever, severe trauma, or infections, diabetics may require appropriate doses of insulin to insure continued control.

Orinase should not be used in patients with severe renal insufficiency.

Pregnancy Warning: The *safety* and the usefulness of *Orinase* (tolbutamide) during pregnancy have not been established at this time, either from the standpoint of the mother or the fetus. In animal studies, tolbutamide has been shown to have feticidal and teratogenic effects at doses of 1000 to 2500 mg per kg of body weight per day [Tuckmann-Duplessis, H., and Mercier-Parot, L., J. Ann. Diab. de l'Hotel Dieu (Paris) **3**:141-149, 1962; DeMeyer, R., 4e Congrèss de la Fédération Internationále du Diabète, Geneva 401-403, July 10-14, 1961; and Smithberg, M., Univ. of Minn. Med. Bull. **33**: 62-72, 1961]. It is not known at the present time whether or not this finding is applicable to human subjects. Clinical studies thus far are quite limited and experimental. Therefore, the use of *Orinase* is not recommended for the management of diabetes when complicated by *pregnancy*.

These facts should be borne in mind whenever the advisability of administering *Orinase* to women of the childbearing age is considered.

Precautions:

1. Those diagnostic and therapeutic measures which are necessary to insure optimal control of the diabetic state with insulin are equally necessary for control with tolbutamide.
2. The patient on *Orinase* (tolbutamide) must receive full and complete instructions about the nature of his disease, what he must do to prevent and detect complications, and how to control his condition.
3. He must understand that he cannot neglect his dietary restrictions, develop a careless attitude, or disregard instructions relative to body weight, exercise, personal hygiene, and avoidance of infection.
4. The patient must know how to recognize and counteract impending hypoglycemia.
5. The patient must know how and when to test for glycosuria and ketonuria.
6. During the trial period when insulin is being withdrawn, care should be taken to avoid ketosis, acidosis, and coma.
7. Caution should be observed in administering the thiazide-type diuretics to diabetic patients on *Orinase* therapy, because the thiazides have been reported to aggravate the diabetic state and to result in increased tolbutamide requirement, temporary loss of control, or even secondary failure. Response to tolbutamide is diminished in patients receiving therapy with *beta* blocking agents.
8. Very close observation and careful adjustment of dosage is mandatory in patients with impaired hepatic and/or renal function and in debilitated, malnourished or semistarved patients. In such patients severe hypoglycemia may occur and may require corrective therapy over a period of several days.
9. Tolbutamide is not an oral insulin nor a substitute for insulin. It has no blood sugar lowering effect in the absence of the pancreatic beta cells and must not be used as sole therapeutic agent in the juvenile type of diabetes.
10. Tolbutamide is of no value in diabetes complicated by acidosis and coma—here insulin is indispensable.
11. Care must be exercised in the presence of severe trauma, infection, or surgical procedures. In these circumstances it may be necessary, temporarily, to return the patient to insulin or to use insulin in addition to *Orinase*.
12. During the initial test period the patient should communicate with the physician daily, and for the first month report at least once weekly for physical examination and definitive evaluation of efficacy of diabetic control. After the first month, the patient should be examined at monthly intervals or as indicated.
13. The patient should be instructed to report immediately to his physician if he does not feel as well as usual.
14. For the protection of both patient and physician, uncooperative individuals should be considered unsuitable for treatment with this agent. Pharmacists should refill prescriptions only on the specific instruction of the physician.
15. As some diabetics are not suitable candidates for management with *Orinase*, it is essential that physicians familiarize themselves with the indications, limits of application, and the criteria for selection of patients for this therapy.
16. Patients must be under continuous medical supervision. *Orinase* therapy does not obviate the necessity for maintaining standard dietary regulation.

Adverse Reactions: Severe hypoglycemia, though uncommon, may occur in patients receiving *Orinase* (tolbutamide) and may mimic acute neurological disorders such as cerebral thrombosis. Certain factors, such as hepatic and renal disease, malnutrition, debility, advanced age, alcohol ingestion, and adrenal and pituitary insufficiency may predispose to hypoglycemia. Also, certain drugs may prolong or enhance the action of tolbutamide and thereby increase the risk of hypoglycemia. These include insulin, sulfonamides, oxyphenbutazone, salicylates, probenecid, monamine oxidase inhibitors, phenylbutazone, bishydroxycoumarin and phenyramidol.

Tolbutamide is mildly goitrogenic in animals in high doses, and in humans it has been reported to cause a reduction of RAI uptake after long term administration, without producing clinical hypothyroidism or thyroid enlargement.

Photosensitivity reactions and disulfiram-like reactions after ingestion of alcohol have been reported in patients taking tolbutamide.

Other untoward reactions are usually not of a serious nature and consist principally of gastrointestinal disturbances, headache, and variable allergic skin manifestations. The gastrointestinal disturbances (nausea, epigastric fullness, heartburn) and headache appear to be related to the size of the dose, and they frequently disappear when dosage is reduced to maintenance levels or the total daily dose is administered in divided portions after meals. The allergic skin manifestations (pruritus, erythema, and urticarial, morbilliform, or maculopapular eruptions) are transient reactions, which frequently disappear with continued drug administration. However, if the skin reactions persist, *Orinase* (tolbutamide) should be discontinued.

While early reports concerning the effect of sulfonylureas on body weight were inconsistent, recent reports have indicated that long-term use of *Orinase* per se has no appreciable effect in this respect.

Orinase appears to be remarkably free from gross clinical toxicity on the basis of experience accumulated during many years of clinical use. Crystalluria or other untoward effects on renal function have not been observed. Long term studies of hepatic function in human subjects and experience in over 1,000,000 diabetics have shown the incidence of tolbutamide-induced liver dysfunction to be remarkably low. Jaundice in association with the administration of tolbutamide has been rare and has cleared up readily upon discontinuance of the drug. Carcinoma of the pancreas or other extrahepatic biliary obstruction should be ruled out in instances of persistent jaundice.

Leukopenia, agranulocytosis, thrombocytopenia, hemolytic anemia, aplastic anemia, pancytopenia, hepatic porphyria and porphyria cutanea tarda have been reported.

Dosage and Administration: ***Institution of therapy and method of administration***—As with insulin therapy, there is no fixed dosage regimen for management of diabetes with *Orinase* (tolbutamide). There is no set dosage for beginning therapy in a candidate whether or not he is receiving insulin.

The average starting dose is 1 to 2 grams daily. This may be increased or decreased, depending on individual patient response. The ideal dose is the smallest amount which will maintain optimum control. This will vary considerably among patients and may be as little as 0.25 gram, particularly in elderly patients, or as much as 3 grams.

Generally, patients who do not respond to 2 grams will not respond to a higher dose; but, as with insulin therapy, dosage changes may be necessary during the course of management of a given case, and temporary increases over the 2 gram level may be required on occasion to maintain control. Maintenance dosage over 2 grams daily is seldom required.

The total daily dose may be taken either in the morning or in divided doses through the day. While either schedule is usually effective, the divided dose system is preferred by some clinicians from the standpoint of digestive tolerance (see **Adverse Reactions**). Occasionally, patients who initially respond are later found to have unsatisfactory control. This may be attributable to dietary indiscretion, emotional stress, secondary failure, or other factors. Often, temporary small increases in dosage restore control. A small percentage of patients may exhibit idiopathic loss of responsiveness after an extended period of good control. Such cases have been termed *secondary failures*.

Patients not receiving insulin—When *Orinase* is indicated, therapy is initiated as described above.

Patients receiving insulin—Patients requiring 20 units or less of insulin daily may be placed directly on *Orinase* and insulin abruptly discontinued. Patients whose insulin requirement is between 20 and 40 units daily may be started on *Orinase* therapy with a concurrent 30 to 50% reduction in insulin dose, with further daily reduction of the insulin as response to tolbutamide is observed. In patients requiring more than 40 units of insulin daily, *Orinase* therapy may be initiated in conjunction with a 20% reduction in insulin dose the first day, with further careful reduction of insulin as response is observed. During the withdrawal period the patient should test his urine for sugar and ketone bodies as frequently as three times daily and report the results to his physician daily. Occasionally, conversion to *Orinase* in the hospital may be advisable in candidates who required more than 40 units of insulin daily. If, during the trial period, ketosis or unsatisfactory blood or urine sugar control results, the patient should be returned to his former insulin therapy.

Continued on next page

Information on these Upjohn products is based on labeling in effect on November 1, 1979. Further information on dosage and administration, side effects, precautions and contraindications for these and other Upjohn products may be obtained from either the package insert or Medical Services, The Upjohn Company, Kalamazoo, Michigan.

Upjohn—Cont.

During the conversion period mild symptoms of hypoglycemia may occur on rare occasions. In these instances symptoms are readily corrected by administration of carbohydrate, and recurrences of hypoglycemic symptoms are avoided by more rapid withdrawal of insulin. Patients who develop ketosis, unsatisfactory lowering or persistent elevation of the blood sugar, or complications other than hypoglycemia within 24 hours after complete withdrawal of insulin should be withdrawn from tolbutamide and their former insulin therapy reinstituted. *The patient should be instructed as to the necessity of reporting to his physician immediately if any feeling of illness develops.*

Combination Therapy with Insulin: Although not universally accepted, use of *Orinase* Tablets (tolbutamide) as a supplement to insulin therapy in insulin-dependent diabetic patients with maturity-onset or growth-onset types of diabetes has been reported to decrease insulin requirements, provide easier regulation and stabilization of the diabetes, and afford an increased feeling of well being. Long term studies on this combined therapy show that the daily insulin requirement may be reduced from 10 to 70% in certain stable patients and from 10 to 50% in certain labile patients.

In insulin-resistant patients, use of the combination may be warranted in an effort to reduce the insulin requirement.

Acute Complications: During the course of intercurrent complications (e.g., ketoacidosis, severe trauma, major surgical procedures, infections, severe diarrhea, or nausea and vomiting) *supportive therapy with insulin may be necessary.* Depending upon the severity of the diabetes, the nature of the complication, and the availability of laboratory facilities, tolbutamide therapy may be continued or withdrawn while insulin is being used. Insulin is indispensable in the management of many acute complications, and all diabetics should be carefully instructed in its use.

How Supplied: Scored tablets are available as follows:

250 mg
- Bottles of 100 — *NDC 0009-0701-01*

0.5 gram
- Bottles of 50 — *NDC 0009-0100-01*
- Bottles of 100 — *NDC 0009-0100-11*
- Bottles of 200 — *NDC 0009-0100-02*
- Bottles of 500 — *NDC 0009-0100-03*
- Bottles of 1000 — *NDC 0009-0100-05*
- Unit Dose Package (100) — *NDC 0009-0100-06*
- Unit of Use Bottles (30) — *NDC 0009-0100-10*

Code LAO-11

[*Shown in Product Identification Section*]

OXYLONE® CREAM ℞
(Fluorometholone Cream, NF)
For External Use

How Supplied: *Oxylone* Cream (fluorometholone) 0.025% is available in the following sizes:

15 Gm tube *NDC 0009-0661-02*
60 Gm tube *NDC 0009-0661-03*
120 Gm jar *NDC 0009-0661-04*

PAMINE® TABLETS ℞
(Methscopolamine Bromide Tablets, NF)

500:s: NSN 6505-00-584-3315 A (VA)

How Supplied: Each tablet contains 2.5 mg methscopolamine bromide.

Bottles of 100 *NDC 0009-0061-01*
Bottles of 500 *NDC 0009-0061-02*
[*Shown in Product Identification Section*]

PANMYCIN® CAPSULES ℞
(Tetracycline Hydrochloride Capsules, USP)

How Supplied: Each capsule contains 250 mg tetracycline hydrochloride.

Bottles of 100 *NDC 0009-0782-01*
Bottles of 1000 *NDC 0009-0782-03*
[*Shown in Product Identification Section*]

PANMYCIN® SYRUP ℞
(Tetracycline Oral Suspension, USP)

How Supplied: Each 5 ml (teaspoonful) contains tetracycline equivalent to 125 mg tetracycline hydrochloride. Preserved with methylparaben 0.075%, propylparaben 0.025% and sodium metabisulfite 0.1%.

2 oz bottles *NDC 0009-0806-01*
Pint bottles *NDC 0009-0806-02*

PANMYCIN® TABLETS ℞
(Tetracycline Hydrochloride Tablets, NF)

How Supplied: Each tablet contains 250 mg or 500 mg tetracycline hydrochloride.

250 mg Bottles of 1000 *NDC 0009-0195-02*
500 mg Bottles of 100 *NDC 0009-0310-01*

PENSYN™ CAPSULES ℞
(Ampicillin Capsules, USP)

How Supplied: In capsules containing ampicillin trihydrate equivalent to 250 mg or 500 mg ampicillin.

250 mg:
Bottles of 100 *NDC 0009-0829-02*
Bottles of 500 *NDC 0009-0829-03*
500 mg:
Bottles of 100 *NDC 0009-0977-02*
[*Shown in Product Identification Section*]

PENSYN™ ORAL POWDER ℞
(Ampicillin for Oral Suspension, USP)

How Supplied: When reconstituted, each 5 ml contains ampicillin trihydrate equivalent to 125 mg or 250 mg ampicillin. Available in the following packages:

125 mg/5 ml:
100 ml bottles *NDC 0009-0261-03*
200 ml bottles *NDC 0009-0261-04*
250 mg/5 ml:
80 ml bottles *NDC 0009-0512-01*
100 ml bottles *NDC 0009-0512-03*
200 ml bottles *NDC 0009-0512-04*

PROVERA® TABLETS ℞
(Medroxyprogesterone Acetate Tablets, USP)
10 mg
10s (unit of use)
NSN 6505-01-071-5605 (VA)
100s (bottle)
NSN 6505-00-890-1355 (M)

WARNING:

THE USE OF PROGESTATIONAL AGENTS DURING THE FIRST FOUR MONTHS OF PREGNANCY IS NOT RECOMMENDED

Progestational agents have been used beginning with the first trimester of pregnancy in an attempt to prevent habitual abortion or treat threatened abortion. There is no adequate evidence that such use is effective and there is evidence of potential harm to the fetus when such drugs are given during the first four months of pregnancy. Furthermore, in the vast majority of women, the cause of abortion is a defective ovum, which progestational agents could not be expected to influence. In addition, the use of progestational agents with their uterine-relaxant properties, in patients with fertilized defective ova may cause a delay in spontaneous abortion. Therefore, the use of such drugs during the first four months of pregnancy is not recommended.

Several reports suggest an association between intrauterine exposure to female sex hormones and congenital anomalies, including congenital heart defects and limb reduction defects[1–5]. One study[4] estimated a 4.7-fold increased risk of limb reduction defects in infants exposed in utero to sex hormones (oral contraceptives, hormone withdrawal tests for pregnancy, or attempted treatment for threatened abortion). Some of these exposures were very short and involved only a few days of treatment. The data suggest that the risk of limb reduction defects in exposed fetuses is somewhat less than 1 in 1,000.

If the patient is exposed to *Provera* Tablets (medroxyprogesterone acetate) during the first four months of pregnancy or if she becomes pregnant while taking this drug, she should be apprised of the potential risks to the fetus.

Description: *Provera* (medroxyprogesterone acetate) is a derivative of progesterone. It is white to off-white, odorless crystalline powder, stable in air, melting between 200 and 210° C. It is freely soluble in chloroform, soluble in acetone and in dioxane, sparingly soluble in alcohol and in methanol, slightly soluble in ether, and insoluble in water.

The chemical name for medroxyprogesterone acetate is Pregn-4-ene-3,20-dione, 17-(acetyloxy)-6-methyl-, (6α)-.

Provera Tablets are available in two strengths, each tablet containing either 2.5 or 10 mg medroxyprogesterone acetate.

Actions: Medroxyprogesterone acetate, administered orally or parenterally in the recommended doses to women with adequate endogenous estrogen, transforms proliferative into secretory endometrium. Androgenic and anabolic effects have been noted, but the drug is apparently devoid of significant estrogenic activity. While parenterally administered medroxyprogesterone acetate inhibits gonadotropin production, which in turn prevents follicular maturation and ovulation, available data indicate that this does not occur when the usually recommended oral dosage is given as single daily doses.

Indications: Secondary amenorrhea; abnormal uterine bleeding due to hormonal imbalance in the absence of organic pathology, such as fibroids or uterine cancer.

Contraindications:
1. Thrombophlebitis, thromboembolic disorders, cerebral apoplexy or patients with a past history of these conditions.
2. Liver dysfunction or disease.
3. Known or suspected malignancy of breast or genital organs.
4. Undiagnosed vaginal bleeding.
5. Missed abortion.
6. As a diagnostic test for pregnancy.
7. Known sensitivity to *Provera* (medroxyprogesterone acetate).

Warnings:
1. The physician should be alert to the earliest manifestations of thrombotic disorders (thrombophlebitis, cerebrovascular disorders, pulmonary embolism, and retinal thrombosis). Should any of these occur or be suspected, the drug should be discontinued immediately.
2. Beagle dogs treated with medroxyprogesterone acetate developed mammary nodules some of which were malignant. Although nodules occasionally appeared in control animals, they were intermittent in nature, whereas the nodules in the drug-treated animals were larger, more numerous, persistent, and there were some breast malignancies with metastases. Their significance with respect to humans has not been established.
3. Discontinue medication pending examination if there is sudden partial or complete loss of vision, or if there is a sudden onset of

proptosis, diplopia or migraine. If examination reveals papilledema or retinal vascular lesions, medication should be withdrawn.

4. Detectable amounts of progestin have been identified in the milk of mothers receiving the drug. The effect of this on the nursing infant has not been determined.
5. Usage in pregnancy is not recommended (See WARNING Box).
6. Retrospective studies of morbidity and mortality in Great Britain and studies of morbidity in the United States have shown a statistically significant association between thrombophlebitis, pulmonary embolism, and cerebral thrombosis and embolism and the use of oral contraceptives.[6–9] The estimate of the relative risk of thromboembolism in the study by Vessey and Doll[8] was about sevenfold, while Sartwell and associates[9] in the United States found a relative risk of 4.4, meaning that the users are several times as likely to undergo thromboembolic disease without evident cause as nonusers. The American study also indicated that the risk did not persist after discontinuation of administration, and that it was not enhanced by long continued administration. The American study was not designed to evaluate a difference between products.

Precautions:

1. The pretreatment physical examination should include special reference to breast and pelvic organs, as well as Papanicolaou smear.
2. Because progestogens may cause some degree of fluid retention, conditions which might be influenced by this factor, such as epilepsy, migraine, asthma, cardiac or renal dysfunction, require careful observation.
3. In cases of breakthrough bleeding, as in all cases of irregular bleeding per vaginum, nonfunctional causes should be borne in mind. In cases of undiagnosed vaginal bleeding, adequate diagnostic measures are indicated.
4. Patients who have a history of psychic depression should be carefully observed and the drug discontinued if the depression recurs to a serious degree.
5. Any possible influence of prolonged progestin therapy on pituitary, ovarian, adrenal, hepatic or uterine functions awaits further study.
6. A decrease in glucose tolerance has been observed in a small percentage of patients on estrogen-progestin combination drugs. The mechanism of this decrease is obscure. For this reason, diabetic patients should be carefully observed while receiving progestin therapy.
7. The age of the patient constitutes no absolute limiting factor although treatment with progestins may mask the onset of the climacteric.
8. The pathologist should be advised of progestin therapy when relevant specimens are submitted.
9. Because of the occasional occurrence of thrombotic disorders, (thrombophlebitis, pulmonary embolism, retinal thrombosis, and cerebrovascular disorders) in patients taking estrogen-progestin combinations and since the mechanism is obscure, the physician should be alert to the earliest manifestation of these disorders.

Information for the Patient

See Patient Information at the end of insert.

Adverse Reactions:

Pregnancy—(See WARNING Box for possible adverse effects on the fetus)

Breast—Breast tenderness or galactorrhea has been reported rarely.

Skin—Sensitivity reactions consisting of urticaria, pruritus, edema and generalized rash have occurred in an occasional patient. Acne, alopecia and hirsutism have been reported in a few cases.

Thromboembolic Phenomena—Thromboembolic phenomena including thrombophlebitis and pulmonary embolism have been reported.

The following adverse reactions have been observed in women taking progestins including *Provera* (medroxyprogesterone acetate):

- breakthrough bleeding
- spotting
- change in menstrual flow
- amenorrhea
- edema
- change in weight (increase or decrease)
- changes in cervical erosion and cervical secretions
- cholestatic jaundice
- rash (allergic) with and without pruritus
- mental depression

A statistically significant association has been demonstrated between use of estrogen-progestin combination drugs and the following serious adverse reactions: thrombophlebitis; pulmonary embolism and cerebral thrombosis and embolism. For this reason patients on progestin therapy should be carefully observed.

Although available evidence is suggestive of an association, such a relationship has been neither confirmed nor refuted for the following serious adverse reactions:

- neuro-ocular lesions, eg, retinal thrombosis and optic neuritis.

The following adverse reactions have been observed in patients receiving estrogen-progestin combination drugs:

- rise in blood pressure in susceptible individuals
- premenstrual-like syndrome
- changes in libido
- changes in appetite
- cystitis-like syndrome
- headache
- nervousness
- dizziness
- fatigue
- backache
- hirsutism
- loss of scalp hair
- erythema multiforme
- erythema nodosum
- hemorrhagic eruption
- itching

In view of these observations, patients on progestin therapy should be carefully observed.

The following laboratory results may be altered by the use of estrogen-progestin combination drugs:

Increased sulfobromophthalein retention and other hepatic function tests.

Coagulation tests: increase in prothrombin factors VII, VIII, IX and X.

Metyrapone test.

Pregnanediol determination.

Thyroid function: increase in PBI, and butanol extractable protein bound iodine and decrease in T^3 uptake values.

Dosage and Administration:

Secondary Amenorrhea—*Provera* (medroxyprogesterone acetate) may be given in dosages of 5 to 10 mg daily for from 5 to 10 days. A dose for inducing an optimum secretory transformation of an endometrium that has been adequately primed with either endogenous or exogenous estrogen is 10 mg of *Provera* daily for 10 days. In cases of secondary amenorrhea, therapy may be started at any time. Progestin withdrawal bleeding usually occurs within three to seven days after discontinuing *Provera* therapy.

Abnormal Uterine Bleeding Due to Hormonal Imbalance in the Absence of Organic Pathology—Beginning on the calculated 16th or 21st day of the menstrual cycle, 5 to 10 mg of *Provera* may be given daily for from 5 to 10 days. To produce an optimum secretory transformation of an endometrium that has been adequately primed with either endogenous or exogenous estrogen, 10 mg of *Provera* daily for 10 days beginning on the 16th day of the cycle is suggested. Progestin withdrawal bleeding usually occurs within three to seven days after discontinuing *Provera* therapy. Patients with a past history of recurrent episodes of abnormal uterine bleeding may benefit from planned menstrual cycling with *Provera*.

How Supplied: *Provera* Tablets (medroxyprogesterone acetate) are available in two strengths:

2.5 mg	—bottles of 25.	NDC 0009-0064-01
10 mg	—bottles of 25.	NDC 0009-0050-01
	bottles of 100.	NDC 0009-0050-02
	Dosepak™ of 10	NDC 0009-0050-07

References:

1. Gal I, Kirman B, Stern J: Hormonal pregnancy tests and congenital malformation. Nature *216*:83, 1967.
2. Levy EP, Cohen A, Fraser FC: Hormone treatment during pregnancy and congenital heart defects. Lancet *1*:611, 1973.
3. Nora JJ, Nora AH: Birth defects and oral contraceptives. Lancet *1*:941–942, 1973.
4. Janerich DT, Piper JM, Glebatis DM: Oral contraceptives and congenital limb-reduction defects. N Engl J Med *291*:697–700, 1974.
5. Heinonen OP, Slone D, Monson RR, et al: Cardiovascular birth defects and antenatal exposure to female sex hormones. N Engl J Med *296*:67–70, 1977.
6. Royal College of General Practitioners: Oral contraception and thromboembolic disease. J Coll Gen Pract *13*:267–279, 1967.
7. Inman WHW, Vessey MP: Investigation of deaths from pulmonary, coronary, and cerebral thrombosis and embolism in women of child-bearing age. Br Med J *2*:193–199, 1968.
8. Vessey MP, Doll R: Investigation of relation between use of oral contraceptives and thromboembolic disease. A further report. Br Med J *2*:651–657, 1969.
9. Sartwell PE, Masi AT, Arthes FG, et al: Thromboembolism and oral contraceptives: An epidemiological case-control study. Am J Epidemiol *90*:365–380, 1969.

The text of the patient insert for progesterone and progesterone-like drugs is set forth below.

Patient Information: *Provera* Tablets contain a progesterone (medroxyprogesterone acetate). The information below is that which the U.S. Food and Drug Administration requires be provided for all patients taking progesterones. The information below relates only to the risk to the unborn child associated with use of progesterone during pregnancy. For further information on the use, side effects and other risks associated with this product, ask your doctor.

WARNING FOR WOMEN

There is an increased risk of birth defects in children whose mothers take this drug during the first four months of pregnancy.

Medroxyprogesterone Acetate is similar to the progesterone hormones naturally produced by the body. Progesterone and progesterone-like drugs are used to treat menstrual disorders, to test if the body is producing certain hormones, and to treat some forms of cancer in women. They have been used as a test for pregnancy but such use is no longer considered safe because of possible damage to a developing baby. Also, more rapid methods for testing for pregnancy are now available.

Continued on next page

Information on these Upjohn products is based on labeling in effect on November 1, 1979. Further information on dosage and administration, side effects, precautions and contraindications for these and other Upjohn products may be obtained from either the package insert or Medical Services, The Upjohn Company, Kalamazoo, Michigan.

Upjohn—Cont.

These drugs have also been used to prevent miscarriage in the first few months of pregnancy. No adequate evidence is available to show that they are effective for this purpose. Furthermore, most cases of early miscarriage are due to causes which could not be helped by these drugs.

There is an increased risk of birth defects, such as heart or limb defects if progesterone and progesterone-like drugs are taken during the first four months of pregnancy. The exact risk of taking this drug early in pregnancy and having a baby with a birth defect is not known. However, one study found that babies born to women who had taken sex hormones (such as progesterone-like drugs) during the first three months of pregnancy were 4 to 5 times more likely to have abnormalities of the arms or legs than if their mothers had not taken such drugs. Some of these women had taken these drugs for only a few days. The chance that an infant whose mother had taken this drug will have this type of defect is about 1 in 1,000.

If you take *Provera* Tablets and later find you were pregnant when you took it, be sure to discuss this with your doctor as soon as possible.

Code NPA

[Shown in Product Identification Section]

SIGTAB® TABLETS

Composition: Each tablet contains:

Vitamin A	5000 IU
Vitamin D	400 IU
Vitamin E	15 IU
Vitamin C	333 mg
Folic Acid	0.4 mg
Thiamine	10.3 mg
Riboflavin	10 mg
Niacin	100 mg
Vitamin B_6	6 mg
Vitamin B_{12}	18 mcg
Pantothenic Acid	20 mg

How Supplied: Coated compressed tablets in the following sizes:

Bottles of 30 *NDC 0009-0461-01*
Bottles of 90 *NDC 0009-0461-02*
Bottles of 500 *NDC 0009-0461-03*

SOLU-B® ℞

Sterile Injectable B Vitamins

Composition: Each 2 ml (when mixed) contains:

Thiamine Hydrochloride	10 mg
Riboflavin	10 mg
Pyridoxine Hydrochloride	5 mg
Calcium Pantothenate	50 mg
Niacinamide	250 mg
Also	
Methylparaben	2.55 mg
Propylparaben	0.29 mg
Water for injection	qs

How Supplied:
NDC 0009-0863-02 (5-pack)

SOLU-B® WITH ASCORBIC ACID STERILE POWDER ℞

Sterile Injectable B and C Vitamins
***Mix-O-Vial* with Transfer Needle**
NSN 6505-00-122-3851A (VA)

Composition: Each 5 ml (when mixed) contains:

Thiamine Hydrochloride	10 mg
Riboflavin (as riboflavin and 5′-phosphate sodium)	10 mg
Niacinamide	250 mg
Pyridoxine Hydrochloride	5 mg
Sodium Pantothenate	50 mg
Ascorbic Acid	500 mg
also	
Methylparaben	4.33 mg
Propylparaben	0.5 mg
Water for Injection	qs

When necessary, pH was adjusted with hydrochloric acid and/or sodium hydroxide.

How Supplied: Available in a 5 ml *Mix-O-Vial*® Two-Compartment Vial with transfer needle.

5 ml vial *NDC 0009-0606-01*
(with transfer needle)

SOLU-B-FORTE® (S-B-F®) STERILE POWDER ℞

Multivitamins for I.M. or I.V. use
***Mix-O-Vial* with Transfer Needle:**
NSN 6505-00-764-3340 (M)
NSN 6505-00-122-3847A (VA)

Composition: Each 10 ml (when mixed) contains:

Thiamine Hydrochloride	250 mg
Riboflavin	50 mg
Ascorbic Acid	1000 mg
Niacinamide	1250 mg
Pyridoxine Hydrochloride	50 mg
Sodium Pantothenate	500 mg
Methylparaben	9.09 mg
Propylparaben	1.04 mg
Water for Injection	qs

When necessary, pH was adjusted with hydrochloric acid and/or sodium hydroxide.

How Supplied: Available in a 10 ml *Mix-O-Vial*® Two-Compartment Vial with transfer needle.

10 ml vial *NDC 0009-0414-01*
(with transfer needle)

SOLU-CORTEF® STERILE POWDER ℞

(Hydrocortisone Sodium Succinate for Injection, USP)
For Intravenous or Intramuscular Administration

100 mg *Mix-O-Vial*®:
NSN 6505-00-753-9609A (M & VA)
250 mg *Mix-O-Vial:*
NSN 6505-00-951-5533A (M & VA)
500 mg *Mix-O-Vial:*
NSN 6505-00-116-5055A (VA)
1000 mg *Mix-O-Vial:*
NSN 6505-00-238-5222A (VA)

	100 mg *Mix-O-Vial* Each 2 ml contains: (when mixed)	250 mg *Mix-O-Vial* Each 2 ml contains: (when mixed)	500 mg *Mix-O-Vial* Each 4 ml contains: (when mixed)	1000 mg *Mix-O-Vial* Each 8 ml contains: (when mixed)
Hydrocortisone sodium succinate	equiv. to 100 mg hydrocortisone	equiv. to 250 mg hydrocortisone	equiv. to 500 mg hydrocortisone	equiv. to 1000 mg hydrocortisone
Sodium biphosphate anhydrous	0.8 mg	2 mg	4 mg	8 mg
Dried sodium phosphate	8.76 mg	21.8 mg	44 mg	88 mg
Benzyl alcohol	10 mg	10 mg	20 mg	40 mg
Water for Injection	qs	qs	qs	qs

When necessary, the pH of each formula was adjusted with sodium hydroxide and/or hydrochloric acid so that the pH of the reconstituted solution is within the USP specified range of 7 to 8.

Description: Hydrocortisone sodium succinate is a white or nearly white, odorless, hygroscopic amorphous solid. It is very soluble in water and in alcohol, very slightly soluble in acetone and insoluble in chloroform. The chemical name is pregn-4-ene-3,20-dione,21-(3-carboxy-1-oxopropoxy)-11,17-dihydroxy-, monosodium salt, (11β)-and its molecular weight is 484.52.

Hydrocortisone sodium succinate is an anti-inflammatory adrenocortical steroid. This highly water-soluble sodium succinate ester of hydrocortisone permits the immediate intravenous administration of high doses of hydrocortisone in a small volume of diluent and is particularly useful where high blood levels of hydrocortisone are required rapidly.

Solu-Cortef Sterile Powder (hydrocortisone sodium succinate) is available in several packages for intravenous or intramuscular administration.

100 mg Plain—Vials containing hydrocortisone sodium succinate equivalent to 100 mg hydrocortisone, also 0.8 mg sodium biphosphate anhydrous, 8.73 mg dried sodium phosphate.

100 mg with Bacteriostatic Water for Injection—Vials containing hydrocortisone sodium succinate equivalent to 100 mg hydrocortisone, also 0.8 mg sodium biphosphate anhydrous, 8.73 mg dried sodium phosphate; each vial accompanied by one 2 ml size ampoule Bacteriostatic Water for Injection with Benzyl Alcohol 0.9% w/v., **and in the *Mix-O-Vial*® Two-Compartment Vial in four strengths:**

[See table below].

Actions: Hydrocortisone sodium succinate has the same metabolic and anti-inflammatory actions as hydrocortisone. When given parenterally and in equimolar quantities, the two compounds are equivalent in biologic activity. Following the intravenous injection of hydrocortisone sodium succinate, demonstrable effects are evident within one hour and persist for a variable period. Excretion of the administered dose is nearly complete within 12 hours. Thus, if constantly high blood levels are required, injections should be made every 4 to 6 hours. This preparation is also rapidly absorbed when administered intramuscularly and is excreted in a pattern similar to that observed after intravenous injection.

Indications: When oral therapy is not feasible, and the strength, dosage form and route of administration of the drug reasonably lend the preparation to the treatment of the condition, *Solu-Cortef* (hydrocortisone sodium succinate) is indicated for intravenous or intramuscular use in the following conditions:

1. **Endocrine Disorders**
   Primary or secondary adrenocortical insufficiency (hydrocortisone or cortisone is the drug of choice; synthetic analogs may be used in conjunction with mineralocorticoids where applicable; in infancy, mineralocorticord supplementation is of particular importance)
   Acute adrenocortical insufficiency (hydrocortisone or cortisone is the drug of choice; mineralocorticoid supplementation may be necessary, particularly when synthetic analogs are used)
   Preoperatively and in the event of serious trauma or illness, in patients with known adrenal insufficiency or when adrenocortical reserve is doubtful
   Shock unresponsive to conventional therapy if adrenocortical insufficiency exists or is suspected
   Congenital adrenal hyperplasia
   Hypercalcemia associated with cancer
   Nonsuppurative thyroiditis
2. **Rheumatic Disorders**
   As adjunctive therapy for short-term administration (to tide the patient over an acute episode or exacerbation) in:

Post-traumatic osteoarthritis
Synovitis of osteoarthritis
Rheumatoid arthritis, including juvenile rheumatoid arthritis (selected cases may require low-dose maintenance therapy)
Acute and subacute bursitis
Epicondylitis
Acute nonspecific tenosynovitis
Acute gouty arthritis
Psoriatic arthritis
Ankylosing spondylitis

3. Collagen Diseases
During an exacerbation or as maintenance therapy in selected cases of:
Systemic lupus erythematosus
Systemic dermatomyositis (polymyositis)
Acute rheumatic carditis

4. Dermatologic Diseases
Pemphigus
Severe erythema multiforme (Stevens-Johnson syndrome)
Exfoliative dermatitis
Bullous dermatitis herpetiformis
Severe seborrheic dermatitis
Severe psoriasis
Mycosis fungoides

5. Allergic States
Control of severe or incapacitating allergic conditions intractable to adequate trials of conventional treatment in:
Bronchial asthma
Contact dermatitis
Atopic dermatitis
Serum sickness
Seasonal or perennial allergic rhinitis
Drug hypersensitivity reactions
Urticarial transfusion reactions
Acute noninfectious laryngeal edema (epinephrine is the drug of first choice)

6. Ophthalmic Diseases
Severe acute and chronic allergic and inflammatory processes involving the eye, such as:
Herpes zoster ophthalmicus
Iritis, iridocyclitis
Chorioretinitis
Diffuse posterior uveitis and choroiditis
Optic neuritis
Sympathetic ophthalmia
Anterior segment inflammation
Allergic conjunctivitis
Allergic corneal marginal ulcers
Keratitis

7. Gastrointestinal Diseases
To tide the patient over a critical period of the disease in:
Ulcerative colitis (systemic therapy)
Regional enteritis (systemic therapy)

8. Respiratory Diseases
Symptomatic sarcoidosis
Berylliosis
Fulminating or disseminated pulmonary tuberculosis when used concurrently with appropriate antituberculous chemotherapy
Loeffler's syndrome not manageable by other means
Aspiration pneumonitis

9. Hematologic Disorders
Acquired (autoimmune) hemolytic anemia
Idiopathic thrombocytopenic purpura in adults (IV only; IM administration is contraindicated)
Secondary thrombocytopenia in adults
Erythroblastopenia (RBC anemia)
Congenital (erythroid) hypoplastic anemia

10. Neoplastic Diseases
For palliative mangement of:
Leukemias and lymphomas in adults
Acute leukemia of childhood

11. Edematous States
To induce diuresis or remission of proteinuria in the nephrotic syndrome, without uremia, of the idiopathic type or that due to lupus erythematosus

12. Nervous System
Acute exacerbations of multiple sclerosis

13. Miscellaneous
Tuberculous meningitis with subarachnoid block or impending block when used concurrently with appropriate antituberculous chemotherapy
Trichinosis with neurologic or myocardial involvement

Contraindications: Systemic fungal infections.

Warnings: In patients on corticosteroid therapy subjected to unusual stress, increased dosage of rapidly acting corticosteroids before, during, and after the stressful situation is indicated.

Corticosteroids may mask some signs of infection, and new infections may appear during their use. There may be decreased resistance and inability to localize infection when corticosteroids are used.

Prolonged use of corticosteroids may produce posterior subcapsular cataracts, glaucoma with possible damage to the optic nerves, and may enhance the establishment of secondary ocular infections due to fungi or viruses.

Usage in pregnancy. Since adequate human reproduction studies have not been done with corticosteroids, the use of these drugs in pregnancy, nursing mothers, or women of childbearing potential requires that the possible benefits of the drug be weighed against the potential hazards to the mother and embryo or fetus. Infants born of mothers who have received substantial doses of corticosteroids during pregnancy should be carefully observed for signs of hypoadrenalism.

Average and large doses of hydrocortisone can cause elevation of blood pressure, salt and water retention, and increased excretion of potassium. These effects are less likely to occur with the synthetic derivatives except when used in large doses. Dietary salt restriction and potassium supplementation may be necessary. All corticosteroids increase calcium excretion.

While on corticosteroid therapy patients should not be vaccinated against smallpox. Other immunization procedures should not be undertaken in patients who are on corticosteroids, especially on high dose, because of possible hazards of neurological complications and a lack of antibody response.

The use of *Solu-Cortef* (hydrocortisone sodium succinate) in active tuberculosis should be restricted to those cases of fulminating or disseminated tuberculosis in which the corticosteroid is used for the management of the disease in conjunction with appropriate antituberculous regimen.

If corticosteroids are indicated in patients with latent tuberculosis or tuberculin reactivity, close observation is necessary as reactivation of the disease may occur. During prolonged corticosteroid therapy, these patients should receive chemoprophylaxis.

Because rare instances of anaphylactoid reactions have occurred in patients receiving parenteral corticosteroid therapy, appropriate precautionary measures should be taken prior to administration, especially when the patient has a history of allergy to any drug.

Precautions: Drug-induced secondary adrenocortical insufficiency may be minimized by gradual reduction of dosage. This type of relative insufficiency may persist for months after discontinuation of therapy; therefore, in any situation of stress occurring during that period, hormone therapy should be reinstituted. Since mineralocorticoid secretion may be impaired, salt and/or a mineralocorticoid should be administered concurrently.

There is an enhanced effect of corticosteroids in patients with hypothyroidism and in those with cirrhosis.

Corticosteroids should be used cautiously in patients with ocular herpes simplex for fear of corneal perforation.

The lowest possible dose of corticosteroid should be used to control the condition under treatment, and when reduction in dosage is possible, the reduction must be gradual.

Psychic derangements may appear when corticosteroids are used, ranging from euphoria, insomnia, mood swings, personality changes, and severe depression to frank psychotic manifestations. Also, existing emotional instability or psychotic tendencies may be aggravated by corticosteroids.

Aspirin should be used cautiously in conjunction with corticosteroids in hypoprothrombinemia.

Steroids should be used with caution in nonspecific ulcerative colitis, if there is a probability of impending perforation, abscess or other pyogenic infection, also in diverticulitis, fresh intestinal anastomoses, active or latent peptic ulcer, renal insufficiency, hypertension, osteoporosis, and myasthenia gravis.

Growth and development of infants and children on prolonged corticosteroid therapy should be carefully followed.

Although controlled clinical trials have shown corticosteroids to be effective in speeding the resolution of acute exacerbations of multiple sclerosis, they do not show that corticosteroids affect the ultimate outcome or natural history of the disease. The studies do show that relatively high doses of corticosteroids are necessary to demonstrate a significant effect. (See **Dosage and Administration**).

Since complications of treatment with glucocorticoides are dependent on the size of the dose and the duration of treatment, a risk/benefit decision must be made in each individual case as to dose and duration of treatment and as to whether daily or intermittent therapy should be used.

Adverse Reactions:

Fluid and Electrolyte Disturbances
Sodium retention
Fluid retention
Congestive heart failure in susceptible patients
Potassium loss
Hypokalemic alkalosis
Hypertension

Musculoskeletal
Muscle weakness
Steroid myopathy
Loss of muscle mass
Osteoporosis
Vertebral compression fractures
Aseptic necrosis of femoral and humeral heads
Pathologic fracture of long bones

Gastrointestinal
Peptic ulcer with possible perforation and hemorrhage
Pancreatitis
Abdominal distention
Ulcerative esophagitis

Dermatologic
Impaired wound healing
Thin fragile skin
Petechiae and ecchymoses
Facial erythema
Increased sweating
May suppress reactions to skin tests

Continued on next page

Information on these Upjohn products is based on labeling in effect on November 1, 1979. Further information on dosage and administration, side effects, precautions and contraindications for these and other Upjohn products may be obtained from either the package insert or Medical Services, The Upjohn Company, Kalamazoo, Michigan.

Upjohn—Cont.

Neurological
- Convulsions
- Increased intracranial pressure with papilledema (pseudotumor cerebri) usually after treatment
- Vertigo
- Headache

Endocrine
- Menstrual irregularities
- Development of Cushingoid state
- Suppression of growth in children
- Secondary adrenocortical and pituitary unresponsiveness, particularly in times of stress, as in trauma, surgery, or illness
- Decreased carbohydrate tolerance
- Manifestations of latent diabetes mellitus
- Increased requirements for insulin or oral hypoglycemic agents in diabetics

Ophthalmic
- Posterior subcapsular cataracts
- Increased intraocular pressure
- Glaucoma
- Exophthalmos

Metabolic
- Negative nitrogen balance due to protein catabolism

The following additional reactions are related to parenteral corticosteroid therapy:
- Hyperpigmentation or hypopigmentation
- Subcutaneous and cutaneous atrophy
- Sterile abscess

Administration and Dosage: This preparation may be administered by intravenous injection, by intravenous infusion, or by intramuscular injection, the preferred method for initial emergency use being intravenous injection. Following the initial emergency period, consideration should be given to employing a longer acting injectable preparation or an oral preparation.

In treating severe shock, there is a tendency in current medical practice to use massive (pharmacologic) doses of corticosteroids. The following are *Solu-Cortef* (hydrocortisone sodium succinate) doses suggested by various authors:

Author	*Dose*	*Repeat*
Melby[1]	0.5 gram	Every 4–6 hours
Oaks[2]	1–2 grams	Every 2–6 hours
Melnick[3]	1 gram	50 mg/kg every 24 hours
Wilson[4]	50 mg/kg	50 mg/kg every 24 hours
Dietzman[5]	50 mg/kg	In four hours if needed

Therapy is initiated by administering *Solu-Cortef* intravenously over a period of one to several minutes. In general, high dose corticosteroid therapy should be continued only until the patient's condition has stabilized—usually not beyond 48 to 72 hours. Although adverse effects associated with high dose, short-term corticoid therapy are uncommon, peptic ulceration may occur. Prophylactic anatacid therapy may be indicated.

When massive hydrocortisone therapy must be continued beyond 48–72 hours, hypernatremia may occur. Under such circumstances it may be desirable to replace *Solu-Cortef* with a corticoid such as methylprednisolone sodium succinate which causes little or no sodium retention.

In other situations in which adequate preparation with intramuscularly administered cortisone or hydrocortisone cannot be accomplished, the initial dose is 100 mg to 500 mg, depending on the severity of the condition, administered by intravenous injection over a period of at least 30 seconds. This dose may be repeated at intervals of 1, 3, 6, and 10 hours as indicated by the patient's response and clinical condition. While the dose may be reduced for infants and children, it is governed more by the severity of the condition and response of the patient than by age or body weight but should not be less than 25 mg daily.

Patients subjected to severe stress following corticosteroid therapy should be observed closely for signs and symptoms of adrenocortical insufficiency.

Corticoid therapy is an adjunct to, and not a replacement for, conventional therapy.

Multiple Sclerosis

In treatment of acute exacerbations of multiple sclerosis daily doses of 200 mg of prednisolone for a week followed by 80 mg every other day for 1 month have been shown to be effective (20 mg of hydrocortisone is equivalent to 5 mg of prednisolone).

Preparation of Solutions

100 mg Plain or with Bacteriostatic Water for Injection—For intravenous or intramuscular injection, prepare solution by aseptically adding **not more than 2 ml** of Bacteriostatic Water for Injection or Bacteriostatic Sodium Chloride Injection to the contents of one vial. **For intravenous infusion,** first prepare solution by adding **not more than 2 ml** of Bacteriostatic Water for Injection to the vial; this solution may then be added to 100 to 1000 ml (but not less than 100 ml) of the following: 5% dextrose in water (or isotonic saline solution or 5% dextrose in isotonic saline solution if patient is not on sodium restriction).

Directions for using *Mix-O-Vial®* *Two-Compartment Vial*

1. Remove protective cap, give the plunger-stopper a quarter-turn and press to force diluent into the lower compartment.
2. Gently agitate to effect solution.
3. Sterilize top of plunger-stopper with a suitable germicide.
4. Insert needle **squarely through center** of plunger-stopper until tip is just visible. Invert vial and withdraw dose.

Further dilution is not necessary for intravenous or intramuscular injection. For intravenous infusion, first prepare solution as just described. The **100 mg** solution may then be added to 100 to 1000 ml (but not less than 100 ml) of 5% dextrose in water (or isotonic saline solution or 5% dextrose in isotonic saline solution if patient is not on sodium restriction). The **250 mg** solution may be added to 250 to 1000 ml (but not less than 250 ml), the **500 mg** solution may be added to 500 to 1000 ml (but not less than 500 ml) and the **1000 mg** solution to not less than 1000 ml of the same diluents.

When reconstituted as directed, pH's of the solutions range from 7 to 8 and the tonicities are: 100 mg *Mix-O-Vial,* .36 osmolar; 250 mg *Mix-O-Vial,* 500 mg *Mix-O-Vial,* and the 1000 mg *Mix-O-Vial,* .57 osmolar. (Isotonic saline=.28 osmolar.)

Storage Conditions: Store unreconstituted product at controlled room temperature 15°–30°C (59°–86°F).

Store solution at controlled room temperature 15°–30°C (59°–86°F) and protect from light. Use solution only if it is clear. Unused solution should be discarded after 3 days.

How Supplied: *Solu-Cortef* Sterile Powder (hydrocortisone sodium succinate) is available in the following packages:

100 mg Plain—NDC 0009-0825-01
100 mg with Bacteriostatic Water for Injection—NDC 0009-0834-01
100 mg *Mix-O-Vial*—NDC 0009-0900-01
250 mg *Mix-O-Vial*—NDC 0009-0909-01
500 mg *Mix-O-Vial*—NDC 0009-0912-01
1000 mg *Mix-O-Vial*—NDC 0009-0920-01

References:

1. Melby, James C.: Corticosteroids in Shock in Man and Animals, *New Phy.* **13**:426-428 (November) 1964. 2. Oaks, Wilbur W. and Cohen, Herbert E.: Endotoxin Shock in the Geriatric Patient, *Geriatrics* **22**:120-130 (March) 1967. 3. Melnick, Irving and Litvak, Austin S.: Gram-Negative Bacteremia: An Evaluation of Fifty-Nine Cases During 1963, *J. Urol.* **96**:257-262 (August) 1966. 4. Wilson, Robert F.: Chiscano, Alfonso D.; Quadros, Everton; et al.: *Anesth. Analg.* **46**:751-763 (Nov.-Dec.) 1967. 5. Dietzman, Ronald H., et al.: Treatment of Shock, *GP* **36**:(3):135-141 (September) 1967.

Code 810 379 000

SOLU-MEDROL® STERILE POWDER ℞

(Methylprednisolone Sodium Succinate for Injection, USP)
For Intravenous or Intramuscular Administration

40 mg (1 ml *Mix-O-Vial®* Two-Compartment Vial):
NSN 6505-00-768-3598A (M & VA)
125 mg (2 ml *Mix-O-Vial*):
NSN 6505-00-943-4380A (M & VA)
500 mg:
NSN 6505-00-432-1124A (VA)
1000 mg:
NSN 6505-00-104-8069A (M & VA)

Description: Methylprednisolone sodium succinate, USP, occurs as a white, or nearly white, odorless hygroscopic, amorphous solid. It is very soluble in water and in alcohol; it is insoluble in chloroform and is very slightly soluble in acetone.

Solu-Medrol Sterile Powder (methylprednisolone sodium succinate) is so extremely soluble in water that it may be administered in a small volume of diluent and is especially well suited for intravenous use in situations in which high blood levels of methylprednisolone are required rapidly. *Solu-Medrol* is available as **40 mg *Mix-O-Vial®*** Two-Compartment Vial—Each ml (when mixed) contains methylprednisolone sodium succinate equiv. to 40 mg methylprednisolone; also 1.6 mg sodium biphosphate anhydrous; 17.46 mg dried sodium phosphate; 25 mg lactose hydrous; 5 mg benzyl alcohol. **125 mg *Mix-O-Vial*** Two-Compartment Vial—Each 2 ml (when mixed) contains methylprednisolone sodium succinate equiv. to 125 mg methylprednisolone; also 1.6 mg sodium biphosphate anhydrous; 17.4 mg dried sodium phosphate; 10 mg benzyl alcohol. **500 mg Vial**—Each 8 ml (when mixed as directed) contains methylprednisolone sodium succinate equiv. to 500 mg methylprednisolone; also 6.4 mg sodium biphosphate anhydrous; 69.6 mg dried sodium phosphate; and 66.8 mg benzyl alcohol. **1000 mg Vial**—Each 16 ml (when mixed as directed) contains methylprednisolone sodium succinate equiv. to 1000 mg methylprednisolone; also 12.8 mg sodium biphosphate anhydrous; 139.2 mg dried sodium phosphate; and 133.6 mg benzyl alcohol. When necessary the pH of the 125 mg, 500 mg and 1000 mg formulas was adjusted with sodium hydroxide and/or hydrochloric acid.

IMPORTANT—Only the accompanying diluent is to be used when dissolving the *Solu-Medrol* in vials.

Use within 48 hours after mixing

When reconstituted as directed, pH's of the solutions range from 7-8 and the tonicities are, for the 40 mg per ml solution, .50 osmolar; for the 125 mg per 2 ml, 500 mg per 8 ml and 1000 mg per 16 ml solutions, .40 osmolar. (Isotonic saline = .28 osmolar).

Actions: Methylprednisolone is a potent anti-inflammatory steroid synthesized in the Research Laboratories of The Upjohn Company. It has a greater anti-inflammatory potency than prednisolone and even less tendency than prednisolone to induce sodium and water retention.

Methylprednisolone sodium succinate has the same metabolic and anti-inflammatory actions as methylprednisolone. When given parenterally and in equimolar quantities, the two compounds are equivalent in biologic activity. The relative potency of *Solu-Medrol* (methylprednisolone sodium succinate) and hydrocortisone sodium succinate, as indicated by depression of eosinophil count, following intravenous administration, is at least four to one. This is in good agreement with the relative oral potency of methylprednisolone and hydrocortisone.

Indications

Based on a review of this drug by the National Academy of Sciences—National Research Council and/or other information, FDA has classified the indications as follows:

Effective:

1. **Endocrine disorders.**
   a. Acute adrenocortical insufficiency (hydrocortisone or cortisone is the drug of choice; mineralocorticoid supplementation may be necessary, particularly when synthetic analogs are used)
2. **Collagen diseases**—During an exacerbation or as maintenance therapy in selected cases of:
   a. Systemic lupus erythematosus
3. **Dermatologic diseases.**
   a. Pemphigus
   b. Severe erythema multiforme (Stevens-Johnson syndrome)
   c. Exfoliative dermatitis
4. **Allergic States**—Control of severe or incapacitating allergic conditions intractable to adequate trials of conventional treatment in:
   a. Bronchial asthma
   b. Contact dermatitis
   c. Serum sickness
   d. Drug hypersensitivity reactions
5. **Gastrointestinal diseases**—To tide the patient over a critical period of disease in:
   a. Ulcerative colitis (systemic therapy)
6. **Nervous System**
   Acute exacerbations of multiple sclerosis

Probably Effective:

a. To control severe or incapacitating allergic conditions intractable to adequate trials of conventional treatment in angioedema and urticaria and as an adjunct to epinephrine in anaphylaxis; as an enema or drip in selected cases to tide the patient over a critical period of disease in ulcerative colitis

Possibly Effective:

a. Generalized neurodermatitis
b. Acute rheumatic fever
c. Severe shock
   Hemorrhagic, traumatic, surgical, septic
   In severe shock adjunctive use of intravenous *Solu-Medrol* (methylprednisolone sodium succinate) may aid in achieving hemodynamic restoration. Corticoid therapy should not replace standard methods of combating shock, but present evidence indicates that concurrent use of large doses of corticoids with other measures may improve survival rates
d. Overwhelming infections with severe toxicity
   In patients moribund from overwhelmingly severe infections for which specific antibiotic therapy is available, intensive therapy with *Solu-Medrol* may permit survival until the antibiotic has had time to take effect. All procedures required for the establishment of a bacterial diagnosis should be carried out and intensive therapy with the indicated antibiotic begun before therapy with methylprednisolone sodium succinate is started. In the presence of infection, therapy with *Solu-Medrol* should be administered for the briefest period necessary for adequate clinical response and must be stopped at least three days before discontinuing antibiotic therapy. In the case of surgical infections (eg, peritonitis secondary to ruptured viscus) definitive surgical therapy should be scheduled as promptly as the patient's condition permits. Clinical improvement resulting from hormonal therapy must not be cause to defer surgical treatment
e. Croup—As adjunctive therapy, some investigators have found corticoids to be of value in the treatment of moderately severe and severe "croup" (acute laryngotracheobronchitis) when administered to infants and children in conjunction with other accepted therapeutic measures. At the present time, however, there are no data concerning the effect of corticoids in the acute epiglottic form of croup due to *H. influenzae.* There is no evidence that the incidence of tracheostomies is decreased by the administration of *Solu-Medrol.* The recommended dose is 40 mg intramuscularly, administered as early in the attack as possible. This therapy has been well tolerated. Transient bradycardia has been reported to occur occasionally in patients treated with this agent
f. Esophageal burns due to ingestion of caustic—Corticosteroid therapy has been associated with a lower incidence of stricture formation and decreased morbidity. In order to be effective, corticoids must be started within 48 hours of the time the burn is sustained. A rapid-acting steroid such as *Solu-Medrol* may be given in conjunction with supportive fluid and antibiotic therapy as initial treatment. After esophagoscopy the drug may be stopped in patients who have no burns. Treatment of those with esophageal damage should be continued with DEPO-MEDROL® (methylprednisolone acetate) or oral MEDROL® (methylprednisolone), if tolerated, antibiotics and bougienage where required

Final classification of the less-than-effective indications requires further investigation.

Contraindications: Systemic fungal infections.

Warnings: In patients on corticosteroid therapy subjected to any unusual stress, increased dosage of rapidly acting corticosteroids before, during, and after the stressful situation is indicated.

Corticosteroids may mask some signs of infection, and new infections may appear during their use. There may be decreased resistance and inability to localize infection when corticosteroids are used.

Prolonged use of corticosteroids may produce posterior subcapsular cataracts, glaucoma with possible damage to the optic nerves, and may enhance the establishment of secondary ocular infections due to fungi or viruses.

Usage in pregnancy. Since adequate human reproduction studies have not been done with corticosteroids, the use of these drugs in pregnancy, nursing mothers, or women of childbearing potential requires that the possible benefits of the drug be weighed against the potential hazards to the mother and embryo or fetus. Infants born of mothers who have received substantial doses of corticosteroids during pregnancy should be carefully observed for signs of hypoadrenalism.

Average and large doses of cortisone or hydrocortisone can cause elevation of blood pressure, salt and water retention, and increased excretion of potassium. These effects are less likely to occur with the synthetic derivatives except when used in large doses. Dietary salt restriction and potassium supplementation may be necessary. All corticosteroids increase calcium excretion.

While on corticosteroid therapy patients should not be vaccinated against smallpox. Other immunization procedures should not be undertaken in patients who are on corticosteroids, especially on high dose, because of possible hazards of neurological complications and a lack of antibody response.

The use of *Solu-Medrol* (methylprednisolone sodium succinate) in active tuberculosis should be restricted to those cases of fulminating or disseminated tuberculosis in which the corticosteroid is used for the management of the disease in conjunction with appropriate antituberculous regimen.

If corticosteroids are indicated in patients with latent tuberculosis or tuberculin reactivity, close observation is necessary as reactivation of the disease may occur. During prolonged corticosteroid therapy, these patients should receive chemoprophylaxis.

Because rare instances of anaphylactoid reactions have occurred in patients receiving parenteral corticosteroid therapy, appropriate precautionary measures should be taken prior to administration, especially when the patient has a history of allergy to any drug.

There are reports of cardiac arrhythmias and/or circulatory collapse following the rapid administration of large IV doses of *Solu-Medrol* (> 0.5 gm). These reactions have occurred primarily in renal transplant recipients and appear to be related, in some instances, to the rate of administration, eg, when the dose is given over a period of less than 10 minutes. The use of *Solu-Medrol* for this condition is not a listed indication, but physicians should be aware of the above possibility.

Precautions: Drug-induced secondary adrenocortical insufficiency may be minimized by gradual reduction of dosage. This type of relative insufficiency may persist for months after discontinuation of therapy; therefore, in any situation of stress occurring during that period, hormone therapy should be reinstituted. Since mineralocorticoid secretion may be impaired, salt and/or a mineralocorticoid should be administered concurrently.

There is an enhanced effect of corticosteroids on patients with hypothyroidism and in those with cirrhosis.

Corticosteroids should be used cautiously in patients with ocular herpes simplex because of possible corneal perforation.

The lowest possible dose of corticosteroid should be used to control the condition under treatment, and when reduction in dosage is possible, the reduction should be gradual.

Psychic derangements may appear when corticosteroids are used, ranging from euphoria, insomnia, mood swings, personality changes, and severe depression, to frank psychotic manifestations. Also, existing emotional instability or psychotic tendencies may be aggravated by corticosteroids.

Aspirin should be used cautiously in conjunction with corticosteroids in hypoprothrombinemia.

Steroids should be used with caution in nonspecific ulcerative colitis, if there is a probability of impending perforation, abscess or other pyo-

Continued on next page

Information on these Upjohn products is based on labeling in effect on November 1, 1979. Further information on dosage and administration, side effects, precautions and contraindications for these and other Upjohn products may be obtained from either the package insert or Medical Services, The Upjohn Company, Kalamazoo, Michigan.

Upjohn—Cont.

genic infection; diverticulitis; fresh intestinal anastomoses; active or latent peptic ulcer; renal insufficiency; hypertension; osteoporosis; and myasthenia gravis.

Growth and development of infants and children on prolonged corticosteroid therapy should be carefully observed.

Although controlled clinical trials have shown corticosteroids to be effective in speeding the resolution of acute exacerbations of multiple sclerosis, they do not show that corticosteroids affect the ultimate outcome or natural history of the disease. The studies do show that relatively high doses of corticosteroids are necessary to demonstrate a significant effect. (See **Dosage and Administration**).

Since complications of treatment with glucocorticoids are dependent on the size of the dose and the duration of treatment, a risk/benefit decision must be made in each individual case as to dose and duration of treatment and as to whether daily or intermittent therapy should be used.

Adverse Reactions:

Fluid and Electrolyte Disturbances
- Sodium retention
- Fluid retention
- Congestive heart failure in susceptible patients
- Potassium loss
- Hypokalemic alkalosis
- Hypertension

Musculoskeletal
- Muscle weakness
- Steroid myopathy
- Loss of muscle mass
- Severe arthralgia
- Osteoporosis
- Vertebral compression fractures
- Aseptic necrosis of femoral and humeral heads
- Pathologic fracture of long bones

Gastrointestinal
- Peptic ulcer with possible perforation and hemorrhage
- Pancreatitis
- Abdominal distention
- Ulcerative esophagitis

Dermatologic
- Impaired wound healing
- Thin fragile skin
- Petechiae and ecchymoses
- Facial erythema
- Increased sweating
- May suppress reactions to skin tests

Neurological
- Increased intracranial pressure with papilledema (pseudo-tumor cerebri) usually after treatment
- Convulsions
- Vertigo
- Headache

Endocrine
- Development of Cushingoid state
- Suppression of growth in children
- Secondary adrenocortical and pituitary unresponsiveness, particularly in times of stress, as in trauma, surgery or illness
- Menstrual irregularities
- Decreased carbohydrate tolerance
- Manifestations of latent diabetes mellitus
- Increased requirements for insulin or oral hypoglycemic agents in diabetics

Ophthalmic
- Posterior subcapsular cataracts
- Increased intraocular pressure
- Glaucoma
- Exophthalmos

Metabolic
- Negative nitrogen balance due to protein catabolism

The following *additional* adverse reactions are related to parenteral corticosteroid therapy:
- Hyperpigmentation or hypopigmentation
- Subcutaneous and cutaneous atrophy
- Sterile abscess

Dosage and Administration: In treating severe shock there is a tendency in current medical practice to use massive (pharmacologic) doses of corticosteroids. The following are *Solu-Medrol* (methylprednisolone sodium succinate) doses suggested by various authors:

Author	*Dose*	*Repeat*
Oaks[1]	100 mg	Every 2 to 6 hours
Weil[2]	200 mg	100 mg every 4 to 6 hours
Melby[3]	250 mg	Every 4 to 6 hours
Cavanagh[4]	15 mg/kg	Every 24 hours
Dietzman[5]	30 mg/kg	in 4 hours if needed

Therapy is initiated by administering *Solu-Medrol* intravenously over a period of one to several minutes. In general, high dose corticosteroid therapy should be continued only until the patient's condition has stabilized; usually not beyond 48 to 72 hours.

Although adverse effects associated with high dose short-term corticoid therapy are uncommon, peptic ulceration may occur. Prophylactic antacid therapy may be indicated.

In other indications initial dosage will vary from 10 to 40 mg of methylprednisolone depending on the clinical problem being treated. The larger doses may be required for short-term management of severe, acute conditions. The initial dose usually should be given intravenously over a period of one to several minutes. Subsequent doses may be given intravenously or intramuscularly at intervals dictated by the patient's response and clinical condition. Corticoid therapy is an adjunct to, and not replacement for, conventional therapy.

Dosage may be reduced for infants and children but should be governed more by the severity of the condition and response of the patient than by age or size. It should not be less than 0.5 mg per kg every 24 hours.

Dosage must be decreased or discontinued gradually when the drug has been administered for more than a few days. If a period of spontaneous remission occurs in a chronic condition, treatment should be discontinued. Routine laboratory studies, such as urinalysis, two-hour postprandial blood sugar, determination of blood pressure and body weight, and a chest X-ray should be made at regular intervals during prolonged therapy. Upper GI X-rays are desirable in patients with an ulcer history or significant dyspepsia.

Solu-Medrol, may be administered by intravenous or intramuscular injection or by intravenous infusion, the preferred method for initial emergency use being intravenous injection. To administer by intravenous (or intramuscular) injection, prepare solution as directed. The desired dose may be administered intravenously over a period of approximately 60 seconds. Subsequent doses may be withdrawn and administered similarly. If desired, the medication may be administered in diluted solutions by adding Water for Injection or other suitable diluent to the *Mix-O-Vial* and withdrawing the indicated dose.

To prepare solutions for intravenous infusion, first prepare the solution for injection as directed. This solution may then be added to indicated amounts of 5% dextrose in water, isotonic saline solution or 5% dextrose in isotonic saline solution.

Doses of 20 to 40 mg administered as retention enemas or by continuous drip three to seven times weekly for periods of two or more weeks have been shown to be a useful adjunct in the treatment of some patients with ulcerative colitis. Many patients can be controlled with 40 mg of methylprednisolone administered in from 1 to 10 fluidounces of water depending on the degree of involvement of the inflamed colonic mucosa. Other accepted therapeutic measures should, of course, be instituted.

Multiple Sclerosis

In treatment of acute exacerbations of multiple sclerosis, daily doses of 200 mg of prednisolone for a week followed by 80 mg every other day for 1 month have been shown to be effective (4 mg of methylpredisolone is equivalent to 5 mg of prednisolone).

Directions for Using the *Mix-O-Vial:*
1. Remove protective cap, give the plunger-stopper a quarter turn and press to force diluent into the lower compartment.
2. Gently agitate to effect solution. Use solution within 48 hours.
3. Sterilize top of plunger-stopper with a suitable germicide.
4. Insert needle **squarely through center** of plunger-stopper until tip is just visible. Invert vial and withdraw dose.

Storage Conditions: Store unreconstituted product at controlled room temperature 15°–30° C (59°–86° F). Store solution at controlled room temperature 15°–30° C (59°–86° F). Use solution within 48 hours after mixing.

How Supplied: *Solu-Medrol* Sterile Powder (methylprednisolone sodium succinate) is available in the following packages:

40 mg *Mix-O-Vial* Two-Compartment Vial
NDC 0009-0113-01

125 mg *Mix-O-Vial* Two-Compartment Vial
NDC 0009-0190-01

500 mg Vial with Diluent
NDC 0009-0887-01

1000 mg Vial with Diluent
NDC 0009-0911-01

References:

1. Oaks, WW, Cohen, HE: Endotoxin Shock in the geriatric patient. Geriatrics **22**:120-130, 1967.
2. Weil, MH, Shubin H, Biddle M: Shock caused by gram-negative microorganisms. Ann Intern Med **60**:384-400, 1964.
3. Melby JC: Corticosteroids in shock in man and animals. New Physician **13**:426-428, 1964.
4. Cavanagh D, Clark PJ, McLeod AG: Septic shock of endotoxin type. Amer J Obstet Gynecol **102**:13-20, 1968.
5. Dietzman RH, Bloch JH, Lillehei RC: Treatment of shock. GP **36**:135-141, 1967.

Code 810 431 000

[*Shown in Product Identification Section*]

TOLINASE® TABLETS ℞
(Tolazamide Tablets, USP)

250 mg (30s)
NSN 6505-01-061-6992 (VA)
250 mg (100s):
NSN 6505-00-159-4990A (VA)
250 mg (1000s):
NSN 6505-00-105-5842A (M & VA)

Tolinase Tablets are an orally effective hypoglycemic agent which has been shown to be effective and safe in over 3,000 diabetic patients in a period of more than four years of clinical trials. It is effective in the mild to moderately severe maturity-onset type of diabetes. It represents the culmination of a seven year search by The Upjohn Company involving over 4,000 compounds to find an oral agent as safe as *Orinase*® Tablets (tolbutamide, Upjohn) which might help fill the therapeutic gap created by sulfonylurea failures. Clinical trials have indicated that *Tolinase* **is effective in approximately one-third of failures to tolbutamide, chlorpropamide or phenformin.** It should be recognized, however, that this "salvage" rate may not be sustained and that some of these patients will also eventually fail on *Tolinase. Tolinase* in **once-a-day therapy** has proven to be as effective in providing satisfactory diabetic control as in multiple daily doses. **Patients must be under continuous medical supervision, particularly during the first six weeks of treatment. They should check their urines daily for sugar and acetone and should see their doctors at least once a week.** ***Tolinase***

is not an oral insulin or an insulin substitute. It is not recommended for the juvenile diabetic or the diabetic under stress of infection, surgery, severe trauma, or in ketoacidosis or coma. It is not recommended for use in the pregnant diabetic patient. Since the primary mechanism of action is the release of endogenous insulin, occasionally hypoglycemic reactions have occurred (verified hypoglycemic reactions were reported in 0.4%). This usually results from the administration of too large a dose for the patient's immediate needs. It is imperative that the physician familiarize himself with the indications and limitations of therapy, as well as the criteria for the proper selection of patients.

Chemistry: *Tolinase* (tolazamide) was synthesized by chemists at The Upjohn Company. It is 1-(hexahydro-1H-azepin-1-yl)-3-(*p*-tolylsulfonyl)urea.

The molecular weight is 311.40. It is a white or creamy white powder with a melting point of 165° to 173° C. The minimum solubility at 37.5° C. in aqueous buffers is 0.09 grams per liter at pH 4.5; the solubility increases logarithmically at higher and lower pH values; for example, the solubility is 1.13 grams per liter at pH 2.0 and 1.97 grams per liter at pH 7.0. Its solubility is between 4 and 5 grams per liter in 95% ethanol.

The solubility of *Tolinase* at pH 6.0 (mean urinary pH) is 27.8 mg per 100 ml. Besides the absence of crystalluria in the extensive clinical trials, the fact that small daily doses are used and that 93% of the pooled urinary extracts of man (following oral ingestion of *Tolinase*) are metabolites which are more soluble than *Tolinase* gives assurance that crystalluria should not occur.

Animal Studies: *Tolinase* (tolazamide) is five to nine and one-half times more potent than *Orinase* (tolbutamide) in glucose-primed, fasted, intact rats and four times as potent as *Orinase* in glucose-primed, fasted, adrenalectomized rats. As is true with other sulfonylurea compounds, *Tolinase* has no hypoglycemic effect in alloxanized diabetic or eviscerate rats.

Animal Toxicology: Acute toxicity is extremely low, as the mouse LD_{50} is 2200 mg per kg intraperitoneally, and the rat LD_{50} is greater than 5 grams per kg orally. One month and six month studies in dogs at doses from 12.5 to 50 mg per kg showed no significant toxicity, nor did one month and one year studies in Sprague-Dawley rats at doses from 25 to 100 mg per kg, although these rats did demonstrate marked beta cell islet hyperplasia with some resultant degeneration and fibrosis of the islet cells. Doses up to 400 mg/kg daily in the rabbit for periods of one year showed no similar changes. Doses of 100 mg/kg daily for periods up to two years in the Wistar rat produced only minimal changes in the pancreatic islets. Drug treatment of pregnant rats produced no reproductive aberrations or drug related fetal anomalies at a daily dose of 14 mg per kg. At the elevated dose of 100 mg per kg, there was a reduction in number of pups born and an increased perinatal mortality.

Absorption, Metabolism and Excretion: Isotopic techniques show that *Tolinase* (tolazamide) is well absorbed with little subject-to-subject variation. Due to slower absorption of *Tolinase* compared with tolbutamide or chlorpropamide, peak blood drug levels occur at four to eight hours following the oral administration of therapeutic doses. An average of 85% of the radioactivity of an oral dose appears in the urine.

Utilizing both chemical and isotopic methods, the average biological half-life is 7.0 hours. The drug does not continue to cumulate in the blood after the first four to six doses are administered. A steady or equilibrium state is reached during which the peak and nadir values do not change from day to day after the fourth to sixth dose.

Actions: As with other sulfonylureas, the primary mechanism of action appears to be stimulation of the beta cells of the pancreas with increased endogenous insulin secretion. Utilizing the immunoassay technique of Yalow and Berson, dog studies have shown *Tolinase* (tolazamide) to produce increased pancreatic venous insulin levels. Further, these levels are maintained longer than with equal doses of *Orinase* (tolbutamide) or chlorpropamide. When normal, nondiabetic, fasting volunteers are given single doses of *Tolinase* orally, the peak hypoglycemic effect occurs in one hour. Following an oral dose of 500 mg of *Tolinase*, a statistically significant hypoglycemic effect was demonstrated in nondiabetic subjects 20 hours following administration. With fasting diabetic patients, the peak hypoglycemic effect occurs at four to six hours. The duration of maximal hypoglycemic effect in fed diabetic patients is about ten hours, with the onset occurring at four to six hours and with the blood sugar levels beginning to rise at fourteen to sixteen hours.

Single-dose potency of *Tolinase* in the normal subject has been shown to be 6.7 times that of tolbutamide on a milligram basis. Clinical experience in diabetic patients has demonstrated *Tolinase* to be approximately five times more potent than tolbutamide.

Tolazamide does not appear to have an antidiuretic effect and a mild diuresis has been observed.

Indications:

1. The primary indication for *Tolinase* (tolazamide) is the stable or maturity-onset type of mild or moderately severe diabetes mellitus.
2. Approximately one-third of diabetic patients purported to be primary or secondary failures with other sulfonylurea agents or with phenformin have been reported to respond satisfactorily to *Tolinase* therapy.
3. Some patients who have developed significant side effects or intolerance to other sulfonylurea drugs or phenformin may subsequently be successfully maintained on *Tolinase*.

Contraindications:

1. *Tolinase* (tolazamide) is not indicated in diabetic patients who have infections, severe trauma or who are undergoing surgery, who have ketosis, acidosis or coma or give a history of repeated bouts of ketoacidosis or coma.
2. It is not indicated in the therapy of juvenile or labile (brittle) diabetes.
3. Since *Tolinase* has not been studied extensively in patients with concurrent liver, renal or endocrine disease, its use is not recommended in these conditions and is contraindicated in subjects with uremia. Nevertheless, no instance of jaundice, renal or endocrine disease attributable solely to therapy with *Tolinase* has occurred.
4. In view of the question of the safety of any new drug in pregnancy, and in view of the fact that the safety and usefulness of *Tolinase* during pregnancy has not been evaluated at this time, *Tolinase* is not recommended for the treatment of the pregnant diabetic patient. Serious consideration should be given to the possible hazards of its use in women of child-bearing age who might become pregnant.

Precautions:

1. The diagnostic and therapeutic measures which are necessary to insure optimal control of the diabetic state with insulin or other sulfonylureas are equally necessary for control with *Tolinase* (tolazamide). No false positive tests for urinary albumin have been reported, as has been occasionally noted with other sulfonylureas.
2. The patient must receive full and complete instructions about the nature of his disease, what he must do to prevent and detect complications and how to control his condition.
3. He must understand that he cannot neglect his dietary restrictions, develop a careless attitude or disregard instructions relative to body weight, exercise, personal hygiene and avoidance of infection.
4. The patient must know how to recognize and counteract impending hypoglycemia.
5. The patient must know how and when to test for glycosuria and ketonuria.
6. During the trial period, when insulin is being withdrawn, care should be taken to avoid ketosis, acidosis and coma.
7. When *Tolinase* is administered as sole therapy to patients who have previously required combination therapy (phenformin plus sulfonylureas), careful observation of the patient is mandatory, particularly during the transitional phase.
8. Caution should be observed in administering the thiazide-type diuretics to diabetic patients on *Tolinase* therapy because the thiazides have been reported to aggravate diabetes mellitus and to result in increased sulfonylurea requirements.
9. Very close observation and careful adjustment of dosage is mandatory in patients who are debilitated, malnourished, semistarved or simply not eating properly. In such patients severe hypoglycemic reactions may occur and may require corrective therapy.
10. Severe hypoglycemia, though uncommon, may occur in patients receiving *Tolinase* and may mimic acute neurological disorders such as cerebral thrombosis. Certain conditions, such as hepatic and renal disease, malnutrition, debility, advanced age, alcoholism, and adrenal and pituitary insufficiency may predispose to hypoglycemia. Also, certain drugs may prolong or enhance the action of *Tolinase* and thereby increase the risk of hypoglycemia. These include insulin, phenformin, sulfonamides, oxyphenbutazone, phenylbutazone, salicylates, probenecid and monamine oxidase inhibitors.

Adverse Reactions: *Tolinase* Tablets (tolazamide) have been generally well tolerated. In 1,784 diabetic patients specially evaluated for incidence of side effects during the clinical studies, 2.1% were discontinued from therapy because of side effects.

The following adverse reactions have been reported in connection with the use of this agent either during the clinical studies or subsequent thereto.

Gastrointestinal—Nausea and vomiting have been reported occasionally. In the clinical studies gastrointestinal symptoms related to *Tolinase* (tolazamide) were noted in 1.0% of the patients, with nausea, vomiting and gas each noted in less than 1% of the patients studied.

Hematopoietic—Rare cases of leukopenia, thrombocytopenia, agranulocytosis, and anemia have been reported.

Hypoglycemia—Hypoglycemia has been reported occasionally. Hypoglycemia is actually a physiological extension of the primary action of the drug and generally represents the result of the administration of a dose larger than that

Continued on next page

Information on these Upjohn products is based on labeling in effect on November 1, 1979. Further information on dosage and administration, side effects, precautions and contraindications for these and other Upjohn products may be obtained from either the package insert or Medical Services, The Upjohn Company, Kalamazoo, Michigan.

Upjohn—Cont.

needed by the subject. Reduction in dose generally will result in alleviation of most of the mild to moderately severe hypoglycemic symptoms. Undernourished or underweight or geriatric patients, or those failing to eat properly are particularly susceptible to hypoglycemia and should be treated cautiously. It is not recommended that patients with chronic liver or kidney disease receive *Tolinase* therapy as they may well metabolize or excrete *Tolinase* poorly and be more susceptible to hypoglycemic reactions.

Liver—Hepatic toxicity as manifested by alterations in liver function tests (bilirubin, cholesterol, SGOT, SGPT, etc.) and by cholestatic jaundice has occasionally been associated with *Tolinase* therapy. Transient elevations in alkaline phosphatase determinations are not uncommon after initiation of sulfonylurea therapy. However, these are not necessarily drug related, inasmuch as fluctuating abnormalities of hepatic function are frequently observed in patients with diabetes mellitus.

Skin and Mucous Membranes—Hematologic and allergic reactions as manifested by urticaria and rash have been reported occasionally.

Miscellaneous—Miscellaneous symptoms of weakness, fatigue, dizziness, vertigo, malaise and headache were reported infrequently, but the relationship to *Tolinase* therapy is difficult to assess.

Photosensitivity reactions and disulfiram-like reactions after ingestion of alcohol have been reported occasionally in patients taking tolazamide.

Selection of Patients: Generally, the basic requirement for *Tolinase* (tolazamide) therapy is that the diabetes be of the maturity-onset (adult) type. The patient has usually developed his diabetes after the age of 30 years. He may be a newly diagnosed diabetic or one taking less than 40 units a day of insulin. He may be one who has developed intolerance or significant side effects to phenformin, chlorpropamide or tolbutamide.

Tolinase is effective in some patients with a history of ketoacidosis or coma. Such patients must be observed very closely, however, particularly during the early transitional period.

In approximately one-third of cases reported as being primary or secondary failures to chlorpropamide, tolbutamide, or phenformin, *Tolinase* has provided satisfactory control as sole therapy in these subjects. It should be recognized, however, that this "salvage" rate may not be sustained and that some of these patients will also eventually fail on *Tolinase.*

The only reliable method of determining responsiveness to *Tolinase* is therapeutic trial, with the patient being evaluated at weekly intervals and the dose regulated according to the patient's response.

Dosage:

The newly diagnosed diabetic subject

No initial loading or priming dose is necessary. The mild to moderately severe, newly diagnosed, adult-onset diabetic should be started on from 100 mg to 250 mg of *Tolinase* (tolazamide) once a day (given with breakfast).

If the patient is malnourished, underweight, elderly, or not eating properly, the initial therapy should be 100 mg once a day.

The following is a suggested initial dose schedule for a newly diagnosed diabetic subject:

If the fasting blood sugar value is less than 200 mg% (True), start with 100 mg per day of *Tolinase* as a single daily dose.

If the fasting blood sugar is greater than 200 mg% (True), start with 250 mg per day of *Tolinase* as a single dose.

Depending upon the results of the patient's urinary glucose test at home, the weekly blood sugar determinations, and the evaluations by the physician, the dose is then either raised or lowered accordingly at weekly intervals by amounts of one tablet (100 mg or 250 mg) per day. If more than 500 mg per day is required, the dose should be divided and given twice daily. Doses larger than 1,000 mg daily doubtfully will result in improved control.

In underweight, undernourished, or geriatric patients, when increments in dosage are required, these should be on the order of ½ tablet (50 mg or 125 mg) daily at weekly intervals to help avoid hypoglycemic reactions.

Patients Receiving Other Oral Hypoglycemic Agents

When transferring patients from other oral hypoglycemic agents to *Tolinase* (tolazamide), no transitional period and no initial or priming dose is necessary. The following dose equivalents are recommended:

Tolbutamide: If receiving 1 gram per day or less, begin *Tolinase* at 100 mg per day as a single dose. If receiving more than 1 gram per day, initiate *Tolinase* at 250 mg per day as a single dose.

Chlorpropamide: 250 mg of chlorpropamide may be considered equivalent to 250 mg of *Tolinase.* The patient should be observed carefully for hypoglycemia during the transition period from chlorpropamide to *Tolinase* (1-2 weeks) due to the prolonged retention of chlorpropamide in the body and subsequent overlapping drug effect.

Acetohexamide: 100 mg of *Tolinase* may be considered equivalent to 250 mg of acetohexamide.

Phenformin: 100 mg of phenformin may be considered equivalent to 250 mg of *Tolinase.*

If necessary, the dose should be adjusted (increased or decreased) weekly with increments of one tablet daily (either 100 mg or 250 mg) depending upon the patient's response. If more than 500 mg a day is required, the dose should be divided and given more often than once a day.

In underweight, undernourished, or geriatric patients, when increments in dosage are required, these should be on the order of ½ tablet (50 mg or 125 mg) daily at weekly intervals to help avoid hypoglycemic reactions.

Patients Receiving Insulin

Many maturity-onset, mild to moderate diabetic patients who have been treated only with insulin may respond satisfactorily to *Tolinase* (tolazamide) therapy.

The following schedule is recommended as based on previous insulin dosage:

Insulin dosage less than 20 units: Place directly on *Tolinase* 100 mg as a single daily dose.

Insulin dosage less than 40 units but more than 20 units: Place directly on *Tolinase* 250 mg as a single daily dose.

Insulin dosage greater than 40 units: Reduce insulin dosage 50% and start *Tolinase* 250 mg daily.

Tolinase dosage should then be adjusted on a weekly basis (or more often in the group previously requiring more than 40 units of insulin).

It is important during insulin withdrawal that the patient test his urine for glucose and acetone at least three times daily and report the results to his physician.

The appearance of significant acetonuria would make discontinuation of *Tolinase* and the return to insulin therapy mandatory.

In the event that the patient cannot be transferred completely to *Tolinase* therapy, *Tolinase* Tablets (tolazamide) should be discontinued and the subject maintained on insulin therapy only.

When doses larger than 500 mg daily are required, a divided dosage regimen is recommended. Doses larger than 1,000 mg daily doubtfully will provide any improvement in diabetic control.

How Supplied: Scored tablets containing tolazamide in the following strengths and package sizes:

100 mg	Bottles of 100	*NDC 0009-0070-02*
250 mg	Bottles of 100	*NDC 0009-0114-05*
	Bottles of 200	*NDC 0009-0114-04*
	Bottles of 1000	*NDC 0009-0114-02*
	Unit Dose Packages (100)	*NDC 0009-0114-06*
	Unit of Use Bottle of 30	*NDC 0009-0114-16*
500 mg	Bottles of 50	*NDC 0009-0477-01*
	Unit of Use Bottle of 30	*NDC 0009-0477-04*

Code KRM-17

[*Shown in Product Identification Section*]

TROBICIN® STERILE POWDER ℞

(Sterile Spectinomycin Hydrochloride, USP)

For Intramuscular Injection

2 Gm vial
NSN 6505-00-079-7611 (M)
4 Gm vial
NSN 6505-00-079-7643 (M)

Description: *Trobicin* Sterile Powder (spectinomycin hydrochloride) is an aminocyclitol antibiotic produced by a species of soil microorganism designated as *Streptomyces spectabilis.* Sterile spectinomycin hydrochloride is the pentahydrated dihydrochloride salt of spectinomycin.

Trobicin is isolated as a white crystalline dihydrochloride pentahydrate, molecular weight 495, and is stable in the dry state for 36 months.

Actions: *Trobicin* (spectinomycin hydrochloride) is an inhibitor of protein synthesis in the bacterial cell; the site of action is the 30S ribosomal subunit.

In vitro studies have shown *Trobicin* to be active against most strains of *Neisseria gonorrhoeae* (minimum inhibitory concentration < 7.5 to 20 mcg/ml).

Definitive *in vitro* studies have shown no cross-resistance of *N. gonorrhoeae* between *Trobicin* and penicillin. The antibiotic is not significantly bound to plasma protein.

Indications: *Trobicin* (spectinomycin hydrochloride) is indicated in the treatment of acute gonorrheal urethritis and proctitis in the male and acute gonorrheal cervicitis and proctitis in the female when due to susceptible strains of *N. gonorrhoeae.* Men and women with known recent exposure to gonorrhea should be treated as those known to have gonorrhea.

The *in vitro* susceptibility of *N. gonorrhoeae* to *Trobicin* can be tested by agar dilution methods. *Trobicin* Susceptibility Powder is available for this purpose, and its package insert should be consulted for details.

Contraindications: The use of *Trobicin* (spectinomycin hydrochloride) is contraindicated in patients previously found hypersensitive to it.

Warnings: *Trobicin* is not effective in the treatment of syphilis. Antibiotics used in high doses for short periods of time to treat gonorrhea may mask or delay the symptoms of incubating syphilis. Since the treatment of syphilis demands prolonged therapy with any effective antibiotic, patients being treated for gonorrhea should be closely observed clinically. All patients with gonorrhea should have a serologic test for syphilis at the time of diagnosis. Patients treated with *Trobicin* should have a follow-up serologic test for syphilis after three months.

Usage in pregnancy: Safety for use in pregnancy has not been established.

Usage in infants and children: Safety for use in infants and children has not been established.

Precautions: The usual precautions should be observed with atopic individuals.

The clinical effectiveness of *Trobicin* (spectinomycin hydrochloride) should be monitored to detect evidence of development of resistance by *N. gonorrhoeae.*

Adverse Reactions: The following reactions were observed during the single dose clinical trials: soreness at the injection site, urticaria, dizziness, nausea, chills, fever and insomnia. During multiple dose subchronic tolerance studies in normal human volunteers, the following were noted: a decrease in hemoglobin, hematocrit and creatinine clearance; elevation of alkaline phosphatase, BUN and SGPT. In single and multiple dose studies in normal volunteers, a reduction in urine output was noted. Extensive renal function studies demonstrated no consistent changes indicative of renal toxicity.

Dosage and Administration:

Preparation of Drug for Intramuscular Injection

2 gram Sterile *Trobicin* (spectinomycin hydrochloride): reconstitute with 3.2 ml of the accompanying diluent.*

4 gram Sterile *Trobicin:* reconstitute with 6.2 ml of the accompanying diluent.*

*Bacteriostatic Water for Injection with Benzyl Alcohol 0.9% w/v.

Shake vials vigorously immediately after adding diluent and before withdrawing dose. Prepared suspension should be stored at room temperature (25° C.) and used within 24 hours. It is recommended that disposable syringes and needles be used to avoid contamination with penicillin residue, especially when treating patients known to be highly sensitive to penicillin. **Use of 20 gauge needle is recommended.**

Dosage

Intramuscular injections should be made deep into the upper outer quadrant of the gluteal muscle.

Adults (Men and Women)—Inject 5 ml intramuscularly for a 2 gram dose. This is also the recommended dose for patients being treated after failure of previous antibiotic therapy.

In geographic areas where antibiotic resistance is known to be prevalent, initial treatment with 4 grams (10 ml) intramuscularly is preferred. The 10 ml injection may be divided between two gluteal injection sites.

How Supplied: *Trobicin* (spectinomycin hydrochloride) is available as:

Sterile *Trobicin,* 2 gram vial—with one ampoule of Bacteriostatic Water for Injection with Benzyl Alcohol 0.9% w/v. When reconstituted with 3.2 ml of the accompanying diluent, each vial yields a sufficient quantity for withdrawal of 5 ml of a suspension containing 400 mg spectinomycin per ml (as the hydrochloride). 5 ml provides 2 Gm spectinomycin. For intramuscular use only.

NDC 0009-0566-01

Sterile *Trobicin,* 4 gram vial—with one ampoule of Bacteriostatic Water for Injection with Benzyl Alcohol 0.9% w/v. When reconstituted with 6.2 ml of the accompanying diluent, each vial yields a sufficient quantity for withdrawal of 10 ml of a suspension containing 400 mg spectinomycin per ml (as the hydrochloride). 10 ml provides 4 Gm spectinomycin. For intramuscular use only.

NDC 0009-0592-01

***Trobicin* Susceptibility Powder**—100 mg. See package insert for *in vitro* testing procedure.

Human Pharmacology: *Trobicin* Sterile Powder (spectinomycin hydrochloride) is rapidly absorbed after intramuscular injection. A single, two-gram injection produces peak serum concentrations averaging about 100 mcg/ml at one hour; a single, four-gram injection produces peak serum concentrations averaging 160 mcg/ml at two hours. Average serum concentrations of 15 mcg/ml for the two-gram dose and 31 mcg/ml for the four-gram dose were present eight hours after dosing.

Code NGB

UTICILLIN VK® FLAVORED GRANULES ℞
(Penicillin V Potassium for Oral Solution, USP)

How Supplied: When reconstituted, each 5 ml contains penicillin V potassium equivalent to 125 or 250 mg penicillin V. Available in the following packages:

125 mg/5 ml (200,000 Units)
100 ml bottles *NDC 0009-0787-03*
200 ml bottles *NDC 0009-0787-04*

250 mg/5 ml (400,000 Units)
100 ml bottles *NDC 0009-0865-03*
150 ml bottles *NDC 0009-0865-02*
200 ml bottles *NDC 0009-0865-04*

UTICILLIN VK® TABLETS ℞
(Penicillin V Potassium Tablets, USP)

How Supplied: Scored tablets containing penicillin V potassium equivalent to 250 mg or 500 mg penicillin V. Available in the following packages:

250 mg tablets (400,000 Units)
Bottles of 100 *NDC 0009-0586-01*
Bottles of 1000 *NDC 0009-0586-02*

500 mg tablets (800,000 Units)
Bottles of 100 *NDC 0009-0671-01*

[*Shown in Product identification Section*]

Upsher-Smith Laboratories, Inc.
14905 23RD AVE., NORTH
MINNEAPOLIS, MINNESOTA 55441

ACETAMINOPHEN UNISERTS® OTC
Rectal Suppositories

Description: Acetaminophen Uniserts suppositories are supplied in 120 mg. (pediatric) and 650 mg. strengths. Acetaminophen Uniserts are foil strip-wrapped and unit dose labeled.

Indications: For the temporary relief of fever, minor aches, pains and headaches.

Dosage: Adults—Two 650 mg. suppositories every 4 to 6 hours. No more than a total of 6 suppositories in any 24-hour period.

Children (over 6)—One 650 mg. suppository every 4 to 6 hours. No more than a total of 4 suppositories in any 24-hour period.

Children (3 to 6)—Two 120 mg. (pediatric) suppositories every 4 to 6 hours. No more than a total of 6 suppositories in any 24-hour period.

Children (under 3)—Consult a physician.

Warning: Severe or recurrent pain or high or continued fever may be indicative of serious illness. Under these conditions, consult a physician. Do not use consistently for more than 10 days except on the advice of a physician.

How Supplied: 120 mg., boxes of 12 and 50. 650 mg., boxes of 12, 50 and 500.

HISTATAPP® ELIXIR ℞

Composition: Each 5cc contains: Brompheniramine Maleate, 4 mg.; Phenylephrine HCl, 5 mg.; Phenylpropanolamine HCl, 5 mg.

How Supplied: Grape flavored elixir in 4 fl. oz., pints and gallons.

HISTATAPP® T.D. TABLETS ℞

Composition: Each timed disintegration tablet contains: Brompheniramine Maleate, 12 mg.; Phenylephrine HCl, 15 mg.; Phenylpropanolamine HCl, 15 mg.

How Supplied: Light blue tablets in bottles of 100 and 500; unit dose boxes of 100.

KLOR-10%™ ℞
(potassium chloride oral solution, USP 10%)

How Supplied: 4 fl. oz., pints and gallons.

KLOR-CON® 20% ℞
(potassium chloride oral solution, USP 20%)

How Supplied: 4 fl. oz., pints and gallons.

KLOR-CON® Powder ℞
(Potassium Chloride)
20 mEq. (1.5g) per packet

Description: Each packet contains 1.5g potassium chloride providing potassium 20 mEq and chloride 20 mEq. Fruit-flavored with artificial color and sweetener (saccharin) added.

Indications: Treatment of potassium deficiency which may occur with long-term diuretic therapy, corticosteroid therapy, digitalis intoxication, low dietary intake of potassium or loss of potassium due to vomiting and diarrhea.

Contraindications: Renal impairment, untreated Addison's disease, dehydration, heat cramps and hyperkalemia. Potassium chloride should not be employed in patients receiving potassium-sparing agents such as aldosterone antagonists and triamterene.

Precautions: Potassium chloride must be administered with caution since the degree of potassium deficiency and the corresponding daily dosage is often not accurately known. Excessive or even therapeutic dosages may result in potassium intoxication. The patient should be checked frequently and periodic ECG and/or plasma potassium levels made. High plasma concentrations of potassium ion may cause cardiac depression, arrhythmias or arrest. Use with caution in the presence of cardiac disease. Patients should be cautioned to adhere to dilution instructions.

Adverse Reactions: Vomiting, diarrhea, nausea and abdominal discomfort may occur. Symptoms and signs of potassium intoxication include mental confusion, listlessness, paresthesias of the extremities, flaccid paralysis, weakness of the legs, fall in blood pressure, cardiac arrhythmias and heart block. Hyperkalemia, when detected, must be treated promptly.

Dosage and Administration: The usual adult dose is 20 to 80 mEq of potassium per day (1 packet 1 to 4 times daily after meals.) The contents of 1 packet should be dissolved in at least 4 oz cold water or fruit juice. This preparation, like other potassium supplements, must be properly diluted to avoid the possibility of gastrointestinal irritation.

How Supplied: KLOR-CON Powder 20 mEq (1.5g) (Potassium Chloride). In cartons of 30 and 100 packets.

SSKI™ ℞
(potassium iodide solution, U.S.P.)

Composition: Each 0.3ml. contains potassium iodide 300 mg.

Action and Uses: An expectorant in the symptomatic treatment of chronic pulmonary diseases where tenacious mucus complicates the problem, including bronchial asthma, bronchitis and pulmonary emphysema.

Contraindications: Contraindicated in patients with hyperthyroidism or known sensitivity to iodides.

Adverse Reactions: May include gastrointestinal upset, metallic taste, minor skin eruptions, nausea, vomiting and epigastric pain. If these symptoms develop, discontinue use.

Precautions: Caution is recommended in patients during pregnancy. In some patients prolonged use of iodides can lead to hypothyroidism.

Administration and Dosage: Adults, 0.3ml. or 0.6ml. diluted in one glassful of water 3 or 4 times daily.

How Supplied: In bottles of 1 oz. (calibrated dropper, marked to deliver 0.3ml. and 0.6ml.) and 8 oz.

Continued on next page

Upsher-Smith—Cont.

TROFAN®
L-Tryptophan Tablets, 0.5 Gm.

Composition: Each white, capsule shaped tablet contains L-Tryptophan, 0.5 Gm. Trofan tablets are dye-free.
How Supplied: Trofan tablets 0.5 Gm. in bottles of 30 and 100.

Vale Chemical Co., Inc., The
1201 LIBERTY ST.
ALLENTOWN, PA 18102

GLYCOTUSS
(Guaifenesin)

Composition: Each 5 ml. teaspoonful and each tablet contains: 100 mg. of Guaifenesin.
Action: Guaifenesin is an effective expectorant which furthers the productivity of cough by stimulating the secretion of fluids of the bronchial tree thereby reducing the viscosity of tenacious mucus. The increased water content of the upper respiratory tract is partly the result of a gastric reflex following ingestion and partly after absorption into the blood stream, presumably by an effect on the brain stem or directly upon the secretory glands of the respiratory tract itself.
Indications: GLYCOTUSS (Guaifenesin) is useful for the symptomatic relief of respiratory conditions associated with dry, unproductive cough, and in the presence of mucus in the respiratory tract. Its long action and efficient stimulation of respiratory tract fluid make it a valuable help in removing the cause of the cough instead of merely suppressing it. GLYCOTUSS (Guaifenesin) finds its greatest usefulness in relief of dry cough associated with the common cold, pertussis, measles, and influenza.
Contraindications: Contraindicated in patients who have a history of sensitivity to guaiacol.
Adverse Reactions: No serious side effects of Guaifenesin have been reported. Occasional drowsiness, gastric disturbance and nausea have been encountered.
Administration and Dosage: *Adults*—one or two tablets, or one or two teaspoonfuls every three or four hours. The suggested adult maximum daily dosage is 800 mg. *Children*—(6 to 12 years)—one-half the adult dosage.
How Supplied: GLYCOTUSS is available as tablets in bottles of 100, 500, and 1,000; also as a pleasant, grape-flavored syrup in pints and gallons.

Vicks Toiletry Products Division
RICHARDSON-MERRELL INC.
TEN WESTPORT ROAD
WILTON, CT 06897

CLEARASIL® Acne Treatment Cream
Vanishing and Tinted

Active Ingredients: Benzoyl Peroxide 10% in an odorless, greaseless cream base, containing water, propylene glycol, bentonite, glyceryl stearate SE, isopropyl myristate, dimethicone, methylparaben, propylparaben and cellulose gum. The tinted formula also contains titanium dioxide and iron oxides.
Indications: For the topical treatment of acne vulgaris.
Actions: CLEARASIL Acne Treatment Cream contains benzoyl peroxide, an antibaterial and keratolytic as well as bentonite an oil absorbant. The product 1) dries and helps heal acne lesions (pimples), 2) reduces comedones (blackheads and whiteheads), 3) kills bacteria associated with acne lesions, 4) helps prevent acne lesions from forming, and 5) absorbs excess skin oil for up to 12 hours.
Warnings: Persons with a known sensitivity to benzoyl peroxide should not use this medication. If itching, redness, burning, swelling or undue dryness occurs, discontinue use. If symptoms persist, consult a physician promptly. For external use only. Keep from eyes, lips, mouth and sensitive areas of the neck. Colored or dyed fabrics may be bleached by the oxidizing action of this product. Keep this and all medicine out of the reach of children.
Symptoms and Treatment of Ingestion: These symptoms are based upon medical judgement, not on actual experience. Theoretically, ingestion of very large amounts may cause nausea, vomiting, abdominal discomfort and diarrhea. Treatment is symptomatic, with bedrest and observation.
Directions For Use:
1. Follow normal skin care and cleansing routine.
2. Some people are sensitive to the active ingredients of acne medications, so try this test: the first three days apply cream sparingly with fingertips to one or two small affected areas. If no discomfort or reaction occurs, apply up to two times daily, wherever acne lesions and oil are a problem.
3. Recap tightly after each use.
4. If bothersome dryness or peeling occurs, reduce dosage to one application per day or every other day.

How Supplied: Available in both Vanishing and Tinted formulas in 1 oz. and .65 oz. squeeze tubes.

CLEARASIL® Antibacterial Acne Lotion

Active Ingredients: Benzoyl Peroxide 5% in a colorless, greaseless lotion which is fragrance-free.
Indications: For the topical treatment of acne vulgaris.
Actions: CLEARASIL ANTIBACTERIAL ACNE LOTION contains benzoyl peroxide an antibacterial and keratolytic. The product 1) dries and helps heal acne lesions (pimples), 2) reduces comedones (blackheads and whiteheads), 3) kills bacteria associated with acne lesions, and 4) helps prevent acne lesions from forming.
Warnings: Persons with a known sensitivity to benzoyl peroxide should not use this medication. If itching, redness, burning, swelling or undue dryness occurs, discontinue use. If symptoms persist, consult a physician promptly. For external use only. Keep from eyes, lips, mouth and sensitive areas of the neck. Colored or dyed fabrics may be bleached by the oxidizing action of this product. Keep this and all medicine out of the reach of children.
Symptoms and Treatment of Ingestion: These symptoms are based upon medical judgement, not on actual experience. Theoretically, ingestion of very large amounts may cause nausea, vomiting, abdominal discomfort and diarrhea. Treatment is symptomatic, with bedrest and observation.
Directions For Use:
1. Follow your normal skin care and cleansing routine.
2. Shake well.
3. Some people are sensitive to the active ingredients of acne medications, so try this test: the first three days apply lotion sparingly with fingertips to one or two small affected areas. If no discomfort or reaction occurs, apply up to two times daily, wherever acne lesions are a problem.
4. Gently rub in lotion until it disappears.
5. If bothersome dryness or peeling occurs, reduce dosage to one application per day or every other day.

How Supplied: Available in a 1 fl. oz. squeeze bottle.

TOPEX® Acne Clearing Medication

Active Ingredient: 10% Benzoyl Peroxide in a colorless, greaseless lotion which is fragrance-free.
Indications: For the topical treatment of acne vulgaris.
Actions: TOPEX Acne Clearing Medication contains benzoyl peroxide an antibacterial and keratolytic. The product 1) dries and helps heal acne lesions (pimples), 2) reduces comedones (blackheads and whiteheads), 3) kills bacteria associated with acne lesions, and 4) helps prevent acne lesions from forming.
Warnings: Persons with a known sensitivity to benzoyl peroxide should not use this medication. If itching, redness, burning, swelling or undue dryness occurs, discontinue use. If symptoms persist, consult a physician promptly. For external use only. Keep from eyes, lips, mouth and sensitive areas of the neck. Colored or dyed fabrics may be bleached by the oxidizing action of this product. Keep this and all medicine out of the reach of children.
Symptoms and Treatment of Ingestion: These symptoms are based upon medical judgement, not on actual experience. Theoretically, ingestion of very large amounts may cause nausea, vomiting, abdominal discomfort and diarrhea. Treatment is symptomatic, with bedrest and observation.
Directions For Use:
1. Follow your normal skin care and cleansing routine.
2. Shake well.
3. Some people are sensitive to the active ingredients of acne medications, so try this test: the first three days apply lotion sparingly with fingertips to one or two small affected areas. If no discomfort or reaction occurs, apply up to two times daily, wherever acne lesions are a problem.
4. Gently rub in lotion until it disappears.
5. If bothersome dryness or peeling occurs, reduce dosage to one application per day or every other day.

How Supplied: Available in a 1 fl. oz. squeeze bottle.

Vicks Health Care Division
RICHARDSON-MERRELL INC.
TEN WESTPORT ROAD
WILTON, CT 06897

DAYCARE®
Daytime Colds Medicine
in oral liquid form

Active Ingredients: Each fluid ounce (2 tbs.) contains Acetaminophen 650 mg., Dextromethorphan Hydrobromide 20 mg., Phenylpropanolamine Hydrochloride 25 mg. in an orange, apricot-flavored, cooling liquid base. Also contains Alcohol 10%.
Indications: For the temporary relief of major colds symptoms, as follows: nasal congestion, coughing, aches and pains, fever, and cough irritated throat of a cold or flu without drowsy side effects.
Actions: VICKS DAYCARE is an antitussive, demulcent, decongestant and analgesic. It helps clear stuffy nose, congested sinus openings. Calms, quiets coughing. Eases headache pain and the ache-all-over feeling. Reduces fever due to colds and flu. Soothes a cough irritated throat. By relieving these symptoms without drowsiness, helps patients get through an active day.

Warning: Do not administer to children under 6 years of age unless directed by a physician. Persistent cough may indicate the presence of a serious condition. Persons with a high fever or persistent cough or with high blood pressure, diabetes, heart or thyroid disease should not use this preparation unless directed by a physician. Do not use more than ten days unless directed by a physician.
Do not exceed recommended dosage unless directed by a physician. As with all medication, keep out of reach of children.
Symptoms and Treatment of Overdosage: These symptoms are based upon medical judgement, not on actual experience, since no significant incidence of overdose has been brought to our attention in clinical or consumer experience. Ingestion of very large amounts may cause dizziness, drowsiness, nausea, diarrhea, insomnia, nervousness, anxiety, tremors, tachycardia, extrasystoles, headache, sweating, confusion and delerium. Treatment is symptomatic, with bedrest and observation.
Dosage: A plastic measuring cup with 1 and 2 tablespoonful gradations is supplied.
Adults (12 and over): one fluid ounce (2 tablespoonfuls)
Children: (6–12): one-half fluid ounce (1 tablespoonful)
May be repeated every four hours as needed. Maximum 4 doses per day.
How Supplied: Available in 6 fl. oz. and 10 fl. oz. bottles.

FORMULA 44® COUGH CONTROL DISCS

Active Ingredients per disc: Dextromethorphan equivalent to Dextromethorphan Hydrobromide 5 mg., Benzocaine 1.25 mg., Special Vicks Medication (menthol, anethole, peppermint oil) 0.35% in a dark brown sugar base.
Indications: Provides temporary relief from coughs and relieves throat irritation caused by colds, flu, bronchitis.
Actions: VICKS FORMULA 44 COUGH CONTROL DISCS are antitussive, local anesthetic and demulcent cough drops. They calm, quiet coughs and help coat and soothe irritated throats.
Warning: Do not exceed recommended dosage. Do not administer to children under 4 unless directed by physician. Persistent cough may indicate presence of a serious condition. Persons with high fever or persistent cough should not use this preparation unless directed by physician. As with all medication, keep out of reach of children.
Symptoms and Treatment of Overdosage: These symptoms are based upon medical judgement, not on actual experience, since no significant incidence of overdose has been brought to our attention in clinical or consumer experience. Though unlikely, ingestion of large amounts may cause dizziness, drowsiness, nausea, vomiting, diarrhea, central excitement and a possibility of cyanosis in young children. Treatment is symptomatic, with bedrest and observation.
Dosage:
ADULTS (12 years and over) 2 discs. Dissolve in mouth. Two additional discs every three hours as needed.
CHILDREN (4 to 12 years) 1 disc. Dissolve in mouth. One additional disc every three hours as needed.
How Supplied: Available as individual foil wrapped portable packets in boxes of 24.

FORMULA 44® COUGH MIXTURE

Active Ingredients per 2 tsp. (10 ml.): Dextromethorphan Hydrobromide 15 mg., Doxylamine Succinate 7.5 mg., Sodium Citrate 500 mg. in a pleasant tasting, dark brown syrup base. Also contains Alcohol 10%.
Indications: For the temporary relief of coughs due to colds, flu, bronchitis.
Actions: VICKS FORMULA 44 COUGH MIXTURE is an antitussive, antihistamine, demulcent and expectorant. Calms and quiets coughs. Reduces sneezing and sniffling. Coats, soothes irritated throat.
Warning: Do not exceed recommended dosage unless directed by a physician. Do not administer to children under 6 years of age unless directed by a physician. Persistent cough may indicate the presence of a serious condition. Persons with a high fever or persistent cough should not use the product unless directed by a physician. FORMULA 44 may cause drowsiness. Do not drive or operate machinery while taking the product. If relief does not occur within three days, discontinue use and consult a physician. As with all medication, keep out of reach of children.
Symptoms and Treatment of Overdosage: These symptoms are based on medical judgement and not on clinical experience, since no significant incidence of overdose has been brought to our attention in clinical or consumer experience. Presenting symptom is drowsiness. Nausea, vomiting, dizziness, ataxia, mydriasis and headache may ensue with ingestion of excessive amounts. Treatment is symptomatic, with bedrest and observation.
Dosage:
Adults: 12 years and over—2 teaspoonfuls
Children: 6 to 12 years: 1 teaspoonful
Repeat every 4 hours as needed.
No more than 6 doses per day.
How Supplied: Available in 3 fl. oz., 6 fl. oz. and 8 fl. oz. bottles.

FORMULA 44D®
DECONGESTANT COUGH MIXTURE

Active Ingredients per 2 tsp. (10 ml): Dextromethorphan Hydrobromide 20 mg., Phenylpropanolamine Hydrochloride 25 mg., Guaifenesin 100 mg. in a red, cherry-flavored, cooling syrup. Also contains Alcohol 10%.
Indications: Relieves coughs, decongests nasal passages and loosens upper chest congestion due to colds, flu, bronchitis.
Actions: VICKS FORMULA 44D is an antitussive, nasal decongestant, expectorant and demulcent. It calms, quiets coughs; relieves nasal congestion; loosens phlegm, mucus; and coats, soothes an irritated throat.
Warning: Do not exceed recommended dosage unless directed by physician. Do not administer to children under 2 years of age unless directed by physician. Persistent cough may indicate the presence of a serious condition. Persons with a high fever or persistent cough or with high blood pressure, diabetes, heart or thyroid disease should not use this preparation unless directed by physician. As with all medication, keep out of reach of children.
Symptoms and Treatment of Overdosage: These symptoms are based upon medical judgement, not on actual experience, since no signifcant incidence of overdose has been brought to our attention in clinical or consumer experience. Ingestion of large amounts may cause drowsiness, dizziness, nausea, vomiting, diarrhea, central excitement, restlessness, anxiety, sweating, tremor, extrasystoles, confusion and delerium. Treatment is symptomatic, with bedrest and observation.
Dosage:
ADULTS (12 years and over): 2 teaspoonfuls
CHILDREN (6–12 years): 1 teaspoonful
(2–6 years): ½ teaspoonful
No more than 6 doses per day. Repeat every 4 hours as needed.
How Supplied: Available in 3 fl. oz., 6 fl. oz. and 8 fl. oz. bottles.

NYQUIL®
Nighttime Colds Medicine in oral liquid form.

Active Ingredients per fluid oz. (2 tbs.): Acetaminophen 600 mg., Doxylamine Succinate 7.5 mg., Ephedrine Sulfate 8.0 mg., and Dextromethorphan Hydrobromide 15.0 mg. Also contains Alcohol 25%.
Indications: For the temporary relief of major colds symptoms, as follows: stuffy nose, sniffles and sneezing, aches and pains, and coughing.
Actions: Decongestant, antihistaminic, antitussive, analgesic. Helps decongest nasal passages and sinus openings, relieves sniffles and sneezing, eases aches and pains, reduces fever, soothes headache, minor sore throat pain, and quiets coughing due to a cold. By relieving these symptoms, also helps patient get to sleep to get the rest he needs.
Warning: This preparation may cause drowsiness. Do not drive or operate machinery while taking this medication. Do not give to children under ten, unless directed by physician. If relief does not occur within three days, discontinue use and consult physician. Reduce dosage if nervousness, restlessness or sleeplessness occurs. Do not use if high blood pressure, heart disease, diabetes or thyroid disease is present unless directed by physician.
Persistent cough may indicate a serious condition. Persons with a high fever or persistent cough should not use this preparation unless directed by a physician. Do not exceed recommended dosage. As with all medication, keep out of reach of children.
Symptoms and Treatment of Overdosage: These symptoms are based on medical judgement and not on actual clinical experience, since no significant incidence of overdose has been brought to our attention in clinical or consumer experience. Presenting symptom of overdosage is drowsiness. Large overdoses may cause emesis, ataxia, nausea, vomiting, restlessness, vertigo, dysuria, palpitations, tinnitus, diaphoresis, insomnia. Treatment is symptomatic, with bedrest and observation.
Dosage and Dosage Form: A green, anise-flavored oral liquid (syrup). A plastic measuring cup with 1 and 2 tablespoonful gradations is supplied.
ADULTS (12 and over): One fluid ounce (2 tablespoonfuls) at bedtime.
CHILDREN 10 to 12: One half ounce (1 tablespoonful) at bedtime.
If confined to bed or at home, a total of 4 doses may be taken per day, each 4 hours apart.
How Supplied: Available in 6 fl. oz. and 10 fl. oz. bottles.

ORACIN®
Cooling Throat Lozenges

Active Ingredients per lozenge: Benzocaine 6.25 mg., Menthol 0.1% in a green, cooling (sugarless) sorbitol base.
Indications: Provides temporary relief of minor sore throat pain.
Actions: VICKS ORACIN is a local anesthetic, demulcent throat lozenge. It soothes and cools to temporarily relieve minor throat irritations and ease pain.
Warning: Do not exceed recommended dosage. Severe or persistent sore throat, or sore throat accompanied by high fever, headache, nausea and vomiting may be serious. Consult physician promptly. Do not use more than 2 days or administer to children under 6 years of age unless directed by a physician. As with all medication, keep out of reach of children. VICKS ORACIN is not a product for diabetics.
Symptoms and Treatment of Overdosage: These symptoms are based upon medical judgement, not on actual experience, since no significant incidence of overdose has

Continued on next page

Vicks Health—Cont.

been brought to our attention in clinical or consumer experience. Presenting symptom after ingesting large amounts would be diarrhea. Theoretically, ingestion of very large amounts may cause nausea, vomiting, gastrointestinal upset, central excitement, and a possibility of cyanosis in young children. Treatment is symptomatic, with bedrest and observation.
Dosage: ADULTS AND CHILDREN (6 years and over): allow one lozenge to dissolve slowly in the mouth. Repeat hourly as needed. Do not take more than 12 lozenges per day.
How Supplied: Available in boxes of 18.

ORACIN®
Cherry Flavor
Cooling Throat Lozenges

Active Ingredients per lozenge: Benzocaine 6.25 mg., Menthol 0.08% in a red, cherry flavored, cooling (sugarless) sorbitol base.
Indications: Provides temporary relief of minor sore throat pain.
Actions: VICKS ORACIN is a local anesthetic, demulcent throat lozenge. It soothes and cools to temporarily relieve minor throat irritations and ease pain.
Warning: Do not exceed recommended dosage. Severe or persistent sore throat, or sore throat accompanied by high fever, headache, nausea and vomiting may be serious. Consult physician promptly. Do not use more than 2 days or administer to children under 6 years of age unless directed by a physician. As with all medication, keep out of reach of children. VICKS ORACIN is not a product for diabetics.
Symptoms and Treatment of Overdosage: These symptoms are based upon medical judgement, not on actual experience, since no significant incidence of overdose has been brought to our attention in clinical or consumer experience. Presenting symptom after ingesting large amounts would be diarrhea. Theoretically, ingestion of very large amounts may cause nausea, vomiting, gastrointestinal upset, central excitement, and a possiblity of cyanosis in young children. Treatment is symptomatic, with bedrest and observation.
Dosage: ADULTS AND CHILDREN (6 years and over): allow one lozenge to dissolve slowly in the mouth. Repeat hourly as needed. Do not take more than 12 lozenges per day.
How Supplied: Available in boxes of 18.

SINEX™
Decongestant Nasal Spray

Active Ingredients: Phenylephrine Hydrochloride 0.5%, Cetylpyridinium Chloride 0.04%, Special Vicks Blend of Aromatics (menthol, eucalyptol, camphor, methyl salicylate). Also contains Thimerosal 0.001% as a preservative.
Indications: To provide temporary relief of nasal and sinus congestion of head colds and hay fever.
Actions: VICKS SINEX is a decongestant nasal spray. The product shrinks swollen membranes to restore freer breathing; gives fast relief of nasal stuffiness and congested sinus openings; allows congested sinuses to drain; and instantly cools irritated nasal passages.
Warning: Do not exceed recommended dosage. Follow directions for use carefully. For children under 6 years, consult your physician. If condition persists consult physician. As with all medication, keep out of reach of children.
Symptoms and Treatment of Ingestion: These symptoms are based upon medical judgement, not on actual experience, since no significant incidence of overdose or ingestion has been brought to our attention in clinical or consumer experience. Though unlikely, ingestion of very large amounts may cause restlessness, anxiety, ventricular arrhythmias, nausea and gastrointestinal upset. Treatment is symptomatic, with bedrest and observation.
Directions For Use: Keep head and dispenser upright. May be used every 3 hours as needed.
ADULTS: Spray quickly, firmly 2 times up each nostril, sniffing the spray upward.
CHILDREN 6 to 12 years: Spray 1 time up each nostril.
How Supplied: Available in ½ fl. oz. and 1 fl. oz. plastic spray bottles.

SINEX™ LONG-ACTING
Decongestant Nasal Spray

Active Ingredient: Xylometazoline Hydrochloride 0.1% in an aqueous solution. Also contains thimerosal 0.001% as a preservative.
Indications: For temporary relief of nasal congestion due to the common cold, hay fever or other upper respiratory allergies or nasal congestion associated with sinusitis.
Actions: Xylometazoline constricts the arterioles of the nasal passages—resulting in a nasal decongestant effect which lasts up to ten hours, restoring freer breathing through the nose. SINEX LONG-ACTING helps decongest sinus openings and sinus passages thus promoting sinus drainage.
Warning: For adult use only. Do not administer the product to children under 12 years except under the advice and supervision of a physician. Do not exceed recommended dosage because symptoms may occur such as burning, stinging, sneezing or increase of nasal discharge. Do not use the product for more than three days. If symptoms persist, consult a physician. The use of this dispenser by more than one person may spread infection. In case of accidental ingestion, seek professional assistance or contact a Poison Control Center immediately. As with all medication, keep out of reach of children.
Symptoms and Treatment of Oral Ingestion: These symptoms are based upon medical judgement, not on actual experience, since no significant incidence of overdose or ingestion has been brought to our attention in clinical or consumer experience. Depending upon the amount of oral ingestion, somnolence, sedation, or deep coma may occur.
With excessive ingestion, profound CNS depression may be accompanied by hypertension, bradycardia, and decreased cardiac output, which may be followed by rebound hypotension and cardiovascular collapse. Prompt gastric evacuation and intensive supportive care is indicated following marked overdosage.
Dosage and Administration: Adults: 2 sprays in each nostril every 8 to 10 hours or as directed by a physician. Spray quickly, firmly, sniffing the spray upward. Keep head and dispenser upright.
How Supplied: Available in ½ fl. oz. and 1 fl. oz. plastic spray bottles.

VAPOSTEAM®
Liquid Medication for Hot Steam Vaporizers.

Active Ingredients: Polyoxyethylene Dodecanol 1.8%, Aromatics (eucalyptus oil, camphor, menthol) 12.4%, Tincture of Benzoin 5%, in a liquid vehicle. Also contains Alcohol 55%.
Indications: For the symptomatic relief of colds, coughs, chest congestion.
Actions: VAPOSTEAM increases the action of steam to help relieve colds symptoms in the following ways: relieves coughs of colds, even croupy coughs, eases stuffy nasal congestion, loosens phlegmy chest congestion, and moistens dry, irritated breathing passages.
Warning: VAPOSTEAM is for hot steam medication only. Do not ingest.
Persistent coughing may indicate the presence of a serious condition. If symptoms persist, discontinue use and consult physician. Persons with high fever or persistent cough should not use this preparation except as directed by a physician. Keep away from open flame or extreme heat. As with all medication, keep out of reach of children.
Symptoms and Treatment of Ingestion: Based on the medical literature and clinical judgement, ingestion of large amounts may cause nausea, vomiting, epigastric pain, discomfort and weakness, coma and death. Treatment should consist of cautious gastric lavage, barbiturates for convulsions, Metrazol for coma and supportive therapy as indicated.
Dosage and Administration: In a hot steam vaporizer: Use one tablespoonful of VAPOSTEAM with each quart of water added to the vaporizer. In an open bowl: Simply add VAPOSTEAM to any ordinary bowl of hot water—2 teaspoonfuls for each pint of water —and breathe in the medicated vapors.
How Supplied: Available in 4 fl. oz. and 6 fl. oz. bottles.

VATRONOL®
Nose Drops

Active Ingredients: Ephedrine Sulfate 0.5%, Special Vicks Aromatic Blend (menthol, eucalyptol, camphor, methyl salicylate) 0.06% in an aqueous base. Also contains Thimerosal 0.001% as a preservative.
Indications: Relieves nasal congestion caused by head colds and hay fever.
Actions: VICKS VATRONOL is a decongestant nose drop. It helps restore freer breathing by relieving nasal stuffiness and congested sinus openings. VATRONOL also cools irritated nasal passages.
Warning: Do not exceed recommended dosage. Overdosage may cause nervousness, restlessness, or sleeplessness. Do not use for more than 4 consecutive days or administer to children under 6, unless directed by a physician. As with all medication, keep out of reach of children.
Symptoms and Treatment of Ingestion: These symptoms are based upon medical judgement, not on actual experience, since no significant incidence of overdose or ingestion has been brought to our attention in clinical or consumer experience. Ingestion of very large quantities may cause restlessness, anxiety, sweating, tremor, rapid pulse, extrasystoles, confusion, delirium, nausea and gastrointestinal upset. Treatment is symptomatic, with bedrest and observation.
Dosage:
ADULTS: Fill dropper to upper mark.
CHILDREN (6–12 years): Fill dropper to lower mark.
Apply up one nostril, repeat in other nostril. Repeat every 4 hours as needed.
How Supplied: Available in ½ fl. oz. and 1 fl. oz. dropper bottles.

VICKS® COUGH SILENCERS
Cough Drops

Active Ingredients per lozenge: Dextromethorphan (expressed as Dextromethorphan Hydrobromide) 2.5 mg., Benzocaine 1 mg., Special Vicks Medication (menthol, anethole, peppermint oil) 0.35% in a cooling green, sugar base.
Indications: Provides all-day relief from coughs of colds, excessive smoking, dry or irritated throats when used as directed.
Actions: VICKS COUGH SILENCERS are antitussive, local anesthetic and demulcent throat lozenges.
Warning: Do not administer to children under 4 years of age unless directed by a physician. Severe or persistent cough, sore throat, or sore throat accompanied by fever, headache, nausea and vomiting may be serious. Consult physician promptly. Persons with a high fever or persistent cough should not use this prepa-

ration unless directed by a physician. As with all medication, keep out of reach of children.
Symptoms and Treatment of Overdosage: These symptoms are based upon medical judgement, not on actual experience, since no significant incidence of overdose has been brought to our attention in clinical or consumer experience. Though unlikely, ingestion of large quantities may cause dizziness, drowsiness, nausea, vomiting, gastrointestinal upset, diarrhea, central excitement, and a possibility of cyanosis in young children. Treatment is symptomatic, with bedrest and observation.
Dosage: Age 12 and over, 2 drops, dissolve in mouth one at a time, then 1 or 2 each hour as needed. Ages 4 to 12, 1 drop, dissolve in mouth then 1 drop each hour as needed. Do not exceed recommended dosage.
How Supplied: Available in boxes of 15's.

VICKS® COUGH SYRUP
Expectorant, Antitussive Cough Syrup

Active Ingredients per 3 tsp. (15 ml.): Dextromethorphan Hydrobromide 10.5 mg., Guaifenesin 75 mg., Sodium Citrate 600 mg. in a red, cherry-flavored, syrup base. Also contains Alcohol 5%.
Indications: Provides temporary relief of coughs due to colds, helps loosen phlegm and rid passageways of bothersome mucus, and soothes a cough-irritated throat.
Actions: VICKS COUGH SYRUP is an antitussive, expectorant and demulcent. It calms, quiets coughs of colds, flu and bronchitis; loosens phlegm, promotes drainage of bronchial tubes; and coats and soothes a cough irritated throat.
Warning: Do not exceed recommended dosage. Do not administer to children under 2 years of age unless directed by a physician. Persistent cough may indicate the presence of a serious condition. Persons with a high fever or persistent cough should not use this preparation unless directed by a physician. As with all medication, keep out of reach of children.
Symptoms and Treatment of Overdosage: These symptoms are based upon medical judgement, not on actual experience, since no significant incidence of overdose has been brought to our attention in clinical or consumer experience. Ingestion of large amounts may cause drowsiness, dizziness, nausea, vomiting, diarrhea, central excitement and alkalosis. Treatment is gastric lavage and symptomatic treatment with bedrest and observation.
Dosage:
ADULTS (12 years and over): 3 teaspoonfuls
CHILDREN (6–12 years): 2 teaspoonfuls
(2–6 years): 1 teaspoonful
Repeat every 4 hours as needed.
How Supplied: Available in 3 fl. oz. and 6 fl. oz. bottles.

VICKS® INHALER
with decongestant action

Active Ingredients per inhaler: l-Desoxyephedrine 50 mg., Special Vicks Medication (menthol, camphor, methyl salicylate, bornyl acetate) 150 mg.
Indications: Provides temporary relief of nasal congestion of colds and hay fever. Decongests sinus openings.
Actions: VICKS INHALER is an intranasal inhaled decongestant. It shrinks swollen membranes and provides fast relief from a stuffy nose.
Warning: As with all medication, keep out of reach of children.
Symptoms and Treatment of Ingestion: These symptoms are based upon medical judgement, not on actual experience, since no significant incidence of overdose or ingestion has been brought to our attention in clinical or consumer experience. Though VICKS INHALER is unlikely to be ingested, consumption of large quantities of its active ingredients may cause dizziness, nervousness, headache, tachycardia, nausea and vomiting. Treatment is symptomatic, with bedrest and observation.
Directions For Use: Inhale medicated vapors through each nostril while blocking off other nostril. Use as often as needed.
VICKS INHALER is medically effective for 3 months after first use.
How Supplied: Available as a cylindrical plastic nasal inhaler (net wt. 0.007 oz.).

VICKS® THROAT LOZENGES

Active Ingredients per lozenge: Benzocaine 5 mg., Cetylpyridinium Chloride 1.66 mg., Special Vicks Medication (menthol, camphor, eucalyptus oil) in a red cooling sugar base.
Indications: For fast-acting temporary relief of minor sore throat pain, cough of colds.
Actions: VICKS THROAT LOZENGES are local anesthetic and demulcent cough drops. They temporarily soothe minor sore throat irritations—ease pain—and relieve irritation and dryness of mouth and throat.
Warning: Do not exceed recommended dosage. Severe or persistent cough, sore throat, or sore throat accompanied by high fever, headache, nausea, and vomiting may be serious. Consult physician promptly. Do not use more than 2 days or administer to children under 3 years of age unless directed by physician. As with all medication, keep out of reach of children.
Symptoms and Treatment of Overdosage: These symptoms are based upon medical judgement, not on actual experience, since no significant incidence of overdose has been brought to our attention in clinical or consumer experience. Though unlikely, ingestion of large amounts may cause nausea, vomiting, gastrointestinal upset, central excitement, and a possiblity of cyanosis in young children. Treatment is symptomatic, with bedrest and observation.
Dosage: ADULTS AND CHILDREN 3 years and over: allow one lozenge to dissolve slowly in mouth. Repeat hourly as needed.
How Supplied: Box of 12's.

VICKS® VAPORUB®
Decongestant Vaporizing Ointment

For use as a rub or in steam.
Active Ingredients: Special Vicks Medication (menthol, spirits of turpentine, eucalyptus oil, camphor, cedar leaf oil, myristica oil, thymol) 14% in a petrolatum base.
Indications: For the symptomatic relief of nasal congestion (up to 8 hours), bronchial mucous congestion, coughs, laryngitis and huskiness, muscular tightness and muscular aches and pains due to colds. Also for chapped hands.
Actions: The inhaled vapors of VICKS VAPORUB have a decongestant, and antitussive effect. Applied externally, the medication acts as a local analgesic. The ointment is soothing to chapped hands and skin.
Warning: For external application and use in steam only. Do not swallow or place in nostrils. If fever is present or cough or other symptoms persist, see your doctor. In case of illness in very young children, it is wise to consult your physician. To avoid possibility of fire, never expose VAPORUB to flame or place VAPORUB in any container in which you are heating water. Do not direct steam from vaporizer toward face. As with all medication, keep out of reach of children.
Symptoms and Treatment of Ingestion: These symptoms are based upon medical judgement, not on actual experience, since no significant incidence of overdose or ingestion has been brought to our attention in clinical or consumer experience. Ingestion of large quantities may cause nausea, vomitimg, abdominal discomfort, diarrhea. Theoretically, very large quantities could cause weakness, vertigo, convulsions and drowsiness. If the extent of accidental ingestion is not known, treatment should consist of cautious gastric lavage. Otherwise, supportive and symptomatic treatment as necessary. If indicated, saline cathartics, demulcents and barbiturates for convulsions. Do not induce emesis.
Dosage:
AS A RUB: For relief of head and chest cold symptoms and coughs due to colds. Rub on throat, chest and back. Cover with a dry warm cloth if desired. Repeat as needed, especially at bedtime for continous breathing relief.
For relief of muscle tightness, apply hot, moist towel to affected area. Remove towel, then massage well with VAPORUB. Cover with a dry, warm cloth if desired.
For chapped hands and skin, apply liberally as a dressing.
IN STEAM: Fill medicine cup of vaporizer with VICKS VAPORUB and follow directions of vaporizer manufacturer. VAPORUB may also be used in a steam bowl. Fill a bowl 3/4 full with steaming water and add 2 teaspoonfuls of VAPORUB (after removing from heat). Then inhale steaming vapors. Add extra steaming water as steam decreases.
How Supplied: Available in 1.5 oz., 3.0 oz. and 6.0 oz. plastic jars.

Viobin Corporation
A subsidiary of A. H. Robins Co.
MONTICELLO, ILLINOIS 61856

VIOKASE® (pancreatin) ℞

Description: VIOKASE is a pancreatic enzyme concentrate of porcine origin containing standardized amylase, protease and lipase activities plus esterases, peptidases, nucleases and elastase.
The enzyme potency of the tablets and powder are:

	Each 325 mg. Tablet	Each 0.75 gram (1/3 teaspoonful)
Lipase, NF Units	6,500	15,000
Protease, NF Units	32,000	75,000
Amylase, NF Units	48,000	112,500

Under conditions of the NF test method (in vitro) VIOKASE has the following total digestive capacity:

	Each 325 mg. Tablet	Each 0.75 g. Powder
Dietary Fat	23	53 grams
Dietary Protein	32	75 grams
Dietary Starch	48	112 grams

VIOKASE Tablets are not enteric coated.
Indications: As a digestive aid in cystic fibrosis and in exocrine pancreatic deficiencies usually due to chronic pancreatitis, pancreatectomy or obstruction in the pancreas caused by malignant growth.
Administration and Dosage:
Powder: Dosage to patients with cystic fibrosis: 1/3 teaspoon (0.75 grams) with meals
Tablets: Dosage to patients with cystic fibrosis or chronic pancreatitis - 1 to 3 tablets with meals. For aiding digestion in patients with pancreatectomy or gastrectomy - 1 to 2 tablets taken at 2-hour intervals, or as directed by physician.
Caution: Federal law prohibits dispensing without prescription
Warnings: Avoid inhalation of powder
Precautions: Use with caution in patients known to be allergic to pork protein.
How Supplied:
Powder: Bottles of 4 ounces and 8 ounces
Tablet: Bottles of 100 and 500
Literature Available: Complete literature available upon request including information on BEEF VIOKASE DERIVED FROM BEEF PANCREAS FOR THOSE EXCEPTIONAL PATIENTS ALLERGIC TO PORK.

Walker, Corp & Co., Inc.
EASTHAMPTON PL. &
N. COLLINGWOOD AVE.
SYRACUSE, NY 13206

EVAC-U-GEN ® OTC

Composition: Each scored tablet contains yellow phenolphthalein.
Action and Uses: A pleasantly flavored laxative designed to be chewed. Because it has a mild action and tends to cause the stool to be soft, Evac-U-Gen is desirable for those sensitive to harsh laxatives, particularly in pregnancy, hemorrhoidal cases and for children.
Administration and Dosage: *Adult* dose: Chew 1 or 2 tablets night or morning. Children, 3 to 10 years, ½ tablet daily.
Side Effects: Discontinue use if skin rash appears.
Precaution: Frequent or prolonged use may result in dependence on laxatives.
Contraindications: Symptoms of appendicitis.
How Supplied: Bottles of 35, 100, 500, 1000, 2000 and 6000 tablets.

Walker Pharmacal Company
4200 LACLEDE AVENUE
ST. LOUIS, MO 63108

SUCCUS CINERARIA MARITIMA ℞
(Senecio Cineraria Compound Solution)
Sterile—Ophthalmic

Description: Succus Cineraria Maritima is an aqueous and glycerin solution of the total extractives of the fresh Senecio Cineraria USPH 7th (Senecio Compositae) with extract of Hamamilis Vulgaris (Witch Hazel) and boric acid USP. The Alkaloids included in the total extract include Senecine and Senecionine. Total nonvolatiles is approximately 20%. The pH is adjusted to 4.1 pH; osmotic pressure is 5.5 osmols.

Actions and Uses: Succus Cineraria Maritima applied locally to the eyes acts as a safe lymphagogue, increasing circulation in the intraocular tissues, also stimulating collateral circulation and normal metabolism, functions so necessary from the standpoint of the physiology of the eye. Clinical observation indicates the definite value of local applications of Succus Cineraria Maritima in checking, or even aborting existing opacities. The benefits attained are obviously more satisfactory when treatment is instituted in the early stage of Cataract. In cases of well advanced opacity, and where pathological changes caused by the deterioration of the Metabolic functions have occurred, as is characteristic in senility, less favorable results can be expected.

The use of Succus Cineraria Maritima, however, is justified in certain cases well past the incipient stage, particularly when an operation is not contemplated or is contraindicated. It gives comfort to the patient to know that something potentially beneficial is being done. Clinical studies of advanced stages of cataract treated with Succus Cineraria Maritima indicated that in 22.5% of these cases beneficial results were obtained. In many of the cases which did not show improvement the process of the opacity was retarded or checked. In certain cases Succus Cineraria Maritima only gives temporary relief or serves to postpone the surgical removal.

Indications: Succus Cineraria Maritima is indicated in the treatment of various cases of optic opacity caused by cataract.

Contraindications: A history of a previous hypersensitivity reaction to any of the Senecio Alkaloids or the Hamamilis Vulgaris is a contraindication.

Warning: The possibility of sensitivity reactions should be considered in patients with a history of Allergy. If excessive irritation occurs it may be advisable to dilute the dosage, or discontinue treatment. (pH of 4.1 may cause minor irritation). For topical ophthalmic use only. If excessive irritation should develop, patient should consult the prescribing physician.

Caution: Federal Law prohibits dispensing without prescription.

Caution: Not intended for use in Glaucoma.

Dosage and Administration: Succus Cineraria Maritima should be instilled in the affected eye, two drops morning and evening, or as directed by physician. Do not touch dropper tip to any surface, since this may contaminate the solution.

Supplied: In sterile ¼ oz. dropper vial (7 cc). NDC 619-4021-38.

MEMORANDUM

Wallace Laboratories

HALF ACRE ROAD
CRANBURY, NJ 08512

AQUATENSEN® ℞

(methyclothiazide, NF 5 mg)
Tablets

Description: AQUATENSEN (methyclothiazide) is a member of the benzothiadiazine (thiazide) family of drugs. It is an analogue of hydrodchlorothiazide.

Clinically, AQUATENSEN is an oral diuretic-antihypertensive agent.

Actions: The diuretic and saluretic effects of AQUATENSEN result from a drug-induced inhibition of the renal tubular reabsorption of electrolytes. The excretion of sodium and chloride is greatly enhanced. Potassium excretion is also enhanced to a variable degree, as it is with the other thiazides. Although urinary excretion of bicarbonate is increased slightly, there is usually no significant change in urinary pH.

Methyclothiazide has a per mg natriuretic activity approximately 100 times that of the prototype thiazide, chlorothiazide. At maximal therapeutic dosages, all thiazides are approximately equal in their diuretic/natriuretic effects.

There is significant natriuresis and diuresis within two hours after administration of a single dose of methyclothiazide. These effects reach a peak in about six hours and persist for 24 hours following oral administration of a single dose.

Like other benzothiadiazines, AQUATENSEN also has antihypertensive properties, and may be used for this purpose either alone or to enhance the antihypertensive action of other drugs. The mechanism by which the benzothiadiazines, including methyclothiazide, produce a reduction of elevated blood pressure is not known. However, sodium depletion appears to be involved.

AQUATENSEN is readily absorbed from the gastrointestinal tract and is excreted unchanged by the kidneys.

Indications: AQUATENSEN is indicated in the management of hypertension either as the sole therapeutic agent or to enhance the effect of other antihypertensive drugs in the more severe forms of hypertension.

AQUATENSEN is indicated as adjunctive therapy in edema associated with congestive heart failure, hepatic cirrhosis, and corticosteroid and estrogen therapy.

AQUATENSEN has also been found useful in edema due to various forms of renal dysfunction such as the nephrotic syndrome, acute glomerulonephritis and chronic renal failure.

Usage in Pregnancy. The routine use of diuretics in an otherwise healthy woman is inappropriate and exposes mother and fetus to unnecessary hazard. Diuretics do not prevent development of toxemia of pregnancy, and there is no satisfactory evidence that they are useful in the treatment of developed toxemia.

Edema during pregnancy may arise from pathological causes or from the physiological and mechanical consequences of pregnancy. Thiazides are indicated in pregnancy when edema is due to pathologic causes, just as they are in the absence of pregnancy (however, see Warnings, below). Dependent edema in pregnancy, resulting from restriction of venous return by the expanded uterus, is properly treated through elevation of the lower extremities and use of support hose; use of diuretics to lower intravascular volume in this case is illogical and unnecessary. There is hypervolemia during normal pregnancy which is harmful to neither the fetus nor the mother (in the absence of cardiovascular disease), but which is associated with edema, including generalized edema, in the majority of pregnant women. If this edema produces discomfort, increased recumbency will often provide relief. In rare instances, this edema may cause extreme discomfort which is not relieved by rest. In these cases, a short course of diuretics may provide relief and may be appropriate.

Contraindications: Renal decompensation. Hypersensitivity to this or other sulfonamide derived drugs.

Warnings: Methyclothiazide shares with other thiazides the propensity to deplete potassium reserves to an unpredictable degree.

Thiazides should be used with caution in patients with renal disease or significant impairment of renal function, since azotemia may be precipitated and cumulative drug effects may occur.

Thiazides should be used with caution in patients with impaired hepatic function or progressive liver disease, since minor alterations of fluid and electrolyte balance may precipitate hepatic coma.

Thiazides may be additive or potentiative of the action of other antihypertensive drugs. Potentiation occurs with ganglionic or pheripheral adrenergic blocking drugs.

Sensitivity reactions may occur in patients with a history of allergy or bronchial asthma.

The possibility of exacerbation or activation of systemic lupus erythematosus has been reported.

Usage in Pregnancy. Thiazides cross the placental barrier and appear in cord blood. The use of thiazides in pregnant women requires that the anticipated benefit be weighed against possible hazards to the fetus. These hazards include fetal or neonatal jaundice, thrombocytopenia, and possibly other adverse reactions, that have occurred in the adult.

Nursing Mothers. Thiazides appear in breast milk. If use of the drug is deemed essential, the patient should stop nursing.

Precautions: Periodic determination of serum electrolytes should be performed at appropriate intervals for the purpose of detecting possible electrolyte imbalances such as hyponatremia, hypochloremic alkalosis, and hypokalemia. Serum and urine electrolyte determinations are particularly important when a patient is vomiting excessively or receiving parenteral fluids. All patients should be observed for other clinical signs of electrolyte imbalances such as dryness of mouth, thirst, weakness, lethargy, drowsiness, restlessness, muscle pains or cramps, muscular fatigue, hypotension, oliguria, tachycardia, and gastrointestinal disturbances such as nausea and vomiting.

Hypokalemia may develop with thiazides as with any other potent diuretic, especially when brisk diuresis occurs, severe cirrhosis is present, or when corticosteroids or ACTH are given concomitantly. Interference with the adequate oral intake of electrolytes will also contribute to the possible development of hypokalemia. Potassium depletion, even of a mild degree, resulting from thiazide use, may sensitize a patient to the effects of cardiac glycosides such as digitalis.

Any chloride deficit is generally mild and usually does not require specific treatment except under extraordinary circumstances (as in liver disease or renal disease). Dilutional hyponatremia may occur in edematous patients in hot weather; appropriate therapy is water restriction, rather than administration of salt except in rare instances when the hyponatremia is life threatening.

In actual salt depletion, appropriate replacement is the therapy of choice.

Hyperuricemia may occur or frank gout may be precipitated in certain patients receiving thiazide therapy.

Insulin requirements in diabetic patients may be increased, decreased, or unchanged. Latent diabetes mellitus may become manifest during thiazide administration.

Thiazide drugs may increase the responsiveness to tubocurarine.

The antihypertensive effects of the drug may be enhanced in the postsympathectomy patient.

Thiazides may decrease arterial responsiveness to nonrepinephrine. This diminution is not sufficient to preclude effectiveness of the pressor agent for therapeutic use.

If progressive renal impairment becomes evident as indicated by a rising nonprotein nitrogen or blood urea nitrogen, a careful reappraisal of therapy is necessary with consideration given to withholding or discontinuing diuretic therapy.

Thiazides may decrease serum PBI levels without signs of thyroid disturbance.

Thiazides have been reported, on rare occasions, to have elevated serum calcium to hypercalcemic levels. The serum calcium levels have returned to normal when the medication has been stopped. This phenomenon may be related to the ability of the thiazide diuretics to lower the amount of calcium excreted in the urine.

Adverse Reactions: *Gastrointestinal system reactions:* Anorexia, gastric irritation, nausea, vomiting, cramping, diarrhea, constipation, jaundice (intrahepatic cholestatic jaundice), pancreatitis.

Central nervous system reactions: Dizziness, vertigo, paresthesia, headache, xanthopsia.

Hematologic reactions: Leukopenia, agranulocytosis, thrombocytopenia, aplastic anemia.

Dermatologic-hypersensitivity reactions: Purpura, photosensitivity, rash, urticaria, necrotizing angiitis (vasculitis) (cutaneous vasculitis).

Cardiovascular reactions: Orthostatic hypotension may occur and may be aggravated by alcohol, barbiturates, or narcotics.

Other: Hyperglycemia, glycosuria, hypercalcemia, hyperuricemia, muscle spasm, weakness, restlessness.

There have been isolated reports that certain nonedematous individuals developed severe fluid and electrolyte derangements after only brief exposure to normal doses of thiazide and non-thiazide diuretics. The condition is usually manifested as severe dilutional hyponatremia, hypokalemia, and hypochloremia. It has been reported to be due to inappropriately increased ADH secretion and appears to be idiosyncratic. Potassium replacement is apparently the most important therapy in the treatment of this syndrome along with removal of the offending drug.

Whenever adverse reactions are severe, treatment should be discontinued.

Dosage and Administration:

AQUATENSEN (methyclothiazide) is administered orally. The usual adult dose ranges from 2.5 to 10 mg once daily.

Therapy should be individualized according to patient response. This therapy should be titrated to gain maximal therapeutic response as well as the minimal dose possible to maintain that therapeutic response.

To maintain an edema-free state or as an adjunct in the management of hypertension, 2.5 to 5.0 mg once daily is often adequate.

Maximum effective single dose is 10 mg; larger single doses do not accomplish greater diuresis, and are not recommended.

In the treatment of hypertension, methyclothiazide may be either employed alone or concurrently with other antihypertensive drugs. Combined therapy may provide adequate control of hypertension with lower dosage of the component drugs and fewer or less severe side effects.

For treatment of moderately severe or severe hypertension, supplemental use of other more potent antihypertensive agents may be indicated.

When other antihypertensive agents are to be added to the regimen, this should be accom-

Continued on next page

Wallace—Cont.

plished gradually. Ganglionic blocking agents should be given at only half the usual dose since their effect is potentiated by pretreatment with AQUATENSEN.

Overdosage: Symptoms of overdosage include electrolyte imbalance and signs of potassium deficiency such as confusion, dizziness, muscular weakness, and gastrointestinal disturbances. General supportive measures including replacement of fluids and electrolytes may be indicated in treatment of overdosage.

How Supplied: AQUATENSEN (methylclothiazide) is supplied as a 5 mg, pink monogrammed, grooved, rectangular-shaped tablet.

NDC 0037-0153-92, bottle of 100.

NDC 0037-0153-96, bottle of 500.

[*Shown in Product Identification Section*]

AVAZYME®/AVAZYME®-100 Tablets ℞
(crystalline chymotrypsin)

Description: AVAZYME: Each yellow tablet contains 20 mg crystalline chymotrypsin equivalent in proteolytic activity to 50,000 Wallace units (20,000 U.S.P. units). AVAZYME-100: Each white tablet contains 40 mg crystalline chymotrypsin equivalent in proteolytic activity to 100,000 Wallace units (40,000 U.S.P. units). Both tablets have a special enteric coating to insure release in the intestine.

Action: A mode of action for AVAZYME has not been established.

INDICATIONS: Based on a review of this drug by the National Academy of Sciences — National Research Council and/or other information, FDA has classified the indications as follows:
"Possibly" effective: Relief of symptoms related to episiotomy.
Lack of substantial evidence of effectiveness: Adjunctive therapy for the resolution of inflammation and edema resulting from serious accidental trauma or surgical trauma.
Final classification of the less-than-effective indications requires further investigation.

Contraindications: This drug is contraindicated in patients with a history of a prior allergic reaction to chymotrypsin.

Warning: USE IN PREGNANCY—Safe use of this drug during pregnancy has not been established.

Precautions: 'AVAZYME' 20 mg Tablets contain FD&C Yellow No. 5 (tartrazine) which may cause allergic-type reactions (including bronchial asthma) in certain susceptible individuals. Although the overall incidence of FD&C Yellow No. 5 (tartrazine) sensitivity in the general population is low, it is frequently seen in patients who also have aspirin hypersensitivity.

Adverse Reactions: An occasional patient may experience nausea, vomiting, diarrhea, or skin rash.

Dosage and Administration: AVAZYME —In mild conditions, one tablet four times daily. For more severe conditions, two tablets four times daily. AVAZYME-100—One tablet four times daily. There are no known incompatibilities.

How Supplied: AVAZYME: 20 mg tablets (yellow enteric coated) in bottles of 48 (NDC 0037-1241-10) and 250 (NDC 0037-1241-20). AVAZYME-100: 40 mg tablets (white enteric coated) in bottles of 48 (NDC 0037-1741-10) and 250 (NDC 0037-1741-20).

Rev. 7/79

DEPEN® Titratabs™ ℞
(Penicillamine, Wallace)

Physicians planning to use penicillamine should thoroughly familiarize themselves with its toxicity, special dosage considerations, and therapeutic benefits. Penicillamine should never be used casually. Each patient should remain constantly under the close supervision of the physician. Patients should be warned to report promptly any symptoms suggesting toxicity.

Description: Penicillamine is the D-isomer of 3-mercaptovaline. It is a white or practically white, crystalline powder, freely soluble in water, slightly soluble in alcohol, and insoluble in ether, acetone, benzene, and carbon tetrachloride. Although its configuration is D, it is levorotatory as usually measured:

$$[\alpha]^{25^\circ}_{D} = -63^\circ \pm 5^\circ \ (C = 1,\ 1N \text{ NaOH}).$$

The empirical formula is $C_5H_{11}NO_2S$, giving it a molecular weight of 149.21.

It reacts readily with formaldehyde or acetone to form a thiazolidine-carboxylic acid.

Clinical Pharmacology: Penicillamine is a chelating agent recommended for the removal of excess copper in patients with Wilson's disease. From *in vitro* studies which indicate that one atom of copper combines with two molecules of penicillamine, it would appear that one gram of penicillamine should be followed by the excretion of about 200 milligrams of copper; however, the actual amount excreted is about one percent of this.

Penicillamine also reduces excess cystine excretion in cystinuria. This is done, at least in part, by disulfide interchange between penicillamine and cystine, resulting in formation of penicillamine-cysteine disulfide, a substance that is much more soluble than cystine and is excreted readily.

Penicillamine interferes with the formation of cross-links between tropocollagen molecules and cleaves them when newly formed. The mechanism of action of penicillamine in rheumatoid arthritis is unknown, although it appears to suppress disease activity. Unlike cytotoxic immunosuppressants, penicillamine markedly lowers IgM rheumatoid factor but produces no significant depression in absolute levels of serum immunoglobulins. Also unlike cytotoxic immunosuppressants, which act on both, penicillamine *in vitro* depresses T-cell activity but not B-cell activity. *In vitro*, penicillamine dissociates macroglobulins (rheumatoid factor) although the relationship of the activity to its effect in rheumatoid arthritis is not known.

In rheumatoid arthritis, the onset of therapeutic response to DEPEN (Penicillamine, Wallace) may not be seen for two or three months. In those patients who respond, however, the first evidence of suppression of symptoms such as pain, tenderness, and swelling usually is apparent within three months. The optimum duration of therapy has not been determined. If remissions occur, they may last from months to years but usually require continued treatment (see DOSAGE AND ADMINISTRATION).

In patients with rheumatoid arthritis, it is important that DEPEN be given on an empty stomach, at least one hour before meals and at least one hour apart from any other drug, food or milk. This permits maximum absorption and reduces the likelihood of metal binding.

Methodology for determining the bioavailability of penicillamine is not available; however, penicillamine is known to be a very soluble substance.

Indications: DEPEN is indicated in the treatment of Wilson's disease, cystinuria, and in patients with severe, active rheumatoid arthritis who have failed to respond to an adequate trial of conventional therapy. Available evidence suggests that DEPEN is not of value in ankylosing spondylitis.

Wilson's Disease—Wilson's disease (hepatolenticular degeneration) results from the interaction of an inherited defect and an abnormality in copper metabolism. The metabolic defect, which is the consequence of the autosomal inheritance of one abnormal gene from each parent, manifests itself in a greater positive copper balance than normal. As a result, copper is deposited in several organs and appears eventually to produce pathologic effects most prominently seen in the brain, where degeneration is widespread; in the liver, where fatty infiltration, inflammation, and hepatocellular damage progress to postnecrotic cirrhosis; in the kidney, where tubular and glomerular dysfunction results; and in the eye, where characteristic corneal copper deposits are known as Kayser-Fleischer rings.

Two types of patients require treatment for Wilson's disease: (1) the symptomatic, and (2) the asymptomatic in whom it can be assumed the disease will develop in the future if the patient is not treated.

Diagnosis, suspected on the basis of family or individual history, physical examination, or a low serum concentration of ceruloplasmin*, is confirmed by the demonstration of Kayser-Fleischer rings or, particularly in the asymptomatic patient, by the quantitative demonstration in a liver biopsy specimen of a concentration of copper in excess of 250 mcg/g dry weight.

Treatment has two objectives:
(1) to minimize dietary intake and absorption of copper.
(2) to promote excretion of copper deposited in tissues.

The first objective is attained by a daily diet that contains no more than one or two milligrams of copper. Such a diet should exclude, most importantly, chocolate, nuts, shellfish, mushrooms, liver, molasses, broccoli, and cereals enriched with copper, and be composed to as great an extent as possible of foods with a low copper content. Distilled or demineralized water should be used if the patient's drinking water contains more than 0.1 mg of copper per liter.

For the second objective, a copper chelating agent is used. Penicillamine is the only one of these agents that is orally effective.

In symptomatic patients, this treatment usually produces marked neurologic improvement, fading of Kayser-Fleischer rings, and gradual amelioration of hepatic dysfunction and psychic disturbances.

Clinical experience to date suggests that life is prolonged with the above regimen.

Noticeable improvement may not occur for one to three months. Occasionally, neurologic symptoms become worse during initiation of therapy with DEPEN. Despite this, the drug should not be discontinued permanently, although temporary interruption may result in clinical improvement of the neurological symptoms but it carries an increased risk of developing a sensitivity reaction upon resumption of therapy (See WARNINGS).

Treatment of asymptomatic patients has been carried out for over ten years. Symptoms and signs of the disease appear to be prevented indefinitely if daily treatment with DEPEN can be continued.

Cystinuria—Cystinuria is characterized by excessive urinary excretion of the dibasic amino acids, arginine, lysine, ornithine, and cystine, and the mixed disulfide of cysteine and homocysteine. The metabolic defect that leads to cystinuria is inherited as an autosomal, recessive trait. Metabolism of the affected amino acids is influenced by at least two abnormal factors: (1) defective gastrointestinal absorption and (2) renal tubular dysfunction.

Arginine, lysine, ornithine, and cysteine are soluble substances, readily excreted. There is no apparent pathology connected with their excretion in excessive quantities.
Cystine, however, is so slightly soluble at the usual range of urinary pH that it is not excreted readily, and so crystallizes and forms stones in the urinary tract. Stone formation is the only known pathology in cystinuria.
Normal daily output of cystine is 40 to 80 mg. In cystinuria, output is greatly increased and may exceed 1 g/day. At 500 to 600 mg/day, stone formation is almost certain. When it is more than 300 mg/day, treatment is indicated.
Conventional treatment is directed at keeping urinary cystine diluted enough to prevent stone formation, keeping the urine alkaline enough to dissolve as much cystine as possible, and minimizing cystine production by a diet low in methionine (the major dietary precursor of cystine). Patients must drink enough fluid to keep urine specific gravity below 1.010, take enough alkali to keep urinary pH at 7.5 to 8, and maintain a diet low in methionine. This diet is not recommended in growing children and probably is contraindicated in pregnancy because of its low protein content (see PRECAUTIONS).
When these measures are inadequate to control recurrent stone formation, DEPEN may be used as additional therapy. When patients refuse to adhere to conventional treatment, DEPEN may be a useful substitute. It is capable of keeping cystine excretion to near normal values, thereby hindering stone formation and the serious consequences of pyelonephritis and impaired renal function that develop in some patients.
Bartter and colleagues depict the process by which penicillamine interacts with cystine to form penicillamine-cysteine mixed disulfide as:

$$\text{CSSC} + \text{PS}' \rightleftharpoons \text{CS}' + \text{CSSP}$$
$$\text{PSSP} + \text{CS}' \rightleftharpoons \text{PS}' + \text{CSSP}$$
$$\text{CSSC} + \text{PSSP} \rightleftharpoons 2\text{CSSP}$$

CSSC = cystine
CS′ = deprotonated cysteine
PSSP = penicillamine
PS′ = deprotonated penicillamine sulfhydryl
CSSP = penicillamine-cysteine mixed disulfide

In this process, it is assumed that the deprotonated form of penicillamine, PS′, is the active factor in bringing about the disulfide interchange.
Rheumatoid Arthritis—Because DEPEN can cause severe adverse reactions, its use in rheumatoid arthritis should be restricted to patients who have severe, active disease and who have failed to respond to an adequate trial of conventional therapy. Even then, benefit-to-risk ratio should be carefully considered. Other measures, such as rest, physiotherapy, salicylates and corticosteroids should be used, when indicated, in conjunction with DEPEN (see PRECAUTIONS).
Contraindications: Penicillamine should not be administered to patients with rheumatoid arthritis who are pregnant (see PRECAUTIONS).
Patients with a history of penicillamine-related aplastic anemia or agranulocytosis should not be restarted on penicillamine (see WARNINGS and ADVERSE REACTIONS).
Because of its potential for causing renal damage, penicillamine should not be administered to rheumatoid arthritis patients with a history or other evidence of renal insufficiency.
Warnings: The use of penicillamine has been associated with fatalities due to certain diseases, such as aplastic anemia, agranulocytosis, thrombocytopenia, Goodpasture's syndrome, and myasthenic syndrome.
Because of the potential for serious hematological and renal adverse reactions, routine urinalysis, white and differential blood cell count, hemoglobin determination, and direct platelet count must be done every two weeks for the first six months of penicillamine therapy and monthly thereafter. Patients should be instructed to report promptly signs and symptoms of granulocytopenia and/or thrombocytopenia such as fever, sore throat, chills, bruising or bleeding and the above laboratory studies should be promptly repeated.
Leukopenia and thrombocytopenia have been reported to occur in up to 5% of patients during penicillamine therapy. Leukopenia is of the granulocytic series and may or may not be associated with an increase in eosinophils. A confirmed reduction in WBC below 3500 mandates discontinuance of penicillamine therapy. Thrombocytopenia may be on an idiosyncratic basis with decreased or absent megakaryocytes in the marrow, when it is part of an aplastic anemia. In other cases the thrombocytopenia is presumably on an immune basis since the number of megakaryocytes in the marrow has been reported to be normal or sometimes increased. The development of a platelet count below 100,000, even in the absence of clinical bleeding, requires at least temporary cessation of penicillamine therapy. A progressive fall in either platelet count or WBC in three successive determinations, even though values are still within the normal range, likewise requires at least temporary cessation.
Proteinuria and/or hematuria may develop during therapy and may be warning signs of membranous glomerulopathy which can progress to a nephrotic syndrome. Close observation of these patients is essential. In some patients the proteinuria disappears with continued therapy; in others penicillamine must be discontinued. When a patient develops proteinuria or hematuria the physician must ascertain whether it is a sign of drug-induced glomerulopathy or is unrelated to penicillamine.
Rheumatoid arthritis patients who develop moderate degrees of proteinuria may be continued cautiously on penicillamine therapy, provided that quantitative 24-hour urinary protein determinations are obtained at intervals of one to two weeks. Penicillamine dosage should not be increased under these circumstances. Proteinuria which exceeds 1 g/24 hours, or proteinuria which is progressively increasing requires either discontinuance of the drug or a reduction in the dosage. In some patients, proteinuria has been reported to clear following reduction in dosage.
In rheumatoid arthritis patients, penicillamine should be discontinued if unexplained gross hematuria or persistent microscopic hematuria develops.
In patients with Wilson's disease or cystinuria the risks of continued penicillamine therapy in patients manifesting potentially serious urinary abnormalities must be weighed against the expected therapeutic benefits.
When penicillamine is used in cystinuria, an annual x-ray for renal stones is advised. Cystine stones form rapidly, sometimes in six months.
Up to one year or more may be required for any urinary abnormalities to disappear after penicillamine has been discontinued.
Because of rare reports of intrahepatic cholestasis and toxic hepatitis, liver function tests are recommended every six months during therapy.
Goodpasture's syndrome has occurred rarely. The development of abnormal urinary findings associated with hemoptysis and pulmonary infiltrates on x-ray requires immediate cessation of penicillamine.
A myasthenic syndrome has been reported. In the majority of cases, symptoms of myasthenia have receded after withdrawal of penicillamine.
Pemphigoid-type reactions characterized by bullous lesions clinically indistinguishable from pemphigus have occurred and have required discontinuation of penicillamine and treatment with corticosteroids.
Once instituted for Wilson's disease or cystinuria, treatment with penicillamine should, as a rule, be continued on a daily basis. Interruptions for even a few days have been followed by sensitivity reactions after reinstitution of therapy.
Precautions: Some patients may experience drug fever, a marked febrile response to penicillamine, usually in the second or third week following initiation of therapy. Drug fever may sometimes be accompanied by a macular cutaneous eruption.
In the case of drug fever in patients with Wilson's disease or cystinuria, because no alternative treatment is available, penicillamine should be temporarily discontinued until the reaction subsides. Then penicillamine should be reinstituted with a small dose that is gradually increased until the desired dosage is attained. Systemic steroid therapy may be necessary, and is usually helpful, in such patients in whom toxic reactions develop a second or third time.
In the case of drug fever in rheumatoid arthritis patients, because other treatments are available, penicillamine should be discontinued and another therapeutic alternative tried, since experience indicates that the febrile reaction will recur in a very high percentage of patients upon readministration of penicillamine.
The skin and mucous membranes should be observed for allergic reactions. Early and late rashes have occurred. Early rash occurs during the first few months of treatment and is more common. It is usually a generalized pruritic, erythematous, maculopapular or morbilliform rash and resembles the allergic rash seen with other drugs. Early rash usually disappears within days after stopping penicillamine and seldom recurs when the drug is restarted at a lower dosage. Pruritus and early rash may often be controlled by the concomitant administration of antihistamines. Less commonly, a late rash may be seen, usually after six months or more of treatment, and requires discontinuation of penicillamine. It is usually on the trunk, is accompanied by intense pruritus, and is usually unresponsive to topical corticosteroid therapy. Late rash may take weeks to disappear after penicillamine is stopped and usually recurs if the drug is restarted.
The appearance of a drug eruption accompanied by fever, arthralgia, lymphadenopathy or other allergic manifestations usually requires discontinuation of penicillamine.
Certain patients will develop a positive antinuclear antibody (ANA) test and some of these may show a lupus erythematosus-like syndrome similar to drug-induced lupus associated with other drugs. The lupus erythematosus-like syndrome is not associated with hypocomplementemia and may be present without nephropathy. The development of a positive ANA test does not mandate discontinuance of the drug; however, the physician should be alerted to the possibility that a lupus erythematosus-like syndrome may develop in the future.
Some patients may develop oral ulcerations which in some cases have the appearance of aphthous stomatitis. The stomatitis usually recurs on rechallenge but often clears on a lower dosage. Although rare, cheilosis, glossitis and gingivostomatitis have also been reported. These oral lesions are frequently dose-related and may preclude further increase in penicillamine dosage or require discontinuation of the drug.
Hypogeusia (a blunting or diminution in taste perception) has occurred in some patients. This may last two to three months or more and may develop into a total loss of taste; however, it is usually self-limited, despite continued penicillamine treatment. Such taste impairment is rare in patients with Wilson's disease.

Continued on next page

Wallace—Cont.

Penicillamine should not be used in patients who are receiving concurrent gold therapy, antimalarial or cytotoxic drugs, oxyphenbutazone or phenylbutazone because these drugs are also associated with similar serious hematologic and/or renal adverse reactions.
Patients who are allergic to penicillin may theoretically have cross-sensitivity to penicillamine. The possibility of reactions from contamination of penicillamine by trace amounts of penicillin has been precluded now that penicillamine is being produced synthetically rather than as a degradation product of penicillin.
Because of their dietary restrictions, patients with Wilson's disease and cystinuria should be given 25 mg/day of pyridoxine during therapy, since penicillamine increases the requirement for this vitamin. Patients also may receive benefit from a multivitamin preparation, although there is no evidence that deficiency of any vitamin other than pyridoxine is associated with penicillamine. In Wilson's disease, multivitamin preparations must be copper-free.
Rheumatoid arthritis patients whose nutrition is impaired should also be given a daily supplement of pyridoxine. Mineral supplements should not be given, since they may block the response to penicillamine.
Iron deficiency may develop, especially in children and in menstruating women. In Wilson's disease, this may be a result of adding the effects of the low copper diet, which is probably also low in iron, and the penicillamine to the effects of blood loss or growth. In cystinuria, a low methionine diet may contribute to iron deficiency, since it is necessarily low in protein. If necessary, iron may be given in short courses, but a period of two hours should elapse between administration of penicillamine and iron, since orally administered iron has been shown to reduce the effects of penicillamine.
Penicillamine causes an increase in the amount of soluble collagen. In the rat this results in inhibition of normal healing and also a decrease in tensile strength of intact skin. In man this may be the cause of increased skin friability at sites especially subject to pressure or trauma, such as shoulders, elbows, knees, toes, and buttocks. Extravasations of blood may occur and may appear as purpuric areas, with external bleeding if the skin is broken, or as vesicles containing dark blood. Neither type is progressive. There is no apparent association with bleeding elsewhere in the body and no associated coagulation defect has been found. Therapy with penicillamine may be continued in the presence of these lesions. They may disappear if dosage is reduced. Other reported effects probably due to the action of penicillamine on collagen are excessive wrinkling of the skin and development of small, white papules at venipuncture and surgical sites.
The effects of penicillamine on collagen and elastin make it advisable to consider a reduction in dosage to 250 mg/day when surgery is contemplated. Reinstitution of full therapy should be delayed until wound healing is complete.
Carcinogenesis—Long-term animal carcinogenicity studies have not been done with penicillamine. There is a report that 5 of 10 autoimmune disease-prone NZB Hybrid mice developed lymphocytic leukemia after 6 months' intraperitoneal treatment with a dose of 400 mg/kg penicillamine 5 days per week.
Usage in Pregnancy—Penicillamine has been shown to be teratogenic in rats when given in doses several times higher than the highest dose recommended for human use. Skeletal defects, cleft palates and fetal toxicity (resorptions) have been reported.
Wilson's disease—There are no controlled studies in pregnant women with Wilson's disease, but experience does not include any positive evidence of adverse effects to the fetus. Reported experience** shows that continued treatment with penicillamine throughout pregnancy protects the mother against relapse of the Wilson's disease, and that discontinuation of penicillamine has deleterious effects on the mother. It indicates that the drug does not increase the risk of fetal abnormalities, but it does not exclude the possibility of infrequent or subtle damage to the fetus.
If penicillamine is administered during pregnancy to patients with Wilson's disease, it is recommended that the daily dosage be limited to 1 g. If Caesarean section is planned, the daily dosage should be limited to 250 mg during the last six weeks of pregnancy and postoperatively until wound healing is complete.
Cystinuria—If possible, penicillamine should not be given during pregnancy to women with cystinuria. There is a report of a woman with cystinuria treated with 2 g/day of penicillamine during pregnancy who gave birth to a child with a generalized connective tissue defect that may have been caused by penicillamine. If stones continue to form in these patients, the benefits of therapy to the mother must be evaluated against the risk to the fetus.
Rheumatoid Arthritis—Penicillamine should not be administered to rheumatoid arthritis patients who are pregnant (see CONTRAINDICATIONS) and should be discontinued promptly in patients in whom pregnancy is suspected or diagnosed. Penicillamine should be used in women of childbearing potential only when the expected benefits outweigh possible hazards. Women of childbearing potential should be informed of the possible hazards of penicillamine to the developing fetus and should be advised to report promptly any missed menstrual periods or other indications of possible pregnancy.
There is a report that a women with rheumatoid arthritis treated with less than 1 g/day of penicillamine during pregnancy gave birth (Caesarean delivery) to an infant with growth retardation, flattened face with broad nasal bridge, low set ears, short neck with loose skin folds, and unusually lax body skin.
Usage in Children
The efficacy of DEPEN in juvenile rheumatoid arthritis has not been established.
Adverse Reactions: Penicillamine is a drug with a high incidence of untoward reactions, some of which are potentially fatal. Therefore, it is mandatory that patients receiving penicillamine therapy remain under close medical supervision throughout the period of drug administration (see WARNINGS and PRECAUTIONS).
Reported incidences (%) for the most commonly occurring adverse reactions in rheumatoid arthritis patients are noted, based on 17 representative clinical trials reported in the literature (1270 patients).
Allergic—Generalized pruritus, early and late rashes (5%), pemphigoid-type reactions and drug eruptions which may be accompanied by fever, arthralgia or lymphadenopathy have occurred (see WARNINGS and PRECAUTIONS). Some patients may show a lupus erythematosus-like syndrome similar to drug induced lupus produced by other pharmacological agents (see PRECAUTIONS).
Urticaria and exfoliative dermatitis have occurred.
Thyroiditis has been reported but is extremely rare.
Some patients may develop a migratory polyarthralgia, often with objective synovitis (see DOSAGE and ADMINISTRATION).
Gastrointestinal—Anorexia, epigastric pain, nausea, vomiting or occasional diarrhea may occur (17%).
Isolated cases of reactivated peptic ulcer have occurred, as have hepatic dysfunction, cholestatic jaundice and pancreatitis. There have been a few reports of increased serum alkaline phosphatase, lactic dehydrogenase, and positive cephalin flocculation and thymol turbidity tests.
Some patients may report a blunting, diminution or total loss of taste perception (12%) or may develop oral ulcerations. Although rare, cheilosis, glossitis and gingivostomatitis have been reported (see PRECAUTIONS).
Gastrointestinal side effects are usually reversible following cessation of therapy.
Hematological—Penicillamine can cause bone marrow depression (see WARNINGS). Leukopenia (2%) and thrombocytopenia (4%) have occurred. Fatalities have been reported as a result of thrombocytopenia, agranulocytosis and aplastic anemia.
Thrombotic thrombocytopenic purpura, hemolytic anemia, red cell aplasia, monocytosis, leukocytosis, eosinophilia and thrombocytosis have also been reported.
Renal—Patients on penicillamine therapy may develop proteinuria (6%) and/or hematuria which, in some, may progress to the development of the nephrotic syndrome as a result of an immune complex membranous glomerulopathy. (See WARNINGS.)
Central Nervous System—Tinnitus has been reported. Reversible optic neuritis has been reported with the administration of the racemic penicillamine (dl-form) and may be related to pyridoxine deficiency.
Other—Adverse reactions that have been reported rarely include thrombophlebitis; hyperpyrexia (see PRECAUTIONS); falling hair or alopecia; myasthenic syndrome (see WARNINGS); polymyositis; mammary hyperplasia; elastosis perforans serpiginosa; toxic epidermal necrolysis; anetoderma (cutaneous macular atrophy); and Goodpasture's syndrome, a severe and ultimately fatal glomerulonephritis associated with intra-alveolar hemorrhage (see WARNINGS). Allergic alveolitis and obliterative bronchiolitis have been reported in patients with severe rheumatoid arthritis, some of whom were receiving penicillamine.
Increased skin friability, excessive wrinkling of skin, and development of small, white papules at venipuncture and surgical sites have been reported (see PRECAUTIONS).
The chelating action of the drug may cause incresed excretion of other heavy metals such as zinc, mercury and lead.
Dosage and Administration:
Wilson's Disease—DEPEN tablets should be given on an empty stomach, four times a day; one-half to one hour before meals and at bedtime—at least two hours after the evening meal.
Optimal dosage can be determined only by measurement of urinary copper excretion. The urine must be collected in copper-free glassware, and should be quantitatively analyzed for copper before and soon after initiation of therapy with DEPEN. Continued therapy should be monitored by doing a 24-hour urinary copper analysis every three months or so for the duration of therapy. Since a low copper diet should keep copper absorption down to less than one milligram a day, the patient probably will be in negative copper balance if 0.5 to one milligram of copper is present in a 24-hour collection of urine.
To achieve this, the suggested initial dosage of DEPEN in the treatment of Wilson's disease is 1 g/day for children or adults. This may be increased, as indicated by the urinary copper analyses, but it is seldom necessary to exceed a dosage of 2 g/day.
In patients who cannot tolerate as much as 1 g/day initially, initiating dosage with 250 mg/day, and increasing gradually to the requisite amount, gives closer control of the effects of the drug and may help to reduce the incidence of adverse reactions.
Cystinuria—It is recommended that DEPEN be used along with conventional therapy. By reducing urinary cystine, it decreases crystalluria and stone formation. In some instances, it

has been reported to decrease the size of, and even to dissolve, stones already formed.
The usual dosage of DEPEN in the treatment of cystinuria is 2 g/day for adults, with a range of 1 to 4 g/day. For children, dosage can be based on 30 mg/kg/day. The total daily amount should be divided into four doses. If four equal doses are not feasible, give the larger portion at bedtime. If adverse reactions necessitate a reduction in dosage, it is important to retain the bedtime dose.
Initiating dosage with 250 mg/day, and increasing gradually to the requisite amount, gives closer control of the effects of the drug and may help to reduce the incidence of adverse reactions.
In addition to taking DEPEN, patients should drink copiously. It is especially important to drink about a pint of fluid at bedtime and another pint once during the night when urine is more concentrated and more acid than during the day. The greater the fluid intake, the lower the required dosage of DEPEN.
Dosage must be individualized to an amount that limits cystine excretion to 100–200 mg/day in those with no history of stones, and below 100 mg/day in those who have had stone formation and/or pain. Thus, in determining dosage, the inherent tubular defect, the patient's size, age, and rate of growth, and his diet and water intake all must be taken into consideration.
The standard nitroprusside cyanide test has been reported useful as a qualitative measure of the effective dose†: Add 2 ml of freshly prepared 5 percent sodium cyanide to 5 ml of a 24-hour aliquot of protein-free urine and let stand ten minutes. Add 5 drops of freshly prepared 5 percent sodium nitroprusside and mix. Cystine will turn the mixture magenta. If the result is negative, it can be assumed that cystine excretion is less than 100 mg/g creatinine.
Although penicillamine is rarely excreted unchanged, it also will turn the mixture magenta. If there is any question as to which substance is causing the reaction, a ferric chloride test can be dose to eliminate doubt: Add 3 percent ferric chloride dropwise to the urine. Penicillamine will turn the urine an immediate and quickly fading blue. Cystine will not produce any change in appearance.
Rheumatoid Arthritis—The principal rule of treatment with DEPEN in rheumatoid arthritis is patience. The onset of therapeutic response is typically delayed. Two or three months may be required before the first evidence of a clinical response is noted (see CLINICAL PHARMACOLOGY).
When treatment with DEPEN has been interrupted because of adverse reactions or other reasons, the drug should be reintroduced cautiously by starting with a lower dosage and increasing slowly.
Initial Therapy—
The currently recommended dosage regimen in rheumatoid arthritis begins with a single daily dose of 125 mg or 250 mg which is thereafter increased at one to three month intervals, by 125 mg or 250 mg/day, as patient response and tolerance indicate. If a satisfactory remission of symptoms is achieved, the dose associated with the remission should be continued (see Maintenance Therapy). If there is no improvement and there are no signs of potentially serious toxicity after two to three months of treatment with doses of 500–750 mg/day, increases of 250 mg/day at two to three month intervals may be continued until a satisfactory remission occurs (see Maintenance Therapy) or signs of toxicity develop (see WARNINGS and PRECAUTIONS). If there is no discernible improvement after three to four months of treatment with 1000 to 1500 mg penicillamine/day, it may be assumed the patient will not respond and DEPEN should be discontinued.
It is important that DEPEN be given on an empty stomach at least one hour before meals and at least one hour apart from any other drug, food or milk (see CLINICAL PHARMACOLOGY).
Maintenance Therapy—
The maintenance dosage of DEPEN must be individualized, and may require adjustment during the course of treatment. Many patients respond satisfactorily to a dosage within the 500–750 mg/day range. Some need less.
Changes in maintenance dosage levels may not be reflected clinically or in the erythrocyte sedimentation rate for two to three months after each dosage adjustment.
Some patients will subsequently require an increase in the maintenance dosage to achieve maximal disease suppression. In those patients who do respond, but who evidence incomplete suppression of their disease after the first six to nine months of treatment, the daily dosage of DEPEN may be increased by 125 mg or 250 mg/day at three-month intervals. It is unusual in current practice to employ a dosage in excess of 1 g/day, but up to 1.5 g/day has sometimes been required.
Management of Exacerbations—
During the course of treatment some patients may experience an exacerbation of disease activity following an initial good response. These may be self-limited and can subside within twelve weeks. They are usually controlled by the addition of non-steroidal anti-inflammatory drugs, and only if the patient has demonstrated a true "escape" phenomenon (as evidenced by failure of the flare to subside within this time period) should an increase in the maintenance dose ordinarily be considered.
In the rheumatoid patient, migratory polyarthralgia due to penicillamine is extremely difficult to differentiate from an exacerbation of the rheumatoid arthritis. Discontinuance or a substantial reduction in the dosage of DEPEN for up to several weeks will usually determine which of these processes is responsible for the arthralgia.
Duration of Therapy—
The optimum duration of DEPEN therapy in rheumatoid arthritis has not been determined. If the patient has been in remission for six months or more, a gradual, stepwise dosage reduction in decrements of 125 mg or 250 mg/day at approximately three month intervals may be attempted.
Concomitant Drug Therapy—
DEPEN should not be used in patients who are receiving gold therapy, antimalarial or cytotoxic drugs, oxyphenbutazone or phenylbutazone (see PRECAUTIONS). Other measures, such as salicylates, other nonsteroidal anti-inflammatory drugs or systemic corticosteroids may be continued when DEPEN is initiated. After improvement commences, analgesic and anti-inflammatory drugs may be slowly discontinued as symptoms permit. Steroid withdrawal must be done gradually, and many months of DEPEN treatment may be required before steroids can be completely eliminated.
Dosage Frequency—
Based on clinical experience, dosages up to 500 mg/day can be given as a single daily dose. Dosages in excess of 500 mg/day should be administered in divided doses.
How Supplied: DEPEN® Titratabs™ (penicillamine, Wallace) 250 mg scored, white tablets available in bottles of 100 (NDC 0037-4401-01).
Manufactured under license from
HOMBURG (Degussa), West Germany
Rev. 2/79

* For quantitative test for serum ceruloplasmin see: Morell, A.G.; Windsor, J.; Sternlieb, I.; Scheinberg, I.H.: Measurement of the concentration of ceruloplasmin in serum by determination of its oxidase activity, in "Laboratory Diagnosis of Liver Disease", F.W. Sunderman; F.W. Sunderman, Jr. (eds.), St. Louis, Warren H. Green, Inc., 1968, pp. 193–195.
** Scheinberg, I.H., Sternlieb, I.: *N Engl J Med 293*:1300–1302, Dec. 18, 1975.
† Lotz, M., Potts, J.T. and Bartter, F.C.: *Brit Med J 2*:521, Aug. 28, 1965 (in Medical Memoranda).

DEPROL® ℞ Ⓒ

(meprobamate 400 mg + benactyzine hydrochloride 1 mg)

Description: 'Deprol' is available as light pink, scored tablets, each containing meprobamate, U.S.P., 400 mg and benactyzine hydrochloride 1 mg.
Actions: 'Deprol' (meprobamate + benactyzine hydrochloride) combines the tranquilizing action of meprobamate with the antidepressant action of benactyzine hydrochloride.
Benactyzine hydrochloride
Benactyzine hydrochloride is a mild antidepressant and anticholinergic agent which in animals has been shown to reduce the autonomic response to emotion-provoking stress.
Meprobamate
Meprobamate is a carbamate derivative which has been shown in animal studies to have effects at multiple sites in the central nervous system, including the thalamus and limbic system.

Indications: Based on a review of this drug by the National Academy of Sciences—National Research Council and/or other information, FDA has classified the indication as follows:
"Possibly" effective: in the management of depression, both acute (reactive) and chronic. It is particularly useful in the less severe depressions and where the depression is accompanied by anxiety, insomnia, agitation, or rumination. It is also useful for management of depression and associated anxiety accompanying or related to organic illnesses.
Final classification of this indication requires further investigation.

Contraindications:
Benactyzine hydrochloride
Glaucoma and allergic or idiosyncratic reactions to benactyzine hydrochloride or related compounds.
Meprobamate
Acute intermittent porphyria as well as allergic or idiosyncratic reactions to meprobamate or related compounds such as carisoprodol, mebutamate, tybamate, or carbromal.
Warnings: The following information on meprobamate pertains to 'Deprol' (meprobamate + benactyzine hydrochloride):
Meprobamate
Drug Dependence—Physical dependence, psychological dependence, and abuse have occurred. When chronic intoxication from prolonged use occurs, it usually involves ingestion of greater than recommended doses and is manifested by ataxia, slurred speech, and vertigo. Therefore, careful supervision of dose and amounts prescribed is advised, as well as avoidance of prolonged administration, especially for alcoholics and other patients with a known propensity for taking excessive quantities of drugs.
Sudden withdrawal of the drug after prolonged and excessive use may precipitate recurrence of pre-existing symptoms, such as anxiety, anorexia, or insomnia, or withdrawal reactions, such as vomiting, ataxia, tremors, muscle twitching, confusional states, hallucinosis, and, rarely, convulsive seizures. Such seizures are more likely to occur in persons with central nervous system damage or pre-existent or latent convulsive disorders. Onset

Continued on next page

Wallace—Cont.

of withdrawal symptoms occurs usually within 12 to 48 hours after discontinuation of meprobamate; symptoms usually cease within the next 12 to 48 hours.
When excessive dosage has continued for weeks or months, dosage should be reduced gradually over a period of one or two weeks rather than abruptly stopped. Alternatively, a short-acting barbiturate may be substituted, then gradually withdrawn.
Potentially Hazardous Tasks—Patients should be warned that this drug may impair the mental and/or physical abilities required for the performance of potentially hazardous tasks such as driving a motor vehicle or operating machinery.
Additive Effects—Since the effects of meprobamate and alcohol or meprobamate and other CNS depressants or psychotropic drugs may be additive, appropriate caution should be exercised with patients who take more than one of these agents simultaneously.

Usage in Pregnancy and Lactation
An increased risk of congenital malformations associated with the use of minor tranquilizers (meprobamate, chlordiazepoxide, and diazepam) during the first trimester of pregnancy has been suggested in several studies. Because use of these drugs is rarely a matter of urgency, their use during this period should almost always be avoided. The possibility that a woman of childbearing potential may be pregnant at the time of institution of therapy should be considered. Patients should be advised that if they become pregnant during therapy or intend to become pregnant they should communicate with their physicians about the desirability of discontinuing the drug.
Meprobamate passes the placental barrier. It is present both in umbilical cord blood at or near maternal plasma levels and in breast milk of lactating mothers at concentrations two to four times that of maternal plasma. When use of meprobamate is contemplated in breast-feeding patients, the drug's higher concentrations in breast milk as compared to maternal plasma levels should be considered.
Usage in Children—This combination is not intended for use in children.
Precautions: This product contains FD&C Yellow No. 5 (tartrazine) which may cause allergic-type reactions (including bronchial asthma) in certain susceptible individuals. Although the overall incidence of FD&C Yellow No. 5 (tartrazine) sensitivity in the general population is low, it is frequently seen in patients who also have aspirin hypersensitivity.
Meprobamate
The lowest effective dose should be administered, particularly to elderly and/or debilitated patients, in order to preclude oversedation.
The possibility of suicide attempts should be considered and the least amount of drug feasible should be dispensed at any one time.
Meprobamate is metabolized in the liver and excreted by the kidney; to avoid its excess accumulation, caution should be exercised in administration to patients with compromised liver or kidney function.
Meprobamate occasionally may precipitate seizures in epileptic patients.
Adverse Reactions: Side effects have included nausea, dryness of mouth, and other gastrointestinal symptoms; syncope; and one case each of severe nervousness and loss of power of concentration.
The following side effects, which have occurred after administration of its components alone, have either occurred or might occur when the combination is taken.
Benactyzine hydrochloride
Benactyzine hydrochloride alone, particularly in high dosage, may produce dizziness, thought-blocking, a sense of depersonalization, aggravation of anxiety, or disturbance of sleep patterns, and a subjective feeling of muscle relaxation. There may also be anticholinergic effects such as blurred vision, dryness of mouth, or failure of visual accommodation. Other reported side effects have included gastric distress, allergic response, ataxia, and euphoria.
Meprobamate
Central Nervous System—Drowsiness, ataxia, dizziness, slurred speech, headache, vertigo, weakness, paresthesias, impairment of visual accommodation, euphoria, overstimulation, paradoxical excitement, fast EEG activity.
Gastrointestinal — Nausea, vomiting, diarrhea.
Cardiovascular — Palpitations, tachycardia, various forms of arrhythmia, transient ECG changes, syncope; also, hypotensive crises (including one fatal case).
Allergic or Idiosyncratic—Allergic or idiosyncratic reactions are usually seen within the period of the first to fourth dose in patients having had no previous contact with the drug. Milder reactions are characterized by an itchy, urticarial, or erythematous maculopapular rash which may be generalized or confined to the groin. Other reactions have included leukopenia, acute nonthrombocytopenic purpura, petechiae, ecchymoses, eosinophilia, peripheral edema, adenopathy, fever, fixed drug eruption with cross reaction to carisoprodol, and cross sensitivity between meprobamate/-mebutamate and meprobamate/carbromal.
More severe hypersensitivity reactions, rarely reported, include hyperpyrexia, chills, angioneurotic edema, bronchospasm, oliguria, and anuria. Also, anaphylaxis, erythema multiforme, exfoliative dermatitis, stomatitis, proctitis, Stevens-Johnson syndrome, and bullous dermatitis, including one fatal case of the latter following administration of meprobamate in combination with prednisolone.
In case of allergic or idiosyncratic reactions to meprobamate, discontinue the drug and initiate appropriate symptomatic therapy, which may include epinephrine, antihistamines, and in severe cases corticosteroids. In evaluating possible allergic reactions, also consider allergy to excipients (information on excipients is available to physicians on request).
Hematologic (See also **Allergic or Idiosyncratic.**)—Agranulocytosis and aplastic anemia have been reported, although no causal relationship has been established. These cases rarely were fatal. Rare cases of thrombocytopenic purpura have been reported.
Other—Exacerbation of porphyric symptoms.
Dosage and Administration: The usual adult starting dosage of 'Deprol' (meprobamate + benactyzine hydrochloride) is one tablet three or four times daily, which may be increased gradually to six tablets daily and gradually reduced to maintenance levels upon establishment of relief. Doses above six tablets daily are not recommended, even though higher doses have been used by some clinicians to control depression, and in chronic psychotic patients.
Overdosage: Overdosage of 'Deprol' (meprobamate + benactyzine hydrochloride) has not differed substantially from meprobamate overdosage:
Meprobamate
Suicidal attempts with meprobamate have resulted in drowsiness, lethargy, stupor, ataxia, coma, shock, vasomotor and respiratory collapse. Some suicidal attempts have been fatal.
The following data on meprobamate tablets have been reported in the literature and from other sources. These data are not expected to correlate with each case (considering factors such as individual susceptibility and length of time from ingestion to treatment), but represent the *usual ranges* reported.
Acute simple overdose (meprobamate alone): Death has been reported with ingestion of as little as 12 gm meprobamate and survival with as much as 40 gm.
Blood Levels:
0.5—2.0 mg% represents the usual blood level range of meprobamate after therapeutic doses. The level may occasionally be as high as 3.0 mg%.
3 —10 mg% usually corresponds to findings of mild to moderate symptoms of overdosage, such as stupor or light coma.
10 —20 mg% usually corresponds to deeper coma, requiring more intensive treatment. Some fatalities occur.
At levels greater than 20 mg%, more fatalities than survivals can be expected.
Acute combined overdose (meprobamate with alcohol or other CNS depressants or psychotropic drugs): Since effects can be additive, a history of ingestion of a low dose of meprobamate plus any of these compounds (or of a relatively low blood or tissue level) cannot be used as a prognostic indicator.
In cases where excessive doses have been taken, sleep ensues rapidly and blood pressure, pulse, and respiratory rates are reduced to basal levels. Any drug remaining in the stomach should be removed and symptomatic therapy given. Should respiration or blood pressure become compromised, respiratory assistance, central nervous system stimulants, and pressor agents should be administered cautiously as indicated. Meprobamate is metabolized in the liver and excreted by the kidney. Diuresis, osmotic (mannitol) diuresis, peritoneal dialysis, and hemodialysis have been used successfully. Careful monitoring of urinary output is necessary and caution should be taken to avoid overhydration. Relapse and death, after initial recovery, have been attributed to incomplete gastric emptying and delayed absorption. Meprobamate can be measured in biological fluids by two methods: colorimetric (Hoffman, A.J. and Ludwig, B.J.: *J Amer Pharm Assn* **48**: 740, 1959) and gas chromatographic (Douglas, J.F. et al: *Anal Chem* **39**: 956, 1967).
How Supplied: Bottles of 100 (NDC 0037-3001-01). Bottles of 500 (NDC 0037-3001-03). Unit Dose: 500 (NDC 0037-3001-05). Unit Dose: 1000 (NDC 0037-3001-04). Rev. 7/79
[*Shown in Product Identification Section*]

DIUTENSEN® TABLETS ℞

Description: Diutensen® is a round, white-blue mottled tablet. Each tablet contains:
Cryptenamine ....2 mg.†
(as tannate salts)
Methyclothiazide.......................................2.5 mg.
†Equivalent to 260 Carotid Sinus Reflex Units.
Actions: Cryptenamine is an alkaloidal fraction obtained from *Veratrum viride* by a nonaqueous extraction procedure. The antihypertensive response to cryptenamine is widely documented. The principal mechanism of action of the drug in reducing the blood pressure involves widespread arteriolar dilatation mediated centrally, without peripheral adrenergic or ganglionic blockade. The major cardiovascular effects are reflex in nature and are mainly due to stimulation of afferent pressor receptors predominantly in the heart and carotid sinus area. These receptors initiate an increase in impulses which are interpreted by areas in the brain stem as denoting a pressure higher than that actually present. As a result, the mechanism concerned with blood pressure homeostasis is activated, sympathetic tone is decreased, vagal tone is increased, and the blood pressure is therefore reduced. Both systolic and diastolic pressures are decreased and the heart is slowed. Atropine abolishes the bradycrotic effect but only partially reverses the hypotensive effect.

Methyclothiazide is a synthetic saluretic-antihypertensive agent. It is a potent analogue of hydrochlorothiazide, being about 20 times as active by weight, as the latter compound. The renal mechanism involved in the diuretic action of methyclothiazide is indistinguishable from that elicited by chlorothiazide or hydrochlorothiazide, but the duration of action of methyclothiazide is longer than that of either of these compounds. The principle mechanism of action of methyclothiazide is the production of diuresis by inhibition of renal tubular reabsorption of electrolytes, resulting in a marked increase in the urinary excretion of sodium, chloride, and water, and moderate increase in the excretion of potassium and bicarbonate.

Indications: Based on a review of this drug by the national Academy of Sciences—National Research Council and/or other information, FDA has classified the indications as follows:
Lacking substantial evidence of effectiveness as a fixed combination for use in basic hypertensive therapy and for essential hypertension of all grades of severity. (See box warning.)
Final classification of less-than-effective indications requires further investigation.

Contraindicaions: DIUTENSEN is contraindicated for patients with known idiosyncrasy to *Veratrum viride* or thiazide compounds and for those who have recently experienced either coronary artery occlusion or cerebral thrombosis. Treatment with thiazide diuretics (including methyclothiazide) is also contraindicated for patients with severe renal or hepatic disease.

Warning: THIS FIXED COMBINATION DRUG IS NOT INDICATED FOR INITIAL THERAPY OF HYPERTENSION. HYPERTENSION REQUIRES THERAPY TITRATED TO THE INDIVIDUAL PATIENT. IF THE FIXED COMBINATION REPRESENTS THE DOSAGE SO DETERMINED, ITS USE MAY BE MORE CONVENIENT IN PATIENT MANAGEMENT. THE TREATMENT OF HYPERTENSION IS NOT STATIC, BUT MUST BE RE-EVALUATED AS CONDITIONS IN EACH PATIENT WARRANT.

Warnings: There have been several reports, published and unpublished, concerning nonspecific small-bowel lesions consisting of stenosis with or without ulceration, associated with the administration of enteric-coated thiazides with potassium salts. These lesions may occur with enteric-coated potassium tablets alone or when they are used with nonenteric-coated thiazides, or certain other oral diuretics. These small-bowel lesions have caused obstruction, hemorrhage, and perforation. Surgery was frequently required and deaths have occurred. Available information tends to implicate enteric-coated potassium salts although lesions of this type also occur spontaneously. Therefore, coated potassium-containing formulations should be administered only when indicated, and should be discontinued immediately if abdominal pain, distention, nausea, vomiting, or gastrointestinal bleeding ocur. Coated potassium tablets should be used only when adequate dietary supplementation is not practical.
Use in Pregnancy: USE OF ANY DRUG IN PREGNANCY, LACTATION, OR IN WOMEN OF CHILDBEARING AGE REQUIRES THAT THE POTENTIAL BENEFITS OF THE DRUG SHOULD BE WEIGHED AGAINST THE POSSIBLE HAZARDS TO THE MOTHER AND CHILD. DIUTENSEN SHOULD BE USED WITH CARE IN PREGNANT AND NURSING MOTHERS SINCE THIAZIDES CROSS THE PLACENTAL BARRIER AND APPEAR IN CORD BLOOD AND BREAST MILK. THIAZIDES MAY RESULT IN FETAL OR NEONATAL JAUNDICE, THROMBOCYTOPENIA, AND POSSIBLY OTHER ADVERSE REACTIONS WHICH HAVE OCCURRED IN THE ADULT.
Thiazides potentiate the action of other antihypertensive drugs. Therefore the dosage of these agents, especially the ganglion blockers, must be reduced by at least 50 percent as soon as thiazides are added to the regimen.
Exacerbation or activation of systemic lupus erythematosus has been reported with sulfonamide derived drugs, including thiazides.
Precautions: Cryptenamine is a potent hypotensive and occasionally bradycrotic drug. Overdosage may produce nausea and vomiting, excessive hypotension and prostration and, rarely, bronchoconstriction. If necessary, atropine sulfate (0.5 to 1.0 mg.) may be administered to reverse the bradycrotic effect. In the event of excessive fall in blood pressure, administer vasopressor drugs, such as ephedrine sulfate (30 to 50 mg.) or phenylephrine hydrochloride (5 mg.) subcutaneously. If left untended, the reaction will gradually disappear within 60 to 90 minutes.
Particular caution is warranted when treating patients with angina pectoris, coronary thrombosis, or cerebrovascular disease. Caution should also be exercised when treating hypertensive patients with chronic renal disease, since they adjust poorly to lowered blood pressure.
Special caution is warranted when treating patients with histories of bronchial asthma who may respond adversely to the cholinergic effect of cryptenamine.
The bradycrotic effect of veratrum alkaloids is additive to, but not synergistic with, that produced by morphine and related drugs.
Methyclothiazide is a potent saluretic drug. After initiation of therapy, the patient should be seen regularly to determine his individual response to therapy. Ordinarily, a total daily dose of 10 mg. (4 DIUTENSEN tablets daily), or less, is not accompanied by significant untoward reactions. However, certain patients may be unusually responsive to the saluretic effect of methyclothiazide and they may experience disturbances in electrolyte balance with subsequent development of hypokalemia. Serum electrolytes should be checked periodically during treatment, particularly in patients receiving relatively large doses of the drug. Patients who are receiving simultaneous treatment either with DIUTENSEN and digitalis or DIUTENSEN and potassium-depleting corticosteriods and those with impending hepatic coma should be carefully watched for signs and symptoms of disturbances in serum electrolyte balance. In the event evidence of electrolyte imbalance with hypokalemia is seen, it may be necessary to give supplemental potassium therapy in the form of fruit juices or direct potassium supplements of one gram, two to four times daily. In severe cases not responding to supplemental potasium therapy, it may be necessary to withdraw the drug.
Hypochloremic alkalosis occurs infrequently with methyclothiazide. Nevertheless, it is a possibility and if this condition develops, it may be treated by the addition of ammonium chloride to the dosage schedule. However, ammonium chloride should not be administered concurrently with a thiazide compound to patients with liver disease because each may cause an elevation in serum ammonia and precipitate onset of coma.
Some elevation of the blood urea nitrogen has been noted occasionally in patients receiving methylothiazide. This reaction occurs more frequently in patients with decreased renal function. If serum nitrogen (BUN, NPN, creatinine) increases progressively, thiazide therapy should be discontinued.
As with other thiazide diuretics, hyperglycemia has been noted during treatment with methyclothiazide. If a significant elevation in blood sugar is noted, the drug should be withdrawn.
As with thiazides in general, serum uric acid has been observed to rise in a few patients treated with methyclothiazide, with overt symptoms of gout appearing in some of these. Symptoms of gout are readily controlled by treatment with colchicine.
Because some patients receiving veratrum alkaloids have experienced marked hypotension when undergoing surgical procedures, it may be advisable to discontinue treatment with DIUTENSEN for a period of approximately two weeks prior to elective surgery. Thiazide drugs may increase the responsiveness of of patients to tubocurarine. Thiazides may decrease arterial responsiveness to norepinephrine and therefore should be withdrawn 48 hours before elective surgery. If emergency surgery is indicated, pre-anesthetic and anesthetic agents should be administered in reduced dosage. Emergency surgery may be carried out with the use, if necessary, of anticholinergic or adrenergic drugs to prevent vagal circulatory responses and of other supportive measures, as indicated.
Thiazides may decrease serum protein bound iodine levels without signs of thyroid disturbance.
The antihypertensive effects of these drugs may be enhanced in the post-sympathectomy patient.
The concurrent use of DIUTENSEN with digitalis may increase the possibility of digitalis intoxication (due chiefly to the saluretic effects of methyclothiazide and perhaps to the vagotonic effects of cryptenamine). If there is evidence of myocardial irritability (extrasystoles, bigeminy, or AV block), dosage of DIUTENSEN should be reduced or discontinued.
Adverse Reactions: THIAZIDES: Varied reactions have been noted in patients treated with thiazides as follows: *Gastrointestinal:* anorexia, gastric irritation, nausea, vomiting, cramping, diarrhea, constipation, jaundice (intra-hepatic cholestatic) and pancreatitis. *Central nervous system:* vertigo, paresthesia, headache and xanthopsia. *Dermatologic-hypersensitivity:* skin rash, photosensitivity, urticaria and cutaneous vasculitis. *Hematologic:* purpura, thrombocytopenia, leukopenia, agranulocytosis and aplastic anemia.
In addition, orthostatic hypotension (aggravated when thiazides were administered in combination with either alcohol, barbiturates or narcotics), hyperglycemia, glycosuria, muscle cramps, dizziness, weakness, and restlessness have been reported.
CRYPTENAMINE: Patients treated with cryptenamine have experienced a variety of reactions as follows: excessive hypotension; prostration; anorexia; nausea and vomiting; epigastric and substernal burning, which may be mistaken for angina pectoris; unpleasant taste; salivation; sweating; hiccough; blurring of vision; mental confusion; cardiac arrhythmias; bradycardia; and, with excessive doses, bronchiolar constriction and respiratory depression.
When adverse reactions occur during treatment with DIUTENSEN, they are usually reversible and disappear when treatment is discontinued.
Dosage and Administration: As determined by individual titration (see box warning). The usual adult dosage of DIUTENSEN is 1 to 4 tablets a day depending on the individual patient response.
How Supplied:
NDC 0037-0272-92, bottle of 100
NDC 0037-0272-96, bottle of 500
[*Shown in Product Identification Section*]

Continued on next page

Wallace—Cont.

DIUTENSEN®-R TABLETS ℞

> **Warning:** THIS FIXED COMBINATION DRUG IS NOT INDICATED FOR INITIAL THERAPY OF HYPERTENSION. HYPERTENSION REQUIRES THERAPY TITRATED TO THE INDIVIDUAL PATIENT. IF THE FIXED COMBINATION REPRESENTS THE DOSAGE SO DETERMINED, ITS USE MAY BE MORE CONVENIENT IN PATIENT MANAGEMENT. THE TREATMENT OF HYPERTENSION IS NOT STATIC, BUT MUST BE RE-EVALUATED AS CONDITIONS IN EACH PATIENT WARRANT.

Description: Diutensen®-R is a two-component system of active ingredients containing 2.5 mg. methyclothiazide and 0.1 mg. reserpine per tablet. DIUTENSEN-R thus provides for easier titration of hypertensive patients than does a three-component system. DIUTENSEN-R tablets are round, white, pink-mottled tablets.
NOTE: DIUTENSEN-R previously contained cryptenamine tannate as a third antihypertensive agent.
Actions: *Methyclothiazide*—The predominant effects of methyclothiazide are diuresis, natriuresis, and chloruresis. The mechanism of action results in an interference with the renal tubular mechanism of electrolyte reabsorption. There is significant natriuresis and diuresis within two hours after administration of a single dose of methyclothiazide. These effects reach a peak in about six hours and persist for 24 hours following oral administration of a single dose.
In nonedematous patients the "peak" (maximum effective) natriuretic single dose of methyclothiazide is 10 mg., whereas the peak kaliuretic dose is 5 mg. Thus, doubling a daily dose of 5 mg. results in an increase of sodium output without significantly increasing potassium excretion.
Like other benzothiadiazines, methyclothiazide also has antihypertensive properties. It also may be used to enhance the antihypertensive action of other drugs. The mechanism by which benzothiadiazines, including methyclothiazide, produce a reduction of elevated blood pressure has not been definitely established. Sodium depletion, however, appears to be of primary importance.
Methyclothiazide is readily absorbed from the gastrointestinal tract and is excreted unchanged by the kidneys.
Reserpine—Reserpine is a pure crystalline alkaloid from the root of *Rauwolfia serpentina*. The drug has mild antihypertensive and bradycrotic effects in addition to sedative and tranquilizing properties.
Reserpine probably produces its antihypertensive effects through depletion of tissue stores of catecholamines (epinephrine and norepinephrine) from peripheral sites. By contrast, its sedative and tranquilizing properties are thought to be due to a depletion of 5-hydroxytryptamine from the brain.
Reserpine is characterized by slow onset of action and sustained effect. Both its cardiovascular and central nervous system effects may persist following withdrawal of the drug.
Indications: Hypertension (see box warning).
Contraindications: *Methyclothiazide*—This compound should not be used in anuric patients or those who exhibit a hypersensitivity to this or other sulfonamide derived drugs.
Reserpine—Reserpine is contraindicated in patients with known hypersensitivity, mental depression especially with suicidal tendencies, active peptic ulcer, and ulcerative colitis. It is also contraindicated in patients receiving electroconvulsive therapy.
Warnings: *Methyclothiazide* — Thiazides should be used with caution in severe renal disease. In patients with renal disease, thiazides may precipitate azotemia. Cumulative effects of the drug may develop in patients with impaired renal function.
Thiazides should be used with caution in patients with impaired hepatic function or progressive liver disease, since minor alterations of fluid and electrolyte balance may precipitate hepatic coma.
Thiazides may be additive or potentiate the action of other antihypertensive drugs. Potentiation occurs with ganglionic or peripheral adrenergic blocking drugs.
Sensitivity reactions may occur in patients with a history of allergy or bronchial asthma.
The possibility of exacerbation or activation of systemic lupus erythematosus has been reported.
Reserpine—Extreme caution should be exercised in treating patients with a history of mental depression. Discontinue the drug at the first sign of despondency, early morning insomnia, loss of appetite, impotence, or self-deprecation. Drug-induced depression may persist for several months after drug withdrawal and may be severe enough to result in suicide.
Electroshock therapy should not be given to patients under treatment with reserpine since severe and even fatal reactions to such therapy have been reported in patients receiving reserpine. Reserpine should be discontinued for two weeks before electroshock therapy is given.
Use in Pregnancy: USE OF ANY DRUG IN PREGNANCY, LACTATION, OR IN WOMEN OF CHILDBEARING AGE REQUIRES THAT THE POTENTIAL BENEFITS OF THE DRUG SHOULD BE WEIGHED AGAINST THE POSSIBLE HAZARDS TO THE MOTHER AND CHILD. DIUTENSEN-R SHOULD BE USED WITH CARE IN PREGNANT AND NURSING MOTHERS SINCE METHYCLOTHIAZIDE AND RESERPINE CROSS THE PLACENTAL BARRIER AND APPEAR IN CORD BLOOD AND BREAST MILK.
THE SAFETY OF RESERPINE FOR USE DURING PREGNANCY OR LACTATION HAS NOT BEEN ESTABLISHED. INCREASED RESPIRATORY SECRETIONS, NASAL CONGESTION, CYANOSIS, AND ANOREXIA MAY OCCUR IN INFANTS BORN TO RESERPINE-TREATED MOTHERS.
THIAZIDES MAY RESULT IN FETAL OR NEONATAL JAUNDICE, THROMBOCYTOPENIA, AND POSSIBLE OTHER ADVERSE REACTIONS WHICH HAVE OCCURRED IN THE ADULT.
Precautions: *Methyclothiazide* — Periodic determination of serum electrolytes to detect possible electrolyte imbalance should be performed at appropriate intervals.
All patients receiving thiazide therapy should be observed for clinical signs of fluid or electrolyte imbalance; namely, hyponatremia, hypochloremic alkalosis, and hypokalemia. Serum and urine electrolyte determinations are particularly important when the patient is vomiting excessively or receiving parenteral fluids. Medication such as digitalis may also influence serum electrolytes. Warning signs, irrespective of cause, are: Dryness of mouth, thirst, weakness, lethargy, drowsiness, restlessness, muscle pains or cramps, muscular fatigue, hypotension, oliguria, tachycardia, and gastrointestinal disturbances such as nausea and vomiting.
Hypokalemia may develop with thiazides as with any other potent diuretic, especially with brisk diuresis, when severe cirrhosis is present, or during concomitant use of corticosteroids or ACTH.
Interference with adequate oral electrolyte intake will also contribute to hypokalemia. Digitalis therapy may exaggerate metabolic effects of hypokalemia especially with reference to myocardial activity.
Any chloride deficit is generally mild and usually does not require specific treatment except under extraordinary circumstances (as in liver disease or renal disease). Dilutional hyponatremia may occur in edematous patients in hot weather; appropriate therapy is water restriction, rather than administration of salt except in rare instances when the hyponatremia is life threatening. In actual salt depletion, appropriate replacement is the therapy of choice.
Hyperuricemia may occur or frank gout may be precipitated in certain patients receiving thiazide therapy.
Insulin requirements in diabetic patients may be increased, decreased, or unchanged. Latent diabetes mellitus may become manifest during thiazide administration.
Thiazide drugs may increase the responsiveness of tubocurarine.
The antihypertensive effects of the drug may be enhanced in the postsympathectomy patient.
Thiazides may decrease arterial responsiveness to norepinephrine. This diminution is not sufficient to preclude effectiveness of the pressor agent for therapeutic use.
If progressive renal impairment becomes evident, as indicated by a rising non-protein nitrogen or blood urea nitrogen, a careful reappraisal of therapy is necessary with consideration given to withholding or discontinuing diuretic therapy.
Thiazides may decrease serum PBI levels without signs of thyroid disturbance.
Reserpine—Because reserpine preparations increase gastrointestinal motility and secretion, this drug should be used cautiously in patients with a history of peptic ulcer, ulcerative colitis, or gallstones, where biliary colic may be precipitated.
Caution should be exercised when treating hypertensive patients with renal insufficiency since they adjust poorly to lowered blood pressure levels.
Use reserpine cautiously with digitalis and quinidine since cardiac arrhythmias have occurred with the concurrent use of rauwolfia preparations.
Preoperative withdrawal of reserpine does not assure that circulatory instability will not occur. It is important that the anesthesiologist be aware of the patient's drug intake and consider this in the overall management, since hypotension has occurred in patients receiving rauwolfia preparations. Anticholinergic and/or adrenergic drugs (metaraminol, norepinephrine) have been employed to treat adverse vagocirculatory effects.
Adverse Reactions: *Methcylothiazide:* The following adverse reactions have been associated with the use of thiazide diuretics.
Gastrointestinal: Anorexia, gastric irritation, nausea, vomiting, cramping, diarrhea, constipation, jaundice (intrahepatic cholestatic jaundice), pancreatitis.
Central nervous system: Dizziness, vertigo, parasthesia, headache, xanthopsia.
Dermatologic-Hypersensitivity: Purpura, photosensitivity, rash, urticaria, necrotizing angiitis (vasculitis) (cutaneous vasculitis).
Hematologic: Leukopenia, agranulocytosis, thrombocytopenia, aplastic anemia.
Cardiovascular: Orthostatic hypotension may occur and may be aggravated by alcohol, barbiturates or narcotics.
Miscellaneous: Hyperglycemia, glycosuria, hyperuricemia, muscle spasm, weakness, restlessness.
Reserpine—Reserpine preparations have caused gastrointestinal reactions including hypersecretion, nausea and vomiting, anorexia, and diarrhea; cardiovascular reactions including angina-like symptoms, arrhythmias particularly when used concurrently with digitalis or quinidine, and bradycardia; and cen-

tral nervous system reactions including drowsiness, depression, nervousness, paradoxical anxiety, nightmares, rare parkinsonian syndrome, C.N.S. sensitization manifested by dull sensorium, deafness, glaucoma, uveitis, and optic atrophy. Nasal congestion is a frequent complaint, and pruritus, rash, dryness of mouth, dizziness, headache, dyspnea, purpura, impotence or decreased libido, dysuria, muscular aches, conjunctival injection, and weight gain have been reported. Extrapyramidal tract symptoms have also occurred. These reactions are usually reversible and disappear when the drug is discontinued.

Whenever DIUTENSEN-R therapy results in adverse reactions which are moderate or severe, dosage should be reduced or therapy withdrawn.

Dosage and Administration: As determined by individual titration (see box warning). The usual adult dosage of DIUTENSEN-R is 1 to 4 tablets a day depending on the individual patient response.

How Supplied:

NDC 0037-0274-92, bottle of 100
NDC 0037-0274-96, bottle of 500
[*Shown in Product Identification Section*]

LUFYLLIN® Elixir ℞
(dyphylline)

How Supplied:

NDC 0037-0515-68, pint bottle
NDC 0037-0515-69, gallon bottle

LUFYLLIN® Injection ℞
(dyphylline, 250 mg/ml)
FOR INTRAMUSCULAR USE ONLY

Description: Dyphylline is chemically 7-(2,3-dihydroxypropyl) theophylline, an alkylated theophylline molecule.

LUFYLLIN® Injection: Clear, colorless sterile solution.

Each ml contains:
Dyphylline .... 250 mg
(pH adjusted with sodium hydroxide)

Actions: As a xanthine derivative, dyphylline possesses the peripheral vasodilator and bronchodilator actions characteristic of theophylline. It has diuretic and myocardial stimulant effects, and is effective orally and by intramuscular injection. Dyphylline may show fewer side effect than aminophylline, but its blood levels and possibly its activity are also lower. The injectable preparation is for intramuscular use only, and is indicated for treatment of an acute asthma attack.

Indications: For relief of acute bronchial asthma and for reversible bronchospasm associated with chronic bronchitis and emphysema.

Contraindications: In individuals who have shown hypersensitivity to any of its components.

Dyphylline should not be administered concurrently with other xanthine preparations.

Warnings: Status asthmaticus is a medical emergency. Excessive doses may be expected to be toxic.

Usage in Pregnancy: Safe use in pregnancy has not been established relative to possible adverse effects on fetal development. Therefore, dyphylline should not be used in pregnant women unless, in the judgment of the physician, the potential benefits outweigh the possible hazards.

Precautions: Use with caution in patients with severe cardiac disease, hypertension, hyperthyroidism, or acute myocardial injury.

Great caution should be used in giving dyphylline to patients in congestive heart failure. Such patients have shown markedly prolonged blood level curves which have persisted for long periods following discontinuation of the drug.

Adverse Reactions: Note: Included in this listing which follows are a few adverse reactions which may not have been reported with this specific drug. However, pharmacological similarities among the xanthine drugs require that each of the reactions be considered when dyphylline is administered.

The most consistent adverse reactions are:

1. Gastrointestinal: irritation, nausea, vomiting, and epigastric pain, generally preceded by headache, hematemesis, diarrhea.
2. Central nervous system: stimulation, irritability, restlessness, insomnia, reflex hyperexcitability, muscle twitching, clonic and tonic generalized convulsions, agitation.
3. Cardiovascular: palpitation, tachycardia, extra systoles, flushing, marked hypotension, and circulatory failure.
4. Respiratory: tachypnea, respiratory arrest.
5. Renal: albuminuria, increased excretion of renal tubule and red blood cells.
6. Others: fever, dehydration.

Overdosage:

Symptoms: In infants and small children: agitation, headache, hyperreflexia, fasiculations, and clonic and tonic convulsions.

In adults: nervousness, insomnia, nausea, vomiting, tachycardia, and extra systoles.

Therapy: Discontinue drug immediately.

No specific treatment.

Avoid sympathomimetics.

Supporting treatment for hypotension, seizure, arrhythmias and dehydration.

Sedatives such as short-acting barbiturates will help control central nervous system stimulation.

Restore the acid-base balance with lactate or bicarbonate.

Oxygen and antibiotics provide supportive treatment as indicated.

Drug Interactions: Toxic synergism with ephedrine and other sympathomimetic bronchodilator drugs may occur.

Recent controlled studies suggest that the addition of ephedrine to adequate dosage regimens of dyphylline produces no increase in effectiveness over that of dyphylline alone, but does produce an increase in toxic effects.

Dosage and Administration: The injectable product is for intramuscular use only and is to be injected very slowly. Preferably the drug is to be given at six-hour intervals.

Adults: Usual Dose—1–2 ml (250–500 mg) may be injected intramuscularly, very slowly; and may be repeated if necessary.

"Therapeutic blood levels are considered to be between 10 mcg/ml and 20 mcg/ml. Levels above 20 mcg/ml may produce toxic effects. There is great variation from patient to patient in dosage needed in order to achieve a therapeutic blood level. Also, the duration of action of oral theophylline preparations varies widely from one patient to another. Because of this wide variation from patient to patient and the relatively narrow therapeutic blood level range, dosage must be individualized with monitoring of theophylline blood levels, particularly when prolonged or repeated use is planned."

Pulmonary function measurements before and after a period of treatment allow an objective assessment of whether or not therapy should be continued in patients with chronic bronchitis and emphysema.

How Supplied:

NDC 0037-0537-01, box of 25 × 2 ml ampuls

Storage: Store at room temperature. Excessive cold may cause the injectable product to precipitate. DO NOT USE if precipitate is present, but clear solution can be achieved by autoclaving for 10 minutes at 250°F.

[*Shown in Product Identification Section*]

LUFYLLIN® Tablets ℞
(dyphylline, 200 mg)
LUFYLLIN®-400 Tablets
(dyphylline, 400 mg)

Description: Dyphylline [7-(2,3-dihydroxypropyl) theophylline] [$C_{10}H_{14}N_4O_4$] is a white, extremely bitter, amorphous solid, freely soluble in water and soluble to the extent of 2 g in 100 ml alcohol. Dyphylline contains the equivalent of about 70 percent of anhydrous theophylline.

Actions: As a xanthine derivative, dyphylline possesses the peripheral vasodilator and bronchodilator actions characteristic of theophylline. It has diuretic and myocardial stimulant effects, and is effective orally. Dyphylline may show fewer side effects than aminophylline, but its blood levels and possibly its activity are also lower.

Indications: For relief of acute bronchial asthma and for reversible bronchospasm associated with chronic bronchitis and emphysema.

Contraindications: In individuals who have shown hypersensitivity to any of its components.

Dyphylline should not be administered concurrently with other xanthine preparations.

Warnings: Status asthmaticus is a medical emergency. Excessive doses may be expected to be toxic.

Usage in Pregnancy: Safe use in pregnancy has not been established relative to possible adverse effects on fetal development. Therefore, dyphylline should not be used in pregnant women unless, in the judgment of the physician, the potential benefits outweigh the possible hazards.

Precautions: Use with caution in patients with severe cardiac disease, hypertension, hyperthyroidism, or acute myocardial injury. Particular caution in dose administration must be exercised in patients with peptic ulcers, since the condition may be exacerbated. Chronic oral administration in high doses (500 to 1,000 mg) is usually associated with gastrointestinal irritation.

Great caution should be used in giving dyphylline to patients in congestive heart failure. Such patients have shown markedly prolonged blood level curves which have persisted for long periods following discontinuation of the drug.

Adverse Reactions: Note: Included in this listing which follows are a few adverse reactions which may not have been reported with this specific drug. However, pharmacological similarities among the xanthine drugs require that each of the reactions be considered when dyphylline is administered.

The most consistent adverse reactions are:

1. **Gastrointestinal:** irritation, nausea, vomiting, and epigastric pain, generally preceded by headache, hematemesis, diarrhea.
2. **Central nervous system:** stimulation, irritability, restlessness, insomnia, reflex hyperexcitability, muscle twitching, clonic and tonic generalized convulsions, agitation.
3. **Cardiovascular:** palpitation, tachycardia, extra systoles, flushing, marked hypotension, and circulatory failure.
4. **Respiratory:** tachypnea, respiratory arrest.
5. **Renal:** albuminuria, increased excretion of renal tubule and red blood cells.
6. **Others:** fever, dehydration.

Overdosage:

Symptoms: In infants and small children: agitation, headache, hyper-reflexia, fasiculations, and clonic and tonic convulsions.

In adults: nervousness, insomnia, nausea, vomiting, tachycardia, and extra systoles.

Continued on next page

Wallace—Cont.

Therapy: Discontinue drug immediately.
No specific treatment.
Ipecac syrup for oral ingestion.
Avoid sympathomimetics.
Supporting treatment for hypotension, seizure, arrhythmias and dehydration.
Sedatives such as short-acting barbiturates will help control central nervous system stimulation.
Restore the acid-base balance with lactate or bicarbonate.
Oxygen and antibiotics provide supportive treatment as indicated.

Drug Interactions: Toxic synergism with ephedrine and other sympathomimetic bronchodilator drugs may occur.
Recent controlled studies suggest that the addition of ephedrine to adequate dosage regimens of dyphylline produces no increase in effectiveness over that of dyphylline alone, but does produce an increase in toxic effects.

Dosage and Administration: When administered orally LUFYLLIN produces less nausea than aminophylline and other alkaline theophylline compounds. Absorption orally appears to be faster on an empty stomach; preferably the drug is to be given at six-hour intervals.

Adults: Usual Dose—15 mg/kg every 6 hours, up to four times a day. The dosage should be individualized by titration to the condition and response of the patient.
"Therapeutic blood levels are considered to be between 10 mcg/ml and 20 mcg/ml. Levels above 20 mcg/ml may produce toxic effects. There is great variation from patient to patient in dosage needed in order to achieve a therapeutic blood level. Also, the duration of action of oral theophylline preparations varies widely from one patient to another. Because of this wide variation from patient to patient and the relatively narrow therapeutic blood level range, dosage must be individualized with monitoring of theophylline blood levels, particularly when prolonged or repeated use is planned."
Pulmonary function measurements before and after a period of treatment allow an objective assessment of whether or not therapy should be continued in patients with chronic bronchitis and emphysema.

How Supplied:
LUFYLLIN Tablets (Each white, rectangular, monogrammed tablet contains 200 mg dyphylline):
NDC 0037-0521-92, bottle of 100
NDC 0037-0521-97, bottle of 1000
LUFYLLIN-400 Tablets (Each white, capsule-shaped, monogrammed tablet contains 400 mg dyphylline):
NDC 0037-0731-92, bottle of 100
NDC 0037-0731-97, bottle of 1000
[*Shown in Product Identification Section*]

LUFYLLIN®-EPG, Tablets and Elixir ℞

Description: LUFYLLIN®-EPG Tablets: Round, pink, monogrammed tablets, scored on one side. Each tablet contains:

Dyphylline	100 mg.
Guaifenesin	200 mg.
Ephedrine Hydrochloride	16 mg.
Phenobarbital	16 mg.

(Warning: May be habit forming)
LUFYLLIN®-EPG Elixir: Clear red liquid with a fruit-like odor and taste. Each 10 ml. (two teaspoonfuls) contains:

Dyphylline	100 mg.
Guaifenesin	200 mg.
Ephedrine Hydrochloride	16 mg.
Phenobarbital	16 mg.
(Warning: May be habit forming)	
Alcohol	5.5%

How Supplied:
LUFYLLIN-EPG Tablets:
NDC 0037-0561-92, bottle of 100
LUFYLLIN-EPG Elixir:
NDC 0037-0565-68, pint bottle

LUFYLLIN®–GG Tablets and Elixir ℞

Description: LUFYLLIN®-GG Tablets: Round, light yellow monogrammed tablets, scored on one side. Each tablet contains:

Dyphylline	200 mg
Guaifenesin	200 mg

LUFYLLIN®-GG Elixir: Clear yellow-orange liquid with a mild wine-like odor and taste. Each 30 ml (two tablespoonfuls) contains:

Dyphylline	200 mg
Guaifenesin	200 mg
Alcohol	17%

Actions: LUFYLLIN (Dyphylline) is 7-(2,3-dihydroxypropyl) theophylline. It exhibits all the pharmacological effects of theophylline, including bronchodilation, vasodilation, myocardial stimulation and mild diuresis.
LUFYLLIN is completely soluble over the physiological pH range. Therapeutic dosages are readily tolerated with little or no gastric distress. LUFYLLIN effectively increases pulmonary function as determined by spirometric measurement. It is tolerated in adequate dosage levels over long periods of time without diminution of effectiveness. LUFYLLIN is neutral and stable.
LUFYLLIN-GG combines the expectorant action of guaifenesin with the bronchodilating properties of dyphylline to relieve acute bronchial asthma and reversible bronchospasm and its associated dyspnea, nonproductive cough and tracheobronchial irritation.

Indications: For relief of acute bronchial asthma and for reversible bronchospasm associated with chronic bronchitis and emphysema.

Precautions: Exercise caution with use in the presence of severe cardiac disease, renal or hepatic malfunction, glaucoma, hyperthroidism, peptic ulcer, and concomitant use of other xanthine-containing formulations or other CNS stimulating drugs.

Adverse Reactions: May cause nausea, headache, cardiac palpitation and CNS stimulation. Postprandial administration may help to avoid gastric discomfort.

Dosage and Administration: These dosage recommendations are meant to offer a range in which one can anticipate a therapeutic response, recognizing that in the therapy of reversible bronchospasm there is considerable patient-to-patient variation; and, therefore, adjustments will probably be necessary based on the severity of symptoms and individual patient response.
Adults:
LUFYLLIN-GG Tablets and Elixir: One tablet or 30 ml (2 tablespoonfuls) four times a day. Larger doses are generally required for the control of acute bronchial asthma.
Children:
Dosages for children have not been established. Therefore, these agents are not recommended for children under six. Older children should be started on low doses which are gradually increased to the lowest effective dosage, not to exceed 5 mg/lb/day of dyphylline. Caution should be exercised in administration to children.

How Supplied:
LUFYLLIN-GG Tablets:
NDC 0037-0541-92, bottle of 100
NDC 0037-0541-97, bottle of 1000
NDC 0037-0541-85, box of 100 unit-dose individually film-sealed tablets.
LUFYLLIN-GG Elixir:
NDC 0037-0545-68, pint bottle
NDC 0037-0545-69, gallon bottle

MALTSUPEX®
(malt soup extract)
Powder, Liquid, Tablets

Composition: 'Maltsupex' is a nondiastatic extract from barley malt, which is available in powder, liquid, and tablet form. 'Maltsupex' has a gentle laxative action and promotes soft, easily passed stools. Each **Tablet** contains 750 mg of 'Maltsupex' and approximately 0.15–0.25 mEq of potassium. Each tablespoonful of **Liquid** (0.5 fl. oz.) and heaping tablespoonful of **Powder** (0.56 oz.) contains 16 grams of 'Maltsupex' and approximately 3.1–5.5 mEq of potassium.

Indications: 'Maltsupex' is indicated for the dietary management and treatment of functional constipation in infants and children. It is also useful in treating constipation in adults, including those with laxative dependence.

Warning: Do not use when abdominal pain, nausea or vomiting malt, present. Keep this and all medications out of the reach of children.

Caution: 'Maltsupex' contains potassium and should not be used by individuals with renal impairment or by persons who must manage the amount of potassium in their diet.

Precautions: In patients with diabetes, allow for carbohydrate content of approximately 14 grams per tablespoonful of liquid (56 calories), 13 grams per tablespoonful of powder (52 calories), and 0.6 grams per tablet (3 calories).

Tablets only: This product contains FD&C Yellow No. 5 (tartrazine) which may cause allergic-type reactions (including bronchial asthma) in certain susceptible individuals. Although the overall incidence of FD&C Yellow No. 5 (tartrazine) sensitivity in the general population is low, it is frequently seen in patients who also have aspirin hypersensitivity.

Dosage and Administration: Powder and Liquid: Use heaping measures of powder. 'Maltsupex' liquid mixes more easily with cold beverages when first stirred with a little hot water.

Adults: 2 heaping tablespoonfuls twice daily for 3 or 4 days, or until relief begins. Then 1 or 2 tablespoonfuls at bedtime to maintain the effect. **Children:** 1 or 2 tablespoonfuls in milk or on cereal once or twice daily. **Bottle-Fed Infants:** (over 1 month) ½ to 2 tablespoonfuls in the day's feeding (or 1 to 2 teaspoonfuls in a single feeding). For daily use in the regular formula to **prevent constipation**, add 1 to 2 teaspoonfuls to each day's feeding as part of the carbohydrate. **To prevent constipation when baby goes on whole milk**, add 1 teaspoonful of 'Maltsupex' to every other bottle or cup. **Breast-Fed Infants:** (over 1 month) dissolve 1 or 2 teaspoonfuls in 2 to 4 ounces of water or fruit juice, and give once or twice a day before nursings.

Tablets: Usual Adult Dosage—Two or three tablets with meals and at bedtime for about four days or until improvement is experienced. Then begin two to four tablets at bedtime for as long as necessary. With severe cases increase dosage to four tablets with meals and at bedtime. With mild cases four tablets at bedtime will usually suffice.

How Supplied: 'Maltsupex' is supplied in 8 ounce (NDC 0037-9101-12) and 16 ounce (NDC 0037-9101-08) jars of 'Maltsupex' Powder; 8 fluid ounce (NDC 0037-9001-12) and 1 pint (NDC 0037-9001-08) bottles of 'Maltsupex' Liquid; and in bottles of 100 'Maltsupex' Tablets (NDC 0037-9201-01). Rev. 7/79

MEPROSPAN® ©
(meprobamate, sustained-release capsules)

Description: Meprobamate is a white powder with a characteristic odor and a bitter taste. It is slightly soluble in water, freely soluble in acetone and alcohol, and sparingly soluble in ether.

Actions: Meprobamate is a carbamate derivative which has been shown in animal studies to have effects at multiple sites in the central nervous system, including the thalamus and limbic system.

Indications: Meprobamate is indicated for the relief of anxiety and tension; as an adjunct in the treatment of various disease states in which anxiety and tension are manifested; and to promote sleep in anxious, tense patients.

The effectiveness of 'Meprospan' in long-term use, that is, more than 4 months, has not been assessed by systematic clinical studies. The physician should periodically reassess the usefulness of the drug for the individual patient.

Contraindications: Acute intermittent porphyria as well as allergic or idiosyncratic reactions to meprobamate or related compounds such as carisoprodol, mebutamate, tybamate, or carbromal.

Warnings:

Drug Dependence

Physical dependence, psychological dependence, and abuse have occurred. When chronic intoxication from prolonged use occurs, it usually involves ingestion of greater than recommended doses and is manifested by ataxia, slurred speech, and vertigo. Therefore, careful supervision of dose and amounts prescribed is advised, as well as avoidance of prolonged administration, especially for alcoholics and other patients with a known propensity for taking excessive quantities of drugs.

Sudden withdrawal of the drug after prolonged and excessive use may precipitate recurrence of preexisting symptoms, such as anxiety, anorexia, or insomnia, or withdrawal reactions, such as vomiting, ataxia, tremors, muscle twitching, confusional states, hallucinosis, and, rarely, convulsive seizures. Such seizures are more likely to occur in persons with central nervous system damage or preexistent or latent convulsive disorders. Onset of withdrawal symptoms occurs usually within 12 to 48 hours after discontinuation of meprobamate; symptoms usually cease within the next 12 to 48 hours.

When excessive dosage has continued for weeks or months, dosage should be reduced gradually over a period of one or two weeks rather than abruptly stopped. Alternatively, a short-acting barbiturate may be substituted, then gradually withdrawn.

Potentially Hazardous Tasks

Patients should be warned that this drug may impair the mental and/or physical abilities required for the performance of potentially hazardous tasks such as driving a motor vehicle or operating machinery.

Additive Effects

Since the effects of meprobamate and alcohol or meprobamate and other CNS depressants or psychotropic drugs may be additive, appropriate caution should be exercised with patients who take more than one of these agents simultaneously.

Usage in Pregnancy and Lactation

An increased risk of congenital malformations associated with the use of minor tranquilizers (meprobamate, chlordiazepoxide, and diazepam), during the first trimester of pregnancy has been suggested in several studies. Because use of these drugs is rarely a matter of urgency, their use during this period should almost always be avoided. The possibility that a woman of childbearing potential may be pregnant at the time of institution of therapy should be considered. Patients should be advised that if they become pregnant during therapy or intend to become pregnant they should communicate with their physicians about the desirability of discontinuing the drug.

Meprobamate passes the placental barrier. It is present both in umbilical cord blood at or near maternal plasma levels and in breast milk of lactating mothers at concentrations two to four times that of maternal plasma. When use of meprobamate is contemplated in breast-feeding patients, the drug's higher concentrations in breast milk as compared to maternal plasma levels should be considered.

Usage in Children

Meprobamate should not be administered to children under age six, since there is a lack of documented evidence for safety and effectiveness in this age group.

Precautions: The lowest effective dose should be administered, particularly to elderly and/or debilitated patients, in order to preclude oversedation.

The possibility of suicide attempts should be considered and the least amount of the drug feasible should be dispensed at any one time.

Meprobamate is metabolized in the liver and excreted by the kidney; to avoid its excess accumulation, caution should be exercised in administration to patients with compromised liver or kidney function.

Meprobamate occasionally may precipitate seizures in epileptic patients.

Adverse Reactions:

Central Nervous System

Drowsiness, ataxia, dizziness, slurred speech, headache, vertigo, weakness, paresthesias, impairment of visual accommodation, euphoria, overstimulation, paradoxical excitement, fast EEG activity.

Gastrointestinal

Nausea, vomiting, diarrhea.

Cardiovascular

Palpitations, tachycardia, various forms of arrhythmia, transient ECG changes, syncope; also, hypotensive crises (including one fatal case).

Allergic or Idiosyncratic

Allergic or idiosyncratic reactions are usually seen within the period of the first to fourth dose in patients having had no previous contact with the drug. Milder reactions are characterized by an itchy, urticarial, or erythematous maculopapular rash which may be generalized or confined to the groin. Other reactions have included leukopenia, acute nonthrombocytopenic purpura, petechiae, ecchymoses, eosinophilia, peripheral edema, adenopathy, fever, fixed drug eruption with cross reaction to carisoprodol, and cross sensitivity between meprobamate/mebutamate and meprobamate/carbromal.

More severe hypersensitivity reactions, rarely reported, include hyperpyrexia, chills, angioneurotic edema, bronchospasm, oliguria, and anuria. Also, anaphylaxis, erythema multiforme, exfoliative dermatitis, stomatitis, proctitis, Stevens-Johnson syndrome, and bullous dermatitis, including one fatal case of the latter following administration of meprobamate in combination with prednisolone.

In case of allergic or idiosyncratic reactions to meprobamate, discontinue the drug and initiate appropriate symptomatic therapy, which may include epinephrine, antihistamines, and in severe cases corticosteroids. In evaluating possible allergic reactions, also consider allergy to excipients (information on excipients is available to physicians on request).

Hematologic

(See also **Allergic or Idiosyncratic.**) Agranulocytosis and aplastic anemia have been reported, although no causal relationship has been established. These cases rarely were fatal. Rare cases of thrombocytopenic purpura have been reported.

Other

Exacerbation of porphyric symptoms.

Dosage and Administration: The usual adult dosage of 'Meprospan' (meprobamate, sustained-release capsules) is one to two 400 mg capsules in the morning and again at bedtime; doses above 2400 mg daily are not recommended. The usual dosage for children ages six to twelve is one 200 mg capsule in the morning and again at bedtime. Meprobamate is not recommended for children under age six.

Overdosage: Suicidal attempts with meprobamate have resulted in drowsiness, lethargy, stupor, ataxia, coma, shock, vasomotor and respiratory collapse. Some suicidal attempts have been fatal.

Overdosage experience with 'Meprospan' (meprobamate, sustained-release capsules) is limited. However, the following data on meprobamate tablets have been reported in the literature and from other sources. These data are not expected to correlate with each case (considering factors such as individual susceptibility and length of time from ingestion to treatment), but represent the *usual ranges* reported.

Acute simple overdose (meprobamate alone): Death has been reported with ingestion of as little as 12 gm meprobamate and survival with as much as 40 gm.

Blood Levels:

0.5 — 2.0 mg% represents the usual blood level range of meprobamate after therapeutic doses. The level may occasionally be as high as 3.0 mg%.

3 — 10 mg% usually corresponds to findings of mild to moderate symptoms of overdosage, such as stupor or light coma.

10 — 20 mg% usually corresponds to deeper coma, requiring more intensive treatment. Some fatalities occur.

At levels greater than 20 mg%, more fatalities than survivals can be expected.

Acute combined overdose (meprobamate with alcohol or other CNS depressants or psychotropic drugs): Since effects can be additive, a history of ingestion of a low dose of meprobamate plus any of these compounds (or of a relatively low blood or tissue level) cannot be used as a prognostic indicator.

In cases where excessive doses have been taken, sleep ensues rapidly and blood pressure, pulse, and respiratory rates are reduced to basal levels. Any drug remaining in the stomach should be removed and symptomatic therapy given. Should respiration or blood pressure become compromised, respiratory assistance, central nervous system stimulants, and pressor agents should be administered cautiously as indicated. Meprobamate is metabolized in the liver and excreted by the kidney. Diuresis, osmotic (mannitol) diuresis, peritoneal dialysis, and hemodialysis have been used successfully. Careful monitoring of urinary output is necessary and caution should be taken to avoid overhydration. Relapse and death, after initial recovery, have been attributed to incomplete gastric emptying and delayed absorption. Meprobamate can be measured in biological fluids by two methods: colorimetric (Hoffman, A.J. and Ludwig, B.J.: *J Amer Pharm Assn* **48:** 740, 1959) and gas chromatographic (Douglas, J.F. et al: *Anal Chem* **39:** 956, 1967).

How Supplied: 'Meprospan' 400: Each sustained-release, blue-topped capsule contains meprobamate, U.S.P., 400 mg in bottles of 100 (NDC 0037-1301-01). 'Meprospan' 200: Each sustained-release yellow-topped capsule contains meprobamate, U.S.P., 200 mg in bottles of 100 (NDC 0037-1401-01). Rev. 2/78

[*Shown in Product Identification Section*]

MICRAININ® Ⓒ

(meprobamate + aspirin)

Description: Each Micrainin® tablet contains 200 mg meprobamate and 325 mg aspirin.

Actions: Meprobamate, a carbamate derivative, is a tranquilizing agent which has been shown in animal studies to have effects at multiple sites in the central nervous system including the thalamus and limbic system.

Acetylsalicylic acid (aspirin) is an analgesic with antipyretic and antiinflammatory properties.

Continued on next page

Wallace—Cont.

Indications: As an adjunct in the short term treatment of pain accompanied by tension and/ or anxiety in patients with musculoskeletal disease. Clinical trials have demonstrated that in these situations, relief of pain is somewhat greater than with aspirin alone.
The effectiveness of 'Micrainin' in long-term use, that is, more than 4 months, has not been assessed by systematic clinical studies. The physician should periodically reassess the usefulness of the drug for the individual patient.
Contraindications: 'Micrainin' should not be given to individuals with acute intermittent porphyria or with a history of sensitivity or severe intolerance to aspirin, meprobamate, or compounds related to meprobamate, such as carisoprodol, mebutamate, tybamate, or carbromal.
Warnings: Salicylates should be used with extreme caution in the presence of peptic ulcer or coagulation abnormalities. In rare instances the use of aspirin in persons allergic to salicylates can result in life-threatening allergic episodes.

Usage in Pregnancy and Lactation
The safety of 'Micrainin' for use during pregnancy or lactation has not been established. Like many compounds with anti-inflammatory activity, extensive testing of aspirin in several animal species has revealed the possibility for a dose responsive teratogenic effect.
An increased risk of congenital malformations associated with the use of minor tranquilizers (meprobamate, chlordiazepoxide, and diazepam) during the first trimester of pregnancy has been suggested in several studies. Because use of these drugs is rarely a matter of urgency, their use during this period should almost always be avoided. The possibility that a woman of childbearing potential may be pregnant at the time of institution of therapy should be considered. Patients should be advised that if they become pregnant during therapy or intend to become pregnant they should communicate with their physicians about the desirability of discontinuing the drug.
Meprobamate and aspirin both cross the placental barrier, and both have been found present in human milk. Meprobamate is present in umbilical cord blood at or near maternal plasma levels and in breast milk of lactating mothers at concentrations two to four times that of maternal plasma. When use of meprobamate is contemplated in breast-feeding patients, the drug's higher concentration in breast milk as compared to maternal plasma levels should be considered.

Drug Dependence
Physical dependence, psychological dependence, and abuse have occurred with meprobamate. When chronic intoxication from prolonged use occurs, it usually involves ingestion of greater than recommended doses and is manifested by ataxia, slurred speech, and vertigo. Therefore, careful supervision of dose and amounts prescribed is advised, as well as avoidance of prolonged administration, especially for alcoholics and other patients with a known propensity for taking excessive quantities of drugs.
Sudden withdrawal of meprobamate after prolonged and excessive use may precipitate recurrence of pre-existing symptoms, such as anxiety, anorexia, or insomnia, or withdrawal reactions such as vomiting, ataxia, tremors, muscle twitching, confusional states, hallucinosis, and rarely, convulsive seizures. Such seizures are more likely to occur in persons with central nervous system damage or pre-existent or latent convulsive disorders. Onset of withdrawal symptoms occurs usually within 12 to 48 hours after discontinuation of meprobamate; symptoms usually cease within the next 12 to 48 hours.
When excessive dosage of meprobamate has continued for weeks or months, dosage should be reduced gradually over a period of one or two weeks rather than abruptly stopped. Alternatively, a short-acting barbiturate may be substituted, then gradually withdrawn.

Potentially Hazardous Tasks
Patients should be warned that the meprobamate component may impair the mental and/ or physical abilities required for the performance of potentially hazardous tasks such as driving a motor vehicle or operating machinery.

Additive Effects
Since the effects of meprobamate and alcohol or meprobamate and other CNS depressants or psychotropic drugs may be additive, appropriate caution should be exercised with patients who take more than one of these agents simultaneously.

Usage in Children
'Micrainin' is not recommended for patients 12 years of age or under.

Precautions: Preparations containing aspirin should be kept out of the reach of children. Careful supervision of dose and amounts of 'Micrainin' prescribed for patients is advised, especially with those patients with a known propensity for taking excessive quantities of drugs. The lowest effective dose should be administered, particularly to elderly and/or debilitated patients, in order to preclude oversedation.
The possibility of suicide attempts should be considered and the least amount of the drug feasible should be dispensed at any one time.
Meprobamate is metabolized in the liver and excreted by the kidney; to avoid its excess accumulation, caution should be exercised in administration to patients with compromised liver or kidney function.
Meprobamate occasionally may precipitate seizures in epileptic patients.

Adverse Reactions:
Central Nervous System—Drowsiness, ataxia, dizziness, slurred speech, headache, vertigo, weakness, paresthesias, impairment of visual accommodation, euphoria, overstimulation, paradoxical excitement, fast EEG activity.
Gastrointestinal—Nausea, vomiting, diarrhea.
Cardiovascular—Palpitations, tachycardia, various forms of arrhythmia, transient ECG changes, syncope; also hypotensive crises (including one fatal case).
Allergic or Idiosyncratic—A clearly related side effect to the administration of meprobamate is the rare occurrence of allergic or idiosyncratic reactions. This response develops, as a rule, in patients who have had only 1–4 doses of meprobamate and have not had a previous contact with the drug. Milder reactions are characterized by an itchy, urticarial, or erythematous maculopapular rash which may be generalized or confined to the groin. Other reactions have included leukopenia, acute nonthrombocytopenic purpura, petechiae, ecchymoses, eosinophilia, peripheral edema, adenopathy, fever, fixed drug eruption with cross sensitivity between meprobamate/mebutamate and meprobamate/carbromal.
More severe hypersensitivity reactions, rarely reported, include hyperpyrexia, chills, angioneurotic edema, bronchospasm, oliguria, and anuria. Also, anaphylaxis, erythema multiforme, exfoliative dermatitis, stomatitis, proctitis, Stevens-Johnson syndrome, and bullous dermatitis, including one fatal case of the latter following administration of meprobamate in combination with prednisolone.
In case of allergic or idiosyncratic reactions to meprobamate, discontinue the drug and initiate appropriate symptomatic therapy, which may include epinephrine, antihistamines, and in severe cases corticosteroids. In evaluating possible allergic reactions, also consider allergy to excipients (information on excipients is available to physicians on request).
Hematologic (See also Allergic or Idiosyncratic.)
Agranulocytosis and aplastic anemia have been reported with meprobamate although no causal relationship has been established. These cases rarely were fatal. Rare cases of thrombocytopenic purpura have been reported.
Other—Exacerbation of porphyric symptoms.

Dosage and Administration: 'Micrainin' is given orally. The usual dose is one or two tablets (each tablet contains meprobamate 200 mg and aspirin 325 mg) three or four times daily as needed for pain when tension or anxiety are present. Doses of meprobamate above 2400 mg daily are not recommended.
'Micrainin' is not recommended for patients 12 years of age or under.

Overdosage: Overdosage with 'Micrainin' would probably produce the usual signs and symptoms of salicylate intoxication combined with those which may occur with meprobamate.
Suicidal attempts with meprobamate have resulted in drowsiness, lethargy, stupor, ataxia, coma, shock, vasomotor and respiratory collapse. Some suicidal attempts have been fatal.
The following data on meprobamate overdosage have been summarized from the literature and other sources. These data are not expected to correlate with each case (considering factors such as individual susceptibility and length of time from ingestion to treatment), but represent the *usual ranges* reported.
Acute Simple Overdosage (meprobamate alone): Death has been reported with ingestion of as little as 12 gm meprobamate and survival with as much as 40 gm.
Blood Levels:
0.5–2.0 mg%: the usual blood level range of meprobamate after therapeutic doses. The level may occasionally be as high as 3.0 mg%.
3–10 mg%: usually corresponds to findings of mild to moderate symptoms of overdosage, such as stupor or light coma.
10–20 mg%: usually corresponds to deeper coma, requiring more intensive treatment. Some fatalities may occur.
20 mg% or greater: more fatalities than survivals can be expected.
Acute Combined Overdosage (meprobamate with alcohol or other CNS depressants or psychotropic drugs): Since effects can be additive, a history of ingestion of a low dose of meprobamate plus any of these compounds (or of a relatively low blood or tissue level) cannot be used as a prognostic indicator.
Treatment
In cases where excessive doses have been taken, sleep ensues rapidly and blood pressure, pulse, and respiratory rates are reduced to basal levels. Any drug remaining in the stomach should be removed and symptomatic therapy given. Should respiration or blood pressure become compromised, respiratory assistance, central nervous system stimulants, and pressor agents should be administered cautiously as indicated. Meprobamate is metabolized in the liver and excreted by the kidney. Diuresis, osmotic (mannitol) diuresis, peritoneal dialysis, and hemodialysis have been used successfully. Careful monitoring of urinary output is necessary and caution should be taken to avoid overhydration. Relapse and death, after initial recovery, have been attributed to incomplete gastric emptying and delayed absorption. Meprobamate can be measured in biological fluids by two methods: colorimetric (Hoffman, A.J. and Ludwig, B.J.: *J Amer Pharm Assn 48*:740, 1959) and gas chromatographic (Douglas, J.F., et al: *Anal Chem 39*:956, 1967).

How Supplied: 'Micrainin' (meprobamate 200 mg + aspirin 325 mg): Capsule-shaped,

orange and white, layered tablets in bottles of 100 (NDC 0037-0120-01).
Manufactured by: ICN Pharmaceuticals
Cincinnati, Ohio 45213
Rev. 3/79

MILPATH® ℞
(meprobamate + tridihexethyl chloride)

Description: 'Milpath' is available in two formulations:
'Milpath'-400 Yellow, scored tablets, each containing:
meprobamate, U.S.P. ....400 mg
tridihexethyl chloride ....25 mg
'Milpath'-200 Yellow, coated tablets, each containing:
meprobamate, U.S.P. ....200 mg
tridihexethyl chloride ....25 mg

Actions: 'Milpath' combines meprobamate, a tranquilizing agent, with tridihexethyl chloride, an anticholinergic agent.

Tridihexethyl chloride
Tridihexethyl chloride possesses antimuscarinic actions. Gastrointestinal actions include reduction in both gastric secretion and gastrointestinal motility.

Meprobamate
Meprobamate is a carbamate derivative which has been shown in animal studies to have effects at multiple sites in the central nervous system, including the thalamus and limbic system.

Indications: Based on a review of this drug by the National Academy of Sciences—National Research Council and/or other information, FDA has classified the indication as follows:
"Possibly" effective: as adjunctive therapy in the treatment of peptic ulcer and in the treatment of the irritable bowel syndrome (irritable colon, spastic colon, mucous colitis) and acute enterocolitis.
Final classification of this indication requires further investigation.

Contraindications:
Tridihexethyl chloride
Allergic or idiosyncratic reactions to tridihexethyl chloride or related compounds; urinary bladder-neck obstructions, such as prostatic obstructions due to hypertrophy; pyloric obstructions because of reduction of motility and tonus; organic cardiospasm (megaesophagus); glaucoma. It may also be contraindicated in stenosing gastric or duodenal ulcers with significant gastric retention.
Meprobamate
Acute intermittent porphyria as well as allergic or idiosyncratic reactions to meprobamate or related compounds such as carisoprodol, mebutamate, tybamate, or carbromal.

Warnings:
Meprobamate
Drug Dependence—Physical dependence, psychological dependence, and abuse have occurred. When chronic intoxication from prolonged use occurs, it usually involves ingestion of greater than recommended doses and is manifested by ataxia, slurred speech, and vertigo. Therefore, careful supervision of dose and amounts prescribed is advised, as well as avoidance of prolonged administration, especially for alcoholics and other patients with a known propensity for taking excessive quantities of drugs. Sudden withdrawal of the drug after prolonged and excessive use may precipitate recurrence of pre-existing symptoms, such as anxiety, anorexia, or insomnia, or withdrawal reactions, such as vomiting, ataxia, tremors, muscle twitching, confusional states, hallucinosis, and, rarely, convulsive seizures. Such seizures are more likely to occur in persons with central nervous system damage or pre-existent or latent convulsive disorders. Onset of withdrawal symptoms occurs usually within 12 to 48 hours after discontinuation of meprobamate; symptoms usually cease within the next 12 to 48 hours.
When excessive dosage has continued for weeks or months, dosage should be reduced gradually over a period of one or two weeks rather than abruptly stopped. Alternatively, a short-acting barbiturate may be substituted, then gradually withdrawn.
Potentially Hazardous Tasks—Patients should be warned that this drug may impair the mental and/or physical abilities required for the performance of potentially hazardous tasks such as driving a motor vehicle or operating machinery.
Additive Effects—Since the effects of meprobamate and alcohol or meprobamate and other CNS depressants or psychotropic drugs may be additive, appropriate caution should be exercised with patients who take more than one of these agents simultaneously.

Usage in Pregnancy and Lactation
An increased risk of congenital malformations associated with the use of minor tranquilizers (meprobamate, chlordiazepoxide, and diazepam) during the first trimester of pregnancy has been suggested in several studies. Because use of these drugs is rarely a matter of urgency, their use during this period should almost always be avoided. The possibility that a woman of childbearing potential may be pregnant at the time of institution of therapy should be considered. Patients should be advised that if they become pregnant during therapy or intend to become pregnant they should communicate with their physicians about the desirability of discontinuing the drug.
Meprobamate passes the placental barrier. It is present both in umbilical cord blood at or near maternal plasma levels and in breast milk of lactating mothers at concentrations two to four times that of maternal plasma. When use of meprobamate is contemplated in breast-feeding patients, the drug's higher concentrations in breast milk as compared to maternal plasma levels should be considered.

Precautions:
Tridihexethyl chloride
Use cautiously in elderly male patients because of the possibility of prostatic hypertrophy.
Meprobamate
The lowest effective dose should be administered, particularly to elderly and/or debilitated patients, in order to preclude oversedation.
The possibility of suicide attempts should be considered and the least amount of drug feasible should be dispensed at any one time.
Meprobamate is metabolized in the liver and excreted by the kidney; to avoid its excess accumulation, caution should be exercised in administration to patients with compromised liver or kidney function.
Meprobamate occasionally may precipitate seizures in epileptic patients.

Adverse Reactions: While few of the following reactions have been reported with 'Milpath' (meprobamate + tridihexethyl chloride) administration, it is possible that side effects which have occurred with the constituents alone might also occur when the combination is taken.
Tridihexethyl chloride
At recommended dosage severe effects are rare; those reported are the occurrences typically related to administration of anticholinergic drugs. Dry mouth is fairly frequent at oral doses of 100 mg. Constipation or a "bloated" feeling sometimes occurs. Other possible anticholinergic side effects include tachycardia, bradycardia, dilation of pupils, increased ocular tension, weakness, nausea, vomiting, headache, drowsiness, urinary hesitancy or retention, and dizziness.
Meprobamate
Central Nervous System—Drowsiness, ataxia, dizziness, slurred speech, headache, vertigo, weakness, paresthesias, impairment of visual accommodation, euphoria, overstimulation, paradoxical excitement, fast EEG activity.
Gastrointestinal — Nausea, vomiting, diarrhea.
Cardiovascular — Palpitations, tachycardia, various forms of arrhythmia, transient ECG changes, syncope; also, hypotensive crises (including one fatal case).
Allergic or Idiosyncratic—Allergic or idiosyncratic reactions are usually seen within the period of the first to fourth dose in patients having had no previous contact with the drug. Milder reactions are characterized by an itchy, urticarial, or erythematous maculopapular rash which may be generalized or confined to the groin. Other reactions have included leukopenia, acute nonthrombocytopenic purpura, petechiae, ecchymoses, eosinophilia, peripheral edema, adenopathy, fever, fixed drug eruption with cross reaction to carisoprodol, and cross sensitivity between meprobamate/-mebutamate and meprobamate/carbromal.
More severe hypersensitivity reactions, rarely reported, include hyperpyrexia, chills, angioneurotic edema, bronchospasm, oliguria, and anuria. Also, anaphylaxis, erythema multiforme, exfoliative dermatitis, stomatitis, proctitis, Stevens-Johnson syndrome, and bullous dermatitis, including one fatal case of the latter following administration of meprobamate in combination with prednisolone.
In case of allergic or idiosyncratic reactions to meprobamate, discontinue the drug and initiate appropriate symptomatic therapy, which may include epinephrine, antihistamines, and in severe cases corticosteroids. In evaluating possible allergic reactions, also consider allergy to excipients (information on excipients is available to physicians on request).
Hematologic (See also **Allergic or Idiosyncratic.**)—Agranulocytosis and aplastic anemia have been reported, although no causal relationship has been established. These cases rarely were fatal. Rare cases of thrombocytopenic purpura have been reported.
Other—Exacerbation of porphyric symptoms.

Dosage and Administration: The usual adult dosage of 'Milpath'-400 (meprobamate 400 mg + tridihexethyl chloride 25 mg) is one tablet three times a day at mealtimes, and two tablets at bedtime. If a greater anticholinergic effect is desired, the usual adult dosage is two 'Milpath'-200 (meprobamate 200 mg + tridihexethyl chloride 25 mg) tablets three times a day at mealtimes, and two tablets at bedtime. Doses of meprobamate above 2400 mg daily are not recommended.
Not for use in children under age 12.

Overdosage: Although no cases of overdosage have been reported with 'Milpath' (meprobamate + tridihexethyl chloride), following is information on the separate components.
Tridihexethyl chloride
Acute overdosage of anticholinergic agents can produce dry mouth, difficulty swallowing, marked thirst; blurred vision, photophobia; flushed, hot, dry skin; rash; hyperthermia; palpitations, tachycardia with weak pulse, elevated blood pressure; urinary urgency with difficulty in micturition; abdominal distention; restlessness, confusion, delirium and other signs suggestive of an acute organic psychosis. Treatment should include removal of remaining drug from stomach after administration of Universal Antidote, and supportive and symptomatic therapy as indicated.
Meprobamate
Suicidal attempts with meprobamate have resulted in drowsiness, lethargy, stupor, ataxia, coma, shock, vasomotor and respira-

Continued on next page

Wallace—Cont.

tory collapse. Some suicidal attempts have been fatal.

The following data on meprobamate tablets have been reported in the literature and from other sources. These data are not expected to correlate with each case (considering factors such as individual susceptibility and length of time from ingestion to treatment), but represent the *usual ranges* reported.

Acute simple overdose (meprobamate alone): Death has been reported with ingestion of as little as 12 gm meprobamate and survival with as much as 40 gm.

Blood Levels:

0.5 — 2.0 mg% represents the usual blood level range of meprobamate after therapeutic doses. The level may occasionally be as high as 3.0 mg%.

3 —10 mg% usually corresponds to findings of mild to moderate symptoms of overdosage, such as stupor or light coma.

10 —20 mg% usually corresponds to deeper coma, requiring more intensive treatment. Some fatalities occur.

At levels greater than 20 mg%, more fatalities than survivals can be expected.

Acute combined overdose (meprobamate with alcohol or other CNS depressants or psychotropic drugs): Since effects can be additive, a history of ingestion of a low dose of meprobamate plus any of these compounds (or of a relatively low blood or tissue level) cannot be used as a prognostic indicator.

In cases where excessive doses have been taken, sleep ensues rapidly and blood pressure, pulse, and respiratory rates are reduced to basal levels. Any drug remaining in the stomach should be removed and symptomatic therapy given. Should respiration or blood pressure become compromised, respiratory assistance, central nervous system stimulants, and pressor agents should be administered cautiously as indicated. Meprobamate is metabolized in the liver and excreted by the kidney. Diuresis, osmotic (mannitol) diuresis, peritoneal dialysis, and hemodialysis have been used successfully. Careful monitoring of urinary output is necessary and caution should be taken to avoid overhydration. Relapse and death, after initial recovery, have been attributed to incomplete gastric emptying and delayed absorption. Meprobamate can be measured in biological fluids by two methods: colorimetric (Hoffman, A.J. and Ludwig, B.J.: *J Amer Pharm Assn* **48:** 740, 1959) and gas chromatographic (Douglas, J.F. et al: *Anal Chem* **39:** 956, 1967).

How supplied: 'Milpath'- 400 Bottles of 100 (NDC 0037-5001-01) and 500 (NDC 0037-5001-03) 'Milpath'-200 Bottles of 100. (NDC 0037-5101-01) Rev. 1/79

[*Shown in Product Identification Section*]

MILPREM® ℞
(meprobamate + conjugated estrogens)

WARNING

1. ESTROGENS HAVE BEEN REPORTED TO INCREASE THE RISK OF ENDOMETRIAL CARCINOMA.

Three independent case control studies have shown an increased risk of endometrial cancer in postmenopausal women exposed to exogenous estrogens for prolonged periods.[1–3] This risk was independent of the other known risk factors for endometrial cancer. These studies are further supported by the finding that incidence rates of endometrial cancer have increased sharply since 1969 in eight different areas of the United States with population-based cancer reporting systems, an increase which may be related to the rapidly expanding use of estrogens during the last decade.[4]

The three case control studies reported that the risk of endometrial cancer in estrogen users was about 4.5 to 13.9 times greater than in nonusers. The risk appears to depend on both duration of treatment[1] and on estrogen dose.[3] In view of these findings, when estrogens are used for the treatment of menopausal symptoms, the lowest dose that will control symptoms should be utilized and medication should be discontinued as soon as possible. When prolonged treatment is medically indicated, the patient should be reassessed on at least a semiannual basis to determine the need for continued therapy. Although the evidence must be considered preliminary, one study suggests that cyclic administration of low doses of estrogen may carry less risk than continuous administration;[3] it therefore appears prudent to utilize such a regimen.

Close clinical surveillance of all women taking estrogens is important. In all cases of undiagnosed persistent or recurring abnormal vaginal bleeding, adequate diagnostic measures should be undertaken to rule out malignancy.

There is no evidence at present that "natural" estrogens are more or less hazardous than "synthetic" estrogens at equiestrogenic doses.

2. ESTROGENS SHOULD NOT BE USED DURING PREGNANCY.

The use of female sex hormones, both estrogens and progestogens, during early pregnancy may seriously damage the offspring. It has been shown that females exposed in utero to diethylstilbestrol, a nonsteroidal estrogen, have an increased risk of developing in later life a form of vaginal or cervical cancer that is ordinarily extremely rare.[5,6] This risk has been estimated as not greater than 4 per 1000 exposures.[7] Furthermore, a high percentage of such exposed women (from 30 to 90 percent) have been found to have vaginal adenosis,[8–12] epithelial changes of the vagina and cervix. Although these changes are histologically benign, it is not known whether they are precursors of malignancy. Although similar data are not available with the use of other estrogens, it cannot be presumed they would not induce similar changes.

Several reports suggest an association between intrauterine exposure to female sex hormones and congenital anomalies, including congenital heart defects and limb reduction defects.[13–16] One case control study[16] estimated a 4.7 fold increased risk of limb reduction defects in infants exposed in utero to sex hormones (oral contraceptives, hormone withdrawal tests for pregnancy, or attempted treatment for threatened abortion). Some of these exposures were very short and involved only a few days of treatment. The data suggest that the risk of limb reduction defects in exposed fetuses is somewhat less than 1 per 1000.

In the past, female sex hormones have been used during pregnancy in an attempt to treat threatened or habitual abortion. There is considerable evidence that estrogens are ineffective for these indications, and there is no evidence from well controlled studies that progestogens are effective for these uses.

If 'Milprem' (meprobamate + conjugated estrogens) is used during pregnancy, or if the patient becomes pregnant while taking this drug, she should be apprised of the potential risks to the fetus, and the advisability of pregnancy continuation.

3. THIS FIXED COMBINATION DRUG IS NOT INDICATED FOR INITIAL THERAPY.

In cases where estrogen given alone has not alleviated anxiety and tension existing as part of the menopausal symptom complex, therapy may then consist of separate administration of estrogen and meprobamate in order to determine the appropriate dosage of each drug for the patient. If this fixed combination represents the dosage so determined, its use may be more convenient in patient management. The treatment of such patients is not static, but must be re-evaluated as conditions in each patient warrant.

Description: 'Milprem' is a combination of meprobamate, a tranquilizing agent, and conjugated estrogens, U.S.P.

'Milprem' is available in two formulations for oral use:

'Milprem'–400	Dark pink, coated tablets, each containing: meprobamate, U.S.P., 400 mg conjugated estrogens, U.S.P., 0.45 mg
'Milprem'–200	Light pink, coated tablets, each containing: meprobamate, U.S.P., 200 mg conjugated estrogens, U.S.P., 0.45 mg

Clinical Pharmacology:

Conjugated Estrogens

Conjugated estrogens are active when taken orally. They are specific for alleviation of symptoms caused by declining ovarian function.

Meprobamate

Meprobamate is a carbamate derivative which has been shown in animal studies to have effects at multiple sites in the central nervous system, including the thalamus and limbic system.

Indications: For the treatment of moderate to severe vasomotor symptoms of the menopause when anxiety and tension are part of the symptom complex and only in those cases in which the use of estrogens alone has not resulted in alleviation of such symptoms.

Contraindications:

Conjugated Estrogens

Estrogens should not be used in women (or men) with any of the following conditions:

1. Known or suspected cancer of the breast except in appropriately selected patients being treated for metastatic disease.
2. Known or suspected estrogen-dependent neoplasia.
3. Known or suspected pregnancy (See Boxed Warning).
4. Undiagnosed abnormal genital bleeding.
5. Active thrombophlebitis or thromboembolic disorders.
6. A past history of thrombophlebitis, thrombosis, or thromboembolic disorders associated with previous estrogen use (except when used in treatment of breast or prostatic malignancy).

Meprobamate

Acute intermittent porphyria as well as allergic or idiosyncratic reactions to meprobamate or related compounds such as carisoprodol, mebutamate, tybamate, or carbromal.

Warnings:

Conjugated Estrogens

1. **Induction of malignant neoplasms.** Long term continuous administration of natural and synthetic estrogens in certain animal species increases the frequency of carcinomas of the breast, cervix, vagina, and liver. There is now evidence that estrogens increase the risk of carcinoma of the endometrium in humans. (See Boxed Warning.)

At the present time there is no satisfactory evidence that estrogens given to postmenopausal women increase the risk of cancer of the breast,[18] although a recent long-term follow-up of a single physician's practice has raised this possibility.[18a] Because of the animal data there is a need for caution, in prescribing estrogens for women with a strong family history of breast cancer or who have breast nodules, fibrocystic disease, or abnormal mammograms.

2. **Gall bladder disease.** A recent study has reported a 2 to 3-fold increase in the risk of surgically confirmed gall bladder disease in women receiving postmenopausal estrogens[18] similar to the 2-fold increase previously noted in users of oral contraceptives.[19,24] In the case of oral contraceptives the increased risk appeared after two years of use.[24]

3. **Effects similar to those caused by estrogen-progestogen oral contraceptives.** There are several serious adverse effects of oral contraceptives, most of which have not, up to now, been documented as consequences of postmenopausal estrogen therapy. This may reflect the comparatively low doses of estrogen used in postmenopausal women. It would be expected that the larger doses of estrogen used to treat prostatic or breast cancer or postpartum breast engorgement are more likely to result in these adverse effects, and, in fact, it has been shown that there is an increased risk of thrombosis in men receiving estrogens for prostatic cancer and women for postpartum breast engorgement.[20–23]

a. **Thromboembolic disease.** It is now well established that users of oral contraceptives have an increased risk of various thromboembolic and thrombotic vascular diseases, such as thrombophlebitis, pulmonary embolism, stroke, and myocardial infarction.[24–31] Cases of retinal thrombosis, mesenteric thrombosis and optic neuritis have been reported in oral contraceptive users. There is evidence that the risk of several of these adverse reactions is related to the dose of the drug.[32,33] An increased risk of post-surgery thromboembolic complications has also been reported in users of oral contraceptives.[34,35] If feasible, estrogen should be discontinued at least 4 weeks before surgery of the type associated with an increased risk of thromboembolism, or during period of prolonged immobilization.

While an increased rate of thromboembolic and thrombotic disease in postmenopausal users of estrogens has not been found,[18,36] this does not rule out the possibility that such an increase may be present or that subgroups of women who have underlying risk factors or who are receiving relatively large doses of estrogen may have an increased risk. Therefore estrogens should not be used in persons with active thrombophlebitis or thromboembolic disorders and they should not be used (except in treatment of malignancy) in persons with a history of such disorders in association with estrogen use. They should be used with caution in patients with cerebral vascular or coronary artery disease and only for those in whom estrogens are clearly needed.

Large doses of estrogen (5 mg conjugated estrogens per day), comparable to those used to treat cancer of the prostate and breast, have been shown in a large prospective clinical trial in men[37] to increase the risk of nonfatal myocardial infarction, pulmonary embolism and thrombophlebitis. When estrogen doses of this size are used, any of the thromboembolic and thrombotic adverse effects associated with oral contraceptive use should be considered a clear risk.

b. **Hepatic adenoma.** Benign hepatic adenomas appear to be associated with the use of oral contraceptives.[38–40] Although benign, and rare, these may rupture and may cause death through intraabdominal hemorrhage. Such lesions have not yet been reported in association with other estrogen or progestogen preparations but should be considered in estrogen users having abdominal pain and tenderness, abdominal mass, or hypovolemic shock. Hepatocellular carcinoma has also been reported in women taking estrogen-containing oral contraceptives.[39] The relationship of this malignancy to these drugs is not known at this time.

c. **Elevated blood pressure.** Increased blood pressure is not uncommon in women using oral contraceptives. There is now a report that this may occur with the use of estrogens in the menopause[41] and blood pressure should be monitored with estrogen use, especially if high doses are used.

d. **Glucose tolerance.** A worsening of glucose tolerance has been observed in a significant percentage of patients on estrogen-containing oral contraceptives. For this reason, diabetic patients should be carefully observed while receiving estrogen.

4. **Hypercalcemia.** Administration of estrogens may lead to severe hypercalcemia in patients with breast cancer and bone metastases. If this occurs, the drug should be stopped and appropriate measures taken to reduce the serum calcium level.

Meprobamate

Drug Dependence—Physical dependence, psychological dependence, and abuse have occurred. When chronic intoxication from prolonged use occurs, it usually involves ingestion of greater than recommended doses and is manifested by ataxia, slurred speech, and vertigo. Therefore, careful supervision of dose and amounts prescribed is advised, as well as avoidance of prolonged administration, especially for alcoholics and other patients with a known propensity for taking excessive quantities of drugs.

Sudden withdrawal of the drug after prolonged and excessive use may precipitate recurrence of preexisting symptoms, such as anxiety, anorexia, or insomnia, or withdrawal reactions, such as vomiting, ataxia, tremors, muscle twitching, confusional states, hallucinosis, and, rarely, convulsive seizures. Such seizures are more likely to occur in persons with central nervous system damage or preexistent or latent convulsive disorders. Onset of withdrawal symptoms occurs usually within 12 to 48 hours after discontinuation of meprobamate; symptoms usually cease within the next 12 to 48 hours.

When excessive dosage has continued for weeks or months, dosage should be reduced gradually over a period of one or two weeks rather than abruptly stopped. Alternatively, a short-acting barbiturate may be substituted, then gradually withdrawn.

Potentially Hazardous Tasks—Patients should be warned that this drug may impair the mental and/or physical abilities required for the performance of potentially hazardous tasks such as driving a motor vehicle or operating machinery.

Additive Effects—Since the effects of meprobamate and alcohol or meprobamate and other CNS depressants of psychotropic drugs may be additive, appropriate caution should be exercised with patients who take more than one of these agents simultaneously.

Usage in Pregnancy and Lactation

An increased risk of congenital malformations associated with the use of minor tranquilizers (meprobamate, chlordiazepoxide, and diazepam) during the first trimester of pregnancy has been suggested in several studies. Because use of these drugs is rarely a matter of urgency, their use during this period should almost always be avoided. The possibility that a woman of childbearing potential may be pregnant at the time of institution of therapy should be considered. Patients should be advised that if they become pregnant during therapy or intend to become pregnant they should communicate with their physicians about the desirability of discontinuing the drug.

Meprobamate passes the placental barrier. It is present both in umbilical cord blood at or near maternal plasma levels and in breast milk of lactating mothers at concentrations two to four times that of maternal plasma. When use of meprobamate is contemplated in breast-feeding patients, the drug's higher concentrations in breast milk as compared to maternal plasma levels should be considered.

Usage in Children—This combination is not intended for use in children.

Precautions:

Conjugated Estrogens

A. General Precautions.

1. A complete medical and family history should be taken prior to the initiation of any estrogen therapy. The pretreatment and periodic physical examination should include special reference to blood pressure, breasts, abdomen, and pelvic organs, and should include a Papanicolau smear. As a general rule, estrogen should not be prescribed for longer than one year without another physical examination being performed.
2. Fluid retention—Because estrogens may cause some degree of fluid retention, conditions which might be influenced by this factor such as epilepsy, migraine, and cardiac or renal dysfunction, require careful observation.
3. Certain patients may develop undesirable manifestations of excessive estrogenic stimulation, such as abnormal or excessive uterine bleeding, mastodynia, etc.
4. Oral contraceptives appear to be associated with an increased incidence of mental depression.[24] Although it is not clear whether this is due to the estrogenic or progestogenic component of the contraceptive, patients with a history of depression should be carefully observed.
5. Preexisting uterine leiomyomata may increase in size during estrogen use.
6. The pathologist should be advised of estrogen therapy when relevant specimens are submitted.
7. Patients with a past history of jaundice during pregnancy have an increased risk of recurrence of jaundice while receiving estrogen-containing oral contraceptive therapy. If jaundice develops in any patient receiving estrogen, the medication should be discontinued while the cause is investigated.
8. Estrogens may be poorly metabolized in patients with impaired liver function and they should be administered with caution in such patients.
9. Because estrogens influence the metabolism of calcium and phosphorus, they should be used with caution in patients with metabolic bone diseases that are associated with hypercalcemia or in patients with renal insufficiency.
10. Because of the effects of estrogens on epiphyseal closure, they should be used judiciously in young patients in whom bone growth is not complete.

Continued on next page

Wallace—Cont.

11. Certain endocrine and liver function tests may be affected by estrogen-containing oral contraceptives. The following similar changes may be expected with larger doses of estrogen:
    a. Increased sulfobromophthalein retention.
    b. Increased prothrombin and factors VII, VIII, IX, and X; decreased antithrombin 3; increased norepinephrine-induced platelet aggregability.
    c. Increased thyroid binding globulin (TBG) leading to increased circulating total thyroid hormone, as measured by PBI, T4 by column, or T4 by radioimmunoassay. Free T3 resin uptake is decreased, reflecting the elevated TBG; free T4 concentration is unaltered.
    d. Impaired glucose tolerance.
    e. Decreased pregnanediol excretion.
    f. Reduced response to metyrapone test.
    g. Reduced serum folate concentration.
    h. Increased serum triglyceride and phospholipid concentration.

B. Information for the Patient. See text of Patient Package Insert which is attached below.

C. Pregnancy Category X (See Contraindications and Boxed Warning).

D. Nursing Mothers. As a general principle, the administration of any drug to nursing mothers should be done only when clearly necessary since many drugs are excreted in human milk.

Meprobamate

The lowest effective dose should be administered, particularly to elderly and/or debilitated patients, in order to preclude oversedation.

The possibility of suicide attempts should be considered and the least amount of drug feasible should be dispensed at any one time.

Meprobamate is metabolized in the liver and excreted by the kidney; to avoid its excess accumulation, caution should be exercised in administration to patients with compromised liver or kidney function.

Meprobamate occasionally may precipitate seizures in epileptic patients.

Adverse Reactions: Side effects with 'Milprem' (meprobamate + conjugated estrogens) have included nausea, drowsiness, withdrawal or breakthrough bleeding, and breast discomfort. While few of the side effects listed below have been reported with 'Milprem' administration, it is possible that any side effect which has occurred with either constituent alone might also occur when they are taken in combination.

Conjugated Estrogens

(See Warnings regarding induction of neoplasia, adverse effects on the fetus, increased incidence of gall bladder disease, and adverse effects similar to those of oral contraceptives, including thromboembolism.) The following additional adverse reactions have been reported with estrogenic therapy, including oral contraceptives:

1. **Genitourinary System** — breakthrough bleeding, spotting, change in menstrual flow; dysmenorrhea; premenstrual-like syndrome; amenorrhea during and after treatment; increase in size of uterine fibromyomata; vaginal candidiasis; change in cervical eversion and in degree of cervical secretion; cystitis-like syndrome.
2. **Breasts**—tenderness, enlargement, secretion.
3. **Gastrointestinal**—nausea, vomiting; abdominal cramps, bloating; cholestatic jaundice.
4. **Skin**—chloasma or melasma which may persist when drug is discontinued; erythema multiforme; erythema nodosum; hemorrhagic eruption; loss of scalp hair; hirsutism.
5. **Eyes**—steepening of corneal curvature; intolerance to contact lenses.
6. **CNS**—headache, migraine, dizziness, mental depression, chorea.
7. **Miscellaneous**—increase or decrease in weight; reduced carbohydrate tolerance; aggravation of porphyria; edema, changes in libido.

Meprobamate

Central Nervous System—drowsiness, ataxia, dizziness, slurred speech, headache, vertigo, weakness, paresthesias, impairment of visual accommodation, euphoria, overstimulation, paradoxical excitement, fast EEG activity.

Gastrointestinal—nausea, vomiting, diarrhea.

Cardiovascular—palpitations, tachycardia, various forms of arrhythmia, transient ECG changes, syncope; also, hypotensive crises (including one fatal case).

Allergic or Idiosyncratic—allergic or idiosyncratic reactions are usually seen within the period of the first to fourth dose in patients having had no previous contact with the drug. Milder reactions are characterized by an itchy, urticarial, or erythematous maculopapular rash which may be generalized or confined to the groin. Other reactions have included leukopenia, acute nonthrombocytopenic purpura, petechiae, ecchymoses, eosinophilia, peripheral edema, adenopathy, fever, fixed drug eruption with cross reaction to carisoprodol, and cross sensitivity between meprobamate/mebutamate and meprobamate/carbromal.

More severe hypersensitivity reactions, rarely reported, include hyperpyrexia, chills, angioneurotic edema, bronchospasm, oliguria, and anuria. Also, anaphylaxis, erythema multiforme, exfoliative dermatitis, stomatitis, proctitis, Stevens-Johnson syndrome, and bullous dermatitis, including one fatal case of the latter following administration of meprobamate in combination with prednisolone.

In case of allergic or idiosyncratic reactions to meprobamate, discontinue the drug and initiate appropriate symptomatic therapy, which may include epinephrine, antihistamines, and in severe cases corticosteroids. In evaluating possible allergic reactions, also consider allergy to excipients (information on excipients is available to physicians on request).

Hematologic (See also **Allergic or Idiosyncratic.**)—Agranulocytosis and aplastic anemia have been reported, although no causal relationship has been established. These cases rarely were fatal. Rare cases of thrombocytopenic purpura have been reported.

Other—Exacerbation of porphyric symptoms.

Acute Overdosage: Two cases of accidental 'Milprem' (meprobamate + conjugated estrogens) ingestion have been reported in children; one adult ingestion of 40 to 90 'Milprem'–400 tablets resulted in coma and hypotension; all three patients recovered completely. Large amounts of estrogen resulting from overdosage could cause sodium retention, requiring diuretic therapy.

Following is overdosage information on the 'Milprem' components:

Conjugated Estrogens

Numerous reports of ingestion of large doses of estrogen-containing oral contraceptives by young children indicate that serious ill effects do not occur. Overdosage of estrogen may cause nausea, and withdrawal bleeding may occur in females.

Meprobamate

Suicidal attempts with meprobamate have resulted in drowsiness, lethargy, stupor, ataxia, coma, shock, vasomotor and respiratory collapse. Some suicidal attempts have been fatal.

The following data on meprobamate tablets have been reported in the literature and from other sources. These data are not expected to correlate with each case (considering factors such as individual susceptibility and length of time from ingestion to treatment), but represent the **usual ranges** reported.

Acute simple overdose (meprobamate alone): Death has been reported with ingestion of as little as 12 gm meprobamate and survival with as much as 40 gm.

Blood Levels:

0.5 - 2.0 mg% represents the usual blood level range of meprobamate after therapeutic doses. The level may occasionally be as high as 3.0 mg%.

3 - 10 mg% usually corresponds to findings of mild to moderate symptoms of overdosage, such as stupor or light coma.

10 - 20 mg% usually corresponds to deeper coma, requiring more intensive treatment. Some fatalities occur.

At levels greater than 20 mg%, more fatalities than survivals can be expected.

Acute combined overdose (meprobamate with alcohol or other CNS depressants or psychotropic drugs): Since effects can be additive a history of ingestion of a low dose of meprobamate plus any of these compounds (or of a relatively low blood or tissue level) cannot be used as a prognostic indicator.

In cases where excessive doses have been taken, sleep ensues rapidly and blood pressure, pulse, and respiratory rates are reduced to basal levels. Any drug remaining in the stomach should be removed and symptomatic therapy given. Should respiration or blood pressure become compromised, respiratory assistance, central nervous system stimulants, and pressor agents should be administered cautiously as indicated. Meprobamate is metabolized in the liver and excreted by the kidney. Diuresis, osmotic (mannitol) diuresis, peritoneal dialysis, and hemodialysis have been used successfully. Careful monitoring of urinary output is necessary and caution should be taken to avoid overhydration. Relapse and death, after initial recovery, have been attributed to incomplete gastric emptying and delayed absorption. Meprobamate can be measured in biological fluid by two methods: colorimetric (Hoffman, A.J. and Ludwig, B.J.: *J Amer Pharm Assn 48:* 740, 1959) and gas chromatographic (Douglas, J.F. et al: *Anal Chem 39:* 956, 1967).

Dosage and Administration: 'Milprem' **should be administered cyclically for short-term use only** in the treatment of moderate to severe **vasomotor** symptoms, atrophic vaginitis, or kraurosis vulvae associated with the menopause when emotional symptoms (i.e., anxiety and tension) are also present and indicate the need for a tranquilizer. The lowest dose that will control symptoms should be chosen and medication should be discontinued as promptly as possible. Attempts to discontinue or taper medication should be made at 3 to 6 month intervals. The usual dosage of conjugated estrogen is 1.25 mg daily. The usual dosage of meprobamate is 1200 to 1600 mg daly.

'Milprem'–200 and 'Milprem'–400:

The usual dosage is one tablet of either strength three times daily administered cyclically (e.g., 3 weeks on and 1 week off). Use of 'Miltown' (meprobamate) alone, in equivalent dosage, during the one-week rest periods, should be considered for patients who have a continuing need for a tranquilizer for their anxiety and tension. Daily dosage should be adjusted to individual requirements and severity of symptoms. The daily dose of meprobamate should not exceed 2400 mg.

Treated patients with an intact uterus should be monitored closely for signs of endometrial cancer and appropriate diagnostic measures should be taken to rule out malignancy in the event of persistent or recurring abnormal vaginal bleeding.

How Supplied: 'Milprem'–200: Bottles of 100 (NDC 0037-5501-01). 'Milprem'–400: Bottles of 100 (NDC 0037-5401-01).

References:

1. Ziel, H. K. and W. D. Finkel, "Increased Risk of Endometrial Carcinoma Among Users of Conjugated Estrogens," *New England Journal of Medicine 293*:1167–1170, 1975.
2. Smith, D. C., R. Prentic, D. J. Thompson, and W. L. Hermann, "Association of Exogenous Estrogen and Endometrial Carcinoma," *New England Journal of Medicine 293*:1164–1167, 1975.
3. Mack, T. M., M. C. Pike, B. E. Henderson, R. I. Pfeffer, V. R. Gerkins, M. Arthur, and S. E. Brown, "Estrogens and Endometrial Cancer in a Retirement Community," *New England Journal of Medicine 294*:1262–1267, 1976.
4. Weiss, N. S., D. R. Szekely and D. F. Austin, "Increasing Incidence of Endometrial Cancer in the United States," *New England Journal of Medicine 294*:1259–1262, 1976.
5. Herbst, A. L., H. Ulfelder and D. C. Poskanzer, "Andenocarcinoma of Vagina," *New England Journal of Medicine 284*:878–881, 1971.
6. Greenwald, P., J. Barlow, P. Nasca, and W. Burnett, "Vaginal Cancer after Maternal Treatment with Synthetic Estrogens," *New England Journal of Medicine 285*:390–392, 1971.
7. Lanier, A., K. Noller, D. Decker, L. Elveback, and L. Kurland, "Cancer and Stilbestrol. A Follow-up of 1719 Persons Exposed to Estrogens In Utero and Born 1943–1959," *Mayo Clinic Proceedings 48*:793–799, 1973.
8. Herbst, A., R. Kurman, and R. Scully, "Vaginal and Cervical Abnormalities After Exposure to Stilbestrol In Utero," *Obstetrics and Gynecology 40*:287–298, 1972.
9. Herbst, A., S. Robboy, G. Macdonald, and R. Scully, "The Effects of Local Progesterone on Stilbestrol-Associated Vaginal Adenosis," *American Journal of Obstetrics and Gynecology 118*:607–615, 1974.
10. Herbst, A., D. Poskanzer, S. Robboy, L. Friedlander, and R. Scully, "Prenatal Exposure to Stilbestrol, A Prospective Comparison of Exposed Female Offspring with Unexposed Controls," *New England Journal of Medicine 292*:334–339, 1975.
11. Stafl, A., R. Mattingly, D. Foley, and W. Fetherston, "Clinical Diagnosis of Vaginal Adenosis," *Obstetrics and Gynecology 43*:118–128, 1974.
12. Sherman, A. I., M. Goldrath, A. Berlin, V. Vakhariya, F. Banooni, W. Michaels, P. Goodman, S. Brown, "Cervical-Vaginal Adenosis After *In Utero* Exposure to Synthetic Estrogens," *Obstetrics and Gynecology 44*:531–545, 1974.
13. Gal, I., B. Kirman, and J. Stern, "Hormone Pregnancy Tests and Congenital Malformation," *Nature 216*:83, 1967.
14. Levy, E. P., A. Cohen, and F. C. Fraser, "Hormone Treatment During Pregnancy and Congenital Heart Defects," *Lancet 1*:611, 1973.
15. Nora, J. and A. Nora, "Birth Defects and Oral Contraceptives," *Lancet 1*:941–942, 1973.
16. Janerich, D. T., J. M. Piper, and D. M. Glebatis, "Oral Contraceptives and Congenital Limb-Reduction Defects," *New England Journal of Medicine 291*:697–700, 1974.
17. "Estrogens for Oral or Parenteral Use," *Federal Register 40*:8212, 1975.
18. Boston Collaborative Drug Surveillance Program "Surgically Confirmed Gall Bladder Disease, Venous Thromboembolism and Breast Tumors in Relation to Post-Menopausal Estrogen Therapy," *New England Journal of Medicine 290*:15–19, 1974.

18a Hoover, R., L. A. Gray, Sr., P. Cole, and B. MacMahon, "Menopausal Estrogens and Breast Cancer," *New England Journal of Medicine 295*:401–405, 1976.

19. Boston Collaborative Drug Surveillance Program, "Oral Contraceptives and Venous Thromboembolic Disease, Surgically Confirmed Gall Bladder Disease, and Breast Tumors," *Lancet 1*:1399–1404, 1973.
20. Daniel, D. G., H. Campbell, and A. C. Turnbull, "Puerperal Thromboembolism and Suppression of Lactation," *Lancet 2*:287–289, 1967.
21. The Veterans Administration Cooperative Urological Research Group, "Carcinoma of the Prostate: Treatment Comparisons," *Journal of Urology 98*:516–522, 1967.
22. Bailar, J. C., "Thromboembolism and Oestrogen Therapy," *Lancet 2*:560, 1967.
23. Blackard, C., R. Doe, G. Mellinger, and D. Byar, "Incidence of Cardiovascular Disease and Death in Patients Receiving Diethylstilbestrol for Carcinoma of the Prostate," *Cancer 26*:249–256, 1970.
24. Royal College of General Practitioners, "Oral Contraception and Thromboembolic Disease," *Journal of the Royal College of General Practitioners 13*:267–279, 1967.
25. Inman, W. H. W. and M. P. Vessey, "Investigation of Deaths from Pulmonary, Coronary, and Cerebral Thrombosis and Embolism in Women of Child-Bearing Age," *British Medical Journal 2*:193–199, 1968.
26. Vessey, M. P. and R. Doll, "Investigation of Relation Between Use of Oral Contraceptives and Thromboembolic Disease. A Further Report," *British Medical Journal 2*:651–657, 1969.
27. Sartwell, P. E., A. T. Masi, F. G. Arthes, G. R. Greene, and H. E. Smith, "Thromboembolism and Oral Contraceptives: An Epidemiological Case Control Study," *American Journal of Epidemiology 90*:365–380, 1969.
28. Collaborative Group for the Study of Stroke in Young Women, "Oral Contraception and Increased Risk of Cerebral Ischemia or Thrombosis," *New England Journal of Medicine 288*:871–878, 1973.
29. Collaborative Group for the Study of Stroke in Young Women, "Oral Contraceptives and Stroke in Young Women: Associated Risk Factors," *Journal of the American Medical Association 231*:718–722, 1975.
30. Mann, J. I. and W. H. W. Inman, "Oral Contraceptives and Death from Myocardial Infarction," *British Medical Journal 2*:245–248, 1975.
31. Mann, J. I., M. P. Vessey, M. Thorogood, and R. Doll, "Myocardial Infarction in Young Women with Special Reference to Oral Contraceptive Practice," *British Medical Journal 2*:241–245, 1975.
32. Inman, W. H. W., V. P. Vessey, B. Westerholm, and A. Engelund, "Thromboembolic Disease and the Steroidal Content of Oral Contraceptives," *British Medical Journal 2*:203–209, 1970.
33. Stolley, P. D., J. A. Tonascia, M. S. Tockman, P. E. Sartwell, A. H. Rutledge, and M. P. Jacobs, "Thrombosis with Low-Estrogen Oral Contraceptives," *American Journal of Epidemiology 102*:197–208, 1975.
34. Vessey, M. P., R. Doll, A. S. Fairbairn, and G. Glober, "Post-Operative Thromboembolism and the Use of the Oral Contraceptives," *British Medical Journal 3*:123–126, 1970.
35. Greene, G. R. and P. E. Sartwell, "Oral Contraceptive Use in Patients with Thromboembolism Following Surgery, Trauma or Infection," *American Journal of Public Health 62*:680–685, 1972.
36. Rosenberg, L., M. B. Armstrong and H. Jick, "Myocardial Infarction and Estrogen Therapy in Postmenopausal Women," *New England Journal of Medicine 294*:1256–1259, 1976.
37. Coronary Drug Project Research Group, "The Coronary Drug Project: Initial Findings Leading to Modifications of Its Research Protocol," *Journal of the American Medical Association 214*:1303–1313, 1970.
38. Baum, J., F. Holtz, J. J. Bookstein, and E. W. Klein, "Possible Association Between Benign Hepatomas and Oral Contraceptives," *Lancet 2*:926–928, 1973.
39. Mays, E. T., W. M. Christopherson, M. M. Mahr, and H. C. Williams, "Hepatic Changes in Young Women Ingesting Contraceptive Steroids, Hepatic Hemorrhage and Primary Hepatic Tumors," *Journal of the American Medical Association 235*:730–782, 1976.
40. Edmondson, H. A., B. Henderson, and B. Benton, "Liver Cell Adenomas Associated with the Use of Oral Contraceptives," *New England Journal of Medicine 294*:470–472, 1976.
41. Pfeffer, R. I. and S. Van Den Noort, "Estrogen Use and Stroke Risk in Postmenopausal Women," *American Journal of Epidemiology 103*:445–456, 1976.

Patient Package Insert
for
MILPREM®
(meprobamate + conjugated estrogens)

Your doctor has prescribed 'Milprem' for the management of certain symptoms of the menopause. Because 'Milprem' contains conjugated estrogens, the information on estrogens set forth below is being made available to you. If you have any questions after reading this information, please consult with your doctor.

What You Should Know About Estrogens: Estrogens are female hormones produced by the ovaries. The ovaries make several different kinds of estrogens. In addition, scientists have been able to make a variety of synthetic estrogens. As far as we know, all these estrogens have similar properties and therefore much the same usefulness, side effects, and risks. This leaflet is intended to help you understand what estrogens are used for, the risks involved in their use, and how to use them as safely as possible.

This leaflet includes the most important informatin about estrogens, but not all the information. If you want to know more, you can ask your doctor or pharmacist to let you read the package insert prepared for the doctor.

Uses of Estrogen: Estrogens are prescribed by doctors for a number of purposes, including:

1. To provide estrogen during a period of adjustment when a woman's ovaries no longer produce it, in order to prevent certain uncomfortable symptoms of estrogen deficiency. (All women normally stop producing estrogens, generally between the ages of 45 and 55; this is called the menopause.)
2. To prevent symptoms of estrogen deficiency when a woman's ovaries have been removed surgically before the natural menopause.
3. To prevent pregnancy. (Estrogens are given along with a progestogen, another female hormone; these combinations are called oral contraceptives or birth control pills. Patient labeling is available to women taking oral contraceptives and they will not be discussed in this leaflet.)
4. To treat certain cancers in women and men.
5. To prevent painful swelling of the breasts after pregnancy in women who choose not to nurse their babies.

THERE IS NO PROPER USE OF ESTROGENS IN A PREGNANT WOMAN.

Estrogens in the Menopause: In the natural course of their lives, all women eventually experience a decrease in estrogen production. This usually occurs between ages 45 and 55 but may occur earlier or later. Sometimes the ovaries may need to be removed before natural

Continued on next page

Wallace—Cont.

menopause by an operation, producing a "surgical menopause".

When the amount of estrogen in the blood begins to decrease, many women may develop typical symptoms: Feelings of warmth in the face, neck, and chest or sudden intense episodes of heat and sweating throughout the body (called "hot flashes" or "hot flushes"). These symptoms are sometimes very uncomfortable. A few women eventually develop changes in the vagina (called "atrophic vaginitis") which cause discomfort, especially during and after intercourse.

Estrogens can be prescribed to treat these symptoms of the menopause. It is estimated that considerably more than half of all women undergoing the menopause have only mild symptoms or no symptoms at all and therefore do not need estrogens. Other women may need estrogens for a few months, while their bodies adjust to lower estrogen levels. Sometimes the need will be for periods longer than six months. In an attempt to avoid over-stimulation of the uterus (womb), estrogens are usually given cyclically during each month of use, that is, three weeks of pills followed by one week without pills.

Sometimes women experience nervous symptoms or depression during menopause. There is no evidence that estrogens are effective for such symptoms and they should not be used to treat them, although other treatment may be needed.

You may have heard that taking estrogens for long periods (years) after the menopause will keep your skin soft and supple and keep you feeling young. There is no evidence that this is so, however, and such long-term treatment carries important risks.

Estrogens To Prevent Swelling of The Breasts After Pregnancy: If you do not breast feed your baby after delivery, your breasts may fill up with milk and become painful and engorged. This usually begins about 3 to 4 days after delivery and may last for a few days to up to a week or more. Sometimes the discomfort is severe, but usually it is not and can be controlled by pain relieving drugs such as aspirin and by binding the breasts up tightly. Estrogens can be used to try to prevent the breasts from filling up. While this treatment is sometimes successful, in many cases the breasts fill up to some degree in spite of treatment. The dose of estrogens needed to prevent pain and swelling of the breasts is much larger than the dose needed to treat symptoms of the menopause and this may increase your chances of developing blood clots in the legs or lungs (see below). Therefore, it is important that you discuss the benefits and the risks of estrogen use with your doctor if you have decided not to breast feed your baby.

The Dangers of Estrogens:

1. **Cancer of the uterus.** If estrogens are used in the postmenopausal period for more than a year, there is an increased risk of **endometrial cancer** (cancer of the uterus). Women taking estrogens have roughly 5 to 10 times as great a chance of getting this cancer as women who take no estrogens. To put this another way, while a postmenopausal woman not taking estrogens has 1 chance in 1,000 each year of getting cancer of the uterus, a woman taking estrogens has 5 to 10 chances in 1,000 each year. For this reason **it is important to take estrogens only when you really need them.** The risk of this cancer is greater the longer estrogens are used and also seems to be greater when larger doses are taken. For this reason **it is important to take the lowest dose of estrogen that will control symptoms and to take it only as long as it is needed.** If estrogens are needed for longer periods of time, your doctor will want to reevaluate your need for estrogens at least every six months.
   Women using estrogens should report any irregular vaginal bleeding to their doctors; such bleeding may be of no importance, but it can be an early warning of cancer of the uterus. If you have undiagnosed vaginal bleeding, you should not use estrogens until a diagnosis is made and you are certain there is no cancer of the uterus.
   If you have had your uterus completely removed (total hysterectomy), there is no danger of developing cancer of the uterus.
2. **Other possible cancers.** Estrogens can cause development of other tumors in animals, such as tumors of the breast, cervix, vagina, or liver, when given for a long time. At present there is no good evidence that women using estrogen in the menopause have an increased risk of such tumors, but there is no way yet to be sure they do not; and one study raises the possibility that use of estrogens in the menopause may increase the risk of breast cancer many years later. This is a further reason to use estrogens only when clearly needed. While you are taking estrogens, it is important that you go to your doctor at least once a year for a physical examination. Also, if members of your family have had breast cancer or if you have breast nodules or abnormal mammograms (breast x-rays), your doctor may wish to carry out more frequent examinations of your breasts.
3. **Gall bladder disease.** Women who use estrogens after menopause are more likely to develop gall bladder disease needing surgery as women who do not use estrogens. Birth control pills have a similar effect.
4. **Abnormal blood clotting.** Oral contraceptives increase the risk of blood clotting in various parts of the body. This can result in a stroke (if the clot is in the brain), a heart attack (clot in a blood vessel of the heart), or a pulmonary embolus (a clot which forms in the legs or pelvis, then breaks off and travels to the lungs). Any of these can be fatal.
   At this time use of estrogens in the menopause is not known to cause such blood clotting, but this has not been fully studied and there could still prove to be such a risk. It is recommended that if you have had clotting in the legs or lungs or a heart attack or stroke while you were using estrogens or birth control pills, you should not use estrogens (unless they are being used to treat cancer of the breast or prostate). If you have had a stroke or heart attack or if you have angina pectoris, estrogens should be used with great caution and only if clearly needed (for example, if you have severe symptoms of the menopause).
   The larger doses of estrogen used to prevent swelling of the breasts after pregnancy have been reported to cause clotting in the legs and lungs.

Special Warning About Pregnancy: You should not receive estrogen if you are pregnant. If this should occur, there is a greater than usual chance that the developing child will be born with a birth defect, although the possibility remains fairly small. A female child may have an increased risk of developing cancer of the vagina or cervix later in life (in the teens or twenties). Every possible effort should be made to avoid exposure to estrogens during pregnancy. If exposure occurs, see your doctor.

Other Effects of Estrogens: In addition to the serious known risks of estrogens described above, estrogens have the following side effects and potential risks:

1. **Nausea and vomiting.** The most common side effect of estrogen therapy is nausea. Vomiting is less common.
2. **Effects on breasts.** Estrogens may cause breast tenderness or enlargement and may cause the breasts to secrete a liquid. These effects are not dangerous.
3. **Effects on the uterus.** Estrogens may cause benign fibroid tumors of the uterus to get larger.
   Some women will have menstrual bleeding when estrogens are stopped. But if the bleeding occurs on days you are still taking estrogens you should report this to your doctor.
4. **Effects on liver.** Women taking oral contraceptives develop on rare occasions a tumor of the liver which can rupture and bleed into the abdomen. So far, these tumors have not been reported in women using estrogens in the menopause, but you should report any swelling or unusual pain or tenderness in the abdomen to your doctor immediately.
   Women with a past history of jaundice (yellowing of the skin and white parts of the eyes) may get jaundice again during estrogen use. If this occurs, stop taking estrogens and see your doctor.
5. **Darkening of the skin.** Estrogens may cause an increase in pigmentation similar to that occurring during pregnancy.
6. **Other effects.** Estrogens may cause excess fluid to be retained in the body. This may make some conditions worse, such as epilepsy, migraine, heart disease, or kidney disease.

Summary: Estrogens have important uses, but they have serious risks as well. You must decide, with your doctor, whether the risks are acceptable to you in view of the benefits of treatment. Except where your doctor has prescribed estrogens for use in special cases of cancer of the breast or prostate, you should not use estrogens if you have cancer of the breast or uterus, are pregnant, have undiagnosed abnormal vaginal bleeding, clotting in the legs or lungs, or have had a stroke, heart attack or angina, or clotting in the legs or lungs in the past while you were taking estrogens.

You can use estrogens as safely as possible by understanding that your doctor will require regular physical examinations while you are taking them and will try to discontinue the drug as soon as possible and use the smallest dose possible. Be alert for signs of trouble including:

1. Abnormal bleeding from the vagina.
2. Pains in the calves or chest or sudden shortness of breath, or coughing blood (indicating possible clots in the legs, heart, or lungs).
3. Severe headache, dizziness, faintness, or changes in vision (indicating possible developing clots in the brain or eye).
4. Breast lumps (you should ask your doctor how to examine your own breasts).
5. Jaundice (yellowing of the skin).
6. Mental depression.

Based on his or her assessment of your medical needs, your doctor has prescribed this drug for you. Do not give the drug to anyone else.

How Supplied:

'Milprem' is available in two formulations for oral use:

'Milprem'-400: dark pink, coated tablets, each containing meprobamate, U.S.P., 400 mg and conjugated estrogens, U.S.P., 0.45 mg.

'Milprem'-200: light pink, coated tablets, each containing meprobamate, U.S.P., 200 mg and conjugated estrogens, U.S.P., 0.45 mg.

WALLACE LABORATORIES, Distribution
Division of
CARTER-WALLACE, INC.
Cranbury, New Jersey 08512

Manufactured by Ayerst Laboratories
Rouses Point, New York

Rev. 6/79

[*Shown in Product Identification Section*]

MILTOWN®/MILTOWN® 600 ℭ
(meprobamate/meprobamate 600 mg)

Description: Meprobamate is a white powder with a characteristic odor and a bitter taste. It is slightly soluble in water, freely soluble in acetone and alcohol, and sparingly soluble in ether.

Actions: Meprobamate is a carbamate derivative which has been shown in animal studies to have effects at multiple sites in the central nervous system, including the thalamus and limbic system.

Indications: Meprobamate is indicated for the relief of anxiety and tension; as an adjunct in the treatment of various disease states in which anxiety and tension are manifested; and to promote sleep in anxious, tense patients.
The effectiveness of 'Miltown' in long-term use, that is, more than 4 months, has not been assessed by systematic clinical studies. The physician should periodically reassess the usefulness of the drug for the individual patient.

Contraindications: Acute intermittent porphyria as well as allergic or idiosyncratic reactions to meprobamate or related compounds such as carisoprodol, mebutamate, tybamate, or carbromal.

Warnings:
Drug Dependence
Physical dependence, psychological dependence, and abuse have occurred. When chronic intoxication from prolonged use occurs, it usually involves ingestion of greater than recommended doses and is manifested by ataxia, slurred speech, and vertigo. Therefore, careful supervision of dose and amounts prescribed is advised, as well as avoidance of prolonged administration, especially for alcoholics and other patients with a known propensity for taking excessive quantities of drugs.
Sudden withdrawal of the drug after prolonged and excessive use may precipitate recurrence of preexisting symptoms, such as anxiety, anorexia, or insomnia, or withdrawal reactions, such as vomiting, ataxia, tremors, muscle twitching, confusional states, hallucinosis, and, rarely, convulsive seizures. Such seizures are more likely to occur in persons with central nervous system damage or preexistent or latent convulsive disorders. Onset of withdrawal symptoms occurs usually within 12 to 48 hours after discontinuation of meprobamate; symptoms usually cease within the next 12 to 48 hours.
When excessive dosage has continued for weeks or months, dosage should be reduced gradually over a period of one or two weeks rather than abruptly stopped. Alternatively, a short-acting barbiturate may be substituted, then gradually withdrawn.

Potentially Hazardous Tasks
Patients should be warned that this drug may impair the mental and/or physical abilities required for the performance of potentially hazardous tasks such as driving a motor vehicle or operating machinery.

Additive Effects
Since the effects of meprobamate and alcohol or meprobamate and other CNS depressants or psychotropic drugs may be additive, appropriate caution should be exercised with patients who take more than one of these agents simultaneously.

Usage in Pregnancy and Lactation
An increased risk of congenital malformations associated with the use of minor tranquilizers (meprobamate, chlordiazepoxide, and diazepam) during the first trimester of pregnancy has been suggested in several studies. Because use of these drugs is rarely a matter of urgency, their use during this period should almost always be avoided. The possibility that a woman of childbearing potential may be pregnant at the time of institution of therapy should be considered. Patients should be advised that if they become pregnant during therapy or intend to become pregnant they should communicate with their physicians about the desirability of discontinuing the drug.
Meprobamate passes the placental barrier. It is present both in umbilical cord blood at or near maternal plasma levels and in breast milk of lactating mothers at concentrations two to four times that of maternal plasma. When use of meprobamate is contemplated in breast-feeding patients, the drug's higher concentrations in breast milk as compared to maternal plasma levels should be considered.

Usage in Children—Meprobamate should not be administered to children under age six, since there is a lack of documented evidence for safety and effectiveness in this age group.
'Miltown' 600 (meprobamate 600 mg)—This dosage form is not intended for use in children.
Precautions: The lowest effective dose should be administered, particularly to elderly and/or debilitated patients, in order to preclude oversedation.
The possibility of suicide attempts should be considered and the least amount of drug feasible should be dispensed at any one time.
Meprobamate is metabolized in the liver and excreted by the kidney; to avoid its excess accumulation, caution should be exercised in administration to patients with compromised liver or kidney function.
Meprobamate occasionally may precipitate seizures in epileptic patients.
Adverse Reactions:
Central Nervous System
Drowsiness, ataxia, dizziness, slurred speech, headache, vertigo, weakness, paresthesias, impairment of visual accommodation, euphoria, overstimulation, paradoxical excitement, fast EEG activity.
Gastrointestinal
Nausea, vomiting, diarrhea.
Cardiovascular
Palpitations, tachycardia, various forms of arrhythmia, transient ECG changes, syncope; also, hypotensive crises (including one fatal case).
Allergic or Idiosyncratic
Allergic or idiosyncratic reactions are usually seen within the period of the first to fourth dose in patients having had no previous contact with the drug. Milder reactions are characterized by an itchy, urticarial, or erythematous maculopapular rash which may be generalized or confined to the groin. Other reactions have included leukopenia, acute nonthrombocytopenic purpura, petachiae, ecchymoses, eosinophilia, peripheral edema, adenopathy, fever, fixed drug eruption with cross reaction to carisoprodol, and cross sensitivity between meprobamate / mebutamate and meprobamate/carbromal.
More severe hypersensitivity reactions, rarely reported, include hyperpyrexia, chills, angioneurotic edema, bronchospasm, oliguria, and anuria. Also, anaphylaxis, erythema multiforme, exfoliative dermatitis, stomatitis, proctitis, Stevens-Johnson syndrome, and bullous dermatitis, including one fatal case of the latter following administration of meprobamate in combination with prednisolone.
In case of allergic or idiosyncratic reactions to meprobamate, discontinue the drug and initiate appropriate symptomatic therapy, which may include epinephrine, antihistamines, and in severe cases corticosteroids. In evaluating possible allergic reactions, also consider allergy to excipients (information on excipients is available to physicians on request).
Hematologic
(See also **Allergic or Idiosyncratic.**) Agranulocytosis and aplastic anemia have been reported, although no causal relationship has been established. These cases rarely were fatal. Rare cases of thrombocytopenic purpura have been reported.
Other
Exacerbation of prophyric symptoms.
Dosage and Administration:
Adults: **'Miltown'** (meprobamate)—the usual dosage is 1200 to 1600 mg daily administered in three or four divided doses.
'Miltown' 600 (meprobamate 600 mg)—the recommended dosage is one tablet twice a day. Doses of meprobamate above 2400 mg daily are not recommended.
Children:
'Miltown' (meprobamate)—the usual dosage for children ages six to twelve is 100 to 200 mg two or three times daily. Meprobamate is not recommended for children under six.
'Miltown' 600 (meprobamate 600 mg)—is not intended for use in children.
Overdosage: Suicidal attempts with meprobamate have resulted in drowsiness, lethargy, stupor, ataxia, coma, shock, vasomotor and respiratory collapse. Some suicidal attempts have been fatal.
The following data on meprobamate tablets have been reported in the literature and from other sources. These data are not expected to correlate with each case (considering factors such as individual susceptibility and length of time from ingestion to treatment), but represent the *usual ranges* reported.
Acute simple overdose (meprobamate alone): Death has been reported with ingestion of as little as 12 gm meprobamate and survival with as much as 40 gm.
Blood Levels
0.5—2.0 mg% represents the usual blood level range of meprobamate after therapeutic doses. The level may occasionally be as high as 3.0 mg%.
3— 10 mg% usually corresponds to findings of mild to moderate symptoms of overdosage, such as stupor or light coma.
10— 20 mg% usually corresponds to deeper coma, requiring more intensive treatment. Some fatalities occur.
At levels greater than 20 mg%, more fatalities than survivals can be expected.
Acute combined overdose (meprobamate with alcohol or other CNS depressants or psychotropic drugs): Since effects can be additive a history of ingestion of a low dose of meprobamate plus any of these compounds (or of a relatively low blood or tissue level) cannot be used as a prognostic indicator.
In cases where excessive doses have been taken, sleep ensues rapidly and blood pressure, pulse, and respiratory rates are reduced to basal levels. Any drug remaining in the stomach should be removed and symptomatic therapy given. Should respiration or blood pressure become compromised, respiratory assistance, central nervous system stimulants, and pressor agents should be administered cautiously as indicated. Meprobamate is metabolized in the liver and excreted by the kidney. Diuresis, osmotic (mannitol) diuresis, peritoneal dialysis, and hemodialysis have been used successfully. Careful monitoring of urinary output is necessary and caution should be taken to avoid overhydration. Relapse and death, after initial recovery, have been attributed to incomplete gastric emptying and delayed absorption. Meprobamate can be measured in biological fluids by two methods: colorimetric (Hoffman, A.J. and Ludwig, B.J.: *J Amer Pharm Assn 48*: 740, 1959) and gas chromatographic (Douglas, J.F. et al: *Anal Chem 39*: 956, 1967).
How Supplied: 'Miltown' (meprobamate, U.S.P.) is available as:

Continued on next page

Wallace—Cont.

—400 mg white, scored tablets in bottles of
100 (NDC 0037-1001-01)
500 (NDC 0037-1001-03)
1000 (NDC 0037-1001-02)

—200 mg white, sugar-coated tablets in bottles of
100 (NDC 0037-1101-01)

'Miltown' 600 is available as white, capsule-shaped tablets, each containing 600 mg meprobamate, U.S.P.—in bottles of
100 (NDC 0037-1601-01)

Rev. 2/78

[*Shown in Product Identification Section*]

MILTRATE® ℞

(meprobamate + pentaerythritol tetranitrate)

Description: 'Miltrate' is available in two formulations:

'Miltrate'—10: White tablets. Each tablet contains:

meprobamate, U.S.P. ....200 mg
pentaerythritol tetranitrate....................10 mg

'Miltrate' — 20: Orange tablets. Each tablet contains:

meprobamate, U.S.P...............................200 mg
pentaerythritol tetranitrate...................20 mg

Actions: 'Miltrate' combines meprobamate, a tranquilizing agent, with pentaerythritol tetranitrate.

Pentaerythritol tetranitrate (PETN)

The mechanism of action of PETN in the relief of angina pectoris is unknown at this time, although the basic pharmacologic action is to relax smooth muscle.

Meprobamate

Meprobamate is a carbamate derivative which has been shown in animal studies to have effects at multiple sites in the central nervous system, including the thalamus and limbic system.

Indications: Based on a review of this drug by the National Academy of Sciences—National Research Council and/or other information, FDA has classified the indication as follows:

"Possibly" effective: for the relief of angina pectoris (pain associated with coronary artery disease). It is not intended to abort the acute anginal episode but is widely regarded as useful in the prophylactic treatment of angina pectoris.

Final classification of this indication requires further investigation.

Contraindications:

Pentaerythritol tetranitrate (PETN)

Allergic or idiosyncratic reactions to PETN or related compounds contraindicate subsequent use. Like all nitrates, pentaerythritol tetranitrate should be avoided or prescribed cautiously for patients with glaucoma.

Meprobamate

Acute intermittent porphyria as well as allergic or idiosyncratic reactions to meprobamate or related compounds such as carisoprodol, mebutamate, tybamate, or carbromal.

Warnings:

Pentaerythritol tetranitrate (PETN)

The safety and efficacy of the nitrates and nitrites as a class in the acute phase of myocardial infarction (i.e., the period during which clinical and laboratory findings are unstable) have not been established.

Meprobamate

Drug Dependence—Physical dependence, psychological dependence, and abuse have occurred. When chronic intoxication from prolonged use occurs, it usually involves ingestion of greater than recommended doses and is manifested by ataxia, slurred speech, and vertigo. Therefore, careful supervision of dose and amounts prescribed is advised, as well as avoidance of prolonged administration, especially for alcoholics and other patients with a known propensity for taking excessive quantities of drugs.

Sudden withdrawal of the drug after prolonged and excessive use may precipitate recurrence of preexisting symptoms, such as anxiety, anorexia, or insomnia, or withdrawal reactions, such as vomiting, ataxia, tremors, muscle twitching, confusional states, hallucinosis, and, rarely, convulsive seizures. Such seizures are more likely to occur in persons with central nervous system damage or preexistent or latent convulsive disorders. Onset of withdrawal symptoms occurs usually within 12 to 48 hours after discontinuation of meprobamate; symptoms usually cease within the next 12 to 48 hours.

When excessive dosage has continued for weeks or months, dosage should be reduced gradually over a period of one or two weeks rather than abruptly stopped. Alternatively, a short-acting barbiturate may be substituted, then gradually withdrawn.

Potentially Hazardous Tasks

Patients should be warned that this drug may impair the mental and/or physical abilities required for the performance of potentially hazardous tasks such as driving a motor vehicle or operating machinery.

Additive Effects

Since the effects of meprobamate and alcohol or meprobamate and other CNS depressants or psychotropic drugs may be additive, appropriate caution should be exercised with patients who take more than one of these agents simultaneously.

Usage in Pregnancy and Lactation

An increased risk of congenital malformations associated with the use of minor tranquilizers (meprobamate, chlordiazepoxide, and diazepam) during the first trimester of pregnancy has been suggested in several studies. Because use of these drugs is rarely a matter of urgency, their use during this period should almost always be avoided. The possibility that a woman of childbearing potential may be pregnant at the time of institution of therapy should be considered. Patients should be advised that if they become pregnant during therapy or intend to become pregnant they should communicate with their physicians about the desirability of discontinuing the drug.

Meprobamate passes the placental barrier. It is present both in umbilical cord blood at or near maternal plasma levels and in breast milk of lactating mothers at concentrations two to four times that of maternal plasma. When use of meprobamate is contemplated in breast-feeding patients, the drug's higher concentrations in breast milk as compared to maternal plasma levels should be considered.

Usage in Children

This combination is not intended for use in children.

Precautions:

'Miltrate' — 20 only: This product contains FD&C Yellow No. 5 (tartrazine) which may cause allergic-type reactions (including bronchial asthma) in certain susceptible individuals. Although the overall incidence of FD&C Yellow No. 5 (tartrazine) sensitivity in the general population is low, it is frequently seen in patients who also have aspirin hypersensitivity.

Pentaerythritol tetranitrate (PETN)

Tolerance to pentaerythritol tetranitrate and cross tolerance to other nitrates may occur.

Meprobamate

The lowest effective dose should be administered, particularly to elderly and/or debilitated patients, in order to preclude oversedation.

The possibility of suicide attempts should be considered and the least amount of drug feasible should be dispensed at any one time.

Meprobamate is metabolized in the liver and excreted by the kidney; to avoid its excess accumulation, caution should be exercised in administration to patients with compromised liver or kidney function.

Meprobamate occasionally may precipitate seizures in epileptic patients.

Adverse Reactions: Side effects have included headache, nausea, sleepiness as well as insomnia, and dizziness. While few of the following reactions have been reported with 'Miltrate' (meprobamate + pentaerythritol tetranitrate) administration, it is possible that side effects which have occurred with the constituents alone might also occur when the combination is taken.

Pentaerythritol tetranitrate

The most common side effects occurring with the use of pentaerythritol tetranitrate are transient headache, nausea, and rash. Weakness, palpitation, flushing, gastrointestinal distress, light-headedness or dizziness, and exfoliative dermatitis have been reported on a few occasions. This drug can act as a physiological antagonist to norepinephrine, acetylcholine, histamine, and many other agents.

An occasional individual exhibits marked sensitivity to the hypotensive effects of nitrites and severe responses (nausea, vomiting, weakness, restlessness, pallor, perspiration, and collapse) can occur even with usual therapeutic doses. Alcohol may enhance this effect.

Meprobamate

Central Nervous System—Drowsiness, ataxia, dizziness, slurred speech, headache, vertigo, weakness, paresthesias, impairment of visual accommodation, euphoria, overstimulation, paradoxical excitement, fast EEG activity.

Gastrointestinal — Nausea, vomiting, diarrhea.

Cardiovascular — Palpitations, tachycardia, various forms of arrhythmia, transient ECG changes, syncope; also, hypotensive crises (including one fatal case).

Allergic or Idiosyncratic—Allergic or idiosyncratic reactions are usually seen within the period of the first to fourth dose in patients having had no previous contact with the drug. Milder reactions are characterized by an itchy, urticarial, or erythematous maculopapular rash which may be generalized or confined to the groin. Other reactions have included leukopenia, acute nonthrombocytopenic purpura, petechiae, ecchymoses, eosinophilia, peripheral edema, adenopathy, fever, fixed drug eruption with cross reaction to carisoprodol, and cross sensitivity between meprobamate/mebutamate and meprobamate/carbromal.

More severe hypersensitivity reactions, rarely reported, include hyperpyrexia, chills, angioneurotic edema, bronchospasm, oliguria, and anuria. Also, anaphylaxis, erythema multiforme, exfoliative dermatitis, stomatitis, proctitis, Stevens-Johnson syndrome, and bullous dermatitis, including one fatal case of the latter following administration of meprobamate in combination with prednisolone.

In case of allergic or idiosyncratic reactions to meprobamate, discontinue the drug and initiate appropriate symptomatic therapy, which may include epinephrine, antihistamines, and in severe cases corticosteroids. In evaluating possible allergic reactions, also consider allergy to excipients (information on excipients is available to physicians on request).

Hematologic (See also **Allergic or Idiosyncratic.**)—Agranulocytosis and aplastic anemia have been reported, although no causal relationship has been established. These cases rarely were fatal. Rare cases of thrombocytopenic purpura have been reported.

Other—Exacerbation of porphyric symptoms.

Dosage and Administration:

The usual adult dosages are:

'Miltrate'-10: One or two tablets before meals and at bedtime.

'Miltrate'-20: One tablet before meals and at bedtime.

Individualization of dosage is required for maximum therapeutic effect.

(NOTE: When titration of the doses of the individual components of 'Miltrate' [meprobamate + pentaerythritol tetranitrate] is desired, meprobamate is available as 'Miltown' [meprobamate] tablets and as 'Meprospan' [meprobamate, sustained release] capsules. The usual dose of meprobamate is 1200 to 1600 mg daily. Doses of meprobamate above 2400 mg per day are not recommended.)

Overdosage: Although no cases of overdosage have been reported with 'Miltrate' (meprobamate + pentaerythritol tetranitrate), following is information on the separate components.

Pentaerythritol tetranitrate

Acute overdosage can produce effects as noted under **Adverse Reactions.** Although organic nitrates do not directly cause methemoglobinemia, the nitrates can be converted to nitrites by intestinal bacteria and it is possible that methemoglobinemia could occur. Infants and children would be more susceptible than adults because of differences in intestinal pH and bacterial flora.

Should methemoglobinemia occur, the recommended treatment is a 1% aqueous solution of methylene blue, 1 to 2 mg/kg body weight, injected intravenously over a period of several minutes. This may be repeated at hourly intervals if cyanosis has not disappeared, but the total dosage should not exceed 7 mg/kg.

Meprobamate

Suicidal attempts with meprobamate have resulted in drowsiness, lethargy, stupor, ataxia, coma, shock, vasomotor and respiratory collapse. Some suicidal attempts have been fatal.

The following data on meprobamate tablets have been reported in the literature and from other sources. These data are not expected to correlate with each case (considering factors such as individual susceptibility and length of time from ingestion to treatment), but represent the *usual ranges* reported.

Acute simple overdose (meprobamate alone): Death has been reported with ingestion of as little as 12 gm meprobamate and survival with as much as 40 gm.

Blood Levels:

0.5 — 2.0 mg% represents the usual blood level range of meprobamate after therapeutic doses. The level may occasionally be as high as 3.0 mg%.

3 —10 mg% usually corresponds to findings of mild to moderate symptoms of overdosage, such as stupor or light coma.

10 —20 mg% usually corresponds to deeper coma, requiring more intensive treatment. Some fatalities occur.

At levels greater than 20 mg%, more fatalities than survivals can be expected.

Acute combined overdose (meprobamate with alcohol or other CNS depressants or psychotropic drugs): Since effects can be additive, a history of ingestion of a low dose of meprobamate plus any of these compounds (or of a relatively low blood or tissue level) cannot be used as a prognostic indicator.

In cases where excessive doses have been taken, sleep ensues rapidly and blood pressure, pulse, and respiratory rates are reduced to basal levels. Any drug remaining in the stomach should be removed and symptomatic therapy given. Should respiration or blood pressure become compromised, respiratory assistance, central nervous system stimulants, and pressor agents should be administered cautiously as indicated. Meprobamate is metabolized in the liver and excreted by the kidney. Diuresis, osmotic (mannitol) diuresis, peritoneal dialysis, and hemodialysis have been used successfully. Careful monitoring of urinary output is necessary and caution should be taken to avoid overhydration. Relapse and death, after initial recovery, have been attributed to incomplete gastric emptying and delayed absorption. Meprobamate can be measured in biological fluids by two methods: colorimetric (Hoffman, A.J. and Ludwig, B.J.: *J Amer Pharm Assn* **48**: 740, 1959) and gas chromatographic (Douglas, J.F. et al: *Anal Chem* **39**: 956, 1967).

How Supplied: 'Miltrate'—10: Bottles of 100 (NDC 0037-5201-01) and 'Miltrate'—20: Bottles of 100 (NDC 0037-5301-01).

Rev. 7/79

[*Shown in Product Identification Section*]

ORGANIDIN® ℞

(iodinated glycerol)
Solution, Tablets, Elixir

Description: Organidin® (iodinated glycerol) is a stable complex formed by the interaction of iodine and glycerol; its active ingredient is iodopropylidene glycerol. Organidin formulations contain virtually no inorganic iodides and no free iodine and are stable in various media, including gastric juice. **Solution:** 5%, containing 50 mg Organidin (25 mg organically bound iodine) per ml. **Tablets:** containing 30 mg Organidin (15 mg organically bound iodine). **Elixir:** 1.2%, containing 60 mg Organidin (30 mg organically bound iodine) per 5 ml teaspoonful. Alcohol, 21.75% by volume.

Actions: Organidin increases the output of thin respiratory tract fluid and helps liquefy tenacious mucus in the bronchial tree.

Indications: Mucolytic-expectorant for adjunctive treatment in respiratory tract conditions, such as: bronchitis, bronchial asthma, pulmonary emphysema, cystic fibrosis, chronic sinusitis, or after surgery to help prevent atelectasis.

Contraindications: History of marked sensitivity to inorganic iodides; hypersensitivity to any of the ingredients or related compounds.

Warnings: Discontinue use if skin rash or other evidence of hypersensitivity appears.

Precautions: Dermatitis and other reversible manifestations of iodism have been reported in patients sensitive to iodine with the chronic use of inorganic iodides and interference with laboratory determinations of PBI has also occurred. Although these have not been reported to be a problem clinically with the use of Organidin, they should be kept in mind in patients receiving these preparations for prolonged periods.

Adverse Reactions: Gastrointestinal irritation, rash and hypersensitivity have rarely been reported.

Dosage and Administration: *Adults*—**Solution:** 20 drops (60 mg) 4 times a day, with liquid. **Tablets:** 2 tablets 4 times a day, with liquid. **Elixir:** 1 teaspoonful 4 times a day.

Children—Up to one-half the adult dosage, based on the child's weight. Each drop is equivalent to approximately 3 mg of Organidin (iodinated glycerol).

How Supplied: Organidin is available as:

Solution: 5%, in 30 ml dropper bottles (NDC 0037-4211-10)

Tablets: 30 mg, in bottles of 100 (NDC 0037-4224-40)

[*Shown in Product Identification Section*]

Elixir: 1.2% in bottles of one pint (NDC 0037-4213-30) and one gallon (NDC 0037-4213-40).

Rev. 7/78

RONDOMYCIN® ℞

(methacycline hydrochloride)

Description: 'Rondomycin' (methacycline HCl) is a broad-spectrum antibiotic synthetically derived from oxytetracycline. Chemical dehydration at the 6-position yields a structural homologue which is a light-yellow crystalline powder with a chemical designation of 6 methylene-5-oxytetracycline.

Actions: The tetracyclines are primarily bacteriostatic and are thought to exert their antimicrobial effect by the inhibition of protein synthesis. Tetracyclines are active against a wide range of gram-negative and gram-positive organisms.

The drugs in the tetracycline class have closely similar antimicrobial spectra, and cross-resistance among them is common. Microorganisms may be considered susceptible if the MIC (minimum inhibitory concentration) is not more than 4.0 mcg/ml and intermediate if the MIC is 4.0 to 12.5 mcg/ml.

Susceptibility plate testing: A tetracycline disc may be used to determine microbial susceptibility to drugs in the tetracycline class. If the Kirby-Bauer method of disc susceptibility testing is used, a 30 mcg tetracycline disc should give a zone of at least 19 mm when tested against a tetracycline-susceptible bacterial strain.

Tetracyclines are readily absorbed and are bound to plasma proteins in varying degree. They are concentrated by the liver in the bile and excreted in the urine and feces at high concentrations and in a biologically active form.

Indications: 'Rondomycin' (methacycline HCl) is indicated in infections caused by the following microorganisms:

Rickettsiae (Rocky Mountain spotted fever, typhus fever and the typhus group, Q fever, rickettsialpox and tick fevers),

Mycoplasma pneumoniae (PPLO, Eaton Agent),

Agents of psittacosis and ornithosis,

Agents of lymphogranuloma venereum and granuloma inguinale,

The spirochetal agent of relapsing fever (*Borrelia recurrentis*).

The following gram-negative microorganisms

Haemophilus ducreyi (chancroid),

Pasteurella pestis and *Pasteurella tularensis,*

Bartonella bacilliformis,

Bacteroides species,

Vibrio comma and *Vibrio fetus,*

Brucella species (in conjunction with streptomycin).

Because many strains of the following groups of microorganisms have been shown to be resistant to tetracyclines, culture and susceptibility testing are recommended.

'Rondomycin' (methacycline HCl) is indicated for treatment of infections caused by the following gram-negative microorganisms, when bacteriologic testing indicates appropriate susceptibility to the drug:

Escherichia coli,

Enterobacter aerogenes (formerly *Aerobacter aerogenes),*

Shigella species,

Mima species and *Herellea* species,

Haemophilus influenzae (respiratory infections),

Klebsiella species (respiratory and urinary infections).

'Rondomycin' (methacycline HCl) is indicated for treatment of infections caused by the following gram-positive microorganisms when bacteriologic testing indicates appropriate susceptibility to the drug:

Streptococcus species: Up to 44 percent of strains of *streptococcus pyogenes* and 74 percent of *streptococcus faecalis* have been found to be resistant to tetracycline drugs. Therefore, tetracyclines should not be used for streptococcal disease unless the organism has been demonstrated to be sensitive.

For upper respiratory infections due to group A beta-hemolytic streptococci, penicillin is the usual drug of choice, including prophylaxis of rheumatic fever.

Continued on next page

Wallace—Cont.

Diplococcus pneumoniae,
Staphylococcus aureus, skin and soft tissue infections. Tetracyclines are not the drugs of choice in the treatment of any type of staphylococcal infections.

When penicillin is contraindicated, tetracyclines are alternative drugs in the treatment of infections due to:
Neisseria gonorrhoeae,
Treponema pallidum and *Treponema pertenue* (syphilis and yaws),
Listeria monocytogenes,
Clostridium species,
Bacillus anthracis,
Fusobacterium fusiforme (Vincent's infection),
Actinomyces species.

In acute intestinal amebiasis, the tetracyclines may be a useful adjunct to amebicides. In severe acne, the tetracyclines may be useful adjunctive therapy.

Tetracyclines are indicated in the treatment of trachoma, although the infectious agent is not always eliminated, as judged by immunofluorescence.

Inclusion conjunctivitis may be treated with oral tetracyclines or with a combination of oral and topical agents.

Contraindications: This drug is contraindicated in persons who have shown hypersensitivity to any of the tetracyclines.

Warnings: THE USE OF DRUGS OF THE TETRACYCLINE CLASS DURING TOOTH DEVELOPMENT (LAST HALF OF PREGNANCY, INFANCY, AND CHILDHOOD TO THE AGE OF 8 YEARS) MAY CAUSE PERMANENT DISCOLORATION OF THE TEETH (YELLOW-GRAY-BROWN). This adverse reaction is more common during long-term use of the drugs but has been observed following repeated short-term courses. Enamel hypoplasia has also been reported. TETRACYCLINE DRUGS, THEREFORE, SHOULD NOT BE USED IN THIS AGE GROUP UNLESS OTHER DRUGS ARE NOT LIKELY TO BE EFFECTIVE OR ARE CONTRAINDICATED.

If renal impairment exists, even usual oral or parenteral doses may lead to excessive systemic accumulation of the drug and possible liver toxicity. Under such conditions, lower than usual total doses are indicated, and, if therapy is prolonged, serum level determinations of the drug may be advisable.

Photosensitivity manifested by an exaggerated sunburn reaction has been observed in some individuals taking tetracyclines. Patients apt to be exposed to direct sunlight or ultraviolet light should be advised that this reaction can occur with tetracycline drugs, and treatment should be discontinued at the first evidence of skin erythema.

The antianabolic action of the tetracyclines may cause an increase in BUN. While this is not a problem in those with normal renal function, in patients with significantly impaired function, higher serum levels of tetracycline may lead to azotemia, hyperphosphatemia, and acidosis.

Usage in pregnancy. (See above **Warnings** about use during tooth development.)

Results of animal studies indicate that tetracyclines cross the placenta, are found in fetal tissues and can have toxic effects on the developing fetus (often related to retardation of skeletal development). Evidence of embryotoxicity has also been noted in animals treated early in pregnancy.

Usage in newborns, infants, and children. (See above **Warnings** about use during tooth development.)

All tetracyclines form a stable calcium complex in any bone-forming tissue. A decrease in the fibula growth rate has been observed in prematures given oral tetracycline in doses of 25 mg/kg every 6 hours. This reaction was shown to be reversible when the drug was discontinued.

Tetracyclines are present in the milk of lactating women who are taking a drug in this class.

Precautions: As with other antibiotic preparations, use of this drug may result in overgrowth of nonsusceptible organisms, including fungi. If superinfection occurs, the antibiotic should be discontinued and appropriate therapy instituted.

In venereal diseases when coexistent syphilis is suspected, darkfield examination should be done before treatment is started and the blood serology repeated monthly for at least 4 months.

Because tetracyclines have been shown to depress plasma prothrombin activity, patients who are on anticoagulant therapy may require downward adjustment of their anticoagulant dosage.

In long-term therapy, periodic laboratory evaluation of organ systems, including hematopoietic, renal and hepatic studies should be performed.

All infections due to Group A beta-hemolytic streptococci should be treated for at least 10 days.

Since bacteriostatic drugs may interfere with the bactericidal action of penicillin, it is advisable to avoid giving tetracycline in conjunction with penicillin.

Adverse Reactions:

Gastrointestinal: Anorexia, nausea, vomiting, diarrhea, glossitis, dysphagia, enterocolitis, and inflammatory lesions (with monilial overgrowth) in the anogenital region. These reactions have been caused by both the oral and parenteral administration of tetracyclines.

Skin: Maculopapular and erythematous rashes. Exfoliative dermatitis has been reported but is uncommon. Photosensitivity is discussed above. (See **Warnings.**)

Renal toxicity: Rise in BUN has been reported and is apparently dose related. (See **Warnings.**)

Hypersensitivity reactions: Urticaria, angioneurotic edema, anaphylaxis, anaphylactoid purpura, pericarditis and exacerbation of systemic lupus erythematosus.

Bulging fontanels in infants and benign intracranial hypertension in adults have been reported in individuals receiving full therapeutic dosages. These conditions disappeared rapidly when the drug was discontinued.

Blood: Hemolytic anemia, thrombocytopenia, neutropenia and eosinophilia have been reported.

When given over prolonged periods, tetracyclines have been reported to produce brown-black microscopic discoloration of thyroid glands. No abnormalities of thyroid function studies are known to occur.

Dosage and Administration: The usual adult dosage of 'Rondomycin' (methacycline HCl) is 600 mg daily. This may be given in four divided doses of 150 mg each or two divided doses of 300 mg each. An initial dose of 300 mg followed by 150 mg every six hours or 300 mg every 12 hours may be used in the management of more severe infections.

In uncomplicated gonorrhea, when penicillin is contraindicated, 'Rondomycin' (methacycline HCl) may be used for treating both males and females in the following clinical dosage schedule: 900 mg initially, followed by 300 mg q.i.d. for a total of 5.4 grams.

For treatment of syphilis, when penicillin is contraindicated, a total of 18 to 24 grams of 'Rondomycin' (methacycline HCl) in equally divided doses over a period of 10-15 days should be given. Close follow-up, including laboratory tests, is recommended.

In Eaton Agent pneumonia, the usual adult dosage is 900 mg daily for 6 days.

The recommended dosage schedule for children above eight years of age is 3 to 6 mg/lb of body weight per day divided into two or four equally spaced doses. Therapy should be continued for at least 24-48 hours after symptoms and fever have subsided. It should be noted, however, that antibacterial serum levels may usually be present from 24 to 36 hours following the discontinuation of 'Rondomycin' (methacycline HCl).

Concomitant therapy: Antacids containing aluminum, calcium, or magnesium impair absorption and should not be given to patients taking oral tetracyclines.

Food and some dairy products also interfere with absorption. Oral forms of tetracycline should be given 1 hour before or 2 hours after meals. Pediatric oral dosage forms should not be given with milk formulas and should be given at least 1 hour prior to feeding.

In patients with renal impairment: (See **Warnings.**) Total dosage should be decreased by reduction of recommended individual doses and/or by extending time intervals between doses.

In the treatment of streptococcal infections, a therapeutic dose of tetracycline should be administered for at least 10 days.

How Supplied: 'Rondomycin'- 300 is available as blue and white capsules, each containing 300 mg methacycline HCl equivalent to 280 mg methacycline base, supplied in bottles of 50 (NDC 0037-4101-06).

'Rondomycin'-150 is available as blue and white capsules, each containing 150 mg methacycline HCl equivalent to 140 mg methacycline base, supplied in bottles of 100 (NDC 0037-4001-01).

[*Shown in Product Identification Section*]

Rev. 10/78

RYNA™ Liquid

Description: Each 5 ml (one teaspoonful) contains:

Chlorpheniramine maleate .... 2 mg
Pseudoephedrine hydrochloride .... 30 mg

in a clear, slightly yellow colored, lemon-vanilla flavored demulcent base containing no sugar, dyes or alcohol.

Actions: RYNA Liquid combines chlorpheniramine maleate, an antihistamine that antagonizes the effects of histamine, with pseudoephedrine hydrochloride, a sympathomimetic nasal decongestant that acts to shrink swollen mucosa of the respiratory tract.

Indications: For the temporary relief of the concurrent symptoms of nasal congestion, sneezing, itchy and watery eyes, and running nose as occur with the common cold or allergic rhinitis.

Directions: ***Adults:*** 2 teaspoonfuls every 4 hours.

Children 6–12 years: 1 teaspoonful every 4 hours.

Children 2–5 years: ½ teaspoonful every 4 hours (see WARNINGS).

Do not exceed 6 doses in 24 hours.

Warnings: Do not give RYNA to children taking other medication or to children under 6 years except under the advice and supervision of a physician. Do not exceed recommended dosage unless directed by a physician because nervousness, dizziness, or sleeplessness may occur at higher doses. If symptoms do not improve within 3 days or are accompanied by high fever, discontinue use and consult a physician. Do not take this product except under the advice and supervision of a physician if you have any of the following symptoms or conditions: high blood pressure; heart disease; thyroid disease; diabetes; asthma; glaucoma; or difficulty in urination due to enlargement of the prostate. This product contains an antihistamine which may cause excitability, especially in children, or drowsiness or may impair mental alertness. Combined use with alcohol, sedatives, or other depressants may have an additive effect. Do not drive motor vehicles, operate machinery, or drink alcoholic beverages while taking this product.

KEEP THIS AND ALL DRUGS OUT OF THE REACH OF CHILDREN. IN CASE OF ACCIDENTAL OVERDOSE, SEEK PROFESSIONAL ASSISTANCE OR CONTACT A POISON CONTROL CENTER IMMEDIATELY.

Drug Interaction Precaution: Do not take this product, except under the advice and supervision of a physician, if you are presently taking a prescription antihypertensive or antidepressant drug containing a monoamine oxidase inhibitor.

How Supplied:
NDC 0037-0638-66, 4 fl oz bottle
NDC 0037-0638-68, pint bottle
NDC 0037-0638-69, gallon bottle

RYNA–C® Liquid Ⓒ

Description: Each 5 ml (one teaspoonful) contains:
Codeine Phosphate....................................10 mg
(WARNING: May be habit forming)
Pseudoephedrine Hydrochloride ....30 mg
Chlorpheniramine Maleate ....2 mg
in a clear, colorless, cinnamon-flavored demulcent base containing no sugar, dyes or alcohol.

Actions: RYNA-C combines the effectiveness of codeine as a centrally acting antitussive, with the sympathomimetic nasal decongestant effects of pseudoephedrine and the antihistaminic effects of chlorpheniramine. The gross therapeutic effect is to inhibit tiresome nonproductive cough, while simultaneously shrinking swollen mucosa of the respiratory tract and antagonizing the effects of histamine.

Indications: For the temporary relief of the concurrent symptoms of cough, nasal congestion, sneezing, itchy and watery eyes, and running nose as occurs with the common cold or allergic rhinitis.

Directions: *Adults:* 2 teaspoonfuls every 4 hours.
Children 6–12 years: 1 teaspoonful every 4 hours.
Children 2–5 years: ½ teaspoonful every 4 hours (see WARNINGS).
Do not exceed 6 doses in 24 hours.

Warnings: Do not give this product to children taking other medications or to children under 6 years except under the advice and supervision of a physician. The codeine component may cause or aggravate constipation. A persistent cough may be a sign of a serious condition. Do not take this product except under the advice and supervision of a physician if you have any of the following symptoms or conditions: cough that persists more than 3 days or tends to recur; chronic cough, such as occurs with smoking, asthma, or emphysema; cough accompanied by excessive secretions, high fever, rash, or persistent headache; chronic pulmonary disease or shortness of breath; high blood pressure; heart disease; thyroid disease; diabetes; asthma; glaucoma; or difficulty in urination due to enlargement of the prostate. Do not exceed recommended dosage unless directed by a physician, because nervousness, dizziness, or sleeplessness may occur at higher doses. If symptoms do not improve within 3 days, discontinue use and consult a physician. Antihistamines may cause excitability, especially in children. They may cause drowsiness or impair mental alertness. Combined use with alcohol, sedatives, or other depressants may have an additive effect. Do not drive motor vehicles, operate machinery, or drink alcoholic beverages while taking this product.
KEEP THIS AND ALL DRUGS OUT OF THE REACH OF CHILDREN. IN CASE OF ACCIDENTAL OVERDOSE, SEEK PROFESSIONAL ASSISTANCE OR CONTACT A POISON CONTROL CENTER IMMEDIATELY.

Drug Interaction Precautions: Do not take this product if you are presently taking a prescription antihypertensive or antidepressant drug containing a monoamine oxidase inhibitor, except under the advice and supervision of a physician.

How Supplied:
NDC 0037-0522-66, 4 fluid ounce bottle.
NDC 0037-0522-68, pint bottle.
NDC 0037-0522-69, gallon bottle.

RYNA–CX® Liquid Ⓒ

Description: Each 5 ml (one teaspoonful) contains:
Codeine Phosphate ....10 mg
(WARNING: May be habit forming)
Pseudoephedrine Hydrochloride ....30 mg
Guaifenesin ....100 mg
in a clear, colorless, cherry-vanilla-menthol flavored demulcent base containing no sugar, dyes or alcohol.

Actions: RYNA CX combines the effectiveness of codeine as a centrally acting antitussive, with the sympathomimetic nasal decongestant effects of pseudoephedrine; and the expectorant action of guaifenesin which relieves irritated membranes in the respiratory passageways by preventing dryness through increased mucus flow.

Indications: For the temporary relief of the concurrent symptoms of dry, nonproductive cough and nasal congestion.

Directions: *Adults:* 2 teaspoonfuls every 4 hours.
Children 6–12 years: 1 teaspoonful every 4 hours.
Children 2–5 years: ½ teaspoonful every 4 hours.
Do not exceed 6 doses in 24 hours.

Warnings: Do not give this product to children taking other medications or to children under 2 years except under the advice and supervision of a physician. The codeine component may cause or aggravate constipation. A persistent cough may be a sign of a serious condition. Do not take this product except under the advice and supervision of a physician if you have any of the following symptoms or conditions: cough that persists more than 3 days or tends to recur; chronic cough, such as occurs with smoking, asthma, or emphysema; cough accompanied by excessive secretions, high fever, rash, or persistent headache; chronic pulmonary disease or shortness of breath; high blood pressure; heart disease; thyroid disease or diabetes. Do not exceed recommended dosage unless directed by a physician, because nervousness, dizziness, or sleeplessness may occur at higher doses. If symptoms do not improve within 3 days, discontinue use and consult a physician.
KEEP THIS AND ALL DRUGS OUT OF THE REACH OF CHILDREN. IN CASE OF ACCIDENTAL OVERDOSE, SEEK PROFESSIONAL ASSISTANCE OR CONTACT A POISON CONTROL CENTER IMMEDIATELY.

Drug Interaction Precaution: Do not take this product if you are presently taking a prescription antihypertensive or antidepressant drug containing a monoamine oxidase inhibitor, except under the advice and supervision of a physician.

How Supplied:
NDC 0037-0801-66, 4 fluid ounce bottle
NDC 0037-0801-68, pint bottle
NDC 0037-0801-69, gallon bottle

RYNATAN® Tablets and Pediatric Suspension ℞

Description: RYNATAN® Tablets are capsule-shaped, buff-colored, compressed tablets. Each tablet contains:
Phenylephrine Tannate ....25 mg.
Chlorpheniramine Tannate ....8 mg.
Pyrilamine Tannate ....25 mg.
RYNATAN® Pediatric Suspension is a dark pink-colored, strawberry-currant flavored liquid. Each 5 ml. (1 teaspoonful) contains:
Phenylephrine Tannate ....5 mg.
Chlorpheniramine
Tannate ....2 mg.
Pyrilamine Tannate ....12.5 mg.

Indications: RYNATAN provides symptomatic relief of the coryza and nasal congestion associated with the common cold, other upper respiratory infections and allergic rhinitis. In sinusitis, drainage from the affected sinuses may be improved. This formulation is based on the well documented precept that the use of two antihistamines in concert affords potentiation of action and broader therapeutic range. Additionally, the reliable nasal decongestant, phenylephrine tannate, is included.

Contraindications: RYNATAN is contraindicated in those patients who are sensitive to sympathomimetic drugs.

Precautions: Use with caution in patients with hypertension, hyperthyroidism, diabetes or coronary artery disease; warn of possible drowsiness in patients who may operate vehicles or machinery.

Adverse Reactions: Drowsiness and dryness of the mouth are occasionally associated with antihistamine therapy in some individuals.

Dosage and Administration:
RYNATAN Tablets:
Adults: 1 or 2 tablets every 12 hours.
RYNATAN Pediatric Suspension: For children over six years of age, 5 to 10 ml. (1 to 2 teaspoonfuls) every 12 hours; for children two to six years of age, 2.5 to 5 ml. (½ to 1 teaspoonful) every 12 hours; for children under two years of age, 1.7 ml. (⅓ teaspoonful) every 12 hours.

How Supplied:
RYNATAN Tablets:
NDC 0037-0713-92, bottle of 100.
NDC 0037-0713-96, bottle of 500.
RYNATAN Pediatric Suspension:
NDC 0037-0715-68, pint bottle.
[Shown in Product Identification Section]

RYNATUSS® Tablets and Pediatric Suspension ℞

Description: RYNATUSS® Tablets are capsule-shaped, lavender-rose colored, compressed tablets. Each tablet contains:
Carbetapentane
Tannate ....60 mg.
Chlorpheniramine
Tannate ....5 mg.
Ephedrine Tannate ....10 mg.
Phenylephrine Tannate ....10 mg.
RYNATUSS® Pediatric Suspension is a pink-colored, strawberry-currant flavored liquid. Each 5 ml. (1 teaspoonful) contains:
Carbetapentane
Tannate ....30 mg.
Chlorpheniramine
Tannate ....4 mg.
Ephedrine Tannate ....5 mg.
Phenylephrine Tannate ....5 mg.

Indications: In the treatment of coughs due to the common cold, asthma, and in acute and chronic bronchitis.
RYNATUSS provides an effective non-narcotic antitussive for inhibition of non-productive cough, in combination with an antihistamine, a sympathomimetic agent for decongestion of mucous membrane and alleviation of postnasal drip. The reliable bronchodilator, ephedrine, is also included.

Contraindications: RYNATUSS is contraindicated in those patients who are sensitive to sympathomimetic drugs.

Precaution: Use with caution in patients with hypertension, hyperthyroidism, diabetes or coronary artery disease; warn of possible drowsiness in patients who may operate vehicles or machinery.

RYNATUSS Suspension Only: This product contains FD&C Yellow No. 5 (tartrazine) which

Continued on next page

Wallace—Cont.

may cause allergic-type reactions (including bronchial asthma) in certain susceptible individuals. Although the overall incidence of FD&C Yellow No. 5 (tartrazine) sensitivity in the general population is low, it is frequently seen in patients who also have aspirin hypersensitivity.

Adverse Reactions: Drowsiness and dryness of the mouth are occasionally associated with antihistamine therapy in some individuals.

Dosage and Administration:

RYNATUSS® Tablets: Adults—1 to 2 tablets every 12 hours.

RYNATUSS® Pediatric Suspension: For children over six years of age, 5 to 10 ml. (1 to 2 teaspoonfuls) every 12 hours; for children two to six years of age, 2.5 to 5 ml. (½ to 1 teaspoonful) every 12 hours; for children under two years of age, 1.7 ml. (⅓ teaspoonful) every 12 hours.

How Supplied:

RYNATUSS® Tablets:

NDC 0037-0717-92, bottle of 100.

NDC 0037-0717-96, bottle of 500.

RYNATUSS® Pediatric Suspension:

NDC 0037-0718-67, 8 fl. oz. bottle.

NDC 0037-0718-68, pint bottle.

[*Shown in Product Identification Section*]

SOMA® ℞

(carisoprodol)

Description: 'Soma' (carisoprodol) is available as 350 mg white tablets. Carisoprodol is N-isopropyl -2- methyl -2- propyl-1,3-propanediol dicarbamate.

Actions: Carisoprodol produces muscle relaxation in animals by blocking interneuronal activity in the descending reticular formation and spinal cord. The onset of action is rapid and effects last four to six hours.

Indications: Carisoprodol is indicated as an adjunct to rest, physical therapy, and other measures for the relief of discomfort associated with acute, painful musculo-skeletal conditions. The mode of action of this drug has not been clearly identified, but may be related to its sedative properties. Carisoprodol does not directly relax tense skeletal muscles in man.

Contraindications: Acute intermittent porphyria as well as allergic or idiosyncratic reactions to carisoprodol or related compounds such as meprobamate, mebutamate, or tybamate.

Warnings:

Idiosyncratic Reactions—On very rare occasions, the first dose of carisoprodol has been followed by idiosyncratic symptoms appearing within minutes or hours. Symptoms reported include: extreme weakness, transient quadriplegia, dizziness, ataxia, temporary loss of vision, diplopia, mydriasis, dysarthria, agitation, euphoria, confusion, and disorientation. Symptoms usually subside over the course of the next several hours. Supportive and symptomatic therapy, including hospitalization, may be necessary.

Usage in Pregnancy and Lactation—Safe usage of this drug in pregnancy or lactation has not been established. Therefore, use of this drug in pregnancy, in nursing mothers, or in women of childbearing potential requires that the potential benefits of the drug be weighed against the potential hazards to mother and child. Carisoprodol is present in breast milk of lactating mothers at concentrations two to four times that of maternal plasma. This factor should be taken into account when use of the drug is contemplated in breast-feeding patients.

Usage in Children—Because of limited clinical experience, 'Soma' is not recommended for use in patients under 12 years of age.

Potentially Hazardous Tasks—Patients should be warned that this drug may impair the mental and/or physical abilities required for the performance of potentially hazardous tasks such as driving a motor vehicle or operating machinery.

Additive Effects—Since the effects of carisoprodol and alcohol or carisoprodol and other CNS depressants or psychotropic drugs may be additive, appropriate caution should be exercised with patients who take more than one of these agents simultaneously.

Drug Dependence—In dogs, no withdrawal symptoms occurred after abrupt cessation of carisoprodol from dosages as high as 1 gm/kg/day. In a study in man, abrupt cessation of 100 mg/kg/day (about five times the recommended daily adult dosage) was followed in some subjects by mild withdrawal symptoms such as abdominal cramps, insomnia, chilliness, headache, and nausea. Delirium and convulsions did not occur. In clinical use, psychological dependence and abuse have been rare, and there have been no reports of significant abstinence signs. Nevertheless, the drug should be used with caution in addiction-prone individuals.

Precautions: Carisoprodol is metabolized in the liver and excreted by the kidney; to avoid its excess accumulation, caution should be exercised in administration to patients with compromised liver or kidney function.

Adverse Reactions: Central Nervous System—Drowsiness and other CNS effects may require dosage reduction. Also observed: dizziness, vertigo, ataxia, tremor, agitation, irritability, headache, depressive reactions, syncope, and insomnia. (See also Idiosyncratic Reactions under "Warnings".)

Allergic or Idiosyncratic—Allergic or idiosyncratic reactions occasionally develop. They are usually seen within the period of the first to fourth dose in patients having had no previous contact with the drug. Skin rash, erythema multiforme, pruritus, eosinophilia, and fixed drug eruption with cross reaction to meprobamate have been reported with carisoprodol. Severe reactions have been manifested by asthmatic episodes, fever, weakness, dizziness, angioneurotic edema, smarting eyes, hypotension, and anaphylactoid shock. (See also Idiosyncratic Reactions under "Warnings".)

In case of allergic or idiosyncratic reactions to carisoprodol, discontinue the drug and initiate appropriate symptomatic therapy, which may include epinephrine, antihistamines, and in severe cases corticosteroids. In evaluating possible allergic reactions, also consider allergy to excipients (information on excipients is available to physicians on request).

Cardiovascular—Tachycardia, postural hypotension, and facial flushing.

Gastrointestinal — Nausea, vomiting, hiccup, and epigastric distress.

Hematologic — Leukopenia, in which other drugs or viral infection may have been responsible, and pancytopenia, attributed to phenylbutazone, have been reported. No serious blood dyscrasias have been attributed to carisoprodol.

Dosage and Administration: The usual adult dosage of 'Soma' (carisoprodol) is one 350 mg tablet, three times daily and at bedtime. Usage in patients under age 12 is not recommended.

Overdosage: Overdosage of carisoprodol has produced stupor, coma, shock, respiratory depression, and, very rarely, death. The effects of an overdosage of carisoprodol and alcohol or other CNS depressants or psychotropic agents can be additive even when one of the drugs has been taken in the usual recommended dosage. Any drug remaining in the stomach should be removed and symptomatic therapy given. Should respiration or blood pressure become compromised, respiratory assistance, central nervous system stimulants, and pressor agents should be administered cautiously as indicated. Carisoprodol is metabolized in the liver and excreted by the kidney. Although carisoprodol overdosage experience is limited, the following types of treatment have been used successfully with the related drug meprobamate: diuresis, osmotic (mannitol) diuresis, peritoneal dialysis, and hemodialysis (carisoprodol is dialyzable). Careful monitoring of urinary output is necessary and caution should be taken to avoid overhydration. Observe for possible relapse due to incomplete gastric emptying and delayed absorption. Carisoprodol can be measured in biological fluids by gas chromatography (Douglas, J.F. et al: *J Pharm Sci 58:* 145, 1969).

How Supplied: 'Soma' 350: Bottles of 100 (NDC 0037-2001-01) and 500 (NDC 0037-2001-03). Rev. 8/74

[*Shown in Product Identification Section*]

SOMA® COMPOUND ℞

(carisoprodol 200 mg + phenacetin 160 mg + caffeine 32 mg)

Description: 'Soma' Compound is available as orange, scored tablets, each containing carisoprodol 200 mg, phenacetin 160 mg, and caffeine 32 mg.

Actions:

Carisoprodol

Carisoprodol produces muscle relaxation in animals by blocking interneuronal activity in the descending reticular formation and spinal cord. The onset of action is rapid and effects last four to six hours.

Phenacetin

The exact nature of the pain-relieving action of phenacetin is not understood. The main site of activity is thought to be the central nervous system.

Caffeine

Caffeine acts as a stimulant of all parts of the central nervous system, affecting first the cortex and then the medulla. Large amounts will stimulate the spinal cord.

Indications: As an adjunct to rest, physical therapy, and other measures for the relief of discomfort associated with acute, painful musculoskeletal conditions. The mode of action of carisoprodol has not been clearly identified, but may be related to its sedative properties. Carisoprodol does not directly relax tense skeletal muscles in man.

Contraindications: Acute intermittent porphyria as well as allergic or idiosyncratic reactions to phenacetin, caffeine, or carisoprodol and related compounds such as meprobamate, mebutamate, or tybamate.

Warnings:

THIS PRODUCT CONTAINS PHENACETIN. PHENACETIN, IF TAKEN IN LARGE DOSES FOR LONG PERIODS IN COMBINATION WITH OTHER ANALGESICS, IS ASSOCIATED WITH SEVERE KIDNEY DISEASE AND WITH CANCER OF THE KIDNEY.

Kidney disease, often irreversible, has been noted with doses of phenacetin of 1 gm or more per day taken for 1-3 years and with total doses of 2 kg or more. It is not known whether prolonged ingestion of doses of phenacetin lower than 1 gm per day might also result in kidney disease.

Idiosyncratic Reactions

On very rare occasions, the first dose of carisoprodol has been followed by idiosyncratic symptoms appearing within minutes or hours. Symptoms reported include: extreme weakness, transient quadriplegia, dizziness, ataxia, temporary loss of vision, diplopia, mydriasis, dysarthria, agitation, euphoria, confusion, and disorientation. Symptoms usually subside over the course of the next several hours. Supportive and symptomatic therapy, including hospitalization, may be necessary.

Usage in Pregnancy and Lactation
Safe usage of this drug in pregnancy or lactation has not been established. Therefore, use of this drug in pregnancy, in nursing mothers, or in women of childbearing potential requires that the potential benefits of the drug be weighed against the potential hazards to mother and child. Carisoprodol is present in breast milk of lactating mothers at concentrations two to four times that of maternal plasma. This factor should be taken into account when use of the drug is contemplated in breast-feeding patients.
Usage in Children Under Age Five
Usage of this drug in children under age five is not recommended.
Potentially Hazardous Tasks
Patients should be warned that this drug may impair the mental and/or physical abilities required for the performance of potentially hazardous tasks such as driving a motor vehicle or operating machinery.
Additive Effects
Since the effects of carisoprodol and alcohol or carisoprodol and other CNS depressants or psychotropic drugs may be additive, appropriate caution should be exercised with patients who take more than one of these agents simultaneously.
Drug Dependence
Phenacetin
Restlessness and excitement may occur when phenacetin has been abruptly discontinued.
Caffeine
Psychological dependence has been reported.
Carisoprodol
In dogs, no withdrawal symptoms occurred after abrupt cessation of carisoprodol from dosages as high as 1 gm/kg/day. In a study in man, abrupt cessation of 100 mg/kg/day (about five times the recommended daily adult dosage) was followed in some subjects by mild withdrawal symptoms such as abdominal cramps, insomnia, chilliness, headache, and nausea. Delirium and convulsions did not occur. In clinical use, psychological dependence and abuse have been rare, and there have been no reports of significant abstinence signs. Nevertheless, the drug should be used with caution in addiction-prone individuals.
Precautions:
Phenacetin
In cases of long-term therapy, phenacetin should be administered with caution to patients with anemia or cardiac, pulmonary, renal, or hepatic disease.
Caffeine
Caffeine should not be given to persons extremely sensitive to its CNS-stimulating action.
Carisoprodol
Carisoprodol is metabolized in the liver and excreted by the kidney; to avoid its excess accumulation, caution should be exercised in administration to patients with compromised liver or kidney function.
Adverse Reactions: Drowsiness, lightheadedness, dizziness, itching, nervousness, palpitations, overdose, and idiosyncratic reactions have been reported. Side effects which have occurred after administration of the constituents alone might also occur when the combination is taken.
Phenacetin
Side effects are extremely rare with short-term use of recommended doses. Usage in large amounts or for long periods may result in gastrointestinal disturbances, anemia, methemoglobinemia, and renal damage. (See **Overdosage** section.)
Caffeine
Average doses of caffeine may rarely cause nausea, nervousness, insomnia, and diuresis. Side effects are almost always the result of overdosage. (See **Overdosage** section.)
Carisoprodol
Central Nervous System—Drowsiness and other CNS effects may require dosage reduction. Also observed: dizziness, vertigo, ataxia, tremor, agitation, irritability, headache, depressive reactions, syncope, and insomnia. (See also Idiosyncratic Reactions under **Warnings.**)
Allergic or Idiosyncratic—Allergic or idiosyncratic reactions occasionally develop. They are usually seen within the period of the first to fourth dose in patients having had no previous contact with the drug. Skin rash, erythema multiforme, pruritus, eosinophilia, and fixed drug eruption with cross reaction to meprobamate have been reported with carisoprodol. Severe reactions have been manifested by asthmatic episodes, fever, weakness, dizziness, angioneurotic edema, smarting eyes, hypotension, and anaphylactoid shock. (See also Idiosyncratic Reactions under **Warnings.**)
In case of allergic or idiosyncratic reactions to carisoprodol, discontinue the drug and initiate appropriate symptomatic therapy, which may include epinephrine, antihistamines, and in severe cases corticosteroids. In evaluating possible allergic reactions, also consider allergy to excipients (information on excipients is available to physicians on request).
Cardiovascular—Tachycardia, postural hypotension, and facial flushing.
Gastrointestinal — Nausea, vomiting, hiccup, and epigastric distress.
Hematologic — Leukopenia, in which other drugs or viral infection may have been responsible, and pancytopenia, attributed to phenylbutazone, have been reported. No serious blood dyscrasias have been attributed to carisoprodol.
Dosage and Administration: The usual adult dosage of 'Soma' Compound (carisoprodol +phenacetin +caffeine) is one or two tablets, three times daily and at bedtime. Usage in children under age five is not recommended.
Overdosage: Diagnosis and treatment are according to component signs and symptoms. Note that symptoms and signs which could develop with one component used alone would be modified in varying degrees by the presence of the other components in the combination.
Phenacetin
Acute overdosage of phenacetin can produce dyspnea, cyanosis (due to methemoglobinemia and sulfhemoglobinemia), hemolytic anemia, skin reactions with or without fever, anorexia, hypothermia, insomnia, and in severe cases: stupor, coma, vascular collapse, and death. Remove any remaining drug from stomach and institute appropriate symptomatic therapy as indicated.
For methemoglobinemia the recommended treatment is a 1% aqueous solution of methylene blue, 1 to 2 mg/kg body weight, injected intravenously over a period of several minutes. This may be repeated at hourly intervals if cyanosis has not disappeared, but the total dose should not exceed 7 mg/kg.
Caffeine
Excessive dosage of caffeine can produce restlessness, nervousness, tolerance, delirium, tinnitus, tremors, scintillating scotomata, diuresis, tachycardia, and cardiac arrhythmias. It is possible that stimulatory signs would be offset by the CNS-depressant overdosage effects of the carisoprodol present in the combination.
Carisoprodol
Overdosage of carisoprodol has produced stupor, coma, shock, respiratory depression, and, very rarely, death. The effects of an overdosage of carisoprodol and alcohol or other CNS depressants or psychotropic agents can be additive, even when one of the drugs has been taken in the usual recommended dosage. Any drug remaining in the stomach should be removed and symptomatic therapy given. Should respiration or blood pressure become compromised, respiratory assistance, central nervous system stimulants, and pressor agents should be administered cautiously as indicated. Carisoprodol is metabolized in the liver and excreted by the kidney. Although carisoprodol overdosage experience is limited, the following types of treatment have been used successfully with the related drug meprobamate: diuresis, osmotic (mannitol) diuresis, peritoneal dialysis, and hemodialysis (carisoprodol is dialyzable). Careful monitoring of urinary output is necessary and caution should be taken to avoid overhydration. Observe for possible relapse due to incomplete gastric emptying and delayed absorption. Carisoprodol can be measured in biological fluids by gas chromatography (Douglas, J.F. et al: *J Pharm Sci* **58**: 145, 1969).
How Supplied: Bottles of 100 (NDC 0037-2101-01) and 500 (NDC 0037-2101-03).
Rev. 5/79
[*Shown in Product Identification Section*]

SOMA® COMPOUND with CODEINE ©℞
(carisoprodol 200 mg+phenacetin 160 mg +caffeine 32 mg +codeine phosphate 16 mg)

WARNING: May be habit-forming.
Description: 'Soma' Compound with Codeine is available as white, capsule-shaped tablets, each containing carisoprodol 200 mg, phenacetin 160 mg, caffeine 32 mg, and codeine phosphate 16 mg.
Actions:
Carisoprodol
Carisoprodol produces muscle relaxation in animals by blocking interneuronal activity in the descending reticular formation and spinal cord. The onset of action is rapid and effects last four to six hours.
Phenacetin
The exact nature of the pain-relieving action of phenacetin is not understood. The main site of activity is thought to be the central nervous system.
Caffeine
Caffeine acts as a stimulant of all parts of the central nervous system, affecting first the cortex and then the medulla. Large amounts will stimulate the spinal cord.
Codeine Phosphate
Codeine phosphate is a narcotic-analgesic whose actions are qualitatively similar to morphine, but whose potency is substantially less.
Indications: As an adjunct to rest, physical therapy, and other measures for the relief of discomfort associated with acute, painful musculo-skeletal conditions when the additional action of codeine is desired. The mode of action of carisoprodol has not been clearly identified, but may be related to its sedative properties. Carisoprodol does not directly relax tense skeletal muscles in man.
Contraindications: Acute intermittent porphyria as well as allergic or idiosyncratic reactions to phenacetin, caffeine, codeine, or carisoprodol and related compounds such as meprobamate, mebutamate, or tybamate.
Warnings:

FOR PRODUCT CONTAINS PHENACETIN. PHENACETIN, IF TAKEN IN LARGE DOSES FOR LONG PERIODS IN COMBINATION WITH OTHER ANALGESICS, IS ASSOCIATED WITH SEVERE KIDNEY DISEASE AND WITH CANCER OF THE KIDNEY.

Kidney disease, often irreversible, has been noted with doses of phenacetin of 1 gm or more per day taken for 1-3 years and with total doses of 2 kg or more. It is not known whether prolonged ingestion of doses of phenacetin lower than 1 gm per day might also result in kidney disease.
Idiosyncratic Reactions
On very rare occasions, the first dose of carisoprodol has been followed by idiosyncratic symptoms appearing within minutes or hours. Symptoms reported include: extreme weak-

Continued on next page

Wallace—Cont.

ness, transient quadriplegia, dizziness, ataxia, temporary loss of vision, diplopia, mydriasis, dysarthria, agitation, euphoria, confusion, and disorientation. Symptoms usually subside over the course of the next several hours. Supportive and symptomatic therapy, including hospitalization, may be necessary.

Usage in Pregnancy and Lactation
Safe usage of this drug in pregnancy or lactation has not been established. Therefore, use of this drug in pregnancy, in nursing mothers, or in women of childbearing potential requires that the potential benefits of the drug be weighed against the potential hazards to mother and child. Carisoprodol is present in breast milk of lactating mothers at concentrations two to four times that of maternal plasma. This factor should be taken into account when use of the drug is contemplated in breast-feeding patients.

Usage in Children Under Age Five
Usage of this drug in children under age five is not recommended.

Potentially Hazardous Tasks
Patients should be warned that this drug may impair the mental and/or physical abilities required for the performance of potentially hazardous tasks such as driving a motor vehicle or operating machinery.

Additive Effects
Since the effects of carisoprodol and alcohol or carisoprodol and other CNS depressants or psychotropic drugs may be additive, appropriate caution should be exercised with patients who take more than one of these agents simultaneously.

Drug Dependence
Phenacetin
Restlessness and excitement may occur when phenacetin has been abruptly discontinued.
Caffeine
Psychological dependence has been reported.
Carisoprodol
In dogs, no withdrawal symptoms occurred after abrupt cessation of carisoprodol from dosages as high as 1 gm/kg/day. In a study in man, abrupt cessation of 100 mg/kg/day (about five times the recommended daily adult dosage) was followed in some subjects by mild withdrawal symptoms such as abdominal cramps, insomnia, chilliness, headache, and nausea. Delirium and convulsions did not occur. In clinical use, psychological dependence and abuse have been rare, and there have been no reports of significant abstinence signs. Nevertheless, the drug should be used with caution in addiction-prone individuals.
Codeine Phosphate
Codeine phosphate should be used with caution since it may result in drug dependence of the morphine type.

Precautions:
Phenacetin
In cases of long-term therapy, phenacetin should be administered with caution to patients with anemia or cardiac, pulmonary, renal or hepatic disease.
Caffeine
Caffeine should not be given to persons extremely sensitive to its CNS-stimulating action.
Carisoprodol
Carisoprodol is metabolized in the liver and excreted by the kidney; to avoid its excess accumulation, caution should be exercised in administration to patients with compromised liver or kidney function.

Adverse Reactions: These have consisted primarily of drowsiness, dizziness, and gastric complaints. Side effects which have occurred after administration of the constituents alone might also occur when the combination is taken.
Phenacetin
Side effects are extremely rare with short-term use of recommended doses. Usage in large amounts or for long periods may result in gastrointestinal disturbances, anemia, methemoglobinemia, and renal damage. (See **Overdosage** section.)
Caffeine
Average doses of caffeine may rarely cause nausea, nervousness, insomnia, and diuresis. Side effects are almost always the result of overdosage. (See **Overdosage** section.)
Codeine Phosphate
Possible side effects associated with the administration of codeine phosphate are nausea, vomiting, constipation, miosis, sedation, and dizziness.
Carisoprodol
Central Nervous System—Drowsiness and other CNS effects may require dosage reduction. Also observed: dizziness, vertigo, ataxia, tremor, agitation, irritability, headache, depressive reactions, syncope, and insomnia. (See also Idiosyncratic Reactions under **Warnings.**)
Allergic or Idiosyncratic—Allergic or idiosyncratic reactions occasionally develop. They are usually seen within the period of the first to fourth dose in patients having had no previous contact with the drug. Skin rash, erythema multiforme, pruritus, eosinophilia, and fixed drug eruption with cross reaction to meprobamate have been reported with carisoprodol. Severe reactions have been manifested by asthmatic episodes, fever, weakness, dizziness, angioneurotic edema, smarting eyes, hypotension, and anaphylactoid shock. (See also Idiosyncratic Reactions under **Warnings.**)
In case of allergic or idiosyncratic reactions to carisoprodol, discontinue the drug and initiate appropriate symptomatic therapy, which may include epinephrine, antihistamines, and in severe cases corticosteroids. In evaluating possible allergic reactions, also consider allergy to excipients (information on excipients is available to physicians on request).
Cardiovascular—Tachycardia, postural hypotension, and facial flushing.
Gastrointestinal — Nausea, vomiting, hiccup, and epigastric distress.
Hematologic — Leukopenia, in which other drugs or viral infection may have been responsible, and pancytopenia, attributed to phenylbutazone, have been reported. No serious blood dyscrasias have been attributed to carisoprodol.

Dosage and Administration: The usual adult dosage of 'Soma' Compound with Codeine (carisoprodol + phenacetin + caffeine + codeine) is one or two tablets, three times daily and at bedtime. Usage in children under age five is not recommended.

Overdosage: Diagnosis and treatment are according to component signs and symptoms. Note that symptoms and signs which could develop with one component used alone would be modified in varying degrees by the presence of the other components in the combination.
Phenacetin
Acute overdosage of phenacetin can produce dyspnea, cyanosis (due to methemoglobinemia and sulfhemoglobinemia), hemolytic anemia, skin reactions with or without fever, anorexia, hypothermia, insomnia, and in severe cases: stupor, coma, vascular collapse, and death. Remove any remaining drug from stomach and institute appropriate symptomatic therapy as indicated.
For methemoglobinemia the recommended treatment is a 1% aqueous solution of methylene blue, 1 to 2 mg/kg body weight, injected intravenously over a period of several minutes. This may be repeated at hourly intervals if cyanosis has not disappeared, but the total dose should not exceed 7 mg/kg.
Caffeine
Excessive dosage of caffeine can produce restlessness, nervousness, tolerance, delirium, tinnitus, tremors, scintillating scotomata, diuresis, tachycardia, and cardiac arrhythmias. It is possible that stimulatory signs would be offset by the CNS-depressant overdosage effect of the carisoprodol present in the combination.
Codeine Phosphate
Overdosage of codeine may produce coma, pinpoint pupils, depressed respiration, and shock. Treat symptomatically, using respiratory assistance as needed, narcotic antagonists such as nalorphine and levallorphan, and pressor agents if indicated for shock.
Carisoprodol
Overdosage of carisoprodol has produced stupor, coma, shock, respiratory depression, and, very rarely, death. Overdosage of carisoprodol plus alcohol or other CNS depressants or psychotropic drugs can be additive. Any drug remaining in the stomach should be removed and symptomatic therapy given. Should respiration or blood pressure become compromised, respiratory assistance, central nervous system stimulants, and pressor agents should be administered cautiously as indicated. Carisoprodol is metabolized in the liver and excreted by the kidney. Although carisoprodol overdosage experience is limited, the following types of treatment have been used successfully with the related drug meprobamate: diuresis, osmotic (mannitol) diuresis, peritoneal dialysis, and hemodialysis (carisoprodol is dialyzable). Careful monitoring of urinary output is necessary and caution should be taken to avoid overhydration. Observe for possible relapse due to incomplete gastric emptying and delayed absorption. Carisoprodol can be measured in biological fluids by gas chromatography (Douglas, J.F. et al: *J Pharm Sci* **58**: 145, 1969).

How Supplied: Bottles of 100 (NDC 0037-2401-01) Rev. 5/79

[*Shown in Product Identification Section*]

SYLLACT® **OTC**
(Powdered Psyllium Seed Husks)

Composition: Each rounded teaspoonful of **'Syllact'** contains 3.3 Gm of powdered psyllium seed husks and an equal amount of dextrose as a dispersing agent in a fruit-flavored preparation, with potassium sorbate, methyl- and propyl-paraben added as preservatives. The bland, non-irritating, bulk-forming action of psyllium makes this preparation a suitable treatment for constipation by promoting natural elimination. The pleasant fruit flavor makes it acceptable to patients. Each dose of 'Syllact' provides about 14 calories and negligible amounts of potassium and sodium.

Indications: 'Syllact' is useful for the treatment of constipation and, when recommended by a physician, in other types of disorders where normal elimination is desired.

Warnings: Drink a full glass (8 oz.) of water or other liquid with each dose. Esophageal, gastric, small intestinal, or rectal obstructions have been extremely rare with the use of bulk-forming agents. In most cases, the underlying causes have been inadequate fluid intake or organic disease with resulting compromised lumen or partial obstruction. Do not use when abdominal pain, nausea and/or vomiting are present. Keep this and all medications out of the reach of children.

Precautions: Bulk forming agents should not be swallowed dry. They should not be used if impaction or gross intestinal pathology is present.

Dosage and Administration: *Usual Adult Dosage*—One rounded teaspoonful of 'Syllact' (7 Gm) in a full glass (8 oz.) of cool water one to three times daily before or after meals.
Children's Dosage—as directed by the physician. The usually recommended dosage for children over 6 years of age is approximately half the adult dosage with the same fluid requirement.
Do not swallow dry. Lower dosage as improvement is experienced. If constipation persists, consult your physician.

How Supplied: 'Syllact' is available as a powder in 10 oz. jars (NDC 0037-9501-13).

Rev. 10/79

THEO-ORGANIDIN™ ℞
(theophylline-iodinated glycerol)
Elixir

Description: Each tablespoonful of Theo-Organidin Elixir contains Organidin® (iodinated glycerol) 30 mg (15 mg organically bound iodine) and anhydrous theophylline 120 mg in a pleasant tasting, hydroalcoholic vehicle, 15% alcohol (by volume).
Actions: Theo-Organidin combines the bronchodilator effects of theophylline, a xanthine alkaloid with minimal CNS stimulation, and the mucolytic-expectorant action of Organidin. Hydro-alcoholic preparations of theophylline provide therapeutic blood levels in approximately 15 minutes and peak blood levels in one hour.
Indications: Theo-Organidin is indicated in the symptomatic treatment of bronchial asthma and other bronchospastic conditions such as bronchitis, bronchiolitis, and pulmonary emphysema; for the relief of wheezing and respiratory distress due to bronchospasm and tenacious mucous secretions; and for daily maintenance therapy of patients with bronchial asthma and other chronic bronchospastic pulmonary disorders.
Contraindications: History of marked sensitivity to inorganic iodides; hypersensitivity to any of the ingredients or related compounds.
Warnings: Discontinue use if rash or other evidence of hypersensitivity appears. Do not exceed recommended dosage. Do not administer more often than every 6 hours or within 12 hours after rectal administration of any preparation containing theophylline or aminophylline. Use with caution or avoid use with other xanthine derivatives or CNS stimulants.
Precautions: Children have been known to exhibit marked sensitivity to the CNS stimulant action of the xanthines. Toxic synergism (i.e., CNS stimulation) may occur with other sympathomimetic bronchodilator agents, particularly in children.
Dermatitis and other reversible manifestations of iodism have been reported in patients sensitive to iodine with the chronic use of inorganic iodides and interference with laboratory determinations of PBI has also occurred. Although these have not been reported to be a problem clinically with the use of Organidin, they should be kept in mind in patients receiving these preparations for long periods.
Adverse Reactions: Side effects sometimes seen with individual ingredients may occur and may be modified by their combination.
Theophylline—Gastric irritation, nausea, and vomiting may occur; these can be minimized by taking Theo-Organidin after meals. Palpitations and mild central nervous system stimulation (e.g., restlessness, sleeplessness) have been reported, particularly in children.
Organidin—Gastrointestinal irritation, rash and hypersensitivity have rarely been reported.
Dosage and Administration: Do not exceed recommended dosage. While the acute attack of asthma is usually terminated fairly rapidly with the recommended dosage of Theo-Organidin, the need for intravenous aminophylline or other regimens should be considered in the management of severe episodes.
Usual Adult Dosage: **For maintenance therapy:** 1–2 tablespoons 3 times a day followed by a glass of water to encourage proper hydration.
For the acute asthmatic attack: 3 tablespoons initially, then reduce dosage to maintenance levels.
Children: 1 teaspoonful (5 ml) per 20 lbs. (9 kg) body weight, 2–3 times daily (children over 100 lbs. (40 kg) may require adult dosage).
In severe attacks or if desirable when initiating treatment, the dosage may be increased by ⅓ for 24 hours.
How Supplied: Theo-Organidin Elixir, bottles of one pint (NDC 0037-4611-10) and one gallon (NDC 0037-4611-20).

Rev. 6/77

TUSSI-ORGANIDIN™ Ⓒ
TUSSI-ORGANIDIN™ DM ℞

Description: **Tussi-Organidin** - each 5 ml teaspoonful contains Organidin® (iodinated glycerol) 30 mg (15 mg organically bound iodine); chlorpheniramine maleate 2 mg; codeine phosphate (**Warning:** May be habit-forming) 10 mg; and alcohol 15%, by volume.
Tussi-Organidin DM - as for Tussi-Organidin except that codeine phosphate is replaced by dextromethorphan hydrobromide 10 mg, a nonnarcotic antitussive.
Actions: **Tussi-Organidin** combines the antitussive action of codeine with the mucolytic-expectorant action of Organidin and the antihistaminic action of chlorpheniramine maleate.
Tussi-Organidin DM combines the nonnarcotic antitussive action of dextromethorphan hydrobromide with the mucolytic-expectorant action of Organidin and the antihistaminic action of chlorpheniramine maleate.
Indications: For the symptomatic relief of irritating, nonproductive cough associated with allergic manifestations of respiratory tract conditions such as allergic bronchitis, bronchial asthma, tracheobronchitis, and the common cold; also for the symptomatic relief of cough accompanying other respiratory tract conditions such as laryngitis, pharyngitis, croup, pertussis and emphysema. Appropriate therapy should be provided for the primary disease.
Contraindications: History of marked sensitivity to inorganic iodides; hypersensitivity to any of the ingredients or related compounds.
Warnings: Discontinue if rash or other evidence of hypersensitivity appears. Antihistamines may produce various degrees of drowsiness and patients should not engage in potentially hazardous activities requiring mental alertness, such as driving or operating machinery until their response has been determined. The central nervous system (CNS) effects of antihistamines and alcohol or other CNS depressants (e.g., hypnotics, sedatives, tranquilizers) may be additive.
Tussi-Organidin only: Codeine may be habit-forming.
Precautions: Antihistamines may produce excitation, particularly in children. Dermatitis and other reversible manifestations of iodism have been reported in patients sensitive to iodine with the chronic use of inorganic iodides and interference with laboratory determinations of PBI has also occurred. Although these have not been reported to be a problem clinically with the use of Organidin, they should be kept in mind in patients receiving these preparations for prolonged periods.
Adverse Reactions: Have generally been uncommon with these preparations, but any of the side effects sometimes seen with the individual ingredients may occur and may be modified in combination.
Organidin - Gastrointestinal irritation, rash and hypersensitivity have rarely been reported.
Chlorpheniramine maleate - The most frequent side effects of antihistamines have been drowsiness, sedation, dry mouth, nausea, restlessness and drying of the mucous membranes. Dizziness, headache, heartburn, dysuria, polyuria, visual disturbances, and excitation, particularly in children, have also been reported with antihistamines.
Codeine phosphate - Nausea, vomiting, constipation, drowsiness, dizziness, and miosis have been reported.
Dextromethorphan hydrobromide - Rarely produces drowsiness or gastrointestinal disturbances. Extremely high doses are required to produce any respiratory depression.
Dosage and Administration: The same dosage recommendations apply to both Tussi-Organidin and Tussi-Organidin DM.
Adults: 1-2 teaspoonfuls every 4 hours.
Children: ½-1 teaspoonful every 4 hours.
How Supplied: **Tussi-Organidin** is available in bottles of one pint (NDC 0037-4811-10) and one gallon (NDC 0037-4811-20).
Tussi-Organidin DM is available in bottles of one pint (NDC 0037-4711-10).

Rev. 6/77

UNITENSEN® AQUEOUS INJECTION ℞
(cryptenamine acetates)

Description: Each ml. of sterile aqueous solution contains 260 CSR (Carotid Sinus Reflex) Units of cryptenamine (as the acetates) with 0.5% chlorobutanol in a 0.8% sodium chloride solution, pH adjusted with sodium bicarbonate.
Actions: Cryptenamine is an alkaloidal fraction obtained from *Veratrum viride* by a nonaqueous extraction procedure. The antihypertensive response to cryptenamine is widely documented. The principal mechanism of action of the drug in reducing the blood pressure involves widespread arteriolar dilatation mediated centrally, without peripheral adrenergic or ganglionic blockade. The major cardiovascular effects are reflex in nature and are mainly due to stimulation of afferent pressor receptors predominantly in the heart and carotid sinus area. These receptors initiate an increase in impulses which are interpreted by areas in the brain stem as denoting a pressure higher than that actually present. As a result, the mechanism concerned with blood pressure homeostasis is activated, sympathetic tone is decreased, vagal tone is increased, and the blood pressure is therefore reduced. Both systolic and diastolic pressure are decreased and the heart is slowed. Atropine abolishes the bradycrotic effect but only partially reverses the hypotensive effect.
Indications: UNITENSEN Aqueous (cryptenamine acetates) is indicated for short-term use in the treatment of hypertensive crises.
Contraindications: UNITENSEN Aqueous is contraindicated for patients with known idiosyncrasy to *Veratrum viride.*
Warning: UNITENSEN AQUEOUS MUST BE DILUTED FOR INTRAVENOUS ADMINISTRATION. The drug may be given undiluted by intramuscular injection. A narrow margin exists between the dose reducing the blood pressure and that producing side effects such as nausea and vomiting. Therefore, it may be difficult to obtain a significant reduction in blood pressure without accompanying side effects.
USE IN PREGNANCY: USE OF ANY DRUG IN PREGNANCY, LACTATION, OR IN WOMEN OF CHILDBEARING AGE REQUIRES THAT THE POTENTIAL BENEFITS OF THE DRUG BE WEIGHED AGAINST THE POSSIBLE HAZARDS TO THE MOTHER AND CHILD.
Precautions: UNITENSEN Aqueous is a potent therapeutic agent. Established practice for the administration and dosage of the drug should be carefully observed. Veratrum alkaloids may increase the heightened cardiac irritability produced by digitalis, and concurrent use of UNITENSEN Aqueous with digitalis may lead to ectopic cardiac rhythms. The bradycrotic effect of Veratrum alkaloids is additive to, but not synergistic with, that produced by morphine and related drugs.
As with other antihypertensive agents, UNITENSEN Aqueous should be used with care in hypertensive patients with angina pectoris or

Continued on next page

Wallace—Cont.

those with extensive cardiovascular disease. The drug should also be used cautiously in patients who have experienced a recent coronary or cerebral thrombosis.

Special caution is warranted when treating patients with histories of bronchial asthma who may respond adversely to the cholinergic effect of cryptenamine. Caution should be exercised when treating hypertensive patients with renal insufficiency or preexisting uremia since they adjust poorly to lowered blood pressure levels.

Clinical studies indicate that concomitant treatment of hypertensive patients with cryptenamine, or its formulations, and a saluretic agent can, in some patients, result in a greater reduction of blood pressure than does treatment with either agent alone. This additive effect should be borne in mind whenever cryptenamine is added to the regimen of patients previously or currently receiving a saluretic agent and lower doses of both agents should be given.

Adverse Reactions: Adverse reactions reported to have occurred in patients treated with Veratrum alkaloids include the following: Excessive hypotension; prostration; anorexia; nausea and vomiting; epigastric and substernal burning, which may be mistaken for angina pectoris; unpleasant taste; salivation; sweating; hiccough; blurring of vision; mental confusion; cardiac arrhythmias; bradycardia; and from excessive doses, bronchiolar constriction and respiratory depression.

When adverse reactions occur during treatment with Veratrum alkaloids, they are usually reversible and disappear when the drug is discontinued.

Dosage and Administration: INTRAMUSCULAR (Impending Hypertensive Crisis, Non-Convulsive Toxemia):

1. Record several blood pressure readings at frequent intervals to establish the control or baseline blood pressure and to estimate the desired blood pressure.
2. Administer 0.5 ml of UNITENSEN Aqueous (cryptenamine acetates) (130 CSR Units) by deep intramuscular injection.
3. Record the blood pressure and pulse rate every 15 to 30 minutes.
4. If there is no hypotensive effect from 0.5 ml of UNITENSEN Aqueous at the end of one hour, the dose may be increased by increments of 0.1 ml (0.6 ml, 0.7 ml, and so on).
5. After a hypotensive response has been observed, intramuscular UNITENSEN Aqueous may be repeated as often as every hour, if necessary, or whenever the blood pressure exceeds the desired level (usually 140/90 to 160/100).
6. If nausea or vomiting occurs, 50 to 100 mg of pentobarbital sodium may be given intravenously.
7. Once the acute hypertensive state is controlled (48–72 hours), if indicated, a long-term program utilizing an effective oral antihypertensive drug should be instituted.

NOTE: Both the amount of the drug needed to control the blood pressure and the interval between doses may vary from patient to patient without relation to the initial blood pressure or severity of condition presented. Therefore, the management of each patient must be individualized by continuing observation of his blood pressure and general evaluation of his clinical status. The effect of intramuscular administration of UNITENSEN Aqueous may last from 1 to 10 hours; it usually lasts 3 to 4 hours.

INTRAVENOUS (Hypertensive Crisis, Convulsive Toxemia):

1. Record several blood pressure readings at frequent intervals to establish the control or baseline blood pressure and to estimate the desired blood pressure.
2. An intravenous injection of 100 mg of pentobarbital sodium may be given if desired for sedation and reduction of the risk of nausea; or, it may be given later, if needed.
3. Dilute 0.5 ml (130 CSR Units) of UNITENSEN Aqueous with 20 ml of sterile 5% solution of glucose in water and administer the diluted solution intravenously at a rate of one ml per minute. Stop injection immediately after the first drop in blood pressure of 20 mm Hg, systolic, or 10 mm Hg, diastolic. Blood pressure should be recorded at intervals of approximately one minute.
4. After the first drop in blood pressure, as above, detach syringe and use needle for intravenous injection of 5% glucose in water.
5. A further drop in blood pressure (which can be precipitous) may occur within the next minute or two. If none occurs during the next five minutes, proceed with the further administration of the diluted solution of UNITENSEN Aqueous through the infusion tubing at the rate of one ml per minute, stopping when the blood pressure is at the desired level (usually about 160/100).
6. After the first hypotensive response has been noted, blood pressure readings should be recorded at intervals of 5 to 15 minutes. One-half the previously effective dose may be given when the blood pressure exceeds the desired level (usually 160/100).
7. When the interval between intravenous administrations of UNITENSEN Aqueous has reached one hour, the drug may be given instead by intramuscular injection using the following procedure: Administer 0.5 ml (130 CSR Units) of the undiluted preparation intramuscularly. Record blood pressure and pulse rate every 30 minutes. Repeat whenever blood pressure exceeds 160/100. The preparation may be administered every hour, if necessary; the duration of effects of intramuscularly administered UNITENSEN Aqueous may be from 1 to 10 hours, they usually last 3 to 4 hours. Dosage may be increased by increments of 0.1 ml (0.6 ml, 0.7 ml, etc.) if 0.5 ml is inadequate.
8. Once the acute hypertensive state is controlled (48–72 hours) a long-term program utilizing an effective oral antihypertensive drug should be instituted, if indicated.

How Supplied:

NDC 0037-0870-01, box of 5 × 2 ml (260 CSR Units per ml) ampuls.

[*Shown in Product Identification Section*]

UNITENSEN® TABLETS ℞
(Cryptenamine Tannates)

Description: Each round, white, scored tablet contains:

Cryptenamine ....2 mg.†
(as tannate salts)

†Equivalant to 260 Carotid Sinus Reflex Units.

Actions: Cryptenamine is an alkaloidal fraction obtained from *Veratrum viride* by a nonaqueous extraction procedure. The antihypertensive response to cryptenamine is widely documented. The principal mechanism of action of the drug in reducing the blood pressure involves widespread arteriolar dilatation mediated centrally, without peripheral adrenergic or ganglionic blockade. The major cardiovascular effects are reflex in nature and are mainly due to stimulation of afferent pressor receptors predominantly in the heart and carotid sinus area. These receptors initiate an increase in impulses which are interpreted by areas in the brain stem as denoting a pressure higher than that actually present. As a result, the mechanism concerned with blood pressure homeostasis is activated, sympathetic tone is decreased, vagal tone is increased, and the blood pressure is therefore reduced. Both systolic and diastolic pressures are decreased and the heart is slowed. Atropine abolishes the bradycrotic effect but only partially reverses the hypotensive effect.

Indications: UNITENSEN (cryptenamine tannates) is indicated for the treatment of mild to moderate hypertension. The efficacy-safety relationship in this preparation is such that the effective and toxic (emetic) dose levels are often approximately the same.

Contraindications: UNITENSEN is contraindicated for patients with known idiosyncrasy to *Veratrum viride* and for patients who have recently experienced either coronary artery occlusion or cerebral thrombosis.

Warnings: USE IN PREGNANCY: USE OF ANY DRUG IN PREGNANCY, LACTATION, OR IN WOMEN OF CHILDBEARING AGE REQUIRES THAT THE POTENTIAL BENEFITS OF THE DRUG BE WEIGHED AGAINST THE POSSIBLE HAZARDS TO THE MOTHER AND CHILD.

Precautions: Cryptenamine is a hypotensive and occasionally bradycrotic drug. Overdosage may produce nausea and vomiting, excessive hypotension and prostration and, rarely, bronchoconstriction. If necessary, atropine sulfate (0.5 to 1.0 mg.) may be administered to reverse the bradycrotic effect. In the event of excessive fall in blood pressure, administer vasopressor drugs, such as ephedrine sulfate (30 to 50 mg.) or phenylephrine hydrochloride (5 mg.) subcutaneously. If left untended, the reaction will gradually disappear within 60 to 90 minutes.

Particular care should be exercised in the use of UNITENSEN for treating hypertensive patients with angina pectoris, coronary thrombosis, or cerebrovascular disease. Caution should also be exercised when treating hypertensive patients with renal insufficiency or pre-existing uremia since they adjust poorly to lowered blood pressure levels.

Veratrum alkaloids may increase the heightened cardiac irritability produced by digitalis, and concurrent use of UNITENSEN with digitalis may lead to ectopic cardiac rhythms. The bradycrotic effect of veratrum alkaloids is additive to, but not synergistic with, that produced by morphine and related drugs.

Special caution is warranted when treating patients with histories of bronchial asthma who may respond adversely to the cholinergic effect of cryptenamine.

Caution must be exercised when this preparation is used in conjunction with surgery because of the additive hypotensive effects of anesthetic and pre-anesthetic agents.

Clinical studies indicate that concomitant treatment of hypertensive patients with cryptenamine and a saluretic agent can result in a greater reduction of blood pressure than does treatment with either agent alone. This additive effect should be borne in mind whenever a saluretic agent is added to the regimen of patients previously or currently receiving cryptenamine and lower doses of both agents should be given.

Adverse Reactions: Adverse reactions reported to have occurred in patients treated with veratrum alkaloids include the following: excessive hypotension; prostration; anorexia; nausea and vomiting; epigastric and substernal burning, which may be mistaken for angina pectoris; unplesant taste; salivation; sweating; hiccough; blurring of vision; mental confusion; cardiac arrhythmias; bradycardia; and from excessive doses, bronchiolar constriction and respiratory depression.

When adverse reactions occur during treatment with cryptenamine, they are usually reversible and disappear when treatment is discontinued.

Dosage And Administration: UNITENSEN (cryptenamine tannates): Usual dose, 2 to 6 tablets daily in divided doses.

Treatment with UNITENSEN should begin with low doses and when indicated, the dosage should be increased gradually either day by day or week by week, depending on whether the patient is hospitalized or ambulant. Careful titration of dosage according to the pa-

tient's response is necessary because gastrointestinal absorption is variable and the drug exerts a cholingergic effect on the gut. For effective control of elevated blood pressure with minimum side effects, UNITENSEN may be administered in the following manner:
Begin treatment with 2 tablets daily, one immediately after breakfast and the other at bedtime. If an increase in dosage is indicated, an additional dose may be given in the afternoon —at 1:00 or 2:00 P.M. The daily dose, as it is increased, should be varied so that the medium dose is taken after breakfast, the smallest dose at 1:00 or 2:00 P.M., and the largest dose at bedtime. For example, if the total dose is increased to 6 tablets daily, the schedule would be: 2 tablets after breakfast, 1 tablet at 2 P.M., and 3 tablets on retiring.
The time intervals between doses in each 24-hour period are very important and the dosage should be adjusted to the patient's daily mealtime routine. The afternoon dose should be the smallest of the day because it is taken at relatively short intervals after the morning dose and before the evening dose. The largest dose should be given at night because the interval between night and morning doses is the longest of the 24-hour period. If the patient refrains from eating for approximately 4 hours after taking the medication, the tendency for nausea and vomiting to occur is lessened.
Concomitant use of this preparation with ganglionic blocking agents, hydralazine, guanethidine, methyldopa, reserpine, chlorthalidone, or thiazides necessitates immediate reduction in dosage of both agents by about 50 percent. Patients receiving combined therapy with UNITENSEN and any other antihypertensive agent must be carefully followed for changes in blood pressure.
NOTE: During periods of excessively hot weather, the dosage may need to be reduced in some patients.
How Supplied:
NDC 0037-0873-92, bottle of 100.
NDC 0037-0873-96, bottle of 500.
[*Shown in Product Identification Section*]

VōSoL® Otic Solution ℞
(acetic acid-nonaqueous 2%)

VōSoL® HC Otic Solution ℞
(hydrocortisone 1%, acetic acid–nonaqueous 2%)

Description: VōSoL is a nonaqueous solution of acetic acid (2%), in a propylene glycol vehicle containing propylene glycol diacetate (3%), benzethonium chloride (0.02%), and sodium acetate (0.015%). VōSoL HC also contains hydrocortisone (1%) and citric acid (0.2%).
Action: VōSoL is antibacterial, antifungal, hydrophilic, has an acid pH and a low surface tension.
VōSoL HC is, in addition, anti-inflammatory and antipruritic.

Indications: (VōSoL only)
Based on a review of this drug by the National Academy of Sciences—National Research Council and/or other information, FDA has classified the indications as follows:
Effective: For the treatment of superficial infections of the external auditory canal caused by organisms susceptible to the action of the antimicrobial.
"Possibly" effective: For prophylaxis of otitis externa in swimmers and susceptible subjects.
Final classification of the less-than-effective indication requires further investigation.

Indications: (VōSoL HC only) For the treatment of superficial infections of the external auditory canal caused by organisms susceptible to the action of the antimicrobial, complicated by inflammation.
Contraindications: These products are contraindicated in those individuals who have shown hypersensitivity to any of their components; perforated tympanic membranes are frequently considered a contraindication to the use of external ear canal medication. VōSoL HC is contraindicated in vaccinia and varicella.
Precautions: VōSoL HC only: As safety of topical steroids during pregnancy has not been confirmed, they should not be used for an extended period during pregnancy. Systemic side effects may occur with extensive use of steroids.
Vōsol and Vōsol HC: If sensitization or irritation occurs, medication should be discontinued promptly.
Dosage and Administration: Carefully remove all cerumen and debris to allow VōSoL (or VōSoL HC) to contact infected surfaces immediately. To promote continuous contact, insert a VōSoL (or VōSoL HC) saturated cotton wick in the ear with instructions to the patient to keep wick moist for the next 24 hours by occasionally adding a few drops on the wick. Remove wick after first 24 hours and continue to instill 5 drops of VōSoL (or VōSoL HC) three or four times daily thereafter.
During treatment, to prevent infection of the other ear, use VōSoL in unaffected ear 3 times daily. To help prevent otitis externa in swimmers and susceptible subjects, instill two drops of VōSoL each morning and evening.
How Supplied: VōSoL Otic Solution, in 15 ml (NDC 0037-3611-10) and 30 ml (NDC 0037-3611-30) measured-drop, safety-tip plastic bottles. VōSoL HC Otic Solution, in 10 ml measured-drop, safety-tip plastic bottle (NDC 0037-3811-12).
Rev. 8/78
[*Shown in Product Identification Section*]

Warner/Chilcott

Warner/Chilcott products are now marketed by Parke-Davis, Division of Warner-Lambert Company.
Please see the Parke-Davis product monographs.

Warren-Teed Laboratories
Division of Adria Laboratories Inc.
582 W. GOODALE STREET
COLUMBUS, OHIO 43215

EVAC-Q-KIT®

Description: Each Evac-Q-Kit® contains:
1. Evac-Q-Mag®—10 fl. oz. Sugar-Free. Ingredients: magnesium citrate, citric acid and potassium citrate in cherry flavored base. Carbonated.
2. Evac-Q-Tabs®—2 tablets. Ingredients: Each tablet contains phenolphthalein—2 grains.
3. Evac-Q-Sert®—2 suppositories. Ingredients: Potassium bitartrate and sodium bicarbonate in polyethylene glycol base.
4. 1 Instruction Sheet (In English and Spanish)

Actions: Bowel Evacuant.
Indications: Preparations of the colon for single and multiple radiology examinations requiring a clean colon.
Contraindications: Evac-Q-Mag is contraindicated in the presence of severe renal insufficiency.
Warnings: Do not use any of these preparations when abdominal pain, nausea, or vomiting are present. Frequent and continued use may cause dependence upon laxatives. Rectal bleeding or failure to respond may indicate a serious condition. Consult physician. KEEP OUT OF REACH OF CHILDREN.
Precautions: If skin rash appears, do not use this or any other preparation containing phenolphthalein.
Dosage and Administration:
Instructions for Patients—early schedule*
Your physician is preparing you for an X-ray examination that requires thorough clearing of the intestinal tract. He is using this EVAC-Q-KIT® routine to make this procedure more comfortable for you.
BE SURE TO FOLLOW EACH STEP AND COMPLETE ALL INSTRUCTIONS OR ENTIRE X-RAY EXAMINATION MAY HAVE TO BE REPEATED.
DAY BEFORE EXAMINATION
IMPORTANT: A high fluid intake is essential to the success of this regimen. You MUST take a large glass (8 oz.) of fluid at specified times. (**= 8 oz. fluid.) Drink only black coffee, plain tea, strained fruit juice, soft drinks or water at the times indicated. NO MILK OR CREAM.**

☐ **Noon.** Light lunch. Clear soup, two hardboiled eggs, plain Jell-O, fluid.
☐ **12:30 P.M.** (or ½ hr. after lunch) Drink entire contents—EVAC-Q-MAG® (#1 in your kit), over Ice.
☐ **1:00 P.M.** + .
☐ **3:00 P.M.** Take two (2) EVAC-Q-TABS® laxative tablets (#2 in your kit) with large glass of water.
☐ **4:00 P.M.** + .
☐ **5:00 P.M.** Liquid dinner. Clear soup, plain Jell-O + .
☐ **6:00 P.M.** + 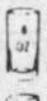.
☐ **9:00 P.M.** + .
☐ **10:00 P.M.** Remove cover from EVAC-Q-SERT® suppository (#3 in your kit). Moisten the suppository in tap water. Insert suppository into rectum. Wait at least 10–15 minutes before evacuating, even if urge is strong.
☐ **BEDTIME:** + .

DAY OF TEST. No breakfast.
☐ **6:00 A.M.** (must be at least 2 hours before test).
Use remaining EVAC-Q-SERT® suppository (#4 in your kit). Follow same directions as 10:00 P.M. night before.

BE SURE TO DRINK ALL THE FLUID SPECIFIED.
NOTE: This product information is for professional use only.
How Supplied: Each Evac-Q-Kit NDC 013-2199 contains:
1. One 10 fl. oz. Evac-Q-Mag
2. Two tablets—Evac-Q-Tabs
3. Two suppositories—Evac-Q-Sert
4. 1 Instruction Sheet

Shipping Unit: 12 Evac-Q-Kit units per carton.

*Late schedule also available. See Instruction Sheet in Evac-Q-Kit. Instruction sheet printed in both English and Spanish.)

EVAC-Q-KWIK®

Description: Each Evac-Q-Kwik® contains:
1. Evac-Q-Mag®—10 fl. oz. Sugar-Free. Ingredients: Magnesium citrate, citric acid and potassium citrate in cherry flavored base. Carbonated.

Continued on next page

Warren-Teed—Cont.

2. Evac-Q-Tabs®—2 tablets. Ingredients: Each tablet contains phenolphthalein = 2 grains (130 mg.).
3. Evac-Q-Kwik Suppository. Suppository contains 10 mg. of bisacodyl.
4. Illustrated Multilingual Instruction Sheet.

Actions: Bowel Evacuant

Indications: Preparation of the colon for single and multiple radiology examinations requiring a clean colon.

Contraindications: Evac-Q-Mag is contraindicated in the presence of severe renal insufficiency.

Warnings: Do not use any laxative preparations when abdominal pain, nausea, or vomiting are present. Frequent and continued use may cause dependence upon laxatives. Rectal bleeding or failure to respond may indicate a serious condition. Consult physician. KEEP OUT OF REACH OF CHILDREN.

Precautions: If skin rash appears, do not use this or any other preparaion containing phenolphthalein.

Dosage and Administration: Your physician is preparing you for an X-ray examination that requires thorough clearing of the intestinal tract. He is using this Evac-Q-Kwik routine to make the procedure more comfortable for you. BE SURE TO FOLLOW EACH STEP AND COMPLETE ALL INSTRUCTIONS OR ENTIRE X-RAY EXAMINATION MAY HAVE TO BE REPEATED.

IMPORTANT: A high fluid intake is essential to the success of this regimen. You MUST take a large glass (8 oz.) of fluid at specified times. Drink only black coffee, plain tea, strained fruit juice, soft drinks or water at the time indicated. NO MILK OR CREAM.

4:00 P.M.	Drink entire contents—EVAC-Q-MAG® (No. 1 in your kit), over ice.
5:00 P.M.	8 oz. of fluid.
6:00 P.M.	Liquid dinner. Clear soup, plain Jell-O. 8 oz. of fluid.
7:00 P.M.	Take two (2) EVAC-Q-TABS® laxative tablets (No. 2 in your kit) with large glass of water.
8:00 P.M.	8 oz. of fluid.
9:00 P.M.	8 oz. of fluid.
10:00 P.M.	Insert one EVAC-Q-KWIK suppository (No. 3 in your kit) into rectum as far as possible, retain as long as comfort will permit—usually 10–15 minutes—before defecating. Nothing by mouth after 10:00 P.M. until X-ray exam.

BE SURE TO DRINK ALL THE FLUID SPECIFIED.

See Illustrated Multilingual Instruction Sheet.

NOTE: This product information is for professional use only.

How Supplied: Each Evac-Q-Kwik® NDC 0013-2189 contains:

1. One 10 fl. oz. Evac-Q-Mag®
2. Two tablets—Evac-Q-Tabs®
3. One Evac-Q-Kwik Suppository
4. Instruction Sheet

Shipping unit: 12 Evac-Q-Kwik units per carton.

ILOPAN® INJECTION ℞

(Dexpanthenol)

Description: Each ml. contains dexpanthenol (d-pantothenyl alcohol), 250 mg. in distilled water. Solution in 10 ml. vials and 2 ml. Stat Pak® (disposable syringe) preserved with not more than 0.5% chlorobutanol.

Actions: Coenzyme A precursor.

Indications: Prophylactic use immediately after major abdominal surgery to minimize the possibility of paralytic ileus. Intestinal atony causing abdominal distention; postoperative or postpartum retention of flatus, or postoperative delay in resumption of intestinal motility; paralytic ileus.

Contraindications: None known.

Warnings: There have been rare instances of allergic reaction of unknown cause during the concomitant use of this drug and other drugs such as antibiotics, narcotics, and barbiturates. Administration of full-strength Ilopan directly into the vein is not advised.

Precautions: Wait 12 hours after neostigmine or other enterokinetic drugs and wait 1 hour after succinylcholine before starting ILOPAN. If there is any evidence of allergic reaction discontinue treatment. If the ileus is mechanical in nature, appropriate measures to eliminate its cause should not be delayed by the use of ILOPAN. Good results cannot be expected if medication is discontinued prematurely, or if patient is hypokalemic.

Dosage and Administration: Adults: (1.) Treatment or prevention of postoperative abdominal distention due to retained flatus: 1 or 2 ml. intramuscularly. Repeat in 2 hours followed by like doses every 6 hours to effect or until all danger of distention has passed. Distention may require treatment for 48 to 72 hours or longer. For dosages less than 2 ml. use Ilopan Injection in 10 ml. vials. (2.) **Treatment of paralytic ileus:** 2 ml. intramuscularly. Repeat in 2 hours followed by like doses every 4 to 6 hours to effect or until all danger of distention has passed. Administration for 48 to 72 hours or longer may be needed. (3.) **Intravenous administration:** The 500 mg. (2 ml.) dose has been intimately mixed with intravenous bulk solutions such as glucose or lactate-Ringer's and slowly infused satisfactorily by intravenous drip.

How Supplied:

Ilopan Injection
NDC 0013-2356-86 Vial, 10 ml.
NDC 0013-2356-93 Ampuls 2 ml., Box of 12
NDC 0013-2356-95 Ampuls 2 ml., Box of 25
NDC 0013-2356-97 Ampuls 2 ml., Box of 100
Ilopan Injection Stat-Pak®
NDC 0013-2366-95 Disposable Syringe 2 ml., Box of 25.

Bibliography: Available upon request.

A.H.F.S. 88:08

ILOPAN®-CHOLINE TABLETS ℞

(Dexpanthenol with Choline Bitartrate)

Description: Each tablet contains: ILOPAN (brand of dexpanthenol) 50 mg. and choline bitartrate 25 mg.

Actions: Antiflatulent.

Indications: May be helpful in relieving patients with gas retention associated with the splenic flexure syndrome, cholecystitis, gastritis, gastric hyperacidity, irritable colon, regional ileitis, post-antibiotic and postoperative gas retention or during laxative withdrawal.

Contraindications: None known.

Precautions: Wait 12 hours after neostigmine or other enterokinetic drugs and 1 hour after succinylcholine before starting Ilopan-Choline. In hypokalemia the effectiveness of Ilopan-Choline may be impaired.

Adverse Reactions: May increase frequency of bowel movements.

Dosage and Administration: Adult dosage—2 to 3 tablets three times daily.

How Supplied:

NDC 0013-2311-17 Bottle of 100 Tablets
NDC 0013-2311-21 Bottle of 500 Tablets
A.H.F.S. 88:08

ILOZYME® TABLETS ℞

(Pancrelipase N.F.)

Description: Each compressed tablet contains Pancrelipase N.F., 400 mg. representing not less than 9600 N.F. units of lipase activity, 40,000 N.F. units of protease activity and 40,000 N.F. units of amylase activity. One tablet hydrolyzes not less than 40 Gm. each of protein (casein) and starch. The lipase in one Ilozyme Tablet liberates 9600 microequivalents of acid per minute at pH 9.0 and 37° C. under the conditions of the N.F. assay for lipase activity. Standardization of lipolytic activity in N.F. XIII lipase units, provides a basis to aid control of steatorrhea where a deficiency of pancreatic exocrine secretion has been diagnosed.

Ilozyme Tablets are not enteric coated.

At simulated physiological conditions prevailing in the upper intestine during digestion—pH 7.0 $\pm$ 0.5 and 37° C. one Ilozyme tablet will digest in one hour: 40 grams of protein (casein); 150 grams of starch (potato starch); 27 grams of fat (olive oil).

Actions: Supplemental pancreatic digestive enzymes.

Indications: Exocrine pancreatic insufficiency, usually due to chronic pancreatitis, pancreatectomy, cystic fibrosis or obstruction caused by cancer of the pancreas.

Warnings: Pancreatic exocrine replacement therapy should not delay or supplant treatment of the primary disorder.

Precautions: Use with caution in patients known to be sensitive to pork or enzymes. Discontinue use in patients with symptoms of sensitivity.

Adverse Reactions: High dosages may cause nausea or diarrhea in certain patients.

Dosage and Administration: 1 to 3 tablets with meals and 1 tablet with any food eaten between meals. In severe deficiencies the frequency of dosage may be increased to hourly intervals if no nausea or diarrhea result.

How Supplied: NDC 0013-2001-19 Bottles of 250.

KAOCHLOR® 10% LIQUID ℞

(Potassium Chloride)
Contains Sugar

Description: Each 15 ml (tablespoonful) supplies 20 mEq each of elemental potassium and chloride (as potassium chloride, 1.5 g) with sugar, saccharin and flavoring. Alcohol 5%.

Actions: Potassium ion is the principal intracellular cation of most body tissues. Potassium ions participate in a number of essential physiological processes including the maintenance of intracellular tonicity, the transmission of nerve impulses, the contraction of cardiac, skeletal, and smooth muscle, and the maintenance of normal renal functions.

Potassium depletion may occur whenever the rate of potassium loss through renal excretion and or loss from the gastrointestinal tract exceeds the rate of potassium intake. Potassium depletion sufficient to cause hypokalemia usually requires the loss of 200 or more mEq of potassium from the total body store. Such depletion usually develops slowly as a consequence of prolonged therapy with oral diuretics, primary or secondary hyperaldosteronism, diabetic ketoacidosis, severe diarrhea, or inadequate replacement of potassium in patients on prolonged parenteral nutrition. Potassium depletion due to these causes is usually accompanied by a concomitant deficiency of chloride and is manifested by hypokalemia and metabolic alkalosis. Potassium depletion may produce weakness, fatique, disturbances of cardiac rhythm (primarily ectopic beats), prominent U-waves in the electrocardiogram, and in advanced cases, flaccid paralysis and or impaired ability to concentrate urine.

Potassium depletion associated with metabolic alkalosis is managed by correcting the fundamental cause of the deficiency whenever possible and administering supplemental potassium chloride, in the form of high potassium food or potassium chloride solution or tablets. In rare circumstances (e.g. patients with renal tubular acidosis) potassium depletion may be associated with metabolic acidosis and hyperchloremia. In such patients potassium replacement should be accomplished with potassium salts other than the chloride, such as potassium bicarbonate, potassium citrate, potassium acetate, or potassium gluconate (Kaon Elixir).

Indications: Kaochlor 10% Liquid is indicated for the treatment of potassium depletion in patients with hypokalemia and metabolic alkalosis, and for the treatment of digitalis intoxication. Kaochlor 10% Liquid is also indicated for the prevention of potassium depletion when the dietary intake of potassium is inadequate for this purpose. The prophylactic administration of potassium ion may be indicated in patients receiving digitalis and diuretics for the treatment of congestive heart failure; hepatic cirrhosis with ascites; patients with hypertension on long-term diuretic therapy; patients on corticosteroid therapy; hyperaldosteronism states with normal renal function; the nephrotic syndrome; and certain diarrheal states.

Contraindications: Potassium supplements are contraindicated in patients with hyperkalemia since a further increase in serum potassium concentration in such patients can produce cardiac arrest. Hyperkalemia may complicate any of the following conditions: Chronic renal failure, systemic acidosis such as diabetic acidosis, acute dehydration, extensive tissue breakdown as in severe burns, adrenal insufficiency, or the administration of a potassium-sparing diuretic (e.g. spironolactone, triamterene).

Warnings: Do not administer full strength. Kaochlor 10% Liquid will cause gastrointestinal irritation if administered undiluted. For details regarding adequate dilution, see Dosage and Administration.

In patients with impaired mechanisms for excreting potassium, the administration of potassium salts can produce hyperkalemia and cardiac arrest. This occurs most commonly in patients given potassium by the intravenous route but may also occur in patients given potassium orally. Potentially fatal hyperkalemia can develop rapidly and be asymptomatic. The use of potassium salts in patients with chronic renal disease, or any other condition which impairs potassium excretion, requires particularly careful monitoring of the serum potassium concentration and appropriate dosage adjustment.

Hypokalemia should not be treated by the concomitant administration of potassium salts and a potassium-sparing diuretic (e.g. spironolactone or triamterene) since the simultaneous administration of these agents can produce severe hyperkalemia.

Potassium chloride tablets have produced stenotic and or ulcerative lesions of the small bowel and deaths. These lesions are caused by a high localized concentration of potassium ion in the region of a rapidly dissolving tablet, which injures the bowel wall and thereby produces obstruction, hemorrhage, or perforation.

Hypokalemia in patients with metabolic acidosis should be treated with an alkalinizing potassium salt such as potassium bicarbonate, potassium citrate, potassium acetate, or potassium gluconate (Kaon Elixir).

Precautions: The diagnosis of potassium depletion is ordinarily made by demonstrating hypokalemia in a patient with a clinical history suggesting some cause for potassium depletion. In interpreting the serum potassium level, the physician should bear in mind that acute alkalosis *per se* can produce hypokalemia in the absence of a deficit in total body potassium while acute acidosis *per se* can increase the serum potassium concentration into the normal range even in the presence of a reduced total body potassium. The treatment of potassium depletion, particularly in the presence of cardiac disease, renal disease, or acidosis requires careful attention to acid-base balance and appropriate monitoring of serum electrolytes, the electrocardiogram, and the clinical status of the patient.

Adverse Reactions: The most common adverse reactions to oral potassium salts are nausea, vomiting, abdominal discomfort and diarrhea. These symptoms are due to irritation of the gastrointestinal tract and are best managed by diluting the preparation further, taking the dose with meals, or reducing the dose. The most severe adverse effects are hyperkalemia (see Contraindications, Warnings, and Overdosage) and gastrointestinal obstruction, bleeding or perforation (see Warnings).

Dosage and Administration: To minimize gastrointestinal irritation, patients must follow directions regarding dilution. Each tablespoonful (15 ml), equivalent to 20 mEq of potassium chloride, should be diluted with three fluid ounces or more of water or other liquid. Dosage must be adjusted to the individual needs of each patient, but is typically in the range of 20 mEq per day for the prevention of hypokalemia, to 40–100 mEq per day or more for the treatment of potassium depletion. During therapy serum potassium levels should be monitored and the dosage titrated to achieve the desired clinical and laboratory effects.

Overdosage: The administration of oral potassium salts to persons with normal excretory mechanisms for potassium rarely causes serious hyperkalemia. However, if excretory mechanisms are impaired or if potassium is administered too rapidly intravenously, potentially fatal hyperkalemia can result (see Contraindications and Warnings). It is important to recognize that hyperkalemia is usually asymptomatic and may be manifested only by an increased serum potassium concentration and characteristic electrocardiographic changes (peaking of T-waves, loss of P-wave, depression of S-T segment, and prolongation of the QT interval). Late manifestations include muscle-paralysis and cardiovascular collapse from cardiac arrest.

Treatment measures for hyperkalemia include the following:

1. Elimination of foods and medications containing potassium and of potassium-sparing diuretics.
2. Intravenous administration of 300 to 500 ml/hr of 10% dextrose solution containing 10–20 units of crystalline insulin per 1,000 ml.
3. Correction of acidosis, if present, with intravenous sodium bicarbonate.
4. Use of exchange resins, hemodialysis, or peritoneal dialysis.

In treating hyperkalemia, it should be recalled that in patients who have been stabilized on digitalis, too rapid a lowering of the serum potassium concentration can produce digitalis toxicity.

How Supplied:
NDC 0013-3103-51 Pint.
NDC 0013-3103-53 Gallon.
NDC 0013-3103-56 Bottle of 4 Fl. Oz. (36's only)
NDC 0013-3103-58 Bottle of 15 ml., Stat-Pak® (Unit Dose), 100's only.

KAOCHLOR-EFF® ℞
Effervescent Tablets
Sugar-Free

Description: Each tablet contains 20 mEq each of potassium chloride supplied by: Potassium chloride 0.60 g; potassium citrate 0.20 g; potassium bicarbonate 1.00 g; betaine hydrochloride 1.84 g; saccharin; artificial citrus fruit flavor and color.

Actions: See KAOCHLOR 10% LIQUID.
Indications: See KAOCHLOR 10% LIQUID.
Contraindications: See KAOCHLOR 10% LIQUID.
Warnings: See KAOCHLOR 10% LIQUID.
Precautions: See KAOCHLOR 10% LIQUID.
Adverse Reactions: See KAOCHLOR 10% LIQUID.
Dosage and Administration: To minimize gastrointestinal irritation, patients must follow directions regarding dilution. One tablet dissolved in three fluid ounces or more of water or other liquid provides 20 mEq of potassium chloride.

Dosage must be adjusted to the individual needs of each patient, but is typically in the range of 20 mEq per day for the prevention of hypokalemia, to 40–100 mEq per day or more for the treatment of potassium depletion. During therapy serum potassium levels should be monitored and the dosage titrated to achieve the desired clinical and laboratory effects.

Overdosage: See KAOCHLOR 10% LIQUID.
Treatment Measures for Hyperkalemia: See KAOCHLOR 10% LIQUID.
How supplied: NDC 0013-3051-16 Dispensing carton of 60 Tablets (Twin-Pack of 30's).
NDC 0013-3051-22 Box of 1000 Tablets

KAOCHLOR® S-F ℞
(Potassium Chloride)
10% LIQUID
Sugar-Free

Description: Each 15 ml (tablespoonful) supplies 20 mEq each of elemental potassium chloride (as potassium chloride, 1.5 g) with saccharin and flavoring. Alcohol 5%.

Actions: See KAOCHLOR 10% LIQUID.
Indications: See KAOCHLOR 10% LIQUID.
Contraindications: See KAOCHLOR 10% LIQUID.
Warnings: See KAOCHLOR 10% LIQUID.
Precautions: See KAOCHLOR 10% LIQUID.
Adverse Reactions: See KAOCHLOR 10% LIQUID.
Dosage and Administration: To minimize gastrointestinal irritation, patients must follow directions regarding dilution. Each tablespoonful (15 ml), equivalent to 20 mEq of potassium chloride, should be diluted with three fluid ounces or more of water or other liquid. Dosage must be adjusted to the individual needs of each patient, but is typically in the range of 20 mEq per day for the prevention of hypokalemia, to 40–100 mEq per day or more for the treatment of potassium depletion. During therapy serum potassium levels should be monitored and the dosage titrated to achieve the desired clinical and laboratory effects.

Overdosage: See KAOCHLOR 10% LIQUID.
Treatment Measures for Hyperkalemia: See KAOCHLOR 10% LIQUID.
How Supplied:
NDC 0013-3093-51 Pint.
NDC 0013-3093-53 Gallon.
NDC 0013-3093-56 Bottle of 4 Fl. Oz. (36's only).
NDC 0013-3093-58 Bottle of 15 ml. Stat-Pak® (Unit Dose) 100's only.

KAON® ELIXIR ℞
(Potassium Gluconate)
Grape or Lemon-Lime Flavors
Sugar-Free

Description: Each 15 ml (tablespoonful) supplies 20 mEq of elemental potassium (as potassium gluconate, 4.68 g) with saccharin and aromatics. Alcohol 5%.

Actions: Potassium ion is the principal intracellular cation of most body tissues. Potassium ions participate in a number of essential

Continued on next page

Warren-Teed—Cont.

physiological processes including the maintenance of intracellular tonicity, the transmission of nerve impulses, the contraction of cardiac, skeletal, and smooth muscle, and the maintenance of normal renal function.

Potassium depletion may occur whenever the rate of potassium loss through renal excretion and/or loss from the gastrointestinal tract exceeds the rate of potassium intake. Potassium depletion sufficient to cause hypokalemia usually requires the loss of 200 or more mEq of potassium from the total body store. Such depletion usually develops slowly as a consequence of prolonged therapy with oral diuretics, primary or secondary hyperaldosteronism, diabetic ketoacidosis, severe diarrhea, or inadequate replacement of potassium in patients on prolonged parenteral nutrition. Potassium depletion may produce weakness, fatigue, disturbances of cardiac rhythm (primarily ectopic beats), prominent U-waves in the electrocardiogram, and in advanced cases, flaccid paralysis and/or imparied ability to concentrate urine.

Indications: See KAOCHLOR 10% LIQUID.

Contraindications: See KAOCHLOR 10% LIQUID.

Warnings: Do not administer full strength. KAON ELIXIR may cause gastrointestinal irritation if administered undiluted. For details regarding adequate dilution, see Dosage and Administration.

In patients with impaired mechanisms for excreting potassium, the administration of potassium salts can produce hyperkalemia and cardiac arrest. This occurs most commonly in patients given potassium by the intravenous route but may also occur in patients given potassium orally. Potentially fatal hyperkalemia can develop rapidly and be asymptomatic. The use of potassium salts in patients with chronic renal disease, or any other condition which impairs potassium excretion, requires particularly careful monitoring of the serum potassium concentration and appropriate dosage adjustment.

Hypokalemia should not be treated by the concomitant administration of potassium salts and a potassium-sparing diuretic (e.g. spironolactone or triamterene) since the simultaneous administration of these agents can produce severe hyperkalemia.

Precautions: The diagnosis of potassium depletion is ordinarily made by demonstrating hypokalemia in a patient with a clinical history suggesting some cause for potassium depletion. In interpreting the serum potassium level, the physician should bear in mind that acute alkalosis per se can produce hypokalemia in the absence of a deficit in total body potassium, while acute acidosis per se can increase the serum potassium concentration into the normal range even in the presence of a reduced total body potassium. The treatment of potassium depletion, particularly in the presence of cardiac disease, renal disease, or acidosis, requires careful attention to acid-base balance and appropriate monitoring of serum electrolytes, the electrocardiogram, and the clinical status of the patient.

In hypokalemic states, especially in patients on a low-salt diet, hypochloremic alkalosis is a possibility that may require chloride as well as potassium supplementation. In these circumstances, potassium replacement with potassium chloride (e.g. KAOCHLOR 10% LIQUID, W-T) may be more advantageous than with other potassium salts. However, KAON can be supplemented with chloride. Amomonium chloride is an excellent source of chloride ion (18.7 mEq per gram) but it should not be used in patients with hepatic cirrhosis where ammonium salts are contraindicated.

Adverse Reactions: Nausea, vomiting, diarrhea, and abdominal discomfort have been reported. The symptoms and signs of potassium intoxication include paresthesias of the extremities, flaccid paralysis, listlessness, mental confusion, weakness and heaviness of the legs, fall in blood pressure, cardiac arrhythmias, and heart block.

Dosage and Administration: To minimize gastrointestinal irritation, patients must follow directions regarding dilution. Each tablespoonful (15 ml), equivalent to 20 mEq of potassium, should be diluted with one fluid ounce or more of water or other liquid.

Dosage must be adjusted to the individual needs of each patient, but is typically in the range of 20 mEq per day for the prevention of hypokalemia, to 40–100 mEq per day or more for the treatment of potassium depletion. During therapy serum potassium levels should be monitored and the dosage titrated to achieve the desired clinical and laboratory effects.

Overdosage: See KAOCHLOR 10% LIQUID.

Treatment Measures for Hyperkalemia: See KAOCHLOR 10% LIQUID.

How Supplied:
KAON Elixir-Grape
NDC 0013-3203-51 Pint.
NDC 0013-3203-53 Gallon.
NDC 0013-3203-56 Bottle of 4 Fl.Oz. (36's only).
NDC 0013-3203-58 Bottle of 15 ml., Stat-Pak® (Unit Dose) 100's only.
KAON Elixir-Lemon-Lime
NDC 0013-3303-51 Pint.
NDC 0013-3303-53 Gallon.
A.H.F.S. 40:12

KAON® TABLETS ℞
(Potassium Gluconate)

Description: Each sugar coated tablet supplies 5 mEq of elemental potassium (as potassium gluconate 1.17 g). Kaon Tablets are sugar coated, not enteric coated, which favors dissolution in the stomach and absorption before reaching the small intestine where the lesions with enteric potassium chloride have occurred. The sugar coating merely adds to palatability and ease of swallowing, not to delay absorption as does the enteric coating.

Indications: Oral potassium therapy for the prevention and treatment of hypokalemia which may occur secondary to diuretic or corticosteroid administration. It may be used in the treatment of cardiac arrhythmias due to digitalis intoxication.

Contraindications: Severe renal impairment with oliguria or azotemia, untreated Addison's disease, adynamia episodica hereditaria, acute dehydration, heat cramps and hyperkalemia from any cause.

Warning: There have been several reports, published and unpublished, concerning nonspecific small-bowel lesions consisting of stenosis, with or without ulceration, associated with the administration of enteric-coated thiazides with potassium salts. These lesions may occur with enteric-coated potassium tablets alone or when they are used with nonenteric-coated thiazides or certain other oral diuretics. These small bowel lesions have caused obstruction, hemorrhage and perforation. Surgery was frequently required and deaths have occurred. Available information tends to implicate enteric-coated potassium salts, although lesions of this type also occur spontaneously. Therefore, coated potassium-containing formulations should be administered only when indicated and should be discontinued immediately if abdominal pain, distention, nausea, vomiting, or gastrointestinal bleeding occur. Coated potassium tablets should be used only when adequate dietary supplementation is not practical.

Precautions: In response to a rise in the concentration of body potassium, renal excretion of the ion is increased. With normal kidney function, it is difficult, therefore, to produce potassium intoxication by oral administration. However, potassium supplements must be administered with caution, since the amount of the deficiency or daily dosage is not accurately known. Frequent checks of the clinical status of the patient, and periodic ECG and/or serum potassium levels should be made. High serum concentrations of potassium ion may cause death through cardiac depression, arrhythmias or arrest. This drug should be used with caution in the presence of cardiac disease.

In hypokalemic states, especially in patients on a salt-free diet, hypochloremic alkalosis is a possibility that may require chloride as well as potassium supplementation. In these circumstances, Kaon (potassium gluconate) should be supplemented with chloride. Ammonium chloride is an excellent source of chloride ion (18.7 mEq per Gram), but it should not be used in patients with hepatic cirrhosis where ammonium salts are contraindicated. Other sources for chloride are sodium chloride and Diluted Hydrochloric Acid, U.S.P. It should also be kept in mind that ammonium cycle cation exchange resin, sometimes used to treat hyperkalemia, should not be administered to patients with hepatic cirrhosis.

Adverse Reactions: Nausea, vomiting, diarrhea and abdominal discomfort have been reported. The symptoms and signs of potassium intoxication include paresthesias of the extremities, flaccid paralysis, listlessness, mental confusion, weakness and heaviness of the legs, fall in blood pressure, cardiac arrhythmias and heart block. Hyperkalemia may exhibit the following electrocardiographic abnormalities: disappearance of the P wave, widening and slurring of QRS complex, changes of the S-T segment, tall peaked T waves, etc.

Dosage and Administration: The usual adult dosage is 2 tablets four times daily (after meals and at bedtime). This supplies 40 mEq of elemental potassium, the approximate minimum adult daily requirement for potassium. Deviations from this recommendation may be indicated, since no average total daily dose can be defined but must be governed by close observation for clinical effects. However, potassium intoxication may result from any therapeutic dosage. See "Overdosage" and "Precautions."

Overdosage: Potassium intoxication may result from overdosage of potassium or from therapeutic dosage in conditions stated under "Contraindications." Hyperkalemia, when detected, must be treated immediately because lethal levels can be reached in a few hours.

Treatment of Hyperkalemia:

1. Dextrose solution, 10 or 25% containing 10 units of crystalline insulin per 20 g dextrose, given I.V. in a dose of 300 to 500 ml in an hour.
2. Adsorption and exchange of potassium using sodium or ammonium cycle cation exchange resin, orally and as retention enema. See "Precautions."
3. Hemodialysis and peritoneal dialysis.
4. The use of potassium-containing foods or medicaments must be eliminated.

In cases of digitalization too rapid a lowering of plasma potassium concentration can cause digitalis toxicity.

How Supplied:
NDC 0013-3121-17 Bottle of 100 Tablets
NDC 0013-3121-21 Bottle of 500 Tablets
NDC 0013-3121-18 Stat-Pak® (Unit Dose) 100's only
A.H.F.S. 40:12

KAON-CL TABS® ℞
(Potassium Chloride)
CONTROLLED RELEASE TABLETS

Description: Kaon-Cl Tabs is a sugar coated (not enteric-coated) tablet containing 500 mg potassium chloride (equivalent to 6.7 mEq potassium chloride) in a wax matrix. This formulation is intended to provide a controlled release of potassium from the matrix to minimize the likelihood of producing high localized concentrations of potassium within the gastrointestinal tract.

Actions: Potassium ion is the principal intracellular cation of most body tissues. Potassium ions participate in a number of essential physiological processes including the maintenance of intracellular tonicity, the transmission of nerve impulses, the contraction of cardiac, skeletal and smooth muscle and the maintenance of normal renal function.

Potassium depletion may occur whenever the rate of potassium loss through renal excretion and/or loss from the gastrointestinal tract exceeds the rate of potassium intake. Such depletion usually develops slowly as a consequence of prolonged therapy with oral diuretics, primary or secondary hyperaldosteronism, diabetic ketoacidosis, severe diarrhea, or inadequate replacement of potassium in patients on prolonged parenteral nutrition. Potassium depletion due to these causes is usually accompanied by a concomitant deficiency of chloride and is manifested by hypokalemia and metabolic alkalosis. Potassium depletion may produce weakness, fatigue, disturbances of cardiac rhythm (primarily ectopic beats), prominent U-waves in the electrocardiogram, and in advanced cases, flaccid paralysis and/or impaired ability to concentrate urine.

Potassium depletion associated with metabolic alkalosis is managed by correcting the fundamental cause of the deficiency whenever possible and administering supplemental potassium chloride, in the form of high potassium food or potassium chloride solution or tablets. In rare circumstances (e.g., patients with renal tubular acidosis) potassium depletion may be associated with metabolic acidosis and hyperchloremia. In such patients potassium replacement should be accomplished with potassium salts other than the chloride, such as potassium bicarbonate, potassium citrate, potassium acetate, or potassium gluconate.

Indications:

BECAUSE OF REPORTS OF INTESTINAL AND GASTRIC ULCERATION AND BLEEDING WITH SLOW RELEASE POTASSIUM CHLORIDE PREPARATIONS, THESE DRUGS SHOULD BE RESERVED FOR THOSE PATIENTS WHO CANNOT TOLERATE OR REFUSE TO TAKE LIQUIDS OR EFFERVESCENT POTASSIUM PREPARATIONS OR FOR PATIENTS IN WHOM THERE IS A PROBLEM OF COMPLIANCE WITH THESE PREPARATIONS.

1. For therapeutic use in patients with hypokalemia with or without metabolic alkalosis, in digitalis intoxication and in patients with hypokalemic familial periodic paralysis.
2. For the prevention of potassium depletion when the dietary intake is inadequate in the following conditions: Patients receiving digitalis and diuretics for congestive heart failure; hepatic cirrhosis with ascites, states of aldosterone excess with normal renal function, potassium-losing nephropathy, and with certain diarrheal states.
3. The use of potassium salts in patients receiving diuretics for uncomplicated essential hypertension is often unnecessary when such patients have a normal dietary pattern. Serum potassium should be checked periodically, however, and if hypokalemia occurs, dietary supplementation with potassium-containing foods may be adequate to control milder cases. In more severe cases supplementation with potassium salts may be indicated.

Contraindications: Potassium supplements are contraindicated in patients with hyperkalemia since a further increase in serum potassium concentration in such patients can produce cardiac arrest. Hyperkalemia may complicate any of the following conditions: Chronic renal failure, systemic acidosis such as diabetic acidosis, acute dehydration, extensive tissue breakdown as in severe burns, adrenal insufficiency, or the administration of a potassium-sparing diuretic (e.g., spironolactone, triamterene).

Wax-matrix potassium chloride preparations have produced esophageal ulceration in certain cardiac patients with esophageal compression due to enlarged left atrium. Potassium supplementation, when indicated in such patients, should be with a liquid preparation.

All solid dosage forms of potassium chloride supplements are contraindicated in any patient in whom there is cause for arrest or delay in tablet passage through the gastrointestinal tract. In these instances. potassium supplementation should be with a liquid preparation.

Warnings:

Hyperkalemia—In patients with impaired mechanisms for excreting potassium, the administration of potassium salts can produce hyperkalemia and cardiac arrest. This occurs most commonly in patients given potassium by the intravenous route but may also occur in patients given potassium orally. Potentially fatal hyperkalemia can develop rapidly and be asymptomatic. The use of potassium salts in patients with chronic renal disease, or any other condition which impairs potassium excretion, requires particularly careful monitoring of the serum potassium concentration and appropriate dosage adjustment.

Interaction with Potassium Sparing Diuretics—Hypokalemia should not be treated by the concomitant administration of potassium salts and a potassium-sparing diuretic (e.g., spironolactone or triamterene) since the simultaneous administration of these agents can produce severe hyperkalemia.

Gastrointestinal Lesions—Potassium chloride tablets have produced stenotic and/or ulcerative lesions of the small bowel and deaths. These lesions are caused by a high localized concentration of potassium ion in the region of a rapidly dissolving tablet, which injures the bowel wall and thereby produces obstruction, hemorrhage, or perforation. Kaon-Cl Tabs (potassium chloride) is a wax-matrix tablet formulated to provide a controlled rate of release of potassium chloride and thus to minimize the possibility of a high local concentration of potassium ion near the bowel wall. While the reported frequency of small bowel lesions is much less with wax-matrix tablets (less than one per 100,000 patient years) than with enteric-coated potassium chloride tablets (40-50 per 100,000 patient years) cases associated with wax-matrix tablets have been reported both in foreign countries and in the United States. In addition, perhaps because the wax-matrix preparations are not enteric-coated and release potassium in the stomach, there have been reports of upper gastrointestinal bleeding associated with these products. The total number of gastrointestinal lesions remains less than one per 100,000 patient years. Kaon-Cl Tabs should be discontinued immediately and the possibility of bowel obstruction or perforation considered if severe vomiting, abdominal pain, distention, or gastrointestinal bleeding occurs.

Metabolic Acidosis—Hypokalemia in patients with metabolic acidosis should be treated with an alkalinizing potassium salt such as potassium bicarbonate, potassium citrate, potassium acetate, or potassium gluconate.

Precautions: The diagnosis of potassium depletion is ordinarily made by demonstrating hypokalemia in a patient with a clinical history suggesting some cause for potassium depletion. In interpreting the serum potassium level, the physician should bear in mind that acute alkalosis *per se* can produce hypokalemia in the absence of a deficit in total body potassium while acute acidosis *per se* can increase the serum potassium concentration into the normal range even in the presence of a reduced total body potassium. The treatment of potassium depletion, particularly in the presence of cardiac disease, renal disease, or acidosis requires careful attention to acid-base balance and appropriate monitoring of serum electrolytes, the electrocardiogram, and the clinical status of the patient.

Adverse Reactions: The most common adverse reactions to oral potassium salts are nausea, vomiting, abdominal discomfort and diarrhea. These symptoms are due to irritation of the gastrointestinal tract and are best managed by diluting the preparation further, taking the dose with meals, or reducing the dose. The most severe adverse effects are hyperkalemia (see Contraindication, Warnings and Overdosage) and gastrointestinal obstruction, bleeding or perforation (see Warnings).

Overdosage: The administration of oral potassium salts to persons with normal excretory mechanisms for potassium rarely causes serious hyperkalemia. However, if excretory mechanisms are impaired or if potassium is administered too rapidly intravenously, potentially fatal hyperkalemia can result (see Contraindications and Warnings). It is important to recognize that hyperkalemia is usually asymptomatic and may be manifested only by an increased serum potassium concentration and characteristic electrocardiographic changes (peaking of T-waves, loss of P-wave, depression of S-T segment, and prolongation of the QT interval). Late manifestations include muscle-paralysis and cardiovascular collapse from cardiac arrest.

Treatment measures for hyperkalemia include the following:

1. Elimination of foods and medications containing potassium and of potassium-sparing diuretics.
2. Intravenous administration of 300 to 500 ml/hr of 10% dextrose solution containing 10–20 units of crystalline insulin per 1,000 ml.
3. Correction of acidosis, if present, with intravenous sodium bicarbonate.
4. Use of exchange resins, hemodialysis, or peritoneal dialysis.

In treating hyperkalemia, it should be recalled that in patients who have been stabilized on digitalis, too rapid a lowering of the serum potassium concentration can produce digitalis toxicity.

Dosage and Administration: The usual dietary intake of potassium by the average adult is 40 to 80 mEq per day. Potassium depletion sufficient to cause hypokalemia usually requires the loss of 200 or more mEq of potassium from the total body store.

Dosage must be adjusted to the individual needs of each patient but is typically in the range of 20 mEq per day for the prevention of hypokalemia to 40–100 mEq per day or more for the treatment of potassium depletion.

One Kaon-Cl Tabs three times daily provides 20 mEq of potassium chloride. Two Kaon-Cl Tabs three times daily provides 40 mEq of potassium chloride.

Tablets should be taken with a glass of water or other liquid.

How Supplied:

NDC 0013-3071-17 Bottle of 100 Tablets.
NDC 0013-3071-19 Bottle of 250 Tablets.
NDC 0013-3071-23 Bottle of 1000 Tablets.
NDC 0013-3071-18 Stat-Pak® Unit Dose Box of 100 Tablets.

KAON-CL 20%® ℞

(Potassium Chloride)
Sugar-Free

Description: Each 15 ml (tablespoonful) supplies 40 mEq each of potassium and chloride (as potassium chloride, 3 g) with saccharin and flavoring. Alcohol 5%.

Continued on next page

Warren-Teed—Cont.

Actions: See KAON-CL TABS®.
Indications: KAON-CL 20% is indicated for the treatment of potassium depletion in patients with hypokalemia and metabolic alkalosis, and for the treatment of digitalis intoxication. During therapy serum potassium levels should be monitored and the dosage titrated to achieve the desired clinical and laboratory effects. KAON-CL 20% is also indicated for the prevention of potassium depletion when the dietary intake of potassium is inadequate for this purpose. The prophylactic administration of potassium ion may be indicated in patients receiving digitalis and diuretics for the treatment of congestive heart failure, hepatic cirrhosis with ascites, patients with hypertension on long-term diuretic therapy, hyperaldosteronism states with normal renal function, the nephrotic syndrome, and certain diarrheal states.
Contraindications: Potassium supplements are contraindicated in patients with hyperkalemia since a further increase in serum potassium concentration in such patients can produce cardiac arrest. Hyperkalemia may complicate any of the following conditions: Chronic renal failure, systemic acidosis such as diabetic acidosis, acute dehydration, extensive tissue breakdown as in severe burns, adrenal insufficiency, or the administration of a potassium-sparing diuretic (e.g., spironolactone, triamterene).
Warnings: Do not administer full strength. Kaon-CL 20% will cause gastrointestinal irritation if administered undiluted. For details regarding adequate dilution, see Dosage and Administration.
In patients with impaired mechanisms for excreting potassium, the administration of potassium salts can produce hyperkalemia and cardiac arrest. This occurs most commonly in patients given potassium by the intravenous route but may also occur in patients given potassium orally. Potentially fatal hyperkalemia can develop rapidly and be asymptomatic. The use of potassium salts in patients with chronic renal disease, or any other condition which impairs potassium excretion, requires particularly careful monitoring of the serum potassium concentration and appropriate dosage adjustment.
Hypokalemia should not be treated by the concomitant administration of potassium salts and a potassium-sparing diuretic (e.g., spironolactone or triamterene) since the simultaneous administration of these agents can produce severe hyperkalemia.
Potassium chloride tablets have produced stenotic and/or ulcerative lesions of the small bowel and deaths. These lesions are caused by a high localized concentration of potassium ion in the region of a rapidly dissolving tablet, which injures the bowel wall and thereby produces obstruction, hemorrhage, or perforation.
Hypokalemia in patients with metabolic *acidosis* should be treated with an alkalinizing potassium salt such as potassium bicarbonate, potassium citrate, potassium acetate, or potassium gluconate.
Precautions: See KAON-CL TABS®
Adverse Reactions: See KAON-CL TABS®
Overdosage: See KAON-CL TABS®
Dosage and Administration: In order to assure against gastrointestinal injury, patients should be reminded to follow directions regarding dilution. The usual dietary intake of potassium by the average adult is 40 to 80 mEq per day. Potassium depletion sufficient to cause hypokalemia usually requires the loss of 200 or more mEq of potassium from the total body store.
Dosage must be adjusted to the individual needs of each patient but is typically in the range of 20 mEq per day for the prevention of hypokalemia to 40–100 mEq per day or more for the treatment of potassium depletion.
One tablespoonful (15 ml) in six fluid ounces or more of water provides 40 mEq of potassium chloride.
One tablespoonful twice a day in six or more fluid ounces of water or other liquid provides 80 mEq potassium chloride.
How Supplied:
NDC 0013-3113-51 Pint.
NDC 0013-3113-53 Gallon.
NDC 0013-3113-56 Bottles of 4 Fl. Oz. (36's only).

MAGAN® ℞
(Magnesium Salicylate)

Description: Each capsule shaped scored tablet contains: 650 mg magnesium salicylate (10 grains).
Actions: Antiarthritic.
Indications: Magan is indicated for the relief of the signs and symptoms of rheumatoid arthritis, osteoarthritis, bursitis and other musculoskeletal disorders.
Contraindications: Magan is contraindicated in patients with advanced chronic renal insufficiency. May counteract the effect of uricosuric agents and should not be prescribed for patients on such drugs.
Warnings: As with all salicylates, Magan should be avoided or administered with caution to patients with liver damage, pre-existing hypoprothrombinemia, vitamin K deficiency, and before surgery.
Precautions: Appropriate precautions should be taken in prescribing Magan for persons known to be sensitive to salicylates, and in patients with erosive gastritis or peptic ulcer. If reaction develops, drug should be discontinued. Magan should be used with caution, if at all, concomitantly with anticoagulants.
Appropriate precautions should be taken in administering Magan to patients with any impairment of renal function including discontinuing other drugs containing magnesium and monitoring serum magnesium levels if dosage levels of Magan are high.
Adverse Reactions: Side effects encountered with aspirin may be encountered with Magan with the exception of asthmatic reactions, and inhibition of platelet aggregation and increased bleeding time.
Dosage and Administration: The dosage for Magan in the treatment of muscular skeletal disorders such as arthritis should be adjusted according to individual patient needs. The recommended initial dosage is six tablets per day, given in divided doses.
Children under 12 years of age: Not recommended since experience is limited.
Overdosage: Symptoms of salicylism resulting from high doses of Magan can be expected to resemble those associated with aspirin intoxication. These may range from dizziness, drowsiness and ringing in the ears to vertigo, convulsions, coma.
How Supplied:
NDC 0013-4111-17 Bottle of 100 Tablets
NDC 0013-4111-21 Bottle of 500 Tablets

MODANE® Bulk

Description: Modane Bulk is a powdered mixture consisting of: Psyllium and dextrose in equal parts.
Actions: Modane Bulk acts to increase the frequency of bowel movements by adding bulk and softens the fecal mass by retaining water.
Indications: Modane Bulk is useful in the treatment of constipation resulting from an inadequate or low residue diet. It is also useful as adjunctive therapy in treating the constipation of diverticular disease and in spastic or irritable colon, as well as in the bowel management of hemorrhoids, pregnancy, convalescence and senility.
Contraindications: Intestinal obstruction, fecal impaction.
Adverse Reactions: Esophageal, gastric, small intestinal and rectal obstruction due to the accumulation of mucilaginous components of psyllium have been reported. Most frequently this results from inadequate water intake or underlying organic disease. The dosage and administration schedule and fluid requirements should be carefully observed, as with other preparations.
Precaution: This product may combine with certain other drugs. Do not take this product if you are presently taking salicylates or a prescription drug.
Dosage and Administration: Adults (over 12 years): one rounded teaspoonful taken 1–3 times a day stirred into an 8 ounce glass of water, juice or other suitable liquids and preferably followed by an equal amount of liquid. Children (6 to 12 years): One-half the adult dosage in 8 ounces of liquid.
The laxative effect usually occurs in 12–24 hours, but up to three days of medication may be necessary to achieve full effect.
This product information is for professional use only.
How Supplied:
NDC 0013-5025-72 14 oz. container.

MODANE® Soft
(Dioctyl Sodium Sulfosuccinate)

Description: Each Modane Soft capsule contains dioctyl sodium sulfosuccinate, 120 mg, in a soft-gelatin capsule.
Actions: Modane Soft is a stool softener which has surface active properties believed to permit water and lipid to penetrate the fecal mass and soften the stool for easier passage.
Indications: Functional constipation caused by dry, hard stools. Modane Soft is useful when painful rectal conditions or other patient conditions require a soft, easily passed stool.
Contraindications: Mineral oil administration, or when abdominal pain, nausea, or vomiting are present.
Dosage and Administration: Adults (over 12 years)—1 to 3 capsules daily. Children (6 to 12 years)—1 capsule daily.
Usually require 1–2 days for full effect.
How Supplied:
NDC 0013-5031-13 Package of 30 capsules.

MODANE®, TABLETS AND LIQUID
(Danthron)

Description: Modane Tablets (yellow)—Each contains danthron 75 mg. Modane Mild Tablets (half-strength, pink)—Each contains danthron 37.5 mg. Modane Liquid—Each 5 ml. (teaspoonful) contains danthron 37.5 mg. and alcohol 5%.
Actions: Laxative.
Indications: A laxative designed for gentle overnight relief of constipation without straining, griping or cramping at optimal dosage. There is usually no tolerance build-up or need for increasing dosage with danthron, the laxative component of MODANE having a selective action on the large bowel. MODANE may be useful in the management of constipation in geriatric, cardiac, surgical, pregnant, post partum and pediatric patients. MODANE has been found useful in the management of constipation which may occur with or during the concomitant use of ganglionic blocking agents, antihistamines, tranquilizers, sympathomimetics and anticholingergics.
Contraindications: Should not be used when abdominal pain, nausea, vomiting or other signs and/or symptoms of appendicitis are present.
Precautions: Frequent or prolonged use of this preparation may result in dependence on laxatives. Pink coloration of urine is harmless and usually signals an alkaline urine (frequently a diagnostic aid). If excessive bowel

activity due to excessive dosage causes perianal irritation, discontinue MODANE temporarily and/or decrease dosage. Hypokalemia may impair the effectiveness of Modane.

Dosage and Administration: Modane Tablet (yellow)—Adults—1 tablet with the evening meal. Modane Mild Tablet (half-strength, pink) - Adults - 1 or 2 tablets with the evening meal. For hypersensitive, diet-restricted and bedfast patients; also children (6 to 12 years of age) - 1 tablet with the evening meal. Modane Liquid - Adults - 1 to 2 teaspoonfuls with the evening meal. For hypersensitive, diet-restricted and bedfast patients; also children (6 to 12 years of age) - 1 teaspoonful with the evening meal. Children (1 to 6 years of age) - 1/4 to 1 teaspoonful, according to age, with the evening meal. Infants (6 to 12 months of age) - 1/5 to 1/4 teaspoonful (20 to 25 drops), according to age, with the evening meal.

How Supplied:
Modane Tablets
NDC 0013-5011-17 Bottle of 100 Tablets
NDC 0013-5011-23 Bottle of 1000 Tablets
NDC 0013-5011-18 Stat-Pak® (Unit Dose of one tablet) 100's only
NDC 0013-5011-07 Package of 10
NDC 0013-5011-13 Package of 30
Modane Mild Tablets
NDC 0013-5021-17 Bottle of 100 Tablets
NDC 0013-5021-23 Bottle of 1000 Tablets
Modane Liquid
NDC 0013-5033-51 Pint
A.H.F.S. 56:12

MYOFLEX® CREME
(Triethanolamine Salicylate)

Description: Triethanolamine salicylate 10% in a non-greasy base. Nonirritating, nonburning, odorless, stainless, readily absorbed.

Actions: Topical Analgesic. Penetration assured with maximal salicylate appearing in urine 5 hours after application.

Indications: An effective analgesic rub for sore muscles, joint attachments, stiffness and strains; a helpful topical adjunct in arthritis and rheumatism. Excellent as a hand cream for patients with minor rheumatic stiffness and soreness of the hands. Excellent for sore feet.

Contraindications: Do not use in patients manifesting idiosyncrasy to salicylates.

Warnings: For external use only. Avoid getting into eyes or on mucous membranes. To be used only according to directions. Keep out of the reach of children.

Precautions: Apply to affected parts only. Do not apply to irritated skin or if excessive irritation develops, consult physician. A 2 oz. tube contains the salicylate equivalent of about 56 grains of aspirin.

Adverse Reactions: None reported, but if applied to large skin areas may cause typical salicylate side effects such as tinnitus, nausea, or vomiting.

Dosage and Administration: Adults—Rub into area of soreness two or three times daily. Wrists, elbows, knees and ankles may be wrapped loosely with 2″ or 3″ elastic bandage after liberal application.

How Supplied:
NDC 0013-5404-61 Tubes, 2 oz.
NDC 0013-5404-74 Jars, 1 lb.

TYMPAGESIC® ℞

Description: Phenylephrine hydrochloride 0.25%, antipyrine 5%, benzocaine 5% in propylene glycol.

Actions: Analgesic and decongestant ear drops.

Indications: To help relieve the pain and reduce the swelling which may occur in patients with acute non-suppurative otitis media and /or otitis externa.

Contraindications: Benzocaine sensitivity.

Adverse Reaction: Dermatitis (rarely).

Dosage and Administration: Fill the ear canal. Plug with cotton. May repeat every four hours as necessary.

How Supplied:
NDC 0013-7363-39 Dropper Bottle, 13 ml.

Webcon Pharmaceuticals
Division of ALCON LABORATORIES (PUERTO RICO), INC.
P.O. BOX 1629
FORT WORTH, TEXAS 76101

SUPPRETTES®, Webcon's identifying trademark for suppository medication in the NEOCERA® BASE, a unique blend of water-soluble Carbowaxes* that release drugs by hydrophilic action.
*TM Union Carbide.

ANESTACON® ℞
(2% lidocaine hydrochloride)

Description: A sterile anesthetic for endourethral use. Each ml contains: Active: Lidocaine Hydrochloride 20 mg (2%). Vehicle: Hydroxypropyl Methylcellulose 10 mg (1%). Preservative: Benzalkonium Chloride 0.1 mg (0.01%). Inactive: Sodium Chloride, Hydrochloric Acid and/or Sodium Hydroxide (to adjust pH), Purified Water. DM-OO

Actions: Acts on surface mucous membranes of the urethra to produce local anesthesia. The anesthetic effect usually begins within two to five minutes and lasts for at least 30 minutes.

Indications: For prevention and control of pain in procedures involving the male and female urethra and for topical treatment of painful urethritis.

Contraindications: Contraindicated in patients with a known sensitivity (allergy) to lidocaine or other drugs of a similar chemical nature.

Warnings: RESUSCITATIVE EQUIPMENT AND DRUGS SHOULD BE IMMEDIATELY AVAILABLE WHEN ANY LOCAL ANESTHETIC IS USED. Lidocaine should be used with extreme caution on traumatized mucosa or in a region of sepsis.

USAGE IN PREGNANCY: Safe use of lidocaine has not been established with respect to possible adverse effects upon fetal development; therefore, it should not be used in women of childbearing potential and particularly during early pregnancy unless in the judgment of the physician the potential benefits outweigh the unknown hazards.

NOTE: After initial use, the remaining contents of the container should be discarded.

Precautions: The smallest volume that will produce effective anesthesia is recommended, and caution should be exercised to avoid overdosage. The safety and effectiveness are dependent on proper dosage, correct technique, adequate precautions, and readiness for emergencies. The debilitated, elderly, acutely ill, and children should be given reduced doses commensurate with their age and physical condition. Use cautiously in persons with known drug sensitivities or allergies.

Adverse Reactions: Adverse reactions result from high plasma levels due to excessive dosage, rapid absorption, or inadvertent intravascular injection. Hypersensitivity, idiosyncrasy, or diminished tolerance may also be the cause of reactions. Reactions due to overdosage (high plasma levels) are systemic and involve the central nervous system and the cardiovascular system.

Reactions involving the central nervous system are characterized by excitation and/or depression. Nervousness, dizziness, blurred vision or tremors may occur, followed by convulsions, unconsciousness, drowsiness, and possible respiratory arrest. Excitement may be transient or absent, and the first manifestations may be drowsiness, merging into unconsciousness and respiratory arrest.

Reactions involving the cardiovascular system include depression of the myocardium, hypotension, bradycardia, and even cardiac arrest. Treatment of a patient with toxic manifestations consists of maintaining an airway, and supporting ventilation using oxygen and assisted or controlled respiration as required. Supportive treatment of the cardiovascular system consists of using vasopressors, preferably those that stimulate the myocardium (e.g. ephedrine, metaraminol, etc.) and intravenous fluids. Convulsions may be controlled by the intravenous administration in small increments of an ultra-short-acting barbiturate (i.e. thiopental, thiamylal) or a short-acting muscle relaxant (succinylcholine), together with oxygen. Muscle relaxants and intravenous barbiturates should only be used by those familiar with their use.

Allergic reactions are characterized by cutaneous lesions of delayed onset, urticaria, edema, or other manifestations of allergy. The detection of sensitivity by skin testing is of doubtful value.

Dosage and Administration: Dosage varies and depends upon the area to be anesthetized, vascularity of the tissues, individual tolerance, and the technique of anesthesia. The least volume of the drug needed to provide effective anesthesia should be administered. For specific techniques and procedures refer to standard texts. THE USUAL DOSE SHOULD NOT EXCEED 600 mg IN ANY TWELVE HOUR PERIOD.

15 ML SINGLE-DOSE CONTAINER: ADULT MALES: Immediately before use, remove the label and cap and firmly insert the sterile tip into the urethral orifice. Slowly instill 5 ml to 15 ml by exerting pressure on opposite sides of the container—the full dose should be administered in a single action without removing the tip. While waiting two to five minutes for induction of anesthesia, the urethra should be occluded with a penile clamp or by manual compression. ADULT FEMALES: The sterile tip may be used to insert about 1 ml.

240 ML CONTAINER: Note: This is for use for only one patient.

ADULT MALES: Instill slowly into the urethra 5 ml to 15 ml and allow two to five minutes for induction of anesthesia. The medication is retained in the urethra by means of a penile clamp or by manual compression of the distal urethra. ADULT FEMALES: Apply liberal amount of medication on a cotton swab and insert into urethra for two to five minutes, or a dropper may be employed to insert about 1 ml.

How Supplied: In 15 ml and 240 ml single-dose disposable containers.
Mfd. for: Alcon Laboratories (Puerto Rico), Inc. Humacao, P.R. 00661
Mfd by: Alcon Laboratories, Inc. Fort Worth, Texas 76134 USA

AQUACHLORAL® SUPPRETTES® Ⓒ ℞
(chloral hydrate suppositories)

Description: Each SUPPRETTE® (suppository) contains: Active: chloral hydrate 5 gr (325 mg) (grooved for 1/2 dosage), 10 gr (650 mg), or 15 gr (1.0 g); Vehicle: NEOCERA® base containing polyethylene glycol 400, polyethylene glycol 1540, polyethylene glycol 6000, polysorbate 60 and color additives including FD&C Yellow No. 5 (tartrazine) in AQUACHLORAL 5 gr. and AQUACHLORAL 15 gr.

AQUACHLORAL® SUPPRETTES® are color-coded for easy identification by the patient and the physician—green for AQUA-

Continued on next page

Webcon—Cont.

CHLORAL 5 gr, blue for AQUACHLORAL 10 gr, and Yellow for AQUACHLORAL 15 gr.
Warning: May be habit forming.
Actions: Since 1953 chloral hydrate in the NEOCERA® suppository base has proven to be very effective rectally as a hypnotic and/or sedative. Irritation has rarely been encountered following correct insertion, a simple procedure which specifies wetting the suppository and the inserting finger with water only before inserting. Absorption of the drug occurs in a short period of time and with therapeutic doses blood pressure and respiration are affected little more than by ordinary sleep. Older patients usually tolerate chloral hydrate even when they are intolerant of barbiturates.
Indications: Hypnotic and/or sedative therapy rectally.
Contraindications: Sensitivity to chloral hydrate and/or the base; large doses in patients with severe heart disease; patients with severe renal or hepatic impairment.
Warnings: Habituation and tolerance do occur. Sudden withdrawal may result in delirium. Chloral hydrate antagonizes the action of some drugs such as coumarin and related anticoagulants.
Precautions: Caution is recommended in combining chloral hydrate with other CNS depressants such as alcohol.
AQUACHLORAL 5 gr and AQUACHLORAL 15 gr contain FD&C Yellow No. 5 (tartrazine) which may cause allergic-type reactions (including bronchial asthma) in certain susceptible individuals. Although the overall incidence of FD&C Yellow No. 5 (tartrazine) sensitivity in the general population is low, it is frequently seen in patients who also have aspirin hypersensitivity.
Adverse Reactions: No significant adverse reactions have been reported with AQUACHLORAL® SUPPRETTES®. Oral administration has resulted in gastric irritation and vomiting. Occasionally allergic skin rashes have been reported.
Dosage and Administration: Adults: Hypnotic Use—15 to 30 grains rectally in a single dose on retiring. Sedative Use—5 to 10 grains rectally three times daily. Total daily dose not to exceed 30 grains. Children: Hypnotic use—5 grains rectally per 40 lbs body weight, three times daily. Sedative use—½ the hypnotic dose. Lubricate the SUPPRETTE® and inserting finger with water only.
How Supplied: In strip-packaged units of 12.

B & O SUPPRETTES® Ⓒ℞
No. 15A and No. 16A
(belladonna and opium suppositories)

Description: Each B & O Supprette® contains (in water-soluble Neocera® Base):
B & O No. 15A: powdered opium* 30 mg (½ gr) and powdered belladonna extract ¼ gr (15 mg) (equivalent to 0.00312 gr alkaloids of belladonna).
B & O No. 16A: powdered opium* 60 mg (1 gr) and powdered belladonna extract ¼ gr (15 mg) (equivalent to 0.00312 gr alkaloids of belladonna).
*WARNING: **May be habit forming.**
Neocera® Base is a blend of polyethylene glycol 400, 1540 and 6000, and polysorbate 60.
Actions: Morphine, an alkaloid of opium, is the predominant active principle of powdered opium. The atropine effect is predominant in belladonna extract and serves to eliminate morphine-induced smooth muscle spasm without affecting the sedative-analgesic action of powdered opium.
Indications: For relief of moderate to severe pain not responsive to non-narcotic analgesics; to space intervals between injections of opiates; relief of pain due to ureteral spasm.
Contraindications: Glaucoma, severe hepatic or renal disease, bronchial asthma, narcotic idiosyncrasies, respiratory depression, convulsive disorders, acute alcoholism, delirium tremens and premature labor. The preparations are not recommended for use in children.
Warning: True addiction may result from opium usage.
Precautions: Administer with caution to persons with a known idiosyncrasy to atropine-like compounds, cardiac disease, incipient glaucoma or prostatic hypertrophy. Caution should be used in administration to old and debilitated patients, and patients with increased intracranial pressure, toxic psychosis, and myxedema.
Adverse Reactions: Belladonna may cause drowsiness, dry mouth, urinary retention, photophobia, rapid pulse, dizziness and blurred vision. Opium usage may result in constipation and nausea and vomiting may occur. Pruritus and urticaria occasionally occur.
Dosage and Administration: Adults: One B & O No. 15A or No. 16A Supprette®, rectally, once or twice daily, or as recommended by the physician. Moisten finger and Supprette® with water before inserting.
Overdosage: As with morphine and related narcotics, overdosage is characterized by respiratory depression, pinpoint pupils and coma. Respiratory depression may be reversed by intravenous administration of naloxone hydrochloride or levallorphan tartrate. In addition, supportive measures such as oxygenation, intravenous fluids and vasopressors should be used as indicated.
How Supplied: In strip-packaged units of 12 (scored for ½ dosage). DEA order required (Schedule II).

CYSTOSPAZ® ℞
Hyoscyamine Tablets, N.F.
CYSTOSPAZ-SR® ℞
hyoscyamine sulfate and butabarbital
CYSTOSPAZ-M® ℞
hyoscyamine sulfate

Description:
CYSTOSPAZ®: Each tablet contains hyoscyamine 0.15 mg.
CYSTOSPAZ-SR®: Each sustained release capsule contains hyoscyamine sulfate 375 mcg with butabarbital* 45 mg. (Warning: may be habit forming).
*Derivative of Barbituric Acid
CYSTOSPAZ-M®: Each sustained release capsule contains hyoscyamine sulfate 375 mcg.
Actions:
CYSTOSPAZ® provides prompt relief of smooth muscle spasm through the anticholinergic action of hyoscyamine.
CYSTOSPAZ-SR® provides prompt and prolonged antispasmodic and sedative action.
CYSTOSPAZ-M® provides prompt and prolonged antispasmodic action.
Indications: Management of disorders of the lower urinary tract associated with hypermotility. Although specific therapy is often required to remove the underlying cause of spasm, CYSTOSPAZ® and CYSTOSPAZ-M® are offered as antispasmodic agents and CYSTOSPAZ-SR® is offered as an antispasmodic-sedative which may be combined with other forms of therapy where indicated.
Contraindications: Glaucoma, urinary bladder neck or pyloric obstruction, duodenal obstruction and cardiospasm. Hypersensitivity to any of the ingredients.
CYSTOSPAZ-SR® because of its barbiturate content is contraindicated in porphyria and in individuals sensitive to barbiturates.
Precautions: Administer with caution to persons with known idiosyncrasy to atropine-like compounds, and to patients suffering from cardiac disease.
Adverse Reactions: Though rarely a problem, the side effects encountered with other antispasmodic - antisecretory agents (drowsiness, dry mouth, photophobia, constipation, urinary retention) may also be seen with these drugs.
If rapid pulse, dizziness, or blurring of vision occurs, discontinue use immediately. Acute urinary retention may be precipitated in prostatic hypertrophy. NOTE: Slight dryness of the mouth is an indication that parasympathetic blockage is effective. The patient should be warned that this may occur.
Dosage and Administration:
CYSTOSPAZ®: Adults: One or two tablets four times daily or fewer if needed. Older Children: Reduce dosage in proportion to age and weight.
CYSTOSPAZ-SR®: One capsule twice daily; every 12 hours.
CYSTOSPAZ-M®: One capsule twice daily; every 12 hours.
How Supplied:
CYSTOSPAZ®: Bottles of 100 light blue tablets.
CYSTOSPAZ-SR®: Bottles of 100 opaque blue and clear yellow sustained release capsules.
CYSTOSPAZ-M®: Bottles of 100 clear blue sustained release capsules.

URISED® ℞

Description: *Each tablet contains active:*

Atropine Sulfate	0.03 mg
Hyoscyamine	0.03 mg
Methenamine	40.8 mg
Methylene Blue	5.4 mg
Phenyl Salicylate	18.1 mg
Benzoic Acid	4.5 mg

Actions: The parasympatholytic action of atropine and hyoscyamine relaxes smooth muscle spasm. Methenamine is a lower urinary tract anti-infective as a result of its conversion to formaldehyde in acid bladder urine.
Indications: URISED® is indicated for the relief of discomfort of the lower urinary tract caused by hypermotility, and in the treatment of cystitis, urethritis, and trigonitis when the offending organisms are susceptible to formaldehyde. URISED® is useful as a prophylactic prior to urinary tract instrumentation or operation, and for relief of lower urinary tract symptoms during diagnostic procedures.
Contraindications: Glaucoma, urinary bladder neck or pyloric obstruction, duodenal obstruction and cardiospasm. Hypersensitivity to any of the ingredients.
Precautions: Administer with caution to persons with known idiosyncrasy to atropine-like compounds, and to patients suffering from cardiac disease. During URISED® therapy, the urine is blue; patients should be so advised to allay apprehension.
Adverse Reactions: If pronounced dryness of the mouth, flushing, or difficulty in initiating micturition occurs, decrease dosage. If rapid pulse, dizziness, or blurring of vision occurs, discontinue use immediately. Acute urinary retention may be precipitated in prostatic hypertrophy.
Dosage and Administration: Adults: Two tablets four times daily, followed by liberal fluid intake. Older Children: Reduce dosage in proportion to age and weight.
How Supplied: Bottles of 100, 500, and 1,000 blue tablets.
Note: Store at room temperature.

WANS® Ⓒ
(ANTI-NAUSEA SUPPRETTES®)
(pyrilamine maleate and pentobarbital sodium)

Description: Each WANS® SUPPRETTE® contains (in water-soluble Neocera® Base):
WANS® Children (blue): pyrilamine maleate 25 mg and pentobarbital sodium* 30 mg; scored for ½ dosage.

WANS® No. 1 (pink): pyrilamine maleate 50 mg and pentobarbital sodium* 50 mg; scored for ½ dosage.
WANS® No. 2 (yellow): pyrilamine maleate 50 mg and pentobarbital sodium* 100 mg; scored ½ dosage.
***Warning: May be habit forming.**
Neocera® Base is a blend of Polyethylene Glycol 400, 1540 and 6000, Polysorbate 60 and coloring.
Actions: Combines the antihistaminic properties of pyrilamine maleate with the sedative effects of pentobarbital sodium.
Indications: Symptomatic treatment of nausea and vomiting.
Contraindications: Acute intermittent porphyria, known hypersensitivity to barbiturates or antihistamines, known previous barbiturate addiction, in senility, severe hepatic impairment, and in the presence of uncontrolled pain, acute head injury associated with vomiting or other signs of CNS injury. Not for use in infants under 6 months of age since they are more sensitive to the central nervous system stimulating effects of pyrilamine maleate than adults. Pyrilamine maleate may cause convulsions in infants, particularly in excessive dosage.
Warnings:

Caution should be exercised when administering WANS® to children for the treatment of vomiting. Antiemetics are not recommended for treatment of uncomplicated vomiting in children and their use should be limited to prolonged vomiting of known etiology. There are three principal reasons for caution:

1. There have been some recent reports of toxic encephalopathy, characterized by a depressed level of consciousness, marked irritability and ataxia, in infants and children following administration of higher-than-recommended doses of pyrilamine maleate and pentobarbital sodium combination products such as WANS®. **The recommended dosage should therefore not be exceeded.**
2. There has been some suspicion that centrally acting antiemetics may contribute, in combination with viral illnesses (a possible cause of vomiting in children), to development of Reye's syndrome, a potentially fatal acute childhood encephalopathy with visceral fatty degeneration, especially involving the liver. Although there is no confirmation of this suspicion, caution is nevertheless recommended.
3. It should also be noted that salicylates and acetaminophen are hepatotoxic at large doses. Although it is not known that at usual doses they would represent a hazard in patients with the underlying hepatic disorder of Reye's syndrome, these drugs should be avoided in children whose signs and symptoms could represent Reye's syndrome, unless alternative methods of controlling fever are not successful.

Barbiturates may be habit forming. Administration in the presence of pre-existing psychologic disturbances may result in confusion, delirium, and accentuation of symptoms. Idiosyncratic reactions may occur and include lassitude, vertigo, nausea, vomiting, and diarrhea. Acquired sensitivity to barbiturates may result in allergic reactions including urticaria, dermatitis, and rarely, exfoliative dermatitis and degenerative changes in the liver and kidney. The safety of WANS® in pregnancy has not been established.
Precautions: WANS® should be administered with caution to patients with a history of drug dependence or suicidal tendencies. Caution should be exercised when the drug is used concurrently with other sedative, hypnotic, or narcotic agents. Patients should also be cautioned against taking alcoholic beverages or other CNS depressants while taking this product. This drug should be given with caution to patients with known acute or chronic hepatic disease, fever, hyperthyroidism, diabetes mellitus, severe anemia, and congestive heart failure. Patients taking WANS® should not drive, operate machinery, or otherwise engage in activities where impairment of alertness and coordination could result in accidents and injury.
Adverse Reactions: Antihistamine side effects include drowsiness, potentiation of the sedative effect of barbiturates, fatigue, vertigo, incoordination, tremor, muscle weakness, dryness of the nose, mouth and throat, tinnitus, pupillary dilatation and blurred vision, urinary retention, impotence, epigastric and intestinal pain, anorexia, nausea, vomiting, diarrhea, excitation, euphoria, insomnia, nervousness, palpitation, tachycardia, hypotension, hypersensitivity reactions such as allergic dermatitis, and rarely, blood dyscrasias. Overdose, particularly in children, may result in hallucinations, excitement, ataxia, incoordination, athetosis, convulsions, and death.
Side effects associated with barbiturates include drowsiness, lethargy, sedation, paradoxic restlessness or excitement in susceptible persons, respiratory depression, coma, and delirium.
Dosage and Administration:
Children: For children 2 to 12 years of age (over 15 kg bodyweight) the usual dose is one WANS® Children, rectally, every 6 to 8 hours as required. Do not exceed three doses in 24 hours. Children 6 months to 2 years of age (less than 15 kg bodyweight) should use not more than ½ the above dosage. **Do not use in infants below the age of 6 months.** In determining the optimum dosage in infants and children, consideration should be given in each case to the age and weight of the patient, the etiology and severity of the condition being treated and the clinical response. **The above recommended dosages should not be exceeded (see "Warnings").**
Adults: Rectally, one WANS® No. 1 to inhibit mild nausea and/or vomiting or one WANS® No. 2 to control prenicious vomiting. Repeat doses for adults should be 4 to 6 hours apart; do not exceed four doses in 24 hours. The optimum dosage must be determined in each case by the clinical response. Moisten finger and SUPPRETTE® with water before inserting.
How Supplied: In strip packaged units of 12 (scored for ½ dosage).

Wesley Pharmacal Company, Inc., The
**4831-33 RISING SUN AVE.
PHILADELPHIA, PA 19120**

P.D.P. LIQUID PROTEIN
Protein Supplement
15 gm. per 30 cc - 60 Calories per 30 cc

P.D.P. PROTEIN CAPSULES
1 gm. per Capsule

P.D.P. is hydrolyzed protein (pre-disgested) in which the protein has been broken down into amino acids and is utilized 100% by the body. No fats or carbohydrates are contained.
How Supplied: 1 Quart Bottles, 100 Capsules.

P.D.P. PROTEIN POWDER
Cream of Chicken Soup
Cream of Vegetable Soup
Soy Base

How Supplied: 1 lb. Containers.

PANITOL TABLETS ℞

Composition: Each Capsule Shaped Tablet contains 15 mg. BUTALBITAL (Warning: May be habit forming) and 300 mg. PANITONE (Wesley brand of Acetaminophen).
Action and Uses: PANITOL Tablets are an anodyne-calmative specifically formulated for tension headaches. PANITOL Tablets contain Butalbital, an intermediate-acting barbituate which produces mild sedation in about 15 minutes and lasts for about 4 hours, and Acetaminophen, an analgesic which rarely causes gastric disturbances.
Administration and Dosage: Adults—one tablet three times daily.
Precautions: May cause drowsiness.
Contraindications: PANITOL is contraindicated in hepatic disease.
How Supplied:

100 Bottles	NDC 0917 0817 01
1000 "	NDC 0917 0817 10

URACID ℞
(dl Methionine)

Description: Each capsule contains:
dl-Methionine..........0.2 gm.
Action and Uses: Management of diaper rash in infants, and the control of odor in incontinent adults. An ammonia-free urine is affected by the acid producing effect of dl-methionine on pH of urine.
Contraindications: Do not use in patients with a history of liver disease because the toxemia of the disease may be exaggerated by large doses of methionine.
Precautions: Prolonged excessive doses of methionine may result in a below-normal weight gain. Adequate protein intake should be assured during long periods of methionine therapy.
Administration and Dosages: Diaper rash in infants, empty contents of one capsule into evening formula, preferably while still warm; or it may be added to orange juice. Odor control in adults: One capsule three times daily with meals.
How Supplied:

100 bottles.	NDC 0917-0240-01
1000 bottles.	NDC 0917-0240-10

Literature Available: Yes.

Western Research Laboratories, Inc.
**301 SOUTH CHEROKEE
DENVER, COLORADO 80223**

MAGNESIUM GLUCONATE
PROD. IDENT. MG

Formula: Each Tablet Contains:
Magnesium Gluconate..........(0.5 Gm.) 500 mg.
(supplying approximate 29 mg. Elemental Magnesium)
Action: Magnesium is the second most abundant interacellular cation. The human body contains 20-30 grams slightly more than half of which is in the skeletal system. Adult fat tissue contains about 43 mg./kg. Magnesium is now known to be required for the activity of a great many enzymes, particularly those concerned with oxidative phosphorylation. Clear cut evidence of magnesium deficiency in man has recently been described. Hypomagnesemic tetany, very similar to hypocalemic tetany, is distinguished by the serum calcium and magnesium levels and prompt response to magnesium administration. Recent evidence leaves no doubt that magnesium deficiency may be a substantial clinical problem. There is no satisfactory evidence of the normal requirement, but values of 150 mg. per day for infants, 400 mg. per day during pregnancy and lactation

Continued on next page

Western Research—Cont.

and 250 mg. per day for adults have been suggested as adequate. Serum magnesium values are 1.5 to 2.5 mEq./L. Magnesium gluconate is a most desirable source of magnesium. Its low toxicity, lack of irritating properties and tolerance during treatment of extended duration are advantageous properties for therapeutic use. It is stable, lacks odor and taste and is readily soluble and is promptly absorbed.
Indications: In hypomagnesemic states; malnutrition, excessive gastro-intestinal losses, renal wasting and hepatic insufficiency, and alcoholic states. In primary dysmenorrhea MG (Magnesium Gluconate) helps diminish the frequency and intensity of uterine contractions and abolishes myometrial hyperexcitability, anoxia and pain. Magnesium deficiency syndrome is characterized by muscle twitching, hyperactive reflexes, tremors, convulsions, coma and anxiety. It is occasionally manifested by delirium, fever, excessive perspiration and mental confusion. Low body magnesium (deficiency) is best indicated by a 24 hour urine value below the normal 14-20 mEq/24 hours.
Contraindications: None observed with prescribed dosage.
Dosage and Administration: Adults, one or two tablets with glass of water 2 or 3 times daily, ½ to ¾ of an hour before meals.
Also Available: Calcium Gluconate, Ferrous Gluconate, Manganese Gluconate, Potassium Gluconate and Zinc Gluconate.

Prod. Ident.	Type Tablet	Color
MG	Uncoated	Natural
MGP	"	Purple

How Supplied: Bottles of 1000 Tablets.

Westwood Pharmaceuticals Inc.
468 DEWITT ST.
BUFFALO, NY 14213

ALPHA KERI®
Therapeutic bath oil

Composition: Contains mineral oil, lanolin oil, PEG-4 dilaurate, benzophenone-3, D&C green 6, fragrance.
Action and Uses: ALPHA KERI is a water-dispersible, antipruritic oil for the care of dry skin. ALPHA KERI effectively deposits a thin, uniform, emulsified film of oil over the skin. This film helps relieve itching, lubricates and softens the skin. ALPHA KERI is valuable as an aid in the treatment of dry, pruritic skin and mild skin irritations such as chronic atopic dermatitis; pruritus senilis and hiemalis; contact dermatitis; "bath-itch"; xerosis or asteatosis; ichthyosis; soap dermatitis; psoriasis.
Administration and Dosage: ALPHA KERI *should always be used with water, either added to water or rubbed on to wet skin.* Because of its inherent cleansing properties it is not necessary to use soap when ALPHA KERI is being used.
For exact dosage, label directions should be followed.
BATH: Added as directed to bathtub of water. For optimum relief: 10 to 20 minute soak.
SHOWER: Small amount is poured into wet washcloth and rubbed on to wet skin. Rinse follows.
SPONGE BATH: Added as directed to a basin of warm water then rubbed over entire body with washcloth.
SITZ BATH: Added as directed to tub water. Soak should last for 10 to 20 minutes.
INFANT BATH: Added as directed to basin or bathinette of water.
SKIN CLEANSING OTHER THAN BATH OR SHOWER: A small amount is rubbed on to wet skin, which is then patted dry.
Precaution: The patient should be warned to guard against slipping in tub or shower.
How Supplied: 4 fl. oz. (NDC 0072-3600-04), 8 fl. oz. (NDC 0072-3600-08) and 16 fl. oz. (NDC 0072-3600-16) plastic bottles. Also available for patients who prefer to shower—ALPHA KERI SPRAY—5 oz. aerosol container (NDC 0072-3600-05), ALPHA KERI SOAP—4 oz. bar (NDC 0072-3500-04).

ALPHA KERI® SOAP
Non-detergent Soap

Composition: Contains therapeutic ALPHA KERI® bath oil in a non-detergent soap.
Action and Uses: ALPHA KERI SOAP, rich in emollient oils, thoroughly cleanses as it soothes and softens the skin.
Indications: Adjunctive use in dry skin care.
Administration and Dosage: To be used as any other soap.
How Supplied: 4 oz. bar (NDC 0072-3500-04).

BALNEOL®
Perianal cleansing lotion

Composition: Contains water, mineral oil, propylene glycol, glyceryl stearate/PEG-100 stearate, PEG-40 stearate, laureth-4, PEG-4 dilaurate, lanolin oil, sodium acetate, carbomer-934, triethanolamine, sorbic acid, dioctyl sodium sulfosuccinate, fragrance, acetic acid.
Action and Uses: BALNEOL is a soothing, emollient cleanser for hygienic cleansing of irritated perianal and external vaginal areas. It helps relieve itching and other discomforts, helps stop irritation due to toilet tissue. BALNEOL gently yet thoroughly cleanses and provides a soothing, protecting film.
Administration and Dosage: For cleansing without discomfort after each bowel movement, a small amount of BALNEOL is spread on tissue or cotton and used to wipe the perianal area. Also used between bowel movements and at bedtime for additional comfort.
For cleansing and soothing the external vaginal area: to be used on clean tissue or cotton as often as necessary.
Caution: In all cases of rectal bleeding, the cause should be sought. If irritation persists or increases, adjust usage or discontinue use.
How Supplied: 4 oz. plastic bottle (NDC 0072-6200-04).

BALNETAR®
Water-dispersible Emollient Tar

Composition: Contains WESTWOOD® TAR (equivalent to 2.5% Coal Tar USP), mineral oil and lanolin oil.
Action and Uses: For temporary relief of itching and scaling due to psoriasis, eczema, and other tar-responsive dermatoses. Tar ingredient is chemically and biologically standardized to insure uniform therapeutic activity. BALNETAR exerts keratoplastic, antieczematous, antipruritic, and emollient actions. It deposits microfine particles of tar over the skin in a lubricant-moisturizing film that helps soften and remove scales and crusts, making the skin smoother and more supple. BALNETAR is an important adjunct in a wide range of dermatoses, including: atopic dermatitis; chronic eczematoid dermatitis; seborrheic dermatitis.
Contraindications: Not indicated when acute inflammation is present.
Administration and Dosage: BALNETAR *should always be used with water... either added to water or rubbed into wet skin.* For exact dosage label directions are to be followed.
IN THE TUB—Add as directed to a bathtub of water. Soap is not used. The patient soaks for 10 to 20 minutes and then pats dry.
FOR DIRECT APPLICATION—A small amount is rubbed into the wet skin. Excess is wiped off with tissue to help prevent staining of clothes or linens.
FOR SCALP APPLICATION —A small amount is rubbed into the wet scalp with fingertips.
Caution: If irritation persists, discontinue use. In rare instances temporary discoloration of blond, bleached or tinted hair may occur. In rare cases BALNETAR may cause allergic irritation attributable to coal tar.
Precaution: After use of BALNETAR, patient should avoid exposure to direct sunlight unless sunlight is being used therapeutically in a supervised, modified Goeckerman regimen. Contact with the eyes should be avoided. Patient should be cautioned against slipping when BALNETAR is used in bathtub. Also advise patient that use in a plastic or fiberglass tub may cause staining of the tub.
How Supplied: 8 fl. oz. plastic shatterproof bottle (NDC 0072-4200-08).

CAPITROL® ℞
(chloroxine 2%)
Cream Shampoo

Description: CAPITROL shampoo provides 2% chloroxine (each gram contains 20 mg. chloroxine) suspended in a shampoo base containing: sodium octoxynol-3 sulfonate, PEG-6 lauramide, dextrin, stearyl alcohol/ceteareth-20, sodium lauryl sulfoacetate, dioctyl sodium sulfosuccinate, magnesium aluminum silicate, PEG-14M, EDTA, citric acid, water, color and fragrance. The pH of the shampoo is 7.0.
The chemical name of chloroxine is 5, 7-dichloro-8-hydroxyquinoline.
Actions: Chloroxine is a synthetic antibacterial compound. It has a structural similarity to a number of substituted 8-hydroxyquinolines that have been in therapeutic use for some years.
Indications: CAPITROL is indicated in the treatment of dandruff and mild to moderately severe seborrheic dermatitis of the scalp.
Contraindications: CAPITROL (chloroxine) may produce allergic contact sensitization reactions in patients who are sensitive to hydroxyquinolines or EDTA. This shampoo should not be used on acutely inflamed (exudative) lesions of the scalp.
Precautions: Patients should be advised to exercise care not to allow CAPITROL to enter the eyes. For external use only.
Adverse Reactions: Irritation and burning of the scalp and adjacent areas have been reported. Allergic type skin eruptions may occur in patients who are sensitive to any component of the shampoo. As with any medicated shampoo, chemical conjunctivitis may result if CAPITROL enters the eyes. Discoloration of light-colored hair (e.g. blond, gray or bleached) may follow use of this preparation. Dryness of the scalp and increased itching have been reported.
Dosage and Administration: CAPITROL (chloroxine) should be massaged thoroughly into the wet scalp, avoiding contact with the eyes. Lather should remain on the scalp for approximately three minutes, then rinsed. The application should be repeated and the scalp rinsed thoroughly. Two treatments per week are usually sufficient.
Caution: Keep this and all drugs out of the reach of children.
How Supplied: CAPITROL (chloroxine shampoo) is supplied in 85 g. plastic tubes (NDC 0072-6800-02).

DESQUAM-X 5® GEL ℞
DESQUAM-X 10® GEL ℞
Benzoyl Peroxide and Laureth-4 Gel

Composition: DESQUAM-X 5 contains 5% Benzoyl Peroxide, 6% laureth-4, carbomer-940, diisopropanolamine, disodium edetate and water.
DESQUAM-X 10 contains 10% Benzoyl Peroxide, 6% laureth-4, carbomer-940, diisopropanolamine, disodium edetate and water.
Indications: A topical aid for the control of acne vulgaris.
Actions: Provides the desirable drying and desquamation needed in the topical treatment of acne. DESQUAM-X has been demonstrated to have anti-bacterial effects, especially against Propionibacterium acnes.
Administration and Dosage: After washing as instructed, DESQUAM-X is rubbed into affected areas twice daily. In fair skinned individuals or under excessively dry atmospheric conditions it is suggested that therapy be initiated with one application daily. The desired degree of drying and peeling can be obtained by modification of the dosage schedule.
Contraindications: Not to be used in patients known to be sensitive to any ingredient of DESQUAM-X.
Precautions: Avoid contact with eyes and mucous membranes. For external use only. Keep this and all drugs out of the reach of children. Store below 75° F. May bleach colored fabrics.
How Supplied: 5% 1.5 oz. (42.5 g.) plastic tubes (NDC 0072-6621-01) 3 oz. (85 g.) (NDC 0072-6621-03). 10% 1.5 oz. (42.5 g.) plastic tubes (NDC 0072-6721-01) 3 oz. (85 g.) (NDC-0072-6721-03).

DESQUAM-X® WASH ℞
4% Benzoyl Peroxide

Composition: DESQUAM-X WASH contains 4% benzoyl peroxide, sodium octoxynol-3 sulfonate, water, dioctyl sodium sulfosuccinate, sodium lauryl sulfoacetate, magnesium aluminum silicate, methylcellulose, EDTA.
Indications: May be used topically alone for mild to moderate acne vulgaris. In severe, complicated acne, DESQUAM-X WASH may be used as an adjunct to therapeutic regimens which might include antibiotics, retinoic acid products, and/or sulfur and salicylic acid containing preparations.
Action: Provides drying and desquamation desirable in the topical treatment of acne. DESQUAM-X WASH has demonstrated antibacterial activity against Propionibacterium acnes. DESQUAM-X WASH has also been shown to reduce the concentration of free fatty acids in the sebum.
Administration and Dosage: Wash with DESQUAM-X WASH once or twice daily, avoiding contact with eyes or mucous membranes. Drying and peeling may be modified by adjusting the dosage schedule.
Contraindications: Not to be used in patients known to be sensitive to benzoyl peroxide or other ingredients.
Precautions: Avoid contact with eyes and mucous membranes. To prevent bleaching, avoid contact with hair. Keep this and all drugs out of the reach of children. For external use only. May bleach colored fabrics. Store below 77° F.
How Supplied: Plastic bottles 5 oz. (141.8 g.) (NDC 0072-6900-05).

ESTAR®
Therapeutic Tar Gel

Composition: Westwood® Tar (biologically equivalent to 5% Coal Tar USP) in a hydroalcoholic gel (29% alcohol).
Actions and Uses: A therapeutic aid in the treatment of eczema, psoriasis, and other tar-responsive dermatoses such as atopic dermatitis, lichen simplex chronicus, and nummular eczema. ESTAR exerts keratoplastic, antieczematous, and antipruritic actions. It is equivalent in its photodynamic activity to 5% crude coal tar in either hydrophilic ointment or petrolatum. ESTAR provides the characteristic benefits of tar therapy in a form that is readily accepted by patients and nursing staff, due to its negligible tar odor and staining potential, and the superior cosmetic qualities of its gel base. ESTAR is suitable for use in a modified Goeckerman regimen, either in the hospital or on an outpatient basis; it also can be used in follow-up treatment to help maintain remissions. Substantivity to the skin can be demonstrated by examination with a Wood's light, which shows residual microfine particles of tar on the skin several days after application.
Contraindications: ESTAR should not be applied to acutely inflamed skin or used by individuals who are known to be sensitive to coal tar.
Administration and Dosage:
Psoriasis: ESTAR can be applied at bedtime in the following manner: the patient should massage ESTAR into affected areas, allowing the gel to remain for five minutes, and then remove excess by patting with tissues. This procedure minimizes staining of skin and clothing, leaving behind an almost invisible layer of the active tar. If any staining of fabric should occur, it can be removed easily by standard laundry procedures.
The same technique of application may be used the following morning. If dryness occurs, an emollient may be applied one hour after ESTAR.
Because of ESTAR's superior substantivity and cosmetic qualities, patients who might otherwise be hospitalized for tar/UV therapy can now be treated as outpatients. The patient can easily apply ESTAR at bedtime and the following morning, then report for UV treatment that day. Laboratory tests and clinical experience to date suggest that it may be advisable to carefully regulate the length of UV exposure.
Chronic atopic dermatitis, Lichen simplex chronicus, Nummular eczema, and Seborrheic dermatitis: One or two applications per day, as described above, are suggested. If dryness occurs, an emollient may be applied one hour after ESTAR and between applications as needed.
Caution: AFTER USING, TREATED AREAS SHOULD BE PROTECTED FROM SUNLIGHT, ESPECIALLY IF ESTAR HAS BEEN USED ON THE FACE. THIS PRECAUTION SHOULD BE TAKEN FOR AT LEAST 24 HOURS AFTER APPLICATION, UNLESS OTHERWISE DIRECTED. ESTAR SHOULD NOT BE USED ON HIGHLY INFLAMED OR BROKEN SKIN. If used on the scalp, temporary discoloration of blond, bleached, or tinted hair may occur. If undue irritation develops or increases, the usage schedule should be changed or ESTAR discontinued. Contact with the eyes should be avoided. In case of contact, flush eyes with water.
Slight staining of clothing may occur. Standard laundry procedures will usually remove stains. For external use only.
How Supplied: 3 oz. plastic tube (NDC 0072-7600-03).

FOSTEX BPO 5%

Composition: Contains benzoyl peroxide 5%.
Action and Uses: FOSTEX BPO 5% Anti-Bacterial Acne Gel is a penetrating, disappearing gel which helps unclog pores, kill bacteria, promote rapid drying of oily skin, and gently desquamates.
Indications: A topical aid for the control of acne vulgaris.
Administration and Dosage: After washing, rub FOSTEX BPO 5% into affected areas twice daily. In fair-skinned individuals or in excessively dry climates it is suggested that therapy be initiated with one application daily. The desired degree of drying and peeling can be obtained by increasing or decreasing frequency of use.
Caution: Avoid contact with eyes, lips and mouth. If undue skin irritation develops or increases, discontinue use and consult physician. For external use only. Store below 75°F.
How Supplied: .65 oz. tube (NDC 0072-3300-01).

FOSTEX® CAKE
Acne Skin Cleanser

Composition: Contains sulfur 2%, salicylic acid 2%, plus a combination of soapless cleansers and wetting agents.
Action and Uses: FOSTEX CAKE is a surface-active, penetrating anti-seborrheic cleanser for therapeutic washing of the skin in the local treatment of acne and other skin conditions characterized by excessive oiliness. Degreases, dries and mildly desquamates.
Administration and Dosage: FOSTEX CAKE is used instead of soap to wash the face and other affected areas, followed by thorough rinse. FOSTEX CAKE is used two to three times a day, or as directed. Frequency of use determines degree of drying.
Caution: If undue skin irritation develops or increases, adjust usage schedule or discontinue use. If necessary, treat with anti-inflammatory measures. For external use only. Contact with the eyes should be avoided. In case of contact, flush eyes thoroughly with water.
How Supplied: 3¾ oz. bar (NDC 0072-3000-01).

FOSTEX® CREAM and MEDICATED CLEANSER
Acne Skin Cleanser and Dandruff Shampoo

Composition: Contains sulfur 2%, salicylic acid 2%, plus a combination of soapless cleansers and wetting agents.
Action and Uses: A penetrating antiseborrheic cleanser for the local treatment of acne, dandruff and other seborrheic skin conditions, characterized by excessive oiliness. Degreases, dries and mildly desquamates.
Administration and Dosage: WASHING THE SKIN—Instead of using soap, the face and other affected areas are washed with FOSTEX, followed by a thorough rinse. FOSTEX is usually used two to three times a day or as directed. Frequency of use determines degree of drying. SHAMPOO—After wetting the hair and scalp a liberal amount of FOSTEX is massaged into the scalp. A thorough shampoo is followed by a rinse. FOSTEX is then used for a repeat shampoo and then a rinse. No other shampoos are required. FOSTEX is used as often as necessary to keep the scalp free from excessive oiliness or scaling, or as often as directed.
Caution: If undue skin irritation develops or increases, adjust the usage schedule or discontinue use. If necessary, after discontinuance anti-inflammatory measures may be used. For external use only. Avoid contact with eyes. In case of contact, flush eyes thoroughly with water.
How Supplied: FOSTEX CREAM in 4 oz. tube (NDC 0072-3200-01) and FOSTEX MEDICATED CLEANSER in 5 oz. (NDC 0072-3400-05) bottle.

FOSTRIL®
Drying Lotion for Acne

Composition: Contains 6% laureth-4, 2% sulfur, in a greaseless base.
Action and Uses: Promotes drying and peeling of the skin in the treatment of acne. Daily use of FOSTRIL should result in a desirable

Continued on next page

Westwood—Cont.

degree of dryness and peeling in about 7 days. FOSTRIL removes excess oil and follicular obstruction, helping to remove comedones. It also helps prevent epithelial closure of pores and formation of new lesions.
Administration and Dosage: A thin film is applied to affected areas once or twice daily, or as directed.
Caution: If undue skin irritation develops or increases, adjust usage schedule or discontinue use. Anti-inflammatory measures may be used if necessary. For external use only. Contact with eyes should be avoided. In case of contact, flush eyes thoroughly with water.
How Supplied: 1 oz. tube (NDC 0072-3800-01).

HALOTEX® CREAM/SOLUTION ℞
(Haloprogin)
Antifungal Agent

Description: HALOTEX (haloprogin) is 3-iodo-2-propynyl 2,4,5-trichlorophenyl ether. HALOTEX cream provides 1% haloprogin in a water-dispersible, semi-solid cream base. Each gram contains 10 mg. haloprogin solubilized in polyethylene glycol 400, polyethylene glycol 4000, diethyl sebacate and polyvinylpyrrolidone.
HALOTEX solution provides 1% (10 mg. per ml.) haloprogin in a homogenous vehicle of diethyl sebacate and alcohol.
Action: HALOTEX is a synthetic antifungal agent for the treatment of superficial fungal infections of the skin.
Indications: HALOTEX cream and solution are indicated for the topical treatment of tinea pedis, tinea cruris, tinea corporis and tinea manuum due to infection with Trichophyton rubrum, Trichophyton tonsurans, Trichophyton mentagrophytes, Microsporum canis, and Epidermophyton floccosum. It is also useful in the topical treatment of tinea versicolor due to Malassezia furfur.
Contraindications: HALOTEX preparations are contraindicated in those individuals who have shown hypersensitivity to any of the components.
Warning: USAGE IN PREGNANCY - Safety for use in pregnancy has not been established.
Precautions: In case of sensitization or irritation due to HALOTEX cream or solution or any of the ingredients, treatment with these preparations should be discontinued and appropriate therapy instituted. If a patient shows no improvement after four weeks of treatment with HALOTEX cream or solution, the diagnosis should be redetermined. In mixed infections where bacteria or nonsusceptible fungi are present, supplementary systemic anti-infective therapy may be indicated.
For external use only: KEEP OUT OF EYES.
Adverse Reactions: Reactions reported include: (1) local irritation, burning sensation, vesicle formation, and; (2) increased maceration, pruritus or exacerbation of pre-existing lesions.
Dosage and Administration: HALOTEX cream and solution should be applied liberally to the affected area twice daily for two to three weeks. Interdigital lesions may require up to four weeks of therapy.
How Supplied:
HALOTEX cream 1% (10 mg.per g.) 15 g. collapsible aluminum tube (NDC 0072-7130-15) and 30 g. collapsible aluminum tube (NDC 0072-7130-02).
HALOTEX solution 1% (10 mg. per ml.) 10 ml. polyethylene bottle with controlled drop tip (NDC 0072-7210-02) and 30 ml. polyethylene bottle with controlled drop tip (NDC 0072-7230-02.)

KERALYT® GEL ℞
Salicylic Acid Gel

Composition: Contains 6% salicylic acid in a gel containing propylene glycol (60%), ethyl alcohol (19.4%), hydroxypropyl cellulose and water.
Indications: *For Dermatological Use:* KERALYT is a topical aid in the removal of excessive keratin in hyperkeratotic skin disorders, including the various ichthyoses (vulgaris, sex-linked and lamellar), keratosis palmaris and plantaris, keratosis pilaris, pityriasis rubra pilaris, psoriasis (including body, scalp, palms and soles). KERALYT has been reported as helpful as adjunctive therapy for fungal infections.
For Podiatric Use: KERALYT is a topical aid in the removal of excessive keratin in dorsal and plantar hyperkeratotic lesions. KERALYT has been reported as helpful as adjunctive therapy for verruca plantaris.
Administration and Dosage: The preferable method of use is to apply thoroughly to the affected area and place under occlusion at night. The skin should be hydrated for at least 5 minutes prior to application. The medication is washed off in the morning, and if excessive drying and/or irritation is observed, a bland cream or lotion may be applied. Once clearing is apparent, the occasional use of KERALYT will usually maintain the remission. In those areas where occlusion is difficult or impossible, application may be made more frequently, and hydration by wet packs or baths prior to application apparently enhances the effect. Unless hands are being treated, they should be rinsed thoroughly following application.
Contraindications: Not to be used in patients known to be sensitive to any ingredient of KERALYT.
Precautions: In view of the salicylic acid content, use in children under 12 years of age should be limited to no more than one tube (1 oz.) in 24 hours. Avoid contact with eyes and mucous membranes. For external use only. Keep this and all medications out of reach of children.
How Supplied: Plastic tube 1 oz. (28.4 g.) (NDC 0072-6500-01).

KERI® CREME
Concentrated Moisturizer—
Nongreasy Emollient

Composition: Contains water, mineral oil, talc, sorbitol, ceresin, lanolin alcohol/mineral oil, magnesium stearate, glyceryl oleate/propylene glycol, isopropyl myristate, methylparaben, propylparaben, fragrance, quaternium-15.
Actions and Uses: KERI CREME is a concentrated moisturizer and nongreasy emollient for problem dry skin—hands, face, elbows, feet, legs. KERI CREME helps retain moisture that makes skin feel soft, smooth, supple. Helps resist the drying effects of soaps, detergents and chemicals.
Administration and Dosage: A small amount is rubbed into dry skin areas as needed.
How Supplied: 2½ oz. tube (NDC 0072-5800-01).

KERI® FACIAL SOAP
Non-detergent Facial Soap

Composition: KERI LOTION® concentrate in a gentle, non-detergent soap.
Action and Uses: KERI FACIAL SOAP helps keep skin soft while thoroughly cleansing.
Administration and Dosage: To be used as facial soap.
How Supplied: 3.25 oz. bar (NDC 0072-4900-03).

KERI® LOTION
Skin Lubricant—Moisturizer

Composition: Contains mineral oil, water, propylene glycol, glyceryl stearate/ PEG-100 stearate, PEG-40 stearate, PEG-4 dilaurate, laureth-4, lanolin oil, methylparaben, propylparaben, fragrance, carbomer-934, triethanolamine, dioctyl sodium sulfosuccinate, quaternium-15.
Action and Uses: KERI LOTION lubricates and helps hydrate the skin, making it soft and smooth. It relieves itching, helps maintain a normal moisture balance and supplements the protective action of skin lipids. Indicated for generalized dryness and itching; detergent hands; chapped or chafed skin; sunburn; "winter-itch"; aging, dry skin; diaper rash; heat rash.
Administration and Dosage: Apply as often as needed. Use particularly after bathing and exposure to sun, water, soaps and detergents.
How Supplied: 6½ oz. (NDC 0072-4600-56), 13 oz. (NDC 0072-4600-63) and 20 oz. (NDC 0072-4600-70 plastic bottles. Also available as KERI LOTION FRESHLY SCENTED—6½ oz. (NDC 0072-4500-56), 13 oz. (NDC 0072-4500-63), and 20 oz. (NDC 0072-4500-70) plastic bottles.

LOWILA® CAKE
Soap-free Skin Cleanser

Composition: Contains dextrin, sodium lauryl sulfoacetate, water, boric acid, urea, sorbitol, mineral oil, PEG-14 M, lactic acid, dioctyl sodium sulfosuccinate, cellulose gum, fragrance.
Action and Uses: LOWILA CAKE is indicated for cleansing skin that is sensitive or irritated, or in dermatitic and eczematous conditions. Used for general bathing, infant bathing, routine washing of hands and face and shampooing. The pH of LOWILA CAKE helps protect the skin's normal acid mantle and create an environment favorable to therapy and healing.
Administration and Dosage: LOWILA CAKE is used in place of soap. Lathers well in both hard and soft water.
How Supplied: 3¾ oz. bar (NDC 0072-2300-01).

PERNOX®
Medicated Lathering Scrub Cleanser for Acne

Composition: Contains 26% polyethylene granules, 2% sulfur, 1.5% salicylic acid, plus a combination of soapless cleansers and wetting agents.
Actions and Uses: A lathering scrub cleanser for acne, oily skin. PERNOX provides microfine, uniform-size scrub particles with a rounded surface area to enable patients to achieve effective and gentle desquamation as they wash their skin. PERNOX helps loosen and remove comedones, dries, peels and degreases acne skin. It lathers abundantly and leaves the skin feeling smooth.
Contraindications: Not indicated when acute inflammation is present or in nodular or cystic acne.
Administration and Dosage: After wetting the skin, PERNOX is applied with the fingertips and massaged into the skin for about one-half to one minute. The skin is then thoroughly rinsed. May be used instead of soap one to two times daily, or as directed.
Caution: If undue skin irritation develops or increases, adjust usage schedule or discontinue use. If necessary, anti-inflammatory measures may be used after discontinuance. For external use only. Contact with eyes should be avoided. In case of contact, flush eyes thoroughly with water.
How Supplied: 2 oz tube (NDC 0072-5200-02), 4 oz. tube (NDC 0072-5200-04), lemon scented: 2 oz. tube (NDC 0072-5300-02), 4 oz. tube (NDC 0072-5300-04).

PERNOX® LOTION
Lathering Abradant Scrub Cleanser for Acne

Composition: Contains 20% polyethylene granules, 2% sulfur, 1.5% salicylic acid, plus a combination of soapless cleansers and wetting agents.
Actions and Uses: PERNOX LOTION is a therapeutic abradant scrub cleanser that is to be used routinely instead of soap. It gently desquamates or peels acne or oily skin. PERNOX LOTION also removes excessive oil from the skin surface and will produce mild drying of the affected skin areas when used regularly. It helps skin feel fresher and smoother with each wash.
Contraindications: Not indicated when acute inflammation is present or in nodular or cystic acne.
Administration and Dosage: To be shaken well before using.
PERNOX may be used instead of soap one or two times daily or as directed. The skin should be wet first and PERNOX applied with the fingertips. The lather should be massaged into skin for ½ to 1 minute. The patient then rinses thoroughly and pats dry.
Caution: If undue skin irritation develops or increases, adjust usage schedule or discontinue use. For external use only. Contact with eyes should be avoided. In case of contact, flush eyes with water.
How Supplied: 6 oz. bottle (NDC 0072-7900-06).

PERNOX® SHAMPOO
For Oily Hair

Composition: A blend of biodegradable cleansers and hair conditioners, containing: sodium laureth sulfate, water, lauramide DEA, quaternium 22, PEG-75 lanolin/hydrolyzed animal protein, sodium chloride, fragrance, lactic acid, sorbic acid, disodium EDTA, FD&C yellow 6, FD&C blue 1.
Actions and Uses: A gentle but thorough shampoo especially formulated to cleanse, control and condition oily hair. Especially suitable for adjunctive use with acne patients. PERNOX SHAMPOO works into a rich, pleasant lather, leaves the hair lustrous and manageable. Its special conditioners help prevent tangles and fly away hair. Gentle enough to be used every day. It contains a refreshing natural scent.
Administration and Dosage: A liberal amount is massaged into wet hair and scalp. A good lather is worked up, massaging thoroughly. This is followed by a rinse and repeat application. A final rinse is used. No other shampoos or hair conditioners are necessary. May be used as needed.
Caution: For external use only. Contact with the eyes should be avoided. In case of contact, flush eyes with water.
How Supplied: 8 fl. oz. (NDC 0072-5500-08) shatter-proof plastic bottles.

PRESUN® 4 SUNSCREEN LOTION
Moderate Sunscreen Protection

Composition: Contains 4% Padimate O, 10% SD alcohol 40, water, mineral oil, PPG-15 stearyl ether, stearyl alcohol, mono- and diglycerides, benzyl alcohol, laureth-23, carbomer 934, ceteth-10, sodium hydroxide.
Action and Uses: PRESUN 4 provides 4 times an individual's natural protection. Liberal and regular use may help reduce the chance of premature aging of the skin and skin cancer from overexposure to the sun. PRESUN 4 provides moderate protection, permits tanning, and reduces the chance of sunburn.
Administration and Dosage: Apply liberally and evenly 30 minutes before exposure. Reapply after swimming or excessive sweating. If used, cosmetics or emollients may be applied after PRESUN.
Caution: For external use only. Keep out of the reach of children. Discontinue use if irritation or rash appears. AVOID CONTACT WITH EYES.
How Supplied: 4 oz. (NDC 0072-5900-04) plastic bottles.

PRESUN® 8; LOTION, CREAMY LOTION, AND GEL
Maximal Sunscreen Protection

Composition: LOTION: Contains 5% (w/w) aminobenzoic acid (PABA), 55% (w/w) SD alcohol 40, water, glycerin, choleth-24, hydroxypropyl cellulose. CREAMY LOTION: 5% Aminobenzoic acid (PABA), 15% SD alcohol 40, water, PEG-8, PPG-15 stearyl ether, glyceryl stearate/PEG-100 stearate, glycerin, mineral oil, magnesium aluminum silicate, titanium dioxide, DEA-cetyl phosphate, benzyl alcohol, mono- and diglycerides, fragrance, cetyl alcohol, cellulose gum, simethicone. GEL: Contains 5% (w/w) aminobenzoic acid (PABA), 55% (w/w) SD alcohol 40, water, animal protein derivative, hydroxyethyl cellulose.
Action and Uses: PRESUN 8 provides 8 times an individual's natural protection. Liberal and regular use may reduce the chance of premature aging of the skin and skin cancer from overexposure to the sun. PRESUN 8 permits limited tanning and reduces the chance of sunburn. It gives maximum protection in the erythemogenic range, screening out the burning rays of the sun.
Contraindications: Do not use if sensitive to aminobenzoic acid, benzocaine, sulfonamides or aniline dyes.
Administration and Dosage: Apply liberally and evenly one hour before exposure. Let dry before dressing. Reapply after swimming or excessive sweating. If used, cosmetics or emollients may be applied after PRESUN.
Caution: For external use only. Keep out of the reach of children. Avoid contact with light-colored fabric, as staining may result. Avoid flame. Discontinue use if irritation or rash appears. AVOID CONTACT WITH EYES.
How Supplied: Lotion: 4 fl. oz. (NDC 0072-5400-04) and 7 fl. oz. (NDC 0072-5400-07) plastic bottles. Creamy Lotion: 4 oz. (NDC 0072-8502-04) plastic bottles. Gel: 3 oz. (NDC 0072-7700-03) plastic tubes.

PRESUN® 15 SUNSCREEN LOTION
Ultra Sunscreen Protection

Composition: 5% Aminobenzoic acid (PABA), 5% Padimate O, 3% oxybenzone, 58% SD alcohol 40, water, PPG-15 stearyl ether, hydroxypropyl cellulose.
Actions and Uses: PRESUN 15 provides 15 times an individual's natural protection. Liberal and regular use may reduce the chance of premature aging of the skin and skin cancer from overexposure to the sun. PRESUN 15 permits no tanning and provides the highest degree of sunburn protection.
Contraindications: Do not use if sensitive to aminobenzoic acid, benzocaine, sulfonamides or aniline dyes.
Administration and Dosage: Apply liberally and evenly one hour before exposure. Let dry before dressing. Reapply after swimming or excessive sweating. If used, cosmetics or emollients may be applied after PRESUN.
Caution: For external use only. Keep out of the reach of children. Avoid contact with light-colored fabric, as staining may result. Avoid flame. Discontinue use if irritation or rash appears. AVOID CONTACT WITH EYES.
How Supplied: 4 oz. (NDC 0072-8800-04) plastic bottles.

SEBUCARE®
Antiseborrheic Scalp Lotion

Contains: 1.8% Salicylic acid, 61% alcohol, water, PPG-40 butyl ether, laureth-4, dihydroabietyl alcohol, fragrance.
Action and Uses: An aid in the treatment of dandruff, seborrhea capitis and other scaling conditions of the scalp. SEBUCARE helps control scaling, oiliness and itching. The unique base helps soften brittle hair and grooms the hair, thus eliminating the need for hair dressing which often impedes antiseborrheic treatment. SEBUCARE should be used every day in conjunction with therapeutic shampoos such as SEBULEX® or FOSTEX® CREAM.
Administration and Dosage: SEBUCARE is applied directly to scalp and massaged thoroughly with fingertips. Comb or brush as usual. Grooms as it medicates. Use once or twice daily or as directed..
Precaution: Volatile—Flame should be avoided. Contact with eyes should be avoided. In case of contact, flush eyes thoroughly with water. For external use only.
How Supplied: 4 fl. oz. plastic bottle (NDC 0072-4800-04).

SEBULEX®
Antiseborrheic Treatment Shampoo

Composition: Contains sulfur 2% and salicylic acid 2% in SEBULYTIC® brand of surface active cleansers and wetting agents.
Action and Uses: A penetrating therapeutic shampoo for the temporary relief of itchy scalp and the scaling of dandruff, SEBULEX helps relieve itching, remove dandruff, excess oil. It penetrates and softens the crusty, matted layers of scales adhering to the scalp, and leaves the hair soft and manageable.
Administration and Dosage: SEBULEX should be shaken before being used. It is to be massaged into wet scalp. Lather should be allowed to remain on scalp for about 5 minutes and then rinsed. Application is repeated, followed by a thorough rinse. Initially, SEBULEX can be used daily, or every other day, or as directed, depending on the condition. Once symptoms are under control, one or two treatments a week usually will maintain control of itching, oiliness and scaling.
Caution: If undue skin irritation develops or increases, discontinue use. Contact with eyes should be avoided. In case of contact, flush eyes thoroughly with water.
How Supplied: SEBULEX in 4 oz. (NDC 0072-2700-04) and 8 oz. (NDC 0072-2700-08) bottles.

SEBULEX® CONDITIONING SHAMPOO WITH PROTEIN
Antiseborrheic Treatment and Conditioning Shampoo

Composition: Contains sulfur 2%, salicylic acid 2%, water, sodium octoxynol-3 sulfonate, sodium lauryl sulfate, lauramide DEA, acetamide MEA, amphoteric-2, hydrolyzed animal protein, magnesium aluminum silicate, propylene glycol, methylcellulose, PEG-14 M, fragrance, disodium EDTA, dioctyl sodium sulfosuccinate, FD & C blue 1, D & C yellow 10.
Action and Uses: SEBULEX CONDITIONING SHAMPOO provides effective temporary control of the scaling and itching of dandruff and seborrheic dermatitis, while adding protein to the hair shaft to increase its manageability.
Administration and Dosage: SEBULEX CONDITIONING SHAMPOO should be shaken before use. It is to be massaged into the wet scalp. For optimum dandruff control and conditioning, lather should be allowed to remain on scalp for about 5 minutes and then rinsed off. Application is repeated, followed by a thorough rinse. Initially, SEBULEX CONDITIONING SHAMPOO may be used daily, or as

Continued on next page

Westwood—Cont.

directed, to achieve control of symptoms. Two or three treatments per week usually will maintain control of oiliness, itching, and scaling.

Caution: If undue skin irritation develops or increases, use should be discontinued. Contact with eyes should be avoided. In cases of contact, eyes should be flushed thoroughly with water.

How Supplied: 4 oz. (NDC 0072-2600-04) and 8 oz. (NDC 0072-2600-08) plastic bottles.

SEBUTONE®
Antiseborrheic Tar Shampoo

Composition: WESTWOOD® TAR (equivalent to 0.5% Coal Tar USP), sulfur 2% and salicylic acid 2% in SEBULYTIC® brand of surface-active cleansers and wetting agents.

Action and Uses: A surface-active, penetrating therapeutic shampoo for the temporary relief of itchy scalp and the scaling of stubborn dandruff and psoriasis. Provides prompt and prolonged relief of itching, helps control oiliness and rid the scalp of scales and crust. Tar ingredient is chemically and biologically standardized to produce uniform therapeutic activity. Wood's light demonstrates residual microfine particles of tar on the scalp several days after a course of SEBUTONE shampoo. In addition to its antipruritic and antiseborrheic actions, SEBUTONE also helps offset excessive scalp dryness with a special moisturizing emollient.

Administration and Dosage: A liberal amount is massaged into the wet scalp for 5 minutes and the scalp is then rinsed. Application is repeated, followed by a thorough rinse. Use as often as necessary to keep the scalp free from itching and scaling or as directed. No other shampoo or soap washings are required.

Caution: If undue skin irritation develops or increases, discontinue use. In rare instances, temporary discoloration of white, blond, bleached or tinted hair may occur. Contact with the eyes is to be avoided. In case of contact flush eyes with water.

How Supplied: SEBUTONE in 4 oz. (NDC 0072-5000-04) and 8 oz. (NDC 0072-5000-08) bottles.

TACARYL Tablets and Syrup ℞
(Methdilazine HCl)
TACARYL Chewable Tablets ℞
(Methdilazine)

Description: TACARYL, available as methdilazine or methdilazine HCl, a phenothiazine derivative, is 10- (1-methyl-3-pyrrolidinyl) methyl phenothiazine.

Actions: TACARYL and TACARYL HCl are phenothiazine derivatives, possessing antipruritic and antihistaminic properties with anticholinergic (drying) and sedative side effects.

Indication: TACARYL and TACARYL HCl are indicated for the symptomatic relief of pruritic symptoms in urticaria.

Contraindications: TACARYL is contraindicated in comatose states, in patients who have received large amounts of central nervous system depressants (alcohol, barbiturates, narcotics, etc.). It is contraindicated in patients who have bone marrow depression, jaundice, or in those who have demonstrated an idiosyncrasy or hypersensitivity to TACARYL or other phenothiazines. This drug is contraindicated in newborn or premature infants. Further, it should not be used in children acutely ill and dehydrated, as there may be an increased susceptibility to dystonias. Because of the higher risk of drugs of this type for infants generally and prematures in particular, TACARYL is contraindicated in nursing mothers.

Warnings: TACARYL may impair the mental and/or physical ability required for the performance of potentially hazardous tasks, such as driving a vehicle or operating machinery. Similarly, it may impair mental alertness in children. The concomitant use of alcohol or other central nervous system depressants may have an additive effect. Patients should be warned accordingly. TACARYL should be used with extreme caution in patients with: asthmatic attack, narrow-angle glaucoma, prostatic hypertrophy, stenosing peptic ulcer, pyloroduodenal obstruction, bladder neck obstruction, as well as in patients receiving monoamine oxidase inhibitors.

Usage in Pregnancy: The safe use of TACARYL has not been established with respect to the possible adverse effects upon fetal development. Therefore, it is recommended that this medication be given to pregnant patients, or women of child-bearing potential, only when in the judgment of the physician the potential benefits outweigh the possible hazards. There are reports of jaundice and prolonged extrapyramidal symptoms in infants whose mothers received phenothiazines during pregnancy.

Use in Children: TACARYL should be used with caution, as administration in the young child may result in excitation. Overdosage may produce hallucinations, convulsions, and sudden death.

Use in the Elderly (60 Years or Older): The elderly are more prone to develop the following side effects from phenothiazines: hypotension; syncope; toxic confusional states; excessive sedation; extrapyramidal signs, especially parkinsonism; akathisia; persistent dyskinesia.

Precautions: TACARYL may significantly affect the actions of other drugs. It may increase, prolong or intensify the sedative action of central nervous system depressants such as anesthetics, barbiturates or alcohol. The dose of a narcotic or barbiturate may be reduced to ¼ or ½ the usual amount when TACARYL is administered concomitantly. Excessive amounts of TACARYL, relative to a narcotic, may lead to restlessness and motor hyperactivity in the patient with pain.

Phenothiazines may block and even reverse some of the actions of epinephrine.

TACARYL should be used cautiously in persons with acute or chronic respiratory impairment, particularly children. The cough reflex can be suppressed.

TACARYL should be used cautiously in persons with cardiovascular disease, impairment of liver function or those with a history of ulcer disease.

Adverse Reactions: This drug may produce adverse reactions common to both phenothiazines and antihistamines.

Note: Not all of the following adverse reactions have been reported with this specific drug; however, pharmacological similarities among the phenothiazine derivatives require that each be considered when TACARYL is administered. There have been occasional reports of sudden death in patients receiving phenothiazine derivatives chronically.

CNS: Drowsiness is the most prominent CNS effect of this drug. Extrapyramidal reactions occur, particularly with high doses. Hyperreflexia has been reported in the newborn when a phenothiazine was used during pregnancy. Other reported reactions include dizziness, lassitude, tinnitus, incoordination, fatigue, blurred vision, euphoria, diplopia, nervousness, insomnia, tremors and grand mal seizures; excitation, catatonic-like states, neuritis and hysteria.

Cardiovascular: Postural hypotension is the most common cardiovascular effect of the phenothiazines. Reflex tachycardia may be seen. Bradycardia, faintness, dizziness and cardiac arrest have been reported. ECG changes, including blunting of T waves and prolongation of the Q-T interval, may be seen.

Gastrointestinal: Anorexia, nausea, vomiting, epigastric distress, constipation and dry mouth may occur. Diarrhea has also been reported as well as increased appetite and weight gain.

Genitourinary: Urinary frequency and dysuria, urinary retention, early menses, induced lactation, gynecomastia, decreased libido, inhibition of ejaculation and false pregnancy tests have been reported.

Respiratory: Thickening of bronchial secretions, tightness of the chest, wheezing and nasal stuffiness may occur.

Allergic Reactions: These include urticaria, dermatitis, asthma, laryngeal edema, photosensitivity, lupus erythematosus-like syndrome and anaphylactoid reactions.

Other Reported Reactions: Leukopenia, agranulocytosis, elevation of plasma cholesterol levels, thrombocytopenic purpura and jaundice of the obstructive type have been reported. The jaundice is usually reversible, but chronic jaundice has been reported. High or prolonged glucose tolerance curves, glycosuria, elevated spinal fluid proteins may also occur.

Long-Term Therapy Considerations: After prolonged administration at high dosage, pigmentation of the skin has occurred, chiefly in the exposed areas. Ocular changes consist of the appearance of lenticular and corneal opacities, epithelial keratopathies and pigmentary retinopathy. Vision may be impaired.

Dosage and Administration:

TACARYL® Hydrochloride Tablets (methdilazine HCl)
- Adults: 1 tablet (8 mg.) 2 to 4 times daily.
- Children over 3 years: ½ tablet (4 mg.) 2 to 4 times daily.

TACARYL® Hydrochloride Syrup (methdilazine HCl)
- Adults: 2 teaspoons (8 mg.) 2 to 4 times daily.
- Children over 3 years: 1 teaspoon (4 mg.) 2 to 4 times daily.

TACARYL® Chewable Tablets (methdilazine)
- Adults: 2 tablets (7.2 mg.) 2 to 4 times daily.
- Children over 3 years: 1 tablet (3.6 mg.) 2 to 4 times daily.
- This product form should be chewed and swallowed promptly.

The above doses should be considered maximal daily doses and every effort should be made to minimize side-effects and adverse reactions, through the use of the minimal effective dosage.

Drug Interactions: MAO inhibitors and thiazide diuretics prolong and intensify the anticholinergic effects of the phenothiazines. Combined use of MAO inhibitors and phenothiazines may result in hypotension and extrapyramidal reactions.

Narcotics: The CNS depressant and analgesic effects of narcotics are potentiated by phenothiazines.

The following drugs result in potentiation of phenothiazine effect: oral contraceptives, progesterone, reserpine, nylidrin hydrochloride.

Management of Overdosage: Signs and symptoms of overdosage range from mild depression of the central nervous system and cardiovascular system, to profound hypotension, respiratory depression and unconsciousness. Stimulation may be evident, especially in children and geriatric patients. Atropine-like signs and symptoms—dry mouth; fixed, dilated pupils; flushing; etc.—as well as gastrointestinal symptoms may occur. The treatment of overdosage is essentially symptomatic and supportive. Early gastric lavage may be beneficial. Centrally acting emetics are of little use. Avoid analeptics, which may cause convulsions. Severe hypotension usually responds to the administration of levarterenol or phenylephrine. EPINEPHRINE SHOULD NOT BE USED, since its use in the patient with partial adrenergic blockade may further lower the blood pressure. Additional measures include oxygen and intravenous fluids. Limited experience with dialysis indicates that it is not helpful.

How Supplied:
TACARYL® Hydrochloride (methdilazine HCl) Tablets 8 mg. each, scored:
NDC 0072-7400-01 Bottles of 100 (with child-resistant closures)
TACARYL® Hydrochloride (methdilazine HCl) Syrup 4 mg./5 ml:
NDC 0072-7500-01 Bottles of 16 fl. oz. (1 pint) (with child-resistant closures)
TACARYL® (methdilazine) Chewable Tablets 3.6 mg. each (equivalent to 4 mg. methdilazine HCl):
NDC 0072-7300-01 Bottles of 100 (with child-resistant closures)

TRANSACT®
Transparent Medicated Acne Gel

Composition: Contains 6% laureth-4, 2% sulfur and 37% alcohol in a greaseless gel base.
Action and Uses: TRANSACT is a transparent, nonstaining and greaseless gel, which leaves a fresh, clean fragrance on the skin. It dries, peels and degreases the skin of acne patients. Its effect is controlled by frequency of application and climatic conditions.
Administration and Dosage: After washing acne skin thoroughly, a thin film is applied to affected areas once daily or as directed. A brief tingling sensation may be expected upon application. Patient should anticipate beneficial drying and peeling in 5 to 7 days. Since TRANSACT is a highly active drying agent it should be used sparingly when initiating therapy, particularly for patients with sensitive skin. 1. Patients with tender skin may best be started on one application every other day. 2. Most other patients can be started on one daily application. 3. When patients develop tolerance, applications may be increased to two and then three times daily to maintain an adequate therapeutic effect. 4. TRANSACT is also for use on the shoulders and back. In dry or cold climates skin is more reactive to TRANSACT and frequency of use should be reduced. During warm, humid months, frequency of use may be increased.
Caution: If undue skin irritation develops, usage schedule should be adjusted or TRANSACT discontinued. For external use only. Contact with the eyes should be avoided. In case of contact, flush eyes with water. Avoid flame.
How Supplied: 1 oz. plastic tube (NDC 0072-5600-01).

WESTCORT® CREAM ℞
(Hydrocortisone Valerate) 0.2%

Description: WESTCORT CREAM contains hydrocortisone valerate, an active, non-fluorinated ester of the corticosteroid hydrocortisone. It has the following chemical name: 11β,21-dihydroxy-17 α-valeryloxy-4-pregnene-3, 20-dione.
Each gram of WESTCORT CREAM contains 2.0 mg hydrocortisone valerate in a hydrophilic base composed of white petrolatum, stearyl alcohol, propylene glycol, amphoteric-9, carbomer-940, dried sodium phosphate, sodium lauryl sulfate, sorbic acid (as preservative) and water.
Actions: WESTCORT (hydrocortisone valerate) CREAM is effective primarily because of its anti-inflammatory, anti-pruritic, and vasoconstrictive actions.
Indications: WESTCORT CREAM is intended for the relief of the inflammatory manifestations of corticosteroid-responsive dermatoses.
Contraindications: Topical steroids are contraindicated in those patients with a history of hypersensitivity to any of the components of the preparation.
Precautions: If irritation develops, the product should be discontinued and appropriate therapy instituted. In the presence of an infection the use of an appropriate antifungal or antibacterial agent should be instituted. If a favorable response does not occur promptly, the corticosteroid should be discontinued until the infection has been adequately controlled.
If extensive areas are treated, or if the occlusive technique is used, there will be increased systemic absorption of the corticosteroid and suitable precautions should be taken, particularly in children and infants.
Although topical steroids have not been reported to have an adverse effect in human pregnancy, the safety of their use in pregnant women has not absolutely been established. In laboratory animals, increases in incidence of fetal abnormalities have been associated with exposure of gestating females to topical corticosteroids, in some cases at rather low dosage levels. Therefore, drugs of this class should not be used extensively on pregnant patients, in large amounts, or for prolonged periods of time.
The product is not for ophthalmic use.
Adverse Reactions: The following local adverse reactions have been reported with topical corticosteroids, especially under occlusive dressings:
1. Burning; 2. Itching; 3. Irritation; 4. Dryness; 5. Folliculitis; 6. Hypertrichosis; 7. Acneiform eruptions; 8. Hypopigmentation; 9. Perioral dermatitis; 10. Allergic contact dermatitis; 11. Maceration of the skin; 12. Secondary infection; 13. Skin atrophy; 14. Striae; 15. Miliaria.
Dosage and Administration: A small amount should be massaged gently into the affected areas 2 or 3 times daily, as needed.
How Supplied: WESTCORT (hydrocortisone valerate) CREAM 0.2% is supplied in 15 g., NDC 0072-8100-15; 45 g., NDC 0072-8100-45; and 60 g., NDC 0072-8100-60 tubes.

Wharton Laboratories, Inc.
Div. U.S. Ethicals Inc.
37-02 FORTY-EIGHTH AVE.
LONG ISLAND CITY, NY 11101

NITRONG® OINTMENT ℞
(Nitroglycerin 2%)

Description: NITRONG® Ointment contains 2% nitroglycerin in a special absorptive lanolin-white petrolatum base. It acts as a prompt vasodilator effective in the relief and prevention of anginal attacks; especially suitable for application at night.
Action: When the ointment is spread on the skin, the active ingredient (nitroglycerin) is continuously absorbed through the skin into the circulation, thus exerting prolonged vasodilator effect. Nitroglycerin ointment is effective in the control of angina pectoris, regardless of the site of application.
Nitroglycerin ointment exhibits a consistently prolonged beneficial effect. After application of nitroglycerin ointment, the effect of the drug can be noted promptly. Exercise capacity is increased significantly. More importantly, exercise capacity continues to show increases in patients studied three hours after treatment. When nitroglycerin ointment is applied, a marked and consistent beneficial effect is observed on the exercise electrocardiogram and on exercise capacity, which persists essentially undiminished three to four hours after application.
Nitroglycerin ointment applied to the chest can be utilized as a slow-release preparation which is especially useful in the treatment of angina decubitus. An application of ointment at bedtime may give the patient a night's sleep without a nocturnal attack.
Indications: Prevention and treatment of angina pectoris attacks especially at night.
Precautions: A headache is a definite sign of overdosage and, therefore, dosage should be reduced. As with sublingual nitroglycerin, transient headaches may occur. In terminating treatment, dosage and frequency of application must be gradually reduced over a period of 4 to 6 weeks to prevent sudden withdrawal reactions, which are characteristic of all vasodilators in the nitrate class.
Contraindications: NITRONG ointment is contraindicated in patients known to be intolerant to the organic nitrates. May be contraindicated in patients with marked anemia, increased intraocular pressure or increased intracranial pressure.
Adverse Reactions: Occasionally elderly patients may have no untoward symptoms while recumbent but may develop postural hypotension with faintness upon suddenly arising.
Dosage and Administration: When applying the ointment, place the specially designed Dose Determining Applicator supplied with the package printed side down, and squeeze the necessary amount of ointment from the tube onto the Dose Determining Applicator, then place the Dose Determining Applicator, ointment side down, on the desired skin area, spreading it in a thin, uniform layer. Cover with plastic wrap which can be held in place with adhesive or transparent tape. The Dose Determining Applicator allows the patient to measure the amount of ointment, which can then be spread onto the skin. At the same time, the ointment is prevented from being absorbed through the fingers while applied to the skin.
Angina Pectoris: NITRONG ointment may be applied every 3 to 4 hours if necessary, but one application at bedtime frequently suffices for the entire night. It may also be used throughout the day, but it is particularly useful in patients who suffer from the fear of nocturnal attacks of angina pectoris.
The usual dose is 1 to 2 inches, (25 to 50 mm) containing 15 mg to 30 mg nitroglycerin as squeezed from the tube, although some patients require as much as 4 or 5 inches (100 to 125 mm). The ointment measured on the Dose Determining Applicator is spread in a thin uniform layer over the chest, abdomen or anterior thighs, without massaging or rubbing it in. The optimal dosage is determined by starting with an application of as little as 1 inch (25 mm) and increasing the dose ½ inch (12.5 mm) at a time until headache occurs, then dropping back to the largest dose which does not cause a headache. The dose should be titrated to the need of the patient in the prevention and treatment of angina pectoris. This ointment is effective in the control of angina pectoris regardless of the skin site of application. Therefore, any convenient skin area may be used, but, psychologically, many patients prefer the chest because anginal pain originates in this area.
Keep the tube tightly closed and store at room temperature (59° to 86°F).
In terminating treatment of anginal patients, the dosage and frequency of application must be gradually reduced over a period of 4 to 6 weeks to prevent sudden withdrawal reactions, which are characteristic of all vasodilators in the nitroglycerin class.
Caution: Federal law prohibits dispensing without prescription.
How Supplied: 60 gram tubes with Dose Determining Applicators.

NITRONG® Tablets ℞
2.6 mg and 6.5 mg
(nitroglycerin, oral, controlled-release)

Description: Each NITRONG 2.6 mg. tablet for oral administration contains 2.6 mg. nitroglycerin in controlled-release form with light green granules. Each NITRONG 6.5 mg. tablet for oral administration contains 6.5 mg. nitroglycerin in controlled-release form with light orange granules.

Continued on next page

Wharton—Cont.

How Supplied: NITRONG is available in bottles of 100 tablets. The tablets are scored and have a mottled appearance.

Willen Drug Company
18 NORTH HIGH STREET
BALTIMORE, MARYLAND 21202

BICITRA®—SUGAR-FREE ℞
(Brand of Sodium Citrate & Citric Acid Solution USP)

Description: BICITRA is a pleasant tasting oral liquid containing Sodium Citrate and Citric Acid in a sugar-free base.
Indications: BICITRA is an effective alkalinizing agent useful in those conditions where long term maintenance of an alkaline urine is desirable, and is of value in the alleviation of chronic metabolic acidosis such as results from chronic renal insufficiency, especially when the administration of potassium salts is undesirable or contraindicated. It is also effective in correcting the acidosis of certain renal tubular disorders. BICITRA is the USP formula for SHOHL'S Solution.
Composition: BICITRA contains in each teaspoonful (5 ml): Sodium Citrate Dihydrate 500 mg and Citric Acid Anhydrous 300 mg. Each ml contains 1 mEq. Sodium ion and is equivalent to 1 mEq. Bicarbonate (HCO_3).
Advantages: BICITRA is concentrated and when administered after meals and before bedtime, allows one to maintain an alkaline urinary pH around the clock, usually without the necessity of a 2 AM dose. BICITRA alkalinizes the urine without producing a systemic alkalosis in the recommended dosage. BICITRA is pleasant tasting and tolerable, even when administered for long periods, and offers these advantages over SHOHL'S Solution while supplying the equivalent sodium content.
Administration and Dosage: BICITRA should be taken diluted in water, followed by additional water, if desired. Palatability is enhanced if chilled before taking. Adults: 10 to 30 ml diluted in 1 to 3 ounces water, after meals and before bedtime, or as directed by physician. Children: 5 to 15 ml diluted in 1 to 3 ounces water after meals and before bedtime, or as directed by physician. Occasional patients will require more or less to achieve the desired alkalizing effect.
Precautions and Side Effects: BICITRA is generally well tolerated without any unpleasant side effects when given in recommended doses to patients with normal renal function and urinary output. However, as with any alkalinizing agent, caution must be used in certain patients with abnormal renal mechanisms to avoid development of alkalosis, especially in the presence of hypocalcemia. Overdosage with sodium salts may cause diarrhea, nausea and vomiting, hypernoea, and convulsions. Sodium salts should be used cautiously in patients with cardiac failure, hypertension, impaired renal function, peripheral and pulmonary edema and toxemia of pregnancy. Periodic examinations and determinations of serum electrolytes, particularly serum bicarbonate level, should be carried out in those patients with renal disease in order to avoid these complications.
How Supplied: 16 fl. oz. (473 ml) (NDC 11414-207-01), 1 gallon (3785 ml) (11414-207-08) and 4 fl. oz. (120 ml) hospital size (NDC 11414-207-04).
Literature Available: Yes.

NEUTRA-PHOS® Powder & Capsules
NEUTRA-PHOS®-K Powder & Capsules
Oral Phosphorus Dietary Supplement

NEUTRA-PHOS and NEUTRA-PHOS-K supply the physiologically important element—PHOSPHORUS—as inorganic orthophosphate, in a well tolerated oral compound. Each contains a chemically balanced combination of readily soluble inorganic phosphates, affording a very high source of elemental Phosphorus. Both products supply equal concentration of elemental Phosphorus.
Composition: NEUTRA-PHOS is a stable powder combination of monobasic and dibasic Sodium and Potassium Phosphates. NEUTRA-PHOS-K is a stable sodium-free powder combination of monobasic and dibasic Potassium Phosphates intended for oral use in low sodium diets. Both products form an oral solution by reconstitution with water and are neutral (pH 7.3), isotonic, pleasant tasting sources of Phosphorus. There is less than 1 calorie per average dose.
Indications: NEUTRA-PHOS and NEUTRA-PHOS-K are recommended as oral Phosphorus supplements, particularly if the diet is low in mineral intake or if needs are increased.
Advantages: NEUTRA-PHOS and NEUTRA-PHOS-K, reconstituted to an oral liquid, provide rapid absorption and utilization from the alimentary tract. This is very advantageous compared to the use of coated or uncoated tablet dosage forms. (The patient ingests a liquid rather than a slowly dissolving tablet which may cause localized irritation or inflamation in sensitive individuals.) Both products are highly concentrated and thus economically provide inorganic Phosphate. They are especially useful for long term maintenance requirements. NEUTRA-PHOS also supplies Sodium and Potassium in equimolar proportions—a decided advantage over products which supply a high amount of sodium and a low amount of potassium per dose. NEUTRA-PHOS-K supplies only Potassium and is recommended when a low sodium diet is indicated.
Electrolytes Supplied: 2-½ fluid ounces (75 ml) of the reconstituted solution or contents of 1 capsule* supplies:
[See table below].
Average Directions for Adults and Children: 4 or more years of age: 2-½ fl. oz. (75 ml) of the oral solution, or contents of 1 capsule, equivalent to 250 mg Phosphorus, taken 4 times a day.
Pediatric Dose: Infants and children under 4 years of age: 2 fl. oz. (60 ml) of the oral solution, equivalent to 200 mg of Phosphorus, taken 4 times a day.
Usual Dose Range: 2-½ fl. oz. to 20 fl. oz. (75 ml to 600 ml) of the oral solution, or contents of 1 to 8 capsules (equivalent from 250 mg to 2 grams of Phosphorus) taken daily in divided doses, after meals and at bedtime.
2-½ fl. oz. (75 ml) or 1 capsule, 4 times a day supplies 1 gm. Phosphorus. 5 fl. oz. (150 ml) or 2 capsules, 3 times a day supplies 1.5 gm. Phosphorus. 5 fl. oz. (150 ml) or 2 capsules, 4 times a day supplies 2 gm. Phosphorus.
Precautions and Side Effects: Occasionally some individuals may experience a mild laxative effect for the first day or two when beginning to use NEUTRA-PHOS. If this persists to an unpleasant degree, reduce the daily intake until this effect subsides or, if necessary, discontinue its use.
How Supplied: Both products are supplied as powder concentrates, to be reconstituted with water by the patient, and are available in multiple dose or unit dose sizes.
Multiple Dose Powder Concentrate: For patient convenience, these powder concentrates are packaged in a size sufficient to make 1 gallon (3.785 Liters) and are intended for use while at home. This económical dosage form is prepared by the patient who is instructed to dissolve the entire contents of 1 bottle in sufficient water to make 1 gallon of solution. This solution is not to be diluted, but can be chilled if desired, to increase palatability. 2-½ fl. oz. (75 ml) of this solution supplies 250 mg Phosphorus (refer to electrolyte chart).
Unit Dose Capsules: These products are also supplied in pre-measured unit-dose capsules which are intended for use if the above multiple dose form precludes transportation of liquid. The contents of 1 capsule makes 2-½ fl. oz. (75 ml) of an oral suspension equal to the oral solution prepared above. To use, empty the contents of 1 capsule into ⅓ glass water (approx. 2-½ fl. oz.) and stir well before taking. Each capsule supplies 250 mg Phosphorus (refer to electrolyte chart).
NEUTRA-PHOS Powder Concentrate—2-¼ oz. (64 gm) bottle. Reconstitutes to 1 gallon Stock No. 201-01.
NEUTRA-PHOS Unit Dose Capsules—1.25 gm powder concentrate per capsule, 48 capsules per bottle Stock No. 202-01.
NEUTRA-PHOS-K Powder Concentrate—2-½ oz. (71 gm) bottle. Reconstitutes to 1 gallon Stock No. 203-01.
NEUTRA-PHOS-K Unit Dose Capsules—1.45 gm powder concentrate per capsule, 48 capsules per bottle Stock No. 204-01.
Is this product O.T.C.: Yes.
Literature Available: Yes.

Electrolyte	NEUTRA-PHOS mg.	NEUTRA-PHOS mEq	NEUTRA-PHOS-K mg.	NEUTRA-PHOS-K mEq
Phosphorus	250	14.25	250	14.25
Phosphate (PO_4)	765	—	765	—
Sodium	164	7.125	none	none
Potassium	278	7.125	556	14.25

(* reconstituted in water as per label directions.)

POLYCITRA® Syrup ℞
POLYCITRA®-LC—SUGAR-FREE
(Brand of Potassium Citrate, Sodium Citrate and Citric Acid Solution—W.D.)

Description: POLYCITRA Syrup and POLYCITRA-LC are stable and pleasant-tasting oral preparations containing Potassium Citrate, Sodium Citrate and Citric Acid. POLYCITRA is a syrup base preparation. POLYCITRA-LC is a sugar-free solution.
Composition: POLYCITRA Syrup and POLYCITRA-LC contains in each teaspoonful (5 ml): Potassium Citrate Monohydrate 550 mg, Sodium Citrate Dihydrate 500 mg, and Citric Acid Monohydrate 334 mg. Each ml contains 1 mEq. Potassium and 1 mEq. Sodium and is equivalent to 2 mEq. Bicarbonate (HCO_3). POLYCITRA Syrup is syrup base and contains approximately 8 calories per 5 ml. POLYCITRA-LC is sugar-free and contains less than 1 calorie per 5 ml.
Indications: POLYCITRA Syrup and POLYCITRA-LC are effective alkalinizing agents useful in those conditions where long term maintenance of an alkaline urine is desirable, such as in patients with uric acid and cystine calculi of the urinary tract. In addition, they are valuable adjuvants when administered with uricosuric agents in gout therapy, since urates tend to crystallize out of an acid urine. They are also effective in correcting the acidosis of certain renal tubular disorders.
Advantages: POLYCITRA Syrup and POLYCITRA-LC are highly concentrated, and when administered after meals and before bedtime, allows one to maintain an alkaline uri-

nary pH around the clock, usually without the necessity of a 2 AM dose. Both alkalinize the urine without producing a systemic alkalosis in recommended dosage. They are pleasant-tasting and tolerable, even when administered for long periods.

Administration and Dosage: POLYCITRA Syrup and POLYCITRA-LC should be taken diluted in water, followed by additional water, if desired. Palatability is enhanced if chilled before taking.

Usual Dosage: Adults: 15 to 30 ml diluted in water, after meals and before bedtime, or as directed by physician. Children: 5 to 15 ml, diluted in water, after meals and before bedtime, or as directed by physician.

Usual Dosage Range: 15 to 20 ml taken 4 times a day has usually maintained a urinary pH of 7.0–7.6 throughout most of 24 hours without unpleasant side effects. 10 to 15 ml taken 4 times a day will usually maintain a urinary pH of 6.5 to 7.4. Occasional patients will require more or less to achieve the desired urinary pH.

Precautions and Side Effects: POLYCITRA Syrup and POLYCITRA-LC are generally well tolerated without any unpleasant side effects when administered to patients with normal renal function and urinary output. However, as with any alkalinizing agent, caution must be used in certain patients with abnormal renal mechanisms to avoid development of hyperkalemia or alkalosis. Periodic examinations and determinations of serum electrolytes should be carried out in those patients with renal disease in order to avoid these complications.

How Supplied: POLYCITRA Syrup—16 fl oz (473 ml) (NDC 11414-205-01) and 4 fl oz (120 ml) hospital size (NDC 11414-205-04).

POLYCITRA-LC—16 fl oz (473 ml) (NDC 11414-208-01) and 4 fl oz (120 ml) hospital size (NDC 11414-208-04).

Literature Available: Yes.

POLYCITRA®-K SYRUP ℞
(Potassium Citrate and Citric Acid Syrup-W.D.)

How Supplied: Each teaspoonful (5 ml) contains: Potassium Citrate Monohydrate 1100 mg and Citric Acid Monohydrate 334 mg. Each ml contains 2 mEq. Potassium and is equivalent to 2 mEq. Bicarbonate (HCO_3). 16 fl. oz. (473 ml) (NDC 11414-206-01) and 4 fl. oz. (120 ml) hospital size (NDC 11414-206-04).

Winthrop Laboratories

90 PARK AVENUE
NEW YORK, NY 10016

AMIPAQUE® ℞
brand of metrizamide

(See Diagnostic Section.)

ARALEN® Hydrochloride ℞
brand of chloroquine hydrochloride injection, USP

For Malaria and Extraintestinal Amebiasis

WARNING: PHYSICIANS SHOULD COMPLETELY FAMILIARIZE THEMSELVES WITH THE COMPLETE CONTENTS OF THIS LEAFLET BEFORE PRESCRIBING ARALEN.

Description: Parenteral solution, each ml containing 50 mg of the dihydrochloride salt equivalent to 40 mg of chloroquine base. ARALEN hydrochloride, a 4-aminoquinoline compound, is chemically 7-(chloro-4-[[4-diethylamino)-1-methylbutyl] amino] quinoline dihydrochloride (1:2), a white, crystalline substance, freely soluble in water.

Actions: The compound is a highly active antimalarial and amebicidal agent.

ARALEN hydrochloride has been found to be highly active against the erythrocytic forms of *Plasmodium vivax* and *malariae* and most strains of *Plasmodium falciparum* (but not the gametocytes of *P. falciparum).* The precise mechanism of action of the drug is not known.

ARALEN hydrochloride does not prevent relapses in patients with vivax or malariae malaria because it is not effective against exoerythrocytic forms of the parasite, nor will it prevent vivax or malariae infection when administered as a prophylactic. It is highly effective as a suppressive agent in patients with vivax or malariae malaria, in terminating acute attacks, and significantly lengthening the interval between treatment and relapse. In patients with falciparum malaria it abolishes the acute attack and effects complete cure of the infection, unless due to a resistant strain of *P. falciparum.*

Indications: ARALEN hydrochloride is indicated for the treatment of extraintestinal amebiasis and for treatment of acute attacks of malaria due to *P. vivax, P. malariae, P. ovale,* and susceptible strains of *P. falciparum* when oral therapy is not feasible.

Contraindications: Use of this drug is contraindicated in the presence of retinal or visual field changes either attributable to 4-aminoquinoline compounds or to any other etiology, and in patients with known hypersensitivity to 4-aminoquinoline compounds. However, in the treatment of acute attacks of malaria caused by susceptible strains of plasmodia, the physician may elect to use this drug after carefully weighing the possible benefits and risks to the patient.

Warnings: *Children and infants are extremely susceptible to adverse effects from an overdose of parenteral ARALEN and sudden deaths have been recorded after such administration. In no instance should the single dose of parenteral ARALEN administered to infants or children exceed 5 mg base per kg.*

In recent years it has been found that certain strains of *P. falciparum* have become resistant to 4-aminoquinoline compounds (including chloroquine and hydroxychloroquine) as shown by the fact that normally adequate doses have failed to prevent or cure clinical malaria or parasitemia. Treatment with quinine or other specific forms of therapy is therefore advised for patients infected with a resistant strain of parasites.

Use of ARALEN should be avoided in patients with psoriasis, for it may precipitate a severe attack of psoriasis. Some authors consider the use of 4-aminoquinoline compounds contraindicated in patients with porphyria since the condition may be exacerbated.

Irreversible retinal damage has been observed in some patients who had received long-term or high-dosage 4-aminoquinoline therapy. Retinopathy has been reported to be dose related. If there is any indication (past or present) of abnormality in the visual acuity, visual field, or retinal macular areas (such as pigmentary changes, loss of foveal reflex), or any visual symptoms (such as light flashes and streaks) which are not fully explainable by difficulties of accommodation or corneal opacities, the drug should be discontinued immediately and the patient closely observed for possible progression. Retinal changes (and visual disturbances) may progress even after cessation of therapy.

Usage in Pregnancy. Usage of this drug during pregnancy should be avoided except in the suppression or treatment of malaria when in the judgment of the physician the benefit outweighs the possible hazard. It should be noted that radioactively tagged chloroquine administered intravenously to pregnant pigmented CBA mice passed rapidly across the placenta, accumulated selectively in the melanin structures of the fetal eyes and was retained in the ocular tissues for five months after the drug had been eliminated from the rest of the body.[1]

Precautions: Since the drug is known to concentrate in the liver, it should be used with caution in patients with hepatic disease or alcoholism or in conjunction with known hepatotoxic drugs.

The drug should be administered with caution to patients having G-6-PD (glucose-6-phosphate dehydrogenase) deficiency.

Adverse Reactions: Respiratory depression, cardiovascular collapse, shock, convulsions, and death have been reported with overdoses of ARALEN hydrochloride, brand of chloroquine hydrochloride injection, especially in infants and children.

Any of the adverse reactions associated with short-term oral administration of chloroquine phosphate must be considered a possibility with chloroquine hydrochloride. Cardiovascular effects, such as hypotension and electrocardiographic changes (particularly inversion or depression of the T-wave, widening of the QRS complex), have rarely been noted in patients receiving usual antimalarial doses of the drug. Mild and transient headache, pruritus, psychic stimulation, visual disturbances (blurring of vision and difficulty of focusing or accommodation), pleomorphic skin eruptions, and gastrointestinal complaints (anorexia, nausea, vomiting, diarrhea, abdominal cramps) have been observed.

Instances of convulsive seizures associated with oral chloroquine therapy in patients with extraintestinal amebiasis have been reported.

A few cases of a nerve type of deafness have been reported after prolonged therapy, usually in high doses. Tinnitus and reduced hearing have been reported, in a patient with preexistent auditory damage, after administration of only 500 mg once a week for a few months. Since neuromyopathy, blood dyscrasias, lichen planus-like eruptions, and skin and mucosal pigmentary changes have been noted during prolonged oral therapy, their occurrence with this dosage form is possible.

Patients with retinal changes may be asymptomatic, especially in early cases, or may complain of nyctalopia and scotomatous vision with field defects of paracentral, pericentral ring types, and typically temporal scotomas, e.g., difficulty in reading with words tending to disappear, seeing only half an object, misty vision, and fog before the eyes. Rarely scotomatous vision may occur without observable retinal changes.

Dosage and Administration: *Malaria—*

Adult Dose. An initial dose of 4 or 5 ml (160 to 200 mg chloroquine base) may be injected intramuscularly and repeated in 6 hours if necessary. The total parenteral dosage in the first 24 hours should not exceed 800 mg chloroquine base. Treatment by mouth should be started as soon as practicable and continued until a course of approximately 1.5 g of base in 3 days is completed.

Pediatric Dose. Infants and children are extremely susceptible to overdosage of parenteral ARALEN. Severe reactions and deaths have occurred. In the pediatric age range, parenteral ARALEN dosage should be calculated in proportion to the adult dose based upon body

Continued on next page

This product information was effective as of November 21, 1979. On these and other products of Winthrop Laboratories, detailed information may be obtained on a current basis by direct inquiry to the Professional Services Department, 90 Park Avenue, New York, N Y 10016 (212) 972-4095.

Winthrop—Cont.

weight. The recommended single dose in infants and children is 5 mg base per kg. This dose may be repeated in 6 hours; however, the total dose in any 24 hour period should not exceed 10 mg base per kg of body weight. Parenteral administration should be terminated and oral therapy instituted as soon as possible.
Extraintestinal Amebiasis—In adult patients not able to tolerate oral therapy, from 4 to 5 ml (160 to 200 mg chloroquine base) may be injected daily for 10 to 12 days. Oral administration should be substituted or resumed as soon as possible.
Overdosage: Inadvertent toxic doses may produce respiratory depression or shock with hypotension. Respiratory depression is treated by artificial respiration and administration of oxygen. In shock with hypotension, a potent vasopressor, such as NEO-SYNEPHRINE® hydrochloride, brand of phenylephrine hydrochloride, USP, should be given intramuscularly in doses of 2 to 5 mg.
How Supplied: Ampuls of 5 ml, boxes of 5.
Reference: 1. Ullberg, S., Lindquist, N. G., and Sjostrand, S. E.: Accumulation of chorio-retinotoxic drugs in the foetal eye, *Nature* *227*:1257, Sept. 19, 1970.

ARALEN® Phosphate ℞
brand of chloroquine phosphate tablets, USP

For Malaria and Extraintestinal Amebiasis

WARNING: PHYSICIANS SHOULD COMPLETELY FAMILIARIZE THEMSELVES WITH THE COMPLETE CONTENTS OF THIS LEAFLET BEFORE PRESCRIBING ARALEN.

Description: ARALEN phosphate, a 4-aminoquinoline compound, is chemically 7-chloro-4-[[4- (diethylamino) -1-methylbutyl]amino]-quinoline phosphate (1:2), a white, crystalline substance, freely soluble in water.
Actions: ARALEN phosphate has been found to be highly active against the erythrocytic forms of *Plasmodium vivax* and *malariae* and most strains of *Plasmodium falciparum* (but not the gametocytes of *P. falciparum*). The precise mechanism of action of the drug is not known.
ARALEN phosphate does not prevent relapses in patients with vivax or malariae malaria because it is not effective against exo-erythrocytic forms of the parasite, nor will it prevent vivax or malariae infection when administered as a prophylactic. It is highly effective as a suppressive agent in patients with vivax or malariae malaria, in terminating acute attacks, and significantly lengthening the interval between treatment and relapse. In patients with falciparum malaria it abolishes the acute attack and effects complete cure of the infection, unless due to a resistant strain of *P. falciparum*.
In vitro studies with trophozoites of *Entamoeba histolytica* have demonstrated that ARALEN phosphate also possesses amebicidal activity comparable to that of emetine.
Indications: ARALEN phosphate is indicated for the suppressive treatment and for acute attacks of malaria due to *P. vivax, P. malariae, P. ovale,* and susceptible strains of *P. falciparum.* The drug is also indicated for treatment of extraintestinal amebiasis.
Contraindications: Use of this drug is contraindicated in the presence of retinal or visual field changes either attributable to 4- aminoquinoline compounds or to any other etiology, and in patients with known hypersensitivity to 4-aminoquinoline compounds. However, in the treatment of acute attacks of malaria caused by susceptible strains of plasmodia, the physician may elect to use this drug after carefully weighing the possible benefits and risks to the patient.
Warnings: In recent years it has been found that certain strains of *P. falciparum* have become resistant to 4-aminoquinoline compounds (including chloroquine and hydroxychloroquine) as shown by the fact that normally adequate doses have failed to prevent or cure clinical malaria or parasitemia. Treatment with quinine or other specific forms of therapy is therefore advised for patients infected with a resistant strain of parasites.
Irreversible retinal damage has been observed in some patients who had received long-term or high-dosage 4-aminoquinoline therapy. Retinopathy has been reported to be dose related. When prolonged therapy with any antimalarial compound is contemplated, initial (base line) and periodic ophthalmologic examinations (including visual acuity, expert slit-lamp, funduscopic, and visual field tests) should be performed.
If there is any indication (past or present) of abnormality in the visual acuity, visual field, or retinal macular areas (such as pigmentary changes, loss of foveal reflex), or any visual symptoms (such as light flashes and streaks) which are not fully explainable by difficulties of accommodation or corneal opacities, the drug should be discontinued immediately and the patient closely observed for possible progression. Retinal changes (and visual disturbances) may progress even after cessation of therapy.
All patients on long-term therapy with this preparation should be questioned and examined periodically, including testing knee and ankle reflexes, to detect any evidence of muscular weakness. If weakness occurs, discontinue the drug.
A number of fatalities have been reported following the accidental ingestion of chloroquine, sometimes in relatively small doses (0.75 or 1 g chloroquine phosphate in one 3-year-old child). Patients should be strongly warned to keep this drug out of the reach of children because they are especially sensitive to the 4- aminoquinoline compounds.
Use of ARALEN phosphate, brand of chloroquine phosphate tablets, in patients with psoriasis may precipitate a severe attack of psoriasis. When used in patients with porphyria the condition may be exacerbated. The drug should not be used in these conditions unless in the judgment of the physician the benefit to the patient outweighs the possible hazard.
Usage in Pregnancy. Usage of this drug during pregnancy should be avoided except in the suppression or treatment of malaria when in the judgment of the physician the benefit outweighs the possible hazard. It should be noted that radioactively tagged chloroquine administered intravenously to pregnant pigmented CBA mice passed rapidly across the placenta, accumulated selectively in the melanin structures of the fetal eyes and was retained in the ocular tissues for five months after the drug had been eliminated from the rest of the body.[1]
Precautions: Since the drug is known to concentrate in the liver, it should be used with caution in patients with hepatic disease or alcoholism or in conjunction with known hepatotoxic drugs.
Complete blood cell counts should be made periodically if patients are given prolonged therapy. If any severe blood disorder appears which is not attributable to the disease under treatment, discontinuance of the drug should be considered. The drug should be administered with caution to patients having G-6-PD (glucose-6-phosphate dehydrogenase) deficiency.
Adverse Reactions: Following the administration of ARALEN phosphate in doses adequate for the treatment of an acute malarial attack or extraintestinal amebiasis, mild and transient headache, pruritus, gastrointestinal complaints (anorexia, nausea, vomiting, diarrhea, abdominal cramps), psychic stimulation, and rarely psychotic episodes or convulsions have been observed. Cardiovascular effects, such as hypotension and electrocardiographic changes (particularly inversion or depression of the T-wave, widening of the QRS complex), have rarely been noted in patients receiving usual antimalarial doses of the drug. A few cases of a nerve type of deafness have been reported after prolonged therapy, usually in high doses. Tinnitus and reduced hearing have been reported, in a patient with preexistent auditory damage, after administration of only 500 mg once a week for a few months. Neuromyopathy, blood dyscrasias, lichen planus-like eruptions, and skin and mucosal pigmentary changes have also been noted during prolonged therapy.
When employed for the indications (malaria and extraintestinal amebiasis) and in the dosages recommended in this leaflet, visual disturbances, consisting of blurring of vision or difficulty in focusing or accommodation, occasionally may be noted; they are reversible and disappear on discontinuation of therapy. Other types of visual disturbances and ocular complications have been reported during the use of chloroquine for long-term therapy usually in daily doses exceeding 250 mg of chloroquine phosphate. These consisted of (1) reversible corneal changes (transient edema or opaque deposits in the epithelium) which may be asymptomatic or cause visual halos, focusing difficulties, or blurred vision and (2) generally irreversible, sometimes progressive, or, rarely delayed, retinal changes, such as narrowing of the arterioles, macular lesions (loss of foveal reflex, areas of edema, atrophy, and abnormal pigmentation), pallor of the optic disc, optic atrophy, and patchy retinal pigmentation.
Patients with retinal changes may be asymptomatic, especially in early cases, or may complain of nyctalopia and scotomatous vision with field defects of paracentral, pericentral ring types, and typically temporal scotomas, e.g., difficulty in reading with words tending to disappear, seeing only half an object, misty vision, and fog before the eyes. Rarely scotomatous vision may occur without observable retinal changes.
Dosage and Administration: The dosage of chloroquine phosphate is often expressed or calculated as the base. Each 500 mg tablet of ARALEN phosphate, brand of chloroquine phosphate tablets, is equivalent to 300 mg base. In infants and children the dosage is preferably calculated on the body weight.
Malaria: Suppression — **In adults,** 500 mg (= 300 mg base) on exactly the same day of each week. **In infants and children** the weekly suppressive dosage is 5 mg, calculated as base, per kg of body weight, but should not exceed the adult dose regardless of weight.
If circumstances permit, suppressive therapy should begin two weeks prior to exposure. However, failing this in adults, an initial double (loading) dose of 1 g (= 600 mg base), or in children 10 mg base/kg may be taken in two divided doses, six hours apart. The suppressive therapy should be continued for eight weeks after leaving the endemic area.
Treatment of the acute attack—**In adults,** an initial dose of 1 g (= 600 mg base) followed by an additional 500 mg (= 300 mg base) after six to eight hours and a single dose of 500 mg (= 300 mg base) on each of two consecutive days. This represents a total dose of 2.5 g chloroquine phosphate or 1.5 g base in three days.
The dosage for adults may also be calculated on the basis of body weight; this method is preferred for infants and children. A total dose representing 25 mg of base per kg of body weight is administered in three days, as follows:

First dose: 10 mg base per kg (but not exceeding a single dose of 600 mg base).
Second dose: 5 mg base per kg (but not exceeding a single dose of 300 mg base) 6 hours after first dose.
Third dose: 5 mg base per kg 18 hours after second dose.
Fourth dose: 5 mg base per kg 24 hours after third dose.
For radical cure of *vivax* and *malariae* malaria concomitant therapy with an 8- aminoquinoline compound is necessary.

Extraintestinal Amebiasis: Adults, 1 g (600 mg base) daily for two days, followed by 500 mg (300 mg base) daily for at least two to three weeks. Treatment is usually combined with an effective intestinal amebicide.

Overdosage: Chloroquine is very rapidly and completely absorbed after ingestion, and in accidental overdosage, or rarely with lower doses in hypersensitive patients, toxic symptoms may occur within thirty minutes. These consist of headache, drowsiness, visual disturbances, cardiovascular collapse, and convulsions followed by sudden and early respiratory and cardiac arrest. The electrocardiogram may reveal atrial standstill, nodal rhythm, prolonged intraventricular conduction time, and progressive bradycardia leading to ventricular fibrillation and/or arrest. Treatment is symptomatic and must be prompt with immediate evacuation of the stomach by emesis (at home, before transportation to the hospital) or gastric lavage until the stomach is completely emptied. If finely powdered, activated charcoal is introduced by stomach tube, after lavage, and within 30 minutes after ingestion of the antimalarial, it may inhibit further intestinal absorption of the drug. To be effective, the dose of activated charcoal should be at least five times the estimated dose of chloroquine ingested.
Convulsions, if present, should be controlled before attempting gastric lavage. If due to cerebral stimulation, cautious administration of an ultrashort-acting barbiturate may be tried but, if due to anoxia, it should be corrected by oxygen administration, artificial respiration or, in shock with hypotension, by vasopressor therapy. Because of the importance of supporting respiration, tracheal intubation or tracheostomy, followed by gastric lavage, may also be necessary. Peritoneal dialysis and exchange transfusions have also been suggested to reduce the level of the drug in the blood.
A patient who survives the acute phase and is asymptomatic should be closely observed for at least six hours. Fluids may be forced, and sufficient ammonium chloride (8 g daily in divided doses for adults) may be administered for a few days to acidify the urine to help promote urinary excretion in cases of both overdosage or sensitivity.

How Supplied: Tablets of 500 mg (= 300 mg base), bottles of 25.

Reference: 1. Ullberg, S., Lindquist, N. G., and Sjostrand, S. E.: Accumulation of chorio-retinotoxic drugs in the foetal eye, *Nature 227:* 1257, Sept. 19, 1970.

[*Shown in Product Identification Section*]

ARALEN® Phosphate ℞
brand of chloroquine phosphate, USP
with
PRIMAQUINE Phosphate, USP

For Malaria Prophylaxis Only

WARNING: PHYSICIANS SHOULD COMPLETELY FAMILIARIZE THEMSELVES WITH THE COMPLETE CONTENTS OF THIS LEAFLET BEFORE PRESCRIBING ARALEN PHOSPHATE WITH PRIMAQUINE PHOSPHATE.

Description: Each tablet contains ARALEN phosphate, brand of chloroquine phosphate, USP, 500 mg (equivalent to 300 mg base) and primaquine phosphate 79 mg (equivalent to 45 mg base).

Actions: ARALEN is a 4-aminoquinoline compound which is highly active against the erythrocytic forms of *Plasmodium vivax* and most strains of *Plasmodium falciparum* (but not the gametocytes of *P. falciparum).*
Primaquine is an 8-aminoquinoline compound which eliminates tissue (exo-erythrocytic) infection. Thereby, it prevents the development of the blood (erythrocytic) forms of the parasite which are responsible for relapses in vivax malaria. Primaquine phosphate is active against gametocytes of *P. falciparum.*
ARALEN phosphate with primaquine phosphate demonstrates antimalarial activity against all stages of human-malaria parasites, except for certain strains of *P. falciparum* resistant to chloroquine.

Indication: ARALEN phosphate with primaquine phosphate is intended solely for use in the prophylaxis of malaria, regardless of species, in all areas where this disease is endemic.

Contraindications: The drug is contraindicated in acutely ill patients suffering from systemic disease manifested by tendency to granulocytopenia, such as rheumatoid arthritis and lupus erythematosus. The drug is also contraindicated in those patients receiving concurrently other potentially hemolytic drugs or depressants of myeloid elements of the bone marrow.
Primaquine should not be administered to patients who have received quinacrine recently, as toxicity is increased.

Warnings: Children are especially sensitive to 4-aminoquinoline compounds. A number of fatalities have been reported following the accidental ingestion of chloroquine, sometimes in relatively small doses (0.75 or 1 g in one 3- year-old child). Patients should be strongly warned to keep these drugs out of the reach of children.
Hemolytic reactions (moderate to severe) may occur after even a weekly dose of this preparation in glucose-6-phosphate dehydrogenase (G-6-PD) deficient Caucasians (particularly, in Sardinians and in individuals with a family or personal history of favism).
Usage in Pregnancy. Safe usage of this preparation in pregnancy has not been established. Therefore, use of it during pregnancy should be avoided except when in the judgment of the physician the benefit outweighs the possible hazard. It should be noted that radioactively tagged chloroquine administered intravenously to pregnant pigmented CBA mice passed rapidly across the placenta, accumulated selectively in the melanin structures of the fetal eyes and was retained in the ocular tissues for five months after the drug had been eliminated from the rest of the body.[1]

Precautions: ARALEN phosphate, brand of chloroquine phosphate, with primaquine phosphate is intended for malaria prophylaxis only; it should not be used for the treatment of clinical malaria. The recommended dosage (one tablet weekly, on the same day each week) should not be exceeded. The drug should not be taken more often than once every seven days to minimize danger of toxicity.
If the combination is prescribed for (1) an individual who has shown a previous idiosyncrasy to either chloroquine or primaquine (as manifested by dermatitis, hemolytic anemia, methemoglobinemia, or leukopenia), (2) an individual with a family or personal history of favism, or (3) an individual with erythrocytic glucose-6-phosphate dehydrogenase (G-6-PD) deficiency or nicotinamide adenine dinucleotide (NADH) methemoglobin reductase deficiency, the person should be observed closely for tolerance. The drug should be discontinued immediately if marked darkening of the urine, sudden decrease in hemoglobin concentration or leukocyte count, or severe skin reaction occurs.
In areas with endemic falciparum malaria due to strains that are resistant to the 4-aminoquinolines (chloroquine, amodiaquine, hydroxychloroquine), chemoprophylaxis with this combination alone may not be effective.

Adverse Reactions: *Gastrointestinal reactions:* anorexia, nausea, vomiting, epigastric distress, and abdominal cramps. *Hematologic reactions:* leukopenia, hemolytic anemia in glucose-6-phosphate dehydrogenase (G-6-PD) deficient individuals, methemoglobinemia in nicotinamide adenine dinucleotide (NADH) methemoglobin reductase deficient individuals.
Cardiovascular effects, such as hypotension and electrocardiographic changes (particularly inversion or depression of the T-wave, widening of the QRS complex), have rarely been noted in patients receiving usual antimalarial doses of the drug.
Visual disturbances, consisting of blurring of vision or difficulty in focusing or accommodation, have occasionally been noted when chloroquine has been employed for malaria. These symptoms are reversible and disappear on discontinuation of therapy. Other types of visual disturbances (reversible corneal changes) and ocular complications including retinal changes (narrowing of the arterioles, macular lesions, pallor of the optic disc, optic atrophy, and patchy retinal pigmentation) have been reported during the use of chloroquine for long-term therapy usually in daily doses exceeding 250 mg of chloroquine phosphate. These changes have not been reported with the use of ARALEN phosphate, brand of chloroquine phosphate, with primaquine phosphate for malaria prophylaxis.
Auditory disturbances: tinnitus and reduced hearing have been reported, in a patient with preexistent auditory damage, after administration of only 500 mg of ARALEN phosphate, brand of chloroquine phosphate, once a week for a few months.

Dosage and Administration:
Adults—Starting at least one day before entering the malarious area, one tablet weekly, taken on the same day each week. This schedule (one tablet weekly) should be continued for eight weeks after leaving the endemic area.
Children—The following dosage, based on body weight, is suggested.

Weight (lb)	ARALEN base (mg)	Primaquine base (mg)	Dose* (ml)
10-15	20	3	2.5
16-25	40	6	5.0
26-35	60	9	7.5
36-45	80	12	10.0
46-55	100	15	12.5
56-100	150	22.5	½ tab.
100+	300	45	1 tab.

*Dose based on liquid containing approximately 40 mg of chloroquine base and 6 mg of primaquine base per 5 ml (1 teaspoon) prepared from ARALEN phosphate, brand of chloroquine phosphate, with primaquine phosphate tablets. Chocolate syrup could be used to prepare a suspension (one tablet crushed and suspended in 40 ml of liquid). Shake well before use.

Overdosage: Symptoms of overdosage are due to the two drug components.

Continued on next page

This product information was effective as of November 21, 1979. On these and other products of Winthrop Laboratories, detailed information may be obtained on a current basis by direct inquiry to the Professional Services Department, 90 Park Avenue, New York, N Y 10016 (212) 972-4095.

Winthrop—Cont.

Chloroquine is very rapidly and completely absorbed after ingestion, and in accidental overdosage, or rarely with lower doses in hypersensitive patients, toxic symptoms may occur within thirty minutes. These consist of headache, drowsiness, visual disturbances, cardiovascular collapse, and convulsions followed by sudden and early respiratory and cardiac arrest. The electrocardiogram may reveal atrial standstill, nodal rhythm, prolonged intraventricular conduction time, and progressive bradycardia leading to ventricular fibrillation and/or arrest.
Symptoms of overdosage of primaquine are similar to those seen after overdosage of pamaquine. They include abdominal cramps, vomiting, burning epigastric distress, central nervous system and cardiovascular disturbances, cyanosis, methemoglobinemia, moderate leukocytosis or leukopenia, and anemia. The most striking symptoms are granulocytopenia and acute hemolytic anemia in sensitive persons. Acute hemolysis occurs, but patients recover completely if the dosage is discontinued.
Treatment is symptomatic and must be prompt with immediate evacuation of the stomach by emesis (at home, before transportation to the hospital) or gastric lavage until the stomach is completely emptied. Finely powdered, activated charcoal in a dose not less than five times the estimated dose of chloroquine ingested, if introduced by the stomach tube after lavage within thirty minutes after ingestion of the antimalarial, may inhibit further intestinal absorption of the drug.
Convulsions, if present, should be controlled before attempting gastric lavage. If due to cerebral stimulation, cautious administration of an ultrashort-acting barbiturate may be tried but, if due to anoxia, it should be corrected by oxygen administration, artificial respiration or, in shock with hypotension, by vasopressor therapy. Because of the importance of supporting respiration, tracheal intubation or tracheostomy, followed by gastric lavage, may also be necessary. Exchange transfusions have also been suggested to reduce the level of the drug in the blood.
The patient should be kept in bed and warm. If methemoglobinemia and cyanosis occur, oxygen may be administered and use of methylene blue may be considered. If collapse and hypotension or shock occur, vasopressors may be used. The patient should be observed for the possible development of leukopenia or hemolytic anemia.
A patient who survives the acute stage and is asymptomatic should be closely observed for at least six hours. Fluids may be forced, and sufficient ammonium chloride (8 g daily in divided doses for adults) may be administered for a few days to acidify the urine to help promote urinary excretion in cases of both overdosage or sensitivity.
How Supplied: Tablets, bottles of 100.
Clinical Studies: On the basis of carefully controlled preliminary clinical trials, Alving and his associates[2] found that the weekly administration of 300 mg chloroquine base and 45 mg primaquine base (administered as the phosphate salts) proved highly effective as a prophylactic against severe *P. vivax* infections with the Chesson strain and did not produce clinical hemolysis even among primaquine-sensitive American Negro adult volunteers. A weekly dose of primaquine phosphate equivalent to 45 mg primaquine base cured 90 per cent of infections.
The studies of these workers indicate that the toxicity of primaquine phosphate, as regards the production of hemolysis, is markedly diminished when administered in weekly doses. When administered with standard suppressive doses of chloroquine phosphate, its therapeutic effectiveness in the radical cure of Chesson vivax malaria is increased. Thus, a weekly dose equivalent to 60 mg of primaquine base is less toxic than 15 mg base administered daily; and a dose equivalent to 45 mg base administered weekly was found to be practically without demonstrable toxicity. A dose equivalent to 45 mg base weekly for 8 weeks was more effective in the radical cure of infections than 15 mg base daily for 14 days.
Wittmer[3] conducted a double-blind study in 24 Caucasian male adults who received ARALEN phosphate, brand of chloroquine phosphate, with primaquine phosphate once each week (Friday) for 15 weeks to determine its safety and suitability for use in Armed Forces flying personnel. The author concluded that there appear to be no contraindications to the long-term use of the combination in flying personnel since there was no effect on vision, time of useful consciousness, or psychomotor performance. No deleterious synergistic effect of the two drugs was demonstrated. Charles[4] investigated the effects of 5 weekly doses of primaquine phosphate (1 to 1.5 mg base per kg body weight) in combination with a 4-aminoquinoline antimalarial agent on the parasitemia and blood picture of 100 Ghanaian children from 2½ to 8 years old. Although the enzyme-deficiency trait (glucose-6-phosphate dehydrogenase deficiency) for primaquine sensitivity occurred in approximately 25 per cent of the group, no general evidence of hemolysis was observed. Eight of the treated subjects were positive for the glucose-6-phosphate dehydrogenase deficiency test but maintained their pretreatment hemoglobin values.
However, Ziai and his associates[5] noted that serious hematologic reactions can occur in persons with a glucose-6-phosphate dehydrogenase (G-6-PD) deficiency with the small weekly doses of chloroquine-primaquine used for malaria suppressive therapy. This has been reported primarily in patients with a family history and/or personal history of favism.
Methemoglobinemia has been discovered in individuals with nicotinamide adenine dinucleotide methemoglobin reductase deficiency.[6]
The susceptibility of primaquine-sensitive children to hemolysis by primaquine phosphate is considered to be of the same order of magnitude as that of adults on an equal drug/body weight basis.

References:

1. Ullberg, S., Lindquist, N. G., and Sjostrand, S. E.: Accumulation of chorio-retinotoxic drugs in the foetal eye, *Nature* *227*:1257, Sept. 19, 1970.
2. Alving, A. S. *et al.:* Mitigation of the haemolytic effect of primaquine and enhancement of its action against exo-erythrocytic forms of the Chesson strain of *Plasmodium vivax* by intermittent regimens of drug administration, *Bull. WHO* *22*:621, 1960.
3. Wittmer, J. F.: Aeromedical aspects of malaria prophylaxis with chloroquine-primaquine, *Aerospace Med. 34:*944, Oct. 1963.
4. Charles, L. J.: Observations on the haemolytic effect of primaquine in 100 Ghanaian children, *Ann. Trop. Med. 54:*460, Dec. 1960.
5. Ziai, M. *et al.:* Malaria prophylaxis and treatment in G-6-PD deficiency, *Clin. Pediat. 6:*242, April 1967.
6. Cohen, R. *et al.*: Methemoglobinemia provoked by malarial chemoprophylaxis in Vietnam, *New Eng. J. Med. 279:*1127-1131, Nov. 21, 1968.

BILOPAQUE® SODIUM ℞
brand of sodium tyropanoate

(See Diagnostic Section.)

DANOCRINE® ℞
brand of danazol

Description: DANOCRINE, brand of danazol, is a synthetic androgen derived from ethisterone. Chemically, danazol is 17α-pregna-2,4-dien-20-yno[2,3-*d*]-isoxazol-17-ol.
Each hard gelatin capsule contains 200 mg of danazol.
Clinical Pharmacology: DANOCRINE suppresses the pituitary-ovarian axis by inhibiting the output of gonadotropins from the pituitary gland. The only other demonstrable hormonal effect is weak androgenic activity which is dose related. Studies have established that the drug is neither estrogenic nor progestational. DANOCRINE depresses the output of both follicle-stimulating hormone (FSH) and luteinizing hormone (LH).
When effective for the treatment of endometriosis, DANOCRINE alters the normal and ectopic endometrial tissue so that it becomes inactive and atrophic. Complete resolution of endometrial lesions occurs in the majority of cases. This regression is due to the suppression of ovarian function, resulting in anovulation with associated amenorrhea. Changes in vaginal cytology and cervical mucus reflect the suppressive effect of DANOCRINE on the pituitary-ovarian axis.
Generally the pituitary-suppressive action of DANOCRINE is reversible. Ovulation and cyclic bleeding usually return within 60 to 90 days when DANOCRINE therapy is discontinued.
Indications and Usage: Until additional studies have been completed which define the lowest clinically effective dose, DANOCRINE is indicated for the treatment of endometriosis amenable to hormonal management and only for those patients 1) who cannot tolerate other drug therapy, 2) in whom other effective drugs are contraindicated, or 3) who fail to respond to other effective drug therapy when given in adequate doses.
DANOCRINE is not indicated in those patients where surgery alone is considered the treatment of choice.
Contraindications: DANOCRINE should not be administered to patients with:
1. Undiagnosed abnormal genital bleeding.
2. Markedly impaired hepatic, renal, or cardiac function.
3. Pregnancy.
4. Breast feeding.

Warnings: Further studies are ongoing to define the lowest clinically effective dose of DANOCRINE, brand of danazol. Consequently, at the present time, DANOCRINE should be limited in its use to the select group of patients mentioned in the INDICATIONS AND USAGE Section. In view of the fact that some cases of endometriosis may be resistant to one specific form of hormone therapy and responsive to another, DANOCRINE may prove to be of benefit in such cases. There are some limited data in support of the use of DANOCRINE in therapy-resistant cases of this type.
Safe use of the drug in pregnancy has not been established clinically. Therefore, a nonhormonal method of contraception should be recommended. If a patient becomes pregnant during treatment, administration of the drug should be discontinued. Continuing treatment may result in an androgenic effect on the fetus. Patients should be watched closely for signs of virilization. Some androgenic effects may not be reversible even when drug administration is stopped.
Precautions: Because DANOCRINE may cause some degree of fluid retention, conditions that might be influenced by this factor, such as epilepsy, migraine, or cardiac or renal dysfunction, require careful observation.
Adverse Reactions: The following androgenic effects have occurred in patients receiving DANOCRINE: acne, edema, mild hirsut-

ism, decrease in breast size, deepening of the voice, oiliness of the skin or hair, weight gain, and rarely, clitoral hypertrophy.

Also hypoestrogenic manifestations such as flushing, sweating, vaginitis including itching, dryness, burning and vaginal bleeding, nervousness, and emotional lability have been reported.

Although the following reactions have also been reported, a causal relationship to the administration of DANOCRINE has neither been confirmed nor refuted: *allergic:* skin rashes and rarely, nasal congestion; *CNS effects:* dizziness, headache, sleep disorders, fatigue, tremor, and rarely, paresthesia in extremities, visual disturbances, changes in appetite, and chills; *gastrointestinal:* gastroenteritis, and rarely, nausea, vomiting, and constipation; *musculoskeletal:* muscle cramps or spasms, and pain in back, neck, or legs; *genitourinary:* rarely, hematuria; *other:* loss of hair, changes in libido, elevation in blood pressure, and rarely, pelvic pain.

Dosage and Administration: The dosage of DANOCRINE, brand of danazol, is 800 mg, divided into two doses per day, until additional studies on the effectiveness of lower doses are completed. **Therapy should begin during menstruation. Otherwise, appropriate tests should be performed to ensure that the patient is not pregnant while on DANOCRINE therapy. It is essential that therapy continue uninterrupted for 3 to 6 months but may be extended to 9 months if necessary.** After termination of therapy, if symptoms recur, treatment can be reinstituted.

How Supplied: Capsules of 200 mg (orange), bottles of 100 (NDC 0024-0305-06).

[*Shown in Product Identification Section*]

DEMEROL® Hydrochloride Ⓒ
brand of meperidine hydrochloride ℞

Description: Meperidine hydrochloride is ethyl 1-methyl-4-phenylisonipecotate hydrochloride, a white crystalline substance with a melting point of 186° to 189° C. It is readily soluble in water and has a neutral reaction and a slightly bitter taste. The solution is not decomposed by a short period of boiling.

The syrup is a pleasant-tasting, nonalcoholic, banana-flavored solution containing 50 mg of DEMEROL hydrochloride, brand of meperidine hydrochloride, per 5 ml teaspoon (25 drops contain 13 mg of DEMEROL hydrochloride). The tablets contain 50 or 100 mg of the analgesic.

DEMEROL hydrochloride, brand of meperidine hydrochloride, 5 per cent solution has a specific gravity of 1.0086 at 20°C and 10 per cent solution, a specific gravity of 1.0165 at 20°C.

Clinical Pharmacology: Meperidine hydrochloride is a narcotic analgesic with multiple actions qualitatively similar to those of morphine; the most prominent of these involve the central nervous system and organs composed of smooth muscle. The principal actions of therapeutic value are analgesia and sedation. There is some evidence which suggests that meperidine may produce less smooth muscle spasm, constipation, and depression of the cough reflex than equianalgesic doses of morphine. Meperidine, in 60 to 80 mg parenteral doses, is approximately equivalent in analgesic effect to 10 mg of morphine. The onset of action is slightly more rapid than with morphine, and the duration of action is slightly shorter. Meperidine is significantly less effective by the oral than by the parenteral route, but the exact ratio of oral to parenteral effectiveness is unknown.

Indications and Usage:

For the relief of moderate to severe pain (parenteral and oral forms)

For preoperative medication (parenteral form only)

For support of anesthesia (parenteral form only)

For obstetrical analgesia (parenteral form only)

Contraindications:

Hypersensitivity to meperidine.

Meperidine is contraindicated in patients who are receiving monoamine oxidase (MAO) inhibitors or those who have recently received such agents. Therapeutic doses of meperidine have occasionally precipitated unpredictable, severe, and occasionally fatal reactions in patients who have received such agents within 14 days. The mechanism of these reactions is unclear, but may be related to a preexisting hyperphenylalaninemia. Some have been characterized by coma, severe respiratory depression, cyanosis, and hypotension, and have resembled the syndrome of acute narcotic overdose. In other reactions the predominant manifestations have been hyperexcitability, convulsions, tachycardia, hyperpyrexia, and hypertension. Although it is not known that other narcotics are free of the risk of such reactions, virtually all of the reported reactions have occurred with meperidine. If a narcotic is needed in such patients, a sensitivity test should be performed in which repeated, small, incremental doses of morphine are administered over the course of several hours while the patient's condition and vital signs are under careful observation. (Intravenous hydrocortisone or prednisolone have been used to treat severe reactions, with the addition of intravenous chlorpromazine in those cases exhibiting hypertension and hyperpyrexia. The usefulness and safety of narcotic antagonists in the treatment of these reactions is unknown.)

Solutions of DEMEROL and barbiturates are chemically incompatible.

Warnings: *Drug Dependence.* Meperidine can produce drug dependence of the morphine type and therefore has the potential for being abused. Psychic dependence, physical dependence, and tolerance may develop upon repeated administration of meperidine, and it should be prescribed and administered with the same degree of caution appropriate to the use of morphine. Like other narcotics, meperidine is subject to the provisions of the Federal narcotic laws.

Interaction with Other Central Nervous System Depressants. Meperidine should be used with great caution and in reduced dosage in patients who are concurrently receiving other narcotic analgesics, general anesthetics, phenothiazines, other tranquilizers (see Dosage and Administration), sedative-hypnotics (including barbiturates), tricyclic antidepressants, and other CNS depressants (including alcohol). Respiratory depression, hypotension, and profound sedation or coma may result.

Head Injury and Increased Intracranial Pressure. The respiratory depressant effects of meperidine and its capacity to elevate cerebrospinal fluid pressure may be markedly exaggerated in the presence of head injury, other intracranial lesions, or a preexisting increase in intracranial pressure. Furthermore, narcotics produce adverse reactions which may obscure the clinical course of patients with head injuries. In such patients, meperidine must be used with extreme caution and only if its use is deemed essential.

Intravenous Use. If necessary, meperidine may be given intravenously, but the injection should be given very slowly, preferably in the form of a diluted solution. Rapid intravenous injection of narcotic analgesics, including meperidine, increases the incidence of adverse reactions; severe respiratory depression, apnea, hypotension, peripheral circulatory collapse, and cardiac arrest have occurred. Meperidine should not be administered intravenously unless a narcotic antagonist and the facilities for assisted or controlled respiration are immediately available. When meperidine is given parenterally, especially intravenously, the patient should be lying down.

Asthma and Other Respiratory Conditions. Meperidine should be used with extreme caution in patients having an acute asthmatic attack, patients with chronic obstructive pulmonary disease or cor pulmonale, patients having a substantially decreased respiratory reserve, and patients with preexisting respiratory depression, hypoxia, or hypercapnia. In such patients, even usual therapeutic doses of narcotics may decrease respiratory drive while simultaneously increasing airway resistance to the point of apnea.

Hypotensive Effect. The administration of meperidine may result in severe hypotension in the postoperative patient or any individual whose ability to maintain blood pressure has been compromised by a depleted blood volume or the administration of drugs such as the phenothiazines or certain anesthetics.

Usage in Ambulatory Patients. Meperidine may impair the mental and/or physical abilities required for the performance of potentially hazardous tasks such as driving a car or operating machinery. The patient should be cautioned accordingly.

Meperidine, like other narcotics, may produce orthostatic hypotension in ambulatory patients.

Usage in Pregnancy and Lactation. Meperidine should not be used in pregnant women prior to the labor period, unless in the judgment of the physician the potential benefits outweigh the possible hazards, because safe use in pregnancy prior to labor has not been established relative to possible adverse effects on fetal development.

When used as an obstetrical analgesic, meperidine crosses the placental barrier and can produce depression of respiration and psychophysiologic functions in the newborn. Resuscitation may be required (see section on **OVERDOSAGE).**

Meperidine appears in the milk of nursing mothers receiving the drug.

Precautions: *Supraventricular Tachycardias.* Meperidine should be used with caution in patients with atrial flutter and other supraventricular tachycardias because of a possible vagolytic action which may produce a significant increase in the ventricular response rate.

Convulsions. Meperidine may aggravate preexisting convulsions in patients with convulsive disorders. If dosage is escalated substantially above recommended levels because of tolerance development, convulsions may occur in individuals without a history of convulsive disorders.

Acute Abdominal Conditions. The administration of meperidine or other narcotics may obscure the diagnosis or clinical course in patients with acute abdominal conditions.

Special Risk Patients. Meperidine should be given with caution and the initial dose should be reduced in certain patients such as the elderly or debilitated, and those with severe impairment of hepatic or renal function, hypothyroidism, Addison's disease, and prostatic hypertrophy or urethral stricture.

Adverse Reactions: The major hazards of meperidine, as with other narcotic analgesics, are respiratory depression and, to a lesser degree, circulatory depression; respiratory arrest, shock, and cardiac arrest have occurred.

Continued on next page

This product information was effective as of November 21, 1979. On these and other products of Winthrop Laboratories, detailed information may be obtained on a current basis by direct inquiry to the Professional Services Department, 90 Park Avenue, New York, N Y 10016 (212) 972-4095.

Winthrop—Cont.

The most frequently observed adverse reactions include lightheadedness, dizziness, sedation, nausea, vomiting, and sweating. These effects seem to be more prominent in ambulatory patients and in those who are not experiencing severe pain. In such individuals, lower doses are advisable. Some adverse reactions in ambulatory patients may be alleviated if the patient lies down.
Other adverse reactions include:
Nervous System. Euphoria, dysphoria, weakness, headache, agitation, tremor, uncoordinated muscle movements, transient hallucinations and disorientation, visual disturbances. Inadvertent injection about a nerve trunk may result in sensory-motor paralysis which is usually, though not always, transitory.
Gastrointestinal. Dry mouth, constipation, biliary tract spasm.
Cardiovascular. Flushing of the face, tachycardia, bradycardia, palpitation, hypotension (see Warnings), syncope, phlebitis following intravenous injection.
Genitourinary. Urinary retention.
Allergic. Pruritus, urticaria, other skin rashes, wheal and flare over the vein with intravenous injection.
Other. Pain at injection site; local tissue irritation and induration following subcutaneous injection, particularly when repeated; antidiuretic effect.

Dosage and Administration:

For Relief of Pain

Dosage should be adjusted according to the severity of the pain and the response of the patient. While subcutaneous administration is suitable for occasional use, intramuscular administration is preferred when repeated doses are required. If intravenous administration is required, dosage should be decreased and the injection made very slowly, preferably utilizing a diluted solution. Meperidine is less effective orally than on parenteral administration. The dose of DEMEROL should be proportionately reduced (usually by 25 to 50 per cent) when administered concomitantly with phenothiazines and many other tranquilizers since they potentiate the action of DEMEROL, brand of meperidine.
Adults. The usual dosage is 50 to 150 mg intramuscularly, subcutaneously, or orally, every 3 or 4 hours as necessary.
Children. The usual dosage is 0.5 to 0.8 mg/lb intramuscularly, subcutaneously, or orally up to the adult dose, every 3 or 4 hours as necessary.
Each dose of the syrup should be taken in one half glass of water, since if taken undiluted, it may exert a slight topical anesthetic effect on mucous membranes.

For Preoperative Medication

Adults. The usual dosage is 50 to 100 mg intramuscularly or subcutaneously, 30 to 90 minutes before the beginning of anesthesia.
Children. The usual dosage is 0.5 to 1 mg/lb intramuscularly or subcutaneously up to the adult dose, 30 to 90 minutes before the beginning of anesthesia.

For Support of Anesthesia

Repeated slow intravenous injections of fractional doses (e.g., 10 mg/ml) or continuous intravenous infusion of a more dilute solution (e.g., 1 mg/ml) should be used. The dose should be titrated to the needs of the patient and will depend on the premedication and type of anesthesia being employed, the characteristics of the particular patient, and the nature and duration of the operative procedure.

For Obstetrical Analgesia

The usual dosage is 50 to 100 mg intramuscularly or subcutaneously when pain becomes regular, and may be repeated at 1- to 3-hour intervals.

Overdosage: *Symptoms.* Serious overdosage with meperidine is characterized by respiratory depression (a decrease in respiratory rate and/or tidal volume, Cheyne-Stokes respiration, cyanosis), extreme somnolence progressing to stupor or coma, skeletal muscle flaccidity, cold and clammy skin, and sometimes bradycardia and hypotension. In severe overdosage, particularly by the intravenous route, apnea, circulatory collapse, cardiac arrest, and death may occur.
Treatment. Primary attention should be given to the reestablishment of adequate respiratory exchange through provision of a patent airway and institution of assisted or controlled ventilation. The narcotic antagonist, naloxone hydrochloride, is a specific antidote against respiratory depression which may result from overdosage or unusual sensitivity to narcotics, including meperidine. Therefore, an appropriate dose of this antagonist should be administered, preferably by the intravenous route, simultaneously with efforts at respiratory resuscitation.
An antagonist should not be administered in the absence of clinically significant respiratory or cardiovascular depression.
Oxygen, intravenous fluids, vasopressors, and other supportive measures should be employed as indicated.
In cases of overdosage with DEMEROL, brand of meperidine, tablets, the stomach should be evacuated by emesis or gastric lavage.
NOTE: In an individual physically dependent on narcotics, the administration of the usual dose of a narcotic antagonist will precipitate an acute withdrawal syndrome. The severity of this syndrome will depend on the degree of physical dependence and the dose of antagonist administered. The use of narcotic antagonists in such individuals should be avoided if possible. If a narcotic antagonist must be used to treat serious respiratory depression in the physically dependent patient, the antagonist should be administered with extreme care and only one-fifth to one-tenth the usual initial dose administered.

How Supplied:

For Parenteral Use

2.5 per cent solution (25 mg per 1 ml), CARPUJECT®, boxes of 10.
5 per cent solution (50 mg per 1 ml), vials of 30 ml; ampuls of 0.5 ml (25 mg), 1 ml (50 mg), 1.5 ml (75 mg), and 2 ml (100 mg), boxes of 25; Uni-Amp®, boxes of 25 and CARPUJECT, boxes of 10.
7.5 per cent solution (75 mg per 1 ml), CARPUJECT, boxes of 10.
10 per cent solution (100 mg per 1 ml), vials of 20 ml; ampuls of 1 ml (100 mg), boxes of 25; Uni-Amp, boxes of 25 and CARPUJECT, boxes of 10.
The half-filled syringes are designed to permit mixture with other compatible medication.
Note: The pH of DEMEROL, brand of meperidine, solutions is adjusted between 3.5 and 6.0 with sodium hydroxide or hydrochloric acid. Multiple-dose vials contain metacresol 0.1 per cent as preservative. No preservatives are added to the ampuls.

For Oral Use

Tablets of 50 and 100 mg, bottles of 100 and 500.
Syrup, nonalcoholic, banana-flavored, 50 mg per 5 ml teaspoon, bottles of 16 fl oz

[*Shown in Product Identification Section*]

HALEY'S M-O® OTC

(See PDR For Nonprescription Drugs)

HYPAQUE® SODIUM ℞
brand of diatrizoate sodium, USP
ORAL POWDER
HYPAQUE SODIUM ORAL SOLUTION
brand of diatrizoate sodium solution, USP

(See Diagnostic Section.)

HYPAQUE® SODIUM 25% ℞
brand of diatrizoate sodium injection, USP

(See Diagnostic Section.)

HYPAQUE-CYSTO® ℞
brand of diatrizoate meglumine injection, USP
Sterile Aqueous Solution

(See Diagnostic Section.)

HYPAQUE® MEGLUMINE 30% ℞
brand of diatrizoate meglumine injection, USP
Sterile Aqueous Solution

(See Diagnostic Section.)

HYPAQUE® SODIUM 50% ℞
brand of diatrizoate sodium injection, USP
Sterile Aqueous Injection

(See Diagnostic Section.)

HYPAQUE® MEGLUMINE 60% ℞
brand of diatrizoate meglumine injection, USP
Sterile Aqueous Injection

(See Diagnostic Section.)

HYPAQUE®-M, 75% ℞
brand of diatrizoate meglumine and diatrizoate sodium injection, USP
Sterile Aqueous Injection

(See Diagnostic Section.)

HYPAQUE®-M, 90% ℞
brand of diatrizoate meglumine and diatrizoate sodium injection, USP
Sterile Aqueous Injection

(See Diagnostic Section.)

NegGram® ℞
brand of nalidixic acid, NF
CAPLETS® and Suspension

Description: Nalidixic acid, an oral antibacterial agent, is 1-ethyl-1,4-dihydro-7-methyl-4-oxo-1,8-naphthyridine-3-carboxylic acid. It is a pale yellow, crystalline substance and a very weak organic acid.
Action: NegGram has marked antibacterial activity against gram-negative bacteria including *Proteus mirabilis, P. morganii, P. vulgaris,* and *P. rettgeri; Escherichia coli;* Enterobacter (Aerobacter), and Klebsiella. Pseudomonas strains are generally resistant to the drug. NegGram is bactericidal and is effective over the entire urinary pH range. Conventional chromosomal resistance to NegGram taken in full dosage has been reported to emerge in approximately 2 to 14 per cent of patients during treatment; however, bacterial resistance to NegGram has not been shown to be transferable via R factor.
Indications: NegGram is indicated for the treatment of urinary tract infections caused by susceptible gram-negative microorganisms, including the majority of Proteus strains, Klebsiella, Enterobacter (Aerobacter), and *E. coli.* Disc susceptibility testing with the 30 μg disc should be performed prior to administration of the drug, and during treatment if clinical response warrants.
Contraindications: NegGram is contraindicated in patients with known hypersensitivity to nalidixic acid and in patients with a history of convulsive disorders.
Warnings: CNS effects including brief convulsions, increased intracranial pressure, and

toxic psychosis have been reported rarely. These have occurred in infants and children or in geriatric patients, usually from overdosage or in patients with predisposing factors, and have been completely and rapidly reversible upon discontinuation of the drug. If these reactions occur, NegGram should be discontinued and appropriate therapeutic measures instituted; only if rapid disappearance of CNS symptoms does not occur within 48 hours should diagnostic procedures involving risk to the patient be undertaken. (See Adverse Reactions and Overdosage.)

Usage in Pregnancy. Safe use of NegGram during the first trimester of pregnancy has not been established. However, the drug has been used during the last two trimesters without producing apparent ill effects in mother or child.

Precautions: Blood counts and renal and liver function tests should be performed periodically if treatment is continued for more than two weeks. NegGram should be used with caution in patients with liver disease, epilepsy, or severe cerebral arteriosclerosis. While caution should be used in patients with severe renal failure, therapeutic concentrations of NegGram in the urine, without increased toxicity due to drug accumulation in the blood, have been observed in patients on full dosage with creatinine clearances as low as 2 to 8 ml/min.

Patients should be cautioned to avoid undue exposure to direct sunlight while receiving NegGram. Therapy should be discontinued if photosensitivity occurs.

If bacterial resistance to NegGram emerges during treatment, it usually does so within 48 hours, permitting rapid change to another antimicrobial. Therefore, if the clinical response is unsatisfactory or if relapse occurs, cultures and sensitivity tests should be repeated. Underdosage with NegGram during initial treatment (with less than 4 g per day for adults) may predispose to emergence of bacterial resistance. (See Dosage and Administration.)

Cross resistance between NegGram and other antimicrobials has been observed only with oxolinic acid.

Nalidixic acid may enhance the effects of oral anticoagulants, warfarin or bishydroxycoumarin, by displacing significant amounts from serum albumin binding sites.

When Benedict's or Fehling's solutions or Clinitest® Reagent Tablets are used to test the urine of patients taking NegGram, a false-positive reaction for glucose may be obtained, due to the liberation of glucuronic acid from the metabolites excreted. However, a colorimetric test for glucose based on an enzyme reaction (e.g., with Clinistix® Reagent Strips or Tes-Tape®) does not give a false-positive reaction to the liberated glucuronic acid.

Incorrect values may be obtained for urinary 17-keto and ketogenic steroids in patients receiving NegGram, brand of nalidixic acid, because of an interaction between the drug and the *m*-dinitrobenzene used in the usual assay method. In such cases, the Porter-Silber test for 17-hydroxycorticoids may be used.

Adverse Reactions: Reactions reported after oral administration of NegGram include *CNS effects:* drowsiness, weakness, headache, and dizziness and vertigo. Reversible subjective visual disturbances without objective findings have occurred infrequently (generally with each dose during the first few days of treatment). These reactions include overbrightness of lights, change in color perception, difficulty in focusing, decrease in visual acuity, and double vision. They usually disappeared promptly when dosage was reduced or therapy was discontinued. Toxic psychosis or brief convulsions have been reported rarely, usually following excessive doses. In general, the convulsions have occurred in patients with predisposing factors such as epilepsy or cerebral arteriosclerosis. In infants and children receiving therapeutic doses of NegGram, increased intracranial pressure with bulging anterior fontanel, papilledema, and headache has occasionally been observed. A few cases of 6th cranial nerve palsy have been reported. Although the mechanisms of these reactions are unknown, the signs and symptoms usually disappeared rapidly with no sequelae when treatment was discontinued. *Gastrointestinal:* abdominal pain, nausea, vomiting, and diarrhea. *Allergic:* rash, pruritus, urticaria, angioedema, eosinophilia, arthralgia with joint stiffness and swelling, and rarely, anaphylactoid reaction. Photosensitivity reactions consisting of erythema and bullae on exposed skin surfaces usually resolve completely in 2 weeks to 2 months after NegGram is discontinued; however, bullae may continue to appear with successive exposures to sunlight or with mild skin trauma for up to 3 months after discontinuation of drug. (See Precautions.) *Other;* rarely, cholestasis, paresthesia, metabolic acidosis, thrombocytopenia, leukopenia, or hemolytic anemia, sometimes associated with glucose-6-phosphate dehydrogenase deficiency.

Dosage and Administration: *Adults.* The recommended dosage for initial therapy in adults is 1 g administered four times daily for one or two weeks (total daily dose, 4 g). For prolonged therapy, the total daily dose may be reduced to 2 g after the initial treatment period. Underdosage during initial treatment may predispose to emergence of bacterial resistance.

Children. Until further experience is gained, NegGram should not be administered to infants younger than three months. Dosage in children 12 years of age and under should be calculated on the basis of body weight. The recommended total daily dosage for initial therapy is 25 mg/lb/day (55 mg/kg/day), administered in four equally divided doses. For prolonged therapy, the total daily dose may be reduced to 15 mg/lb/day (33 mg/kg/day). NegGram Suspension or NegGram CAPLETS of 250 mg may be used. One 250 mg tablet is equivalent to one teaspoon (5 ml) of the Suspension.

Overdosage: *Manifestations:* Toxic psychosis, convulsions, increased intracranial pressure, or metabolic acidosis may occur in patients taking more than the recommended dosage. Vomiting, nausea, and lethargy may also occur following overdosage.

Treatment: Reactions are short-lived (two to three hours) because the drug is rapidly excreted. If overdosage is noted early, gastric lavage is indicated. If absorption has occurred, increased fluid administration is advisable and supportive measures such as oxygen and means of artificial respiration should be available. Although anticonvulsant therapy has not been used in the few instances of overdosage reported, it may be indicated in a severe case.

How Supplied:

Suspension (250 mg/5 ml tsp), raspberry flavored, bottles of 1 pint
CAPLETS of 1 Gram, scored, bottles of 100
CAPLETS of 500 mg, scored, bottles of 56, 500, and 1000
CAPLETS of 250 mg, scored, bottles of 56
Unit Dose Pack of 100 (10 strips of ten-500 mg CAPLETS each)

Pharmacology: Following oral administration, NegGram, brand of nalidixic acid, is rapidly absorbed from the gastrointestinal tract, partially metabolized in the liver, and rapidly excreted through the kidneys. Unchanged nalidixic acid appears in the urine along with an active metabolite, hydroxynalidixic acid, which has antibacterial activity similar to that of nalidixic acid. Other metabolites include glucuronic acid conjugates of nalidixic acid and hydroxynalidixic acid, and the dicarboxylic acid derivative. The hydroxy metabolite represents 30 per cent of the biologically active drug in the blood and 85 per cent in the urine. Peak serum levels of active drug average approximately 20 to 40 μg per ml (90 per cent protein bound), one to two hours after administration of a 1 g dose to a fasting normal individual, with a half-life of about 90 minutes. Peak urine levels of active drug average approximately 150 to 200 μg per ml, three to four hours after administration, with a half-life of about six hours. Approximately four per cent of NegGram is excreted in the feces. Traces of nalidixic acid were found in blood and urine of an infant whose mother had received the drug during the last trimester of pregnancy.

[*Shown in Product Identification Section*]

Long Acting
NEO-SYNEPHRINE® II **OTC**
brand of xylometazoline hydrochloride

(See PDR For Nonprescription Drugs)

NEO-SYNEPHRINE® Hydrochloride ℞
brand of phenylephrine hydrochloride injection, USP
1% INJECTION

Well-Tolerated Vasoconstrictor and Pressor

WARNING: PHYSICIANS SHOULD COMPLETELY FAMILIARIZE THEMSELVES WITH THE COMPLETE CONTENTS OF THIS LEAFLET BEFORE PRESCRIBING NEO-SYNEPHRINE.

Description: NEO-SYNEPHRINE hydrochloride is a vasoconstrictor and pressor drug chemically related to epinephrine and ephedrine.

Actions: When applied topically or infiltrated into the tissues, NEO-SYNEPHRINE hydrochloride produces vasoconstriction that lasts longer than that of epinephrine and ephedrine. Its action on the heart contrasts sharply with that of epinephrine and ephedrine, in that it slows the heart rate and increases the stroke output, inducing no disturbance in the rhythm of the pulse.

In therapeutic doses, it produces little if any stimulation of either the spinal cord or cerebrum. A singular advantage of this drug is the fact that repeated injections produce comparable effects.

Indications: NEO-SYNEPHRINE is intended for the maintenance of an adequate level of blood pressure during spinal and inhalation anesthesia and for the treatment of vascular failure in shock, shocklike states, and drug-induced hypotension, or hypersensitivity. It is also employed to overcome paroxysmal supraventricular tachycardia, to prolong spinal anesthesia, and as a vasoconstrictor in regional analgesia.

Precautions: Parenteral administration of NEO-SYNEPHRINE may be contraindicated in patients with hypertension or ventricular tachycardia and should be employed only with extreme caution in elderly patients or in patients with hyperthyroidism, bradycardia, partial heart block, myocardial disease, or severe arteriosclerosis.

When NEO-SYNEPHRINE is administered intravenously in the treatment of patients with paroxysmal supraventricular tachycardia, overdosage may induce ventricular ex-

Continued on next page

This product information was effective as of November 21, 1979. On these and other products of Winthrop Laboratories, detailed information may be obtained on a current basis by direct inquiry to the Professional Services Department, 90 Park Avenue, New York, N Y 10016 (212) 972-4095.

Winthrop—Cont.

trasystoles and short paroxysms of ventricular tachycardia, a sensation of fullness in the head, and tingling of the extremities.
Vasopressors, particularly metaraminol, may cause serious cardiac arrhythmias during halothane anesthesia and therefore should be used only with great caution or not at all.
Oxytocics—In obstetrics, if vasopressor drugs are either used to correct hypotension or added to the local anesthetic solution, the obstetrician should be warned that some oxytocic drugs may cause severe persistent hypertension and that even a rupture of a cerebral blood vessel may occur during the postpartum period.
MAO Inhibitors—The pressor effect of sympathomimetic pressor amines is markedly potentiated in patients receiving a monoamine oxidase (MAO) inhibitor. Therefore, when initiating pressor therapy in these patients, the initial dose should be small and used with due caution.
The pressor response of adrenergic agents may also be potentiated by tricyclic antidepressants.
Should an excessive elevation of blood pressure occur, it may be immediately relieved by an α-adrenergic blocking agent, e.g., phentolamine.

Dosage and Administration:
NEO-SYNEPHRINE is generally injected subcutaneously, intramuscularly, slowly intravenously, or in dilute solution as a continuous intravenous infusion. In patients with paroxysmal supraventricular tachycardia and, if indicated, in case of emergency, NEO-SYNEPHRINE is administered directly intravenously. The dose should be adjusted according to the pressor response.

Dosage Calculations

Dose Required	***Use NEO-SYNEPHRINE 1%***
10 mg	1 ml
5 mg	0.5 ml
1 mg	0.1 ml

For convenience in intermittent intravenous administration, dilute 1 ml NEO-SYNEPHRINE 1% with 9 ml Sterile Water for Injection, USP, to yield 0.1% NEO-SYNEPHRINE.

Dose Required	***Use Diluted NEO-SYNEPHRINE (0.1%)***
0.1 mg	0.1 ml
0.2 mg	0.2 ml
0.5 mg	0.5 ml

Mild or Moderate Hypotension
Subcutaneously or Intramuscularly: Usual dose, from 2 to 5 mg. Range, from 1 to 10 mg. Initial dose should not exceed 5 mg.
Intravenously: Usual dose, 0.2 mg. Range, from 0.1 to 0.5 mg. Initial dose should not exceed 0.5 mg.
Injections should not be repeated more often than every 10 to 15 minutes. A 5 mg intramuscular dose should raise blood pressure for one to two hours. A 0.5 mg intravenous dose should elevate the pressure for about 15 minutes.

Severe Hypotension and Shock—Including Drug-Related Hypotension
Blood volume depletion should always be corrected as fully as possible before any vasopressor is administered. When, as an emergency measure, intraaortic pressures must be maintained to prevent cerebral or coronary artery ischemia, NEO-SYNEPHRINE hydrochloride, brand of phenylephrine hydrochloride injection, can be administered before and concurrently with blood volume replacement.
Hypotension and occasionally severe shock may result from overdosage or idiosyncrasy following the administration of certain drugs, especially adrenergic and ganglionic blocking agents, rauwolfia and veratrum alkaloids, and phenothiazine tranquilizers. Patients who receive a phenothiazine derivative as preoperative medication are especially susceptible to these reactions. As an adjunct in the management of such episodes, NEO-SYNEPHRINE hydrochloride is a suitable agent for restoring blood pressure.
Higher initial and maintenance doses of NEO-SYNEPHRINE are required in patients with persistent or untreated severe hypotension or shock. Hypotension produced by powerful peripheral adrenergic blocking agents, chlorpromazine, or pheochromocytomectomy may also require more intensive therapy.
Continuous Infusion—Add 10 mg of the drug (1 ml of 1 per cent solution) to 500 ml of Dextrose Injection, USP, or Sodium Chloride Injection, USP (providing a 1:50,000 solution). To raise the blood pressure rapidly, start the infusion at about 100 to 180 drops per minute. When the blood pressure is stabilized (at a low normal level for the individual), a maintenance rate of 40 to 60 drops per minute usually suffices. If a prompt initial pressor response is not obtained, additional increments of NEO-SYNEPHRINE (10 mg or more) are added to the infusion bottle. The rate of flow is then adjusted until the desired blood pressure level is obtained. (In some cases, a more potent vasopressor, such as levarterenol bitartrate, may be required.) Hypertension should be avoided. The blood pressure should be checked frequently. Headache and/ or bradycardia may indicate hypertension. Arrhythmias are rare.

Spinal Anesthesia—Hypotension
Routine parenteral use of NEO-SYNEPHRINE has been recommended for the prophylaxis and treatment of hypotension during spinal anesthesia. It is best administered subcutaneously or intramuscularly three or four minutes before injection of the spinal anesthetic. The total requirement for high anesthetic levels is usually 3 mg, and for lower levels, 2 mg. For hypotensive emergencies during spinal anesthesia, NEO-SYNEPHRINE may be injected intravenously, using an initial dose of 0.2 mg. Any subsequent dose should not exceed the previous dose by more than 0.1 to 0.2 mg and no more than 0.5 mg should be administered in a single dose. To combat hypotension during spinal anesthesia in children, a dose of 0.5 to 1 mg per 25 pounds of body weight, administered subcutaneously or intramuscularly, is recommended.

Prolongation of Spinal Anesthesia
The addition of 2 to 5 mg of NEO-SYNEPHRINE hydrochloride to the anesthetic solution increases the duration of motor block by as much as approximately 50 per cent without any increase in the incidence of complications such as nausea, vomiting, or blood pressure disturbances.

Vasoconstrictor for Regional Analgesia
Concentrations about ten times those employed when epinephrine is used as a vasoconstrictor are recommended. The optimum strength is 1:20,000 (made by adding 1 mg of NEO-SYNEPHRINE hydrochloride to every 20 ml. of local anesthetic solution). Some pressor responses can be expected when 2 mg or more are injected.

Paroxysmal Supraventricular Tachycardia
Rapid intravenous injection (within 20 to 30 seconds) is recommended; the initial dose should not exceed 0.5 mg, and subsequent doses, which are determined by the initial blood pressure response, should not exceed the preceding dose by more than 0.1 to 0.2 mg, and should never exceed 1 mg.

How Supplied:
Solution 1 per cent
Ampuls—Each 1 ml contains 10 mg of NEO-SYNEPHRINE hydrochloride, 3.5 mg of sodium chloride, 4 mg of sodium citrate, 1 mg of citric acid monohydrate, and not more than 2 mg of sodium bisulfite. The pH is adjusted between 3.0 and 5.5 with sodium citrate or citric acid. Ampuls of 1 ml, boxes of 25.
The air in all ampuls has been displaced by nitrogen gas.

NEO-SYNEPHRINE® Hydrochloride ℞
brand of phenylephrine hydrochloride ophthalmic solution, USP
Vasoconstrictor and Mydriatic
SOLUTIONS 2.5% AND 10%
VISCOUS SOLUTION 10%

For Use in Ophthalmology

WARNING: PHYSICIANS SHOULD COMPLETELY FAMILIARIZE THEMSELVES WITH THE COMPLETE CONTENTS OF THIS LEAFLET BEFORE PRESCRIBING NEO-SYNEPHRINE.

Description: NEO-SYNEPHRINE hydrochloride is a synthetic sympathomimetic compound structurally similar to epinephrine and ephedrine.

Clinical Pharmacology:
NEO-SYNEPHRINE hydrochloride is used for disorders of the eye because of its vasoconstrictor and mydriatic action.
The ophthalmologic usefulness of NEO-SYNEPHRINE hydrochloride is due to its rapid effect and moderately prolonged action, as well as to the fact that it produces no compensatory vasodilatation. In addition, undesirable systemic effects are rare.
The action of different concentrations of ophthalmic solutions of NEO-SYNEPHRINE hydrochloride is shown in the following table:

Strength of solution (%)	Mydriasis		Paralysis of accommodation
	Maximal (minutes)	Recovery time (hours)	
2.5	15-60	3	trace
10	10-60	6	slight

Indications and Usage: NEO-SYNEPHRINE hydrochloride is recommended for use as a decongestant and vasoconstrictor and for pupil dilatation in uveitis (posterior synechiae), wide angle glaucoma, surgery, refraction, ophthalmoscopic examination, and diagnostic procedures.

Contraindications: Ophthalmic solutions of NEO-SYNEPHRINE hydrochloride are contraindicated in persons with narrow angle glaucoma. NEO-SYNEPHRINE hydrochloride 10 per cent ophthalmic solutions are contraindicated in infants and in patients with aneurysms.

Warnings: As with all other adrenergic drugs, when NEO-SYNEPHRINE 10 per cent ophthalmic solutions or 2.5 per cent ophthalmic solution is administered simultaneously with, or up to 21 days after, administration of monoamine oxidase (MAO) inhibitors, careful supervision and adjustment of dosages are required since exaggerated adrenergic effects may occur. The pressor response of adrenergic agents may also be potentiated by tricyclic antidepressants, propranolol, reserpine, guanethidine, methyldopa, and atropine-like drugs.
Exceeding recommended dosages or applying NEO-SYNEPHRINE hydrochloride ophthalmic solutions to the instrumented, traumatized, diseased or post surgical eye or adnexae, or to patients with suppressed lacrimation as during anesthesia, may result in the absorption of sufficient quantities of phenylephrine to produce a systemic vasopressor response.
Certain rare individuals may demonstrate an increased sensitivity to sympathomimetic agents.

There have been rare reports associating the use of NEO-SYNEPHRINE 10 per cent ophthalmic solutions with the development of serious cardiovascular reactions, including ventricular arrhythmias and myocardial infarctions. These episodes, some ending fatally, have usually occurred in elderly patients with preexisting cardiovascular diseases.

Precautions: A significant elevation in blood pressure is rare but has been reported following conjunctival instillation of recommended doses of NEO-SYNEPHRINE 10 per cent ophthalmic solutions. Caution, therefore, should be exercised in administering the 10 per cent solutions to children of low body weight (see Contraindications), the elderly, and patients with insulin-dependent diabetes, hypertension, hyperthyroidism, generalized arteriosclerosis, or cardiovascular disease (see Warnings). The post treatment blood pressure of these patients, and any patients who develop symptoms, should be carefully monitored.

Ordinarily, any mydriatic, including NEO-SYNEPHRINE hydrochloride, is contraindicated in patients with glaucoma, since it may occasionally raise intraocular pressure. However, when temporary dilatation of the pupil may free adhesions or when vasoconstriction of intrinsic vessels may lower intraocular tension, these advantages may temporarily outweigh the danger from coincident dilatation of the pupil.

Rebound miosis has been reported in older persons one day after receiving NEO-SYNEPHRINE hydrochloride ophthalmic solutions, and reinstillation of the drug produced a reduction in mydriasis. This may be of clinical importance in dilating the pupils of older subjects prior to retinal detachment or cataract surgery.

Due to a strong action of the drug on the dilator muscle, older individuals may also develop transient pigment floaters in the aqueous humor 30 to 45 minutes following the administration of NEO-SYNEPHRINE hydrochloride ophthalmic solutions. The appearance may be similar to anterior uveitis or to a microscopic hyphema.

To prevent pain, a drop of suitable topical anesthetic may be applied before using the 10 per cent ophthalmic solution.

Dosage and Administration: Prolonged exposure to air or strong light may cause oxidation and discoloration. Do not use if solution is brown or contains a precipitate.

Vasoconstriction and Pupil Dilatation

NEO-SYNEPHRINE hydrochloride 10 per cent ophthalmic solutions is especially useful when rapid and powerful dilatation of the pupil and reduction of congestion in the capillary bed are desired. A drop of a suitable topical anesthetic may be applied, followed in a few minutes by 1 drop of the NEO-SYNEPHRINE hydrochloride 10 per cent ophthalmic solution on the upper limbus. The anesthetic prevents stinging and consequent dilution of the solution by lacrimation. It may occasionally be necessary to repeat the instillation after one hour, again preceded by the use of the topical anesthetic.

Uveitis: Posterior Synechiae

NEO-SYNEPHRINE hydrochloride 10 per cent ophthalmic solutions may be used in patients with uveitis when synechiae are present or may develop. The formation of synechiae may be prevented by the use of the 10 per cent ophthalmic solutions and atropine to produce wide dilatation of the pupil. It should be emphasized, however, that the vasoconstrictor effect of NEO-SYNEPHRINE hydrochloride may be antagonistic to the increase of local blood flow in uveal infection.

To free recently formed posterior synechiae, 1 drop of the 10 per cent ophthalmic solutions may be applied to the upper surface of the cornea. On the following day, treatment may be continued if necessary. In the interim, hot compresses should be applied for five or ten minutes three times a day, with 1 drop of a 1 or 2 per cent solution of atropine sulfate before and after each series of compresses.

Glaucoma

In certain patients with glaucoma, temporary reduction of intraocular tension may be attained by producing vasoconstriction of the intraocular vessels; this may be accomplished by placing 1 drop of the 10 per cent ophthalmic solutions on the upper surface of the cornea. This treatment may be repeated as often as necessary.

NEO-SYNEPHRINE hydrochloride, brand of phenylephrine hydrochloride ophthalmic solution, may be used with miotics in patients with wide angle glaucoma. It reduces the difficulties experienced by the patient because of the small field produced by miosis, and still it permits and often supports the effect of the miotic in lowering the intraocular pressure. Hence, there may be marked improvement in visual acuity after using NEO-SYNEPHRINE hydrochloride in conjunction with miotic drugs.

Surgery

When a short-acting mydriatic is needed for wide dilatation of the pupil before intraocular surgery, the 10 per cent ophthalmic solutions or 2.5 per cent ophthalmic solution may be applied topically from 30 to 60 minutes before the operation.

Refraction

Prior to determination of refractive errors, NEO-SYNEPHRINE hydrochloride 2.5 per cent ophthalmic solution may be used effectively with homatropine hydrobromide, atropine sulfate, or a combination of homatropine and cocaine hydrochloride.

For *adults*, a drop of the preferred cycloplegic is placed in each eye, followed in five minutes by 1 drop of NEO-SYNEPHRINE hydrochloride 2.5 per cent ophthalmic solution and in ten minutes by another drop of the cycloplegic. In 50 to 60 minutes, the eyes are ready for refraction.

For *children*, a drop of atropine sulfate 1 per cent is placed in each eye, followed in 10 to 15 minutes by 1 drop of NEO-SYNEPHRINE hydrochloride 2.5 per cent ophthalmic solution and in five to ten minutes by a second drop of atropine sulfate 1 per cent. In one to two hours, the eyes are ready for refraction.

For a "one application method," NEO-SYNEPHRINE hydrochloride 2.5 per cent ophthalmic solution may be combined with a cycloplegic to elicit synergistic action. The additive effect varies depending on the patient. Therefore, when using a "one application method," it may be desirable to increase the concentration of the cycloplegic.

Ophthalmoscopic Examination

One drop of NEO-SYNEPHRINE hydrochloride 2.5 per cent ophthalmic solution is placed in each eye. Sufficient mydriasis to permit examination is produced in 15 to 30 minutes. Dilatation lasts from one to three hours.

Diagnostic Procedures

Provocative Test for Angle Block in Patients with Glaucoma: The 2.5 per cent ophthalmic solution may be used as a provocative test when latent increased intraocular pressure is suspected. Tension is measured before application of NEO-SYNEPHRINE hydrochloride and again after dilatation. A 3 to 5 mm of mercury rise in pressure suggests the presence of angle block in patients with glaucoma; however, failure to obtain such a rise does not preclude the presence of glaucoma from other causes.

Shadow Test (Retinoscopy): When dilatation of the pupil without cycloplegic action is desired for the shadow test, the 2.5 per cent ophthalmic solution may be used alone.

Blanching Test: One or 2 drops of the 2.5 per cent ophthalmic solution should be applied to the injected eye. After five minutes, examine for perilimbal blanching. If blanching occurs, the congestion is superficial and probably does not indicate iritis.

Overdosage: The hypertensive effects of phenylephrine may be treated with an alpha-adrenergic blocking agent such as phentolamine mesylate, 5 to 10 mg intravenously, repeated as necessary.

How Supplied: *In MONO-DROP® (plastic dropper) bottle:*

Low surface tension solutions

2.5 per cent ophthalmic solution —NEO-SYNEPHRINE hydrochloride, brand of phenylephrine hydrochloride ophthalmic solution, 2.5 per cent in a sterile, isotonic, buffered, low surface tension vehicle with sodium phosphate, sodium biphosphate, boric acid, and, as antiseptic preservative, benzalkonium chloride, USP, 1:7500. The pH is adjusted with phosphoric acid or sodium hydroxide.
Bottles of 15 ml (NDC 0024-1358-01)

10 per cent ophthalmic solution —NEO-SYNEPHRINE hydrochloride 10 per cent in a sterile, buffered, low surface tension vehicle with sodium phosphate, sodium biphosphate, and, as antiseptic preservative, benzalkonium chloride 1:10,000. The pH is adjusted with phosphoric acid or sodium hydroxide.
Bottles of 5 ml (NDC 0024-1359-01)

Viscous solution

10 per cent ophthalmic solution —NEO-SYNEPHRINE hydrochloride 10 per cent in a sterile, buffered, viscous vehicle with sodium phosphate, sodium biphosphate, methylcellulose, and, as antiseptic preservative, benzalkonium chloride 1:10,000. The pH is adjusted with phosphoric acid or sodium hydroxide.
Bottles of 5 ml (NDC 0024-1362-01)

NEO-SYNEPHRINE® Hydrochloride OTC
brand of phenylephrine hydrochloride, USP

(See PDR For Nonprescription Drugs)

NTZ® SOLUTION OTC

(See PDR For Nonprescription Drugs)

pHisoDerm® OTC

(See PDR For Nonprescription Drugs)

pHisoHex® ℞
brand of hexachlorophene detergent cleanser
sudsing antibacterial soapless skin cleanser

Description: pHisoHex is an antibacterial sudsing emulsion. It contains a colloidal dispersion of hexachlorophene 3% (w/w) in a stable emulsion consisting of entsufon sodium, petrolatum, lanolin cholesterols, methylcellulose, polyethylene glycol, polyethylene glycol monostearate, lauryl myristyl diethanolamide, sodium benzoate, and water. pH is adjusted with hydrochloric acid. Entsufon sodium is a synthetic detergent (sodium octylphenoxyethoxyethyl ether sulfonate).

Clinical Pharmacology: pHisoHex is a bacteriostatic cleansing agent. It cleanses the skin thoroughly and has bacteriostatic action against staphylococci and other gram-positive bacteria. Cumulative antibacterial action develops with repeated use. This antibacterial residue is resistant to removal by many solvents, soaps, and detergents for several days.

Continued on next page

This product information was effective as of November 21, 1979. On these and other products of Winthrop Laboratories, detailed information may be obtained on a current basis by direct inquiry to the Professional Services Department, 90 Park Avenue, New York, N Y 10016 (212) 972-4095.

Winthrop—Cont.

pHisoHex has the same slight acidity as normal skin (pH value 5.0 to 6.0).

Indications and Usage: pHisoHex is indicated for use as a surgical scrub and a bacteriostatic skin cleanser. It may also be used to control an outbreak of gram-positive infection where other infection control procedures have been unsuccessful. Use only as long as necessary for infection control.

Contraindications: pHisoHex should not be used on burned or denuded skin.

It should not be used as an occlusive dressing, wet pack, or lotion.

It should not be used routinely for prophylactic total body bathing.

It should not be used as a vaginal pack or tampon, or on any mucous membranes.

pHisoHex should not be used on persons with sensitivity to any of its components. It should not be used on persons who have demonstrated primary light sensitivity to halogenated phenol derivatives because of the possibility of cross-sensitivity to hexachlorophene.

Warnings: RINSE THOROUGHLY AFTER USE, especially from sensitive areas such as the scrotum and perineum.

Rapid absorption of hexachlorophene may occur with resultant toxic blood levels when preparations containing hexachlorophene are applied to skin lesions such as ichthyosis congenita, the dermatitis of Letterer-Siwe's syndrome, or other generalized dermatological conditions. Application to burns has also produced neurotoxicity and death.

PHISOHEX SHOULD BE DISCONTINUED PROMPTLY IF SIGNS OR SYMPTOMS OF CEREBRAL IRRITABILITY OCCUR.

Infants, especially premature infants or those with dermatoses, are particularly susceptible to hexachlorophene absorption. Systemic toxicity may be manifested by signs of stimulation (irritation) of the central nervous system, sometimes with convulsions.

Infants have developed dermatitis, irritability, generalized clonic muscular contractions and decerebrate rigidity following application of a 6 per cent hexachlorophene powder. Examination of brainstems of those infants revealed vacuolization like that which can be produced in newborn experimental animals following repeated topical application of 3 per cent hexachlorophene. Moreover, a study of histologic sections of premature infants who died of unrelated causes has shown a positive correlation between hexachlorophene baths and lesions in white matter of brains.

pHisoHex is intended for *external use only.* If swallowed, pHisoHex is harmful, especially to infants and children. **pHisoHex, brand of hexachlorophene detergent cleanser, should not be poured into measuring cups, medicine bottles, or similar containers since it may be mistaken for baby formula or other medications.**

Precaution: pHisoHex suds that get into the eyes accidentally during washing should be rinsed out promptly and thoroughly with water.

Adverse Reactions: Adverse reactions to pHisoHex may include dermatitis and photosensitivity. Sensitivity to hexachlorophene is rare; however, persons who have developed photoallergy to similar compounds also may become sensitive to hexachlorophene.

In persons with highly sensitive skin, the use of pHisoHex may at times produce a reaction characterized by redness and/or mild scaling or dryness, especially when it is combined with such mechanical factors as excessive rubbing or exposure to heat or cold.

Directions for Surgical Wash—(Without Brush): From 1/4 to 1 teaspoon (1 to 4 ml) of pHisoHex is sufficient for cleansing the hands and forearms if the following directions are followed:

(1.) The preliminary washing. A few drops are spread over the wet hands. Suds are developed by repeatedly adding small amounts of water while thoroughly rubbing the suds over all areas. This should take from 20 to 30 seconds.

(2.) Clean under nails carefully.

(3.) The second washing. After the preliminary washing 1 teaspoon or less of pHisoHex is rubbed over hands and worked into copious suds by adding small amounts of water from time to time. Wash for the allotted time of two to four minutes and *rinse thoroughly* under running water.

Directions for Surgical Scrub—(With Brush): Following the preliminary washing, rinsing, and nail cleansing, a teaspoon or less of the emulsion is applied to a wet brush which is then used for scrubbing during the prescribed period.

Rinse and repeat if necessary.

Scrub with the brush and include every area of the skin. Each area should receive the number of completed brush strokes (forward and back) indicated, as follows:

(1.) Those who scrub at intervals of more than three days, 30 brush strokes to the skin; 50 to the nails.

(2.) Those who scrub daily, 15 strokes to the skin; 25 to the nails.

(3.) Those who use pHisoHex routinely and exclusively for washing the hands, 9 strokes to the skin; 15 to the nails.

(4.) *Rinse thoroughly* under running water.

The wash-rinse-scrub method need consume no more time or material than does one continuous scrubbing.

Directions for Bacteriostatic Cleansing: Squeeze 1/2 to 1 teaspoon of pHisoHex into the palm, work up a lather with water and apply to area to be cleansed.

Rinse thoroughly after each washing.

INFANT CARE: pHisoHex should not be used routinely for bathing infants. See section on **WARNINGS.**

PREMATURE INFANTS: See section on **WARNINGS.**

Use of baby skin products containing alcohol may decrease the antibacterial action of pHisoHex, brand of hexachlorophene detergent cleanser.

Treatment of Accidental Ingestion: The accidental ingestion of pHisoHex in amounts from 1 to 4 oz has caused anorexia, vomiting, abdominal cramps, diarrhea, dehydration, convulsions, hypotension and shock, and in several reported instances, fatalities.

If patients are seen early, the stomach should be evacuated by emesis or gastric lavage. Olive oil or vegetable oil (60 ml or 2 fl oz) may then be given to delay absorption of hexachlorophene, followed by a saline cathartic to hasten removal. Treatment is symptomatic and supportive; intravenous fluids (5 per cent dextrose in physiologic saline solution) may be given for dehydration. Any other electrolyte derangement should be corrected. If marked hypotension occurs, vasopressor therapy is indicated. Use of opiates may be considered if gastrointestinal symptoms (cramping, diarrhea) are severe. Scheduled medical or surgical procedures should be postponed until the patient's condition has been evaluated and stabilized.

How Supplied: pHisoHex is available in unbreakable plastic squeeze bottles of 5 ounces (refillable) (NDC 0024-1535-02) and 1 pint (NDC 0024-1535-06), and in plastic bottles of 1 gallon (NDC 0024-1536-08).

Also available—1/4 oz (8 ml) unit packets, boxes of 50 (NDC 0024-1535-05).

The following, specially constructed, refillable dispensers made with metals and plastics compatible with pHisoHex can also be supplied: 16 oz hand operated wall dispensers; 30 oz pedal operated wall dispensers; 30 oz pedal operated wall dispenser with stand; portable stand with two 30 oz pedal operated dispensers.

Prolonged direct exposure of pHisoHex to strong light may cause brownish surface discoloration but does not affect its antibacterial or detergent properties. Shaking will disperse the color. If pHisoHex is spilled or splashed on porous surfaces, rinse off to avoid discoloration. pHisoHex should not be dispensed from, or stored in, containers with ordinary metal parts. A special type of stainless steel must be used or undesirable discoloration of the product or oxidation of metal may occur. Specially designed dispensers for hospital or office use may be obtained through your local dealer.

Directions for Cleaning Dispensers: Remove dispenser and pour off remainder of pHisoHex emulsion. Rinse empty dispenser with water. Run water through the working parts by operating the dispenser. Glass parts may be boiled if necessary. Run an antiseptic, such as an aqueous solution of benzalkonium chloride, USP, 1:500 to 1:750, or alcohol, through the working parts; rinse with sterile water. Dispensers should be cleaned every 1 or 2 weeks.

PLAQUENIL® Sulfate ℞

brand of hydroxychloroquine sulfate tablets, USP

WARNING

PHYSICIANS SHOULD COMPLETELY FAMILIARIZE THEMSELVES WITH THE COMPLETE CONTENTS OF THIS LEAFLET BEFORE PRESCRIBING HYDROXYCHLOROQUINE.

Description: The compound is a colorless crystalline solid, soluble in water to at least 20 per cent; chemically the drug is 2-[[4-[(7-chloro-4-quinolyl)amino] pentyl] ethylamino] ethanol sulfate (1:1).

Actions: The drug possesses antimalarial actions and also exerts a beneficial effect in lupus erythematosus (chronic discoid or systemic) and acute or chronic rheumatoid arthritis. The precise mechanism of action is not known.

Indications: PLAQUENIL is indicated for the suppressive treatment and treatment of acute attacks of malaria due to *Plasmodium vivax, P. malariae, P. ovale,* and susceptible strains of *P. falciparum.* It is also indicated for the treatment of discoid and systemic lupus erythematosus, and rheumatoid arthritis.

Contraindications: Use of this drug is contraindicated (1) in the presence of retinal or visual field changes attributable to any 4-aminoquinoline compound, (2) in patients with known hypersensitivity to 4-aminoquinoline compounds and (3) for long-term therapy in children.

Warnings, General: PLAQUENIL is not effective against chloroquine-resistant strains of *P. falciparum.*

Children are especially sensitive to the 4-aminoquinoline compounds. A number of fatalities have been reported following the accidental ingestion of chloroquine, sometimes in relatively small doses (0.75 or 1 g in one 3-year-old child). Patients should be strongly warned to keep these drugs out of the reach of children.

Use of PLAQUENIL in patients with psoriasis may precipitate a severe attack of psoriasis. When used in patients with porphyria the condition may be exacerbated. The preparation should not be used in these conditions unless in the judgment of the physician the benefit to the patient outweighs the possible hazard.

Usage in Pregnancy—Usage of this drug during pregnancy should be avoided except in the suppression or treatment of malaria when in the judgment of the physician the benefit outweighs the possible hazard. It should be noted that radioactively-tagged chloroquine administered intravenously to pregnant, pigmented CBA mice passed rapidly across the placenta. It accumulated selectively in the melanin structures of the fetal eyes and was retained in the ocular tissues for five months after the drug had been eliminated from the rest of the body.[1]

Precautions, General: Antimalarial compounds should be used with caution in patients with hepatic disease or alcoholism or in conjunction with known hepatotoxic drugs.

Periodic blood cell counts should be made if patients are given prolonged therapy. If any severe blood disorder appears which is not attributable to the disease under treatment, discontinuation of the drug should be considered. The drug should be administered with caution in patients having G-6-PD (glucose-6-phosphate dehydrogenase) deficiency.

Overdosage: The 4-aminoquinoline compounds are very rapidly and completely absorbed after ingestion, and in accidental overdosage, or rarely with lower doses in hypersensitive patients, toxic symptoms may occur within 30 minutes. These consist of headache, drowsiness, visual disturbances, cardiovascular collapse, and convulsions, followed by sudden and early respiratory and cardiac arrest. The electrocardiogram may reveal atrial standstill, nodal rhythm, prolonged intraventricular conduction time, and progressive bradycardia leading to ventricular fibrillation and/or arrest. Treatment is symptomatic and must be prompt with immediate evacuation of the stomach by emesis (at home, before transportation to the hospital) or gastric lavage until the stomach is completely emptied. If finely powdered, activated charcoal is introduced by the stomach tube, after lavage, and within 30 minutes after ingestion of the tablets, it may inhibit further intestinal absorption of the drug. To be effective, the dose of activated charcoal should be at least five times the estimated dose of hydroxychloroquine ingested. Convulsions, if present, should be controlled before attempting gastric lavage. If due to cerebral stimulation, cautious administration of an ultrashort-acting barbiturate may be tried but, if due to anoxia, it should be corrected by oxygen administration, artificial respiration or, in shock with hypotension, by vasopressor therapy. Because of the importance of supporting respiration, tracheal intubation or tracheostomy, followed by gastric lavage, may also be necessary. Exchange transfusions have been used to reduce the level of 4-aminoquinoline drug in the blood.

A patient who survives the acute phase and is asymptomatic should be closely observed for at least six hours. Fluids may be forced, and sufficient ammonium chloride (8 g daily in divided doses for adults) may be administered for a few days to acidify the urine to help promote urinary excretion in cases of both overdosage and sensitivity.

MALARIA

Actions: Like chloroquine phosphate, USP, PLAQUENIL sulfate is highly active against the erythrocytic forms of *P. vivax* and *malariae* and most strains of *P. falciparum* (but not the gametocytes of *P. falciparum*).

PLAQUENIL sulfate does not prevent relapses in patients with *vivax* or *malariae* malaria because it is not effective against exo-erythrocytic forms of the parasite, nor will it prevent *vivax* or *malariae* infection when administered as a prophylactic. It is highly effective as a suppressive agent in patients with *vivax* or *malariae* malaria, in terminating acute attacks, and significantly lengthening the interval between treatment and relapse. In patients with *falciparum* malaria, it abolishes the acute attack and effects complete cure of the infection, unless due to a resistant strain of *P. falciparum*.

Indications: PLAQUENIL sulfate, brand of hydroxychloroquine sulfate tablets, is indicated for the treatment of acute attacks and suppression of malaria.

Warning: In recent years, it has been found that certain strains of *P. falciparum* have become resistant to 4-aminoquinoline compounds (including hydroxychloroquine) as shown by the fact that normally adequate doses have failed to prevent or cure clinical malaria or parasitemia. Treatment with quinine or other specific forms of therapy is therefore advised for patients infected with a resistant strain of parasites.

Adverse Reactions: Following the administration in doses adequate for the treatment of an acute malarial attack, mild and transient headache, dizziness, and gastrointestinal complaints (diarrhea, anorexia, nausea, abdominal cramps and, on rare occasions, vomiting) may occur.

Dosage and Administration: One tablet of 200 mg of hydroxychloroquine sulfate is equivalent to 155 mg base.

Malaria: Suppression—*In adults,* 400 mg (=310 mg base) on exactly the same day of each week. *In infants and children,* the weekly suppressive dosage is 5 mg, calculated as base, per kg of body weight, but should not exceed the adult dose regardless of weight.

If circumstances permit, suppressive therapy should begin two weeks prior to exposure. However, failing this, in adults an initial double (loading) dose of 800 mg (= 620 mg base), or in children 10 mg base/kg may be taken in two divided doses, six hours apart. The suppressive therapy should be continued for eight weeks after leaving the endemic area.

Treatment of the acute attack—*In adults,* an initial dose of 800 mg (= 620 mg base) followed by 400 mg (= 310 mg base) in six to eight hours and 400 mg (310 mg base) on each of two consecutive days (total 2 g hydroxychloroquine sulfate or 1.55 g base). An alternative method, employing a single dose of 800 mg (= 620 mg base), has also proved effective.

The dosage for adults may also be calculated on the basis of body weight; this method is preferred for infants and children. A total dose representing 25 mg of base per kg of body weight is administered in three days, as follows:

First dose: 10 mg base per kg (but not exceeding a single dose of 620 mg base).

Second dose: 5 mg base per kg (but not exceeding a single dose of 310 mg base) 6 hours after first dose.

Third dose: 5 mg base per kg 18 hours after second dose.

Fourth dose: 5 mg base per kg 24 hours after third dose.

For radical cure of *vivax* and *malariae* malaria concomitant therapy with an 8-aminoquinoline compound is necessary.

LUPUS ERYTHEMATOSUS AND RHEUMATOID ARTHRITIS

Indications: PLAQUENIL is useful in patients with the following disorders who have not responded satisfactorily to drugs with less potential for serious side effects: lupus erythematosus (chronic discoid and systemic) and acute or chronic rheumatoid arthritis.

Warnings: PHYSICIANS SHOULD COMPLETELY FAMILIARIZE THEMSELVES WITH THE COMPLETE CONTENTS OF THIS LEAFLET BEFORE PRESCRIBING PLAQUENIL.

Irreversible retinal damage has been observed in some patients who had received long-term or high-dosage 4-aminoquinoline therapy for discoid and systemic lupus erythematosus, or rheumatoid arthritis. Retinopathy has been reported to be dose related.

When prolonged therapy with any antimalarial compound is contemplated, initial (base line) and periodic (every three months) ophthalmologic examinations (including visual acuity, expert slit-lamp, funduscopic, and visual field tests) should be performed.

If there is any indication of abnormality in the visual acuity, visual field, or retinal macular areas (such as pigmentary changes, loss of foveal reflex), or any visual symptoms (such as light flashes and streaks) which are not fully explainable by difficulties of accommodation or corneal opacities, the drug should be discontinued immediately and the patient closely observed for possible progression. Retinal changes (and visual disturbances) may progress even after cessation of therapy.

All patients on long-term therapy with this preparation should be questioned and examined periodically, including the testing of knee and ankle reflexes, to detect any evidence of muscular weakness. If weakness occurs, discontinue the drug.

In the treatment of rheumatoid arthritis, if objective improvement (such as reduced joint swelling, increased mobility) does not occur within six months, the drug should be discontinued. Safe use of the drug in the treatment of juvenile arthritis has not been established.

Precautions: Dermatologic reactions to PLAQUENIL sulfate, brand of hydroxychloroquine sulfate tablets, may occur and, therefore, proper care should be exercised when it is administered to any patient receiving a drug with a significant tendency to produce dermatitis.

The methods recommended for early diagnosis of "chloroquine retinopathy" consist of (1) funduscopic examination of the macula for fine pigmentary disturbances or loss of the foveal reflex and (2) examination of the central visual field with a small red test object for pericentral or paracentral scotoma or determination of retinal thresholds to red. Any unexplained visual symptoms, such as light flashes or streaks should also be regarded with suspicion as possible manifestations of retinopathy.[2-6]

If serious toxic symptoms occur from overdosage or sensitivity, it has been suggested that ammonium chloride (8 g daily in divided doses for adults) be administered orally three or four days a week for several months after therapy has been stopped, as acidification of the urine increases renal excretion of the 4- aminoquinoline compounds by 20 to 90 per cent. However, caution must be exercised in patients with impaired renal function and/or metabolic acidosis.

Adverse Reactions: Not all of the following reactions have been observed with every 4-aminoquinoline compound during long-term therapy, but they have been reported with one or more and should be borne in mind when drugs of this class are administered. Adverse effects with different compounds vary in type and frequency.

CNS Reactions: irritability, nervousness, emotional changes, nightmares, psychosis, headache, dizziness, vertigo, tinnitus, nystagmus, nerve deafness, convulsions, ataxia.

Neuromuscular Reactions: extraocular muscle palsies, skeletal muscle weakness, absent or hypoactive deep tendon reflexes.

Ocular Reactions:

A. *Ciliary body:* disturbance of accommodation with symptoms of blurred vision. This reaction is dose related and reversible with cessation of therapy.

B. *Cornea:* transient edema, punctate to lineal opacities, decreased corneal sensitivity. The corneal changes, with or without accompanying symptoms (blurred vision, halos around lights, photophobia), are fairly common, but

Continued on next page

This product information was effective as of November 21, 1979. On these and other products of Winthrop Laboratories, detailed information may be obtained on a current basis by direct inquiry to the Professional Services Department, 90 Park Avenue, New York, N Y 10016 (212) 972-4095.

Winthrop—Cont.

reversible. Corneal deposits may appear as early as three weeks following initiation of therapy.
The incidence of corneal changes and visual side effects appears to be considerably lower with hydroxychloroquine than with chloroquine.
C. *Retina:*
Macula: Edema, atrophy, abnormal pigmentation (mild pigment stippling to a "bull's-eye" appearance), loss of foveal reflex, increased macular recovery time following exposure to a bright light (photo-stress test), elevated retinal threshold to red light in macular, paramacular and peripheral retinal areas.
Other fundus changes include optic disc pallor and atrophy, attenuation of retinal arterioles, fine granular pigmentary disturbances in the peripheral retina and prominent choroidal patterns in advanced stage.
D. *Visual field defects:* pericentral or paracentral scotoma, central scotoma with decreased visual acuity, rarely field constriction.
The most common visual symptoms attributed to the retinopathy are: reading and seeing difficulties (words, letters, or parts of objects missing), photophobia, blurred distance vision, missing or blacked out areas in the central or peripheral visual field, light flashes and streaks.
Retinopathy appears to be dose related and has occurred within several months (rarely) to several years of daily therapy; a small number of cases have been reported several years after antimalarial drug therapy was discontinued. It has not been noted during prolonged use of weekly doses of the 4-aminoquinoline compounds for suppression of malaria.
Patients with retinal changes may have visual symptoms or may be asymptomatic (with or without visual field changes). Rarely scotomatous vision or field defects may occur without obvious retinal change.
Retinopathy may progress even after the drug is discontinued. In a number of patients, early retinopathy (macular pigmentation sometimes with central field defects) diminished or regressed completely after therapy was discontinued. Paracentral scotoma to red targets (sometimes called "premaculopathy") is indicative of early retinal dysfunction which is usually reversible with cessation of therapy.
A small number of cases of retinal changes have been reported as occurring in patients who received only hydroxychloroquine. These usually consisted of alteration in retinal pigmentation which was detected on periodic ophthalmologic examination; visual field defects were also present in some instances. A case of delayed retinopathy has been reported with loss of vision starting one year after administration of hydroxychloroquine had been discontinued.
Dermatologic Reactions: Bleaching of hair, alopecia, pruritus, skin and mucosal pigmentation, skin eruptions (urticarial, morbilliform, lichenoid, maculopapular, purpuric, erythema annulare centrifugum and exfoliative dermatitis).
Hematologic Reactions: Various blood dyscrasias such as aplastic anemia, agranulocytosis, leukopenia, thrombocytopenia (hemolysis in individuals with glucose-6- phosphate dehydrogenase (G-6-PD) deficiency).
Gastrointestinal Reactions: Anorexia, nausea, vomiting, diarrhea, and abdominal cramps.
Miscellaneous Reactions: Weight loss, lassitude, exacerbation or precipitation of porphyria and nonlight-sensitive psoriasis.
Dosage and Administration: One tablet of hydroxychloroquine sulfate, 200 mg, is equivalent to 155 mg base.
Lupus erythematosus—Initially, the average *adult* dose is 400 mg (=310 mg base) once or twice daily. This may be continued for several weeks or months, depending on the response of the patient. For prolonged maintenance therapy, a smaller dose, from 200 to 400 mg (=155 to 310 mg base) daily will frequently suffice. The incidence of retinopathy has been reported to be higher when this maintenance dose is exceeded.
Rheumatoid arthritis—The compound is cumulative in action and will require several weeks to exert its beneficial therapeutic effects, whereas minor side effects may occur relatively early. Several months of therapy may be required before maximum effects can be obtained. If objective improvement (such as reduced joint swelling, increased mobility) does not occur within six months, the drug should be discontinued. Safe use of the drug in the treatment of juvenile rheumatoid arthritis has not been established.
Initial dosage—In ***adults,*** from 400 to 600 mg (=310 to 465 mg base) daily, each dose to be taken with a meal or a glass of milk. In a small percentage of patients, troublesome side effects may require temporary reduction of the initial dosage. Later (usually from five to ten days), the dose may gradually be increased to the optimum response level, often without return of side effects.
Maintenance dosage—When a good response is obtained (usually in four to twelve weeks), the dosage is reduced by 50 per cent and continued at a usual maintenance level of 200 to 400 mg (=155 to 310 mg base) daily, each dose to be taken with a meal or a glass of milk. The incidence of retinopathy has been reported to be higher when this maintenance dose is exceeded.
Should a relapse occur after medication is withdrawn, therapy may be resumed or continued on an intermittent schedule if there are no ocular contraindications.
Corticosteroids and salicylates may be used in conjunction with this compound, and they can generally be decreased gradually in dosage or eliminated after the drug has been used for several weeks. When gradual reduction of steroid dosage is indicated, it may be done by reducing every four to five days the dose of cortisone by no more than from 5 to 15 mg; of hydrocortisone from 5 to 10 mg; of prednisolone and prednisone from 1 to 2.5 mg; of methylprednisolone and triamcinolone from 1 to 2 mg; and of dexamethasone from 0.25 to 0.5 mg.
How Supplied: Tablets of 200 mg (equivalent to 155 mg of base), bottles of 100.
References:

1. Ullberg, S., Lindquist, N.G., and Sjostrand, S. E.: Accumulation of chorio-retinotoxic drugs in the foetal eye, *Nature 227:*1257, Sept. 19, 1970.
2. Carr, R. E., Gouras, P., and Gunkel, R. D.: Chloroquine retinopathy. Early detection by retinal threshold test, *Arch. Ophthal. 75:*171, Feb. 1966.
3. Bernstein, H. N.: Chloroquine ocular toxicity, *Survey Ophthal. 12:*415, October 1967.
4. Percival, S. P. B. and Meanock, I.: Chloroquine: Ophthalmological safety and clinical assessment in rheumatoid arthritis, *Brit. Med. J. 3:*579, September 1968.
5. Carr, R. E., Henkind, P., Rothfield, Naomi, and Siegel, I. M.: Ocular toxicity of antimalarial drugs, *Amer. J. Ophthal. 66:*738, October 1968.
6. Young, P., White, G., and Fry, J.: Measurement of red light perception as a practical means of detecting retinal toxicity to antimalarials before it is irreversible. Paper presented at Interim Meeting of American Rheumatism Association, Atlanta, Georgia, Dec. 5-8, 1968; abstr. *Arthritis Rheum. 11:*850, December 1968.

[*Shown in Product Identification Section*]

SULFAMYLON® Cream ℞
brand of mafenide acetate cream, USP

Topical Antibacterial Agent for Adjunctive Therapy in Second- and Third-Degree Burns

Description: SULFAMYLON Cream is a soft, white, nonstaining, water-miscible cream containing the antibacterial agent, mafenide acetate (α-amino-*p*-toluenesulfonamide monoacetate).
SULFAMYLON Cream spreads easily, and can be washed off readily with water. It has a slight acetic odor. Each gram of SULFAMYLON Cream contains mafenide acetate equivalent to 85 mg of the base. The cream vehicle consists of cetyl alcohol, stearyl alcohol, spermaceti, polyoxyl 40 stearate, polyoxyl 8 stearate, glycerin, and water, with methylparaben, propylparaben, sodium bisulfite, and edetate disodium as preservatives.
Actions: SULFAMYLON Cream, applied topically, produces a marked reduction in the bacterial population present in the avascular tissues of second- and third-degree burns. Reduction in bacterial growth after application of SULFAMYLON Cream has also been reported to permit spontaneous healing of deep partial-thickness burns, and thus prevent conversion of burn wounds from partial thickness to full thickness. It should be noted, however, that delayed eschar separation has occurred in some cases.
Absorption and Metabolism. Applied topically, SULFAMYLON Cream diffuses through devascularized areas, is absorbed, and rapidly converted to a metabolite (*p*-carboxybenzenesulfonamide) which is cleared through the kidneys. SULFAMYLON is active in the presence of pus and serum, and its activity is not altered by changes in the acidity of the environment.
Antibacterial Activity. SULFAMYLON exerts bacteriostatic action against many gram-negative and gram-positive organisms, including *Pseudomonas aeruginosa* and certain strains of anaerobes.
Indication: SULFAMYLON Cream is a topical antibacterial agent indicated for adjunctive therapy of patients with second- and third-degree burns.
Warnings: SULFAMYLON Cream should be administered with caution to patients with history of hypersensitivity to mafenide. It is not known whether there is cross sensitivity to other sulfonamides.
Fungal colonization in and below the eschar may occur concomitantly with reduction of bacterial growth in the burn wound. However, fungal dissemination through the infected burn wound is rare.
Usage in Pregnancy. Safe use of SULFAMYLON Cream during pregnancy has not been established. Therefore, the preparation is not recommended for the treatment of women of childbearing potential, *unless* the burned area covers more than 20 per cent of the total body surface, or the need for the therapeutic benefit of SULFAMYLON Cream is, in the physician's judgment, greater than the possible risk to the fetus.
Precautions: SULFAMYLON and its metabolite, *p*-carboxybenzenesulfonamide, inhibit carbonic anhydrase, which may result in metabolic acidosis, usually compensated by hyperventilation. In the presence of impaired renal function, high blood levels of SULFAMYLON and its metabolite may exaggerate the carbonic anhydrase inhibition. Therefore, close monitoring of acid-base balance is necessary, particularly in patients with extensive second-degree or partial thickness burns and in those with pulmonary or renal dysfunction. Some burn patients treated with SULFAMYLON Cream have also been reported to manifest an unexplained syndrome

of marked hyperventilation with resulting respiratory alkalosis (slightly alkaline blood pH, low arterial pCO_2 and decreased total CO_2); change in arterial pO_2 is variable. The etiology and significance of these findings are unknown.

Mafenide acetate cream should be used with caution in burn patients with acute renal failure.

Adverse Reactions: It is frequently difficult to distinguish between an adverse reaction to SULFAMYLON Cream and the effect of a severe burn. The most frequently reported reaction was pain or a burning sensation. Allergic manifestations included rash, itching, facial edema, swelling, hives, blisters, erythema, and eosinophilia. Other reactions, which have rarely occurred, are tachypnea or hyperventilation, acidosis, increase in serum chloride, decrease in arterial pCO_2, excoriation of new skin, and bleeding of skin. A single case of bone marrow depression and a single case of an acute attack of porphyria have been reported following SULFAMYLON Cream therapy. Fatal hemolytic anemia with disseminated intravascular coagulation, presumably related to a glucose-6-phosphate dehydrogenase deficiency, has been reported following SULFAMYLON Cream therapy. Accidental ingestion of SULFAMYLON Cream has been reported to cause diarrhea.

Administration: Prompt institution of appropriate measures for controlling shock and pain is of prime importance. The burn wounds are then cleansed and debrided, and SULFAMYLON Cream, brand of mafenide acetate cream, is applied with a sterile gloved hand. Satisfactory results can be achieved with application of the cream once or twice daily, to a thickness of approximately 1/16 inch; thicker application is not recommended. The burned areas should be covered with SULFAMYLON Cream at all times. Therefore, whenever necessary, the cream should be reapplied to any areas from which it has been removed (e.g., by patient activity). The routine of administration can be accomplished in minimal time, since dressings usually are not required. If individual patient demands make them necessary, however, only a thin layer of dressing should be used.

When feasible, the patient should be bathed daily, to aid in debridement. A whirlpool bath is particularly helpful, but the patient may be bathed in bed or in a shower.

The duration of therapy with SULFAMYLON Cream depends on each patient's requirements. Treatment is usually continued until healing is progressing well or until the burn site is ready for grafting. *SULFAMYLON Cream should not be withdrawn from the therapeutic regimen while there is the possibility of infection.* However, if allergic manifestations occur during treatment with SULFAMYLON Cream, discontinuation of treatment should be considered.

If acidosis occurs and becomes difficult to control, particularly in patients with pulmonary dysfunction, discontinuing SULFAMYLON Cream therapy for 24 to 48 hours while continuing fluid therapy may aid in restoring acid-base balance.

How Supplied:
Cans of 14.5 ounces (411 g)
Collapsible tubes of 4 ounces (113.4 g)
Collapsible tubes of 2 ounces (56.7 g)

TALWIN® Lactate © ℞
brand of pentazocine lactate injection, NF

Analgesic for Parenteral Use

Description: TALWIN lactate, brand of pentazocine lactate injection, is a member of the benzazocine series (also known as the benzomorphan series). Chemically, pentazocine lactate is 1,2,3,4,5,6-hexahydro - 6, 11 - dimethyl-3-(3-methyl-2-butenyl) -2,6-methano-3-benzazocin-8-ol lactate, a white, crystalline substance soluble in acidic aqueous solutions.

Actions: TALWIN is a potent analgesic and 30 mg is usually as effective an analgesic as morphine 10 mg or meperidine 75 to 100 mg; however, a few studies suggest the TALWIN to morphine ratio may range from 20 to 40 mg TALWIN to 10 mg morphine. The duration of analgesia may sometimes be less than that of morphine. Analgesia usually occurs within 15 to 20 minutes after intramuscular or subcutaneous injection and within 2 to 3 minutes after intravenous injection. TALWIN weakly antagonizes the analgesic effects of morphine, meperidine, and phenazocine; in addition, it produces incomplete reversal of cardiovascular, respiratory, and behavioral depression induced by morphine and meperidine. TALWIN has about 1/50 the antagonistic activity of nalorphine. It also has sedative activity.

Indications: For the relief of moderate to severe pain. TALWIN may also be used for preoperative or preanesthetic medication and as a supplement to surgical anesthesia.

Contraindication: TALWIN should not be administered to patients who are hypersensitive to it.

Warnings: Drug Dependence. *Special care should be exercised in prescribing pentazocine for emotionally unstable patients and for those with a history of drug misuse. Such patients should be closely supervised when long-term therapy is contemplated. There have been instances of psychological and physical dependence on TALWIN in patients with such a history and, rarely, in patients without such a history. Abrupt discontinuance following the extended use of parenteral TALWIN has resulted in symptoms such as abdominal cramps, elevated temperature, rhinorrhea, restlessness, anxiety, and lacrimation. Even when these occurred, discontinuance has been accomplished with minimal difficulty. In the rare patient in whom more than minor difficulty has been encountered, reinstitution of parenteral TALWIN with gradual withdrawal has ameliorated the patient's symptoms. Substituting methadone or other narcotics for TALWIN in the treatment of the pentazocine abstinence syndrome should be avoided. There have been rare reports of possible abstinence syndromes in newborns after prolonged use of TALWIN during pregnancy.*

In prescribing parenteral TALWIN for chronic use, particularly if the drug is to be self-administered, the physician should take precautions to avoid increases in dose and frequency of injection by the patient and to prevent the use of the drug in anticipation of pain rather than for the relief of pain.

Just as with all medication, the oral form of TALWIN is preferable for chronic administration.

Tissue Damage at Injection Sites. Severe sclerosis of the skin, subcutaneous tissues, and underlying muscle have occurred at the injection sites of patients who have received multiple doses of pentazocine lactate. Constant rotation of injection sites is, therefore, essential. In addition, animal studies have demonstrated that TALWIN is tolerated less well subcutaneously than intramuscularly. (See DOSAGE AND ADMINISTRATION.)

Head Injury and Increased Intracranial Pressure. As in the case of other potent analgesics, the potential of TALWIN lactate for elevating cerebrospinal fluid pressure may be attributed to CO_2 retention due to the respiratory depressant effects of the drug. These effects may be markedly exaggerated in the presence of head injury, other intracranial lesions, or a preexisting increase in intracranial pressure. Furthermore, TALWIN can produce effects which may obscure the clinical course of patients with head injuries. In such patients, TALWIN must be used with extreme caution and only if its use is deemed essential.

Usage in Pregnancy. Safe use of TALWIN during pregnancy (other than labor) has not been established. Animal reproduction studies have not demonstrated teratogenic or embryotoxic effects. However, TALWIN should be administered to pregnant patients (other than labor) only when, in the judgment of the physician, the potential benefits outweigh the possible hazards. Patients receiving TALWIN during labor have experienced no adverse effects other than those that occur with commonly used analgesics. TALWIN should be used with caution in women delivering premature infants.

Acute CNS Manifestations. Patients receiving therapeutic doses of TALWIN have experienced, in rare instances, hallucinations (usually visual), disorientation, and confusion which have cleared spontaneously within a period of hours. The mechanism of this reaction is not known. Such patients should be very closely observed and vital signs checked. If the drug is reinstituted, it should be done with caution since the acute CNS manifestations may recur.

Usage in Children. Because clinical experience in children under twelve years of age is limited, the use of TALWIN in this age group is not recommended.

Ambulatory Patients. Since sedation, dizziness, and occasional euphoria have been noted, ambulatory patients should be warned not to operate machinery, drive cars, or unnecessarily expose themselves to hazards.

Myocardial Infarction. Caution should be exercised in the intravenous use of pentazocine for patients with acute myocardial infarction accompanied by hypertension or left ventricular failure. Data suggest that intravenous administration of pentazocine increases systemic and pulmonary arterial pressure and systemic vascular resistance in patients with acute myocardial infarction.

Precautions: Certain Respiratory Conditions. The possibility that TALWIN may cause respiratory depression should be considered in treatment of patients with bronchial asthma. TALWIN lactate, brand of pentazocine lactate injection, should be administered only with caution and in low dosage to patients with respiratory depression (e.g., from other medication, uremia, or severe infection), severely limited respiratory reserve, obstructive respiratory conditions, or cyanosis.

Impaired Renal or Hepatic Function. Although laboratory tests have not indicated that TALWIN causes or increases renal or hepatic impairment, the drug should be administered with caution to patients with such impairment. Extensive liver disease appears to predispose to greater side effects (e.g., marked apprehension, anxiety, dizziness, sleepiness) from the usual clinical dose, and may be the result of decreased metabolism of the drug by the liver.

Biliary Surgery. As with all strong analgesics, TALWIN should be used with caution in patients about to undergo surgery of the biliary tract since it may cause spasm of the sphincter of Oddi.

Patients Receiving Narcotics. TALWIN is a mild narcotic antagonist. Some patients previously given narcotics, including methadone for the daily treatment of narcotic dependence, have experienced withdrawal symptoms after receiving TALWIN.

Continued on next page

This product information was effective as of November 21, 1979. On these and other products of Winthrop Laboratories, detailed information may be obtained on a current basis by direct inquiry to the Professional Services Department, 90 Park Avenue, New York, N Y 10016 (212) 972-4095.

Winthrop—Cont.

CNS Effect. Caution should be used when TALWIN is administered to patients prone to seizures; seizures have occurred in a few such patients in association with the use of TALWIN although no cause and effect relationship has been established.

Adverse Reactions: The most commonly occurring reactions are: nausea, dizziness or lightheadedness, vomiting, euphoria.

Dermatologic Reactions. Soft tissue induration, nodules, and cutaneous depression can occur at injection sites. Ulceration (sloughing) and severe sclerosis of the skin and subcutaneous tissues (and, rarely, underlying muscle) have been reported after multiple doses.

Infrequently occurring reactions are—*respiratory:* respiratory depression, dyspnea, transient apnea in a small number of newborn infants whose mothers received TALWIN during labor; *cardiovascular:* circulatory depression, shock, hypertension; *CNS effects:* sedation, alteration of mood (nervousness, apprehension, depression, floating feeling), dreams; *gastrointestinal:* constipation, dry mouth; *dermatologic including local:* diaphoresis, sting on injection, flushed skin including plethora, dermatitis including pruritus; *other:* urinary retention, headache, paresthesia, alterations in rate or strength of uterine contractions during labor.

Rarely reported reactions include—*neuromuscular and psychiatric:* muscle tremor, insomnia, disorientation, hallucinations; *gastrointestinal:* taste alteration, diarrhea and cramps; *ophthalmic:* blurred vision, nystagmus, diplopia, miosis; *hematologic:* depression of white blood cells (especially granulocytes), which is usually reversible, moderate transient eosinophilia; *other:* tachycardia, weakness or faintness, chills, allergic reactions including edema of the face, toxic epidermal necrolysis.

See **Acute CNS Manifestations** and **Drug Dependence** under **WARNINGS.**

Dosage and Administration: Adults, Excluding Patients in Labor. The recommended single parenteral dose is 30 mg by intramuscular, subcutaneous, or intravenous route. This may be repeated every 3 to 4 hours. Doses in excess of 30 mg intravenously or 60 mg intramuscularly or subcutaneously are not recommended. Total daily dosage should not exceed 360 mg. The subcutaneous route of administration should be used only when necessary because of possible severe tissue damage at injection sites (see WARNINGS). When frequent injections are needed, the drug should be administered intramuscularly. In addition, constant rotation of injection sites (e.g., the upper outer quadrants of the buttocks, mid-lateral aspects of the thighs, and the deltoid areas) is essential.

Patients in Labor. A single, intramuscular 30 mg dose has been most commonly administered. An intravenous 20 mg dose has given adequate pain relief to some patients in labor when contractions become regular, and this dose may be given two or three times at two-to three-hour intervals, as needed.

Children Under 12 Years of Age. Since clinical experience in children under twelve years of age is limited, the use of TALWIN in this age group is not recommended.

CAUTION. TALWIN should not be mixed in the same syringe with soluble barbiturates because precipitation will occur.

Overdosage: Manifestations: Clinical experience with TALWIN overdosage has been insufficient to define the signs of this condition.

Treatment: Oxygen, intravenous fluids, vasopressors, and other supportive measures should be employed as indicated. Assisted or controlled ventilation should also be considered. For respiratory depression due to overdosage or unusual sensitivity to TALWIN, parenteral naloxone (Narcan®, available through Endo Laboratories) is a specific and effective antagonist.

How Supplied: *Uni-Amp®—Individual unit dose ampuls of 1 ml (30 mg)* **NDC 0024-1924-04**, *1½ ml (45 mg)* **NDC 0024-1925-04**, *and 2 ml (60 mg)* **NDC 0024-1926-04** in boxes of 25.

Uni-Nest™ ampuls of 1 ml (30 mg) **NDC 0024-1924-14**, *1½ ml (45 mg)* **NDC 0024-1925-14**, *and 2 ml (60 mg)* **NDC 0024-1926-14** in boxes of 25.

Each 1 ml contains pentazocine lactate equivalent to 30 mg base and 2.8 mg sodium chloride, in water for injection.

Carpuject® **Sterile Cartridge-Needle Units**, *1 ml (30 mg)* **NDC 0024-1917-02**, *1½ ml (45 mg)* **NDC 0024-1918-02**, *and 2 ml (60 mg)* **NDC 0024-1919-02, all in 2 ml cartridge, boxes of 10.** Each 1 ml contains pentazocine lactate equivalent to 30 mg base, 1 mg acetone sodium bisulfite, and 2.2 mg sodium chloride, in water for injection.

Multiple-dose vials of 10 ml **NDC 0024-1916-01**, boxes of 1. Each 1 ml contains pentazocine lactate equivalent to 30 mg base, 2 mg acetone sodium bisulfite, 1.5 mg sodium chloride, and 1 mg methylparaben as preservative, in water for injection.

The pH of TALWIN solutions is adjusted between 4 and 5 with lactic acid or sodium hydroxide. The air in the ampuls and vials has been displaced by nitrogen gas.

TALWIN® 50 Ⓒ ℞

brand of pentazocine hydrochloride tablets, NF

Analgesic for Oral Use

Description: TALWIN 50, brand of pentazocine hydrochloride tablets, is a member of the benzazocine series (also known as the benzomorphan series). Chemically, pentazocine hydrochloride is 1,2,3,4,5,6 - hexahydro - 6, 11-dimethyl-3- (3-methyl-2-butenyl)-2, 6-methano-3-benzazocin-8-ol hydrochloride, a white, crystalline substance soluble in acidic aqueous solutions.

Clinical Pharmacology: TALWIN 50 is a potent analgesic which when administered orally in a 50 mg dose appears equivalent in analgesic effect to 60 mg (1 gr) of codeine. Onset of significant analgesia usually occurs between 15 and 30 minutes after oral administration, and duration of action is usually three hours or longer. Onset and duration of action and the degree of pain relief are related both to dose and the severity of pretreatment pain. TALWIN 50 weakly antagonizes the analgesic effects of morphine, meperidine, and phenazocine; in addition, it produces incomplete reversal of cardiovascular, respiratory, and behavioral depression induced by morphine and meperidine. TALWIN 50 has about 1/50 the antagonistic activity of nalorphine. It also has sedative activity.

Indications and Usage: For the relief of moderate to severe pain

Contraindication: TALWIN 50 should not be administered to patients who are hypersensitive to it.

Warnings: *Drug Dependence. There have been instances of psychological and physical dependence on parenteral pentazocine in patients with a history of drug abuse and, rarely, in patients without such a history. Abrupt discontinuance following the extended use of parenteral pentazocine has resulted in withdrawal symptoms. There have been a few reports of dependence and of withdrawal symptoms with orally administered TALWIN 50. Patients with a history of drug dependence should be under close supervision while receiving TALWIN 50 orally. There have been rare reports of possible abstinence syndromes in newborns after prolonged use of TALWIN 50 during pregnancy.*

In prescribing TALWIN 50 for chronic use, the physician should take precautions to avoid increases in dose by the patient and to prevent the use of the drug in anticipation of pain rather than for the relief of pain.

Head Injury and Increased Intracranial Pressure. As in the case of other potent analgesics, the potential of TALWIN 50 for elevating cerebrospinal fluid pressure may be attributed to CO_2 retention due to the respiratory depressant effects of the drug. These effects may be markedly exaggerated in the presence of head injury, other intracranial lesions, or a preexisting increase in intracranial pressure. Furthermore, TALWIN 50 can produce effects which may obscure the clinical course of patients with head injuries. In such patients, TALWIN 50 must be used with extreme caution and only if its use is deemed essential.

Usage in Pregnancy. Safe use of TALWIN 50 during pregnancy (other than labor) has not been established. Animal reproduction studies have not demonstrated teratogenic or embryotoxic effects. However, TALWIN 50 should be administered to pregnant patients (other than labor) only when, in the judgment of the physician, the potential benefits outweigh the possible hazards. Patients receiving TALWIN 50 during labor have experienced no adverse effects other than those that occur with commonly used analgesics. TALWIN 50 should be used with caution in women delivering premature infants.

Acute CNS Manifestations. Patients receiving therapeutic doses of TALWIN 50 have experienced, in rare instances, hallucinations (usually visual), disorientation, and confusion which have cleared spontaneously within a period of hours. The mechanism of this reaction is not known. Such patients should be very closely observed and vital signs checked. If the drug is reinstituted, it should be done with caution since the acute CNS manifestations may recur.

Usage in Children. Because clinical experience in children under 12 years of age is limited, administration of TALWIN 50 in this age group is not recommended.

Ambulatory Patients. Since sedation, dizziness, and occasional euphoria have been noted, ambulatory patients should be warned not to operate machinery, drive cars, or unnecessarily expose themselves to hazards.

Precautions: *Certain Respiratory Conditions.* Although respiratory depression has rarely been reported after oral administration of TALWIN 50, the drug should be administered with caution to patients with respiratory depression from any cause, severely limited respiratory reserve, severe bronchial asthma and other obstructive respiratory conditions, or cyanosis.

Impaired Renal or Hepatic Function. Decreased metabolism of the drug by the liver in extensive liver disease may predispose to accentuation of side effects. Although laboratory tests have not indicated that TALWIN 50 causes or increases renal or hepatic impairment, the drug should be administered with caution to patients with such impairment.

Myocardial Infarction. As with all drugs, TALWIN 50 should be used with caution in patients with myocardial infarction who have nausea or vomiting.

Biliary Surgery. As with all strong analgesics, TALWIN 50 should be used with caution in patients about to undergo surgery of the biliary tract since it may cause spasm of the sphincter of Oddi.

Patients Receiving Narcotics. TALWIN 50 is a mild narcotic antagonist. Some patients previously given narcotics, including methadone for the daily treatment of narcotic dependence, have experienced withdrawal symptoms after receiving TALWIN 50.

CNS Effect. Caution should be used when TALWIN 50 is administered to patients prone to seizures; seizures have occurred in a few such patients in association with the use of TALWIN 50 although no cause and effect relationship has been established.

Adverse Reactions: Reactions reported after oral administration of TALWIN 50 include *gastrointestinal:* nausea, vomiting; infrequently constipation; and rarely abdominal distress, anorexia, diarrhea. *CNS effects:* dizziness, lightheadedness, sedation, euphoria, headache; infrequently weakness, disturbed dreams, insomnia, syncope, visual blurring and focusing difficulty, hallucinations (see *Acute CNS Manifestations* under **WARNINGS**); and rarely tremor, irritability, excitement, tinnitus. *Autonomic:* sweating; infrequently flushing; and rarely chills. *Allergic:* infrequently rash; and rarely urticaria, edema of the face. *Cardiovascular:* infrequently decrease in blood pressure, tachycardia. *Hematologic:* rarely depression of white blood cells (especially granulocytes), which is usually reversible, moderate transient eosinophilia. *Other:* rarely respiratory depression, urinary retention, paresthesia, toxic epidermal necrolysis.

Dosage and Administration: *Adults.* The usual initial adult dose is 1 tablet (50 mg) every three or four hours. This may be increased to 2 tablets (100 mg) when needed. Total daily dosage should not exceed 600 mg.

When antiinflammatory or antipyretic effects are desired in addition to analgesia, aspirin can be administered concomitantly with TALWIN 50, brand of pentazocine hydrochloride tablets.

Children Under 12 Years of Age. Since clinical experience in children under 12 years of age is limited, administration of TALWIN 50 in this age group is not recommended.

Duration of Therapy. Patients with chronic pain who receive TALWIN 50 orally for prolonged periods have only rarely been reported to experience withdrawal symptoms when administration was abruptly discontinued (see WARNINGS). Tolerance to the analgesic effect has also been reported only rarely. Significant abnormalities of liver and kidney function tests have not been reported, even after prolonged administration of TALWIN 50.

Overdosage: *Manifestations:* Clinical experience with TALWIN 50 overdosage has been insufficient to define the signs of this condition.

Treatment: Oxygen, intravenous fluids, vasopressors, and other supportive measures should be employed as indicated. Assisted or controlled ventilation should also be considered. For respiratory depression due to overdosage or unusual sensitivity to TALWIN 50, parenteral naloxone (Narcan®, available through Endo Laboratories) is a specific and effective antagonist.

How Supplied: Tablets, peach color, scored, each equivalent to 50 mg base.

Bottles of 100 (NDC 0024-1921-04)

Unit Dose Pack of 100, 20 strips of 5 tablets each (NDC 0024-1921-14)

Distributed by
Winthrop Laboratories
Division of Sterling Drug Inc.
New York, NY 10016
Manufactured by
Winthrop Laboratories Inc. Barceloneta,
Puerto Rico 00617

[*Shown in Product Identification Section*]

TALWIN® Compound ©̷ ℞

Pentazocine hydrochloride, NF, equivalent to 12.5 mg base and aspirin 325 mg.

Description: Pentazocine is a member of the benzazocine series (also known as the benzomorphan series). Chemically, pentazocine is 1, 2, 3, 4, 5, 6 - hexahydro - 6, 11-dimethyl-3-(3-methyl-2-butenyl)-2, 6-methano-3-benzazocin-8-ol, a white, crystalline substance soluble in acidic aqueous solutions. TALWIN Compound is a combination of pentazocine hydrochloride equivalent to 12.5 mg base and aspirin 325 mg.

Clinical Pharmacology: Pentazocine is a potent analgesic which when administered orally is approximately equivalent, on a mg for mg basis, in analgesic effect to codeine. Two Caplets® of TALWIN Compound when administered orally have the additive analgesic effect equivalent to 25 mg of TALWIN plus 650 mg of aspirin. TALWIN Compound provides the analgesic effects of pentazocine and the analgesic, antiinflammatory, and antipyretic actions of aspirin.

Onset of significant analgesia usually occurs between 15 and 30 minutes after oral administration, and duration of action is usually three hours or longer. Onset and duration of action and the degree of pain relief are related both to dose and the severity of pretreatment pain. Pentazocine weakly antagonizes the analgesic effects of morphine, meperidine, and phenazocine; in addition, it produces incomplete reversal of cardiovascular, respiratory, and behavioral depression induced by morphine and meperidine. Pentazocine has about $\frac{1}{50}$ the antagonistic activity of nalorphine. It also has sedative activity.

Indication and Usage: For the relief of moderate pain

Contraindications: TALWIN Compound should not be administered to patients who are hypersensitive to either pentazocine or salicylates, or in any situation where aspirin is contraindicated.

Warnings: *Drug Dependence. There have been instances of psychological and physical dependence on parenteral pentazocine in patients with a history of drug abuse and, rarely, in patients without such a history. Abrupt discontinuance following the extended use of parenteral pentazocine has resulted in withdrawal symptoms. There have been a few reports of dependence and of withdrawal symptoms with orally administered pentazocine. Patients with a history of drug dependence should be under close supervision while receiving TALWIN Compound orally. There have been rare reports of possible abstinence syndromes in newborns after prolonged use of pentazocine during pregnancy. In prescribing TALWIN Compound for chronic use, the physician should take precautions to avoid increases in dose by the patient and to prevent the use of the drug in anticipation of pain rather than for the relief of pain.*

Head Injury and Increased Intracranial Pressure. The respiratory depressant effects of pentazocine and its potential for elevating cerebrospinal fluid pressure may be markedly exaggerated in the presence of head injury, other intracranial lesions, or a preexisting increase in intracranial pressure. Furthermore, pentazocine can produce effects which may obscure the clinical course of patients with head injuries. In such patients, TALWIN Compound must be used with extreme caution and only if its use is deemed essential.

Usage in Pregnancy. Safe use of pentazocine during pregnancy (other than labor) has not been established. Animal reproduction studies have not demonstrated teratogenic or embryotoxic effects. However, TALWIN Compound should be administered to pregnant patients (other than labor) only when, in the judgment of the physician, the potential benefits outweigh the possible hazards. Patients receiving pentazocine during labor have experienced no adverse effects other than those that occur with commonly used analgesics. TALWIN Compound should be used with caution in women delivering premature infants.

Acute CNS Manifestations. Patients receiving therapeutic doses of pentazocine have experienced, in rare instances, hallucinations (usually visual), disorientation, and confusion which have cleared spontaneously within a period of hours. The mechanism of this reaction is not known. Such patients should be very closely observed and vital signs checked. If the drug is reinstituted it should be done with caution since the acute CNS manifestations may recur.

Usage in Children. Because clinical experience in children under 12 years of age is limited, administration of TALWIN Compound in this age group is not recommended.

Ambulatory Patients. Since sedation, dizziness, and occasional euphoria have been noted, ambulatory patients should be warned not to operate machinery, drive cars, or unnecessarily expose themselves to hazards.

Other. Because of its aspirin content, TALWIN Compound should be used with caution in the presence of peptic ulcer, in conjunction with anticoagulant therapy, or in any situation where the effects of aspirin may be deleterious.

Precautions: *Certain Respiratory Conditions.* Although respiratory depression has rarely been reported after oral administration of pentazocine, TALWIN Compound should be administered with caution to patients with respiratory depression from any cause, severely limited respiratory reserve, severe bronchial asthma and other obstructive respiratory conditions, or cyanosis.

Impaired Renal or Hepatic Function. Decreased metabolism of the drug by the liver in extensive liver disease may predispose to accentuation of side effects. Although laboratory tests have not indicated that pentazocine causes or increases renal or hepatic impairment, TALWIN Compound should be administered with caution to patients with such impairment.

Myocardial Infarction. As with all drugs, TALWIN Compound should be used with caution in patients with myocardial infarction who have nausea or vomiting.

Biliary Surgery. As with all strong analgesics, TALWIN Compound should be used with caution in patients about to undergo surgery of the biliary tract since it may cause spasm of the sphincter of Oddi.

Patients Receiving Narcotics. Pentazocine is a mild narcotic antagonist. Some patients previously given narcotics, including methadone for the daily treatment of narcotic dependence, have experienced withdrawal symptoms after receiving pentazocine.

CNS Effect. Caution should be used when pentazocine is administered to patients prone to seizures. Seizures have occurred in a few such patients in association with the use of pentazocine although no cause and effect relationship has been established.

Adverse Reactions: Reactions reported after oral administration of pentazocine or TALWIN Compound include *gastrointestinal:* nausea, vomiting; infrequently constipation; and rarely abdominal distress, anorexia, diarrhea. *CNS Effects:* dizziness, lightheadedness, sedation, euphoria, headache; infrequently weakness, disturbed dreams, insomnia, syncope, visual blurring and focusing difficulty, depression, hallucinations (see *Acute CNS Manifestations* under **WARNINGS**); and rarely confusion, tremor, irritability, excitement, tinnitus. *Autonomic:* sweating, infrequently flushing, and rarely chills. *Allergic:* infrequently rash; and rarely urticaria, edema of the face. *Cardiovascular:* infrequently decrease in blood pressure, tachycardia. *Hematologic:* rarely depression of white blood cells (especially granulocytes), which is usually reversible, moderate transient eosinophilia. *Other:* rarely respiratory depression, urinary retention, paresthesia, toxic epidermal necrolysis.

Continued on next page

This product information was effective as of November 21, 1979. On these and other products of Winthrop Laboratories, detailed information may be obtained on a current basis by direct inquiry to the Professional Services Department, 90 Park Avenue, New York, N Y 10016 (212) 972-4095.

Winthrop—Cont.

Dosage and Administration: *Adults.* The usual adult dose is 2 CAPLETS three or four times a day.
Children Under 12 Years of Age. Since clinical experience in children under 12 years of age is limited, administration of TALWIN Compound in this age group is not recommended.
Duration of Therapy. Patients with chronic pain who receive pentazocine orally for prolonged periods have only rarely been reported to experience withdrawal symptoms when administration was abruptly discontinued (see WARNINGS). Tolerance to the analgesic effect of pentazocine has also been reported only rarely. Significant abnormalities of liver and kidney function tests have not been reported, even after prolonged administration of pentazocine.
Overdosage: *Manifestations:* Clinical experience with pentazocine overdosage has been insufficient to define the signs of this condition. Signs of salicylate overdosage include headache, dizziness, confusion, tinnitus, diaphoresis, thirst, nausea, vomiting, diarrhea, tachycardia, tachypnea, Kussmaul breathing, convulsions, and coma. Death is usually from respiratory failure.
Treatment: Treatment for overdosage of TALWIN Compound should include treatment for salicylate poisoning as outlined in standard references.
Oxygen, intravenous fluids, vasopressors, and other supportive measures should be employed as indicated. Assisted or controlled ventilation should also be considered. For respiratory depression due to overdosage or unusual sensitivity to pentazocine, parenteral naloxone (Narcan®, available through Endo Laboratories) is a specific and effective antagonist.
How Supplied: CAPLETS, white, each containing pentazocine hydrochloride equivalent to 12.5 mg base and aspirin, 325 mg. Bottles of 100 (NDC 0024-1927-04).
Distributed by Winthrop Laboratories Division of Sterling Drug Inc., New York, NY 10016, Manufactured by Winthrop Laboratories Inc., Barceloneta, Puerto Rico 00617

[*Shown in Product Identification Section*]

TELEPAQUE® ℞
brand of iopanoic acid tablets, USP

(See Diagnostic Section.)

WinGel® OTC

(See PDR For Nonprescription Drugs)

WINSTROL® ℞
brand of stanozolol tablets, NF

ANABOLIC STEROID

Description: WINSTROL, brand of stanozolol tablets, is 17-methyl-2′*H*-5α-androst -2- eno [3, 2- c] pyrazol -17β-ol.It is a heterocyclic steroid.
Clinical Pharmacology: Anabolic steroids are synthetic derivatives of testosterone. WINSTROL is primarily used for its protein anabolic effect and its catabolic inhibiting effect on tissue. Nitrogen balance is improved with anabolic agents but only when there is sufficient intake of calories and protein. Whether this positive nitrogen balance is of primary benefit in the utilization of protein-building dietary substances has not been established.
Increases in hemoglobin levels have occurred in some patients with aplastic anemia receiving anabolic steroids.
Certain clinical effects and adverse reactions demonstrate the androgenic properties of this class of drugs. Complete dissociation of anabolic and androgenic effects has not been achieved. The actions of anabolic steroids are therefore similar to those of male sex hormones with the possibility of causing serious disturbances of growth and sexual development if given to young children. They suppress the gonadotropic functions of the pituitary and may exert a direct effect upon the testes.
Indications and Usage: WINSTROL has been effective in increasing hemoglobin levels in some patients with aplastic (congenital and idiopathic) anemia. WINSTROL should be used only after diagnosis has been established.

> Based on a review of WINSTROL by the National Academy of Sciences—National Research Council and/or other information, FDA has classified the other indications as follows:
> "Probably" effective: as adjunctive but not primary therapy in senile and postmenopausal osteoporosis. Equal or greater consideration should be given to diet, calcium balance, physiotherapy, and good general health-promoting measures. Anabolic steroids are without value as primary therapy. In pituitary dwarfism anabolic agents may be used with care until growth hormone is more available.
> Final classification of less-than-effective indications requires further investigation.

Contraindications: The use of WINSTROL is contraindicated in the following:

1. Carcinoma of the prostate or breast in male patients.
2. Carcinoma of the breast in some females.
3. Pregnancy (because of masculinization of the fetus).
4. Nephrosis or the nephrotic phase of nephritis.

Warning: Anabolic steroids do not enhance athletic ability.
Precautions: Hypercalcemia may develop, both spontaneously and as a result of hormonal therapy, in women with disseminated breast carcinoma. If it develops during anabolic steroid therapy, the drug should be stopped.
Caution is required in administering anabolic steroids to patients with cardiac, renal, or hepatic disease. Edema may occur occasionally. Concomitant administration with adrenal steroids or ACTH may add to the edema.
If amenorrhea or menstrual irregularities develop during treatment with an anabolic steroid, the drug should be discontinued until the cause is determined.
Anabolic steroids may increase sensitivity to anticoagulants; therefore, dosage of an anticoagulant may have to be decreased in order to maintain the prothrombin time at the desired therapeutic level.
Anabolic steroids have been shown to alter glucose tolerance tests. Diabetics should be carefully observed and the insulin or oral hypoglycemic dosage adjusted accordingly.
Since WINSTROL, brand of stanozolol tablets, contains a 17-alkyl group, liver function should be checked at regular intervals in patients receiving this drug.
Anabolic steroids should be used with caution in patients with benign prostatic hypertrophy.
Serum cholesterol levels may increase or decrease during therapy with anabolic steroids. Therefore, caution is required in administering these agents to patients with a history of myocardial infarction or coronary artery disease. Serial determinations of serum cholesterol levels should be made and therapy adjusted accordingly.
Anabolic agents may accelerate epiphyseal maturation more rapidly than linear growth in children, and the effect may continue for 6 months after the drug has been stopped. Therefore, therapy should be monitored by x-ray studies at 3 to 6 month intervals and the drug discontinued well before the bone age reaches the norm for chronological age, in order to avoid the risk of compromising the adult height.
Adverse Reactions: Reactions to oral anabolic steroids include nausea and vomiting; diarrhea; increased or decreased libido; acne (especially in females and prepubertal males); habituation; excitation and insomnia; chills; bleeding in patients on concomitant anticoagulant therapy; premature closure of epiphyses in children; and jaundice with, rarely, hepatic necrosis and death.
There have been rare reports of hepatocellular neoplasms and peliosis hepatis in association with long-term androgenic-anabolic steroid therapy.
Phallic enlargement and increased frequency of erections have occurred in prepubertal males. Inhibition of testicular function, testicular atrophy and oligospermia, impotence, chronic priapism, gynecomastia, and epididymitis and bladder irritability have occurred in postpubertal males.
In females, hirsutism, male pattern baldness, deepening of the voice, and clitoral enlargement have occurred. These changes are usually irreversible even after prompt discontinuance of therapy, and are not prevented by concomitant use of estrogens. Menstrual irregularities have also occurred.
Therapy with anabolic steroids has caused alterations in these clinical laboratory tests: the metyrapone test; the fasting blood sugar and glucose tolerance test; thyroid function tests [decrease in protein-bound iodine (PBI), thyroxine-binding capacity, and radioactive iodine (RAI) uptake, and increase in T_3 uptake by the red blood cells or resin. Free thyroxine is normal. The altered tests usually persist for 2 to 3 weeks after anabolic therapy has been stopped.]; liver function tests [increased Bromsulphalein (BSP) retention, increased or decreased serum cholesterol, increased serum glutamic oxaloacetic transaminase (SGOT), increased serum bilirubin, and increased alkaline phosphatase]; serum electrolytes [retention of sodium, chloride, potassium, phosphate, calcium, and water]; blood clotting tests [suppression of clotting factors II, V, VII, and X]; increased creatine and creatinine excretion lasting up to two weeks after discontinuance of therapy; and decreased 17-ketosteroid excretion.
Dosage and Administration: The suggested initial dosage for adults is 1 tablet (2 mg) three times daily just before or with meals. Although considerably smaller doses have produced a response in some patients, consistently better results have been obtained with a daily dose of 6 mg. Higher doses have been employed in patients with bone marrow damage and patients on corticosteroid therapy.
The dosage for children should be adjusted according to age. The following routine is suggested: ½ tablet twice daily for children under 6 years and up to 1 tablet three times daily for children from 6 to 12. (See Precautions.)
For young women who appear particularly susceptible to the androgenic effects of the drug, 1 tablet twice daily appears adequate for long-term administration. If this amount does not produce the desired results, the dosage may be raised to 1 tablet three times daily.
WINSTROL, brand of stanozolol tablets, should not be given to pregnant women. (See Contraindications.)
To obtain the maximal therapeutic effect, a well-balanced diet should accompany the administration of WINSTROL.
Duration of therapy will depend on the response of the condition and the appearance of adverse reactions. Therapy should be intermittent.
Duration of therapy with WINSTROL has, in most cases, varied from several weeks to one year.

TABLE 2
Correct Use of ZEPHIRAN Chloride

ZEPHIRAN Chloride solutions must be prepared, stored, and used correctly to achieve and maintain their antiseptic action. Serious inactivation and contamination of ZEPHIRAN Chloride solutions may occur with misuse.

CORRECT DILUENTS	INCOMPATIBILITIES	PREFERRED FORM
Sterile Water for Injection is recommended for irrigation of body cavities.	Anionic detergents and soaps should be thoroughly rinsed from the skin or other areas prior to use of ZEPHIRAN Chloride solutions because they reduce the antibacterial activity of the solutions.	ZEPHIRAN Chloride Tinted Tincture 1:750 is recommended for preoperative skin preparation because it contains alcohol and acetone which enhance its cleansing action and promote rapid drying.
Sterile distilled water is recommended for irrigating traumatized tissue and in the eye.		
Freshly distilled water is recommended for skin antisepsis.	Serum and protein material also decrease the activity of ZEPHIRAN Chloride solutions.	ZEPHIRAN Chloride Tinted Tincture 1:750, containing acetone, is recommended when it is desirable to outline the operative site. (Aqueous solutions of ZEPHIRAN Chloride used in skin preparation have a tendency to "run off" the skin.)
Resin deionized water should not be used because the deionizing resins can carry pathogens (especially gram-negative bacteria); they also inactivate quaternary ammonium compounds.	Corks should not be used to stopper bottles containing ZEPHIRAN Chloride solutions.	
Stored water is not recommended since it may contain many organisms.	Fibers of fabrics when stored in ZEPHIRAN Chloride solutions adsorb ZEPHIRAN from the surrounding liquid. Examples are: Cotton, Gauze sponges Wool, Rayon Rubber materials	Caution: Because of the flammable organic solvents in ZEPHIRAN Chloride Tinted Tincture 1:750 and Spray, these products should be kept away from open flame or cautery.
Saline should not be used since it may decrease the antibacterial potency of ZEPHIRAN Chloride solutions.	Applicators or sponges, intended for a skin prep, should be stored separately and dipped in ZEPHIRAN Chloride solutions immediately before use.	
	Under certain circumstances the following commonly encountered substances are incompatible with ZEPHIRAN Chloride solutions: Iodine, Aluminum Silver nitrate, Caramel Fluorescein, Kaolin Nitrates, Pine oil Peroxide, Zinc sulfate Lanolin, Zinc oxide Potassium permanganate, Yellow oxide of mercury	

How Supplied: Tablets of 2 mg, scored
bottles of 100 (NDC 0024-2253-04)
bottles of 1000 (NDC 0024-2253-08)
[*Shown in Product Identification Section*]

ZEPHIRAN® CHLORIDE OTC
brand of benzalkonium chloride

ANTISEPTIC

AQUEOUS SOLUTION 1:750
TINTED TINCTURE 1:750
SPRAY—TINTED TINCTURE 1:750

Description: ZEPHIRAN Chloride, brand of benzalkonium chloride, USP, a mixture of alkylbenzyldimethylammonium chlorides, is a cationic quaternary ammonium surface-acting agent. It is very soluble in water, alcohol, and acetone. Aqueous solutions of ZEPHIRAN Chloride are neutral to slightly alkaline, generally colorless, and nonstaining. They have a bitter taste, aromatic odor, and foam when shaken. ZEPHIRAN Chloride Tinted Tincture 1:750 contains alcohol 50 per cent and acetone 10 per cent by volume. ZEPHIRAN Chloride Spray—Tinted Tincture 1:750 contains alcohol 92 per cent. The Tinted Tincture and Spray also contain an orange-red coloring agent.

Clinical Pharmacology: ZEPHIRAN Chloride solutions are rapidly acting antiinfective agents with a moderately long duration of action. They are active against bacteria and some viruses, fungi, and protozoa. Bacterial spores are considered to be resistant. Solutions are bacteriostatic or bactericidal according to their concentration. The exact mechanism of bactericidal action is unknown but is thought to be due to enzyme inactivation. Activity generally increases with increasing temperature and pH. Gram-positive bacteria are more susceptible than gram-negative bacteria (TABLE 1).

TABLE 1
Highest Dilution of ZEPHIRAN Chloride Aqueous Solution Destroying the Organism in 10 but not in 5 Minutes

Organisms	**20 C**
Streptococcus pyogenes	1:75,000
Staphylococcus aureus	1:52,500
Salmonella typhosa	1:37,500
Escherichia coli	1:10,500

Pseudomonas is the most resistant gram-negative genus. Using the AOAC Use-Dilution Confirmation Method, no growth was obtained when *Staphylococcus aureus, Salmonella choleraesuis,* and *Pseudomonas aeruginosa* (strain PRD-10) were exposed for ten minutes at 20 C to ZEPHIRAN Chloride Aqueous Solution 1:750 and Tinted Tincture 1:750.

ZEPHIRAN Chloride Aqueous Solution 1:750 has been shown to retain its bactericidal activity following autoclaving for 30 minutes at 15 lb pressure, freezing, and then thawing.

The tubercle bacillus may be resistant to aqueous ZEPHIRAN Chloride solutions but is susceptible to the 1:750 tincture (AOAC Method, 10 minutes at 20 C).

ZEPHIRAN Chloride solutions also demonstrate deodorant, wetting, detergent, keratolytic, and emulsifying activity.

Indications and Usage: ZEPHIRAN Chloride aqueous solutions in appropriate dilutions (see Recommended Dilutions) are indicated for the antisepsis of skin, mucous membranes, and wounds. They are used for preoperative preparation of the skin, surgeons' hand and arm soaks, treatment of wounds, preservation of ophthalmic solutions, irrigations of the eye, body cavities, bladder, urethra, and vaginal douching.

ZEPHIRAN Chloride Tinted Tincture 1:750 and Spray are indicated for preoperative preparation of the skin and for treatment of minor skin wounds and abrasions.

Contraindication: The use of ZEPHIRAN Chloride solutions in occlusive dressings, casts, and anal or vaginal packs is inadvisable, as they may produce irritation or chemical burns.

Warnings: Sterile Water for Injection, USP, should be used as diluent in preparing diluted aqueous solutions intended for use on deep wounds or for irrigation of body cavities. Otherwise, freshly distilled water should be used. Tap water, containing metallic ions and organic matter, may reduce antibacterial potency. Resin deionized water should not be used since it may contain pathogenic bacteria. Organic, inorganic, and synthetic materials and surfaces may adsorb sufficient quantities of ZEPHIRAN Chloride to significantly reduce its antibacterial potency in solutions. This has

Continued on next page

This product information was effective as of November 21, 1979. On these and other products of Winthrop Laboratories, detailed information may be obtained on a current basis by direct inquiry to the Professional Services Department, 90 Park Avenue, New York, N Y 10016 (212) 972-4095.

Winthrop—Cont.

resulted in serious contamination of solutions of ZEPHIRAN Chloride with viable pathogenic bacteria. Solutions should not be stored in bottles stoppered with cork closures, but rather in those equipped with appropriate screw-caps. Cotton, wool, rayon, and other materials should not be stored in ZEPHIRAN Chloride solutions. Gauze sponges and fiber pledgets used to apply solutions of ZEPHIRAN Chloride to the skin should be sterilized and stored in separate containers. Only immediately prior to application should they be immersed in ZEPHIRAN Chloride solutions.

Since ZEPHIRAN Chloride solutions are inactivated by soaps and anionic detergents, thorough rinsing is necessary if these agents are employed prior to their use.

Antiseptics such as ZEPHIRAN Chloride solutions must not be relied upon to achieve complete sterilization, because they do not destroy bacterial spores and certain viruses, including the etiologic agent of infectious hepatitis, and may not destroy *Mycobacterium tuberculosis* and other rare bacterial strains.

ZEPHIRAN Chloride Tinted Tincture 1:750 and Spray contain flammable organic solvents and should not be used near an open flame or cautery.

If solutions stronger than 1:3000 enter the eyes, irrigate immediately and repeatedly with water. Prompt medical attention should then be obtained. Concentrations greater than 1:5000 should not be used on mucous membranes, with the exception of the vaginal mucosa (see Recommended Dilutions).

Precautions: In preoperative antisepsis of the skin, ZEPHIRAN Chloride solutions should not be permitted to remain in prolonged contact with the patient's skin. Avoid pooling of the solution on the operating table.

ZEPHIRAN Chloride solutions that are used on inflamed or irritated tissues must be more dilute than those used on normal tissues (see Recommended Dilutions). ZEPHIRAN Chloride Tinted Tincture 1:750 and Spray, which contain irritating organic solvents, should be kept away from the eyes or other mucous membranes.

Adverse Reactions: ZEPHIRAN Chloride solutions in normally used concentrations have low systemic and local toxicity and are generally well tolerated, although a rare individual may exhibit hypersensitivity.

Directions for Use:

General: For most surgical applications, the recommended concentration of ZEPHIRAN Chloride Aqueous Solution or ZEPHIRAN Chloride Tinted Tincture is 1:750 (0.13 per cent). Liberal use of the solution is recommended to compensate for any adsorption of ZEPHIRAN Chloride by cotton or other materials.

To use ZEPHIRAN Chloride Spray—Tinted Tincture 1:750, remove protective cap, hold in an UPRIGHT position several inches away from the surgical field or injured area (to prevent chilling), and apply by spraying freely.

Preoperative preparation of skin: ZEPHIRAN Chloride solutions 1:750 are recommended as an antiseptic for use on unbroken skin in the preoperative preparation of the surgical field.

Detergents and soaps should be thoroughly rinsed from the skin before applying ZEPHIRAN Chloride solutions. The detergent action of ZEPHIRAN Chloride solutions, particularly when used alternately with alcohol, leaves the skin smooth and clean. When ZEPHIRAN Chloride solutions are applied by friction (using several changes of sponges), dirt, skin fats, desquamating epithelium, and superficial bacteria are effectively removed, thus exposing the underlying skin to the antiseptic activity of the solutions.

The following procedure has been found satisfactory for preparation of the surgical field. On the day prior to surgery, the operative site is shaved and then scrubbed thoroughly with ZEPHIRAN Chloride Aqueous Solution 1:750. Immediately before surgery, ZEPHIRAN Chloride Tinted Tincture 1:750 or Spray is applied to the site in the usual manner (see Precautions). If the red tinted solution turns yellow during the preparation of patient's skin for surgery, it usually indicates the presence of soap (alkali) residue which is incompatible with ZEPHIRAN solutions. Therefore, rinse thoroughly and reapply the antiseptic. Because ZEPHIRAN Chloride Tinted Tincture 1:750 contains alcohol and acetone, its cleansing action on the skin is particularly effective and it dries more rapidly than the aqueous solution. The Tinted Tincture is recommended when it is desirable to outline the operative site.

Recommended Dilutions: For specific directions, see Tables 2 and 3.

Surgery

Preoperative preparation of skin: Aqueous solution 1:750 and Tinted Tincture 1:750 or Spray

Surgeons' hand and arm soaks: Aqueous solution 1:750

Treatment of minor wounds and lacerations: Tinted Tincture 1:750 or Spray

Irrigation of deep infected wounds: Aqueous solution 1:3000 to 1:20,000

Denuded skin and mucous membranes: Aqueous solution 1:5000 to 1:10,000

Obstetrics and Gynecology

Preoperative preparation of skin: Aqueous solution 1:750 and Tinted Tincture 1:750 or Spray

Vaginal douche and irrigation: Aqueous solution 1:2000 to 1:5000

Postepisiotomy care: Aqueous solution 1:5000 to 1:10,000

Breast and nipple hygiene: Aqueous solution 1:1000 to 1:2000

Urology

Bladder and urethral irrigation: Aqueous solution 1:5000 to 1:20,000

Bladder retention lavage: Aqueous solution 1:20,000 to 1:40,000

Dermatology

Oozing and open infections: Aqueous solution 1:2000 to 1:5000

Wet dressings by irrigation or open dressing (Use in occlusive dressings is inadvisable.): Aqueous solution 1:5000 or less

Ophthalmology

Eye irrigation: Aqueous solution 1:5000 to 1:10,000

Preservation of ophthalmic solutions: Aqueous solution 1:5000 to 1:7500

[See table on preceding page].

Table 3
Dilutions of ZEPHIRAN Chloride
Aqueous Solution 1:750

Final Dilution	ZEPHIRAN Chloride Aqueous Solution 1:750 (parts)	Distilled Water (parts)
1:1000	3	1
1:2000	3	5
1:2500	3	7
1:3000	3	9
1:4000	3	13
1:5000	3	17
1:10,000	3	37
1:20,000	3	77
1:40,000	3	157

Accidental Ingestion: If ZEPHIRAN Chloride solution, particularly a concentrated solution, is ingested, marked local irritation of the gastrointestinal tract, manifested by nausea and vomiting, may occur. Signs of systemic toxicity include restlessness, apprehension, weakness, confusion, dyspnea, cyanosis, collapse, convulsions, and coma. Death occurs as a result of paralysis of the respiratory muscles.
Treatment: Immediate administration of several glasses of a mild soap solution, milk, or egg whites beaten in water is recommended. This may be followed by gastric lavage with a mild soap solution. Alcohol should be avoided as it promotes absorption.

To support respiration, the airway should be clear and oxygen should be administered, employing artificial respiration if necessary. If convulsions occur, a short-acting barbiturate may be given parenterally with caution.

How Supplied:
ZEPHIRAN Chloride Aqueous Solution 1:750
Bottles of 8 fl oz (NDC 0024-2521-04)
and 1 gallon (NDC 0024-2521-08)

ZEPHIRAN Chloride Tinted Tincture 1:750
(*flammable*)
Bottles of 1 gallon (NDC 0024-2523-08)

ZEPHIRAN Chloride Spray—Tinted Tincture 1:750
(*flammable*)
Bottles of
1 fl oz (NDC 0024-2527-01) and
6 fl oz (NDC 0024-2527-03)

Wyeth Laboratories

Division of American Home Products Corporation
P.O. BOX 8299
PHILADELPHIA, PA 19101

Product Identification Codes

The process of imprinting all oral solid dosage forms manufactured by Wyeth with their respective National Drug Code (NDC) numbers is at present incomplete. In the future that portion of the number indicating product and strength will appear on each tablet and capsule, together with the name Wyeth. The following is a numerical list of NDC code numbers with their corresponding product names.

Numerical Listing

Product Ident. Code	Product
1	Equanil® (meprobamate) Tablet 400 mg. Ⓒ
2	Equanil® (meprobamate) Tablet 200 mg. Ⓒ
5	Equagesic® (meprobamate and ethoheptazine citrate with aspirin) Tablet
6	Serax® (oxazepam) Capsule 15 mg. Ⓒ
13	Amphojel® (dried aluminum hydroxide gel) Tablet 0.6 Gm.
16	Purodigin® (crystalline digitoxin) Tablet 0.1 mg.
19	Phenergan® (promethazine HCl) Tablet 12.5 mg.
22	Aludrox® (alumina and magnesia) Tablet

27 Phenergan® (promethazine HCl) Tablet 25 mg.
28 Sparine® (promazine HCl) Tablet 50 mg.
29 Sparine® (promazine HCl) Tablet 25 mg.
30 Zactirin® (ethoheptazine citrate with aspirin) Tablet
33 Equanil® (meprobamate) Tablet Wyseals® 400 mg. Ⓒ
35 Equanitrate® 10 (meprobamate and pentaerythritol tetranitrate) Tablet
39 Equanitrate® 20 (meprobamate and pentaerythritol tetranitrate) Tablet
44 Equanil® (meprobamate) Capsule 400 mg. Ⓒ
49 Zactirin® Compound-100 (ethoheptazine citrate with aspirin, phenacetin and caffeine) Tablet
51 Serax® (oxazepam) Capsule 10 mg. Ⓒ
52 Serax® (oxazepam) Capsule 30 mg. Ⓒ
53 Omnipen® (ampicillin) Capsule 250 mg.
56 Ovral® (each tablet contains 0.5 mg. norgestrel with 0.05 mg. ethinyl estradiol) Tablet, white
57 Unipen® [(nafcillin sodium) as the monohydrate] Capsule 250 mg.
58 Pen•Vee® K (penicillin V potassium) Tablet 125 mg.
59 Pen•Vee® K (penicillin V potassium) Tablet 250 mg.
62 Ovrette® (norgestrel) Tablet
64 Ativan® (lorazepam) Tablet 1 mg. Ⓒ
65 Ativan® (lorazepam) Tablet 2 mg. Ⓒ
78 Lo/Ovral® (each tablet contains 0.3 mg. norgestrel with 0.03 mg. ethinyl estradiol) Tablet, white
81 Ativan® (lorazepam) Tablet 0.5 mg. Ⓒ
85 Wygesic® (each tablet contains 65 mg. propoxyphene HCl, U.S.P., and 650 mg. acetaminophen, U.S.P.) Tablet Ⓒ
114 Purodigin® (crystalline digitoxin) Tablet 0.2 mg.
119 Amphojel® (dried aluminum hydroxide gel) Tablet 0.3 Gm.
127 Purodigin® (crystalline digitoxin) Tablet 0.15 mg.
138 A-M-T® (alumina magnesium trisilicate) Tablet
141 Sulfose® (trisulfapyrimidines) Tablet 0.5 Gm.
165 Bicillin® (penicillin G benzathine) Tablet 200,000 units
177 Ethobral® (triple barbiturate) Capsule 2 gr. Ⓒ
200 Sparine® (promazine HCl) Tablet 100 mg.
202 Sparine® (promazine HCl) Tablet 10 mg.
225 Zactane® (ethoheptazine citrate) Tablet 75 mg.
227 Phenergan® (promethazine HCl) Tablet 50 mg.
251 Proketazine® (carphenazine maleate) Tablet 12.5 mg.
252 Proketazine® (carphenazine maleate) Tablet 25 mg.
253 Proketazine® (carphenazine maleate) Tablet 50 mg.
255 Penicillin G Potassium Tablet 200,000 units
256 Penicillin G Potassium Tablet 250,000 units
261 Mepergan® Fortis (meperidine HCl and promethazine HCl) Capsule Ⓒ
266 Secobarbital Sodium Capsule 100 mg. Ⓒ
267 Phenobarbital Tablet 15 mg. Ⓒ
268 Phenobarbital Tablet 30 mg. Ⓒ
269 Phenobarbital Tablet 100 mg. Ⓒ
272 Penicillin G Potassium Tablet 400,000 units
285 Pentobarbital Sodium Capsule 100 mg. Ⓒ
308 Meperidine HCl Tablet 50 mg. Ⓒ
309 Omnipen® (ampicillin) Capsule 500 mg.
310 A.P.C. w/Codeine Phosphate 15 mg. Tablet Ⓒ
311 A.P.C. w/Codeine Phosphate 30 mg. Tablet Ⓒ
312 A.P.C. w/Meperidine HCl 30 mg. Tablet Ⓒ
313 Aspirin Tablet 300 mg.
314 A.P.C. Tablet
317 Serax® (oxazepam) Tablet 15 mg. Ⓒ
320 Phenobarbital Tablet 60 mg. Ⓒ
322 Chloral Hydrate Capsule 500 mg. Ⓒ
325 Codeine Sulfate Tablet 15 mg. Ⓒ
326 Codeine Sulfate Tablet 30 mg. Ⓒ
327 Codeine Sulfate Tablet 60 mg. Ⓒ
360 Pathocil® (dicloxacillin sodium monohydrate) Capsule 250 mg.
389 Tetracycline HCl Capsule 250 mg.
390 Pen•Vee® K (penicillin V potassium) Tablet 500 mg.
433 Phenergan® Compound (promethazine HCl and pseudoephedrine HCl with aspirin) Tablets
434 Phenergan®-D (promethazine HCl with pseudoephedrine HCl) Tablet
443 Polymagma® Plain Tablet (each tablet contains Claysorb® [activated attapulgite] 500 mg., pectin 45 mg., hydrated alumina powder 50 mg.)
464 Unipen® [(nafcillin sodium) as the monohydrate] 500 mg. Tablet
469 Wyamycin® S (erythromycin stearate) Tablet 250 mg.
470 Wyamycin® S (erythromycin stearate) Tablet 500 mg.
471 Tetracycline HCl Capsule 500 mg.
472 Basaljel® (dried basic aluminum carbonate gel) Capsules
473 Basaljel® (dried basic aluminum carbonate gel) Swallow Tablets
512 Cyclapen® (cyclacillin) Tablet 250 mg.
517 Cyclapen® (cyclacillin) Tablet 500 mg.
559 Wymox® (amoxicillin) 250 mg. Capsule
560 Wymox® (amoxicillin) 500 mg. Capsule
2511 Ovral®-28 (21 white tablets each containing 0.5 mg. norgestrel with 0.05 mg. ethinyl estradiol and 7 pink inert tablets)
2514 Lo/Ovral®-28 (21 white tablets each containing 0.3 mg. norgestrel with 0.03 mg. ethinyl estradiol and 7 pink inert tablets)

ALUDROX® OTC
(alumina and magnesia)
ORAL SUSPENSION • TABLETS

Composition: Nonconstipating, noncathartic, effective and palatable antacid containing, in each 5 ml. teaspoonful of suspension, 307 mg. of aluminum hydroxide as a gel, and 103 mg. of magnesium hydroxide. Each tablet contains 233 mg. aluminum hydroxide as a dried gel and 83 mg. magnesium hydroxide. Sodium content is 0.07 mEq per tablet and 0.05 mEq per 5 ml suspension.
Indications: For the symptomatic relief of hyperacidity associated with the diagnosis of peptic ulcer, gastritis, peptic esophagitis, gastric hyperacidity, and hiatal hernia.
Dosage and Administration: Two tablets or 2 teaspoonfuls (10 ml.) of suspension every four hours, or as required. Suspension may be followed by a sip of water if desired. Tablets are designed to be chewed with or without water. Two ALUDROX tablets have the capacity to neutralize 23 mEq of acid; 10 ml. of ALUDROX suspension have the capacity to neutralize 28 mEq of acid.
Drug Interaction Precautions: This product must not be taken if the patient is presently taking a prescription antibiotic drug containing any form of tetracycline.
How Supplied: *Oral Suspension,* bottles of 12 fluidounces.
Tablets, boxes of 100; each tablet is sealed in cellophane so that a day's supply can be conveniently carried.

AMPHOJEL® OTC
(aluminum hydroxide gel)
SUSPENSION • TABLETS

Composition: *Suspension*—Each 5 ml. teaspoonful contains 320 mg. of aluminum hydroxide as a gel, and not more than 0.3 mEq of sodium. *Tablets* contain a dried gel. The 0.3 Gm. (5 grain) strength is equivalent to about 1 teaspoonful of the suspension and the 0.6 Gm. (10 grain) strength is equivalent to about 2 teaspoonfuls.
Indications: For the symptomatic relief of hyperacidity associated with the diagnosis of peptic ulcer, gastritis, peptic esophagitis, gastric hyperacidity, and hiatal hernia.
Dosage: *Suspension*—two teaspoonfuls followed by a sip of water if desired, five or six times daily, between meals and at bedtime. 2 teaspoonfuls have the capacity to neutralize 13 mEq of acid. *Tablets*—Two tablets of the 0.3 Gm. strength, or one tablet of the 0.6 Gm. strength, five or six times daily between meals and at bedtime. 2 tablets have the capacity to neutralize 18 mEq of acid.
Precaution: May cause constipation.
Drug Interaction Precautions: This product must not be taken if the patient is presently taking a prescription antibiotic drug containing any form of tetracycline.
How Supplied: *Suspension*—Peppermint flavored; without flavor; and with 10% by volume mineral oil—bottles of 12 fluidounces. *Tablets*—a convenient auxiliary dosage form—0.3 Gm. (5 gr.), bottles of 100; 0.6 Gm. (10 gr.), boxes of 100.

ATIVAN® Ⓒ ℞
(lorazepam)

Description: Ativan (lorazepam), an antianxiety agent, has the chemical formula, 7-chloro-5-(o-chlorophenyl)-1, 3-dihydro-3-hydroxy-2H-1,4-benzodiazepin-2-one.
It is a nearly white powder almost insoluble in water. Each Ativan (lorazepam) tablet, to be taken orally, contains 0.5 mg, 1 mg or 2 mg of lorazepam.
Clinical Pharmacology: Studies in healthy volunteers show that in single high doses Ativan (lorazepam) has a tranquilizing action on the central nervous system with no appreciable effect on the respiratory or cardiovascular systems.
Ativan (lorazepam) is readily absorbed with an absolute bioavailability of 90 percent. Peak concentrations in plasma occur approximately 2 hours following administration. The peak plasma level of lorazepam from a 2 mg dose is approximately 20 ng/ml.
The mean half-life of unconjugated lorazepam in human plasma is about 12 hours and for its major metabolite, lorazepam glucuronide, about 18 hours. At clinically relevant concentrations, lorazepam is approximately 85% bound to plasma proteins. Ativan (lorazepam) is rapidly conjugated at its 3-hydroxy group into lorazepam glucuronide which is then excreted in the urine. Lorazepam glucuronide has no demonstrable CNS activity in animals. The plasma levels of lorazepam are proportional to the dose given. There is no evidence of accumulation of lorazepam on administration up to six months.
Indications and Usage: Ativan (lorazepam) is indicated for the symptomatic relief of anxiety, tension, agitation, irritability, and insomnia associated with anxiety neuroses and transient situational disturbances; anxiety associated with depressive symptoms and as a treatment for symptoms of anxiety if such symptoms are a significant feature of functional or organic disorders, particularly gastrointestinal or cardiovascular.
The effectiveness of Ativan (lorazepam) in long-term use, that is, more than 4 months, has

Continued on next page

Wyeth—Cont.

not been assessed by systematic clinical studies. The physician should periodically reassess the usefulness of the drug for the individual patient.

Contraindications: Ativan (lorazepam) is contraindicated in patients with known sensitivity to the benzodiazepines or with acute narrow-angle glaucoma.

Warnings: Ativan (lorazepam) is not recommended for use in patients with a primary depressive disorder or psychosis. As with all patients on CNS-acting drugs, patients receiving lorazepam should be warned not to operate dangerous machinery or motor vehicles and that their tolerance for alcohol and other CNS depressants will be diminished.

Physical and Psychological Dependence: Withdrawal symptoms similar in character to those noted with barbiturates and alcohol have occurred following abrupt discontinuance of benzodiazepine drugs. These symptoms include convulsions, tremor, abdominal and muscle cramps, vomiting and sweating. Addiction-prone individuals, such as drug addicts and alcoholics, should be under careful surveillance when receiving benzodiazepines because of the predisposition of such patients to habituation and dependence.

Precautions: In patients with depression accompanying anxiety, a possibility for suicide should be borne in mind.

For elderly or debilitated patients, the initial daily dosage should not exceed 2 mg in order to avoid oversedation.

Ativan® (lorazepam) dosage should be terminated gradually, since abrupt withdrawal of any anti-anxiety agent may result in symptoms similar to those for which patients are being treated: anxiety, agitation, irritability, tension, insomnia, and occasional convulsions. The usual precautions for treating patients with impaired renal or hepatic function should be observed.

In patients where gastrointestinal or cardiovascular disorders coexist with anxiety, it should be noted that lorazepam has not been shown to be of significant benefit in treating the gastrointestinal or cardiovascular component.

Esophageal dilation occurred in rats treated with lorazepam for more than one year at 6 mg/kg/day. The no-effect dose was 1.25 mg/kg/day (approximately 6 times the maximum human therapeutic dose of 10 mg per day). The effect was reversible only when the treatment was withdrawn within two months of first observation of the phenomenon. The clinical significance of this is unknown. However, use of lorazepam for prolonged periods and in geriatric patients requires caution, and there should be frequent monitoring for symptoms of upper G.I. disease.

Safety and effectiveness of Ativan (lorazepam) in children of less than 12 years have not been established.

ESSENTIAL LABORATORY TESTS: Some patients on Ativan (lorazepam) have developed leukopenia, and some have had elevations of LDH. As with other benzodiazepines, periodic blood counts and liver-function tests are recommended for patients on long-term therapy.

CLINICALLY SIGNIFICANT DRUG INTERACTIONS: The benzodiazepines, including Ativan (lorazepam), produce CNS depressant effects when administered with such medications as barbiturates or alcohol.

CARCINOGENESIS AND MUTAGENESIS: No evidence of carcinogenic potential emerged in rats during an 18-month study with Ativan (lorazepam). No studies regarding mutagenesis have been performed.

PREGNANCY: Reproductive studies in animals were performed in mice, rats, and two strains of rabbits. Occasional anomalies (reduction of tarsals, tibia, metatarsals, malrotated limbs, gastroschisis, malformed skull, and microphthalmia) were seen in drug-treated rabbits without relationship to dosage. Although all of these anomalies were not present in the concurrent control group, they have been reported to occur randomly in historical controls. At doses of 40 mg/kg and higher, there was evidence of fetal resorption and increased fetal loss in rabbits which was not seen at lower doses.

The clinical significance of the above findings is not known. However, an increased risk of congenital malformations associated with the use of minor tranquilizers (chlordiazepoxide, diazepam, and meprobamate) during the first trimester of pregnancy has been suggested in several studies. Because the use of these drugs is rarely a matter of urgency, the use of lorazepam during this period should almost always be avoided. The possibility that a woman of childbearing potential may be pregnant at the time of institution of therapy should be considered. Patients should be advised that if they become pregnant, they should communicate with their physician about the desirability of discontinuing the drug.

In humans, blood levels obtained from umbilical cord blood indicate placental transfer of lorazepam and lorazepam glucuronide.

NURSING MOTHERS: It is not known whether oral lorazepam is excreted in human milk like the other benzodiazepine tranquilizers. As a general rule, nursing should not be undertaken while a patient is on a drug, since many drugs are excreted in human milk.

Adverse Reactions: Adverse reactions, if they occur, are usually observed at the beginning of therapy and generally disappear on continued medication or upon decreasing the dose. In a sample of about 3,500 anxious patients, the most frequent adverse reaction to Ativan® (lorazepam) is sedation (15.9%), followed by dizziness (6.9%), weakness (4.2%), and unsteadiness (3.4%). Less frequent adverse reactions are disorientation, depression, nausea, change in appetite, headache, sleep disturbance, agitation, dermatological symptoms, eye function disturbance, together with various gastrointestinal symptoms and autonomic manifestations. The incidence of sedation and unsteadiness increased with age.

Small decreases in blood pressure have been noted but are not clinically significant, probably being related to the relief of anxiety produced by Ativan (lorazepam).

Overdosage: In the management of overdosage with any drug, it should be borne in mind that multiple agents may have been taken.

Manifestations of Ativan (lorazepam) overdosage include somnolence, confusion, and coma. Induced vomiting and/or gastric lavage should be undertaken, followed by general supportive care, monitoring of vital signs, and close observation of the patient. Hypotension, though unlikely, usually may be controlled with Levarterenol Bitartrate Injection, USP. Caffeine and Sodium Benzoate Injection, USP, may be used to counteract CNS depressant effects. The usefulness of dialysis has not been determined.

Dosage and Administration: Ativan® (lorazepam) is administered orally. For optimal results, dose, frequency of administration, and duration of therapy should be individualized according to patient response. To facilitate this, 0.5 mg, 1 mg and 2 mg tablets are available.

The usual range is 2 to 6 mg/day given in divided doses, the largest dose being taken before bedtime, but the daily dosage may vary from 1 to 10 mg/day.

For anxiety, most patients require an initial dose of 2 to 3 mg/day given b.i.d. or t.i.d.

For insomnia due to anxiety or transient situational stress, a single daily dose of 2 to 4 mg may be given, usually at bedtime.

For elderly or debilitated patients, an initial dosage of 1 to 2 mg/day in divided doses is recommended, to be adjusted as needed and tolerated.

The dosage of Ativan (lorazepam) should be increased gradually when needed to help avoid adverse effects. When higher dosage is indicated, the evening dose should be increased before the daytime doses.

How Supplied: Tablets—0.5 mg (white), bottles of 100; 1.0 mg (scored, white), bottles of 100, 500 and Redipak® (Strip Pack), boxes of 25. 2.0 mg. (scored, white), bottles of 100 and Redipak® (Strip Pack), boxes of 25.

Tablets should be stored at controlled room temperature.

[*Shown in Product Identification Section*]

BASALJEL® OTC
(basic aluminum carbonate gel)
SUSPENSION •CAPSULES •SWALLOW TABLETS

Composition: Suspension—each 5 ml teaspoonful contains basic aluminum carbonate gel equivalent to 400 mg aluminum hydroxide. Extra Strength Suspension—each 5 ml teaspoonful contains basic aluminum carbonate gel equivalent to 1000 mg aluminum hydroxide. Capsule contains dried basic aluminum carbonate gel equivalent to 608 mg of dried aluminum hydroxide gel or 500 mg aluminum hydroxide. Tablet contains dried basic aluminum carbonate gel equivalent to 608 mg of dried aluminum hydroxide gel or 500 mg aluminum hydroxide.

Indications: For the symptomatic relief of hyperacidity associated with the diagnosis of peptic ulcer, gastritis, peptic esophagitis, gastric hyperacidity and hiatal hernia.

Warnings: No more than 24 tablets/capsules/teaspoonfuls of BASALJEL, and no more than 12 teaspoonfuls of BASALJEL Extra Strength Suspension should be taken in a 24-hour period. Dosage should be carefully supervised since continued overdosage, in conjunction with restriction of dietary phosphorous and calcium, may produce a persistently lowered serum phosphate and a mildly elevated alkaline phosphatase. A usually transient hypercalciuria of mild degree may be associated with the early weeks of therapy.

Dosage and Administration: Suspension—two teaspoonfuls (10 ml) in water or fruit juice taken as often as every two hours up to twelve times daily. Two teaspoonfuls have the capacity to neutralize 28 mEq of acid. Extra Strength Suspension—one teaspoonful (5 ml) as often as every two hours up to twelve times daily. One teaspoonful is equivalent to two capsules or tablets and has the capacity to neutralize 22 mEq of acid. Capsules—two capsules as often as every two hours up to twelve times daily. Two capsules have the capacity to neutralize 26 mEq of acid. Swallow Tablets—two tablets as often as every two hours up to twelve times daily. Two tablets have the capacity to neutralize 28 mEq of acid. The sodium content of each dosage form is as follows: 0.1 mEq/5 ml for the suspension, 1.0 mEq/5 ml for the extra strength suspension, 0.12 mEq per capsule, and 0.09 mEq per tablet.

Precautions: May cause constipation. Adequate fluid intake should be maintained in addition to the specific medical or surgical management indicated by the patient's condition.

Drug Interaction Precautions: Alumina-containing antacids should not be used concomitantly with any form of tetracycline therapy.

How Supplied: Suspension—bottles of 12 fluidounces.

Extra Strength Suspension—bottles of 12 fluidounces.

Capsules and Swallow Tablets (scored)—available in bottles of 100.

BICILLIN® C-R ℞
(penicillin G benzathine and penicillin G procaine suspension)
INJECTION

Description: Multiple dose vials of *300,000 units per ml.* contain in each ml. 150,000 units penicillin G benzathine and 150,000 units penicillin G procaine in a stabilized aqueous suspension with sodium citrate buffer, approximately 6 mg. lecithin, 3 mg. povidone, 1 mg. carboxymethylcellulose, 0.5 mg. sorbitan monopalmitate, 0.5 mg. polyoxyethylene sorbitan monopalmitate, 1.2 mg. methylparaben and 0.14 mg. propylparaben.
TUBEX® Sterile Cartridge-Needle Units and disposable syringes of *600,000 units per ml.* contain in each ml. 300,000 units penicillin G benzathine and 300,000 units penicillin G procaine in a stabilized aqueous suspension with sodium citrate buffer; and as w/v, approximately 0.5% lecithin, 0.55% carboxymethylcellulose, 0.55% povidone, 0.1% methylparaben and 0.01% propylparaben.
Each disposable syringe (4 ml. size) contains 2,400,000 units of penicillin comprising: 1,200,000 units penicillin G benzathine and 1,200,000 units penicillin G procaine in a stabilized aqueous suspension with sodium citrate buffer, and as w/v, approximately 0.5% lecithin, 0.55% carboxymethylcellulose, 0.55% povidone, 0.1% methylparaben and 0.01% propylparaben.
FOR DEEP INTRAMUSCULAR INJECTION ONLY
Actions and Pharmacology: Penicillin G exerts a bactericidal action against penicillin-sensitive microorganisms during the stage of active multiplication. It acts through the inhibition of biosynthesis of cell-wall mucopeptide. It is not active against the penicillinase-producing bacteria, which include many strains of staphylococci. Penicillin G exerts high *in vitro* activity against staphylococci (except penicillinase-producing strains), streptococci (groups A, C, G, H, L and M) and pneumococci. Other organisms sensitive to penicillin G are *Neisseria gonorrhoeae, Corynebacterium diphtheriae, Bacillus anthracis,* Clostridia, *Actinomyces bovis, Streptobacillus moniliformis, Listeria monocytogenes* and Leptospira. *Treponema pallidum* is extremely sensitive to the bactericidal action of penicillin G.
Sensitivity plate testing: If the Kirby-Bauer method of disc sensitivity is used, a 10-unit penicillin disc should give a zone greater than 28 mm. when tested against a penicillin-sensitive bacterial strain.
Intramuscular penicillin G benzathine is absorbed very slowly into the blood stream from the intramuscular site and converted by hydrolysis to penicillin G. This combination of hydrolysis and slow absorption results in blood serum levels much lower but much more prolonged than other parenteral penicillins.
Penicillin G procaine is an equimolecular compound of procaine and penicillin G administered intramuscularly as a suspension. It dissolves slowly at the site of injection, giving a plateau type of blood level at about 4 hours which falls slowly over a period of the next 15–20 hours.
Approximately 60% of penicillin G is bound to serum protein. The drug is distributed throughout the body tissues in widely varying amounts. Highest levels are found in the kidneys with lesser amounts in the liver, skin and intestines. Penicillin G penetrates into all other tissues and the spinal fluid to a lesser degree. With normal kidney function the drug is excreted rapidly by tubular excretion. In neonates and young infants and in individuals with impaired kidney function, excretion is considerably delayed.
Indications: This drug is indicated in the treatment of moderately severe infections due to penicillin G-susceptible microorganisms that are susceptible to serum levels common to this particular dosage form. Therapy should be guided by bacteriological studies (including susceptibility testing) and by clinical response.
NOTE: When high, sustained serum levels are required, penicillin G sodium or potassium either IM or IV, should be used. This drug should *not* be used in the treatment of venereal diseases, including syphilis, gonorrhea, yaws, bejel, and pinta.
The following infections will usually respond to adequate dosages of this drug:
Streptococcal infections Group A (without bacteremia). Moderately severe to severe infections of the upper respiratory tract, skin and soft tissue infections, scarlet fever, and erysipelas.
NOTE: Streptococci in Groups A, C, G, H, L, and M are very sensitive to penicillin G. Other groups, including Group D (enterococci), are resistant. Penicillin G sodium or potassium is recommended for streptococcal infections with bacteremia.
Pneumococcal infections: Moderately severe pneumonia and otitis media.
NOTE: Severe pneumonia, empyema, bacteremia, pericarditis, meningitis, peritonitis, and arthritis of pneumococcal etiology are better treated with penicillin G sodium or potassium during the acute stage.
Contraindications: A previous hypersensitivity reaction to any penicillin or to procaine is a contraindication.
Warnings: Serious and occasionally fatal hypersensitivity (anaphylactoid) reactions have been reported in patients on penicillin therapy. Although anaphylaxis is more frequent following parenteral therapy it has occurred in patients on oral penicillins. These reactions are more apt to occur in individuals with a history of sensitivity to multiple allergens.
There have been well-documented reports of individuals with a history of penicillin hypersensitivity reactions who have experienced severe hypersensitivity reactions when treated with a cephalosporin. Before therapy with a penicillin, careful inquiry should be made concerning previous hypersensitivity reactions to penicillins, cephalosporins, and other allergens. If an allergic reaction occurs, the drug should be discontinued and the patient treated with the usual agents e.g., pressor amines, antihistamines and corticosteroids.
Precautions: Penicillin should be used with caution in individuals with histories of significant allergies and/or asthma.
Care should be taken to avoid intravenous or intra-arterial administration, or injection into or near major peripheral nerves or blood vessels, since such injections may produce neurovascular damage.
In streptococcal infections, therapy must be sufficient to eliminate the organism; otherwise the sequelae of streptococcal disease may occur. Cultures should be taken following completion of treatment to determine whether streptococci have been eradicated.
A small percentage of patients are sensitive to procaine. If there is a history of sensitivity make the usual test: Inject intradermally 0.1 ml. of a 1 to 2 percent procaine solution. Development of an erythema, wheal, flare or eruption indicates procaine sensitivity. Sensitivity should be treated by the usual methods, including barbiturates, and procaine penicillin preparations should not be used. Antihistaminics appear beneficial in treatment of procaine reactions.
The use of antibiotics may result in overgrowth of nonsusceptible organisms. Constant observation of the patient is essential. If new infections due to bacteria or fungi appear during therapy, the drug should be discontinued and appropriate measures taken.
Whenever allergic reactions occur, penicillin should be withdrawn unless, in the opinion of the physician, the condition being treated is life-threatening and amenable only to penicillin therapy.
In prolonged therapy with penicillin, and particularly with high-dosage schedules, periodic evaluation of the renal and hematopoietic systems is recommended.
Adverse Reactions: Penicillin is a substance of low toxicity but does possess a significant index of sensitization. The following hypersensitivity reactions associated with use of penicillin have been reported: Skin rashes, ranging from maculopapular eruptions to exfoliative dermatitis; urticaria; serum sickness-like reactions, including chills, fever, edema, arthralgia and prostration. Severe and often fatal anaphylaxis has been reported (see "Warnings").
Dosage and Administration: Administer by **DEEP INTRAMUSCULAR INJECTION** in the upper outer quadrant of the buttock. In infants and small children, the midlateral aspect of the thigh may be preferable. When doses are repeated, vary the injection site. Before injecting the dose, aspirate to be sure needle bevel is not in a blood vessel.
The Wyeth disposable syringe for this product incorporates several new features that are designed to facilitate its use.
A single small indentation, or "dot", has been punched into the metal ring that surrounds the neck of the syringe near the base of the needle. It is important that this "dot" be placed in a position so that it can be easily visualized by the operator following the intramuscular insertion of the syringe needle. Once the needle has been inserted, aspiration should be carried out in accordance with good medical technic before the medication is injected. During the process of aspiration the barrel of the syringe immediately proximal to the location of the "dot" should be closely observed by the operator, since this is the area in which blood that may have entered the needle is most likely to appear.
When using the TUBEX or the disposable syringe, if blood or any suspicious discoloration is apparent, the needle should be withdrawn without injecting any of the medication, the syringe and its contents discarded, and the process repeated using a new syringe at a different site.
Streptococcal infections Group A—Infections of the upper respiratory tract, skin and soft tissue infections, scarlet fever and erysipelas.
The following doses are recommended:
Adults and children over 60 lbs. in weight: 2,400,000 units. Children from 30–60 lbs.: 900,000 units to 1,200,000 units. Infants and children under 30 lbs.: 600,000 units.
NOTE: Treatment with the recommended dosage is usually given at a single session using multiple IM sites when indicated. An alternative dosage schedule may be used giving one half (½) the total dose on day 1 and one half (½) on day 3. This will also insure the penicillinemia required over a 10-day period; however, this alternate schedule should be used only when the physician can be assured of the patient's cooperation.
Pneumococcal infections (except pneumococcal meningitis): 600,000 units in children and 1,200,000 units in adults repeated every 2 or 3 days until the temperature is normal for 48 hours. Other forms of penicillin may be necessary for severe cases.
Shake multiple dose vial vigorously before withdrawing the desired dose. Shake Tubex® and disposable syringe well before using.
How Supplied: *300,000 units per ml.*—multiple-dose vials of 10 ml. *600,000 units per ml.*—1 ml. Tubex® Sterile Cartridge-Needle Units, packages of 10 and 50; 2 ml. Tubex Sterile Cartridge-Needle Units (1,200,000 units per Tubex), packages of 10 and 50; 2 ml. single-dose (1,200,000 units) disposable syringes, packages of 10; 4 ml. single-dose (2,400,000 units) disposable syringes, packages of 10.

Continued on next page

Wyeth—Cont.

BICILLIN® C-R 900/300 ℞
(penicillin G benzathine and penicillin G procaine suspension) for deep IM injection only

Description: Each TUBEX® cartridge (2 ml size) contains 1,200,000 units of penicillin comprising: 900,000 units penicillin G benzathine and 300,000 units penicillin G procaine in a stabilized aqueous suspension with sodium citrate buffer; and as w/v, approximately 0.5% lecithin, 0.55% carboxymethylcellulose, 0.55% povidone, 0.1% methylparaben, and 0.01% propylparaben.
Actions and Pharmacology: Penicillin G exerts a bactericidal action against penicillin-sensitive microorganisms during the stage of active multiplication. It acts through the inhibition of biosynthesis of cell-wall mucopeptide. It is not active against the penicillinase-producing bacteria, which include many strains of staphylococci. Penicillin G exerts high *in vitro* activity against staphylococci (except penicillinase-producing strains), streptococci (groups A, C, G, H, L, and M), and pneumococci. Other organisms sensitive to penicillin G are *Neisseria gonorrhoeae, Corynebacterium diphtheriae, Bacillus anthracis,* Clostridia, *Actinomyces bovis, Streptobacillus moniliformis, Listeria monocytogenes,* and Leptospira. *Treponema pallidum* is extremely sensitive to the bactericidal action of penicillin G.
Sensitivity plate testing: If the Kirby-Bauer method of disc sensitivity is used, a 10-unit penicillin disc should give a zone greater than 28 mm. when tested against a penicillin-sensitive bacterial strain.
Intramuscular penicillin G benzathine is absorbed very slowly into the bloodstream from the intramuscular site and converted by hydrolysis to penicillin G. This combination of hydrolysis and slow absorption results in blood serum levels much lower but much more prolonged than other parenteral penicillins.
Penicillin G procaine is an equimolecular compound of procaine and penicillin G, administered intramuscularly as a suspension. It dissolves slowly at the site of injection, giving a plateau type of blood level at about 4 hours which falls slowly over a period of the next 15–20 hours.
Approximately 60% of penicillin G is bound to serum protein. The drug is distributed throughout the body tissues in widely varying amounts. Highest levels are found in the kidneys with lesser amounts in the liver, skin, and intestines. Penicillin G penetrates into all other tissues and the spinal fluid to a lesser degree. With normal kidney function the drug is excreted rapidly by tubular excretion. In neonates and young infants and in individuals with impaired kidney function, excretion is considerably delayed.
Indications: This drug is indicated for use in children of all ages in the treatment of moderately severe infections due to penicillin G-susceptible microorganisms that are susceptible to serum levels common to this particular dosage form. Therapy should be guided by bacteriological studies (including susceptibility testing) and by clinical response.
NOTE: When high-sustained serum levels are required, penicillin G sodium or potassium, either IM or IV, should be used. This drug should *not* be used in the treatment of venereal diseases, including syphilis, gonorrhea, yaws, bejel, and pinta.
The following infections will usually respond to adequate dosages of this drug:
Streptococcal infections Group A (without bacteremia). Moderately severe to severe infections of the upper respiratory tract, skin and soft tissue infections, scarlet fever, and erysipelas.
NOTE: Streptococci in groups A, C, G, H, L, and M are very sensitive to penicillin G. Other groups, including group D (enterococci), are resistant. Penicillin G sodium or potassium is recommended for streptococcal infections with bacteremia.
Pneumococcal infections. Moderately severe pneumonia and otitis media.
NOTE: Severe pneumonia, empyema, bacteremia, pericarditis, meningitis, peritonitis, and arthritis of pneumococcal etiology are better treated with penicillin G sodium or potassium during the acute stage.
Contraindications: A previous hypersensitivity reaction to any penicillin or to procaine is a contraindication.
Warnings: Serious and occasionally fatal hypersensitivity (anaphylactoid) reactions have been reported in patients on penicillin therapy. Although anaphylaxis is more frequent following parenteral therapy, it has occurred in patients on oral penicillins. These reactions are more apt to occur in individuals with a history of sensitivity to multiple allergens.
There have been well-documented reports of individuals with a history of penicillin hypersensitivity reactions who have experienced severe hypersensitivity reactions when treated with a cephalosporin. Before therapy with a penicillin, careful inquiry should be made concerning previous hypersensitivity reactions to penicillins, cephalosporins, and other allergens. If an allergic reaction occurs, the drug should be discontinued and the patient treated with the usual agents, e.g., pressor amines, antihistamines, and corticosteroids.
Precautions: Penicillin should be used with caution in individuals with histories of significant allergies and/or asthma.
Care should be taken to avoid intravenous or intra-arterial administration, or injection into or near major peripheral nerves or blood vessels, since such injections may produce neurovascular damage.
In streptococcal infections, therapy must be sufficient to eliminate the organism; otherwise the sequelae of streptococcal disease may occur. Cultures should be taken following completion of treatment to determine whether streptococci have been eradicated.
A small percentage of patients are sensitive to procaine. If there is a history of sensitivity make the usual test: Inject intradermally 0.1 ml of a 1 to 2 percent procaine solution. Development of an erythema, wheal, flare, or eruption indicates procaine sensitivity. Sensitivity should be treated by the usual methods, including barbiturates, and procaine penicillin preparations should not be used. Antihistaminics appear beneficial in treatment of procaine reactions.
The use of antibiotics may result in overgrowth of nonsusceptible organisms. Constant observation of the patient is essential. If new infections due to bacteria or fungi appear during therapy, the drug should be discontinued and appropriate measures taken.
Whenever allergic reactions occur, penicillin should be withdrawn unless, in the opinion of the physician, the condition being treated is life-threatening and amenable only to penicillin therapy.
In prolonged therapy with penicillin, and particularly with high-dosage schedules, periodic evaluation of the renal and hematopoietic systems is recommended.
Adverse reactions: Penicillin is a substance of low toxicity but does possess a significant index of sensitization. The following hypersensitivity reactions associated with use of penicillin have been reported: skin rashes, ranging from maculopapular eruptions to exfoliative dermatitis; urticaria; serum sickness-like reactions, including chills, fever, edema, arthralgia, and prostration. Severe and often fatal anaphylaxis has been reported (see "Warnings").
Dosage and Administration: Administer by DEEP INTRAMUSCULAR INJECTION in the upper, outer quadrant of the buttock. In infants and small children, the midlateral aspect of the thigh may be preferable. When doses are repeated, vary the injection site. Before injecting the dose, aspirate to be sure needle bevel is not in a blood vessel. If blood or any suspicious discoloration is apparent, the needle should be withdrawn without injecting any of the medication, the syringe and its contents discarded, and the process repeated using a new syringe at a different site.
Streptococcal infections Group A—Infections of the upper respiratory tract, skin and soft tissue infections, scarlet fever, and erysipelas.
A single injection of Bicillin C-R 900/300 is usually sufficient for the treatment of Group A streptococcal infections in children of all ages.
Pneumococcal infections (except pneumococcal meningitis): One TUBEX Bicillin C-R 900/300 repeated at 2- or 3-day intervals until the temperature is normal for 48 hours. Other forms of penicillin may be necessary for severe cases.
How Supplied: Bicillin® C-R 900/300 is supplied in 2 ml TUBEX® (Sterile Cartridge-Needle Unit) in packages of 10.

BICILLIN® L-A ℞
(sterile penicillin G benzathine suspension) INJECTION

Description: Each Tubex® sterile cartridge-needle unit or disposable syringe contains penicillin G benzathine in aqueous suspension with sodium citrate buffer; and as w/v, approximately 0.5% lecithin, 0.6% carboxymethylcellulose, 0.6% povidone, 0.1% methylparaben and 0.01% propylparaben.
Each multiple-dose vial contains in each milliliter 300,000 units penicillin G benzathine with sodium citrate buffer and approx. 6 mg. lecithin, 3 mg. povidone, 1 mg. carboxymethylcellulose, 0.5 mg. sorbitan monopalmitate, 0.5 mg. polyoxyethylene sorbitan monopalmitate, 1.2 mg. methylparaben and 0.14 mg. propylparaben.
FOR DEEP INTRAMUSCULAR INJECTION ONLY
Actions and Pharmacology: Penicillin G exerts a bactericidal action against penicillin-sensitive microorganisms during the stage of active multiplication. It acts through the inhibition of biosynthesis of cell-wall mucopeptide. It is not active against the penicillinase-producing bacteria, which include many strains of staphylococci. Penicillin G exerts high *in vitro* activity against staphylococci (except penicillinase-producing strains), streptococci (groups A, C, G, H, L and M), and pneumococci. Other organisms sensitive to penicillin G are: *Neisseria gonorrhoeae, Corynebacterium diphtheriae, Bacillus anthracis,* Clostridia, *Actinomyces bovis, Streptobacillus moniliformis, Listeria monocytogenes,* and Leptospira. *Treponema pallidum* is extremely sensitive to the bactericidal action of penicillin G.
Intramuscular penicillin G benzathine is absorbed very slowly into the bloodstream from the intramuscular site and converted by hydrolysis to penicillin G. This combination of hydrolysis and slow absorption results in blood serum levels much lower but much more prolonged than other parenteral penicillins.
Approximately 60% of penicillin G is bound to serum protein. The drug is distributed throughout the body tissues in widely varying amounts. Highest levels are found in the kidneys with lesser amounts in the liver, skin and intestines. Penicillin G penetrates into all other tissues and the spinal fluid to a lesser degree. With normal kidney function the drug is excreted rapidly by tubular excretion. In neonates and young infants and in individuals with impaired kidney function, excretion is considerably delayed.
Indications: Intramuscular penicillin G benzathine is indicated in the treatment of infec-

tions due to penicillin G sensitive microorganisms that are susceptible to the low and very prolonged serum levels common to this particular dosage form. Therapy should be guided by bacteriological studies (including sensitivity tests) and by clinical response.
The following infections will usually respond to adequate dosage of intramuscular penicillin G benzathine.
Streptococcal infections (group A—without bacteremia). Mild-to-moderate infections of the upper respiratory tract (e.g. pharyngitis).
Venereal infections—Syphilis, yaws, bejel, and pinta.
Medical Conditions in Which Penicillin G Benzathine Therapy Is Indicated as Prophylaxis: Rheumatic fever and/or chorea—Prophylaxis with penicillin G benzathine has proven effective in preventing recurrence of these conditions. It has also been used as follow-up prophylactic therapy for rheumatic heart disease and acute glomerulonephritis.
Contraindications: A history of a previous hypersensitivity reaction to any of the penicillins is a contraindication.
Warnings: Serious and occasionally fatal hypersensitivity (anaphylactoid) reactions have been reported in patients on penicillin therapy. Although anaphylaxis is more frequent following parenteral therapy it has occurred in patients on oral penicillins. These reactions are more apt to occur in individuals with a history of sensitivity to multiple allergens.
There have been well-documented reports of individuals with a history of penicillin hypersensitivity reactions who have experienced severe hypersensitivity reactions when treated with a cephalosporin. Before therapy with a penicillin, careful inquiry should be made concerning previous hypersensitivity reactions to penicillins, cephalosporins, and other allergens. If an allergic reaction occurs, the drug should be discontinued and the patient treated with the usual agents e.g., pressor amines, antihistamines and corticosteroids.
Precautions: Penicillin should be used with caution in individuals with histories of significant allergies and/or asthma.
Care should be taken to avoid intravenous or intra-arterial administration, or injection into or near major peripheral nerves or blood vessels, since such injection may produce neurovascular damage.
In streptococcal infections, therapy must be sufficient to eliminate the organism; otherwise the sequelae of streptococcal disease may occur. Cultures should be taken following completion of treatment to determine whether streptococci have been eradicated.
Prolonged use of antibiotics may promote the overgrowth of nonsusceptible organisms, including fungi. Should superinfection occur, appropriate measures should be taken.
Adverse Reactions: The hypersensitivity reactions reported are skin eruptions (maculopapular to exfoliative dermatitis), urticaria and other serum sickness-like reactions, laryngeal edema and anaphylaxis. Fever and eosinophilia may frequently be the only reaction observed. Hemolytic anemia, leukopenia, thrombocytopenia, neuropathy and nephropathy are infrequent reactions and usually associated with high doses of parenteral penicillin.
As with other treatments for syphilis, the Jarisch-Herxheimer reaction has been reported.
Dosage and Administration:
Streptococcal (Group A) upper respiratory infections (for example, pharyngitis).
A single injection of 1,200,000 units for adults.
A single injection of 900,000 units for older children.
A single injection of 300,000 to 600,000 units for infants and for children under 60 pounds.
Venereal infections—
Syphilis—Primary, secondary and latent—2.4 million units (1 dose). Late (tertiary and neurosyphilis)—2.4 million units at 7-day intervals for three doses.
Congenital—under 2 years of age: 50,000 units/kg./body weight; ages 2-12 years: adjust dosage based on adult dosage schedule.
Yaws, Bejel and Pinta—1.2 million units (1 injection).
Prophylaxis—for rheumatic fever and glomerulonephritis.
Following an acute attack, penicillin G benzathine (parenteral) may be given in doses of 1,200,000 units once a month or 600,000 units every 2 weeks.
Administer by **deep intramuscular injection** in the upper outer quadrant of the buttock. In infants and small children, the midlateral aspect of the thigh may be preferable. When doses are repeated, vary the injection site. Before injecting the dose, aspirate to be sure needle bevel is not in a blood vessel.
The Wyeth disposable syringe for this product incorporates several new features that are designed to facilitate its use.
A single small indentation, or "dot", has been punched into the metal ring that surrounds the neck of the syringe near the base of the needle. It is important that this "dot" be placed in a position so that it can be easily visualized by the operator following the intramuscular insertion of the syringe needle. Once the needle has been inserted, aspiration should be carried out in accordance with good medical technic before the medication is injected. During the process of aspiration the barrel of the syringe immediately proximal to the location of the "dot" should be closely observed by the operator, since this is the area in which blood that may have entered the needle is most likely to appear.
When using the TUBEX or the disposable syringe, if blood or any suspicious discoloration is apparent, the needle should be withdrawn without injecting any of the medication, the syringe and its contents discarded, and the process repeated using a new syringe at a different site.
Some TUBEX cartridges and disposable syringes may contain a small air bubble which may be disregarded since it does not affect administration of the product. Because of the high concentration of suspended material in this product, the needle may be blocked if the injection is not made at a slow, steady rate.
Shake multiple dose vial vigorously before withdrawing the desired dose.
How Supplied: BICILLIN® L-A (sterile penicillin G benzathine suspension) Injection: *300,000 units per ml.*—vials of 10 ml.; *600,000 units per 1 ml.* TUBEX® sterile cartridge needle unit, packages of 10; *900,000 units per* TUBEX—1.5 ml. fill in 2 ml. size, packages of 10; *1,200,000 units per 2 ml.* disposable syringe or TUBEX, packages of 10; *2,400,000 units per 4 ml.* disposable syringe, packages of 10.

BIOLOGICALS

ANTIVENIN (CROTALIDAE) POLYVALENT (equine origin) ℞

Composition: Each combination package contains: One vacuum vial to yield 10 ml of serum—to be used immediately after reconstitution—(with preservatives: phenol 0.25% and thimerosal mercury derivative 0.005%). One vial containing 10 ml of Bacteriostatic Water for Injection, USP (with preservative: phenylmercuric nitrate 0.001%). One 1 ml vial of normal horse serum (diluted 1:10) as sensitivity testing material with preservatives: thimerosal (mercury derivative) 0.005% and phenol 0.35%.
How Supplied: Combination packages as described (not returnable).

ANTIVENIN (Micrurus fulvius) (equine origin) ℞

Composition: Each combination package contains one vial of lyophilized Antivenin (Micrurus fulvius) with 0.25% phenol and 0.005% thimerosal (mercury derivative) as preservatives (before lyophilization); one vial of diluent containing 10 ml. of Bacteriostatic Water for Injection, U.S.P., with phenylmercuric nitrate (1:100,000) as preservative.
How Supplied: Combination packages as described (not returnable).

CHOLERA VACCINE, U.S.P. ℞

Description: Each ml. contains 8 units each serotype antigen (Ogawa and Inaba). The preservative is 0.5% phenol.
How Supplied: Vials of 1.5 ml. and 20 ml.

DIPHTHERIA AND TETANUS TOXOIDS ADSORBED (PEDIATRIC) aluminum phosphate adsorbed, ULTRAFINED® ℞

Description: Antigens adsorbed on aluminum phosphate. Preservative is 0.01% thimerosal (mercury derivative).
How Supplied: Vials of 5 ml.; and 0.5-ml. TUBEX® Sterile Cartridge-Needle Units, packages of 10.

DIPHTHERIA AND TETANUS TOXOIDS AND PERTUSSIS VACCINE ADSORBED aluminum phosphate adsorbed ULTRAFINED® Triple Antigen ℞

Description: Triple Antigen Adsorbed (Diphtheria and Tetanus Toxoids and Pertussis Vaccine Adsorbed), Wyeth, is a combination of diphtheria toxoid adsorbed, tetanus toxoid adsorbed, and pertussis vaccine. The diphtheria toxoid is prepared by cultivating a suitable strain of *Corynebacterium diphtheriae* on a modified Mueller's casein hydrolysate medium (J. Immunology *37:*103, 1939). The tetanus toxoid is prepared by growing a suitable strain of *Clostridium tetani* on a protein-free semisynthetic medium (Appl. Microbiol. *10:*146, 1962). Formaldehyde is used as the toxoiding (detoxifying) agent for both diphtheria and tetanus toxins. The final product contains no more than 0.02 percent free formaldehyde. The pertussis vaccine component is prepared by growing suitable strains of Phase I B. pertussis on a modified Cohen and Wheeler medium: casein hydrolysate medium with yeast dialyzate (Wadsworth:Standard Methods, 3rd. Ed., p. 200, Williams and Wilkins Co., 1947) supplemented with 5% agar and 4% charcoal. The preservative in the final product is 0.01% thimerosal (mercury derivative).
The aluminum content of the final product does not exceed 0.85 mg per 0.5 ml dose. During processing, hydrochloric acid and sodium hydroxide are used to adjust the pH. Sodium chloride is added to the final product to control isotonicity.
The total primary immunizing dose (1.5 ml) contains 12 protective units of pertussis vaccine.
Indication: Triple Antigen, Aluminum Phosphate Adsorbed, Wyeth, is indicated for active immunization of infants and children through 6 years of age against diphtheria, tetanus, and pertussis.[1]
Contraindications: An acute respiratory infection or other active infection is reason for deferring administration.
Occurrence of any of the following signs, symptoms, or conditions following administration is a contraindication to further use of this product and/or pertussis vaccine as the single anti-

Continued on next page

Wyeth—Cont.

gen: fever over 103° F (39° C); convulsion(s) with or without accompanying fever; alterations of consciousness; focal neurologic signs; screaming episodes (also called screaming fits); shock; collapse; thrombocytopenic purpura.[2]
The presence of an evolving or changing neurologic disorder is a contraindication to use.
Immunosuppressive therapy, including irradiation, corticosteroids, antimetabolites, alkylating agents, and cytotoxic agents may result in aberrant responses to active immunization procedures.
Administration should be deferred in individuals receiving such therapy.

Precautions: This product should be used for the age group between two months and the seventh birthday.
When an infant or child is returned for the next dose in the series, the parent should be questioned concerning occurrence of any symptoms and/or signs of a severe adverse reaction after the previous dose (See Contraindications; Side Effects and Adverse Reactions). If such are reported, further doses of Triple Antigen are contraindicated and active immunization against diphtheria and tetanus should be completed with Diphtheria and Tetanus Toxoids Adsorbed **(Pediatric)**.
If the vial is used, rather than the TUBEX® Sterile Cartridge-Needle Unit, a separate syringe and needle which have been adequately cleaned and sterilized should be used for each patient to prevent transmission of hepatitis B virus and other infectious agents from one person to another.
Before the injection of any biological, the physician should take all precautions known for prevention of allergic or any other side reactions. This should include: A review of the patient's history regarding possible sensitivity; the ready availability of epinephrine 1:1000 and other appropriate agents used for control of immediate allergic reactions; and a knowledge of the recent literature pertaining to use of the biological concerned, including the nature of side effects and adverse reactions that may follow its use.

Side Effects and Adverse Reactions: Local reactions, manifested by erythema and induration with or without tenderness, are common after administration of Triple Antigen Adsorbed.[3] Such local reactions are usually self-limited and require no therapy. A nodule may be palpable at the injection site for a few weeks. Abscess formation at the site of injection has been reported.
Mild-to-moderate temperature elevations, accompanied by malaise occurring within several hours of administration and persisting for one to two days, occur frequently.[3]
The below-listed serious, and occasionally fatal, adverse reactions have been reported following administration of pertussis-vaccine-containing preparations. The incidence of these reactions is unknown, but they seem to be exceedingly rare. Should such reactions occur, further immunization against pertussis is contraindicated.[2] See also Contraindications and Precautions.

1. Severe temperature elevations—105° F or higher.
2. Collapse with rapid recovery.
3. Collapse followed by prolonged prostration and a shock-like state.
4. Screaming episodes characterized by a prolonged period of peculiar crying during which the infant cannot be comforted.
5. Isolated convulsion(s) with or without fever.
6. Frank encephalopathy with changes in the level of consciousness, focal neurological signs, and convulsions with or without permanent neurological and/or mental deficit.[4–9]
7. Thrombocytopenic purpura.

The occurrence of sudden-infant-death syndrome (SIDS) has been reported following administration of DTP.[10,11] The significance of these reports is unclear. It should be kept in mind that the three primary immunizing doses of DTP are usually administered to infants between the age of 2 and 6 months and that approximately 85 percent of SIDS cases occur in the period 1 through 6 months of age, with the peak incidence at age 2 to 4 months.[12,13]

Dosage and Administration: The basic immunizing course for infants and children through 6 years of age consists of three (primary) doses of 0.5 ml each at 4- to 8-week intervals, followed by a fourth (reinforcing) dose of 0.5 ml approximately one year after the third primary dose. The fourth (reinforcing) dose is an integral part of the basic immunizing course; basic immunization cannot be considered completed until the reinforcing dose has been given.
Interruption of the recommended schedule with a delay between doses does not interfere with the final immunity achieved; nor does it necessitate starting the series over again, regardless of the length of time elapsed between doses.[2] All doses should be injected intramuscularly, preferably into the midlateral muscles of the thigh or deltoid, with care to avoid major peripheral nerve trunks. The same muscle site should not be injected more than once during the course of basic immunization. It is recommended that active immunization against diphtheria, tetanus, and pertussis be started at 2 months of age.[1,2]
A routine recall (booster) dose of 0.5 ml is indicated at age 4–6 years, preferably prior to entrance into kindergarten or elementary school.
If a child less than 6 years of age who has received fewer than 4 properly spaced doses of a DTP preparation is exposed to diphtheria or pertussis or suffers a wound which might possibly be contaminated with Cl. tetani spores or bacilli, it may be advisable to administer a 0.5 ml dose of this product (or the appropriate single active immunizing antigen) AND: 1. an adequate dose of the appropriate passive immunizing agent (at a different site with a different syringe); 2. an adequate course of the prophylactic therapy with an appropriate antibiotic, depending, among other factors, on the number of doses of DTP received in the past and the interval since the last dose, the duration and intimacy of exposure, and the interval between exposure and initiation of specific prophylactic measures.
For basic or recall (booster) immunization against tetanus and diphtheria of individuals over 6 years of age, the use of Tetanus and Diphtheria Toxoids Adsorbed, Aluminum Phosphate Adsorbed **(For Adult Use)** is recommended.

How Supplied: Diphtheria and Tetanus Toxoids and Pertussis Vaccine Adsorbed, Aluminum Phosphate Adsorbed, Ultrafined®, Triple Antigen, is available in vials of 7.5 ml and 0.5 ml TUBEX® Sterile Cartridge-Needle Units in packages of 10 TUBEX.

Technic for Injection: Before injection, the skin over the site to be injected should be cleansed and prepared with a suitable germicide. After insertion of the needle, aspirate to help avoid inadvertent injection into a blood vessel. Expel the antigen slowly and terminate the dose with a small bubble of air (0.1 to 0.2 ml). Do not inject intracutaneously or into superficial subcutaneous structures.

Directions for Use of Vials

Shake the vial vigorously before withdrawing each dose.

Before injection, the rubber diaphragm of the vial should be cleansed and prepared with a suitable germicide. Injections from the vial must be administered promptly to prevent settling of the material in the syringe. Flush the syringe after injection to prevent the remaining material from drying within the syringe.

References:

1. Recommendation of the Public Health Service Advisory Committee on Immunization Practices. Morbidity and Mortality Weekly Report 26 (No. 49): 401, 1977.
2. Report of the Committee on Infectious Diseases, American Academy of Pediatrics (Red Book), 1977.
3. BARKIN, R., PICHICHERO, M.: Diphtheria-pertussis-tetanus vaccine: Reactogenicity of commercial products. Pediatrics *63:*256, 1979.
4. TOOMEY, J. A.: Reactions to pertussis vaccine. J. Am. Med. Assoc. *139:*448, 1949.
5. BYERS, B. K., MOLL, F. C.: Encephalopathies following prophylactic pertussis vaccine. Pediatrics *1:*437, 1948.
6. BERG, J.: Neurological complications of pertussis immunization. Brit. Med. J. *2:*24, 1958.
7. STROM, J.: Further experience of reactions, especially of a cerebral nature, in conjunction with triple vaccination: A study based on vaccinations in Sweden. 1959–65. Brit. Med. J. *4:*320, 1967.
8. STEWART, G.: Vaccination against whooping cough. Efficacy versus risks. Lancet *1:*234, 1977.
9. KULENKAMPFF, M. et al.: Neurological complications of pertussis inoculation. Arch. Dis. Child. *49:*46, 1974.
10. Morbidity and Mortality Weekly Report: DTP vaccination and sudden infant deaths—Tennessee. *28* (No. 11):131, 1979.
11. Morbidity and Mortality Weekly Report: Follow-up on DTP vaccination and sudden infant deaths—Tennessee. *28* (No. 12):134, 1979.
12. STANDFAST, S., et al.: The epidemiology of sudden infant death in upstate New York. JAMA *241:*1127, 1979.
13. KRAUS, J., BORHANI, N.: Post-neonatal sudden unexplained death in California: A cohort study. Am. J. Epidemiol. *95:*497, 1972.

DRYVAX® ℞
(dried smallpox vaccine) calf lymph type

For complete prescribing information, see alphabetical product monograph.

IMMUNE SERUM GLOBULIN ℞
(human), U.S.P.

Description: Immune Serum Globulin (human), U.S.P. is a sterile concentrated solution containing 16.5% (±1.5%) immunoglobulin stabilized with 0.3M glycine and containing 1:10,000 thimerosal (mercury derivative) as preservative.

How Supplied: Vials of 10 ml; and 2 ml Tubex® Sterile Cartridge-Needle Units, packages of 1.

INFLUENZA VIRUS VACCINE, SUBVIRION TYPE ℞

For current information about formulation, dosage and recommended use, consult product direction circular which can be obtained through your Wyeth representative or by writing Professional Service, Wyeth Laboratories, P.O. Box 8299, Phila., Pa. 19101.

SMALLPOX VACCINE, DRIED
calf lymph type
(*See* DRYVAX® [dried smallpox vaccine])

TETANUS AND DIPHTHERIA TOXOIDS ADSORBED ℞
(for adult use)
aluminum phosphate adsorbed
ULTRAFINED®

Description: A combination of refined tetanus and diphtheria toxoids for adult use, in which the fully potent antigens are adsorbed on aluminum phosphate. The preservative is 0.01% thimerosal (mercury derivative). Each dose

contains no more than 2 Lf of purified diphtheria toxoid.
How Supplied: Vials of 5 ml.; and 0.5-ml. TUBEX® Sterile Cartridge-Needle Units, packages of 10.

TETANUS IMMUNE GLOBULIN ℞
(human)

Description: A sterile 16.5% (± 1.5%) solution of human gamma globulin, prepared by Cohn cold ethanol fractionation of plasma from donors hyperimmunized with tetanus toxoid. The final product contains 0.3 molar glycine as a diluent and stabilizer and 0.01% thimerosal (mercury derivative) as a preservative. Prepared from blood that was nonreactive when tested for hepatitis B surface antigen (HB_s Ag).
How Supplied: 1 ml TUBEX® Sterile Cartridge-Needle Unit, packages of 10.

TETANUS TOXOID ADSORBED ℞
aluminum phosphate adsorbed, ULTRAFINED®

Description: A refined toxoid, in which the fully potent antigen is adsorbed on aluminum phosphate. The preservative is 0.01% thimerosal (mercury derivative).
How Supplied: Vials of 5 ml.; and 0.5-ml. TUBEX® Sterile Cartridge-Needle Units, packages of 10.

TETANUS TOXOID, fluid ℞
purified, ULTRAFINED®

Description: A refined tetanus toxoid. The preservative is 0.01% thimerosal (mercury derivative).
How Supplied: Vials of 7.5 ml.; and 0.5-ml. TUBEX® Sterile Cartridge-Needle Units, packages of 10.

TYPHOID VACCINE, U.S.P. ℞

Description: Each ml. contains not more than 1000 million Salmonella typhosa (Ty-2 strain) organisms, killed and suspended in buffered sodium chloride injection. The preservative is 0.5% phenol. Contains 8 units per ml.
How Supplied: Vials of 5 ml., 10 ml., and 20 ml.

Full prescribing information on the Biological Products listed above is available on request.

Smallpox Vaccine
Dried
Calf Lymph Type
DRYVAX® ℞
dried smallpox vaccine

Composition: DRYVAX, SMALLPOX VACCINE, DRIED, is prepared from calf lymph. The calf lymph is purified, concentrated, and dried by lyophilization. During processing, not more than 100 units of polymyxin B sulfate, 200 micrograms of dihydrostreptomycin sulfate, 200 micrograms of chlortetracycline hydrochloride, and 100 micrograms of neomycin sulfate per ml are added, and trace amounts of these antibiotics may be present in the final product. The reconstituted vaccine has been shown by appropriate test methods to contain not more than 200 organisms per ml.
The Diluent for DRYVAX, SMALLPOX VACCINE, DRIED, contains 50% glycerine, 0.25% phenol in Sterile Water for Injection, USP, with 0.005% brilliant green.
Storage: Store DRYVAX in the refrigerator (2-8° C, 35-46° F). RECONSTITUTED DRYVAX may be used for 3 months if stored in the coldest part of the refrigerator, preferably below 0° C (32° F), when not in actual use. At time of reconstitution, record date in space provided on vial label.
DRYVAX should not be used after the expiration date regardless of whether it is in the dry or reconstituted form.
Indications: Smallpox vaccine is indicated for and should only be used for immunization against smallpox.
The PHS Advisory Committee on Immunization Practices recommends that use of smallpox vaccine in the United States be limited to:
1. Travelers to countries that require valid International Certificates of Vaccination.
2. Travelers to or from countries in which smallpox is occurring.
3. Personnel of laboratories working with variola virus.
For those in the above special-risk categories, revaccination is recommended at appropriate intervals (approximately every three years).
Directions for Reconstitution: Complete directions for reconstitution and use of reconstituted vaccine are given in the package Literature.
Interpretation of Responses: The vaccination site should be inspected 6 to 8 days after vaccination. The response should be interpreted as follows:
PRIMARY VACCINATION
A primary vaccination which is successful should show a typical Jennerian vesicle. If none is observed, vaccination procedures should be checked and vaccination repeated with another lot of vaccine until a successful result is obtained.
REVACCINATION
Following revaccination, two responses are defined by the WHO Expert Committee on Smallpox, eliminating use of older terms such as "accelerated", "vaccinoid", and "immune".
a. "MAJOR REACTION"
A vesicular or pustular lesion or an area of definite palpable induration or congestion surrounding a central lesion which may be a crust or ulcer. This reaction indicates that virus multiplication has most likely taken place and that the revaccination is successful.
b. "EQUIVOCAL REACTION"
Any other reaction should be regarded as equivocal. These responses may be the consequence of immunity adequate to suppress virus multiplication or may represent only allergic reactions to an inactive vaccine. If an equivocal reaction is observed, revaccination procedures should be checked and revaccination repeated with another lot of vaccine.
Precautions: Smallpox vaccine should NOT be used for treatment of warts or prevention of recurrent herpes simplex infections.
Blot off any vaccine remaining on skin at vaccination site with clean, dry gauze or cotton.
The vaccine vial, its stopper, and the needle used for administration should be burned, boiled, or autoclaved before disposal.
In the past, it has been generally recommended that there be an interval of no less than one month between administrations of live virus vaccines, whenever possible. However, simultaneous administration of various live virus vaccines offers some obvious advantages, particularly when there is a threat of concomitant exposure, when the individual to be immunized may be inaccessible for further immunization, or when a one-month interval would disrupt immunization programs. Such situations are valid reasons for simultaneous administration of poliovirus, measles, smallpox, and yellow fever vaccines, provided no contraindication is present to use of any of the individual vaccines. If the theoretically desirable one-month interval is not feasible, the vaccines should be given on the same day—at different sites for parenteral products. An interval of about two days to two weeks between live-virus-vaccine administrations should always be avoided.
Contraindications: Primary AND revaccination with smallpox vaccine are contraindicated:
1. For infants manifesting failure to thrive.
2. For individuals of any age with eczema, other skin conditions, wounds, or burns or for siblings or other household contacts of such individuals.
3. For persons of any age receiving therapy with X ray, ACTH, corticosteroids, or immunosuppressive drugs.
4. For individuals with known or suspected disorders of gamma globulin synthesis.
5. For individuals with leukemia, lymphomas of any type, or other malignant neoplasms affecting the bone marrow or lymphatic systems.
6. During pregnancy.
In endemic areas or in direct contacts of smallpox cases, there are no absolute contraindications.
Side Effects and Complications: Complications that may follow either primary or revaccination include: encephalitis, encephalomyelitis, encephalopathy, transverse myelitis, acute infectious polyneuritis; vaccinia necrosum; eczema vaccinatum; generalized vaccinia; accidental infection (autoinoculation); generalized rashes (erythematous, urticarial, nonspecific); and secondary pyogenic infections at the site of vaccine application. Such complications may result in severe disability, permanent neurological sequelae, and/or death. Accidental infection (autoinoculation) of the eye may result in blindness. Lane and Millar[1] have analyzed the available data and estimated the risks of occurrence of complications after primary vaccination as follows:
[See table on next page].
How Supplied: Combination package of 1 vial of Dried Smallpox Vaccine, 1 container of Diluent (0.15 ml, sufficient for 25 vaccinations), and 25 sterile bifurcated needles.
Combination package of 1 vial of Dried Smallpox Vaccine, 1 container of Diluent (0.25 ml, sufficient for 100 vaccinations), and 100 sterile bifurcated needles.
Reference:
1. LANE, J. & MILLAR, J.: Risks of smallpox vaccination complications in the United States. Am. J. Epidemiol *93:*238, 1971.

EQUAGESIC® • © ℞
(meprobamate and ethoheptazine citrate with aspirin)

Description: Each tablet contains 150 mg meprobamate, 75 mg ethoheptazine citrate, and 250 mg aspirin.

Indications:
Based on a review of this drug by the National Academy of Sciences—National Research Council and/or other information, FDA has classified the indication as follows:
"Possibly" effective: for the treatment of pain accompanied by tension and/or anxiety in patients with musculoskeletal disease or tension headache.
Final classification of the less-than-effective indications requires further investigation.
The effectiveness of Equagesic (meprobamate and ethoheptazine citrate with aspirin) in long-term use, that is, more than 4 months, has not been assessed by systematic clinical studies. The physician should periodically reassess the usefulness of the drug for the individual patient.

Contraindications: Equagesic should not be given to individuals with a history of sensitivity or severe intolerance to aspirin, meprobamate, or ethoheptazine citrate.
Warnings: Careful supervision of dose and amounts prescribed for patients is advised, especially with those patients with a known propensity for taking excessive quantities of

Continued on next page

Wyeth—Cont.

drugs. Excessive and prolonged use in susceptible persons, for example, alcoholics, former addicts, and other severe psychoneurotics, has been reported to result in dependence on or habituation to the drug. Where excessive dosage has continued for weeks or months, dosage should be reduced gradually rather than abruptly stopped, since withdrawal of a "crutch" may precipitate withdrawal reaction of greater proportions than that for which the drug was originally prescribed. Abrupt discontinuance of doses in excess of the recommended dose has resulted in some cases in the occurrence of epileptiform seizures.
Special care should be taken to warn patients taking meprobamate that their tolerance to alcohol may be lowered with resultant slowing of reaction time and impairment of judgment and coordination.

USAGE IN PREGNANCY AND LACTATION

An increased risk of congenital malformations associated with the use of minor tranquilizers (meprobamate, chlordiazepoxide, and diazepam) during the first trimester of pregnancy has been suggested in several studies. Because use of these drugs is rarely a matter of urgency, their use during this period should almost always be avoided. The possibility that a woman of childbearing potential may be pregnant at the time of institution of therapy should be considered. Patients should be advised that if they become pregnant during therapy or intend to become pregnant they should communicate with their physicians about the desirability of discontinuing the drug.
Meprobamate passes the placental barrier. It is present both in umbilical-cord blood at or near maternal plasma levels and in breast milk of lactating mothers at concentrations two to four times that of maternal plasma. When use of meprobamate is contemplated in breast-feeding patients, the drug's higher concentrations in breast milk as compared to maternal plasma levels should be considered.
Preparations containing aspirin should be kept out of the reach of children. Equagesic is not recommended for patients 12 years of age and under.
Precautions: Should drowsiness, ataxia, or visual disturbance occur, the dose should be reduced. If the symptoms continue, the patient should not operate a motor vehicle or any dangerous machinery.
Suicidal attempts with meprobamate have resulted in coma, shock, vasomotor and respiratory collapse, and anuria. Very few suicidal attempts were fatal, although some patients ingested very large amounts of the drug (20 to 40 gram). These doses are much greater than those recommended. The drug should be given cautiously, and in small amounts, to patients who have suicidal tendencies. In cases where excessive doses have been taken, sleep ensues rapidly and blood pressure, pulse, and respiratory rates are reduced to basal levels. Hyperventilation has been reported occasionally. Any drug remaining in the stomach should be removed and symptomatic treatment given. Should respiration become very shallow and slow, central-nervous-system stimulants, such as caffeine, metrazol, or amphetamine, may be cautiously administered. If severe hypotension develops, pressor amines should be used parenterally to restore blood pressure to normal levels.
Adverse Reactions: A small percentage of patients may experience nausea with or without vomiting and epigastric distress. Dizziness occurs but rarely when meprobamate and ethoheptazine citrate with aspirin is administered in the recommended dosage. The meprobamate may cause drowsiness but, as a rule, this disappears as the therapy is continued. Should drowsiness persist and be associated with ataxia, this symptom can usually be controlled by decreasing the dose, but occasionally it may be desirable to administer central stimulants such as amphetamine or mephentermine sulfate concomitantly to control drowsiness.
A clearly related side effect to the administration of meprobamate is the rare occurrence of allergic or idiosyncratic reactions. This response develops, as a rule, in patients who have had only 1–4 doses of meprobamate and have not had a previous contact with the drug. Previous history of allergy may or may not be related to the incidence of reactions.
Mild reactions are characterized by an itchy urticarial or erythematous, maculopapular rash which may be generalized or confined to the groin. Acute nonthrombocytopenic purpura with cutaneous petechiae, ecchymoses, peripheral edema, and fever have also been reported.
The more severe cases, observed only very rarely, may also have other allergic responses, including fever, fainting spells, angioneurotic edema, bronchial spasms, hypotensive crises (1 fatal case), anaphylaxis, stomatitis and proctitis (1 case), and hyperthermia. Treatment should be symptomatic, such as the administration of epinephrine, antihistamine, and possibly hydrocortisone. Meprobamate should be stopped, and reinstitution of therapy should not be attempted.

Complication rates per million primary smallpox vaccinations in the United States by age and diagnosis

	Age at vaccination (in years)			
	1	1-4	5-19	20+
Death (from all complications)	5	0.5	0.5	unknown
Postvaccinial encephalitis	6	2	2.5	4
Vaccinia necrosum	1	0.5	1	7
Eczema vaccinatum	14	44	35	30
Generalized vaccinia	394	233	140	212
Accidental infection	507	577	371	606
Erythematous urticarial reactions	unknown	9,600	unknown	unknown

The risk associated with revaccination is extremely low but, as stated above, such complications have occurred, especially in patients with underlying diseases or receiving therapy which impairs immunologic competence or in subjects who have not been vaccinated for many years. Subjects who have not been vaccinated for many years may respond as primary vaccinees as regards both the local and systemic reaction to vaccine administration and risk of occurrence of the above-mentioned serious complications.

Rare cases have been reported where patients receiving meprobamate suffered from aplastic anemia (1 fatal case), thrombocytopenic purpura, agranulocytosis, and hemolytic anemia. In nearly every instance reported, other toxic agents known to have caused these conditions have been associated with the administration of meprobamate. A few cases of leukopenia during the continuous administration of meprobamate are reported; most of these returned to normal without discontinuation of the drug. Impairment of accommodation and visual acuity have been reported in rare instances.
Dosage and Administration: The usual dosage of Equagesic® (meprobamate and ethoheptazine citrate with aspirin) is one to two tablets 3 or 4 times daily as needed for the relief of pain and accompanying tension or anxiety.
Equagesic is not recommended for patients 12 years of age and under.
Overdose: Two instances of accidental or intentional significant overdosage with ethoheptazine citrate combined with aspirin have been reported. These were accompanied by symptoms of central-nervous-system depression, including drowsiness and a feeling of lightheadedness, with uneventful recovery. However, on the basis of pharmacological data, it may be anticipated that CNS stimulation could occur. Other anticipated symptoms would include nausea and vomiting. Appropriate therapy of the signs and symptoms as they appear is the only recommendation possible at this time. Overdosage with ethoheptazine combined with aspirin would probably produce the usual symptoms and signs of salicylate intoxication. Observation and treatment should include induced vomiting or gastric lavage, specific parenteral electrolyte therapy for ketoacidosis and dehydration, watching for evidence of hemorrhagic manifestations due to hypoprothrombinemia which, if it occurs, usually requires whole-blood transfusions.
How Supplied: Bottles of 50 scored tablets, and REDIPAK® (strip pack), Wyeth, boxes of 25 and 100.

[*Shown in Product Identification Section*]

EQUANIL® Ⓒ ℞
(meprobamate)
Capsules • Tablets

How Supplied: Tablets (white, scored)—200 mg and 400 mg, bottles of 50, 100, 500, 1000, and REDIPAK® (Strip Pack), boxes of 25; REDIPAK® (Unit Dose Medication), boxes of 100 (individually wrapped). WYSEALS® EQUANIL (meprobamate), especially coated for easy swallowing, sealed yellow tablets with no distinctive markings, 400 mg, bottles of 50 and 500. Capsules—400 mg, bottles of 50.
For prescribing information write to Professional Service, Wyeth Laboratories, Box 8299, Philadelphia, PA, 19101, or contact your local Wyeth representative.
[*Shown in Product Identification Section*]

LO/OVRAL® ℞
Tablets

Description: Each LO/OVRAL® tablet contains 0.3 mg of norgestrel (dl-13-beta-ethyl-17-alpha-ethinyl-17-beta-hydroxygon- 4-en-3-one), a totally synthetic progestogen, and 0.03 mg of ethinyl estradiol (19-Nor-17α-pregna-1,3,5 (10)-trien-20-yne-3,17-diol).
Clinical Pharmacology: Combination oral contraceptives act primarily through the mechanism of gonadotropin suppression due to the estrogenic and progestational activity of the ingredients. Although the primary mechanism of action is inhibition of ovulation, alterations in the genital tract, including changes in the cervical mucus (which increase the difficulty of sperm penetration) and the endometrium (which reduce the likelihood of implan-

tation), may also contribute to contraceptive effectiveness.

Indications and Usage: LO/OVRAL® is indicated for the prevention of pregnancy in women who elect to use oral contraceptives as a method of contraception.

Oral contraceptives are highly effective. The pregnancy rate in women using conventional combination oral contraceptives (containing 35 mcg or more of ethinyl estradiol or 50 mcg or more of mestranol) is generally reported as less than one pregnancy per 100 woman-years of use. Slightly higher rates (somewhat more than 1 pregnancy per 100 woman-years of use) are reported for some combination products containing 35 mcg or less of ethinyl estradiol, and rates on the order of 3 pregnancies per 100 woman-years are reported for the progestogen-only oral contraceptives.

These rates are derived from separate studies conducted by different investigators in several population groups and cannot be compared precisely. Furthermore, pregnancy rates tend to be lower as clinical studies are continued, possibly due to selective retention in the longer studies of those patients who accept the treatment regimen and do not discontinue as a result of adverse reactions, pregnancy, or other reasons.

In clinical trials with LO/OVRAL®, 1,700 patients completed 22,489 cycles, and a total of two pregnancies were reported. This represents a pregnancy rate of 0.12 per 100 woman-years.

Table 1 gives ranges of pregnancy rates reported in the literature[1] for other means of contraception. The efficacy of these means of contraception (except the IUD) depends upon the degree of adherence to the method.

TABLE 1

PREGNANCIES PER 100 WOMAN-YEARS

IUD, less than 1–6; Diaphragm with spermicidal products (creams or jellies), 2–20; Condom, 3–36; Aerosol foams, 2–29; Jellies and creams, 4–36;

Periodic abstinence (rhythm) all types, less than 1–47:

1. Calendar method, 14–47;
2. Temperature method, 1–20;
3. Temperature method—intercourse only in postovulatory phase, less than 1–7;
4. Mucus method, 1–25;

No contraception, 60–80.

Dose-Related Risk of Thromboembolism from Oral Contraceptives: Two studies have shown a positive association between the dose of estrogens in oral contraceptives and the risk of thromboembolism.[2,3] For this reason, it is prudent and in keeping with good principles of therapeutics to minimize exposure to estrogen. The oral-contraceptive product prescribed for any given patient should be that product which contains the least amount of estrogen that is compatible with an acceptable pregnancy rate and patient acceptance. It is recommended that new acceptors of oral contraceptives be started on preparations containing 0.05 mg or less of estrogen.

Contraindications: Oral contraceptives should not be used in women with any of the following conditions:

1. Thrombophlebitis or thromboembolic disorders.
2. A past history of deep-vein thrombophlebitis or thromboembolic disorders.
3. Cerebral-vascular or coronary-artery disease.
4. Known or suspected carcinoma of the breast.
5. Known or suspected estrogen-dependent neoplasia.
6. Undiagnosed abnormal genital bleeding.
7. Known or suspected pregnancy (see Warning No. 5).

Warnings:

Cigarette smoking increases the risk of serious cardiovascular side effects from oral-contraceptive use. This risk increases with age and with heavy smoking (15 or more cigarettes per day) and is quite marked in women over 35 years of age. Women who use oral contraceptives should be strongly advised not to smoke.

The use of oral contraceptives is associated with increased risk of several serious conditions, including thromboembolism, stroke, myocardial infarction, hepatic adenoma, gallbladder disease, hypertension. Practitioners prescribing oral contraceptives should be familiar with the following information relating to these risks.

1. *Thromboembolic Disorders and Other Vascular Problems:* An increased risk of thromboembolic and thrombotic disease associated with the use of oral contraceptives is well-established. Three principal studies in Great Britain[4–6] and three in the United States[7–10] have demonstrated an increased risk of fatal and nonfatal venous thromboembolism and stroke, both hemorrhagic and thrombotic.

These studies estimate that users of oral contraceptives are 4 to 11 times more likely than nonusers to develop these diseases without evident cause (Table 2).

CEREBROVASCULAR DISORDERS

In a collaborative American study[9,10] of cerebrovascular disorders in women with and without predisposing causes, it was estimated that the risk of hemorrhagic stroke was 2.0 times greater in users than nonusers and the risk of thrombotic stroke was 4 to 9.5 times greater in users than in nonusers (Table 2).

TABLE 2

SUMMARY OF RELATIVE RISK OF THROMBOEMBOLIC DISORDERS AND OTHER VASCULAR PROBLEMS IN ORAL-CONTRACEPTIVE USERS COMPARED TO NONUSERS

	Relative risk, times greater
Idiopathic thromboembolic disease	4–11
Postsurgery thromboembolic complications	4–6
Thrombotic stroke	4–9.5
Hemorrhagic stroke	2
Myocardial infarction	2–12

MYOCARDIAL INFARCTION

An increased risk of myocardial infarction associated with the use of oral contraceptives has been reported,[11,12,13] confirming a previously suspected association. These studies, conducted in the United Kingdom, found, as expected, that the greater the number of underlying risk factors for coronary-artery disease (cigarette smoking, hypertension, hypercholesterolemia, obesity, diabetes, history of preeclamptic toxemia) the higher the risk of developing myocardial infarction, regardless of whether the patient was an oral-contraceptive user or not. Oral contraceptives, however, were found to be a clear additional risk factor.

In terms of relative risk, it has been estimated[52] that oral-contraceptive users who do not smoke (smoking is considered a major predisposing condition to myocardial infarction) are about twice as likely to have a fatal myocardial infarction as nonusers who do not smoke. Oral-contraceptive users who are also smokers have about a 5-fold increased risk of fatal infarction compared to users who do not smoke, but about a 10- to 12-fold increased risk compared to non-users who do not smoke. Furthermore, the amount of smoking is also an important factor. In determining the importance of these relative risks, however, the baseline rates for various age groups, as shown in Table 3, must be given serious consideration. The importance of other predisposing conditions mentioned above in determining relative and absolute risks has not as yet been quantified; it is quite likely that the same synergistic action exists, but perhaps to a lesser extent.

TABLE 3

Estimated annual mortality rate per 100,000 women from myocardial infarction by use of oral contraceptives, smoking habits, and age (in years):

	Myocardial infarction			
	Women aged 30–39		Women aged 40–44	
Smoking habits	Users	Non-users	Users	Non-users
All smokers	10.2	2.6	62.0	15.9
Heavy*	13.0	5.1	78.7	31.3
Light	4.7	0.9	28.6	5.7
Nonsmokers	1.8	1.2	10.7	7.4
Smokers and nonsmokers	5.4	1.9	32.8	11.7

*Heavy smoker: 15 or more cigarettes per day.

From JAIN, A.K., *Studies in Family Planning, 8*:50, 1977

RISK OF DOSE

In an analysis of data derived from several national adverse-reaction reporting systems,[2] British investigators concluded that the risk of thromboembolism, including coronary thrombosis, is directly related to the dose of estrogen used in oral contraceptives. Preparations containing 100 mcg or more of estrogen were associated with a higher risk of thromboembolism than those containing 50–80 mcg of estrogen. Their analysis did suggest, however, that the quantity of estrogen may not be the sole factor involved. This finding has been confirmed in the United States.[3] Careful epidemiological studies to determine the degree of thromboembolic risk associated with progestogen-only oral contraceptives have not been performed. Cases of thromboembolic disease have been reported in women using these products, and they should not be presumed to be free of excess risk.

ESTIMATE OF EXCESS MORTALITY FROM CIRCULATORY DISEASES

A large prospective study[53] carried out in the U.K. estimated the mortality rate per 100,000 women per year from diseases of the circulatory system for users and nonusers of oral contraceptives according to age, smoking habits, and duration of use. The overall excess death rate annually from circulatory diseases for oral-contraceptive users was estimated to be 20 per 100,000 (ages 15–34—5/100,000; ages 35–44—33/100,000; ages 45–49—140/100,000), the risk being concentrated in older women, in those with a long duration of use, and in cigarette smokers. It was not possible, however, to examine the interrelationships of age, smoking, and duration of use, nor to compare the effects of continuous vs. intermittent use. Although the study showed a 10-fold increase in death due to circulatory diseases in users for 5 or more years, all of these deaths occurred in women 35 or older. Until larger numbers of women under 35 with continuous use for 5 or more years are available, it is not possible to assess the magnitude of the relative risk for this younger age group.

The available data from a variety of sources have been analyzed[14] to estimate the risk of death associated with various methods of contraception. The estimates of risk of death for each method include the combined risk of the contraceptive method (e.g., thromboembolic and thrombotic disease in the case of oral contraceptives) plus the risk attributable to pregnancy or abortion in the event of method failure. This latter risk varies with the effectiveness of the contraceptive method. The findings

Continued on next page

Wyeth—Cont.

of this analysis are shown in Figure 1 below.[14] The study concluded that the mortality associated with all methods of birth control is low and below that associated with childbirth, with the exception of oral contraceptives in women over 40 who smoke. (The rates given for Pill only/smokers for each age group are for smokers as a class. For "heavy" smokers (more than 15 cigarettes a day), the rates given would be about double; for "light" smokers (less than 15 cigarettes a day), about 50 percent. The lowest mortality is associated with the condom or diaphragm backed up by early abortion. The risk of thromboembolic and thrombotic disease associated with oral contraceptives increases with age after approximately age 30 and, for myocardial infarction, is further increased by hypertension, hypercholesterolemia, obesity, diabetes, or history of preeclamptic toxemia and especially by cigarette smoking.

Based on the data currently available, the following chart gives a gross estimate of the risk of death from circulatory disorders associated with the use of oral contraceptives:

SMOKING HABITS AND OTHER PREDISPOSING CONDITIONS—
RISK ASSOCIATED WITH USE OF ORAL CONTRACEPTIVES

Age	Below 30	30–39	40+
Heavy smokers	C	B	A
Light smokers	D	C	B
Nonsmokers (no predisposing conditions)	D	C,D	C
Nonsmokers (other predisposing conditions)	C	C,B	B,A

A—Use associated with very high risk.
B—Use associated with high risk.
C—Use associated with moderate risk.
D—Use associated with low risk.

The physician and the patient should be alert to the earliest manifestations of thromboembolic and thrombotic disorders (e.g., thrombophlebitis, pulmonary embolism, cerebrovascular insufficiency, coronary occlusion, retinal thrombosis, and mesenteric thrombosis). Should any of these occur or be suspected, the drug should be discontinued immediately.

A four- to six-fold increased risk of postsurgery thromboembolic complications has been reported in oral-contraceptive users.[15,16]

If feasible, oral contraceptives should be discontinued at least 4 weeks before surgery of a type associated with an increased risk of thromboembolism or prolonged immobilization.

2. *Ocular Lesions:*
There have been reports of neuro-ocular lesions such as optic neuritis or retinal thrombosis associated with the use of oral contraceptives. Discontinue oral-contraceptive medication if there is unexplained, sudden or gradual, partial or complete loss of vision; onset of proptosis or diplopia; papilledema; or retinal-vascular lesions, and institute appropriate diagnostic and therapeutic measures.

3. *Carcinoma:*
Long-term continuous administration of either natural or synthetic estrogen in certain animal species increases the frequency of carcinoma of the breast, cervix, vagina, and liver. Certain synthetic progestogens, none currently contained in oral contraceptives, have been noted to increase the incidence of mammary nodules, benign and malignant, in dogs.

In humans, three case-control studies have reported an increased risk of endometrial carcinoma associated with the prolonged use of exogenous estrogen in postmenopausal women.[17,18,19] One publication[20] reported on the first 21 cases submitted by physicians to a registry of cases of adenocarcinoma of the endometrium in women under 40 on oral contraceptives. Of the cases found in women without predisposing risk factors for adenocarcinoma of the endometrium (e.g., irregular bleeding at the time oral contraceptives were first given, polycystic ovaries), nearly all occurred in women who had used a sequential oral contraceptive. These products are no longer marketed. No evidence has been reported suggesting an increased risk of endometrial cancer in users of conventional combination or progestogen-only oral contraceptives.

Several studies[8,21–24] have found no increase in breast cancer in women taking oral contraceptives or estrogen. One study,[25] however, while also noting no overall increased risk of breast cancer in women treated with oral contraceptives, found an excess risk in the subgroups of oral-contraceptive users with documented benign breast disease. A reduced occurrence of benign breast tumors in users of oral contraceptives has been well-documented.[8,21,25,26,27]

Figure 1. Estimated annual number of deaths associated with control of fertility and no control per 100,000 nonsterile women, by regimen of control and age of woman.

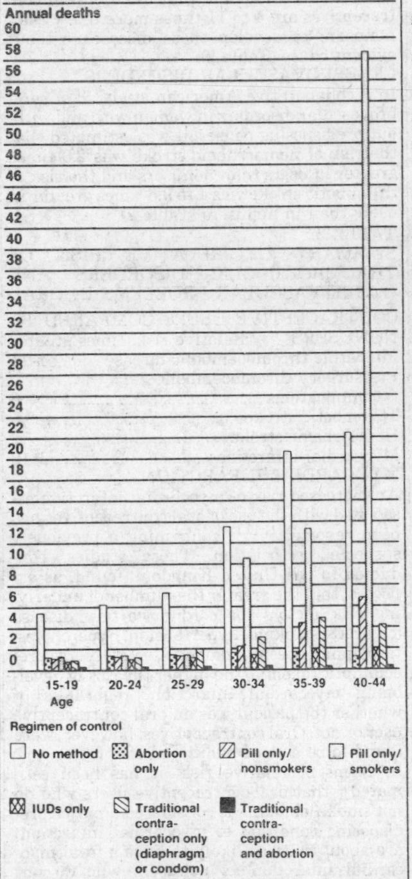

In summary, there is at present no confirmed evidence from human studies of an increased risk of cancer associated with oral contraceptives. Close clinical surveillance of all women taking oral contraceptives is, nevertheless, essential. In all cases of undiagnosed persistent or recurrent abnormal vaginal bleeding, appropriate diagnostic measures should be taken to rule out malignancy. Women with a strong family history of breast cancer or who have breast nodules, fibrocystic disease, or abnormal mammograms should be monitored with particular care if they elect to use oral contraceptives instead of other methods of contraception.

4. *Hepatic Tumors:*
Benign hepatic adenomas have been found to be associated with the use of oral contraceptives.[28,29,30,46] One study[46] showed that oral contraceptive formulations with high hormonal potency were associated with a higher risk than lower potency formulations. Although benign, hepatic adenomas may rupture and may cause death through intra-abdominal hemorrhage. This has been reported in short-term as well as long-term users of oral contraceptives. Two studies relate risk with duration of use of the contraceptive, the risk being much greater after 4 or more years of oral-contraceptive use.[30,46] While hepatic adenoma is a rare lesion, it should be considered in women presenting abdominal pain and tenderness, abdominal mass or shock. A few cases of hepatocellular carcinoma have been reported in women taking oral contraceptives. The relationship of these drugs to this type of malignancy is not known at this time.

5. *Use in or Immediately Preceding Pregnancy, Birth Defects in Offspring, and Malignancy in Female Offspring:*
The use of female sex hormones—both estrogenic and progestational agents—during early pregnancy may seriously damage the offspring. It has been shown that females exposed in utero to diethylstilbestrol, a nonsteroidal estrogen, have an increased risk of developing in later life a form of vaginal or cervical cancer that is ordinarily extremely rare.[31,32] This risk has been estimated to be of the order of 1 in 1,000 exposures or less.[33,47] Although there is no evidence at the present time that oral contraceptives further enhance the risk of developing this type of malignancy, such patients should be monitored with particular care if they elect to use oral contraceptives instead of other methods of contraception. Furthermore, a high percentage of such exposed women (from 30 to 90%) have been found to have epithelial changes of the vagina and cervix.[34–38] Although these changes are histologically benign, it is not known whether this condition is a precursor of vaginal malignancy. Male children so exposed may develop abnormalities of the urogenital tract.[48,49,50] Although similar data are not available with the use of other estrogens, it cannot be presumed that they would not induce similar changes.

An increased risk of congenital anomalies, including heart defects and limb defects, has been reported with the use of sex hormones, including oral contraceptives, in pregnancy.[39–42,51] One case-control study[42] has estimated a 4.7-fold increase in risk of limb-reduction defects in infants exposed in utero to sex hormones (oral contraceptives, hormonal withdrawal tests for pregnancy, or attempted treatment for threatened abortion). Some of these exposures were very short and involved only a few days of treatment. The data suggest that the risk of limb-reduction defects in exposed fetuses is somewhat less than one in 1,000 live births.

In the past, female sex hormones have been used during pregnancy in an attempt to treat threatened or habitual abortion. There is considerable evidence that estrogens are ineffective for these indications, and there is no evidence from well-controlled studies that progestogens are effective for these uses.

There is some evidence that triploidy and possibly other types of polyploidy are increased among abortuses from women who become pregnant soon after ceasing oral contraceptives.[43] Embryos with these anomalies are virtually always aborted spontaneously. Whether there is an overall increase in spontaneous abortion of pregnancies conceived soon after stopping oral contraceptives is unknown.

It is recommended that, for any patient who has missed two consecutive periods, pregnancy should be ruled out before continuing the contraceptive regimen. If the patient has not adhered to the prescribed schedule, the possibility of pregnancy should be considered at the time of the first missed period (or after 45 days from the last menstrual period if the progestogen-only oral contraceptives are used), and further use of oral contraceptives should be withheld until pregnancy has been ruled out. If pregnancy is confirmed, the patient should be apprised of the potential risks to the fetus, and the advisability of continuation of the pregnancy should be discussed in the light of these risks.

It is also recommended that women who discontinue oral contraceptives with the intent of becoming pregnant use an alternate form of contraception for a period of time before attempting to conceive.

Many clinicians recommend 3 months, although no precise information is available on which to base this recommendation.

The administration of progestogen-only or progestogen-estrogen combinations to induce withdrawal bleeding should not be used as a test of pregnancy.

6. *Gallbladder Disease:*

Studies [8,23,26] report an increased risk of surgically confirmed gallbladder disease in users of oral contraceptives and estrogens. In one study, an increased risk appeared after 2 years of use and doubled after 4 or 5 years of use. In one of the other studies, an increased risk was apparent between 6 and 12 months of use.

7. *Carbohydrate and Lipid Metabolic Effects:*

A decrease in glucose tolerance has been observed in a significant percentage of patients on oral contraceptives. For this reason, prediabetic and diabetic patients should be carefully observed while receiving oral contraceptives.

An increase in triglycerides and total phospholipids has been observed in patients receiving oral contraceptives.[44] The clinical significance of this finding remains to be defined.

8. *Elevated Blood Pressure:*

An increase in blood pressure has been reported in patients receiving oral contraceptives.[26] In some women, hypertension may occur within a few months of beginning oral-contraceptive use. In the first year of use, the prevalence of women with hypertension is low in users and may be no higher than that of a comparable group of nonusers. The prevalence in users increases, however, with longer exposure, and in the fifth year of use is two-and-a-half to three times the reported prevalence in the first year. Age is also strongly correlated with the development of hypertension in oral-contraceptive users. Women who previously have had hypertension during pregnancy may be more likely to develop elevation of blood pressure when given oral contraceptives. Hypertension that develops as a result of taking oral contraceptives usually returns to normal after discontinuing the drug.

9. *Headache:*

The onset or exacerbation of migraine or development of headache of a new pattern which is recurrent, persistent, or severe, requires discontinuation of oral contraceptives and evaluation of the cause.

10. *Bleeding Irregularities:*

Breakthrough bleeding, spotting, and amenorrhea are frequent reasons for patients discontinuing oral contraceptives. In breakthrough bleeding, as in all cases of irregular bleeding from the vagina, nonfunctional causes should be borne in mind. In undiagnosed persistent or recurrent abnormal bleeding from the vagina, adequate diagnostic measures are indicated to rule out pregnancy or malignancy. If pathology has been excluded, time or a change to another formulation may solve the problem. Changing to an oral contraceptive with a higher estrogen content, while potentially useful in minimizing menstrual irregularity, should be done only if necessary, since this may increase the risk of thromboembolic disease.

Women with a past history of oligomenorrhea or secondary amenorrhea or young women without regular cycles may have a tendency to remain anovulatory or to become amenorrheic after discontinuation of oral contraceptives. Women with these preexisting problems should be advised of this possibility and encouraged to use other contraceptive methods. Post-use anovulation, possibly prolonged, may also occur in women without previous irregularities.

11. *Ectopic Pregnancy:*

Ectopic as well as intrauterine pregnancy may occur in contraceptive failures. However, in progestogen-only oral contraceptive failures, the ratio of ectopic to intrauterine pregnancies is higher than in women who are not receiving oral contraceptives, since the drugs are more effective in preventing intrauterine than ectopic pregnancies.

12. *Breast-feeding:*

Oral contraceptives given in the postpartum period may interfere with lactation. There may be a decrease in the quantity and quality of the breast milk. Furthermore, a small fraction of the hormonal agents in oral contraceptives has been identified in the milk of mothers receiving these drugs.[45] The effects, if any, on the breast-fed child have not been determined. If feasible, the use of oral contraceptives should be deferred until the infant has been weaned.

Precautions:

GENERAL

1. A complete medical and family history should be taken prior to initiation of oral contraceptives. The pretreatment and periodic physical examinations should include special reference to blood pessure, breasts, abdomen and pelvic organs, including Papanicolaou smear and relevant laboratory tests. As a general rule, oral contraceptives should not be prescribed for longer than 1 year without another physical examination being performed.
2. Under the influence of estrogen-progestogen preparations, pre-existing uterine leiomyomata may increase in size.
3. Patients with a history of psychic depression should be carefully observed and the drug discontinued if depression recurs to a serious degree. Patients becoming significantly depressed while taking oral contraceptives should stop the medication and use an alternate method of contraception in an attempt to determine whether the symptom is drug-related.
4. Oral contraceptives may cause some degree of fluid retention. They should be prescribed with caution, and only with careful monitoring, in patients with conditions which might be aggravated by fluid retention, such as convulsive disorders, migraine syndrome, asthma, or cardiac or renal insufficiency.
5. Patients with a past history of jaundice during pregnancy have an increased risk of recurrence of jaundice while receiving oral-contraceptive therapy. If jaundice develops in any patient receiving such drugs, the medication should be discontinued.
6. Steroid hormones may be poorly metabolized in patients with impaired liver function and should be administered with caution in such patients.
7. Oral-contraceptive users may have disturbances in normal tryptophan metabolism which may result in a relative pyridoxine deficiency. The clinical significance of this is yet to be determined.
8. Serum folate levels may be depressed by oral-contraceptive therapy. Since the pregnant woman is predisposed to the development of folate deficiency and the incidence of folate deficiency increases with increasing gestation, it is possible that if a woman becomes pregnant shortly after stopping oral contraceptives, she may have a greater chance of developing folate deficiency and complications attributed to this deficiency.
9. The pathologist should be advised of oral-contraceptive therapy when relevant specimens are submitted.
10. Certain endocrine- and liver-function tests and blood components may be affected by estrogen-containing oral contraceptives:

a. Increased sulfobromophthalein retention.
b. Increased prothrombin and factors VII, VIII, IX, and X; decreased antithrombin 3; increased norepinephrine-induced platelet aggregability.
c. Increased thyroid-binding globulin (TBG) leading to increased circulating total-thyroid hormone, as measured by protein-bound iodine (PBI), T4 by column, or T4 by radioimmunoassay. Free T3 resin uptake is decreased, reflecting the elevated TBG; free T4 concentration is unaltered.
d. Decreased pregnanediol excretion.
e. Reduced response to metyrapone test.

Informaton for the Patient: (See Patient Labeling Printed Below.)

Drug Interactions: Reduced efficacy and increased incidence of breakthrough bleeding have been associated with concomitant use of rifampin. A similar association has been suggested with barbiturates, phenylbutazone, phenytoin sodium, and ampicillin.

Carcinogenesis: See Warnings section for information on the carcinogenic potential of oral contraceptives.

Pregnancy: Pregnancy category X. See Contraindications and Warnings.

Nursing Mothers: See Warnings.

Adverse Reactions: An increased risk of the following serious adverse reactions has been associated with the use of oral contraceptives (see Warnings):

- Thrombophlebitis.
- Pulmonary embolism.
- Coronary thrombosis.
- Cerebral thrombosis.
- Cerebral hemorrhage.
- Hypertension.
- Gallbladder disease.
- Benign hepatomas.
- Congenital anomalies.

There is evidence of an association between the following conditions and the use of oral contraceptives, although additional confirmatory studies are needed:

- Mesenteric thrombosis.
- Neuro-ocular lesions, e.g., retinal thrombosis and optic neuritis.

The following adverse reactions have been reported in patients receiving oral contraceptives and are believed to be drug-related:

- Nausea and/or vomiting, usually the most common adverse reactions, occur in approximately 10% or less of patients during the first cycle. Other reactions, as a general rule, are seen much less frequently or only occasionally.
- Gastrointestinal symptoms (such as abdominal cramps and bloating).
- Breakthrough bleeding.
- Spotting.
- Change in menstrual flow.
- Dysmenorrhea.
- Amenorrhea during and after treatment.
- Temporary infertility after discontinuance of treatment.
- Edema.
- Chloasma or melasma which may persist.
- Breast changes: tenderness, enlargement, and secretion.
- Change in weight (increase or decrease).
- Change in cervical erosion and cervical secretion.

Continued on next page

Wyeth—Cont.

Possible diminution in lactation when given immediately post-partum.
Cholestatic jaundice.
Migraine.
Increase in size of uterine leiomyomata.
Rash (allergic).
Mental depression.
Reduced tolerance to carbohydrates.
Vaginal candidiasis.
Change in corneal curvature (steepening).
Intolerance to contact lenses.

The following adverse reactions have been reported in users of oral contraceptives, and the association has been neither confirmed nor refuted:

Premenstrual-like syndrome.
Cataracts.
Changes in libido.
Chorea.
Changes in appetite.
Cystitis-like syndrome.
Headache.
Nervousness.
Dizziness.
Hirsutism.
Loss of scalp hair.
Erythema multiforme.
Erythema nodosum.
Hemorrhagic eruption.
Vaginitis.
Porphyria.

Acute Overdose: Serious ill effects have not been reported following acute ingestion of large doses of oral contraceptives by young children. Overdosage may cause nausea, and withdrawal bleeding may occur in females.

Dosage and Administration: To achieve maximum contraceptive effectiveness, LO/OVRAL® must be taken exactly as directed and at intervals not exceeding 24 hours. The dosage of LO/OVRAL® is one tablet daily for 21 consecutive days per menstrual cycle according to prescribed schedule. Tablets are then discontinued for 7 days (three weeks on, one week off).

It is recommended that LO/OVRAL® tablets be taken at the same time each day, preferably after the evening meal or at bedtime.

During the first cycle of medication, the patient is instructed to take one LO/OVRAL® tablet daily for twenty-one consecutive days beginning on day five of her menstrual cycle. (The first day of menstruation is day one.) The tablets are then discontinued for one week (7 days). Withdrawal bleeding should usually occur within three days following discontinuation of LO/OVRAL®.

(If LO/OVRAL® is first taken later than the fifth day of the first menstrual cycle of medication or postpartum, contraceptive reliance should not be placed on LO/OVRAL® until after the first seven consecutive days of administration. The possibility of ovulation and conception prior to initiation of medication should be considered.)

The patient begins her next and all subsequent 21-day courses of LO/OVRAL® tablets on the same day of the week that she began her first course, following the same schedule: 21 days on—7 days off. She begins taking her tablets on the 8th day after discontinuance regardless of whether or not a menstrual period has occurred or is still in progress. Any time a new cycle of LO/OVRAL® is started later than the 8th day the patient should be protected by another means of contraception until she has taken a tablet daily for seven consecutive days.

If spotting or breakthrough bleeding occurs, the patient is instructed to continue on the same regimen. This type of bleeding is usually transient and without significance; however, if the bleeding is persistent or prolonged the patient is advised to consult her physician.

Although the occurrence of pregnancy is highly unlikely if LO/OVRAL® is taken according to directions, if withdrawal bleeding does not occur, the possibility of pregnancy must be considered. If the patient has not adhered to the prescribed schedule (missed one or more tablets or started taking them on a day later than she should have) the probability of pregnancy should be considered at the time of the first missed period and appropriate diagnostic measures taken before the medication is resumed. If the patient has adhered to the prescribed regimen and misses two consecutive periods, pregnancy should be ruled out before continuing the contraceptive regimen.

The patient should be instructed to take a missed tablet as soon as it is remembered. If two consecutive tablets are missed they should both be taken as soon as remembered. The next tablet should be taken at the usual time.

Any time the patient misses one or two tablets she should also use another method of contraception until she has taken a tablet daily for seven consecutive days. If breakthrough bleeding occurs following missed tablets it will usually be transient and of no consequence.

While there is little likelihood of ovulation occurring if only one or two tablets are missed, the possibility of ovulation increases with each successive day that scheduled tablets are missed. If three consecutive tablets are missed, all medication should be discontinued and the remainder of the package discarded. A new tablet cycle should be started on the 8th day after the last tablet was taken, and an alternate means of contraception should be prescribed during the seven days without tablets and until the patient has taken a tablet daily for seven consecutive days. In the nonlactating mother LO/OVRAL® may be prescribed in the postpartum period either immediately or at the first postpartum examination whether or not menstruation has resumed.

How Supplied: LO/OVRAL® tablets (0.3 mg norgestrel + 0.03 mg ethinyl estradiol) are available in containers of 21 tablets.

References:

1. "Population Reports," Series H, Number 2, May 1974; Series I, Number 1, June 1974; Series B, Number 2, January 1975; Series H, Number 3, 1975; Series H, Number 4, January 1976 (published by the Population Information Program, The George Washington University Medical Center, 2001 S St. NW., Washington, D.C.).

2. Inman, W. H. W., Vessey, M. P., Westerholm, B., and Engelund, A., "Thromboembolic disease and the steroidal content of oral contraceptives. A report to the Committee on Safety of Drugs," Brit Med J *2*:203–209, 1970.

3. Stolley, P. D., Tonascia, J. A., Tockman, M. S., Sartwell, P. E., Rutledge, A. H., and Jacobs, M. P., "Thrombosis with low-estrogen oral contraceptives," Am J Epidemiol *102*:197–208, 1975.

4. Royal College of General Practitioners, "Oral contraception and thromboembolic disease," J Coll Gen Pract *13*:267–279, 1967.

5. Inman, W. H. W., and Vessey, M. P., "Investigation of deaths from pulmonary, coronary and cerebral thrombosis and embolism in women of childbearing age," Brit Med J *2*:193–199, 1968.

6. Vessey, M. P., and Doll, R., "Investigation of relation between use of oral contraceptives and thromboembolic disease. A further report," Brit Med J *2*:651–657, 1969.

7. Sartwell, P. E., Masi, A. T., Arthes, F. G., Greene, G. R., and Smith, H. E., "Thromboembolism and oral contraceptives: an epidemiological case control study," Am J Epidemiol *90*:365–380, 1969.

8. Boston Collaborative Drug Surveillance Program, "Oral contraceptives and venous thromboembolic disease, surgically confirmed gallbladder disease and breast tumors," Lancet *1*:1399–1404, 1973.

9. Collaborative Group for the Study of Stroke in Young Women, "Oral contraception and increased risk of cerebral ischemia or thrombosis," N Engl J Med *288*:871–878, 1973.

10. Collaborative Group for the Study of Stroke in Young Women, "Oral contraceptives and stroke in young women: associated risk factors," JAMA *231*:718–722, 1975.

11. Mann, J. I., and Inman, W. H. W., "Oral contraceptives and death from myocardial infarction," Brit Med J *2*:245–248, 1975.

12. Mann, J. I., Inman, W. H. W., and Thorogood, M., "Oral contraceptive use in older women and fatal myocardial infarction," Brit Med J *2*:445–447, 1976.

13. Mann, J. I., Vessey, M. P., Thorogood, M., and Doll, R., "Myocardial infarction in young women with special reference to oral contraceptive practice," Brit Med J *2*:241–245, 1975.

14. Tietze, C., "New Estimates of Mortality Associated with Fertility Control," Family Planning Perspectives, *9*:74–76, 1977.

15. Vessey, M. P., Doll, R., Fairbairn, A. S., and Glober, G., "Post-operative thromboembolism and the use of oral contraceptives," Brit Med J *3*:123–126, 1970.

16. Greene, G. R., Sartwell, P. E., "Oral contraceptive use in patients with thromboembolism following surgery, trauma, or infection," Am J Pub Health *62*:680–685, 1972.

17. Smith, D. C., Prentice, R., Thompson, D. J., and Herrmann, W. L., "Association of exogenous estrogen and endometrial carcinoma," N Engl J Med *293*:1164–1167, 1975.

18. Ziel, H. K., and Finkle, W. D., "Increased risk of endometrial carcinoma among users of conjugated estrogens," N Engl J Med *293*:1167–1170, 1975.

19. Mack, T. N., Pike, M. C., Henderson, B. E., Pfeffer, R. I., Gerkins, V. R., Arthur, M., and Brown, S. E., "Estrogens and endometrial cancer in a retirement community," N Engl J Med *294*:1262–1267, 1976.

20. Silverberg, S. G., and Makowski, E. L., "Endometrial carcinoma in young women taking oral contraceptive agents," Obstet Gynecol *46*:503–506, 1975.

21. Vessey, M. P., Doll, R., and Sutton, P. M., "Oral contraceptives and breast neoplasia: a retrospective study," Brit Med J *3*:719–724, 1972.

22. Vessey, M. P., Doll, R., and Jones K., "Oral contraceptives and breast cancer. Progress report of an epidemiological study," Lancet *1*:941–943, 1975.

23. Boston Collaborative Drug Surveillance Program, "Surgically confirmed gallbladder disease, venous thromboembolism and breast tumors in relation to postmenopausal estrogen therapy," N Engl J Med *290*:15–19, 1974.

24. Arthes, F. G., Sartwell, P. E., and Lewison, E. F., "The pill, estrogens, and the breast. Epidemiologic aspects," Cancer *28*:1391–1394, 1971.

25. Fasal, E., and Paffenbarger, R. S., "Oral contraceptives as related to cancer and benign

lesions of the breast," J Natl Cancer Inst *55*:767–773. 1975.

26. Royal College of General Practitioners, "Oral Contraceptives and Health," London, Pitman, 1974.

27. Ory, H., Cole P., MacMahon, B., and Hoover, R., "Oral contraceptives and reduced risk of benign breast diseases," N Engl J Med *294*:419–422, 1976.

28. Baum, J., Holtz, F., Bookstein, J. J., and Klein, E. W., "Possible association between benign hepatomas and oral contraceptives," Lancet *2*:926–928, 1973.

29. Mays, E. T., Christopherson, W. M., Mahr, M. M., and Williams, H. C., "Hepatic changes in young women ingesting contraceptive steroids. Hepatic hemorrhage and primary hepatic tumors," JAMA *235*:730–732, 1976.

30. Edmondson, H. A., Henderson, B., and Benton, B., "Liver-cell adenomas associated with use of oral contraceptives," N Engl J Med *294*:470–472, 1976.

31. Herbst, A. L., Ulfedler, H., and Poskanzer, D. C., "Adenocarcinoma of the vagina," N Engl J Med *284*:878–881, 1971.

32. Greenwald, P., Barlow, J. J., Nasca, P. C., and Burnett, W., "Vaginal cancer after maternal treatment with synthetic estrogens," N Engl J Med *285*:390–392, 1971.

33. Lanier, A. P., Noller, K. L., Decker, D. G., Elveback, L., and Kurland, L. T., "Cancer and stilbestrol. A follow-up of 1719 persons exposed to estrogens in utero and born 1943–1959," Mayo Clin Pro *48*:793–799, 1973.

34. Herbst, A. L., Kurman, R. J., and Scully, R. E., "Vaginal and cervical abnormalities after exposure to stilbestrol in utero," Obstet Gynecol *40*:287–298, 1972.

35. Herbst, A. L., Robboy, S. J., Macdonald, G. J., and Scully, R. E., "The effects of local progesterone on stilbestrol-associated vaginal adenosis," Am J Obstet Gynecol *118*:607–615, 1974.

36. Herbst, A. L., Poskanzer, D. C., Robboy, S. J., Friedlander, L., and Scully, R. E., "Prenatal exposure to stilbestrol: a prospective comparison of exposed female offspring with unexposed controls," N Engl J Med *292*:334–339, 1975.

37. Stafl, A., Mattingly, R. F., Foley, D. V., Fetherston, W., "Clinical diagnosis of vaginal adenosis," Obstet Gynecol *43*:118–128, 1974.

38. Sherman, A. I., Goldrath, M., Berlin, A., Vakhariya, V., Banooni, F., Michaels, W., Goodman, P., and Brown, S., "Cervical-vaginal adenosis after in utero exposure to synthetic estrogens," Obstet Gynecol *44*:531–545, 1974.

39. Gal, I., Kirman, B., and Stern, J., "Hormone pregnancy tests and congenital malformation," Nature *216*:83. 1967.

40. Levy, E. P., Cohen, A., and Fraser, F. C., "Hormone treatment during pregnancy and congenital heart defects," Lancet *1*:611. 1973.

41. Nora, J. J., and Nora, A. H., "Birth defects and oral contraceptives," Lancet *1*:941–942, 1973.

42. Janerich, D. T., Piper, J. M., and Glebatis, D. M., "Oral contraceptives and congenital limb-reduction defects," N Engl J Med *291*:697–700, 1974.

43. Carr, D. H., "Chromosome studies in selected spontaneous abortions: I. Conception after oral contraceptives," Canad Med Assoc J *103*:343–348, 1970.

44. Wynn, V., Doar, J. W. H., and Mills, G. L., "Some effects of oral contraceptives on serum-lipid and lipoprotein levels," Lancet *2*:720–723, 1966.

45. Laumas, K. R., Malkani, P. K., Bhatnagar, S., and Laumas, V., "Radioactivity in the breast milk of lactating women after oral administration of 3 H-norethynodrel," Amer J Obstet Gynecol *98*:411–413, 1967.

46. Center for Disease Control, "Increased Risk of Hepatocellular Adenoma in Women with Long-term use of Oral Contraceptives," Morbidity and Mortality Weekly Report, *26*:293–294, 1977.

47. Herbst, A. L., Cole, P., Colton, T., Robboy, S. J., Scully, R. E., "Age-incidence and Risk of Diethylstilbestrol-related Clear Cell Adenocarcinoma of the Vagina and Cervix," Am. J. Obstet. Gynecol., *128*:43–50, 1977.

48. Bibbo, M., Al-Naqeeb, M., Baccarini, I., Gill, W., Newton, M., Sleeper, K. M., Sonek, M., Wied, G. L., "Follow-up Study of Male and Female Offspring of DES-treated Mothers. A Preliminary Report," Jour. of Repro. Med., *15*:29–32, 1975.

49. Gill, W. B., Schumacher, G. F. B., Bibbo, M., "Structural and Functional Abnormalities in the Sex Organs of Male Offspring of Mothers Treated with Diethylstilbestrol (DES)," Jour. of Repro. Med., *16*:147–153, 1976.

50. Henderson, B. E., Senton, B., Cosgrove, M., Baptista, J., Aldrich, J., Townsend, D., Hart, W., Mack, T., "Urogenital Tract Abnormalities in Sons of Women Treated with Diethylstilbestrol," Pediatrics, *58*:505–507, 1976.

51. Heinonen, O. P., Slone, D., Nonson, R. R., Hook, E. B., Shapiro, S., "Cardiovascular Birth Defects and Antenatal Exposure to Female Sex Hormones," N. Engl. J. Med., *296*:67–70, 1977.

52. Jain, A. K., "Mortality Risk Associated with the Use of Oral Contraceptives," Studies in Family Planning, *8*:50–54, 1977.

53. Beral, V., "Mortality Among Oral Contraceptive Users," Lancet, *2*:727–731, 1977.

The patient labeling for oral-contraceptive drug products is set forth below:

Brief Summary Patient Package Insert

Cigarette smoking increases the risk of serious adverse effects on the heart and blood vessels from oral-contraceptive use. This risk increases with age and with heavy smoking (15 or more cigarettes per day) and is quite marked in women over 35 years of age. Women who use oral contraceptives should not smoke.

Oral contraceptives taken as directed are about 99% effective in preventing pregnancy. (The mini-pill, however, is somewhat less effective.) Forgetting to take your pills increases the chance of pregnancy. Women who have or have had clotting disorders, cancer of the breast or sex organs, unexplained vaginal bleeding, a stroke, heart attack, angina pectoris, or who suspect they may be pregnant should not use oral contraceptives.

Most side effects of the pill are not serious. The most common side effects are nausea, vomiting, bleeding between menstrual periods, weight gain, and breast tenderness. However, proper use of oral contraceptives requires that they be taken under your doctor's continuous supervision, because they can be associated with serious side effects which may be fatal. Fortunately, these occur very infrequently. The serious side effects are:

1. Blood clots in the legs, lungs, brain, heart, or other organs, and hemorrhage into the brain due to bursting of a blood vessel.
2. Liver tumors, which may rupture and cause severe bleeding.
3. Birth defects if the pill is taken while you are pregnant.
4. High blood pressure.
5. Gallbladder disease.

The symptoms associated with these serious side effects are discussed in the detailed leaflet given you with your supply of pills. Notify your doctor if you notice any unusual physical disturbance while taking the pill.

The estrogen in oral contraceptives has been found to cause breast cancer and other cancers in certain animals. These findings suggest that oral contraceptives may also cause cancer in humans. However, studies to date in women taking currently marketed oral contraceptives have not confirmed that oral contraceptives cause cancer in humans.

The detailed leaflet describes more completely the benefits and risks of oral contraceptives. It also provides information on other forms of contraception. Read it carefully. If you have any questions, consult your doctor.

Caution: Oral contraceptives are of no value in the prevention or treatment of venereal disease.

[*Shown in Product Identification Section*]

MEPERGAN® Ⓒ ℞
(meperidine HCl and promethazine HCl) Injection

Description: This product is available in concentration providing 25 mg each of meperidine hydrochloride and promethazine hydrochloride per ml with 0.1 mg edetate disodium, 0.04 mg calcium chloride, and not more than 0.75 mg sodium formaldehyde sulfoxylate, 0.25 mg sodium metabisulfite, and 5 mg phenol with sodium acetate buffer.

Actions: Meperidine hydrochloride is a narcotic analgesic with multiple actions qualitatively similar to those of morphine. Phenergan® (promethazine HCl) is a phenothiazine derivative that has several different pharmacologic properties including antihistaminic, sedative, and antiemetic actions.

Indications: As a preanesthetic medication when analgesia and sedation are indicated. As an adjunct to local and general anesthesia.

Contraindications: Hypersensitivity to meperidine or promethazine.

Under no circumstances should Mepergan be given by intra-arterial injection, due to the likelihood of severe arteriospasm and the possiblity of resultant gangrene (see Warnings).

Mepergan should not be given by the subcutaneous route; evidence of chemical irritation has been noted and necrotic lesions have resulted on rare occasions following subcutaneous injection. The preferred parenteral route of administration is by deep intramuscular injection.

Meperidine is contraindicated in patients who are receiving monoamine oxidase inhibitors (MAOI) or those who have received such agents within 14 days.

Therapeutic doses of meperidine have inconsistently precipitated unpredictable, severe, and occasionally fatal reactions in patients who have received such agents within 14 days. The mechanism of these reactions is unclear. Some have been characterized by coma, severe respiratory depression, cyanosis, and hypotension, and have resembled the syndrome of acute narcotic overdose. In other reactions the predominant manifestations have been hyperexcitability, convulsions, tachycardia, hyperpyrexia, and hypertension. Although it is not known that other narcotics are free of the risk of such reactions, virtually all of the reported reactions have occurred with meperidine. If a narcotic is needed in such patients, a sensitivity test should be performed in which repeated,

Continued on next page

Wyeth—Cont.

small, incremental doses of morphine are administered over the course of several hours while the patient's condition and vital signs are under careful observation.
(Intravenous hydrocortisone or prednisolone have been used to treat severe reactions, with the addition of intravenous chlorpromazine in those cases exhibiting hypertension and hyperpyrexia. The usefulness and safety of narcotic antagonists in the treatment of these reactions is unknown.)

Warnings: Tolerance and Addiction Liability

Warning—may be habit forming
DRUG DEPENDENCE: Meperidine can produce drug dependence of the morphine-type and therefore has the potential for being abused. Psychic dependence, physical dependence, and tolerance may develop upon repeated administration of meperidine, and it should be prescribed and administered with the same degree of caution appropriate to the use of morphine. Like other narcotics, meperidine is subject to the provisions of the Federal narcotic laws.
INTERACTION WITH OTHER CENTRAL-NERVOUS-SYSTEM DEPRESSANTS: Meperidine should be used with great caution and in reduced dosage in patients who are concurrently receiving other narcotic analgesics, general anesthetics, phenothiazines, other tranquilizers, sedative-hypnotics, tricyclic antidepressants, and other CNS depressants (including alcohol). Respiratory depression, hypotension, and profound sedation or coma may result.
The sedative action of promethazine hydrochloride is additive to the sedative effects of central-nervous-system depressants; therefore, agents such as alcohol, barbiturates, and narcotic analgesics should either be eliminated or given in reduced dosage in the presence of promethazine hydrochloride. When given concomitantly with promethazine hydrochloride the dose of barbiturates should be reduced by at least one-half and the dose of analgesic depressants, such as morphine or meperidine, should be reduced by one-quarter to one-half.
HEAD INJURY AND INCREASED INTRACRANIAL PRESSURE: The respiratory depressant effects of meperidine and its capacity to elevate cerebrospinal-fluid pressure may be markedly exaggerated in the presence of head injury, other intracranial lesions, or a preexisting increase in intracranial pressure. Furthermore, narcotics produce adverse reactions which may obscure the clinical course of patients with head injuries. In such patients, meperidine must be used with extreme caution and only if its use is deemed essential.
INADVERTENT INTRA-ARTERIAL INJECTION: Due to the close proximity of arteries and veins in the areas most commonly used for intravenous injection, extreme care should be exercised to avoid perivascular extravasation or inadvertent intra-arterial injection of Mepergan. Reports compatible with inadvertent intra-arterial injection suggest that pain, severe chemical irritation, severe spasm of distal vessels, and resultant gangrene requiring amputation is likely under such circumstances. Intravenous injection was intended in all the cases reported, but perivascular extravasation or arterial placement of the needle is now suspect. There is no proven successful management of this condition after it occurs, although sympathetic block and heparinization are commonly employed during the acute management because of the results of animal experiments with other known arteriolar irritants. Aspiration of dark blood does not preclude intra-arterial needle placement, because blood is discolored upon contact with promethazine. Use of syringes with rigid plungers or of small bore needles might obscure typical arterial backflow if this is relied upon alone.
INTRAVENOUS USE: If necessary, meperidine may be given intravenously, but the injection should be given very slowly, preferably in the form of a diluted solution. Rapid intravenous injection of narcotic analgesics, including meperidine, increases the incidence of adverse reactions; severe respiratory depression, apnea, hypotension, peripheral circulatory collapse, and cardiac arrest have occurred. Meperidine should not be administered intravenously unless a narcotic antagonist and the facilities for assisted or controlled respiration are immediately available. When meperidine is given parenterally, especially intravenously, the patient should be lying down.
When used intravenously, Mepergan® should be given at a rate not to exceed 1 ml (25 mg of each component) per minute. When administering any irritant drug intravenously it is usually preferable to inject it through the tubing of an intravenous infusion set that is known to be functioning satisfactorily. In the event that a patient complains of pain during intended intravenous injection of Mepergan, the injection should immediately be stopped to provide for evaluation of possible arterial placement or perivascular extravasation.
ASTHMA AND OTHER RESPIRATORY CONDITIONS: Meperidine should be used with extreme caution in patients having an acute asthmatic attack, patients with chronic obstructive pulmonary disease or cor pulmonale, patients having a substantially decreased respiratory reserve, and patients with preexisting respiratory depression, hypoxia, or hypercapnia. In such patients, even usual therapeutic doses of narcotics may decrease respiratory drive while simultaneously increasing airway resistance to the point of apnea.
HYPOTENSIVE EFFECT: The administration of meperidine may result in severe hypotension in an individual whose ability to maintain his blood pressure has already been compromised by a depleted blood volume or concurrent administration of drugs such as the phenothiazines or certain anesthetics.
USAGE IN AMBULATORY PATIENTS: Meperidine may impair the mental and/or physical abilities required for the performance of potentially hazardous tasks such as driving a car or operating machinery. The patient should be cautioned accordingly.
Meperidine, like other narcotics, may produce orthostatic hypotension in ambulatory patients.
USAGE IN PREGNANCY AND LACTATION: Meperidine should not be used in pregnant women prior to the labor period, unless in the judgment of the physician the potential benefits outweigh the possible hazards, because safe use in pregnancy prior to labor has not been established relative to possible adverse effects on fetal development.
When used as an obstetrical analgesic, meperidine crosses the placental barrier and can produce respiratory depression in the newborn; resuscitation may be required (see section on Overdosage).
Meperidine appears in the milk of nursing mothers receiving the drug.

Precautions: SUPRAVENTRICULAR TACHYCARDIAS: Meperidine should be used with caution in patients with atrial flutter and other supraventricular tachycardias because of a possible vagolytic action which may produce a significant increase in the ventricular response rate.
CONVULSIONS: Meperidine may aggravate preexisting convulsions in patients with convulsive disorders. If dosage is escalated substantially above recommended levels because of tolerance development, convulsions may occur in individuals without a history of convulsive disorders.
ACUTE ABDOMINAL CONDITIONS: The administration of meperidine or other narcotics may obscure the diagnosis or clinical course in patients with acute abdominal conditions.
SPECIAL-RISK PATIENTS: Meperidine should be given with caution and the initial dose should be reduced in certain patients such as the elderly or debilitated, and those with severe impairment of hepatic or renal function, hypothyroidism, Addison's disease, and prostatic hypertrophy or urethral stricture.
Antiemetics may mask the symptoms of an unrecognized disease and thereby interfere with diagnosis.
Patients in pain who have received inadequate or no analgesia have been noted to develop "athetoid-like" movements of the upper extremities following the parenteral administration of promethazine. These symptoms usually disappear upon adequate control of the pain.
Ambulatory patients should be cautioned against driving automobiles or operating dangerous machinery until it is known that they do not become drowsy or dizzy from promethazine hydrochloride therapy.

Adverse Reactions: The major hazards of meperidine, as with other narcotic analgesics, are respiratory depression and, to a lessor degree, circulatory depression; respiratory arrest, shock, and cardiac arrest have occurred.
The most frequently observed adverse reactions include light-headedness, dizziness, sedation, nausea, vomiting, and sweating. These effects seem to be more prominent in ambulatory patients and in those who are not experiencing severe pain. In such individuals, lower doses are advisable. Some adverse reactions in ambulatory patients may be alleviated if the patient lies down.
Other adverse reactions include:
CENTRAL NERVOUS SYSTEM: Euphoria, dysphoria, weakness, headache, agitation, tremor, uncoordinated muscle movements, transient hallucinations and disorientation, visual disturbances and, rarely, extrapyramidal reactions.
GASTROINTESTINAL: Dry mouth, constipation, biliary-tract spasm.
CARDIOVASCULAR: Flushing of the face, tachycardia, bradycardia, palpitation, faintness, syncope.
Cardiovascular effects from promethazine have been rare. Minor increases in blood pressure and occasional mild hypotension have been reported. Venous thrombosis at the injection site has been reported. Intraarterial injection of Mepergan may result in gangrene of the affected extremity (see Warnings).
GENITOURINARY: Urinary retention.
ALLERGIC: Pruritus, urticaria, other skin rashes, wheal and flare over the vein with IV injection.
Photosensitivity, although extremely rare, has been reported. Occurrence of photosensitivity may be a contraindication to further treatment with promethazine or related drugs.
OTHER: Pain at injection site; local tissue irritation and induration following subcutaneous injection, particularly when repeated; antidiuretic effect.
Patients may occasionally complain of autonomic reactions such as dryness of the mouth, blurring of vision and, rarely, dizziness following the use of promethazine.
Very rare cases have been reported where patients receiving promethazine have developed leukopenia. In one instance agranulocytosis has been reported. In nearly every instance reported, other toxic agents known to have caused these conditions have been associated with the administration of promethazine.

Dosage and Administration: WARNING—BARBITURATES ARE NOT CHEMICALLY COMPATIBLE IN SOLUTION WITH MEPERGAN® (MEPERIDINE HYDROCHLORIDE AND PROMETHAZINE HYDROCHLORIDE), AND SHOULD NOT BE MIXED IN THE SAME SYRINGE.
The TUBEX® (Sterile Cartridge-Needle Unit) is designed for single-dose use. VIALS should

be used when required doses are fractions of a milliliter, as indicated below.
Mepergan® is usually administered intramuscularly. However, in certain specific situations, the intravenous route may be employed. INADVERTENT INTRA-ARTERIAL INJECTION CAN RESULT IN GANGRENE OF THE AFFECTED EXTREMITY (see Warnings). SUBCUTANEOUS ADMINISTRATION IS CONTRAINDICATED, AS IT MAY RESULT IN TISSUE NECROSIS (see Contraindications). INJECTION INTO OR NEAR PERIPHERAL NERVES MAY RESULT IN PERMANENT NEUROLOGICAL DEFICIT.
When used intravenously, the rate should not be greater than 1 ml of Mepergan (25 mg of each component) per minute; it is preferable to inject through the tubing of an intravenous infusion set that is known to be functioning satisfactorily.
ADULT DOSE: 1-2 ml (25-50 mg of each component) per single injection, which can be repeated every 3 to 4 hours.
CHILDREN 12 YEARS OF AGE AND UNDER: 0.5 mg of each component per pound of body weight. The dosage may be repeated every 3 to 4 hours as necessary. For preanesthetic medication the usual adult dose is 2 ml (50 mg of each component) intramuscularly with or without appropriate atropine-like drug. Atropine sulfate 0.3 to 0.4 mg or scopolamine hydrobromide 0.25 to 0.4 mg in sterile solution may be mixed in the same syringe with Mepergan. Repeat doses of 50 mg or less of both promethazine and meperidine may be administered by either route at 3- to 4-hour intervals, as necessary. As an adjunct to local or general anesthesia the usual dose is 2 ml (50 mg each of meperidine and promethazine).
Overdosage: SYMPTOMS: Serious overdose with meperidine is characterized by respiratory depression (a decrease in respiratory rate and/or tidal volume, Cheyne-Stokes respiration, cyanosis), extreme somnolence progressing to stupor or coma, skeletal muscle flaccidity, cold and clammy skin, and sometimes bradycardia and hypotension. In severe overdosage, particularly by the intravenous route, apnea, circulatory collapse, cardiac arrest, and death may occur.
TREATMENT: Primary attention should be given to the reestablishment of adequate respiratory exchange through provision of a patent airway and institution of assisted or controlled ventilation. The narcotic antagonists, naloxone hydrochloride, nalorphine hydrochloride, and levallorphan tartrate, are specific antidotes against respiratory depression which may result from overdosage or unusual sensitivity to narcotics, including meperidine. Therefore, an appropriate dose of one of these antagonists should be administered, preferably by the intravenous route, simultaneously with efforts at respiratory resuscitation.
An antagonist should not be administered in absence of clinically significant respiratory or cardiovascular depression.
Oxygen, intravenous fluids, vasopressors, and other supportive measures should be employed as indicated.
NOTE: In an individual physically dependent on narcotics, the administration of the usual dose of a narcotic antagonist will precipitate an acute withdrawal syndrome. The severity of this syndrome will depend on the degree of physical dependence and the dose of antagonist administered. The use of narcotic antagonists in such individuals should be avoided if possible. If a narcotic antagonist must be used to treat serious respiratory depression in the physically dependent patient, the antagonist should be administered with extreme care and only one-fifth to one-tenth the usual initial dose administered.
Attempted suicides with promethazine have resulted in deep sedation, coma, rarely convulsions and cardiorespiratory symptoms compatible with the depth of sedation present. Extrapyramidal reactions may be treated with anticholinergic antiparkinson agents, diphenhydramine, or barbiturates.
If severe hypotension occurs, levarterenol or phenylephrine may be indicated. Epinephrine is probably best avoided, since it has been suggested that promethazine overdosage could produce a partial alphaadrenergic blockade.
A paradoxical reaction, characterized by hyperexcitability and nightmares, has been reported in children receiving large single doses of promethazine.
How Supplied: Mepergan® (meperidine hydrochloride and promethazine hydrochloride) is supplied in 10 ml vials and TUBEX® Sterile Cartridge-Needle Units.
Subject to Regulations of Federal Bureau Narcotics and Dangerous Drugs.

OMNIPEN® ℞
(ampicillin)
ORAL SUSPENSION

Description: Omnipen (ampicillin) is a semisynthetic penicillin derived from the basic penicillin nucleus, 6-amino-penicillanic acid. For concentrations see under "How Supplied."
Actions
MICROBIOLOGY:
In vitro studies have shown sensitivity of the following microorganisms to ampicillin:
GRAM-POSITIVE: Alpha- and beta-hemolytic streptococci, *Diplococcus pneumoniae*, staphylococci (nonpenicillinase-producing), *Bacillus anthracis*, clostridia spp., *Corynebacterium xerose*, and most strains of enterococci.
The drug does not resist destruction by penicillinase; hence, it is not effective against penicillin G-resistant staphylococci.
GRAM-NEGATIVE: *Hemophilus influenzae, Neisseria gonorrhoeae, Neisseria meningitidis, Proteus mirabilis,* and many strains of Salmonella (including *S. typhosa*), Shigella, and *Escherichia coli.*
TESTING FOR SUSCEPTIBILITY: The invading organism should be cultured and its sensitivity demonstrated as a guide to therapy. If the Kirby-Bauer method of disc sensitivity is used, a 10 mcg. ampicillin disc should be used to determine the relative *in vitro* susceptibility.
HUMAN PHARMACOLOGY:
Ampicillin is stable in the presence of gastric acid and is well absorbed from the gastrointestinal tract. It diffuses readily into most body tissues and fluids. However, penetration into the cerebrospinal fluid and brain occurs only with meningeal inflammation. Ampicillin is excreted largely unchanged in the urine. Its excretion can be delayed by concurrent administration of probenecid. Ampicillin is the least serum-bound of all the penicillins, averaging 20% compared to 60–90% for other penicillins.
Blood-level determinations were made in 60 normal male volunteers receiving a total of 116 separate dosages with anhydrous ampicillin. Of these volunteers 57 also received ampicillin trihydrate in crossover studies. Results show statistically significant higher blood levels at the ½, 1- and 2-hour periods with the anhydrous form. After the first two hours, the same high and persistent blood levels were observed with both forms. The studies utilized oral suspensions given as a single 250 mg. dose of each drug. Assay was performed against sarcina lutea. MIC of the test organism was 0.005 mcg. per ml.

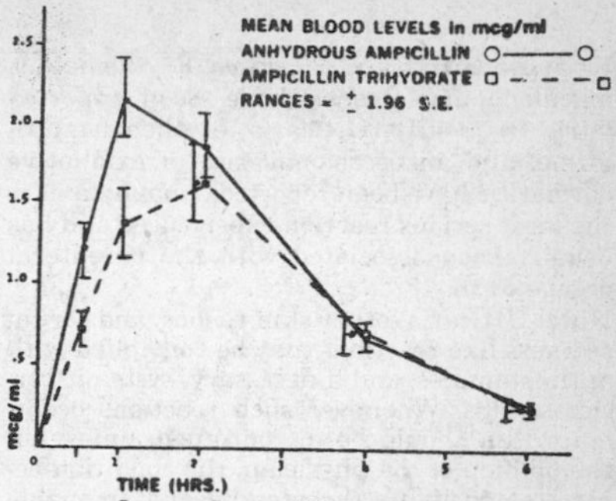

Source: Poole, J.W., et. al, CURR. THERAP. Res.; 10:292 (June) 1968.

Indications: Ampicillin is indicated primarily in the treatment of infections caused by susceptible strains of the following microorganisms: Shigella, Salmonella (including *S. typhosa*), *E. coli, H. influenzae, P. mirabilis, N. gonorrhoeae,* and enterococci. Ampicillin is also indicated in certain infections caused by susceptible gram-positive organisms: penicillin G-sensitive staphylococci, streptococci and pneumococci. Bacteriology studies to determine the causative organisms and their sensitivity to ampicillin should be performed. Therapy may be instituted prior to the results of sensitivity testing.
Contraindications: Ampicillin is contraindicated in patients with a history of a hypersensitivity reaction to the penicillins.
Warnings: Serious and occasionally fatal hypersensitivity (anaphylactic) reactions have been reported in patients on penicillin therapy. Although anaphylaxis is more frequent following parenteral therapy, it has occurred in patients on oral penicillins. These reactions are more apt to occur in individuals with a history of sensitivity to multiple allergens.
There have been reports of individuals with a history of penicillin hypersensitivity who experienced severe reactions when treated with cephalosporins. Before therapy with any penicillin, careful inquiry should be made concerning previous hypersensitivity reactions to penicillins, cephalosporins, or other allergens. If an allergic reaction occurs, appropriate therapy should be instituted and discontinuance of ampicillin therapy considered. The usual agents (antihistamines, pressor amines, corticosteroids) should be readily available. Serious anaphylactic reactions require the immediate use of these agents.
Usage in Pregnancy: Safety for use in pregnancy has not been established.
Precautions: As with any potent drug, periodic assessment of renal, hepatic, and hematopoietic function should be made during prolonged therapy.
The possibility of superinfections with mycotic or bacterial pathogens should be kept in mind during therapy. If superinfections occur, appropriate therapy should be instituted.
Adverse Reactions: As with other penicillins, it may be expected that untoward reactions will be essentially limited to sensitivity phenomena. They are more likely to occur in individuals who have previously demonstrated hypersensitivity to penicillins and in those with a history of allergy, asthma, hay fever, or urticaria.
The following adverse reactions have been reported as associated with the use of ampicillin:
Gastrointestinal: Glossitis, stomatitis, nausea, vomiting, enterocolitis, pseudomembranous colitis, and diarrhea. (These reactions are usually associated with oral-dosage forms.)

Continued on next page

Wyeth—Cont.

Hypersensitivity Reactions: Erythematous maculopapular rashes have been reported fairly frequently. Urticaria, erythema multiforme, and an occasional case of exfoliative dermatitis have been reported. Anaphylaxis is the most serious reaction experienced and has usually been associated with the parenteral dosage form.
Note: Urticaria, other skin rashes, and serum sickness-like reactions may be controlled with antihistamines, and if necessary, systemic corticosteroids. Whenever such reactions occur, ampicillin should be discontinued, unless, in the opinion of the physician, the condition being treated is life threatening and amenable only to ampicillin therapy. Serious anaphylactic reactions require the immediate use of epinephrine, oxygen, and intravenous steroids.
Liver: A moderate rise in serum glutamic-oxaloacetic transaminase (SGOT) has been noted, particularly in infants, but the significance of this finding is unknown.
Hemic and Lymphatic Systems: Anemia, thrombocytopenia, thrombocytopenic purpura, eosinophilia, leukopenia, and agranulocytosis have been reported during therapy with the penicillins. These reactions are usually reversible on discontinuation of therapy and are believed to be hypersensitivity phenomena.
Dosage and Administration: See Chart.

OMNIPEN (ampicillin)
ORAL SUSPENSION

Dosage and Administration

Infection	Adults*	Children*†
Respiratory tract	250 mg. q. 6 h.	50 mg/kg/day in equal doses q. 6-8 h.
Gastrointestinal tract	500 mg. q. 6 h.	100 mg/kg/day in equal doses q. 6-8 h.
Genitourinary tract	500 mg. q. 6 h.	100 mg/kg/day in equal doses q. 6-8 h.

*Larger doses may be needed for severe infections.
*†Children's dosage recommendations are intended for those whose weight will not result in a dosage higher than the adult.

N. gonorrhoeae infections: Urethral, cervical, rectal, and pharyngeal infections in adults should be treated with a single oral dose of 3.5 grams with 1 gram of probenecid given simultaneously. Follow-up cultures should be performed in males within 4-7 days and in females from 7-14 days post therapy.
All gonorrhea patients should have a serologic test for syphilis at the time of diagnosis. Patients with negative serology and no suspected lesions of syphilis should have a follow-up test for syphilis monthly for 4 months to detect possible syphilis masked by gonorrhea therapy.
Patients with gonorrhea who also have syphilis should be given additional treatment appropriate to the stage of syphilis.
Patients should continue the medication at least 48 to 72 hours after all symptoms have subsided or cultures have become negative.
Infections due to hemolytic streptococci require a minimum of 10 days' therapy to help prevent acute rheumatic fever or glomerulonephritis.
For chronic infections of the genitourinary and gastrointestinal tracts, frequent bacteriologic and clinical appraisal is necessary, with follow-up of several months after cessation of therapy.
How Supplied: OMNIPEN (ampicillin) for Oral Suspension: 125 mg. per 5 ml., bottles of 2, 2.5, 3.75, or 5 Gm. ampicillin to be reconstituted with water to make 80 ml., 100 ml., 150 ml., or 200 ml. of suspension; 250 mg. per 5 ml., bottles of 4, 5, 7.5, or 10 Gm. ampicillin to be reconstituted with water to make 80 ml., 100 ml., 150 ml., or 200 ml. of suspension; 250 mg. per pouch (REDIPAK®) for individual dose, carton of 20, to be reconstituted with water; 500 mg. per 5 ml., bottles of 10 Gm. ampicillin to be reconstituted with water to make 100 ml. of suspension.

OMNIPEN® ℞
(ampicillin)
CAPSULES

Description: Omnipen (ampicillin) is a semisynthetic penicillin derived from the basic penicillin nucleus, 6-amino-penicillanic acid.
Actions
MICROBIOLOGY:
In vitro studies have shown sensitivity of the following microorganisms to ampicillin:
GRAM-POSITIVE: Alpha- and beta-hemolytic streptococci, *Diplococcus pneumoniae*, staphylococci (nonpenicillinase-producing), *Bacillus anthracis*, clostridia spp., *Corynebacterium xerose*, and most strains of enterococci.
The drug does not resist destruction by penicillinase; hence, it is not effective against penicillin G-resistant staphylococci.
GRAM-NEGATIVE: *Hemophilus influenzae, Neisseria gonorrhoeae, Neisseria meningitidis, Proteus mirabilis,* and many strains of Salmonella (including *S. typhosa*), Shigella, and *Escherichia coli.*
TESTING FOR SUSCEPTIBILITY: The invading organism should be cultured and its sensitivity demonstrated as a guide to therapy. If the Kirby-Bauer method of disc sensitivity is used, a 10 mcg ampicillin disc should be used to determine the relative *in vitro* susceptibility.
HUMANPHARMACOLOGY:
Ampicillin is stable in the presence of gastric acid and is well-absorbed from the gastrointestinal tract. It diffuses readily into most body tissues and fluids. However, penetration into the cerebrospinal fluid and brain occurs only with meningeal inflammation. Ampicillin is excreted largely unchanged in the urine. Its excretion can be delayed by concurrent administration of probenicid. Ampicillin is the least serum-bound of all the penicillins, averaging 20% compared to 60–90% for other penicillins. Blood-serum levels of approximately 2 mcg/ml are attained within 1–2 hours following a 250 mg oral dose given to fasting adults. Detectable amounts persist for about 6 hours.
Indications: Ampicillin is indicated primarily in the treatment of infections caused by susceptible strains of the following microorganisms: Shigella, Salmonella (including *S. typhosa*), *E. coli, H. influenzae, P. mirabilis, N. gonorrhoeae* and enterococci. Ampicillin is also indicated in certain infections caused by susceptible gram-positive organisms: penicillin G-sensitive staphylococci, streptococci and pneumococci.
Bacteriology studies to determine the causative organisms and their sensitivity to ampicillin should be performed. Therapy may be instituted prior to the results of sensitivity testing.
Contraindications: The use of this drug is contraindicated in individuals with a history of an allergic reaction to the penicillins.
Warnings: Serious and occasionally fatal hypersensitivity (anaphylactic) reactions have been reported in patients on penicillin therapy. Although anaphylaxis is more frequent following parenteral therapy, it has occurred in patients on oral penicillins. These reactions are more apt to occur in individuals with a history of sensitivity to multiple allergens.
There have been reports of individuals with a history of penicillin hypersensitivity who experienced severe reactions when treated with cephalosporins. Before therapy with any penicillin, careful inquiry should be made concerning previous hypersensitivity reactions to penicillins, cephalosporins, or other allergens. If an allergic reaction occurs, appropriate therapy should be instituted and discontinuance of ampicillin therapy considered. The usual agents (antihistamines, pressor amines, corticosteroids) should be readily available. Serious anaphylactic reactions require the immediate use of these agents.
Usage in Pregnancy: Safety for use in pregnancy has not been established.
Precautions: As with any potent drug, periodic assessment of renal, hepatic, and hematopoietic function should be made during prolonged therapy.
The possibility of superinfections with mycotic or bacterial pathogens should be kept in mind during therapy. If superinfections occur, appropriate therapy should be instituted.
Adverse Reactions: As with other penicillins, it may be expected that untoward reactions will be essentially limited to sensitivity phenomena. They are more likely to occur in individuals who have previously demonstrated hypersensitivity to penicillins and in those with a history of allergy, asthma, hay fever, or urticaria.
The following adverse reactions have been reported as associated with the use of ampicillin:
Gastrointestinal: Glossitis, stomatitis, nausea, vomiting, enterocolitis, pseudomembranous colitis, and diarrhea. (These reactions are usually associated with oral-dosage forms.)
Hypersensitivity Reactions: Erythematous maculopapular rashes have been reported fairly frequently. Urticaria, erythema multiforme, and an occasional case of exfoliative dermatitis have been reported. Anaphylaxis is the most serious reaction experienced and has usually been associated with the parenteral-dosage form.
Note: Urticaria, other skin rashes, and serum sickness-like reactions may be controlled with antihistamines, and if necessary, systemic corticosteroids. Whenever such reactions occur, ampicillin should be discontinued, unless, in the opinion of the physician, the condition being treated is life-threatening and amenable only to ampicillin therapy. Serious anaphylactic reactions require the immediate use of epinephrine, oxygen and intravenous steroids.
Liver: A moderate rise in the serum glutamic-oxaloacetic transaminase (SGOT) has been noted, particularly in infants, but the significance of this finding is unknown.
Hemic and Lymphatic Systems: Anemia, thrombocytopenia, thrombocytopenic purpura, eosinophilia, leukopenia, and agranulocytosis have been reported during therapy with the penicillins. These reactions are usually reversible on discontinuation of therapy and are believed to be hypersensitivity phenomena.
Dosage and Administration: Infections of the ear, nose, throat and lower respiratory tract due to streptococci, pneumococci, and nonpenicillinase-producing staphylococci; and also those infections of the upper and lower respiratory tract due to *H. influenzae.*
Adults: 250 mg every 6 hours.
Children: 50 mg./kg./day in divided doses every 6 or 8 hours.
Infections of the genitourinary tract caused by sensitive gram-negative and gram-positive bacteria.
Adults: 500 mg. every 6 hours. Larger doses may be required for severe infections.
Children: 100 mg./kg./day in divided doses every 6 hours.
N. gonorrhoeae infections: urethral, cervical, rectal, and pharyngeal infections in adults should be treated with a single oral dose of 3.5 grams with 1 gram of probenecid given simultaneously. Follow-up cultures should be performed in males within 4-7 days and in females from 7-14 days post therapy.
All gonorrhea patients should have a serologic test for syphilis at the time of diagnosis. Patients with negative serology and no suspected lesions of syphilis should have a follow-up test

for syphilis monthly for 4 months to detect possible syphilis masked by gonorrhea therapy.
Patients with gonorrhea who also have syphilis should be given additional treatment appropriate to the stage of syphilis.
Infections of the gastrointestinal tract.
Adults: 500 mg. every 6 hours.
Children: 100 mg./kg./day in divided doses every 6 hours.
Larger doses may be required for stubborn or severe infections.
The children's dosage is intended for individuals whose weight will not cause a dosage to be calculated greater than that recommended for adults. Children weighing more than 20 kg should be dosed according to the adult recommendations.
It should be recognized that in the treatment of chronic urinary-tract and intestinal infections, frequent bacteriological and clinical appraisal are necessary. Smaller doses than those recommended above should not be used. Even higher doses may be needed at times. In stubborn infections, therapy may be required for several weeks. It may be necessary to continue clinical and/or bacteriological follow-up for several months after cessation of therapy.
Treatment should be continued for a minimum of 48 to 72 hours beyond the time that the patient becomes asymptomatic or evidence of bacterial eradication has been obtained. It is recommended that there be at least 10 days' treatment for any infection caused by hemolytic streptococci, to prevent the occurrence of acute rheumatic fever or glomerulonephritis.
How Supplied: OMNIPEN® (ampicillin) Capsules—250 mg. ampicillin anhydrous, bottles of 100 and 500 capsules; 500 mg., bottles of 100 and 500 capsules. REDIPAK® Unit Dose Medication, 250 mg. and 500 mg., boxes of 100 capsules (individually wrapped).

[*Shown in Product Identification Section*]

OMNIPEN®-N ℞

(ampicillin sodium)
INJECTION

FOR INTRAMUSCULAR OR INTRAVENOUS INJECTION

Description: Omnipen-N (ampicillin sodium) for Injection is a semisynthetic penicillin derived from the basic penicillin nucleus, 6-amino penicillanic acid.
NOTE: Omnipen-N contains 3.1 milliequivalents of sodium per gram of ampicillin as the sodium salt.

Actions

MICROBIOLOGY:
In vitro studies have shown sensitivity of the following microorganisms to ampicillin:
GRAM-POSITIVE: Alpha- and beta-hemolytic streptococci, *Diplococcus pneumoniae,* staphylococci (nonpenicillinase-producing), *Bacillus anthracis,* clostridia spp., *Corynebacterium xerosis,* and most strains of enterococci.
The drug does not resist destruction by penicillinase; hence, it is not effective against penicillin G-resistant staphylococci.
GRAM-NEGATIVE: *Hemophilus influenzae, Neisseria gonorrhoeae, Neisseria meningitidis, Proteus mirabilis,* and many strains of Salmonella (including *Salmonella typhosa),* Shigella, and *Escherichia coli.*
TESTING FOR SUSCEPTIBILITY: The invading organism should be cultured and its sensitivity demonstrated as a guide to therapy. If the Kirby-Bauer method of disc sensitivity is used, a 10-mcg ampicillin disc should be used to determine the relative *in vitro* susceptibility.
HUMAN PHARMACOLOGY:
Ampicillin is stable in the presence of gastric acid and is well-absorbed from the gastrointestinal tract. It diffuses readily into most body tissues and fluids. However, penetration into the cerebrospinal fluid and brain occurs only with meningeal inflammation.
Ampicillin is excreted largely unchanged in the urine. Its excretion can be delayed by concurrent administration of probenecid. Ampicillin is the least serum-bound of all the penicillins, averaging 20% compared to 60–90% for other penicillins.
Blood serum levels obtained on IM injection are proportionate to the dose administered. Levels of approximately 40 mcg/ml per 1-gram IM dose are attained at one-half hour. Higher levels are attainable with IV injection, depending on the dose and rate of administration.
Indications: Ampicillin is indicated primarily in the treatment of infections caused by susceptible strains of the following microorganisms: Shigella, Salmonella (including *S. typhosa), E. coli, H. influenzae, P. mirabilis, N. gonorrhoeae,* and enterococci. It is also effective in the treatment of meningitis due to *N. meningitidis.* Since it is effective against the commonest pathogens causing meningitis, it may be used intravenously as initial therapy before the results of bacteriology are available. Ampicillin is also indicated in certain infections caused by susceptible gram-positive organisms: penicillin G-sensitive staphylococci, streptococci, and pneumococci. Bacteriologic studies to determine the causative organisms and their sensitivity to ampicillin should be performed. Therapy may be instituted prior to the results of culture and sensitivity testing.
It is advisable to reserve the parenteral form of this drug for moderately severe and severe infections and for patients who are unable to take the oral forms (capsules, oral suspension, or pediatric drops). A change to oral Omnipen (ampicillin) may be made as soon as appropriate.
Contraindications: Ampicillin is contraindicated in patients with a history of a hypersensitivity reaction to the penicillins.
Warnings: Serious and occasionally fatal hypersensitivity (anaphylactoid) reactions have been reported in patients on penicillin therapy. Although anaphylaxis is more frequent following parenteral therapy, it has occurred in patients on oral penicillins. These reactions are more apt to occur in individuals with a history of sensitivity to multiple allergens.
There have been reports of individuals with a history of penicillin hypersensitivity who experienced severe reactions when treated with cephalosporins. Before therapy with any penicillin, careful inquiry should be made concerning previous hypersensitivity reactions to penicillins, cephalosporins, or other allergens. If an allergic reaction occurs, appropriate therapy should be instituted and discontinuation of ampicillin therapy considered. **Serious anaphylactoid reactions require immediate emergency treatment with epinephrine. Oxygen, intravenous steroids, and airway management, including intubation, should be administered as indicated.**
Usage in Pregnancy: Safety for use in pregnancy has not been established.
Precautions: As with any potent drug, periodic assessment of renal, hepatic, and hematopoietic function should be made during prolonged therapy.
The possibility of superinfections with mycotic or bacterial pathogens should be kept in mind during therapy. If superinfections occur, appropriate therapy should be instituted.
Adverse Reactions: As with other penicillins, it may be expected that untoward reactions will be essentially limited to sensitivity phenomena. They are more likely to occur in individuals who have previously demonstrated hypersensitivity to penicillins and in those with a history of allergy, asthma, hay fever, or urticaria.
The following adverse reactions have been reported in association with ampicillin uses:
Gastrointestinal: Glossitis, stomatitis, nausea, vomiting, diarrhea. (These reactions are usually associated with oral dosage forms.)
Hypersensitivity: Erythematous maculopapular rashes have been reported fairly frequently. Urticaria, erythema multiforme, and an occasional case of exfoliative dermatitis have been reported. Anaphylaxis is the most serious reaction experienced and has usually been associated with the parenteral dosage form.
NOTE: Urticaria, other skin rashes, and serum-sicknesslike reactions may be controlled with antihistamines and, if necessary, systemic corticosteroids. Whenever such reactions occur, ampicillin should be discontinued, unless, in the opinion of the physician, the condition being treated is life-threatening and amenable only to ampicillin therapy. Serious anaphylactoid reactions require the immediate use of epinephrine, oxygen, and intravenous steroids.
Hepatic: A moderate rise in serum glutamic-oxalocetic transaminase (SGOT) has been noted, particularly in infants, but the significance of this finding is unknown.
Hemic and Lymphatic Systems: anemia, thrombocytopenia, thrombocytopenic purpura, eosinophilia, leukopenia, and agranulocytosis have been reported during therapy with the penicillins. These reactions are usually reversible on discontinuation of therapy and are believed to be hypersensitivity phenomena.
Dosage:
[See table on next page].
Smaller doses than those recommended in the table above should not be used. In stubborn or severe infections, therapy may be required for several weeks, and even higher doses may be needed. In treatment of chronic urinary or intestinal infections, frequent bacteriological and clinical appraisal is necessary, with follow-up for several months after cessation of therapy.
The treatment of gram-negative infections is often complicated by the emergence of resistant organisms *(A. aerogenes, Ps. aeruginosa* and others) which may cause superinfections. The possibility of such an occurrence should be kept in mind with use of ampicillin sodium.
Treatment should be continued at least 48 to 72 hours after the patient becomes asymptomatic or evidence of bacterial eradication is obtained. A minimum of 10 days' treatment is recommended for beta-hemolytic streptococcal infections to help prevent acute rheumatic fever or glomerulonephritis.
A change to oral OMNIPEN (ampicillin) may be made as soon as appropriate.

Administration

VIALS—125 mg, 250 mg, 500 mg, 1 gram, and 2 gram.
Intramuscular Use: 125 mg. vial: Add 1 ml Sterile Water for Injection, USP, or Bacteriostatic Water for Injection, USP (TUBEX® Sterile Cartridge-Needle Unit) to give a final concentration of 125 mg. per ml. For fractional doses, withdraw the ampicillin sodium solution as follows:

Dose	Withdraw
25 mg	0.2 ml
50 mg	0.4 ml
75 mg	0.6 ml
100 mg	0.8 ml
125 mg	1 ml

250 mg vial: Add 0.9 ml Sterile Water for Injection, USP, or Bacteriostatic Water for Injection, USP (TUBEX) to give a final concentration of 250 mg./ml. For fractional doses, withdraw the ampicillin sodium solution as follows:

Dose	Withdraw
125 mg	0.5 ml
150 mg	0.6 ml
175 mg	0.7 ml
200 mg	0.8 ml
225 mg	0.9 ml
250 mg	1 ml

For dilution of 500-mg, 1-gram, and 2-gram vials, dissolve contents of a vial with the

Continued on next page

Wyeth—Cont.

amount of Sterile Water for Injection, USP, or Bacteriostatic Water for Injection, USP, listed in the table below:

Label Claim	Recommended Amount of Diluent	Withdrawable Volume	Concentration in mg/ml
500 mg	1.8 ml	2.0 ml	250 mg
1.0 gram	3.4 ml	4.0 ml	250 mg
2.0 gram	6.8 ml	8.0 ml	250 mg

While the 1-gram and 2-gram vials are primarily for intravenous use, they may be administered intramuscularly when the 250-mg or 500-mg vials are unavailable. In such instances, dissolve in 3.4 or 6.8 ml Sterile Water for Injection, USP, or Bacteriostatic Water for Injection, USP, to give a final concentration of 250 mg/ml.

The above solutions must be used within one hour after reconstitution.

Direct Intravenous Use: 125-mg, 250-mg, and 500-mg vials: Add 5 ml Sterile Water for Injection, USP, or Bacteriostatic Water for Injection, USP (TUBEX®), and withdraw the entire contents; the dose should be injected over a period of 3 to 5 minutes.

1-gram and 2-gram vials: Add 10 ml Sterile Water for Injection, USP or Bacteriostatic Water for Injection, USP (TUBEX) and withdraw the entire contents; administer slowly over a period of at least 10 to 15 minutes. CAUTION: More rapid administration may result in convulsive seizures. The above solutions should be used within one hour after reconstitution.

To reconstitute for continuous intravenous infusion, dissolve the contents of 125-mg, 250-mg, 500-mg vials in 5 ml and the 1-gram and 2-gram vials in 10 ml Sterile Water for Injection, USP, or Bacteriostatic Water for Injection, USP (TUBEX), and transfer directly to acceptable large-volume IV fluids. Stability of the resulting solution at room temperature or under refrigeration will vary with the bulk fluid. (See tables.)

For Administration by Intravenous Drip: Stability studies on ampicillin sodium in various intravenous solutions indicate the drug will lose less than 10% activity at room temperature (70°F) for the time periods and concentrations stated:

IV Solution	Concentrations	Stability Periods
Sterile Water for Injection	Up to 30 mg/ml	8 hours
Isotonic Sodium Chloride	Up to 30 mg/ml	8 hours
M/6 Sodium Lactate Solution	Up to 30 mg/ml	8 hours
5% Dextrose in Water	10 to 20 mg/ml	2 hours
5% Dextrose in Water	Up to 2 mg/ml	4 hours
5% Dextrose in 0.45% Sodium Chloride	Up to 2 mg/ml	4 hours
10% Invert Sugar	Up to 2 mg/ml	4 hours
Lactated Ringer's Solution	Up to 30 mg/ml	8 hours

If the solutions below are stored under refrigeration, they will remain stable for the time periods indicated:

IV Solution	Concentrations	Stability Periods
Sterile Water for Injection	30 mg/ml	48 hours
Sterile Water for Injection	Up to 20 mg/ml	72 hours
Isotonic Sodium Chloride	30 mg/ml	48 hours
Isotonic Sodium Chloride	Up to 20 mg/ml	72 hours
Lactated Ringer's Solution	Up to 30 mg/ml	24 hours
M/6 Sodium Lactate Solution	Up to 30 mg/ml	8 hours
5% Dextrose in Water	Up to 20 mg/ml	4 hours
5% Dextrose in 0.4% Sodium Chloride	Up to 10 mg/ml	4 hours
10% Invert Sugar	Up to 20 mg/ml	3 hours

Piggyback Units (for Intravenous Drip Use)—Use Sterile Water for Injection or Isotonic Sodium Chloride.

500-MG BOTTLE:

Add a minimum of 50 ml water or saline, and shake well. If lower concentrations are desired, the solution could be further diluted with up to a total of 100 ml of diluent.

Diluent Amount	Solution Concentration
50 ml	10 mg/ml
100 ml	5 mg/ml

ONE-GRAM BOTTLE:

Add a minimum of 49 ml water or saline, and shake well. If lower concentrations are desired, the solution could be further diluted with up to a total of 99 ml of diluent.

Diluent Amount	Solution Concentration
49 ml	20 mg/ml
99 ml	10 mg/ml

TWO-GRAM BOTTLE:

Add 99 ml water or saline, and shake well. The resulting solution will contain 20 mg/ml.

Caution: Administer slowly by intravenous route over a period of at least 10–15 minutes. More rapid administration may result in convulsive seizures. The solution should be used within 8 hours after reconstitution if kept at room temperature.

To reconstitute for continuous intravenous infusion, dissolve the contents of the 500-mg, 1-gram or 2-gram piggyback unit in 10 ml Sterile Water for Injection, USP, or Bacteriostatic Water for Injection, USP (TUBEX®), and transfer directly to acceptable large-volume IV fluids. Stability of the resulting solution at room temperature or under refrigeration will vary with the bulk fluid used. (See tables.)

How Supplied: Omnipen®-N (ampicillin sodium) for Injection: Ampicillin sodium equivalent to 125 mg, 250 mg, 500 mg, 1 gram or 2 gram ampicillin per standard vial and **Piggyback Units:** Supplied in single units equivalent to 1 gram or 2 gram ampicillin per unit, packed in 10 vials per package.

OMNIPEN®-N
(ampicillin sodium)

Infection	Organisms	Dosage (IM or IV) Adults	Dosage (IM or IV) Children*
Respiratory tract	streptococci, pneumococci, nonpenicillinase-producing staphylococci, *H. influenzae*	250-500 mg. q. 6 h.	25-50 mg/kg/day in equal doses q. 6 h.
Gastrointestinal tract	susceptible pathogens	500 mg. q. 6 h.	50 mg/kg/day in equal doses q. 6 h.
Genitourinary tract	susceptible gram-negative or gram-positive pathogens	500 mg. q. 6 h.	50 mg/kg/day in equal doses q. 6 h.
Urethritis (acute) in adult males	*N. gonorrhoeae*	500 mg. b.i.d. for 1 day (IM)	
	(In complications such as prostatitis and epididymitis, prolonged and intensive therapy is recommended. Gonorrhea cases with suspected primary lesion of syphilis should have dark-field examinations before treatment. In any case suspected of concomitant syphilis, monthly serologic tests for at least 4 months are necessary.)		
Bacterial meningitis	*N. meningitidis* *H. influenzae*	8-14 gm/day	100-200 mg/kg/day
	(Initial treatment is usually by IV drip, followed by frequent [q. 3-4 h.] IM injections.)		

***Children's dosage recommendations are intended for those whose weight will not result in a dosage higher than the adult.**

OVRAL® TABLETS ℞

Description: Each Ovral® tablet contains 0.5 mg of norgestrel (dl-13-beta-ethyl-17-alpha-ethinyl-17-beta-hydroxygon-4-en-3-one), a totally synthetic progestogen, and 0.05 mg of ethinyl estradiol (19-Nor-17α-pregna-1,3,5 (10)-trien-20-yne-3,17-diol).

Clinical Pharmacology: See LO/OVRAL®.

Indications and Usage: Ovral® is indicated for the prevention of pregnancy in women who elect to use oral contraceptives as a method of contraception.

Oral contraceptives are highly effective. The pregnancy rate in women using conventional combination oral contraceptives (containing 35 mcg or more of ethinyl estradiol or 50 mcg or more of mestranol) is generally reported as less than one pregnancy per 100 woman-years of use. Slightly higher rates (somewhat more than 1 pregnancy per 100 woman-years of use) are reported for some combination products containing 35 mcg or less of ethinyl estradiol, and rates on the order of 3 pregnancies per 100 woman-years are reported for the progestogen-only oral contraceptives.

These rates are derived from separate studies conducted by different investigators in several population groups and cannot be compared precisely. Furthermore, pregnancy rates tend to be lower as clinical studies are continued possibly due to selective retention in the longer studies of those patients who accept the treatment regimen and do not discontinue as a result of adverse reactions, pregnancy, or other reasons.

In clinical trials with Ovral®, 6,806 patients completed 127,872 cycles, and a total of 19 pregnancies were reported. This represents a pregnancy rate of 0.19 per 100 woman-years. All of the pregnancies reported in these trials were the result of patient failure.

Table 1 gives ranges of pregnancy rates reported in the literature[1] for other means of contraception. The efficacy of these means of contraception (except the IUD) depends upon the degree of adherence to the method.

TABLE 1

PREGNANCIES PER 100 WOMAN-YEARS

IUD, less than 1–6; Diaphragm with spermicidal products (creams or jellies), 2–20; Con-

dom, 3–36; Aerosol foams, 2–29; Jellies and creams, 4–36;
Periodic abstinence (rhythm) all types, less than 1–47:
1. Calendar method, 14–47;
2. Temperature method, 1–20;
3. Temperature method—intercourse only in postovulatory phase, less than 1–7;
4. Mucus method, 1–25;
No contraception, 60–80.

Dose-Related Risk of Thromboembolism from Oral Contraceptives: See LO/OVRAL.
Contraindications: See LO/OVRAL.
Warnings: See LO/OVRAL.
Precautions: See LO/OVRAL.
Information for the Patient: See LO/OVRAL.
Drug Interactions: See LO/OVRAL.
Carcinogenesis: See LO/OVRAL.
Pregnancy: See LO/OVRAL.
Nursing Mothers: See LO/OVRAL.
Adverse Reactions: See LO/OVRAL.
Acute Overdose: See LO/OVRAL.
Dosage and Administration: To achieve maximum contraceptive effectiveness, Ovral® must be taken exactly as directed and at intervals not exceeding 24 hours. The dosage of Ovral® is one tablet daily for 21 consecutive days per menstrual cycle according to prescribed schedule. Tablets are then discontinued for 7 days (three weeks on, one week off). It is recommended that Ovral® tablets be taken at the same time each day, preferably after the evening meal or at bedtime.
During the first cycle of medication, the patient is instructed to take one Ovral® tablet daily for twenty-one consecutive days beginning on day five of her menstrual cycle. (The first day of menstruation is day one.) The tablets are then discontinued for one week (7 days). Withdrawal bleeding should usually occur within three days following discontinuation of Ovral®. (If Ovral® is first taken later than the fifth day of the first menstrual cycle of medication or postpartum, contraceptive reliance should not be placed on Ovral® until after the first seven consecutive days of administration. The possibility of ovulation and conception prior to initiation of medication should be considered.) The patient begins her next and all subsequent 21-days courses of Ovral® tablets on the same day of the week that she began her first course, following the same schedule: 21 days on—7 days off.
She begins taking her tablets on the 8th day after discontinuance regardless of whether or not a menstrual period has occurred or is still in progress. Any time a new cycle of Ovral® is started later than the 8th day the patient should be protected by another means of contraception until she has taken a tablet daily for seven consecutive days.
If spotting or breakthrough bleeding occurs, the patient is instructed to continue on the same regimen. This type of bleeding is usually transient and without significance; however, if the bleeding is persistent or prolonged the patient is advised to consult her physician. Although the occurrence of pregnancy is highly unlikely if Ovral® is taken according to directions, if withdrawal bleeding does not occur, the possibility of pregnancy must be considered. If the patient has not adhered to the prescribed schedule (missed one or more tablets or started taking them on a day later than she should have) the probability of pregnancy should be considered at the time of the first missed period and appropriate diagnostic measures taken before the medication is resumed. If the patient has adhered to the prescribed regimen and misses two consecutive periods, pregnancy should be ruled out before continuing the contraceptive regimen.
The patient should be instructed to take a missed tablet as soon as it is remembered. If two consecutive tablets are missed they should both be taken as soon a remembered. The next tablet should be taken at the usual time.
Any time the patient misses one or two tablets she should also use another method of contraception until she has taken a tablet daily for seven consecutive days. If breakthrough bleeding occurs following missed tablets it will usually be transient and of no consequence. While there is little likelihood of ovulation occuring if only one or two tablets are missed, the possibility of ovulation increases with each successive day that scheduled tablets are missed. If three consecutive tablets are missed, all medication should be discontinued and the remainder of the package discarded. A new tablet cycle should be started on the 8th day after the last tablet was taken, and an alternate means of contraception should be prescribed during the seven days without tablets and until the patient has taken a tablet daily for seven consecutive days. In the nonlactating mother Ovral® may be prescribed in the postpartum period either immediately or at the first postpartum examination whether or not menstruation has resumed.
How Supplied: Ovral® tablets (0.5 mg norgestrel + 0.05 mg ethinyl estradiol) are available in containers of 21 tablets.
References: See LO/OVRAL®.
Brief Summary Patient Package Insert: See LO/OVRAL®.
[Shown in Product Identification Section]

OVRETTE® (norgestrel) TABLETS ℞

Each OVRETTE® tablet contains 0.075 mg of norgestrel (dl-13-beta-ethyl-17-alpha-ethinyl-17-beta-hydroxygon-4-en-3-one).
Description: Each OVRETTE® tablet contains 0.075 mg of a single active steroid ingredient, norgestrel, a totally synthetic progestogen. The available data suggest that the *d*-enantiomeric form of norgestrel is the biologically active portion. This form amounts to 0.0375 mg per OVRETTE® tablet.
Clinical Pharmacology: The primary mechanism through which OVRETTE® prevents conception is not known, but progestogen-only contraceptives are known to alter the cervical mucus, exert a progestational effect on the endometrium, interfering with implantation, and, in some patients, suppress ovulation.
Indications and Usage: OVRETTE® is indicated for the prevention of pregnancy in women who elect to use oral contraceptives as a method of contraception. Oral contraceptives are highly effective. The pregnancy rate in women using conventional combination oral contraceptives (containing 35 mcg or more of ethinyl estradiol or 50 mcg or more of mestranol) is generally reported as less than one pregnancy per 100 woman-years of use. Slightly higher rates (somewhat more than 1 pregnancy per 100 woman-years of use) are reported for some combination products containing 35 mcg or less of ethinyl estradiol, and rates on the order of 3 pregnancies per 100 woman-years are reported for the progestogen-only oral contraceptives.
These rates are derived from separate studies conducted by different investigators in several population groups and cannot be compared precisely. Furthermore, pregnancy rates tend to be lower as clinical studies are continued, possibly due to selective retention in the longer studies of those patients who accept the treatment regimen and do not discontinue as a result of adverse reactions, pregnancy, or other reasons.
In clinical trials with OVRETTE®, 2,752 patients completed 38,245 cycles, and a total of 78 pregnancies were reported. This represents a pregnancy rate of 2.45 per 100 woman-years. Approximately one-half of the pregnancies reported in these trials were due to method failure, and the other half were due to patient failure.
Table 1 gives ranges of pregnancy rates reported in the literature[1] for other means of contraception. The efficacy of these means of contraception (except the IUD) depends upon the degree of adherence to the method.

TABLE 1
PREGNANCIES PER 100 WOMAN-YEARS
IUD, less than 1–6; Diaphragm with spermicidal products (creams or jellies), 2–20; Condom, 3–36; Aerosol foams, 2–29; Jellies and creams, 4–36;
Periodic abstinence (rhythm) all types, less than 1–47:
1. Calendar method, 14–47;
2. Temperature method, 1–20;
3. Temperature method—intercourse only in postovulatory phase, less than 1–7;
4. Mucus method, 1–25;
No contraception, 60–80.

Dose-Related Risk of Thromboembolism from Oral Contraceptives: Two studies have shown a positive association between the dose of estrogens in oral contraceptives and the risk of thromboembolism.[2,3] For this reason, it is prudent and in keeping with good principles of therapeutics to minimize exposure to estrogen. The oral-contraceptive product prescribed for any given patient should be that product which contains the least amount of estrogen that is compatible with an acceptable pregnancy rate and patient acceptance. It is recommended that new acceptors of oral contraceptives be started on preparations containing 0.05 mg or less of estrogen.
Contraindications: Oral contraceptives should not be used in women with any of the following conditions:
1. Thrombophlebitis or thromboembolic disorders.
2. A past history of deep-vein thrombophlebitis or thromboembolic disorders.
3. Cerebral-vascular or coronary-artery disease.
4. Known or suspected carcinoma of the breast.
5. Known or suspected estrogen-dependent neoplasia.
6. Undiagnosed abnormal genital bleeding.
7. Known or suspected pregnancy (see Warning No. 5).

Warnings

Cigarette smoking increases the risk of serious cardiovascular side effects from oral-contraceptive use. This risk increases with age and with heavy smoking (15 or more cigarettes per day) and is quite marked in women over 35 years of age. Women who use oral contraceptives should be strongly advised not to smoke.
The use of oral contraceptives is associated with increased risk of several serious conditions, including thromboembolism, stroke, myocardial infarction, hepatic adenoma, gallbladder disease, hypertension. Practitioners prescribing oral contraceptives should be familiar with the following information relating to these risks.

1. *Thromboembolic Disorders and Other Vascular Problems:* An increased risk of thromboembolic and thrombotic disease associated with the use of oral contraceptives is well-established. Three principal studies in Great Britain[4–6] and three in the United States[7–10] have demonstrated an increased risk of fatal and nonfatal venous thromboembolism and stroke, both hemorrhagic and thrombotic. These studies estimate that users of oral contaceptives are 4 to 11 times more likely than nonusers to develop these diseases without evident cause (Table 2).

Continued on next page

Wyeth—Cont.

CEREBROVASCULAR DISORDERS
In a collaborative American study[9,10] of cerebrovascular disorders in women with and without predisposing causes, it was estimated that the risk of hemorrhagic stroke was 2.0 times greater in users than nonusers and the risk of thrombotic stroke was 4 to 9.5 times greater in users than in nonusers (Table 2).

TABLE 2
SUMMARY OF RELATIVE RISK OF THROMBOEMBOLIC DISORDERS AND OTHER VASCULAR PROBLEMS IN ORAL-CONTRACEPTIVE USERS COMPARED TO NONUSERS

	Relative risk, times greater
Idiopathic thromboembolic disease	4–11
Postsurgery thromboembolic complications	4–6
Thrombotic stroke	4–9.5
Hemorrhagic stroke	2
Myocardial infarction	2–12

MYOCARDIAL INFARCTION
An increased risk of myocardial infarction associated with the use of oral contraceptives has been reported,[11,12,13] confirming a previously suspected association. These studies, conducted in the United Kingdom, found, as expected, that the greater the number of underlying risk factors for coronary-artery disease (cigarette smoking, hypertension, hypercholesterolemia, obesity, diabetes, history of preeclamptic toxemia) the higher the risk of developing myocardial infarction, regardless of whether the patient was an oral-contraceptive user or not. Oral contraceptives, however, were found to be a clear additional risk factor.
In terms of relative risk, it has been estimated[52] that oral-contraceptive users who do not smoke (smoking is considered a major predisposing condition to myocardial infarction) are about twice as likely to have a fatal myocardial infarction as nonusers who do not smoke. Oral-contraceptive users who are also smokers have about a 5-fold increased risk of fatal infarction compared to users who do not smoke, but about a 10- to 12-fold increased risk compared to nonusers who do not smoke. Furthermore, the amount of smoking is also an important factor. In determining the importance of these relative risks, however, the baseline rates for various age groups, as shown in Table 3, must be given serious consideration. The importance of other predisposing conditions mentioned above in determining relative and absolute risks has not as yet been quantified; it is quite likely that the same synergistic action exists, but perhaps to a lesser extent.

TABLE 3
Estimated annual mortality rate per 100,000 women from myocardial infarction by use of oral contraceptives, smoking habits, and age (in years):

	Myocardial infarction			
	Women aged 30–39		Women aged 40–44	
Smoking habits	Users	Non-users	Users	Non-users
All smokers	10.2	2.6	62.0	15.9
Heavy*	13.0	5.1	78.7	31.3
Light	4.7	0.9	28.6	5.7
Nonsmokers	1.8	1.2	10.7	7.4
Smokers and nonsmokers	5.4	1.9	32.8	11.7

*Heavy smoker: 15 or more cigarettes per day.
From JAIN, A.K., *Studies in Family Planning, 8*:50, 1977

RISK OF DOSE
In an analysis of data derived from several national adverse-reaction reporting systems,[2] British investigators concluded that the risk of thromboembolism, including coronary thrombosis, is directly related to the dose of estrogen used in oral contraceptives. Preparations containing 100 mcg or more of estrogen were associated with a higher risk of thromboembolism than those containing 50–80 mcg of estrogen. Their analysis did suggest, however, that the quantity of estrogen may not be the sole factor involved. This finding has been confirmed in the United States.[3] Careful epidemiological studies to determine the degree of thromboembolic risk associated with progestogen-only oral contraceptives have not been performed. Cases of thromboembolic disease have been reported in women using these products, and they should not be presumed to be free of excess risk.

ESTIMATE OF EXCESS MORTALITY FROM CIRCULATORY DISEASES

A large prospective study[53] carried out in the U.K. estimated the mortality rate per 100,000 women per year from diseases of the circulatory system for users and nonusers of oral contraceptives according to age, smoking habits, and duration of use. The overall excess death rate annually from circulatory diseases for oral-contraceptive users was estimated to be 20 per 100,000 (ages 15–34—5/100,000; ages 35–44—33/100,000; ages 45–49—140/100,000), the risk being concentrated in older women, in those with a long duration of use, and in cigarette smokers. It was not possible, however, to examine the interrelationships of age, smoking, and duration of use, nor to compare the effects of continuous vs. intermittent use. Although the study showed a 10-fold increase in death due to circulatory diseases in users for 5 or more years, all of these deaths occurred in women 35 or older. Until larger numbers of women under 35 with continuous use for 5 or more years are available, it is not possible to assess the magnitude of the relative risk for this younger age group.

The available data from a variety of sources have been analyzed[14] to estimate the risk of death associated with various methods of contraception. The estimates of risk of death for each method include the combined risk of the contraceptive method (e.g., thromboembolic and thrombotic disease in the case of oral contraceptives) plus the risk attributable to pregnancy or abortion in the event of method failure. This latter risk varies with the effectiveness of the contraceptive method. The findings of this analysis are shown in Figure 1 below.[14] The study concluded that the mortality associated with all methods of birth control is low and below that associated with childbirth, with the exception of oral contraceptives in women over 40 who smoke. (The rates given for Pill only/smokers for each age group are for smokers as a class. For "heavy" smokers (more than 15 cigarettes a day), the rates given would be about double; for "light" smokers (less than 15 cigarettes a day), about 50 percent. The lowest mortality is associated with the condom or diaphragm backed up by early abortion. The risk of thromboembolic and thrombotic disease associated with oral contraceptives increases with age after approximately age 30 and, for myocardial infarction, is further increased by hypertension, hypercholesterolemia, obesity, diabetes, or history of preeclamptic toxemia and especially by cigarette smoking.

Based on the data currently available, the following chart gives a gross estimate of the risk of death from circulatory disorders associated with the use of oral contraceptives:

SMOKING HABITS AND OTHER PREDISPOSING CONDITIONS— RISK ASSOCIATED WITH USE OF ORAL CONTRACEPTIVES

Age	Below 30	30–39	40+
Heavy smokers	C	B	A
Light smokers	D	C	B
Nonsmokers (no predisposing conditions)	D	C,D	C
Nonsmokers (other predisposing conditions)	C	C,B	B,A

A—Use associated with very high risk.
B—Use associated with high risk.
C—Use associated with moderate risk.
D—Use associated with low risk.

The physician and the patient should be alert to the earliest manifestations of thromboembolic and thrombotic disorders (e.g., thrombophlebitis, pulmonary embolism, cerebrovascular insufficiency, coronary occlusion, retinal thrombosis, and mesenteric thrombosis). Should any of these occur or be suspected, the drug should be discontinued immediately.
A four- to six-fold increased risk of postsurgery thromboembolic complications has been reported in oral-contraceptive users.[15,16] If feasible, oral contraceptives should be discontinued at least 4 weeks before surgery of a type associated with an increased risk of thromboembolism or prolonged immobilization.

2. *Ocular Lesions:*
There have been reports of neuro-ocular lesions such as optic neuritis or retinal thrombosis associated with the use of oral contraceptives. Discontinue oral-contraceptive medication if there is unexplained, sudden or gradual, partial or complete loss of vision; onset of proptosis or diplopia; papilledema; or retinal-vascular lesions, and institute appropriate diagnostic and therapeutic measures.

3. *Carcinoma:*
Long-term continuous administration of either natural or synthetic estrogen in certain animal species increases the frequency of carcinoma of the breast, cervix, vagina, and liver. Certain synthetic progestogens, none currently contained in oral contraceptives, have been noted to increase the incidence of mammary nodules, benign and malignant, in dogs.
In humans, three case-control studies have reported an increased risk of endometrial carcinoma associated with the prolonged use of exogenous estrogen in postmenopausal women.[17,18,19] One publication[20] reported on the first 21 cases submitted by physicians to a registry of cases of adenocarcinoma of the endometrium in women under 40 on oral contraceptives. Of the cases found in women without predisposing risk factors for adenocarcinoma of the endometrium (e.g, irregular bleeding at the time oral contraceptives were first given, polycystic ovaries), nearly all occurred in women who had used a sequential oral contraceptive. These products are no longer marketed. No evidence has been reported suggesting an increased risk of endometrial cancer in users of conventional combination or progestogen-only oral contraceptives.

Figure 1. Estimated annual number of deaths associated with control of fertility and no control per 100,000 nonsterile women, by regimen of control and age of woman.

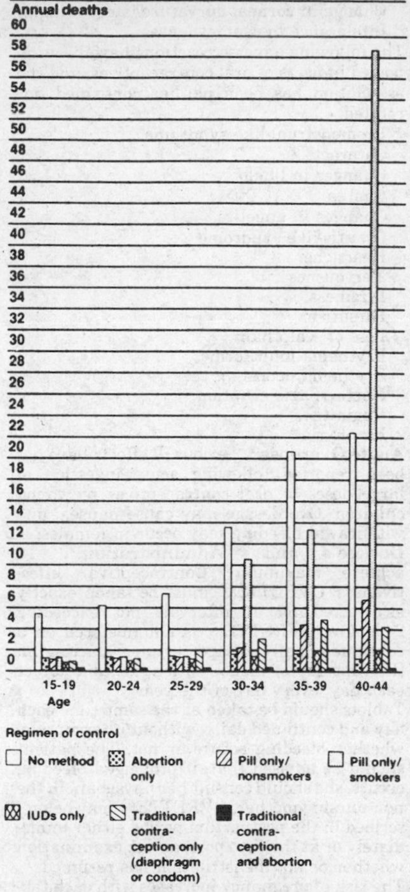

Several studies[8,21–24] have found no increase in breast cancer in women taking oral contraceptives or estrogens. One study,[25] however, while also noting no overall increased risk of breast cancer in women treated with oral contraceptives, found an excess risk in the subgroups of oral-contraceptive users with documented benign breast disease. A reduced occurrence of benign breast tumors in users of oral contraceptives has been well-documented.[8,21,25,26,27] In summary, there is at present no confirmed evidence from human studies of an increased risk of cancer associated with oral contraceptives. Close clinical surveillance of all women taking oral contraceptives is, nevertheless, essential. In all cases of undiagnosed persistent or recurrent abnormal vaginal bleeding, appropriate diagnostic measures should be taken to rule out malignancy. Women with a strong family history of breast cancer or who have breast nodules, fibrocystic disease, or abnormal mammograms should be monitored with particular care if they elect to use oral contraceptives instead of other methods of contraception.

4. *Hepatic Tumors:*
Benign hepatic adenomas have been found to be associated with the use of oral contraceptives.[28,29,30,46] One study[46] showed that oral contraceptive formulations with high hormonal potency were associated with a higher risk than lower potency formulations. Although benign, hepatic adenomas may rupture and may cause death through intra-abdominal hemorrhage. This has been reported in short-term as well as long-term users of oral contraceptives. Two studies relate risk with duration of use of the contraceptive, the risk being much greater after 4 or more years of oral-contraceptive use.[30,46] While hepatic adenoma is a rare lesion, it should be considered in women presenting abdominal pain and tenderness, abdominal mass or shock. A few cases of hepatocellular carcinoma have been reported in women taking oral contraceptives. The relationship of these drugs to this type of malignancy is not known at this time.

5. *Use in or Immediately Preceding Pregnancy, Birth Defects in Offspring, and Malignancy in Female Offspring:*
The use of female sex hormones—both estrogenic and progestational agents—during early pregnancy may seriously damage the offspring. It has been shown that females exposed in utero to diethylstilbestrol, a nonsteroidal estrogen, have an increased risk of developing in later life a form of vaginal or cervical cancer that is ordinarily extremely rare.[31,32] This risk has been estimated to be of the order of 1 in 1,000 exposures or less.[33,47] Although there is no evidence at the present time that oral contraceptives further enhance the risk of developing this type of malignancy, such patients should be monitored with particular care if they elect to use oral contraceptives instead of other methods of contraception. Furthermore, a high percentage of such exposed women (from 30 to 90%) have been found to have epithelial changes of the vagina and cervix.[34–38] Although these changes are histologically benign, it is not known whether this condition is a precursor of vaginal malignancy. Male children so exposed may develop abnormalities of the urogenital tract.[48,49,50] Although similar data are not available with the use of other estrogens, it cannot be presumed that they would not induce similar changes.
An increased risk of congenital anomalies, including heart defects and limb defects, has been reported with the use of sex hormones, including oral contraceptives, in pregnancy.[39–42,51] One case-control study[42] has estimated a 4.7-fold increase in risk of limb-reduction defects in infants exposed in utero to sex hormones (oral contraceptives, hormonal withdrawal tests for pregnancy, or attempted treatment for threatened abortion). Some of these exposures were very short and involved only a few days of treatment. The data suggest that the risk of limb-reduction defects in exposed fetuses is somewhat less than one in 1,000 live births.
In the past, female sex hormones have been used during pregnancy in an attempt to treat threatened or habitual abortion. There is considerable evidence that estrogens are ineffective for these indications, and there is no evidence from well-controlled studies that progestogens are effective for these uses.
There is some evidence that triploidy and possibly other types of polyploidy are increased among abortuses from women who become pregnant soon after ceasing oral contraceptives.[43] Embryos with these anomalies are virtually always aborted spontaneously. Whether there is an overall increase in spontaneous abortion of pregnancies conceived soon after stopping oral contraceptives is unknown.
It is recommended that, for any patient who has missed two consecutive periods, pregnancy should be ruled out before continuing the contraceptive regimen. If the patient has not adhered to the prescribed schedule, the possibility of pregnancy should be considered at the time of the first missed period (or after 45 days from the last menstrual period if the progestogen-only oral contraceptives are used), and further use of oral contraceptives should be withheld until pregnancy has been ruled out. If pregnancy is confirmed, the patient should be apprised of the potential risks to the fetus, and the advisability of continuation of the pregnancy should be discussed in the light of these risks.
It is also recommended that women who discontinue oral contraceptives with the intent of becoming pregnant use an alternate form of contraception for a period of time before attempting to conceive. Many clinicians recommend 3 months, although no precise information is available on which to base this recommendation.
The administration of progestogen-only or progestogen-estrogen combinations to induce withdrawal bleeding should not be used as a test of pregnancy.

6. *Gallbladder Disease:*
Studies[8,23,26] report an increased risk of surgically confirmed gallbladder disease in users of oral contraceptives and estrogens. In one study, an increased risk appeared after 2 years of use and doubled after 4 or 5 years of use. In one of the other studies, an increased risk was apparent between 6 and 12 months of use.

7. *Carbohydrate and Lipid Metabolic Effects:*
A decrease in glucose tolerance has been observed in a significant percentage of patients on oral contraceptives. For this reason, prediabetic and diabetic patients should be carefully observed while receiving oral contraceptives.
An increase in triglycerides and total phospholipids has been observed in patients receiving oral contraceptives.[44] The clinical significance of this finding remains to be defined.

8. *Elevated Blood Pressure:*
An increase in blood pressure has been reported in patients receiving oral contraceptives.[26] In some women, hypertension may occur within a few months of beginning oral-contraceptive use. In the first year of use, the prevalence of women with hypertension is low in users and may be no higher than that of a comparable group of nonusers. The prevalence in users increases, however, with longer exposure, and in the fifth year of use is two-and-a-half to three times the reported prevalence in the first year. Age is also strongly correlated with the development of hypertension in oral-contraceptive users. Women who previously have had hypertension during pregnancy may be more likely to develop elevation of blood pressure when given oral contraceptives. Hypertension that develops as a result of taking oral contraceptives usually returns to normal after discontinuing the drug.

9. *Headache:*
The onset or exacerbation of migraine or development of headache of a new pattern which is recurrent, persistent, or severe, requires discontinuation of oral contraceptives and evaluation of the cause.

10. *Bleeding Irregularities:*
Breakthrough bleeding, spotting, and amenorrhea are frequent reasons for patients discontinuing oral contraceptives. In breakthrough bleeding, as in all cases of irregular bleeding from the vagina, nonfunctional causes should be borne in mind. In undiagnosed persistent or recurrent abnormal bleeding from the vagina, adequate diagnostic measures are indicated to rule out pregnancy or malignancy. If pathology has been excluded, time or a change to another formulation may solve the problem. Changing to an oral contraceptive with a higher estrogen content, while potentially useful in minimizing menstrual irregularity, should be done only if necessary, since this may increase the risk of thromboembolic disease.
An alteration in menstrual patterns is likely to occur in women using progestogen-only oral contraceptives. The amount and duration of flow, cycle length, breakthrough bleeding, spotting, and amenorrhea will probably be quite variable. Bleeding irregularities occur more frequently with the use of progestogen-only oral contraceptives than with the combinations, and the dropout rate due to such conditions is higher.

Continued on next page

Wyeth—Cont.

Women with a past history of oligomenorrhea or secondary amenorrhea or young women without regular cycles may have a tendency to remain anovulatory or to become amenorrheic after discontinuation of oral contraceptives. Women with these preexisting problems should be advised of this possibility and encouraged to use other contraceptive methods. Post-use anovulation, possibly prolonged, may also occur in women without previous irregularities.

11. *Ectopic Pregnancy:*
Ectopic as well as intrauterine pregnancy may occur in contraceptive failures. However, in progestogen-only oral contraceptive failures, the ratio of ectopic to intrauterine pregnancies is higher than in women who are not receiving oral contraceptives, since the drugs are more effective in preventing intrauterine than ectopic pregnancies.

12. *Breast-feeding:*
Oral contraceptives given in the postpartum period may interfere with lactation. There may be a decrease in the quantity and quality of the breast milk. Furthermore, a small fraction of the hormonal agents in oral contraceptives has been identified in the milk of mothers receiving these drugs.[45] The effects, if any, on the breast-fed child have not been determined. If feasible, the use of oral contraceptives should be deferred until the infant has been weaned.

Precautions

GENERAL

1. A complete medical and family history should be taken prior to initiation of oral contraceptives. The pretreatment and periodic physical examinations should include special reference to blood pressure, breasts, abdomen and pelvic organs, including Papanicolaou smear and relevant laboratory tests. As a general rule, oral contraceptives should not be prescribed for longer than 1 year without another physical examination being performed.
2. Under the influence of estrogen-progestogen preparations, preexisting uterine leiomyomata may increase in size.
3. Patients with a history of psychic depression should be carefully observed and the drug discontinued if depression recurs to a serious degree. Patients becoming significantly depressed while taking oral contraceptives should stop the medication and use an alternate method of contraception in an attempt to determine whether the symptom is drug-related.
4. Oral contraceptives may cause some degree of fluid retention. They should be prescribed with caution, and only with careful monitoring, in patients with conditions which might be aggravated by fluid retention, such as convulsive disorders, migraine syndrome, asthma, or cardiac or renal insufficiency.
5. Patients with a past history of jaundice during pregnancy have an increased risk of recurrence of jaundice while receiving oral-contraceptive therapy. If jaundice develops in any patient receiving such drugs, the medication should be discontinued.
6. Steroid hormones may be poorly metabolized in patients with impaired liver function and should be administered with caution in such patients.
7. Oral-contraceptive users may have disturbances in normal tryptophan metabolism which may result in a relative pyridoxine deficiency. The clinical significance of this is yet to be determined.
8. Serum folate levels may be depressed by oral-contraceptive therapy. Since the pregnant woman is predisposed to the development of folate deficiency and the incidence of folate deficiency increases with increasing gestation, it is possible that if a woman becomes pregnant shortly after stopping oral contraceptives, she may have a greater chance of developing folate deficiency and complications attributed to this deficiency.
9. The pathologist should be advised of oral-contraceptive therapy when relevant specimens are submitted.
10. Certain endocrine- and liver-function tests and blood components may be affected by estrogen-containing oral contraceptives:

a. Increased sulfobromophthalein retention.
b. Increased prothrombin and factors VII, VIII, IX, and X; decreased antithrombin 3; increased norepinephrine-induced platelet aggregability.
c. Increased thyroid-binding globulin (TBG) leading to increased circulating total-thyroid hormone, as measured by protein-bound iodine (PBI), T4 by column, or T4 by radioimmunoassay. Free T3 resin uptake is decreased, reflecting the elevated TBG; free T4 concentration is unaltered.
d. Decreased pregnanediol excretion.
e. Reduced response to metyrapone test.

Information for the Patient: (See Patient Labeling Printed Below.)

Drug Interactions: Reduced efficacy and increased incidence of breakthrough bleeding have been associated with concomitant use of rifampin. A similar association has been suggested with barbiturates, phenylbutazone, phenytoin sodium, and ampicillin.

Carcinogenesis: See Warnings section for information on the carcinogenic potential of oral contraceptives.

Pregnancy: Pregnancy category X. See Contraindications and Warnings.

Nursing Mothers: See Warnings.

Adverse Reactions: An increased risk of the following serious adverse reactions has been associated with the use of oral contraceptives (see Warnings):

Thrombophlebitis.
Pulmonary embolism.
Coronary thrombosis.
Cerebral thrombosis.
Cerebral hemorrhage.
Hypertension.
Gallbladder disease.
Benign hepatomas.
Congenital anomalies.

There is evidence of an association between the following conditions and the use of oral contraceptives, although additional confirmatory studies are needed;

Mesenteric thrombosis.
Neuro-ocular lesions, e.g., retinal thrombosis and optic neuritis.

The following adverse reactions have been reported in patients receiving oral contraceptives and are believed to be drug-related:

Nausea and/or vomiting, usually the most common adverse reactions, occur in approximately 10% or less of patients during the first cycle. Other reactions, as a general rule, are seen much less frequently or only occasionally.
Gastrointestinal symptoms (such as abdominal cramps and bloating).
Breakthrough bleeding.
Spotting.
Change in menstrual flow.
Dysmenorrhea.
Amenorrhea during and after treatment.
Temporary infertility after discontinuance of treatment.
Edema
Chloasma or melasma which may persist.
Breast changes: tenderness, enlargement, and secretion.
Change in weight (increase or decrease)
Change in cervical erosion and cervical secretion.
Possible diminution in lactation when given immediately postpartum.
Cholestatic jaundice.
Migraine.
Increase in size of uterine leiomyomata.
Rash (allergic).
Mental depression.
Reduced tolerance to carbohydrates.
Vaginal candidiasis.
Change in corneal curvature (steepening).
Intolerance to contact lenses.

The following adverse reactions have been reported in users of oral contraceptives, and the association has been neither confirmed nor refuted:

Premenstrual-like syndrome.
Cataracts.
Changes in libido.
Chorea.
Changes in appetite.
Cystitis-like syndrome.
Headache.
Nervousness.
Dizziness.
Hirsutism.
Loss of scalp hair.
Erythema multiforme.
Erythema nodosum.
Hemorrhagic eruption.
Vaginitis.
Porphyria.

Acute Overdose: Serious ill effects have not been reported following acute ingestion of large doses of oral contraceptives by young children. Overdosage may cause nausea, and withdrawal bleeding may occur in females.

Dosage and Administration: To achieve maximum Contraceptive effectiveness, OVRETTE® must be taken exactly as directed and at intervals not exceeding 24 hours. OVRETTE® is administered on a continuous daily dosage regimen starting on the first day of menstruation, i.e., one tablet each day, every day of the year.

Tablets should be taken at the same time each day and continued daily, without interruption, whether bleeding occurs or not. The patient should be advised that, if prolonged bleeding occurs, she should consult her physician. In the non-nursing mother, OVRETTE® may be prescribed in the postpartum period either immediately or at the first postpartum examination whether or not menstruation has resumed.

The risk of pregnancy increases with each tablet missed. If the patient misses one tablet, she should be instructed to take it as soon as she remembers and to also take her next tablet at the regular time. If she misses two tablets, she should take one of the missed tablets as soon as she remembers, as well as taking her regular tablet for that day at the proper time. Furthermore, she should use a method of non-hormonal contraception in addition to taking OVRETTE® until fourteen tablets have been taken. If more than 2 tablets have been missed, OVRETTE® should be discontinued immediately and a method of nonhormonal contraception should be used until menses has appeared or pregnancy has been excluded. If menses does not appear within 45 days from the last period, a method of nonhormonal contraception should be substituted until the start of the next menstrual period or an appropriate diagnostic procedure is performed to rule out pregnancy.

How Supplied: OVRETTE® (as yellow, round tablets) is available in 28-tablet dispensers.

References:

1. "*Population Reports,*" Series H, Number 2, May 1974; Series I, Number 1, June 1974; Series B, Number 2, January 1975; Series H, Number 3, 1975; Series H, Number 4, January 1976 (published by the Population Information Program, The George Washington University Medical Center, 2001 S St. NW., Washington, D.C.).
2. Inman, W. H. W., Vessey, M. P., Westerholm, B., and Engelund, A., "Thromboembolic disease and the steroidal content of oral contraceptives. A report to the Committee on Safety of Drugs," Brit Med J *2*:203-209, 1970.

3. Stolley, P. D., Tonascia, J. A., Tockman, M. S., Sartwell, P. E., Rutledge, A. H., and Jacobs, M. P., "Thrombosis with low-estrogen oral contraceptives," Am J Epidemiol *102*:197–208, 1975.
4. Royal College of General Practitioners, "Oral contraception and thromboembolic disease," J Coll Gen Pract *13*:267–279, 1967.
5. Inman, W. H. W., and Vessey, M. P., "Investigation of deaths from pulmonary, coronary and cerebral thrombosis and embolism in women of childbearing age," Brit Med J *2*:193–199, 1968.
6. Vessey, M.P., and Doll, R., "Investigation of relation between use of oral contraceptives and thromboembolic disease. A further report," Brit Med J *2*:651–657, 1969.
7. Sartwell, P.E., Masi, A. T., Arthes, F. G., Greene, G. R., and Smith, H. E., "Thromboembolism and oral contraceptives: an epidemiological case control study," Am J Epidemiol *90*:365–380, 1969.
8. Boston Collaborative Drug Surveillance Program, "Oral contraceptives and venous thromboembolic disease, surgically confirmed gallbladder disease and breast tumors," Lancet *1*:1399–1404, 1973.
9. Collaborative Group for the Study of Stroke in Young Women, "Oral contraception and increased risk of cerebral ischemia or thrombosis," N Engl J Med *288*:871–878, 1973.
10. Collaborative Group for the Study of Stroke in Young Women. "Oral contraceptives and stroke in young women: associated risk factors," JAMA *231*:718–722, 1975.
11. Mann, J. I., and Inman, W. H. W., "Oral contraceptives and death from myocardial infarction," Brit Med J *2*:245–248, 1975.
12. Mann, J. I., Inman, W. H. W., and Thorogood, M., "Oral contraceptive use in older women and fatal myocardial infarction," Brit Med J *2*:445–447, 1976.
13. Mann, J. I., Vessey, M. P., Thorogood, M., and Doll, R., "Myocardial infarction in young women with special reference to oral contraceptive practice," Brit Med J *2*:241–245, 1975.
14. Tietze, C., "New Estimates of Mortality Associated with Fertility Control," Family Planning Perspectives, *9*:74–76, 1977.
15. Vessey, M. P., Doll, R., Fairbairn, A. S., and Glober, G., "Post-operative thromboembolism and the use of oral contraceptives," Brit Med J *3*:123–126, 1970.
16. Greene, G. R., Sartwell, P. E., "Oral contraceptive use in patients with thromboembolism following surgery, trauma, or infection," Am J Pub Health *62*:680–685, 1972.
17. Smith, D. C., Prentice, R., Thompson, D. J., and Herrmann, W. L., "Association of exogenous estrogen and endometrial carcinoma," N Eng J Med *293*:1164–1167, 1975.
18. Ziel, H. K., and Finkle, W. D., "Increased risk of endometrial carcinoma among users of conjugated estrogens," N Engl J Med *293*:1167–1170, 1975.
19. Mack, T. N., Pike, M. C., Henderson, B. E., Pfeffer, R. I., Gerkins, V. R., Arthur, M., and Brown, S. E., "Estrogens and endometrial cancer in a retirement community,"N Engl J Med *294*:1262–1267, 1976.
20. Silverberg, S. G., and Makowski, E. L., "Endometrial carcinoma in young women taking oral contraceptive agents," Obstet Gynecol *46*:503–506, 1975.
21. Vessey, M. P., Doll, R., and Sutton, P. M., "Oral contraceptives and breast neoplasia: a retrospective study," Brit Med J *3*:719–724, 1972.
22. Vessey, M.P., Doll, R., and Jones, K., "Oral contraceptives and breast cancer. Progress report of an epidemiological study," Lancet *1*:941–943, 1975.
23. Boston Collaborative Drug Surveillance Program, "Surgically confirmed gallbladder disease, venous thromboembolism and breast tumors in relation to postmenopausal estrogen therapy," N Engl J Med *290*:15–19, 1974.
24. Arthes, F. G., Sartwell, P. E., and Lewison, E. F., "The pill, estrogens, and the breast. Epidemiologic aspects," Cancer *28*:1391–1394, 1971.
25. Fasal, E., and Paffenbarger, R. S., "Oral contraceptives as related to cancer and benign lesions of the breast," J Natl Cancer Inst *55*:767–773, 1975.
26. Royal College of General Practitioners, "Oral Contraceptives and Health," London, Pitman, 1974.
27. Ory, H., Cole, P., MacMahon, B., and Hoover, R., "Oral contraceptives and reduced risk of benign breast diseases," N Engl J Med *294*:419–422, 1976.
28. Baum, J., Holtz, F., Bookstein, J. J., and Klein, E. W., "Possible association between benign hepatomas and oral contraceptives," Lancet *2*:926–928, 1973.
29. Mays, E. T., Christopherson, W. M., Mahr, M. M., and Williams, H. C., "Hepatic changes in young women ingesting contraceptive steroids. Hepatic hemorrhage and primary hepatic tumors," JAMA *235*:730–732, 1976.
30. Edmondson, H. A., Henderson, B., and Benton, B., "Liver-cell adenomas associated with use of oral contraceptives," N Engl J Med *294*:470–472, 1976.
31. Herbst, A. L., Ulfedler, H., and Poskanzer, D. C., "Adenocarcinoma of the vagina," N Engl J Med *284*:878–881, 1971.
32. Greenwald, P., Barlow, J. J., Nasca, P. C., and Burnett, W., "Vaginal cancer after maternal treatment with synthetic estrogens," N Engl J Med *285*:390–392, 1971.
33. Lanier, A. P., Noller, K. L., Decker, D. G., Elveback, L., and Kurland, L. T., "Cancer and stilbestrol. A follow-up of 1719 persons exposed to estrogens in utero and born 1943–1959," Mayo Clin Pro *48*: 793–799, 1973.
34. Herbst, A. L., Kurman, R. J., and Scully, R. E., "Vaginal and cervical abnormalities after exposure to stilbestrol in utero," Obstet Gynecol *40*:287–298, 1972.
35. Herbst, A. L., Robboy, S. J., Macdonald, G. J., and Scully, R. E., "The effects of local progesterone on stilbestrol-associated vaginal adenosis," Am J Obstet Gynecol *118*:607–615, 1974.
36. Herbst, A. L., Poskanzer, D. C., Robboy, S. J., Friedlander, L., and Scully, R. E., "Prenatal exposure to stilbestrol: a prospective comparison of exposed female offspring with unexposed controls," N Engl J. Med *292*:334–339, 1975.
37. Stafl, A., Mattingly, R. F., Foley, D. V., Fetherston, W., "Clinical diagnosis of vaginal adenosis," Obstet Gynecol *43*:118–128, 1974.
38. Sherman, A. I., Goldrath, M., Berlin, A., Vakhariya, V., Banooni, F., Michaels, W., Goodman, P., and Brown, S., "Cervical-vaginal adenosis after in utero exposure to synthetic estrogens," Obstet Gynecol *44*:531–545, 1974.
39. Gal, I., Kirman, B., and Stern, J., "Hormone pregnancy tests and congenital malformation," Nature *216*:83, 1967.
40. Levy, E. P., Cohen, A., and Fraser, F. C., "Hormone treatment during pregnancy and congenital heart defects," Lancet *1*:611, 1973.
41. Nora, J. J., and Nora, A. H., "Birth defects and oral contraceptives," Lancet *1*:941–942, 1973.
42. Janerich, D. T., Piper, J. M., and Glebatis, D. M., "Oral contraceptives and congenital limb-reduction defects," N Engl J Med *291*:697–700, 1974.
43. Carr, D. H., "Chromosome studies in selected spontaneous abortions: I. Conception after oral contraceptives," Canad Med Assoc J *103*:343–348, 1970.
44. Wynn, V., Doar, J. W. H., and Mills, G. L., "Some effects of oral contraceptives on serum-lipid and lipoprotein levels," Lancet *2*:720–723, 1966.
45. Laumas, K. R., Malkani, P. K., Bhatnager, S., and Laumas, V., "Radioactivity in the breast milk of lactating women after oral administration of 3 H-norethynodrel," Amer J Obstet Gynecol *98*:411–413, 1967.
46. Center for Disease Control, "Increased Risk of Hepatocellular Adenoma in Women with Long-term use of Oral contraceptives," Morbidity and Mortality Weekly Report, *26*:293–294, 1977.
47. Herbst, A. L., Cole, P., Colton, T., Robboy, S. J., Scully, R. E., "Age-incidence and Risk of Diethylstilbestrol-related Clear Cell Adenocarcinoma of the Vagina and Cervix," Am. J. Obstet. Gynecol., *128*:43–50, 1977.
48. Bibbo, M., Al-Naqeeb, M., Baccarini, I., Gill, W., Newton, M., Sleeper, K. M., Sonek, M., Wied, G. L., "Follow-up Study of Male and Female Offspring of DES-treated Mothers. A Preliminary Report," Jour. of Repro. Med., *15*:29–32, 1975.
49. Gill, W. B., Schumacher, G. F. B., Bibbo, M., "Structural and Functional Abnormalities in the Sex Organs of Male Offspring of Mothers Treated with Diethylstilbestrol (DES)," Jour. of Repro. Med., *16*:147–153, 1976.
50. Henderson, B. E., Senton, B., Cosgrove, M., Baptista, J., Aldrich, J., Townsend, D., Hart, W., Mack., T., "Urogenital Tract Abnormalities in Sons of Women Treated with Diethylstilbestrol," Pediatrics, *58*:505–507, 1976.
51. Heinonen, O. P., Slone, D., Nonson, R. R., Hook, E. B., Shapiro, S., "Cardiovascular Birth Defects and Antenatal Exposure to Female Sex Hormones," N. Eng. J. Med., *296*:67–70, 1977.
52. Jain, A. K., "Mortality Risk Associated with the Use of Oral Contraceptives," Studies in Family Planning, *8*:50–54, 1977.
53. Beral, V., "Mortality Among Oral Contraceptive Users," Lancet, *2*:727–731, 1977.

The patient labeling for oral-contraceptive drug products is set forth below:

Brief Summary Patient Package Insert

Cigarette smoking increases the risk of serious adverse effects on the heart and blood vessels from oral-contraceptive use. This risk increases with age and with heavy smoking (15 or more cigarettes per day) and is quite marked in women over 35 years of age. Women who use oral contraceptives should not smoke.

Oral contraceptives taken as directed are about 99% effective in preventing pregnancy. (The mini-pill, however, is somewhat less effective.) Forgetting to take your pills increases the chance of pregnancy. Women who have or have had clotting disorders, cancer of the breast or sex organs, unexplained vaginal bleeding, a stroke, heart attack, angina pectoris, or who suspect they may be pregnant should not use oral contraceptives.

Most side effects of the pill are not serious. The most common side effects are nausea, vomiting, bleeding between menstrual periods, weight gain, and breast tenderness. However, proper use of oral contraceptives requires that they be taken under your doctor's continuous supervision, because they can be associated with serious side effects which may be fatal. Fortunately, these occur very infrequently. The serious side effects are:

1. Blood clots in the legs, lungs, brain, heart, or other organs, and hemorrhage into the brain due to bursting of a blood vessel.
2. Liver tumors, which may rupture and cause severe bleeding.
3. Birth defects if the pill is taken while you are pregnant.
4. High blood pressure.
5. Gallbladder disease.

The symptoms associated with these serious side effects are discussed in the detailed leaflet given you with your supply of pills. Notify your doctor if you notice any unusual physical disturbance while taking the pill.

Continued on next page

Wyeth—Cont.

The estrogen in oral contraceptives has been found to cause breast cancer and other cancers in certain animals. These findings suggest that oral contraceptives may also cause cancer in humans. However, studies to date in women taking currently marketed oral contraceptives have not confirmed that oral contraceptives cause cancer in humans.
The detailed leaflet describes more completely the benefits and risks of oral contraceptives. It also provides information on other forms of contraception. Read it carefully. If you have any questions, consult your doctor.
Caution: Oral contraceptives are of no value in the prevention or treatment of venereal disease.

[*Shown in Product Identification Section*]

PATHOCIL® ℞
(dicloxacillin sodium monohydrate)
CAPSULES • ORAL SUSPENSION

Description: Dicloxacillin sodium monohydrate is an isoxazolyl penicillin which resists destruction by the enzyme penicillinase (beta-lactamase). It is the monohydrate sodium salt of 6-[3-(2,6- Dichlorophenyl) -5- methyl-4-isoxazolecarboxamido]-3, 3-dimethyl-7-oxo-4-thia - 1-azabicyclo [3.2.0] heptane-2-carboxylic acid.
Actions:
Pharmacology
Dicloxacillin sodium monohydrate is resistant to destruction by acid and is exceptionally well absorbed from the gastrointestinal tract. Oral administration of dicloxacillin sodium monohydrate gives blood levels considerably higher than those obtained with equivalent doses of any other presently available oral penicillin.
Microbiology
In vitro dicloxacillin is active against certain gram-positive cocci, including most strains of beta-hemolytic streptococci, pneumococci, penicillin G-sensitive staphylococci and, because of its resistance to penicillinase, penicillin G-resistant staphylococci. Dicloxacillin has less intrinsic antibacterial activity and a narrower spectrum than penicillin G.
Disc Susceptibility Tests
Quantitative methods that require measurement of zone diameters give the most precise estimates of antibiotic susceptibility. One such procedure* has been recommended for use with discs for testing susceptibility to penicillinase-resistant penicillin-class antibiotics. Interpretations correlate diameters on the disc test with MIC values for penicillinase-resistant penicillins. With this procedure, a report from the laboratory of "susceptible" indicates that the infecting organism is likely to respond to therapy. A report of "resistant" indicates that the infecting organism is not likely to respond to therapy. A report of "intermediate susceptibility" suggests that the organism would be susceptible if high dosage is used, or if the infection is confined to tissues and fluids (e.g., urine), in which high antibiotic levels are attained.
Indications: Although the principal indication for dicloxacillin is in the treatment of infections due to penicillinase-producing staphylococci, it may be used to initiate therapy in such patients in whom a staphylococcal infection is suspected. (See Important Note.)
Bacteriologic studies to determine the causative organisms and their sensitivity to dicloxacillin should be performed.
In serious, life-threatening infections, oral preparations of the penicillinase-resistant penicillins should not be relied on for initial therapy.
Important Note: When it is judged necessary that treatment be initiated before definitive culture and sensitivity results are known, the choice of dicloxacillin should take into consideration the fact that it has been shown to be effective only in the treatment of infections caused by pneumococci, Group A beta-hemolytic streptococci, and penicillin G-resistant and penicillin G-sensitive staphylococci. If the bacteriology report later indicates the infection is due to an organism other than a penicillin G-resistant staphylococcus sensitive to dicloxacillin, the physician is advised to continue therapy with a drug other than dicloxacillin or any other penicillinase-resistant penicillin.
Recent studies have reported that the percentage of staphylococcal isolates resistant to penicillin G outside the hospital is increasing, approximating the high percentage of resistant staphylococcal isolates found in the hospital. For this reason, it is recommended that a penicillinase-resistant penicillin be used as initial therapy for any suspected staphylococcal infection until culture and sensitivity results are known.
Dicloxacillin acts through a mechanism similar to that of methicillin against penicillin G-resistant staphylococci. Strains of staphylococci resistant to methicillin have existed in nature and it is known that the number of these strains reported has been increasing. Such strains of staphylococci have been capable of producing serious disease, in some instances resulting in fatality. Because of this, there is concern that widespread use of the penicillinase-resistant penicillins may result in the appearance of an increasing number of staphylococcal strains which are resistant to these penicillins.
Methicillin-resistant strains are almost always resistant to all other penicillinase-resistant penicillins (cross-resistance with cephalosporin derivatives also occurs frequently). Resistance to any penicillinase-resistant penicillin should be interpreted as evidence of clinical resistance to all in spite of the fact that minor variations in *in vitro* sensitivity may be encountered when more than one penicillinase-resistant penicillin is tested against the same strain of staphylococcus.
Contraindications: A history of a previous hypersensitivity reaction to any of the penicillins is a contraindication.
Warnings: Serious and occasionally fatal hypersensitivity (anaphylactoid) reactions have been reported in patients on penicillin therapy. Although anaphylaxis is more frequent following parenteral therapy, it has occurred in patients on oral penicillins. These reactions are more apt to occur in individuals with a history of sensitivity to multiple allergens.
There have been reports of individuals with a history of penicillin hypersensitivity reactions who experienced severe hypersensitivity reactions when treated with cephalosporins. Before therapy with a penicillin, careful inquiry should be made concerning previous hypersensitivity reactions to penicillins, cephalosporins, and other allergens. If an allergic reaction occurs, appropriate therapy should be instituted and discontinuance of dicloxacillin therapy considered. The usual agents (antihistamines, pressor amines, corticosteroids) should be readily available.
Usage in pregnancy
Safety for use in pregnancy has not been established.
Precautions: As with any potent drug, periodic assessment of organ-system function, including renal, hepatic, and hematopoietic, should be made during prolonged therapy.
The possibility of bacterial and fungal superinfection should be kept in mind during long-term therapy. If overgrowth of resistant organisms occurs, appropriate measures should be taken.
This oral preparation should not be relied upon in patients with severe illness or with nausea, vomiting, gastric dilatation, cardiospasm or intestinal hypermotility.
Since experience in neonates is limited, a dose for the newborn is not recommended at this time.
Adverse Reactions: Gastrointestinal disturbances such as nausea, vomiting, epigastric discomfort, flatulence, and loose stools have been noted in some patients receiving dicloxacillin. As with other penicillins, pruritus, urticaria, skin rashes, eosinophilia, anaphylactic reactions, and other allergic symptoms have been occasionally encountered.
Minor changes in the results of liver-function tests such as transient elevation of SGOT and changes in cephalin flocculation tests have been reported. The clinical significance of these changes is unknown.
Dosage and Administration: For mild-to-moderate upper respiratory and localized skin and soft tissue infections due to sensitive organisms:
Adults and children weighing 40 Kg (88 lbs.) or more: 125 mg q. 6h.
Children weighing less than 40 Kg (88 lbs.): 12.5 mg/Kg/day in equally-divided doses q. 6h.
For more severe infections such as those of the lower respiratory tract or disseminated infections:
Adults and children weighing 40 Kg (88 lbs.) or more: 250 mg q. 6h or higher.
Children weighing less than 40 Kg (88 lbs.): 25 mg/Kg/day or higher in equally-divided doses q. 6h.
Since experience in neonates is limited, a dose for the newborn is not recommended at this time.
Dicloxacillin sodium monohydrate is best absorbed when taken on an empty stomach, preferably one to two hours before meals.
N.B.: INFECTIONS CAUSED BY GROUP A BETA-HEMOLYTIC STREPTOCOCCI SHOULD BE TREATED FOR AT LEAST 10 DAYS TO HELP PREVENT THE OCCURRENCE OF ACUTE RHEUMATIC FEVER OR ACUTE GLOMERULONEPHRITIS.
How Supplied: Capsules equivalent to 250 mg. dicloxacillin, bottles of 100.
Powder for Oral Suspension containing dicloxacillin sodium monohydrate equivalent to 62.5 mg. dicloxacillin per 5 ml, bottles to yield 80 ml.

*Bauer, A.W., Kirby, W.M.M., Sherris, J.C., and Turck, M.: Antibiotic Testing by a Standardized Single Discs Method, Am. J. Clin. Pathol., 45:493, 1966; Standardized Disc Susceptibility Test, FEDERAL REGISTER 37:20527-29, 1972.

[*Shown in Product Identification Section*]

PEN • VEE® K ℞
(penicillin V potassium)
TABLETS • FOR ORAL SOLUTION

Description: Penicillin V is the phenoxymethyl analog of penicillin G.
Penicillin V potassium is the potassium salt of penicillin V.
Action and Pharmacology: Penicillin V exerts a bactericidal action against penicillin-sensitive microorganisms during the stage of active multiplication. It acts through the inhibition of biosynthesis of cell-wall mucopeptide. It is not active against the penicillinase-producing bacteria, which include many strains of staphylococci. The drug exerts high *in vitro* activity against staphylococci (except penicillinase-producing strains), streptococci (groups A, C, G, H, L, and M) and pneumococci. Other organisms sensitive *in vitro* to penicillin V are *Corynebacterium diphtheriae, Bacillus anthracis,* Clostridia, *Actinomyces bovis, Streptobacillus moniliformis, Listeria monocytogenes,* Leptospira and *Neisseria gonorrhoeae. Treponema pallidum* is extremely sensitive.
The potassium salt of penicillin V has the distinct advantage over penicillin G in resistance to inactivation by gastric acid. It may be given with meals; however, blood levels are slightly higher when the drug is given on an empty

stomach. Average blood levels are two to five times higher than the levels following the same dose of oral penicillin G and also show much less individual variation.
Once absorbed, penicillin V is about 80% bound to serum protein. Tissue levels are highest in the kidneys, with lesser amounts in the liver, skin and intestines. Small amounts are found in all other body tissues and the cerebrospinal fluid. The drug is excreted as rapidly as it is absorbed in individuals with normal kidney function; however, recovery of the drug from the urine indicates that only about 25% of the dose given is absorbed. In neonates, young infants, and individuals with impaired kidney function, excretion is considerably delayed.

Indications: Penicillin V potassium is indicated in the treatment of mild to moderately severe infections due to penicillin-G sensitive microorganisms. Therapy should be guided by bacteriological studies (including sensitivity tests) and by clinical response.

NOTE: Severe pneumonia, empyema, bacteremia, pericarditis, meningitis, and arthritis should not be treated with penicillin V during the acute stage.

Indicated surgical procedures should be performed.

The following infections will usually respond to adequate dosage of penicillin V.

Streptococcal infections (without bacteremia). Mild to moderate infections of the upper respiratory tract, scarlet fever, and mild erysipelas.

NOTE: Streptococci in groups A, C, G, H, L, and M are very sensitive to penicillin. Other groups, including group D (enterococcus), are resistant.

Pneumococcal infections. Mild to moderately severe infections of the respiratory tract.

Staphylococcal Infections—penicillin G-sensitive. Mild infections of the skin and soft tissues.

NOTE: Reports indicate an increasing number of strains of staphylococci resistant to penicillin G, emphasizing the need for culture and sensitivity studies in treating suspected staphylococcal infections.

Fusospirochetosis(Vincent's gingivitis and pharyngitis)—Mild to moderately severe infections of the oropharynx usually respond to therapy with oral penicillin.

NOTE: Necessary dental care should be accomplished in infections involving the gum tissue.

Medical conditions in which oral penicillin therapy is indicated as prophylaxis:

For the prevention of recurrence following rheumatic fever and/or chorea: Prophylaxis with oral penicillin on a continuing basis has proven effective in preventing recurrence of these conditions.

To prevent bacterial endocarditis in patients with congenital and/or rheumatic heart lesions in patients to undergo dental procedures or minor upper-respiratory-tract surgery or instrumentation. Prophylaxis should be instituted the day of the procedure and for 2 or more days following. Patients who have a past history of rheumatic fever and are receiving continuous prophylaxis may harbor increased numbers of penicillin-resistant organisms; use of another prophylactic anti-infective agent should be considered. If penicillin is to be used in these patients at surgery, the regular rheumatic fever program should be interrupted 1 week prior to the contemplated surgery. At the time of surgery, penicillin may be reinstituted as a prophylactic measure against the hazards of surgically induced bacteremia.

NOTE: Oral penicillin should not be used as adjunctive prophylaxis for genitourinary instrumentation or surgery, lower-intestinal tract surgery, sigmoidoscopy, and childbirth.

Contraindications: A previous hypersensitivity reaction to any penicillin is a contraindication.

Warnings: Serious and occasionally fatal hypersensitivity (anaphylactoid) reactions have been reported in patients on penicillin therapy. Although anaphylaxis is more frequent following parenteral therapy, it has occurred in patients on oral penicillins. These reactions are more apt to occur in individuals with a history of sensitivity to multiple allergens.

There have been well-documented reports of individuals with a history of penicillin hypersensitivity reactions who have experienced severe hypersensitivity reactions when treated with a cephalosporin. Before therapy with a penicillin, careful inquiry should be made concerning previous hypersensitivity reactions to penicillins, cephalosporins, and other allergens. If an allergic reaction occurs, the drug should be discontinued and the patient treated with the usual agents, e.g., pressor amines, antihistamines, and corticosteroids.

Precautions: Penicillin should be used with caution in individuals with histories of significant allergies and/or asthma.

The oral route of administration should not be relied upon in patients with severe illness, or with nausea, vomiting, gastric dilatation, cardiospasm, or intestinal hypermotility.

Occasional patients will not absorb therapeutic amounts of orally administered penicillin.

In streptococcal infections, therapy must be sufficient to eliminate the organism (10-day minimum); otherwise the sequelae of streptococcal disease may occur. Cultures should be taken following completion of treatment to determine whether streptococci have been eradicated.

Prolonged use of antibiotics may promote the overgrowth of nonsusceptible organisms, including fungi. Should superinfection occur, appropriate measures should be taken.

Adverse Reactions: Although the incidence of reactions to oral penicillins has been reported with much less frequency than following parenteral therapy, it should be remembered that all degrees of hypersensitivity, including fatal anaphylaxis, have been reported with oral penicillin.

The most common reactions to oral penicillin are nausea, vomiting, epigastric distress, diarrhea, and black hairy tongue. The hypersensitivity reactions reported are skin eruptions (maculopapular to exfoliative dermatitis), urticaria and other serum sickness like reactions, laryngeal edema, and anaphylaxis. Fever and eosinophilia may frequently be the only reaction observed. Hemolytic anemia, leukopenia, thrombocytopenia, neuropathy, and nephropathy are infrequent reactions and usually associated with high doses of parenteral penicillin.

Dosage and Administration: The dosage of penicillin V should be determined according to the sensitivity of the causative microorganisms and the severity of infection, and adjusted to the clinical response of the patient.

The usual dosage recommendations for adults and children 12 years and over are as follows:

Streptococcal infections—mild to moderately severe—of the upper respiratory tract and including scarlet fever and erysipelas: 125-250 mg (200,000-400,000 units) every 6-8 hours for 10 days.

Pneumococcal infections—mild to moderately severe—of the respiratory tract, including otitis media: 250-500 mg. (400,000-800,000 units) every 6 hours until the patient has been afebrile for at least 2 days.

Staphylococcal infections—mild infections of skin and soft tissue (culture and sensitivity tests should be performed): 250-500 mg. (400,000-800,000 units) every 6-8 hours.

Fusospirochetosis (Vincent's infection) of the oropharynx. Mild to moderately severe infections: 250-500 mg. (400,000-800,000 units) every 6-8 hours.

For the prevention of recurrence following rheumatic fever and/or chorea: 125-250 mg. (200,000-400,000 units) twice daily on a continuing basis.

To prevent bacterial endocarditis in patients with rheumatic or congenital heart lesions who are to undergo dental or upper-respiratory-tract surgery or instrumentation:

ADULTS—2 gram (3,200,000 units) orally 30 minutes to 1 hour prior to the procedure and then 500 mg (800,000 units) orally every 6 hours for 8 doses.

CHILDREN—For those weighing 60 lbs. or more, use adult dose recommendations (see above). For those weighing less than 60 lbs., use 1 gram (1,600,000 units) orally 30 minutes to 1 hour prior to the procedure and then 250 mg (400,000 units) orally every 6 hours for 8 doses.

How Supplied: *Tablets* (scored, white)—**125 mg.** (200,000 units), bottles of 36; **250 mg.** (400,000 units), bottles of 100 and 500, REDIPAK®, Unit Dose Medication, boxes of 100 (individually wrapped); **500 mg.** (800,000 units) bottles of 25, 100 and 500, and REDIPAK® Unit Dose Medication, boxes of 100 (individually wrapped). *Powder, for Oral Solution*—125 mg. (200,000 units) per 5-ml teaspoonful, bottles of powder to make 100 ml and 200 ml; 250 mg. (400,000 units) per 5-ml teaspoonful, bottles of powder to make 100 ml, 150 ml and 200 ml liquid; 250 mg. per pouch (REDIPAK®) for individual dose, carton of 20, to be reconstituted with water.

[*Shown in Product Identification Section*]

PHENERGAN® ℞
(promethazine hydrochloride)
INJECTION

Description: Each ml of TUBEX® (Sterile Cartridge-Needle Unit) contains either 25 or 50 mg promethazine hydrochloride with 0.1 mg edetate disodium, 0.04 mg calcium chloride, not more than 5 mg monothioglycerol and 5 mg phenol with sodium acetate-acetic acid buffer. Each Ampul of injection contains either 25 mg or 50 mg promethazine hydrochloride with 0.1 mg edetate disodium, 0.04 mg calcium chloride, not more than 0.25 mg sodium metabisulfite and 5 mg phenol with sodium acetate-acetic acid buffer.

Actions: Promethazine hydrochloride, a phenothiazine derivative, possesses antihistaminic, sedative, antimotion-sickness, antiemetic, and anticholinergic effects. The duration of action is generally from four to six hours. The major side reaction of this drug is sedation. As an antihistamine it acts by competitive antagonism, but does not block the release of histamine. It antagonizes in varying degrees most but not all of the pharmacological effects of histamine.

Indications: The injectable form of promethazine hydrochloride is indicated for the following conditions:

1. Amelioration of allergic reactions to blood or plasma.
2. In anaphylaxis as an adjunct to epinephrine and other standard measures after the acute symptoms have been controlled.
3. For other uncomplicated allergic conditions of the immediate type when oral therapy is impossible or contraindicated.
4. Active treatment of motion sickness.
5. Preoperative, postoperative, and obstetric (during labor) sedation.
6. Prevention and control of nausea and vomiting associated with certain types of anesthesia and surgery.
7. As an adjunct to analgesics for the control of postoperative pain.
8. For sedation and relief of apprehension and to produce light sleep from which the patient can be easily aroused.
9. Intravenously in special surgical situations, such as repeated bronchoscopy, ophthalmic surgery, and poor-risk patients, with reduced amounts of meperidine or other narcotic analgesic as an adjunct to anesthesia and analgesia.

Contraindications: Promethazine is contraindicated in comatose states, in patients who

Continued on next page

Wyeth—Cont.

have received large amounts of central-nervous-system depressants (alcohol, barbiturates, narcotics, etc.) and in patients who have demonstrated an idiosyncrasy or hypersensitivity to promethazine.

Under no circumstances should promethazine be given by intra-arterial injection due to the likelihood of severe arteriospasm and the possibility of resultant gangrene (see Warnings). Phenergan injection should not be given by the subcutaneous route; evidence of chemical irritation has been noted and necrotic lesions have resulted on rare occasions following subcutaneous injection. The preferred parenteral route of administration is by deep intramuscular injection.

Warnings: Promethazine may impair the mental and/or physical abilities required for the performance of potentially hazardous tasks such as driving a vehicle or operating machinery. The concomitant use of alcohol or other central-nervous-system depressants may have an additive effect. Patients should be warned accordingly.

USAGE IN PREGNANCY: The safe use of promethazine has not been established with respect to the possible adverse effects upon fetal development. Therefore, the need for the use of this drug during pregnancy should be weighed against the possible but unknown hazards to the developing fetus.

USE IN CHILDREN: Excessively large dosages of antihistamines, including promethazine, in children may cause hallucinations, convulsions, and sudden death. In children who are acutely ill associated with dehydration, there is an increased susceptibility to dystonias with the use of promethazine hydrochloride injection.

CAUTION SHOULD BE EXERCISED WHEN ADMINISTERING PHENERGAN TO CHILDREN. ANTIEMETICS ARE NOT RECOMMENDED FOR TREATMENT OF UNCOMPLICATED VOMITING IN CHILDREN, AND THEIR USE SHOULD BE LIMITED TO PROLONGED VOMITING OF KNOWN ETIOLOGY. THE EXTRAPYRAMIDAL SYMPTOMS WHICH CAN OCCUR SECONDARY TO PHENERGAN® ADMINISTRATION MAY BE CONFUSED WITH THE CNS SIGNS OF UNDIAGNOSED PRIMARY DISEASE, e.g., ENCEPHALOPATHY OR REYE'S SYNDROME. THE USE OF PHENERGAN SHOULD BE AVOIDED IN CHILDREN WHOSE SIGNS AND SYMPTOMS MAY SUGGEST REYE'S SYNDROME, OR OTHER HEPATIC DISEASES.

USE IN THE ELDERLY (APPROXIMATELY 60 YEARS OR OLDER): Since therapeutic requirements for sedative drugs tend to be less in elderly patients, the dosage of Phenergan should be reduced for these patients.

OTHER CONSIDERATIONS: Drugs having anticholinergic properties should be used with caution in patients with asthmatic attack, narrow-angle glaucoma, prostatic hypertrophy, stenosing peptic ulcer, pyloroduodenal obstruction, and bladder-neck obstruction.

Phenergan should be used with caution in patients with bone-marrow depression. Leukopenia and agranulocytosis have been reported, usually when Phenergan has been used in association with other known toxic agents.

INADVERTENT INTRA-ARTERIAL INJECTION: Due to the close proximity of arteries and veins in the areas most commonly used for intravenous injection, extreme care should be exercised to avoid perivascular extravasation or inadvertent intra-arterial injection. Reports compatible with inadvertent intra-arterial injection of promethazine, usually in conjunction with other drugs intended for intravenous use, suggest that pain, severe chemical irritation, severe spasm of distal vessels, and resultant gangrene requiring amputation are likely under such circumstances. Intravenous injection was intended in all the cases reported but perivascular extravasation or arterial placement of the needle is now suspect. There is no proven successful management of this condition after it occurs, although sympathetic block and heparinization are commonly employed during the acute management because of the results of animal experiments with other known arteriolar irritants. Aspiration of dark blood does not preclude intra-arterial needle placement, because blood is discolored upon contact with promethazine. Use of syringes with rigid plungers or of small bore needles might obscure typical arterial backflow if this is relied upon alone.

When used intravenously promethazine hydrochloride should be given in a concentration no greater than 25 mg per ml and at a rate not to exceed 25 mg per minute. When administering any irritant drug intravenously it is usually preferable to inject it through the tubing of an intravenous infusion set that is known to be functioning satisfactorily. In the event that a patient complains of pain during intended intravenous injection of promethazine, the injection should immediately be stopped to provide for evaluation of possible arterial placement or perivascular extravasation.

Precautions: Promethazine may significantly affect the actions of other drugs. It may increase, prolong, or intensify the sedative action of central-nervous-system depressants, such as anesthetics, barbiturates, or alcohol. When given concomitantly with promethazine hydrochloride, the dose of barbiturates should be reduced by at least one-half, and the dose of narcotics should be reduced by one-quarter to one-half. Dosage must be individualized. Excessive amounts of promethazine relative to a narcotic may lead to restlessness and motor hyperactivity in the patient with pain; these symptoms usually disappear with adequate control of the pain. Promethazine should be used cautiously in persons with cardiovascular disease or impairment of liver function.

Although reversal of the vasopressor effect of epinephrine has not been reported with promethazine, the possibility should be considered in case of promethazine overdose.

Adverse Reactions: CNS EFFECTS: Drowsiness is the most prominent CNS effect of this drug. Extrapyramidal reactions may occur with high doses; this is almost always responsive to a reduction in dosage. Other reported reactions include dizziness, lassitude, tinnitus, incoordination, fatigue, blurred vision, euphoria, diplopia, nervousness, insomnia, tremors, convulsive seizures, oculogyric crises, excitation, catatonic-like states, and hysteria.

CARDIOVASCULAR EFFECTS: Tachycardia, bradycardia, faintness, dizziness, and increases and decreases in blood pressure have been reported following the use of promethazine hydrochloride injection. Venous thrombosis at the injection site has been reported. INTRA-ARTERIAL INJECTION MAY RESULT IN GANGRENE OF THE AFFECTED EXTREMITY (see Warnings).

GASTROINTESTINAL: Nausea and vomiting have been reported, usually in association with surgical procedures and combination drug therapy.

ALLERGIC REACTIONS: These include urticaria, dermatitis, asthma, and photosensitivity. Angioneurotic edema has been reported.

OTHER REPORTED REACTIONS: Leukopenia and agranulocytosis, usually when Phenergan® has been used in association with other known toxic agents, have been reported. Thrombocytopenic purpura and jaundice of the obstructive type have been associated with the use of promethazine. The jaundice is usually reversible on discontinuation of the drug. Subcutaneous injection has resulted in tissue necrosis. Nasal stuffiness may occur. Dry mouth has been reported.

LABORATORY TESTS: The following laboratory tests may be affected in patients who are receiving therapy with promethazine hydrochloride:

Pregnancy Tests—Diagnostic pregnancy tests based on immunological reactions between HCG and anti-HCG may result in false-negative or false-positive interpretations.

Glucose Tolerance Test—An increase in glucose tolerance has been reported in patients receiving promethazine hydrochloride.

PARADOXICAL REACTIONS (OVERDOSAGE): Hyperexcitability and abnormal movements which have been reported in children following a single administration of promethazine may be manifestations of relative overdosage, in which case, consideration should be given to the discontinuation of the promethazine and to the use of other drugs. Respiratory depression, nightmares, delirium, and agitated behavior have also been reported in some of these patients.

Drug Interactions: NARCOTICS AND BARBITURATES: The CNS depressant effects of narcotics and barbiturates are additive with promethazine hydrochloride.

MAO INHIBITORS: Drug interactions, including an increased incidence of extra-pyramidal effects, have been reported when some MAO inhibitors and phenothiazines are used concomitantly. Although such a reaction has not been reported with promethazine, the possibility should be considered.

Dosage and Administration: The preferred parenteral route of administration for promethazine hydrochloride is by deep intramuscular injection. The proper intravenous administration of this product is well-tolerated, but use of this route is not without some hazard.

INADVERTENT INTRA-ARTERIAL INJECTION CAN RESULT IN GANGRENE OF THE AFFECTED EXTREMITY (see Warnings). SUBCUTANEOUS INJECTION IS CONTRAINDICATED AS IT MAY RESULT IN TISSUE NECROSIS (see Contraindications). When used intravenously, promethazine hydrochloride should be given in concentration no greater than 25 mg/ml at a rate not to exceed 25 mg per minute; it is preferable to inject through the tubing of an intravenous infusion set that is known to be functioning satisfactorily.

ALLERGIC CONDITIONS: The average adult dose is 25 mg. This dose may be repeated within two hours if necessary, but continued therapy, if indicated, should be via the oral route as soon as existing circumstances permit. After initiation of treatment, dosage should be adjusted to the smallest amount adequate to relieve symptoms. The average adult dose for amelioration of allergic reactions to blood or plasma is 25 mg.

SEDATION: In hospitalized adult patients, nighttime sedation may be achieved by a dose of 25 to 50 mg of promethazine hydrochloride.

PRE-AND POST-OPERATIVE USE:

As an adjunct to pre- or post-operative medication, 25 to 50 mg of promethazine hydrochloride in adults may be combined with appropriately reduced doses of analgesics and atropine-like drugs as desired. Dosage of concomitant analgesic or hypnotic medication should be reduced accordingly.

NAUSEA AND VOMITING: For control of nausea and vomiting the usual adult dose is 12.5 to 25 mg, not to be repeated more frequently than every four hours. When used for control of post-operative nausea and vomiting, the medication may be administered either intramuscularly or intravenously and dosage of analgesics and barbiturates reduced accordingly.

OBSTETRICS: Phenergan® in doses of 50 mg will provide sedation and relieve apprehension in the early stages of labor. When labor is definitely established, 25 to 75 mg (average dose, 50 mg) promethazine hydrochloride may be given intramuscularly or intravenously with an appropriately reduced dose of any desired narcotic. Amnesic agents may be administered as necesssary. If necessary, Phenergan with a reduced dose of analgesic may be repeated once or twice at four-hour intervals in the course of a normal labor. A maximum total dose of 100 mg of Phenergan may be administered during a 24-hour period to patients in labor.

CHILDREN: In children under the age of 12 years the dosage should not exceed half that of the suggested adult dose. As an adjunct to premedication the suggested dose is 0.5 mg per lb. of body weight in combination with an equal dose of narcotic or barbiturate and the appropriate dose of an atropine-like drug. Antiemetics should not be used in vomiting of unknown etiology in children.

Management of Overdosage: Signs and symptoms of overdosage range from mild depression of the central nervous system and cardiovascular system, to profound hypotension, respiratory depression, and unconsciousness. Stimulation may be evident, especially in children and geriatric patients. Atropine-like signs and symptoms—dry mouth, fixed, dilated pupils, flushing, etc., as well as gastrointestinal symptoms, may occur. The treatment of overdosage is essentially symptomatic and supportive. Early gastric lavage may be beneficial if promethazine has been taken orally. Centrally acting emetics are of little use.

Avoid analeptics, which may cause convulsions. Severe hypotension usually responds to the administration of levarterenol or phenylephrine. EPINEPHRINE SHOULD NOT BE USED, since its use in a patient with partial adrenergic blockade may further lower the blood pressure. Extrapyramidal reactions may be treated with anticholinergic antiparkinson agents, diphenhydramine, or barbiturates. Additional measures include oxygen and intravenous fluids. Limited experience with dialysis indicates that it is not helpful.

How Supplied: Phenergan® (promethazine hydrochloride) Injection as TUBEX® (Sterile Cartridge-Needle Unit), either 25 or 50 mg per ml, in packages of 10 TUBEX, and Ampuls of 1 ml, either 25 or 50 mg per ml, in packages of 5 and 25 Ampuls.

PHENERGAN® ℞

(promethazine hydrochloride)
TABLETS • SYRUP •
RECTAL SUPPOSITORIES

Description: Each tablet contains 12.5 mg., 25 mg., or 50 mg. promethazine hydrochloride; the syrup contains 6.25 mg. or 25 mg. promethazine hydrochloride per 5 ml.; each rectal suppository contains 12.5 mg., 25 mg. or 50 mg. promethazine hydrochloride with ascorbyl palmitate, silicon dioxide, white wax and cocoa butter.

Actions: Phenergan® is a phenothiazine derivative that has several different types of pharmacologic properties. In addition to its antihistaminic action, which is of marked potency and prolonged duration, it also provides antiemetic as well as sedative actions, so that it is useful in a variety of clinical situations.

Indications: Phenergan, either orally or by suppository, is useful in the management of the following conditions:

Perennial and seasonal allergic rhinitis.
Vasomotor rhinitis.
Allergic conjunctivitis due to inhalant allergens and foods.
Mild, uncomplicated allergic skin manifestations of urticaria and angioedema.
Amelioration of allergic reactions to blood or plasma.
Dermographism.
As therapy for anaphylactic reactions adjunctive to epinephrine and other standard measures after the acute manifestations have been controlled.
Preoperative, postoperative, or obstetric sedation.
Prevention and control of nausea and vomiting associated with certain types of anesthesia and surgery.
Therapy adjunctive to meperidine or other analgesics for control of postoperative pain.
Sedation in both children and adults as well as relief of apprehension and production of light sleep from which the patient can be easily aroused.
Active and prophylactic treatment of motion sickness.
Antiemetic effect in postoperative patients.

Contraindications: Phenergan is contraindicated in individuals with a known hypersensitivity to the drug.

Warnings: The sedative action of promethazine hydrochloride is additive to the sedative effects of central-nervous-system depressants; therefore, agents such as alcohol, barbiturates and narcotic analgesics should either be eliminated or given in reduced dosage in the presence of promethazine hydrochloride. When given concomitantly with promethazine hydrochloride the dose of barbiturates should be reduced by at least one-half and the dose of analgesic depressants, such as morphine or meperidine, should be reduced by one-quarter to one-half.

Precautions: Ambulatory patients should be cautioned against driving automobiles or operating dangerous machinery until it is known that they do not become drowsy or dizzy from promethazine hydrochloride therapy.

Antiemetics may mask the symptoms of an unrecognized disease and thereby interfere with diagnosis.

Adverse Reactions: Patients may occasionally complain of autonomic reactions such as dryness of the mouth, blurring of vision and, rarely, dizziness.

Very rare cases have been reported where patients receiving promethazine have developed leukopenia. In one instance agranulocytosis has been reported. In nearly every instance reported, other toxic agents known to have caused these conditions have been associated with the administration of promethazine.

Cardiovascular by-effects from promethazine have been rare. Minor increases in blood pressure and occasional mild hypotension have been reported.

Photosensitivity, although extremely rare, has been reported. Occurrence of photosensitivity may be a contraindication to further treatment with promethazine or related drugs. In the presence of abraded or denuded rectal lesions the patient may experience initial local discomfort following administration of promethazine hydrochloride suppositories.

Attempted suicides with promethazine have resulted in deep sedation, coma, rarely convulsions and cardiorespiratory symptoms compatible with the depth of sedation present. A paradoxical reaction has been reported in children receiving single doses of 75 mg. to 125 mg. orally, characterized by hyperexcitability and nightmares.

Dosage and Administration: Allergy: The average oral dose is 25 mg. taken before retiring; however, 12.5 mg. may be taken before meals and on retiring, if necessary. Children tolerate this product well. Single 25 mg. doses at bedtime or 6.25 to 12.5 mg. taken three times daily will usually suffice. After initiation of treatment, in children or adults, dosage should be adjusted to the smallest amount adequate to relieve symptoms. When the oral route is not feasible, Phenergan HCl Rectal Suppositories in 25 mg. doses may be used. The dose may be repeated within two hours if necessary, but oral therapy should be resumed if indicated and existing circumstances permit. The administration of promethazine hydrochloride in 25 mg. doses will control minor transfusion reactions of an allergic nature.

Motion Sickness: The average adult dose is 25 mg. taken twice daily. The initial dose should be taken one-half to one hour before anticipated travel and be repeated eight to twelve hours later if necessary. On succeeding days of travel, it is recommended that 25 mg. be given on arising and again before the evening meal. For children, Phenergan Tablets, Syrup, or Rectal Suppositories, 12.5 to 25 mg., twice daily, may be administered.

Nausea and Vomiting: The average effective dose of Phenergan for the active therapy of nausea and vomiting in children or adults is 25 mg. When oral medication cannot be tolerated, the dose should be given parenterally (cf. Phenergan Injection) or by rectal suppository. 12.5 to 25 mg. doses may be repeated as necessary at four- to six-hour intervals.

For nausea and vomiting in children the dose should be adjusted to the age and weight of the patient and the severity of the condition being treated.

For prophylaxis of nausea and vomiting, as during surgery and the postoperative period, the average dose is 25 mg. repeated at four- to six-hour intervals as necessary.

Sedation: This product relieves apprehension and induces a quiet sleep from which the patient can be easily aroused. Administration of 12.5 to 25 mg. Phenergan by the oral route or by rectal suppository at bedtime will provide sedation in children. Adults usually require 25 to 50 mg. for nighttime, presurgical or obstetrical sedation.

Pre- and Postoperative Use: Phenergan in 12.5 to 25 mg. doses for children and 50 mg. doses for adults the night before surgery relieves apprehension and produces a quiet sleep.

For preoperative medication, children require doses of 0.5 mg. per pound of body weight in combination with an equal dose of meperidine and the appropriate dose of an atropine-like drug. Phenergan Suppositories, 25 mg., in children up to three years, and 50 mg. suppositories in older children, may be used in lieu of oral or parenteral medication. Usual adult dosage is 50 mg. Phenergan with an equal amount of meperidine and the required amount of a belladonna alkaloid.

Postoperative sedation and adjunctive use with analgesics may be obtained by the administration of 12.5 to 25 mg. in children and 25 to 50 mg. doses in adults.

How Supplied: *Tablets*—**12.5 mg.** (orange, scored), bottles of 100 and 1000, and REDIPAK® Unit Dose Medication, boxes of 100 (individually wrapped); **25 mg.** (white, scored), bottles of 100 and 1000, REDIPAK® Strip Pack, boxes of 25, and REDIPAK® Unit Dose Medication, boxes of 100 (individually wrapped); **50 mg.** (pink), bottles of 100. *Syrup*—6.25 mg. per 5 ml. (alcohol 1.5%), pint bottles. *Syrup Fortis*—25 mg. per 5 ml. (alcohol 1.5%), pint bottles. *Rectal Suppositories*—12.5 mg., 25 mg. and 50 mg., boxes of 12; 25 mg. and 50 mg. also available in REDIPAK® (Unit of Use Suppository Pack), boxes of 25.

[*Shown in Product Identification Section*]

Continued on next page

Wyeth—Cont.

PHENERGAN® Expectorant with Codeine © ℞

PHENERGAN® Expectorant PLAIN (without Codeine) ℞

PHENERGAN® VC Expectorant with Codeine © ℞

PHENERGAN® VC Expectorant PLAIN (without Codeine) ℞

PHENERGAN® Expectorant with Dextromethorphan PEDIATRIC ℞

For prescribing information write to Professional Service, Wyeth Laboratories, Box 8299, Philadelphia, Pa., 19101, or contact your local Wyeth representative.

SMA®
Iron fortified infant formula
READY-TO-FEED
CONCENTRATED LIQUID
POWDER

SMA® is unique among prepared formulas for its fat blend, whey-dominated protein composition, amino acid pattern and mineral content. SMA®, utilizing a hybridized safflower (oleic) oil, became the first infant formula offering fat and calcium absorption equal to that of human milk, with a physiologic level of linoleic acid. Thus, the fat blend in SMA® provides a ready source of energy, helps protect infants against neonatal tetany and produces a ratio of Vitamin E to polyunsaturated fatty acids (linoleic acid) more than adequate to prevent hemolytic anemia.

By combining demineralized whey with skimmed cow's milk, SMA® adjusts the protein content to within the range of human milk, reverses the lactalbumin-casein ratio of cow's milk so that it is identical to that of human milk, and reduces the mineral content to a physiologic level.

The resultant 60:40 lactalbumin-casein ratio provides protein nutrition superior to a casein-dominated formula. In addition, the essential amino acids, including cystine, are present in amounts close to those of human milk. So the protein in SMA® is of high biologic value.

The physiologic mineral content makes possible a low renal solute load which helps protect the functionally immature infant kidney, increases expendable water reserves and helps protect against dehydration.

Use of lactose as the carbohydrate results in a physiologic stool flora and a low stool pH, decreasing the incidence of perianal dermatitis.

Ingredients: SMA® Concentrated Liquid or Ready-to-Feed. Water; nonfat milk; demineralized (electrodialyzed) whey; lactose; oleo, coconut, oleic (safflower), and soybean oils; soy lecithin, calcium carrageenan. *Minerals:* Potassium bicarbonate; calcium chloride and citrate; potassium chloride; sodium citrate; ferrous sulfate; sodium bicarbonate; zinc, cupric, and manganese sulfates. *Vitamins:* Ascorbic acid, d-alpha tocopheryl acetate, niacinamide, vitamin A palmitate, calcium pantothenate, thiamine hydrochloride, riboflavin, pyridoxine hydrochloride, beta-carotene, folic acid, phytonadione, activated 7-dehydrocholesterol, biotin, cyanocobalamin.

SMA® Powder. Nonfat milk; demineralized (electrodialyzed) whey; lactose; oleo, coconut, oleic (safflower), and soybean oils; soy lecithin. *Minerals:* Calcium chloride; sodium bicarbonate; calcium citrate; ferrous sulfate; potassium hydroxide and bicarbonate; potassium chloride; zinc, cupric, and manganese sulfates. *Vitamins:* Ascorbic acid, d-alpha tocopheryl acetate, niacinamide, vitamin A palmitate, calcium pantothenate, thiamine hydrochloride, riboflavin, pyridoxine hydrochloride, beta-carotene, folic acid, phytonadione, activated 7-dehydrocholesterol, biotin, cyanocobalamin.

PROXIMATE ANALYSIS at 20 calories per fluidounce READY-TO-FEED, POWDER, and CONCENTRATED LIQUID:

	(w/v)
Fat	3.6%
Carbohydrate	7.2%
Protein	1.5%
60% Lactalbumin (whey protein)	0.9%
40% Casein	0.6%
Ash	0.25%
Crude Fiber	None
Total Solids	12.6%
Calories/fl. oz.	20

Vitamins, Minerals: In normal dilution, each quart contains 2500 I.U. vitamin A, 400 I.U. vitamin D_3, 9 I.U. vitamin E, 55 mcg. Vitamin K_1, 0.67 mg. vitamin B_1 (thiamine), 1 mg. vitamin B_2 (riboflavin), 55 mg. vitamin C (ascorbic acid), 0.4 mg. vitamin B_6 (pyridoxine hydrochloride), 1 mcg. vitamin B_{12}, 9.5 mg. equivalents niacin, 2 mg. pantothenic acid, 50 mcg. folic acid, 14 mcg. biotin, 130 mg. choline, 420 mg. calcium, 312 mg. phosphorus, 50 mg. magnesium, 142 mg. sodium, 530 mg. potassium, 350 mg. chloride, 12 mg. iron, 0.45 mg. copper, 3.5 mg. zinc, 150 mcg. manganese, 65 mcg. iodine.

Preparation: *Ready-to-Feed* (8 and 32 fl. oz. cans of 20 calories per fluidounce formula)—shake can, open and pour into previously sterilized nursing bottle; attach nipple and feed. Cover opened can and store in refrigerator. Use contents of can within 48 hours of opening.

Powder—For normal dilution supplying 20 calories per fluidounce, use 1 scoop (or 1 standard tablespoonful) of powder, packed and leveled, to 2 fluidounces of water. For larger amount of formula, use 1/4 standard measuring cup of powder, packed and leveled, to 8 fluidounces (1 cup) of water. Three of these portions make 26 fluidounces of formula.

Concentrated Liquid—For normal dilution supplying 20 calories per fluidounce, use equal amounts of SMA® liquid and water.

How Supplied: *Ready-to-Feed*—presterilized and premixed, 32 fluidounce (1 quart) cans, cases of 6; 8 fluidounce cans, case of 24 (4 carriers of 6 cans). *Powder*—1 pound cans with measuring scoop, cases of 12. *Concentrated Liquid*—13 fluidounce cans, cases of 24.

For Hospital Nursery Use—an infant feeding system which provides premixed, presterilized, ready-to-feed items, thus saving space, time and equipment. It eliminates washing, measuring, mixing, sterilizing, refrigerating and heating.

The system is offered in a choice of two forms:

1. Prefilled and presterilized 4 oz. glass bottles for which sterile nipple assemblies are available, to be attached before feeding. These units may be used again after resterilizing or may be discarded, as desired.
2. The E-Z NURSER™ (single unit nurser), also prefilled and presterilized, consists of a 4 oz. glass bottle with sterile nipple already attached; the entire unit is designed to be discarded after use.

The following items are supplied in both the forms described above:

SMA® Ready-to-Feed	
13 calories/oz.	48 bottles of 4 fl. oz.
20 calories/oz.	48 bottles of 4 fl. oz.
24 calories/oz.	48 bottles of 4 fl. oz.
27 calories/oz.	48 bottles of 4 fl. oz.
Distilled Water	48 bottles of 4 fl. oz.
Glucose, 5% in Distilled Water, 6 calories/oz.	48 bottles of 4 fl. oz.
Glucose, 10% in Distilled Water, 12 calories/oz.	48 bottles of 4 fl. oz.
NURSOY® (soy protein formula) 20 calories/oz.	48 bottles of 4 fl. oz.

(Not available in the E-Z NURSER™)

Supplied only in 8 oz. bottles, to which sterile nipple assemblies must be attached before feeding, are the following:

SMA® Ready-to-Feed 20 calories/oz.	24 bottles of 8 fl. oz.
Oral Electrolyte Solution	24 bottles of 8 fl. oz.
Distilled Water	24 bottles of 8 fl. oz.
Whole Milk	24 bottles of 8 fl. oz.
Skim Milk	24 bottles of 8 fl. oz.

Presterilized nipple assemblies, for both premature and term infants, single-hole and cross-cut, suitable for use with all ready-to-feed products requiring them, cartons of 288 nipple units.

Also Available: NURSOY® (soy protein formula), for infants with special feeding needs, soy protein replaces the cow's milk protein in the formula. Does not contain corn syrup solids.

Concentrated Liquid, 13 fl. oz. cans, cases of 24.
Ready-to-Feed, 32 fl. oz. cans, cases of 6.

Preparation of the standard 20 calories per fluidounce formula of NURSOY Ready-to-Feed and Concentrated Liquid is the same as for SMA® Ready-to-Feed and Concentrated Liquid respectively given above.

SERAX® © ℞
(oxazepam)
CAPSULES • TABLETS

Description: A therapeutic agent providing versatility and flexibility in control of common emotional disturbances, this product exerts prompt action in a wide variety of disorders associated with anxiety, tension, agitation and irritability, and anxiety associated with depression. In tolerance and toxicity studies on several animal species, this product reveals significantly greater safety factors than related compounds (chlordiazepoxide and diazepam) and manifests a wide separation of effective doses and doses inducing side effects.

Serax is 7 chloro-1,3-dihydro-3-hydroxy-5-phenyl-2*H*-1,4-benzodiazepin-2-one.

Animal Pharmacology and Toxicology: In mice, SERAX exerts an anticonvulsant (anti-Metrazol®) activity at 50 percent effective doses of about 0.6 mg. per kg. orally. (Such anticonvulsant activity of benzodiazepines correlates with their tranquilizing properties.) To produce ataxia (rotabar test) and sedation (abolition of spontaneous motor activity), the 50 percent effective doses of this product are greater than 5 mg. per kg. orally. Thus about ten times the therapeutic (anticonvulsant) dose must be given before ataxia ensues, indicating a wide separation of effective doses and doses inducing side effects.

In evaluation of antianxiety activity of compounds, conflict behavioral tests in rats differentiate continuous response for food in the presence of anxiety-provoking stress (shock) from drug-induced motor incoordination. This product shows significant separation of doses required to relieve anxiety and doses producing sedation or ataxia. Ataxia-producing doses exceed those of related CNS-acting drugs.

Acute oral LD_{50} in mice is greater than 5000 mg. per kg., compared to 800 mg. per kg. for a related compound (chlordiazepoxide).

Subacute toxicity studies in dogs for four weeks at 480 mg. per kg. daily showed no specific changes; at 960 mg. per kg. two out of eight died with evidence of circulatory collapse. This wide margin of safety is significant compared to chlordiazepoxide HCl, which showed non-specific changes in six dogs at 80 mg. per kg. On chlordiazepoxide, two out of six died with evidence of circulatory collapse at 127 mg. per kg., and six out of six died at 200 mg. per kg. daily. Chronic toxicity studies of Serax in dogs at 120 mg. per kg. per day for 52 weeks produced no toxic manifestation.

Fatty metamorphosis of the liver has been noted in six-week toxicity studies in rats given this product at 0.5% of the diet. Such accumulations of fat are considered reversible as there is no liver necrosis or fibrosis.
Breeding studies in rats through two successive litters did not produce fetal abnormality.
This product has a single major metabolite in man, a glucuronide excreted in the urine.
Indications: SERAX (oxazepam) is indicated for the management and control of anxiety, tension, agitation, irritability and related symptoms. Such symptoms are commonly seen in patients with a diagnosis of psychoneurotic reaction, psychophysiological reaction, personality disorder, or in patients with underlying organic disease.
Anxiety associated with depression is also responsive to SERAX (oxazepam) therapy.
This product has been found particularly useful in the management of anxiety, tension, agitation and irritability in older patients.
Alcoholics with acute tremulousness, inebriation, or with anxiety associated with alcohol withdrawal are responsive to therapy.
The effectiveness of Serax in long-term use, that is, more than 4 months, has not been assessed by systematic clinical studies. The physician should reassess periodically the usefulness of the drug for the individual patient.
Contraindications: History of previous hypersensitivity reaction to oxazepam. Oxazepam is not indicated in psychoses.

Warning: Use in Pregnancy: An increased risk of congenital malformations associated with the use of minor tranquilizers (chlordiazepoxide, diazepam, and meprobamate) during the first trimester of pregnancy has been suggested in several studies. Serax, a benzodiazepine derivative, has not been studied adequately to determine whether it, too, may be associated with an increased risk of fetal abnormality. Because use of these drugs is rarely a matter of urgency, their use during this period should almost always be avoided. The possibility that a woman of childbearing potential may be pregnant at the time of institution of therapy should be considered. Patients should be advised that if they become pregnant during therapy or intend to become pregnant they should communicate with their physician about the desirability of discontinuing the drug.

Precautions: Although hypotension has occurred only rarely, oxazepam should be administered with caution to patients in whom a drop in blood pressure might lead to cardiac complications. This is particularly true in the elderly patient.
In some patients exhibiting drug dependency through chronic overdose with SERAX (oxazepam) withdrawal symptoms have been noted on discontinuance of drug administration. Careful supervision of dose and amounts prescribed for patients is advised, especially with those patients with a known propensity for taking excessive quantities of drugs. Excessive and prolonged use in susceptible persons, for example, alcoholics, former addicts, and others, may result in dependence on or habituation to the drug. Where excessive dosage is continued for weeks or months, dosage should be reduced gradually rather than abruptly stopped. Abrupt discontinuance of doses in excess of the recommended dose may result in some cases in the occurrence of epileptiform seizures. Withdrawal symptoms following abrupt discontinuance are similar to those seen with barbiturates.
As with other CNS-acting drugs, patients should be cautioned against driving automobiles or operating dangerous machinery until it is known that they do not become drowsy or dizzy on oxazepam therapy.
Care should be taken to warn patients taking oxazepam that their tolerance to alcohol may be lowered.

SERAX (oxazepam)

	Usual Dose
Mild to moderate anxiety, with associated tension, irritability, agitation or related symptoms of functional origin or secondary to organic disease.	10 to 15 mg, 3 or 4 times daily
Severe anxiety syndromes, agitation or anxiety associated with depression.	15 to 30 mg, 3 or 4 times daily
Older patients with anxiety, tension, irritability and agitation.	Initial dosage: 10 mg, 3 times daily. If necessary, increase cautiously to 15 mg, 3 or 4 times daily
Alcoholics with acute inebriation, tremulousness, or anxiety on withdrawal.	15 to 30 mg, 3 or 4 times daily

Adverse Reactions: The necessity for discontinuation of therapy due to undesirable effects has been rare. Transient mild drowsiness is commonly seen in the first few days of therapy. If it persists, the dosage should be reduced. In few instances, dizziness, vertigo, headache and rarely syncope have occurred either alone or together with drowsiness. Mild paradoxical reactions, i.e., excitement, stimulation of affect, have been reported in psychiatric patients; these reactions may be secondary to relief of anxiety and usually appear in the first two weeks of therapy.
Other side effects occurring during oxazepam therapy include rare instances of minor diffuse skin rashes—morbilliform, urticarial and maculopapular—nausea, lethargy, edema, slurred speech, tremor and altered libido. Such side effects have been infrequent and are generally controlled with reduction of dosage.
Although rare, leukopenia and hepatic dysfunction including jaundice have been reported during therapy. Periodic blood counts and liver function tests are advisable.
Ataxia with oxazepam has been reported in rare instances and does not appear to be specifically related to dose or age.
Although the following side reactions have not as yet been reported with oxazepam, they have occurred with related compounds (chlordiazepoxide and diazepam): paradoxical excitation with severe rage reactions, hallucinations, menstrual irregularities, change in EEG pattern, blood dyscrasias including agranulocytosis, blurred vision, diplopia, incontinence, stupor, disorientation, fever and euphoria.
Dosage and Administration: Because of the flexibility of this product and the range of emotional disturbances responsive to it, dosage should be individualized for maximum beneficial effects.
[See table above].

This product is not indicated in children under 6 years of age. Absolute dosage for children 6–12 years of age is not established.
How Supplied: Capsules—10 mg. (pink and white), 15 mg. (red and white), 30 mg. (maroon and white), bottles of 100 and 500, and REDIPAK® (Strip Pack), boxes of 25; 15 and 30 mg. capsules also in REDIPAK® Unit Dose Medication, boxes of 100, (individually wrapped).
Tablets—15 mg. (yellow), bottles of 100.

[Shown in Product Identification Section]

SIMECO® OTC
(aluminum hydroxide gel, magnesium hydroxide, simethicone)
SUSPENSION

Composition: Each teaspoonful (5 ml) contains aluminum hydroxide gel equivalent to 365 mg of dried gel, USP, 300 mg of magnesium hydroxide and 30 mg of simethicone. Sodium content is 0.3 mEq-0.6 mEq per teaspoonful. High potency and low dose are provided by high concentration of antacid per teaspoonful.
Indications: For the symptomatic relief of hyperacidity associated with the diagnosis of peptic ulcer, gastritis, peptic esophagitis, gastric hyperacidity and hiatal hernia. To relieve the symptoms of gas.
Dosage and Administration: Usually: 1 or 2 teaspoonfuls undiluted or with a little water to be taken 3 or 4 times daily between meals and at bedtime. 5 ml SIMECO suspension neutralizes 22 mEq of acid.
Drug Interaction Precautions: Alumina-containing antacids should not be used concomitantly with any form of tetracycline therapy.
How Supplied: Suspension—Cool mint flavor available in 12 fl. oz. plastic bottles.

THIOMERIN® ℞
(mercaptomerin sodium)
INJECTION

Description: Injection THIOMERIN is available in a ready-to-use solution provided both in vials and in TUBEX® (Sterile Cartridge-Needle Unit) Wyeth.
Each ml contains 125 mg. mercaptomerin sodium equivalent to approximately 40 mg mercury in Water for Injection, U.S.P. and 0.1 mg. edetate disodium.
The disodium salt of N-(3-carboxymethylmercaptomercuri-2-methoxy) propylcamphoramic acid ($C_{16}H_{25}HgNNa_2O_6S$: molecular weight, 606.03), Thiomerin is a mercaptide, an organomercurial compound in which the xanthine has been replaced by sodium thioglycolate —one of the monothiols. (These substances, in therapeutic doses, have been shown to reduce, in laboratory animals, the cardiotoxic effects of organic mercury while preserving the diuretic action.) The reduction in local irritation is attributed to this structural modification.
Action: The primary action of mercaptomerin is to depress the tubular reabsorption of sodium and fixed anion. The increase it produces in water excretion is secondary to this decreased electrolyte reabsorption. Mercaptomerin is rapidly and completely absorbed from its parenteral sites of administration and rapidly excreted by the kidney; 95% of injected mercury can be recovered from the urine within 24 hours of administration. This large and rapid excretion by the kidney makes it possible for mercaptomerin, as opposed to inorganic mercurials, to produce reversible functional changes in the renal tubule with minimal danger of producing anatomical changes in the kidney or other organs.
Indications: This drug is indicated for the treatment of edema secondary to congestive heart failure, the nephrotic syndrome, the nephrotic stage of glomerulonephritis, and hepatic cirrhosis or portal obstruction.
Contraindications: Mercurial compounds should be withheld from patients with acute and subacute nephritis, ulcerative colitis, evidence of dehydration or hypersensitivity to the mercury ion.
In any case wherein a patient does not respond to initial therapy with Thiomerin the agent

Continued on next page

Wyeth—Cont.

should be discontinued until the overall regimen and indications are reassessed. If refractoriness is due to hypochloremic alkalosis, a normal response may be achieved when the electrolyte abnormality is corrected. The intravenous route of administration should not be employed with the organic mercurial diuretics.

Precautions: Maintain sufficient sodium intake to avoid salt deficiency, especially in hot weather. Dietary sodium should be reduced but not too severely restricted.

Instruct the patient carefully in symptoms of salt depletion. Muscle cramps may indicate sodium deficiency from too rapid diuresis. If leg cramps persist, reduce dose of the mercurial or lengthen the intervals between injections; in such cases serum electrolytes should be determined and supplements administered, as sodium deficiency may result in failure of diuretic action despite presence of edema. Excessive dehydration following mercurials is more likely to occur in elderly than in young patients, particularly in long-standing cases treated with prolonged salt restriction and frequent diuresis. Shock also may develop.

Various factors leading to sodium retention in congestive failure (as impaired cardiovascular-renal hemodynamics, elevated venous pressure, altered serum electrolytes, increased adrenocortical activity, stimulation of volume receptors, and other variables) may contribute to the failure of certain cardiac patients to respond to mercurial diuretics. No single explanation will apply to all cases.

In view of the potential electrolyte and volume disturbances common to all effective diuretic agents, it is recommended that serum electrolytes (Na, K, Cl) be determined periodically in all patients receiving repeated doses of diuretic drugs. In such patients the possibility of hyponatremia, hypokaliemia and hypochloremia should be kept in mind. The hypokaliemia produced by the action of diuretics can sensitize or exaggerate the response of the heart to the toxic effects of digitalis (e.g., increased ventricular irritability).

Adverse Reactions: Rarely, an idiosyncrasy to the mercurials may occur as indicated by flushing of the face, fever, chills, gastrointestinal disturbances, cutaneous eruptions, pruritus and urticaria. These symptoms are often on an allergic basis and are not in themselves serious, but serve as warning signals of more serious reactions that may develop if mercury is continued; administration of mercurials should be discontinued in the presence of such symptoms. Weakness, somnolence, muscle pains and shock secondary to depletion of extracellular electrolytes have occurred following excessive or injudicious use of diuretics.

Dosage and Administration: Use of any diuretic is an individual problem in every patient. Thiomerin (mercaptomerin sodium) may be injected subcutaneously in most cases and is uniformly well-tolerated when properly given by this route. Such injections should avoid edematous or adipose tissue and areas of poor circulation, while changing the site with each injection.

The *intramuscular* route may be better tolerated in the obese, the extremely emaciated, and patients whose skin is abnormally susceptible to trauma. (No local anesthetic is required for intramuscular injection of this product.) For intramuscular injection of mercurials, the gluteus maximus is the preferred site.

DIGITALIZE the patient, if required, with a digitalis preparation such as Purodigin® (crystalline digitoxin) Wyeth, before start of mercurial diuretic therapy.

DOSAGE: Use the smallest effective dose of Thiomerin at intervals which best maintain the "dry" (normal) weight of the patient. From 0.2 to 2 ml daily by subcutaneous injection is usually recommended.

In the presence of edema accompanying congestive heart failure, if there is associated dyspnea or orthopnea, moist rales in lung bases, prolonged circulation time, enlarged liver, or elevated venous pressure, this product is administered in 1 or 2 ml doses as required.

To potentiate diuresis an *acidifying agent,* as ammonium chloride, may be administered, as 2 to 3 gram in oral tablets three or four times daily for two days before injection of a mercurial.

Technic for Injection: When the ready-to-use solution in vials is used, the needle for injection should always be the *rustless* type. Syringe and needle should be sterilized. In injection of any medication beneath the skin, it is essential to employ an *absolutely accurate technic.*

Select a site on the thigh or upper arm. Cleanse injection site.

For *subcutaneous* injection the technic is the same as for administration of insulin. Pick up the skin of the selected site in a fold between the fingers of one hand and pull backward on the skin below it with the hand holding the syringe, thus stretching the skin between the two hands. Insert needle, at this point, into the empty space underneath the lifted skin. The needle will penetrate the stretched skin with practically no pain.

For *intramuscular* injection, shift the skin of the injection site away from its normal position; stretch the skin, do not pick it up in a fold. Insert needle straight (not slantwise) through the skin and underlying fat, well into muscle mass, meanwhile maintaining light lateral pressure of the plunger against the barrel of the syringe to keep the plunger from descending before the needle tip is properly placed for the injection.

To make sure the needle tip does not lie within a blood vessel, draw back on plunger. If blood is aspirated, withdraw the needle and insert at another point.

Following administration of the solution, very gentle massage of the area immediately after injection is desirable.

Do not inject Thiomerin (mercaptomerin sodium) intracutaneously, intravenously, or intra-arterially.

Stability: Store the ready-to-use solution (vials and TUBEX) in the refrigerator, preferably below 10°C (50°F). (Freezing should be avoided since the container might break.) Protect from light. Carton may be used to protect contents from light. Do not use if solution has color or precipitate. (When the ready-to-use solution in vials is used, rust or other foreign material present in the needle cannula or barrel of the syringe used for injection may introduce sufficient contamination into a multiple-dose vial to cause decomposition of the solution in a few days after a dose is withdrawn.)

How Supplied: This product is available in a ready-to-use solution. Each ml of injection contains 125 mg mercaptomerin sodium equivalent to approximately 40 mg mercury in water for injection, and 0.1 mg disodium edetate.

Solution—2-ml TUBEX® sterile cartridge-needle units, packages of 10; vials of 2 ml, boxes of 25; single vials of 10 ml.

TUBEX® Closed Injection System

The TUBEX® closed injection system delivers injectable medication in accurately machine-measured doses with each sterile, prefilled cartridge-needle unit permanently identified up to the moment of injection. Precisely calibrated single-use cartridge-needle units eliminate cross contamination and minimize dosage errors. Super-sharp, siliconized needles minimize penetration pressure. Medication is easily delivered via the sturdy, stainless TUBEX® hypodermic syringe.

TUBEX sterile cartridge-needle units are ready for instant use, fit easily into the physician's bag, and are readily stored and inventoried in the office.

TAMP-R-TEL® (tamper resistant package) — a clear, sturdy plastic package for all TUBEX narcotics and barbiturates — adds a new dimension to the handling and record keeping of these controlled drugs. In TAMP-R-TEL, each TUBEX® sterile cartridge-needle unit is locked into an individual slot within the package by its own end-lock tab, which is easily broken to release the unit for use. Once the end-lock tab is broken, it is almost impossible to replace it. TAMP-R-TEL thus enhances package integrity, discourages pilferage and facilitates "at a glance" drug count.

The following products are currently available in TUBEX® closed injection system:

Product and Needle Size Units Per Pkg	NDC 0008-
NARCOTICS in TAMP-R-TEL® **(tamper resistant package)**	
ATROPINE SULFATE AND MEPERIDINE HYDROCHLORIDE Ⓒ●	
0.4 mg Atropine SO_4 and 50 mg Meperidine HCl (22 G × 1¼″) 10—1 ml	0504-01
0.4 mg Atropine SO_4 and 75 mg Meperidine HCl (22 G × 1¼″) 10—1 ml	0505-01
0.4 mg Atropine SO_4 and 100 mg Meperidine HCl (22 G × 1¼″) 10—1 ml	0506-01
CODEINE PHOSPHATE, USP Ⓒ●	
30 mg (½ gr.) (25 G × ⅝″) 10—1 ml	0208-01
60 mg (1 gr.) (25 G × ⅝″) 10—1 ml	0209-01
HYDROMORPHONE HYDROCHLORIDE, NF Ⓒ●	
1 mg (1/60 gr.) (25 G × ⅝″) 10—1 ml fill in 2 ml	0387-01
1 mg (1/60 gr.) (22 G × 1¼″) 10—1 ml fill in 2 ml	0387-03
2 mg (1/30 gr.) (25 G × ⅝″) 10—1 ml fill in 2 ml	0295-02
2 mg (1/30 gr.) (22 G × 1¼″) 10—1 ml fill in 2 ml	0295-01
3 mg (1/20 gr.) (25 G × ⅝″) 10—1 ml fill in 2 ml	0388-01
4 mg (1/15 gr.) (25 G × ⅝″) 10—1 ml fill in 2 ml	0296-02
4 mg (1/15 gr.) (22 G × 1¼″) 10—1 ml fill in 2 ml	0296-01
MEPERGAN® (Meperidine HCl and Promethazine HCl) 25 mg each/ml Ⓒ● (22 G × 1¼″) 10—2 ml	0235-01
MEPERIDINE HYDROCHLORIDE, USP Ⓒ●	
25 mg (25 G × ⅝″) 10—1 ml fill in 2 ml	0525-03
25 mg (22 G × 1¼″) 10—1 ml fill in 2 ml	0525-02
50 mg (22 G × 1¼″) 10—1 ml	0258-04
50 mg (25 G × ⅝″) 10—1 ml fill in 2 ml	0258-03
50 mg (22 G × 1¼″) 10—1 ml fill in 2 ml	0258-02

75 mg (22 G × 1¼″)
10—1 ml 0526-04

75 mg (25 G × ⅝″)
10—1 ml fill in 2 ml 0526-03

75 mg (22 G × 1¼″)
10—1 ml fill in 2 ml 0526-02

100 mg (22 G × 1¼″)
10—1 ml 0259-04

100 mg (25 G × ⅝″)
10—1 ml fill in 2 ml 0259-03

100 mg (22 G × 1¼″)
10—1 ml fill in 2 ml 0259-02

MORPHINE SULFATE, USP ©•
2 mg (1/30 gr.) (25 G × ⅝″)
10—1 ml 0532-01

4 mg (1/15 gr.) (25 G × ⅝″)
10—1 ml 0533-01

8 mg (1/8 gr.) (25 G × ⅝″)
10—1 ml 0205-02

8 mg (1/8 gr.) (25 G × ⅝″)
10—1 ml fill in 2 ml 0205-01

8 mg (1/8 gr.) (22 G × 1¼″)
10—1 ml fill in 2 ml 0205-03

10 mg (1/6 gr.) (25 G × ⅝″)
10—1 ml 0206-03

10 mg (1/6 gr.) (25 G × ⅝″)
10—1 ml fill in 2 ml 0206-02

10 mg (1/6 gr.) (22 G × 1¼″)
10—1 ml fill in 2 ml 0206-01

15 mg (¼ gr.) (25 G × ⅝″)
10—1 ml 0207-03

15 mg (¼ gr.) (25 G × ⅝″)
10—1 ml fill in 2 ml 0207-02

15 mg (¼ gr.) (22 G × 1¼″)
10—1 ml fill in 2 ml 0207-01

BARBITURATES in TAMP-R-TEL®

PENTOBARBITAL SODIUM, USP ©•
50 mg (¾ gr.) (22 G × 1¼″)
10—1 ml 0303-01

100 mg (1½ gr.) (22 G × 1¼″)
10—2 ml 0303-02

PHENOBARBITAL SODIUM, USP ©
30 mg (½ gr.) (22 G × 1¼″)
10—1 ml 0499-01

60 mg (1 gr.) (22 G × 1¼″)
10—1 ml 0457-01

130 mg (2 gr.) (22 G × 1¼″)
10—1 ml 0304-01

SECOBARBITAL SODIUM, USP ©•
50 mg (¾ gr.) (22 G × 1¼″)
10—1 ml 0305-01

100 mg (1½ gr.) (22 G × 1¼″)
10—2 ml 0305-02

• Narcotic order blank required.

ANTIBIOTICS

BICILLIN® C-R (Penicillin G Benzathine and Penicillin G Procaine Suspension) 300,000 U each/ml
600,000 U (20 G × 1¼″)
10—1 ml 0026-17

600,000 U (20 G × 1¼″)
50—1 ml 0026-13

600,000 U (20 G × 1″)
10—1 ml 0026-18

1,200,000 U (20 G × 1¼″)
10—2 ml 0026-16

1,200,000 U (20 G × 1¼″)
50—2 ml 0026-14

1,200,00 U (20 G × 1″)
10—2 ml 0026-19

1,200,000 U (20 G × 1¼″)
10—2 ml 0026-21
(disposable syringe)

2,400,000 U (18 G × 2″)
10—4 ml 0026-22
(disposable syringe)

BICILLIN C-R 900/300
(900,000 units Penicillin G Benzathine and 300,000 units Penicillin G Procaine in suspension)
1,200,000 U (20 G × 1¼″)
10—2 ml 0079-01

BICILLIN LONG-ACTING (Sterile Penicillin G Benzathine Suspension)
600,000 U (20 G × 1¼″)
10—1 ml 0021-08

900,000 U (20 G × 1¼″)
10—1.5 ml fill in 2 ml 0021-13

1,200,000 U (20 G × 1¼″)
10—2 ml 0021-07

1,200,000 U (20 G × 1¼″)
10—2 ml 0021-11
(disposable syringe)

2,400,000 U (18 G × 2″)
10—4 ml 0021-12
(disposable syringe)

WYCILLIN® (Sterile Penicillin G Procaine Suspension)
300,000 U (22 G × 1¼″)
10—1 ml 0134-02

600,000 U (20 G × 1¼″)
10—1 ml 0018-10

600,000 U (20 G × 1¼″)
50—1 ml 0018-07

1,200,000 U (20 G × 1¼″)
10—2 ml 0018-08

2,400,000 U (18 G × 2″)
10—4 ml 0018-12
(disposable syringe)

WYCILLIN Injection and PROBENECID Tablets
(Sterile Penicillin G Procaine Suspension and Probenecid Tablets)
2,400,000 U (18 G × 2″)
2—4 ml 2517-01
(package contains two disposable syringes and two 0.5 gram Probenecid tablets)

BIOLOGICALS

DIPHTHERIA and TETANUS TOXOIDS ADSORBED (PEDIATRIC)
(25 G × ⅝″)
10—0.5 ml 0338-01

IMMUNE SERUM GLOBULIN (HUMAN), USP
(20 G × 1¼″)
1—2 ml 0437-02

INFLUENZA VIRUS VACCINE (purified subvirion)
(25 G × ⅝″)
10—0.5 ml 0568-02

TETANUS and DIPHTHERIA TOXOIDS ADSORBED (ADULT)
(25 G × ⅝″)
10—0.5 ml 0341-01

TETANUS IMMUNE GLOBULIN (HUMAN)
250 U (20 G × 1¼″)
10—1 ml 0408-02

TETANUS TOXOID ADSORBED
(25 G × ⅝″)
10—0.5 ml 0339-01

TETANUS TOXOID FLUID
(25 G × ⅝″)
10—0.5 ml 0340-01

TRIPLE ANTIGEN (Diphtheria and Tetanus Toxoids and Pertussis Vaccine Adsorbed)
(25 G × ⅝″)
10—0.5 ml 0358-01

VITAMINS

CYANOCOBALAMIN, USP
100 mcg (22 G × 1¼″)
10—1 ml 0265-01

1,000 mcg (25 G × ⅝″)
10—1 ml 0264-03

1,000 mcg (22 G × 1¼″)
10—1 ml 0264-01

1,000 mcg (22 G × 1¼″)
10—1 ml fill in 2 ml 0264-02

THIAMINE HYDROCHLORIDE, USP
100 mg (22 G × 1¼″)
10—1 ml fill in 2 ml 0302-01

VITAMIN B COMPLEX WITH B_{12}
Each ml contains:

Thiamine HCl	10 mg	Pyridoxine HCl	5 mg
Riboflavin	5 mg	d-Pantothenyl alcohol	5 mg
Niacinamide	100 mg	Cyanocobalamin	7.5 mcg

(22 G × 1¼″)
10—1 ml 0301-01

VITAMIN B COMPLEX WITH VITAMIN C
Each ml contains:

Thiamine HCl	10 mg	Pyridoxine HCl	2.5 mg
Riboflavin	2.5 mg	d-Pantothenyl alcohol	2.5 mg
Niacinamide	50 mg	Ascorbic acid (as acid and sodium ascorbate)	75 mg

(22 G × 1¼″)
10—2 ml 0300-01

CARDIOVASCULAR AGENTS

DIGOXIN, USP
0.25 mg (22 G × 1¼″)
10—1 ml 0480-02

0.5 mg (22 G × 1¼″)
10—2 ml 0480-01

EPINEPHRINE, USP (1:1000)
(25 G × ⅝″)
10—1 ml 0263-01

HEPARIN SODIUM, USP
1,000 USP units (22 G × 1¼″)
10—1 ml 0275-01

2,500 USP units (25 G × ⅝″)
10—1 ml 0482-01

Continued on next page

Wyeth—Cont.

5,000 USP units (25 G × 5/8″)
10—0.5 ml 0277-02

5,000 USP units (25 G × 5/8″)
10—1 ml 0278-02

5,000 USP units (22 G × 1¼″)
10—1 ml 0278-01

7,500 USP units (25 G × 5/8″)
10—1 ml 0293-01

10,000 USP units (25 G × 5/8″)
10—1 ml 0277-01

15,000 USP units (25 G × 5/8″)
10—1 ml 0279-01

20,000 USP units (25 G × 5/8″)
10—1 ml 0276-01

HEPARIN LOCK FLUSH Solution, USP
10 USP units (25 G × 5/8″)
50—1 ml 0523-01

100 USP units (25 G × 5/8″)
50—1 ml 0487-01

THIOMERIN®(Mercaptomerin Sodium)
250 mg (22 G × 1¼″)
10—2 ml 0294-02

WYAMINE® SULFATE (Mephentermine Sulfate)
30 mg (22 G × 1¼″)
10—1 ml 0239-01

SPECIAL AGENTS

CHLORPROMAZINE HYDROCHLORIDE, USP
25 mg (22 G × 1¼″)
10—1 ml 0435-01

50 mg (22 G × 1¼″)
10—2 ml 0435-03

DEXAMETHASONE SODIUM PHOSPHATE, USP
4 mg (22 G × 1¼″)
10—1 ml 0546-01

DIMENHYDRINATE, USP
50 mg (22 G × 1¼″)
10—1 ml 0485-01

DIPHENHYDRAMINE HYDROCHLORIDE, USP
50 mg (22 G × 1¼″)
10—1 ml 0384-01

ERGONOVINE MALEATE, NF
0.2 mg (1/300 gr.) (22 G × 1¼″)
10—1 ml 0307-01

LARGON® (Propiomazine HCl) (1678CB)
20 mg (22 G × 1¼″)
10—1 ml 0260-01

LIDOCAINE HYDROCHLORIDE, USP
1% 10 mg (25 G × 5/8″)
10—2.5 ml 0454-01

2% 20 mg (25 G × 5/8″)
10—2.5 ml 0460-01

OXYTOCIN, USP (Synthetic)
10 USP units (22 G × 1¼″)
10—1 ml 0406-01

PHENERGAN® (Promethazine HCl)
25 mg (22 G × 1¼″)
10—1 ml 0416-01

50 mg (22 G × 1¼″)
10—1 ml 0417-01

PROCHLORPERAZINE EDISYLATE, USP
5 mg (22 G × 1¼″)
10—1 ml 0542-01

10 mg (22 G × 1¼″)
10—2 ml 0542-02

SPARINE® (Promazine HCl)
25 mg (22 G × 1¼″)
10—1 ml 0232-01

50 mg (22 G ×1¼″)
10—1 ml 0236-01

100 mg (22 G × 1¼″)
10—2 ml 0236-02

SODIUM CHLORIDE, USP (Bacteriostatic)
(22 G × 1¼″)
50—2.5 ml 0333-05

TUBEX, EMPTY, STERILE CARTRIDGE-NEEDLE UNITS
(25 G × 5/8″)
50—1 ml 9103-02

(22 G × 1¼″)
50—1 ml 9103-01

(25 G × 5/8″)
50—2 ml 9103-04

(22 G × 1¼″)
50—2 ml 9103-03

UNIPEN® ℞
(nafcillin sodium) as the monohydrate
INJECTION • CAPSULES • POWDER FOR ORAL SOLUTION • TABLETS

Description: UNIPEN (nafcillin sodium) is a semisynthetic penicillin developed by Wyeth research. Although primarily designed as an antistaphylococcal penicillin, in limited clinical trials it has been shown to be effective in the treatment of infections caused by pneumococci and Group A beta-hemolytic streptococci. Because of this wide gram-positive spectrum, this product is particularly suitable for *Initial Therapy* in severe or potentially severe infections before definitive culture results are known and in which staphylococci are suspected.
This product is readily soluble and can be conveniently administered in both oral and parenteral dosage forms. It is resistant to inactivation by staphylococcal penicillinase. Following intramuscular administration in humans, it rapidly appears in the plasma, penetrates body tissues in high concentration, and diffuses well into pleural, pericardial, and synovial fluids.
NOTE: Unipen contains 2.9 milliequivalents of sodium per gram of nafcillin as the sodium salt.

Microbiology: UNIPEN is a bactericidal penicillin which has shown activity *in vitro* against both penicillin G-sensitive and penicillin G-resistant strains of *Staphylococcus aureus* as well as against pneumococcus, beta-hemolytic streptococcus, and alpha streptococcus (viridans).
In experimental mouse infections induced with pneumococci, beta-hemolytic streptococci, and both penicillin G-susceptible and penicillin G-resistant strains of *Staph. aureus*, nafcillin sodium was compared with methicillin and oxacillin. Regardless of the route of drug administration (intramuscular or oral), nafcillin sodium was consistently and significantly more effective than the other two penicillins. The fate of a penicillin G-resistant strain of *Staph. aureus* was determined in the kidneys of mice treated with penicillin G, methicillin, and nafcillin sodium. Animals injected with the nafcillin sodium showed negative cultures after the fourteenth day, whereas positive kidney cultures were obtained during the entire 28-day period from mice treated with penicillin G and methicillin.

Pharmacology: UNIPEN is relatively nontoxic for animals. The acute LD_{50} of this product by oral administration in rats and mice was greater than 5 g./kg; by intramuscular administration in rats 2800 mg./kg; by intraperitoneal administration in rats, 1240 mg./kg; and by intravenous administration in mice, 1140 mg/kg. The intraperitoneal LD_{50} in dogs is 600 mg/kg. Animal studies indicated that local tissue responses following intramuscular administration of 25% solutions were minimal and resembled those of penicillin G rather than methicillin.
Animal studies indicate that antibacterial amounts are concentrated in the bile, kidney, lung, heart, spleen, and liver. Eighty-four percent of an intravenously administered dose can be recovered by biliary cannulation and 13 percent by renal excretion in 24 hours. High and prolonged tissue levels can be demonstrated by both biological activity assays and C^{14} distribution patterns.
At comparable dosage, intramuscular absorption of this product is nearly equivalent to that of intramuscular methicillin, and oral absorption to that of oral oxacillin. Blood concentrations may be tripled by the concurrent use of probenecid. Clinical studies with nafcillin sodium monohydrate in infants under three days of age and prematures have revealed higher blood levels and slower rates of urinary excretion than in older children and adults.
Studies of the effect of this product on reproduction in rats and rabbits have been completed and reveal no fetal or maternal abnormalities. These studies include the observation of the effects of administration of the drug before conception and continuously through weaning (one generation).

Disc Susceptibility Tests: Quantitative methods that require measurement of zone diameters give the most precise estimates of antibiotic susceptibility. One such procedure* has been recommended for use with discs for testing susceptibility to penicillinase-resistant penicillin-class antibiotics. Interpretations correlate diameters on the disc test with MIC values for penicillinase-resistant penicillins. With this procedure, a report from the laboratory of "susceptible" indicates that the infecting organism is likely to respond to therapy. A report of "resistant" indicates that the infecting organism is not likely to respond to therapy. A report of "intermediate susceptibility" suggests that the organism would be susceptible if high dosage is used, or if the infection is confined to tissues and fluids (e.g., urine) in which high antibiotic levels are attained.

*Bauer, A.W., Kirby, W.M.M., Sherris, J.C., and Turck, M.: Antibiotic Testing by a Standardized Single Disc Method, Am. J. Clin. Pathol., *45*:493, 1966; Standardized Disc Susceptibility Test, FEDERAL REGISTER *37*:20527–29, 1972.

Indications: Although the principal indication for nafcillin sodium is in the treatment of infections due to penicillinase-producing staphylococci, it may be used to initiate therapy in such patients in whom a staphylococcal infection is suspected. (See Important Note below.)
Bacteriologic studies to determine the causative organisms and their sensitivity to nafcillin sodium should be performed.
In serious, life-threatening infections, oral preparations of the penicillinase-resistant penicillins should not be relied on for initial therapy.

Important Note: When it is judged necessary that treatment be initiated before definitive culture and sensitivity results are known, the choice of nafcillin sodium should take into consideration the fact that it has been shown to be effective only in the treatment of infections caused by pneumococci, Group A beta-hemolytic streptococci, and penicillin G-resistant and penicillin G-sensitive staphylococci. If the bacteriology report later indicates the infection is due to an organism other than a penicillin G-resistant staphylococcus sensitive to nafcillin sodium, the physician is advised to continue therapy with a drug other than nafcillin sodium or any other penicillinase-resistant, semisynthetic penicillin.

Recent studies have reported that the percentage of staphylococcal isolates resistant to penicillin G outside the hospital is increasing, approximating the high percentage of resistant staphylococcal isolates found in the hospital. For this reason, it is recommended that a penicillinase-resistant penicillin be used as initial therapy for any suspected staphylococcal infection until culture and sensitivity results are known.

Methicillin is a compound that acts through a mechanism similar to that of nafcillin sodium against penicillin G-resistant staphylococci. Strains of staphylococci resistant to methicillin have existed in nature, and it is known that the number of these strains reported has been increasing. Such strains of staphylococci have been capable of producing serious disease, in some instances resulting in fatality. Because of this there is concern that widespread use of the penicillinase-resistant penicillins may result in the appearance of an increasing number of staphylococcal strains which are resistant to these penicillins.

Methicillin-resistant strains are almost always resistant to all other penicillinase-resistant penicillins (cross-resistance with cephalosporin derivatives also occurs frequently). Resistance to any penicillinase-resistant penicillin should be interpreted as evidence of clinical resistance to all, in spite of the fact that minor variations in *in vitro* sensitivity may be encountered when more than one penicillinase-resistant penicillin is tested against the same strain of staphylococcus.

Contraindications: A history of allergic reaction to any of the penicillins is a contraindication.

Warnings: Serious and occasionally fatal hypersensitivity (anaphylactoid) reactions have been reported in patients on penicillin therapy. Although anaphylaxis is more frequent following parenteral therapy, it has occurred in patients on oral penicillins. These reactions are more apt to occur in individuals with a history of sensitivity to multiple allergens.

There have been reports of individuals with a history of penicillin hypersensitivity reactions who have experienced severe hypersensitivity reactions when treated with a cephalosporin. Before therapy with a penicillin, careful inquiry should be made concerning previous hypersensitivity reactions to penicillins, cephalosporins, and other allergens. If an allergic reaction occurs, appropriate therapy should be instituted, and discontinuation of nafcillin therapy considered. The usual agents (antihistamines, pressor amines, corticosteroids) should be readily available.

Precautions: As with any potent drug, periodic assessment of organ-system function, including renal, hepatic and hematopoietic, should be made during prolonged therapy.

The possibility of bacterial and fungal overgrowth should be kept in mind during long-term therapy. If overgrowth of resistant organisms occurs, appropriate measures should be taken.

The oral route of administration should not be relied upon in patients with severe illness, or with nausea, vomiting, gastric dilatation, cardiospasm, or intestinal hypermotility.

Safety for use in pregnancy has not been established.

Particular care should be taken with intravenous administration because of the possibility of thrombophlebitis.

Adverse Reactions: Reactions to nafcillin sodium have been infrequent and mild in nature. As with other penicillins, the possibility of an anaphylactic reaction or serum-sickness-like reactions should be considered. A careful history should be taken. Patients with histories of hay fever, asthma, urticaria, or previous sensitivity to penicillin are more likely to react adversely.

Transient leukopenia, neutropenia with evidence of granulocytopenia or thrombocytopenia are infrequent and usually associated with prolonged therapy with high doses of penicillin. These alteration have been noted to return to normal after cessation of therapy.

The few reactions associated with the intramuscular use of nafcillin sodium have been skin rash, pruritus, and possible drug fever. As with other penicillins, reactions from oral use of the drug have included nausea, vomiting, diarrhea, urticaria, and pruritus.

Dosage and Administration: It is recommended that parenteral therapy be used initially in severe infections. The patient should be placed on oral therapy with this product as soon as the clinical condition warrants. Very severe infections may require very high doses.

Intravenous route: 500 mg every 4 hours; double the dose if necessary in very severe infections.

The required amount of drug should be diluted in 15 to 30 ml of Sterile Water for Injection, U.S.P., or Sodium Chloride Injection, U.S.P., and injected over a 5- to 10-minute period. This may be accomplished through the tubing of an intravenous infusion if desirable.

Stability studies on nafcillin sodium at concentrations of 2 mg/ml to 40 mg/ml in the following intravenous solutions indicate the drug will lose less than 10% activity at room temperature (70°F.) or, if kept under refrigeration, during the time period stipulated:

Stability at	Room Temperature	Refrigerated
Sterile Water for Injection	24 hours	96 hours
Isotonic sodium chloride	24 hours	96 hours
5% dextrose in water	24 hours	96 hours
5% dextrose in 0.4% sodium chloride solution	24 hours	96 hours
Ringer's solution	24 hours	96 hours
M/6 sodium lactate solution	24 hours	96 hours

Discard any unused portions of intravenous solutions after 24 hours if kept at room temperature or after 96 hours if kept under refrigeration.

Only those solutions listed above should be used for the intravenous infusion of UNIPEN (nafcillin sodium). The concentration of the antibiotic should fall within the range of 2 to 40 mg/ml. The drug concentrate and the rate and volume of the infusion should be adjusted so that the total dose of nafcillin is administered before the drug loses its stability in the solution in use.

There is no clinical experience available on the use of this agent in neonates or infants for this route of administration.

This route of administration should be used for relatively short-term therapy (24-48 hours) because of the occasional occurrence of thrombophlebitis, particularly in elderly patients.

Piggyback Units (for Intravenous Drip Use)—Use Sterile Water for Injection or Isotonic Sodium Chloride.

ONE-GRAM BOTTLE:

Add a minimum of 49 ml water or saline, and shake well. If lower concentrations are desired, the solution could be further diluted with up to a total of 99 ml of diluent.

Amount of Diluent	Solution Concentration
49 ml	20 mg/ml
99 ml	10 mg/ml

TWO-GRAM BOTTLE:

Add a minimum of 49 ml water or saline, and shake well. If lower concentrations are desired, the solution could be further diluted with up to a total of 99 ml of diluent.

Amount of Diluent	Solution Concentration
49 ml	40 mg/ml
99 ml	20 mg/ml

FOUR-GRAM BOTTLE:

Add 97 ml water or saline, and shake well. The resulting solution will contain 40 mg/ml.

The resulting solutions may then be administered alone or with the intravenous solutions listed above. Discard unused solution after 24 hours at room temperature (70°F) or 96 hours if kept under refrigeration. Administer piggyback through an IV tubing very slowly (at least 30–60 minutes) to avoid vein irritation.

At times it may be desired to use the contents of the piggyback bottles for addition to large-volume IV fluids. In this case the entire vial contents should be dissolved in not less than 25 ml of Sterile Water for Injection. Use the resulting concentration within 24 hours when kept at room temperature or within 96 hours when kept under refrigeration.

Intramuscular Route: 500 mg every 6 hours in adults; decrease the interval to 4 hours if necessary in severe infections. In infants and children a dose of 25 mg/kg (about 12 mg per pound) twice daily is usually adequate.

For neonates, 10 mg/kg is recommended twice daily.

To reconstitute, see directions and table below. The clear solution should be administered by deep intragluteal injection immediately after reconstitution. After reconstitution, keep refrigerated (2°–8° C) and use within 7 days or keep at room temperature (25° C) and use within 3 days.

Oral Route: In adults a dose of 250 to 500 mg every 4 to 6 hours is sufficient for mild-to-moderate infections. In severe infections 1 gram every 4 to 6 hours may be necessary.

In children, streptococcal pharyngitis cases have responded to a dosage of 250 mg t.i.d. Beta-hemolytic streptococcal infections should be treated for at least ten days to prevent development of acute rheumatic fever or glomerulonephritis.

Children and infants with scarlet fever and pneumonia should receive 25 mg/kg/day in four divided doses. For staphylococcal infections, 50 mg/kg/day in four divided doses is recommended. For neonates, 10 mg/kg three to four times daily is recommended. If inadequate, resort to parenteral UNIPEN® (nafcillin sodium) Wyeth.

To reconstitute the powder for oral solution, add the water in two separate portions. Shake well after each addition. After reconstitution the solution must be refrigerated. Discard any unused portion after one week.

How Supplied: *Capsules*—containing nafcillin sodium, as the monohydrate, equivalent to 250 mg. nafcillin buffered with calcium carbonate, bottles of 100, and REDIPAK® Unit Dose Medication boxes of 100 (individually wrapped).

Tablets (film-coated)—containing nafcillin sodium, as the monohydrate, equivalent to 500 mg. nafcillin buffered with calcium carbonate, bottles of 50.

Oral Solution: Supplied as a powder for oral solution. When reconstituted with water each 5 ml will contain nafcillin sodium equivalent to 250 mg nafcillin, bottle to make 100 ml.

Continued on next page

Wyeth—Cont.

For Parenteral Administration—(intravenous or intramuscular)

Vials: Supplied in vial sizes of 500 mg., 1 gram, and 2 gram nafcillin sodium as the monohydrate, buffered. When reconstituted as recommended (see table below) with Sterile Water for Injection, U.S.P., Bacteriostatic Water for Injection, U.S.P., (with parabens), or Bacteriostatic Water for Injection, U.S.P., with benzyl alcohol, the contents of each vial provides, respectively, 2-, 4- or 8-ml. of nafcillin sodium solution equivalent **per ml.** to 250 mg. nafcillin buffered with 10 mg. sodium citrate.

Vial Size	Amount of Diluent	Nafcillin Sodium Solution*
500 mg.	1.7 ml.	2 ml.
1 gram	3.4 ml.	4 ml.
2 gram	6.8 ml.	8 ml.

*Contents of each vial provides the specified amount of solution containing the equivalent of 250 mg. nafcillin and 10 mg. sodium citrate in each ml.

FOR INTRAVENOUS USE ONLY

Piggyback Units: Supplied in single units equivalent to 1, 2 or 4 gram nafcillin per unit buffered with 40 mg sodium citrate per gram.

[*Shown in Product Identification Section*]

WYAMYCIN® E ℞
Liquid
(erythromycin ethylsuccinate oral suspension)

Description: Erythromycin is produced by a strain of *Streptomyces erythraeus* and belongs to the macrolide group of antibiotics. It is basic and readily forms salts with acids. The base, the stearate salt, and the esters are poorly soluble in water. Erythromycin ethylsuccinate is an ester of erythromycin suitable for oral administration.

The pleasant-tasting, fruit-flavored liquids are supplied ready for oral administration.

The ready-made suspensions are intended primarily for pediatric use but can also be used in adults.

Actions: The mode of action of erythromycin is by inhibition of protein synthesis without affecting nucleic acid synthesis. Resistance to erythromycin of some strains of *Hemophilus influenzae* and staphylococci has been demonstrated. Culture and susceptibility testing should be done. If the Kirby-Bauer method of disc susceptibility is used, a 15 mcg erythromycin disc should give a zone diameter of at least 18 mm when tested against an erythromycin-susceptible organism.

Orally administered erythromycin ethylsuccinate suspensions are readily and reliably absorbed. Serum levels are comparable when the drug is administered in either the fasting or nonfasting state.

After absorption, erythromycin diffuses readily into most body fluids. In the absence of meningeal inflammation low concentrations are normally achieved in the spinal fluid, but passage of the drug across the blood-brain barrier increases in meningitis. In the presence of normal hepatic function, erythromycin is concentrated in the liver and excreted in the bile; the effect of hepatic dysfunction on excretion of erythromycin by the liver into the bile is not known. After oral administration, less than 5 percent of the activity of the administered dose can be recovered in the urine.

Erythromycin crosses the placental barrier, but fetal plasma levels are generally low.

Indications: *Streptococcus Pyogenes* (Group A beta-hemolytic streptococcus):

Upper- and lower-respiratory-tract, skin, and soft tissue infections of mild-to-moderate severity.

Injectable penicillin G benzathine is considered by the American Heart Association to be the drug of choice in the treatment and prevention of streptococcal pharyngitis and in long-term prophylaxis of rheumatic fever.

When oral medication is preferred for treatment of the above conditions, penicillin G, V, or erythromycin are alternate drugs of choice. When oral medication is given, the importance of strict adherence by the patient to the prescribed dosage regimen must be stressed. A therapeutic dose should be administered for at least 10 days.

Alpha-hemolytic Streptococci (viridans group): Short-term prophylaxis of bacterial endocarditis prior to dental or other operative procedures in patients with a history of rheumatic fever or congenital heart disease who are hypersensitive to penicillin. (Erythromycin is not suitable prior to genitourinary surgery where the organisms likely to lead to bacteremia are gram-negative bacilli or the enterococcus group of streptococci.)

Staphylococcus Aureus: Acute infections of skin and soft tissue of mild-to-moderate severity. Resistant organisms may emerge during treatment.

Streptococcus Pneumoniae (Diplococcus pneumoniae): Upper-respiratory-tract infections (e.g., otitis media, pharyngitis) and lower-respiratory-tract infections (e.g., pneumonia) of mild-to-moderate degree.

Mycoplasma Pneumoniae (Eaton agent, PPLO): For respiratory infections due to this organism.

Hemophilus Influenzae: For upper-respiratory-tract infections of mild-to-moderate severity when used concomitantly with adequate doses of sulfonamides. Not all strains of this organism are susceptible at the erythromycin concentrations ordinarily achieved (see appropriate sulfonamide labeling for prescribing information).

Treponema Pallidum: Erythromycin is an alternate choice of treatment for primary syphilis in patients allergic to the penicillins. In treatment of primary syphilis, spinal-fluid examinations should be done before treatment and as part of follow-up after therapy.

Corynebacterium Diphtheriae and *C. Minutissimum:* As an adjunct to antitoxin, to prevent establishment of carriers, and to eradicate the organism in carriers.

In the treatment of erythrasma.

Entamoeba Histolytica: In the treatment of intestinal amebiasis only. Extra-enteric amebiasis requires treatment with other agents.

Listeria Monocytogenes: Infections due to this organism.

Legionnaires' Disease: Although no controlled clinical efficacy studies have been conducted, *in vitro* and limited preliminary clinical data suggest that erythromycin may be effective in treating Legionnaires' Disease.

Contraindications: Erythromycin is contraindicated in patients with known hypersensitivity to this antibiotic.

Warnings: USAGE IN PREGNANCY: Safety for use in pregnancy has not been established.

Precautions: Erythromycin is principally excreted by the liver. Caution should be exercised in administering the antibiotic to patients with impaired hepatic function. There have been reports of hepatic dysfunction, with or without jaundice, occurring in patients receiving oral erythromycin products.

Recent data from studies of erythromycin reveal that its use in patients who are receiving high doses of theophylline may be associated with an increase of serum theophylline levels and potential theophylline toxicity. In case of theophylline toxicity and/or elevated serum theophylline levels, the dose of theophylline should be reduced while the patient is receiving concomitant erythromycin therapy.

Surgical procedures should be performed when indicated.

Adverse Reactions: The most frequent side effects of erythromycin preparations are gastrointestinal, such as abdominal cramping and discomfort, and are dose-related. Nausea, vomiting, and diarrhea occur infrequently with usual oral doses.

During prolonged or repeated therapy, there is a possibility of overgrowth of nonsusceptible bacteria or fungi. If such infections occur, the drug should be discontinued and appropriate therapy instituted.

Mild allergic reactions such as urticaria and other skin rashes have occurred. Serious allergic reactions, including anaphylaxis, have been reported.

Dosage and Administration: Erythromycin ethylsuccinate suspensions may be administered without regard to meals.

Children: Age, weight, and severity of the infecton are important factors in determining the proper dosage. In mild-to-moderate infections the usual dosage of erythromycin ethylsuccinate for children is 30 to 50 mg/kg/day in divided doses. For more severe infections this dosage may be doubled.

The following dosage schedule is suggested for mild-to-moderate infections:

Body Weight	Total Daily Dose
Under 10 lbs.	30-50 mg/kg/day 15-25 mg/lb/day
10 to 15 lbs.	200 mg
16 to 25 lbs.	400 mg
26 to 50 lbs.	800 mg
51 to 100 lbs.	1200 mg
over 100 lbs.	1600 mg

The total daily dosage must be administered in divided doses.

Adults: 400 mg erythromycin ethylsuccinate every 6 hours is the usual dose. Dosage may be increased up to 4 gram per day according to the severity of the infection.

If twice-a-day dosage is desired in either adults or children, one-half of the total daily dose may be given every 12 hours.

In the treatment of streptococcal infections, a therapeutic dosage of erythromycin ethylsuccinate should be administered for at least 10 days. In continuous prophylaxis against recurrences of streptococcal infections in persons with a history of rheumatic heart disease, the usual dosage is 400 mg twice a day.

When used prior to surgery to prevent endocarditis (see *alpha-hemolytic streptococci*), a recommended schedule for adults is 800 mg erythromycin ethylsuccinate before the procedure and 400 mg every 6 hours for 4 doses after the procedure. For small children, 30 to 50 mg/kg/day divided into 3 or 4 evenly spaced doses.

For Treatment of Primary Syphilis:

Adults—48 to 64 gram, given in divided doses over a period of 10 to 15 days.

For Intestinal Amebiasis:

Adults—400 mg four times daily for 10 to 14 days.

Children—30 to 50 mg/kg/day in divided doses for 10 to 14 days.

For treatment of Legionnaires' Disease:

Although optimal doses have not been established, doses utilized in reported clinical data were those recommended above, 1.6 to 4 gram daily in divided doses.

How Supplied: Wyamycin® E 200 (erythromycin ethylsuccinate oral suspension) is supplied in 1-pint bottles. Each 5 ml teaspoonful of fruit-flavored suspension contains activity equivalent to 200 mg of erythromycin.

Wyamycin® E 400 (erythromycin ethylsuccinate oral suspension) is supplied in 1-pint bottles. Each 5 ml teaspoonful of fruit-flavored suspension contains activity equivalent to 400 mg of erythromycin.

Also Available: Wyamycin® S (erythromycin stearate) tablets, containing the equivalent of 250 mg erythromycin, are available in bottles of 100 and 500 film-coated tablets. Wyamycin® S (erythromycin stearate) tablets, containing the equivalent of 500 mg erythromycin, are available in bottles of 100 film-coated tablets.

[*Shown in Production Identification Section*]

WYANOIDS® HC ℞

Rectal Suppositories
(with hydrocortisone)

Description: Each suppository contains 10 mg. hydrocortisone acetate, 15 mg. extract belladonna (0.19 mg. equiv. total alkaloids), 3 mg. ephedrine sulfate, 176 mg. zinc oxide, 543 mg. boric acid, 30 mg. bismuth oxyiodide, 146 mg. bismuth subcarbonate, 30 mg. peruvian balsam in cocoa butter and beeswax.

Action: Hydrocortisone, an active adrenal cortical hormone and the chief corticosteroid in human plasma, appears to act directly on the tissues of the body and reduces the tissue response to acute inflammation. In the management of severe inflammatory anorectal disorders, it has proved to be a significant advance over spasmolytics, astringents, and emollients which formerly were often the only therapy available.

The combination of hydrocortisone and the soothing ingredients of the Wyanoids base relieves itching, burning, and soreness and tends to reduce inflammation and edema.

Indications

Based on a review of this drug by the National Academy of Sciences—National Research Council and/or other information, FDA has classified the indication as follows:

"Possibly" effective: Treatment of proctitis secondary to ulcerative colitis.

Final classification of the less-than-effective indications requires further investigation.

Dosage: One suppository inserted rectally twice daily for six days or as required.

WARNING: Hydrocortisone should not be used until an adequate proctologic examination is completed and a diagnosis made. Other specific measures against infections, allergy, and other causal factors must not be neglected.

Belladonna should not be used in patients with glaucoma or organic pyloric stenosis. It should be used with caution in prostatism, urinary retention, elderly persons, and children under six years of age. If eye pain occurs, the drug should be discontinued since this may indicate undiagnosed glaucoma.

Patients should be cautioned not to exceed the prescribed dose, to decrease dose if dryness of the mouth occurs, and to discontinue use if rapid pulse, blurring of vision, or dizziness occurs.

Frequent or prolonged use of preparations containing belladonna should be avoided.

How Supplied: Wyanoids® HC Suppositories are available in boxes of 12 suppositories; and Redipak®, Unit of Use Suppository Pack, as combination packages of one Wyanoids HC Suppository, one finger cot, and one 0.5 gram packet of lubricant (White Petrolatum, U.S.P.) in packages of 25 combination packages.

Also available: WYANOID Ointment and WYANOIDS hemorrhoidal suppositories. The ointment contains zinc oxide, boric acid, ephedrine sulfate, benzocaine and peruvian balsam in a soothing emollient base. Each suppository contains 15 mg extract belladonna (0.19 mg equiv. total alkaloids), 3 mg ephedrine sulfate, zinc oxide, boric acid, bismuth oxyiodide, bismuth subcarbonate, and peruvian balsam in cocoa butter and beeswax.

How Supplied: *Ointment*—Tube of 1 ounce with applicator.

Suppositories—Boxes of 12. Each combination package contains one WYANOIDS Suppository, one finger cot and one 0.5 gram packet of lubricant (White Petrolatum, U.S.P.).

[*Shown in Product Identification Section*]

WYCILLIN® ℞

(sterile penicillin G procaine suspension)
INJECTION

FOR DEEP INTRAMUSCULAR INJECTION ONLY

Description: This product is designed to provide a stable aqueous suspension of sterile penicillin G procaine, ready for immediate use. This eliminates the necessity for addition of any diluent, required for the usual dry formulation of injectable penicillin.

Each TUBEX® (Sterile Cartridge-Needle Unit, Wyeth), 1,200,000 units (2 ml. size) or 600,000 units (1 ml. size) or disposable syringe 2,400,000 units (4 ml. size) contains penicillin G procaine in a stabilized aqueous suspension with sodium citrate buffer; and as w/v, approximately 0.5% lecithin, 0.5% carboxymethylcellulose, 0.5% povidone, 0.1% methylparaben and 0.01% propylparaben.

Each TUBEX, 300,000 units (1 ml. size), contains penicillin G procaine in a stabilized aqueous suspension with sodium citrate buffer; and as w/v, approximately 0.3% lecithin, 0.9% carboxymethylcellulose, 0.9% povidone, 0.14% methylparaben, and 0.015% propylparaben.

The multiple dose vial contains per ml. 300,000 units penicillin G procaine in a stabilized aqueous suspension with sodium citrate buffer, and approximately 7 mg. lecithin, 2 mg. carboxymethylcellulose, 3 mg. povidone, 0.5 mg. sorbitan monopalmitate, 0.5 mg. polyoxyethylene sorbitan monopalmitate, 1.2 mg. methylparaben and 0.14 mg. propylparaben.

WYCILLIN (sterile penicillin G procaine suspension) must be stored in a refrigerator. Keep from freezing. This will prevent deterioration and assure that no significant loss of potency occurs within the expiration date.

Actions and Pharmacology: Penicillin G exerts a bactericidal action against penicillin-sensitive microorganisms during the stage of active multiplication. It acts through the inhibition of biosynthesis of cell-wall mucopeptide. It is not active against the penicillinase-producing bacteria, which include many strains of staphylococci. Penicillin G exerts high *in vitro* activity against staphylococci (except penicillinase-producing strains), streptococci (groups A, C, G, H, L, and M) and pneumococci. Other organisms sensitive to penicillin G are *Neisseria gonorrhoeae, Corynebacterium diphtheriae, Bacillus anthracis,* Clostridia, *Actinomyces bovis, Streptobacillus moniliformis, Listeria monocytogenes* and Leptospira. *Treponema pallidum* is extremely sensitive to the bactericidal action of penicillin G.

Sensitivity plate testing: If the Kirby-Bauer method of disc sensitivity is used, a 10-unit penicillin disc should give a zone greater than 28 mm. when tested against a penicillin-sensitive bacterial strain.

Penicillin G procaine is an equimolecular compound of procaine and penicillin G, administered intramuscularly as a suspension. It dissolves slowly at the site of injection, giving a plateau type of blood level at about 4 hours which falls slowly over a period of the next 15–20 hours.

Approximately 60% of penicillin G is bound to serum protein. The drug is distributed throughout the body tissues in widely varying amounts. Highest levels are found in the kidneys with lesser amounts in the liver, skin and intestines. Penicillin G penetrates into all other tissues to a lesser degree with a very small level found in the cerebrospinal fluid. With normal kidney function the drug is excreted rapidly by tubular excretion. In neonates and young infants and in individuals with impaired kidney functions, excretion is considerably delayed. Approximately 60–90 percent of a dose of parenteral penicillin G is excreted in the urine within 24–36 hours.

Indications: Penicillin G procaine is indicated in the treatment of moderately severe infections due to penicillin G-sensitive microorganisms that are sensitive to the low and persistent serum levels common to this particular dosage form. Therapy should be guided by bacteriological studies (including sensitivity tests) and by clinical response.

NOTE: When high, sustained serum levels are required, aqueous penicillin G, either IM or IV, should be used.

The following infections will usually respond to adequate dosages of intramuscular penicillin G procaine:

Streptococcal infections (Group A—without bacteremia). Moderately severe to severe infections of the upper respiratory tract, skin and soft tissue infections, scarlet fever, and erysipelas.

NOTE: Streptococci in Groups A, C, G, H, L, and M are very sensitive to penicillin G. Other groups, including Group D (enterococcus), are resistant. Aqueous penicillin is recommended for streptococcal infections with bacteremia.

Pneumococcal infections. Moderately severe infections of the respiratory tract.

NOTE: Severe pneumonia, empyema, bacteremia, pericarditis, meningitis, peritonitis, and arthritis of pneumococcal etiology are better treated with aqueous penicillin G during the acute stage.

Staphylococcal infections—penicillin G-sensitive. Moderately severe infections of the skin and soft tissues.

NOTE: Reports indicate an increasing number of strains of staphylococci resistant to penicillin G, emphasizing the need for culture and sensitivity studies in treating suspected staphylococcal infections.

Indicated surgical procedures should be performed.

Fusospirochetosis (Vincent's gingivitis and pharyngitis). Moderately severe infections of the oropharynx respond to therapy with penicillin G procaine.

NOTE: Necessary dental care should be accomplished in infections involving the gum tissue.

Treponema pallidum (syphilis); all stages.

N. gonorrhoeae; acute and chronic (without bacteremia).

Yaws, Bejel, Pinta.

C. diphtheriae—penicillin G procaine as an adjunct to antitoxin for prevention of the carrier stage.

Anthrax.

Streptobacillus moniliformis and *Spirillum minus* infections (rat-bite fever).

Erysipeloid.

Subacute bacterial endocarditis (Group A streptococcus), only in extremely sensitive infections.

Prophylaxis Against Bacterial Endocarditis—Penicillin G procaine may be given to patients with congenital and/or rheumatic heart lesions who are to undergo dental or upper-respiratory-tract surgery or instrumentation. Prophylaxis should be instituted the day of the procedure and continued for 2 or more days following.

NOTE: Since patients who have a past history of rheumatic fever and are receiving continuous prophylaxis may harbor increased numbers of penicillin-resistant organisms, use of another prophylactic anti-infective agent should be considered. If penicillin is to be used in these patients at surgery, the regular rheumatic fever program should be interrupted 1 week prior to the contemplated surgery. At the time of surgery, penicillin may be reinstituted as a prophylactic measure against the hazards of surgically-induced bacteremia.

Continued on next page

Wyeth—Cont.

Contraindications: A previous hypersensitivity reaction to any penicillin is a contraindication.

Warnings: Serious and occasionally fatal hypersensitivity (anaphylactoid) reactions have been reported in patients on penicillin therapy.

Serious anaphylactoid reactions require immediate emergency treatment with epinephrine. Oxygen and intravenous corticosteroids should also be administered as indicated.

Although anaphylaxis is more frequent following parenteral therapy, it has occurred in patients on oral penicillins. These reactions are more apt to occur in individuals with a history of sensitivity to multiple allergens.

There have been well-documented reports of individuals with a history of penicillin hypersensitivity reactions who have experienced severe hypersensitivity reactions when treated with a cephalosporin. Before therapy with a penicillin, careful inquiry should be made concerning previous hypersensitivity reactions to penicillins, cephalosporins, and other allergens. If an allergic reaction occurs, the drug should be discontinued and the patient treated with the usual agents, e.g., pressor amines, antihistamines and corticosteroids.

Immediate toxic reactions to procaine may occur in some individuals, particularly when a large single dose is administered in the treatment of gonorrhea (4.8 million units). These reactions may be manifested by mental disturbances, including anxiety, confusion, agitation, depression, weakness, seizures, hallucinations, combativeness, and expressed "fear of impending death". The reactions noted in carefully controlled studies occurred in approximately one in 500 patients treated for gonorrhea. Reactions are transient, lasting from 15–30 minutes.

Precautions: Penicillin should be used with caution in individuals with histories of significant allergies and/or asthma.

Care should be taken to avoid intravenous or intra-arterial administration, or injection into or near major peripheral nerves or blood vessels, since such injections may produce neurovascular damage.

In suspected staphylococcal infections, proper laboratory studies, including sensitivity tests, should be performed.

A small percentage of patients are sensitive to procaine. If there is a history of sensitivity make the usual test: Inject intradermally 0.1 ml of a 1 to 2 percent procaine solution. Development of an erythema, wheal, flare or eruption indicates procaine sensitivity. Sensitivity should be treated by the usual methods, including barbiturates, and procaine penicillin preparations should not be used. Antihistaminics appear beneficial in treatment of procaine reactions.

The use of antibiotics may result in overgrowth of nonsusceptible organisms. Constant observation of the patient is essential. If new infections due to bacteria or fungi appear during therapy, the drug should be discontinued and appropriate measures taken.

Whenever allergic reactions occur, penicillin should be withdrawn unless, in the opinion of the physician, the condition being treated is life-threatening and amenable only to penicillin therapy.

In prolonged therapy with penicillin, and particularly with high-dosage schedules, periodic evaluation of the renal and hematopoietic systems is recommended.

When treating gonococcal infections in which primary or secondary syphilis may be suspected, proper diagnostic procedures, including dark-field examinations, should be done. In all cases in which concomitant syphilis is suspected, monthly serological tests should be made for at least four months.

Adverse Reactions: Penicillin is a substance of low toxicity but does possess a significant index of sensitization. The following hypersensitivity reactions associated with use of penicillin have been reported: Skin rashes, ranging from maculopapular eruptions to exfoliative dermatitis; urticaria; serum sickness-like reactions, including chills, fever, edema, arthralgia, and prostration. Severe and often fatal anaphylaxis has been reported (see "Warnings"). As with other treatments for syphilis, the Jarisch-Herxheimer reaction has been reported.

Procaine toxicity manifestations have been reported (see "Warnings"). Although procaine hypersensitivity reactions have not been reported with this drug, there are patients who are sensitive to procaine (see "Precautions").

Dosage and Administration: Penicillin G procaine (aqueous) is for intramuscular injection only.

Administer by **DEEP INTRAMUSCULAR INJECTION** in the upper, outer quadrant of the buttock. In infants and small children, the midlateral aspect of the thigh may be preferable. When doses are repeated, vary the injection site. Before injecting the dose, aspirate to be sure needle bevel is not in a blood vessel.

The Wyeth disposable syringe for this product incorporates several new features that are designed to facilitate its use.

A single small indentation, or "dot", has been punched into the metal ring that surrounds the neck of the syringe near the base of the needle. It is important that this "dot" be placed in a position so that it can be easily visualized by the operator following the intramuscular insertion of the syringe needle. Once the needle has been inserted, aspiration should be carried out in accordance with good medical technic before the medication is injected. During the process of aspiration the barrel of the syringe immediately proximal to the location of the "dot" should be closely observed by the operator, since this is the area in which blood that may have entered the needle is most likely to appear.

When using the TUBEX or the disposable syringe, if blood or any suspicious discoloration is apparent, the needle should be withdrawn without injecting any of the medication, the syringe and its contents discarded, and the process repeated using a new syringe at a different site.

Pneumonia (pneumococcal), moderately severe (uncomplicated): 600,000-1,000,000 units daily.

Streptococcal infections (Group A), moderately severe to severe tonsillitis, erysipelas, scarlet fever, upper respiratory tract, skin and soft tissue: 600,000-1,000,000 units daily for 10-day minimum.

Staphylococcal infections, moderately severe to severe: 600,000-1,000,000 units daily.

In pneumonia, streptococcal (Group A) and staphylococcal infections in children under 60 pounds: 300,000 units daily.

Bacterial endocarditis (Group A streptococci) only in extremely sensitive infections: 600,000-1,000,000 units daily.

To prevent bacterial endocarditis in patients with rheumatic or congenital heart lesions who are to undergo dental or upper-respiratory-tract surgery or instrumentation:

600,000 units penicillin G procaine aqueous the day of the procedure.

600,000 units penicillin G aqueous 1-2 hours before surgery.

600,000 units penicillin G procaine aqueous daily for 2 days following surgery.

Syphilis—

Primary, secondary and latent with a negative spinal fluid in adults and children over 12 years of age: 600,000 units daily for 8 days—total 4,800,000 units.

Late (tertiary, neurosyphilis and latent syphilis with positive spinal-fluid examination or no spinal-fluid examination): 600,000 units daily for 10-15 days—total 6-9 million units.

Congenital syphilis under 70-lb. body weight: 10,000 units/kg./day for 10 days.

Yaws, Bejel, and Pinta: Treatment as syphilis in corresponding stage of disease.

Gonorrhea—

Although some isolates of *Neisseria gonorrhoeae* have decreased susceptibility to penicillin, this inherent resistance is relative, not absolute, and penicillin in large doses remains the drug of choice for these strains. Strains producing penicillinase, however, are resistant to penicillin G, and a drug other than penicillin G should be used. Physicians are cautioned not to use less than recommended doses.

Gonorrheal infections (uncomplicated)—Men or Women: Aqueous penicillin G procaine, 4.8 million units intramuscularly, divided into at least two doses and injected at different sites at one visit, together with 1 gram of oral probenecid, preferably given just before the injection.

NOTE: Treatment of severe complications of gonorrhea should be individualized, using large amounts of short-acting penicillin. Gonorrheal endocarditis should be treated intensively with aqueous penicillin G. Prophylactic or epidemiologic treatment for gonorrhea (male and female) is accomplished with the same treatment schedules as for the uncomplicated gonorrhea.

Retreatment

The National Center for Disease Control, Venereal Disease Branch, U.S. Department of Health, Education and Welfare, Atlanta, Georgia, recommends:

Test of cure procedures at approximately 7-14 days after therapy. In the male, a gram-stained smear is adequate if positive; otherwise, a culture specimen should be obtained from the anterior urethra. In the female, culture specimens should be obtained from both the endocervical and anal canal sites.

Retreatment in the male is indicated if the urethral discharge persists for three or more days following initial therapy and the smear or culture remains positive. Follow-up treatment consists of 4,800,000 units of aqueous penicillin G procaine intramuscularly, divided in two injection sites at a single visit.

In uncomplicated gonorrhea in the female, retreatment is indicated if follow-up cervical or rectal cultures remain positive for *N. gonorrhoeae.* Follow-up treatment consists of 4,800,000 units of aqueous penicillin G procaine daily on two successive days.

Syphilis: All gonorrhea patients should have a serologic test for syphilis at the time of diagnosis. Patients with gonorrhea who also have syphilis should be given additional treatment appropriate to the stage of syphilis.

Diphtheria—adjunctive therapy with antitoxin: 300,000-600,000 units daily.

Diphtheria carrier state: 300,000 units daily for 10 days.

Anthrax-cutaneous: 600,000-1,000,000 units/day.

Vincent's infection (fusospirochetosis): 600,000-1,000,000 units/day.

Erysipeloid: 600,000-1,000,000 units/day.

Streptobacillus moniliformis and Spirillum minus (rat bite fever): 600,000-1,000,000 units/-day.

How Supplied: *300,000 units per ml.*—1 ml. TUBEX® sterile cartridge-needle unit, packages of 10, vials of 10 ml.; *600,000 units per ml.*—1 ml. TUBEX sterile cartridge-needle unit, packages of 10 and 50; *1,200,000 units in 2 ml.* TUBEX, packages of 10; *2,400,000 units in 4 ml.* single-dose disposable syringe, packages of 10.

WYCILLIN® and PROBENECID ℞

(sterile penicillin G procaine suspension and probenecid tablets)

Description: The Wycillin disposable syringe is designed to provide a stable aqueous suspension of sterile penicillin G procaine,

ready for immediate use. This eliminates the necessity for addition of any diluent, required for the usual dry formulation of injectable penicillin.
Each syringe, 2,400,000 units (4 ml size), contains penicillin G procaine in a stabilized aqueous suspension with sodium citrate buffer; and as w/v, approximately 0.5% lecithin, 0.5% carboxymethylcellulose, 0.5% povidone, 0.1% methylparaben, and 0.01% propylparaben.
Wycillin must be stored in a refrigerator. Keep from freezing. This will prevent deterioration and assure that no significant loss of potency occurs within the expiration date.
Probenecid is a uricosuric and renal tubular-blocking agent.
Actions: Penicillin G exerts a bactericidal action against penicillin-sensitive microorganisms during the stage of active multiplication. It acts through the inhibition of biosynthesis of cell-wall mucopeptide. It is not active against the penicillinase-producing bacteria, which include many strains of staphylococci. *Neisseria gonorrhoeae* are included among the various organisms which are sensitive to penicillin G. Penicillin G procaine is an equimolecular salt of procaine and penicillin G, administered intramuscularly as a suspension. It dissolves slowly at the site of injection, giving a plateau type of blood level at about 4 hours which falls slowly over a period of the next 15–20 hours. Approximately 60% to 90% of a dose of penicillin G is excreted in the urine within 24 to 36 hours.
Approximately 60% of penicillin G is bound to serum protein. The drug is distributed throughout the body tissues in widely varying amounts, with highest levels found in the kidneys and lesser amounts in the liver, skin, and intestines. Penicillin G penetrates into all other tissues to a lesser degree, with a very small level found in the cerebrospinal fluid. With normal kidney function the drug is excreted rapidly by tubular excretion. In neonates and young infants and in individuals with impaired kidney function, excretion is considerably delayed.
Probenecid inhibits the tubular reabsorption of urate, thus increasing the urinary excretion of uric acid and decreasing serum uric acid levels. It also inhibits the tubular excretion of penicillin and usually increases penicillin-plasma levels, regardless of the route by which the antibiotic is given. A 2-fold to 4-fold elevation has been demonstrated for various penicillins. Probenecid does not influence plasma concentrations of salicylates, nor the excretion of streptomycin, chloramphenicol, chlortetracycline, oxytetracycline, or neomycin.
Indications: Wycillin and Probenecid is indicated for the single-dose treatment of uncomplicated (without bacteremia) urethral, cervical, rectal, or pharyngeal infections caused by *Neisseria gonorrhoeae* (gonorrhea) in men and women.
Susceptibility studies should be performed when recurrent infections or resistant strains are encountered. Urethritis and the presence of gram-negative diplococci in urethral smears are strong presumptive evidence of gonorrhea. Culture or fluorescent antibody studies will confirm the diagnosis. Therapy may be instituted prior to obtaining results of susceptibility testing.
Contraindications: A history of a previous hypersensitivity reaction to any of the penicillins or to Probenecid is a contraindication.
Probenecid is not recommended in persons with known blood dyscrasias or uric acid kidney stones or during an acute attack of gout. It is not recommended in conjunction with penicillin G procaine suspension in the presence of known renal impairment.
Warnings: **PENICILLIN G PROCAINE: Serious and occasionally fatal hypersensitivity (anaphylactoid) reactions have been reported in patients on penicillin therapy. Serious anaphylactoid reactions require immediate emergency treatment with epinephrine. Oxygen and intravenous corticosteroids should also be administered as indicated. Although anaphylaxis is more frequent following parenteral therapy, it has occurred in patients on oral penicillins. These reactions are more apt to occur in individuals with a history of sensitivity to multiple allergens.**
There have been well-documented reports of individuals with a history of penicillin-hypersensitivity reactions who have experienced severe hypersensitivity reactions when treated with a cephalosporin. Before therapy with a penicillin, careful inquiry should be made concerning previous hypersensitivity reactions to penicillins, cephalosporins, and other allergens. If an allergic reaction occurs, the drug should be discontinued and the patient treated with the usual agents, e.g., pressor amines, antihistamines, and corticosteroids.
Immediate toxic reactions to procaine may occur in some individuals, particularly when a large single dose is administered in the treatment of gonorrhea (4.8 million units). These reactions may be manifested by mental disturbances, including anxiety, confusion, agitation, depression, weakness, seizures, hallucinations, combativeness, and expressed "fear of impending death". The reactions noted in carefully controlled studies occurred in approximately one in 500 patients treated for gonorrhea. Reactions are transient, lasting from 15–30 minutes.
PROBENECID: Exacerbation of gout following therapy with Probenecid may occur; in such cases colchicine therapy is advisable.
In patients on Probenecid, the use of salicylates in either small or large doses is not recommended because it antagonizes the uricosuric action of Probenecid. Patients on Probenecid who require a mild analgesic agent should receive acetaminophen rather than salicylates, even in small doses.
USAGE IN PREGNANCY: The safety of these drugs for use in pregnancy has not been established.
Precautions: PENICILLIN G PROCAINE: When treating gonococcal infections in which primary or secondary syphilis may be suspected, proper diagnostic procedures, including dark-field examinations, should be done. In all cases in which concomitant syphilis is suspected, monthly serological tests should be made for at least four months. Patients with gonorrhea, who also have syphilis, should be given additional appropriate parenteral-penicillin treatment.
Penicillin should be used with caution in individuals with histories of significant allergies and/or asthma. When administering Wycillin, care should be taken to avoid intravenous or intra-arterial administration, or injection into or near major peripheral nerves or blood vessels, since such injections may produce neurovascular damage.
A small percentage of patients are sensitive to procaine. If there is a history of sensitivity make the usual test: Inject intradermally 0.1 ml of a 1- to 2-percent procaine solution. Development of an erythema, wheal, flare, or eruption indicates procaine sensitivity. Sensitivity should be treated by the usual methods, including barbiturates, and procaine penicillin preparations should not be used. Antihistaminics appear beneficial in treatment of procaine reactions.
PROBENECID: Use Probenecid with caution in patients with a history of peptic ulcer. A reducing substance may appear in the urine of patients receiving Probenecid. Although this disappears with discontinuance of therapy, a false diagnosis of glycosuria may be made because of a false-positive Benedict's test.
Adverse Reactions: WYCILLIN®: Penicillin is a substance of low toxicity but does possess a significant index of sensitization. The following hypersensitivity reactions associated with use of penicillin have been reported: Skin rashes, ranging from maculopapular eruptions to exfoliative dermatitis; urticaria; serum sickness-like reactions, including chills, fever, edema, arthralgia, and prostration. Severe and often fatal anaphylaxis has been reported (see "Warnings"). As with other treatments for syphilis, the Jarisch-Herxheimer reaction has been reported.
Procaine toxicity manifestations have been reported (see "Warnings"). Although procaine hypersensitivity reactions have not been reported with this drug, there are patients who are sensitive to procaine (see "Precautions").
PROBENECID: The following are the principal adverse reactions which have been reported as associated with the use of Probenecid, generally with more prolonged or repeated administration: Hypersensitivity reactions (including anaphylaxis), nephrotic syndrome, hepatic necrosis, aplastic anemia; also other anemias, including hemolytic anemia related to genetic deficiency of glucose-6-phosphate dehydrogenase.
Dosage and Administration: Penicillin G procaine (aqueous) is for intramuscular injection only.
Administer by DEEP INTRAMUSCULAR INJECTION in the upper, outer quadrant of the buttock. When doses are repeated, vary the injection site. Before injecting the dose, aspirate to be sure needle bevel is not in a blood vessel.
The Wyeth disposable syringe for this product incorporates several new features that are designed to facilitate its use.
A single small indentation, or "dot", has been punched into the metal ring that surrounds the neck of the syringe near the base of the needle. It is important that this "dot" be placed in a position so that it can be easily visualized by the operator following the intramuscular insertion of the syringe needle. Once the needle has been inserted, aspiration should be carried out in accordance with good medical technic before the medication is injected.
During the process of aspiration the barrel of the syringe immediately proximal to the location of the "dot" should be closely observed by the operator, since this is the area in which blood that may have entered the needle is most likely to appear. If blood or any suspicious discoloration is apparent, the needle should be withdrawn without injecting any of the medication, the syringe and its contents discarded, and the process repeated using a new syringe at a different site.
Although some isolates of *Neisseria gonorrhoeae* have decreased susceptibility to penicillin, this inherent resistance is relative, not absolute, and penicillin in large doses remains the drug of choice for these strains. Strains producing penicillinase, however, are resistant to Penicillin G, and a drug other than penicillin G should be used.
GONORRHEAL INFECTIONS (UNCOMPLICATED) MEN OR WOMEN: Aqueous penicillin G procaine, 4.8 million units intramuscularly, divided into at least two doses and injected at different sites at one visit, together with 1 gram (2 tablets, 0.5 gram each) of Probenecid orally, given just before the injections. Physicians are cautioned to use no less than the recommended dosages.
NOTE: Treatment of severe complications of gonorrhea should be individualized using large amounts of short-acting penicillin. Gonorrheal endocarditis should be treated intensively with aqueous penicillin G. Prophylactic or epidemiologic treatment for gonorrhea (male and female) is accomplished with the same treatment schedules as for the uncomplicated gonorrhea.
RETREATMENT: The National Center for Disease Control, Venereal Disease Branch,

Continued on next page

Wyeth—Cont.

U.S. Department of Health, Education and Welfare, Atlanta, Georgia, recommends:
Test of cure procedures at approximately 7–14 days after therapy. In the male, a gram-stained smear is adequate if positive; otherwise, a culture specimen should be obtained from the anterior urethra. In the female, culture specimens should be obtained from both the endocervical and anal canal sites.
Retreatment in the male is indicated if the urethral discharge persists for three or more days following initial therapy and the smear or culture remains positive. Follow-up treatment consists of 4,800,000 units of aqueous penicillin G procaine, intramuscular, divided in two injection sites at a single visit.
In uncomplicated gonorrhea in the female, retreatment is indicated if follow-up cervical or rectal cultures remain positive for *N. gonorrhoeae*.
Follow-up treatment consists of 4,800,000 units of aqueous penicillin G procaine daily on two successive days.
Syphilis: All gonorrhea patients should have a serologic test for syphilis at the time of diagnosis. Patients with gonorrhea who also have syphilis should be given additional treatment appropriate to the stage of syphilis.
How Supplied: Supplied as a combination package containing two disposable syringes of Wycillin® (2,400,000 units each) and two tablets Probenecid (0.5 gram each).

WYDASE® ℞
(hyaluronidase)
INJECTION

Description: This product, a preparation of highly purified bovine testicular hyaluronidase, is available in two dosage forms, as follows: WYDASE LYOPHILIZED: Hyaluronidase, dehydrated in the frozen state under high vacuum, with lactose and thimerosal (mercury derivative).
Reconstitute with Sodium Chloride Injection, U.S.P., before use, usually in the proportion of one milliliter per 150 N.F. Units of Hyaluronidase (WYDASE LYOPHILIZED).
Each vial of 1500 N.F. units contains 13.3 mg. lactose and 0.1 mg. thimerosal (mercury derivative). Each vial of 150 N.F. units contains 2.66 mg. lactose and 0.02 mg. thimerosal (mercury derivative).
WYDASE SOLUTION (Stabilized): An injection solution ready for use, containing 150 N.F. units of hyaluronidase per milliliter with 8.5 mg. sodium chloride, 1 mg. edetate disodium, 0.4 mg. calcium chloride, sodium biphosphate buffer, and not more than 0.1 mg. thimerosal (mercury derivative).
The N.F. Hyaluronidase Unit is equivalent to the turbidity-reducing (TR) unit and the International Unit.
Action: The enzymatic action of hyaluronidase hydrolyzes hyaluronic acid, a viscous polysaccharide found in the interstices of the tissues, where it normally obstructs diffusion of invasive substances. Thus hyaluronidase promotes diffusion and consequently absorption of fluids in the tissues, and has the action of the spreading factor of Duran-Reynals. When no spreading factor is present, material injected subcutaneously spreads very slowly; but hyaluronidase causes rapid spreading, provided local interstitial pressure is adequate to furnish the necessary mechanical impulse. Such an impulse is normally initiated by injected solutions. The rate of diffusion is proportionate to the amount of enzyme, and the extent is proportionate to the volume of solution.
Intravenous administration of even 75,000 N.F. units (500 times the maximal therapeutic dose) of hyaluronidase in animals causes no significant change in blood pressure, respiration, body temperature, or kidney function, and no histological changes in the tissues. Results from an experimental study on the influence of hyaluronidase in bone repair supports the conclusion that this enzyme alone, in the usual clinical dosage, does not deter bone healing. Hyaluronidase has no effect on the spread of localized infection provided it is not injected into the infected area, and seems to have no deleterious effect on bacterial or viral infections. But when crude testicular extracts which contained tissue irritants as well as "spreading factor" were used, an increase in area and virulence of the infection was observed.
Indications: This drug is indicated as an adjuvant to increase the absorption and dispersion of other injected drugs, for hypodermoclysis, and as an adjunct in subcutaneous urography for improving resorption of radiopaque agents.
Contraindications: Do not inject hyaluronidase into acutely inflamed or cancerous areas.
Precautions: Discontinue hyaluronidase if sensitization occurs. Sensitivity to hyaluronidase occurs infrequently. A preliminary test for sensitivity should be conducted. The skin test is made by an intradermal injection of approximately 0.02 ml. of the solution. A positive reaction consists of a wheal with pseudopods appearing within five minutes and persisting for 20 to 30 minutes and accompanied by localized itching. Transient vasodilation at the site of the test, i.e., erythema, is not a positive reaction.
When epinephrine is injected along with hyaluronidase the usual precautions for the use of epinephrine in cardiovascular disease, thyroid disease, diabetes, digital nerve block, ischemia of the fingers and toes, etc., should be observed.
Dosage and Administration: WYDASE® (hyaluronidase) should be administered only as discussed below, since its effects relative to the absorption and dispersion of other drugs are not produced when it is administered intravenously.
ABSORPTION AND DISPERSION OF INJECTED DRUGS. Absorption and dispersion of other injected drugs may be enhanced by adding 150 units hyaluronidase to the menstruum containing the other medication.
HYPODERMOCLYSIS. Insert needle with aseptic precautions. With tip lying free and movable between skin and muscle, begin clysis; fluid should start in readily without pain or lump. Then inject Solution Wydase into rubber tubing close to needle. An alternate method is to inject Wydase under skin prior to clysis. 150 units will facilitate absorption of 1000 ml. or more of solution. As with all parenteral fluid therapy, observe effect closely, with same precautions for restoring fluid and electrolyte balance as in intravenous injections. The dose, the rate of injection, and the type of solution (saline, glucose, Ringer's, etc.) must be adjusted carefully to the individual patient. When solutions devoid of inorganic electrolytes are given by hypodermoclysis, hypovolemia may occur. This may be prevented by using solutions containing adequate amounts of inorganic electrolytes and/or controlling the volume and speed of administration.
Hyaluronidase may be added to small volumes of solution (up to 200 ml.), such as a small clysis for infants or solutions of drugs for subcutaneous injection. **For children less than 3 years old the volume of a single clysis should be limited to 200 ml.; and in premature infants or during the neonatal period, the daily dosage should not exceed 25 ml. per kilogram of body weight; the rate of administration should not be greater than 2 ml. per minute. For older patients the rate and volume of administration should not exceed those employed for intravenous infusion.**
SUBCUTANEOUS UROGRAPHY. The subcutaneous route of administration of urographic contrast media is indicated when intravenous administration cannot be successfully accomplished, particularly in infants and small children. With the patient prone, 75 units of Wydase® (hyaluronidase) Wyeth is injected subcutaneously over each scapula, followed by injection of the contrast medium at the same sites.
How Supplied:
WYDASE® LYOPHILIZED:
150 N.F. (TR) units, vials of 1 ml.;
1500 N.F. (TR) units, vials of 10 ml.
WYDASE® SOLUTION (Stabilized):
150 N.F. (TR) units per ml., vials of 1 ml. and 10 ml.

WYGESIC® Ⓒ ℞

Each tablet contains: 65 mg propoxyphene HCl and 650 mg acetaminophen.
Description: Propoxyphene hydrochloride is an odorless white crystalline powder with a bitter taste. It is freely soluble in water. Chemically, it is alpha-(+)-4-(Dimethylamino)-3-methyl-1,2-diphenyl-2-butanol Propionate Hydrochloride.
Acetaminophen is a white, crystalline powder, possessing a slightly bitter taste.
Actions: Propoxyphene hydrochloride is a mild analgesic structurally related to the narcotic analgesic, methadone; though propoxyphene's general pharmacologic properties are those of the narcotics as a group, it does not compare with them in analgesic potency.
In addition to propoxyphene hydrochloride these tablets contain the nonnarcotic antipyretic analgesic acetaminophen.
Indications: For the relief of mild-to-moderate pain.
Contraindication: Hypersensitivity to propoxyphene or to acetaminophen.
Warnings: CNS ADDITIVE EFFECTS AND OVERDOSAGE: Propoxyphene in combination with alcohol, tranquilizers, sedative-hypnotics, or other central-nervous-system depressants has an additive depressant effect. Patients taking this drug should be advised of the additive effect and warned not to exceed the dosage recommended by their physician. Toxic effects and fatalities have occurred following overdoses of propoxyphene alone or in combination with other central-nervous-system depressants. The majority of these patients have had histories of emotional disturbances or suicidal ideation or attempts, as well as histories of misuse of tranquilizers, alcohol, or other CNS-active drugs. Caution should be exercised in prescribing unnecessarily large amounts of propoxyphene for such patients (see **Management of Overdosage).**
DRUG DEPENDENCE: Propoxyphene can produce drug dependence characterized by psychic dependence and, less frequently, physical dependence and tolerance. Propoxyphene will only partially suppress the withdrawal syndrome in individuals physically dependent on morphine or other narcotics. The abuse liability of propoxyphene is qualitatively similar to that of codeine although quantitatively less, and propoxyphene should be prescribed with the same degree of caution appropriate to the use of codeine.
USAGE IN AMBULATORY PATIENTS: Propoxyphene may impair the mental and/or physical abilities required for the performance of potentially hazardous tasks such as driving a car or operating machinery. The patient should be cautioned accordingly.
USAGE IN PREGNANCY: Safe use in pregnancy has not been established relative to possible adverse effects on fetal development. INSTANCES OF WITHDRAWAL SYMPTOMS IN THE NEONATE HAVE BEEN REPORTED FOLLOWING USAGE DURING PREGNANCY.
Therefore, propoxphene should not be used in pregnant women unless, in the judgment of the physician, the potential benefits outweigh the possible hazards.

USAGE IN CHILDREN: Propoxyphene is not recommended for use in children because documented clinical experience has been insufficient to establish safety and a suitable dosage regimen in the pediatric age group.
Precautions: Confusion, anxiety, and tremors have been reported in a few patients receiving propoxyphene concomitantly with orphenadrine.
The central-nervous-system depressant effect of propoxyphene may be additive with that of other CNS depressants, including alcohol.
Adverse Reactions: The most frequent adverse reactions are dizziness, sedation, nausea, and vomiting. These effects seem to be more prominent in ambulatory than in nonambulatory patients, and some of these adverse reactions may be alleviated if the patient lies down. Other adverse reactions include constipation, abdominal pain, skin rashes, light-headedness, headache, weakness, euphoria, dysphoria, and minor visual disturbances.
The chronic ingestion of propoxyphene in doses exceeding 800 mg per day has caused toxic psychoses and convulsions.
Cases of liver dysfunction have been reported.
Dosage and Administration: Propoxyphene hydrochloride and acetaminophen tablets are given orally. The usual dosage is one tablet, which contains 65 mg propoxyphene hydrochloride and 650 mg acetaminophen, every 4 hours as needed for pain.
Drug Interactions: Propoxyphene in combination with alcohol, tranquilizers, sedative-hypnotics, and other central-nervous-system depressants has an additive depressant effect. Patients taking this drug should be advised of the additive effect and warned not to exceed the dosage recommended by their physician (see **Warnings**).
Confusion, anxiety, and tremors have been reported in a few patients receiving propoxyphene concomitantly with orphenadrine.
Management of Overdosage: SYMPTOMS: The manifestations of serious overdosage with propoxyphene are similar to those of narcotic overdosage and include respiratory depression (a decrease in respiratory rate and/or tidal volume, Cheyne-Stokes respiration, cyanosis), extreme somnolence progressing to stupor or coma, pupillary constriction, and circulatory collapse. In addition to these characteristics, which are reversed by treatment with narcotic antagonists such as naloxone, there may be other effects. Overdoses of propoxyphene can cause delay of cardiac conduction as well as focal or generalized convulsions, which constitute a prominent feature in most cases of severe poisoning. Cardiac arrhythmias and pulmonary edema have occasionally been reported, and apnea, cardiac arrest, and death have occurred.
Symptoms of massive overdosage with acetaminophen may include nausea, vomiting, anorexia, and abdominal pain, beginning shortly after ingestion and lasting for a period of 12 to 24 hours. However, early recognition may be difficult since early symptoms may be mild and nonspecific. Evidence of liver damage is usually delayed. After the initial symptoms, the patient may feel less ill; however, laboratory determinations are likely to show a rapid rise in liver enzymes and bilirubin. In case of serious hepatotoxicity, jaundice, coagulation defects, hypoglycemia, encephalopathy, coma, and death may follow. Renal failure due to tubular necrosis, and myocardiopathy, have also been reported.
Ingestion of 10 grams or more of acetaminophen may produce hepatotoxicity. A 13-gram dose has reportedly been fatal.
TREATMENT: Primary attention should be given to the reestablishment of adequate respiratory exchange through provision of a patent airway and institution of assisted or controlled ventilation. The narcotic antagonists, naloxone, nalorphine, and levallorphan, are specific antidotes against the respiratory depression produced by propoxyphene. An appropriate dose of one of these antagonists should be administered, preferably by the intravenous route, simultaneously with efforts at respiratory resuscitation, and the antagonist should be repeated as necessary until the patient's condition remains satisfactory. In addition to the use of a narcotic antagonist, the patient may require careful titration with an anticonvulsant to control seizures. Analeptic drugs (for example, caffeine or amphetamine) should not be used because of their tendency to precipitate convulsions.
Oxygen, intravenous fluids, vasopressors, and other supportive measures should be employed as indicated.
Gastric lavage may be helpful. Activated charcoal can absorb a significant amount of ingested propoxyphene. Dialysis is of little value in poisoning by propoxyphene alone.
Acetaminophen is rapidly absorbed, and efforts to remove the drug from the body should not be delayed. Copious gastric lavage and/or induction of emesis may be indicated. Activated charcoal is probably ineffective unless administered almost immediately after acetaminophen ingestion.
Neither forced diuresis nor hemodialysis appear to be effective in removing acetaminophen. Since acetaminophen in overdose may have an antidiuretic effect and may produce renal damage, administration of fluids should be carefully monitored to avoid overload.
It has been reported that mercaptamine (cysteamine) or other thiol compounds may protect against liver damage if given soon after overdosage (8-10 hours). N-acetyl-cysteine is under investigation as a less toxic alternative to mercaptamine, which may cause anorexia, nausea, vomiting, and drowsiness. Appropriate literature should be consulted for further information. (JAMA *237:*2406-2407, 1977.)
Clinical and laboratory evidence of hepatotoxicity may be delayed up to one week. Acetaminophen plasma levels and half-life may be useful in assessing the likelihood of hepatotoxicity. Serial hepatic enzyme determinations are also recommended.
How Supplied: Wygesic® tablets, containing 65 mg propoxyphene hydrochloride and 650 mg acetaminophen per scored tablet, are supplied in bottles of 100 and 500 tablets and in Redipak® Strip Pack, Wyeth, boxes of 100 (10 strips of 10).
[*Shown in Product Identification Section*]

WYMOX® ℞
(amoxicillin)
Capsules and Oral Suspension

How Supplied: Capsules contain 250 mg or 500 mg amoxicillin as the trihydrate, and are supplied in bottles of 100 for the 250 mg capsules and bottles of 50 for the 500 mg capsules. WYMOX Oral Suspension is supplied in bottles of powder for reconstitution. When reconstituted with water, it will make a palatable suspension containing amoxicillin trihydrate equivalent to 125 mg or 250 mg amoxicillin per 5 ml.
For prescribing information write to Professional Service, Wyeth Laboratories, Box 8299, Philadelphia, PA, 19101, or contact your local Wyeth representative.
[*Shown in Product Identification System*]

Directory of Poison Control Centers

The Directory of Poison Control Centers has been compiled from information furnished by the National Clearinghouse for Poison Control Centers, Bureau of Drugs, 5600 Fishers Lane, Rockville, Md. 20857.

It includes those facilities which provide for the medical profession, on a 24-hour basis, information concerning the prevention and treatment of accidents involving ingestion of poisonous and potentially poisonous substances. Unless otherwise noted, address inquiries to: Poison Control Center

ALABAMA

STATE COORDINATOR
Department of Public Health 832-3914
Montgomery 36117

Anniston
N.E. Alabama Regional Medical Center 237-5421 Ext. 307
400 E. 10th St. 36201

Auburn
Auburn University 826-4037
School of Pharmacy 36830

Birmingham
Children's Hospital 933-4000
1601 6th Ave., S. 35233

Dothan
Southeast Alabama General Hospital 36301 794-3131

Florence
Eliza Coffee Memorial Hospital 767-1111
P.O. Box 1079 Ext. 2045
600 W. Alabama St. 35630 Ext. 2045, 2046

Gadsden
Baptist Memorial Hospital 492-8111
1007 Goodyear Avenue 35903

Huntsville
Huntsville Hospital 539-6320
101 Sivley Road 35801

Mobile
University of So. Alabama Medical Center 473-3325
2451 Fillingim St. 36617

Opelika
Lee County Hospital 749-3411
2000 Pepperill Parkway 36801

Tuskegee
John A. Andrew Hospital 727-8583
Tuskegee Institute 36088

ALASKA

STATE COORDINATOR for Administration
Department of Health & Social Services 465-3100
Juneau 99811

Anchorage
Providence Hospital 274-6535
3200 Providence Dr. 99504

ARIZONA

STATE COORDINATOR
College of Pharmacy 882-6300
University of Arizona
Tucson 85721

Douglas
Cochise County Hospital 364-7931
Rural Route #1 85607

Flagstaff
Flagstaff Hospital 744-5233
1215 N. Beaver St. 86001 Ext. 255

Ganado
Navajo Health Foundation 755-3411
Sage Memorial Hospital
Box 457 86505

Kingman
Mohave General Hospital 757-2101
3269 Stockton Hill Rd. 86401 Ext. 247

Nogales
St. Joseph's Hospital 287-2771
Target Range Road Ext. 200
P.O. Box 1809 85621

Phoenix
Good Samaritan Hospital 257-4545
1033 E. McDowell Rd. 85006

Maricopa County General Hospital 267-5011
2601 E. Roosevelt 85008 Ext. 5411

Memorial Hospital 252-5911
1201 S. 7th Ave. 85007 Ext. 391

St. Joseph's Hospital 277-6611
350 W. Thomas Rd. 85013 Ext. 3581

St. Luke's Hospital Medical Center 253-3334
525 N. 18th St. 85006

Prescott
Yavapai Community Hospital 445-2700
1003 Willow Creek Rd. 86301 Ext. 25, 28

Tucson
Kino Community Hospital 624-2721
(Pima County General) Ext. 220
2800 E. Ajo Way 85713

St. Mary's Hospital 622-5833
1601 W. St. Mary's Rd. 85703 Ext. 724

Tucson General Hospital 327-5431
3838 N. Campbell Ave. 85719 Ext. 111

Tucson Medical Center 327-5461
E. Grant Rd. and Ext. 428
Beverly Blvd. 85716

Arizona Hlth. Sciences Ctr. 626-6016
University of Arizona 85721

Winslow
Winslow Memorial Hospital 289-4691
1500 Williamson Ave. 86047

Yuma
Yuma Regional Med. Center 344-2000
Avenue A and 24th St. 85364 Ext. 321

ARKANSAS

STATE COORDINATOR
Department of Health 661-2397
Little Rock 72201

El Dorado
Warner Brown Hospital 863-2266
460 West Oak St. 71730

Fort Smith
St. Edward's Mercy Medical Center 452-5100
7301 Rogers Avenue 72903 Ext. 2043

Sparks Regional Med. Center 441-5011
1311 S. Eye St. 72901

Harrison
Boone County Hospital 741-6141
620 N. Willow St. 72601 Ext. 275, 276

Helena
Helena Hospital 338-6411
Hospital Drive 72342 Ext. 340

Little Rock
Univ. of Arkansas Medical Center 661-6161
4301 W. Markham St. 72201

Osceola
Osceola Memorial Hospital 563-7180
611 Lee Ave. West 72370

Pine Bluff
Jefferson Hospital 535-6800
1515 W. 42nd Ave. 71601 Ext. 4706

CALIFORNIA

STATE COORDINATOR
Department of Health Services 322-2300
Sacramento 95814

Fresno
Fresno Community Hospital 442-6000
Fresno & R Sts. Ext. 3131
P.O. Box 1232 93715

Los Angeles
Thos. J. Fleming Memorial Ctr. 664-2121
Children's Hosp. of Los Angeles 669-2401
P.O. Box 54700
4650 Sunset Blvd. 90054

Oakland
Alameda-Contra Costa Medical Association 652-8171
6230 Claremont Ave. 94619

Children's Hosp. Medical Center 547-2928
51st & Grove St. 94609

Orange
University of California 634-5988
Irvine Medical Center
101 City Drive South 92668

Sacramento
Emergency Medical Services 453-3692
Sacramento Medical Center
Univ. of California, Davis
2315 Stockton Blvd. 95817

San Diego
University of California 294-6000
San Diego Medical Center
225 W. Dickinson St. 92103

San Francisco
San Francisco Bay Area Poison Center 666-2845
San Francisco General Hosp.
1001 Potrero Ave. Room 1E-6 94110

San Jose
Santa Clara Valley Medical Center 279-5112
751 S. Bascom Ave., 95128

CANAL ZONE

Balboa Heights
Gorgas Hospital 52-7500
Box O

COLORADO

STATE COORDINATOR
Department of Health; EMS Div. 320-8476
Denver 80220
Denver
Rocky Mountain Poison Center 629-1123
Denver General Hospital
W. 8th Ave. & Cherokee St.
80204

CONNECTICUT

STATE COORDINATOR
University of Connecticut 674-2782
Health Center
Farmington 06032
Bridgeport
Bridgeport Hospital 384-3566
267 Grant St. 06602
St. Vincent's Hospital 576-5178
2820 Main St. 06606
Danbury
Danbury Hospital 797-7300
95 Locust Ave. 06810
Farmington
University of Connecticut 674-2782
Health Center 06032
Middletown
Middlesex Memorial Hospital 347-9471
28 Crescent St. 06457
New Haven
The Hosp. of St. Raphael 789-3464
1450 Chapel St. 06511
Yale-New Haven Hospital 436-1960
789 Howard Ave. 06504
Norwalk
Norwalk Hospital 852-2160
24 Stevens St. 06852
Waterbury
St. Mary's Hospital 574-6011
56 Franklin St. 06702

DELAWARE

Wilmington
Poison Information Service 655-3389
501 W. 14th St. 19899

DISTRICT OF COLUMBIA

STATE COORDINATOR
Department of Human Resources 673-6694
Washington, D.C. 20009
Washington, D.C.
Children's Hospital National 745-2000
Medical Center
111 Michigan Ave., N.W. 20010

FLORIDA

STATE COORDINATOR
Department of Health and 487-1566
Rehabilitative Services
Tallahassee 32301
Apalachicola
George E. Weems Memorial 653-8853
Hospital P.O. Box 610
Franklin Square 32320
Bartow
PolkG eneral Hospital 533-1111
2010 E. Georgia St. Ext. 204-237
P.O. Box 81 33830
Bradenton
Manatee Memorial Hospital 746-5111
206 2nd St. E. 33505 Ext. 466
Daytona Beach
Halifax Hospital Med. Ctr. 258-1515
Clyde Morris Blvd.
P.O. Box 1990 32014
Ft. Lauderdale
Broward General Medical Center 463-3131
1600 S. Andrews Ave. 33316 Ext. 1511
Fort Myers
Lee Memorial Hospital 332-1111
2776 Cleveland Ave.
P.O. Drawer 2218 33902
Ft. Walton Beach
General Hospital of 242-1111
Ft. Walton Beach Ext. 106
1000 Mar-Walt Drive 32548
Gainesville
Shands Teaching Hosp. 392-3746
and Clinics
University of Florida 33610
Jacksonville
St. Vincent's Medical Center 389-7751
Barrs St. & St. Johns Ave. 32204 Ext. 8315
Key West
Florida Keys Mem. Hospital 294-5531
600 Junior College Rd.
Stock Island 33040
Lakeland
Lakeland General Hospital 686-4913
Lakeland Hills Blvd.
P.O. Box 480 33802
Leesburg
Leesburg General Hospital 787-7222
600 E. Dixie 32748 Ext.381
Melbourne
James E. Holmes Regional 727-7000
Medical Center Ext. 675
1350 S. Hickory St. 32901
Miami
Jackson Memorial Hospital 325-6799
Attn: Pharmacy
1611 N.W. 12th Ave. 33136
Naples
Naples Community Hospital 262-3131
350 7th St. N. 33940 Ext. 2221
Ocala
Munroe Memorial Hospital 732-1111
140 S.E. Orange St. 32670 Ext. 15
Orlando
Orlando Reg. Med. Ctr. 841-5222
Orange Memorial Hospital
1416 S. Orange Ave. 32806
Panama City
Bay Memorial Med. Ctr. 769-1511
600 N. MacArthur Ave. 32401 Ext. 415-416
Pensacola
Baptist Hospital 434-4811
1000 W. Moreno St. 32501
Punta Gorda
Medical Center 639-3131
809 E. Marion Ave. 33950
Rockledge
Wuesthoff Memorial Hospital 636-2211
110 Longwood Ave. 32955 Ext. 108
St. Petersburg
Bayfront Medical Center, Inc. 821-5858
701 6th St., S. 33701
Sarasota
Memorial Hospital 953-1332
1901 Arlington Ave. 33579
Tallahassee
Tallahassee Mem. Regional 599-5100
Medical Center
Magnolia Drive and
Miccouskee 32304
Tampa
Tampa General Hospital 251-6995
Davis Islands 33606
Titusville
Jess Parrish Mem. Hospital 269-1100
951 N. Washington Ave. 32780 Ext. 194
West Palm Beach
Good Samaritan Hospital 655-5511
Flagler Dr. at Ext. 4250
Palm Beach Lakes Blvd. 33402
Winter Haven
Winter Haven Hospital, Inc. 299-9701
200 Avenue F., N.E. 33880

GEORGIA

STATE COORDINATOR
Department of Human Resources 894-5068
Atlanta 30308
Albany
Phoebe Putney Memorial Hosp. 883-1800
417 Third Avenue 31705 Ext. 158
Athens
Athens General Hospital 549-9977
797 Cobb St. 30601 Ext. 446
Atlanta
Grady Memorial Hospital 588-4400
80 Butler St., S.E. 30303
Augusta
University Hospital 722-9011
1350 Walton Way 30902 Ext. 2440
Columbus
The Medical Center 324-4711
710 Center Street 31902 Ext. 6431
Macon
Medical Center of Central Georgia 742-1122
777 Hemlock St. 31201 Ext. 3144
Rome
Floyd Hospital 232-1541
P.O. Box 233 30161 Ext. 747
Savannah
Memorial Medical Center 355-5228
P.O. Box 23089 31403
Thomasville
John D. Archbold 226-4121
Memorial Hospital Ext. 169
900 Gordon Ave. 31792
Valdosta
S. Georgia Medical Center 242-3450
P.O. Box 1727 31601 Ext. 717
Waycross
Memorial Hospital 283-3030
410 Darling Ave. 31501 Ext. 170

GUAM

STATE COORDINATOR
Guam Memorial Hospital 646-5801
P.O. Box AX
Agana 96910
Agana
Pharmacy Service, Box 7696 344-9265
U.S. Naval Regional Medical 344-9354
Center (GUAM)
FPO San Francisco, CA 96630

HAWAII

STATE COORDINATOR
Department of Health 531-7776
Honolulu 96801
Honolulu
Kapiolani-Childrens Medical Center 941-4411
1319 Punahou St. 96826
Emergency 911

IDAHO

STATE COORDINATOR
Department of Health and Welfare 384-2125
Boise 83701
Boise
St. Alphonsus Hospital 376-1211
1055 N. Curtis Rd. 83704 Ext. 707
Idaho Falls
Idaho Falls Hospital 522-3620
Emergency Department Ext. 208
900 Memorial Dr. 83401
Pocatello
St. Anthony Hospital 232-2733
650 North 7th St. 83201 Ext. 244

ILLINOIS

STATE COORDINATOR	
Division of Emergency Medical Services and Highway Safety, Springfield 62761	785-2080
Chicago	
Rush-Presbyterian-St. Lukes Medical Center, 1753 W. Congress Parkway 60612	942-5969
Peoria	
St. Francis Hospital & Medical Center, 530 N.E. Glen Oak Avenue 61637	1-800 322-5330
Springfield	
St. John's Hospital, 800 East Carpenter 62702	753-3330

INDIANA

STATE COORDINATOR	
State Board of Health, Indianapolis 46206	633-0332
Anderson	
Community Hospital, 1515 N. Madison Ave. 46012	646-5198
St. John's Hickey Memorial Hospital, 2015 Jackson St. 46014	646-8251
Angola	
Cameron Memorial Hospital, 416 East Maumee St. 46703	665-2141 Ext. 42; 665-2166
Columbus	
Bartholomew County Hosp., 2400 East 17th St., 47201	376-5277
Crown Point	
St. Anthony Medical Ctr., Main at Franciscan Rd. 46307	738-2100
East Chicago	
St. Catherine Hospital, 4321 Fir Street 46312	392-1700; 392-7203
Elkhart	
Elkhart General Hospital, 600 East Blvd. 46514	294-2621
Evansville	
Deaconess Hospital, 600 Mary St. 47710	426-3405
St. Mary's Hospital, 3700 Washington Ave. 47715	477-6261
Welborn Memorial Baptist Hospital, 401 S.E. 6th St. 47713	426-8000
Fort Wayne	
Lutheran Hospital Emergency Dept., 3024 Fairfield Ave. 46807	458-2211
Parkview Memorial Hospital, 220 Randalia Dr. 46805	484-6636 Ext. 7800
St. Joseph's Hospital, 700 Boradway 46802	423-2614
Frankfort	
Clinton County Hospital, 1300 S. Jackson St. 46041	654-4451
Gary	
Methodist Hospital of Gary, Inc., 600 Grant St. 46402	886-4710
Goshen	
Goshen General Hospital, 200 High Park Ave. 46526	533-2141 Ext. 462
Hammond	
St. Margaret Hospital, 25 Douglas St. 46320	932-2300 Ext. 700
Huntington	
Huntington Memorial Hospital, 1215 Etna Ave. 46750	356-3000
Indianapolis	
Methodist Hospital of Indiana, Inc., 1604 N. Capitol Ave. 46202	927-3033
Wishard Memorial Hospital, 1001 West 10th St. 46202	630-7351
Kendallville	
McCray Memorial Hospital, Hospital Drive 46755	347-1100
Kokomo	
Howard Community Hospital, 3500 S. LaFountain St. 46901	453-0702 Ext. 444
Lafayette	
Lafayette Home Hospital, 2400 South Street 47902	447-6811
St. Elizabeth Hospital, 1501 Hartfort St. 47904	423-6271
LaGrange	
LaGrange County Hospital, Route #1 46761	463-2144
LaPorte	
LaPorte Hospital, Inc., 1007 Lincolnway 46350	362-7541 Ext. 212
Lebanon	
Witham Memorial Hospital, 1124 N. Lebanon St. 46052	482-2700 Ext. 44
Madison	
King's Daughter's Hospital, 112 Presbyterian Ave., P.O. Box 447 47250	265-5211 Ext. 14
Marion	
Marion General Hospital, Wabash & Euclid Ave. 46952	662-4694
Mishawaka	
St. Joseph's Hospital, 215 W. 4th St. 46544	259-2431
Muncie	
Ball Memorial Hospital, 2401 University Ave. 47303	747-3241
Portland	
Jay County Hospital, 505 W. Arch St. 47371	726-7131 Ext. 159
Richmond	
Reid Memorial Hospital, 1401 Chester Blvd. 47374	692-7010 Ext. 622
Shelbyville	
Wm. S. Major Hospital, 150 W. Washington St. 46176	392-3211 Ext. 52
South Bend	
St. Joseph's Hospital, 811 E. Madison St. 46622	234-2151 Ext. 253; Ext. 264
Terre Haute	
Union Hospital, Inc., 1606 N. 7th St. 47804	238-7000 Ext. 7523
Valparaiso	
Porter Memorial Hosp., 814 LaPorte Ave. 46383	464-8611 Ext. 232, 312, 334
Vincennes	
The Good Samaritan Hospital, 520 S. 7th St. 47591	885-3348

IOWA

STATE COORDINATOR	
Department of Health, Des Moines 50319	281-4964
Des Moines	
Iowa Methodist Hospital, 1200 Pleasant St. 50308	283-6212
Dubuque	
Mercy Medical Center, Mercy Drive 52001	588-8210
Fort Dodge	
Trinity Regional Hospital, Dept. of Pharmacy, Kenyon Rd. 50501	573-3101
Iowa City	
Univ. of Iowa Hospital and Clinics, Pharmacy Department 52240	356-2922
Waterloo	
Allen Memorial Hospital, 1825 Logan Avenue 50703	235-3893

KANSAS

STATE COORDINATOR	
Department of Health & Environment, Topeka 66620	862-9360 Ext. 542
Atchison	
Atchison Hospital, 1301 N. 2nd St. 66002	367-2131
Dodge City	
Dodge City Reg. Hosp., PO Box 1478, Ross & Ave. "A" 67801	225-2036
Emporia	
Newman Memorial Hospital, 12th & Chestnut Sts. 66801	343-6800 Ext. 545
Fort Riley	
Irwin Army Hospital 66442	239-2323
Fort Scott	
Mercy Hospital, 821 Burke St. 66701	223-2200; Night: 223-0476
Great Bend	
Central Kansas Medical Center, 3515 Broadway 67530	793-3523; Night: 792-2511
Hays	
Hadley Regional Medical Center, 201 E. 7th St. 67601	628-8251
Kansas City	
University of Kansas Medical Center, 39th & Rainbow Blvd. 66103	588-6633
Bethany Medical Center, 51 N. 12th St. 66102	281-8880
Lawrence	
Lawrence Memorial Hospital, 325 Main St. 66044	843-3680 Ext. 162, 163
Parsons	
Labette County Medical Center, S. 21st St. 67357	421-4880 Ext. 320
Salina	
St. John's Hospital, 139 N. Penn St. 67401	827-5591 Ext. 112
Topeka	
Stormont-Vail Hospital, 10th & Washburn Sts. 66606	354-6100
Wichita	
Wesley Medical Center, 550 N. Hillside Ave. 67214	685-2151 Ext. 7515

KENTUCKY

STATE COORDINATOR	
Department For Human Resources, Frankfort 40601	564-4935
Ashland	
King's Daughters Hospital, 2201 Lexington Ave. 41101	324-2222
Berea	
Porter Moore Drug, Inc., 124 Main St. 40403	986-3061
Fort Thomas	
St. Lukes Hospital, 85 N. Grand Ave. 41075	292-3215
Lexington	
Central Baptist Hospital, 1740 S. Limestone St. 40503	278-3411 Ext. 152
Drug Information Center, University of Kentucky Medical Center 40536	233-5320
Louisville	
Norton-Children's Hospital, Pharmacy Dept., 200 E. Chestnut St. 40202	589-8222
Murray	
Murray-Calloway County Hospital, 803 Popular 42071	753-7588

Owensboro
Owensboro-Daviess County Hospital — 926-3030 Ext. 180
811 Hospital Court 42301 — Night: Ext. 174
Paducah
Western Baptist Hospital — 444-6361
2501 Kentucky Ave. 42001 — Ext. 105, Night: Ext. 199
Prestonsburg
Poison Control Center — 886-8511
Highland Reg. Med. Ctr 41653

LOUISIANA

STATE COORDINATOR
Emergency Medical Services of Louisiana — 342-2600
Baton Rouge 70801
Alexandria
Rapides General Hospital — 487-8111
Emergency Dept.
P.O. Box 7146 71301
Baton Rouge
Doctors Hospital — 927-9050
2414 Bunker Hill Dr. 70808
Lafayette
Our Lady of Lourdes Hosp. — 234-7381
611 St. Landry St. 70501
Lake Charles
Lake Charles Memorial Hosp. — 478-6800
P.O. Drawer M 70601
Monroe
Northeast University — 342-3008
Department of Pharmacology
700 University Ave. 70201
St. Francis Hospital — 325-6454
P.O. Box 1901 71301
New Orleans
Charity Hospital — 568-5222
1532 Tulane Ave. 71040
Shreveport
LSU Medical Center — 425-1524
P.O. Box 33932 71130

MAINE

STATE COORDINATOR
Maine Poison Control Center — 1-800 442-6305
Portland 04102
Portland
Maine Medical Center — 871-2950
Emergency Division
22 Bramhall St. 04102

MARYLAND

STATE COORDINATOR
Maryland Poison Information Center — 528-7604
University of Maryland School of Pharmacy
Baltimore 21201
Baltimore
Maryland Poison Information Center
University of Maryland School of Pharmacy — 528-7701
636 W. Lombard St. 21201
Cumberland
Sacred Heart Hospital — 722-6677
900 Seton Drive 21502

MASSACHUSETTS

STATE COORDINATOR
Department of Public Health — 727-2670
Boston 02111
Boston
Massachusetts Poison Control System — 232-2120
300 Longwood Ave. 02115

MICHIGAN

STATE COORDINATOR
Division of Emergency Medical Services — 373-1406
Lansing 48909
Adrian
Emma L. Bixby Hospital — 263-2412
818 Riverside Ave. 49221
Ann Arbor
University Hospital — 764-5102
1405 E. Ann St. 48104
Battle Creek
Community Hospital — 963-5521
183 West St. 49016
Bay City
Bay Medical Center — 892-6589
100 15th St. 48706
Berrien Center
Berrien General Hospital — 471-7761
Dean's Hill Rd. 49102
Coldwater
Community Health Center of Branch County — 278-7361
274 E. Chicago St. 49036
Detroit
Children's Hospital of Michigan — 494-5711
3901 Beaubien 48201
Mount Carmel Mercy Hosp. — 864-5400
6071 W. Outer Dr. 48235 — Ext. 416
Eloise
Wayne County General — Day: 722-3748
30712 Michigan Ave. 48132 — Night: 274-3000
Flint
Hurley Hospital — 766-0111
6th Ave. & Begole 48502
Grand Rapids
St. Mary's Hospital — 774-6794
201 Lafayette, S.E. 49503
Western Michigan Poison Center — 442-4571, 632-2727
1840 Wealthy, S.E. 49506
Hancock
Portage View Hospital — 482-1122
200-210 Michigan Ave. 49930 — Ext. 209
Holland
Holland Community Hospital — 396-4661
602 Michigan Ave. 49423
Jackson
W.A. Foote Memorial Hosp. — 788-4816
205 N. East St. 49201
Kalamazoo
Borgess Hospital — 383-4815
Ambulatory Care Svc.
1521 Gull Rd. 49001
Bronson Methodist Hospital — 383-6409
252 E. Lovell St. 49006
Lansing
St. Lawrence Hospital — 372-5112
1210 W. Saginaw St. 48914 — 372-5113
Marquette
Marquette General Hospital — 562-9723
420 Magnetic Dr. 49855
Midland
Midland Hospital — 631-7700
4005 Orchard 48640 — Ext. 304
Petoskey
Little Traverse Hospital — 347-7373
416 Connable 49770
Pontiac
St. Joseph Mercy Hospital — 858-7373
900 Woodward Ave. 48053 — 858-7374
Port Huron
Port Huron Hospital — 987-5555
1001 Kearney St. 48060 — 987-5000
Saginaw
Saginaw General Hospital — 755-1111
1447 N. Harrison 48602
Traverse City
Munson Medical Center — 947-6140
Sixth St. 49684

MINNESOTA

STATE COORDINATOR
State Department of Health — 296-5276
Minneapolis 55415
Bemidji
Bemidji Hospital 56601 — 751-5430
Brainerd
St. Joseph's Hospital 56401 — 829-2861 Ext. 211
Crookston
Riverview Hospital — 281-4682
320 S. Hubbard 56716
Duluth
St. Luke's Hospital — 727-6636
Emergency Department
915 E. First St. 55805
St. Mary's Hospital — 727-4551
407 E. 3rd St. 55805 — Ext. 359
Edina
Fairview-Southdale Hospital — 920-4400
6401 France Ave., S. 55435
Fergus Falls
Lake Region Hospital 56537 — 736-5475
Fridley
Unity Hospital — 786-2200
550 Osborne Rd. 55432
Mankato
Immanual - St. Joseph's Hospital — 387-4031
325 Garden Blvd. 56001
Marshall
Louis Weiner Memorial Hospital 56258 — 532-9661
Minneapolis
Fairview Hospital — 371-6402
Outpatient Department
2312 S. 6th St. 55406
Hennepin County Medical Center — 347-3141
701 Park Ave. 55415
North Memorial Hospital — 588-0616
3220 Lowry North 55422
Northwestern Hospital — 874-4233
810 E. 27th St. 55407
Morris
Stevens County Memorial Hospital 56267 — 589-1313
Rochester
St. Mary's Hospital — 285-5123
1216 Second St., S.W. 55901
St. Cloud
St. Cloud Hospital — 251-2700
1406 6th Avenue, N. 56301 — Ext. 221
St. Paul
Bethesda Lutheran Hospital — 221-2301
559 Capitol Blvd. 55103
The Children's Hospital, Inc. — 227-6521
311 Pleasant Ave. 55102
St. John's Hospital — 228-3132
403 Maria Ave. 55106
St. Joseph's Hospital — 291-3348
69 W. Exchange 55102 — 291-3139
United Hospitals, Inc. — 298-8402
St. Luke's Division
300 Pleasant Ave. 55102
St. Paul-Ramsey Hospital — 221-2113
640 Jackson St. 55101
Willmar
Rice Memorial Hospital — 235-4543
402 W. 3rd St. 56201
Worthington
Worthington Regional Hosp. — 372-2941
1016 6th Ave. 56187

MISSISSIPPI

STATE COORDINATOR
State Board of Health — 354-6650
Jackson 39205

Biloxi
Gulf Coast Community Hospital — 388-1919
4642 West Beach Blvd. 39531

USAF Hospital Keesler — 377-2516
Keesler Air Force Base — 377-6555
39534 — 377-6556

Brandon
Rankin General Hospital — 825-2811
350 Crossgates Blvd. 39042 — Ext. 487
Ext. 488

Columbia
Marion County General — 736-6303
Hospital 39429 — Ext. 217

Greenwood
Greenwood-LeFlore Hosp. — 453-9751
River Road 38930 — Ext. 633

Hattiesburg
Forrest Couty General Hosp. — 264-4235
400 S. 28th Ave. 39401

Jackson
Mississippi Baptist — 968-1704
Medical Center
1225 N. State St. 39201

St. Dominic-Jackson — 982-0121
Memorial Hospital — Ext. 345
969 Lakeland Dr. 39216

State Board of Health — 354-6650
Bureau of Disease
Control 39205

University Medical Center — 354-7660
2500 N. State St. 39216

Laurel
Jones County Community — 649-4000
Hospital — Ext. 207
Jefferson St. at 13th Ave. — Ext. 218
39440 — Ext. 220
Ext. 248

Meridian
St. Joseph's Hospital — 483-6211
Highway 39, North 39301 — Ext. 54
Ext. 71

Pascagoula
Singing River Hospital — 938-5162
Highway 90 East 39567

University
School of Pharmacy — 234-1522
University of Mississippi
38677

Vicksburg
Mercy Regional Medical — 636-2131
Center — Ext. 250
100 McAuley Dr. 39181 — Ext. 276

MISSOURI

STATE COORDINATOR
Missouri Division of Health — 751-2713
Jefferson City 65102

Cape Girardeau
St. Francis Medical Ctr. — 335-1251
St. Francis Drive — Ext. 217

Columbia
University of Missouri — 442-5111
Medical Center
807 Stadium Blvd. 65201

Hannibal
St. Elizabeth Hospital — 221-0414
109 Virginia St. 63401 — Ext. 101,183

Jefferson City
Charles E. Still — 635-7141
Osteopathic Hospital — Ext. 215
1125 S. Madison 65101

Joplin
St. John's Medical Center — 781-2727
2727 McClelland Blvd. 64801 — Ext. 393

Kansas City
Children's Mercy Hospital — 471-0626
24th & Gillham Rd. 64108 — Ext. 383, 384

Kirksville
Kirksville Osteopathic — 626-2266
Hospital
800 W. Jefferson St. 63501

Poplar Bluff
Lucy Lee Hospital — 785-7721
330 N. 2nd St. 63901

Rolla
Phelps County Memorial Hosp. — 364-3100
1000 W. 10th St. 65401 — Ext. 136,137

St. Joseph
Methodist — 271-7580
Medical Center — 232-8481
Seventh to Ninth on Faraon Sts. 64501 — Ext. 277

St. Louis
Cardinal Glennon Children's — 772-5200
Hospital
1465 S. Grand Ave. 63104

St. Louis Children's Hosp. — 367-2034
500 S. Kingshighway 63110

Springfield
Lester E. Cox Medical Center — 831-9746
1423 N. Jefferson St. 65802

St. John's Hospital — 885-2115
1235 E. Cherokee 65802

West Plains
West Plains Memorial Hosp. — 256-9111
1103 Alaska Ave. 65775 — Ext. 258
Ext. 259

MONTANA

STATE COORDINATOR
Department of Health and — 1-800-525-5042
Environmental Sciences
Helena 59601

NEBRASKA

STATE COORDINATOR
Department of Health — 471-2122
Lincoln 68502

Omaha
Children's Memorial Hospital — 553-5400
44th & Dewey Sts. 68105

NEVADA

STATE COORDINATOR
Department of Human Resources — 885-4750
Carson City 89710

Las Vegas
Southern Nevada Memorial Hosp. — 385-1277
1800 W. Charleston Blvd.
89102

Sunrise Hospital Med. Ctr. — 731-8000
3186 South Maryland Parkway
89109

Reno
St. Mary's Hospital — 323-2041
235 W. 6th 89503

Washoe Medical Center — 785-4129
77 Pringle Way 89502 — Night: 785-4140

NEW HAMPSHIRE

Hanover
Mary Hitchcock Hospital — 643-4000
2 Maynard St. 03755

NEW JERSEY

STATE COORDINATOR
Department of Health — 292-5666
Trenton 08625

Atlantic City
Atlantic City Medical Center — 344-4081
1925 Pacific Ave. 08401

Belleville
Clara Maass Memorial Hosp. — 751-1000
1A Franklin Ave. 07109 — Ext 781
Ext. 782
Ext. 783

Boonton
Riverside Hospital — 334-5000
Powerville Rd. 07055 — Ext. 186,187

Bridgeton
Bridgeton Hospital — 451-6600
Irving Ave. 08302

Camden
West Jersey Hospital — 795-5554
Evesham Ave. and
Voorhees Tnpk. 08104

Denville
St. Clare's Hospital — 627-3000
Pocono Rd. 07834 — Ext. 6063

East Orange
East Orange General — 672-8400
Hospital — Ext. 223
300 Central Ave. 07019

Elizabeth
St. Elizabeth Hospital — 527-5059
225 Williamson St. 07207

Englewood
Englewood Hospital — 568-3400
350 Engle St. 07631

Flemington
Hunterdon Medical Center — 782-2121
Route #31 08822

Livingston
St. Barnabas Medical Center — 992-5161
Old Short Hills Rd. 07039

Long Branch
Monmouth Medical Center — 222-2210
Dunbar & 2nd Ave. 07740

Montclair
Mountainside Hospital — 746-6000
Bay & Highland Ave. 07042

Mount Holly
Burlington County Memorial — 267-7877
175 Madison Ave. 08060

Neptune
Jersey Shore Medical Center- — 988-1818
Fitkin Hospital
1945 Corlies Ave. 07753

Newark
Newark Beth Israel — 926-7240
Medical Center — 926-7241
201 Lyons Ave. 07112 — 926-7242
926-7243

St. James Hospital — 589-1300
155 Jefferson Street 07105

New Brunswick
Middlesex General Hospital — 828-3000
180 Somerset St. 08903

St. Peter's Medical Center — 745-8526
254 Easton Ave. 08903

Newton
Newton Memorial Hospital — 383-2121
175 High St. 07860 — Ext.270, 1,2
Ext. 273

Orange
Hospital Center at Orange — 678-1100
188 S. Essex Ave. 07051 — Ext. 231

Passaic
St. Mary's Hospital — 473-1000
211 Pennington Ave. 07055

Perth Amboy
Perth Amboy General Hosp. — 442-3700
530 New Brunswick Ave. — Ext. 2500
08861

Phillipsburg
Warren Hospital — 859-1500
185 Roseberry St. 08865 — Ext. 280

Point Pleasant
Point Pleasant Hospital — 892-1100
Osborn Ave. & River Front — Ext. 385
08742

Princeton
Medical Center at Princeton 921-7700
253 Witherspoon St. 08540 Ext. 241
Saddle Brook
Saddle Brook General Hosp. 368-6023
300 Market St. 07662
Somers Point
Shore Memorial Hospital 653-3515
Brighton & Sunny Aves. 08244
Somerville
Somerset Medical Center 725-4000
Rehill Ave. 08876 Ext. 431, 432
Summit
Overlook Hospital 522-2232
193 Morris Ave. 07901
Teaneck
Holy Name Hospital 837-3070
718 Teaneck Rd. 07666
Trenton
Helene Fuld Med. Ctr. 396-1077
750 Brunswick Ave. 08607
Union
Memorial General Hospital 687-1900
1000 Galloping Hill Rd. 07083 Ext. 237
Wayne
Greater Paterson General Hospital 684-6900
Ext. 224
224 Hamburg Tnpk. 07470 Ext. 225
Ext. 226

NEW MEXICO

STATE COORDINATOR
The University of New Mexico 843-2551
N.M. Poison, Drug Inf. & Med. Crisis Center
Albuquerque 87131

NEW YORK

STATE COORDINATOR
Department of Health 474-3664
Albany 12210
Binghamton
Binghamton General Hospital 772-1100
Mitchell & Lark Sts. 13903 Ext. 431
Our Lady of Lourdes Memorial Hospital 798-5231
169 Riverside Drive 13905
Buffalo
Children's Hospital 878-7654
219 Bryant St. 14222
Dunkirk
Brooks Memorial Hospital 366-1111
10 West 6th St. 14048 Ext. 414
Ext. 415
East Meadow
Nassau County Medical Ctr. 542-2323
2201 Hempstead Tpk. 11554 542-2324
542-2325
Elmira
Arnot Ogden Memorial Hosp. 737-4194
Roe Ave. & Grove 14901
St. Joseph's Hospital Health Center 734-2662
555 E. Market St. 14901
Endicott
Ideal Hospital 754-7171
600 High Ave. 13760
Glens Falls
Glens Falls Hospital 792-3151
100 Park St. 12801 Ext. 456
Jamestown
W.C.A. Hospital 487-0141
207 Foote Ave. 14707 484-8648
Johnson City
Wilson Memorial Hospital 773-6611
33-57 Harrison St. 14707
Kingston
Kingston Hospital 331-3131
396 Broadway 12401

New York
N.Y. City, Dept. of Health 340-4494
Bureau of Laboratories 340-4495
455 First Ave. 10016
Niagara Falls
Niagara Falls Memorial Medical Center 278-4511
621 Tenth St. 14302
Nyack
Nyack Hospital (Pharmacy) 358-5581
North Midland Ave. 358-6200
10960 Ext. 451
Ext. 452
Rochester
Strong Memorial Hospital 275-5151
260 Crittenden Blvd. 14620
Schenectady
Ellis Hospital 382-4039
1101 Nott Street 382-4121
Syracuse
Onondaga County Health Dept.
Upstate Medical Center 476-7529
750 E. Adams St. 13210
Watertown
House of the Good Samaritan Hospital 788-8700
Corner Washington & Pratt Sts. 13602

NORTH CAROLINA

STATE COORDINATOR
Duke University Medical Center 684-8111
Durham 27710
Asheville
Memorial Mission Hospital 255-4660
509 Biltmore Ave. 28801
Charlotte
Mercy Hospital 372-5100
Durham
Duke University Medical Ctr. 684-8111
Box 3007 27710
Greensboro
Moses Cone Hospital 379-4105
1200 N. Elm St. 27401
Hendersonville
Margaret R. Pardee Hospital 693-6522
Fleming St. 28739 Ext.222
Hickory
Catawba Memorial Hospital 322-6649
Fairgrove-Church Rd. 28601
Jacksonville
Onslow Memorial Hospital 353-1234
Western Blvd. 28540 Ext. 240
Wilmington
New Hanover Memorial Hosp. 343-7046
2131 S. 17th St. 28401

NORTH DAKOTA

STATE COORDINATOR
Department of Health 224-2388
Bismarck 58505
Bismarck
Bismarck Hospital 223-4357
300 N. 7th St. 58501
Fargo
St. Luke's Hospital 280-5575
Fifth St. at Mills Ave. 58102
Grand Forks
United Hospital 780-5000
1200 S. Columbia Rd. 58201
Minot
St. Joseph's Hospital 857-2553
Third St. & Fourth Ave., S.E. 58701
Williston
Mercy Hospital 572-7661
1301 15th Ave. 58801

OHIO

STATE COORDINATOR
Department of Health 466-2544
Columbus 43216
Akron
Children's Hospital 379-8562
Buchtel at Bowery 44308
Canton
Aultman Hospital 452-9911
Emergency Room Ext. 203
2600 Sixth St., S.W. 44710
Cincinnati
Drug & Poison Inf. Ctr.
Univ. of Cincinnati 872-5111
Medical Center, Rm. 7701
Bridge 45267
Cleveland
Academy of Medicine 231-4455
11001 Cedar Ave. 44106
Columbus
Children's Hospital 228-1323
700 Children's Dr. 43205
Dayton
Children's Medical Center 222-2227
1735 Chapel St. 45404
Lorain
Lorain Community Hospital 282-2220
3700 Kolbe Rd. 44053
Mansfield
Mansfield General Hospital 522-3411
335 Glessner Ave. 44903 Ext. 545
Springfield
Community Hospital 325-1255
2615 E. High St. 44505
Toledo
Medical College Hospital 381-3897
P.O. Box 6190 43699
Youngstown
Mahoning Valley Poison Control Center
St. Elizabeth Hospital & Med Ctr. 746-2222
1044 Belmont Ave. 44505
Zanesville
Bethesda Hospital 454-4221
Poison Information Center
2951 Maple Ave. 43701

OKLAHOMA

STATE COORDINATOR
Oklahoma Children's Memorial Hospital 271-5454
P.O. Box 26307
Oklahoma City 73126
Ada
Valley View Hospital 322-2323
1300 E. 6th St. 74820 Ext. 200
Ardmore
Memorial Hospital of Southern Oklahoma 223-5400
1011-14th Ave. 73401
Lawton
Comanche County Memorial Hospital 355-8620
3401 Gore Blvd. 73501
McAlester
McAlester General Hospital, West 426-1800
P.O. Box 669 74501 Ext. 240
Oklahoma City
Oklahoma Children's Memorial Hospital 271-5454
P.O. Box 26307
940 N.E. 13th
73126
Ponca City
St. Joseph Medical Center 765-3321
14th & Hartford 74601
Tulsa
Hillcrest Medical Center 584-1351
1653 East 12th 74104 Ext. 6165

OREGON

Portland
Oregon Poison Control and Drug Info. Center
University of Oregon Hlth Sciences Center 225-8500
3181 S.W. Sam Jackson Park Rd. 97201

PENNSYLVANIA

STATE COORDINATOR
Department of Health 787-2307
Harrisburg 17120
Allentown
Lehigh Valley Poison Center 921-2121
17th & Chew St. 18102
Altoona
Altoona Region Poison Center 946-3711
Mercy Hospital of Altoona
2500 Seventh Ave. 16603
Bethlehem
St. Luke's Hospital 691-4141
800 Ostrum St. 18015
Bloomsburg
The Bloomsburg Hospital 784-7121
549 E. Fair St. 17815
Bradford
Bradford Hospital 368-4143
Interstate Pkwy 16701
Bryn Mawr
The Bryn Mawr Hospital 527-0600
19010
Chambersburg
The Chambersburg Hospital 264-5171
7th and King St. 17201 Ext. 431
Chester
Sacred Heart General Hosp. 494-0721
9th and Wilson St. 19013 Ext. 232
Clearfield
Clearfield Hospital 765-5341
809 Turnpike Ave. 16830
Coaldale
Coaldale State General Hospital 18218 645-2131
Coudersport
Charles Cole Memorial Hospital 274-9300
RD #3, Route 6 16915
Danville
Susquehanna Poison Center 275-6116
Geisinger Medical Center
North Academy Ave. 17821
Doylestown
Doylestown Hospital 345-2281
595 W. State St. 18901
Drexel Hill
Delaware County Memorial Hospital 259-3800
Lansdowne & Keystone Ave 19026
East Stroudsburg
Pocono Hospital 421-4000
206 E. Brown St. 18301
Easton
Easton Hospital 258-6221
21st & Lehigh St. 18042
Erie
Doctors Osteopathic 455-3961
252 W. 11th St. 16501

Erie Osteopathic Hospital 864-4031
5515 Peach St. 16509

Hamot Medical Center 455-6711
4 E. Second St. 16512 Ext. 521

Northwest Poison Center 452-3232
St. Vincent Health Center
P.O. Box 740 16512
Gettysburg
Annie M. Warner Hospital 334-2121
S. Washington St. 17325
Greensburg
Westmoreland Hosp. Assn. 837-0100
532 W. Pittsburgh St. 15601
Hanover
Hanover General Hospital 637-3711
300 Highland Ave. 17331
Harrisburg
Harrisburg Hospital 782-3639
S. Front & Mulberry St. 17101

Polyclinic Hospital 782-4141
3rd & Polyclinic Ave. 17105 Ext. 4132
Hershey
Milton S. Hershey Medical Center 534-6111
University Dr. 17033
Jeannete
Jeannete District Memorial Hospital 527-3551
600 Jefferson Ave. 15644
Jersey Shore
Jersey Shore Hospital 398-0100
Thompson St. 17740
Johnstown
Conemaugh Valley Memorial Hospital 536-5351
1086 Franklin St. 15905

Lee Hospital 535-7541
320 Main St. 15901

Mercy Hospital 536-5353
1020 Franklin St. 15905
Lancaster
Lancaster General Hospital 299-5511
555 North Duke St. 17604

St. Joseph's Hospital 299-4546
250 College Ave. 17604
Lansdale
North Penn Hospital 368-2100
7th & Broad St. 19446
Lebanon
Good Samaritan Hospital 272-7611
4th & Walnut Sts. 17042
Lehighton
Gnaden-Huetten Memorial Hospital 377-1300
11th & Hamilton St. 18235
Lewistown
Lewistown Hospital 248-5411
Highland Ave. 17044
Muncy
Muncy Valley Hospital 546-8282
P.O. Box 340 17756
Nanticoke
Nanticoke State Hospital 735-5000
W. Washington St. 18634
Paoli
Paoli Memorial Hospital 19301 647-2200
Philadelphia
Philadelphia Poison Information 922-5523
922-5524
321 University Ave. 19104
Phillipsburg
Phillipsburg State General Hospital 16866 342-3320
Pittsburgh
Children's Hospital 681-6669
125 DeSoto St. 15213
Pittston
Pittston Hospital 654-3341
Oregon Heights 18640
Pottstown
Pottstown Memorial Medical Center 327-1000
High St. & Firestone Blvd. 19464
Pottsville
Good Samaritan Hospital 622-3400
E. Norwegian and Tremont St. 17901
Reading
Community General Hospital 376-4881
145 N. 6th St. 19601

Reading Hospital and Medical Center 19603 378-6218
Sayre
The Robert Packer Hospital 888-6666
Guthrie Square 18840
Sellersville
Grandview Hospital 18960 257-3611
Somerset
Somerset Community Hospital 443-2626
225 South Center Ave. 15501
State College
Centre Community Hospital 238-4351
16801
Titusville
Titusville Hospital 827-1851
406 W. Oak St. 16354
Tunkhannock
Tyler Memorial Hospital 836-2161
RD #1 18657
York
Memorial Osteopathic Hospital 843-8623
325 S. Belmont St. 17403

York Hospital 771-2311
1001 S. George St. 17405

PUERTO RICO

STATE COORDINATOR
University of Puerto Rico 765-4880
Rio Piedras 765-0615
Arecibo
District Hospital of 878-7272
Arecibo 00613 Ext. 7459
7510
Fajardo
District Hospital of 863-3792
Fajardo 00649 863-0939
Mayaguez
Mayaguez Medical Center 832-8686
Department of Health Ext. 1224
P.O. Box 1868 00709
Ponce
District Hospital of 842-8364
Ponce 00731
Rio Piedras
Medical Center of 764-3515
Puerto Rico 00936

RHODE ISLAND

STATE COORDINATOR
Department of Health 277-2401
Providence 02908
Kingston
College of Pharmacy 792-2775
University of Rhode Island 02881 792-2762
Pawtucket
Memorial Hospital 724-1230
Prospect St. 02860
Providence
Rhode Island Hospital 277-4000
593 Eddy St. 02902

Roger Williams General Hospital 521-5055
825 Chalkstone Ave. 02907

SOUTH CAROLINA

STATE COORDINATOR
Department of Health & Environmental Control 758-5625
Columbia 29201
Charleston
Poison Information Serv. 792-4201
Medical University of South Carolina
171 Ashley Ave. 29403
Columbia
Poison & Drug Inf. Ctr. 765-7359
College of Pharmacy
Room 313 Coker Life Science Bldg.
University of S.C. 29208

SOUTH DAKOTA

STATE COORDINATOR
Department of Health 773-3361
Pierre 57501

Rapid City
West River Poison Ctr. 343-3333
Rapid City Regional
Hospital East 57701

Sioux Falls
McKennan Hospital 336-3894
800 East 21st St. 57101

TENNESSEE

STATE COORDINATOR
Department of Public Health 741-2407
Nashville 37219

Chattanooga
T.C. Thompson Children's 755-6100
Hospital
910 Blackford St. 37403

Cookeville
Cookeville General Hospital 528-2541
142 W. 5th St. 38501

Jackson
Madison General Hospital 424-0424
708 W. Forest 38301

Johnson City
Memorial Hospital 926-1131
Boone & Fairview Ave. 37601

Knoxville
Memorial Research Center 971-3261
and Hospital
1924 Alcoa Highway 37920

Memphis
University of Tennessee 528-6048
College of Pharmacy
874 Union Avenue 38163

Nashville
Vanderbilt University Hospital 322-3391
21st & Garland 37232

TEXAS

STATE COORDINATOR
Department of Health 458-7254
Austin 78756

Abilene
Hendrick Hospital 677-3551
19th & Hickory Sts. 79601 Ext. 266
Ext. 267

Amarillo
Amarillo Hospital District 376-4431
Amarillo Emergency Receiving Ext. 501
Center Ext. 502
P.O. Box 1110 Ext. 503
2203 W. 6th St. 79175 Ext. 504

Austin
Brackenridge Hospital 478-4490
14th & Sabine Sts. 78701

Beaumont
Baptist Hospital of 833-7409
Southeast Texas
P.O. Box 1591
College & 11th St. 77701

Corpus Christi
Memorial Medical Center 884-4511
P.O. Box 5280 Ext. 556
2606 Hospital Blvd. 78405 Ext. 557

El Paso
R.E. Thomason General 544-1200
Hospital
P.O. Box 20009
4815 Alameda Ave. 79905

Fort Worth
W.I. Cook Children's 336-5521
Hospital Ext. 17
1212 W. Lancaster 76102 336-6611

Galveston
Southeast Texas Poison 765-1420
Control Center 765-1561
8th & Mechanic Sts. 77550

Grand Prairie
Grand Prairie Community 647-1141
Hospital
2709 Hospital Blvd. 75051

Harlingen
Valley Baptist Hospital 423-1224
P.O. Box 2558 Ext. 283
2101 S. Commerce St. 78550

Laredo
Mercy Hospital 722-2431
1515 Logan St. 78040 Ext. 29

Lubbock
Methodist Hospital 792-1011
Pharmacy Ext. 315
3615 19th St. 79410

Midland
Midland Memorial Hospital 684-8257
1908 W. Wall 79701

Odessa
Medical Center Hospital 337-7311
P.O. Box 633 79760 Ext. 250, 252

Plainview
Plainview Hospital 296-9601
2404 Yonkers St. 79072

San Angelo
Shannon West Texas 653-6741
Memorial Hospital Ext. 210
P.O. Box 1879
9 S. Magdalen St. 76901

San Antonio
Bexar County Hospital 223-1481
District
c/o Department of Pediatrics
Univ. of Texas Medical
School at San Antonio
7703 Floyd Dr. 78229

Tyler
Medical Center Hospital 597-0351
1000 S. Beckham St. 75701 Ext. 255

Waco
Hillcrest Baptist Hosp. 753-1412
3000 Herring Ave. 76708 756-6111

Wichita Falls
Wichita General Hospital 322-6771
Emergency Room
1600 8th St. 76301

UTAH

STATE COORDINATOR
Division of Health 533-6191
Salt Lake City 84113 533-6131

Salt Lake City
Intermountain Regional 581-2151
Poison Control Center
50 N. Medical Drive 84132

VIRGIN ISLANDS

STATE COORDINATOR
Department of Health 774-1321
St. Thomas 00801 Ext. 275

St. Croix
Charles Harwood Memorial 773-1212
Hospital 773-1311
Christiansted 00820 Ext. 221
Ingeborg Nesbitt Clinic 772-0260
Fredericksted 00840 772-0212

St. John
Morris F. DeCastro Clinic 776-1469
Cruz Bay 00830

St. Thomas
Knud-Hansen Memorial 774-1321
Hospital 00801 Ext. 224, 225

VIRGINIA

STATE COORDINATOR
Bureau of Emergency 786-5188
Medical Services
Richmond 23219

Alexandria
Alexandria Hospital 370-9000
4320 Seminary Rd. 22314 Ext. 555

Arlington
Arlington Hospital 558-6161
5129 N. 16th St. 22205

Blacksburg
Montgomery County 951-1111
Community Hospital
Rt. 460, S. 24060

Charlottesville
Blue Ridge Poison Center
Univ. of Virginia Hospital 924-5543
22903

Danville
Danville Memorial Hospital 799-2100
142 S. Main St. 22201 Ext. 3869

Falls Church
Fairfax Hospital 698-3600
3300 Gallows Rd. 22046 698-3111

Hampton
Hampton General Hospital 722-1131
3120 Victoria Blvd. 23661

Harrisonburg
Rockingham Memorial Hospital 434-4421
738 S. Mason St. 22801 Ext. 225

Lexington
Stonewall Jackson Hosp. 463-9141
22043

Lynchburg
Lynchburg Gen. Marshall 528-2066
Lodge Hosp., Inc.
Tate Springs Rd. 24504

Nassawadox
Northampton-Accomack 442-8000
Memorial Hospital 23413

Norfolk
DePaul Hospital 489-5111
Granby St. at Kingsley
Lane 23505

Petersburg
Petersburg General Hospital 861-2992
801 South Adams Street 23803

Portsmouth
U.S. Naval Hospital 397-6541
23708 Ext. 418

Richmond
Virginia Poison Center 786-9123
Virginia Commonwealth Univ.
Box 763 MCV Station 23298

Roanoke
Roanoke Memorial Hospital 981-7336
Belleview at Jefferson St.
P.O. Box 13367 24033

Staunton
King's Daughters' Hospital 885-0361
P.O. Box 2007 24401 Ext. 209
Ext. 247

Waynesboro
Waynesboro Community 942-8355
Hospital Ext. 440
501 Oak Ave. 22980 Ext. 500

Williamsburg
Williamsburg Community Hosp. 229-1120
Mt. Vernon Ave. Ext. 65
Drawer H 23185

WASHINGTON

STATE COORDINATOR
Department of Social & 633-0505
Health Services
Olympia 98105

Aberdeen
St. Joseph's Hospital 533-0450
1006 North H. St. 98520 Ext. 277

Bellingham
St. Luke's General Hospital 676-8400
809 E. Chestnut St. 98225 676-8401

Longview
St. John's Hospital 636-5252
1614 E. Kessler 98632

Madigan
Madigan Army Medical 967-6792
Center Emergency Room
98431

Olympia
St. Peter's Hospital 491-0222
413 N. Lilly Rd. 98506
Seattle
Children's Orthopedic Hosp. & Med. Center 634-5252
4800 Sandpoint Way, N.E. 98105
Spokane
Deaconess Hospital 747-1077
W. 800 5th Ave. 99210
Tacoma
Mary Bridge Children's Hospital 272-1281 Ext. 259
311 S. L St. 98405
Vancouver
St. Joseph Community Hospital 256-2067
600 N.E. 92nd St. 98664
Yakima
Yakima Valley Memorial Hospital 248-4400
2811 Tieton Dr. 98902

WEST VIRGINIA

STATE COORDINATOR
Department of Health 348-2971
Charleston 25305
Beckley
Beckley Hospital 252-6431
1007 S. Oakwood Ave. 25801 Ext. 10
Belle
E.I. DuPont de Nemours and Co. 25015 949-4313 Ext. 261
Charleston
Charleston Area Medical Center Memorial Division 348-4211
3200 Noyes Ave. 25304
Clarksburg
United Hospital Center Inc. 623-3444
Downtown Division Ext. 251
Washington & Chestnut Sts. 26301
Huntington
Cabell-Huntington Hospital 696-6160
1340 16th St. 25701
St. Mary's Hospital 696-3760
2900 1st Ave. 25701
Martinsburg
City Hospital 263-8971
Dry Run Rd. 25401
Morgantown
West Virginia University Medical Center 26506 293-5341
Parkersburg
Camden-Clark Hospital 428-8011 Ext. 28 Ext. 130
717 Ann St. 26101
St. Joseph's Hospital 422-8535 Ext. 251
19th St. & Murdoch Ave. 26101
Pt. Pleasant
Pleasant Valley Hospital 696-6160
Valley Drive 25550 696-3762
Ronceverte
Greenbrier Valley Hospital 647-4411 647-4412 647-4413 Ext. 33
608 Greenbrier Ave. 24970
Weirton
Weirton General Hospital 748-3232 Ext. 208
St. John's Rd. 26062
Weston
Stonewall Jackson Hospital 269-3000 Ext. 201 Ext. 228
507 Main Ave. 26452
Wheeling
Wheeling Hospital 233-4455 Ext. 224
109 Main St. 26003

WISCONSIN

STATE COORDINATOR
Department of Health & Social Services, Div. of Health 266-0923
Madison 53701
Eau Claire
Luther Hospital 835-1511
310 Chestnut St. 54701
Green Bay
St. Vincent Hospital 432-8621
835 S. Van Buren St. 54305
LaCrosse
St. Francis Hospital 784-3971
709 S. Tenth St. 54601
Madison
University Hospitals and Clinics 262-3702
600 Highland Ave. 53792
Milwaukee
Milwaukee Children's Hospital 931-1010
1700 W. Wisconsin 53233

WYOMING

STATE COORDINATOR
Department of Health & Social Services 777-7955
Cheyenne 82001
Cheyenne
Wyoming Poison Center 635-9256
De Paul Hospital
2600 East 18th St. 82001

PDR
34
EDITION
SECTION 7

Diagnostic Product Information

This section is intended to reflect the increased use of diagnostic products in the practice of medicine. It is intended for the use of all practitioners and is included in this format to make it easier for the physician to find the information which he seeks about these products.

Products described in PHYSICIANS' DESK REFERENCE® which have official package circulars must be in full compliance with Food & Drug Administration regulations pertaining to labeling for prescription drugs. These regulations require that for PDR copy, "indications, effects, dosages, routes, methods, and frequency and duration of administration, and any relevant warnings, hazards, contraindications, side effects, and precautions" must be the "same in language and emphasis" as the approved labeling for the product. FDA regards the words "same in language and emphasis" as requiring verbatim use of the approved labeling providing such information. For products which do not have official package circulars, the Publisher emphasized to manufacturers the necessity of describing such products comprehensively so that physicians would have access to all information essential for intelligent and informed prescribing. In organizing and presenting the material in PHYSICIANS' DESK REFERENCE, the Publisher is providing all the information made available to PDR by manufacturers.

This edition of PHYSICIANS' DESK REFERENCE contains the latest product information available at press-time. During the year, however, new and revised information about the products described herein may be furnished us. This information will be published in the PDR Supplement. Therefore, before prescribing or administering any product described in the following pages, you should first consult the PDR Supplement.

In presenting the following material to the medical profession, the Publisher is not necessarily advocating the use of any product listed.

Abbott Laboratories
DIAGNOSTICS DIVISION
ABBOTT PARK 6C4, DEPT. 49B
NORTH CHICAGO, ILL. 60064

THYPINONE® ℞
(Protirelin)

Description: Chemically, Thypinone® (protirelin) is identified as 5-oxo-L-prolyl-L-histidyl-L-proline amide. It is a synthetic tripeptide which is believed to be structurally identical with the naturally-occurring thyrotropin-releasing hormone produced by the hypothalamus.

Thypinone (protirelin) is supplied as 1 ml ampules. Each ampule contains 500 mcg protirelin in a sterile non-pyrogenic isotonic saline solution having a pH of approximately 5.6. In addition, each ampule contains sodium chloride, 9.0 mg, Water for Injection, and hydrochloric acid as needed to adjust pH. Thypinone (protirelin) is intended for intravenous administration.

Clinical Pharmacology: Pharmacologically, Thypinone increases the release of the thyroid stimulating hormone (TSH) from the anterior pituitary. With the exception of prolactin release, which is also increased, Thypinone (protirelin) has no clinically significant effect on the release of other pituitary hormones. Following intravenous administration, the mean plasma half-life of protirelin in normal subjects is approximately five minutes. TSH levels rise rapidly and reach a peak at 20 to 30 minutes. The decline in TSH levels takes place more slowly, approaching baseline levels after approximately three hours.

Indications and Usage: Thypinone (protirelin) is indicated as an adjunctive agent in the diagnostic assessment of thyroid function. As an adjunct to other diagnostic procedures, testing with Thypinone may yield useful information in patients with pituitary or hypothalamic dysfunction.

Warnings: Transient changes in blood pressure occur frequently following administration of Thypinone (protirelin). The patient should be in the supine position when the drug is administered and blood pressure should be monitored during the first 15 minutes. Increased systolic pressure (usually less than 30 mm Hg) and/or increased diastolic pressure (usually less than 20 mm Hg) have been observed more frequently than decreased pressure. When blood pressure changes have occurred, they have not ordinarily persisted for more than 15 minutes, and have not required therapy. In patients in whom such changes would be hazardous, the benefit versus risk ratio should be carefully weighed.

Precautions: Thyroid hormones reduce the TSH response to Thypinone (protirelin). Accordingly, patients in whom Thypinone is to be used diagnostically should be taken off liothyronine (T3) approximately seven days prior to testing and should be taken off thyroid medications containing levothyroxine (T4), e.g., desiccated thyroid, thyroglobulin, or liotrix, at least 14 days before testing.

Chronic administration of levodopa has been reported to inhibit the TSH response to Thypinone.

It is not advisable to withdraw maintenance doses of adrenocortical drugs used in the therapy of known hypopituitarism. Several published reports have shown that prolonged treatment with glucocorticoids at physiologic doses has no significant effect on the TSH response to thyrotropin releasing hormone, but that the administration of pharmacologic doses of steroids reduces the TSH response.

Pregnancy: Reproduction studies have been performed in rats and rabbits. At doses 1-½ and 6 times the human dose, there was an increase in the number of resorption sites in the pregnant rabbit. There are no studies in pregnant women which bear on the safety of Thypinone for the human fetus. Thypinone should be used in pregnant women only when clearly needed.

Adverse Reactions: Side effects have been reported in about 50 percent of those tested with Thypinone (protirelin). Generally, the side effects are minor, have occurred promptly, and have persisted for only a few minutes following injection. The adverse effects most frequently reported were (in decreasing order of occurrence) nausea, urge to urinate, flushed sensation, lightheadedness, bad taste, abdominal discomfort, headache, and dry mouth. Less frequently reported complaints were anxiety, sweating, tightness in the throat, pressure in the chest, a tingling sensation and drowsiness. Thypinone has been reported to cause breast engorgement and leakage in lactating women for up to two or three days.

Dosage and Administration: Thypinone (protirelin) is intended for intravenous administration with the patient in the supine position. The drug is administered as a bolus over a period of 15 to 30 seconds, with the patient remaining supine for an additional 15 minutes during which time the blood pressure is monitored.

Dosage:

Adults: 500 mcg. Doses between 200 and 500 mcg have been used. 500 mcg is considered the optimum dose to give the maximum response in the greatest number of patients. Doses greater than 500 mcg are unlikely to elicit a greater TSH response.

Children age 6 to 16 years: 7 mcg/kg body weight up to 500 mcg.

Infants and children up to 6 years: Experience is limited in this age group; doses of 7 mcg/kg have been administered.

One blood sample for TSH assay should be drawn immediately prior to the injection of Thypinone, and a second sample should be obtained 30 minutes after injection.

The TSH response to Thypinone (protirelin) is reduced by repetitive administration of the drug. Accordingly, if the Thypinone test is repeated, an interval of seven days before testing is recommended.

Elevated serum lipids may interfere with the TSH assay. Thus, fasting (except in patients with hypopituitarism) or a low-fat meal is recommended prior to the test.

Interpretation of Test Results: Interpretation of the TSH response to Thypinone (protirelin) requires an understanding of thyroid-pituitary-hypothalamic physiology and knowledge of the clinical status of the individual patient. Because the TSH test results may vary with the laboratory, the physician should be familiar with the TSH assay method used and the normal range for the laboratory performing the assay.

TSH response 30 minutes after Thypinone administration in normal subjects and in patients with hyperthyroidism and hypothyroidism are presented in Figure 1. The diagnoses were established prior to the administration of Thypinone on the basis of the clinical history, physical examination, and the results of other thyroid and/or pituitary function tests.

Among the normal euthyroid subjects, women and children were found to have higher levels of TSH at 30 minutes than men. Among the patients with hyperthyroidism or primary (thyroidal), secondary (pituitary) or tertiary (hypothalamic) hypothyroidism, no significant differences in TSH levels by age or sex were found.

Normal: Baseline TSH levels of less than 10 microunits/ml (μU/ml) were observed in 97% of euthyroid normal subjects tested. Thirty minutes after Thypinone (protirelin), the serum TSH increased by 2.0 μU/ml or more in 95% of euthyroid subjects.

Hyperthyroidism: All hyperthyroid patients tested had baseline TSH levels of less than 10 μU/ml and a rise of less than 2 μU/ml 30 minutes after Thypinone. (See Table 1)

Primary (thyroidal) hypothyroidism: The diagnosis of primary hypothyroidism is frequently supported by finding clearly elevated baseline TSH levels; 93% of patients tested had levels above 10 μU/ml. Thypinone (protirelin) administration to these patients generally would not be expected to yield additional useful information. Ninety-four percent of patients with primary hypothyroidism given Thypinone in clinical trials responded with a rise in TSH of 2.0 μU/ml or greater; since this response is also found in normal subjects. Thypinone testing does not differentiate primary hypothyroidism from normal.

Secondary (pituitary) and tertiary (hypothalamic) hypothyroidism: In the presence of clinical and other laboratory evidence of hypothyroidism, the finding of a baseline TSH level less than 10 μU/ml should suggest secondary or tertiary hypothyroidism. In this situation, a response to Thypinone of less than 2 μU/ml suggests secondary hypothyroidism since this response was observed in about 60% of patients with secondary hypothyroidism and only approximately 5% of patients with tertiary hypothyroidism. A TSH response to Thypinone greater than 2 μU/ml is not helpful in differentiating between secondary and tertiary hypothyroidism since this response was noted in about 40% of the former and about 95% of the latter.

Establishing the diagnosis of secondary or tertiary hypothyroidism requires a careful his-

Table 1
Characterization Based on Serum TSH Levels at Baseline and 30 Minutes after Thypinone

	Baseline Serum TSH (μU/ml)	Change of Serum TSH (μU/ml) at 30 Minutes
Euthyroidism (normal thyroid function)	10 or less (usually 6 or less; 20% have <1.5 μU/ml)	2 or more (usually 6 to 30)
Hyperthyroidism	10 or less (usually 4 or less)	less than 2
Primary Hypothyroidism (thyroidal)	more than 10 (usually 15 to 200)	2 or more (usually 20 or more)
Secondary Hypothyroidism (pituitary)	10 or less (usually 6 or less)	less than 2 (59%) 2 to 50 (41%)
Tertiary Hypothyroidism (hypothalamic)	10 or less (often less than 2)	2 or more

Figure 1

Mean ± One Standard Deviation of TSH levels Observed at Baseline and 30 Minutes After Thypinone (μ U/ml)

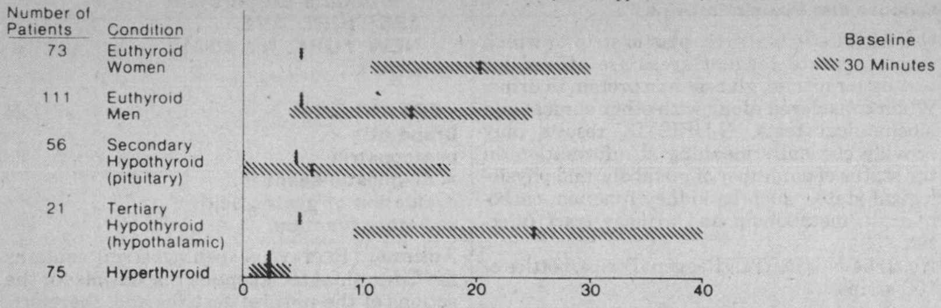

tory and physical examination along with appropriate tests of anterior pituitary and/or target gland function. The Thypinone test should not be used as the only laboratory determinant for establishing these diagnoses. (See Figure 1)

How Supplied: As 1 ml ampules—boxes of 5 (NDC 0074-8971-05). Each ml contains Thypinone (protirelin) 0.50 mg (500 mcg), sodium chloride 9.0 mg for isotonicity, and pH adjusted with hydrochloric acid.

Ames Division

Miles Laboratories, Inc.
P.O. BOX 70
ELKHART, INDIANA 46515

N-MULTISTIX®
Reagent Strips

Designed for testing of urine specimens for protein, glucose, ketones, bilirubin, occult blood, urobilinogen, nitrite, and to indicate urinary pH. N-MULTISTIX provides significant information in 60 seconds which relates to urinary tract status, renal function, carbohydrate metabolism, liver function, biliary tract status, and is an aid in differential diagnosis of liver disease.

No. 2829—N-MULTISTIX Reagent Strips, bottles of 100.

(See table at right)

Ordering/Pricing Information:
(219) 264-8645
Customer Services: (219) 264-8901

DIASTIX®
Reagent Strips
KETO-DIASTIX®
Reagent Strips

DIASTIX is a clear, flexible plastic strip to which is affixed a reagent area for the quantitative, 30-second determination of glucose in urine. KETO-DIASTIX is designed for the determination of ketones and glucose in urine. Results are read by comparison with color chart (on containers): ketones in 15 seconds, glucose in 30 seconds.

No. 2806–DIASTIX Reagent Strips, plastic vials of 50.

No. 2803—DIASTIX Reagent Strips, bottles of 100.

No. 2882—KETO-DIASTIX Reagent Strips, bottles of 100.

No. 2883—KETO-DIASTIX Reagent Strips, bottles of 50.

TEK-CHEK®
Controls for Routine Urinalysis

A convenient quality control system to help determine if AMES urinalysis tests are properly performed and interpreted. Particularly valuable in instituting a quality control system, or making an existing system more convenient by the use of ready-made controls.

No. 1301—TEK-CHEK #1, package of 4 vials, negative reactions for all AMES urine tests.*

No. 1302—TEK-CHEK #2, package of 4 vials, positive for protein and nitrite; all other AMES tests negative.*

No. 1303—TEK-CHEK #3, package of 4 vials, positive for glucose all other AMES tests negative.*

No. 1304—TEK-CHEK #4, package of 4 vials, positive reactions for protein, glucose, ketones, bilirubin, and blood.*

*pH and specific gravity values specified in package insert.

DEXTROSTIX®
Reagent Strips

DEXTROSTIX is a firm plastic strip with an impregnated reagent area that contains a reagent system for determination of blood-glucose levels with the use of fingertip or venous blood. DEXTROSTIX is a convenient 60-second test which can be read qualitatively by comparison with color chart (on bottle label) or quantitatively with the EYETONE® Reflectance Colorimeter or AMES™ Reflectance Meter.

No. 2888—DEXTROSTIX Reagent Strips, bottles of 25.

No. 2895—DEXTROSTIX Reagent Strips, bottles of 100.

No. 2893—DEXTROSTIX Reagent Strips, individually foil wrapped-Package of 10.

OTHER AVAILABLE REAGENT STRIPS AND/OR TABLETS

	Glucose	Protein	pH	Blood	Ketones	Bilirubin	Urobilinogen	Phenylketones (PKU)	Nitrite
CLINISTIX®	X								
*CLINITEST®	X								
DIASTIX®	X								
URISTIX®	X	X							
ALBUSTIX®		X							
BUMINTEST®		X							
COMBISTIX®	X	X	X						
HEMA-COMBISTIX®	X	X	X	X					
HEMASTIX®				X					
LABSTIX®	X	X	X	X	X				
KETO-DIASTIX®	X				X				
KETOSTIX®					X				
ACETEST®					X				
BILI-LABSTIX®	X	X	X	X	X	X			
ICTOTEST®						X			
MULTISTIX®	X	X	X	X	X	X	X		
N-MULTISTIX®	X	X	X	X	X	X	X		X
UROBILISTIX®							X		
PHENISTIX®								X	
N-URISTIX®	X	X							X
MICROSTIX®-NITRITE (test for Nitrite)									X

*Available as 5-drop or 2-drop methods.

Continued on next page

Ames—Cont.

MICROCULT®-GC
Miniaturized Culture Test for the Detection of Neisseria Gonorrhoeae

MICROCULT-GC test system consists of a plastic Culture Slide containing two dry culture areas, a bottle of Rehydration Fluid, a CO_2 Generating Tablet to provide the proper environment during incubation, and Cytochrome Oxidase Detection Strips to visualize growth locations after culture. The culture areas use a modified Thayer-Martin medium which provides nutrients for *Neisseria gonorrhoeae* while inhibiting growth of other flora normally found in the lower reproductive tract. The foil pouch used to store the Culture Slide also serves as an incubation pouch. The CO_2 atmosphere needed during incubation is provided by a TABCO$_2$® tablet. After incubation, colonies producing cytochrome oxidase are visualized by using the detection strips.
MICROCULT-GC is stable in the dry state and ready for use on removal from the foil pouch. The test does not require refrigerated storage and possesses much longer stability than conventional agar or other culture tests.
MICROCULT-GC culture tests are available in kits of 10 culture slides (#3025). Also available Ames MICROSTIX® Incubator (#3056).

MICROSTIX®-3
Reagent Strips

A bacteriuria testing system consisting of a firm plastic strip with three separate reagent areas—a chemical test area for immediate recognition of nitrite in urine, and two culture areas for semiquantitation of bacterial growth after 18-24 hours incubation. One culture area supports total bacterial (both Gram-positive and Gram-negative) growth; the other, only Gram-negative organisms. The dry-reagent microbiologic technology provides a unique growth vehicle which does not require refrigeration and is more stable than agar plates. A compact MICROSTIX Incubator is available at nominal cost.
No. 3009—MICROSTIX-3 Reagent Strips, box of 25 foil-wrapped strips, and 25 incubation pouches and labels.
No. 3056—MICROSTIX Incubator/Adapter.
No. 3007—MICROSTIX®-Nitrite Reagent Strips, 3 foil wrapped strips per catch cover, ten catch covers per box. Test detects nitrite in urine, and indicator of bacteriuria. Designed as a patient take-home self-test.

MICROSTIX®-CANDIDA
Miniaturized Culture Test for the Detection of Candida Species in Vaginal Specimens

MICROSTIX®-CANDIDA is a culture test which contains a selective growth medium for *Candida* species and is intended as an aid to diagnosis of *Candida.*
The MICROSTIX-CANDIDA test system consists of a firm, plastic strip to which is affixed a dry culture area, a bottle of water for rehydration, and a plastic pouch which provides a suitable environment for the strip during incubation. The test area uses a modified Nickerson's medium which contains a support nutrient along with agents to inhibit bacterial growth, and is a selective isolation medium for *Candida* species. The dry-reagent microbiological technology provides a unique culture vehicle which does not require refrigeration, and possesses much longer stability than conventional agar plates or slide tests.
No. 3004—MICROSTIX-CANDIDA culture tests are available in kits of 25 strips.
No. 3056—MICROSTIX Incubator.

N-URISTIX®
Reagent Strips
Dip-and Read Test for Nitrite, Glucose and Protein in Urine

N-URISTIX® is a firm, plastic strip to which three separate reagent areas are affixed for testing for nitrite, glucose and protein in urine. When considered along with other clinical and biochemical tests, N-URISTIX results may provide clinically meaningful information on the status of a number of metabolic and physiological states, such as kidney function, carbohydrate metabolism and urinary tract infection.
No. 2854-N-URISTIX Reagent Strips, bottles of 100 strips.

AMES INSTRUMENTS

AMES™
Blood Analyzer

AMES Blood Analyzer performs up to 14 in-office blood-chemistry determinations to aid diagnosis. Particularly compact, the instrument gives reliable readings for albumin, alkaline phosphatase, bilirubin (total and direct), BUN, cholesterol, creatinine, cyanmethemoglobin, oxyhemoglobin, triglyceride, SGOT, SGPT, total protein, globulin by derivation, true glucose, and uric acid.
No. 6200—AMES Blood Analyzer.

EYETONE®
Reflectance Colorimeter

A small, lightweight, portable, line-operated instrument with a built-in light source for quantitative measurement of glucose using fingertip or venous blood when used with DEXTROSTIX® Reagent Strips. The EYETONE/DEXTROSTIX System provides results with greater accuracy and reproducibility than can be obtained solely by reading DEXTROSTIX visually. Rapid and accurate single and multiple determinations of blood-glucose levels are easily read on a precisely calibrated meter that covers the range of 10–400 mg. glucose per 100 ml. of whole blood.
No. 5551—EYETONE® Reflectance Colorimeter.

URIN-TEK®
System for Urine Specimen Collection

The system consists of a disposable plastic tube (15 ml. capacity) with an easy-on, easy-off plastic cap, a self-adhesive identification label, a flat-bottom 3 oz. paper collection cup, and a 10-tube disposable tube holder for easy specimen collection, transport and testing.
No. 4202—URIN-TEK System with 5 twist-top plastic bags, each containing 100 tubes, caps, labels, and collection cups, and 1 disposable tube holder.
No. 4204—URIN-TEK Tubes Only (500).
No. 4205—URIN-TEK Caps Only (500).
No. 4221—URIN-TEK Urine Tube Rack-each.

IDENTIFICATION PROBLEM?

Consult PDR's

Product Identification Section

where you'll find over 900

products pictured actual size

and in full color.

Ayerst Laboratories
Division of American Home Products Corporation
685 THIRD AVE.
NEW YORK, NY 10017

PEPTAVLON® ℞
Brand of pentagastrin
A diagnostic agent for evaluation of gastric acid secretory function.

Actions: PEPTAVLON (pentagastrin) contains the C-terminal tetrapeptide responsible for the actions of the natural gastrins and, therefore, acts as a physiologic gastric acid secretagogue. The recommended dose of 6 mcg/kg subcutaneously produces a peak acid output which is reproducible when used in the same individual.
PEPTAVLON stimulates gastric acid secretion approximately ten minutes after subcutaneous injection, with peak responses occurring in most cases twenty to thirty minutes after administration. Duration of activity is usually between sixty and eighty minutes.
Indications: PEPTAVLON is used as a diagnostic agent to evaluate gastric acid secretory function. It is useful in testing for:
Anacidity:—as a diagnostic aid in patients with suspected pernicious anemia, atrophic gastritis, or gastric carcinoma.
Hypersecretion:—as a diagnostic aid in patients with suspected duodenal ulcer or postoperative stomal ulcer, and for the diagnosis of Zollinger-Ellison tumor.
PEPTAVLON (pentagastrin) is also useful in determining the adequacy of acid-reducing operations for peptic ulcer.
Contraindications: Hypersensitivity or idiosyncrasy to pentagastrin.
Warnings: *Use in Pregnancy*—The use of pentagastrin in pregnancy has NOT been studied, and the benefit of administration of the drug must be weighed against any possible risk to the mother and/or fetus.
Use in Children—There are insufficient data to recommend the use of, or establish a dosage, in children.

****

In amounts in excess of the recommended dose, pentagastrin may cause inhibition of gastric acid secretion.
Precautions: Use with caution in patients with pancreatic, hepatic, or biliary disease. Like gastrin, pentagastrin could, in some cases, have the physiologic effect of stimulating pancreatic enzyme and bicarbonate secretion, as well as biliary flow.
Adverse Reactions: Pentagastrin causes fewer and less severe cardiovascular and other adverse reactions than histamine or betazole. The majority of reactions to pentagastrin are related to the gastrointestinal tract.
The following reactions associated with the use of pentagastrin have been reported.
Gastrointestinal: abdominal pain, desire to defecate, nausea, vomiting, borborygmi, blood-tinged mucus
Cardiovascular: flushing, tachycardia
Central Nervous System: dizziness, faintness or lightheadedness, drowsiness, sinking feeling, transient blurring of vision, tiredness, headache
Allergic and Hypersensitivity Reactions: May occur in some patients.
Miscellaneous: shortness of breath, heavy sensation in arms and legs, tingling in fingers, chills, sweating, generalized burning sensation, warmth, pain at site of injection, bile in collected specimens
Dosage and Administration: *Adults:* 6 mcg/kg subcutaneously. Effect begins in about ten minutes; peak response usually occurs in twenty to thirty minutes. (For discussion of the test and explicit directions, consult Baron,

J.H.: Gastric Function Tests, in Wastell, C.: Chronic Duodenal Ulcer, New York, Appleton-Century-Crofts, 1972, pp. 82–114.)

Note: Data are inadequate to recommend the use of, or establish a dosage, in children.

Overdosage: In case of overdosage or idiosyncrasy, symptomatic treatment should be administered as required.

How Supplied: PEPTAVLON—In 2 ml ampuls. Each ml contains 0.25 mg (250 mcg) pentagastrin. Also contains 0.88% sodium chloride, and Water for Injection U.S.P. The pH is adjusted with ammonium hydroxide. Cartons of 10 (NDC 0046-3290-10).

Bio-Dynamics/bmc
9115 HAGUE ROAD
INDIANAPOLIS, INDIANA 46250

CHEMSTRIP® bG BLOOD GLUCOSE TEST
Dip-and-Read Test Strips for Semi-Quantitative Determination of Glucose in Whole Blood

Summary and Explanation: CHEMSTRIP bG is a sensitive and specific test strip which facilitates accurate semi-quantitative determination of blood glucose within 2 minutes.
CHEMSTRIP bG is the only glucose test strip with 2 separate test zones whose different reagent concentrations optimize sensitivity and colorimetric accuracy of semi-quantitative values from 20 mg/dl to 800 mg/dl. A wider range of test values than other test strips permits wider use of CHEMSTRIP bG—for **stat** semi-quantitative assays of hypo- and hyperglycemia in neonatal, surgical, and cardiac care, as well as in emergency diagnosis of coma, mass screening of metabolic status and monitoring of diabetes mellitus.

Specimen Collection and Preparation: CHEMSTRIP bG is free from interference when used with fresh capillary blood. It is specific for D-glucose in whole blood and nonreactive to fructose, lactose, galactose, and pentose sugars. Hematocrit values between 30–70% have no significant effect, and neither physiologic concentrations of uric or ascorbic acid, nor therapy with heparin, EDTA or the usual plasma expanders, affect test results with CHEMSTRIP bG.

Procedure for *In Vitro* Diagnostic Use: Two-minute test procedure with CHEMSTRIP bG requires only 3 steps—fewer than any other blood-glucose test strip: (1) Place a large enough drop of whole blood on the reagent area to cover both test zones completely. (2) After 60 seconds, wipe off the blood with a dry cotton ball and then rewipe the strip 2 more times. **Do not use water**; unlike other strips, CHEMSTRIP bG needs no washing. (3) After another 60 seconds, read test results by comparing test-zone colors with the vial label's color values for 20, 40, 80, 120, 180, and 240 mg/dl. (For colors **darker** than those for 240 mg/dl, wait an extra minute before reading 400 or 800 mg/dl.) The 8 clearly separate, precalibrated color values facilitate reproducible reading and permit practical estimation of intermediate values.

How Supplied: Nonbreakable aluminum vials of 25 test strips, moisture-protected by drying agent in vial cap. Cat. No. 318728.

Ordering/Pricing/Technical Information: Call (317) 845-2000 or toll-free (800) 428-5074.

CHEMSTRIP® URINE TESTING SYSTEM
Dip and Read Test Strips for Nitrite-pH-Protein-Glucose-Ketones-Urobilinogen-Bilirubin-Blood in Urine

Summary and Explanation: CHEMSTRIP is a uniquely constructed test strip of inert plastic to which a nylon mesh bonds, without glue, 1 to 8 reagent papers to determine nitrite, pH, protein, glucose, ketones, urobilinogen, bilirubin, and blood in urine. The nylon mesh holds each reagent paper in place, protects it and promotes rapid and even urine-diffusion in each complete test area. To prevent the "run-over" phenomenon, certain test papers also have an inert absorbent paper between the reagent paper and the plastic strip.
[See table above].

	Nitrite	pH	Protein	Glucose	Ketones	Urobilinogen	Bilirubin	Blood	Catalog No.	Strips Per Vial
CHEMSTRIP® 8	X	X	X	X	X	X	X	X	200697	100
CHEMSTRIP® 7		X	X	X	X	X	X	X	200719	100
CHEMSTRIP® 6		X	X	X	X		X	X	200727	100
CHEMSTRIP® 5		X	X	X	X			X	200735	100
CHEMSTRIP® 4		X	X	X				X	203840	100
CHEMSTRIP® 3		X	X	X					274232	100
CHEMSTRIP® GP			X	X					200743	100
CHEMSTRIP® GK				X	X				221279	100
CHEMSTRIP® K					X				200760	100
CHEMSTRIP® G				X					221244	100

CHEMSTRIPS are packaged in an aluminum vial with a tight-fitting cap which contains a drying agent. Each CHEMSTRIP is stable and ready for use when removed from the vial. No additional equipment or instrumentation is required.

Specimen Collection and Preparation: CHEMSTRIPS may be used on any freshly voided urine specimen or on urines collected under special conditions, such as first-morning specimens and postprandial urines. The urine must be collected in a clean container and should be tested as soon as possible after collection (do not centrifuge). It is of particular importance to use fresh urine to obtain the best results with the test for urine bilirubin because this compound is very unstable when exposed to room temperature and daylight. If testing cannot be performed within an hour after collection, the specimen should be refrigerated immediately 2 to 8° C and returned to room temperature before testing. Mix thoroughly before use.

Procedure for *In Vitro* Diagnostic Use. For convenience, all values on the strip may be read at 60 seconds (during the second minute) after immersion in the urine. Color changes occurring more than 2 minutes after strip immersion are not of diagnostic value. (Semi-quantitative assay of abnormally high glucose concentrations may require 4–5 minutes, however.) Color changes that occur only along the edge of the test area should be ignored. Careful removal of excess urine should eliminate this effect.
Calibration of the CHEMSTRIP during use is not required. Color blocks on vial label are previously calibrated by use of precise standards during the manufacturing process.

Ordering/Pricing/Technical Information: Call (317) 845-2000 or toll free (800) 428-5074

FECSCAN™ FECAL BLOOD TEST
30-Second Screen and Monitor of Occult Blood in Feces

Summary and Explanation: FECSCAN is a specimen-collecting and testing kit especially developed for practical sensitivity, convenience, and compliance when screening or monitoring patients with colorectal cancer or other causes of rectal bleeding.

Test Principle: The FECSCAN indicator is a guaiac resin fraction chromatographically purified for uniform color reactivity. Hemoglobin catalyzes oxidation of this color-indicator by hydrogen peroxide in the reagent developer. Blue coloration of test paper reveals fecal blood within 30 seconds.
FECSCAN covers the full range of pathologic occult blood values, without the excessive or erratic sensitivity of benzidine or orthotolidine tests, and reduces risk of interference by foreign peroxidases and ascorbic acid.

Indications: *Routine Screening*—at first and annual examination of patients over 40–50 years of age—for rectal bleeding due to colon or rectal cancer, hemorrhoids, polyps, gastrointestinal ulceration or inflammation and systemic hemolysis. *Problem-Oriented Screening*—selectively, with patients of any age—for occult bleeding due to gastrointestinal disease, Meckel's diverticulum, intussusception and trauma, as well as hemolytic or neoplastic conditions. *Periodic Monitoring*—at regular intervals—to monitor conditions and chemotherapy with risk of gastrointestinal bleeding or blood dyscrasias—e.g., in patients with peptic ulcer or ulcerative colitis and during therapy with salicylates, thiazide diuretics and many other anti-inflammatory and anti-hypertensive drugs.

Specimen Collection and Test Procedure: (1) The patient is given a FECSCAN envelope containing 3 two-window test folders, 6 spatulas, and instructions for collecting fecal specimens. (2) With 2 disposable spatulas, the patient collects specimens from different parts of the stool and places them in different windows of the test folder. After specimens are collected in the same way for the next two stools, the patient returns the specimen-containing folders to the physician's office or laboratory. (3) The technologist puts 2 drops of FECSCAN reagent-developer on the 6 fecal specimens in the 3 test folders. Blue coloration around any specimen within 30 seconds is a positive finding for fecal blood. Observing test-reaction differences also may yield clues to bleeding's volume and source.

How Supplied: FECSCAN Kit, with bottle of reagent-developer and specimen-collection envelopes for 50 patients. Cat. No. 192451. Also supplied in bulk size for 150 patients. Cat. No. 292460.

Ordering/Pricing/Technical Information: Call (317) 845-2000 or toll-free (800) 428-5074.

Cutter Biological
DIV. CUTTER LABORATORIES, INC.
4TH & PARKER STS.
BERKELEY, CA 94710

THROMBOSCREEN™ ℞
(Antithrombin III Assay)
50 determinations

THROMBOSCREEN™ ℞
(Heparin Assay)
50 determinations

Ethical Data, Inc.
POST OFFICE BOX 263
WEST CHICAGO, IL 60185

HAIR ANALYSIS (TMA-H)

Description: Trace mineral analysis of hair (TMA-H) by atomic absorption and emission is a diagnostic aid which indicates levels and ratios, singly or by panel, of essential and/or potentially toxic body minerals.
Special Environmental Use: TMA-H screening is ideal for the detection of toxic, heavy metals in individual patients, industrial employees or population groups.
Information and Data Supplied: A computerized report of each hair sample is returned to the requesting physician providing the mineral levels and ratios in parts per million. The standard panel includes Calcium, Magnesium, Phosphorus, Sodium, Potassium, Zinc, Iron, Copper, Manganese, Chromium, Molybdenum, Lead, Cadmium, Mercury and Aluminum. Additional elements are available on request such as Lithium, Nickel, Selenium, Arsenic, etc.
Contraindications: None. TMA-H is a noninvasive, easy to use diagnostic technique.
How Supplied: A hair test kit containing an envelope and cutting instructions is furnished to the ordering physician for each sample.
Literature available on request.

Lederle Laboratories
A Division of American Cyanamid Co.
WAYNE, NEW JERSEY 07470

TUBERCULIN, OLD, TINE TEST® ℞

The TUBERCULIN, OLD, TINE TEST® is a sterile, simple, multiple-puncture, disposable intradermal test device for the detection of tuberculin reactivity. These convenient devices are especially useful in mass tuberculosis screening programs.
Each test unit consists of a stainless steel disc attached to a plastic handle. Projecting from the disc are four triangular-shaped prongs (tines) which are 2 mm long and approximately 4 mm apart. The tines have been mechanically dipped in a solution of Old Tuberculin, containing 7% Acacia (Gum Arabic) and 8.5% Lactose as stabilizers, and then dried. The entire unit has been sterilized by ethylene oxide gas. No preservative has been added. The unit is disposable and there is no need for syringes, needles, and other equipment necessary for the standard intradermal tests.
TUBERCULIN, OLD, TINE TEST® UNITS have been standardized by clinical evaluation in human subjects to give reactions equivalent to or more potent than 5 T.U.* of standard old tuberculin administered intradermally in the Mantoux test. However, all multiple puncture-type devices must be regarded as screening tools and other appropriate diagnostic procedures such as the Mantoux test should be utilized for retesting reactors.

*U.S. (International) tuberculin units.
Indications: TUBERCULIN, OLD, TINE TEST® is indicated to detect tuberculin-sensitive individuals. Tine Test units are also useful in programs to determine priorities for additional testing (i.e., chest x-rays) and in epidemiological surveys to identify those areas having high levels of infection.
The frequency of repeated tuberculin tests depends on risk of exposure of the child and on the prevalence of tuberculosis in the population group. For the pediatrician's office or outpatient clinic, an annual or biennial tuberculin test, unless local circumstances clearly indicate otherwise, is appropriate. The initial test should be done at the time of, or preceding, the measles immunization.[1] The repeated testing of uninfected individuals does not sensitize to tuberculin. Among individuals with waning sensitivity to homologous or heterologous mycobacterial antigens, however, the stimulus of a tuberculin test may "boost" or increase the size of the reaction to a second test, even causing an apparent development of sensitivity in some cases.[2]
Directions for Use: Site: the volar surface of the upper one-third of the forearm, over a muscle belly, is the preferred site. Hairy areas, and areas without adequate subcutaneous tissue, e.g. concavities over a tendon or bone should be avoided.
Method of Application: Alcohol, acetone, ether, or soap and water may be used to cleanse the skin. The area must be clean and thoroughly dry before application of the TUBERCULIN, OLD, TINE TEST. Expose the four impregnated tines by removing the protective cap while holding the plastic handle. Grasp the patient's forearm firmly, since the sharp momentary sting may cause the patient to jerk his arm, resulting in scratching. Stretch the skin of the forearm tightly and apply the disc with the other hand. ***Hold at least one second.*** Release tension grip on forearm. Withdraw tine unit.
Sufficient pressure should be exerted so that the four puncture sites, and a circular depression of the skin from the plastic base are visible. Local care of the skin is not necessary.
TUBERCULIN, OLD, TINE TEST® Unit must never be re-used.
Reading the Reaction: Tests should be read at 48–72 hours. Vesiculation or the extent of induration are the determining factors; erythema without induration is of no significance. Readings should be made in a good light with the forearm slightly flexed. The size of the induration in millimeters should be determined by inspection, measuring and palpation with gentle finger stroking. Identification of the application site is usually easy because of the distinct four-point pattern. The diameter of the largest single reaction around one of the puncture sites should be measured. With pronounced reactions the areas of induration around the puncture sites may coalesce.
Vesiculation: Positive Reaction. If vesiculation is present, the test may be interpreted as positive, in which case the management of the patient is the same as that for one classified as positive to the Mantoux test.[3]
Induration, 2 mm or greater: *Interpretation.* The criterion for classifying a tuberculin skin test as positive or negative is determined by the incidence of sensitivity to the antigens of the so-called atypical mycobacteria. Induration as small as 5 mm in the PPD-S Mantoux test (5 T.U.) may be accepted as positive in areas in which such incidence is low or nonexistent. The size of induration to the TUBERCULIN, OLD, TINE TEST® which corresponds to a 5 mm induration to the Mantoux test is 2 mm. In clinical studies covering various geographical areas of the U.S. and all age groups, with a total of 30,588 test subjects, which include studies with a more potent tine test, there were 911 (4%) false positive reactors among 26,236 subjects who were Mantoux negative, and 342 (8%) false negative reactors among 4,352 subjects who were Mantoux positive.
Induration less than 2 mm: *Negative Reaction.* There is no need for retesting unless the person is a contact of a patient with tuberculosis or there is clinical evidence suggestive of the disease.[3]
Descriptive literature illustrating typical reactions is available on request.
Precautions: Tuberculin testing should be done with caution in individuals with active tuberculosis. Although activation of quiescent lesions is rare, if a patient has a history of occurrence of vesiculation and necrosis with a previous tuberculin test by any method, tuberculin testing should be avoided.
Although clinical allergy to acacia is very rare, this product contains some acacia as a stabilizer and should be used with caution in patients with known allergy to this component.
Reactivity to the test may be suppressed in patients who are receiving corticosteroids or immunosuppressive agents, or those who have recently been vaccinated with live virus vaccine such as measles, mumps, rubella, polio, etc. With a doubtful or positive reaction (vesiculation), further diagnostic procedures must be considered. These may include x-ray of the chest, microbiologic examinations of sputa and other specimens, and confirmation of the positive TINE TEST reaction (except vesiculation reactions) using the Mantoux method. In general, the TINE TEST does not need to be repeated. Antituberculous chemotherapy should not be instituted solely on the basis of a single positive TINE TEST.
When vesiculation occurs, the reaction is to be interpreted as strongly positive and a repeat test by the Mantoux method must not be attempted. Similar or more severe vesiculation with or without necrosis is likely to occur.
Adverse Reactions: Vesiculation (positive reaction), ulceration, or necrosis may occur at the test site in highly sensitive persons. Pain, pruritus and discomfort at the test site may be relieved by cold packs or by a topical glucocorticoid ointment or cream. Transient bleeding may be observed at a puncture site and is of no significance.
References:
1. Report of the Committee on the Control of Infectious Diseases. American Academy of Pediatrics, 1977.
2. Comstock, G.W., et al., The Tuberculin Skin Test, Amer. Rev. Respiratory Disease 104:769–775, No. 5 (Nov) 1971.
3. Committee on Diagnostic Skin Testing of the American Thoracic Society, The Tuberculin Test (Revised 1974), New York, American Lung Association, 1974.

How Supplied: Tuberculin, Old, Tine Test® is supplied as follows:
5 individual tests
25 individual tests in a jar
100 individual tests
250 individual tests
Storage: Tuberculin, Old, Tine Test® Units should be stored unrefrigerated below 30°C (86°F).
Military Depot and USPHS Depots
25 Tests—NSN 6505-00-890-1534

TUBERCULIN PURIFIED PROTEIN DERIVATIVE TINE TEST® (PPD) ℞

Description: The Tuberculin, Purified Protein Derivative (PPD) Tine Test® is a sterile, simple, multiple-puncture, disposable intradermal test device for the detection of tuberculin reactivity. These convenient devices are especially useful in mass tuberculosis screening programs.
Each test unit consists of a stainless steel disc attached to a light blue plastic handle. Projecting from the disc are four triangular-shaped prongs (tines) which are 2 mm long and approx-

imately 4 mm apart. The tines have been mechanically dipped into a concentrated solution of PPD. The PPD concentrate is prepared by the Seibert Process[1,2] and is stabilized with seven percent acacia (gum Arabic), thirty percent dextrose and five percent glycerol. The glycerol also acts as a humectant preventing the film on the tines from becoming brittle-dry. The final PPD concentrate is standardized against U.S. Standard PPD. The tines are dipped into concentrated PPD, capped and sterilized with ethylene oxide. The Tine Test (PPD) unit is disposable, and there is no need for syringes, needles, and other equipment necessary for the standard intradermal tests.

The Tine Test (PPD) units have been standardized by clinical evaluation in human subjects to give reactions equivalent to or more potent than 5 T.U.* of standard PPD administered intradermally in the Mantoux test. However, all multiple puncture-type devices must be regarded as screening tools and other appropriate diagnostic procedures such as the Mantoux test should be utilized for retesting reactors.

---

*(International) tuberculin units.

Data obtained from clinical studies with a total of 3,062 volunteer subjects (males and females), ranging in age from 4 to 96 years, of which 47.5% (1,443) were Mantoux positive, clearly demonstrates that Tine Test PPD, when used as a screening test to determine tuberculin reactivity is associated with very little, if any, adverse reactivity. Other than the skin test reaction itself, slight vesiculation and slight ulceration were the only adverse experiences reported. The slight to mild vesiculation was equally divided between the two tests (Tine Test, 54/3062, 1.78%, and PPD-T Mantoux, 55/3062, 1.81%). The slight ulceration observed with one subject at 72 hours was associated with the Tine Test site. Of the subjects classified as positive or intermediate by PPD-T Mantoux, 93.8% were classified similarly with the Tine Test. The results of the clinical trials revealed a 72-hour false positive rate of 10.9% and a false negative rate of 6.2%.

Indications: Tuberculin, Purified Protein Derivative Tine Test® PPD is indicated to detect tuberculin-sensitive individuals. Tine Test units are also useful in programs to determine priorities for additional testing (i.e., chest x-rays) and in epidemiological surveys to identify those areas having high levels of infection.

The frequency of repeated tuberculin tests depends on risk of exposure of the child and on the prevalence of tuberculosis in the population group. For the pediatrician's office or outpatient clinic, an annual or biennial tuberculin test, unless local circumstances clearly indicate otherwise, is appropriate. The initial test should be done at the time of, or preceding, the measles immunization.[3] The repeated testing of uninfected individuals does not sensitize to tuberculin. Among individuals with waning sensitivity to homologous or heterologous mycobacterial antigens, however, the stimulus of a tuberculin test may "boost" or increase the size of the reaction to a second test, even causing an apparent development of sensitivity in some cases.[4]

Directions For Use: Site: The volar surface of the upper one-third of the forearm, over a muscle belly, is the preferred site. Hairy areas, and areas without adequate subcutaneous tissue, e.g., concavities over a tendon or bone should be avoided.

Method of Application: Alcohol, acetone, ether, or soap and water may be used to cleanse the skin. The area must be clean and thoroughly dry before application of the Tine Test PPD.

Expose the four coated tines by removing the protective cap while holding the plastic handle. Grasp the patient's forearm firmly, since the sharp momentary sting may cause the patient to jerk his or her arm, resulting in scratching. Stretch the skin of the forearm tightly and apply the disc with the other hand. ***Hold at least one second.*** Release tension grip on forearm. Withdraw tine unit.

Sufficient pressure should be exerted so that the four puncture sites, and a circular depression of the skin from the plastic base are visible.

Local care of the skin is not necessary.

Tuberculin, Purified Protein Derivative Tine Test® PPD Unit *must never be re-used.*

Reading Reactions: Tests should be read at *72 hours.* Vesiculation or the extent of induration are the determining factors; erythema without induration is of no significance. Readings should be made in good light with the forearm slightly flexed. The size of the induration in millimeters should be determined by inspection, measuring, and palpation with gentle finger stroking. Identification of the application site is usually easy because of the distinct four-point pattern. The diameter of the largest single reaction around one of the puncture sites should be measured. With pronounced reactions, the areas of induration around the puncture sites may coalesce.

Vesiculation: *Positive Reaction.* If vesiculation is present, the test may be interpreted as positive, in which case the management of the patient is the same as that for one classified as positive to the Mantoux test.[5]

Induration, 2 mm or greater: *Interpretation.* The criterion for classifying a tuberculin skin test as positive or negative is determind by the incidence of sensitivity to the antigens of the so-called atypical mycobacteria.

Induration as small as 5 mm in the PPD-S Mantoux test (5 T.U.) may be accepted as positive in areas in which such incidence is low or non-existent. The size of induration to the Tine Test PPD which corresponds to a 5 mm induration to the Mantoux test is 2 mm. In clinical studies in which the above criteria for both tests were applied, of more than 1,800 Mantoux positive subjects only 6.3% gave negative Tine Test PPD reactions at 72 hours; of more than 1,900 Tine Test PPD positive tests, less than 11% gave negative Mantoux results.

Induration less than 2 mm: *Negative Reaction.* There is no need for retesting unless the person is a contact of a patient with tuberculosis or there is clinical evidence suggestive of the disease.[5]

Descriptive literature illustrating typical reactions is available upon request.

Precautions: Tuberculin testing should be done with caution in individuals with active tuberculosis. However, activation of quiescent lesions is rare. If a patient has a history of occurrence of vesiculation and necrosis with a previous tuberculin test by any method, tuberculin testing should be avoided.

Although clinical allergy to acacia is very rare, this product contains some acacia as stabilizer and should be used with caution in patients with known allergy to this component.

Reactivity to the test may be suppressed in patients who are receiving corticosteroids or immunosuppressive agents, or those who have recently been vaccinated with live virus vaccines such as measles, mumps, rubella, polio, etc.

With a positive reaction (vesiculation), further diagnostic procedures must be considered. These may include x-ray of the chest, microbiologic examinations of sputa and other specimens, and confirmation of the positive Tine Test reaction (except vesiculation reactions) using the Mantoux method. In general, the Tine Test does not need to be repeated. Antituberculous chemotherapy should not be instituted solely on the basis of a single positive Tine Test.

When vesiculation occurs, the reaction is to be interpreted as strongly positive and a repeat test by the Mantoux method must not be attempted. Similar or more severe vesiculation with or without necrosis is likely to occur.

Adverse Reactions: Vesiculation (positive reaction), ulceration, or necrosis may occur at the test site in highly sensitive persons. Pain, pruritis, and discomfort at the test site may be relieved by cold packs or by topical glucocorticoid ointment or cream. Transient bleeding may be observed at a puncture site and is of no significance.

How Supplied: Tuberculin, Purified Protein Derivative Tine Test® PPD is supplied as follows:

25 Individual tests in a jar
100 Individual tests

Storage: Tine Test PPD Units should be stored unrefrigerated below 30° C (86° F).

References:

1. Seibert, F. B. "Isolation and Properties of Purified Protein Derivative of Tuberculin." *Am. Rev. Tuberc.*, 30 (1934) 713.
2. Seibert, F.B., and Glenn, J.F. "Tuberculin Purified Protein Derivative—Preparation and Analysis of a Large Quantity for Standard." *Amer. Rev. Tuberc.*, 44 (1941) 9.
3. Report of the Committee on the Control of Infectious Diseases. American Academy of Pediatrics, 1977.
4. Comstock, G.W., et. al., The Tuberculin Skin Test, *Amer. Rev. Respiratory Disease* 104:769-775, No. 5 (Nov) 1971.
5. Committee on Diagnostic Skin Testing of the American Thoracic Society, The Tuberculin Test (Revised 1974), New York, American Lung Association 1974.

Lilly and Company, Eli

307 E. McCARTY ST.
INDIANAPOLIS, IN 46206

HISTALOG™ ℞

(betazole hydrochloride)
Injection, USP
For Gastric Test

Description: Histalog™ (betazole hydrochloride, Lilly) is 3-beta-aminoethylpyrazole dihydrochloride, an analog of histamine. Each ampoule contains 50 mg of Histalog in 1 ml of solution. The solution is stable and does not require refrigeration. Sodium hydroxide may have been added during manufacture to adjust the *p*H.

Actions: Histalog is similar to histamine in respect to its effect on blood pressure, gastric acid secretion, and smooth muscle. However, unlike histamine, Histalog is selective in its actions. Its primary effect is to stimulate production of gastric acid. This is much more prominent than are its other histamine-like actions.

Antihistaminic drugs do not affect the stimulation of gastric secretion produced by Histalog (or histamine).

Indications: Histalog™ (betazole hydrochloride, Lilly) is indicated in the clinical testing of gastric secretion. In the recommended dosage, it will produce stimulation of gastric secretion equal to that obtained with the usual dosage of histamine, but it has minimum effects on other organs and, as a result, produces less severe side effects.

Histalog is not recommended for use in other conditions in which histamine is used clinically.

Warnings: Patients with an allergic diathesis may react severely to Histalog™ (betazole hydrochloride, Lilly). The drug should be used with caution in patients with moderate to severe allergic disease.

Use in Pregnancy—The safety of the use of this agent during pregnancy has not been established. The potential hazards of the drug must be weighed against the possible benefits.

Precautions: Weakness and syncope may occur (*see* Overdosage and Toxic Reactions).

Continued on next page

Lilly—Cont.

Adverse Reactions: The most commonly observed side effect is flushing of the face accompanied by a sense of warmth. Headache and urticaria may also occur.
Overdosage and Toxic Reactions: Should hypotension or acute asthma follow accidental overdosage, the administration of epinephrine would be indicated.
Urticaria has been improved with the use of antihistaminics.
Administration and Dosage: Histalog™ (betazole hydrochloride, Lilly) is administered intramuscularly or subcutaneously. The dose of Histalog comparable to the usually employed dose of histamine in fractional gastric analyses (0.01 mg histamine base or 0.0275 mg histamine phosphate per kilogram of body weight) is 0.5 mg per kilogram of body weight. Therefore, the minimum effective dosage may be calculated on the basis of 0.5 mg per kilogram of body weight. If a simplified procedure is desired, a fixed amount of 50 mg (one ampoule) may be given to all adult patients of nearly average weight. This will provide a slightly higher dosage on a weight basis for most patients, but the side effects will not be significantly greater. There is a wide margin of safety in dosage, and amounts of 200 mg have been given without apparent harm but have been associated with a higher incidence and increased severity of side effects.
Histalog has been administered orally in experimental studies. The gastric and secretory response to a 100-mg oral dose of Histalog (suspended in 30 ml of water and administered through the gastric tube) was slightly greater than the response to the 50-mg subcutaneous dose of Histalog. The response to a 50-mg oral dose was significantly less than that following both the 100-mg oral and the 50-mg subcutaneous doses. Until further studies have been made, however, the oral route is not recommended for routine use.
Technique of Fractional Gastric Analysis—Testing of gastric secretion is usually performed clinically either to determine whether achlorhydria is present, as in patients suspected of having pernicious anemia, or to measure the secretory capacity of the gastric glands, as in patients suspected of having carcinoma of the stomach or peptic ulcer. Various methods are used, but only one procedure will be described.
The fasting patient is intubated with a Levin tube or a Rehfuss stomach tube, and the stomach contents are aspirated by continuous suction with a syringe. The aspirate is fractionated into 15-minute specimens. After the first 15 minutes, Histalog™ (betazole hydrochloride, Lilly) is injected. Fractional specimens are usually collected for one hour following the injection. Their acidity is determined by titration with a standard solution of sodium hydroxide or by a pH meter. In addition, the volume and the concentrations of blood, bile, and mucus in each specimen may be determined; this depends on the information desired from the procedure.
Interpretation of Results of Fractional Gastric Analysis—The gastric secretory response to the administration of Histalog™ (betazole hydrochloride, Lilly) is the same as that obtained with histamine, and the results have the same clinical significance. The response varies according to the age and general state of health of the patient, being highest in robust young adult males. In general, the fasting specimen may normally contain 0 to 2 milliequivalents of free hydrochloric acid and 1 additional milliequivalent of total hydrochloric acid in a volume up to 50 ml of gastric juice.
The maximum secretory response to Histalog begins about 45 minutes after administration and lasts approximately two and one-half hours. The secretory volume and acidity are usually increased 100 to 200 percent in the normal patient. A specimen obtained over a period of 15 minutes during the interval of maximum response will usually contain 3 to 13 milliequivalents (average 8.5) of free acid. High values are often associated with duodenal ulcer and pyloric obstruction. Low values may be found with gastric ulcer, carcinoma of the stomach, and chronic gastritis and in chronic diseases and debilitated states. Absence of free hydrochloric acid is always found in patients with pernicious anemia. Normal persons may have achlorhydria, the frequency being low in children and young adults and reaching approximately 30 percent beyond the age of 50. Normal amounts of mucus and pepsin may be found in the gastric secretion of such patients, but they are absent or nearly absent in patients with pernicious anemia.
How Supplied: (℞) *Ampoules No. 639, Histalog™ (Betazole Hydrochloride Injection, USP),* 50 mg, 1 ml, in packages of 6.

[072872A]

HISTAMINE PHOSPHATE ℞
Injection, USP
For Gastric Histamine Test

Description: Histamine is a basic substance which may be obtained by decarboxylation of the amino acid histidine. It is usually administered as the stable, water-soluble acid phosphate. Two molecules of phosphoric acid are attached to each molecule of histamine. Since the molecular weight of histamine phosphate is 307.15 and that of histamine itself is 111.15, 2.75 mg of the salt are required to obtain 1 mg of the active principle.
Actions: Histamine acts on the vascular system, smooth muscle, and exocrine glands. Histamine increases the volume and acidity of the gastric juice.
Indication: Histamine phosphate solution is intended for subcutaneous administration to test the ability of the gastric mucosa to produce hydrochloric acid.
Contraindications: The gastric histamine test is contraindicated in patients with a history of hypersensitivity to histamine products. It is contraindicated in patients with hypotension, severe hypertension, vasomotor instability, bronchial asthma (past or present), urticaria (past or present), or severe cardiac, pulmonary, or renal disease.
Warnings: Attacks of severe asthma or other serious allergic conditions may be precipitated by the administration of histamine phosphate. The possible benefit that may be derived from the gastric histamine test should be carefully weighed against the serious untoward reactions that may develop in patients with allergic diseases. Small doses by any route of administration may precipitate asthma in patients with bronchial disease. The utmost caution is advised in using histamine in such patients.
When histamine phosphate is administered, pull back on the syringe plunger before the injection is made to be sure the end of the needle is not in a blood vessel. Care should be taken to avoid accidental introduction into a vein or artery. Epinephrine, 1:1000, should be immediately available to counteract the effects of histamine.
Use in Pregnancy—The safety of this agent for use during pregnancy or lactation has not been established; therefore, the benefits must be weighed against its possible hazards to the mother and child.
The physician must carefully weigh the risk/benefit ratio when considering the use of the gastric histamine test in patients with pheochromocytoma.
Precautions: Average or large doses of histamine may cause flushing, dizziness, headache, nervousness, local or generalized allergic manifestations, marked hypertension or hypotension, tachycardia, and abdominal cramps. These reactions may be alarming and are potentially dangerous. Local reactions at the site of injection may include erythema and edema. Histamine increases the acid of the gastric juice and may cause symptoms of peptic ulcer. A large subcutaneous dose of histamine may cause severe occipital headache, blurred vision, anginal pain, a rapid drop in blood pressure, and cyanosis of the face. Overdosage may cause severe symptoms, including circulatory collapse, shock, and even death. The blood pressure and pulse should be carefully monitored during injection of histamine.
Use with caution in patients with any cardiac abnormality.
Adverse Reactions: Following the injection of an average or large dose of histamine, side effects may include such local reactions as erythema and edema and/or such systemic reactions as flushing, dizziness, headache, bronchial constriction, dyspnea, visual disturbances, faintness, syncope, urticaria, asthma, marked hypertension or hypotension, weakness, palpitation, tachycardia, nervousness, abdominal cramps, diarrhea, nausea, vomiting, metallic taste, local or generalized allergic manifestations, or collapse with convulsions.
Administration and Dosage—Gastric Histamine Test: *Histamine Test*—After the basal gastric secretion has been collected, histamine phosphate is given subcutaneously. The dose is 0.0275 mg of histamine phosphate (or 0.01 mg of the histamine base) per kg of body weight. The gastric contents are then collected in four 15-minute specimens for one hour and analyzed for volume, acidity, pH, and acid output.
Augmented Histamine Test—Initially, a suitable dose of antihistamine is administered intramuscularly, e.g., 10 mg chlorpheniramine maleate, 50 mg pyrilamine maleate, or 50 mg diphenhydramine hydrochloride.
After the conclusion of the basal secretion study, histamine phosphate is given subcutaneously in a dose of 0.04 mg per kg of body weight.
Before undertaking these procedures, the physician should thoroughly familiarize himself with the technique or methodology of performing the gastric histamine test or the augmented histamine test and with the interpretation of the results from standard reference texts.
Overdosage: Overdosage of Histamine Phosphate Injection may cause severe symptoms, including circulatory collapse, shock, and even death (*see* Warnings, Precautions, and Adverse Reactions). If accidental overdosage is discovered early, temporary application of a tourniquet proximally to the injection site may be tried to slow down the absorption of the drug.
Antidotes to histamine are the following:

Epinephrine hydrochloride, 0.1–0.5 ml of a 1:1000 aqueous solution, given subcutaneously in case of emergency due to severe reactions.

An antihistamine preparation, given orally in case of mild allergic reactions caused by the usual dose of the drug.

How Supplied: (℞) *Histamine Phosphate Injection, USP: Ampoules (Vials) No. 328,* 2.75 mg (equivalent to 1 mg histamine base) in 5 ml, 5 ml, rubber-stoppered, in singles (10 per carton); 1 ml contains 0.55 mg histamine phosphate (equivalent to 0.2 mg histamine base), with 16 mg glycerin and 2 mg phenol. Phosphoric acid may have been added to adjust the pH. *Ampoules No. 269,* 2.75 mg (equivalent to 1 mg histamine base), 1 ml, in packages of 6 and 100.

[062679]

HISTAMINE PHOSPHATE ℞
Injection, USP
Histamine Test for Pheochromocytoma

Description: Histamine is a basic substance which may be obtained by decarboxylation of the amino acid histidine. It is usually administered as the stable, water-soluble acid phosphate. Two molecules of phosphoric acid are attached to each molecule of histamine.
Since the molecular weight of histamine phosphate is 307.15 and that of histamine itself is 111.15, 2.75 mg of the salt are required to obtain 1 mg of the active principle.
Each ml of Ampoules No. 338, Histamine Phosphate Injection, USP (histamine test for pheochromocytoma), contains 0.275 mg histamine phosphate (equivalent to 0.1 mg histamine) and 9 mg sodium chloride.
Indication: Histamine Phosphate Injection may be used intravenously for the presumptive diagnosis of pheochromocytoma.
Contraindications: The histamine test for pheochromocytoma is contraindicated in the elderly or in the presence of severe hypertension.
Warnings: Attacks of severe asthma or other serious allergic conditions may be precipitated by the administration of histamine phosphate. The possible benefit that may be derived from the histamine test for pheochromocytoma should be carefully weighed against the serious untoward reactions that may develop in patients with severe allergic diseases.
Precautions: Average or large doses of histamine may cause flushing, dizziness, headache, nervousness, local or generalized allergic manifestations, marked hypertension or hypotension, tachycardia, and abdominal cramps. These reactions may be alarming and are potentially dangerous. Histamine increases the acid of the gastric juice and may cause symptoms of peptic ulcer. Small doses by any route of administration may precipitate asthma in patients with bronchial disease. The utmost caution is advised in using histamine in such patients and in those with a history of bronchial asthma.
Frequent checks of the blood pressure and pulse should be made during intravenous injections of histamine. If there is a dangerous fall in blood pressure, a prompt injection of epinephrine should be given.
A large dose of histamine may cause severe occipital headache, blurred vision, anginal pain, a rapid drop in blood pressure, and cyanosis of the face. Overdosage by the intravenous route may cause severe symptoms, including vasomotor collapse, shock, and even death.
Adverse Reactions: Following the injection of an average or large dose of histamine, side effects may include such systemic reactions as flushing, dizziness, headache, bronchial constriction, dyspnea, visual disturbances, faintness, syncope, urticaria, asthma, marked hypertension or hypotension, palpitation, tachycardia, nervousness, abdominal cramps, diarrhea, vomiting, metallic taste, local or generalized allergic manifestations, or collapse with convulsions.
Administration and Dosage—Histamine Test for Pheochromocytoma: Antihypertensive drugs, sympathomimetic agents, sedatives, and narcotics should be withheld from the patient for at least 24 hours, preferably 72 hours, before the histamine test is performed. *Food should not be withheld.*
The histamine test for pheochromocytoma is a provocative test and, therefore, is indicated only for the occasional patient who has paroxysmal signs of excessive catecholamine secretion and who has normal urinary values for assays of catecholamines and metabolites during periods when he is asymptomatic.
A well-conducted test provides information on the symptomatic and physiologic responses and changes in urinary catecholamine levels. This test is to be used only in patients in whom resting blood pressure does not exceed 150/110.
Epinephrine should be available in case a severe hypotensive response is produced. Phentolamine should be on hand to depress any alarming increase in blood pressure.
The patient rests in bed while a slow intravenous infusion of either 5 percent dextrose or isotonic saline solution is established. The blood pressure is recorded until it is stable. At that time, a two-hour period of urine collection for catecholamine assay is started. At the end of this period, histamine is rapidly administered through the infusion, and another two-hour urine collection is started.
The first dose of histamine should be 0.01 mg, or 10 mcg. This dose is provided in 0.1 ml of Ampoules No. 338 (0.275 mg histamine phosphate, or 0.1 mg histamine, in 1 ml of solution). If no response is observed within five minutes, a dose of 0.05 mg (50 mcg) should be administered. The blood pressure and pulse are to be recorded every 30 seconds for 15 minutes. The expected responses in both positive and negative tests are headache, flushing, and a decrease in blood pressure followed within two minutes by an increase.
Positive tests have been defined as—
1. An increase in blood pressure of at least 20/10 mm Hg greater than that obtained with the cold pressor test.
2. An increase in blood pressure of at least 60/40 mm Hg above the base line and greater than that with the cold pressor test.

An increase in urinary catecholamine levels from normal during the pretest control period to abnormally high during the test lessens the possibility of false-positive tests.
How Supplied: (℞) *Ampoules No. 338, Histamine Phosphate Injection, USP,* 0.275 mg (equivalent to 0.1 mg histamine), 1 ml, in packages of 6.

[111276]

TES-TAPE® OTC
(glucose enzymatic test strip)
USP

For In Vitro Diagnostic Use in Testing for the Presence and Semiquantitative Measurement of Glucose in Human Urine

Tes-Tape has been used since 1956, when Dr. A. S. Keston described the novel idea of using two enzymes simultaneously to test for glucose and Dr. J. P. Comer published data on the specificity and accuracy of Tes-Tape for the semiquantitative analysis of urine glucose.
During the development and testing of this urine test method, Tes-Tape was found to be an accurate and reliable semiquantitative method for determining urine glucose. To date, relatively few instances of faulty results have occurred with the use of Tes-Tape. Problems associated with the product are usually due to improper techniques or exposure of the tape to adverse conditions or due to drugs which have an inhibitory effect on the enzyme reaction. Considerable data may be found in the published scientific documents.
Tes-Tape is impregnated with the enzymes glucose oxidase and peroxidase and an oxidizable substrate, orthotolidine. When the tape is dipped into urine containing glucose, the glucose oxidase catalyzes the reaction of glucose in the urine with oxygen from the air to form gluconic acid and hydrogen peroxide. The enzyme peroxidase (from horseradish) then catalyzes the reaction of hydrogen peroxide and orthotolidine to form a blue color. With the addition of a yellow dye (FDC Yellow No. 5) to the paper, the possible color range of the test is extended from yellow to light green to deep blue. If no glucose is present, the tape maintains its yellow color.

Reactive Ingredient	Approximate Amount per 1.5 Inches of Tape
Glucose oxidase	3.78 units
Horseradish peroxidase	2.82 PZ units
O-tolidine	0.136 mg

Nonreactive ingredients include filter paper, FDC Yellow No. 5 coloring, buffers, stabilizers, and wetting agents.
For in vitro diagnostic use. Store below 86°F (30°C). Protect from high humidity and light. Do not use if the tape becomes dark yellow or yellowish-brown or if a 2 percent reading is not obtained when the reliability is tested, as described under the heading **Important**.
The urine should be collected in a container free of chemicals and glucose.
If the freshly voided specimen is not to be tested within four hours, it should be refrigerated.
Drugs that are known to have an inhibitory effect on the enzyme reactions include ascorbic acid (vitamin C), dipyrone, gentisic acid (a metabolite of aspirin), homogentisic acid (present in alkaptonuria), levodopa, meralluride injection, and methyldopa. The inhibiting effect is notable on the dipped part of the tape, but accurate readings may be obtained by observing the narrow band of color at the junction of the dry and wet portions. A separation of glucose from the inhibitory substances occurs as the urine travels along the dry portion of the tape.
Ingestion of more than 1.5 gm of ascorbic acid may produce urine with inhibitory action on Tes-Tape.
Specimens for storage or shipment should be refrigerated or preserved with up to 0.37 percent formaldehyde.
All materials are provided for the test and include dispenser, tape, and color chart.
Results on the color chart are expressed in percent of glucose (urine sugar) and by a corresponding arbitrary system of 0, +, + +, + + +, + + + +, representing 0, 1/10, 1/4, 1/2, 2 (or more) percent of glucose respectively.
When testing, do not place the tape on the lavatory or on paper or allow moistened portion to contact fingers. Contamination of the tape by glucose from other sources (e.g., perspiration, tears, and saliva) or with a residue of chlorine from lavatory cleansing agents can cause false-positive results.
Patients who are receiving high doses of ascorbic acid or whose urine contains dipyrone, meralluride, homogentisic acid, gentisic acid, levodopa, or methyldopa should read only the very narrow band of color in the moist portion of the tape above the level to which it was dipped into the specimen.
Very high doses of ascorbic acid may cause a false-negative test even with the above precaution. (Urinary levels of ascorbic acid in excess of 0.1 percent are necessary to block the test completely. This concentration is most likely to appear within three to seven hours after a single dose of 1.5 gm or more.)
Normal urine should test 0 percent with Tes-Tape. Persons using Tes-Tape for a screening test should report all values above 0 percent to their physician. Diabetic urine values in the range of the color chart should also be recorded and reported to the patient's physician. Measured values of 2 percent should be reported as 2 percent or more.
The overall semiquantitative accuracy of Tes-Tape originally reported in 1956 on 1000 determinations was 96 percent. This was confirmed in 1973 on 14,000 determinations over a two-year period. These data were obtained on urine samples containing concentrations of glucose at each increment shown to be measurable on the color chart. The color chart provided is based on the average color perception of many observers. Patients who have difficulty in dif-

Continued on next page

Lilly—Cont.

ferentiating color should seek the advice of their physician before using Tes-Tape.
Numerous other clinical and laboratory studies have shown that Tes-Tape is accurate in qualitative and semiquantitative determination of urine sugar. Tes-Tape is specific for glucose in urine sugar testing. Except for instances involving contamination of the tape or urine receptacle with glucose from other sources (e.g., perspiration, tears, and saliva) or with a residue of chlorine from cleansing agents, there is no known clinical situation in which a false-positive test for glucose occurs with Tes-Tape. The sensitivity of Tes-Tape is such that it will react with concentrations of 0.05 percent glucose or more. Trace reactions shown by the development of a very light yellow-green color may be observed with less than this amount of glucose.
After opening plastic wrapper, use tape within four months. It must be used prior to expiration date.
Important: The reliability of a roll of Tes-Tape may easily be checked by dipping a piece into a properly prepared glucose solution.* The tape should be removed immediately, as one would when testing a urine specimen. After two minutes have elapsed, the reading obtained when the tape is compared with the color chart should be approximately + + + + (2 percent). If such a reading is not obtained, the tape has apparently deteriorated and should not be used.
Measurements for the amount of glucose present (semiquantitative) should not be made after two minutes because the colors gradually change as the tape dries. Screening tests for the presence of glucose (qualitative) in urine may be made for several hours after the tape has dried.
The patient should consult the package insert in regard to Procedure, What to Do If Tape Breaks, and a record chart for urine sugar tests with Tes-Tape.

*If a properly prepared glucose solution is not available, any nationally known *sugar (glucose)-containing* beverage from a freshly opened bottle or can is satisfactory. (Diet cola beverages would not be satisfactory.)

How Supplied: *M-73, Tes-Tape® (Glucose Enzymatic Test Strip, USP),* dispenser package, approximately 100 tests, in single packages.
[080179]

M-73—100 tests—6505-00-559-6859A

Lincoln Laboratories, Inc.
HICKORY POINT ROAD
DECATUR, IL 62526

MULTI-TEST ℞

Multi-Test is a sterile, disposable, multiple test head applicator used to administer allergenic extracts and other skin test substances. Stock No. MH-6, Box of 6
Complete information on request. (217) 877-2531

TUBERCULIN, MONO-VACC® TEST ℞
(old tuberculin)
(U.S. 3,062,212; 3,136,314; and Re. 25,637)
25 Tests—NSN 6505-00-142-8868

Description: The TUBERCULIN, OLD, MONO-VACC® TEST is an intradermal test for the detection of tuberculin sensitivity. The TUBERCULIN, MONO-VACC® TEST provides a convenient and reliable method for determining tuberculin sensitivity of individuals in mass tuberculosis screening programs or in office, ward or clinic use. The TUBERCULIN, MONO-VACC® TEST unit consists of a sterile, disposable, multiple puncture plastic scarifier with liquid old tuberculin on the points. A plastic tube provides an airtight seal around the circular platform of the unit, assuring the sterility of the points and the test liquid until the tube is removed. The preloaded test unit is disposable, eliminating the need for special syringes, needles and syringe trays. No preservative has been added. The TUBERCULIN, MONO-VACC TEST provides the following advantages:

1. The TUBERCULIN, MONO-VACC TEST employs liquid tuberculin for instantaneous administration, eliminating two variables associated with dried tuberculin—the length of time tines are held in the skin, and the moisture content of the skin.
2. The uniform presence of liquid tuberculin on each TUBERCULIN, MONO-VACC TEST is visually assured by the user.
3. The TUBERCULIN, MONO-VACC TEST has consistently shown a high level of sensitivity when compared to intradermal PPD (5 TU). The risk of false negative results from the TUBERCULIN, MONO-VACC TEST is not statistically significant. In contrast, reported false negative results from multiple puncture tests containing tuberculin dried on the tines have ranged from a low to significant incidence.
4. The TUBERCULIN, MONO-VACC TEST produces a well defined single, usually circular reaction that is easy to read. A multiple puncture test utilizing tuberculin dried on the tines may produce 1, 2, 3, or 4 separate reactions of varying size, or two or more reactions may coalesce.
5. The TUBERCULIN, MONO-VACC TEST utilizes old tuberculin because it is generally believed that concentrated old tuberculin is very stable under ordinary conditions of storage. There are no reliable data supporting greater specificity of purified protein derivative (PPD) over old tuberculin (OT).
6. The TUBERCULIN, MONO-VACC TEST rarely produces bleeding upon administration and is well accepted by patients.

Indications: The detection of tuberculin sensitivity in individuals and mass screening for tuberculin sensitivity in large population groups. Routine tuberculin testing is recommended at 12 to 15 months of age, preferably just before measles vaccination. The frequency of repeated tuberculin tests depends on the risk of exposure and the prevalence of tuberculosis in the population group. There is a common misconception that most adults have been infected, whereas in truth, many have not. The tuberculin test is now as useful in adults as in children. Repeated testing of the uninfected individual does not sensitize to tuberculin. Repeated testing, however, may have a "booster" effect in persons with low degrees of sensitivity to homologous or heterologous mycobacterial antigens.
Warning: Discard MONO-VACC ring and tube containing tuberculin after use. DO NOT REUSE.
Precautions: Tuberculin testing should be done with caution in persons with active tuberculosis. However, activation of quiescent lesions is not to be expected.
Do not apply the MONO-VACC TEST on acnic skin, hairy areas or areas without adequate subcutaneous tissue.
Tuberculin sensitivity may decrease or disappear temporarily as a result of: febrile illness; measles and other exanthemas; live virus vaccination; sarcoidosis; overwhelming miliary or pulmonary tuberculosis; the administration of adrenal corticosteroids or immunosuppressive drugs.
Adverse Reactions: Vesiculation, ulceration, or necrosis may occur in highly sensitive subjects at site of test. Pain or pruritis at test site may be relieved by topical glucocorticoid ointment or ice packs.
Dosage and Administration: The activity per test is comparable to or greater than 5 tuberculin units (5 TU) administered by the Mantoux method.
Cleanse volar surface of mid-forearm with alcohol, ether, or acetone. Remove plastic tube that surrounds the points. With skin taut, press loaded points firmly into cleansed site.
Reading the Reaction: The test should be read 48 to 96 hours following administration. With a positive reaction, local erythema may or may not be observed. Erythema should be disregarded. The sole criterion for a positive reaction is palpable induration. The presence of palpable induration (even 1 to 2 mm.) indicates a positive reaction. A negative reaction is indicated by complete absence of induration.
As with all screening procedures, positive MONO-VACC reactions should be confirmed by a standard Mantoux (PPD, 5 TU) Test and possibly other diagnostic test procedures such as chest x-ray and microbiological examination of sputa and other specimens.
Descriptive literature illustrating typical reactions is available on request.
How Supplied: Box of 25 tests, Stock No. MT-25.
NDC 0289-7724-25.
Store at 15°–30° C. (59°–86° F.).

Parke-Davis
DIVISION OF WARNER-LAMBERT COMPANY
201 TABOR ROAD
MORRIS PLAINS, NJ 07950

APLISOL® ℞
(tuberculin purified protein derivative, diluted)
Stabilized Solution

Description: Aplisol (tuberculin PPD, diluted) is an aqueous solution of a purified protein fraction isolated from culture filtrates of human-type strains of *Mycobacterium tuberculosis* by the method of F B Seibert. This product is made from a single master lot (No. 974777) to eliminate lot-to-lot variation inherent in manufacturing. The solution is stabilized with polysorbate (Tween) 80, buffered with potassium and sodium phosphates, and contains approximately 0.35% phenol as a preservative.
The product is clinically equivalent in potency to the standard PPD-S* (5 TU† per 0.1 ml) of the U S Public Health Service, National Center for Disease Control, and is ready for immediate use without further dilution. The 5-TU dose of tuberculin PPD intradermally (Mantoux) is recommended as the standard tuberculin test, and tuberculin PPD is recommended by the American Lung Association as an aid in the detection of infection with *M tuberculosis.* Reactions to the Mantoux test are interpreted on the basis of a quantitative measurement of the response to a specific dose (5 TU PPD-S or equivalent) of tuberculin PPD. Other dosages are regarded as having no demonstrable usefulness in ordinary practice. Accordingly, Aplisol is available in only one potency (5 TU equivalent) and the use of this potency only is recommended. The selection of 5 TU as the test dose is based upon data indicating that (1) the 5-TU dose gives measurable reactions in over 95% of the known tuberculous infected; (2) doses larger than 5 TU might elicit reactions not caused by tuberculous infection; and (3) nonreactors to doses considerably less than 5 TU are not accepted as negative but are retested with a stronger dose.
This product meets all applicable standards.
Indications: Tuberculin PPD is recommended by the American Lung Association as an aid in the detection of infection with *M tuberculosis.* The standard tuberculin test recommended employs the intradermal (Mantoux)

test using a 5-TU dose of tuberculin PPD. The 0.1-ml test dose of Aplisol (tuberculin PPD, diluted) is equivalent to the 5-TU dose recommended as clinically established and standardized with PPD-S.

Warnings: Tuberculin should not be administered to known tuberculin-positive reactors because of the severity of reactions (eg, vesiculation, ulceration, or necrosis) that may occur at the test site in very highly sensitive individuals.

Avoid injecting tuberculin subcutaneously. If this occurs, no local reaction develops, but a general febrile reaction and/or acute inflammation around old tuberculous lesions may occur in highly sensitive individuals.

Precautions: A separate, heat-sterilized syringe and needle, or a sterile, disposable unit should be used for each individual patient to prevent possible transmission of homologous serum hepatitis virus and other infectious agents from one person to another.

Syringes that have previously been used with histoplasmin, blastomycin, and other antigens should not be used for tuberculin.

As with any biological product, epinephrine should be immediately available in case an anaphylactoid or acute hypersensitivity reaction occurs.

Adverse Reactions: In highly sensitive individuals, strongly positive reactions including vesiculation, ulceration, or necrosis may occur at the test site. Cold packs or topical steroid preparations may be employed for symptomatic relief of the associated pain, pruritis, and discomfort.

Strongly positive test reactions may result in scarring at the test site.

Dosage and Administration:

Standard Method (Mantoux Test)

The Mantoux test is performed by intradermally injecting with a syringe and needle exactly 0.1 ml of tuberculin PPD, diluted. The result is read 48 to 72 hours later and induration only is considered in interpreting the test.

The standard test is performed as follows.

1. The site of the test is usually the flexor or dorsal surface of the forearm about 4 inches below the elbow. Other skin sites may be used, but the flexor surface of the forearm is preferred.
2. The skin at the injection site is cleansed with 70% alcohol and allowed to dry.
3. The test material is administered with a tuberculin syringe (0.5 or 1.0 ml) fitted with a short (½ inch) 26- or 27-gauge needle.
4. The syringe and needle should be of a sterile, disposable, single-use type or should have been sterilized by autoclaving, boiling, or by the use of dry heat. A separate, sterile unit should be used for each person tested.
5. The diaphragm of the vial stopper should be wiped with 70% alcohol.
6. The needle is inserted through the stopper diaphragm of the inverted vial. Exactly 0.1 ml is filled into the syringe, with care being taken to exclude air bubbles and to maintain the lumen of the needle filled.
7. The point of the needle is inserted into the most superficial layers of the skin with the needle bevel pointing upward. As the tuberculin solution is injected, a pale bleb 6 to 10 mm in size (⅜ inch) will rise over the point of the needle. This is quickly absorbed and no dressing is required.

In the event the injection is delivered subcutaneously (ie, no bleb will form), or if a significant part of the dose leaks from the injection site, the test should be repeated immediately at another site at least 5 cm (2 inches) removed.

The Mantoux test is the standard of comparison for all other tuberculin tests.

Aplisol is a stabilized solution of tuberculin PPD. Data indicates that Aplisol is stable when prefilled into syringes and stored in a refrigerator for up to 30 days. However, the practice of storing such prefilled syringes is not recommended as good practice because of the increased potential for contamination.

Interpretation of Tuberculin Reaction

Readings of Mantoux reactions should be made during the period from 48 to 72 hours after the injection. Induration only should be considered in interpreting the test. The diameter of induration should be measured transversely to the long axis of the forearm and recorded in millimeters. Erythema of less than 10 mm should be disregarded. If the area of erythema is greater than 10 mm and induration is absent, the injection may have been made too deeply and retesting is indicated.

Reactions should be interpreted as follows.

Positive—Induration measuring 10 mm or more. This indicates hypersensitivity to tuberculoprotein and should be interpreted as positive for past or present infection with *M tuberculosis.*

Doubtful—Induration measuring 5 to 9 mm. Retesting is indicated using a different site of injection. Evaluation to rule out cross-reaction from other mycobacterial infection should be considered.

Negative—Induration of less than 5 mm. This indicates a lack of hypersensitivity to tuberculoprotein and tuberculosis infection is highly unlikely.

It should be noted that reactivity to tuberculin may be depressed or suppressed for as long as four weeks by viral infections, live virus vaccines (ie, measles, smallpox, polio, rubella, and mumps), or by the administration of corticosteroids. Malnutrition may also have a similar effect. When of diagnostic importance, a negative test should be accepted as proof that hypersensitivity is absent only after normal reactivity to nonspecific irritants has been demonstrated.

A child who is known to have been exposed to a tuberculous adult must not be adjudged free of infection until he has a negative tuberculin reaction at least 10 weeks after contact with the tuberculous person has ceased.

A positive tuberculin reaction does not necessarily signify the presence of active disease. Further diagnostic procedures should be carried out before a diagnosis of tuberculosis is made.

How Supplied:

N 0071-4525-03 (Bio 1525)
1 ml (10 tests)—rubber
diaphragm-capped vial
(NSN 6505-00-117-8783)

N 0071-4525-08 (Bio 1607)
5 ml (50 tests)—rubber
diaphragm-capped vial
(NSN 6505-00-105-0102)

This product should be stored at 2 to 8 C (36 to 46 F), and protected from light.

AHFS 36:84 **WA**

---

*PPD-S (No. 49608) World Health Organization International PPD-Tuberculin Standard (PPD-S is a dried powder from which WHO and U S Standard tuberculin solutions are made.)
†U S Tuberculin Unit

APLITEST® ℞

(tuberculin purified protein derivative)
Multiple-Puncture Device

Description: Aplitest (tuberculin PPD) is a sterile, single-use, multiple-puncture type device for use in determining the tuberculin sensitivity status of individuals. These convenient, disposable devices are especially useful in mass tuberculosis screening programs. The product packaging also facilitates the use of Aplitest units for testing of individual patients in office, ward, or clinic settings.

Each Aplitest unit consists of a cylindrical plastic holder bearing four equally spaced stainless steel tines at one end. The tines have been coated by dipping in a solution of tuberculin PPD and dried.

These devices are designed so that the narrow (tine-bearing) end of each unit fits into the hollow, handle portion of the adjacent unit (or into a protective cap) to protect the tines and maintain their sterility.

The purified tuberculin protein fraction is isolated from culture filtrates of human-type strains of *Mycobacterium tuberculosis* by the method of Florence B Seibert. Purified tuberculin protein solution is prepared from a single master lot (No. 975302) to eliminate lot-to-lot variation.

The tuberculin solution which is applied to the tines is buffered with potassium and sodium phosphates and contains approximately 0.5% phenol as a preservative.

Tuberculin PPD is employed as the diagnostic reagent because, in studies by Parke-Davis, it was demonstrated to offer greater negative and overall test agreement with the Mantoux tests than did Old Tuberculin. In clinical trials comparing multiple-puncture devices with Old Tuberculin-coated tines to those coated with tuberculin PPD, the Old Tuberculin devices engendered a significantly greater incidence of false-positive reactions than did the tuberculin PPD devices.

Aplitest has been standardized by clinical studies in human subjects against 5 TU* of PPD-S administered intradermally by the Mantoux test and guidelines relating response to the two treatments have been formulated. (See Interpretation of Response section.)

The incidence of false-positive reactions engendered by Aplitest is significantly reduced relative to the rate associated with the OT-coated tine. However, all multiple-puncture type devices should be regarded as screening tools and appropriate diagnostic procedures (eg, Mantoux test with tuberculin PPD diluted, Aplisol®), should be employed for retesting "doubtful" reactors.

Indications: Aplitest is indicated to detect tuberculin-sensitive individuals. Aplitest units are also useful in programs to establish priorities for additional testing (ie, chest x-rays) and in epidemiological surveys to identify areas with high levels of infection.

Regular periodic (annual) testing of tuberculin-negative persons is recommended and is especially valuable because the conversion of an individual from negative to positive is highly indicative of recent tuberculosis infection. Repeated testing of the uninfected individual does not sensitize to tuberculin. In persons with waning sensitivity to homologous or heterologous mycobacterial antigens, however, the stimulus of a tuberculin test may boost or increase the size of reaction to a second test, even causing an apparent development of sensitivity in some instances.

Warning: Tuberculin should not be administered to known tuberculin-positive reactors because of the severity of reactions (eg, vesiculation, ulceration, or necrosis) that may occur at the test site in very highly sensitive individuals.

Precautions: A separate, sterile unit must be used for each individual patient and disposed of after use.

As with any biological product, epinephrine should be immediately available in case an anaphylactoid or acute hypersensitivity reaction occurs.

Continued on next page

This product information was prepared in October, 1978. On these and other Parke-Davis Products, detailed information may be obtained by addressing PARKE-DAVIS, Division of Warner-Lambert Company, Morris Plains, NJ 07950.

Parke-Davis—Cont.

Sensitivity may decrease or disappear temporarily during or immediately following severe febrile illness, measles, and other exanthemas, live virus vaccination, sarcoidosis, overwhelming miliary or pulmonary tuberculosis, and the administration of corticosteroids or immunosuppressive drugs. Severe malnutrition may also have a similar effect.
A positive tuberculin reaction does not necessarily signify the presence of active disease. Further diagnostic procedures should be carried out before a diagnosis of tuberculosis is made.
Adverse Reactions: In highly sensitive individuals, strongly positive reactions including vesiculation, ulceration, or necrosis may occur at the test site. Cold packs or topical steroid preparations may be employed for symptomatic relief of the associated pain, pruritis, and discomfort.
Strongly positive test reactions may result in scarring at the test site.
Minimal bleeding may be experienced at a puncture site. This occurs infrequently and does not affect the interpretation of the test.
Dosage and Administration: Each Aplitest unit provides for the intradermal administration of one test-dose of tuberculin PPD.
Method of Application
1. The preferred site of the test is the flexor surface of the forearm about 4 inches below the elbow. Other suitable skin sites, such as the dorsal surface of the forearm, may be used. Areas without adequate subcutaneous tissue, such as over a tendon, should be avoided.
2. The skin at the test site should be cleansed with 70% alcohol, or other suitable agents, and allowed to dry thoroughly.
3. To expose the four impregnated tines, grasp the device (top one if stacked) and twist to break the perforated label seal. To prevent loss of sterility of the other units in a stack, the top unit must always be removed first and the remaining ones in sequence. Care should be taken to avoid breaking the seals on the remaining units when the end unit is removed.
4. Grasp the patient's forearm firmly to stretch the skin taut at the test site and to prevent any jerking motion of the arm that could cause scratching with the tines.
5. Apply the Aplitest unit firmly and without twisting to the test area for approximately one second. Sufficient pressure should be exerted to assure that all four tines have penetrated the skin of the test area.
6. Dispose of used units in a manner to avoid accidents. Do not re-use.
Interpretation of Response: Reading of reactions should be made during the period from 48 to 72 hours after application of Aplitest and should be conducted under good lighting conditions. Induration only should be considered in interpreting the test. Erythema should be disregarded. The diameter of the induration of the greatest response at any of the four puncture points should be determined by visual inspection and palpation. If there is coalescence of reaction, the largest diameter of coalescent induration should be measured and recorded.
The American Thoracic Society recommendeds that responses to all multiple-puncture tuberculin skin test devices be interpreted as follows. If vesiculation is present, the test may be interpreted as positive. If vesiculation is not present, induration of 2 mm or more is considered as a doubtful reaction and should be confirmed by Mantoux testing. Induration of less than 2 mm and/or erythema of any size is a negative test and there is no need for re-testing.
In clinical studies with Aplitest, it has been determined that coalescence of the induration around two or more puncture sites corresponds more than 90% of the time to 10 mm or more of induration in the same individual tested by Mantoux at the 5-TU level with PPD-S.†
Thus, the following criteria of interpretation have been established.
Vesiculation—Positive Reaction
The test should be interpreted as positive and the management of the subject is the same as that for one classified as positive by Mantoux test.
Coalescence of induration from two or more puncture points—Doubtful Reaction
A subject with a coalescent reaction may be considered for Mantoux retest.
However, more than 90% of the time this reaction was equivalent to a reaction of 10 mm or more of induration with PPD-S (5 TU) administered by Mantoux test. Other criteria, such as contact with tuberculosis patients and case history, should be considered to determine the likelihood that such a reaction is considered positive.
2 mm or more of induration without coalescence—Doubtful Reaction
Reactions of this size range reflect sensitivity that can result from infection with either atypical mycobacteria or *M tuberculosis;* hence, they are classified as doubtful. A standard Mantoux test should be done on all subjects in this group. Management should be based on the reaction to the Mantoux test, as well as other clinical considerations.
Less than 2 mm of induration—Negative Reaction
There is no need for retesting unless the individual is in contact with a case of tuberculosis or there is clinical evidence suggestive of the disease.
Selection of the appropriate criteria for interpretation of response to the tuberculin PPD Aplitest should be made in accordance with the objectives of the specific testing program and with consideration of the history and clinical status of the individuals.
How Supplied:
N 0071-4589-03 (Bio 1589) 25-test package, five stacks of five Aplitest units
N 0071-4589-01 (Bio 1590) 25-test package, 25 individually capped Aplitest units in a dispensing package
Aplitest (tuberculin PPD, multiple-puncture device) units should be stored at no warmer than 30 C (86 F).
AHFS 36:84 **UE**

*US (International) Tuberculin Units

†Purified Protein Derivative (Seibert). Lot No. 49608, the standard adopted by the World Health Organization in 1952 as International PPD Tuberculin and used to prepare the official US Public Health Service 5-TU solution of tuberculin for skin testing known as PPD-S.

HISTOPLASMIN, DILUTED ℞
(Stabilized Solution)

Description: Histoplasmin is an aqueous solution containing standardized, sterile culture filtrates of *Histoplasma capsulatum* grown on liquid synthetic medium described by Emmons et al.
The solution is stabilized with 8 ppm polysorbate (Tween) 80, buffered with potassium and sodium phosphates and contains 0.5% phenol as a preservative. The product is clinically equivalent in potency to the US Reference Standard, Lot H-42(1:100), of the US Public Health Service, National Center for Disease Control, and is ready for immediate use without further dilution. The vial contains sufficient excess to allow withdrawal of 10 doses of 0.1 ml.
This product meets all applicable standards.
Indications: Histoplasmin is employed as an aid in the diagnosis of histoplasmosis and the differentiation of possible histoplasmosis from coccidioidomycosis, sarcoidosis, and other mycotic or bacterial infections, and in the interpretation of roentgenographic plates showing pulmonary infiltration and calcification.
Precautions: Inject intradermally only.
Doses greater than that recommended may produce severe erythema and induration followed by necrosis and ulceration that may last for several weeks.
A separate, sterile syringe and needle should be used for each individual patient to prevent transmission of hepatitis B virus and other infectious agents from one person to another.
As with any biological product, epinephrine should be immediately available in case an anaphylactoid or acute hypersensitivity reaction occurs.
Adverse Reactions: Hypersensitivity reactions, such as urticaria, shortness of breath, and excessive perspiration, may occur.
In highly sensitive individuals, strongly positive reactions including vesiculation, ulceration, or necrosis may occur at the test site. Cold packs or topical steroid preparations may be employed for symptomatic relief of the associated pain, pruritis, and discomfort. Strongly positive test reactions may result in scarring at the test site.
Dosage and Administration: The skin test is performed by injecting 0.1 ml intradermally into the flexor surface of the forearm. The site of injection is first cleansed with 70% alcohol and allowed to dry. A tuberculin syringe (one that has not been used for tuberculin) and a 26-gauge x ⅜ inch or 27- gauge x ½ inch needle is used. If injections are correctly made, a small bleb will rise over the needle point. The reactions should be read in a well-lighted room 48 to 72 hours after injection.
If serological studies are clinically indicated, the blood sample should preferably be drawn prior to administering the skin test. If not obtained prior to skin testing, the sample may be obtained within 48 to 96 hours following the skin test injection. After the forementioned time period, a rise in titer, as associated with a positive skin test, may occur.
Interpretation of Reaction: The reaction should be described and measured in terms of mm of induration and degree of reaction (from slight induration to vesiculation and necrosis). In many studies reported in the literature, a reaction of 5 mm or greater induration is considered to be positive. In case of doubt, and if clinically indicated, the test should be repeated but only after obtaining serum for antibody titer.
A positive histoplasmin reaction may be indicative of a past infection or a mild, subacute, or chronic infection with *H capsulatum* or immunologically related organisms, such as *Blastomyces* or *Coccidioides* species. Reaction may also denote improvement in cases of serious illness of symptomatic histoplasmosis that previously may have been histoplasmin-negative. Histoplasmin is of little value in diagnosing acute fulminating infections because a negative reaction usually occurs in such cases. In mild infections, repeatedly negative reactions may suggest the exclusion of *Histoplasma* as the causative agent. It is advised that the tuberculin test be employed in conjunction with histoplasmin in order to exclude the possibility of tuberculosis. The histoplasmin skin test sometimes causes elevation of serum antibody titers to histoplasmin.
Furcolow et al employed three criteria to distinguish lesions associated with histoplasmin sensitivity from those due to other causes. These are: (1) the individual has skin sensitivity to histoplasmin but not tuberculin; (2) lesions must persist for two months (to exclude transient pneumonic lesions); and (3) laboratory and clinical examinations to exclude tuberculosis, Boeck's sarcoid, sarcoidosis, Hodgkins' disease, etc. These criteria might be helpful in the interpretation of roentgenographic findings.

How Supplied: N 0071-4499-03 (Bio 4499)—rubber diaphragm-capped vial
Each vial contains sufficient Histoplasmin, Diluted (stabilized solution), to deliver ten 0.1 ml doses.
AHFS 36:32 **WB**

Roche Laboratories

Division of Hoffmann-La Roche Inc.
NUTLEY, NEW JERSEY 07110

PROSTIGMIN® INJECTABLE ℞

(neostigmine methylsulfate/Roche)
Ampuls • Vials

The following text is complete prescribing information based on official labeling in effect August 1, 1979.

Description: Prostigmin (neostigmine methylsulfate/Roche), a cholinergic stimulant, enhances cholinergic action by facilitating the transmission of impulses across the myoneural junction. It inhibits the destruction of acetylcholine by acetylcholinesterase. Its effect is similar to that of physostigmine (eserine) but, in therapeutic doses, it is less likely to cause disturbing side effects. It also has a direct effect on voluntary muscle fibers[1] and possibly on autonomic ganglion cells and neurons of the central nervous system.[2]

Chemically, neostigmine methylsulfate is the dimethylcarbamate of (*m*-hydroxyphenyl) trimethylammonium methylsulfate. It has a molecular weight of 334.4.

Animal Pharmacology: The drug has been studied in many species of animals but most extensively in the cat. These studies indicate that it inhibits or inactivates acetylcholine esterases and thus allows the accumulation of acetylcholine at cholinergic sites. Neostigmine labeled with ^{14}C in one of the methyl groups of the quaternary nitrogen has been used to investigate the excretion and metabolism of neostigmine after administration to cats by stomach tube. About 10% of the dose is excreted in the urine in 5 hours and 20% after 24 hours. Approximately 50% was detected in the intestinal contents and feces 24 hours after administration. The peak concentration in the liver occurs about 2 hours after injection and is equivalent to 2% of the dose.[3]

The LD_{50} of neostigmine methylsulfate in mice is 0.3 ± 0.02 mg/kg intravenously, 0.54 ± 0.03 mg/kg subcutaneously, and 0.395 ± 0.025 mg/kg intramuscularly; in rats the LD_{50} is 0.315 ± 0.019 mg/kg intravenously, 0.445 ± 0.032 mg/kg subcutaneously, and 0.423 ± 0.032 mg/kg intramuscularly.

Indications: Prostigmin is indicated in the prevention and treatment of postoperative distention and urinary retention. It may be utilized as a screening test for early pregnancy. It is of use in the treatment of delayed menstruation. Prostigmin is of particular use in the symptomatic control of myasthenia gravis. It can be used as a diagnostic test for myasthenia gravis; however, Tensilon® (edrophonium chloride/Roche) is usually recommended as a diagnostic test for myasthenia gravis because of its more rapid onset and brief duration of action. Prostigmin can also be used as an antidote for tubocurarine.

Contraindications: Prostigmin is contraindicated in mechanical intestinal or urinary obstruction. It is contraindicated in patients with known sensitivity to the drug.

Precautions: Prostigmin should be used with caution in asthmatic patients. When large doses of Prostigmin are administered, the prior or simultaneous injection of atropine sulfate may be advisable. Separate syringes should be used for Prostigmin and atropine. Because of the possibility of hypersensitivity in an occasional patient, atropine and antishock medication should always be readily available.

As is true of all cholinergic drugs, overdosage of Prostigmin may result in cholinergic crisis, a state characterized by increasing muscle weakness which, through involvement of the muscles of respiration, may lead to death. Myasthenic crisis due to an increase in the severity of the disease is also accompanied by extreme muscle weakness and thus may be difficult to distinguish from cholinergic crisis on a symptomatic basis. Such differentiation is extremely important, since increases in doses of Prostigmin or other drugs in this class in the presence of cholinergic crisis or of a refractory or "insensitive" state could have grave consequences. Osserman and Genkins[4] indicate that the two types of crises may be differentiated by the use of Tensilon® (edrophonium chloride/Roche) as well as by clinical judgment. The treatment of the two conditions obviously differs radically. Whereas the presence of *myasthenic crisis* requires more intensive anticholinesterase therapy, *cholinergic crisis,* according to Osserman and Genkins,[4] calls for the prompt withdrawal of all drugs of this type. The immediate use of atropine in cholinergic crisis is also recommended.

Atropine may also be used to abolish or obtund gastrointestinal side effects or other muscarinic reactions; but such use, by masking signs of overdosage, can lead to inadvertent induction of cholinergic crisis.

For detailed information on the management of patients with myasthenia gravis, the physician is referred to one of the excellent reviews such as those by Osserman and Genkins[5] or Grob.[6]

Adverse Reactions: The side effects of Prostigmin are most commonly related to overdosage and generally are of two varieties, muscarinic and nicotinic. Among the former group are nausea, vomiting, diarrhea, abdominal cramps, increased salivation, increased bronchial secretions, miosis, and diaphoresis. Nicotinic side effects are comprised chiefly of muscle cramps, fasciculation, and weakness. Muscarinic side effects can usually be counteracted by atropine.

Dosage: *Prevention of postoperative distention and urinary retention:* One ml of the 1:4000 solution (0.25 mg) subcutaneously or intramuscularly as soon as possible after operation; repeat every 4 to 6 hours for two or three days.

Treatment of postoperative distention: One ml of the 1:2000 solution (0.5 mg) subcutaneously or intramuscularly, as required.

Treatment of urinary retention: One ml of the 1:2000 solution (0.5 mg) subcutaneously or intramuscularly. If urination does not occur within an hour, the patient should be catheterized. After the patient has voided, or the bladder has been emptied, continue the 0.5 mg injections every three hours for at least 5 injections.

Screening test for early pregnancy and treatment of delayed menstruation: One ml of the 1:1000 solution (1 mg) injected intramuscularly daily for three successive days. The patient may be assumed to be pregnant if bleeding does not occur within 72 hours after the third injection, providing pelvic lesions, systemic disease, the menopause and endocrine disorders have been ruled out.

Symptomatic control of myasthenia gravis: One ml of the 1:2000 solution (0.5 mg) subcutaneously or intramuscularly. Subsequent doses should be based on the individual patient's response. In most patients, however, oral treatment with Prostigmin tablets, 15 mg each, is adequate for control of symptoms.

As an antidote for tubocurarine: When Prostigmin is administered intravenously, it is recommended that atropine sulfate (0.6 to 1.2 mg) also be given intravenously using separate syringes. Some authorities have recommended that the atropine be injected several minutes before the Prostigmin rather than concomitantly. The usual dose is 0.5 to 2 mg Prostigmin given by *slow* intravenous injection, repeated as required; however, only in exceptional cases should the total dose of Prostigmin exceed 5 mg. It is recommended that the patient be well ventilated and a patent airway maintained until complete recovery of normal respiration is assured. The optimum time to administer the drug is when the patient is being hyperventilated and the carbon dioxide level of the blood is low. It should never be administered in the presence of high concentrations of halothane or cyclopropane. In small children, cardiac cases, and severely ill patients it is advisable to titrate the exact dose of Prostigmin required, using a peripheral nerve stimulator device. In the presence of a bradycardia, the pulse rate should be increased to about 80/minute with atropine before administering neostigmine.

How Supplied: *Prostigmin 1:2000, 1-ml ampuls (boxes of 10)*—Each ml contains 0.5 mg neostigmine methylsulfate/Roche compounded with 0.2% parabens (methyl and propyl) as preservatives and pH adjusted to approximately 5.9 with sodium hydroxide.

Prostigmin 1:4000, 1-ml ampuls (boxes of 10)—Each ml contains 0.25 mg neostigmine methylsulfate/Roche compounded with 0.2% parabens (methyl and propyl) as preservatives and pH adjusted to approximately 5.9 with sodium hydroxide.

Prostigmin 1:1000, 10-ml multiple dose vials—Each ml contains 1 mg neostigmine methylsulfate/Roche compounded with 0.45% phenol as preservative, 0.2 mg sodium acetate, and pH adjusted to approximately 5.9 with acetic acid and sodium hydroxide.

Prostigmin 1:2000, 10-ml multiple dose vials—Each ml contains 0.5 mg neostigmine methylsulfate/Roche compounded with 0.45% phenol as preservative, 0.2 mg sodium acetate, and pH adjusted to approximately 5.9 with acetic acid and sodium hydroxide.

References:

1. Riker, W. F., and Wescoe, W. C.: *J. Pharmacol. & Exper. Therap. 88*:58, 1946.
2. Goodman, L. S., and Gilman, A.: *The Pharmacological Basis of Therapeutics,* 3rd ed., New York, Macmillan, 1965, p. 459.
3. Roberts, J. B., *et al.*: *Biochem. Pharm. 15*:71, 1966.
4. Osserman, K. E. and Genkins, G.: *J.A.M.A. 183*:97, 1963.
5. Osserman, K. E. and Genkins, G.: *New York J. Med. 61*:2076, 1961.
6. Grob, D.: *Arch. Int. Med. 108*:615, 1961.

TENSILON® ℞

(edrophonium chloride/Roche)
Injectable Solution
ampuls • vials

The following text is complete prescribing information based on official labeling in effect August 1, 1979.

Description: Tensilon is a short and rapid-acting cholinergic drug. Chemically, edrophonium chloride is ethyl (*m*-hydroxyphenyl)-dimethylammonium chloride.

10-ml vials: Each ml contains, in a sterile solution, 10 mg edrophonium chloride/Roche compounded with 0.45% phenol and 0.2% sodium sulfite as preservatives, buffered with sodium citrate and citric acid, and pH adjusted to approximately 5.4.

1-ml ampuls: Each ml contains, in a sterile solution, 10 mg edrophonium chloride/Roche compounded with 0.2% sodium sulfite, buffered with sodium citrate and citric acid, and pH adjusted to approximately 5.4.

Actions: Tensilon is an anticholinesterase drug. Its pharmacological action is due primarily to the inhibition or inactivation of acetylcholinesterase at sites of cholinergic transmission. Its effect is manifest within 30 to 60 seconds after injection and lasts an average of 10 minutes.

Continued on next page

Roche—Cont.

Indications: Tensilon is recommended for the differential diagnosis of myasthenia gravis and as an adjunct in the evaluation of treatment requirements in this disease. It may also be used for evaluating emergency treatment in myasthenic crises. Because of its brief duration of action, it is not recommended for maintenance therapy in myasthenia gravis.
Tensilon is also useful whenever a curare antagonist is needed to reverse the neuromuscular block produced by curare, tubocurarine, gallamine triethiodide or dimethyl-tubocurarine. It is *not* effective against decamethonium bromide and succinylcholine chloride. It may be used adjunctively in the treatment of respiratory depression caused by curare overdosage.
Contraindications: Known hypersensitivity to anticholinesterase agents; intestinal and urinary obstructions of mechanical type.
Warnings: Whenever anticholinesterase drugs are used for testing, a syringe containing 1 mg of atropine sulfate should be immediately available to be given in aliquots intravenously to counteract severe cholinergic reactions which may occur in the hypersensitive individual, whether he is normal or myasthenic. Tensilon should be used with caution in patients with bronchial asthma or cardiac dysrhythmias. The transient bradycardia which sometimes occurs can be relieved by atropine sulfate. Isolated instances of cardiac and respiratory arrest following administration of Tensilon have been reported. It is postulated that these are vagotonic effects.
Usage in Pregnancy: The safety of Tensilon during pregnancy or lactation in humans has not been established. Therefore, use of Tensilon in women who may become pregnant requires weighing the drug's potential benefits against its possible hazards to mother and child.
Precautions: Patients may develop "anticholinesterase insensitivity" for brief or prolonged periods. During these periods the patients should be carefully monitored and may need respiratory assistance. Dosages of anticholinesterase drugs should be reduced or withheld until patients again become sensitive to them.
Adverse Reactions: Careful observation should be made for severe cholinergic reactions in the hyperreactive individual. The myasthenic patient in crisis who is being tested with Tensilon should be observed for bradycardia or cardiac standstill and cholinergic reactions if an overdose is given. The following reactions common to anticholinesterase agents may occur, although not all of these reactions have been reported with the administration of Tensilon, probably because of its short duration of action and limited indications: **Eye:** Increased lacrimation, pupillary constriction, spasm of accommodation, diplopia, conjunctival hyperemia. **CNS:** Convulsions, dysarthria, dysphonia, dysphagia. **Respiratory:** Increased tracheobronchial secretions, laryngospasm, bronchiolar constriction, paralysis of muscles of respiration, central respiratory paralysis. **Cardiac:** Arrhythmias (especially bradycardia), fall in cardiac output leading to hypotension. **G.I.:** Increased salivary, gastric and intestinal secretion, nausea, vomiting, increased peristalsis, diarrhea, abdominal cramps. **Skeletal Muscle:** Weakness, fasciculations. **Miscellaneous:** Increased urinary frequency and incontinence, diaphoresis.
Dosage and Administration: *Tensilon Test in the Differential Diagnosis of Myasthenia Gravis:*[1-8]
Intravenous Dosage (Adults): A tuberculin syringe containing 1 ml (10 mg) of Tensilon is prepared with an intravenous needle, and 0.2 ml (2 mg) is injected intravenously within 15 to 30 seconds. The needle is left *in situ*. *Only* if no reaction occurs after 45 seconds is the remaining 0.8 ml (8 mg) injected. If a cholinergic reaction (muscarinic side effects, skeletal muscle fasciculations and increased muscle weakness) occurs after injection of 0.2 ml (2 mg), the test is discontinued and atropine sulfate 0.4 mg to 0.5 mg is administered intravenously. After one-half hour the test may be repeated.
Intramuscular Dosage (Adults): In adults with inaccessible veins, dosage for intramuscular injection is 1 ml (10 mg) of Tensilon. Subjects who demonstrate hyperreactivity to this injection (cholinergic reaction), should be retested after one-half hour with 0.2 ml (2 mg) of Tensilon intramuscularly to rule out false-negative reactions.
Dosage (Children): The intravenous testing dose of Tensilon in children weighing up to 75 lbs is 0.1 ml (1 mg); above this weight, the dose is 0.2 ml (2 mg). If there is no response after 45 seconds, it may be titrated up to 0.5 ml (5 mg) in children under 75 lbs, given in increments of 0.1 ml (1 mg) every 30 to 45 seconds and up to 1 ml (10 mg) in heavier children. In infants, the recommended dose is 0.05 ml (0.5 mg). Because of technical difficulty with intravenous injection in children, the intramuscular route may be used. In children weighing up to 75 lbs, 0.2 ml (2 mg) is injected intramuscularly. In children weighing more than 75 lbs, 0.5 ml (5 mg) is injected intramuscularly. All signs which would appear with the intravenous test appear with the intramuscular test except that there is a delay of two to ten minutes before a reaction is noted.
Tensilon Test for Evaluation of Treatment Requirements in Myasthenia Gravis: The recommended dose is 0.1 ml to 0.2 ml (1 mg to 2 mg) of Tensilon, administered intravenously one hour after oral intake of the drug being used in treatment.[1-5] Response will be myasthenic in the undertreated patient, adequate in the controlled patient, and cholinergic in the overtreated patient. Responses to Tensilon in myasthenic and nonmyasthenic individuals are summarized in the accompanying chart.[2]
Tensilon Test in Crisis: The term *crisis* is applied to the myasthenic whenever severe respiratory distress with objective ventilatory inadequacy occurs and the response to medication is not predictable. This state may be secondary to a sudden increase in severity of myasthenia gravis (myasthenic crisis), or to overtreatment with anticholinesterase drugs (cholinergic crisis).
When a patient is apneic, controlled ventilation must be secured immediately in order to avoid cardiac arrest and irreversible central nervous system damage. No attempt is made to test with Tensilon until respiratory exchange is adequate. *Dosage used at this time is most important:* If the patient is cholinergic, Tensilon will cause increased oropharyngeal secretions and further weakness in the muscles of respiration. If the crisis is myasthenic, the test clearly improves respiration and the patient can be treated with longer-acting intravenous anticholinesterase medication. When the test is performed, there should not be more than 0.2 ml (2 mg) Tensilon in the syringe. An intravenous dose of 0.1 ml (1 mg) is given initially. The patient's heart action is carefully observed. If, after an interval of one minute, this dose does not further impair the patient, the remaining 0.1 ml (1 mg) can be injected. If no clear improvement of respiration occurs after 0.2 ml (2 mg) dose, it is usually wisest to discontinue all anticholinesterase drug therapy and secure controlled ventilation by tracheostomy with assisted respiration.[5]
For Use as a Curare Antagonist: Tensilon should be administered by intravenous injection in 1 ml (10 mg) doses given slowly over a period of 30 to 45 seconds so that the onset of cholinergic reaction can be detected. This dosage may be repeated whenever necessary. The maximal dose for any one patient should be 4 ml (40 mg). Because of its brief effect, Tensilon should not be given prior to the administration of curare, tubocurarine, gallamine triethiodide or dimethyl-tubocurarine; it should be used at the time when its effect is needed. When given to counteract curare overdosage, the effect of each dose on the respiration should be carefully observed before it is repeated, and assisted ventilation should always be employed.
Drug Interactions: Care should be given when administering this drug to patients with symptoms of myasthenic weakness who are also on anticholinesterase drugs. Since symptoms of anticholinesterase overdose (cholinergic crisis) may mimic underdosage (myasthenic weakness), their condition may be worsened by the use of this drug. (See OVERDOSAGE section for treatment.)
Overdosage: With drugs of this type, muscarine-like symptoms (nausea, vomiting, diarrhea, sweating, increased bronchial and salivary secretions and bradycardia) often appear with overdosage (cholinergic crisis). An important complication that can arise is obstruction of the airway by bronchial secretions. These may be managed with suction (especially if tracheostomy has been performed) and by the use of atropine. Many experts have advocated a wide range of dosages of atropine *(for Tensilon, see atropine dosage below),* but if there are copious secretions, up to 1.2 mg intravenously may be given initially and repeated every 20 minutes until secretions are controlled. Signs of atropine overdosage such as dry mouth, flush and tachycardia should be avoided as tenacious secretions and bronchial plugs may form. A total dose of atropine of 5 to 10 mg or even more may be required. The following steps should be taken in the management of overdosage of Tensilon:

1. Adequate respiratory exchange should be maintained by assuring an open airway, and the use of assisted respiration augmented by oxygen.
2. Cardiac function should be monitored until complete stabilization has been achieved.
3. Atropine sulfate in doses of 0.4 to 0.5 mg should be administered intravenously. This may be repeated every 3 to 10 minutes. Because of the short duration of action of Ten-

	Myasthenic*	Adequate**	Cholinergic***
Muscle Strength . . . (ptosis, diplopia, dysphonia, dysphagia, dysarthria, respiration, limb strength)	Increased	No change	Decreased
Fasciculations . . . (orbicularis oculi, facial muscles, limb muscles)	Absent	Present or absent	Present or absent
Side reactions . . . (lacrimation, diaphoresis, salivation, abdominal cramps, nausea, vomiting, diarrhea)	Absent	Minimal	Severe

*Myasthenic Response—occurs in untreated myasthenics and may serve to establish diagnosis; in patients under treatment, indicates that therapy is inadequate.
**Adequate Response—observed in treated patients when therapy is stabilized; a typical response in normal individuals. In addition to this response in nonmyasthenics, the phenomenon of forced lid closure is often observed in psychoneurotics.[1]
***Cholinergic Response—seen in myasthenics who have been overtreated with anticholinesterase drugs.

silon the total dose required will seldom exceed 2 mg.

4. Pralidoxime chloride (a cholinesterase reactivator) may be given intravenously at the rate of 50 to 100 mg per minute; usually the total dose does not exceed 1000 mg. Extreme caution should be exercised in the use of pralidoxime chloride when the cholinergic symptoms are induced by double-bond phosphorous anticholinesterase drugs.[9]
5. If convulsions or shock is present, appropriate measures should be instituted.

How Supplied: *Multiple Dose Vials,* 10 ml. *Ampuls,* 1 ml, boxes of 10.

References:

1. Osserman, K.E. and Kaplan, L.I., *J.A.M.A., 150:*265, 1952.
2. Osserman, K.E., Kaplan, L.I. and Besson, G., *J. Mt. Sinai Hosp., 20:*165, 1953.
3. Osserman, K.E. and Kaplan, L.I., *Arch. Neurol. & Psychiat., 70:*385, 1953.
4. Osserman, K.E. and Teng, P., *J.A.M.A., 160:*153, 1956.
5. Osserman, K.E. and Genkins, G., *Ann. N.Y. Acad. Sci., 135:*312, 1966.
6. Tether, J.E., Second International Symposium Proceedings, Myasthenia Gravis, 1961, p. 444.
7. Tether, J.E., in H.F. Conn: *Current Therapy 1960,* Philadelphia, W. B. Saunders Company, p. 551.
8. Tether, J.E., in H.F. Conn: *Current Therapy 1965,* Philadelphia, W. B. Saunders Company, p. 556.
9. Grob, D. and Johns, R.J., *J.A.M.A., 166:*1855, 1958.

Sclavo Inc.

5 MANSARD COURT
WAYNE, NEW JERSEY 07470

SclavoTest®-PPD ℞

Tuberculin Purified Protein Derivative (PPD) Multiple Puncture Device

Composition/Description: SclavoTest-PPD is a sterile multiple-puncture device containing a tuberculin PPD used for the identification of individuals who have a delayed hypersensitivity to tuberculin. SclavoTest-PPD is an easy-to-use, self-contained, unit-dose disposable system which minimizes waste and can be stored at room temperature. No needles, syringes, or vials are needed.

The SclavoTest-PPD device is composed of a plastic handle with four sharp stainless steel points to which has been affixed and dried a tuberculin PPD solution. The retracted points are projected, after the device is placed upon the skin, by gentle pressure applied through a spring inside the handle. SclavoTest-PPD is stored at room temperature until the moment of use in a hermetically sealed unit-dose blister pack, which is designed to impede the passage of moisture and maintain sterility.

Warnings and Precautions: Dispose of safely after use—never reuse. Intensity of reaction may be diminished by delayed hypersensitivity caused by such factors as acute viral infection, vaccination with live virus vaccine, immunosuppression by disease or medication, anergic status (e.g., sarcoidosis, malignancy), malnutrition (especially in children), overwhelming infections, advancing age. Also, some individuals with tuberculosis infection but with none of the above conditions do not react to ordinary doses of tuberculin. In patients seriously ill with tuberculosis, test usually becomes positive after a few weeks of treatment. Antituberculosis chemotherapy should not be started solely on basis of one positive test but only after further diagnosis (e.g., chest X rays, bacteriologic examination of sputa). Consider INH treatment for recent converters and other high-risk groups without evidence of active disease.

Adverse Reactions: Vesiculation, occasionally necrosis, ulceration.

How Supplied: 2, 20 or 250 units individually blister-sealed in strips of 2.

Squibb & Sons, Inc., E.R.

GENERAL OFFICES
P.O. BOX 4000
PRINCETON, NJ 08540

CARDIOGRAFIN® ℞

(Diatrizoate Meglumine Injection USP 85%)

Description: Cardiografin is a radiopaque contrast agent for use in roentgenography of the heart and major vessels, including the aorta. It is supplied as a sterile, aqueous solution for intravascular administration. Each ml. provides 850 mg. diatrizoate meglumine, 3.2 mg. sodium citrate as a buffer and 0.4 mg. edetate disodium as a sequestering agent. *Each ml. of solution also contains approximately 0.91 mg. (0.04 mEq.) sodium (45.5 mg./50 ml.)* and 400 mg. (20 g./50 ml.) organically bound iodine. At the time of manufacture, the air in the container is replaced by nitrogen.

Actions: Following introduction into a vessel or directly into the heart, diatrizoate meglumine is rapidly diffused through the vascular system and is excreted by the kidneys. As the contrast medium enters the cardiac chambers, the vessels and the aorta, lesions or malformations of the heart and obstruction or anomalies of the major thoracic vessels are visualized.

Indications: Cardiografin (Diatrizoate Meglumine Injection USP 85%) is indicated for adult angiocardiography and thoracic aortography.

Contraindications: This preparation is contraindicated in patients with a hypersensitivity to salts of diatrizoic acid or with advanced uremia.

Warnings: A definite risk exists in the use of intravascular contrast agents in patients who are known to have multiple myeloma. In such instances there has been anuria resulting in progressive uremia, renal failure, and eventually death. Although neither the contrast agent nor dehydration has separately proved to be the cause of anuria in myeloma, it has been speculated that the combination of both may be the causative factor. The risk in myelomatous patients is not a contraindication to the procedures; however, partial dehydration in the preparation of these patients for the examination is not recommended since this may predispose for the precipitation of myeloma protein in the renal tubules. No form of therapy, including dialysis, has been successful in reversing this effect. Myeloma, which occurs most commonly in persons over age 40, should be considered before instituting intravascular administration of contrast agents.

Administration of radiopaque materials to patients known or suspected to have pheochromocytoma should be performed with extreme caution. If, in the opinion of the physician, the possible benefits of such procedures outweigh the considered risks, the procedures may be performed; however, the amount of radiopaque medium injected should be kept to an absolute minimum. The blood pressure should be assessed throughout the procedure and measures for treatment of a hypertensive crisis should be available.

The inherent risks of *angiocardiography* in patients with chronic pulmonary emphysema must be weighed against the necessity for performing the procedure.

Contrast media have been shown to promote the phenomenon of sickling in individuals who are homozygous for sickle cell disease when the material is injected intravenously or intra-arterially.

Since iodine-containing contrast agents may alter the results of thyroid function tests, such tests, if indicated, should be performed prior to the administration of this preparation.

A history of sensitivity to iodine *per se* or to contrast media other than salts of diatrizoic acid is not an absolute contraindication to the use of diatrizoate meglumine, but calls for extreme caution in administration.

Precautions: Diagnostic procedures which involve the use of radiopaque contrast agents should be carried out under the direction of personnel with the prerequisite training and with a thorough knowledge of the particular procedure to be performed (see ADVERSE REACTIONS).

Severe, life-threatening reactions suggest hypersensitivity to the radiopaque agent, which has prompted the use of several pretesting methods, none of which can be relied upon to predict severe reactions. Many authorities question the value of any pretest. A history of bronchial asthma or allergy, a family history of allergy, or a previous reaction to a contrast agent warrant special attention. Such a history, by suggesting histamine sensitivity and a consequent proneness to reactions, may be more accurate than pretesting in predicting the likelihood of a reaction, although not necessarily the severity or type of reaction in the individual case.

The sensitivity test most often performed is the slow injection of 0.5 to 1.0 ml. of the radiopaque medium, administered intravenously, prior to injection of the full diagnostic dose. It should be noted that the absence of a reaction to the test dose does not preclude the possibility of a reaction to the full diagnostic dose. If the test dose causes an untoward response of any kind, the necessity for continuing with the examination should be carefully reevaluated and, if it is deemed essential, the examination should be conducted with all possible caution. In rare instances, reactions to the test dose itself may be extremely severe; therefore, close observation of the patient and facilities for emergency treatment appear indicated.

Renal toxicity has been reported in a few patients with liver dysfunction who were given oral cholecystographic agents followed by intravascular contrast agents. Administration of Cardiografin (Diatrizoate Meglumine Injection USP 85%) should therefore be postponed in any patient with a known or suspected hepatic or biliary disorder who has recently taken a cholecystographic contrast agent.

Caution should be exercised with the use of radiopaque media in severely debilitated patients, in those with marked hypertension, and in cases of congestive heart failure.

When any percutaneous technique is employed the possibility of thrombosis or of other complications due to the mechanical trauma of the procedure should be borne in mind.

Consideration must be given to the functional ability of the kidneys before injecting this preparation. Decreased excretion of the contrast material due to impaired renal function increases the possibility of renal damage or other adverse reactions. Combined renal and hepatic disease present an additional hazard.

Acute renal failure has been reported with the use of contrast agents in patients with diabetic nephropathy and susceptible nondiabetic patients (often elderly with preexisting renal disease).

Contrast agents may interfere with some chemical determinations made on urine specimens; therefore, urine should be collected before administration of the contrast medium or two or three days afterwards.

Continued on next page

Squibb—Cont.

Repeated intra-aortic injections may be hazardous.

Usage in Pregnancy: The safety of diatrizoate meglumine for use during pregnancy has not been established with respect to adverse effects upon fetal development; therefore, this preparation should be used in pregnant patients only when, in the judgment of the physician, its use is deemed essential to the welfare of the patient.

Adverse Reactions: Adverse reactions accompanying the use of iodine-containing intravascular contrast agents are usually mild and transient although severe and life-threatening reactions, including fatalities, have occurred. Because of the possibility of severe reactions to the procedure and/or the radiopaque medium, appropriate emergency facilities and well-trained personnel should be available to treat both conditions. Emergency facilities and personnel should remain available for 30 to 60 minutes following the procedure since severe delayed reactions have been known to occur.

Nausea, vomiting, flushing, or a generalized feeling of warmth are the reactions seen most frequently with intravascular injection. Symptoms which may occur are chills, fever, sweating, headache, dizziness, pallor, weakness, severe retching and choking, wheezing, a rise or fall in blood pressure, ventricular fibrillation, cardiac arrest, facial or conjunctival petechiae, urticaria, pruritus, rash and other eruptions, edema, cramps, tremors, itching, sneezing, lacrimation, etc. Antihistaminic agents may be of benefit; rarely such reactions may be severe enough to require discontinuation of dosage. Pulmonary edema, spasm, seizures, hemiparesis, and impairment of vision have occurred with parenteral injection of diatrizoates.

Severe reactions which may require emergency measures may take the form of a cardiovascular reaction characterized by peripheral vasodilatation with resultant hypotension and reflex tachycardia, apnea, dyspnea, agitation, confusion, and cyanosis progressing to unconsciousness. Or, the histamine-liberating effect of these compounds may induce an allergic-like reaction which may range in severity from rhinitis or angioneurotic edema to laryngeal or bronchial spasm or anaphylactoid shock.

Temporary renal shutdown or other nephropathy may occur.

Although local tissue tolerance is usually good, there have been a few reports of a burning or stinging sensation or numbness and of venospasm or venous pain, and partial collapse of the injected vein. Neutropenia or thrombophlebitis may occur.

Adverse reactions may also occur as a consequence of the procedure for which the contrast agent is used. Adverse reactions due to *angiocardiography* in adults have included arrhythmia and death. In *thoracic aortography,* the risks of the procedure include injury to the aorta and neighboring organs, pleural puncture, renal damage including infarction and acute tubular necrosis with oliguria and anuria, accidental selective filling of the right renal artery during the translumbar procedure in the presence of preexistent renal disease, retroperitoneal hemorrhage from the translumbar approach, spinal cord injury and pathology associated with the syndrome of transverse myelitis, generalized petechiae, and death following hypotension, arrhythmia and anaphylactoid reactions.

Dosage and Administration: The vial should be warmed in a water bath to 37° to 40° C. before use, thereby minimizing the viscosity of the solution. Since the contrast medium is given by rapid injection, the patient should be watched for untoward reactions during the injection.

In the preparation of the patient, preanesthetic medication should be given.

Angiocardiography: Normally, patients not under general anesthesia experience a feeling of bodily warmth in the area injected. This sensation is of short duration. Transient nausea and vomiting, tightness of the chest, or headache may occur in some patients. The contrast agent may be administered by injection into a large peripheral vein or, to increase the density, by catheter, approximating the catheter tip to the right heart or other area where pathology is suspected. Mechanical injectors permit a faster injection rate and greater bolus density.

The suggested dose for adults is 40 to 50 ml. This dose may be repeated once if necessary.

A preliminary control film may be made in the usual manner. After the medium has been injected, serial films are usually taken in rapid sequence and continued until the desired information is obtained.

Thoracic Aortography: The contrast agent may be injected into the aorta by translumbar or retrograde methods of administration. Unless general anesthesia is employed, patients should be warned that they may feel some transient pain or burning during the injection followed by a feeling of warmth immediately afterward.

The suggested adult dose is 15 to 20 ml. as a single injection and repeated if indicated.

A scout film may be made before the preparation is administered.

How Supplied: Cardiografin (Diatrizoate Meglumine Injection USP 85%) is available in 50 ml. single-dose vials. An excess volume (1 ml.) is available in each container for sensitivity testing.

Storage: When kept in the syringe for prolonged periods of time prior to injection, the preparation should be protected from exposure to strong light.

Note: Prolonged standing may result in the separation of solids. To obtain a clear solution, place vial in boiling water and shake gently until solids redissolve. Allow solution to cool to 37° to 40° C. before use. The preparation should be injected promptly after withdrawal into the syringe, and the syringe should be rinsed as soon as possible after injection to prevent freezing of the plunger.

CHOLOGRAFIN® MEGLUMINE ℞
(Iodipamide Meglumine Injection USP 52%)
FOR INTRAVENOUS USE ONLY

Description: Cholografin Meglumine is a radiopaque medium for rapid intravenous cholangiography and cholecystography, supplied as a sterile, aqueous solution providing 52% iodipamide meglumine. The bound iodine content of the solution is about 26% (5.2 grams per 20 ml.). Cholografin Meglumine also contains 0.32% sodium citrate as a buffer and 0.04% edetate disodium as a sequestering agent. *The solution contains approximately 0.91 mg. (0.039 mEq.) sodium per ml. (18.2 mg./20 ml.).* At the time of manufacture, the air in the container is replaced by nitrogen. Sufficient excess for sensitivity testing is included in the vials.

The appearance of the solution may vary from essentially colorless to light amber. Solutions which have become substantially darker, however, should not be used.

Actions: Following intravenous administration of Cholografin Meglumine, iodipamide is carried to the liver where it is rapidly secreted. The contrast medium appears in the bile within 10 to 15 minutes after injection, thus permitting visualization of the hepatic and common bile ducts, even in cholecystectomized patients. The biliary ducts are readily visualized within about 25 minutes after administration, except in patients with impaired liver function. The gallbladder begins to fill within an hour after injection; maximum filling is reached after two to two and one-half hours. The contrast medium is finally eliminated in the feces without passing through the enterohepatic circulation, except for approximately 10 percent of the intravenously administered dose which is excreted through the kidneys.

The LD_{50} for intravenous administration of a 52% iodipamide meglumine solution in mice is 6.2 plus or minus 0.3 ml./kg. (equivalent to 3224 plus or minus 156 mg. iodipamide meglumine/kg.).

Indications: Cholografin Meglumine (Iodipamide Meglumine Injection USP 52%) is indicated for intravenous cholangiography and cholecystography as follows: (a) visualization of the gallbladder and biliary ducts in the differential diagnosis of acute abdominal conditions, (b) visualization of the biliary ducts, especially in patients with symptoms after cholecystectomy, and (c) visualization of the gallbladder in patients unable to take oral contrast media or to absorb contrast media from the gastrointestinal tract.

Contraindications: Iodipamide meglumine is contraindicated in patients with a hypersensitivity to salts of iodipamide or who exhibit sensitivity reactions to the test dose. It is also contraindicated in patients with concomitant severe impairment of renal and liver function.

Warnings: Administration of radiopaque materials to patients known or suspected to have pheochromocytoma should be performed with extreme caution. If, in the opinion of the physician, the possible benefits of such procedures outweigh the considered risks, the procedures may be performed; however, the amount of radiopaque medium injected should be kept to an absolute minimum. The blood pressure should be assessed throughout the procedure and measures for treatment of a hypertensive crisis should be available.

Contrast media have been shown to promote the phenomenon of sickling in individuals who are homozygous for sickle cell disease when the material is injected intravenously or intra-arterially.

Since iodine-containing contrast agents may alter the results of thyroid function tests, such tests, if indicated, should be performed prior to the administration of this preparation.

A history of sensitivity to iodine *per se* or to other contrast agents is not an absolute contraindication to the use of iodipamide meglumine, but calls for extreme caution in administration.

Usage in Pregnancy: The safety of iodipamide meglumine for use during pregnancy has not been established; therefore, it should be used in pregnant patients only when, in the judgment of the physician, its use is deemed essential to the welfare of the patient.

Precautions: Diagnostic procedures which involve the use of radiopaque contrast agents should be carried out under the direction of personnel with the prerequisite training and with a thorough knowledge of the particular procedure to be performed. Appropriate facilities should be available for coping with situations which may arise as a result of the procedure, as well as for emergency treatment of severe reactions to the contrast agent itself.

After intravascular administration of a radiopaque agent, competent personnel and emergency facilities should be available for at least 30 to 60 minutes, since severe delayed reactions have been known to occur.

These severe, life-threatening reactions suggest hypersensitivity to the radiopaque agent, which has prompted the use of several pretesting methods, none of which can be relied upon to predict severe reactions. Many authorities question the value of any pretest. A history of bronchial asthma or allergy, a family history of allergy, or a previous reaction to a contrast agent warrant special attention. Such a history, by suggesting histamine sensitivity and a consequent proneness to reactions, may be more accurate than pretesting in predicting the likelihood of a reaction, although not nec-

essarily the severity or type of reaction in the individual case.
The sensitivity test most often performed is the slow injection of 0.5 to 1.0 ml. of the radiopaque medium, administered intravenously, prior to injection of the full diagnostic dose. It should be noted that the absence of a reaction to the test dose does not preclude the possibility of a reaction to the full diagnostic dose. If the test dose causes an untoward response of any kind, the neccessity for continuing with the examination should be carefully reevaluated and, if it is deemed essential, the examination should be conducted with all possible caution. In rare instances reactions to the test dose itself may be extremely severe; therefore, close observation of the patient, and facilities for emergency treatment, appear indicated.
Caution should be exercised with the use of radiopaque media in severely debilitated patients and in those with marked hypertension. The possibility of thrombosis should be borne in mind when intravenous techniques are employed.
Contrast agents may interfere with some chemical determinations made on urine specimens; therefore, urine should be collected before administration of the contrast medium or two or more days afterwards.
Some clinicians feel it may be advisable to have a continuous intravenous infusion running prior to and during administration of the drug.
The admixture of Benadryl® (Diphenhydramine Hydrochloride Injection) with Cholografin Meglumine (Iodipamide Meglumine Injection USP 52%) may cause a precipitate which may form in the syringe or tubing. If antihistamines are administered concomitantly, they should not be mixed with the contrast agent but administered at another site.
Adverse Reactions: Local reactions at the site of injection are not observed, unless excessive amounts are extravasated during injection. After too rapid administration, mild transient symptoms such as restlessness, sensations of warmth, sneezing, perspiration, salivation, flushing, pressure in the upper abdomen, dizziness, nausea, vomiting, chills, fever, headache, pallor and tremors may occur. These symptoms disappear when the injection has been completed. Rarely, swollen eyelids, laryngospasm, respiratory difficulties, hypotension, cardiac reactions and cyanosis have been reported. Hypersensitivity reactions may occur. In rare instances, despite the most careful sensitivity testing, anaphylactoid reactions may occur.
Renal function tests may be altered and renal failure may occur.
Dosage and Administration: Cholografin Meglumine is for intravenous use only.
Directions for Use: *Preparation of the Patient:* For best results, the usual preliminary measures for cholecystography are recommended, particularly in cholecystectomized patients, i.e., a low residue diet on the day before examination and administration of castor oil the night before or neostigmine at the time of examination to dispel excess intestinal gas. Cholecystography is preferably carried out in the morning with the patient fasting.
Dose: The usual adult dose is 20 ml. For infants and children, the suggested dose is 0.3 to 0.6 ml./kg. of body weight; the dosage for infants and children should not exceed 20 ml.
Note: The dose should not be repeated for 24 hours.
Administration: After warming to body temperature, Cholografin Meglumine (Iodipamide Meglumine Injection USP 52%) should be given by slow intravenous injection, following the usual precautions of intravenous administration. *It is important that the preparation be injected slowly over a period of 10 minutes.* Use of a narrow bore hypodermic needle will ensure a slow rate of injection. During the injection, the patient should be watched for untoward reactions such as a feeling of warmth, flushing and occasionally nausea. Nausea indicates that the injection rate is too rapid.
Radiography: A scout film should be exposed routinely before the intravenous injection is made.
Position of the patient: With the patient prone and right side elevated, radiographs are made in the posterior-anterior projection. Some radiologists prefer the supine position with the left side elevated. Serial 10-minute exposures should be started 10 minutes after the injection is made and continued until optimal visualization of the *biliary ducts* is obtained. Wet films should be examined immediately by the radiologist. In some cases a 15-degree rotation or the upright position may prove helpful. Depending on the situation revealed by the roentgenograms in which the duct is first seen, the position of the subject should be changed to displace the shadow of the common bile duct from that of the spine. Tomography is a useful technique for enhancing bile duct visualization after administration of the radiopaque medium.
Examination of the *gallbladder* should be started about two hours after administration. The standard positions in routine examination of the gallbladder should be used unless otherwise indicated. There is no need for the patient to remain quiet awaiting the time for the gallbladder film to be exposed. Moderate activity on the part of the patient will, in most cases, preclude "stratification" of the contrast agent in the gallbladder. If the contrast medium should stratify in the gallbladder, decubitus as well as upright films should be obtained. Additional exposures may be made after the ingestion of a fatty meal.
If visualization is not achieved after two and one-half hours, the patient should be returned for a 24-hour film, whenever possible. Occasionally, delayed opacification of the gallbladder will occur in 24 hours.
In infants and children, gallbladder visualization may be expected to occur 30 minutes to four hours after administration.
Note: In the presence of liver disease (BSP retention greater than 30 to 40 percent), the contrast medium is not excreted efficiently by the liver and visualization is usually not achieved. Visualization is rarely achieved in the presence of a serum bilirubin of 3.0 mg. per 100 ml. if the elevated bilirubin level is due to mechanical obstruction or hepatocellular damage. In the presence of severe liver damage, the contrast agent is excreted by the kidneys.
Interpretation: When intravenous cholecystography and cholangiography are used as an aid in the differential diagnosis of acute abdominal conditions, visualization of the gallbladder is considered strong evidence against a diagnosis of acute cholecystitis, while nonvisualization of the gallbladder two and one-half hours after administration *with* visualization of the bile ducts is considered strong evidence in favor of a diagnosis of acute cholecystitis (if the bile ducts are only faintly visualized, gallbladder films four hours after administration may occasionally show visualization of the gallbladder). When neither the bile ducts nor the gallbladder is visualized, the study provides no definitive information with regard to determining the presence or absence of acute cholecystitis.
How Supplied: In single dose vials of 20 ml. (Military Depot Item, NSN6505-00-926-9109; V.A. Depot Item, NSN6505-00-926-9109A.)
Storage: Protect from light; store at room temperature; avoid excessive heat.
In the event that crystallization occurs, the solution may be clarified by placing the vial in hot water and shaking gently for several minutes or until the solids redissolve. If cloudiness persists, discard the preparation. Allow the solution to cool to body temperature before administering.

CYSTOGRAFIN® ℞

(Diatrizoate Meglumine Injection USP 30%)
For retrograde cystourethrography
Not intended for intravascular injection

Description: Cystografin is a radiopaque contrast agent supplied as a sterile, aqueous solution. Each ml. provides 300 mg. diatrizoate meglumine with 0.4 mg. edetate disodium as a sequestering agent. Each ml. of solution also contains approximately 141 mg. organically bound iodine. At the time of manufacture, the air in the container is replaced by nitrogen. The preparation should be protected from strong light.
Indication: Cystografin (Diatrizoate Meglumine Injection USP 30%) is indicated for retrograde cystourethrography.
Contraindications: This preparation is contraindicated in patients with a hypersensitivity to salts of diatrizoic acid.
Warnings: Severe sensitivity reactions are more likely to occur in patients with a personal or family history of bronchial asthma, significant allergies, or previous reactions to contrast agents.
A history of sensitivity to iodine *per se* or to other contrast agents is not an absolute contraindication to the use of diatrizoate meglumine, but calls for extreme caution in administration.
Precautions: Safe and effective use of this preparation depends upon proper dosage, correct technique, adequate precautions, and readiness for emergencies.
Retrograde cystourethrography should be performed with caution in patients with a known active infectious process of the urinary tract. Sterile technique should be employed in administration. During administration, care should be taken to avoid excessive pressure, rapid or acute distention of the bladder, and trauma.
Contrast agents may interfere with some chemical determinations made on urine specimens; therefore, urine should be collected before administration of the contrast medium or two or more days afterwards.
Usage in Pregnancy: The safety of diatrizoate meglumine for use during pregnancy has not been established; therefore, it should be used in pregnant patients only when, in the judgment of the physician, its use is deemed essential to the welfare of the patient.
Adverse Reactions: Retrograde genitourinary procedures may cause such complications as hematuria, perforation of the urethra or bladder, introduction of infection into the genitourinary tract, and oliguria or anuria.
If intravasation of this drug occurs, the reactions which may be associated with intravenous administration may possibly be encountered. Hypersensitivity or anaphylactoid reactions may occur. Severe reactions may be manifested by edema of the face and glottis, respiratory distress, convulsions or shock; such reactions may prove fatal unless promptly controlled by such emergency measures as maintenance of a clear airway and immediate use of oxygen and resuscitative drugs.
Dosage and Administration: Preparation of the patient—Appropriate preparation is desirable for optimal results. A laxative the night before the examination and a low residue diet the day before the procedure are recommended.
Dosage—The dose for retrograde use in cystography and voiding cystourethrography ranges from 25 to 300 ml. depending on the age of the patient and the degree of bladder irritability; amounts greater than 300 ml. may be used if the bladder capacity allows. Best results are obtained when the bladder is filled with the contrast agent. If desired, the preparation may be diluted with sterile water or sterile saline as indicated below.

Continued on next page

Squibb—Cont.

Administration—After sterile catheterization, the bladder should be filled to capacity with Cystografin (Diatrizoate Meglumine Injection USP 30%) using a suitable sterile administration set. Care should be taken to avoid using excessive pressure. The presence of bladder discomfort or reflux and/or spontaneous voiding usually indicates that the bladder is full.
Radiography—The commonly employed radiographic techniques should be used. A scout film is recommended before the contrast agent is administered.
Dilution directions—USE DILUTED SOLUTIONS IMMEDIATELY. Use sterile water or sterile saline as a diluent.
Using the **100 ml. bottle:** For a 30% (w/v) diatrizoate meglumine solution, use the 100 ml. bottle undiluted [100 ml. total volume, 14.1% (w/v) organically bound iodine]; for a 24% (w/v) diatrizoate meglumine solution, add 25 ml. diluent to the 100 ml. bottle [125 ml. total volume, 11.3% (w/v) organically bound iodine]; for a 20% (w/v) diatrizoate meglumine solution, add 50 ml. diluent to the 100 ml. bottle [150 ml. total volume, 9.4% (w/v) organically bound iodine]; for an 18% (w/v) diatrizoate meglumine solution, add 67 ml. diluent to the 100 ml. bottle [167 ml. total volume, 8.5% (w/v) organically bound iodine].
Using the **300 ml. bottle:** For a 30% (w/v) diatrizoate meglumine solution, use the 300 ml. bottle undiluted [300 ml. total volume, 14.1% (w/v) organically bound iodine]; for a 25.7% (w/v) diatrizoate meglumine solution, add 50 ml. diluent to the 300 ml. bottle [350 ml. total volume, 12.1% (w/v) organically bound iodine]; for a 22.5% (w/v) diatrizoate meglumine solution, add 100 ml. diluent to the 300 ml. bottle [400 ml. total volume, 10.6% (w/v) organically bound iodine]; for a 20% (w/v) diatrizoate meglumine solution, add 150 ml. diluent to the 300 ml. bottle [450 ml. total volume, 9.4% (w/v) organically bound iodine]; for an 18% (w/v) diatrizoate meglumine solution, add 200 ml. diluent to the 300 ml. bottle [500 ml. total volume, 8.5% (w/v) organically bound iodine].
How Supplied: Cystografin (Diatrizoate Meglumine Injection USP 30%) is available in 200 ml. and 500 ml. bottles containing 100 ml. and 300 ml. diatrizoate meglumine respectively with sufficient capacity for dilution up to 167 ml. and 500 ml. respectively.
Storage: Store at room temperature; protect from light.

GASTROGRAFIN® ℞
(Diatrizoate Meglumine and Diatrizoate Sodium Solution USP)

Description: Gastrografin is a water-soluble, oral radiopaque medium for radiographic examination of the gastrointestinal tract. Each ml. contains 660 mg. diatrizoate meglumine and 100 mg. diatrizoate sodium. Each 30 ml. contains approximately 11 g. organically bound iodine (367 mg./ml.).
Clinical Pharmacology: Gastrografin is an oral contrast medium for the radiographic examination of the gastrointestinal tract; it is water-soluble, of medium viscosity, and provides uniform radiopacity; it is not absorbed from the gastrointestinal tract in significant amounts; it is non-irritating, well tolerated and, unlike barium, it is relatively nontoxic when accidentally introduced into body cavities; it is palatable, readily miscible with gastrointestinal fluids and with blood and it is not affected by retained food particles. Because it is not particulate, there is no hazard of inspissation. Accidental aspiration into the bronchi or into a tracheobronchial fistula is not of serious consequence since the medium is promptly expectorated by the patient.
Indications and Usage: Gastrografin is indicated for radiography of the gastrointestinal tract following oral or rectal administration. The preparation is particularly indicated where the use of barium is not feasible or is potentially dangerous.
Contraindications: This preparation is contraindicated in patients with a hypersensitivity to salts of diatrizoic acid.
Warnings: A history of sensitivity to iodine *per se* or to contrast media other than salts of diatrizoic acid is not an absolute contraindication to the use of Gastrografin but calls for extreme caution in administration.
Iodine-containing contrast agents may alter the results of thyroid function tests; therefore, if such tests are indicated, they should be performed prior to the administration of Gastrogafin (Diatrizoate Meglumine and Diatrizoate Sodium Solution USP).
Precautions: Oral administration in children may cause a decrease in circulating plasma volume due to osmosis when the contrast agent passes through the stomach and small intestine. In the very young child (weighing less than 21 lbs.) and the debilitated child, the loss of plasma fluid may be sufficient to cause a shock-like state which, if left untreated, could be life-threatening. This hazard can be avoided by dilution of the contrast medium with water before administration, and by the adequate hydration of the child before and after the procedure. The same considerations may possibly apply in elderly cachectic individuals as well.
Usage in Pregnancy—Safety for use during pregnancy has not been established; therefore, the preparation should be used in pregnant patients only when, in the judgment of the physician, its use is deemed essential to the welfare of the patient.
Adverse Reactions: Orally administered salts of diatrizoic acid are usually well tolerated.
Occasionally, some degree of diarrhea may be encountered due to the osmotic activity of the preparation when it is used as an enema. In young children fluids should be administered intravenously or by clysis to prevent dehydration.
Dosage and Administration: Not for parenteral use.
Preparation of the patient: The routine preparatory measures employed for barium studies are also indicated for Gastrografin. Adequate preparation is desirable for optimal results.
Dosage: Adult oral dosage may range from 30 to 90 ml., depending on the nature of the examination and the size of the patient. For infants and children up to 5 years of age, 30 ml. are usually adequate; for children 5 to 10 years of age, the suggested dose is 60 ml.
For the very young child (weighing less than 21 lbs.) and the debilitated child, *the dose should be diluted:* 1 part Gastrografin in 3 parts water is recommended. For other infants and children, the dose may be diluted 1:1, if desired, with water, carbonated beverages, milk or mineral oil. A 1:1 dilution is also recommended when the contrast medium is used in elderly cachectic individuals.
The preparation should also be diluted when it is used for enemas and enterostomy instillations. When used as an enema, the suggested dilution for adults is 240 ml. in 1,000 ml. of tap water. For children under 5 years of age, a 1:5 dilution in tap water is suggested; for children over 5 years of age, 90 ml. in 500 ml. of tap water is a suitable dilution.
Administration: Gastrografin (Diatrizoate Meglumine and Diatrizoate Sodium Solution USP) may be ingested directly or given by tube. When used in infants, it may be given in a nursing bottle.
How Supplied: As an aqueous, flavored solution in bottles of 120 ml. [V.A. Depot Item, NSN6505-01-008-3323A.]
Storage: Store at room temperature; avoid excessive heat.

KINEVAC® ℞
(Sincalide for Injection)

Description: Kinevac is a sterile, lyophilized, white powder of the synthetic C-terminal octapeptide of cholecystokinin. Each vial provides 5 mcg. sincalide with 45 mg. sodium chloride as a carrier; sodium hydroxide or hydrochloric acid may be added during manufacture to adjust the pH to 5.5 to 6.5. When reconstituted with 5 ml. of Sterile Water for Injection USP, each ml. contains 1 mcg. sincalide and 9 mg. sodium chloride. At the time of manufacture, the air in the vial is replaced by nitrogen.
Actions: When injected intravenously, sincalide produces a substantial reduction in gallbladder size by causing this organ to contract. The evacuation of bile that results is similar to that which occurs physiologically in response to endogenous cholecystokinin. The intravenous (bolus) administration of sincalide causes a prompt contraction of the gallbladder that becomes maximal in 5 to 15 minutes, as compared with the stimulus of a fatty meal which causes a progressive contraction that becomes maximal after approximately 40 minutes. Generally, a 40 percent reduction in radiographic area of the gallbladder is considered satisfactory contraction.
Like cholecystokinin, sincalide, when given in conjunction with secretin stimulates pancreatic secretion; concurrent administration increases the volume of pancreatic secretion and the output of bicarbonate and protein (enzymes) by the gland. This combined effect of secretin and sincalide permits the assessment of specific pancreatic function through measurement and analysis of the duodenal aspirate. The parameters usually determined are: volume of the secretion; bicarbonate concentration; and amylase content (which parallels the content of trypsin and total protein).
Indications: Kinevac (Sincalide for Injection) is a diagnostic agent which may be used: (1) to provide a sample of gallbladder bile that may be aspirated from the duodenum for analysis of its composition, e.g., to determine the degree of cholesterol saturation, (2) in conjunction with secretin (see DOSAGE AND ADMINISTRATION) to stimulate pancreatic secretion for analysis of its composition and examination of cytology, e.g., in suspected cancer of the pancreas, (3) for postevacuation cholecystography, where the physician deems this procedure indicated but wishes to avoid the fatty meal.
Contraindications: The preparation is contraindicated in patients sensitive to sincalide.
Warnings:
Usage in Pregnancy: Although no teratogenic or antifertility effects were seen in animal studies, data are inadequate to determine the safety of sincalide in human pregnancy. Accordingly, sincalide should be used in pregnant women only when, in the judgment of the physician, the benefits outweigh the possible risk to the fetus.
Usage in Children: The safety of sincalide for use in children has not been established.
Precautions: The possiblity exists that stimulation of gallbladder contraction in patients with small gallbladder stones could lead to the evacuation of the stones from the gallbladder, resulting in their lodging in the cystic duct or in the common bile duct. The risk of such an event is considered to be minimal because sincalide, when given as directed, does not ordinarily cause complete contraction of the gallbladder.
Adverse Reactions: Gastrointestinal symptoms such as abdominal discomfort or pain, and an urge to defecate, frequently accompany the injection of sincalide. These phenomena are usually manifestations of the physiologic action of the drug, which include delayed gastric emptying and increased intestinal motil-

ity, and are not to be construed as necessarily indicating an abnormality of the biliary tract unless there is other clinical or radiologic evidence of disease. Nausea, dizziness, and flushing occur occasionally.

Dosage and Administration: For prompt contraction of the gallbladder, a dose of 0.02 mcg. sincalide per kg. (1.4 mcg. per 70 kg.) is injected intravenously over a 30- to 60-second interval; if satisfactory contraction of the gallbladder does not occur in 15 minutes, a second dose, 0.04 mcg. sincalide per kg., may be administered. When Kinevac (Sincalide for Injection) is used in cholecystography, roentgenograms are usually taken at five-minute intervals after the injection. For visualization of the cystic duct, it may be necessary to take roentgenograms at one-minute intervals during the first five minutes after the injection.

For the Secretin-Kinevac test of pancreatic function, the patient receives a dose of 0.25 units secretin per kg. infused intravenously over a 60-minute period. Thirty minutes after the initiation of the secretin infusion, a separate I.V. infusion of Kinevac at a total dose of 0.02 mcg. per kg. is administered over a 30-minute interval. For example, the total dose for a 70 kg. patient is 1.4 mcg. of sincalide; therefore, dilute 1.4 ml. of reconstituted Kinevac solution to 30 ml. with Sodium Chloride Injection USP and administer at a rate of 1 ml. per minute.

Reconstitution and Storage: Kinevac (Sincalide for Injection) may be stored at room temperature prior to reconstitution.

To reconstitute, aseptically add 5 ml. Sterile Water for Injection USP to the vial; the solution may be kept at room temperature and should be used within 24 hours of reconstitution, after which time any unused portion should be discarded.

How Supplied: In vials containing 5 mcg. of sincalide.

MEDOTOPES® ℞
(Radiopharmaceuticals)

Medotopes represent the latest developments in nuclear medicine. They are available only to those physicians who are qualified by training and experience in the safe use and handling of radionuclides and whose experience and training have been approved by the appropriate government agency authorized to license the use of radionuclides. Medotopes are supplied in a variety of forms intended for diagnostic or therapeutic use. (For a partial list of available radiopharmaceutical products see Alphabetical Index by Manufacturer Section of the PDR.)

All Medotopes have appropriate packaging safeguard to protect against unnecessary exposure.

Each order is custom-handled, each delivery custom-routed by Squibb Traffic Service. Access to three major airports expedites shipment.

For information on preparations currently available, write Medotopes Customer Services. P.O. Box 4000, Princeton, N.J. 08540

ORAGRAFIN® CALCIUM GRANULES ℞
(Ipodate Calcium for Oral Suspension USP)

ORAGRAFIN® SODIUM CAPSULES ℞
(Ipodate Sodium Capsules USP)

Description: Oragrafin Calcium Granules (Ipodate Calcium for Oral Suspension USP) and Oragrafin Sodium Capsules (Ipodate Sodium Capsules USP) are oral radiopaque media for cholangiography and cholecystography. Ipodate *calcium* is available in single-dose foil packets providing 3 g. ipodate calcium as granules dispersed in flavored sucrose. When mixed with water, the granules produce a pleasantly-flavored suspension. Ipodate *sodium* is available in capsules providing 500 mg. ipodate sodium per capsule. The capsules contain FD&C Yellow No. 5 (tartrazine).

The organically bound iodine content of ipodate calcium and ipodate sodium is 61.7% (approximately 1.85 g./packet) and 61.4% (approximately 307 mg./capsule), respectively.

Clinical Pharmacology: Ipodate calcium and ipodate sodium are absorbed from the gastrointestinal tract, excreted by the liver into the bile, and stored and concentrated in the gallbladder. The calcium salt, which is absorbed somewhat faster than the sodium salt, appears in the ducts as early as 30 minutes after ingestion. Optimal concentration of either salt in the hepatic and biliary ducts occurs within one to three hours after ingestion in nearly all cases; rarely, maximal opacification may be delayed for as much as five hours. Adequate opacification of the ducts usually persists for about 45 minutes. The ducts may be visualized in patients who have undergone cholecystectomy.

The gallbladder is optimally opacified approximately 10 hours after ingestion of either salt. Diagnostically adequate filling, however, often takes place within five hours or less after ingestion, particularly with the calcium salt. Thus, studies of ducts and gallbladder may be carried out in as little as five hours when necessary or desirable. In this connection, it should be pointed out that both salts have been administered to unprepared patients as well as to previously prepared patients, with no significant difference in results.

Indications and Usage: Ipodate calcium and ipodate sodium are indicated for cholecystography. They may also be used for cholangiography, although they are not considered the drugs of choice.

Contraindications: Both preparations are contraindicated in patients who are hypersensitive to ipodate salts.

Warnings: A history of sensitivity to iodine *per se* or to other iodinated compounds is not an absolute contraindication to the use of these preparations, but calls for extreme caution in administration.

Usage in Pregnancy—The safety of these preparations for use during pregnancy has not been established; therefore, they should be used in pregnant patients only when, in the judgment of the physician, their use is deemed essential to the welfare of the patient.

Precautions: Increasing the dosage above that recommended increases the possibility of hypotension.

Anuria may result when these preparations are administered to patients with combined renal and hepatic disease or severe renal impairment.

Renal toxicity has been reported in a few patients with liver dysfunction who were given oral cholecystographic agents followed by urographic agents. Administration of urographic agents should therefore be postponed in any patient with a known or suspected hepatic or biliary disorder who has recently taken a cholecystographic contrast agent.

Gastrointestinal disorders which interfere with absorption, liver disorders which interfere with excretion, or obstruction of the biliary duct may result in nonvisualization of the hepatic and biliary ducts and the gallbladder.

Contrast agents may interfere with some chemical determinations made on urine specimens; therefore, urine should be collected before administration of the contrast medium or two or more days afterwards.

Thyroid function tests, if indicated, should be performed prior to the administration of these preparations since iodine-containing contrast agents may alter the results of these tests.

Oragrafin Sodium Capsules (Ipodate Sodium Capsules USP) contain FD&C Yellow No. 5 (tartrazine) which may cause allergic-type reactions (including bronchial asthma) in certain susceptible individuals. Although the overall incidence of FD&C Yellow No. 5 (tartrazine) sensitivity in the general population is low, it is frequently seen in patients who also have aspirin hypersensitivity.

Adverse Reactions: Ipodate calcium and ipodate sodium are usually well tolerated. Unwanted effects such as mild and transient nausea, vomiting, or diarrhea sometimes occur but the incidence can be reduced by restricting the dosage to 3 g. and administering only the granules to patients who may be prone to gastrointestinal reactions. Headache, dysuria, or abdominal pains may occur infrequently as transient disturbances.

Hypersensitivity reactions may include urticaria, serum sickness-like reactions (fever, rash, arthralgia), other skin rashes, and, rarely, anaphylactoid shock. They are more likely to occur in individuals with a history of allergy, asthma, hay fever, or urticaria, and in those who have previously demonstrated hypersensitivity to iodine compounds.

Dosage and Administration: The capsules should be taken with as little water as possible. They may be swallowed in rapid succession or slowly over the course of ½ hour or more, depending on patient preference.

The granules should be stirred vigorously into a small amount of water (¼ glass or less) and swallowed immediately. If lukewarm rather than cold water is used, the patient will find the suspension quite palatable and there will be less likelihood of nausea.

A total dose of 6 g. (12 capsules or two packets of granules) per 24 hour period should not be exceeded.

When an upper gastrointestinal barium study is scheduled, prior administration of either salt will not interfere. Either salt may also be used in conjunction with an intravenous cholangiographic agent.

The recommended dosage and patient preparation for cholangiography and/or cholecystography are as follows:

Routine Cholecystography: On the day before the examination, the patient may, if feasible, eat a high-fat lunch so that the gallbladder will evacuate and refill with opacified bile. The evening meal should be eaten two hours before the contrast medium is taken; there is no need to change the patient's customary diet, whether low-fat or routine. The contrast agent should be administered 10 to 12 hours before the roentgenologic examination. The usual dose is six capsules (providing 3 g. ipodate sodium), although up to 12 capsules may be given; one to two packets of granules may be used instead. No other food or drink except small amounts of water should be taken before the examination. A mild laxative or other cathartic may be given, but is not generally necessary.

Roentgenologic examination of the gallbladder is performed the next morning in the usual manner, employing the standard positions. An immediate study of the wet films will determine any need for repositioning of the patient. Administration of a fat meal or other cholecystokinetic agent provides good dynamic studies of gallbladder function. If a barium meal examination is also to be performed, the fat meal may be given simultaneously with or following the barium meal. Gallbladder function studies are then made after the barium meal examination is completed.

Repeat Examination: To minimize the possibility of diagnostic error, it may be desirable to repeat the study when the initial examination results in nonvisualization or is nondiagnostic. If the repeat examination also results in nonvisualization, gallbladder disease may be inferred although it should be recognized that nonvisualization may be due to other factors (see PRECAUTIONS); also, a small proportion of normal gallbladders may fail to visualize.

Continued on next page

Squibb—Cont.

Reexamination can be performed on the same day if the usual dose (3 g.) was administered initially; administer 3 g. (one packet) of the granules or, alternatively, 3 g. ipodate sodium (six capsules).

At least five days should intervene between the initial and repeat examinations when the total dose will exceed 6 g.

A total dose of 6 g. per 24-hour period should not be exceeded.

Cholangiography: No prior preparation of the patient is necessary. For this procedure, the granules should be used. They are administered one hour before cholangiography. Although only one packet (providing 3 g. ipodate calcium) may suffice, two packets (6 g.) are usually necessary for visualization of the ducts.

Beginning one hour after ingestion of the granules, and at 15-minute intervals thereafter, films should be taken, preferably with the aid of tomography or laminography. With proper positioning of the patient, residual contrast medium in the gastrointestinal tract is not likely to be a problem, particularly with the more rapidly absorbed calcium salt. Optimal visualization of the ducts is generally achieved between 1½ and 2½ hours after ingestion of the medium.

Combined Cholangiography and Cholecystography: Preparation of the patient and administration of dosage should be as outlined under *Routine Cholecystography,* with a dose of six capsules or, if preferred, one packet of granules taken on the evening before examination. On the following morning, one hour before the examination, one additional packet of granules should be administered.

Beginning one hour after the morning dose, and at 15-minute intervals thereafter, films should be made, preferably with the use of tomography or laminography. While the gallbladder will have concentrated the evening dose of the medium, the additional morning dose will provide opacification of the ducts, and simultaneous visualization may be achieved. When satisfactory films have been obtained, a fat meal may be administered to provide gallbladder function studies.

Rapid Combined Cholangiography and Cholecystography: No prior preparation of the patient is necessary. On the day of examination, the patient should be given two packets of granules. Beginning one hour later, examination of the ducts should be performed as described above under *Cholangiography.* If the gallbladder has not opacified sufficiently by the time the cholangiographic examination is completed, further cholecystograms may be taken after two or three hours. Dynamic studies of gallbladder function may be carried out in the usual manner.

How Supplied: Oragrafin Calcium Granules (Ipodate Calcium for Oral Suspension USP) are supplied in single-dose foil packets providing 3 g. ipodate calcium per packet; boxes of 25 packets.

*Oragrafin Sodium Capsules (Ipodate Sodium Capsules USP) are available for oral use providing 500 mg. ipodate sodium per capsule; boxes of 25 vials (6 capsules in each vial), bottles of 100, and Unimatic® cartons of 100.

Storage: Store the Granules at room temperature. Store the Capsules at room temperature; avoid excessive heat.

*[*Shown in Product Identification Section*]

RENOGRAFIN®-60 ℞

(Diatrizoate Meglumine and Diatrizoate Sodium Injection USP)

Description: Renografin-60 is a radiopaque contrast agent supplied as a sterile, aqueous solution. Each ml. provides 520 mg. diatrizoate meglumine and 80 mg. diatrizoate sodium with 3.2 mg. sodium citrate, and 0.4 mg. edetate disodium; pH has been adjusted between 7.0 and 7.6 with sodium hydroxide. *Each ml. of solution also contains approximately 3.76 mg. (0.16 mEq.) sodium* and 292.5 mg. organically bound iodine. At the time of manufacture, the air in the container is replaced by nitrogen.

Clinical Pharmacology: Following intravascular injection, Renografin-60 (Diatrizoate Meglumine and Diatrizoate Sodium Injection USP) is rapidly transported through the bloodstream to the kidneys and is excreted unchanged in the urine by glomerular filtration. When urinary tract obstruction is severe enough to block glomerular filtration, the agent appears to be excreted by the tubular epithelium.

Certain applications of the contrast agent make use of the natural physiologic mechanism of excretion. Thus, the intravenous injection of the agent permits visualization of the kidneys and urinary passages.

Renal accumulation is sufficiently rapid that the period of maximal opacification of the renal passages may begin as early as five minutes after injection. In infants and small children excretion takes place somewhat more promptly than in adults, so that maximal opacification occurs more rapidly and is less sustained. The normal kidney eliminates the contrast medium almost immediately. In nephropathic conditions, particularly when excretory capacity has been altered, the rate of excretion varies unpredictably, and opacification may be delayed for 30 minutes or more after injection; with severe impairment opacification may not occur. Generally, however, the medium is concentrated in sufficient amounts and promptly enough to permit a thorough evaluation of the anatomy and physiology of the urinary tract. After intramuscular injection, the contrast agent is promptly absorbed and normally reaches the renal passages within 20 to 60 minutes.

Intravascular injection of diatrizoate also opacifies those vessels in the path of flow of the medium, permitting visualization until the circulating blood dilutes the concentration of the medium. Thus selective angiography may be performed following injection directly into veins or arteries such as the carotid, the vertebral, or the vessels of the extremities.

Under certain circumstances, specific parts of the body which do not concentrate the contrast agent physiologically may be visualized by injecting the agent directly into the region to be studied. The biliary tract is one organ system which may be visualized in this manner. In operative cholangiography, injection of the radiopaque medium into the cystic duct or choledochal lumen, at laparotomy, opacifies the intra- and extra-hepatic biliary ductal system, revealing the nature and location of obstructions such as stones or strictures. Injection of the medium through an in-place T-tube, immediately after exploration of the common duct, permits the visualization of retained stones. A repetition of "T-tube cholangiography," performed as part of the postoperative follow-up, insures the patency of the ductal system before removal of the T-tube. The biliary ductal system may also be opacified by the percutaneous-transhepatic route. In relatively long-standing biliary obstruction, the biliary ducts are usually enlarged sufficiently to be located promptly by percutaneous transhepatic probing, permitting injection of the contrast agent directly into the biliary ductal system.

If the contrast agent is injected directly into the splenic pulp, significant opacification of the splenic and portal veins is obtained. Because of gravity, the dependent portions of the portal system are better opacified than the superior portions. The agent is carried from the portal vein into the hepatic veins, and a diffuse opacification of the liver results. In patients with portal hypertension, collateral pathways caused by the change in portal blood flow may be visualized and esophageal varices are often delineated. The procedure may reveal the site of portal obstruction.

Injection of Renografin-60 (Diatrizoate Meglumine and Diatrizoate Sodium Injection USP) directly into a joint space provides visual information about joint derangements.

A small amount of the radiopaque agent injected into a normal cervical or lumbar disk will, under optimal conditions, concentrate within the nucleus pulposus. In the presence of disk pathology the injected agent may reveal significant bulging or disruption of the annulus beyond its normal confines and may identify disk degeneration, retropulsion, or rupture.

Computed Tomography—Renografin-60 enhances computed tomographic brain scanning through augmentation of radiographic efficiency. The degree of enhancement of visualization of tissue density is directly related to the iodine content in an administered dose; peak iodine blood levels occur immediately following rapid injection of the dose. These levels fall rapidly within five to ten minutes. This can be accounted for by the dilution in the vascular and extracellular fluid compartments which causes an initial sharp fall in plasma concentration. Equilibration with the extracellular compartments is reached in about ten minutes; thereafter, the fall becomes exponential. Maximum contrast enhancement frequently occurs after peak blood iodine levels are reached. The delay in maximum contrast enhancement can range from five to forty minutes, depending on the peak iodine levels achieved and the cell type of the lesion. This lag suggests that radiographic contrast enhancement is at least in part dependent on the accumulation of iodine within the lesion and outside the blood pool although the mechanism by which this occurs is not clear. The radiographic enhancement of nontumoral lesions, such as arteriovenous malformations and aneurysms, is probably dependent on the iodine content of the circulating blood pool.

Indications: Renografin-60 is indicated in excretion urography (by direct I.V. or drip infusion); cerebral angiography; peripheral arteriography; venography; operative, T-tube, or percutaneous transhepatic cholangiography; splenoportography; arthrography; and discography.

Computed Tomography: Renografin-60 (Diatrizoate Meglumine and Diatrizoate Sodium Injection USP) is also indicated for radiographic contrast enhancement in computed tomography (CT) of the brain. Contrast enhancement is advantageous in delineating or ruling out disease in suspicious areas which may otherwise not have been satisfactorily visualized.

Tumors—Renografin-60 may be useful to demonstrate the presence and extent of certain malignancies such as: gliomas including malignant gliomas, glioblastomas, astrocytomas, oligodendrogliomas and gangliomas; ependymomas; medulloblastomas; meningiomas; neuromas; pinealomas; pituitary adenomas; craniopharyngiomas; germinomas; and metastatic lesions.

The usefulness of contrast enhancement for the investigation of the retrobulbar space and in cases of low grade or infiltrative glioma has not been demonstrated. In cases where lesions have calcified, there is less likelihood of enhancement. Following therapy, tumors may show decreased or no enhancement.

Non-Neoplastic Conditions—The use of Renografin-60 may be beneficial in the enhancement of images of lesions not due to neoplasms. Cerebral infarctions of recent onset may be better visualized with the contrast enhancement, while some infarctions are obscured if a contrast medium is used. The use of Renografin-60 (Diatrizoate Meglumine and Diatrizoate Sodium Injection USP) improved the contrast enhancement in approximately 60 percent of cerebral infarctions studied from one week to four weeks from the onset of symptoms.

Sites of active infection also will produce contrast enhancement following contrast medium administration.

Arteriovenous malformations and aneurysms will show contrast enhancement. In the case of these vascular lesions, the enhancement is probably dependent on the iodine content of the circulating blood pool.

Hematomas and intraparenchymal bleeders seldom demonstrate any contrast enhancement. However, in cases of intraparenchymal clot, for which there is no obvious clinical explanation, contrast medium administration may be helpful in ruling out the possibility of associated arteriovenous malformation.

The opacification of the inferior vermis following contrast medium administration has resulted in false-positive diagnoses in a number of normal studies.

Contraindications: This preparation is contraindicated in patients with a hypersensitivity to salts of diatrizoic acid.

Urography is contraindicated in patients with anuria.

Specific contraindications to **percutaneous transhepatic cholangiography** include a prothrombin time below 50 percent and evidence of coagulation defects.

Splenoportography should not be performed on any patient for whom splenectomy is contraindicated, since complications of the procedure at times make splenectomy necessary. Other contraindications include prothrombin time below 50 percent, significant thrombocytopenia or coagulation defect, and any condition which may increase the possibility of rupture of the spleen.

Arthrography should not be performed if infection is present in or near the joint.

Discography should not be performed in patients with an infection or open injury near the region to be examined.

Warnings: A definite risk exists in the use of intravascular contrast agents in patients who are known to have multiple myeloma. In such instances there has been anuria resulting in progressive uremia, renal failure and eventually death. Although neither the contrast agent nor dehydration has separately proved to be the cause of anuria in myeloma, it has been speculated that the combination of both may be the causative factor. The risk in myelomatous patients is not a contraindication to the procedures; however, partial dehydration in the preparation of these patients for the examination is not recommended since this may predispose to the precipitation of myeloma protein in the renal tubules. No form of therapy, including dialysis, has been successful in reversing this effect. Myeloma, which occurs most commonly in persons over age 40, should be considered before intravascular administration of a contrast agent.

Administration of radiopaque materials to patients known or suspected to have pheochromocytoma should be performed with extreme caution. If, in the opinion of the physician, the possible benefits of such procedures outweigh the considered risks, the procedures may be performed; however, the amount of radiopaque medium injected should be kept to an absolute minimum. The blood pressure should be assessed throughout the procedure and measures for treatment of a hypertensive crisis should be available.

Cerebral angiography should be undertaken with special caution in extreme age, poor clinical condition, advanced arteriosclerosis, severe arterial hypertension, cardiac decompensation, recent cerebral embolism, or thrombosis.

Urography should be performed with extreme caution in patients with severe concomitant hepatic and renal disease.

Contrast media have been shown to promote the phenomenon of sickling in individuals who are homozygous for sickle cell disease when the material is injected intravenously or intra-arterially.

Since iodine-containing contrast agents may alter the results of thyroid function tests, such tests, if indicated, should be performed prior to the administration of this preparation.

A history of sensitivity to iodine *per se* or to other contrast agents is not an absolute contraindication to the use of diatrizoate, but calls for extreme caution in administration.

Avoid accidental introduction of this preparation into the subarachnoid space since even small amounts may produce convulsions and possible fatal reactions.

Precautions: Diagnostic procedures which involve the use of radiopaque contrast agents should be carried out under the direction of personnel with the prerequisite training and with a thorough knowledge of the particular procedure to be performed (see ADVERSE REACTIONS).

Severe, life-threatening reactions suggest hypersensitivity to the radiopaque agent, which has prompted the use of several pretesting methods, none of which can be relied upon to predict severe reactions. Many authorities question the value of any pretest. A history of bronchial asthma or allergy, a family history of allergy, or a previous reaction to a contrast agent warrant special attention. Such a history, by suggesting histamine sensitivity and a consequent proneness to reactions, may be more accurate than pretesting in predicting the likelihood of a reaction, although not necessarily the severity or type of reaction in the individual case.

The sensitivity test most often performed is the slow injection of 0.5 to 1.0 ml. of the radiopaque medium, administered intravenously, prior to injection of the full diagnostic dose. It should be noted that the absence of a reaction to the test dose does not preclude the possibility of a reaction to the full diagnostic dose. If the test dose causes an untoward response of any kind, the necessity for continuing with the examination should be carefully reevaluated and, if it is deemed essential, the examination should be conducted with all possible caution. In rare instances, reactions to the test dose itself may be extremely severe; therefore, close observation of the patient, and facilities for emergency treatment, appear indicated.

Renal toxicity has been reported in a few patients with liver dysfunction who were given oral cholecystographic agents followed by urographic agents. Administration of Renografin-60 (Diatrizoate Meglumine and Diatrizoate Sodium Injection USP) should therefore be postponed in any patient with a known or suspected hepatic or biliary disorder who has recently taken a cholecystographic contrast agent.

Caution should be exercised with the use of radiopaque media in severely debilitated patients and in those with marked hypertension. The possibility of thrombosis should be borne in mind when percutaneous techniques are employed.

Consideration must be given to the functional ability of the kidneys before injecting this preparation.

Contrast agents may interfere with some chemical determinations made on urine specimens; therefore, urine should be collected before administration of the contrast medium or two or more days afterwards.

The following precautions pertain to specific procedures:

Peripheral arteriography: Hypotension or moderate decreases in blood pressure seem to occur frequently with intra-arterial (brachial) injections; therefore, the blood pressure should be monitored during the immediate ten minutes after injection; this blood pressure change is transient and usually requires no treatment.

Excretion urography: Adequate visualization may be difficult or impossible to attain in uremic patients or others with severely impaired renal function (see CONTRAINDICATIONS). The increased osmotic load associated with drip infusion pyelography should be considered in patients with congestive heart failure. The diuretic effect of the drip infusion pyelography procedure may hinder assessment of residual urine in the bladder. The recommended rate of infusion should not be exceeded.

Acute renal failure has been reported in diabetic patients with diabetic nephropathy and susceptible nondiabetic patients (often elderly with preexisting renal disease) following excretion urography. Therefore, careful consideration should be given before performing this procedure in these patients.

Operative and T-tube cholangiography: Injection should be made slowly to prevent extravasation of the medium into the peritoneal cavity, and to minimize reflux flow into the pancreatic duct which may result in pancreatic irritation.

Percutaneous transhepatic cholangiography: To reduce the possibility of bile leakage and consequent peritonitis, as much of the contrast agent as possible should be aspirated on completion of successful films. All patients should be carefully and constantly monitored for 24 hours after the procedure for signs of internal hemorrhage or bile leakage; if these complications are recognized immediately, remedial measures can be instituted promptly with minimal increase in morbidity. Percutaneous transhepatic cholangiography is not without risk and should therefore be reserved for special circumstances when ordinary studies of the biliary system have failed to provide the requisite information in jaundiced patients who are not good candidates for surgery. The procedure should only be attempted when competent surgical intervention can be promptly obtained if needed.

Splenoportography: It is best to avoid manipulations which would prolong the time the needle is in the spleen since they may contribute to subcapsular extravasation of the contrast agent and also to postpuncture bleeding. Following splenoportography, the patient should lie on his left side for several hours and should be closely observed for 24 hours for signs of internal bleeding, which is the most common complication of the procedure. Fatal hemorrhage has occurred on rare occasion, but leakage of up to 300 ml. of blood from the spleen is apparently not uncommon. Blood transfusions may be required, and rarely splenectomy.

Discography: To minimize the possibility of introducing infection, discography should be postponed in any patient with an infection or open injury near the region to be examined, including upper respiratory infections in the case of cervical discography. All possible care should be taken to preclude contamination and resultant infection of the disk, which has been reported after discography. In cervical discography, particular care is needed to avoid puncturing the esophagus and thereby introducing contamination into the disk. Rupture of the disk is highly unlikely if care in performance is observed, but may occur if the point of the needle has been barbed by contact with bone; use of the two-needle technique should help reduce this hazard.

Usage in Pregnancy: Safety for use during pregnancy has not been established; therefore, the preparation should be used in pregnant patients only when, in the judgment of the physician, its use is deemed essential to the welfare of the patient.

Adverse Reactions: Adverse reactions accompanying the use of iodine-containing intravascular contrast agents are usually mild and

Continued on next page

Squibb—Cont.

transient although severe and life-threatening reactions, including fatalities, have occurred. Because of the possibility of severe reactions to the procedure and/or the radiopaque medium, appropriate emergency facilities and well-trained personnel should be available to treat both conditions. Emergency facilities and personnel should remain available for 30 to 60 minutes following the procedure since severe delayed reactions have been known to occur.

Nausea, vomiting, flushing, or a generalized feeling of warmth are the reactions seen most frequently with intravascular injection. Symptoms which may occur are chills, fever, sweating, headache, dizziness, pallor, weakness, severe retching and choking, wheezing, a rise or fall in blood pressure, facial or conjunctival petechiae, urticaria, pruritus, rash and other eruptions, edema, cramps, tremors, itching, sneezing, lacrimation, etc. Antihistaminic agents may be of benefit; rarely such reactions may be severe enough to require discontinuation of dosage.

Severe reactions which may require emergency measures may take the form of a cardiovascular reaction characterized by peripheral vasodilatation with resultant hypotension and reflex tachycardia, dyspnea, agitation, confusion, and cyanosis progressing to unconsciousness. Or, the histamine-liberating effect of these compounds may induce an allergic-like reaction which may range in severity from rhinitis or angioneurotic edema to laryngeal or bronchial spasm or anaphylactoid shock.

Temporary renal shutdown or other nephropathy may occur. Temporary neurologic effects of varying severity have occurred in a few instances, particularly when the medium was used for angiography in the diagnosis of cerebral pathology. Although local tissue tolerance is usually good, there have been a few reports of a burning or stinging sensation or numbness and of venospasm or venous pain, and partial collapse of the injected vein. Neutropenia or thrombophlebitis may occur.

Adverse effects may sometimes occur as a consequence of the procedure for which the contrast agent is used. Adverse reactions in **excretion urography** have included cardiac arrest, ventricular fibrillation, anaphylaxis with severe asthmatic reaction, and flushing due to generalized vasodilation. **Cerebral angiography** has been known to cause temporary neurologic complications such as induction of seizures, particularly in patients with convulsive disorders; confusional states or drowsiness; transient paresis; coma; temporary disturbances in vision; or seventh nerve weakness. During **peripheral arteriography,** complications have occurred including hemorrhage from the puncture site, thrombosis of the vessel, and brachial plexus palsy following axillary artery injections.

Complications of **percutaneous transhepatic cholangiography** have been estimated to occur in four to six percent of cases and have included bile leakage and biliary peritonitis, gallbladder perforation, internal bleeding, septicemia involving gram-negative organisms, and tension pneumothorax from inadvertent puncture of the diaphragm and lung. Bile leakage may be more likely in patients with complete obstruction due to carcinoma.

During **splenoportography,** intraperitoneal extravasation of the contrast medium may cause transient diaphragmatic irritation or mild to moderate transient pain which may sometimes be referred to the shoulder, the periumbilical region, or other areas. Because of the proximity of the pleural cavity, accidental pneumothorax has been known to occur. Inadvertent injection of the medium into other nearby structures is not likely to cause untoward consequences.

Arthrography may induce joint pain or increase existing pain, particularly if a large dose is used and the medium extravasates into surrounding soft tissue. Pain or discomfort is usually immediate and transient but may be delayed or of extended duration (up to 24 hours). Lipid-filled histiocytes have been found in tissue removed following arthrography. The technique of **discography** may be painful, particularly when disk pathology exists. Pain on injection may also be related to the volume of the dose. The nature of the disk pathology or extravasation of contrast agent may cause referred pain.

When any percutaneous technique is employed, the possibility of thrombosis or of other complications due to the mechanical trauma of the procedure should be borne in mind.

Dosage and Administration: Renografin-60 (Diatrizoate Meglumine and Diatrizoate Sodium Injection USP) should be at body temperature when injected and may need to be warmed before use. If kept in a syringe for prolonged periods before injection, it should be protected from exposure to strong light.

Dilution and withdrawal of the contrast agent should be accomplished under aseptic conditions with sterile syringe.

Excretion Urography—Appropriate preparation of the patient is desirable for optimal results. In adults and older children, a laxative the night before the examination, a low residue diet the day before, and low liquid intake for 12 hours prior to the procedure may be used to clear the gastrointestinal tract and to induce a partial dehydration which is believed to increase the urinary concentration of the contrast medium. Preparatory partial dehydration is not recommended in infants, young children, the elderly, or azotemic patients (especially those with polyuria, oliguria, diabetes, advanced vascular disease, or preexisting dehydration). The undesirable dehydration in these patients may be accentuated by the osmotic diuretic action of the medium.

In uremic patients partial dehydration is not necessary and maintenance of adequate fluid intake is particularly desirable.

Direct I.V. Injection—The dose range for adults is 25 to 50 ml.; the usual dose is 25 ml.; children require proportionately less. Suggested dosages are as follows: Under 6 months—5 ml.; 6 to 12 months—8 ml.; 1 to 2 years—10 ml.; 2 to 5 years—12 ml.; 5 to 7 years—15 ml.; 8 to 10 years—18 ml.; 11 to 15 years—20 ml.; adults (16 years and older)—25 to 50 ml. In adults, when the smaller dose has provided inadequate visualization, or when poor visualization is anticipated, the 50 ml. dose may be given. Drip infusion may be used when direct I.V. pyelography is not expected to be or has not been satisfactory (see below).

The preparation is given by intravenous injection. If flushing or nausea occurs during administration, injection should be slowed or briefly interrupted until the side effects have disappeared.

A scout film should be made before the contrast medium is administered. To allow for individual variation, several films should be exposed beginning approximately five minutes after injection. In patients with renal dysfunction, optimal visualization may be delayed until 30 minutes or more after injection.

NOTE: In infants and children and in certain adults, the medium may be injected intramuscularly. The suggested dose is 25 ml. for adults and proportionately less for children, divided and given bilaterally in the gluteal muscles. Radiographs should be taken at 20, 40, and 60 minutes after the medium is injected.

Drip Infusion Pyelography—In drip infusion pyelography, the recommended dose of Renografin-60 is calculated on the basis of 1 ml. of Renografin-60 (Diatrizoate Meglumine and Diatrizoate Sodium Injection USP) per pound of body weight diluted with an equal volume of Sterile Water for Injection USP. The diluted preparation (30%) is given by I.V. infusion through a large bore (17- to 18-gauge) needle at a rate of 40 ml. per minute. The recommended rate of infusion should not be exceeded and the total volume administered should generally not exceed 300 ml. In older patients and in patients with known or suspected cardiac decompensation, a slower rate of infusion is probably wise.

If nausea or flushing occurs during administration, the infusion should be slowed or briefly interrupted.

Films are taken before the onset of the infusion and at the desired intervals following its completion. When renal function is normal, a nephrogram may be taken as soon as the infusion is completed, and films of the collecting system at 10 and 20 minutes thereafter. Voiding cystourethrograms are usually optimal at 20 minutes after the infusion is completed. In hypertensive patients, early minute sequence films may be taken during the course of infusion, in addition to subsequent pyelograms. In patients with renal dysfunction, optimal visualization is usually delayed, and late films are taken as indicated.

The nephrogram obtained by the drip infusion procedure may be dense enough to obscure the pelvocalyceal system in some cases. The presence of gas in the bowel may hamper early visualization of the renal collecting system. Tomographic "cuts" may help to overcome such difficulties.

Nephrotomography may begin when the infusion is completed. The sustained contrast achieved by the drip infusion technique eliminates the need for precise timing and teamwork that is necessary with ordinary nephrotomography. Thus, if nephrograms taken after infusion of the medium suggest the need for sectional films, or if preselected tomographic "cuts" are not sufficient, additional tomograms may be obtained at once, and without repetition of dosage.

Cerebral Angiography—Appropriate preparation of the patient is indicated, including suitable premedication. The average single dose for adults is 10 ml. repeated as indicated. Children require less in proportion to weight.

Either the percutaneous or operative method of administration may be used. For visualization of the cerebral vessels, the contrast medium is injected into the common carotid artery; for angiography of the vessels in the posterior fossa or the occipital lobes, the medium is injected into the vertebral artery. Since the medium is given by rapid injection, the patient should be watched for untoward reactions. Unless general anesthesia is used, patients should be warned that the medium may provoke movement and that they may feel transient pain, flushing, or burning during the injection.

A scout film should be made routinely before the contrast medium is injected. Serial films begun while the last few ml. are being injected should permit visualization of the arterial, intermediate, and venous phases.

Peripheral Arteriography—Appropriate preparation of the patient is indicated, including suitable premedication. For visualization of an entire extremity, a single dose of 20 to 40 ml. is suggested; for the upper or lower half of the extremity only, 10 to 20 ml. is usually sufficient.

Injection is made into the femoral or subclavian artery by the percutaneous or operative method. Because the contrast agent is given by rapid injection, flushing of the skin may occur. Patients not under general anesthesia may experience nausea and vomiting or a transient feeling of warmth. Vascular spasm is not likely to occur.

A scout film should be made routinely before administering the contrast medium. Radiograms of the upper half of the extremity are taken while the last few ml. are being injected, followed by radiograms of the lower half of the extremity a few seconds later.

minutes following the procedure since severe delayed reactions have been known to occur.
Nausea, vomiting, flushing, or a generalized feeling of warmth are the reactions seen most frequently with intravascular injection. Symptoms which may occur are chills, fever, sweating, headache, dizziness, pallor, weakness, severe retching and choking, wheezing, a rise or fall in blood pressure, facial or conjunctival petechiae, urticaria, pruritus, rash and other eruptions, edema, cramps, tremors, itching, sneezing, lacrimation, etc. Antihistaminic agents may be of benefit; rarely, such reactions may be severe enough to require discontinuation of dosage.
Although local tissue tolerance is usually good, there have been a few reports of a burning or stinging sensation or numbness and of venospasm or venous pain, and partial collapse of the injected vein. Neutropenia or thrombophlebitis may occur.
Severe reactions which may require emergency measures may take the form of a cardiovascular reaction characterized by peripheral vasodilatation with resultant hypotension and reflex tachycardia, dyspnea, agitation, confusion, and cyanosis progressing to unconsciousness. Or, the histamine-liberating effect of these compounds may induce an allergic-like reaction which may range in severity from rhinitis or angioneurotic edema to laryngeal or bronchial spasm or anaphylactoid shock.
Temporary renal shutdown or other nephropathy may occur.
Adverse reactions may sometimes occur as a consequence of the procedure for which the contrast agent is used. Adverse reactions in *excretion urography* have included cardiac arrest, ventricular fibrillation, anaphylaxis with severe asthmatic reaction, and flushing due to generalized vasodilatation. In *aortography*, the risks of procedures include injury to the aorta and neighboring organs, pleural puncture, renal damage including infarction and acute tubular necrosis with oliguria and anuria, accidental selective filling of the right renal artery during the translumbar procedure in the presence of preexistent renal disease, retroperitoneal hemorrhage from the translumbar approach, spinal cord injury and pathology associated with the syndrome of transverse myelitis, generalized petechiae, and death following hypotension, arrhythmia, and anaphylactoid reactions. Adverse reactions in *pediatric angiocardiography* have included arrhythmia and death. During *peripheral arteriography*, complications have occurred including hemorrhage from the puncture site, thrombosis of the vessel, and brachial plexus palsy following axillary artery injections. During *selective coronary arteriography* and *selective coronary arteriography combined with left ventriculography*, most patients will have transient ECG changes. Transient arrhythmias may occur infrequently. Ventricular fibrillation may result from manipulation of the catheter during the procedure or administration of the medium. Other reactions may include hypotension, chest pain, and myocardial infarction. Transient elevation of CPK (creatine phosphokinase) has occurred in approximately 30 percent of the patients tested. Fatalities have been reported. Complications due to the procedure include hemorrhage, thrombosis, pseudoaneurysms at the puncture site, and dislodgment of arteriosclerotic plaques. Dissection of the coronary vessels and transient sinus arrest have occurred rarely.
Adverse reactions in *selective renal arteriography* include nausea, vomiting, hypotension and hypertension. Post-arteriographic changes in laboratory studies include transient elevations in BUN, serum creatinine and glucose.
Complications due to the procedure during *selective visceral arteriography* include hematomas, thrombosis, pseudoaneurysms at injection site, and dislodgment of arteriosclerotic plaques. Other reactions may include urticaria, hypotension, hypertension, and insignificant changes in renal function and liver chemistry tests.

Dosage and Administration: Renografin-76 (Diatrizoate Meglumine and Diatrizoate Sodium Injection USP) should be at body temperature when injected, and may need to be warmed before use. Syringes should be rinsed as soon as possible after injection to prevent freezing of the plunger.

Withdrawal of the contrast agent should be accomplished under aseptic conditions with sterile syringe.

Excretion Urography

Appropriate preparation of the patient is desirable for optimal results. A laxative the night before the examination, a low residue diet the day before, and low liquid intake for 12 hours prior to the procedure may be used to clear the gastrointestinal tract and to induce a partial dehydration which is believed to increase the urinary concentration of the contrast medium. Enemas are to be avoided to prevent rehydration.
Preparatory partial dehydration is not recommended in infants, young children, the elderly, or azotemic patients (especially those with polyuria, oliguria, diabetes, advanced vascular disease, or preexisting dehydration). The undesirable dehydration in these patients may be accentuated by the osmotic diuretic action of the medium.
In uremic patients partial dehydration is not necessary and maintenance of adequate fluid intake is particularly desirable.
The usual intravenous dose for patients aged 16 years or more is 20 ml., but 30 or 40 ml. have been used. Children require less in proportion to weight: Under 6 months of age—4 ml.; 6 to 12 months—6 ml.; 1 to 2 years—8 ml.; 2 to 5 years—10 ml.; 5 to 7 years—12 ml.; 8 to 10 years—14 ml.; 11 to 15 years—16 ml.
The preparation is given by intravenous injection. If flushing or nausea occurs during administration, injection should be slowed or briefly interrupted until the side effects have disappeared.
A scout film should be made before the contrast medium is administered. To allow for individual variation, several films should be exposed beginning approximately five minutes after injection. In patients with renal dysfunction, optimal visualization may be delayed until 30 minutes or more after injection.
NOTE: In infants and children and in certain adults, the medium may be injected intramuscularly. The suggested dose is the same as the intravenous dose divided and given bilaterally in the gluteal muscles. Radiographs should be taken at 20, 40, and 60 minutes after the medium is injected.

Aortography

Renografin-76 (Diatrizoate Meglumine and Diatrizoate Sodium Injection USP) injected into the aorta by the translumbar or retrograde method of administration permits radiographic visualization of the aorta, its major branches and the abdominal arteries. An incidental nephrogram is obtained as the contrast medium travels through the renal vasculature, provided it has been injected above the renal artery.
Patients should be prepared in a manner similar to that used for intravenous urography. Premedication with a suitable barbiturate is generally indicated.
As in any form of surgery, certain hazards accompany aortographic procedures (see ADVERSE REACTIONS).
For adults and children over 16 years of age, the usual dose is 15 to 40 ml. as a single injection, repeated if indicated. Children require less in proportion to weight. Doses up to a total of 160 ml. have been given safely.
Since the medium is given by rapid injection in this procedure, patients should be watched for untoward reactions during the injection. Unless general anesthesia is employed, patients should be warned that they may feel some transient pain or burning during the injection followed by a feeling of warmth immediately afterward.
A scout film should be made before the contrast agent is administered. The first radiogram should be taken as the last few ml. of the contrast medium are being injected.

Pediatric Angiocardiography

Angiocardiography with Renografin-76 (Diatrizoate Meglumine and Diatrizoate Sodium Injection USP) may be performed by injection into a large peripheral vein or by direct catheterization of the heart. An excretory urogram can be obtained 10 to 15 minutes after injection of the contrast medium since it is concentrated in and eliminated by the kidneys.
Patients should be prepared in a manner similar to that used for intravenous urography. Appropriate preanesthetic medication should be given.
Clinical studies in man and related animal experiments have suggested that the hypertonicity of diatrizoate contrast agents produces significant hemodynamic effects, especially in right-sided injections. Large volumes of such agents cause a drop in peripheral arterial and systemic pressures and cardiac output, a rise in pulmonary arterial and right-heart pressures, bradycardia, and regular ectopic beats. Resulting effects on peripheral arterial and pulmonary arterial pressures are postulated to be due to mechanical blockage of the pulmonary vascular bed and clumping of red cells.
Hypertonic solutions cause a decrease in hematocrit *in vitro* and *in vivo*, and shrinkage of red blood cells.
It is suggested that hemodynamic changes be monitored and that pressures considered abnormal under roentgenographic conditions be allowed to return to a preangiographic level before continuation of radiopaque injection; this usually takes 15 minutes.
The suggested single dose for children *under* five years of age is 10 to 20 ml., depending on the size of the child. For children 5 to 10 years of age, single doses of 20 to 30 ml. are recommended. Doses up to a total of 100 ml. have been given safely.
Since the contrast medium is given by rapid injection, the patient should be watched for untoward reactions during the injection. Some patients not under general anesthesia may experience a feeling of bodily warmth, tightness of the chest and throbbing headache. All these sensations are of short duration. Transient nausea and vomiting may occur in some patients.
A preliminary control film should be made in the usual manner.

Peripheral Arteriography

Appropriate preparation of the patient is indicated, including suitable premedication. For visualization of an entire extremity, a single dose of 20 to 40 ml. is suggested; for the upper or lower half of the extremity only, 10 to 20 ml. is usually sufficient.
Injection is made into the femoral or subclavian artery by the percutaneous or operative method. Because the contrast agent is given by rapid injection, flushing of the skin may occur. Patients not under general anesthesia may experience nausea and vomiting or a transient feeling of warmth. Vascular spasm is not likely to occur.
A scout film should be made routinely before administering the contrast medium. Radiograms of the upper half of the extremity are taken while the last few ml. are being injected, followed by radiograms of the lower half of the extremity a few seconds later.

Selective Renal Arteriography

The usual dose is 5 to 10 ml. injected into either or both renal arteries via femoral artery

Continued on next page

Squibb—Cont.

catheterization. This dose may be repeated as necessary; doses up to 60 ml. have been given.

Selective Visceral Arteriography
The usual dose is 30 to 50 ml. injected into the appropriate visceral artery (celiac axis and its branches, superior mesenteric artery, or inferior mesenteric artery) via femoral artery catheterization. This may be repeated as necessary. It is recommended that the combined total dose not exceed 250 ml.

Selective Coronary Arteriography
The usual dose is 4 to 10 ml. injected into a coronary artery. This dose, repeated as necessary, may be administered into each coronary artery; doses up to a total of 150 ml. have been given. Patients should be monitored continuously by ECG throughout the procedure.

Selective Coronary Arteriography Combined with Left Ventriculography
For left ventriculography the usual dose is 35 to 50 ml. injected into the left ventricle. This may be repeated as necessary. It is recommended that the total dose for combined selective coronary arteriography and left ventriculography not exceed 200 ml.

Computed Tomography
The suggested dose is 50 to 125 ml. by intravenous administration; scanning may be performed immediately after completion of administration. Doses for children should be proportionately less, depending on age and weight.

Patient Preparation—No special patient preparation is required for contrast enhancement of CT brain scanning. However, it is advisable to insure that patients are well hydrated prior to examination.

How Supplied: Single dose vials of 20 ml. and 50 ml. and single dose bottles of 100 ml. and 200 ml. An excess volume (1 ml.) is available in each container for sensitivity testing. [50 ml. vials—Military Depot Item, NSN6505-00-159-5008 and V.A. Depot Item, NSN6505-00-605-8942A; 200 ml. bottle—Military Depot Item, NSN6505-00-138-7344 and V.A. Depot Item, NSN6505-00-330-7505A].

Storage: The preparation should be stored at room temperature, protected from light. If precipitation or solidification has occurred due to storage in the cold, immerse the container in hot water and shake intermittently to redissolve any solids.

RENO-M-30® ℞

(Diatrizoate Meglumine Injection USP 30%)
For retrograde pyelography
Not intended for intravascular injection

Description: Reno-M-30 is a radiopaque contrast agent for retrograde pyelography supplied as a sterile, aqueous solution. Each ml. provides 300 mg. diatrizoate meglumine with 3.2 mg. sodium citrate as a buffer, 0.4 mg. edetate disodium as a sequestering agent, and 1 mg. methylparaben and 0.3 mg. propylparaben as preservatives. Each ml. of solution also contains approximately 141 mg. organically bound iodine. At the time of manufacture, the air in the container is replaced by nitrogen.

Indications: Reno-M-30 (Diatrizoate Meglumine Injection USP 30%) is intended for retrograde or ascending pyelography. This procedure may be used if intravenous excretion urography is contraindicated and it is also useful in complementing other diagnostic information.

Contraindications: Contraindications pertain to the procedure of retrograde pyelography rather than to the administration of the medium *per se*. Retrograde pyelography should not be performed in those conditions which do not allow for the successful catheterizaton of the ureters such as extensive urinary tuberculosis, tumors of the bladder, impassable obstructions of the ureters, or marked enlargement of the prostate gland.

Warning: Apart from the possible adverse effects of diatrizoate meglumine, the hazards of the performance of a retrograde genitourinary procedure exist. These include such complications as hematuria, perforation of the ureter or bladder, introduction of infection into the genitourinary tract, and oliguria or anuria.

Precautions: Because of the possibility of inducing temporary suppression of urine, it is wise to avoid repetition of retrograde pyelography within 48 hours in patients with reduced renal function.

Retrograde pyelography should be performed with caution in patients with a known active infectious process of the urinary tract.

Contrast agents may interfere with some chemical determinations made on urine specimens; therefore, urine should be collected before administration of the contrast medium or two or more days afterwards.

Adverse Reactions: The incidence of adverse reactions with diatrizoate meglumine is very low. Costovertebral angle tenderness, elevated temperature and flank pain have been reported in a few patients following use of the preparation for retrograde pyelography, as have nausea, sweating and flushing.

Irritation of the urinary tract mucosa attributable to the contrast agent itself is not likely to occur. However, the technique of retrograde pyelography may be painful and may initiate pelvic, caliceal, or ureteral spasms with consequent renal colic.

Since retrograde pyelography does not involve systemic administration of a contrast agent, the risk of severe reactions, which may occur with intravenous administration, is extremely remote. However, they should be kept in mind whenever a contrast agent is administered. Severe reactions may be manifested by edema of the face and glottis, respiratory distress, convulsions, or shock; such reactions may prove fatal unless promptly controlled by such emergency measures as maintenance of a clear airway and immediate use of oxygen and resuscitative drugs. Like other sensitivity phenomena, severe reactions are more likely to occur in patients with a personal or family history of bronchial asthma, significant allergies, drug reactions, or previous reactions to contrast agents.

Dosage and Administration: Preparation of the patient: Appropriate preparation is desirable for optimal results. A laxative the night before the examination and a low residue diet the day before the procedure are recommended.

Dosage: The usual dose for patients aged 16 years or more is 15 ml. for unilateral and appropriately increased volumes for bilateral pyelograms. Approximately 5 to 6 ml. will generally be required for each exposure. The dosage for children should be proportionately smaller than the adult dose.

As supplied, the preparation provides maximum opacification. If a lesser contrast is desired, it may be diluted with sterile distilled water.

Administration: Reno-M-30 (Diatrizoate Meglumine Injection USP 30%) may be introduced by a gravity flow system or by syringe. When the syringe method is used, the injection should be made slowly and care should be exercised to use as little manual pressure as possible. Regardless of the system used, injection of the contrast medium should be terminated as soon as the patient complains of a sense of fullness or pain in the renal region.

Radiography: The commonly employed radiographic techniques should be used. A scout film is recommended before the contrast agent is administered.

How Supplied: Available in multiple-dose vials of 50 ml. and 100 ml.

Storage: The preparation should be protected from strong light and stored at room temperature; avoid freezing.

RENO-M-60® ℞

(Diatrizoate Meglumine Injection USP 60%)

Description: Reno-M-60 is a radiopaque contrast agent supplied as a sterile, aqueous solution for parenteral use. Each ml. provides 600 mg. diatrizoate meglumine with 3.2 mg. sodium citrate as a buffer and 0.4 mg. edetate disodium as a sequestering agent; pH has been adjusted between 6.5 and 7.7 with meglumine or diatrizoic acid. *Each ml. of solution also contains appoximately 0.91 mg. (0.04 mEq.) sodium* and 282 mg. organically bound iodine. At the time of manufacture, the air in the container is replaced by nitrogen.

Clinical Pharmacology: Following intravascular injection, Reno-M-60 (Diatrizoate Meglumine Injection USP 60%) is rapidly transported through the bloodstream to the kidneys and is excreted unchanged in the urine by glomerular filtration. When urinary tract obstruction is severe enough to block glomerular filtration, the agent appears to be excreted by the tubular epithelium.

Certain applications of the contrast agent make use of the natural physiologic mechanism of excretion. Thus, the intravenous injection of the agent permits visualization of the kidneys and urinary passages.

Renal accumulation is sufficiently rapid that the period of maximal opacification of the renal passages may begin as early as five minutes after injection. In infants and small children excretion takes place somewhat more promptly than in adults, so that maximal opacification occurs more rapidly and is less sustained. The normal kidney eliminates the contrast medium almost immediately. In nephropathic conditions, particularly when excretory capacity has been altered, the rate of excretion varies unpredictably, and opacification may be delayed for 30 minutes or more after injection; with severe impairment opacification may not occur. Generally, however, the medium is concentrated in sufficient amounts and promptly enough to permit a thorough evaluation of the anatomy and physiology of the urinary tract.

After intramuscular injection, the contrast agent is promptly absorbed and normally reaches the renal passages within 20 to 60 minutes.

Intravascular injection of diatrizoate meglumine also opacifies those vessels in the path of flow of the medium, permitting visualization until the circulating blood dilutes the concentration of the medium. Thus selective angiography may be performed following injection directly into veins or arteries such as the carotid, the vertebral, or the vessels of the extremities.

Under certain circumstances, specific parts of the body which do not concentrate the contrast agent physiologically may be visualized by injecting the agent directly into the region to be studied. The biliary tract is one organ system which may be visualized in this manner. In operative cholangiography, injection of the radiopaque medium into the cystic duct or choledochal lumen, at laparotomy, opacifies the intra- and extra-hepatic biliary ductal system, revealing the nature and location of obstructions such as stones or strictures. Injection of the medium through an in-place T-tube, immediately after exploration of the common duct, permits the visualization of retained stones. A repetition of "T-tube cholangiography," performed as part of the postoperative follow-up, insures the patency of the ductal system before removal of the T-tube. The biliary ductal system may also be opacified by the percutaneous-transhepatic route. In relatively long-standing biliary obstruction, the biliary ducts are usually enlarged sufficiently to be located promptly by percutaneous transhepatic probing, permitting injection of the contrast agent directly into the biliary ductal system.

If the contrast agent is injected directly into the splenic pulp, significant opacification of the splenic and portal veins is obtained. Because of gravity, the dependent portions of the portal system are better opacified than the superior portions. The agent is carried from the portal vein into the hepatic veins, and a diffuse opacification of the liver results. In patients with portal hypertension, collateral pathways caused by the change in portal blood flow may be visualized and esophageal varices are often delineated. The procedure may reveal the site of portal obstruction.

Injection of Reno-M-60 (Diatrizoate Meglumine Injection USP 60%) directly into a joint space provides visual information about joint derangements.

A small amount of the radiopaque agent injected into a normal cervical or lumbar disk will, under optimal conditions, concentrate within the nucleus pulposus. In the presence of disk pathology the injected agent may reveal significant bulging or disruption of the annulus beyond its normal confines and may identify disk degeneration, retropulsion, or rupture.

Indications: Reno-M-60 (Diatrizoate Meglumine Injection USP 60%) is indicated in excretion urography (by direct I.V. or drip infusion); cerebral angiography; peripheral arteriography; venography; operative, T-tube, or percutaneous transhepatic cholangiography; splenoportography; arthrography; and discography.

Contraindications: This preparation is contraindicated in patients with a hypersensitivity to salts of diatrizoic acid.

Urography is contraindicated in patients with anuria.

Specific contraindications to **percutaneous transhepatic cholangiography** include a prothrombin time below 50 percent and evidence of coagulation defects.

Splenoportography should not be performed on any patient for whom splenectomy is contraindicated since complications of the procedure at times make splenectomy necessary. Other contraindications include prothrombin time below 50 percent, significant thrombocytopenia or coagulation defect, and any condition which may increase the possibility of rupture of the spleen.

Arthrography should not be performed if infection is present in or near the joint.

Discography should not be performed in patients with an infection or open injury near the region to be examined.

Warnings: A definite risk exists in the use of intravascular contrast agents in patients who are known to have multiple myeloma. In such instances there has been anuria resulting in progressive uremia, renal failure, and eventually death. Although neither the contrast agent nor dehydration has separately proved to be the cause of anuria in myeloma, it has been speculated that the combination of both may be the causative factor. The risk in myelomatous patients is not a contraindication to the procedures; however, partial dehydration in the preparation of these patients for the examination is not recommended since this may predispose to the precipitation of myeloma protein in the renal tubules. No form of therapy, including dialysis, has been successful in reversing this effect. Myeloma, which occurs most commonly in persons over age 40, should be considered before intravascular administration of a contrast agent.

Administration of radiopaque materials to patients known or suspected to have pheochromocytoma should be performed with extreme caution. If, in the opinion of the physician, the possible benefits of such procedures outweigh the considered risks, the procedures may be performed; however, the amount of radiopaque medium injected should be kept to an absolute minimum. The blood pressure should be assessed throughout the procedure and measures for treatment of a hypertensive crisis should be available.

Cerebral angiography should be undertaken with special caution in extreme age, poor clinical condition, advanced arteriosclerosis, severe arterial hypertension, cardiac decompensation, recent cerebral embolism, or thrombosis.

Urography should be performed with extreme caution in patients with severe concomitant hepatic and renal disease.

Contrast media have been shown to promote the phenomenon of sickling in individuals who are homozygous for sickle cell disease when the material is injected intravenously or intra-arterially.

Since iodine-containing contrast agents may alter the results of thyroid function tests, such tests, if indicated, should be performed prior to the administration of this preparation.

A history of sensitivity to iodine *per se* or to other contrast agents is not an absolute contraindication to the use of diatrizoate meglumine, but calls for extreme caution in administration.

Avoid accidental introduction of this preparation into the subarachnoid space since even small amounts may produce convulsions and possible fatal reactions.

Precautions: Diagnostic procedures which involve the use of radiopaque contrast agents should be carried out under the direction of personnel with the prerequisite training and with a thorough knowledge of the particular procedure to be performed (see ADVERSE REACTIONS).

Severe, life-threatening reactions suggest hypersensitivity to the radiopaque agent, which has prompted the use of several pretesting methods, none of which can be relied upon to predict severe reactions. Many authorities question the value of any pretest. A history of bronchial asthma or allergy, a family history of allergy, or a previous reaction to a contrast agent warrant special attention. Such a history, by suggesting histamine sensitivity and a consequent proneness to reactions, may be more accurate than pretesting in predicting the likelihood of a reaction, although not necessarily the severity or type of reaction in the individual case.

The sensitivity test most often performed is the slow injection of 0.5 to 1.0 ml. of the radiopaque medium, administered intravenously, prior to injection of the full diagnostic dose. It should be noted that the absence of a reaction to the test dose does not preclude the possibility of a reaction to the full diagnostic dose. If the test dose causes an untoward response of any kind, the necessity for continuing with the examination should be carefully reevaluated and, if it is deemed essential, the examination should be conducted with all possible caution. In rare instances, reactions to the test dose itself may be extremely severe; therefore, close observation of the patient, and facilities for emergency treatment, appear indicated.

Renal toxicity has been reported in a few patients with liver dysfunction who were given oral cholecystographic agents followed by urographic agents. Administration of Reno-M-60 (Diatrizoate Meglumine Injection USP 60%) should therefore be postponed in any patient with a known or suspected hepatic or biliary disorder who has recently taken a cholecystographic contrast agent.

Caution should be exercised with the use of radiopaque media in severely debilitated patients and in those with marked hypertension. The possibility of thrombosis should be borne in mind when percutaneous techniques are employed.

Consideration must be given to the functional ability of the kidneys before injecting diatrizoate meglumine.

Contrast agents may interfere with some chemical determinations made on urine specimens; therefore, urine should be collected before administration of the contrast medium or two or more days afterwards.

The following precautions pertain to specific procedures:

Peripheral arteriography: Hypotension or moderate decreases in blood pressure seem to occur frequently with intra-arterial (brachial) injections; therefore, the blood pressure should be monitored during the immediate ten minutes after injection; this blood pressure change is transient and usually requires no treatment.

Excretion urography: Adequate visualization may be difficult or impossible to attain in uremic patients or others with severely impaired renal function (see CONTRAINDICATIONS). The increased osmotic load associated with drip infusion pyelography should be considered in patients with congestive heart failure. The diuretic effect of the drip infusion pyelography procedure may hinder assessment of residual urine in the bladder. The recommended rate of infusion should not be exceeded.

Acute renal failure has been reported in diabetic patients with diabetic nephropathy and susceptible nondiabetic patients (often elderly with preexisting renal disease) following excretion urography. Therefore, careful consideration should be given before performing this procedure in these patients.

Operative and T-tube cholangiography: Injection should be made slowly to prevent extravasation of the medium into the peritoneal cavity, and to minimize reflux flow into the pancreatic duct which may result in pancreatic irritation.

Percutaneous transhepatic cholangiography: To reduce the possibility of bile leakage and consequent peritonitis, as much of the contrast agent as possible should be aspirated on completion of successful films. All patients should be carefully and constantly monitored for 24 hours after the procedure for signs of internal hemorrhage or bile leakage; if these complications are recognized immediately, remedial measures can be instituted promptly with minimal increase in morbidity. Percutaneous transhepatic cholangiography is not without risk and should therefore be reserved for special circumstances when ordinary studies of the biliary system have failed to provide the requisite information in jaundiced patients who are not good candidates for surgery. The procedure should only be attempted when competent surgical intervention can be promptly obtained if needed.

Splenoportography: It is best to avoid manipulations which would prolong the time the needle is in the spleen since they may contribute to subcapsular extravasation of the contrast agent and also to postpuncture bleeding. Following splenoportography, the patient should lie on his left side for several hours and should be closely observed for 24 hours for signs of internal bleeding, which is the most common complication of the procedure. Fatal hemorrhage has occurred on rare occasion, but leakage of up to 300 ml. of blood from the spleen is apparently not uncommon. Blood transfusions may be required, and rarely splenectomy.

Discography: To minimize the possibility of introducing infection, discography should be postponed in any patient with an infection or open injury near the region to be examined, including upper respiratory infections in the case of cervical discography. All possible care should be taken to preclude contamination and resultant infection of the disk, which has been reported after discography. In cervical discography, particular care is needed to avoid puncturing the esophagus and thereby introducing contamination into the disk. Rupture of the

Continued on next page

Squibb—Cont.

disk is highly unlikely if care in performance is observed, but may occur if the point of the needle has been barbed by contact with bone; use of the two-needle technique should help reduce this hazard.

Usage in Pregnancy: The safety of diatrizoate meglumine for use during pregnancy has not been established; therefore, this preparation should be used in pregnant patients only when, in the judgment of the physician, its use is deemed essential to the welfare of the patient.

Adverse Reactions: Adverse reactions accompanying the use of iodine-containing intravascular contrast agents are usually mild and transient although severe and life-threatening reactions, including fatalities, have occurred. Because of the possibility of severe reactions to the procedure and/or the radiopaque medium, appropriate emergency facilities and well-trained personnel should be available to treat both conditions. Emergency facilities and personnel should remain available for 30 to 60 minutes following the procedure since severe delayed reactions have been known to occur.

Nausea, vomiting, flushing, or a generalized feeling of warmth are the reactions seen most frequently with intravascular injection. Symptoms which may occur are chills, fever, sweating, headache, dizziness, pallor, weakness, severe retching and choking, wheezing, a rise or fall in blood pressure, facial or conjunctival petechiae, urticaria, pruritus, rash and other eruptions, edema, cramps, tremors, itching, sneezing, lacrimation, etc. Antihistaminic agents may be of benefit; rarely such reactions may be severe enough to require discontinuation of dosage.

Severe reactions which may require emergency measures may take the form of a cardiovascular reaction characterized by peripheral vasodilatation with resultant hypotension and reflex tachycardia, dyspnea, agitation, confusion, and cyanosis progressing to unconsciousness. Or, the histamine-liberating effect of these compounds may induce an allergic-like reaction which may range in severity from rhinitis or angioneurotic edema to laryngeal or bronchial spasm or anaphylactoid shock.

Temporary renal shutdown or other nephropathy may occur. Temporary neurologic effects of varying severity have occurred in a few instances, particularly when the medium was used for angiography in the diagnosis of cerebral pathology. Although local tissue tolerance is usually good, there have been a few reports of a burning or stinging sensation or numbness and of venospasm or venous pain, and partial collapse of the injected vein. Neutropenia or thrombophlebitis may occur.

Adverse effects may sometimes occur as a consequence of the procedure for which the contrast agent is used. Adverse reactions in **excretion urography** have included cardiac arrest, ventricular fibrillation, anaphylaxis with severe asthmatic reaction, and flushing due to generalized vasodilation. **Cerebral angiography** has been known to cause temporary neurologic complications such as induction of seizures, particularly in patients with convulsive disorders; confusional states or drowsiness; transient paresis; coma; temporary disturbances in vision; or seventh nerve weakness. During **peripheral arteriography,** complications have occurred including hemorrhage from the puncture site, thrombosis of the vessel, and brachial plexus palsy following axillary artery injections.

Complications of **percutaneous transhepatic cholangiography** have been estimated to occur in four to six percent of cases and have included bile leakage and biliary peritonitis, gallbladder perforation, internal bleeding, septicemia involving gram-negative organisms, and tension pneumothorax from inadvertent puncture of the diaphragm and lung. Bile leakage may be more likely in patients with complete obstruction due to carcinoma.

During **splenoportography,** intraperitoneal extravasation of the contrast medium may cause transient diaphragmatic irritation or mild to moderate transient pain which may sometimes be referred to the shoulder, the periumbilical region, or other areas. Because of the proximity of the pleural cavity, accidental pneumothorax has been known to occur. Inadvertent injection of the medium into other nearby structures is not likely to cause untoward consequences.

Arthrography may induce joint pain or increase existing pain, particularly if a large dose is used and the medium extravasates into surrounding soft tissue. Pain or discomfort is usually immediate and transient but may be delayed or of extended duration (up to 24 hours). Lipid-filled histiocytes have been found in tissue removed following arthrography. The technique of **discography** may be painful, particularly when disk pathology exists. Pain on injection may also be related to the volume of the dose. The nature of the disk pathology or extravasation of contrast agent may cause referred pain.

When any percutaneous technique is employed, the possibility of thrombosis or of other complications due to the mechanical trauma of the procedure should be borne in mind.

Dosage and Administration: Reno-M-60 (Diatrizoate Meglumine Injection USP 60%) should be at body temperature when injected and may need to be warmed before use. If kept in a syringe for prolonged periods before injection, it should be protected from exposure to strong light.

Dilution and withdrawal of the contrast agent should be accomplished under aseptic conditions with sterile needle and syringe.

Excretion Urography—Appropriate preparation of the patient is desirable for optimal results. In adults and older children, a laxative the night before the examination, a low residue diet the day before, and low liquid intake for 12 hours prior to the procedure may be used to clear the gastrointestinal tract and to induce a partial dehydration which is believed to increase the urinary concentration of the contrast medium. Preparatory partial dehydration is not recommended in infants, young children, the elderly, or azotemic patients (especially those with polyuria, oliguria, diabetes, advanced vascular disease, or preexisting dehydration). The undesirable dehydration in these patients may be accentuated by the osmotic diuretic action of the medium.

In uremic patients partial dehydration is not necessary and maintenance of adequate fluid intake is particularly desirable.

Direct I.V. Injection—The dose range for adults is 25 to 50 ml.; the usual dose is 25 ml.; children require proportionately less. Suggested dosages are as follows: Under 6 months—5 ml.; 6 to 12 months—8 ml.; 1 to 2 years—10 ml.; 2 to 5 years—12 ml.; 5 to 7 years—15 ml.; 8 to 10 years—18 ml.; 11 to 15 years—20 ml.; adults (16 years and older)—25 to 50 ml. In adults, when the smaller dose has provided inadequate visualization or when poor visualization is anticipated, the 50 ml. dose may be given. Drip infusion may be used when direct I.V. pyelography is not expected to be or has not been satisfactory (see below).

The preparation is given by intravenous injection. If flushing or nausea occurs during administration, injection should be slowed or briefly interrupted until the side effects have disappeared.

A scout film should be made before the contrast medium is administered. To allow for individual variation, several films should be exposed beginning approximately five minutes after injection. In patients with renal dysfunction, optimal visualization may be delayed until 30 minutes or more after injection.

NOTE: In infants and children and in certain adults, the medium may be injected intramuscularly. The suggested dose is 25 ml. for adults and proportionately less for children, divided and given bilaterally in the gluteal muscles. Radiographs should be taken at 20, 40, and 60 minutes after the medium is injected.

Drip Infusion Pyelography—In drip infusion pyelography, the recommended dose of Reno-M-60 is calculated on the basis of 1 ml. of Reno-M-60 (Diatrizoate Meglumine Injection USP 60%) per pound of body weight diluted with an equal volume of Sterile Water for Injection USP. The diluted preparation (30%) is given by I.V. infusion through a large bore (17- to 18-gauge) needle at a rate of 40 ml. per minute. The recommended rate of infusion should not be exceeded and the total volume administered should generally not exceed 300 ml. In older patients and in patients with known or suspected cardiac decompensation, a slower rate of infusion is probably wise.

If nausea or flushing occurs during administration, the infusion should be slowed or briefly interrupted.

Films are taken before the onset of the infusion and at the desired intervals following its completion. When renal function is normal, a nephrogram may be taken as soon as the infusion is completed, and films of the collecting system at 10 and 20 minutes thereafter. Voiding cystourethrograms are usually optimal at 20 minutes after the infusion is completed. In hypertensive patients, early minute sequence films may be taken during the course of infusion, in addition to subsequent pyelograms. In patients with renal dysfunction, optimal visualization is usually delayed, and late films are taken as indicated.

The nephrogram obtained by the drip infusion procedure may be dense enough to obscure the pelvocalyceal system in some cases. The presence of gas in the bowel may hamper early visualization of the renal collecting system. Tomographic "cuts" may help to overcome such difficulties.

Nephrotomography may begin when the infusion is completed. The sustained contrast achieved by the drip infusion technique eliminates the need for precise timing and teamwork that is necessary with ordinary nephrotomography. Thus, if nephrograms taken after infusion of the medium suggest the need for sectional films, or if preselected tomographic "cuts" are not sufficient, additional tomograms may be obtained at once, and without repetition of dosage.

Cerebral Angiography—Appropriate preparation of the patient is indicated, including suitable premedication. The average single dose for adults is 10 ml., repeated as indicated. Children require less in proportion to weight.

Either the percutaneous or operative method of administration may be used. For visualization of the cerebral vessels, the contrast medium is injected into the common carotid artery; for angiography of the vessels in the posterior fossa or the occipital lobes, the medium is injected into the vertebral artery. Since the medium is given by rapid injection, the patient should be watched for untoward reactions. Unless general anesthesia is used, patients should be warned that the medium may provoke movement and that they may feel transient pain, flushing, or burning during the injection. A scout film should be made routinely before the contrast medium is injected. Serial films begun while the last few ml. are being injected should permit visualization of the arterial, intermediate, and venous phases.

Peripheral Arteriography—Appropriate preparation of the patient is indicated, including suitable premedication. For visualization of an entire extremity, a single dose of 20 to 40 ml. is suggested; for the upper or lower half of the

extremity only, 10 to 20 ml. is usually sufficient.
Injection is made into the femoral or subclavian artery by the percutaneous or operative method. Because the contrast agent is given by rapid injection, flushing of the skin may occur. Patients not under general anesthesia may experience nausea and vomiting or a transient feeling of warmth. Vascular spasm is not likely to occur.
A scout film should be made routinely before administering the contrast medium. Radiograms of the upper half of the extremity are taken while the last few ml. are being injected, followed by radiograms of the lower half of the extremity a few seconds later.
Venography—For visualization of veins in the upper extremities, a single dose of 10 ml. per extremity is suggested. For veins in the lower extremities, doses of 20 to 40 ml. per extremity are suggested. In exceptional circumstances, larger doses may be necessary; visualization of the iliac vein, extensive varicosities or large veins may require 50 ml. or more. Total doses up to 100 ml. per lower extremity have been used safely.
For visualization of an upper extremity, the medium may be given by percutaneous injection into any convenient superficial vein of the forearm or hand. For the visualization of a lower extremity, it should be injected into a superficial vein on the lateral side of the foot. The medium is injected rapidly; patients should be observed for untoward reactions.
Radiograms are taken when injection is completed; sufficient time should be allowed to permit diffusion of the contrast medium.
Operative and Postoperative Cholangiography—Operative cholangiography is performed as soon as the gallbladder and ducts have been exposed surgically. The usual dose is 10 ml., but as much as 25 ml. may be needed, depending on the caliber of the ducts. If desired, the contrast agent may be diluted 1:1 with Sodium Chloride Injection USP under strict aseptic procedures.
The contrast medium is instilled slowly through the stump of the cystic duct or directly into the choledochal lumen. Following surgical exploration of the ductal system, repeat studies may be performed before closure of the abdomen, using the same dose as before.
Postoperatively, the ductal system may be examined by injection of the contrast agent through an in-place T-tube. "T-tube cholangiography" is usually performed eight to ten days after operation; the usual dose is the same as for operative cholangiography.
For each procedure, films are taken immediately after instillation of the medium and are read immediately. Additional films are then taken if necessary.
Percutaneous Transhepatic Cholangiography—Facilities for emergency surgery should be available whenever this examination is performed. Appropriate premedication of the patient is recommended; drugs which are likely to cause spasm, such as morphine, should be avoided.
Depending on the caliber of the biliary tree, a dose of 20 to 40 ml. is generally sufficient to opacify the entire ductal system. The contrast agent may be diluted 1:1 with Sodium Chloride Injection USP, if desired, under strict aseptic procedures.
Injection is made into a biliary duct by the percutaneous transhepatic method. Before the dose is administered, as much bile as possible is aspirated. The medium is then slowly injected into the duct under very slight pressure. If a duct is not located promptly, successive small doses of 1 to 2 ml. are injected into the liver as the needle is gradually withdrawn, until a duct is visualized by x-ray. If no duct can be located after three or four attempts, the procedure is abandoned.
Serial films are taken rapidly during and after injection of the medium into the biliary ducts. Repositioning of the patient, if necessary, should be done with care.
In hepatocellular disease, the biliary ducts are generally not enlarged and cannot successfully be opacified by this method. Thus, in the presence of long-standing jaundice, failure to obtain a successful percutaneous transhepatic cholangiogram by a person experienced in the technique is generally considered to be strongly suggestive of nonobstructive or hepatocellular-type jaundice.
Splenoportography—Prior gastrointestinal x-ray examination should include particular attention to the lower esophageal area. A hematologic survey, including prothrombin time and platelet count, should be performed. The patient should have no food for several hours and should be mildly sedated. Splenoportography is usually performed under local anesthesia.
Approximately 20 to 25 ml. of the contrast agent is usually adequate. The dose is injected rapidly, following radiologic location and percutaneous puncture of the spleen.
Preliminary films are taken to locate the spleen before the injection is begun. Rapid serial films are then started simultaneously with injection of the dose. Serial films are necessary since the entire portal system cannot be captured on a single film and also because of individual variations in portal circulation time.
Arthrography—The amount of contrast agent required is dependent on the size of the joint to be injected. For an adult, the following doses are generally suitable: Knee—5 to 15 ml.; shoulder or hip—5 to 10 ml.; other joints—1 to 4 ml. Dosage for children should be suitably reduced.
The injection site should be prepared aseptically. Excessive synovial fluid should be aspirated to minimize pain and to reduce intra-articular dilution of the contrast agent. If indicated, the agent may be administered under local anesthesia. After injection of the medium, the joint should be manipulated gently in order to spread the medium throughout the joint space. In some instances, double contrast arthrography, injecting both air and contrast medium, has been of value.
Films are taken from several angles; stereoscopic films may be advantageous.
When the contrast agent is used to opacify a joint space, much of the agent may be aspirated at the end of the procedure.
Discography—No prior preparation of the patient is required, although administration of an analgesic or sedative 20 minutes before the procedure may be helpful. Discography is performed under local anesthesia using the usual aseptic precautions.
Dosage is generally determined by the amount of contrast agent which can easily be injected into the disk without force. A cervical disk will normally accept up to 0.5 ml. and a lumbar disk 1 or 2 ml. The amount may vary, and injection should be discontinued when resistance is felt. The rate of injection may influence the amount which can be injected. To reduce the probability of extravasation and to minimize unnecessary pain, injection should be made slowly and not more than 2 ml. should be injected into any one disk.
A two-needle technique may be used to administer the contrast medium, with a large-gauge needle to locate the disk and a small-gauge needle within the larger one to puncture the disk and administer the medium. The correct position of the two needles is established radiologically before the medium is injected.
Spot roentgenograms should be taken anteroposteriorly, obliquely, and laterally as soon as disks have been injected.
When the contrast agent is used for discography, it need not be aspirated at the end of the procedure.
How Supplied: Single dose vials of 10 ml., 30 ml. and 50 ml., and single dose bottles of 100 ml. An excess volume (1 ml.) is available in each container for sensitivity testing.
Storage: The preparation should be stored at room temperature, protected from light. If precipitation or solidification has occurred due to storage in the cold, immerse the container in hot water and shake intermittently to redissolve any solids.

RENO–M–DIP® ℞

(Diatrizoate Meglumine Injection USP 30%)
For Intravenous Drip Infusion

Description: Reno-M-DIP is a radiopaque contrast agent supplied as a sterile, aqueous solution for intravenous drip infusion, in 300 ml. bottles. Each ml. provides 300 mg. diatrizoate meglumine with 0.4 mg. edetate disodium as a sequestering agent; pH has been adjusted between 6.5 and 7.7 with meglumine or diatrizoic acid. *Each ml. of solution also contains approximately 0.054 mg. (0.002 mEq.) sodium (16.2 mg./300 ml.)* and 141 mg. (42.3 g./300 ml.) organically bound iodine.
Clinical Pharmacology: Following intravenous administration, diatrizoate meglumine is rapidly transported through the bloodstream to the kidneys and is excreted unchanged in the urine by glomerular filtration. When urinary tract obstruction is severe enough to block glomerular filtration, the agent appears to be excreted by the tubular epithelium.
Diuresis commonly occurs, due primarily to the osmotic effects of the contrast agent.
Drip Infusion Pyelography—When a large volume of the contrast agent is administered in dilute form by intravenous drip infusion, the nephrographic phase of renal excretion is enhanced, and a dense, sustained nephrogram is usually obtained.
Following drip infusion of the contrast agent, the upper and lower urinary tract is opacified. Anatomically complete pyelograms and voiding cystograms may be obtained, and the entire course of the ureter may be seen on a single film. Filling defects may be visualized and the site of an obstruction may be clearly localized. Renal accumulation is sufficiently rapid that optimal opacification of the kidney normally is reached by the time the infusion is completed, while filling of the collecting system is maximal within 20 or 30 minutes after the start of the infusion. Impairment of renal function commonly delays accumulation and excretion of the contrast agent, so that opacification may be delayed until three or more hours after the infusion; with severe impairment adequate opacification may not occur.
Because transport of the contrast agent is slowed by renal dysfunction, the ischemic kidney of renal vascular hypertension may be distinguished from the normal kidney. Renal ischemia produces a nephrogram which is slower to appear, less dense, and sustained for a markedly prolonged period of time.
Computed Tomography—Reno-M-DIP (Diatrizoate Meglumine Injection USP 30%) enhances computed tomographic brain scanning through augmentation of radiographic efficiency. The degree of enhancement of visualization of tissue density is directly related to the iodine content in an administered dose; peak iodine blood levels occur immediately following rapid infusion of the dose. These levels fall rapidly within five to ten minutes. This can be accounted for by the dilution in the vascular and extracellular fluid compartments which causes an initial sharp fall in plasma concentration. Equilibration with the extracellular compartments is reached in about ten minutes; thereafter, the fall becomes exponential. Maximum contrast enhancement frequently occurs after peak blood iodine levels are reached. The delay in maximum contrast enhancement can range from five to forty minutes, depending on the peak iodine levels

Continued on next page

Squibb—Cont.

achieved and the cell type of the lesion. This lag suggests that radiographic contrast enhancement is at least in part dependent on the accumulation of iodine within the lesion and outside the blood pool although the mechanism by which this occurs is not clear. The radiographic enhancement of nontumoral lesions, such as arteriovenous malformations and aneurysms, is probably dependent on the iodine content of the circulating blood pool.

Indications and Usage:

Drip Infusion Pyelography—Reno-M-DIP is indicated for use in those patients in whom routine pyelography would not be expected to be, or has not been, satisfactory for diagnosis. It is not intended to replace retrograde pyelography where this procedure is indicated.

Computed Tomography—Reno-M-DIP is also indicated for radiographic contrast enhancement in computed tomography (CT) of the brain. Contrast enhancement is advantageous in delineating or ruling out disease in suspicious areas which may otherwise not have been satisfactorily visualized.

Tumors—Reno-M-DIP may be useful to demonstrate the presence and extent of certain malignancies such as: gliomas including malignant gliomas, glioblastomas, astrocytomas, oligodendrogliomas and gangliomas; ependymomas; medulloblastomas; meningiomas; neuromas; pinealomas; pituitary adenomas; craniopharyngiomas; germinomas; and metastatic lesions.

The usefulness of contrast enhancement for the investigation of the retrobulbar space and in cases of low grade or infiltrative glioma has not been demonstrated. In cases where lesions have calcified, there is less likelihood of enhancement. Following therapy, tumors may show decreased or no enhancement.

Non-Neoplastic Conditions—The use of Reno-M-DIP (Diatrizoate Meglumine Injection USP 30%) may be beneficial in the enhancement of images of lesions not due to neoplasms. Cerebral infarctions of recent onset may be better visualized with the contrast enhancement, while some infarctions are obscured if a contrast medium is used. The use of Reno-M-DIP (Diatrizoate Meglumine Injection USP 30%) improved the contrast enhancement in approximately 60 percent of cerebral infarctions studied from one week to four weeks from the onset of symptoms.

Sites of active infection also will produce contrast enhancement following contrast medium administration.

Arteriovenous malformations and aneurysms will show contrast enhancement. In the case of these vascular lesions, the enhancement is probably dependent on the iodine content of the circulating blood pool.

Hematomas and intraparenchymal bleeders seldom demonstrate any contrast enhancement. However, in cases of intraparenchymal clot, for which there is no obvious clinical explanation, contrast medium administration may be helpful in ruling out the possibility of associated arteriovenous malformation.

The opacification of the inferior vermis following contrast medium administration has resulted in false-positive diagnoses in a number of normal studies.

Contraindications: This preparation is contraindicated in patients with a hypersensitivity to salts of diatrizoic acid.

The administration of diatrizoate meglumine is contraindicated in patients with anuria.

Warnings: A definite risk exists in the use of intravascular contrast agents in patients who are known to have multiple myeloma. In such instances there has been anuria resulting in progressive uremia, renal failure and eventually death. Although neither the contrast agent nor dehydration has separately proved to be the cause of anuria in myeloma, it has been speculated that the combination of both may be the causative factor. The risk in myelomatous patients is not a contraindication to the procedures; however, partial dehydration in the preparation of these patients for the examination is not recommended since this may predispose to the precipitation of myeloma protein in the renal tubules. No form of therapy, including dialysis, has been successful in reversing this effect. Myeloma, which occurs most commonly in persons over age 40, should be considered before intravascular administration of a contrast agent.

Administration of radiopaque materials to patients known or suspected to have pheochromocytoma should be performed with extreme caution. If, in the opinion of the physician, the possible benefits of such procedures outweigh the considered risks, the procedures may be performed; however, the amount of radiopaque medium injected should be kept to an absolute minimum. The blood pressure should be assessed throughout the procedure and measures for treatment of a hypertensive crisis should be available.

Contrast media have been shown to promote the phenomenon of sickling in individuals who are homozygous for sickle cell disease when the material is injected intravenously or intra-arterially.

Diatrizoate meglumine should be used with extreme caution in patients with severe concomitant hepatic and renal disease.

Since iodine-containing contrast agents may alter the results of thyroid function tests, such tests, if indicated, should be performed prior to the administration of this preparation.

A history of sensitivity to iodine *per se* or to other contrast media is not an absolute contraindication to the use of diatrizoate meglumine but calls for extreme caution in administration.

Precautions: Diagnostic procedures which involve the use of radiopaque contrast agents should be carried out under the direction of personnel with the prerequisite training and with a thorough knowledge of the particular procedure to be performed (see ADVERSE REACTIONS).

Severe, life-threatening reactions suggest hypersensitivity to the radiopaque agent, which has prompted the use of several pretesting methods, none of which can be relied upon to predict severe reactions. Many authorities question the value of any pretest. A history of bronchial asthma or allergy, a family history of allergy, or a previous reaction to a contrast agent warrant special attention. Such a history, by suggesting histamine sensitivity and a consequent proneness to reactions, may be more accurate than pretesting in predicting the likelihood of a reaction, although not necessarily the severity or type of reaction in the individual case.

The sensitivity test most often performed is the slow injection of 0.5 to 1.0 ml. of the radiopaque medium, administered intravenously, prior to injection of the full diagnostic dose. It should be noted that the absence of a reaction to the test dose does not preclude the possibility of a reaction to the full diagnostic dose. If the test dose causes an untoward response of any kind, the necessity for continuing with the examination should be carefully reevaluated and, if it is deemed essential, the examination should be conducted with all possible caution. In rare instances, reactions to the test dose itself may be extremely severe; therefore, close observation of the patient and facilities for emergency treatment appear indicated.

The recommended rate of infusion should not be exceeded.

Renal toxicity has been reported in a few patients with liver dysfunction who were given oral cholecystographic agents followed by urographic agents. Diagnostic infusion studies should therefore be postponed in any patient with a known or suspected hepatic or biliary disorder who has recently taken a cholecystographic contrast agent.

The diuretic effect of the drip infusion procedure may hinder an assessment of residual urine in the bladder.

Consideration must be given to the functional ability of the kidneys before injecting diatrizoate meglumine. Adequate visualization may be difficult or impossible to attain in uremic patients or others with severely impaired renal function.

Acute renal failure has been reported with the use of contrast agents in patients with diabetic nephropathy and susceptible nondiabetic patients (often elderly with preexisting renal disease).

Contrast agents may interfere with some chemical determinations made on urine specimens; therefore, urine should be collected before administration of the contrast medium or two or more days afterwards.

Usage in Pregnancy: The safety of diatrizoate meglumine for use during pregnancy has not been established; therefore, it should be used in pregnant patients only when, in the judgment of the physician, its use is deemed essential to the welfare of the patient.

Adverse Reactions: Adverse reactions accompanying the use of iodine-containing intravascular contrast agents are usually mild and transient although severe and life-threatening reactions, including fatalities, have occurred. Because of the possibility of severe reactions to the procedure and/or the radiopaque medium, appropriate emergency facilities and well-trained personnel should be available to treat both conditions. Emergency facilities and personnel should remain available for 30 to 60 minutes following the procedure since severe delayed reactions have been known to occur.

Nausea and urticaria have been the reactions most frequently encountered with administration of contrast agents by drip infusion. Such symptoms as chills, metallic taste, vomiting, dizziness, a rise or fall in blood pressure, itching, flushing, or generalized feeling of warmth, sneezing, etc., may occur. Rarely, such reactions may be severe enough to require discontinuation of dosage.

Severe reactions which may require emergency measures may take the form of a cardiovascular reaction characterized by peripheral vasodilatation with resultant hypotension and reflex tachycardia, dyspnea, and confusion and cyanosis progressing to unconsciousness. Or, the histamine-liberating effect of these compounds may induce an allergic-like reaction which may range in severity from rhinitis or angioneurotic edema to laryngeal or bronchial spasm or anaphylactoid shock.

Temporary renal shutdown or other nephropathy may occur.

Although local tissue tolerance to diatrizoate meglumine is usually good, intravenous injection of the medium in a more concentrated formulation has produced a few instances of a burning or stinging sensation and of venospasm or venous pain.

Dosage and Administration:

Drip Infusion Pyelography—While preparation of the patient is not essential for drip infusion pyelography, it is advocated by some investigators. If desired, adults and older children may be given a laxative the night before the examination and a low residue diet the day before, to clear the gastrointestinal tract. Clinicians who feel that partial dehydration enhances radiographic contrast recommend a low liquid intake for 12 hours prior to the procedure; however, adequate hydration has improved the quality of films for other investigators. Preparatory partial dehydration is not recommended in infants, young children, the elderly, or azotemic patients (especially those with polyuria, oliguria, diabetes, advanced vascular disease, or preexisting dehydration). The undesirable dehydration in these patients may be accentuated by the osmotic diuretic action of the medium.

In uremic patients partial dehydration is not necessary and maintenance of adequate fluid intake is particularly desirable.

Cleansing enemas are not recommended since they may increase residual gas in the bowel.

The recommended dose is 2 ml. per pound of body weight. The preparation is given by continuous intravenous infusion, over a period of 8 minutes or longer (see PRECAUTIONS), through a needle with a large bore, usually a 17- or 18-gauge needle. In older patients and in patients with known or suspected cardiac decompensation, a slower rate of infusion is probably wise.

If nausea or flushing occurs during administration, the infusion should be slowed or briefly interrupted.

Films are taken before the onset of the infusion and at the desired intervals following its completion. When renal function is normal, a nephrogram may be taken as soon as the infusion is completed, and films of the collecting system at 10 and 20 minutes thereafter. Voiding cystourethrograms are usually optimal at 20 minutes after the infusion is completed. In hypertensive patients, early minute sequence films may be taken during the course of infusion, in addition to subsequent pyelograms. In patients with renal dysfunction, optimal visualization is usually delayed, and the late films are taken as indicated.

The nephrogram obtained by the drip infusion procedure may be dense enough to obscure the pelvocalyceal system in some cases. The presence of gas in the bowel may hamper early visualization of the renal collecting system. Tomographic "cuts" may help to overcome such difficulties.

Nephrotomography may begin when the infusion is completed. The sustained contrast achieved by the drip infusion technique eliminates the need for precise timing and teamwork that is necessary with ordinary nephrotomography. Thus, if nephrograms taken after infusion of the medium suggest the need for sectional films, or if preselected tomographic "cuts" are not sufficient, additional tomograms may be obtained at once, and without repetition of dosage.

Computed Tomography—The suggested dose is 2 ml. per pound of body weight by intravenous drip over a period of eight minutes or longer; scanning may be performed during administration and/or immediately afterwards.

Patient Preparation—No special patient preparation is required for contrast enhancement of CT brain scanning. However, it is advisable to insure that patients are well hydrated prior to examination.

How Supplied: Available in single-dose bottles of 300 ml. and in single-dose bottles of 300 ml. with Solution Administration Set. An excess volume (1 ml.) is available in each container for sensitivity testing.

Storage: The preparation should be protected from strong light and stored at room temperature.

RENOVIST® ℞

(Diatrizoate Meglumine and Diatrizoate Sodium Injection USP)

Description: Renovist is a radiopaque contrast agent supplied in vials as a sterile, aqueous solution. Each ml. provides 343 mg. diatrizoate meglumine and 350 mg. diatrizoate sodium with 3.2 mg. sodium citrate and 0.4 mg. edetate disodium; pH has been adjusted to 6.5 to 7.7 with sodium hydroxide. *Each ml. of solution also contains approximately 13.5 mg. (0.58 mEq.) sodium (675 mg./50 ml.)* and 370.5 mg. (18.5 g./50 ml.) organically bound iodine. At the time of manufacture, the air in the container is replaced by nitrogen.

Clinical Pharmacology: Following intravascular injection, Renovist is rapidly transported through the bloodstream to the kidneys and is excreted unchanged in the urine by glomerular filtration. When urinary tract obstruction is severe enough to block glomerular filtration, the agent appears to be excreted by the tubular epithelium.

Renal accumulation is sufficiently rapid so that the period of maximal opacification of the renal passages may begin as early as five minutes after injection. In infants and small children, excretion takes place somewhat more promptly than in adults, so that maximal opacification occurs more rapidly and is less sustained. The normal kidney eliminates the contrast medium almost immediately. In nephropathic conditions, particularly when excretory capacity has been altered, the rate of excretion varies unpredictably, and opacification may be delayed for 30 minutes or more after injection; with severe impairment opacification may not occur. Generally, however, the medium is concentrated in sufficient amounts and promptly enough to permit a thorough evaluation of the anatomy and physiology of the urinary tract.

After intramuscular injection, the contrast agent is promptly absorbed and normally reaches the renal passages within 20 to 60 minutes.

Intravascular injection of diatrizoate also opacifies those vessels in the path of the flow of the medium, permitting visualization until the circulating blood dilutes the concentration of the medium. Thus selective angiography may be performed following injection directly into veins or arteries.

Indications: Renovist (Diatrizoate Meglumine and Diatrizoate Sodium Injection USP) is indicated for use in excretion urography, aortography, angiocardiography, peripheral arteriography, peripheral venography, and venocavography.

Contraindications: This preparation is contraindicated in patients with a hypersensitivity to salts of diatrizoic acid.

Urography is contraindicated in patients with anuria.

Warnings: A definite risk exists in the use of intravascular contrast agents in patients who are known to have multiple myeloma. In such instances there has been anuria resulting in progressive uremia, renal failure, and eventually death. Although neither the contrast agent nor dehydration has separately proved to be the cause of anuria in myeloma, it has been speculated that the combination of both may be the causative factor. The risk in myelomatous patients is not a contraindication to the procedures; however, partial dehydration in the preparation of these patients for the examination is not recommended since this may predispose to the precipitation of myeloma protein in the renal tubules. No form of therapy, including dialysis, has been successful in reversing this effect. Myeloma, which occurs most commonly in persons over age 40, should be considered before intravascular administration of a contrast agent.

Administration of radiopaque materials to patients known or suspected to have pheochromocytoma should be performed with extreme caution. If, in the opinion of the physician, the possible benefits of such procedures outweigh the considered risks, the procedures may be performed; however, the amount of radiopaque medium injected should be kept to an absolute minimum. The blood pressure should be assessed throughout the procedure and measures for treatment of a hypertensive crisis should be available.

The inherent risks of angiocardiography in cyanotic infants and patients with chronic pulmonary emphysema must be weighed against the necessity for performing this procedure. In pediatric angiocardiography, a dose of 10 to 20 ml. may be particularly hazardous in infants weighing less than 7 kg. This risk is probably significantly increased if these infants have preexisting right heart "strain," right heart failure, and effectively decreased or obliterated pulmonary vascular beds.

Contrast media have been shown to promote the phenomenon of sickling in individuals who are homozygous for sickle cell disease when the material is injected intravenously or intraarterially.

Urography should be performed with extreme caution in patients with severe concomitant hepatic and renal disease.

Since iodine-containing contrast agents may alter the results of thyroid function tests, such tests, if indicated, should be performed prior to the administration of this preparation.

A history of sensitivity to iodine *per se* or to other contrast agents is not an absolute contraindication to the use of diatrizoate, but calls for extreme caution in administration.

Precautions: Diagnostic procedures which involve the use of radiopaque contrast agents should be carried out under the direction of personnel with the prerequisite training and with a thorough knowledge of the particular procedure to be performed (see ADVERSE REACTIONS).

Severe, life-threatening reactions suggest hypersensitivity to the radiopaque agent, which has prompted the use of several pretesting methods, none of which can be relied upon to predict severe reactions. Many authorities question the value of any pretest. A history of bronchial asthma or allergy, a family history of allergy, or a previous reaction to a contrast agent warrant special attention. Such a history, by suggesting histamine sensitivity and a consequent proneness to reactions, may be more accurate than pretesting in predicting the likelihood of a reaction, although not necessarily the severity or type of reaction in the individual case.

The sensitivity test most often performed is the slow injection of 0.5 to 1.0 ml. of the radiopaque medium, administered intravenously, prior to injection of the full diagnostic dose. It should be noted that the absence of a reaction to the test dose does not preclude the possibility of a reaction to the full diagnostic dose. If the test dose causes an untoward response of any kind, the necessity for continuing with the examination should be carefully reevaluated and, if it is deemed essential, the examination should be conducted with all possible caution. In rare instances, reactions to the test dose itself may be extremely severe; therefore, close observation of the patient, and facilities for emergency treatment, appear indicated.

Renal toxicity has been reported in a few patients with liver dysfunction who were given oral cholecystographic agents followed by urographic agents. Administration of Renovist (Diatrizoate Meglumine and Diatrizoate Sodium Injection USP) should therefore be postponed in any patient with a known or suspected hepatic or biliary disorder who has recently taken a cholecystographic contrast agent.

Caution should be exercised with the use of radiopaque media in severely debilitated patients and in those with marked hypertension.

The possibility of thrombosis should be borne in mind when percutaneous techniques are employed.

Consideration must be given to the functional ability of the kidneys before injecting this preparation.

Contrast agents may interfere with some chemical determinations made on urine specimens; therefore, urine should be collected before administration of the contrast medium or two or more days afterwards.

Continued on next page

Squibb—Cont.

The following precautions pertain to specific procedures:
Excretion urography: Adequate visualization may be difficult or impossible to obtain in uremic patients or others with severely impaired renal function (see CONTRAINDICATIONS).
Acute renal failure has been reported in diabetic patients with diabetic nephropathy and susceptible nondiabetic patients (often elderly with preexisting renal disease) following excretion urography. Therefore, careful consideration should be given before performing this procedure in these patients.
Aortography: Repeated intra-aortic injections may be hazardous.
Angiocardiography: Repeated injections may be hazardous particularly in infants weighing less than 7 kg. (see WARNINGS).
Peripheral arteriography: Hypotension or moderate decreases in blood pressure seem to occur frequently with intra-arterial (brachial) injections; therefore, the blood pressure should be monitored during the immediate ten minutes after injection; this blood pressure change is transient and usually requires no treatment.
Peripheral venography: Caution should be exercised in the presence of thrombosis or phlebitis.
Usage in Pregnancy: Safety for use during pregnancy has not been established with respect to adverse effects upon fetal development; therefore, this preparation should be used in pregnant patients only when, in the judgment of the physician, its use is deemed essential to the welfare of the patient.
Adverse Reactions: Adverse reactions accompanying the use of iodine-containing intravascular contrast agents are usually mild and transient although severe and life-threatening reactions, including fatalities, have occurred. Because of the possibility of severe reactions to the procedure and/or the radiopaque medium, appropriate emergency facilities and well-trained personnel should be available to treat both conditions. Emergency facilities and personnel should remain available for 30 to 60 minutes following the procedure since severe delayed reactions have been known to occur.
Nausea, vomiting, flushing, or a generalized feeling of warmth are the reactions seen most frequently with intravascular injection. Symptoms which may occur are chills, fever, sweating, headache, dizziness, pallor, weakness, severe retching and choking, wheezing, a rise or fall in blood pressure, ventricular fibrillation, cardiac arrest, facial or conjunctival petechiae, urticaria, pruritus, rash and other eruptions, edema, cramps, tremors, itching, sneezing, lacrimation, etc. Antihistaminic agents may be of benefit; rarely, such reactions may be severe enough to require discontinuation of dosage. Pulmonary edema, spasm, seizures, hemiparesis, and impairment of vision have occurred.
Although local tissue tolerance is usually good, there have been a few reports of a burning or stinging sensation or numbness and of venospasm or venous pain, and partial collapse of the injected vein. Neutropenia or thrombophlebitis may occur.
Severe reactions are a possibility. Such reactions which may require emergency measures may take the form of a cardiovascular reaction characterized by peripheral vasodilatation with resultant hypotension and reflex tachycardia, apnea, dyspnea, agitation, confusion, and cyanosis progressing to unconsciousness. Or, the histamine-liberating effect of these compounds may induce an allergic-like reaction which may range in severity from rhinitis or angioneurotic edema to laryngeal or bronchial spasm or anaphylactoid shock.
Temporary renal shutdown or other nephropathy may occur.
Adverse reactions may sometimes occur as a consequence of the procedure for which the contrast agent is used. Adverse reactions in **excretion urography** have included cardiac arrest, ventricular fibrillation, anaphylaxis with severe asthmatic reaction, and flushing due to generalized vasodilatation. In **aortography**, the risks of procedures include injury to the aorta and neighboring organs, pleural puncture, renal damage including infarction and acute tubular necrosis with oliguria and anuria, accidental selective filling of the right renal artery during the translumbar procedure in the presence of preexistent renal disease, retroperitoneal hemorrhage from the translumbar approach, spinal cord injury and pathology associated with the syndrome of transverse myelitis, generalized petechiae, and death following hypotension, arrhythmia, and anaphylactoid reactions. Adverse reactions in **angiocardiography** have included arrhythmia and death. During **peripheral arteriography**, complications have occurred including hemorrhage from the puncture site, thrombosis of the vessel, and brachial plexus palsy following axillary artery injections.
Dosage and Administration: Renovist (Diatrizoate Meglumine and Diatrizoate Sodium Injection USP) should be at body temperature when injected, and may need to be warmed before use. The preparation should be used as promptly as possible following withdrawal into the syringe, and syringes should be rinsed as soon as possible after injection to prevent freezing of the plunger.
Note: In the event crystallization occurs, the solution may be clarified by placing the vial in a water bath at 40° to 50° C. and shaking gently for two to three minutes or until the solids redissolve.
Withdrawal of the contrast agent should be accomplished under aseptic conditions with sterile needle and syringe.
Excretion Urography: Appropriate preparation of the patient is desirable for optimal results. A laxative the night before the examination, a low residue diet the day before, and low liquid intake for 12 hours prior to the procedure are recommended. The partial dehydration so induced is believed to effect a greater urinary concentration of the contrast medium. Enemas are to be avoided to prevent rehydration.
Preparatory partial dehydration is not recommended in infants, young children, the elderly, or azotemic patients (especially those with polyuria, oliguria, diabetes, advanced vascular disease, or preexisting dehydration). The undesirable dehydration in these patients may be accentuated by the osmotic action of the medium.
For many patients aged 16 years or older, an intravenous dose of 25 ml. is sufficient; alternatively, in instances where inadequate visualization may be anticipated, a higher dose may be administered on a weight basis (0.36 to 0.45 ml./lb.). Children under 16 require proportionately less: Under 6 months of age—5 ml.; 6 to 12 months—8 ml.; 1 to 2 years—10 ml.; 2 to 5 years—12 ml.; 5 to 7 years—15 ml.; 7 to 10 years—18 ml.; 10 to 15 years—20 ml.
Use of a 20- or 21-gauge needle is recommended. During the injection, the patient should be watched for untoward reactions. If flushing or nausea occurs, the rate of injection should be slowed or administration briefly interrupted until the side effects have disappeared.
A scout film should be made before Renovist is administered. Since maximal opacification of the urinary tract usually occurs between 5 to 15 minutes after injection of the contrast agent, radiographs are best taken during this period. To allow for individual variation, several films should be exposed. In infants and children maximal opacification occurs more rapidly after injection and is sustained over a shorter period of time. In patients with renal dysfunction, optimal opacification may be delayed for 30 minutes or more after injection.
Aortography: Renovist (Diatrizoate Meglumine and Diatrizoate Sodium Injection USP) injected into the aorta by the translumbar or retrograde method of administration permits radiographic visualization of the aorta, its major branches, and the abdominal arteries. An incidental nephrogram is obtained as the contrast medium travels through the renal vasculature, provided it has been injected above the renal artery.
Patients should be prepared in a manner similar to that used for intravenous urography. Premedication with a suitable barbiturate is generally indicated.
As in any form of surgery, certain hazards accompany aortographic procedures (see ADVERSE REACTIONS).
For adults and children over 16 years of age, the usual dose is 15 to 25 ml. as a single injection, repeated if indicated. Children require less in proportion to age and weight.
Since the medium is given by rapid injection in this procedure, patients should be watched for untoward reactions during the injection. Unless general anesthesia is employed, patients should be warned that they may feel some transient pain or burning during the injection followed by a feeling of warmth immediately afterward.
A scout film should be made before the contrast agent is administered. The first radiogram should be taken as the last few ml. of the contrast medium are being injected.
Angiocardiography: Angiocardiography with Renovist (Diatrizoate Meglumine and Diatrizoate Sodium Injection USP) may be performed by injection into a large peripheral vein or by direct catheterization of the heart. An excretory urogram can be obtained 10 to 15 minutes after injection of the contrast medium since it is concentrated in and eliminated by the kidneys.
Patients should be prepared in a manner similar to that used for intravenous urography. Appropriate preanesthetic medication should be given.
Clincal studies in man, and related animal experiments, have suggested that the hypertonicity of diatrizoate contrast agents produces significant hemodynamic effects, especially in right-sided injections. Large volumes of such agents cause a drop in peripheral arterial and systemic pressures and cardiac output, a rise in pulmonary arterial and right-heart pressures, bradycardia, and regular ectopic beats. Resulting effects on peripheral arterial and pulmonary arterial pressures are postulated to be due to mechanical blockage of the pulmonary vascular bed and clumping of red cells.
Hypertonic solutions cause a decrease in hematocrit *in vitro* and *in vivo*, and shrinkage of red blood cells.
It is suggested that hemodynamic changes be monitored and that pressures considered abnormal under roentgenographic conditions be allowed to return to a preangiographic level before continuation of radiopaque injection; this usually takes 15 minutes.
For adults the suggested single dose is 50 ml.; doses up to a total of 200 ml. have been given safely. Children under 16 require proportionally less. The suggested single dose for children under 2 years of age is 10 to 15 ml., depending upon the weight of the child; the smallest amount necessary to obtain adequate visualization should be used. For children 2 to 4 years of age, single doses of 15 to 20 ml. are recommended; for children 4 to 10 years of age, 20 to 30 ml. Doses up to 100 ml. have been given safely. For children 10 to 15 years of age, dosage depends on the size of the patient.
Since the contrast medium is given by rapid injection, the patient should be watched for untoward reactions during the injection. Some

patients not under general anesthesia may experience a feeling of bodily warmth, tightness of the chest, and throbbing headache. All these sensations are of short duration. Transient nausea and vomiting may occur in some patients.
The roentgenograms should be taken immediately at the beginning of the injection and continued for 5 to 10 seconds or longer, depending upon the desired roentgenographic information.

Peripheral Arteriography: Renovist is injected into the femoral or subclavian artery by the percutaneous or operative method. If only the lower half of the extremity is to be studied, Renovist is injected into the brachial or popliteal artery.
Appropriate preparation of the patient is indicated, including suitable premedication.
For visualization of an entire extremity, a single dose of 20 to 40 ml. is suggested. For arteriography of the upper half or the lower half of the extremity only, a single dose of 10 to 20 ml. is sufficient.
Because the contrast medium is given by rapid injection, flushing of the skin may occur. Patients not under general anesthesia may experience a feeling of warmth and, rarely, nausea and vomiting.
A scout film should be made routinely before administering the contrast medium. Radiograms of the upper half should be taken while the last 2 ml. of Renovist (Diatrizoate Meglumine and Diatrizoate Sodium Injection USP) are being injected, followed by radiograms of the lower half of the extremity a few seconds later.

Peripheral Venography: For visualization of an upper extremity, Renovist may be given by percutaneous injection into any convenient superficial vein of the forearm or hand. For visualization of a lower extremity, it should be injected into a superficial vein on the lateral side of the foot.
Appropriate preparation of the patient is indicated, including suitable premedication.
For the visualization of an upper extremity in adults, a single dose of 20 ml. is suggested; a single dose of 20 ml. is sufficient for the visualization of a lower extremity. Children require less in proportion to age and weight.
The contrast medium is administered rapidly in this procedure.
The radiographs are taken at the termination of the injection.

Venocavography: Inferior venocavography may be performed with Renovist injected into the saphenous, femoral, or iliac veins by percutaneous injection, either directly or by catheterization procedures.
Appropriate preparation of the patient is indicated, including suitable premedication.
For adults the suggested average single dose is 30 to 60 ml. The dosage for children depends upon age and weight.
Renovist (Diatrizoate Meglumine and Diatrizoate Sodium Injection USP) is injected as rapidly as possible via the saphenous vein and roentgenograms are taken immediately. A repeat injection is given if an additional view is desired. An alternate technique is to catheterize both femoral veins and to place the catheter in each common iliac vein immediately caudad to their junction. Bilateral injection gives better filling than the unilateral injection.
Roentgenograms are taken immediately after injection of the medium. They are taken in a supine position and in the right posterior oblique or lateral position.

How Supplied: Available in 50 ml. single-dose vials. An excess volume (1 ml.) is available in each container for sensitivity testing.

Storage: Protect from light. Store at room temperature.

RENOVIST® II ℞

(Diatrizoate Meglumine and Diatrizoate Sodium Injection USP)

Description: Renovist II is a radiopaque contrast agent supplied in vials as a sterile, aqueous solution. Each ml. provides 285 mg. diatrizoate meglumine and 291 mg. diatrizoate sodium with 3.2 mg. sodium citrate as a buffer, and 0.4 mg. edetate disodium as a sequestering agent; pH has been adjusted between 6.5 and 7.7 with sodium hydroxide. *Each ml. of solution also contains approximately 11.39 mg. (0.49 mEq.) sodium* and 309 mg. organically bound iodine. At the time of manufacture, the air in the container is replaced by nitrogen.

Clinical Pharmacology: Following intravascular injection, Renovist II is rapidly transported through the bloodstream to the kidneys and is excreted unchanged in the urine by glomerular filtration. When urinary tract obstruction is severe enough to block glomerular filtration, the agent appears to be excreted by the tubular epithelium.
Renal accumulation is sufficiently rapid so that the period of maximal opacification of the renal passages may begin as early as 5 minutes after injection. In infants and small children excretion takes place somewhat more promptly than in adults, so that maximal opacification occurs more rapidly and is less sustained. The normal kidney eliminates the contrast medium almost immediately. In nephropathic conditions, particularly when excretory capacity has been altered, the rate of excretion varies unpredictably, and opacification may be delayed for 30 minutes or more after injection; with severe impairment, opacification may not occur. Generally, however, the medium is concentrated in sufficient amounts and promptly enough to permit a thorough evaluation of the anatomy and physiology of the urinary tract.
After intramuscular injection, the contrast agent is promptly absorbed and normally reaches the renal passages within 20 to 60 minutes.
Intravascular injection of diatrizoate also opacifies those vessels in the path of the flow of the medium, permitting visualization until the circulating blood dilutes the concentration of the medium. Thus, selective angiography may be performed following injection directly into veins or arteries.

Indications: Renovist II (Diatrizoate Meglumine and Diatrizoate Sodium Injection USP) is indicated for use in excretion urography, aortography, angiocardiography, peripheral arteriography, peripheral venography, and venocavography.

Contraindications: This preparation is contraindicated in patients with a hypersensitivity to salts of diatrizoic acid.
Urography is contraindicated in patients with anuria.

Warnings: A definite risk exists in the use of intravascular contrast agents in patients who are known to have multiple myeloma. In such instances there has been anuria resulting in progressive uremia, renal failure, and eventually death. Although neither the contrast agent nor dehydration has separately proved to be the cause of anuria in myeloma, it has been speculated that the combination of both may be the causative factor. The risk in myelomatous patients is not a contraindication to the procedures; however, partial dehydration in the preparation of these patients for the examination is not recommended since this may predispose to the precipitation of myeloma protein in the renal tubules. No form of therapy, including dialysis, has been successful in reversing this effect. Myeloma, which occurs most commonly in persons over age 40, should be considered before intravascular administration of a contrast agent.
Administration of radiopaque materials to patients known or suspected to have pheochromocytoma should be performed with extreme caution. If, in the opinion of the physician, the possible benefits of such procedures outweigh the considered risks, the procedures may be performed; however, the amount of radiopaque medium injected should be kept to an absolute minimum. The blood pressure should be assessed throughout the procedure and measures for treatment of a hypertensive crisis should be available.
The inherent risks of angiocardiography in cyanotic infants and patients with chronic pulmonary emphysema must be weighed against the necessity for performing this procedure. In pediatric angiocardiography, a dose of 10 to 20 ml. may be particularly hazardous in infants weighing less than 7 kg. This risk is probably significantly increased if these infants have preexisting right heart "strain," right heart failure, and effectively decreased or obliterated pulmonary vascular beds.
Contrast media have been shown to promote the phenomenon of sickling in individuals who are homozygous for sickle cell disease when the material is injected intravenously or intra-arterially.
Urography should be performed with extreme caution in patients with severe concomitant hepatic and renal disease.
Since iodine-containing contrast agents may alter the results of thyroid function tests, such tests, if indicated, should be performed prior to the administration of this preparation.
A history of sensitivity to iodine *per se* or to other contrast agents is not an absolute contraindication to the use of diatrizoate, but calls for extreme caution in administration.

Precautions: Diagnostic procedures which involve the use of radiopaque contrast agents should be carried out under the direction of personnel with the prerequisite training and with a thorough knowledge of the particular procedure to be performed (see ADVERSE REACTIONS).
Severe, life-threatening reactions suggest hypersensitivity to the radiopaque agent, which has prompted the use of several pretesting methods, none of which can be relied upon to predict severe reactions. Many authorities question the value of any pretest. A history of bronchial asthma or allergy, a family history of allergy, or a previous reaction to a contrast agent warrant special attention. Such a history, by suggesting histamine sensitivity and a consequent proneness to reactions, may be more accurate than pretesting in predicting the likelihood of a reaction, although not necessarily the severity or type of reaction in the individual case.
The sensitivity test most often performed is the slow injection of 0.5 to 1.0 ml. of the radiopaque medium, administered intravenously, prior to injection of the full diagnostic dose. It should be noted that the absence of a reaction to the test dose does not preclude the possibility of a reaction to the full diagnostic dose. If the test dose causes an untoward response of any kind, the necessity for continuing with the examination should be carefully reevaluated and, if it is deemed essential, the examination should be conducted with all possible caution. In rare instances, reactions to the test dose itself may be extremely severe; therefore, close observation of the patient, and facilities for emergency treatment, appear indicated.
Renal toxicity has been reported in a few patients with liver dysfunction who were given oral cholecystographic agents followed by urographic agents. Administration of Renovist II (Diatrizoate Meglumine and Diatrizoate Sodium Injection USP) should therefore be postponed in any patient with a known or suspected hepatic or biliary disorder who has recently taken a cholecystographic contrast agent.

Continued on next page

Squibb—Cont.

Caution should be exercised with the use of radiopaque media in severely debilitated patients and in those with marked hypertension. The possibility of thrombosis should be borne in mind when percutaneous techniques are employed.
Consideration must be given to the functional ability of the kidneys before injecting this preparation.
Contrast agents may interfere with some chemical determinations made on urine specimens; therefore, urine should be collected before administration of the contrast medium or two or more days afterwards.
The following precautions pertain to specific procedures:
Excretion urography: Adequate visualization may be difficult or impossible to obtain in uremic patients or others with severely impaired renal function (see CONTRAINDICATIONS).
Acute renal failure has been reported in diabetic patients with diabetic nephropathy and susceptible nondiabetic patients (often elderly with preexisting renal disease) following excretion urography. Therefore, careful consideration should be given before performing this procedure in these patients.
Aortography: Repeated intra-aortic injections may be hazardous.
Angiocardiography: Repeated injections may be hazardous particularly in infants weighing less than 7 kg. (see WARNINGS).
Peripheral arteriography: Hypotension or moderate decreases in blood pressure seem to occur frequently with intra-arterial (brachial) injections; therefore, the blood pressure should be monitored during the immediate ten minutes after injection; this blood pressure change is transient and usually requires no treatment.
Peripheral venography: Caution should be exercised in the presence of thrombosis or phlebitis.
Usage in Pregnancy: Safety for use during pregnancy has not been established with respect to adverse effects upon fetal development; therefore, this preparation should be used in pregnant patients only when, in the judgment of the physician, its use is deemed essential to the welfare of the patient.
Adverse Reactions: Adverse reactions accompanying the use of iodine-containing intravascular contrast agents are usually mild and transient although severe and life-threatening reactions, including fatalities, have occurred. Because of the possibility of severe reactions to the procedure and/or the radiopaque medium, appropriate emergency facilities and well-trained personnel should be available to treat both conditions. Emergency facilities and personnel should remain available for 30 to 60 minutes following the procedure since severe delayed reactions have been known to occur.
Nausea, vomiting, flushing, or a generalized feeling of warmth are the reactions seen most frequently with intravascular injection. Symptoms which may occur are chills, fever, sweating, headache, dizziness, pallor, weakness, severe retching and choking, wheezing, a rise or fall in blood pressure, ventricular fibrillation, cardiac arrest, facial or conjunctival petechiae, urticaria, pruritus, rash and other eruptions, edema, cramps, tremors, itching, sneezing, lacrimation, etc. Antihistaminic agents may be of benefit; rarely, such reactions may be severe enough to require discontinuation of dosage. Pulmonary edema, spasm, seizures, hemiparesis, and impairment of vision have occurred.
Although local tissue tolerance is usually good, there have been a few reports of a burning or stinging sensation or numbness and of venospasm or venous pain, and partial collapse of the injected vein. Neutropenia or thrombophlebitis may occur.
Severe reactions which may require emergency measures (see PRECAUTIONS) may take the form of a cardiovascular reaction characterized by peripheral vasodilatation with resultant hypotenson and reflex tachycardia, apnea, dyspnea, agitation, confusion, and cyanosis progressing to unconsciousness. Or, the histamine-liberating effect of these compounds may induce an allergic-like reaction which may range in severity from rhinitis or angioneurotic edema to laryngeal or bronchial spasm or anaphylactoid shock.
Temporary renal shutdown or other nephropathy may occur.
Adverse reactions may sometimes occur as a consequence of the procedure for which the contrast agent is used. Adverse reactions in **excretion urography** have included cardiac arrest, ventricular fibrillation, anaphylaxis with severe asthmatic reaction, and flushing due to generalized vasodilatation. In **aortography,** the risks of procedures include injury to the aorta and neighboring organs, pleural puncture, renal damage including infarction and acute tubular necrosis with oliguria and anuria, accidental selective filling of the right renal artery during the translumbar procedure in the presence of preexistent renal disease, retroperitoneal hemorrhage from the translumbar approach, spinal cord injury and pathology associated with the syndrome of transverse myelitis, generalized petechiae, and death following hypotension, arrhythmia and anaphylactoid reactions. Adverse reactions in **angiocardiography** have included arrhythmia and death. During **peripheral arteriography,** complications have occurred including hemorrhage from the puncture site, thrombosis of the vessel, and brachial plexus palsy following axillary artery injections.
Dosage and Administration: Renovist II (Diatrizoate Meglumine and Diatrizoate Sodium Injection USP) should be at body temperature when injected, and may need to be warmed before use. Renovist II should be used as promptly as possible following withdrawal into the syringe, and syringes should be rinsed as soon as possible after injection to prevent freezing of the plunger.
Since Renovist II does not usually crystallize in storage even at low temperatures, the need for heating of the preparation to effect re-solution is reduced.
Note: In the event crystallization does occur, the solution may be clarified by placing the vial in a water bath at 40° to 50° C. and shaking gently for two to three minutes or until the solids redissolve.
Withdrawal of the contrast agent should be accomplished under aseptic conditions with sterile needle and syringe.
Excretion Urography: Appropriate preparation of the patient is desirable for optimal results. A laxative the night before the examination, a low residue diet the day before, and low liquid intake for 12 hours prior to the procedure are recommended. The partial dehydration so induced is believed to effect a greater urinary concentration of the contrast medium. Enemas are to be avoided to prevent rehydration.
Preparatory partial dehydration is not recommended in infants, young children, the elderly, or azotemic patients (especially those with polyuria, oliguria, diabetes, advanced vascular disease, or preexisting dehydration). The undesirable dehydration in these patients may be accentuated by the osmotic action of the medium.
The usual intravenous dose for patients aged 16 or more is 30 ml. Children under 16 require proportionately less: Under 6 months of age—6 ml.; 6 to 12 months—10 ml.; 1 to 2 years—12 ml.; 2 to 5 years—15 ml.; 5 to 7 years—18 ml.; 7 to 10 years—22 ml.; 10 to 15 years—24 ml.; 16 years and over—30 ml.
Use of a 20- or 21-gauge needle is recommended. During the injection, the patient should be watched for untoward reactions. If flushing or nausea occurs, the rate of injection should be slowed or administration briefly interrupted until the side effects have disappeared.
A scout film should be made before Renovist II is administered. Since maximal opacification of the urinary tract usually occurs between 5 to 15 minutes after injection of this contrast agent, radiographs are best taken during this period. To allow for individual variation, several films should be exposed. In infants and children, maximal opacification occurs more rapidly after injection and is sustained over a shorter period of time. In patients with renal dysfunction, optimal opacification may be delayed for 30 minutes or more after injection.
Aortography: Renovist II injected into the aorta by the translumbar or retrograde method of administration permits radiographic visualization of the aorta, its major branches and the abdominal arteries. An incidental nephrogram is obtained as the contrast medium travels through the renal vasculature, provided it has been injected above the renal artery.
Patients should be prepared in a manner similar to that used for intravenous urography. Premedication with a suitable barbiturate is generally indicated.
As in any form of surgery, certain hazards accompany aortographic procedures (see ADVERSE REACTIONS).
For adults and children over 16 years of age, the usual dose is 20 to 30 ml. as a single injection, repeated if indicated. Chidren require less in proportion to age and weight.
Since the medium is given by rapid injection in this procedure, patients should be watched for untoward reactions during the injection. Unless general anesthesia is employed, patients should be warned that they may feel some transient pain or burning during the injection followed by a feeling of warmth immediately afterward.
A scout film should be made before the contrast agent is administered. The first radiogram should be taken as the last few ml. of the contrast medium are being injected.
Angiocardiography: Angiocardiography with Renovist II (Diatrizoate Meglumine and Diatrizoate Sodium Injection USP) may be performed by injection into a large peripheral vein or by direct catheterization of the heart. An excretory urogram can be obtained 10 to 15 minutes after injection of the contrast medium since it is concentrated in and eliminated by the kidneys.
Patients should be prepared in a manner similar to that used for intravenous urography. Appropriate preanesthetic medication should be given.
Clinical studies in man, and related animal experiments, have suggested that the hypertonicity of diatrizoate contrast agents produces significant hemodynamic effects, especially in right-sided injections. Large volumes of such agents cause a drop in peripheral arterial and systemic pressures and cardiac output, a rise in pulmonary arterial and right-heart pressures, bradycardia, and regular ectopic beats. Resulting effects on peripheral arterial and pulmonary arterial pressures are postulated to be due to mechanical blockage of the pulmonary vascular bed and clumping of red cells.
Hypertonic solutions cause a decrease in hematocrit *in vitro* and *in vivo*, and shrinkage of red blood cells.
It is suggested that hemodynamic changes be monitored and that pressures considered abnormal under roentgenographic conditions be allowed to return to a preangiographic level before continuation of radiopaque injection; this usually takes 15 minutes.
For adults the suggested single dose is 50 ml.; doses up to a total of 200 ml. have been given

safely. Children under 16 require proportionally less. The suggested single dose for children under 2 years of age is 10 to 20 ml., depending upon the weight of the child; the smallest amount necessary to obtain adequate visualization should be used. For children 2 to 4 years of age, single doses of 20 to 30 ml. are recommended; for children 4 to 10 years of age, 30 to 40 ml. Doses up to 100 ml. have been given safely. For children 10 to 15 years of age, dosage depends on the size of the patient.

Since the contrast medium is given by rapid injection, the patient should be watched for untoward reactions during the injection. Some patients not under general anesthesia may experience a feeling of bodily warmth, tightness of the chest and throbbing headache. All these sensations are of short duration. Transient nausea and vomiting may occur in some patients.

The roentgenograms should be taken immediately at the beginning of the injection and continued for 5 to 10 seconds or longer, depending upon the desired roentgenographic information.

Peripheral Arteriography: Renovist II is injected into the femoral or subclavian artery by the percutaneous or operative method. If only the lower half of the extremity is to be studied, Renovist II is injected into the brachial or popliteal artery.

Appropriate preparation of the patient is indicated, including suitable premedication.

For visualization of an entire extremity, a single dose of 30 to 50 ml. is suggested. For arteriography of the upper half or the lower half of the extremity only, a single dose of 20 to 30 ml. is sufficient.

Because the contrast medium is given by rapid injection, flushing of the skin may occur. Patients not under general anesthesia may experience a feeling of warmth and, rarely, nausea and vomiting.

A scout film should be made routinely before administering the contrast medium. Radiograms of the upper half should be taken while the last 2 ml. of Renovist II are being injected, followed by radiograms of the lower half of the extremity a few seconds later.

Peripheral Venography: For visualization of an upper extremity, Renovist II (Diatrizoate Meglumine and Diatrizoate Sodium Injection USP) may be given by percutaneous injection into any convenient superficial vein of the forearm or hand. For visualization of a lower extremity, it should be injected into a superficial vein on the lateral side of the foot.

Appropriate preparation of the patient is indicated, including suitable premedication.

For the visualization of an upper extremity in adults, a single dose of 20 ml. is suggested; a single dose of 20 ml. is sufficient for the visualization of a lower extremity. Children require less in proportion to age and weight.

The contrast medium is administered rapidly in this procedure.

The radiographs are taken at the termination of the injection.

Venocavography: Inferior venocavography may be performed with Renovist II injected into the saphenous, femoral or iliac veins by percutaneous injection, either directly or by catheterization procedures.

Appropriate preparation of the patient is indicated, including suitable premedication.

For adults the suggested average single dose is 30 to 60 ml. The dosage for children depends upon age and weight.

Renovist II (Diatrizoate Meglumine and Diatrizoate Sodium Injection USP) is injected as rapidly as possible via the saphenous vein and roentgenograms are taken immediately. A repeat injection is given if an additional view is desired. An alternate technique is to catheterize both femoral veins and to place the catheter in each common iliac vein immediately caudad to their junction. Bilateral injection gives better filling than the unilateral injection.

Roentgenograms are taken immediately after injection of the medium. They are taken in a supine position and in the right posterior oblique or lateral position.

How Supplied: Available in 30 ml. and 60 ml. single-dose vials. An excess volume (1 ml.) is available in each container for sensitivity testing.

Storage: Protect from light. Store at room temperature.

RENOVUE®-65 ℞

(Iodamide Meglumine Injection)

Description: Renovue-65 is a radiopaque urographic contrast agent supplied as a sterile, nonpyrogenic, aqueous, intravenous solution providing 65% iodamide meglumine with approximately 30% (300 mg./ml.) organically bound iodine; the solution also contains 0.01% edetate disodium as a sequestering stabilizing agent. The clear, colorless to pale yellow solution has a viscosity of 6.4 cps. at 37° C. and 8.6 cps. at 25° C.; the pH has been adjusted to 6.5 to 7.7 with iodamide. The solution has an osmolarity of approximately 1.59 mOsm per ml. at 37° C. *Renovue-65 contains approximately 0.0124 mg. (0.0005 mEq.) sodium per ml.* At the time of manufacture, the air in the container is replaced with nitrogen.

Chemically, iodamide meglumine is 3-(acetylamino)-5 [(acetylamino)methyl] -2,4,6-triiodobenzoic acid, N-methylglucamine salt.

Clinical Pharmacology: Following intravenous injection, Renovue-65 is rapidly transported through the bloodstream to the kidneys and is excreted essentially unchanged in the urine, principally by glomerular filtration. However, at least one-third of the intravenous dose is secreted by the renal tubules.

After injection, the contrast agent permits visualization of the kidneys and urinary passages through the natural physiologic mechanism of excretion.

Renal accumulation is sufficiently rapid so that the period of maximal opacification of the renal passages may begin as early as one minute after injection. Normal kidneys rapidly eliminate the contrast medium. In nephropathic conditions, particularly when excretory capacity has been altered, the rate of excretion varies unpredictably, and opacification may be delayed for 30 minutes or more after injection; with severe renal impairment, opacification may not occur. Generally the medium is concentrated sufficiently and promptly enough to permit satisfactory visualization of the urinary tract.

Indications and Usage: Renovue-65 is a diagnostic agent for intravenous excretory urography.

Contraindications: There are no absolute contraindications to the use of Renovue-65 (Iodamide Meglumine Injection) (see WARNINGS).

Warnings: A definite risk exists in the performance of excretion urography in patients who are known to have multiple myeloma, because of the great possibility of producing transient to fatal renal failure. The risk of excretion urography in myelomatous patients is not a contraindication to the procedure; however, dehydration in the preparation of these patients should be avoided, since this may predispose to the precipitation of protein in the renal tubules.

Administration of radiopaque materials to patients known or suspected to have pheochromocytoma should be performed only if the physician deems that the possible benefits outweigh the considered risks; the procedure should then be performed with extreme caution and the volume of radiopaque medium injected should be kept to an absolute minimum. The blood pressure should be assessed throughout the procedure and measures for treatment of a hypertensive crisis should be available.

Contrast media administered intravenously have been shown to promote the phenomenon of sickling in individuals who are homozygous for sickle cell disease.

Urography should be performed with extreme caution in patients with severe concomitant hepatic and renal disease, or anuria.

A history of sensitivity to iodine *per se* or to any contrast agent is not an absolute contraindication to the use of iodamide meglumine, but calls for extreme caution in administration.

Precautions: *General*—All procedures utilizing contrast media carry a definite risk of producing adverse reactions. While most reactions may be minor, life-threatening and fatal reactions may occur without warning. The risk-benefit factor should always be carefully evaluated before such a procedure is undertaken. At all times a fully equipped emergency cart, or equivalent supplies and equipment, and personnel competent in recognizing and treating adverse reactions of all severity or situations which may arise as a result of the procedure should be immediately available. If a serious reaction should occur, administration should be discontinued immediately.

Since severe delayed reactions have been known to occur, emergency facilities and competent personnel should be available for at least 30 to 60 minutes after administration.

Renal toxicity has been reported in a few patients with liver dysfunction who were given oral cholecystographic agents followed by urographic agents. Administration of Iodamide Meglumine Injection should therefore be postponed in any patient with a known or suspected hepatic or biliary disorder who has recently taken a cholecystographic contrast agent.

Caution should be exercised with the use of radiopaque media in severely debilitated patients and in those with marked hypertension.

Consideration must be given to the functional ability of the kidneys before injecting this preparation.

When any intravenous injection technique is employed, the possibility of thrombosis or of other complications due to the mechanical trauma of the procedure should be borne in mind.

Contrast agents may interfere with some chemical determinations made on urine specimens; therefore, urine should be collected before administration of the contrast medium or two or more days afterwards.

Since iodine-containing contrast agents may alter the results of thyroid function tests depending on iodine estimations (e.g., PBI and radioactive iodine uptake studies), such tests, if indicated, should be performed prior to administration of this preparation. However, measurements of serum thyroxine concentration involving use of tests such as the Resin Triiodothyronine Uptake test, "RT_3U," or the Thyroxine (Displacement) assay, "$T_4(D)$," are not affected.

Premedication with antihistamines to avoid or minimize possible allergic reactions, or their use in the management of adverse reactions, may be considered; however, admixture of an antihistamine with a contrast agent may result in a precipitate (see DOSAGE AND ADMINISTRATION).

Use of a diuretic prior to the examination in order to increase the urinary concentration of the contrast medium is not desirable (see DOSAGE AND ADMINISTRATION); dehydration may predispose to a greater incidence of, or more severe, reactions.

Sensitivity Testing—Severe, life-threatening reactions to radiopaque agents often resemble hypersensitivity phenomena. This has prompted the use of several pretesting methods, none of which can be relied on to predict severe reactions. Many authorities question

Continued on next page

Squibb—Cont.

the value of any pretest. A history of bronchial asthma or allergy, a family history of allergy, or a previous reaction to a contrast agent warrant special attention. Such a history, by suggesting histamine sensitivity and a consequent proneness to reactions may be more accurate than pretesting in predicting the likelihood of a reaction, although it will not necessarily indicate the severity or type of reaction in the individual case.

The sensitivity test most often performed is the slow intravenous injection of 0.5 to 1.0 ml. of the radiopaque medium prior to injection of the full diagnostic dose. It should be noted that the absence of a reaction to the test dose does not preclude the possibility of a reaction to the full diagnostic dose. If the test dose causes an untoward response of any kind, the necessity for continuing with the examination should be carefully reevaluated and, if it is deemed essential, the examination should be conducted with all possible caution. In rare instances reactions to the test dose itself may be extremely severe; therefore, close observation of the patient and facilities for emergency treatment are essential.

Usage in Pregnancy—No teratogenic effects attributable to the Iodamide Meglumine Injection have been observed in reproduction studies performed in mice, rats, and rabbits. Safety for use during pregnancy in humans has not been established. Although there is no clearly defined risk, the possibility of infrequent or subtle damage to the fetus cannot be excluded. Iodamide Meglumine Injection should be used in pregnant women only when clearly needed.

Pediatric Use—Safety and effectiveness for pediatric use have not been established.

Adverse Reactions: In clinical studies with iodamide meglumine, adverse reactions occurred in approximately 9.5 to 13 percent of patients. The most frequently seen reactions were nausea and/or vomiting, urticaria, pruritus, a rise or fall in blood pressure, sneezing, and sensation of warmth, individually occurring at a frequency of approximately one to five percent. Reactions were usually mild. Reactions occurring less frequently are: generalized flushing, lacrimation, headache, edema of the eyelids, coughing, retching, bitter or metallic taste, pharyngeal burning sensation, nasal congestion, hoarseness, sweating and weakness, malaise, perianal burning sensation, pain and erythema around the injection site due to faulty technique, bradycardia, hyperpnea, and shock.

Other reactions to iodinated contrast media may occur including chills, fever, pulse rate increase, shortness of breath, dizziness, syncope, restlessness, lightheadedness, pallor, choking, chest pain, tachycardia, laryngeal or pulmonary edema, dysphagia, facial or conjunctival petechiae, rash and other eruptions, wheezing, asthmatic reaction, cramps, tremors, anxiety, hemiparesis, hematomas and ecchymoses due to technique, vein cramp, partial collapse of the injected vein, thrombophlebitis and cellulitis following injection, neutropenia, transient proteinuria, hysterical reaction and numbness of head and neck, and convulsions. "Iodism" (salivary gland swelling) has been reported infrequently; immediate or delayed rigors sometimes with hyperpyrexia has occurred rarely.

Antihistaminic agents may be of benefit in the event of adverse reactions. Adverse reactions may be severe enough to require discontinuation of injection.

Severe reactions to contrast agents, which may require emergency measures (see PRECAUTIONS), may take the form of a cardiovascular reaction characterized by peripheral vasodilatation with resultant hypotension and reflex tachycardia, dyspnea, agitation, confusion, and cyanosis progressing to unconsciousness. Rare cases of cardiac arrest, ventricular fibrillation, cardiac arrhythmias, and hypertension may occur. The histamine-liberating effect of these compounds may induce an allergic-like reaction which may range in severity from rhinitis or angioneurotic edema to laryngeal or bronchial spasm and, rarely, anaphylactoid shock.

Rarely, temporary renal shutdown or other nephropathy may occur.

Dosage and Administration: Renovue-65 (Iodamide Meglumine Injection) should be at body temperature when injected, and may need to be warmed before use. If kept in a syringe for prolonged periods before injection, it should be protected from exposure to strong light.

Appropriate preparation of the patient is desirable for optimal results. A laxative the night before the examination and a low residue diet the day before the procedure may be used to clear the gastrointestinal tract. However, a normal liquid intake during this time is desirable.

Renovue-65 is administered by intravenous injection. The recommended adult dose is 0.8 ml. per kg. of body weight, up to a maximum total dose of 50 ml., administered within one to two minutes. If flushing or nausea occurs during administration, injection should be slowed or briefly interrupted until the side effects have disappeared. If a serious reaction should occur, administration should be discontinued immediately.

The admixture of Benadryl® (Diphenhydramine Hydrochloride Injection) with Renovue-65 may cause a precipitate to form in the syringe. If antihistamines are administered concomitantly (see PRECAUTIONS), they should *not* be mixed with the contrast agent and should be administered at another site.

Roentgenographic Procedure: A scout film should be made before the contrast medium is administered. Several films should be exposed after injection to allow for individual variation and to insure visualization of the desired sites of the urinary tract. Times at which optimal opacification may be observed in most patients are as follows: renal parenchyma at 1 minute after injection; calyces, pelves, and ureters at 10 minutes; and urinary bladder at 20 minutes. In patients with renal dysfunction, optimal visualization may be delayed until 30 minutes or more after injection.

How Supplied: Available in 50 ml. single-dose vials containing sufficient excess for sensitivity testing.

Storage: The preparation should be stored at room temperature, protected from light and excessive heat. If precipitation or solidification has occurred due to storage in the cold, immerse the container in hot water and shake intermittently to dissolve any solids.

RENOVUE®-DIP ℞
(Iodamide Meglumine Injection 24%)
For Drip Infusion Pyelography

Description: Renovue-DIP is a radiopaque contrast agent for drip infusion pyelography supplied as a sterile, nonpyrogenic, aqueous, intravenous solution providing 24% iodamide meglumine with approximately 11.1% (111 mg./ml.) organically bound iodine. The solution also contains 0.00368% edetate disodium as a sequestering agent. The clear, colorless to pale yellow solution has a viscosity of 1.8 cps. at 37° C. and 2.0 cps. at 25° C.; the pH has been adjusted to 6.5 to 7.7 with iodamide. The solution has an osmolarity of approximately 0.5 mOsm per ml. at 37° C. *Renovue-DIP contains approximately 0.0046 mg. (0.0002 mEq.) sodium per ml.* At the time of manufacture, the air in the container is replaced with nitrogen.

Chemically, iodamide meglumine is 3-(acetylamino)-5 [(acetylamino)methyl] -2,4,6-triiodobenzoic acid, N-methylglucamine salt.

Clinical Pharmacology: Following intravenous infusion, Renovue-DIP is rapidly transported through the bloodstream to the kidneys and is excreted essentially unchanged in the urine, principally by glomerular filtration. However, at least one-third of the intravenous dose is secreted by the renal tubules.

After infusion, the contrast agent permits visualization of the kidneys and urinary passages through the natural physiologic mechanism of excretion.

Renal accumulation is sufficiently rapid so that the period of maximal opacification of the renal passages may begin within five minutes after start of infusion. Normal kidneys rapidly eliminate the contrast medium. In nephropathic conditions, particularly when excretory capacity has been altered, the rate of excretion varies unpredictably, and opacification may be delayed for 60 minutes or more after start of infusion; with severe renal impairment, opacification may not occur. Generally the medium is concentrated sufficiently and promptly enough to permit satisfactory visualization of the urinary tract.

Indications and Usage: Renovue-DIP is a diagnostic agent for excretion urography by intravenous infusion.

Contraindications: There are no absolute contraindications to the use of Renovue-DIP (Iodamide Meglumine Injection 24%) (see WARNINGS).

Warnings: A definite risk exists in the performance of excretion urography in patients who are known to have multiple myeloma, because of the great possibility of producing transient to fatal renal failure. The risk of excretion urography in myelomatous patients is not a contraindication to the procedure; however, dehydration in the preparation of these patients should be avoided, since this may predispose to the precipitation of protein in the renal tubules.

Administration of radiopaque materials to patients known or suspected to have pheochromocytoma should be performed only if the physician deems that the possible benefits outweigh the considered risks; the procedure should then be performed with extreme caution and the volume of radiopaque medium injected should be kept to an absolute minimum. The blood pressure should be assessed throughout the procedure and measures for treatment of a hypertensive crisis should be available.

Contrast media administered intravenously have been shown to promote the phenomenon of sickling in individuals who are homozygous for sickle cell disease.

Urography should be performed with extreme caution in patients with severe concomitant hepatic and renal disease, or anuria.

A history of sensitivity to iodine *per se* or to any contrast agent is not an absolute contraindication to the use of iodamide meglumine, but calls for extreme caution in administration.

Precautions: *General*—All procedures utilizing contrast media carry a definite risk of producing adverse reactions. While most reactions may be minor, life-threatening and fatal reactions may occur without warning. The risk-benefit factor should always be carefully evaluated before such a procedure is undertaken. At all times a fully equipped emergency cart, or equivalent supplies and equipment, and personnel competent in recognizing and treating adverse reactions of all severity (or situations which may arise as a result of the procedure) should be immediately available. If a serious reaction should occur, administration should be discontinued immediately.

Since severe delayed reactions have been known to occur, emergency facilities and competent personnel should be available for at least 30 to 60 minutes after administration.

Renal toxicity has been reported in a few patients with liver dysfunction who were given oral choleystographic agents followed by urographic agents. Administration of Iodamide Meglumine Injection 24% should therefore be postponed in any patient with a known or suspected hepatic or biliary disorder who has recently taken a cholecystographic contrast agent.
Caution should be exercised with the use of radiopaque media in severely debilitated patients and in those with marked hypertension.
The increased osmotic load associated with drip infusion pyelography should also be considered in patients with congestive heart failure.
Consideration must be given to the functional ability of the kidneys before infusing this preparation.
The diuretic effect of the drip infusion pyelography procedure may hinder assessment of residual urine in the bladder.
When any intravenous infusion technique is employed, the possibility of thrombosis or of other complications due to the mechanical trauma of the procedure should be borne in mind.
The recommended rate of infusion should not be exceeded.
Contrast agents may interfere with some chemical determinations made on urine specimens; therefore, urine should be collected before administration of the contrast medium or two or more days afterwards.
Since iodine-containing contrast agents may alter the results of thyroid function tests which depend on iodine estimations (e.g., PBI and radioactive iodine uptake studies), such tests, if indicated, should be performed prior to the administration of this preparation. However, measurements of serum thyroxine concentration involving use of tests such as the Resin Triiodothyronine Uptake test, "RT_3U," or the Thyroxine (Displacement) assay, "$T_4(D)$," are not affected.
Premedication with antihistamines to avoid or minimize possible allergic reactions, or their use in the management of adverse reactions, may be considered; however, admixture of an antihistamine with a contrast agent may result in a precipitate (see DOSAGE AND ADMINISTRATION).
Use of a diuretic prior to the examination in order to increase the urinary concentration of the contrast medium is not desirable (see DOSAGE AND ADMINISTRATION); dehydration may predispose to a greater incidence of, or more severe, reactions.
Sensitivity Testing: Severe, life-threatening reactions to radiopaque agents often resemble hypersensitivity phenomena. This has prompted the use of several pretesting methods, none of which can be relied on to predict severe reactions. Many authorities question the value of any pretest. A history of bronchial asthma or allergy, a family history of allergy, or a previous reaction to a contrast agent warrant special attention. Such a history, by suggesting histamine sensitivity and a consequent proneness to reactions may be more accurate than pretesting in predicting the likelihood of a reaction, although it will not necessarily indicate the severity or type of reaction in the individual case.
The sensitivity test most often performed is the slow intravenous injection of 0.5 to 1.0 ml. of the radiopaque medium, prior to infusion of the full diagnostic dose. It should be noted that the absence of a reaction to the test dose does not preclude the possibility of a reaction to the full diagnostic dose. If the test dose causes an untoward response of any kind, the necessity for continuing with the examination should be carefully reevaluated and, if it is deemed essential, the examination should be conducted with all possible caution. In rare instances reactions to the test dose itself may be extremely severe; therefore, close observation of the patient, and facilities for emergency treatment, are essential.
Usage in Pregnancy: No teratogenic effects attributable to Iodamide Meglumine Injection 24% have been observed in reproduction studies performed in mice, rats, and rabbits. Safety for use during pregnancy in humans has not been established. Although there is no clearly defined risk, the possibility of infrequent or subtle damage to the fetus cannot be excluded. Iodamide Meglumine Injection 24% should be used in pregnant women only when clearly needed.
Pediatric Use: Safety and effectiveness for pediatric use have not been established.
Adverse Reactions: In clinical studies with iodamide meglumine, adverse reactions occurred in approximately 9.5 to 13 percent of patients. The most frequently seen adverse reactions were nausea and/or vomiting, urticaria, pruritus, and a rise or fall in blood pressure, individually occurring at a frequency of approximately one to five percent. Reactions were usually mild. Reactions occurring less frequently are generalized flushing, retching, nasal congestion, sneezing, flank tenderness, chills, syncope, pulse rate increase, hyperpnea, shortness of breath, chest pain, tachycardia, and hemiparesis.
Other reactions to iodinated contrast media may occur including fever; dizziness; headache; lacrimation; sweating and weakness; lightheadedness; restlessness; pallor; coughing; choking; hoarseness; laryngeal or pulmonary edema; dysphagia; malaise; edema of the eyelids; bitter or metallic taste; pharyngeal burning sensation; facial or conjunctival petechiae; rash and other eruptions; perianal burning sensation; wheezing; asthmatic reaction; cramps; tremors; anxiety; pain, erythema, hematomas, and ecchymoses around injection site due to faulty technique; warmth or burning sensation; vein cramp; partial collapse of the injected vein; thrombophlebitis and cellulitis following injection; neutropenia; transient proteinuria; hysterical reaction and numbness of head and neck; bradycardia; shock; and convulsions. "Iodism" (salivary gland swelling) has been reported infrequently; immediate or delayed rigors sometimes with hyperpyrexia has occurred rarely.
Antihistaminic agents may be of benefit in the event of adverse reactions. Adverse reactions may be severe enough to require discontinuation of injection.
Severe reactions to contrast agents, which may require emergency measures (see PRECAUTIONS), may take the form of a cardiovascular reaction characterized by peripheral vasodilatation with resultant hypotension and reflex tachycardia, dyspnea, agitation, confusion, and cyanosis progressing to unconsciousness. Rare cases of cardiac arrest, ventricular fibrillation, cardiac arrhythmias, and hypertension may occur. The histamine-liberating effect of these compounds may induce an allergic-like reaction which may range in severity from rhinitis or angioneurotic edema to laryngeal or bronchial spasm and, rarely, anaphylactoid shock.
Rarely, temporary renal shutdown or other nephropathy may occur.
Dosage and Administration: Renovue-DIP (Iodamide Meglumine Injection 24%) should be at body temperature when infused, and may need to be warmed before use.
Appropriate preparation of the patient is desirable for optimal results. A laxative the night before the examination and a low residue diet the day before the procedure may be used to clear the gastrointestinal tract. However, a normal liquid intake during this time is desirable.
The recommended adult dose is 4.5 ml. per kg. of body weight, administered intravenously by continuous infusion, with a maximum total dose of 300 ml.; the appropriate volume should be infused in approximately 10 minutes (about 30 ml. per minute for a 147 lb. or heavier patient), through a large-bore (usually 17- or 18-gauge) needle. In older patients and in patients with known or suspected cardiac decompensation, a slower rate of infusion is probably wise. If flushing or nausea occurs during administration, infusion should be slowed or briefly interrupted until the side effects have disappeared. If a serious reaction should occur, administration should be discontinued immediately.
The admixture of Benadryl® (Diphenhydramine Hydrochloride Injection) with Renovue-DIP may cause a precipitate to form in the tubing. If antihistamines are administered concomitantly (see PRECAUTIONS), they should *not* be mixed with the contrast agent and should be administered at another site.
Roentgenographic Procedure: A scout film should be made before the contrast medium is administered. Several films should be exposed after infusion to allow for individual variation and to insure visualization of the desired sites of the urinary tract. Times at which optimal opacification may be first observed in the majority of patients are as follows: renal parenchyma at 10 minutes after start of infusion, calyces and pelves at 20 minutes, and ureters and bladder at 30 minutes. In patients with renal dysfunction, optimal visualization may be delayed until 60 minutes or more after the start of infusion.
How Supplied: Available in calibrated 300 ml. infusion bottles (designed to be suspended from an I.V. stand), containing sufficient excess for sensitivity testing.
Storage: The preparation should be stored at room temperature, protected from light and excessive heat. If precipitation or solidification has occurred due to storage in the cold, immerse the container in hot water and shake intermittently to dissolve any solids.

SINOGRAFIN® ℞
(Diatrizoate Meglumine and Iodipamide Meglumine Injection)

Description: Sinografin is available as a sterile, aqueous solution for intrauterine instillation. Each ml. provides 527 mg. diatrizoate meglumine and 268 mg. iodipamide meglumine with 3.2 mg. sodium citrate as a buffer, and 0.4 mg. edetate disodium. Each vial contains approximately 3.8 g. organically bound iodine (380 mg./ml.). At the time of manufacture, the air in the container is replaced by nitrogen.
Actions: Following intrauterine administration, immediate visualization of the uterus and tubes is achieved. Present evidence indicates that any medium spilled into the peritoneal cavity as a result of the procedure is absorbed within 20 to 60 minutes. A 24-hour film has shown complete absorption even in cases of large hydrosalpinx.
Indications: Sinografin is indicated for use in hysterosalpingography.
Contraindications: This preparation is contraindicated during pregnancy or in the presence of acute pelvic inflammatory disease. Hysterosalpingography should not be attempted within 30 days following curettage or conization. Sinografin should not be administered to patients with a hypersensitivity to iodipamide or salts of diatrizoic acid.
Warnings: Since iodine-containing contrast agents may alter the results of thyroid function tests, such tests, if indicated, should be performed prior to the administration of this drug.
A history of sensitivity to iodine *per se* or to contrast media other than iodipamide or salts of diatrizoic acid is not an absolute contraindication to the use of Sinografin but calls for extreme caution in administration.
Precautions: Hypersensitivity reactions have occurred and are more likely in patients

Continued on next page

Squibb—Cont.

with a personal or familial history of allergy. These may be manifested by reactions such as urticaria, respiratory symptoms and circulatory collapse. Facilities for treatment of circulatory collapse and respiratory distress should be immediately available, and patients should be carefully observed during performance of the examination and for at least 30 to 60 minutes thereafter.

When performing radiography, serial x-ray pictures should be taken where possible in preference to fluoroscopic visualization to minimize radiation exposure.

Adverse Reactions: Hypersensitivity reactions, which include sweating, flushing, pruritus, urticaria, skin rashes, arthralgia, respiratory distress, and circulatory collapse have occurred. Chills, fever, nausea, vomiting, and abdominal pain and tenderness are occasionally seen following instillation of the contrast material.

Dosage and Administration: *Dosage:* 3 to 4 ml. of Sinografin are usually adequate to visualize the uterus, and an additional 3 to 4 ml. will demonstrate the tubes. Total dosage varying from 1.5 to 10 ml. has been employed with satisfactory results.

Preparation of the patient: Hysterosalpingography should be performed three to five days after the cessation of the patient's menstrual period as a precautionary measure. An enema and vaginal douche one hour before the examination are helpful, but not essential. The patient should empty her bladder before the examination. Since the procedure is remarkably free of pain when Sinografin is used, the use of a narcotic or anesthesia is unnecessary.

Administration: The patient is placed in the lithotomy position and the vulva is cleansed with a suitable antiseptic solution. A Graves-type vaginal speculum is introduced, the cervix is exposed, and the vaginal vault is sponged with antiseptic solution.

A tenaculum is placed on the cervical lip, usually the anterior lip. A sterile sound may be passed to determine the position of the uterus and the direction of the cervical canal, and, when necessary, the cervical canal may be dilated. (Sounding the uterine cavity and dilatation of the canal are not usually required when a flexible cannula tip is used.)

A sterile syringe containing the Sinografin is attached by Luer-Lok to a uterine cannula. The two-way cannula valve is opened and all air bubbles in the cannula and syringe are expressed. About 1.5 to 2 ml. of Sinografin are required to fill the cannula. (If preferred, a tubal insufflator under controlled pressure with a salpingogram attachment may be used instead of the syringe.)

The cannula tip is inserted into the cervical canal so that the adjustable rubber acorn obturator fits snugly at the external os. Careful placement of the cannula is important to avoid trauma and pain. Squeezing the trigger of the cannula to provide simultaneous traction on the tenaculum and forward pressure on the cannula should give a nonleaking cervical seal. Sinografin flows freely so that only gentle pressure on the plunger is necessary.

The connection at the external os is checked for leakage. If the acorn obturator is inadequate, an inflatable balloon-obturator may be used to seal the cervical canal. When the equipment has been positioned satisfactorily, the tenaculum and cannula may be fixed in position until the procedure is terminated.

Radiography: Sinografin is administered in fractional doses of approximately 1 ml. A scout film may be made before the medium is administered. After the initial injection, a film should be made using a Bucky diaphragm. After each successive injection of 1 ml., a film is taken, developed immediately, and inspected in the dark room before the next fractional dose of Sinografin is given, until the procedure is completed. Further injection and subsequent films can be made as required using posterior-anterior or oblique angles.

Clinical experience indicates that tubal patency, if present, will be demonstrable at the time of the injection and delayed films have not been required. The medium is completely absorbed within one hour, unless there is an obstruction and dilatation of the tubes, in which case absorption is generally complete within 24 hours. Any residual Sinografin within the uterine cavity is usually expelled immediately upon removal of the cannula.

How Supplied: Available in single-dose vials of 10 ml.

Storage: Store at room temperature (20° to 25°C.) and protect against exposure to strong light. The Sinografin solution may vary in color from essentially colorless to light amber; however, solutions which have become strongly discolored should not be used. Sinografin should be used as promptly as possible following withdrawal into the syringe, and the syringe should be rinsed as soon as possible after injection to prevent freezing of the plunger.

For information on Squibb products, write to: Squibb Professional Services Department, Lawrenceville-Princeton Road, Princeton, N.J. 08540.

United States Packaging Corporation

Medical Products Division
506 CLAY STREET
LA PORTE, IN 46350

GONODECTEN® TEST KIT ℞

Intended Use of the Product: GONODECTEN® is an *in vitro* diagnostic system used as a **presumptive test** for the diagnosis of gonorrhea in the urethral exudate from the male without the use of conventional culture or gram stain.

Summary and Explanation of the Test: The principal mechanism utilized by the GONODECTEN® TEST KIT is based upon oxidase technology.[1,2,3] This oxidase reaction is an enzymatic reaction that involves cytochrome oxidase catalyzing the oxidation of reduced cytochrome by molecular oxygen which acts as the terminal state in electron transfer. The active ingredient of the kit, N,N,N',N' -Tetramethyl-p-phenylenediamine Dihydrochloride at a 1% concentration undergoes a color change and becomes a distinct purple color when it comes into contact with an oxidase positive organism, e.g.: *N. gonorrhoeae.*

The purpose of the GONODECTEN® TEST KIT is a procedure to detect an oxidizing enzyme which is associated with certain bacteria such as *N. gonorrhoeae.*

The Principles of the Procedure: The principal mechanism on which the GONODECTEN® TEST KIT is based depends upon catalyzing the oxidation of reduced cytochrome by molecular oxygen which acts as the terminal state in electron transfer.

N,N,N',N' -Tetramethyl-p-phenylenediamine (Wurster's reagent) ($C_{16}H_{16}N_2$). The dihydrochloride form of this salt reacts with cytochrome oxidase from *N. gonorrhoeae* forming a purple color.

Reagents: N,N,N',N'-Tetramethyl-p- phenylenediamine Dihydrochloride at a 1% concentration is the reactive ingredient.

Warnings and Precautions: GONODECTEN® is for *in vitro* diagnostic use. As the urethral exudate may contain pathogens, usual aseptic procedures should be taken by the user and/or accompanying assisting personnel. No part or portion of the GONODECTEN® TEST KIT is to be inserted into any body orifice.

Storage Instructions: The GONODECTEN® TEST KIT can be stored at 72°F ± 30°. Discoloration (brownish color of the pledget) can occur at the upper temperature within the expiration date of the product. However, this will not affect the test results. Theoretically, the stability of the active ingredient is enhanced at lower temperatures in a darkened area.

Physical, Biological, or Chemical Indications of Instability or Deterioration: Frangible glass ampul must not be broken. Turbidity of saline in ampul due to occasional long term storage of the saline in the presence of the alkaline glass ampul does not affect the test. Discoloration of the pledget may occur after long term storage but does not affect the test.

Special Collection and Preparation for Analysis: Special precautions regarding specimen collection:

The test is not to be used if urination has occurred until after one hour has elapsed.

The urethral specimen should be expressed onto the side of the dacron sterile swab.

After the swab is wetted by crushing the ampul, pull swab back from the Webril® pledget and observe if purple coloration occurs at the **site of the exudate** on the swab.

Avoid overwetting the swab by repeated squeezing of the wetted Webril® pledget.

ONLY READ TEST RESULTS FROM INOCULUM SITE ON SWAB.

Interfering Substances: If pledget is wetted, oxidase positive organisms and iron containing substances will eventually result in an even, light purple (dependent upon length of time) coloration.

Procedure: The procedure for the use of the GONODECTEN® TEST KIT is as follows:

1. Open package and remove sterile swab from its envelope.
2. Apply expressed specimen of the urethral exudate to the side of the sterile swab.
3. This test is not to be used if urination has occurred until after one hour has elapsed.
4. Remove white cap and insert swab with exudate into tube.
5. Replace white cap on plastic tube.
6. Squeeze the tube below Webril® pledget to crush the ampul and push down on white cap, bringing swab into contact with wetted Webril® pledget. After swab is wetted, withdraw swab a few millimeters away breaking contact from the pledget.
7. Pull swab back from the Webril® pledget and observe if a purple color has developed **on the swab** at the **site of the exudate.** Allow **up to** a maximum of 3 minutes for color development to occur.
8. Development of a purple color on the swab at the site of the exudate within a 3 minute time interval is a presumptive positive test for *Neisseria gonorrhoeae.* Observation of a color change is best noted if the specimen is placed on the side of the dacron portion of the sterile swab. Also, overwetting of the swab can dilute the color intensity.

List of all Materials Provided:

- plastic envelope containing system
- label
- package insert
- sterile swab in paper container
- plastic tube containing frangible ampul with ½ ml physiological saline, pH buffered to 7.2, Webril® pledget impregnated with reactive agent and cardboard cap.

Stability of Final Reaction to be Measured and Time within which it shall be Measured to assure Accurate Results: Allow up to a maximum of 3 minutes for color development to occur.

Reference Material: Verification of a GONODECTEN® TEST KIT may be done using a known culture of *N. gonorrhoeae* and following directions for use as stated in the package insert with the exception that the *N. gonor-*

rhoeae colonies in the culture media are used instead of an urethral exudate.

Results: Procedure for calculating the value of the unknown: The "unknown" specimen relative to the absence or presence of *N. gonorrhoeae* is related to the color development in the described test.

Limitation of the Procedure: No part or portion of the GONODECTEN® TEST KIT is to be inserted into any body orifice. This test kit is not suitable for use on specimens other than a male urethral discharge. Test kit is not to be used if urination has occurred until after one hour has elapsed. This kit is positive in the presence of oxidase positive organisms which will yield a dark blue to purple coloration on the swab at the site of the specimen collection. Normally oxidase positive organisms are not found in the male urethra.[4] There are a number of bacterial urethretides in the male that may produce an exudate. These bacteria may be either oxidase positive, e.g.: *N. gonorrhoeae, Mima polymorpha V. oxidans, Pseudomonas aeruginosa*, etc., or oxidase negative, e.g.: *Staphylococcus aureus, Staphylococcus epidermidis*, etc. This test only determines oxidase positive organisms. The likelihood of other oxidase positive organisms present in the male urethral discharge other than gonorrhea is unlikely. The test results are valid only within a 3-minute time interval in the presence of a male urethral discharge. Should the GONODECTEN® TEST KIT yield a negative result, additional tests should be performed such as: gram staining, culture, sugar fermentations, etc. for diagnosis. DO NOT USE if frangible glass ampul is broken. Iron containing substances will react with the wetted Webril® pledget yielding a purple color.

Expected Values: The purple color reaction is an all or none process. The color depth is unaltered except that more colored area will be produced if the positive specimen area is increased.

Specific Performance Characteristics: 518 patients were evaluated at venereal disease and hospital associated clinics. No data was obtained from private physicians' offices although there is no reason to believe that the data would be different. Of the 518 patients, 323 were positive and 91 negative, respectively, for *N. gonorrhoeae* by the GONODECTEN® TEST KIT, gram stain and culture. GONODECTEN® was positive for *N. gonorrhoeae* in 31 patients whereby both the gram and culture were negative, and negative in 25 patients where the gram stain and culture were positive. 397 patients were identified as having gonorrhea by gram stain or culture. GONODECTEN® identified 395 patients resulting in a sensitivity of 99.5%. There were 121 specimens negative by both gram stain and culture. GONODECTEN® was negative for 91 of these 121 specimens resulting in a specificity of 74.2%.

Data collected from 6 venereal centers support the conclusion that the sensitivities of the GONODECTEN® TEST KIT and gram stain are similar within a Center. Both test procedures have higher sensitivities than culture sensitivities. The largest number of cases (201 of 518) were conducted at the N.Y.C. Health Department whereby there appeared to be no evidence of a difference between the test kit and gram stain procedures with respect to sensitivity or specificity. Additionally, the N.Y.C.H.D. data suggest the test kit and gram stain results are much superior to culture in detecting *N. gonorrhoeae* when it is in fact present. When both the test kit and gram stain indicate a presumptive diagnosis of *N. gonorrhoeae* they are equal despite a negative culture, in which it is assumed that the subject does not have *N. gonorrhoeae*.

Availability: GONODECTEN® TEST KIT is available in boxes of 25 kits/box; 4 boxes/carton.

Bibliography:

1. Steel, K. J., The oxidase reaction as a taxonomic tool, *J. Gen. Microbiol. 25*, 297–306, 1961.
2. Gordon, J. and McLeod, J. W., The practical application of the direct oxidase reaction in bacteriology. *J. Path. Bact. 31*, 185, 1928.
3. Rein, Michael, F., Practice of Medicine, Vol. III, Chapter 19, 1975, pg. 2.
4. Smith, A. L., Microbiology and Pathology, 9th ed., 1968.

Manufactured By:
United States Packaging Corporation, Medical Products Division, 506 Clay Street, LaPorte, IN 46350 U.S.A.
GONODECTEN®—Registered Trademark of United States Packaging Corporation, La-Porte, Indiana
Webril®—Registered Trademark of The Kendall Company, Walpole, Massachusetts

Printed in U.S.A.
U.S. Patent Nos. 3,876,503; 4,018,653
Part No. 11 Revised 5/79

PHYSICIANS INSERT (Above)

GONODECTEN®
FOR IN VITRO DIAGNOSTIC USE
A presumptive test for the diagnosis of gonorrhea in the urethral exudate from the male

Reactive Ingredient: N,N,N',N'-Tetramethyl-p-phenylenediamine Dihydrochloride—1% concentration.

Contents: One sterile swab and one plastic tube containing a diagnostic system.

Precautions: GONODECTEN® is for *in vitro* diagnostic use. No part or portion of the GONODECTEN® TEST KIT is to be inserted into any body orifice. This test kit is not suitable for use on specimens other than a male urethral discharge. Test kit not to be used if urination has occurred until after one hour has elapsed. This test is positive in the presence of oxidase positive organisms which will yield a dark blue to purple coloration on the swab at the site of the specimen collection. Normally oxidase positive organisms are not found in the male urethra. There are a number of bacterial urethretides in the male that can produce an exudate. These bacteria may be either oxidase positive, e.g.: *N. gonorrhoeae, Mima polymorpha V. oxidans, Pseudomonas aeruginosa*, etc., or oxidase negative, e.g.: *Staphylococcus aureus, Staphylococcus epidermidis*, etc. This test only determines oxidase positive organisms. The likelihood of other oxidase positive organisms present in the male urethral discharge other than gonorrhea is unlikely. The test results are valid only within a 3 minute time interval. In the presence of a male urethral discharge whereby the GONODECTEN® TEST KIT yields a negative result, additional tests should be performed such as gram staining, culture, sugar fermentations, etc., for diagnosis. As the urethral exudate may contain pathogens, usual aseptic procedures should be taken. DO NOT USE if frangible glass ampul is broken. Turbidity of saline in ampul will not affect the test results. Verification of a GONODECTEN® TEST KIT may be done using a known culture of *N. gonorrhoeae* and following directions for use as stated in the package insert.

Store at 72°F ± 30°
Pledget discoloration may occur without affecting test results

Manufactured by: United States Packaging Corporation, Medical Products Division, La-Porte, Indiana 46350 U.S.A.

U.S. Patent Nos. 3,876,503; 4,018,653
Part No. 10 Revised 5/79

LABEL (Above)

Winthrop Laboratories
90 PARK AVENUE
NEW YORK, NY 10016

AMIPAQUE® ℞
brand of metrizamide

Description: Metrizamide, 2-[3-Acetamido-2, 4, 6-triiodo-5-(N-methylacetamido) benzamido]-2-deoxy-D-glucopyranose, is a compound derived from metrizoic acid and glucosamine. It is a nonionic water-soluble contrast medium with a molecular weight of 789 (iodine content: 48.25%).

AMIPAQUE is provided as a sterile, white lyophilized powder. Each 3.75 g/20 ml vial contains 3.75 g metrizamide (1.81 g organically-bound iodine) and 1.2 mg edetate calcium disodium. Each 6.75 g/50 ml vial contains 6.75 g metrizamide (3.26 g organically-bound iodine) and 2.16 mg edetate calcium disodium.

Each 20 ml vial of sterile aqueous diluent contains 0.05 mg/ml sodium bicarbonate in water for injection. pH is adjusted with carbon dioxide, USP, if necessary.

When AMIPAQUE is reconstituted to the lowest recommended concentration (170 mg I/ml) it has a specific gravity of 1.184 at 37°C, is hyperbaric to cerebrospinal fluid, is isotonic with CSF, and has a pH of approximately 7.4. AMIPAQUE solution and powder is sensitive to heat or light and, therefore, should be protected from exposure.

Clinical Pharmacology: AMIPAQUE is absorbed from cerebrospinal fluid into the blood stream. Approximately 60 per cent of the administered dose is excreted unchanged through the kidneys within 48 hours.

The initial concentration and volume of the medium, in conjunction with appropriate patient manipulation, will determine the extent of the diagnostic contrast that can be achieved. This can be monitored by fluoroscopy.

Following spinal subarachnoid injection, conventional radiography will continue to provide diagnostic contrast for approximately an hour. At 4 to 5 hours contrast is hazy and none is detectable at 24 hours.

Following subarachnoid placement, irrespective of the position the patient has maintained, upward diffusion of AMIPAQUE takes place through the CSF.

After introduction into the lumbar subarachnoid space, computerized tomography (CT) shows CSF contrast enhancement in the thoracic region in about one hour, in the cervical region in about 2 hours, and in the basal cisterns in 3 to 4 hours.

When low doses of AMIPAQUE (see DOSAGE AND ADMINISTRATION) are introduced into the lumbar CSF and moved cephalad under gravity control and examined by CT scanning, they will provide immediate CSF contrast in the basal cisterns. Depending on the specific technique used, the lateral, third, and fourth ventricles may also be visualized. The contrast in this area will markedly diminish at 6 hours and disappear by 24 hours. CSF enhancement will be evident at the cortical sulci and interhemispheric fissures at 6 hours. Between 12 and 24 hours the surfaces of the cerebrum and cerebellum, in contact with the subarachnoid spaces, will develop a "blush" effect on the scan which will normally disappear in 36 to 48 hours. The rate, time, extent of diffusion, and the disappearance or stasis of AMIPAQUE as demonstrated with CT scanning, can be used to detect or infer the presence of CNS abnormalities.

Indications and Usage: AMIPAQUE is indicated for lumbar, thoracic, cervical, and total columnar myelography and for use in computerized tomography of the intracranial subarachnoid spaces following spinal subarachnoid injection.

Continued on next page

Winthrop—Cont.

Contraindications: AMIPAQUE should not be administered to patients with a known hypersensitivity to metrizamide.

Warnings: If grossly bloody CSF is encountered, the possible benefits of a myelographic procedure should be considered in terms of the risk to the patient.

Usage in pregnancy. No teratogenic effects attributable to AMIPAQUE have been observed in reproduction studies in animals. However, before administration of AMIPAQUE to women during pregnancy, the benefit to the patient should be carefully weighed against the possible risk to the fetus.

Until further experience is gained in children younger than 12 years, administration of AMIPAQUE, brand of metrizamide, in this age group is not recommended.

Fatal reactions have been associated with the administration of water-soluble contrast media. Although no fatal reactions have been associated with AMIPAQUE, it is of utmost importance that a course of action be carefully planned in advance for the immediate treatment of serious reactions, and that adequate and appropriate facilities and personnel be readily available in case of a severe reaction.

Precautions: Caution is advised in patients with a history of epilepsy, severe cardiovascular disease, chronic alcoholism, multiple sclerosis, or with a history of bronchial asthma or other allergic manifestations.

Before a contrast medium is injected, the patient should be questioned for a history of allergy. Although a history of allergy, including asthma, may imply a greater than usual risk, it does not arbitrarily contraindicate the use of the medium. No conclusive relationship between severe reactions and antigen-antibody reactions or other manifestations of allergy has been established.

Patients who are receiving anticonvulsants should be maintained on this therapy. Should a seizure occur, intravenous diazepam or sodium phenobarbital is recommended.

The intrathecal administration of corticosteroids with AMIPAQUE is not indicated and may be contraindicated.

Care is required in patient management to prevent inadvertent intracranial entry of a large dose or concentrated bolus of the medium. Direct intracisternal or ventricular administration for standard radiography (not CT) is not recommended.

Prophylactic anticonvulsant treatment with barbiturates or diazepam orally for 24 to 48 hours should be considered in patients with evidence of inadvertent intracranial entry of a large or concentrated bolus of the contrast medium since there is an increased risk of seizures in such cases.

Drugs which lower the seizure threshold, especially phenothiazine derivatives, should not be used with AMIPAQUE. Others include: MAO inhibitors, tricyclic antidepressants, antihistamines, CNS stimulants, psychoactive drugs described as analeptics, major tranquilizers, or antipsychotic drugs. Such medication should be discontinued at least 24 hours before myelography, should not be used for the control of nausea and vomiting, and should not be resumed for at least 24 hours postprocedure.

In patients with severe renal insufficiency or failure, the drug is excreted by the liver into the bile at a much slower rate. Patients with hepatorenal insufficiency should not be examined unless the possibility of benefit clearly outweighs the additional risk. Reexamination should be delayed for 5 to 7 days.

Adverse Reactions: In general, the adverse reactions following subarachnoid injection of AMIPAQUE are not substantially different from those seen after lumbar puncture alone. The most frequently occurring adverse reactions are headache, nausea, and vomiting. These reactions occur 3 to 8 hours postinjection, almost all occurring within 24 hours. They are usually mild to moderate in degree lasting for a few hours and usually disappearing within 24 hours. Rarely, headaches may be severe or persist for days.

Backache, neck stiffness, numbness and paresthesias, leg or sciatic-type pain occurred less frequently, often in the form of a transient exacerbation of preexisting symptomatology. Temperature elevations and dizziness have also been reported.

Rarely, muscle spasm or generalized convulsions have occurred 4 to 8 hours following injection and in some cases were attributed to a history of epilepsy, medication with neuroleptic drugs, or inadvertent overdose. In all cases, treatment with intravenous diazepam or sodium phenobarbital has provided rapid control.

Transient alterations in vital signs may occur, the significance of which is difficult to assess since these parameters may be affected by the procedure or the patient's physical or emotional state.

Other rarely occurring adverse reactions include the following:

Allergy or Idiosyncrasy: chills, pruritus, urticaria, nasal congestion, and dyspnea.

CNS Irritation: mild and transitory perceptual aberrations such as hallucinations, depersonalization, anxiety, depression, hyperesthesia, visual, auditory, or speech disturbances, confusion and disorientation. In addition, malaise, weakness, EEG changes, and meningismus have occurred.

Cardiovascular: chest pain, tachycardia, bradycardia, and arrhythmia.

Other: diarrhea.

Dosage and Administration: The dosage and concentration of AMIPAQUE will depend on the degree and extent of contrast required in the area(s) under examination and on the equipment and technique employed. Concentrations which are approximately isotonic (170 to 190 mg I/ml) are recommended for examination in the lumbar region. For movement of the medium to distant target areas, higher concentrations are recommended to compensate for dilution of AMIPAQUE with CSF.

A total dose of 3000 mg iodine or a concentration of 300 mg I/ml should not be exceeded.

It is recommended that an interval of at least 48 hours should elapse, whenever possible, before repeat examination.

The recommended usual and maximum doses of AMIPAQUE, brand of metrizamide, are summarized in the following table:

(See table below)

DOSAGE TABLE

Procedure	Conc. of Solution (mg I/ml)	Usual Recommended Dose* (ml)	Max. Dose Total (mg I)
Lumbar myelogram	170–190	10–15	2850
Thoracic myelogram	220	12	2640
Cervical myelogram (via lumbar injection)	250–300	10	3000
Cervical myelogram (via lat. cervical inj.)	220	10	2200
Total columnar myelography	250–280	10	2800
CT cisternography (via lumbar inj.)	170–190	4–6	1140

* Refer to RECONSTITUTION TABLE for preparation of Solution.

Patient Management.

PREPROCEDURE—Anesthesia is not necessary. Premedication sedatives or tranquilizers are usually not needed (see PRECAUTIONS). Patients should be well hydrated. Epileptic patients should be maintained on their anticonvulsant medication.

INSTRUCTIONS FOR PREPARATION OF THE SOLUTION—Contents under vacuum. Use only if vacuum is present as evidenced by diluent being drawn into vial when stopper is punctured.

1. Fill a sterile syringe with the exact volume of diluent as indicated in the following RECONSTITUTION TABLE to obtain the desired iodine concentration.

Examples:
- a. For vials containing 3.75 g AMIPAQUE:
  - To obtain 170 mg I/ml, use 8.9 ml of diluent.
  - To obtain 190 mg I/ml, use 7.8 ml of diluent.
- b. For vials containing 6.75 g AMIPAQUE:
  - To obtain 170 mg I/ml, use 16.1 ml of diluent.
  - To obtain 190 mg I/ml, use 14.0 ml of diluent.

(See table above)

RECONSTITUTION TABLE

Conc. of Solution (mg I/ml)	Volume of Diluent to be Added: 3.75 g Vial (ml)	6.75 g Vial (ml)
170	8.9	16.1
180	8.3	15.0
190	7.8	14.0
220	6.5	11.7
250	5.5	10.0
260	5.2	9.4
270	5.0	9.0
280	4.7	8.5
290	4.5	8.1
300	4.3	7.8
	The volume of the final solution will equal the volume of the diluent + 1.7 ml	The volume of the final solution will equal the volume of the diluent + 3.1 ml

The volume of the final solution will exceed the amount required to achieve the recommended dosage. For precise volume for injection refer to DOSAGE TABLE.

2. Inject the diluent into the vial, and leave the syringe and needle in place.
3. Gently swirl the vial (without shaking) until its contents are dissolved (approximately 3 to 10 minutes). The solution should be clear and colorless to slightly yellow.

Use immediately after reconstitution (see DOSAGE AND ADMINISTRATION). Discard any unused portion.

As with any lumbar puncture, sterile technique must be employed. The lumbar puncture is usually made between L3 and L4, but if pathology is suspected at this level the interspace immediately above or below may be selected. A lateral cervical puncture may also be used.

POSTPROCEDURE—The lumbar puncture needle may be removed immediately following injection since it is not necessary to remove AMIPAQUE, brand of metrizamide, after injection into subarachnoid spaces.

Management of the patient is similar to that used following simple lumbar puncture. Maintaining the patient recumbent in bed with the head raised 15 to 30° for 8 hours may reduce the rate of upward dispersion of the medium. The patient may then remain horizontal for a further 16 hours at the discretion of the physician.

How Supplied:
Kits, each containing
One-3.75 g/20 ml single-dose vial of AMIPAQUE with 1 vial of diluent (NDC 0024-0044-01); or
One-6.75 g/50 ml single-dose vial of AMIPAQUE with 1 vial of diluent (NDC 0024-0046-01).
Combination packs, each containing
Five-3.75 g/20 ml single-dose vials of AMIPAQUE with 5 vials of diluent (NDC 0024-0044-12); or
Five-6.75 g/50 ml single-dose vials of AMIPAQUE with 5 vials of diluent (NDC 0024-0046-12).
Protect vials of AMIPAQUE from light.

Distributed by
Winthrop Laboratories
Division of Sterling Drug Inc.
New York, NY 10016
Manufactured by
Nyegaard & Co • AS
Nycoveien 2, Oslo 4, Norway

BILOPAQUE® SODIUM ℞
brand of sodium tyropanoate

ORAL CHOLECYSTOGRAPHIC MEDIUM

Description: BILOPAQUE sodium, brand of sodium tyropanoate, is sodium 2-(3-butyramido-2,4, 6-triiodobenzyl)-butanoate. BILOPAQUE sodium is an off-white, odorless, hygroscopic solid containing 57.4 per cent iodine. The molecular weight is 663.1. BILOPAQUE sodium is soluble in water to 14.7 per cent.

Clinical Pharmacology: After ingestion, BILOPAQUE is absorbed from the duodenum into the bloodstream. The liver converts it primarily into radiopaque glucuronic acid conjugates, which are concentrated by the functioning gallbladder. These conjugates provide visualization of the gallbladder and may, upon contraction of the gallbladder, provide visualization of the extrahepatic ducts.

Indication and Usage: BILOPAQUE is indicated for radiographic delineation of the gallbladder.

Contraindications: BILOPAQUE should not be administered to patients with advanced hepatorenal disease, severe impairment of renal function, or severe gastrointestinal disorders that prevent absorption.

Warnings: Usage in Pregnancy. Although no teratogenic effects attributable to BILOPAQUE have been observed in animals, safe use of the agent in pregnant women has not been established. Before cholecystography with BILOPAQUE is performed in women of childbearing potential, the benefit should be weighed against the possible risk to the patient or child. In addition, most authorities consider elective contrast radiography of the abdomen contraindicated during pregnancy.

The use of BILOPAQUE in children under 12 years is not recommended, since no clinical trials have been performed in this age group.

Elevation of protein-bound iodine for several months and false-positive urine albumin tests for several days may occur after ingestion of cholecystographic media.

Precautions: Caution should be exercised in administration of BILOPAQUE to patients with known iodine sensitivity.

Severe, advanced liver disease may interfere with metabolism of the radiopaque medium, and therefore, a greater amount of unchanged BILOPAQUE may be diverted to the kidney. Renal function in patients with severe, advanced liver disease should be assessed before cholecystography, and renal output and hepatic function should be observed for a few days after the procedure.

The recommended dose of BILOPAQUE should not be exceeded in patients with preexisting renal disease. Possible renal irritation in susceptible individuals could result in reflex vascular spasm with partial or complete renal shutdown.

Patients with renal or hepatic diseases should not be dehydrated beforehand and should drink liberal amounts of fluids after taking the capsules.

The uricosuric effect of BILOPAQUE should be considered when it is administered to patients with evidence of impaired renal function.

Caution is advised in patients with symptoms of coronary artery disease.

Adverse Reactions: The most common reactions after administration of BILOPAQUE have been mild and transient *gastrointestinal disturbances* including nausea, abdominal cramps, diarrhea, vomiting, and weakness and abdominal discomfort. *Allergic type reactions affecting* skin, mucous membrane, and systemic hypersensitivity reactions are unusual and include urticaria with or without pruritus, erythema, morbilliform rash, and localized areas of edema. Very rarely a systemic serum sickness-type reaction with fever, rash, and arthralgia has been reported. *Other reactions,* which have occurred infrequently, include dysuria, dyspnea, difficulty in swallowing, headache, perspiration, dizziness, fatigue, lightheadedness, pain or cramps in limbs, and rarely, laryngotracheal edema.

Very rarely disturbances in hepatic, renal, or cardiovascular function have been reported with cholecystographic media, usually in patients with preexisting disease (see Precautions).

Dosage and Administration: A single oral dose of 3 g (4 capsules) is recommended for adults. The optimal time interval between administration of BILOPAQUE and cholecystography is 10 to 12 hours, although satisfactory results have been reported as early as 4 to 6 hours.

The use of BILOPAQUE in children under 12 years is not recommended, since no clinical trials have been performed in this age group.

If no visualization occurs after administration of BILOPAQUE, repeat examination with a 3 g dose may be performed the following day. *Increasing the amount of the repeat dose is not recommended.*

Cholestasis is a common cause of nonvisualization in patients who have been on almost completely fat-free diets. To reduce the incidence of false-negative nonvisualization, such patients should eat a diet containing some fat for one or two days before cholecystographic examination. Fat is a long-acting cholecystagogue, and will stimulate emptying of the gallbladder and prepare it to receive the radiopaque medium. *The meal immediately before ingestion of the BILOPAQUE capsules should be fat free.*

Preparatory dehydration is unnecessary and undesirable, especially in elderly patients. After the fat-free evening meal, the patient should swallow 4 BILOPAQUE capsules (3 g) with water. Between ingestion of BILOPAQUE and cholecystographic examination, the patient should take nothing by mouth except water, and should not smoke or chew gum.

Many physicians believe that the quality of gallbladder visualization is enhanced when the intestine is relatively free of residue. This may be achieved with an enema the morning of the examination, or a laxative the day before.

For observation of gallbladder contractility, the patient may be given a fatty meal or a cholecystagogue after the initial x-ray examination. Additional exposures may be made 5 to 30 minutes later.

Nonvisualization

Nonvisualization in routine cholecystography with BILOPAQUE, brand of sodium tyropanoate, usually implies substantial loss of gallbladder function. However, nonvisualization may also result on occasion from other factors not related to disease of the biliary tract.

Repeat Examination

When adequate visualization is not obtained initially, repeat cholecystography with the recommended dose of 3 g helps reduce the possibility of diagnostic error. A larger dose is not recommended. Disease may be inferred with reasonable certainty if the gallbladder does not visualize on repeat examination.

How Supplied: Capsules of 750 mg—Envelopes of 4 capsules (3 g, the recommended dose), in boxes of 5 (NDC 0024-0134-01) and 25 (NDC 0024-0134-03). Bottles of 500 capsules with 150 dispensing envelopes (NDC 0024-0134-06).

[*Shown in Product Identification Section*]

HYPAQUE® SODIUM ℞
brand of diatrizoate sodium, USP
ORAL POWDER
HYPAQUE® SODIUM ORAL SOLUTION
brand of diatrizoate sodium solution, USP

For Examination of the Gastrointestinal Tract

Description: HYPAQUE sodium, brand of diatrizoate sodium, is sodium 3,5-diacetamido-2,4,6-triiodobenzoate ($C_{11}H_8I_3N_2NaO_4$) and contains 59.87 per cent iodine. It is available as a powder and a liquid. The powder (for preparing radiopaque solutions) provides about 600 mg organically-bound iodine per gram of powder and contains caramel as a coloring agent. The 41.66 per cent oral solution is supplied as a thin, slightly viscous, colorless to light brown solution of diatrizoate sodium in water. Each ml contains 249 mg of organically-bound iodine.

Clinical Pharmacology: When administered orally or given as an enema, the medium produces excellent opacification and delineation of the upper and lower gastrointestinal tract; however, because of dilution, contrast in the small bowel may be unsatisfactory. HYPAQUE solutions are particularly valuable when a more viscous agent, such as barium sulfate which is not water soluble, is unsuitable or potentially harmful.

From 0.04 to 1.2 per cent of the medium may be absorbed from the gastrointestinal tract after

Continued on next page

Winthrop—Cont.

oral administration. In some patients, particularly in infants and patients with engorgement of the intestinal mucosa, sufficient absorption to cause some visualization of the urinary tract may occur occasionally. HYPAQUE is also absorbed across the peritoneum and pleura.

Indications and Usage: This medium is indicated for radiographic examination of the gastrointestinal tract following oral or rectal administration.

Warnings: Serious or fatal reactions have been associated with the parenteral administration of radiopaque media. It is important that a course of action be carefully planned in advance for the treatment of possible serious reactions with oral use of HYPAQUE solutions. (See Precautions.)

Usage in Pregnancy. The safety of orally administered HYPAQUE solutions during pregnancy has not been established. Therefore, before administration of the drug to women of childbearing potential, the benefit to the patient should be carefully weighed against the possible risk to the fetus. In addition, most authorities consider elective contrast radiography of the abdomen contraindicated during pregnancy.

Precautions: A 10 per cent solution of the medium in water is isotonic. Hence, the solutions generally employed clinically (i.e., from 15 to 40 per cent) are hypertonic. Highly hypertonic solutions may draw excessive amounts of fluid into the intestine and may lead to hypovolemia. In very young or debilitated children, and in elderly cachectic persons, the loss of plasma fluid may be sufficient to cause a shock-like state which, if untreated, could be dangerous to the patient. Wherever possible, the use of the lower concentrations is advised for infants and young children (under 10 kg) and for dehydrated or debilitated patients. The higher concentrations should be used in such patients only when necessary and with great caution.
It is advisable to correct any electrolyte disturbances before using solutions that are extremely hypertonic.
Bronchial entry of the medium causes a copious osmotic effusion. Therefore, pulmonary entry by aspiration or by use in patients with esophagotracheal fistula should be avoided.
Caution is also advised in patients with severe renal or hepatic disease.

Adverse Reactions: There have been few reported cases of adverse reactions with orally administered solutions of water-soluble contrast agents. Because of their osmotic effect, such solutions tend to exert cathartic action, but this is generally considered an advantage. Nausea, vomiting, or slight diarrhea may occasionally occur, particularly when the medium is used in a high concentration or large volume. Urticaria has been observed in a few patients; presumably the condition was caused by allergy to the contrast medium and it was readily alleviated by antihistamine therapy.
Because small amounts of the medium may be absorbed, the possibility of systemic reactions should be considered, particularly in cases of perforation.

Dosage and Administration:
Adults: ***Oral,*** from 90 to 180 ml of a 25 to 40 per cent solution.
Enema, from 500 to 1000 ml of a 15 to 25 per cent solution.
Infants and Children: ***Oral,*** from 30 to 75 ml of a 20 to 40 per cent solution.
Enema, from 100 to 500 ml of a 10 to 15 per cent solution, depending on weight of patient.
Warning: Neither the powder nor the liquid is to be used for the preparation of solutions for parenteral injection. [See table.]

Directions for Measurement and Dilution

A. *Using powder*

Solution (%)	Measuring spoons* of powder (per 100 ml diluent†)
10	1
15	1½
20	2
25	2½
40	4

* One level measuring spoon is equal to approximately 10 g of powder.
† Solutions may be sweetened or flavored (e.g., with vanilla, lemon, chocolate); the diluent may be water, milk, or a carbonated drink.

B. *Using liquid* (Approximate Values)

Solution (%)	Dilution Required
40	Use undiluted
25	Dilute each 60 ml to 100 ml
20	Dilute each 50 ml to 100 ml
15	Dilute each 40 ml to 100 ml
10	Dilute each 25 ml to 100 ml

How Supplied: Powder—cans of 250 g with measuring spoon (approximately 10 g capacity), NDC 0024-0769-01
Liquid—bottles of 120 ml, each containing 50 g of diatrizoate sodium, NDC 0024-0768-01

HYPAQUE® Sodium 25% ℞
brand of diatrizoate sodium injection, USP
Sterile Aqueous Solution

INTRAVENOUS INFUSION FOR UROGRAPHY AND CT SCAN ENHANCEMENT

Description: HYPAQUE sodium, brand of diatrizoate sodium, is monosodium 3, 5-diacetamido-2, 4, 6-triiodobenzoate ($C_{11}H_8I_3N_2NaO_4$), which contains 59.87 per cent organically-bound iodine.
The 25 per cent solution (w/v) contains 150 mg iodine per ml and 0.4 mEq (9.05 mg) sodium per ml. It has an osmolarity of approximately 657 mOs per liter (0.657 mOs per ml) at 25°C and is, therefore, hypertonic. The viscosity (cps) is about 1.59 at 25°C and 1.19 at 37°C. Sodium carbonate or hydrochloric acid has been added to adjust pH between 6.5 and 7.7. The sterile, aqueous solution is clear and nearly colorless. It is relatively thermostable and may be autoclaved once. It does not contain an antibacterial preservative. The 25 per cent solution contains edetate calcium disodium 1:10,000 as a sequestering stabilizing agent.

Clinical Pharmacology: HYPAQUE sodium 25 per cent is a diagnostic radiopaque medium which provides visualization of internal structures. In urography, the infusion technique facilitates the administration of the larger dose of contrast medium for improved diagnostic visualization of the entire urinary system.
Infusion of HYPAQUE sodium 25 per cent will increase density differentials of intracranial structures during computed tomographic scanning, often providing additional diagnostic information.

Infusion urography. Infusion urography is a method of excretion urography utilizing a relatively large volume of HYPAQUE sodium 25 per cent by rapid intravenous infusion. The medium is carried rapidly to the kidneys where it is excreted unchanged in the urine. If renal function is normal, excretion begins almost immediately.
Intravenous infusion of a large volume of dilute contrast material has been shown to give consistently excellent pyelograms, dense nephrograms, and satisfactory cystograms and voiding urethrograms.
A more anatomically complete visualization of the urinary tract is generally attainable with the infusion technique than with conventional urographic techniques. It may be particularly useful when indeterminate or unsatisfactory results have been obtained with conventional urographic studies. The infusion technique may be utilized prior to retrograde pyelography when this procedure is being considered as it may obviate the need for a retrograde study.
Nephrotomography following infusion urography will frequently provide an accurate differential diagnosis between renal tumors and cysts. Infusion nephrotomography has also been successfully utilized in the localization of adrenal tumors. Nephrotomographic sections are usually made immediately following the completion of the infusion urogram. However, adequate tomograms may be obtained for as long as 40 minutes following the completion of the infusion.

Indications and Usage: HYPAQUE sodium 25 per cent is indicated for use in intravenous urography and contrast enhancement of computerized axial tomography for cerebral imaging.

Warnings: Serious or fatal reactions have been associated with the administration of radiopaque media. It is of utmost importance that a course of action be carefully planned in advance for the immediate treatment of serious reactions, and that adequate and appropriate facilities and personnel be readily available in case a severe reaction occurs.
Intravascular administration of contrast media may promote sickling in patients who are homozygous for sickle cell disease. Therefore, fluid restriction is not advised.
The results of PBI and RAI uptake studies, which depend on iodine estimations, will not reflect thyroid function for up to 16 days following administration of iodinated urographic media. However, function tests not depending on iodine estimations, e.g., T_3 resin uptake or free thyroxine assays, are not affected.

Precautions: Before injecting a contrast medium, the patient should be questioned for a history of allergy. Although a history of allergy may imply a greater than usual risk, it does not arbitrarily contraindicate the use of the medium. Premedication with antihistamines to avoid or minimize possible allergic reactions may be considered. **Benadryl® (brand of diphenhydramine hydrochloride), however, may cause precipitation when mixed with HYPAQUE sodium.** The intravenous injection of a test dose of 0.5 to 1 ml of the contrast agent before injection of the full dose has been employed in an attempt to predict severe or fatal adverse reactions. The preponderance of recent scientific literature, however, now demonstrates that this provocative test procedure is not reliably predictive of serious or fatal reactions. Severe reactions and fatalities have occurred with the test dose alone, with the full dose after a nonreactive test dose, and with or without a history of allergy. No conclusive relationship between severe or fatal reactions and antigen-antibody reactions or other manifestations of allergy has been established. A history of allergy may be useful in predicting reactions of a mild or intermediate nature.

Usage in pregnancy. Safe use of HYPAQUE sodium, brand of diatrizoate sodium injection, 25 per cent during pregnancy has not been established. Therefore, before administration of the drug to women of childbearing potential, the benefit to the patient should be carefully weighed against the possible risk to the fetus. In addition, most authorities consider elective contrast radiography of the abdomen contraindicated during pregnancy.
Caution is advised in patients with severe cardiovascular disease and in patients with a history of bronchial asthma or other allergic manifestations or of sensitivity to iodine.

In myelomatosis, urography should only be performed with caution. If a weak protein-binding agent such as a diatrizoate is used for the procedure, it is essential to omit preparatory dehydration, administer fluids, and attempt to alkalinize the urine.

Immediate adverse reactions to infusion urography have not been reported to occur at a higher frequency or greater severity than with routine excretory urography. However, sequelae of this procedure are possible some hours after the examination. The infusion imposes not only a sudden osmotic load, but also may present as much as 160 mEq of sodium (3.7 g) to patients with established, decreased glomerular filtration and renal tubular damage. In addition, these patients may also have coexisting or associated cardiovascular disease. Therefore, the possibility of the development of congestive heart failure hours after the procedure should be considered.

Because of the possibility of inducing temporary suppression of urine, it is wise to allow an interval of at least 48 hours to pass before repeating infusion urography in patients with unilateral or bilateral reduction of normal renal function.

Preparatory dehydration or abdominal compression may not be necessary in infusion urography. Preparatory dehydration may be dangerous in infants, young children, the elderly, and azotemic patients (especially those with polyuria, oliguria, diabetes, advanced vascular disease, or preexisting dehydration). The undersirable dehydration in these patients may be accentuated by the osmotic diuretic action of the medium.

Adverse Reactions: Reactions accompanying the use of contrast media may vary directly with the concentration of the substance, the amount used, the technique used, and the underlying pathology.

The following adverse reactions, usually of a minor nature, have occurred in 10 to 14 per cent of patients who have received diatrizoate solutions and similar contrast media. *Cardiovascular reactions:* rare cases of cardiac arrhythmias (including ventricular fibrillation), hypertension, hypotension, shock, and cardiac arrest; vein cramp, thrombophlebitis, vasodilatation with flushing. *Renal reactions:* occasionally, transient proteinuria, and rarely, oliguria and anuria which may be secondary to hypotension. *Allergic reactions:* asthmatic attacks, nasal and conjunctival symptoms, dermal reactions such as urticaria, and rarely, anaphylactic shock, sometimes with fatal outcome. Infrequently, immediate or delayed chills can occur, sometimes accompanied by fever. *Respiratory reactions:* pulmonary or laryngeal edema, bronchospasm, laryngospasm, dyspnea, cyanosis, coughing. *CNS reactions:* restlessness, confusion, convulsions. *Other reactions:* pain on injection, hematomas, ecchymoses, warmth, fever, nausea, vomiting, anxiety, headache, dizziness, excessive salivation. Infrequently, "iodism" (salivary gland swelling) from organic iodinated compounds appears two days after exposure and subsides by the sixth day.

Dosage and Administration:

Infusion urography. The recommended dose is calculated on the basis of 2 ml of HYPAQUE sodium, brand of diatrizoate sodium injection, 25 per cent per pound of body weight. The average dose of the solution for adults is 300 ml; for optimum results, a minimum dose of 250 ml should be used. A maximum dose of 400 ml is generally sufficient for the largest of subjects. The solution is administered intravenously through an 18-gauge needle over a period of three to ten minutes. Pyelographic films are taken at 10, 20, and 30 minutes from the beginning of the infusion. Early 2, 3, 4, and 5 minute films are obtained when indicated for the evaluation of hypertension. Nephrotomographic sections are best taken just at the end of the infusion, and voiding cystourethrograms when desired are usually made at 30 minutes.

CT scanning. The dose and administration will depend on the technique and equipment used. The usual dose in adults is 300 ml of HYPAQUE sodium 25 per cent, infused over 10 to 20 minutes.

The solution should be protected from strong light. *Discard any unused portion remaining in the container.*

How Supplied:

Calibrated bottles of 300 ml (NDC 0024-0758-03)

Calibrated bottles of 300 ml with intravenous infusion set (NDC 0024-0757-03)

HYPAQUE-CYSTO® ℞

brand of diatrizoate meglumine injection, USP
Sterile Aqueous Solution

FOR RETROGRADE CYSTOURETHROGRAPHY

Description: HYPAQUE-CYSTO is a radiopaque medium which contains approximately 141 mg organically-bound iodine per ml. It is a 30 per cent (weight/volume) sterile aqueous solution of the meglumine salt of 3, 5-diacetamido-2, 4, 6-triiodobenzoic acid ($C_{18}H_{26}I_3N_3O_9$). The viscosity is 1.94 cps at 25°C and 1.42 cps at 37°C. The pH is adjusted with hydrochloric acid or meglumine solution. HYPAQUE-CYSTO is clear and colorless to pale yellow. It should be protected from strong light. The solution is relatively thermostable and may be autoclaved. Edetate calcium disodium 1:10,000 has been added as a sequestering stabilizing agent.

Action: HYPAQUE-CYSTO is a diagnostic radiopaque medium which provides visualization of the lower urinary tract.

Indication: HYPAQUE-CYSTO is indicated for retrograde cystourethrography.

Adverse Reactions: No irritation or other undesirable effects have been reported following the administration of HYPAQUE-CYSTO in clinical investigations.

Dosage and Administration: After the bladder is emptied, HYPAQUE-CYSTO is gently instilled without force, often beyond the first desire to micturate, but not beyond the point of urgency or mild discomfort. The volume required to fill the bladder to slightly less than capacity may vary from patient to patient.

Bladder capacity in normal adults is generally 200 to 300 ml, and rarely, up to 600 ml. Capacity at birth is 20 to 50 ml, and increases about 400 per cent in the first year. In children 3 to 5 years old, bladder capacity is 150 to 180 ml. In children older than 8 years, it is in the low adult range.

In disease, bladder capacity in adults may vary from 50 ml in a hypertonic reflex bladder to over 1000 ml in an atonic or sensory paralytic bladder or chronic lower urinary tract obstruction.

Repeat examination may be required to detect reflux, or in function studies.

The concentration varies with technique and equipment used. HYPAQUE-CYSTO may be diluted with sterile water or 5 per cent dextrose solution, as indicated in the following tables.

STANDARD PACKAGE
(250 ml of HYPAQUE-CYSTO in 500 ml bottle)

TO MAKE		ADD	FINAL SOLUTION CONTAINS
Final conc.	Final volume	Sterile water or 5% dextrose solution	Iodine
30 %	250 ml	—	141 mg/ml
25 %	300 ml	50 ml	118 mg/ml
21.4%	350 ml	100 ml	101 mg/ml
20 %	375 ml	125 ml	94 mg/ml
18.8%	400 ml	150 ml	88 mg/ml
16.7%	450 ml	200 ml	78 mg/ml
15 %	500 ml	250 ml	71 mg/ml

PEDIATRIC PACKAGE
(100 ml of HYPAQUE-CYSTO in 300 ml bottle)

TO MAKE		ADD	FINAL SOLUTION CONTAINS
Final conc.	Final volume	Sterile water or 5% dextrose solution	Iodine
30%	100 ml	—	141 mg/ml
24%	125 ml	25 ml	113 mg/ml
20%	150 ml	50 ml	94 mg/ml
15%	200 ml	100 ml	71 mg/ml
12%	250 ml	150 ml	56 mg/ml
10%	300 ml	200 ml	47 mg/ml

How Supplied:

STANDARD PACKAGE—Calibrated 500 ml dilution bottles containing 250 ml HYPAQUE-CYSTO; rubber stoppered, with inner removable seal and screw neck.

PEDIATRIC PACKAGE—Calibrated 300 ml dilution bottles containing 100 ml HYPAQUE-CYSTO, brand of diatrizoate meglumine injection; rubber stoppered, with inner removable seal and screw neck.

HYPAQUE® MEGLUMINE 30% ℞

brand of diatrizoate meglumine injection, USP
Sterile Aqueous Solution

INTRAVENOUS INFUSION FOR UROGRAPHY AND CT SCAN ENHANCEMENT

Description: HYPAQUE meglumine 30 per cent is a solution of 1-Deoxy-1-(methylamino)-D-glucitol 3, 5-diacetamido-2, 4, 6-triiodobenzoate (salt), with a molecular formula of $C_7H_{17}NO_5 \cdot C_{11}H_9I_3N_2O_4$.

The 30 per cent solution (w/v) contains approximately 141 mg of organically-bound iodine per ml. It has a viscosity of 1.94 cps at 25°C and 1.42 cps at 37°C. The pH is adjusted with hydrochloric acid or meglumine solution. Edetate calcium disodium 1:10,000 has been added as a sequestering stabilizing agent. The sterile aqueous solution is clear and colorless to pale yellow. HYPAQUE meglumine 30 per cent is relatively thermostable and may be autoclaved once. It does not contain an antibacterial preservative.

Clinical Pharmacology: HYPAQUE meglumine 30 per cent is a diagnostic radiopaque medium which provides visualization of internal structures. In urography, the infusion technique facilitates the administration of the larger dose of contrast medium for improved diagnostic visualization of the entire urinary system.

Infusion of HYPAQUE meglumine 30 per cent will increase density differentials of intracranial structures during computed tomographic scanning, often providing additional diagnostic information.

Indications and Usage: HYPAQUE meglumine 30 per cent is indicated for use in intravenous urography and contrast enhancement of computerized axial tomography for cerebral imaging.

Warnings: Serious or fatal reactions have been associated with the administration of radiopaque media. It is of utmost importance that a course of action be carefully planned in

Continued on next page

Winthrop—Cont.

advance for the immediate treatment of serious reactions, and that adequate and appropriate facilities and personnel be readily available in case a severe reaction occurs.
Intravascular administration of contrast media may promote sickling in patients who are homozygous for sickle cell disease. Therefore, fluid restriction is not advised.
The results of PBI and RAI uptake studies, which depend on iodine estimations, will not reflect thyroid function for up to 16 days following administration of iodinated urographic media. However, function tests not depending on iodine estimations, e.g., T_3 resin uptake or free thyroxine assays, are not affected.
Precautions: Before injecting a contrast medium, the patient should be questioned for a history of allergy. Although a history of allergy may imply a greater than usual risk, it does not arbitrarily contraindicate the use of the medium. Premedication with antihistamines to avoid or minimize possible allergic reactions may be considered. **Benadryl® (brand of diphenhydramine hydrochloride), however, may cause precipitation when mixed with HYPAQUE meglumine 30 per cent.** The intravenous injection of a test dose of 0.5 to 1 ml of the contrast agent before infusion of the full dose has been employed in an attempt to predict severe or fatal adverse reactions. The preponderance of recent scientific literature, however, now demonstrates that this provocative test procedure is not reliably predictive of serious or fatal reactions. Severe reactions and fatalities have occurred with the test dose alone, with the full dose after a nonreactive test dose, and with or without a history of allergy. No conclusive relationship between severe or fatal reactions and antigen-antibody reactions or other manifestations of allergy has been established. A history of allergy may be useful in predicting reactions of a mild or intermediate nature.
Usage in pregnancy. No teratogenic effects attributable to a 60 per cent solution of HYPAQUE meglumine have been observed in reproduction studies in animals. However, before administration of HYPAQUE meglumine, brand of diatrizoate meglumine injection, 30 per cent to women of childbearing potential, the benefit to the patient should be carefully weighed against the possible risk to the fetus. In addition, most authorities consider elective contrast radiography of the abdomen contraindicated during pregnancy.
Caution is advised in patients with severe cardiovascular disease and in patients with a history of bronchial asthma or other allergic manifestations, or of sensitivity to iodine. Transient ECG changes have been reported in older patients with evidence of heart disease. In myelomatosis, urography should only be performed with caution. If a weak protein-binding agent such as a diatrizoate is used for the procedure, it is essential to omit preparatory dehydration, to administer fluids, and attempt to alkalinize the urine.
Immediate adverse reactions to infusion urography have not been reported to occur at a higher frequency or with greater severity than with routine excretory urography. However, sequelae of this procedure are possible some hours after the examination. The infusion imposes a sudden osmotic load. This should be considered in patients with established, decreased glomerular filtration and renal tubular damage. In addition, these patients may also have coexisting or associated cardiovascular disease. Therefore, there is a possibility of the development of congestive heart failure hours after the procedure.
Because of the possibility of inducing temporary suppression of urine, it is wise to allow an interval of at least 48 hours to pass before repeating infusion urography in patients with unilateral or bilateral reduction of normal renal function.
Preparatory dehydration or abdominal compression may not be necessary in infusion urography. Preparatory dehydration may be dangerous in infants, young children, the elderly, and azotemic patients (especially those with polyuria, oliguria, diabetes, advanced vascular disease, or preexisting dehydration). The undesirable dehydration in these patients may be accentuated by the osmotic diuretic action of the medium.
Adverse Reactions: Reactions accompanying the use of contrast media may vary directly with the concentration of the substance, the amount used, the technique used, and the underlying pathology.
The following adverse reactions, usually of a minor nature, have occurred in 10 to 14 per cent of patients who have received diatrizoate solutions and similar iodinated contrast media. *Cardiovascular reactions:* rare cases of cardiac arrhythmias (including ventricular fibrillation), hypertension, hypotension, shock, and cardiac arrest; vein cramp, thrombophlebitis, vasodilatation with flushing. *Renal reactions:* occasionally, transient proteinuria, and rarely, oliguria and anuria which may be secondary to hypotension. *Allergic reactions:* asthmatic attacks, nasal and conjunctival symptoms, dermal reactions such as urticaria, and rarely, anaphylactic shock, sometimes with fatal outcome. Infrequently, immediate or delayed chills can occur, sometimes accompanied by fever. *Respiratory reactions:* pulmonary or laryngeal edema, bronchospasm, laryngospasm, dyspnea, cyanosis, coughing. *CNS reactions:* restlessness, confusion, convulsions. *Other reactions:* pain on injection, hematomas, ecchymoses, warmth, fever, nausea, vomiting, anxiety, headache, dizziness, excessive salivation. Infrequently, "iodism" (salivary gland swelling) from organic iodinated compounds appears two days after exposure and subsides by the sixth day.
Dosage and Administration:
Infusion urography. The recommended dose for infusion urography is calculated on the basis of 2 ml of HYPAQUE meglumine 30 per cent per pound of body weight. The average dose of the solution for adults is 300 ml; for optimal results, a minimum dose of 250 ml should be used. A maximum dose of 400 ml is generally sufficient for the largest of subjects.
The solution is infused over a period of three to ten minutes. Radiographs are usually taken at 10, 20, and 30 minutes from the beginning of the infusion. Earlier films may be obtained for the evaluation of hypertension. Nephrograms are usually obtained at the end of the infusion, and voiding cystourethrograms are usually obtained 30 minutes after the beginning of the infusion.
CT scanning. The dose and administration will depend on the technique and equipment used. The usual dose in adults is 300 ml of HYPAQUE meglumine, brand of diatrizoate meglumine injection, 30 per cent, infused over 10 to 20 minutes.
The solution should be protected from strong light. *Discard any unused portion remaining in the container.*
How Supplied:
Calibrated bottles of 300 ml (NDC 0024-0739-03)
Calibrated bottles of 300 ml with intravenous infusion set (NDC 0024-0740-03)

HYPAQUE® SODIUM 50% ℞
brand of diatrizoate sodium injection, USP
Sterile Aqueous Injection

Description: HYPAQUE sodium, brand of diatrizoate sodium, is monosodium 3,5-diacetamido-2,4,6-triiodobenzoate ($C_{11}H_8I_3N_2NaO_4$), that contains 59.87 per cent iodine. HYPAQUE sodium 50 per cent (w/v) contains 300 mg iodine per ml, 0.8 mEq (18.1 mg) sodium per ml, and has an osmolarity of approximately 1270 mOs per liter (1.27 mOs per ml) with a viscosity (cps) of about 3.25 at 25°C and 2.34 at 37°C. All dilutions of HYPAQUE sodium are hypertonic. Sodium carbonate and either sodium hydroxide or hydrochloric acid have been added to adjust the pH between 6.5 and 7.7. If a solution of this medium is chilled, crystals may form but readily dissolve if the vial is placed in moderately hot water before use; cool to body temperature before injecting. The sterile aqueous solution is clear and nearly colorless. It is relatively thermostable and may be autoclaved without harmful effects. It should be protected from strong light. The 50 per cent solution contains edetate calcium disodium 1:10,000 as a sequestering stabilizing agent.
Action: A radiopaque medium used to delineate internal structures.
Indication: HYPAQUE sodium 50 per cent is indicated for excretory urography.
Contraindications, General: **Do not use HYPAQUE sodium 50 per cent for myelography or for examination of dorsal cysts or sinuses which might communicate with the subarachnoid space.** Even a small amount of the medium in the subarachnoid space may produce convulsions and result in fatality. Epidural injection is also contraindicated.
Warnings, General: Serious or fatal reactions have been associated with the administration of radiopaque media. It is of utmost importance that a course of action be carefully planned in advance for the immediate treatment of serious reactions, and that adequate and appropriate facilities be readily available in case a severe reaction occurs.
Selective spinal arteriography or arteriography of trunks providing spinal branches can cause mild to severe muscle spasm. However, serious neurologic sequelae, including permanent paralysis, have occasionally been reported. (See also Aortography, Precautions, in PDR for Radiology and Nuclear Medicine.)
Usage in Pregnancy. Safe use of HYPAQUE sodium 50 per cent during pregnancy has not been established. Therefore, before administration of the drug to women of childbearing potential, the benefit to the patient should be carefully weighed against the possible risk to the fetus. In addition, most authorities consider elective contrast radiography of the abdomen contraindicated during pregnancy.
Intravascular administration of contrast media may promote sickling in patients who are homozygous for sickle cell disease.
The results of PBI and RAI uptake studies, which depend on iodine estimations, will not reflect thyroid function for up to 16 days following administration of iodinated urographic media. However, function tests not depending on iodine estimations, e.g., T_3 resin uptake or direct thyroxine assays, are not affected.
Precautions, General: Before injecting a contrast medium, the patient should be questioned for a history of allergy. Although a history of allergy may imply a greater than usual risk, it does not arbitrarily contraindicate the use of the medium. Premedication with antihistamines to avoid or minimize possible allergic reactions may be considered. **Benadryl®, brand of diphenhydramine hydrochloride, however, may cause precipitation when mixed in the same syringe with HYPAQUE sodium.** The intravenous injection of a test dose of 0.5 to 1 ml of the contrast agent before injection of the full dose has been employed in an attempt to predict severe or fatal adverse reactions. The preponderance of recent scientific literature, however, now demonstrates that this provocative test procedure is not reliably predictive of serious or fatal reactions. Severe reactions and fatalities have occurred with the test dose alone, with the full dose after a nonreactive test dose, and with or without a history of allergy. No conclusive relationship

between severe or fatal reactions and antigen-antibody reactions or other manifestations of allergy has been established. A history of allergy may be useful in predicting reactions of a mild or intermediate nature.
Caution is advised in patients with severe cardiovascular disease and in patients with a history of bronchial asthma or other allergic manifestations, or of sensitivity to iodine.
Adverse Reactions, General: Reactions accompanying the use of contrast media may vary directly with the concentration of the substance, the amount used, the technique used, and the underlying pathology.
Adverse reactions, usually of a minor nature, have occurred in 10 to 14 per cent of patients who have received HYPAQUE sodium, brand of diatrizoate sodium, 50% intravenously. Rarely, atheromatous or other embolic phenomena can occur in angiography. *Cardiovascular reactions* include vasodilatation with flushing, hypotension, and vein cramp (occasionally thrombosis or, rarely, thrombophlebitis) in the injected vein. Serious reactions include rare cases of cardiac arrhythmias (e.g., ventricular fibrillation), shock, and cardiac arrest. Transient proteinuria may occur occasionally following the injection of radiopaques and, rarely, oliguria and anuria (renal shutdown) have been reported as a secondary effect of a hypotensive reaction. *Allergic reactions* include asthmatic attacks, nasal and conjunctival symptoms, dermal reactions such as urticaria and, rarely, anaphylactoid shock. Rare fatalities have been reported, due to this or unknown causes. Severe reactions may also be manifested by signs and symptoms relating to the *respiratory system* (dyspnea, cyanosis, pulmonary or laryngeal edema), or to the *nervous system* (restlessness, confusion, or convulsions). Infrequently, immediate or delayed rigors can occur, sometimes accompanied by hyperpyrexia. *Other reactions* include nausea, vomiting, excessive salivation, anxiety, headache, and dizziness. Infrequently, "iodism" (salivary gland swelling) from organic compounds appears two days after exposure and subsides by the sixth day.
Subcutaneous extravasation, chiefly because of hypertonicity of the medium, causes transitory stinging. If the volume is small, ill effects are very unlikely. However, if subcutaneous extravasation is extensive, especially in the foot, the physician should consider infiltration with Sterile Water for Injection, USP, or injection of spreading agents. (See also Subcutaneous and Intramuscular Dosage in section on Excretory Urography.)
Diffuse petechiae have been described and, in several instances, were traced to contamination of syringes, gloves with talc, or fine lint.

EXCRETORY UROGRAPHY

When injected intravenously, the medium is carried rapidly to the kidneys where it is eliminated unchanged in the urine. If the kidneys are functioning normally, the substance is excreted almost immediately.
Precautions: Because of the possibility of inducing temporary suppression of urine, it is wise to allow an interval of at least 48 hours to pass before repeating excretory or retrograde pyelography in patients with unilateral or bilateral reduction of normal renal function.
In myelomatosis, urography should only be performed with caution. If a weak protein-binding agent such as a diatrizoate is used for the procedure, it is essential to omit preparatory dehydration, administer fluids, and attempt to alkalinize the urine.
Preparatory dehydration may be dangerous in infants, young children, the elderly, and azotemic patients (especially those with polyuria, oliguria, diabetes, advanced vascular disease, or preexisting dehydration). The undesirable dehydration in these patients may be accentuated by the osmotic diuretic action of the medium.

Dosage and Administration:
Preliminary Preparation of Patient
Clear shadows are often obtained with the radiopaque medium in patients who have had no preliminary preparation for urography. However, the largest precentage of satisfactory films is secured by following a routine that assures the highest possible concentration of the opaque material in the urinary tract at the time of the x-ray exposure. This is accomplished by directing the patient to abstain from fluids for 12 to 15 hours before the intravenous injection so that partial dehydration results. (See Precautions concerning dehydration.) Unless contraindicated, a laxative is taken at bedtime to eliminate gas from the intestine.
Intravenous Dosage. Adults: A dose of 30 ml of the 50 per cent solution administered intravenously with or without compression produces diagnostic shadows in the majority of adults subjected to partial dehydration and to effective purgation. If the administration of 30 ml does not provide satisfactory visualization, this dose may be repeated in 15 to 30 minutes. In persons of slight build, 20 ml may produce adequate shadows.
Larger doses ranging from 50 to 60 ml of the 50 per cent solution may be used for routine excretory urography in adults. The increased dosage offers better and more complete visualization of the urinary tract. This technique requires neither compression nor dehydration and is more effective in obese patients. Adverse reactions to the larger dose are similar to those encountered with lower doses without an increase in incidence, severity, or type of reaction. Voiding cystourethrograms may be obtained when desired. For the best results and minimal side effects, it is advisable to inject the total amount of solution intravenously in one to three minutes.
Children: The dosage of the 50 per cent solution for children under 6 months of age is 5 ml; for children 6 to 12 months of age, 6 to 8 ml; for children 1 to 2 years of age, 8 to 10 ml; for children 2 to 5 years of age, 10 to 12 ml; for children 5 to 7 years of age, 12 to 15 ml; for children 7 to 11 years of age, 15 to 18 ml, and for children 11 to 15 years of age, 18 to 20 ml.
Subcutaneous Dosage. The compound may be given subcutaneously, diluted with equal quantities of sterile water for injection. Although not necessary, hyaluronidase (150 turbidity units) may be given simultaneously if desired. The total volume is divided into two equal doses and injected over each scapula. A large, rounded mass appears after the injection has been completed. A piece of cotton saturated with collodion may be applied over each injection point to prevent seepage of the contrast medium.
Adults and older children: The usual dose is 20 to 30 ml of the 50 per cent solution diluted with equal quantities of sterile water for injection.
Infants and young children: The dose ranges from 5 ml of the 50 per cent solution for smaller infants up to 15 ml for older children and should be diluted with equal quantities of sterile water for injection.
Intramuscular Dosage. The 50 per cent solution may also be injected intramuscularly undiluted or diluted with an equal quantity of sterile water for injection. Generally, the total volume is introduced into the gluteal muscles in two separate, equal doses. Hyaluronidase also may be injected if desired.
Generally, doses of 5 to 15 ml of the 50 per cent solution may be administered to **children**; the usual 20 to 30 ml dose is suggested for **adults.**
Roentgenography
Intravenous Technique. A film should be exposed routinely before the intravenous injection is made. If the plain film shows evidence of gas accumulation, it may be best to defer the examination to some other day.
Excellent shadows can often be obtained immediately after administration of the radiopaque medium (within a five-minute period). If preliminary preparation has been carried out, the urinary organs are usually best visualized on films exposed 5, 10, or 15 minutes after intravenous injection. If a film of the bladder is required, it generally is taken 25 or 35 minutes after injection.
In patients with impaired renal function, the best shadows may not be obtainable until later (30 minutes or more) because of delayed excretion, and additional film may have to be exposed.
Subcutaneous Technique. The excretion of the drug occurs promptly so that films may be exposed at intervals of 10, 20, and 30 minutes.
Intramuscular Technique. Diagnostically, visualization of the upper urinary tract following the intramuscular administration of the 50 per cent solution has been found almost to equal that achieved with intravenous injections. Since excretion of the medium is rapid, it may be evident within five minutes after intramuscular injection. The time for obtaining the best filling and contrast varies, but the first exposure is generally made after a 10-minute interval.

For other uses, see latest package insert and PDR for Radiology and Nuclear Medicine.

How Supplied: Vials of 20 and 30 ml, rubber stoppered, boxes of 25.
Vials of 50 ml, rubber stoppered, boxes of 10.

HYPAQUE® MEGLUMINE 60% ℞
brand of diatrizoate meglumine injection, USP
Sterile Aqueous Injection

FOR EXCRETORY UROGRAPHY
For other uses, see latest package insert and PDR for Radiology and Nuclear Medicine.

Description: HYPAQUE meglumine, brand of diatrizoate meglumine, is meglumine 3, 5-diacetamido-2, 4, 6-triiodobenzoate ($C_{18}H_{26}I_3N_3O_9$), which contains 47.06 per cent iodine. It is a colorless, microcrystalline solid that is readily soluble in water.
HYPAQUE meglumine 60 per cent (w/v) is a sterile aqueous solution containing 60 g of the meglumine salt of diatrizoic acid per 100 ml of solution. It was specifically designed for those indications in which the physician does not desire to use a sodium-containing radiopaque medium. The solution is a clear, colorless to pale yellow liquid, and the pH is adjusted between 6.5 and 7.7 with diatrizoic acid or meglumine solution. It is a relatively thermostable solution and may be autoclaved without harmful effects, although it should be protected from strong light. The 60 per cent solution contains edetate calcium disodium 1:10,000 as a sequestering stabilizing agent. Each 1 ml contains approximately 282 mg of organically-bound iodine. The viscosity of the solution is 6.17 cps at 25°C and 4.12 cps at 37°C.
Action: A radiopaque medium used to delineate internal structures.
Indication: HYPAQUE meglumine 60 per cent is indicated for excretory urography.
Contraindications, General: Do not use HYPAQUE meglumine 60 per cent solution for myelography or for examination of dorsal cysts or sinuses which might communicate with the subarachnoid space. Injection of even a small amount into the subarachnoid space may produce convulsions and result in fatality. Epidural injection is also contraindicated.

Continued on next page

Winthrop—Cont.

Warnings, General: Serious or fatal reactions have been associated with the administration of radiopaque media. It is of utmost importance that a course of action be carefully planned in advance for the immediate treatment of serious reactions, and that adequate and appropriate facilities be readily available in case a severe reaction occurs.

Selective spinal arteriography or arteriography of trunks providing spinal branches can cause mild to severe muscle spasm. However, serious neurologic sequelae, including permanent paralysis, have occasionally been reported. (See also Angiography, Precaution, in PDR for Radiology and Nuclear Medicine.)

Usage in Pregnancy. No teratogenic effects attributable to HYPAQUE meglumine 60 per cent have been observed in reproduction studies in animals. However, before administration of HYPAQUE meglumine 60 per cent to women of childbearing potential, the benefit to the patient should be carefully weighed against the possible risk to the fetus. In addition, most authorities consider elective contrast radiography of the abdomen contraindicated during pregnancy.

Administration of radiopaque materials to patients known or suspected to have **pheochromocytoma** should be performed with extreme caution. If, in the opinion of the physician, the possible benefits of such procedures outweigh the considered risk, the amount of radiopaque material injected should be kept to an absolute minimum. The blood pressure should be assessed throughout the procedure, and measures for treatment of a hypertensive crisis should be available.

Contrast media have been shown to promote the phenomenon of sickling in individuals who are homozygous for sickle cell disease when the material is injected intravenously or intraarterially.

Precautions, General: Before a contrast medium is injected, the patient should be questioned for a history of allergy. Although a history of allergy may imply a greater than usual risk, it does not arbitrarily contraindicate the use of the medium. Premedication with antihistamines to avoid or minimize possible allergic reactions may be considered. **Benadryl®, brand of diphenhydramine hydrochloride, however, may cause precipitation when mixed in the same syringe with HYPAQUE meglumine, brand of diatrizoate meglumine.** The intravenous injection of a test dose of 0.5 to 1 ml of the contrast agent before injection of the full dose has been employed in an attempt to predict severe or fatal adverse reactions. The preponderance of recent scientific literature, however, now demonstrates that this provocative test procedure is not reliably predictive of serious or fatal reactions. Severe reactions and fatalities have occurred with the test dose alone, with the full dose after a nonreactive test dose, and with or without a history of allergy. No conclusive relationship between severe or fatal reactions and antigen-antibody reactions or other manifestations of allergy has been established. A history of allergy may be useful in predicting reactions of a mild or intermediate nature.

Caution is advised in patients with severe cardiovascular disease, hyperthyroidism, extreme senility (but not old age *per se*), and in patients with a history of bronchial asthma or other allergic manifestations, or of sensitivity to iodine.

The results of PBI and RAI uptake studies, which depend on iodine estimations, will not reflect thyroid function for up to 16 days following administration of iodinated urographic media. However, function tests not depending on iodine estimations, e.g., T_3 resin uptake or direct thyroxine assays, are not affected.

Adverse Reactions, General: Reactions accompanying the use of contrast media may vary directly with the concentration of the substance, the amount used, the technique used, and the underlying pathology.

The following have been reported after administration of diatrizoates and other iodinated contrast media. *Reactions due to technique:* hematomas and ecchymoses. *Hemodynamic reactions:* vein cramp and thrombophlebitis following intravenous injection. *Cardiovascular reactions:* rare cases of cardiac arrhythmias, hypertension, hypotension and shock, and cardiac arrest. Occasionally, transient proteinuria, and rarely, oliguria or anuria. *Allergic reactions:* asthmatic attacks, nasal and conjunctival symptoms, dermal reactions such as urticaria, and rarely, anaphylactic reactions. Signs and symptoms related to the *respiratory system:* pulmonary or laryngeal edema, bronchospasm; or to the *nervous system:* restlessness, convulsions. *Other reactions:* flushing, pain, warmth, nausea, vomiting, anxiety, headache, and dizziness. Rarely, immediate or delayed rigors can occur, sometimes accompanied by hyperpyrexia. Infrequently, "iodism" (salivary gland swelling) from organic iodinated compounds appears two days after exposure and subsides by the sixth day.

Subcutaneous extravasation, chiefly because of hypertonicity of the medium, causes transitory stinging. If the volume is small, ill effects are very unlikely. However, if subcutaneous extravasation is extensive, especially in the foot, the physician should consider infiltration with Sterile Water for Injection, USP, or injection of spreading agents.

Diffuse petechiae have been described and, in several instances, were traced to contamination of syringes, gloves with talc, or fine lint.

EXCRETORY UROGRAPHY

Indication: Since HYPAQUE meglumine, brand of diatrizoate meglumine injection, 60 per cent is rapidly eliminated by the kidneys in radiopaque concentration, its use is indicated for excretory urography.

Precautions: See section on Precautions, General.

Some clinicians consider multiple myeloma a contraindication to excretory urography because of the great possibility of producing transient to fatal renal failure. Others believe that the risk of causing anuria is definite but small. If excretory urography is performed in the presence of multiple myeloma, dehydration should be avoided since it favors protein precipitation in renal tubules.

Because of the possibility of temporary suppression of urine, it is wise to allow an interval of at least 48 hours before excretory urography is repeated in patients with unilateral or bilateral reduction of normal renal function.

Preparatory dehydration may be dangerous in infants, young children, the elderly, and azotemic patients (especially those with polyuria, oliguria, diabetes, advanced vascular disease, or preexisting dehydration). The undesirable dehydration in these patients may be accentuated by the osmotic diuretic action of the medium.

Adverse Reactions: See section on Adverse Reactions, General.

Dosage and Administration:

Intravenous Dosage

Adults. A dose of 30 to 60 ml produces excellent shadows in the majority of adults subjected to partial dehydration and effective purgation. In persons of slight build, 20 ml produces adequate shadows. For best results and minimal reactions, the total 30 to 60 ml should be injected in one to three minutes and compression may be used. A small intravenous test dose may be administered as a possible aid in determining sensitivity to the medium. (See Precautions, General.)

Children. The suggested dosage for children up to 12 years old is presented in the table. Children older than 12 years may be given an adult dose.

[See table below].

Preliminary Preparation of Patient

Although clear shadows are often seen in patients who have had no preliminary preparation for urography, the largest percentage of satisfactory films is obtained in patients who abstain from fluids for 12 to 15 hours before the intravenous injection so that partial dehydration results. (See Precautions concerning dehydration.) Unless contraindicated, a laxative may be taken at bedtime to eliminate gas from the intestine.

Roentgenographic Technique

A preliminary scout film may be obtained before the intravenous injection. Excellent shadows can often be obtained immediately after administration of the radiopaque medium (within a five-minute period). If preliminary preparation has been carried out, the urinary organs are usually best visualized on films exposed 5, 10, or 15 minutes after intravenous injection. If a film of the bladder is required, it is generally taken 25 or 35 minutes after injection.

In patients with impaired renal function, the best shadows may not be obtainable until later (30 minutes or more) because of delayed excretion, and additional film may have to be exposed.

Most urologists and roentgenologists believe that compression immediately above the symphysis (obtained by application of a small hollow rubber ball about the size of a grapefruit or by the rolled bed sheet technique) assures adequate filling of the pelves and ureters, and hence is of great value. Although compression undoubtedly improves the urogram, it also seems to increase the possibility of pyelorenal backflow or reflux by raising the pressure within the urinary tract.

How Supplied:

Vials of 20 and 30 ml, rubber stoppered, boxes of 25.

Vials of 50 and 100 ml, rubber stoppered, boxes of 10.

Pediatric Dosage for Excretory Urography

Age	Body Weight	Dosage
Under 2 years	up to 10 lb	5 to 10 ml
	10 to 30 lb	10 to 15 ml
2 to 12 years	30 to 60 lb	15 to 30 ml
	over 60 lb	30 ml

HYPAQUE®-M, 75% ℞

brand of diatrizoate meglumine and diatrizoate sodium injection, USP

Sterile Aqueous Injection

See latest package insert and PDR for Radiology and Nuclear Medicine for complete prescribing information.

How Supplied: HYPAQUE-M, 75 per cent is supplied in vials of 20 and 50 ml, boxes of 10.

HYPAQUE®-M, 90% ℞

brand of diatrizoate meglumine and diatrizoate sodium injection, USP
Sterile Aqueous Injection

> **See latest package insert and PDR for Radiology and Nuclear Medicine for complete prescribing information.**

How Supplied: HYPAQUE-M, 90 per cent is supplied in vials of 50 ml, boxes of 10.

TELEPAQUE® ℞

brand of iopanoic acid tablets, USP

Description: TELEPAQUE, brand of iopanoic acid tablets, is 3-amino-α-ethyl-2,4,6-triiodohydrocinnamic acid ($C_{11}H_{12}I_3NO_2$). It is a cream-colored solid which is insoluble in water. It contains 66.68 per cent organically-bound iodine and has a molecular weight of 570.93. TELEPAQUE is an oral radiopaque medium for cholecystography and cholangiography. Each off-white, scored tablet contains 500 mg iopanoic acid.

Clinical Pharmacology: TELEPAQUE is absorbed from the duodenum, excreted by the liver as a glucuronide, and stored and concentrated in the gallbladder. This conjugate provides visualization of the gallbladder and may, upon contraction of the gallbladder, provide visualization of the extrahepatic ducts. Approximately 50 per cent of the administered dose is excreted within 24 hours, and each day thereafter, 50 per cent of the remainder; excretion is complete in about five days. Partition of excretion is approximately two thirds through the gastrointestinal tract and one third through the kidneys. The glucuronide of TELEPAQUE is not reabsorbed to any extent; thus, there is no enterohepatic recycling. The glucuronide is visible in the intestinal tract as discrete radiopacities.

The healthy gallbladder concentrates TELEPAQUE; faint contrast becomes apparent in about four hours, and maximum contrast in about 14 hours. In substantial gallbladder disease, concentration does not take place and no contrast is apparent.

Indications and Usage: TELEPAQUE is indicated for use in oral cholecystography. It may also be used for oral cholangiography, although it is not considered the method of choice.

Contraindications: Administration of TELEPAQUE is contraindicated in severe impairment of renal function and particularly in advanced hepatorenal disease. It is also contraindicated in severe gastrointestinal disorders that prevent absorption, and in some patients sensitive to iodinated compounds.

Warning: Usage in Pregnancy. Reproduction studies have not been performed in animals. Before cholecystography in women who are of childbearing potential, the benefits should be weighed against the possible risk to the fetus.

Precautions: *Cholecystography in Liver Disease.* TELEPAQUE is generally well tolerated by patients with impaired liver function, and adequate gallbladder visualization can often be achieved in the presence of hepatic disease. However, severe, advanced liver disease (e.g., bilirubin exceeding 5 mg per 100 ml) very frequently results in nonvisualization of the gallbladder.

Severe, advanced liver disease may interfere with metabolism of the radiopaque medium, and therefore, a greater amount of unchanged TELEPAQUE will be diverted for renal excretion, increasing the load on the kidneys. Although renal difficulty has rarely been attributed to TELEPAQUE, renal function in patients with severe, advanced liver disease should be assessed before cholecystography, and renal output and hepatic function should be observed for a few days after the procedure.

Renal Disease. Patients with preexisting renal disease should not receive high doses of cholecystographic media. Possible renal irritation in susceptible individuals could result in reflex vascular spasm with partial or complete renal shutdown.

Dehydration. Patients with renal or hepatic diseases should not be dehydrated beforehand and should drink liberal amounts of fluids after taking the tablets.

Uricosuric Effect. It has been shown that TELEPAQUE has uricosuric activity. This fact should be taken into consideration when the product is administered to patients with evidence of impaired renal function.

Coronary Disease. Caution is advised in patients with coronary disorders, especially those with recent symptoms of coronary artery disease. Blood pressure should be observed after administration of cholecystographic media to these patients.

Elderly Patients. For elderly patients, see Dosage.

Effect on Laboratory Tests

Thyroid Function Tests. The results of PBI and RAI uptake studies, which depend on iodine estimations, will not reflect thyroid function for several months following administration of cholecystographic media. However, function tests not depending on iodine estimations, e.g., T_3 resin uptake or free thyroxine assays, are not affected.

Liver Function Tests. Bilirubin, thymol turbidity, cephalin flocculation, and serum enzyme values are unaffected but TELEPAQUE may delay BSP clearance values for up to two days.

Pseudoalbuminuria may be present for three days in response to certain chemical protein precipitation tests. Positive reactions should be verified by the heat-and-acetic acid or colorimetric dip-strip methods.

Uricosuric Effect. TELEPAQUE may increase the rate of excretion of uric acid, lowering blood levels and raising urinary excretion values for a few days.

Adverse Reactions: Most reactions are mild and transitory; a very low incidence of serious side effects has been attributed to TELEPAQUE.

Most frequently reported have been mild and transitory nausea, vomiting, cramps, and diarrhea (usually occurring as a few loose stools). Frank diarrhea and cramps have been noted in only a small number of patients, and severe diarrhea with prostration is rare. A mild stinging sensation during urination may occur. Skin, mucous membrane, and systemic hypersensitivity reactions are unusual and include urticaria with or without pruritus, erythema, morbilliform rash, and localized areas of edema. Very rarely a systemic serum sickness-type reaction with fever, rash, and arthralgia has been reported. A few cases of transitory thrombocytopenia with petechiae have been reported. Miscellaneous subjective complaints are dryness of the throat, burning on swallowing, heartburn, sore throat, dizziness, and headache.

Very rarely disturbances in hepatic, renal, or cardiovascular function have been reported, usually in patients with preexisting disease (see Precautions).

Dosage and Administration:

Adult Dosage

The standard adult dose of 3 g (six tablets) is usually ingested with water in the evening after a fat-free dinner, about 14 hours before the cholecystography. In some instances, double doses of 6 g (12 tablets) may be ingested, e.g., for duct visualization or for some repeat examinations made over 7 days later. Many radiologists prefer that the patient take a laxative (e.g., castor oil) about four to six hours before ingesting TELEPAQUE, brand of iopanoic acid tablets. (See also Repeat Examination.) Preparatory dehydration is unnecessary and undesirable, especially in elderly patients. The use of large or repeated doses over a number of days to force visualization of a poorly functioning gallbladder *in elderly patients* is not recommended.

Diet before Cholecystography

A normal diet (containing some fat) is advised at least one or two days before TELEPAQUE cholecystography. The meal immediately before ingestion of TELEPAQUE, however, should be *strictly fat free:* e.g., fruit or fruit juice; vegetables *cooked without fat;* bread with jelly; coffee or tea with sugar but *no milk or cream. No meats are permitted.*

During the interval between ingestion of TELEPAQUE and the morning of cholecystographic examination the patient should take *nothing by mouth* except water, and should not smoke or chew gum. In the morning, before the radiologic examination, the patient may take an enema in order to remove accumulated gas which might interfere with visualization.

Fatty Meal after Cholecystography

After the gallbladder has been visualized the patient may be given a fat-containing meal or a commercially available cholecystagogue, for determining the extent and duration of gallbladder contractility (thus, the degree of function), to help identify small radiolucent stones or to visualize the bile ducts.

Duct Visualization

Occasionally, the bile ducts may be visualized on the original film during cholecystography. However, in a substantial percentage of patients, administration of a fat is necessary. The more frequent the roentgenographic exposures, the greater the probability of visualization of the ducts; however, the best time intervals are usually 20 and 30 minutes after the fatty meal. Some investigators believe contrast in the ducts is enhanced by an increased dose of TELEPAQUE (up to 6 g).

Repeat Examination

Most radiologists consider repeat examination desirable when the gallbladder does not visualize initially, in order to reduce the possibility of false diagnosis. If the second cholecystographic examination also results in nonvisualization, gallbladder disease may be inferred with reasonable certainty.

For repeat examination on the same day as the initial cholecystographic procedure, an additional 3 g (six tablets) may be given. However, if repeat cholecystography is to be performed with a double dose, a period of at least five to seven days should intervene between the first and the repeat examinations. No more than a total of 6 g (12 tablets) should be ingested during a 24-hour period.

How Supplied:

Tablets of 500 mg,
- envelopes of 6 tablets, boxes of 5 (NDC 0024-1931-01)
- envelopes of 6 tablets, boxes of 25 (NDC 0024-1931-03)
- bottles of 500 tablets with dispensing envelopes (NDC 0024-1931-06)

[*Shown in Product Identification Section*]

Important Notice

Before prescribing or administering any product described in Physicians' Desk Reference always consult the PDR Supplement for possible new or revised information.

GUIDE TO MANAGEMENT OF DRUG OVERDOSE

Prepared by:
Institute of Clinical Toxicology
Eric G. Comstock, M.D., Director
Houston, Texas

INTRODUCTION . . . The following discussion is designed for use in adult patients. In the pediatric age group, the general principles apply, but volumes of fluid or suggested medication must be adjusted to be appropriate for body size. Symptomatic and supportive care is the approach to drug overdose upon which primary reliance should be placed. All other approaches to treatment are secondary to the support of vital function. Procedures directed toward the offending substance, such as the performance of gastric lavage or the administration of specific pharmacologic antagonist, should be undertaken only after adequate vital function has been assured. Procedures to facilitate excretion of toxic substances, such as peritoneal or extracorporeal dialysis and forced diuresis are required infrequently, and never should be relied upon as the primary approach to treatment. For sedative, hypnotic, and tranquilizer drugs, alone or in combination, supportive care is sufficent as outlined in the following discussion.

INITIAL ASSESSMENT . . . the initial assessment of a drug overdosed patient should determine whether the patient is asymptomatic or symptomatic. If the patient is symptomatic, determine the adequacy of respiration and cardiac function and note reflex activity, such as pupillary, corneal, gag and deep tendon. If vital function is compromised, or consciousness is impaired, proceed immediately to supportive measures.

THE ASYMPTOMATIC PATIENT . . . The drug overdosed patient may be asymptomatic because he has not ingested a sufficient dose of the drugs, or because a sufficient quantity of the drug has not been absorbed to produce symptoms. After the ingestion of a life threatening quantity of drugs, symptoms may be delayed as long as six hours, although ordinarily symptoms are manifested within thirty (30) minutes to two (2) hours. Ingestion of alcohol simultaneously with drugs may result in symptoms as early as ten to fifteen minutes with compromise of vital function within thirty minutes. Vomiting should be induced only during the asymptomatic interval. If significant central nervous system depression intervenes between the administration of emetic and the occurrence of vomiting, then the airway should be protected by insertion of a cuffed endotracheal tube. The delay between the administration of emetic and the occurrence of emesis can be avoided by the use of apomorphine. Fluids must be forced orally to obtain satisfactory results from any effort to induce vomiting. An alternate approach to the asymptomatic patient alleged to have ingested drugs, is the administration by mouth of a slurry of activated charcoal containing no less than 100 grams of activated charcoal powder (USP) in water. Gastric lavage with a large caliber tube (34 French) may be performed in the asymptomatic patient. Any patient whose consciousness is impaired to the point where a cuffed endotracheal tube will be tolerated should be intubated prior to the performance of gastric lavage.

THE SYMPTOMATIC PATIENT . . . If the patient is symptomatic all treatment procedures directed toward the toxic substance are secondary to appraisal and support of the vital function. If the patient is in deep coma, attention to respiratory support and cardiac function should proceed immediately and simultaneously.

RESPIRATORY SUPPORT . . . Examine the mouth. Remove all foreign material including dentures. Position the head so that respiration is not sonorous and so that regurgitated stomach contents are not readily aspirated. If respiration is not present, provide mechanical ventilation by mouth-to-mouth, ambu bag, or positive pressure respirator until the patient is adequately oxygenated. Insert an oropharyngeal airway and suction excess excretions while preparing to insert an endotracheal tube. A cuffed endotracheal tube should be inserted and the cuff inflated. Bronchial suction should be administered to clear mucus and foreign material from the major bronchi. Determine that the chest is being inflated symmetrically and that breath sounds are audible bilaterally. After the acute emergency, determine placement of the endotracheal tube by x-ray. Monitor adequacy of ventilation using arterial blood gases.

IV ACCESS AND CARDIAC FUNCTION . . . While one member of the treatment team is assuring adequate ventilation, a second member of the team should be assuring adequate IV access by insertion of an 18 gauge venous catheter and initiation of IV fluid administration, such as Ringers Lactate, at a maintenance rate in adults of 150 ml. per hour. Since hypotension from sedative drug intoxication results from relative hypovolemia complicated frequently by dehydration, the rate of intravenous infusion should be increased to 10-20 cc per minute if the systolic pressure is under 80 mm of mercury. When the systolic pressure returns to 80 mm, the rate of infusion should be reduced to 2-3 cc per minute. A central venous pressure catheter and monitoring of central venous pressure is required if the continuous high rate infusion reaches one (1) liter or if the positive fluid balance exceeds two (2) liters during the first two hours. Intermittent monitoring of central venous pressure should continue throughout the period of intensive supportive care. A baseline electrocardiogram should be obtained as soon as procedures for support of vital function have been implemented. An abnormal electrocardiogram should result in reduction in the rate of IV infusion to baseline of 2 ml per minute until the cardiac abnormality has been evaluated. The appearance of conduction defects should lead to suspicion of drugs with direct cardiac effects, such as the tricyclic antidepressants. In uncomplicated sedative drug overdose, the central venous pressure will be under ten centimeters of water and will not change appreciably with high volume fluid infusion. If the central venous pressure increases abruptly in excess of five centimeters of water, or if the CVP exceeds 16 centimenters of water, high rate fluid infusion should be stopped pending evaluation of cardiac status. Adequate tissue perfusion is obtained with a systolic pressure in the range of 80 to 100 milliliters of mercury. A systolic pressure higher than this is required only in the patient with pre-existing hypertension. The formation of urine is an indication that tissue perfusion is adequate.

URINARY CATHETERIZATION . . . An in-dwelling urinary catheter should be inserted early in the course of treatment of any unconscious drug overdose patient. Upon insertion of the catheter, the volume of residual urine should be measured and the specimen should be saved separately for urinalysis including specific gravity, labeled for drug analysis, and sent to the laboratory to be retained for 24 hours. The specific gravity of the initial urine will help identify patients who are severely dehydrated at the time of admission and influence the amount of positive fluid balance which should be tolerated during the initial few hours of treatment. Recording of urine output hourly is necessary to maintain fluid balance records. Continuing urine formation is a guide to the adequacy of tissue perfusion. Abrupt cessation of urine output most frequently is due to an obstructed catheter, but deserves immediate appraisal. Anuria for a period in excess of one hour should lead to reduction of high rate intravascular volume infusion until cardiac and renal status has been reappraised. Failure to achieve adequate urinary output after initial emptying of the bladder may reflect uncompensated